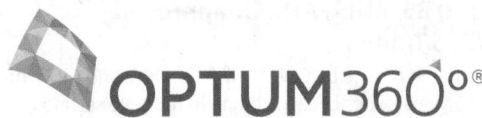

EXPERT

ICD-10-CM Expert for Hospitals

The complete official code set

Codes valid from October 1, 2020
through September 30, 2021

**Value-Added Content —
Just For Our Customers**

Scan the QR code below
with your phone or tablet to
access value-added content.

Check back often for new content
that supports and expands on the
details in this ICD-10 code set.

Can't scan?

Then go to

optum360coding.com/icd-10-extra/

Publisher's Notice

The *ICD-10-CM Expert for Hospitals: The Complete Official Code Set* is designed to be an accurate and authoritative source regarding coding and every reasonable effort has been made to ensure accuracy and completeness of the content. However, Optum360 makes no guarantee, warranty, or representation that this publication is accurate, complete or without errors. It is understood that Optum360 is not rendering any legal or other professional services or advice in this publication and that Optum360 bears no liability for any results or consequences that may arise from the use of this book.

Acknowledgments

Marianne Randall, CPC, *Product Manager*
Anita Schmidt, BS, RHIA, AHIMA-approved ICD-10-CM/PCS Trainer, *Subject Matter Expert*
Karen Krawzik, RHIT, CCS, AHIMA-approved ICD-10-CM/PCS Trainer, *Subject Matter Expert*
Leanne Patterson, CPC, *Subject Matter Expert*
LaJuana Green, RHIA, CCS, *Subject Matter Expert*
Jacqueline R. Petersen, RHIA, CHDA, CPC, *Subject Matter Expert*
Stacy Perry, *Manager, Desktop Publishing*
Tracy Betzler, *Senior Desktop Publishing Specialist*
Hope M. Dunn, *Senior Desktop Publishing Specialist*
Katie Russell, *Desktop Publishing Specialist*
Kate Holden, *Editor*

Our Commitment to Accuracy

Optum360 is committed to producing accurate and reliable materials.

To report corrections, please email accuracy@optum.com. You can also reach customer service by calling 1.800.464.3649, option 1.

Copyright

Property of Optum360, LLC. Optum360 and the Optum360 logo are trademarks of Optum360, LLC. All other brand or product names are trademarks or registered trademarks of their respective owner.

© 2020 Optum360, LLC. All rights reserved.

Made in the USA
ISBN 978-1-62254-523-0

Anita Schmidt, BS, RHIA, AHIMA-approved ICD-10-CM/PCS Trainer

Ms. Schmidt has expertise in ICD-10-CM/PCS, DRG, and CPT with more than 15 years' experience in coding in multiple settings, including inpatient, observation, and same-day surgery. Her experience includes analysis of medical record documentation, assignment of ICD-10-CM and PCS codes, and DRG validation. She has conducted training for ICD-10-CM/PCS and electronic health record. She has also collaborated with clinical documentation specialists to identify documentation needs and potential areas for physician education. Most recently she has been developing content for resource and educational products related to ICD-10-CM, ICD-10-PCS, DRG, and CPT. Ms. Schmidt is an AHIMA-approved ICD-10-CM/PCS trainer and is an active member of the American Health Information Management Association (AHIMA) and the Minnesota Health Information Management Association.

Karen Krawzik, RHIT, CCS, AHIMA-approved ICD-10-CM/PCS Trainer

Ms. Krawzik has expertise in ICD-10-CM, ICD-9-CM, CPT/HCPCS, DRG, and data quality and analytics, with more than 30 years' experience coding in multiple settings, including inpatient, observation, ambulatory surgery, ancillary, and emergency room. She has served as a DRG analyst and auditor of commercial and government payer claims, as a contract administrator, and worked on a team providing enterprise-wide conversion of the ICD-9-CM code set to ICD-10. More recently, she has been developing print and electronic content related to ICD-10-CM and ICD-10-PCS coding systems, MS-DRGs, and HCCs. Ms. Krawzik is credentialed by the American Health Information Management Association (AHIMA) as a Registered Health Information Technician (RHIT) and a Certified Coding Specialist (CCS) and is an AHIMA-approved ICD-10-CM/PCS trainer. She is an active member of AHIMA and the Missouri Health Information Management Association.

2021 ICD-10-CM Official Guidelines for Coding and Reporting

Optum360 is pleased to provide you with this 2021 ICD-10-CM code book that INCLUDES the 2021 Official Guidelines for Coding and Reporting.

Welcome to 25 years of **coding expertise.**

Every medical organization knows that medical documentation and coding accuracy are vital to the revenue cycle. As a leading health services business, Optum360® has proudly created industry-leading coding, billing and reimbursement solutions for more than 25 years. Serving the broad health market, including physicians, health care organizations, payers and government, we help health systems reduce costs and achieve timely and accurate revenue.

You'll find ICD-10-CM/PCS, CPT®, HCPCS, DRG, specialty and reference content across our full suite of medical coding, billing and reimbursement products. And to ensure you have expert insight and the right information at your fingertips, our subject matter experts have incorporated proprietary features into these resources. These include supplementary edits and notations, coding tips and tools, and appendixes — making each product comprehensive and easy to use. Think of it as coding resources built by coders, for coders like you.

Your coding, billing and reimbursement product team,

Ryan   Nichole   Greg   LaJuana
Ken   Julie
Regina   Marianne   Denise   Leanne
Jacqui   Anita   Debbie   Elizabeth   Nann
Karen

Put Optum360 medical coding, billing and reimbursement content at your fingertips today. Choose what works for you.

- Print books
- Online coding tools
- Data files
- Web services

Visit us at **optum360coding.com** to browse our products, or call us at **1-800-464-3649, option 1** for more information.

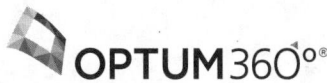

At our core, we're about coding.

Essential medical code sets are just that — essential to your revenue cycle. In our ICD-10-CM/PCS, CPT®, HCPCS and DRG coding tools, we apply our collective coding expertise to present these code sets in a way that is comprehensive, plus easy to use and apply. Print books are inexpensive and easily referenced, created with intuitive features and formats, such as visual alerts, color-coding and symbols to identify important coding notes and instructions — plus great coding tips.

Find the same content, tips and features in a variety of formats. Choose from print products, online coding tools, data files or web services, as well as from various educational opportunities.

Your coding, billing and reimbursement product team,

Ryan   Nichole   Greg   LaJuana
Regina   Ken   Julie
Jacqui   Marianne   Denise   Leanne
   Anita   Debbie   Elizabeth   Nann
         Karen

Put Optum360 medical coding, billing and reimbursement content at your fingertips today. Choose what works for you.

Print books

Online coding tools

Data files

Web services

Visit us at **optum360coding.com** to browse our products, or call us at **1-800-464-3649, option 1** for more information.

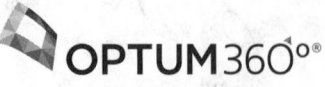

What if you could go back in time?

How much time do you think you spend researching elusive codes? Too much, probably. Time you would like to have back. We can't give time back, but we can help you save it. Our all-in-one coding solutions consolidate specialty coding processes so you can find information more easily and quickly. Each specialty-specific procedure code includes its official and lay descriptions, coding tips, cross-coding to common ICD-10-CM codes, relative value units, Medicare edit guidance, *CPT Assistant®* references, CCI edits and, when relevant, specific reimbursement and documentation tips.

With tools available for 30 specialties, we're sure you'll find the right resource to meet your organization's unique needs, even if those needs are allergy, anesthesia/pain management, behavioral health, cardiology, cardiothoracic surgery, dental, dermatology, emergency medicine, ENT, gastroenterology, general surgery, hematology, laboratory/pathology, nephrology, neurology, neurosurgery, OB/GYN, OMS, oncology, ophthalmology, orthopaedics, pediatrics, physical therapy, plastics, podiatry, primary care, pulmonology, radiology, urology or vascular surgery.

Say good-bye to time wasted digging for those elusive codes.

Your coding, billing and reimbursement product team,

Ryan Nichole Greg LaJuana
Ken Julie
Regina Marianne Denise Leanne
Jacqui Anita Debbie Elizabeth Nann
Karen

Put Optum360 medical coding, billing and reimbursement content at your fingertips today. Choose what works for you.

- Print books
- Online coding tools
- Data files
- Web services

Visit us at **optum360coding.com** to browse our products, or call us at **1-800-464-3649, option 1** for more information.

A lot goes into coding resources.
We know.

Most think that coding, billing and reimbursement includes only your essential code sets, but that leaves out reference products. An important part of the revenue cycle, reference tools provide clarity — along with coding and billing tips — to deepen medical coding knowledge, make the coding process more efficient and help reduce errors on claims. Optum360 offers reference tools for facility, physician and post-acute markets, in addition to physicians-only fee products that inform the best business decisions possible for practices.

There's a lot that goes into coding, billing and reimbursement. Make sure your organization isn't leaving anything to chance.

Your coding, billing and reimbursement product team,

Ryan Nichole Greg LaJuana
Ken Julie
Regina Denise Leanne
Marianne
Jacqui Anita Debbie Elizabeth Nann
Karen

Put Optum360 medical coding, billing and reimbursement content at your fingertips today. Choose what works for you.

 Print books

 Online coding tools

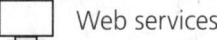 Data files

Web services

Visit us at **optum360coding.com** to browse our products, or call us at **1-800-464-3649, option 1** for more information.

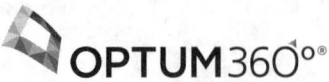 OPTUM360°®

Contents

Preface

ICD-10-CM Official Preface

This FY 2021 update of the International Statistical Classification of Diseases and Related Health Problems, 10th revision, Clinical Modification (ICD-10-CM) is being published by the United States government in recognition of its responsibility to promulgate this classification throughout the United States for morbidity coding. The International Statistical Classification of Diseases and Related Health Problems, 10th Revision (ICD-10), published by the World Health Organization (WHO), is the foundation of ICD-10-CM. ICD-10 continues to be the classification used in cause-of-death coding in the United States. The ICD-10-CM is comparable with the ICD-10. The WHO Collaborating Center for the Family of International Classifications in North America, housed at the Centers for Disease Control and Prevention's National Center for Health Statistics (NCHS), has responsibility for the implementation of ICD and other WHO-FIC classifications and serves as a liaison with the WHO, fulfilling international obligations for comparable classifications and the national health data needs of the United States. The historical background of ICD and ICD-10 can be found in the Introduction to the International Classification of Diseases and Related Health Problems (ICD-10), 2010, World Health Organization, Geneva, Switzerland.

ICD-10-CM is the United States' clinical modification of the World Health Organization's ICD-10. The term "clinical" is used to emphasize the modification's intent: to serve as a useful tool in the area of classification of morbidity data for indexing of health records, medical care review, and ambulatory and other health care programs, as well as for basic health statistics. To describe the clinical picture of the patient the codes must be more precise than those needed only for statistical groupings and trend analysis.

Characteristics of ICD-10-CM

ICD-10-CM far exceeds its predecessors in the number of concepts and codes provided. The disease classification has been expanded to include health-related conditions and to provide greater specificity at the sixth and seventh character level. The sixth and seventh characters are not optional and are intended for use in recording the information documented in the clinical record.

ICD-10-CM extensions, interpretations, modifications, addenda, or errata other than those approved by the Centers for Disease Control and Prevention are not to be considered official and should not be utilized. Continuous maintenance of the ICD-10-CM is the responsibility of the aforementioned agencies. However, because the ICD-10-CM represents the best in contemporary thinking of clinicians, nosologists, epidemiologists, and statisticians from both public and private sectors, when future modifications are considered, advice will be sought from all stakeholders.

All official authorized addenda since the last complete update (October 1, 2020) have been included in this revision. For more detailed information please see the complete official authorized addenda to ICD-10-CM, including the "ICD-10-CM Official Guidelines for Coding and Reporting," and a description of the ICD-10-CM updating and maintenance process.

How to Use ICD-10-CM Expert for Hospitals 2021

Introduction

ICD-10-CM Expert for Hospitals: The Complete Official Code Set is your definitive coding resource, combining the work of the National Center for Health Statistics (NCHS), Centers for Medicare and Medicaid Services (CMS), American Hospital Association (AHA), and Optum360 experts to provide the information you need for coding accuracy.

The International Classification of Diseases, 10th Revision, Clinical Modification (ICD-10-CM), is an adaptation of ICD-10, copyrighted by the World Health Organization (WHO). The development and maintenance of this clinical modification (CM) is the responsibility of the NCHS as authorized by WHO. Any new concepts added to ICD-10-CM are based on an established update process through the collaboration of WHO's Update and Revision Committee and the ICD-10-CM Coordination and Maintenance Committee.

In addition to the ICD-10-CM classification, other official government source information has been included in this manual. Depending on the source, updates to information may be annual or quarterly. This manual provides the most current information that was available at the time of publication. For updates to the source documents that may have occurred after this manual was published, please refer to the following:

- **NCHS, International Classification of Diseases, Tenth Revision, Clinical Modification (ICD-10-CM)**

  https://www.cdc.gov/nchs/icd/icd10cm.htm

  https://www.cms.gov/medicare/icd-10/2021-icd-10-cm

- **CMS Inpatient Prospective Payment System Proposed Rule, FY2021**

  https://www.cms.gov/medicare/acute-inpatient-pps/fy-2021-ipps-proposed-rule-home-page

- **CMS Inpatient Prospective Payment System Proposed Rule, FY 2021 — Proposed, version 38, MS-DRG grouper software, Definitions Manual files and Medicare Code Editor (MCE) Files**

  https://www.cms.gov/Medicare/Medicare-Fee-for-Service-Payment/AcuteInpatientPPS/MS-DRG-Classifications-and-Software

- **CMS Risk Adjustment Model, version 24**

  https://www.cms.gov/Medicare/Health-Plans/MedicareAdvtgSpecRateStats/Risk-Adjustors.html

- **CMS Long-term Care Hospital Prospective Payment System Proposed Rule and Data Files, FY 2021**

  https://www.cms.gov/medicaremedicare-fee-service-paymentlongtermcarehospitalppsltchpps-regulations-and-notices/cms-1735-p

- **AHA Coding Clinics**

  https://www.codingclinicadvisor.com/

- **Additional specialty-specific resources will also be provided on our product updates page at Optum360coding.com, which can be accessed at the following:**

  https://www.optum360coding.com/ProductUpdates/

  Password: Hospital21

The official NCHS ICD-10-CM classification includes three main sections: the guidelines, the indexes, and the tabular list, all of which make up the bulk of this coding manual. To complement the classification, Optum360's coding experts have incorporated Medicare-related coding edits and proprietary features, such as supplementary notations, coding tools, and appendixes, into a comprehensive and easy-to-use reference. This publication is organized as follows:

What's New for 2021

This section provides a high-level overview of the changes made to the ICD-10-CM official code set for fiscal 2021, identifying codes that have been added and deleted from the classification, codes that had validity changes as a result of these additions and deletions, as well as codes that had revisions to their descriptions. All changes are based on the 2021 official addendum, posted June 30, 2020, by the National Center for Health Statistics (NCHS), the agency charged with maintaining and updating ICD-10-CM. NCHS is part of the Centers for Disease Control and Prevention (CDC).

Conversion Table

The conversion table was developed by National Center for Healthcare Statistics (NCHS) to help facilitate data retrieval as new codes are added to the ICD-10-CM classification. This table provides a crosswalk from each FY 2021 new code to the equivalent code(s) assigned prior to October 1, 2020, for that particular diagnosis or condition. For the full conversion table, including code crosswalks before October 1, 2020, refer to the 2021 Conversion Table zip file at https://www.cms.gov/medicare/icd-10/2021-icd-10-cm.

10 Steps to Correct Coding

This step-by-step tutorial walks the coder through the process of finding the correct code — from locating the code in the official indexes to verifying the code in the tabular section — while following applicable conventions, guidelines, and instructional notes. Specific examples are provided with detailed explanations of each coding step along with advice for proper sequencing.

Official ICD-10-CM Guidelines for Coding and Reporting

This section provides the full official conventions and guidelines regulating the appropriate assignment and reporting of ICD-10-CM codes. These conventions and guidelines are published by the U.S. Department of Health and Human Services (DHHS) and approved by the cooperating parties (American Health Information Management Association [AHIMA], National Center for Health Statistics [NCHS], Centers for Disease Control and Prevention [CDC], and the American Hospital Association [AHA]).

Indexes

Index to Diseases and Injuries

The Index to Diseases and Injuries is arranged in alphabetic order by terms specific to a disease, condition, illness, injury, eponym, or abbreviation as well as terms that describe circumstances other than a disease or injury that may require attention from a health care professional.

Neoplasm Table

The Neoplasm Table is arranged in alphabetic order by anatomical site. Codes are then listed in individual columns based upon the histological behavior (malignant, in situ, benign, uncertain, or unspecified) of the neoplasm.

Table of Drugs and Chemicals

The Table of Drugs and Chemicals is arranged in alphabetic order by the specific drug or chemical name. Codes are listed in individual columns based upon the associated intent (poisoning, adverse effect, or underdosing).

External Causes Index

The External Causes Index is arranged in alphabetic order by main terms that describe the cause, the intent, the place of occurrence, the activity, and the status of the patient at the time the injury occurred or health condition arose.

Index Notations

With

The word "with" or "in" should be interpreted to mean "associated with" or "due to." The classification presumes a causal relationship between the two conditions linked by these terms in the index. These conditions should be coded as related even in the absence of provider documentation explicitly linking them unless the documentation clearly states the conditions are unrelated or when another guideline specifically requires a documented linkage between two conditions (e.g., the sepsis guideline for "acute organ dysfunction that is not clearly associated with the sepsis"). For conditions not specifically linked by these relational terms in the classification or when a guideline requires explicit documentation of a linkage between two conditions, provider documentation must link the conditions to code them as related.

The word "with" in the index is sequenced immediately following the main term, not in alphabetical order.

> **Dermatopolymyositis** M33.9Ø
>   with
>   myopathy M33.92
>   respiratory involvement M33.91
>   specified organ involvement NEC M33.99
>   in neoplastic disease — *see also* Neoplasm D49.9 *[M36.Ø]*

See

When the instruction "see" follows a term in the index, it indicates that another term must be referenced to locate the correct code.

> **Hematoperitoneum** — *see* Hemoperitoneum

See Also

The instructional note "see also" simply provides alternative terms the coder may reference that may be useful in determining the correct code but are not necessary to follow if the main term supplies the appropriate code.

> **Hematinuria** — *see also* Hemaglobinuria
>   malarial B5Ø.8

Default Codes

In the index, the default code is the code listed next to the main term and represents the condition most commonly associated with that main term. This code may be assigned when documentation does not support reporting a more specific code. Alternatively, it may provide an unspecified code for the condition.

> **Hemiatrophy** R68.89
>   cerebellar G31.9
>   face, facial, progressive (Romberg) G51.8
>   tongue K14.8

Parentheses

Parentheses in the indexes enclose nonessential modifiers, supplementary words that may be present or absent in the statement of a disease without affecting the code.

> **Pseudomeningocele** (cerebral) (infective) (post-traumatic) G96.198
>   postprocedural (spinal) G97.82

Brackets

ICD-10-CM has a coding convention addressing code assignment for manifestations that occur as a result of an underlying condition. This convention requires the underlying condition to be sequenced first, followed by the code or codes for the associated manifestation. In the index, italicized codes in brackets identify manifestation codes.

> **Polyneuropathy** (peripheral) G62.9
>   alcoholic G62.1
>   amyloid (Portuguese) E85.1 *[G63]*
>   transthyretin-related (ATTR) familial E85.1 *[G63]*

Shaded Guides

Exclusive vertical shaded guides in the Index to Diseases and Injuries and External Causes Index help the user easily follow the indent levels for the subentries under a main term. Sequencing rules may apply depending on the level of indent for separate subentries.

> **Hemicrania**
>   congenital malformation QØØ.Ø
>   continua G44.51
>   meaning migraine — *see also* Migraine G43.9Ø9
>   paroxysmal G44.Ø39
>   chronic G44.Ø49
>   intractable G44.Ø41
>   not intractable G44.Ø49
>   episodic G44.Ø39
>   intractable G44.Ø31
>   not intractable G44.Ø39
>   intractable G44.Ø31
>   not intractable G44.Ø39

Following References

The Index to Diseases and Injuries includes following references to assist in locating out-of-sequence codes in the tabular list. Out-of-sequence codes contain an alphabetic character (letter) in the third- or fourth-character position. These codes are placed according to the classification rules — according to condition — not according to alphabetic or numeric sequencing rules.

> **Carcinoma** (malignant) — *see also* Neoplasm, by site, malignant
>   neuroendocrine — *see also* Tumor, neuroendocrine
>   high grade, any site C7A.1 (*following* C75)
>   poorly differentiated, any site C7A.1 (*following* C75)

Additional Character Required

The Index to Diseases and Injuries, Neoplasm Table, and External Causes Index provide an icon after certain codes to signify to the user that additional characters are required to make the code valid. The tabular list should be consulted for appropriate character selection.

> **Fall, falling** (accidental) W19 ☑
>   building W2Ø.1 ☑

Tabular List of Diseases

ICD-10-CM codes and descriptions are arranged numerically within the tabular list of diseases with 19 separate chapters providing codes associated with a particular body system or nature of injury or disease. There is also a chapter providing codes for external causes of an injury or health conditions, a chapter for codes that address encounters with healthcare facilities for circumstances other than a disease or injury, and finally a chapter for codes that capture special circumstances such as new diseases of uncertain etiology or emergency use codes.

Code and Code Descriptions

ICD-10-CM is an alphanumeric classification system that contains categories, subcategories, and valid codes. The first character is always a letter with any additional characters represented by either a letter or number. A three-character category without further subclassification is equivalent to a valid three-character code. Valid codes may be three, four, five, six, or seven characters in length, with each level of subdivision after a three-character category representing a subcategory. The final level of subdivision is a valid code.

Boldface

Boldface type is used for all codes and descriptions in the tabular list.

Italics

Italicized type is used to identify manifestation codes, those codes that should not be reported as first-listed diagnoses.

Deleted Text

~~Strikethrough~~ on a code and code description indicates a deletion from the classification for the current year.

Key Word

Green font is used throughout the Tabular List of Diseases to differentiate the key words that appear in similar code descriptions in a given category or subcategory. The key word convention is used only in those categories in which there are multiple codes with very similar descriptions with only a few words that differentiate them.

For example, refer to the list of codes below from category H55:

✓4ᵗʰ	**H55**	**Nystagmus and other** irregular eye movements
✓5ᵗʰ	**H55.0**	**Nystagmus**
	H55.00	**Unspecified nystagmus**
	H55.01	**Congenital nystagmus**
	H55.02	**Latent nystagmus**
	H55.03	**Visual deprivation nystagmus**
	H55.04	**Dissociated nystagmus**
	H55.09	**Other forms of nystagmus**

The portion of the code description that appears in green font in the tabular list helps the coder quickly identify the key terms and the correct code. This convention is especially useful when the codes describe laterality, such as the following codes from subcategory H40.22:

✓6ᵗʰ	**H40.22**	**Chronic angle-closure glaucoma**
		Chronic primary angle-closure glaucoma
✓7ᵗʰ	**H40.221**	**Chronic angle-closure glaucoma, right eye**
✓7ᵗʰ	**H40.222**	**Chronic angle-closure glaucoma, left eye**
✓7ᵗʰ	**H40.223**	**Chronic angle-closure glaucoma, bilateral**
✓7ᵗʰ	**H40.229**	**Chronic angle-closure glaucoma, unspecified eye**

Tabular Notations

Official parenthetical notes as well as Optum360's supplementary notations are provided at the chapter, code block, category, subcategory, and individual code level to help the user assign proper codes. The information in the notation can apply to one or more codes depending on where the citation is placed.

Official Notations

Includes Notes

The word INCLUDES appears immediately under certain categories to further define, clarify, or give examples of the content of a code category.

Inclusion Terms

Lists of inclusion terms are included under certain codes. These terms indicate some of the conditions for which that code number may be used. Inclusion terms may be synonyms with the code title, or, in the case of "other specified" codes, the terms may also provide a list of various conditions included within a classification code. The inclusion terms are not exhaustive. The index may provide additional terms that may also be assigned to a given code.

Excludes Notes

ICD-10-CM has two types of excludes notes. Each note has a different definition for use. However, they are similar in that they both indicate that codes excluded from each other are independent of each other.

Excludes 1

An EXCLUDES 1 note is a "pure" excludes. It means "NOT CODED HERE!" An Excludes 1 note indicates mutually exclusive codes: two conditions that cannot be reported together. An Excludes1 note indicates that the code excluded should never be used at the same time as the code above the Excludes1 note. An Excludes1 is used when two conditions cannot occur together, such as a congenital form versus an acquired form of the same condition.

An exception to the Excludes 1 definition is when the two conditions are unrelated to each other. If it is not clear whether the two conditions involving an Excludes 1 note are related or not, query the provider. For example, code F45.8 Other somatoform disorders, has an Excludes 1 note for "sleep related teeth grinding (G47.63)" because "teeth grinding" is an inclusion term under F45.8. Only one of these two codes should be assigned for teeth grinding. However, psychogenic dysmenorrhea is also an inclusion term under F45.8, and a patient could have both this condition and sleep-related teeth grinding. In this case, the two conditions are clearly unrelated to each other, so it would be appropriate to report F45.8 and G47.63 together.

Excludes 2

An EXCLUDES 2 note means "NOT INCLUDED HERE." An Excludes 2 note indicates that although the excluded condition is not part of the condition it is excluded from, a patient may have both conditions at the same time. Therefore, when an Excludes 2 note appears under a code, it may be acceptable to use both the code and the excluded code together if supported by the medical documentation.

Note

The term "NOTE" appears as an icon and precedes the instructional information. These notes function as alerts to highlight coding instructions within the text.

Code First/Use additional code

These instructional notes provide sequencing instruction. They may appear independently of each other or to designate certain etiology/manifestation paired codes. These instructions signal the coder that an additional code should be reported to provide a more complete picture of that diagnosis.

In etiology/manifestation coding, ICD-10-CM requires the underlying condition to be sequenced first, followed by the manifestation. In these situations, codes with "In diseases classified elsewhere" in the code description are never permitted as a first-listed or principal diagnosis code and must be sequenced following the underlying condition code.

Code Also

A "code also" note alerts the coder that more than one code may be required to fully describe the condition. The sequencing depends on the circumstances of the encounter. Factors that may determine sequencing include severity and reason for the encounter.

Revised Text

The revised text ►◄ "bow ties" alert the user to changes in official notations for the current year. Revised text may include the following:

- A change in a current parenthetical description

- A change in the code(s) associated with a current parenthetical note

- A change in how a current parenthetical note is classified (e.g., an Excludes 1 note that changed to an Excludes 2 note)

- Addition of a new parenthetical note(s) to a code

Deleted Text

~~Strikethrough~~ on official notations indicate a deletion from the classification for the current year.

Optum360 Notations

AHA Coding Clinic Citations

Coding Clinics are official American Hospital Association (AHA) publications that provide coding advice specific to ICD-10-CM and ICD-10-PCS.

Coding Clinic citations included in this manual are current up to the second quarter of 2020.

These citations identify the year, quarter, and page number of one or more *Coding Clinic* publications that may have coding advice relevant to a particular code or group of codes. With the most current citation listed first, these notations are preceded by the symbol **AHA:** and appear in purple type.

> **I15.1 Hypertension secondary to other renal disorders**
> **AHA:** 2016, 3Q, 22

Definitions

Definitions explain a specific term, condition, or disease process in layman's terms. These notations are preceded by the symbol **DEF:** and appear in purple type.

> ✓5ᵗʰ **M51.4 Schmorl's nodes**
> **DEF:** Irregular bone defect in the margin of the vertebral body that causes herniation into the end plate of the vertebral body.

Coding Tips

The tips in the tabular list offer coding advice that is not readily available within the ICD-10-CM classification. It may relate official coding guidelines, indexing nuances, or advice from *AHA's Coding Clinic for ICD-10-CM/PCS*. These notations are preceded by the symbol **TIP:** and appear in brown type.

> ✓5ᵗʰ **B97.2 Coronavirus as the cause of diseases classified elsewhere**
> **TIP:** Do not report a code from this subcategory for COVID-19; refer to U07.1.

Icons

Note: The following icons are placed to the left of the code.

● **New Code**
    Codes that have been added to the classification system for the current year.

▲ **Revised Code Title**
    Codes that have had a change to their description or validity change for the current year. For additional information on codes with validity changes, see the "What's New" section.

☑ **Additional Characters Required**

    ✓4ᵗʰ This symbol indicates that the code requires a 4th character.

    ✓5ᵗʰ This symbol indicates that the code requires a 5th character.

    ✓6ᵗʰ This symbol indicates that the code requires a 6th character.

    ✓7ᵗʰ This symbol indicates that the code requires a 7th character.

> ✓5ᵗʰ **H60.3 Other infective otitis externa**
>   ✓6ᵗʰ **H60.31 Diffuse otitis externa**
>   **H60.311 Diffuse otitis externa, right ear**
>   **H60.312 Diffuse otitis externa, left ear**
>   **H60.313 Diffuse otitis externa, bilateral**
>   **H60.319 Diffuse otitis externa, unspecified ear**

✓x7ᵗʰ **Placeholder Alert**

This symbol indicates that the code requires a 7th character following the placeholder "X". Codes with fewer than six characters that require a 7th character must contain placeholder "X" to fill in the empty character(s).

> ✓x7ᵗʰ **T16.1 Foreign body in right ear**

This manual provides the most current information that was available at the time of publication. Except where otherwise noted, the icons and/or color bars reflect edits associated with the inpatient prospective payment system (IPPS). Because the fiscal 2021 IPPS final rule was not available at the time this book was printed, the edits in this manual are based on the proposed, version 38, MS-DRG grouper software, Definitions Manual files, and Medicare Code Editor (MCE) files, published with the fiscal 2021 IPPS proposed rule.

In an effort to provide the most current edit information, Optum360 has provided a searchable data file that includes the final edit designations for all ICD-10-CM codes based on the fiscal 2021 IPPS final rule official files, effective October 1, 2020. The edits included in the data file are as follows:

- Age

- Sex

- Hospital-acquired condition (HAC)

- CC

- MCC

- HIV

- Manifestation code

- Unacceptable diagnosis

- Questionable diagnosis

This data file can be accessed at the following:

https://www.optum360coding.com/ProductUpdates/
Title: "2021 ICD-10-CM for Hospital IPPS Data File"
Password: Hospital21

Note: The following icons are placed at the end of the code description.

Age Edits

Ⓝ **Newborn Age: 0**
    These diagnoses are intended for newborns and neonates and the patient's age must be 0 years.

> **N47.0 Adherent prepuce, newborn**   Ⓝ♂

Ⓟ **Pediatric Age: 0-17**
    These diagnoses are intended for children and the patient's age must be between 0 and 17 years.

> **L21.1 Seborrheic infantile dermatitis**   Ⓟ

M Maternity Age: 9-64

These diagnoses are intended for childbearing patients between the age of 9 and 64 years.

| O02.9 | Abnormal product of conception, unspecified | M ♀ |

A Adult Age: 15-124

These diagnoses are intended for patients between the age of 15 and 124 years.

R54	Age-related physical debility	A
	Frailty	
	Old age	
	Senescence	
	Senile asthenia	
	Senile debility	
	EXCLUDES 1 age-related cognitive decline (R41.81)	
	sarcopenia (M62.84)	
	senile psychosis (F03)	
	senility NOS (R41.81)	

Sex Edits

♂ **Male diagnosis only**

| Q98.0 | Klinefelter syndrome karyotype 47, XXY | ♂ |

♀ **Female diagnosis only**

| N35.12 | Postinfective urethral stricture, not elsewhere classified, female | ♀ |

H1 - H14 Hospital Acquired Condition (HAC)

These codes identify conditions that are high cost or high volume or both, are either a complication or comorbidity (CC) or major complication or comorbidity (MCC) that as a secondary diagnosis results in assignment of a case to a higher-paying MS-DRG. These conditions are reasonably preventable through the application of evidence-based guidelines. If the condition is not present on admission (meaning it developed during the hospital admission), the case will not group to the higher-paying MS-DRG based solely upon the reporting of the HAC code. Many of these HACs are conditional, and are based on reporting the specific diagnosis code(s) in combination with certain procedure codes.

Note: Hospital-acquired conditions do not impact MS-LTC-DRG assignment.

The comprehensive list of HAC tables that coincide with these icon numbers appears in appendix G of this book.

| N15.1 | Renal and perinephric abscess | MCC H6 |

CC CC Condition

This symbol designates a complication or comorbidity diagnosis that may affect DRG assignment. A complication or comorbidity diagnosis, CC condition, is defined as a significant acute disease, a significant acute manifestation of a chronic disease, an advanced or end-stage chronic disease, or a chronic disease associated with systemic physiological decompensation and debility that have consistently greater impact on hospital resources.

A comprehensive list of ICD-10-CM codes considered a CC appears in appendix E of this book.

| G90.59 | Complex regional pain syndrome I of other specified site | CC |

MCC MCC Condition

This symbol designates a major complication or comorbidity diagnosis that may affect DRG assignment. An MCC condition meets the same criteria as a CC condition but is associated with a higher acuity level and hospital resource consumption is expected to be higher than that for a CC condition. There are fewer conditions that meet the criteria as an MCC than those for a CC condition.

A comprehensive list of ICD-10-CM codes considered an MCC appears in appendix D of this book.

| ✓7ᵗʰ S35.238 | Other injury of inferior mesenteric artery | MCC |

Note: The assignment of an MS-DRG or MS-LTC-DRG often depends on the presence or absence of a secondary diagnosis code that is designated as an MCC or CC. However, in some instances the MCC or CC designation for that secondary diagnosis code is negated due to its relationship with the principal diagnosis; this is referred to as CC exclusion. The ICD-10 MS-DRG Definitions Manual included with the IPPS final rule provides a list of all principal diagnosis codes that would render ineffective the MCC/CC designation for a particular ICD-10-CM code when used as a secondary diagnosis. Optum360 has provided this CC exclusion list in an easily searchable data file, which can be accessed at the following:

https://www.optum360coding.com/ProductUpdates/
Title: "2021 ICD-10-CM for Hospitals CC Excludes Data File"
Password: Hospital21

HIV HIV-related Condition

This symbol indicates that the condition is considered a major HIV-related diagnosis. When the condition is coded in combination with a diagnosis of human immunodeficiency virus (HIV), code B20, the case will move from MS-DRG/MS-LTC-DRG 977 to MS-DRGs/MS-LTC-DRGs 974-976.

| G96.9 | Disorder of central nervous system, unspecified | HIV |

HCC CMS-HCC Condition

Identify conditions that are considered a CMS-HCC (hierarchical condition category) diagnosis.

The HCC codes represented in this manual have been updated to reflect the 2021 Initial ICD-10-CM Mappings for CMS-HCC Model v24. Midyear final mappings were not available at the time this publication went to print; refer to the following CMS website for final mappings: https://www.cms.gov/Medicare/Health-Plans/MedicareAdvtgSpecRateStats/Risk-Adjustors.html.

| Y62.2 | Failure of sterile precautions during kidney dialysis and other perfusion | HCC |

SW Severe Wound Diagnosis

This symbol indicates that the condition is considered a severe wound diagnosis. Depending on the facility from which the patient is discharged, these conditions may not require that the payment rate for that admission be adjusted.

A comprehensive list of ICD-10-CM codes considered a severe wound diagnosis appears in appendix K of this book.

| L89.014 | Pressure ulcer of right elbow, stage 4 | MCC H4 HCC SW |

Color Bars

Manifestation Code

Codes defined as manifestation codes appear in italic type, with a blue color bar over the code description. A manifestation cannot be reported as a first-listed code; it is sequenced as a secondary diagnosis with the underlying disease code listed first.

> **G32.89** *Other specified degenerative disorders of nervous system in diseases classified elsewhere*
> Degenerative encephalopathy in diseases classified elsewhere

Unacceptable Principal Diagnoses

Unacceptable principal diagnoses will appear with a purple color bar over the code description. These codes do not describe a current illness or injury, but a circumstance which influences a patient's health status. They are considered an unacceptable principal diagnosis for *inpatient* admission.

> ✓7ᵗʰ **T48.5X5** Adverse effect of other anti-common-cold drugs

Questionable Admission Diagnoses

Questionable admission diagnoses will appear with a yellow color bar over the code description. These codes, although not unacceptable as a PDx, may be considered a "questionable admission" when used as PDx in an acute care hospital.

> **E66.09** Other obesity due to excess calories

Wrong Procedure Performed Edit

An orange color bar over the code title indicates the Wrong Procedure Performed edit. This edit was created to identify cases in which wrong surgeries occurred. Any claim with a code from Y65.51-Y65.53 will be denied and returned to the provider. A surgical or other invasive procedure is considered to be a wrong procedure if one of the following is true:

- The procedure was performed on the wrong site.

- The procedure was performed on the wrong patient.

- The incorrect procedure was performed on a patient.

> **Y65.51** Performance of wrong procedure (operation) on correct patient
> Wrong device implanted into correct surgical site
> **EXCLUDES 1** *performance of correct procedure (operation) on wrong side or body part (Y65.53)*

Unspecified Diagnosis

Codes that appear with a gray color bar over the alphanumeric code identify unspecified diagnoses. These codes should be used in limited circumstances, when neither the diagnostic statement nor the documentation provides enough information to assign a more specific diagnosis code. The abbreviation NOS, "not otherwise specified," in the tabular list may be interpreted as "unspecified."

> **G03.9** Meningitis, unspecified   **MCC**
> Arachnoiditis (spinal) NOS

Footnotes

Certain codes in the tabular section have a numerical superscript located to the upper left of the code. This numerical superscript corresponds to a specific footnote description.

For example:

> [1] **R57.1** Hypovolemic shock   **MCC** **HCC**

For convenience, the footnote descriptions are provided on the front cover.

The following list also provides the footnote descriptions of all numerical superscripts found in the Tabular List of Diseases:

1 These codes are considered major complication/comorbidity (MCC) conditions only if the patient is discharged alive.

2 This condition is considered an MCC only when reported as an initial encounter for an open fracture (7th character B or C specific to category).

3 This condition is considered a CC only when reported as an initial encounter for a fracture (7th character A, B, or C specific to category) or a subsequent encounter for nonunion or malunion fracture (7th character K, M, N, P, Q, or R specific to category).

4 This condition is considered a CC only when reported as a subsequent encounter for a nonunion or malunion fracture (7th character K, M, N, P, Q, or R specific to category).

5 This condition is considered a CC only when reported as an initial encounter or subsequent encounter (7th character A or D).

6 This condition is considered an HCC when reported as initial encounter (7th character A, B, or C specific to category).

7 This condition is considered an HCC when reported as initial encounter (7th character A or B specific to category) or as a sequela.

8 This condition is considered an HCC when reported as a sequela.

Chapter-Level Notations

Chapter-Specific Guidelines with Coding Examples

Each chapter begins with the Official Guidelines for Coding and Reporting specific to that chapter, where provided. Coding examples specific to inpatient care settings have been provided to illustrate the coding and/or sequencing guidance in these guidelines.

Muscle and Tendon Table

ICD-10-CM categorizes certain muscles and tendons in the upper and lower extremities by their action (e.g., extension or flexion) as well as their anatomical location. The Muscle/Tendon table is provided at the beginning of chapter 13 and chapter 19 to help users when code selection depends on the action of the muscle and/or tendon.

Note: This table is not all-inclusive, and proper code assignment should be based on the provider's documentation.

Appendixes

The additional resources described below have been included as appendixes for the *ICD-10-CM Expert for Hospitals*. These resources further instruct the professional coder on the appropriate application of the ICD-10-CM code set.

Appendix A: Valid 3-character ICD-10-CM Codes

The user may consult this table to confirm that no further specificity, such as the use of 4th, 5th, 6th, or 7th characters or placeholders (X), is necessary. All ICD-10-CM codes that are valid at the three-character level are listed.

Appendix B: Pharmacology List 2021

This reference is a comprehensive but not all-inclusive list of pharmacological agents used to treat acute and/or chronic conditions. Drugs are listed in alphabetical order by their brand and/or generic names along with their drug action and indications for which they may commonly be prescribed. Some drugs have also been mapped to their appropriate long-term drug use Z code.

Appendix C: Z Codes for Long-Term Drug Use with Associated Drugs

This resource correlates Z codes that are used to identify current long-term drug use with a list of drugs that are typically categorized to that class of drug.

Note: These tables are not all-inclusive but list some of the more commonly used drugs.

Appendix D: Major Complication and Comorbidity (MCC) Code List

This is a full listing of conditions considered to be major complications and/or comorbidities that when present as a secondary diagnosis may affect DRG assignment under the Medicare Severity DRG (MS-DRG) system.

Note: This resource provides the most current MCC information that was available at the time of publication using the proposed, version 38, MS-DRG grouper software and Definitions Manual files published with the fiscal 2021 IPPS proposed rule.

Appendix E: Complication and Comorbidity (CC) Code List

This is a full listing of conditions considered to be complications and/or comorbidities that when present as a secondary diagnosis may affect DRG assignment under the MS-DRG system.

Note: This resource provides the most current CC information that was available at the time of publication using the proposed, version 38, MS-DRG Grouper software and Definitions Manual files published with the fiscal 2021 IPPS proposed rule.

Appendix F: Present on Admission (POA) Tutorial

This tutorial walks the coder through the process of assigning the appropriate present-on-admission (POA) indicator for inpatient codes based on the POA reporting guidelines. Detailed scenarios for a variety of situations are provided and discussed.

Appendix G: Hospital Acquired Conditions

This comprehensive table displays codes that identify conditions that are considered reasonably preventable when occurring during the hospital admission and may prevent the case from grouping to a higher-paying MS-DRG. Many of these HACs are conditional and are based on reporting the specific diagnosis code(s) in combination with certain procedure codes, which are also noted in this table.

Note: This resource provides the most current HAC information that was available at the time of publication using the proposed, version 38, MS-DRG Grouper software and Definitions Manual files published with the fiscal 2021 IPPS proposed rule.

Appendix H: Centers for Medicare & Medicaid Services (CMS) Hierarchical Condition Categories (HCC) (CMS-HCC)

This resource provides the framework behind CMS's Medicare Advantage (MA) program, a risk-adjustment model developed as a means of compensating health care plans with large numbers of Medicare Part C beneficiaries. It includes a brief synopsis of the evolution of the program from its inception; insight into the various elements needed to predict risk, including the principles used to develop the hierarchical condition categories (HCCs), one of the fundamental components of the risk adjustment model; and a description of the audit process used to ensure the accuracy of payments made to MA plans.

Appendix I: Long-term Care Hospital Prospective Payment System Overview

The long-term care hospital prospective payment system (LTCH PPS) provides payment rates for LTCH facilities certified by Medicare as LTCH with an average length of stay (LOS) of 25 days or longer. This resource summarizes the certification qualifications for LTCH facilities, payment methodology, and current fiscal year PPS updates.

Appendix J: Long-Term Care Hospital Quality Reporting Program

The LTCH QRP is a mandatory reporting component for LTCH facilities certified by Medicare as LTCH with an average LOS of 25 days or longer. Much of the current QRP for LTCH, like other post-acute care providers, is based upon the requirements of the 2014 IMPACT Act. This resource summarizes the current QRP requirements for facilities certified as LTCH under Medicare, including required data set items and market-basket payment impact.

Appendix K: Severe Wound Diagnosis Codes by Category

This resource includes a full listing of codes identified as severe wound diagnoses that may allow certain discharges from LTCHs a temporary exception from the site-neutral payment rate.

Illustrations

This section includes illustrations of normal anatomy with ICD-10-CM-specific terminology.

What's New for 2021

Official Updates

The official ICD-10-CM addendum identifies changes to the ICD-10-CM code set for fiscal 2021, effective October 1, 2020, to September 30, 2021. These changes were made by the agency charged with maintaining and updating the ICD-10-CM code set, the National Center for Health Statistics (NCHS), a section of the Centers for Disease Control and Prevention (CDC). A summary of the changes is provided below:

39 Codes with a Change in Validity

Note: Validity changes are the result of codes being added to or deleted from the classification. Codes that change from valid to invalid allow the creation of a new subcategory to which new codes can be assigned that provide greater detail about the condition. Codes that change from invalid to valid are the result of codes being deleted from a subcategory in the classification, when the detail provided in those codes is no longer required.

Valid to Invalid

A84.8	B60.0	D59.1	D72.1	D84.8	E70.8	E74.8
G11.1	G71.2	G96.0	G96.19	G96.8	H18.50	H18.51
H18.52	H18.53	H18.54	H18.55	H18.59	J82	J84.17
K20.8	K20.9	K21.0	K59.8	K74.0	M92.50	M92.51
M92.52	N18.3	O99.89	R51	R74.0	T86.840	T86.841
T86.842	T86.848	T86.849	Y77.1			

Invalid to Valid
No applicable codes

19 Codes Deleted from the Classification

Q51.20	Other doubling of uterus, unspecified
T40.4X1A	Poisoning by other synthetic narcotics, accidental (unintentional), initial encounter
T40.4X1D	Poisoning by other synthetic narcotics, accidental (unintentional), subsequent encounter
T40.4X1S	Poisoning by other synthetic narcotics, accidental (unintentional), sequela
T40.4X2A	Poisoning by other synthetic narcotics, intentional self-harm, initial encounter
T40.4X2D	Poisoning by other synthetic narcotics, intentional self-harm, subsequent encounter
T40.4X2S	Poisoning by other synthetic narcotics, intentional self-harm, sequela
T40.4X3A	Poisoning by other synthetic narcotics, assault, initial encounter
T40.4X3D	Poisoning by other synthetic narcotics, assault, subsequent encounter
T40.4X3S	Poisoning by other synthetic narcotics, assault, sequela
T40.4X4A	Poisoning by other synthetic narcotics, undetermined, initial encounter
T40.4X4D	Poisoning by other synthetic narcotics, undetermined, subsequent encounter
T40.4X4S	Poisoning by other synthetic narcotics, undetermined, sequela
T40.4X5A	Adverse effect of other synthetic narcotics, initial encounter
T40.4X5D	Adverse effect of other synthetic narcotics, subsequent encounter
T40.4X5S	Adverse effect of other synthetic narcotics, sequela
T40.4X6A	Underdosing of other synthetic narcotics, initial encounter
T40.4X6D	Underdosing of other synthetic narcotics, subsequent encounter
T40.4X6S	Underdosing of other synthetic narcotics, sequela

490 New Codes Added to the Classification

A84.81	Powassan virus disease
A84.89	Other tick-borne viral encephalitis
B60.00	Babesiosis, unspecified
B60.01	Babesiosis due to Babesia microti
B60.02	Babesiosis due to Babesia duncani
B60.03	Babesiosis due to Babesia divergens
B60.09	Other babesiosis
D57.03	Hb-SS disease with cerebral vascular involvement
D57.09	Hb-SS disease with crisis with other specified complication
D57.213	Sickle-cell/Hb-C disease with cerebral vascular involvement
D57.218	Sickle-cell/Hb-C disease with crisis with other specified complication
D57.413	Sickle-cell thalassemia, unspecified, with cerebral vascular involvement
D57.418	Sickle-cell thalassemia, unspecified, with crisis with other specified complication
D57.42	Sickle-cell-thalassemia beta zero without crisis
D57.431	Sickle-cell thalassemia beta zero with acute chest syndrome
D57.432	Sickle-cell thalassemia beta zero with splenic sequestration
D57.433	Sickle-cell thalassemia beta zero with cerebral vascular involvement
D57.438	Sickle-cell thalassemia beta zero with crisis with other specified complication
D57.439	Sickle-cell thalassemia beta zero with crisis, unspecified
D57.44	Sickle-cell thalassemia beta plus without crisis
D57.451	Sickle-cell thalassemia beta plus with acute chest syndrome
D57.452	Sickle-cell thalassemia beta plus with splenic sequestration
D57.453	Sickle-cell thalassemia beta plus with cerebral vascular involvement
D57.458	Sickle-cell thalassemia beta plus with crisis with other specified complication
D57.459	Sickle-cell thalassemia beta plus with crisis, unspecified
D57.813	Other sickle-cell disorders with cerebral vascular involvement
D57.818	Other sickle-cell disorders with crisis with other specified complication
D59.10	Autoimmune hemolytic anemia, unspecified
D59.11	Warm autoimmune hemolytic anemia
D59.12	Cold autoimmune hemolytic anemia
D59.13	Mixed type autoimmune hemolytic anemia
D59.19	Other autoimmune hemolytic anemia
D72.10	Eosinophilia, unspecified
D72.110	Idiopathic hypereosinophilic syndrome [IHES]
D72.111	Lymphocytic Variant Hypereosinophilic Syndrome [LHES]

D72.118	Other hypereosinophilic syndrome
D72.119	Hypereosinophilic syndrome [HES], unspecified
D72.12	Drug rash with eosinophilia and systemic symptoms syndrome
D72.18	Eosinophilia in diseases classified elsewhere
D72.19	Other eosinophilia
D84.81	Immunodeficiency due to conditions classified elsewhere
D84.821	Immunodeficiency due to drugs
D84.822	Immunodeficiency due to external causes
D84.89	Other immunodeficiencies
D89.831	Cytokine release syndrome, grade 1
D89.832	Cytokine release syndrome, grade 2
D89.833	Cytokine release syndrome, grade 3
D89.834	Cytokine release syndrome, grade 4
D89.835	Cytokine release syndrome, grade 5
D89.839	Cytokine release syndrome, grade unspecified
E70.81	Aromatic L-amino acid decarboxylase deficiency
E70.89	Other disorders of aromatic amino-acid metabolism
E74.810	Glucose transporter protein type 1 deficiency
E74.818	Other disorders of glucose transport
E74.819	Disorders of glucose transport, unspecified
E74.89	Other specified disorders of carbohydrate metabolism
F10.130	Alcohol abuse with withdrawal, uncomplicated
F10.131	Alcohol abuse with withdrawal delirium
F10.132	Alcohol abuse with withdrawal with perceptual disturbance
F10.139	Alcohol abuse with withdrawal, unspecified
F10.930	Alcohol use, unspecified with withdrawal, uncomplicated
F10.931	Alcohol use, unspecified with withdrawal delirium
F10.932	Alcohol use, unspecified with withdrawal with perceptual disturbance
F10.939	Alcohol use, unspecified with withdrawal, unspecified
F11.13	Opioid abuse with withdrawal
F12.13	Cannabis abuse with withdrawal
F13.130	Sedative, hypnotic or anxiolytic abuse with withdrawal, uncomplicated
F13.131	Sedative, hypnotic or anxiolytic abuse with withdrawal delirium
F13.132	Sedative, hypnotic or anxiolytic abuse with withdrawal with perceptual disturbance
F13.139	Sedative, hypnotic or anxiolytic abuse with withdrawal, unspecified
F14.13	Cocaine abuse, unspecified with withdrawal
F14.93	Cocaine use, unspecified with withdrawal
F15.13	Other stimulant abuse with withdrawal
F19.130	Other psychoactive substance abuse with withdrawal, uncomplicated
F19.131	Other psychoactive substance abuse with withdrawal delirium
F19.132	Other psychoactive substance abuse with withdrawal with perceptual disturbance
F19.139	Other psychoactive substance abuse with withdrawal, unspecified
G11.10	Early-onset cerebellar ataxia, unspecified
G11.11	Friedreich ataxia
G11.19	Other early-onset cerebellar ataxia
G40.42	Cyclin-Dependent Kinase-Like 5 Deficiency Disorder
G40.833	Dravet syndrome, intractable, with status epilepticus
G40.834	Dravet syndrome, intractable, without status epilepticus
G71.20	Congenital myopathy, unspecified
G71.21	Nemaline myopathy
G71.220	X-linked myotubular myopathy
G71.228	Other centronuclear myopathy
G71.29	Other congenital myopathy
G96.00	Cerebrospinal fluid leak, unspecified
G96.01	Cranial cerebrospinal fluid leak, spontaneous
G96.02	Spinal cerebrospinal fluid leak, spontaneous
G96.08	Other cranial cerebrospinal fluid leak
G96.09	Other spinal cerebrospinal fluid leak
G96.191	Perineural cyst
G96.198	Other disorders of meninges, not elsewhere classified
G96.810	Intracranial hypotension, unspecified
G96.811	Intracranial hypotension, spontaneous
G96.819	Other intracranial hypotension
G96.89	Other specified disorders of central nervous system
G97.83	Intracranial hypotension following lumbar cerebrospinal fluid shunting
G97.84	Intracranial hypotension following other procedure
H18.501	Unspecified hereditary corneal dystrophies, right eye
H18.502	Unspecified hereditary corneal dystrophies, left eye
H18.503	Unspecified hereditary corneal dystrophies, bilateral
H18.509	Unspecified hereditary corneal dystrophies, unspecified eye
H18.511	Endothelial corneal dystrophy, right eye
H18.512	Endothelial corneal dystrophy, left eye
H18.513	Endothelial corneal dystrophy, bilateral
H18.519	Endothelial corneal dystrophy, unspecified eye
H18.521	Epithelial (juvenile) corneal dystrophy, right eye
H18.522	Epithelial (juvenile) corneal dystrophy, left eye
H18.523	Epithelial (juvenile) corneal dystrophy, bilateral
H18.529	Epithelial (juvenile) corneal dystrophy, unspecified eye
H18.531	Granular corneal dystrophy, right eye
H18.532	Granular corneal dystrophy, left eye
H18.533	Granular corneal dystrophy, bilateral
H18.539	Granular corneal dystrophy, unspecified eye
H18.541	Lattice corneal dystrophy, right eye
H18.542	Lattice corneal dystrophy, left eye
H18.543	Lattice corneal dystrophy, bilateral
H18.549	Lattice corneal dystrophy, unspecified eye
H18.551	Macular corneal dystrophy, right eye
H18.552	Macular corneal dystrophy, left eye
H18.553	Macular corneal dystrophy, bilateral
H18.559	Macular corneal dystrophy, unspecified eye
H18.591	Other hereditary corneal dystrophies, right eye
H18.592	Other hereditary corneal dystrophies, left eye
H18.593	Other hereditary corneal dystrophies, bilateral
H18.599	Other hereditary corneal dystrophies, unspecified eye
H55.82	Deficient smooth pursuit eye movements

J82.81	Chronic eosinophilic pneumonia
J82.82	Acute eosinophilic pneumonia
J82.83	Eosinophilic asthma
J82.89	Other pulmonary eosinophilia, not elsewhere classified
J84.17Ø	Interstitial lung disease with progressive fibrotic phenotype in diseases classified elsewhere
J84.178	Other interstitial pulmonary diseases with fibrosis in diseases classified elsewhere
K2Ø.8Ø	Other esophagitis without bleeding
K2Ø.81	Other esophagitis with bleeding
K2Ø.9Ø	Esophagitis, unspecified without bleeding
K2Ø.91	Esophagitis, unspecified with bleeding
K21.ØØ	Gastro-esophageal reflux disease with esophagitis, without bleeding
K21.Ø1	Gastro-esophageal reflux disease with esophagitis, with bleeding
K59.81	Ogilvie syndrome
K59.89	Other specified functional intestinal disorders
K74.ØØ	Hepatic fibrosis, unspecified
K74.Ø1	Hepatic fibrosis, early fibrosis
K74.Ø2	Hepatic fibrosis, advanced fibrosis
MØ5.7A	Rheumatoid arthritis with rheumatoid factor of other specified site without organ or systems involvement
MØ5.8A	Other rheumatoid arthritis with rheumatoid factor of other specified site
MØ6.ØA	Rheumatoid arthritis without rheumatoid factor, other specified site
MØ6.8A	Other specified rheumatoid arthritis, other specified site
MØ8.ØA	Unspecified juvenile rheumatoid arthritis, other specified site
MØ8.2A	Juvenile rheumatoid arthritis with systemic onset, other specified site
MØ8.4A	Pauciarticular juvenile rheumatoid arthritis, other specified site
MØ8.9A	Juvenile arthritis, unspecified, other specified site
M19.Ø9	Primary osteoarthritis, other specified site
M19.19	Post-traumatic osteoarthritis, other specified site
M19.29	Secondary osteoarthritis, other specified site
M24.19	Other articular cartilage disorders, other specified site
M24.29	Disorder of ligament, other specified site
M24.39	Pathological dislocation of other specified joint, not elsewhere classified
M24.49	Recurrent dislocation, other specified joint
M24.59	Contracture, other specified joint
M24.69	Ankylosis, other specified joint
M24.89	Other specific joint derangement of other specified joint, not elsewhere classified
M25.39	Other instability, other specified joint
M25.59	Pain in other specified joint
M25.69	Stiffness of other specified joint, not elsewhere classified
M26.641	Arthritis of right temporomandibular joint
M26.642	Arthritis of left temporomandibular joint
M26.643	Arthritis of bilateral temporomandibular joint
M26.649	Arthritis of unspecified temporomandibular joint
M26.651	Arthropathy of right temporomandibular joint

M26.652	Arthropathy of left temporomandibular joint
M26.653	Arthropathy of bilateral temporomandibular joint
M26.659	Arthropathy of unspecified temporomandibular joint
M8Ø.ØAXA	Age-related osteoporosis with current pathological fracture, other site, initial encounter for fracture
M8Ø.ØAXD	Age-related osteoporosis with current pathological fracture, other site, subsequent encounter for fracture with routine healing
M8Ø.ØAXG	Age-related osteoporosis with current pathological fracture, other site, subsequent encounter for fracture with delayed healing
M8Ø.ØAXK	Age-related osteoporosis with current pathological fracture, other site, subsequent encounter for fracture with nonunion
M8Ø.ØAXP	Age-related osteoporosis with current pathological fracture, other site, subsequent encounter for fracture with malunion
M8Ø.ØAXS	Age-related osteoporosis with current pathological fracture, other site, sequela
M8Ø.8AXA	Other osteoporosis with current pathological fracture, other site, initial encounter for fracture
M8Ø.8AXD	Other osteoporosis with current pathological fracture, other site, subsequent encounter for fracture with routine healing
M8Ø.8AXG	Other osteoporosis with current pathological fracture, other site, subsequent encounter for fracture with delayed healing
M8Ø.8AXK	Other osteoporosis with current pathological fracture, other site, subsequent encounter for fracture with nonunion
M8Ø.8AXP	Other osteoporosis with current pathological fracture, other site, subsequent encounter for fracture with malunion
M8Ø.8AXS	Other osteoporosis with current pathological fracture, other site, sequela
M92.5Ø1	Unspecified juvenile osteochondrosis, right leg
M92.5Ø2	Unspecified juvenile osteochondrosis, left leg
M92.5Ø3	Unspecified juvenile osteochondrosis, bilateral leg
M92.5Ø9	Unspecified juvenile osteochondrosis, unspecified leg
M92.511	Juvenile osteochondrosis of proximal tibia, right leg
M92.512	Juvenile osteochondrosis of proximal tibia, left leg
M92.513	Juvenile osteochondrosis of proximal tibia, bilateral
M92.519	Juvenile osteochondrosis of proximal tibia, unspecified leg
M92.521	Juvenile osteochondrosis of tibia tubercle, right leg
M92.522	Juvenile osteochondrosis of tibia tubercle, left leg
M92.523	Juvenile osteochondrosis of tibia tubercle, bilateral
M92.529	Juvenile osteochondrosis of tibia tubercle, unspecified leg
M92.591	Other juvenile osteochondrosis of tibia and fibula, right leg
M92.592	Other juvenile osteochondrosis of tibia and fibula, left leg
M92.593	Other juvenile osteochondrosis of tibia and fibula, bilateral
M92.599	Other juvenile osteochondrosis of tibia and fibula, unspecified leg
NØØ.A	Acute nephritic syndrome with C3 glomerulonephritis
NØ1.A	Rapidly progressive nephritic syndrome with C3 glomerulonephritis
NØ2.A	Recurrent and persistent hematuria with C3 glomerulonephritis

Code	Description
N03.A	Chronic nephritic syndrome with C3 glomerulonephritis
N04.A	Nephrotic syndrome with C3 glomerulonephritis
N05.A	Unspecified nephritic syndrome with C3 glomerulonephritis
N06.A	Isolated proteinuria with C3 glomerulonephritis
N07.A	Hereditary nephropathy, not elsewhere classified with C3 glomerulonephritis
N18.30	Chronic kidney disease, stage 3 unspecified
N18.31	Chronic kidney disease, stage 3a
N18.32	Chronic kidney disease, stage 3b
N61.20	Granulomatous mastitis, unspecified breast
N61.21	Granulomatous mastitis, right breast
N61.22	Granulomatous mastitis, left breast
N61.23	Granulomatous mastitis, bilateral breast
O34.218	Maternal care for other type scar from previous cesarean delivery
O34.22	Maternal care for cesarean scar defect (isthmocele)
O99.891	Other specified diseases and conditions complicating pregnancy
O99.892	Other specified diseases and conditions complicating childbirth
O99.893	Other specified diseases and conditions complicating puerperium
P91.821	Neonatal cerebral infarction, right side of brain
P91.822	Neonatal cerebral infarction, left side of brain
P91.823	Neonatal cerebral infarction, bilateral
P91.829	Neonatal cerebral infarction, unspecified side
R51.0	Headache with orthostatic component, not elsewhere classified
R51.9	Headache, unspecified
R74.01	Elevation of levels of liver transaminase levels
R74.02	Elevation of levels of lactic acid dehydrogenase [LDH]
S20.213A	Contusion of bilateral front wall of thorax, initial encounter
S20.213D	Contusion of bilateral front wall of thorax, subsequent encounter
S20.213S	Contusion of bilateral front wall of thorax, sequela
S20.214A	Contusion of middle front wall of thorax, initial encounter
S20.214D	Contusion of middle front wall of thorax, subsequent encounter
S20.214S	Contusion of middle front wall of thorax, sequela
S20.223A	Contusion of bilateral back wall of thorax, initial encounter
S20.223D	Contusion of bilateral back wall of thorax, subsequent encounter
S20.223S	Contusion of bilateral back wall of thorax, sequela
S20.224A	Contusion of middle back wall of thorax, initial encounter
S20.224D	Contusion of middle back wall of thorax, subsequent encounter
S20.224S	Contusion of middle back wall of thorax, sequela
S20.303A	Unspecified superficial injuries of bilateral front wall of thorax, initial encounter
S20.303D	Unspecified superficial injuries of bilateral front wall of thorax, subsequent encounter
S20.303S	Unspecified superficial injuries of bilateral front wall of thorax, sequela
S20.304A	Unspecified superficial injuries of middle front wall of thorax, initial encounter
S20.304D	Unspecified superficial injuries of middle front wall of thorax, subsequent encounter
S20.304S	Unspecified superficial injuries of middle front wall of thorax, sequela
S20.313A	Abrasion of bilateral front wall of thorax, initial encounter
S20.313D	Abrasion of bilateral front wall of thorax, subsequent encounter
S20.313S	Abrasion of bilateral front wall of thorax, sequela
S20.314A	Abrasion of middle front wall of thorax, initial encounter
S20.314D	Abrasion of middle front wall of thorax, subsequent encounter
S20.314S	Abrasion of middle front wall of thorax, sequela
S20.323A	Blister (nonthermal) of bilateral front wall of thorax, initial encounter
S20.323D	Blister (nonthermal) of bilateral front wall of thorax, subsequent encounter
S20.323S	Blister (nonthermal) of bilateral front wall of thorax, sequela
S20.324A	Blister (nonthermal) of middle front wall of thorax, initial encounter
S20.324D	Blister (nonthermal) of middle front wall of thorax, subsequent encounter
S20.324S	Blister (nonthermal) of middle front wall of thorax, sequela
S20.343A	External constriction of bilateral front wall of thorax, initial encounter
S20.343D	External constriction of bilateral front wall of thorax, subsequent encounter
S20.343S	External constriction of bilateral front wall of thorax, sequela
S20.344A	External constriction of middle front wall of thorax, initial encounter
S20.344D	External constriction of middle front wall of thorax, subsequent encounter
S20.344S	External constriction of middle front wall of thorax, sequela
S20.353A	Superficial foreign body of bilateral front wall of thorax, initial encounter
S20.353D	Superficial foreign body of bilateral front wall of thorax, subsequent encounter
S20.353S	Superficial foreign body of bilateral front wall of thorax, sequela
S20.354A	Superficial foreign body of middle front wall of thorax, initial encounter
S20.354D	Superficial foreign body of middle front wall of thorax, subsequent encounter
S20.354S	Superficial foreign body of middle front wall of thorax, sequela
S20.363A	Insect bite (nonvenomous) of bilateral front wall of thorax, initial encounter
S20.363D	Insect bite (nonvenomous) of bilateral front wall of thorax, subsequent encounter
S20.363S	Insect bite (nonvenomous) of bilateral front wall of thorax, sequela
S20.364A	Insect bite (nonvenomous) of middle front wall of thorax, initial encounter
S20.364D	Insect bite (nonvenomous) of middle front wall of thorax, subsequent encounter
S20.364S	Insect bite (nonvenomous) of middle front wall of thorax, sequela

S20.373A	Other superficial bite of bilateral front wall of thorax, initial encounter
S20.373D	Other superficial bite of bilateral front wall of thorax, subsequent encounter
S20.373S	Other superficial bite of bilateral front wall of thorax, sequela
S20.374A	Other superficial bite of middle front wall of thorax, initial encounter
S20.374D	Other superficial bite of middle front wall of thorax, subsequent encounter
S20.374S	Other superficial bite of middle front wall of thorax, sequela
T40.411A	Poisoning by fentanyl or fentanyl analogs, accidental (unintentional), initial encounter
T40.411D	Poisoning by fentanyl or fentanyl analogs, accidental (unintentional), subsequent encounter
T40.411S	Poisoning by fentanyl or fentanyl analogs, accidental (unintentional), sequela
T40.412A	Poisoning by fentanyl or fentanyl analogs, intentional self-harm, initial encounter
T40.412D	Poisoning by fentanyl or fentanyl analogs, intentional self-harm, subsequent encounter
T40.412S	Poisoning by fentanyl or fentanyl analogs, intentional self-harm, sequela
T40.413A	Poisoning by fentanyl or fentanyl analogs, assault, initial encounter
T40.413D	Poisoning by fentanyl or fentanyl analogs, assault, subsequent encounter
T40.413S	Poisoning by fentanyl or fentanyl analogs, assault, sequela
T40.414A	Poisoning by fentanyl or fentanyl analogs, undetermined, initial encounter
T40.414D	Poisoning by fentanyl or fentanyl analogs, undetermined, subsequent encounter
T40.414S	Poisoning by fentanyl or fentanyl analogs, undetermined, sequela
T40.415A	Adverse effect of fentanyl or fentanyl analogs, initial encounter
T40.415D	Adverse effect of fentanyl or fentanyl analogs, subsequent encounter
T40.415S	Adverse effect of fentanyl or fentanyl analogs, sequela
T40.416A	Underdosing of fentanyl or fentanyl analogs, initial encounter
T40.416D	Underdosing of fentanyl or fentanyl analogs, subsequent encounter
T40.416S	Underdosing of fentanyl or fentanyl analogs, sequela
T40.421A	Poisoning by tramadol, accidental (unintentional), initial encounter
T40.421D	Poisoning by tramadol, accidental (unintentional), subsequent encounter
T40.421S	Poisoning by tramadol, accidental (unintentional), sequela
T40.422A	Poisoning by tramadol, intentional self-harm, initial encounter
T40.422D	Poisoning by tramadol, intentional self-harm, subsequent encounter
T40.422S	Poisoning by tramadol, intentional self-harm, sequela
T40.423A	Poisoning by tramadol, assault, initial encounter
T40.423D	Poisoning by tramadol, assault, subsequent encounter
T40.423S	Poisoning by tramadol, assault, sequela

T40.424A	Poisoning by tramadol, undetermined, initial encounter
T40.424D	Poisoning by tramadol, undetermined, subsequent encounter
T40.424S	Poisoning by tramadol, undetermined, sequela
T40.425A	Adverse effect of tramadol, initial encounter
T40.425D	Adverse effect of tramadol, subsequent encounter
T40.425S	Adverse effect of tramadol, sequela
T40.426A	Underdosing of tramadol, initial encounter
T40.426D	Underdosing of tramadol, subsequent encounter
T40.426S	Underdosing of tramadol, sequela
T40.491A	Poisoning by other synthetic narcotics, accidental (unintentional), initial encounter
T40.491D	Poisoning by other synthetic narcotics, accidental (unintentional), subsequent encounter
T40.491S	Poisoning by other synthetic narcotics, accidental (unintentional), sequela
T40.492A	Poisoning by other synthetic narcotics, intentional self-harm, initial encounter
T40.492D	Poisoning by other synthetic narcotics, intentional self-harm, subsequent encounter
T40.492S	Poisoning by other synthetic narcotics, intentional self-harm, sequela
T40.493A	Poisoning by other synthetic narcotics, assault, initial encounter
T40.493D	Poisoning by other synthetic narcotics, assault, subsequent encounter
T40.493S	Poisoning by other synthetic narcotics, assault, sequela
T40.494A	Poisoning by other synthetic narcotics, undetermined, initial encounter
T40.494D	Poisoning by other synthetic narcotics, undetermined, subsequent encounter
T40.494S	Poisoning by other synthetic narcotics, undetermined, sequela
T40.495A	Adverse effect of other synthetic narcotics, initial encounter
T40.495D	Adverse effect of other synthetic narcotics, subsequent encounter
T40.495S	Adverse effect of other synthetic narcotics, sequela
T40.496A	Underdosing of other synthetic narcotics, initial encounter
T40.496D	Underdosing of other synthetic narcotics, subsequent encounter
T40.496S	Underdosing of other synthetic narcotics, sequela
T86.8401	Corneal transplant rejection, right eye
T86.8402	Corneal transplant rejection, left eye
T86.8403	Corneal transplant rejection, bilateral
T86.8409	Corneal transplant rejection, unspecified eye
T86.8411	Corneal transplant failure, right eye
T86.8412	Corneal transplant failure, left eye
T86.8413	Corneal transplant failure, bilateral
T86.8419	Corneal transplant failure, unspecified eye
T86.8421	Corneal transplant infection, right eye
T86.8422	Corneal transplant infection, left eye
T86.8423	Corneal transplant infection, bilateral
T86.8429	Corneal transplant infection, unspecified eye
T86.8481	Other complications of corneal transplant, right eye
T86.8482	Other complications of corneal transplant, left eye

T86.8483	Other complications of corneal transplant, bilateral
T86.8489	Other complications of corneal transplant, unspecified eye
T86.8491	Unspecified complication of corneal transplant, right eye
T86.8492	Unspecified complication of corneal transplant, left eye
T86.8493	Unspecified complication of corneal transplant, bilateral
T86.8499	Unspecified complication of corneal transplant, unspecified eye
U07.0	Vaping-related disorder
U07.1	COVID-19
V00.031A	Pedestrian on foot injured in collision with rider of standing electric scooter, initial encounter
V00.031D	Pedestrian on foot injured in collision with rider of standing electric scooter, subsequent encounter
V00.031S	Pedestrian on foot injured in collision with rider of standing electric scooter, sequela
V00.038A	Pedestrian on foot injured in collision with rider of other standing micro-mobility pedestrian conveyance, initial encounter
V00.038D	Pedestrian on foot injured in collision with rider of other standing micro-mobility pedestrian conveyance, subsequent encounter
V00.038S	Pedestrian on foot injured in collision with rider of other standing micro-mobility pedestrian conveyance, sequela
V00.841A	Fall from standing electric scooter, initial encounter
V00.841D	Fall from standing electric scooter, subsequent encounter
V00.841S	Fall from standing electric scooter, sequela
V00.842A	Pedestrian on standing electric scooter colliding with stationary object, initial encounter
V00.842D	Pedestrian on standing electric scooter colliding with stationary object, subsequent encounter
V00.842S	Pedestrian on standing electric scooter colliding with stationary object, sequela
V00.848A	Other accident with standing micro-mobility pedestrian conveyance, initial encounter
V00.848D	Other accident with standing micro-mobility pedestrian conveyance, subsequent encounter
V00.848S	Other accident with standing micro-mobility pedestrian conveyance, sequela
V01.031A	Pedestrian on standing electric scooter injured in collision with pedal cycle in nontraffic accident, initial encounter
V01.031D	Pedestrian on standing electric scooter injured in collision with pedal cycle in nontraffic accident, subsequent encounter
V01.031S	Pedestrian on standing electric scooter injured in collision with pedal cycle in nontraffic accident, sequela
V01.038A	Pedestrian on other standing micro-mobility pedestrian conveyance injured in collision with pedal cycle in nontraffic accident, initial encounter
V01.038D	Pedestrian on other standing micro-mobility pedestrian conveyance injured in collision with pedal cycle in nontraffic accident, subsequent encounter
V01.038S	Pedestrian on other standing micro-mobility pedestrian conveyance injured in collision with pedal cycle in nontraffic accident, sequela
V01.131A	Pedestrian on standing electric scooter injured in collision with pedal cycle in traffic accident, initial encounter
V01.131D	Pedestrian on standing electric scooter injured in collision with pedal cycle in traffic accident, subsequent encounter
V01.131S	Pedestrian on standing electric scooter injured in collision with pedal cycle in traffic accident, sequela
V01.138A	Pedestrian on other standing micro-mobility pedestrian conveyance injured in collision with pedal cycle in traffic accident, initial encounter
V01.138D	Pedestrian on other standing micro-mobility pedestrian conveyance injured in collision with pedal cycle in traffic accident, subsequent encounter
V01.138S	Pedestrian on other standing micro-mobility pedestrian conveyance injured in collision with pedal cycle in traffic accident, sequela
V01.931A	Pedestrian on standing electric scooter injured in collision with pedal cycle, unspecified whether traffic or nontraffic accident, initial encounter
V01.931D	Pedestrian on standing electric scooter injured in collision with pedal cycle, unspecified whether traffic or nontraffic accident, subsequent encounter
V01.931S	Pedestrian on standing electric scooter injured in collision with pedal cycle, unspecified whether traffic or nontraffic accident, sequela
V01.938A	Pedestrian on other standing micro-mobility pedestrian conveyance injured in collision with pedal cycle, unspecified whether traffic or nontraffic accident, initial encounter
V01.938D	Pedestrian on other standing micro-mobility pedestrian conveyance injured in collision with pedal cycle, unspecified whether traffic or nontraffic accident, subsequent encounter
V01.938S	Pedestrian on other standing micro-mobility pedestrian conveyance injured in collision with pedal cycle, unspecified whether traffic or nontraffic accident, sequela
V02.031A	Pedestrian on standing electric scooter injured in collision with two- or three-wheeled motor vehicle in nontraffic accident, initial encounter
V02.031D	Pedestrian on standing electric scooter injured in collision with two- or three-wheeled motor vehicle in nontraffic accident, subsequent encounter
V02.031S	Pedestrian on standing electric scooter injured in collision with two- or three-wheeled motor vehicle in nontraffic accident, sequela
V02.038A	Pedestrian on other standing micro-mobility pedestrian conveyance injured in collision with two- or three-wheeled motor vehicle in nontraffic accident, initial encounter
V02.038D	Pedestrian on other standing micro-mobility pedestrian conveyance injured in collision with two- or three-wheeled motor vehicle in nontraffic accident, subsequent encounter
V02.038S	Pedestrian on other standing micro-mobility pedestrian conveyance injured in collision with two- or three-wheeled motor vehicle in nontraffic accident, sequela
V02.131A	Pedestrian on standing electric scooter injured in collision with two- or three-wheeled motor vehicle in traffic accident, initial encounter
V02.131D	Pedestrian on standing electric scooter injured in collision with two- or three-wheeled motor vehicle in traffic accident, subsequent encounter
V02.131S	Pedestrian on standing electric scooter injured in collision with two- or three-wheeled motor vehicle in traffic accident, sequela
V02.138A	Pedestrian on other standing micro-mobility pedestrian conveyance injured in collision with two- or three-wheeled motor vehicle in traffic accident, initial encounter

V02.138D Pedestrian on other standing micro-mobility pedestrian conveyance injured in collision with two- or three-wheeled motor vehicle in traffic accident, subsequent encounter

V02.138S Pedestrian on other standing micro-mobility pedestrian conveyance injured in collision with two- or three-wheeled motor vehicle in traffic accident, sequela

V02.931A Pedestrian on standing electric scooter injured in collision with two- or three wheeled motor vehicle, unspecified whether traffic or nontraffic accident, initial encounter

V02.931D Pedestrian on standing electric scooter injured in collision with two- or three wheeled motor vehicle, unspecified whether traffic or nontraffic accident, subsequent encounter

V02.931S Pedestrian on standing electric scooter injured in collision with two- or three wheeled motor vehicle, unspecified whether traffic or nontraffic accident, sequela

V02.938A Pedestrian on other standing micro-mobility pedestrian conveyance injured in collision with two- or three wheeled motor vehicle, unspecified whether traffic or nontraffic accident, initial encounter

V02.938D Pedestrian on other standing micro-mobility pedestrian conveyance injured in collision with two- or three wheeled motor vehicle, unspecified whether traffic or nontraffic accident, subsequent encounter

V02.938S Pedestrian on other standing micro-mobility pedestrian conveyance injured in collision with two- or three wheeled motor vehicle, unspecified whether traffic or nontraffic accident, sequela

V03.031A Pedestrian on standing electric scooter injured in collision with car, pick-up or van in nontraffic accident, initial encounter

V03.031D Pedestrian on standing electric scooter injured in collision with car, pick-up or van in nontraffic accident, subsequent encounter

V03.031S Pedestrian on standing electric scooter injured in collision with car, pick-up or van in nontraffic accident, sequela

V03.038A Pedestrian on other standing micro-mobility pedestrian conveyance injured in collision with car, pick-up or van in nontraffic accident, initial encounter

V03.038D Pedestrian on other standing micro-mobility pedestrian conveyance injured in collision with car, pick-up or van in nontraffic accident, subsequent encounter

V03.038S Pedestrian on other standing micro-mobility pedestrian conveyance injured in collision with car, pick-up or van in nontraffic accident, sequela

V03.131A Pedestrian on standing electric scooter injured in collision with car, pick-up or van in traffic accident, initial encounter

V03.131D Pedestrian on standing electric scooter injured in collision with car, pick-up or van in traffic accident, subsequent encounter

V03.131S Pedestrian on standing electric scooter injured in collision with car, pick-up or van in traffic accident, sequela

V03.138A Pedestrian on other standing micro-mobility pedestrian conveyance injured in collision with car, pick-up or van in traffic accident, initial encounter

V03.138D Pedestrian on other standing micro-mobility pedestrian conveyance injured in collision with car, pick-up or van in traffic accident, subsequent encounter

V03.138S Pedestrian on other standing micro-mobility pedestrian conveyance injured in collision with car, pick-up or van in traffic accident, sequela

V03.931A Pedestrian on standing electric scooter injured in collision with car, pick-up or van, unspecified whether traffic or nontraffic accident, initial encounter

V03.931D Pedestrian on standing electric scooter injured in collision with car, pick-up or van, unspecified whether traffic or nontraffic accident, subsequent encounter

V03.931S Pedestrian on standing electric scooter injured in collision with car, pick-up or van, unspecified whether traffic or nontraffic accident, sequela

V03.938A Pedestrian on other standing micro-mobility pedestrian conveyance injured in collision with car, pick-up or van, unspecified whether traffic or nontraffic accident, initial encounter

V03.938D Pedestrian on other standing micro-mobility pedestrian conveyance injured in collision with car, pick-up or van, unspecified whether traffic or nontraffic accident, subsequent encounter

V03.938S Pedestrian on other standing micro-mobility pedestrian conveyance injured in collision with car, pick-up or van, unspecified whether traffic or nontraffic accident, sequela

V04.031A Pedestrian on standing electric scooter injured in collision with heavy transport vehicle or bus in nontraffic accident, initial encounter

V04.031D Pedestrian on standing electric scooter injured in collision with heavy transport vehicle or bus in nontraffic accident, subsequent encounter

V04.031S Pedestrian on standing electric scooter injured in collision with heavy transport vehicle or bus in nontraffic accident, sequela

V04.038A Pedestrian on other standing micro-mobility pedestrian conveyance injured in collision with heavy transport vehicle or bus in nontraffic accident, initial encounter

V04.038D Pedestrian on other standing micro-mobility pedestrian conveyance injured in collision with heavy transport vehicle or bus in nontraffic accident, subsequent encounter

V04.038S Pedestrian on other standing micro-mobility pedestrian conveyance injured in collision with heavy transport vehicle or bus in nontraffic accident, sequela

V04.131A Pedestrian on standing electric scooter injured in collision with heavy transport vehicle or bus in traffic accident, initial encounter

V04.131D Pedestrian on standing electric scooter injured in collision with heavy transport vehicle or bus in traffic accident, subsequent encounter

V04.131S Pedestrian on standing electric scooter injured in collision with heavy transport vehicle or bus in traffic accident, sequela

V04.138A Pedestrian on other standing micro-mobility pedestrian conveyance injured in collision with heavy transport vehicle or bus in traffic accident, initial encounter

V04.138D Pedestrian on other standing micro-mobility pedestrian conveyance injured in collision with heavy transport vehicle or bus in traffic accident, subsequent encounter

V04.138S Pedestrian on other standing micro-mobility pedestrian conveyance injured in collision with heavy transport vehicle or bus in traffic accident, sequela

V04.931A Pedestrian on standing electric scooter injured in collision with heavy transport vehicle or bus, unspecified whether traffic or nontraffic accident, initial encounter

V04.931D Pedestrian on standing electric scooter injured in collision with heavy transport vehicle or bus, unspecified whether traffic or nontraffic accident, subsequent encounter

V04.931S Pedestrian on standing electric scooter injured in collision with heavy transport vehicle or bus, unspecified whether traffic or nontraffic accident, sequela

V04.938A Pedestrian on other standing micro-mobility pedestrian conveyance injured in collision with heavy transport vehicle or bus, unspecified whether traffic or nontraffic accident, initial encounter

V04.938D Pedestrian on other standing micro-mobility pedestrian conveyance injured in collision with heavy transport vehicle or bus, unspecified whether traffic or nontraffic accident, subsequent encounter

V04.938S Pedestrian on other standing micro-mobility pedestrian conveyance injured in collision with heavy transport vehicle or bus, unspecified whether traffic or nontraffic accident, sequela

V05.031A Pedestrian on standing electric scooter injured in collision with railway train or railway vehicle in nontraffic accident, initial encounter

V05.031D Pedestrian on standing electric scooter injured in collision with railway train or railway vehicle in nontraffic accident, subsequent encounter

V05.031S Pedestrian on standing electric scooter injured in collision with railway train or railway vehicle in nontraffic accident, sequela

V05.038A Pedestrian on other standing micro-mobility pedestrian conveyance injured in collision with railway train or railway vehicle in nontraffic accident, initial encounter

V05.038D Pedestrian on other standing micro-mobility pedestrian conveyance injured in collision with railway train or railway vehicle in nontraffic accident, subsequent encounter

V05.038S Pedestrian on other standing micro-mobility pedestrian conveyance injured in collision with railway train or railway vehicle in nontraffic accident, sequela

V05.131A Pedestrian on standing electric scooter injured in collision with railway train or railway vehicle in traffic accident, initial encounter

V05.131D Pedestrian on standing electric scooter injured in collision with railway train or railway vehicle in traffic accident, subsequent encounter

V05.131S Pedestrian on standing electric scooter injured in collision with railway train or railway vehicle in traffic accident, sequela

V05.138A Pedestrian on other standing micro-mobility pedestrian conveyance injured in collision with railway train or railway vehicle in traffic accident, initial encounter

V05.138D Pedestrian on other standing micro-mobility pedestrian conveyance injured in collision with railway train or railway vehicle in traffic accident, subsequent encounter

V05.138S Pedestrian on other standing micro-mobility pedestrian conveyance injured in collision with railway train or railway vehicle in traffic accident, sequela

V05.931A Pedestrian on standing electric scooter injured in collision with railway train or railway vehicle, unspecified whether traffic or nontraffic accident, initial encounter

V05.931D Pedestrian on standing electric scooter injured in collision with railway train or railway vehicle, unspecified whether traffic or nontraffic accident, subsequent encounter

V05.931S Pedestrian on standing electric scooter injured in collision with railway train or railway vehicle, unspecified whether traffic or nontraffic accident, sequela

V05.938A Pedestrian on other standing micro-mobility pedestrian conveyance injured in collision with railway train or railway vehicle, unspecified whether traffic or nontraffic accident, initial encounter

V05.938D Pedestrian on other standing micro-mobility pedestrian conveyance injured in collision with railway train or railway vehicle, unspecified whether traffic or nontraffic accident, subsequent encounter

V05.938S Pedestrian on other standing micro-mobility pedestrian conveyance injured in collision with railway train or railway vehicle, unspecified whether traffic or nontraffic accident, sequela

V06.031A Pedestrian on standing electric scooter injured in collision with other nonmotor vehicle in nontraffic accident, initial encounter

V06.031D Pedestrian on standing electric scooter injured in collision with other nonmotor vehicle in nontraffic accident, subsequent encounter

V06.031S Pedestrian on standing electric scooter injured in collision with other nonmotor vehicle in nontraffic accident, sequela

V06.038A Pedestrian on other standing micro-mobility pedestrian conveyance injured in collision with other nonmotor vehicle in nontraffic accident, initial encounter

V06.038D Pedestrian on other standing micro-mobility pedestrian conveyance injured in collision with other nonmotor vehicle in nontraffic accident, subsequent encounter

V06.038S Pedestrian on other standing micro-mobility pedestrian conveyance injured in collision with other nonmotor vehicle in nontraffic accident, sequela

V06.131A Pedestrian on standing electric scooter injured in collision with other nonmotor vehicle in traffic accident, initial encounter

V06.131D Pedestrian on standing electric scooter injured in collision with other nonmotor vehicle in traffic accident, subsequent encounter

V06.131S Pedestrian on standing electric scooter injured in collision with other nonmotor vehicle in traffic accident, sequela

V06.138A Pedestrian on other standing micro-mobility pedestrian conveyance injured in collision with other nonmotor vehicle in traffic accident, initial encounter

V06.138D Pedestrian on other standing micro-mobility pedestrian conveyance injured in collision with other nonmotor vehicle in traffic accident, subsequent encounter

V06.138S Pedestrian on other standing micro-mobility pedestrian conveyance injured in collision with other nonmotor vehicle in traffic accident, sequela

V06.931A Pedestrian on standing electric scooter injured in collision with other nonmotor vehicle, unspecified whether traffic or nontraffic accident, initial encounter

V06.931D Pedestrian on standing electric scooter injured in collision with other nonmotor vehicle, unspecified whether traffic or nontraffic accident, subsequent encounter

V06.931S Pedestrian on standing electric scooter injured in collision with other nonmotor vehicle, unspecified whether traffic or nontraffic accident, sequela

V06.938A Pedestrian on other standing micro-mobility pedestrian conveyance injured in collision with other nonmotor vehicle, unspecified whether traffic or nontraffic accident, initial encounter

V06.938D　Pedestrian on other standing micro-mobility pedestrian conveyance injured in collision with other nonmotor vehicle, unspecified whether traffic or nontraffic accident, subsequent encounter

V06.938S　Pedestrian on other standing micro-mobility pedestrian conveyance injured in collision with other nonmotor vehicle, unspecified whether traffic or nontraffic accident, sequela

Y77.11　Contact lens associated with adverse incidents

Y77.19　Other therapeutic (nonsurgical) and rehabilitative ophthalmic devices associated with adverse incidents

Z03.821　Encounter for observation for suspected ingested foreign body ruled out

Z03.822　Encounter for observation for suspected aspirated (inhaled) foreign body ruled out

Z03.823　Encounter for observation for suspected inserted (injected) foreign body ruled out

47 Code Descriptions Revised
Note: Each code is listed with its revised description only. Please refer to the full FY 2021 official addenda code files at Conversion Table zip file at https://www.cms.gov/medicare/icd-10/2021-icd-10-cm for the specific changes made to the codes listed.

D57.411　Sickle-cell thalassemia, unspecified, with acute chest syndrome

D57.412　Sickle-cell thalassemia, unspecified, with splenic sequestration

D57.419　Sickle-cell thalassemia, unspecified, with crisis

H55.81　Deficient saccadic eye movements

Q51.21　Complete doubling of uterus

Q51.22　Partial doubling of uterus

Q51.28　Other and unspecified doubling of uterus

Y92.002　Bathroom of unspecified non-institutional (private) residence as the place of occurrence of the external cause

Z68.1　Body mass index [BMI] 19.9 or less, adult

Z68.20　Body mass index [BMI] 20.0-20.9, adult

Z68.21　Body mass index [BMI] 21.0-21.9, adult

Z68.22　Body mass index [BMI] 22.0-22.9, adult

Z68.23　Body mass index [BMI] 23.0-23.9, adult

Z68.24　Body mass index [BMI] 24.0-24.9, adult

Z68.25　Body mass index [BMI] 25.0-25.9, adult

Z68.26　Body mass index [BMI] 26.0-26.9, adult

Z68.27　Body mass index [BMI] 27.0-27.9, adult

Z68.28　Body mass index [BMI] 28.0-28.9, adult

Z68.29　Body mass index [BMI] 29.0-29.9, adult

Z68.30　Body mass index [BMI] 30.0-30.9, adult

Z68.31　Body mass index [BMI] 31.0-31.9, adult

Z68.32　Body mass index [BMI] 32.0-32.9, adult

Z68.33　Body mass index [BMI] 33.0-33.9, adult

Z68.34　Body mass index [BMI] 34.0-34.9, adult

Z68.35　Body mass index [BMI] 35.0-35.9, adult

Z68.36　Body mass index [BMI] 36.0-36.9, adult

Z68.37　Body mass index [BMI] 37.0-37.9, adult

Z68.38　Body mass index [BMI] 38.0-38.9, adult

Z68.39　Body mass index [BMI] 39.0-39.9, adult

Z68.41　Body mass index [BMI] 40.0-44.9, adult

Z68.42　Body mass index [BMI] 45.0-49.9, adult

Z68.43　Body mass index [BMI] 50.0-59.9, adult

Z68.44　Body mass index [BMI] 60.0-69.9, adult

Z68.45　Body mass index [BMI] 70 or greater, adult

Z68.51　Body mass index [BMI] pediatric, less than 5th percentile for age

Z68.52　Body mass index [BMI] pediatric, 5th percentile to less than 85th percentile for age

Z68.53　Body mass index [BMI] pediatric, 85th percentile to less than 95th+percentile for age

Z68.54　Body mass index [BMI] pediatric, greater than or equal to 95th percentile for age

Z88.1　Allergy status to other antibiotic agents

Z88.2　Allergy status to sulfonamides

Z88.3　Allergy status to other anti-infective agents

Z88.4　Allergy status to anesthetic agent

Z88.5　Allergy status to narcotic agent

Z88.6　Allergy status to analgesic agent

Z88.7　Allergy status to serum and vaccine

Z88.8　Allergy status to other drugs, medicaments and biological substances

Z88.9　Allergy status to unspecified drugs, medicaments and biological substances

Proprietary Updates
The following proprietary features have also been added:

- New definitions that describe, in lay terms, a specific condition or disease process
- New coding tips that provide coding advice beyond the code classification
- Updated *AHA Coding Clinic* references through second quarter 2020

Conversion Table of ICD-10-CM Codes

At the time of printing, the Centers for Medicare and Medicaid Services (CMS) had not released the 2021 conversion table. Please see the product update page on optum360coding.com for a PDF of the 2021 conversion table. The password for obtaining your update is: **Hospital21**

10 Steps to Correct Coding

Follow the 10 steps below to correctly code encounters for health care services.

Step 1: Identify the reason for the visit or encounter (i.e., a sign, symptom, diagnosis and/or condition).

The medical record documentation should accurately reflect the patient's condition, using terminology that includes specific diagnoses and symptoms or clearly states the reasons for the encounter.

Choosing the main term that best describes the reason chiefly responsible for the service provided is the most important step in coding. If symptoms are present and documented but a definitive diagnosis has not yet been determined, code the symptoms. *For outpatient cases, do not code conditions that are referred to as "rule out," "suspected," "probable," or "questionable."* Diagnoses often are not established at the time of the initial encounter/visit and may require two or more visits to be established. Code only what is documented in the available outpatient records and only to the highest degree of certainty known at the time of the patient's visit. For inpatient medical records, uncertain diagnoses may be reported if documented at the time of discharge.

Step 2: After selecting the reason for the encounter, consult the alphabetic index.

The most critical rule is to begin code selection in the alphabetic index. Never turn first to the tabular list. The index provides cross-references, essential and nonessential modifiers, and other instructional notations that may not be found in the tabular list.

Step 3: Locate the main term entry.

The alphabetic index lists conditions, which may be expressed as nouns or eponyms, with critical use of adjectives. Some conditions known by several names have multiple main entries. Reasons for encounters may be located under general terms such as admission, encounter, and examination. Other general terms such as history, status (post), or presence (of) can be used to locate other factors influencing health.

Step 4: Scan subterm entries.

Scan the subterm entries, as appropriate, being sure to review continued lines and additional subterms that may appear in the next column or on the next page. Shaded vertical guidelines in the index indicate the indentation level for each subterm in relation to the main terms.

Step 5: Pay close attention to index instructions.

- Parentheses ( ) enclose nonessential modifiers, terms that are supplementary words or explanatory information that may or may not appear in the diagnostic statement and do not affect code selection.

- Brackets [ ] enclose manifestation codes that can be used only as secondary codes to the underlying condition code immediately preceding it. If used, manifestation codes must be reported with the appropriate etiology codes.

- Default codes are listed next to the main term and represent the condition most commonly associated with the main term or the unspecified code for the main term.

- *"See"* cross-references, identified by italicized type and "code by" cross-references indicate that another term *must be referenced* to locate the correct code.

- *"See also"* cross-references, identified by italicized type, provide alternative terms that may be useful to look up but *are not mandatory*.

- "Omit code" cross-references identify instances when a code is not applicable depending on the condition being coded.

- "With" subterms are listed out of alphabetic order and identify a presumed causal relationship between the two conditions they link.

- "Due to" subterms identify a relationship between the two conditions they link.

- "NEC," abbreviation for "not elsewhere classified," follows some main terms or subterms and indicates that there is no specific code for the condition even though the medical documentation may be very specific.

- "NOS," abbreviation for "not otherwise specified," follows some main terms or subterms and is the equivalent of unspecified; NOS signifies that the information in the medical record is insufficient for assigning a more specific code.

- *Following* references help coders locate alphanumeric codes that are out of sequence in the tabular section.

- Check-additional-character symbols flag codes that require additional characters to make the code valid; the characters available to complete the code should be verified in the tabular section.

Step 6: Choose a potential code and locate it in the tabular list.

To prevent coding errors, always use both the alphabetic index (to identify a code) and the tabular list (to verify a code), as the index does not include the important instructional notes found in the tabular list. An added benefit of using the tabular list, which groups like things together, is that while looking at one code in the list, a coder might see a more specific one that would have been missed had the coder relied solely on the alphabetic index. Additionally, many of the codes require a fourth, fifth, sixth, or seventh character to be valid, and many of these characters can be found only in the tabular list.

Step 7: Read all instructional material in the tabular section.

The coder must follow any Includes, Excludes 1 and Excludes 2 notes, and other instructional notes, such as "Code first" and "Use additional code," listed in the tabular list for the chapter, category, subcategory, and subclassification levels of code selection that direct the coder to use a different or additional code. Any codes in the tabular range A00.0- through T88.9- may be used to identify the diagnostic reason for the encounter. The tabular list encompasses many codes describing disease and injury classifications (e.g., infectious and parasitic diseases, neoplasms, symptoms, nervous and circulatory system etc.).

Codes that describe symptoms and signs, as opposed to definitive diagnoses, should be reported when an established diagnosis has not been made (confirmed) by the physician. Chapter 18 of the ICD-10-CM code book, "Symptoms, Signs, and Abnormal Clinical and Laboratory Findings, Not Elsewhere Classified" (codes R00.--R99), contains many, but not all, codes for symptoms.

ICD-10-CM classifies encounters with health care providers for circumstances other than a disease or injury in chapter 21, "Factors Influencing Health Status and Contact with Health Services" (codes Z00–Z99). Circumstances other than a disease or injury often are recorded as chiefly responsible for the encounter.

A code is invalid if it does not include the full number of characters (greatest level of specificity) required. Codes in ICD-10-CM can contain from three to seven alphanumeric characters. A three-character code is to be used only if the category is not further subdivided into four-, five-, six-, or seven-character codes. Placeholder character X is used as part of an alphanumeric code to allow for future expansion and as a placeholder for empty characters in a code that requires a seventh character but has no fourth, fifth, or sixth character. Note that certain categories require seventh characters that apply to all codes in that category. Always check the category level for applicable seventh characters for that category.

Step 8: Consult the official ICD-10-CM conventions and guidelines.

The *ICD-10-CM Official Guidelines for Coding and Reporting* govern the use of certain codes. These guidelines provide both general and chapter-specific coding guidance.

Step 9: Confirm and assign the code.

Having reviewed all relevant information concerning the possible code choices, assign the code that most completely describes the condition.

Repeat steps 1 through 9 for all additional documented conditions that meet the following criteria:

- They exist at the time of the visit *AND*
- They require or affect patient care, treatment, or management

Step 10: Sequence codes correctly.

Sequencing is the order in which the codes are listed on the claim. List first the ICD-10-CM code for the diagnosis, condition, problem, or other reason for the encounter/visit that is shown in the medical record to be chiefly responsible for the services provided. List additional codes that describe any coexisting conditions. Follow the official coding guidelines (see the guidelines, section II, "Selection of Principal Diagnosis"; section III, "Reporting Additional Diagnoses"; and section IV, "Diagnostic Coding and Reporting Guidelines for Outpatient Services") on proper sequencing of codes.

Coding Examples

Diagnosis: Anorexia

Step 1: The reason for the encounter was the condition, anorexia.

Step 2: Consult the alphabetic index.

Step 3: Locate the main term "Anorexia."

Step 4: Two possible subterms are available, "hysterical" and "nervosa." Neither is documented in this instance, however, so they cannot be used in code selection.

Step 5: The code listed next to the main term is called the default code selection. Because the two subentries (essential modifiers) do not apply in this instance, the default code (R63.0) should be used.

Step 6: Turn to code R63.0 in the tabular list and read all instructional notes.

Step 7: The Excludes 1 note at code R63.0 indicates that anorexia nervosa and loss of appetite determined to be of nonorganic origin should be reported with a code from chapter 5. The diagnostic statement does not describe the condition as anorexia nervosa, however, and does not indicate that the anorexia is of a nonorganic origin. There is no further division of the category past the fourth-character subcategory. Therefore, code R63.0 is at the highest level of specificity.

Step 8: Review of official guideline I.C.18 indicates that a symptom code is appropriate when a more definitive diagnosis is not documented.

Step 9: The default code, R63.0 Anorexia, is the correct code selection.

Repeat steps 1 through 9 for any concomitant diagnoses.

Step 10: Since anorexia is listed as the chief reason for the health care encounter, the first-listed, or principal, diagnosis is R63.0. Note that this is a chapter 18 symptom code but can be assigned for both inpatient and outpatient records since the provider did not establish a more definitive diagnosis, according to sections II.A and IV.D.

Diagnosis: Acute bronchitis

Step 1: The reason for the encounter was the condition, acute bronchitis.

Step 2: Consult the alphabetic index.

Step 3: Locate the main term "Bronchitis."

Step 4: There is a subterm for "acute or subacute." Additional subterms are not included in the diagnostic statement.

Step 5: Review the instructional notes. Nonessential modifiers (with bronchospasm or obstruction) are terms that do not affect code assignment. Since no other subterms indented under "acute" apply here, the code listed next to this subentry—in this case J20.9—should be chosen.

Step 6: Turn to code J20.9 in the tabular list and read all instructional notes.

Step 7: The Includes note under category J20 lists alternative terms for acute bronchitis. Note that the list is not exhaustive but is only a representative selection of diagnoses that are included in the subcategory. The Excludes 1 note refers to category J40 for bronchitis and tracheobronchitis NOS. There are several conditions in the Excludes 2 notes that, if applicable, can be coded in addition to this code.

Note that the codes included in J20 represent acute bronchitis due to various infectious organisms that could be selected if identified in the documentation. In this case, the organism was not identified and there is no further division of the category past the fourth character subcategory. Therefore, code J20.9 is at the highest level of specificity.

Step 8: Review of official guideline I.C.10 provides no additional information affecting the code selected.

Step 9: Assign code J20.9 Acute bronchitis, unspecified.

Repeat steps 1 through 9 for any concomitant diagnoses.

Step 10: In the absence of additional diagnoses that may affect sequencing, code J20.9 should be sequenced as the first-listed, or principal, diagnosis.

Diagnosis: Cerebellar ataxia in myxedema

Step 1: The reason for the encounter was the condition, cerebellar ataxia.

Step 2: Consult the alphabetic index.

Step 3: Locate the main term "Ataxia."

Step 4: Available subterms include "cerebellar (hereditary)," with additional indented subterms for "in" and "myxedema," all essential modifiers that are included in the diagnostic statement. Two codes are provided, E03.9 and G13.2, the latter of which is in brackets.

Step 5: Note the nonessential modifier (in parentheses) after the subterm cerebellar includes the term "hereditary." Because it is in parentheses, this term is not required in the diagnostic statement for this subentry to apply. The brackets around G13.2 identify this code as a manifestation of the condition described by code E03.9 and indicate that the two must be reported together and sequencing rules apply.

Step 6: Locate codes E03.9 and G13.2 in the tabular list, and read all instructional notes.

Step 7: For code E03.9, there are no instructional notes in the tabular list at the category E03 or code level that indicate that this condition should be coded elsewhere in the classification or that additional codes are required. Without further information from the diagnostic statement, myxedema, not otherwise specified (NOS), is appropriately reported with code E03.9 Hypothyroidism, unspecified, according to the inclusion term at this code.

Code G13.2 in the tabular list has an instructional note to "Code first underlying disease," which includes conditions found in category E03.-. Based on this note, codes E03.9 and G13.2 are to be coded together, with G13.2 listed only as a secondary diagnosis. This correlates with what the alphabetic index indicated. As there is no further division of codes in category G13 beyond the fourth character, G13.2 is at the highest level of specificity.

Step 8: Although there are some general conventions, such as how to interpret brackets in the alphabetic index, no chapter-specific guidelines apply to this coding scenario.

Step 9: Assign codes E03.9 Hypothyroidism, unspecified, and G13.2 Systemic atrophy primarily affecting the central nervous system in myxedema.

Repeat steps 1 through 9 for any concomitant diagnoses.

Step 10: Based on the alphabetic index and tabular instructional notations, code E03.9 should be sequenced as the first-listed, or principal, diagnosis followed by G13.2 as a secondary diagnosis.

Diagnosis: Decubitus ulcer of right elbow with skin loss and necrosis of subcutaneous tissue

Step 1: The reason for the encounter was the condition, decubitus ulcer.

Step 2: Consult the alphabetic index.

Step 3: Locate the main term "Ulcer."

Step 4: For the subterm "decubitus," there is no code provided or additional subterms indented, but a cross-reference is listed.

Step 5: The italicized cross-reference instructs the coder to "*see* Ulcer, pressure, by site."

Repeat steps 3 through 5 for the cross-reference.

Step 3: Locate the main term "Ulcer."

Step 4: Review the subentries for the subterm "pressure." The next level of indent lists either the site of the ulcer or the specific stage of the ulcer (stage 1–4, unstageable, and unspecified stages). The diagnostic statement provides the site, right elbow, and the extent of tissue damage (skin loss and necrosis of subcutaneous tissue) but does not specifically state that the ulcer is stage 1, stage 2, etc. Nonessential modifiers (in parentheses) at each stage include a description of the typical extent of damage at each stage. For example, stage 1 describes "pre-ulcer skin changes limited to persistent focal edema." Based on the documentation in the record, the coder can correlate the documentation to the nonessential modifiers and choose the specific stage from the index. The coder can also go directly to the body site, choosing the stage of the ulcer after reviewing the code options and instructional notations in the tabular list.

The diagnostic statement indicates that the extent of the damage to the elbow includes skin loss and necrosis of subcutaneous tissue, coinciding with the nonessential modifier next to the subentry "stage 3." The body site of elbow (L89.0-) is listed as another level of indent with other body sites.

Step 5: Note that code L89.0 is followed by a dash and an additional-character-required icon, which indicate that more characters are needed to complete the code. From here, the tabular listing for L89.0- can be consulted.

Step 6: Locate code L89.0- in the tabular list and read all instructional notes.

Step 7: The tabular listing at category L89 has an Includes note for "decubitus ulcer," which confirms that category L89 is the appropriate category to represent what is documented in the diagnostic statement.

Several Excludes 2 notes are also listed at the category level. Excludes 2 notes represent conditions that can occur concomitantly with the decubitus ulcer and can be coded in addition to code L89, if supported by the documentation.

The subcategory codes under L89.0 indicate that the fifth character describes laterality. Locate the right elbow at subcategory L89.01. See that an additional sixth character to specify the stage of the ulcer is now needed to complete the code. The stage can be determined either by the specific documentation of the stage (e.g., stage 1, stage 2) or, in this case, a description that matches one of the inclusion terms that follow

each stage code. For example, the diagnostic description in this case of "skin loss and necrosis of the subcutaneous tissue" matches the inclusion term under L89.013 Pressure ulcer of right elbow, stage 3. No additional characters are required because code L89.013 is at its highest level of specificity.

Step 8: The official guidelines contain quite a bit of information relating to pressure ulcers in chapter-specific guideline I.C.12 as well as information in general guideline I.B.14. These and any other pertinent guidelines should be reviewed to ensure appropriate code assignment.

Step 9: Assign code L89.013 Pressure ulcer of right elbow, stage 3.

Repeat steps 1 through 9 for any concomitant diagnoses.

Step 10: Since the decubitus ulcer is listed as the chief reason for the health care encounter, the first-listed, or principal, diagnosis is L89.013. However, according to the code first instructional note at the L89 category level, gangrene (I96) would be sequenced before the pressure ulcer if it were documented.

Diagnosis: Emergency department visit for bimalleolar fracture of the right ankle due to trauma

Step 1: The reason for the encounter was the condition, bimalleolar fracture.

Step 2: Consult the alphabetic index.

Step 3: Locate the main term "Fracture." Note that many main terms represent fractures: "Fracture, burst," "Fracture, chronic," "Fracture, insufficiency," "Fracture, nontraumatic NEC," "Fracture, pathological," and "Fracture, traumatic." Since the diagnostic statement specifically states that this fracture was the result of trauma, the main term "Fracture, traumatic" should be used.

Step 4: Subterms that should be referenced are "ankle" and "bimalleolar (displaced)," which lists code S82.84-.

Step 5: A nonessential modifier (in parentheses) next to the term bimalleolar for "displaced" indicates that S82.84- is the default category unless the fracture is specifically identified as "nondisplaced."

Note that code S82.84- is followed by a dash and an additional-character icon, both of which indicate that more characters are required. From here, the tabular list can be consulted.

Step 6: Locate code S82.84- in the tabular list and read all instructional notes.

Step 7 The instructional notes at category S82 indicate that fractures not specified as displaced or nondisplaced default to displaced and that fractures not designated as open or closed default to closed. Additional instructional notes can be found at the category level but none pertain to the current scenario.

Read through the subcategory codes under S82.84, and note that the sixth character specifies displaced or nondisplaced and laterality. Based on the index nonessential modifier (displaced) and the code note at category S82, code selection should identify a displaced fracture of the right side. A displaced bimalleolar fracture of the right lower leg is coded to S82.841.

To complete the code, a seventh character must be assigned to identify the type of encounter (initial, subsequent, or sequela) and whether the fracture is open or closed. Most of the codes in category S82 require a seventh character represented in the list at the category level. However, it is important to note that some subcategories have their own specific set of seventh characters. In this instance, subcategory S82.84- does not have a unique set of seventh characters and the list provided at the category level should be used. Without documentation of the fracture being open, the tabular notation indicates that the default is closed. Character A, representing "initial encounter for closed fracture," listed in the box at the category level is the most appropriate option.

Step 8: Assign code S82.841A Displaced bimalleolar fracture of right lower leg, initial encounter for closed fracture.

Repeat steps 1 through 9 for any concomitant diagnoses.

Step 9: Review chapter-specific guideline I.C.19. and any other official conventions or guidelines to ensure appropriate code assignment.

Step 10: Additional codes can be applied to relate the specific cause of the injury, the place of occurrence, the activity of the patient at the time of the injury, and the patient's status, when this information is available in the record. However, coding this information is voluntary and reporting requirements depend on state mandates and/or facility-specific reporting requirements. If assigned, the external cause codes should be reported as secondary diagnoses only with the injury (fracture) sequenced first. Most codes in chapter 20, "External Causes of Morbidity," require a seventh character to identify the type of encounter. The seventh character assigned to an external cause code should match the seventh character of the code assigned for the associated injury or condition for the encounter.

2021 ICD-10-CM Official Guidelines for Coding and Reporting

Narrative changes appear in **bold** text

Items <u>underlined</u> have been moved within the guidelines since the FY 2020 version

Italics are used to indicate revisions to heading changes

The Centers for Medicare and Medicaid Services (CMS) and the National Center for Health Statistics (NCHS), two departments within the U.S. Federal Government's Department of Health and Human Services (DHHS) provide the following guidelines for coding and reporting using the International Classification of Diseases, 10th Revision, Clinical Modification (ICD-10-CM). These guidelines should be used as a companion document to the official version of the ICD-10-CM as published on the NCHS website. The ICD-10-CM is a morbidity classification published by the United States for classifying diagnoses and reason for visits in all health care settings. The ICD-10-CM is based on the ICD-10, the statistical classification of disease published by the World Health Organization (WHO).

These guidelines have been approved by the four organizations that make up the Cooperating Parties for the ICD-10-CM: the American Hospital Association (AHA), the American Health Information Management Association (AHIMA), CMS, and NCHS.

These guidelines are a set of rules that have been developed to accompany and complement the official conventions and instructions provided within the ICD-10-CM itself. The instructions and conventions of the classification take precedence over guidelines. These guidelines are based on the coding and sequencing instructions in the Tabular List and Alphabetic Index of ICD-10-CM, but provide additional instruction. Adherence to these guidelines when assigning ICD-10-CM diagnosis codes is required under the Health Insurance Portability and Accountability Act (HIPAA). The diagnosis codes (Tabular List and Alphabetic Index) have been adopted under HIPAA for all healthcare settings. A joint effort between the healthcare provider and the coder is essential to achieve complete and accurate documentation, code assignment, and reporting of diagnoses and procedures. These guidelines have been developed to assist both the healthcare provider and the coder in identifying those diagnoses that are to be reported. The importance of consistent, complete documentation in the medical record cannot be overemphasized. Without such documentation accurate coding cannot be achieved. The entire record should be reviewed to determine the specific reason for the encounter and the conditions treated.

The term encounter is used for all settings, including hospital admissions. In the context of these guidelines, the term provider is used throughout the guidelines to mean physician or any qualified health care practitioner who is legally accountable for establishing the patient's diagnosis. Only this set of guidelines, approved by the Cooperating Parties, is official.

The guidelines are organized into sections. Section I includes the structure and conventions of the classification and general guidelines that apply to the entire classification, and chapter-specific guidelines that correspond to the chapters as they are arranged in the classification. Section II includes guidelines for selection of principal diagnosis for non-outpatient settings. Section III includes guidelines for reporting additional diagnoses in non-outpatient settings. Section IV is for outpatient coding and reporting. It is necessary to review all sections of the guidelines to fully understand all of the rules and instructions needed to code properly.

Section I. Conventions, general coding guidelines and chapter specific guidelines

The conventions, general guidelines and chapter-specific guidelines are applicable to all health care settings unless otherwise indicated. The conventions and instructions of the classification take precedence over guidelines.

A. Conventions for the ICD-10-CM

The conventions for the ICD-10-CM are the general rules for use of the classification independent of the guidelines. These conventions are incorporated within the Alphabetic Index and Tabular List of the ICD-10-CM as instructional notes.

1. **The Alphabetic Index and Tabular List**

   The ICD-10-CM is divided into the Alphabetic Index, an alphabetical list of terms and their corresponding code, and the Tabular List, a structured list of codes divided into chapters based on body system or condition. The Alphabetic Index consists of the following parts: the Index of Diseases and Injury, the Index of External Causes of Injury, the Table of Neoplasms and the Table of Drugs and Chemicals.

   See Section I.C2. General guidelines

   See Section I.C.19. Adverse effects, poisoning, underdosing and toxic effects

2. **Format and Structure:**

   The ICD-10-CM Tabular List contains categories, subcategories and codes. Characters for categories, subcategories and codes may be either a letter or a number. All categories are 3 characters. A three-character category that has no further subdivision is equivalent to a code. Subcategories are either 4 or 5 characters. Codes may be 3, 4, 5, 6 or 7 characters. That is, each level of subdivision after a category is a subcategory. The final level of subdivision is a code. Codes that have applicable 7th characters are still referred to as codes, not subcategories. A code that has an applicable 7th character is considered invalid without the 7th character.

   The ICD-10-CM uses an indented format for ease in reference.

3. **Use of codes for reporting purposes**

   For reporting purposes only codes are permissible, not categories or subcategories, and any applicable 7th character is required.

4. **Placeholder character**

   The ICD-10-CM utilizes a placeholder character "X". The "X" is used as a placeholder at certain codes to allow for future expansion. An example of this is at the poisoning, adverse effect and underdosing codes, categories T36-T50.

   Where a placeholder exists, the X must be used in order for the code to be considered a valid code.

5. **7th Characters**

   Certain ICD-10-CM categories have applicable 7th characters. The applicable 7th character is required for all codes within the category, or as the notes in the Tabular List instruct. The 7th character must always be the 7th character in the data field. If a code that requires a 7th character is not 6 characters, a placeholder X must be used to fill in the empty characters.

6. **Abbreviations**

   a. **Alphabetic Index abbreviations**

   NEC "Not elsewhere classifiable"

   This abbreviation in the Alphabetic Index represents "other specified." When a specific code is not available for a condition, the Alphabetic Index directs the coder to the "other specified" code in the Tabular List.

   NOS "Not otherwise specified"

   This abbreviation is the equivalent of unspecified.

   b. **Tabular List abbreviations**

   NEC "Not elsewhere classifiable"

   This abbreviation in the Tabular List represents "other specified". When a specific code is not available for a condition, the Tabular List includes an NEC entry under a code to identify the code as the "other specified" code.

   NOS "Not otherwise specified"

This abbreviation is the equivalent of unspecified.

7. **Punctuation**

   [ ]   Brackets are used in the Tabular List to enclose synonyms, alternative wording or explanatory phrases. Brackets are used in the Alphabetic Index to identify manifestation codes.

   ( )   Parentheses are used in both the Alphabetic Index and Tabular List to enclose supplementary words that may be present or absent in the statement of a disease or procedure without affecting the code number to which it is assigned. The terms within the parentheses are referred to as nonessential modifiers. The nonessential modifiers in the Alphabetic Index to Diseases apply to subterms following a main term except when a nonessential modifier and a subentry are mutually exclusive, the subentry takes precedence. For example, in the ICD-10-CM Alphabetic Index under the main term Enteritis, "acute" is a nonessential modifier and "chronic" is a subentry. In this case, the nonessential modifier "acute" does not apply to the subentry "chronic".

   :   Colons are used in the Tabular List after an incomplete term which needs one or more of the modifiers following the colon to make it assignable to a given category.

8. **Use of "and"**

   See Section I.A.14. Use of the term "And"

9. **Other and Unspecified codes**

   a. **"Other" codes**

   Codes titled "other" or "other specified" are for use when the information in the medical record provides detail for which a specific code does not exist. Alphabetic Index entries with NEC in the line designate "other" codes in the Tabular List. These Alphabetic Index entries represent specific disease entities for which no specific code exists, so the term is included within an "other" code.

   b. **"Unspecified" codes**

   Codes titled "unspecified" are for use when the information in the medical record is insufficient to assign a more specific code. For those categories for which an unspecified code is not provided, the "other specified" code may represent both other and unspecified.

   See Section I.B.18 Use of Signs/Symptom/Unspecified Codes

10. **Includes Notes**

    This note appears immediately under a three-character code title to further define, or give examples of, the content of the category.

11. **Inclusion terms**

    List of terms is included under some codes. These terms are the conditions for which that code is to be used. The terms may be synonyms of the code title, or, in the case of "other specified" codes, the terms are a list of the various conditions assigned to that code. The inclusion terms are not necessarily exhaustive. Additional terms found only in the Alphabetic Index may also be assigned to a code.

12. **Excludes Notes**

    The ICD-10-CM has two types of excludes notes. Each type of note has a different definition for use but they are all similar in that they indicate that codes excluded from each other are independent of each other.

    a. **Excludes1**

    A type 1 Excludes note is a pure excludes note. It means "NOT CODED HERE!" An Excludes1 note indicates that the code excluded should never be used at the same time as the code above the Excludes1 note. An Excludes1 is used when two conditions cannot occur together, such as a congenital form versus an acquired form of the same condition.

    An exception to the Excludes1 definition is the circumstance when the two conditions are unrelated to each other. If it is not clear whether the two conditions involving an Excludes1 note are related or not, query the provider. For example, code F45.8, Other somatoform disorders, has an Excludes1 note for "sleep related teeth grinding (G47.63)," because "teeth grinding" is an inclusion term under F45.8. Only one of these two codes should be assigned for teeth grinding. However psychogenic dysmenorrhea is also an inclusion term under F45.8, and a patient could have both this condition and sleep related teeth grinding. In this case, the two conditions are clearly unrelated to each other, and so it would be appropriate to report F45.8 and G47.63 together.

    b. **Excludes2**

    A type 2 Excludes note represents "Not included here." An excludes2 note indicates that the condition excluded is not part of the condition represented by the code, but a patient may have both conditions at the same time. When an Excludes2 note appears under a code, it is acceptable to use both the code and the excluded code together, when appropriate.

13. Etiology/manifestation convention ("code first", "use additional code" and "in diseases classified elsewhere" notes)

Certain conditions have both an underlying etiology and multiple body system manifestations due to the underlying etiology. For such conditions, the ICD-10-CM has a coding convention that requires the underlying condition be sequenced first, if applicable, followed by the manifestation. Wherever such a combination exists, there is a "use additional code" note at the etiology code, and a "code first" note at the manifestation code. These instructional notes indicate the proper sequencing order of the codes, etiology followed by manifestation.

In most cases the manifestation codes will have in the code title, "in diseases classified elsewhere." Codes with this title are a component of the etiology/ manifestation convention. The code title indicates that it is a manifestation code. "In diseases classified elsewhere" codes are never permitted to be used as first listed or principal diagnosis codes. They must be used in conjunction with an underlying condition code and they must be listed following the underlying condition. See category F02, Dementia in other diseases classified elsewhere, for an example of this convention.

There are manifestation codes that do not have "in diseases classified elsewhere" in the title. For such codes, there is a "use additional code" note at the etiology code and a "code first" note at the manifestation code, and the rules for sequencing apply.

In addition to the notes in the Tabular List, these conditions also have a specific Alphabetic Index entry structure. In the Alphabetic Index both conditions are listed together with the etiology code first followed by the manifestation codes in brackets. The code in brackets is always to be sequenced second.

An example of the etiology/manifestation convention is dementia in Parkinson's disease. In the Alphabetic Index, code G20 is listed first, followed by code F02.80 or F02.81 in brackets. Code G20 represents the underlying etiology, Parkinson's disease, and must be sequenced first, whereas code F02.80 and F02.81 represent the manifestation of dementia in diseases classified elsewhere, with or without behavioral disturbance.

"Code first" and "Use additional code" notes are also used as sequencing rules in the classification for certain codes that are not part of an etiology/manifestation combination.

See Section I.B.7. Multiple coding for a single condition.

14. "And"

The word "and" should be interpreted to mean either "and" or "or" when it appears in a title.

For example, cases of "tuberculosis of bones", "tuberculosis of joints" and "tuberculosis of bones and joints" are classified to subcategory A18.0, Tuberculosis of bones and joints.

15. "With"

The word "with" or "in" should be interpreted to mean "associated with" or "due to" when it appears in a code title, the Alphabetic Index (either under a main term or subterm), or an instructional note in the Tabular List. The classification presumes a causal relationship between the two conditions linked by these terms in the Alphabetic Index or Tabular List. These conditions should be coded as related even in the absence of provider documentation explicitly linking them, unless the documentation clearly states the conditions are unrelated or when another guideline exists that specifically requires a documented linkage between two conditions (e.g., sepsis guideline for "acute organ dysfunction that is not clearly associated with the sepsis").

For conditions not specifically linked by these relational terms in the classification or when a guideline requires that a linkage between two conditions be explicitly documented, provider documentation must link the conditions in order to code them as related.

The word "with" in the Alphabetic Index is sequenced immediately following the main term or subterm, not in alphabetical order.

16. "See" and "See Also"

The "see" instruction following a main term in the Alphabetic Index indicates that another term should be referenced. It is necessary to go to the main term referenced with the "see" note to locate the correct code.

A "see also" instruction following a main term in the Alphabetic Index instructs that there is another main term that may also be referenced that may provide additional Alphabetic Index entries that may be useful. It is not necessary to follow the "see also" note when the original main term provides the necessary code.

17. "Code also" note

A "code also" note instructs that two codes may be required to fully describe a condition, but this note does not provide sequencing direction. The sequencing depends on the circumstances of the encounter.

18. Default codes

A code listed next to a main term in the ICD-10-CM Alphabetic Index is referred to as a default code. The default code represents that condition that is most commonly associated with the main term, or is the unspecified code for the condition. If a condition is documented in a medical record (for example, appendicitis) without any additional information, such as acute or chronic, the default code should be assigned.

19. Code assignment and Clinical Criteria

The assignment of a diagnosis code is based on the provider's diagnostic statement that the condition exists. The provider's statement that the patient has a particular condition is sufficient. Code assignment is not based on clinical criteria used by the provider to establish the diagnosis.

B. General Coding Guidelines

1. Locating a code in the ICD-10-CM

To select a code in the classification that corresponds to a diagnosis or reason for visit documented in a medical record, first locate the term in the Alphabetic Index, and then verify the code in the Tabular List. Read and be guided by instructional notations that appear in both the Alphabetic Index and the Tabular List.

It is essential to use both the Alphabetic Index and Tabular List when locating and assigning a code. The Alphabetic Index does not always provide the full code. Selection of the full code, including laterality and any applicable 7th character can only be done in the Tabular List. A dash (-) at the end of an Alphabetic Index entry indicates that additional characters are required. Even if a dash is not included at the Alphabetic Index entry, it is necessary to refer to the Tabular List to verify that no 7th character is required.

2. Level of Detail in Coding

Diagnosis codes are to be used and reported at their highest number of characters available.

ICD-10-CM diagnosis codes are composed of codes with 3, 4, 5, 6 or 7 characters. Codes with three characters are included in ICD-10-CM as the heading of a category of codes that may be further subdivided by the use of fourth and/or fifth characters and/or sixth characters, which provide greater detail.

A three-character code is to be used only if it is not further subdivided. A code is invalid if it has not been coded to the full number of characters required for that code, including the 7th character, if applicable.

3. Code or codes from A00.0 through T88.9, Z00-Z99.8

The appropriate code or codes from A00.0 through T88.9, Z00-Z99.8 must be used to identify diagnoses, symptoms, conditions, problems, complaints or other reason(s) for the encounter/visit.

4. Signs and symptoms

Codes that describe symptoms and signs, as opposed to diagnoses, are acceptable for reporting purposes when a related definitive diagnosis has not been established (confirmed) by the provider. Chapter 18 of ICD-10-CM, Symptoms, Signs, and Abnormal Clinical and Laboratory Findings, Not Elsewhere Classified (codes R00.0 - R99) contains many, but not all, codes for symptoms.

See Section I.B.18 Use of Signs/Symptom/Unspecified Codes

5. Conditions that are an integral part of a disease process

Signs and symptoms that are associated routinely with a disease process should not be assigned as additional codes, unless otherwise instructed by the classification.

6. Conditions that are not an integral part of a disease process

Additional signs and symptoms that may not be associated routinely with a disease process should be coded when present.

7. Multiple coding for a single condition

In addition to the etiology/manifestation convention that requires two codes to fully describe a single condition that affects multiple body systems, there are other single conditions that also require more than one code. "Use additional code" notes are found in the Tabular List at codes that are not part of an etiology/manifestation pair where a secondary code is useful to fully describe a condition. The sequencing rule is the same as the etiology/manifestation pair, "use additional code" indicates that a secondary code should be added, if known.

For example, for bacterial infections that are not included in chapter 1, a secondary code from category B95, Streptococcus, Staphylococcus, and Enterococcus, as the cause of diseases classified elsewhere, or B96, Other bacterial agents as the cause of diseases classified elsewhere, may be required to identify the bacterial organism causing the infection. A "use additional code" note will normally be found at the infectious disease code, indicating a need for the organism code to be added as a secondary code.

"Code first" notes are also under certain codes that are not specifically manifestation codes but may be due to an underlying cause. When there is a "code first" note and an underlying condition is present, the underlying condition should be sequenced first, if known.

"Code, if applicable, any causal condition first" notes indicate that this code may be assigned as a principal diagnosis when the causal condition is unknown or not applicable. If a causal condition is known, then the code for that condition should be sequenced as the principal or first-listed diagnosis.

Multiple codes may be needed for sequela, complication codes and obstetric codes to more fully describe a condition. See the specific guidelines for these conditions for further instruction.

8. **Acute and Chronic Conditions**
   If the same condition is described as both acute (subacute) and chronic, and separate subentries exist in the Alphabetic Index at the same indentation level, code both and sequence the acute (subacute) code first.

9. **Combination Code**
   A combination code is a single code used to classify:
   > Two diagnoses, or
   > A diagnosis with an associated secondary process (manifestation)
   > A diagnosis with an associated complication

   Combination codes are identified by referring to subterm entries in the Alphabetic Index and by reading the inclusion and exclusion notes in the Tabular List.

   Assign only the combination code when that code fully identifies the diagnostic conditions involved or when the Alphabetic Index so directs. Multiple coding should not be used when the classification provides a combination code that clearly identifies all of the elements documented in the diagnosis. When the combination code lacks necessary specificity in describing the manifestation or complication, an additional code should be used as a secondary code.

10. **Sequela (Late Effects)**
    A sequela is the residual effect (condition produced) after the acute phase of an illness or injury has terminated. There is no time limit on when a sequela code can be used. The residual may be apparent early, such as in cerebral infarction, or it may occur months or years later, such as that due to a previous injury. Examples of sequela include: scar formation resulting from a burn, deviated septum due to a nasal fracture, and infertility due to tubal occlusion from old tuberculosis. Coding of sequela generally requires two codes sequenced in the following order: the condition or nature of the sequela is sequenced first. The sequela code is sequenced second.

    An exception to the above guidelines are those instances where the code for the sequela is followed by a manifestation code identified in the Tabular List and title, or the sequela code has been expanded (at the fourth, fifth or sixth character levels) to include the manifestation(s). The code for the acute phase of an illness or injury that led to the sequela is never used with a code for the late effect.

    See Section I.C.9. Sequelae of cerebrovascular disease

    See Section I.C.15. Sequelae of complication of pregnancy, childbirth and the puerperium

    See Section I.C.19. Application of 7th characters for Chapter 19

11. **Impending or Threatened Condition**
    Code any condition described at the time of discharge as "impending" or "threatened" as follows:
    > If it did occur, code as confirmed diagnosis.
    > If it did not occur, reference the Alphabetic Index to determine if the condition has a subentry term for "impending" or "threatened" and also reference main term entries for "Impending" and for "Threatened."
    > If the subterms are listed, assign the given code.
    > If the subterms are not listed, code the existing underlying condition(s) and not the condition described as impending or threatened.

12. **Reporting Same Diagnosis Code more than Once**
    Each unique ICD-10-CM diagnosis code may be reported only once for an encounter. This applies to bilateral conditions when there are no distinct codes identifying laterality or two different conditions classified to the same ICD-10-CM diagnosis code.

13. **Laterality**
    Some ICD-10-CM codes indicate laterality, specifying whether the condition occurs on the left, right or is bilateral. If no bilateral code is provided and the condition is bilateral, assign separate codes for both the left and right side. If the side is not identified in the medical record, assign the code for the unspecified side.

    When a patient has a bilateral condition and each side is treated during separate encounters, assign the "bilateral" code (as the condition still exists on both sides), including for the encounter to treat the first side. For the second encounter for treatment after one side has previously been treated and the condition no longer exists on that side, assign the appropriate unilateral code for the side where the condition still exists (e.g., cataract surgery performed on each eye in separate encounters). The bilateral code would not be assigned for the subsequent encounter, as the patient no longer has the condition in the previously-treated site. If the treatment on the first side did not completely resolve the condition, then the bilateral code would still be appropriate.

14. **Documentation by *Clinicians Other than the Patient's Provider***
    Code assignment is based on the documentation by patient's provider (i.e., physician or other qualified healthcare practitioner legally accountable for establishing the patient's diagnosis). There are a few exceptions, such as codes for the Body Mass Index (BMI), depth of non-pressure chronic ulcers, pressure ulcer stage, coma scale, and NIH stroke scale (NIHSS) codes, code assignment may be based on medical record documentation from clinicians who are not the patient's provider (i.e., physician or other qualified healthcare practitioner legally accountable for establishing the patient's diagnosis), since this information is typically documented by other clinicians involved in the care of the patient (e.g., a dietitian often documents the BMI, a nurse often documents the pressure ulcer stages, and an emergency medical technician often documents the coma scale). However, the associated diagnosis (such as overweight, obesity, acute stroke, or pressure ulcer) must be documented by the patient's provider. If there is conflicting medical record documentation, either from the same clinician or different clinicians, the patient's attending provider should be queried for clarification.

    For social determinants of health, such as information found in categories Z55-Z65, Persons with potential health hazards related to socioeconomic and psychosocial circumstances, code assignment may be based on medical record documentation from clinicians involved in the care of the patient who are not the patient's provider since this information represents social information, rather than medical diagnoses. **Patient self-reported documentation may also be used to assign codes for social determinants of health, as long as the patient self-reported information is signed-off by and incorporated into the health record by either a clinician or provider.**

    The BMI, coma scale, NIHSS codes and categories Z55-Z65 should only be reported as secondary diagnoses.

15. **Syndromes**
    Follow the Alphabetic Index guidance when coding syndromes. In the absence of Alphabetic Index guidance, assign codes for the documented manifestations of the syndrome. Additional codes for manifestations that are not an integral part of the disease process may also be assigned when the condition does not have a unique code.

16. **Documentation of Complications of Care**
    Code assignment is based on the provider's documentation of the relationship between the condition and the care or procedure, unless otherwise instructed by the classification. The guideline extends to any complications of care, regardless of the chapter the code is located in. It is important to note that not all conditions that occur during or following medical care or surgery are classified as complications. There must be a cause-and-effect relationship between the care provided and the condition, and an indication in the documentation that it is a complication. Query the provider for clarification, if the complication is not clearly documented.

17. **Borderline Diagnosis**
    If the provider documents a "borderline" diagnosis at the time of discharge, the diagnosis is coded as confirmed, unless the classification provides a specific entry (e.g., borderline diabetes). If a borderline condition has a specific index entry in ICD-10-CM, it should be coded as such. Since borderline conditions are not uncertain diagnoses, no distinction is made between the care setting (inpatient versus outpatient). Whenever the documentation is unclear regarding a borderline condition, coders are encouraged to query for clarification.

18. **Use of Sign/Symptom/Unspecified Codes**

Sign/symptom and "unspecified" codes have acceptable, even necessary, uses. While specific diagnosis codes should be reported when they are supported by the available medical record documentation and clinical knowledge of the patient's health condition, there are instances when signs/symptoms or unspecified codes are the best choices for accurately reflecting the healthcare encounter. Each healthcare encounter should be coded to the level of certainty known for that encounter.

If a definitive diagnosis has not been established by the end of the encounter, it is appropriate to report codes for sign(s) and/or symptom(s) in lieu of a definitive diagnosis. When sufficient clinical information isn't known or available about a particular health condition to assign a more specific code, it is acceptable to report the appropriate "unspecified" code (e.g., a diagnosis of pneumonia has been determined, but not the specific type). Unspecified codes should be reported when they are the codes that most accurately reflect what is known about the patient's condition at the time of that particular encounter. It would be inappropriate to select a specific code that is not supported by the medical record documentation or conduct medically unnecessary diagnostic testing in order to determine a more specific code.

19. **Coding for Healthcare Encounters in Hurricane Aftermath**
    a. **Use of External Cause of Morbidity Codes**

    An external cause of morbidity code should be assigned to identify the cause of the injury(ies) incurred as a result of the hurricane. The use of external cause of morbidity codes is supplemental to the application of ICD-10-CM codes. External cause of morbidity codes are never to be recorded as a principal diagnosis (first-listed in non-inpatient settings). The appropriate injury code should be sequenced before any external cause codes. The external cause of morbidity codes capture how the injury or health condition happened (cause), the intent (unintentional or accidental; or intentional, such as suicide or assault), the place where the event occurred, the activity of the patient at the time of the event, and the person's status (e.g., civilian, military). They should not be assigned for encounters to treat hurricane victims' medical conditions when no injury, adverse effect or poisoning is involved. External cause of morbidity codes should be assigned for each encounter for care and treatment of the injury. External cause of morbidity codes may be assigned in all health care settings. For the purpose of capturing complete and accurate ICD-10-CM data in the aftermath of the hurricane, a healthcare setting should be considered as any location where medical care is provided by licensed healthcare professionals.

    b. **Sequencing of External Causes of Morbidity Codes**

    Codes for cataclysmic events, such as a hurricane, take priority over all other external cause codes except child and adult abuse and terrorism and should be sequenced before other external cause of injury codes. Assign as many external cause of morbidity codes as necessary to fully explain each cause. For example, if an injury occurs as a result of a building collapse during the hurricane, external cause codes for both the hurricane and the building collapse should be assigned, with the external causes code for hurricane being sequenced as the first external cause code. For injuries incurred as a direct result of the hurricane, assign the appropriate code(s) for the injuries, followed by the code X37.0-, Hurricane (with the appropriate 7th character), and any other applicable external cause of injury codes. Code X37.0- also should be assigned when an injury is incurred as a result of flooding caused by a levee breaking related to the hurricane. Code X38.-, Flood (with the appropriate 7th character), should be assigned when an injury is from flooding resulting directly from the storm. Code X36.0.-, Collapse of dam or man-made structure, should not be assigned when the cause of the collapse is due to the hurricane. Use of code X36.0- is limited to collapses of man-made structures due to earth surface movements, not due to storm surges directly from a hurricane.

    c. **Other External Causes of Morbidity Code Issues**

    For injuries that are not a direct result of the hurricane, such as an evacuee that has incurred an injury as a result of a motor vehicle accident, assign the appropriate external cause of morbidity code(s) to describe the cause of the injury, but do not assign code X37.0-, Hurricane. If it is not clear whether the injury was a direct result of the hurricane, assume the injury is due to the hurricane and assign code X37.0-, Hurricane, as well as any other applicable external cause of morbidity codes. In addition to code X37.0-, Hurricane, other possible applicable external cause of morbidity codes include:

    W54.0-, Bitten by dog

    X30-, Exposure to excessive natural heat

    X31-, Exposure to excessive natural cold

    X38-, Flood

    d. **Use of Z codes**

    Z codes (other reasons for healthcare encounters) may be assigned as appropriate to further explain the reasons for presenting for healthcare services, including transfers between healthcare facilities. The ICD-10-CM Official Guidelines for Coding and Reporting identify which codes maybe assigned as principal or first-listed diagnosis only, secondary diagnosis only, or principal/first-listed or secondary (depending on the circumstances). Possible applicable Z codes include:

    Z59.0, Homelessness

    Z59.1, Inadequate housing

    Z59.5, Extreme poverty

    Z75.1, Person awaiting admission to adequate facility elsewhere

    Z75.3, Unavailability and inaccessibility of health-care facilities

    Z75.4, Unavailability and inaccessibility of other helping agencies

    Z76.2, Encounter for health supervision and care of other healthy infant and child

    Z99.12, Encounter for respirator [ventilator] dependence during power failure

    The external cause of morbidity codes and the Z codes listed above are not an all-inclusive list. Other codes may be applicable to the encounter based upon the documentation. Assign as many codes as necessary to fully explain each healthcare encounter. Since patient history information may be very limited, use any available documentation to assign the appropriate external cause of morbidity and Z codes.

C. Chapter-Specific Coding Guidelines

In addition to general coding guidelines, there are guidelines for specific diagnoses and/or conditions in the classification. Unless otherwise indicated, these guidelines apply to all health care settings. Please refer to Section II for guidelines on the selection of principal diagnosis.

1. **Chapter 1: Certain Infectious and Parasitic Diseases (A00-B99), *U07.1***
   a. **Human Immunodeficiency Virus (HIV) Infections**
      1) **Code only confirmed cases**

      Code only confirmed cases of HIV infection/illness. This is an exception to the hospital inpatient guideline Section II, H.

      In this context, "confirmation" does not require documentation of positive serology or culture for HIV; the provider's diagnostic statement that the patient is HIV positive, or has an HIV-related illness is sufficient.

      2) **Selection and sequencing of HIV codes**
         (a) **Patient admitted for HIV-related condition**

         If a patient is admitted for an HIV-related condition, the principal diagnosis should be B20, Human immunodeficiency virus [HIV] disease followed by additional diagnosis codes for all reported HIV-related conditions.

         (b) **Patient with HIV disease admitted for unrelated condition**

         If a patient with HIV disease is admitted for an unrelated condition (such as a traumatic injury), the code for the unrelated condition (e.g., the nature of injury code) should be the principal diagnosis. Other diagnoses would be B20 followed by additional diagnosis codes for all reported HIV-related conditions.

         (c) **Whether the patient is newly diagnosed**

         Whether the patient is newly diagnosed or has had previous admissions/encounters for HIV conditions is irrelevant to the sequencing decision.

         (d) **Asymptomatic human immunodeficiency virus**

         Z21, Asymptomatic human immunodeficiency virus [HIV] infection status, is to be applied when the patient without any documentation of symptoms is listed as being "HIV positive," "known HIV," "HIV test positive," or similar terminology. Do not use this code if the term "AIDS" is used or if the patient is treated for any HIV-related illness or is described as having any condition(s) resulting from his/her HIV positive status; use B20 in these cases.

(e) **Patients with inconclusive HIV serology**
Patients with inconclusive HIV serology, but no definitive diagnosis or manifestations of the illness, may be assigned code R75, Inconclusive laboratory evidence of human immunodeficiency virus [HIV].

(f) **Previously diagnosed HIV-related illness**
Patients with any known prior diagnosis of an HIV-related illness should be coded to B20. Once a patient has developed an HIV-related illness, the patient should always be assigned code B20 on every subsequent admission/encounter. Patients previously diagnosed with any HIV illness (B20) should never be assigned to R75 or Z21, Asymptomatic human immunodeficiency virus [HIV] infection status.

(g) **HIV Infection in Pregnancy, Childbirth and the Puerperium**
During pregnancy, childbirth or the puerperium, a patient admitted (or presenting for a health care encounter) because of an HIV-related illness should receive a principal diagnosis code of O98.7-, Human immunodeficiency [HIV] disease complicating pregnancy, childbirth and the puerperium, followed by B20 and the code(s) for the HIV-related illness(es). Codes from Chapter 15 always take sequencing priority.

Patients with asymptomatic HIV infection status admitted (or presenting for a health care encounter) during pregnancy, childbirth, or the puerperium should receive codes of O98.7- and Z21.

(h) **Encounters for testing for HIV**
If a patient is being seen to determine his/her HIV status, use code Z11.4, Encounter for screening for human immunodeficiency virus [HIV]. Use additional codes for any associated high-risk behavior.

If a patient with signs or symptoms is being seen for HIV testing, code the signs and symptoms. An additional counseling code Z71.7, Human immunodeficiency virus [HIV] counseling, may be used if counseling is provided during the encounter for the test.

When a patient returns to be informed of his/her HIV test results and the test result is negative, use code Z71.7, Human immunodeficiency virus [HIV] counseling.

If the results are positive, see previous guidelines and assign codes as appropriate.

b. **Infectious agents as the cause of diseases classified to other chapters**
Certain infections are classified in chapters other than Chapter 1 and no organism is identified as part of the infection code. In these instances, it is necessary to use an additional code from Chapter 1 to identify the organism. A code from category B95, Streptococcus, Staphylococcus, and Enterococcus as the cause of diseases classified to other chapters, B96, Other bacterial agents as the cause of diseases classified to other chapters, or B97, Viral agents as the cause of diseases classified to other chapters, is to be used as an additional code to identify the organism. An instructional note will be found at the infection code advising that an additional organism code is required.

c. **Infections resistant to antibiotics**
Many bacterial infections are resistant to current antibiotics. It is necessary to identify all infections documented as antibiotic resistant. Assign a code from category Z16, Resistance to antimicrobial drugs, following the infection code only if the infection code does not identify drug resistance.

d. **Sepsis, Severe Sepsis, and Septic Shock**
1) **Coding of Sepsis and Severe Sepsis**
(a) **Sepsis**
For a diagnosis of sepsis, assign the appropriate code for the underlying systemic infection. If the type of infection or causal organism is not further specified, assign code A41.9, Sepsis, unspecified organism.

A code from subcategory R65.2, Severe sepsis, should not be assigned unless severe sepsis or an associated acute organ dysfunction is documented.

(i) **Negative or inconclusive blood cultures and sepsis**
Negative or inconclusive blood cultures do not preclude a diagnosis of sepsis in patients with clinical evidence of the condition; however, the provider should be queried.

(ii) **Urosepsis**
The term urosepsis is a nonspecific term. It is not to be considered synonymous with sepsis. It has no default code in the Alphabetic Index. Should a provider use this term, he/she must be queried for clarification.

(iii) **Sepsis with organ dysfunction**
If a patient has sepsis and associated acute organ dysfunction or multiple organ dysfunction (MOD), follow the instructions for coding severe sepsis.

(iv) **Acute organ dysfunction that is not clearly associated with the sepsis**
If a patient has sepsis and an acute organ dysfunction, but the medical record documentation indicates that the acute organ dysfunction is related to a medical condition other than the sepsis, do not assign a code from subcategory R65.2, Severe sepsis. An acute organ dysfunction must be associated with the sepsis in order to assign the severe sepsis code. If the documentation is not clear as to whether an acute organ dysfunction is related to the sepsis or another medical condition, query the provider.

(b) **Severe sepsis**
The coding of severe sepsis requires a minimum of 2 codes: first a code for the underlying systemic infection, followed by a code from subcategory R65.2, Severe sepsis. If the causal organism is not documented, assign code A41.9, Sepsis, unspecified organism, for the infection. Additional code(s) for the associated acute organ dysfunction are also required.

Due to the complex nature of severe sepsis, some cases may require querying the provider prior to assignment of the codes.

2) **Septic shock**
(a) **Septic shock generally refers to circulatory failure associated with severe sepsis, and therefore, it represents a type of acute organ dysfunction.**
For cases of septic shock, the code for the systemic infection should be sequenced first, followed by code R65.21, Severe sepsis with septic shock or code T81.12, Postprocedural septic shock. Any additional codes for the other acute organ dysfunctions should also be assigned. As noted in the sequencing instructions in the Tabular List, the code for septic shock cannot be assigned as a principal diagnosis.

3) **Sequencing of severe sepsis**
If severe sepsis is present on admission, and meets the definition of principal diagnosis, the underlying systemic infection should be assigned as principal diagnosis followed by the appropriate code from subcategory R65.2 as required by the sequencing rules in the Tabular List. A code from subcategory R65.2 can never be assigned as a principal diagnosis.

When severe sepsis develops during an encounter (it was not present on admission), the underlying systemic infection and the appropriate code from subcategory R65.2 should be assigned as secondary diagnoses.

Severe sepsis may be present on admission, but the diagnosis may not be confirmed until sometime after admission. If the documentation is not clear whether severe sepsis was present on admission, the provider should be queried.

4) **Sepsis or severe sepsis with a localized infection**
If the reason for admission is sepsis or severe sepsis and a localized infection, such as pneumonia or cellulitis, a code(s) for the underlying systemic infection should be assigned first and the code for the localized infection should be assigned as a secondary diagnosis. If the patient has severe sepsis, a code from subcategory R65.2 should also be assigned as a secondary diagnosis. If the patient is admitted with a localized infection, such as pneumonia, and sepsis/severe sepsis doesn't develop until after admission, the localized infection should be assigned first, followed by the appropriate sepsis/severe sepsis codes.

5) Sepsis due to a postprocedural infection

(a) Documentation of causal relationship

As with all postprocedural complications, code assignment is based on the provider's documentation of the relationship between the infection and the procedure.

(b) Sepsis due to a postprocedural infection

For infections following a procedure, a code from T81.40, to T81.43 Infection following a procedure, or a code from O86.00 to O86.03, Infection of obstetric surgical wound, that identifies the site of the infection should be coded first, if known. Assign an additional code for sepsis following a procedure (T81.44) or sepsis following an obstetrical procedure (O86.04). Use an additional code to identify the infectious agent. If the patient has severe sepsis, the appropriate code from subcategory R65.2 should also be assigned with the additional code(s) for any acute organ dysfunction.

For infections following infusion, transfusion, therapeutic injection, or immunization, a code from subcategory T80.2, Infections following infusion, transfusion, and therapeutic injection, or code T88.0-, Infection following immunization, should be coded first, followed by the code for the specific infection. If the patient has severe sepsis, the appropriate code from subcategory R65.2 should also be assigned, with the additional codes(s) for any acute organ dysfunction.

(c) Postprocedural infection and postprocedural septic shock

If a postprocedural infection has resulted in postprocedural septic shock, assign the codes indicated above for sepsis due to a postprocedural infection, followed by code T81.12-, Postprocedural septic shock. Do not assign code R65.21, Severe sepsis with septic shock. Additional code(s) should be assigned for any acute organ dysfunction.

6) Sepsis and severe sepsis associated with a noninfectious process (condition)

In some cases, a noninfectious process (condition) such as trauma, may lead to an infection which can result in sepsis or severe sepsis. If sepsis or severe sepsis is documented as associated with a noninfectious condition, such as a burn or serious injury, and this condition meets the definition for principal diagnosis, the code for the noninfectious condition should be sequenced first, followed by the code for the resulting infection. If severe sepsis is present, a code from subcategory R65.2 should also be assigned with any associated organ dysfunction(s) codes. It is not necessary to assign a code from subcategory R65.1, Systemic inflammatory response syndrome (SIRS) of non-infectious origin, for these cases.

If the infection meets the definition of principal diagnosis, it should be sequenced before the non-infectious condition. When both the associated non-infectious condition and the infection meet the definition of principal diagnosis, either may be assigned as principal diagnosis.

Only one code from category R65, Symptoms and signs specifically associated with systemic inflammation and infection, should be assigned. Therefore, when a non-infectious condition leads to an infection resulting in severe sepsis, assign the appropriate code from subcategory R65.2, Severe sepsis. Do not additionally assign a code from subcategory R65.1, Systemic inflammatory response syndrome (SIRS) of non-infectious origin.

See Section I.C.18. SIRS due to non-infectious process

7) Sepsis and septic shock complicating abortion, pregnancy, childbirth, and the puerperium

See Section I.C.15. Sepsis and septic shock complicating abortion, pregnancy, childbirth and the puerperium

8) Newborn sepsis

See Section I.C.16. f. Bacterial sepsis of Newborn

e. Methicillin Resistant Staphylococcus aureus (MRSA) Conditions

1) Selection and sequencing of MRSA codes

(a) Combination codes for MRSA infection

When a patient is diagnosed with an infection that is due to methicillin resistant *Staphylococcus aureus* (MRSA), and that infection has a combination code that includes the causal organism (e.g., sepsis, pneumonia) assign the appropriate combination code for the condition (e.g., code A41.02, Sepsis due to Methicillin resistant Staphylococcus aureus or code

J15.212, Pneumonia due to Methicillin resistant Staphylococcus aureus). Do not assign code B95.62, Methicillin resistant Staphylococcus aureus infection as the cause of diseases classified elsewhere, as an additional code, because the combination code includes the type of infection and the MRSA organism. Do not assign a code from subcategory Z16.11, Resistance to penicillins, as an additional diagnosis.

See Section C.1. for instructions on coding and sequencing of sepsis and severe sepsis.

(b) Other codes for MRSA infection

When there is documentation of a current infection (e.g., wound infection, stitch abscess, urinary tract infection) due to MRSA, and that infection does not have a combination code that includes the causal organism, assign the appropriate code to identify the condition along with code B95.62, Methicillin resistant Staphylococcus aureus infection as the cause of diseases classified elsewhere for the MRSA infection. Do not assign a code from subcategory Z16.11, Resistance to penicillins.

(c) Methicillin susceptible Staphylococcus aureus (MSSA) and MRSA colonization

The condition or state of being colonized or carrying MSSA or MRSA is called colonization or carriage, while an individual person is described as being colonized or being a carrier. Colonization means that MSSA or MSRA is present on or in the body without necessarily causing illness. A positive MRSA colonization test might be documented by the provider as "MRSA screen positive" or "MRSA nasal swab positive".

Assign code Z22.322, Carrier or suspected carrier of Methicillin resistant Staphylococcus aureus, for patients documented as having MRSA colonization. Assign code Z22.321, Carrier or suspected carrier of Methicillin susceptible Staphylococcus aureus, for patients documented as having MSSA colonization. Colonization is not necessarily indicative of a disease process or as the cause of a specific condition the patient may have unless documented as such by the provider.

(d) MRSA colonization and infection

If a patient is documented as having both MRSA colonization and infection during a hospital admission, code Z22.322, Carrier or suspected carrier of Methicillin resistant Staphylococcus aureus, and a code for the MRSA infection may both be assigned.

f. Zika virus infections

1) Code only confirmed cases

Code only a confirmed diagnosis of Zika virus (A92.5, Zika virus disease) as documented by the provider. This is an exception to the hospital inpatient guideline Section II, H. In this context, "confirmation" does not require documentation of the type of test performed; the provider's diagnostic statement that the condition is confirmed is sufficient. This code should be assigned regardless of the stated mode of transmission.

If the provider documents "suspected", "possible" or "probable" Zika, do not assign code A92.5. Assign a code(s) explaining the reason for encounter (such as fever, rash, or joint pain) or Z20.821, Contact with and (suspected) exposure to Zika virus.

g. Coronavirus infections

1) COVID-19 infections (Infections due to SARS-CoV-2)

a) Code only confirmed cases

Code only a confirmed diagnosis of the 2019 novel coronavirus disease (COVID-19) as documented by the provider or documentation of a positive COVID-19 test result. For a confirmed diagnosis, assign code U07.1, COVID-19. This is an exception to the hospital inpatient guideline Section II, H. In this context, "confirmation" does not require documentation of a positive test result for COVID-19; the provider's documentation that the individual has COVID-19 is sufficient.

If the provider documents "suspected," "possible," "probable," or "inconclusive" COVID-19, do not assign code U07.1. Instead, code the signs and symptoms reported. See guideline I.C.1.g.1.g.

b) **Sequencing of codes**
When COVID-19 meets the definition of principal diagnosis, code U07.1, COVID-19, should be sequenced first, followed by the appropriate codes for associated manifestations, except when another guideline requires that certain codes be sequenced first, such as obstetrics, sepsis, or transplant complications.

For a COVID-19 infection that progresses to sepsis, see Section I.C.1.d. Sepsis, Severe Sepsis, and Septic Shock

See Section I.C.15.s. for COVID-19 infection in pregnancy, childbirth, and the puerperium

See Section I.C.16.h. for COVID-19 infection in newborn

For a COVID-19 infection in a lung transplant patient, see Section I.C.19.g.3.a. Transplant complications other than kidney.

c) **Acute respiratory manifestations of COVID-19**
When the reason for the encounter/admission is a respiratory manifestation of COVID-19, assign code U07.1, COVID-19, as the principal/first-listed diagnosis and assign code(s) for the respiratory manifestation(s) as additional diagnoses.

The following conditions are examples of common respiratory manifestations of COVID-19.

(i) **Pneumonia**
For a patient with pneumonia confirmed as due to COVID-19, assign codes U07.1, COVID-19, and J12.89, Other viral pneumonia.

(ii) **Acute bronchitis**
For a patient with acute bronchitis confirmed as due to COVID-19, assign codes U07.1, and J20.8, Acute bronchitis due to other specified organisms.

Bronchitis not otherwise specified (NOS) due to COVID-19 should be coded using code U07.1 and J40, Bronchitis, not specified as acute or chronic.

(iii) **Lower respiratory infection**
If the COVID-19 is documented as being associated with a lower respiratory infection, not otherwise specified (NOS), or an acute respiratory infection, NOS, codes U07.1 and J22, Unspecified acute lower respiratory infection, should be assigned.

If the COVID-19 is documented as being associated with a respiratory infection, NOS, codes U07.1 and J98.8, Other specified respiratory disorders, should be assigned.

(iv) **Acute respiratory distress syndrome**
For acute respiratory distress syndrome (ARDS) due to COVID-19, assign codes U07.1, and J80, Acute respiratory distress syndrome.

(v) **Acute respiratory failure**
For acute respiratory failure due to COVID-19, assign code U07.1, and code J96.0-, Acute respiratory failure.

d) **Non-respiratory manifestations of COVID-19**
When the reason for the encounter/admission is a non-respiratory manifestation (e.g., viral enteritis) of COVID-19, assign code U07.1, COVID-19, as the principal/first-listed diagnosis and assign code(s) for the manifestation(s) as additional diagnoses.

e) **Exposure to COVID-19**
For asymptomatic individuals with actual or suspected exposure to COVID-19, assign code Z20.828, Contact with and (suspected) exposure to other viral communicable diseases.

For symptomatic individuals with actual or suspected exposure to COVID-19 and the infection has been ruled out, or test results are inconclusive or unknown, assign code Z20.828, Contact with and (suspected) exposure to other viral communicable diseases. See guideline I.C.21.c.1, Contact/Exposure, for additional guidance regarding the use of category Z20 codes.

If COVID-19 is confirmed, see guideline I.C.1.g.1.a.

f) **Screening for COVID-19**
During the COVID-19 pandemic, a screening code is generally not appropriate. For encounters for COVID-19 testing, including preoperative testing, code as exposure to COVID-19 (guideline I.C.1.g.1.e).

Coding guidance will be updated as new information concerning any changes in the pandemic status becomes available.

g) **Signs and symptoms without definitive diagnosis of COVID-19**
For patients presenting with any signs/symptoms associated with COVID-19 (such as fever, etc.) but a definitive diagnosis has not been established, assign the appropriate code(s) for each of the presenting signs and symptoms such as:

- R05 Cough
- R06.02 Shortness of breath
- R50.9 Fever, unspecified

If a patient with signs/symptoms associated with COVID-19 also has an actual or suspected contact with or exposure to COVID-19, assign Z20.828, Contact with and (suspected) exposure to other viral communicable diseases, as an additional code.

h) **Asymptomatic individuals who test positive for COVID-19**
For asymptomatic individuals who test positive for COVID-19, see guideline I.C.1.g.1.a. Although the individual is asymptomatic, the individual has tested positive and is considered to have the COVID-19 infection.

i) **Personal history of COVID-19**
For patients with a history of COVID-19, assign code Z86.19, Personal history of other infectious and parasitic diseases.

j) **Follow-up visits after COVID-19 infection has resolved**
For individuals who previously had COVID-19 and are being seen for follow-up evaluation, and COVID-19 test results are negative, assign codes Z09, Encounter for follow-up examination after completed treatment for conditions other than malignant neoplasm, and Z86.19, Personal history of other infectious and parasitic diseases.

k) **Encounter for antibody testing**
For an encounter for antibody testing that is not being performed to confirm a current COVID-19 infection, nor is a follow-up test after resolution of COVID-19, assign Z01.84, Encounter for antibody response examination.

Follow the applicable guidelines above if the individual is being tested to confirm a current COVID-19 infection.

For follow-up testing after a COVID-19 infection, see guideline I.C.1.g.1.j.

2. **Chapter 2: Neoplasms (C00-D49)**
General guidelines
Chapter 2 of the ICD-10-CM contains the codes for most benign and all malignant neoplasms. Certain benign neoplasms, such as prostatic adenomas, may be found in the specific body system chapters. To properly code a neoplasm, it is necessary to determine from the record if the neoplasm is benign, in-situ, malignant, or of uncertain histologic behavior. If malignant, any secondary (metastatic) sites should also be determined.

Primary malignant neoplasms overlapping site boundaries

A primary malignant neoplasm that overlaps two or more contiguous (next to each other) sites should be classified to the subcategory/code .8 ('overlapping lesion'), unless the combination is specifically indexed elsewhere. For multiple neoplasms of the same site that are not contiguous such as tumors in different quadrants of the same breast, codes for each site should be assigned.

Malignant neoplasm of ectopic tissue

Malignant neoplasms of ectopic tissue are to be coded to the site of origin mentioned, e.g., ectopic pancreatic malignant neoplasms involving the stomach are coded to malignant neoplasm of pancreas, unspecified (C25.9).

The neoplasm table in the Alphabetic Index should be referenced first. However, if the histological term is documented, that term should be referenced first, rather than going immediately to the Neoplasm Table, in order to determine which column in the Neoplasm Table is appropriate. For example, if the documentation indicates "adenoma," refer to the term in the Alphabetic Index to review the entries under this term and the instructional note to "see also neoplasm, by site, benign." The table provides the proper code based on the type of neoplasm and the site. It is important to select the proper column in the table that corresponds to the type of neoplasm. The Tabular List should then be referenced to verify that the correct code has been selected from the table and that a more specific site code does not exist.

See Section I.C.21. Factors influencing health status and contact with health services, Status, for information regarding Z15.0, codes for genetic susceptibility to cancer.

a. Treatment directed at the malignancy

If the treatment is directed at the malignancy, designate the malignancy as the principal diagnosis.

The only exception to this guideline is if a patient admission/encounter is solely for the administration of chemotherapy, immunotherapy or external beam radiation therapy, assign the appropriate Z51.-- code as the first-listed or principal diagnosis, and the diagnosis or problem for which the service is being performed as a secondary diagnosis.

b. Treatment of secondary site

When a patient is admitted because of a primary neoplasm with metastasis and treatment is directed toward the secondary site only, the secondary neoplasm is designated as the principal diagnosis even though the primary malignancy is still present.

c. Coding and sequencing of complications

Coding and sequencing of complications associated with the malignancies or with the therapy thereof are subject to the following guidelines:

1) Anemia associated with malignancy

When admission/encounter is for management of an anemia associated with the malignancy, and the treatment is only for anemia, the appropriate code for the malignancy is sequenced as the principal or first-listed diagnosis followed by the appropriate code for the anemia (such as code D63.0, Anemia in neoplastic disease).

2) Anemia associated with chemotherapy, immunotherapy and radiation therapy

When the admission/encounter is for management of an anemia associated with an adverse effect of the administration of chemotherapy or immunotherapy and the only treatment is for the anemia, the anemia code is sequenced first followed by the appropriate codes for the neoplasm and the adverse effect (T45.1X5-, Adverse effect of antineoplastic and immunosuppressive drugs).

When the admission/encounter is for management of an anemia associated with an adverse effect of radiotherapy, the anemia code should be sequenced first, followed by the appropriate neoplasm code and code Y84.2, Radiological procedure and radiotherapy as the cause of abnormal reaction of the patient, or of later complication, without mention of misadventure at the time of the procedure.

3) Management of dehydration due to the malignancy

When the admission/encounter is for management of dehydration due to the malignancy and only the dehydration is being treated (intravenous rehydration), the dehydration is sequenced first, followed by the code(s) for the malignancy.

4) Treatment of a complication resulting from a surgical procedure

When the admission/encounter is for treatment of a complication resulting from a surgical procedure, designate the complication as the principal or first-listed diagnosis if treatment is directed at resolving the complication.

d. Primary malignancy previously excised

When a primary malignancy has been previously excised or eradicated from its site and there is no further treatment directed to that site and there is no evidence of any existing primary malignancy at that site, a code from category Z85, Personal history of malignant neoplasm, should be used to indicate the former site of the malignancy. Any mention of extension, invasion, or metastasis to another site is coded as a secondary malignant neoplasm to that site. The secondary site

may be the principal or first-listed diagnosis with the Z85 code used as a secondary code.

e. Admissions/Encounters involving chemotherapy, immunotherapy and radiation therapy

1) Episode of care involves surgical removal of neoplasm

When an episode of care involves the surgical removal of a neoplasm, primary or secondary site, followed by adjunct chemotherapy or radiation treatment during the same episode of care, the code for the neoplasm should be assigned as principal or first-listed diagnosis.

2) Patient admission/encounter solely for administration of chemotherapy, immunotherapy and radiation therapy

If a patient admission/encounter is solely for the administration of chemotherapy, immunotherapy or external beam radiation therapy assign code Z51.0, Encounter for antineoplastic radiation therapy, or Z51.11, Encounter for antineoplastic chemotherapy, or Z51.12, Encounter for antineoplastic immunotherapy as the first-listed or principal diagnosis. If a patient receives more than one of these therapies during the same admission more than one of these codes may be assigned, in any sequence.

The malignancy for which the therapy is being administered should be assigned as a secondary diagnosis.

If a patient admission/encounter is for the insertion or implantation of radioactive elements (e.g., brachytherapy) the appropriate code for the malignancy is sequenced as the principal or first-listed diagnosis. Code Z51.0 should not be assigned.

3) Patient admitted for radiation therapy, chemotherapy or immunotherapy and develops complications

When a patient is admitted for the purpose of external beam radiotherapy, immunotherapy or chemotherapy and develops complications such as uncontrolled nausea and vomiting or dehydration, the principal or first-listed diagnosis is Z51.0, Encounter for antineoplastic radiation therapy, or Z51.11, Encounter for antineoplastic chemotherapy, or Z51.12, Encounter for antineoplastic immunotherapy followed by any codes for the complications.

When a patient is admitted for the purpose of insertion or implantation of radioactive elements (e.g., brachytherapy) and develops complications such as uncontrolled nausea and vomiting or dehydration, the principal or first-listed diagnosis is the appropriate code for the malignancy followed by any codes for the complications.

f. Admission/encounter to determine extent of malignancy

When the reason for admission/encounter is to determine the extent of the malignancy, or for a procedure such as paracentesis or thoracentesis, the primary malignancy or appropriate metastatic site is designated as the principal or first-listed diagnosis, even though chemotherapy or radiotherapy is administered.

g. Symptoms, signs, and abnormal findings listed in Chapter 18 associated with neoplasms

Symptoms, signs, and ill-defined conditions listed in Chapter 18 characteristic of, or associated with, an existing primary or secondary site malignancy cannot be used to replace the malignancy as principal or first-listed diagnosis, regardless of the number of admissions or encounters for treatment and care of the neoplasm.

See section I.C.21. Factors influencing health status and contact with health services, Encounter for prophylactic organ removal.

h. Admission/encounter for pain control/management

See Section I.C.6. for information on coding admission/encounter for pain control/management.

i. Malignancy in two or more noncontiguous sites

A patient may have more than one malignant tumor in the same organ. These tumors may represent different primaries or metastatic disease, depending on the site. Should the documentation be unclear, the provider should be queried as to the status of each tumor so that the correct codes can be assigned.

j. Disseminated malignant neoplasm, unspecified

Code C80.0, Disseminated malignant neoplasm, unspecified, is for use only in those cases where the patient has advanced metastatic disease and no known primary or secondary sites are specified. It should not be used in place of assigning codes for the primary site and all known secondary sites.

k. **Malignant neoplasm without specification of site**
   Code C80.1, Malignant (primary) neoplasm, unspecified, equates to Cancer, unspecified. This code should only be used when no determination can be made as to the primary site of a malignancy. This code should rarely be used in the inpatient setting.

l. **Sequencing of neoplasm codes**
   1) **Encounter for treatment of primary malignancy**
      If the reason for the encounter is for treatment of a primary malignancy, assign the malignancy as the principal/first-listed diagnosis. The primary site is to be sequenced first, followed by any metastatic sites.

   2) **Encounter for treatment of secondary malignancy**
      When an encounter is for a primary malignancy with metastasis and treatment is directed toward the metastatic (secondary) site(s) only, the metastatic site(s) is designated as the principal/first-listed diagnosis. The primary malignancy is coded as an additional code.

   3) **Malignant neoplasm in a pregnant patient**
      When a pregnant woman has a malignant neoplasm, a code from subcategory O9A.1-, Malignant neoplasm complicating pregnancy, childbirth, and the puerperium, should be sequenced first, followed by the appropriate code from Chapter 2 to indicate the type of neoplasm.

   4) **Encounter for complication associated with a neoplasm**
      When an encounter is for management of a complication associated with a neoplasm, such as dehydration, and the treatment is only for the complication, the complication is coded first, followed by the appropriate code(s) for the neoplasm.

      The exception to this guideline is anemia. When the admission/encounter is for management of an anemia associated with the malignancy, and the treatment is only for anemia, the appropriate code for the malignancy is sequenced as the principal or first-listed diagnosis followed by code D63.0, Anemia in neoplastic disease.

   5) **Complication from surgical procedure for treatment of a neoplasm**
      When an encounter is for treatment of a complication resulting from a surgical procedure performed for the treatment of the neoplasm, designate the complication as the principal/first-listed diagnosis. See the guideline regarding the coding of a current malignancy versus personal history to determine if the code for the neoplasm should also be assigned.

   6) **Pathologic fracture due to a neoplasm**
      When an encounter is for a pathological fracture due to a neoplasm, and the focus of treatment is the fracture, a code from subcategory M84.5, Pathological fracture in neoplastic disease, should be sequenced first, followed by the code for the neoplasm.

      If the focus of treatment is the neoplasm with an associated pathological fracture, the neoplasm code should be sequenced first, followed by a code from M84.5 for the pathological fracture.

m. **Current malignancy versus personal history of malignancy**
   When a primary malignancy has been excised but further treatment, such as an additional surgery for the malignancy, radiation therapy or chemotherapy is directed to that site, the primary malignancy code should be used until treatment is completed.

   When a primary malignancy has been previously excised or eradicated from its site, there is no further treatment (of the malignancy) directed to that site, and there is no evidence of any existing primary malignancy at that site, a code from category Z85, Personal history of malignant neoplasm, should be used to indicate the former site of the malignancy.

   Codes from subcategories Z85.0 – Z85.85 should only be assigned for the former site of a primary malignancy, not the site of a secondary malignancy. **Code Z85.89** may be assigned for the former site(s) of either a primary or secondary malignancy.

   See Section I.C.21. Factors influencing health status and contact with health services, History (of)

n. **Leukemia, Multiple Myeloma, and Malignant Plasma Cell Neoplasms in remission versus personal history**
   The categories for leukemia, and category C90, Multiple myeloma and malignant plasma cell neoplasms, have codes indicating whether or not the leukemia has achieved remission. There are also codes Z85.6, Personal history of leukemia, and Z85.79, Personal history of other

malignant neoplasms of lymphoid, hematopoietic and related tissues. If the documentation is unclear as to whether the leukemia has achieved remission, the provider should be queried.

See Section I.C.21. Factors influencing health status and contact with health services, History (of)

o. **Aftercare following surgery for neoplasm**
   See Section I.C.21. Factors influencing health status and contact with health services, Aftercare

p. **Follow-up care for completed treatment of a malignancy**
   See Section I.C.21. Factors influencing health status and contact with health services, Follow-up

q. **Prophylactic organ removal for prevention of malignancy**
   See Section I.C. 21, Factors influencing health status and contact with health services, Prophylactic organ removal

r. **Malignant neoplasm associated with transplanted organ**
   A malignant neoplasm of a transplanted organ should be coded as a transplant complication. Assign first the appropriate code from category T86.-, Complications of transplanted organs and tissue, followed by code C80.2, Malignant neoplasm associated with transplanted organ. Use an additional code for the specific malignancy.

3. **Chapter 3: Disease of the blood and blood-forming organs and certain disorders involving the immune mechanism (D50-D89)**
   Reserved for future guideline expansion

4. **Chapter 4: Endocrine, Nutritional, and Metabolic Diseases (E00-E89)**
   a. **Diabetes mellitus**
      The diabetes mellitus codes are combination codes that include the type of diabetes mellitus, the body system affected, and the complications affecting that body system. As many codes within a particular category as are necessary to describe all of the complications of the disease may be used. They should be sequenced based on the reason for a particular encounter. Assign as many codes from categories E08 – E13 as needed to identify all of the associated conditions that the patient has.

      1) **Type of diabetes**
         The age of a patient is not the sole determining factor, though most type 1 diabetics develop the condition before reaching puberty. For this reason type 1 diabetes mellitus is also referred to as juvenile diabetes.

      2) **Type of diabetes mellitus not documented**
         If the type of diabetes mellitus is not documented in the medical record the default is E11.-, Type 2 diabetes mellitus.

      3) **Diabetes mellitus and the use of insulin, oral hypoglycemics, and injectable non-insulin drugs**
         If the documentation in a medical record does not indicate the type of diabetes but does indicate that the patient uses insulin, code E11-, Type 2 diabetes mellitus, should be assigned. An additional code should be assigned from category Z79 to identify the long-term (current) use of insulin or oral hypoglycemic drugs. If the patient is treated with both oral medications and insulin, only the code for long-term (current) use of insulin should be assigned. **If the patient is treated with both insulin and an injectable non-insulin antidiabetic drug, assign codes Z79.4, Long-term (current) use of insulin, and Z79.899, Other long term (current) drug therapy. If the patient is treated with both oral hypoglycemic drugs and an injectable non-insulin antidiabetic drug, assign codes Z79.84, Long-term (current) use of oral hypoglycemic drugs, and Z79.899, Other long-term (current) drug therapy.** Code Z79.4 should not be assigned if insulin is given temporarily to bring a type 2 patient's blood sugar under control during an encounter.

      4) **Diabetes mellitus in pregnancy and gestational diabetes**
         See Section I.C.15. Diabetes mellitus in pregnancy.
         See Section I.C.15. Gestational (pregnancy induced) diabetes

      5) **Complications due to insulin pump malfunction**
         (a) **Underdose of insulin due to insulin pump failure**
            An underdose of insulin due to an insulin pump failure should be assigned to a code from subcategory T85.6, Mechanical complication of other specified internal and external prosthetic devices, implants and grafts, that specifies the type of pump malfunction, as the principal or first-listed code, followed by code T38.3X6-, Underdosing of insulin and oral hypoglycemic [antidiabetic] drugs.

Additional codes for the type of diabetes mellitus and any associated complications due to the underdosing should also be assigned.

(b) Overdose of insulin due to insulin pump failure

The principal or first-listed code for an encounter due to an insulin pump malfunction resulting in an overdose of insulin, should also be T85.6-, Mechanical complication of other specified internal and external prosthetic devices, implants and grafts, followed by code T38.3X1-, Poisoning by insulin and oral hypoglycemic [antidiabetic] drugs, accidental (unintentional).

6) Secondary diabetes mellitus

Codes under categories E08, Diabetes mellitus due to underlying condition, E09, Drug or chemical induced diabetes mellitus, and E13, Other specified diabetes mellitus, identify complications/manifestations associated with secondary diabetes mellitus. Secondary diabetes is always caused by another condition or event (e.g., cystic fibrosis, malignant neoplasm of pancreas, pancreatectomy, adverse effect of drug, or poisoning).

(a) Secondary diabetes mellitus and the use of insulin or oral hypoglycemic drugs

For patients with secondary diabetes mellitus who routinely use insulin or oral hypoglycemic drugs, an additional code from category Z79 should be assigned to identify the long-term (current) use of insulin or oral hypoglycemic drugs. If the patient is treated with both oral medications and insulin, only the code for long-term (current) use of insulin should be assigned. **If the patient is treated with both insulin and an injectable non-insulin antidiabetic drug, assign codes Z79.4, Long-term (current) use of insulin, and Z79.899, Other long term (current) drug therapy. If the patient is treated with both oral hypoglycemic drugs and an injectable non-insulin antidiabetic drug, assign codes Z79.84, Long-term (current) use of oral hypoglycemic drugs, and Z79.899, Other long-term (current) drug therapy.** Code Z79.4 should not be assigned if insulin is given temporarily to bring a secondary diabetic patient's blood sugar under control during an encounter.

(b) Assigning and sequencing secondary diabetes codes and its causes

The sequencing of the secondary diabetes codes in relationship to codes for the cause of the diabetes is based on the Tabular List instructions for categories E08, E09 and E13.

(i) Secondary diabetes mellitus due to pancreatectomy

For postpancreatectomy diabetes mellitus (lack of insulin due to the surgical removal of all or part of the pancreas), assign code E89.1, Postprocedural hypoinsulinemia. Assign a code from category E13 and a code from subcategory Z90.41, Acquired absence of pancreas, as additional codes.

(ii) Secondary diabetes due to drugs

Secondary diabetes may be caused by an adverse effect of correctly administered medications, poisoning or sequela of poisoning.

See section I.C.19.e for coding of adverse effects and poisoning, and section I.C.20 for external cause code reporting.

5. Chapter 5: Mental, Behavioral and Neurodevelopmental disorders (F01-F99)

a. Pain disorders related to psychological factors

Assign code F45.41, for pain that is exclusively related to psychological disorders. As indicated by the Excludes 1 note under category G89, a code from category G89 should not be assigned with code F45.41.

Code F45.42, Pain disorders with related psychological factors, should be used with a code from category G89, Pain, not elsewhere classified, if there is documentation of a psychological component for a patient with acute or chronic pain.

See Section I.C.6. Pain

b. Mental and behavioral disorders due to psychoactive substance use

1) In Remission

Selection of codes for "in remission" for categories F10-F19, Mental and behavioral disorders due to psychoactive substance use (categories F10-F19 with -.11, -.21) requires the provider's clinical judgment. The appropriate codes for "in remission" are assigned only on the basis of provider documentation (as defined in the Official Guidelines for Coding and Reporting), unless otherwise instructed by the classification.

Mild substance use disorders in early or sustained remission are classified to the appropriate codes for substance abuse in remission, and moderate or severe substance use disorders in early or sustained remission are classified to the appropriate codes for substance dependence in remission.

2) Psychoactive Substance Use, Abuse and Dependence

When the provider documentation refers to use, abuse and dependence of the same substance (e.g. alcohol, opioid, cannabis, etc.), only one code should be assigned to identify the pattern of use based on the following hierarchy:

- If both use and abuse are documented, assign only the code for abuse
- If both abuse and dependence are documented, assign only the code for dependence
- If use, abuse and dependence are all documented, assign only the code for dependence
- If both use and dependence are documented, assign only the code for dependence.

3) Psychoactive Substance Use, Unspecified

As with all other unspecified diagnoses, the codes for unspecified psychoactive substance use (F10.9-, F11.9-, F12.9-, F13.9-, F14.9-, F15.9-, F16.9-, F18.9-, F19.9-) should only be assigned based on provider documentation and when they meet the definition of a reportable diagnosis (see Section III, Reporting Additional Diagnoses). These codes are to be used only when the psychoactive substance use is associated with a physical **disorder included in chapter 5 (such as sexual dysfunction and sleep disorder), or a** mental or behavioral disorder, and such a relationship is documented by the provider.

c. Factitious Disorder

Factitious disorder imposed on self or Munchausen's syndrome is a disorder in which a person falsely reports or causes his or her own physical or psychological signs or symptoms. For patients with documented factitious disorder on self or Munchausen's syndrome, assign the appropriate code from subcategory F68.1-, Factitious disorder imposed on self.

Munchausen's syndrome by proxy (MSBP) is a disorder in which a caregiver (perpetrator) falsely reports or causes an illness or injury in another person (victim) under his or her care, such as a child, an elderly adult, or a person who has a disability. The condition is also referred to as "factitious disorder imposed on another" or "factitious disorder by proxy." The perpetrator, not the victim, receives this diagnosis. Assign code F68.A, Factitious disorder imposed on another, to the perpetrator's record. For the victim of a patient suffering from MSBP, assign the appropriate code from categories T74, Adult and child abuse, neglect and other maltreatment, confirmed, or T76, Adult and child abuse, neglect and other maltreatment, suspected.

See Section I.C.19.f. Adult and child abuse, neglect and other maltreatment

6. Chapter 6: Diseases of the Nervous System (G00-G99)

a. Dominant/nondominant side

Codes from category G81, Hemiplegia and hemiparesis, and subcategories G83.1, Monoplegia of lower limb, G83.2, Monoplegia of upper limb, and G83.3, Monoplegia, unspecified, identify whether the dominant or nondominant side is affected. Should the affected side be documented, but not specified as dominant or nondominant, and the classification system does not indicate a default, code selection is as follows:

- For ambidextrous patients, the default should be dominant.
- If the left side is affected, the default is non-dominant.
- If the right side is affected, the default is dominant.

b. **Pain - Category G89**
1) **General coding information**

Codes in category G89, Pain, not elsewhere classified, may be used in conjunction with codes from other categories and chapters to provide more detail about acute or chronic pain and neoplasm-related pain, unless otherwise indicated below.

If the pain is not specified as acute or chronic, post-thoracotomy, postprocedural, or neoplasm-related, do not assign codes from category G89.

A code from category G89 should not be assigned if the underlying (definitive) diagnosis is known, unless the reason for the encounter is pain control/ management and not management of the underlying condition.

When an admission or encounter is for a procedure aimed at treating the underlying condition (e.g., spinal fusion, kyphoplasty), a code for the underlying condition (e.g., vertebral fracture, spinal stenosis) should be assigned as the principal diagnosis. No code from category G89 should be assigned.

(a) **Category G89 Codes as Principal or First-Listed Diagnosis**

Category G89 codes are acceptable as principal diagnosis or the first-listed code:

- When pain control or pain management is the reason for the admission/encounter (e.g., a patient with displaced intervertebral disc, nerve impingement and severe back pain presents for injection of steroid into the spinal canal). The underlying cause of the pain should be reported as an additional diagnosis, if known.

- When a patient is admitted for the insertion of a neurostimulator for pain control, assign the appropriate pain code as the principal or first-listed diagnosis. When an admission or encounter is for a procedure aimed at treating the underlying condition and a neurostimulator is inserted for pain control during the same admission/encounter, a code for the underlying condition should be assigned as the principal diagnosis and the appropriate pain code should be assigned as a secondary diagnosis.

(b) **Use of Category G89 Codes in Conjunction with Site Specific Pain Codes**

(i) **Assigning Category G89 and Site-Specific Pain Codes**

Codes from category G89 may be used in conjunction with codes that identify the site of pain (including codes from chapter 18) if the category G89 code provides additional information. For example, if the code describes the site of the pain, but does not fully describe whether the pain is acute or chronic, then both codes should be assigned.

(ii) **Sequencing of Category G89 Codes with Site-Specific Pain Codes**

The sequencing of category G89 codes with site-specific pain codes (including chapter 18 codes), is dependent on the circumstances of the encounter/admission as follows:

- If the encounter is for pain control or pain management, assign the code from category G89 followed by the code identifying the specific site of pain (e.g., encounter for pain management for acute neck pain from trauma is assigned code G89.11, Acute pain due to trauma, followed by code M54.2, Cervicalgia, to identify the site of pain).

- If the encounter is for any other reason except pain control or pain management, and a related definitive diagnosis has not been established (confirmed) by the provider, assign the code for the specific site of pain first, followed by the appropriate code from category G89.

2) **Pain due to devices, implants and grafts**
See Section I.C.19. Pain due to medical devices

3) **Postoperative Pain**

The provider's documentation should be used to guide the coding of postoperative pain, as well as *Section III. Reporting*

Additional Diagnoses and Section IV. Diagnostic Coding and Reporting in the Outpatient Setting.

The default for post-thoracotomy and other postoperative pain not specified as acute or chronic is the code for the acute form.

Routine or expected postoperative pain immediately after surgery should not be coded.

(a) **Postoperative pain not associated with specific postoperative complication**

Postoperative pain not associated with a specific postoperative complication is assigned to the appropriate postoperative pain code in category G89.

(b) **Postoperative pain associated with specific postoperative complication**

Postoperative pain associated with a specific postoperative complication (such as painful wire sutures) is assigned to the appropriate code(s) found in Chapter 19, Injury, poisoning, and certain other consequences of external causes. If appropriate, use additional code(s) from category G89 to identify acute or chronic pain (G89.18 or G89.28).

4) **Chronic pain**

Chronic pain is classified to subcategory G89.2. There is no time frame defining when pain becomes chronic pain. The provider's documentation should be used to guide use of these codes.

5) **Neoplasm Related Pain**

Code G89.3 is assigned to pain documented as being related, associated or due to cancer, primary or secondary malignancy, or tumor. This code is assigned regardless of whether the pain is acute or chronic.

This code may be assigned as the principal or first-listed code when the stated reason for the admission/encounter is documented as pain control/pain management. The underlying neoplasm should be reported as an additional diagnosis.

When the reason for the admission/encounter is management of the neoplasm and the pain associated with the neoplasm is also documented, code G89.3 may be assigned as an additional diagnosis. It is not necessary to assign an additional code for the site of the pain.

See Section I.C.2 for instructions on the sequencing of neoplasms for all other stated reasons for the admission/encounter (except for pain control/pain management).

6) **Chronic pain syndrome**

Central pain syndrome (G89.0) and chronic pain syndrome (G89.4) are different than the term "chronic pain," and therefore codes should only be used when the provider has specifically documented this condition.

See Section I.C.5. Pain disorders related to psychological factors

7. **Chapter 7: Diseases of the Eye and Adnexa (H00-H59)**
a. **Glaucoma**
1) **Assigning Glaucoma Codes**

Assign as many codes from category H40, Glaucoma, as needed to identify the type of glaucoma, the affected eye, and the glaucoma stage.

2) **Bilateral glaucoma with same type and stage**

When a patient has bilateral glaucoma and both eyes are documented as being the same type and stage, and there is a code for bilateral glaucoma, report only the code for the type of glaucoma, bilateral, with the seventh character for the stage.

When a patient has bilateral glaucoma and both eyes are documented as being the same type and stage, and the classification does not provide a code for bilateral glaucoma (i.e. subcategories H40.10 and H40.20) report only one code for the type of glaucoma with the appropriate seventh character for the stage.

3) **Bilateral glaucoma stage with different types or stages**

When a patient has bilateral glaucoma and each eye is documented as having a different type or stage, and the classification distinguishes laterality, assign the appropriate code for each eye rather than the code for bilateral glaucoma.

When a patient has bilateral glaucoma and each eye is documented as having a different type, and the classification does not distinguish laterality (i.e. subcategories H40.10 and H40.20), assign one code for each type of glaucoma with the appropriate seventh character for the stage.

When a patient has bilateral glaucoma and each eye is documented as having the same type, but different stage, and the classification does not distinguish laterality (i.e. subcategories H40.10 and H40.20), assign a code for the type of glaucoma for each eye with the seventh character for the specific glaucoma stage documented for each eye.

4) Patient admitted with glaucoma and stage evolves during the admission

If a patient is admitted with glaucoma and the stage progresses during the admission, assign the code for highest stage documented.

5) Indeterminate stage glaucoma

Assignment of the seventh character "4" for "indeterminate stage" should be based on the clinical documentation. The seventh character "4" is used for glaucomas whose stage cannot be clinically determined. This seventh character should not be confused with the seventh character "0", unspecified, which should be assigned when there is no documentation regarding the stage of the glaucoma.

b. Blindness

If "blindness" or "low vision" of both eyes is documented but the visual impairment category is not documented, assign code H54.3, Unqualified visual loss, both eyes. If "blindness" or "low vision" in one eye is documented but the visual impairment category is not documented, assign a code from H54.6-, Unqualified visual loss, one eye. If "blindness" or "visual loss" is documented without any information about whether one or both eyes are affected, assign code H54.7, Unspecified visual loss.

8. Chapter 8: Diseases of the Ear and Mastoid Process (H60-H95)

Reserved for future guideline expansion

9. Chapter 9: Diseases of the Circulatory System (I00-I99)

a. Hypertension

The classification presumes a causal relationship between hypertension and heart involvement and between hypertension and kidney involvement, as the two conditions are linked by the term "with" in the Alphabetic Index. These conditions should be coded as related even in the absence of provider documentation explicitly linking them, unless the documentation clearly states the conditions are unrelated.

For hypertension and conditions not specifically linked by relational terms such as "with," "associated with" or "due to" in the classification, provider documentation must link the conditions in order to code them as related.

1) Hypertension with Heart Disease

Hypertension with heart conditions classified to I50.- or I51.4-I51.7, I51.89, I51.9, are assigned to a code from category I11, Hypertensive heart disease. Use additional code(s) from category I50, Heart failure, to identify the type(s) of heart failure in those patients with heart failure.

The same heart conditions (I50.-, I51.4-I51.7, I51.89, I51.9) with hypertension are coded separately if the provider has documented they are unrelated to the hypertension. Sequence according to the circumstances of the admission/encounter.

2) Hypertensive Chronic Kidney Disease

Assign codes from category I12, Hypertensive chronic kidney disease, when both hypertension and a condition classifiable to category N18, Chronic kidney disease (CKD), are present. CKD should not be coded as hypertensive if the provider indicates the CKD is not related to the hypertension.

The appropriate code from category N18 should be used as a secondary code with a code from category I12 to identify the stage of chronic kidney disease.

See Section I.C.14. Chronic kidney disease.

If a patient has hypertensive chronic kidney disease and acute renal failure, the acute renal failure should also be coded. Sequence according to the circumstances of the admission/encounter.

3) Hypertensive Heart and Chronic Kidney Disease

Assign codes from combination category I13, Hypertensive heart and chronic kidney disease, when there is hypertension with both heart and kidney involvement. If heart failure is present, assign an additional code from category I50 to identify the type of heart failure.

The appropriate code from category N18, Chronic kidney disease, should be used as a secondary code with a code from category I13 to identify the stage of chronic kidney disease.

See Section I.C.14. Chronic kidney disease.

The codes in category I13, Hypertensive heart and chronic kidney disease, are combination codes that include hypertension, heart disease and chronic kidney disease. The Includes note at I13 specifies that the conditions included at I11 and I12 are included together in I13. If a patient has hypertension, heart disease and chronic kidney disease, then a code from I13 should be used, not individual codes for hypertension, heart disease and chronic kidney disease, or codes from I11 or I12.

For patients with both acute renal failure and chronic kidney disease, **the** acute renal failure **should also be coded. Sequence according to the circumstances of the admission/encounter.**

4) Hypertensive Cerebrovascular Disease

For hypertensive cerebrovascular disease, first assign the appropriate code from categories I60-I69, followed by the appropriate hypertension code.

5) Hypertensive Retinopathy

Subcategory H35.0, Background retinopathy and retinal vascular changes, should be used with a code from category I10- I15, Hypertensive disease to include the systemic hypertension. The sequencing is based on the reason for the encounter.

6) Hypertension, Secondary

Secondary hypertension is due to an underlying condition. Two codes are required: one to identify the underlying etiology and one from category I15 to identify the hypertension. Sequencing of codes is determined by the reason for admission/encounter.

7) Hypertension, Transient

Assign code R03.0, Elevated blood pressure reading without diagnosis of hypertension, unless patient has an established diagnosis of hypertension. Assign code O13.-, Gestational [pregnancy-induced] hypertension without significant proteinuria, or O14.-, Pre-eclampsia, for transient hypertension of pregnancy.

8) Hypertension, Controlled

This diagnostic statement usually refers to an existing state of hypertension under control by therapy. Assign the appropriate code from categories I10-I15, Hypertensive diseases.

9) Hypertension, Uncontrolled

Uncontrolled hypertension may refer to untreated hypertension or hypertension not responding to current therapeutic regimen. In either case, assign the appropriate code from categories I10-I15, Hypertensive diseases.

10) Hypertensive Crisis

Assign a code from category I16, Hypertensive crisis, for documented hypertensive urgency, hypertensive emergency or unspecified hypertensive crisis. Code also any identified hypertensive disease (I10-I15). The sequencing is based on the reason for the encounter.

11) Pulmonary Hypertension

Pulmonary hypertension is classified to category I27, Other pulmonary heart diseases. For secondary pulmonary hypertension (I27.1, I27.2-), code also any associated conditions or adverse effects of drugs or toxins. The sequencing is based on the reason for the encounter, except for adverse effects of drugs (See Section I.C.19.e.).

b. Atherosclerotic Coronary Artery Disease and Angina

ICD-10-CM has combination codes for atherosclerotic heart disease with angina pectoris. The subcategories for these codes are I25.11, Atherosclerotic heart disease of native coronary artery with angina pectoris and I25.7, Atherosclerosis of coronary artery bypass graft(s) and coronary artery of transplanted heart with angina pectoris.

When using one of these combination codes it is not necessary to use an additional code for angina pectoris. A causal relationship can be assumed in a patient with both atherosclerosis and angina pectoris, unless the documentation indicates the angina is due to something other than the atherosclerosis.

If a patient with coronary artery disease is admitted due to an acute myocardial infarction (AMI), the AMI should be sequenced before the coronary artery disease.

See Section I.C.9. Acute myocardial infarction (AMI)

c. **Intraoperative and Postprocedural Cerebrovascular Accident**

Medical record documentation should clearly specify the cause-and-effect relationship between the medical intervention and the cerebrovascular accident in order to assign a code for intraoperative or postprocedural cerebrovascular accident.

Proper code assignment depends on whether it was an infarction or hemorrhage and whether it occurred intraoperatively or postoperatively. If it was a cerebral hemorrhage, code assignment depends on the type of procedure performed.

d. **Sequelae of Cerebrovascular Disease**

1) **Category I69, Sequelae of Cerebrovascular disease**

Category I69 is used to indicate conditions classifiable to categories I60-I67 as the causes of sequela (neurologic deficits), themselves classified elsewhere. These "late effects" include neurologic deficits that persist after initial onset of conditions classifiable to categories I60-I67. The neurologic deficits caused by cerebrovascular disease may be present from the onset or may arise at any time after the onset of the condition classifiable to categories I60-I67.

Codes from category I69, Sequelae of cerebrovascular disease, that specify hemiplegia, hemiparesis and monoplegia identify whether the dominant or nondominant side is affected. Should the affected side be documented, but not specified as dominant or nondominant, and the classification system does not indicate a default, code selection is as follows:

- For ambidextrous patients, the default should be dominant.
- If the left side is affected, the default is non-dominant.
- If the right side is affected, the default is dominant.

2) **Codes from category I69 with codes from I60-I67**

Codes from category I69 may be assigned on a health care record with codes from I60-I67, if the patient has a current cerebrovascular disease and deficits from an old cerebrovascular disease.

3) **Codes from category I69 and Personal history of transient ischemic attack (TIA) and cerebral infarction (Z86.73)**

Codes from category I69 should not be assigned if the patient does not have neurologic deficits.

See Section I.C.21. 4. History (of) for use of personal history codes

e. **Acute myocardial infarction (AMI)**

1) **Type 1 ST elevation myocardial infarction (STEMI) and non-ST elevation myocardial infarction (NSTEMI)**

The ICD-10-CM codes for type 1 acute myocardial infarction (AMI) identify the site, such as anterolateral wall or true posterior wall. Subcategories I21.0-I21.2 and code I21.3 are used for type 1 ST elevation myocardial infarction (STEMI). Code I21.4, Non-ST elevation (NSTEMI) myocardial infarction, is used for type 1 non-ST elevation myocardial infarction (NSTEMI) and nontransmural MIs.

If a type 1 NSTEMI evolves to STEMI, assign the STEMI code. If a type 1 STEMI converts to NSTEMI due to thrombolytic therapy, it is still coded as STEMI.

For encounters occurring while the myocardial infarction is equal to, or less than, four weeks old, including transfers to another acute setting or a postacute setting, and the myocardial infarction meets the definition for "other diagnoses" (see Section III, Reporting Additional Diagnoses), codes from category I21 may continue to be reported. For encounters after the 4 week time frame and the patient is still receiving care related to the myocardial infarction, the appropriate aftercare code should be assigned, rather than a code from category I21. For old or healed myocardial infarctions not requiring further care, code I25.2, Old myocardial infarction, may be assigned.

2) **Acute myocardial infarction, unspecified**

Code I21.9, Acute myocardial infarction, unspecified, is the default for unspecified acute myocardial infarction or unspecified type. If only type 1 STEMI or transmural MI without the site is documented, assign code I21.3, ST elevation (STEMI) myocardial infarction of unspecified site.

3) **AMI documented as nontransmural or subendocardial but site provided**

If an AMI is documented as nontransmural or subendocardial, but the site is provided, it is still coded as a subendocardial AMI.

See Section I.C.21.3 for information on coding status post administration of tPA in a different facility within the last 24 hours.

4) **Subsequent acute myocardial infarction**

A code from category I22, Subsequent ST elevation (STEMI) and non-ST elevation (NSTEMI) myocardial infarction, is to be used when a patient who has suffered a type 1 or unspecified AMI has a new AMI within the 4 week time frame of the initial AMI. A code from category I22 must be used in conjunction with a code from category I21. The sequencing of the I22 and I21 codes depends on the circumstances of the encounter.

Do not assign code I22 for subsequent myocardial infarctions other than type 1 or unspecified. For subsequent type 2 AMI assign only code I21.A1. For subsequent type 4 or type 5 AMI, assign only code I21.A9.

If a subsequent myocardial infarction of one type occurs within 4 weeks of a myocardial infarction of a different type, assign the appropriate codes from category I21 to identify each type. Do not assign a code from category I22. Codes from category I22 should only be assigned if both the initial and subsequent myocardial infarctions are type 1 or unspecified.

5) **Other Types of Myocardial Infarction**

The ICD-10-CM provides codes for different types of myocardial infarction. Type 1 myocardial infarctions are assigned to codes I21.0-I21.4.

Type 2 myocardial infarction (myocardial infarction due to demand ischemia or secondary to ischemic imbalance), is assigned to code I21.A1, Myocardial infarction type 2 with the underlying cause coded first. Do not assign code I24.8, Other forms of acute ischemic heart disease, for the demand ischemia. If a type 2 AMI is described as NSTEMI or STEMI, only assign code I21.A1. Codes I21.01-I21.4 should only be assigned for type 1 AMIs.

Acute myocardial infarctions type 3, 4a, 4b, 4c and 5 are assigned to code I21.A9, Other myocardial infarction type.

The "Code also" and "Code first" notes should be followed related to complications, and for coding of postprocedural myocardial infarctions during or following cardiac surgery.

10. **Chapter 10: Diseases of the Respiratory System (J00-J99), U07.0**

a. **Chronic Obstructive Pulmonary Disease [COPD] and Asthma**

1) **Acute exacerbation of chronic obstructive bronchitis and asthma**

The codes in categories J44 and J45 distinguish between uncomplicated cases and those in acute exacerbation. An acute exacerbation is a worsening or a decompensation of a chronic condition. An acute exacerbation is not equivalent to an infection superimposed on a chronic condition, though an exacerbation may be triggered by an infection.

b. **Acute Respiratory Failure**

1) **Acute respiratory failure as principal diagnosis**

A code from subcategory J96.0, Acute respiratory failure, or subcategory J96.2, Acute and chronic respiratory failure, may be assigned as a principal diagnosis when it is the condition established after study to be chiefly responsible for occasioning the admission to the hospital, and the selection is supported by the Alphabetic Index and Tabular List. However, chapter-specific coding guidelines (such as obstetrics, poisoning, HIV, newborn) that provide sequencing direction take precedence.

2) **Acute respiratory failure as secondary diagnosis**

Respiratory failure may be listed as a secondary diagnosis if it occurs after admission, or if it is present on admission, but does not meet the definition of principal diagnosis.

3) **Sequencing of acute respiratory failure and another acute condition**

When a patient is admitted with respiratory failure and another acute condition, (e.g., myocardial infarction, cerebrovascular accident, aspiration pneumonia), the principal diagnosis will not be the same in every situation. This applies whether the other acute condition is a respiratory or nonrespiratory condition. Selection of the principal diagnosis will be dependent on the circumstances of admission. If both the respiratory failure and the other acute condition are equally responsible for occasioning the admission to the hospital, and there are no chapter-specific sequencing rules, the guideline regarding two or more diagnoses that equally meet the definition for principal diagnosis (Section II, C.) may be applied in these situations.

If the documentation is not clear as to whether acute respiratory failure and another condition are equally responsible for occasioning the admission, query the provider for clarification.

c. Influenza due to certain identified influenza viruses

Code only confirmed cases of influenza due to certain identified influenza viruses (category J09), and due to other identified influenza virus (category J10). This is an exception to the hospital inpatient guideline Section II, H. (Uncertain Diagnosis).

In this context, "confirmation" does not require documentation of positive laboratory testing specific for avian or other novel influenza A or other identified influenza virus. However, coding should be based on the provider's diagnostic statement that the patient has avian influenza, or other novel influenza A, for category J09, or has another particular identified strain of influenza, such as H1N1 or H3N2, but not identified as novel or variant, for category J10.

If the provider records "suspected" or "possible" or "probable" avian influenza, or novel influenza, or other identified influenza, then the appropriate influenza code from category J11, Influenza due to unidentified influenza virus, should be assigned. A code from category J09, Influenza due to certain identified influenza viruses, should not be assigned nor should a code from category J10, Influenza due to other identified influenza virus.

d. Ventilator associated Pneumonia

1) Documentation of Ventilator associated Pneumonia

As with all procedural or postprocedural complications, code assignment is based on the provider's documentation of the relationship between the condition and the procedure.

Code J95.851, Ventilator associated pneumonia, should be assigned only when the provider has documented ventilator associated pneumonia (VAP). An additional code to identify the organism (e.g., Pseudomonas aeruginosa, code B96.5) should also be assigned. Do not assign an additional code from categories J12-J18 to identify the type of pneumonia.

Code J95.851 should not be assigned for cases where the patient has pneumonia and is on a mechanical ventilator and the provider has not specifically stated that the pneumonia is ventilator-associated pneumonia. If the documentation is unclear as to whether the patient has a pneumonia that is a complication attributable to the mechanical ventilator, query the provider.

2) Ventilator associated Pneumonia Develops after Admission

A patient may be admitted with one type of pneumonia (e.g., code J13, Pneumonia due to Streptococcus pneumonia) and subsequently develop VAP. In this instance, the principal diagnosis would be the appropriate code from categories J12-J18 for the pneumonia diagnosed at the time of admission. Code J95.851, Ventilator associated pneumonia, would be assigned as an additional diagnosis when the provider has also documented the presence of ventilator associated pneumonia.

e. Vaping-related disorders

For patients presenting with condition(s) related to vaping, assign code U07.0, Vaping-related disorder, as the principal diagnosis. For lung injury due to vaping, assign only code U07.0. Assign additional codes for other manifestations, such as acute respiratory failure (subcategory J96.0-) or pneumonitis (code J68.0).

Associated respiratory signs and symptoms due to vaping, such as cough, shortness of breath, etc., are not coded separately, when a definitive diagnosis has been established. However, it would be appropriate to code separately any gastrointestinal symptoms, such as diarrhea and abdominal pain.

11. Chapter 11: Diseases of the Digestive System (K00-K95)
Reserved for future guideline expansion

12. Chapter 12: Diseases of the Skin and Subcutaneous Tissue (L00-L99)

a. Pressure ulcer stage codes

1) Pressure ulcer stages

Codes in category L89, Pressure ulcer, identify the site and stage of the pressure ulcer.

The ICD-10-CM classifies pressure ulcer stages based on severity, which is designated by stages 1-4, deep tissue pressure injury, unspecified stage and unstageable.

Assign as many codes from category L89 as needed to identify all the pressure ulcers the patient has, if applicable.

See Section I.B.14 for pressure ulcer stage documentation by clinicians other than patient's provider

2) Unstageable pressure ulcers

Assignment of the code for unstageable pressure ulcer (L89.--0) should be based on the clinical documentation. These codes are used for pressure ulcers whose stage cannot be clinically determined (e.g., the ulcer is covered by eschar or has been treated with a skin or muscle graft). This code should not be confused with the codes for unspecified stage (L89.--9). When there is no documentation regarding the stage of the pressure ulcer, assign the appropriate code for unspecified stage (L89.--9).

3) Documented pressure ulcer stage

Assignment of the pressure ulcer stage code should be guided by clinical documentation of the stage or documentation of the terms found in the Alphabetic Index. For clinical terms describing the stage that are not found in the Alphabetic Index, and there is no documentation of the stage, the provider should be queried.

4) Patients admitted with pressure ulcers documented as healed

No code is assigned if the documentation states that the pressure ulcer is completely healed at the time of admission.

5) Pressure ulcers documented as healing

Pressure ulcers described as healing should be assigned the appropriate pressure ulcer stage code based on the documentation in the medical record. If the documentation does not provide information about the stage of the healing pressure ulcer, assign the appropriate code for unspecified stage.

If the documentation is unclear as to whether the patient has a current (new) pressure ulcer or if the patient is being treated for a healing pressure ulcer, query the provider.

For ulcers that were present on admission but healed at the time of discharge, assign the code for the site and stage of the pressure ulcer at the time of admission.

6) Patient admitted with pressure ulcer evolving into another stage during the admission

If a patient is admitted to an inpatient hospital with a pressure ulcer at one stage and it progresses to a higher stage, two separate codes should be assigned: one code for the site and stage of the ulcer on admission and a second code for the same ulcer site and the highest stage reported during the stay.

7) Pressure-induced deep tissue damage

For pressure-induced deep tissue damage or deep tissue pressure injury, assign only the appropriate code for pressure-induced deep tissue damage (L89.--6).

b. Non-Pressure Chronic Ulcers

1) Patients admitted with non-pressure ulcers documented as healed

No code is assigned if the documentation states that the non-pressure ulcer is completely healed at the time of admission.

2) Non-pressure ulcers documented as healing

Non-pressure ulcers described as healing should be assigned the appropriate non-pressure ulcer code based on the documentation in the medical record. If the documentation does not provide information about the severity of the healing non-pressure ulcer, assign the appropriate code for unspecified severity.

If the documentation is unclear as to whether the patient has a current (new) non-pressure ulcer or if the patient is being treated for a healing non-pressure ulcer, query the provider.

For ulcers that were present on admission but healed at the time of discharge, assign the code for the site and severity of the non-pressure ulcer at the time of admission.

3) Patient admitted with non-pressure ulcer that progresses to another severity level during the admission

If a patient is admitted to an inpatient hospital with a non-pressure ulcer at one severity level and it progresses to a higher severity level, two separate codes should be assigned: one code for the site and severity level of the ulcer on admission and a second code for the same ulcer site and the highest severity level reported during the stay.

See Section I.B.14 for pressure ulcer stage documentation by clinicians other than patient's provider

13. Chapter 13: Diseases of the Musculoskeletal System and Connective Tissue (M00-M99)

a. Site and laterality

Most of the codes within Chapter 13 have site and laterality designations. The site represents the bone, joint or the muscle involved. For some conditions where more than one bone, joint or muscle is usually involved, such as osteoarthritis, there is a "multiple sites" code available. For categories where no multiple site code is provided and more than one bone, joint or muscle is involved, multiple codes should be used to indicate the different sites involved.

1) Bone versus joint

For certain conditions, the bone may be affected at the upper or lower end, (e.g., avascular necrosis of bone, M87, Osteoporosis, M80, M81). Though the portion of the bone affected may be at the joint, the site designation will be the bone, not the joint.

b. Acute traumatic versus chronic or recurrent musculoskeletal conditions

Many musculoskeletal conditions are a result of previous injury or trauma to a site, or are recurrent conditions. Bone, joint or muscle conditions that are the result of a healed injury are usually found in chapter 13. Recurrent bone, joint or muscle conditions are also usually found in chapter 13. Any current, acute injury should be coded to the appropriate injury code from chapter 19. Chronic or recurrent conditions should generally be coded with a code from chapter 13. If it is difficult to determine from the documentation in the record which code is best to describe a condition, query the provider.

c. Coding of Pathologic Fractures

7th character A is for use as long as the patient is receiving active treatment for the fracture. While the patient may be seen by a new or different provider over the course of treatment for a pathological fracture, assignment of the 7th character is based on whether the patient is undergoing active treatment and not whether the provider is seeing the patient for the first time.

7th character D is to be used for encounters after the patient has completed active treatment for the fracture and is receiving routine care for the fracture during the healing or recovery phase. The other 7th characters, listed under each subcategory in the Tabular List, are to be used for subsequent encounters for treatment of problems associated with the healing, such as malunions, nonunions, and sequelae.

Care for complications of surgical treatment for fracture repairs during the healing or recovery phase should be coded with the appropriate complication codes.

See Section I.C.19. Coding of traumatic fractures.

d. Osteoporosis

Osteoporosis is a systemic condition, meaning that all bones of the musculoskeletal system are affected. Therefore, site is not a component of the codes under category M81, Osteoporosis without current pathological fracture. The site codes under category M80, Osteoporosis with current pathological fracture, identify the site of the fracture, not the osteoporosis.

1) Osteoporosis without pathological fracture

Category M81, Osteoporosis without current pathological fracture, is for use for patients with osteoporosis who do not currently have a pathologic fracture due to the osteoporosis, even if they have had a fracture in the past. For patients with a history of osteoporosis fractures, status code Z87.310, Personal history of (healed) osteoporosis fracture, should follow the code from M81.

2) Osteoporosis with current pathological fracture

Category M80, Osteoporosis with current pathological fracture, is for patients who have a current pathologic fracture at the time of an encounter. The codes under M80 identify the site of the fracture. A code from category M80, not a traumatic fracture code, should be used for any patient with known osteoporosis who suffers a fracture, even if the patient had a minor fall or trauma, if that fall or trauma would not usually break a normal, healthy bone.

14. Chapter 14: Diseases of Genitourinary System (N00-N99)

a. Chronic kidney disease

1) Stages of chronic kidney disease (CKD)

The ICD-10-CM classifies CKD based on severity. The severity of CKD is designated by stages 1-5. Stage 2, code N18.2, equates to mild CKD; stage 3, **codes N18.30-N18.32, equate** to moderate CKD; and stage 4, code N18.4, equates to severe CKD. Code N18.6,

End stage renal disease (ESRD), is assigned when the provider has documented end-stage-renal disease (ESRD).

If both a stage of CKD and ESRD are documented, assign code N18.6 only.

2) Chronic kidney disease and kidney transplant status

Patients who have undergone kidney transplant may still have some form of chronic kidney disease (CKD) because the kidney transplant may not fully restore kidney function. Therefore, the presence of CKD alone does not constitute a transplant complication. Assign the appropriate N18 code for the patient's stage of CKD and code Z94.0, Kidney transplant status. If a transplant complication such as failure or rejection or other transplant complication is documented, see section I.C.19.g for information on coding complications of a kidney transplant. If the documentation is unclear as to whether the patient has a complication of the transplant, query the provider.

3) Chronic kidney disease with other conditions

Patients with CKD may also suffer from other serious conditions, most commonly diabetes mellitus and hypertension. The sequencing of the CKD code in relationship to codes for other contributing conditions is based on the conventions in the Tabular List.

See I.C.9. Hypertensive chronic kidney disease.

See I.C.19. Chronic kidney disease and kidney transplant complications.

15. Chapter 15: Pregnancy, Childbirth, and the Puerperium (O00-O9A)

a. General Rules for Obstetric Cases

1) Codes from chapter 15 and sequencing priority

Obstetric cases require codes from chapter 15, codes in the range O00-O9A, Pregnancy, Childbirth, and the Puerperium. Chapter 15 codes have sequencing priority over codes from other chapters. Additional codes from other chapters may be used in conjunction with chapter 15 codes to further specify conditions. Should the provider document that the pregnancy is incidental to the encounter, then code Z33.1, Pregnant state, incidental, should be used in place of any chapter 15 codes. It is the provider's responsibility to state that the condition being treated is not affecting the pregnancy.

2) Chapter 15 codes used only on the maternal record

Chapter 15 codes are to be used only on the maternal record, never on the record of the newborn.

3) Final character for trimester

The majority of codes in Chapter 15 have a final character indicating the trimester of pregnancy. The timeframes for the trimesters are indicated at the beginning of the chapter. If trimester is not a component of a code, it is because the condition always occurs in a specific trimester, or the concept of trimester of pregnancy is not applicable. Certain codes have characters for only certain trimesters because the condition does not occur in all trimesters, but it may occur in more than just one.

Assignment of the final character for trimester should be based on the provider's documentation of the trimester (or number of weeks) for the current admission/encounter. This applies to the assignment of trimester for pre-existing conditions as well as those that develop during or are due to the pregnancy. The provider's documentation of the number of weeks may be used to assign the appropriate code identifying the trimester.

Whenever delivery occurs during the current admission, and there is an "in childbirth" option for the obstetric complication being coded, the "in childbirth" code should be assigned.

4) Selection of trimester for inpatient admissions that encompass more than one trimester

In instances when a patient is admitted to a hospital for complications of pregnancy during one trimester and remains in the hospital into a subsequent trimester, the trimester character for the antepartum complication code should be assigned on the basis of the trimester when the complication developed, not the trimester of the discharge. If the condition developed prior to the current admission/encounter or represents a pre-existing condition, the trimester character for the trimester at the time of the admission/encounter should be assigned.

5) Unspecified trimester

Each category that includes codes for trimester has a code for "unspecified trimester." The "unspecified trimester" code should rarely be used, such as when the documentation in the record is insufficient to determine the trimester and it is not possible to obtain clarification.

6) **7th character for Fetus Identification**

Where applicable, a 7th character is to be assigned for certain categories (O31, O32, O33.3 - O33.6, O35, O36, O40, O41, O60.1, O60.2, O64, and O69) to identify the fetus for which the complication code applies.

Assign 7th character "0":

- For single gestations
- When the documentation in the record is insufficient to determine the fetus affected and it is not possible to obtain clarification.
- When it is not possible to clinically determine which fetus is affected.

b. **Selection of OB Principal or First-listed Diagnosis**

1) **Routine outpatient prenatal visits**

For routine outpatient prenatal visits when no complications are present, a code from category Z34, Encounter for supervision of normal pregnancy, should be used as the first-listed diagnosis. These codes should not be used in conjunction with chapter 15 codes.

2) **Supervision of High-Risk Pregnancy**

Codes from category O09, Supervision of high-risk pregnancy, are intended for use only during the prenatal period. For complications during the labor or delivery episode as a result of a high-risk pregnancy, assign the applicable complication codes from Chapter 15. If there are no complications during the labor or delivery episode, assign code O80, Encounter for full-term uncomplicated delivery.

For routine prenatal outpatient visits for patients with high-risk pregnancies, a code from category O09, Supervision of high-risk pregnancy, should be used as the first-listed diagnosis. Secondary chapter 15 codes may be used in conjunction with these codes if appropriate.

3) **Episodes when no delivery occurs**

In episodes when no delivery occurs, the principal diagnosis should correspond to the principal complication of the pregnancy which necessitated the encounter. Should more than one complication exist, all of which are treated or monitored, any of the complication codes may be sequenced first.

4) **When a delivery occurs**

When an obstetric patient is admitted and delivers during that admission, the condition that prompted the admission should be sequenced as the principal diagnosis. If multiple conditions prompted the admission, sequence the one most related to the delivery as the principal diagnosis. A code for any complication of the delivery should be assigned as an additional diagnosis. In cases of cesarean delivery, if the patient was admitted with a condition that resulted in the performance of a cesarean procedure, that condition should be selected as the principal diagnosis. If the reason for the admission was unrelated to the condition resulting in the cesarean delivery, the condition related to the reason for the admission should be selected as the principal diagnosis.

5) **Outcome of delivery**

A code from category Z37, Outcome of delivery, should be included on every maternal record when a delivery has occurred. These codes are not to be used on subsequent records or on the newborn record.

c. **Pre-existing conditions versus conditions due to the pregnancy**

Certain categories in Chapter 15 distinguish between conditions of the mother that existed prior to pregnancy (pre-existing) and those that are a direct result of pregnancy. When assigning codes from Chapter 15, it is important to assess if a condition was pre-existing prior to pregnancy or developed during or due to the pregnancy in order to assign the correct code.

Categories that do not distinguish between pre-existing and pregnancy-related conditions may be used for either. It is acceptable to use codes specifically for the puerperium with codes complicating pregnancy and childbirth if a condition arises postpartum during the delivery encounter.

d. **Pre-existing hypertension in pregnancy**

Category O10, Pre-existing hypertension complicating pregnancy, childbirth and the puerperium, includes codes for hypertensive heart disease and hypertensive chronic kidney disease. When assigning one of the O10 codes that includes hypertensive heart disease or hypertensive chronic kidney disease, it is necessary to add a secondary code from the appropriate hypertension category to specify the type of heart failure or chronic kidney disease.

See Section I.C.9. Hypertension.

e. **Fetal Conditions Affecting the Management of the Mother**

1) **Codes from categories O35 and O36**

Codes from categories O35, Maternal care for known or suspected fetal abnormality and damage, and O36, Maternal care for other fetal problems, are assigned only when the fetal condition is actually responsible for modifying the management of the mother, i.e., by requiring diagnostic studies, additional observation, special care, or termination of pregnancy. The fact that the fetal condition exists does not justify assigning a code from this series to the mother's record.

2) **In utero surgery**

In cases when surgery is performed on the fetus, a diagnosis code from category O35, Maternal care for known or suspected fetal abnormality and damage, should be assigned identifying the fetal condition. Assign the appropriate procedure code for the procedure performed.

No code from Chapter 16, the perinatal codes, should be used on the mother's record to identify fetal conditions. Surgery performed in utero on a fetus is still to be coded as an obstetric encounter.

f. **HIV Infection in Pregnancy, Childbirth and the Puerperium**

During pregnancy, childbirth or the puerperium, a patient admitted because of an HIV-related illness should receive a principal diagnosis from subcategory O98.7-, Human immunodeficiency [HIV] disease complicating pregnancy, childbirth and the puerperium, followed by the code(s) for the HIV-related illness(es).

Patients with asymptomatic HIV infection status admitted during pregnancy, childbirth, or the puerperium should receive codes of O98.7- and Z21, Asymptomatic human immunodeficiency virus [HIV] infection status.

g. **Diabetes mellitus in pregnancy**

Diabetes mellitus is a significant complicating factor in pregnancy. Pregnant women who are diabetic should be assigned a code from category O24, Diabetes mellitus in pregnancy, childbirth, and the puerperium, first, followed by the appropriate diabetes code(s) (E08-E13) from Chapter 4.

h. **Long term use of insulin and oral hypoglycemics**

See section I.C.4.a.3 for information on the long-term use of insulin and oral hypoglycemics.

i. **Gestational (pregnancy induced) diabetes**

Gestational (pregnancy induced) diabetes can occur during the second and third trimester of pregnancy in women who were not diabetic prior to pregnancy. Gestational diabetes can cause complications in the pregnancy similar to those of pre-existing diabetes mellitus. It also puts the woman at greater risk of developing diabetes after the pregnancy. Codes for gestational diabetes are in subcategory O24.4, Gestational diabetes mellitus. No other code from category O24, Diabetes mellitus in pregnancy, childbirth, and the puerperium, should be used with a code from O24.4.

The codes under subcategory O24.4 include diet controlled, insulin controlled, and controlled by oral hypoglycemic drugs. If a patient with gestational diabetes is treated with both diet and insulin, only the code for insulin-controlled is required. If a patient with gestational diabetes is treated with both diet and oral hypoglycemic medications, only the code for "controlled by oral hypoglycemic drugs" is required. Code Z79.4, Long-term (current) use of insulin or code Z79.84, Long-term (current) use of oral hypoglycemic drugs, should not be assigned with codes from subcategory O24.4.

An abnormal glucose tolerance in pregnancy is assigned a code from subcategory O99.81, Abnormal glucose complicating pregnancy, childbirth, and the puerperium.

j. **Sepsis and septic shock complicating abortion, pregnancy, childbirth and the puerperium**

When assigning a chapter 15 code for sepsis complicating abortion, pregnancy, childbirth, and the puerperium, a code for the specific type of infection should be assigned as an additional diagnosis. If severe sepsis is present, a code from subcategory R65.2, Severe sepsis, and code(s) for associated organ dysfunction(s) should also be assigned as additional diagnoses.

k. Puerperal sepsis

Code O85, Puerperal sepsis, should be assigned with a secondary code to identify the causal organism (e.g., for a bacterial infection, assign a code from category B95-B96, Bacterial infections in conditions classified elsewhere). A code from category A40, Streptococcal sepsis, or A41, Other sepsis, should not be used for puerperal sepsis. If applicable, use additional codes to identify severe sepsis (R65.2-) and any associated acute organ dysfunction.

Code O85 should not be assigned for sepsis following an obstetrical procedure (See Section I.C.1.d.5.b., Sepsis due to a postprocedural infection).

l. Alcohol, tobacco and drug use during pregnancy, childbirth and the puerperium

1) Alcohol use during pregnancy, childbirth and the puerperium

Codes under subcategory O99.31, Alcohol use complicating pregnancy, childbirth, and the puerperium, should be assigned for any pregnancy case when a mother uses alcohol during the pregnancy or postpartum. A secondary code from category F10, Alcohol related disorders, should also be assigned to identify manifestations of the alcohol use.

2) Tobacco use during pregnancy, childbirth and the puerperium

Codes under subcategory O99.33, Smoking (tobacco) complicating pregnancy, childbirth, and the puerperium, should be assigned for any pregnancy case when a mother uses any type of tobacco product during the pregnancy or postpartum. A secondary code from category F17, Nicotine dependence, should also be assigned to identify the type of nicotine dependence.

3) Drug use during pregnancy, childbirth and the puerperium

Codes under subcategory O99.32, Drug use complicating pregnancy, childbirth, and the puerperium, should be assigned for any pregnancy case when a mother uses drugs during the pregnancy or postpartum. This can involve illegal drugs, or inappropriate use or abuse of prescription drugs. Secondary code(s) from categories F11-F16 and F18-F19 should also be assigned to identify manifestations of the drug use.

m. Poisoning, toxic effects, adverse effects and underdosing in a pregnant patient

A code from subcategory O9A.2, Injury, poisoning and certain other consequences of external causes complicating pregnancy, childbirth, and the puerperium, should be sequenced first, followed by the appropriate injury, poisoning, toxic effect, adverse effect or underdosing code, and then the additional code(s) that specifies the condition caused by the poisoning, toxic effect, adverse effect or underdosing.

See Section I.C.19. Adverse effects, poisoning, underdosing and toxic effects.

n. Normal Delivery, Code O80

1) Encounter for full term uncomplicated delivery

Code O80 should be assigned when a woman is admitted for a full-term normal delivery and delivers a single, healthy infant without any complications antepartum, during the delivery, or postpartum during the delivery episode. Code O80 is always a principal diagnosis. It is not to be used if any other code from chapter 15 is needed to describe a current complication of the antenatal, delivery, or postnatal period. Additional codes from other chapters may be used with code O80 if they are not related to or are in any way complicating the pregnancy.

2) Uncomplicated delivery with resolved antepartum complication

Code O80 may be used if the patient had a complication at some point during the pregnancy, but the complication is not present at the time of the admission for delivery.

3) Outcome of delivery for O80

Z37.0, Single live birth, is the only outcome of delivery code appropriate for use with O80.

o. The Peripartum and Postpartum Periods

1) Peripartum and Postpartum periods

The postpartum period begins immediately after delivery and continues for six weeks following delivery. The peripartum period is defined as the last month of pregnancy to five months postpartum.

2) Peripartum and postpartum complication

A postpartum complication is any complication occurring within the six-week period.

3) Pregnancy-related complications after 6-week period

Chapter 15 codes may also be used to describe pregnancy-related complications after the peripartum or postpartum period if the provider documents that a condition is pregnancy related.

4) Admission for routine postpartum care following delivery outside hospital

When the mother delivers outside the hospital prior to admission and is admitted for routine postpartum care and no complications are noted, code Z39.0, Encounter for care and examination of mother immediately after delivery, should be assigned as the principal diagnosis.

5) Pregnancy associated cardiomyopathy

Pregnancy associated cardiomyopathy, code O90.3, is unique in that it may be diagnosed in the third trimester of pregnancy but may continue to progress months after delivery. For this reason, it is referred to as peripartum cardiomyopathy. Code O90.3 is only for use when the cardiomyopathy develops as a result of pregnancy in a woman who did not have pre-existing heart disease.

p. Code O94, Sequelae of complication of pregnancy, childbirth, and the puerperium

1) Code O94

Code O94, Sequelae of complication of pregnancy, childbirth, and the puerperium, is for use in those cases when an initial complication of a pregnancy develops a sequelae requiring care or treatment at a future date.

2) After the initial postpartum period

This code may be used at any time after the initial postpartum period.

3) Sequencing of Code O94

This code, like all sequela codes, is to be sequenced following the code describing the sequelae of the complication.

q. Termination of Pregnancy and Spontaneous abortions

1) Abortion with Liveborn Fetus

When an attempted termination of pregnancy results in a liveborn fetus, assign code Z33.2, Encounter for elective termination of pregnancy and a code from category Z37, Outcome of Delivery.

2) Retained Products of Conception following an abortion

Subsequent encounters for retained products of conception following a spontaneous abortion or elective termination of pregnancy, without complications are assigned O03.4, Incomplete spontaneous abortion without complication, or code O07.4, Failed attempted termination of pregnancy without complication. This advice is appropriate even when the patient was discharged previously with a discharge diagnosis of complete abortion. If the patient has a specific complication associated with the spontaneous abortion or elective termination of pregnancy in addition to retained products of conception, assign the appropriate complication code (e.g., O03.-, O04.-, O07.-) instead of code O03.4 or O07.4

3) Complications leading to abortion

Codes from Chapter 15 may be used as additional codes to identify any documented complications of the pregnancy in conjunction with codes in categories in O04, O07 and O08.

r. Abuse in a pregnant patient

For suspected or confirmed cases of abuse of a pregnant patient, a code(s) from subcategories O9A.3, Physical abuse complicating pregnancy, childbirth, and the puerperium, O9A.4, Sexual abuse complicating pregnancy, childbirth, and the puerperium, and O9A.5, Psychological abuse complicating pregnancy, childbirth, and the puerperium, should be sequenced first, followed by the appropriate codes (if applicable) to identify any associated current injury due to physical abuse, sexual abuse, and the perpetrator of abuse.

See Section I.C.19. Adult and child abuse, neglect and other maltreatment.

s. **COVID-19 infection in pregnancy, childbirth, and the puerperium**
During pregnancy, childbirth or the puerperium, when COVID-19 is the reason for admission/encounter, code O98.5-, Other viral diseases complicating pregnancy, childbirth and the puerperium, should be sequenced as the principal/first-listed diagnosis, and code U07.1, COVID-19, and the appropriate codes for associated manifestation(s) should be assigned as additional diagnoses. Codes from Chapter 15 always take sequencing priority.

If the reason for admission/encounter is unrelated to COVID-19 but the patient tests positive for COVID-19 during the admission/encounter, the appropriate code for the reason for admission/encounter should be sequenced as the principal/first-listed diagnosis, and codes O98.5- and U07.1, as well as the appropriate codes for associated COVID-19 manifestations, should be assigned as additional diagnoses.

16. **Chapter 16: Certain Conditions Originating in the Perinatal Period (P00-P96)**
For coding and reporting purposes the perinatal period is defined as before birth through the 28th day following birth. The following guidelines are provided for reporting purposes.

a. **General Perinatal Rules**
1) **Use of Chapter 16 Codes**
Codes in this chapter are <u>never</u> for use on the maternal record. Codes from Chapter 15, the obstetric chapter, are never permitted on the newborn record. Chapter 16 codes may be used throughout the life of the patient if the condition is still present.

2) **Principal Diagnosis for Birth Record**
When coding the birth episode in a newborn record, assign a code from category Z38, Liveborn infants according to place of birth and type of delivery, as the principal diagnosis. A code from category Z38 is assigned only once, to a newborn at the time of birth. If a newborn is transferred to another institution, a code from category Z38 should not be used at the receiving hospital.

A code from category Z38 is used only on the newborn record, not on the mother's record.

3) **Use of Codes from other Chapters with Codes from Chapter 16**
Codes from other chapters may be used with codes from chapter 16 if the codes from the other chapters provide more specific detail. Codes for signs and symptoms may be assigned when a definitive diagnosis has not been established. If the reason for the encounter is a perinatal condition, the code from chapter 16 should be sequenced first.

4) **Use of Chapter 16 Codes after the Perinatal Period**
Should a condition originate in the perinatal period, and continue throughout the life of the patient, the perinatal code should continue to be used regardless of the patient's age.

5) **Birth process or community acquired conditions**
If a newborn has a condition that may be either due to the birth process or community acquired and the documentation does not indicate which it is, the default is due to the birth process and the code from Chapter 16 should be used. If the condition is community-acquired, a code from Chapter 16 should not be assigned.

<u>For COVID-19 infection in a newborn, see guideline I.C.16.h.</u>

6) **Code all clinically significant conditions**
All clinically significant conditions noted on routine newborn examination should be coded. A condition is clinically significant if it requires:

- clinical evaluation; or
- therapeutic treatment; or
- diagnostic procedures; or
- extended length of hospital stay; or
- increased nursing care and/or monitoring; or
- has implications for future health care needs

Note: The perinatal guidelines listed above are the same as the general coding guidelines for "additional diagnoses," except for the final point regarding implications for future health care needs. Codes should be assigned for conditions that have been specified by the provider as having implications for future health care needs.

b. **Observation and Evaluation of Newborns for Suspected Conditions not Found**
1) **Use of Z05 codes**
Assign a code from category Z05, Observation and evaluation of newborns and infants for suspected conditions ruled out, to identify those instances when a healthy newborn is evaluated for a suspected condition that is determined after study not to be present. Do not use a code from category Z05 when the patient has identified signs or symptoms of a suspected problem; in such cases code the sign or symptom.

2) **Z05 on other than the birth record**
A code from category Z05 may also be assigned as a principal or first-listed code for readmissions or encounters when the code from category Z38 code no longer applies. Codes from category Z05 are for use only for healthy newborns and infants for which no condition after study is found to be present.

3) **Z05 on a birth record**
A code from category Z05 is to be used as a secondary code after the code from category Z38, Liveborn infants according to place of birth and type of delivery.

c. **Coding Additional Perinatal Diagnoses**
1) **Assigning codes for conditions that require treatment**
Assign codes for conditions that require treatment or further investigation, prolong the length of stay, or require resource utilization.

2) **Codes for conditions specified as having implications for future health care needs**
Assign codes for conditions that have been specified by the provider as having implications for future health care needs.
Note: This guideline should not be used for adult patients.

d. **Prematurity and Fetal Growth Retardation**
Providers utilize different criteria in determining prematurity. A code for prematurity should not be assigned unless it is documented. Assignment of codes in categories P05, Disorders of newborn related to slow fetal growth and fetal malnutrition, and P07, Disorders of newborn related to short gestation and low birth weight, not elsewhere classified, should be based on the recorded birth weight and estimated gestational age.

When both birth weight and gestational age are available, two codes from category P07 should be assigned, with the code for birth weight sequenced before the code for gestational age.

e. **Low birth weight and immaturity status**
Codes from category P07, Disorders of newborn related to short gestation and low birth weight, not elsewhere classified, are for use for a child or adult who was premature or had a low birth weight as a newborn and this is affecting the patient's current health status.

See Section I.C.21. Factors influencing health status and contact with health services, Status.

f. **Bacterial Sepsis of Newborn**
Category P36, Bacterial sepsis of newborn, includes congenital sepsis. If a perinate is documented as having sepsis without documentation of congenital or community acquired, the default is congenital and a code from category P36 should be assigned. If the P36 code includes the causal organism, an additional code from category B95, Streptococcus, Staphylococcus, and Enterococcus as the cause of diseases classified elsewhere, or B96, Other bacterial agents as the cause of diseases classified elsewhere, should not be assigned. If the P36 code does not include the causal organism, assign an additional code from category B96. If applicable, use additional codes to identify severe sepsis (R65.2-) and any associated acute organ dysfunction.

g. **Stillbirth**
Code P95, Stillbirth, is only for use in institutions that maintain separate records for stillbirths. No other code should be used with P95. Code P95 should not be used on the mother's record.

h. **COVID-19 Infection in Newborn**
For a newborn that tests positive for COVID-19, assign code U07.1, COVID-19, and the appropriate codes for associated manifestation(s) in neonates/newborns in the absence of documentation indicating a specific type of transmission. For a newborn that tests positive for COVID-19 and the provider documents the condition was contracted in utero or during the birth process, assign codes P35.8, Other congenital viral diseases, and U07.1, COVID-19. When coding the birth episode in a newborn record, the appropriate code from category Z38,

Liveborn infants according to place of birth and type of delivery, should be assigned as the principal diagnosis.

17. **Chapter 17: Congenital malformations, deformations, and chromosomal abnormalities (Q00-Q99)**

Assign an appropriate code(s) from categories Q00-Q99, Congenital malformations, deformations, and chromosomal abnormalities when a malformation/deformation or chromosomal abnormality is documented. A malformation/deformation/or chromosomal abnormality may be the principal/first-listed diagnosis on a record or a secondary diagnosis.

When a malformation/deformation or chromosomal abnormality does not have a unique code assignment, assign additional code(s) for any manifestations that may be present.

When the code assignment specifically identifies the malformation/deformation or chromosomal abnormality, manifestations that are an inherent component of the anomaly should not be coded separately. Additional codes should be assigned for manifestations that are not an inherent component.

Codes from Chapter 17 may be used throughout the life of the patient. If a congenital malformation or deformity has been corrected, a personal history code should be used to identify the history of the malformation or deformity. Although present at birth, a malformation/deformation/or chromosomal abnormality may not be identified until later in life. Whenever the condition is diagnosed by the provider, it is appropriate to assign a code from codes Q00-Q99. For the birth admission, the appropriate code from category Z38, Liveborn infants, according to place of birth and type of delivery, should be sequenced as the principal diagnosis, followed by any congenital anomaly codes, Q00- Q99.

18. **Chapter 18: Symptoms, signs, and abnormal clinical and laboratory findings, not elsewhere classified (R00-R99)**

Chapter 18 includes symptoms, signs, abnormal results of clinical or other investigative procedures, and ill-defined conditions regarding which no diagnosis classifiable elsewhere is recorded. Signs and symptoms that point to a specific diagnosis have been assigned to a category in other chapters of the classification.

a. **Use of symptom codes**

Codes that describe symptoms and signs are acceptable for reporting purposes when a related definitive diagnosis has not been established (confirmed) by the provider.

b. **Use of a symptom code with a definitive diagnosis code**

Codes for signs and symptoms may be reported in addition to a related definitive diagnosis when the sign or symptom is not routinely associated with that diagnosis, such as the various signs and symptoms associated with complex syndromes. The definitive diagnosis code should be sequenced before the symptom code.

Signs or symptoms that are associated routinely with a disease process should not be assigned as additional codes, unless otherwise instructed by the classification.

c. **Combination codes that include symptoms**

ICD-10-CM contains a number of combination codes that identify both the definitive diagnosis and common symptoms of that diagnosis.

When using one of these combination codes, an additional code should not be assigned for the symptom.

d. **Repeated falls**

Code R29.6, Repeated falls, is for use for encounters when a patient has recently fallen and the reason for the fall is being investigated.

Code Z91.81, History of falling, is for use when a patient has fallen in the past and is at risk for future falls. When appropriate, both codes R29.6 and Z91.81 may be assigned together.

e. **Coma scale**

The coma scale codes (R40.2-) can be used in conjunction with traumatic brain injury codes. These codes are primarily for use by trauma registries, but they may be used in any setting where this information is collected. The coma scale codes should be sequenced after the diagnosis code(s).

These codes, one from each subcategory, are needed to complete the scale. The 7th character indicates when the scale was recorded. The 7th character should match for all three codes.

At a minimum, report the initial score documented on presentation at your facility. This may be a score from the emergency medicine technician (EMT) or in the emergency department. If desired, a facility may choose to capture multiple coma scale scores.

Assign code R40.24, Glasgow coma scale, total score, when only the total score is documented in the medical record and not the individual score(s).

Do not report codes for individual or total Glasgow coma scale scores for a patient with a medically induced coma or a sedated patient.

See Section I.B.14 for coma scale documentation by clinicians other than patient's provider

f. **Functional quadriplegia**

GUIDELINE HAS BEEN DELETED EFFECTIVE OCTOBER 1, 2017

g. **SIRS due to Non-Infectious Process**

The systemic inflammatory response syndrome (SIRS) can develop as a result of certain non-infectious disease processes, such as trauma, malignant neoplasm, or pancreatitis. When SIRS is documented with a noninfectious condition, and no subsequent infection is documented, the code for the underlying condition, such as an injury, should be assigned, followed by code R65.10, Systemic inflammatory response syndrome (SIRS) of non-infectious origin without acute organ dysfunction, or code R65.11, Systemic inflammatory response syndrome (SIRS) of non-infectious origin with acute organ dysfunction. If an associated acute organ dysfunction is documented, the appropriate code(s) for the specific type of organ dysfunction(s) should be assigned in addition to code R65.11. If acute organ dysfunction is documented, but it cannot be determined if the acute organ dysfunction is associated with SIRS or due to another condition (e.g., directly due to the trauma), the provider should be queried.

h. **Death NOS**

Code R99, Ill-defined and unknown cause of mortality, is only for use in the very limited circumstance when a patient who has already died is brought into an emergency department or other healthcare facility and is pronounced dead upon arrival. It does not represent the discharge disposition of death.

i. **NIHSS Stroke Scale**

The NIH stroke scale (NIHSS) codes (R29.7- -) can be used in conjunction with acute stroke codes (I63) to identify the patient's neurological status and the severity of the stroke. The stroke scale codes should be sequenced after the acute stroke diagnosis code(s).

At a minimum, report the initial score documented. If desired, a facility may choose to capture multiple stroke scale scores.

See Section I.B.14 for NIHSS stroke scale documentation by clinicians other than patient's provider

19. **Chapter 19: Injury, poisoning, and certain other consequences of external causes (S00-T88)**

a. **Application of 7th Characters in Chapter 19**

Most categories in chapter 19 have a 7th character requirement for each applicable code. Most categories in this chapter have three 7th character values (with the exception of fractures): A, initial encounter, D, subsequent encounter and S, sequela. Categories for traumatic fractures have additional 7th character values. While the patient may be seen by a new or different provider over the course of treatment for an injury, assignment of the 7th character is based on whether the patient is undergoing active treatment and not whether the provider is seeing the patient for the first time.

For complication codes, active treatment refers to treatment for the condition described by the code, even though it may be related to an earlier precipitating problem. For example, code T84.50XA, Infection and inflammatory reaction due to unspecified internal joint prosthesis, initial encounter, is used when active treatment is provided for the infection, even though the condition relates to the prosthetic device, implant or graft that was placed at a previous encounter.

7th character "A", initial encounter is used for each encounter where the patient is receiving active treatment for the condition.

7th character "D" subsequent encounter is used for encounters after the patient has completed active treatment of the condition and is receiving routine care for the condition during the healing or recovery phase.

The aftercare Z codes should not be used for aftercare for conditions such as injuries or poisonings, where 7th characters are provided to identify subsequent care. For example, for aftercare of an injury, assign the acute injury code with the 7th character "D" (subsequent encounter).

7th character "S", sequela, is for use for complications or conditions that arise as a direct result of a condition, such as scar formation after a burn. The scars are sequelae of the burn. When using 7th character "S", it is necessary to use both the injury code that precipitated the sequela and the code for the sequela itself. The "S" is added only to the injury code, not the sequela code. The 7th character "S" identifies the injury responsible for the sequela. The specific type of sequela (e.g. scar) is sequenced first, followed by the injury code.

See Section I.B.10 Sequelae, (Late Effects)

b. Coding of Injuries

When coding injuries, assign separate codes for each injury unless a combination code is provided, in which case the combination code is assigned. Codes from category T07, Unspecified multiple injuries should not be assigned in the inpatient setting unless information for a more specific code is not available. Traumatic injury codes (S00-T14.9) are not to be used for normal, healing surgical wounds or to identify complications of surgical wounds.

The code for the most serious injury, as determined by the provider and the focus of treatment, is sequenced first.

1) Superficial injuries

Superficial injuries such as abrasions or contusions are not coded when associated with more severe injuries of the same site.

2) Primary injury with damage to nerves/blood vessels

When a primary injury results in minor damage to peripheral nerves or blood vessels, the primary injury is sequenced first with additional code(s) for injuries to nerves and spinal cord (such as category S04), and/or injury to blood vessels (such as category S15). When the primary injury is to the blood vessels or nerves, that injury should be sequenced first.

3) Iatrogenic injuries

Injury codes from Chapter 19 should not be assigned for injuries that occur during, or as a result of, a medical intervention. Assign the appropriate complication code(s).

c. Coding of Traumatic Fractures

The principles of multiple coding of injuries should be followed in coding fractures. Fractures of specified sites are coded individually by site in accordance with both the provisions within categories S02, S12, S22, S32, S42, S49, S52, S59, S62, S72, S79, S82, S89, S92 and the level of detail furnished by medical record content.

A fracture not indicated as open or closed should be coded to closed. A fracture not indicated whether displaced or not displaced should be coded to displaced.

More specific guidelines are as follows:

1) Initial vs. subsequent encounter for fractures

Traumatic fractures are coded using the appropriate 7th character for initial encounter (A, B, C) for each encounter where the patient is receiving active treatment for the fracture. The appropriate 7th character for initial encounter should also be assigned for a patient who delayed seeking treatment for the fracture or nonunion.

Fractures are coded using the appropriate 7th character for subsequent care for encounters after the patient has completed active treatment of the fracture and is receiving routine care for the fracture during the healing or recovery phase.

Care for complications of surgical treatment for fracture repairs during the healing or recovery phase should be coded with the appropriate complication codes.

Care of complications of fractures, such as malunion and nonunion, should be reported with the appropriate 7th character for subsequent care with nonunion (K, M, N,) or subsequent care with malunion (P, Q, R).

Malunion/nonunion: The appropriate 7th character for initial encounter should also be assigned for a patient who delayed seeking treatment for the fracture or nonunion.

The open fracture designations in the assignment of the 7th character for fractures of the forearm, femur and lower leg, including ankle are based on the Gustilo open fracture classification. When the Gustilo classification type is not specified for an open fracture, the 7th character for open fracture type I or II should be assigned (B, E, H, M, Q).

A code from category M80, not a traumatic fracture code, should be used for any patient with known osteoporosis who suffers a fracture, even if the patient had a minor fall or trauma, if that fall or trauma would not usually break a normal, healthy bone.

See Section I.C.13. Osteoporosis.

The aftercare Z codes should not be used for aftercare for traumatic fractures. For aftercare of a traumatic fracture, assign the acute fracture code with the appropriate 7th character.

2) Multiple fractures sequencing

Multiple fractures are sequenced in accordance with the severity of the fracture.

3) Physeal fractures

For physeal fractures, assign only the code identifying the type of physeal fracture. Do not assign a separate code to identify the specific bone that is fractured.

d. Coding of Burns and Corrosions

The ICD-10-CM makes a distinction between burns and corrosions. The burn codes are for thermal burns, except sunburns, that come from a heat source, such as a fire or hot appliance. The burn codes are also for burns resulting from electricity and radiation. Corrosions are burns due to chemicals. The guidelines are the same for burns and corrosions.

Current burns (T20-T25) are classified by depth, extent and by agent (X code). Burns are classified by depth as first degree (erythema), second degree (blistering), and third degree (full-thickness involvement). Burns of the eye and internal organs (T26-T28) are classified by site, but not by degree.

1) Sequencing of burn and related condition codes

Sequence first the code that reflects the highest degree of burn when more than one burn is present.

a. When the reason for the admission or encounter is for treatment of external multiple burns, sequence first the code that reflects the burn of the highest degree.

b. When a patient has both internal and external burns, the circumstances of admission govern the selection of the principal diagnosis or first-listed diagnosis.

c. When a patient is admitted for burn injuries and other related conditions such as smoke inhalation and/or respiratory failure, the circumstances of admission govern the selection of the principal or first-listed diagnosis.

2) Burns of the same anatomic site

Classify burns of the same anatomic site and on the same side but of different degrees to the subcategory identifying the highest degree recorded in the diagnosis (e.g., for second and third degree burns of right thigh, assign only code T24.311-).

3) Non-healing burns

Non-healing burns are coded as acute burns.

Necrosis of burned skin should be coded as a non-healed burn.

4) Infected burn

For any documented infected burn site, use an additional code for the infection.

5) Assign separate codes for each burn site

When coding burns, assign separate codes for each burn site. Category T30, Burn and corrosion, body region unspecified is extremely vague and should rarely be used.

Codes for burns of "multiple sites" should only be assigned when the medical record documentation does not specify the individual sites.

6) Burns and corrosions classified according to extent of body surface involved

Assign codes from category T31, Burns classified according to extent of body surface involved, or T32, Corrosions classified according to extent of body surface involved, when the site of the burn is not specified or when there is a need for additional data. It is advisable to use category T31 as additional coding when needed to provide data for evaluating burn mortality, such as that needed by burn units. It is also advisable to use category T31 as an additional code for reporting purposes when there is mention of a third-degree burn involving 20 percent or more of the body surface.

Categories T31 and T32 are based on the classic "rule of nines" in estimating body surface involved: head and neck are assigned nine percent, each arm nine percent, each leg 18 percent, the anterior trunk 18 percent, posterior trunk 18 percent, and genitalia one percent. Providers may change these percentage assignments where necessary to accommodate infants and children who have proportionately larger heads than adults, and patients who have large buttocks, thighs, or abdomen that involve burns.

7) Encounters for treatment of sequela of burns
Encounters for the treatment of the late effects of burns or corrosions (i.e., scars or joint contractures) should be coded with a burn or corrosion code with the 7th character "S" for sequela.

8) Sequelae with a late effect code and current burn
When appropriate, both a code for a current burn or corrosion with 7th character "A" or "D" and a burn or corrosion code with 7th character "S" may be assigned on the same record (when both a current burn and sequelae of an old burn exist). Burns and corrosions do not heal at the same rate and a current healing wound may still exist with sequela of a healed burn or corrosion.
See Section I.B.10 Sequela (Late Effects)

9) Use of an external cause code with burns and corrosions
An external cause code should be used with burns and corrosions to identify the source and intent of the burn, as well as the place where it occurred.

e. Adverse Effects, Poisoning, Underdosing and Toxic Effects
Codes in categories T36-T65 are combination codes that include the substance that was taken as well as the intent. No additional external cause code is required for poisonings, toxic effects, adverse effects and underdosing codes.

1) Do not code directly from the Table of Drugs
Do not code directly from the Table of Drugs and Chemicals. Always refer back to the Tabular List.

2) Use as many codes as necessary to describe
Use as many codes as necessary to describe completely all drugs, medicinal or biological substances.

3) If the same code would describe the causative agent
If the same code would describe the causative agent for more than one adverse reaction, poisoning, toxic effect or underdosing, assign the code only once.

4) If two or more drugs, medicinal or biological substances
If two or more drugs, medicinal or biological substances are taken, code each individually unless a combination code is listed in the Table of Drugs and Chemicals.

If multiple unspecified drugs, medicinal or biological substances were taken, assign the appropriate code from subcategory T50.91, Poisoning by, adverse effect of and underdosing of multiple unspecified drugs, medicaments and biological substances.

5) The occurrence of drug toxicity is classified in ICD-10-CM as follows:

(a) Adverse Effect
When coding an adverse effect of a drug that has been correctly prescribed and properly administered, assign the appropriate code for the nature of the adverse effect followed by the appropriate code for the adverse effect of the drug (T36-T50). The code for the drug should have a 5th or 6th character "5" (for example T36.0X5-) Examples of the nature of an adverse effect are tachycardia, delirium, gastrointestinal hemorrhaging, vomiting, hypokalemia, hepatitis, renal failure, or respiratory failure.

(b) Poisoning
When coding a poisoning or reaction to the improper use of a medication (e.g., overdose, wrong substance given or taken in error, wrong route of administration), first assign the appropriate code from categories T36-T50. The poisoning codes have an associated intent as their 5th or 6th character (accidental, intentional self-harm, assault and undetermined. If the intent of the poisoning is unknown or unspecified, code the intent as accidental intent. The undetermined intent is only for use if the documentation in the record specifies that the intent cannot be determined. Use additional code(s) for all manifestations of poisonings.

If there is also a diagnosis of abuse or dependence of the substance, the abuse or dependence is assigned as an additional code.

Examples of poisoning include:

(i) Error was made in drug prescription
Errors made in drug prescription or in the administration of the drug by provider, nurse, patient, or other person.

(ii) Overdose of a drug intentionally taken
If an overdose of a drug was intentionally taken or administered and resulted in drug toxicity, it would be coded as a poisoning.

(iii) Nonprescribed drug taken with correctly prescribed and properly administered drug
If a nonprescribed drug or medicinal agent was taken in combination with a correctly prescribed and properly administered drug, any drug toxicity or other reaction resulting from the interaction of the two drugs would be classified as a poisoning.

(iv) Interaction of drug(s) and alcohol
When a reaction results from the interaction of a drug(s) and alcohol, this would be classified as poisoning.

See Section I.C.4. if poisoning is the result of insulin pump malfunctions.

(c) Underdosing
Underdosing refers to taking less of a medication than is prescribed by a provider or a manufacturer's instruction. Discontinuing the use of a prescribed medication on the patient's own initiative (not directed by the patient's provider) is also classified as an underdosing. For underdosing, assign the code from categories T36-T50 (fifth or sixth character "6").

Codes for underdosing should never be assigned as principal or first-listed codes. If a patient has a relapse or exacerbation of the medical condition for which the drug is prescribed because of the reduction in dose, then the medical condition itself should be coded.

Noncompliance (Z91.12-, Z91.13- and Z91.14-) or complication of care (Y63.6-Y63.9) codes are to be used with an underdosing code to indicate intent, if known.

(d) Toxic Effects
When a harmful substance is ingested or comes in contact with a person, this is classified as a toxic effect. The toxic effect codes are in categories T51-T65.

Toxic effect codes have an associated intent: accidental, intentional self-harm, assault and undetermined.

f. Adult and child abuse, neglect and other maltreatment
Sequence first the appropriate code from categories T74, Adult and child abuse, neglect and other maltreatment, confirmed) or T76, Adult and child abuse, neglect and other maltreatment, suspected) for abuse, neglect and other maltreatment, followed by any accompanying mental health or injury code(s).

If the documentation in the medical record states abuse or neglect it is coded as confirmed (T74.-). It is coded as suspected if it is documented as suspected (T76.-).

For cases of confirmed abuse or neglect an external cause code from the assault section (X92-Y09) should be added to identify the cause of any physical injuries. A perpetrator code (Y07) should be added when the perpetrator of the abuse is known. For suspected cases of abuse or neglect, do not report external cause or perpetrator code.

If a suspected case of abuse, neglect or mistreatment is ruled out during an encounter code Z04.71, Encounter for examination and observation following alleged physical adult abuse, ruled out, or code Z04.72, Encounter for examination and observation following alleged child physical abuse, ruled out, should be used, not a code from T76.

If a suspected case of alleged rape or sexual abuse is ruled out during an encounter code Z04.41, Encounter for examination and observation following alleged adult rape or code Z04.42, Encounter for examination and observation following alleged child rape, should be used, not a code from T76.

If a suspected case of forced sexual exploitation or forced labor exploitation is ruled out during an encounter, code Z04.81, Encounter for examination and observation of victim following forced sexual exploitation, or code Z04.82, Encounter for examination and observation of victim following forced labor exploitation, should be used, not a code from T76.

See Section I.C.15. Abuse in a pregnant patient.

g. Complications of care

1) General guidelines for complications of care

(a) Documentation of complications of care
See Section I.B.16. for information on documentation of complications of care.

2) **Pain due to medical devices**

Pain associated with devices, implants or grafts left in a surgical site (for example painful hip prosthesis) is assigned to the appropriate code(s) found in Chapter 19, Injury, poisoning, and certain other consequences of external causes. Specific codes for pain due to medical devices are found in the T code section of the ICD-10-CM. Use additional code(s) from category G89 to identify acute or chronic pain due to presence of the device, implant or graft (G89.18 or G89.28).

3) **Transplant complications**

(a) **Transplant complications other than kidney**

Codes under category T86, Complications of transplanted organs and tissues, are for use for both complications and rejection of transplanted organs. A transplant complication code is only assigned if the complication affects the function of the transplanted organ. Two codes are required to fully describe a transplant complication: the appropriate code from category T86 and a secondary code that identifies the complication.

Pre-existing conditions or conditions that develop after the transplant are not coded as complications unless they affect the function of the transplanted organs.

See I.C.21. for transplant organ removal status

See I.C.2. for malignant neoplasm associated with transplanted organ.

(b) **Kidney transplant complications**

Patients who have undergone kidney transplant may still have some form of chronic kidney disease (CKD) because the kidney transplant may not fully restore kidney function. Code T86.1- should be assigned for documented complications of a kidney transplant, such as transplant failure or rejection or other transplant complication. Code T86.1- should not be assigned for post kidney transplant patients who have chronic kidney (CKD) unless a transplant complication such as transplant failure or rejection is documented. If the documentation is unclear as to whether the patient has a complication of the transplant, query the provider.

Conditions that affect the function of the transplanted kidney, other than CKD, should be assigned a code from subcategory T86.1, Complications of transplanted organ, Kidney, and a secondary code that identifies the complication.

For patients with CKD following a kidney transplant, but who do not have a complication such as failure or rejection, *see section I.C.14. Chronic kidney disease and kidney transplant status.*

4) **Complication codes that include the external cause**

As with certain other T codes, some of the complications of care codes have the external cause included in the code. The code includes the nature of the complication as well as the type of procedure that caused the complication. No external cause code indicating the type of procedure is necessary for these codes.

5) **Complications of care codes within the body system chapters**

Intraoperative and postprocedural complication codes are found within the body system chapters with codes specific to the organs and structures of that body system. These codes should be sequenced first, followed by a code(s) for the specific complication, if applicable.

Complication codes from the body system chapters should be assigned for intraoperative and postprocedural complications (e.g., the appropriate complication code from chapter 9 would be assigned for a vascular intraoperative or postprocedural complication) unless the complication is specifically indexed to a T code in chapter 19.

20. **Chapter 20: External Causes of Morbidity (V00-Y99)**

The external causes of morbidity codes should never be sequenced as the first-listed or principal diagnosis.

External cause codes are intended to provide data for injury research and evaluation of injury prevention strategies. These codes capture how the injury or health condition happened (cause), the intent (unintentional or accidental; or intentional, such as suicide or assault), the place where the event occurred the activity of the patient at the time of the event, and the person's status (e.g., civilian, military).

There is no national requirement for mandatory ICD-10-CM external cause code reporting. Unless a provider is subject to a state-based external cause code reporting mandate or these codes are required by a particular payer, reporting of ICD-10-CM codes in Chapter 20, External Causes of Morbidity, is not required. In the absence of a mandatory reporting requirement, providers are encouraged to voluntarily report external cause codes, as they provide valuable data for injury research and evaluation of injury prevention strategies.

a. **General External Cause Coding Guidelines**

1) **Used with any code in the range of A00.0-T88.9 Z00-Z99**

An external cause code may be used with any code in the range of A00.0-T88.9, Z00-Z99, classification that represents a health condition due to an external cause. Though they are most applicable to injuries, they are also valid for use with such things as infections or diseases due to an external source, and other health conditions, such as a heart attack that occurs during strenuous physical activity.

2) **External cause code used for length of treatment**

Assign the external cause code, with the appropriate 7th character (initial encounter, subsequent encounter or sequela) for each encounter for which the injury or condition is being treated.

Most categories in chapter 20 have a 7th character requirement for each applicable code. Most categories in this chapter have three 7th character values: A, initial encounter, D, subsequent encounter and S, sequela. While the patient may be seen by a new or different provider over the course of treatment for an injury or condition, assignment of the 7th character for external cause should match the 7th character of the code assigned for the associated injury or condition for the encounter.

3) **Use the full range of external cause codes**

Use the full range of external cause codes to completely describe the cause, the intent, the place of occurrence, and if applicable, the activity of the patient at the time of the event, and the patient's status, for all injuries, and other health conditions due to an external cause.

4) **Assign as many external cause codes as necessary**

Assign as many external cause codes as necessary to fully explain each cause. If only one external code can be recorded, assign the code most related to the principal diagnosis.

5) **The selection of the appropriate external cause code**

The selection of the appropriate external cause code is guided by the Alphabetic Index of External Causes and by Inclusion and Exclusion notes in the Tabular List.

6) **External cause code can never be a principal diagnosis**

An external cause code can never be a principal (first-listed) diagnosis.

7) **Combination external cause codes**

Certain of the external cause codes are combination codes that identify sequential events that result in an injury, such as a fall which results in striking against an object. The injury may be due to either event or both. The combination external cause code used should correspond to the sequence of events regardless of which caused the most serious injury.

8) **No external cause code needed in certain circumstances**

No external cause code from Chapter 20 is needed if the external cause and intent are included in a code from another chapter (e.g. T36.0X1- Poisoning by penicillins, accidental (unintentional)).

b. **Place of Occurrence Guideline**

Codes from category Y92, Place of occurrence of the external cause, are secondary codes for use after other external cause codes to identify the location of the patient at the time of injury or other condition.

Generally, a place of occurrence code is assigned only once, at the initial encounter for treatment. However, in the rare instance that a new injury occurs during hospitalization, an additional place of occurrence code may be assigned. No 7th characters are used for Y92.

Do not use place of occurrence code Y92.9 if the place is not stated or is not applicable.

c. **Activity Code**

Assign a code from category Y93, Activity code, to describe the activity of the patient at the time the injury or other health condition occurred.

An activity code is used only once, at the initial encounter for treatment. Only one code from Y93 should be recorded on a medical record.

The activity codes are not applicable to poisonings, adverse effects, misadventures or sequela.

Do not assign Y93.9, Unspecified activity, if the activity is not stated.

A code from category Y93 is appropriate for use with external cause and intent codes if identifying the activity provides additional information about the event.

d. **Place of Occurrence, Activity, and Status Codes Used with other External Cause Code**

When applicable, place of occurrence, activity, and external cause status codes are sequenced after the main external cause code(s). Regardless of the number of external cause codes assigned, generally there should be only one place of occurrence code, one activity code, and one external cause status code assigned to an encounter. However, in the rare instance that a new injury occurs during hospitalization, an additional place of occurrence code may be assigned.

e. **If the Reporting Format Limits the Number of External Cause Codes**

If the reporting format limits the number of external cause codes that can be used in reporting clinical data, report the code for the cause/intent most related to the principal diagnosis. If the format permits capture of additional external cause codes, the cause/intent, including medical misadventures, of the additional events should be reported rather than the codes for place, activity, or external status.

f. **Multiple External Cause Coding Guidelines**

More than one external cause code is required to fully describe the external cause of an illness or injury. The assignment of external cause codes should be sequenced in the following priority:

If two or more events cause separate injuries, an external cause code should be assigned for each cause. The first-listed external cause code will be selected in the following order:

External codes for child and adult abuse take priority over all other external cause codes.

See Section I.C.19., Child and Adult abuse guidelines.

External cause codes for terrorism events take priority over all other external cause codes except child and adult abuse.

External cause codes for cataclysmic events take priority over all other external cause codes except child and adult abuse and terrorism.

External cause codes for transport accidents take priority over all other external cause codes except cataclysmic events, child and adult abuse and terrorism.

Activity and external cause status codes are assigned following all causal (intent) external cause codes.

The first-listed external cause code should correspond to the cause of the most serious diagnosis due to an assault, accident, or self-harm, following the order of hierarchy listed above.

g. **Child and Adult Abuse Guideline**

Adult and child abuse, neglect and maltreatment are classified as assault. Any of the assault codes may be used to indicate the external cause of any injury resulting from the confirmed abuse.

For confirmed cases of abuse, neglect and maltreatment, when the perpetrator is known, a code from Y07, Perpetrator of maltreatment and neglect, should accompany any other assault codes.

See Section I.C.19. Adult and child abuse, neglect and other maltreatment

h. **Unknown or Undetermined Intent Guideline**

If the intent (accident, self-harm, assault) of the cause of an injury or other condition is unknown or unspecified, code the intent as accidental intent. All transport accident categories assume accidental intent.

1) **Use of undetermined intent**

External cause codes for events of undetermined intent are only for use if the documentation in the record specifies that the intent cannot be determined.

i. **Sequelae (Late Effects) of External Cause Guidelines**

1) **Sequelae external cause codes**

Sequela are reported using the external cause code with the 7th character "S" for sequela. These codes should be used with any report of a late effect or sequela resulting from a previous injury.

See Section I.B.10 Sequela (Late Effects)

2) **Sequela external cause code with a related current injury**

A sequela external cause code should never be used with a related current nature of injury code.

3) **Use of sequela external cause codes for subsequent visits**

Use a late effect external cause code for subsequent visits when a late effect of the initial injury is being treated. Do not use a late effect external cause code for subsequent visits for follow-up care (e.g., to assess healing, to receive rehabilitative therapy) of the injury when no late effect of the injury has been documented.

j. **Terrorism Guidelines**

1) **Cause of injury identified by the Federal Government (FBI) as terrorism**

When the cause of an injury is identified by the Federal Government (FBI) as terrorism, the first-listed external cause code should be a code from category Y38, Terrorism. The definition of terrorism employed by the FBI is found at the inclusion note at the beginning of category Y38. Use additional code for place of occurrence (Y92.-). More than one Y38 code may be assigned if the injury is the result of more than one mechanism of terrorism.

2) **Cause of an injury is suspected to be the result of terrorism**

When the cause of an injury is suspected to be the result of terrorism a code from category Y38 should not be assigned. Suspected cases should be classified as assault.

3) **Code Y38.9, Terrorism, secondary effects**

Assign code Y38.9, Terrorism, secondary effects, for conditions occurring subsequent to the terrorist event. This code should not be assigned for conditions that are due to the initial terrorist act.

It is acceptable to assign code Y38.9 with another code from Y38 if there is an injury due to the initial terrorist event and an injury that is a subsequent result of the terrorist event.

k. **External Cause Status**

A code from category Y99, External cause status, should be assigned whenever any other external cause code is assigned for an encounter, including an Activity code, except for the events noted below. Assign a code from category Y99, External cause status, to indicate the work status of the person at the time the event occurred. The status code indicates whether the event occurred during military activity, whether a non-military person was at work, whether an individual including a student or volunteer was involved in a non-work activity at the time of the causal event.

A code from Y99, External cause status, should be assigned, when applicable, with other external cause codes, such as transport accidents and falls. The external cause status codes are not applicable to poisonings, adverse effects, misadventures or late effects.

Do not assign a code from category Y99 if no other external cause codes (cause, activity) are applicable for the encounter.

An external cause status code is used only once, at the initial encounter for treatment. Only one code from Y99 should be recorded on a medical record.

Do not assign code Y99.9, Unspecified external cause status, if the status is not stated.

21. **Chapter 21: Factors influencing health status and contact with health services (Z00-Z99)**

Note: The chapter specific guidelines provide additional information about the use of Z codes for specified encounters.

a. **Use of Z Codes in Any Healthcare Setting**

Z codes are for use in any healthcare setting. Z codes may be used as either a first-listed (principal diagnosis code in the inpatient setting) or secondary code, depending on the circumstances of the encounter. Certain Z codes may only be used as first-listed or principal diagnosis.

b. **Z Codes Indicate a Reason for an Encounter**

Z codes are not procedure codes. A corresponding procedure code must accompany a Z code to describe any procedure performed.

c. **Categories of Z Codes**

1) **Contact/Exposure**

Category Z20 indicates contact with, and suspected exposure to, communicable diseases. These codes are for patients who are suspected to have been exposed to **a disease** by close personal contact with an infected individual or are in an area where a disease is epidemic.

Category Z77, Other contact with and (suspected) exposures hazardous to health, indicates contact with and suspected exposures hazardous to health.

Contact/exposure codes may be used as a first-listed code to explain an encounter for testing, or, more commonly, as a secondary code to identify a potential risk.

2) **Inoculations and vaccinations**

Code Z23 is for encounters for inoculations and vaccinations. It indicates that a patient is being seen to receive a prophylactic inoculation against a disease. Procedure codes are required to identify the actual administration of the injection and the type(s) of immunizations given. Code Z23 may be used as a secondary code if the inoculation is given as a routine part of preventive health care, such as a well-baby visit.

3) **Status**

Status codes indicate that a patient is either a carrier of a disease or has the sequelae or residual of a past disease or condition. This includes such things as the presence of prosthetic or mechanical devices resulting from past treatment. A status code is informative, because the status may affect the course of treatment and its outcome. A status code is distinct from a history code. The history code indicates that the patient no longer has the condition.

A status code should not be used with a diagnosis code from one of the body system chapters, if the diagnosis code includes the information provided by the status code. For example, code Z94.1, Heart transplant status, should not be used with a code from subcategory T86.2, Complications of heart transplant. The status code does not provide additional information. The complication code indicates that the patient is a heart transplant patient.

For encounters for weaning from a mechanical ventilator, assign a code from subcategory J96.1, Chronic respiratory failure, followed by code Z99.11, Dependence on respirator [ventilator] status.

The status Z codes/categories are:

Z14　Genetic carrier

Genetic carrier status indicates that a person carries a gene, associated with a particular disease, which may be passed to offspring who may develop that disease. The person does not have the disease and is not at risk of developing the disease.

Z15　Genetic susceptibility to disease

Genetic susceptibility indicates that a person has a gene that increases the risk of that person developing the disease.

Codes from category Z15 should not be used as principal or first-listed codes. If the patient has the condition to which he/she is susceptible, and that condition is the reason for the encounter, the code for the current condition should be sequenced first. If the patient is being seen for follow-up after completed treatment for this condition, and the condition no longer exists, a follow-up code should be sequenced first, followed by the appropriate personal history and genetic susceptibility codes. If the purpose of the encounter is genetic counseling associated with procreative management, code Z31.5, Encounter for genetic counseling, should be assigned as the first-listed code, followed by a code from category Z15. Additional codes should be assigned for any applicable family or personal history.

Z16　Resistance to antimicrobial drugs

This code indicates that a patient has a condition that is resistant to antimicrobial drug treatment. Sequence the infection code first.

Z17　Estrogen receptor status

Z18　Retained foreign body fragments

Z19　Hormone sensitivity malignancy status

Z21　Asymptomatic HIV infection status

This code indicates that a patient has tested positive for HIV but has manifested no signs or symptoms of the disease.

Z22　Carrier of infectious disease

Carrier status indicates that a person harbors the specific organisms of a disease without manifest symptoms and is capable of transmitting the infection.

Z28.3　Underimmunization status

Z33.1　Pregnant state, incidental

This code is a secondary code only for use when the pregnancy is in no way complicating the reason for visit. Otherwise, a code from the obstetric chapter is required.

Z66　Do not resuscitate

This code may be used when it is documented by the provider that a patient is on do not resuscitate status at any time during the stay.

Z67　Blood type

Z68　Body mass index (BMI)

BMI codes should only be assigned when there is an associated, reportable diagnosis (such as obesity). Do not assign BMI codes during pregnancy.

See Section I.B.14 for BMI documentation by clinicians other than the patient's provider.

Z74.Ø1　Bed confinement status

Z76.82　Awaiting organ transplant status

Z78　Other specified health status

Code Z78.1, Physical restraint status, may be used when it is documented by the provider that a patient has been put in restraints during the current encounter. Please note that this code should not be reported when it is documented by the provider that a patient is temporarily restrained during a procedure.

Z79　Long-term (current) drug therapy

Codes from this category indicate a patient's continuous use of a prescribed drug (including such things as aspirin therapy) for the long-term treatment of a condition or for prophylactic use. It is not for use for patients who have addictions to drugs. This subcategory is not for use of medications for detoxification or maintenance programs to prevent withdrawal symptoms (e.g., methadone maintenance for opiate dependence). Assign the appropriate code for the drug **use, abuse, or** dependence instead.

Assign a code from Z79 if the patient is receiving a medication for an extended period as a prophylactic measure (such as for the prevention of deep vein thrombosis) or as treatment of a chronic condition (such as arthritis) or a disease requiring a lengthy course of treatment (such as cancer). Do not assign a code from category Z79 for medication being administered for a brief period of time to treat an acute illness or injury (such as a course of antibiotics to treat acute bronchitis).

Z88　Allergy status to drugs, medicaments and biological substances

Except: Z88.9, Allergy status to unspecified drugs, medicaments and biological substances status

Z89　Acquired absence of limb

Z9Ø　Acquired absence of organs, not elsewhere classified

Z91.Ø-　Allergy status, other than to drugs and biological substances

Z92.82　Status post administration of tPA (rtPA) in a different facility within the last 24 hours prior to admission to a current facility

Assign code Z92.82, Status post administration of tPA (rtPA) in a different facility within the last 24 hours prior to admission to current facility, as a secondary diagnosis when a patient is received by transfer into a facility and documentation indicates they were administered tissue plasminogen activator (tPA) within the last 24 hours prior to admission to the current facility.

This guideline applies even if the patient is still receiving the tPA at the time they are received into the current facility.

The appropriate code for the condition for which the tPA was administered (such as cerebrovascular disease or myocardial infarction) should be assigned first.

Code Z92.82 is only applicable to the receiving facility record and not to the transferring facility record.

Z93   Artificial opening status

Z94   Transplanted organ and tissue status

Z95   Presence of cardiac and vascular implants and grafts

Z96   Presence of other functional implants

Z97   Presence of other devices

Z98   Other postprocedural states

Assign code Z98.85, Transplanted organ removal status, to indicate that a transplanted organ has been previously removed. This code should not be assigned for the encounter in which the transplanted organ is removed. The complication necessitating removal of the transplant organ should be assigned for that encounter.

See section I.C19. for information on the coding of organ transplant complications.

Z99   Dependence on enabling machines and devices, not elsewhere classified

Note: Categories Z89-Z90 and Z93-Z99 are for use only if there are no complications or malfunctions of the organ or tissue replaced, the amputation site or the equipment on which the patient is dependent.

4) History (of)

There are two types of history Z codes, personal and family. Personal history codes explain a patient's past medical condition that no longer exists and is not receiving any treatment, but that has the potential for recurrence, and therefore may require continued monitoring.

Family history codes are for use when a patient has a family member(s) who has had a particular disease that causes the patient to be at higher risk of also contracting the disease.

Personal history codes may be used in conjunction with follow-up codes and family history codes may be used in conjunction with screening codes to explain the need for a test or procedure. History codes are also acceptable on any medical record regardless of the reason for visit. A history of an illness, even if no longer present, is important information that may alter the type of treatment ordered.

The history Z code categories are:

Z80   Family history of primary malignant neoplasm

Z81   Family history of mental and behavioral disorders

Z82   Family history of certain disabilities and chronic diseases (leading to disablement)

Z83   Family history of other specific disorders

Z84   Family history of other conditions

Z85   Personal history of malignant neoplasm

Z86   Personal history of certain other diseases

Z87   Personal history of other diseases and conditions

Z91.4-   Personal history of psychological trauma, not elsewhere classified

Z91.5   Personal history of self-harm

Z91.81   History of falling

Z91.82   Personal history of military deployment

Z92   Personal history of medical treatment

Except: Z92.0, Personal history of contraception

Except: Z92.82, Status post administration of tPA (rtPA) in a different facility within the last 24 hours prior to admission to a current facility

5) Screening

Screening is the testing for disease or disease precursors in seemingly well individuals so that early detection and treatment can be provided for those who test positive for the disease (e.g., screening mammogram).

The testing of a person to rule out or confirm a suspected diagnosis because the patient has some sign or symptom is a diagnostic examination, not a screening. In these cases, the sign or symptom is used to explain the reason for the test.

A screening code may be a first-listed code if the reason for the visit is specifically the screening exam. It may also be used as an additional code if the screening is done during an office visit for other health problems. A screening code is not necessary if the screening is inherent to a routine examination, such as a pap smear done during a routine pelvic examination.

Should a condition be discovered during the screening then the code for the condition may be assigned as an additional diagnosis.

The Z code indicates that a screening exam is planned. A procedure code is required to confirm that the screening was performed.

The screening Z codes/categories:

Z11   Encounter for screening for infectious and parasitic diseases

Z12   Encounter for screening for malignant neoplasms

Z13   Encounter for screening for other diseases and disorders

Except: Z13.9, Encounter for screening, unspecified

Z36   Encounter for antenatal screening for mother

6) Observation

There are three observation Z code categories. They are for use in very limited circumstances when a person is being observed for a suspected condition that is ruled out. The observation codes are not for use if an injury or illness or any signs or symptoms related to the suspected condition are present. In such cases the diagnosis/symptom code is used with the corresponding external cause code.

The observation codes are **primarily** to be used as a principal/**first-listed** diagnosis. **An observation code may be assigned as a secondary diagnosis code when the patient is being observed for a condition that is ruled out and is unrelated to the principal/first-listed diagnosis (e.g., patient presents for treatment following injuries sustained in a motor vehicle accident and is also observed for suspected COVID-19 infection that is subsequently ruled out). Also,** when the principal diagnosis is required to be a code from category Z38, Liveborn infants according to place of birth and type of delivery, **then** a code from category Z05, Encounter for observation and evaluation of newborn for suspected diseases and conditions ruled out, is sequenced after the Z38 code. Additional codes may be used in addition to the observation code, but only if they are unrelated to the suspected condition being observed.

Codes from subcategory Z03.7, Encounter for suspected maternal and fetal conditions ruled out, may either be used as a first-listed or as an additional code assignment depending on the case. They are for use in very limited circumstances on a maternal record when an encounter is for a suspected maternal or fetal condition that is ruled out during that encounter (for example, a maternal or fetal condition may be suspected due to an abnormal test result). These codes should not be used when the condition is confirmed. In those cases, the confirmed condition should be coded. In addition, these codes are not for use if an illness or any signs or symptoms related to the suspected condition or problem are present. In such cases the diagnosis/symptom code is used.

Additional codes may be used in addition to the code from subcategory Z03.7, but only if they are unrelated to the suspected condition being evaluated.

Codes from subcategory Z03.7 may not be used for encounters for antenatal screening of mother. *See Section I.C.21. Screening.*

For encounters for suspected fetal condition that are inconclusive following testing and evaluation, assign the appropriate code from category O35, O36, O40 or O41.

The observation Z code categories:

Z03   Encounter for medical observation for suspected diseases and conditions ruled out

Z04   Encounter for examination and observation for other reasons

Except: Z04.9, Encounter for examination and observation for unspecified reason

Z05   Encounter for observation and evaluation of newborn for suspected diseases and conditions ruled out

7) Aftercare

Aftercare visit codes cover situations when the initial treatment of a disease has been performed and the patient requires continued care during the healing or recovery phase, or for the long-term consequences of the disease. The aftercare Z code should not be used if treatment is directed at a current, acute disease. The diagnosis code is to be used in these cases. Exceptions to this rule are codes Z51.Ø, Encounter for antineoplastic radiation therapy, and codes from subcategory Z51.1, Encounter for antineoplastic chemotherapy and immunotherapy. These codes are to be first listed, followed by the diagnosis code when a patient's encounter is solely to receive radiation therapy, chemotherapy, or immunotherapy for the treatment of a neoplasm. If the reason for the encounter is more than one type of antineoplastic therapy, code Z51.Ø and a code from subcategory Z51.1 may be assigned together, in which case one of these codes would be reported as a secondary diagnosis.

The aftercare Z codes should also not be used for aftercare for injuries. For aftercare of an injury, assign the acute injury code with the appropriate 7th character (for subsequent encounter).

The aftercare codes are generally first listed to explain the specific reason for the encounter. An aftercare code may be used as an additional code when some type of aftercare is provided in addition to the reason for admission and no diagnosis code is applicable. An example of this would be the closure of a colostomy during an encounter for treatment of another condition.

Aftercare codes should be used in conjunction with other aftercare codes or diagnosis codes to provide better detail on the specifics of an aftercare encounter visit, unless otherwise directed by the classification. The sequencing of multiple aftercare codes depends on the circumstances of the encounter.

Certain aftercare Z code categories need a secondary diagnosis code to describe the resolving condition or sequelae. For others, the condition is included in the code title.

Additional Z code aftercare category terms include fitting and adjustment, and attention to artificial openings.

Status Z codes may be used with aftercare Z codes to indicate the nature of the aftercare. For example, code Z95.1, Presence of aortocoronary bypass graft, may be used with code Z48.812, Encounter for surgical aftercare following surgery on the circulatory system, to indicate the surgery for which the aftercare is being performed. A status code should not be used when the aftercare code indicates the type of status, such as using Z43.Ø, Encounter for attention to tracheostomy, with Z93.Ø, Tracheostomy status.

The aftercare Z category/codes:

Z42   Encounter for plastic and reconstructive surgery following medical procedure or healed injury

Z43   Encounter for attention to artificial openings

Z44   Encounter for fitting and adjustment of external prosthetic device

Z45   Encounter for adjustment and management of implanted device

Z46   Encounter for fitting and adjustment of other devices

Z47   Orthopedic aftercare

Z48   Encounter for other postprocedural aftercare

Z49   Encounter for care involving renal dialysis

Z51   Encounter for other aftercare and medical care

8) Follow-up

The follow-up codes are used to explain continuing surveillance following completed treatment of a disease, condition, or injury. They imply that the condition has been fully treated and no longer exists. They should not be confused with aftercare codes, or injury codes with a 7th character for subsequent encounter, that explain ongoing care of a healing condition or its sequelae. Follow-up codes may be used in conjunction with history codes to provide the full picture of the healed condition and its treatment. The follow-up code is sequenced first, followed by the history code.

A follow-up code may be used to explain multiple visits. Should a condition be found to have recurred on the follow-up visit, then the diagnosis code for the condition should be assigned in place of the follow-up code.

The follow-up Z code categories:

ZØ8   Encounter for follow-up examination after completed treatment for malignant neoplasm

ZØ9   Encounter for follow-up examination after completed treatment for conditions other than malignant neoplasm

Z39   Encounter for maternal postpartum care and examination

9) Donor

Codes in category Z52, Donors of organs and tissues, are used for living individuals who are donating blood or other body tissue. These codes are only for individuals donating for others, not for self-donations. They are not used to identify cadaveric donations.

10) Counseling

Counseling Z codes are used when a patient or family member receives assistance in the aftermath of an illness or injury, or when support is required in coping with family or social problems.

The counseling Z codes/categories:

Z30.Ø-   Encounter for general counseling and advice on contraception

Z31.5   Encounter for procreative genetic counseling

Z31.6-   Encounter for general counseling and advice on procreation

Z32.2   Encounter for childbirth instruction

Z32.3   Encounter for childcare instruction

Z69   Encounter for mental health services for victim and perpetrator of abuse

Z70   Counseling related to sexual attitude, behavior and orientation

Z71   Persons encountering health services for other counseling and medical advice, not elsewhere classified

Note: Code Z71.84, Encounter for health counseling related to travel, is to be used for health risk and safety counseling for future travel purposes.

Z76.81   Expectant mother prebirth pediatrician visit

11) Encounters for Obstetrical and Reproductive Services

See Section I.C.15. Pregnancy, Childbirth, and the Puerperium, for further instruction on the use of these codes.

Z codes for pregnancy are for use in those circumstances when none of the problems or complications included in the codes from the Obstetrics chapter exist (a routine prenatal visit or postpartum care). Codes in category Z34, Encounter for supervision of normal pregnancy, are always first listed and are not to be used with any other code from the OB chapter.

Codes in category Z3A, Weeks of gestation, may be assigned to provide additional information about the pregnancy. Category Z3A codes should not be assigned for pregnancies with abortive outcomes (categories OØØ-OØ8), elective termination of pregnancy (code Z33.2), nor for postpartum conditions, as category Z3A is not applicable to these conditions. The date of the admission should be used to determine weeks of gestation for inpatient admissions that encompass more than one gestational week.

The outcome of delivery, category Z37, should be included on all maternal delivery records. It is always a secondary code. Codes in category Z37 should not be used on the newborn record.

Z codes for family planning (contraceptive) or procreative management and counseling should be included on an obstetric record either during the pregnancy or the postpartum stage, if applicable.

Z codes/categories for obstetrical and reproductive services:

Z30   Encounter for contraceptive management

Z31   Encounter for procreative management

Z32.2   Encounter for childbirth instruction

Z32.3   Encounter for childcare instruction

Z33   Pregnant state

Z34   Encounter for supervision of normal pregnancy

Z36   Encounter for antenatal screening of mother

Z3A	Weeks of gestation
Z37	Outcome of delivery
Z39	Encounter for maternal postpartum care and examination
Z76.81	Expectant mother prebirth pediatrician visit

12) Newborns and Infants

See Section I.C.16. Newborn (Perinatal) Guidelines, for further instruction on the use of these codes.

Newborn Z codes/categories:

Z76.1	Encounter for health supervision and care of foundling
Z00.1-	Encounter for routine child health examination
Z38	Liveborn infants according to place of birth and type of delivery

13) Routine and Administrative Examinations

The Z codes allow for the description of encounters for routine examinations, such as, a general check-up, or, examinations for administrative purposes, such as, a pre-employment physical. The codes are not to be used if the examination is for diagnosis of a suspected condition or for treatment purposes. In such cases the diagnosis code is used. During a routine exam, should a diagnosis or condition be discovered, it should be coded as an additional code. Pre-existing and chronic conditions and history codes may also be included as additional codes as long as the examination is for administrative purposes and not focused on any particular condition.

Some of the codes for routine health examinations distinguish between "with" and "without" abnormal findings. Code assignment depends on the information that is known at the time the encounter is being coded. For example, if no abnormal findings were found during the examination, but the encounter is being coded before test results are back, it is acceptable to assign the code for "without abnormal findings." When assigning a code for "with abnormal findings," additional code(s) should be assigned to identify the specific abnormal finding(s).

Pre-operative examination and pre-procedural laboratory examination Z codes are for use only in those situations when a patient is being cleared for a procedure or surgery and no treatment is given.

The Z codes/categories for routine and administrative examinations:

Z00	Encounter for general examination without complaint, suspected or reported diagnosis
Z01	Encounter for other special examination without complaint, suspected or reported diagnosis
Z02	Encounter for administrative examination
	Except: Z02.9, Encounter for administrative examinations, unspecified
Z32.0-	Encounter for pregnancy test

14) Miscellaneous Z Codes

The miscellaneous Z codes capture a number of other health care encounters that do not fall into one of the other categories. Certain of these codes identify the reason for the encounter; others are for use as additional codes that provide useful information on circumstances that may affect a patient's care and treatment.

Prophylactic Organ Removal

For encounters specifically for prophylactic removal of an organ (such as prophylactic removal of breasts due to a genetic susceptibility to cancer or a family history of cancer), the principal or first-listed code should be a code from category Z40, Encounter for prophylactic surgery, followed by the appropriate codes to identify the associated risk factor (such as genetic susceptibility or family history).

If the patient has a malignancy of one site and is having prophylactic removal at another site to prevent either a new primary malignancy or metastatic disease, a code for the malignancy should also be assigned in addition to a code from subcategory Z40.0, Encounter for prophylactic surgery for risk factors related to malignant neoplasms. A Z40.0 code should not be assigned if the patient is having organ removal for treatment of a malignancy, such as the removal of the testes for the treatment of prostate cancer.

Miscellaneous Z codes/categories:

Z28	Immunization not carried out
	Except: Z28.3, Underimmunization status
Z29	Encounter for other prophylactic measures
Z40	Encounter for prophylactic surgery
Z41	Encounter for procedures for purposes other than remedying health state
	Except: Z41.9, Encounter for procedure for purposes other than remedying health state, unspecified
Z53	Persons encountering health services for specific procedures and treatment, not carried out
Z55	Problems related to education and literacy
Z56	Problems related to employment and unemployment
Z57	Occupational exposure to risk factors
Z58	Problems related to physical environment
Z59	Problems related to housing and economic circumstances
Z60	Problems related to social environment
Z62	Problems related to upbringing
Z63	Other problems related to primary support group, including family circumstances
Z64	Problems related to certain psychosocial circumstances
Z65	Problems related to other psychosocial circumstances
Z72	Problems related to lifestyle
	Note: These codes should be assigned only when the documentation specifies that the patient has an associated problem
Z73	Problems related to life management difficulty
Z74	Problems related to care provider dependency
	Except: Z74.01, Bed confinement status
Z75	Problems related to medical facilities and other health care
Z76.0	Encounter for issue of repeat prescription
Z76.3	Healthy person accompanying sick person
Z76.4	Other boarder to healthcare facility
Z76.5	Malingerer [conscious simulation]
Z91.1-	Patient's noncompliance with medical treatment and regimen
Z91.83	Wandering in diseases classified elsewhere
Z91.84-	Oral health risk factors
Z91.89	Other specified personal risk factors, not elsewhere classified

See Section I.B.14 for Z55-Z65 Persons with potential health hazards related to socioeconomic and psychosocial circumstances, documentation by clinicians other than the patient's provider.

15) Nonspecific Z Codes

Certain Z codes are so non-specific, or potentially redundant with other codes in the classification, that there can be little justification for their use in the inpatient setting. Their use in the outpatient setting should be limited to those instances when there is no further documentation to permit more precise coding. Otherwise, any sign or symptom or any other reason for visit that is captured in another code should be used.

Nonspecific Z codes/categories:

Z02.9	Encounter for administrative examinations, unspecified
Z04.9	Encounter for examination and observation for unspecified reason
Z13.9	Encounter for screening, unspecified
Z41.9	Encounter for procedure for purposes other than remedying health state, unspecified
Z52.9	Donor of unspecified organ or tissue
Z86.59	Personal history of other mental and behavioral disorders
Z88.9	Allergy status to unspecified drugs, medicaments and biological substances status
Z92.0	Personal history of contraception

16) Z Codes That May Only be Principal/First-Listed Diagnosis

The following Z codes/categories may only be reported as the principal/first-listed diagnosis, except when there are multiple encounters on the same day and the medical records for the encounters are combined:

Z00	Encounter for general examination without complaint, suspected or reported diagnosis
	Except: Z00.6
Z01	Encounter for other special examination without complaint, suspected or reported diagnosis
Z02	Encounter for administrative examination
Z04	Encounter for examination and observation for other reasons
Z33.2	Encounter for elective termination of pregnancy
Z31.81	Encounter for male factor infertility in female patient
Z31.83	Encounter for assisted reproductive fertility procedure cycle
Z31.84	Encounter for fertility preservation procedure
Z34	Encounter for supervision of normal pregnancy
Z39	Encounter for maternal postpartum care and examination
Z38	Liveborn infants according to place of birth and type of delivery
Z40	Encounter for prophylactic surgery
Z42	Encounter for plastic and reconstructive surgery following medical procedure or healed injury
Z51.0	Encounter for antineoplastic radiation therapy
Z51.1-	Encounter for antineoplastic chemotherapy and immunotherapy
Z52	Donors of organs and tissues
	Except: Z52.9, Donor of unspecified organ or tissue
Z76.1	Encounter for health supervision and care of foundling
Z76.2	Encounter for health supervision and care of other healthy infant and child
Z99.12	Encounter for respirator [ventilator] dependence during power failure

22. **Chapter 22: Codes for Special Purposes (U00-U85)**
    U07.0 Vaping-related disorder (see Section I.C.10.e., Vaping-related disorders)
    U07.1 COVID-19 (see Section I.C.1.g.1., COVID-19 infection)

Section II. Selection of Principal Diagnosis

The circumstances of inpatient admission always govern the selection of principal diagnosis. The principal diagnosis is defined in the Uniform Hospital Discharge Data Set (UHDDS) as "that condition established after study to be chiefly responsible for occasioning the admission of the patient to the hospital for care."

The UHDDS definitions are used by hospitals to report inpatient data elements in a standardized manner. These data elements and their definitions can be found in the July 31, 1985, Federal Register (Vol. 50, No, 147), pp. 31038-40.

Since that time, the application of the UHDDS definitions has been expanded to include all non-outpatient settings (acute care, short term, long term care and psychiatric hospitals; home health agencies; rehab facilities; nursing homes, etc.). The UHDDS definitions also apply to hospice services (all levels of care).

In determining principal diagnosis, coding conventions in the ICD-10-CM, the Tabular List and Alphabetic Index take precedence over these official coding guidelines.

(See Section I.A., Conventions for the ICD-10-CM)

The importance of consistent, complete documentation in the medical record cannot be overemphasized. Without such documentation the application of all coding guidelines is a difficult, if not impossible, task.

A. **Codes for symptoms, signs, and ill-defined conditions**
   Codes for symptoms, signs, and ill-defined conditions from Chapter 18 are not to be used as principal diagnosis when a related definitive diagnosis has been established.

B. **Two or more interrelated conditions, each potentially meeting the definition for principal diagnosis.**
   When there are two or more interrelated conditions (such as diseases in the same ICD-10-CM chapter or manifestations characteristically associated with a certain disease) potentially meeting the definition of principal diagnosis, either condition may be sequenced first, unless the circumstances of the admission, the therapy provided, the Tabular List, or the Alphabetic Index indicate otherwise.

C. **Two or more diagnoses that equally meet the definition for principal diagnosis**
   In the unusual instance when two or more diagnoses equally meet the criteria for principal diagnosis as determined by the circumstances of admission, diagnostic workup and/or therapy provided, and the Alphabetic Index, Tabular List, or another coding guidelines does not provide sequencing direction, any one of the diagnoses may be sequenced first.

D. **Two or more comparative or contrasting conditions**
   In those rare instances when two or more contrasting or comparative diagnoses are documented as "either/or" (or similar terminology), they are coded as if the diagnoses were confirmed and the diagnoses are sequenced according to the circumstances of the admission. If no further determination can be made as to which diagnosis should be principal, either diagnosis may be sequenced first.

E. **A symptom(s) followed by contrasting/comparative diagnoses**
   GUIDELINE HAS BEEN DELETED EFFECTIVE OCTOBER 1, 2014

F. **Original treatment plan not carried out**
   Sequence as the principal diagnosis the condition, which after study occasioned the admission to the hospital, even though treatment may not have been carried out due to unforeseen circumstances.

G. **Complications of surgery and other medical care**
   When the admission is for treatment of a complication resulting from surgery or other medical care, the complication code is sequenced as the principal diagnosis. If the complication is classified to the T80-T88 series and the code lacks the necessary specificity in describing the complication, an additional code for the specific complication should be assigned.

H. **Uncertain Diagnosis**
   If the diagnosis documented at the time of discharge is qualified as "probable," "suspected," "likely," "questionable," "possible," or "still to be ruled out," "compatible with," "consistent with," or other similar terms indicating uncertainty, code the condition as if it existed or was established. The bases for these guidelines are the diagnostic workup, arrangements for further workup or observation, and initial therapeutic approach that correspond most closely with the established diagnosis.

   Note: This guideline is applicable only to inpatient admissions to short-term, acute, long-term care and psychiatric hospitals.

I. **Admission from Observation Unit**
   1. **Admission Following Medical Observation**
      When a patient is admitted to an observation unit for a medical condition, which either worsens or does not improve, and is subsequently admitted as an inpatient of the same hospital for this same medical condition, the principal diagnosis would be the medical condition which led to the hospital admission.

   2. **Admission Following Post-Operative Observation**
      When a patient is admitted to an observation unit to monitor a condition (or complication) that develops following outpatient surgery, and then is subsequently admitted as an inpatient of the same hospital, hospitals should apply the Uniform Hospital Discharge Data Set (UHDDS) definition of principal diagnosis as "that condition established after study to be chiefly responsible for occasioning the admission of the patient to the hospital for care."

J. **Admission from Outpatient Surgery**
   When a patient receives surgery in the hospital's outpatient surgery department and is subsequently admitted for continuing inpatient care at the same hospital, the following guidelines should be followed in selecting the principal diagnosis for the inpatient admission:
   - If the reason for the inpatient admission is a complication, assign the complication as the principal diagnosis.
   - If no complication, or other condition, is documented as the reason for the inpatient admission, assign the reason for the outpatient surgery as the principal diagnosis.
   - If the reason for the inpatient admission is another condition unrelated to the surgery, assign the unrelated condition as the principal diagnosis.

K. **Admissions/Encounters for Rehabilitation**
   When the purpose for the admission/encounter is rehabilitation, sequence first the code for the condition for which the service is being performed. For example, for an admission/encounter for rehabilitation for right-sided dominant hemiplegia following a cerebrovascular infarction, report code I69.351, Hemiplegia and hemiparesis following cerebral infarction affecting right dominant side, as the first-listed or principal diagnosis.

If the condition for which the rehabilitation service is being provided is no longer present, report the appropriate aftercare code as the first-listed or principal diagnosis, unless the rehabilitation service is being provided following an injury. For rehabilitation services following active treatment of an injury, assign the injury code with the appropriate seventh character for subsequent encounter as the first-listed or principal diagnosis. For example, if a patient with severe degenerative osteoarthritis of the hip, underwent hip replacement and the current encounter/admission is for rehabilitation, report code Z47.1, Aftercare following joint replacement surgery, as the first-listed or principal diagnosis. If the patient requires rehabilitation post hip replacement for right intertrochanteric femur fracture, report code S72.141D, Displaced intertrochanteric fracture of right femur, subsequent encounter for closed fracture with routine healing, as the first-listed or principal diagnosis.

See Section I.C.21.c.7, Factors influencing health states and contact with health services, Aftercare.

See Section I.C.19.a, for additional information about the use of 7th characters for injury codes.

Section III. Reporting Additional Diagnoses

GENERAL RULES FOR OTHER (ADDITIONAL) DIAGNOSES

For reporting purposes, the definition for "other diagnoses" is interpreted as additional conditions that affect patient care in terms of requiring:

    clinical evaluation; or
    therapeutic treatment; or
    diagnostic procedures; or
    extended length of hospital stay; or
    increased nursing care and/or monitoring.

The UHDDS item #11-b defines Other Diagnoses as "all conditions that coexist at the time of admission, that develop subsequently, or that affect the treatment received and/or the length of stay. Diagnoses that relate to an earlier episode which have no bearing on the current hospital stay are to be excluded." UHDDS definitions apply to inpatients in acute care, short-term, long term care and psychiatric hospital setting. The UHDDS definitions are used by acute care short-term hospitals to report inpatient data elements in a standardized manner. These data elements and their definitions can be found in the July 31, 1985, Federal Register (Vol. 50, No, 147), pp. 31038-40.

Since that time, the application of the UHDDS definitions has been expanded to include all non-outpatient settings (acute care, short term, long term care and psychiatric hospitals; home health agencies; rehab facilities; nursing homes, etc.). The UHDDS definitions also apply to hospice services (all levels of care).

The following guidelines are to be applied in designating "other diagnoses" when neither the Alphabetic Index nor the Tabular List in ICD-10-CM provide direction. The listing of the diagnoses in the patient record is the responsibility of the attending provider.

A. Previous conditions
If the provider has included a diagnosis in the final diagnostic statement, such as the discharge summary or the face sheet, it should ordinarily be coded. Some providers include in the diagnostic statement resolved conditions or diagnoses and status-post procedures from previous admissions that have no bearing on the current stay. Such conditions are not to be reported and are coded only if required by hospital policy.

However, history codes (categories Z80-Z87) may be used as secondary codes if the historical condition or family history has an impact on current care or influences treatment.

B. Abnormal findings
Abnormal findings (laboratory, x-ray, pathologic, and other diagnostic results) are not coded and reported unless the provider indicates their clinical significance. If the findings are outside the normal range and the attending provider has ordered other tests to evaluate the condition or prescribed treatment, it is appropriate to ask the provider whether the abnormal finding should be added.

Please note: This differs from the coding practices in the outpatient setting for coding encounters for diagnostic tests that have been interpreted by a provider.

C. Uncertain Diagnosis
If the diagnosis documented at the time of discharge is qualified as "probable," "suspected," "likely," "questionable," "possible," or "still to be ruled out," "compatible with," "consistent with," or other similar terms indicating uncertainty, code the condition as if it existed or was

established. The bases for these guidelines are the diagnostic workup, arrangements for further workup or observation, and initial therapeutic approach that correspond most closely with the established diagnosis.

Note: This guideline is applicable only to inpatient admissions to short-term, acute, long-term care and psychiatric hospitals.

Section IV. Diagnostic Coding and Reporting Guidelines for Outpatient Services

These coding guidelines for outpatient diagnoses have been approved for use by hospitals/ providers in coding and reporting hospital-based outpatient services and provider-based office visits. Guidelines in Section I, Conventions, general coding guidelines and chapter-specific guidelines, should also be applied for outpatient services and office visits.

Information about the use of certain abbreviations, punctuation, symbols, and other conventions used in the ICD-10-CM Tabular List (code numbers and titles), can be found in Section IA of these guidelines, under "Conventions Used in the Tabular List." Section I.B. contains general guidelines that apply to the entire classification. Section I.C. contains chapter-specific guidelines that correspond to the chapters as they are arranged in the classification. Information about the correct sequence to use in finding a code is also described in Section I.

The terms encounter and visit are often used interchangeably in describing outpatient service contacts and, therefore, appear together in these guidelines without distinguishing one from the other.

Though the conventions and general guidelines apply to all settings, coding guidelines for outpatient and provider reporting of diagnoses will vary in a number of instances from those for inpatient diagnoses, recognizing that:

The Uniform Hospital Discharge Data Set (UHDDS) definition of principal diagnosis does not apply to hospital-based outpatient services and provider-based office visits.

Coding guidelines for inconclusive diagnoses (probable, suspected, rule out, etc.) were developed for inpatient reporting and do not apply to outpatients.

A. Selection of first-listed condition
In the outpatient setting, the term first-listed diagnosis is used in lieu of principal diagnosis.

In determining the first-listed diagnosis the coding conventions of ICD-10-CM, as well as the general and disease specific guidelines take precedence over the outpatient guidelines.

Diagnoses often are not established at the time of the initial encounter/visit. It may take two or more visits before the diagnosis is confirmed.

The most critical rule involves beginning the search for the correct code assignment through the Alphabetic Index. Never begin searching initially in the Tabular List as this will lead to coding errors.

1. Outpatient Surgery
When a patient presents for outpatient surgery (same day surgery), code the reason for the surgery as the first-listed diagnosis (reason for the encounter), even if the surgery is not performed due to a contraindication.

2. Observation Stay
When a patient is admitted for observation for a medical condition, assign a code for the medical condition as the first-listed diagnosis.

When a patient presents for outpatient surgery and develops complications requiring admission to observation, code the reason for the surgery as the first reported diagnosis (reason for the encounter), followed by codes for the complications as secondary diagnoses.

B. Codes from A00.0 through T88.9, Z00-Z99
The appropriate code(s) from A00.0 through T88.9, Z00-Z99 must be used to identify diagnoses, symptoms, conditions, problems, complaints, or other reason(s) for the encounter/visit.

C. Accurate reporting of ICD-10-CM diagnosis codes
For accurate reporting of ICD-10-CM diagnosis codes, the documentation should describe the patient's condition, using terminology which includes specific diagnoses as well as symptoms, problems, or reasons for the encounter. There are ICD-10-CM codes to describe all of these.

D. Codes that describe symptoms and signs
Codes that describe symptoms and signs, as opposed to diagnoses, are acceptable for reporting purposes when a diagnosis has not been established (confirmed) by the provider. Chapter 18 of ICD-10-CM, Symptoms, Signs, and Abnormal Clinical and Laboratory Findings Not Elsewhere Classified (codes R00-R99) contain many, but not all codes for symptoms.

E. Encounters for circumstances other than a disease or injury

ICD-10-CM provides codes to deal with encounters for circumstances other than a disease or injury. The Factors Influencing Health Status and Contact with Health Services codes (Z00-Z99) are provided to deal with occasions when circumstances other than a disease or injury are recorded as diagnosis or problems.

See Section I.C.21. Factors influencing health status and contact with health services.

F. Level of Detail in Coding

1. **ICD-10-CM codes with 3, 4, 5, 6 or 7 characters**

   ICD-10-CM is composed of codes with 3, 4, 5, 6 or 7 characters. Codes with three characters are included in ICD-10-CM as the heading of a category of codes that may be further subdivided by the use of fourth, fifth, sixth or seventh characters to provide greater specificity.

2. **Use of full number of characters required for a code**

   A three-character code is to be used only if it is not further subdivided. A code is invalid if it has not been coded to the full number of characters required for that code, including the 7th character, if applicable.

G. ICD-10-CM code for the diagnosis, condition, problem, or other reason for encounter/visit

List first the ICD-10-CM code for the diagnosis, condition, problem, or other reason for encounter/visit shown in the medical record to be chiefly responsible for the services provided. List additional codes that describe any coexisting conditions. In some cases the first-listed diagnosis may be a symptom when a diagnosis has not been established (confirmed) by the provider.

H. Uncertain diagnosis

Do not code diagnoses documented as "probable", "suspected," "questionable," "rule out," "compatible with," "consistent with," or "working diagnosis" or other similar terms indicating uncertainty. Rather, code the condition(s) to the highest degree of certainty for that encounter/visit, such as symptoms, signs, abnormal test results, or other reason for the visit.

Please note: This differs from the coding practices used by short-term, acute care, long-term care and psychiatric hospitals.

I. Chronic diseases

Chronic diseases treated on an ongoing basis may be coded and reported as many times as the patient receives treatment and care for the condition(s)

J. Code all documented conditions that coexist

Code all documented conditions that coexist at the time of the encounter/visit, and require or affect patient care treatment or management. Do not code conditions that were previously treated and no longer exist. However, history codes (categories Z80-Z87) may be used as secondary codes if the historical condition or family history has an impact on current care or influences treatment.

K. Patients receiving diagnostic services only

For patients receiving diagnostic services only during an encounter/visit, sequence first the diagnosis, condition, problem, or other reason for encounter/visit shown in the medical record to be chiefly responsible for the outpatient services provided during the encounter/visit. Codes for other diagnoses (e.g., chronic conditions) may be sequenced as additional diagnoses.

For encounters for routine laboratory/radiology testing in the absence of any signs, symptoms, or associated diagnosis, assign Z01.89, Encounter for other specified special examinations. If routine testing is performed during the same encounter as a test to evaluate a sign, symptom, or diagnosis, it is appropriate to assign both the Z code and the code describing the reason for the non-routine test.

For outpatient encounters for diagnostic tests that have been interpreted by a physician, and the final report is available at the time of coding, code any confirmed or definitive diagnosis(es) documented in the interpretation. Do not code related signs and symptoms as additional diagnoses.

Please note: This differs from the coding practice in the hospital inpatient setting regarding abnormal findings on test results.

L. Patients receiving therapeutic services only

For patients receiving therapeutic services only during an encounter/visit, sequence first the diagnosis, condition, problem, or other reason for encounter/visit shown in the medical record to be chiefly responsible for the outpatient services provided during the encounter/visit. Codes for other diagnoses (e.g., chronic conditions) may be sequenced as additional diagnoses.

The only exception to this rule is that when the primary reason for the admission/encounter is chemotherapy or radiation therapy, the appropriate Z code for the service is listed first, and the diagnosis or problem for which the service is being performed listed second.

M. Patients receiving preoperative evaluations only

For patients receiving preoperative evaluations only, sequence first a code from subcategory Z01.81, Encounter for pre-procedural examinations, to describe the pre-op consultations. Assign a code for the condition to describe the reason for the surgery as an additional diagnosis. Code also any findings related to the pre-op evaluation.

N. Ambulatory surgery

For ambulatory surgery, code the diagnosis for which the surgery was performed. If the postoperative diagnosis is known to be different from the preoperative diagnosis at the time the diagnosis is confirmed, select the postoperative diagnosis for coding, since it is the most definitive.

O. Routine outpatient prenatal visits

See Section I.C.15. Routine outpatient prenatal visits.

P. Encounters for general medical examinations with abnormal findings

The subcategories for encounters for general medical examinations, Z00.0- and encounter for routine child health examination, Z00.12-, provide codes for with and without abnormal findings. Should a general medical examination result in an abnormal finding, the code for general medical examination with abnormal finding should be assigned as the first-listed diagnosis. An examination with abnormal findings refers to a condition/diagnosis that is newly identified or a change in severity of a chronic condition (such as uncontrolled hypertension, or an acute exacerbation of chronic obstructive pulmonary disease) during a routine physical examination. A secondary code for the abnormal finding should also be coded.

Q. Encounters for routine health screenings

See Section I.C.21. Factors influencing health status and contact with health services, Screening

Appendix I. Present on Admission Reporting Guidelines

Introduction

These guidelines are to be used as a supplement to the *ICD-10-CM Official Guidelines for Coding and Reporting* to facilitate the assignment of the Present on Admission (POA) indicator for each diagnosis and external cause of injury code reported on claim forms (UB-04 and 837 Institutional).

These guidelines are not intended to replace any guidelines in the main body of the *ICD-10-CM Official Guidelines for Coding and Reporting*. The POA guidelines are not intended to provide guidance on when a condition should be coded, but rather, how to apply the POA indicator to the final set of diagnosis codes that have been assigned in accordance with Sections I, II, and III of the official coding guidelines. Subsequent to the assignment of the ICD-10-CM codes, the POA indicator should then be assigned to those conditions that have been coded.

As stated in the Introduction to the *ICD-10-CM Official Guidelines for Coding and Reporting,* a joint effort between the healthcare provider and the coder is essential to achieve complete and accurate documentation, code assignment, and reporting of diagnoses and procedures. The importance of consistent, complete documentation in the medical record cannot be overemphasized. Medical record documentation from any provider involved in the care and treatment of the patient may be used to support the determination of whether a condition was present on admission or not. In the context of the official coding guidelines, the term "provider" means a physician or any qualified healthcare practitioner who is legally accountable for establishing the patient's diagnosis.

These guidelines are not a substitute for the provider's clinical judgment as to the determination of whether a condition was/was not present on admission. The provider should be queried regarding issues related to the linking of signs/symptoms, timing of test results, and the timing of findings.

Please see the CDC website for the detailed list of ICD-10-CM codes that do not require the use of a POA indicator (https://www.cdc.gov/nchs/icd/icd10cm.htm). The codes and categories on this exempt list are for circumstances regarding the healthcare encounter or factors influencing health status that do not represent a current disease or injury or that describe conditions that are always present on admission.

General Reporting Requirements

All claims involving inpatient admissions to general acute care hospitals or other facilities that are subject to a law or regulation mandating collection of present on admission information.

Present on admission is defined as present at the time the order for inpatient admission occurs -- conditions that develop during an outpatient encounter, including emergency department, observation, or outpatient surgery, are considered as present on admission.

POA indicator is assigned to principal and secondary diagnoses (as defined in Section II of the Official Guidelines for Coding and Reporting) and the external cause of injury codes.

Issues related to inconsistent, missing, conflicting or unclear documentation must still be resolved by the provider.

If a condition would not be coded and reported based on UHDDS definitions and current official coding guidelines, then the POA indicator would not be reported.

Reporting Options

Y - Yes

N - No

U - Unknown

W – Clinically undetermined

Unreported/Not used – (Exempt from POA reporting)

Reporting Definitions

Y = present at the time of inpatient admission

N = not present at the time of inpatient admission

U = documentation is insufficient to determine if condition is present on admission

W = provider is unable to clinically determine whether condition was present on admission or not

Timeframe for POA Identification and Documentation

There is no required timeframe as to when a provider (per the definition of "provider" used in these guidelines) must identify or document a condition to be present on admission. In some clinical situations, it may not be possible for a provider to make a definitive diagnosis (or a condition may not be recognized or reported by the patient) for a period of time after admission. In some cases, it may be several days before the provider arrives at a definitive diagnosis. This does not mean that the condition was not present on admission. Determination of whether the condition was present on admission or not will be based on the applicable POA guideline as identified in this document, or on the provider's best clinical judgment.

If at the time of code assignment the documentation is unclear as to whether a condition was present on admission or not, it is appropriate to query the provider for clarification.

Assigning the POA Indicator

Condition is on the "Exempt from Reporting" list

Leave the "present on admission" field blank if the condition is on the list of ICD-10-CM codes for which this field is not applicable. This is the only circumstance in which the field may be left blank.

POA Explicitly Documented

Assign Y for any condition the provider explicitly documents as being present on admission.

Assign N for any condition the provider explicitly documents as not present at the time of admission.

Conditions diagnosed prior to inpatient admission

Assign "Y" for conditions that were diagnosed prior to admission (example: hypertension, diabetes mellitus, asthma)

Conditions diagnosed during the admission but clearly present before admission

Assign "Y" for conditions diagnosed during the admission that were clearly present but not diagnosed until after admission occurred.

Diagnoses subsequently confirmed after admission are considered present on admission if at the time of admission they are documented as suspected, possible, rule out, differential diagnosis, or constitute an underlying cause of a symptom that is present at the time of admission.

Condition develops during outpatient encounter prior to inpatient admission

Assign Y for any condition that develops during an outpatient encounter prior to a written order for inpatient admission.

Documentation does not indicate whether condition was present on admission

Assign "U" when the medical record documentation is unclear as to whether the condition was present on admission. "U" should not be routinely assigned and used only in very limited circumstances. Coders are encouraged to query the providers when the documentation is unclear.

Documentation states that it cannot be determined whether the condition was or was not present on admission

Assign "W" when the medical record documentation indicates that it cannot be clinically determined whether or not the condition was present on admission.

Chronic condition with acute exacerbation during the admission

If a single code identifies both the chronic condition and the acute exacerbation, see POA guidelines pertaining to codes that contain multiple clinical concepts.

If a single code only identifies the chronic condition and not the acute exacerbation (e.g., acute exacerbation of chronic leukemia), assign "Y."

Conditions documented as possible, probable, suspected, or rule out at the time of discharge

If the final diagnosis contains a possible, probable, suspected, or rule out diagnosis, and this diagnosis was based on signs, symptoms or clinical findings suspected at the time of inpatient admission, assign "Y."

If the final diagnosis contains a possible, probable, suspected, or rule out diagnosis, and this diagnosis was based on signs, symptoms or clinical findings that were not present on admission, assign "N".

Conditions documented as impending or threatened at the time of discharge

If the final diagnosis contains an impending or threatened diagnosis, and this diagnosis is based on symptoms or clinical findings that were present on admission, assign "Y".

If the final diagnosis contains an impending or threatened diagnosis, and this diagnosis is based on symptoms or clinical findings that were not present on admission, assign "N".

Acute and Chronic Conditions

Assign "Y" for acute conditions that are present at time of admission and N for acute conditions that are not present at time of admission.

Assign "Y" for chronic conditions, even though the condition may not be diagnosed until after admission.

If a single code identifies both an acute and chronic condition, see the POA guidelines for codes that contain multiple clinical concepts.

Codes That Contain Multiple Clinical Concepts

Assign "N" if at least one of the clinical concepts included in the code was not present on admission (e.g., COPD with acute exacerbation and the exacerbation was not present on admission; gastric ulcer that does not start bleeding until after admission; asthma patient develops status asthmaticus after admission).

Assign "Y" if all of the clinical concepts included in the code were present on admission (e.g., duodenal ulcer that perforates prior to admission).

For infection codes that include the causal organism, assign "Y" if the infection (or signs of the infection) were present on admission, even though the culture results may not be known until after admission (e.g., patient is admitted with pneumonia and the provider documents Pseudomonas as the causal organism a few days later).

Same Diagnosis Code for Two or More Conditions

When the same ICD-10-CM diagnosis code applies to two or more conditions during the same encounter (e.g. two separate conditions classified to the same ICD-10-CM diagnosis code):

Assign "Y" if all conditions represented by the single ICD-10-CM code were present on admission (e.g. bilateral unspecified age-related cataracts).

Assign "N" if any of the conditions represented by the single ICD-10-CM code was not present on admission (e.g. traumatic secondary and recurrent hemorrhage and seroma is assigned to a single code T79.2, but only one of the conditions was present on admission).

Obstetrical conditions

Whether or not the patient delivers during the current hospitalization does not affect assignment of the POA indicator. The determining factor for POA assignment is whether the pregnancy complication or obstetrical condition described by the code was present at the time of admission or not.

If the pregnancy complication or obstetrical condition was present on admission (e.g., patient admitted in preterm labor), assign "Y."

If the pregnancy complication or obstetrical condition was not present on admission (e.g., 2nd degree laceration during delivery, postpartum hemorrhage that occurred during current hospitalization, fetal distress develops after admission), assign "N".

If the obstetrical code includes more than one diagnosis and any of the diagnoses identified by the code were not present on admission assign "N". (e.g., Category O11, Pre-existing hypertension with pre-eclampsia)

Perinatal conditions

Newborns are not considered to be admitted until after birth. Therefore, any condition present at birth or that developed in utero is considered present at admission and should be assigned "Y". This includes conditions that occur during delivery (e.g., injury during delivery, meconium aspiration, exposure to streptococcus B in the vaginal canal).

Congenital conditions and anomalies

Assign "Y" for congenital conditions and anomalies except for categories Q00-Q99, Congenital anomalies, which are on the exempt list. Congenital conditions are always considered present on admission.

External cause of injury codes

Assign "Y" for any external cause code representing an external cause of morbidity that occurred prior to inpatient admission (e.g., patient fell out of bed at home, patient fell out of bed in emergency room prior to admission)

Assign "N" for any external cause code representing an external cause of morbidity that occurred during inpatient hospitalization (e.g., patient fell out of hospital bed during hospital stay, patient experienced an adverse reaction to a medication administered after inpatient admission).

A

Aarskog's syndrome Q87.19
Abandonment — *see* Maltreatment
Abasia (-astasia) (hysterical) F44.4
Abderhalden-Kaufmann-Lignac syndrome (cystinosis) E72.04
Abdomen, abdominal — *see also* condition
  muscle deficiency syndrome Q79.4
    angina K55.1
    acute R10.0
Abdominalgia — *see* Pain, abdominal
Abduction contracture, hip or other joint — *see* Contraction, joint
Aberrant (congenital) — *see also* Malposition, congenital
  adrenal gland Q89.1
  artery (peripheral) Q27.8
    basilar NEC Q28.1
    cerebral Q28.3
    coronary Q24.5
    digestive system Q27.8
    eye Q15.8
    lower limb Q27.8
    precerebral Q28.1
    pulmonary Q25.79
    renal Q27.2
    retina Q14.1
    specified site NEC Q27.8
    subclavian Q27.8
    upper limb Q27.8
    vertebral Q28.1
  breast Q83.8
  endocrine gland NEC Q89.2
  hepatic duct Q44.5
  pancreas Q45.3
  parathyroid gland Q89.2
  pituitary gland Q89.2
  sebaceous glands, mucous membrane, mouth, congenital Q38.6
  spleen Q89.09
  subclavian artery Q27.8
  thymus (gland) Q89.2
  thyroid gland Q89.2
  vein (peripheral) NEC Q27.8
    cerebral Q28.3
    digestive system Q27.8
    lower limb Q27.8
    precerebral Q28.1
    specified site NEC Q27.8
    upper limb Q27.8
Aberration
  distantial — *see* Disturbance, visual
  mental F99
Abetalipoproteinemia E78.6
Abiotrophy R68.89
Ablatio, ablation
  retinae — *see* Detachment, retina
Ablepharia, ablepharon Q10.3
Abnormal, abnormality, abnormalities — *see also* Anomaly
  acid-base balance (mixed) E87.4
  albumin R77.0
  alphafetoprotein R77.2
  alveolar ridge K08.9
  anatomical relationship Q89.9
  apertures, congenital, diaphragm Q79.1
  auditory perception H93.29- ☑
    diplacusis — *see* Diplacusis
    hyperacusis — *see* Hyperacusis
    recruitment — *see* Recruitment, auditory
    threshold shift — *see* Shift, auditory threshold
  autosomes Q99.9
    fragile site Q95.5
  basal metabolic rate R94.8
  biosynthesis, testicular androgen E29.1
  bleeding time R79.1
  blood-gas level R79.81
  blood level (of)
    cobalt R79.0
    copper R79.0
    iron R79.0
    lithium R78.89

Abnormal, abnormality, abnormalities — *continued*
  blood level — *continued*
    magnesium R79.0
    mineral NEC R79.0
    zinc R79.0
  blood pressure
    elevated R03.0
    low reading (nonspecific) R03.1
  blood sugar R73.09
  bowel sounds R19.15
    absent R19.11
    hyperactive R19.12
  brain scan R94.02
  breathing R06.9
  caloric test R94.138
  cerebrospinal fluid R83.9
    cytology R83.6
    drug level R83.2
    enzyme level R83.0
    hormones R83.1
    immunology R83.4
    microbiology R83.5
    nonmedicinal level R83.3
    specified type NEC R83.8
  chemistry, blood R79.9
    C-reactive protein R79.82
    drugs — *see* Findings, abnormal, in blood
    gas level R79.81
    minerals R79.0
    pancytopenia D61.818
    PTT R79.1
    specified NEC R79.89
    toxins — *see* Findings, abnormal, in blood
  chest sounds (friction) (rales) R09.89
  chromosome, chromosomal Q99.9
    with more than three X chromosomes, female Q97.1
    analysis result R89.8
      bronchial washings R84.8
      cerebrospinal fluid R83.8
      cervix uteri NEC R87.89
      nasal secretions R84.8
      nipple discharge R89.8
      peritoneal fluid R85.89
      pleural fluid R84.8
      prostatic secretions R86.8
      saliva R85.89
      seminal fluid R86.8
      sputum R84.8
      synovial fluid R89.8
      throat scrapings R84.8
      vagina R87.89
      vulva R87.89
      wound secretions R89.8
    dicentric replacement Q93.2
    ring replacement Q93.2
    sex Q99.8
      female phenotype Q97.9
        specified NEC Q97.8
      male phenotype Q98.9
        specified NEC Q98.8
      structural male Q98.6
    specified NEC Q99.8
  clinical findings NEC R68.89
  coagulation D68.9
    newborn, transient P61.6
    profile R79.1
    time R79.1
  communication — *see* Fistula
  conjunctiva, vascular H11.41- ☑
  coronary artery Q24.5
  cortisol-binding globulin E27.8
  course, eustachian tube Q17.8
  creatinine clearance R94.4
  cytology
    anus R85.619
      atypical squamous cells cannot exclude high grade squamous intraepithelial lesion (ASC-H) R85.611
      atypical squamous cells of undetermined significance (ASC-US) R85.610
      cytologic evidence of malignancy R85.614

Abnormal, abnormality, abnormalities — *continued*
  cytology — *continued*
    anus — *continued*
      high grade squamous intraepithelial lesion (HGSIL) R85.613
      human papillomavirus (HPV) DNA test
        high risk positive R85.81
        low risk postive R85.82
      inadequate smear R85.615
      low grade squamous intraepithelial lesion (LGSIL) R85.612
      satisfactory anal smear but lacking transformation zone R85.616
      specified NEC R85.618
      unsatisfactory smear R85.615
    female genital organs — *see* Abnormal, Papanicolaou (smear)
  dark adaptation curve H53.61
  dentofacial NEC — *see* Anomaly, dentofacial
  development, developmental Q89.9
    central nervous system Q07.9
  diagnostic imaging
    abdomen, abdominal region NEC R93.5
    biliary tract R93.2
    bladder R93.41
    breast R92.8
    central nervous system NEC R90.89
    cerebrovascular NEC R90.89
    coronary circulation R93.1
    digestive tract NEC R93.3
    gastrointestinal (tract) R93.3
    genitourinary organs R93.89
    head R93.0
    heart R93.1
    intrathoracic organ NEC R93.89
    kidney R93.42- ☑
    limbs R93.6
    liver R93.2
    lung (field) R91.8
    musculoskeletal system NEC R93.7
    renal pelvis R93.41
    retroperitoneum R93.5
    site specified NEC R93.89
    skin and subcutaneous tissue R93.89
    skull R93.0
    testis R93.81- ☑
    ureter R93.41
    urinary organs specified NEC R93.49
  direction, teeth, fully erupted M26.30
  ear ossicles, acquired NEC H74.39- ☑
    ankylosis — *see* Ankylosis, ear ossicles
    discontinuity — *see* Discontinuity, ossicles, ear
    partial loss — *see* Loss, ossicles, ear (partial)
  Ebstein Q22.5
  echocardiogram R93.1
  echoencephalogram R90.81
  echogram — *see* Abnormal, diagnostic imaging
  electrocardiogram [ECG] [EKG] R94.31
  electroencephalogram [EEG] R94.01
  electrolyte — *see* Imbalance, electrolyte
  electromyogram [EMG] R94.131
  electro-oculogram [EOG] R94.110
  electrophysiological intracardiac studies R94.39
  electroretinogram [ERG] R94.111
  erythrocytes
    congenital, with perinatal jaundice D58.9
  feces (color) (contents) (mucus) R19.5
  finding — *see* Findings, abnormal, without diagnosis
  fluid
    amniotic — *see* Abnormal, specimen, specified
    cerebrospinal — *see* Abnormal, cerebrospinal fluid
    peritoneal — *see* Abnormal, specimen, digestive organs
    pleural — *see* Abnormal, specimen, respiratory organs
    synovial — *see* Abnormal, specimen, specified
    thorax (bronchial washings) (pleural fluid) — *see* Abnormal, specimen, respiratory organs
    vaginal — *see* Abnormal, specimen, female genital organs
  form
    teeth K00.2

Abnormal, abnormality, abnormalities — *continued*

form — *continued*
uterus — *see* Anomaly, uterus
function studies
auditory R94.120
bladder R94.8
brain R94.09
cardiovascular R94.30
ear R94.128
endocrine NEC R94.7
eye NEC R94.118
kidney R94.4
liver R94.5
nervous system
central NEC R94.09
peripheral NEC R94.138
pancreas R94.8
placenta R94.8
pulmonary R94.2
special senses NEC R94.128
spleen R94.8
thyroid R94.6
vestibular R94.121
gait — *see* Gait
hysterical F44.4
gastrin secretion E16.4
globulin R77.1
cortisol-binding E27.8
thyroid-binding E07.89
glomerular, minor — *see also* N00-N07 with fourth
character .0 N05.0
glucagon secretion E16.3
glucose tolerance (test) (non-fasting) R73.09
gravitational (G) forces or states (effect of) T75.81 ☑
hair (color) (shaft) L67.9
specified NEC L67.8
hard tissue formation in pulp (dental) K04.3
head movement R25.0
heart
rate R00.9
specified NEC R00.8
shadow R93.1
sounds NEC R01.2
hemoglobin (disease) — *see also* Disease, hemoglobin
D58.2
trait — *see* Trait, hemoglobin, abnormal
histology NEC R89.7
immunological findings R89.4
in serum R76.9
specified NEC R76.8
increase in appetite R63.2
involuntary movement — *see* Abnormal, movement,
involuntary
jaw closure M26.51
karyotype R89.8
kidney function test R94.4
knee jerk R29.2
leukocyte (cell) (differential) NEC D72.9
liver function test R94.5
loss of
height R29.890
weight R63.4
mammogram NEC R92.8
calcification (calculus) R92.1
microcalcification R92.0
Mantoux test R76.11
movement (disorder) — *see also* Disorder, movement
head R25.0
involuntary R25.9
fasciculation R25.3
of head R25.0
spasm R25.2
specified type NEC R25.8
tremor R25.1
myoglobin (Aberdeen) (Annapolis) R89.7
neonatal screening P09
oculomotor study R94.113
palmar creases Q82.8
Papanicolaou (smear)
anus R85.619
atypical squamous cells cannot exclude high
grade squamous intraepithelial lesion
(ASC-H) R85.611
atypical squamous cells of undetermined significance (ASC-US) R85.610
cytologic evidence of malignancy R85.614

Abnormal, abnormality, abnormalities — *continued*

Papanicolaou — *continued*
anus — *continued*
high grade squamous intraepithelial lesion
(HGSIL) R85.613
human papillomavirus (HPV) DNA test
high risk positive R85.81
low risk postive R85.82
inadequate smear R85.615
low grade squamous intraepithelial lesion (LGSIL)
R85.612
satisfactory anal smear but lacking transformation zone R85.616
specified NEC R85.618
unsatisfactory smear R85.615
bronchial washings R84.6
cerebrospinal fluid R83.6
cervix R87.619
atypical squamous cells cannot exclude high
grade squamous intraepithelial lesion
(ASC-H) R87.611
atypical squamous cells of undetermined significance (ASC-US) R87.610
cytologic evidence of malignancy R87.614
high grade squamous intraepithelial lesion
(HGSIL) R87.613
inadequate smear R87.615
low grade squamous intraepithelial lesion (LGSIL)
R87.612
non-atypical endometrial cells R87.618
satisfactory cervical smear but lacking transformation zone R87.616
specified NEC R87.618
thin preparaton R87.619
unsatisfactory smear R87.615
nasal secretions R84.6
nipple discharge R89.6
peritoneal fluid R85.69
pleural fluid R84.6
prostatic secretions R86.6
saliva R85.69
seminal fluid R86.6
sites NEC R89.6
sputum R84.6
synovial fluid R89.6
throat scrapings R84.6
vagina R87.629
atypical squamous cells cannot exclude high
grade squamous intraepithelial lesion
(ASC-H) R87.621
atypical squamous cells of undetermined significance (ASC-US) R87.620
cytologic evidence of malignancy R87.624
high grade squamous intraepithelial lesion
(HGSIL) R87.623
inadequate smear R87.625
low grade squamous intraepithelial lesion (LGSIL)
R87.622
specified NEC R87.628
thin preparation R87.629
unsatisfactory smear R87.625
vulva R87.69
wound secretions R89.6
partial thromboplastin time (PTT) R79.1
pelvis (bony) — *see* Deformity, pelvis
percussion, chest (tympany) R09.89
periods (grossly) — *see* Menstruation
phonocardiogram R94.39
plantar reflex R29.2
plasma
protein R77.9
specified NEC R77.8
viscosity R70.1
pleural (folds) Q34.0
posture R29.3
product of conception O02.9
specified type NEC O02.89
prothrombin time (PT) R79.1
pulmonary
artery, congenital Q25.79
function, newborn P28.89
test results R94.2
pulsations in neck R00.2
pupillary H21.56- ☑
function (reaction) (reflex) — *see* Anomaly, pupil,
function
radiological examination — *see* Abnormal, diagnostic
imaging

Abnormal, abnormality, abnormalities — *continued*

red blood cell(s) (morphology) (volume) R71.8
reflex — *see* Reflex
renal function test R94.4
response to nerve stimulation R94.130
retinal correspondence H53.31
retinal function study R94.111
rhythm, heart — *see also* Arrhythmia
saliva — *see* Abnormal, specimen, digestive organs
scan
kidney R94.4
liver R93.2
thyroid R94.6
secretion
gastrin E16.4
glucagon E16.3
semen, seminal fluid — *see* Abnormal, specimen, male
genital organs
serum level (of)
acid phosphatase R74.8
alkaline phosphatase R74.8
amylase R74.8
enzymes R74.9
specified NEC R74.8
lipase R74.8
triacylglycerol lipase R74.8
shape
gravid uterus — *see* Anomaly, uterus
sinus venosus Q21.1
size, tooth, teeth K00.2
spacing, tooth, teeth, fully erupted M26.30
specimen
digestive organs (peritoneal fluid) (saliva) R85.9
cytology R85.69
drug level R85.2
enzyme level R85.0
histology R85.7
hormones R85.1
immunology R85.4
microbiology R85.5
nonmedicinal level R85.3
specified type NEC R85.89
female genital organs (secretions) (smears) R87.9
cytology R87.69
cervix R87.619
human papillomavirus (HPV) DNA test
high risk positive R87.810
low risk positive R87.820
inadequate (unsatisfactory) smear
R87.615
non-atypical endometrial cells R87.618
specified NEC R87.618
vagina R87.629
human papillomavirus (HPV) DNA test
high risk positive R87.811
low risk positive R87.821
inadequate (unsatisfactory) smear
R87.625
vulva R87.69
drug level R87.2
enzyme level R87.0
histological R87.7
hormones R87.1
immunology R87.4
microbiology R87.5
nonmedicinal level R87.3
specified type NEC R87.89
male genital organs (prostatic secretions) (semen)
R86.9
cytology R86.6
drug level R86.2
enzyme level R86.0
histological R86.7
hormones R86.1
immunology R86.4
microbiology R86.5
nonmedicinal level R86.3
specified type NEC R86.8
nipple discharge — *see* Abnormal, specimen, specified
respiratory organs (bronchial washings) (nasal secretions) (pleural fluid) (sputum) R84.9
cytology R84.6
drug level R84.2
enzyme level R84.0
histology R84.7
hormones R84.1
immunology R84.4

Abnormal, abnormality, abnormalities — *continued*
  specimen — *continued*
    respiratory organs — *continued*
      microbiology R84.5
      nonmedicinal level R84.3
      specified type NEC R84.8
    specified organ, system and tissue NOS R89.9
      cytology R89.6
      drug level R89.2
      enzyme level R89.0
      histology R89.7
      hormones R89.1
      immunology R89.4
      microbiology R89.5
      nonmedicinal level R89.3
      specified type NEC R89.8
    synovial fluid — *see* Abnormal, specimen, specified
    thorax (bronchial washings) (pleural fluids) — *see* Abnormal, specimen, respiratory organs
    vagina (secretion) (smear) R87.629
    vulva (secretion) (smear) R87.69
    wound secretion — *see* Abnormal, specimen, specified
  spermatozoa — *see* Abnormal, specimen, male genital organs
  sputum (amount) (color) (odor) R09.3
  stool (color) (contents) (mucus) R19.5
    bloody K92.1
    guaiac positive R19.5
  synchondrosis Q78.8
  thermography — *see also* Abnormal, diagnostic imaging R93.89
  thyroid-binding globulin E07.89
  tooth, teeth (form) (size) K00.2
  toxicology (findings) R78.9
  transport protein E88.09
  tumor marker NEC R97.8
  ultrasound results — *see* Abnormal, diagnostic imaging
  umbilical cord complicating delivery O69.9 ☑
  urination NEC R39.198
  urine (constituents) R82.90
    bile R82.2
    cytological examination R82.89
    drugs R82.5
    fat R82.0
    glucose R81
    heavy metals R82.6
    hemoglobin R82.3
    histological examination R82.89
    ketones R82.4
    microbiological examination (culture) R82.79
    myoglobin R82.1
    positive culture R82.79
    protein — *see* Proteinuria
    specified substance NEC R82.998
      chromoabnormality NEC R82.91
    substances nonmedical R82.6
  uterine hemorrhage — *see* Hemorrhage, uterus
  vectorcardiogram R94.39
  visually evoked potential (VEP) R94.112
  white blood cells D72.9
    specified NEC D72.89
  X-ray examination — *see* Abnormal, diagnostic imaging
Abnormity (any organ or part) — *see* Anomaly
Abocclusion M26.29
  hemolytic disease (newborn) P55.1
  incompatibility reaction ABO — *see* Complication(s), transfusion, incompatibility reaction, ABO
Abolition, language R48.8
Aborter, habitual or recurrent — *see* Loss (of), pregnancy, recurrent
Abortion (complete) (spontaneous) O03.9
  with
    retained products of conception — *see* Abortion, incomplete
  attempted (elective) (failed) O07.4
    complicated by O07.30
      afibrinogenemia O07.1
      cardiac arrest O07.36
      chemical damage of pelvic organ(s) O07.34
      circulatory collapse O07.31
      cystitis O07.38
      defibrination syndrome O07.1
      electrolyte imbalance O07.33
      embolism (air) (amniotic fluid) (blood clot) (fat) (pulmonary) (septic) (soap) O07.2
      endometritis O07.0

Abortion — *continued*
  attempted — *continued*
    complicated by — *continued*
      genital tract and pelvic infection O07.0
      hemolysis O07.1
      hemorrhage (delayed) (excessive) O07.1
      infection
        genital tract or pelvic O07.0
        urinary tract tract O07.38
      intravascular coagulation O07.1
      laceration of pelvic organ(s) O07.34
      metabolic disorder O07.33
      oliguria O07.32
      oophoritis O07.0
      parametritis O07.0
      pelvic peritonitis O07.0
      perforation of pelvic organ(s) O07.34
      renal failure or shutdown O07.32
      salpingitis or salpingo-oophoritis O07.0
      sepsis O07.37
      shock O07.31
      specified condition NEC O07.39
      tubular necrosis (renal) O07.32
      uremia O07.32
      urinary tract infection O07.38
      venous complication NEC O07.35
        embolism (air) (amniotic fluid) (blood clot) (fat) (pulmonary) (septic) (soap) O07.2
  complicated (by) (following) O03.80
    afibrinogenemia O03.6
    cardiac arrest O03.86
    chemical damage of pelvic organ(s) O03.84
    circulatory collapse O03.81
    cystitis O03.88
    defibrination syndrome O03.6
    electrolyte imbalance O03.83
    embolism (air) (amniotic fluid) (blood clot) (fat) (pulmonary) (septic) (soap) O03.7
    endometritis O03.5
    genital tract and pelvic infection O03.5
    hemolysis O03.6
    hemorrhage (delayed) (excessive) O03.6
    infection
      genital tract or pelvic O03.5
      urinary tract O03.88
    intravascular coagulation O03.6
    laceration of pelvic organ(s) O03.84
    metabolic disorder O03.83
    oliguria O03.82
    oophoritis O03.5
    parametritis O03.5
    pelvic peritonitis O03.5
    perforation of pelvic organ(s) O03.84
    renal failure or shutdown O03.82
    salpingitis or salpingo-oophoritis O03.5
    sepsis O03.87
    shock O03.81
    specified condition NEC O03.89
    tubular necrosis (renal) O03.82
    uremia O03.82
    urinary tract infection O03.88
    venous complication NEC O03.85
      embolism (air) (amniotic fluid) (blood clot) (fat) (pulmonary) (septic) (soap) O03.7
  failed — *see* Abortion, attempted
  habitual or recurrent N96
    with current abortion — *see* categories O03-O04
    without current pregnancy N96
    care in current pregnancy O26.2- ☑
  incomplete (spontaneous) O03.4
    complicated (by) (following) O03.30
      afibrinogenemia O03.1
      cardiac arrest O03.36
      chemical damage of pelvic organ(s) O03.34
      circulatory collapse O03.31
      cystitis O03.38
      defibrination syndrome O03.1
      electrolyte imbalance O03.33
      embolism (air) (amniotic fluid) (blood clot) (fat) (pulmonary) (septic) (soap) O03.2
      endometritis O03.0
      genital tract and pelvic infection O03.0
      hemolysis O03.1
      hemorrhage (delayed) (excessive) O03.1
      infection
        genital tract or pelvic O03.0
        urinary tract O03.38
      intravascular coagulation O03.1
      laceration of pelvic organ(s) O03.34

Abortion — *continued*
  incomplete — *continued*
    complicated — *continued*
      metabolic disorder O03.33
      oliguria O03.32
      oophoritis O03.0
      parametritis O03.0
      pelvic peritonitis O03.0
      perforation of pelvic organ(s) O03.34
      renal failure or shutdown O03.32
      salpingitis or salpingo-oophoritis O03.0
      sepsis O03.37
      shock O03.31
      specified condition NEC O03.39
      tubler necrosis (renal) O03.32
      uremia O03.32
      urinary infection O03.38
      venous complication NEC O03.35
        embolism (air) (amniotic fluid) (blood clot) (fat) (pulmonary) (septic) (soap) O03.2
  induced (encounter for) Z33.2
    complicated by O04.80
      afibrinogenemia O04.6
      cardiac arrest O04.86
      chemical damage of pelvic organ(s) O04.84
      circulatory collapse O04.81
      cystitis O04.88
      defibrination syndrome O04.6
      electrolyte imbalance O04.83
      embolism (air) (amniotic fluid) (blood clot) (fat) (pulmonary) (septic) (soap) O04.7
      endometritis O04.5
      genital tract and pelvic infection O04.5
      hemolysis O04.6
      hemorrhage (delayed) (excessive) O04.6
      infection
        genital tract or pelvic O04.5
        urinary tract O04.88
      intravascular coagulation O04.6
      laceration of pelvic organ(s) O04.84
      metabolic disorder O04.83
      oliguria O04.82
      oophoritis O04.5
      parametritis O04.5
      pelvic peritonitis O04.5
      perforation of pelvic organ(s) O04.84
      renal failure or shutdown O04.82
      salpingitis or salpingo-oophoritis O04.5
      sepsis O04.87
      shock O04.81
      specified condition NEC O04.89
      tubular necrosis (renal) O04.82
      uremia O04.82
      urinary tract infection O04.88
      venous complication NEC O04.85
        embolism (air) (amniotic fluid) (blood clot) (fat) (pulmonary) (septic) (soap) O04.7
  inevitable O03.4
  missed O02.1
  spontaneous — *see* Abortion (complete) (spontaneous)
    threatened O20.0
  threatened (spontaneous) O20.0
  tubal O00.10- ☑
    with intrauterine pregnancy O00.11- ☑
Abortus fever A23.1
Aboulomania F60.7
Abrami's disease D59.8
Abramov-Fiedler myocarditis (acute isolated myocarditis) I40.1
Abrasion T14.8 ☑
  abdomen, abdominal (wall) S30.811 ☑
  alveolar process S00.512 ☑
  ankle S90.51- ☑
  antecubital space — *see* Abrasion, elbow
  anus S30.817 ☑
  arm (upper) S40.81- ☑
  auditory canal — *see* Abrasion, ear
  auricle — *see* Abrasion, ear
  axilla — *see* Abrasion, arm
  back, lower S30.810 ☑
  breast S20.11- ☑
  brow S00.81 ☑
  buttock S30.810 ☑
  calf — *see* Abrasion, leg
  canthus — *see* Abrasion, eyelid
  cheek S00.81 ☑
    internal S00.512 ☑
  chest wall — *see* Abrasion, thorax

Abrasion — continued
- chin S00.81 ☑
- clitoris S30.814 ☑
- cornea S05.0- ☑
- costal region — see Abrasion, thorax
- dental K03.1
- digit(s)
  - foot — see Abrasion, toe
  - hand — see Abrasion, finger
- ear S00.41- ☑
- elbow S50.31- ☑
- epididymis S30.813 ☑
- epigastric region S30.811 ☑
- epiglottis S10.11 ☑
- esophagus (thoracic) S27.818 ☑
  - cervical S10.11 ☑
- eyebrow — see Abrasion, eyelid
- eyelid S00.21- ☑
- face S00.81 ☑
- finger(s) S60.41- ☑
  - index S60.41- ☑
  - little S60.41- ☑
  - middle S60.41- ☑
  - ring S60.41- ☑
- flank S30.811 ☑
- foot (except toe(s) alone) S90.81- ☑
  - toe — see Abrasion, toe
- forearm S50.81- ☑
  - elbow only — see Abrasion, elbow
- forehead S00.81 ☑
- genital organs, external
  - female S30.816 ☑
  - male S30.815 ☑
- groin S30.811 ☑
- gum S00.512 ☑
- hand S60.51- ☑
- head S00.91 ☑
  - ear — see Abrasion, ear
  - eyelid — see Abrasion, eyelid
  - lip S00.511 ☑
  - nose S00.31 ☑
  - oral cavity S00.512 ☑
  - scalp S00.01 ☑
  - specified site NEC S00.81 ☑
- heel — see Abrasion, foot
- hip S70.21- ☑
- inguinal region S30.811 ☑
- interscapular region S20.419 ☑
- jaw S00.81 ☑
- knee S80.21- ☑
- labium (majus) (minus) S30.814 ☑
- larynx S10.11 ☑
- leg (lower) S80.81- ☑
  - knee — see Abrasion, knee
  - upper — see Abrasion, thigh
- lip S00.511 ☑
- lower back S30.810 ☑
- lumbar region S30.810 ☑
- malar region S00.81 ☑
- mammary — see Abrasion, breast
- mastoid region S00.81 ☑
- mouth S00.512 ☑
- nail
  - finger — see Abrasion, finger
  - toe — see Abrasion, toe
- nape S10.81 ☑
- nasal S00.31 ☑
- neck S10.91 ☑
  - specified site NEC S10.81 ☑
  - throat S10.11 ☑
- nose S00.31 ☑
- occipital region S00.01 ☑
- oral cavity S00.512 ☑
- orbital region — see Abrasion, eyelid
- palate S00.512 ☑
- palm — see Abrasion, hand
- parietal region S00.01 ☑
- pelvis S30.810 ☑
- penis S30.812 ☑
- perineum
  - female S30.814 ☑
  - male S30.810 ☑
- periocular area — see Abrasion, eyelid
- phalanges
  - finger — see Abrasion, finger
  - toe — see Abrasion, toe

Abrasion — continued
- pharynx S10.11 ☑
- pinna — see Abrasion, ear
- popliteal space — see Abrasion, knee
- prepuce S30.812 ☑
- pubic region S30.810 ☑
- pudendum
  - female S30.816 ☑
  - male S30.815 ☑
- sacral region S30.810 ☑
- scalp S00.01 ☑
- scapular region — see Abrasion, shoulder
- scrotum S30.813 ☑
- shin — see Abrasion, leg
- shoulder S40.21- ☑
- skin NEC T14.8 ☑
- sternal region S20.319 ☑
- submaxillary region S00.81 ☑
- submental region S00.81 ☑
- subungual
  - finger(s) — see Abrasion, finger
  - toe(s) — see Abrasion, toe
- supraclavicular fossa S10.81 ☑
- supraorbital S00.81 ☑
- temple S00.81 ☑
- temporal region S00.81 ☑
- testis S30.813 ☑
- thigh S70.31- ☑
- thorax, thoracic (wall) S20.91 ☑
  - back S20.41- ☑
  - front S20.31- ☑
- throat S10.11 ☑
- thumb S60.31- ☑
- toe(s) (lesser) S90.416 ☑
  - great S90.41- ☑
- tongue S00.512 ☑
- tooth, teeth (dentifrice) (habitual) (hard tissues) (occupational) (ritual) (traditional) K03.1
- trachea S10.11 ☑
- tunica vaginalis S30.813 ☑
- tympanum, tympanic membrane — see Abrasion, ear
- uvula S00.512 ☑
- vagina S30.814 ☑
- vocal cords S10.11 ☑
- vulva S30.814 ☑
- wrist S60.81- ☑

Abrism — see Poisoning, food, noxious, plant
Abruptio placentae O45.9- ☑
- with
  - afibrinogenemia O45.01- ☑
  - coagulation defect O45.00- ☑
    - specified NEC O45.09- ☑
  - disseminated intravascular coagulation O45.02- ☑
  - hypofibrinogenemia O45.01- ☑
- specified NEC O45.8- ☑

Abruption, placenta — see Abruptio placentae
Abscess (connective tissue) (embolic) (fistulous) (infective) (metastatic) (multiple) (pernicious) (pyogenic) (septic) L02.91
- with
  - diverticular disease (intestine) K57.80
    - with bleeding K57.81
    - large intestine K57.20
      - with
        - bleeding K57.21
        - small intestine K57.40
          - with bleeding K57.41
      - small intestine K57.00
        - with
          - bleeding K57.01
          - large intestine K57.40
            - with bleeding K57.41
  - lymphangitis — code by site under Abscess
- abdomen, abdominal
  - cavity K65.1
  - wall L02.211
- abdominopelvic K65.1
- accessory sinus — see Sinusitis
- adrenal (capsule) (gland) E27.8
- alveolar K04.7
  - with sinus K04.6
- amebic A06.4
  - brain (and liver or lung abscess) A06.6
  - genitourinary tract A06.82
  - liver (without mention of brain or lung abscess) A06.4

Abscess — continued
- amebic — continued
  - lung (and liver) (without mention of brain abscess) A06.5
    - specified site NEC A06.89
    - spleen A06.89
- anerobic A48.0
- ankle — see Abscess, lower limb
- anorectal K61.2
- antecubital space — see Abscess, upper limb
- antrum (chronic) (Highmore) — see Sinusitis, maxillary
- anus K61.0
- apical (tooth) K04.7
  - with sinus (alveolar) K04.6
- appendix K35.33
- areola (acute) (chronic) (nonpuerperal) N61.1
  - puerperal, postpartum or gestational — see Infection, nipple
- arm (any part) — see Abscess, upper limb
- artery (wall) I77.89
- atheromatous I77.2
- auricle, ear — see Abscess, ear, external
- axilla (region) L02.41- ☑
  - lymph gland or node L04.2
- back (any part, except buttock) L02.212
- Bartholin's gland N75.1
  - with
    - abortion — see Abortion, by type complicated by, sepsis
    - ectopic or molar pregnancy O08.0
  - following ectopic or molar pregnancy O08.0
- Bezold's — see Mastoiditis, acute
- bilharziasis B65.1
- bladder (wall) — see Cystitis, specified type NEC
- bone (subperiosteal) — see also Osteomyelitis, specified type NEC
  - accessory sinus (chronic) — see Sinusitis
  - chronic or old — see Osteomyelitis, chronic
  - jaw (lower) (upper) M27.2
  - mastoid — see Mastoiditis, acute, subperiosteal
  - petrous — see Petrositis
  - spinal (tuberculous) A18.01
    - nontuberculous — see Osteomyelitis, vertebra
- bowel K63.0
- brain (any part) (cystic) (otogenic) G06.0
  - amebic (with abscess of any other site) A06.6
  - gonococcal A54.82
  - pheomycotic (chromomycotic) B43.1
  - tuberculous A17.81
- breast (acute) (chronic) (nonpuerperal) N61.1
  - newborn P39.0
  - puerperal, postpartum, gestational — see Mastitis, obstetric, purulent
- broad ligament N73.2
  - acute N73.0
  - chronic N73.1
- Brodie's (localized) (chronic) M86.8X- ☑
- bronchi J98.09
- buccal cavity K12.2
- bulbourethral gland N34.0
- bursa M71.00
  - ankle M71.07- ☑
  - elbow M71.02- ☑
  - foot M71.07- ☑
  - hand M71.04- ☑
  - hip M71.05- ☑
  - knee M71.06- ☑
  - multiple sites M71.09
  - pharyngeal J39.1
  - shoulder M71.01- ☑
  - specified site NEC M71.08
  - wrist M71.03- ☑
- buttock L02.31
- canthus — see Blepharoconjunctivitis
- cartilage — see Disorder, cartilage, specified type NEC
- cecum K35.33
- cerebellum, cerebellar G06.0
  - sequelae G09
- cerebral (embolic) G06.0
  - sequelae G09
- cervical (meaning neck) L02.11
  - lymph gland or node L04.0
- cervix (stump) (uteri) — see Cervicitis
- cheek (external) L02.01
  - inner K12.2
- chest J86.9
  - with fistula J86.0
  - wall L02.213

☑ Additional Character Required — Refer to the Tabular List for Character Selection   ⓥ Subterms under main terms may continue to next column or page

Abscess — *continued*
  chin L02.01
  choroid — *see* Inflammation, chorioretinal
  circumtonsillar J36
  cold (lung) (tuberculous) — *see also* Tuberculosis, abscess, lung
    articular — *see* Tuberculosis, joint
  colon (wall) K63.0
  colostomy K94.02
  conjunctiva — *see* Conjunctivitis, acute
  cornea H16.31- ☑
  corpus
    cavernosum N48.21
    luteum — *see* Oophoritis
  Cowper's gland N34.0
  cranium G06.0
  cul-de-sac (Douglas') (posterior) — *see* Peritonitis, pelvic, female
  cutaneous — *see* Abscess, by site
  dental K04.7
    with sinus (alveolar) K04.6
  dentoalveolar K04.7
    with sinus K04.6
  diaphragm, diaphragmatic K65.1
  Douglas' cul-de-sac or pouch — *see* Peritonitis, pelvic, female
  Dubois A50.59
  ear (middle) — *see also* Otitis, media, suppurative
    acute — *see* Otitis, media, suppurative, acute
    external H60.0- ☑
  entamebic — *see* Abscess, amebic
  enterostomy K94.12
  epididymis N45.4
  epidural G06.2
    brain G06.0
    spinal cord G06.1
  epiglottis J38.7
  epiploon, epiploic K65.1
  erysipelatous — *see* Erysipelas
  esophagus K20.80
  ethmoid (bone) (chronic) (sinus) J32.2
  external auditory canal — *see* Abscess, ear, external
  extradural G06.2
    brain G06.0
      sequelae G09
    spinal cord G06.1
  extraperitoneal K68.19
  eye — *see* Endophthalmitis, purulent
  eyelid H00.03- ☑
  face (any part, except ear, eye and nose) L02.01
  fallopian tube — *see* Salpingitis
  fascia M72.8
  fauces J39.1
  fecal K63.0
  femoral (region) — *see* Abscess, lower limb
  filaria, filarial — *see* Infestation, filarial
  finger (any) — *see also* Abscess, hand
    nail — *see* Cellulitis, finger
  foot L02.61- ☑
  forehead L02.01
  frontal sinus (chronic) J32.1
  gallbladder K81.0
  genital organ or tract
    female (external) N76.4
    male N49.9
      multiple sites N49.8
      specified NEC N49.8
  gestational mammary O91.11- ☑
  gestational subareolar O91.11- ☑
  gingival — *see* Periodontitis, localized
  gland, glandular (lymph) (acute) — *see* Lymphadenitis, acute
  gluteal (region) L02.31
  gonorrheal — *see* Gonococcus
  groin L02.214
  gum — *see* Periodontitis, localized
  hand L02.51- ☑
  head NEC L02.811
    face (any part, except ear, eye and nose) L02.01
  heart — *see* Carditis
  heel — *see* Abscess, foot
  helminthic — *see* Infestation, helminth
  hepatic (cholangitic) (hematogenic) (lymphogenic) (pylephlebitic) K75.0
    amebic A06.4
  hip (region) — *see* Abscess, lower limb
  horseshoe K61.31
  ileocecal K35.33

Abscess — *continued*
  ileostomy (bud) K94.12
  iliac (region) L02.214
    fossa K35.33
  infraclavicular (fossa) — *see* Abscess, upper limb
  inguinal (region) L02.214
    lymph gland or node L04.1
  intersphincteric K61.4
  intestine, intestinal NEC K63.0
    rectal K61.1
  intra-abdominal — *see also* Abscess, peritoneum K65.1
    following procedure T81.43 ☑
      obstetrical O86.03
    postprocedural T81.43 ☑
    retroperitoneal K68.11
  intracranial G06.0
  intramammary — *see* Abscess, breast
  intramuscular, following procedure T81.42 ☑
    obstetrical O86.02
  intraorbital — *see* Abscess, orbit
  intraperitoneal K65.1
  intrasphincteric (anus) K61.4
  intraspinal G06.1
  intratonsillar J36
  ischiorectal (fossa) (specified NEC) K61.39
  jaw (bone) (lower) (upper) M27.2
  joint — *see* Arthritis, pyogenic or pyemic
    spine (tuberculous) A18.01
      nontuberculous — *see* Spondylopathy, infective
  kidney N15.1
    with calculus N20.0
      with hydronephrosis N13.6
    puerperal (postpartum) O86.21
  knee — *see also* Abscess, lower limb
    joint M00.9
  labium (majus) (minus) N76.4
  lacrimal
    caruncle — *see* Inflammation, lacrimal, passages, acute
    gland — *see* Dacryoadenitis
    passages (duct) (sac) — *see* Inflammation, lacrimal, passages, acute
  lacunar N34.0
  larynx J38.7
  lateral (alveolar) K04.7
    with sinus K04.6
  leg (any part) — *see* Abscess, lower limb
  lens H27.8
  lingual K14.0
    tonsil J36
  lip K13.0
  Littre's gland N34.0
  liver (cholangitic) (hematogenic) (lymphogenic) (pylephlebitic) (pyogenic) K75.0
    amebic (due to Entamoeba histolytica) (dysenteric) (tropical) A06.4
      with
        brain abscess (and liver or lung abscess) A06.6
        lung abscess A06.5
  loin (region) L02.211
  lower limb L02.41- ☑
  lumbar (tuberculous) A18.01
    nontuberculous L02.212
  lung (miliary) (putrid) J85.2
    with pneumonia J85.1
      due to specified organism (see Pneumonia, in (due to))
    amebic (with liver abscess) A06.5
      with
        brain abscess A06.6
        pneumonia A06.5
  lymph, lymphatic, gland or node (acute) — *see also* Lymphadenitis, acute
  mesentery I88.0
  malar M27.2
  mammary gland — *see* Abscess, breast
  marginal, anus K61.0
  mastoid — *see* Mastoiditis, acute
  maxilla, maxillary M27.2
    molar (tooth) K04.7
      with sinus K04.6
    premolar K04.7
    sinus (chronic) J32.0
  mediastinum J85.3
  meibomian gland — *see* Hordeolum
  meninges G06.2
  mesentery, mesenteric K65.1
  mesosalpinx — *see* Salpingitis

Abscess — *continued*
  mons pubis L02.215
  mouth (floor) K12.2
  muscle — *see* Myositis, infective
  myocardium I40.0
  nabothian (follicle) — *see* Cervicitis
  nasal J32.9
  nasopharyngeal J39.1
  navel L02.216
    newborn P38.9
      with mild hemorrhage P38.1
      without hemorrhage P38.9
  neck (region) L02.11
    lymph gland or node L04.0
  nephritic — *see* Abscess, kidney
  nipple N61.1
    associated with
      lactation — *see* Pregnancy, complicated by
      pregnancy — *see* Pregnancy, complicated by
  nose (external) (fossa) (septum) J34.0
    sinus (chronic) — *see* Sinusitis
  omentum K65.1
  operative wound T81.49 ☑
  orbit, orbital — *see* Cellulitis, orbit
  otogenic G06.0
  ovary, ovarian (corpus luteum) — *see* Oophoritis
  oviduct — *see* Oophoritis
  palate (soft) K12.2
    hard M27.2
  palmar (space) — *see* Abscess, hand
  pancreas (duct) — *see* Pancreatitis, acute
  parafrenal N48.21
  parametric, parametrium N73.2
    acute N73.0
    chronic N73.1
  paranephric N15.1
  parapancreatic — *see* Pancreatitis, acute
  parapharyngeal J39.0
  pararectal K61.1
  parasinus — *see* Sinusitis
  parauterine — *see also* Disease, pelvis, inflammatory N73.2
  paravaginal — *see* Vaginitis
  parietal region (scalp) L02.811
  parodontal — *see* Periodontitis, aggressive, localized
  parotid (duct) (gland) K11.3
    region K12.2
  pectoral (region) L02.213
  pelvis, pelvic
    female — *see* Disease, pelvis, inflammatory
    male, peritoneal K65.1
  penis N48.21
    gonococcal (accessory gland) (periurethral) A54.1
  perianal K61.0
  periapical K04.7
    with sinus (alveolar) K04.6
  periappendicular K35.33
  pericardial I30.1
  pericecal K35.33
  pericemental — *see* Periodontitis, aggressive, localized
  pericholecystic — *see* Cholecystitis, acute
  pericoronal — *see* Periodontitis, aggressive, localized
  peridental — *see* Periodontitis, aggressive, localized
  perimetric — *see also* Disease, pelvis, inflammatory N73.2
  perinephric, perinephritic — *see* Abscess, kidney
  perineum, perineal (superficial) L02.215
    urethra N34.0
  periodontal (parietal) — *see* Periodontitis, aggressive, localized
    apical K04.7
  periosteum, periosteal — *see also* Osteomyelitis, specified type NEC
    with osteomyelitis — *see also* Osteomyelitis, specified type NEC
      acute — *see* Osteomyelitis, acute
      chronic — *see* Osteomyelitis, chronic
  peripharyngeal J39.0
  peripleuritic J86.9
    with fistula J86.0
  periprostatic N41.2
  perirectal K61.1
  perirenal (tissue) — *see* Abscess, kidney
  perisinuous (nose) — *see* Sinusitis
  peritoneum, peritoneal (perforated) (ruptured) K65.1
    with appendicitis — *see also* Appendicitis K35.33
    pelvic
      female — *see* Peritonitis, pelvic, female

Abscess — *continued*
  peritoneum, peritoneal — *continued*
    pelvic — *continued*
      male K65.1
    postoperative T81.49 ☑
    puerperal, postpartum, childbirth O85
    tuberculous A18.31
  peritonsillar J36
  perityphlic K35.33
  periureteral N28.89
  periurethral N34.0
    gonococcal (accessory gland) (periurethral) A54.1
  periuterine — *see also* Disease, pelvis, inflammatory N73.2
  perivesical — *see* Cystitis, specified type NEC
  petrous bone — *see* Petrositis
  phagedenic NOS L02.91
    chancroid A57
  pharynx, pharyngeal (lateral) J39.1
  pilonidal L05.01
  pituitary (gland) E23.6
  pleura J86.9
    with fistula J86.0
  popliteal — *see* Abscess, lower limb
  postcecal K35.33
  postlaryngeal J38.7
  postnasal J34.0
  postoperative (any site) — *see also* Infection, postoperative wound T81.49 ☑
    retroperitoneal K68.11
  postpharyngeal J39.0
  posttonsillar J36
  post-typhoid A01.09
  pouch of Douglas — *see* Peritonitis, pelvic, female
  premammary — *see* Abscess, breast
  prepatellar — *see* Abscess, lower limb
  prostate N41.2
    gonococcal (acute) (chronic) A54.22
  psoas muscle K68.12
  puerperal — *code by* site under Puerperal, abscess
  pulmonary — *see* Abscess, lung
  pulp, pulpal (dental) K04.01
    irreversible K04.02
    reversible K04.01
  rectovaginal septum K63.0
  rectovesical — *see* Cystitis, specified type NEC
  rectum K61.1
  renal — *see* Abscess, kidney
  retina — *see* Inflammation, chorioretinal
  retrobulbar — *see* Abscess, orbit
  retrocecal K65.1
  retrolaryngeal J38.7
  retromammary — *see* Abscess, breast
  retroperitoneal NEC K68.19
    postprocedural K68.11
  retropharyngeal J39.0
  retrouterine — *see* Peritonitis, pelvic, female
  retrovesical — *see* Cystitis, specified type NEC
  root, tooth K04.7
    with sinus (alveolar) K04.6
  round ligament — *see also* Disease, pelvis, inflammatory N73.2
  rupture (spontaneous) NOS L02.91
  sacrum (tuberculous) A18.01
    nontuberculous M46.28
  salivary (duct) (gland) K11.3
  scalp (any part) L02.811
  scapular — *see* Osteomyelitis, specified type NEC
  sclera — *see* Scleritis
  scrofulous (tuberculous) A18.2
  scrotum N49.2
  seminal vesicle N49.0
  septal, dental K04.7
    with sinus (alveolar) K04.6
  serous — *see* Periostitis
  shoulder (region) — *see* Abscess, upper limb
  sigmoid K63.0
  sinus (accessory) (chronic) (nasal) — *see also* Sinusitis
    intracranial venous (any) G06.0
  Skene's duct or gland N34.0
  skin — *see* Abscess, by site
  specified site NEC L02.818
  spermatic cord N49.1
  sphenoidal (sinus) (chronic) J32.3
  spinal cord (any part) (staphylococcal) G06.1
    tuberculous A17.81
  spine (column) (tuberculous) A18.01
    epidural G06.1

Abscess — *continued*
  spine — *continued*
    nontuberculous — *see* Osteomyelitis, vertebra
  spleen D73.3
    amebic A06.89
  stitch T81.41 ☑
    following an obstetrical procedure O86.01
  subarachnoid G06.2
    brain G06.0
    spinal cord G06.1
  subareolar — *see* Abscess, breast
  subcecal K35.33
  subcutaneous — *see also* Abscess, by site
    following procedure T81.41 ☑
      obstetrical O86.01
    pheomycotic (chromomycotic) B43.2
  subdiaphragmatic K65.1
  subdural G06.2
    brain G06.0
      sequelae G09
    spinal cord G06.1
  sub-fascial, following an obstetrical procedure O86.02
  subgaleal L02.811
  subhepatic K65.1
  sublingual K12.2
    gland K11.3
  submammary — *see* Abscess, breast
  submandibular (region) (space) (triangle) K12.2
    gland K11.3
  submaxillary (region) L02.01
    gland K11.3
  submental L02.01
    gland K11.3
  subperiosteal — *see* Osteomyelitis, specified type NEC
  subphrenic K65.1
    following an obstetrical procedure O86.03
    postoperative T81.43 ☑
  suburethral N34.0
  sudoriparous L75.8
  supraclavicular (fossa) — *see* Abscess, upper limb
  supralevator K61.5
  suprapelvic, acute N73.0
  suprarenal (capsule) (gland) E27.8
  sweat gland L74.8
  tear duct — *see* Inflammation, lacrimal, passages, acute
  temple L02.01
  temporal region L02.01
  temporosphenoidal G06.0
  tendon (sheath) M65.00
    ankle M65.07- ☑
    foot M65.07- ☑
    forearm M65.03- ☑
    hand M65.04- ☑
    lower leg M65.06- ☑
    pelvic region M65.05- ☑
    shoulder region M65.01- ☑
    specified site NEC M65.08
    thigh M65.05- ☑
    upper arm M65.02- ☑
  testis N45.4
  thigh — *see* Abscess, lower limb
  thorax J86.9
    with fistula J86.0
  throat J39.1
  thumb — *see also* Abscess, hand
    nail — *see* Cellulitis, finger
  thymus (gland) E32.1
  thyroid (gland) E06.0
  toe (any) — *see also* Abscess, foot
    nail — *see* Cellulitis, toe
  tongue (staphylococcal) K14.0
  tonsil(s) (lingual) J36
  tonsillopharyngeal J36
  tooth, teeth (root) K04.7
    with sinus (alveolar) K04.6
    supporting structures NEC — *see* Periodontitis, aggressive, localized
  trachea J39.8
  trunk L02.219
    abdominal wall L02.211
    back L02.212
    chest wall L02.213
    groin L02.214
    perineum L02.215
    umbilicus L02.216
  tubal — *see* Salpingitis
  tuberculous — *see* Tuberculosis, abscess
  tubo-ovarian — *see* Salpingo-oophoritis

Abscess — *continued*
  tunica vaginalis N49.1
  umbilicus L02.216
  upper
    limb L02.41- ☑
    respiratory J39.8
  urethral (gland) N34.0
  urinary N34.0
  uterus, uterine (wall) — *see also* Endometritis
    ligament — *see also* Disease, pelvis, inflammatory N73.2
    neck — *see* Cervicitis
  uvula K12.2
  vagina (wall) — *see* Vaginitis
  vaginorectal — *see* Vaginitis
  vas deferens N49.1
  vermiform appendix K35.33
  vertebra (column) (tuberculous) A18.01
    nontuberculous — *see* Osteomyelitis, vertebra
  vesical — *see* Cystitis, specified type NEC
  vesico-uterine pouch — *see* Peritonitis, pelvic, female
  vitreous (humor) — *see* Endophthalmitis, purulent
  vocal cord J38.3
  von Bezold's — *see* Mastoiditis, acute
  vulva N76.4
  vulvovaginal gland N75.1
  web space — *see* Abscess, hand
  wound T81.49 ☑
  wrist — *see* Abscess, upper limb
Absence (of) (organ or part) (complete or partial)
  adrenal (gland) (congenital) Q89.1
    acquired E89.6
  albumin in blood E88.09
  alimentary tract (congenital) Q45.8
    upper Q40.8
  alveolar process (acquired) — *see* Anomaly, alveolar
  ankle (acquired) Z89.44- ☑
  anus (congenital) Q42.3
    with fistula Q42.2
  aorta (congenital) Q25.41
  appendix, congenital Q42.8
  arm (acquired) Z89.20- ☑
    above elbow Z89.22- ☑
      congenital (with hand present) — *see* Agenesis, arm, with hand present
      and hand — *see* Agenesis, forearm, and hand
    below elbow Z89.21- ☑
      congenital (with hand present) — *see* Agenesis, arm, with hand present
      and hand — *see* Agenesis, forearm, and hand
    congenital — *see* Defect, reduction, upper limb
    shoulder (following explantation of shoulder joint prosthesis) (joint) (with or without presence of antibiotic-impregnated cement spacer) Z89.23- ☑
    congenital (with hand present) — *see* Agenesis, arm, with hand present
  artery (congenital) (peripheral) Q27.8
    brain Q28.3
    coronary Q24.5
    pulmonary Q25.79
    specified NEC Q27.8
    umbilical Q27.0
  atrial septum (congenital) Q21.1
  auditory canal (congenital) (external) Q16.1
  auricle (ear), congenital Q16.0
  bile, biliary duct, congenital Q44.5
  bladder (acquired) Z90.6
    congenital Q64.5
  bowel sounds R19.11
  brain Q00.0
    part of Q04.3
  breast(s) (and nipple(s)) (acquired) Z90.1- ☑
    congenital Q83.8
  broad ligament Q50.6
  bronchus (congenital) Q32.4
  canaliculus lacrimalis, congenital Q10.4
  cerebellum (vermis) Q04.3
  cervix (acquired) (with uterus) Z90.710
    with remaining uterus Z90.712
    congenital Q51.5
  chin, congenital Q18.8
  cilia (congenital) Q10.3
    acquired — *see* Madarosis
  clitoris (congenital) Q52.6
  coccyx, congenital Q76.49
  cold sense R20.8

Absence — *continued*
  congenital
    lumen — *see* Atresia
    organ or site NEC — *see* Agenesis
    septum — *see* Imperfect, closure
  corpus callosum Q04.0
  cricoid cartilage, congenital Q31.8
  diaphragm (with hernia), congenital Q79.1
  digestive organ(s) or tract, congenital Q45.8
    acquired NEC Z90.49
    upper Q40.8
  ductus arteriosus Q28.8
  duodenum (acquired) Z90.49
    congenital Q41.0
  ear, congenital Q16.9
    acquired H93.8- ☑
    auricle Q16.0
    external Q16.0
    inner Q16.5
    lobe, lobule Q17.8
    middle, except ossicles Q16.4
      ossicles Q16.3
    ossicles Q16.3
  ejaculatory duct (congenital) Q55.4
  endocrine gland (congenital) NEC Q89.2
    acquired E89.89
  epididymis (congenital) Q55.4
    acquired Z90.79
  epiglottis, congenital Q31.8
  esophagus (congenital) Q39.8
    acquired (partial) Z90.49
  eustachian tube (congenital) Q16.2
  extremity (acquired) Z89.9
    congenital Q73.0
    knee (following explantation of knee joint prosthe-sis) (joint) (with or without presence of antibi-otic-impregnated cement spacer) Z89.52- ☑
    lower (above knee) Z89.619
      below knee Z89.51- ☑
    upper — *see* Absence, arm
  eye (acquired) Z90.01
    congenital Q11.1
    muscle (congenital) Q10.3
  eyeball (acquired) Z90.01
    congenital Q11.1
  eyelid (fold) (congenital) Q10.3
    acquired Z90.01
  face, specified part NEC Q18.8
  fallopian tube(s) (acquired) Z90.79
    congenital Q50.6
  family member (causing problem in home) NEC — *see also* Disruption, family Z63.32
  femur, congenital — *see* Defect, reduction, lower limb, longitudinal, femur
  fibrinogen (congenital) D68.2
    acquired D65
  finger(s) (acquired) Z89.02- ☑
    congenital — *see* Agenesis, hand
  foot (acquired) Z89.43- ☑
    congenital — *see* Agenesis, foot
  forearm (acquired) — *see* Absence, arm, below elbow
  gallbladder (acquired) Z90.49
    congenital Q44.0
  gamma globulin in blood D80.1
    hereditary D80.0
  genital organs
    acquired (female) (male) Z90.79
    female, congenital Q52.8
      external Q52.71
      internal NEC Q52.8
    male, congenital Q55.8
  genitourinary organs, congenital NEC
    female Q52.8
    male Q55.8
  globe (acquired) Z90.01
    congenital Q11.1
  glottis, congenital Q31.8
  hand and wrist (acquired) Z89.11- ☑
    congenital — *see* Agenesis, hand
  head, part (acquired) NEC Z90.09
  heat sense R20.8
  hip (following explantation of hip joint prosthesis) (joint) (with or without presence of antibiotic-impregnated cement spacer) Z89.62- ☑
  hymen (congenital) Q52.4
  ileum (acquired) Z90.49
    congenital Q41.2
  immunoglobulin, isolated NEC D80.3
    IgA D80.2

Absence — *continued*
  immunoglobulin, isolated — *continued*
    IgG D80.3
    IgM D80.4
  incus (acquired) — *see* Loss, ossicles, ear
    congenital Q16.3
  inner ear, congenital Q16.5
  intestine (acquired) (small) Z90.49
    congenital Q41.9
      specified NEC Q41.8
    large Z90.49
      congenital Q42.9
        specified NEC Q42.8
  iris, congenital Q13.1
  jejunum (acquired) Z90.49
    congenital Q41.1
  joint
    acquired
      hip (following explantation of hip joint prosthe-sis) (with or without presence of antibiotic-impregnated cement spacer) Z89.62- ☑
      knee (following explantation of knee joint pros-thesis) (with or without presence of antibi-otic-impregnated cement spacer) Z89.52- ☑
      shoulder (following explantation of shoulder joint prosthesis) (with or without presence of antibiotic-impregnated cement spacer) Z89.23- ☑
    congenital NEC Q74.8
  kidney(s) (acquired) Z90.5
    congenital Q60.2
      bilateral Q60.1
      unilateral Q60.0
  knee (following explantation of knee joint prosthesis) (joint) (with or without presence of antibiotic-impregnated cement spacer) Z89.52- ☑
  labyrinth, membranous Q16.5
  larynx (congenital) Q31.8
    acquired Z90.02
  leg (acquired) (above knee) Z89.61- ☑
    below knee (acquired) Z89.51- ☑
    congenital — *see* Defect, reduction, lower limb
  lens (acquired) — *see also* Aphakia
    congenital Q12.3
    post cataract extraction Z98.4- ☑
  limb (acquired) — *see* Absence, extremity
  lip Q38.6
  liver (congenital) Q44.7
  lung (fissure) (lobe) (bilateral) (unilateral) (congenital) Q33.3
    acquired (any part) Z90.2
  menstruation — *see* Amenorrhea
  muscle (congenital) (pectoral) Q79.8
    ocular Q10.3
  neck, part Q18.8
  neutrophil — *see* Agranulocytosis
  nipple(s) (with breast(s)) (acquired) Z90.1- ☑
    congenital Q83.2
  nose (congenital) Q30.1
    acquired Z90.09
  organ
    of Corti, congenital Q16.5
    or site, congenital NEC Q89.8
      acquired NEC Z90.89
  osseous meatus (ear) Q16.4
  ovary (acquired)
    bilateral Z90.722
    congenital
      bilateral Q50.02
      unilateral Q50.01
    unilateral Z90.721
  oviduct (acquired)
    bilateral Z90.722
    congenital Q50.6
    unilateral Z90.721
  pancreas (congenital) Q45.0
    acquired Z90.410
      complete Z90.410
      partial Z90.411
      total Z90.410
  parathyroid gland (acquired) E89.2
    congenital Q89.2
  patella, congenital Q74.1
  penis (congenital) Q55.5
    acquired Z90.79
  pericardium (congenital) Q24.8
  pituitary gland (congenital) Q89.2

Absence — *continued*
  pituitary gland — *continued*
    acquired E89.3
  prostate (acquired) Z90.79
    congenital Q55.4
  pulmonary valve Q22.0
  punctum lacrimale (congenital) Q10.4
  radius, congenital — *see* Defect, reduction, upper limb, longitudinal, radius
  rectum (congenital) Q42.1
    with fistula Q42.0
    acquired Z90.49
  respiratory organ NOS Q34.9
  rib (acquired) Z90.89
    congenital Q76.6
  sacrum, congenital Q76.49
  salivary gland(s), congenital Q38.4
  scrotum, congenital Q55.29
  seminal vesicles (congenital) Q55.4
    acquired Z90.79
  septum
    atrial (congenital) Q21.1
    between aorta and pulmonary artery Q21.4
    ventricular (congenital) Q20.4
  sex chromosome
    female phenotype Q97.8
    male phenotype Q98.8
  skull bone (congenital) Q75.8
    with
      anencephaly Q00.0
      encephalocele — *see* Encephalocele
      hydrocephalus Q03.9
        with spina bifida — *see* Spina bifida, by site, with hydrocephalus
      microcephaly Q02
  spermatic cord, congenital Q55.4
  spine, congenital Q76.49
  spleen (congenital) Q89.01
    acquired Z90.81
  sternum, congenital Q76.7
  stomach (acquired) (partial) Z90.3
    congenital Q40.2
  superior vena cava, congenital Q26.8
  teeth, tooth (congenital) K00.0
    acquired (complete) K08.109
      class I K08.101
      class II K08.102
      class III K08.103
      class IV K08.104
      due to
        caries K08.139
          class I K08.131
          class II K08.132
          class III K08.133
          class IV K08.134
        periodontal disease K08.129
          class I K08.121
          class II K08.122
          class III K08.123
          class IV K08.124
        specified NEC K08.199
          class I K08.191
          class II K08.192
          class III K08.193
          class IV K08.194
        trauma K08.119
          class I K08.111
          class II K08.112
          class III K08.113
          class IV K08.114
    partial K08.409
      class I K08.401
      class II K08.402
      class III K08.403
      class IV K08.404
      due to
        caries K08.439
          class I K08.431
          class II K08.432
          class III K08.433
          class IV K08.434
        periodontal disease K08.429
          class I K08.421
          class II K08.422
          class III K08.423
          class IV K08.424
        specified NEC K08.499
          class I K08.491
          class II K08.492

Absence — *continued*
  teeth, tooth — *continued*
    acquired — *continued*
      partial — *continued*
        due to — *continued*
          specified — *continued*
            class III K08.493
            class IV K08.494
            trauma K08.419
              class I K08.411
              class II K08.412
              class III K08.413
              class IV K08.414
  tendon (congenital) Q79.8
  testis (congenital) Q55.0
    acquired Z90.79
  thumb (acquired) Z89.01- ☑
    congenital — *see* Agenesis, hand
  thymus gland Q89.2
  thyroid (gland) (acquired) E89.0
    cartilage, congenital Q31.8
    congenital E03.1
  toe(s) (acquired) Z89.42- ☑
    with foot — *see* Absence, foot and ankle
    congenital — *see* Agenesis, foot
    great Z89.41- ☑
  tongue, congenital Q38.3
  trachea (cartilage), congenital Q32.1
  transverse aortic arch, congenital Q25.49
  tricuspid valve Q22.4
  umbilical artery, congenital Q27.0
  upper arm and forearm with hand present, congenital — *see* Agenesis, arm, with hand present
  ureter (congenital) Q62.4
    acquired Z90.6
  urethra, congenital Q64.5
  uterus (acquired) Z90.710
    with cervix Z90.710
    with remaining cervical stump Z90.711
    congenital Q51.0
  uvula, congenital Q38.5
  vagina, congenital Q52.0
  vas deferens (congenital) Q55.4
    acquired Z90.79
  vein (peripheral) congenital NEC Q27.8
    cerebral Q28.3
    digestive system Q27.8
    great Q26.8
    lower limb Q27.8
    portal Q26.5
    precerebral Q28.1
    specified site NEC Q27.8
    upper limb Q27.8
  vena cava (inferior) (superior), congenital Q26.8
  ventricular septum Q20.4
  vertebra, congenital Q76.49
  vulva, congenital Q52.71
  wrist (acquired) Z89.12- ☑

Absorbent system disease I87.8

Absorption
  carbohydrate, disturbance K90.49
  chemical — *see* Table of Drugs and Chemicals
    through placenta (newborn) P04.9
      environmental substance P04.6
      nutritional substance P04.5
      obstetric anesthetic or analgesic drug P04.0
  drug NEC — *see* Table of Drugs and Chemicals
    addictive
      through placenta (newborn) — *see also* Newborn, affected by, maternal, use of P04.40
        cocaine P04.41
        hallucinogens P04.42
        specified drug NEC P04.49
    medicinal
      through placenta (newborn) P04.19
    through placenta (newborn) P04.19
      obstetric anesthetic or analgesic drug P04.0
  fat, disturbance K90.49
    pancreatic K90.3
  noxious substance — *see* Table of Drugs and Chemicals
  protein, disturbance K90.49
  starch, disturbance K90.49
  toxic substance — *see* Table of Drugs and Chemicals
  uremic — *see* Uremia

Abstinence symptoms, syndrome
  alcohol F10.239
    with delirium F10.231
  cocaine F14.23

Abstinence symptoms, syndrome — *continued*
  neonatal P96.1
  nicotine — *see* Dependence, drug, nicotine, with, withdrawal
  opioid F11.93
    with dependence F11.23
  psychoactive NEC F19.939
    with
      delirium F19.931
      dependence F19.239
        with
          delirium F19.231
          perceptual disturbance F19.232
        uncomplicated F19.230
      perceptual disturbance F19.932
    uncomplicated F19.930
  sedative F13.939
    with
      delirium F13.931
      dependence F13.239
        with
          delirium F13.231
          perceptual disturbance F13.232
        uncomplicated F13.230
      perceptual disturbance F13.932
    uncomplicated F13.930
  stimulant NEC F15.93
    with dependence F15.23

Abulia R68.89

Abulomania F60.7

Abuse
  adult — *see* Maltreatment, adult
    as reason for
      couple seeking advice (including offender) Z63.0
  alcohol (non-dependent) F10.10
    with
      anxiety disorder F10.180
      intoxication F10.129
        with delirium F10.121
        uncomplicated F10.120
      mood disorder F10.14
      other specified disorder F10.188
      psychosis F10.159
        delusions F10.150
        hallucinations F10.151
      sexual dysfunction F10.181
      sleep disorder F10.182
      unspecified disorder F10.19
      withdrawal F10.139
        with
          perceptual disturbance F10.132
        delirium F10.131
        uncomplicated F10.130
    counseling and surveillance Z71.41
    in remission (early) (sustained) F10.11
  amphetamine (or related substance) — *see also* Abuse, drug, stimulant NEC
    stimulant NEC F15.10
      with
        anxiety disorder F15.180
        intoxication F15.129
          with
            delirium F15.121
            perceptual disturbance F15.122
        withdrawal F15.13
  analgesics (non-prescribed) (over the counter) F55.8
  antacids F55.0
  antidepressants — *see* Abuse, drug, psychoactive NEC
  anxiolytic — *see* Abuse, drug, sedative
  barbiturates — *see* Abuse, drug, sedative
  caffeine — *see* Abuse, drug, stimulant NEC
  cannabis, cannabinoids — *see* Abuse, drug, cannabis
  child — *see* Maltreatment, child
  cocaine — *see* Abuse, drug, cocaine
  drug NEC (non-dependent) F19.10
    with sleep disorder F19.182
    amphetamine type — *see* Abuse, drug, stimulant NEC
    analgesics (non-prescribed) (over the counter) F55.8
    antacids F55.0
    antidepressants — *see* Abuse, drug, psychoactive NEC
    anxiolytics — *see* Abuse, drug, sedative
    barbiturates — *see* Abuse, drug, sedative
    caffeine — *see* Abuse, drug, stimulant NEC
    cannabis F12.10
      with
        anxiety disorder F12.180

Abuse — *continued*
  drug — *continued*
    cannabis — *continued*
      with — *continued*
        intoxication F12.129
          with
            delirium F12.121
            perceptual disturbance F12.122
          uncomplicated F12.120
        other specified disorder F12.188
        psychosis F12.159
          delusions F12.150
          hallucinations F12.151
        unspecified disorder F12.19
        withdrawal F12.13
      in remission (early) (sustained) F12.11
    cocaine F14.10
      with
        anxiety disorder F14.180
        intoxication F14.129
          with
            delirium F14.121
            perceptual disturbance F14.122
          uncomplicated F14.120
        mood disorder F14.14
        other specified disorder F14.188
        psychosis F14.159
          delusions F14.150
          hallucinations F14.151
        sexual dysfunction F14.181
        sleep disorder F14.182
        unspecified disorder F14.19
        withdrawal F14.13
      in remission (early) (sustained) F14.11
    counseling and surveillance Z71.51
    hallucinogen F16.10
      with
        anxiety disorder F16.180
        flashbacks F16.183
        intoxication F16.129
          with
            delirium F16.121
            perceptual disturbance F16.122
          uncomplicated F16.120
        mood disorder F16.14
        other specified disorder F16.188
        perception disorder, persisting F16.183
        psychosis F16.159
          delusions F16.150
          hallucinations F16.151
        unspecified disorder F16.19
      in remission (early) (sustained) F16.11
    hashish — *see* Abuse, drug, cannabis
    herbal or folk remedies F55.1
    hormones F55.3
    hypnotics — *see* Abuse, drug, sedative
    in remission (early) (sustained) F19.11
    inhalant F18.10
      with
        anxiety disorder F18.180
        dementia, persisting F18.17
        intoxication F18.129
          with delirium F18.121
          uncomplicated F18.120
        mood disorder F18.14
        other specified disorder F18.188
        psychosis F18.159
          delusions F18.150
          hallucinations F18.151
        unspecified disorder F18.19
      in remission (early) (sustained) F18.11
    laxatives F55.2
    LSD — *see* Abuse, drug, hallucinogen
    marihuana — *see* Abuse, drug, cannabis
    morphine type (opioids) — *see* Abuse, drug, opioid
    opioid F11.10
      with
        intoxication F11.129
          with
            delirium F11.121
            perceptual disturbance F11.122
          uncomplicated F11.120
        mood disorder F11.14
        other specified disorder F11.188
        psychosis F11.159
          delusions F11.150
          hallucinations F11.151
        sexual dysfunction F11.181
        sleep disorder F11.182

Abuse — *continued*
  drug — *continued*
    opioid — *continued*
      with — *continued*
        unspecified disorder F11.19
        withdrawal F11.13
      in remission (early) (sustained) F11.11
    PCP (phencyclidine) (or related substance) — *see* Abuse, drug, hallucinogen
    psychoactive NEC F19.10
      with
        amnestic disorder F19.16
        anxiety disorder F19.180
        dementia F19.17
        intoxication F19.129
          with
            delirium F19.121
            perceptual disturbance F19.122
          uncomplicated F19.120
        mood disorder F19.14
        other specified disorder F19.188
        psychosis F19.159
          delusions F19.150
          hallucinations F19.151
        sexual dysfunction F19.181
        sleep disorder F19.182
        unspecified disorder F19.19
        withdrawal F19.139
          with
            perceptual disturbance F19.132
          delirium F19.131
          uncomplicated F19.130
    sedative, hypnotic or anxiolytic F13.10
      with
        anxiety disorder F13.180
        intoxication F13.129
          with delirium F13.121
          uncomplicated F13.120
        mood disorder F13.14
        other specified disorder F13.188
        psychosis F13.159
          delusions F13.150
          hallucinations F13.151
        sexual dysfunction F13.181
        sleep disorder F13.182
        unspecified disorder F13.19
        withdrawal F13.139
          with
            perceptual disturbance F13.132
          delirium F13.131
          uncomplicated F13.130
      in remission (early) (sustained) F13.11
    solvent — *see* Abuse, drug, inhalant
    steroids F55.3
    stimulant NEC F15.10
      with
        anxiety disorder F15.180
        intoxication F15.129
          with
            delirium F15.121
            perceptual disturbance F15.122
          uncomplicated F15.120
        mood disorder F15.14
        other specified disorder F15.188
        psychosis F15.159
          delusions F15.150
          hallucinations F15.151
        sexual dysfunction F15.181
        sleep disorder F15.182
        unspecified disorder F15.19
        withdrawal F15.13
      in remission (early) (sustained) F15.11
    tranquilizers — *see* Abuse, drug, sedative
    vitamins F55.4
  hallucinogens — *see* Abuse, drug, hallucinogen
  hashish — *see* Abuse, drug, cannabis
  herbal or folk remedies F55.1
  hormones F55.3
  hypnotic — *see* Abuse, drug, sedative
  inhalant — *see* Abuse, drug, inhalant
  laxatives F55.2
  LSD — *see* Abuse, drug, hallucinogen
  marihuana — *see* Abuse, drug, cannabis
  morphine type (opioids) — *see* Abuse, drug, opioid
  non-psychoactive substance NEC F55.8
    antacids F55.0
    folk remedies F55.1
    herbal remedies F55.1

Abuse — *continued*
  non-psychoactive substance — *continued*
    hormones F55.3
    laxatives F55.2
    steroids F55.3
    vitamins F55.4
  opioids — *see* Abuse, drug, opioid
  PCP (phencyclidine) (or related substance) — *see* Abuse, drug, hallucinogen
  physical (adult) (child) — *see* Maltreatment
  psychoactive substance — *see* Abuse, drug, psychoactive NEC
  psychological (adult) (child) — *see* Maltreatment
  sedative — *see* Abuse, drug, sedative
  sexual — *see* Maltreatment
  solvent — *see* Abuse, drug, inhalant
  steroids F55.3
  vitamins F55.4
Acalculia R48.8
  developmental F81.2
Acanthamebiasis (with) B60.10
  conjunctiva B60.12
  keratoconjunctivitis B60.13
  meningoencephalitis B60.11
  other specified B60.19
Acanthocephaliasis B83.8
Acanthocheilonemiasis B74.4
Acanthocytosis E78.6
Acantholysis L11.9
Acanthosis (acquired) (nigricans) L83
  benign Q82.8
  congenital Q82.8
  seborrheic L82.1
    inflamed L82.0
  tongue K14.3
Acapnia E87.3
Acarbia E87.2
Acardia, acardius Q89.8
Acardiacus amorphus Q89.8
Acardiotrophia I51.4
Acariasis B88.0
  scabies B86
Acarodermatitis (urticarioides) B88.0
Acarophobia F40.218
Acatalasemia, acatalasia E80.3
Acathisia (drug induced) G25.71
Accelerated atrioventricular conduction I45.6
Accentuation of personality traits (type A) Z73.1
Accessory (congenital)
  adrenal gland Q89.1
  anus Q43.4
  appendix Q43.4
  atrioventricular conduction I45.6
  auditory ossicles Q16.3
  auricle (ear) Q17.0
  biliary duct or passage Q44.5
  bladder Q64.79
  blood vessels NEC Q27.9
    coronary Q24.5
  bone NEC Q79.8
  breast tissue, axilla Q83.1
  carpal bones Q74.0
  cecum Q43.4
  chromosome(s) NEC (nonsex) Q92.9
    with complex rearrangements NEC Q92.5
      seen only at prometaphase Q92.8
    13 — *see* Trisomy, 13
    18 — *see* Trisomy, 18
    21 — *see* Trisomy, 21
    partial Q92.9
    sex
      female phenotype Q97.8
  coronary artery Q24.5
  cusp(s), heart valve NEC Q24.8
    pulmonary Q22.3
  cystic duct Q44.5
  digit(s) Q69.9
  ear (auricle) (lobe) Q17.0
  endocrine gland NEC Q89.2
  eye muscle Q10.3
  eyelid Q10.3
  face bone(s) Q75.8
  fallopian tube (fimbria) (ostium) Q50.6
  finger(s) Q69.0
  foreskin N47.8
  frontonasal process Q75.8
  gallbladder Q44.1

Accessory — *continued*
  genital organ(s)
    female Q52.8
      external Q52.79
      internal NEC Q52.8
    male Q55.8
  genitourinary organs NEC Q89.8
    female Q52.8
    male Q55.8
  hallux Q69.2
  heart Q24.8
    valve NEC Q24.8
      pulmonary Q22.3
  hepatic ducts Q44.5
  hymen Q52.4
  intestine (large) (small) Q43.4
  kidney Q63.0
  lacrimal canal Q10.6
  leaflet, heart valve NEC Q24.8
  ligament, broad Q50.6
  liver Q44.7
    duct Q44.5
  lobule (ear) Q17.0
  lung (lobe) Q33.1
  muscle Q79.8
  navicular of carpus Q74.0
  nervous system, part NEC Q07.8
  nipple Q83.3
  nose Q30.8
  organ or site not listed — *see* Anomaly, by site
  ovary Q50.31
  oviduct Q50.6
  pancreas Q45.3
  parathyroid gland Q89.2
  parotid gland (and duct) Q38.4
  pituitary gland Q89.2
  preauricular appendage Q17.0
  prepuce N47.8
  renal arteries (multiple) Q27.2
  rib Q76.6
    cervical Q76.5
  roots (teeth) K00.2
  salivary gland Q38.4
  sesamoid bones Q74.8
    foot Q74.2
    hand Q74.0
  skin tags Q82.8
  spleen Q89.09
  sternum Q76.7
  submaxillary gland Q38.4
  tarsal bones Q74.2
  teeth, tooth K00.1
  tendon Q79.8
  thumb Q69.1
  thymus gland Q89.2
  thyroid gland Q89.2
  toes Q69.2
  tongue Q38.3
  tooth, teeth K00.1
  tragus Q17.0
  ureter Q62.5
  urethra Q64.79
  urinary organ or tract NEC Q64.8
  uterus Q51.28
  vagina Q52.10
  valve, heart NEC Q24.8
    pulmonary Q22.3
  vertebra Q76.49
  vocal cords Q31.8
  vulva Q52.79
Accident
  birth — *see* Birth, injury
  cardiac — *see* Infarct, myocardium
  cerebral I63.9
  cerebrovascular (embolic) (ischemic) (thrombotic) I63.9
    aborted I63.9
    hemorrhagic — *see* Hemorrhage, intracranial, intracerebral
    old (without sequelae) Z86.73
      with sequelae (of) — *see* Sequelae, infarction, cerebral
  coronary — *see* Infarct, myocardium
  craniovascular I63.9
  vascular, brain I63.9
Accidental — *see* condition
Accommodation (disorder) — *see also* condition
  hysterical paralysis of F44.89
  insufficiency of H52.4

Accommodation — *continued*
  paresis — *see* Paresis, of accommodation
  spasm — *see* Spasm, of accommodation
Accouchement — *see* Delivery
Accreta placenta O43.21- ☑
Accretio cordis (nonrheumatic) I31.0
Accretions, tooth, teeth K03.6
Acculturation difficulty Z60.3
Accumulation secretion, prostate N42.89
Acephalia, acephalism, acephalus, acephaly Q00.0
Acephalobrachia monster Q89.8
Acephalochirus monster Q89.8
Acephalogaster Q89.8
Acephalostomus monster Q89.8
Acephalothorax Q89.8
Acerophobia F40.298
Acetonemia R79.89
  in Type 1 diabetes E10.10
    with coma E10.11
Acetonuria R82.4
Achalasia (cardia) (esophagus) K22.0
  congenital Q39.5
  pylorus Q40.0
  sphincteral NEC K59.89
Ache(s) — *see* Pain
Acheilia Q38.6
Achillobursitis — *see* Tendinitis, Achilles
Achillodynia — *see* Tendinitis, Achilles
Achlorhydria, achlorhydric (neurogenic) K31.83
  anemia D50.8
  diarrhea K31.83
  psychogenic F45.8
  secondary to vagotomy K91.1
Achluophobia F40.228
Acholia K82.8
Acholuric jaundice (familial) (splenomegalic) — *see also* Spherocytosis
  acquired D59.8
Achondrogenesis Q77.0
Achondroplasia (osteosclerosis congenita) Q77.4
Achroma, cutis L80
Achromat (ism), achromatopsia (acquired) (congenital) H53.51
Achromia, congenital — *see* Albinism
Achromia parasitica B36.0
Achylia gastrica K31.89
  psychogenic F45.8
Acid
  burn — *see* Corrosion
  deficiency
    amide nicotinic E52
    ascorbic E54
    folic E53.8
    nicotinic E52
    pantothenic E53.8
  intoxication E87.2
  peptic disease K30
  phosphatase deficiency E83.39
  stomach K30
    psychogenic F45.8
Acidemia E87.2
  argininosuccinic E72.22
  isovaleric E71.110
  metabolic (newborn) P19.9
    first noted before onset of labor P19.0
    first noted during labor P19.1
    noted at birth P19.2
  methylmalonic E71.120
  pipecolic E72.3
  propionic E71.121
Acidity, gastric (high) K30
  psychogenic F45.8
Acidocytopenia — *see* Agranulocytosis
Acidocytosis D72.10
Acidopenia — *see* Agranulocytosis
Acidosis (lactic) (respiratory) E87.2
  in Type 1 diabetes E10.10
    with coma E10.11
  kidney, tubular N25.89
  lactic E87.2
  metabolic NEC E87.2
    with respiratory acidosis E87.4
    hyperchloremic, of newborn P74.421
    late, of newborn P74.0
  mixed metabolic and respiratory, newborn P84
  newborn P84
  renal (hyperchloremic) (tubular) N25.89

Acidosis — *continued*
  respiratory E87.2
    complicated by
      metabolic
        acidosis E87.4
        alkalosis E87.4
Aciduria
  4-hydroxybutyric E72.81
  argininosuccinic E72.22
  gamma-hydroxybutyric E72.81
  glutaric (type I) E72.3
    type II E71.313
    type III E71.5- ☑
  orotic (congenital) (hereditary) (pyrimidine deficiency) E79.8
    anemia D53.0
Acladiosis (skin) B36.0
Aclasis, diaphyseal Q78.6
Acleistocardia Q21.1
Aclusion — *see* Anomaly, dentofacial, malocclusion
Acne L70.9
  artificialis L70.8
  atrophica L70.2
  cachecticorum (Hebra) L70.8
  conglobata L70.1
  cystic L70.0
  decalvans L66.2
  excoriée (des jeunes filles) L70.5
  frontalis L70.2
  indurata L70.0
  infantile L70.4
  keloid L73.0
  lupoid L70.2
  necrotic, necrotica (miliaris) L70.2
  neonatal L70.4
  nodular L70.0
  occupational L70.8
  picker's L70.5
  pustular L70.0
  rodens L70.2
  rosacea L71.9
  specified NEC L70.8
  tropica L70.3
  varioliformis L70.2
  vulgaris L70.0
Acnitis (primary) A18.4
Acosta's disease T70.29 ☑
Acoustic — *see* condition
Acousticophobia F40.298
ACPO (acute colonic pseudo-obstruction) K59.81
Acquired — *see also* condition
  immunodeficiency syndrome (AIDS) B20
Acrania Q00.0
Acroangiodermatitis I78.9
Acroasphyxia, chronic I73.89
Acrobystitis N47.7
Acrocephalopolysyndactyly Q87.0
Acrocephalosyndactyly Q87.0
Acrocephaly Q75.0
Acrochondrohyperplasia — *see* Syndrome, Marfan's
Acrocyanosis I73.89
  newborn P28.2
    meaning transient blue hands and feet — *omit code*
Acrodermatitis L30.8
  atrophicans (chronica) L90.4
  continua (Hallopeau) L40.2
  enteropathica (hereditary) E83.2
  Hallopeau's L40.2
  infantile papular L44.4
  perstans L40.2
  pustulosa continua L40.2
  recalcitrant pustular L40.2
Acrodynia — *see* Poisoning, mercury
Acromegaly, acromegalia E22.0
Acromelalgia I73.81
Acromicria, acromikria Q79.8
Acronyx L60.0
Acropachy, thyroid — *see* Thyrotoxicosis
Acroparesthesia (simple) (vasomotor) I73.89
Acropathy, thyroid — *see* Thyrotoxicosis
Acrophobia F40.241
Acroposthitis N47.7
Acroscleriasis, acroscleroderma, acrosclerosis — *see* Sclerosis, systemic
Acrosphacelus I96
Acrospiroma, eccrine — *see* Neoplasm, skin, benign
Acrostealgia — *see* Osteochondropathy

Acrotrophodynia — *see* Immersion
ACTH ectopic syndrome E24.3
Actinic — *see* condition
Actinobacillosis, actinobacillus A28.8
  mallei A24.0
  muris A25.1
Actinomyces israelii (infection) — *see* Actinomycosis
Actinomycetoma (foot) B47.1
Actinomycosis, actinomycotic A42.9
  with pneumonia A42.0
  abdominal A42.1
  cervicofacial A42.2
  cutaneous A42.89
  gastrointestinal A42.1
  pulmonary A42.0
  sepsis A42.7
  specified site NEC A42.89
Actinoneuritis G62.82
Action, heart
  disorder I49.9
  irregular I49.9
    psychogenic F45.8
Activated protein C resistance D68.51
Activation
  mast cell (disorder) (syndrome) D89.40
    idiopathic D89.42
    monoclonal D89.41
    secondary D89.43
    specified type NEC D89.49
Active — *see* condition
Acute — *see also* condition
  abdomen R10.0
  gallbladder — *see* Cholecystitis, acute
Acyanotic heart disease (congenital) Q24.9
Acystia Q64.5
Adair-Dighton syndrome (brittle bones and blue sclera, deafness) Q78.0
Adamantinoblastoma — *see* Ameloblastoma
Adamantinoma — *see also* Cyst, calcifying odontogenic
  long bones C40.90
    lower limb C40.2- ☑
    upper limb C40.0- ☑
  malignant C41.1
    jaw (bone) (lower) C41.1
      upper C41.0
  tibial C40.2- ☑
Adamantoblastoma — *see* Ameloblastoma
Adams-Stokes (-Morgagni) disease or syndrome I45.9
Adaption reaction — *see* Disorder, adjustment
Addiction — *see also* Dependence F19.20
  alcohol, alcoholic (ethyl) (methyl) (wood) (without remission) F10.20
    with remission F10.21
  drug — *see* Dependence, drug
  ethyl alcohol (without remission) F10.20
    with remission F10.21
  heroin — *see* Dependence, drug, opioid
  methyl alcohol (without remission) F10.20
    with remission F10.21
  methylated spirit (without remission) F10.20
    with remission F10.21
  morphine (-like substances) — *see* Dependence, drug, opioid
  nicotine — *see* Dependence, drug, nicotine
  opium and opioids — *see* Dependence, drug, opioid
  tobacco — *see* Dependence, drug, nicotine
Addison-Biermer anemia (pernicious) D51.0
Addisonian crisis E27.2
Addison's
  anemia (pernicious) D51.0
  disease (bronze) or syndrome E27.1
    tuberculous A18.7
  keloid L94.0
Addison-Schilder complex E71.528
Additional — *see also* Accessory
  chromosome(s) Q99.8
    21 — *see* Trisomy, 21
    sex — *see* Abnormal, chromosome, sex
Adduction contracture, hip or other joint — *see* Contraction, joint
Adenitis — *see also* Lymphadenitis
  acute, unspecified site L04.9
  axillary I88.9
    acute L04.2
    chronic or subacute I88.1
  Bartholin's gland N75.8
  bulbourethral gland — *see* Urethritis

Accommodation — Adenitis

10

☑ **Additional Character Required** — Refer to the Tabular List for Character Selection   ▽ **Subterms under main terms may continue to next column or page**

Adenitis — *continued*
  cervical I88.9
    acute L04.0
    chronic or subacute I88.1
  chancroid (Hemophilus ducreyi) A57
  chronic, unspecified site I88.1
  Cowper's gland — *see* Urethritis
  due to Pasteurella multocida (P. septica) A28.0
  epidemic, acute B27.09
  gangrenous L04.9
  gonorrheal NEC A54.89
  groin I88.9
    acute L04.1
    chronic or subacute I88.1
  infectious (acute) (epidemic) B27.09
  inguinal I88.9
    acute L04.1
    chronic or subacute I88.1
  lymph gland or node, except mesenteric I88.9
    acute — *see* Lymphadenitis, acute
    chronic or subacute I88.1
  mesenteric (acute) (chronic) (nonspecific) (subacute)
      I88.0
  parotid gland (suppurative) — *see* Sialoadenitis
  salivary gland (any) (suppurative) — *see* Sialoadenitis
  scrofulous (tuberculous) A18.2
  Skene's duct or gland — *see* Urethritis
  strumous, tuberculous A18.2
  subacute, unspecified site I88.1
  sublingual gland (suppurative) — *see* Sialoadenitis
  submandibular gland (suppurative) — *see* Sialoadenitis
  submaxillary gland (suppurative) — *see* Sialoadenitis
  tuberculous — *see* Tuberculosis, lymph gland
  urethral gland — *see* Urethritis
  Wharton's duct (suppurative) — *see* Sialoadenitis
Adenoacanthoma — *see* Neoplasm, malignant, by site
Adenoameloblastoma — *see* Cyst, calcifying odonto-
    genic
Adenocarcinoid (tumor) — *see* Neoplasm, malignant,
    by site
Adenocarcinoma — *see also* Neoplasm, malignant, by
    site
  acidophil
    specified site — *see* Neoplasm, malignant, by site
    unspecified site C75.1
  adrenal cortical C74.0- ☑
  alveolar — *see* Neoplasm, lung, malignant
  apocrine
    breast — *see* Neoplasm, breast, malignant
    in situ
      breast D05.8- ☑
      specified site NEC — *see* Neoplasm, skin, in situ
      unspecified site D04.9
    specified site NEC — *see* Neoplasm, skin, malignant
    unspecified site C44.99
  basal cell
    specified site — *see* Neoplasm, skin, malignant
    unspecified site C08.9
  basophil
    specified site — *see* Neoplasm, malignant, by site
    unspecified site C75.1
  bile duct type C22.1
    liver C22.1
    specified site NEC — *see* Neoplasm, malignant, by
      site
    unspecified site C22.1
  bronchiolar — *see* Neoplasm, lung, malignant
  bronchioloalveolar — *see* Neoplasm, lung, malignant
  ceruminous C44.29- ☑
  cervix, in situ — *see also* Carcinoma, cervix uteri, in situ
      D06.9
  chromophobe
    specified site — *see* Neoplasm, malignant, by site
    unspecified site C75.1
  diffuse type
    specified site — *see* Neoplasm, malignant, by site
    unspecified site C16.9
  duct
    infiltrating
      with Paget's disease — *see* Neoplasm, breast,
        malignant
      specified site — *see* Neoplasm, malignant, by
        site
      unspecified site (female) C50.91- ☑
        male C50.92- ☑
    specified site — *see* Neoplasm, malignant, by site
    unspecified site
      female C56.9

Adenocarcinoma — *continued*
  duct — *continued*
    unspecified site — *continued*
      male C61
  eosinophil
    specified site — *see* Neoplasm, malignant, by site
    unspecified site C75.1
  follicular
    with papillary C73
    moderately differentiated C73
    specified site — *see* Neoplasm, malignant, by site
    trabecular C73
    unspecified site C73
    well differentiated C73
  Hurthle cell C73
  in
    adenomatous
      polyposis coli C18.9
  infiltrating duct
    with Paget's disease — *see* Neoplasm, breast, ma-
        lignant
    specified site — *see* Neoplasm, by site, malignant
    unspecified site (female) C50.91- ☑
      male C50.92- ☑
  inflammatory
    specified site — *see* Neoplasm, by site, malignant
    unspecified site (female) C50.91- ☑
      male C50.92- ☑
  intestinal type
    specified site — *see* Neoplasm, by site, malignant
    unspecified site C16.9
  intracystic papillary
  intraductal
    breast D05.1- ☑
    noninfiltrating
      breast D05.1- ☑
      papillary
        with invasion
          specified site — *see* Neoplasm, by site,
            malignant
          unspecified site (female) C50.91- ☑
            male C50.92- ☑
        breast D05.1- ☑
        specified site NEC — *see* Neoplasm, in situ,
          by site
        unspecified site D05.1- ☑
      specified site NEC — *see* Neoplasm, in situ, by
        site
      unspecified site D05.1- ☑
    papillary
      with invasion
        specified site — *see* Neoplasm, malignant, by
          site
        unspecified site (female) C50.91- ☑
          male C50.92- ☑
      breast D05.1- ☑
      specified site — *see* Neoplasm, in situ, by site
      unspecified site D05.1- ☑
    specified site NEC — *see* Neoplasm, in situ, by site
    unspecified site D05.1- ☑
  islet cell
    with exocrine, mixed
      specified site — *see* Neoplasm, malignant, by
        site
      unspecified site C25.9
    pancreas C25.4
    specified site NEC — *see* Neoplasm, malignant, by
      site
    unspecified site C25.4
  lobular
    in situ
      breast D05.0- ☑
      specified site NEC — *see* Neoplasm, in situ, by
        site
      unspecified site D05.0- ☑
    specified site — *see* Neoplasm, malignant, by site
    unspecified site (female) C50.91- ☑
      male C50.92- ☑
  mucoid — *see also* Neoplasm, malignant, by site
    cell
      specified site — *see* Neoplasm, malignant, by
        site
      unspecified site C75.1
  nonencapsulated sclerosing C73
  papillary
    with follicular C73
    follicular variant C73

Adenocarcinoma — *continued*
  papillary — *continued*
    intraductal (noninfiltrating)
      with invasion
        specified site — *see* Neoplasm, malignant, by
          site
        unspecified site (female) C50.91- ☑
          male C50.92- ☑
      breast D05.1- ☑
      specified site NEC — *see* Neoplasm, in situ, by
        site
      unspecified site D05.1- ☑
    serous
      specified site — *see* Neoplasm, malignant, by
        site
      unspecified site C56.9
  papillocystic
    specified site — *see* Neoplasm, malignant, by site
    unspecified site C56.9
  pseudomucinous
    specified site — *see* Neoplasm, malignant, by site
    unspecified site C56.9
  renal cell C64- ☑
  sebaceous — *see* Neoplasm, skin, malignant
  serous — *see also* Neoplasm, malignant, by site
    papillary
      specified site — *see* Neoplasm, malignant, by
        site
      unspecified site C56.9
  sweat gland — *see* Neoplasm, skin, malignant
  water-clear cell C75.0
Adenocarcinoma-in-situ — *see also* Neoplasm, in situ,
    by site
  breast D05.9- ☑
Adenofibroma
  clear cell — *see* Neoplasm, benign, by site
  endometrioid D27.9
    borderline malignancy D39.10
    malignant C56- ☑
  mucinous
    specified site — *see* Neoplasm, benign, by site
    unspecified site D27.9
  papillary
    specified site — *see* Neoplasm, benign, by site
    unspecified site D27.9
  prostate — *see* Enlargement, enlarged, prostate
  serous
    specified site — *see* Neoplasm, benign, by site
    unspecified site D27.9
  specified site — *see* Neoplasm, benign, by site
  unspecified site D27.9
Adenofibrosis
  breast — *see* Fibroadenosis, breast
  endometrioid N80.0
Adenoiditis (chronic) J35.02
  with tonsillitis J35.03
  acute J03.90
    recurrent J03.91
    specified organism NEC J03.80
      recurrent J03.81
    staphylococcal J03.80
      recurrent J03.81
    streptococcal J03.00
      recurrent J03.01
Adenoids — *see* condition
Adenolipoma — *see* Neoplasm, benign, by site
Adenolipomatosis, Launois-Bensaude E88.89
Adenolymphoma
  specified site — *see* Neoplasm, benign, by site
  unspecified site D11.9
Adenoma — *see also* Neoplasm, benign, by site
  acidophil
    specified site — *see* Neoplasm, benign, by site
    unspecified site D35.2
  acidophil-basophil, mixed
    specified site — *see* Neoplasm, benign, by site
    unspecified site D35.2
  adrenal (cortical) D35.00
    clear cell D35.00
    compact cell D35.00
    glomerulosa cell D35.00
    heavily pigmented variant D35.00
    mixed cell D35.00
  alpha-cell
    pancreas D13.7
    specified site NEC — *see* Neoplasm, benign, by site
    unspecified site D13.7
  alveolar D14.30

Adenoma — Adhesions, adhesive

Adenoma — *continued*
apocrine
breast D24- ☑
specified site NEC — *see* Neoplasm, skin, benign, by site
unspecified site D23.9
basal cell D11.9
basophil
specified site — *see* Neoplasm, benign, by site
unspecified site D35.2
basophil-acidophil, mixed
specified site — *see* Neoplasm, benign, by site
unspecified site D35.2
beta-cell
pancreas D13.7
specified site NEC — *see* Neoplasm, benign, by site
unspecified site D13.7
bile duct D13.4
common D13.5
extrahepatic D13.5
intrahepatic D13.4
specified site NEC — *see* Neoplasm, benign, by site
unspecified site D13.4
black D35.00
bronchial D38.1
cylindroid type — *see* Neoplasm, lung, malignant
ceruminous D23.2- ☑
chief cell D35.1
chromophobe
specified site — *see* Neoplasm, benign, by site
unspecified site D35.2
colloid
specified site — *see* Neoplasm, benign, by site
unspecified site D34
duct
eccrine, papillary — *see* Neoplasm, skin, benign
endocrine, multiple
single specified site — *see* Neoplasm, uncertain behavior, by site
two or more specified sites D44- ☑
unspecified site D44.9
endometrioid — *see also* Neoplasm, benign
borderline malignancy — *see* Neoplasm, uncertain behavior, by site
eosinophil
specified site — *see* Neoplasm, benign, by site
unspecified site D35.2
fetal
specified site — *see* Neoplasm, benign, by site
unspecified site D34
follicular
specified site — *see* Neoplasm, benign, by site
unspecified site D34
hepatocellular D13.4
Hurthle cell D34
islet cell
pancreas D13.7
specified site NEC — *see* Neoplasm, benign, by site
unspecified site D13.7
liver cell D13.4
macrofollicular
specified site — *see* Neoplasm, benign, by site
unspecified site D34
malignant, malignum — *see* Neoplasm, malignant, by site
microcystic
pancreas D13.6
specified site NEC — *see* Neoplasm, benign, by site
unspecified site D13.6
microfollicular
specified site — *see* Neoplasm, benign, by site
unspecified site D34
mucoid cell
specified site — *see* Neoplasm, benign, by site
unspecified site D35.2
multiple endocrine
single specified site — *see* Neoplasm, uncertain behavior, by site
two or more specified sites D44- ☑
unspecified site D44.9
nipple D24- ☑
papillary — *see also* Neoplasm, benign, by site
eccrine — *see* Neoplasm, skin, benign, by site
Pick's tubular
specified site — *see* Neoplasm, benign, by site
unspecified site
female D27.9
male D29.20

Adenoma — *continued*
pleomorphic
carcinoma in — *see* Neoplasm, salivary gland, malignant
specified site — *see* Neoplasm, malignant, by site
unspecified site C08.9
polypoid — *see also* Neoplasm, benign
adenocarcinoma in — *see* Neoplasm, malignant, by site
adenocarcinoma in situ — *see* Neoplasm, in situ, by site
prostate — *see* Neoplasm, benign, prostate
rete cell D29.20
sebaceous — *see* Neoplasm, skin, benign
Sertoli cell
specified site — *see* Neoplasm, benign, by site
unspecified site
female D27.9
male D29.20
skin appendage — *see* Neoplasm, skin, benign
sudoriferous gland — *see* Neoplasm, skin, benign
sweat gland — *see* Neoplasm, skin, benign
testicular
specified site — *see* Neoplasm, benign, by site
unspecified site
female D27.9
male D29.20
tubular — *see also* Neoplasm, benign, by site
adenocarcinoma in — *see* Neoplasm, malignant, by site
adenocarcinoma in situ — *see* Neoplasm, in situ, by site
Pick's
specified site — *see* Neoplasm, benign, by site
unspecified site
female D27.9
male D29.20
tubulovillous — *see also* Neoplasm, benign, by site
adenocarcinoma in — *see* Neoplasm, malignant, by site
adenocarcinoma in situ — *see* Neoplasm, in situ, by site
villous — *see* Neoplasm, uncertain behavior, by site
adenocarcinoma in — *see* Neoplasm, malignant, by site
adenocarcinoma in situ — *see* Neoplasm, in situ, by site
water-clear cell D35.1
Adenomatosis
endocrine (multiple) E31.20
single specified site — *see* Neoplasm, uncertain behavior, by site
erosive of nipple D24- ☑
pluriendocrine — *see* Adenomatosis, endocrine
pulmonary D38.1
malignant — *see* Neoplasm, lung, malignant
specified site — *see* Neoplasm, benign, by site
unspecified site D12.6
Adenomatous
goiter (nontoxic) E04.9
with hyperthyroidism — *see* Hyperthyroidism, with, goiter, nodular
toxic — *see* Hyperthyroidism, with, goiter, nodular
Adenomyoma — *see also* Neoplasm, benign, by site
prostate — *see* Enlarged, prostate
Adenomyometritis N80.0
Adenomyosis N80.0
Adenopathy (lymph gland) R59.9
generalized R59.1
inguinal R59.0
localized R59.0
mediastinal R59.0
mesentery R59.0
syphilitic (secondary) A51.49
tracheobronchial R59.0
tuberculous A15.4
primary (progressive) A15.7
tuberculous — *see also* Tuberculosis, lymph gland
tracheobronchial A15.4
primary (progressive) A15.7
Adenosalpingitis — *see* Salpingitis
Adenosarcoma — *see* Neoplasm, malignant, by site
Adenosclerosis I88.8
Adenosis (sclerosing) breast — *see* Fibroadenosis, breast
Adenovirus, as cause of disease classified elsewhere B97.0

Adentia (complete) (partial) — *see* Absence, teeth
Adherent — *see also* Adhesions
labia (minora) N90.89
pericardium (nonrheumatic) I31.0
rheumatic I09.2
placenta (with hemorrhage) O72.0
without hemorrhage O73.0
prepuce, newborn N47.0
scar (skin) L90.5
tendon in scar L90.5
Adhesions, adhesive (postinfective) K66.0
with intestinal obstruction K56.50
complete K56.52
incomplete K56.51
partial K56.51
abdominal (wall) — *see* Adhesions, peritoneum
appendix K38.8
bile duct (common) (hepatic) K83.8
bladder (sphincter) N32.89
bowel — *see* Adhesions, peritoneum
cardiac I31.0
rheumatic I09.2
cecum — *see* Adhesions, peritoneum
cervicovaginal N88.1
congenital Q52.8
postpartal O90.89
old N88.1
cervix N88.1
ciliary body NEC — *see* Adhesions, iris
clitoris N90.89
colon — *see* Adhesions, peritoneum
common duct K83.8
congenital — *see also* Anomaly, by site
fingers — *see* Syndactylism, complex, fingers
omental, anomalous Q43.3
peritoneal Q43.3
tongue (to gum or roof of mouth) Q38.3
conjunctiva (acquired) H11.21- ☑
congenital Q15.8
cystic duct K82.8
diaphragm — *see* Adhesions, peritoneum
due to foreign body — *see* Foreign body
duodenum — *see* Adhesions, peritoneum
ear
middle H74.1- ☑
epididymis N50.89
epidural — *see* Adhesions, meninges
epiglottis J38.7
eyelid H02.59
female pelvis N73.6
gallbladder K82.8
globe H44.89
heart I31.0
rheumatic I09.2
ileocecal (coil) — *see* Adhesions, peritoneum
ileum — *see* Adhesions, peritoneum
intestine — *see also* Adhesions, peritoneum
with obstruction K56.50
complete K56.52
incomplete K56.51
partial K56.51
intra-abdominal — *see* Adhesions, peritoneum
iris H21.50- ☑
anterior H21.51- ☑
goniosynechiae H21.52- ☑
posterior H21.54- ☑
to corneal graft T85.898 ☑
joint — *see* Ankylosis
knee M23.8X ☑
temporomandibular M26.61- ☑
labium (majus) (minus), congenital Q52.5
liver — *see* Adhesions, peritoneum
lung J98.4
mediastinum J98.59
meninges (cerebral) (spinal) G96.12
congenital Q07.8
tuberculous (cerebral) (spinal) A17.0
mesenteric — *see* Adhesions, peritoneum
nasal (septum) (to turbinates) J34.89
ocular muscle — *see* Strabismus, mechanical
omentum — *see* Adhesions, peritoneum
ovary N73.6
congenital (to cecum, kidney or omentum) Q50.39
paraovarian N73.6
pelvic (peritoneal)
female N73.6
postprocedural N99.4
male — *see* Adhesions, peritoneum

☑ **Additional Character Required — Refer to the Tabular List for Character Selection**   ▽ **Subterms under main terms may continue to next column or page**

Adhesions, adhesive — *continued*
  pelvic — *continued*
   postpartal (old) N73.6
   tuberculous A18.17
  penis to scrotum (congenital) Q55.8
  periappendiceal — *see also* Adhesions, peritoneum
  pericardium (nonrheumatic) I31.0
   focal I31.8
   rheumatic I09.2
   tuberculous A18.84
  pericholecystic K82.8
  perigastric — *see* Adhesions, peritoneum
  periovarian N73.6
  periprostatic N42.89
  perirectal — *see* Adhesions, peritoneum
  perirenal N28.89
  peritoneum, peritoneal (postinfective) K66.0
   with obstruction (intestinal) K56.50
    complete K56.52
    incomplete K56.51
    partial K56.51
   congenital Q43.3
   pelvic, female N73.6
    postprocedural N99.4
   postpartal, pelvic N73.6
   postprocedural K66.0
   to uterus N73.6
  peritubal N73.6
  periureteral N28.89
  periuterine N73.6
  perivesical N32.89
  perivesicular (seminal vesicle) N50.89
  pleura, pleuritic J94.8
   tuberculous NEC A15.6
  pleuropericardial J94.8
  postoperative (gastrointestinal tract) K66.0
   with obstruction — *see also* Obstruction, intestine, postoperative K91.30
   due to foreign body accidentally left in wound — *see* Foreign body, accidentally left during a procedure
   pelvic peritoneal N99.4
   urethra — *see* Stricture, urethra, postprocedural
   vagina N99.2
  postpartal, old (vulva or perineum) N90.89
  preputial, prepuce N47.5
  pulmonary J98.4
  pylorus — *see* Adhesions, peritoneum
  sciatic nerve — *see* Lesion, nerve, sciatic
  seminal vesicle N50.89
  shoulder (joint) — *see* Capsulitis, adhesive
  sigmoid flexure — *see* Adhesions, peritoneum
  spermatic cord (acquired) N50.89
   congenital Q55.4
  spinal canal G96.12
  stomach — *see* Adhesions, peritoneum
  subscapular — *see* Capsulitis, adhesive
  temporomandibular M26.61- ☑
  tendinitis (*see also* Tenosynovitis, specified type NEC)
   shoulder — *see* Capsulitis, adhesive
  testis N44.8
  tongue, congenital (to gum or roof of mouth) Q38.3
   acquired K14.8
  trachea J39.8
  tubo-ovarian N73.6
  tunica vaginalis N44.8
  uterus N73.6
   internal N85.6
   to abdominal wall N73.6
  vagina (chronic) N89.5
   postoperative N99.2
  vitreomacular H43.82- ☑
  vitreous H43.89
  vulva N90.89
Adiaspiromycosis B48.8
Adie (-Holmes) **pupil or syndrome** — *see* Anomaly, pupil, function, tonic pupil
Adiponecrosis neonatorum P83.88
Adiposis — *see also* Obesity
  cerebralis E23.6
  dolorosa E88.2
Adiposity — *see also* Obesity
  heart — *see* Degeneration, myocardial
  localized E65
Adiposogenital dystrophy E23.6
Adjustment
  disorder — *see* Disorder, adjustment

Adjustment — *continued*
  implanted device — *see* Encounter (for), adjustment (of)
  prosthesis, external — *see* Fitting
  reaction — *see* Disorder, adjustment
Administration of tPA (rtPA) in a different facility within the last 24 hours prior to admission to current facility Z92.82
Admission (for) — *see also* Encounter (for)
  adjustment (of)
   artificial
    arm Z44.00- ☑
     complete Z44.01- ☑
     partial Z44.02- ☑
    eye Z44.2 ☑
    leg Z44.10- ☑
     complete Z44.11- ☑
     partial Z44.12- ☑
   brain neuropacemaker Z46.2
    implanted Z45.42
   breast
    implant Z45.81 ☑
    prosthesis (external) Z44.3 ☑
   colostomy belt Z46.89
   contact lenses Z46.0
   cystostomy device Z46.6
   dental prosthesis Z46.3
   device NEC
    abdominal Z46.89
    implanted Z45.89
     cardiac Z45.09
      defibrillator (with synchronous cardiac pacemaker) Z45.02
      pacemaker (cardiac resynchronization therapy (CRT-P)) Z45.018
       pulse generator Z45.010
      resynchronization therapy defibrillator (CRT-D) Z45.02
     hearing device Z45.328
      bone conduction Z45.320
      cochlear Z45.321
     infusion pump Z45.1
     nervous system Z45.49
      CSF drainage Z45.41
      hearing device — *see* Admission, adjustment, device, implanted, hearing device
      neuropacemaker Z45.42
      visual substitution Z45.31
     specified NEC Z45.89
     vascular access Z45.2
     visual substitution Z45.31
   nervous system Z46.2
    implanted — *see* Admission, adjustment, device, implanted, nervous system
   orthodontic Z46.4
   prosthetic Z44.9
    arm — *see* Admission, adjustment, artificial, arm
    breast Z44.3 ☑
    dental Z46.3
    eye Z44.2 ☑
    leg — *see* Admission, adjustment, artificial, leg
    specified type NEC Z44.8
   substitution
    auditory Z46.2
     implanted — *see* Admission, adjustment, device, implanted, hearing device
    nervous system Z46.2
     implanted — *see* Admission, adjustment, device, implanted, nervous system
    visual Z46.2
     implanted Z45.31
   urinary Z46.6
  hearing aid Z46.1
   implanted — *see* Admission, adjustment, device, implanted, hearing device
  ileostomy device Z46.89
  intestinal appliance or device NEC Z46.89
  neuropacemaker (brain) (peripheral nerve) (spinal cord) Z46.2
   implanted Z45.42
  orthodontic device Z46.4
  orthopedic (brace) (cast) (device) (shoes) Z46.89
  pacemaker (cardiac resynchronization therapy (CRT-P))
   cardiac Z45.018

Admission — *continued*
  adjustment — *continued*
   pacemaker — *continued*
    cardiac — *continued*
     pulse generator Z45.010
    nervous system Z46.2
     implanted Z45.42
   portacath (port-a-cath) Z45.2
   prosthesis Z44.9
    arm — *see* Admission, adjustment, artificial, arm
    breast Z44.3 ☑
    dental Z46.3
    eye Z44.2 ☑
    leg — *see* Admission, adjustment, artificial, leg
    specified NEC Z44.8
   spectacles Z46.0
  aftercare — *see also* Aftercare Z51.89
   postpartum
    immediately after delivery Z39.0
    routine follow-up Z39.2
   radiation therapy (antineoplastic) Z51.0
  attention to artificial opening (of) Z43.9
   artificial vagina Z43.7
   colostomy Z43.3
   cystostomy Z43.5
   enterostomy Z43.4
   gastrostomy Z43.1
   ileostomy Z43.2
   jejunostomy Z43.4
   nephrostomy Z43.6
   specified site NEC Z43.8
    intestinal tract Z43.4
    urinary tract Z43.6
   tracheostomy Z43.0
   ureterostomy Z43.6
   urethrostomy Z43.6
  breast augmentation or reduction Z41.1
  breast reconstruction following mastectomy Z42.1
  change of
   dressing (nonsurgical) Z48.00
   neuropacemaker device (brain) (peripheral nerve) (spinal cord) Z46.2
    implanted Z45.42
   surgical dressing Z48.01
  circumcision, ritual or routine (in absence of diagnosis) Z41.2
  clinical research investigation (control) (normal comparison) (participant) Z00.6
  contraceptive management Z30.9
  cosmetic surgery NEC Z41.1
  counseling — *see also* Counseling
   dietary Z71.3
   gestational carrier Z31.7
   HIV Z71.7
   human immunodeficiency virus Z71.7
   nonattending third party Z71.0
   procreative management NEC Z31.69
  delivery, full-term, uncomplicated O80
   cesarean, without indication O82
  desensitization to allergens Z51.6
  dietary surveillance and counseling Z71.3
  ear piercing Z41.3
  examination at health care facility (adult) — *see also* Examination Z00.00
   with abnormal findings Z00.01
   clinical research investigation (control) (normal comparison) (participant) Z00.6
   dental Z01.20
    with abnormal findings Z01.21
   donor (potential) Z00.5
   ear Z01.10
    with abnormal findings NEC Z01.118
   eye Z01.00
    with abnormal findings Z01.01
    following failed vision screening Z01.020
     with abnormal findings Z01.021
   general, specified reason NEC Z00.8
   hearing Z01.10
    with abnormal findings NEC Z01.118
    infant or child (over 28 days old) Z00.129
     with abnormal findings Z00.121
   postpartum checkup Z39.2
   psychiatric (general) Z00.8
    requested by authority Z04.6
   vision Z01.00
    with abnormal findings Z01.01
    following failed vision screening Z01.020
     with abnormal findings Z01.021

Admission — *continued*
  examination at health care facility — *see also* Examination — *continued*
    vision — *continued*
      infant or child (over 28 days old) Z00.129
        with abnormal findings Z00.121
  fitting (of)
    artificial
      arm — *see* Admission, adjustment, artificial, arm
      eye Z44.2 ☑
      leg — *see* Admission, adjustment, artificial, leg
    brain neuropacemaker Z46.2
      implanted Z45.42
    breast prosthesis (external) Z44.3 ☑
    colostomy belt Z46.89
    contact lenses Z46.0
    cystostomy device Z46.6
    dental prosthesis Z46.3
    dentures Z46.3
    device NEC
      abdominal Z46.89
      nervous system Z46.2
        implanted — *see* Admission, adjustment, device, implanted, nervous system
      orthodontic Z46.4
      prosthetic Z44.9 ☑
        breast Z44.3 ☑
        dental Z46.3
        eye Z44.2 ☑
    substitution
      auditory Z46.2
        implanted — *see* Admission, adjustment, device, implanted, hearing device
      nervous system Z46.2
        implanted — *see* Admission, adjustment, device, implanted, nervous system
      visual Z46.2
        implanted Z45.31
    hearing aid Z46.1
    ileostomy device Z46.89
    intestinal appliance or device NEC Z46.89
    neuropacemaker (brain) (peripheral nerve) (spinal cord) Z46.2
      implanted Z45.42
    orthodontic device Z46.4
    orthopedic device (brace) (cast) (shoes) Z46.89
    prosthesis Z44.9
      arm — *see* Admission, adjustment, artificial, arm
      breast Z44.3 ☑
      dental Z46.3
      eye Z44.2 ☑
      leg — *see* Admission, adjustment, artificial, leg
      specified type NEC Z44.8
    spectacles Z46.0
  follow-up examination Z09
  intrauterine device management Z30.431
    initial prescription Z30.014
  mental health evaluation Z00.8
    requested by authority Z04.6
  observation — *see* Observation
  Papanicolaou smear, cervix Z12.4
    for suspected malignant neoplasm Z12.4
  plastic and reconstructive surgery following medical procedure or healed injury NEC Z42.8
  plastic surgery, cosmetic NEC Z41.1
  postpartum observation
    immediately after delivery Z39.0
    routine follow-up Z39.2
  poststerilization (for restoration) Z31.0
    aftercare Z31.42
  procreative management Z31.9
  prophylactic (measure) — *see also* Encounter, prophylactic measures
    organ removal Z40.00
      breast Z40.01
      fallopian tube(s) Z40.03
        with ovary(s) Z40.02
      ovary(s) Z40.02
      specified organ NEC Z40.09
      testes Z40.09
    vaccination Z23
  psychiatric examination (general) Z00.8
    requested by authority Z04.6
  radiation therapy (antineoplastic) Z51.0
  reconstructive surgery following medical procedure or healed injury NEC Z42.8
  removal of
    cystostomy catheter Z43.5

Admission — *continued*
  removal of — *continued*
    drains Z48.03
    dressing (nonsurgical) Z48.00
    implantable subdermal contraceptive Z30.46
    intrauterine contraceptive device Z30.432
    neuropacemaker (brain) (peripheral nerve) (spinal cord) Z46.2
      implanted Z45.42
    staples Z48.02
    surgical dressing Z48.01
    sutures Z48.02
    ureteral stent Z46.6
  respirator [ventilator] use during power failure Z99.12
  restoration of organ continuity (poststerilization) Z31.0
    aftercare Z31.42
  sensitivity test — *see also* Test, skin
    allergy NEC Z01.82
    Mantoux Z11.1
  tuboplasty following previous sterilization Z31.0
    aftercare Z31.42
  vasoplasty following previous sterilization Z31.0
    aftercare Z31.42
  vision examination Z01.00
    with abnormal findings Z01.01
      following failed vision screening Z01.020
        with abnormal findings Z01.021
    infant or child (over 28 days old) Z00.129
      with abnormal findings Z00.121
  waiting period for admission to other facility Z75.1
Adnexitis (suppurative) — *see* Salpingo-oophoritis
Adolescent X-linked adrenoleukodystrophy E71.521
Adrenal (gland) — *see* condition
Adrenalism, tuberculous A18.7
Adrenalitis, adrenitis E27.8
  autoimmune E27.1
  meningococcal, hemorrhagic A39.1
Adrenarche, premature E27.0
Adrenocortical syndrome — *see* Cushing's, syndrome
Adrenogenital syndrome E25.9
  acquired E25.8
  congenital E25.0
  salt loss E25.0
Adrenogenitalism, congenital E25.0
Adrenoleukodystrophy E71.529
  neonatal E71.511
  X-linked E71.529
    Addison only phenotype E71.528
    Addison-Schilder E71.528
    adolescent E71.521
    adrenomyeloneuropathy E71.522
    childhood cerebral E71.520
    other specified E71.528
Adrenomyeloneuropathy E71.522
Adventitious bursa — *see* Bursopathy, specified type NEC
Adverse effect — *see* Table of Drugs and Chemicals, categories T36-T50, with 6th character 5
Advice — *see* Counseling
Adynamia (episodica) (hereditary) (periodic) G72.3
Aeration lung imperfect, newborn — *see* Atelectasis
Aerobullosis T70.3 ☑
Aerocele — *see* Embolism, air
Aerodermectasia
  subcutaneous (traumatic) T79.7 ☑
Aerodontalgia T70.29 ☑
Aeroembolism T70.3 ☑
Aerogenes capsulatus infection A48.0
Aero-otitis media T70.0 ☑
Aerophagy, aerophagia (psychogenic) F45.8
Aerophobia F40.228
Aerosinusitis T70.1 ☑
Aerotitis T70.0 ☑
Affection — *see* Disease
Afibrinogenemia — *see also* Defect, coagulation D68.8
  acquired D65
  congenital D68.2
  following ectopic or molar pregnancy O08.1
  in abortion — *see* Abortion, by type, complicated by, afibrinogenemia
  puerperal O72.3
African
  sleeping sickness B56.9
  tick fever A68.1
  trypanosomiasis B56.9
    gambian B56.0
    rhodesian B56.1
Aftercare — *see also* Care Z51.89

Aftercare — *continued*
  following surgery (for) (on)
    amputation Z47.81
    attention to
      drains Z48.03
      dressings (nonsurgical) Z48.00
        surgical Z48.01
      sutures Z48.02
    circulatory system Z48.812
    delayed (planned) wound closure Z48.1
    digestive system Z48.815
    explantation of joint prosthesis (staged procedure)
      hip Z47.32
      knee Z47.33
      shoulder Z47.31
    genitourinary system Z48.816
    joint replacement Z47.1
    neoplasm Z48.3
    nervous system Z48.811
    oral cavity Z48.814
    organ transplant
      bone marrow Z48.290
      heart Z48.21
      heart-lung Z48.280
      kidney Z48.22
      liver Z48.23
      lung Z48.24
      multiple organs NEC Z48.288
      specified NEC Z48.298
    orthopedic NEC Z47.89
    planned wound closure Z48.1
    removal of internal fixation device Z47.2
    respiratory system Z48.813
    scoliosis Z47.82
    sense organs Z48.810
    skin and subcutaneous tissue Z48.817
    specified body system
      circulatory Z48.812
      digestive Z48.815
      genitourinary Z48.816
      nervous Z48.811
      oral cavity Z48.814
      respiratory Z48.813
      sense organs Z48.810
      skin and subcutaneous tissue Z48.817
      teeth Z48.814
    specified NEC Z48.89
    spinal Z47.89
    teeth Z48.814
  fracture — *code to* fracture with seventh character D
  involving
    removal of
      drains Z48.03
      dressings (nonsurgical) Z48.00
      staples Z48.02
      surgical dressings Z48.01
      sutures Z48.02
    neuropacemaker (brain) (peripheral nerve) (spinal cord) Z46.2
      implanted Z45.42
    orthopedic NEC Z47.89
    postprocedural — *see* Aftercare, following surgery
After-cataract — *see* Cataract, secondary
Agalactia (primary) O92.3
  elective, secondary or therapeutic O92.5
Agammaglobulinemia (acquired (secondary) (nonfamilial) D80.1
  with
    immunoglobulin-bearing B-lymphocytes D80.1
    lymphopenia D81.9
  autosomal recessive (Swiss type) D80.0
  Bruton's X-linked D80.0
  common variable (CVAgamma) D80.1
  congenital sex-linked D80.0
  hereditary D80.0
  lymphopenic D81.9
  Swiss type (autosomal recessive) D80.0
  X-linked (with growth hormone deficiency) (Bruton) D80.0
Aganglionosis (bowel) (colon) Q43.1
Age (old) — *see* Senility
Agenesis
  adrenal (gland) Q89.1
  alimentary tract (complete) (partial) NEC Q45.8
    upper Q40.8
  anus, anal (canal) Q42.3
    with fistula Q42.2
  aorta Q25.41

Agenesis — continued
- appendix Q42.8
- arm (complete) Q71.0- ☑
  - with hand present Q71.1- ☑
- artery (peripheral) Q27.9
  - brain Q28.3
  - coronary Q24.5
  - pulmonary Q25.79
  - specified NEC Q27.8
  - umbilical Q27.0
- auditory (canal) (external) Q16.1
- auricle (ear) Q16.0
- bile duct or passage Q44.5
- bladder Q64.5
- bone Q79.9
- brain Q00.0
  - part of Q04.3
- breast (with nipple present) Q83.8
  - with absent nipple Q83.0
- bronchus Q32.4
- canaliculus lacrimalis Q10.4
- carpus — see Agenesis, hand
- cartilage Q79.9
- cecum Q42.8
- cerebellum Q04.3
- cervix Q51.5
- chin Q18.8
- cilia Q10.3
- circulatory system, part NOS Q28.9
- clavicle Q74.0
- clitoris Q52.6
- coccyx Q76.49
- colon Q42.9
  - specified NEC Q42.8
- corpus callosum Q04.0
- cricoid cartilage Q31.8
- diaphragm (with hernia) Q79.1
- digestive organ(s) or tract (complete) (partial) NEC Q45.8
  - upper Q40.8
- ductus arteriosus Q28.8
- duodenum Q41.0
- ear Q16.9
  - auricle Q16.0
  - lobe Q17.8
- ejaculatory duct Q55.4
- endocrine (gland) NEC Q89.2
- epiglottis Q31.8
- esophagus Q39.8
- eustachian tube Q16.2
- eye Q11.1
  - adnexa Q15.8
- eyelid (fold) Q10.3
- face
  - bones NEC Q75.8
  - specified part NEC Q18.8
- fallopian tube Q50.6
- femur — see Defect, reduction, lower limb, longitudinal, femur
- fibula — see Defect, reduction, lower limb, longitudinal, fibula
- finger (complete) (partial) — see Agenesis, hand
- foot (and toes) (complete) (partial) Q72.3- ☑
- forearm (with hand present) — see Agenesis, arm, with hand present
  - and hand Q71.2- ☑
- gallbladder Q44.0
- gastric Q40.2
- genitalia, genital (organ(s))
  - female Q52.8
    - external Q52.71
    - internal NEC Q52.8
  - male Q55.8
- glottis Q31.8
- hair Q84.0
- hand (and fingers) (complete) (partial) Q71.3- ☑
- heart Q24.8
  - valve NEC Q24.8
    - pulmonary Q22.0
- hepatic Q44.7
- humerus — see Defect, reduction, upper limb
- hymen Q52.4
- ileum Q41.2
- incus Q16.3
- intestine (small) Q41.9
  - large Q42.9
    - specified NEC Q42.8
- iris (dilator fibers) Q13.1

Agenesis — continued
- jaw M26.09
- jejunum Q41.1
- kidney(s) (partial) Q60.2
  - bilateral Q60.1
  - unilateral Q60.0
- labium (majus) (minus) Q52.71
- labyrinth, membranous Q16.5
- lacrimal apparatus Q10.4
- larynx Q31.8
- leg (complete) Q72.0- ☑
  - with foot present Q72.1- ☑
  - lower leg (with foot present) — see Agenesis, leg, with foot present
  - and foot Q72.2- ☑
- lens Q12.3
- limb (complete) Q73.0
  - lower — see Agenesis, leg
  - upper — see Agenesis, arm
- lip Q38.0
- liver Q44.7
- lung (fissure) (lobe) (bilateral) (unilateral) Q33.3
- mandible, maxilla M26.09
- metacarpus — see Agenesis, hand
- metatarsus — see Agenesis, foot
- muscle Q79.8
  - eyelid Q10.3
  - ocular Q15.8
- musculoskeletal system NEC Q79.8
- nail(s) Q84.3
- neck, part Q18.8
- nerve Q07.8
- nervous system, part NEC Q07.8
- nipple Q83.2
- nose Q30.1
- nuclear Q07.8
- organ
  - of Corti Q16.5
  - or site not listed — see Anomaly, by site
- osseous meatus (ear) Q16.1
- ovary
  - bilateral Q50.02
  - unilateral Q50.01
- oviduct Q50.6
- pancreas Q45.0
- parathyroid (gland) Q89.2
- parotid gland(s) Q38.4
- patella Q74.1
- pelvic girdle (complete) (partial) Q74.2
- penis Q55.5
- pericardium Q24.8
- pituitary (gland) Q89.2
- prostate Q55.4
- punctum lacrimale Q10.4
- radioulnar — see Defect, reduction, upper limb
- radius — see Defect, reduction, upper limb, longitudinal, radius
- rectum Q42.1
  - with fistula Q42.0
- renal Q60.2
  - bilateral Q60.1
  - unilateral Q60.0
- respiratory organ NEC Q34.8
- rib Q76.6
- roof of orbit Q75.8
- round ligament Q52.8
- sacrum Q76.49
- salivary gland Q38.4
- scapula Q74.0
- scrotum Q55.29
- seminal vesicles Q55.4
- septum
  - atrial Q21.1
  - between aorta and pulmonary artery Q21.4
  - ventricular Q20.4
- shoulder girdle (complete) (partial) Q74.0
- skull (bone) Q75.8
  - with
    - anencephaly Q00.0
    - encephalocele — see Encephalocele
    - hydrocephalus Q03.9
      - with spina bifida — see Spina bifida, by site, with hydrocephalus
    - microcephaly Q02
- spermatic cord Q55.4
- spinal cord Q06.0
- spine Q76.49
- spleen Q89.01

Agenesis — continued
- sternum Q76.7
- stomach Q40.2
- submaxillary gland(s) (congenital) Q38.4
- tarsus — see Agenesis, foot
- tendon Q79.8
- testicle Q55.0
- thymus (gland) Q89.2
- thyroid (gland) E03.1
  - cartilage Q31.8
- tibia — see Defect, reduction, lower limb, longitudinal, tibia
- tibiofibular — see Defect, reduction, lower limb, specified type NEC
- toe (and foot) (complete) (partial) — see Agenesis, foot
- tongue Q38.3
- trachea (cartilage) Q32.1
- ulna — see Defect, reduction, upper limb, longitudinal, ulna
- upper limb — see Agenesis, arm
- ureter Q62.4
- urethra Q64.5
- urinary tract NEC Q64.8
- uterus Q51.0
- uvula Q38.5
- vagina Q52.0
- vas deferens Q55.4
- vein(s) (peripheral) Q27.9
  - brain Q28.3
  - great NEC Q26.8
  - portal Q26.5
- vena cava (inferior) (superior) Q26.8
- vermis of cerebellum Q04.3
- vertebra Q76.49
- vulva Q52.71

Ageusia R43.2
Agitated — see condition
Agitation R45.1
Aglossia (congenital) Q38.3
Aglossia-adactylia syndrome Q87.0
Aglycogenosis E74.00
Agnosia (body image) (other senses) (tactile) R48.1
- developmental F88
- verbal R48.1
  - auditory R48.1
    - developmental F80.2
  - developmental F80.2
- visual (object) R48.3
Agoraphobia F40.00
- with panic disorder F40.01
- without panic disorder F40.02
Agrammatism R48.8
Agranulocytopenia — see Agranulocytosis
Agranulocytosis (chronic) (cyclical) (genetic) (infantile) (periodic) (pernicious) — see also Neutropenia D70.9
- congenital D70.0
- cytoreductive cancer chemotherapy sequela D70.1
- drug-induced D70.2
  - due to cytoreductive cancer chemotherapy D70.1
- due to infection D70.3
- secondary D70.4
  - drug-induced D70.2
    - due to cytoreductive cancer chemotherapy D70.1
Agraphia (absolute) R48.8
- with alexia R48.0
- developmental F81.81
Ague (dumb) — see Malaria
Agyria Q04.3
Ahumada-del Castillo syndrome E23.0
Aichomophobia F40.298
AIDS (related complex) B20
Ailment heart — see Disease, heart
Ailurophobia F40.218
AIN — see Neoplasia, intraepithelial, anal
Ainhum (disease) L94.6
AIPHI (acute idiopathic pulmonary hemorrhage in infants (over 28 days old)) R04.81
Air
- anterior mediastinum J98.2
- compressed, disease T70.3 ☑
- conditioner lung or pneumonitis J67.7
- embolism (artery) (cerebral) (any site) T79.0 ☑
  - with ectopic or molar pregnancy O08.2
  - due to implanted device NEC — see Complications, by site and type, specified NEC

Air — *continued*
  embolism — *continued*
    following
      abortion — *see* Abortion by type, complicated by, embolism
      ectopic or molar pregnancy O08.2
      infusion, therapeutic injection or transfusion T80.0 ☑
    in pregnancy, childbirth or puerperium — *see* Embolism, obstetric
    traumatic T79.0 ☑
  hunger, psychogenic F45.8
  rarefied, effects of — *see* Effect, adverse, high altitude
  sickness T75.3 ☑
Airplane sickness T75.3 ☑
Akathisia (drug-induced) (treatment-induced) G25.71
  neuroleptic induced (acute) G25.71
  tardive G25.71
Akinesia R29.898
Akinetic mutism R41.89
Akureyri's disease G93.3
Alactasia, congenital E73.0
Alagille's syndrome Q44.7
Alastrim B03
Albers-Schönberg syndrome Q78.2
Albert's syndrome — *see* Tendinitis, Achilles
Albinism, albino E70.30
  with hematologic abnormality E70.339
    Chédiak-Higashi syndrome E70.330
    Hermansky-Pudlak syndrome E70.331
    other specified E70.338
  I E70.320
  II E70.321
  ocular E70.319
    autosomal recessive E70.311
    other specified E70.318
    X-linked E70.310
  oculocutaneous E70.329
    other specified E70.328
    tyrosinase (ty) negative E70.320
    tyrosinase (ty) positive E70.321
  other specified E70.39
Albinismus E70.30
Albright (-McCune)(-Sternberg) syndrome Q78.1
Albuminous — *see* condition
Albuminuria, albuminuric (acute) (chronic) (subacute) — *see also* Proteinuria R80.9
  complicating pregnancy — *see* Proteinuria, gestational
  with
    gestational hypertension — *see* Pre-eclampsia
    pre-existing hypertension — *see* Hypertension, complicating pregnancy, pre-existing, with, pre-eclampsia
  gestational — *see* Proteinuria, gestational
    with
      gestational hypertension — *see* Pre-eclampsia
      pre-existing hypertension — *see* Hypertension, complicating pregnancy, pre-existing, with, pre-eclampsia
  orthostatic R80.2
  postural R80.2
  pre-eclamptic — *see* Pre-eclampsia
  scarlatinal A38.8
Albuminurophobia F40.298
Alcaptonuria E70.29
Alcohol, alcoholic, alcohol-induced
  addiction (without remission) F10.20
    with remission F10.21
  amnestic disorder, persisting F10.96
    with dependence F10.26
  anxiety disorder F10.980
  bipolar and related disorder F10.94
  brain syndrome, chronic F10.97
    with dependence F10.27
  cardiopathy I42.6
  counseling and surveillance Z71.41
    family member Z71.42
  delirium (acute) (tremens) (withdrawal) F10.231
    with intoxication F10.921
      in
        abuse F10.121
        dependence F10.221
  dementia F10.97
    with dependence F10.27
  depressive disorder F10.94
  deterioration F10.97
    with dependence F10.27
  hallucinosis (acute) F10.951

Alcohol, alcoholic, alcohol-induced — *continued*
  hallucinosis — *continued*
    in
      abuse F10.151
      dependence F10.251
  insanity F10.959
  intoxication (acute) (without dependence) F10.129
    with
      delirium F10.121
      dependence F10.229
        with delirium F10.221
        uncomplicated F10.220
      uncomplicated F10.120
  jealousy F10.988
  Korsakoff's, Korsakov's, Korsakow's F10.26
  liver K70.9
    acute — *see* Disease, liver, alcoholic, hepatitis
  major neurocognitive disorder, amnestic-confabulatory type F10.96
  major neurocognitive disorder, nonamnestic-confabulatory type F10.97
  mania (acute) (chronic) F10.959
  mild neurocognitive disorder F10.988
  paranoia, paranoid (type) psychosis F10.950
  pellagra E52
  poisoning, accidental (acute) NEC — *see* Table of Drugs and Chemicals, alcohol, poisoning
  psychosis — *see* Psychosis, alcoholic
  psychotic disorder F10.959
  sexual dysfunction F10.981
  sleep disorder F10.982
  withdrawal (without convulsions) F10.239
    with delirium F10.231
Alcoholism (chronic) (without remission) F10.20
  with
    psychosis — *see* Psychosis, alcoholic
    remission F10.21
  Korsakov's F10.96
  with dependence F10.26
Alder (-Reilly) **anomaly or syndrome** (leukocyte granulation) D72.0
Aldosteronism E26.9
  familial (type I) E26.02
  glucocorticoid-remediable E26.02
  primary (due to) (bilateral) adrenal hyperplasia) E26.09
  primary NEC E26.09
  secondary E26.1
  specified NEC E26.89
Aldosteronoma D44.10
Aldrich (-Wiskott) **syndrome** (eczema-thrombocytopenia) D82.0
Alektorophobia F40.218
Aleppo boil B55.1
Aleukemic — *see* condition
Aleukia
  congenital D70.0
  hemorrhagica D61.9
    congenital D61.09
  splenica D73.1
Alexia R48.0
  developmental F81.0
  secondary to organic lesion R48.0
Algoneurodystrophy M89.00
  ankle M89.07- ☑
  foot M89.07- ☑
  forearm M89.03- ☑
  hand M89.04- ☑
  lower leg M89.06- ☑
  multiple sites M89.0- ☑
  shoulder M89.01- ☑
  specified site NEC M89.08
  thigh M89.05- ☑
  upper arm M89.02- ☑
Algophobia F40.298
Alienation, mental — *see* Psychosis
Alkalemia E87.3
Alkalosis E87.3
  metabolic E87.3
    with respiratory acidosis E87.4
    of newborn P74.41
  respiratory E87.3
Alkaptonuria E70.29
Allen-Masters syndrome N83.8
Allergy, allergic (reaction) (to) T78.40 ☑
  air-borne substance NEC (rhinitis) J30.89
  alveolitis (extrinsic) J67.9
    due to
      Aspergillus clavatus J67.4

Allergy, allergic — *continued*
  alveolitis — *continued*
    due to — *continued*
      Cryptostroma corticale J67.6
      organisms (fungal, thermophilic actinomycete) growing in ventilation (air conditioning) systems J67.7
      specified type NEC J67.8
  anaphylactic reaction or shock T78.2 ☑
  angioneurotic edema T78.3 ☑
  animal (dander) (epidermal) (hair) (rhinitis) J30.81
  bee sting (anaphylactic shock) — *see* Toxicity, venom, arthropod, bee
  biological — *see* Allergy, drug
  colitis — *see also* Colitis, allergic K52.29
  dander (animal) (rhinitis) J30.81
  dandruff (rhinitis) J30.81
  dental restorative material (existing) K08.55
  dermatitis — *see* Dermatitis, contact, allergic
  diathesis — *see* History, allergy
  drug, medicament & biological (any) (external) (internal) T78.40 ☑
    correct substance properly administered — *see* Table of Drugs and Chemicals, by drug, adverse effect
    wrong substance given or taken NEC (by accident) — *see* Table of Drugs and Chemicals, by drug, poisoning
  due to pollen J30.1
  dust (house) (stock) (rhinitis) J30.89
    with asthma — *see* Asthma, allergic extrinsic
  eczema — *see* Dermatitis, contact, allergic
  epidermal (animal) (rhinitis) J30.81
  feathers (rhinitis) J30.89
  food (any) (ingested) NEC T78.1 ☑
    anaphylactic shock — *see* Shock, anaphylactic, due to food
    dermatitis — *see* Dermatitis, due to, food
    dietary counseling and surveillance Z71.3
    in contact with skin L23.6
    rhinitis J30.5
    status (without reaction) Z91.018
      eggs Z91.012
      milk products Z91.011
      peanuts Z91.010
      seafood Z91.013
      specified NEC Z91.018
  gastrointestinal — *see also* specific type of allergic reaction
    meaning colitis — *see also* Colitis, allergic K52.29
    meaning gastroenteritis — *see also* Gastroenteritis, allergic K52.29
    meaning other adverse food reaction not elsewhere classified T78.1 ☑
  grain J30.1
  grass (hay fever) (pollen) J30.1
    asthma — *see* Asthma, allergic extrinsic
  hair (animal) (rhinitis) J30.81
  history (of) — *see* History, allergy
  horse serum — *see* Allergy, serum
  inhalant (rhinitis) J30.89
    pollen J30.1
  kapok (rhinitis) J30.89
  medicine — *see* Allergy, drug
  milk protein — *see also* Allergy, food Z91.011
    anaphylactic reaction T78.07 ☑
    dermatitis L27.2
    enterocolitis syndrome K52.21
    enteropathy K52.22
    gastroenteritis K52.29
    gastroesophageal reflux — *see also* Reaction, adverse, food K21.9
      with esophagitis (without bleeding) K21.00
        with bleeding K21.01
    proctocolitis K52.82
  nasal, seasonal due to pollen J30.1
  pneumonia J82.89
  pollen (any) (hay fever) J30.1
    asthma — *see* Asthma, allergic extrinsic
  primrose J30.1
  primula J30.1
  proctocolitis K52.82
  purpura D69.0
  ragweed (hay fever) (pollen) J30.1
    asthma — *see* Asthma, allergic extrinsic
  rose (pollen) J30.1
  seasonal NEC J30.2
  Senecio jacobae (pollen) J30.1

Allergy, allergic — *continued*
  serum — *see also* Reaction, serum T80.69 ☑
    anaphylactic shock T80.59 ☑
  shock (anaphylactic) T78.2 ☑
    due to
      administration of blood and blood products
        T80.51 ☑
      adverse effect of correct medicinal substance
        properly administered T88.6 ☑
      immunization T80.52 ☑
      serum NEC T80.59 ☑
      vaccination T80.52 ☑
  specific NEC T78.49 ☑
  tree (any) (hay fever) (pollen) J30.1
    asthma — *see* Asthma, allergic extrinsic
  upper respiratory J30.9
  urticaria L50.0
  vaccine — *see* Allergy, serum
  wheat — *see* Allergy, food
Allescheriasis B48.2
Alligator skin disease Q80.9
Allocheiria, allochiria R20.8
Almeida's disease — *see* Paracoccidioidomycosis
Alopecia (hereditaria) (seborrheica) L65.9
  androgenic L64.9
    drug-induced L64.0
    specified NEC L64.8
  areata L63.9
    ophiasis L63.2
    specified NEC L63.8
    totalis L63.0
    universalis L63.1
  cicatricial L66.9
    specified NEC L66.8
  circumscripta L63.9
  congenital, congenitalis Q84.0
  due to cytotoxic drugs NEC L65.8
  mucinosa L65.2
  postinfective NEC L65.8
  postpartum L65.0
  premature L64.8
  specific (syphilitic) A51.32
  specified NEC L65.8
  syphilitic (secondary) A51.32
  totalis (capitis) L63.0
  universalis (entire body) L63.1
  X-ray L58.1
Alpers' disease G31.81
Alpine sickness T70.29 ☑
Alport syndrome Q87.81
ALTE (apparent life threatening event) **in newborn and infant** R68.13
Alteration (of), **Altered**
  awareness
    transient R40.4
    unintended under general anesthesia, during procedure T88.53 ☑
  mental status R41.82
  pattern of family relationships affecting child Z62.898
  sensation
    following
      cerebrovascular disease I69.998
        cerebral infarction I69.398
        intracerebral hemorrhage I69.198
        nontraumatic intracranial hemorrhage NEC I69.298
        specified disease NEC I69.898
        subarachnoid hemorrhage I69.098
Alternating — *see* condition
Altitude, high (effects) — *see* Effect, adverse, high altitude
Aluminosis (of lung) J63.0
Alveolitis
  allergic (extrinsic) — *see* Pneumonitis, hypersensitivity
  due to
    Aspergillus clavatus J67.4
    Cryptostroma corticale J67.6
  fibrosing (cryptogenic) (idiopathic) J84.112
  jaw M27.3
  sicca dolorosa M27.3
Alveolus, alveolar — *see* condition
Alymphocytosis D72.810
  thymic (with immunodeficiency) D82.1
Alymphoplasia, thymic D82.1
Alzheimer's disease or sclerosis — *see* Disease, Alzheimer's
Amastia (with nipple present) Q83.8
  with absent nipple Q83.0

Amathophobia F40.228
Amaurosis (acquired) (congenital) — *see also* Blindness
  fugax G45.3
  hysterical F44.6
  Leber's congenital H35.50
  uremic — *see* Uremia
Amaurotic idiocy (infantile) (juvenile) (late) E75.4
Amaxophobia F40.248
Ambiguous genitalia Q56.4
Amblyopia (congenital) (ex anopsia) (partial) (suppression) H53.00-
  anisometropic — *see* Amblyopia, refractive
  deprivation H53.01-
  hysterical F44.6
  nocturnal — *see also* Blindness, night
    vitamin A deficiency E50.5
  refractive H53.02- ☑
  strabismic H53.03- ☑
  suspect H53.04- ☑
  tobacco H53.8
  toxic NEC H53.8
  uremic — *see* Uremia
Ameba, amebic (histolytica) — *see also* Amebiasis
  abscess (liver) A06.4
Amebiasis A06.9
  with abscess — *see* Abscess, amebic
  acute A06.0
  chronic (intestine) A06.1
    with abscess — *see* Abscess, amebic
  cutaneous A06.7
  cutis A06.7
  cystitis A06.81
  genitourinary tract NEC A06.82
  hepatic — *see* Abscess, liver, amebic
  intestine A06.0
  nondysenteric colitis A06.2
  skin A06.7
  specified site NEC A06.89
Ameboma (of intestine) A06.3
Amelia Q73.0
  lower limb — *see* Agenesis, leg
  upper limb — *see* Agenesis, arm
Ameloblastoma — *see also* Cyst, calcifying odontogenic
  long bones C40.9-
    lower limb C40.2- ☑
    upper limb C40.0- ☑
  malignant C41.1
    jaw (bone) (lower) C41.1
      upper C41.0
  tibial C40.2-
Amelogenesis imperfecta K00.5
  nonhereditaria (segmentalis) K00.4
Amenorrhea N91.2
  hyperhormonal E28.8
  primary N91.0
  secondary N91.1
Amentia — *see* Disability, intellectual
  Meynert's (nonalcoholic) F04
American
  leishmaniasis B55.2
  mountain tick fever A93.2
Ametropia — *see* Disorder, refraction
AMH (asymptomatic microscopic hematuria) R31.21
Amianthosis J61
Amimia R48.8
Amino-acid disorder E72.9
  anemia D53.0
Aminoacidopathy E72.9
Aminoaciduria E72.9
Amnesia R41.3
  anterograde R41.1
  auditory R48.8
  dissociative F44.0
    with dissociative fugue F44.1
  hysterical F44.0
  postictal in epilepsy — *see* Epilepsy
  psychogenic F44.0
  retrograde R41.2
  transient global G45.4
Amnes(t)ic syndrome (post-traumatic) F04
  induced by
    alcohol F10.96
      with dependence F10.26
    psychoactive NEC F19.96
      with
        abuse F19.16
        dependence F19.26

Amnes(t)ic syndrome — *continued*
  induced by — *continued*
    sedative F13.96
      with dependence F13.26
Amnion, amniotic — *see* condition
Amnionitis — *see* Pregnancy, complicated by
Amok F68.8
Amoral traits F60.89
Amphetamine (or other stimulant) **-induced**
  anxiety disorder F15.980
  bipolar and related disorder F15.94
  delirium F15.921
  depressive disorder F15.94
  obsessive-compulsive and related disorder F15.988
  psychotic disorder F15.959
  sexual dysfunction F15.981
  sleep disorder F15.982
  stimulant withdrawal F15.23
Ampulla
  lower esophagus K22.8
  phrenic K22.8
Amputation — *see also* Absence, by site, acquired
  neuroma (postoperative) (traumatic) — *see* Complications, amputation stump, neuroma
  stump (surgical)
    abnormal, painful, or with complication (late) — *see* Complications, amputation stump
    healed or old NOS Z89.9
  traumatic (complete) (partial)
    arm (upper) (complete) S48.91- ☑
      at
        elbow S58.01- ☑
          partial S58.02- ☑
        shoulder joint (complete) S48.01- ☑
          partial S48.02- ☑
      between
        elbow and wrist (complete) S58.11- ☑
          partial S58.12- ☑
        shoulder and elbow (complete) S48.11- ☑
          partial S48.12- ☑
      partial S48.92- ☑
    breast (complete) S28.21- ☑
      partial S28.22- ☑
    clitoris (complete) S38.211 ☑
      partial S38.212 ☑
    ear (complete) S08.11- ☑
      partial S08.12- ☑
    finger (complete) (metacarpophalangeal) S68.11- ☑
      index S68.11- ☑
      little S68.11- ☑
      middle S68.11- ☑
      partial S68.12- ☑
        index S68.12- ☑
        little S68.12- ☑
        middle S68.12- ☑
        ring S68.12- ☑
      ring S68.11- ☑
      thumb — *see* Amputation, traumatic, thumb
      transphalangeal (complete) S68.61- ☑
        index S68.61- ☑
        little S68.61- ☑
        middle S68.61- ☑
        partial S68.62- ☑
          index S68.62- ☑
          little S68.62- ☑
          middle S68.62- ☑
          ring S68.62- ☑
        ring S68.61- ☑
    foot (complete) S98.91- ☑
      at ankle level S98.01- ☑
        partial S98.02- ☑
      midfoot S98.31- ☑
        partial S98.32- ☑
      partial S98.92- ☑
    forearm (complete) S58.91- ☑
      at elbow level (complete) S58.01- ☑
        partial S58.02- ☑
      between elbow and wrist (complete) S58.11- ☑
        partial S58.12- ☑
      partial S58.92- ☑
    genital organ(s) (external)
      female (complete) S38.211 ☑
        partial S38.212 ☑
      male
        penis (complete) S38.221 ☑
          partial S38.222 ☑

Amputation — *continued*
traumatic — *continued*
genital organ(s) — *continued*
male — *continued*
scrotum (complete) S38.231 ☑
partial S38.232 ☑
testes (complete) S38.231 ☑
partial S38.232 ☑
hand (complete) (wrist level) S68.41- ☑
finger(s) alone — *see* Amputation, traumatic, finger
partial S68.42- ☑
thumb alone — *see* Amputation, traumatic, thumb
transmetacarpal (complete) S68.71- ☑
partial S68.72- ☑
head
ear — *see* Amputation, traumatic, ear
nose (partial) S08.812 ☑
complete S08.811 ☑
part S08.89 ☑
scalp S08.0 ☑
hip (and thigh) (complete) S78.91- ☑
at hip joint (complete) S78.01- ☑
partial S78.02- ☑
between hip and knee (complete) S78.11- ☑
partial S78.12- ☑
partial S78.92- ☑
labium (majus) (minus) (complete) S38.21- ☑
partial S38.21- ☑
leg (lower) S88.91- ☑
at knee level S88.01- ☑
partial S88.02- ☑
between knee and ankle S88.11- ☑
partial S88.12- ☑
partial S88.92- ☑
nose (partial) S08.812 ☑
complete S08.811 ☑
penis (complete) S38.221 ☑
partial S38.222 ☑
scrotum (complete) S38.231 ☑
partial S38.232 ☑
shoulder — *see* Amputation, traumatic, arm
at shoulder joint — *see* Amputation, traumatic, arm, at shoulder joint
testes (complete) S38.231 ☑
partial S38.232 ☑
thigh — *see* Amputation, traumatic, hip
thorax, part of S28.1 ☑
breast — *see* Amputation, traumatic, breast
thumb (complete) (metacarpophalangeal) S68.01- ☑
partial S68.02- ☑
transphalangeal (complete) S68.51- ☑
partial S68.52- ☑
toe (lesser) S98.13- ☑
great S98.11- ☑
partial S98.12- ☑
more than one S98.21- ☑
partial S98.22- ☑
partial S98.14- ☑
vulva (complete) S38.211 ☑
partial S38.212 ☑
Amputee (bilateral) (old) Z89.9
Amsterdam dwarfism Q87.19
Amusia R48.8
developmental F80.89
Amyelencephalus, amyelencephaly Q00.0
Amyelia Q06.0
Amygdalitis — *see* Tonsillitis
Amygdalolith J35.8
Amyloid heart (disease) E85.4 *[I43]*
Amyloidosis (generalized) (primary) E85.9
with lung involvement E85.4 *[J99]*
familial E85.2
genetic E85.2
heart E85.4 *[I43]*
hemodialysis-associated E85.3
light chain (AL) E85.81
liver E85.4 *[K77]*
localized E85.4
neuropathic heredofamilial E85.1
non-neuropathic heredofamilial E85.0
organ limited E85.4
Portuguese E85.1
pulmonary E85.4 *[J99]*

Amyloidosis — *continued*
secondary systemic E85.3
senile systemic (SSA) E85.82
skin (lichen) (macular) E85.4 *[L99]*
specified NEC E85.89
subglottic E85.4 *[J99]*
wild-type transthyretin-related (ATTR) E85.82
Amylopectinosis (brancher enzyme deficiency) E74.03
Amylophagia — *see* Pica
Amyoplasia congenita Q79.8
Amyotonia M62.89
congenita G70.2
Amyotrophia, amyotrophy, amyotrophic G71.8
congenita Q79.8
diabetic — *see* Diabetes, amyotrophy
lateral sclerosis G12.21
neuralgic G54.5
spinal progressive G12.25
Anacidity, gastric K31.83
psychogenic F45.8
Anaerosis of newborn P28.89
Analbuminemia E88.09
Analgesia — *see* Anesthesia
Analphalipoproteinemia E78.6
Anaphylactic
purpura D69.0
shock or reaction — *see* Shock, anaphylactic
Anaphylactoid shock or reaction — *see* Shock, anaphylactic
Anaphylactoid syndrome of pregnancy O88.01- ☑
Anaphylaxis — *see* Shock, anaphylactic
Anaplasia cervix — *see also* Dysplasia, cervix N87.9
Anaplasmosis, human A77.49
Anarthria R47.1
Anasarca R60.1
cardiac — *see* Failure, heart, congestive
lung J18.2
newborn P83.2
nutritional E43
pulmonary J18.2
renal N04.9
Anastomosis
aneurysmal — *see* Aneurysm
arteriovenous ruptured brain I60.8
intracerebral I61.8
intraparenchymal I61.8
intraventricular I61.5
subarachnoid I60.8
intestinal K63.89
complicated NEC K91.89
involving urinary tract N99.89
retinal and choroidal vessels (congenital) Q14.8
Anatomical narrow angle H40.03- ☑
Ancylostoma, ancylostomiasis (braziliense) (caninum) (ceylanicum) (duodenale) B76.0
Necator americanus B76.1
Andersen's disease (glycogen storage) E74.09
Anderson-Fabry disease E75.21
Andes disease T70.29
Andrews' disease (bacterid) L08.89
Androblastoma
benign
specified site — *see* Neoplasm, benign, by site
unspecified site
female D27.9
male D29.20
malignant
specified site — *see* Neoplasm, malignant, by site
unspecified site
female C56.9
male C62.90
specified site — *see* Neoplasm, uncertain behavior, by site
tubular
with lipid storage
specified site — *see* Neoplasm, benign, by site
unspecified site
female D27.9
male D29.20
specified site — *see* Neoplasm, benign, by site
unspecified site
female D27.9
male D29.20
unspecified site
female D39.10
male D40.10

Androgen insensitivity syndrome — *see also* Syndrome, androgen insensitivity E34.50
Androgen resistance syndrome — *see also* Syndrome, androgen insensitivity E34.50
Android pelvis Q74.2
with disproportion (fetopelvic) O33.3 ☑
causing obstructed labor O65.3
Androphobia F40.290
Anectasis, pulmonary (newborn) — *see* Atelectasis
Anemia (essential) (general) (hemoglobin deficiency) (infantile) (primary) (profound) D64.9
with (due to) (in)
disorder of
anaerobic glycolysis D55.2
pentose phosphate pathway D55.1
koilonychia D50.9
achlorhydric D50.8
achrestic D53.1
Addison (-Biermer) (pernicious) D51.0
agranulocytic — *see* Agranulocytosis
amino-acid-deficiency D53.0
aplastic D61.9
congenital D61.09
drug-induced D61.1
due to
drugs D61.1
external agents NEC D61.2
infection D61.2
radiation D61.2
idiopathic D61.3
red cell (pure) D60.9
chronic D60.0
congenital D61.01
specified type NEC D60.8
transient D60.1
specified type NEC D61.89
toxic D61.2
aregenerative
congenital D61.09
asiderotic D50.9
atypical (primary) D64.9
Baghdad spring D55.0
Balantidium coli A07.0
Biermer's (pernicious) D51.0
blood loss (chronic) D50.0
acute D62
bothriocephalus B70.0 *[D63.8]*
brickmaker's B76.9 *[D63.8]*
cerebral I67.89
childhood D58.9
chlorotic D50.8
chronic
blood loss D50.0
hemolytic D58.9
idiopathic D59.9
simple D53.9
chronica congenita aregenerativa D61.09
combined system disease NEC D51.0 *[G32.0]*
due to dietary vitamin B12 deficiency D51.3 *[G32.0]*
complicating pregnancy, childbirth or puerperium — *see* Pregnancy, complicated by (management affected by), anemia
congenital P61.4
aplastic D61.09
due to isoimmunization NOS P55.9
dyserythropoietic, dyshematopoietic D64.4
following fetal blood loss P61.3
Heinz body D58.2
hereditary hemolytic NOS D58.9
pernicious D51.0
spherocytic D58.0
Cooley's (erythroblastic) D56.1
cytogenic D51.0
deficiency D53.9
2, 3 diphosphoglycurate mutase D55.2
2, 3 PG D55.2
6 phosphogluconate dehydrogenase D55.1
6-PGD D55.1
amino-acid D53.0
combined B12 and folate D53.1
enzyme D55.9
drug-induced (hemolytic) D59.2
glucose-6-phosphate dehydrogenase (G6PD) D55.0
glycolytic D55.2
nucleotide metabolism D55.3
related to hexose monophosphate (HMP) shunt pathway NEC D55.1

☑ **Additional Character Required — Refer to the Tabular List for Character Selection**   ▽ **Subterms under main terms may continue to next column or page**

Anemia — *continued*
deficiency — *continued*
  enzyme — *continued*
    specified type NEC D55.8
  erythrocytic glutathione D55.1
  folate D52.9
    dietary D52.0
    drug-induced D52.1
  folic acid D52.9
    dietary D52.0
    drug-induced D52.1
  G SH D55.1
  G6PD D55.0
  GGS-R D55.1
  glucose-6-phosphate dehydrogenase D55.0
  glutathione reductase D55.1
  glyceraldehyde phosphate dehydrogenase D55.2
  hexokinase D55.2
  iron D50.9
    secondary to blood loss (chronic) D50.0
  nutritional D53.9
    with
      poor iron absorption D50.8
      specified deficiency NEC D53.8
  phosphofructo-aldolase D55.2
  phosphoglycerate kinase D55.2
  PK D55.2
  protein D53.0
  pyruvate kinase D55.2
  transcobalamin II D51.2
  triose-phosphate isomerase D55.2
  vitamin B12 NOS D51.9
    dietary D51.3
    due to
      intrinsic factor deficiency D51.0
      selective vitamin B12 malabsorption with
        proteinuria D51.1
    pernicious D51.0
    specified type NEC D51.8
Diamond-Blackfan (congenital hypoplastic) D61.01
dibothriocephalus B70.0 *[D63.8]*
dimorphic D53.1
diphasic D53.1
Diphyllobothrium (Dibothriocephalus) B70.0 *[D63.8]*
due to (in) (with)
  antineoplastic chemotherapy D64.81
  blood loss (chronic) D50.0
    acute D62
  chemotherapy, antineoplastic D64.81
  chronic disease classified elsewhere NEC D63.8
  chronic kidney disease D63.1
  deficiency
    amino-acid D53.0
    copper D53.8
    folate (folic acid) D52.9
      dietary D52.0
      drug-induced D52.1
    molybdenum D53.8
    protein D53.0
    zinc D53.8
  dietary vitamin B12 deficiency D51.3
  disorder of
    glutathione metabolism D55.1
    nucleotide metabolism D55.3
  drug — *see* Anemia, by type — *see also* Table of
    Drugs and Chemicals
  end stage renal disease D63.1
  enzyme disorder D55.9
  fetal blood loss P61.3
  fish tapeworm (D.latum) infestation B70.0 *[D63.8]*
  hemorrhage (chronic) D50.0
    acute D62
  impaired absorption D50.9
  loss of blood (chronic) D50.0
    acute D62
  myxedema E03.9 *[D63.8]*
  Necator americanus B76.1 *[D63.8]*
  prematurity P61.2
  selective vitamin B12 malabsorption with protein-
    uria D51.1
  transcobalamin II deficiency D51.2
Dyke-Young type (secondary) (symptomatic) D59.19
dyserythropoietic (congenital) D64.4
dyshematopoietic (congenital) D64.4
Egyptian B76.9 *[D63.8]*
elliptocytosis — *see* Elliptocytosis
enzyme-deficiency, drug-induced D59.2
epidemic — *see also* Ancylostomiasis B76.9 *[D63.8]*

Anemia — *continued*
erythroblastic
  familial D56.1
  newborn — *see also* Disease, hemolytic P55.9
  of childhood D56.1
erythrocytic glutathione deficiency D55.1
erythropoietin-resistant anemia (EPO resistant anemia)
  D63.1
Faber's (achlorhydric anemia) D50.9
factitious (self-induced blood letting) D50.0
familial erythroblastic D56.1
Fanconi's (congenital pancytopenia) D61.09
favism D55.0
fish tapeworm (D. latum) infestation B70.0 *[D63.8]*
folate (folic acid) deficiency D52.9
glucose-6-phosphate dehydrogenase (G6PD) deficiency
  D55.0
glutathione-reductase deficiency D55.1
goat's milk D52.0
granulocytic — *see* Agranulocytosis
Heinz body, congenital D58.2
hemolytic D58.9
  acquired D59.9
    with hemoglobinuria NEC D59.6
    autoimmune NEC D59.19
    infectious D59.4
    specified type NEC D59.8
    toxic D59.4
  acute D59.9
    due to enzyme deficiency specified type NEC
      D55.8
    Lederer's D59.19
  autoimmune D59.10
    cold D59.12
    drug-induced D59.0
    mixed D59.13
    warm D59.11
  chronic D58.9
    idiopathic D59.9
  cold type (primary) (secondary) (symptomatic)
    D59.12
  congenital (spherocytic) — *see* Spherocytosis
  due to
    cardiac conditions D59.4
    drugs (nonautoimmune) D59.2
      autoimmune D59.0
    enzyme disorder D55.9
      drug-induced D59.2
    presence of shunt or other internal prosthetic
      device D59.4
  familial D58.9
  hereditary D58.9
    due to enzyme disorder D55.9
      specified type NEC D55.8
    specified type NEC D58.8
  idiopathic (chronic) D59.9
  mechanical D59.4
  microangiopathic D59.4
  mixed type (primary) (secondary) (symptomatic)
    D59.13
  nonautoimmune D59.4
    drug-induced D59.2
  nonspherocytic
    congenital or hereditary NEC D55.8
      glucose-6-phosphate dehydrogenase deficien-
        cy D55.0
      pyruvate kinase deficiency D55.2
      type
        I D55.1
        II D55.2
    type
      I D55.1
      II D55.2
  primary
    autoimmune
      cold type D59.12
      mixed type D59.13
      warm type D59.11
  secondary D59.4
    autoimmune
      cold type D59.12
      mixed type D59.13
      warm type D59.11
  specified (hereditary) type NEC D58.8
  Stransky-Regala type — *see also* Hemoglobinopathy
    D58.8
  symptomatic D59.4
    autoimmune
      cold type D59.12

Anemia — *continued*
hemolytic — *continued*
  symptomatic — *continued*
    autoimmune — *continued*
      mixed type D59.13
      warm type D59.11
    toxic D59.4
    warm type (primary) (secondary) (symptomatic)
      D59.11
hemorrhagic (chronic) D50.0
  acute D62
Herrick's D57.1
hexokinase deficiency D55.2
hookworm B76.9 *[D63.8]*
hypochromic (idiopathic) (microcytic) (normoblastic)
  D50.9
  due to blood loss (chronic) D50.0
    acute D62
  familial sex-linked D64.0
  pyridoxine-responsive D64.3
  sideroblastic, sex-linked D64.0
hypoplasia, red blood cells D61.9
  congenital or familial D61.01
hypoplastic (idiopathic) D61.9
  congenital or familial (of childhood) D61.01
hypoproliferative (refractive) D61.9
idiopathic D64.9
  aplastic D61.3
  hemolytic, chronic D59.9
in (due to) (with)
  chronic kidney disease D63.1
  end stage renal disease D63.1
  failure, kidney (renal) D63.1
  neoplastic disease — *see also* Neoplasm D63.0
intertropical — *see also* Ancylostomiasis D63.8
iron deficiency D50.9
  secondary to blood loss (chronic) D50.0
    acute D62
  specified type NEC D50.8
Joseph-Diamond-Blackfan (congenital hypoplastic)
  D61.01
Lederer's (hemolytic) D59.19
leukoerythroblastic D61.82
macrocytic D53.9
  nutritional D52.0
  tropical D52.8
malarial — *see also* Malaria B54 *[D63.8]*
malignant (progressive) D51.0
malnutrition D53.9
marsh — *see also* Malaria B54 *[D63.8]*
Mediterranean (with other hemoglobinopathy) D56.9
megaloblastic D53.1
  combined B12 and folate deficiency D53.1
  hereditary D51.1
  nutritional D52.0
  orotic aciduria D53.0
  refractory D53.1
  specified type NEC D53.1
megalocytic D53.1
microcytic (hypochromic) D50.9
  due to blood loss (chronic) D50.0
    acute D62
  familial D56.8
microdrepanocytosis D57.40
microelliptopoikilocytic (Rietti-Greppi- Micheli) D56.9
miner's B76.9 *[D63.8]*
myelodysplastic D46.9
myelofibrosis D75.81
myelogenous D64.89
myelopathic D64.89
myelophthisic D61.82
myeloproliferative D47.Z9 (*following* D47.4)
newborn P61.4
  due to
    ABO (antibodies, isoimmunization, maternal/fetal
      incompatibility) P55.1
    Rh (antibodies, isoimmunization, maternal/fetal
      incompatibility) P55.0
    following fetal blood loss P61.3
    posthemorrhagic (fetal) P61.3
nonspherocytic hemolytic — *see* Anemia, hemolytic,
  nonspherocytic
normocytic (infectional) D64.9
  due to blood loss (chronic) D50.0
    acute D62
  myelophthisic D61.82
nutritional (deficiency) D53.9

Anemia — *continued*
nutritional — *continued*
with
poor iron absorption D50.8
specified deficiency NEC D53.8
megaloblastic D52.0
of prematurity P61.2
orotaciduric (congenital) (hereditary) D53.0
osteosclerotic D64.89
ovalocytosis (hereditary) — *see* Elliptocytosis
paludal — *see also* Malaria B54 [D63.8]
pernicious (congenital) (malignant) (progressive) D51.0
pleochromic D64.89
of sprue D52.8
posthemorrhagic (chronic) D50.0
acute D62
newborn P61.3
postoperative (postprocedural)
due to (acute) blood loss D62
chronic blood loss D50.0
specified NEC D64.9
postpartum O90.81
pressure D64.89
progressive D64.9
malignant D51.0
pernicious D51.0
protein-deficiency D53.0
pseudoleukemica infantum D64.89
pure red cell D60.9
congenital D61.01
pyridoxine-responsive D64.3
pyruvate kinase deficiency D55.2
refractory D46.4
with
excess of blasts D46.20
1 (RAEB 1) D46.21
2 (RAEB 2) D46.22
in transformation (RAEB T) — *see* Leukemia,
acute myeloblastic
hemochromatosis D46.1
sideroblasts (ring) (RARS) D46.1
megaloblastic D53.1
sideroblastic D46.1
sideropenic D50.9
without ring sideroblasts, so stated D46.0
without sideroblasts without excess of blasts D46.0
Rietti-Greppi-Micheli D56.9
scorbutic D53.2
secondary to
blood loss (chronic) D50.0
acute D62
hemorrhage (chronic) D50.0
acute D62
semiplastic D61.89
sickle-cell — *see* Disease, sickle-cell
sideroblastic D64.3
hereditary D64.0
hypochromic, sex-linked D64.0
pyridoxine-responsive NEC D64.3
refractory D46.1
secondary (due to)
disease D64.1
drugs and toxins D64.2
specified type NEC D64.3
sideropenic (refractory) D50.9
due to blood loss (chronic) D50.0
acute D62
simple chronic D53.9
specified type NEC D64.89
spherocytic (hereditary) — *see* Spherocytosis
splenic D64.89
splenomegalic D64.89
stomatocytosis D58.8
syphilitic (acquired) (late) A52.79 [D63.8]
target cell D64.89
thalassemia D56.9
thrombocytopenic — *see* Thrombocytopenia
toxic D61.2
tropical B76.9 [D63.8]
macrocytic D52.8
tuberculous A18.89 [D63.8]
vegan D51.3
vitamin
B12 deficiency (dietary) pernicious D51.0
B6-responsive D64.3
von Jaksch's D64.89
Witts' (achlorhydric anemia) D50.8
Anemophobia F40.228

Anencephalus, anencephaly Q00.0
Anergasia — *see* Psychosis, organic
Anesthesia, anesthetic R20.0
complication or reaction NEC — *see also* Complications,
anesthesia T88.59 ☑
due to
correct substance properly administered — *see*
Table of Drugs and Chemicals, by drug,
adverse effect
overdose or wrong substance given — *see* Table
of Drugs and Chemicals, by drug, poisoning
unintended awareness under general anesthesia
during procedure T88.53 ☑
personal history of Z92.84
cornea H18.81- ☑
dissociative F44.6
functional (hysterical) F44.6
hyperesthetic, thalamic G89.0
hysterical F44.6
local skin lesion R20.0
sexual (psychogenic) F52.1
shock (due to) T88.2 ☑
skin R20.0
testicular N50.9
Anetoderma (maculosum) (of) L90.8
Jadassohn-Pellizzari L90.2
Schweniger-Buzzi L90.1
Aneurin deficiency E51.9
Aneurysm (anastomotic) (artery) (cirsoid) (diffuse) (false)
(fusiform) (multiple) (saccular) I72.9
abdominal (aorta) I71.4
ruptured I71.3
syphilitic A52.01
aorta, aortic (nonsyphilitic) I71.9
abdominal I71.4
ruptured I71.3
arch I71.2
ruptured I71.1
arteriosclerotic I71.9
ruptured I71.8
ascending I71.2
ruptured I71.1
congenital Q25.43
descending I71.9
abdominal I71.4
ruptured I71.3
ruptured I71.8
thoracic I71.2
ruptured I71.1
root Q25.43
ruptured I71.8
sinus, congenital Q25.43
syphilitic A52.01
thoracic I71.2
ruptured I71.1
thoracoabdominal I71.6
ruptured I71.5
thorax, thoracic (arch) I71.2
ruptured I71.1
transverse I71.2
ruptured I71.1
valve (heart) — *see also* Endocarditis, aortic I35.8
arteriosclerotic I72.9
cerebral I67.1
ruptured — *see* Hemorrhage, intracranial, subarachnoid
arteriovenous (congenital) — *see also* Malformation,
arteriovenous
acquired I77.0
brain I67.1
ruptured — *see* Aneurysm, arteriovenous,
brain, ruptured
coronary I25.41
pulmonary I28.0
brain Q28.2
ruptured I60.8
intracerebral I61.8
intraparenchymal I61.8
intraventricular I61.5
subarachnoid I60.8
peripheral — *see* Malformation, arteriovenous, peripheral
precerebral vessels Q28.0
specified site NEC — *see also* Malformation, arteriovenous
acquired I77.0
basal — *see* Aneurysm, brain

Aneurysm — *continued*
basilar (trunk) I72.5
berry (congenital) (nonruptured) I67.1
ruptured I60.7
brain I67.1
arteriosclerotic I67.1
ruptured — *see* Hemorrhage, intracranial, subarachnoid
arteriovenous (congenital) (nonruptured) Q28.2
acquired I67.1
ruptured — *see* Aneurysm, arteriovenous,
brain, ruptured I60.8-
ruptured — *see* Aneurysm, arteriovenous, brain,
ruptured I60.8-
berry (congenital) (nonruptured) I67.1
ruptured — *see also* Hemorrhage, intracranial,
subarachnoid I60.7
congenital Q28.3
ruptured I60.7
meninges I67.1
ruptured I60.8
miliary (congenital) (nonruptured) I67.1
ruptured — *see also* Hemorrhage, intracranial,
subarachnoid I60.7
mycotic I33.0
ruptured — *see* Aneurysm, arteriovenous, brain,
ruptured I60.8
syphilitic (hemorrhage) A52.05
cardiac (false) — *see also* Aneurysm, heart I25.3
carotid artery (common) (external) I72.0
internal (intracranial) I67.1
extracranial portion I72.0
ruptured into brain I60.0- ☑
syphilitic A52.09
intracranial A52.05
cavernous sinus I67.1
arteriovenous (congenital) (nonruptured) Q28.3
ruptured I60.8
celiac I72.8
central nervous system, syphilitic A52.05
cerebral — *see* Aneurysm, brain
chest — *see* Aneurysm, thorax
circle of Willis I67.1
congenital Q28.3
ruptured I60.6
ruptured I60.6
common iliac artery I72.3
congenital (peripheral) Q27.8
aorta (root) (sinus) Q25.43
brain Q28.3
ruptured I60.7
coronary Q24.5
digestive system Q27.8
lower limb Q27.8
pulmonary Q25.79
retina Q14.1
specified site NEC Q27.8
upper limb Q27.8
conjunctiva — *see* Abnormality, conjunctiva, vascular
conus arteriosus — *see* Aneurysm, heart
coronary (arteriosclerotic) (artery) I25.41
arteriovenous, congenital Q24.5
congenital Q24.5
ruptured — *see* Infarct, myocardium
syphilitic A52.06
vein I25.89
cylindroid (aorta) I71.9
ruptured I71.8
syphilitic A52.01
ductus arteriosus Q25.0
endocardial, infective (any valve) I33.0
femoral (artery) (ruptured) I72.4
gastroduodenal I72.8
gastroepiploic I72.8
heart (wall) (chronic or with a stated duration of over
4 weeks) I25.3
valve — *see* Endocarditis
hepatic I72.8
iliac (common) (artery) (ruptured) I72.3
infective I72.9
endocardial (any valve) I33.0
innominate (nonsyphilitic) I72.8
syphilitic A52.09
interauricular septum — *see* Aneurysm, heart
interventricular septum — *see* Aneurysm, heart
intrathoracic (nonsyphilitic) I71.2
ruptured I71.1
syphilitic A52.01

☑ **Additional Character Required — Refer to the Tabular List for Character Selection** ▽ **Subterms under main terms may continue to next column or page**

Aneurysm — *continued*
lower limb I72.4
lung (pulmonary artery) I28.1
mediastinal (nonsyphilitic) I72.8
syphilitic A52.09
miliary (congenital) I67.1
ruptured — *see* Hemorrhage, intracerebral, subarachnoid, intracranial
mitral (heart) (valve) I34.8
mural — *see* Aneurysm, heart
mycotic I72.9
endocardial (any valve) I33.0
ruptured, brain — *see* Hemorrhage, intracerebral,
subarachnoid
myocardium — *see* Aneurysm, heart
neck I72.0
pancreaticoduodenal I72.8
patent ductus arteriosus Q25.0
peripheral NEC I72.8
congenital Q27.8
digestive system Q27.8
lower limb Q27.8
specified site NEC Q27.8
upper limb Q27.8
popliteal (artery) (ruptured) I72.4
precerebral
congenital (nonruptured) Q28.1
specified site, NEC I72.5
pulmonary I28.1
arteriovenous Q25.72
acquired I28.0
syphilitic A52.09
valve (heart) — *see* Endocarditis, pulmonary
racemose (peripheral) I72.9
congenital — *see* Aneurysm, congenital
radial I72.1
Rasmussen NEC A15.0
renal (artery) I72.2
retina — *see also* Disorder, retina, microaneurysms
congenital Q14.1
diabetic — *see* E08-E13 with .3-
sinus of Valsalva Q25.49
specified NEC I72.8
spinal (cord) I72.8
syphilitic (hemorrhage) A52.09
splenic I72.8
subclavian (artery) (ruptured) I72.8
syphilitic A52.09
superior mesenteric I72.8
syphilitic (aorta) A52.01
central nervous system A52.05
congenital (late) A50.54 [I79.0]
spine, spinal A52.09
thoracoabdominal (aorta) I71.6
ruptured I71.5
syphilitic A52.01
thorax, thoracic (aorta) (arch) (nonsyphilitic) I71.2
ruptured I71.1
syphilitic A52.01
traumatic (complication) (early), specified site — *see*
Injury, blood vessel
tricuspid (heart) (valve) I07.8
ulnar I72.1
upper limb (ruptured) I72.1
valve, valvular — *see* Endocarditis
venous — *see also* Varix I86.8
congenital Q27.8
digestive system Q27.8
lower limb Q27.8
specified site NEC Q27.8
upper limb Q27.8
ventricle — *see* Aneurysm, heart
vertebral artery I72.6
visceral NEC I72.8
Angelman syndrome Q93.51
Anger R45.4
Angiectasis, angiectopia I99.8
Angiitis I77.6
allergic granulomatous M30.1
hypersensitivity M31.0
necrotizing M31.9
specified NEC M31.8
nervous system, granulomatous I67.7
Angina (attack) (cardiac) (chest) (heart) (pectoris) (syndrome) (vasomotor) I20.9
with
atherosclerotic heart disease — *see* Arteriosclerosis,
coronary (artery),

Angina — *continued*
with — *continued*
documented spasm I20.1
abdominal K55.1
accelerated — *see* Angina, unstable
agranulocytic — *see* Agranulocytosis
angiospastic — *see* Angina, with documented spasm
aphthous B08.5
crescendo — *see* Angina, unstable
croupous J05.0
cruris I73.9
de novo effort — *see* Angina, unstable
diphtheritic, membranous A36.0
equivalent I20.8
exudative, chronic J37.0
following acute myocardial infarction I23.7
gangrenous diphtheritic A36.0
intestinal K55.1
Ludovici K12.2
Ludwig's K12.2
malignant diphtheritic A36.0
membranous J05.0
diphtheritic A36.0
Vincent's A69.1
mesenteric K55.1
monocytic — *see* Mononucleosis, infectious
of effort — *see* Angina, specified NEC
phlegmonous J36
diphtheritic A36.0
post-infarctional I23.7
pre-infarctional — *see* Angina, unstable
Prinzmetal — *see* Angina, with documented spasm
progressive — *see* Angina, unstable
pseudomembranous A69.1
pultaceous, diphtheritic A36.0
spasm-induced — *see* Angina, with documented spasm
specified NEC I20.8
stable I20.8
stenocardia — *see* Angina, specified NEC
stridulous, diphtheritic A36.2
tonsil J36
trachealis J05.0
unstable I20.0
variant — *see* Angina, with documented spasm
Vincent's A69.1
worsening effort — *see* Angina, unstable
Angioblastoma — *see* Neoplasm, connective tissue,
uncertain behavior
Angiocholecystitis — *see* Cholecystitis, acute
Angiocholitis — *see also* Cholecystitis, acute K83.09
Angiodysgenesis spinalis G95.19
Angiodysplasia (cecum) (colon) K55.20
with bleeding K55.21
duodenum (and stomach) K31.819
with bleeding K31.811
stomach (and duodenum) K31.819
with bleeding K31.811
Angioedema (allergic) (any site) (with urticaria) T78.3 ☑
episodic, with eosinophilia D72.118
hereditary D84.1
Angioendothelioma — *see* Neoplasm, uncertain behavior, by site
benign D18.00
intra-abdominal D18.03
intracranial D18.02
skin D18.01
specified site NEC D18.09
bone — *see* Neoplasm, bone, malignant
Ewing's — *see* Neoplasm, bone, malignant
Angioendotheliomatosis C85.8- ☑
Angiofibroma — *see also* Neoplasm, benign, by site
juvenile
specified site — *see* Neoplasm, benign, by site
unspecified site D10.6
Angiohemophilia (A) (B) D68.0
Angioid streaks (choroid) (macula) (retina) H35.33
Angiokeratoma — *see* Neoplasm, skin, benign
corporis diffusum E75.21
Angioleiomyoma — *see* Neoplasm, connective tissue,
benign
Angiolipoma — *see also* Lipoma
infiltrating — *see* Lipoma
Angioma — *see also* Hemangioma, by site
capillary I78.1
hemorrhagicum hereditaria I78.0
intra-abdominal D18.03
intracranial D18.02

Angioma — *continued*
malignant — *see* Neoplasm, connective tissue, malignant
plexiform D18.00
intra-abdominal D18.03
intracranial D18.02
skin D18.01
specified site NEC D18.09
senile I78.1
serpiginosum L81.7
skin D18.01
specified site NEC D18.09
spider I78.1
stellate I78.1
venous Q28.3
Angiomatosis Q82.8
bacillary A79.89
encephalotrigeminal Q85.8
hemorrhagic familial I78.0
hereditary familial I78.0
liver K76.4
Angiomyolipoma — *see* Lipoma
Angiomyoliposarcoma — *see* Neoplasm, connective
tissue, malignant
Angiomyoma — *see* Neoplasm, connective tissue, benign
Angiomyosarcoma — *see* Neoplasm, connective tissue,
malignant
Angiomyxoma — *see* Neoplasm, connective tissue, uncertain behavior
Angioneurosis F45.8
Angioneurotic edema (allergic) (any site) (with urticaria)
T78.3 ☑
hereditary D84.1
Angiopathia, angiopathy I99.9
cerebral I67.9
amyloid E85.4 [I68.0]
diabetic (peripheral) — *see* Diabetes, angiopathy
peripheral I73.9
diabetic — *see* Diabetes, angiopathy
specified type NEC I73.89
retinae syphilitica A52.05
retinalis (juvenilis)
diabetic — *see* Diabetes, retinopathy
proliferative — *see* Retinopathy, proliferative
Angiosarcoma — *see also* Neoplasm, connective tissue,
malignant
liver C22.3
Angiosclerosis — *see* Arteriosclerosis
Angiospasm (peripheral) (traumatic) (vessel) I73.9
brachial plexus G54.0
cerebral G45.9
cervical plexus G54.2
nerve
arm — *see* Mononeuropathy, upper limb
axillary G54.0
median — *see* Lesion, nerve, median
ulnar — *see* Lesion, nerve, ulnar
axillary G54.0
leg — *see* Mononeuropathy, lower limb
median — *see* Lesion, nerve, median
plantar — *see* Lesion, nerve, plantar
ulnar — *see* Lesion, nerve, ulnar
Angiospastic disease or edema I73.9
Angiostrongyliasis
due to
Parastrongylus
cantonensis B83.2
costaricensis B81.3
intestinal B81.3
Anguillulosis — *see* Strongyloidiasis
Angulation
cecum — *see* Obstruction, intestine
coccyx (acquired) — *see also* subcategory M43.8 ☑
congenital NEC Q76.49
femur (acquired) — *see also* Deformity, limb, specified
type NEC, thigh
congenital Q74.2
intestine (large) (small) — *see* Obstruction, intestine
sacrum (acquired) — *see also* subcategory M43.8 ☑
congenital NEC Q76.49
sigmoid (flexure) — *see* Obstruction, intestine
spine — *see* Dorsopathy, deforming, specified NEC
tibia (acquired) — *see also* Deformity, limb, specified
type NEC, lower leg
congenital Q74.2
ureter N13.5
with infection N13.6

Angulation — *continued*
  wrist (acquired) — *see also* Deformity, limb, specified
    type NEC, forearm
    congenital Q74.0
Angulus infectiosus (lips) K13.0
Anhedonia R45.84
  sexual F52.0
Anhidrosis L74.4
Anhydration E86.0
Anhydremia E86.0
Anidrosis L74.4
Aniridia (congenital) Q13.1
Anisakiasis (infection) (infestation) B81.0
Anisakis larvae infestation B81.0
Aniseikonia H52.32
Anisocoria (pupil) H57.02
  congenital Q13.2
Anisocytosis R71.8
Anisometropia (congenital) H52.31
Ankle — *see* condition
Ankyloblepharon (eyelid) (acquired) — *see also* Blepharophimosis
  filiforme (adnatum) (congenital) Q10.3
  total Q10.3
Ankyloglossia Q38.1
Ankylosis (fibrous) (osseous) (joint) M24.60
  ankle M24.67- ☑
  arthrodesis status Z98.1
  cricoarytenoid (cartilage) (joint) (larynx) J38.7
  dental K03.5
  ear ossicles H74.31- ☑
  elbow M24.62- ☑
  foot M24.67- ☑
  hand M24.64- ☑
  hip M24.65- ☑
  incostapedial joint (infectional) — *see* Ankylosis, ear
    ossicles
  jaw (temporomandibular) M26.61- ☑
  knee M24.66- ☑
  lumbosacral (joint) M43.27
  postoperative (status) Z98.1
  produced by surgical fusion, status Z98.1
  sacro-iliac (joint) M43.28
  shoulder M24.61- ☑
  specified site NEC M24.69
  spine (joint) — *see also* Fusion, spine
    spondylitic — *see* Spondylitis, ankylosing
  surgical Z98.1
  temporomandibular M26.61- ☑
  tooth, teeth (hard tissues) K03.5
  wrist M24.63- ☑
Ankylostoma — *see* Ancylostoma
Ankylostomiasis — *see* Ancylostomiasis
Ankylurethria — *see* Stricture, urethra
Annular — *see also* condition
  detachment, cervix N88.8
  organ or site, congenital NEC — *see* Distortion
  pancreas (congenital) Q45.1
Anodontia (complete) (partial) (vera) K00.0
  acquired K08.10 ☑
Anomaly, anomalous (congenital) (unspecified type)
    Q89.9
  abdominal wall NEC Q79.59
  acoustic nerve Q07.8
  adrenal (gland) Q89.1
  Alder (-Reilly) (leukocyte granulation) D72.0)
  alimentary tract Q45.9
    upper Q40.9
  alveolar M26.70
    hyperplasia M26.79
      mandibular M26.72
      maxillary M26.71
    hypoplasia M26.79
      mandibular M26.74
      maxillary M26.73
    ridge (process) M26.79
    specified NEC M26.79
  ankle (joint) Q74.2
  anus Q43.9
  aorta (arch) NEC Q25.40
    coarctation (preductal) (postductal) Q25.1
  aortic cusp or valve Q23.9
  appendix Q43.8
  apple peel syndrome Q41.1
  aqueduct of Sylvius Q03.0
    with spina bifida — *see* Spina bifida, with hydrocephalus

Anomaly, anomalous — *continued*
  arm Q74.0
  arteriovenous NEC
    coronary Q24.5
    gastrointestinal Q27.33
      acquired — *see* Angiodysplasia
  artery (peripheral) Q27.9
    basilar NEC Q28.1
    cerebral Q28.3
    coronary Q24.5
    digestive system Q27.8
    eye Q15.8
    great Q25.9
      specified NEC Q25.8
    lower limb Q27.8
    peripheral Q27.9
      specified NEC Q27.8
    pulmonary NEC Q25.79
    renal Q27.2
    retina Q14.1
    specified site NEC Q27.8
    subclavian Q27.8
      origin Q25.48
    umbilical Q27.0
    upper limb Q27.8
    vertebral NEC Q28.1
  aryteno-epiglottic folds Q31.8
  atrial
    bands or folds Q20.8
    septa Q21.1
  atrioventricular
    excitation I45.6
    septum Q21.0
  auditory canal Q17.8
  auricle
    ear Q17.8
      causing impairment of hearing Q16.9
    heart Q20.8
  Axenfeld's Q15.0
  back Q89.9
  band
    atrial Q20.8
    heart Q24.8
    ventricular Q24.8
  Bartholin's duct Q38.4
  biliary duct or passage Q44.5
  bladder Q64.70
    absence Q64.5
    diverticulum Q64.6
    exstrophy Q64.10
      cloacal Q64.12
      extroversion Q64.19
      specified type NEC Q64.19
      supravesical fissure Q64.11
    neck obstruction Q64.31
    specified type NEC Q64.79
  bone Q79.9
    arm Q74.0
    face Q75.9
    leg Q74.2
    pelvic girdle Q74.2
    shoulder girdle Q74.0
    skull Q75.9
      with
        anencephaly Q00.0
        encephalocele — *see* Encephalocele
        hydrocephalus Q03.9
          with spina bifida — *see* Spina bifida, by
          site, with hydrocephalus
        microcephaly Q02
  brain (multiple) Q04.9
    vessel Q28.3
  breast Q83.9
  broad ligament Q50.6
  bronchus Q32.4
  bulbus cordis Q21.9
  bursa Q79.9
  canal of Nuck Q52.4
  canthus Q10.3
  capillary Q27.9
  cardiac Q24.9
    chambers Q20.9
      specified NEC Q20.8
    septal closure Q21.9
      specified NEC Q21.8
    valve NEC Q24.8
      pulmonary Q22.3
  cardiovascular system Q28.8
  carpus Q74.0

Anomaly, anomalous — *continued*
  caruncle, lacrimal Q10.6
  cascade stomach Q40.2
  cauda equina Q06.3
  cecum Q43.9
  cerebral Q04.9
    vessels Q28.3
  cervix Q51.9
  Chédiak-Higashi (-Steinbrinck) (congenital gigantism
    of peroxidase granules) E70.330
  cheek Q18.9
  chest wall Q67.8
    bones Q76.9
  chin Q18.9
  chordae tendineae Q24.8
  choroid Q14.3
    plexus Q07.8
  chromosomes, chromosomal Q99.9
    D (1) — *see* condition, chromosome 13
    E (3) — *see* condition, chromosome 18
    G — *see* condition, chromosome 21
    sex
      female phenotype Q97.8
      gonadal dysgenesis (pure) Q99.1
      Klinefelter's Q98.4
      male phenotype Q98.9
      Turner's Q96.9
    specified NEC Q99.8
  cilia Q10.3
  circulatory system Q28.9
  clavicle Q74.0
  clitoris Q52.6
  coccyx Q76.49
  colon Q43.9
  common duct Q44.5
  communication
    coronary artery Q24.5
    left ventricle with right atrium Q21.0
  concha (ear) Q17.3
  connection
    portal vein Q26.5
    pulmonary venous Q26.4
      partial Q26.3
      total Q26.2
    renal artery with kidney Q27.2
  cornea (shape) Q13.4
  coronary artery or vein Q24.5
  cranium — *see* Anomaly, skull
  cricoid cartilage Q31.8
  cystic duct Q44.5
  dental
    alveolar — *see* Anomaly, alveolar
    arch relationship M26.20
      specified NEC M26.29
  dentofacial M26.9
    alveolar — *see* Anomaly, alveolar
    dental arch relationship M26.20
      specified NEC M26.29
    functional M26.50
      specified NEC M26.59
    jaw size M26.00
      macrogenia M26.05
      mandibular
        hyperplasia M26.03
        hypoplasia M26.04
      maxillary
        hyperplasia M26.01
        hypoplasia M26.02
      microgenia M26.06
      specified type NEC M26.09
    jaw-cranial base relationship M26.10
      asymmetry M26.12
        maxillary M26.11
      specified type NEC M26.19
    malocclusion M26.4
      dental arch relationship NEC M26.29
      jaw size — *see* Anomaly, dentofacial, jaw size
      jaw-cranial base relationship — *see* Anomaly,
        dentofacial, jaw-cranial base relationship
    specified type NEC M26.89
    temporomandibular joint M26.60- ☑
      adhesions M26.61- ☑
      ankylosis M26.61- ☑
      arthralgia M26.62- ☑
      articular disc M26.63- ☑
      specified type NEC M26.69
    tooth position, fully erupted M26.30
      specified NEC M26.39

Anomaly, anomalous — *continued*
  dermatoglyphic Q82.8
  diaphragm (apertures) NEC Q79.1
  digestive organ(s) or tract Q45.9
    lower Q43.9
    upper Q40.9
  distance, interarch (excessive) (inadequate) M26.25
  distribution, coronary artery Q24.5
  ductus
    arteriosus Q25.0
    botalli Q25.0
  duodenum Q43.9
  dura (brain) Q04.9
    spinal cord Q06.9
  ear (external) Q17.9
    causing impairment of hearing Q16.9
    inner Q16.5
    middle (causing impairment of hearing) Q16.4
      ossicles Q16.3
  Ebstein's (heart) (tricuspid valve) Q22.5
  ectodermal Q82.9
  ejaculatory duct Q55.4
  elbow Q74.0
  endocrine gland NEC Q89.2
  epididymis Q55.4
  epiglottis Q31.8
  esophagus Q39.9
  eustachian tube Q17.8
  eye Q15.9
    anterior segment Q13.9
      specified NEC Q13.89
    posterior segment Q14.9
      specified NEC Q14.8
    ptosis (eyelid) Q10.0
    specified NEC Q15.8
  eyebrow Q18.8
  eyelid Q10.3
    ptosis Q10.0
  face Q18.9
    bone(s) Q75.9
  fallopian tube Q50.6
  fascia Q79.9
  femur NEC Q74.2
  fibula NEC Q74.2
  finger Q74.0
  fixation, intestine Q43.3
  flexion (joint) NOS Q74.9
    hip or thigh Q65.89
  foot NEC Q74.2
    varus (congenital) Q66.3- ☑
  foramen
    Botalli Q21.1
    ovale Q21.1
  forearm Q74.0
  forehead Q75.8
  form, teeth K00.2
  fovea centralis Q14.1
  frontal bone — *see* Anomaly, skull
  gallbladder (position) (shape) (size) Q44.1
  Gartner's duct Q52.4
  gastrointestinal tract Q45.9
  genitalia, genital organ(s) or system
    female Q52.9
      external Q52.70
      internal NOS Q52.9
    male Q55.9
      hydrocele P83.5
      specified NEC Q55.8
  genitourinary NEC
    female Q52.9
    male Q55.9
  Gerbode Q21.0
  glottis Q31.8
  granulation or granulocyte, genetic (constitutional) (leukocyte) D72.0
  gum Q38.6
  gyri Q07.9
  hair Q84.2
  hand Q74.0
  hard tissue formation in pulp K04.3
  head — *see* Anomaly, skull
  heart Q24.9
    auricle Q20.8
    bands or folds Q24.8
    fibroelastosis cordis I42.4
    obstructive NEC Q22.6
    patent ductus arteriosus (Botalli) Q25.0
    septum Q21.9

Anomaly, anomalous — *continued*
  heart — *continued*
    septum — *continued*
      auricular Q21.1
      interatrial Q21.1
      interventricular Q21.0
        with pulmonary stenosis or atresia, dextraposition of aorta and hypertrophy of right ventricle Q21.3
      specified NEC Q21.8
      ventricular Q21.0
        with pulmonary stenosis or atresia, dextraposition of aorta and hypertrophy of right ventricle Q21.3
    tetralogy of Fallot Q21.3
    valve NEC Q24.8
      aortic
        bicuspid valve Q23.1
        insufficiency Q23.1
        stenosis Q23.0
          subaortic Q24.4
      mitral
        insufficiency Q23.3
        stenosis Q23.2
      pulmonary Q22.3
        atresia Q22.0
        insufficiency Q22.2
        stenosis Q22.1
          infundibular Q24.3
          subvalvular Q24.3
      tricuspid
        atresia Q22.4
        stenosis Q22.4
    ventricle Q20.8
  heel NEC Q74.2
  Hegglin's D72.0
  hemianencephaly Q00.0
  hemicephaly Q00.0
  hemicrania Q00.0
  hepatic duct Q44.5
  hip NEC Q74.2
  hourglass stomach Q40.2
  humerus Q74.0
  hydatid of Morgagni
    female Q50.5
    male (epididymal) Q55.4
      testicular Q55.29
  hymen Q52.4
  hypersegmentation of neutrophils, hereditary D72.0
  hypophyseal Q89.2
  ileocecal (coil) (valve) Q43.9
  ileum Q43.9
  ilium NEC Q74.2
  integument Q84.9
    specified NEC Q84.8
  interarch distance (excessive) (inadequate) M26.25
  intervertebral cartilage or disc Q76.49
  intestine (large) (small) Q43.9
    with anomalous adhesions, fixation or malrotation Q43.3
  iris Q13.2
  ischium NEC Q74.2
  jaw — *see* Anomaly, dentofacial
    alveolar — *see* Anomaly, alveolar
  jaw-cranial base relationship — *see* Anomaly, dentofacial, jaw-cranial base relationship
  jejunum Q43.8
  joint Q74.9
    specified NEC Q74.8
  Jordan's D72.0
  kidney(s) (calyx) (pelvis) Q63.9
    artery Q27.2
    specified NEC Q63.8
  Klippel-Feil (brevicollis) Q76.1
  knee Q74.1
  labium (majus) (minus) Q52.70
  labyrinth, membranous Q16.5
  lacrimal apparatus or duct Q10.6
  larynx, laryngeal (muscle) Q31.9
    web (bed) Q31.0
  lens Q12.9
  leukocytes, genetic D72.0
    granulation (constitutional) D72.0
  lid (fold) Q10.3
  ligament Q79.9
    broad Q50.6
    round Q52.8
  limb Q74.9
    lower NEC Q74.2

Anomaly, anomalous — *continued*
  limb — *continued*
    lower — *continued*
      reduction deformity — *see* Defect, reduction, lower limb
    upper Q74.0
  lip Q38.0
  liver Q44.7
    duct Q44.5
  lower limb NEC Q74.2
  lumbosacral (joint) (region) Q76.49
    kyphosis — *see* Kyphosis, congenital
    lordosis — *see* Lordosis, congenital
  lung (fissure) (lobe) Q33.9
  mandible — *see* Anomaly, dentofacial
  maxilla — *see* Anomaly, dentofacial
  May (-Hegglin) D72.0
  meatus urinarius NEC Q64.79
  meningeal bands or folds Q07.9
    constriction of Q07.8
    spinal Q06.9
  meninges Q07.9
    cerebral Q04.8
    spinal Q06.9
  meningocele Q05.9
  mesentery Q45.9
  metacarpus Q74.0
  metatarsus NEC Q74.2
  middle ear Q16.4
    ossicles Q16.3
  mitral (leaflets) (valve) Q23.9
    insufficiency Q23.3
    specified NEC Q23.8
    stenosis Q23.2
  mouth Q38.6
  Müllerian — *see also* Anomaly, by site
    uterus NEC Q51.818
  multiple NEC Q89.7
  muscle Q79.9
    eyelid Q10.3
  musculoskeletal system, except limbs Q79.9
  myocardium Q24.8
  nail Q84.6
  narrowness, eyelid Q10.3
  nasal sinus (wall) Q30.8
  neck (any part) Q18.9
  nerve Q07.9
    acoustic Q07.8
    optic Q07.8
  nervous system (central) Q07.9
  nipple Q83.9
  nose, nasal (bones) (cartilage) (septum) (sinus) Q30.9
    specified NEC Q30.8
  ocular muscle Q15.8
  omphalomesenteric duct Q43.0
  opening, pulmonary veins Q26.4
  optic
    disc Q14.2
    nerve Q07.8
  opticociliary vessels Q13.2
  orbit (eye) Q10.7
  organ Q89.9
    of Corti Q16.5
  origin
    artery
      innominate Q25.8
      pulmonary Q25.79
      renal Q27.2
      subclavian Q25.48
  osseous meatus (ear) Q16.1
  ovary Q50.39
  oviduct Q50.6
  palate (hard) (soft) NEC Q38.5
  pancreas or pancreatic duct Q45.3
  papillary muscles Q24.8
  parathyroid gland Q89.2
  paraurethral ducts Q64.79
  parotid (gland) Q38.4
  patella Q74.1
  Pelger-Huët (hereditary hyposegmentation) D72.0
  pelvic girdle NEC Q74.2
  pelvis (bony) NEC Q74.2
    rachitic E64.3
  penis (glans) Q55.69
  pericardium Q24.8
  peripheral vascular system Q27.9
  Peter's Q13.4
  pharynx Q38.8
  pigmentation L81.9

Anomaly, anomalous — *continued*
  pigmentation — *continued*
    congenital Q82.8
  pituitary (gland) Q89.2
  pleural (folds) Q34.0
  portal vein Q26.5
    connection Q26.5
  position, tooth, teeth, fully erupted M26.30
    specified NEC M26.39
  precerebral vessel Q28.1
  prepuce Q55.69
  prostate Q55.4
  pulmonary Q33.9
    artery NEC Q25.79
    valve Q22.3
      atresia Q22.0
      insufficiency Q22.2
      specified type NEC Q22.3
      stenosis Q22.1
        infundibular Q24.3
        subvalvular Q24.3
    venous connection Q26.4
      partial Q26.3
      total Q26.2
  pupil Q13.2
    function H57.00
      anisocoria H57.02
      Argyll Robertson pupil H57.01
      miosis H57.03
      mydriasis H57.04
      specified type NEC H57.09
      tonic pupil H57.05- ☑
  pylorus Q40.3
  radius Q74.0
  rectum Q43.9
  reduction (extremity) (limb)
    femur (longitudinal) — *see* Defect, reduction, lower limb, longitudinal, femur
    fibula (longitudinal) — *see* Defect, reduction, lower limb, longitudinal, fibula
    lower limb — *see* Defect, reduction, lower limb
    radius (longitudinal) — *see* Defect, reduction, upper limb, longitudinal, radius
    tibia (longitudinal) — *see* Defect, reduction, lower limb, longitudinal, tibia
    ulna (longitudinal) — *see* Defect, reduction, upper limb, longitudinal, ulna
    upper limb — *see* Defect, reduction, upper limb
  refraction — *see* Disorder, refraction
  renal Q63.9
    artery Q27.2
    pelvis Q63.9
      specified NEC Q63.8
  respiratory system Q34.9
    specified NEC Q34.8
  retina Q14.1
  rib Q76.6
    cervical Q76.5
  Rieger's Q13.81
  rotation — *see* Malrotation
    hip or thigh Q65.89
  round ligament Q52.8
  sacroiliac (joint) NEC Q74.2
  sacrum NEC Q76.49
    kyphosis — *see* Kyphosis, congenital
    lordosis — *see* Lordosis, congenital
  saddle nose, syphilitic A50.57
  salivary duct or gland Q38.4
  scapula Q74.0
  scrotum — *see* Malformation, testis and scrotum
  sebaceous gland Q82.9
  seminal vesicles Q55.4
  sense organs NEC Q07.8
  sex chromosomes NEC — *see also* Anomaly, chromosomes
    female phenotype Q97.8
    male phenotype Q98.9
  shoulder (girdle) (joint) Q74.0
  sigmoid (flexure) Q43.9
  simian crease Q82.8
  sinus of Valsalva Q25.49
  skeleton generalized Q78.9
  skin (appendage) Q82.9
  skull Q75.9
    with
      anencephaly Q00.0
      encephalocele — *see* Encephalocele
      hydrocephalus Q03.9

Anomaly, anomalous — *continued*
  skull — *continued*
    with — *continued*
      hydrocephalus — *continued*
        with spina bifida — *see* Spina bifida, by site, with hydrocephalus
      microcephaly Q02
  specified organ or site NEC Q89.8
  spermatic cord Q55.4
  spine, spinal NEC Q76.49
    column NEC Q76.49
      kyphosis — *see* Kyphosis, congenital
      lordosis — *see* Lordosis, congenital
    cord Q06.9
    nerve root Q07.8
  spleen Q89.09
    agenesis Q89.01
  stenonian duct Q38.4
  sternum NEC Q76.7
  stomach Q40.3
  submaxillary gland Q38.4
  tarsus NEC Q74.2
  tendon Q79.9
  testis — *see* Malformation, testis and scrotum
  thigh NEC Q74.2
  thorax (wall) Q67.8
    bony Q76.9
  throat Q38.8
  thumb Q74.0
  thymus gland Q89.2
  thyroid (gland) Q89.2
    cartilage Q31.8
  tibia NEC Q74.2
    saber A50.56
  toe Q74.0
  tongue Q38.3
  tooth, teeth K00.9
    eruption K00.6
    position, fully erupted M26.30
    spacing, fully erupted M26.30
  trachea (cartilage) Q32.1
  tragus Q17.9
  tricuspid (leaflet) (valve) Q22.9
    atresia or stenosis Q22.4
    Ebstein's Q22.5
  Uhl's (hypoplasia of myocardium, right ventricle) Q24.8
  ulna Q74.0
  umbilical artery Q27.0
  union
    cricoid cartilage and thyroid cartilage Q31.8
    thyroid cartilage and hyoid bone Q31.8
    trachea with larynx Q31.8
  upper limb Q74.0
  urachus Q64.4
  ureter Q62.8
    obstructive NEC Q62.39
      cecoureterocele Q62.32
      orthotopic ureterocele Q62.31
  urethra Q64.70
    absence Q64.5
    double Q64.74
    fistula to rectum Q64.73
    obstructive Q64.39
      stricture Q64.32
    prolapse Q64.71
    specified type NEC Q64.79
  urinary tract Q64.9
  uterus Q51.9
    with only one functioning horn Q51.4
  uvula Q38.5
  vagina Q52.4
  valleculae Q31.8
  valve (heart) NEC Q24.8
    coronary sinus Q24.5
    inferior vena cava Q24.8
    pulmonary Q22.3
    sinus coronario Q24.5
    venae cavae inferioris Q24.8
  vas deferens Q55.4
  vascular Q27.9
    brain Q28.3
    ring Q25.45
  vein(s) (peripheral) Q27.9
    brain Q28.3
    cerebral Q28.3
    coronary Q24.5
    developmental Q28.3
    great Q26.9
      specified NEC Q26.8

Anomaly, anomalous — *continued*
  vena cava (inferior) (superior) Q26.9
  venous — *see* Anomaly, vein(s)
  venous return Q26.8
  ventricular
    bands or folds Q24.8
    septa Q21.0
  vertebra Q76.49
    kyphosis — *see* Kyphosis, congenital
    lordosis — *see* Lordosis, congenital
  vesicourethral orifice Q64.79
  vessel(s) Q27.9
    optic papilla Q14.2
    precerebral Q28.1
  vitelline duct Q43.0
  vitreous body or humor Q14.0
  vulva Q52.70
  wrist (joint) Q74.0
Anomia R48.8
Anonychia (congenital) Q84.3
  acquired L60.8
Anophthalmos, anophthalmus (congenital) (globe) Q11.1
  acquired Z90.01
Anopia, anopsia H53.46- ☑
  quadrant H53.46- ☑
Anorchia, anorchism, anorchidism Q55.0
Anorexia R63.0
  hysterical F44.89
  nervosa F50.00
    atypical F50.9
    binge-eating type F50.2
      with purging F50.02
    restricting type F50.01
Anorgasmy, psychogenic (female) F52.31
  male F52.32
Anosmia R43.0
  hysterical F44.6
  postinfectional J39.8
Anosognosia R41.89
Anosteoplasia Q78.9
Anovulatory cycle N97.0
Anoxemia R09.02
  newborn P84
Anoxia (pathological) R09.02
  altitude T70.29 ☑
  cerebral G93.1
    complicating
      anesthesia (general) (local) or other sedation T88.59 ☑
        in labor and delivery O74.3
        in pregnancy O29.21- ☑
        postpartum, puerperal O89.2
      delivery (cesarean) (instrumental) O75.4
    during a procedure G97.81
    newborn P84
    resulting from a procedure G97.82
    due to
      drowning T75.1 ☑
      high altitude T70.29 ☑
  heart — *see* Insufficiency, coronary
  intrauterine P84
  myocardial — *see* Insufficiency, coronary
  newborn P84
  spinal cord G95.11
  systemic (by suffocation) (low content in atmosphere) — *see* Asphyxia, traumatic
Anteflexion — *see* Anteversion
Antenatal
  care (normal pregnancy) Z34.90
  screening (encounter for) of mother — *see also* Encounter, antenatal screening Z36.9
Antepartum — *see* condition
Anterior — *see* condition
Antero-occlusion M26.220
Anteversion
  cervix — *see* Anteversion, uterus
  femur (neck), congenital Q65.89
  uterus, uterine (cervix) (postinfectional) (postpartal, old) N85.4
    congenital Q51.818
    in pregnancy or childbirth — *see* Pregnancy, complicated by
Anthophobia F40.228
Anthracosilicosis J60
Anthracosis (lung) (occupational) J60
  lingua K14.3

Anthrax A22.9
  with pneumonia A22.1
  cerebral A22.8
  colitis A22.2
  cutaneous A22.0
  gastrointestinal A22.2
  inhalation A22.1
  intestinal A22.2
  meningitis A22.8
  pulmonary A22.1
  respiratory A22.1
  sepsis A22.7
  specified manifestation NEC A22.8
Anthropoid pelvis Q74.2
  with disproportion (fetopelvic) O33.0
Anthropophobia F40.10
  generalized F40.11
Antibodies, maternal (blood group) — *see* Isoimmuniza-
    tion, affecting management of pregnancy
  anti-D — *see* Isoimmunization, affecting management
    of pregnancy, Rh
  newborn P55.0
Antibody
  anticardiolipin R76.0
    with
      hemorrhagic disorder D68.312
      hypercoagulable state D68.61
  antiphosphatidylglycerol R76.0
    with
      hemorrhagic disorder D68.312
      hypercoagulable state D68.61
  antiphosphatidylinositol R76.0
    with
      hemorrhagic disorder D68.312
      hypercoagulable state D68.61
  antiphosphatidylserine R76.0
    with
      hemorrhagic disorder D68.312
      hypercoagulable state D68.61
  antiphospholipid R76.0
    with
      hemorrhagic disorder D68.312
      hypercoagulable state D68.61
Anticardiolipin syndrome D68.61
Anticoagulant, circulating (intrinsic) — *see also* Disor-
    der, hemorrhagic D68.318
  drug-induced (extrinsic) — *see also* Disorder, hemor-
    rhagic D68.32
  iatrogenic D68.32
Antidiuretic hormone syndrome E22.2
Antimonial cholera — *see* Poisoning, antimony
Antiphospholipid
  antibody
    with hemorrhagic disorder D68.312
    syndrome D68.61
Antisocial personality F60.2
Antithrombinemia — *see* Circulating anticoagulants
Antithromboplastinemia D68.318
Antithromboplastinogenemia D68.318
Antitoxin complication or reaction — *see* Complica-
    tions, vaccination
Antlophobia F40.228
Antritis J32.0
  maxilla J32.0
    acute J01.00
      recurrent J01.01
  stomach K29.60
    with bleeding K29.61
Antrum, antral — *see* condition
Anuria R34
  calculous (impacted) (recurrent) — *see also* Calculus,
    urinary N20.9
  following
    abortion — *see* Abortion by type complicated by,
      renal failure
    ectopic or molar pregnancy O08.4
  newborn P96.0
  postprocedural N99.0
  postrenal N13.8
  traumatic (following crushing) T79.5 ☑
Anus, anal — *see* condition
Anusitis K62.89
Anxiety F41.9
  depression F41.8
  episodic paroxysmal F41.0
  generalized F41.1
  hysteria F41.8
  neurosis F41.1

Anxiety — *continued*
  panic type F41.0
  reaction F41.1
  separation, abnormal (of childhood) F93.0
  specified NEC F41.8
  state F41.1
Aorta, aortic — *see* condition
Aortectasia — *see* Ectasia, aorta
  with aneurysm — *see* Aneurysm, aorta
Aortitis (nonsyphilitic) (calcific) I77.6
  arteriosclerotic I70.0
  Doehle-Heller A52.02
  luetic A52.02
  rheumatic — *see* Endocarditis, acute, rheumatic
  specific (syphilitic) A52.02
  syphilitic A52.02
    congenital A50.54 *[I79.1]*
Apathetic thyroid storm — *see* Thyrotoxicosis
Apathy R45.3
Apeirophobia F40.228
Apepsia K30
  psychogenic F45.8
Aperistalsis, esophagus K22.0
Apertognathia M26.29
Apert's syndrome Q87.0
Aphagia R13.0
  psychogenic F50.9
Aphakia (acquired) (postoperative) H27.0- ☑
  congenital Q12.3
Aphasia (amnestic) (global) (nominal) (semantic) (syntac-
    tic) R47.01
  acquired, with epilepsy (Landau-Kleffner syndrome)
    — *see* Epilepsy, specified NEC
  auditory (developmental) F80.2
  developmental (receptive type) F80.2
    expressive type F80.1
    Wernicke's F80.2
  following
    cerebrovascular disease I69.920
      cerebral infarction I69.320
      intracerebral hemorrhage I69.120
      nontraumatic intracranial hemorrhage NEC
        I69.220
      specified disease NEC I69.820
      subarachnoid hemorrhage I69.020
  primary progressive G31.01 *[F02.80]*
    with behavioral disturbance G31.01 *[F02.81]*
  progressive isolated G31.01 *[F02.80]*
    with behavioral disturbance G31.01 *[F02.81]*
  sensory F80.2
  syphilis, tertiary A52.19
  Wernicke's (developmental) F80.2
Aphonia (organic) R49.1
  hysterical F44.4
  psychogenic F44.4
Aphthae, aphthous — *see also* condition
  Bednar's K12.0
  cachectic K14.0
  epizootic B08.8
  fever B08.8
  oral (recurrent) K12.0
  stomatitis (major) (minor) K12.0
  thrush B37.0
  ulcer (oral) (recurrent) K12.0
    genital organ(s) NEC
      female N76.6
      male N50.89
    larynx J38.7
Apical — *see* condition
Apiphobia F40.218
Aplasia — *see also* Agenesis
  abdominal muscle syndrome Q79.4
  alveolar process (acquired) — *see* Anomaly, alveolar
    congenital Q38.6
  aorta (congenital) Q25.41
  axialis extracorticalis (congenita) E75.29
  bone marrow (myeloid) D61.9
    congenital D61.01
  brain Q00.0
    part of Q04.3
  bronchus Q32.4
  cementum K00.4
  cerebellum Q04.3
  cervix (congenital) Q51.5
  congenital pure red cell D61.01
  corpus callosum Q04.0
  cutis congenita Q84.8
  erythrocyte congenital D61.01

Aplasia — *continued*
  extracortical axial E75.29
  eye Q11.1
  fovea centralis (congenital) Q14.1
  gallbladder, congenital Q44.0
  iris Q13.1
  labyrinth, membranous Q16.5
  limb (congenital) Q73.8
    lower — *see* Defect, reduction, lower limb
    upper — *see* Agenesis, arm
  lung, congenital (bilateral) (unilateral) Q33.3
  pancreas Q45.0
  parathyroid-thymic D82.1
  Pelizaeus-Merzbacher E75.29
  penis Q55.5
  prostate Q55.4
  red cell (with thymoma) D60.9
    acquired D60.9
      due to drugs D60.9
    adult D60.9
    chronic D60.0
    congenital D61.01
    constitutional D61.01
    due to drugs D60.9
    hereditary D61.01
    of infants D61.01
    primary D61.01
    pure D61.01
      due to drugs D60.9
    specified type NEC D60.8
    transient D60.1
  round ligament Q52.8
  skin Q84.8
  spermatic cord Q55.4
  spleen Q89.01
  testicle Q55.0
  thymic, with immunodeficiency D82.1
  thyroid (congenital) (with myxedema) E03.1
  uterus Q51.0
  ventral horn cell Q06.1
Apnea, apneic (of) (spells) R06.81
  newborn NEC P28.4
    obstructive P28.4
    sleep (central) (obstructive) (primary) P28.3
  prematurity P28.4
  sleep G47.30
    central (primary) G47.31
      idiopathic G47.31
      in conditions classified elsewhere G47.37
    obstructive (adult) (pediatric) G47.33
      hypopnea G47.33
    primary central G47.31
    specified NEC G47.39
Apneumatosis, newborn P28.0
Apocrine metaplasia (breast) — *see* Dysplasia, mamma-
    ry, specified type NEC
Apophysitis (bone) — *see also* Osteochondropathy
  calcaneus M92.8
  juvenile M92.9
Apoplectiform convulsions (cerebral ischemia) I67.82
Apoplexia, apoplexy, apoplectic
  adrenal A39.1
  heart (auricle) (ventricle) — *see* Infarct, myocardium
  heat T67.01 ☑
  hemorrhagic (stroke) — *see* Hemorrhage, intracranial
  meninges, hemorrhagic — *see* Hemorrhage, intracra-
    nial, subarachnoid
  uremic N18.9 *[I68.8]*
Appearance
  bizarre R46.1
  specified NEC R46.89
  very low level of personal hygiene R46.0
Appendage
  epididymal (organ of Morgagni) Q55.4
  intestine (epiploic) Q43.8
  preauricular Q17.0
  testicular (organ of Morgagni) Q55.29
Appendicitis (pneumococcal) (retrocecal) K37
  with
    gangrene K35.891
    perforation NOS K35.32
    peritoneal abscess K35.33
    peritonitis NEC K35.33
      generalized (with perforation or rupture) K35.20
        with abscess K35.21
      localized K35.30
        with
          gangrene K35.31

Appendicitis — *continued*
  with — *continued*
    peritonitis — *continued*
      localized — *continued*
        with — *continued*
          perforation K35.32
            and abscess K35.33
        rupture (with localized peritonitis) K35.32
  acute (catarrhal) (fulminating) (gangrenous) (obstructive) (retrocecal) (suppurative) K35.80
    with
      gangrene K35.891
      peritoneal abscess K35.33
      peritonitis NEC K35.33
        generalized (with perforation or rupture) K35.20
          with abscess K35.21
        localized K35.30
          with
            gangrene K35.31
            perforation K35.32
              and abscess K35.33
      specified NEC K35.890
        with gangrene K35.891
  amebic A06.89
  chronic (recurrent) K36
  exacerbation — *see* Appendicitis, acute
  gangrenous — *see* Appendicitis, acute
  healed (obliterative) K36
  interval K36
  neurogenic K36
  obstructive K36
  recurrent K36
  relapsing K36
  ruptured NOS (with localized peritonitis) K35.32
  subacute (adhesive) K36
  subsiding K36
  suppurative — *see* Appendicitis, acute
  tuberculous A18.32
Appendicopathia oxyurica B80
Appendix, appendicular — *see also* condition
  epididymis Q55.4
  Morgagni
    female Q50.5
    male (epididymal) Q55.4
      testicular Q55.29
  testis Q55.29
Appetite
  depraved — *see* Pica
  excessive R63.2
  lack or loss — *see also* Anorexia R63.0
    nonorganic origin F50.89
    psychogenic F50.89
  perverted (hysterical) — *see* Pica
Apple peel syndrome Q41.1
Apprehension state F41.1
Apprehensiveness, abnormal F41.9
Approximal wear K03.0
Apraxia (classic) (ideational) (ideokinetic) (ideomotor) (motor) (verbal) R48.2
  following
    cerebrovascular disease I69.990
      cerebral infarction I69.390
      intracerebral hemorrhage I69.190
      nontraumatic intracranial hemorrhage NEC I69.290
      specified disease NEC I69.890
      subarachnoid hemorrhage I69.090
  oculomotor, congenital H51.8
Aptyalism K11.7
Apudoma — *see* Neoplasm, uncertain behavior, by site
Aqueous misdirection H40.83- ☑
Arabicum elephantiasis — *see* Infestation, filarial
Arachnitis — *see* Meningitis
Arachnodactyly — *see* Syndrome, Marfan's
Arachnoiditis (acute) (adhesive) (basal) (brain) (cerebrospinal) — *see* Meningitis
Arachnophobia F40.210
Arboencephalitis, Australian A83.4
Arborization block (heart) I45.5
ARC (AIDS-related complex) B20
Arch
  aortic Q25.49
  bovine Q25.49
Arches — *see* condition
Arcuate uterus Q51.810
Arcuatus uterus Q51.810
Arcus (cornea) senilis — *see* Degeneration, cornea, senile

Arc-welder's lung J63.4
Areflexia R29.2
Areola — *see* condition
Argentaffinoma — *see also* Neoplasm, uncertain behavior, by site
  malignant — *see* Neoplasm, malignant, by site
  syndrome E34.0
Argininemia E72.21
Arginosuccinic aciduria E72.22
Argyll Robertson phenomenon, pupil or syndrome (syphilitic) A52.19
  atypical H57.09
  nonsyphilitic H57.09
Argyria, argyriasis
  conjunctival H11.13- ☑
  from drug or medicament — *see* Table of Drugs and Chemicals, by substance
Argyrosis, conjunctival H11.13- ☑
Arhinencephaly Q04.1
Ariboflavinosis E53.0
Arm — *see* condition
Arnold-Chiari disease, obstruction or syndrome (type II) Q07.00
  with
    hydrocephalus Q07.02
      with spina bifida Q07.03
    spina bifida Q07.01
      with hydrocephalus Q07.03
  type III — *see* Encephalocele
  type IV Q04.8
Aromatic amino-acid metabolism disorder E70.9
  specified NEC E70.89
Arousals, confusional G47.51
Arrest, arrested
  cardiac I46.9
    complicating
      abortion — *see* Abortion, by type, complicated by, cardiac arrest
      anesthesia (general) (local) or other sedation — *see* Table of Drugs and Chemicals, by drug
        in labor and delivery O74.2
        in pregnancy O29.11- ☑
        postpartum, puerperal O89.1
      delivery (cesarean) (instrumental) O75.4
    due to
      cardiac condition I46.2
      specified condition NEC I46.8
    intraoperative I97.71- ☑
    newborn P29.81
    personal history, successfully resuscitated Z86.74
    postprocedural I97.12- ☑
      obstetric procedure O75.4
  cardiorespiratory — *see* Arrest, cardiac
  circulatory — *see* Arrest, cardiac
  deep transverse O64.0 ☑
  development or growth
    bone — *see* Disorder, bone, development or growth
    child R62.50
    tracheal rings Q32.1
  epiphyseal
    complete
      femur M89.15- ☑
      humerus M89.12- ☑
      tibia M89.16- ☑
      ulna M89.13- ☑
      forearm M89.13- ☑
        specified NEC M89.13- ☑
        ulna — *see* Arrest, epiphyseal, by type, ulna
      lower leg M89.16- ☑
        specified NEC M89.168
        tibia — *see* Arrest, epiphyseal, by type, tibia
    partial
      femur M89.15- ☑
      humerus M89.12- ☑
      tibia M89.16- ☑
      ulna M89.13- ☑
    specified NEC M89.18
  granulopoiesis — *see* Agranulocytosis
  growth plate — *see* Arrest, epiphyseal
  heart — *see* Arrest, cardiac
  legal, anxiety concerning Z65.3
  physeal — *see* Arrest, epiphyseal
  respiratory R09.2
    newborn P28.81
  sinus I45.5
  spermatogenesis (complete) — *see* Azoospermia
    incomplete — *see* Oligospermia

Arrest, arrested — *continued*
  transverse (deep) O64.0 ☑
Arrhenoblastoma
  benign
    specified site — *see* Neoplasm, benign, by site
    unspecified site
      female D27.9
      male D29.20
  malignant
    specified site — *see* Neoplasm, malignant, by site
    unspecified site
      female C56.9
      male C62.90
  specified site — *see* Neoplasm, uncertain behavior, by site
  unspecified site
    female D39.10
    male D40.10
Arrhythmia (auricle) (cardiac) (juvenile) (nodal) (reflex) (supraventricular) (transitory) (ventricle) I49.9
  block I45.9
  extrasystolic I49.49
  newborn
    bradycardia P29.12
    occurring before birth P03.819
      before onset of labor P03.810
      during labor P03.811
    tachycardia P29.11
  psychogenic F45.8
  sinus I49.8
  specified NEC I49.8
  vagal R55
  ventricular re-entry I47.0
Arrillaga-Ayerza syndrome (pulmonary sclerosis with pulmonary hypertension) I27.0
Arsenical pigmentation L81.8
  from drug or medicament — *see* Table of Drugs and Chemicals
Arsenism — *see* Poisoning, arsenic
Arterial — *see* condition
Arteriofibrosis — *see* Arteriosclerosis
Arteriolar sclerosis — *see* Arteriosclerosis
Arteriolith — *see* Arteriosclerosis
Arteriolitis I77.6
  necrotizing, kidney I77.5
  renal — *see* Hypertension, kidney
Arteriolosclerosis — *see* Arteriosclerosis
Arterionephrosclerosis — *see* Hypertension, kidney
Arteriopathy I77.9
  cerebral autosomal dominant, with subcortical infarcts and leukoencephalopathy (CADASIL) I67.850
Arteriosclerosis, arteriosclerotic (diffuse) (obliterans) (of) (senile) (with calcification) I70.90
  with
    chronic limb-threatening ischemia — *see* Arteriosclerosis, with critical limb ischemia
    critical limb ischemia
      bypass graft I70.329
        autologous vein graft I70.429
          leg I70.429
            with
              gangrene (and intermittent claudication, rest pain, and ulcer) I70.469
              rest pain (and intermittent claudication) I70.429
          bilateral I70.423
            with
              gangrene (and intermittent claudication, rest pain, and ulcer) I70.463
              rest pain (and intermittent claudication) I70.423
          left I70.422
            with
              gangrene (and intermittent claudication, rest pain, and ulcer) I70.462
              rest pain (and intermittent claudication) I70.422
              ulceration (and intermittent claudication and rest pain) I70.449
                ankle I70.443
                calf I70.442
                foot site NEC I70.445
                heel I70.444
                lower leg NEC I70.448

26

☑ **Additional Character Required** — Refer to the Tabular List for Character Selection   ▽ Subterms under main terms may continue to next column or page

Arteriosclerosis, arteriosclerotic — *continued*
  with — *continued*
    critical limb ischemia — *continued*
      bypass graft — *continued*
        autologous vein graft — *continued*
          leg — *continued*
            left — *continued*
              with — *continued*
                ulceration — *continued*
                  mid foot I70.444
                  thigh I70.441
            right I70.421
              with
                gangrene (and intermittent claudication, rest pain, and ulcer) I70.461
                rest pain (and intermittent claudication) I70.421
                ulceration (and intermittent claudication and rest pain) I70.439
                  ankle I70.433
                  calf I70.432
                  foot site NEC I70.435
                  heel I70.434
                  lower leg NEC I70.438
                  midfoot I70.434
                  thigh I70.431
          leg I70.329
            with
              gangrene (and intermittent claudication, rest pain, and ulcer) I70.369
              rest pain (and intermittent claudication) I70.329
            bilateral I70.323
              with
                gangrene (and intermittent claudication, rest pain, and ulcer) I70.363
                rest pain (and intermittent claudication) I70.323
            left I70.322
              with
                gangrene (and intermittent claudication, rest pain, and ulcer) I70.362
                rest pain (and intermittent claudication) I70.322
                ulceration (and intermittent claudication and rest pain) I70.349
                  ankle I70.343
                  calf I70.342
                  foot site NEC I70.345
                  heel I70.344
                  lower leg NEC I70.348
                  midfoot I70.344
                  thigh I70.341
            right I70.321
              with
                gangrene (and intermittent claudication, rest pain, and ulcer) I70.361
                rest pain (and intermittent claudication) I70.321
                ulceration (and intermittent claudication and rest pain) I70.339
                  ankle I70.333
                  calf I70.332
                  foot site NEC I70.335
                  heel I70.334
                  lower leg NEC I70.338
                  midfoot I70.334
                  thigh I70.331
        nonautologous biological graft I70.529
          leg I70.529
            with
              gangrene (and intermittent claudication, rest pain, and ulcer) I70.569
              rest pain (and intermittent claudication) I70.529
            bilateral I70.523
              with
                gangrene (and intermittent claudication, rest pain, and ulcer) I70.563
                rest pain (and intermittent claudication) I70.523

Arteriosclerosis, arteriosclerotic — *continued*
  with — *continued*
    critical limb ischemia — *continued*
      bypass graft — *continued*
        nonautologous biological graft — *continued*
          leg — *continued*
            left I70.522
              with
                gangrene (and intermittent claudication, rest pain, and ulcer) I70.562
                rest pain (and intermittent claudication) I70.522
                ulceration (and intermittent claudication and rest pain) I70.549
                  ankle I70.543
                  calf I70.542
                  foot site NEC I70.545
                  heel I70.544
                  lower leg NEC I70.548
                  midfoot I70.544
                  thigh I70.541
            right I70.521
              with
                gangrene (and intermittent claudication, rest pain, and ulcer) I70.561
                rest pain (and intermittent claudication) I70.521
                ulceration (and intermittent claudication and rest pain) I70.539
                  ankle I70.533
                  calf I70.532
                  foot site NEC I70.535
                  heel I70.534
                  lower leg NEC I70.538
                  midfoot I70.534
                  thigh I70.531
        nonbiological graft I70.629
          leg I70.629
            with
              gangrene (and intermittent claudication, rest pain, and ulcer) I70.669
              rest pain (and intermittent claudication) I70.629
            bilateral I70.623
              with
                gangrene (and intermittent claudication, rest pain, and ulcer) I70.663
                rest pain (intermittent claudication) I70.623
            left I70.622
              with
                gangrene (and intermittent claudication, rest pain, and ulcer) I70.662
                rest pain (and intermittent claudication) I70.622
                ulceration (and intermittent claudication and rest pain) I70.649
                  ankle I70.643
                  calf I70.642
                  foot site NEC I70.645
                  heel I70.644
                  lower leg NEC I70.648
                  midfoot I70.644
                  thigh I70.641
            right I70.621
              with
                gangrene (and intermittent claudication, rest pain, and ulcer) I70.661
                rest pain (and intermittent claudication) I70.621
                ulceration (and intermittent claudication and rest pain) I70.639
                  ankle I70.633
                  calf I70.632
                  foot site NEC I70.635
                  heel I70.634
                  lower leg NEC I70.638
                  midfoot I70.634

Arteriosclerosis, arteriosclerotic — *continued*
  with — *continued*
    critical limb ischemia — *continued*
      bypass graft — *continued*
        nonbiological graft — *continued*
          leg — *continued*
            right — *continued*
              with — *continued*
                ulceration — *continued*
                  thigh I70.631
        specified graft NEC I70.729
          leg I70.729
            with
              gangrene (and intermittent claudication, rest pain, and ulcer) I70.769
              rest pain (and intermittent claudication) I70.729
            bilateral I70.723
              with
                gangrene (and intermittent claudication, rest pain, and ulcer) I70.763
                rest pain (and intermittent claudication) I70.723
            left I70.722
              with
                gangrene (and intermittent claudication, rest pain, and ulcer) I70.762
                rest pain (and intermittent claudication) I70.722
                ulceration (and intermittent claudication and rest pain) I70.749
                  ankle I70.743
                  calf I70.742
                  foot site NEC I70.745
                  heel I70.744
                  lower leg NEC I70.748
                  midfoot I70.744
                  thigh I70.741
            right I70.721
              with
                gangrene (and intermittent claudication, rest pain, and ulcer) I70.761
                rest pain (and intermittent claudication) I70.721
                ulceration (and intermittent claudication and rest pain) I70.739
                  ankle I70.733
                  calf I70.732
                  foot site NEC I70.735
                  heel I70.734
                  lower leg NEC I70.738
                  midfoot I70.734
                  thigh I70.731
      leg I70.229
        with
          gangrene (and intermittent claudication, rest pain, and ulcer) I70.269
          rest pain (and intermittent claudication) I70.229
        bilateral I70.223
          with
           gangrene (and intermittent claudication, rest pain, and ulcer) I70.263
           rest pain (and intermittent claudication) I70.223
        left I70.222
          with
           gangrene (and intermittent claudication, rest pain, and ulcer) I70.262
           rest pain (and intermittent claudication) I70.222
           ulceration (and intermittent claudication and rest pain) I70.249
             ankle I70.243
             calf I70.242
             foot site NEC I70.245
             heel I70.244
             lower leg NEC I70.248
             midfoot I70.244
             thigh I70.241
        right I70.221

Arteriosclerosis, arteriosclerotic — *continued*
- with — *continued*
  - critical limb ischemia — *continued*
    - leg — *continued*
      - right — *continued*
        - with
          - gangrene (and intermittent claudication, rest pain, and ulcer) I70.261
          - rest pain (and intermittent claudication) I70.221
          - ulceration (and intermittent claudication and rest pain) I70.239
            - ankle I70.233
            - calf I70.232
            - foot site NEC I70.235
            - heel I70.234
            - lower leg NEC I70.238
            - midfoot I70.234
            - thigh I70.231
- aorta I70.0
- arteries of extremities — *see* Arteriosclerosis, extremities
  - with
    - chronic limb-threatening ischemia — *see* Arteriosclerosis, with critical limb ischemia
    - critical limb ischemia — *see* Arteriosclerosis, with critical limb ischemia
- brain I67.2
- bypass graft
  - with
    - chronic limb-threatening ischemia — *see* Arteriosclerosis, with critical limb ischemia
    - critical limb ischemia — *see* Arteriosclerosis, with critical limb ischemia
    - coronary — *see* Arteriosclerosis, coronary, bypass graft
    - extremities — *see* Arteriosclerosis, extremities, bypass graft
- cardiac — *see* Disease, heart, ischemic, atherosclerotic
- cardiopathy — *see* Disease, heart, ischemic, atherosclerotic
- cardiorenal — *see* Hypertension, cardiorenal
- cardiovascular — *see* Disease, heart, ischemic, atherosclerotic
- carotid — *see also* Occlusion, artery, carotid I65.2- ☑
- central nervous system I67.2
- cerebral I67.2
- cerebrovascular I67.2
- coronary (artery)
  - due to
    - calcified coronary lesion (severely) I25.84
    - lipid rich plaque I25.83
  - bypass graft I25.810
    - with
      - angina pectoris I25.709
        - with documented spasm I25.701
        - specified type NEC I25.708
        - unstable I25.700
      - ischemic chest pain I25.709
    - autologous artery I25.810
      - with
        - angina pectoris I25.729
          - with documented spasm I25.721
          - specified type I25.728
          - unstable I25.720
        - ischemic chest pain I25.729
    - autologous vein I25.810
      - with
        - angina pectoris I25.719
          - with documented spasm I25.711
          - specified type I25.718
          - unstable I25.710
        - ischemic chest pain I25.719
    - nonautologous biological I25.810
      - with
        - angina pectoris I25.739
          - with documented spasm I25.731
          - specified type I25.738
          - unstable I25.730
        - ischemic chest pain I25.739
    - specified type NEC I25.810
      - with
        - angina pectoris I25.799
          - with documented spasm I25.791
          - specified type I25.798
          - unstable I25.790
        - ischemic chest pain I25.799

Arteriosclerosis, arteriosclerotic — *continued*
- coronary — *continued*
  - native vessel
    - with
      - angina pectoris I25.119
        - with documented spasm I25.111
        - specified type NEC I25.118
        - unstable I25.110
      - ischemic chest pain I25.119
  - transplanted heart I25.811
    - bypass graft I25.812
      - with
        - angina pectoris I25.769
          - with documented spasm I25.761
          - specified type I25.768
          - unstable I25.760
        - ischemic chest pain I25.769
    - native coronary artery I25.811
      - with
        - angina pectoris I25.759
          - with documented spasm I25.751
          - specified type I25.758
          - unstable I25.750
        - ischemic chest pain I25.759
- extremities (native arteries) I70.209
  - with
    - chronic limb-threatening ischemia — *see* Arteriosclerosis, with critical limb ischemia
    - critical limb ischemia — *see* Arteriosclerosis, with critical limb ischemia
  - bypass graft I70.309
    - with
      - chronic limb-threatening ischemia — *see* Arteriosclerosis, with critical limb ischemia
      - critical limb ischemia — *see* Arteriosclerosis, with critical limb ischemia
    - autologous vein graft I70.409
      - leg I70.409
        - with
          - gangrene (and intermittent claudication, rest pain and ulcer) I70.469
          - intermittent claudication I70.419
          - rest pain (and intermittent claudication) I70.429
        - bilateral I70.403
          - with
            - gangrene (and intermittent claudication, rest pain and ulcer) I70.463
            - intermittent claudication I70.463
            - rest pain (and intermittent claudication) I70.423
          - specified type NEC I70.493
        - left I70.402
          - with
            - gangrene (and intermittent claudication, rest pain and ulcer) I70.462
            - intermittent claudication I70.412
            - rest pain (and intermittent claudication) I70.422
            - ulceration (and intermittent claudication and rest pain) I70.449
              - ankle I70.443
              - calf I70.442
              - foot site NEC I70.445
              - heel I70.444
              - lower leg NEC I70.448
              - midfoot I70.444
              - thigh I70.441
          - specified type NEC I70.492
        - right I70.401
          - with
            - gangrene (and intermittent claudication, rest pain and ulcer) I70.461
            - intermittent claudication I70.411
            - rest pain (and intermittent claudication) I70.421
            - ulceration (and intermittent claudication and rest pain) I70.439
              - ankle I70.433
              - calf I70.432
              - foot site NEC I70.435
              - heel I70.434
              - lower leg NEC I70.438
              - midfoot I70.434
              - thigh I70.431
          - specified type NEC I70.491

Arteriosclerosis, arteriosclerotic — *continued*
- extremities — *continued*
  - bypass graft — *continued*
    - autologous vein graft — *continued*
      - leg — *continued*
        - specified type NEC I70.499
        - specified NEC I70.408
          - with
            - gangrene (and intermittent claudication, rest pain and ulcer) I70.468
            - intermittent claudication I70.418
            - rest pain (and intermittent claudication) I70.428
            - ulceration (and intermittent claudication and rest pain) I70.45
          - specified type NEC I70.498
      - leg I70.309
        - with
          - gangrene (and intermittent claudication, rest pain and ulcer) I70.369
          - intermittent claudication I70.319
          - rest pain (and intermittent claudication) I70.329
        - bilateral I70.303
          - with
            - gangrene (and intermittent claudication, rest pain and ulcer) I70.363
            - intermittent claudication I70.313
            - rest pain (and intermittent claudication) I70.323
          - specified type NEC I70.393
        - left I70.302
          - with
            - gangrene (and intermittent claudication, rest pain and ulcer) I70.362
            - intermittent claudication I70.312
            - rest pain (and intermittent claudication) I70.322
            - ulceration (and intermittent claudication and rest pain) I70.349
              - ankle I70.343
              - calf I70.342
              - foot site NEC I70.345
              - heel I70.344
              - lower leg NEC I70.348
              - midfoot I70.344
              - thigh I70.341
          - specified type NEC I70.392
        - right I70.301
          - with
            - gangrene (and intermittent claudication, rest pain and ulcer) I70.361
            - intermittent claudication I70.311
            - rest pain (and intermittent claudication) I70.321
            - ulceration (and intermittent claudication and rest pain I70.339
              - ankle I70.333
              - calf I70.332
              - foot site NEC I70.335
              - heel I70.334
              - lower leg NEC I70.338
              - midfoot I70.334
              - thigh I70.331
          - specified type NEC I70.391
        - specified type NEC I70.399
    - nonautologous biological graft I70.509
      - leg I70.509
        - with
          - gangrene (and intermittent claudication, rest pain and ulcer) I70.569
          - intermittent claudication I70.519
          - rest pain (and intermittent claudication) I70.529
        - bilateral I70.503
          - with
            - gangrene (and intermittent claudication, rest pain and ulcer) I70.563
            - intermittent claudication I70.513
            - rest pain (and intermittent claudication) I70.523
          - specified type NEC I70.593
        - left I70.502
          - with
            - gangrene (and intermittent claudication, rest pain and ulcer) I70.562
            - intermittent claudication I70.512

Arteriosclerosis, arteriosclerotic — *continued*
  extremities — *continued*
    bypass graft — *continued*
      nonautologous biological graft — *continued*
        leg — *continued*
          left — *continued*
            with — *continued*
              rest pain (and intermittent claudication) I70.522
              ulceration (and intermittent claudication and rest pain) I70.549
                ankle I70.543
                calf I70.542
                foot site NEC I70.545
                heel I70.544
                lower leg NEC I70.548
                midfoot I70.544
                thigh I70.541
              specified type NEC I70.592
          right I70.501
            with
              gangrene (and intermittent claudication, rest pain and ulcer) I70.561
              intermittent claudication I70.511
              rest pain (and intermittent claudication) I70.521
              ulceration (and intermittent claudication and rest pain) I70.539
                ankle I70.533
                calf I70.532
                foot site NEC I70.535
                heel I70.534
                lower leg NEC I70.538
                midfoot I70.534
                thigh I70.531
              specified type NEC I70.591
          specified type NEC I70.599
        specified NEC I70.508
          with
            gangrene (and intermittent claudication, rest pain and ulcer) I70.568
            intermittent claudication I70.518
            rest pain (and intermittent claudication) I70.528
            ulceration (and intermittent claudication and rest pain) I70.55
          specified type NEC I70.598
      nonbiological graft I70.609
        leg I70.609
          with
            gangrene (and intermittent claudication, rest pain and ulcer) I70.669
            intermittent claudication I70.619
            rest pain (and intermittent claudication) I70.629
          bilateral I70.603
            with
              gangrene (and intermittent claudication, rest pain and ulcer) I70.663
              intermittent claudication I70.613
              rest pain (and intermittent claudication) I70.623
            specified type NEC I70.693
          left I70.602
            with
              gangrene (and intermittent claudication, rest pain and ulcer) I70.662
              intermittent claudication I70.612
              rest pain (and intermittent claudication) I70.622
              ulceration (and intermittent claudication and rest pain) I70.649
                ankle I70.643
                calf I70.642
                foot site NEC I70.645
                heel I70.644
                lower leg NEC I70.648
                midfoot I70.644
                thigh I70.641
              specified type NEC I70.692
          right I70.601
            with
              gangrene (and intermittent claudication, rest pain and ulcer) I70.661
              intermittent claudication I70.611

Arteriosclerosis, arteriosclerotic — *continued*
  extremities — *continued*
    bypass graft — *continued*
      nonbiological graft — *continued*
        leg — *continued*
          right — *continued*
            with — *continued*
              rest pain (and intermittent claudication) I70.621
              ulceration (and intermittent claudication and rest pain) I70.639
                ankle I70.633
                calf I70.632
                foot site NEC I70.635
                heel I70.634
                lower leg NEC I70.638
                midfoot I70.634
                thigh I70.631
              specified type NEC I70.691
          specified type NEC I70.699
        specified NEC I70.608
          with
            gangrene (and intermittent claudication, rest pain and ulcer) I70.668
            intermittent claudication I70.618
            rest pain (and intermittent claudication) I70.628
            ulceration (and intermittent claudication and rest pain) I70.65
          specified type NEC I70.698
      specified graft NEC I70.709
        leg I70.709
          with
            gangrene (and intermittent claudication, rest pain and ulcer) I70.769
            intermittent claudication I70.719
            rest pain (and intermittent claudication) I70.729
          bilateral I70.703
            with
              gangrene (and intermittent claudication, rest pain and ulcer) I70.763
              intermittent claudication I70.713
              rest pain (and intermittent claudication) I70.723
            specified type NEC I70.793
          left I70.702
            with
              gangrene (and intermittent claudication, rest pain and ulcer) I70.762
              intermittent claudication I70.712
              rest pain (and intermittent claudication) I70.722
              ulceration (and intermittent claudication and rest pain) I70.749
                ankle I70.743
                calf I70.742
                foot site NEC I70.745
                heel I70.744
                lower leg NEC I70.748
                midfoot I70.744
                thigh I70.741
              specified type NEC I70.792
          right I70.701
            with
              gangrene (and intermittent claudication, rest pain and ulcer) I70.761
              intermittent claudication I70.711
              rest pain (and intermittent claudication) I70.721
              ulceration (and intermittent claudication and rest pain) I70.739
                ankle I70.733
                calf I70.732
                foot site NEC I70.735
                heel I70.734
                lower leg NEC I70.738
                midfoot I70.734
                thigh I70.731
              specified type NEC I70.791
          specified type NEC I70.799
        specified NEC I70.708
          with
            gangrene (and intermittent claudication, rest pain and ulcer) I70.768
            intermittent claudication I70.718

Arteriosclerosis, arteriosclerotic — *continued*
  extremities — *continued*
    bypass graft — *continued*
      specified graft — *continued*
        specified — *continued*
          with — *continued*
            rest pain (and intermittent claudication) I70.728
            ulceration (and intermittent claudication and rest pain) I70.75
          specified type NEC I70.798
        specified NEC I70.308
          with
            gangrene (and intermittent claudication, rest pain and ulcer) I70.368
            intermittent claudication I70.318
            rest pain (and intermittent claudication) I70.328
            ulceration (and intermittent claudication and rest pain) I70.35
          specifiec type NEC I70.398
      leg I70.209
        with
          gangrene (and intermittent claudication, rest pain and ulcer) I70.269
          intermittent claudication I70.219
          rest pain (and intermittent claudication) I70.229
        bilateral I70.203
          with
           gangrene (and intermittent claudication, rest pain and ulcer) I70.263
           intermittent claudication I70.213
           rest pain (and intermittent claudication) I70.223
          specified type NEC I70.293
        left I70.202
          with
           gangrene (and intermittent claudication, rest pain and ulcer) I70.262
           intermittent claudication I70.212
           rest pain (and intermittent claudication) I70.222
           ulceration (and intermittent claudication and rest pain) I70.249
            ankle I70.243
            calf I70.242
            foot site NEC I70.245
            heel I70.244
            lower leg NEC I70.248
            midfoot I70.244
            thigh I70.241
          specified type NEC I70.292
        right I70.201
          with
           gangrene (and intermittent claudication, rest pain and ulcer) I70.261
           intermittent claudication I70.211
           rest pain (and intermittent claudication) I70.221
           ulceration (and intermittent claudication and rest pain) I70.239
            ankle I70.233
            calf I70.232
            foot site NEC I70.235
            heel I70.234
            lower leg NEC I70.238
            midfoot I70.234
            thigh I70.231
          specified type NEC I70.291
      specified type NEC I70.299
    specified site NEC I70.208
      with
        gangrene (and intermittent claudication, rest pain and ulcer) I70.268
        intermittent claudication I70.218
        rest pain (and intermittent claudication) I70.228
        ulceration (and intermittent claudication and rest pain) I70.25
      specified type NEC I70.298
  generalized I70.91
  heart (disease) — *see* Arteriosclerosis, coronary (artery),
  kidney — *see* Hypertension, kidney
  medial — *see* Arteriosclerosis, extremities
  mesenteric (artery) K55.1
  Mönckeberg's — *see* Arteriosclerosis, extremities
  myocarditis I51.4

Arteriosclerosis, arteriosclerotic — *continued*
   peripheral (of extremities) — *see* Arteriosclerosis, extremities
   pulmonary (idiopathic) I27.0
   renal (arterioles) — *see also* Hypertension, kidney
      artery I70.1
   retina (vascular) I70.8 *[H35.0-]* ☑
   specified artery NEC I70.8
   spinal (cord) G95.19
   vertebral (artery) I67.2
Arteriospasm I73.9
Arteriovenous — *see* condition
Arteritis I77.6
   allergic M31.0
   aorta (nonsyphilitic) I77.6
      syphilitic A52.02
   aortic arch M31.4
   brachiocephalic M31.4
   brain I67.7
      syphilitic A52.04
   cerebral I67.7
      in systemic lupus erythematosus M32.19
      listerial A32.89
      syphilitic A52.04
      tuberculous A18.89
   coronary (artery) I25.89
      rheumatic I01.8
         chronic I09.89
      syphilitic A52.06
   cranial (left) (right), giant cell M31.6
   deformans — *see* Arteriosclerosis
   giant cell NEC M31.6
      with polymyalgia rheumatica M31.5
   necrosing or necrotizing M31.9
      specified NEC M31.8
   nodosa M30.0
   obliterans — *see* Arteriosclerosis
   pulmonary I28.8
   rheumatic — *see* Fever, rheumatic
   senile — *see* Arteriosclerosis
   suppurative I77.2
   syphilitic (general) A52.09
      brain A52.04
      coronary A52.06
      spinal A52.09
   temporal, giant cell M31.6
   young female aortic arch syndrome M31.4
Artery, arterial — *see also* condition
   abscess I77.89
   single umbilical Q27.0
Arthralgia (allergic) — *see also* Pain, joint
   in caisson disease T70.3 ☑
   temporomandibular M26.62- ☑
Arthritis, arthritic (acute) (chronic) (nonpyogenic) (subacute) M19.90
   allergic — *see* Arthritis, specified form NEC
   ankylosing (crippling) (spine) — *see also* Spondylitis, ankylosing
      sites other than spine — *see* Arthritis, specified form NEC
   atrophic — *see* Osteoarthritis
      spine — *see* Spondylitis, ankylosing
   back — *see* Spondylopathy, inflammatory
   blennorrhagic (gonococcal) A54.42
   Charcot's — *see* Arthropathy, neuropathic
      diabetic — *see* Diabetes, arthropathy, neuropathic
      syringomyelic G95.0
   chylous (filarial) — *see also* category M01 B74.9
   climacteric (any site) NEC — *see* Arthritis, specified form NEC
   crystal (-induced) — *see* Arthritis, in, crystals
   deformans — *see* Osteoarthritis
   degenerative — *see* Osteoarthritis
   due to or associated with
      acromegaly E22.0
      brucellosis — *see* Brucellosis
      caisson disease T70.3 ☑
      diabetes — *see* Diabetes, arthropathy
      dracontiasis — *see also* category M01 B72
      enteritis NEC
         regional — *see* Enteritis, regional
      erysipelas — *see also* category M01 A46
      erythema
         epidemic A25.1
         nodosum L52
      filariasis NOS B74.9
      glanders A24.0
      helminthiasis — *see also* category M01 B83.9

Arthritis, arthritic — *continued*
   due to or associated with — *continued*
      hemophilia D66 *[M36.2]*
      Henoch- (Schönlein) purpura D69.0 *[M36.4]*
      human parvovirus — *see also* category M01 B97.6
      infectious disease NEC M01 ☑
      leprosy (see also category M01) — *see also* Leprosy A30.9
      Lyme disease A69.23
      mycobacteria — *see also* category M01 A31.8
      parasitic disease NEC — *see also* category M01 B89
      paratyphoid fever (see also category M01) — *see also* Fever, paratyphoid A01.4
      rat bite fever — *see also* category M01 A25.1
      regional enteritis — *see* Enteritis, regional
      respiratory disorder NOS J98.9
      serum sickness — *see also* Reaction, serum T80.69 ☑
      syringomyelia G95.0
      typhoid fever A01.04
   epidemic erythema A25.1
   febrile — *see* Fever, rheumatic
   gonococcal A54.42
   gouty (acute) — *see* Gout
   in (due to)
      acromegaly — *see also* subcategory M14.8- E22.0
      amyloidosis — *see also* subcategory M14.8- E85.4
      bacterial disease — *see also* subcategory M01 A49.9
      Behçet's syndrome M35.2
      caisson disease — *see also* subcategory M14.8- T70.3 ☑
      coliform bacilli (Escherichia coli) — *see* Arthritis, in, pyogenic organism NEC
      crystals M11.9
         dicalcium phosphate — *see* Arthritis, in, crystals, specified type NEC
         hydroxyapatite M11.0- ☑
         pyrophosphate — *see* Arthritis, in, crystals, specified type NEC
         specified type NEC M11.80
            ankle M11.87- ☑
            elbow M11.82- ☑
            foot joint M11.87- ☑
            hand joint M11.84- ☑
            hip M11.85- ☑
            knee M11.86- ☑
            multiple sites M11.8- ☑
            shoulder M11.81- ☑
            vertebrae M11.88
            wrist M11.83- ☑
      dermatoarthritis, lipoid E78.81
      dracontiasis (dracunculiasis) — *see also* category M01 B72
      endocrine disorder NEC — *see also* subcategory M14.8- E34.9
      enteritis, infectious NEC — *see also* category M01 A09
         specified organism NEC — *see also* category M01 A08.8
      erythema
         multiforme — *see also* subcategory M14.8- L51.9
         nodosum — *see also* subcategory M14.8- L52
      gout — *see* Gout
      helminthiasis NEC — *see also* category M01 B83.9
      hemochromatosis — *see also* subcategory M14.8- E83.118
      hemoglobinopathy NEC D58.2 *[M36.3]*
      hemophilia NEC D66 *[M36.2]*
      Hemophilus influenzae M00.8- ☑ *[B96.3]*
      Henoch (-Schönlein) purpura D69.0 *[M36.4]*
      hyperparathyroidism NEC — *see also* subcategory M14.8- E21.3
      hypersensitivity reaction NEC T78.49 ☑ *[M36.4]*
      hypogammaglobulinemia — *see also* subcategory M14.8- D80.1
      hypothyroidism NEC — *see also* subcategory M14.8- E03.9
      infection — *see* Arthritis, pyogenic or pyemic
         spine — *see* Spondylopathy, infective
      infectious disease NEC M01 ☑
      leprosy — *see also* category M01 A30.9
      leukemia NEC C95.9- ☑ *[M36.1]*
      lipoid dermatoarthritis E78.81
      Lyme disease A69.23
      Mediterranean fever, familial — *see also* subcategory M14.8- M04.1
      Meningococcus A39.83

Arthritis, arthritic — *continued*
   in — *continued*
      metabolic disorder NEC — *see also* subcategory M14.8- E88.9
      multiple myelomatosis C90.0- ☑ *[M36.1]*
      mumps B26.85
      mycosis NEC — *see also* category M01 B49
      myelomatosis (multiple) C90.0- ☑ *[M36.1]*
      neurological disorder NEC G98.0
      ochronosis — *see also* subcategory M14.8- E70.29
      O'nyong-nyong — *see also* category M01 A92.1
      parasitic disease NEC — *see also* category M01 B89
      paratyphoid fever — *see also* category M01 A01.4
      Pseudomonas — *see* Arthritis, pyogenic, bacterial NEC
      psoriasis L40.50
      pyogenic organism NEC — *see* Arthritis, pyogenic, bacterial NEC
      Reiter's disease — *see* Reiter's disease
      respiratory disorder NEC — *see also* subcategory M14.8- J98.9
      reticulosis, malignant — *see also* subcategory M14.8- C86.0
      rubella B06.82
      Salmonella (arizonae) (cholerae-suis) (enteritidis) (typhimurium) A02.23
      sarcoidosis D86.86
      specified bacteria NEC — *see* Arthritis, pyogenic, bacterial NEC
      sporotrichosis B42.82
      syringomyelia G95.0
      thalassemia NEC D56.9 *[M36.3]*
      tuberculosis — *see* Tuberculosis, arthritis
      typhoid fever A01.04
      urethritis, Reiter's — *see* Reiter's disease
      viral disease NEC — *see also* category M01 B34.9
   infectious or infective — *see also* Arthritis, pyogenic or pyemic
      spine — *see* Spondylopathy, infective
   juvenile M08.90
      with systemic onset — *see* Still's disease
      ankle M08.97- ☑
      elbow M08.92- ☑
      foot joint M08.97- ☑
      hand joint M08.94- ☑
      hip M08.95- ☑
      knee M08.96- ☑
      multiple site M08.99
      pauciarticular M08.40
         ankle M08.47- ☑
         elbow M08.42- ☑
         foot joint M08.47- ☑
         hand joint M08.44- ☑
         hip M08.45- ☑
         knee M08.46- ☑
         shoulder M08.41- ☑
         specified site NEC M08.4A
         vertebrae M08.48
         wrist M08.43- ☑
      psoriatic L40.54
      rheumatoid — *see* Arthritis, rheumatoid, juvenile
      shoulder M08.91- ☑
      specified site NEC M08.9A
      specified type NEC M08.80
         ankle M08.87- ☑
         elbow M08.82- ☑
         foot joint M08.87- ☑
         hand joint M08.84- ☑
         hip M08.85- ☑
         knee M08.86- ☑
         multiple site M08.89
         shoulder M08.81- ☑
         specified joint NEC M08.88
         vertebrae M08.88
         wrist M08.83- ☑
      wrist M08.93- ☑
   meaning osteoarthritis — *see* Osteoarthritis
   meningococcal A39.83
   menopausal (any site) NEC — *see* Arthritis, specified form NEC
   mutilans (psoriatic) L40.52
   mycotic NEC — *see also* category M01 B49
   neuropathic (Charcot) — *see* Arthropathy, neuropathic
      diabetic — *see* Diabetes, arthropathy, neuropathic
      nonsyphilitic NEC G98.0
      syringomyelic G95.0
   ochronotic — *see also* subcategory M14.8- E70.29

☑ **Additional Character Required** — Refer to the Tabular List for Character Selection   ▽ Subterms under main terms may continue to next column or page

Arthritis, arthritic — *continued*
  palindromic (any site) — *see* Rheumatism, palindromic
  pneumococcal M00.10
    ankle M00.17- ☑
    elbow M00.12- ☑
    foot joint — *see* Arthritis, pneumococcal, ankle
    hand joint M00.14- ☑
    hip M00.15- ☑
    knee M00.16- ☑
    multiple site M00.19
    shoulder M00.11- ☑
    vertebra M00.18
    wrist M00.13- ☑
  postdysenteric — *see* Arthropathy, postdysenteric
  postmeningococcal A39.84
  postrheumatic, chronic — *see* Arthropathy, postrheumatic, chronic
  primary progressive — *see also* Arthritis, specified form NEC
    spine — *see* Spondylitis, ankylosing
  psoriatic L40.50
  purulent (any site except spine) — *see* Arthritis, pyogenic or pyemic
    spine — *see* Spondylopathy, infective
  pyogenic or pyemic (any site except spine) M00.9
    bacterial NEC M00.80
      ankle M00.87- ☑
      elbow M00.82- ☑
      foot joint — *see* Arthritis, pyogenic, bacterial NEC, ankle
      hand joint M00.84- ☑
      hip M00.85- ☑
      knee M00.86- ☑
      multiple site M00.89
      shoulder M00.81- ☑
      vertebra M00.88
      wrist M00.83- ☑
    pneumococcal — *see* Arthritis, pneumococcal
    spine — *see* Spondylopathy, infective
    staphylococcal — *see* Arthritis, staphylococcal
    streptococcal — *see* Arthritis, streptococcal NEC
      pneumococcal — *see* Arthritis, pneumococcal
  reactive — *see* Reiter's disease
  rheumatic — *see also* Arthritis, rheumatoid
    acute or subacute — *see* Fever, rheumatic
  rheumatoid M06.9
    with
      carditis — *see* Rheumatoid, carditis
      endocarditis — *see* Rheumatoid, carditis
      heart involvement NEC — *see* Rheumatoid, carditis
      lung involvement — *see* Rheumatoid, lung
      myocarditis — *see* Rheumatoid, carditis
      myopathy — *see* Rheumatoid, myopathy
      pericarditis — *see* Rheumatoid, carditis
      polyneuropathy — *see* Rheumatoid, polyneuropathy
      rheumatoid factor — *see* Arthritis, rheumatoid, seropositive
      splenoadenomegaly and leukopenia — *see* Felty's syndrome
      vasculitis — *see* Rheumatoid, vasculitis
      visceral involvement NEC — *see* Rheumatoid, arthritis, with involvement of organs NEC
    juvenile (with or without rheumatoid factor) M08.00
      with systemic onset — *see* Still's disease
      ankle M08.07- ☑
      elbow M08.02- ☑
      foot joint M08.07- ☑
      hand joint M08.04- ☑
      hip M08.05- ☑
      knee M08.06- ☑
      multiple site M08.09
      shoulder M08.01- ☑
      specified site NEC M08.0A
      vertebra M08.08
      wrist M08.03- ☑
    seronegative M06.00
      ankle M06.07- ☑
      elbow M06.02- ☑
      foot joint M06.07- ☑
      hand joint M06.04- ☑
      hip M06.05- ☑
      knee M06.06- ☑
      multiple site M06.09
      shoulder M06.01- ☑
      specified site NEC M06.0A

Arthritis, arthritic — *continued*
  rheumatoid — *continued*
    seronegative — *continued*
      vertebra M06.08
      wrist M06.03- ☑
    seropositive M05.9
      specified NEC M05.80
        ankle M05.87- ☑
        elbow M05.82- ☑
        foot joint M05.87- ☑
        hand joint M05.84- ☑
        hip M05.85- ☑
        knee M05.86- ☑
        multiple sites M05.89
        shoulder M05.81- ☑
        specified site NEC M05.8A
        vertebra — *see* Spondylitis, ankylosing
        wrist M05.83- ☑
      without organ involvement M05.70
        ankle M05.77- ☑
        elbow M05.72- ☑
        foot joint M05.77- ☑
        hand joint M05.74- ☑
        hip M05.75- ☑
        knee M05.76- ☑
        multiple sites M05.79
        shoulder M05.71- ☑
        specified site NEC M05.7A
        vertebra — *see* Spondylitis, ankylosing
        wrist M05.73- ☑
    specified type NEC M06.80
      ankle M06.87- ☑
      elbow M06.82- ☑
      foot joint M06.87- ☑
      hand joint M06.84- ☑
      hip M06.85- ☑
      knee M06.86- ☑
      multiple site M06.89
      shoulder M06.81- ☑
      specified site NEC M06.8A
      vertebra M06.88
      wrist M06.83- ☑
    spine — *see* Spondylitis, ankylosing
  rubella B06.82
  scorbutic — *see also* subcategory M14.8- E54
  senile or senescent — *see* Osteoarthritis
  septic (any site except spine) — *see* Arthritis, pyogenic or pyemic
    spine — *see* Spondylopathy, infective
  serum (nontherapeutic) (therapeutic) — *see* Arthropathy, postimmunization
  specified form NEC M13.80
    ankle M13.87- ☑
    elbow M13.82- ☑
    foot joint M13.87- ☑
    hand joint M13.84- ☑
    hip M13.85- ☑
    knee M13.86- ☑
    multiple site M13.89
    shoulder M13.81- ☑
    specified joint NEC M13.88
    wrist M13.83- ☑
  spine — *see also* Spondylosis
    infectious or infective NEC — *see* Spondylopathy, infective
    Marie-Strümpell — *see* Spondylitis, ankylosing
    pyogenic — *see* Spondylopathy, infective
    rheumatoid — *see* Spondylitis, ankylosing
    traumatic (old) — *see* Spondylopathy, traumatic
    tuberculous A18.01
  staphylococcal M00.00
    ankle M00.07- ☑
    elbow M00.02- ☑
    foot joint — *see* Arthritis, staphylococcal, ankle
    hand joint M00.04- ☑
    hip M00.05- ☑
    knee M00.06- ☑
    multiple site M00.09
    shoulder M00.01- ☑
    vertebra M00.08
    wrist M00.03- ☑
  streptococcal NEC M00.20
    ankle M00.27- ☑
    elbow M00.22- ☑
    foot joint — *see* Arthritis, streptococcal, ankle
    hand joint M00.24- ☑

Arthritis, arthritic — *continued*
  streptococcal — *continued*
    hip M00.25- ☑
    knee M00.26- ☑
    multiple site M00.29
    shoulder M00.21- ☑
    vertebra M00.28
    wrist M00.23- ☑
  suppurative — *see* Arthritis, pyogenic or pyemic
  syphilitic (late) A52.16
    congenital A50.55 *[M12.80]*
  syphilitica deformans (Charcot) A52.16
  temporomandibular joint M26.64- ☑
  toxic of menopause (any site) — *see* Arthritis, specified form NEC
  transient — *see* Arthropathy, specified form NEC
  traumatic (chronic) — *see* Arthropathy, traumatic
  tuberculous A18.02
    spine A18.01
  uratic — *see* Gout
  urethritica (Reiter's) — *see* Reiter's disease
  vertebral — *see* Spondylopathy, inflammatory
  villous (any site) — *see* Arthropathy, specified form NEC
Arthrocele — *see* Effusion, joint
Arthrodesis status Z98.1
Arthrodynia — *see also* Pain, joint
Arthrodysplasia Q74.9
Arthrofibrosis, joint — *see* Ankylosis
Arthrogryposis (congenital) Q68.8
  multiplex congenita Q74.3
Arthrokatadysis M24.7
Arthropathy — *see also* Arthritis M12.9
  Charcot's — *see* Arthropathy, neuropathic
    diabetic — *see* Diabetes, arthropathy, neuropathic
    syringomyelic G95.0
  cricoarytenoid J38.7
  crystal (-induced) — *see* Arthritis, in, crystals
  diabetic NEC — *see* Diabetes, arthropathy
  distal interphalangeal, psoriatic L40.51
  enteropathic M07.60
    ankle M07.67- ☑
    elbow M07.62- ☑
    foot joint M07.67- ☑
    hand joint M07.64- ☑
    hip M07.65- ☑
    knee M07.66- ☑
    multiple site M07.69
    shoulder M07.61- ☑
    vertebra M07.68
    wrist M07.63- ☑
  following intestinal bypass M02.00
    ankle M02.07- ☑
    elbow M02.02- ☑
    foot joint M02.07- ☑
    hand joint M02.04- ☑
    hip M02.05- ☑
    knee M02.06- ☑
    multiple site M02.09
    shoulder M02.01- ☑
    vertebra M02.08
    wrist M02.03- ☑
  gouty — *see also* Gout
    in (due to)
      Lesch-Nyhan syndrome E79.1 *[M14.8-]* ☑
      sickle-cell disorders D57- *[M14.8-]* ☑
  hemophilic NEC D66 *[M36.2]*
    in (due to)
      hyperparathyroidism NEC E21.3 *[M14.8-]* ☑
      metabolic disease NOS E88.9 *[M14.8-]* ☑
  in (due to)
    acromegaly E22.0 *[M14.8-]* ☑
    amyloidosis E85.4 *[M14.8-]* ☑
    blood disorder NOS D75.9 *[M36.3]*
    diabetes — *see* Diabetes, arthropathy
    endocrine disease NOS E34.9 *[M14.8-]* ☑
    erythema
      multiforme L51.9 *[M14.8-]* ☑
      nodosum L52 *[M14.8-]* ☑
    hemochromatosis E83.118 *[M14.8-]* ☑
    hemoglobinopathy NEC D58.2 *[M36.3]*
    hemophilia NEC D66 *[M36.2]*
    Henoch-Schönlein purpura D69.0 *[M36.4]*
    hyperthyroidism E05.90 *[M14.8-]* ☑
    hypothyroidism E03.9 *[M14.8-]* ☑
    infective endocarditis I33.0 *[M12.80]*

Arthritis, arthritic — Arthropathy

Arthropathy — *continued*
  in — *continued*
    leukemia NEC C95.9- ☑ *[M36.1]*
    malignant histiocytosis C96.A *[M36.1]*
    metabolic disease NOS E88.9 *[M14.8-]* ☑
    multiple myeloma C90.0- ☑ *[M36.1]*
    neoplastic disease NOS (*see also* Neoplasm)
      D49.9 *[M36.1]*
    nutritional deficiency — *see also* subcategory
      M14.8- E63.9
    psoriasis NOS L40.50
    sarcoidosis D86.86
    syphilis (late) A52.77
      congenital A50.55 *[M12.80]*
    thyrotoxicosis — *see also* subcategory M14.8-
      E05.90
    ulcerative colitis K51.90 *[M07.60]*
    viral hepatitis (postinfectious) NEC B19.9 *[M12.80]*
    Whipple's disease — *see also* subcategory M14.8-
      K90.81
  Jaccoud — *see* Arthropathy, postrheumatic, chronic
  juvenile — *see* Arthritis, juvenile
    psoriatic L40.54
  mutilans (psoriatic) L40.52
  neuropathic (Charcot) M14.60
    ankle M14.67- ☑
    diabetic — *see* Diabetes, arthropathy, neuropathic
    elbow M14.62- ☑
    foot joint M14.67- ☑
    hand joint M14.64- ☑
    hip M14.65- ☑
    knee M14.66- ☑
    multiple site M14.69
    nonsyphilitic NEC G98.0
    shoulder M14.61- ☑
    syringomyelic G95.0
    vertebra M14.68
    wrist M14.63- ☑
  osteopulmonary — *see* Osteoarthropathy, hyper-
    trophic, specified NEC
  postdysenteric M02.10
    ankle M02.17- ☑
    elbow M02.12- ☑
    foot joint M02.17- ☑
    hand joint M02.14- ☑
    hip M02.15- ☑
    knee M02.16- ☑
    multiple site M02.19
    shoulder M02.11- ☑
    vertebra M02.18
    wrist M02.13- ☑
  postimmunization M02.20
    ankle M02.27- ☑
    elbow M02.22- ☑
    foot joint M02.27- ☑
    hand joint M02.24- ☑
    hip M02.25- ☑
    knee M02.26- ☑
    multiple site M02.29
    shoulder M02.21- ☑
    vertebra M02.28
    wrist M02.23- ☑
  postinfectious NEC B99 ☑ *[M12.80]*
    in (due to)
      enteritis due to Yersinia enterocolitica
        A04.6 *[M12.80]*
      syphilis A52.77
      viral hepatitis NEC B19.9 *[M12.80]*
  postrheumatic, chronic (Jaccoud) M12.00
    ankle M12.07- ☑
    elbow M12.02- ☑
    foot joint M12.07- ☑
    hand joint M12.04- ☑
    hip M12.05- ☑
    knee M12.06- ☑
    multiple site M12.09
    shoulder M12.01- ☑
    specified joint NEC M12.08
    vertebrae M12.08
    wrist M12.03- ☑
  psoriatic NEC L40.59
    interphalangeal, distal L40.51
  reactive M02.9
    in (due to)
      infective endocarditis I33.0 *[M02.9]*
    specified type NEC M02.80
      ankle M02.87- ☑

Arthropathy — *continued*
  reactive — *continued*
    specified type — *continued*
      elbow M02.82- ☑
      foot joint M02.87- ☑
      hand joint M02.84- ☑
      hip M02.85- ☑
      knee M02.86- ☑
      multiple site M02.89
      shoulder M02.81- ☑
      vertebra M02.88
      wrist M02.83- ☑
  specified form NEC M12.80
    ankle M12.87- ☑
    elbow M12.82- ☑
    foot joint M12.87- ☑
    hand joint M12.84- ☑
    hip M12.85- ☑
    knee M12.86- ☑
    multiple site M12.89
    shoulder M12.81- ☑
    specified joint NEC M12.88
    vertebrae M12.88
    wrist M12.83- ☑
  syringomyelic G95.0
  tabes dorsalis A52.16
  tabetic A52.16
  temporomandibular joint M26.65- ☑
  transient — *see* Arthropathy, specified form NEC
  traumatic M12.50
    ankle M12.57- ☑
    elbow M12.52- ☑
    foot joint M12.57- ☑
    hand joint M12.54- ☑
    hip M12.55- ☑
    knee M12.56- ☑
    multiple site M12.59
    shoulder M12.51- ☑
    specified joint NEC M12.58
    vertebrae M12.58
    wrist M12.53- ☑
Arthropyosis — *see* Arthritis, pyogenic or pyemic
Arthrosis (deformans) (degenerative) (localized) — *see also* Osteoarthritis M19.90
  spine — *see* Spondylosis
Arthus' phenomenon or reaction T78.41 ☑
  due to
    drug — *see* Table of Drugs and Chemicals, by drug
Articular — *see* condition
Articulation, reverse (teeth) M26.24
Artificial
  insemination complication — *see* Complications, arti-
    ficial, fertilization
  opening status (functioning) (without complication)
    Z93.9
    anus (colostomy) Z93.3
    colostomy Z93.3
    cystostomy Z93.50
      appendico-vesicostomy Z93.52
      cutaneous Z93.51
      specified NEC Z93.59
    enterostomy Z93.4
    gastrostomy Z93.1
    ileostomy Z93.2
    intestinal tract NEC Z93.4
    jejunostomy Z93.4
    nephrostomy Z93.6
    specified site NEC Z93.8
    tracheostomy Z93.0
    ureterostomy Z93.6
    urethrostomy Z93.6
    urinary tract NEC Z93.6
    vagina Z93.8
  vagina status Z93.8
Arytenoid — *see* condition
Asbestosis (occupational) J61
Ascariasis B77.9
  with
    complications NEC B77.89
    intestinal complications B77.0
    pneumonia, pneumonitis B77.81
Ascaridosis, ascaridiasis — *see* Ascariasis
Ascaris (infection) (infestation) (lumbricoides) — *see* As-
  cariasis
Ascending — *see* condition

ASC-H (atypical squamous cells cannot exclude high grade
  squamous intraepithelial lesion on cytologic smear)
  anus R85.611
  cervix R87.611
  vagina R87.621
Aschoff's bodies — *see* Myocarditis, rheumatic
Ascites (abdominal) R18.8
  cardiac — *see also* Failure, heart, right I50.810
  chylous (nonfilarial) I89.8
    filarial — *see* Infestation, filarial
  due to
    cirrhosis, alcoholic K70.31
    hepatitis
      alcoholic K70.11
      chronic active K71.51
    S. japonicum B65.2
  heart — *see also* Failure, heart, right I50.810
  malignant R18.0
  pseudochylous R18.8
  syphilitic A52.74
  tuberculous A18.31
ASC-US (atypical squamous cells of undetermined signif-
  icance on cytologic smear)
  anus R85.610
  cervix R87.610
  vagina R87.620
Aseptic — *see* condition
Asherman's syndrome N85.6
Asialia K11.7
Asiatic cholera — *see* Cholera
Asimultagnosia (simultanagnosia) R48.3
Askin's tumor — *see* Neoplasm, connective tissue, malignant
Asocial personality F60.2
Asomatognosia R41.4
Aspartylglucosaminuria E77.1
Asperger's disease or syndrome F84.5
Aspergilloma — *see* Aspergillosis
Aspergillosis (with pneumonia) B44.9
  bronchopulmonary, allergic B44.81
  disseminated B44.7
  generalized B44.7
  pulmonary NEC B44.1
    allergic B44.81
    invasive B44.0
  specified NEC B44.89
  tonsillar B44.2
Aspergillus (flavus) (fumigatus) (infection) (terreus) —
  see Aspergillosis
Aspermatogenesis — *see* Azoospermia
Aspermia (testis) — *see* Azoospermia
Asphyxia, asphyxiation (by) R09.01
  antenatal P84
  birth P84
  bunny bag — *see* Asphyxia, due to, mechanical threat
    to breathing, trapped in bed clothes
  crushing S28.0 ☑
  drowning T75.1 ☑
  gas, fumes, or vapor — *see* Table of Drugs and Chemi-
    cals
  inhalation — *see* Inhalation
  intrauterine P84
  local I73.00
    with gangrene I73.01
  mucus — *see also* Foreign body, respiratory tract,
    causing asphyxia
  newborn P84
  pathological R09.01
  postnatal P84
    mechanical — *see* Asphyxia, due to, mechanical
      threat to breathing
  prenatal P84
  reticularis R23.1
  strangulation — *see* Asphyxia, due to, mechanical
    threat to breathing
  submersion T75.1 ☑
  traumatic T71.9 ☑
    due to
      crushed chest S28.0 ☑
      foreign body (in) — *see* Foreign body, respiratory
        tract, causing asphyxia
      low oxygen content of ambient air T71.20 ☑
        due to
          being trapped in
            low oxygen environment T71.29 ☑
            in car trunk T71.221 ☑

Asphyxia, asphyxiation — *continued*
  traumatic — *continued*
    due to — *continued*
      low oxygen content of ambient air — *continued*
        due to — *continued*
          being trapped in — *continued*
            low oxygen environment — *continued*
              in car trunk — *continued*
                circumstances undetermined T71.224 ☑
                done with intent to harm by
                  another person T71.223 ☑
                  self T71.222 ☑
              in refrigerator T71.231 ☑
                circumstances undetermined T71.234 ☑
                done with intent to harm by
                  another person T71.233 ☑
                  self T71.232 ☑
        cave-in T71.21 ☑
      mechanical threat to breathing (accidental) T71.191 ☑
        circumstances undetermined T71.194 ☑
        done with intent to harm by
          another person T71.193 ☑
          self T71.192 ☑
        hanging T71.161 ☑
        circumstances undetermined T71.164 ☑
        done with intent to harm by
          another person T71.163 ☑
          self T71.162 ☑
        plastic bag T71.121 ☑
        circumstances undetermined T71.124 ☑
        done with intent to harm by
          another person T71.123 ☑
          self T71.122 ☑
      smothering
        in furniture T71.151 ☑
          circumstances undetermined T71.154 ☑
          done with intent to harm by
           another person T71.153 ☑
           self T71.152 ☑
        under
          another person's body T71.141 ☑
           circumstances undetermined T71.144 ☑
           done with intent to harm T71.143 ☑
          pillow T71.111 ☑
           circumstances undetermined T71.114 ☑
           done with intent to harm by
            another person T71.113 ☑
            self T71.112 ☑
        trapped in bed clothes T71.131 ☑
        circumstances undetermined T71.134 ☑
        done with intent to harm by
          another person T71.133 ☑
          self T71.132 ☑
  vomiting, vomitus — *see* Foreign body, respiratory tract, causing asphyxia

Aspiration
  amniotic (clear) fluid (newborn) P24.10
    with
      pneumonia (pneumonitis) P24.11
      respiratory symptoms P24.11
  blood
    newborn (without respiratory symptoms) P24.20
      with
        pneumonia (pneumonitis) P24.21
        respiratory symptoms P24.21
    specified age NEC — *see* Foreign body, respiratory tract
  bronchitis J69.0
  food or foreign body (with asphyxiation) — *see* Asphyxia, food
  liquor (amnii) (newborn) P24.10
    with
      pneumonia (pneumonitis) P24.11
      respiratory symptoms P24.11
  meconium (newborn) (without respiratory symptoms) P24.00
    with
      pneumonitis (pneumonitis) P24.01
      respiratory symptoms P24.01

Aspiration — *continued*
  milk (newborn) (without respiratory symptoms) P24.30
    with
      pneumonia (pneumonitis) P24.31
      respiratory symptoms P24.31
    specified age NEC — *see* Foreign body, respiratory tract
  mucus — *see also* Foreign body, by site, causing asphyxia
    newborn P24.10
      with
        pneumonia (pneumonitis) P24.11
        respiratory symptoms P24.11
  neonatal P24.9
    specific NEC (without respiratory symptoms) P24.80
      with
        pneumonia (pneumonitis) P24.81
        respiratory symptoms P24.81
  newborn P24.9
    specific NEC (without respiratory symptoms) P24.80
      with
        pneumonia (pneumonitis) P24.81
        respiratory symptoms P24.81
  pneumonia J69.0
  pneumonitis J69.0
  syndrome of newborn — *see* Aspiration, by substance, with pneumonia
  vernix caseosa (newborn) P24.80
    with
      pneumonia (pneumonitis) P24.81
      respiratory symptoms P24.81
  vomitus — *see also* Foreign body, respiratory tract
    newborn (without respiratory symptoms) P24.30
      with
        pneumonia (pneumonitis) P24.31
        respiratory symptoms P24.31
Asplenia (congenital) Q89.01
  postsurgical Z90.81
Assam fever B55.0
Assault, sexual — *see* Maltreatment
Assmann's focus NEC A15.0
Astasia (-abasia) (hysterical) F44.4
Asteatosis cutis L85.3
Astereognosia, astereognosis R48.1
Asterixis R27.8
  in liver disease K71.3
Asteroid hyalitis — *see* Deposit, crystalline
Asthenia, asthenic R53.1
  cardiac — *see also* Failure, heart I50.9
    psychogenic F45.8
  cardiovascular — *see also* Failure, heart I50.9
    psychogenic F45.8
  heart — *see also* Failure, heart I50.9
    psychogenic F45.8
  hysterical F44.4
  myocardial — *see also* Failure, heart I50.9
    psychogenic F45.8
  nervous F48.8
  neurocirculatory F45.8
  neurotic F48.8
  psychogenic F48.8
  psychoneurotic F48.8
  psychophysiologic F48.8
  reaction (psychophysiologic) F48.8
  senile R54
Asthenopia — *see also* Discomfort, visual
  hysterical F44.6
  psychogenic F44.6
Asthenospermia — *see* Abnormal, specimen, male genital organs
Asthma, asthmatic (bronchial) (catarrh) (spasmodic) J45.909
  with
    chronic obstructive bronchitis J44.9
      with
        acute lower respiratory infection J44.0
        exacerbation (acute) J44.1
    chronic obstructive pulmonary disease J44.9
      with
        acute lower respiratory infection J44.0
        exacerbation (acute) J44.1
    exacerbation (acute) J45.901
    hay fever — *see* Asthma, allergic extrinsic
    rhinitis, allergic — *see* Asthma, allergic extrinsic
    status asthmaticus J45.902
  allergic extrinsic J45.909
    with
      exacerbation (acute) J45.901

Asthma, asthmatic — *continued*
  allergic extrinsic — *continued*
    with — *continued*
      status asthmaticus J45.902
  atopic — *see* Asthma, allergic extrinsic
  cardiac — *see* Failure, ventricular, left
  cardiobronchial I50.1
  childhood J45.909
    with
      exacerbation (acute) J45.901
      status asthmaticus J45.902
  chronic obstructive J44.9
    with
      acute lower respiratory infection J44.0
      exacerbation (acute) J44.1
  collier's J60
  cough variant J45.991
  detergent J69.8
  due to
    detergent J69.8
    inhalation of fumes J68.3
  eosinophilic J82.83
  extrinsic, allergic — *see* Asthma, allergic extrinsic
  grinder's J62.8
  hay — *see* Asthma, allergic extrinsic
  heart I50.1
  idiosyncratic — *see* Asthma, nonallergic
  intermittent (mild) J45.20
    with
      exacerbation (acute) J45.21
      status asthmaticus J45.22
  intrinsic, nonallergic — *see* Asthma, nonallergic
  Kopp's E32.8
  late-onset J45.909
    with
      exacerbation (acute) J45.901
      status asthmaticus J45.902
  mild intermittent J45.20
    with
      exacerbation (acute) J45.21
      status asthmaticus J45.22
  mild persistent J45.30
    with
      exacerbation (acute) J45.31
      status asthmaticus J45.32
  Millar's (laryngismus stridulus) J38.5
  miner's J60
  mixed J45.909
    with
      exacerbation (acute) J45.901
      status asthmaticus J45.902
  moderate persistent J45.40
    with
      exacerbation (acute) J45.41
      status asthmaticus J45.42
  nervous — *see* Asthma, nonallergic
  nonallergic (intrinsic) J45.909
    with
      exacerbation (acute) J45.901
      status asthmaticus J45.902
  persistent
    mild J45.30
      with
        exacerbation (acute) J45.31
        status asthmaticus J45.32
    moderate J45.40
      with
        exacerbation (acute) J45.41
        status asthmaticus J45.42
    severe J45.50
      with
        exacerbation (acute) J45.51
        status asthmaticus J45.52
  platinum J45.998
  pneumoconiotic NEC J64
  potter's J62.8
  predominantly allergic J45.909
  psychogenic F54
  pulmonary eosinophilic J82.83
  red cedar J67.8
  Rostan's I50.1
  sandblaster's J62.8
  sequoiosis J67.8
  severe persistent J45.50
    with
      exacerbation (acute) J45.51
      status asthmaticus J45.52
  specified NEC J45.998

▽ Subterms under main terms may continue to next column or page   ☑ Additional Character Required — Refer to the Tabular List for Character Selection   33

Asphyxia, asphyxiation — Asthma, asthmatic

Asthma, asthmatic — *continued*
  stonemason's J62.8
  thymic E32.8
  tuberculous — *see* Tuberculosis, pulmonary
  Wichmann's (laryngismus stridulus) J38.5
  wood J67.8
Astigmatism (compound) (congenital) H52.20- ☑
  irregular H52.21- ☑
  regular H52.22- ☑
Astraphobia F40.220
Astroblastoma
  specified site — *see* Neoplasm, malignant, by site
  unspecified site C71.9
Astrocytoma (cystic)
  anaplastic
    specified site — *see* Neoplasm, malignant, by site
    unspecified site C71.9
  fibrillary
    specified site — *see* Neoplasm, malignant, by site
    unspecified site C71.9
  fibrous
    specified site — *see* Neoplasm, malignant, by site
    unspecified site C71.9
  gemistocytic
    specified site — *see* Neoplasm, malignant, by site
    unspecified site C71.9
  juvenile
    specified site — *see* Neoplasm, malignant, by site
    unspecified site C71.9
  pilocytic
    specified site — *see* Neoplasm, malignant, by site
    unspecified site C71.9
  piloid
    specified site — *see* Neoplasm, malignant, by site
    unspecified site C71.9
  protoplasmic
    specified site — *see* Neoplasm, malignant, by site
    unspecified site C71.9
  specified site NEC — *see* Neoplasm, malignant, by site
  subependymal D43.2
    giant cell
      specified site — *see* Neoplasm, uncertain behavior, by site
      unspecified site D43.2
    specified site — *see* Neoplasm, uncertain behavior, by site
    unspecified site C71.9
Astroglioma
  specified site — *see* Neoplasm, malignant, by site
  unspecified site C71.9
Asymbolia R48.8
Asymmetry — *see also* Distortion
  between native and reconstructed breast N65.1
  face Q67.0
  jaw (lower) — *see* Anomaly, dentofacial, jaw-cranial base relationship, asymmetry
Asynergia, asynergy R27.8
  ventricular I51.89
Asystole (heart) — *see* Arrest, cardiac
At risk
  for
    dental caries Z91.849
      high Z91.843
      low Z91.841
      moderate Z91.842
    falling Z91.81
Ataxia, ataxy, ataxic R27.0
  acute R27.8
  autosomal recessive Friedreich G11.11
  brain (hereditary) G11.9
  cerebellar (hereditary) G11.9
    with defective DNA repair G11.3
    alcoholic G31.2
    early-onset G11.10
    with
      essential tremor G11.19
      myoclonus [Hunt's ataxia] G11.19
      retained tendon reflexes G11.19
    in
      alcoholism G31.2
      myxedema E03.9 *[G13.2]*
      neoplastic disease — *see also* Neoplasm D49.9 *[G32.81]*
      specified disease NEC G32.81
    late-onset (Marie's) G11.2
  cerebral (hereditary) G11.9
  congenital nonprogressive G11.0

Ataxia, ataxy, ataxic — *continued*
  family, familial — *see* Ataxia, hereditary
  following
    cerebrovascular disease I69.993
      cerebral infarction I69.393
      intracerebral hemorrhage I69.193
      nontraumatic intracranial hemorrhage NEC I69.293
      specified disease NEC I69.893
      subarachnoid hemorrhage I69.093
  Friedreich's (heredofamilial) (cerebellar) (spinal) (with retained reflexes) G11.11
  gait R26.0
    hysterical F44.4
  general R27.8
  gluten M35.9 *[G32.81]*
    with celiac disease K90.0 *[G32.81]*
  hereditary G11.9
    with neuropathy G60.2
    cerebellar — *see* Ataxia, cerebellar
    spastic G11.4
    specified NEC G11.8
    spinal (Friedreich's) G11.11
  heredofamilial — *see* Ataxia, hereditary
  Hunt's G11.19
  hysterical F44.4
  locomotor (progressive) (syphilitic) (partial) (spastic) A52.11
    diabetic — *see* Diabetes, ataxia
  Marie's (cerebellar) (heredofamilial) (late- onset) G11.2
  nonorganic origin F44.4
  nonprogressive, congenital G11.0
  psychogenic F44.4
  Roussy-Lévy G60.0
  Sanger-Brown's (hereditary) G11.2
  spastic hereditary G11.4
  spinal
    hereditary (Friedreich's) G11.11
    progressive (syphilitic) A52.11
  spinocerebellar, X-linked recessive G11.19
  telangiectasia (Louis-Bar) G11.3
Ataxia-telangiectasia (Louis-Bar) G11.3
Atelectasis (massive) (partial) (pressure) (pulmonary) J98.11
  newborn P28.10
    due to resorption P28.11
    partial P28.19
    primary P28.0
    secondary P28.19
  primary (newborn) P28.0
  tuberculous — *see* Tuberculosis, pulmonary
Atelocardia Q24.9
Atelomyelia Q06.1
Atheroembolism
  of
    extremities
      lower I75.02- ☑
      upper I75.01- ☑
    kidney I75.81
    specified NEC I75.89
Atheroma, atheromatous — *see also* Arteriosclerosis I70.90
  aorta, aortic I70.0
    valve — *see also* Endocarditis, aortic I35.8
  aorto-iliac I70.0
  artery — *see* Arteriosclerosis
  basilar (artery) I67.2
  carotid (artery) (common) (internal) I67.2
  cerebral (arteries) I67.2
  coronary (artery) I25.10
    with angina pectoris — *see* Arteriosclerosis, coronary (artery),
  degeneration — *see* Arteriosclerosis
  heart, cardiac — *see* Disease, heart, ischemic, atherosclerotic
  mitral (valve) I34.8
  myocardium, myocardial — *see* Disease, heart, ischemic, atherosclerotic
  pulmonary valve (heart) — *see also* Endocarditis, pulmonary I37.8
  tricuspid (heart) (valve) I36.8
  valve, valvular — *see* Endocarditis
  vertebral (artery) I67.2
Atheromatosis — *see* Arteriosclerosis
Atherosclerosis — *see also* Arteriosclerosis
  coronary
    artery I25.10

Atherosclerosis — *continued*
  coronary — *continued*
    artery — *continued*
      with angina pectoris — *see* Arteriosclerosis, coronary (artery),
      due to
        calcified coronary lesion (severely) I25.84
        lipid rich plaque I25.83
  transplanted heart I25.811
    bypass graft I25.812
      with angina pectoris — *see* Arteriosclerosis, coronary (artery),
    native coronary artery I25.811
      with angina pectoris — *see* Arteriosclerosis, coronary (artery),
Athetosis (acquired) R25.8
  bilateral (congenital) G80.3
  congenital (bilateral) (double) G80.3
  double (congenital) G80.3
  unilateral R25.8
Athlete's
  foot B35.3
  heart I51.7
Athrepsia E41
Athyrea (acquired) — *see also* Hypothyroidism
  congenital E03.1
Atonia, atony, atonic
  bladder (sphincter) (neurogenic) N31.2
  capillary I78.8
  cecum K59.89
    psychogenic F45.8
  colon — *see* Atony, intestine
  congenital P94.2
  esophagus K22.8
  intestine K59.89
    psychogenic F45.8
  stomach K31.89
    neurotic or psychogenic F45.8
  uterus (during labor) O62.2
    with hemorrhage (postpartum) O72.1
    postpartum (with hemorrhage) O72.1
      without hemorrhage O75.89
Atopy — *see* History, allergy
Atransferrinemia, congenital E88.09
Atresia, atretic
  alimentary organ or tract NEC Q45.8
    upper Q40.8
  ani, anus, anal (canal) Q42.3
    with fistula Q42.2
  aorta (ring) Q25.29
  aortic (orifice) (valve) Q23.0
    arch Q25.21
      congenital with hypoplasia of ascending aorta and defective development of left ventricle (with mitral stenosis) Q23.4
    in hypoplastic left heart syndrome Q23.4
  aqueduct of Sylvius Q03.0
    with spina bifida — *see* Spina bifida, with hydrocephalus
  artery NEC Q27.8
    cerebral Q28.3
    coronary Q24.5
    digestive system Q27.8
    eye Q15.8
    lower limb Q27.8
    pulmonary Q25.5
    specified site NEC Q27.8
    umbilical Q27.0
    upper limb Q27.8
  auditory canal (external) Q16.1
  bile duct (common) (congenital) (hepatic) Q44.2
    acquired — *see* Obstruction, bile duct
  bladder (neck) Q64.39
    obstruction Q64.31
  bronchus Q32.4
  cecum Q42.8
  cervix (acquired) N88.2
    congenital Q51.828
      in pregnancy or childbirth — *see* Anomaly, cervix, in pregnancy or childbirth
        causing obstructed labor O65.5
  choana Q30.0
  colon Q42.9
    specified NEC Q42.8
  common duct Q44.2
  cricoid cartilage Q31.8
  cystic duct Q44.2
    acquired K82.8

☑ **Additional Character Required** — Refer to the Tabular List for Character Selection   ▽ **Subterms under main terms may continue to next column or page**

Atresia, atretic — *continued*
  cystic duct — *continued*
    acquired — *continued*
      with obstruction K82.0
  digestive organs NEC Q45.8
  duodenum Q41.0
  ear canal Q16.1
  ejaculatory duct Q55.4
  epiglottis Q31.8
  esophagus Q39.0
    with tracheoesophageal fistula Q39.1
  eustachian tube Q17.8
  fallopian tube (congenital) Q50.6
    acquired N97.1
  follicular cyst N83.0- ☑
  foramen of
    Luschka Q03.1
      with spina bifida — *see* Spina bifida, with hydro-
        cephalus
    Magendie Q03.1
      with spina bifida — *see* Spina bifida, with hydro-
        cephalus
  gallbladder Q44.1
  genital organ
    external
      female Q52.79
      male Q55.8
    internal
      female Q52.8
      male Q55.8
  glottis Q31.8
  gullet Q39.0
    with tracheoesophageal fistula Q39.1
  heart valve NEC Q24.8
    pulmonary Q22.0
    tricuspid Q22.4
  hymen Q52.3
    acquired (postinfective) N89.6
  ileum Q41.2
  intestine (small) Q41.9
    large Q42.9
      specified NEC Q42.8
  iris, filtration angle Q15.0
  jejunum Q41.1
  lacrimal apparatus Q10.4
  larynx Q31.8
  meatus urinarius Q64.33
  mitral valve Q23.2
    in hypoplastic left heart syndrome Q23.4
  nares (anterior) (posterior) Q30.0
  nasopharynx Q34.8
  nose, nostril Q30.0
    acquired J34.89
  organ or site NEC Q89.8
  osseous meatus (ear) Q16.1
  oviduct (congenital) Q50.6
    acquired N97.1
  parotid duct Q38.4
    acquired K11.8
  pulmonary (artery) Q25.5
    valve Q22.0
  pulmonic Q22.0
  pupil Q13.2
  rectum Q42.1
    with fistula Q42.0
  salivary duct Q38.4
    acquired K11.8
  sublingual duct Q38.4
    acquired K11.8
  submandibular duct Q38.4
    acquired K11.8
  submaxillary duct Q38.4
    acquired K11.8
  thyroid cartilage Q31.8
  trachea Q32.1
  tricuspid valve Q22.4
  ureter Q62.10
    pelvic junction Q62.11
    vesical orifice Q62.12
  ureteropelvic junction Q62.11
  ureterovesical orifice Q62.12
  urethra (valvular) Q64.39
    stricture Q64.32
  urinary tract NEC Q64.8
  uterus Q51.818
    acquired N85.8
  vagina (congenital) Q52.4
    acquired (postinfectional) (senile) N89.5
  vas deferens Q55.3

Atresia, atretic — *continued*
  vascular NEC Q27.8
    cerebral Q28.3
    digestive system Q27.8
    lower limb Q27.8
    specified site NEC Q27.8
    upper limb Q27.8
  vein NEC Q27.8
    digestive system Q27.8
    great Q26.8
    lower limb Q27.8
    portal Q26.5
    pulmonary Q26.4
      partial Q26.3
      total Q26.2
    specified site NEC Q27.8
    upper limb Q27.8
  vena cava (inferior) (superior) Q26.8
  vesicourethral orifice Q64.31
  vulva Q52.79
    acquired N90.5
Atrichia, atrichosis — *see* Alopecia
Atrophia — *see also* Atrophy
  cutis senilis L90.8
    due to radiation L57.8
  gyrata of choroid and retina H31.23
  senilis R54
    dermatological L90.8
      due to radiation (nonionizing) (solar) L57.8
  unguium L60.3
    congenita Q84.6
Atrophie blanche (en plaque) (de Milian) L95.0
Atrophoderma, atrophodermia (of) L90.9
  diffusum (idiopathic) L90.4
  maculatum L90.8
    et striatum L90.8
      due to syphilis A52.79
    syphilitic A51.39
  neuriticum L90.8
  Pasini and Pierini L90.3
  pigmentosum Q82.1
  reticulatum symmetricum faciei L66.4
  senile L90.8
    due to radiation (nonionizing) (solar) L57.8
  vermiculata (cheeks) L66.4
Atrophy, atrophic (of)
  adrenal (capsule) (gland) E27.49
    primary (autoimmune) E27.1
  alveolar process or ridge (edentulous) K08.20
  anal sphincter (disuse) N81.84
  appendix K38.8
  arteriosclerotic — *see* Arteriosclerosis
  bile duct (common) (hepatic) K83.8
  bladder N32.89
    neurogenic N31.8
  blanche (en plaque) (of Milian) L95.0
  bone (senile) NEC — *see also* Disorder, bone, specified
    type NEC
    due to
      tabes dorsalis (neurogenic) A52.11
  brain (cortex) (progressive) G31.9
    frontotemporal circumscribed G31.01 *[F02.80]*
      with behavioral disturbance G31.01 *[F02.81]*
    senile NEC G31.1
  breast N64.2
    obstetric — *see* Disorder, breast, specified type NEC
  buccal cavity K13.79
  cardiac — *see* Degeneration, myocardial
  cartilage (infectional) (joint) — *see* Disorder, cartilage,
    specified NEC
  cerebellar — *see* Atrophy, brain
  cerebral — *see* Atrophy, brain
  cervix (mucosa) (senile) (uteri) N88.8
    menopausal N95.8
  Charcot-Marie-Tooth G60.0
  choroid (central) (macular) (myopic) (retina) H31.10- ☑
    diffuse secondary H31.12- ☑
    gyrate H31.23
    senile H31.11- ☑
  ciliary body — *see* Atrophy, iris
  conjunctiva (senile) H11.89
  corpus cavernosum N48.89
  cortical — *see* Atrophy, brain
  cystic duct K82.8
  Déjérine-Thomas G23.8
  disuse NEC — *see* Atrophy, muscle
  Duchenne-Aran G12.21
  ear H93.8- ☑

Atrophy, atrophic — *continued*
  edentulous alveolar ridge K08.20
  endometrium (senile) N85.8
    cervix N88.8
  enteric K63.89
  epididymis N50.89
  eyeball — *see* Disorder, globe, degenerated condition,
    atrophy
  eyelid (senile) — *see* Disorder, eyelid, degenerative
  facial (skin) L90.9
  fallopian tube (senile) N83.32- ☑
    with ovary N83.33- ☑
  fascioscapulohumeral (Landouzy- Déjérine) G71.02
  fatty, thymus (gland) E32.8
  gallbladder K82.8
  gastric K29.40
    with bleeding K29.41
  gastrointestinal K63.89
  glandular I89.8
  globe H44.52- ☑
  gum — *see* Recession, gingival
  hair L67.8
  heart (brown) — *see* Degeneration, myocardial
  hemifacial Q67.4
    Romberg G51.8
  infantile E41
    paralysis, acute — *see* Poliomyelitis, paralytic
  intestine K63.89
  iris (essential) (progressive) H21.26- ☑
    specified NEC H21.29
  kidney (senile) (terminal) — *see also* Sclerosis, renal
    N26.1
    congenital or infantile Q60.5
      bilateral Q60.4
      unilateral Q60.3
    hydronephrotic — *see* Hydronephrosis
  lacrimal gland (primary) H04.14- ☑
    secondary H04.15- ☑
  Landouzy-Déjérine G71.02
  laryngitis, infective J37.0
  larynx J38.7
  Leber's optic (hereditary) H47.22
  lip K13.0
  liver (yellow) K72.90
    with coma K72.91
    acute, subacute K72.00
      with coma K72.01
    chronic K72.10
      with coma K72.11
  lung (senile) J98.4
  macular (dermatological) L90.8
    syphilitic, skin A51.39
      striated A52.79
  mandible (edentulous) K08.20
    minimal K08.21
    moderate K08.22
    severe K08.23
  maxilla K08.20
    minimal K08.24
    moderate K08.25
    severe K08.26
  muscle, muscular (diffuse) (general) (idiopathic) (prima-
    ry) M62.50
    ankle M62.57- ☑
    Duchenne-Aran G12.21
    foot M62.57- ☑
    forearm M62.53- ☑
    hand M62.54- ☑
    infantile spinal G12.0
    lower leg M62.56- ☑
    multiple sites M62.59
    myelopathic — *see* Atrophy, muscle, spinal
    myotonic G71.11
    neuritic G58.9
    neuropathic (peroneal) (progressive) G60.0
    pelvic (disuse) N81.84
    peroneal G60.0
    progressive (bulbar) G12.21
      adult G12.1
      infantile (spinal) G12.0
      spinal G12.25
        adult G12.1
        infantile G12.0
    pseudohypertrophic G71.02
    shoulder region M62.51- ☑
    specified site NEC M62.58
    spinal G12.9
      adult form G12.1

▽ **Subterms under main terms may continue to next column or page**   ☑ **Additional Character Required** — **Refer to the Tabular List for Character Selection**   **35**

Atresia, atretic — Atrophy, atrophic

Atrophy, atrophic — *continued*
  muscle, muscular — *continued*
    spinal — *continued*
      Aran-Duchenne G12.21
      childhood form, type II G12.1
      distal G12.1
      hereditary NEC G12.1
      infantile, type I (Werdnig-Hoffmann) G12.0
      juvenile form, type III (Kugelberg- Welander) G12.1
      progressive G12.25
      scapuloperoneal form G12.1
      specified NEC G12.8
    syphilitic A52.78
    thigh M62.55- ☑
    upper arm M62.52- ☑
  myocardium — *see* Degeneration, myocardial
  myometrium (senile) N85.8
    cervix N88.8
  myopathic NEC — *see* Atrophy, muscle
  myotonia G71.11
  nail L60.3
  nasopharynx J31.1
  nerve — *see also* Disorder, nerve
    abducens — *see* Strabismus, paralytic, sixth nerve
    accessory G52.8
    acoustic or auditory H93.3 ☑
    cranial G52.9
      eighth (auditory) H93.3 ☑
      eleventh (accessory) G52.8
      fifth (trigeminal) G50.8
      first (olfactory) G52.0
      fourth (trochlear) — *see* Strabismus, paralytic, fourth nerve
      second (optic) H47.20
      sixth (abducens) — *see* Strabismus, paralytic, sixth nerve
      tenth (pneumogastric) (vagus) G52.2
      third (oculomotor) — *see* Strabismus, paralytic, third nerve
      twelfth (hypoglossal) G52.3
    hypoglossal G52.3
    oculomotor — *see* Strabismus, paralytic, third nerve
    olfactory G52.0
    optic (papillomacular bundle)
      syphilitic (late) A52.15
        congenital A50.44
    pneumogastric G52.2
    trigeminal G50.8
    trochlear — *see* Strabismus, paralytic, fourth nerve
    vagus (pneumogastric) G52.2
  neurogenic, bone, tabetic A52.11
  nutritional E41
  old age R54
  olivopontocerebellar G23.8
  optic (nerve) H47.20
    glaucomatous H47.23- ☑
    hereditary H47.22
    primary H47.21- ☑
    specified type NEC H47.29- ☑
    syphilitic (late) A52.15
      congenital A50.44
  orbit H05.31- ☑
  ovary (senile) N83.31- ☑
    with fallopian tube N83.33- ☑
  oviduct (senile) — *see* Atrophy, fallopian tube
  palsy, diffuse (progressive) G12.22
  pancreas (duct) (senile) K86.89
  parotid gland K11.0
  pelvic muscle N81.84
  penis N48.89
  pharynx J39.2
  pluriglandular E31.8
    autoimmune E31.0
  polyarthritis M15.9
  prostate N42.89
  pseudohypertrophic (muscle) G71.02
  renal — *see also* Sclerosis, renal N26.1
  retina, retinal (postinfectional) H35.89
  rhinitis J31.0
  salivary gland K11.0
  scar L90.5
  sclerosis, lobar (of brain) G31.09 *[F02.80]*
    with behavioral disturbance G31.09 *[F02.81]*
  scrotum N50.89
  seminal vesicle N50.89
  senile R54
    due to radiation (nonionizing) (solar) L57.8

Atrophy, atrophic — *continued*
  skin (patches) (spots) L90.9
    degenerative (senile) L90.8
    due to radiation (nonionizing) (solar) L57.8
    senile L90.8
  spermatic cord N50.89
  spinal (acute) (cord) G95.89
    muscular — *see* Atrophy, muscle, spinal
    paralysis G12.20
      acute — *see* Poliomyelitis, paralytic
      meaning progressive muscular atrophy G12.25
  spine (column) — *see* Spondylopathy, specified NEC
  spleen (senile) D73.0
  stomach K29.40
    with bleeding K29.41
  striate (skin) L90.6
    syphilitic A52.79
  subcutaneous L90.9
  sublingual gland K11.0
  submandibular gland K11.0
  submaxillary gland K11.0
  Sudeck's — *see* Algoneurodystrophy
  suprarenal (capsule) (gland) E27.49
    primary E27.1
  systemic affecting central nervous system in
    myxedema E03.9 *[G13.2]*
    neoplastic disease — *see also* Neoplasm D49.9 *[G13.1]*
    specified disease NEC G13.8
  tarso-orbital fascia, congenital Q10.3
  testis N50.0
  thenar, partial — *see* Syndrome, carpal tunnel
  thymus (fatty) E32.8
  thyroid (gland) (acquired) E03.4
    with cretinism E03.1
    congenital (with myxedema) E03.1
  tongue (senile) K14.8
    papillae K14.4
  trachea J39.8
  tunica vaginalis N50.89
  turbinate J34.89
  tympanic membrane (nonflaccid) H73.82- ☑
    flaccid H73.81- ☑
  upper respiratory tract J39.8
  uterus, uterine (senile) N85.8
    cervix N88.8
    due to radiation (intended effect) N85.8
      adverse effect or misadventure N99.89
  vagina (senile) N95.2
  vas deferens N50.89
  vascular I99.8
  vertebra (senile) — *see* Spondylopathy, specified NEC
  vulva (senile) N90.5
  Werdnig-Hoffmann G12.0
  yellow — *see* Failure, hepatic

Attack, attacks
  with alteration of consciousness (with automatisms) — *see* Epilepsy, localization-related, symptomatic, with complex partial seizures
  Adams-Stokes I45.9
  akinetic — *see* Epilepsy, generalized, specified NEC
  angina — *see* Angina
  atonic — *see* Epilepsy, generalized, specified NEC
  benign shuddering G25.83
  cataleptic — *see* Catalepsy
  coronary — *see* Infarct, myocardium
  cyanotic, newborn P28.2
  drop NEC R55
  epileptic — *see* Epilepsy
  heart — *see* infarct, myocardium
  hysterical F44.9
  jacksonian — *see* Epilepsy, localization-related, symptomatic, with simple partial seizures
  myocardium, myocardial — *see* Infarct, myocardium
  myoclonic — *see* Epilepsy, generalized, specified NEC
  panic F41.0
  psychomotor — *see* Epilepsy, localization-related, symptomatic, with complex partial seizures
  salaam — *see* Epilepsy, spasms
  schizophreniform, brief F23
  shuddering, benign G25.83
  Stokes-Adams I45.9
  syncope R55
  transient ischemic (TIA) G45.9
    specified NEC G45.8
  unconsciousness R55
    hysterical F44.89

Attack, attacks — *continued*
  vasomotor R55
  vasovagal (paroxysmal) (idiopathic) R55
  without alteration of consciousness — *see* Epilepsy, localization-related, symptomatic, with simple partial seizures

Attention (to)
  artificial
    opening (of) Z43.9
      digestive tract NEC Z43.4
        colon Z43.3
        ilium Z43.2
        stomach Z43.1
      specified NEC Z43.8
      trachea Z43.0
      urinary tract NEC Z43.6
        cystostomy Z43.5
        nephrostomy Z43.6
        ureterostomy Z43.6
        urethrostomy Z43.6
      vagina Z43.7
  colostomy Z43.3
  cystostomy Z43.5
  deficit disorder or syndrome F98.8
    with hyperactivity — *see* Disorder, attention-deficit hyperactivity
  gastrostomy Z43.1
  ileostomy Z43.2
  jejunostomy Z43.4
  nephrostomy Z43.6
  surgical dressings Z48.01
  sutures Z48.02
  tracheostomy Z43.0
  ureterostomy Z43.6
  urethrostomy Z43.6

Attrition
  gum — *see* Recession, gingival
  tooth, teeth (excessive) (hard tissues) K03.0

Atypical, atypism — *see also* condition
  cells (on cytolgocial smear) (endocervical) (endometrial) (glandular)
    cervix R87.619
    vagina R87.629
  cervical N87.9
  endometrium N85.9
    hyperplasia N85.00
  parenting situation Z62.9

Auditory — *see* condition
Aujeszky's disease B33.8
Aurantiasis, cutis E67.1
Auricle, auricular — *see also* condition
  cervical Q18.2
Auriculotemporal syndrome G50.8
Austin Flint murmur (aortic insufficiency) I35.1
Australian
  Q fever A78
  X disease A83.4
Autism, autistic (childhood) (infantile) F84.0
  atypical F84.9
  spectrum disorder F84.0
Autodigestion R68.89
Autoerythrocyte sensitization (syndrome) D69.2
Autographism L50.3
Autoimmune
  disease (systemic) M35.9
  inhibitors to clotting factors D68.311
  lymphoproliferative syndrome [ALPS] D89.82
  thyroiditis E06.3
Autointoxication R68.89
Automatism G93.89
  with temporal sclerosis G93.81
  epileptic — *see* Epilepsy, localization-related, symptomatic, with complex partial seizures
  paroxysmal, idiopathic — *see* Epilepsy, localization-related, symptomatic, with complex partial seizures
Autonomic, autonomous
  bladder (neurogenic) N31.2
  hysteria seizure F44.5
Autosensitivity, erythrocyte D69.2
Autosensitization, cutaneous L30.2
Autosome — *see* condition by chromosome involved
Autotopagnosia R48.1
Autotoxemia R68.89
Autumn — *see* condition
Avellis' syndrome G46.8
Aversion
  oral R63.3

Aversion — *continued*
  oral — *continued*
    newborn P92.- ☑
    nonorganic origin F98.2 ☑
  sexual F52.1
Aviator's
  disease or sickness — *see* Effect, adverse, high altitude
  ear T70.0 ☑
Avitaminosis (multiple) — *see also* Deficiency, vitamin
  E56.9
  B E53.9
    with
      beriberi E51.11
      pellagra E52
  B2 E53.0
  B6 E53.1
  B12 E53.8
  D E55.9
    with rickets E55.0
  G E53.0
  K E56.1
  nicotinic acid E52
AVNRT (atrioventricular nodal re-entrant tachycardia)
  I47.1
AVRT (atrioventricular nodal re-entrant tachycardia) I47.1
Avulsion (traumatic)
  blood vessel — *see* Injury, blood vessel
  bone — *see* Fracture, by site
  cartilage — *see also* Dislocation, by site
    symphyseal (inner), complicating delivery O71.6
  external site other than limb — *see* Wound, open, by
    site
  eye S05.7- ☑
  head (intracranial)
    external site NEC S08.89 ☑
    scalp S08.0 ☑
  internal organ or site — *see* Injury, by site
  joint — *see also* Dislocation, by site
    capsule — *see* Sprain, by site
  kidney S37.06- ☑
  ligament — *see* Sprain, by site
  limb — *see also* Amputation, traumatic, by site
    skin and subcutaneous tissue — *see* Wound, open,
      by site
  muscle — *see* Injury, muscle
  nerve (root) — *see* Injury, nerve
  scalp S08.0 ☑
  skin and subcutaneous tissue — *see* Wound, open, by
    site
  spleen S36.032 ☑
  symphyseal cartilage (inner), complicating delivery
    O71.6
  tendon — *see* Injury, muscle
  tooth S03.2 ☑
Awareness of heart beat R00.2
Axenfeld's
  anomaly or syndrome Q15.0
  degeneration (calcareous) Q13.4
Axilla, axillary — *see also* condition
  breast Q83.1
Axonotmesis — *see* Injury, nerve
Ayerza's disease or syndrome (pulmonary artery sclerosis with pulmonary hypertension) I27.0
Azoospermia (organic) N46.01
  due to
    drug therapy N46.021
    efferent duct obstruction N46.023
    infection N46.022
    radiation N46.024
    specified cause NEC N46.029
    systemic disease N46.025
Azotemia R79.89
  meaning uremia N19
Aztec ear Q17.3
Azygos
  continuation inferior vena cava Q26.8
  lobe (lung) Q33.1

B

Baastrup's disease — *see* Kissing spine
Babesiosis B60.00
  due to
    Babesia
      divergens B60.03
      duncani B60.02
      KO-1 B60.09

Babesiosis — *continued*
  due to — *continued*
    Babesia — *continued*
      microti B60.01
      MO-1 B60.03
      species
        unspecified B60.00
      venatorum B60.09
    specified NEC B60.09
Babington's disease (familial hemorrhagic telangiectasia) I78.0
Babinski's syndrome A52.79
Baby
  crying constantly R68.11
  floppy (syndrome) P94.2
Bacillary — *see* condition
Bacilluria R82.71
Bacillus — *see also* Infection, bacillus
  abortus infection A23.1
  anthracis infection A22.9
  coli infection — *see also* Escherichia coli B96.20
  Flexner's A03.1
  mallei infection A24.0
  Shiga's A03.0
  suipestifer infection — *see* Infection, salmonella
Back — *see* condition
Backache (postural) M54.9
  sacroiliac M53.3
  specified NEC M54.89
Backflow — *see* Reflux
Backward reading (dyslexia) F81.0
Bacteremia R78.81
  with sepsis — *see* Sepsis
Bactericholia — *see* Cholecystitis, acute
Bacterid, bacteride (pustular) L40.3
Bacterium, bacteria, bacterial
  agent NEC, as cause of disease classified elsewhere
    B96.89
  in blood — *see* Bacteremia
  in urine — *see* Bacteriuria
Bacteriuria, bacteruria R82.71
  asymptomatic R82.71
Bacteroides
  fragilis, as cause of disease classified elsewhere B96.6
Bad
  heart — *see* Disease, heart
  trip
    due to drug abuse — *see* Abuse, drug, hallucinogen
    due to drug dependence — *see* Dependence, drug,
      hallucinogen
Baelz's disease (cheilitis glandularis apostematosa) K13.0
Baerensprung's disease (eczema marginatum) B35.6
Bagasse disease or pneumonitis J67.1
Bagassosis J67.1
Baker's cyst — *see* Cyst, Baker's
Bakwin-Krida syndrome (metaphyseal dysplasia) Q78.5
Balancing side interference M26.56
Balanitis (circinata) (erosiva) (gangrenosa) (phagedenic)
  (vulgaris) N48.1
  amebic A06.82
  candidal B37.42
  due to Haemophilus ducreyi A57
  gonococcal (acute) (chronic) A54.23
  xerotica obliterans N48.0
Balanoposthitis N47.6
  gonococcal (acute) (chronic) A54.23
  ulcerative (specific) A63.8
Balanorrhagia — *see* Balanitis
Balantidiasis, balantidiosis A07.0
Bald tongue K14.4
Baldness — *see also* Alopecia
  male-pattern — *see* Alopecia, androgenic
Balkan grippe A78
Balloon disease — *see* Effect, adverse, high altitude
Balo's disease (concentric sclerosis) G37.5
Bamberger-Marie disease — *see* Osteoarthropathy,
  hypertrophic, specified type NEC
Bancroft's filariasis B74.0
Band(s)
  adhesive — *see* Adhesions, peritoneum
  anomalous or congenital — *see also* Anomaly, by site
    heart (atrial) (ventricular) Q24.8
    intestine Q43.3
    omentum Q43.3
  cervix N88.1
  constricting, congenital Q79.8
  gallbladder (congenital) Q44.1

Band(s) — *continued*
  intestinal (adhesive) — *see* Adhesions, peritoneum
  obstructive
    intestine K56.50
      complete K56.52
      incomplete K56.51
      partial K56.51
    peritoneum K56.50
      complete K56.52
      incomplete K56.51
      partial K56.51
  periappendiceal, congenital Q43.3
  peritoneal (adhesive) — *see* Adhesions, peritoneum
  uterus N73.6
    internal N85.6
  vagina N89.5
Bandemia D72.825
Bandl's ring (contraction), complicating delivery O62.4
Bangkok hemorrhagic fever A91
Bang's disease (brucella abortus) A23.1
Bankruptcy, anxiety concerning Z59.8
Bannister's disease T78.3 ☑
  hereditary D84.1
Banti's disease or syndrome (with cirrhosis) (with portal
  hypertension) K76.6
Bar, median, prostate — *see* Enlargement, enlarged,
  prostate
Barcoo disease or rot — *see* Ulcer, skin
Barlow's disease E54
Barodontalgia T70.29 ☑
Baron Münchausen syndrome — *see* Disorder, facti-
  tious
Barosinusitis T70.1 ☑
Barotitis T70.0 ☑
Barotrauma T70.29 ☑
  odontalgia T70.29 ☑
  otitic T70.0 ☑
  sinus T70.1 ☑
Barraquer (-Simons) **disease or syndrome** (progressive
  lipodystrophy) E88.1
Barré-Guillain disease or syndrome G61.0
Barrel chest M95.4
Barré-Liéou syndrome (posterior cervical sympathetic)
  M53.0
Barrett's
  disease — *see* Barrett's, esophagus
  esophagus K22.70
    with dysplasia K22.719
      high grade K22.711
      low grade K22.710
    without dysplasia K22.70
  syndrome — *see* Barrett's, esophagus
  ulcer K22.10
    with bleeding K22.11
    without bleeding K22.10
Bársony (-Polgár) (-Teschendorf) **syndrome** (corkscrew
  esophagus) K22.4
Barth syndrome E78.71
Bartholinitis (suppurating) N75.8
  gonococcal (acute) (chronic) (with abscess) A54.1
Bartonellosis A44.9
  cutaneous A44.1
  mucocutaneous A44.1
  specified NEC A44.8
  systemic A44.0
Barton's fracture S52.56- ☑
Bartter's syndrome E26.81
Basal — *see* condition
Basan's (hidrotic) ectodermal dysplasia Q82.4
Baseball finger — *see* Dislocation, finger
Basedow's disease (exophthalmic goiter) — *see* Hyper-
  thyroidism, with, goiter
Basic — *see* condition
Basilar — *see* condition
Bason's (hidrotic) ectodermal dysplasia Q82.4
Basopenia — *see* Agranulocytosis
Basophilia D72.824
Basophilism (cortico-adrenal) (Cushing's) (pituitary) E24.0
Bassen-Kornzweig disease or syndrome E78.6
Bat ear Q17.5
Bateman's
  disease B08.1
  purpura (senile) D69.2
Bathing cramp T75.1 ☑
Bathophobia F40.248
Batten (-Mayou) **disease** E75.4
  retina E75.4 *[H36]*

Batten-Steinert syndrome G71.11
Battered — *see* Maltreatment
Battey Mycobacterium infection A31.0
Battle exhaustion F43.0
Battledore placenta O43.19- ☑
Baumgarten-Cruveilhier cirrhosis, disease or syndrome K74.69
Bauxite fibrosis (of lung) J63.1
Bayle's disease (general paresis) A52.17
Bazin's disease (primary) (tuberculous) A18.4
Beach ear — *see* Swimmer's, ear
Beaded hair (congenital) Q84.1
Béal conjunctivitis or syndrome B30.2
Beard's disease (neurasthenia) F48.8
Beat(s)
  atrial, premature I49.1
  ectopic I49.49
  elbow — *see* Bursitis, elbow
  escaped, heart I49.49
  hand — *see* Bursitis, hand
  knee — *see* Bursitis, knee
  premature I49.40
    atrial I49.1
    auricular I49.1
    supraventricular I49.1
Beau's
  disease or syndrome — *see* Degeneration, myocardial
  lines (transverse furrows on fingernails) L60.4
Bechterev's syndrome — *see* Spondylitis, ankylosing
Becker's
  cardiomyopathy I42.8
  disease
    idiopathic mural endomyocardial disease I42.3
    myotonia congenita, recessive form G71.12
  dystrophy G71.01
  pigmented hairy nevus D22.5
Beck's syndrome (anterior spinal artery occlusion) I65.8
Beckwith-Wiedemann syndrome Q87.3
Bed confinement status Z74.01
Bed sore — *see* Ulcer, pressure, by site
Bedbug bite(s) — *see* Bite(s), by site, superficial, insect
Bedclothes, asphyxiation or suffocation by — *see* Asphyxia, traumatic, due to, mechanical, trapped
Bednar's
  aphthae K12.0
  tumor — *see* Neoplasm, malignant, by site
Bedridden Z74.01
Bedsore — *see* Ulcer, pressure, by site
Bedwetting — *see* Enuresis
Bee sting (with allergic or anaphylactic shock) — *see* Toxicity, venom, arthropod, bee
Beer drinker's heart (disease) I42.6
Begbie's disease (exophthalmic goiter) — *see* Hyperthyroidism, with, goiter
Behavior
  antisocial
    adult Z72.811
    child or adolescent Z72.810
  disorder, disturbance — *see* Disorder, conduct
  disruptive — *see* Disorder, conduct
  drug seeking Z76.5
  inexplicable R46.2
  marked evasiveness R46.5
  obsessive-compulsive R46.81
  overactivity R46.3
  poor responsiveness R46.4
  self-damaging (life-style) Z72.89
  sleep-incompatible Z72.821
  slowness R46.4
  specified NEC R46.89
  strange (and inexplicable) R46.2
  suspiciousness R46.5
  type A pattern Z73.1
  undue concern or preoccupation with stressful events R46.6
  verbosity and circumstantial detail obscuring reason for contact R46.7
Behçet's disease or syndrome M35.2
Behr's disease — *see* Degeneration, macula
Beigel's disease or morbus (white piedra) B36.2
Bejel A65
Bekhterev's syndrome — *see* Spondylitis, ankylosing
Belching — *see* Eructation
Bell's
  mania F30.8
  palsy, paralysis G51.0
    infant or newborn P11.3

Bell's — *continued*
  spasm G51.3- ☑
Bence Jones albuminuria or proteinuria NEC R80.3
Bends T70.3 ☑
Benedikt's paralysis or syndrome G46.3
Benign — *see also* condition
  prostatic hyperplasia — *see* Hyperplasia, prostate
Bennett's fracture (displaced) S62.21- ☑
Benson's disease — *see* Deposit, crystalline
Bent
  back (hysterical) F44.4
  nose M95.0
    congenital Q67.4
Bereavement (uncomplicated) Z63.4
Bergeron's disease (hysterical chorea) F44.4
Berger's disease — *see* Nephropathy, IgA
Beriberi (dry) E51.11
  heart (disease) E51.12
  polyneuropathy E51.11
  wet E51.12
    involving circulatory system E51.11
Berlin's disease or edema (traumatic) S05.8X- ☑
Berlock (berloque) **dermatitis** L56.2
Bernard-Horner syndrome G90.2
Bernard-Soulier disease or thrombopathia D69.1
Bernhardt (-Roth) **disease** — *see* Mononeuropathy, lower limb, meralgia paresthetica
Bernheim's syndrome — *see* Failure, heart, right
Bertielliasis B71.8
Berylliosis (lung) J63.2
Besnier-Boeck (-Schaumann) **disease** — *see* Sarcoidosis
Besnier's
  lupus pernio D86.3
  prurigo L20.0
Bestiality F65.89
Best's disease H35.50
Betalipoproteinemia, broad or floating E78.2
Beta-mercaptolactate-cysteine disulfiduria E72.09
Betting and gambling Z72.6
  pathological (compulsive) F63.0
Bezoar T18.9 ☑
  intestine T18.3 ☑
  stomach T18.2 ☑
Bezold's abscess — *see* Mastoiditis, acute
Bianchi's syndrome R48.8
Bicornate or bicornis uterus Q51.3
  in pregnancy or childbirth O34.00
    causing obstructed labor O65.5
Bicuspid aortic valve Q23.1
Biedl-Bardet syndrome Q87.89
Bielschowsky (-Jansky) disease E75.4
Biermer's (pernicious) anemia or disease D51.0
Biett's disease L93.0
Bifid (congenital)
  apex, heart Q24.8
  clitoris Q52.6
  kidney Q63.8
  nose Q30.2
  patella Q74.1
  scrotum Q55.29
  toe NEC Q74.2
  tongue Q38.3
  ureter Q62.8
  uterus Q51.3
  uvula Q35.7
Biforis uterus (suprasimplex) Q51.3
Bifurcation (congenital)
  gallbladder Q44.1
  kidney pelvis Q63.8
  renal pelvis Q63.8
  rib Q76.6
  tongue, congenital Q38.3
  trachea Q32.1
  ureter Q62.8
  urethra Q64.74
  vertebra Q76.49
Big spleen syndrome D73.1
Bigeminal pulse R00.8
Bilateral — *see* condition
Bile
  duct — *see* condition
  pigments in urine R82.2
Bilharziasis — *see also* Schistosomiasis
  chyluria B65.0
  cutaneous B65.3
  galacturia B65.0
  hematochyluria B65.0

Bilharziasis — *continued*
  intestinal B65.1
  lipemia B65.9
  lipuria B65.0
  oriental B65.2
  piarhemia B65.9
  pulmonary NOS B65.9 *[J99]*
    pneumonia B65.9 *[J17]*
  tropical hematuria B65.0
  vesical B65.0
Biliary — *see* condition
Bilirubin metabolism disorder E80.7
  specified NEC E80.6
Bilirubinemia, familial nonhemolytic E80.4
Bilirubinuria R82.2
Biliuria R82.2
Bilocular stomach K31.2
Binswanger's disease I67.3
Biparta, bipartite
  carpal scaphoid Q74.0
  patella Q74.1
  vagina Q52.10
Bird
  face Q75.8
  fancier's disease or lung J67.2
Birth
  complications in mother — *see* Delivery, complicated
  compression during NOS P15.9
  defect — *see* Anomaly
  immature (less than 37 completed weeks) — *see* Preterm, newborn
    extremely (less than 28 completed weeks) — *see* Immaturity, extreme
  inattention, at or after — *see* Maltreatment, child, neglect
  injury NOS P15.9
    basal ganglia P11.1
    brachial plexus NEC P14.3
    brain (compression) (pressure) P11.2
    central nervous system NOS P11.9
    cerebellum P11.1
    cerebral hemorrhage P10.1
    external genitalia P15.5
    eye P15.3
    face P15.4
    fracture
      bone P13.9
        specified NEC P13.8
      clavicle P13.4
      femur P13.2
      humerus P13.3
      long bone, except femur P13.3
      radius and ulna P13.3
      skull P13.0
      spine P11.5
      tibia and fibula P13.3
    intracranial P11.2
      laceration or hemorrhage P10.9
        specified NEC P10.8
    intraventricular hemorrhage P10.2
    laceration
      brain P10.1
      by scalpel P15.8
      peripheral nerve P14.9
    liver P15.0
    meninges
      brain P11.1
      spinal cord P11.5
    nerve
      brachial plexus P14.3
      cranial NEC (except facial) P11.4
      facial P11.3
      peripheral P14.9
      phrenic (paralysis) P14.2
    paralysis
      facial nerve P11.3
      spinal P11.5
    penis P15.5
    rupture
      spinal cord P11.5
    scalp P12.9
    scalpel wound P15.8
    scrotum P15.5
    skull NEC P13.1
      fracture P13.0
    specified type NEC P15.8
    spinal cord P11.5
    spine P11.5

Birth — *continued*
  injury — *continued*
    spleen P15.1
    sternomastoid (hematoma) P15.2
    subarachnoid hemorrhage P10.3
    subcutaneous fat necrosis P15.6
    subdural hemorrhage P10.0
    tentorial tear P10.4
    testes P15.5
    vulva P15.5
  lack of care, at or after — *see* Maltreatment, child, neglect
  neglect, at or after — *see* Maltreatment, child, neglect
  palsy or paralysis, newborn, NOS (birth injury) P14.9
  premature (infant) — *see* Preterm, newborn
  shock, newborn P96.89
  trauma — *see* Birth, injury
  weight
    low (2499 grams or less) — *see* Low, birthweight
      extremely (999 grams or less) — *see* Low, birthweight, extreme
    4000 grams to 4499 grams P08.1
    4500 grams or more P08.0
Birthmark Q82.5
Birt-Hogg-Dube syndrome Q87.89
Bisalbuminemia E88.09
Biskra's button B55.1
Bite(s) (animal) (human)
  abdomen, abdominal
    wall S31.159 ☑
      with penetration into peritoneal cavity S31.659 ☑
      epigastric region S31.152 ☑
        with penetration into peritoneal cavity S31.652 ☑
      left
        lower quadrant S31.154 ☑
          with penetration into peritoneal cavity S31.654 ☑
        upper quadrant S31.151 ☑
          with penetration into peritoneal cavity S31.651 ☑
      periumbilic region S31.155 ☑
        with penetration into peritoneal cavity S31.655 ☑
      right
        lower quadrant S31.153 ☑
          with penetration into peritoneal cavity S31.653 ☑
        upper quadrant S31.150 ☑
          with penetration into peritoneal cavity S31.650 ☑
      superficial NEC S30.871 ☑
        insect S30.861 ☑
  alveolar (process) — *see* Bite, oral cavity
  amphibian (venomous) — *see* Venom, bite, amphibian
  animal — *see also* Bite, by site
    venomous — *see* Venom
  ankle S91.05- ☑
    superficial NEC S90.57- ☑
      insect S90.56- ☑
  antecubital space — *see* Bite, elbow
  anus S31.835 ☑
    superficial NEC S30.877 ☑
      insect S30.867 ☑
  arm (upper) S41.15- ☑
    lower — *see* Bite, forearm
    superficial NEC S40.87- ☑
      insect S40.86- ☑
  arthropod NEC — *see* Venom, bite, arthropod
  auditory canal (external) (meatus) — *see* Bite, ear
  auricle, ear — *see* Bite, ear
  axilla — *see* Bite, arm
  back — *see also* Bite, thorax, back
    lower S31.050 ☑
      with penetration into retroperitoneal space S31.051 ☑
      superficial NEC S30.870 ☑
        insect S30.860 ☑
  bedbug — *see* Bite(s), by site, superficial, insect
  breast S21.05- ☑
    superficial NEC S20.17- ☑
      insect S20.16- ☑
  brow — *see* Bite, head, specified site NEC
  buttock S31.805 ☑
    left S31.825 ☑
    right S31.815 ☑

Bite(s) — *continued*
  buttock — *continued*
    superficial NEC S30.870 ☑
      insect S30.860 ☑
  calf — *see* Bite, leg
  canaliculus lacrimalis — *see* Bite, eyelid
  canthus, eye — *see* Bite, eyelid
  centipede — *see* Toxicity, venom, arthropod, centipede
  cheek (external) S01.45- ☑
    internal — *see* Bite, oral cavity
    superficial NEC S00.87 ☑
      insect S00.86 ☑
  chest wall — *see* Bite, thorax
  chigger B88.0
  chin — *see* Bite, head, specified site NEC
  clitoris — *see* Bite, vulva
  costal region — *see* Bite, thorax
  digit(s)
    hand — *see* Bite, finger
    toe — *see* Bite, toe
  ear (canal) (external) S01.35- ☑
    superficial NEC S00.47- ☑
      insect S00.46- ☑
  elbow S51.05- ☑
    superficial NEC S50.37- ☑
      insect S50.36- ☑
  epididymis — *see* Bite, testis
  epigastric region — *see* Bite, abdomen
  epiglottis — *see* Bite, neck, specified site NEC
  esophagus, cervical S11.25 ☑
    superficial NEC S10.17 ☑
      insect S10.16 ☑
  eyebrow — *see* Bite, eyelid
  eyelid S01.15- ☑
    superficial NEC S00.27- ☑
      insect S00.26- ☑
  face NEC — *see* Bite, head, specified site NEC
  finger(s) S61.259 ☑
    with
      damage to nail S61.359 ☑
    index S61.258 ☑
      with
        damage to nail S61.358 ☑
      left S61.251 ☑
        with
          damage to nail S61.351 ☑
      right S61.250 ☑
        with
          damage to nail S61.350 ☑
      superficial NEC S60.478 ☑
        insect S60.46- ☑
    little S61.25- ☑
      with
        damage to nail S61.35- ☑
      superficial NEC S60.47- ☑
        insect S60.46- ☑
    middle S61.25- ☑
      with
        damage to nail S61.35- ☑
      superficial NEC S60.47- ☑
        insect S60.46- ☑
    ring S61.25- ☑
      with
        damage to nail S61.35- ☑
      superficial NEC S60.47- ☑
        insect S60.46- ☑
    superficial NEC S60.479 ☑
      insect S60.469 ☑
    thumb — *see* Bite, thumb
  flank — *see* Bite, abdomen, wall
  flea — *see* Bite, by site, superficial, insect
  foot (except toe(s) alone) S91.35- ☑
    superficial NEC S90.87- ☑
      insect S90.86- ☑
    toe — *see* Bite, toe
  forearm S51.85- ☑
    elbow only — *see* Bite, elbow
    superficial NEC S50.87- ☑
      insect S50.86- ☑
  forehead — *see* Bite, head, specified site NEC
  genital organs, external
    female S31.552 ☑
      superficial NEC S30.876 ☑
        insect S30.866 ☑
      vagina and vulva — *see* Bite, vulva
    male S31.551 ☑

Bite(s) — *continued*
  genital organs, external — *continued*
    male — *continued*
      penis — *see* Bite, penis
      scrotum — *see* Bite, scrotum
      superficial NEC S30.875 ☑
        insect S30.865 ☑
      testes — *see* Bite, testis
  groin — *see* Bite, abdomen, wall
  gum — *see* Bite, oral cavity
  hand S61.45- ☑
    finger — *see* Bite, finger
    superficial NEC S60.57- ☑
      insect S60.56- ☑
    thumb — *see* Bite, thumb
  head S01.95 ☑
    cheek — *see* Bite, cheek
    ear — *see* Bite, ear
    eyelid — *see* Bite, eyelid
    lip — *see* Bite, lip
    nose — *see* Bite, nose
    oral cavity — *see* Bite, oral cavity
    scalp — *see* Bite, scalp
    specified site NEC S01.85 ☑
      superficial NEC S00.87 ☑
        insect S00.86 ☑
    superficial NEC S00.97 ☑
      insect S00.96 ☑
    temporomandibular area — *see* Bite, cheek
  heel — *see* Bite, foot
  hip S71.05- ☑
    superficial NEC S70.27- ☑
      insect S70.26- ☑
  hymen S31.45 ☑
  hypochondrium — *see* Bite, abdomen, wall
  hypogastric region — *see* Bite, abdomen, wall
  inguinal region — *see* Bite, abdomen, wall
  insect — *see* Bite, by site, superficial, insect
  instep — *see* Bite, foot
  interscapular region — *see* Bite, thorax, back
  jaw — *see* Bite, head, specified site NEC
  knee S81.05- ☑
    superficial NEC S80.27- ☑
      insect S80.26- ☑
  labium (majus) (minus) — *see* Bite, vulva
  lacrimal duct — *see* Bite, eyelid
  larynx S11.015 ☑
    superficial NEC S10.17 ☑
      insect S10.16 ☑
  leg (lower) S81.85- ☑
    ankle — *see* Bite, ankle
    foot — *see* Bite, foot
    knee — *see* Bite, knee
    superficial NEC S80.87- ☑
      insect S80.86- ☑
    toe — *see* Bite, toe
    upper — *see* Bite, thigh
  lip S01.551 ☑
    superficial NEC S00.571 ☑
      insect S00.561 ☑
  lizard (venomous) — *see* Venom, bite, reptile
  loin — *see* Bite, abdomen, wall
  lower back — *see* Bite, back, lower
  lumbar region — *see* Bite, back, lower
  malar region — *see* Bite, head, specified site NEC
  mammary — *see* Bite, breast
  marine animals (venomous) — *see* Toxicity, venom, marine animal
  mastoid region — *see* Bite, head, specified site NEC
  mouth — *see* Bite, oral cavity
  nail
    finger — *see* Bite, finger
    toe — *see* Bite, toe
  nape — *see* Bite, neck, specified site NEC
  nasal (septum) (sinus) — *see* Bite, nose
  nasopharynx — *see* Bite, head, specified site NEC
  neck S11.95 ☑
    involving
      cervical esophagus — *see* Bite, esophagus, cervical
      larynx — *see* Bite, larynx
      pharynx — *see* Bite, pharynx
      thyroid gland S11.15 ☑
      trachea — *see* Bite, trachea
    specified site NEC S11.85 ☑
    superficial NEC S10.87 ☑

☞ Subterms under main terms may continue to next column or page   ☑ Additional Character Required — Refer to the Tabular List for Character Selection   39

Birth — Bite

Index

Bite(s) — *continued*
  neck — *continued*
    specified site — *continued*
      superficial — *continued*
        insect S10.86 ☑
      superficial NEC S10.97 ☑
        insect S10.96 ☑
      throat S11.85 ☑
        superficial NEC S10.17 ☑
          insect S10.16 ☑
  nose (septum) (sinus) S01.25 ☑
    superficial NEC S00.37 ☑
      insect S00.36 ☑
  occipital region — *see* Bite, scalp
  oral cavity S01.552 ☑
    superficial NEC S00.572 ☑
      insect S00.562 ☑
  orbital region — *see* Bite, eyelid
  palate — *see* Bite, oral cavity
  palm — *see* Bite, hand
  parietal region — *see* Bite, scalp
  pelvis S31.050 ☑
    with penetration into retroperitoneal space
      S31.051 ☑
    superficial NEC S30.870 ☑
      insect S30.860 ☑
  penis S31.25 ☑
    superficial NEC S30.872 ☑
      insect S30.862 ☑
  perineum
    female — *see* Bite, vulva
    male — *see* Bite, pelvis
  periocular area (with or without lacrimal passages) —
    see Bite, eyelid
  phalanges
    finger — *see* Bite, finger
    toe — *see* Bite, toe
  pharynx S11.25 ☑
    superficial NEC S10.17 ☑
      insect S10.16 ☑
  pinna — *see* Bite, ear
  poisonous — *see* Venom
  popliteal space — *see* Bite, knee
  prepuce — *see* Bite, penis
  pubic region — *see* Bite, abdomen, wall
  rectovaginal septum — *see* Bite, vulva
  red bug B88.0
  reptile NEC — *see also* Venom, bite, reptile
    nonvenomous — *see* Bite, by site
    snake — *see* Venom, bite, snake
  sacral region — *see* Bite, back, lower
  sacroiliac region — *see* Bite, back, lower
  salivary gland — *see* Bite, oral cavity
  scalp S01.05 ☑
    superficial NEC S00.07 ☑
      insect S00.06 ☑
  scapular region — *see* Bite, shoulder
  scrotum S31.35 ☑
    superficial NEC S30.873 ☑
      insect S30.863 ☑
  sea-snake (venomous) — *see* Toxicity, venom, snake,
    sea snake
  shin — *see* Bite, leg
  shoulder S41.05- ☑
    superficial NEC S40.27- ☑
      insect S40.26- ☑
  snake — *see also* Venom, bite, snake
    nonvenomous — *see* Bite, by site
  spermatic cord — *see* Bite, testis
  spider (venomous) — *see* Toxicity, venom, spider
    nonvenomous — *see* Bite, by site, superficial, insect
  sternal region — *see* Bite, thorax, front
  submaxillary region — *see* Bite, head, specified site
    NEC
  submental region — *see* Bite, head, specified site NEC
  subungual
    finger(s) — *see* Bite, finger
    toe — *see* Bite, toe
  superficial — *see* Bite, by site, superficial
  supraclavicular fossa S11.85 ☑
  supraorbital — *see* Bite, head, specified site NEC
  temple, temporal region — *see* Bite, head, specified
    site NEC
  temporomandibular area — *see* Bite, cheek
  testis S31.35 ☑
    superficial NEC S30.873 ☑

Bite(s) — *continued*
  testis — *continued*
    superficial — *continued*
      insect S30.863 ☑
  thigh S71.15- ☑
    superficial NEC S70.37- ☑
      insect S70.36- ☑
  thorax, thoracic (wall) S21.95 ☑
    back S21.25- ☑
      with penetration into thoracic cavity S21.45- ☑
    breast — *see* Bite, breast
    front S21.15- ☑
      with penetration into thoracic cavity S21.35- ☑
    superficial NEC S20.97 ☑
      back S20.47- ☑
      front S20.37- ☑
      insect S20.96 ☑
        back S20.46- ☑
        front S20.36- ☑
  throat — *see* Bite, neck, throat
  thumb S61.05- ☑
    with
      damage to nail S61.15- ☑
    superficial NEC S60.37- ☑
      insect S60.36- ☑
  thyroid S11.15 ☑
    superficial NEC S10.87 ☑
      insect S10.86 ☑
  toe(s) S91.15- ☑
    with
      damage to nail S91.25- ☑
    great S91.15- ☑
      with
        damage to nail S91.25- ☑
    lesser S91.15- ☑
      with
        damage to nail S91.25- ☑
    superficial NEC S90.47- ☑
      great S90.47- ☑
      insect S90.46- ☑
        great S90.46- ☑
  tongue S01.552 ☑
  trachea S11.025 ☑
    superficial NEC S10.17 ☑
      insect S10.16 ☑
  tunica vaginalis — *see* Bite, testis
  tympanum, tympanic membrane — *see* Bite, ear
  umbilical region S31.155 ☑
  uvula — *see* Bite, oral cavity
  vagina — *see* Bite, vulva
  venomous — *see* Venom
  vocal cords S11.035 ☑
    superficial NEC S10.17 ☑
      insect S10.16 ☑
  vulva S31.45 ☑
    superficial NEC S30.874 ☑
      insect S30.864 ☑
  wrist S61.55- ☑
    superficial NEC S60.87- ☑
      insect S60.86- ☑
Biting, cheek or lip K13.1
Biventricular failure (heart) I50.82
Björck (-Thorson) **syndrome** (malignant carcinoid) E34.0
Black
  death A20.9
  eye S00.1- ☑
  hairy tongue K14.3
  heel (foot) S90.3- ☑
  lung (disease) J60
  palm (hand) S60.22- ☑
Blackfan-Diamond anemia or syndrome (congenital
  hypoplastic anemia) D61.01
Blackhead L70.0
Blackout R55
Bladder — *see* condition
Blast (air) (hydraulic) (immersion) (underwater)
  blindness S05.8X- ☑
  injury
    abdomen or thorax — *see* Injury, by site
    ear (acoustic nerve trauma) — *see* Injury, nerve,
      acoustic, specified type NEC
    syndrome NEC T70.8 ☑
Blastoma — *see* Neoplasm, malignant, by site
  pulmonary — *see* Neoplasm, lung, malignant
Blastomycosis, blastomycotic B40.9
  Brazilian — *see* Paracoccidioidomycosis

Blastomycosis, blastomycotic — *continued*
  cutaneous B40.3
  disseminated B40.7
  European — *see* Cryptococcosis
  generalized B40.7
  keloidal B48.0
  North American B40.9
  primary pulmonary B40.0
  pulmonary B40.2
    acute B40.0
    chronic B40.1
  skin B40.3
  South American — *see* Paracoccidioidomycosis
  specified NEC B40.89
Bleb(s) R23.8
  emphysematous (lung) (solitary) J43.9
  endophthalmitis H59.43
  filtering (vitreous), after glaucoma surgery Z98.83
  inflamed (infected), postprocedural H59.40
    stage 1 H59.41
    stage 2 H59.42
    stage 3 H59.43
  lung (ruptured) J43.9
    congenital — *see* Atelectasis
    newborn P25.8
  subpleural (emphysematous) J43.9
Blebitis, postprocedural H59.40
  stage 1 H59.41
  stage 2 H59.42
  stage 3 H59.43
Bleeder (familial) (hereditary) — *see* Hemophilia
Bleeding — *see also* Hemorrhage
  anal K62.5
  anovulatory N97.0
  atonic, following delivery O72.1
  capillary I78.8
    puerperal O72.2
  contact (postcoital) N93.0
  due to uterine subinvolution N85.3
  ear — *see* Otorrhagia
  excessive, associated with menopausal onset N92.4
  familial — *see* Defect, coagulation
  following intercourse N93.0
  gastrointestinal K92.2
  hemorrhoids — *see* Hemorrhoids
  intermenstrual (regular) N92.3
    irregular N92.1
  intraoperative — *see* Complication, intraoperative,
    hemorrhage
  irregular N92.6
  menopausal N92.4
  newborn, intraventricular — *see* Newborn, affected
    by, hemorrhage, intraventricular
  nipple N64.59
  nose R04.0
  ovulation N92.3
  perimenopausal N92.4
  postclimacteric N95.0
  postcoital N93.0
  postmenopausal N95.0
  postoperative — *see* Complication, postprocedural,
    hemorrhage
  preclimacteric N92.4
  pre-pubertal vaginal N93.1
  puberty (excessive, with onset of menstrual periods)
    N92.2
  rectum, rectal K62.5
    newborn P54.2
  tendencies — *see* Defect, coagulation
  throat R04.1
  tooth socket (post-extraction) K91.840
  umbilical stump P51.9
  uterus, uterine NEC N93.9
    climacteric N92.4
    dysfunctional or functional N93.8
    menopausal N92.4
    preclimacteric or premenopausal N92.4
    unrelated to menstrual cycle N93.9
  vagina, vaginal (abnormal) N93.9
    dysfunctional or functional N93.8
    newborn P54.6
    pre-pubertal N93.1
  vicarious N94.89
Blennorrhagia, blennorrhagic — *see* Gonorrhea
Blennorrhea (acute) (chronic) — *see also* Gonorrhea
  inclusion (neonatal) (newborn) P39.1
  lower genitourinary tract (gonococcal) A54.00
  neonatorum (gonococcal ophthalmia) A54.31

Blepharelosis — *see* Entropion
Blepharitis (angularis) (ciliaris) (eyelid) (marginal)
   (nonulcerative) H01.009
  herpes zoster B02.39
  left H01.006
    lower H01.005
    upper H01.004
    upper and lower H01.00B
  right H01.003
    lower H01.002
    upper H01.001
    upper and lower H01.00A
  squamous R01.029
    left H01.026
      lower H01.025
      upper H01.024
      upper and lower H01.02B
    right H01.023
      lower H01.022
      upper H01.021
      upper and lower H01.02A
  ulcerative H01.019
    left H01.016
      lower H01.015
      upper H01.014
      upper and lower H01.01B
    right H01.013
      lower H01.012
      upper H01.011
      upper and lower H01.01A
Blepharochalasis H02.30
  congenital Q10.0
  left H02.36
    lower H02.35
    upper H02.34
  right H02.33
    lower H02.32
    upper H02.31
Blepharoclonus H02.59
Blepharoconjunctivitis H10.50- ☑
  angular H10.52- ☑
  contact H10.53- ☑
  ligneous H10.51- ☑
Blepharophimosis (eyelid) H02.529
  congenital Q10.3
  left H02.526
    lower H02.525
    upper H02.524
  right H02.523
    lower H02.522
    upper H02.521
Blepharoptosis H02.40- ☑
  congenital Q10.0
  mechanical H02.41- ☑
  myogenic H02.42- ☑
  neurogenic H02.43- ☑
  paralytic H02.43- ☑
Blepharopyorrhea, gonococcal A54.39
Blepharospasm G24.5
  drug induced G24.01
Blighted ovum O02.0
Blind — *see also* Blindness
  bronchus (congenital) Q32.4
  loop syndrome K90.2
    congenital Q43.8
  sac, fallopian tube (congenital) Q50.6
  spot, enlarged — *see* Defect, visual field, localized,
    scotoma, blind spot area
  tract or tube, congenital NEC — *see* Atresia, by site
Blindness (acquired) (congenital) (both eyes) H54.0X- ☑
  blast S05.8X- ☑
  color — *see* Deficiency, color vision
  concussion S05.8X- ☑
  cortical H47.619
    left brain H47.612
    right brain H47.611
  day H53.11
  due to injury (current episode) S05.9- ☑
    sequelae — *code to* injury with seventh character
      S
  eclipse (total) — *see* Retinopathy, solar
  emotional (hysterical) F44.6
  face H53.16
  hysterical F44.6
  legal (both eyes) (USA definition) H54.8
  mind R48.8
  night H53.60
    abnormal dark adaptation curve H53.61

Blindness — *continued*
  night — *continued*
    acquired H53.62
    congenital H53.63
    specified type NEC H53.69
    vitamin A deficiency E50.5
  one eye (other eye normal) H54.40
    left (normal vision on right) H54.42- ☑
      low vision on right H54.12- ☑
    low vision, other eye H54.10
    right (normal vision on left) H54.41- ☑
      low vision on left H54.11- ☑
  psychic R48.8
  river B73.01
  snow — *see* Photokeratitis
  sun, solar — *see* Retinopathy, solar
  transient — *see* Disturbance, vision, subjective, loss,
    transient
  traumatic (current episode) S05.9- ☑
  word (developmental) F81.0
    acquired R48.0
    secondary to organic lesion R48.0
Blister (nonthermal)
  abdominal wall S30.821 ☑
  alveolar process S00.522 ☑
  ankle S90.52- ☑
  antecubital space — *see* Blister, elbow
  anus S30.827 ☑
  arm (upper) S40.82- ☑
  auditory canal — *see* Blister, ear
  auricle — *see* Blister, ear
  axilla — *see* Blister, arm
  back, lower S30.820 ☑
  beetle dermatitis L24.89
  breast S20.12- ☑
  brow S00.82 ☑
  calf — *see* Blister, leg
  canthus — *see* Blister, eyelid
  cheek S00.82 ☑
    internal S00.522 ☑
  chest wall — *see* Blister, thorax
  chin S00.82 ☑
  costal region — *see* Blister, thorax
  digit(s)
    foot — *see* Blister, toe
    hand — *see* Blister, finger
  due to burn — *see* Burn, by site, second degree
  ear S00.42- ☑
  elbow S50.32- ☑
  epiglottis S10.12 ☑
  esophagus, cervical S10.12 ☑
  eyebrow — *see* Blister, eyelid
  eyelid S00.22- ☑
  face S00.82 ☑
  fever B00.1
  finger(s) S60.429 ☑
    index S60.42- ☑
    little S60.42- ☑
    middle S60.42- ☑
    ring S60.42- ☑
  foot (except toe(s) alone) S90.82- ☑
    toe — *see* Blister, toe
  forearm S50.82- ☑
    elbow only — *see* Blister, elbow
  forehead S00.82 ☑
  fracture — *omit code*
  genital organ
    female S30.826 ☑
    male S30.825 ☑
  gum S00.522 ☑
  hand S60.52- ☑
  head S00.92 ☑
    ear — *see* Blister, ear
    eyelid — *see* Blister, eyelid
    lip S00.521 ☑
    nose S00.32 ☑
    oral cavity S00.522 ☑
    scalp S00.02 ☑
    specified site NEC S00.82 ☑
  heel — *see* Blister, foot
  hip S70.22- ☑
  interscapular region S20.429 ☑
  jaw S00.82 ☑
  knee S80.22- ☑
  larynx S10.12 ☑
  leg (lower) S80.82- ☑

Blister — *continued*
  leg — *continued*
    knee — *see* Blister, knee
    upper — *see* Blister, thigh
  lip S00.521 ☑
  malar region S00.82 ☑
  mammary — *see* Blister, breast
  mastoid region S00.82 ☑
  mouth S00.522 ☑
  multiple, skin, nontraumatic R23.8
  nail
    finger — *see* Blister, finger
    toe — *see* Blister, toe
  nasal S00.32 ☑
  neck S10.92 ☑
    specified site NEC S10.82 ☑
    throat S10.12 ☑
  nose S00.32 ☑
  occipital region S00.02 ☑
  oral cavity S00.522 ☑
  orbital region — *see* Blister, eyelid
  palate S00.522 ☑
  palm — *see* Blister, hand
  parietal region S00.02 ☑
  pelvis S30.820 ☑
  penis S30.822 ☑
  periocular area — *see* Blister, eyelid
  phalanges
    finger — *see* Blister, finger
    toe — *see* Blister, toe
  pharynx S10.12 ☑
  pinna — *see* Blister, ear
  popliteal space — *see* Blister, knee
  scalp S00.02 ☑
  scapular region — *see* Blister, shoulder
  scrotum S30.823 ☑
  shin — *see* Blister, leg
  shoulder S40.22- ☑
  sternal region S20.329 ☑
  submaxillary region S00.82 ☑
  submental region S00.82 ☑
  subungual
    finger(s) — *see* Blister, finger
    toe(s) — *see* Blister, toe
  supraclavicular fossa S10.82 ☑
  supraorbital S00.82 ☑
  temple S00.82 ☑
  temporal region S00.82 ☑
  testis S30.823 ☑
  thermal — *see* Burn, second degree, by site
  thigh S70.32- ☑
  thorax, thoracic (wall) S20.92 ☑
    back S20.42- ☑
    front S20.32- ☑
  throat S10.12 ☑
  thumb S60.32- ☑
  toe(s) S90.42- ☑
    great S90.42- ☑
  tongue S00.522 ☑
  trachea S10.12 ☑
  tympanum, tympanic membrane — *see* Blister, ear
  upper arm — *see* Blister, arm (upper)
  uvula S00.522 ☑
  vagina S30.824 ☑
  vocal cords S10.12 ☑
  vulva S30.824 ☑
  wrist S60.82- ☑
Bloating R14.0
Bloch-Sulzberger disease or syndrome Q82.3
Block, blocked
  alveolocapillary J84.10
  arborization (heart) I45.5
  arrhythmic I45.9
  atrioventricular (incomplete) (partial) I44.30
    with atrioventricular dissociation I44.2
    complete I44.2
      congenital Q24.6
    congenital Q24.6
    first degree I44.0
    second degree (types I and II) I44.1
    specified NEC I44.39
    third degree I44.2
    types I and II I44.1
  auriculoventricular — *see* Block, atrioventricular
  bifascicular (cardiac) I45.2
  bundle-branch (complete) (false) (incomplete) I45.4

Block, blocked — continued
 bundle-branch — continued
  bilateral I45.2
  left I44.7
   with right bundle branch block I45.2
   hemiblock I44.60
    anterior I44.4
    posterior I44.5
   incomplete I44.7
    with right bundle branch block I45.2
  right I45.10
   with
    left bundle branch block I45.2
    left fascicular block I45.2
   specified NEC I45.19
   Wilson's type I45.19
 cardiac I45.9
 conduction I45.9
  complete I44.2
 fascicular (left) I44.60
  anterior I44.4
  posterior I44.5
  right I45.0
  specified NEC I44.69
 foramen Magendie (acquired) G91.1
  congenital Q03.1
   with spina bifida — *see* Spina bifida, by site, with
    hydrocephalus
 heart I45.9
  bundle branch I45.4
   bilateral I45.2
  complete (atrioventricular) I44.2
  congenital Q24.6
  first degree (atrioventricular) I44.0
  second degree (atrioventricular) I44.1
  specified type NEC I45.5
  third degree (atrioventricular) I44.2
 hepatic vein I82.0
 intraventricular (nonspecific) I45.4
  bundle branch
   bilateral I45.2
 kidney N28.9
  postcystoscopic or postprocedural N99.0
 Mobitz (types I and II) I44.1
 myocardial — *see* Block, heart
 nodal I45.5
 organ or site, congenital NEC — *see* Atresia, by site
 portal (vein) I81
 second degree (types I and II) I44.1
 sinoatrial I45.5
 sinoauricular I45.5
 third degree I44.2
 trifascicular I45.3
 tubal N97.1
 vein NOS I82.90
 Wenckebach (types I and II) I44.1
Blockage — *see* Obstruction
Blocq's disease F44.4
Blood
 constituents, abnormal R78.9
 disease D75.9
 donor — *see* Donor, blood
 dyscrasia D75.9
  with
   abortion — *see* Abortion, by type, complicated
    by, hemorrhage
   ectopic pregnancy O08.1
   molar pregnancy O08.1
  following ectopic or molar pregnancy O08.1
  newborn P61.9
  puerperal, postpartum O72.3
 flukes NEC — *see* Schistosomiasis
 in
  feces K92.1
   occult R19.5
  urine — *see* Hematuria
 mole O02.0
 occult in feces R19.5
 pressure
  decreased, due to shock following injury T79.4 ☑
  examination only Z01.30
  fluctuating I99.8
  high — *see* Hypertension
   borderline R03.0
   incidental reading, without diagnosis of hyper-
    tension R03.0
  low — *see also* Hypotension

Blood — continued
 pressure — continued
  low — *see also* Hypotension — continued
   incidental reading, without diagnosis of hypoten-
    sion R03.1
 spitting — *see* Hemoptysis
 staining cornea — *see* Pigmentation, cornea, stromal
 transfusion
  reaction or complication — *see* Complications,
   transfusion
 type
  A (Rh positive) Z67.10
   Rh negative Z67.11
  AB (Rh positive) Z67.30
   Rh negative Z67.31
  B (Rh positive) Z67.20
   Rh negative Z67.21
  O (Rh positive) Z67.40
   Rh negative Z67.41
  Rh (positive) Z67.90
   negative Z67.91
 vessel rupture — *see* Hemorrhage
 vomiting — *see* Hematemesis
Blood-forming organs, disease D75.9
Bloodgood's disease — *see* Mastopathy, cystic
Bloom (-Machacek)(-Torre) **syndrome** Q82.8
Blount disease or osteochondrosis M92.51- ☑
Blue
 baby Q24.9
 diaper syndrome E72.09
 dome cyst (breast) — *see* Cyst, breast
 dot cataract Q12.0
 nevus D22.9
 sclera Q13.5
  with fragility of bone and deafness Q78.0
 toe syndrome I75.02- ☑
Blueness — *see* Cyanosis
Blues, postpartal O90.6
 baby O90.6
Blurring, visual H53.8
Blushing (abnormal) (excessive) R23.2
BMI — *see* Body, mass index
Boarder, hospital NEC Z76.4
 accompanying sick person Z76.3
 healthy infant or child Z76.2
  foundling Z76.1
Bockhart's impetigo L01.02
Bodechtel-Guttman disease (subacute sclerosing panencephalitis) A81.1
Boder-Sedgwick syndrome (ataxia-telangiectasia) G11.3
Body, bodies
 Aschoff's — *see* Myocarditis, rheumatic
 asteroid, vitreous — *see* Deposit, crystalline
 cytoid (retina) — *see* Occlusion, artery, retina
 drusen (degenerative) (macula) (retinal) — *see also*
  Degeneration, macula, drusen
  optic disc — *see* Drusen, optic disc
 foreign — *see* Foreign body
 loose
  joint, except knee — *see* Loose, body, joint
   knee M23.4- ☑
  sheath, tendon — *see* Disorder, tendon, specified
   type NEC
 mass index (BMI)
  adult
   19.9 or less Z68.1
   20.0-20.9 Z68.20
   21.0-21.9 Z68.21
   22.0-22.9 Z68.22
   23.0-23.9 Z68.23
   24.0-24.9 Z68.24
   25.0-25.9 Z68.25
   26.0-26.9 Z68.26
   27.0-27.9 Z68.27
   28.0-28.9 Z68.28
   29.0-29.9 Z68.29
   30.0-30.9 Z68.30
   31.0-31.9 Z68.31
   32.0-32.9 Z68.32
   33.0-33.9 Z68.33
   34.0-34.9 Z68.34
   35.0-35.9 Z68.35
   36.0-36.9 Z68.36
   37.0-37.9 Z68.37
   38.0-38.9 Z68.38
   39.0-39.9 Z68.39
   40.0-44.9 Z68.41
   45.0-49.9 Z68.42

Body, bodies — continued
 mass index — continued
  adult — continued
   50.0-59.9 Z68.43
   60.0-69.9 Z68.44
   70 and over Z68.45
  pediatric
   5th percentile to less than 85th percentile for
    age Z68.52
   85th percentile to less than 95th percentile for
    age Z68.53
   greater than or equal to ninety-fifth percentile
    for age Z68.54
   less than fifth percentile for age Z68.51
 Mooser's A75.2
 rice — *see also* Loose, body, joint
  knee M23.4- ☑
 rocking F98.4
Boeck's
 disease or sarcoid — *see* Sarcoidosis
 lupoid (miliary) D86.3
Boerhaave's syndrome (spontaneous esophageal rupture) K22.3
Boggy
 cervix N88.8
 uterus N85.8
Boil — *see also* Furuncle, by site
 Aleppo B55.1
 Baghdad B55.1
 Delhi B55.1
 lacrimal
  gland — *see* Dacryoadenitis
  passages (duct) (sac) — *see* Inflammation, lacrimal,
   passages, acute
 Natal B55.1
 orbit, orbital — *see* Abscess, orbit
 tropical B55.1
Bold hives — *see* Urticaria
Bombé, iris — *see* Membrane, pupillary
Bone — *see* condition
Bonnevie-Ullrich syndrome — *see also* Turner's syn-
 drome Q87.19
Bonnier's syndrome H81.8 ☑
Bonvale dam fever T73.3 ☑
Bony block of joint — *see* Ankylosis
BOOP (bronchiolitis obliterans organized pneumonia)
 J84.89
Borderline
 diabetes mellitus R73.03
 hypertension R03.0
 osteopenia M85.8- ☑
 pelvis, with obstruction during labor O65.1
 personality F60.3
Borna disease A83.9
Bornholm disease B33.0
Boston exanthem A88.0
Botalli, ductus (patent) (persistent) Q25.0
Bothriocephalus latus infestation B70.0
Botulism (foodborne intoxication) A05.1
 infant A48.51
 non-foodborne A48.52
 wound A48.52
Bouba — *see* Yaws
Bouchard's nodes (with arthropathy) M15.2
Bouffée délirante F23
Bouillaud's disease or syndrome (rheumatic heart
 disease) I01.9
Bourneville's disease Q85.1
Boutonniere deformity (finger) — *see* Deformity, finger,
 boutonniere
Bouveret (-Hoffmann) **syndrome** (paroxysmal tachycardia) I47.9
Bovine heart — *see* Hypertrophy, cardiac
Bowel — *see* condition
Bowen's
 dermatosis (precancerous) — *see* Neoplasm, skin, in
  situ
 disease — *see* Neoplasm, skin, in situ
 epithelioma — *see* Neoplasm, skin, in situ
 type
  epidermoid carcinoma-in-situ — *see* Neoplasm,
   skin, in situ
  intraepidermal squamous cell carcinoma — *see*
   Neoplasm, skin, in situ
Bowing
 femur — *see also* Deformity, limb, specified type NEC,
  thigh

Bowing — *continued*
  femur — *see also* Deformity, limb, specified type, thigh — *continued*
    congenital Q68.3
  fibula — *see also* Deformity, limb, specified type NEC, lower leg
    congenital Q68.4
  forearm — *see* Deformity, limb, specified type NEC, forearm
  leg(s), long bones, congenital Q68.5
  radius — *see* Deformity, limb, specified type NEC, forearm
  tibia — *see also* Deformity, limb, specified type NEC, lower leg
    congenital Q68.4
Bowleg(s) (acquired) M21.16- ☑
  congenital Q68.5
  rachitic E64.3
Boyd's dysentery A03.2
Brachial — *see* condition
Brachycardia R00.1
Brachycephaly Q75.0
Bradley's disease A08.19
Bradyarrhythmia, cardiac I49.8
Bradycardia (sinoatrial) (sinus) (vagal) R00.1
  neonatal P29.12
  reflex G90.09
  tachycardia syndrome I49.5
Bradykinesia R25.8
Bradypnea R06.89
Bradytachycardia I49.5
Brailsford's disease or osteochondrosis — *see* Osteochondrosis, juvenile, radius
Brain — *see also* condition
  death G93.82
  syndrome — *see* Syndrome, brain
Branched-chain amino-acid disorder E71.2
Branchial — *see* condition
  cartilage, congenital Q18.2
Branchiogenic remnant (in neck) Q18.0
Brandt's syndrome (acrodermatitis enteropathica) E83.2
Brash (water) R12
Bravais-jacksonian epilepsy — *see* Epilepsy, localization-related, symptomatic, with simple partial seizures
Braxton Hicks contractions — *see* False, labor
Brazilian leishmaniasis B55.2
BRBPR K62.5
Break, retina (without detachment) H33.30- ☑
  with retinal detachment — *see* Detachment, retina
  horseshoe tear H33.31- ☑
  multiple H33.33- ☑
  round hole H33.32- ☑
Breakdown
  device, graft or implant — *see also* Complications, by site and type, mechanical T85.618 ☑
    arterial graft NEC — *see* Complication, cardiovascular device, mechanical, vascular
    breast (implant) T85.41 ☑
    catheter NEC T85.618 ☑
      cystostomy T83.010 ☑
      dialysis (renal) T82.41 ☑
        intraperitoneal T85.611 ☑
      Hopkins T83.018 ☑
      ileostomy T83.018 ☑
      infusion NEC T82.514 ☑
        cranial T85.610- ☑
        epidural T85.610 ☑
        intrathecal T85.610 ☑
        spinal T85.610 ☑
        subarachnoid T85.610 ☑
        subdural T85.610 ☑
      nephrostomy T83.012 ☑
      urethral indwelling T83.011 ☑
      urinary NEC T83.018 ☑
      urostomy T83.018 ☑
    electronic (electrode) (pulse generator) (stimulator)
      bone T84.310 ☑
      cardiac T82.119 ☑
        electrode T82.110 ☑
        pulse generator T82.111 ☑
        specified type NEC T82.118 ☑
      nervous system — *see* Complication, prosthetic device, mechanical, electronic nervous system stimulator
    urinary — *see* Complication, genitourinary, device, urinary, mechanical

Breakdown — *continued*
  device, graft or implant — *see also* Complications, by site and type, mechanical — *continued*
    fixation, internal (orthopedic) NEC — *see* Complication, fixation device, mechanical
    gastrointestinal — *see* Complications, prosthetic device, mechanical, gastrointestinal device
    genital NEC T83.418 ☑
      intrauterine contraceptive device T83.31 ☑
      penile prosthesis (cylinder) (implanted) (pump) (resevoir) T83.410 ☑
      testicular prosthesis T83.411 ☑
    heart NEC — *see* Complication, cardiovascular device, mechanical
    intrathecal infusion pump T85.615 ☑
    joint prosthesis — *see* Complications..., joint prosthesis,internal, mechanical, by site
    nervous system, specified device NEC T85.615 ☑
    ocular NEC — *see* Complications, prosthetic device, mechanical, ocular device
    orthopedic NEC — *see* Complication, orthopedic, device, mechanical
    specified NEC T85.618 ☑
    subcutaneous device pocket
      nervous system prosthetic device, implant, or graft T85.890 ☑
      other internal prosthetic device, implant, or graft T85.898 ☑
    sutures, permanent T85.612 ☑
      used in bone repair — *see* Complications, fixation device, internal (orthopedic), mechanical
    urinary NEC T83.118 ☑
      graft T83.21 ☑
      sphincter, implanted T83.111 ☑
      stent (ileal conduit) (nephroureteral) T83.113 ☑
      ureteral indwelling T83.112 ☑
    vascular NEC — *see* Complication, cardiovascular device, mechanical
    ventricular intracranial shunt T85.01 ☑
  nervous F48.8
  perineum O90.1
  respirator J95.850
    specified NEC J95.859
  ventilator J95.850
    specified NEC J95.859
Breast — *see also* condition
  buds E30.1
    in newborn P96.89
  dense R92.2
  nodule — *see also* Lump, breast N63.0
Breath
  foul R19.6
  holder, child R06.89
  holding spell R06.89
  shortness R06.02
Breathing
  labored — *see* Hyperventilation
  mouth R06.5
    causing malocclusion M26.5 ☑
  periodic R06.3
    high altitude G47.32
Breathlessness R06.81
Breda's disease — *see* Yaws
Breech presentation (mother) O32.1 ☑
  causing obstructed labor O64.1 ☑
  footling O32.8 ☑
    causing obstructed labor O64.8 ☑
  incomplete O32.8 ☑
    causing obstructed labor O64.8 ☑
Breisky's disease N90.4
Brennemann's syndrome I88.0
Brenner
  tumor (benign) D27.9
    borderline malignancy D39.1- ☑
    malignant C56 ☑
    proliferating D39.1- ☑
Bretonneau's disease or angina A36.0
Breus' mole O02.0
Brevicollis Q76.49
Brickmakers' anemia B76.9 *[D63.8]*
Bridge, myocardial Q24.5
Bright red blood per rectum (BRBPR) K62.5
Bright's disease — *see also* Nephritis
  arteriosclerotic — *see* Hypertension, kidney
Brill (-Zinsser) **disease** (recrudescent typhus) A75.1
Brill-Symmers' disease C82.90
Brion-Kayser disease — *see* Fever, parathyroid

Briquet's disorder or syndrome F45.0
Brissaud's
  infantilism or dwarfism E23.0
  motor-verbal tic F95.2
Brittle
  bones disease Q78.0
  nails L60.3
    congenital Q84.6
Broad — *see also* condition
  beta disease E78.2
  ligament laceration syndrome N83.8
Broad- or floating-betalipoproteinemia E78.2
Brock's syndrome (atelectasis due to enlarged lymph nodes) J98.19
Brocq-Duhring disease (dermatitis herpetiformis) L13.0
Brodie's abscess or disease M86.8X- ☑
Broken
  arches — *see also* Deformity, limb, flat foot
  arm (meaning upper limb) — *see* Fracture, arm
  back — *see* Fracture, vertebra
  bone — *see* Fracture
  implant or internal device — *see* Complications, by site and type, mechanical
  leg (meaning lower limb) — *see* Fracture, leg
  nose S02.2 ☑
  tooth, teeth — *see* Fracture, tooth
Bromhidrosis, bromidrosis L75.0
Bromidism, bromism G92
  due to
    correct substance properly administered — *see* Table of Drugs and Chemicals, by drug, adverse effect
    overdose or wrong substance given or taken — *see* Table of Drugs and Chemicals, by drug, poisoning
  chronic (dependence) F13.20
Bromidrosiphobia F40.298
Bronchi, bronchial — *see* condition
Bronchiectasis (cylindrical) (diffuse) (fusiform) (localized) (saccular) J47.9
  with
    acute
      bronchitis J47.0
      lower respiratory infection J47.0
    exacerbation (acute) J47.1
  congenital Q33.4
  tuberculous NEC — *see* Tuberculosis, pulmonary
Bronchiolectasis — *see* Bronchiectasis
Bronchiolitis (acute) (infective) (subacute) J21.9
  with
    bronchospasm or obstruction J21.9
    influenza, flu or grippe — *see* Influenza, with, respiratory manifestations NEC
  chemical (chronic) J68.4
    acute J68.0
  chronic (fibrosing) (obliterative) J44.9
  due to
    external agent — *see* Bronchitis, acute, due to
    human metapneumovirus J21.1
    respiratory syncytial virus (RSV) J21.0
    specified organism NEC J21.8
  fibrosa obliterans J44.9
  influenzal — *see* Influenza, with, respiratory manifestations NEC
  obliterans J42
    with organizing pneumonia (BOOP) J84.89
  obliterative (chronic) (subacute) J44.9
    due to fumes or vapors J68.4
    due to chemicals, gases, fumes or vapors (inhalation) J68.4
  respiratory, interstitial lung disease J84.115
Bronchitis (diffuse) (fibrinous) (hypostatic) (infective) (membranous) J40
  with
    influenza, flu or grippe — *see* Influenza, with, respiratory manifestations NEC
    obstruction (airway) (lung) J44.9
    tracheitis (15 years of age and above) J40
      acute or subacute J20.9
      chronic J42
      under 15 years of age J20.9
  acute or subacute (with bronchospasm or obstruction) J20.9
    with
      bronchiectasis J47.0
      chronic obstructive pulmonary disease J44.0
      chemical (due to gases, fumes or vapors) J68.0

▼ **Subterms under main terms may continue to next column or page**   ☑ **Additional Character Required — Refer to the Tabular List for Character Selection**   **43**

Bowing — Bronchitis

Bronchitis — *continued*
  acute or subacute — *continued*
    due to
      fumes or vapors J68.0
      Haemophilus influenzae J20.1
      Mycoplasma pneumoniae J20.0
      radiation J70.0
      specified organism NEC J20.8
      Streptococcus J20.2
      virus
        coxsackie J20.3
        echovirus J20.7
        parainfluenzae J20.4
        respiratory syncytial (RSV) J20.5
        rhinovirus J20.6
      viral NEC J20.8
  allergic (acute) J45.909
    with
      exacerbation (acute) J45.901
      status asthmaticus J45.902
  arachidic T17.528 ☑
  aspiration (due to food and vomit) J69.0
  asthmatic J45.9 ☑
    chronic J44.9
      with
        acute lower respiratory infection J44.0
        exacerbation (acute) J44.1
  capillary — *see* Pneumonia, broncho
  caseous (tuberculous) A15.5
  Castellani's A69.8
  catarrhal (15 years of age and above) J40
    acute — *see* Bronchitis, acute
    chronic J41.0
    under 15 years of age J20.9
  chemical (acute) (subacute) J68.0
    chronic J68.4
    due to fumes or vapors J68.0
      chronic J68.4
  chronic J42
    with
      airways obstruction J44.9
      tracheitis (chronic) J42
    asthmatic (obstructive) J44.9
    catarrhal J41.0
    chemical (due to fumes or vapors) J68.4
    due to
      chemicals, gases, fumes or vapors (inhalation) J68.4
      radiation J70.1
      tobacco smoking J41.0
    emphysematous J44.9
    mucopurulent J41.1
    non-obstructive J41.0
    obliterans J44.9
    obstructive J44.9
    purulent J41.1
    simple J41.0
  croupous — *see* Bronchitis, acute
  due to gases, fumes or vapors (chemical) J68.0
  emphysematous J44.9
  exudative — *see* Bronchitis, acute
  fetid J41.1
  grippal — *see* Influenza, with, respiratory manifestations NEC
  in those under 15 years age — *see* Bronchitis, acute
    chronic — *see* Bronchitis, chronic
  influenzal — *see* Influenza, with, respiratory manifestations NEC
  mixed simple and mucopurulent J41.8
  moulder's J62.8
  mucopurulent (chronic) (recurrent) J41.1
    acute or subacute J20.9
    simple (mixed) J41.8
  obliterans (chronic) J44.9
  obstructive (chronic) (diffuse) J44.9
  pituitous J41.1
  pneumococcal, acute or subacute J20.2
  pseudomembranous, acute or subacute — *see* Bronchitis, acute
  purulent (chronic) (recurrent) J41.1
    acute or subacute — *see* Bronchitis, acute
  putrid J41.1
  senile (chronic) J42
  simple and mucopurulent (mixed) J41.8
  smokers' J41.0
  spirochetal NEC A69.8
  subacute — *see* Bronchitis, acute
  suppurative (chronic) J41.1

Bronchitis — *continued*
  suppurative — *continued*
    acute or subacute — *see* Bronchitis, acute
  tuberculous A15.5
  under 15 years of age — *see* Bronchitis, acute
    chronic — *see* Bronchitis, chronic
  viral NEC, acute or subacute — *see also* Bronchitis, acute J20.8
Bronchoalveolitis J18.0
Bronchoaspergillosis B44.1
Bronchocele meaning goiter E04.0
Broncholithiasis J98.09
  tuberculous NEC A15.5
Bronchomalacia J98.09
  congenital Q32.2
Bronchomycosis NOS B49 [J99]
  candidal B37.1
Bronchopleuropneumonia — *see* Pneumonia, broncho
Bronchopneumonia — *see* Pneumonia, broncho
Bronchopneumonitis — *see* Pneumonia, broncho
Bronchopulmonary — *see* condition
Bronchopulmonitis — *see* Pneumonia, broncho
Bronchorrhagia (see Hemoptysis)
Bronchorrhea J98.09
  acute J20.9
  chronic (infective) (purulent) J42
Bronchospasm (acute) J98.01
  with
    bronchiolitis, acute J21.9
    bronchitis, acute (conditions in J20) — *see* Bronchitis, acute
  due to external agent — *see* condition, respiratory, acute, due to
  exercise induced J45.990
Bronchospirochetosis A69.8
  Castellani A69.8
Bronchostenosis J98.09
Bronchus — *see* condition
Brontophobia F40.220
Bronze baby syndrome P83.88
Brooke's tumor — *see* Neoplasm, skin, benign
Brown enamel of teeth (hereditary) K00.5
Brown's sheath syndrome H50.61- ☑
Brown-Séquard disease, paralysis or syndrome G83.81
Bruce sepsis A23.0
Brucellosis (infection) A23.9
  abortus A23.1
  canis A23.3
  dermatitis A23.9
  melitensis A23.0
  mixed A23.8
  sepsis A23.9
    melitensis A23.0
    specified NEC A23.8
  suis A23.2
Bruck-de Lange disease Q87.19
Bruck's disease — *see* Deformity, limb
BRUE (brief resolved unexplained event) R68.13
Brugsch's syndrome Q82.8
Bruise (skin surface intact) — *see also* Contusion
  with
    open wound — *see* Wound, open
  internal organ — *see* Injury, by site
  newborn P54.5
  scalp, due to birth injury, newborn P12.3
  umbilical cord O69.5 ☑
Bruit (arterial) R09.89
  cardiac R01.1
Brush burn — *see* Abrasion, by site
Bruton's X-linked agammaglobulinemia D80.0
Bruxism
  psychogenic F45.8
  sleep related G47.63
Bubbly lung syndrome P27.0
Bubo I88.8
  blennorrhagic (gonococcal) A54.89
  chancroidal A57
  climatic A55
  due to Haemophilus ducreyi A57
  gonococcal A54.89
  indolent (nonspecific) I88.8
  inguinal (nonspecific) I88.8
    chancroidal A57
    climatic A55
    due to H. ducreyi A57
    infective I88.8

Bubo — *continued*
  scrofulous (tuberculous) A18.2
  soft chancre A57
  suppurating — *see* Lymphadenitis, acute
  syphilitic (primary) A51.0
    congenital A50.07
  tropical A55
  virulent (chancroidal) A57
Bubonic plague A20.0
Bubonocele — *see* Hernia, inguinal
Buccal — *see* condition
Buchanan's disease or osteochondrosis M91.0
Buchem's syndrome (hyperostosis corticalis) M85.2
Bucket-handle fracture or tear (semilunar cartilage) — *see* Tear, meniscus
Budd-Chiari syndrome (hepatic vein thrombosis) I82.0
Budgerigar fancier's disease or lung J67.2
Buds
  breast E30.1
    in newborn P96.89
Buerger's disease (thromboangiitis obliterans) I73.1
Bulbar — *see* condition
Bulbus cordis (left ventricle) (persistent) Q21.8
Bulimia (nervosa) F50.2
  atypical F50.9
  normal weight F50.9
Bulky
  stools R19.5
  uterus N85.2
Bulla (e) R23.8
  lung (emphysematous) (solitary) J43.9
    newborn P25.8
Bullet wound — *see also* Wound, open
  fracture — *code as* Fracture, by site
  internal organ — *see* Injury, by site
Bundle
  branch block (complete) (false) (incomplete) — *see* Block, bundle-branch
  of His — *see* condition
Bunion M21.61- ☑
  tailor's M21.62- ☑
Bunionette M21.62- ☑
Buphthalmia, buphthalmos (congenital) Q15.0
Burdwan fever B55.0
Bürger-Grütz disease or syndrome E78.3
Buried
  penis (congenital) Q55.64
    acquired N48.83
  roots K08.3
Burke's syndrome K86.89
Burkitt
  cell leukemia C91.0- ☑
  lymphoma (malignant) C83.7- ☑
    small noncleaved, diffuse C83.7- ☑
    spleen C83.77
    undifferentiated C83.7- ☑
  tumor C83.7- ☑
  type
    acute lymphoblastic leukemia C91.0- ☑
    undifferentiated C83.7- ☑
Burn (electricity) (flame) (hot gas, liquid or hot object) (radiation) (steam) (thermal) T30.0
  abdomen, abdominal (muscle) (wall) T21.02 ☑
    first degree T21.12 ☑
    second degree T21.22 ☑
    third degree T21.32 ☑
  above elbow T22.039 ☑
    first degree T22.139 ☑
    left T22.032 ☑
      first degree T22.132 ☑
      second degree T22.232 ☑
      third degree T22.332 ☑
    right T22.031 ☑
      first degree T22.131 ☑
      second degree T22.231 ☑
      third degree T22.331 ☑
    second degree T22.239 ☑
    third degree T22.339 ☑
  acid (caustic) (external) (internal) — *see* Corrosion, by site
  alimentary tract NEC T28.2 ☑
    esophagus T28.1 ☑
    mouth T28.0 ☑
    pharynx T28.0 ☑
  alkaline (caustic) (external) (internal) — *see* Corrosion, by site

☑ Additional Character Required — Refer to the Tabular List for Character Selection   Subterms under main terms may continue to next column or page

Burn — *continued*
ankle T25.019 ☑
  first degree T25.119 ☑
  left T25.012 ☑
    first degree T25.112 ☑
    second degree T25.212 ☑
    third degree T25.312 ☑
  multiple with foot — *see* Burn, lower, limb, multiple, ankle and foot
  right T25.011 ☑
    first degree T25.111 ☑
    second degree T25.211 ☑
    third degree T25.311 ☑
  second degree T25.219 ☑
  third degree T25.319 ☑
anus — *see* Burn, buttock
arm (lower) (upper) — *see* Burn, upper, limb
axilla T22.049 ☑
  first degree T22.149 ☑
  left T22.042 ☑
    first degree T22.142 ☑
    second degree T22.242 ☑
    third degree T22.342 ☑
  right T22.041 ☑
    first degree T22.141 ☑
    second degree T22.241 ☑
    third degree T22.341 ☑
  second degree T22.249 ☑
  third degree T22.349 ☑
back (lower) T21.04 ☑
  first degree T21.14 ☑
  second degree T21.24 ☑
  third degree T21.34 ☑
  upper T21.03 ☑
    first degree T21.13 ☑
    second degree T21.23 ☑
    third degree T21.33 ☑
blisters — *code as* Burn, second degree, by site
breast(s) — *see* Burn, chest wall
buttock(s) T21.05 ☑
  first degree T21.15 ☑
  second degree T21.25 ☑
  third degree T21.35 ☑
calf T24.039 ☑
  first degree T24.139 ☑
  left T24.032 ☑
    first degree T24.132 ☑
    second degree T24.232 ☑
    third degree T24.332 ☑
  right T24.031 ☑
    first degree T24.131 ☑
    second degree T24.231 ☑
    third degree T24.331 ☑
  second degree T24.239 ☑
  third degree T24.339 ☑
canthus (eye) — *see* Burn, eyelid
caustic acid or alkaline — *see* Corrosion, by site
cervix T28.3 ☑
cheek T20.06 ☑
  first degree T20.16 ☑
  second degree T20.26 ☑
  third degree T20.36 ☑
chemical (acids) (alkalines) (caustics) (external) (internal) — *see* Corrosion, by site
chest wall T21.01 ☑
  first degree T21.11 ☑
  second degree T21.21 ☑
  third degree T21.31 ☑
chin T20.03 ☑
  first degree T20.13 ☑
  second degree T20.23 ☑
  third degree T20.33 ☑
colon T28.2 ☑
conjunctiva (and cornea) — *see* Burn, cornea
cornea (and conjunctiva) T26.1- ☑
  chemical — *see* Corrosion, cornea
corrosion (external) (internal) — *see* Corrosion, by site
deep necrosis of underlying tissue — *code as* Burn, third degree, by site
dorsum of hand T23.069 ☑
  first degree T23.169 ☑
  left T23.062 ☑
    first degree T23.162 ☑
    second degree T23.262 ☑
    third degree T23.362 ☑
  right T23.061 ☑

Burn — *continued*
dorsum of hand — *continued*
  right — *continued*
    first degree T23.161 ☑
    second degree T23.261 ☑
    third degree T23.361 ☑
  second degree T23.269 ☑
  third degree T23.369 ☑
due to ingested chemical agent — *see* Corrosion, by site
ear (auricle) (external) (canal) T20.01 ☑
  first degree T20.11 ☑
  second degree T20.21 ☑
  third degree T20.31 ☑
elbow T22.029 ☑
  first degree T22.129 ☑
  left T22.022 ☑
    first degree T22.122 ☑
    second degree T22.222 ☑
    third degree T22.322 ☑
  right T22.021 ☑
    first degree T22.121 ☑
    second degree T22.221 ☑
    third degree T22.321 ☑
  second degree T22.229 ☑
  third degree T22.329 ☑
epidermal loss — *code as* Burn, second degree, by site
erythema, erythematous — *code as* Burn, first degree, by site
esophagus T28.1 ☑
extent (percentage of body surface)
  less than 10 percent T31.0
  10-19 percent T31.10
    with 0-9 percent third degree burns T31.10
    with 10-19 percent third degree burns T31.11
  20-29 percent T31.20
    with 0-9 percent third degree burns T31.20
    with 10-19 percent third degree burns T31.21
    with 20-29 percent third degree burns T31.22
  30-39 percent T31.30
    with 0-9 percent third degree burns T31.30
    with 10-19 percent third degree burns T31.31
    with 20-29 percent third degree burns T31.32
    with 30-39 percent third degree burns T31.33
  40-49 percent T31.40
    with 0-9 percent third degree burns T31.40
    with 10-19 percent third degree burns T31.41
    with 20-29 percent third degree burns T31.42
    with 30-39 percent third degree burns T31.43
    with 40-49 percent third degree burns T31.44
  50-59 percent T31.50
    with 0-9 percent third degree burns T31.50
    with 10-19 percent third degree burns T31.51
    with 20-29 percent third degree burns T31.52
    with 30-39 percent third degree burns T31.53
    with 40-49 percent third degree burns T31.54
    with 50-59 percent third degree burns T31.55
  60-69 percent T31.60
    with 0-9 percent third degree burns T31.60
    with 10-19 percent third degree burns T31.61
    with 20-29 percent third degree burns T31.62
    with 30-39 percent third degree burns T31.63
    with 40-49 percent third degree burns T31.64
    with 50-59 percent third degree burns T31.65
    with 60-69 percent third degree burns T31.66
  70-79 percent T31.70
    with 0-9 percent third degree burns T31.70
    with 10-19 percent third degree burns T31.71
    with 20-29 percent third degree burns T31.72
    with 30-39 percent third degree burns T31.73
    with 40-49 percent third degree burns T31.74
    with 50-59 percent third degree burns T31.75
    with 60-69 percent third degree burns T31.76
    with 70-79 percent third degree burns T31.77
  80-89 percent T31.80
    with 0-9 percent third degree burns T31.80
    with 10-19 percent third degree burns T31.81
    with 20-29 percent third degree burns T31.82
    with 30-39 percent third degree burns T31.83
    with 40-49 percent third degree burns T31.84
    with 50-59 percent third degree burns T31.85
    with 60-69 percent third degree burns T31.86
    with 70-79 percent third degree burns T31.87
    with 80-89 percent third degree burns T31.88
  90 percent or more T31.90
    with 0-9 percent third degree burns T31.90
    with 10-19 percent third degree burns T31.91
    with 20-29 percent third degree burns T31.92

Burn — *continued*
extent — *continued*
  90 percent or more — *continued*
    with 30-39 percent third degree burns T31.93
    with 40-49 percent third degree burns T31.94
    with 50-59 percent third degree burns T31.95
    with 60-69 percent third degree burns T31.96
    with 70-79 percent third degree burns T31.97
    with 80-89 percent third degree burns T31.98
    with 90 percent or more third degree burns T31.99
extremity — *see* Burn, limb
eye(s) and adnexa T26.4-
  with resulting rupture and destruction of eyeball T26.2-
  conjunctival sac — *see* Burn, cornea
  cornea — *see* Burn, cornea
  lid — *see* Burn, eyelid
  periocular area — *see* Burn, eyelid
  specified site NEC T26.3-
eyeball — *see* Burn, eye
eyelid(s) T26.0- ☑
  chemical — *see* Corrosion, eyelid
face — *see* Burn, head
finger T23.029 ☑
  first degree T23.129 ☑
  left T23.022 ☑
    first degree T23.122 ☑
    second degree T23.222 ☑
    third degree T23.322 ☑
  multiple sites (without thumb) T23.039 ☑
    with thumb T23.049 ☑
      first degree T23.149 ☑
      left T23.042 ☑
        first degree T23.142 ☑
        second degree T23.242 ☑
        third degree T23.342 ☑
      right T23.041 ☑
        first degree T23.141 ☑
        second degree T23.241 ☑
        third degree T23.341 ☑
      second degree T23.249 ☑
      third degree T23.349 ☑
    first degree T23.139 ☑
    left T23.032 ☑
      first degree T23.132 ☑
      second degree T23.232 ☑
      third degree T23.332 ☑
    right T23.031 ☑
      first degree T23.131 ☑
      second degree T23.231 ☑
      third degree T23.331 ☑
    second degree T23.239 ☑
    third degree T23.339 ☑
  right T23.021 ☑
    first degree T23.121 ☑
    second degree T23.221 ☑
    third degree T23.321 ☑
  second degree T23.229 ☑
  third degree T23.329 ☑
flank — *see* Burn, abdominal wall
foot T25.029 ☑
  first degree T25.129 ☑
  left T25.022 ☑
    first degree T25.122 ☑
    second degree T25.222 ☑
    third degree T25.322 ☑
  multiple with ankle — *see* Burn, lower, limb, multiple, ankle and foot
  right T25.021 ☑
    first degree T25.121 ☑
    second degree T25.221 ☑
    third degree T25.321 ☑
  second degree T25.229 ☑
  third degree T25.329 ☑
forearm T22.019 ☑
  first degree T22.119 ☑
  left T22.012 ☑
    first degree T22.112 ☑
    second degree T22.212 ☑
    third degree T22.312 ☑
  right T22.011 ☑
    first degree T22.111 ☑
    second degree T22.211 ☑
    third degree T22.311 ☑
  second degree T22.219 ☑

☒ Subterms under main terms may continue to next column or page   ☑ Additional Character Required — Refer to the Tabular List for Character Selection   45

Burn — Burn

Burn — *continued*
  forearm — *continued*
    third degree T22.319 ☑
  forehead T20.06 ☑
    first degree T20.16 ☑
    second degree T20.26 ☑
    third degree T20.36 ☑
  fourth degree — *code as* Burn, third degree, by site
  friction — *see* Burn, by site
  from swallowing caustic or corrosive substance NEC
    — *see* Corrosion, by site
  full thickness skin loss — *code as* Burn, third degree,
    by site
  gastrointestinal tract NEC T28.2 ☑
    from swallowing caustic or corrosive substance
      T28.7 ☑
  genital organs
    external
      female T21.07 ☑
        first degree T21.17 ☑
        second degree T21.27 ☑
        third degree T21.37 ☑
      male T21.06 ☑
        first degree T21.16 ☑
        second degree T21.26 ☑
        third degree T21.36 ☑
    internal T28.3 ☑
      from caustic or corrosive substance T28.8 ☑
  groin — *see* Burn, abdominal wall
  hand(s) T23.009 ☑
    back — *see* Burn, dorsum of hand
    finger — *see* Burn, finger
    first degree T23.109 ☑
    left T23.002 ☑
      first degree T23.102 ☑
      second degree T23.202 ☑
      third degree T23.302 ☑
    multiple sites with wrist T23.099 ☑
      first degree T23.199 ☑
      left T23.092 ☑
        first degree T23.192 ☑
        second degree T23.292 ☑
        third degree T23.392 ☑
      right T23.091 ☑
        first degree T23.191 ☑
        second degree T23.291 ☑
        third degree T23.391 ☑
      second degree T23.299 ☑
      third degree T23.399 ☑
    palm — *see* Burn, palm
    right T23.001 ☑
      first degree T23.101 ☑
      second degree T23.201 ☑
      third degree T23.301 ☑
    second degree T23.209 ☑
    third degree T23.309 ☑
    thumb — *see* Burn, thumb
  head (and face) (and neck) T20.00 ☑
    cheek — *see* Burn, cheek
    chin — *see* Burn, chin
    ear — *see* Burn, ear
    eye(s) only — *see* Burn, eye
    first degree T20.10 ☑
    forehead — *see* Burn, forehead
    lip — *see* Burn, lip
    multiple sites T20.09 ☑
      first degree T20.19 ☑
      second degree T20.29 ☑
      third degree T20.39 ☑
    neck — *see* Burn, neck
    nose — *see* Burn, nose
    scalp — *see* Burn, scalp
    second degree T20.20 ☑
    third degree T20.30 ☑
  hip(s) — *see* Burn, thigh
  inhalation — *see* Burn, respiratory tract
    caustic or corrosive substance (fumes) — *see* Corro-
      sion, respiratory tract
  internal organ(s) T28.40 ☑
    alimentary tract T28.2 ☑
      esophagus T28.1 ☑
    eardrum T28.41 ☑
    esophagus T28.1 ☑
    from caustic or corrosive substance (swallowing)
      NEC — *see* Corrosion, by site
    genitourinary T28.3 ☑

Burn — *continued*
  internal organ(s) — *continued*
    mouth T28.0 ☑
    pharynx T28.0 ☑
    respiratory tract — *see* Burn, respiratory tract
    specified organ NEC T28.49 ☑
  interscapular region — *see* Burn, back, upper
  intestine (large) (small) T28.2 ☑
  knee T24.029 ☑
    first degree T24.129 ☑
    left T24.022 ☑
      first degree T24.122 ☑
      second degree T24.222 ☑
      third degree T24.322 ☑
    right T24.021 ☑
      first degree T24.121 ☑
      second degree T24.221 ☑
      third degree T24.321 ☑
    second degree T24.229 ☑
    third degree T24.329 ☑
  labium (majus) (minus) — *see* Burn, genital organs,
    external, female
  lacrimal apparatus, duct, gland or sac — *see* Burn, eye,
    specified site NEC
  larynx T27.0 ☑
    with lung T27.1 ☑
  leg(s) (lower) (upper) — *see* Burn, lower, limb
  lightning — *see* Burn, by site
  limb(s)
    lower (except ankle or foot alone) — *see* Burn,
      lower, limb
    upper — *see* Burn, upper limb
  lip(s) T20.02 ☑
    first degree T20.12 ☑
    second degree T20.22 ☑
    third degree T20.32 ☑
  lower
    back — *see* Burn, back
    limb T24.009 ☑
      ankle — *see* Burn, ankle
      calf — *see* Burn, calf
      first degree T24.109 ☑
      foot — *see* Burn, foot
      hip — *see* Burn, thigh
      knee — *see* Burn, knee
      left T24.002 ☑
        first degree T24.102 ☑
        second degree T24.202 ☑
        third degree T24.302 ☑
      multiple sites, except ankle and foot T24.099 ☑
        ankle and foot T25.099 ☑
          first degree T25.199 ☑
          left T25.092 ☑
            first degree T25.192 ☑
            second degree T25.292 ☑
            third degree T25.392 ☑
          right T25.091 ☑
            first degree T25.191 ☑
            second degree T25.291 ☑
            third degree T25.391 ☑
          second degree T25.299 ☑
          third degree T25.399 ☑
        first degree T24.199 ☑
        left T24.092 ☑
          first degree T24.192 ☑
          second degree T24.292 ☑
          third degree T24.392 ☑
        right T24.091 ☑
          first degree T24.191 ☑
          second degree T24.291 ☑
          third degree T24.391 ☑
        second degree T24.299 ☑
        third degree T24.399 ☑
      right T24.001 ☑
        first degree T24.101 ☑
        second degree T24.201 ☑
        third degree T24.301 ☑
      second degree T24.209 ☑
      thigh — *see* Burn, thigh
      third degree T24.309 ☑
      toe — *see* Burn, toe
  lung (with larynx and trachea) T27.1 ☑
  mouth T28.0 ☑
  neck T20.07 ☑
    first degree T20.17 ☑
    second degree T20.27 ☑

Burn — *continued*
  neck — *continued*
    third degree T20.37 ☑
  nose (septum) T20.04 ☑
    first degree T20.14 ☑
    second degree T20.24 ☑
    third degree T20.34 ☑
  ocular adnexa — *see* Burn, eye
  orbit region — *see* Burn, eyelid
  palm T23.059 ☑
    first degree T23.159 ☑
    left T23.052 ☑
      first degree T23.152 ☑
      second degree T23.252 ☑
      third degree T23.352 ☑
    right T23.051 ☑
      first degree T23.151 ☑
      second degree T23.251 ☑
      third degree T23.351 ☑
    second degree T23.259 ☑
    third degree T23.359 ☑
  partial thickness — *code as* Burn, degree, by site
  pelvis — *see* Burn, trunk
  penis — *see* Burn, genital organs, external, male
  perineum
    female — *see* Burn, genital organs, external, female
    male — *see* Burn, genital organs, external, male
  periocular area — *see* Burn, eyelid
  pharynx T28.0 ☑
  rectum T28.2 ☑
  respiratory tract T27.3 ☑
    larynx — *see* Burn, larynx
    specified part NEC T27.2 ☑
    trachea — *see* Burn, trachea
  sac, lacrimal — *see* Burn, eye, specified site NEC
  scalp T20.05 ☑
    first degree T20.15 ☑
    second degree T20.25 ☑
    third degree T20.35 ☑
  scapular region T22.069 ☑
    first degree T22.169 ☑
    left T22.062 ☑
      first degree T22.162 ☑
      second degree T22.262 ☑
      third degree T22.362 ☑
    right T22.061 ☑
      first degree T22.161 ☑
      second degree T22.261 ☑
      third degree T22.361 ☑
    second degree T22.269 ☑
    third degree T22.369 ☑
  sclera — *see* Burn, eye, specified site NEC
  scrotum — *see* Burn, genital organs, external, male
  shoulder T22.059 ☑
    first degree T22.159 ☑
    left T22.052 ☑
      first degree T22.152 ☑
      second degree T22.252 ☑
      third degree T22.352 ☑
    right T22.051 ☑
      first degree T22.151 ☑
      second degree T22.251 ☑
      third degree T22.351 ☑
    second degree T22.259 ☑
    third degree T22.359 ☑
  stomach T28.2 ☑
  temple — *see* Burn, head
  testis — *see* Burn, genital organs, external, male
  thigh T24.019 ☑
    first degree T24.119 ☑
    left T24.012 ☑
      first degree T24.112 ☑
      second degree T24.212 ☑
      third degree T24.312 ☑
    right T24.011 ☑
      first degree T24.111 ☑
      second degree T24.211 ☑
      third degree T24.311 ☑
    second degree T24.219 ☑
    third degree T24.319 ☑
  thorax (external) — *see* Burn, trunk
  throat (meaning pharynx) T28.0 ☑
  thumb(s) T23.019 ☑
    first degree T23.119 ☑
    left T23.012 ☑
      first degree T23.112 ☑

46

☑ Additional Character Required — Refer to the Tabular List for Character Selection   ▽ Subterms under main terms may continue to next column or page

Index

Burn — *continued*
  thumb(s) — *continued*
    left — *continued*
      second degree T23.212 ☑
      third degree T23.312 ☑
    multiple sites with fingers T23.049 ☑
      first degree T23.149 ☑
      left T23.042 ☑
        first degree T23.142 ☑
        second degree T23.242 ☑
        third degree T23.342 ☑
      right T23.041 ☑
        first degree T23.141 ☑
        second degree T23.241 ☑
        third degree T23.341 ☑
      second degree T23.249 ☑
      third degree T23.349 ☑
    right T23.011 ☑
      first degree T23.111 ☑
      second degree T23.211 ☑
      third degree T23.311 ☑
    second degree T23.219 ☑
    third degree T23.319 ☑
  toe T25.039 ☑
    first degree T25.139 ☑
    left T25.032 ☑
      first degree T25.132 ☑
      second degree T25.232 ☑
      third degree T25.332 ☑
    right T25.031 ☑
      first degree T25.131 ☑
      second degree T25.231 ☑
      third degree T25.331 ☑
    second degree T25.239 ☑
    third degree T25.339 ☑
  tongue T28.0 ☑
  tonsil(s) T28.0 ☑
  trachea T27.0 ☑
    with lung T27.1 ☑
  trunk T21.00 ☑
    abdominal wall — *see* Burn, abdominal wall
    anus — *see* Burn, buttock
    axilla — *see* Burn, upper limb
    back — *see* Burn, back
    breast — *see* Burn, chest wall
    buttock — *see* Burn, buttock
    chest wall — *see* Burn, chest wall
    first degree T21.10 ☑
    flank — *see* Burn, abdominal wall
    genital
      female — *see* Burn, genital organs, external, female
      male — *see* Burn, genital organs, external, male
    groin — *see* Burn, abdominal wall
    interscapular region — *see* Burn, back, upper
    labia — *see* Burn, genital organs, external, female
    lower back — *see* Burn, back
    penis — *see* Burn, genital organs, external, male
    perineum
      female — *see* Burn, genital organs, external, female
      male — *see* Burn, genital organs, external, male
    scapula region — *see* Burn, scapular region
    scrotum — *see* Burn, genital organs, external, male
    second degree T21.20 ☑
    specified site NEC T21.09 ☑
      first degree T21.19 ☑
      second degree T21.29 ☑
      third degree T21.39 ☑
    testes — *see* Burn, genital organs, external, male
    third degree T21.30 ☑
    upper back — *see* Burn, back, upper
    vulva — *see* Burn, genital organs, external, female
  unspecified site with extent of body surface involved
    specified
      less than 10 percent T31.0
      10-19 percent (0-9 percent third degree) T31.10
        with 10-19 percent third degree T31.11
      20-29 percent (0-9 percent third degree) T31.20
        with
          10-19 percent third degree T31.21
          20-29 percent third degree T31.22
      30-39 percent (0-9 percent third degree) T31.30
        with
          10-19 percent third degree T31.31
          20-29 percent third degree T31.32

Burn — *continued*
  unspecified site with extent of body surface involved
    specified — *continued*
      30-39 percent — *continued*
        with — *continued*
          30-39 percent third degree T31.33
      40-49 percent (0-9 percent third degree) T31.40
        with
          10-19 percent third degree T31.41
          20-29 percent third degree T31.42
          30-39 percent third degree T31.43
          40-49 percent third degree T31.44
      50-59 percent (0-9 percent third degree) T31.50
        with
          10-19 percent third degree T31.51
          20-29 percent third degree T31.52
          30-39 percent third degree T31.53
          40-49 percent third degree T31.54
          50-59 percent third degree T31.55
      60-69 percent (0-9 percent third degree) T31.60
        with
          10-19 percent third degree T31.61
          20-29 percent third degree T31.62
          30-39 percent third degree T31.63
          40-49 percent third degree T31.64
          50-59 percent third degree T31.65
          60-69 percent third degree T31.66
      70-79 percent (0-9 percent third degree) T31.70
        with
          10-19 percent third degree T31.71
          20-29 percent third degree T31.72
          30-39 percent third degree T31.73
          40-49 percent third degree T31.74
          50-59 percent third degree T31.75
          60-69 percent third degree T31.76
          70-79 percent third degree T31.77
      80-89 percent (0-9 percent third degree) T31.80
        with
          10-19 percent third degree T31.81
          20-29 percent third degree T31.82
          30-39 percent third degree T31.83
          40-49 percent third degree T31.84
          50-59 percent third degree T31.85
          60-69 percent third degree T31.86
          70-79 percent third degree T31.87
          80-89 percent third degree T31.88
      90 percent or more (0-9 percent third degree) T31.90
        with
          10-19 percent third degree T31.91
          20-29 percent third degree T31.92
          30-39 percent third degree T31.93
          40-49 percent third degree T31.94
          50-59 percent third degree T31.95
          60-69 percent third degree T31.96
          70-79 percent third degree T31.97
          80-89 percent third degree T31.98
          90-99 percent third degree T31.99
  upper limb T22.00 ☑
    above elbow — *see* Burn, above elbow
    axilla — *see* Burn, axilla
    elbow — *see* Burn, elbow
    first degree T22.10 ☑
    forearm — *see* Burn, forearm
    hand — *see* Burn, hand
    interscapular region — *see* Burn, back, upper
    multiple sites T22.099 ☑
      first degree T22.199 ☑
      left T22.092 ☑
        first degree T22.192 ☑
        second degree T22.292 ☑
        third degree T22.392 ☑
      right T22.091 ☑
        first degree T22.191 ☑
        second degree T22.291 ☑
        third degree T22.391 ☑
      second degree T22.299 ☑
      third degree T22.399 ☑
    scapular region — *see* Burn, scapular region
    second degree T22.20 ☑
    shoulder — *see* Burn, shoulder
    third degree T22.30 ☑
    wrist — *see* Burn, wrist
  uterus T28.3 ☑
  vagina T28.3 ☑
  vulva — *see* Burn, genital organs, external, female
  wrist T23.079 ☑
    first degree T23.179 ☑
    left T23.072 ☑

Burn — *continued*
  wrist — *continued*
    left — *continued*
      first degree T23.172 ☑
      second degree T23.272 ☑
      third degree T23.372 ☑
    multiple sites with hand T23.099 ☑
      first degree T23.199 ☑
      left T23.092 ☑
        first degree T23.192 ☑
        second degree T23.292 ☑
        third degree T23.392 ☑
      right T23.091 ☑
        first degree T23.191 ☑
        second degree T23.291 ☑
        third degree T23.391 ☑
      second degree T23.299 ☑
      third degree T23.399 ☑
    right T23.071 ☑
      first degree T23.171 ☑
      second degree T23.271 ☑
      third degree T23.371 ☑
    second degree T23.279 ☑
    third degree T23.379 ☑
Burnett's syndrome E83.52
Burning
  feet syndrome E53.9
  sensation R20.8
  tongue K14.6
Burn-out (state) Z73.0
Burns' disease or osteochondrosis — *see* Osteochondrosis, juvenile, ulna
Bursa — *see* condition
Bursitis M71.9
  Achilles — *see* Tendinitis, Achilles
  adhesive — *see* Bursitis, specified NEC
  ankle — *see* Enthesopathy, lower limb, ankle, specified type NEC
  calcaneal — *see* Enthesopathy, foot, specified type NEC
  collateral ligament, tibial — *see* Bursitis, tibial collateral
  due to use, overuse, pressure — *see also* Disorder, soft tissue, due to use, specified type NEC
    specified NEC — *see* Disorder, soft tissue, due to use, specified NEC
  Duplay's M75.0 ☑
  elbow NEC M70.3- ☑
    olecranon M70.2- ☑
  finger — *see* Disorder, soft tissue, due to use, specified type NEC, hand
  foot — *see* Enthesopathy, foot, specified type NEC
  gonococcal A54.49
  gouty — *see* Gout
  hand M70.1- ☑
  hip NEC M70.7- ☑
    trochanteric M70.6- ☑
  infective NEC M71.10
    abscess — *see* Abscess, bursa
    ankle M71.17- ☑
    elbow M71.12- ☑
    foot M71.17- ☑
    hand M71.14- ☑
    hip M71.15- ☑
    knee M71.16- ☑
    multiple sites M71.19
    shoulder M71.11- ☑
    specified site NEC M71.18
    wrist M71.13- ☑
  ischial — *see* Bursitis, hip
  knee NEC M70.5- ☑
    prepatellar M70.4- ☑
  occupational NEC — *see also* Disorder, soft tissue, due to, use
  olecranon — *see* Bursitis, elbow, olecranon
  pharyngeal J39.1
  popliteal — *see* Bursitis, knee
  prepatellar M70.4- ☑
  radiohumeral M77.8
  rheumatoid M06.20
    ankle M06.27- ☑
    elbow M06.22- ☑
    foot joint M06.27- ☑
    hand joint M06.24- ☑
    hip M06.25- ☑
    knee M06.26- ☑
    multiple site M06.29
    shoulder M06.21- ☑

Burn — Bursitis

Bursitis — *continued*
  rheumatoid — *continued*
    vertebra M06.28
    wrist M06.23- ☑
  scapulohumeral — *see* Bursitis, shoulder
  semimembranous muscle (knee) — *see* Bursitis, knee
  shoulder M75.5- ☑
    adhesive — *see* Capsulitis, adhesive
  specified NEC M71.50
    ankle M71.57- ☑
    due to use, overuse or pressure — *see* Disorder, soft
      tissue, due to, use
    elbow M71.52- ☑
    foot M71.57- ☑
    hand M71.54- ☑
    hip M71.55- ☑
    knee M71.56- ☑
    shoulder — *see* Bursitis, shoulder
    specified site NEC M71.58
    tibial collateral M76.4- ☑
    wrist M71.53- ☑
  subacromial — *see* Bursitis, shoulder
  subcoracoid — *see* Bursitis, shoulder
  subdeltoid — *see* Bursitis, shoulder
  syphilitic A52.78
  Thornwaldt, Tornwaldt J39.2
  tibial collateral M76.4- ☑
  toe — *see* Enthesopathy, foot, specified type NEC
  trochanteric (area) — *see* Bursitis, hip, trochanteric
  wrist — *see* Bursitis, hand
Bursopathy M71.9
  specified type NEC M71.80
    ankle M71.87- ☑
    elbow M71.82- ☑
    foot M71.87- ☑
    hand M71.84- ☑
    hip M71.85- ☑
    knee M71.86- ☑
    multiple sites M71.89
    shoulder M71.81- ☑
    specified site NEC M71.88
    wrist M71.83- ☑
Burst stitches or sutures (complication of surgery)
  T81.31 ☑
  external operation wound T81.31 ☑
  internal operation wound T81.32 ☑
Buruli ulcer A31.1
Bury's disease L95.1
Buschke's
  disease — *see* Cryptococcosis by site
  scleredema — *see* Sclerosis, systemic
Busse-Buschke disease — *see* Cryptococcosis by site
Buttock — *see* condition
Button
  Biskra B55.1
  Delhi B55.1
  oriental B55.1
Buttonhole deformity (finger) — *see* Deformity, finger,
  boutonniere
Bwamba fever A92.8
Byssinosis J66.0
Bywaters' syndrome T79.5 ☑

C

Cachexia R64
  cancerous R64
  cardiac — *see* Disease, heart
  dehydration E86.0
  due to malnutrition R64
  exophthalmic — *see* Hyperthyroidism
  heart — *see* Disease, heart
  hypophyseal E23.0
  hypopituitary E23.0
  lead — *see* Poisoning, lead
  malignant R64
  marsh — *see* Malaria
  nervous F48.8
  old age R54
  paludal — *see* Malaria
  pituitary E23.0
  renal N28.9
  saturnine — *see* Poisoning, lead
  senile R54
  Simmonds' E23.0
  splenica D73.0
  strumipriva E03.4

Cachexia — *continued*
  tuberculous NEC — *see* Tuberculosis
CADASIL (cerebral autosomal dominant arteriopathy with
  subcortical infarcts and leukoencephalopathy)
  I67.850
Café, au lait spots L81.3
Caffeine-induced
  anxiety disorder F15.980
  sleep disorder F15.982
Caffey's syndrome Q78.8
Caisson disease T70.3 ☑
Cake kidney Q63.1
Caked breast (puerperal, postpartum) O92.79
Calabar swelling B74.3
Calcaneal spur — *see* Spur, bone, calcaneal
Calcaneo-apophysitis M92.8
Calcareous — *see* condition
Calcicosis J62.8
Calciferol (vitamin D) deficiency E55.9
  with rickets E55.0
Calcification
  adrenal (capsule) (gland) E27.49
    tuberculous E35 *[B90.8]*
  aorta I70.0
  artery (annular) — *see* Arteriosclerosis
  auricle (ear) — *see* Disorder, pinna, specified type NEC
  basal ganglia G23.8
  bladder N32.89
    due to Schistosoma hematobium B65.0
  brain (cortex) — *see* Calcification, cerebral
  bronchus J98.09
  bursa M71.40
    ankle M71.47- ☑
    elbow M71.42- ☑
    foot M71.47- ☑
    hand M71.44- ☑
    hip M71.45- ☑
    knee M71.46- ☑
    multiple sites M71.49
    shoulder M75.3- ☑
    specified site NEC M71.48
    wrist M71.43- ☑
  cardiac — *see* Degeneration, myocardial
  cerebral (cortex) G93.89
    artery I67.2
  cervix (uteri) N88.8
  choroid plexus G93.89
  conjunctiva — *see* Concretion, conjunctiva
  corpora cavernosa (penis) N48.89
  cortex (brain) — *see* Calcification, cerebral
  dental pulp (nodular) K04.2
  dentinal papilla K00.4
  fallopian tube N83.8
  falx cerebri G96.198
  gallbladder K82.8
  general E83.59
  heart — *see also* Degeneration, myocardial
    valve — *see* Endocarditis
  idiopathic infantile arterial (IIAC) Q28.8
  intervertebral cartilage or disc (postinfective) — *see*
    Disorder, disc, specified NEC
  intracranial — *see* Calcification, cerebral
  joint — *see* Disorder, joint, specified type NEC
  kidney N28.89
    tuberculous N29 *[B90.1]*
  larynx (senile) J38.7
  lens — *see* Cataract, specified NEC
  lung (active) (postinfectional) J98.4
    tuberculous B90.9
  lymph gland or node (postinfectional) I89.8
    tuberculous — *see also* Tuberculosis, lymph gland
      B90.8
  mammographic R92.1
  massive (paraplegic) — *see* Myositis, ossificans, in,
    quadriplegia
  medial — *see* Arteriosclerosis, extremities
  meninges (cerebral) (spinal) G96.198
  metastatic E83.59
  Mönckeberg's — *see* Arteriosclerosis, extremities
  muscle M61.9
    due to burns — *see* Myositis, ossificans, in, burns
    paralytic — *see* Myositis, ossificans, in, quadriplegia
    specified type NEC M61.40
      ankle M61.47- ☑
      foot M61.47- ☑
      forearm M61.43- ☑
      hand M61.44- ☑

Calcification — *continued*
  muscle — *continued*
    specified type — *continued*
      lower leg M61.46- ☑
      multiple sites M61.49
      pelvic region M61.45- ☑
      shoulder region M61.41- ☑
      specified site NEC M61.48
      thigh M61.45- ☑
      upper arm M61.42- ☑
  myocardium, myocardial — *see* Degeneration, myocar-
    dial
  ovary N83.8
  pancreas K86.89
  penis N48.89
  periarticular — *see* Disorder, joint, specified type NEC
  pericardium — *see also* Pericarditis I31.1
  pineal gland E34.8
  pleura J94.8
    postinfectional J94.8
    tuberculous NEC B90.9
  pulpal (dental) (nodular) K04.2
  sclera H15.89
  spleen D73.89
  subcutaneous L94.2
  suprarenal (capsule) (gland) E27.49
  tendon (sheath) — *see also* Tenosynovitis, specified
    type NEC
    with bursitis, synovitis or tenosynovitis — *see* Ten-
      dinitis, calcific
  trachea J39.8
  ureter N28.89
  uterus N85.8
  vitreous — *see* Deposit, crystalline
Calcified — *see* Calcification
Calcinosis (interstitial) (tumoral) (universalis) E83.59
  with Raynaud's phenomenon, esophageal dysfunction,
    sclerodactyly, telangiectasia (CREST syndrome)
    M34.1
  circumscripta (skin) L94.2
  cutis L94.2
Calciphylaxis — *see also* Calcification, by site E83.59
Calcium
  deposits — *see* Calcification, by site
  metabolism disorder E83.50
  salts or soaps in vitreous — *see* Deposit, crystalline
Calciuria R82.994
Calculi — *see* Calculus
Calculosis, intrahepatic — *see* Calculus, bile duct
Calculus, calculi, calculous
  ampulla of Vater — *see* Calculus, bile duct
  anuria (impacted) (recurrent) — *see also* Calculus, uri-
    nary N20.9
  appendix K38.1
  bile duct (common) (hepatic) K80.50
    with
      calculus of gallbladder — *see* Calculus, gallblad-
        der and bile duct
      cholangitis K80.30
        with
          cholecystitis — *see* Calculus, bile duct,
            with cholecystitis
          obstruction K80.31
        acute K80.32
          with
            chronic cholangitis K80.36
              with obstruction K80.37
            obstruction K80.33
        chronic K80.34
          with
            acute cholangitis K80.36
              with obstruction K80.37
            obstruction K80.35
      cholecystitis (with cholangitis) K80.40
        with obstruction K80.41
        acute K80.42
          with
            chronic cholecystitis K80.46
              with obstruction K80.47
            obstruction K80.43
        chronic K80.44
          with
            acute cholecystitis K80.46
              with obstruction K80.47
            obstruction K80.45
  biliary — *see also* Calculus, gallbladder
    specified NEC K80.80
      with obstruction K80.81

48

☑ Additional Character Required — Refer to the Tabular List for Character Selection   ▽ Subterms under main terms may continue to next column or page

Calculus, calculi, calculous — *continued*
　bilirubin, multiple — *see* Calculus, gallbladder
　bladder (encysted) (impacted) (urinary) (diverticulum)
　　　N21.0
　bronchus J98.09
　calyx (kidney) (renal) — *see* Calculus, kidney
　cholesterol (pure) (solitary) — *see* Calculus, gallbladder
　common duct (bile) — *see* Calculus, bile duct
　conjunctiva — *see* Concretion, conjunctiva
　cystic N21.0
　　duct — *see* Calculus, gallbladder
　dental (subgingival) (supragingival) K03.6
　diverticulum
　　bladder N21.0
　　kidney N20.0
　epididymis N50.89
　gallbladder K80.20
　　with
　　　bile duct calculus — *see* Calculus, gallbladder
　　　　and bile duct
　　　cholecystitis K80.10
　　　　with obstruction K80.11
　　　　acute K80.00
　　　　　with
　　　　　　chronic cholecystitis K80.12
　　　　　　　with obstruction K80.13
　　　　　　　obstruction K80.01
　　　　　chronic K80.10
　　　　　　with
　　　　　　　acute cholecystitis K80.12
　　　　　　　　with obstruction K80.13
　　　　　　　　obstruction K80.11
　　　　specified NEC K80.18
　　　　　with obstruction K80.19
　　　obstruction K80.21
　gallbladder and bile duct K80.70
　　with
　　　cholecystitis K80.60
　　　　with obstruction K80.61
　　　　acute K80.62
　　　　　with
　　　　　　chronic cholecystitis K80.66
　　　　　　　with obstruction K80.67
　　　　　　　obstruction K80.63
　　　　　chronic K80.64
　　　　　　with
　　　　　　　acute cholecystitis K80.66
　　　　　　　　with obstruction K80.67
　　　　　　　　obstruction K80.65
　　　obstruction K80.71
　hepatic (duct) — *see* Calculus, bile duct
　ileal conduit N21.8
　intestinal (impaction) (obstruction) K56.49
　kidney (impacted) (multiple) (pelvis) (recurrent)
　　　(staghorn) N20.0
　　with calculus, ureter N20.2
　　congenital Q63.8
　lacrimal passages — *see* Dacryolith
　liver (impacted) — *see* Calculus, bile duct
　lung J98.4
　mammographic R92.1
　nephritic (impacted) (recurrent) — *see* Calculus, kidney
　nose J34.89
　pancreas (duct) K86.89
　parotid duct or gland K11.5
　pelvis, encysted — *see* Calculus, kidney
　prostate N42.0
　pulmonary J98.4
　pyelitis (impacted) (recurrent) N20.0
　　with hydronephrosis N13.6
　pyelonephritis (impacted) (recurrent) — *see* category
　　　N20
　　with hydronephrosis N13.6
　renal (impacted) (recurrent) — *see* Calculus, kidney
　salivary (duct) (gland) K11.5
　seminal vesicle N50.89
　staghorn — *see* Calculus, kidney
　Stensen's duct K11.5
　stomach K31.89
　sublingual duct or gland K11.5
　　congenital Q38.4
　submandibular duct, gland or region K11.5
　submaxillary duct, gland or region K11.5
　suburethral N21.8
　tonsil J35.8
　tooth, teeth (subgingival) (supragingival) K03.6
　tunica vaginalis N50.89
　ureter (impacted) (recurrent) N20.1

Calculus, calculi, calculous — *continued*
　ureter — *continued*
　　with calculus, kidney N20.2
　　　with hydronephrosis N13.2
　　　　with infection N13.6
　　ureteropelvic junction N20.1
　urethra (impacted) N21.1
　urinary (duct) (impacted) (passage) (tract) N20.9
　　with hydronephrosis N13.2
　　　with infection N13.6
　　in (due to)
　　　lower N21.9
　　　　specified NEC N21.8
　vagina N89.8
　vesical (impacted) N21.0
　Wharton's duct K11.5
　xanthine E79.8 *[N22]*
Calicectasis N28.89
Caliectasis N28.89
California
　disease B38.9
　encephalitis A83.5
Caligo cornea — *see* Opacity, cornea, central
Callositas, callosity (infected) L84
Callus (infected) L84
　bone — *see* Osteophyte
　excessive, following fracture — *code as* Sequelae
　　　of fracture
CALME (childhood asymmetric labium majus enlarge-
　　ment) N90.61
Calorie deficiency or malnutrition — *see also* Malnu-
　　trition E46
Calvé-Perthes disease — *see* Legg-Calvé-Perthes dis-
　　ease
Calvé's disease — *see* Osteochondrosis, juvenile, spine
Calvities — *see* Alopecia, androgenic
Cameroon fever — *see* Malaria
Camptocormia (hysterical) F44.4
Camurati-Engelmann syndrome Q78.3
Canal — *see also* condition
　atrioventricular common Q21.2
Canaliculitis (lacrimal) (acute) (subacute) H04.33- ☑
　Actinomyces A42.89
　chronic H04.42- ☑
Canavan's disease E75.29
Canceled procedure (surgical) Z53.9
　because of
　　contraindication Z53.09
　　　smoking Z53.01
　　left against medical advice (AMA) Z53.29
　　patient's decision Z53.20
　　　for reasons of belief or group pressure Z53.1
　　　specified reason NEC Z53.29
　　specified reason NEC Z53.8
Cancer — *see also* Neoplasm, by site, malignant
　bile duct type liver C22.1
　blood — *see* Leukemia
　breast — *see also* Neoplasm, breast, malignant
　　　C50.91- ☑
　hepatocellular C22.0
　lung — *see also* Neoplasm, lung, malignant C34.90
　ovarian — *see also* Neoplasm ovary, malignant C56.9
　unspecified site (primary) C80.1
Cancer (o)phobia F45.29
Cancerous — *see* Neoplasm, malignant, by site
Cancrum oris A69.0
Candidiasis, candidal B37.9
　balanitis B37.42
　bronchitis B37.1
　cheilitis B37.83
　congenital P37.5
　cystitis B37.41
　disseminated B37.7
　endocarditis B37.6
　enteritis B37.82
　esophagitis B37.81
　intertrigo B37.2
　lung B37.1
　meningitis B37.5
　mouth B37.0
　nails B37.2
　neonatal P37.5
　onychia B37.2
　oral B37.0
　osteomyelitis B37.89
　otitis externa B37.84
　paronychia B37.2
　perionyxis B37.2

Candidiasis, candidal — *continued*
　pneumonia B37.1
　proctitis B37.82
　pulmonary B37.1
　pyelonephritis B37.49
　sepsis B37.7
　skin B37.2
　specified site NEC B37.89
　stomatitis B37.0
　systemic B37.7
　urethritis B37.41
　urogenital site NEC B37.49
　vagina B37.3
　vulva B37.3
　vulvovaginitis B37.3
Candidid L30.2
Candidosis — *see* Candidiasis
Candiru infection or infestation B88.8
Canities (premature) L67.1
　congenital Q84.2
Canker (mouth) (sore) K12.0
　rash A38.9
Cannabinosis J66.2
Cannabis induced
　anxiety disorder F12.980
　psychotic disorder F12.959
　sleep disorder F12.988
Canton fever A75.9
Cantrell's syndrome Q87.89
Capillariasis (intestinal) B81.1
　hepatic B83.8
Capillary — *see* condition
Caplan's syndrome — *see* Rheumatoid, lung
Capsule — *see* condition
Capsulitis (joint) — *see also* Enthesopathy
　adhesive (shoulder) M75.0- ☑
　hepatic K65.8
　labyrinthine — *see* Otosclerosis, specified NEC
　thyroid E06.9
Caput
　crepitus Q75.8
　medusae I86.8
　succedaneum P12.81
Car sickness T75.3 ☑
Carapata (disease) A68.0
Carate — *see* Pinta
Carbon lung J60
Carbuncle L02.93
　abdominal wall L02.231
　anus K61.0
　auditory canal, external — *see* Abscess, ear, external
　auricle ear — *see* Abscess, ear, external
　axilla L02.43- ☑
　back (any part) L02.232
　breast N61.1
　buttock L02.33
　cheek (external) L02.03
　chest wall L02.233
　chin L02.03
　corpus cavernosum N48.21
　ear (any part) (external) (middle) — *see* Abscess, ear,
　　　external
　external auditory canal — *see* Abscess, ear, external
　eyelid — *see* Abscess, eyelid
　face NEC L02.03
　femoral (region) — *see* Carbuncle, lower limb
　finger — *see* Carbuncle, hand
　flank L02.231
　foot L02.63- ☑
　forehead L02.03
　genital — *see* Abscess, genital
　gluteal (region) L02.33
　groin L02.234
　hand L02.53- ☑
　head NEC L02.831
　heel — *see* Carbuncle, foot
　hip — *see* Carbuncle, lower limb
　kidney — *see* Abscess, kidney
　knee — *see* Carbuncle, lower limb
　labium (majus) (minus) N76.4
　lacrimal
　　gland — *see* Dacryoadenitis
　　passages (duct) (sac) — *see* Inflammation, lacrimal,
　　　passages, acute
　leg — *see* Carbuncle, lower limb
　lower limb L02.43- ☑
　malignant A22.0

Carbuncle — *continued*
navel L02.236
neck L02.13
nose (external) (septum) J34.0
orbit, orbital — *see* Abscess, orbit
palmar (space) — *see* Carbuncle, hand
partes posteriores L02.33
pectoral region L02.233
penis N48.21
perineum L02.235
pinna — *see* Abscess, ear, external
popliteal — *see* Carbuncle, lower limb
scalp L02.831
seminal vesicle N49.0
shoulder — *see* Carbuncle, upper limb
specified site NEC L02.838
temple (region) L02.03
thumb — *see* Carbuncle, hand
toe — *see* Carbuncle, foot
trunk L02.239
abdominal wall L02.231
back L02.232
chest wall L02.233
groin L02.234
perineum L02.235
umbilicus L02.236
umbilicus L02.236
upper limb L02.43- ☑
urethra N34.0
vulva N76.4
Carbunculus — *see* Carbuncle
Carcinoid (tumor) — *see* Tumor, carcinoid
Carcinoidosis E34.0
Carcinoma (malignant) — *see also* Neoplasm, by site, malignant
acidophil
specified site — *see* Neoplasm, malignant, by site
unspecified site C75.1
acidophil-basophil, mixed
specified site — *see* Neoplasm, malignant, by site
unspecified site C75.1
adnexal (skin) — *see* Neoplasm, skin, malignant
adrenal cortical C74.0- ☑
alveolar — *see* Neoplasm, lung, malignant
cell — *see* Neoplasm, lung, malignant
ameloblastic C41.1
upper jaw (bone) C41.0
apocrine
breast — *see* Neoplasm, breast, malignant
specified site NEC — *see* Neoplasm, skin, malignant
unspecified site C44.99
basal cell (pigmented) (*see also* Neoplasm, skin, malignant) C44.91
fibro-epithelial — *see* Neoplasm, skin, malignant
morphea — *see* Neoplasm, skin, malignant
multicentric — *see* Neoplasm, skin, malignant
basaloid
basal-squamous cell, mixed — *see* Neoplasm, skin, malignant
basophil
specified site — *see* Neoplasm, malignant, by site
unspecified site C75.1
basophil-acidophil, mixed
specified site — *see* Neoplasm, malignant, by site
unspecified site C75.1
basosquamous — *see* Neoplasm, skin, malignant
bile duct
with hepatocellular, mixed C22.0
liver C22.1
specified site NEC — *see* Neoplasm, malignant, by site
unspecified site C22.1
branchial or branchiogenic C10.4
bronchial or bronchogenic — *see* Neoplasm, lung, malignant
bronchiolar — *see* Neoplasm, lung, malignant
bronchioloalveolar — *see* Neoplasm, lung, malignant
C cell
specified site — *see* Neoplasm, malignant, by site
unspecified site C73
ceruminous C44.29- ☑
cervix uteri
in situ D06.9
endocervix D06.0
exocervix D06.1
specified site NEC D06.7
chorionic
specified site — *see* Neoplasm, malignant, by site

Carcinoma — *continued*
chorionic — *continued*
unspecified site
female C58
male C62.90
chromophobe
specified site — *see* Neoplasm, malignant, by site
unspecified site C75.1
cloacogenic
specified site — *see* Neoplasm, malignant, by site
unspecified site C21.2
diffuse type
specified site — *see* Neoplasm, malignant, by site
unspecified site C16.9
duct (cell)
with Paget's disease — *see* Neoplasm, breast, malignant
infiltrating
with lobular carcinoma (in situ)
specified site — *see* Neoplasm, malignant, by site
unspecified site (female) C50.91- ☑
male C50.92- ☑
specified site — *see* Neoplasm, malignant, by site
unspecified site (female) C50.91- ☑
male C50.92- ☑
ductal
with lobular
specified site — *see* Neoplasm, malignant, by site
unspecified site (female) C50.91- ☑
male C50.92- ☑
ductular, infiltrating
specified site — *see* Neoplasm, malignant, by site
unspecified site (female) C50.91- ☑
male C50.92- ☑
embryonal
liver C22.7
endometrioid
specified site — *see* Neoplasm, malignant, by site
unspecified site
female C56.9
male C61
eosinophil
specified site — *see* Neoplasm, malignant, by site
unspecified site C75.1
epidermoid — *see also* Neoplasm, skin, malignant
in situ, Bowen's type — *see* Neoplasm, skin, in situ
fibroepithelial, basal cell — *see* Neoplasm, skin, malignant
follicular
with papillary (mixed) C73
moderately differentiated C73
pure follicle C73
specified site — *see* Neoplasm, malignant, by site
trabecular C73
unspecified site C73
well differentiated C73
generalized, with unspecified primary site C80.0
glycogen-rich — *see* Neoplasm, breast, malignant
granulosa cell C56- ☑
hepatic cell C22.0
hepatocellular C22.0
with bile duct, mixed C22.0
fibrolamellar C22.0
hepatocholangiolitic C22.0
Hurthle cell C73
in
adenomatous
polyposis coli C18.9
pleomorphic adenoma — *see* Neoplasm, salivary glands, malignant
situ — *see* Carcinoma-in-situ
infiltrating
duct
with lobular
specified site — *see* Neoplasm, malignant, by site
unspecified site (female) C50.91- ☑
male C50.92- ☑
with Paget's disease — *see* Neoplasm, breast, malignant
specified site — *see* Neoplasm, malignant
unspecified site (female) C50.91- ☑
male C50.92- ☑
ductular
specified site — *see* Neoplasm, malignant

Carcinoma — *continued*
infiltrating — *continued*
ductular — *continued*
unspecified site (female) C50.91- ☑
male C50.92- ☑
lobular
specified site — *see* Neoplasm, malignant
unspecified site (female) C50.91- ☑
male C50.92- ☑
inflammatory
specified site — *see* Neoplasm, malignant
unspecified site (female) C50.91- ☑
male C50.92- ☑
intestinal type
specified site — *see* Neoplasm, malignant, by site
unspecified site C16.9
intracystic
noninfiltrating — *see* Neoplasm, in situ, by site
intraductal (noninfiltrating)
with Paget's disease — *see* Neoplasm, breast, malignant
breast D05.1- ☑
papillary
with invasion
specified site — *see* Neoplasm, malignant, by site
unspecified site (female) C50.91- ☑
male C50.92- ☑
breast D05.1- ☑
specified site NEC — *see* Neoplasm, in situ, by site
unspecified site (female) D05.1- ☑
specified site NEC — *see* Neoplasm, in situ, by site
unspecified site (female) D05.1- ☑
intraepidermal — *see* Neoplasm, in situ
squamous cell, Bowen's type — *see* Neoplasm, skin, in situ
intraepithelial — *see* Neoplasm, in situ, by site
squamous cell — *see* Neoplasm, in situ, by site
intraosseous C41.1
upper jaw (bone) C41.0
islet cell
with exocrine, mixed
specified site — *see* Neoplasm, malignant, by site
unspecified site C25.9
pancreas C25.4
specified site NEC — *see* Neoplasm, malignant, by site
unspecified site C25.4
juvenile, breast — *see* Neoplasm, breast, malignant
large cell
small cell
specified site — *see* Neoplasm, malignant, by site
unspecified site C34.90
Leydig cell (testis)
specified site — *see* Neoplasm, malignant, by site
unspecified site
female C56.9
male C62.90
lipid-rich (female) C50.91- ☑
male C50.92- ☑
liver cell C22.0
liver NEC C22.7
lobular (infiltrating)
with intraductal
specified site — *see* Neoplasm, malignant, by site
unspecified site (female) C50.91- ☑
male C50.92- ☑
noninfiltrating
breast D05.0- ☑
specified site NEC — *see* Neoplasm, in situ, by site
unspecified site D05.0- ☑
specified site — *see* Neoplasm, malignant, by site
unspecified site (female) C50.91- ☑
male C50.92- ☑
medullary
with
amyloid stroma
specified site — *see* Neoplasm, malignant, by site
unspecified site C73

☑ Additional Character Required — Refer to the Tabular List for Character Selection   Subterms under main terms may continue to next column or page

Carcinoma — *continued*
  medullary — *continued*
    with — *continued*
      lymphoid stroma
        specified site — *see* Neoplasm, malignant, by site
        unspecified site (female) C50.91- ☑
          male C50.92- ☑
  Merkel cell C4A.9 (*following* C43)
    anal margin C4A.51 (*following* C43)
    anal skin C4A.51 (*following* C43)
    canthus C4A.1- ☑ (*following* C43)
    ear and external auricular canal C4A.2- ☑ (*following* C43)
    external auricular canal C4A.2- ☑ (*following* C43)
    eyelid, including canthus C4A.1- ☑ (*following* C43)
    face C4A.30 (*following* C43)
      specified NEC C4A.39 (*following* C43)
    hip C4A.7- ☑ (*following* C43)
    lip C4A.0 (*following* C43)
    lower limb, including hip C4A.7- ☑ (*following* C43)
    neck C4A.4 (*following* C43)
    nodal presentation C7B.1 (*following* C75)
    nose C4A.31 (*following* C43)
    overlapping sites C4A.8 (*following* C43)
    perianal skin C4A.51 (*following* C43)
    scalp C4A.4 (*following* C43)
    secondary C7B.1 (*following* C75)
    shoulder C4A.6- ☑ (*following* C43)
    skin of breast C4A.52 (*following* C43)
    trunk NEC C4A.59 (*following* C43)
    upper limb, including shoulder C4A.6- ☑ (*following* C43)
    visceral metastatic C7B.1 (*following* C75)
  metastatic — *see* Neoplasm, secondary, by site
  metatypical — *see* Neoplasm, skin, malignant
  morphea, basal cell — *see* Neoplasm, skin, malignant
  mucoid
    cell
      specified site — *see* Neoplasm, malignant, by site
      unspecified site C75.1
  neuroendocrine — *see also* Tumor, neuroendocrine
    high grade, any site C7A.1 (*following* C75)
    poorly differentiated, any site C7A.1 (*following* C75)
  nonencapsulated sclerosing C73
  noninfiltrating
    intracystic — *see* Neoplasm, in situ, by site
    intraductal
      breast D05.1- ☑
      papillary
        breast D05.1- ☑
        specified site NEC — *see* Neoplasm, in situ, by site
        unspecified site D05.1- ☑
      specified site — *see* Neoplasm, in situ, by site
      unspecified site D05.1- ☑
    lobular
      breast D05.0- ☑
      specified site NEC — *see* Neoplasm, in situ, by site
      unspecified site (female) D05.0- ☑
  oat cell
    specified site — *see* Neoplasm, malignant, by site
    unspecified site C34.90
  odontogenic C41.1
    upper jaw (bone) C41.0
  papillary
    with follicular (mixed) C73
    follicular variant C73
    intraductal (noninfiltrating)
      with invasion
        specified site — *see* Neoplasm, malignant, by site
        unspecified site (female) C50.91- ☑
          male C50.92- ☑
      breast D05.1- ☑
      specified site NEC — *see* Neoplasm, in situ, by site
      unspecified site D05.1- ☑
    serous
      specified site — *see* Neoplasm, malignant, by site
      surface
        specified site — *see* Neoplasm, malignant, by site
        unspecified site C56.9

Carcinoma — *continued*
  papillary — *continued*
    serous — *continued*
      unspecified site C56.9
  papillocystic
    specified site — *see* Neoplasm, malignant, by site
    unspecified site C56.9
  parafollicular cell
    specified site — *see* Neoplasm, malignant, by site
    unspecified site C73
  pilomatrix — *see* Neoplasm, skin, malignant
  pseudomucinous
    specified site — *see* Neoplasm, malignant, by site
    unspecified site C56.9
  renal cell C64- ☑
  Schmincke — *see* Neoplasm, nasopharynx, malignant
  Schneiderian
    specified site — *see* Neoplasm, malignant, by site
    unspecified site C30.0
  sebaceous — *see* Neoplasm, skin, malignant
  secondary — *see also* Neoplasm, secondary, by site
    Merkel cell C7B.1 (*following* C75)
  secretory, breast — *see* Neoplasm, breast, malignant
  serous
    papillary
      specified site — *see* Neoplasm, malignant, by site
      unspecified site C56.9
    surface, papillary
      specified site — *see* Neoplasm, malignant, by site
      unspecified site C56.9
  Sertoli cell
    specified site — *see* Neoplasm, malignant, by site
    unspecified site C62.90
      female C56.9
      male C62.90
  skin appendage — *see* Neoplasm, skin, malignant
  small cell
    fusiform cell
      specified site — *see* Neoplasm, malignant, by site
      unspecified site C34.90
    intermediate cell
      specified site — *see* Neoplasm, malignant, by site
      unspecified site C34.90
    large cell
      specified site — *see* Neoplasm, malignant, by site
      unspecified site C34.90
  solid
    with amyloid stroma
      specified site — *see* Neoplasm, malignant, by site
      unspecified site C73
    microinvasive
      specified site — *see* Neoplasm, malignant, by site
      unspecified site C53.9
  sweat gland — *see* Neoplasm, skin, malignant
  theca cell C56.- ☑
  thymic C37
  unspecified site (primary) C80.1
  water-clear cell C75.0
Carcinoma-in-situ — *see also* Neoplasm, in situ, by site
  breast NOS D05.9- ☑
    specified type NEC D05.8- ☑
  epidermoid — *see also* Neoplasm, in situ, by site
    with questionable stromal invasion
      cervix D06.9
      specified site NEC — *see* Neoplasm, in situ, by site
      unspecified site D06.9
    Bowen's type — *see* Neoplasm, skin, in situ
  intraductal
    breast D05.1- ☑
    specified site NEC — *see* Neoplasm, in situ, by site
    unspecified site D05.1- ☑
  lobular
    with
      infiltrating duct
        breast (female) C50.91- ☑
          male C50.92- ☑
        specified site NEC — *see* Neoplasm, malignant
        unspecified site (female) C50.91- ☑
          male C50.92- ☑

Carcinoma-in-situ — *continued*
  lobular — *continued*
    with — *continued*
      intraductal
        breast D05.8- ☑
        specified site NEC — *see* Neoplasm, in situ, by site
        unspecified site (female) D05.8- ☑
    breast D05.0- ☑
    specified site NEC — *see* Neoplasm, in situ, by site
    unspecified site D05.0- ☑
  squamous cell — *see also* Neoplasm, in situ, by site
    with questionable stromal invasion
      cervix D06.9
      specified site NEC — *see* Neoplasm, in situ, by site
      unspecified site D06.9
Carcinomaphobia F45.29
Carcinomatosis C80.0
  peritonei C78.6
  unspecified site (primary) (secondary) C80.0
Carcinosarcoma — *see* Neoplasm, malignant, by site
  embryonal — *see* Neoplasm, malignant, by site
Cardia, cardial — *see* condition
Cardiac — *see also* condition
  death, sudden — *see* Arrest, cardiac
  pacemaker
    in situ Z95.0
    management or adjustment Z45.018
  tamponade I31.4
Cardialgia — *see* Pain, precordial
Cardiectasis — *see* Hypertrophy, cardiac
Cardiochalasia K21.9
Cardiomalacia I51.5
Cardiomegalia glycogenica diffusa E74.02 *[I43]*
Cardiomegaly — *see also* Hypertrophy, cardiac
  congenital Q24.8
  glycogen E74.02 *[I43]*
  idiopathic I51.7
Cardiomyoliposis I51.5
Cardiomyopathy (familial) (idiopathic) I42.9
  alcoholic I42.6
  amyloid E85.4 *[I43]*
    transthyretin-related (ATTR) familial E85.4 *[I43]*
  arteriosclerotic — *see* Disease, heart, ischemic, atherosclerotic
  beriberi E51.12
  cobalt-beer I42.6
  congenital I42.4
  congestive I42.0
  constrictive NOS I42.5
  dilated I42.0
  due to
    alcohol I42.6
    beriberi E51.12
    cardiac glycogenosis E74.02 *[I43]*
    drugs I42.7
    external agents NEC I42.7
    Friedreich's ataxia G11.11
    myotonia atrophica G71.11 *[I43]*
    progressive muscular dystrophy G71.09 *[I43]*
  glycogen storage E74.02 *[I43]*
  hypertensive — *see* Hypertension, heart
  hypertrophic (nonobstructive) I42.2
    obstructive I42.1
      congenital Q24.8
  in
    Chagas' disease (chronic) B57.2
      acute B57.0
    sarcoidosis D86.85
  ischemic I25.5
  metabolic E88.9 *[I43]*
    thyrotoxic E05.90 *[I43]*
      with thyroid storm E05.91 *[I43]*
  newborn I42.8
    congenital I42.4
  non-ischemic — *see also* by cause I42.8
  nutritional E63.9 *[I43]*
    beriberi E51.12
  obscure of Africa I42.8
  peripartum O90.3
  postpartum O90.3
  restrictive NEC I42.5
  rheumatic I09.0
  secondary I42.9
  specified NEC I42.8
  stress induced I51.81
  takotsubo I51.81

▽ Subterms under main terms may continue to next column or page   ☑ Additional Character Required — Refer to the Tabular List for Character Selection   **51**

Carcinoma — Cardiomyopathy

Cardiomyopathy — *continued*
  thyrotoxic E05.90 *[I43]*
    with thyroid storm E05.91 *[I43]*
  toxic NEC I42.7
  transthyretin-related (ATTR) familial amyloid E85.4
  tuberculous A18.84
  viral B33.24
Cardionephritis — *see* Hypertension, cardiorenal
Cardionephropathy — *see* Hypertension, cardiorenal
Cardionephrosis — *see* Hypertension, cardiorenal
Cardiopathia nigra I27.0
Cardiopathy — *see also* Disease, heart I51.9
  idiopathic I42.9
  mucopolysaccharidosis E76.3 *[I52]*
Cardiopericarditis — *see* Pericarditis
Cardiophobia F45.29
Cardiorenal — *see* condition
Cardiorrhexis — *see* Infarct, myocardium
Cardiosclerosis — *see* Disease, heart, ischemic, atherosclerotic
Cardiosis — *see* Disease, heart
Cardiospasm (esophagus) (reflex) (stomach) K22.0
  congenital Q39.5
    with megaesophagus Q39.5
Cardiostenosis — *see* Disease, heart
Cardiosymphysis I31.0
Cardiovascular — *see* condition
Carditis (acute) (bacterial) (chronic) (subacute) I51.89
  meningococcal A39.50
  rheumatic — *see* Disease, heart, rheumatic
  rheumatoid — *see* Rheumatoid, carditis
  viral B33.20
Care (of) (for) (following)
  child (routine) Z76.2
  family member (handicapped) (sick)
    creating problem for family Z63.6
    provided away from home for holiday relief Z75.5
    unavailable, due to
      absence (person rendering care) (sufferer) Z74.2
      inability (any reason) of person rendering care Z74.2
  foundling Z76.1
  holiday relief Z75.5
  improper — *see* Maltreatment
  lack of (at or after birth) (infant) — *see* Maltreatment, child, neglect
  lactating mother Z39.1
  palliative Z51.5
  postpartum
    immediately after delivery Z39.0
    routine follow-up Z39.2
  respite Z75.5
  unavailable, due to
    absence of person rendering care Z74.2
    inability (any reason) of person rendering care Z74.2
  well-baby Z76.2
Caries
  bone NEC A18.03
  dental (dentino enamel junction) (early childhood) (of dentine) (pre-eruptive) (recurrent) (to the pulp) K02.9
    arrested (coronal) (root) K02.3
    chewing surface
      limited to enamel K02.51
      penetrating into dentin K02.52
      penetrating into pulp K02.53
    coronal surface
      chewing surface
        limited to enamel K02.51
        penetrating into dentin K02.52
        penetrating into pulp K02.53
      pit and fissure surface
        limited to enamel K02.51
        penetrating into dentin K02.52
        penetrating into pulp K02.53
      smooth surface
        limited to enamel K02.61
        penetrating into dentin K02.62
        penetrating into pulp K02.63
    pit and fissure surface
      limited to enamel K02.51
      penetrating into dentin K02.52
      penetrating into pulp K02.53
    primary, cervical origin K02.52
    root K02.7
    smooth surface
      limited to enamel K02.61
      penetrating into dentin K02.62

Caries — *continued*
  dental — *continued*
    smooth surface — *continued*
      penetrating into pulp K02.63
  external meatus — *see* Disorder, ear, external, specified type NEC
  hip (tuberculous) A18.02
  initial (tooth)
    chewing surface K02.51
    pit and fissure surface K02.51
    smooth surface K02.61
  knee (tuberculous) A18.02
  labyrinth H83.8 ☑
  limb NEC (tuberculous) A18.03
  mastoid process (chronic) — *see* Mastoiditis, chronic
    tuberculous A18.03
  middle ear H74.8 ☑
  nose (tuberculous) A18.03
  orbit (tuberculous) A18.03
  ossicles, ear — *see* Abnormal, ear ossicles
  petrous bone — *see* Petrositis
  root (dental) (tooth) K02.7
  sacrum (tuberculous) A18.01
  spine, spinal (column) (tuberculous) A18.01
  syphilitic A52.77
    congenital (early) A50.02 *[M90.80]*
  tooth, teeth — *see* Caries, dental
  tuberculous A18.03
  vertebra (column) (tuberculous) A18.01
Carious teeth — *see* Caries, dental
Carneous mole O02.0
Carnitine insufficiency E71.40
Carotenemia (dietary) E67.1
Carotenosis (cutis) (skin) E67.1
Carotid body or sinus syndrome G90.01
Carotidynia G90.01
Carpal tunnel syndrome — *see* Syndrome, carpal tunnel
Carpenter's syndrome Q87.0
Carpopedal spasm — *see* Tetany
Carr-Barr-Plunkett syndrome Q97.1
Carrier (suspected) of
  amebiasis Z22.1
  bacterial disease NEC Z22.39
    diphtheria Z22.2
    intestinal infectious NEC Z22.1
      typhoid Z22.0
    meningococcal Z22.31
    sexually transmitted Z22.4
    specified NEC Z22.39
    staphylococcal (Methicillin susceptible) Z22.321
      Methicillin resistant Z22.322
    streptococcal Z22.338
      group B Z22.330
        complicating pregnancy or delivery O99.82- ☑
    typhoid Z22.0
  cholera Z22.1
  diphtheria Z22.2
  gastrointestinal pathogens NEC Z22.1
  genetic Z14.8
    cystic fibrosis Z14.1
    hemophilia A (asymptomatic) Z14.01
      symptomatic Z14.02
  gestational, pregnant Z33.1
  gonorrhea Z22.4
  HAA (hepatitis Australian-antigen) B18.8
  HB (c)(s)-AG B18.1
  hepatitis (viral) B18.9
    Australia-antigen (HAA) B18.8
    B surface antigen (HBsAg) B18.1
      with acute delta- (super)infection B17.0
    C B18.2
    specified NEC B18.8
  human T-cell lymphotropic virus type-1 (HTLV-1) infection Z22.6
  infectious organism Z22.9
    specified NEC Z22.8
  meningococci Z22.31
  Salmonella typhosa Z22.0
  serum hepatitis — *see* Carrier, hepatitis
  staphylococci (Methicillin susceptible) Z22.321
    Methicillin resistant Z22.322
  streptococci Z22.338
    group B Z22.330
      complicating pregnancy or delivery O99.82- ☑
  syphilis Z22.4
  typhoid Z22.0
  venereal disease NEC Z22.4

Carrion's disease A44.0
Carter's relapsing fever (Asiatic) A68.1
Cartilage — *see* condition
Caruncle (inflamed)
  conjunctiva (acute) — *see* Conjunctivitis, acute
  labium (majus) (minus) N90.89
  lacrimal — *see* Inflammation, lacrimal, passages
  myrtiform N89.8
  urethral (benign) N36.2
Cascade stomach K31.2
Caseation lymphatic gland (tuberculous) A18.2
Cassidy (-Scholte) syndrome (malignant carcinoid) E34.0
Castellani's disease A69.8
Castration, traumatic, male S38.231 ☑
Casts in urine R82.998
Cat
  cry syndrome Q93.4
  ear Q17.3
  eye syndrome Q92.8
Catabolism, senile R54
Catalepsy (hysterical) F44.2
  schizophrenic F20.2
Cataplexy (idiopathic) — *see* Narcolepsy
Cataract (cortical) (immature) (incipient) H26.9
  with
    neovascularization — *see* Cataract, complicated
  age-related — *see* Cataract, senile
  anterior
    and posterior axial embryonal Q12.0
    pyramidal Q12.0
  associated with
    galactosemia E74.21 *[H28]*
    myotonic disorders G71.19 *[H28]*
  blue Q12.0
  central Q12.0
  cerulean Q12.0
  complicated H26.20
    with
      neovascularization H26.21- ☑
      ocular disorder H26.22- ☑
      glaucomatous flecks H26.23- ☑
  congenital Q12.0
  coraliform Q12.0
  coronary Q12.0
  crystalline Q12.0
  diabetic — *see* Diabetes, cataract
  drug-induced H26.3- ☑
  due to
    ocular disorder — *see* Cataract, complicated
    radiation H26.8
  electric H26.8
  extraction status Z98.4- ☑
  glass-blower's H26.8
  heat ray H26.8
  heterochromic — *see* Cataract, complicated
  hypermature — *see* Cataract, senile, morgagnian type
  in (due to)
    chronic iridocyclitis — *see* Cataract, complicated
    diabetes — *see* Diabetes, cataract
    endocrine disease E34.9 *[H28]*
    eye disease — *see* Cataract, complicated
    hypoparathyroidism E20.9 *[H28]*
    malnutrition-dehydration E46 *[H28]*
    metabolic disease E88.9 *[H28]*
    myotonic disorders G71.19 *[H28]*
    nutritional disease E63.9 *[H28]*
  infantile — *see* Cataract, presenile
  irradiational — *see* Cataract, specified NEC
  juvenile — *see* Cataract, presenile
  malnutrition-dehydration E46 *[H28]*
  morgagnian — *see* Cataract, senile, morgagnian type
  myotonic G71.19 *[H28]*
  myxedema E03.9 *[H28]*
  nuclear
    embryonal Q12.0
    sclerosis — *see* Cataract, senile, nuclear
  presenile H26.00- ☑
    combined forms H26.06- ☑
    cortical H26.01- ☑
    lamellar — *see* Cataract, presenile, cortical
    nuclear H26.03- ☑
    specified NEC H26.09
    subcapsular polar (anterior) H26.04- ☑
      posterior H26.05- ☑
    zonular — *see* Cataract, presenile, cortical
  secondary H26.40
    Soemmering's ring H26.41- ☑

Cataract — *continued*
  secondary — *continued*
    specified NEC H26.49- ☑
    to eye disease — *see* Cataract, complicated
  senile H25.9
    brunescens — *see* Cataract, senile, nuclear
    combined forms H25.81- ☑
    coronary — *see* Cataract, senile, incipient
    cortical H25.01- ☑
    hypermature — *see* Cataract, senile, morgagnian
      type
    incipient (mature) (total) H25.09- ☑
      cortical — *see* Cataract, senile, cortical
      subcapsular — *see* Cataract, senile, subcapsular
    morgagnian type (hypermature) H25.2- ☑
    nuclear (sclerosis) H25.1- ☑
    polar subcapsular (anterior) (posterior) — *see*
      Cataract, senile, incipient
    punctate — *see* Cataract, senile, incipient
    specified NEC H25.89
    subcapsular polar (anterior) H25.03- ☑
      posterior H25.04- ☑
  snowflake — *see* Diabetes, cataract
  specified NEC H26.8
  toxic — *see* Cataract, drug-induced
  traumatic H26.10- ☑
    localized H26.11- ☑
    partially resolved H26.12- ☑
    total H26.13- ☑
  zonular (perinuclear) Q12.0
Cataracta — *see also* Cataract
  brunescens — *see* Cataract, senile, nuclear
  centralis pulverulenta Q12.0
  cerulea Q12.0
  complicata — *see* Cataract, complicated
  congenita Q12.0
  coralliformis Q12.0
  coronaria Q12.0
  diabetic — *see* Diabetes, cataract
  membranacea
    accreta — *see* Cataract, secondary
    congenita Q12.0
  nigra — *see* Cataract, senile, nuclear
  sunflower — *see* Cataract, complicated
Catarrh, catarrhal (acute) (febrile) (infectious) (inflammation) — *see also* condition J00
  bronchial — *see* Bronchitis
  chest — *see* Bronchitis
  chronic J31.0
  due to congenital syphilis A50.03
  enteric — *see* Enteritis
  eustachian H68.009
  fauces — *see* Pharyngitis
  gastrointestinal — *see* Enteritis
  gingivitis K05.00
    nonplaque induced K05.01
    plaque induced K05.00
  hay — *see* Fever, hay
  intestinal — *see* Enteritis
  larynx, chronic J37.0
  liver B15.9
    with hepatic coma B15.0
  lung — *see* Bronchitis
  middle ear, chronic — *see* Otitis, media, nonsuppurative, chronic, serous
  mouth K12.1
  nasal (chronic) — *see* Rhinitis
  nasobronchial J31.1
  nasopharyngeal (chronic) J31.1
    acute J00
  pulmonary — *see* Bronchitis
  spring (eye) (vernal) — *see* Conjunctivitis, acute, atopic
  summer (hay) — *see* Fever, hay
  throat J31.2
  tubotympanal — *see also* Otitis, media, nonsuppurative
    chronic — *see* Otitis, media, nonsuppurative, chronic, serous
Catatonia (schizophrenic) F20.2
Catatonic
  disorder due to known physiologic condition F06.1
  schizophrenia F20.2
  stupor R40.1
Cat-scratch — *see also* Abrasion
  disease or fever A28.1
Cauda equina — *see* condition
Cauliflower ear M95.1-
Causalgia (upper limb) G56.4- ☑

Causalgia — *continued*
  lower limb G57.7- ☑
Cause
  external, general effects T75.89 ☑
Caustic burn — *see* Corrosion, by site
Cavare's disease (familial periodic paralysis) G72.3
Cave-in, injury
  crushing (severe) — *see* Crush
  suffocation — *see* Asphyxia, traumatic, due to low oxygen, due to cave-in
Cavernitis (penis) N48.29
Cavernositis N48.29
Cavernous — *see* condition
Cavitation of lung — *see also* Tuberculosis, pulmonary
  nontuberculous J98.4
Cavities, dental — *see* Caries, dental
Cavity
  lung — *see* Cavitation of lung
  optic papilla Q14.2
  pulmonary — *see* Cavitation of lung
Cavovarus foot, congenital Q66.1- ☑
Cavus foot (congenital) Q66.7- ☑
  acquired — *see* Deformity, limb, foot, specified NEC
Cazenave's disease L10.2
CDKL5 (Cyclin-Dependent Kinase-Like 5 Deficiency Disorder) G40.42
Cecitis K52.9
  with perforation, peritonitis, or rupture K65.8
Cecoureterocele Q62.32
Cecum — *see* condition
Celiac
  artery compression syndrome I77.4
  disease (with steatorrhea) K90.0
  infantilism K90.0
Cell(s), **cellular** — *see also* condition
  in urine R82.998
Cellulitis (diffuse) (phlegmonous) (septic) (suppurative) L03.90
  abdominal wall L03.311
  anaerobic A48.0
  ankle — *see* Cellulitis, lower limb
  anus K61.0
  arm — *see* Cellulitis, upper limb
  auricle (ear) — *see* Cellulitis, ear
  axilla L03.11- ☑
  back (any part) L03.312
  breast (acute) (nonpuerperal) (subacute) N61.0
    nipple N61.0
  broad ligament
    acute N73.0
  buttock L03.317
  cervical (meaning neck) L03.221
  cervix (uteri) — *see* Cervicitis
  cheek (external) L03.211
    internal K12.2
  chest wall L03.313
  chronic L03.90
  clostridial A48.0
  corpus cavernosum N48.22
  digit
    finger — *see* Cellulitis, finger
    toe — *see* Cellulitis, toe
  Douglas' cul-de-sac or pouch
    acute N73.0
  drainage site (following operation) T81.49 ☑
  ear (external) H60.1- ☑
  eosinophilic (granulomatous) L98.3
  erysipelatous — *see* Erysipelas
  external auditory canal — *see* Cellulitis, ear
  eyelid — *see* Abscess, eyelid
  face NEC L03.211
  finger (intrathecal) (periosteal) (subcutaneous) (subcuticular) L03.01- ☑
  foot — *see* Cellulitis, lower limb
  gangrenous — *see* Gangrene
  genital organ NEC
    female (external) N76.4
    male N49.9
      multiple sites N49.8
      specified NEC N49.8
  gluteal (region) L03.317
  gonococcal A54.89
  groin L03.314
  hand — *see* Cellulitis, upper limb
  head NEC L03.811
    face (any part, except ear, eye and nose) L03.211
  heel — *see* Cellulitis, lower limb

Cellulitis — *continued*
  hip — *see* Cellulitis, lower limb
  jaw (region) L03.211
  knee — *see* Cellulitis, lower limb
  labium (majus) (minus) — *see* Vulvitis
  lacrimal passages — *see* Inflammation, lacrimal, passages
  larynx J38.7
  leg — *see* Cellulitis, lower limb
  lip K13.0
  lower limb L03.11- ☑
    toe — *see* Cellulitis, toe
  mouth (floor) K12.2
  multiple sites, so stated L03.90
  nasopharynx J39.1
  navel L03.316
    newborn P38.9
      with mild hemorrhage P38.1
      without hemorrhage P38.9
  neck (region) L03.221
  nipple (acute) (nonpuerperal) (subacute) N61.0
  nose (septum) (external) J34.0
  orbit, orbital H05.01- ☑
  palate (soft) K12.2
  pectoral (region) L03.313
  pelvis, pelvic (chronic)
    female — *see also* Disease, pelvis, inflammatory N73.2
      acute N73.0
    following ectopic or molar pregnancy O08.0
    male K65.0
  penis N48.22
  perineal, perineum L03.315
  periorbital L03.213
  perirectal K61.1
  peritonsillar J36
  periurethral N34.0
  periuterine — *see also* Disease, pelvis, inflammatory N73.2
    acute N73.0
  pharynx J39.1
  preseptal L03.213
  rectum K61.1
  retroperitoneal K68.9
  round ligament
    acute N73.0
  scalp (any part) L03.811
  scrotum N49.2
  seminal vesicle N49.0
  shoulder — *see* Cellulitis, upper limb
  specified site NEC L03.818
  submandibular (region) (space) (triangle) K12.2
    gland K11.3
  submaxillary (region) K12.2
    gland K11.3
  thigh — *see* Cellulitis, lower limb
  thumb (intrathecal) (periosteal) (subcutaneous) (subcuticular) — *see* Cellulitis, finger
  toe (intrathecal) (periosteal) (subcutaneous) (subcuticular) L03.03- ☑
  tonsil J36
  trunk L03.319
    abdominal wall L03.311
    back (any part) L03.312
    buttock L03.317
    chest wall L03.313
    groin L03.314
    perineal, perineum L03.315
    umbilicus L03.316
  tuberculous (primary) A18.4
  umbilicus L03.316
  upper limb L03.11- ☑
    axilla — *see* Cellulitis, axilla
    finger — *see* Cellulitis, finger
    thumb — *see* Cellulitis, finger
  vaccinal T88.0 ☑
  vocal cord J38.3
  vulva — *see* Vulvitis
  wrist — *see* Cellulitis, upper limb
Cementoblastoma, benign — *see* Cyst, calcifying odontogenic
Cementoma — *see* Cyst, calcifying odontogenic
Cementoperiostitis — *see* Periodontitis
Cementosis K03.4
Central auditory processing disorder H93.25
Central pain syndrome G89.0
Cephalematocele, cephal (o)hematocele
  newborn P52.8

Cephalematocele, cephalhematocele — *continued*
  newborn — *continued*
    birth injury P10.8
  traumatic — *see* Hematoma, brain
Cephalematoma, cephalhematoma (calcified)
  newborn (birth injury) P12.0
  traumatic — *see* Hematoma, brain
Cephalgia, cephalalgia — *see also* Headache
  histamine G44.009
    intractable G44.001
    not intractable G44.009
  trigeminal autonomic (TAC) NEC G44.099
    intractable G44.091
    not intractable G44.099
Cephalic — *see* condition
Cephalitis — *see* Encephalitis
Cephalocele — *see* Encephalocele
Cephalomenia N94.89
Cephalopelvic — *see* condition
Cerclage (with cervical incompetence) in pregnancy —
  see Incompetence, cervix, in pregnancy
Cerebellitis — *see* Encephalitis
Cerebellum, cerebellar — *see* condition
Cerebral — *see* condition
Cerebritis — *see* Encephalitis
Cerebro-hepato-renal syndrome Q87.89
Cerebromalacia — *see* Softening, brain
  sequelae of cerebrovascular disease I69.398
Cerebroside lipidosis E75.22
Cerebrospasticity (congenital) G80.1
Cerebrospinal — *see* condition
Cerebrum — *see* condition
Ceroid-lipofuscinosis, neuronal E75.4
Cerumen (accumulation) (impacted) H61.2- ☑
Cervical — *see also* condition
  auricle Q18.2
  dysplasia in pregnancy — *see* Abnormal, cervix, in
    pregnancy or childbirth
  erosion in pregnancy — *see* Abnormal, cervix, in
    pregnancy or childbirth
  fibrosis in pregnancy — *see* Abnormal, cervix, in preg-
    nancy or childbirth
  fusion syndrome Q76.1
  rib Q76.5
  shortening (complicating pregnancy) O26.87- ☑
Cervicalgia M54.2
Cervicitis (acute) (chronic) (nonvenereal) (senile (atrophic)) (subacute) (with ulceration) N72
  with
    abortion — *see* Abortion, by type complicated by
      genital tract and pelvic infection
    ectopic pregnancy O08.0
    molar pregnancy O08.0
  chlamydial A56.09
  gonococcal A54.03
  herpesviral A60.03
  puerperal (postpartum) O86.11
  syphilitic A52.76
  trichomonal A59.09
  tuberculous A18.16
Cervicocolpitis (emphysematosa) — *see also* Cervicitis
  N72
Cervix — *see* condition
Cesarean delivery, previous, affecting management
  of pregnancy O34.219
  classical (vertical) scar O34.212
  isthmocele O34.22
  low transverse scar O34.211
  mid-transverse T incision O34.218
  scar
    defect (isthmocele) O34.22
    specified type NEC O34.218
Céstan (-Chenais) paralysis or syndrome G46.3
Céstan-Raymond syndrome I65.8
Cestode infestation B71.9
  specified type NEC B71.8
Cestodiasis B71.9
Chabert's disease A22.9
Chacaleh E53.8
Chafing L30.4
Chagas' (-Mazza) disease (chronic) B57.2
  with
    cardiovascular involvement NEC B57.2
    digestive system involvement B57.30
      megacolon B57.32
      megaesophagus B57.31
      other specified B57.39

Chagas' disease — *continued*
  with — *continued*
    megacolon B57.32
    megaesophagus B57.31
    myocarditis B57.2
    nervous system involvement B57.40
      meningitis B57.41
      meningoencephalitis B57.42
      other specified B57.49
    specified organ involvement NEC B57.5
  acute (with) B57.1
    cardiovascular NEC B57.0
    myocarditis B57.0
Chagres fever B50.9
Chairridden Z74.09
Chalasia (cardiac sphincter) K21.9
Chalazion H00.19
  left H00.16
    lower H00.15
    upper H00.14
  right H00.13
    lower H00.12
    upper H00.11
Chalcosis — *see also* Disorder, globe, degenerative,
  chalcosis
  cornea — *see* Deposit, cornea
  crystalline lens — *see* Cataract, complicated
  retina H35.89
Chalicosis (pulmonum) J62.8
Chancre (any genital site) (hard) (hunterian) (mixed)
  (primary) (seronegative) (seropositive) (syphilitic)
  A51.0
  congenital A50.07
  conjunctiva NEC A51.2
  Ducrey's A57
  extragenital A51.2
  eyelid A51.2
  lip A51.2
  nipple A51.2
  Nisbet's A57
  of
    carate A67.0
    pinta A67.0
    yaws A66.0
  palate, soft A51.2
  phagedenic A57
  simple A57
  soft A57
    bubo A57
    palate A51.2
  urethra A51.0
  yaws A66.0
Chancroid (anus) (genital) (penis) (perineum) (rectum)
  (urethra) (vulva) A57
Chandler's disease (osteochondritis dissecans, hip) —
  see Osteochondritis, dissecans, hip
Change(s) (in) (of) — *see also* Removal
  arteriosclerotic — *see* Arteriosclerosis
  bone — *see also* Disorder, bone
    diabetic — *see* Diabetes, bone change
  bowel habit R19.4
  cardiorenal (vascular) — *see* Hypertension, cardiorenal
  cardiovascular — *see* Disease, cardiovascular
  circulatory I99.9
  cognitive (mild) (organic) R41.89
  color, tooth, teeth
    during formation K00.8
    posteruptive K03.7
  contraceptive device Z30.433
  corneal membrane H18.30
    Bowman's membrane fold or rupture H18.31- ☑
    Descemet's membrane
      fold H18.32- ☑
      rupture H18.33- ☑
  coronary — *see* Disease, heart, ischemic
  degenerative, spine or vertebra — *see* Spondylosis
  dental pulp, regressive K04.2
  dressing (nonsurgical) Z48.00
    surgical Z48.01
  heart — *see* Disease, heart
  hip joint — *see* Derangement, joint, hip
  hyperplastic larynx J38.7
  hypertrophic
    nasal sinus J34.89
    turbinate, nasal J34.3
    upper respiratory tract J39.8
  indwelling catheter Z46.6
  inflammatory — *see also* Inflammation

Change(s) — *continued*
  inflammatory — *see also* Inflammation — *contin-*
    ued
    sacroiliac M46.1
  job, anxiety concerning Z56.1
  joint — *see* Derangement, joint
  life — *see* Menopause
  mental status R41.82
  minimal (glomerular) — *see also* N00-N07 with fourth
    character .0 N05.0
  myocardium, myocardial — *see* Degeneration, myocar-
    dial
  of life — *see* Menopause
  pacemaker Z45.018
    pulse generator Z45.010
  personality (enduring) F68.8
    due to (secondary to)
      general medical condition F07.0
    secondary (nonspecific) F60.89
  regressive, dental pulp K04.2
  renal — *see* Disease, renal
  retina H35.9
    myopic — *see also* Myopia, degenerative H44.2- ☑
  sacroiliac joint M53.3
  senile — *see also* condition R54
  sensory R20.8
  skin R23.9
    acute, due to ultraviolet radiation L56.9
      specified NEC L56.8
    chronic, due to nonionizing radiation L57.9
      specified NEC L57.8
    cyanosis R23.0
    flushing R23.2
    pallor R23.1
    petechiae R23.3
    specified change NEC R23.8
    swelling — *see* Mass, localized
    texture R23.4
  trophic
    arm — *see* Mononeuropathy, upper limb
    leg — *see* Mononeuropathy, lower limb
  vascular I99.9
  vasomotor I73.9
  voice R49.9
    psychogenic F44.4
    specified NEC R49.8
Changing sleep-work schedule, affecting sleep
  G47.26
Changuinola fever A93.1
Chapping skin T69.8 ☑
Charcot-Marie-Tooth disease, paralysis or syndrome
  G60.0
Charcot's
  arthropathy — *see* Arthropathy, neuropathic
  cirrhosis K74.3
  disease (tabetic arthropathy) A52.16
  joint (disease) (tabetic) A52.16
    diabetic — *see* Diabetes, with, arthropathy
    syringomyelic G95.0
  syndrome (intermittent claudication) I73.9
CHARGE association Q89.8
Charley-horse (quadriceps) M62.831
  traumatic (quadriceps) S76.11- ☑
Charlouis' disease — *see* Yaws
Cheadle's disease E54
Checking (of)
  cardiac pacemaker (battery) (electrode(s)) Z45.018
    pulse generator Z45.010
  implantable subdermal contraceptive Z30.46
  intrauterine contraceptive device Z30.431
  wound Z48.0- ☑
    due to injury — code to Injury, by site, using appro-
      priate seventh character for subsequent en-
      counter
Check-up — *see* Examination
Chédiak-Higashi (-Steinbrinck) **syndrome** (congenital
  gigantism of peroxidase granules) E70.330
Cheek — *see* condition
Cheese itch B88.0
Cheese-washer's lung J67.8
Cheese-worker's lung J67.8
Cheilitis (acute) (angular) (catarrhal) (chronic) (exfoliative)
  (gangrenous) (glandular) (infectional) (suppurative)
  (ulcerative) (vesicular) K13.0
  actinic (due to sun) L56.8
    other than from sun L59.8
  candidal B37.83
Cheilodynia K13.0

Cheiloschisis — *see* Cleft, lip
Cheilosis (angular) K13.0
  with pellagra E52
  due to
    vitamin B2 (riboflavin) deficiency E53.0
Cheiromegaly M79.89
Cheiropompholyx L30.1
Cheloid — *see* Keloid
Chemical burn — *see* Corrosion, by site
Chemodectoma — *see* Paraganglioma, nonchromaffin
Chemosis, conjunctiva — *see* Edema, conjunctiva
Chemotherapy (session) (for)
  cancer Z51.11
  neoplasm Z51.11
Cherubism M27.8
Chest — *see* condition
Cheyne-Stokes breathing (respiration) R06.3
Chiari's
  disease or syndrome (hepatic vein thrombosis) I82.0
  malformation
    type I G93.5
    type II — *see* Spina bifida
  net Q24.8
Chicago disease B40.9
Chickenpox — *see* Varicella
Chiclero ulcer or sore B55.1
Chigger (infestation) B88.0
Chignon (disease) B36.8
  newborn (from vacuum extraction) (birth injury) P12.1
Chilaiditi's syndrome (subphrenic displacement, colon)
  Q43.3
Chilblain(s) (lupus) T69.1 ☑
Child
  custody dispute Z65.3
Childbirth — *see* Delivery
Childhood
  cerebral X-linked adrenoleukodystrophy E71.520
  period of rapid growth Z00.2
Chill(s) R68.83
  with fever R50.9
  congestive in malarial regions B54
  without fever R68.83
Chilomastigiasis A07.8
Chimera 46,XX/46,XY Q99.0
Chin — *see* condition
Chinese dysentery A03.9
Chionophobia F40.228
Chitral fever A93.1
Chlamydia, chlamydial A74.9
  cervicitis A56.09
  conjunctivitis A74.0
  cystitis A56.01
  endometritis A56.11
  epididymitis A56.19
  female
    pelvic inflammatory disease A56.11
    pelviperitonitis A56.11
  orchitis A56.19
  peritonitis A74.81
  pharyngitis A56.4
  proctitis A56.3
  psittaci (infection) A70
  salpingitis A56.11
  sexually-transmitted infection NEC A56.8
  specified NEC A74.89
  urethritis A56.01
  vulvovaginitis A56.02
Chlamydiosis — *see* Chlamydia
Chloasma (skin) (idiopathic) (symptomatic) L81.1
  eyelid H02.719
    hyperthyroid E05.90 *[H02.719]*
      with thyroid storm E05.91 *[H02.719]*
    left H02.716
      lower H02.715
      upper H02.714
    right H02.713
      lower H02.712
      upper H02.711
Chloroma C92.3- ☑
Chlorosis D50.9
  Egyptian B76.9 *[D63.8]*
  miner's B76.9 *[D63.8]*
Chlorotic anemia D50.8
Chocolate cyst (ovary) N80.1
Choked
  disc or disk — *see* Papilledema

Choked — *continued*
  on food, phlegm, or vomitus NOS — *see* Foreign body,
    by site
  while vomiting NOS — *see* Foreign body, by site
Chokes (resulting from bends) T70.3 ☑
Choking sensation R09.89
Cholangiectasis K83.8
Cholangiocarcinoma
  with hepatocellular carcinoma, combined C22.0
  liver C22.1
  specified site NEC — *see* Neoplasm, malignant, by site
  unspecified site C22.1
Cholangiohepatitis K83.8
  due to fluke infestation B66.1
Cholangiohepatoma C22.0
Cholangiolitis (acute) (chronic) (extrahepatic) (gangrenous) (intrahepatic) K83.09
  paratyphoidal — *see* Fever, paratyphoid
  typhoidal A01.09
Cholangioma D13.4
  malignant — *see* Cholangiocarcinoma
Cholangitis (ascending) (recurrent) (secondary) (stenosing) (suppurative) K83.09
  with calculus, bile duct — *see* Calculus, bile duct, with
    cholangitis
  chronic nonsuppurative destructive K74.3
  primary K83.09
    sclerosing K83.01
  sclerosing K83.09
Cholecystectasia K82.8
Cholecystitis K81.9
  with
    calculus, stones in
      bile duct (common) (hepatic) — *see* Calculus,
        bile duct, with cholecystitis
      cystic duct — *see* Calculus, gallbladder, with
        cholecystitis
      gallbladder — *see* Calculus, gallbladder, with
        cholecystitis
    choledocholithiasis — *see* Calculus, bile duct, with
      cholecystitis
    cholelithiasis — *see* Calculus, gallbladder, with
      cholecystitis
    gangrene of gallbladder K82.A1
    perforation of gallbladder K82.A2
  acute (emphysematous) (gangrenous) (suppurative)
    K81.0
    with
      calculus, stones in
        cystic duct — *see* Calculus, gallbladder, with
          cholecystitis, acute
        gallbladder — *see* Calculus, gallbladder, with
          cholecystitis, acute
        choledocholithiasis — *see* Calculus, bile duct,
          with cholecystitis, acute
        cholelithiasis — *see* Calculus, gallbladder, with
          cholecystitis, acute
    chronic cholecystitis K81.2
      with gallbladder calculus K80.12
        with obstruction K80.13
  chronic K81.1
    with acute cholecystitis K81.2
      with gallbladder calculus K80.12
        with obstruction K80.13
  emphysematous (acute) — *see* Cholecystitis, acute
  gangrenous — *see* Cholecystitis, acute
  paratyphoidal, current A01.4
  suppurative — *see* Cholecystitis, acute
  typhoidal A01.09
Cholecystolithiasis — *see* Calculus, gallbladder
Choledochitis (suppurative) K83.09
Choledocholith — *see* Calculus, bile duct
Choledocholithiasis (common duct) (hepatic duct) —
  see Calculus, bile duct
  cystic — *see* Calculus, gallbladder
  typhoidal A01.09
Cholelithiasis (cystic duct) (gallbladder) (impacted)
  (multiple) — *see* Calculus, gallbladder
  bile duct (common) (hepatic) — *see* Calculus, bile duct
  hepatic duct — *see* Calculus, bile duct
  specified NEC K80.80
    with obstruction K80.81
Cholemia — *see also* Jaundice
  familial (simple) (congenital) E80.4
  Gilbert's E80.4
Choleperitoneum, choleperitonitis K65.3
Cholera (Asiatic) (epidemic) (malignant) A00.9

Cholera — *continued*
  antimonial — *see* Poisoning, antimony
  classical A00.0
  due to Vibrio cholerae 01 A00.9
    biovar cholerae A00.0
    biovar eltor A00.1
    el tor A00.1
  el tor A00.1
Cholerine — *see* Cholera
Cholestasis NEC K83.1
  with hepatocyte injury K71.0
  due to total parenteral nutrition (TPN) K76.89
  pure K71.0
Cholesteatoma (ear) (middle) (with reaction) H71.9- ☑
  attic H71.0- ☑
  external ear (canal) H60.4- ☑
  mastoid H71.2- ☑
  postmastoidectomy cavity (recurrent) — *see* Complica-
    tions, postmastoidectomy, recurrent
    cholesteatoma
  recurrent (postmastoidectomy) — *see* Complications,
    postmastoidectomy, recurrent cholesteatoma
  tympanum H71.1- ☑
Cholesteatosis, diffuse H71.3- ☑
Cholesteremia E78.00
Cholesterin in vitreous — *see* Deposit, crystalline
Cholesterol
  deposit
    retina H35.89
    vitreous — *see* Deposit, crystalline
  elevated (high) E78.00
    with elevated (high) triglycerides E78.2
    screening for Z13.220
  imbibition of gallbladder K82.4
Cholesterolemia (essential) (pure) E78.00
  familial E78.01
  hereditary E78.01
Cholesterolosis, cholesterosis (gallbladder) K82.4
  cerebrotendinous E75.5
Cholocolic fistula K82.3
Choluria R82.2
Chondritis M94.8X9
  aurical H61.03- ☑
  costal (Tietze's) M94.0
  external ear H61.03- ☑
  patella, posttraumatic — *see* Chondromalacia, patella
  pinna H61.03- ☑
  purulent M94.8X- ☑
  tuberculous NEC A18.02
    intervertebral A18.01
Chondroblastoma — *see also* Neoplasm, bone, benign
  malignant — *see* Neoplasm, bone, malignant
Chondrocalcinosis M11.20
  ankle M11.27- ☑
  elbow M11.22- ☑
  familial M11.10
    ankle M11.17- ☑
    elbow M11.12- ☑
    foot joint M11.17- ☑
    hand joint M11.14- ☑
    hip M11.15- ☑
    knee M11.16- ☑
    multiple site M11.19
    shoulder M11.11- ☑
    vertebrae M11.18
    wrist M11.13- ☑
  foot joint M11.27- ☑
  hand joint M11.24- ☑
  hip M11.25- ☑
  knee M11.26- ☑
  multiple site M11.29
  shoulder M11.21- ☑
  specified type NEC M11.20
    ankle M11.27- ☑
    elbow M11.22- ☑
    foot joint M11.27- ☑
    hand joint M11.24- ☑
    hip M11.25- ☑
    knee M11.26- ☑
    multiple site M11.29
    shoulder M11.21- ☑
    vertebrae M11.28
    wrist M11.23- ☑
  vertebrae M11.28
  wrist M11.23- ☑
Chondrodermatitis nodularis helicis or anthelicis —
  see Perichondritis, ear

Chondrodysplasia Q78.9
　with hemangioma Q78.4
　calcificans congenita Q77.3
　fetalis Q77.4
　metaphyseal (Jansen's) (McKusick's) (Schmid's) Q78.8
　punctata Q77.3
Chondrodystrophy, chondrodystrophia (familial) (fetalis) (hypoplastic) Q78.9
　calcificans congenita Q77.3
　myotonic (congenital) G71.13
　punctata Q77.3
Chondroectodermal dysplasia Q77.6
Chondrogenesis imperfecta Q77.4
Chondrolysis M94.35-
Chondroma — see also Neoplasm, cartilage, benign
　juxtacortical — see Neoplasm, bone, benign
　periosteal — see Neoplasm, bone, benign
Chondromalacia (systemic) M94.20
　acromioclavicular joint M94.21- ☑
　ankle M94.27- ☑
　elbow M94.22- ☑
　foot joint M94.27- ☑
　glenohumeral joint M94.21- ☑
　hand joint M94.24- ☑
　hip M94.25- ☑
　knee M94.26- ☑
　　patella M22.4- ☑
　multiple sites M94.29
　patella M22.4- ☑
　rib M94.28
　sacroiliac joint M94.259
　shoulder M94.21- ☑
　sternoclavicular joint M94.21- ☑
　vertebral joint M94.28
　wrist M94.23- ☑
Chondromatosis — see also Neoplasm, cartilage, uncertain behavior
　internal Q78.4
Chondromyxosarcoma — see Neoplasm, cartilage, malignant
Chondro-osteodysplasia (Morquio-Brailsford type) E76.219
Chondro-osteodystrophy E76.29
Chondro-osteoma — see Neoplasm, bone, benign
Chondropathia tuberosa M94.0
Chondrosarcoma — see Neoplasm, cartilage, malignant
　juxtacortical — see Neoplasm, bone, malignant
　mesenchymal — see Neoplasm, connective tissue, malignant
　myxoid — see Neoplasm, cartilage, malignant
Chordee (nonvenereal) N48.89
　congenital Q54.4
　gonococcal A54.09
Chorditis (fibrinous) (nodosa) (tuberosa) J38.2
Chordoma — see Neoplasm, vertebral (column), malignant
Chorea (chronic) (gravis) (posthemiplegic) (senile) (spasmodic) G25.5
　with
　　heart involvement I02.0
　　　active or acute (conditions in I01-) I02.0
　　　　rheumatic I02.9
　　　　　with valvular disorder I02.0
　　　rheumatic heart disease (chronic) (inactive)(quiescent) — code to rheumatic heart condition involved
　drug-induced G25.4
　habit F95.8
　hereditary G10
　Huntington's G10
　hysterical F44.4
　minor I02.9
　　with heart involvement I02.0
　progressive G25.5
　　hereditary G10
　rheumatic (chronic) I02.9
　　with heart involvement I02.0
　Sydenham's I02.9
　　with heart involvement — see Chorea, with rheumatic heart disease
　　nonrheumatic G25.5
Choreoathetosis (paroxysmal) G25.5
Chorioadenoma (destruens) D39.2
Chorioamnionitis O41.12- ☑
Chorioangioma D26.7
Choriocarcinoma — see Neoplasm, malignant, by site

Choriocarcinoma — continued
　combined with
　　embryonal carcinoma — see Neoplasm, malignant, by site
　　other germ cell elements — see Neoplasm, malignant, by site
　　teratoma — see Neoplasm, malignant, by site
　specified site — see Neoplasm, malignant, by site
　unspecified site
　　female C58
　　male C62.90
Chorioencephalitis (acute) (lymphocytic) (serous) A87.2
Chorioepithelioma — see Choriocarcinoma
Choriomeningitis (acute) (lymphocytic) (serous) A87.2
Chorionepithelioma — see Choriocarcinoma
Chorioretinitis — see also Inflammation, chorioretinal
　disseminated — see also Inflammation, chorioretinal, disseminated
　　in neurosyphilis A52.19
　Egyptian B76.9 [D63.8]
　focal — see also Inflammation, chorioretinal, focal
　histoplasmic B39.9 [H32]
　in (due to)
　　histoplasmosis B39.9 [H32]
　　syphilis (secondary) A51.43
　　　late A52.71
　　toxoplasmosis (acquired) B58.01
　　　congenital (active) P37.1 [H32]
　　tuberculosis A18.53
　juxtapapillary, juxtapapillaris — see Inflammation, chorioretinal, focal, juxtapapillary
　leprous A30.9 [H32]
　miner's B76.9 [D63.8]
　progressive myopia (degeneration) — see also Myopia, degenerative H44.2- ☑
　syphilitic (secondary) A51.43
　　congenital (early) A50.01 [H32]
　　　late A50.32
　　late A52.71
　tuberculous A18.53
Chorioretinopathy, central serous H35.71- ☑
Choroid — see condition
Choroideremia H31.21
Choroiditis — see Chorioretinitis
Choroidopathy — see Disorder, choroid
Choroidoretinitis — see Chorioretinitis
Choroidoretinopathy, central serous — see Chorioretinopathy, central serous
Christian-Weber disease M35.6
Christmas disease D67
Chromaffinoma — see also Neoplasm, benign, by site
　malignant — see Neoplasm, malignant, by site
Chromatopsia — see Deficiency, color vision
Chromhidrosis, chromidrosis L75.1
Chromoblastomycosis — see Chromomycosis
Chromoconversion R82.91
Chromomycosis B43.9
　brain abscess B43.1
　cerebral B43.1
　cutaneous B43.0
　skin B43.0
　specified NEC B43.8
　subcutaneous abscess or cyst B43.2
Chromophytosis B36.0
Chromosome — see Anomaly, by chromosome involved
　D (1) — see Anomaly, chromosome 13
　E (3) — see Anomaly, chromosome 18
　G — see Anomaly, chromosome 21
Chromotrichomycosis B36.8
Chronic — see condition
　fracture — see Fracture, pathological
Churg-Strauss syndrome M30.1
Chyle cyst, mesentery I89.8
Chylocele (nonfilarial) I89.8
　filarial — see also Infestation, filarial B74.9 [N51]
　tunica vaginalis N50.89
　　filarial — see also Infestation, filarial B74.9 [N51]
Chylomicronemia (fasting) (with hyperprebetalipoproteinemia) E78.3
Chylopericardium I31.3
　acute I30.9
Chylothorax (nonfilarial) I89.8
　filarial — see also Infestation, filarial B74.9 [J91.8]
Chylous — see condition
Chyluria (nonfilarial) R82.0
　due to
　　bilharziasis B65.0

Chyluria — continued
　due to — continued
　　Brugia (malayi) B74.1
　　　timori B74.2
　　schistosomiasis (bilharziasis) B65.0
　　Wuchereria (bancrofti) B74.0
　filarial — see Infestation, filarial
Cicatricial (deformity) — see Cicatrix
Cicatrix (adherent) (contracted) (painful) (vicious) — see also Scar L90.5
　adenoid (and tonsil) J35.8
　alveolar process M26.79
　anus K62.89
　auricle — see Disorder, pinna, specified type NEC
　bile duct (common) (hepatic) K83.8
　bladder N32.89
　bone — see Disorder, bone, specified type NEC
　brain G93.89
　cervix (postoperative) (postpartal) N88.1
　common duct K83.8
　cornea H17.9
　　tuberculous A18.59
　duodenum (bulb), obstructive K31.5
　esophagus K22.2
　eyelid — see Disorder, eyelid function
　hypopharynx J39.2
　lacrimal passages — see Obstruction, lacrimal
　larynx J38.7
　lung J98.4
　middle ear H74.8 ☑
　mouth K13.79
　muscle M62.89
　　with contracture — see Contraction, muscle NEC
　nasopharynx J39.2
　palate (soft) K13.79
　penis N48.89
　pharynx J39.2
　prostate N42.89
　rectum K62.89
　retina — see Scar, chorioretinal
　semilunar cartilage — see Derangement, meniscus
　seminal vesicle N50.89
　skin L90.5
　　infected L08.89
　　postinfective L90.5
　　tuberculous B90.8
　specified site NEC L90.5
　throat J39.2
　tongue K14.8
　tonsil (and adenoid) J35.8
　trachea J39.8
　tuberculous NEC B90.9
　urethra N36.8
　uterus N85.8
　vagina N89.8
　　postoperative N99.2
　vocal cord J38.3
　wrist, constricting (annular) L90.5
CIDP (chronic inflammatory demyelinating polyneuropathy) G61.81
CIN — see Neoplasia, intraepithelial, cervix
CINCA (chronic infantile neurological, cutaneous and articular syndrome) M04.2
Cinchonism — see Deafness, ototoxic
　correct substance properly administered — see Table of Drugs and Chemicals, by drug, adverse effect
　overdose or wrong substance given or taken — see Table of Drugs and Chemicals, by drug, poisoning
Circle of Willis — see condition
Circular — see condition
Circulating anticoagulants — see also Disorder, hemorrhagic D68.318
　due to drugs — see also Disorder, hemorrhagic D68.32
　following childbirth O72.3
Circulation
　collateral, any site I99.8
　defective (lower extremity) I99.9
　　congenital Q28.9
　embryonic Q28.9
　failure (peripheral) R57.9
　　newborn P29.89
　fetal, persistent P29.38
　heart, incomplete Q28.9
Circulatory system — see condition
Circulus senilis (cornea) — see Degeneration, cornea, senile
Circumcision (in absence of medical indication) (ritual) (routine) Z41.2

☑ Additional Character Required — Refer to the Tabular List for Character Selection　　　☝ Subterms under main terms may continue to next column or page

Circumscribed — *see* condition
Circumvallate placenta O43.11- ☑
Cirrhosis, cirrhotic (hepatic) (liver) K74.60
  alcoholic K70.30
    with ascites K70.31
  atrophic — *see* Cirrhosis, liver
  Baumgarten-Cruveilhier K74.69
  biliary (cholangiolitic) (cholangitic) (hypertrophic)
      (obstructive) (pericholangiolitic) K74.5
    due to
      Clonorchiasis B66.1
      flukes B66.3
    primary K74.3
    secondary K74.4
  cardiac (of liver) K76.1
  Charcot's K74.3
  cholangiolitic, cholangitic, cholostatic (primary) K74.3
  congestive K76.1
  Cruveilhier-Baumgarten K74.69
  cryptogenic (liver) K74.69
  due to
    hepatolenticular degeneration E83.01
    Wilson's disease E83.01
    xanthomatosis E78.2
  fatty K76.0
    alcoholic K70.30
  Hanot's (hypertrophic) K74.3
  hepatic — *see* Cirrhosis, liver
  hypertrophic K74.3
  Indian childhood K74.69
  kidney — *see* Sclerosis, renal
  Laennec's K70.30
    with ascites K70.31
    alcoholic K70.30
      with ascites K70.31
    nonalcoholic K74.69
  liver K74.60
    alcoholic K70.30
      with ascites K70.31
    fatty K70.0
    congenital P78.81
    syphilitic A52.74
  lung (chronic) J84.10
  macronodular K74.69
    alcoholic K70.30
      with ascites K70.31
  micronodular K74.69
    alcoholic K70.30
      with ascites K70.31
  mixed type K74.69
  monolobular K74.3
  nephritis — *see* Sclerosis, renal
  nutritional K74.69
    alcoholic K70.30
      with ascites K70.31
  obstructive — *see* Cirrhosis, biliary
  ovarian N83.8
  pancreas (duct) K86.89
  pigmentary E83.110
  portal K74.69
    alcoholic K70.30
      with ascites K70.31
  postnecrotic K74.69
    alcoholic K70.30
      with ascites K70.31
  pulmonary J84.10
  renal — *see* Sclerosis, renal
  spleen D73.2
  stasis K76.1
  Todd's K74.3
  unilobar K74.3
  xanthomatous (biliary) K74.5
    due to xanthomatosis (familial) (metabolic) (primary) E78.2
Cistern, subarachnoid R93.0
Citrullinemia E72.23
Citrullinuria E72.23
Civatte's disease or poikiloderma L57.3
Clam digger's itch B65.3
Clammy skin R23.1
Clap — *see* Gonorrhea
Clarke-Hadfield syndrome (pancreatic infantilism)
    K86.89
Clark's paralysis G80.9
Clastothrix L67.8
Claude Bernard-Horner syndrome G90.2
  traumatic — *see* Injury, nerve, cervical sympathetic
Claude's disease or syndrome G46.3

Claudicatio venosa intermittens I87.8
Claudication (intermittent) I73.9
  cerebral (artery) G45.9
  spinal cord (arteriosclerotic) G95.19
    syphilitic A52.09
  venous (axillary) I87.8
Claustrophobia F40.240
Clavus (infected) L84
Clawfoot (congenital) Q66.89
  acquired — *see* Deformity, limb, clawfoot
Clawhand (acquired) — *see also* Deformity, limb, claw-
    hand
  congenital Q68.1
Clawtoe (congenital) Q66.89
  acquired — *see* Deformity, toe, specified NEC
Clay eating — *see* Pica
Cleansing of artificial opening — *see* Attention to, ar-
    tificial, opening
Cleft (congenital) — *see also* Imperfect, closure
  alveolar process M26.79
  branchial (persistent) Q18.2
    cyst Q18.0
      fistula Q18.0
      sinus Q18.0
  cricoid cartilage, posterior Q31.8
  cyst Q18.0
    fistula Q18.0
    sinus Q18.0
  foot Q72.7 ☑
  hand Q71.6 ☑
  lip (unilateral) Q36.9
    with cleft palate Q37.9
      hard Q37.1
        with soft Q37.5
      soft Q37.3
        with hard Q37.5
    bilateral Q36.0
      with cleft palate Q37.8
        hard Q37.0
          with soft Q37.4
        soft Q37.2
          with hard Q37.4
    median Q36.1
  nose Q30.2
  palate Q35.9
    with cleft lip (unilateral) Q37.9
      bilateral Q37.8
    hard Q35.1
      with
        cleft lip (unilateral) Q37.1
          bilateral Q37.0
        soft Q35.5
          with cleft lip (unilateral) Q37.5
            bilateral Q37.4
    medial Q35.5
    soft Q35.3
      with
        cleft lip (unilateral) Q37.3
          bilateral Q37.2
        hard Q35.5
          with cleft lip (unilateral) Q37.5
            bilateral Q37.4
  penis Q55.69
  scrotum Q55.29
  thyroid cartilage Q31.8
  uvula Q35.7
Cleidocranial dysostosis Q74.0
Cleptomania F63.2
Clicking hip (newborn) R29.4
Climacteric (female) — *see also* Menopause
  arthritis (any site) NEC — *see* Arthritis, specified form
    NEC
  depression (single episode) F32.89
    recurrent episode F33.8
  male (symptoms) (syndrome) NEC N50.89
  melancholia (single episode) F32.89
    recurrent episode F33.8
  paranoid state F22
  polyarthritis NEC — *see* Arthritis, specified form NEC
  symptoms (female) N95.1
Clinical research investigation (clinical trial) (control
    subject) (normal comparison) (participant) Z00.6
Clitoris — *see* condition
Cloaca (persistent) Q43.7
Clonorchiasis, clonorchis infection (liver) B66.1
Clonus R25.8
Closed bite M26.29

Clostridium (C.) **perfringens, as cause of disease
    classified elsewhere** B96.7
Closure
  congenital, nose Q30.0
  cranial sutures, premature Q75.0
  defective or imperfect NEC — *see* Imperfect, closure
  fistula, delayed — *see* Fistula
  foramen ovale, imperfect Q21.1
  hymen N89.6
  interauricular septum, defective Q21.1
  interventricular septum, defective Q21.0
  lacrimal duct — *see also* Stenosis, lacrimal, duct
    congenital Q10.5
  nose (congenital) Q30.0
    acquired M95.0
  of artificial opening — *see* Attention to, artificial,
    opening
  vagina N89.5
  valve — *see* Endocarditis
  vulva N90.5
Clot (blood) — *see also* Embolism
  artery (obstruction) (occlusion) — *see* Embolism
  bladder N32.89
  brain (intradural or extradural) — *see* Occlusion, artery,
    cerebral
  circulation I74.9
  heart — *see also* Infarct, myocardium
    not resulting in infarction I51.3
  vein — *see* Thrombosis
Clouded state R40.1
  epileptic — *see* Epilepsy, specified NEC
  paroxysmal — *see* Epilepsy, specified NEC
Cloudy antrum, antra J32.0
Clouston's (hidrotic) **ectodermal dysplasia** Q82.4
Clubbed nail pachydermoperiostosis M89.40 *[L62]*
Clubbing of finger(s) (nails) R68.3
Clubfinger R68.3
  congenital Q68.1
Clubfoot (congenital) Q66.89
  acquired — *see* Deformity, limb, clubfoot
  equinovarus Q66.0- ☑
  paralytic — *see* Deformity, limb, clubfoot
Clubhand (congenital) (radial) Q71.4- ☑
  acquired — *see* Deformity, limb, clubhand
Clubnail R68.3
  congenital Q84.6
Clump, kidney Q63.1
Clumsiness, clumsy child syndrome F82
Cluttering F80.81
Clutton's joints A50.51 *[M12.80]*
Coagulation, intravascular (diffuse) (disseminated) —
    see also Defibrination syndrome
  complicating abortion — *see* Abortion, by type, com-
      plicated by, intravascular coagulation
  following ectopic or molar pregnancy O08.1
Coagulopathy — *see also* Defect, coagulation
  consumption D65
  intravascular D65
  newborn P60
Coalition
  calcaneo-scaphoid Q66.89
  tarsal Q66.89
Coalminer's
  elbow — *see* Bursitis, elbow, olecranon
  lung or pneumoconiosis J60
Coalworker's lung or pneumoconiosis J60
Coarctation
  aorta (preductal) (postductal) Q25.1
  pulmonary artery Q25.71
Coated tongue K14.3
Coats' disease (exudative retinopathy) — *see* Retinopa-
    thy, exudative
Cocaine-induced
  anxiety disorder F14.980
  bipolar and related disorder F14.94
  depressive disorder F14.94
  obsessive-compulsive and related disorder F14.988
  psychotic disorder F14.959
  sexual dysfunction F14.981
  sleep disorder F14.982
Cocainism — *see* Disorder, cocaine use
Coccidioidomycosis B38.9
  cutaneous B38.3
  disseminated B38.7
  generalized B38.7
  meninges B38.4
  prostate B38.81

Coccidioidomycosis — continued
- pulmonary B38.2
  - acute B38.0
  - chronic B38.1
- skin B38.3
- specified NEC B38.89

Coccidioidosis — see Coccidioidomycosis
Coccidiosis (intestinal) A07.3
Coccydynia, coccygodynia M53.3
Coccyx — see condition
Cochin-China diarrhea K90.1
Cockayne's syndrome Q87.19
Cocked up toe — see Deformity, toe, specified NEC
Cock's peculiar tumor L72.3
Codman's tumor — see Neoplasm, bone, benign
Coenurosis B71.8
Coffee-worker's lung J67.8
Cogan's syndrome H16.32- ☑
- oculomotor apraxia H51.8

Coitus, painful (female) N94.10
- male N53.12
- psychogenic F52.6

Cold J00
- with influenza, flu, or grippe — see Influenza, with, respiratory manifestations NEC
- agglutinin disease or hemoglobinuria (chronic) D59.12
- bronchial — see Bronchitis
- chest — see Bronchitis
- common (head) J00
- effects of T69.9 ☑
  - specified effect NEC T69.8 ☑
- excessive, effects of T69.9 ☑
  - specified effect NEC T69.8 ☑
- exhaustion from T69.8 ☑
- exposure to T69.9 ☑
  - specified effect NEC T69.8 ☑
- head J00
- injury syndrome (newborn) P80.0
- on lung — see Bronchitis
- rose J30.1
- sensitivity, auto-immune D59.12
- symptoms J00
- virus J00

Coldsore B00.1
Colibacillosis A49.8
- as the cause of other disease — see also Escherichia coli B96.20
- generalized A41.50

Colic (bilious) (infantile) (intestinal) (recurrent) (spasmodic) R10.83
- abdomen R10.83
  - psychogenic F45.8
- appendix, appendicular K38.8
- bile duct — see Calculus, bile duct
- biliary — see Calculus, bile duct
- common duct — see Calculus, bile duct
- cystic duct — see Calculus, gallbladder
- Devonshire NEC — see Poisoning, lead
- gallbladder — see Calculus, gallbladder
- gallstone — see Calculus, gallbladder
  - gallbladder or cystic duct — see Calculus, gallbladder
- hepatic (duct) — see Calculus, bile duct
- hysterical F45.8
- kidney N23
- lead NEC — see Poisoning, lead
- mucous K58.9
  - with diarrhea K58.0
  - psychogenic F54
- nephritic N23
- painter's NEC — see Poisoning, lead
- pancreas K86.89
- psychogenic F45.8
- renal N23
- saturnine NEC — see Poisoning, lead
- ureter N23
- urethral N36.8
  - due to calculus N21.1
- uterus NEC N94.89
  - menstrual — see Dysmenorrhea
- worm NOS B83.9

Colicystitis — see Cystitis
Colitis (acute) (catarrhal) (chronic) (noninfective) (hemorrhagic) — see also Enteritis K52.9
- allergic K52.29

Colitis — continued
- allergic — continued
  - with
    - food protein-induced enterocolitis syndrome K52.21
    - proctocolitis K52.82
- amebic (acute) — see also Amebiasis A06.0
  - nondysenteric A06.2
- anthrax A22.2
- bacillary — see Infection, Shigella
- balantidial A07.0
- Clostridium difficile
  - not specified as recurrent A04.72
  - recurrent A04.71
- coccidial A07.3
- collagenous K52.831
- cystica superficialis K52.89
- dietary counseling and surveillance (for) Z71.3
- dietetic — see also Colitis, allergic K52.29
- drug-induced K52.1
- due to radiation K52.0
- eosinophilic K52.82
- food hypersensitivity — see also Colitis, allergic K52.29
- giardial A07.1
- granulomatous — see Enteritis, regional, large intestine
- indeterminate, so stated K52.3
- infectious — see Enteritis, infectious
- ischemic K55.9
  - acute (subacute) — see also Ischemia, intestine, acute K55.039
  - chronic K55.1
  - due to mesenteric artery insufficiency K55.1
  - fulminant (acute) — see also Ischemia, intestine, acute K55.039
- left sided K51.50
  - with
    - abscess K51.514
    - complication K51.519
      - specified NEC K51.518
    - fistula K51.513
    - obstruction K51.512
    - rectal bleeding K51.511
- lymphocytic K52.832
- membranous
  - psychogenic F54
- microscopic K52.839
  - specified NEC K52.838
- mucous — see Syndrome, irritable, bowel
  - psychogenic F54
- noninfective K52.9
  - specified NEC K52.89
- polyposa — see Polyp, colon, inflammatory
- protozoal A07.9
- pseudomembranous
  - not specified as recurrent A04.72
  - recurrent A04.71
- pseudomucinous — see Syndrome, irritable, bowel
- regional — see Enteritis, regional, large intestine
  - infectious A09
- segmental — see Enteritis, regional, large intestine
- septic — see Enteritis, infectious
- spastic K58.9
  - with diarrhea K58.0
  - psychogenic F54
- staphylococcal A04.8
  - foodborne A05.0
- subacute ischemic — see also Ischemia, intestine, acute K55.039
- thromboulcerative — see also Ischemia, intestine, acute K55.039
- toxic NEC K52.1
  - due to Clostridium difficile
    - not specified as recurrent A04.72
    - recurrent A04.71
- transmural — see Enteritis, regional, large intestine
- trichomonal A07.8
- tuberculous (ulcerative) A18.32
- ulcerative (chronic) K51.90
  - with
    - complication K51.919
      - abscess K51.914
      - fistula K51.913
      - obstruction K51.912
      - rectal bleeding K51.911
      - specified complication NEC K51.918
  - enterocolitis — see Enterocolitis, ulcerative
  - ileocolitis — see Ileocolitis, ulcerative
  - mucosal proctocolitis — see Proctocolitis, mucosal

Colitis — continued
- ulcerative — continued
  - proctitis — see Proctitis, ulcerative
  - pseudopolyposis — see Polyp, colon, inflammatory
  - psychogenic F54
  - rectosigmoiditis — see Rectosigmoiditis, ulcerative
  - specified type NEC K51.80
    - with
      - complication K51.819
        - abscess K51.814
        - fistula K51.813
        - obstruction K51.812
        - rectal bleeding K51.811
        - specified complication NEC K51.818

Collagenosis, collagen disease (nonvascular) (vascular) M35.9
- cardiovascular I42.8
- reactive perforating L87.1
- specified NEC M35.8

Collapse R55
- adrenal E27.2
- cardiorespiratory R57.0
- cardiovascular R57.0
  - newborn P29.89
- circulatory (peripheral) R57.9
  - during or after labor and delivery O75.1
  - following ectopic or molar pregnancy O08.3
  - newborn P29.89
- during or
  - after labor and delivery O75.1
  - resulting from a procedure, not elsewhere classified T81.10 ☑
- external ear canal — see Stenosis, external ear canal
- general R55
- heart — see Disease, heart
- heat T67.1 ☑
- hysterical F44.89
- labyrinth, membranous (congenital) Q16.5
- lung (massive) — see also Atelectasis J98.19
  - pressure due to anesthesia (general) (local) or other sedation T88.2 ☑
    - during labor and delivery O74.1
    - in pregnancy O29.02- ☑
    - postpartum, puerperal O89.09
- myocardial — see Disease, heart
- nervous F48.8
- neurocirculatory F45.8
- nose M95.0
- postoperative T81.10 ☑
- pulmonary — see also Atelectasis J98.19
  - newborn — see Atelectasis
- trachea J39.8
- tracheobronchial J98.09
- valvular — see Endocarditis
- vascular (peripheral) R57.9
  - during or after labor and delivery O75.1
  - following ectopic or molar pregnancy O08.3
  - newborn P29.89
- vertebra M48.50- ☑
  - cervical region M48.52- ☑
  - cervicothoracic region M48.53- ☑
  - in (due to)
    - metastasis — see Collapse, vertebra, in, specified disease NEC
    - osteoporosis — see also Osteoporosis M80.88 ☑
      - cervical region M80.88 ☑
      - cervicothoracic region M80.88 ☑
      - lumbar region M80.88 ☑
      - lumbosacral region M80.88 ☑
      - multiple sites M80.88 ☑
      - occipito-atlanto-axial region M80.88 ☑
      - sacrococcygeal region M80.88 ☑
      - thoracic region M80.88 ☑
      - thoracolumbar region M80.88 ☑
    - specified disease NEC M48.50- ☑
      - cervical region M48.52- ☑
      - cervicothoracic region M48.53- ☑
      - lumbar region M48.56- ☑
      - lumbosacral region M48.57- ☑
      - occipito-atlanto-axial region M48.51- ☑
      - sacrococcygeal region M48.58- ☑
      - thoracic region M48.54- ☑
      - thoracolumbar region M48.55- ☑
  - lumbar region M48.56- ☑
  - lumbosacral region M48.57- ☑
  - occipito-atlanto-axial region M48.51- ☑
  - sacrococcygeal region M48.58- ☑

Collapse — continued
  vertebra — continued
    thoracic region M48.54- ☑
    thoracolumbar region M48.55- ☑
Collateral — see also condition
  circulation (venous) I87.8
  dilation, veins I87.8
Colles' fracture S52.53- ☑
Collet (-Sicard) syndrome G52.7
Collier's asthma or lung J60
Collodion baby Q80.2
Colloid nodule (of thyroid) (cystic) E04.1
Coloboma (iris) Q13.0
  eyelid Q10.3
  fundus Q14.8
  lens Q12.2
  optic disc (congenital) Q14.2
    acquired H47.31- ☑
Coloenteritis — see Enteritis
Colon — see condition
Colonization
  MRSA (Methicillin resistant Staphylococcus aureus)
    Z22.322
  MSSA (Methicillin susceptible Staphylococcus aureus)
    Z22.321
  status — see Carrier (suspected) of
Coloptosis K63.4
Color blindness — see Deficiency, color vision
Colostomy
  attention to Z43.3
  fitting or adjustment Z46.89
  malfunctioning K94.03
  status Z93.3
Colpitis (acute) — see Vaginitis
Colpocele N81.5
Colpocystitis — see Vaginitis
Colpospasm N94.2
Column, spinal, vertebral — see condition
Coma R40.20
  with
    motor response (none) R40.231 ☑
      abnormal extensor posturing to pain or noxious
        stimuli (< 2 years of age) R40.232 ☑
      abnormal flexure posturing to pain or noxious
        stimuli (0-5 years of age) R40.233 ☑
      extensor posturing to pain or noxious stimuli (2-
        5 years of age) R40.232 ☑
      flexion/decorticate posturing (< 2 years of age)
        R40.233 ☑
      localizes pain (2-5 years of age) R40.235 ☑
      normal or spontaneous movement (< 2 years of
        age) R40.236 ☑
      obeys commands (2-5 years of age) R40.236 ☑
      score of
        1 R40.231 ☑
        2 R40.232 ☑
        3 R40.233 ☑
        4 R40.234 ☑
        5 R40.235 ☑
        6 R40.236 ☑
      withdraws from pain or noxious stimuli (0-5 years
        of age) R40.234 ☑
      withdraws to touch (< 2 years of age) R40.235 ☑
    opening of eyes (never) R40.211 ☑
      in response to
        pain R40.212 ☑
        sound R40.213 ☑
      score of
        1 R40.211 ☑
        2 R40.212 ☑
        3 R40.213 ☑
        4 R40.214 ☑
      spontaneous R40.214 ☑
    verbal response (none) R40.221 ☑
      confused conversation R40.224 ☑
      cooing or babbling or crying appropriately (<2
        years of age) R40.225 ☑
      inappropriate crying or screaming (< 2 years of
        age) R40.223 ☑
      inappropriate words (2-5 years of age)
        R40.224 ☑
      incomprehensible sounds (2-5 years of age)
        R40.222 ☑
      incomprehensible words R40.222 ☑
      irritable cries (< 2 years of age) R40.224 ☑
      moans/grunts to pain; restless (< 2 years old)
        R40.222 ☑

Coma — continued
  with — continued
    verbal response — continued
      oriented R40.225 ☑
      score of
        1 R40.221 ☑
        2 R40.222 ☑
        3 R40.223 ☑
        4 R40.224 ☑
        5 R40.225 ☑
      screaming (2-5 years of age) R40.223 ☑
      uses appropriate words (2-5 years of age)
        R40.225 ☑
  eclamptic — see Eclampsia
  epileptic — see Epilepsy
  Glasgow, scale score — see Glasgow coma scale
  hepatic — see Failure, hepatic, by type, with coma
  hyperglycemic (diabetic) — see Diabetes, by type, with
    hyperosmolarity, with coma
  hyperosmolar (diabetic) — see Diabetes, by type, with
    hyperosmolarity, with coma
  hypoglycemic (diabetic) — see Diabetes, by type, with
    hypoglycemia, with coma
    nondiabetic E15
  in diabetes — see Diabetes, coma
  insulin-induced — see Coma, hypoglycemic
  ketoacidotic (diabetic) — see Diabetes, by type, with
    ketoacidosis, with coma
  myxedematous E03.5
  newborn P91.5
  persistent vegetative state R40.3
  specified NEC, without documented Glasgow coma
    scale score, or with partial Glasgow coma scale
    score reported R40.244 ☑
Comatose — see Coma
Combat fatigue F43.0
Combined — see condition
Comedo, comedones (giant) L70.0
Comedocarcinoma — see also Neoplasm, breast, malignant
  noninfiltrating
    breast D05.8- ☑
    specified site — see Neoplasm, in situ, by site
    unspecified site D05.8- ☑
Comedomastitis — see Ectasia, mammary duct
Comminuted fracture — code as Fracture, closed
Common
  arterial trunk Q20.0
  atrioventricular canal Q21.2
  atrium Q21.1
  cold (head) J00
  truncus (arteriosus) Q20.0
  variable immunodeficiency — see Immunodeficiency,
    common variable
  ventricle Q20.4
Commotio, commotion (current)
  brain — see Injury, intracranial, concussion
  cerebri — see Injury, intracranial, concussion
  retinae S05.8X- ☑
  spinal cord — see Injury, spinal cord, by region
  spinalis — see Injury, spinal cord, by region
Communication
  between
    base of aorta and pulmonary artery Q21.4
    left ventricle and right atrium Q20.5
    pericardial sac and pleural sac Q34.8
    pulmonary artery and pulmonary vein, congenital
      Q25.72
  congenital between uterus and digestive or urinary
    tract Q51.7
Compartment syndrome (deep) (posterior) (traumatic)
  T79.A0 ☑ (following T79.7)
  abdomen T79.A3 ☑ (following T79.7)
  lower extremity (hip, buttock, thigh, leg, foot, toes)
    T79.A2 ☑ (following T79.7)
  nontraumatic
    abdomen M79.A3 (following M79.7)
    lower extremity (hip, buttock, thigh, leg, foot, toes)
      M79.A2- ☑ (following M79.7)
    specified site NEC M79.A9 (following M79.7)
    upper extremity (shoulder, arm, forearm, wrist,
      hand, fingers) M79.A1- ☑ (following M79.7)
  specified site NEC T79.A9 ☑ (following T79.7)
  upper extremity (shoulder, arm, forearm, wrist, hand,
    fingers) T79.A1- ☑ (following T79.7)
Compensation
  failure — see Disease, heart

Compensation — continued
  neurosis, psychoneurosis — see Disorder, factitious
Complaint — see also Disease
  bowel, functional K59.9
    psychogenic F45.8
  intestine, functional K59.9
    psychogenic F45.8
  kidney — see Disease, renal
  miners' J60
Complete — see condition
Complex
  Addison-Schilder E71.528
  cardiorenal — see Hypertension, cardiorenal
  Costen's M26.69
  disseminated mycobacterium avium- intracellulare
    (DMAC) A31.2
  Eisenmenger's (ventricular septal defect) I27.83
  hypersexual F52.8
  jumped process, spine — see Dislocation, vertebra
  primary, tuberculous A15.7
  Schilder-Addison E71.528
  subluxation (vertebral) M99.19
    abdomen M99.19
    acromioclavicular M99.17
    cervical region M99.11
    cervicothoracic M99.11
    costochondral M99.18
    costovertebral M99.18
    head region M99.10
    hip M99.15
    lower extremity M99.16
    lumbar region M99.13
    lumbosacral M99.13
    occipitocervical M99.10
    pelvic region M99.15
    pubic M99.15
    rib cage M99.18
    sacral region M99.14
    sacrococcygeal M99.14
    sacroiliac M99.14
    specified NEC M99.19
    sternochondral M99.18
    sternoclavicular M99.17
    thoracic region M99.12
    thoracolumbar M99.12
    upper extremity M99.17
  Taussig-Bing (transposition, aorta and overriding pul-
    monary artery) Q20.1
Complication(s) (from) (of)
  accidental puncture or laceration during a procedure
    (of) — see Complications, intraoperative (in-
    traprocedural), puncture or laceration
  amputation stump (surgical) (late) NEC T87.9
    dehiscence T87.81
    infection or inflammation T87.40
      lower limb T87.4- ☑
      upper limb T87.4- ☑
    necrosis T87.50
      lower limb T87.5- ☑
      upper limb T87.5- ☑
    neuroma T87.30
      lower limb T87.3- ☑
      upper limb T87.3- ☑
    specified type NEC T87.89
  anastomosis (and bypass) — see also Complications,
    prosthetic device or implant
    intestinal (internal) NEC K91.89
      involving urinary tract N99.89
    urinary tract (involving intestinal tract) N99.89
    vascular — see Complications, cardiovascular device
      or implant
  anesthesia, anesthetic — see also Anesthesia, compli-
    cation T88.59 ☑
    brain, postpartum, puerperal O89.2
    cardiac
      in
        labor and delivery O74.2
        pregnancy O29.19- ☑
      postpartum, puerperal O89.1
    central nervous system
      in
        labor and delivery O74.3
        pregnancy O29.29- ☑
      postpartum, puerperal O89.2
    difficult or failed intubation T88.4 ☑
      in pregnancy O29.6- ☑
    failed sedation (conscious) (moderate) during pro-
      cedure T88.52 ☑

▽ **Subterms under main terms may continue to next column or page**   ☑ **Additional Character Required — Refer to the Tabular List for Character Selection**   **59**

Collapse — Complication

Complication(s) — *continued*
 anesthesia, anesthetic — *see also* Anesthesia, complication — *continued*
  general, unintended awareness during procedure T88.53 ☑
  hyperthermia, malignant T88.3
  hypothermia T88.51 ☑
  intubation failure T88.4
  malignant hyperthermia T88.3
  pulmonary
   in
    labor and delivery O74.1
    pregnancy NEC O29.09-
   postpartum, puerperal O89.09
  shock T88.2 ☑
  spinal and epidural
   in
    labor and delivery NEC O74.6
     headache O74.5
    pregnancy NEC O29.5X-
   postpartum, puerperal NEC O89.5
    headache O89.4
  unintended awareness under general anesthesia during procedure T88.53 ☑
 anti-reflux device — *see* Complications, esophageal anti-reflux device
 aortic (bifurcation) graft — *see* Complications, graft, vascular
 aortocoronary (bypass) graft — *see* Complications, coronary artery (bypass) graft
 aortofemoral (bypass) graft — *see* Complications, extremity artery (bypass) graft
 arteriovenous
  fistula, surgically created T82.9 ☑
   embolism T82.818 ☑
   fibrosis T82.828 ☑
   hemorrhage T82.838 ☑
   infection or inflammation T82.7 ☑
   mechanical
    breakdown T82.510 ☑
    displacement T82.520 ☑
    leakage T82.530 ☑
    malposition T82.520 ☑
    obstruction T82.590 ☑
    perforation T82.590 ☑
    protrusion T82.590 ☑
   pain T82.848 ☑
   specified type NEC T82.898 ☑
   stenosis T82.858 ☑
   thrombosis T82.868 ☑
  shunt, surgically created T82.9 ☑
   embolism T82.818 ☑
   fibrosis T82.828 ☑
   hemorrhage T82.838 ☑
   infection or inflammation T82.7 ☑
   mechanical
    breakdown T82.511 ☑
    displacement T82.521 ☑
    leakage T82.531 ☑
    malposition T82.521 ☑
    obstruction T82.591 ☑
    perforation T82.591 ☑
    protrusion T82.591 ☑
   pain T82.848 ☑
   specified type NEC T82.898 ☑
   stenosis T82.858 ☑
   thrombosis T82.868 ☑
 arthroplasty — *see* Complications, joint prosthesis
 artificial
  fertilization or insemination N98.9
   attempted introduction (of)
    embryo in embryo transfer N98.3
    ovum following in vitro fertilization N98.2
   hyperstimulation of ovaries N98.1
   infection N98.0
   specified NEC N98.8
  heart T82.9 ☑
   embolism T82.817 ☑
   fibrosis T82.827 ☑
   hemorrhage T82.837 ☑
   infection or inflammation T82.7 ☑
   mechanical
    breakdown T82.512 ☑
    displacement T82.522 ☑
    leakage T82.532 ☑
    malposition T82.522 ☑
    obstruction T82.592 ☑

Complication(s) — *continued*
 artificial — *continued*
  heart — *continued*
   mechanical — *continued*
    perforation T82.592 ☑
    protrusion T82.592 ☑
   pain T82.847 ☑
   specified type NEC T82.897 ☑
   stenosis T82.857 ☑
   thrombosis T82.867 ☑
  opening
   cecostomy — *see* Complications, colostomy
   colostomy — *see* Complications, colostomy
   cystostomy — *see* Complications, cystostomy
   enterostomy — *see* Complications, enterostomy
   gastrostomy — *see* Complications, gastrostomy
   ileostomy — *see* Complications, enterostomy
   jejunostomy — *see* Complications, enterostomy
   nephrostomy — *see* Complications, stoma, urinary tract
   tracheostomy — *see* Complications, tracheostomy
   ureterostomy — *see* Complications, stoma, urinary tract
   urethrostomy — *see* Complications, stoma, urinary tract
 balloon implant or device
  gastrointestinal T85.9 ☑
   embolism T85.818 ☑
   fibrosis T85.828 ☑
   hemorrhage T85.838 ☑
   infection and inflammation T85.79 ☑
   pain T85.848 ☑
   specified type NEC T85.898 ☑
   stenosis T85.858 ☑
   thrombosis T85.868 ☑
  vascular (counterpulsation) T82.9 ☑
   embolism T82.818 ☑
   fibrosis T82.828 ☑
   hemorrhage T82.838 ☑
   infection or inflammation T82.7 ☑
   mechanical
    breakdown T82.513 ☑
    displacement T82.523 ☑
    leakage T82.533 ☑
    malposition T82.523 ☑
    obstruction T82.593 ☑
    perforation T82.593 ☑
    protrusion T82.593 ☑
   pain T82.848 ☑
   specified type NEC T82.898 ☑
   stenosis T82.858 ☑
   thrombosis T82.868 ☑
 bariatric procedure
  gastric band procedure K95.09
   infection K95.01
  specified procedure NEC K95.89
   infection K95.81
 bile duct implant (prosthetic) T85.9 ☑
  embolism T85.818 ☑
  fibrosis T85.828 ☑
  hemorrhage T85.838 ☑
  infection and inflammation T85.79 ☑
  mechanical
   breakdown T85.510 ☑
   displacement T85.520 ☑
   malfunction T85.510 ☑
   malposition T85.520 ☑
   obstruction T85.590 ☑
   perforation T85.590 ☑
   protrusion T85.590 ☑
   specified NEC T85.590 ☑
  pain T85.848 ☑
  specified type NEC T85.898 ☑
  stenosis T85.858 ☑
  thrombosis T85.868 ☑
 bladder device (auxiliary) — *see* Complications, genitourinary, device or implant, urinary system
 bleeding (postoperative) — *see* Complication, postoperative, hemorrhage
  intraoperative — *see* Complication, intraoperative, hemorrhage
 blood vessel graft — *see* Complications, graft, vascular
 bone
  device NEC T84.9 ☑
   embolism T84.81 ☑

Complication(s) — *continued*
 bone — *continued*
  device — *continued*
   fibrosis T84.82 ☑
   hemorrhage T84.83 ☑
   infection or inflammation T84.7 ☑
   mechanical
    breakdown T84.318 ☑
    displacement T84.328 ☑
    malposition T84.328 ☑
    obstruction T84.398 ☑
    perforation T84.398 ☑
    protrusion T84.398 ☑
   pain T84.84 ☑
   specified type NEC T84.89 ☑
   stenosis T84.85 ☑
   thrombosis T84.86 ☑
  graft — *see* Complications, graft, bone
  growth stimulator (electrode) — *see* Complications, electronic stimulator device, bone
  marrow transplant — *see* Complications, transplant, bone, marrow
 brain neurostimulator (electrode) — *see* Complications, electronic stimulator device, brain
 breast implant (prosthetic) T85.9 ☑
  capsular contracture T85.44 ☑
  embolism T85.818 ☑
  fibrosis T85.828 ☑
  hemorrhage T85.838 ☑
  infection and inflammation T85.79 ☑
  mechanical
   breakdown T85.41 ☑
   displacement T85.42 ☑
   leakage T85.43 ☑
   malposition T85.42 ☑
   obstruction T85.49 ☑
   perforation T85.49 ☑
   protrusion T85.49 ☑
   specified NEC T85.49 ☑
  pain T85.848 ☑
  specified type NEC T85.898 ☑
  stenosis T85.858 ☑
  thrombosis T85.868 ☑
 bypass — *see also* Complications, prosthetic device or implant
  aortocoronary — *see* Complications, coronary artery (bypass) graft
  arterial — *see also* Complications, graft, vascular
   extremity — *see* Complications, extremity artery (bypass) graft
 cardiac — *see also* Disease, heart
  device, implant or graft T82.9 ☑
   embolism T82.817 ☑
   fibrosis T82.827 ☑
   hemorrhage T82.837 ☑
   infection or inflammation T82.7 ☑
    valve prosthesis T82.6 ☑
   mechanical
    breakdown T82.519 ☑
     specified device NEC T82.518 ☑
    displacement T82.529 ☑
     specified device NEC T82.528 ☑
    leakage T82.539 ☑
     specified device NEC T82.538 ☑
    malposition T82.529 ☑
     specified device NEC T82.528 ☑
    obstruction T82.599 ☑
     specified device NEC T82.598 ☑
    perforation T82.599 ☑
     specified device NEC T82.598 ☑
    protrusion T82.599 ☑
     specified device NEC T82.598 ☑
   pain T82.847 ☑
   specified type NEC T82.897 ☑
   stenosis T82.857 ☑
   thrombosis T82.867 ☑
 cardiovascular device, graft or implant T82.9 ☑
  aortic graft — *see* Complications, graft, vascular
  arteriovenous
   fistula, artificial — *see* Complication, arteriovenous, fistula, surgically created
   shunt — *see* Complication, arteriovenous, shunt, surgically created
  artificial heart — *see* Complication, artificial, heart
  balloon (counterpulsation) device — *see* Complication, balloon implant, vascular

☑ **Additional Character Required** — Refer to the Tabular List for Character Selection 　☝ Subterms under main terms may continue to next column or page

Complication(s) — *continued*
　cardiovascular device, graft or implant — *continued*
　　carotid artery graft — *see* Complications, graft, vascular
　　coronary bypass graft — *see* Complication, coronary artery (bypass) graft
　　dialysis catheter (vascular) — *see* Complication, catheter, dialysis
　　electronic T82.9 ☑
　　　electrode T82.9 ☑
　　　　embolism T82.817 ☑
　　　　fibrosis T82.827 ☑
　　　　hemorrhage T82.837 ☑
　　　　infection T82.7 ☑
　　　　mechanical
　　　　　breakdown T82.110 ☑
　　　　　displacement T82.120 ☑
　　　　　leakage T82.190 ☑
　　　　　obstruction T82.190 ☑
　　　　　perforation T82.190 ☑
　　　　　protrusion T82.190 ☑
　　　　　specified type NEC T82.190 ☑
　　　　pain T82.847 ☑
　　　　specified NEC T82.897 ☑
　　　　stenosis T82.857 ☑
　　　　thrombosis T82.867 ☑
　　　embolism T82.817 ☑
　　　fibrosis T82.827 ☑
　　　hemorrhage T82.837 ☑
　　　infection T82.7 ☑
　　　mechanical
　　　　breakdown T82.119 ☑
　　　　displacement T82.129 ☑
　　　　leakage T82.199 ☑
　　　　obstruction T82.199 ☑
　　　　perforation T82.199 ☑
　　　　protrusion T82.199 ☑
　　　　specified type NEC T82.199 ☑
　　　pain T82.847 ☑
　　　pulse generator T82.9 ☑
　　　　embolism T82.817 ☑
　　　　fibrosis T82.827 ☑
　　　　hemorrhage T82.837 ☑
　　　　infection T82.7 ☑
　　　　mechanical
　　　　　breakdown T82.111 ☑
　　　　　displacement T82.121 ☑
　　　　　leakage T82.191 ☑
　　　　　obstruction T82.191 ☑
　　　　　perforation T82.191 ☑
　　　　　protrusion T82.191 ☑
　　　　　specified type NEC T82.191 ☑
　　　　pain T82.847 ☑
　　　　specified NEC T82.897 ☑
　　　　stenosis T82.857 ☑
　　　　thrombosis T82.867 ☑
　　　specified condition NEC T82.897 ☑
　　　specified device NEC T82.9 ☑
　　　　embolism T82.817 ☑
　　　　fibrosis T82.827 ☑
　　　　hemorrhage T82.837 ☑
　　　　infection T82.7 ☑
　　　　mechanical
　　　　　breakdown T82.118 ☑
　　　　　displacement T82.128 ☑
　　　　　leakage T82.198 ☑
　　　　　obstruction T82.198 ☑
　　　　　perforation T82.198 ☑
　　　　　protrusion T82.198 ☑
　　　　　specified type NEC T82.198 ☑
　　　　pain T82.847 ☑
　　　　specified NEC T82.897 ☑
　　　　stenosis T82.857 ☑
　　　　thrombosis T82.867 ☑
　　　stenosis T82.857 ☑
　　　thrombosis T82.867 ☑
　　extremity artery graft — *see* Complication, extremity artery (bypass) graft
　　femoral artery graft — *see* Complication, extremity artery (bypass) graft
　　heart
　　　transplant — *see* Complication, transplant, heart
　　　valve — *see* Complication, prosthetic device, heart valve
　　　　graft — *see* Complication, heart, valve, graft

Complication(s) — *continued*
　cardiovascular device, graft or implant — *continued*
　　heart-lung transplant — *see* Complication, transplant, heart, with lung
　　infection or inflammation T82.7 ☑
　　umbrella device — *see* Complication, umbrella device, vascular
　　vascular graft (or anastomosis) — *see* Complication, graft, vascular
　carotid artery (bypass) graft — *see* Complications, graft, vascular
　catheter (device) NEC — *see also* Complications, prosthetic device or implant
　　cranial infusion
　　　infection and inflammation T85.735 ☑
　　　mechanical
　　　　breakdown T85.610 ☑
　　　　displacement T85.620 ☑
　　　　leakage T85.630 ☑
　　　　malfunction T85.690 ☑
　　　　malposition T85.620 ☑
　　　　obstruction T85.690 ☑
　　　　perforation T85.690 ☑
　　　　protrusion T85.690 ☑
　　　　specified NEC T85.690 ☑
　　cystostomy T83.9 ☑
　　　embolism T83.81 ☑
　　　fibrosis T83.82 ☑
　　　hemorrhage T83.83 ☑
　　　infection and inflammation T83.510 ☑
　　　mechanical
　　　　breakdown T83.010 ☑
　　　　displacement T83.020 ☑
　　　　leakage T83.030 ☑
　　　　malposition T83.020 ☑
　　　　obstruction T83.090 ☑
　　　　perforation T83.090 ☑
　　　　protrusion T83.090 ☑
　　　　specified NEC T83.090 ☑
　　　pain T83.84 ☑
　　　specified type NEC T83.89 ☑
　　　stenosis T83.85 ☑
　　　thrombosis T83.86 ☑
　　dialysis (vascular) T82.9 ☑
　　　embolism T82.818 ☑
　　　fibrosis T82.828 ☑
　　　hemorrhage T82.838 ☑
　　　infection and inflammation T82.7 ☑
　　　intraperitoneal — *see* Complications, catheter, intraperitoneal
　　　mechanical
　　　　breakdown T82.41 ☑
　　　　displacement T82.42 ☑
　　　　leakage T82.43 ☑
　　　　malposition T82.42 ☑
　　　　obstruction T82.49 ☑
　　　　perforation T82.49 ☑
　　　　protrusion T82.49 ☑
　　　pain T82.848 ☑
　　　specified type NEC T82.898 ☑
　　　stenosis T82.858 ☑
　　　thrombosis T82.868 ☑
　　epidural infusion T85.9 ☑
　　　embolism T85.810 ☑
　　　fibrosis T85.820 ☑
　　　hemorrhage T85.830 ☑
　　　infection and inflammation T85.735 ☑
　　　mechanical
　　　　breakdown T85.610 ☑
　　　　displacement T85.620 ☑
　　　　leakage T85.630 ☑
　　　　malfunction T85.610 ☑
　　　　malposition T85.620 ☑
　　　　obstruction T85.690 ☑
　　　　perforation T85.690 ☑
　　　　protrusion T85.690 ☑
　　　　specified NEC T85.690 ☑
　　　pain T85.840 ☑
　　　specified type NEC T85.890 ☑
　　　stenosis T85.850 ☑
　　　thrombosis T85.860 ☑
　　intraperitoneal dialysis T85.9 ☑
　　　embolism T85.818 ☑
　　　fibrosis T85.828 ☑
　　　hemorrhage T85.838 ☑
　　　infection and inflammation T85.71

Complication(s) — *continued*
　catheter — *see also* Complications, prosthetic device or implant — *continued*
　　intraperitoneal dialysis — *continued*
　　　mechanical
　　　　breakdown T85.611 ☑
　　　　displacement T85.621 ☑
　　　　leakage T85.631 ☑
　　　　malfunction T85.611 ☑
　　　　malposition T85.621 ☑
　　　　obstruction T85.691 ☑
　　　　perforation T85.691 ☑
　　　　protrusion T85.691 ☑
　　　　specified NEC T85.691 ☑
　　　pain T85.848 ☑
　　　specified type NEC T85.898 ☑
　　　stenosis T85.858 ☑
　　　thrombosis T85.868 ☑
　　intrathecal infusion
　　　infection and inflammation T85.735 ☑
　　　mechanical
　　　　breakdown T85.610 ☑
　　　　displacement T85.620 ☑
　　　　leakage T85.630 ☑
　　　　malfunction T85.690 ☑
　　　　malposition T85.620 ☑
　　　　obstruction T85.690 ☑
　　　　perforation T85.690 ☑
　　　　protrusion T85.690 ☑
　　　　specified NEC T85.690 ☑
　　intravenous infusion T82.9 ☑
　　　embolism T82.818 ☑
　　　fibrosis T82.828 ☑
　　　hemorrhage T82.838 ☑
　　　infection or inflammation T82.7 ☑
　　　mechanical
　　　　breakdown T82.514 ☑
　　　　displacement T82.524 ☑
　　　　leakage T82.534 ☑
　　　　malposition T82.524 ☑
　　　　obstruction T82.594 ☑
　　　　perforation T82.594 ☑
　　　　protrusion T82.594 ☑
　　　pain T82.848 ☑
　　　specified type NEC T82.898 ☑
　　　stenosis T82.858 ☑
　　　thrombosis T82.868 ☑
　　spinal infusion
　　　infection and inflammation T85.735 ☑
　　　mechanical
　　　　breakdown T85.610 ☑
　　　　displacement T85.620 ☑
　　　　leakage T85.630 ☑
　　　　malfunction T85.690 ☑
　　　　malposition T85.620 ☑
　　　　obstruction T85.690 ☑
　　　　perforation T85.690 ☑
　　　　protrusion T85.690 ☑
　　　　specified NEC T85.690 ☑
　　subarachnoid infusion
　　　infection and inflammation T85.735 ☑
　　　mechanical
　　　　breakdown T85.610 ☑
　　　　displacement T85.620 ☑
　　　　leakage T85.630 ☑
　　　　malfunction T85.690 ☑
　　　　malposition T85.620 ☑
　　　　obstruction T85.690 ☑
　　　　perforation T85.690 ☑
　　　　protrusion T85.690 ☑
　　　　specified NEC T85.690 ☑
　　subdural infusion T85.9 ☑
　　　embolism T85.810 ☑
　　　fibrosis T85.820 ☑
　　　hemorrhage T85.830 ☑
　　　infection and inflammation T85.735 ☑
　　　mechanical
　　　　breakdown T85.610 ☑
　　　　displacement T85.620 ☑
　　　　leakage T85.630 ☑
　　　　malfunction T85.610 ☑
　　　　malposition T85.620 ☑
　　　　obstruction T85.690 ☑
　　　　perforation T85.690 ☑
　　　　protrusion T85.690 ☑
　　　　specified NEC T85.690 ☑

Complication(s) — *continued*
- catheter — *see also* Complications, prosthetic device or implant — *continued*
  - subdural infusion — *continued*
    - pain T85.840 ☑
    - specified type NEC T85.890 ☑
    - stenosis T85.850 ☑
    - thrombosis T85.860 ☑
  - urethral T83.9
    - displacement T83.028 ☑
    - embolism T83.81
    - fibrosis T83.82 ☑
    - hemorrhage T83.83 ☑
    - indwelling
      - breakdown T83.011 ☑
      - displacement T83.021 ☑
      - infection and inflammation T83.511 ☑
      - leakage T83.031 ☑
      - specified complication NEC T83.091 ☑
    - infection and inflammation T83.511 ☑
    - leakage T83.038 ☑
    - malposition T83.028 ☑
    - mechanical
      - breakdown T83.011 ☑
    - obstruction (mechanical) T83.091 ☑
    - pain T83.84 ☑
    - perforation T83.091 ☑
    - protrusion T83.091 ☑
    - specified type NEC T83.091 ☑
    - stenosis T83.85 ☑
    - thrombosis T83.86 ☑
  - urinary NEC
    - breakdown T83.018 ☑
    - displacement T83.028 ☑
    - infection and inflammation T83.518 ☑
    - leakage T83.038 ☑
    - specified complication NEC T83.098 ☑
- cecostomy (stoma) — *see* Complications, colostomy
- cesarean delivery wound NEC O90.89
  - disruption O90.0
  - hematoma O90.2
  - infection (following delivery) O86.00
- chemotherapy (antineoplastic) NEC T88.7 ☑
- chin implant (prosthetic) — *see* Complication, prosthetic device or implant, specified NEC
- circulatory system I99.8
  - intraoperative I97.88
  - postprocedural I97.89
    - following cardiac surgery — *see also* Infarct, myocardium, associated with revascularization procedure I97.19- ☑
      - postcardiotomy syndrome I97.0
    - hypertension I97.3
    - lymphedema after mastectomy I97.2
    - postcardiotomy syndrome I97.0
    - specified NEC I97.89
- colostomy (stoma) K94.00
  - hemorrhage K94.01
  - infection K94.02
  - malfunction K94.03
  - mechanical K94.03
  - specified complication NEC K94.09
- contraceptive device, intrauterine — *see* Complications, intrauterine, contraceptive device
- cord (umbilical) — *see* Complications, umbilical cord
- corneal graft — *see* Complications, graft, cornea
- coronary artery (bypass) graft T82.9 ☑
  - atherosclerosis — *see* Arteriosclerosis, coronary (artery),
  - embolism T82.818 ☑
  - fibrosis T82.828 ☑
  - hemorrhage T82.838 ☑
  - infection and inflammation T82.7 ☑
  - mechanical
    - breakdown T82.211 ☑
    - displacement T82.212 ☑
    - leakage T82.213 ☑
    - malposition T82.212 ☑
    - obstruction T82.218 ☑
    - perforation T82.218 ☑
    - protrusion T82.218 ☑
    - specified NEC T82.218 ☑
  - pain T82.848 ☑
  - specified type NEC T82.898 ☑
  - stenosis T82.858 ☑
  - thrombosis T82.868 ☑

Complication(s) — *continued*
- counterpulsation device (balloon), intra- aortic — *see* Complications, balloon implant, vascular
- cystostomy (stoma) N99.518
  - catheter — *see* Complications, catheter, cystostomy
  - hemorrhage N99.510
  - infection N99.511
  - malfunction N99.512
  - specified type NEC N99.518
- delivery — *see also* Complications, obstetric O75.9
  - procedure (instrumental) (manual) (surgical) O75.4
  - specified NEC O75.89
- dialysis (peritoneal) (renal) — *see also* Complications, infusion
  - catheter (vascular) — *see* Complication, catheter, dialysis
    - peritoneal, intraperitoneal — *see* Complications, catheter, intraperitoneal
- dorsal column (spinal) neurostimulator — *see* Complications, electronic stimulator device, spinal cord
- drug NEC T88.7 ☑
- ear procedure — *see also* Disorder, ear
  - intraoperative H95.88
    - hematoma — *see* Complications, intraoperative, hemorrhage (hematoma) (of), ear
    - hemorrhage — *see* Complications, intraoperative, hemorrhage (hematoma) (of), ear
    - laceration — *see* Complications, intraoperative, puncture or laceration…, ear
    - specified NEC H95.88
  - postoperative H95.89
    - external ear canal stenosis H95.81- ☑
    - hematoma — *see* Complications, postprocedural, hematoma (of), ear
    - hemorrhage — *see* Complications, postprocedural, hemorrhage (of), ear
    - postmastoidectomy — *see* Complications, postmastoidectomy
    - seroma — *see* Complications, postprocedural, seroma (of), mastoid process
    - specified NEC H95.89
- ectopic pregnancy O08.9
  - damage to pelvic organs O08.6
  - embolism O08.2
  - genital infection O08.0
  - hemorrhage (delayed) (excessive) O08.1
  - metabolic disorder O08.5
  - renal failure O08.4
  - shock O08.3
  - specified type NEC O08.0
  - venous complication NEC O08.7
- electronic stimulator device
  - bladder (urinary) — *see* Complications, electronic stimulator device, urinary
  - bone T84.9 ☑
    - breakdown T84.310 ☑
    - displacement T84.320 ☑
    - embolism T84.81 ☑
    - fibrosis T84.82 ☑
    - hemorrhage T84.83 ☑
    - infection or inflammation T84.7 ☑
    - malfunction T84.310 ☑
    - malposition T84.320 ☑
    - mechanical NEC T84.390 ☑
    - obstruction T84.390 ☑
    - pain T84.84 ☑
    - perforation T84.390 ☑
    - protrusion T84.390 ☑
    - specified type NEC T84.89 ☑
    - stenosis T84.85 ☑
    - thrombosis T84.86 ☑
  - brain T85.9 ☑
    - embolism T85.810 ☑
    - fibrosis T85.820 ☑
    - hemorrhage T85.830 ☑
    - infection and inflammation T85.731 ☑
    - mechanical
      - breakdown T85.110 ☑
      - displacement T85.120 ☑
      - leakage T85.190 ☑
      - malposition T85.120 ☑
      - obstruction T85.190 ☑
      - perforation T85.190 ☑
      - protrusion T85.190 ☑
      - specified NEC T85.190 ☑
    - pain T85.840 ☑
    - specified type NEC T85.890 ☑

Complication(s) — *continued*
- electronic stimulator device — *continued*
  - brain — *continued*
    - stenosis T85.850 ☑
    - thrombosis T85.860 ☑
  - cardiac (defibrillator) (pacemaker) — *see* Complications, cardiovascular device or implant, electronic
  - generator (brain) (gastric) (peripheral) (sacral) (spinal)
    - breakdown T85.113 ☑
    - displacement T85.123 ☑
    - leakage T85.193 ☑
    - malposition T85.123 ☑
    - obstruction T85.193 ☑
    - perforation T85.193 ☑
    - protrusion T85.193 ☑
    - specified type NEC T85.193 ☑
  - muscle T84.9 ☑
    - breakdown T84.418 ☑
    - displacement T84.428 ☑
    - embolism T84.81 ☑
    - fibrosis T84.82 ☑
    - hemorrhage T84.83 ☑
    - infection or inflammation T84.7 ☑
    - mechanical NEC T84.498 ☑
    - pain T84.84 ☑
    - specified type NEC T84.89 ☑
    - stenosis T84.85 ☑
    - thrombosis T84.86 ☑
  - nervous system T85.9 ☑
    - brain — *see* Complications, electronic stimulator device, brain
    - cranial nerve — *see* Complications, electronic stimulator device, peripheral nerve
    - embolism T85.810 ☑
    - fibrosis T85.820 ☑
    - gastric nerve — *see* Complications, electronic stimulator device, peripheral nerve
    - hemorrhage T85.830 ☑
    - infection and inflammation T85.738 ☑
    - mechanical
      - breakdown T85.118 ☑
      - displacement T85.128 ☑
      - leakage T85.199 ☑
      - malposition T85.128 ☑
      - obstruction T85.199 ☑
      - perforation T85.199 ☑
      - protrusion T85.199 ☑
      - specified NEC T85.199 ☑
    - pain T85.840 ☑
    - peripheral nerve — *see* Complications, electronic stimulator device, peripheral nerve
    - sacral nerve — *see* Complications, electronic stimulator device, peripheral nerve
    - specified type NEC T85.890 ☑
    - spinal cord — *see* Complications, electronic stimulator device, spinal cord
    - stenosis T85.850 ☑
    - thrombosis T85.860 ☑
    - vagal nerve — *see* Complications, electronic stimulator device, peripheral nerve
  - peripheral nerve T85.9 ☑
    - embolism T85.810 ☑
    - fibrosis T85.820 ☑
    - hemorrhage T85.830 ☑
    - infection and inflammation T85.732 ☑
    - mechanical
      - breakdown T85.111 ☑
      - displacement T85.121 ☑
      - leakage T85.191 ☑
      - malposition T85.121 ☑
      - obstruction T85.191 ☑
      - perforation T85.191 ☑
      - protrusion T85.191 ☑
      - specified NEC T85.191 ☑
    - pain T85.840 ☑
    - specified type NEC T85.890 ☑
    - stenosis T85.850 ☑
    - thrombosis T85.860 ☑
  - spinal cord T85.9 ☑
    - embolism T85.810 ☑
    - fibrosis T85.820 ☑
    - hemorrhage T85.830 ☑
    - infection and inflammation T85.733 ☑

☑ Additional Character Required — Refer to the Tabular List for Character Selection
🔻 Subterms under main terms may continue to next column or page

Complication(s) — *continued*
  electronic stimulator device — *continued*
    spinal cord — *continued*
      mechanical
        breakdown T85.112 ☑
        displacement T85.122 ☑
        leakage T85.192 ☑
        malposition T85.122 ☑
        obstruction T85.192 ☑
        perforation T85.192 ☑
        protrusion T85.192 ☑
        specified NEC T85.192 ☑
      pain T85.840 ☑
      specified type NEC T85.890 ☑
      stenosis T85.850 ☑
      thrombosis T85.860 ☑
  urinary T83.9 ☑
    embolism T83.81 ☑
    fibrosis T83.82 ☑
    hemorrhage T83.83 ☑
    infection and inflammation T83.598 ☑
    mechanical
      breakdown T83.110 ☑
      displacement T83.120 ☑
      malposition T83.120 ☑
      perforation T83.190 ☑
      protrusion T83.190 ☑
      specified NEC T83.190 ☑
    pain T83.84 ☑
    specified type NEC T83.89 ☑
    stenosis T83.85 ☑
    thrombosis T83.86 ☑
  electroshock therapy T88.9 ☑
    specified NEC T88.8 ☑
  endocrine E34.9
    postprocedural
      adrenal hypofunction E89.6
      hypoinsulinemia E89.1
      hypoparathyroidism E89.2
      hypopituitarism E89.3
      hypothyroidism E89.0
      ovarian failure E89.40
        asymptomatic E89.40
        symptomatic E89.41
      specified NEC E89.89
      testicular hypofunction E89.5
  endodontic treatment NEC M27.59
  enterostomy (stoma) K94.10
    hemorrhage K94.11
    infection K94.12
    malfunction K94.13
    mechanical K94.13
    specified complication NEC K94.19
  episiotomy, disruption O90.1
  esophageal anti-reflux device T85.9 ☑
    embolism T85.818 ☑
    fibrosis T85.828 ☑
    hemorrhage T85.838 ☑
    infection and inflammation T85.79 ☑
    mechanical
      breakdown T85.511 ☑
      displacement T85.521 ☑
      malfunction T85.511 ☑
      malposition T85.521 ☑
      obstruction T85.591 ☑
      perforation T85.591 ☑
      protrusion T85.591 ☑
      specified NEC T85.591 ☑
    pain T85.848 ☑
    specified type NEC T85.898 ☑
    stenosis T85.858 ☑
    thrombosis T85.868 ☑
  esophagostomy K94.30
    hemorrhage K94.31
    infection K94.32
    malfunction K94.33
    mechanical K94.33
    specified complication NEC K94.39
  extracorporeal circulation T80.90 ☑
  extremity artery (bypass) graft T82.9 ☑
    arteriosclerosis — *see* Arteriosclerosis, extremities, bypass graft
    embolism T82.818 ☑
    fibrosis T82.828 ☑
    hemorrhage T82.838 ☑
    infection and inflammation T82.7 ☑

Complication(s) — *continued*
  extremity artery graft — *continued*
    mechanical
      breakdown T82.318 ☑
        femoral artery T82.312 ☑
      displacement T82.328 ☑
        femoral artery T82.322 ☑
      leakage T82.338 ☑
        femoral artery T82.332 ☑
      malposition T82.328 ☑
        femoral artery T82.322 ☑
      obstruction T82.398 ☑
        femoral artery T82.392 ☑
      perforation T82.398 ☑
        femoral artery T82.392 ☑
      protrusion T82.398 ☑
        femoral artery T82.392 ☑
    pain T82.848 ☑
    specified type NEC T82.898 ☑
    stenosis T82.858 ☑
    thrombosis T82.868 ☑
  eye H57.9
    corneal graft — *see* Complications, graft, cornea
    implant (prosthetic) T85.9 ☑
      embolism T85.818 ☑
      fibrosis T85.828 ☑
      hemorrhage T85.838 ☑
      infection and inflammation T85.79 ☑
      mechanical
        breakdown T85.318 ☑
        displacement T85.328 ☑
        leakage T85.398 ☑
        malposition T85.328 ☑
        obstruction T85.398 ☑
        perforation T85.398 ☑
        protrusion T85.398 ☑
        specified NEC T85.398 ☑
      pain T85.848 ☑
      specified type NEC T85.898 ☑
      stenosis T85.858 ☑
      thrombosis T85.868 ☑
    intraocular lens — *see* Complications, intraocular lens
    orbital prosthesis — *see* Complications, orbital prosthesis
  female genital N94.9
    device, implant or graft NEC — *see* Complications, genitourinary, device or implant, genital tract
  femoral artery (bypass) graft — *see* Complication, extremity artery (bypass) graft
  fixation device, internal (orthopedic) T84.9 ☑
    infection and inflammation T84.60 ☑
      arm T84.61- ☑
        humerus T84.61- ☑
        radius T84.61- ☑
        ulna T84.61- ☑
      leg T84.629 ☑
        femur T84.62- ☑
        fibula T84.62- ☑
        tibia T84.62- ☑
      specified site NEC T84.89 ☑
      spine T84.63 ☑
    mechanical
      breakdown
        limb T84.119 ☑
          carpal T84.210 ☑
          femur T84.11- ☑
          fibula T84.11- ☑
          humerus T84.11- ☑
          metacarpal T84.210 ☑
          metatarsal T84.213 ☑
          phalanx
            foot T84.213 ☑
            hand T84.210 ☑
          radius T84.11- ☑
          tarsal T84.213 ☑
          tibia T84.11- ☑
          ulna T84.11- ☑
        specified bone NEC T84.218 ☑
        spine T84.216 ☑
      displacement
        limb T84.129 ☑
          carpal T84.220 ☑
          femur T84.12- ☑
          fibula T84.12- ☑
          humerus T84.12- ☑

Complication(s) — *continued*
  fixation device, internal — *continued*
    mechanical — *continued*
      displacement — *continued*
        limb — *continued*
          metacarpal T84.220 ☑
          metatarsal T84.223 ☑
          phalanx
            foot T84.223 ☑
            hand T84.220 ☑
          radius T84.12- ☑
          tarsal T84.223 ☑
          tibia T84.12- ☑
          ulna T84.12- ☑
        specified bone NEC T84.228 ☑
        spine T84.226 ☑
      malposition — *see* Complications, fixation device, internal, mechanical, displacement
      obstruction — *see* Complications, fixation device, internal, mechanical, specified type NEC
      perforation — *see* Complications, fixation device, internal, mechanical, specified type NEC
      protrusion — *see* Complications, fixation device, internal, mechanical, specified type NEC
      specified type NEC
        limb T84.199 ☑
          carpal T84.290 ☑
          femur T84.19- ☑
          fibula T84.19- ☑
          humerus T84.19- ☑
          metacarpal T84.290 ☑
          metatarsal T84.293 ☑
          phalanx
            foot T84.293 ☑
            hand T84.290 ☑
          radius T84.19- ☑
          tarsal T84.293 ☑
          tibia T84.19- ☑
          ulna T84.19- ☑
        specified bone NEC T84.298 ☑
        vertebra T84.296 ☑
    specified type NEC T84.89 ☑
      embolism T84.81 ☑
      fibrosis T84.82 ☑
      hemorrhage T84.83 ☑
      pain T84.84 ☑
      specified complication NEC T84.89 ☑
      stenosis T84.85 ☑
      thrombosis T84.86 ☑
  following
    acute myocardial infarction NEC I23.8
      aneurysm (false) (of cardiac wall) (of heart wall) (ruptured) I23.3
      angina I23.7
      atrial
        septal defect I23.1
        thrombosis I23.6
      cardiac wall rupture I23.3
      chordae tendinae rupture I23.4
      defect
        septal
          atrial (heart) I23.1
          ventricular (heart) I23.2
      hemopericardium I23.0
      papillary muscle rupture I23.5
      rupture
        cardiac wall I23.3
          with hemopericardium I23.0
        chordae tendineae I23.4
        papillary muscle I23.5
      specified NEC I23.8
      thrombosis
        atrium I23.6
        auricular appendage I23.6
        ventricle (heart) I23.6
      ventricular
        septal defect I23.2
        thrombosis I23.6
    ectopic or molar pregnancy O08.9
      cardiac arrest O08.81
      sepsis O08.82
      specified type NEC O08.89
      urinary tract infection O08.83
    termination of pregnancy — *see* Abortion
  gastrointestinal K92.9
    bile duct prosthesis — *see* Complications, bile duct implant

Complication(s) — *continued*
  gastrointestinal — *continued*
    esophageal anti-reflux device — *see* Complications,
      esophageal anti-reflux device
    postoperative
      colostomy — *see* Complications, colostomy
      dumping syndrome K91.1
      enterostomy — *see* Complications, enterostomy
      gastrostomy — *see* Complications, gastrostomy
      malabsorption NEC K91.2
      obstruction — *see also* Obstruction, intestine,
        postoperative K91.30
      postcholecystectomy syndrome K91.5
      specified NEC K91.89
      vomiting after GI surgery K91.0
    prosthetic device or implant
      bile duct prosthesis — *see* Complications, bile
        duct implant
      esophageal anti-reflux device — *see* Complica-
        tions, esophageal anti-reflux device
      specified type NEC
        embolism T85.818 ☑
        fibrosis T85.828 ☑
        hemorrhage T85.838 ☑
        mechanical
          breakdown T85.518 ☑
          displacement T85.528 ☑
          malfunction T85.518 ☑
          malposition T85.528 ☑
          obstruction T85.598 ☑
          perforation T85.598 ☑
          protrusion T85.598 ☑
          specified NEC T85.598 ☑
        pain T85.848 ☑
        specified complication NEC T85.898 ☑
        stenosis T85.858 ☑
        thrombosis T85.868 ☑
  gastrostomy (stoma) K94.20
    hemorrhage K94.21
    infection K94.22
    malfunction K94.23
    mechanical K94.23
    specified complication NEC K94.29
  genitourinary
    device or implant T83.9 ☑
      genital tract T83.9 ☑
        infection or inflammation T83.69 ☑
        intrauterine contraceptive device — *see*
          Complications, intrauterine, contracep-
          tive device
        mechanical — *see* Complications, by device,
          mechanical
        mesh — *see* Complications, prosthetic device
          or implant, mesh
        penile prosthesis — *see* Complications, pros-
          thetic device, penile
        specified type NEC T83.89 ☑
          embolism T83.81 ☑
          fibrosis T83.82 ☑
          hemorrhage T83.83 ☑
          pain T83.84 ☑
          specified complication NEC T83.89 ☑
          stenosis T83.85 ☑
          thrombosis T83.86 ☑
        vaginal mesh — *see* Complications, prosthetic
          device or implant, mesh
      urinary system T83.9 ☑
        cystostomy catheter — *see* Complication,
          catheter, cystostomy
        electronic stimulator — *see* Complications,
          electronic stimulator device, urinary
        indwelling urethral catheter — *see* Complica-
          tions, catheter, urethral, indwelling
        infection or inflammation T83.598 ☑
          indwelling urethral catheter T83.511 ☑
        kidney transplant — *see* Complication,
          transplant, kidney
        organ graft — *see* Complication, graft, urinary
          organ
        specified type NEC T83.89 ☑
          embolism T83.81 ☑
          fibrosis T83.82 ☑
          hemorrhage T83.83 ☑
          mechanical T83.198 ☑
            breakdown T83.118 ☑
            displacement T83.128 ☑
            malfunction T83.118 ☑

Complication(s) — *continued*
  genitourinary — *continued*
    device or implant — *continued*
      urinary system — *continued*
        specified type — *continued*
          mechanical — *continued*
            malposition T83.128 ☑
            obstruction T83.198 ☑
            perforation T83.198 ☑
            protrusion T83.198 ☑
            specified NEC T83.198 ☑
        sphincter implant — *see* Complications, im-
          plant, urinary sphincter
        sphincter, implanted T83.191 ☑
        stent (ileal conduit) (nephroureteral)
          T83.193 ☑
          pain T83.84 ☑
          specified complication NEC T83.89 ☑
          stenosis T83.85 ☑
          thrombosis T83.86 ☑
          ureteral indwelling T83.192 ☑
    postprocedural
      pelvic peritoneal adhesions N99.4
      renal failure N99.0
      specified NEC N99.89
      stoma — *see* Complications, stoma, urinary tract
      urethral stricture — *see* Stricture, urethra, post-
        procedural
      vaginal
        adhesions N99.2
        vault prolapse N99.3
  graft (bypass) (patch) — *see also* Complications, pros-
    thetic device or implant
    aorta — *see* Complications, graft, vascular
    arterial — *see* Complication, graft, vascular
    bone T86.839
      failure T86.831
      infection T86.832
      mechanical T84.318 ☑
        breakdown T84.318 ☑
        displacement T84.328 ☑
        protrusion T84.398 ☑
        specified type NEC T84.398 ☑
      rejection T86.830
      specified type NEC T86.838
    carotid artery — *see* Complications, graft, vascular
    cornea T86.849- ☑
      failure T86.841- ☑
      infection T86.842- ☑
      mechanical T85.398 ☑
        breakdown T85.318 ☑
        displacement T85.328 ☑
        protrusion T85.398 ☑
        specified type NEC T85.398 ☑
      rejection T86.840- ☑
      retroprosthetic membrane T85.398 ☑
      specified type NEC T86.848- ☑
    femoral artery (bypass) — *see* Complication, extrem-
      ity artery (bypass) graft
    genital organ or tract — *see* Complications, geni-
      tourinary, device or implant, genital tract
    muscle T84.9 ☑
      breakdown T84.410 ☑
      displacement T84.420 ☑
      embolism T84.81 ☑
      fibrosis T84.82 ☑
      hemorrhage T84.83 ☑
      infection and inflammation T84.7 ☑
      mechanical NEC T84.490 ☑
      pain T84.84 ☑
      specified type NEC T84.89 ☑
      stenosis T84.85 ☑
      thrombosis T84.86 ☑
    nerve — *see* Complication, prosthetic device or im-
      plant, specified NEC
    skin — *see* Complications, prosthetic device or im-
      plant, skin graft
    tendon T84.9 ☑
      breakdown T84.410 ☑
      displacement T84.420 ☑
      embolism T84.81 ☑
      fibrosis T84.82 ☑
      hemorrhage T84.83 ☑
      infection and inflammation T84.7 ☑
      mechanical NEC T84.490 ☑
      pain T84.84 ☑

Complication(s) — *continued*
  graft — *see also* Complications, prosthetic device or
    implant — *continued*
    tendon — *continued*
      specified type NEC T84.89 ☑
      stenosis T84.85 ☑
      thrombosis T84.86 ☑
    urinary organ T83.9 ☑
      embolism T83.81 ☑
      fibrosis T83.82 ☑
      hemorrhage T83.83 ☑
      infection and inflammation T83.598 ☑
        indwelling urethral catheter T83.511 ☑
      mechanical
        breakdown T83.21 ☑
        displacement T83.22 ☑
        erosion T83.24 ☑
        exposure T83.25 ☑
        leakage T83.23 ☑
        malposition T83.22 ☑
        obstruction T83.29 ☑
        perforation T83.29 ☑
        protrusion T83.29 ☑
        specified NEC T83.29 ☑
      pain T83.84 ☑
      specified type NEC T83.89 ☑
      stenosis T83.85 ☑
      thrombosis T83.86 ☑
    vascular T82.9 ☑
      embolism T82.818 ☑
      femoral artery — *see* Complication, extremity
        artery (bypass) graft
      fibrosis T82.828 ☑
      hemorrhage T82.838 ☑
      mechanical
        breakdown T82.319 ☑
          aorta (bifurcation) T82.310 ☑
          carotid artery T82.311 ☑
          specified vessel NEC T82.318 ☑
        displacement T82.329 ☑
          aorta (bifurcation) T82.320 ☑
          carotid artery T82.321 ☑
          specified vessel NEC T82.328 ☑
        leakage T82.339 ☑
          aorta (bifurcation) T82.330 ☑
          carotid artery T82.331 ☑
          specified vessel NEC T82.338 ☑
        malposition T82.329 ☑
          aorta (bifurcation) T82.320 ☑
          carotid artery T82.321 ☑
          specified vessel NEC T82.328 ☑
        obstruction T82.399 ☑
          aorta (bifurcation) T82.390 ☑
          carotid artery T82.391 ☑
          specified vessel NEC T82.398 ☑
        perforation T82.399 ☑
          aorta (bifurcation) T82.390 ☑
          carotid artery T82.391 ☑
          specified vessel NEC T82.398 ☑
        protrusion T82.399 ☑
          aorta (bifurcation) T82.390 ☑
          carotid artery T82.391 ☑
          specified vessel NEC T82.398 ☑
      pain T82.848 ☑
      specified complication NEC T82.898 ☑
      stenosis T82.858 ☑
      thrombosis T82.868 ☑
  heart I51.9
    assist device
      infection and inflammation T82.7 ☑
    following acute myocardial infarction — *see* Com-
      plications, following, acute myocardial infarc-
      tion
    postoperative — *see* Complications, circulatory
      system
    transplant — *see* Complication, transplant, heart
      and lung(s) — *see* Complications, transplant,
      heart, with lung
    valve
      graft (biological) T82.9 ☑
        embolism T82.817 ☑
        fibrosis T82.827 ☑
        hemorrhage T82.837 ☑
        infection and inflammation T82.7 ☑
        mechanical T82.228 ☑
          breakdown T82.221 ☑

Complication(s) — *continued*
  heart — *continued*
    valve — *continued*
      graft — *continued*
        mechanical — *continued*
          displacement T82.222 ☑
          leakage T82.223 ☑
          malposition T82.222 ☑
          obstruction T82.228 ☑
          perforation T82.228 ☑
          protrusion T82.228 ☑
        pain T82.847 ☑
        specified type NEC T82.897 ☑
        stenosis T82.857 ☑
        thrombosis T82.867 ☑
    prosthesis T82.9 ☑
      embolism T82.817 ☑
      fibrosis T82.827 ☑
      hemorrhage T82.837 ☑
      infection or inflammation T82.6 ☑
      mechanical T82.09 ☑
        breakdown T82.01 ☑
        displacement T82.02 ☑
        leakage T82.03 ☑
        malposition T82.02 ☑
        obstruction T82.09 ☑
        perforation T82.09 ☑
        protrusion T82.09 ☑
      pain T82.847 ☑
      specified type NEC T82.897 ☑
        mechanical T82.09
      stenosis T82.857 ☑
      thrombosis T82.867 ☑
  hematoma
    intraoperative — *see* Complication, intraoperative, hemorrhage
    postprocedural — *see* Complication, postprocedural, hematoma
  hemodialysis — *see* Complications, dialysis
  hemorrhage
    intraoperative — *see* Complication, intraoperative, hemorrhage
    postprocedural — *see* Complication, postprocedural, hemorrhage
  ileostomy (stoma) — *see* Complications, enterostomy
  immunization (procedure) — *see* Complications, vaccination
  implant — *see also* Complications, by site and type
    urinary sphincter T83.9 ☑
      embolism T83.81 ☑
      fibrosis T83.82 ☑
      hemorrhage T83.83 ☑
      infection and inflammation T83.591 ☑
      mechanical
        breakdown T83.111 ☑
        displacement T83.121 ☑
        leakage T83.191 ☑
        malposition T83.121 ☑
        obstruction T83.191 ☑
        perforation T83.191 ☑
        protrusion T83.191 ☑
        specified NEC T83.191 ☑
      pain T83.84 ☑
      specified type NEC T83.89 ☑
      stenosis T83.85 ☑
      thrombosis T83.86 ☑
  infusion (procedure) T80.90 ☑
    air embolism T80.0 ☑
    blood — *see* Complications, transfusion
    catheter — *see* Complications, catheter
    infection T80.29 ☑
    pump — *see* Complications, cardiovascular, device or implant
    sepsis T80.29 ☑
    serum reaction — *see also* Reaction, serum T80.69 ☑
      anaphylactic shock — *see also* Shock, anaphylactic T80.59 ☑
    specified type NEC T80.89 ☑
  inhalation therapy NEC T81.81 ☑
  injection (procedure) T80.90 ☑
    drug reaction — *see* Reaction, drug
    infection T80.29 ☑
    sepsis T80.29 ☑
    serum (prophylactic) (therapeutic) — *see* Complications, vaccination

Complication(s) — *continued*
  injection — *continued*
    specified type NEC T80.89 ☑
    vaccine (any) — *see* Complications, vaccination
  inoculation (any) — *see* Complications, vaccination
  insulin pump
    infection and inflammation T85.72 ☑
    mechanical
      breakdown T85.614 ☑
      displacement T85.624 ☑
      leakage T85.633 ☑
      malposition T85.624 ☑
      obstruction T85.694 ☑
      perforation T85.694 ☑
      protrusion T85.694 ☑
      specified NEC T85.694 ☑
  intestinal pouch NEC K91.858
  intraocular lens (prosthetic) T85.9 ☑
    embolism T85.818 ☑
    fibrosis T85.828 ☑
    hemorrhage T85.838 ☑
    infection and inflammation T85.79 ☑
    mechanical
      breakdown T85.21 ☑
      displacement T85.22 ☑
      malposition T85.22 ☑
      obstruction T85.29 ☑
      perforation T85.29 ☑
      protrusion T85.29 ☑
      specified NEC T85.29 ☑
    pain T85.848 ☑
    specified type NEC T85.898 ☑
    stenosis T85.858 ☑
    thrombosis T85.868 ☑
  intraoperative (intraprocedural)
    cardiac arrest — *see also* Infarct, myocardium, associated with revascularization procedure
      during cardiac surgery I97.710
      during other surgery I97.711
    cardiac functional disturbance NEC — *see also* Infarct, myocardium, associated with revascularization procedure
      during cardiac surgery I97.790
      during other surgery I97.791
    hemorrhage (hematoma) (of)
      circulatory system organ or structure
        during cardiac bypass I97.411
        during cardiac catheterization I97.410
        during other circulatory system procedure I97.418
        during other procedure I97.42
      digestive system organ
        during procedure on digestive system K91.61
        during procedure on other organ K91.62
      ear
        during procedure on ear and mastoid process H95.21
        during procedure on other organ H95.22
      endocrine system organ or structure
        during procedure on endocrine system organ or structure E36.01
        during procedure on other organ E36.02
      eye and adnexa
        during ophthalmic procedure H59.11- ☑
        during other procedure H59.12- ☑
      genitourinary organ or structure
        during procedure on genitourinary organ or structure N99.61
        during procedure on other organ N99.62
      mastoid process
        during procedure on ear and mastoid process H95.21
        during procedure on other organ H95.22
      musculoskeletal structure
        during musculoskeletal surgery M96.810
        during non-orthopedic surgery M96.811
        during orthopedic surgery M96.810
      nervous system
        during a nervous system procedure G97.31
        during other procedure G97.32
      respiratory system
        during other procedure J95.62
        during procedure on respiratory system organ or structure J95.61
      skin and subcutaneous tissue
        during a dermatologic procedure L76.01
        during a procedure on other organ L76.02

Complication(s) — *continued*
  intraoperative — *continued*
    hemorrhage — *continued*
      spleen
        during a procedure on other organ D78.02
        during a procedure on the spleen D78.01
    puncture or laceration (accidental) (unintentional) (of)
      brain
        during a nervous system procedure G97.48
        during other procedure G97.49
      circulatory system organ or structure
        during circulatory system procedure I97.51
        during other procedure I97.52
      digestive system
        during procedure on digestive system K91.71
        during procedure on other organ K91.72
      ear
        during procedure on ear and mastoid process H95.31
        during procedure on other organ H95.32
      endocrine system organ or structure
        during procedure on endocrine system organ or structure E36.11
        during procedure on other organ E36.12
      eye and adnexa
        during ophthalmic procedure H59.21- ☑
        during other procedure H59.22- ☑
      genitourinary organ or structure
        during procedure on genitourinary organ or structure N99.71
        during procedure on other organ N99.72
      mastoid process
        during procedure on ear and mastoid process H95.31
        during procedure on other organ H95.32
      musculoskeletal structure
        during musculoskeletal surgery M96.820
        during non-orthopedic surgery M96.821
        during orthopedic surgery M96.820
      nervous system
        during a nervous system procedure G97.48
        during other procedure G97.49
      respiratory system
        during other procedure J95.72
        during procedure on respiratory system organ or structure J95.71
      skin and subcutaneous tissue
        during a dermatologic procedure L76.11
        during a procedure on other organ L76.12
      spleen
        during a procedure on other organ D78.12
        during a procedure on the spleen D78.11
    specified NEC
      circulatory system I97.88
      digestive system K91.81
      ear H95.88
      endocrine system E36.8
      eye and adnexa H59.88
      genitourinary system N99.81
      mastoid process H95.88
      musculoskeletal structure M96.89
      nervous system G97.81
      respiratory system J95.88
      skin and subcutaneous tissue L76.81
      spleen D78.81
  intraperitoneal catheter (dialysis) (infusion) — *see* Complications, catheter, intraperitoneal
  intrathecal infusion pump
    infection and inflammation T85.738 ☑
    mechanical
      breakdown T85.615 ☑
      displacement T85.625 ☑
      leakage T85.635 ☑
      malfunction T85.695 ☑
      malposition T85.625 ☑
      obstruction T85.695 ☑
      perforation T85.695 ☑
      protrusion T85.695 ☑
      specified NEC T85.695 ☑
  intrauterine
    contraceptive device
      embolism T83.81 ☑
      fibrosis T83.82 ☑
      hemorrhage T83.83 ☑
      infection and inflammation T83.69 ☑
      mechanical
        breakdown T83.31 ☑

Complication(s) — *continued*
  intrauterine — *continued*
    contraceptive device — *continued*
      mechanical — *continued*
        displacement T83.32 ✓
        malposition T83.32 ✓
        obstruction T83.39 ✓
        perforation T83.39 ✓
        protrusion T83.39 ✓
        specified NEC T83.39 ✓
      pain T83.84 ✓
      specified type NEC T83.89 ✓
      stenosis T83.85 ✓
      thrombosis T83.86 ✓
    procedure (fetal), to newborn P96.5
  jejunostomy (stoma) — *see* Complications, enterostomy
  joint prosthesis, internal T84.9 ✓
    breakage (fracture) T84.01- ✓
    dislocation T84.02- ✓
    fracture T84.01- ✓
    infection or inflammation T84.50 ✓
      hip T84.5- ✓
      knee T84.5- ✓
      specified joint NEC T84.59 ✓
    instability T84.02- ✓
    malposition — *see* Complications, joint prosthesis, mechanical, displacement
    mechanical
      breakage, broken T84.01- ✓
      dislocation T84.02- ✓
      fracture T84.01- ✓
      instability T84.02- ✓
      leakage — *see* Complications, joint prosthesis, mechanical, specified NEC
      loosening T84.039 ✓
        hip T84.03- ✓
        knee T84.03- ✓
        specified joint NEC T84.038 ✓
      obstruction — *see* Complications, joint prosthesis, mechanical, specified NEC
      perforation — *see* Complications, joint prosthesis, mechanical, specified NEC
      osteolysis T84.059 ✓
        hip T84.05- ✓
        knee T84.05- ✓
        other specified joint T84.058 ✓
      periprosthetic T84.059 ✓
      protrusion — *see* Complications, joint prosthesis, mechanical, specified NEC
      specified complication NEC T84.099 ✓
        hip T84.09- ✓
        knee T84.09- ✓
        other specified joint T84.098 ✓
      subluxation T84.02- ✓
      wear of articular bearing surface T84.069 ✓
        hip T84.06- ✓
        knee T84.06- ✓
        other specified joint T84.068 ✓
    specified joint NEC T84.89 ✓
      embolism T84.81 ✓
      fibrosis T84.82 ✓
      hemorrhage T84.83 ✓
      pain T84.84 ✓
      specified complication NEC T84.89 ✓
      stenosis T84.85 ✓
      thrombosis T84.86 ✓
    subluxation T84.02- ✓
  kidney transplant — *see* Complications, transplant, kidney
  labor O75.9
    specified NEC O75.89
  liver transplant (immune or nonimmune) — *see* Complications, transplant, liver
  lumbar puncture G97.1
    cerebrospinal fluid leak G97.0
    headache or reaction G97.1
  lung transplant — *see* Complications, transplant, lung
  lung and heart — *see* Complications, transplant, lung, with heart
  male genital N50.9
    device, implant or graft — *see* Complications, genitourinary, device or implant, genital tract
    postprocedural or postoperative — *see* Complications, genitourinary, postprocedural
    specified NEC N99.89

Complication(s) — *continued*
  mastoid (process) procedure
    intraoperative H95.88
      hematoma — *see* Complications, intraoperative, hemorrhage (hematoma) (of), mastoid process
      hemorrhage — *see* Complications, intraoperative, hemorrhage (hematoma) (of), mastoid process
      laceration — *see* Complications, intraoperative, puncture or laceration, mastoid process
      specified NEC H95.88
    postmastoidectomy — *see* Complications, postmastoidectomy
    postoperative H95.89
      external ear canal stenosis H95.81 ✓
      hematoma — *see* Complications, postprocedural, hematoma (of), mastoid process
      hemorrhage — *see* Complications, postprocedural, hemorrhage (of), mastoid process
      postmastoidectomy — *see* Complications, postmastoidectomy
      seroma — *see* Complications, postprocedural, seroma (of), mastoid process
      specified NEC H95.89
  mastoidectomy cavity — *see* Complications, postmastoidectomy
  mechanical — *see* Complications, by site and type, mechanical
  medical procedures — *see also* Complication(s), intraoperative T88.9 ✓
  metabolic E88.9
    postoperative E89.89
      specified NEC E89.89
  molar pregnancy NOS O08.9
    damage to pelvic organs O08.6
    embolism O08.2
    genital infection O08.0
    hemorrhage (delayed) (excessive) O08.1
    metabolic disorder O08.5
    renal failure O08.4
    shock O08.3
    specified type NEC O08.0
    venous complication NEC O08.7
  musculoskeletal system — *see also* Complication, intraoperative (intraprocedural), by site
    device, implant or graft NEC — *see* Complications, orthopedic, device or implant
    internal fixation (nail) (plate) (rod) — *see* Complications, fixation device, internal
    joint prosthesis — *see* Complications, joint prosthesis
    post radiation M96.89
      kyphosis M96.2
      scoliosis M96.5
      specified complication NEC M96.89
    postoperative (postprocedural) M96.89
      with osteoporosis — *see* Osteoporosis
      fracture following insertion of device — *see* Fracture, following insertion of orthopedic implant, joint prosthesis or bone plate
      joint instability after prosthesis removal M96.89
      lordosis M96.4
      postlaminectomy syndrome NEC M96.1
        kyphosis M96.3
      pseudarthrosis M96.0
      specified complication NEC M96.89
  nephrostomy (stoma) — *see* Complications, stoma, urinary tract, external NEC
  nervous system G98.8
    central G96.9
    device, implant or graft — *see also* Complication, prosthetic device or implant, specified NEC
      electronic stimulator (electrode(s)) — *see* Complications, electronic stimulator device
      specified NEC
        infection and inflammation T85.738 ✓
        mechanical T85.695 ✓
          breakdown T85.615 ✓
          displacement T85.625 ✓
          leakage T85.635 ✓
          malfunction T85.695 ✓
          malposition T85.625 ✓
          obstruction T85.695 ✓
          perforation T85.695 ✓
          protrusion T85.695 ✓
          specified NEC T85.695 ✓

Complication(s) — *continued*
  nervous system — *continued*
    device, implant or graft — *see also* Complication, prosthetic device or implant, specified — *continued*
      ventricular shunt — *see* Complications, ventricular shunt
    electronic stimulator (electrode(s)) — *see* Complications, electronic stimulator device
    postprocedural G97.82
      intracranial hypotension G97.2
      specified NEC G97.82
      spinal fluid leak G97.0
  newborn, due to intrauterine (fetal) procedure P96.5
  nonabsorbable (permanent) sutures — *see* Complication, sutures, permanent
  obstetric O75.9
    procedure (instrumental) (manual) (surgical) specified NEC O75.4
    specified NEC O75.89
    surgical wound NEC O90.89
      hematoma O90.2
      infection O86.00
  ocular lens implant — *see* Complications, intraocular lens
  ophthalmologic
    postprocedural bleb — *see* Blebitis
  orbital prosthesis T85.9 ✓
    embolism T85.818 ✓
    fibrosis T85.828 ✓
    hemorrhage T85.838 ✓
    infection and inflammation T85.79 ✓
    mechanical
      breakdown T85.31- ✓
      displacement T85.32- ✓
      malposition T85.32- ✓
      obstruction T85.39- ✓
      perforation T85.39- ✓
      protrusion T85.39- ✓
      specified NEC T85.39- ✓
    pain T85.848 ✓
    specified type NEC T85.898 ✓
    stenosis T85.858 ✓
    thrombosis T85.868 ✓
  organ or tissue transplant (partial) (total) — *see* Complications, transplant
  orthopedic — *see also* Disorder, soft tissue
    device or implant T84.9 ✓
      bone
        device or implant — *see* Complication, bone, device NEC
        graft — *see* Complication, graft, bone
      breakdown T84.418 ✓
      displacement T84.428 ✓
      electronic bone stimulator — *see* Complications, electronic stimulator device, bone
      embolism T84.81 ✓
      fibrosis T84.82 ✓
      fixation device — *see* Complication, fixation device, internal
      hemorrhage T84.83 ✓
      infection or inflammation T84.7 ✓
      joint prosthesis — *see* Complication, joint prosthesis, internal
      malfunction T84.418 ✓
      malposition T84.428 ✓
      mechanical NEC T84.498 ✓
      muscle graft — *see* Complications, graft, muscle
      obstruction T84.498 ✓
      pain T84.84 ✓
      perforation T84.498 ✓
      protrusion T84.498 ✓
      specified complication NEC T84.89 ✓
      stenosis T84.85 ✓
      tendon graft — *see* Complications, graft, tendon
      thrombosis T84.86 ✓
    fracture (following insertion of device) — *see* Fracture, following insertion of orthopedic implant, joint prosthesis or bone plate
    postprocedural M96.89
      fracture — *see* Fracture, following insertion of orthopedic implant, joint prosthesis or bone plate
      postlaminectomy syndrome NEC M96.1
        kyphosis M96.3
        lordosis M96.4

✓ **Additional Character Required** — Refer to the Tabular List for Character Selection   ꟽ **Subterms under main terms may continue to next column or page**

Complication(s) — *continued*
  orthopedic — *see also* Disorder, soft tissue — *continued*
    postprocedural — *continued*
      postradiation
        kyphosis M96.2
        scoliosis M96.5
      pseudarthrosis post-fusion M96.0
      specified type NEC M96.89
  pacemaker (cardiac) — *see* Complications, cardiovascular device or implant, electronic
  pancreas transplant — *see* Complications, transplant, pancreas
  penile prosthesis (implant) — *see* Complications, prosthetic device, penile
  perfusion NEC T80.90 ☑
  perineal repair (obstetrical) NEC O90.89
    disruption O90.1
    hematoma O90.2
    infection (following delivery) O86.09
  phototherapy T88.9 ☑
    specified NEC T88.8 ☑
  postmastoidectomy NEC H95.19- ☑
    cyst, mucosal H95.13- ☑
    granulation H95.12- ☑
    inflammation, chronic H95.11- ☑
    recurrent cholesteatoma H95.0- ☑
  postoperative — *see* Complications, postprocedural
    circulatory — *see* Complications, circulatory system
    ear — *see* Complications, ear
    endocrine — *see* Complications, endocrine
    eye — *see* Complications, eye
    lumbar puncture G97.1
      cerebrospinal fluid leak G97.0
    nervous system (central) (peripheral) — *see* Complications, nervous system
    respiratory system — *see* Complications, respiratory system
  postprocedural — *see also* Complications, surgical procedure
    cardiac arrest — *see also* Infarct, myocardium, associated with revascularization procedure
      following cardiac surgery I97.120
      following other surgery I97.121
    cardiac functional disturbance NEC — *see also* Infarct, myocardium, associated with revascularization procedure
      following cardiac surgery I97.190
      following other surgery I97.191
    cardiac insufficiency
      following cardiac surgery I97.110
      following other surgery I97.111
    chorioretinal scars following retinal surgery H59.81- ☑
    following cataract surgery
      cataract (lens) fragments H59.02- ☑
      cystoid macular edema H59.03- ☑
      specified NEC H59.09- ☑
      vitreous (touch) syndrome H59.01- ☑
    heart failure
      following cardiac surgery I97.130
      following other surgery I97.131
    hematoma (of)
      circulatory system organ or structure
        following cardiac bypass I97.631
        following cardiac catheterization I97.630
        following other circulatory system procedure I97.638
        following other procedure I97.621
      digestive system
        following procedure on digestive system K91.870
        following procedure on other organ K91.871
      ear
        following other procedure H95.52
        following procedure on ear and mastoid process H95.51
      endocrine system
        following endocrine system procedure E89.820
        following other procedure E89.821
      eye and adnexa
        following ophthalmic procedure H59.33- ☑
        following other procedure H59.34- ☑
      genitourinary organ or structure
        following procedure on genitourinary organ or structure N99.840
        following procedure on other organ N99.841

Complication(s) — *continued*
  postprocedural — *see also* Complications, surgical procedure — *continued*
    hematoma — *continued*
      mastoid process
        following other procedure H95.52
        following procedure on ear and mastoid process H95.51
      musculoskeletal structure
        following musculoskeletal surgery M96.840
        following a non-orthopedic surgery M96.841
        following orthopedic surgery M96.840
      nervous system
        following nervous system procedure G97.61
        following other procedure G97.62
      respiratory system
        following other procedure J95.861
        following procedure on respiratory system organ or structure J95.860
      skin and subcutaneous tissue
        following dermatologic procedure L76.31
        following procedure on other organ L76.32
      spleen
        following procedure on other organ D78.32
        following procedure on the spleen D78.31
    hemorrhage (of)
      circulatory system organ or structure
        following cardiac bypass I97.611
        following cardiac catheterization I97.610
        following other circulatory system procedure I97.618
        following other procedure I97.620
      digestive system
        following procedure on digestive system K91.840
        following procedure on other organ K91.841
      ear
        following other procedure H95.42
        following procedure on ear and mastoid process H95.41
      endocrine system
        following endocrine system procedure E89.810
        following other procedure E89.811
      eye and adnexa
        following ophthalmic procedure H59.31- ☑
        following other procedure H59.32- ☑
      genitourinary organ or structure
        following procedure on genitourinary organ or structure N99.820
        following procedure on other organ N99.821
      mastoid process
        following other procedure H95.42
        following procedure on ear and mastoid process H95.41
      musculoskeletal structure
        following musculoskeletal surgery M96.830
        following non-orthopedic surgery M96.831
        following orthopedic surgery M96.830
      nervous system
        following nervous system procedure G97.51
        following other procedure G97.52
      respiratory system
        following a respiratory system procedure J95.830
        following other procedure J95.831
      skin and subcutaneous tissue
        following a procedure on other organ L76.22
        following dermatologic procedure L76.21
      spleen
        following procedure on other organ D78.22
        following procedure on the spleen D78.21
    seroma (of)
      circulatory system organ or structure
        following cardiac bypass I97.641
        following cardiac catheterization I97.640
        following other circulatory system procedure I97.648
        following other procedure I97.622
      digestive system
        following procedure on digestive system K91.872
        following procedure on other organ K91.873
      ear
        following other procedure H95.54
        following procedure on ear and mastoid process H95.53

Complication(s) — *continued*
  postprocedural — *see also* Complications, surgical procedure — *continued*
    seroma — *continued*
      endocrine system
        following endocrine system procedure E89.822
        following other procedure E89.823
      eye and adnexa
        following ophthalmic procedure H59.35- ☑
        following other procedure H59.36- ☑
      genitourinary organ or structure
        following procedure on genitourinary organ or structure N99.842
        following procedure on other organ N99.843
      mastoid process
        following other procedure H95.54
        following procedure on ear and mastoid process H95.53
      musculoskeletal structure
        following musculoskeletal surgery M96.842
        following non-orthopedic surgery M96.843
        following orthopedic surgery M96.842
      nervous system
        following nervous system procedure G97.63
        following other procedure G97.64
      respiratory system
        following other procedure J95.863
        following procedure on respiratory system organ or structure J95.862
      skin and subcutaneous tissue
        following dermatologic procedure L76.33
        following procedure on other organ L76.34
      spleen
        following procedure on other organ D78.34
        following procedure on the spleen D78.33
    specified NEC
      circulatory system I97.89
      digestive K91.89
      ear H95.89
      endocrine E89.89
      eye and adnexa H59.89
      genitourinary N99.89
      mastoid process H95.89
      metabolic E89.89
      musculoskeletal structure M96.89
      nervous system G97.82
      respiratory system J95.89
      skin and subcutaneous tissue L76.82
      spleen D78.89
  pregnancy NEC — *see* Pregnancy, complicated by
  prosthetic device or implant T85.9 ☑
    bile duct — *see* Complications, bile duct implant
    breast — *see* Complications, breast implant
    bulking agent
      ureteral
        erosion T83.714 ☑
        exposure T83.724 ☑
      urethral
        erosion T83.713 ☑
        exposure T83.723 ☑
    cardiac and vascular NEC — *see* Complications, cardiovascular device or implant
    corneal transplant — *see* Complications, graft, cornea
    electronic nervous system stimulator — *see* Complications, electronic stimulator device
    epidural infusion catheter — *see* Complications, catheter, epidural
    esophageal anti-reflux device — *see* Complications, esophageal anti-reflux device
    genital organ or tract — *see* Complications, genitourinary, device or implant, genital tract
    specified NEC T83.79- ☑
    heart valve — *see* Complications, heart, valve, prosthesis
    infection or inflammation T85.79 ☑
      intestine transplant T86.892
      liver transplant T86.43
      lung transplant T86.812
      pancreas transplant T86.892
      skin graft T86.822
    intraocular lens — *see* Complications, intraocular lens
    intraperitoneal (dialysis) catheter — *see* Complications, catheter, intraperitoneal
    joint — *see* Complications, joint prosthesis, internal
    mechanical NEC T85.698 ☑

Complication(s) — *continued*
 prosthetic device or implant — *continued*
  mechanical — *continued*
   dialysis catheter (vascular) — *see also* Complica-
    tion, catheter, dialysis, mechanical
    peritoneal — *see* Complication, catheter, in-
     traperitoneal, mechanical
   gastrointestinal device T85.598 ☑
   ocular device T85.398 ☑
   subdural (infusion) catheter T85.690 ☑
   suture, permanent T85.692 ☑
    that for bone repair — *see* Complications,
     fixation device, internal (orthopedic),
     mechanical
   ventricular shunt
    breakdown T85.01 ☑
    displacement T85.02 ☑
    leakage T85.03 ☑
    malposition T85.02 ☑
    obstruction T85.09 ☑
    perforation T85.09 ☑
    protrusion T85.09 ☑
    specified NEC T85.09 ☑
  mesh
   erosion (to surrounding organ or tissue)
    T83.718 ☑
    urethral (into pelvic floor muscles) T83.712 ☑
    vaginal (into pelvic floor muscles) T83.711 ☑
   exposure (into surrounding organ or tissue)
    T83.728 ☑
    urethral (through urethral wall) T83.722 ☑
    vaginal (into vagina) (through vaginal wall)
     T83.721 ☑
  orbital — *see* Complications, orbital prosthesis
  penile T83.9 ☑
   embolism T83.81 ☑
   fibrosis T83.82 ☑
   hemorrhage T83.83 ☑
   infection and inflammation T83.61 ☑
   mechanical
    breakdown T83.410 ☑
    displacement T83.420 ☑
    leakage T83.490 ☑
    malposition T83.420 ☑
    obstruction T83.490 ☑
    perforation T83.490 ☑
    protrusion T83.490 ☑
    specified NEC T83.490 ☑
   pain T83.84 ☑
   specified type NEC T83.89 ☑
   stenosis T83.85 ☑
   thrombosis T83.86 ☑
  prosthetic materials NEC
   erosion (to surrounding organ or tissue)
    T83.718 ☑
   exposure (into surrounding organ or tissue)
    T83.728 ☑
  skin graft T86.829
   artificial skin or decellularized allodermis
    embolism T85.818 ☑
    fibrosis T85.828 ☑
    hemorrhage T85.838 ☑
    infection and inflammation T85.79 ☑
    mechanical
     breakdown T85.613 ☑
     displacement T85.623 ☑
     malfunction T85.613 ☑
     malposition T85.623 ☑
     obstruction T85.693 ☑
     perforation T85.693 ☑
     protrusion T85.693 ☑
     specified NEC T85.693 ☑
    pain T85.848 ☑
    specified type NEC T85.898 ☑
    stenosis T85.858 ☑
    thrombosis T85.868 ☑
   failure T86.821
   infection T86.822
   rejection T86.820
   specified NEC T86.828
  sling
   urethral (female) (male)
    erosion T83.712 ☑
    exposure T83.722 ☑
  specified NEC T85.9 ☑
   embolism T85.818 ☑

Complication(s) — *continued*
 prosthetic device or implant — *continued*
  specified — *continued*
   fibrosis T85.828 ☑
   hemorrhage T85.838 ☑
   infection and inflammation T85.79 ☑
   mechanical
    breakdown T85.618 ☑
    displacement T85.628 ☑
    leakage T85.638 ☑
    malfunction T85.618 ☑
    malposition T85.628 ☑
    obstruction T85.698 ☑
    perforation T85.698 ☑
    protrusion T85.698 ☑
    specified NEC T85.698 ☑
   pain T85.848 ☑
   specified type NEC T85.898 ☑
   stenosis T85.858 ☑
   thrombosis T85.868 ☑
  subdural infusion catheter — *see* Complications,
   catheter, subdural
  sutures — *see* Complications, sutures
  urinary organ or tract NEC — *see* Complications,
   genitourinary, device or implant, urinary system
  vascular — *see* Complications, cardiovascular device
   or implant
  ventricular shunt — *see* Complications, ventricular
   shunt (device)
 puerperium — *see* Puerperal
 puncture, spinal G97.1
  cerebrospinal fluid leak G97.0
  headache or reaction G97.1
 pyelogram N99.89
 radiation
  kyphosis M96.2
  scoliosis M96.5
 reattached
  extremity (infection) (rejection)
   lower T87.1X- ☑
   upper T87.0X- ☑
  specified body part NEC T87.2
 reconstructed breast
  asymmetry between native and reconstructed
   breast N65.1
  deformity N65.0
  disproportion between native and reconstructed
   breast N65.1
  excess tissue N65.0
  misshappen N65.0
 reimplant NEC — *see also* Complications, prosthetic
  device or implant
  limb (infection) (rejection) — *see* Complications,
   reattached, extremity
  organ (partial) (total) — *see* Complications, transplant
  prosthetic device NEC — *see* Complications, prosthetic device
 renal N28.9
  allograft — *see* Complications, transplant, kidney
  dialysis — *see* Complications, dialysis
 respirator
  mechanical J95.850
   specified NEC J95.859
 respiratory system J98.9
  device, implant or graft — *see* Complication, prosthetic device or implant, specified NEC
  lung transplant — *see* Complications, prosthetic
   device or implant, lung transplant
  postoperative J95.89
   air leak J95.812
   Mendelson's syndrome (chemical pneumonitis)
    J95.4
   pneumothorax J95.811
   pulmonary insufficiency (acute) (after nontho-
    racic surgery) J95.2
    chronic J95.3
    following thoracic surgery J95.1
   respiratory failure (acute) J95.821
    acute and chronic J95.822
   specified NEC J95.89
   subglottic stenosis J95.5
   tracheostomy complication — *see* Complica-
    tions, tracheostomy
 therapy T81.89 ☑
 sedation during labor and delivery O74.9

Complication(s) — *continued*
 sedation during labor and delivery — *continued*
  cardiac O74.2
  central nervous system O74.3
  pulmonary NEC O74.1
 shunt — *see also* Complications, prosthetic device or
  implant
  arteriovenous — *see* Complications, arteriovenous,
   shunt
  ventricular (communicating) — *see* Complications,
   ventricular shunt
 skin
  graft T86.829
   failure T86.821
   infection T86.822
   rejection T86.820
   specified type NEC T86.828
 spinal
  anesthesia — *see* Complications, anesthesia, spinal
  catheter (epidural) (subdural) — *see* Complications,
   catheter
  puncture or tap G97.1
   cerebrospinal fluid leak G97.0
   headache or reaction G97.1
 stent
  bile duct — *see* Complications, bile duct prosthesis
  ureteral indwelling
   breakdown T83.112 ☑
   displacement T83.122 ☑
   leakage T83.192 ☑
   malposition T83.122 ☑
   obstruction T83.192 ☑
   perforation T83.192 ☑
   protrusion T83.192 ☑
   specified NEC T83.192 ☑
  urinary NEC (ileal conduit) (nephroureteral)
   T83.193 ☑
   embolism T83.81 ☑
   fibrosis T83.82 ☑
   hemorrhage T83.83 ☑
   infection and inflammation T83.593 ☑
   mechanical
    breakdown T83.113 ☑
    displacement T83.123 ☑
    leakage T83.193 ☑
    malposition T83.123 ☑
    obstruction T83.193 ☑
    perforation T83.193 ☑
    protrusion T83.193 ☑
    specified NEC T83.193 ☑
   pain T83.84 ☑
   specified type NEC T83.89 ☑
   stenosis T83.85 ☑
   thrombosis T83.86 ☑
  vascular
   end stent stenosis — *see* Restenosis, stent
   in stent stenosis — *see* Restenosis, stent
 stoma
  digestive tract
   colostomy — *see* Complications, colostomy
   enterostomy — *see* Complications, enterostomy
   esophagostomy — *see* Complications,
    esophagostomy
   gastrostomy — *see* Complications, gastrostomy
  urinary tract N99.528
   continent N99.538
    hemorrhage N99.530
    herniation N99.533
    infection N99.531
    malfunction N99.532
    specified type NEC N99.538
    stenosis N99.534
   cystostomy — *see* Complications, cystostomy
   external NOS N99.528
   hemorrhage N99.520
   herniation N99.523
   incontinent N99.528
    hemorrhage N99.520
    herniation N99.523
    infection N99.521
    malfunction N99.522
    specified type NEC N99.528
    stenosis N99.524
   infection N99.521
   malfunction N99.522
   specified type NEC N99.528
   stenosis N99.524

☑ **Additional Character Required — Refer to the Tabular List for Character Selection**   ᵂ Subterms under main terms may continue to next column or page

Complication(s) — *continued*
    stomach banding — *see* Complication(s), bariatric
        procedure
    stomach stapling — *see* Complication(s), bariatric
        procedure
    surgical material, nonabsorbable — *see* Complication,
        suture, permanent
    surgical procedure (on) T81.9 ☑
        amputation stump (late) — *see* Complications,
            amputation stump
        cardiac — *see* Complications, circulatory system
        cholesteatoma, recurrent — *see* Complications,
            postmastoidectomy, recurrent cholesteatoma
        circulatory (early) — *see* Complications, circulatory
            system
        digestive system — *see* Complications, gastrointesti-
            nal
        dumping syndrome (postgastrectomy) K91.1
        ear — *see* Complications, ear
        elephantiasis or lymphedema I97.89
            postmastectomy I97.2
        emphysema (surgical) T81.82 ☑
        endocrine — *see* Complications, endocrine
        eye — *see* Complications, eye
        fistula (persistent postoperative) T81.83 ☑
        foreign body inadvertently left in wound (sponge)
            (suture) (swab) — *see* Foreign body, acciden-
            tally left during a procedure
        gastrointestinal — *see* Complications, gastrointesti-
            nal
        genitourinary NEC N99.89
        hematoma
            intraoperative — *see* Complication, intraopera-
                tive, hemorrhage
            postprocedural — *see* Complication, postproce-
                dural, hematoma
        hemorrhage
            intraoperative — *see* Complication, intraopera-
                tive, hemorrhage
            postprocedural — *see* Complication, postproce-
                dural, hemorrhage
        hepatic failure K91.82
        hyperglycemia (postpancreatectomy) E89.1
        hypoinsulinemia (postpancreatectomy) E89.1
        hypoparathyroidism (postparathyroidectomy) E89.2
        hypopituitarism (posthypophysectomy) E89.3
        hypothyroidism (post-thyroidectomy) E89.0
        intestinal obstruction — *see also* Obstruction, intes-
            tine, postoperative K91.30
        intracranial hypotension following ventricular
            shunting (ventriculostomy) G97.2
        lymphedema I97.89
            postmastectomy I97.2
        malabsorption (postsurgical) NEC K91.2
            osteoporosis — *see* Osteoporosis, postsurgical
                malabsorption
        mastoidectomy cavity NEC — *see* Complications,
            postmastoidectomy
        metabolic E89.89
            specified NEC E89.89
        musculoskeletal — *see* Complications, musculoskele-
            tal system
        nervous system (central) (peripheral) — *see* Compli-
            cations, nervous system
        ovarian failure E89.40
            asymptomatic E89.40
            symptomatic E89.41
        peripheral vascular — *see* Complications, surgical
            procedure, vascular
        postcardiotomy syndrome I97.0
        postcholecystectomy syndrome K91.5
        postcommissurotomy syndrome I97.0
        postgastrectomy dumping syndrome K91.1
        postlaminectomy syndrome NEC M96.1
            kyphosis M96.3
        postmastectomy lymphedema syndrome I97.2
        postmastoidectomy cholesteatoma — *see* Compli-
            cations, postmastoidectomy, recurrent
            cholesteatoma
        postvagotomy syndrome K91.1
        postvalvulotomy syndrome I97.0
        pulmonary insufficiency (acute) J95.2
            chronic J95.3
            following thoracic surgery J95.1
        reattached body part — *see* Complications, reat-
            tached
        respiratory — *see* Complications, respiratory system
        shock (hypovolemic) T81.19 ☑

Complication(s) — *continued*
    surgical procedure — *continued*
        spleen (postoperative) D78.89
            intraoperative D78.81
        stitch abscess T81.41 ☑
        subglottic stenosis (postsurgical) J95.5
        testicular hypofunction E89.5
        transplant — *see* Complications, organ or tissue
            transplant
        urinary NEC N99.89
        vaginal vault prolapse (posthysterectomy) N99.3
        vascular (peripheral)
            artery T81.719 ☑
                mesenteric T81.710 ☑
                renal T81.711 ☑
                specified NEC T81.718 ☑
            vein T81.72 ☑
        wound infection T81.49 ☑
    suture, permanent (wire) NEC T85.9 ☑
        with repair of bone — *see* Complications, fixation
            device, internal
        embolism T85.818 ☑
        fibrosis T85.828 ☑
        hemorrhage T85.838 ☑
        infection and inflammation T85.79 ☑
        mechanical
            breakdown T85.612 ☑
            displacement T85.622 ☑
            malfunction T85.612 ☑
            malposition T85.622 ☑
            obstruction T85.692 ☑
            perforation T85.692 ☑
            protrusion T85.692 ☑
            specified NEC T85.692 ☑
        pain T85.848 ☑
        specified type NEC T85.898 ☑
        stenosis T85.858 ☑
        thrombosis T85.868 ☑
    tracheostomy J95.00
        granuloma J95.09
        hemorrhage J95.01
        infection J95.02
        malfunction J95.03
        mechanical J95.03
        obstruction J95.03
        specified type NEC J95.09
        tracheo-esophageal fistula J95.04
    transfusion (blood) (lymphocytes) (plasma) T80.92 ☑
        air emblism T80.0 ☑
        circulatory overload E87.71
        febrile nonhemolytic transfusion reaction R50.84
        hemochromatosis E83.111
        hemolysis T80.89 ☑
        hemolytic reaction (antigen unspecified) T80.919 ☑
        incompatibility reaction (antigen unspecified)
            T80.919 ☑
            ABO T80.30 ☑
                delayed serologic (DSTR) T80.39 ☑
                hemolytic transfusion reaction (HTR) (unspec-
                    ified time after transfusion) T80.319 ☑
                    acute (AHTR) (less than 24 hours after
                        transfusion) T80.310 ☑
                    delayed (DHTR) (24 hours or more after
                        transfusion) T80.311 ☑
                specified NEC T80.39 ☑
            acute (antigen unspecified) T80.910 ☑
            delayed (antigen unspecified) T80.911 ☑
            delayed serologic (DSTR) T80.89 ☑
            non-ABO (minor antigens (Duffy) (K) (Kell) (Kidd)
                (Lewis) (M) (N) (P) (S)) T80.A0 ☑ (*following*
                T80.4)
                delayed serologic (DSTR) T80.A9 ☑ (*following*
                    T80.4)
                hemolytic transfusion reaction (HTR) (unspec-
                    ified time after transfusion) T80.A19 ☑
                    (*following* T80.4)
                    acute (AHTR) (less than 24 hours after
                        transfusion) T80.A10 ☑ (*following*
                        T80.4)
                    delayed (DHTR) (24 hours or more after
                        transfusion) T80.A11 ☑ (*following*
                        T80.4)
                specified NEC T80.A9 ☑ (*following* T80.4)
            Rh (antigens (C) (c) (D) (E) (e)) (factor) T80.40 ☑
                delayed serologic (DSTR) T80.49 ☑
                hemolytic transfusion reaction (HTR) (unspec-
                    ified time after transfusion) T80.419 ☑

Complication(s) — *continued*
    transfusion — *continued*
        incompatibility reaction — *continued*
            Rh — *continued*
                hemolytic transfusion reaction — *contin-
                    ued*
                    acute (AHTR) (less than 24 hours after
                        transfusion) T80.410 ☑
                    delayed (DHTR) (24 hours or more after
                        transfusion) T80.411 ☑
                specified NEC T80.49 ☑
        infection T80.29 ☑
            acute T80.22- ☑
        reaction NEC T80.89 ☑
        sepsis T80.29 ☑
        shock T80.89 ☑
    transplant T86.90
        bone T86.839
            failure T86.831
            infection T86.832
            rejection T86.830
            specified type NEC T86.838
        bone marrow T86.00
            failure T86.02
            infection T86.03
            rejection T86.01
            specified type NEC T86.09
        cornea T86.849- ☑
            failure T86.841- ☑
            infection T86.842- ☑
            rejection T86.840- ☑
            specified type NEC T86.848- ☑
        failure T86.92
        heart T86.20
            with lung T86.30
            cardiac allograft vasculopathy T86.290
                failure T86.32
                infection T86.33
                rejection T86.31
                specified type NEC T86.39
            failure T86.22
            infection T86.23
            rejection T86.21
            specified type NEC T86.298
        infection T86.93
        intestine T86.859
            failure T86.851
            infection T86.852
            rejection T86.850
            specified type NEC T86.858
        kidney T86.10
            failure T86.12
            infection T86.13
            rejection T86.11
            specified type NEC T86.19
        liver T86.40
            failure T86.42
            infection T86.43
            rejection T86.41
            specified type NEC T86.49
        lung T86.819
            with heart T86.30
                failure T86.32
                infection T86.33
                rejection T86.31
                specified type NEC T86.39
            failure T86.811
            infection T86.812
            rejection T86.810
            specified type NEC T86.818
        malignant neoplasm C80.2
        pancreas T86.899
            failure T86.891
            infection T86.892
            rejection T86.890
            specified type NEC T86.898
        peripheral blood stem cells T86.5
        post-transplant lymphoproliferative disorder (PTLD)
            D47.Z1 (*following* D47.4)
        rejection T86.91
        skin T86.829
            failure T86.821
            infection T86.822
            rejection T86.820
            specified type NEC T86.828
        specified
            tissue T86.899
                failure T86.891

Complication(s) — *continued*
transplant — *continued*
  specified — *continued*
    tissue — *continued*
      infection T86.892
      rejection T86.890
      specified type NEC T86.898
      type NEC T86.99
  stem cell (from peripheral blood) (from umbilical cord) T86.5
  umbilical cord stem cells T86.5
trauma (early) T79.9 ☑
  specified NEC T79.8 ☑
ultrasound therapy NEC T88.9 ☑
umbilical cord NEC
  complicating delivery O69.9 ☑
    specified NEC O69.89 ☑
umbrella device, vascular T82.9 ☑
  embolism T82.818 ☑
  fibrosis T82.828 ☑
  hemorrhage T82.838 ☑
  infection or inflammation T82.7 ☑
  mechanical
    breakdown T82.515 ☑
    displacement T82.525 ☑
    leakage T82.535 ☑
    malposition T82.525 ☑
    obstruction T82.595 ☑
    perforation T82.595 ☑
    protrusion T82.595 ☑
  pain T82.848 ☑
  specified type NEC T82.898 ☑
  stenosis T82.858 ☑
  thrombosis T82.868 ☑
urethral catheter — *see* Complications, catheter, urethral, indwelling
vaccination T88.1 ☑
  anaphylaxis NEC T80.52 ☑
  arthropathy — *see* Arthropathy, postimmunization
  cellulitis T88.0 ☑
  encephalitis or encephalomyelitis G04.02
  infection (general) (local) NEC T88.0 ☑
  meningitis G03.8
  myelitis G04.02
  protein sickness T80.62 ☑
  rash T88.1 ☑
  reaction (allergic) T88.1 ☑
    serum T80.62 ☑
  sepsis T88.0 ☑
  serum intoxication, sickness, rash, or other serum reaction NEC T80.62 ☑
    anaphylactic shock T80.52 ☑
  shock (allergic) (anaphylactic) T80.52 ☑
  vaccinia (generalized) (localized) T88.1 ☑
vas deferens device or implant — *see* Complications, genitourinary, device or implant, genital tract
vascular I99.9
  device or implant T82.9 ☑
    embolism T82.818 ☑
    fibrosis T82.828 ☑
    hemorrhage T82.838 ☑
    infection or inflammation T82.7 ☑
    mechanical
      breakdown T82.519 ☑
        specified device NEC T82.518 ☑
      displacement T82.529 ☑
        specified device NEC T82.528 ☑
      leakage T82.539 ☑
        specified device NEC T82.538 ☑
      malposition T82.529 ☑
        specified device NEC T82.528 ☑
      obstruction T82.599 ☑
        specified device NEC T82.598 ☑
      perforation T82.599 ☑
        specified device NEC T82.598 ☑
      protrusion T82.599 ☑
        specified device NEC T82.598 ☑
    pain T82.848 ☑
    specified type NEC T82.898 ☑
    stenosis T82.858 ☑
    thrombosis T82.868 ☑
  dialysis catheter — *see* Complication, catheter, dialysis
  following infusion, therapeutic injection or transfusion T80.1 ☑
  graft T82.9 ☑

Complication(s) — *continued*
vascular — *continued*
  graft — *continued*
    embolism T82.818 ☑
    fibrosis T82.828 ☑
    hemorrhage T82.838 ☑
    mechanical
      breakdown T82.319 ☑
        aorta (bifurcation) T82.310 ☑
        carotid artery T82.311 ☑
        specified vessel NEC T82.318 ☑
      displacement T82.329 ☑
        aorta (bifurcation) T82.320 ☑
        carotid artery T82.321 ☑
        specified vessel NEC T82.328 ☑
      leakage T82.339 ☑
        aorta (bifurcation) T82.330 ☑
        carotid artery T82.331 ☑
        specified vessel NEC T82.338 ☑
      malposition T82.329 ☑
        aorta (bifurcation) T82.320 ☑
        carotid artery T82.321 ☑
        specified vessel NEC T82.328 ☑
      obstruction T82.399 ☑
        aorta (bifurcation) T82.390 ☑
        carotid artery T82.391 ☑
        specified vessel NEC T82.398 ☑
      perforation T82.399 ☑
        aorta (bifurcation) T82.390 ☑
        carotid artery T82.391 ☑
        specified vessel NEC T82.398 ☑
      protrusion T82.399 ☑
        aorta (bifurcation) T82.390 ☑
        carotid artery T82.391 ☑
        specified vessel NEC T82.398 ☑
    pain T82.848 ☑
    specified complication NEC T82.898 ☑
    stenosis T82.858 ☑
    thrombosis T82.868 ☑
  postoperative — *see* Complications, postoperative, circulatory
vena cava device (filter) (sieve) (umbrella) — *see* Complications, umbrella device, vascular
ventilation therapy NEC T81.81 ☑
ventilator
  mechanical J95.850
  specified NEC J95.859
ventricular (communicating) shunt (device) T85.9 ☑
  embolism T85.810 ☑
  fibrosis T85.820 ☑
  hemorrhage T85.830 ☑
  infection and inflammation T85.730 ☑
  mechanical
    breakdown T85.01 ☑
    displacement T85.02 ☑
    leakage T85.03 ☑
    malposition T85.02 ☑
    obstruction T85.09 ☑
    perforation T85.09 ☑
    protrusion T85.09 ☑
    specified NEC T85.09 ☑
  pain T85.840 ☑
  specified type NEC T85.890 ☑
  stenosis T85.850 ☑
  thrombosis T85.860 ☑
wire suture, permanent (implanted) — *see* Complications, suture, permanent
Compressed air disease T70.3 ☑
Compression
with injury — *code by* Nature of injury
artery I77.1
  celiac, syndrome I77.4
brachial plexus G54.0
brain (stem) G93.5
  due to
    contusion (diffuse) — *see* Injury, intracranial, diffuse
      focal — *see* Injury, intracranial, focal
    injury NEC — *see* Injury, intracranial, diffuse
    traumatic — *see* Injury, intracranial, diffuse
bronchus J98.09
cauda equina G83.4
celiac (artery) (axis) I77.4
cerebral — *see* Compression, brain
cervical plexus G54.2

Compression — *continued*
cord
  spinal — *see* Compression, spinal
  umbilical — *see* Compression, umbilical cord
cranial nerve G52.9
  eighth H93.3 ☑
  eleventh G52.8
  fifth G50.8
  first G52.0
  fourth — *see* Strabismus, paralytic, fourth nerve
  ninth G52.1
  second — *see* Disorder, nerve, optic
  seventh G51.8
  sixth — *see* Strabismus, paralytic, sixth nerve
  tenth G52.2
  third — *see* Strabismus, paralytic, third nerve
  twelfth G52.3
diver's squeeze T70.3 ☑
during birth (newborn) P15.9
esophagus K22.2
eustachian tube — *see* Obstruction, eustachian tube, cartilaginous
facies Q67.1
fracture
  nontraumatic NOS — *see* Collapse, vertebra
  pathological — *see* Fracture, pathological
  traumatic — *see* Fracture, traumatic
heart — *see* Disease, heart
intestine — *see* Obstruction, intestine
laryngeal nerve, recurrent G52.2
  with paralysis of vocal cords and larynx J38.00
    bilateral J38.02
    unilateral J38.01
lumbosacral plexus G54.1
lung J98.4
lymphatic vessel I89.0
medulla — *see* Compression, brain
nerve — *see also* Disorder, nerve G58.9
  arm NEC — *see* Mononeuropathy, upper limb
  axillary G54.0
  cranial — *see* Compression, cranial nerve
  leg NEC — *see* Mononeuropathy, lower limb
  median (in carpal tunnel) — *see* Syndrome, carpal tunnel
  optic — *see* Disorder, nerve, optic
  plantar — *see* Lesion, nerve, plantar
  posterior tibial (in tarsal tunnel) — *see* Syndrome, tarsal tunnel
  root or plexus NOS (in) G54.9
    intervertebral disc disorder NEC — *see* Disorder, disc, with, radiculopathy
      with myelopathy — *see* Disorder, disc, with, myelopathy
    neoplastic disease — *see also* Neoplasm D49.9 *[G55]*
    spondylosis — *see* Spondylosis, with radiculopathy
  sciatic (acute) — *see* Lesion, nerve, sciatic
  sympathetic G90.8
  traumatic — *see* Injury, nerve
  ulnar — *see* Lesion, nerve, ulnar
  upper extremity NEC — *see* Mononeuropathy, upper limb
spinal (cord) G95.20
  by displacement of intervertebral disc NEC — *see also* Disorder, disc, with, myelopathy
  nerve root NOS G54.9
    due to displacement of intervertebral disc NEC — *see* Disorder, disc, with, radiculopathy
      with myelopathy — *see* Disorder, disc, with, myelopathy
  specified NEC G95.29
  spondylogenic (cervical) (lumbar, lumbosacral) (thoracic) — *see* Spondylosis, with myelopathy NEC
    anterior — *see* Syndrome, anterior, spinal artery, compression
  traumatic — *see* Injury, spinal cord, by region
subcostal nerve (syndrome) — *see* Mononeuropathy, upper limb, specified NEC
sympathetic nerve NEC G90.8
syndrome T79.5 ☑
trachea J39.8
ulnar nerve (by scar tissue) — *see* Lesion, nerve, ulnar
umbilical cord
  complicating delivery O69.2 ☑
    cord around neck O69.1 ☑

Compression — *continued*
umbilical cord — *continued*
complicating delivery — *continued*
prolapse O69.0 ☑
specified NEC O69.2 ☑
ureter N13.5
vein I87.1
vena cava (inferior) (superior) I87.1
Compulsion, compulsive
gambling F63.0
neurosis F42.8
personality F60.5
states F42.8
swearing F42.8
in Gilles de la Tourette's syndrome F95.2
tics and spasms F95.9
Concato's disease (pericardial polyserositis) A19.9
nontubercular I31.1
pleural — *see* Pleurisy, with effusion
Concavity chest wall M95.4
Concealed penis Q55.64
Concern (normal) **about sick person in family** Z63.6
Concrescence (teeth) K00.2
Concretio cordis I31.1
rheumatic I09.2
Concretion — *see also* Calculus
appendicular K38.1
canaliculus — *see* Dacryolith
clitoris N90.89
conjunctiva H11.12- ☑
eyelid — *see* Disorder, eyelid, specified type NEC
lacrimal passages — *see* Dacryolith
prepuce (male) N47.8
salivary gland (any) K11.5
seminal vesicle N50.89
tonsil J35.8
Concussion (brain) (cerebral) (current) S06.0X9 ☑
with
loss of consciousness of 30 minutes or less
S06.0X1 ☑
loss of consciousness of unspecified duration
S06.0X9 ☑
blast (air) (hydraulic) (immersion) (underwater)
abdomen or thorax — *see* Injury, blast, by site
ear with acoustic nerve injury — *see* Injury, nerve,
acoustic, specified type NEC
cauda equina S34.3 ☑
conus medullaris S34.02 ☑
ocular S05.8X- ☑
spinal (cord)
cervical S14.0 ☑
lumbar S34.01 ☑
sacral S34.02 ☑
thoracic S24.0 ☑
syndrome F07.81
without loss of consciousness S06.0X0 ☑
Condition — *see* Disease
Conditions arising in the perinatal period — *see*
Newborn, affected by
Conduct disorder — *see* Disorder, conduct
Condyloma A63.0
acuminatum A63.0
gonorrheal A54.09
latum A51.31
syphilitic A51.31
congenital A50.07
venereal, syphilitic A51.31
Conflagration — *see also* Burn
asphyxia (by inhalation of gases, fumes or vapors) —
see also Table of Drugs and Chemicals T59.9- ☑
Conflict (with) — *see also* Discord
family Z73.9
marital Z63.0
involving divorce or estrangement Z63.5
parent-child Z62.820
parent-adopted child Z62.821
parent-biological child Z62.820
parent-foster child Z62.822
social role NEC Z73.5
Confluent — *see* condition
Confusion, confused R41.0
epileptic F05
mental state (psychogenic) F44.89
psychogenic F44.89
reactive (from emotional stress, psychological trauma)
F44.89
Confusional arousals G47.51

Congelation T69.9 ☑
Congenital — *see also* condition
aortic septum Q25.49
intrinsic factor deficiency D51.0
malformation — *see* Anomaly
Congestion, congestive
bladder N32.89
bowel K63.89
brain G93.89
breast N64.59
bronchial J98.09
catarrhal J31.0
chest R09.89
chill, malarial — *see* Malaria
circulatory NEC I99.8
duodenum K31.89
eye — *see* Hyperemia, conjunctiva
facial, due to birth injury P15.4
general R68.89
glottis J37.0
heart — *see* Failure, heart, congestive
hepatic K76.1
hypostatic (lung) — *see* Edema, lung
intestine K63.89
kidney N28.89
labyrinth H83.8 ☑
larynx J37.0
liver K76.1
lung R09.89
active or acute — *see* Pneumonia
malaria, malarial — *see* Malaria
nasal R09.81
nose R09.81
orbit, orbital — *see also* Exophthalmos
inflammatory (chronic) — *see* Inflammation, orbit
ovary N83.8
pancreas K86.89
pelvic, female N94.89
pleural J94.8
prostate (active) N42.1
pulmonary — *see* Congestion, lung
renal N28.89
retina H35.81
seminal vesicle N50.1
spinal cord G95.19
spleen (chronic) D73.2
stomach K31.89
trachea — *see* Tracheitis
urethra N36.8
uterus N85.8
with subinvolution N85.3
venous (passive) I87.8
viscera R68.89
Congestive — *see* Congestion
Conical
cervix (hypertrophic elongation) N88.4
cornea — *see* Keratoconus
teeth K00.2
Conjoined twins Q89.4
Conjugal maladjustment Z63.0
involving divorce or estrangement Z63.5
Conjunctiva — *see* condition
Conjunctivitis (staphylococcal) (streptococcal) NOS H10.9
Acanthamoeba B60.12
acute H10.3- ☑
atopic H10.1- ☑
chemical — *see also* Corrosion, cornea H10.21- ☑
mucopurulent H10.02- ☑
follicular H10.01- ☑
pseudomembranous H10.22- ☑
serous except viral H10.23- ☑
viral — *see* Conjunctivitis, viral
toxic H10.21- ☑
adenoviral (acute) (follicular) B30.1
allergic (acute) — *see also* Conjunctivitis, acute, atopic
chronic H10.45
vernal H10.44
anaphylactic — *see* Conjunctivitis, acute, atopic
Apollo B30.3
atopic (acute) — *see* Conjunctivitis, acute, atopic
Béal's B30.2
blennorrhagic (gonococcal) (neonatorum) A54.31
chemical (acute) — *see also* Corrosion, cornea
H10.21- ☑
chlamydial A74.0
due to trachoma A71.1
neonatal P39.1

Conjunctivitis — *continued*
chronic (nodosa) (petrificans) (phlyctenular) H10.40- ☑
allergic H10.45
vernal H10.44
follicular H10.43- ☑
giant papillary H10.41- ☑
simple H10.42- ☑
vernal H10.44
coxsackievirus 24 B30.3
diphtheritic A36.86
due to
dust — *see* Conjunctivitis, acute, atopic
filariasis B74.9
mucocutaneous leishmaniasis B55.2
enterovirus type 70 (hemorrhagic) B30.3
epidemic (viral) B30.9
hemorrhagic B30.3
gonococcal (neonatorum) A54.31
granular (trachomatous) A71.1
sequelae (late effect) B94.0
hemorrhagic (acute) (epidemic) B30.3
herpes zoster B02.31
in (due to)
Acanthamoeba B60.12
adenovirus (acute) (follicular) B30.1
Chlamydia A74.0
coxsackievirus 24 B30.3
diphtheria A36.86
enterovirus type 70 (hemorrhagic) B30.3
filariasis B74.9
gonococci A54.31
herpes (simplex) virus B00.53
zoster B02.31
infectious disease NEC B99 ☑
meningococci A39.89
mucocutaneous leishmaniasis B55.2
rosacea H10.82- ☑
syphilis (late) A52.71
zoster B02.31
inclusion A74.0
infantile P39.1
gonococcal A54.31
Koch-Weeks' — *see* Conjunctivitis, acute, mucopurulent
light — *see* Conjunctivitis, acute, atopic
ligneous — *see* Blepharoconjunctivitis, ligneous
meningococcal A39.89
mucopurulent — *see* Conjunctivitis, acute, mucopurulent
neonatal P39.1
gonococcal A54.31
Newcastle B30.8
of Béal B30.2
parasitic
filariasis B74.9
mucocutaneous leishmaniasis B55.2
Parinaud's H10.89
petrificans H10.89
rosacea H10.82- ☑
specified NEC H10.89
swimming-pool B30.1
trachomatous A71.1
acute A71.0
sequelae (late effect) B94.0
traumatic NEC H10.89
tuberculous A18.59
tularemic A21.1
tularensis A21.1
viral B30.9
due to
adenovirus B30.1
enterovirus B30.3
specified NEC B30.8
Conjunctivochalasis H11.82- ☑
Connective tissue — *see* condition
Conn's syndrome E26.01
Conradi (-Hunermann) **disease** Q77.3
Consanguinity Z84.3
counseling Z71.89
Conscious simulation (of illness) Z76.5
Consecutive — *see* condition
Consolidation lung (base) — *see* Pneumonia, lobar
Constipation (atonic) (neurogenic) (simple) (spastic)
K59.00
chronic K59.09
idiopathic K59.04
drug-induced K59.03
functional K59.04
outlet dysfunction K59.02

Constipation — *continued*
  psychogenic F45.8
  slow transit K59.01
  specified NEC K59.09
Constitutional — *see also* condition
  substandard F60.7
Constitutionally substandard F60.7
Constriction — *see also* Stricture
  auditory canal — *see* Stenosis, external ear canal
  bronchial J98.09
  duodenum K31.5
  esophagus K22.2
  external
    abdomen, abdominal (wall) S30.841 ☑
    alveolar process S00.542 ☑
    ankle S90.54- ☑
    antecubital space — *see* Constriction, external, forearm
    arm (upper) S40.84- ☑
    auricle — *see* Constriction, external, ear
    axilla — *see* Constriction, external, arm
    back, lower S30.840 ☑
    breast S20.14- ☑
    brow S00.84 ☑
    buttock S30.840 ☑
    calf — *see* Constriction, external, leg
    canthus — *see* Constriction, external, eyelid
    cheek S00.84 ☑
      internal S00.542 ☑
    chest wall — *see* Constriction, external, thorax
    chin S00.84 ☑
    clitoris S30.844 ☑
    costal region — *see* Constriction, external, thorax
    digit(s)
      foot — *see* Constriction, external, toe
      hand — *see* Constriction, external, finger
    ear S00.44- ☑
    elbow S50.34- ☑
    epididymis S30.843 ☑
    epigastric region S30.841 ☑
    esophagus, cervical S10.14 ☑
    eyebrow — *see* Constriction, external, eyelid
    eyelid S00.24- ☑
    face S00.84 ☑
    finger(s) S60.44- ☑
      index S60.44- ☑
      little S60.44- ☑
      middle S60.44- ☑
      ring S60.44- ☑
    flank S30.841 ☑
    foot (except toe(s) alone) S90.84- ☑
      toe — *see* Constriction, external, toe
    forearm S50.84- ☑
      elbow only — *see* Constriction, external, elbow
    forehead S00.84 ☑
    genital organs, external
      female S30.846 ☑
      male S30.845 ☑
    groin S30.841 ☑
    gum S00.542 ☑
    hand S60.54- ☑
    head S00.94 ☑
      ear — *see* Constriction, external, ear
      eyelid — *see* Constriction, external, eyelid
      lip S00.541 ☑
      nose S00.34 ☑
      oral cavity S00.542 ☑
      scalp S00.04 ☑
      specified site NEC S00.84 ☑
    heel — *see* Constriction, external, foot
    hip S70.24- ☑
    inguinal region S30.841 ☑
    interscapular region S20.449 ☑
    jaw S00.84 ☑
    knee S80.24- ☑
    labium (majus) (minus) S30.844 ☑
    larynx S10.14 ☑
    leg (lower) S80.84- ☑
      knee — *see* Constriction, external, knee
      upper — *see* Constriction, external, thigh
    lip S00.541 ☑
    lower back S30.840 ☑
    lumbar region S30.840 ☑
    malar region S00.84 ☑
    mammary — *see* Constriction, external, breast
    mastoid region S00.84 ☑

Constriction — *continued*
  external — *continued*
    mouth S00.542 ☑
    nail
      finger — *see* Constriction, external, finger
      toe — *see* Constriction, external, toe
    nasal S00.34 ☑
    neck S10.94 ☑
      specified site NEC S10.84 ☑
      throat S10.14 ☑
    nose S00.34 ☑
    occipital region S00.04 ☑
    oral cavity S00.542 ☑
    orbital region — *see* Constriction, external, eyelid
    palate S00.542 ☑
    palm — *see* Constriction, external, hand
    parietal region S00.04 ☑
    pelvis S30.840 ☑
    penis S30.842 ☑
    perineum
      female S30.844 ☑
      male S30.840 ☑
    periocular area — *see* Constriction, external, eyelid
    phalanges
      finger — *see* Constriction, external, finger
      toe — *see* Constriction, external, toe
    pharynx S10.14 ☑
    pinna — *see* Constriction, external, ear
    popliteal space — *see* Constriction, external, knee
    prepuce S30.842 ☑
    pubic region S30.840 ☑
    pudendum
      female S30.846 ☑
      male S30.845 ☑
    sacral region S30.840 ☑
    scalp S00.04 ☑
    scapular region — *see* Constriction, external, shoulder
    scrotum S30.843 ☑
    shin — *see* Constriction, external, leg
    shoulder S40.24- ☑
    sternal region S20.349 ☑
    submaxillary region S00.84 ☑
    submental region S00.84 ☑
    subungual
      finger(s) — *see* Constriction, external, finger
      toe(s) — *see* Constriction, external, toe
    supraclavicular fossa S10.84 ☑
    supraorbital S00.84 ☑
    temple S00.84 ☑
    temporal region S00.84 ☑
    testis S30.843 ☑
    thigh S70.34- ☑
    thorax, thoracic (wall) S20.94 ☑
      back S20.44- ☑
      front S20.34- ☑
    throat S10.14 ☑
    thumb S60.34- ☑
    toe(s) (lesser) S90.44- ☑
      great S90.44- ☑
    tongue S00.542 ☑
    trachea S10.14 ☑
    tunica vaginalis S30.843 ☑
    uvula S00.542 ☑
    vagina S30.844 ☑
    vulva S30.844 ☑
    wrist S60.84- ☑
  gallbladder — *see* Obstruction, gallbladder
  intestine — *see* Obstruction, intestine
  larynx J38.6
    congenital Q31.8
      specified NEC Q31.8
      subglottic Q31.1
  organ or site, congenital NEC — *see* Atresia, by site
  prepuce (acquired) (congenital) N47.1
  pylorus (adult hypertrophic) K31.1
    congenital or infantile Q40.0
    newborn Q40.0
  ring dystocia (uterus) O62.4
  spastic — *see also* Spasm
    ureter N13.5
  ureter N13.5
    with infection N13.6
  urethra — *see* Stricture, urethra
  visual field (peripheral) (functional) — *see* Defect, visual field

Constrictive — *see* condition
Consultation
  medical — *see* Counseling, medical
  religious Z71.81
  specified reason NEC Z71.89
  spiritual Z71.81
  without complaint or sickness Z71.9
    feared complaint unfounded Z71.1
    specified reason NEC Z71.89
Consumption — *see* Tuberculosis
Contact (with) — *see also* Exposure (to)
  acariasis Z20.7
  AIDS virus Z20.6
  air pollution Z77.110
  algae and algae toxins Z77.121
  algae bloom Z77.121
  anthrax Z20.810
  aromatic amines Z77.020
  aromatic (hazardous) compounds NEC Z77.028
  aromatic dyes NOS Z77.028
  arsenic Z77.010
  asbestos Z77.090
  bacterial disease NEC Z20.818
  benzene Z77.021
  blue-green algae bloom Z77.121
  body fluids (potentially hazardous) Z77.21
  brown tide Z77.121
  chemicals (chiefly nonmedicinal) (hazardous) NEC Z77.098
  cholera Z20.09
  chromium compounds Z77.018
  communicable disease Z20.9
    bacterial NEC Z20.818
    specified NEC Z20.89
    viral NEC Z20.828
    Zika virus Z20.821
  cyanobacteria bloom Z77.121
  dyes Z77.098
  Escherichia coli (E. coli) Z20.01
  fiberglass — *see* Table of Drugs and Chemicals, fiberglass
  German measles Z20.4
  gonorrhea Z20.2
  hazardous metals NEC Z77.018
  hazardous substances NEC Z77.29
  hazards in the physical environment NEC Z77.128
  hazards to health NEC Z77.9
  HIV Z20.6
  HTLV-III/LAV Z20.6
  human immunodeficiency virus (HIV) Z20.6
  infection Z20.9
    specified NEC Z20.89
  infestation (parasitic) NEC Z20.7
  intestinal infectious disease NEC Z20.09
    Escherichia coli (E. coli) Z20.01
  lead Z77.011
  meningococcus Z20.811
  mold (toxic) Z77.120
  nickel dust Z77.018
  noise Z77.122
  parasitic disease Z20.7
  pediculosis Z20.7
  pfiesteria piscicida Z77.121
  poliomyelitis Z20.89
  pollution
    air Z77.110
    environmental NEC Z77.118
    soil Z77.112
    water Z77.111
  polycyclic aromatic hydrocarbons Z77.028
  rabies Z20.3
  radiation, naturally occurring NEC Z77.123
  radon Z77.123
  red tide (Florida) Z77.121
  rubella Z20.4
  sexually-transmitted disease Z20.2
  smallpox (laboratory) Z20.89
  syphilis Z20.2
  tuberculosis Z20.1
  uranium Z77.012
  varicella Z20.820
  venereal disease Z20.2
  viral disease NEC Z20.828
  viral hepatitis Z20.5
  water pollution Z77.111
  Zika virus Z20.821
Contamination, food — *see* Intoxication, foodborne

☑ **Additional Character Required** — Refer to the Tabular List for Character Selection   ▽ Subterms under main terms may continue to next column or page

Contraception, contraceptive
advice Z30.09
counseling Z30.09
device (intrauterine) (in situ) Z97.5
  causing menorrhagia T83.83 ☑
  checking Z30.431
  complications — see Complications, intrauterine,
    contraceptive device
  in place Z97.5
  initial prescription Z30.014
  reinsertion Z30.433
  removal Z30.432
  replacement Z30.433
emergency (postcoital) Z30.012
initial prescription Z30.019
  barrier Z30.018
  diaphragm Z30.018
  injectable Z30.013
  intrauterine device Z30.014
  pills Z30.011
  postcoital (emergency) Z30.012
  specified type NEC Z30.018
  subdermal implantable Z30.017
  transdermal patch hormonal Z30.016
  vaginal ring hormonal Z30.015
maintenance Z30.40
  barrier Z30.49
  diaphragm Z30.49
  examination Z30.8
  injectable Z30.42
  intrauterine device Z30.431
  pills Z30.41
  specified type NEC Z30.49
  subdermal implantable Z30.46
  transdermal patch hormonal Z30.45
  vaginal ring hormonal Z30.44
management Z30.9
  specified NEC Z30.8
postcoital (emergency) Z30.012
prescription Z30.019
  repeat Z30.40
sterilization Z30.2
surveillance (drug) — see Contraception, maintenance

Contraction(s), contracture, contracted
Achilles tendon — see also Short, tendon, Achilles
  congenital Q66.89
amputation stump (surgical) (flexion) (late) (next
  proximal joint) T87.89
anus K59.89
bile duct (common) (hepatic) K83.8
bladder N32.89
  neck or sphincter N32.0
bowel, cecum, colon or intestine, any part — see Obstruction, intestine
Braxton Hicks — see False, labor
breast implant, capsular T85.44 ☑
bronchial J98.09
burn (old) — see Cicatrix
cervix — see Stricture, cervix
cicatricial — see Cicatrix
conjunctiva, trachomatous, active A71.1
  sequelae (late effect) B94.0
Dupuytren's M72.0
eyelid — see Disorder, eyelid function
fascia (lata) (postural) M72.8
  Dupuytren's M72.0
  palmar M72.0
  plantar M72.2
finger NEC — see also Deformity, finger
  congenital Q68.1
  joint — see Contraction, joint, hand
flaccid — see Contraction, paralytic
gallbladder K82.0
heart valve — see Endocarditis
hip — see Contraction, joint, hip
hourglass
  bladder N32.89
    congenital Q64.79
  gallbladder K82.0
    congenital Q44.1
  stomach K31.89
    congenital Q40.2
    psychogenic F45.8
  uterus (complicating delivery) O62.4
hysterical F44.4
internal os — see Stricture, cervix
joint (abduction) (acquired) (adduction) (flexion) (rotation) M24.50

Contraction(s), contracture, contracted — continued
joint — continued
  ankle M24.57- ☑
  congenital NEC Q68.8
    hip Q65.89
  elbow M24.52- ☑
  foot joint M24.57- ☑
  hand joint M24.54- ☑
  hip M24.55- ☑
    congenital Q65.89
  hysterical F44.4
  knee M24.56- ☑
  shoulder M24.51- ☑
  specified site NEC M24.59
  wrist M24.53- ☑
kidney (granular) (secondary) N26.9
  congenital Q63.8
  hydronephritic — see Hydronephrosis
  Page N26.2
  pyelonephritic — see Pyelitis, chronic
  tuberculous A18.11
ligament — see also Disorder, ligament
  congenital Q79.8
muscle (postinfective) (postural) NEC M62.40
  with contracture of joint — see Contraction, joint
  ankle M62.47- ☑
  congenital Q79.8
    sternocleidomastoid Q68.0
  extraocular — see Strabismus
  eye (extrinsic) — see Strabismus
  foot M62.47- ☑
  forearm M62.43- ☑
  hand M62.44- ☑
  hysterical F44.4
  ischemic (Volkmann's) T79.6 ☑
  lower leg M62.46- ☑
  multiple sites M62.49
  pelvic region M62.45- ☑
  posttraumatic — see Strabismus, paralytic
  psychogenic F45.8
    conversion reaction F44.4
  shoulder region M62.41- ☑
  specified site NEC M62.48
  thigh M62.45- ☑
  upper arm M62.42- ☑
neck — see Torticollis
ocular muscle — see Strabismus
organ or site, congenital NEC — see Atresia, by site
outlet (pelvis) — see Contraction, pelvis
palmar fascia M72.0
paralytic
  joint — see Contraction, joint
  muscle — see also Contraction, muscle NEC
    ocular — see Strabismus, paralytic
pelvis (acquired) (general) M95.5
  with disproportion (fetopelvic) O33.1
    causing obstructed labor O65.1
    inlet O33.2
    mid-cavity O33.3 ☑
    outlet O33.3 ☑
plantar fascia M72.2
premature
  atrium I49.1
  auriculoventricular I49.49
  heart I49.49
  junctional I49.2
  supraventricular I49.1
  ventricular I49.3
prostate N42.89
pylorus NEC — see also Pylorospasm
  psychogenic F45.8
rectum, rectal (sphincter) K59.89
ring (Bandl's) (complicating delivery) O62.4
scar — see Cicatrix
spine — see Dorsopathy, deforming
sternocleidomastoid (muscle), congenital Q68.0
stomach K31.89
  hourglass K31.89
    congenital Q40.2
    psychogenic F45.8
  psychogenic F45.8
tendon (sheath) M62.40
  with contracture of joint — see Contraction, joint
  Achilles — see Short, tendon, Achilles
  ankle M62.47- ☑
    Achilles — see Short, tendon, Achilles

Contraction(s), contracture, contracted — continued
tendon — continued
  foot M62.47- ☑
  forearm M62.43- ☑
  hand M62.44- ☑
  lower leg M62.46- ☑
  multiple sites M62.49
  neck M62.48
  pelvic region M62.45- ☑
  shoulder region M62.41- ☑
  specified site NEC M62.48
  thigh M62.45- ☑
  thorax M62.48
  trunk M62.48
  upper arm M62.42- ☑
toe — see Deformity, toe, specified NEC
ureterovesical orifice (postinfectional) N13.5
  with infection N13.6
urethra — see also Stricture, urethra
  orifice N32.0
uterus N85.8
  abnormal NEC O62.9
  clonic (complicating delivery) O62.4
  dyscoordinate (complicating delivery) O62.4
  hourglass (complicating delivery) O62.4
  hypertonic O62.4
  hypotonic NEC O62.2
  inadequate
    primary O62.0
    secondary O62.1
  incoordinate (complicating delivery) O62.4
  poor O62.2
  tetanic (complicating delivery) O62.4
vagina (outlet) N89.5
vesical N32.89
  neck or urethral orifice N32.0
visual field — see Defect, visual field, generalized
Volkmann's (ischemic) T79.6 ☑

Contusion (skin surface intact) T14.8 ☑
abdomen, abdominal (muscle) (wall) S30.1 ☑
adnexa, eye NEC S05.8X- ☑
adrenal gland S37.812 ☑
alveolar process S00.532 ☑
ankle S90.0- ☑
antecubital space — see Contusion, forearm
anus S30.3 ☑
arm (upper) S40.02- ☑
  lower (with elbow) — see Contusion, forearm
auditory canal — see Contusion, ear
auricle — see Contusion, ear
axilla — see Contusion, arm, upper
back — see also Contusion, thorax, back
  lower S30.0 ☑
bile duct S36.13 ☑
bladder S37.22 ☑
bone NEC T14.8 ☑
brain (diffuse) — see Injury, intracranial, diffuse
  focal — see Injury, intracranial, focal
brainstem S06.38- ☑
breast S20.0- ☑
broad ligament S37.892 ☑
brow S00.83 ☑
buttock S30.0 ☑
canthus, eye S00.1- ☑
cauda equina S34.3 ☑
cerebellar, traumatic S06.37- ☑
cerebral S06.33- ☑
  left side S06.32- ☑
  right side S06.31- ☑
cheek S00.83 ☑
  internal S00.532 ☑
chest (wall) — see Contusion, thorax
chin S00.83 ☑
clitoris S30.23 ☑
colon — see Injury, intestine, large, contusion
common bile duct S36.13 ☑
conjunctiva S05.1- ☑
  with foreign body (in conjunctival sac) — see For-
    eign body, conjunctival sac
conus medullaris (spine) S34.139 ☑
cornea — see Contusion, eyeball
  with foreign body — see Foreign body, cornea
corpus cavernosum S30.21 ☑
cortex (brain) (cerebral) — see Injury, intracranial, diffuse
  focal — see Injury, intracranial, focal

Contusion — *continued*
- costal region — *see* Contusion, thorax
- cystic duct S36.13 ☑
- diaphragm S27.802 ☑
- duodenum S36.420 ☑
- ear S00.43- ☑
- elbow S50.0- ☑
  - with forearm — *see* Contusion, forearm
- epididymis S30.22 ☑
- epigastric region S30.1 ☑
- epiglottis S10.0 ☑
- esophagus (thoracic) S27.812 ☑
  - cervical S10.0 ☑
- eyeball S05.1- ☑
- eyebrow S00.1- ☑
- eyelid (and periocular area) S00.1- ☑
- face NEC S00.83 ☑
- fallopian tube S37.529 ☑
  - bilateral S37.522 ☑
  - unilateral S37.521 ☑
- femoral triangle S30.1 ☑
- finger(s) S60.00 ☑
  - with damage to nail (matrix) S60.10 ☑
  - index S60.02- ☑
    - with damage to nail S60.12- ☑
  - little S60.05- ☑
    - with damage to nail S60.15- ☑
  - middle S60.03- ☑
    - with damage to nail S60.13- ☑
  - ring S60.04- ☑
    - with damage to nail S60.14- ☑
  - thumb — *see* Contusion, thumb
- flank S30.1 ☑
- foot (except toe(s) alone) S90.3- ☑
  - toe — *see* Contusion, toe
- forearm S50.1- ☑
  - elbow only — *see* Contusion, elbow
- forehead S00.83 ☑
- gallbladder S36.122 ☑
- genital organs, external
  - female S30.202 ☑
  - male S30.201 ☑
- globe (eye) — *see* Contusion, eyeball
- groin S30.1 ☑
- gum S00.532 ☑
- hand S60.22- ☑
  - finger(s) — *see* Contusion, finger
  - wrist — *see* Contusion, wrist
- head S00.93 ☑
  - ear — *see* Contusion, ear
  - eyelid — *see* Contusion, eyelid
  - lip S00.531 ☑
  - nose S00.33 ☑
  - oral cavity S00.532 ☑
  - scalp S00.03 ☑
  - specified part NEC S00.83 ☑
- heart — *see also* Injury, heart S26.91 ☑
- heel — *see* Contusion, foot
- hepatic duct S36.13 ☑
- hip S70.0- ☑
- ileum S36.428 ☑
- iliac region S30.1 ☑
- inguinal region S30.1 ☑
- interscapular region S20.229 ☑
- intra-abdominal organ S36.92 ☑
  - colon — *see* Injury, intestine, large, contusion
  - liver S36.112 ☑
  - pancreas — *see* Contusion, pancreas
  - rectum S36.62 ☑
  - small intestine — *see* Injury, intestine, small, contusion
  - specified organ NEC S36.892 ☑
  - spleen — *see* Contusion, spleen
  - stomach S36.32 ☑
- iris (eye) — *see* Contusion, eyeball
- jaw S00.83 ☑
- jejunum S36.428 ☑
- kidney S37.01- ☑
  - major (greater than 2 cm) S37.02- ☑
  - minor (less than 2 cm) S37.01- ☑
- knee S80.0- ☑
- labium (majus) (minus) S30.23 ☑
- lacrimal apparatus, gland or sac S05.8X- ☑
- larynx S10.0 ☑
- leg (lower) S80.1- ☑
  - knee — *see* Contusion, knee

Contusion — *continued*
- lens — *see* Contusion, eyeball
- lip S00.531 ☑
- liver S36.112 ☑
- lower back S30.0 ☑
- lumbar region S30.0 ☑
- lung S27.329 ☑
  - bilateral S27.322 ☑
  - unilateral S27.321 ☑
- malar region S00.83 ☑
- mastoid region S00.83 ☑
- membrane, brain — *see* Injury, intracranial, diffuse
  - focal — *see* Injury, intracranial, focal
- mesentery S36.892 ☑
- mesosalpinx S37.892 ☑
- mouth S00.532 ☑
- muscle — *see* Contusion, by site
- nail
  - finger — *see* Contusion, finger, with damage to nail
  - toe — *see* Contusion, toe, with damage to nail
- nasal S00.33 ☑
- neck S10.93 ☑
  - specified site NEC S10.83 ☑
  - throat S10.0 ☑
- nerve — *see* Injury, nerve
- newborn P54.5
- nose S00.33 ☑
- occipital
  - lobe (brain) — *see* Injury, intracranial, diffuse
    - focal — *see* Injury, intracranial, focal
  - region (scalp) S00.03 ☑
- orbit (region) (tissues) S05.1- ☑
- ovary S37.429 ☑
  - bilateral S37.422 ☑
  - unilateral S37.421 ☑
- palate S00.532 ☑
- pancreas S36.229 ☑
  - body S36.221 ☑
  - head S36.220 ☑
  - tail S36.222 ☑
- parietal
  - lobe (brain) — *see* Injury, intracranial, diffuse
    - focal — *see* Injury, intracranial, focal
  - region (scalp) S00.03 ☑
- pelvic organ S37.92 ☑
  - adrenal gland S37.812 ☑
  - bladder S37.22 ☑
  - fallopian tube — *see* Contusion, fallopian tube
  - kidney — *see* Contusion, kidney
  - ovary — *see* Contusion, ovary
  - prostate S37.822 ☑
  - specified organ NEC S37.892 ☑
  - ureter S37.12 ☑
  - urethra S37.32 ☑
  - uterus S37.62 ☑
- pelvis S30.0 ☑
- penis S30.21 ☑
- perineum
  - female S30.23 ☑
  - male S30.0 ☑
- periocular area S00.1- ☑
- peritoneum S36.81 ☑
- periurethral tissue — *see* Contusion, urethra
- pharynx S10.0 ☑
- pinna — *see* Contusion, ear
- popliteal space — *see* Contusion, knee
- prepuce S30.21 ☑
- prostate S37.822 ☑
- pubic region S30.1 ☑
- pudendum
  - female S30.202 ☑
  - male S30.201 ☑
- quadriceps femoris — *see* Contusion, thigh
- rectum S36.62 ☑
- retroperitoneum S36.892 ☑
- round ligament S37.892 ☑
- sacral region S30.0 ☑
- scalp S00.03 ☑
  - due to birth injury P12.3
- scapular region — *see* Contusion, shoulder
- sclera — *see* Contusion, eyeball
- scrotum S30.22 ☑
- seminal vesicle S37.892 ☑
- shoulder S40.01- ☑
- skin NEC T14.8 ☑
- small intestine — *see* Injury, intestine, small, contusion

Contusion — *continued*
- spermatic cord S30.22 ☑
- spinal cord — *see* Injury, spinal cord, by region
  - cauda equina S34.3 ☑
  - conus medullaris S34.139 ☑
- spleen S36.029 ☑
  - major S36.021 ☑
  - minor S36.020 ☑
- sternal region S20.219 ☑
- stomach S36.32 ☑
- subconjunctival S05.1- ☑
- subcutaneous NEC T14.8 ☑
- submaxillary region S00.83 ☑
- submental region S00.83 ☑
- subperiosteal NEC T14.8 ☑
- subungual
  - finger — *see* Contusion, finger, with damage to nail
  - toe — *see* Contusion, toe, with damage to nail
- supraclavicular fossa S10.83 ☑
- supraorbital S00.83 ☑
- suprarenal gland S37.812 ☑
- temple (region) S00.83 ☑
- temporal
  - lobe (brain) — *see* Injury, intracranial, diffuse
    - focal — *see* Injury, intracranial, focal
  - region S00.83 ☑
- testis S30.22 ☑
- thigh S70.1- ☑
- thorax (wall) S20.20 ☑
  - back S20.22- ☑
  - front S20.21- ☑
- throat S10.0 ☑
- thumb S60.01- ☑
  - with damage to nail S60.11- ☑
- toe(s) (lesser) S90.12- ☑
  - with damage to nail S90.22- ☑
  - great S90.11- ☑
    - with damage to nail S90.21- ☑
- tongue S00.532 ☑
- trachea (cervical) S10.0 ☑
  - thoracic S27.52 ☑
- tunica vaginalis S30.22 ☑
- tympanum, tympanic membrane — *see* Contusion, ear
- ureter S37.12 ☑
- urethra S37.32 ☑
- urinary organ NEC S37.892 ☑
- uterus S37.62 ☑
- uvula S00.532 ☑
- vagina S30.23 ☑
- vas deferens S37.892 ☑
- vesical S37.22 ☑
- vocal cord(s) S10.0 ☑
- vulva S30.23 ☑
- wrist S60.21- ☑

Conus (congenital) (any type) Q14.8
- cornea — *see* Keratoconus
- medullaris syndrome G95.81

Conversion hysteria, neurosis or reaction F44.9

Converter, tuberculosis (test reaction) R76.11

Conviction (legal), **anxiety concerning** Z65.0
- with imprisonment Z65.1

Convulsions (idiopathic) — *see also* Seizure(s) R56.9
- apoplectiform (cerebral ischemia) I67.82
- dissociative F44.5
- epileptic — *see* Epilepsy
- epileptiform, epileptoid — *see* Seizure, epileptiform
- ether (anesthetic) — *see* Table of Drugs and Chemicals, by drug
- febrile R56.00
  - with status epilepticus G40.901
  - complex R56.01
    - with status epilepticus G40.901
  - simple R56.00
- hysterical F44.5
- infantile P90
  - epilepsy — *see* Epilepsy
- jacksonian — *see* Epilepsy, localization-related, symptomatic, with simple partial seizures
- myoclonic G25.3
- newborn P90
- obstetrical (nephritic) (uremic) — *see* Eclampsia
- paretic A52.17
- post traumatic R56.1
- psychomotor — *see* Epilepsy, localization-related, symptomatic, with complex partial seizures

☑ **Additional Character Required** — Refer to the Tabular List for Character Selection   ▽ **Subterms under main terms may continue to next column or page**

Convulsions — *continued*
  recurrent R56.9
  reflex R25.8
  scarlatinal A38.8
  tetanus, tetanic — *see* Tetanus
  thymic E32.8
Convulsive — *see also* Convulsions
Cooley's anemia D56.1
Coolie itch B76.9
Cooper's
  disease — *see* Mastopathy, cystic
  hernia — *see* Hernia, abdomen, specified site NEC
Copra itch B88.0
Coprophagy F50.89
Coprophobia F40.298
Coproporphyria, hereditary E80.29
Cor
  biloculare Q20.8
  bovis, bovinum — *see* Hypertrophy, cardiac
  pulmonale (chronic) I27.81
    acute I26.09
  triatriatum, triatrium Q24.2
  triloculare Q20.8
    biatrium Q20.4
    biventriculare Q21.1
Corbus' disease (gangrenous balanitis) N48.1
Cord — *see also* condition
  around neck
    complicating delivery O69.81 ✓
      with compression O69.1 ✓
  bladder G95.89
    tabetic A52.19
Cordis ectopia Q24.8
Corditis (spermatic) N49.1
Corectopia Q13.2
Cori's disease (glycogen storage) E74.03
Corkhandler's disease or lung J67.3
Corkscrew esophagus K22.4
Corkworker's disease or lung J67.3
Corn (infected) L84
Cornea — *see also* condition
  donor Z52.5
  plana Q13.4
Cornelia de Lange syndrome Q87.19
Cornu cutaneum L85.8
Cornual gestation or pregnancy O00.80
  with intrauterine pregnancy O00.81
Coronary (artery) — *see* condition
Coronavirus (infection)
  as cause of diseases classified elsewhere B97.29
  coronavirus-19 U07.1
  COVID-19 U07.1
  SARS-associated B97.21
Corpora — *see also* condition
  amylacea, prostate N42.89
  cavernosa — *see* condition
Corpulence — *see* Obesity
Corpus — *see* condition
Corrected transposition Q20.5
Corrosion (injury) (acid) (caustic) (chemical) (lime) (external) (internal) T30.4
  abdomen, abdominal (muscle) (wall) T21.42 ✓
    first degree T21.52 ✓
    second degree T21.62 ✓
    third degree T21.72 ✓
  above elbow T22.439 ✓
    first degree T22.539 ✓
    left T22.432 ✓
      first degree T22.532 ✓
      second degree T22.632 ✓
      third degree T22.732 ✓
    right T22.431 ✓
      first degree T22.531 ✓
      second degree T22.631 ✓
      third degree T22.731 ✓
    second degree T22.639 ✓
    third degree T22.739 ✓
  alimentary tract NEC T28.7 ✓
  ankle T25.419 ✓
    first degree T25.519 ✓
    left T25.412 ✓
      first degree T25.512 ✓
      second degree T25.612 ✓
      third degree T25.712 ✓
    multiple with foot — *see* Corrosion, lower, limb, multiple, ankle and foot
    right T25.411 ✓

Corrosion — *continued*
  ankle — *continued*
    right — *continued*
      first degree T25.511 ✓
      second degree T25.611 ✓
      third degree T25.711 ✓
    second degree T25.619 ✓
    third degree T25.719 ✓
  anus — *see* Corrosion, buttock
  arm(s) (meaning upper limb(s)) — *see* Corrosion, upper limb
  axilla T22.449 ✓
    first degree T22.549 ✓
    left T22.442 ✓
      first degree T22.542 ✓
      second degree T22.642 ✓
      third degree T22.742 ✓
    right T22.441 ✓
      first degree T22.541 ✓
      second degree T22.641 ✓
      third degree T22.741 ✓
    second degree T22.649 ✓
    third degree T22.749 ✓
  back (lower) T21.44 ✓
    first degree T21.54 ✓
    second degree T21.64 ✓
    third degree T21.74 ✓
    upper T21.43 ✓
      first degree T21.53 ✓
      second degree T21.63 ✓
      third degree T21.73 ✓
  blisters — *code as* Corrosion, second degree, by site
  breast(s) — *see* Corrosion, chest wall
  buttock(s) T21.45 ✓
    first degree T21.55 ✓
    second degree T21.65 ✓
    third degree T21.75 ✓
  calf T24.439 ✓
    first degree T24.539 ✓
    left T24.432 ✓
      first degree T24.532 ✓
      second degree T24.632 ✓
      third degree T24.732 ✓
    right T24.431 ✓
      first degree T24.531 ✓
      second degree T24.631 ✓
      third degree T24.731 ✓
    second degree T24.639 ✓
    third degree T24.739 ✓
  canthus (eye) — *see* Corrosion, eyelid
  cervix T28.8 ✓
  cheek T20.46 ✓
    first degree T20.56 ✓
    second degree T20.66 ✓
    third degree T20.76 ✓
  chest wall T21.41 ✓
    first degree T21.51 ✓
    second degree T21.61 ✓
    third degree T21.71 ✓
  chin T20.43 ✓
    first degree T20.53 ✓
    second degree T20.63 ✓
    third degree T20.73 ✓
  colon T28.7 ✓
  conjunctiva (and cornea) — *see* Corrosion, cornea
  cornea (and conjunctiva) T26.6- ✓
  deep necrosis of underlying tissue — *code as* Corrosion, third degree, by site
  dorsum of hand T23.469 ✓
    first degree T23.569 ✓
    left T23.462 ✓
      first degree T23.562 ✓
      second degree T23.662 ✓
      third degree T23.762 ✓
    right T23.461 ✓
      first degree T23.561 ✓
      second degree T23.661 ✓
      third degree T23.761 ✓
    second degree T23.669 ✓
    third degree T23.769 ✓
  ear (auricle) (external) (canal) T20.41 ✓
    drum T28.91 ✓
    first degree T20.51 ✓
    second degree T20.61 ✓
    third degree T20.71 ✓
  elbow T22.429 ✓

Corrosion — *continued*
  elbow — *continued*
    first degree T22.529 ✓
    left T22.422 ✓
      first degree T22.522 ✓
      second degree T22.622 ✓
      third degree T22.722 ✓
    right T22.421 ✓
      first degree T22.521 ✓
      second degree T22.621 ✓
      third degree T22.721 ✓
    second degree T22.629 ✓
    third degree T22.729 ✓
  entire body — *see* Corrosion, multiple body regions
  epidermal loss — *code as* Corrosion, second degree, by site
  epiglottis T27.4 ✓
  erythema, erythematous — *code as* Corrosion, first degree, by site
  esophagus T28.6 ✓
  extent (percentage of body surface)
    less than 10 percent T32.0
    10-19 percent (0-9 percent third degree) T32.10
      with 10-19 percent third degree T32.11
    20-29 percent (0-9 percent third degree) T32.20
      with
        10-19 percent third degree T32.21
        20-29 percent third degree T32.22
    30-39 percent (0-9 percent third degree) T32.30
      with
        10-19 percent third degree T32.31
        20-29 percent third degree T32.32
        30-39 percent third degree T32.33
    40-49 percent (0-9 percent third degree) T32.40
      with
        10-19 percent third degree T32.41
        20-29 percent third degree T32.42
        30-39 percent third degree T32.43
        40-49 percent third degree T32.44
    50-59 percent (0-9 percent third degree) T32.50
      with
        10-19 percent third degree T32.51
        20-29 percent third degree T32.52
        30-39 percent third degree T32.53
        40-49 percent third degree T32.54
        50-59 percent third degree T32.55
    60-69 percent (0-9 percent third degree) T32.60
      with
        10-19 percent third degree T32.61
        20-29 percent third degree T32.62
        30-39 percent third degree T32.63
        40-49 percent third degree T32.64
        50-59 percent third degree T32.65
        60-69 percent third degree T32.66
    70-79 percent (0-9 percent third degree) T32.70
      with
        10-19 percent third degree T32.71
        20-29 percent third degree T32.72
        30-39 percent third degree T32.73
        40-49 percent third degree T32.74
        50-59 percent third degree T32.75
        60-69 percent third degree T32.76
        70-79 percent third degree T32.77
    80-89 percent (0-9 percent third degree) T32.80
      with
        10-19 percent third degree T32.81
        20-29 percent third degree T32.82
        30-39 percent third degree T32.83
        40-49 percent third degree T32.84
        50-59 percent third degree T32.85
        60-69 percent third degree T32.86
        70-79 percent third degree T32.87
        80-89 percent third degree T32.88
    90 percent or more (0-9 percent third degree) T32.90
      with
        10-19 percent third degree T32.91
        20-29 percent third degree T32.92
        30-39 percent third degree T32.93
        40-49 percent third degree T32.94
        50-59 percent third degree T32.95
        60-69 percent third degree T32.96
        70-79 percent third degree T32.97
        80-89 percent third degree T32.98
        90-99 percent third degree T32.99
  extremity — *see* Corrosion, limb
  eye(s) and adnexa T26.9- ✓
    with resulting rupture and destruction of eyeball T26.7- ✓

Corrosion — *continued*
eye(s) and adnexa — *continued*
   conjunctival sac — *see* Corrosion, cornea
   cornea — *see* Corrosion, cornea
   lid — *see* Corrosion, eyelid
   periocular area — *see* Corrosion eyelid
   specified site NEC T26.8- ☑
eyeball — *see* Corrosion, eye
eyelid(s) T26.5- ☑
face — *see* Corrosion, head
finger T23.429 ☑
  first degree T23.529 ☑
  left T23.422 ☑
    first degree T23.522 ☑
    second degree T23.622 ☑
    third degree T23.722 ☑
  multiple sites (without thumb) T23.439 ☑
    with thumb T23.449 ☑
      first degree T23.549 ☑
      left T23.442 ☑
        first degree T23.542 ☑
        second degree T23.642 ☑
        third degree T23.742 ☑
      right T23.441 ☑
        first degree T23.541 ☑
        second degree T23.641 ☑
        third degree T23.741 ☑
      second degree T23.649 ☑
      third degree T23.749 ☑
    first degree T23.539 ☑
    left T23.432 ☑
      first degree T23.532 ☑
      second degree T23.632 ☑
      third degree T23.732 ☑
    right T23.431 ☑
      first degree T23.531 ☑
      second degree T23.631 ☑
      third degree T23.731 ☑
    second degree T23.639 ☑
    third degree T23.739 ☑
  right T23.421 ☑
    first degree T23.521 ☑
    second degree T23.621 ☑
    third degree T23.721 ☑
  second degree T23.629 ☑
  third degree T23.729 ☑
flank — *see* Corrosion, abdomen
foot T25.429 ☑
  first degree T25.529 ☑
  left T25.422 ☑
    first degree T25.522 ☑
    second degree T25.622 ☑
    third degree T25.722 ☑
  multiple with ankle — *see* Corrosion, lower, limb, multiple, ankle and foot
  right T25.421 ☑
    first degree T25.521 ☑
    second degree T25.621 ☑
    third degree T25.721 ☑
  second degree T25.629 ☑
  third degree T25.729 ☑
forearm T22.419 ☑
  first degree T22.519 ☑
  left T22.412 ☑
    first degree T22.512 ☑
    second degree T22.612 ☑
    third degree T22.712 ☑
  right T22.411 ☑
    first degree T22.511 ☑
    second degree T22.611 ☑
    third degree T22.711 ☑
  second degree T22.619 ☑
  third degree T22.719 ☑
forehead T20.46 ☑
  first degree T20.56 ☑
  second degree T20.66 ☑
  third degree T20.76 ☑
fourth degree — *code as* Corrosion, third degree, by site
full thickness skin loss — *code as* Corrosion, third degree, by site
gastrointestinal tract NEC T28.7 ☑
genital organs
  external
    female T21.47 ☑
      first degree T21.57 ☑

Corrosion — *continued*
genital organs — *continued*
  external — *continued*
    female — *continued*
      second degree T21.67 ☑
      third degree T21.77 ☑
    male T21.46 ☑
      first degree T21.56 ☑
      second degree T21.66 ☑
      third degree T21.76 ☑
  internal T28.8 ☑
groin — *see* Corrosion, abdominal wall
hand(s) T23.409 ☑
  back — *see* Corrosion, dorsum of hand
  finger — *see* Corrosion, finger
  first degree T23.509 ☑
  left T23.402 ☑
    first degree T23.502 ☑
    second degree T23.602 ☑
    third degree T23.702 ☑
  multiple sites with wrist T23.499 ☑
    first degree T23.599 ☑
    left T23.492 ☑
      first degree T23.592 ☑
      second degree T23.692 ☑
      third degree T23.792 ☑
    right T23.491 ☑
      first degree T23.591 ☑
      second degree T23.691 ☑
      third degree T23.791 ☑
    second degree T23.699 ☑
    third degree T23.799 ☑
  palm — *see* Corrosion, palm
  right T23.401 ☑
    first degree T23.501 ☑
    second degree T23.601 ☑
    third degree T23.701 ☑
  second degree T23.609 ☑
  third degree T23.709 ☑
  thumb — *see* Corrosion, thumb
head (and face) (and neck) T20.40 ☑
  cheek — *see* Corrosion, cheek
  chin — *see* Corrosion, chin
  ear — *see* Corrosion, ear
  eye(s) only — *see* Corrosion, eye
  first degree T20.50 ☑
  forehead — *see* Corrosion, forehead
  lip — *see* Corrosion, lip
  multiple sites T20.49 ☑
    first degree T20.59 ☑
    second degree T20.69 ☑
    third degree T20.79 ☑
  neck — *see* Corrosion, neck
  nose — *see* Corrosion, nose
  scalp — *see* Corrosion, scalp
  second degree T20.60 ☑
  third degree T20.70 ☑
hip(s) — *see* Corrosion, lower, limb
inhalation — *see* Corrosion, respiratory tract
internal organ(s) — *see also* Corrosion, by site
  T28.90 ☑
  alimentary tract T28.7 ☑
    esophagus T28.6 ☑
  esophagus T28.6 ☑
  genitourinary T28.8 ☑
  mouth T28.5 ☑
  pharynx T28.5 ☑
  specified organ NEC T28.99 ☑
interscapular region — *see* Corrosion, back, upper
intestine (large) (small) T28.7 ☑
knee T24.429 ☑
  first degree T24.529 ☑
  left T24.422 ☑
    first degree T24.522 ☑
    second degree T24.622 ☑
    third degree T24.722 ☑
  right T24.421 ☑
    first degree T24.521 ☑
    second degree T24.621 ☑
    third degree T24.721 ☑
  second degree T24.629 ☑
  third degree T24.729 ☑
labium (majus) (minus) — *see* Corrosion, genital organs, external, female
lacrimal apparatus, duct, gland or sac — *see* Corrosion, eye, specified site NEC

Corrosion — *continued*
larynx T27.4 ☑
  with lung T27.5 ☑
leg(s) (meaning lower limb(s)) — *see* Corrosion, lower limb
limb(s)
  lower — *see* Corrosion, lower, limb
  upper — *see* Corrosion, upper limb
lip(s) T20.42 ☑
  first degree T20.52 ☑
  second degree T20.62 ☑
  third degree T20.72 ☑
lower
  back — *see* Corrosion, back
  limb T24.409 ☑
    ankle — *see* Corrosion, ankle
    calf — *see* Corrosion, calf
    first degree T24.509 ☑
    foot — *see* Corrosion, foot
    knee — *see* Corrosion, knee
    left T24.402 ☑
      first degree T24.502 ☑
      second degree T24.602 ☑
      third degree T24.702 ☑
    multiple sites, except ankle and foot T24.499 ☑
      ankle and foot T25.499 ☑
        first degree T25.599 ☑
        left T25.492 ☑
          first degree T25.592 ☑
          second degree T25.692 ☑
          third degree T25.792 ☑
        right T25.491 ☑
          first degree T25.591 ☑
          second degree T25.691 ☑
          third degree T25.791 ☑
        second degree T25.699 ☑
        third degree T25.799 ☑
      first degree T24.599 ☑
      left T24.492 ☑
        first degree T24.592 ☑
        second degree T24.692 ☑
        third degree T24.792 ☑
      right T24.491 ☑
        first degree T24.591 ☑
        second degree T24.691 ☑
        third degree T24.791 ☑
      second degree T24.699 ☑
      third degree T24.799 ☑
    right T24.401 ☑
      first degree T24.501 ☑
      second degree T24.601 ☑
      third degree T24.701 ☑
    second degree T24.609 ☑
    thigh — *see* Corrosion, thigh
    third degree T24.709 ☑
lung (with larynx and trachea) T27.5 ☑
mouth T28.5 ☑
neck T20.47 ☑
  first degree T20.57 ☑
  second degree T20.67 ☑
  third degree T20.77 ☑
nose (septum) T20.44 ☑
  first degree T20.54 ☑
  second degree T20.64 ☑
  third degree T20.74 ☑
ocular adnexa — *see* Corrosion, eye
orbit region — *see* Corrosion, eyelid
palm T23.459 ☑
  first degree T23.559 ☑
  left T23.452 ☑
    first degree T23.552 ☑
    second degree T23.652 ☑
    third degree T23.752 ☑
  right T23.451 ☑
    first degree T23.551 ☑
    second degree T23.651 ☑
    third degree T23.751 ☑
  second degree T23.659 ☑
  third degree T23.759 ☑
partial thickness — *code as* Corrosion, unspecified degree, by site
pelvis — *see* Corrosion, trunk
penis — *see* Corrosion, genital organs, external, male
perineum
  female — *see* Corrosion, genital organs, external, female

Corrosion — *continued*
  perineum — *continued*
    male — *see* Corrosion, genital organs, external, male
  periocular area — *see* Corrosion, eyelid
  pharynx T28.5 ☑
  rectum T28.7 ☑
  respiratory tract T27.7 ☑
    larynx — *see* Corrosion, larynx
    specified part NEC T27.6 ☑
    trachea — *see* Corrosion, larynx
  sac, lacrimal — *see* Corrosion, eye, specified site NEC
  scalp T20.45 ☑
    first degree T20.55 ☑
    second degree T20.65 ☑
    third degree T20.75 ☑
  scapular region T22.469 ☑
    first degree T22.569 ☑
    left T22.462 ☑
      first degree T22.562 ☑
      second degree T22.662 ☑
      third degree T22.762 ☑
    right T22.461 ☑
      first degree T22.561 ☑
      second degree T22.661 ☑
      third degree T22.761 ☑
    second degree T22.669 ☑
    third degree T22.769 ☑
  sclera — *see* Corrosion, eye, specified site NEC
  scrotum — *see* Corrosion, genital organs, external, male
  shoulder T22.459 ☑
    first degree T22.559 ☑
    left T22.452 ☑
      first degree T22.552 ☑
      second degree T22.652 ☑
      third degree T22.752 ☑
    right T22.451 ☑
      first degree T22.551 ☑
      second degree T22.651 ☑
      third degree T22.751 ☑
    second degree T22.659 ☑
    third degree T22.759 ☑
  stomach T28.7 ☑
  temple — *see* Corrosion, head
  testis — *see* Corrosion, genital organs, external, male
  thigh T24.419 ☑
    first degree T24.519 ☑
    left T24.412 ☑
      first degree T24.512 ☑
      second degree T24.612 ☑
      third degree T24.712 ☑
    right T24.411 ☑
      first degree T24.511 ☑
      second degree T24.611 ☑
      third degree T24.711 ☑
    second degree T24.619 ☑
    third degree T24.719 ☑
  thorax (external) — *see* Corrosion, trunk
  throat (meaning pharynx) T28.5 ☑
  thumb(s) T23.419 ☑
    first degree T23.519 ☑
    left T23.412 ☑
      first degree T23.512 ☑
      second degree T23.612 ☑
      third degree T23.712 ☑
    multiple sites with fingers T23.449 ☑
      first degree T23.549 ☑
      left T23.442 ☑
        first degree T23.542 ☑
        second degree T23.642 ☑
        third degree T23.742 ☑
      right T23.441 ☑
        first degree T23.541 ☑
        second degree T23.641 ☑
        third degree T23.741 ☑
      second degree T23.649 ☑
      third degree T23.749 ☑
    right T23.411 ☑
      first degree T23.511 ☑
      second degree T23.611 ☑
      third degree T23.711 ☑
    second degree T23.619 ☑
    third degree T23.719 ☑
  toe T25.439 ☑
    first degree T25.539 ☑
    left T25.432 ☑

Corrosion — *continued*
  toe — *continued*
    left — *continued*
      first degree T25.532 ☑
      second degree T25.632 ☑
      third degree T25.732 ☑
    right T25.431 ☑
      first degree T25.531 ☑
      second degree T25.631 ☑
      third degree T25.731 ☑
    second degree T25.639 ☑
    third degree T25.739 ☑
  tongue T28.5 ☑
  tonsil(s) T28.5 ☑
  total body — *see* Corrosion, multiple body regions
  trachea T27.4 ☑
    with lung T27.5 ☑
  trunk T21.40 ☑
    abdominal wall — *see* Corrosion, abdominal wall
    anus — *see* Corrosion, buttock
    axilla — *see* Corrosion, upper limb
    back — *see* Corrosion, back
    breast — *see* Corrosion, chest wall
    buttock — *see* Corrosion, buttock
    chest wall — *see* Corrosion, chest wall
    first degree T21.50 ☑
    flank — *see* Corrosion, abdominal wall
    genital
      female — *see* Corrosion, genital organs, external, female
      male — *see* Corrosion, genital organs, external, male
    groin — *see* Corrosion, abdominal wall
    interscapular region — *see* Corrosion, back, upper
    labia — *see* Corrosion, genital organs, external, female
    lower back — *see* Corrosion, back
    penis — *see* Corrosion, genital organs, external, male
    perineum
      female — *see* Corrosion, genital organs, external, female
      male — *see* Corrosion, genital organs, external, male
    scapular region — *see* Corrosion, upper limb
    scrotum — *see* Corrosion, genital organs, external, male
    second degree T21.60 ☑
    shoulder — *see* Corrosion, upper limb
    specified site NEC T21.49 ☑
      first degree T21.59 ☑
      second degree T21.69 ☑
      third degree T21.79 ☑
    testes — *see* Corrosion, genital organs, external, male
    third degree T21.70 ☑
    upper back — *see* Corrosion, back, upper
    vagina T28.8 ☑
    vulva — *see* Corrosion, genital organs, external, female
  unspecified site with extent of body surface involved specified
    less than 10 percent T32.0
    10-19 percent (0-9 percent third degree) T32.10
      with 10-19 percent third degree T32.11
    20-29 percent (0-9 percent third degree) T32.20
      with
        10-19 percent third degree T32.21
        20-29 percent third degree T32.22
    30-39 percent (0-9 percent third degree) T32.30
      with
        10-19 percent third degree T32.31
        20-29 percent third degree T32.32
        30-39 percent third degree T32.33
    40-49 percent (0-9 percent third degree) T32.40
      with
        10-19 percent third degree T32.41
        20-29 percent third degree T32.42
        30-39 percent third degree T32.43
        40-49 percent third degree T32.44
    50-59 percent (0-9 percent third degree) T32.50
      with
        10-19 percent third degree T32.51
        20-29 percent third degree T32.52
        30-39 percent third degree T32.53
        40-49 percent third degree T32.54
        50-59 percent third degree T32.55

Corrosion — *continued*
  unspecified site with extent of body surface involved specified — *continued*
    60-69 percent (0-9 percent third degree) T32.60
      with
        10-19 percent third degree T32.61
        20-29 percent third degree T32.62
        30-39 percent third degree T32.63
        40-49 percent third degree T32.64
        50-59 percent third degree T32.65
        60-69 percent third degree T32.66
    70-79 percent (0-9 percent third degree) T32.70
      with
        10-19 percent third degree T32.71
        20-29 percent third degree T32.72
        30-39 percent third degree T32.73
        40-49 percent third degree T32.74
        50-59 percent third degree T32.75
        60-69 percent third degree T32.76
        70-79 percent third degree T32.77
    80-89 percent (0-9 percent third degree) T32.80
      with
        10-19 percent third degree T32.81
        20-29 percent third degree T32.82
        30-39 percent third degree T32.83
        40-49 percent third degree T32.84
        50-59 percent third degree T32.85
        60-69 percent third degree T32.86
        70-79 percent third degree T32.87
        80-89 percent third degree T32.88
    90 percent or more (0-9 percent third degree) T32.90
      with
        10-19 percent third degree T32.91
        20-29 percent third degree T32.92
        30-39 percent third degree T32.93
        40-49 percent third degree T32.94
        50-59 percent third degree T32.95
        60-69 percent third degree T32.96
        70-79 percent third degree T32.97
        80-89 percent third degree T32.98
        90-99 percent third degree T32.99
  upper limb (axilla) (scapular region) T22.40 ☑
    above elbow — *see* Corrosion, above elbow
    axilla — *see* Corrosion, axilla
    elbow — *see* Corrosion, elbow
    first degree T22.50 ☑
    forearm — *see* Corrosion, forearm
    hand — *see* Corrosion, hand
    interscapular region — *see* Corrosion, back, upper
    multiple sites T22.499 ☑
      first degree T22.599 ☑
      left T22.492 ☑
        first degree T22.592 ☑
        second degree T22.692 ☑
        third degree T22.792 ☑
      right T22.491 ☑
        first degree T22.591 ☑
        second degree T22.691 ☑
        third degree T22.791 ☑
      second degree T22.699 ☑
      third degree T22.799 ☑
    scapular region — *see* Corrosion, scapular region
    second degree T22.60 ☑
    shoulder — *see* Corrosion, shoulder
    third degree T22.70 ☑
    wrist — *see* Corrosion, hand
  uterus T28.8 ☑
  vagina T28.8 ☑
  vulva — *see* Corrosion, genital organs, external, female
  wrist T23.479 ☑
    first degree T23.579 ☑
    left T23.472 ☑
      first degree T23.572 ☑
      second degree T23.672 ☑
      third degree T23.772 ☑
    multiple sites with hand T23.499 ☑
      first degree T23.599 ☑
      left T23.492 ☑
        first degree T23.592 ☑
        second degree T23.692 ☑
        third degree T23.792 ☑
      right T23.491 ☑
        first degree T23.591 ☑
        second degree T23.691 ☑
        third degree T23.791 ☑
      second degree T23.699 ☑
      third degree T23.799 ☑

Corrosion — *continued*
 wrist — *continued*
  right T23.471 ☑
   first degree T23.571 ☑
   second degree T23.671 ☑
   third degree T23.771 ☑
  second degree T23.679 ☑
  third degree T23.779 ☑
Corrosive burn — *see* Corrosion
Corsican fever — *see* Malaria
Cortical — *see* condition
Cortico-adrenal — *see* condition
Coryza (acute) J00
 with grippe or influenza — *see* Influenza, with, respiratory manifestations NEC
 syphilitic
  congenital (chronic) A50.05
Costen's syndrome or complex M26.69
Costiveness — *see* Constipation
Costochondritis M94.0
Cot death R99
Cotard's syndrome F22
Cotia virus B08.8
Cotton wool spots (retinal) H35.81
Cotungo's disease — *see* Sciatica
Cough (affected) (chronic) (epidemic) (nervous) R05
 with hemorrhage — *see* Hemoptysis
 bronchial R05
  with grippe or influenza — *see* Influenza, with, respiratory manifestations NEC
 functional F45.8
 hysterical F45.8
 laryngeal, spasmodic R05
 psychogenic F45.8
 smokers' J41.0
 tea taster's B49
Counseling (for) Z71.9
 abuse NEC
  perpetrator Z69.82
  victim Z69.81
 alcohol abuser Z71.41
  family Z71.42
 child abuse
  nonparental
   perpetrator Z69.021
   victim Z69.020
  parental
   perpetrator Z69.011
   victim Z69.010
 consanguinity Z71.89
 contraceptive Z30.09
 dietary Z71.3
 drug abuser Z71.51
  family member Z71.52
 exercise Z71.82
 family Z71.89
 fertility preservation (prior to cancer therapy) (prior to removal of gonads) Z31.62
 for non-attending third party Z71.0
  related to sexual behavior or orientation Z70.2
 genetic
  nonprocreative Z71.83
  procreative NEC Z31.5
 gestational carrier Z31.7
 health (advice) (education) (instruction) — *see* Counseling, medical
  risk for travel (international) Z71.84
 human immunodeficiency virus (HIV) Z71.7
 impotence Z70.1
 insulin pump use Z46.81
 medical (for) Z71.9
  boarding school resident Z59.3
  consanguinity Z71.89
  feared complaint and no disease found Z71.1
  human immunodeficiency virus (HIV) Z71.7
  institutional resident Z59.3
  on behalf of another Z71.0
   related to sexual behavior or orientation Z70.2
  person living alone Z60.2
  specified reason NEC Z71.89
 natural family planning
  procreative Z31.61
  to avoid pregnancy Z30.02
 perpetrator (of)
  abuse NEC Z69.82
  child abuse
   non-parental Z69.021
   parental Z69.011

Counseling — *continued*
 perpetrator — *continued*
  rape NEC Z69.82
  spousal abuse Z69.12
 procreative NEC Z31.69
  fertility preservation (prior to cancer therapy) (prior to removal of gonads) Z31.62
  using natural family planning Z31.61
 promiscuity Z70.1
 rape victim Z69.81
 religious Z71.81
 safety for travel (international) Z71.84
 sex, sexual (related to) Z70.9
  attitude(s) Z70.0
  behavior or orientation Z70.1
  combined concerns Z70.3
  non-responsiveness Z70.1
  on behalf of third party Z70.2
  specified reason NEC Z70.8
 specified reason NEC Z71.89
 spiritual Z71.81
 spousal abuse (perpetrator) Z69.12
  victim Z69.11
 substance abuse Z71.89
  alcohol Z71.41
  drug Z71.51
  tobacco Z71.6
 tobacco use Z71.6
 travel (international) Z71.84
 use (of)
  insulin pump Z46.81
 victim (of)
  abuse Z69.81
  child abuse
   by parent Z69.010
   non-parental Z69.020
  rape NEC Z69.81
Coupled rhythm R00.8
Couvelaire syndrome or uterus (complicating delivery) O45.8X- ☑
Cowperitis — *see* Urethritis
Cowper's gland — *see* condition
Cowpox B08.010
 due to vaccination T88.1 ☑
Coxa
 magna M91.4- ☑
 plana M91.2- ☑
 valga (acquired) — *see also* Deformity, limb, specified type NEC, thigh
  congenital Q65.81
  sequelae (late effect) of rickets E64.3
 vara (acquired) — *see also* Deformity, limb, specified type NEC, thigh
  congenital Q65.82
  sequelae (late effect) of rickets E64.3
Coxalgia, coxalgic (nontuberculous) — *see also* Pain, joint, hip
 tuberculous A18.02
Coxitis — *see* Monoarthritis, hip
Coxsackie (virus) (infection) B34.1
 as cause of disease classified elsewhere B97.11
 carditis B33.20
 central nervous system NEC A88.8
 endocarditis B33.21
 enteritis A08.39
 meningitis (aseptic) A87.0
 myocarditis B33.22
 pericarditis B33.23
 pharyngitis B08.5
 pleurodynia B33.0
 specific disease NEC B33.8
Crabs, meaning pubic lice B85.3
Crack baby P04.41
Cracked nipple N64.0
 associated with
  lactation O92.13
  pregnancy O92.11- ☑
  puerperium O92.12
Cracked tooth K03.81
Cradle cap L21.0
Craft neurosis F48.8
Cramp(s) R25.2
 abdominal — *see* Pain, abdominal
 bathing T75.1 ☑
 colic R10.83
  psychogenic F45.8
 due to immersion T75.1 ☑
 fireman T67.2 ☑

Cramp(s) — *continued*
 heat T67.2 ☑
 immersion T75.1 ☑
 intestinal — *see* Pain, abdominal
  psychogenic F45.8
 leg, sleep related G47.62
 limb (lower) (upper) NEC R25.2
  sleep related G47.62
 linotypist's F48.8
  organic G25.89
 muscle (limb) (general) R25.2
  due to immersion T75.1 ☑
  psychogenic F45.8
 occupational (hand) F48.8
  organic G25.89
 salt-depletion E87.1
 sleep related, leg G47.62
 stoker's T67.2 ☑
 swimmer's T75.1 ☑
 telegrapher's F48.8
  organic G25.89
 typist's F48.8
  organic G25.89
 uterus N94.89
  menstrual — *see* Dysmenorrhea
 writer's F48.8
  organic G25.89
Cranial — *see* condition
Craniocleidodysostosis Q74.0
Craniofenestria (skull) Q75.8
Craniolacunia (skull) Q75.8
Craniopagus Q89.4
Craniopathy, metabolic M85.2
Craniopharyngeal — *see* condition
Craniopharyngioma D44.4
Craniorachischisis (totalis) Q00.1
Cranioschisis Q75.8
Craniostenosis Q75.0
Craniosynostosis Q75.0
Craniotabes (cause unknown) M83.8
 neonatal P96.3
 rachitic E64.3
 syphilitic A50.56
Cranium — *see* condition
Craw-craw — *see* Onchocerciasis
Creaking joint — *see* Derangement, joint, specified type NEC
Creeping
 eruption B76.9
 palsy or paralysis G12.22
Crenated tongue K14.8
Creotoxism A05.9
Crepitus
 caput Q75.8
 joint — *see* Derangement, joint, specified type NEC
Crescent or conus choroid, congenital Q14.3
CREST syndrome M34.1
Cretin, cretinism (congenital) (endemic) (nongoitrous) (sporadic) E00.9
 pelvis
  with disproportion (fetopelvic) O33.0
   causing obstructed labor O65.0
 type
  hypothyroid E00.1
  mixed E00.2
  myxedematous E00.0
  neurological E00.0
Creutzfeldt-Jakob disease or syndrome (with dementia) A81.00
 familial A81.09
 iatrogenic A81.09
 specified NEC A81.09
 sporadic A81.09
 variant (vCJD) A81.01
Crib death R99
Cribriform hymen Q52.3
Cri-du-chat syndrome Q93.4
Crigler-Najjar disease or syndrome E80.5
Crime, victim of Z65.4
Crimean hemorrhagic fever A98.0
Criminalism F60.2
Crisis
 abdomen R10.0
 acute reaction F43.0
 addisonian E27.2
 adrenal (cortical) E27.2
 celiac K90.0

Crisis — *continued*
  Dietl's N13.8
  emotional — *see also* Disorder, adjustment
    acute reaction to stress F43.0
    specific to childhood and adolescence F93.8
  glaucomatocyclitic — *see* Glaucoma, secondary, inflammation
  heart — *see* Failure, heart
  nitritoid I95.2
    correct substance properly administered — *see* Table of Drugs and Chemicals, by drug, adverse effect
    overdose or wrong substance given or taken — *see* Table of Drugs and Chemicals, by drug, poisoning
  oculogyric H51.8
    psychogenic F45.8
  Pel's (tabetic) A52.11
  psychosexual identity F64.2
  renal N28.0
  sickle-cell D57.00
    with
      acute chest syndrome D57.01
      cerebral vascular involvement D57.03
      crisis (painful) D57.00
        with complication specified NEC D57.09
      splenic sequestration D57.02
      vasoocclusive pain D57.00
  state (acute reaction) F43.0
  tabetic A52.11
  thyroid — *see* Thyrotoxicosis with thyroid storm
  thyrotoxic — *see* Thyrotoxicosis with thyroid storm
Crocq's disease (acrocyanosis) I73.89
Crohn's disease — *see* Enteritis, regional
Crooked septum, nasal J34.2
Cross syndrome E70.328
Crossbite (anterior) (posterior) M26.24
Cross-eye — *see* Strabismus, convergent concomitant
Croup, croupous (catarrhal) (infectious) (inflammatory) (nondiphtheritic) J05.0
  bronchial J20.9
  diphtheritic A36.2
  false J38.5
  spasmodic J38.5
    diphtheritic A36.2
  stridulous J38.5
    diphtheritic A36.2
Crouzon's disease Q75.1
Crowding, tooth, teeth, fully erupted M26.31
CRST syndrome M34.1
Cruchet's disease A85.8
Cruelty in children — *see also* Disorder, conduct
Crural ulcer — *see* Ulcer, lower limb
Crush, crushed, crushing T14.8 ☑
  abdomen S38.1 ☑
  ankle S97.0- ☑
  arm (upper) (and shoulder) S47.- ☑
  axilla — *see* Crush, arm
  back, lower S38.1 ☑
  buttock S38.1 ☑
  cheek S07.0 ☑
  chest S28.0 ☑
  cranium S07.1 ☑
  ear S07.0 ☑
  elbow S57.0- ☑
  extremity
    lower
      ankle — *see* Crush, ankle
      below knee — *see* Crush, leg
      foot — *see* Crush, foot
      hip — *see* Crush, hip
      knee — *see* Crush, knee
      thigh — *see* Crush, thigh
      toe — *see* Crush, toe
    upper
      below elbow S67.9- ☑
      elbow — *see* Crush, elbow
      finger — *see* Crush, finger
      forearm — *see* Crush, forearm
      hand — *see* Crush, hand
      thumb — *see* Crush, thumb
      upper arm — *see* Crush, arm
      wrist — *see* Crush, wrist
  face S07.0 ☑
  finger(s) S67.1- ☑
    with hand (and wrist) — *see* Crush, hand, specified site NEC

Crush, crushed, crushing — *continued*
  finger(s) — *continued*
    index S67.19- ☑
    little S67.19- ☑
    middle S67.19- ☑
    ring S67.19- ☑
    thumb — *see* Crush, thumb
  foot S97.8- ☑
    toe — *see* Crush, toe
  forearm S57.8- ☑
  genitalia, external
    female S38.002 ☑
      vagina S38.03 ☑
      vulva S38.03 ☑
    male S38.001 ☑
      penis S38.01 ☑
      scrotum S38.02 ☑
      testis S38.02 ☑
  hand (except fingers alone) S67.2- ☑
    with wrist S67.4- ☑
  head S07.9 ☑
    specified NEC S07.8 ☑
  heel — *see* Crush, foot
  hip S77.0- ☑
    with thigh S77.2- ☑
  internal organ (abdomen, chest, or pelvis) NEC T14.8 ☑
  knee S87.0- ☑
  labium (majus) (minus) S38.03 ☑
  larynx S17.0 ☑
  leg (lower) S87.8- ☑
    knee — *see* Crush, knee
  lip S07.0 ☑
  lower
    back S38.1 ☑
    leg — *see* Crush, leg
  neck S17.9 ☑
  nerve — *see* Injury, nerve
  nose S07.0 ☑
  pelvis S38.1 ☑
  penis S38.01 ☑
  scalp S07.8 ☑
  scapular region — *see* Crush, arm
  scrotum S38.02 ☑
  severe, unspecified site T14.8 ☑
  shoulder (and upper arm) — *see* Crush, arm
  skull S07.1 ☑
  syndrome (complication of trauma) T79.5 ☑
  testis S38.02 ☑
  thigh S77.1- ☑
    with hip S77.2- ☑
  throat S17.8 ☑
  thumb S67.0- ☑
    with hand (and wrist) — *see* Crush, hand, specified site NEC
  toe(s) S97.10- ☑
    great S97.11- ☑
    lesser S97.12- ☑
  trachea S17.0 ☑
  vagina S38.03 ☑
  vulva S38.03 ☑
  wrist S67.3- ☑
    with hand S67.4- ☑
Crusta lactea L21.0
Crusts R23.4
Crutch paralysis — *see* Injury, brachial plexus
Cruveilhier-Baumgarten cirrhosis, disease or syndrome K74.69
Cruveilhier's atrophy or disease G12.8
Crying (constant) (continuous) (excessive)
  child, adolescent, or adult R45.83
  infant (baby) (newborn) R68.11
Cryofibrinogenemia D89.2
Cryoglobulinemia (essential) (idiopathic) (mixed) (primary) (purpura) (secondary) (vasculitis) D89.1
  with lung involvement D89.1 *[J99]*
Cryptitis (anal) (rectal) K62.89
Cryptococcosis, cryptococcus (infection) (neoformans) B45.9
  bone B45.3
  cerebral B45.1
  cutaneous B45.2
  disseminated B45.7
  generalized B45.7
  meningitis B45.1
  meningocerebralis B45.1
  osseous B45.3

Cryptococcosis, cryptococcus — *continued*
  pulmonary B45.0
  skin B45.2
  specified NEC B45.8
Cryptopapillitis (anus) K62.89
Cryptophthalmos Q11.2
  syndrome Q87.0
Cryptorchid, cryptorchism, cryptorchidism Q53.9
  bilateral Q53.20
    abdominal Q53.211
    perineal Q53.22
  unilateral Q53.10
    abdominal Q53.111
    perineal Q53.12
Cryptosporidiosis A07.2
  hepatobiliary B88.8
  respiratory B88.8
Cryptostromosis J67.6
Crystalluria R82.998
Cubitus
  congenital Q68.8
  valgus (acquired) M21.0- ☑
    congenital Q68.8
    sequelae (late effect) of rickets E64.3
  varus (acquired) M21.1- ☑
    congenital Q68.8
    sequelae (late effect) of rickets E64.3
Cultural deprivation or shock Z60.3
Curling esophagus K22.4
Curling's ulcer — *see* Ulcer, peptic, acute
Curschmann (-Batten) (-Steinert) **disease or syndrome** G71.11
Curse, Ondine's — *see* Apnea, sleep
Curvature
  organ or site, congenital NEC — *see* Distortion
  penis (lateral) Q55.61
  Pott's (spinal) A18.01
  radius, idiopathic, progressive (congenital) Q74.0
  spine (acquired) (angular) (idiopathic) (incorrect) (postural) — *see* Dorsopathy, deforming
    congenital Q67.5
    due to or associated with
      Charcot-Marie-Tooth disease — *see also* subcategory M49.8 G60.0
      osteitis
        deformans M88.88
        fibrosa cystica — *see also* subcategory M49.8 E21.0
      tuberculosis (Pott's curvature) A18.01
    sequelae (late effect) of rickets E64.3
    tuberculous A18.01
Cushingoid due to steroid therapy E24.2
  correct substance properly administered — *see* Table of Drugs and Chemicals, by drug, adverse effect
  overdose or wrong substance given or taken — *see* Table of Drugs and Chemicals, by drug, poisoning
Cushing's
  syndrome or disease E24.9
    drug-induced E24.2
    iatrogenic E24.2
    pituitary-dependent E24.0
    specified NEC E24.8
  ulcer — *see* Ulcer, peptic, acute
Cusp, Carabelli — *omit code*
Cut (external) — *see also* Laceration
  muscle — *see* Injury, muscle
Cutaneous — *see also* condition
  hemorrhage R23.3
  larva migrans B76.9
Cutis — *see also* condition
  hyperelastica Q82.8
    acquired L57.4
  laxa (hyperelastica) — *see* Dermatolysis
  marmorata R23.8
  osteosis L94.2
  pendula — *see* Dermatolysis
  rhomboidalis nuchae L57.2
  verticis gyrata Q82.8
    acquired L91.8
Cyanosis R23.0
  due to
    patent foramen botalli Q21.1
    persistent foramen ovale Q21.1
  enterogenous D74.8
  paroxysmal digital — *see* Raynaud's disease
    with gangrene I73.01
  retina, retinal H35.89
Cyanotic heart disease I24.9

Cyanotic heart disease — *continued*
congenital Q24.9
Cycle
anovulatory N97.0
menstrual, irregular N92.6
Cyclencephaly Q04.9
Cyclical vomiting, in migraine — *see also* Vomiting, cyclical G43.A0 (*following* G43.7)
psychogenic F50.89
Cyclitis — *see also* Iridocyclitis H20.9
chronic — *see* Iridocyclitis, chronic
Fuchs' heterochromic H20.81- ☑
granulomatous — *see* Iridocyclitis, chronic
lens-induced — *see* Iridocyclitis, lens-induced
posterior H30.2- ☑
Cycloid personality F34.0
Cyclophoria H50.54
Cyclopia, cyclops Q87.0
Cyclopism Q87.0
Cyclosporiasis A07.4
Cyclothymia F34.0
Cyclothymic personality F34.0
Cyclotropia H50.41- ☑
Cylindroma — *see also* Neoplasm, malignant, by site
eccrine dermal — *see* Neoplasm, skin, benign
skin — *see* Neoplasm, skin, benign
Cylindruria R82.998
Cynanche
diphtheritic A36.2
tonsillaris J36
Cynophobia F40.218
Cynorexia R63.2
Cyphosis — *see* Kyphosis
Cyprus fever — *see* Brucellosis
Cyst (colloid) (mucous) (simple) (retention)
adenoid (infected) J35.8
adrenal gland E27.8
congenital Q89.1
air, lung J98.4
allantoic Q64.4
alveolar process (jaw bone) M27.40
amnion, amniotic O41.8X- ☑
aneurysmal M27.49
anterior
chamber (eye) — *see* Cyst, iris
nasopalatine K09.1
antrum J34.1
anus K62.89
apical (tooth) (periodontal) K04.8
appendix K38.8
arachnoid, brain (acquired) G93.0
congenital Q04.6
arytenoid J38.7
Baker's M71.2- ☑
ruptured M66.0
tuberculous A18.02
Bartholin's gland N75.0
bile duct (common) (hepatic) K83.5
bladder (multiple) (trigone) N32.89
blue dome (breast) — *see* Cyst, breast
bone (local) NEC M85.60
aneurysmal M85.50
ankle M85.57- ☑
foot M85.57- ☑
forearm M85.53- ☑
hand M85.54- ☑
jaw M27.49
lower leg M85.56- ☑
multiple site M85.59
neck M85.58
rib M85.58
shoulder M85.51- ☑
skull M85.58
specified site NEC M85.58
thigh M85.55- ☑
toe M85.57- ☑
upper arm M85.52- ☑
vertebra M85.58
solitary M85.40
ankle M85.47- ☑
fibula M85.46- ☑
foot M85.47- ☑
hand M85.44- ☑
humerus M85.42- ☑
jaw M27.49
neck M85.48
pelvis M85.45- ☑

Cyst — *continued*
bone — *continued*
solitary — *continued*
radius M85.43- ☑
rib M85.48
shoulder M85.41- ☑
skull M85.48
specified site NEC M85.48
tibia M85.46- ☑
toe M85.47- ☑
ulna M85.43- ☑
vertebra M85.48
specified type NEC M85.60
ankle M85.67- ☑
foot M85.67- ☑
forearm M85.63- ☑
hand M85.64- ☑
jaw M27.40
developmental (nonodontogenic) K09.1
odontogenic K09.0
latent M27.0
lower leg M85.66- ☑
multiple site M85.69
neck M85.68
rib M85.68
shoulder M85.61- ☑
skull M85.68
specified site NEC M85.68
thigh M85.65- ☑
toe M85.67- ☑
upper arm M85.62- ☑
vertebra M85.68
brain (acquired) G93.0
congenital Q04.6
hydatid B67.99 *[G94]*
third ventricle (colloid), congenital Q04.6
branchial (cleft) Q18.0
branchiogenic Q18.0
breast (benign) (blue dome) (pedunculated) (solitary) N60.0- ☑
involution — *see* Dysplasia, mammary, specified type NEC
sebaceous — *see* Dysplasia, mammary, specified type NEC
broad ligament (benign) N83.8
bronchogenic (mediastinal) (sequestration) J98.4
congenital Q33.0
buccal K09.8
bulbourethral gland N36.8
bursa, bursal NEC M71.30
with rupture — *see* Rupture, synovium
ankle M71.37- ☑
elbow M71.32- ☑
foot M71.37- ☑
hand M71.34- ☑
hip M71.35- ☑
multiple sites M71.39
pharyngeal J39.2
popliteal space — *see* Cyst, Baker's
shoulder M71.31- ☑
specified site NEC M71.38
wrist M71.33- ☑
calcifying odontogenic D16.5
upper jaw (bone) (maxilla) D16.4
canal of Nuck (female) N94.89
congenital Q52.4
canthus — *see* Cyst, conjunctiva
carcinomatous — *see* Neoplasm, malignant, by site
cauda equina G95.89
cavum septi pellucidi — *see* Cyst, brain
celomic (pericardium) Q24.8
cerebellopontine (angle) — *see* Cyst, brain
cerebellum — *see* Cyst, brain
cerebral — *see* Cyst, brain
cervical lateral Q18.0
cervix NEC N88.8
embryonic Q51.6
nabothian N88.8
chiasmal optic NEC — *see* Disorder, optic, chiasm
chocolate (ovary) N80.1
choledochus, congenital Q44.4
chorion O41.8X- ☑
choroid plexus G93.0
congenital Q04.6
ciliary body — *see* Cyst, iris
clitoris N90.7
colon K63.89

Cyst — *continued*
common (bile) duct K83.5
congenital NEC Q89.8
adrenal gland Q89.1
epiglottis Q31.8
esophagus Q39.8
fallopian tube Q50.4
kidney Q61.00
more than one (multiple) Q61.02
specified as polycystic Q61.3
adult type Q61.2
infantile type NEC Q61.19
collecting duct dilation Q61.11
solitary Q61.01
larynx Q31.8
liver Q44.6
lung Q33.0
mediastinum Q34.1
ovary Q50.1
oviduct Q50.4
periurethral (tissue) Q64.79
prepuce Q55.69
salivary gland (any) Q38.4
sublingual Q38.6
submaxillary gland Q38.6
thymus (gland) Q89.2
tongue Q38.3
ureterovesical orifice Q62.8
vulva Q52.79
conjunctiva H11.44- ☑
cornea H18.89- ☑
corpora quadrigemina G93.0
corpus
albicans N83.29- ☑
luteum (hemorrhagic) (ruptured) N83.1- ☑
Cowper's gland (benign) (infected) N36.8
cranial meninges G93.0
craniobuccal pouch E23.6
craniopharyngeal pouch E23.6
cystic duct K82.8
Cysticercus — *see* Cysticercosis
Dandy-Walker Q03.1
with spina bifida — *see* Spina bifida
dental (root) K04.8
developmental K09.0
eruption K09.0
primordial K09.0
dentigerous (mandible) (maxilla) K09.0
dermoid — *see* Neoplasm, benign, by site
with malignant transformation C56.- ☑
implantation
external area or site (skin) NEC L72.0
iris — *see* Cyst, iris, implantation
vagina N89.8
vulva N90.7
mouth K09.8
oral soft tissue K09.8
sacrococcygeal — *see* Cyst, pilonidal
developmental K09.1
odontogenic K09.0
oral region (nonodontogenic) K09.1
ovary, ovarian Q50.1
dura (cerebral) G93.0
spinal G96.198
ear (external) Q18.1
echinococcal — *see* Echinococcus
embryonic
cervix uteri Q51.6
fallopian tube Q50.4
vagina Q52.4
endometrium, endometrial (uterus) N85.8
ectopic — *see* Endometriosis
enterogenous Q43.8
epidermal, epidermoid (inclusion) (*see also* Cyst, skin) L72.0
mouth K09.8
oral soft tissue K09.8
epididymis N50.3
epiglottis J38.7
epiphysis cerebri E34.8
epithelial (inclusion) L72.0
epoophoron Q50.5
eruption K09.0
esophagus K22.8
ethmoid sinus J34.1
external female genital organs NEC N90.7
eyelid (sebaceous) H02.829
infected — *see* Hordeolum

☑ **Additional Character Required** — Refer to the Tabular List for Character Selection   ▽ Subterms under main terms may continue to next column or page

Cyst — *continued*
  eyelid — *continued*
    left H02.826
      lower H02.825
      upper H02.824
    right H02.823
      lower H02.822
      upper H02.821
  eye NEC H57.89
    congenital Q15.8
  fallopian tube N83.8
    congenital Q50.4
  fimbrial (twisted) Q50.4
  fissural (oral region) K09.1
  follicle (graafian) (hemorrhagic) N83.0- ☑
    nabothian N88.8
  follicular (atretic) (hemorrhagic) (ovarian) N83.0- ☑
    dentigerous K09.0
    odontogenic K09.0
    skin L72.9
      specified NEC L72.8
  frontal sinus J34.1
  gallbladder K82.8
  ganglion — *see* Ganglion
  Gartner's duct Q52.4
  gingiva K09.0
  gland of Moll — *see* Cyst, eyelid
  globulomaxillary K09.1
  graafian follicle (hemorrhagic) N83.0- ☑
  granulosal lutein (hemorrhagic) N83.1- ☑
  hemangiomatous D18.00
    intra-abdominal D18.03
    intracranial D18.02
    skin D18.01
    specified site NEC D18.09
  hemorrhagic M27.49
  hydatid — *see also* Echinococcus B67.90
    brain B67.99 *[G94]*
    liver — *see also* Cyst, liver, hydatid B67.8
    lung NEC B67.99 *[J99]*
    Morgagni
      female Q50.5
      male (epididymal) Q55.4
        testicular Q55.29
    specified site NEC B67.99
  hymen N89.8
    embryonic Q52.4
  hypopharynx J39.2
  hypophysis, hypophyseal (duct) (recurrent) E23.6
    cerebri E23.6
  implantation (dermoid)
    external area or site (skin) NEC L72.0
    iris — *see* Cyst, iris, implantation
    vagina N89.8
    vulva N90.7
  incisive canal K09.1
  inclusion (epidermal) (epithelial) (epidermoid) (squamous) L72.0
    not of skin — *code under* Cyst, by site
  intestine (large) (small) K63.89
  intracranial — *see* Cyst, brain
  intraligamentous — *see also* Disorder, ligament
    knee — *see* Derangement, knee
  intrasellar E23.6
  iris H21.309
    exudative H21.31- ☑
    idiopathic H21.30- ☑
    implantation H21.32- ☑
    parasitic H21.33- ☑
    pars plana (primary) H21.34- ☑
      exudative H21.35- ☑
  jaw (bone) M27.40
    aneurysmal M27.49
    developmental (odontogenic) K09.0
    fissural K09.1
    hemorrhagic M27.49
    traumatic M27.49
  joint NEC — *see* Disorder, joint, specified type NEC
  kidney (acquired) N28.1
    calyceal — *see* Hydronephrosis
    congenital Q61.00
    more than one (multiple) Q61.02
      specified as polycystic Q61.3
        adult type (autosomal dominant) Q61.2
        infantile type (autosomal recessive) NEC Q61.19
          collecting duct dilation Q61.11
    pyelogenic — *see* Hydronephrosis

Cyst — *continued*
  kidney — *continued*
    simple N28.1
    solitary (single) Q61.01
      acquired N28.1
  labium (majus) (minus) N90.7
    sebaceous N90.7
  lacrimal — *see also* Disorder, lacrimal system, specified NEC
    gland H04.13- ☑
    passages or sac — *see* Disorder, lacrimal system, specified NEC
  larynx J38.7
  lateral periodontal K09.0
  lens H27.8
    congenital Q12.8
  lip (gland) K13.0
  liver (idiopathic) (simple) K76.89
    congenital Q44.6
    hydatid B67.8
      granulosus B67.0
      multilocularis B67.5
  lung J98.4
    congenital Q33.0
    giant bullous J43.9
  lutein N83.1- ☑
  lymphangiomatous D18.1
  lymphoepithelial, oral soft tissue K09.8
  macula — *see* Degeneration, macula, hole
  malignant — *see* Neoplasm, malignant, by site
  mammary gland — *see* Cyst, breast
  mandible M27.40
    dentigerous K09.0
    radicular K04.8
  maxilla M27.40
    dentigerous K09.0
    radicular K04.8
  medial, face and neck Q18.8
  median
    anterior maxillary K09.1
    palatal K09.1
  mediastinum, congenital Q34.1
  meibomian (gland) — *see* Chalazion
    infected — *see* Hordeolum
  membrane, brain G93.0
  meninges (cerebral) G93.0
    spinal G96.198
  meniscus, knee — *see* Derangement, knee, meniscus, cystic
  mesentery, mesenteric K66.8
    chyle I89.8
  mesonephric duct
    female Q50.5
    male Q55.4
  milk N64.89
  Morgagni (hydatid)
    female Q50.5
    male (epididymal) Q55.4
      testicular Q55.29
  mouth K09.8
  Müllerian duct Q50.4
    appendix testis Q55.29
    cervix Q51.6
    fallopian tube Q50.4
    female Q50.4
    male Q55.29
    prostatic utricle Q55.4
    vagina (embryonal) Q52.4
  multilocular (ovary) D39.10
    benign — *see* Neoplasm, benign, by site
  myometrium N85.8
  nabothian (follicle) (ruptured) N88.8
  nasoalveolar N09.1
  nasolabial K09.1
  nasopalatine (anterior) (duct) K09.1
  nasopharynx J39.2
  neoplastic — *see* Neoplasm, uncertain behavior, by site
    benign — *see* Neoplasm, benign, by site
  nerve root
    cervical G96.191
    lumbar G96.191
    sacral G96.191
    thoracic G96.191
  nervous system NEC G96.89
  neuroenteric (congenital) Q06.8
  nipple — *see* Cyst, breast
  nose (turbinates) J34.1

Cyst — *continued*
  nose — *continued*
    sinus J34.1
  odontogenic, developmental K09.0
  omentum (lesser) K66.8
    congenital Q45.8
  ora serrata — *see* Cyst, retina, ora serrata
  oral
    region K09.9
      developmental (nonodontogenic) K09.1
      specified NEC K09.8
    soft tissue K09.9
      specified NEC K09.8
  orbit H05.81- ☑
  ovary, ovarian (twisted) N83.20- ☑
    adherent N83.20- ☑
    chocolate N80.1
    corpus
      albicans N83.29- ☑
      luteum (hemorrhagic) N83.1- ☑
    dermoid D27.9
    developmental Q50.1
    due to failure of involution NEC N83.20- ☑
    endometrial N80.1
    follicular (graafian) (hemorrhagic) N83.0- ☑
    hemorrhagic N83.20- ☑
    in pregnancy or childbirth O34.8- ☑
      with obstructed labor O65.5
    multilocular D39.10
    pseudomucinous D27.9
    retention N83.29- ☑
    serous N83.20- ☑
    specified NEC N83.29- ☑
    theca lutein (hemorrhagic) N83.1- ☑
    tuberculous A18.18
  oviduct N83.8
  palate (median) (fissural) K09.1
  palatine papilla (jaw) K09.1
  pancreas, pancreatic (hemorrhagic) (true) K86.2
    congenital Q45.2
    false K86.3
  paralabral
    hip M24.85- ☑
    shoulder S43.43- ☑
  paramesonephric duct Q50.4
    female Q50.4
    male Q55.29
  paranephric N28.1
  paraphysis, cerebri, congenital Q04.6
  parasitic B89
  parathyroid (gland) E21.4
  paratubal N83.8
  paraurethral duct N36.8
  paroophoron Q50.5
  parotid gland K11.6
  parovarian Q50.5
  pelvis, female N94.89
    in pregnancy or childbirth O34.8- ☑
      causing obstructed labor O65.5
  penis (sebaceous) N48.89
  periapical K04.8
  pericardial (congenital) Q24.8
    acquired (secondary) I31.8
  pericoronal K09.0
  perineural G96.191
  periodontal K04.8
    lateral K09.0
  peripelvic (lymphatic) N28.1
  peritoneum K66.8
    chylous I89.8
  periventricular, acquired, newborn P91.1
  pharynx (wall) J39.2
  pilar L72.11
  pilonidal (infected) (rectum) L05.91
    with abscess L05.01
    malignant C44.59- ☑
  pituitary (duct) (gland) E23.6
  placenta O43.19- ☑
  pleura J94.8
  popliteal — *see* Cyst, Baker's
  porencephalic Q04.6
    acquired G93.0
  postanal (infected) — *see* Cyst, pilonidal
  postmastoidectomy cavity (mucosal) — *see* Complications, postmastoidectomy, cyst
  preauricular Q18.1
  prepuce N47.4
    congenital Q55.69

Cyst — *continued*
  primordial (jaw) K09.0
  prostate N42.83
  pseudomucinous (ovary) D27.9
  pupillary, miotic H21.27- ☑
  radicular (residual) K04.8
  radiculodental K04.8
  ranular K11.8
  Rathke's pouch E23.6
  rectum (epithelium) (mucous) K62.89
  renal — *see* Cyst, kidney
  residual (radicular) K04.8
  retention (ovary) N83.29- ☑
    salivary gland K11.6
  retina H33.19- ☑
    ora serrata H33.11- ☑
    parasitic H33.12- ☑
  retroperitoneal K68.9
  sacrococcygeal (dermoid) — *see* Cyst, pilonidal
  salivary gland or duct (mucous extravasation or retention) K11.6
  Sampson's N80.1
  sclera H15.89
  scrotum L72.9
    sebaceous L72.3
  sebaceous (duct) (gland) L72.3
    breast — *see* Dysplasia, mammary, specified type NEC
    eyelid — *see* Cyst, eyelid
    genital organ NEC
      female N94.89
      male N50.89
    scrotum L72.3
  semilunar cartilage (knee) (multiple) — *see* Derangement, knee, meniscus, cystic
  seminal vesicle N50.89
  serous (ovary) N83.20- ☑
  sinus (accessory) (nasal) J34.1
  Skene's gland N36.8
  skin L72.9
    breast — *see* Dysplasia, mammary, specified type NEC
    epidermal, epidermoid L72.0
    epithelial L72.0
    eyelid — *see* Cyst, eyelid
    genital organ NEC
      female N90.7
      male N50.89
    inclusion L72.0
    scrotum L72.9
    sebaceous L72.3
    sweat gland or duct L74.8
  solitary
    bone — *see* Cyst, bone, solitary
    jaw M27.40
    kidney N28.1
  spermatic cord N50.89
  sphenoid sinus J34.1
  spinal meninges G96.198
  spleen NEC D73.4
    congenital Q89.09
    hydatid — *see also* Echinococcus B67.99 *[D77]*
  Stafne's M27.0
  subarachnoid intrasellar R93.0
  subcutaneous, pheomycotic (chromomycotic) B43.2
  subdural (cerebral) G93.0
    spinal cord G96.198
  sublingual gland K11.6
  submandibular gland K11.6
  submaxillary gland K11.6
  suburethral N36.8
  suprarenal gland E27.8
  suprasellar — *see* Cyst, brain
  sweat gland or duct L74.8
  synovial — *see also* Cyst, bursa
    ruptured — *see* Rupture, synovium
  Tarlov G96.191
  tarsal — *see* Chalazion
  tendon (sheath) — *see* Disorder, tendon, specified type NEC
  testis N44.2
    tunica albuginea N44.1
  theca lutein (ovary) N83.1- ☑
  Thornwaldt's J39.2
  thymus (gland) E32.8
  thyroglossal duct (infected) (persistent) Q89.2
  thyroid (gland) E04.1
  thyrolingual duct (infected) (persistent) Q89.2

Cyst — *continued*
  tongue K14.8
  tonsil J35.8
  tooth — *see* Cyst, dental
  Tornwaldt's J39.2
  trichilemmal (proliferating) L72.12
  trichodermal L72.12
  tubal (fallopian) N83.8
    inflammatory — *see* Salpingitis, chronic
  tubo-ovarian N83.8
    inflammatory N70.13
  tunica
    albuginea testis N44.1
    vaginalis N50.89
  turbinate (nose) J34.1
  Tyson's gland N48.89
  urachus, congenital Q64.4
  ureter N28.89
  ureterovesical orifice N28.89
  urethra, urethral (gland) N36.8
  uterine ligament N83.8
  uterus (body) (corpus) (recurrent) N85.8
    embryonic Q51.818
      cervix Q51.6
  vagina, vaginal (implantation) (inclusion) (squamous cell) (wall) N89.8
    embryonic Q52.4
  vallecula, vallecular (epiglottis) J38.7
  vesical (orifice) N32.89
  vitreous body H43.89
  vulva (implantation) (inclusion) N90.7
    congenital Q52.79
    sebaceous gland N90.7
  vulvovaginal gland N90.7
  wolffian
    female Q50.5
    male Q55.4

Cystadenocarcinoma — *see* Neoplasm, malignant, by site
  bile duct C22.1
  endometrioid — *see* Neoplasm, malignant, by site
    specified site — *see* Neoplasm, malignant, by site
    unspecified site
      female C56.9
      male C61
  mucinous
    papillary
      specified site — *see* Neoplasm, malignant, by site
      unspecified site C56.9
    specified site — *see* Neoplasm, malignant, by site
    unspecified site C56.9
  papillary
    mucinous
      specified site — *see* Neoplasm, malignant, by site
      unspecified site C56.9
    pseudomucinous
      specified site — *see* Neoplasm, malignant, by site
      unspecified site C56.9
    serous
      specified site — *see* Neoplasm, malignant, by site
      unspecified site C56.9
    specified site — *see* Neoplasm, malignant, by site
    unspecified site C56.9
  pseudomucinous
    papillary
      specified site — *see* Neoplasm, malignant, by site
      unspecified site C56.9
    specified site — *see* Neoplasm, malignant, by site
    unspecified site C56.9
  serous
    papillary
      specified site — *see* Neoplasm, malignant, by site
      unspecified site C56.9
    specified site — *see* Neoplasm, malignant, by site
    unspecified site C56.9

Cystadenofibroma
  clear cell — *see* Neoplasm, benign, by site
  endometrioid D27.9
    borderline malignancy D39.1- ☑
    malignant C56.- ☑
  mucinous
    specified site — *see* Neoplasm, benign, by site

Cystadenofibroma — *continued*
  mucinous — *continued*
    unspecified site D27.9
  serous
    specified site — *see* Neoplasm, benign, by site
    unspecified site D27.9
  specified site — *see* Neoplasm, benign, by site
  unspecified site D27.9

Cystadenoma — *see also* Neoplasm, benign, by site
  bile duct D13.4
  endometrioid — *see* Neoplasm, benign, by site
    borderline malignancy — *see* Neoplasm, uncertain behavior, by site
  malignant — *see* Neoplasm, malignant, by site
  mucinous
    borderline malignancy
      ovary C56.- ☑
      specified site NEC — *see* Neoplasm, uncertain behavior, by site
      unspecified site C56.9
    papillary
      borderline malignancy
        ovary C56.- ☑
        specified site NEC — *see* Neoplasm, uncertain behavior, by site
        unspecified site C56.9
      specified site — *see* Neoplasm, benign, by site
      unspecified site D27.9
    specified site — *see* Neoplasm, benign, by site
    unspecified site D27.9
  papillary
    borderline malignancy
      ovary C56.- ☑
      specified site NEC — *see* Neoplasm, uncertain behavior, by site
      unspecified site C56.9
    lymphomatosum
      specified site — *see* Neoplasm, benign, by site
      unspecified site D11.9
    mucinous
      borderline malignancy
        ovary C56.- ☑
        specified site NEC — *see* Neoplasm, uncertain behavior, by site
        unspecified site C56.9
      specified site — *see* Neoplasm, benign, by site
      unspecified site D27.9
    pseudomucinous
      borderline malignancy
        ovary C56.- ☑
        specified site NEC — *see* Neoplasm, uncertain behavior, by site
        unspecified site C56.9
      specified site — *see* Neoplasm, benign, by site
      unspecified site D27.9
    serous
      borderline malignancy
        ovary C56.- ☑
        specified site NEC — *see* Neoplasm, uncertain behavior, by site
        unspecified site C56.9
      specified site — *see* Neoplasm, benign, by site
      unspecified site D27.9
    specified site — *see* Neoplasm, benign, by site
    unspecified site D27.9
  pseudomucinous
    borderline malignancy
      ovary C56.- ☑
      specified site NEC — *see* Neoplasm, uncertain behavior, by site
      unspecified site C56.9
    papillary
      borderline malignancy
        ovary C56.- ☑
        specified site NEC — *see* Neoplasm, uncertain behavior, by site
        unspecified site C56.9
      specified site — *see* Neoplasm, benign, by site
      unspecified site D27.9
    specified site — *see* Neoplasm, benign, by site
    unspecified site D27.9
  serous
    borderline malignancy
      ovary C56.- ☑
      specified site NEC — *see* Neoplasm, uncertain behavior, by site
      unspecified site C56.9

Cystadenoma — *continued*
  serous — *continued*
    papillary
      borderline malignancy
        ovary C56.- ☑
        specified site NEC — *see* Neoplasm, uncertain behavior, by site
        unspecified site C56.9
      specified site — *see* Neoplasm, benign, by site
      unspecified site D27.9
    specified site — *see* Neoplasm, benign, by site
    unspecified site D27.9
Cystathionine synthase deficiency E72.11
Cystathioninemia E72.19
Cystathioninuria E72.19
Cystic — *see also* condition
  breast (chronic) — *see* Mastopathy, cystic
  corpora lutea (hemorrhagic) N83.1- ☑
  duct — *see* condition
  eyeball (congenital) Q11.0
  fibrosis — *see* Fibrosis, cystic
  kidney (congenital) Q61.9
    adult type Q61.2
    infantile type NEC Q61.19
      collecting duct dilatation Q61.11
    medullary Q61.5
  liver, congenital Q44.6
  lung disease J98.4
    congenital Q33.0
  mastitis, chronic — *see* Mastopathy, cystic
  medullary, kidney Q61.5
  meniscus — *see* Derangement, knee, meniscus, cystic
  ovary N83.20- ☑
Cysticercosis, cysticerciasis B69.9
  with
    epileptiform fits B69.0
    myositis B69.81
  brain B69.0
  central nervous system B69.0
  cerebral B69.0
  ocular B69.1
  specified NEC B69.89
Cysticercus cellulose infestation — *see* Cysticercosis
Cystinosis (malignant) E72.04
Cystinuria E72.01
Cystitis (exudative) (hemorrhagic) (septic) (suppurative) N30.90
  with
    fibrosis — *see* Cystitis, chronic, interstitial
    hematuria N30.91
    leukoplakia — *see* Cystitis, chronic, interstitial
    malakoplakia — *see* Cystitis, chronic, interstitial
    metaplasia — *see* Cystitis, chronic, interstitial
    prostatitis N41.3

Cystitis — *continued*
  acute N30.00
    with hematuria N30.01
    of trigone N30.30
      with hematuria N30.31
  allergic — *see* Cystitis, specified type NEC
  amebic A06.81
  bilharzial B65.9 *[N33]*
  blennorrhagic (gonococcal) A54.01
  bullous — *see* Cystitis, specified type NEC
  calculous N21.0
  chlamydial A56.01
  chronic N30.20
    with hematuria N30.21
    interstitial N30.10
      with hematuria N30.11
    of trigone N30.30
      with hematuria N30.31
    specified NEC N30.20
      with hematuria N30.21
  cystic (a) — *see* Cystitis, specified type NEC
  diphtheritic A36.85
  echinococcal
    granulosus B67.39
    multilocularis B67.69
  emphysematous — *see* Cystitis, specified type NEC
  encysted — *see* Cystitis, specified type NEC
  eosinophilic — *see* Cystitis, specified type NEC
  follicular — *see* Cystitis, of trigone
  gangrenous — *see* Cystitis, specified type NEC
  glandularis — *see* Cystitis, specified type NEC
  gonococcal A54.01
  incrusted — *see* Cystitis, specified type NEC
  interstitial (chronic) — *see* Cystitis, chronic, interstitial
  irradiation N30.40
    with hematuria N30.41
  irritation — *see* Cystitis, specified type NEC
  malignant — *see* Cystitis, specified type NEC
  of trigone N30.30
    with hematuria N30.31
  panmural — *see* Cystitis, chronic, interstitial
  polyposa — *see* Cystitis, specified type NEC
  prostatic N41.3
  puerperal (postpartum) O86.22
  radiation — *see* Cystitis, irradiation
  specified type NEC N30.80
    with hematuria N30.81
  subacute — *see* Cystitis, chronic
  submucous — *see* Cystitis, chronic, interstitial
  syphilitic (late) A52.76
  trichomonal A59.03
  tuberculous A18.12
  ulcerative — *see* Cystitis, chronic, interstitial

Cystocele (-urethrocele)
  female N81.10
    with prolapse of uterus — *see* Prolapse, uterus
    lateral N81.12
    midline N81.11
    paravaginal N81.12
  in pregnancy or childbirth O34.8- ☑
    causing obstructed labor O65.5
  male N32.89
Cystolithiasis N21.0
Cystoma — *see also* Neoplasm, benign, by site
  endometrial, ovary N80.1
  mucinous
    specified site — *see* Neoplasm, benign, by site
    unspecified site D27.9
  serous
    specified site — *see* Neoplasm, benign, by site
    unspecified site D27.9
  simple (ovary) N83.29- ☑
Cystoplegia N31.2
Cystoptosis N32.89
Cystopyelitis — *see* Pyelonephritis
Cystorrhagia N32.89
Cystosarcoma phyllodes D48.6- ☑
  benign D24- ☑
  malignant — *see* Neoplasm, breast, malignant
Cystostomy
  attention to Z43.5
  complication — *see* Complications, cystostomy
  status Z93.50
    appendico-vesicostomy Z93.52
    cutaneous Z93.51
    specified NEC Z93.59
Cystourethritis — *see* Urethritis
Cystourethrocele — *see also* Cystocele
  female N81.10
    with uterine prolapse — *see* Prolapse, uterus
    lateral N81.12
    midline N81.11
    paravaginal N81.12
  male N32.89
Cytomegalic inclusion disease
  congenital P35.1
Cytomegalovirus infection B25.9
Cytomycosis (reticuloendothelial) B39.4
Cytopenia D75.9
  refractory
    with multilineage dysplasia D46.A (*following* D46.2)
      and ring sideroblasts (RCMD RS) D46.B (*following* D46.2)
Czerny's disease (periodic hydrarthrosis of the knee) — *see* Effusion, joint, knee

D

Da Costa's syndrome F45.8
Daae (-Finsen) **disease** (epidemic pleurodynia) B33.0
Dabney's grip B33.0
Dacryoadenitis, dacryadenitis H04.00- ☑
  acute H04.01- ☑
  chronic H04.02- ☑
Dacryocystitis H04.30- ☑
  acute H04.32- ☑
  chronic H04.41- ☑
  neonatal P39.1
  phlegmonous H04.31- ☑
  syphilitic A52.71
    congenital (early) A50.01
  trachomatous, active A71.1
    sequelae (late effect) B94.0
Dacryocystoblenorrhea — *see* Inflammation, lacrimal, passages, chronic
Dacryocystocele — *see* Disorder, lacrimal system, changes
Dacryolith, dacryolithiasis H04.51- ☑
Dacryoma — *see* Disorder, lacrimal system, changes
Dacryopericystitis — *see* Dacryocystitis
Dacryops H04.11- ☑
Dacryostenosis — *see also* Stenosis, lacrimal
  congenital Q10.5
Dactylitis
  bone — *see* Osteomyelitis
  sickle-cell D57.00
    Hb C D57.219
    Hb SS D57.00
    specified NEC D57.819
  skin L08.9
  syphilitic A52.77
  tuberculous A18.03
Dactylolysis spontanea (ainhum) L94.6
Dactylosymphysis Q70.9
  fingers — *see* Syndactylism, complex, fingers
  toes — *see* Syndactylism, complex, toes
Damage
  arteriosclerotic — *see* Arteriosclerosis
  brain (nontraumatic) G93.9
    anoxic, hypoxic G93.1
      resulting from a procedure G97.82
    child NEC G80.9
    due to birth injury P11.2
  cardiorenal (vascular) — *see* Hypertension, cardiorenal
  cerebral NEC — *see* Damage, brain
  coccyx, complicating delivery O71.6
  coronary — *see* Disease, heart, ischemic
  deep tissue, pressure-induced — *see also* L89 with final character .6
  eye, birth injury P15.3
  liver (nontraumatic) K76.9
    alcoholic K70.9
    due to drugs — *see* Disease, liver, toxic
    toxic — *see* Disease, liver, toxic
  lung
    dabbing (related) U07.0
    electronic cigarette (related) U07.0
    vaping (associated) (device) (product) (use) U07.0
  medication T88.7 ☑
  organ
    dabbing (related) U07.0
    electronic cigarette (related) U07.0
    vaping (associated) (device) (product) (use) U07.0
  pelvic
    joint or ligament, during delivery O71.6
    organ NEC
      during delivery O71.5
      following ectopic or molar pregnancy O08.6
  renal — *see* Disease, renal
  subendocardium, subendocardial — *see* Degeneration, myocardial
  vascular I99.9
Dana-Putnam syndrome (subacute combined sclerosis with pernicious anemia) — *see* Degeneration, combined
Danbolt (-Cross) **syndrome** (acrodermatitis enteropathica) E83.2
Dandruff L21.0
Dandy-Walker syndrome Q03.1
  with spina bifida — *see* Spina bifida
Danlos' syndrome — *see also* Syndrome, Ehlers-Danlos Q79.60

Darier (-White) **disease** (congenital) Q82.8
  meaning erythema annulare centrifugum L53.1
Darier-Roussy sarcoid D86.3
Darling's disease or histoplasmosis B39.4
Darwin's tubercle Q17.8
Dawson's (inclusion body) **encephalitis** A81.1
De Beurmann (-Gougerot) **disease** B42.1
De la Tourette's syndrome F95.2
De Lange's syndrome Q87.19
De Morgan's spots (senile angiomas) I78.1
De Quervain's
  disease (tendon sheath) M65.4
  syndrome E34.51
  thyroiditis (subacute granulomatous thyroiditis) E06.1
De Toni-Fanconi (-Debré) **syndrome** E72.09
  with cystinosis E72.04
Dead
  fetus, retained (mother) O36.4 ☑
    early pregnancy O02.1
  labyrinth H83.2 ☑
  ovum, retained O02.0
Deaf nonspeaking NEC H91.3
Deafmutism (acquired) (congenital) NEC H91.3
  hysterical F44.6
  syphilitic, congenital — *see also* subcategory H94.8 A50.09
Deafness (acquired) (complete) (hereditary) (partial) H91.9- ☑
  with blue sclera and fragility of bone Q78.0
  auditory fatigue — *see* Deafness, specified type NEC
  aviation T70.0 ☑
    nerve injury — *see* Injury, nerve, acoustic, specified type NEC
  boilermaker's H83.3 ☑
  central — *see* Deafness, sensorineural
  conductive H90.2
    and sensorineural
      mixed H90.8
        bilateral H90.6
    bilateral H90.0
    unilateral H90.1- ☑
      with restricted hearing on the contralateral side H90.A- ☑
  congenital H90.5
    with blue sclera and fragility of bone Q78.0
  due to toxic agents — *see* Deafness, ototoxic
  emotional (hysterical) F44.6
  functional (hysterical) F44.6
  high frequency H91.9- ☑
  hysterical F44.6
  low frequency H91.9- ☑
  mental R48.8
  mixed conductive and sensorineural H90.8
    bilateral H90.6
    unilateral H90.7- ☑
  nerve — *see* Deafness, sensorineural
  neural — *see* Deafness, sensorineural
  noise-induced — *see also* subcategory H83.3 ☑
    nerve injury — *see* Injury, nerve, acoustic, specified type NEC
  nonspeaking H91.3
  ototoxic H91.0 ☑
  perceptive — *see* Deafness, sensorineural
  psychogenic (hysterical) F44.6
  sensorineural H90.5
    and conductive
      bilateral H90.6
      mixed H90.8
        bilateral H90.6
    bilateral H90.3
    unilateral H90.4- ☑
      with restricted hearing on the contralateral side H90.A- ☑
  sensory — *see* Deafness, sensorineural
  specified type NEC H91.8 ☑
  sudden (idiopathic) H91.2- ☑
  syphilitic A52.15
  transient ischemic H93.01- ☑
  traumatic — *see* Injury, nerve, acoustic, specified type NEC
  word (developmental) H93.25
Death (cause unknown) (of) (unexplained) (unspecified cause) R99
  brain G93.82
  cardiac (sudden) (with successful resuscitation) — *code to* underlying disease
    family history of Z82.41

Death — *continued*
  cardiac — *code to* underlying disease — *continued*
    personal history of Z86.74
    family member (assumed) Z63.4
Debility (chronic) (general) (nervous) R53.81
  congenital or neonatal NOS P96.9
  nervous R53.81
  old age R54
  senile R54
Débove's disease (splenomegaly) R16.1
Decalcification
  bone — *see* Osteoporosis
  teeth K03.89
Decapsulation, kidney N28.89
Decay
  dental — *see* Caries, dental
  senile R54
  tooth, teeth — *see* Caries, dental
Deciduitis (acute)
  following ectopic or molar pregnancy O08.0
Decline (general) — *see* Debility
  cognitive, age-associated R41.81
Decompensation
  cardiac (acute) (chronic) — *see* Disease, heart
  cardiovascular — *see* Disease, cardiovascular
  heart — *see* Disease, heart
  hepatic — *see* Failure, hepatic
  myocardial (acute) (chronic) — *see* Disease, heart
  respiratory J98.8
Decompression sickness T70.3 ☑
Decrease (d)
  absolute neutrophil count — *see* Neutropenia
  blood
    platelets — *see* Thrombocytopenia
    pressure R03.1
      due to shock following
        injury T79.4 ☑
        operation T81.19 ☑
  estrogen E28.39
    postablative E89.40
      asymptomatic E89.40
      symptomatic E89.41
  fragility of erythrocytes D58.8
  function
    lipase (pancreatic) K90.3
    ovary in hypopituitarism E23.0
    parenchyma of pancreas K86.89
    pituitary (gland) (anterior) (lobe) E23.0
      posterior (lobe) E23.0
  functional activity R68.89
  glucose R73.09
  hematocrit R71.0
  hemoglobin R71.0
  leukocytes D72.819
    specified NEC D72.818
  libido R68.82
  lymphocytes D72.810
  platelets D69.6
  respiration, due to shock following injury T79.4 ☑
  sexual desire R68.82
  tear secretion NEC — *see* Syndrome, dry eye
  tolerance
    fat K90.49
    glucose R73.09
    pancreatic K90.3
    salt and water E87.8
  vision NEC H54.7
  white blood cell count D72.819
    specified NEC D72.818
Decubitus (ulcer) — *see* Ulcer, pressure, by site
  cervix N86
Deepening acetabulum — *see* Derangement, joint, specified type NEC, hip
Defect, defective Q89.9
  3-beta-hydroxysteroid dehydrogenase E25.0
  11-hydroxylase E25.0
  21-hydroxylase E25.0
  abdominal wall, congenital Q79.59
  antibody immunodeficiency D80.9
  aorticopulmonary septum Q21.4
  atrial septal (ostium secundum type) Q21.1
    following acute myocardial infarction (current complication) I23.1
    ostium primum type Q21.2
  atrioventricular
    canal Q21.2
    septum Q21.2
  auricular septal Q21.1

☑ **Additional Character Required** — Refer to the Tabular List for Character Selection
▽ **Subterms under main terms may continue to next column or page**

Defect, defective — *continued*
  bilirubin excretion NEC E80.6
  biosynthesis, androgen (testicular) E29.1
  bulbar septum Q21.0
  catalase E80.3
  cell membrane receptor complex (CR3) D71
  circulation I99.9
    congenital Q28.9
    newborn Q28.9
  coagulation (factor) — *see also* Deficiency, factor D68.9
    with
      ectopic pregnancy O08.1
      molar pregnancy O08.1
    acquired D68.4
    antepartum with hemorrhage — *see* Hemorrhage,
        antepartum, with coagulation defect
    due to
      liver disease D68.4
      vitamin K deficiency D68.4
    hereditary NEC D68.2
    intrapartum O67.0
    newborn, transient P61.6
    postpartum O99.13
      with hemorrhage O72.3
    specified type NEC D68.8
  complement system D84.1
  conduction (heart) I45.9
    bone — *see* Deafness, conductive
  congenital, organ or site not listed — *see* Anomaly, by
    site
  coronary sinus Q21.1
  cushion, endocardial Q21.2
  degradation, glycoprotein E77.1
  dental bridge, crown, fillings — *see* Defect, dental
    restoration
  dental restoration K08.50
    specified NEC K08.59
  dentin (hereditary) K00.5
  Descemet's membrane, congenital Q13.89
  developmental — *see also* Anomaly
    cauda equina Q06.3
  diaphragm
    with elevation, eventration or hernia — *see* Hernia,
        diaphragm
    congenital Q79.1
      with hernia Q79.0
      gross (with hernia) Q79.0
  ectodermal, congenital Q82.9
  Eisenmenger's Q21.8
  enzyme
    catalase E80.3
    peroxidase E80.3
  esophagus, congenital Q39.9
  extensor retinaculum M62.89
  fibrin polymerization D68.2
  filling
    bladder R93.41
    kidney R93.42- ☑
    renal pelvis R93.41
    stomach R93.3
    ureter R93.41
    urinary organs, specified NEC R93.49
  GABA (gamma aminobutyric acid) metabolic E72.81
  Gerbode Q21.0
  glucose transport, blood-brain barrier E74.810
  glycoprotein degradation E77.1
  Hageman (factor) D68.2
  hearing — *see* Deafness
  high grade F70
  interatrial septal Q21.1
  interauricular septal Q21.1
  interventricular septal Q21.0
    with dextroposition of aorta, pulmonary stenosis
        and hypertrophy of right ventricle Q21.3
    in tetralogy of Fallot Q21.3
  learning (specific) — *see* Disorder, learning
  lymphocyte function antigen-1 (LFA-1) D84.0
  lysosomal enzyme, post-translational modification
    E77.0
  major osseous M89.70
    ankle M89.77- ☑
    carpus M89.74- ☑
    clavicle M89.71- ☑
    femur M89.75- ☑
    fibula M89.76- ☑
    fingers M89.74- ☑
    foot M89.77- ☑
    forearm M89.73- ☑

Defect, defective — *continued*
  major osseous — *continued*
    hand M89.74- ☑
    humerus M89.72- ☑
    lower leg M89.76- ☑
    metacarpus M89.74- ☑
    metatarsus M89.77- ☑
    multiple sites M89.79
    pelvic region M89.75- ☑
    pelvis M89.75- ☑
    radius M89.73- ☑
    scapula M89.71- ☑
    shoulder region M89.71- ☑
    specified NEC M89.78
    tarsus M89.77- ☑
    thigh M89.75- ☑
    tibia M89.76- ☑
    toes M89.77- ☑
    ulna M89.73- ☑
  mental — *see* Disability, intellectual
  modification, lysosomal enzymes, post-translational
    E77.0
  obstructive, congenital
    renal pelvis Q62.39
    ureter Q62.39
      atresia — *see* Atresia, ureter
      cecoureterocele Q62.32
      megaureter Q62.2
      orthotopic ureterocele Q62.31
  osseous, major M89.70
    ankle M89.77- ☑
    carpus M89.74- ☑
    clavicle M89.71- ☑
    femur M89.75- ☑
    fibula M89.76- ☑
    fingers M89.74- ☑
    foot M89.77- ☑
    forearm M89.73- ☑
    hand M89.74- ☑
    humerus M89.72- ☑
    lower leg M89.76- ☑
    metacarpus M89.74- ☑
    metatarsus M89.77- ☑
    multiple sites M89.9
    pelvic region M89.75- ☑
    pelvis M89.75- ☑
    radius M89.73- ☑
    scapula M89.71- ☑
    shoulder region M89.71- ☑
    specified NEC M89.78
    tarsus M89.77- ☑
    thigh M89.75- ☑
    tibia M89.76- ☑
    toes M89.77- ☑
    ulna M89.73- ☑
  osteochondral NEC — *see also* Deformity M95.8
  ostium
    primum Q21.2
    secundum Q21.1
  peroxidase E80.3
  placental blood supply — *see* Insufficiency, placental
  platelets, qualitative D69.1
    constitutional D68.0
  postural NEC, spine — *see* Dorsopathy, deforming
  reduction
    limb Q73.8
      lower Q72.9- ☑
        absence — *see* Agenesis, leg
          foot — *see* Agenesis, foot
        longitudinal
          femur Q72.4- ☑
          fibula Q72.6- ☑
          tibia Q72.5- ☑
        specified type NEC Q72.89- ☑
        split foot Q72.7- ☑
      specified type NEC Q73.8
      upper Q71.9- ☑
        absence — *see* Agenesis, arm
          forearm — *see* Agenesis, forearm
          hand — *see* Agenesis, hand
        lobster-claw hand Q71.6- ☑
        longitudinal
          radius Q71.4- ☑
          ulna Q71.5- ☑
        specified type NEC Q71.89- ☑
  renal pelvis Q63.8

Defect, defective — *continued*
  renal pelvis — *continued*
    obstructive Q62.39
  respiratory system, congenital Q34.9
  restoration, dental K08.50
    specified NEC K08.59
  retinal nerve bundle fibers H35.89
  septal (heart) NOS Q21.9
    acquired (atrial) (auricular) (ventricular) (old) I51.0
    atrial Q21.1
      concurrent with acute myocardial infarction —
        see Infarct, myocardium
      following acute myocardial infarction (current
        complication) I23.1
    ventricular — *see also* Defect, ventricular septal
      Q21.0
  sinus venosus Q21.1
  speech — *see* Disorder, speech
    developmental F80.9
    specified NEC R47.89
  Taussig-Bing (aortic transposition and overriding pul-
    monary artery) Q20.1
  teeth, wedge K03.1
  vascular (local) I99.9
    congenital Q27.9
  ventricular septal Q21.0
    concurrent with acute myocardial infarction — *see*
      Infarct, myocardium
    following acute myocardial infarction (current
      complication) I23.2
    in tetralogy of Fallot Q21.3
  vision NEC H54.7
  visual field H53.40
    bilateral
      heteronymous H53.47
      homonymous H53.46- ☑
    generalized contraction H53.48- ☑
    localized
      arcuate H53.43- ☑
      scotoma (central area) H53.41- ☑
        blind spot area H53.42- ☑
      sector H53.43- ☑
      specified type NEC H53.45- ☑
  voice R49.9
    specified NEC R49.8
  wedge, tooth, teeth (abrasion) K03.1
Deferentitis N49.1
  gonorrheal (acute) (chronic) A54.23
Defibrination (syndrome) D65
  antepartum — *see* Hemorrhage, antepartum, with
    coagulation defect, disseminated intravascular
    coagulation
  following ectopic or molar pregnancy O08.1
  intrapartum O67.0
  newborn P60
  postpartum O72.3
Deficiency, deficient
  3-beta hydroxysteroid dehydrogenase E25.0
  5-alpha reductase (with male pseudohermaphroditism)
    E29.1
  11-hydroxylase E25.0
  21-hydroxylase E25.0
  AADC (aromatic L-amino acid decarboxylase) E70.81
  abdominal muscle syndrome Q79.4
  AC globulin (congenital) (hereditary) D68.2
    acquired D68.4
  accelerator globulin (Ac G) (blood) D68.2
  acid phosphatase E83.39
  activating factor (blood) D68.2
  ADA2 (adenosine deaminase 2) D81.32
  adenosine deaminase (ADA) D81.30
    with severe combined immunodeficiency (SCID)
      D81.31
    partial (type 1) D81.39
    specified NEC D81.39
    type 1 (without SCID) (without severe combined
      immunodeficiency) D81.39
    type 2 D81.32
  aldolase (hereditary) E74.19
  alpha-1-antitrypsin E88.01
  amino-acids E72.9
  anemia — *see* Anemia
  aneurin E51.9
  antibody with
    hyperimmunoglobulinemia D80.6
    near-normal immunoglobins D80.6
  antidiuretic hormone E23.2

Deficiency, deficient — *continued*
anti-hemophilic
  factor (A) D66
    B D67
    C D68.1
  globulin (AHG) NEC D66
antithrombin (antithrombin III) D68.59
aromatic L-amino acid decarboxylase (AADC) E70.81
ascorbic acid E54
attention (disorder) (syndrome) F98.8
  with hyperactivity — *see* Disorder, attention-deficit
    hyperactivity
autoprothrombin
  I D68.2
  II D67
  C D68.2
beta-glucuronidase E76.29
biotin E53.8
biotin-dependent carboxylase D81.819
biotinidase D81.810
brancher enzyme (amylopectinosis) E74.03
C1 esterase inhibitor (C1-INH) D84.1
calciferol E55.9
  with
    adult osteomalacia M83.8
    rickets — *see* Rickets
calcium (dietary) E58
calorie, severe E43
  with marasmus E41
    and kwashiorkor E42
cardiac — *see* Insufficiency, myocardial
carnitine E71.40
  due to
    hemodialysis E71.43
    inborn errors of metabolism E71.42
    Valproic acid therapy E71.43
  iatrogenic E71.43
  muscle palmityltransferase E71.314
  primary E71.41
  secondary E71.448
carotene E50.9
central nervous system G96.89
ceruloplasmin (Wilson) E83.01
choline E53.8
Christmas factor D67
chromium E61.4
clotting (blood) — *see also* Deficiency, coagulation
    factor D68.9
clotting factor NEC (hereditary) — *see also* Deficiency,
    factor D68.2
coagulation NOS D68.9
  with
    ectopic pregnancy O08.1
    molar pregnancy O08.1
  acquired (any) D68.4
  antepartum hemorrhage — *see* Hemorrhage, an-
    tepartum, with coagulation defect
  clotting factor NEC — *see also* Deficiency, factor
    D68.2
  due to
    hyperprothrombinemia D68.4
    liver disease D68.4
    vitamin K deficiency D68.4
  newborn, transient P61.6
  postpartum O72.3
  specified NEC D68.8
cognitive F09
color vision H53.50
  achromatopsia H53.51
  acquired H53.52
  deuteranomaly H53.53
  protanomaly H53.54
  specified type NEC H53.59
  tritanomaly H53.55
combined glucocorticoid and mineralocorticoid E27.49
contact factor D68.2
copper (nutritional) E61.0
corticoadrenal E27.40
  primary E27.1
craniofacial axis Q75.0
cyanocobalamin E53.8
debrancher enzyme (limit dextrinosis) E74.03
dehydrogenase
  long chain/very long chain acyl CoA E71.310
  medium chain acyl CoA E71.311
  short chain acyl CoA E71.312
diet E63.9
dihydropyrimidine dehydrogenase (DPD) E88.89

Deficiency, deficient — *continued*
disaccharidase E73.9
edema — *see* Malnutrition, severe
endocrine E34.9
energy-supply — *see* Malnutrition
enzymes, circulating NEC E88.09
ergosterol E55.9
  with
    adult osteomalacia M83.8
    rickets — *see* Rickets
essential fatty acid (EFA) E63.0
eye movements
  saccadic H55.81
  smooth pursuit H55.82
factor — *see also* Deficiency, coagulation
  Hageman D68.2
  I (congenital) (hereditary) D68.2
  II (congenital) (hereditary) D68.2
  IX (congenital) (functional) (hereditary) (with func-
    tional defect) D67
  multiple (congenital) D68.8
    acquired D68.4
  V (congenital) (hereditary) D68.2
  VII (congenital) (hereditary) D68.2
  VIII (congenital) (functional) (hereditary) (with
    functional defect) D66
    with vascular defect D68.0
  X (congenital) (hereditary) D68.2
  XI (congenital) (hereditary) D68.1
  XII (congenital) (hereditary) D68.2
  XIII (congenital) (hereditary) D68.2
femoral, proximal focal (congenital) — *see* Defect, re-
    duction, lower limb, longitudinal, femur
fibrinase D68.2
fibrinogen (congenital) (hereditary) D68.2
  acquired D65
fibrin-stabilizing factor (congenital) (hereditary) D68.2
  acquired D68.4
folate E53.8
folic acid E53.8
foreskin N47.3
fructokinase E74.11
fructose 1,6-diphosphatase E74.19
fructose-1-phosphate aldolase E74.19
GABA (gamma aminobutyric acid) transaminase E72.81
GABA-T (gamma aminobutyric acid transaminase)
    E72.81
galactokinase E74.29
galactose-1-phosphate uridyl transferase E74.29
gammaglobulin in blood D80.1
  hereditary D80.0
glass factor D68.2
glucocorticoid E27.49
  mineralocorticoid E27.49
glucose transporter protein type 1 E74.810
glucose-6-phosphatase E74.01
glucose-6-phosphate dehydrogenase
  anemia D55.0
  without anemia D75.A
glucuronyl transferase E80.5
Glut1 E74.810
glycogen synthetase E74.09
gonadotropin (isolated) E23.0
growth hormone (idiopathic) (isolated) E23.0
Hageman factor D68.2
hemoglobin D64.9
hepatophosphorylase E74.09
homogentisate 1,2-dioxygenase E70.29
hormone
  anterior pituitary (partial) NEC E23.0
    growth E23.0
  growth (isolated) E23.0
  pituitary E23.0
  testicular E29.1
hypoxanthine- (guanine)-phosphoribosyltransferase
    (HG- PRT) (total H-PRT) E79.1
immunity D84.9
  cell-mediated D84.89
    with thrombocytopenia and eczema D82.0
  combined D81.9
  humoral D80.9
  IgA (secretory) D80.2
  IgG D80.3
  IgM D80.4
immuno — *see* Immunodeficiency
immunoglobulin, selective
  A (IgA) D80.2
  G (IgG) (subclasses) D80.3
  M (IgM) D80.4

Deficiency, deficient — *continued*
inositol (B complex) E53.8
intrinsic
  factor (congenital) D51.0
  sphincter N36.42
    with urethral hypermobility N36.43
iodine E61.8
  congenital syndrome — *see* Syndrome, iodine-defi-
    ciency, congenital
iron E61.1
  anemia D50.9
kalium E87.6
kappa-light chain D80.8
labile factor (congenital) (hereditary) D68.2
  acquired D68.4
lacrimal fluid (acquired) — *see also* Syndrome, dry eye
  congenital Q10.6
lactase
  congenital E73.0
  secondary E73.1
Laki-Lorand factor D68.2
lecithin cholesterol acyltransferase E78.6
lipocaic K86.89
lipoprotein (familial) (high density) E78.6
liver phosphorylase E74.09
lysosomal alpha-1, 4 glucosidase E74.02
magnesium E61.2
major histocompatibility complex
  class I D81.6
  class II D81.7
manganese E61.3
menadione (vitamin K) E56.1
  newborn P53
mental (familial) (hereditary) — *see* Disability, intellec-
    tual
methylenetetrahydrofolate reductase (MTHFR) E72.12
mevalonate kinase M04.1
mineralocorticoid E27.49
  with glucocorticoid E27.49
mineral NEC E61.8
molybdenum (nutritional) E61.5
moral F60.2
multiple nutrient elements E61.7
multiple sulfatase (MSD) E75.26
muscle
  carnitine (palmityltransferase) E71.314
  phosphofructokinase E74.09
myoadenylate deaminase E79.2
myocardial — *see* Insufficiency, myocardial
myophosphorylase E74.04
NADH diaphorase or reductase (congenital) D74.0
NADH-methemoglobin reductase (congenital) D74.0
natrium E87.1
niacin (amide) (-tryptophan) E52
nicotinamide E52
nicotinic acid E52
number of teeth — *see* Anodontia
nutrient element E61.9
  multiple E61.7
  specified NEC E61.8
nutrition, nutritional E63.9
  sequelae — *see* Sequelae, nutritional deficiency
  specified NEC E63.8
of interleukin 1 receptor antagonist [DIRA] M04.8
ornithine transcarbamylase E72.4
ovarian E28.39
oxygen — *see* Anoxia
pantothenic acid E53.8
parathyroid (gland) E20.9
perineum (female) N81.89
phenylalanine hydroxylase E70.1
phosphoenolpyruvate carboxykinase E74.4
phosphofructokinase E74.19
phosphomannomutase E74.818
phosphomannose isomerase E74.818
phosphomannosyl mutase E74.818
phosphorylase kinase, liver E74.09
pituitary hormone (isolated) E23.0
plasma thromboplastin
  antecedent (PTA) D68.1
  component (PTC) D67
plasminogen (type 1) (type 2) E88.02
platelet NEC D69.1
  constitutional D68.0
polyglandular E31.8
  autoimmune E31.0
potassium (K) E87.6
prepuce N47.3

☑ **Additional Character Required** — Refer to the Tabular List for Character Selection   ▽ Subterms under main terms may continue to next column or page

Deficiency, deficient — *continued*
- proaccelerin (congenital) (hereditary) D68.2
  - acquired D68.4
- proconvertin factor (congenital) (hereditary) D68.2
  - acquired D68.4
- protein — *see also* Malnutrition E46
  - anemia D53.0
  - C D68.59
  - S D68.59
- prothrombin (congenital) (hereditary) D68.2
  - acquired D68.4
- Prower factor D68.2
- pseudocholinesterase E88.09
- PTA (plasma thromboplastin antecedent) D68.1
- PTC (plasma thromboplastin component) D67
- purine nucleoside phosphorylase (PNP) D81.5
- pyracin (alpha) (beta) E53.1
- pyridoxal E53.1
- pyridoxamine E53.1
- pyridoxine (derivatives) E53.1
- pyruvate
  - carboxylase E74.4
  - dehydrogenase E74.4
- riboflavin (vitamin B2) E53.0
- salt E87.1
- secretion
  - ovary E28.39
  - salivary gland (any) K11.7
  - urine R34
- selenium (dietary) E59
- serum antitrypsin, familial E88.01
- short stature homeobox gene (SHOX)
  - with
    - dyschondrosteosis Q78.8
    - short stature (idiopathic) E34.3
    - Turner's syndrome Q96.9
- sodium (Na) E87.1
- SPCA (factor VII) D68.2
- sphincter, intrinsic N36.42
  - with urethral hypermobility N36.43
- stable factor (congenital) (hereditary) D68.2
  - acquired D68.4
- Stuart-Prower (factor X) D68.2
- succinic semialdehyde dehydrogenase E72.81
- sucrase E74.39
- sulfatase E75.26
- sulfite oxidase E72.19
- thiamin, thiaminic (chloride) E51.9
  - beriberi (dry) E51.11
    - wet E51.12
- thrombokinase D68.2
  - newborn P53
- thyroid (gland) — *see* Hypothyroidism
- tocopherol E56.0
- tooth bud K00.0
- transcobalamine II (anemia) D51.2
- vanadium E61.6
- vascular I99.9
- vasopressin E23.2
- vertical ridge K06.8
- viosterol — *see* Deficiency, calciferol
- vitamin (multiple) NOS E56.9
  - A E50.9
    - with
      - Bitot's spot (corneal) E50.1
      - follicular keratosis E50.8
      - keratomalacia E50.4
      - manifestations NEC E50.8
      - night blindness E50.5
      - scar of cornea, xerophthalmic E50.6
      - xeroderma E50.8
      - xerophthalmia E50.7
      - xerosis
        - conjunctival E50.0
          - and Bitot's spot E50.1
        - cornea E50.2
          - and ulceration E50.3
    - sequelae E64.1
  - B (complex) NOS E53.9
    - with
      - beriberi (dry) E51.11
        - wet E51.12
      - pellagra E52
  - B1 NOS E51.9
    - beriberi (dry) E51.11
      - with circulatory system manifestations E51.11
        - wet E51.12
  - B12 E53.8
  - B2 (riboflavin) E53.0

Deficiency, deficient — *continued*
- vitamin — *continued*
  - B6 E53.1
  - C E54
    - sequelae E64.2
  - D E55.9
    - with
      - adult osteomalacia M83.8
      - rickets — *see* Rickets
    - 25-hydroxylase E83.32
  - E E56.0
  - folic acid E53.8
  - G E53.0
  - group B E53.9
    - specified NEC E53.8
  - H (biotin) E53.8
  - K E56.1
    - of newborn P53
  - nicotinic E52
  - P E56.8
  - PP (pellagra-preventing) E52
  - specified NEC E56.8
  - thiamin E51.9
    - beriberi — *see* Beriberi
- zinc, dietary E60

Deficit — *see also* Deficiency
- attention and concentration R41.840
  - disorder — *see* Attention, deficit
  - following
    - cerebral infarction I69.310
    - cerebrovascular disease I69.910
      - specified disease NEC I69.810
    - nontraumatic
      - intracerebral hemorrhage I69.110
      - specified intracranial hemorrhage NEC I69.210
      - subarachnoid hemorrhage I69.010
- cognitive
  - communication R41.841
  - emotional
    - following
      - cerebral infarction I69.315
      - cerebrovascular disease I69.915
        - specified disease NEC I69.815
      - nontraumatic
        - intracerebral hemorrhage I69.115
        - specified intracranial hemorrhage NEC I69.215
        - subarachnoid hemorrhage I69.015
  - following
    - cerebral infarction I69.319
    - cerebrovascular disease I69.919
      - specified disease NEC I69.819
    - nontraumatic
      - intracerebral hemorrhage I69.119
      - specified intracranial hemorrhage NEC I69.219
      - subarachnoid hemorrhage I69.019
  - social
    - following
      - cerebral infarction I69.315
      - cerebrovascular disease I69.915
        - specified disease NEC I69.815
      - nontraumatic
        - intracerebral hemorrhage I69.115
        - specified intracranial hemorrhage NEC I69.215
        - subarachnoid hemorrhage I69.015
- cognitive NEC R41.89
  - following
    - cerebral infarction I69.318
    - cerebrovascular disease I69.918
      - specified disease NEC I69.818
    - nontraumatic
      - intracerebral hemorrhage I69.118
      - specified intracranial hemorrhage NEC I69.218
      - subarachnoid hemorrhage I69.018
- concentration R41.840
- executive function R41.844
  - following
    - cerebral infarction I69.314
    - cerebrovascular disease I69.914
      - specified disease NEC I69.814
    - nontraumatic
      - intracerebral hemorrhage I69.114
      - specified intracranial hemorrhage NEC I69.214
      - subarachnoid hemorrhage I69.014
- frontal lobe R41.844
  - following
    - cerebral infarction I69.314
    - cerebrovascular disease I69.914

Deficit — *continued*
- frontal lobe — *continued*
  - following — *continued*
    - cerebrovascular disease — *continued*
      - specified disease NEC I69.814
    - nontraumatic
      - intracerebral hemorrhage I69.114
      - specified intracranial hemorrhage NEC I69.214
      - subarachnoid hemorrhage I69.014
  - memory
    - following
      - cerebral infarction I69.311
      - cerebrovascular disease I69.911
        - specified disease NEC I69.811
      - nontraumatic
        - intracerebral hemorrhage I69.111
        - specified intracranial hemorrhage NEC I69.211
        - subarachnoid hemorrhage I69.011
  - neurologic NEC R29.818
    - ischemic
      - reversible (RIND) I63.9
        - prolonged (PRIND) I63.9
  - oxygen R09.02
  - prolonged reversible ischemic neurologic (PRIND) I63.9
  - psychomotor R41.843
    - following
      - cerebral infarction I69.313
      - cerebrovascular disease I69.913
        - specified disease NEC I69.813
      - nontraumatic
        - intracerebral hemorrhage I69.113
        - specified intracranial hemorrhage NEC I69.213
        - subarachnoid hemorrhage I69.013
  - visuospatial R41.842
    - following
      - cerebral infarction I69.312
      - cerebrovascular disease I69.912
        - specified disease NEC I69.812
      - nontraumatic
        - intracerebral hemorrhage I69.112
        - specified intracranial hemorrhage NEC I69.212
        - subarachnoid hemorrhage I69.012

Deflection
- radius — *see* Deformity, limb, specified type NEC, forearm
- septum (acquired) (nasal) (nose) J34.2
- spine — *see* Curvature, spine
- turbinate (nose) J34.2

Defluvium
- capillorum — *see* Alopecia
- ciliorum — *see* Madarosis
- unguium L60.8

Deformity Q89.9
- abdomen, congenital Q89.9
- abdominal wall
  - acquired M95.8
  - congenital Q79.59
- acquired (unspecified site) M95.9
- adrenal gland Q89.1
- alimentary tract, congenital Q45.9
  - upper Q40.9
- ankle (joint) (acquired) — *see also* Deformity, limb, lower leg
  - abduction — *see* Contraction, joint, ankle
  - congenital Q68.8
  - contraction — *see* Contraction, joint, ankle
  - specified type NEC — *see* Deformity, limb, foot, specified NEC
- anus (acquired) K62.89
  - congenital Q43.9
- aorta (arch) (congenital) Q25.40
  - acquired I77.89
- aortic
  - arch, acquired I77.89
  - cusp or valve (congenital) Q23.8
    - acquired — *see also* Endocarditis, aortic I35.8
- arm (acquired) (upper) — *see also* Deformity, limb, upper arm
  - congenital Q68.8
  - forearm — *see* Deformity, limb, forearm
- artery (congenital) (peripheral) NOS Q27.9
  - acquired I77.89
  - coronary (acquired) I25.9
    - congenital Q24.5
  - umbilical Q27.0
- atrial septal Q21.1
- auditory canal (external) (congenital) — *see also* Malformation, ear, external

Deformity — *continued*
auditory canal — *see also* Malformation, ear, external
— *continued*
    acquired — *see* Disorder, ear, external, specified
      type NEC
  auricle
    ear (congenital) — *see also* Malformation, ear, exter-
      nal
      acquired — *see* Disorder, pinna, deformity
  back — *see* Dorsopathy, deforming
  bile duct (common) (congenital) (hepatic) Q44.5
    acquired K83.8
  biliary duct or passage (congenital) Q44.5
    acquired K83.8
  bladder (neck) (trigone) (sphincter) (acquired) N32.89
    congenital Q64.79
  bone (acquired) NOS M95.9
    congenital Q79.9
    turbinate M95.0
  brain (congenital) Q04.9
    acquired G93.89
    reduction Q04.3
  breast (acquired) N64.89
    congenital Q83.9
    reconstructed N65.0
  bronchus (congenital) Q32.4
    acquired NEC J98.09
  bursa, congenital Q79.9
  canaliculi (lacrimalis) (acquired) — *see also* Disorder,
    lacrimal system, changes
    congenital Q10.6
  canthus, acquired — *see* Disorder, eyelid, specified
    type NEC
  capillary (acquired) I78.8
  cardiovascular system, congenital Q28.9
  caruncle, lacrimal (acquired) — *see also* Disorder,
    lacrimal system, changes
    congenital Q10.6
  cascade, stomach K31.2
  cecum (congenital) Q43.9
    acquired K63.89
  cerebral, acquired G93.89
    congenital Q04.9
  cervix (uterus) (acquired) NEC N88.8
    congenital Q51.9
  cheek (acquired) M95.2
    congenital Q18.9
  chest (acquired) (wall) M95.4
    congenital Q67.8
    sequelae (late effect) of rickets E64.3
  chin (acquired) M95.2
    congenital Q18.9
  choroid (congenital) Q14.3
    acquired H31.8
    plexus Q07.8
      acquired G96.198
  cicatricial — *see* Cicatrix
  cilia, acquired — *see* Disorder, eyelid, specified type
    NEC
  clavicle (acquired) M95.8
    congenital Q68.8
  clitoris (congenital) Q52.6
    acquired N90.89
  clubfoot — *see* Clubfoot
  coccyx (acquired) — *see* subcategory M43.8 ☑
  colon (congenital) Q43.9
    acquired K63.89
  concha (ear), congenital — *see also* Malformation, ear,
    external
    acquired — *see* Disorder, pinna, deformity
  cornea (acquired) H18.70
    congenital Q13.4
    descemetocele — *see* Descemetocele
    ectasia — *see* Ectasia, cornea
    specified NEC H18.79- ☑
    staphyloma — *see* Staphyloma, cornea
  coronary artery (acquired) I25.9
    congenital Q24.5
  cranium (acquired) — *see* Deformity, skull
  cricoid cartilage (congenital) Q31.8
    acquired J38.7
  cystic duct (congenital) Q44.5
    acquired K82.8
  Dandy-Walker Q03.1
    with spina bifida — *see* Spina bifida
  diaphragm (congenital) Q79.1
    acquired J98.6
  digestive organ NOS Q45.9

Deformity — *continued*
ductus arteriosus Q25.0
duodenal bulb K31.89
duodenum (congenital) Q43.9
  acquired K31.89
dura — *see* Deformity, meninges
ear (acquired) — *see also* Disorder, pinna, deformity
  congenital (external) Q17.9
    internal Q16.5
    middle Q16.4
      ossicles Q16.3
    ossicles Q16.3
ectodermal (congenital) NEC Q84.9
ejaculatory duct (congenital) Q55.4
  acquired N50.89
elbow (joint) (acquired) — *see also* Deformity, limb,
  upper arm
  congenital Q68.8
  contraction — *see* Contraction, joint, elbow
endocrine gland NEC Q89.2
epididymis (congenital) Q55.4
  acquired N50.89
epiglottis (congenital) Q31.8
  acquired J38.7
esophagus (congenital) Q39.9
  acquired K22.8
eustachian tube (congenital) NEC Q17.8
eye, congenital Q15.9
eyebrow (congenital) Q18.8
eyelid (acquired) — *see also* Disorder, eyelid, specified
  type NEC
  congenital Q10.3
face (acquired) M95.2
  congenital Q18.9
fallopian tube, acquired N83.8
femur (acquired) — *see* Deformity, limb, specified type
  NEC, thigh
fetal
  with fetopelvic disproportion O33.7 ☑
  causing obstructed labor O66.3
finger (acquired) M20.00- ☑
  boutonniere M20.02- ☑
  congenital Q68.1
  flexion contracture — *see* Contraction, joint, hand
  mallet finger M20.01- ☑
  specified NEC M20.09- ☑
  swan-neck M20.03- ☑
flexion (joint) (acquired) — *see also* Deformity, limb,
  flexion M21.20
  congenital NOS Q74.9
    hip Q65.89
foot (acquired) — *see also* Deformity, limb, lower leg
  cavovarus (congenital) Q66.1- ☑
  congenital NOS Q66.9-
    specified type NEC Q66.89
  specified type NEC — *see* Deformity, limb, foot,
    specified NEC
  valgus (congenital) Q66.6
    acquired — *see* Deformity, valgus, ankle
  varus (congenital) NEC Q66.3- ☑
    acquired — *see* Deformity, varus, ankle
forearm (acquired) — *see also* Deformity, limb, forearm
  congenital Q68.8
forehead (acquired) M95.2
  congenital Q75.8
frontal bone (acquired) M95.2
  congenital Q75.8
gallbladder (congenital) Q44.1
  acquired K82.8
gastrointestinal tract (congenital) NOS Q45.9
  acquired K63.89
genitalia, genital organ(s) or system NEC
  female (congenital) Q52.9
    acquired N94.89
    external Q52.70
  male (congenital) Q55.9
    acquired N50.89
globe (eye) (congenital) Q15.8
  acquired H44.89
gum, acquired NEC K06.8
hand (acquired) — *see* Deformity, limb, hand
  congenital Q68.1
head (acquired) M95.2
  congenital Q75.8
heart (congenital) Q24.9
  septum Q21.9
    auricular Q21.1
    ventricular Q21.0

Deformity — *continued*
heart — *continued*
  valve (congenital) NEC Q24.8
    acquired — *see* Endocarditis
heel (acquired) — *see* Deformity, foot
hepatic duct (congenital) Q44.5
  acquired K83.8
hip (joint) (acquired) (*see also* Deformity, limb, thigh)
  congenital Q65.9
  due to (previous) juvenile osteochondrosis — *see*
    Coxa, plana
  flexion — *see* Contraction, joint, hip
hourglass — *see* Contraction, hourglass
humerus (acquired) M21.82- ☑
  congenital Q74.0
hypophyseal (congenital) Q89.2
ileocecal (coil) (valve) (acquired) K63.89
  congenital Q43.9
ileum (congenital) Q43.9
  acquired K63.89
ilium (acquired) M95.5
  congenital Q74.2
integument (congenital) Q84.9
intervertebral cartilage or disc (acquired) — *see* Disorder, disc, specified NEC
intestine (large) (small) (congenital) NOS Q43.9
  acquired K63.89
intrinsic minus or plus (hand) — *see* Deformity, limb,
  specified type NEC, forearm
iris (acquired) H21.89
  congenital Q13.2
ischium (acquired) M95.5
  congenital Q74.2
jaw (acquired) (congenital) M26.9
joint (acquired) NEC M21.90
  congenital Q68.8
  elbow M21.92- ☑
  hand M21.94- ☑
  hip M21.95- ☑
  knee M21.96- ☑
  shoulder M21.92- ☑
  wrist M21.93- ☑
kidney(s) (calyx) (pelvis) (congenital) Q63.9
  acquired N28.89
  artery (congenital) Q27.2
    acquired I77.89
Klippel-Feil (brevicollis) Q76.1
knee (acquired) NEC — *see* Deformity, limb, lower
  leg
  congenital Q68.2
labium (majus) (minus) (congenital) Q52.79
  acquired N90.89
lacrimal passages or duct (congenital) NEC Q10.6
  acquired — *see* Disorder, lacrimal system, changes
larynx (muscle) (congenital) Q31.8
  acquired J38.7
  web (glottic) Q31.0
leg (upper) (acquired) NEC — *see also* Deformity, limb,
  thigh
  congenital Q68.8
  lower leg — *see* Deformity, limb, lower leg
lens (acquired) H27.8
  congenital Q12.9
lid (fold) (acquired) — *see also* Disorder, eyelid, specified type NEC
  congenital Q10.3
ligament (acquired) — *see* Disorder, ligament
  congenital Q79.9
limb (acquired) M21.90
  clawfoot M21.53- ☑
  clawhand M21.51- ☑
  clubfoot M21.54- ☑
  clubhand M21.52- ☑
  congenital, except reduction deformity Q74.9
  flat foot M21.4- ☑
  flexion M21.20
    ankle M21.27- ☑
    elbow M21.22- ☑
    finger M21.24- ☑
    hip M21.25- ☑
    knee M21.26- ☑
    shoulder M21.21- ☑
    toe M21.27- ☑
    wrist M21.23- ☑
  foot
    claw — *see* Deformity, limb, clawfoot
    club — *see* Deformity, limb, clubfoot

☑ **Additional Character Required** — **Refer to the Tabular List for Character Selection**   ▽ Subterms under main terms may continue to next column or page

Deformity — *continued*
  limb — *continued*
    foot — *continued*
      drop M21.37- ☑
      flat — *see* Deformity, limb, flat foot
      specified NEC M21.6X- ☑
    forearm M21.93- ☑
    hand M21.94- ☑
    lower leg M21.96- ☑
    specified type NEC M21.80
      forearm M21.83- ☑
      lower leg M21.86- ☑
      thigh M21.85- ☑
      upper arm M21.82- ☑
    thigh M21.95- ☑
    unequal length M21.70
      short site is
        femur M21.75- ☑
        fibula M21.76- ☑
        humerus M21.72- ☑
        radius M21.73- ☑
        tibia M21.76- ☑
        ulna M21.73- ☑
    upper arm M21.92- ☑
    valgus — *see* Deformity, valgus
    varus — *see* Deformity, varus
    wrist drop M21.33- ☑
  lip (acquired) NEC K13.0
    congenital Q38.0
  liver (congenital) Q44.7
    acquired K76.89
  lumbosacral (congenital) (joint) (region) Q76.49
    acquired — *see* subcategory M43.8 ☑
    kyphosis — *see* Kyphosis, congenital
    lordosis — *see* Lordosis, congenital
  lung (congenital) Q33.9
    acquired J98.4
  lymphatic system, congenital Q89.9
  Madelung's (radius) Q74.0
  mandible (acquired) (congenital) M26.9
  maxilla (acquired) (congenital) M26.9
  meninges or membrane (congenital) Q07.9
    cerebral Q04.8
      acquired G96.198
    spinal cord (congenital) G96.198
      acquired G96.198
  metacarpus (acquired) — *see* Deformity, limb, forearm
    congenital Q74.0
  metatarsus (acquired) — *see* Deformity, foot
    congenital Q66.9- ☑
  middle ear (congenital) Q16.4
    ossicles Q16.3
  mitral (leaflets) (valve) I05.8
    parachute Q23.2
    stenosis, congenital Q23.2
  mouth (acquired) K13.79
    congenital Q38.6
  multiple, congenital NEC Q89.7
  muscle (acquired) M62.89
    congenital Q79.9
      sternocleidomastoid Q68.0
  musculoskeletal system (acquired) M95.9
    congenital Q79.9
    specified NEC M95.8
  nail (acquired) L60.8
    congenital Q84.6
  nasal — *see* Deformity, nose
  neck (acquired) M95.3
    congenital Q18.9
      sternocleidomastoid Q68.0
  nervous system (congenital) Q07.9
  nipple (congenital) Q83.9
    acquired N64.89
  nose (acquired) (cartilage) M95.0
    bone (turbinate) M95.0
    congenital Q30.9
      bent or squashed Q67.4
    saddle M95.0
      syphilitic A50.57
    septum (acquired) J34.2
      congenital Q30.8
    sinus (wall) (congenital) Q30.8
      acquired M95.0
    syphilitic (congenital) A50.57
      late A52.73
  ocular muscle (congenital) Q10.3
    acquired — *see* Strabismus, mechanical
  opticociliary vessels (congenital) Q13.2

Deformity — *continued*
  orbit (eye) (acquired) H05.30
    atrophy — *see* Atrophy, orbit
    congenital Q10.7
    due to
      bone disease NEC H05.32- ☑
      trauma or surgery H05.33- ☑
    enlargement — *see* Enlargement, orbit
    exostosis — *see* Exostosis, orbit
  organ of Corti (congenital) Q16.5
  ovary (congenital) Q50.39
    acquired N83.8
  oviduct, acquired N83.8
  palate (congenital) Q38.5
    acquired M27.8
    cleft (congenital) — *see* Cleft, palate
  pancreas (congenital) Q45.3
    acquired K86.89
  parathyroid (gland) Q89.2
  parotid (gland) (congenital) Q38.4
    acquired K11.8
  patella (acquired) — *see* Disorder, patella, specified
    NEC
  pelvis, pelvic (acquired) (bony) M95.5
    with disproportion (fetopelvic) O33.0
      causing obstructed labor O65.0
    congenital Q74.2
    rachitic sequelae (late effect) E64.3
  penis (glans) (congenital) Q55.69
    acquired N48.89
  pericardium (congenital) Q24.8
    acquired — *see* Pericarditis
  pharynx (congenital) Q38.8
    acquired J39.2
  pinna, acquired — *see also* Disorder, pinna, deformity
    congenital Q17.9
  pituitary (congenital) Q89.2
  posture — *see* Dorsopathy, deforming
  prepuce (congenital) Q55.69
    acquired N47.8
  prostate (congenital) Q55.4
    acquired N42.89
  pupil (congenital) Q13.2
    acquired — *see* Abnormality, pupillary
  pylorus (congenital) Q40.3
    acquired K31.89
  rachitic (acquired), old or healed E64.3
  radius (acquired) — *see also* Deformity, limb, forearm
    congenital Q68.8
  rectum (congenital) Q43.9
    acquired K62.89
  reduction (extremity) (limb), congenital — *see also*
      condition and site Q73.8
    brain Q04.3
    lower — *see* Defect, reduction, lower limb
    upper — *see* Defect, reduction, upper limb
  renal — *see* Deformity, kidney
  respiratory system (congenital) Q34.9
  rib (acquired) M95.4
    congenital Q76.6
    cervical Q76.5
  rotation (joint) (acquired) — *see* Deformity, limb,
      specified site NEC
    congenital Q74.9
    hip — *see* Deformity, limb, specified type NEC, thigh
      congenital Q65.89
  sacroiliac joint (congenital) — *see* subcategory Q74.2
    acquired — *see* subcategory M43.8 ☑
  sacrum (acquired) — *see* subcategory M43.8 ☑
  saddle
    back — *see* Lordosis
    nose M95.0
      syphilitic A50.57
  salivary gland or duct (congenital) Q38.4
    acquired K11.8
  scapula (acquired) M95.8
    congenital Q68.8
  scrotum (congenital) — *see also* Malformation, testis
      and scrotum
    acquired N50.89
  seminal vesicles (congenital) Q55.4
    acquired N50.89
  septum, nasal (acquired) J34.2
  shoulder (joint) (acquired) — *see* Deformity, limb, up-
      per arm
    congenital Q74.9
    contraction — *see* Contraction, joint, shoulder
  sigmoid (flexure) (congenital) Q43.9

Deformity — *continued*
  sigmoid — *continued*
    acquired K63.89
  skin (congenital) Q82.9
  skull (acquired) M95.2
    congenital Q75.8
    with
      anencephaly Q00.0
      encephalocele — *see* Encephalocele
      hydrocephalus Q03.9
        with spina bifida — *see* Spina bifida, by
          site, with hydrocephalus
      microcephaly Q02
  soft parts, organs or tissues (of pelvis)
    in pregnancy or childbirth NEC O34.8- ☑
    causing obstructed labor O65.5
  spermatic cord (congenital) Q55.4
    acquired N50.89
    torsion — *see* Torsion, spermatic cord
  spinal — *see* Dorsopathy, deforming
    column (acquired) — *see* Dorsopathy, deforming
      congenital Q67.5
    cord (congenital) Q06.9
      acquired G95.89
    nerve root (congenital) Q07.9
  spine (acquired) — *see also* Dorsopathy, deforming
    congenital Q67.5
    rachitic E64.3
    specified NEC — *see* Dorsopathy, deforming, speci-
        fied NEC
  spleen
    acquired D73.89
    congenital Q89.09
  Sprengel's (congenital) Q74.0
  sternocleidomastoid (muscle), congenital Q68.0
  sternum (acquired) M95.4
    congenital NEC Q76.7
  stomach (congenital) Q40.3
    acquired K31.89
  submandibular gland (congenital) Q38.4
  submaxillary gland (congenital) Q38.4
    acquired K11.8
  talipes — *see* Talipes
  testis (congenital) — *see also* Malformation, testis and
      scrotum
    acquired N44.8
    torsion — *see* Torsion, testis
  thigh (acquired) — *see also* Deformity, limb, thigh
    congenital NEC Q68.8
  thorax (acquired) (wall) M95.4
    congenital Q67.8
    sequelae of rickets E64.3
  thumb (acquired) — *see also* Deformity, finger
    congenital NEC Q68.1
  thymus (tissue) (congenital) Q89.2
  thyroid (gland) (congenital) Q89.2
    cartilage Q31.8
      acquired J38.7
  tibia (acquired) — *see also* Deformity, limb, specified
      type NEC, lower leg
    congenital NEC Q68.8
    saber (syphilitic) A50.56
  toe (acquired) M20.6- ☑
    congenital Q66.9- ☑
    hallux rigidus M20.2- ☑
    hallux valgus M20.1- ☑
    hallux varus M20.3- ☑
    hammer toe M20.4- ☑
    specified NEC M20.5X- ☑
  tongue (congenital) Q38.3
    acquired K14.8
  tooth, teeth K00.2
  trachea (rings) (congenital) Q32.1
    acquired J39.8
  transverse aortic arch (congenital) Q25.49
  tricuspid (leaflets) (valve) I07.8
    atresia or stenosis Q22.4
    Ebstein's Q22.5
  trunk (acquired) M95.8
    congenital Q89.9
  ulna (acquired) — *see also* Deformity, limb, forearm
    congenital NEC Q68.8
  urachus, congenital Q64.4
  ureter (opening) (congenital) Q62.8
    acquired N28.89
  urethra (congenital) Q64.79
    acquired N36.8
  urinary tract (congenital) Q64.9

Index

Deformity — Degeneration, degenerative

Deformity — *continued*
  urinary tract — *continued*
    urachus Q64.4
  uterus (congenital) Q51.9
    acquired N85.8
  uvula (congenital) Q38.5
  vagina (acquired) N89.8
    congenital Q52.4
  valgus NEC M21.00
    ankle M21.07- ☑
    elbow M21.02- ☑
    hip M21.05- ☑
    knee M21.06- ☑
  valve, valvular (congenital) (heart) Q24.8
    acquired — *see* Endocarditis
  varus NEC M21.10
    ankle M21.17- ☑
    elbow M21.12- ☑
    hip M21.15 ☑
    knee M21.16- ☑
    tibia — *see* Osteochondrosis, juvenile, tibia
  vas deferens (congenital) Q55.4
    acquired N50.89
  vein (congenital) Q27.9
    great Q26.9
  vertebra — *see* Dorsopathy, deforming
  vertical talus (congenital) Q66.80
    left foot Q66.82
    right foot Q66.81
  vesicourethral orifice (acquired) N32.89
    congenital NEC Q64.79
  vessels of optic papilla (congenital) Q14.2
  visual field (contraction) — *see* Defect, visual field
  vitreous body, acquired H43.89
  vulva (congenital) Q52.79
    acquired N90.89
  wrist (joint) (acquired) — *see also* Deformity, limb, forearm
    congenital Q68.8
    contraction — *see* Contraction, joint, wrist

Degeneration, degenerative
  adrenal (capsule) (fatty) (gland) (hyaline) (infectional) E27.8
  amyloid — *see also* Amyloidosis E85.9
  anterior cornua, spinal cord G12.29
  anterior labral S43.49- ☑
  aorta, aortic I70.0
    fatty I77.89
  aortic valve (heart) — *see* Endocarditis, aortic
  arteriovascular — *see* Arteriosclerosis
  artery, arterial (atheromatous) (calcareous) — *see also* Arteriosclerosis
    cerebral, amyloid E85.4 *[I68.0]*
    medial — *see* Arteriosclerosis, extremities
  articular cartilage NEC — *see* Derangement, joint, articular cartilage, by site
  atheromatous — *see* Arteriosclerosis
  basal nuclei or ganglia G23.9
    specified NEC G23.8
  bone NEC — *see* Disorder, bone, specified type NEC
  brachial plexus G54.0
  brain (cortical) (progressive) G31.9
    alcoholic G31.2
    arteriosclerotic I67.2
    childhood G31.9
      specified NEC G31.89
    cystic G31.89
      congenital Q04.6
    in
      alcoholism G31.2
      beriberi E51.2
      cerebrovascular disease I67.9
      congenital hydrocephalus Q03.9
        with spina bifida — *see also* Spina bifida
      Fabry-Anderson disease E75.21
      Gaucher's disease E75.22
      Hunter's syndrome E76.1
      lipidosis
        cerebral E75.4
        generalized E75.6
      mucopolysaccharidosis — *see* Mucopolysaccharidosis
      myxedema E03.9 *[G32.89]*
      neoplastic disease — *see also* Neoplasm D49.6 *[G32.89]*
      Niemann-Pick disease E75.249 *[G32.89]*
      sphingolipidosis E75.3 *[G32.89]*
      vitamin B12 deficiency E53.8 *[G32.89]*

Degeneration, degenerative — *continued*
  brain — *continued*
    senile NEC G31.1
  breast N64.89
  Bruch's membrane — *see* Degeneration, choroid
  capillaries (fatty) I78.8
    amyloid E85.89 *[I79.8]*
  cardiac — *see also* Degeneration, myocardial
    valve, valvular — *see* Endocarditis
  cardiorenal — *see* Hypertension, cardiorenal
  cardiovascular — *see also* Disease, cardiovascular
    renal — *see* Hypertension, cardiorenal
  cerebellar NOS G31.9
    alcoholic G31.2
    primary (hereditary) (sporadic) G11.9
  cerebral — *see* Degeneration, brain
  cerebrovascular I67.9
    due to hypertension I67.4
  cervical plexus G54.2
  cervix N88.8
    due to radiation (intended effect) N88.8
      adverse effect or misadventure N99.89
  chamber angle H21.21- ☑
  changes, spine or vertebra — *see* Spondylosis
  chorioretinal — *see also* Degeneration, choroid
    hereditary H31.20
  choroid (colloid) (drusen) H31.10- ☑
    atrophy — *see* Atrophy, choroidal
    hereditary — *see* Dystrophy, choroidal, hereditary
  ciliary body H21.22- ☑
  cochlear — *see* subcategory H83.8 ☑
  combined (spinal cord) (subacute) E53.8 *[G32.0]*
    with anemia (pernicious) D51.0 *[G32.0]*
      due to dietary vitamin B12 deficiency D51.3 *[G32.0]*
    in (due to)
      vitamin B12 deficiency E53.8 *[G32.0]*
        anemia D51.9 *[G32.0]*
  conjunctiva H11.10
    concretions — *see* Concretion, conjunctiva
    deposits — *see* Deposit, conjunctiva
    pigmentations — *see* Pigmentation, conjunctiva
    pinguecula — *see* Pinguecula
    xerosis — *see* Xerosis, conjunctiva
  cornea H18.40
    calcerous H18.43
      band keratopathy H18.42- ☑
    familial, hereditary — *see* Dystrophy, cornea
    hyaline (of old scars) H18.49
    keratomalacia — *see* Keratomalacia
    nodular H18.45- ☑
    peripheral H18.46- ☑
    senile H18.41- ☑
    specified type NEC H18.49
  cortical (cerebellar) (parenchymatous) G31.89
    alcoholic G31.2
    diffuse, due to arteriopathy I67.2
  corticobasal G31.85
  cutis L98.8
    amyloid E85.4 *[L99]*
  dental pulp K04.2
  disc disease — *see* Degeneration, intervertebral disc NEC
  dorsolateral (spinal cord) — *see* Degeneration, combined
  extrapyramidal G25.9
  eye, macular — *see also* Degeneration, macula
    congenital or hereditary — *see* Dystrophy, retina
  facet joints — *see* Spondylosis
  fatty
    liver NEC K76.0
      alcoholic K70.0
  grey matter (brain) (Alpers') G31.81
  heart — *see also* Degeneration, myocardial
    amyloid E85.4 *[I43]*
    atheromatous — *see* Disease, heart, ischemic, atherosclerotic
    ischemic — *see* Disease, heart, ischemic
  hepatolenticular (Wilson's) E83.01
  hepatorenal K76.7
  hyaline (diffuse) (generalized)
    localized — *see* Degeneration, by site
  infrapatellar fat pad M79.4
  intervertebral disc NOS
    with
      myelopathy — *see* Disorder, disc, with, myelopathy

Degeneration, degenerative — *continued*
  intervertebral disc — *continued*
    with — *continued*
      radiculitis or radiculopathy — *see* Disorder, disc, with, radiculopathy
    cervical, cervicothoracic — *see* Disorder, disc, cervical, degeneration
      with
        myelopathy — *see* Disorder, disc, cervical, with myelopathy
        neuritis, radiculitis or radiculopathy — *see* Disorder, disc, cervical, with neuritis
    lumbar region M51.36
      with
        myelopathy M51.06
        neuritis, radiculitis, radiculopathy or sciatica M51.16
    lumbosacral region M51.37
      with
        neuritis, radiculitis, radiculopathy or sciatica M51.17
    sacrococcygeal region M53.3
    thoracic region M51.34
      with
        myelopathy M51.04
        neuritis, radiculitis, radiculopathy M51.14
    thoracolumbar region M51.35
      with
        myelopathy M51.05
        neuritis, radiculitis, radiculopathy M51.15
  intestine, amyloid E85.4
  iris (pigmentary) H21.23- ☑
  ischemic — *see* Ischemia
  joint disease — *see* Osteoarthritis
  kidney N28.89
    amyloid E85.4 *[N29]*
    cystic, congenital Q61.9
    fatty N28.89
    polycystic Q61.3
      adult type (autosomal dominant) Q61.2
      infantile type (autosomal recessive) NEC Q61.19
        collecting duct dilatation Q61.11
  Kuhnt-Junius — *see also* Degeneration, macula H35.32- ☑
  lens — *see* Cataract
  lenticular (familial) (progressive) (Wilson's) (with cirrhosis of liver) E83.01
  liver (diffuse) NEC K76.89
    amyloid E85.4 *[K77]*
    cystic K76.89
      congenital Q44.6
    fatty NEC K76.0
      alcoholic K70.0
    hypertrophic K76.89
    parenchymatous, acute or subacute K72.00
      with coma K72.01
    pigmentary K76.89
    toxic (acute) K71.9
  lung J98.4
  lymph gland I89.8
    hyaline I89.8
  macula, macular (acquired) (age-related) (senile) H35.30
    angioid streaks H35.33
    atrophic age-related H35.31- ☑
    congenital or hereditary — *see* Dystrophy, retina
    cystoid H35.35- ☑
    drusen H35.36- ☑
    dry age-related H35.31- ☑
    exudative H35.32- ☑
    hole H35.34- ☑
    nonexudative H35.31- ☑
    puckering H35.37- ☑
    toxic H35.38- ☑
    wet age-related H35.32- ☑
  membranous labyrinth, congenital (causing impairment of hearing) Q16.5
  meniscus — *see* Derangement, meniscus
  mitral — *see* Insufficiency, mitral
  Mönckeberg's — *see* Arteriosclerosis, extremities
  motor centers, senile G31.1
  multi-system G90.3
  mural — *see also* Degeneration, myocardial
  muscle (fatty) (fibrous) (hyaline) (progressive) M62.89
    heart — *see* Degeneration, myocardial
  myelin, central nervous system G37.9
  myocardial, myocardium (fatty) (hyaline) (senile) I51.5
    with rheumatic fever (conditions in I00) I09.0

90

☑ **Additional Character Required** — Refer to the Tabular List for Character Selection   ▽ **Subterms under main terms may continue to next column or page**

Degeneration, degenerative — *continued*
  myocardial, myocardium — *continued*
    with rheumatic fever — *continued*
      active, acute or subacute I01.2
        with chorea I02.0
      inactive or quiescent (with chorea) I09.0
    hypertensive — *see* Hypertension, heart
    rheumatic — *see* Degeneration, myocardial, with
      rheumatic fever
    syphilitic A52.06
  nasal sinus (mucosa) J32.9
    frontal J32.1
    maxillary J32.0
  nerve — *see* Disorder, nerve
  nervous system G31.9
    alcoholic G31.2
    amyloid E85.4 *[G99.8]*
    autonomic G90.9
    fatty G31.89
    specified NEC G31.89
  nipple N64.89
  olivopontocerebellar (hereditary) (familial) G23.8
  osseous labyrinth — *see* subcategory H83.8 ☑
  ovary N83.8
    cystic N83.20- ☑
    microcystic N83.20- ☑
  pallidal pigmentary (progressive) G23.0
  pancreas K86.89
    tuberculous A18.83
  penis N48.89
  pigmentary (diffuse) (general)
    localized — *see* Degeneration, by site
    pallidal (progressive) G23.0
  pineal gland E34.8
  pituitary (gland) E23.6
  popliteal fat pad M79.4
  posterolateral (spinal cord) — *see* Degeneration,
    combined
  pulmonary valve (heart) I37.8
  pulp (tooth) K04.2
  pupillary margin H21.24- ☑
  renal — *see* Degeneration, kidney
  retina H35.9
    hereditary (cerebroretinal) (congenital) (juvenile)
      (macula) (peripheral) (pigmentary) — *see*
      Dystrophy, retina
    Kuhnt-Junius — *see also* Degeneration, macula
      H35.32- ☑
    macula (cystic) (exudative) (hole) (nonexudative)
      (pseudohole) (senile) (toxic) — *see* Degener-
      ation, macula
    peripheral H35.40
      lattice H35.41- ☑
      microcystoid H35.42- ☑
      paving stone H35.43- ☑
      secondary
        pigmentary H35.45- ☑
        vitreoretinal H35.46- ☑
      senile reticular H35.44- ☑
    pigmentary (primary) — *see also* Dystrophy, retina
      secondary — *see* Degeneration, retina, peripher-
      al, secondary
    posterior pole — *see* Degeneration, macula
  saccule, congenital (causing impairment of hearing)
    Q16.5
  senile R54
    brain G31.1
    cardiac, heart or myocardium — *see* Degeneration,
      myocardial
    motor centers G31.1
    vascular — *see* Arteriosclerosis
  sinus (cystic) — *see also* Sinusitis
    polypoid J33.1
  skin L98.8
    amyloid E85.4 *[L99]*
    colloid L98.8
  spinal (cord) G31.89
    amyloid E85.4 *[G32.89]*
    combined (subacute) — *see* Degeneration, com-
      bined
    dorsolateral — *see* Degeneration, combined
    familial NEC G31.89
    fatty G31.89
    funicular — *see* Degeneration, combined
    posterolateral — *see* Degeneration, combined
    subacute combined — *see* Degeneration, combined
    tuberculous A17.81
  spleen D73.0

Degeneration, degenerative — *continued*
  spleen — *continued*
    amyloid E85.4 *[D77]*
  stomach K31.89
  striatonigral G23.2
  suprarenal (capsule) (gland) E27.8
  synovial membrane (pulpy) — *see* Disorder, synovium,
    specified type NEC
  tapetoretinal — *see* Dystrophy, retina
  thymus (gland) E32.8
    fatty E32.8
  thyroid (gland) E07.89
  tricuspid (heart) (valve) I07.9
  tuberculous NEC — *see* Tuberculosis
  turbinate J34.89
  uterus (cystic) N85.8
  vascular (senile) — *see* Arteriosclerosis
    hypertensive — *see* Hypertension
  vitreoretinal, secondary — *see* Degeneration, retina,
    peripheral, secondary, vitreoretinal
  vitreous (body) H43.81- ☑
  Wallerian — *see* Disorder, nerve
  Wilson's hepatolenticular E83.01
Deglutition
  paralysis R13.0
    hysterical F44.4
  pneumonia J69.0
Degos' disease I77.89
Dehiscence (of)
  amputation stump T87.81
  cesarean wound O90.0
  closure of
    cornea T81.31 ☑
    craniotomy T81.32 ☑
    fascia (muscular) (superficial) T81.32 ☑
    internal organ or tissue T81.32 ☑
    laceration (external) (internal) T81.33 ☑
    ligament T81.32 ☑
    mucosa T81.31 ☑
    muscle or muscle flap T81.32 ☑
    ribs or rib cage T81.32 ☑
    skin and subcutaneous tissue (full-thickness) (super-
      ficial) T81.31 ☑
    skull T81.32 ☑
    sternum (sternotomy) T81.32 ☑
    tendon T81.32 ☑
    traumatic laceration (external) (internal) T81.33 ☑
  episiotomy O90.1
  operation wound NEC T81.31 ☑
    external operation wound (superficial) T81.31 ☑
    internal operation wound (deep) T81.32 ☑
  perineal wound (postpartum) O90.1
  traumatic injury wound repair T81.33 ☑
  wound T81.30 ☑
    traumatic repair T81.33 ☑
Dehydration E86.0
  newborn P74.1
Déjérine-Roussy syndrome G89.0
Déjérine-Sottas disease or neuropathy (hypertrophic)
  G60.0
Déjérine-Thomas atrophy G23.8
Delay, delayed
  any plane in pelvis
    complicating delivery O66.9
  birth or delivery NOS O63.9
  closure, ductus arteriosus (Botalli) P29.38
  coagulation — *see* Defect, coagulation
  conduction (cardiac) (ventricular) I45.9
  delivery, second twin, triplet, etc O63.2
  development R62.50
    global F88
    intellectual (specific) F81.9
    language F80.9
      due to hearing loss F80.4
    learning F81.9
    pervasive F84.9
    physiological R62.50
      specified stage NEC R62.0
    reading F81.0
    sexual E30.0
    speech F80.9
      due to hearing loss F80.4
    spelling F81.81
  ejaculation F52.32
  gastric emptying K30
  menarche E30.0
  menstruation (cause unknown) N91.0

Delay, delayed — *continued*
  milestone R62.0
  passage of meconium (newborn) P76.0
  primary respiration P28.9
  puberty (constitutional) E30.0
  separation of umbilical cord P96.82
  sexual maturation, female E30.0
  sleep phase syndrome G47.21
  union, fracture — *see* Fracture, by site
  vaccination Z28.9
Deletion(s)
  autosome Q93.9
    identified by fluorescence in situ hybridization (FISH)
      Q93.89
    identified by in situ hybridization (ISH) Q93.89
  chromosome
    with complex rearrangements NEC Q93.7
    part of NEC Q93.59
    seen only at prometaphase Q93.89
    short arm
      22q11.2 Q93.81
      4 Q93.3
      5p Q93.4
    specified NEC Q93.89
  long arm chromosome 18 or 21 Q93.89
    with complex rearrangements NEC Q93.7
  microdeletions NEC Q93.88
Delhi boil or button B55.1
Delinquency (juvenile) (neurotic) F91.8
  group Z72.810
Delinquent immunization status Z28.3
Delirium, delirious (acute or subacute) (not alcohol- or
  drug-induced) (with dementia) R41.0
  alcoholic (acute) (tremens) (withdrawal) F10.921
    with intoxication F10.921
      in
        abuse F10.121
        dependence F10.221
  due to (secondary to)
    alcohol
      intoxication F10.921
        in
          abuse F10.121
          dependence F10.221
      withdrawal F10.231
    amphetamine intoxication F15.921
      in
        abuse F15.121
        dependence F15.221
    anxiolytic
      intoxication F13.921
        in
          abuse F13.121
          dependence F13.221
      withdrawal F13.231
    cannabis intoxication (acute) F12.921
      in
        abuse F12.121
        dependence F12.221
    cocaine intoxication (acute) F14.921
      in
        abuse F14.121
        dependence F14.221
    general medical condition F05
    hallucinogen intoxication F16.921
      in
        abuse F16.121
        dependence F16.221
    hypnotic
      intoxication F13.921
        in
          abuse F13.121
          dependence F13.221
      withdrawal F13.231
    inhalant intoxication (acute) F18.921
      in
        abuse F18.121
        dependence F18.221
    multiple etiologies F05
    opioid intoxication (acute) F11.921
      in
        abuse F11.121
        dependence F11.221
    other (or unknown) substance F19.921
    phencyclidine intoxication (acute) F16.921
      in
        abuse F16.121
        dependence F16.221

Index

Delirium, delirious — *continued*
due to — *continued*
psychoactive substance NEC intoxication (acute)
F19.921
in
abuse F19.121
dependence F19.221
sedative
intoxication F13.921
in
abuse F13.121
dependence F13.221
withdrawal F13.231
unknown etiology R41.0
exhaustion F43.0
hysterical F44.89
postprocedural (postoperative) F05
puerperal F05
thyroid — *see* Thyrotoxicosis with thyroid storm
traumatic — *see* Injury, intracranial
tremens (alcohol-induced) F10.231
sedative-induced F13.231
Delivery (childbirth) (labor)
arrested active phase O62.1
cesarean (for)
abnormal
pelvis (bony) (deformity) (major) NEC with disproportion (fetopelvic) O33.0
with obstructed labor O65.0
presentation or position O32.9 ☑
abruptio placentae — *see also* Abruptio placentae
O45.9- ☑
acromion presentation O32.2 ☑
atony, uterus O62.2
breech presentation O32.1 ☑
incomplete O32.8 ☑
brow presentation O32.3 ☑
cephalopelvic disproportion O33.9
cerclage O34.3- ☑
chin presentation O32.3 ☑
cicatrix of cervix O34.4- ☑
contracted pelvis (general)
inlet O33.2
outlet O33.3 ☑
cord presentation or prolapse O69.0 ☑
cystocele O34.8- ☑
deformity (acquired) (congenital)
pelvic organs or tissues NEC O34.8- ☑
pelvis (bony) NEC O33.0
disproportion NOS O33.9
eclampsia — *see* Eclampsia
face presentation O32.3 ☑
failed
forceps O66.5
induction of labor O61.9
instrumental O61.1
mechanical O61.1
medical O61.0
specified NEC O61.8
surgical O61.1
trial of labor NOS O66.40
following previous cesarean delivery O66.41
vacuum extraction O66.5
ventouse O66.5
fetal-maternal hemorrhage O43.01- ☑
hemorrhage (intrapartum) O67.9
with coagulation defect O67.0
specified cause NEC O67.8
high head at term O32.4 ☑
hydrocephalic fetus O33.6 ☑
incarceration of uterus O34.51- ☑
incoordinate uterine action O62.4
increased size, fetus O33.5 ☑
inertia, uterus O62.2
primary O62.0
secondary O62.1
isthmocele O34.22
lateroversion, uterus O34.59- ☑
mal lie O32.9 ☑
malposition
fetus O32.9 ☑
pelvic organs or tissues NEC O34.8- ☑
uterus NEC O34.59- ☑
malpresentation NOS O32.9 ☑
oblique presentation O32.2 ☑
occurring after 37 completed weeks of gestation
but before 39 completed weeks gestation due
to (spontaneous) onset of labor O75.82

Delivery — *continued*
cesarean — *continued*
oversize fetus O33.5 ☑
pelvic tumor NEC O34.8- ☑
placenta previa O44.0- ☑
complete O44.0- ☑
with hemorrhage O44.1- ☑
placental insufficiency O36.51- ☑
planned, occurring after 37 completed weeks of
gestation but before 39 completed weeks
gestation due to (spontaneous) onset of labor
O75.82
polyp, cervix O34.4- ☑
causing obstructed labor O65.5
poor dilatation, cervix O62.0
pre-eclampsia O14.94
mild O14.04
moderate O14.04
severe O14.14
with hemolysis, elevated liver enzymes and
low platelet count (HELLP) O14.24
previous
cesarean delivery O34.219
classical (vertical) scar O34.212
isthmocele O34.22
low transverse scar O34.211
mid-transverse T incision O34.218
scar
defect (isthmocele) O34.22
specified type NEC O34.218
surgery (to)
cervix O34.4- ☑
gynecological NEC O34.8- ☑
rectum O34.7- ☑
uterus O34.29
vagina O34.6- ☑
prolapse
arm or hand O32.2 ☑
uterus O34.52- ☑
prolonged labor NOS O63.9
rectocele O34.8- ☑
retroversion
uterus O34.53- ☑
rigid
cervix O34.4- ☑
pelvic floor O34.8- ☑
perineum O34.7- ☑
vagina O34.6- ☑
vulva O34.7- ☑
sacculation, pregnant uterus O34.59- ☑
scar(s)
cervix O34.4- ☑
cesarean delivery O34.219
classical (vertical) O34.212
isthmocele O34.22
low transverse O34.211
mid-transverse T incision O34.218
scar
defect (isthmocele) O34.22
specified type NEC O34.218
defect (isthmocele) O34.22
transmural uterine O34.29
uterus O34.29
Shirodkar suture in situ O34.3- ☑
shoulder presentation O32.2 ☑
stenosis or stricture, cervix O34.4- ☑
streptococcus group B (GBS) carrier state O99.824
transmural uterine scar O34.29
transverse presentation or lie O32.2 ☑
tumor, pelvic organs or tissues NEC O34.8- ☑
cervix O34.4- ☑
umbilical cord presentation or prolapse O69.0 ☑
without indication O82
completely normal case O80
complicated O75.9
by
abnormal, abnormality (of)
forces of labor O62.9
specified type NEC O62.8
glucose O99.814
uterine contractions NOS O62.9
abruptio placentae — *see also* Abruptio placentae O45.9- ☑
abuse
physical O9A.32 (*following* O99)
psychological O9A.52 (*following* O99)
sexual O9A.42 (*following* O99)

Delivery — *continued*
complicated — *continued*
by — *continued*
adherent placenta O72.0
without hemorrhage O73.0
alcohol use O99.314
anemia (pre-existing) O99.02
anesthetic death O74.8
annular detachment of cervix O71.3
atony, uterus O62.2
attempted vacuum extraction and forceps O66.5
Bandl's ring O62.4
bariatric surgery status O99.844
biliary tract disorder O26.62
bleeding — *see* Delivery, complicated by, hemorrhage
blood disorder NEC O99.12
cervical dystocia (hypotonic) O62.2
primary O62.0
secondary O62.1
circulatory system disorder O99.42
compression of cord (umbilical) NEC O69.2 ☑
condition NEC O99.892
contraction, contracted ring O62.4
cord (umbilical)
around neck
with compression O69.1 ☑
without compression O69.81 ☑
bruising O69.5 ☑
complication O69.9 ☑
specified NEC O69.89 ☑
compression NEC O69.2 ☑
entanglement O69.2 ☑
without compression O69.82 ☑
hematoma O69.5 ☑
presentation O69.0 ☑
prolapse O69.0 ☑
short O69.3 ☑
thrombosis (vessels) O69.5 ☑
vascular lesion O69.5 ☑
Couvelaire uterus O45.8X- ☑
damage to (injury to) NEC
perineum O71.82
periurethral tissue O71.82
vulva O71.82
delay following rupture of membranes (spontaneous) — *see* Pregnancy, complicated by,
premature rupture of membranes
depressed fetal heart tones O76
diabetes O24.92
gestational O24.429
diet controlled O24.420
insulin controlled O24.424
oral drug controlled (antidiabetic) (hypoglycemic) O24.425
pre-existing O24.32
specified NEC O24.82
type 1 O24.02
type 2 O24.12
diastasis recti (abdominis) O71.89
dilatation
bladder O66.8
cervix incomplete, poor or slow O62.0
disease NEC O99.892
disruptio uteri — *see* Delivery, complicated by,
rupture, uterus
drug use O99.324
dysfunction, uterus NOS O62.9
hypertonic O62.4
hypotonic O62.2
primary O62.0
secondary O62.1
incoordinate O62.4
eclampsia O15.1
embolism (pulmonary) — *see* Embolism, obstetric
endocrine, nutritional or metabolic disease NEC
O99.284
failed
attempted vaginal birth after previous cesarean delivery O66.41
induction of labor O61.9
instrumental O61.1
mechanical O61.1
medical O61.0
specified NEC O61.8
surgical O61.1
trial of labor O66.40

Delirium, delirious — Delivery

☑ **Additional Character Required** — **Refer to the Tabular List for Character Selection**   ▽ **Subterms under main terms may continue to next column or page**

Delivery — continued
  complicated — continued
    by — continued
      female genital mutilation O65.5
      fetal
        abnormal acid-base balance O68
        acidemia O68
        acidosis O68
        alkalosis O68
        death, early O02.1
        deformity O66.3
        heart rate or rhythm (abnormal) (non-reassuring) O76
        hypoxia O77.8
        stress O77.9
          due to drug administration O77.1
          electrocardiographic evidence of O77.8
          specified NEC O77.8
          ultrasound evidence of O77.8
      fever during labor O75.2
      gastric banding status O99.844
      gastric bypass status O99.844
      gastrointestinal disease NEC O99.62
      gestational
        diabetes O24.429
          diet controlled O24.420
          insulin (and diet) controlled O24.424
          oral drug controlled (antidiabetic) (hypoglycemic) O24.425
        edema O12.04
          with proteinuria O12.24
        proteinuria O12.14
      gonorrhea O98.22
      hematoma O71.7
        ischial spine O71.7
        pelvic O71.7
        vagina O71.7
        vulva or perineum O71.7
      hemorrhage (uterine) O67.9
        associated with
          afibrinogenemia O67.0
          coagulation defect O67.0
          hyperfibrinolysis O67.0
          hypofibrinogenemia O67.0
        due to
          low implantation of placenta O44.5- ☑
          low-lying placenta O44.5- ☑
          placenta previa O44.1- ☑
            marginal O44.3- ☑
            partial O44.3- ☑
          premature separation of placenta (normally implanted) — see also Abruptio placentae O45.9- ☑
          retained placenta O72.0
          uterine leiomyoma O67.8
        placenta NEC O67.8
        postpartum NEC (atonic) (immediate) O72.1
          with retained or trapped placenta O72.0
          delayed O72.2
          secondary O72.2
          third stage O72.0
      hourglass contraction, uterus O62.4
      hypertension, hypertensive (pre-existing) — see Hypertension, complicated by, childbirth (labor)
      hypotension O26.5- ☑
      incomplete dilatation (cervix) O62.0
      incoordinate uterus contractions O62.4
      inertia, uterus O62.2
        during latent phase of labor O62.0
        primary O62.0
        secondary O62.1
      infection (maternal) O98.92
        carrier state NEC O99.834
        gonorrhea O98.22
        human immunodeficiency virus (HIV) O98.72
        sexually transmitted NEC O98.32
        specified NEC O98.82
        syphilis O98.12
        tuberculosis O98.02
        viral hepatitis O98.42
        viral NEC O98.52
      injury (to mother) — see also Delivery, complicated, by, damage to O71.9
      nonobstetric O9A.22 (following O99)
          caused by abuse — see Delivery, complicated by, abuse
      intrauterine fetal death, early O02.1

Delivery — continued
  complicated — continued
    by — continued
      inversion, uterus O71.2
      laceration (perineal) O70.9
        anus (sphincter) O70.4
          with third degree laceration — see also Delivery, complicated, by, laceration, perineum, third degree O70.20
            with mucosa O70.3
          without third degree laceration O70.2 ☑
        bladder (urinary) O71.5
        bowel O71.5
        cervix (uteri) O71.3
        fourchette O70.0
        hymen O70.0
        labia O70.0
        pelvic
          floor O70.1
          organ NEC O71.5
        perineum, perineal O70.9
          first degree O70.0
          fourth degree O70.3
          muscles O70.1
          second degree O70.1
          skin O70.0
          slight O70.0
          third degree O70.20
            with
              both external anal sphincter (EAS) and internal anal sphincter (IAS) torn (IIIc) O70.23
              less than 50% of external anal sphincter (EAS) thickness torn (IIIa) O70.21
              more than 50% external anal sphincter (EAS) thickness torn (IIIb) O70.22
            IIIa O70.21
            IIIb O70.22
            IIIc O70.23
        peritoneum (pelvic) O71.5
        rectovaginal (septum) (without perineal laceration) O71.4
          with perineum — see also Delivery, complicated, by, laceration, perineum, third degree O70.20
          with anal or rectal mucosa O70.3
        specified NEC O71.89
        sphincter ani — see Delivery, complicated, by, laceration, anus (sphincter)
        urethra O71.5
        uterus O71.81
          before labor O71.81
        vagina, vaginal (deep) (high) (without perineal laceration) O71.4
          with perineum O70.0
          muscles, with perineum O70.1
        vulva O70.0
      liver disorder O26.62
      malignancy O9A.12 (following O99)
      malnutrition O25.2
      malposition, malpresentation
        uterus or cervix O65.5
        placenta O44.0- ☑
          with hemorrhage O44.1- ☑
        without obstruction — see also Delivery, complicated by, obstruction O32.9 ☑
          breech O32.1 ☑
          compound O32.6 ☑
          face (brow) (chin) O32.3 ☑
          footling O32.8 ☑
          high head O32.4 ☑
          oblique O32.2 ☑
          specified NEC O32.8 ☑
          transverse O32.2 ☑
          unstable lie O32.0 ☑
      meconium in amniotic fluid O77.0
      mental disorder NEC O99.344
      metrorrhexis — see Delivery, complicated by, rupture, uterus
      nervous system disorder O99.354
      obesity (pre-existing) O99.214
      obesity surgery status O99.844
      obstetric trauma O71.9
        specified NEC O71.89

Delivery — continued
  complicated — continued
    by — continued
      obstructed labor
        due to
          breech (complete) (frank) presentation O64.1 ☑
            incomplete O64.8 ☑
          brow presentation O64.3 ☑
          buttock presentation O64.1 ☑
          chin presentation O64.2 ☑
          compound presentation O64.5 ☑
          contracted pelvis O65.1
          deep transverse arrest O64.0 ☑
          deformed pelvis O65.0
          dystocia (fetal) O66.9
            due to
              conjoined twins O66.3
              fetal
                abnormality NEC O66.3
                ascites O66.3
                hydrops O66.3
                meningomyelocele O66.3
                sacral teratoma O66.3
                tumor O66.3
              hydrocephalic fetus O66.3
            shoulder O66.0
          face presentation O64.2 ☑
          fetopelvic disproportion O65.4
          footling presentation O64.8 ☑
          impacted shoulders O66.0
          incomplete rotation of fetal head O64.0 ☑
          large fetus O66.2
          locked twins O66.1
          malposition O64.9 ☑
            specified NEC O64.8 ☑
          malpresentation O64.9 ☑
            specified NEC O64.8 ☑
          multiple fetuses NEC O66.6
          pelvic
            abnormality (maternal) O65.9
              organ O65.5
              specified NEC O65.8
            contraction
              inlet O65.2
              mid-cavity O65.3
              outlet O65.3
          persistent (position)
            occipitoiliac O64.0 ☑
            occipitoposterior O64.0 ☑
            occipitosacral O64.0 ☑
            occipitotransverse O64.0 ☑
          prolapsed arm O64.4 ☑
          shoulder presentation O64.4 ☑
        specified NEC O66.8
      pathological retraction ring, uterus O62.4
      penetration, pregnant uterus by instrument O71.1
      perforation — see Delivery, complicated by, laceration
      placenta, placental
        ablatio — see also Abruptio placentae O45.9- ☑
        abnormality O43.9- ☑
          specified NEC O43.89- ☑
        abruptio — see also Abruptio placentae O45.9- ☑
        accreta O43.21- ☑
        adherent (with hemorrhage) O72.0
          without hemorrhage O73.0
        detachment (premature) — see also Abruptio placentae O45.9- ☑
        disorder O43.9- ☑
          specified NEC O43.89- ☑
        hemorrhage NEC O67.8
        increta O43.22- ☑
        low (implantation) (lying) O44.4- ☑
          with hemorrhage O44.5- ☑
        malformation O43.10- ☑
        malposition O44.0- ☑
          without hemorrhage O44.1- ☑
        percreta O43.23- ☑
        previa (central) (complete) (lateral) (total) O44.0- ☑
          with hemorrhage O44.1- ☑
          marginal O44.2- ☑

Subterms under main terms may continue to next column or page   ☑ Additional Character Required — Refer to the Tabular List for Character Selection   93

Delivery — Delivery

Delivery — *continued*
  complicated — *continued*
    by — *continued*
      placenta, placental — *continued*
        previa — *continued*
          marginal — *continued*
            with hemorrhage O44.3- ☑
          partial O44.2- ☑
            with hemorrhage O44.3- ☑
        retained (with hemorrhage) O72.0
          without hemorrhage O73.0
        separation (premature) O45.9- ☑
          specified NEC O45.8X- ☑
        vicious insertion O44.1- ☑
      precipitate labor O62.3
      premature rupture, membranes — *see also*
          Pregnancy, complicated by, premature
          rupture of membranes O42.90
      prolapse
        arm or hand O32.2 ☑
        cord (umbilical) O69.0 ☑
        foot or leg O32.8 ☑
        uterus O34.52- ☑
      prolonged labor O63.9
        first stage O63.0
        second stage O63.1
      protozoal disease (maternal) O98.62
      respiratory disease NEC O99.52
      retained membranes or portions of placenta
          O72.2
        without hemorrhage O73.1
      retarded birth O63.9
      retention of secundines (with hemorrhage) O72.0
        without hemorrhage O73.0
        partial O72.2
          without hemorrhage O73.1
      rupture
        bladder (urinary) O71.5
        cervix O71.3
        pelvic organ NEC O71.5
        urethra O71.5
        uterus (during or after labor) O71.1
          before labor O71.0- ☑
      separation, pubic bone (symphysis pubis) O71.6
      shock O75.1
      shoulder presentation O64.4 ☑
      skin disorder NEC O99.72
      spasm, cervix O62.4
      stenosis or stricture, cervix O65.5
      streptococcus group B (GBS) carrier state O99.824
      subluxation of symphysis (pubis) O26.72
      syphilis (maternal) O98.12
      tear — *see* Delivery, complicated by, laceration
      tetanic uterus O62.4
      trauma (obstetrical) — *see also* Delivery, compli-
          cated, by, damage to O71.9
        non-obstetric O9A.22 (*following* O99)
        periurethral O71.82
        specified NEC O71.89
      tuberculosis (maternal) O98.02
      tumor, pelvic organs or tissues NEC O65.5
      umbilical cord around neck
        with compression O69.1 ☑
        without compression O69.81 ☑
      uterine inertia O62.2
        during latent phase of labor O62.0
        primary O62.0
        secondary O62.1
      vasa previa O69.4 ☑
      velamentous insertion of cord O43.12- ☑
    specified complication NEC O75.89
  delayed NOS O63.9
    following rupture of membranes
      artificial O75.5
    second twin, triplet, etc. O63.2
  forceps, low following failed vacuum extraction O66.5
  missed (at or near term) O36.4 ☑
  normal O80
  obstructed — *see* Delivery, complicated by, obstructed
      labor
  precipitate O62.3
  preterm — *see also* Pregnancy, complicated by,
      preterm labor O60.10 ☑
  spontaneous O80
  term pregnancy NOS O80
  uncomplicated O80
  vaginal, following previous cesarean delivery O34.219
    classical (vertical) scar O34.212

Delivery — *continued*
  vaginal, following previous cesarean delivery — *contin-*
      ued
    low transverse scar O34.211
    mid-transverse T incision O34.218
    scar
      defect (isthmocele) O34.22
      specified type NEC O34.218
Delusions (paranoid) — *see* Disorder, delusional
Dementia (degenerative (primary)) (old age) (persisting)
    F03.90
  with
    aggressive behavior F03.91
    behavioral disturbance F03.91
    combative behavior F03.91
    Lewy bodies G31.83 *[F02.80]*
      with behavioral disturbance G31.83 *[F02.81]*
    Parkinsonism G31.83 *[F02.80]*
      with behavioral disturbance G31.83 *[F02.81]*
    Parkinson's disease G20 *[F02.80]*
      with behavioral disturbance G20 *[F02.81]*
    violent behavior F03.91
  alcoholic F10.97
    with dependence F10.27
  Alzheimer's type — *see* Disease, Alzheimer's
  arteriosclerotic — *see* Dementia, vascular
  atypical, Alzheimer's type — *see* Disease, Alzheimer's,
      specified NEC
  congenital — *see* Disability, intellectual
  frontal (lobe) G31.09 *[F02.80]*
    with behavioral disturbance G31.09 *[F02.81]*
  frontotemporal G31.09 *[F02.80]*
    with behavioral disturbance G31.09 *[F02.81]*
    specified NEC G31.09 *[F02.80]*
      with behavioral disturbance G31.09 *[F02.81]*
  in (due to)
    alcohol F10.97
      with dependence F10.27
    Alzheimer's disease — *see* Disease, Alzheimer's
    arteriosclerotic brain disease — *see* Dementia, vas-
        cular
    cerebral lipidoses E75.- ☑ *[F02.80]*
      with behavioral disturbance E75.- ☑ *[F02.81]*
    Creutzfeldt-Jakob disease — *see also* Creutzfeldt-
        Jakob disease or syndrome (with dementia)
        A81.00
    epilepsy G40.- ☑ *[F02.80]*
      with behavioral disturbance G40.- ☑ *[F02.81]*
    hepatolenticular degeneration E83.01 *[F02.80]*
      with behavioral disturbance E83.01 *[F02.81]*
    human immunodeficiency virus (HIV) disease
        B20 *[F02.80]*
      with behavioral disturbance B20 *[F02.81]*
    Huntington's disease or chorea G10 *[F02.80]*
      with behavioral disturbance G10 *[F02.81]*
    hypercalcemia E83.52 *[F02.80]*
      with behavioral disturbance E83.52 *[F02.81]*
    hypothyroidism, acquired E03.9 *[F02.80]*
      with behavioral disturbance E03.9 *[F02.81]*
      due to iodine deficiency E01.8 *[F02.80]*
        with behavioral disturbance E01.8 *[F02.81]*
    inhalants F18.97
      with dependence F18.27
    multiple
      etiologies F03 ☑
      sclerosis G35 *[F02.80]*
        with behavioral disturbance G35 *[F02.81]*
    neurosyphilis A52.17 *[F02.80]*
      with behavioral disturbance A52.17 *[F02.81]*
      juvenile A50.49 *[F02.80]*
        with behavioral disturbance A50.49 *[F02.81]*
    niacin deficiency E52 *[F02.80]*
      with behavioral disturbance E52 *[F02.81]*
    paralysis agitans G20 *[F02.80]*
      with behavioral disturbance G20 *[F02.81]*
    Parkinson's disease G20 *[F02.80]*
    pellagra E52 *[F02.80]*
      with behavioral disturbance E52 *[F02.81]*
    Pick's G31.01 *[F02.80]*
      with behavioral disturbance G31.01 *[F02.81]*
    polyarteritis nodosa M30.0 *[F02.80]*
      with behavioral disturbance M30.0 *[F02.81]*
    psychoactive drug F19.97
      with dependence F19.27
      inhalants F18.97
        with dependence F18.27
      sedatives, hypnotics or anxiolytics F13.97

Dementia — *continued*
  in — *continued*
    psychoactive drug — *continued*
      sedatives, hypnotics or anxiolytics — *contin-*
          ued
        with dependence F13.27
      sedatives, hypnotics or anxiolytics F13.97
        with dependence F13.27
    systemic lupus erythematosus M32.- ☑ *[F02.80]*
      with behavioral disturbance M32.- ☑ *[F02.81]*
    trypanosomiasis
      African B56.9 *[F02.80]*
        with behavioral disturbance B56.9 *[F02.81]*
    unknown etiology F03 ☑
    vitamin B12 deficiency E53.8 *[F02.80]*
      with behavioral disturbance E53.8 *[F02.81]*
    volatile solvents F18.97
      with dependence F18.27
      with behavioral disturbance G31.83 *[F02.81]*
  infantile, infantilis F84.3
  Lewy body G31.83 *[F02.80]*
    with behavioral disturbance G31.83 *[F02.81]*
  multi-infarct — *see* Dementia, vascular
  paralytica, paralytic (syphilitic) A52.17 *[F02.80]*
    with behavioral disturbance A52.17 *[F02.81]*
    juvenilis A50.45
  paretic A52.17
  praecox — *see* Schizophrenia
  presenile F03 ☑
    Alzheimer's type — *see* Disease, Alzheimer's, early
        onset
  primary degenerative F03 ☑
  progressive, syphilitic A52.17
  senile F03 ☑
    with acute confusional state F05
    Alzheimer's type — *see* Disease, Alzheimer's, late
        onset
    depressed or paranoid type F03 ☑
  vascular (acute onset) (mixed) (multi-infarct) (subcorti-
      cal) F01.50
    with behavioral disturbance F01.51
Demineralization, bone — *see* Osteoporosis
Demodex folliculorum (infestation) B88.0
Demophobia F40.248
Demoralization R45.3
Demyelination, demyelinization
  central nervous system G37.9
    specified NEC G37.8
  corpus callosum (central) G37.1
  disseminated, acute G36.9
    specified NEC G36.8
  global G35
  in optic neuritis G36.0
Dengue (classical) (fever) A90
  hemorrhagic A91
  sandfly A93.1
Dennie-Marfan syphilitic syndrome A50.45
Dens evaginatus, in dente or invaginatus K00.2
Dense breasts R92.2
Density
  increased, bone (disseminated) (generalized) (spotted)
      — *see* Disorder, bone, density and structure,
      specified type NEC
  lung (nodular) J98.4
Dental — *see also* condition
  examination Z01.20
    with abnormal findings Z01.21
  restoration
    aesthetically inadequate or displeasing K08.56
    defective K08.50
      specified NEC K08.59
    failure of marginal integrity K08.51
    failure of periodontal anatomical integrity K08.54
Dentia praecox K00.6
Denticles (pulp) K04.2
Dentigerous cyst K09.0
Dentin
  irregular (in pulp) K04.3
  opalescent K00.5
  secondary (in pulp) K04.3
  sensitive K03.89
Dentinogenesis imperfecta K00.5
Dentinoma — *see* Cyst, calcifying odontogenic
Dentition (syndrome) K00.7
  delayed K00.6
  difficult K00.7
  precocious K00.6

Dentition — *continued*
  premature K00.6
  retarded K00.6
Dependence (on) (syndrome) F19.20
  with remission F19.21
  alcohol (ethyl) (methyl) (without remission) F10.20
    with
      amnestic disorder, persisting F10.26
      anxiety disorder F10.280
      dementia, persisting F10.27
      intoxication F10.229
        with delirium F10.221
        uncomplicated F10.220
      mood disorder F10.24
      psychotic disorder F10.259
        with
          delusions F10.250
          hallucinations F10.251
      remission F10.21
      sexual dysfunction F10.281
      sleep disorder F10.282
      specified disorder NEC F10.288
      withdrawal F10.239
        with
          delirium F10.231
          perceptual disturbance F10.232
        uncomplicated F10.230
    counseling and surveillance Z71.41
  amobarbital — *see* Dependence, drug, sedative
  amphetamine(s) (type) — *see* Dependence, drug, stimulant NEC
  amytal (sodium) — *see* Dependence, drug, sedative
  analgesic NEC F55.8
  anesthetic (agent) (gas) (general) (local) NEC — *see* Dependence, drug, psychoactive NEC
  anxiolytic NEC — *see* Dependence, drug, sedative
  barbital(s) — *see* Dependence, drug, sedative
  barbiturate(s) (compounds) (drugs classifiable to T42) — *see* Dependence, drug, sedative
  benzedrine — *see* Dependence, drug, stimulant NEC
  bhang — *see* Dependence, drug, cannabis
  bromide(s) NEC — *see* Dependence, drug, sedative
  caffeine — *see* Dependence, drug, stimulant NEC
  cannabis (sativa) (indica) (resin) (derivatives) (type) — *see* Dependence, drug, cannabis
  chloral (betaine) (hydrate) — *see* Dependence, drug, sedative
  chlordiazepoxide — *see* Dependence, drug, sedative
  coca (leaf) (derivatives) — *see* Dependence, drug, cocaine
  cocaine — *see* Dependence, drug, cocaine
  codeine — *see* Dependence, drug, opioid
  combinations of drugs F19.20
  dagga — *see* Dependence, drug, cannabis
  demerol — *see* Dependence, drug, opioid
  dexamphetamine — *see* Dependence, drug, stimulant NEC
  dexedrine — *see* Dependence, drug, stimulant NEC
  dextromethorphan — *see* Dependence, drug, opioid
  dextromoramide — *see* Dependence, drug, opioid
  dextro-nor-pseudo-ephedrine — *see* Dependence, drug, stimulant NEC
  dextrorphan — *see* Dependence, drug, opioid
  diazepam — *see* Dependence, drug, sedative
  dilaudid — *see* Dependence, drug, opioid
  D-lysergic acid diethylamide — *see* Dependence, drug, hallucinogen
  drug NEC F19.20
    with sleep disorder F19.282
    cannabis F12.20
      with
        anxiety disorder F12.280
        intoxication F12.229
          with
            delirium F12.221
            perceptual disturbance F12.222
          uncomplicated F12.220
        other specified disorder F12.288
        psychosis F12.259
          delusions F12.250
          hallucinations F12.251
        unspecified disorder F12.29
        withdrawal F12.23
      in remission F12.21
    cocaine F14.20
      with
        anxiety disorder F14.280
        intoxication F14.229

Dependence — *continued*
  drug — *continued*
    cocaine — *continued*
      with — *continued*
        intoxication — *continued*
          with
            delirium F14.221
            perceptual disturbance F14.222
          uncomplicated F14.220
        mood disorder F14.24
        other specified disorder F14.288
        psychosis F14.259
          delusions F14.250
          hallucinations F14.251
        sexual dysfunction F14.281
        sleep disorder F14.282
        unspecified disorder F14.29
        withdrawal F14.23
      in remission F14.21
      withdrawal symptoms in newborn P96.1
    counseling and surveillance Z71.51
    hallucinogen F16.20
      with
        anxiety disorder F16.280
        flashbacks F16.283
        intoxication F16.229
          with delirium F16.221
          uncomplicated F16.220
        mood disorder F16.24
        other specified disorder F16.288
        perception disorder, persisting F16.283
        psychosis F16.259
          delusions F16.250
          hallucinations F16.251
        unspecified disorder F16.29
      in remission F16.21
    in remission F19.21
    inhalant F18.20
      with
        anxiety disorder F18.280
        dementia, persisting F18.27
        intoxication F18.229
          with delirium F18.221
          uncomplicated F18.220
        mood disorder F18.24
        other specified disorder F18.288
        psychosis F18.259
          delusions F18.250
          hallucinations F18.251
        unspecified disorder F18.29
      in remission F18.21
    nicotine F17.200
      with disorder F17.209
        in remission F17.201
        specified disorder NEC F17.208
        withdrawal F17.203
      chewing tobacco F17.220
        with disorder F17.229
          in remission F17.221
          specified disorder NEC F17.228
          withdrawal F17.223
      cigarettes F17.210
        with disorder F17.219
          in remission F17.211
          specified disorder NEC F17.218
          withdrawal F17.213
      specified product NEC F17.290
        with disorder F17.299
          remission F17.291
          specified disorder NEC F17.298
          withdrawal F17.293
    opioid F11.20
      with
        intoxication F11.229
          with
            delirium F11.221
            perceptual disturbance F11.222
          uncomplicated F11.220
        mood disorder F11.24
        other specified disorder F11.288
        psychosis F11.259
          delusions F11.250
          hallucinations F11.251
        sexual dysfunction F11.281
        sleep disorder F11.282
        unspecified disorder F11.29
        withdrawal F11.23
      in remission F11.21
    psychoactive NEC F19.20

Dependence — *continued*
  drug — *continued*
    psychoactive — *continued*
      with
        amnestic disorder F19.26
        anxiety disorder F19.280
        dementia F19.27
        intoxication F19.229
          with
            delirium F19.221
            perceptual disturbance F19.222
          uncomplicated F19.220
        mood disorder F19.24
        other specified disorder F19.288
        psychosis F19.259
          delusions F19.250
          hallucinations F19.251
        sexual dysfunction F19.281
        sleep disorder F19.282
        unspecified disorder F19.29
        withdrawal F19.239
          with
            delirium F19.231
            perceptual disturbance F19.232
          uncomplicated F19.230
    sedative, hypnotic or anxiolytic F13.20
      with
        amnestic disorder F13.26
        anxiety disorder F13.280
        dementia, persisting F13.27
        intoxication F13.229
          with delirium F13.221
          uncomplicated F13.220
        mood disorder F13.24
        other specified disorder F13.288
        psychosis F13.259
          delusions F13.250
          hallucinations F13.251
        sexual dysfunction F13.281
        sleep disorder F13.282
        unspecified disorder F13.29
        withdrawal F13.239
          with
            delirium F13.231
            perceptual disturbance F13.232
          uncomplicated F13.230
      in remission F13.21
    stimulant NEC F15.20
      with
        anxiety disorder F15.280
        intoxication F15.229
          with
            delirium F15.221
            perceptual disturbance F15.222
          uncomplicated F15.220
        mood disorder F15.24
        other specified disorder F15.288
        psychosis F15.259
          delusions F15.250
          hallucinations F15.251
        sexual dysfunction F15.281
        sleep disorder F15.282
        unspecified disorder F15.29
        withdrawal F15.23
      in remission F15.21
  ethyl
    alcohol (without remission) F10.20
      with remission F10.21
    bromide — *see* Dependence, drug, sedative
    carbamate F19.20
    chloride F19.20
    morphine — *see* Dependence, drug, opioid
  ganja — *see* Dependence, drug, cannabis
  glue (airplane) (sniffing) — *see* Dependence, drug, inhalant
  glutethimide — *see* Dependence, drug, sedative
  hallucinogenics — *see* Dependence, drug, hallucinogen
  hashish — *see* Dependence, drug, cannabis
  hemp — *see* Dependence, drug, cannabis
  heroin (salt) (any) — *see* Dependence, drug, opioid
  hypnotic NEC — *see* Dependence, drug, sedative
  Indian hemp — *see* Dependence, drug, cannabis
  inhalants — *see* Dependence, drug, inhalant
  khat — *see* Dependence, drug, stimulant NEC
  laudanum — *see* Dependence, drug, opioid
  LSD (-25) (derivatives) — *see* Dependence, drug, hallucinogen
  luminal — *see* Dependence, drug, sedative

Dependence — continued
  lysergic acid — see Dependence, drug, hallucinogen
  maconha — see Dependence, drug, cannabis
  marihuana — see Dependence, drug, cannabis
  meprobamate — see Dependence, drug, sedative
  mescaline — see Dependence, drug, hallucinogen
  methadone — see Dependence, drug, opioid
  methamphetamine(s) — see Dependence, drug, stimulant NEC
  methaqualone — see Dependence, drug, sedative
  methyl
    alcohol (without remission) F10.20
      with remission F10.21
    bromide — see Dependence, drug, sedative
    morphine — see Dependence, drug, opioid
    phenidate — see Dependence, drug, stimulant NEC
    sulfonal — see Dependence, drug, sedative
  morphine (sulfate) (sulfite) (type) — see Dependence, drug, opioid
  narcotic (drug) NEC — see Dependence, drug, opioid
  nembutal — see Dependence, drug, sedative
  neraval — see Dependence, drug, sedative
  neravan — see Dependence, drug, sedative
  neurobarb — see Dependence, drug, sedative
  nicotine — see Dependence, drug, nicotine
  nitrous oxide F19.20
  nonbarbiturate sedatives and tranquilizers with similar effect — see Dependence, drug, sedative
  on
    artificial heart (fully implantable) (mechanical) Z95.812
    aspirator Z99.0
    care provider (because of) Z74.9
      impaired mobility Z74.09
      need for
        assistance with personal care Z74.1
        continuous supervision Z74.3
      no other household member able to render care Z74.2
      specified reason NEC Z74.8
    machine Z99.89
      enabling NEC Z99.89
      specified type NEC Z99.89
    renal dialysis (hemodialysis) (peritoneal) Z99.2
    respirator Z99.11
    ventilator Z99.11
    wheelchair Z99.3
  opiate — see Dependence, drug, opioid
  opioids — see Dependence, drug, opioid
  opium (alkaloids) (derivatives) (tincture) — see Dependence, drug, opioid
  oxygen (long-term) (supplemental) Z99.81
  paraldehyde — see Dependence, drug, sedative
  paregoric — see Dependence, drug, opioid
  PCP (phencyclidine) (or related substance) — see Dependence, drug, hallucinogen
  pentobarbital — see Dependence, drug, sedative
  pentobarbitone (sodium) — see Dependence, drug, sedative
  pentothal — see Dependence, drug, sedative
  peyote — see Dependence, drug, hallucinogen
  phencyclidine (PCP) (or related substance) — see Dependence, drug, hallucinogen
  phenmetrazine — see Dependence, drug, stimulant NEC
  phenobarbital — see Dependence, drug, sedative
  polysubstance F19.20
  psilocibin, psilocin, psilocyn, psilocyline — see Dependence, drug, hallucinogen
  psychostimulant NEC — see Dependence, drug, stimulant NEC
  secobarbital — see Dependence, drug, sedative
  seconal — see Dependence, drug, sedative
  sedative NEC — see Dependence, drug, sedative
  specified drug NEC — see Dependence, drug
  stimulant NEC — see Dependence, drug, stimulant NEC
  substance NEC — see Dependence, drug
  supplemental oxygen Z99.81
  tobacco — see Dependence, drug, nicotine
    counseling and surveillance Z71.6
  tranquilizer NEC — see Dependence, drug, sedative
  vitamin B6 E53.1
  volatile solvents — see Dependence, drug, inhalant
Dependency
  care-provider Z74.9
  passive F60.7
  reactions (persistent) F60.7

Depersonalization (in neurotic state) (neurotic) (syndrome) F48.1
Depletion
  extracellular fluid E86.9
  plasma E86.1
  potassium E87.6
    nephropathy N25.89
  salt or sodium E87.1
    causing heat exhaustion or prostration T67.4 ☑
    nephropathy N28.9
  volume NOS E86.9
Deployment (current) (military) status Z56.82
  in theater or in support of military war, peacekeeping and humanitarian operations Z56.82
  personal history of Z91.82
    military war, peacekeeping and humanitarian deployment (current or past conflict) Z91.82
  returned from Z91.82
Depolarization, premature I49.40
  atrial I49.1
  junctional I49.2
  specified NEC I49.49
  ventricular I49.3
Deposit
  bone in Boeck's sarcoid D86.89
  calcareous, calcium — see Calcification
  cholesterol
    retina H35.89
    vitreous (body) (humor) — see Deposit, crystalline
  conjunctiva H11.11- ☑
  cornea H18.00- ☑
    argentous H18.02- ☑
    due to metabolic disorder H18.03- ☑
    Kayser-Fleischer ring H18.04- ☑
    pigmentation — see Pigmentation, cornea
  crystalline, vitreous (body) (humor) H43.2- ☑
  hemosiderin in old scars of cornea — see Pigmentation, cornea, stromal
  metallic in lens — see Cataract, specified NEC
  skin R23.8
  tooth, teeth (betel) (black) (green) (materia alba) (orange) (tobacco) K03.6
  urate, kidney — see Calculus, kidney
Depraved appetite — see Pica
Depressed
  HDL cholesterol E78.6
Depression (acute) (mental) F32.9
  agitated (single episode) F32.2
  anaclitic — see Disorder, adjustment
  anxiety F41.8
    persistent F34.1
  arches — see also Deformity, limb, flat foot
  atypical (single episode) F32.89
    recurrent episode F33.8
  basal metabolic rate R94.8
  bone marrow D75.89
  central nervous system R09.2
  cerebral R29.818
    newborn P91.4
  cerebrovascular I67.9
  chest wall M95.4
  climacteric (single episode) F32.89
    recurrent episode F33.8
  endogenous (without psychotic symptoms) F33.2
    with psychotic symptoms F33.3
  functional activity R68.89
  hysterical F44.89
  involutional (single episode) F32.89
    recurrent episode F33.8
  major F32.9
    with psychotic symptoms F32.3
    recurrent — see Disorder, depressive, recurrent
  manic-depressive — see Disorder, depressive, recurrent
  masked (single episode) F32.89
  medullary G93.89
  menopausal (single episode) F32.89
    recurrent episode F33.8
  metatarsus — see Depression, arches
  monopolar F33.9
  nervous F34.1
  neurotic F34.1
  nose M95.0
  postnatal (NOS) F53.0
  postpartum (NOS) F53.0
  post-psychotic of schizophrenia F32.89
  post-schizophrenic F32.89
  psychogenic (reactive) (single episode) F32.9
  psychoneurotic F34.1

Depression — continued
  psychotic (single episode) F32.3
    recurrent F33.3
  reactive (psychogenic) (single episode) F32.9
    psychotic (single episode) F32.3
  recurrent — see Disorder, depressive, recurrent
  respiratory center G93.89
  seasonal — see Disorder, depressive, recurrent
  senile F03 ☑
  severe, single episode F32.2
  situational F43.21
  skull Q67.4
  specified NEC (single episode) F32.89
  sternum M95.4
  visual field — see Defect, visual field
  vital (recurrent) (without psychotic symptoms) F33.2
    with psychotic symptoms F33.3
    single episode F32.2
Deprivation
  cultural Z60.3
  effects NOS T73.9 ☑
    specified NEC T73.8 ☑
  emotional NEC Z65.8
    affecting infant or child — see Maltreatment, child, psychological
  food T73.0 ☑
  protein — see Malnutrition
  sleep Z72.820
  social Z60.4
    affecting infant or child — see Maltreatment, child, psychological
  specified NEC T73.8 ☑
  vitamins — see Deficiency, vitamin
  water T73.1 ☑
Derangement
  ankle (internal) — see Derangement, joint, ankle
  cartilage (articular) NEC — see Derangement, joint, articular cartilage, by site
    recurrent — see Dislocation, recurrent
  cruciate ligament, anterior, current injury — see Sprain, knee, cruciate, anterior
  elbow (internal) — see Derangement, joint, elbow
  hip (joint) (internal) (old) — see Derangement, joint, hip
  joint (internal) M24.9
    ankylosis — see Ankylosis
    articular cartilage M24.10
      ankle M24.17- ☑
      elbow M24.12- ☑
      foot M24.17- ☑
      hand M24.14- ☑
      hip M24.15- ☑
      knee NEC M23.9- ☑
      loose body — see Loose, body
      shoulder M24.11- ☑
      specified site NEC M24.19
      wrist M24.13- ☑
    contraction — see Contraction, joint
    current injury — see also Dislocation
      knee, meniscus or cartilage — see Tear, meniscus
    dislocation
      pathological — see Dislocation, pathological
      recurrent — see Dislocation, recurrent
    knee — see Derangement, knee
    ligament — see Disorder, ligament
    loose body — see Loose, body
    recurrent — see Dislocation, recurrent
    specified type NEC M24.80
      ankle M24.87- ☑
      elbow M24.82- ☑
      foot joint M24.87- ☑
      hand joint M24.84- ☑
      hip M24.85- ☑
      shoulder M24.81- ☑
      specified site NEC M24.89
      wrist M24.83- ☑
    temporomandibular M26.69
  knee (recurrent) M23.9- ☑
    ligament disruption, spontaneous M23.60- ☑
      anterior cruciate M23.61- ☑
      capsular M23.67- ☑
      instability, chronic M23.5- ☑
      lateral collateral M23.64- ☑
      medial collateral M23.63- ☑
      posterior cruciate M23.62- ☑
    loose body M23.4- ☑
    meniscus M23.30- ☑

Derangement — *continued*
  knee — *continued*
    meniscus — *continued*
      cystic M23.00- ☑
        lateral M23.002
          anterior horn M23.04- ☑
          posterior horn M23.05- ☑
          specified NEC M23.06- ☑
        medial M23.005
          anterior horn M23.01- ☑
          posterior horn M23.02- ☑
          specified NEC M23.03- ☑
      degenerate — *see* Derangement, knee, meniscus, specified NEC
      detached — *see* Derangement, knee, meniscus, specified NEC
      due to old tear or injury M23.20- ☑
        lateral M23.20- ☑
          anterior horn M23.24- ☑
          posterior horn M23.25- ☑
          specified NEC M23.26- ☑
        medial M23.20- ☑
          anterior horn M23.21- ☑
          posterior horn M23.22- ☑
          specified NEC M23.23- ☑
      retained — *see* Derangement, knee, meniscus, specified NEC
      specified NEC M23.30- ☑
        lateral M23.30- ☑
          anterior horn M23.34- ☑
          posterior horn M23.35- ☑
          specified NEC M23.36- ☑
        medial M23.30- ☑
          anterior horn M23.31- ☑
          posterior horn M23.32- ☑
          specified NEC M23.33- ☑
    old M23.8X- ☑
    specified NEC — *see* subcategory M23.8 ☑
  low back NEC — *see* Dorsopathy, specified NEC
  meniscus — *see* Derangement, knee, meniscus
  mental — *see* Psychosis
  patella, specified NEC — *see* Disorder, patella, derangement NEC
  semilunar cartilage (knee) — *see* Derangement, knee, meniscus, specified NEC
  shoulder (internal) — *see* Derangement, joint, shoulder
Dercum's disease E88.2
Derealization (neurotic) F48.1
Dermal — *see* condition
Dermaphytid — *see* Dermatophytosis
Dermatitis (eczematous) L30.9
  ab igne L59.0
  acarine B88.0
  actinic (due to sun) L57.8
    other than from sun L59.8
  allergic — *see* Dermatitis, contact, allergic
  ambustionis, due to burn or scald — *see* Burn
  amebic A06.7
  ammonia L22
  arsenical (ingested) L27.8
  artefacta L98.1
    psychogenic F54
  atopic L20.9
    psychogenic F54
    specified NEC L20.89
  autoimmune progesterone L30.8
  berlock, berloque L56.2
  blastomycotic B40.3
  blister beetle L24.89
  bullous, bullosa L13.9
    mucosynechial, atrophic L12.1
    seasonal L30.8
    specified NEC L13.8
  calorica L59.0
    due to burn or scald — *see* Burn
  caterpillar L24.89
  cercarial B65.3
  combustionis L59.0
    due to burn or scald — *see* Burn
  congelationis T69.1 ☑
  contact (occupational) L25.9
    allergic L23.9
      due to
        adhesives L23.1
        cement L23.5
        chemical products NEC L23.5
        chromium L23.0

Dermatitis — *continued*
  contact — *continued*
    allergic — *continued*
      due to — *continued*
        cosmetics L23.2
        dander (cat) (dog) L23.81
        drugs in contact with skin L23.3
        dyes L23.4
        food in contact with skin L23.6
        hair (cat) (dog) L23.81
        insecticide L23.5
        metals L23.0
        nickel L23.0
        plants, non-food L23.7
        plastic L23.5
        rubber L23.5
        specified agent NEC L23.89
    due to
      cement L25.3
      chemical products NEC L25.3
      cosmetics L25.0
      dander (cat) (dog) L23.81
      drugs in contact with skin L25.1
      dyes L25.2
      food in contact with skin L25.4
      hair (cat) (dog) L23.81
      plants, non-food L25.5
      specified agent NEC L25.8
    irritant L24.9
      due to
        cement L24.5
        chemical products NEC L24.5
        cosmetics L24.3
        detergents L24.0
        drugs in contact with skin L24.4
        food in contact with skin L24.6
        oils and greases L24.1
        plants, non-food L24.7
        solvents L24.2
        specified agent NEC L24.89
  contusiformis L52
  desquamative L30.8
  diabetic — *see* E08-E13 with .620
  diaper L22
  diphtheritica A36.3
  dry skin L85.3
  due to
    acetone (contact) (irritant) L24.2
    acids (contact) (irritant) L24.5
    adhesive(s) (allergic) (contact) (plaster) L23.1
      irritant L24.5
    alcohol (irritant) (skin contact) (substances in category T51) L24.2
      taken internally L27.8
    alkalis (contact) (irritant) L24.5
    arsenic (ingested) L27.8
    carbon disulfide (contact) (irritant) L24.2
    caustics (contact) (irritant) L24.5
    cement (contact) L25.3
    cereal (ingested) L27.2
    chemical(s) NEC L25.3
      taken internally L27.8
    chlorocompounds L24.2
    chromium (contact) (irritant) L24.81
    coffee (ingested) L27.2
    cold weather L30.8
    cosmetics (contact) L25.0
      allergic L23.2
      irritant L24.3
    cyclohexanes L24.2
    dander (cat) (dog) L23.81
    Demodex species B88.0
    Dermanyssus gallinae B88.0
    detergents (contact) (irritant) L24.0
    dichromate L24.81
    drugs and medicaments (generalized) (internal use) L27.0
      external — *see* Dermatitis, due to, drugs, in contact with skin
      in contact with skin L25.1
        allergic L23.3
        irritant L24.4
      localized skin eruption L27.1
      specified substance — *see* Table of Drugs and Chemicals
    dyes (contact) L25.2
      allergic L23.4
      irritant L24.89
    epidermophytosis — *see* Dermatophytosis

Dermatitis — *continued*
  due to — *continued*
    esters L24.2
    external irritant NEC L24.9
    fish (ingested) L27.2
    flour (ingested) L27.2
    food (ingested) L27.2
      in contact with skin L25.4
    fruit (ingested) L27.2
    furs (allergic) (contact) L23.81
    glues — *see* Dermatitis, due to, adhesives
    glycols L24.2
    greases NEC (contact) (irritant) L24.1
    hair (cat) (dog) L23.81
    hot
      objects and materials — *see* Burn
      weather or places L59.0
    hydrocarbons L24.2
    infrared rays L59.8
    ingestion, ingested substance L27.9
      chemical NEC L27.8
      drugs and medicaments — *see* Dermatitis, due to, drugs
      food L27.2
      specified NEC L27.8
    insecticide in contact with skin L24.5
    internal agent L27.9
      drugs and medicaments (generalized) — *see* Dermatitis, due to, drugs
      food L27.2
    irradiation — *see* Dermatitis, due to, radioactive substance
    ketones L24.2
    lacquer tree (allergic) (contact) L23.7
    light (sun) NEC L57.8
      acute L56.8
      other L59.8
    Liponyssoides sanguineus B88.0
    low temperature L30.8
    meat (ingested) L27.2
    metals, metal salts (contact) (irritant) L24.81
    milk (ingested) L27.2
    nickel (contact) (irritant) L24.81
    nylon (contact) (irritant) L24.5
    oils NEC (contact) (irritant) L24.1
    paint solvent (contact) (irritant) L24.2
    petroleum products (contact) (irritant) (substances in T52.0) L24.2
    plants NEC (contact) L25.5
      allergic L23.7
      irritant L24.7
    plasters (adhesive) (any) (allergic) (contact) L23.1
      irritant L24.5
    plastic (contact) L25.3
    preservatives (contact) — *see* Dermatitis, due to, chemical, in contact with skin
    primrose (allergic) (contact) L23.7
    primula (allergic) (contact) L23.7
    radiation L59.8
      nonionizing (chronic exposure) L57.8
      sun NEC L57.8
        acute L56.8
    radioactive substance L58.9
      acute L58.0
      chronic L58.1
    radium L58.9
      acute L58.0
      chronic L58.1
    ragweed (allergic) (contact) L23.7
    Rhus (allergic) (contact) (diversiloba) (radicans) (toxicodendron) (venenata) (verniciflua) L23.7
    rubber (contact) L24.5
    Senecio jacobaea (allergic) (contact) L23.7
    solvents (contact) (irritant) (substances in category T52) L24.2
    specified agent NEC (contact) L25.8
      allergic L23.89
      irritant L24.89
    sunshine NEC L57.8
      acute L56.8
    tetrachlorethylene (contact) (irritant) L24.2
    toluene (contact) (irritant) L24.2
    turpentine (contact) L24.2
    ultraviolet rays (sun NEC) (chronic exposure) L57.8
      acute L56.8
    vaccine or vaccination L27.0
      specified substance — *see* Table of Drugs and Chemicals

Dermatitis — *continued*
  due to — *continued*
    varicose veins — *see* Varix, leg, with, inflammation
    X-rays L58.9
      acute L58.0
      chronic L58.1
  dyshydrotic L30.1
  dysmenorrheica N94.6
  escharotica — *see* Burn
  exfoliative, exfoliativa (generalized) L26
    neonatorum L00
  eyelid — *see also* Dermatosis, eyelid
    allergic H01.119
      left H01.116
        lower H01.115
        upper H01.114
      right H01.113
        lower H01.112
        upper H01.111
    contact — *see* Dermatitis, eyelid, allergic
    due to
      Demodex species B88.0
      herpes (zoster) B02.39
        simplex B00.59
    eczematous H01.139
      left H01.136
        lower H01.135
        upper H01.134
      right H01.133
        lower H01.132
        upper H01.131
  facta, factitia, factitial L98.1
    psychogenic F54
  flexural NEC L20.82
  friction L30.4
  fungus B36.9
    specified type NEC B36.8
  gangrenosa, gangrenous infantum L08.0
  harvest mite B88.0
  heat L59.0
  herpesviral, vesicular (ear) (lip) B00.1
  herpetiformis (bullous) (erythematous) (pustular)
      (vesicular) L13.0
    juvenile L12.2
    senile L12.0
  hiemalis L30.8
  hypostatic, hypostatica — *see* Varix, leg, with, inflam-
      mation
  infectious eczematoid L30.3
  infective L30.3
  irritant — *see* Dermatitis, contact, irritant
  Jacquet's (diaper dermatitis) L22
  Leptus B88.0
  lichenified NEC L28.0
  medicamentosa (generalized) (internal use) — *see*
      Dermatitis, due to drugs
  mite B88.0
  multiformis L13.0
    juvenile L12.2
  napkin L22
  neurotica L13.0
  nummular L30.0
  papillaris capillitii L73.0
  pellagrous E52
  perioral L71.0
  photocontact L56.2
  polymorpha dolorosa L13.0
  pruriginosa L13.0
  pruritic NEC L30.8
  psychogenic F54
  purulent L08.0
  pustular
    contagious B08.02
    subcorneal L13.1
  pyococcal L08.0
  pyogenica L08.0
  repens L40.2
  Ritter's (exfoliativa) L00
  Schamberg's L81.7
  schistosome B65.3
  seasonal bullous L30.8
  seborrheic L21.9
    infantile L21.1
    specified NEC L21.8
  sensitization NOS L23.9
  septic L08.0
  solare L57.8
  specified NEC L30.8

Dermatitis — *continued*
  stasis I87.2
    with
      varicose ulcer — *see* Varix, leg, with ulcer, with
          inflammation
      varicose veins — *see* Varix, leg, with, inflamma-
          tion
    due to postthrombotic syndrome — *see* Syndrome,
        postthrombotic
  suppurative L08.0
  traumatic NEC L30.4
  trophoneurotica L13.0
  ultraviolet (sun) (chronic exposure) L57.8
    acute L56.8
  varicose — *see* Varix, leg, with, inflammation
  vegetans L10.1
  verrucosa B43.0
  vesicular, herpesviral B00.1
Dermatoarthritis, lipoid E78.81
Dermatochalasis, eyelid H02.839
  left H02.836
    lower H02.835
    upper H02.834
  right H02.833
    lower H02.832
    upper H02.831
Dermatofibroma (lenticulare) — *see* Neoplasm, skin,
    benign
  protuberans — *see* Neoplasm, skin, uncertain behavior
Dermatofibrosarcoma (pigmented) (protuberans) —
    see Neoplasm, skin, malignant
Dermatographia L50.3
Dermatolysis (exfoliativa) (congenital) Q82.8
  acquired L57.4
  eyelids — *see* Blepharochalasis
  palpebrarum — *see* Blepharochalasis
  senile L57.4
Dermatomegaly NEC Q82.8
Dermatomucosomyositis M33.10
  with
    myopathy M33.12
    respiratory involvement M33.11
    specified organ involvement NEC M33.19
Dermatomycosis B36.9
  furfuracea B36.0
  specified type NEC B36.8
Dermatomyositis (acute) (chronic) — *see also* Der-
    matopolymyositis
  adult — *see also* Dermatomyositis, specified NEC
      M33.10
  in (due to) neoplastic disease — *see also* Neoplasm
      D49.9 [M36.0]
  juvenile M33.00
    with
      myopathy M33.02
      respiratory involvement M33.01
      specified organ involvement NEC M33.09
    without myopathy M33.03
  specified NEC M33.10
    with
      myopathy M33.12
      respiratory involvement M33.11
      specified organ involvement NEC M33.19
    without myopathy M33.13
Dermatoneuritis of children — *see* Poisoning, mercury
Dermatophilosis A48.8
Dermatophytid L30.2
Dermatophytide — *see* Dermatophytosis
Dermatophytosis (epidermophyton) (infection) (Mi-
    crosporum) (tinea) (Trichophyton) B35.9
  beard B35.0
  body B35.4
  capitis B35.0
  corporis B35.4
  deep-seated B35.8
  disseminated B35.8
  foot B35.3
  granulomatous B35.8
  groin B35.6
  hand B35.2
  nail B35.1
  perianal (area) B35.6
  scalp B35.0
  specified NEC B35.8
Dermatopolymyositis M33.90
  with
    myopathy M33.92
    respiratory involvement M33.91

Dermatopolymyositis — *continued*
  with — *continued*
    specified organ involvement NEC M33.99
  in neoplastic disease — *see also* Neoplasm
      D49.9 [M36.0]
  juvenile M33.00
    with
      myopathy M33.02
      respiratory involvement M33.01
      specified organ involvement NEC M33.09
  specified NEC M33.10
    myopathy M33.12
    respiratory involvement M33.11
    specified organ involvement NEC M33.19
  without myopathy M33.93
Dermatopolyneuritis — *see* Poisoning, mercury
Dermatorrhexis — *see also* Syndrome, Ehlers-Danlos
    Q79.60
  acquired L57.4
Dermatosclerosis — *see also* Scleroderma
  localized L94.0
Dermatosis L98.9
  Andrews' L08.89
  Bowen's — *see* Neoplasm, skin, in situ
  bullous L13.9
    specified NEC L13.8
  exfoliativa L26
  eyelid (noninfectious)
    dermatitis — *see* Dermatitis, eyelid
    discoid lupus erythematosus — *see* Lupus, erythe-
        matosus, eyelid
    xeroderma — *see* Xeroderma, acquired, eyelid
  factitial L98.1
  febrile neutrophilic L98.2
  gonococcal A54.89
  herpetiformis L13.0
    juvenile L12.2
  linear IgA L13.8
  menstrual NEC L98.8
  neutrophilic, febrile L98.2
  occupational — *see* Dermatitis, contact
  papulosa nigra L82.1
  pigmentary L81.9
    progressive L81.7
    Schamberg's L81.7
  psychogenic F54
  purpuric, pigmented L81.7
  pustular, subcorneal L13.1
  transient acantholytic L11.1
Dermographia, dermographism L50.3
Dermoid (cyst) — *see also* Neoplasm, benign, by site
  with malignant transformation C56- ☑
  due to radiation (nonionizing) L57.8
Dermopathy
  infiltrative with thyrotoxicosis — *see* Thyrotoxicosis
  nephrogenic fibrosing L90.8
Dermophytosis — *see* Dermatophytosis
Descemetocele H18.73- ☑
Descemet's membrane — *see* condition
Descending — *see* condition
Descensus uteri — *see* Prolapse, uterus
Desert
  rheumatism B38.0
  sore — *see* Ulcer, skin
Desertion (newborn) — *see* Maltreatment
Desmoid (extra-abdominal) (tumor) — *see* Neoplasm,
    connective tissue, uncertain behavior
  abdominal D48.1
Despondency F32.9
Desquamation, skin R23.4
Destruction, destructive — *see also* Damage
  articular facet — *see also* Derangement, joint, specified
      type NEC
    knee M23.8X- ☑
    vertebra — *see* Spondylosis
  bone — *see also* Disorder, bone, specified type NEC
    syphilitic A52.77
  joint — *see also* Derangement, joint, specified type
      NEC
    sacroiliac M53.3
  rectal sphincter K62.89
  septum (nasal) J34.89
  tuberculous NEC — *see* Tuberculosis
  tympanum, tympanic membrane (nontraumatic) —
      see Disorder, tympanic membrane, specified NEC
  vertebral disc — *see* Degeneration, intervertebral disc
Destructiveness — *see also* Disorder, conduct

☑ **Additional Character Required** — **Refer to the Tabular List for Character Selection**   ▽ **Subterms under main terms may continue to next column or page**

Destructiveness — *continued*
  adjustment reaction — *see* Disorder, adjustment
Desultory labor O62.2
Detachment
  cartilage — *see* Sprain
  cervix, annular N88.8
    complicating delivery O71.3
  choroid (old) (postinfectional) (simple) (spontaneous)
    H31.40- ☑
    hemorrhagic H31.41- ☑
    serous H31.42- ☑
  ligament — *see* Sprain
  meniscus (knee) — *see also* Derangement, knee,
    meniscus, specified NEC
    current injury — *see* Tear, meniscus
    due to old tear or injury — *see* Derangement, knee,
      meniscus, due to old tear
  retina (without retinal break) (serous) H33.2- ☑
    with retinal:
      break H33.00- ☑
        giant H33.03- ☑
        multiple H33.02- ☑
        single H33.01- ☑
      dialysis H33.04- ☑
    pigment epithelium — *see* Degeneration, retina,
      separation of layers, pigment epithelium de-
      tachment
    rhegmatogenous — *see* Detachment, retina, with
      retinal, break
    specified NEC H33.8
    total H33.05- ☑
    traction H33.4- ☑
  vitreous (body) H43.81 ☑
Detergent asthma J69.8
Deterioration
  epileptic F06.8
  general physical R53.81
  heart, cardiac — *see* Degeneration, myocardial
  mental — *see* Psychosis
  myocardial, myocardium — *see* Degeneration, myocar-
    dial
  senile (simple) R54
Deuteranomaly (anomalous trichromat) H53.53
Deuteranopia (complete) (incomplete) H53.53
Development
  abnormal, bone O79.9
  arrested R62.50
    bone — *see* Arrest, development or growth, bone
    child R62.50
    due to malnutrition E45
  defective, congenital — *see also* Anomaly, by site
    cauda equina Q06.3
    left ventricle Q24.8
      in hypoplastic left heart syndrome Q23.4
    valve Q24.8
      pulmonary Q22.3
  delayed — *see also* Delay, development R62.50
    arithmetical skills F81.2
    language (skills) (expressive) F80.1
    learning skill F81.9
    mixed skills F88
    motor coordination F82
    reading F81.0
    specified learning skill NEC F81.89
    speech F80.9
    spelling F81.81
    written expression F81.81
  imperfect, congenital — *see also* Anomaly, by site
    heart Q24.9
    lungs Q33.6
  incomplete
    bronchial tree Q32.4
    organ or site not listed — *see* Hypoplasia, by site
    respiratory system Q34.9
    sexual, precocious NEC E30.1
  tardy, mental — *see also* Disability, intellectual F79
Developmental — *see* condition
  testing, infant or child — *see* Examination, child
Devergie's disease (pityriasis rubra pilaris) L44.0
Deviation (in)
  conjugate palsy (eye) (spastic) H51.0
  esophagus (acquired) K22.8
  eye, skew H51.8
  midline (jaw) (teeth) (dental arch) M26.29
    specified site NEC — *see* Malposition
  nasal septum J34.2
    congenital Q67.4

Deviation — *continued*
  opening and closing of the mandible M26.53
  organ or site, congenital NEC — *see* Malposition, con-
    genital
  septum (nasal) (acquired) J34.2
    congenital Q67.4
  sexual F65.9
    bestiality F65.89
    erotomania F52.8
    exhibitionism F65.2
    fetishism, fetishistic F65.0
      transvestism F65.1
    frotteurism F65.81
    masochism F65.51
    multiple F65.89
    necrophilia F65.89
    nymphomania F52.8
    pederosis F65.4
    pedophilia F65.4
    sadism, sadomasochism F65.52
    satyriasis F52.8
    specified type NEC F65.89
    transvestism F64.1
    voyeurism F65.3
  teeth, midline M26.29
  trachea J39.8
  ureter, congenital Q62.61
Device
  cerebral ventricle (communicating) in situ Z98.2
  contraceptive — *see* Contraceptive, device
  drainage, cerebrospinal fluid, in situ Z98.2
Devic's disease G36.0
Devil's
  grip B33.0
  pinches (purpura simplex) D69.2
Devitalized tooth K04.99
Devonshire colic — *see* Poisoning, lead
Dextraposition, aorta Q20.3
  in tetralogy of Fallot Q21.3
Dextrinosis, limit (debrancher enzyme deficiency) E74.03
Dextrocardia (true) Q24.0
  with
    complete transposition of viscera Q89.3
    situs inversus Q89.3
Dextrotransposition, aorta Q20.3
d-glycericacidemia E72.59
Dhat syndrome F48.8
Dhobi itch B35.6
Di George's syndrome D82.1
Di Guglielmo's disease C94.0- ☑
Diabetes, diabetic (mellitus) (sugar) E11.9
  with
    amyotrophy E11.44
    arthropathy NEC E11.618
    autonomic (poly)neuropathy E11.43
    cataract E11.36
    Charcot's joints E11.610
    chronic kidney disease E11.22
    circulatory complication NEC E11.59
    complication E11.8
      specified NEC E11.69
    dermatitis E11.620
    foot ulcer E11.621
    gangrene E11.52
    gastroparalysis E11.43
    gastroparesis E11.43
    glomerulonephrosis, intracapillary E11.21
    glomerulosclerosis, intercapillary E11.21
    hyperglycemia E11.65
    hyperosmolarity E11.00
      with coma E11.01
    hypoglycemia E11.649
      with coma E11.641
    ketoacidosis E11.10
      with coma E11.11
    kidney complications NEC E11.29
    Kimmelstiel-Wilson disease E11.21
    loss of protective sensation (LOPS) — *see* Diabetes,
      by type, with neuropathy
    mononeuropathy E11.41
    myasthenia E11.44
    necrobiosis lipoidica E11.620
    nephropathy E11.21
    neuralgia E11.42
    neurologic complication NEC E11.49
    neuropathic arthropathy E11.610
    neuropathy E11.40
    ophthalmic complication NEC E11.39

Diabetes, diabetic — *continued*
  with — *continued*
    oral complication NEC E11.638
    osteomyelitis E11.69
    periodontal disease E11.630
    peripheral angiopathy E11.51
      with gangrene E11.52
    polyneuropathy E11.42
    renal complication NEC E11.29
    renal tubular degeneration E11.29
    retinopathy E11.319
      with macular edema E11.311
        resolved following treatment E11.37- ☑
      nonproliferative E11.329 ☑
        with macular edema E11.321 ☑
        mild E11.329 ☑
          with macular edema E11.321 ☑
        moderate E11.339 ☑
          with macular edema E11.331 ☑
        severe E11.349 ☑
          with macular edema E11.341 ☑
      proliferative E11.359 ☑
        with
          combined traction retinal detachment
            and rhegmatogenous retinal de-
            tachment E11.354 ☑
          macular edema E11.351 ☑
          stable proliferative diabetic retinopathy
            E11.355 ☑
          traction retinal detachment involving the
            macula E11.352 ☑
          traction retinal detachment not involving
            the macula E11.353 ☑
      resolved following treatment E09.37 ☑
    skin complication NEC E11.628
    skin ulcer NEC E11.622
  brittle — *see* Diabetes, type 1
  bronzed E83.110
  complicating pregnancy — *see* Pregnancy, complicated
    by, diabetes
  dietary counseling and surveillance Z71.3
  due to
    autoimmune process — *see* Diabetes, type 1
    immune mediated pancreatic islet beta-cell destruc-
      tion — *see* Diabetes, type 1
  due to drug or chemical E09.9
    with
      amyotrophy E09.44
      arthropathy NEC E09.618
      autonomic (poly)neuropathy E09.43
      cataract E09.36
      Charcot's joints E09.610
      chronic kidney disease E09.22
      circulatory complication NEC E09.59
      complication E09.8
        specified NEC E09.69
      dermatitis E09.620
      foot ulcer E09.621
      gangrene E09.52
      gastroparalysis E09.43
      gastroparesis E09.43
      glomerulonephrosis, intracapillary E09.21
      glomerulosclerosis, intercapillary E09.21
      hyperglycemia E09.65
      hyperosmolarity E09.00
        with coma E09.01
      hypoglycemia E09.649
        with coma E09.641
      ketoacidosis E09.10
        with coma E09.11
      kidney complications NEC E09.29
      Kimmelstiel-Wilson disease E09.21
      mononeuropathy E09.41
      myasthenia E09.44
      necrobiosis lipoidica E09.620
      nephropathy E09.21
      neuralgia E09.42
      neurologic complication NEC E09.49
      neuropathic arthropathy E09.610
      neuropathy E09.40
      ophthalmic complication NEC E09.39
      oral complication NEC E09.638
      periodontal disease E09.630
      peripheral angiopathy E09.51
        with gangrene E09.52
      polyneuropathy E09.42
      renal complication NEC E09.29
      renal tubular degeneration E09.29

Diabetes, diabetic — *continued*
  due to drug or chemical — *continued*
    with — *continued*
      retinopathy E09.319
        with macular edema E09.311
        resolved following treatment E09.37 ☑
        nonproliferative E09.329 ☑
          with macular edema E09.321 ☑
          mild E09.329 ☑
            with macular edema E09.321 ☑
          moderate E09.339 ☑
            with macular edema E09.331 ☑
          severe E09.349 ☑
            with macular edema E09.341 ☑
        proliferative E09.359 ☑
          with
            combined traction retinal detachment and rhegmatogenous retinal detachment E09.354 ☑
            macular edema E09.351 ☑
            stable proliferative diabetic retinopathy E09.355 ☑
            traction retinal detachment involving the macula E09.352 ☑
            traction retinal detachment not involving the macula E09.353 ☑
      skin complication NEC E09.628
      skin ulcer NEC E09.622
  due to underlying condition E08.9
    with
      amyotrophy E08.44
      arthropathy NEC E08.618
      autonomic (poly)neuropathy E08.43
      cataract E08.36
      Charcot's joints E08.610
      chronic kidney disease E08.22
      circulatory complication NEC E08.59
      complication E08.8
        specified NEC E08.69
      dermatitis E08.620
      foot ulcer E08.621
      gangrene E08.52
      gastroparalysis E08.43
      gastroparesis E08.43
      glomerulonephrosis, intracapillary E08.21
      glomerulosclerosis, intercapillary E08.21
      hyperglycemia E08.65
      hyperosmolarity E08.00
        with coma E08.01
      hypoglycemia E08.649
        with coma E08.641
      ketoacidosis E08.10
        with coma E08.11
      kidney complications NEC E08.29
      Kimmelstiel-Wilson disease E08.21
      mononeuropathy E08.41
      myasthenia E08.44
      necrobiosis lipoidica E08.620
      nephropathy E08.21
      neuralgia E08.42
      neurologic complication NEC E08.49
      neuropathic arthropathy E08.610
      neuropathy E08.40
      ophthalmic complication NEC E08.39
      oral complication NEC E08.638
      periodontal disease E08.630
      peripheral angiopathy E08.51
        with gangrene E08.52
      polyneuropathy E08.42
      renal complication NEC E08.29
      renal tubular degeneration E08.29
      retinopathy E08.319
        with macular edema E08.311
        resolved following treatment E08.37 ☑
        nonproliferative E08.329 ☑
          with macular edema E08.321 ☑
          mild E08.329 ☑
            with macular edema E08.321 ☑
          moderate E08.339 ☑
            with macular edema E08.331 ☑
          severe E08.349 ☑
            with macular edema E08.341 ☑
        proliferative E08.359 ☑
          with
            combined traction retinal detachment and rhegmatogenous retinal detachment E08.354 ☑
            macular edema E08.351 ☑

Diabetes, diabetic — *continued*
  due to underlying condition — *continued*
    with — *continued*
      retinopathy — *continued*
        proliferative — *continued*
          with — *continued*
            stable proliferative diabetic retinopathy E08.355 ☑
            traction retinal detachment involving the macula E08.352 ☑
            traction retinal detachment not involving the macula E08.353 ☑
      skin complication NEC E08.628
      skin ulcer NEC E08.622
  gestational (in pregnancy) O24.419
    affecting newborn P70.0
    diet controlled O24.410
    in childbirth O24.429
      diet controlled O24.420
      insulin (and diet) controlled O24.424
      oral drug controlled (antidiabetic) (hypoglycemic) O24.425
    insulin (and diet) controlled O24.414
    oral drug controlled (antidiabetic) (hypoglycemic) O24.415
    puerperal O24.439
      diet controlled O24.430
      insulin (and diet) controlled O24.434
      oral drug controlled (antidiabetic) (hypoglycemic) O24.435
  hepatogenous E13.9
  idiopathic — *see* Diabetes, type 1
  inadequately controlled — *code to* Diabetes, by type, with hyperglycemia
  insipidus E23.2
    nephrogenic N25.1
    pituitary E23.2
    vasopressin resistant N25.1
  insulin dependent — *code to* type of diabetes
  juvenile-onset — *see* Diabetes, type 1
  ketosis-prone — *see* Diabetes, type 1
  latent R73.03
  neonatal (transient) P70.2
  non-insulin dependent — *code to* type of diabetes
  out of control — *code to* Diabetes, by type, with hyperglycemia
  phosphate E83.39
  poorly controlled — *code to* Diabetes, by type, with hyperglycemia
  postpancreatectomy — *see* Diabetes, specified type NEC
  postprocedural — *see* Diabetes, specified type NEC
  secondary diabetes mellitus NEC — *see* Diabetes, specified type NEC
  specified type NEC E13.9
    with
      amyotrophy E13.44
      arthropathy NEC E13.618
      autonomic (poly)neuropathy E13.43
      cataract E13.36
      Charcot's joints E13.610
      chronic kidney disease E13.22
      circulatory complication NEC E13.59
      complication E13.8
        specified NEC E13.69
      dermatitis E13.620
      foot ulcer E13.621
      gangrene E13.52
      gastroparalysis E13.43
      gastroparesis E13.43
      glomerulonephrosis, intracapillary E13.21
      glomerulosclerosis, intercapillary E13.21
      hyperglycemia E13.65
      hyperosmolarity E13.00
        with coma E13.01
      hypoglycemia E13.649
        with coma E13.641
      ketoacidosis E13.10
        with coma E13.11
      kidney complications NEC E13.29
      Kimmelstiel-Wilson disease E13.21
      mononeuropathy E13.41
      myasthenia E13.44
      necrobiosis lipoidica E13.620
      nephropathy E13.21
      neuralgia E13.42
      neurologic complication NEC E13.49
      neuropathic arthropathy E13.610

Diabetes, diabetic — *continued*
  specified type — *continued*
    with — *continued*
      neuropathy E13.40
      ophthalmic complication NEC E13.39
      oral complication NEC E13.638
      periodontal disease E13.630
      peripheral angiopathy E13.51
        with gangrene E13.52
      polyneuropathy E13.42
      renal complication NEC E13.29
      renal tubular degeneration E13.29
      retinopathy E13.319
        with macular edema E13.311
        resolved following treatment E13.37 ☑
        nonproliferative E13.329 ☑
          with macular edema E13.321 ☑
          mild E13.329 ☑
            with macular edema E13.321 ☑
          moderate E13.339 ☑
            with macular edema E13.331 ☑
          severe E13.349 ☑
            with macular edema E13.341 ☑
        proliferative E13.359 ☑
          with
            combined traction retinal detachment and rhegmatogenous retinal detachment E13.354 ☑
            macular edema E13.351 ☑
            stable proliferative diabetic retinopathy E13.355 ☑
            traction retinal detachment involving the macula E13.352 ☑
            traction retinal detachment not involving the macula E13.353 ☑
      skin complication NEC E13.628
      skin ulcer NEC E13.622
  steroid-induced — *see* Diabetes, due to, drug or chemical
  type 1 E10.9
    with
      amyotrophy E10.44
      arthropathy NEC E10.618
      autonomic (poly)neuropathy E10.43
      cataract E10.36
      Charcot's joints E10.610
      chronic kidney disease E10.22
      circulatory complication NEC E10.59
      complication E10.8
        specified NEC E10.69
      dermatitis E10.620
      foot ulcer E10.621
      gangrene E10.52
      gastroparalysis E10.43
      gastroparesis E10.43
      glomerulonephrosis, intracapillary E10.21
      glomerulosclerosis, intercapillary E10.21
      hyperglycemia E10.65
      hypoglycemia E10.649
        with coma E10.641
      ketoacidosis E10.10
        with coma E10.11
      kidney complications NEC E10.29
      Kimmelstiel-Wilson disease E10.21
      mononeuropathy E10.41
      myasthenia E10.44
      necrobiosis lipoidica E10.620
      nephropathy E10.21
      neuralgia E10.42
      neurologic complication NEC E10.49
      neuropathic arthropathy E10.610
      neuropathy E10.40
      ophthalmic complication NEC E10.39
      oral complication NEC E10.638
      osteomyelitis E10.69
      periodontal disease E10.630
      peripheral angiopathy E10.51
        with gangrene E10.52
      polyneuropathy E10.42
      renal complication NEC E10.29
      renal tubular degeneration E10.29
      retinopathy E10.319
        with macular edema E10.311
        resolved following treatment E10.37 ☑
        nonproliferative E10.329 ☑
          with macular edema E10.321 ☑
          mild E10.329 ☑
            with macular edema E10.321 ☑

Diabetes, diabetic — *continued*
  type 1 — *continued*
    with — *continued*
      retinopathy — *continued*
        nonproliferative — *continued*
          moderate E10.339 ☑
            with macular edema E10.331 ☑
          severe E10.349 ☑
            with macular edema E10.341 ☑
        proliferative E10.359 ☑
          with
            combined traction retinal detachment
              and rhegmatogenous retinal
              detachment E10.354 ☑
            macular edema E10.351 ☑
            stable proliferative diabetic retinopa-
              thy E10.355 ☑
            traction retinal detachment involving
              the macula E10.352 ☑
            traction retinal detachment not involv-
              ing the macula E10.353 ☑
    skin complication NEC E10.628
    skin ulcer NEC E10.622
  type 2 E11.9
    with
      amyotrophy E11.44
      arthropathy NEC E11.618
      autonomic (poly)neuropathy E11.43
      cataract E11.36
      Charcot's joints E11.610
      chronic kidney disease E11.22
      circulatory complication NEC E11.59
      complication E11.8
        specified NEC E11.69
      dermatitis E11.620
      foot ulcer E11.621
      gangrene E11.52
      gastroparalysis E11.43
      gastroparesis E11.43
      glomerulonephrosis, intracapillary E11.21
      glomerulosclerosis, intercapillary E11.21
      hyperglycemia E11.65
      hyperosmolarity E11.00
        with coma E11.01
      hypoglycemia E11.649
        with coma E11.641
      ketoacidosis E11.10
        with coma E11.11
      kidney complications NEC E11.29
      Kimmelstiel-Wilson disease E11.21
      mononeuropathy E11.41
      myasthenia E11.44
      necrobiosis lipoidica E11.620
      nephropathy E11.21
      neuralgia E11.42
      neurologic complication NEC E11.49
      neuropathic arthropathy E11.610
      neuropathy E11.40
      ophthalmic complication NEC E11.39
      oral complication NEC E11.638
      osteomyelitis E11.69
      periodontal disease E11.630
      peripheral angiopathy E11.51
        with gangrene E11.52
      polyneuropathy E11.42
      renal complication NEC E11.29
      renal tubular degeneration E11.29
      retinopathy E11.319
        with macular edema E11.311
        resolved following treatment E11.37 ☑
        nonproliferative E11.329 ☑
          with macular edema E11.321 ☑
          mild E11.329 ☑
            with macular edema E11.321 ☑
          moderate E11.339 ☑
            with macular edema E11.331 ☑
          severe E11.349 ☑
            with macular edema E11.341 ☑
        proliferative E11.359 ☑
          with
            combined traction retinal detachment
              and rhegmatogenous retinal
              detachment E11.354 ☑
            macular edema E11.351 ☑
            stable proliferative diabetic retinopa-
              thy E11.355 ☑
            traction retinal detachment involving
              the macula E11.352 ☑

Diabetes, diabetic — *continued*
  type 2 — *continued*
    with — *continued*
      retinopathy — *continued*
        proliferative — *continued*
          with — *continued*
            traction retinal detachment not involv-
              ing the macula E11.353 ☑
      skin complication NEC E11.628
      skin ulcer NEC E11.622
    uncontrolled
      meaning
        hyperglycemia — *see* Diabetes, by type, with,
          hyperglycemia
        hypoglycemia — *see* Diabetes, by type, with,
          hypoglycemia
Diacyclothrombopathia D69.1
Diagnosis deferred R69
Dialysis (intermittent) (treatment)
  noncompliance (with) Z91.15
  renal (hemodialysis) (peritoneal), status Z99.2
  retina, retinal — *see* Detachment, retina, with retinal,
    dialysis
Diamond-Blackfan anemia (congenital hypoplastic)
  D61.01
Diamond-Gardener syndrome (autoerythrocyte sensi-
  tization) D69.2
Diaper rash L22
Diaphoresis (excessive) R61
Diaphragm — *see* condition
Diaphragmalgia R07.1
Diaphragmatitis, diaphragmitis J98.6
Diaphysial aclasis Q78.6
Diaphysitis — *see* Osteomyelitis, specified type NEC
Diarrhea, diarrheal (disease) (infantile) (inflammatory)
  R19.7
  achlorhydric K31.83
  allergic K52.29
    due to
      colitis — *see* Colitis, allergic
      enteritis — *see* Enteritis, allergic
  amebic — *see also* Amebiasis A06.0
    with abscess — *see* Abscess, amebic
    acute A06.0
    chronic A06.1
    nondysenteric A06.2
  bacillary — *see* Dysentery, bacillary
  balantidial A07.0
  cachectic NEC K52.89
  Chilomastix A07.8
  choleriformis A00.1
  chronic (noninfectious) K52.9
  coccidial A07.3
  Cochin-China K90.1
    strongyloidiasis B78.0
  Dientamoeba A07.8
  dietetic — *see also* Diarrhea, allergic K52.29
  drug-induced K52.1
  due to
    bacteria A04.9
      specified NEC A04.8
    Campylobacter A04.5
    Capillaria philippinensis B81.1
    Clostridium difficile
      not specified as recurrent A04.72
      recurrent A04.71
    Clostridium perfringens (C) (F) A04.8
    Cryptosporidium A07.2
    drugs K52.1
    Escherichia coli A04.4
      enteroaggregative A04.4
      enterohemorrhagic A04.3
      enteroinvasive A04.2
      enteropathogenic A04.0
      enterotoxigenic A04.1
      specified NEC A04.4
    food hypersensitivity — *see also* Diarrhea, allergic
      K52.29
    Necator americanus B76.1
    S. japonicum B65.2
    specified organism NEC A08.8
      bacterial A04.8
      viral A08.39
    Staphylococcus A04.8
    Trichuris trichiuria B79
    virus — *see* Enteritis, viral
    Yersinia enterocolitica A04.6
  dysenteric A09

Diarrhea, diarrheal — *continued*
  endemic A09
  epidemic A09
  flagellate A07.9
  Flexner's (ulcerative) A03.1
  functional K59.1
    following gastrointestinal surgery K91.89
    psychogenic F45.8
  Giardia lamblia A07.1
  giardial A07.1
  hill K90.1
  infectious A09
  malarial — *see* Malaria
  mite B88.0
  mycotic NEC B49
  neonatal (noninfectious) P78.3
  nervous F45.8
  neurogenic K59.1
  noninfectious K52.9
  postgastrectomy K91.1
  postvagotomy K91.1
  protozoal A07.9
    specified NEC A07.8
  psychogenic F45.8
  specified
    bacterium NEC A04.8
    virus NEC A08.39
  strongyloidiasis B78.0
  toxic K52.1
  trichomonal A07.8
  tropical K90.1
  tuberculous A18.32
  viral — *see* Enteritis, viral
Diastasis
  cranial bones M84.88
    congenital NEC Q75.8
  joint (traumatic) — *see* Dislocation
  muscle M62.00
    ankle M62.07- ☑
    congenital Q79.8
    foot M62.07- ☑
    forearm M62.03- ☑
    hand M62.04- ☑
    lower leg M62.06- ☑
    pelvic region M62.05- ☑
    shoulder region M62.01- ☑
    specified site NEC M62.08
    thigh M62.05- ☑
    upper arm M62.02- ☑
  recti (abdomen)
    complicating delivery O71.89
    congenital Q79.59
Diastema, tooth, teeth, fully erupted M26.32
Diastematomyelia Q06.2
Diataxia, cerebral G80.4
Diathesis
  allergic — *see* History, allergy
  bleeding (familial) D69.9
  cystine (familial) E72.00
  gouty — *see* Gout
  hemorrhagic (familial) D69.9
    newborn NEC P53
  spasmophilic R29.0
Diaz's disease or osteochondrosis (juvenile) (talus) —
  see Osteochondrosis, juvenile, tarsus
Dibothriocephalus, dibothriocephaliasis (latus) (infection) (infestation) B70.0
  larval B70.1
Dicephalus, dicephaly Q89.4
Dichotomy, teeth K00.2
Dichromat, dichromatopsia (congenital) — *see* Deficiency, color vision
Dichuchwa A65
Dicroceliasis B66.2
Didelphia, didelphys — *see* Double uterus
Didymytis N45.1
  with orchitis N45.3
Dietary
  inadequacy or deficiency E63.9
  surveillance and counseling Z71.3
Dietl's crisis N13.8
Dieulafoy lesion (hemorrhagic)
  duodenum K31.82
  esophagus K22.8
  intestine (colon) K63.81
  stomach K31.82
Difficult, difficulty (in)
  acculturation Z60.3

▽ Subterms under main terms may continue to next column or page   ☑ Additional Character Required — Refer to the Tabular List for Character Selection   **101**

Diabetes, diabetic — Difficult, difficulty

Difficult, difficulty — *continued*
feeding R63.3
newborn P92.9
breast P92.5
specified NEC P92.8
nonorganic (infant or child) F98.29
intubation, in anesthesia T88.4 ☑
mechanical, gastroduodenal stoma K91.89
causing obstruction — *see also* Obstruction, intestine, postoperative K91.30
micturition
need to immediately re-void R39.191
position dependent R39.192
specified NEC R39.198
reading (developmental) F81.0
secondary to emotional disorders F93.9
spelling (specific) F81.81
with reading disorder F81.89
due to inadequate teaching Z55.8
swallowing — *see* Dysphagia
walking R26.2
work
conditions NEC Z56.5
schedule Z56.3
Diffuse — *see* condition
Digestive — *see* condition
Dihydropyrimidine dehydrogenase disease (DPD) E88.89
Diktyoma — *see* Neoplasm, malignant, by site
Dilaceration, tooth K00.4
Dilatation
anus K59.89
venule — *see* Hemorrhoids
aorta (focal) (general) — *see* Ectasia, aorta
with aneuysm — *see* Aneurysm, aorta
congenital Q25.44
artery — *see* Aneurysm
bladder (sphincter) N32.89
congenital Q64.79
blood vessel I99.8
bronchial J47.9
with
exacerbation (acute) J47.1
lower respiratory infection J47.0
calyx (due to obstruction) — *see* Hydronephrosis
capillaries I78.8
cardiac (acute) (chronic) — *see also* Hypertrophy, cardiac
congenital Q24.8
valve NEC Q24.8
pulmonary Q22.3
valve — *see* Endocarditis
cavum septi pellucidi Q06.8
cervix (uteri) — *see also* Incompetency, cervix
incomplete, poor, slow complicating delivery O62.0
colon K59.39
congenital Q43.1
psychogenic F45.8
toxic K59.31
common duct (acquired) K83.8
congenital Q44.5
cystic duct (acquired) K82.8
congenital Q44.5
duct, mammary — *see* Ectasia, mammary duct
duodenum K59.89
esophagus K22.8
congenital Q39.5
due to achalasia K22.0
eustachian tube, congenital Q17.8
gallbladder K82.8
gastric — *see* Dilatation, stomach
heart (acute) (chronic) — *see also* Hypertrophy, cardiac
congenital Q24.8
valve — *see* Endocarditis
ileum K59.89
psychogenic F45.8
jejunum K59.89
psychogenic F45.8
kidney (calyx) (collecting structures) (cystic) (parenchyma) (pelvis) (idiopathic) N28.89
lacrimal passages or duct — *see* Disorder, lacrimal system, changes
lymphatic vessel I89.0
mammary duct — *see* Ectasia, mammary duct
Meckel's diverticulum (congenital) Q43.0
malignant — *see* Table of Neoplasms, small intestine, malignant

Dilatation — *continued*
myocardium (acute) (chronic) — *see* Hypertrophy, cardiac
organ or site, congenital NEC — *see* Distortion
pancreatic duct K86.89
pericardium — *see* Pericarditis
pharynx J39.2
prostate N42.89
pulmonary
artery (idiopathic) I28.8
valve, congenital Q22.3
pupil H57.04
rectum K59.39
saccule, congenital Q16.5
salivary gland (duct) K11.8
sphincter ani K62.89
stomach K31.89
acute K31.0
psychogenic F45.8
submaxillary duct K11.8
trachea, congenital Q32.1
ureter (idiopathic) N28.82
congenital Q62.2
due to obstruction N13.4
urethra (acquired) N36.8
vasomotor I73.9
vein I86.8
ventricular, ventricle (acute) (chronic) — *see also* Hypertrophy, cardiac
cerebral, congenital Q04.8
venule NEC I86.8
vesical orifice N32.89
Dilated, dilation — *see* Dilatation
Diminished, diminution
hearing (acuity) — *see* Deafness
sense or sensation (cold) (heat) (tactile) (vibratory) R20.8
vision NEC H54.7
vital capacity R94.2
Diminuta taenia B71.0
Dimitri-Sturge-Weber disease Q85.8
Dimple
congenital sacral Q82.6
parasacral Q82.6
pilonidal or postanal — *see* Cyst, pilonidal
Dioctophyme renalis (infection) (infestation) B83.8
Dipetalonemiasis B74.4
Diphallus Q55.69
Diphtheria, diphtheritic (gangrenous) (hemorrhagic) A36.9
carrier (suspected) Z22.2
cutaneous A36.3
faucial A36.0
infection of wound A36.3
laryngeal A36.2
myocarditis A36.81
nasal, anterior A36.89
nasopharyngeal A36.1
neurological complication A36.89
pharyngeal A36.0
specified site NEC A36.89
tonsillar A36.0
Diphyllobothriasis (intestine) B70.0
larval B70.1
Diplacusis H93.22- ☑
Diplegia (upper limbs) G83.0
congenital (cerebral) G80.8
facial G51.0
lower limbs G82.20
spastic G80.1
Diplococcus, diplococcal — *see* condition
Diplopia H53.2
Dipsomania F10.20
with
psychosis — *see* Psychosis, alcoholic
remission F10.21
Dipylidiasis B71.1
DIRA (deficiency of interleukin 1 receptor antagonist) M04.8
Direction, teeth, abnormal, fully erupted M26.30
Dirofilariasis B74.8
Dirt-eating child F98.3
Disability, disabilities
heart — *see* Disease, heart
intellectual F79
with
autistic features F84.9
mild (I.Q. 50-69) F70

Disability, disabilities — *continued*
intellectual — *continued*
moderate (I.Q. 35-49) F71
profound (I.Q. under 20) F73
severe (I.Q. 20-34) F72
specified level NEC F78
knowledge acquisition F81.9
learning F81.9
limiting activities Z73.6
spelling, specific F81.81
Disappearance of family member Z63.4
Disarticulation — *see* Amputation
meaning traumatic amputation — *see* Amputation, traumatic
Discharge (from)
abnormal finding in — *see* Abnormal, specimen
breast (female) (male) N64.52
diencephalic autonomic idiopathic — *see* Epilepsy, specified NEC
ear — *see also* Otorrhea
blood — *see* Otorrhagia
excessive urine R35.8
nipple N64.52
penile R36.9
postnasal R09.82
prison, anxiety concerning Z65.2
urethral R36.9
without blood R36.0
hematospermia R36.1
vaginal N89.8
Discitis, diskitis M46.40
cervical region M46.42
cervicothoracic region M46.43
lumbar region M46.46
lumbosacral region M46.47
multiple sites M46.49
occipito-atlanto-axial region M46.41
pyogenic — *see* Infection, intervertebral disc, pyogenic
sacrococcygeal region M46.48
thoracic region M46.44
thoracolumbar region M46.45
Discoid
meniscus (congenital) Q68.6
semilunar cartilage (congenital) — *see* Derangement, knee, meniscus, specified NEC
Discoloration
nails L60.8
teeth (posteruptive) K03.7
during formation K00.8
Discomfort
chest R07.89
visual H53.14- ☑
Discontinuity, ossicles, ear H74.2- ☑
Discord (with)
boss Z56.4
classmates Z55.4
counselor Z64.4
employer Z56.4
family Z63.8
fellow employees Z56.4
in-laws Z63.1
landlord Z59.2
lodgers Z59.2
neighbors Z59.2
probation officer Z64.4
social worker Z64.4
teachers Z55.4
workmates Z56.4
Discordant connection
atrioventricular (congenital) Q20.5
ventriculoarterial Q20.3
Discrepancy
centric occlusion maximum intercuspation M26.55
leg length (acquired) — *see* Deformity, limb, unequal length
congenital — *see* Defect, reduction, lower limb
uterine size date O26.84- ☑
Discrimination
ethnic Z60.5
political Z60.5
racial Z60.5
religious Z60.5
sex Z60.5
Disease, diseased — *see also* Syndrome
absorbent system I87.8
acid-peptic K30
Acosta's T70.29 ☑

Disease, diseased — *continued*
  Adams-Stokes (-Morgagni) (syncope with heart block) I45.9
  Addison's anemia (pernicious) D51.0
  adenoids (and tonsils) J35.9
  adrenal (capsule) (cortex) (gland) (medullary) E27.9
    hyperfunction E27.0
    specified NEC E27.8
  ainhum L94.6
  airway
    obstructive, chronic J44.9
      due to
        cotton dust J66.0
        specific organic dusts NEC J66.8
    reactive — *see* Asthma
  akamushi (scrub typhus) A75.3
  Albers-Schönberg (marble bones) Q78.2
  Albert's — *see* Tendinitis, Achilles
  alimentary canal K63.9
  alligator-skin Q80.9
    acquired L85.0
  alpha heavy chain C88.3
  alpine T70.29 ☑
  altitude T70.20 ☑
  alveolar ridge
    edentulous K06.9
      specified NEC K06.8
  alveoli, teeth K08.9
  Alzheimer's G30.9 *[F02.80]*
    with behavioral disturbance G30.9 *[F02.81]*
    early onset G30.0 *[F02.80]*
      with behavioral disturbance G30.0 *[F02.81]*
    late onset G30.1 *[F02.80]*
      with behavioral disturbance G30.1 *[F02.81]*
    specified NEC G30.8 *[F02.80]*
      with behavioral disturbance G30.8 *[F02.81]*
  amyloid — *see* Amyloidosis
  Andersen's (glycogenosis IV) E74.09
  Andes T70.29 ☑
  Andrews' (bacterid) L08.89
  angiospastic I73.9
    cerebral G45.9
    vein I87.8
  anterior
    chamber H21.9
    horn cell G12.29
  antiglomerular basement membrane (anti- GBM) anti-body M31.0
    tubulo-interstitial nephritis N12
  antral — *see* Sinusitis, maxillary
  anus K62.9
    specified NEC K62.89
  aorta (nonsyphilitic) I77.9
    syphilitic NEC A52.02
  aortic (heart) (valve) I35.9
    rheumatic I06.9
  Apollo B30.3
  aponeuroses — *see* Enthesopathy
  appendix K38.9
    specified NEC K38.8
  aqueous (chamber) H21.9
  Arnold-Chiari — *see* Arnold-Chiari disease
  arterial I77.9
    occlusive — *see* Occlusion, by site
      due to stricture or stenosis I77.1
    peripheral I73.9
  arteriocardiorenal — *see* Hypertension, cardiorenal
  arteriolar (generalized) (obliterative) I77.9
  arteriorenal — *see* Hypertension, kidney
  arteriosclerotic — *see also* Arteriosclerosis
    cardiovascular — *see* Disease, heart, ischemic, atherosclerotic
    coronary (artery) — *see* Disease, heart, ischemic, atherosclerotic
    heart — *see* Disease, heart, ischemic, atherosclerotic
  artery I77.9
    cerebral I67.9
    coronary I25.10
      with angina pectoris — *see* Arteriosclerosis, coronary (artery)
    peripheral I73.9
  arthropod-borne NOS (viral) A94
    specified type NEC A93.8
  atticoantral, chronic H66.20
    left H66.22
      with right H66.23
    right H66.21
      with left H66.23

Disease, diseased — *continued*
  auditory canal — *see* Disorder, ear, external
  auricle, ear NEC — *see* Disorder, pinna
  Australian X A83.4
  autoimmune (systemic) NOS M35.9
    hemolytic D59.10
      cold type (primary) (secondary) (symptomatic) D59.12
      drug-induced D59.0
      mixed type (primary) (secondary) (symptomatic) D59.13
      warm type (primary) (secondary) (symptomatic) D59.11
    thyroid E06.3
  autoinflammatory M04.9
    NOD2-associated M04.8
    specified type NEC M04.8
  aviator's — *see* Effect, adverse, high altitude
  Ayerza's (pulmonary artery sclerosis with pulmonary hypertension) I27.0
  Babington's (familial hemorrhagic telangiectasia) I78.0
  bacterial A49.9
    specified NEC A48.8
    zoonotic A28.9
      specified type NEC A28.8
  Baelz's (cheilitis glandularis apostematosa) K13.0
  bagasse J67.1
  balloon — *see* Effect, adverse, high altitude
  Bang's (brucella abortus) A23.1
  Bannister's T78.3 ☑
  barometer makers' — *see* Poisoning, mercury
  Barraquer (-Simons') (progressive lipodystrophy) E88.1
  Barrett's — *see* Barrett's, esophagus
  Bartholin's gland N75.9
  basal ganglia G25.9
    degenerative G23.9
      specified NEC G23.8
    specified NEC G25.89
  Basedow's (exophthalmic goiter) — *see* Hyperthyroidism, with, goiter (diffuse)
  Bateman's B08.1
  Batten-Steinert G71.11
  Battey A31.0
  Beard's (neurasthenia) F48.8
  Becker
    idiopathic mural endomyocardial I42.3
    myotonia congenita G71.12
  Begbie's (exophthalmic goiter) — *see* Hyperthyroidism, with, goiter (diffuse)
  behavioral, organic F07.9
  Beigel's (white piedra) B36.2
  Benson's — *see* Deposit, crystalline
  Bernard-Soulier (thrombopathy) D69.1
  Bernhardt (-Roth) — *see* Mononeuropathy, lower limb, meralgia paresthetica
  Biermer's (pernicious anemia) D51.0
  bile duct (common) (hepatic) K83.9
    with calculus, stones — *see* Calculus, bile duct
    specified NEC K83.8
  biliary (tract) K83.9
    specified NEC K83.8
  Billroth's — *see* Spina bifida
  bird fancier's J67.2
  black lung J60
  bladder N32.9
    in (due to)
      schistosomiasis (bilharziasis) B65.0 *[N33]*
    specified NEC N32.89
  bleeder's D66
  blood D75.9
    forming organs D75.9
    vessel I99.9
  Bloodgood's — *see* Mastopathy, cystic
  Blount M92.51- ☑
  Bodechtel-Guttmann (subacute sclerosing panencephalitis) A81.1
  bone — *see also* Disorder, bone
    aluminum M83.4
    fibrocystic NEC
      jaw M27.49
  bone-marrow D75.9
  Borna A83.9
  Bornholm (epidemic pleurodynia) B33.0
  Bouchard's (myopathic dilatation of the stomach) K31.0
  Bouillaud's (rheumatic heart disease) I01.9
  Bourneville (-Brissaud) (tuberous sclerosis) Q85.1
  Bouveret (-Hoffmann) (paroxysmal tachycardia) I47.9
  bowel K63.9

Disease, diseased — *continued*
  bowel — *continued*
    functional K59.9
      psychogenic F45.8
  brain G93.9
    arterial, artery I67.9
    arteriosclerotic I67.2
    congenital Q04.9
    degenerative — *see* Degeneration, brain
    inflammatory — *see* Encephalitis
    organic G93.9
      arteriosclerotic I67.2
    parasitic NEC B71.9 *[G94]*
    senile NEC G31.1
    specified NEC G93.89
  breast — *see also* Disorder, breast N64.9
    cystic (chronic) — *see* Mastopathy, cystic
    fibrocystic — *see* Mastopathy, cystic
    Paget's
      female, unspecified side C50.91- ☑
      male, unspecified side C50.92- ☑
    specified NEC N64.89
  Breda's — *see* Yaws
  Bretonneau's (diphtheritic malignant angina) A36.0
  Bright's — *see* Nephritis
    arteriosclerotic — *see* Hypertension, kidney
  Brill's (recrudescent typhus) A75.1
  Brill-Zinsser (recrudescent typhus) A75.1
  Brion-Kayser — *see* Fever, paratyphoid
  broad
    beta E78.2
    ligament (noninflammatory) N83.9
      inflammatory — *see* Disease, pelvis, inflammatory
      specified NEC N83.8
  Brocq-Duhring (dermatitis herpetiformis) L13.0
  Brocq's
    meaning
      dermatitis herpetiformis L13.0
      prurigo L28.2
  bronchopulmonary J98.4
  bronchus NEC J98.09
  bronze Addison's E27.1
    tuberculous A18.7
  budgerigar fancier's J67.2
  Buerger's (thromboangiitis obliterans) I73.1
  bullous L13.9
    chronic of childhood L12.2
    specified NEC L13.8
  Bürger-Grütz (essential familial hyperlipemia) E78.3
  bursa — *see* Bursopathy
  caisson T70.3 ☑
  California — *see* Coccidioidomycosis
  capillaries I78.9
    specified NEC I78.8
  Carapata A68.0
  cardiac — *see* Disease, heart
  cardiopulmonary, chronic I27.9
  cardiorenal (hepatic) (hypertensive) (vascular) — *see* Hypertension, cardiorenal
  cardiovascular (atherosclerotic) I25.10
    with angina pectoris — *see* Arteriosclerosis, coronary (artery),
    congenital Q28.9
    hypertensive — *see* Hypertension, heart
    newborn P29.9
      specified NEC P29.89
    renal (hypertensive) — *see* Hypertension, cardiorenal
    syphilitic (asymptomatic) A52.00
  cartilage — *see* Disorder, cartilage
  Castellani's A69.8
  Castleman (unicentric) (multicentric) D47.Z2
    HHV-8-associated — *see also* Herpesvirus, human, 8 D47.Z2
  cat-scratch A28.1
  Cavare's (familial periodic paralysis) G72.3
  cecum K63.9
  celiac (adult) (infantile) (with steatorrhea) K90.0
  cellular tissue L98.9
  central core G71.29
  cerebellar, cerebellum — *see* Disease, brain
  cerebral — *see also* Disease, brain
    degenerative — *see* Degeneration, brain
  cerebrospinal G96.9
  cerebrovascular I67.9
    acute I67.89
      embolic I63.4- ☑

Disease, diseased — *continued*
 cerebrovascular — *continued*
  acute — *continued*
   thrombotic I63.3- ☑
  arteriosclerotic I67.2
  hereditary NEC I67.858
  specified NEC I67.89
 cervix (uteri) (noninflammatory) N88.9
  inflammatory — *see* Cervicitis
  specified NEC N88.8
 Chabert's A22.9
 Chandler's (osteochondritis dissecans, hip) — *see* Osteochondritis, dissecans, hip
 Charlouis — *see* Yaws
 Chédiak-Steinbrinck (-Higashi) (congenital gigantism of peroxidase granules) E70.330
 chest J98.9
 Chiari's (hepatic vein thrombosis) I82.0
 Chicago B40.9
 Chignon B36.8
 chigo, chigoe B88.1
 childhood granulomatous D71
 Chinese liver fluke B66.1
 chlamydial A74.9
  specified NEC A74.89
 cholecystic K82.9
 choroid H31.9
  specified NEC H31.8
 Christmas D67
 chronic bullous of childhood L12.2
 chylomicron retention E78.3
 ciliary body H21.9
  specified NEC H21.89
 circulatory (system) NEC I99.8
  newborn P29.9
  syphilitic A52.00
   congenital A50.54
 coagulation factor deficiency (congenital) — *see* Defect, coagulation
 coccidioidal — *see* Coccidioidomycosis
 cold
  agglutinin or hemoglobinuria D59.12
   paroxysmal D59.6
  hemagglutinin (chronic) D59.12
 collagen NOS (nonvascular) (vascular) M35.9
  specified NEC M35.8
 colon K63.9
  functional K59.9
   congenital Q43.2
  ischemic — *see also* Ischemia, intestine, acute K55.039
 colonic inflammatory bowel, unclassified (IBDU) K52.3
 combined system — *see* Degeneration, combined
 compressed air T70.3 ☑
 Concato's (pericardial polyserositis) A19.9
  nontubercular I31.1
  pleural — *see* Pleurisy, with effusion
 conjunctiva H11.9
  chlamydial A74.0
  specified NEC H11.89
  viral B30.9
   specified NEC B30.8
 connective tissue, systemic (diffuse) M35.9
  in (due to)
   hypogammaglobulinemia D80.1 *[M36.8]*
   ochronosis E70.29 *[M36.8]*
  specified NEC M35.8
 Conor and Bruch's (boutonneuse fever) A77.1
 Cooper's — *see* Mastopathy, cystic
 Cori's (glycogenosis III) E74.03
 corkhandler's or corkworker's J67.3
 cornea H18.9
  specified NEC H18.89- ☑
 coronary (artery) — *see* Disease, heart, ischemic, atherosclerotic
  congenital Q24.5
  ostial, syphilitic (aortic) (mitral) (pulmonary) A52.03
 corpus cavernosum N48.9
  specified NEC N48.89
 Cotugno's — *see* Sciatica
 COVID-19 U07.1
 coxsackie (virus) NEC B34.1
 cranial nerve NOS G52.9
 Creutzfeldt-Jakob — *see* Creutzfeldt-Jakob disease or syndrome
 Crocq's (acrocyanosis) I73.89
 Crohn's — *see* Enteritis, regional
 Curschmann G71.11

Disease, diseased — *continued*
 cystic
  breast (chronic) — *see* Mastopathy, cystic
  kidney, congenital Q61.9
  liver, congenital Q44.6
  lung J98.4
   congenital Q33.0
 cytomegalic inclusion (generalized) B25.9
  with pneumonia B25.0
  congenital P35.1
 cytomegaloviral B25.9
  specified NEC B25.8
 Czerny's (periodic hydrarthrosis of the knee) — *see* Effusion, joint, knee
 Daae (-Finsen) (epidemic pleurodynia) B33.0
 Darling's — *see* Histoplasmosis capsulati
 de Quervain's (tendon sheath) M65.4
  thyroid (subacute granulomatous thyroiditis) E06.1
 Débove's (splenomegaly) R16.1
 deer fly — *see* Tularemia
 Degos' I77.89
 demyelinating, demyelinizing (nervous system) G37.9
  multiple sclerosis G35
  specified NEC G37.8
 dense deposit — *see also* N00-N07 with fourth character .6 N05.6
 deposition, hydroxyapatite — *see* Disease, hydroxyapatite deposition
 Devergie's (pityriasis rubra pilaris) L44.0
 Devic's G36.0
 diaphorase deficiency D74.0
 diaphragm J98.6
 diarrheal, infectious NEC A09
 digestive (system) K92.9
  specified NEC K92.89
 disc, degenerative — *see* Degeneration, intervertebral disc
 discogenic — *see also* Displacement, intervertebral disc NEC
  with myelopathy — *see* Disorder, disc, with, myelopathy
 diverticular — *see* Diverticula
 Dubois (thymus) A50.59 *[E35]*
 Duchenne-Griesinger G71.01
 Duchenne's
  muscular dystrophy G71.01
  pseudohypertrophy, muscles G71.01
 ductless glands E34.9
 Duhring's (dermatitis herpetiformis) L13.0
 duodenum K31.9
  specified NEC K31.89
 Dupré's (meningism) R29.1
 Dupuytren's (muscle contracture) M72.0
 Durand-Nicholas-Favre (climatic bubo) A55
 Duroziez's (congenital mitral stenosis) Q23.2
 ear — *see* Disorder, ear
 Eberth's — *see* Fever, typhoid
 Ebola (virus) A98.4
 Ebstein's heart Q22.5
 Echinococcus — *see* Echinococcus
 echovirus NEC B34.1
 Eddowes' (brittle bones and blue sclera) Q78.0
 edentulous (alveolar) ridge K06.9
  specified NEC K06.8
 Edsall's T67.2 ☑
 Eichstedt's (pityriasis versicolor) B36.0
 Eisenmenger's (irreversible) I27.83
 Ellis-van Creveld (chondroectodermal dysplasia) Q77.6
 end stage renal (ESRD) N18.6
  due to hypertension I12.0
 endocrine glands or system NEC E34.9
 endomyocardial (eosinophilic) I42.3
 English (rickets) E55.0
 enteroviral, enterovirus NEC B34.1
  central nervous system NEC A88.8
 epidemic B99.9
  specified NEC B99.8
 epididymis N50.9
 Erb (-Landouzy) G71.02
 Erdheim-Chester (ECD) E88.89
 esophagus K22.9
  functional K22.4
  psychogenic F45.8
  specified NEC K22.8
 Eulenburg's (congenital paramyotonia) G71.19
 eustachian tube — *see* Disorder, eustachian tube
 external
  auditory canal — *see* Disorder, ear, external

Disease, diseased — *continued*
 external — *continued*
  ear — *see* Disorder, ear, external
 extrapyramidal G25.9
  specified NEC G25.89
 eye H57.9
  anterior chamber H21.9
  inflammatory NEC H57.89
  muscle (external) — *see* Strabismus
  specified NEC H57.89
  syphilitic — *see* Oculopathy, syphilitic
 eyeball H44.9
  specified NEC H44.89
 eyelid — *see* Disorder, eyelid
  specified NEC — *see* Disorder, eyelid, specified type NEC
 eyeworm of Africa B74.3
 facial nerve (seventh) G51.9
  newborn (birth injury) P11.3
 Fahr (of brain) G23.8
 Fahr Volhard (of kidney) I12.- ☑
 fallopian tube (noninflammatory) N83.9
  inflammatory — *see* Salpingo-oophoritis
  specified NEC N83.8
 familial periodic paralysis G72.3
 Fanconi's (congenital pancytopenia) D61.09
 fascia NEC — *see also* Disorder, muscle
  inflammatory — *see* Myositis
  specified NEC M62.89
 Fauchard's (periodontitis) — *see* Periodontitis
 Favre-Durand-Nicolas (climatic bubo) A55
 Fede's K14.0
 Feer's — *see* Poisoning, mercury
 female pelvic inflammatory — *see also* Disease, pelvis, inflammatory N73.9
  syphilitic (secondary) A51.42
  tuberculous A18.17
 Fernels' (aortic aneurysm) I71.9
 fibrocaseous of lung — *see* Tuberculosis, pulmonary
 fibrocystic — *see* Fibrocystic disease
 Fiedler's (leptospiral jaundice) A27.0
 fifth B08.3
 file-cutter's — *see* Poisoning, lead
 fish-skin Q80.9
  acquired L85.0
 Flajani (-Basedow) (exophthalmic goiter) — *see* Hyperthyroidism, with, goiter (diffuse)
 flax-dresser's J66.1
 fluke — *see* Infestation, fluke
 foot and mouth B08.8
 foot process N04.9
 Forbes' (glycogenosis III) E74.03
 Fordyce-Fox (apocrine miliaria) L75.2
 Fordyce's (ectopic sebaceous glands) (mouth) Q38.6
 Forestier's (rhizomelic pseudopolyarthritis) M35.3
  meaning ankylosing hyperostosis — *see* Hyperostosis, ankylosing
 Fothergill's
  neuralgia — *see* Neuralgia, trigeminal
  scarlatina anginosa A38.9
 Fournier (gangrene) N49.3
  female N76.89
 fourth B08.8
 Fox (-Fordyce) (apocrine miliaria) L75.2
 Francis' — *see* Tularemia
 Franklin C88.2
 Frei's (climatic bubo) A55
 Friedreich's
  combined systemic or ataxia G11.11
  myoclonia G25.3
 frontal sinus — *see* Sinusitis, frontal
 fungus NEC B49
 Gaisböck's (polycythemia hypertonica) D75.1
 gallbladder K82.9
  calculus — *see* Calculus, gallbladder
  cholecystitis — *see* Cholecystitis
  cholesterolosis K82.4
  fistula — *see* Fistula, gallbladder
  hydrops K82.1
  obstruction — *see* Obstruction, gallbladder
  perforation K82.2
  specified NEC K82.8
 gamma heavy chain C88.2
 Gamna's (siderotic splenomegaly) D73.2
 Gamstorp's (adynamia episodica hereditaria) G72.3
 Gandy-Nanta (siderotic splenomegaly) D73.2
 ganister J62.8
 gastric — *see* Disease, stomach

Disease, diseased — *continued*
gastroesophageal reflux (GERD) K21.9
  with esophagitis (without bleeding) K21.00
    with bleeding K21.01
gastrointestinal (tract) K92.9
  amyloid E85.4
  functional K59.9
    psychogenic F45.8
  specified NEC K92.89
Gee (-Herter) (-Heubner) (-Thaysen) (nontropical sprue)
  K90.0
genital organs
  female N94.9
  male N50.9
Gerhardt's (erythromelalgia) I73.81
Gibert's (pityriasis rosea) L42
Gierke's (glycogenosis I) E74.01
Gilles de la Tourette's (motor-verbal tic) F95.2
gingiva K06.9
  plaque induced K05.00
  specified NEC K06.8
gland (lymph) I89.9
Glanzmann's (hereditary hemorrhagic thrombasthenia)
  D69.1
glass-blower's (cataract) — *see* Cataract, specified NEC
  salivary gland hypertrophy K11.1
Glisson's — *see* Rickets
globe H44.9
  specified NEC H44.89
glomerular — *see also* Glomerulonephritis
  with edema — *see* Nephrosis
  acute — *see* Nephritis, acute
  chronic — *see* Nephritis, chronic
  minimal change N05.0
  rapidly progressive N01.9
glycogen storage E74.00
  Andersen's E74.09
  Cori's E74.03
  Forbes' E74.03
  generalized E74.00
  glucose-6-phosphatase deficiency E74.01
  heart E74.02 *[143]*
  hepatorenal E74.09
  Hers' E74.09
  liver and kidney E74.09
  McArdle's E74.04
  muscle phosphofructokinase E74.09
  myocardium E74.02 *[143]*
  Pompe's E74.02
  Tauri's E74.09
  type 0 E74.09
  type I E74.01
  type II E74.02
  type III E74.03
  type IV E74.09
  type V E74.04
  type VI-XI E74.09
  Von Gierke's E74.01
Goldstein's (familial hemorrhagic telangiectasia) I78.0
gonococcal NOS A54.9
graft-versus-host (GVH) D89.813
  acute D89.810
  acute on chronic D89.812
  chronic D89.811
grainhandler's J67.8
granulomatous (childhood) (chronic) D71
Graves' (exophthalmic goiter) — *see* Hyperthyroidism,
  with, goiter (diffuse)
Griesinger's — *see* Ancylostomiasis
Grisel's M43.6
Gruby's (tinea tonsurans) B35.0
Guillain-Barré G61.0
Guinon's (motor-verbal tic) F95.2
gum K06.9
gynecological N94.9
H (Hartnup's) E72.02
Haff — *see* Poisoning, mercury
Hageman (congenital factor XII deficiency) D68.2
hair (color) (shaft) L67.9
  follicles L73.9
    specified NEC L73.8
Hamman's (spontaneous mediastinal emphysema)
  J98.2
hand, foot and mouth B08.4
Hansen's — *see* Leprosy
Hantavirus, with pulmonary manifestations B33.4
  with renal manifestations A98.5
Harada's H30.81- ☑

Disease, diseased — *continued*
Hartnup (pellagra-cerebellar ataxia-renal
  aminoaciduria) E72.02
Hart's (pellagra-cerebellar ataxia-renal aminoaciduria)
  E72.02
Hashimoto's (struma lymphomatosa) E06.3
Hb — *see* Disease, hemoglobin
heart (organic) I51.9
  with
    pulmonary edema (acute) — *see also* Failure,
      ventricular, left I50.1
    rheumatic fever (conditions in I00)
      active I01.9
        with chorea I02.0
        specified NEC I01.8
      inactive or quiescent (with chorea) I09.9
        specified NEC I09.89
  amyloid E85.4 *[143]*
  aortic (valve) I35.9
  arteriosclerotic or sclerotic (senile) — *see* Disease,
    heart, ischemic, atherosclerotic
  artery, arterial — *see* Disease, heart, ischemic,
    atherosclerotic
  beer drinkers' I42.6
  beriberi (wet) E51.12
  black I27.0
  congenital Q24.9
    cyanotic Q24.9
    specified NEC Q24.8
  coronary — *see* Disease, heart, ischemic
  cryptogenic I51.9
  fibroid — *see* Myocarditis
  functional I51.89
    psychogenic F45.8
  glycogen storage E74.02 *[143]*
  gonococcal A54.83
  hypertensive — *see* Hypertension, heart
  hyperthyroid — *see also* Hyperthyroidism
    E05.90 *[143]*
    with thyroid storm E05.91 *[143]*
  ischemic (chronic or with a stated duration of over
    4 weeks) I25.9
    atherosclerotic (of) I25.10
      with angina pectoris — *see* Arteriosclerosis,
        coronary (artery)
      coronary artery bypass graft — *see* Arterioscle-
        rosis, coronary (artery),
        cardiomyopathy I25.5
    diagnosed on ECG or other special investigation,
      but currently presenting no symptoms
      I25.6
    silent I25.6
    specified form NEC I25.89
  kyphoscoliotic I27.1
  meningococcal A39.50
    endocarditis A39.51
    myocarditis A39.52
    pericarditis A39.53
  mitral I05.9
    specified NEC I05.8
  muscular — *see* Degeneration, myocardial
  psychogenic (functional) F45.8
  pulmonary (chronic) I27.9
    in schistosomiasis B65.9 *[152]*
    specified NEC I27.89
  rheumatic (chronic) (inactive) (old) (quiescent) (with
    chorea) I09.9
    active or acute I01.9
      with chorea (acute) (rheumatic) (Sydenham's)
        I02.0
    specified NEC I09.89
  senile — *see* Myocarditis
  syphilitic A52.06
    aortic A52.03
      aneurysm A52.01
    congenital A50.54 *[152]*
  thyrotoxic — *see also* Thyrotoxicosis E05.90 *[143]*
    with thyroid storm E05.91 *[143]*
  valve, valvular (obstructive) (regurgitant) — *see also*
    Endocarditis
    congenital NEC Q24.8
    pulmonary Q22.3
  vascular — *see* Disease, cardiovascular
heavy chain NEC C88.2
  alpha C88.3
  gamma C88.2
  mu C88.2

Disease, diseased — *continued*
Hebra's
  pityriasis
    maculata et circinata L42
    rubra pilaris L44.0
  prurigo L28.2
hematopoietic organs D75.9
hemoglobin or Hb
  abnormal (mixed) NEC D58.2
    with thalassemia D56.9
  AS genotype D57.3
  Bart's D56.0
  C (Hb-C) D58.2
    with other abnormal hemoglobin NEC D58.2
    elliptocytosis D58.1
    Hb-S D57.2- ☑
    sickle-cell D57.2- ☑
    thalassemia D56.8
  Constant Spring D58.2
  D (Hb-D) D58.2
  E (Hb-E) D58.2
  E-beta thalassemia D56.5
  elliptocytosis D58.1
  H (Hb-H) (thalassemia) D56.0
    with other abnormal hemoglobin NEC D56.9
    Constant Spring D56.0
  I thalassemia D56.9
  M D74.0
  S or SS D57.1
    with
      acute chest syndrome D57.01
      cerebral vascular involvement D57.03
      crisis (painful) D57.00
        with complication specified NEC D57.09
      splenic sequestration D57.02
      vasoocclusive pain D57.00
    beta plus D57.44
      with
        acute chest syndrome D57.451
        cerebral vascular involvement D57.453
        crisis D57.459
          with specified complication NEC
            D57.458
        splenic sequestration D57.452
        vasoocclusive pain D57.459
      without crisis D57.44
    beta zero D57.42
      with
        acute chest syndrome D57.431
        cerebral vascular involvement D57.433
        crisis D57.439
          with specified complication NEC
            D57.438
        splenic sequestration D57.432
        vasoocclusive pain
      without crisis D57.42
  SC D57.2- ☑
  SD D57.8- ☑
  SE D57.8- ☑
  spherocytosis D58.0
  unstable, hemolytic D58.2
hemolytic (newborn) P55.9
  autoimmune D59.10
    cold type (primary) (secondary) (symptomatic)
      D59.12
    mixed type (primary) (secondary) (symptomatic)
      D59.13
    warm type (primary) (secondary) (symptomatic)
      D59.11
  drug-induced D59.0
  due to or with
    incompatibility
      ABO (blood group) P55.1
      blood (group) (Duffy) (K) (Kell) (Kidd) (Lewis)
        (M) (S) NEC P55.8
      Rh (blood group) (factor) P55.0
    Rh negative mother P55.0
  specified type NEC P55.8
  unstable hemoglobin D58.2
hemorrhagic D69.9
  newborn P53
Henoch (-Schönlein) (purpura nervosa) D69.0
hepatic — *see* Disease, liver
hepatolenticular E83.01
heredodegenerative NEC
  spinal cord G95.89
herpesviral, disseminated B00.7
Hers' (glycogenosis VI) E74.09
Herter (-Gee) (-Heubner) (nontropical sprue) K90.0

Disease, diseased — *continued*
  Heubner-Herter (nontropical sprue) K90.0
  high fetal gene or hemoglobin thalassemia D56.9
  Hildenbrand's — *see* Typhus
  hip (joint) M25.9
    congenital Q65.89
    suppurative M00.9
    tuberculous A18.02
  His (-Werner) (trench fever) A79.0
  Hodgson's I71.2
    ruptured I71.1
  Holla — *see* Spherocytosis
  hookworm B76.9
    specified NEC B76.8
  host-versus-graft D89.813
    acute D89.810
    acute on chronic D89.812
    chronic D89.811
  human immunodeficiency virus (HIV) B20
  Huntington's G10
    with dementia G10 [F02.80]
  Hutchinson's (cheiropompholyx) — *see* Hutchinson's
      disease
  hyaline (diffuse) (generalized)
    membrane (lung) (newborn) P22.0
      adult J80
  hydatid — *see* Echinococcus
  hydroxyapatite deposition M11.00
    ankle M11.07- ☑
    elbow M11.02- ☑
    foot joint M11.07- ☑
    hand joint M11.04- ☑
    hip M11.05- ☑
    knee M11.06- ☑
    multiple site M11.09
    shoulder M11.01- ☑
    vertebra M11.08
    wrist M11.03- ☑
  hyperkinetic — *see* Hyperkinesia
  hypertensive — *see* Hypertension
  hypophysis E23.7
  Iceland G93.3
  I-cell E77.0
  immune D89.9
  immunoproliferative (malignant) C88.9
    small intestinal C88.3
    specified NEC C88.8
  inclusion B25.9
    salivary gland B25.9
  infectious, infective B99.9
    congenital P37.9
      specified NEC P37.8
    viral P35.9
      specified type NEC P35.8
    specified NEC B99.8
  inflammatory
    penis N48.29
      abscess N48.21
      cellulitis N48.22
    prepuce N47.7
      balanoposthitis N47.6
    tubo-ovarian — *see* Salpingo-oophoritis
  intervertebral disc — *see also* Disorder, disc
    with myelopathy — *see* Disorder, disc, with,
        myelopathy
    cervical, cervicothoracic — *see* Disorder, disc, cervi-
        cal
      with
        myelopathy — *see* Disorder, disc, cervical,
            with myelopathy
        neuritis, radiculitis or radiculopathy — *see*
            Disorder, disc, cervical, with neuritis
        specified NEC — *see* Disorder, disc, cervical,
            specified type NEC
    lumbar (with)
      myelopathy M51.06
      neuritis, radiculitis, radiculopathy or sciatica
          M51.16
      specified NEC M51.86
    lumbosacral (with)
      neuritis, radiculitis, radiculopathy or sciatica
          M51.17
      specified NEC M51.87
    specified NEC — *see* Disorder, disc, specified NEC
    thoracic (with)
      myelopathy M51.04
      neuritis, radiculitis or radiculopathy M51.14
      specified NEC M51.84

Disease, diseased — *continued*
  intervertebral disc — *see also* Disorder, disc — *contin-
      ued*
    thoracolumbar (with)
      myelopathy M51.05
      neuritis, radiculitis or radiculopathy M51.15
      specified NEC M51.85
  intestine K63.9
    functional K59.9
      psychogenic F45.8
      specified NEC K59.89
    organic K63.9
    protozoal A07.9
    specified NEC K63.89
  iris H21.9
    specified NEC H21.89
  iron metabolism or storage E83.10
  island (scrub typhus) A75.3
  itai-itai — *see* Poisoning, cadmium
  Jakob-Creutzfeldt — *see* Creutzfeldt-Jakob disease or
      syndrome
  jaw M27.9
    fibrocystic M27.49
    specified NEC M27.8
  jigger B88.1
  joint — *see also* Disorder, joint
    Charcot's — *see* Arthropathy, neuropathic (Charcot)
    degenerative — *see* Osteoarthritis
      multiple M15.9
      spine — *see* Spondylosis
    hypertrophic — *see* Osteoarthritis
    sacroiliac M53.3
    specified NEC — *see* Disorder, joint, specified type
        NEC
    spine NEC — *see* Dorsopathy
    suppurative — *see* Arthritis, pyogenic or pyemic
  Jourdain's (acute gingivitis) K05.00
    nonplaque induced K05.01
    plaque induced K05.00
  Kaschin-Beck (endemic polyarthritis) M12.10
    ankle M12.17- ☑
    elbow M12.12- ☑
    foot joint M12.17- ☑
    hand joint M12.14- ☑
    hip M12.15- ☑
    knee M12.16- ☑
    multiple site M12.19
    shoulder M12.11- ☑
    vertebra M12.18
    wrist M12.13- ☑
  Katayama B65.2
  Kedani (scrub typhus) A75.3
  Keshan E59
  kidney (functional) (pelvis) N28.9
    chronic N18.9
      hypertensive — *see* Hypertension, kidney
      stage 1 N18.1
      stage 2 (mild) N18.2
      stage 3 (moderate) N18.30
      stage 3a N18.31
      stage 3b N18.32
      stage 4 (severe) N18.4
      stage 5 N18.5
    complicating pregnancy — *see* Pregnancy, compli-
        cated by, renal disease
    cystic (congenital) Q61.9
    fibrocystic (congenital) Q61.8
    hypertensive — *see* Hypertension, kidney
    in (due to)
      schistosomiasis (bilharziasis) B65.9 [N29]
    multicystic Q61.4
    polycystic Q61.3
      adult type Q61.2
      childhood type NEC Q61.19
        collecting duct dilatation Q61.11
  Kimmelstiel (-Wilson) (intercapillary polycystic (congen-
      ital) glomerulosclerosis) — *see* E08-E13 with .21
  Kinnier Wilson's (hepatolenticular degeneration) E83.01
  kissing — *see* Mononucleosis, infectious
  Klebs' — *see also* Glomerulonephritis N05- ☑
  Klippel-Feil (brevicollis) Q76.1
  Köhler-Pellegrini-Stieda (calcification, knee joint) —
      see Bursitis, tibial collateral
  Kok Q89.8
  König's (osteochondritis dissecans) — *see* Osteochon-
      dritis, dissecans
  Korsakoff's (nonalcoholic) F04
    alcoholic F10.96

Disease, diseased — *continued*
  Korsakoff's — *continued*
    alcoholic — *continued*
      with dependence F10.26
  Kostmann's (infantile genetic agranulocytosis) D70.0
  kuru A81.81
  Kyasanur Forest A98.2
  labyrinth, ear — *see* Disorder, ear, inner
  lacrimal system — *see* Disorder, lacrimal system
  Lafora's — *see* Epilepsy, generalized, idiopathic
  Lancereaux-Mathieu (leptospiral jaundice) A27.0
  Landry's G61.0
  Larrey-Weil (leptospiral jaundice) A27.0
  larynx J38.7
  legionnaires' A48.1
    nonpneumonic A48.2
  Lenegre's I44.2
  lens H27.9
    specified NEC H27.8
  Lev's (acquired complete heart block) I44.2
  Lewy body (dementia) G31.83 [F02.80]
    with behavioral disturbance G31.83 [F02.81]
  Lichtheim's (subacute combined sclerosis with perni-
      cious anemia) D51.0
  Lightwood's (renal tubular acidosis) N25.89
  Lignac's (cystinosis) E72.04
  lip K13.0
  lipid-storage E75.6
    specified NEC E75.5
  Lipschütz's N76.6
  liver (chronic) (organic) K76.9
    alcoholic (chronic) K70.9
      acute — *see* Disease, liver, alcoholic, hepatitis
      cirrhosis K70.30
        with ascites K70.31
      failure K70.40
        with coma K70.41
      fatty liver K70.0
      fibrosis K70.2
      hepatitis K70.10
        with ascites K70.11
      sclerosis K70.2
    cystic, congenital Q44.6
    drug-induced (idiosyncratic) (toxic) (predictable)
        (unpredictable) — *see* Disease, liver, toxic
    end stage K72.90
      due to hepatitis — *see* Hepatitis
    fatty, nonalcoholic (NAFLD) K76.0
      alcoholic K70.0
    fibrocystic (congenital) Q44.6
    fluke
      Chinese B66.1
      oriental B66.1
      sheep B66.3
    gestational alloimmune (GALD) P78.84
    glycogen storage E74.09 [K77]
    in (due to)
      schistosomiasis (bilharziasis) B65.9 [K77]
    inflammatory K75.9
      alcoholic K70.1 ☑
      specified NEC K75.89
    polycystic (congenital) Q44.6
    toxic K71.9
      with
        cholestasis K71.0
        cirrhosis (liver) K71.7
        fibrosis (liver) K71.7
        focal nodular hyperplasia K71.8
        hepatic granuloma K71.8
        hepatic necrosis K71.10
          with coma K71.11
        hepatitis NEC K71.6
          acute K71.2
          chronic
            active K71.50
              with ascites K71.51
            lobular K71.4
            persistent K71.3
            lupoid K71.50
              with ascites K71.51
        peliosis hepatis K71.8
        veno-occlusive disease (VOD) of liver K71.8
      veno-occlusive K76.5
  Lobo's (keloid blastomycosis) B48.0
  Lobstein's (brittle bones and blue sclera) Q78.0
  Ludwig's (submaxillary cellulitis) K12.2
  lumbosacral region M53.87
  lung J98.4

Disease, diseased — *continued*
lung — *continued*
  black J60
  congenital Q33.9
  cystic J98.4
    congenital Q33.0
  dabbing (related) U07.0
  electronic cigarette (related) U07.0
  fibroid (chronic) — *see* Fibrosis, lung
  fluke B66.4
    oriental B66.4
  in
    amyloidosis E85.4 *[J99]*
    sarcoidosis D86.0
    Sjögren's syndrome M35.02
    systemic
      lupus erythematosus M32.13
      sclerosis M34.81
  interstitial J84.9
    of childhood, specified NEC J84.848
    respiratory bronchiolitis J84.115
    specified NEC J84.89
    with progressive fibrotic phenotype, in diseases
      classified elsewhere J84.170
  obstructive (chronic) J44.9
    with
      acute
        bronchitis J44.0
        exacerbation NEC J44.1
        lower respiratory infection J44.0
      alveolitis, allergic J67.9
      asthma J44.9
      bronchiectasis J47.9
        with
          exacerbation (acute) J47.1
          lower respiratory infection J47.0
      bronchitis J44.9
        with
          exacerbation (acute) J44.1
          lower respiratory infection J44.0
      emphysema J43.9
      hypersensitivity pneumonitis J67.9
    decompensated J44.1
      with
        exacerbation (acute) J44.1
  polycystic J98.4
    congenital Q33.0
  rheumatoid (diffuse) (interstitial) — *see* Rheuma-
    toid, lung
  vaping (associated) (device) (product) (use) U07.0
Lutembacher's (atrial septal defect with mitral stenosis)
  Q21.1
Lyme A69.20
lymphatic (gland) (system) (channel) (vessel) I89.9
lymphoproliferative D47.9
  specified NEC D47.Z9 *(following* D47.4)
  T-gamma D47.Z9 *(following* D47.4)
  X-linked D82.3
Magitot's M27.2
malarial — *see* Malaria
malignant — *see also* Neoplasm, malignant, by site
Manson's B65.1
maple bark J67.6
maple-syrup-urine E71.0
Marburg (virus) A98.3
Marion's (bladder neck obstruction) N32.0
Marsh's (exophthalmic goiter) — *see* Hyperthyroidism,
  with, goiter (diffuse)
mastoid (process) — *see* Disorder, ear, middle
Mathieu's (leptospiral jaundice) A27.0
Maxcy's A75.2
McArdle (-Schmid-Pearson) (glycogenosis V) E74.04
mediastinum J98.59
medullary center (idiopathic) (respiratory) G93.89
Meige's (chronic hereditary edema) Q82.0
meningococcal — *see* Infection, meningococcal
mental F99
  organic F09
mesenchymal M35.9
mesenteric embolic — *see also* Ischemia, intestine,
  acute K55.039
metabolic, metabolism E88.9
  bilirubin E80.7
metal-polisher's J62.8
metastatic — *see also* Neoplasm, secondary, by site
  C79.9

Disease, diseased — *continued*
microvascular - code to condition
microvillus
  atrophy Q43.8
  inclusion (MVD) Q43.8
middle ear — *see* Disorder, ear, middle
Mikulicz' (dryness of mouth, absent or decreased
  lacrimation) K11.8
Milroy's (chronic hereditary edema) Q82.0
Minamata — *see* Poisoning, mercury
minicore G71.29
Minor's G95.19
Minot's (hemorrhagic disease, newborn) P53
Minot-von Willebrand-Jürgens (angiohemophilia) D68.0
Mitchell's (erythromelalgia) I73.81
mitral (valve) I05.9
  nonrheumatic I34.9
mixed connective tissue M35.1
moldy hay J67.0
Monge's T70.29 ☑
Morgagni-Adams-Stokes (syncope with heart block)
  I45.9
Morgagni's (syndrome) (hyperostosis frontalis interna)
  M85.2
Morton's (with metatarsalgia) — *see* Lesion, nerve,
  plantar
Morvan's G60.8
motor neuron (bulbar) (mixed type) (spinal) G12.20
  amyotrophic lateral sclerosis G12.21
  familial G12.24
  progressive bulbar palsy G12.22
  specified NEC G12.29
moyamoya I67.5
mu heavy chain disease C88.2
multicore G71.29
multiminicore G71.29
muscle — *see also* Disorder, muscle
  inflammatory — *see* Myositis
  ocular (external) — *see* Strabismus
musculoskeletal system, soft tissue — *see also* Disorder,
  soft tissue
  specified NEC — *see* Disorder, soft tissue, specified
    type NEC
mushroom workers' J67.5
mycotic B49
myelodysplastic, not classified C94.6
myeloproliferative, not classified C94.6
  chronic D47.1
myocardium, myocardial — *see also* Degeneration,
  myocardial I51.5
  primary (idiopathic) I42.9
myoneural G70.9
Naegeli's D69.1
nails L60.9
  specified NEC L60.8
Nairobi (sheep virus) A93.8
nasal J34.9
nemaline body G71.21
nerve — *see* Disorder, nerve
nervous system G98.8
  autonomic G90.9
  central G96.9
    specified NEC G96.89
  congenital Q07.9
  parasympathetic G90.9
  specified NEC G98.8
  sympathetic G90.9
  vegetative G90.9
neuromuscular system G70.9
Newcastle B30.8
Nicolas (-Durand)-Favre (climatic bubo) A55
nipple N64.9
  Paget's C50.01- ☑
    female C50.01- ☑
    male C50.02- ☑
Nishimoto (-Takeuchi) I67.5
nonarthropod-borne NOS (viral) B34.9
  enterovirus NEC B34.1
nonautoimmune hemolytic D59.4
  drug-induced D59.2
Nonne-Milroy-Meige (chronic hereditary edema) Q82.0
nose J34.9
nucleus pulposus — *see* Disorder, disc
nutritional E63.9
oast-house-urine E72.19
  ocular
    herpesviral B00.50
    zoster B02.30

Disease, diseased — *continued*
obliterative vascular I77.1
Ohara's — *see* Tularemia
Opitz's (congestive splenomegaly) D73.2
Oppenheim-Urbach (necrobiosis lipoidica diabetico-
  rum) — *see* E08-E13 with .620
optic nerve NEC — *see* Disorder, nerve, optic
orbit — *see* Disorder, orbit
organ
  dabbing (related) U07.0
  electronic cigarette (related) U07.0
  vaping (associated) (device) (product) (use) U07.0
Oriental liver fluke B66.1
Oriental lung fluke B66.4
Ormond's N13.5
Oropouche virus A93.0
Osler-Rendu (familial hemorrhagic telangiectasia) I78.0
osteofibrocystic E21.0
Otto's M24.7
outer ear — *see* Disorder, ear, external
ovary (noninflammatory) N83.9
  cystic N83.20- ☑
  inflammatory — *see* Salpingo-oophoritis
  polycystic E28.2
  specified NEC N83.8
Owren's (congenital) — *see* Defect, coagulation
pancreas K86.9
  cystic K86.2
  fibrocystic E84.9
  specified NEC K86.89
panvalvular I08.9
  specified NEC I08.8
parametrium (noninflammatory) N83.9
parasitic B89
  cerebral NEC B71.9 *[G94]*
  intestinal NOS B82.9
  mouth B37.0
  skin NOS B88.9
  specified type — *see* Infestation
  tongue B37.0
parathyroid (gland) E21.5
  specified NEC E21.4
Parkinson's G20
parodontal K05.6
Parrot's (syphilitic osteochondritis) A50.02
Parry's (exophthalmic goiter) — *see* Hyperthyroidism,
  with, goiter (diffuse)
Parson's (exophthalmic goiter) — *see* Hyperthyroidism,
  with, goiter (diffuse)
Paxton's (white piedra) B36.2
pearl-worker's — *see* Osteomyelitis, specified type NEC
Pellegrini-Stieda (calcification, knee joint) — *see* Bursitis, tibial collateral
pelvis, pelvic
  female NOS N94.9
    specified NEC N94.89
  gonococcal (acute) (chronic) A54.24
  inflammatory (female) N73.9
    acute N73.0
    chlamydial A56.11
    chronic N73.1
    specified NEC N73.8
    syphilitic (secondary) A51.42
      late A52.76
    tuberculous A18.17
  organ, female N94.9
  peritoneum, female NEC N94.89
penis N48.9
  inflammatory N48.29
    abscess N48.21
    cellulitis N48.22
  specified NEC N48.89
periapical tissues NOS K04.90
periodontal K05.6
  specified NEC K05.5
periosteum — *see* Disorder, bone, specified type NEC
peripheral
  arterial I73.9
  autonomic nervous system G90.9
  nerves — *see* Polyneuropathy
  vascular NOS I73.9
peritoneum K66.9
  pelvic, female NEC N94.89
  specified NEC K66.8
persistent mucosal (middle ear) H66.20
  left H66.22
    with right H66.23
  right H66.21

Disease, diseased — *continued*
  persistent mucosal — *continued*
    right — *continued*
      with left H66.23
  Petit's — *see* Hernia, abdomen, specified site NEC
  pharynx J39.2
    specified NEC J39.2
  Phocas' — *see* Mastopathy, cystic
  photochromogenic (acid-fast bacilli) (pulmonary) A31.0
    nonpulmonary A31.9
  Pick's G31.01 *[F02.80]*
    with behavioral disturbance G31.01 *[F02.81]*
      brain G31.01 *[F02.80]*
        with behavioral disturbance G31.01 *[F02.81]*
      of pericardium (pericardial pseudocirrhosis of liver)
        I31.1
  pigeon fancier's J67.2
  pineal gland E34.8
  pink — *see* Poisoning, mercury
  Pinkus' (lichen nitidus) L44.1
  pinworm B80
  Piry virus A93.8
  pituitary (gland) E23.7
  pituitary-snuff-taker's J67.8
  pleura (cavity) J94.9
    specified NEC J94.8
  pneumatic drill (hammer) T75.21 ☑
  Pollitzer's (hidradenitis suppurativa) L73.2
  polycystic
    kidney or renal Q61.3
      adult type Q61.2
      childhood type NEC Q61.19
        collecting duct dilatation Q61.11
    liver or hepatic Q44.6
    lung or pulmonary J98.4
      congenital Q33.0
    ovary, ovaries E28.2
    spleen Q89.09
  polyethylene T84.05- ☑
  Pompe's (glycogenosis II) E74.02
  Posadas-Wernicke B38.9
  Potain's (pulmonary edema) — *see* Edema, lung
  prepuce N47.8
    inflammatory N47.7
      balanoposthitis N47.6
  Pringle's (tuberous sclerosis) Q85.1
  prion, central nervous system A81.9
    specified NEC A81.89
  prostate N42.9
    specified NEC N42.89
  protozoal B64
    acanthamebiasis — *see* Acanthamebiasis
    African trypanosomiasis — *see* African trypanosomi-
      asis
    babesiosis — *see also* Babesiosis B60.00
    Chagas disease — *see* Chagas disease
    intestine, intestinal A07.9
    leishmaniasis — *see* Leishmaniasis
    malaria — *see* Malaria
    naegleriasis B60.2
    pneumocystosis B59
    specified organism NEC B60.8
    toxoplasmosis — *see* Toxoplasmosis
  pseudo-Hurler's E77.0
  psychiatric F99
  psychotic — *see* Psychosis
  Puente's (simple glandular cheilitis) K13.0
  puerperal — *see also* Puerperal O90.89
  pulmonary — *see also* Disease, lung
    artery I28.9
    chronic obstructive J44.9
      with
        acute bronchitis J44.0
        exacerbation (acute) J44.1
        lower respiratory infection (acute) J44.0
      decompensated J44.1
        with
          exacerbation (acute) J44.1
    heart I27.9
      specified NEC I27.89
    hypertensive (vascular) — *see also* Hypertension,
      pulmonary I27.20
      NEC I27.2 ☑
      primary (idiopathic) I27.0
    valve I37.9
      rheumatic I09.89
  pulp (dental) NOS K04.90
  pulseless M31.4

Disease, diseased — *continued*
  Putnam's (subacute combined sclerosis with pernicious
    anemia) D51.0
  Pyle (-Cohn) (metaphyseal dysplasia) Q78.5
  ragpicker's or ragsorter's A22.1
  Raynaud's — *see* Raynaud's disease
  reactive airway — *see* Asthma
  Reclus' (cystic) — *see* Mastopathy, cystic
  rectum K62.9
    specified NEC K62.89
  Refsum's (heredopathia atactica polyneuritiformis)
    G60.1
  renal (functional) (pelvis) — *see also* Disease, kidney
    N28.9
    with
      edema — *see* Nephrosis
      glomerular lesion — *see* Glomerulonephritis
        with edema — *see* Nephrosis
      interstitial nephritis N12
    acute N28.9
    chronic — *see also* Disease, kidney, chronic N18.9
    cystic, congenital Q61.9
    diabetic — *see* E08-E13 with .22
    end-stage (failure) N18.6
      due to hypertension I12.0
    fibrocystic (congenital) Q61.8
    hypertensive — *see* Hypertension, kidney
    lupus M32.14
    phosphate-losing (tubular) N25.0
    polycystic (congenital) Q61.3
      adult type Q61.2
      childhood type NEC Q61.19
        collecting duct dilatation Q61.11
    rapidly progressive N01.9
    subacute N01.9
  Rendu-Osler-Weber (familial hemorrhagic telangiecta-
    sia) I78.0
  renovascular (arteriosclerotic) — *see* Hypertension,
    kidney
  respiratory (tract) J98.9
    acute or subacute NOS J06.9
      due to
        chemicals, gases, fumes or vapors (inhalation)
          J68.3
        external agent J70.9
          specified NEC J70.8
        radiation J70.0
        smoke inhalation J70.5
      noninfectious J39.8
    chronic NOS J98.9
      due to
        chemicals, gases, fumes or vapors J68.4
        external agent J70.9
          specified NEC J70.8
        radiation J70.1
      newborn P27.9
        specified NEC P27.8
    due to
      chemicals, gases, fumes or vapors J68.9
        acute or subacute NEC J68.3
        chronic J68.4
      external agent J70.9
        specified NEC J70.8
    newborn P28.9
      specified type NEC P28.89
    upper J39.9
      acute or subacute J06.9
      noninfectious NEC J39.8
      specified NEC J39.8
      streptococcal J06.9
  retina, retinal H35.9
    Batten's or Batten-Mayou E75.4 *[H36]*
    specified NEC H35.89
  rheumatoid — *see* Arthritis, rheumatoid
  rickettsial NOS A79.9
    specified type NEC A79.89
  Riga (-Fede) (cachectic aphthae) K14.0
  Riggs' (compound periodontitis) — *see* Periodontitis
  Ritter's L00
  Rivalta's (cervicofacial actinomycosis) A42.2
  Robles' (onchocerciasis) B73.01
  rod body G71.21
  Roger's (congenital interventricular septal defect) Q21.0
  Rosenthal's (factor XI deficiency) D68.1
  Ross River B33.1
  Rossbach's (hyperchlorhydria) K31.89
    psychogenic F45.8
  Rotes Quérol — *see* Hyperostosis, ankylosing

Disease, diseased — *continued*
  Roth (-Bernhardt) — *see* Mononeuropathy, lower limb,
    meralgia paresthetica
  Runeberg's (progressive pernicious anemia) D51.0
  sacroiliac NEC M53.3
  salivary gland or duct K11.9
    inclusion B25.9
    specified NEC K11.8
    virus B25.9
  sandworm B76.9
  Schimmelbusch's — *see* Mastopathy, cystic
  Schmorl's — *see* Schmorl's disease or nodes
  Schönlein (-Henoch) (purpura rheumatica) D69.0
  Schottmüller's — *see* Fever, paratyphoid
  Schultz's (agranulocytosis) — *see* Agranulocytosis
  Schwalbe-Ziehen-Oppenheim G24.1
  Schwartz-Jampel G71.13
  sclera H15.9
    specified NEC H15.89
  scrofulous (tuberculous) A18.2
  scrotum N50.9
  sebaceous glands L73.9
  semilunar cartilage, cystic — *see also* Derangement,
    knee, meniscus, cystic
  seminal vesicle N50.9
  serum NEC — *see also* Reaction, serum T80.69 ☑
  sexually transmitted A64
    anogenital
      herpesviral infection — *see* Herpes, anogenital
      warts A63.0
    chancroid A57
    chlamydial infection — *see* Chlamydia
    gonorrhea — *see* Gonorrhea
    granuloma inguinale A58
    specified organism NEC A63.8
    syphilis — *see* Syphilis
    trichomoniasis — *see* Trichomoniasis
  Sézary C84.1- ☑
  shimamushi (scrub typhus) A75.3
  shipyard B30.0
  sickle-cell D57.1
    with
      acute chest syndrome D57.01
      cerebral vascular involvement D57.03
      crisis (painful) D57.00
        with complication specified NEC D57.09
      splenic sequestration D57.02
      vasoocclusive pain D57.00
    elliptocytosis D57.8- ☑
    Hb-C D57.20
      with
        acute chest syndrome D57.211
        cerebral vascular involvement D57.213
        crisis D57.219
          with specified complication NEC D57.218
        splenic sequestration D57.212
        vasoocclusive pain D57.219
      without crisis D57.20
    Hb-SD D57.80
      with
        acute chest syndrome D57.811
        cerebral vascular involvement D57.813
        crisis D57.819
          with complication specified NEC D57.818
        splenic sequestration D57.812
        vasoocclusive pain D57.819
      without crisis D57.80
    Hb-SE D57.80
      with
        acute chest syndrome D57.811
        cerebral vascular involvement D57.813
        crisis D57.819
          with complication specified NEC D57.818
        splenic sequestration D57.812
        vasoocclusive pain D57.819
      without crisis D57.80
    specified NEC D57.80
      with
        acute chest syndrome D57.811
        cerebral vascular involvement D57.813
        crisis D57.819
          with complication specified NEC D57.818
        splenic sequestration D57.812
        vasoocclusive pain D57.819
      without crisis D57.80
    spherocytosis D57.80
      with
        acute chest syndrome D57.811

Disease, diseased — *continued*
  sickle-cell — *continued*
    spherocytosis — *continued*
      with — *continued*
        cerebral vascular involvement D57.813
        crisis D57.819
          with complication specified NEC D57.818
        splenic sequestration D57.812
        vasoocclusive pain D57.819
      without crisis D57.80
    thalassemia D57.40
      with
        acute chest syndrome D57.411
        cerebral vascular involvement D57.413
        crisis (painful) D57.419
          with specified complication NEC D57.418
        splenic sequestration D57.412
        vasoocclusive pain D57.419
      beta plus D57.44
        with
          acute chest syndrome D57.451
          cerebral vascular involvement D57.453
          crisis D57.459
            with specified complication NEC D57.458
          splenic sequestration D57.452
          vasoocclusive pain D57.459
        without crisis D57.44
      beta zero D57.42
        with
          acute chest syndrome D57.431
          cerebral vascular involvement D57.433
          crisis D57.439
            with specified complication NEC D57.438
          splenic sequestration D57.432
          vasoocclusive pain D57.439
        without crisis D57.42
  silo-filler's J68.8
    bronchitis J68.0
    pneumonitis J68.0
    pulmonary edema J68.1
  simian B B00.4
  Simons' (progressive lipodystrophy) E88.1
  sin nombre virus B33.4
  sinus — *see* Sinusitis
  Sirkari's B55.0
  sixth B08.20
    due to human herpesvirus 6 B08.21
    due to human herpesvirus 7 B08.22
  skin L98.9
    due to metabolic disorder NEC E88.9 *[L99]*
    specified NEC L98.8
  slim (HIV) B20
  small vessel I73.9
  Sneddon-Wilkinson (subcorneal pustular dermatosis)
      L13.1
  South African creeping B88.0
  spinal (cord) G95.9
    congenital Q06.9
    specified NEC G95.89
  spine — *see also* Spondylopathy
    joint — *see* Dorsopathy
    tuberculous A18.01
  spinocerebellar (hereditary) G11.9
    specified NEC G11.8
  spleen D73.9
    amyloid E85.4 *[D77]*
    organic D73.9
    polycystic Q89.09
    postinfectional D73.89
  sponge-diver's — *see* Toxicity, venom, marine animal,
      sea anemone
  Startle Q89.8
  Steinert's G71.11
  Sticker's (erythema infectiosum) B08.3
  Stieda's (calcification, knee joint) — *see* Bursitis, tibial
      collateral
  Stokes' (exophthalmic goiter) — *see* Hyperthyroidism,
      with, goiter (diffuse)
  Stokes-Adams (syncope with heart block) I45.9
  stomach K31.9
    functional, psychogenic F45.8
    specified NEC K31.89
  stonemason's J62.8
  storage
    glycogen — *see* Disease, glycogen storage
    mucopolysaccharide — *see* Mucopolysaccharidosis

Disease, diseased — *continued*
  striatopallidal system NEC G25.89
  Stuart-Prower (congenital factor X deficiency) D68.2
  Stuart's (congenital factor X deficiency) D68.2
  subcutaneous tissue — *see* Disease, skin
  supporting structures of teeth K08.9
    specified NEC K08.89
  suprarenal (capsule) (gland) E27.9
    hyperfunction E27.0
    specified NEC E27.8
  sweat glands L74.9
    specified NEC L74.8
  Sweeley-Klionsky E75.21
  Swift (-Feer) — *see* Poisoning, mercury
  swimming-pool granuloma A31.1
  Sylvest's (epidemic pleurodynia) B33.0
  sympathetic nervous system G90.9
  synovium — *see* Disorder, synovium
  syphilitic — *see* Syphilis
  systemic tissue mast cell D47.02
  tanapox (virus) B08.71
  Tangier E78.6
  Tarral-Besnier (pityriasis rubra pilaris) L44.0
  Tauri's E74.09
  tear duct — *see* Disorder, lacrimal system
  tendon, tendinous — *see also* Disorder, tendon
    nodular — *see* Trigger finger
  terminal vessel I73.9
  testis N50.9
  thalassemia Hb-S — *see* Disease, sickle-cell, thalassemia
  Thaysen-Gee (nontropical sprue) K90.0
  Thomsen G71.12
  throat J39.2
    septic J02.0
  thromboembolic — *see* Embolism
  thymus (gland) E32.9
    specified NEC E32.8
  thyroid (gland) E07.9
    heart — *see also* Hyperthyroidism E05.90 *[I43]*
      with thyroid storm E05.91 *[I43]*
    specified NEC E07.89
  Tietze's M94.0
  tongue K14.9
    specified NEC K14.8
  tonsils, tonsillar (and adenoids) J35.9
  tooth, teeth K08.9
    hard tissues K03.9
      specified NEC K03.89
    pulp NEC K04.99
    specified NEC K08.89
  Tourette's F95.2
  trachea NEC J39.8
  tricuspid I07.9
    nonrheumatic I36.9
  triglyceride-storage E75.5
  trophoblastic — *see* Mole, hydatidiform
  tsutsugamushi A75.3
  tube (fallopian) (noninflammatory) N83.9
    inflammatory — *see* Salpingitis
    specified NEC N83.8
  tuberculous NEC — *see* Tuberculosis
  tubo-ovarian (noninflammatory) N83.9
    inflammatory — *see* Salpingo-oophoritis
    specified NEC N83.8
  tubotympanic, chronic — *see* Otitis, media, suppura-
      tive, chronic, tubotympanic
  tubulo-interstitial N15.9
    specified NEC N15.8
  tympanum — *see* Disorder, tympanic membrane
  Uhl's Q24.8
  Underwood's (sclerema neonatorum) P83.0
  Unverricht (-Lundborg) — *see* Epilepsy, generalized,
      idiopathic
  Urbach-Oppenheim (necrobiosis lipoidica diabetico-
      rum) — *see* E08-E13 with .620
  ureter N28.9
    in (due to)
      schistosomiasis (bilharziasis) B65.0 *[N29]*
  urethra N36.9
    specified NEC N36.8
  urinary (tract) N39.9
    bladder N32.9
      specified NEC N32.89
    specified NEC N39.8
  uterus (noninflammatory) N85.9
    infective — *see* Endometritis
    inflammatory — *see* Endometritis
    specified NEC N85.8

Disease, diseased — *continued*
  uveal tract (anterior) H21.9
    posterior H31.9
  vagabond's B85.1
  vagina, vaginal (noninflammatory) N89.9
    inflammatory NEC N76.89
    specified NEC N89.8
  valve, valvular I38
    multiple I08.9
      specified NEC I08.8
  van Creveld-von Gierke (glycogenosis I) E74.01
  vas deferens N50.9
  vascular I99.9
    arteriosclerotic — *see* Arteriosclerosis
    ciliary body NEC — *see* Disorder, iris, vascular
    hypertensive — *see* Hypertension
    iris NEC — *see* Disorder, iris, vascular
    obliterative I77.1
      peripheral I73.9
    occlusive I99.8
    peripheral (occlusive) I73.9
      in diabetes mellitus — *see* E08-E13 with .51
  vasomotor I73.9
  vasospastic I73.9
  vein I87.9
  venereal — *see also* Disease, sexually transmitted A64
    chlamydial NEC A56.8
      anus A56.3
      genitourinary NOS A56.2
      pharynx A56.4
      rectum A56.3
    fifth A55
    sixth A55
    specified nature or type NEC A63.8
  vertebra, vertebral — *see also* Spondylopathy
    disc — *see* Disorder, disc
  vibration — *see* Vibration, adverse effects
  viral, virus — *see also* Disease, by type of virus B34.9
    arbovirus NOS A94
    arthropod-borne NOS A94
    congenital P35.9
      specified NEC P35.8
    Hanta (with renal manifestations) (Dobrava) (Pu-
        umala) (Seoul) A98.5
      with pulmonary manifestations (Andes) (Bayou)
          (Bermejo) (Black Creek Canal) (Choclo)
          (Juquitiba) (Laguna negra) (Lechiguanas)
          (New York) (Oran) (Sin nombre) B33.4
    Hantaan (Korean hemorrhagic fever) A98.5
    human immunodeficiency (HIV) B20
    Kunjin A83.4
    nonarthropod-borne NOS B34.9
    Powassan A84.81
    Rocio (encephalitis) A83.6
    Sin nombre (Hantavirus) (cardio)-pulmonary syn-
        drome) B33.4
    Tahyna B33.8
    vesicular stomatitis A93.8
  vitreous H43.9
    specified NEC H43.89
  vocal cord J38.3
  Volkmann's, acquired T79.6 ☑
  von Eulenburg's (congenital paramyotonia) G71.19
  von Gierke's (glycogenosis I) E74.01
  von Graefe's — *see* Strabismus, paralytic, ophthalmo-
      plegia, progressive
  von Willebrand (-Jürgens) (angiohemophilia) D68.0
  Vrolik's (osteogenesis imperfecta) Q78.0
  vulva (noninflammatory) N90.9
    inflammatory NEC N76.89
    specified NEC N90.89
  Wallgren's (obstruction of splenic vein with collateral
      circulation) I87.8
  Wassilieff's (leptospiral jaundice) A27.0
  wasting NEC R64
    due to malnutrition E41
  Waterhouse-Friderichsen A39.1
  Wegner's (syphilitic osteochondritis) A50.02
  Weil's (leptospiral jaundice of lung) A27.0
  Weir Mitchell's (erythromelalgia) I73.81
  Werdnig-Hoffmann G12.0
  Wermer's E31.21
  Werner-His (trench fever) A79.0
  Werner-Schultz (neutropenic splenomegaly) D73.81
  Wernicke-Posadas B38.9
  whipworm B79
  white blood cells D72.9
    specified NEC D72.89

Index

Disease, diseased — *continued*
  white matter R90.82
  white-spot, meaning lichen sclerosus et atrophicus
      L90.0
    penis N48.0
    vulva N90.4
  Wilkie's K55.1
  Wilkinson-Sneddon (subcorneal pustular dermatosis)
      L13.1
  Willis' — *see* Diabetes
  Wilson's (hepatolenticular degeneration) E83.01
  woolsorter's A22.1
  yaba monkey tumor B08.72
  yaba pox (virus) B08.72
  Zika virus A92.5
    congenital P35.4
  zoonotic, bacterial A28.9
    specified type NEC A28.8
Disfigurement (due to scar) L90.5
Disgerminoma — *see* Dysgerminoma
DISH (diffuse idiopathic skeletal hyperostosis) — *see* Hyperostosis, ankylosing
Disinsertion, retina — *see* Detachment, retina
Dislocatable hip, congenital Q65.6
Dislocation (articular)
  with fracture — *see* Fracture
  acromioclavicular (joint) S43.10- ☑
    with displacement
      100%-200% S43.12- ☑
      more than 200% S43.13- ☑
    inferior S43.14- ☑
    posterior S43.15- ☑
  ankle S93.0- ☑
  astragalus — *see* Dislocation, ankle
  atlantoaxial S13.121 ☑
  atlantooccipital S13.111 ☑
  atloidooccipital S13.111 ☑
  breast bone S23.29 ☑
  capsule, joint — *code by* site under Dislocation
  carpal (bone) — *see* Dislocation, wrist
  carpometacarpal (joint) NEC S63.05- ☑
    thumb S63.04- ☑
  cartilage (joint) — *code by* site under Dislocation
  cervical spine (vertebra) — *see* Dislocation, vertebra, cervical
  chronic — *see* Dislocation, recurrent
  clavicle — *see* Dislocation, acromioclavicular joint
  coccyx S33.2 ☑
  congenital NEC Q68.8
  coracoid — *see* Dislocation, shoulder
  costal cartilage S23.29 ☑
  costochondral S23.29 ☑
  cricoarytenoid articulation S13.29 ☑
  cricothyroid articulation S13.29 ☑
  dorsal vertebra — *see* Dislocation, vertebra, thoracic
  ear ossicle — *see* Discontinuity, ossicles, ear
  elbow S53.10- ☑
    congenital Q68.8
    pathological — *see* Dislocation, pathological NEC, elbow
    radial head alone — *see* Dislocation, radial head
    recurrent — *see* Dislocation, recurrent, elbow
    traumatic S53.10- ☑
      anterior S53.11- ☑
      lateral S53.14- ☑
      medial S53.13- ☑
      posterior S53.12- ☑
      specified type NEC S53.19- ☑
  eye, nontraumatic — *see* Luxation, globe
  eyeball, nontraumatic — *see* Luxation, globe
  femur
    distal end — *see* Dislocation, knee
    proximal end — *see* Dislocation, hip
  fibula
    distal end — *see* Dislocation, ankle
    proximal end — *see* Dislocation, knee
  finger S63.25- ☑
    index S63.25- ☑
    interphalangeal S63.27- ☑
      distal S63.29- ☑
        index S63.29- ☑
        little S63.29- ☑
        middle S63.29- ☑
        ring S63.29- ☑
      index S63.27- ☑
      little S63.27- ☑
      middle S63.27- ☑

Dislocation — *continued*
  finger — *continued*
    interphalangeal — *continued*
      proximal S63.28- ☑
        index S63.28- ☑
        little S63.28- ☑
        middle S63.28- ☑
        ring S63.28- ☑
      ring S63.27- ☑
    little S63.25- ☑
    metacarpophalangeal S63.26- ☑
      index S63.26- ☑
      little S63.26- ☑
      middle S63.26- ☑
      ring S63.26- ☑
    middle S63.25- ☑
    recurrent — *see* Dislocation, recurrent, finger
    ring S63.25- ☑
    thumb — *see* Dislocation, thumb
  foot S93.30- ☑
    recurrent — *see* Dislocation, recurrent, foot
    specified site NEC S93.33- ☑
    tarsal joint S93.31- ☑
    tarsometatarsal joint S93.32- ☑
    toe — *see* Dislocation, toe
  fracture — *see* Fracture
  glenohumeral (joint) — *see* Dislocation, shoulder
  glenoid — *see* Dislocation, shoulder
  habitual — *see* Dislocation, recurrent
  hip S73.00- ☑
    anterior S73.03- ☑
      obturator S73.02- ☑
    central S73.04- ☑
    congenital (total) Q65.2
      bilateral Q65.1
      partial Q65.5
        bilateral Q65.4
        unilateral Q65.3-
      unilateral Q65.0- ☑
    developmental M24.85- ☑
    pathological — *see* Dislocation, pathological NEC, hip
    posterior S73.01- ☑
    recurrent — *see* Dislocation, recurrent, hip
  humerus, proximal end — *see* Dislocation, shoulder
  incomplete — *see* Subluxation, by site
  incus — *see* Discontinuity, ossicles, ear
  infracoracoid — *see* Dislocation, shoulder
  innominate (pubic junction) (sacral junction) S33.39 ☑
    acetabulum — *see* Dislocation, hip
  interphalangeal (joint(s))
    finger S63.279 ☑
      distal S63.29- ☑
        index S63.29- ☑
        little S63.29- ☑
        middle S63.29- ☑
        ring S63.29- ☑
      index S63.27- ☑
      little S63.27- ☑
      middle S63.27- ☑
      proximal S63.28- ☑
        index S63.28- ☑
        little S63.28- ☑
        middle S63.28- ☑
        ring S63.28- ☑
      ring S63.27- ☑
    foot or toe — *see* Dislocation, toe
    thumb S63.12- ☑
  jaw (cartilage) (meniscus) S03.0- ☑
  joint prosthesis — *see* Complications, joint prosthesis, mechanical, displacement, by site
  knee S83.106 ☑
    cap — *see* Dislocation, patella
    congenital Q68.2
    old M23.8X- ☑
    patella — *see* Dislocation, patella
    pathological — *see* Dislocation, pathological NEC, knee
    proximal tibia
      anteriorly S83.11- ☑
      laterally S83.14- ☑
      medially S83.13- ☑
      posteriorly S83.12- ☑
    recurrent — *see also* Derangement, knee, specified NEC
    specified type NEC S83.19- ☑

Dislocation — *continued*
  lacrimal gland H04.16- ☑
  lens (complete) H27.10
    anterior H27.12- ☑
    congenital Q12.1
    ocular implant — *see* Complications, intraocular lens
    partial H27.11- ☑
    posterior H27.13- ☑
    traumatic S05.8X- ☑
  ligament — *code by* site under Dislocation
  lumbar (vertebra) — *see* Dislocation, vertebra, lumbar
  lumbosacral (vertebra) — *see also* Dislocation, vertebra, lumbar
    congenital Q76.49
  mandible S03.0- ☑
  meniscus (knee) — *see* Tear, meniscus
    other sites - code by site under Dislocation
  metacarpal (bone)
    distal end — *see* Dislocation, finger
    proximal end S63.06- ☑
  metacarpophalangeal (joint)
    finger S63.26- ☑
      index S63.26- ☑
      little S63.26- ☑
      middle S63.26- ☑
      ring S63.26- ☑
    thumb S63.11- ☑
  metatarsal (bone) — *see* Dislocation, foot
  metatarsophalangeal (joint(s)) — *see* Dislocation, toe
  midcarpal (joint) S63.03- ☑
  midtarsal (joint) — *see* Dislocation, foot
  neck S13.20 ☑
    specified site NEC S13.29 ☑
    vertebra — *see* Dislocation, vertebra, cervical
  nose (septal cartilage) S03.1 ☑
  occipitoatloid S13.111 ☑
  old — *see* Derangement, joint, specified type NEC
  ossicles, ear — *see* Discontinuity, ossicles, ear
  partial — *see* Subluxation, by site
  patella S83.006 ☑
    congenital Q74.1
    lateral S83.01- ☑
    recurrent (nontraumatic) M22.0- ☑
      incomplete M22.1- ☑
    specified type NEC S83.09- ☑
  pathological NEC M24.30
    ankle M24.37- ☑
    elbow M24.32- ☑
    foot joint M24.37- ☑
    hand joint M24.34- ☑
    hip M24.35- ☑
    knee M24.36- ☑
    lumbosacral joint — *see* subcategory M53.2 ☑
    pelvic region — *see* Dislocation, pathological, hip
    sacroiliac — *see* subcategory M53.2 ☑
    shoulder M24.31- ☑
    specified site NEC M24.39
    wrist M24.33- ☑
  pelvis NEC S33.30 ☑
    specified NEC S33.39 ☑
  phalanx
    finger or hand — *see* Dislocation, finger
    foot or toe — *see* Dislocation, toe
  prosthesis, internal — *see* Complications, prosthetic device, by site, mechanical
  radial head S53.006 ☑
    anterior S53.01- ☑
    posterior S53.02- ☑
    specified type NEC S53.09- ☑
  radiocarpal (joint) S63.02- ☑
  radiohumeral (joint) — *see* Dislocation, radial head
  radioulnar (joint)
    distal S63.01- ☑
    proximal — *see* Dislocation, elbow
  radius
    distal end — *see* Dislocation, wrist
    proximal end — *see* Dislocation, radial head
  recurrent M24.40
    ankle M24.47- ☑
    elbow M24.42- ☑
    finger M24.44- ☑
    foot joint M24.47- ☑
    hand joint M24.44- ☑
    hip M24.45- ☑
    knee M24.46- ☑

Disease, diseased — Dislocation

Dislocation — *continued*
  recurrent — *continued*
    knee — *continued*
      patella — *see* Dislocation, patella, recurrent
    patella — *see* Dislocation, patella, recurrent
    sacroiliac — *see* subcategory M53.2 ☑
    shoulder M24.41- ☑
    specified site NEC M24.49
    toe M24.47- ☑
    vertebra — *see also* subcategory M43.5 ☑
      atlantoaxial M43.4
        with myelopathy M43.3
    wrist M24.43- ☑
  rib (cartilage) S23.29 ☑
  sacrococcygeal S33.2 ☑
  sacroiliac (joint) (ligament) S33.2 ☑
    congenital Q74.2
    recurrent — *see* subcategory M53.2 ☑
  sacrum S33.2 ☑
  scaphoid (bone) (hand) (wrist) — *see* Dislocation, wrist
    foot — *see* Dislocation, foot
  scapula — *see* Dislocation, shoulder, girdle, scapula
  semilunar cartilage, knee — *see* Tear, meniscus
  septal cartilage (nose) S03.1 ☑
  septum (nasal) (old) J34.2
  sesamoid bone — *code by* site under Dislocation
  shoulder (blade) (ligament) (joint) (traumatic)
    S43.006 ☑
    acromioclavicular — *see* Dislocation, acromioclavic-
      ular
    chronic — *see* Dislocation, recurrent, shoulder
    congenital Q68.8
    girdle S43.30- ☑
      scapula S43.31- ☑
      specified site NEC S43.39- ☑
    humerus S43.00- ☑
      anterior S43.01- ☑
      inferior S43.03- ☑
      posterior S43.02- ☑
    pathological — *see* Dislocation, pathological NEC,
      shoulder
    recurrent — *see* Dislocation, recurrent, shoulder
    specified type NEC S43.08- ☑
  spine
    cervical — *see* Dislocation, vertebra, cervical
    congenital Q76.49
    due to birth trauma P11.5
    lumbar — *see* Dislocation, vertebra, lumbar
    thoracic — *see* Dislocation, vertebra, thoracic
  spontaneous — *see* Dislocation, pathological
  sternoclavicular (joint) S43.206 ☑
    anterior S43.21- ☑
    posterior S43.22- ☑
  sternum S23.29 ☑
  subglenoid — *see* Dislocation, shoulder
  symphysis pubis S33.4 ☑
  talus — *see* Dislocation, ankle
  tarsal (bone(s)) (joint(s)) — *see* Dislocation, foot
  tarsometatarsal (joint(s)) — *see* Dislocation, foot
  temporomandibular (joint) S03.0- ☑
  thigh, proximal end — *see* Dislocation, hip
  thorax S23.20 ☑
    specified site NEC S23.29 ☑
    vertebra — *see* Dislocation, vertebra
  thumb S63.10- ☑
    interphalangeal joint — *see* Dislocation, interpha-
      langeal (joint), thumb
    metacarpophalangeal joint — *see* Dislocation,
      metacarpophalangeal (joint), thumb
  thyroid cartilage S13.29 ☑
  tibia
    distal end — *see* Dislocation, ankle
    proximal end — *see* Dislocation, knee
  tibiofibular (joint)
    distal — *see* Dislocation, ankle
    superior — *see* Dislocation, knee
  toe(s) S93.106 ☑
    great S93.10- ☑
      interphalangeal joint S93.11- ☑
      metatarsophalangeal joint S93.12- ☑
    interphalangeal joint S93.119 ☑
    lesser S93.106 ☑
      interphalangeal joint S93.11- ☑
      metatarsophalangeal joint S93.12- ☑
    metatarsophalangeal joint S93.12- ☑
  tooth S03.2 ☑

Dislocation — *continued*
  trachea S23.29 ☑
  ulna
    distal end S63.07- ☑
    proximal end — *see* Dislocation, elbow
  ulnohumeral (joint) — *see* Dislocation, elbow
  vertebra (articular process) (body) (traumatic)
    cervical S13.101 ☑
      atlantoaxial joint S13.121 ☑
      atlantooccipital joint S13.111 ☑
      atloidooccipital joint S13.111 ☑
      joint between
        C0 and C1 S13.111 ☑
        C1 and C2 S13.121 ☑
        C2 and C3 S13.131 ☑
        C3 and C4 S13.141 ☑
        C4 and C5 S13.151 ☑
        C5 and C6 S13.161 ☑
        C6 and C7 S13.171 ☑
        C7 and T1 S13.181 ☑
      occipitoatloid joint S13.111 ☑
    congenital Q76.49
    lumbar S33.101 ☑
      joint between
        L1 and L2 S33.111 ☑
        L2 and L3 S33.121 ☑
        L3 and L4 S33.131 ☑
        L4 and L5 S33.141 ☑
    nontraumatic — *see* Displacement, intervertebral
      disc
    partial — *see* Subluxation, by site
    recurrent NEC — *see* subcategory M43.5 ☑
    thoracic S23.101 ☑
      joint between
        T1 and T2 S23.111 ☑
        T2 and T3 S23.121 ☑
        T3 and T4 S23.123 ☑
        T4 and T5 S23.131 ☑
        T5 and T6 S23.133 ☑
        T6 and T7 S23.141 ☑
        T7 and T8 S23.143 ☑
        T8 and T9 S23.151 ☑
        T9 and T10 S23.153 ☑
        T10 and T11 S23.161 ☑
        T11 and T12 S23.163 ☑
        T12 and L1 S23.171 ☑
  wrist (carpal bone) S63.006 ☑
    carpometacarpal joint — *see* Dislocation, car-
      pometacarpal (joint)
    distal radioulnar joint — *see* Dislocation, radioulnar
      (joint), distal
    metacarpal bone, proximal — *see* Dislocation,
      metacarpal (bone), proximal end
    midcarpal — *see* Dislocation, midcarpal (joint)
    radiocarpal joint — *see* Dislocation, radiocarpal
      (joint)
    recurrent — *see* Dislocation, recurrent, wrist
    specified site NEC S63.09- ☑
    ulna — *see* Dislocation, ulna, distal end
  xiphoid cartilage S23.29 ☑
Disorder (of) — *see also* Disease
  acantholytic L11.9
    specified NEC L11.8
  acute
    psychotic — *see* Psychosis, acute
    stress F43.0
  adjustment (grief) F43.20
    with
      anxiety F43.22
        with depressed mood F43.23
      conduct disturbance F43.24
        with emotional disturbance F43.25
      depressed mood F43.21
        with anxiety F43.23
      other specified symptom F43.29
  adrenal (capsule) (gland) (medullary) E27.9
    specified NEC E27.8
  adrenogenital E25.9
    drug-induced E25.8
    iatrogenic E25.8
    idiopathic E25.8
  adult personality (and behavior) F69
    specified NEC F68.8
  affective (mood) — *see* Disorder, mood
  aggressive, unsocialized F91.1
  alcohol use
    mild F10.10

Disorder — *continued*
  alcohol use — *continued*
    mild — *continued*
      with
        alcohol intoxication F10.129
          delirium F10.121
        alcohol-induced
          anxiety disorder F10.180
          bipolar and related disorder F10.14
          depressive disorder F10.14
          psychotic disorder F10.159
          sexual dysfunction F10.181
          sleep disorder F10.182
      in remission (early) (sustained) F10.11
    moderate or severe F10.20
      with
        alcohol intoxication F10.229
          delirium F10.221
        alcohol-induced
          anxiety disorder F10.280
          bipolar and related disorder F10.24
          depressive disorder F10.24
          major neurocognitive disorder, amnestic-
            confabulatory type F10.26
          major neurocognitive disorder, non-
            amnestic-confabulatory type
            F10.27
          mild neurocognitive disorder F10.288
          psychotic disorder F10.259
          sexual dysfunction F10.281
          sleep disorder F10.282
      in remission (early) (sustained) F10.21
  alcohol-related F10.99
    with
      amnestic disorder, persisting F10.96
      anxiety disorder F10.980
      dementia, persisting F10.97
      intoxication F10.929
        with delirium F10.921
        uncomplicated F10.920
      mood disorder F10.94
      other specified F10.988
      psychotic disorder F10.959
        with
          delusions F10.950
          hallucinations F10.951
      sexual dysfunction F10.981
      sleep disorder F10.982
  allergic — *see* Allergy
  alveolar NEC J84.09
  amino-acid
    cystathioninuria E72.19
    cystinosis E72.04
    cystinuria E72.01
    glycinuria E72.09
    homocystinuria E72.11
    metabolism — *see* Disturbance, metabolism, amino-
      acid
    specified NEC E72.89
    neonatal, transitory P74.8
    renal transport NEC E72.09
    transport NEC E72.09
  amnesic, amnestic
    alcohol-induced F10.96
      with dependence F10.26
    due to (secondary to) general medical condition F04
    psychoactive NEC-induced F19.96
      with
        abuse F19.16
        dependence F19.26
    sedative, hypnotic or anxiolytic-induced F13.96
      with dependence F13.26
  amphetamine (or other stimulant) use
    mild
      with
        amphetamine, cocaine, or other stimulant
          intoxication
          with perceptual disturbances F15.122
          without perceptual disturbances F15.129
        amphetamine (or other stimulant) -induced
          anxiety disorder F15.180
          bipolar and related disorder F15.14
          depressive disorder F15.14
          obsessive-compulsive and related disor-
            der F15.188
          psychotic disorder F15.159
          sexual dysfunction F15.181
        intoxication delirium F15.121

Disorder — continued
- amphetamine use — continued
  - moderate or severe
    - with
      - amphetamine, cocaine, or other stimulant intoxication
        - with perceptual disturbances F15.222
        - without perceptual disturbances F15.229
      - amphetamine (or other stimulant) -induced
        - anxiety disorder F15.280
        - bipolar and related disorder F15.24
        - depressive disorder F15.24
        - obsessive-compulsive and related disorder F15.288
        - psychotic disorder F15.259
        - sexual dysfunction F15.281
      - intoxication delirium F15.221
- amphetamine-type substance use
  - mild F15.10
    - in remission (early) (sustained) F15.11
  - moderate F15.20
    - in remission (early) (sustained) F15.21
  - severe F15.20
    - in remission (early) (sustained) F15.21
- anaerobic glycolysis with anemia D55.2
- anxiety F41.9
  - due to (secondary to)
    - alcohol F10.980
      - in
        - abuse F10.180
        - dependence F10.280
    - amphetamine F15.980
      - in
        - abuse F15.180
        - dependence F15.280
    - anxiolytic F13.980
      - in
        - abuse F13.180
        - dependence F13.280
    - caffeine F15.980
      - in
        - abuse F15.180
        - dependence F15.280
    - cannabis F12.980
      - in
        - abuse F12.180
        - dependence F12.280
    - cocaine F14.980
      - in
        - abuse F14.180
        - dependence F14.180
    - general medical condition F06.4
    - hallucinogen F16.980
      - in
        - abuse F16.180
        - dependence F16.280
    - hypnotic F13.980
      - in
        - abuse F13.180
        - dependence F13.280
    - inhalant F18.980
      - in
        - abuse F18.180
        - dependence F18.280
    - phencyclidine F16.980
      - in
        - abuse F16.180
        - dependence F16.280
    - psychoactive substance NEC F19.980
      - in
        - abuse F19.180
        - dependence F19.280
    - sedative F13.980
      - in
        - abuse F13.180
        - dependence F13.280
    - volatile solvents F18.980
      - in
        - abuse F18.180
        - dependence F18.280
  - generalized F41.1
  - illness F45.21
  - mixed
    - with depression (mild) F41.8
    - specified NEC F41.3
  - organic F06.4
  - phobic F40.9
    - of childhood F40.8
  - specified NEC F41.8

Disorder — continued
- aortic valve — see Endocarditis, aortic
- aromatic amino-acid metabolism E70.9
  - specified NEC E70.89
- arteriole NEC I77.89
- artery NEC I77.89
- articulation — see Disorder, joint
- attachment (childhood)
  - disinhibited F94.2
  - reactive F94.1
- attention-deficit hyperactivity (adolescent) (adult) (child) F90.9
  - combined
    - presentation F90.2
    - type F90.2
  - hyperactive
    - impulsive presentation F90.1
    - type F90.1
  - inattentive
    - presentation F90.0
    - type F90.0
  - specified type NEC F90.8
- attention-deficit without hyperactivity (adolescent) (adult) (child) F98.8
- auditory processing (central) H93.25
- autism spectrum F84.0
- autistic F84.0
- autoimmune D89.89
- autonomic nervous system G90.9
  - specified NEC G90.8
- avoidant
  - child or adolescent F40.10
  - restrictive food intake F50.82
- balance
  - acid-base E87.8
    - mixed E87.4
  - electrolyte E87.8
  - fluid NEC E87.8
- behavioral (disruptive) — see Disorder, conduct
- beta-amino-acid metabolism E72.89
- bile acid and cholesterol metabolism E78.70
  - Barth syndrome E78.71
  - other specified E78.79
  - Smith-Lemli-Opitz syndrome E78.72
- bilirubin excretion E80.6
- binge eating F50.81
- binocular
  - movement H51.9
    - convergence
      - excess H51.12
      - insufficiency H51.11
    - internuclear ophthalmoplegia — see Ophthalmoplegia, internuclear
    - palsy of conjugate gaze H51.0
    - specified type NEC H51.8
  - vision NEC — see Disorder, vision, binocular
- bipolar (I) (type I) F31.9
  - and related due to a known physiological condition
    - with
      - manic features F06.33
      - manic- or hypomanic-like episodes F06.33
      - mixed features F06.34
  - current (or most recent) episode
    - depressed F31.9
      - with psychotic features F31.5
      - without psychotic features F31.30
        - mild F31.31
        - moderate F31.32
        - severe (without psychotic features) F31.4
          - with psychotic features F31.5
    - hypomanic F31.0
    - manic F31.9
      - with psychotic features F31.2
      - without psychotic features F31.10
        - mild F31.11
        - moderate F31.12
        - severe (without psychotic features) F31.13
          - with psychotic features F31.2
    - mixed F31.60
      - mild F31.61
      - moderate F31.62
      - severe (without psychotic features) F31.63
        - with psychotic features F31.64
    - severe depression (without psychotic features) F31.4
      - with psychotic features F31.5
  - in remission (currently) F31.70

Disorder — continued
- bipolar — continued
  - in remission — continued
    - in full remission
      - most recent episode
        - depressed F31.76
        - hypomanic F31.72
        - manic F31.74
        - mixed F31.78
    - in partial remission
      - most recent episode
        - depressed F31.75
        - hypomanic F31.71
        - manic F31.73
        - mixed F31.77
  - organic F06.30
  - single manic episode F30.9
    - mild F30.11
    - moderate F30.12
    - severe (without psychotic symptoms) F30.13
      - with psychotic symptoms F30.2
  - specified NEC F31.89
- bipolar II (type 2) F31.81
- bladder N32.9
  - functional NEC N31.9
  - in schistosomiasis B65.0 [N33]
  - specified NEC N32.89
- bleeding D68.9
- blood D75.9
  - in congenital early syphilis A50.09 [D77]
- body dysmorphic F45.22
- bone M89.9
  - continuity M84.9
    - specified type NEC M84.80
      - ankle M84.87- ☑
      - fibula M84.86- ☑
      - foot M84.87- ☑
      - hand M84.84- ☑
      - humerus M84.82- ☑
      - neck M84.88
      - pelvis M84.859
      - radius M84.83- ☑
      - rib M84.88
      - shoulder M84.81- ☑
      - skull M84.88
      - thigh M84.85- ☑
      - tibia M84.86- ☑
      - ulna M84.83- ☑
      - vertebra M84.88
  - density and structure M85.9
    - cyst — see also Cyst, bone, specified type NEC
      - aneurysmal — see Cyst, bone, aneurysmal
      - solitary — see Cyst, bone, solitary
    - diffuse idiopathic skeletal hyperostosis — see Hyperostosis, ankylosing
    - fibrous dysplasia (monostotic) — see Dysplasia, fibrous, bone
    - fluorosis — see Fluorosis, skeletal
    - hyperostosis of skull M85.2
    - osteitis condensans — see Osteitis, condensans
    - specified type NEC M85.8- ☑
      - ankle M85.87- ☑
      - foot M85.87- ☑
      - forearm M85.83- ☑
      - hand M85.84- ☑
      - lower leg M85.86- ☑
      - multiple sites M85.89
      - neck M85.88
      - rib M85.88
      - shoulder M85.81- ☑
      - skull M85.88
      - thigh M85.85- ☑
      - upper arm M85.82- ☑
      - vertebra M85.88
  - development and growth NEC M89.20
    - carpus M89.24- ☑
    - clavicle M89.21- ☑
    - femur M89.25- ☑
    - fibula M89.26- ☑
    - finger M89.24- ☑
    - humerus M89.22- ☑
    - ilium M89.259
    - ischium M89.259
    - metacarpus M89.24- ☑
    - metatarsus M89.27- ☑
    - multiple sites M89.29
    - neck M89.28

☑ **Additional Character Required** — Refer to the Tabular List for Character Selection   ▽ **Subterms under main terms may continue to next column or page**

Disorder — *continued*
　bone — *continued*
　　development and growth — *continued*
　　　radius M89.23- ☑
　　　rib M89.28
　　　scapula M89.21- ☑
　　　skull M89.28
　　　tarsus M89.27- ☑
　　　tibia M89.26- ☑
　　　toe M89.27- ☑
　　　ulna M89.23- ☑
　　　vertebra M89.28
　　　specified type NEC M89.8X- ☑
　brachial plexus G54.0
　branched-chain amino-acid metabolism E71.2
　　specified NEC E71.19
　breast N64.9
　　agalactia — *see* Agalactia
　　associated with
　　　lactation O92.70
　　　　specified NEC O92.79
　　　pregnancy O92.20
　　　　specified NEC O92.29
　　　puerperium O92.20
　　　　specified NEC O92.29
　　cracked nipple — *see* Cracked nipple
　　galactorrhea — *see* Galactorrhea
　　hypogalactia O92.4
　　lactation disorder NEC O92.79
　　mastitis — *see* Mastitis
　　nipple infection — *see* Infection, nipple
　　retracted nipple — *see* Retraction, nipple
　　specified type NEC N64.89
　Briquet's F45.0
　bullous, in diseases classified elsewhere L14
　caffeine use
　　mild
　　　with
　　　　caffeine-induced
　　　　　anxiety disorder F15.180
　　　　　sleep disorder F15.182
　　moderate or severe
　　　with
　　　　caffeine-induced
　　　　　anxiety disorder F15.280
　　　　　sleep disorder F15.282
　cannabis use
　　mild F12.10
　　　with
　　　　cannabis intoxication delirium F12.121
　　　　　with perceptual disturbances F12.122
　　　　　without perceptual disturbances F12.129
　　　　cannabis-induced
　　　　　anxiety disorder F12.180
　　　　　psychotic disorder F12.159
　　　　　sleep disorder F12.188
　　　　in remission (early) (sustained) F12.11
　　moderate or severe F12.20
　　　with
　　　　cannabis intoxication
　　　　　with perceptual disturbances F12.222
　　　　　without perceptual disturbances F12.229
　　　　cannabis-induced
　　　　　anxiety disorder F12.280
　　　　　psychotic disorder F12.259
　　　　　sleep disorder F12.288
　　　　delirium F12.221
　　　　in remission (early) (sustained) F12.21
　carbohydrate
　　absorption, intestinal NEC E74.39
　　metabolism (congenital) E74.9
　　　specified NEC E74.89
　cardiac, functional I51.89
　carnitine metabolism E71.40
　cartilage M94.9
　　articular NEC — *see* Derangement, joint, articular
　　　cartilage
　　chondrocalcinosis — *see* Chondrocalcinosis
　　specified type NEC M94.8X- ☑
　　　articular — *see* Derangement, joint, articular
　　　cartilage
　　　multiple sites M94.8X0
　catatonia (due to known physiological condition) (with
　　another mental disorder) F06.1
　catatonic
　　due to (secondary to) known physiological condition
　　　F06.1
　　organic F06.1

Disorder — *continued*
　central auditory processing H93.25
　cervical
　　region NEC M53.82
　　root (nerve) NEC G54.2
　character NOS F60.9
　childhood disintegrative NEC F84.3
　cholesterol and bile acid metabolism E78.70
　　Barth syndrome E78.71
　　other specified E78.79
　　Smith-Lemli-Opitz syndrome E78.72
　choroid H31.9
　　atrophy — *see* Atrophy, choroid
　　degeneration — *see* Degeneration, choroid
　　detachment — *see* Detachment, choroid
　　dystrophy — *see* Dystrophy, choroid
　　hemorrhage — *see* Hemorrhage, choroid
　　rupture — *see* Rupture, choroid
　　scar — *see* Scar, chorioretinal
　　solar retinopathy — *see* Retinopathy, solar
　　specified type NEC H31.8
　ciliary body — *see* Disorder, iris
　　degeneration — *see* Degeneration, ciliary body
　coagulation (factor) — *see also* Defect, coagulation
　　D68.9
　　newborn, transient P61.6
　cocaine use
　　mild F14.10
　　　with
　　　　amphetamine, cocaine, or other stimulant
　　　　　intoxication
　　　　　　with perceptual disturbances F14.122
　　　　　　without perceptual disturbances F14.129
　　　　cocaine intoxication delirium F14.121
　　　　cocaine-induced
　　　　　anxiety disorder F14.180
　　　　　bipolar and related disorder F14.14
　　　　　depressive disorder F14.14
　　　　　obsessive-compulsive and related disor-
　　　　　　der F14.188
　　　　　psychotic disorder F14.159
　　　　　sexual dysfunction F14.181
　　　　　sleep disorder F14.182
　　　　in remission (early) (sustained) F14.11
　　moderate or severe F14.20
　　　with
　　　　amphetamine, cocaine, or other stimulant
　　　　　intoxication
　　　　　　with perceptual disturbances F14.222
　　　　　　without perceptual disturbances F14.229
　　　　cocaine intoxication delirium F14.221
　　　　cocaine-induced
　　　　　anxiety disorder F14.280
　　　　　bipolar and related disorder F14.24
　　　　　depressive disorder F14.24
　　　　　obsessive-compulsive and related disor-
　　　　　　der F14.288
　　　　　psychotic disorder F14.259
　　　　　sexual dysfunction F14.281
　　　　　sleep disorder F14.282
　　　　in remission (early) (sustained) F14.21
　coccyx NEC M53.3
　cognitive F09
　　due to (secondary to) general medical condition F09
　　persisting R41.89
　　　due to
　　　　alcohol F10.97
　　　　　with dependence F10.27
　　　　anxiolytics F13.97
　　　　　with dependence F13.27
　　　　hypnotics F13.97
　　　　　with dependence F13.27
　　　　sedatives F13.97
　　　　　with dependence F13.27
　　　　specified substance NEC F19.97
　　　　　with
　　　　　　abuse F19.17
　　　　　　dependence F19.27
　communication F80.9
　　social pragmatic F80.82
　conduct (childhood) F91.9
　　adjustment reaction — *see* Disorder, adjustment
　　adolescent onset type F91.2
　　childhood onset type F91.1
　　compulsive F63.9
　　confined to family context F91.0
　　depressive F91.8
　　group type F91.2

Disorder — *continued*
　conduct — *continued*
　　hyperkinetic — *see* Disorder, attention-deficit hy-
　　　peractivity
　　oppositional defiance F91.3
　　socialized F91.2
　　solitary aggressive type F91.1
　　specified NEC F91.8
　　unsocialized (aggressive) F91.1
　conduction, heart I45.9
　congenital glycosylation (CDG) E74.89
　conjunctiva H11.9
　　infection — *see* Conjunctivitis
　connective tissue, localized L94.9
　　specified NEC L94.8
　conversion (functional neurological symptom disorder)
　　with
　　　abnormal movement F44.4
　　　anesthesia or sensory loss F44.6
　　　attacks or seizures F44.5
　　　mixed symptoms F44.7
　　　special sensory symptoms F44.6
　　　speech symptoms F44.4
　　　swallowing symptoms F44.4
　　　weakness or paralysis F44.4
　convulsive (secondary) — *see* Convulsions
　cornea H18.9
　　deformity — *see* Deformity, cornea
　　degeneration — *see* Degeneration, cornea
　　deposits — *see* Deposit, cornea
　　due to contact lens H18.82- ☑
　　　specified as edema — *see* Edema, cornea
　　edema — *see* Edema, cornea
　　keratitis — *see* Keratitis
　　keratoconjunctivitis — *see* Keratoconjunctivitis
　　membrane change — *see* Change, corneal mem-
　　　brane
　　neovascularization — *see* Neovascularization,
　　　cornea
　　scar — *see* Opacity, cornea
　　specified type NEC H18.89- ☑
　　ulcer — *see* Ulcer, cornea
　corpus cavernosum N48.9
　cranial nerve — *see* Disorder, nerve, cranial
　Cyclin-Dependent Kinase-Like 5 Deficiency (CDKL5)
　　G40.42
　cyclothymic F34.0
　defiant oppositional F91.3
　delusional (persistent) (systematized) F22
　　induced F24
　depersonalization F48.1
　depressive F32.9
　　due to known physiological condition
　　　with
　　　　depressive features F06.31
　　　　major depressive-like episode F06.32
　　　　mixed features F06.34
　　major F32.9
　　　with psychotic symptoms F32.3
　　　in remission (full) F32.5
　　　　partial F32.4
　　　recurrent F33.9
　　　　with psychotic features F33.3
　　　single episode F32.9
　　　　mild F32.0
　　　　moderate F32.1
　　　　severe (without psychotic symptoms) F32.2
　　　　　with psychotic symptoms F32.3
　　organic F06.31
　　persistent F34.1
　　recurrent F33.9
　　　current episode
　　　　mild F33.0
　　　　moderate F33.1
　　　　severe (without psychotic symptoms) F33.2
　　　　　with psychotic symptoms F33.3
　　　in remission F33.40
　　　　full F33.42
　　　　partial F33.41
　　　specified NEC F33.8
　　single episode — *see* Episode, depressive
　　specified NEC F32.89
　developmental F89
　　arithmetical skills F81.2
　　coordination (motor) F82
　　expressive writing F81.81
　　language F80.9
　　　expressive F80.1

Disorder — Disorder

Disorder — *continued*
- developmental — *continued*
  - language — *continued*
    - mixed receptive and expressive F80.2
    - receptive type F80.2
    - specified NEC F80.89
  - learning F81.9
    - arithmetical F81.2
    - reading F81.0
  - mixed F88
  - motor coordination or function F82
  - pervasive F84.9
    - specified NEC F84.8
  - phonological F80.0
  - reading F81.0
  - scholastic skills — *see also* Disorder, learning
    - mixed F81.89
  - specified NEC F88
  - speech F80.9
    - articulation F80.0
    - specified NEC F80.89
  - written expression F81.81
- diaphragm J98.6
- digestive (system) K92.9
  - newborn P78.9
    - specified NEC P78.89
  - postprocedural — *see* Complication, gastrointestinal
  - psychogenic F45.8
- disc (intervertebral) M51.9
  - with
    - myelopathy
      - cervical region M50.00
      - cervicothoracic region M50.03
      - high cervical region M50.01
      - lumbar region M51.06
      - mid-cervical region M50.020
      - sacrococcygeal region M53.3
      - thoracic region M51.04
      - thoracolumbar region M51.05
    - radiculopathy
      - cervical region M50.10
      - cervicothoracic region M50.13
      - high cervical region M50.11
      - lumbar region M51.16
      - lumbosacral region M51.17
      - mid-cervical region M50.120
      - sacrococcygeal region M53.3
      - thoracic region M51.14
      - thoracolumbar region M51.15
  - cervical M50.90
    - with
      - myelopathy M50.00
        - C2-C3 M50.01
        - C3-C4 M50.01
        - C4-C5 M50.021
        - C5-C6 M50.022
        - C6-C7 M50.023
        - C7-T1 M50.03
        - cervicothoracic region M50.03
        - high cervical region M50.01
        - mid-cervical region M50.020
      - neuritis, radiculitis or radiculopathy M50.10
        - C2-C3 M50.11
        - C3-C4 M50.11
        - C4-C5 M50.121
        - C5-C6 M50.122
        - C6-C7 M50.123
        - C7-T1 M50.13
        - cervicothoracic region M50.13
        - high cervical region M50.11
        - mid-cervical region M50.120
    - C2-C3 M50.91
    - C3-C4 M50.91
    - C4-C5 M50.921
    - C5-C6 M50.922
    - C6-C7 M50.923
    - C7-T1 M50.93
    - cervicothoracic region M50.93
    - degeneration M50.30
      - C2-C3 M50.31
      - C3-C4 M50.31
      - C4-C5 M50.321
      - C5-C6 M50.322
      - C6-C7 M50.323
      - C7-T1 M50.33
      - cervicothoracic region M50.33
      - high cervical region M50.31
      - mid-cervical region M50.320
    - displacement M50.20

Disorder — *continued*
- disc — *continued*
  - cervical — *continued*
    - displacement — *continued*
      - C2-C3 M50.21
      - C3-C4 M50.21
      - C4-C5 M50.221
      - C5-C6 M50.222
      - C6-C7 M50.223
      - C7-T1 M50.23
      - cervicothoracic region M50.23
      - high cervical region M50.21
      - mid-cervical region M50.220
    - high cervical region M50.91
    - mid-cervical region M50.920
    - specified type NEC M50.80
      - C2-C3 M50.81
      - C3-C4 M50.81
      - C4-C5 M50.821
      - C5-C6 M50.822
      - C6-C7 M50.823
      - C7-T1 M50.83
      - cervicothoracic region M50.83
      - high cervical region M50.81
      - mid-cervical region M50.820
  - specified NEC
    - lumbar region M51.86
    - lumbosacral region M51.87
    - sacrococcygeal region M53.3
    - thoracic region M51.84
    - thoracolumbar region M51.85
- disinhibited attachment (childhood) F94.2
- disintegrative, childhood NEC F84.3
- disruptive F91.9
  - mood dysregulation F34.81
  - specified NEC F91.8
- disruptive behavior — *see* Disorder, conduct
- dissocial personality F60.2
- dissociative F44.9
  - affecting
    - motor function F44.4
      - and sensation F44.7
    - sensation F44.6
      - and motor function F44.7
  - brief reactive F43.0
  - due to (secondary to) general medical condition F06.8
  - mixed F44.7
  - organic F06.8
  - other specified NEC F44.89
- double heterozygous sickling — *see* Disease, sickle-cell
- dream anxiety F51.5
- drug induced hemorrhagic D68.32
- drug related F19.99
  - abuse — *see* Abuse, drug
  - dependence — *see* Dependence, drug
- dysmorphic body F45.22
- dysthymic F34.1
- ear H93.9- ☑
  - bleeding — *see* Otorrhagia
  - deafness — *see* Deafness
  - degenerative H93.09- ☑
  - discharge — *see* Otorrhea
  - external H61.9- ☑
    - auditory canal stenosis — *see* Stenosis, external ear canal
    - exostosis — *see* Exostosis, external ear canal
    - impacted cerumen — *see* Impaction, cerumen
    - otitis — *see* Otitis, externa
    - perichondritis — *see* Perichondritis, ear
    - pinna — *see* Disorder, pinna
    - specified type NEC H61.89- ☑
  - inner H83.9- ☑
    - vestibular dysfunction — *see* Disorder, vestibular function
  - middle H74.9- ☑
    - adhesive H74.1- ☑
    - ossicle — *see* Abnormal, ear ossicles
    - polyp — *see* Polyp, ear (middle)
    - specified NEC, in diseases classified elsewhere H75.8- ☑
  - postprocedural — *see* Complications, ear, procedure
  - specified NEC, in diseases classified elsewhere H94.8- ☑
- eating (adult) (psychogenic) F50.9
  - anorexia — *see* Anorexia
  - binge F50.81
  - bulimia F50.2

Disorder — *continued*
- eating — *continued*
  - child F98.29
    - pica F98.3
    - rumination disorder F98.21
  - pica F50.89
    - childhood F98.3
- electrolyte (balance) NEC E87.8
  - with
    - abortion — *see* Abortion by type complicated by specified condition NEC
    - ectopic pregnancy O08.5
    - molar pregnancy O08.5
  - acidosis (metabolic) (respiratory) E87.2
  - alkalosis (metabolic) (respiratory) E87.3
- elimination, transepidermal L87.9
  - specified NEC L87.8
- emotional (persistent) F34.9
  - of childhood F93.9
    - specified NEC F93.8
- endocrine E34.9
  - postprocedural E89.89
  - specified NEC E89.89
- erectile (male) (organic) — *see also* Dysfunction, sexual, male, erectile N52.9
  - nonorganic F52.21
- erythematous — *see* Erythema
- esophagus K22.9
  - functional K22.4
  - psychogenic F45.8
- eustachian tube H69.9- ☑
  - infection — *see* Salpingitis, eustachian
  - obstruction — *see* Obstruction, eustachian tube
  - patulous — *see* Patulous, eustachian tube
  - specified NEC H69.8- ☑
- exhibitionistic F65.2
- extrapyramidal G25.9
  - in deseases classified elsewhere — *see* category G26
  - specified type NEC G25.89
- eye H57.9
  - postprocedural — *see* Complication, postprocedural, eye
- eyelid H02.9
  - cyst — *see* Cyst, eyelid
  - degenerative H02.70
    - chloasma — *see* Chloasma, eyelid
    - madarosis — *see* Madarosis
    - specified type NEC H02.79
    - vitiligo — *see* Vitiligo, eyelid
    - xanthelasma — *see* Xanthelasma
  - dermatochalasis — *see* Dermatochalasis
  - edema — *see* Edema, eyelid
  - elephantiasis — *see* Elephantiasis, eyelid
  - foreign body, retained — *see* Foreign body, retained, eyelid
  - function H02.59
    - abnormal innervation syndrome — *see* Syndrome, abnormal innervation
    - blepharochalasis — *see* Blepharochalasis
    - blepharoclonus — *see* Blepharoclonus
    - blepharophimosis — *see* Blepharophimosis
    - blepharoptosis — *see* Blepharoptosis
    - lagophthalmos — *see* Lagophthalmos
    - lid retraction — *see* Retraction, lid
  - hypertrichosis — *see* Hypertrichosis, eyelid
  - specified type NEC H02.89
  - vascular H02.879
    - left H02.876
      - lower H02.875
      - upper H02.874
    - right H02.873
      - lower H02.872
      - upper H02.871
- factitious
  - by proxy F68.A
  - imposed on another F68.A
  - imposed on self F68.10
    - with predominantly
      - psychological symptoms F68.11
        - with physical symptoms F68.13
      - physical symptoms F68.12
        - with psychological symptoms F68.13
- factor, coagulation — *see* Defect, coagulation
- fatty acid
  - metabolism E71.30
    - specified NEC E71.39

☑ **Additional Character Required — Refer to the Tabular List for Character Selection**   ▽ Subterms under main terms may continue to next column or page

Disorder — *continued*
  fatty acid — *continued*
    oxidation
      LCAD E71.310
      MCAD E71.311
      SCAD E71.312
      specified deficiency NEC E71.318
  feeding (infant or child) — *see also* Disorder, eating
    R63.3
    or eating disorder F50.9
    specified NEC F50.9
  feigned (with obvious motivation) Z76.5
    without obvious motivation — *see* Disorder, factitious
  female
    hypoactive sexual desire F52.0
    orgasmic F52.31
    sexual interest/arousal F52.22
  fetishistic F65.0
  fibroblastic M72.9
    specified NEC M72.8
  fluency
    adult onset F98.5
    childhood onset F80.81
    following
      cerebral infarction I69.323
      cerebrovascular disease I69.923
        specified disease NEC I69.823
      intracerebral hemorrhage I69.123
      nontraumatic intracranial hemorrhage NEC
        I69.223
      subarachnoid hemorrhage I69.023
    in conditions classified elsewhere R47.82
  fluid balance E87.8
  follicular (skin) L73.9
    specified NEC L73.8
  frotteuristic F65.81
  fructose metabolism E74.10
    essential fructosuria E74.11
    fructokinase deficiency E74.11
    fructose-1, 6-diphosphatase deficiency E74.19
    hereditary fructose intolerance E74.12
    other specified E74.19
  functional polymorphonuclear neutrophils D71
  gallbladder, biliary tract and pancreas in diseases classified elsewhere K87
  gambling F63.0
  gamma aminobutyric acid (GABA) metabolism E72.81
  gamma-glutamyl cycle E72.89
  gastric (functional) K31.9
    motility K30
    psychogenic F45.8
    secretion K30
  gastrointestinal (functional) NOS K92.9
    newborn P78.9
    psychogenic F45.8
  gender-identity or -role F64.9
    childhood F64.2
    effect on relationship F66
    of adolescence or adulthood F64.0
      nontranssexual F64.8
    specified NEC F64.8
    uncertainty F66
  genito-pelvic pain penetration F52.6
  genitourinary system
    female N94.9
    male N50.9
    psychogenic F45.8
  globe H44.9
    degenerated condition H44.50
      absolute glaucoma H44.51- ☑
      atrophy H44.52- ☑
      leucocoria H44.53- ☑
    degenerative H44.30
      chalcosis H44.31- ☑
      myopia — *see also* Myopia, degenerative
        H44.2- ☑
      siderosis H44.32- ☑
      specified type NEC H44.39- ☑
    endophthalmitis — *see* Endophthalmitis
    foreign body, retained — *see* Foreign body, intraocular, old, retained
    hemophthalmos — *see* Hemophthalmos
    hypotony H44.40
      due to
        ocular fistula H44.42- ☑
        specified disorder NEC H44.43- ☑
      flat anterior chamber H44.41- ☑

Disorder — *continued*
  globe — *continued*
    hypotony — *continued*
      primary H44.44- ☑
    luxation — *see* Luxation, globe
    specified type NEC H44.89
  glomerular (in) N05.9
    amyloidosis E85.4 *[N08]*
    cryoglobulinemia D89.1 *[N08]*
    disseminated intravascular coagulation D65 *[N08]*
    Fabry's disease E75.21 *[N08]*
    familial lecithin cholesterol acyltransferase deficiency E78.6 *[N08]*
    Goodpasture's syndrome M31.0
    hemolytic-uremic syndrome D59.3
    Henoch (-Schönlein) purpura D69.0 *[N08]*
    malariae malaria B52.0
    microscopic polyangiitis M31.7 *[N08]*
    multiple myeloma C90.0- ☑ *[N08]*
    mumps B26.83
    schistosomiasis B65.9 *[N08]*
    sepsis NEC A41.- ☑ *[N08]*
      streptococcal A40.- ☑ *[N08]*
    sickle-cell disorders D57.- ☑ *[N08]*
    strongyloidiasis B78.9 *[N08]*
    subacute bacterial endocarditis I33.0 *[N08]*
    syphilis A52.75
    systemic lupus erythematosus M32.14
    thrombotic thrombocytopenic purpura M31.1 *[N08]*
    Waldenström macroglobulinemia C88.0 *[N08]*
    Wegener's granulomatosis M31.31
  gluconeogenesis E74.4
  glucosaminoglycan metabolism — *see* Disorder,
    metabolism, glucosaminoglycan
  gluecose transport E74.819
    specified NEC E74.818
  glycine metabolism E72.50
    d-glycericacidemia E72.59
    hyperhydroxyprolinemia E72.59
    hyperoxaluria R82.992
      primary E72.53
    hyperprolinemia E72.59
    non-ketotic hyperglycinemia E72.51
    oxalosis E72.53
    oxaluria E72.53
    sarcosinemia E72.59
    trimethylaminuria E72.52
  glycoprotein metabolism E77.9
    specified NEC E77.8
  habit (and impulse) F63.9
    involving sexual behavior NEC F65.9
    specified NEC F63.89
  hallucinogen use
    mild F16.10
      with
        hallucinogen intoxication delirium F16.121
        hallucinogen-induced
          anxiety disorder F16.180
          bipolar and related disorder F16.14
          depressive disorder F16.14
          psychotic disorder F16.159
        other hallucinogen intoxication F16.129
      in remission (early) (sustained) F16.11
    moderate or severe F16.20
      with
        hallucinogen intoxication delirium F16.221
        hallucinogen-induced
          anxiety disorder F16.280
          bipolar and related disorder F16.24
          depressive disorder F16.24
          psychotic disorder F16.259
        other hallucinogen intoxication F16.229
      in remission (early) (sustained) F16.21
  heart action I49.9
  hematological D75.9
    newborn (transient) P61.9
      specified NEC P61.8
  hematopoietic organs D75.9
  hemorrhagic NEC D69.9
    drug-induced D68.32
    due to
      extrinsic circulating anticoagulants D68.32
      increase in
        anti-IIa D68.32
        anti-Xa D68.32
      intrinsic
        circulating anticoagulants D68.318

Disorder — *continued*
  hemorrhagic — *continued*
    due to — *continued*
      intrinsic — *continued*
        increase in
          anti-IXa D68.318
          antithrombin D68.318
          anti-VIIIa D68.318
          anti-XIa D68.318
    following childbirth O72.3
  hemostasis — *see* Defect, coagulation
  histidine metabolism E70.40
    histidinemia E70.41
    other specified E70.49
  hoarding F42.3
  hyperkinetic — *see* Disorder, attention-deficit hyperactivity
  hyperleucine-isoleucinemia E71.19
  hypervalinemia E71.19
  hypoactive sexual desire F52.0
  hypochondriacal F45.20
    body dysmorphic F45.22
    neurosis F45.21
    other specified F45.29
  identity
    dissociative F44.81
    illness anxiety F45.21
    of childhood F93.8
  immune mechanism (immunity) D89.9
    specified type NEC D89.89
  impaired renal tubular function N25.9
    specified NEC N25.89
  impulse (control) F63.9
  inflammatory
    pelvic, in diseases classified elsewhere — *see* category N74
    penis N48.29
      abscess N48.21
      cellulitis N48.22
  inhalant use
    mild F18.10
      with
        inhalant intoxication F18.129
        inhalant intoxication delirium F18.121
        inhalant-induced
          anxiety disorder F18.180
          depressive disorder F18.14
          major neurocognitive disorder F18.17
          mild neurocognitive disorder F18.188
          psychotic disorder F18.159
      in remission (early) (sustained) F18.11
    moderate or severe F18.20
      with
        inhalant intoxication F18.229
        inhalant intoxication delirium F18.221
        inhalant-induced
          anxiety disorder F18.280
          depressive disorder F18.24
          major neurocognitive disorder F18.27
          mild neurocognitive disorder F18.288
          psychotic disorder F18.259
      in remission (early) (sustained) F18.21
  integument, newborn P83.9
    specified NEC P83.88
  intermittent explosive F63.81
  internal secretion pancreas — *see* Increased, secretion, pancreas, endocrine
  intestine, intestinal
    carbohydrate absorption NEC E74.39
      postoperative K91.2
    functional NEC K59.9
      postoperative K91.89
    psychogenic F45.8
    vascular K55.9
      chronic K55.1
      specified NEC K55.8
  intraoperative (intraprocedural) — *see* Complications, intraoperative
  involuntary emotional expression (IEED) F07.89
  iris H21.9
    adhesions — *see* Adhesions, iris
    atrophy — *see* Atrophy, iris
    chamber angle recession — *see* Recession, chamber angle
    cyst — *see* Cyst, iris
    degeneration — *see* Degeneration, iris
    in diseases classified elsewhere H22
    iridodialysis — *see* Iridodialysis

Disorder — *continued*
  iris — *continued*
    iridoschisis — *see* Iridoschisis
    miotic pupillary cyst — *see* Cyst, pupillary
    pupillary
      abnormality — *see* Abnormality, pupillary
      membrane — *see* Membrane, pupillary
    specified type NEC H21.89
    vascular NEC H21.1X- ☑
  iron metabolism E83.10
    specified NEC E83.19
  isovaleric acidemia E71.110
  jaw, developmental M27.0
    temporomandibular — *see also* Anomaly, dentofa-
      cial, temporomandibular joint M26.60- ☑
  joint M25.9
    derangement — *see* Derangement, joint
    effusion — *see* Effusion, joint
    fistula — *see* Fistula, joint
    hemarthrosis — *see* Hemarthrosis
    instability — *see* Instability, joint
    osteophyte — *see* Osteophyte
    pain — *see* Pain, joint
    psychogenic F45.8
    specified type NEC M25.80
      ankle M25.87- ☑
      elbow M25.82- ☑
      foot joint M25.87- ☑
      hand joint M25.84- ☑
      hip M25.85- ☑
      knee M25.86- ☑
      shoulder M25.81- ☑
      wrist M25.83- ☑
    stiffness — *see* Stiffness, joint
  ketone metabolism E71.32
  kidney N28.9
    functional (tubular) N25.9
    in
      schistosomiasis B65.9 [N29]
    tubular function N25.9
    specified NEC N25.89
  lacrimal system H04.9
    changes H04.69
      fistula — *see* Fistula, lacrimal
    gland H04.19
      atrophy — *see* Atrophy, lacrimal gland
      cyst — *see* Cyst, lacrimal, gland
      dacryops — *see* Dacryops
      dislocation — *see* Dislocation, lacrimal gland
      dry eye syndrome — *see* Syndrome, dry eye
      infection — *see* Dacryoadenitis
    granuloma — *see* Granuloma, lacrimal
    inflammation — *see* Inflammation, lacrimal
    obstruction — *see* Obstruction, lacrimal
    specified NEC H04.89
  lactation NEC O92.79
  language (developmental) F80.9
    expressive F80.1
    mixed receptive and expressive F80.2
    receptive F80.2
  late luteal phase dysphoric N94.89
  learning (specific) F81.9
    acalculia R48.8
    alexia R48.0
    mathematics F81.2
    reading F81.0
    specified
      with impairment in
        mathematics F81.2
        reading F81.0
        written expression F81.81
    specified NEC F81.89
    spelling F81.81
    written expression F81.81
  lens H27.9
    aphakia — *see* Aphakia
    cataract — *see* Cataract
    dislocation — *see* Dislocation, lens
    specified type NEC H27.8
  ligament M24.20
    ankle M24.27- ☑
    attachment, spine — *see* Enthesopathy, spinal
    elbow M24.22- ☑
    foot joint M24.27- ☑
    hand joint M24.24- ☑
    hip M24.25- ☑
    knee — *see* Derangement, knee, specified NEC

Disorder — *continued*
  ligament — *continued*
    shoulder M24.21- ☑
    specified site NEC M24.29
    vertebra M24.28
    wrist M24.23- ☑
  ligamentous attachments — *see also* Enthesopathy
    spine — *see* Enthesopathy, spinal
  lipid
    metabolism, congenital E78.9
    storage E75.6
      specified NEC E75.5
  lipoprotein
    deficiency (familial) E78.6
    metabolism E78.9
      specified NEC E78.89
  liver K76.9
    malarial B54 [K77]
  low back — *see also* Dorsopathy, specified NEC
  lumbosacral
    plexus G54.1
    root (nerve) NEC G54.4
  lung, interstitial, drug-induced J70.4
    acute J70.2
    chronic J70.3
    dabbing (related) U07.0
    e-cigarette (related) U07.0
    electronic cigarette (related) U07.0
    vaping (associated) (device) (product) (related) (use)
      U07.0
  lymphoproliferative, post-transplant (PTLD) D47.Z1
    (*following* D47.4)
  lysine and hydroxylysine metabolism E72.3
  major neurocognitive — *see* Dementia, in (due to)
  male
    erectile (organic) — *see also* Dysfunction, sexual,
      male, erectile N52.9
      nonorganic F52.21
    hypoactive sexual desire F52.0
    orgasmic F52.32
  manic F30.9
    organic F06.33
  mast cell activation — *see* Activation, mast cell
  mastoid — *see also* Disorder, ear, middle
    postprocedural — *see* Complications, ear, procedure
  meninges, specified type NEC G96.198
  meniscus — *see* Derangement, knee, meniscus
  menopausal N95.9
    specified NEC N95.8
  menstrual N92.6
    psychogenic F45.8
    specified NEC N92.5
  mental (or behavioral) (nonpsychotic) F99
    due to (secondary to)
      amphetamine
        due to drug abuse — *see* Abuse, drug, stimu-
          lant
        due to drug dependence — *see* Dependence,
          drug, stimulant
      brain disease, damage and dysfunction F09
      caffeine use
        due to drug abuse — *see* Abuse, drug, stimu-
          lant
        due to drug dependence — *see* Dependence,
          drug, stimulant
      cannabis use
        due to drug abuse — *see* Abuse, drug,
          cannabis
        due to drug dependence — *see* Dependence,
          drug, cannabis
      general medical condition F09
      sedative or hypnotic use
        due to drug abuse — *see* Abuse, drug, seda-
          tive
        due to drug dependence — *see* Dependence,
          drug, sedative
      tobacco (nicotine) use — *see* Dependence, drug,
        nicotine
    following organic brain damage F07.9
      frontal lobe syndrome F07.0
      personality change F07.0
      postconcussional syndrome F07.81
      specified NEC F07.89
    infancy, childhood or adolescence F98.9
    neurotic — *see* Neurosis
    organic or symptomatic F09
    presenile, psychotic F03 ☑

Disorder — *continued*
  mental — *continued*
    problem NEC
    psychoneurotic — *see* Neurosis
    psychotic — *see* Psychosis
    puerperal F53.0
    senile, psychotic NEC F03 ☑
  metabolic, amino acid, transitory, newborn P74.8
  metabolism NOS E88.9
    amino-acid E72.9
      aromatic E70.9
        albinism — *see* Albinism
        histidine E70.40
          histidinemia E70.41
          other specified E70.49
        hyperphenylalaninemia E70.1
          classical phenylketonuria E70.0
        other specified E70.89
        tryptophan E70.5
        tyrosine E70.20
          hypertyrosinemia E70.21
          other specified E70.29
      branched chain E71.2
        3-methylglutaconic aciduria E71.111
        hyperleucine-isoleucinemia E71.19
        hypervalinemia E71.19
        isovaleric acidemia E71.110
        maple syrup urine disease E71.0
        methylmalonic acidemia E71.120
        organic aciduria NEC E71.118
        other specified E71.19
        proprionate NEC E71.128
        proprionic acidemia E71.121
      glycine E72.50
        d-glycericacidemia E72.59
        hyperhydroxyprolinemia E72.59
        hyperoxaluria R82.992
          primary E72.53
        hyperprolinemia E72.59
        non-ketotic hyperglycinemia E72.51
        other specified E72.59
        sarcosinemia E72.59
        trimethylaminuria E72.52
      hydroxylysine E72.3
      lysine E72.3
      ornithine E72.4
      other specified E72.89
        beta-amino acid E72.89
        gamma-glutamyl cycle E72.89
      straight-chain E72.89
      sulfur-bearing E72.10
        homocystinuria E72.11
        methylenetetrahydrofolate reductase deficien-
          cy E72.12
        other specified E72.19
    bile acid and cholesterol metabolism E78.70
    bilirubin E80.7
      specified NEC E80.6
    calcium E83.50
      hypercalcemia E83.52
      hypocalcemia E83.51
      other specified E83.59
    carbohydrate E74.9
      specified NEC E74.89
    cholesterol and bile acid metabolism E78.70
    congenital E88.9
    copper E83.00
      specified type NEC E83.09
      Wilson's disease E83.01
    cystinuria E72.01
    fructose E74.10
    galactose E74.20
    glucosaminoglycan E76.9
      mucopolysaccharidosis — *see* Mucopolysaccha-
        ridosis
      specified NEC E76.8
    glutamine E72.89
    glycine E72.50
    glycogen storage (hepatorenal) E74.09
    glycoprotein E77.9
      specified NEC E77.8
    glycosaminoglycan E76.9
      specified NEC E76.8
    in labor and delivery O75.89
    iron E83.10
    isoleucine E71.19
    leucine E71.19
    lipoid E78.9
    lipoprotein E78.9

☑ Additional Character Required — Refer to the Tabular List for Character Selection   ▽ Subterms under main terms may continue to next column or page

Disorder — *continued*
  metabolism — *continued*
    lipoprotein — *continued*
      specified NEC E78.89
    magnesium E83.40
      hypermagnesemia E83.41
      hypomagnesemia E83.42
      other specified E83.49
    mineral E83.9
      specified NEC E83.89
    mitochondrial E88.40
      MELAS syndrome E88.41
      MERRF syndrome (myoclonic epilepsy associated
        with ragged-red fibers) E88.42
      other specified E88.49
    ornithine E72.4
    phosphatases E83.30
    phosphorus E83.30
      acid phosphatase deficiency E83.39
      hypophosphatasia E83.39
      hypophosphatemia E83.39
        familial E83.31
      other specified E83.39
      pseudovitamin D deficiency E83.32
    plasma protein NEC E88.09
    porphyrin — *see* Porphyria
    postprocedural E89.89
      specified NEC E89.89
    purine E79.9
      specified NEC E79.8
    pyrimidine E79.9
      specified NEC E79.8
    pyruvate E74.4
    serine E72.89
    sodium E87.8
    specified NEC E88.89
    threonine E72.89
    valine E71.19
    zinc E83.2
  methylmalonic acidemia E71.120
  micturition NEC — *see also* Difficulty, micturition
    R39.198
    feeling of incomplete emptying R39.14
    hesitancy R39.11
    poor stream R39.12
    psychogenic F45.8
    split stream R39.13
    straining R39.16
    urgency R39.15
  mild neurocognitive G31.84
  mitochondrial metabolism E88.40
  mitral (valve) — *see* Endocarditis, mitral
  mixed
    anxiety and depressive F41.8
    of scholastic skills (developmental) F81.89
    receptive expressive language F80.2
  mood F39
    bipolar — *see* Disorder, bipolar
    depressive — *see* Disorder, depressive
    due to (secondary to)
      alcohol F10.94
      amphetamine F15.94
        in
          abuse F15.14
          dependence F15.24
      anxiolytic F13.94
        in
          abuse F13.14
          dependence F13.24
      cocaine F14.94
        in
          abuse F14.14
          dependence F14.24
      general medical condition F06.30
      hallucinogen F16.94
        in
          abuse F16.14
          dependence F16.24
      hypnotic F13.94
        in
          abuse F13.14
          dependence F13.24
      inhalant F18.94
        in
          abuse F18.14
          dependence F18.24
      opioid F11.94
        in
          abuse F11.14

Disorder — *continued*
  mood — *continued*
    due to — *continued*
      opioid — *continued*
        in — *continued*
          dependence F11.24
      phencyclidine (PCP) F16.94
        in
          abuse F16.14
          dependence F16.24
      physiological condition F06.30
        with
          depressive features F06.31
          major depressive-like episode F06.32
          manic features F06.33
          mixed features F06.34
      psychoactive substance NEC F19.94
        in
          abuse F19.14
          dependence F19.24
      sedative F13.94
        in
          abuse F13.14
          dependence F13.24
      volatile solvents F18.94
        in
          abuse F18.14
          dependence F18.24
    manic episode F30.9
      with psychotic symptoms F30.2
      in remission (full) F30.4
        partial F30.3
      specified type NEC F30.8
      without psychotic symptoms F30.10
        mild F30.11
        moderate F30.12
        severe F30.13
    organic F06.30
      right hemisphere F07.89
    persistent F34.9
      cyclothymia F34.0
      dysthymia F34.1
      specified type NEC F34.89
    recurrent F39
    right hemisphere organic F07.89
  movement G25.9
    drug-induced G25.70
      akathisia G25.71
      specified NEC G25.79
    hysterical F44.4
    in diseases classified elsewhere — *see* category G26
    periodic limb G47.61
      sleep related G47.61
    sleep related NEC G47.69
    specified NEC G25.89
    stereotyped F98.4
    treatment-induced G25.9
  multiple personality F44.81
  muscle M62.9
    attachment, spine — *see* Enthesopathy, spinal
    in trichinellosis — *see* Trichinellosis, with muscle
      disorder
    psychogenic F45.8
    specified type NEC M62.89
    tone, newborn P94.9
      specified NEC P94.8
  muscular
    attachments — *see also* Enthesopathy
      spine — *see* Enthesopathy, spinal
    urethra N36.44
  musculoskeletal system, soft tissue — *see* Disorder,
    soft tissue
    postprocedural M96.89
    psychogenic F45.8
  myoneural G70.9
    due to lead G70.1
    specified NEC G70.89
    toxic G70.1
  myotonic NEC G71.19
  nail, in diseases classified elsewhere L62
  neck region NEC — *see* Dorsopathy, specified NEC
  neonatal onset multisystemic inflammatory (NOMID)
    M04.2
  nerve G58.9
    abducent NEC — *see* Strabismus, paralytic, sixth
      nerve
    accessory G52.8
    acoustic — *see* subcategory H93.3 ☑

Disorder — *continued*
  nerve — *continued*
    auditory — *see* subcategory H93.3 ☑
    auriculotemporal G50.8
    axillary G54.8
    cerebral — *see* Disorder, nerve, cranial
    cranial G52.9
      eighth — *see* subcategory H93.3 ☑
      eleventh G52.8
      fifth G50.9
      first G52.0
      fourth NEC — *see* Strabismus, paralytic, fourth
        nerve
      multiple G52.7
      ninth G52.1
      second NEC — *see* Disorder, nerve, optic
      seventh NEC G51.8
      sixth NEC — *see* Strabismus, paralytic, sixth nerve
      specified NEC G52.8
      tenth G52.2
      third NEC — *see* Strabismus, paralytic, third nerve
      twelfth G52.3
    entrapment — *see* Neuropathy, entrapment
    facial G51.9
      specified NEC G51.8
    femoral — *see* Lesion, nerve, femoral
    glossopharyngeal NEC G52.1
    hypoglossal G52.3
    intercostal G58.0
    lateral
      cutaneous of thigh — *see* Mononeuropathy,
        lower limb, meralgia paresthetica
      popliteal — *see* Lesion, nerve, popliteal
    lower limb — *see* Mononeuropathy, lower limb
    medial popliteal — *see* Lesion, nerve, popliteal,
      medial
    median NEC — *see* Lesion, nerve, median
    multiple G58.7
    oculomotor NEC — *see* Strabismus, paralytic, third
      nerve
    olfactory G52.0
    optic NEC H47.09- ☑
      hemorrhage into sheath — *see* Hemorrhage,
        optic nerve
      ischemic H47.01- ☑
    peroneal — *see* Lesion, nerve, popliteal
    phrenic G58.8
    plantar — *see* Lesion, nerve, plantar
    pneumogastric G52.2
    posterior tibial — *see* Syndrome, tarsal tunnel
    radial — *see* Lesion, nerve, radial
    recurrent laryngeal G52.2
    root G54.9
      cervical G54.2
      lumbosacral G54.1
      specified NEC G54.8
      thoracic G54.3
    sciatic NEC — *see* Lesion, nerve, sciatic
    specified NEC G58.8
      lower limb — *see* Mononeuropathy, lower limb,
        specified NEC
      upper limb — *see* Mononeuropathy, upper limb,
        specified NEC
    sympathetic G90.9
    tibial — *see* Lesion, nerve, popliteal, medial
    trigeminal G50.9
      specified NEC G50.8
    trochlear NEC — *see* Strabismus, paralytic, fourth
      nerve
    ulnar — *see* Lesion, nerve, ulnar
    upper limb — *see* Mononeuropathy, upper limb
    vagus G52.2
  nervous system G98.8
    autonomic (peripheral) G90.9
      specified NEC G90.8
    central G96.9
      specified NEC G96.89
    parasympathetic G90.9
    specified NEC G98.8
    sympathetic G90.9
    vegetative G90.9
  neurocognitive R41.9
    major
      with
        aggressive behavior F01.51
        combative behavior F01.51
        violent behavior F01.51

⬛ **Subterms under main terms may continue to next column or page**   ☑ **Additional Character Required** — Refer to the Tabular List for Character Selection   **117**

Disorder — Disorder

Disorder — *continued*
  neurocognitive — *continued*
    major — *continued*
      due to vascular disease, with behavioral distur-
        bance F01.51
      in (due to) (other diseases classified elsewhere)
        — *see also* Dementia, in (due to) F02.80
        with
          aggressive behavior F02.81
          combative behavior F02.81
          violent behavior F02.81
        without behavioral disturbance F01.50
      mild G31.84
  neurodevelopmental F89
    specified NEC F88
  neurohypophysis NEC E23.3
  neurological NEC R29.818
  neuromuscular G70.9
    hereditary NEC G71.9
    specified NEC G70.89
    toxic G70.1
  neurotic F48.9
    specified NEC F48.8
  neutrophil, polymorphonuclear D71
  nicotine use — *see* Dependence, drug, nicotine
  nightmare F51.5
  non-rapid eye movement sleep arousal
    sleep terror type F51.4
    sleepwalking type F51.3
  nose J34.9
    specified NEC J34.89
  obsessive-compulsive F42.9
    and related disorder due to a known physiological
      condition F06.8
  odontogenesis NOS K00.9
  opioid use
    with
      opioid-induced psychotic disorder F11.959
        with
          delusions F11.950
          hallucinations F11.951
    due to drug abuse — *see* Abuse, drug, opioid
    due to drug dependence — *see* Dependence, drug,
      opioid
    mild F11.10
      with
        opioid-induced
          anxiety disorder F11.188
          depressive disorder F11.14
          sexual dysfunction F11.181
        opioid intoxication
          with perceptual disturbances F11.122
          delirium F11.121
          without perceptual disturbances F11.129
      in remission (early) (sustained) F11.11
    moderate or severe F11.20
      with
        opioid-induced
          anxiety disorder F11.288
          anxiety disorder F11.988
          depressive disorder F11.24
          depressive disorder F11.94
          sexual dysfunction F11.281
          sexual dysfunction F11.981
        opioid intoxication
          with perceptual disturbances F11.222
          delirium F11.221
          without perceptual disturbances F11.229
      in remission (early) (sustained) F11.21
  oppositional defiant F91.3
  optic
    chiasm H47.49
      due to
        inflammatory disorder H47.41
        neoplasm H47.42
        vascular disorder H47.43
    disc H47.39- ☑
      coloboma — *see* Coloboma, optic disc
      drusen — *see* Drusen, optic disc
      pseudopapilledema — *see* Pseudopapilledema
    radiations — *see* Disorder, visual, pathway
    tracts — *see* Disorder, visual, pathway
  orbit H05.9
    cyst — *see* Cyst, orbit
    deformity — *see* Deformity, orbit
    edema — *see* Edema, orbit
    enophthalmos — *see* Enophthalmos
    exophthalmos — *see* Exophthalmos

Disorder — *continued*
  orbit — *continued*
    hemorrhage — *see* Hemorrhage, orbit
    inflammation — *see* Inflammation, orbit
    myopathy — *see* Myopathy, extraocular muscles
    retained foreign body — *see* Foreign body, orbit,
      old
    specified type NEC H05.89
  organic
    anxiety F06.4
    catatonic F06.1
    delusional F06.2
    dissociative F06.8
    emotionally labile (asthenic) F06.8
    mood (affective) F06.30
    schizophrenia-like F06.2
  orgasmic (female) F52.31
    male F52.32
  ornithine metabolism E72.4
  overanxious F41.1
    of childhood F93.8
  pain
    with related psychological factors F45.42
    exclusively related to psychological factors F45.41
    genito-pelvic penetration disorder F52.6
  pancreatic internal secretion E16.9
    specified NEC E16.8
  panic F41.0
    with agoraphobia F40.01
  papulosquamous L44.9
    in diseases classified elsewhere L45
    specified NEC L44.8
  paranoid F22
    induced F24
    shared F24
  paraphilic F65.9
    specified NEC F65.89
  parathyroid (gland) E21.5
    specified NEC E21.4
  parietoalveolar NEC J84.09
  paroxysmal, mixed R56.9
  patella M22.9- ☑
    chondromalacia — *see* Chondromalacia, patella
    derangement NEC M22.3X- ☑
    recurrent
      dislocation — *see* Dislocation, patella, recurrent
      subluxation — *see* Dislocation, patella, recurrent,
        incomplete
    specified NEC M22.8X- ☑
  patellofemoral M22.2X- ☑
  pedophilic F65.4
  pentose phosphate pathway with anemia D55.1
  perception, due to hallucinogens F16.983
    in
      abuse F16.183
      dependence F16.283
  peripheral nervous system NEC G64
  peroxisomal E71.50
    biogenesis
      neonatal adrenoleukodystrophy E71.511
      specified disorder NEC E71.518
      Zellweger syndrome E71.510
    rhizomelic chondrodysplasia punctata E71.540
    specified form NEC E71.548
      group 1 E71.518
      group 2 E71.53
      group 3 E71.542
    X-linked adrenoleukodystrophy E71.529
      adolescent E71.521
      adrenomyeloneuropathy E71.522
      childhood E71.520
      specified form NEC E71.528
    Zellweger-like syndrome E71.541
  persistent
    (somatoform) pain F45.41
    affective (mood) F34.9
  personality — *see also* Personality F60.9
    affective F34.0
    aggressive F60.3
    amoral F60.2
    anankastic F60.5
    antisocial F60.2
    anxious F60.6
    asocial F60.2
    asthenic F60.7
    avoidant F60.6
    borderline F60.3

Disorder — *continued*
  personality — *see also* Personality — *continued*
    change (secondary) due to general medical condi-
      tion F07.0
    compulsive F60.5
    cyclothymic F34.0
    dependent (passive) F60.7
    depressive F34.1
    dissocial F60.2
    emotional instability F60.3
    expansive paranoid F60.0
    explosive F60.3
    following organic brain damage F07.9
    histrionic F60.4
    hyperthymic F34.0
    hypothymic F34.1
    hysterical F60.4
    immature F60.89
    inadequate F60.7
    labile F60.3
    mixed (nonspecific) F60.89
    moral deficiency F60.2
    narcissistic F60.81
    negativistic F60.89
    obsessional F60.5
    obsessive (-compulsive) F60.5
    organic F07.0
    overconscientious F60.5
    paranoid F60.0
    passive (-dependent) F60.7
    passive-aggressive F60.89
    pathological NEC F60.9
    pseudosocial F60.2
    psychopathic F60.2
    schizoid F60.1
    schizotypal F21
    self-defeating F60.7
    specified NEC F60.89
    type A F60.5
    unstable (emotional) F60.3
  pervasive, developmental F84.9
  phencyclidine use
    mild F16.10
      with
        phencyclidine intoxication F16.129
        phencyclidine intoxication delirium F16.121
        phencyclidine-induced
          anxiety disorder F16.180
          bipolar and related disorder F16.14
          depressive disorder F16.14
          psychotic disorder F16.159
      in remission (early) (sustained) F16.11
    moderate or severe F16.20
      with
        phencyclidine intoxication F16.229
        phencyclidine intoxication delirium F16.221
        phencyclidine-induced
          anxiety disorder F16.280
          bipolar and related disorder F16.14
          depressive disorder F16.24
          psychotic disorder F16.259
      in remission (early) (sustained) F16.21
  phobic anxiety, childhood F40.8
  phosphate-losing tubular N25.0
  pigmentation L81.9
    choroid, congenital Q14.3
    diminished melanin formation L81.6
    iron L81.8
    specified NEC L81.8
  pinna (noninfective) H61.10- ☑
    deformity, acquired H61.11- ☑
    hematoma H61.12- ☑
    perichondritis — *see* Perichondritis, ear
    specified type NEC H61.19- ☑
  pituitary gland E23.7
    iatrogenic (postprocedural) E89.3
    specified NEC E23.6
  platelets D69.1
  plexus G54.9
    specified NEC G54.8
  polymorphonuclear neutrophils D71
  porphyrin metabolism — *see* Porphyria
  postconcussional F07.81
  posthallucinogen perception F16.983
    in
      abuse F16.183
      dependence F16.283
  postmenopausal N95.9

☑ **Additional Character Required — Refer to the Tabular List for Character Selection**   Subterms under main terms may continue to next column or page

Disorder — Disorder

Disorder — *continued*
  postmenopausal — *continued*
    specified NEC N95.8
  postprocedural (postoperative) — *see* Complications, postprocedural
  post-transplant lymphoproliferative D47.Z1 (*following* D47.4)
  post-traumatic stress (PTSD) F43.10
    acute F43.11
    chronic F43.12
  premenstrual dysphoric (PMDD) F32.81
  prepuce N47.8
  propionic acidemia E71.121
  prostate N42.9
    specified NEC N42.89
  psychogenic NOS — *see also* condition F45.9
    anxiety F41.8
    appetite F50.9
    asthenic F48.8
    cardiovascular (system) F45.8
    compulsive F42.8
    cutaneous F54
    depressive F32.9
    digestive (system) F45.8
    dysmenorrheic F45.8
    dyspneic F45.8
    endocrine (system) F54
    eye NEC F45.8
    feeding — *see* Disorder, eating
    functional NEC F45.8
    gastric F45.8
    gastrointestinal (system) F45.8
    genitourinary (system) F45.8
    heart (function) (rhythm) F45.8
    hyperventilatory F45.8
    hypochondriacal — *see* Disorder, hypochondriacal
    intestinal F45.8
    joint F45.8
    learning F81.9
    limb F45.8
    lymphatic (system) F45.8
    menstrual F45.8
    micturition F45.8
    monoplegic NEC F44.4
    motor F44.4
    muscle F45.8
    musculoskeletal F45.8
    neurocirculatory F45.8
    obsessive F42.8
    occupational F48.8
    organ or part of body NEC F45.8
    paralytic NEC F44.4
    phobic F40.9
    physical NEC F45.8
    rectal F45.8
    respiratory (system) F45.8
    rheumatic F45.8
    sexual (function) F52.9
    skin (allergic) (eczematous) F54
    sleep F51.9
    specified part of body NEC F45.8
    stomach F45.8
  psychological F99
    associated with
      disease classified elsewhere F54
      sexual
        development F66
        relationship F66
      uncertainty about gender identity F64.9
  psychomotor NEC F44.4
    hysterical F44.4
  psychoneurotic — *see also* Neurosis
    mixed NEC F48.8
  psychophysiologic — *see* Disorder, somatoform
  psychosexual F65.9
    development F66
    identity of childhood F64.2
  psychosomatic NOS — *see* Disorder, somatoform
    multiple F45.0
    undifferentiated F45.1
  psychotic — *see* Psychosis
    transient (acute) F23
  puberty E30.9
    specified NEC E30.8
  pulmonary (valve) — *see* Endocarditis, pulmonary
  purine metabolism E79.9
  pyrimidine metabolism E79.9
  pyruvate metabolism E74.4

Disorder — *continued*
  reactive attachment (childhood) F94.1
  reading R48.0
    developmental (specific) F81.0
  receptive language F80.2
  receptor, hormonal, peripheral — *see also* Syndrome, androgen insensitivity E34.50
  recurrent brief depressive F33.8
  reflex R29.2
  refraction H52.7
    aniseikonia H52.32
    anisometropia H52.31
    astigmatism — *see* Astigmatism
    hypermetropia — *see* Hypermetropia
    myopia — *see* Myopia
    presbyopia H52.4
    specified NEC H52.6
  relationship F68.8
    due to sexual orientation F66
  REM sleep behavior G47.52
  renal function, impaired (tubular) N25.9
  resonance R49.9
    specified NEC R49.8
  respiratory function, impaired — *see also* Failure, respiration
    postprocedural — *see* Complication, postoperative, respiratory system
    psychogenic F45.8
  retina H35.9
    angioid streaks H35.33
    changes in vascular appearance H35.01- ☑
    degeneration — *see* Degeneration, retina
    dystrophy (hereditary) — *see* Dystrophy, retina
    edema H35.81
    hemorrhage — *see* Hemorrhage, retina
    ischemia H35.82
    macular degeneration — *see* Degeneration, macula
    microaneurysms H35.04- ☑
    microvascular abnormality NEC H35.09
    neovascularization — *see* Neovascularization, retina
    retinopathy — *see* Retinopathy
    separation of layers H35.70
      central serous chorioretinopathy H35.71- ☑
      pigment epithelium detachment (serous) H35.72- ☑
        hemorrhagic H35.73- ☑
    specified type NEC H35.89
    telangiectasis — *see* Telangiectasis, retina
    vasculitis — *see* Vasculitis, retina
  retroperitoneal K68.9
  right hemisphere organic affective F07.89
  rumination (infant or child) F98.21
  sacrum, sacrococcygeal NEC M53.3
  schizoaffective F25.9
    bipolar type F25.0
    depressive type F25.1
    manic type F25.0
    mixed type F25.0
    specified NEC F25.8
  schizoid of childhood F84.5
  schizophrenia spectrum and other psychotic disorder F29
    specified NEC F28
  schizophreniform F20.81
    brief F23
  schizotypal (personality) F21
  secretion, thyrocalcitonin E07.0
  sedative, hypnotic, or anxiolytic use
    mild F13.10
      with
        sedative, hypnotic, or anxiolytic intoxication F13.129
        sedative, hypnotic, or anxiolytic intoxication delirium F13.121
        sedative, hypnotic, or anxiolytic-induced
          anxiety disorder F13.180
          bipolar and related disorder F13.14
          depressive disorder F13.14
          psychotic disorder F13.159
          sexual dysfunction F13.181
      in remission (early) (sustained) F13.11
    moderate or severe F13.20
      with
        sedative, hypnotic, or anxiolytic intoxication F13.229
        sedative, hypnotic, or anxiolytic intoxication delirium F13.221

Disorder — *continued*
  sedative, hypnotic, or anxiolytic use — *continued*
    moderate or severe — *continued*
      with — *continued*
        sedative, hypnotic, or anxiolytic-induced
          anxiety disorder F13.280
          bipolar and related disorder F13.24
          depressive disorder F13.24
          major neurocognitive disorder F13.27
          mild neurocognitive disorder F13.288
          psychotic disorder F13.259
          sexual dysfunction F13.281
      in remission (early) (sustained) F13.21
  seizure — *see also* Epilepsy G40.909
    intractable G40.919
      with status epilepticus G40.911
  semantic pragmatic F80.89
    with autism F84.0
  sense of smell R43.1
    psychogenic F45.8
  separation anxiety, of childhood F93.0
  sexual
    aversion F52.1
    function, psychogenic F52.9
    interest/arousal, female F52.22
    masochism F65.51
    maturation F66
    nonorganic F52.9
    preference — *see also* Deviation, sexual F65.9
      fetishistic transvestism F65.1
    relationship F66
    sadism F65.52
  shyness, of childhood and adolescence F40.10
  sibling rivalry F93.8
  sickle-cell (sickling) (homozygous) — *see* Disease, sickle-cell
    heterozygous D57.3
    specified type NEC D57.8- ☑
    trait D57.3
  sinus (nasal) J34.9
    specified NEC J34.89
  skin L98.9
    atrophic L90.9
      specified NEC L90.8
    granulomatous L92.9
      specified NEC L92.8
    hypertrophic L91.9
      specified NEC L91.8
    infiltrative NEC L98.6
    newborn P83.9
      specified NEC P83.88
    picking F42.4
    psychogenic (allergic) (eczematous) F54
  sleep G47.9
    breathing-related — *see* Apnea, sleep
    circadian rhythm G47.20
      advance sleep phase type G47.22
      delayed sleep phase type G47.21
      due to
        alcohol
          abuse F10.182
          dependence F10.282
          use F10.982
        amphetamines
          abuse F15.182
          dependence F15.282
          use F15.982
        caffeine
          abuse F15.182
          dependence F15.282
          use F15.982
        cocaine
          abuse F14.182
          dependence F14.282
          use F14.982
        drug NEC
          abuse F19.182
          dependence F19.282
          use F19.982
        opioid
          abuse F11.182
          dependence F11.282
          use F11.982
        psychoactive substance NEC
          abuse F19.182
          dependence F19.282
          use F19.982
        sedative, hypnotic, or anxiolytic
          abuse F13.182

Disorder — *continued*
  sleep — *continued*
    circadian rhythm — *continued*
      due to — *continued*
        sedative, hypnotic, or anxiolytic — *continued*
          dependence F13.282
          use F13.982
        stimulant NEC
          abuse F15.182
          dependence F15.282
          use F15.982
      free running type G47.24
      in conditions classified elsewhere G47.27
      irregular sleep wake type G47.23
      jet lag type G47.25
      non-24-hour sleep-wake type G47.24
      shift work type G47.26
      specified NEC G47.29
    due to
      alcohol
        abuse F10.182
        dependence F10.282
        use F10.982
      amphetamine
        abuse F15.182
        dependence F15.282
        use F15.982
      anxiolytic
        abuse F13.182
        dependence F13.282
        use F13.982
      caffeine
        abuse F15.182
        dependence F15.282
        use F15.982
      cocaine
        abuse F14.182
        dependence F14.282
        use F14.982
      drug NEC
        abuse F19.182
        dependence F19.282
        use F19.982
      hypnotic
        abuse F13.182
        dependence F13.282
        use F13.982
      opioid
        abuse F11.182
        dependence F11.282
        use F11.982
      psychoactive substance NEC
        abuse F19.182
        dependence F19.282
        use F19.982
      sedative
        abuse F13.182
        dependence F13.282
        use F13.982
      stimulant NEC
        abuse F15.182
        dependence F15.282
        use F15.982
    emotional F51.9
    excessive somnolence — *see* Hypersomnia
    hypersomnia type — *see* Hypersomnia
    initiating or maintaining — *see* Insomnia
    nightmares F51.5
    nonorganic F51.9
      specified NEC F51.8
    parasomnia type G47.50
    specified NEC G47.8
    terrors F51.4
    walking F51.3
  sleep-wake pattern or schedule — *see also* Disorder, sleep, circadian rhythm G47.9
    specified NEC G47.8
  social
    anxiety (of childhood) F40.10
      generalized F40.11
    functioning in childhood F94.9
      specified NEC F94.8
    pragmatic F80.82
  soft tissue M79.9
    ankle M79.9
    due to use, overuse and pressure M70.90
      ankle M70.97- ☑
      bursitis — *see* Bursitis

Disorder — *continued*
  soft tissue — *continued*
    due to use, overuse and pressure — *continued*
      foot M70.97- ☑
      forearm M70.93- ☑
      hand M70.94- ☑
      lower leg M70.96- ☑
      multiple sites M70.99
      pelvic region M70.95- ☑
      shoulder region M70.91- ☑
      specified site NEC M70.98
      specified type NEC M70.80
        ankle M70.87- ☑
        foot M70.87- ☑
        forearm M70.83- ☑
        hand M70.84- ☑
        lower leg M70.86- ☑
        multiple sites M70.89
        pelvic region M70.85- ☑
        shoulder region M70.81- ☑
        specified site NEC M70.88
        thigh M70.85- ☑
        upper arm M70.82- ☑
      thigh M70.95- ☑
      upper arm M70.92- ☑
    foot M79.9
    forearm M79.9
    hand M79.9
    lower leg M79.9
    multiple sites M79.9
    occupational — *see* Disorder, soft tissue, due to use, overuse and pressure
    pelvic region M79.9
    shoulder region M79.9
    specified type NEC M79.89
    thigh M79.9
    upper arm M79.9
  somatic symptom F45.1
  somatization F45.0
  somatoform F45.9
    pain (persistent) F45.41
    somatization (multiple) (long-lasting) F45.0
    specified NEC F45.8
    undifferentiated F45.1
  somnolence, excessive — *see* Hypersomnia
  specific
    arithmetical F81.2
    developmental, of motor F82
    reading F81.0
    speech and language F80.9
    spelling F81.81
    written expression F81.81
  speech R47.9
    articulation (functional) (specific) F80.0
    developmental F80.9
    specified NEC R47.89
  speech-sound F80.0
  spelling (specific) F81.81
  spine — *see also* Dorsopathy
    ligamentous or muscular attachments, peripheral — *see* Enthesopathy, spinal
    specified NEC — *see* Dorsopathy, specified NEC
  stereotyped, habit or movement F98.4
  stimulant use (other) (unspecified)
    mild F15.10
      in remission (early) (sustained) F15.11
    moderate or severe F15.20
      in remission (early) (sustained) F15.21
  stomach (functional) — *see* Disorder, gastric
  stress F43.9
    acute F43.0
    post-traumatic F43.10
      acute F43.11
      chronic F43.12
  substance use (other) (unknown)
    mild F19.10
      with substance-induced
        anxiety disorder F19.180
        bipolar and related disorder F19.14
        depressive disorder F19.14
        major neurocognitive disorder F19.17
        mild neurocognitive disorder F19.188
        obsessive-compulsive and related disorder F19.188
        sexual dysfunction F19.181
      substance intoxication F19.129
      substance intoxication delirium F19.121
    moderate or severe F19.20

Disorder — *continued*
  substance use — *continued*
    moderate or severe — *continued*
      with substance-induced
        anxiety disorder F19.280
        bipolar and related disorder F19.24
        depressive disorder F19.24
        major neurocognitive disorder F19.27
        mild neurocognitive disorder F19.288
        obsessive-compulsive and related disorder F19.288
        sexual dysfunction F19.281
      in remission (early) (sustained) F19.21
      substance intoxication F19.229
      substance intoxication delirium F19.221
  sulfur-bearing amino-acid metabolism E72.10
  sweat gland (eccrine) L74.9
    apocrine L75.9
      specified NEC L75.8
    specified NEC L74.8
  synovium M67.90
    acromioclavicular M67.91- ☑
    ankle M67.97- ☑
    elbow M67.92- ☑
    foot M67.97- ☑
    forearm M67.93- ☑
    hand M67.94- ☑
    hip M67.95- ☑
    knee M67.96- ☑
    multiple sites M67.99
    rupture — *see* Rupture, synovium
    shoulder M67.91- ☑
    specified type NEC M67.80
      acromioclavicular M67.81- ☑
      ankle M67.87- ☑
      elbow M67.82- ☑
      foot M67.87- ☑
      hand M67.84- ☑
      hip M67.85- ☑
      knee M67.86- ☑
      multiple sites M67.89
      wrist M67.83- ☑
    synovitis — *see* Synovitis
    upper arm M67.92- ☑
    wrist M67.93- ☑
  temperature regulation, newborn P81.9
    specified NEC P81.8
  temporomandibular joint M26.60- ☑
  tendon M67.90
    acromioclavicular M67.91- ☑
    ankle M67.97- ☑
    contracture — *see* Contracture, tendon
    elbow M67.92- ☑
    foot M67.97- ☑
    forearm M67.93- ☑
    hand M67.94- ☑
    hip M67.95- ☑
    knee M67.96- ☑
    multiple sites M67.99
    rupture — *see* Rupture, tendon
    shoulder M67.91- ☑
    specified type NEC M67.80
      acromioclavicular M67.81- ☑
      ankle M67.87- ☑
      elbow M67.82- ☑
      foot M67.87- ☑
      hand M67.84- ☑
      hip M67.85- ☑
      knee M67.86- ☑
      multiple sites M67.89
      trunk M67.88
      wrist M67.83- ☑
    synovitis — *see* Synovitis
    tendinitis — *see* Tendinitis
    tenosynovitis — *see* Tenosynovitis
    trunk M67.98
    upper arm M67.92- ☑
    wrist M67.93- ☑
  thoracic root (nerve) NEC G54.3
  thyrocalcitonin hypersecretion E07.0
  thyroid (gland) E07.9
    function NEC, neonatal, transitory P72.2
    iodine-deficiency related E01.8
    specified NEC E07.89
  tic — *see* Tic

☑ **Additional Character Required** — Refer to the Tabular List for Character Selection
▽ Subterms under main terms may continue to next column or page

Disorder — *continued*
  tobacco use
    chewing tobacco (mild) (moderate) (severe)
      in remission (early) (sustained) F17.221
    cigarettes (mild) (moderate) (severe)
      in remission (early) (sustained) F17.211
    mild F17.200
      in remission (early) (sustained) F17.201
    moderate F17.200
      in remission (early) (sustained) F17.201
    severe F17.200
      in remission (early) (sustained) F17.201
    specified product NEC (mild) (moderate) (severe)
      in remission (early) (sustained) F17.291
  tooth K08.9
    development K00.9
      specified NEC K00.8
    eruption K00.6
  Tourette's F95.2
  trance and possession F44.89
  transvestic F65.1
  trauma and stressor-related F43.9
    other specified F43.8
  tricuspid (valve) — *see* Endocarditis, tricuspid
  tryptophan metabolism E70.5
  tubular, phosphate-losing N25.0
  tubulo-interstitial (in)
    brucellosis A23.9 *[N16]*
    cystinosis E72.04
    diphtheria A36.84
    glycogen storage disease E74.00 *[N16]*
    leukemia NEC C95.9- ☑ *[N16]*
    lymphoma NEC C85.9- ☑ *[N16]*
    mixed cryoglobulinemia D89.1 *[N16]*
    multiple myeloma C90.0- ☑ *[N16]*
    Salmonella infection A02.25
    sarcoidosis D86.84
    sepsis A41.9 *[N16]*
      streptococcal A40.9 *[N16]*
    systemic lupus erythematosus M32.15
    toxoplasmosis B58.83
    transplant rejection T86.91 *[N16]*
    Wilson's disease E83.01 *[N16]*
  tubulo-renal function, impaired N25.9
    specified NEC N25.89
  tympanic membrane H73.9- ☑
    atrophy — *see* Atrophy, tympanic membrane
    infection — *see* Myringitis
    perforation — *see* Perforation, tympanum
    specified NEC H73.89- ☑
  unsocialized aggressive F91.1
  urea cycle metabolism E72.20
    argininemia E72.21
    arginosuccinic aciduria E72.22
    citrullinemia E72.23
    ornithine transcarbamylase deficiency E72.4
    other specified E72.29
  ureter (in) N28.9
    schistosomiasis B65.0 *[N29]*
    tuberculosis A18.11
  urethra N36.9
    specified NEC N36.8
  urinary system N39.9
    specified NEC N39.8
  valve, heart
    aortic — *see* Endocarditis, aortic
    mitral — *see* Endocarditis, mitral
    pulmonary — *see* Endocarditis, pulmonary
    rheumatic
      aortic — *see* Endocarditis, aortic, rheumatic
      mitral — *see* Endocarditis, mitral
      pulmonary — *see* Endocarditis, pulmonary, rheumatic
      tricuspid — *see* Endocarditis, tricuspid
    tricuspid — *see* Endocarditis, tricuspid
  vestibular function H81.9- ☑
    specified NEC — *see* subcategory H81.8 ☑
      in diseases classified elsewhere H82.- ☑
    vertigo — *see* Vertigo
  vision, binocular H53.30
    abnormal retinal correspondence H53.31
    diplopia H53.2
    fusion with defective stereopsis H53.32
    simultaneous perception H53.33
    suppression H53.34
  visual
    cortex
      blindness H47.619

Disorder — *continued*
  visual — *continued*
    cortex — *continued*
      blindness — *continued*
        left brain H47.612
        right brain H47.611
      due to
        inflammatory disorder H47.629
          left brain H47.622
          right brain H47.621
        neoplasm H47.639
          left brain H47.632
          right brain H47.631
        vascular disorder H47.649
          left brain H47.642
          right brain H47.641
    pathway H47.9
      due to
        inflammatory disorder H47.51- ☑
        neoplasm H47.52- ☑
        vascular disorder H47.53- ☑
    optic chiasm — *see* Disorder, optic, chiasm
  vitreous body H43.9
    crystalline deposits — *see* Deposit, crystalline
    degeneration — *see* Degeneration, vitreous
    hemorrhage — *see* Hemorrhage, vitreous
    opacities — *see* Opacity, vitreous
    prolapse — *see* Prolapse, vitreous
    specified type NEC H43.89
  voice R49.9
    specified type NEC R49.8
  volatile solvent use
    due to drug abuse — *see* Abuse, drug, inhalant
    due to drug dependence — *see* Dependence, drug, inhalant
  voyeuristic F65.3
  white blood cells D72.9
    specified NEC D72.89
  withdrawing, child or adolescent F40.10
Disorientation R41.0
Displacement, displaced
  acquired traumatic of bone, cartilage, joint, tendon NEC — *see* Dislocation
  adrenal gland (congenital) Q89.1
  appendix, retrocecal (congenital) Q43.8
  auricle (congenital) Q17.4
  bladder (acquired) N32.89
    congenital Q64.19
  brachial plexus (congenital) Q07.8
  brain stem, caudal (congenital) Q04.8
  canaliculus (lacrimalis), congenital Q10.6
  cardia through esophageal hiatus (congenital) Q40.1
  cerebellum, caudal (congenital) Q04.8
  cervix — *see* Malposition, uterus
  colon (congenital) Q43.3
  device, implant or graft — *see also* Complications, by site and type, mechanical T85.628 ☑
    arterial graft NEC — *see* Complication, cardiovascular device, mechanical, vascular
    breast (implant) T85.42 ☑
    catheter NEC T85.628 ☑
      dialysis (renal) T82.42 ☑
        intraperitoneal T85.621 ☑
      infusion NEC T82.524 ☑
        spinal (epidural) (subdural) T85.620 ☑
      urinary
        cystostomy T83.020 ☑
        Hopkins T83.028 ☑
        ileostomy T83.028 ☑
        indwelling T83.021 ☑
        nephrostomy T83.022 ☑
        specified NEC T83.028 ☑
        urostomy T83.028 ☑
    electronic (electrode) (pulse generator) (stimulator) — *see* Complication, electronic stimulator
    fixation, internal (orthopedic) NEC — *see* Complication, fixation device, mechanical
    gastrointestinal — *see* Complications, prosthetic device, mechanical, gastrointestinal device
    genital NEC T83.428 ☑
      intrauterine contraceptive device (string) T83.32 ☑
      penile prosthesis (cylinder) (implanted) (pump) (reservoir) T83.420 ☑
      testicular prosthesis T83.421 ☑
    heart NEC — *see* Complication, cardiovascular device, mechanical

Displacement, displaced — *continued*
  device, implant or graft — *see also* Complications, by site and type, mechanical — *continued*
    joint prosthesis — *see* Complications, joint prosthesis, mechanical
    ocular — *see* Complications, prosthetic device, mechanical, ocular device
    orthopedic NEC — *see* Complication, orthopedic, device or graft, mechanical
    specified NEC T85.628 ☑
    urinary NEC T83.128 ☑
      graft T83.22 ☑
      sphincter, implanted T83.121 ☑
      stent (ileal conduit) (nephroureteral) T83.123 ☑
        ureteral indwelling T83.122 ☑
    vascular NEC — *see* Complication, cardiovascular device, mechanical
    ventricular intracranial shunt T85.02 ☑
  electronic stimulator
    bone T84.320 ☑
    cardiac — *see* Complications, cardiac device, electronic
    nervous system — *see* Complication, prosthetic device, mechanical, electronic nervous system stimulator
    urinary — *see* Complications, electronic stimulator, urinary
  esophageal mucosa into cardia of stomach, congenital Q39.8
  esophagus (acquired) K22.8
    congenital Q39.8
  eyeball (acquired) (lateral) (old) — *see* Displacement, globe
    congenital Q15.8
    current — *see* Avulsion, eye
  fallopian tube (acquired) N83.4- ☑
    congenital Q50.6
    opening (congenital) Q50.6
  gallbladder (congenital) Q44.1
  gastric mucosa (congenital) Q40.2
  globe (acquired) (old) (lateral) H05.21- ☑
    current — *see* Avulsion, eye
  heart (congenital) Q24.8
    acquired I51.89
  hymen (upward) (congenital) Q52.4
  intervertebral disc NEC
    with myelopathy — *see* Disorder, disc, with, myelopathy
    cervical, cervicothoracic (with) M50.20
      myelopathy — *see* Disorder, disc, cervical, with myelopathy
      neuritis, radiculitis or radiculopathy — *see* Disorder, disc, cervical, with neuritis
    due to trauma — *see* Dislocation, vertebra
    lumbar region M51.26
      with
        myelopathy M51.06
        neuritis, radiculitis, radiculopathy or sciatica M51.16
    lumbosacral region M51.27
      with
        neuritis, radiculitis, radiculopathy or sciatica M51.17
    sacrococcygeal region M53.3
    thoracic region M51.24
      with
        myelopathy M51.04
        neuritis, radiculitis, radiculopathy M51.14
    thoracolumbar region M51.25
      with
        myelopathy M51.05
        neuritis, radiculitis, radiculopathy M51.15
  intrauterine device (string) T83.32 ☑
  kidney (acquired) N28.83
    congenital Q63.2
  lachrymal, lacrimal apparatus or duct (congenital) Q10.6
  lens, congenital Q12.1
  macula (congenital) Q14.1
  Meckel's diverticulum Q43.0
    malignant — *see* Table of Neoplasms, small intestine, malignant
  nail (congenital) Q84.6
    acquired L60.8
  opening of Wharton's duct in mouth Q38.4
  organ or site, congenital NEC — *see* Malposition, congenital
  ovary (acquired) N83.4- ☑
    congenital Q50.39

Displacement, displaced — *continued*
ovary — *continued*
free in peritoneal cavity (congenital) Q50.39
into hernial sac N83.4- ☑
oviduct (acquired) N83.4- ☑
congenital Q50.6
parathyroid (gland) E21.4
parotid gland (congenital) Q38.4
punctum lacrimale (congenital) Q10.6
sacro-iliac (joint) (congenital) Q74.2
current injury S33.2 ☑
old — *see* subcategory M53.2 ☑
salivary gland (any) (congenital) Q38.4
spleen (congenital) Q89.09
stomach, congenital Q40.2
sublingual duct Q38.4
tongue (downward) (congenital) Q38.3
tooth, teeth, fully erupted M26.30
horizontal M26.33
vertical M26.34
trachea (congenital) Q32.1
ureter or ureteric opening or orifice (congenital) Q62.62
uterine opening of oviducts or fallopian tubes Q50.6
uterus, uterine — *see* Malposition, uterus
ventricular septum Q21.0
with rudimentary ventricle Q20.4
Disproportion
between native and reconstructed breast N65.1
fiber-type G71.20
congenital G71.29
Disruptio uteri — *see* Rupture, uterus
Disruption (of)
ciliary body NEC H21.89
closure of
cornea T81.31 ☑
craniotomy T81.32 ☑
fascia (muscular) (superficial) T81.32 ☑
internal organ or tissue T81.32 ☑
laceration (external) (internal) T81.33 ☑
ligament T81.32 ☑
mucosa T81.31 ☑
muscle or muscle flap T81.32 ☑
ribs or rib cage T81.32 ☑
skin and subcutaneous tissue (full-thickness) (superficial) T81.31 ☑
skull T81.32 ☑
sternum (sternotomy) T81.32 ☑
tendon T81.32 ☑
traumatic laceration (external) (internal) T81.33 ☑
family Z63.8
due to
absence of family member due to military deployment Z63.31
absence of family member NEC Z63.32
alcoholism and drug addiction in family Z63.72
bereavement Z63.4
death (assumed) or disappearance of family
member Z63.4
divorce or separation Z63.5
drug addiction in family Z63.72
return of family member from military deployment (current or past conflict) Z63.71
stressful life events NEC Z63.79
iris NEC H21.89
ligament(s) — *see also* Sprain
knee
current injury — *see* Dislocation, knee
old (chronic) — *see* Derangement, knee, instability
spontaneous NEC — *see* Derangement, knee,
disruption ligament
ossicular chain — *see* Discontinuity, ossicles, ear
pelvic ring (stable) S32.810 ☑
unstable S32.811 ☑
traumatic injury wound repair T81.33 ☑
wound T81.30 ☑
episiotomy O90.1
operation T81.31 ☑
cesarean O90.0
external operation wound (superficial) T81.31 ☑
internal operation wound (deep) T81.32 ☑
perineal (obstetric) O90.1
traumatic injury repair T81.33 ☑
Dissatisfaction with
employment Z56.9
school environment Z55.4
Dissecting — *see* condition

Dissection
aorta I71.00
abdominal I71.02
thoracic I71.01
thoracoabdominal I71.03
artery I77.70
basilar (trunk) I77.75
carotid I77.71
cerebral (nonruptured) I67.0
ruptured — *see* Hemorrhage, intracranial, subarachnoid
coronary I25.42
extremity
lower I77.77
upper I77.76
iliac I77.72
precerebral
congenital (nonruptured) Q28.1
specified site NEC I77.75
renal I77.73
specified NEC I77.79
vertebral I77.74
precerebral artery, congenital (nonruptured) Q28.1
Heartland A93.8
traumatic — *see* Wound, open, by site
vascular I99.8
wound — *see* Wound, open
Disseminated — *see* condition
Dissociation
auriculoventricular or atrioventricular (AV) (any degree)
(isorhythmic) I45.89
with heart block I44.2
interference I45.89
Dissociative reaction, state F44.9
Dissolution, vertebra — *see* Osteoporosis
Distension, distention
abdomen R14.0
bladder N32.89
cecum K63.89
colon K63.89
gallbladder K82.8
intestine K63.89
kidney N28.89
liver K76.89
seminal vesicle N50.89
stomach K31.89
acute K31.0
psychogenic F45.8
ureter — *see* Dilatation, ureter
uterus N85.8
Distoma hepaticum infestation B66.3
Distomiasis B66.9
bile passages B66.3
hemic B65.9
hepatic B66.3
due to Clonorchis sinensis B66.1
intestinal B66.5
liver B66.3
due to Clonorchis sinensis B66.1
lung B66.4
pulmonary B66.4
Distomolar (fourth molar) K00.1
Disto-occlusion (Division I) (Division II) M26.212
Distortion(s) (congenital)
adrenal (gland) Q89.1
arm NEC Q68.8
bile duct or passage Q44.5
bladder Q64.79
brain Q04.9
cervix (uteri) Q51.9
chest (wall) Q67.8
bones Q76.8
clavicle Q74.0
clitoris Q52.6
coccyx Q76.49
common duct Q44.5
coronary Q24.5
cystic duct Q44.5
ear (auricle) (external) Q17.3
inner Q16.5
middle Q16.4
ossicles Q16.3
endocrine NEC Q89.2
eustachian tube Q17.8
eye (adnexa) Q15.8
face bone(s) NEC Q75.8
fallopian tube Q50.6
femur NEC Q68.8

Distortion(s) — *continued*
fibula NEC Q68.8
finger(s) Q68.1
foot Q66.9- ☑
genitalia, genital organ(s)
female Q52.8
external Q52.79
internal NEC Q52.8
gyri Q04.8
hand bone(s) Q68.1
heart (auricle) (ventricle) Q24.8
valve (cusp) Q24.8
hepatic duct Q44.5
humerus NEC Q68.8
hymen Q52.4
intrafamilial communications Z63.8
jaw NEC M26.89
labium (majus) (minus) Q52.79
leg NEC Q68.8
lens Q12.8
liver Q44.7
lumbar spine Q76.49
with disproportion O33.8
causing obstructed labor O65.0
lumbosacral (joint) (region) Q76.49
kyphosis — *see* Kyphosis, congenital
lordosis — *see* Lordosis, congenital
nerve Q07.8
nose Q30.8
organ
of Corti Q16.5
or site not listed — *see* Anomaly, by site
ossicles, ear Q16.3
oviduct Q50.6
pancreas Q45.3
parathyroid (gland) Q89.2
pituitary (gland) Q89.2
radius NEC Q68.8
sacroiliac joint Q74.2
sacrum Q76.49
scapula Q74.0
shoulder girdle Q74.0
skull bone(s) NEC Q75.8
with
anencephalus Q00.0
encephalocele — *see* Encephalocele
hydrocephalus Q03.9
with spina bifida — *see* Spina bifida, with
hydrocephalus
microcephaly Q02
spinal cord Q06.8
spine Q76.49
kyphosis — *see* Kyphosis, congenital
lordosis — *see* Lordosis, congenital
spleen Q89.09
sternum NEC Q76.7
thorax (wall) Q67.8
bony Q76.8
thymus (gland) Q89.2
thyroid (gland) Q89.2
tibia NEC Q68.8
toe(s) Q66.9- ☑
tongue Q38.3
trachea (cartilage) Q32.1
ulna NEC Q68.8
ureter Q62.8
urethra Q64.79
causing obstruction Q64.39
uterus Q51.9
vagina Q52.4
vertebra Q76.49
kyphosis — *see* Kyphosis, congenital
lordosis — *see* Lordosis, congenital
visual — *see also* Disturbance, vision
shape and size H53.15
vulva Q52.79
wrist (bones) (joint) Q68.8
Distress
abdomen — *see* Pain, abdominal
acute respiratory R06.03
syndrome (adult) (child) J80
epigastric R10.13
fetal P84
complicating pregnancy — *see* Stress, fetal
gastrointestinal (functional) K30
psychogenic F45.8
intestinal (functional) NOS K59.9
psychogenic F45.8

122

☑ **Additional Character Required** — Refer to the Tabular List for Character Selection
▽ **Subterms under main terms may continue to next column or page**

Distress — *continued*
  maternal, during labor and delivery O75.0
  relationship, with spouse or intimate partner Z63.0
  respiratory (adult) (child) R06.03
    newborn P22.9
      specified NEC P22.8
    orthopnea R06.01
    psychogenic F45.8
    shortness of breath R06.02
    specified type NEC R06.09
Distribution vessel, atypical Q27.9
  coronary artery Q24.5
  precerebral Q28.1
Districhiasis L68.8
Disturbance(s) — *see also* Disease
  absorption K90.9
    calcium E58
    carbohydrate K90.49
    fat K90.49
      pancreatic K90.3
    protein K90.49
    starch K90.49
    vitamin — *see* Deficiency, vitamin
  acid-base equilibrium E87.8
    mixed E87.4
  activity and attention (with hyperkinesis) — *see* Disorder, attention-deficit hyperactivity
  amino acid transport E72.00
  assimilation, food K90.9
  auditory nerve, except deafness — *see* subcategory H93.3 ☑
  behavior — *see* Disorder, conduct
  blood clotting (mechanism) — *see also* Defect, coagulation D68.9
  cerebral
    nerve — *see* Disorder, nerve, cranial
    status, newborn P91.9
      specified NEC P91.88
  circulatory I99.9
  conduct — *see also* Disorder, conduct F91.9
    adjustment reaction — *see* Disorder, adjustment
    compulsive F63.9
    disruptive F91.9
    hyperkinetic — *see* Disorder, attention-deficit hyperactivity
    socialized F91.2
    specified NEC F91.8
    unsocialized F91.1
  coordination R27.8
  cranial nerve — *see* Disorder, nerve, cranial
  deep sensibility — *see* Disturbance, sensation
  digestive K30
    psychogenic F45.8
  electrolyte — *see also* Imbalance, electrolyte
    newborn, transitory P74.49
      hyperammonemia P74.6
      hyperchloremia P74.421
      hyperchloremic metabolic acidosis P74.421
      hypochloremia P74.422
      potassium balance
        hyperkalemia P74.31
        hypokalemia P74.32
      sodium balance
        hypernatremia P74.21
        hyponatremia P74.22
      specified type NEC P74.49
  emotions specific to childhood and adolescence F93.9
    with
      anxiety and fearfulness NEC F93.8
      elective mutism F94.0
      oppositional disorder F91.3
      sensitivity (withdrawal) F40.10
      shyness F40.10
      social withdrawal F40.10
    involving relationship problems F93.8
    mixed F93.8
    specified NEC F93.8
  endocrine (gland) E34.9
    neonatal, transitory P72.9
      specified NEC P72.8
  equilibrium R42
  fructose metabolism E74.10
  gait — *see* Gait
    hysterical F44.4
    psychogenic F44.4
  gastrointestinal (functional) K30
    psychogenic F45.8
  habit, child F98.9

Disturbance(s) — *continued*
  hearing, except deafness and tinnitus — *see* Abnormal, auditory perception
  heart, functional (conditions in I44-I50)
    due to presence of (cardiac) prosthesis I97.19- ☑
    postoperative I97.89
      cardiac surgery — *see also* Infarct, myocardium, associated with revascularization procedure I97.19- ☑
  hormones E34.9
  innervation uterus (parasympathetic) (sympathetic) N85.8
  keratinization NEC
    gingiva K05.10
      nonplaque induced K05.11
      plaque induced K05.10
    lip K13.0
    oral (mucosa) (soft tissue) K13.29
    tongue K13.29
  learning (specific) — *see* Disorder, learning
  memory — *see* Amnesia
    mild, following organic brain damage F06.8
  mental F99
    associated with diseases classified elsewhere F54
  metabolism E88.9
    with
      abortion — *see* Abortion, by type with other specified complication
      ectopic pregnancy O08.5
      molar pregnancy O08.5
    amino-acid E72.9
      aromatic E70.9
      branched-chain E71.2
      straight-chain E72.89
      sulfur-bearing E72.10
    ammonia E72.20
    arginine E72.21
    arginosuccinic acid E72.22
    carbohydrate E74.9
    cholesterol E78.9
    citrulline E72.23
    cystathionine E72.19
    general E88.9
    glutamine E72.89
    histidine E70.40
    homocystine E72.19
    hydroxylysine E72.3
    in labor or delivery O75.89
    iron E83.10
    lipoid E78.9
    lysine E72.3
    methionine E72.19
    neonatal, transitory P74.9
      calcium and magnesium P71.9
        specified type NEC P71.8
      carbohydrate metabolism P70.9
        specified type NEC P70.8
      specified NEC P74.8
    ornithine E72.4
    phosphate E83.39
    sodium NEC E87.8
    threonine E72.89
    tryptophan E70.5
    tyrosine E70.20
    urea cycle E72.20
  motor R29.2
  nervous, functional R45.0
  neuromuscular mechanism (eye), due to syphilis A52.15
  nutritional E63.9
    nail L60.3
  ocular motion H51.9
    psychogenic F45.8
  oculogyric H51.8
    psychogenic F45.8
  oculomotor H51.9
    psychogenic F45.8
  olfactory nerve R43.1
  optic nerve NEC — *see* Disorder, nerve, optic
  oral epithelium, including tongue NEC K13.29
  perceptual due to
    alcohol withdrawal F10.232
    amphetamine intoxication F15.922
      in
        abuse F15.122
        dependence F15.222
    anxiolytic withdrawal F13.232
    cannabis intoxication (acute) F12.922

Disturbance(s) — *continued*
  perceptual due to — *continued*
    cannabis intoxication — *continued*
      in
        abuse F12.122
        dependence F12.222
    cocaine intoxication (acute) F14.922
      in
        abuse F14.122
        dependence F14.222
    hypnotic withdrawal F13.232
    opioid intoxication (acute) F11.922
      in
        abuse F11.122
        dependence F11.222
    phencyclidine intoxication (acute) F16.122
    sedative withdrawal F13.232
  personality (pattern) (trait) — *see also* Disorder, personality F60.9
    following organic brain damage F07.9
  polyglandular E31.9
    specified NEC E31.8
  potassium balance, newborn
    hyperkalemia P74.31
    hypokalemia P74.32
  psychogenic F45.9
  psychomotor F44.4
  psychophysical visual H53.16
  pupillary — *see* Anomaly, pupil, function
  reflex R29.2
  rhythm, heart I49.9
  salivary secretion K11.7
  sensation (cold) (heat) (localization) (tactile discrimination) (texture) (vibratory) NEC R20.9
    hysterical F44.6
    skin R20.9
      anesthesia R20.0
      hyperesthesia R20.3
      hypoesthesia R20.1
      paresthesia R20.2
      specified type NEC R20.8
    smell R43.9
      and taste (mixed) R43.8
      anosmia R43.0
      parosmia R43.1
      specified NEC R43.8
    taste R43.9
      and smell (mixed) R43.8
      parageusia R43.2
      specified NEC R43.8
  sensory — *see* Disturbance, sensation
  situational (transient) — *see also* Disorder, adjustment
    acute F43.0
  sleep G47.9
    nonorganic origin F51.9
  smell — *see* Disturbance, sensation, smell
  sociopathic F60.2
  sodium balance, newborn
    hypernatremia P74.21
    hyponatremia P74.22
  speech R47.9
    developmental F80.9
    specified NEC R47.89
  stomach (functional) K31.9
  sympathetic (nerve) G90.9
  taste — *see* Disturbance, sensation, taste
  temperature
    regulation, newborn P81.9
      specified NEC P81.8
    sense R20.8
      hysterical F44.6
  tooth
    eruption K00.6
    formation K00.4
    structure, hereditary NEC K00.5
  touch — *see* Disturbance, sensation
  vascular I99.9
    arteriosclerotic — *see* Arteriosclerosis
  vasomotor I73.9
  vasospastic I73.9
  vision, visual H53.9
    following
      cerebral infarction I69.398
      cerebrovascular disease I69.998
        specified NEC I69.898
      intracerebral hemorrhage I69.198
      nontraumatic intracranial hemorrhage NEC I69.298

Disturbance(s) — continued
  vision, visual — continued
    following — continued
      specified disease NEC I69.898
      subarachnoid hemorrhage I69.098
    psychophysical H53.16
    specified NEC H53.8
    subjective H53.10
      day blindness H53.11
      discomfort H53.14- ☑
      distortions of shape and size H53.15
      loss
        sudden H53.13- ☑
        transient H53.12- ☑
      specified type NEC H53.19
  voice R49.9
    psychogenic F44.4
    specified NEC R49.8
Diuresis R35.8
Diver's palsy, paralysis or squeeze T70.3 ☑
Diverticulitis (acute) K57.92
  bladder — see Cystitis
  ileum — see Diverticulitis, intestine, small
  intestine K57.92
    with
      abscess, perforation K57.80
        with bleeding K57.81
      bleeding K57.93
    congenital Q43.8
    large K57.32
      with
        abscess, perforation K57.20
          with bleeding K57.21
        bleeding K57.33
        small intestine K57.52
          with
            abscess, perforation K57.40
              with bleeding K57.41
            bleeding K57.53
    small K57.12
      with
        abscess, perforation K57.00
          with bleeding K57.01
        bleeding K57.13
        large intestine K57.52
          with
            abscess, perforation K57.40
              with bleeding K57.41
            bleeding K57.53
Diverticulosis K57.90
  with bleeding K57.91
  large intestine K57.30
    with
      bleeding K57.31
      small intestine K57.50
        with bleeding K57.51
  small intestine K57.10
    with
      bleeding K57.11
      large intestine K57.50
        with bleeding K57.51
Diverticulum, diverticula (multiple) K57.90
  appendix (noninflammatory) K38.2
  bladder (sphincter) N32.3
    congenital Q64.6
  bronchus (congenital) Q32.4
    acquired J98.09
  calyx, calyceal (kidney) N28.89
  cardia (stomach) K31.4
  cecum — see Diverticulosis, intestine, large
    congenital Q43.8
  colon — see Diverticulosis, intestine, large
    congenital Q43.8
  duodenum — see Diverticulosis, intestine, small
    congenital Q43.8
  epiphrenic (esophagus) K22.5
  esophagus (congenital) Q39.6
    acquired (epiphrenic) (pulsion) (traction) K22.5
  eustachian tube — see Disorder, eustachian tube,
    specified NEC
  fallopian tube N83.8
  gastric K31.4
  heart (congenital) Q24.8
  ileum — see Diverticulosis, intestine, small
  jejunum — see Diverticulosis, intestine, small
  kidney (pelvis) (calyces) N28.89
    with calculus — see Calculus, kidney
  Meckel's (displaced) (hypertrophic) Q43.0

Diverticulum, diverticula — continued
  Meckel's — continued
    malignant — see Table of Neoplasms, small intes-
      tine, malignant
  midthoracic K22.5
  organ or site, congenital NEC — see Distortion
  pericardium (congenital) (cyst) Q24.8
    acquired I31.8
  pharyngoesophageal (congenital) Q39.6
    acquired K22.5
  pharynx (congenital) Q38.7
  rectosigmoid — see Diverticulosis, intestine, large
    congenital Q43.8
  rectum — see Diverticulosis, intestine, large
  Rokitansky's K22.5
  seminal vesicle N50.89
  sigmoid — see Diverticulosis, intestine, large
    congenital Q43.8
  stomach (acquired) K31.4
    congenital Q40.2
  trachea (acquired) J39.8
  ureter (acquired) N28.89
    congenital Q62.8
  ureterovesical orifice N28.89
  urethra (acquired) N36.1
    congenital Q64.79
  ventricle, left (congenital) Q24.8
  vesical N32.3
    congenital Q64.6
  Zenker's (esophagus) K22.5
Division
  cervix uteri (acquired) N88.8
  glans penis Q55.69
  labia minora (congenital) Q52.79
  ligament (partial or complete) (current) — see also
    Sprain
    with open wound — see Wound, open
  muscle (partial or complete) (current) — see also Injury,
    muscle
    with open wound — see Wound, open
  nerve (traumatic) — see Injury, nerve
  spinal cord — see Injury, spinal cord, by region
  vein I87.8
Divorce, causing family disruption Z63.5
Dix-Hallpike neurolabyrinthitis — see Neuronitis,
  vestibular
Dizziness R42
  hysterical F44.89
  psychogenic F45.8
DMAC (disseminated mycobacterium avium-intracellulare
  complex) A31.2
DNR (do not resuscitate) Z66
Doan-Wiseman syndrome (primary splenic neutropenia)
  — see Agranulocytosis
Doehle-Heller aortitis A52.02
Dog bite — see Bite
Dohle body panmyelopathic syndrome D72.0
Dolichocephaly Q67.2
Dolichocolon Q43.8
Dolichostenomelia — see Syndrome, Marfan's
Donohue's syndrome E34.8
Donor (organ or tissue) Z52.9
  blood (whole) Z52.000
    autologous Z52.010
    specified component (lymphocytes) (platelets) NEC
      Z52.008
      autologous Z52.018
      specified donor NEC Z52.098
    specified donor NEC Z52.090
    stem cells Z52.001
      autologous Z52.011
      specified donor NEC Z52.091
  bone Z52.20
    autologous Z52.21
    marrow Z52.3
    specified type NEC Z52.29
  cornea Z52.5
  egg (Oocyte) Z52.819
    age 35 and over Z52.812
      anonymous recipient Z52.812
      designated recipient Z52.813
    under age 35 Z52.810
      anonymous recipient Z52.810
      designated recipient Z52.811
  kidney Z52.4
  liver Z52.6
  lung Z52.89

Donor — continued
  lymphocyte — see Donor, blood, specified components
    NEC
  Oocyte — see Donor, egg
  platelets Z52.008
  potential, examination of Z00.5
  semen Z52.89
  skin Z52.10
    autologous Z52.11
    specified type NEC Z52.19
  specified organ or tissue NEC Z52.89
  sperm Z52.89
Donovanosis A58
Dorsalgia M54.9
  psychogenic F45.41
  specified NEC M54.89
Dorsopathy M53.9
  deforming M43.9
    specified NEC — see subcategory M43.8 ☑
  specified NEC M53.80
    cervical region M53.82
    cervicothoracic region M53.83
    lumbar region M53.86
    lumbosacral region M53.87
    occipito-atlanto-axial region M53.81
    sacrococcygeal region M53.88
    thoracic region M53.84
    thoracolumbar region M53.85
Double
  albumin E88.09
  aortic arch Q25.45
  auditory canal Q17.8
  auricle (heart) Q20.8
  bladder Q64.79
  cervix Q51.820
    with doubling of uterus (and vagina) Q51.10
      with obstruction Q51.11
  inlet ventricle Q20.4
  kidney with double pelvis (renal) Q63.0
  meatus urinarius Q64.75
  monster Q89.4
  outlet
    left ventricle Q20.2
    right ventricle Q20.1
  pelvis (renal) with double ureter Q62.5
  tongue Q38.3
  ureter (one or both sides) Q62.5
    with double pelvis (renal) Q62.5
  urethra Q64.74
  urinary meatus Q64.75
  uterus Q51.28
    with
      doubling of cervix (and vagina) Q51.10
        with obstruction Q51.11
      complete Q51.21
      in pregnancy or childbirth O34.0- ☑
        causing obstructed labor O65.5
      partial Q51.22
      specified NEC Q51.28
  vagina Q52.10
    with doubling of uterus (and cervix) Q51.10
      with obstruction Q51.11
  vision H53.2
  vulva Q52.79
Douglas' pouch, cul-de-sac — see condition
Down syndrome Q90.9
  meiotic nondisjunction Q90.0
  mitotic nondisjunction Q90.1
  mosaicism Q90.1
  translocation Q90.2
DPD (dihydropyrimidine dehydrogenase deficiency)
  E88.89
Dracontiasis B72
Dracunculiasis, dracunculosis B72
Dream state, hysterical F44.89
Drepanocytic anemia — see Disease, sickle-cell
Dresbach's syndrome (elliptocytosis) D58.1
Dreschlera (hawaiiensis) (infection) B43.8
Dressler's syndrome I24.1
Drift, ulnar — see Deformity, limb, specified type NEC,
  forearm
Drinking (alcohol)
  excessive, to excess NEC (without dependence) F10.10
    habitual (continual) (without remission) F10.20
      with remission F10.21
Drip, postnasal (chronic) R09.82
  due to
    allergic rhinitis — see Rhinitis, allergic

☑ Additional Character Required — Refer to the Tabular List for Character Selection   ⟱ Subterms under main terms may continue to next column or page

Drip, postnasal — *continued*
  due to — *continued*
    common cold J00
    gastroesophageal reflux — *see* Reflux, gastroe-
      sophageal
    nasopharyngitis — *see* Nasopharyngitis
    other known condition — *code to* condition
    sinusitis — *see* Sinusitis
Droop
  facial R29.810
    cerebrovascular disease I69.992
      cerebral infarction I69.392
      intracerebral hemorrhage I69.192
      nontraumatic intracranial hemorrhage NEC
        I69.292
      specified disease NEC I69.892
      subarachnoid hemorrhage I69.092
Drop (in)
  attack NEC R55
  finger — *see* Deformity, finger
  foot — *see* Deformity, limb, foot, drop
  hematocrit (precipitous) R71.0
  hemoglobin R71.0
  toe — *see* Deformity, toe, specified NEC
  wrist — *see* Deformity, limb, wrist drop
Dropped heart beats I45.9
Dropsy, dropsical — *see also* Hydrops
  abdomen R18.8
  brain — *see* Hydrocephalus
  cardiac, heart — *see* Failure, heart, congestive
  gangrenous — *see* Gangrene
  heart — *see* Failure, heart, congestive
  kidney — *see* Nephrosis
  lung — *see* Edema, lung
  newborn due to isoimmunization P56.0
  pericardium — *see* Pericarditis
Drowned, drowning (near) T75.1 ☑
Drowsiness R40.0
Drug
  abuse counseling and surveillance Z71.51
  addiction — *see* Dependence
  dependence — *see* Dependence
  habit — *see* Dependence
  harmful use — *see* Abuse, drug
  induced fever R50.2
  overdose — *see* Table of Drugs and Chemicals, by drug,
    poisoning
  poisoning — *see* Table of Drugs and Chemicals, by
    drug, poisoning
  resistant organism infection — *see also* Resistant, or-
    ganism, to, drug Z16.30
  therapy
    long term (current) (prophylactic) — *see* Therapy,
      drug long-term (current) (prophylactic)
    short term — *omit code*
  wrong substance given or taken in error — *see* Table
    of Drugs and Chemicals, by drug, poisoning
Drunkenness (without dependence) F10.129
  acute in alcoholism F10.229
  chronic (without remission) F10.20
    with remission F10.21
  pathological (without dependence) F10.129
    with dependence F10.229
  sleep F51.9
Drusen
  macula (degenerative) (retina) — *see* Degeneration,
    macula, drusen
  optic disc H47.32- ☑
Dry, dryness — *see also* condition
  larynx J38.7
  mouth R68.2
    due to dehydration E86.0
  nose J34.89
  socket (teeth) M27.3
  throat J39.2
DSAP L56.5
Duane's syndrome H50.81- ☑
Dubin-Johnson disease or syndrome E80.6
Dubois' disease (thymus gland) A50.59 *[E35]*
Dubowitz' syndrome Q87.19
Duchenne-Aran muscular atrophy G12.21
Duchenne-Griesinger disease G71.01
Duchenne's
  disease or syndrome
    motor neuron disease G12.22
    muscular dystrophy G71.01
  locomotor ataxia (syphilitic) A52.11

Duchenne's — *continued*
  paralysis
    birth injury P14.0
    due to or associated with
      motor neuron disease G12.22
      muscular dystrophy G71.01
Ducrey's chancre A57
Duct, ductus — *see* condition
Duhring's disease (dermatitis herpetiformis) L13.0
Dullness, cardiac (decreased) (increased) R01.2
Dumb ague — *see* Malaria
Dumbness — *see* Aphasia
Dumdum fever B55.0
Dumping syndrome (postgastrectomy) K91.1
Duodenitis (nonspecific) (peptic) K29.80
  with bleeding K29.81
Duodenocholangitis — *see* Cholangitis
Duodenum, duodenal — *see* condition
Duplay's bursitis or periarthritis — *see* Tendinitis,
  calcific, shoulder
Duplication, duplex — *see also* Accessory
  alimentary tract Q45.8
  anus Q43.4
  appendix (and cecum) Q43.4
  biliary duct (any) Q44.5
  bladder Q64.79
  cecum (and appendix) Q43.4
  cervix Q51.820
  chromosome NEC
    with complex rearrangements NEC Q92.5
    seen only at prometaphase Q92.8
  cystic duct Q44.5
  digestive organs Q45.8
  esophagus Q39.8
  frontonasal process Q75.8
  intestine (large) (small) Q43.4
  kidney Q63.0
  liver Q44.7
  pancreas Q45.3
  penis Q55.69
  respiratory organs NEC Q34.8
  salivary duct Q38.4
  spinal cord (incomplete) Q06.2
  stomach Q40.2
Dupré's disease (meningism) R29.1
Dupuytren's contraction or disease M72.0
Durand-Nicolas-Favre disease A55
Durotomy (inadvertent) (incidental) G97.41
Duroziez's disease (congenital mitral stenosis) Q23.2
Dutton's relapsing fever (West African) A68.1
Dwarfism E34.3
  achondroplastic Q77.4
  congenital E34.3
  constitutional E34.3
  hypochondroplastic Q77.4
  hypophyseal E23.0
  infantile E34.3
  Laron-type E34.3
  Lorain (-Levi) type E23.0
  metatropic Q77.8
  nephrotic-glycosuric (with hypophosphatemic rickets)
    E72.09
  nutritional E45
  pancreatic K86.89
  pituitary E23.0
  renal N25.0
  thanatophoric Q77.1
Dyke-Young anemia (secondary) (symptomatic) D59.19
Dysacusis — *see* Abnormal, auditory perception
Dysadrenocortism E27.9
  hyperfunction E27.0
Dysarthria R47.1
  following
    cerebral infarction I69.322
    cerebrovascular disease I69.922
      specified disease NEC I69.822
    intracerebral hemorrhage I69.122
    nontraumatic intracranial hemorrhage NEC I69.222
    subarachnoid hemorrhage I69.022
Dysautonomia (familial) G90.1
Dysbarism T70.3 ☑
Dysbasia R26.2
  angiosclerotica intermittens I73.9
  hysterical F44.4
  lordotica (progressiva) G24.1
  nonorganic origin F44.4
  psychogenic F44.4
Dysbetalipoproteinemia (familial) E78.2

Dyscalculia R48.8
  developmental F81.2
Dyschezia K59.00
Dyschondroplasia (with hemangiomata) Q78.4
Dyschromia (skin) L81.9
Dyscollagenosis M35.9
Dyscranio-pygo-phalangy Q87.0
Dyscrasia
  blood (with) D75.9
    antepartum hemorrhage — *see* Hemorrhage, an-
      tepartum, with coagulation defect
    intrapartum hemorrhage O67.0
    newborn P61.9
      specified type NEC P61.8
    puerperal, postpartum O72.3
  polyglandular, pluriglandular E31.9
Dysendocrinism E34.9
Dysentery, dysenteric (catarrhal) (diarrhea) (epidemic)
  (hemorrhagic) (infectious) (sporadic) (tropical) A09
  abscess, liver A06.4
  amebic — *see also* Amebiasis A06.0
    with abscess — *see* Abscess, amebic
    acute A06.0
    chronic A06.1
  arthritis — *see also* category M01 A09
    bacillary (*see also* category M01) A03.9
  bacillary A03.9
    arthritis — *see also* category M01 A03.9
    Boyd A03.2
    Flexner A03.1
    Schmitz (-Stutzer) A03.0
    Shiga (-Kruse) A03.0
    Shigella A03.9
      boydii A03.2
      dysenteriae A03.0
      flexneri A03.1
      group A A03.0
      group B A03.1
      group C A03.2
      group D A03.3
      sonnei A03.3
      specified type NEC A03.8
    Sonne A03.3
    specified type NEC A03.8
  balantidial A07.0
  Balantidium coli A07.0
  Boyd's A03.2
  candidal B37.82
  Chilomastix A07.8
  Chinese A03.9
  coccidial A07.3
  Dientamoeba (fragilis) A07.8
  Embadomonas A07.8
  Entamoeba, entamebic — *see* Dysentery, amebic
  Flexner-Boyd A03.2
  Flexner's A03.1
  Giardia lamblia A07.1
  Hiss-Russell A03.1
  Lamblia A07.1
  leishmanial B55.0
  malarial — *see* Malaria
  metazoal B82.0
  monilial B37.82
  protozoal A07.9
  Salmonella A02.0
  schistosomal B65.1
  Schmitz (-Stutzer) A03.0
  Shiga (-Kruse) A03.0
  Shigella NOS — *see* Dysentery, bacillary
  Sonne A03.3
  strongyloidiasis B78.0
  trichomonal A07.8
  viral — *see also* Enteritis, viral A08.4
Dysequilibrium R42
Dysesthesia R20.8
  hysterical F44.6
Dysfibrinogenemia (congenital) D68.2
Dysfunction
  adrenal E27.9
    hyperfunction E27.0
  autonomic
    due to alcohol G31.2
    somatoform F45.8
  bladder N31.9
    neurogenic NOS — *see* Dysfunction, bladder, neu-
      romuscular
    neuromuscular NOS N31.9
      atonic (motor) (sensory) N31.2

Dysfunction — *continued*
  bladder — *continued*
    neuromuscular — *continued*
      autonomous N31.2
      flaccid N31.2
      nonreflex N31.2
      reflex N31.1
      specified NEC N31.8
      uninhibited N31.0
    bleeding, uterus N93.8
  cerebral G93.89
  colon K59.9
    psychogenic F45.8
  colostomy K94.03
  cystic duct K82.8
  cystostomy (stoma) — *see* Complications, cystostomy
  ejaculatory N53.19
    anejaculatory orgasm N53.13
    painful N53.12
    premature F52.4
    retarded N53.11
  endocrine NOS E34.9
  endometrium N85.8
  enterostomy K94.13
  erectile — *see* Dysfunction, sexual, male, erectile
  gallbladder K82.8
  gastrostomy (stoma) K94.23
  gland, glandular NOS E34.9
    meibomian, of eyelid — *see* Dysfunction, meibomian gland
  heart I51.89
  hemoglobin D75.89
  hepatic K76.89
  hypophysis E23.7
  hypothalamic NEC E23.3
  ileostomy (stoma) K94.13
  jejunostomy (stoma) K94.13
  kidney — *see* Disease, renal
  labyrinthine — *see* subcategory H83.2 ☑
  left ventricular, following sudden emotional stress I51.81
  liver K76.89
  male — *see* Dysfunction, sexual, male
  meibomian gland, of eyelid H02.889
    left H02.886
      lower H02.885
      upper H02.884
      upper and lower eyelids H02.88B
    right H02.883
      lower H02.882
      upper H02.881
      upper and lower eyelids H02.88A
  orgasmic (female) F52.31
    male F52.32
  ovary E28.9
    specified NEC E28.8
  papillary muscle I51.89
  parathyroid E21.4
  physiological NEC R68.89
    psychogenic F59
  pineal gland E34.8
  pituitary (gland) E23.3
  platelets D69.1
  polyglandular E31.9
    specified NEC E31.8
  psychophysiologic F59
  psychosexual F52.9
    with
      dyspareunia F52.6
      premature ejaculation F52.4
      vaginismus F52.5
  pylorus K31.9
  rectum K59.9
    psychogenic F45.8
  reflex (sympathetic) — *see* Syndrome, pain, complex regional I
  segmental — *see* Dysfunction, somatic
  senile R54
  sexual (due to) R37
    alcohol F10.981
    amphetamine F15.981
      in
        abuse F15.181
        dependence F15.281
    anxiolytic F13.981
      in
        abuse F13.181
        dependence F13.281

Dysfunction — *continued*
  sexual — *continued*
    cocaine F14.981
      in
        abuse F14.181
        dependence F14.281
    excessive sexual drive F52.8
    failure of genital response (male) F52.21
      female F52.22
    female N94.9
      aversion F52.1
      dyspareunia N94.10
        psychogenic F52.6
      frigidity F52.22
      nymphomania F52.8
      orgasmic F52.31
      psychogenic F52.9
        aversion F52.1
        dyspareunia F52.6
        frigidity F52.22
        nymphomania F52.8
        orgasmic F52.31
        vaginismus F52.5
      vaginismus N94.2
        psychogenic F52.5
    hypnotic F13.981
      in
        abuse F13.181
        dependence F13.281
    inhibited orgasm (female) F52.31
      male F52.32
    lack
      of sexual enjoyment F52.1
      or loss of sexual desire F52.0
    male N53.9
      anejaculatory orgasm N53.13
      ejaculatory N53.19
        painful N53.12
        premature F52.4
        retarded N53.11
      erectile N52.9
        drug induced N52.2
        due to
          disease classified elsewhere N52.1
          drug N52.2
          postoperative (postprocedural) N52.39
            following
              cryotherapy N52.37
              interstitial seed therapy N52.36
              prostate ablative therapy N52.37
              prostatectomy N52.34
                radical N52.31
              radiation therapy N52.35
              radical cystectomy N52.32
              ultrasound ablative therapy N52.37
              urethral surgery N52.33
        psychogenic F52.21
        specified cause NEC N52.8
        vasculogenic
          arterial insufficiency N52.01
            with corporo-venous occlusive N52.03
          corporo-venous occlusive N52.02
            with arterial insufficiency N52.03
      impotence — *see* Dysfunction, sexual, male, erectile
      psychogenic F52.9
        aversion F52.1
        erectile F52.21
        orgasmic F52.32
        premature ejaculation F52.4
        satyriasis F52.8
        specified type NEC F52.8
      specified type NEC N53.8
    nonorganic F52.9
      specified NEC F52.8
    opioid F11.981
      in
        abuse F11.181
        dependence F11.281
    orgasmic dysfunction (female) F52.31
      male F52.32
    premature ejaculation F52.4
    psychoactive substances NEC F19.981
      in
        abuse F19.181
        dependence F19.281
    psychogenic F52.9
    sedative F13.981

Dysfunction — *continued*
  sexual — *continued*
    sedative — *continued*
      in
        abuse F13.181
        dependence F13.281
    sexual aversion F52.1
    vaginismus (nonorganic) (psychogenic) F52.5
  sinoatrial node I49.5
  somatic M99.09
    abdomen M99.09
    acromioclavicular M99.07
    cervical region M99.01
    cervicothoracic M99.01
    costochondral M99.08
    costovertebral M99.08
    head region M99.00
    hip M99.05
    lower extremity M99.06
    lumbar region M99.03
    lumbosacral M99.03
    occipitocervical M99.00
    pelvic region M99.05
    pubic M99.05
    rib cage M99.08
    sacral region M99.04
    sacrococcygeal M99.04
    sacroiliac M99.04
    specified NEC M99.09
    sternochondral M99.08
    sternoclavicular M99.07
    thoracic region M99.02
    thoracolumbar M99.02
    upper extremity M99.07
  somatoform autonomic F45.8
  stomach K31.89
    psychogenic F45.8
  suprarenal E27.9
    hyperfunction E27.0
  symbolic R48.9
    specified type NEC R48.8
  temporomandibular (joint) M26.69
    joint-pain syndrome M26.62- ☑
  testicular (endocrine) E29.9
    specified NEC E29.8
  thymus E32.9
  thyroid E07.9
  ureterostomy (stoma) — *see* Complications, stoma, urinary tract
  urethrostomy (stoma) — *see* Complications, stoma, urinary tract
  uterus, complicating delivery O62.9
    hypertonic O62.4
    hypotonic O62.2
      primary O62.0
      secondary O62.1
  ventricular I51.9
    with congestive heart failure — *see also* Failure, heart I50.9
    left, reversible, following sudden emotional stress I51.81

Dysgenesis
  gonadal (due to chromosomal anomaly) Q96.9
    pure Q99.1
  renal Q60.5
    bilateral Q60.4
    unilateral Q60.3
  reticular D72.0
  tidal platelet D69.3

Dysgerminoma
  specified site — *see* Neoplasm, malignant, by site
  unspecified site
    female C56.9
    male C62.90

Dysgeusia R43.2

Dysgraphia R27.8

Dyshidrosis, dysidrosis L30.1

Dyskaryotic cervical smear R87.619

Dyskeratosis L85.8
  cervix — *see* Dysplasia, cervix
  congenital Q82.8
  uterus NEC N85.8

Dyskinesia G24.9
  biliary (cystic duct or gallbladder) K82.8
  drug induced
    orofacial G24.01
  esophagus K22.4
  hysterical F44.4

Dyskinesia — *continued*
  intestinal K59.89
  nonorganic origin F44.4
  orofacial (idiopathic) G24.4
    drug induced G24.01
  psychogenic F44.4
  subacute, drug induced G24.01
  tardive G24.01
    neuroleptic induced G24.01
  trachea J39.8
  tracheobronchial J98.09
Dyslalia (developmental) F80.0
Dyslexia R48.0
  developmental F81.0
Dyslipidemia E78.5
  depressed HDL cholesterol E78.6
  elevated fasting triglycerides E78.1
Dysmaturity — *see also* Light for dates
  pulmonary (newborn) (Wilson-Mikity) P27.0
Dysmenorrhea (essential) (exfoliative) N94.6
  congestive (syndrome) N94.6
  primary N94.4
  psychogenic F45.8
  secondary N94.5
Dysmetabolic syndrome X E88.81
Dysmetria R27.8
Dysmorphism (due to)
  alcohol Q86.0
  exogenous cause NEC Q86.8
  hydantoin Q86.1
  warfarin Q86.2
Dysmorphophobia (nondelusional) F45.22
  delusional F22
Dysnomia R47.01
Dysorexia R63.0
  psychogenic F50.89
Dysostosis
  cleidocranial, cleidocranialis Q74.0
  craniofacial Q75.1
  Fairbank's (idiopathic familial generalized osteophytosis) Q78.9
  mandibulofacial (incomplete) Q75.4
  multiplex E76.01
  oculomandibular Q75.5
Dyspareunia (female) N94.10
  deep N94.12
  male N53.12
  nonorganic F52.6
  psychogenic F52.6
  secondary N94.19
  specified NEC N94.19
  superficial (introital) N94.11
Dyspepsia R10.13
  atonic K30
  functional (allergic) (congenital) (gastrointestinal) (occupational) (reflex) K30
  intestinal K59.89
  nervous F45.8
  neurotic F45.8
  psychogenic F45.8
Dysphagia R13.10
  cervical R13.19
  following
    cerebral infarction I69.391
    cerebrovascular disease I69.991
      specified NEC I69.891
    intracerebral hemorrhage I69.191
    nontraumatic intracranial hemorrhage NEC I69.291
    specified disease NEC I69.891
    subarachnoid hemorrhage I69.091
  functional (hysterical) F45.8
  hysterical F45.8
  nervous (hysterical) F45.8
  neurogenic R13.19
  oral phase R13.11
  oropharyngeal phase R13.12
  pharyngeal phase R13.13
  pharyngoesophageal phase R13.14
  psychogenic F45.8
  sideropenic D50.1
  spastica K22.4
  specified NEC R13.19
Dysphagocytosis, congenital D71
Dysphasia R47.02
  developmental
    expressive type F80.1
    receptive type F80.2

Dysphasia — *continued*
  following
    cerebrovascular disease I69.921
      cerebral infarction I69.321
      intracerebral hemorrhage I69.121
      nontraumatic intracranial hemorrhage NEC I69.221
      specified disease NEC I69.821
      subarachnoid hemorrhage I69.021
Dysphonia R49.0
  functional F44.4
  hysterical F44.4
  psychogenic F44.4
  spastica J38.3
Dysphoria
  gender F64.9
    in
      adolescence and adulthood F64.0
      children F64.2
    specified NEC F64.8
  postpartal O90.6
Dyspituitarism E23.3
Dysplasia — *see also* Anomaly
  acetabular, congenital Q65.89
  alveolar capillary, with vein misalignment J84.843
  anus (histologically confirmed) (mild) (moderate) K62.82
    severe D01.3
  arrhythmogenic right ventricular I42.8
  arterial, fibromuscular I77.3
  asphyxiating thoracic (congenital) Q77.2
  brain Q07.9
  bronchopulmonary, perinatal P27.1
  cervix (uteri) N87.9
    mild N87.0
    moderate N87.1
    severe D06.9
  chondroectodermal Q77.6
  colon D12.6
  craniometaphyseal Q78.8
  dentinal K00.5
  diaphyseal, progressive Q78.3
  dystrophic Q77.5
  ectodermal (anhidrotic) (congenital) (hereditary) Q82.4
    hydrotic Q82.8
  epithelial, uterine cervix — *see* Dysplasia, cervix
  eye (congenital) Q11.2
  fibrous
    bone NEC (monostotic) M85.00
      ankle M85.07- ☑
      foot M85.07- ☑
      forearm M85.03- ☑
      hand M85.04- ☑
      lower leg M85.06- ☑
      multiple site M85.09
      neck M85.08
      rib M85.08
      shoulder M85.01- ☑
      skull M85.08
      specified site NEC M85.08
      thigh M85.05- ☑
      toe M85.07- ☑
      upper arm M85.02- ☑
      vertebra M85.08
    diaphyseal, progressive Q78.3
    jaw M27.8
    polyostotic Q78.1
  florid osseous — *see also* Cyst, calcifying odontogenic
  high grade, focal D12.6
  hip, congenital Q65.89
  joint, congenital Q74.8
  kidney Q61.4
    multicystic Q61.4
  leg Q74.2
  lung, congenital (not associated with short gestation) Q33.6
  mammary (gland) (benign) N60.9- ☑
    cyst (solitary) — *see* Cyst, breast
    cystic — *see* Mastopathy, cystic
    duct ectasia — *see* Ectasia, mammary duct
    fibroadenosis — *see* Fibroadenosis, breast
    fibrosclerosis — *see* Fibrosclerosis, breast
    specified type NEC N60.8- ☑
  metaphyseal Q78.5
  muscle Q79.8
  oculodentodigital Q87.0
  periapical (cemental) (cemento-osseous) — *see* Cyst, calcifying odontogenic

Dysplasia — *continued*
  periosteum — *see* Disorder, bone, specified type NEC
  polyostotic fibrous Q78.1
  prostate — *see also* Neoplasia, intraepithelial, prostate N42.30
    severe D07.5
    specified NEC N42.39
  renal Q61.4
    multicystic Q61.4
  retinal, congenital Q14.1
  right ventricular, arrhythmogenic I42.8
  septo-optic Q04.4
  skin L98.8
  spinal cord Q06.1
  spondyloepiphyseal Q77.7
  thymic, with immunodeficiency D82.1
  vagina N89.3
    mild N89.0
    moderate N89.1
    severe NEC D07.2
  vulva N90.3
    mild N90.0
    moderate N90.1
    severe NEC D07.1
Dysplasminogenemia E88.02
Dyspnea (nocturnal) (paroxysmal) R06.00
  asthmatic (bronchial) J45.909
    with
      bronchitis J45.909
        with
          exacerbation (acute) J45.901
          status asthmaticus J45.902
        chronic J44.9
      exacerbation (acute) J45.901
      status asthmaticus J45.902
  cardiac — *see* Failure, ventricular, left
  cardiac — *see* Failure, ventricular, left
  functional F45.8
  hyperventilation R06.4
  hysterical F45.8
  newborn P28.89
  orthopnea R06.01
  psychogenic F45.8
  shortness of breath R06.02
  specified type NEC R06.09
Dyspraxia R27.8
  developmental (syndrome) F82
Dysproteinemia E88.09
Dysreflexia, autonomic G90.4
Dysrhythmia
  cardiac I49.9
    newborn
      bradycardia P29.12
        occurring before birth P03.819
          before onset of labor P03.810
          during labor P03.811
      tachycardia P29.11
    postoperative I97.89
  cerebral or cortical — *see* Epilepsy
Dyssomnia — *see* Disorder, sleep
Dyssynergia
  biliary K83.8
  bladder sphincter N36.44
  cerebellaris myoclonica (Hunt's ataxia) G11.19
Dysthymia F34.1
Dysthyroidism E07.9
Dystocia O66.9
  affecting newborn P03.1
  cervical (hypotonic) O62.2
    affecting newborn P03.6
    primary O62.0
    secondary O62.1
  contraction ring O62.4
  fetal O66.9
    abnormality NEC O66.3
    conjoined twins O66.3
    oversize O66.2
  maternal O66.9
  positional O64.9 ☑
  shoulder (girdle) O66.0
    causing obstructed labor O66.0
  uterine NEC O62.4
Dystonia G24.9
  cervical G24.3
  deformans progressiva G24.1
  drug induced NEC G24.09
    acute G24.02
    specified NEC G24.09

☝ **Subterms under main terms may continue to next column or page**   ☑ **Additional Character Required** — **Refer to the Tabular List for Character Selection**

Dystonia — *continued*
  familial G24.1
  idiopathic G24.1
    familial G24.1
    nonfamilial G24.2
    orofacial G24.4
  lenticularis G24.8
  musculorum deformans G24.1
  neuroleptic induced (acute) G24.02
  orofacial (idiopathic) G24.4
  oromandibular G24.4
    due to drug G24.01
  specified NEC G24.8
  torsion (familial) (idiopathic) G24.1
    acquired G24.8
    genetic G24.1
    symptomatic (nonfamilial) G24.2
Dystonic movements R25.8
Dystrophy, dystrophia
  adiposogenital E23.6
  autosomal recessive, childhood type, muscular dystro-
    phy resembling Duchenne or Becker G71.01
  Becker's type G71.01
  cervical sympathetic G90.2
  choroid (hereditary) H31.20
    central areolar H31.22
    choroideremia H31.21
    gyrate atrophy H31.23
    specified type NEC H31.29
  cornea (hereditary) H18.50- ☑
    endothelial H18.51- ☑
    epithelial H18.52- ☑
    granular H18.53- ☑
    lattice H18.54- ☑
    macular H18.55- ☑
    specified type NEC H18.59- ☑
  Duchenne's type G71.01
  due to malnutrition E45
  Erb's G71.02
  Fuchs' H18.51- ☑
  Gower's muscular G71.01
  hair L67.8
  infantile neuraxonal G31.89
  Landouzy-Déjérine G71.02
  Leyden-Möbius G71.09
  muscular G71.00
    autosomal recessive, childhood type, muscular
      dystrophy resembling Duchenne or Becker
      G71.01
    benign (Becker type) G71.01
      scapuloperoneal with early contractures [Emery-
      Dreifuss] G71.09
    congenital (hereditary) (progressive) (with specific
      morphological abnormalities of the muscle
      fiber) G71.09
      myotonic G71.11
    distal G71.09
    Duchenne type G71.01
    Emery-Dreifuss G71.09
    Erb type G71.02
    facioscapulohumeral G71.02
    Gower's G71.01
    hereditary (progressive) G71.09
    Landouzy-Déjérine type G71.02
    limb-girdle G71.09
    myotonic G71.11
    progressive (hereditary) G71.09
      Charcot-Marie (-Tooth) type G60.0
    pseudohypertrophic (infantile) G71.01
    scapulohumeral G71.02
    scapuloperoneal G71.09
    severe (Duchenne type) G71.01
    specified type NEC G71.09
  myocardium, myocardial — *see* Degeneration, myocar-
    dial
  nail L60.3
    congenital Q84.6
  nutritional E45
  ocular G71.09
  oculocerebrorenal E72.03
  oculopharyngeal G71.09
  ovarian N83.8
  polyglandular E31.8
  reflex (neuromuscular) (sympathetic) — *see* Syndrome,
    pain, complex regional I
  retinal (hereditary) H35.50
    in
      lipid storage disorders E75.6 [H36]

Dystrophy, dystrophia — *continued*
  retinal — *continued*
    in — *continued*
      systemic lipidoses E75.6 [H36]
    involving
      pigment epithelium H35.54
      sensory area H35.53
    pigmentary H35.52
    vitreoretinal H35.51
  Salzmann's nodular — *see* Degeneration, cornea,
    nodular
  scapuloperoneal G71.09
  skin NEC L98.8
  sympathetic (reflex) — *see* Syndrome, pain, complex
    regional I
    cervical G90.2
  tapetoretinal H35.54
  thoracic, asphyxiating Q77.2
  unguium L60.3
    congenital Q84.6
  vitreoretinal H35.51
  vulva N90.4
  yellow (liver) — *see* Failure, hepatic
Dysuria R30.0
  psychogenic F45.8

E

Eales' disease H35.06- ☑
Ear — *see also* condition
  piercing Z41.3
  tropical NEC B36.9 [H62.40]
    in
      aspergillosis B44.89
      candidiasis B37.84
      moniliasis B37.84
  wax (impacted) H61.20
    left H61.22
      with right H61.23
    right H61.21
      with left H61.23
Earache — *see* subcategory H92.0 ☑
Early satiety R68.81
Eaton-Lambert syndrome — *see* Syndrome, Lambert-
  Eaton
Eberth's disease (typhoid fever) A01.00
Ebola virus disease A98.4
Ebstein's anomaly or syndrome (heart) Q22.5
Eccentro-osteochondrodysplasia E76.29
Ecchondroma — *see* Neoplasm, bone, benign
Ecchondrosis D48.0
Ecchymosis R58
  conjunctiva — *see* Hemorrhage, conjunctiva
  eye (traumatic) — *see* Contusion, eyeball
  eyelid (traumatic) — *see* Contusion, eyelid
  newborn P54.5
  spontaneous R23.3
  traumatic — *see* Contusion
Echinococciasis — *see* Echinococcus
Echinococcosis — *see* Echinococcus
Echinococcus (infection) B67.90
  granulosus B67.4
    bone B67.2
    liver B67.0
    lung B67.1
    multiple sites B67.32
    specified site NEC B67.39
    thyroid B67.31
  liver NOS B67.8
    granulosus B67.0
    multilocularis B67.5
  lung NEC B67.99
    granulosus B67.1
    multilocularis B67.69
  multilocularis B67.7
    liver B67.5
    multiple sites B67.61
    specified site NEC B67.69
  specified site NEC B67.99
    granulosus B67.39
    multilocularis B67.69
  thyroid NEC B67.99
    granulosus B67.31
    multilocularis B67.69 [E35]
Echinorhynchiasis B83.8
Echinostomiasis B66.8
Echolalia R48.8

Echovirus, as cause of disease classified elsewhere
  B97.12
Eclampsia, eclamptic (coma) (convulsions) (delirium)
  (with hypertension) NEC O15.9
  complicating
    labor and delivery O15.1
    postpartum O15.2
    pregnancy O15.0- ☑
    puerperium O15.2
Economic circumstances affecting care Z59.9
Economo's disease A85.8
Ectasia, ectasis
  annuloaortic I35.8
  aorta I77.819
    with aneurysm — *see* Aneurysm, aorta
    abdominal I77.811
    thoracic I77.810
    thoracoabdominal I77.812
  breast — *see* Ectasia, mammary duct
  capillary I78.8
  cornea H18.71- ☑
  gastric antral vascular (GAVE) K31.819
    with hemorrhage K31.811
    without hemorrhage K31.819
  mammary duct N60.4- ☑
  salivary gland (duct) K11.8
  sclera — *see* Sclerectasia
Ecthyma L08.0
  contagiosum B08.02
  gangrenosum L08.0
  infectiosum B08.02
Ectocardia Q24.8
Ectodermal dysplasia (anhidrotic) Q82.4
Ectodermosis erosiva pluriorificialis L51.1
Ectopic, ectopia (congenital)
  abdominal viscera Q45.8
    due to defect in anterior abdominal wall Q79.59
  ACTH syndrome E24.3
  adrenal gland Q89.1
  anus Q43.5
  atrial beats I49.1
  beats I49.49
    atrial I49.1
    ventricular I49.3
  bladder Q64.10
  bone and cartilage in lung Q33.5
  brain Q04.8
  breast tissue Q83.8
  cardiac Q24.8
  cerebral Q04.8
  cordis Q24.8
  endometrium — *see* Endometriosis
  gastric mucosa Q40.2
  gestation — *see* Pregnancy, by site
  heart Q24.8
  hormone secretion NEC E34.2
  kidney (crossed) (pelvis) Q63.2
  lens, lentis Q12.1
  mole — *see* Pregnancy, by site
  organ or site NEC — *see* Malposition, congenital
  pancreas Q45.3
  pregnancy — *see* Pregnancy, ectopic
  pupil — *see* Abnormality, pupillary
  renal Q63.2
  sebaceous glands of mouth Q38.6
  spleen Q89.09
  testis Q53.00
    bilateral Q53.02
    unilateral Q53.01
  thyroid Q89.2
  tissue in lung Q33.5
  ureter Q62.63
  ventricular beats I49.3
  vesicae Q64.10
Ectromelia Q73.8
  lower limb — *see* Defect, reduction, limb, lower, spec-
    ified type NEC
  upper limb — *see* Defect, reduction, limb, upper,
    specified type NEC
Ectropion H02.109
  cervix N86
    with cervicitis N72
  congenital Q10.1
  eyelid H02.109
    cicatricial H02.119
      left H02.116
        lower H02.115
        upper H02.114

Ectropion — *continued*
  eyelid — *continued*
    cicatricial — *continued*
      right H02.113
        lower H02.112
        upper H02.111
    congenital Q10.1
    left H02.106
      lower H02.105
      upper H02.104
    mechanical H02.129
      left H02.126
        lower H02.125
        upper H02.124
      right H02.123
        lower H02.122
        upper H02.121
    paralytic H02.159
      left H02.156
        lower H02.155
        upper H02.154
      right H02.153
        lower H02.152
        upper H02.151
    right H02.103
      lower H02.102
      upper H02.101
    senile H02.139
      left H02.136
        lower H02.135
        upper H02.134
      right H02.133
        lower H02.132
        upper H02.131
    spastic H02.149
      left H02.146
        lower H02.145
        upper H02.144
      right H02.143
        lower H02.142
        upper H02.141
  iris H21.89
  lip (acquired) K13.0
    congenital Q38.0
  urethra N36.8
  uvea H21.89
Eczema (acute) (chronic) (erythematous) (fissum)
    (rubrum) (squamous) — *see also* Dermatitis L30.9
  contact — *see* Dermatitis, contact
  dyshydrotic L30.1
  external ear — *see* Otitis, externa, acute, eczematoid
  flexural L20.82
  herpeticum B00.0
  hypertrophicum L28.0
  hypostatic — *see* Varix, leg, with, inflammation
  impetiginous L01.1
  infantile (due to any substance) L20.83
    intertriginous L21.1
    seborrheic L21.1
  intertriginous NEC L30.4
    infantile L21.1
  intrinsic (allergic) L20.84
  lichenified NEC L28.0
  marginatum (hebrae) B35.6
  pustular L30.3
  stasis I87.2
    with varicose veins — *see* Varix, leg, with, inflamma-
      tion
  vaccination, vaccinatum T88.1 ☑
  varicose — *see* Varix, leg, with, inflammation
Eczematid L30.2
Eddowes (-Spurway) **syndrome** Q78.0
Edema, edematous (infectious) (pitting) (toxic) R60.9
  with nephritis — *see* Nephrosis
  allergic T78.3 ☑
  amputation stump (surgical) (sequelae (late effect))
    T87.89
  angioneurotic (allergic) (any site) (with urticaria)
    T78.3 ☑
    hereditary D84.1
  angiospastic I73.9
  Berlin's (traumatic) S05.8X- ☑
  brain (cytotoxic) (vasogenic) G93.6
    due to birth injury P11.0
    newborn (anoxia or hypoxia) P52.4
      birth injury P11.0
    traumatic — *see* Injury, intracranial, cerebral edema
  cardiac — *see* Failure, heart, congestive

Edema, edematous — *continued*
  cardiovascular — *see* Failure, heart, congestive
  cerebral — *see* Edema, brain
  cerebrospinal — *see* Edema, brain
  cervix (uteri) (acute) N88.8
    puerperal, postpartum O90.89
  chronic hereditary Q82.0
  circumscribed, acute T78.3 ☑
    hereditary D84.1
  conjunctiva H11.42- ☑
  cornea H18.2- ☑
    idiopathic H18.22- ☑
    secondary H18.23- ☑
      due to contact lens H18.21- ☑
  due to
    lymphatic obstruction I89.0
    salt retention E87.0
  epiglottis — *see* Edema, glottis
  essential, acute T78.3 ☑
    hereditary D84.1
  extremities, lower — *see* Edema, legs
  eyelid NEC H02.849
    left H02.846
      lower H02.845
      upper H02.844
    right H02.843
      lower H02.842
      upper H02.841
  familial, hereditary Q82.0
  famine — *see* Malnutrition, severe
  generalized R60.1
  glottis, glottic, glottidis (obstructive) (passive) J38.4
    allergic T78.3 ☑
      hereditary D84.1
  heart — *see* Failure, heart, congestive
  heat T67.7 ☑
  hereditary Q82.0
  inanition — *see* Malnutrition, severe
  intracranial G93.6
  iris H21.89
  joint — *see* Effusion, joint
  larynx — *see* Edema, glottis
  legs R60.0
    due to venous obstruction I87.1
    hereditary Q82.0
  localized R60.0
    due to venous obstruction I87.1
  lower limbs — *see* Edema, legs
  lung J81.1
    with heart condition or failure — *see* Failure, ven-
      tricular, left
    acute J81.0
      chemical (acute) J68.1
        chronic J68.1
    chronic J81.1
      due to
        chemicals, gases, fumes or vapors (inhalation)
          J68.1
        external agent J70.9
          specified NEC J70.8
        radiation J70.1
    due to
      chemicals, fumes or vapors (inhalation) J68.1
      external agent J70.9
        specified NEC J70.8
      high altitude T70.29 ☑
      near drowning T75.1 ☑
      radiation J70.0
    meaning failure, left ventricle I50.1
  lymphatic I89.0
    due to mastectomy I97.2
  macula H35.81
    cystoid, following cataract surgery — *see* Complica-
      tions, postprocedural, following cataract
      surgery
    diabetic — *see* Diabetes, by type, with, retinopathy,
      with macular edema
  malignant — *see* Gangrene, gas
  Milroy's Q82.0
  nasopharynx J39.2
  newborn P83.30
    hydrops fetalis — *see* Hydrops, fetalis
    specified NEC P83.39
  nutritional — *see also* Malnutrition, severe
    with dyspigmentation, skin and hair E40
  optic disc or nerve — *see* Papilledema
  orbit H05.22- ☑
  pancreas K86.89

Edema, edematous — *continued*
  papilla, optic — *see* Papilledema
  penis N48.89
  periodic T78.3 ☑
    hereditary D84.1
  pharynx J39.2
  pulmonary — *see* Edema, lung
  Quincke's T78.3 ☑
    hereditary D84.1
  renal — *see* Nephrosis
  retina H35.81
    diabetic — *see* Diabetes, by type, with, retinopathy,
      with macular edema
  salt E87.0
  scrotum N50.89
  seminal vesicle N50.89
  spermatic cord N50.89
  spinal (cord) (vascular) (nontraumatic) G95.19
  starvation — *see* Malnutrition, severe
  stasis — *see* Hypertension, venous, (chronic)
  subglottic — *see* Edema, glottis
  supraglottic — *see* Edema, glottis
  testis N44.8
  tunica vaginalis N50.89
  vas deferens N50.89
  vulva (acute) N90.89
Edentulism — *see* Absence, teeth, acquired
Edsall's disease T67.2 ☑
Educational handicap Z55.9
  specified NEC Z55.8
Edward's syndrome — *see* Trisomy, 18
Effect(s) (of) (from) — *see* Effect, adverse NEC
Effect, adverse
  abnormal gravitational (G) forces or states T75.81 ☑
  abuse — *see* Maltreatment
  air pressure T70.9 ☑
    specified NEC T70.8 ☑
  altitude (high) — *see* Effect, adverse, high altitude
  anesthesia — *see also* Anesthesia T88.59 ☑
    in labor and delivery O74.9
    local, toxic
      in labor and delivery O74.4
      in pregnancy NEC O29.3- ☑
      postpartum, puerperal O89.3
    postpartum, puerperal O89.9
    specified NEC T88.59 ☑
      in labor and delivery O74.8
      postpartum, puerperal O89.8
    spinal and epidural T88.59 ☑
      headache T88.59 ☑
        in labor and delivery O74.5
        postpartum, puerperal O89.4
      specified NEC
        in labor and delivery O74.6
        postpartum, puerperal O89.5
  antitoxin — *see* Complications, vaccination
  atmospheric pressure T70.9 ☑
    due to explosion T70.8 ☑
    high T70.3 ☑
    low — *see* Effect, adverse, high altitude
    specified effect NEC T70.8 ☑
  biological, correct substance properly administered —
    see Effect, adverse, drug
  blood (derivatives) (serum) (transfusion) — *see* Com-
    plications, transfusion
  chemical substance — *see* Table of Drugs and Chemi-
    cals
  cold (temperature) (weather) T69.9 ☑
    chilblains T69.1 ☑
    frostbite — *see* Frostbite
    specified effect NEC T69.8 ☑
  drugs and medicaments T88.7 ☑
    specified drug — *see* Table of Drugs and Chemicals,
      by drug, adverse effect
    specified effect — *code to* condition
  electric current, electricity (shock) T75.4 ☑
    burn — *see* Burn
  exertion (excessive) T73.3 ☑
  exposure — *see* Exposure
  external cause NEC T75.89 ☑
  foodstuffs T78.1 ☑
    allergic reaction — *see* Allergy, food
      causing anaphylaxis — *see* Shock, anaphylactic,
        due to food
    noxious — *see* Poisoning, food, noxious
  gases, fumes, or vapors T59.9- ☑
    specified agent — *see* Table of Drugs and Chemicals

Effect, adverse — *continued*
glue (airplane) sniffing
due to drug abuse — *see* Abuse, drug, inhalant
due to drug dependence — *see* Dependence, drug, inhalant
heat — *see* Heat
high altitude NEC T70.29 ☑
anoxia T70.29 ☑
on
ears T70.0 ☑
sinuses T70.1 ☑
polycythemia D75.1
high pressure fluids T70.4 ☑
hot weather — *see* Heat
hunger T73.0 ☑
immersion, foot — *see* Immersion
immunization — *see* Complications, vaccination
immunological agents — *see* Complications, vaccination
infrared (radiation) (rays) NOS T66 ☑
dermatitis or eczema L59.8
infusion — *see* Complications, infusion
lack of care of infants — *see* Maltreatment, child
lightning — *see* Lightning
medical care T88.9 ☑
specified NEC T88.8 ☑
medicinal substance, correct, properly administered — *see* Effect, adverse, drug
motion T75.3 ☑
noise, on inner ear — *see* subcategory H83.3 ☑
overheated places — *see* Heat
psychosocial, of work environment Z56.5
radiation (diagnostic) (infrared) (natural source) (therapeutic) (ultraviolet) (X-ray) NOS T66 ☑
dermatitis or eczema — *see* Dermatitis, due to, radiation
fibrosis of lung J70.1
pneumonitis J70.0
pulmonary manifestations
acute J70.0
chronic J70.1
skin L59.9
radioactive substance NOS
dermatitis or eczema — *see* Radiodermatitis
reduced temperature T69.9 ☑
immersion foot or hand — *see* Immersion
specified effect NEC T69.8 ☑
serum NEC — *see also* Reaction, serum T80.69 ☑
specified NEC T78.8 ☑
external cause NEC T75.89 ☑
strangulation — *see* Asphyxia, traumatic
submersion T75.1 ☑
thirst T73.1 ☑
toxic — *see* Toxicity
transfusion — *see* Complications, transfusion
ultraviolet (radiation) (rays) NOS T66 ☑
burn — *see* Burn
dermatitis or eczema — *see* Dermatitis, due to, ultraviolet rays
acute L56.8
vaccine (any) — *see* Complications, vaccination
vibration — *see* Vibration, adverse effects
water pressure NEC T70.9 ☑
specified NEC T70.8 ☑
weightlessness T75.82 ☑
whole blood — *see* Complications, transfusion
work environment Z56.5
Effects, late — *see* Sequelae
Effluvium
anagen L65.1
telogen L65.0
Effort syndrome (psychogenic) F45.8
Effusion
amniotic fluid — *see* Pregnancy, complicated by, prematue rupture of membranes
brain (serous) G93.6
bronchial — *see* Bronchitis
cerebral G93.6
cerebrospinal — *see also* Meningitis
vessel G93.6
chest — *see* Effusion, pleura
chylous, chyliform (pleura) J94.0
intracranial G93.6
joint M25.40
ankle M25.47- ☑
elbow M25.42- ☑
foot joint M25.47- ☑

Effusion — *continued*
joint — *continued*
hand joint M25.44- ☑
hip M25.45- ☑
knee M25.46- ☑
shoulder M25.41- ☑
specified joint NEC M25.48
wrist M25.43- ☑
malignant pleural J91.0
meninges — *see* Meningitis
pericardium, pericardial (noninflammatory) I31.3
acute — *see* Pericarditis, acute
peritoneal (chronic) R18.8
pleura, pleurisy, pleuritic, pleuropericardial J90
chylous, chyliform J94.0
due to systemic lupus erythematosis M32.13
in conditions classified elsewhere J91.8
influenzal — *see* Influenza, with, respiratory manifestations NEC
malignant J91.0
newborn P28.89
tuberculous NEC A15.6
primary (progressive) A15.7
spinal — *see* Meningitis
thorax, thoracic — *see* Effusion, pleura
Egg shell nails L60.3
congenital Q84.6
EGPA (eosinophilic granulomatosis with polyangiitis) M30.1
Egyptian splenomegaly B65.1
Ehlers-Danlos syndrome — *see also* Syndrome, Ehlers-Danlos Q79.60
Ehrlichiosis A77.40
due to
E. chafeensis A77.41
E. ewingii A77.49
E. muris euclairensis A77.49
E. sennetsu A79.81
specified organism NEC A77.49
Eichstedt's disease B36.0
Eisenmenger's
complex or syndrome I27.83
defect Q21.8
Ejaculation
delayed F52.32
painful N53.12
premature F52.4
retarded N53.11
retrograde N53.14
semen, painful N53.12
psychogenic F52.6
Ekbom's syndrome (restless legs) G25.81
Ekman's syndrome (brittle bones and blue sclera) Q78.0
Elastic skin Q82.8
acquired L57.4
Elastofibroma — *see* Neoplasm, connective tissue, benign
Elastoma (juvenile) Q82.8
Miescher's L87.2
Elastomyofibrosis I42.4
Elastosis
actinic, solar L57.8
atrophicans (senile) L57.4
perforans serpiginosa L87.2
senilis L57.4
Elbow — *see* condition
Electric current, electricity, effects (concussion) (fatal) (nonfatal) (shock) T75.4 ☑
burn — *see* Burn
Electric feet syndrome E53.8
Electrocution T75.4 ☑
from electroshock gun (taser) T75.4 ☑
Electrolyte imbalance E87.8
with
abortion — *see* Abortion by type, complicated by, electrolyte imbalance
ectopic pregnancy O08.5
molar pregnancy O08.5
Elephantiasis (nonfilarial) I89.0
arabicum — *see* Infestation, filarial
bancroftian B74.0
congenital (any site) (hereditary) Q82.0
due to
Brugia (malayi) B74.1
timori B74.2
mastectomy I97.2
Wuchereria (bancrofti) B74.0
eyelid H02.859

Elephantiasis — *continued*
eyelid — *continued*
left H02.856
lower H02.855
upper H02.854
right H02.853
lower H02.852
upper H02.851
filarial, filariensis — *see* Infestation, filarial
glandular I89.0
graecorum A30.9
lymphangiectatic I89.0
lymphatic vessel I89.0
due to mastectomy I97.2
scrotum (nonfilarial) I89.0
streptococcal I89.0
surgical I97.89
postmastectomy I97.2
telangiectodes I89.0
vulva (nonfilarial) N90.89
Elevated, elevation
alanine transaminase (ALT) R74.01
ALT (alanine transaminase) R74.01
antibody titer R76.0
aspartate transaminase (AST) R74.01
AST (aspartate transaminase) R74.01
basal metabolic rate R94.8
blood pressure — *see also* Hypertension
reading (incidental) (isolated) (nonspecific), no diagnosis of hypertension R03.0
blood sugar R73.9
body temperature (of unknown origin) R50.9
cancer antigen 125 [CA 125] R97.1
carcinoembryonic antigen [CEA] R97.0
cholesterol E78.00
with high triglycerides E78.2
conjugate, eye H51.0
C-reactive protein (CRP) R79.82
diaphragm, congenital Q79.1
erythrocyte sedimentation rate R70.0
fasting glucose R73.01
fasting triglycerides E78.1
finding on laboratory examination — *see* Findings, abnormal, inconclusive, without diagnosis, by type of exam
GFR (glomerular filtration rate) — *see* Findings, abnormal, inconclusive, without diagnosis, by type of exam
glucose tolerance (oral) R73.02
immunoglobulin level R76.8
indoleacetic acid R82.5
lactic acid dehydrogenase (LDH) level R74.02
leukocytes D72.829
lipoprotein a (Lp(a)) level E78.41
liver function
study R94.5
test R79.89
alkaline phosphatase R74.8
aminotransferase R74.01
bilirubin R17
hepatic enzyme R74.8
lactate dehydrogenase R74.02
Lp(a) (lipoprotein(a)) E78.41
lymphocytes D72.820
prostate specific antigen [PSA] R97.20
Rh titer — *see* Complication(s), transfusion, incompatibility reaction, Rh (factor)
scapula, congenital Q74.0
sedimentation rate R70.0
SGOT R74.01
SGPT R74.01
transaminase level R74.01
triglycerides E78.1
with high cholesterol E78.2
troponin R77.8
tumor associated antigens [TAA] NEC R97.8
tumor specific antigens [TSA] NEC R97.8
urine level of
17-ketosteroids R82.5
catecholamine R82.5
indoleacetic acid R82.5
steroids R82.5
vanillylmandelic acid (VMA) R82.5
venous pressure I87.8
white blood cell count D72.829
specified NEC D72.828
Elliptocytosis (congenital) (hereditary) D58.1
Hb C (disease) D58.1

☑ **Additional Character Required — Refer to the Tabular List for Character Selection** ▽ Subterms under main terms may continue to next column or page

Elliptocytosis — *continued*
  hemoglobin disease D58.1
  sickle-cell (disease) D57.8- ☑
    trait D57.3
Ellison-Zollinger syndrome E16.4
Ellis-van Creveld syndrome (chondroectodermal dysplasia) Q77.6
Elongated, elongation (congenital) — *see also* Distortion
  bone Q79.9
  cervix (uteri) Q51.828
    acquired N88.4
    hypertrophic N88.4
  colon Q43.8
  common bile duct Q44.5
  cystic duct Q44.5
  frenulum, penis Q55.69
  labia minora (acquired) N90.69
  ligamentum patellae Q74.1
  petiolus (epiglottidis) Q31.8
  tooth, teeth K00.2
  uvula Q38.6
Eltor cholera A00.1
Emaciation (due to malnutrition) E43
Embadomoniasis A07.8
Embedded tooth, teeth K01.0
  root only K08.3
Embolic — *see* condition
Embolism (multiple) (paradoxical) I74.9
  air (any site) (traumatic) T79.0 ☑
    following
      abortion — *see* Abortion by type complicated by embolism
      ectopic pregnancy O08.2
      infusion, therapeutic injection or transfusion T80.0 ☑
      molar pregnancy O08.2
      procedure NEC
        artery T81.719 ☑
          mesenteric T81.710 ☑
          renal T81.711 ☑
          specified NEC T81.718 ☑
        vein T81.72 ☑
    in pregnancy, childbirth or puerperium — *see* Embolism, obstetric
  amniotic fluid (pulmonary) — *see also* Embolism, obstetric
    following
      abortion — *see* Abortion by type complicated by embolism
      ectopic pregnancy O08.2
      molar pregnancy O08.2
  aorta, aortic I74.10
    abdominal I74.09
      saddle I74.01
    bifurcation I74.09
    saddle I74.01
    thoracic I74.11
  artery I74.9
    auditory, internal I65.8
    basilar — *see* Occlusion, artery, basilar
    carotid (common) (internal) — *see* Occlusion, artery, carotid
    cerebellar (anterior inferior) (posterior inferior) (superior) I66.3
    cerebral — *see* Occlusion, artery, cerebral
    choroidal (anterior) I65.8
    communicating posterior I65.8
    coronary — *see also* Infarct, myocardium
      not resulting in infarction I24.0
    extremity I74.4
      lower I74.3
      upper I74.2
    hypophyseal I65.8
    iliac I74.5
    limb I74.4
      lower I74.3
      upper I74.2
    mesenteric (with gangrene) — *see also* Ischemia, intestine, acute K55.059
    ophthalmic — *see* Occlusion, artery, retina
    peripheral I74.4
    pontine I65.8
    precerebral — *see* Occlusion, artery, precerebral
    pulmonary — *see* Embolism, pulmonary
    renal N28.0
    retinal — *see* Occlusion, artery, retina
    septic I76

Embolism — *continued*
  artery — *continued*
    specified NEC I74.8
    vertebral — *see* Occlusion, artery, vertebral
  basilar (artery) I65.1
  blood clot
    following
      abortion — *see* Abortion by type complicated by embolism
      ectopic or molar pregnancy O08.2
    in pregnancy, childbirth or puerperium — *see* Embolism, obstetric
  brain — *see also* Occlusion, artery, cerebral
    following
      abortion — *see* Abortion by type complicated by embolism
      ectopic or molar pregnancy O08.2
    puerperal, postpartum, childbirth — *see* Embolism, obstetric
  capillary I78.8
  cardiac — *see also* Infarct, myocardium
    not resulting in infarction I51.3
  carotid (artery) (common) (internal) — *see* Occlusion, artery, carotid
  cavernous sinus (venous) — *see* Embolism, intracranial venous sinus
  cerebral — *see* Occlusion, artery, cerebral
  cholesterol — *see* Atheroembolism
  coronary (artery or vein) (systemic) — *see* Occlusion, coronary
  due to device, implant or graft — *see also* Complications, by site and type, specified NEC
    arterial graft NEC T82.818 ☑
    breast (implant) T85.818 ☑
    catheter NEC T85.818 ☑
      dialysis (renal) T82.818 ☑
        intraperitoneal T85.818 ☑
      infusion NEC T82.818 ☑
        spinal (epidural) (subdural) T85.810 ☑
      urinary (indwelling) T83.81 ☑
    electronic (electrode) (pulse generator) (stimulator)
      bone T84.81 ☑
      cardiac T82.817 ☑
      nervous system (brain) (peripheral nerve) (spinal) T85.810 ☑
      urinary T83.81 ☑
    fixation, internal (orthopedic) NEC T84.81 ☑
    gastrointestinal (bile duct) (esophagus) T85.818 ☑
    genital NEC T83.81 ☑
    heart (graft) (valve) T82.817 ☑
    joint prosthesis T84.81 ☑
    ocular (corneal graft) (orbital implant) T85.818 ☑
    orthopedic (bone graft) NEC T86.838
    specified NEC T85.818 ☑
    urinary (graft) NEC T83.81 ☑
    vascular NEC T82.818 ☑
    ventricular intracranial shunt T85.810 ☑
  extremities
    lower — *see* Embolism, vein, lower extremity
      arterial I74.3
    upper I74.2
  eye H34.9
  fat (cerebral) (pulmonary) (systemic) T79.1 ☑
    complicating delivery — *see* Embolism, obstetric
    following
      abortion — *see* Abortion by type complicated by embolism
      ectopic or molar pregnancy O08.2
  following
    abortion — *see* Abortion by type complicated by embolism
    ectopic or molar pregnancy O08.2
    infusion, therapeutic injection or transfusion
      air T80.0 ☑
  heart (fatty) — *see also* Infarct, myocardium
    not resulting in infarction I51.3
  hepatic (vein) I82.0
  in pregnancy, childbirth or puerperium — *see* Embolism, obstetric
  intestine (artery) (vein) (with gangrene) — *see also* Ischemia, intestine, acute K55.039
  intracranial — *see also* Occlusion, artery, cerebral
    venous sinus (any) G08
      nonpyogenic I67.6
  intraspinal venous sinuses or veins G08
    nonpyogenic G95.19
  kidney (artery) N28.0

Embolism — *continued*
  lateral sinus (venous) — *see* Embolism, intracranial, venous sinus
  leg — *see* Embolism, vein, lower extremity
    arterial I74.3
  longitudinal sinus (venous) — *see* Embolism, intracranial, venous sinus
  lung (massive) — *see* Embolism, pulmonary
  meninges I66.8
  mesenteric (artery) (vein) (with gangrene) — *see also* Ischemia, intestine, acute K55.059
  obstetric (in) (pulmonary)
    childbirth O88.22
      air O88.02
      amniotic fluid O88.12
      blood clot O88.22
      fat O88.82
      pyemic O88.32
      septic O88.32
      specified type NEC O88.82
    pregnancy O88.21- ☑
      air O88.01- ☑
      amniotic fluid O88.11- ☑
      blood clot O88.21- ☑
      fat O88.81- ☑
      pyemic O88.31- ☑
      septic O88.31- ☑
      specified type NEC O88.81- ☑
    puerperal O88.23
      air O88.03
      amniotic fluid O88.13
      blood clot O88.23
      fat O88.83
      pyemic O88.33
      septic O88.33
      specified type NEC O88.83
  ophthalmic — *see* Occlusion, artery, retina
  penis N48.81
  peripheral artery NOS I74.4
  pituitary E23.6
  popliteal (artery) I74.3
  portal (vein) I81
  postoperative, postprocedural
    artery T81.719 ☑
      mesenteric T81.710 ☑
      renal T81.711 ☑
      specified NEC T81.718 ☑
    vein T81.72 ☑
  precerebral artery — *see* Occlusion, artery, precerebral
  puerperal — *see* Embolism, obstetric
  pulmonary (acute) (artery) (vein) I26.99
    with acute cor pulmonale I26.09
    chronic I27.82
    following
      abortion — *see* Abortion by type complicated by embolism
      ectopic or molar pregnancy O08.2
    healed or old Z86.711
    in pregnancy, childbirth or puerperium — *see* Embolism, obstetric
    multiple subsegmental without acute cor pulmonale I26.94
    personal history of Z86.711
    saddle I26.92
      with acute cor pulmonale I26.02
    septic I26.90
      with acute cor pulmonale I26.01
    single subsegmental without acute cor pulmonale I26.93
    subsegmental NOS I26.93
  pyemic (multiple) I76
    following
      abortion — *see* Abortion by type complicated by embolism
      ectopic or molar pregnancy O08.2
    Hemophilus influenzae A41.3
    pneumococcal A40.3
      with pneumonia J13
    puerperal, postpartum, childbirth (any organism) — *see* Embolism, obstetric
    specified organism NEC A41.89
    staphylococcal A41.2
    streptococcal A40.9
  renal (artery) N28.0
    vein I82.3
  retina, retinal — *see* Occlusion, artery, retina
  saddle
    abdominal aorta I74.01

☒ Subterms under main terms may continue to next column or page   ☑ Additional Character Required — Refer to the Tabular List for Character Selection   **131**

Elliptocytosis — Embolism

Embolism — *continued*
  saddle — *continued*
    pulmonary artery I26.92
      with acute cor pulmonale I26.02
  septic (arterial) I76
    complicating abortion — *see* Abortion, by type, complicated by, embolism
  sinus — *see* Embolism, intracranial, venous sinus
  soap complicating abortion — *see* Abortion, by type, complicated by, embolism
  spinal cord G95.19
    pyogenic origin G06.1
  spleen, splenic (artery) I74.8
  upper extremity I74.2
  vein (acute) I82.90
    antecubital I82.61- ☑
      chronic I82.71- ☑
    axillary I82.A1- ☑ (*following* I82.7)
      chronic I82.A2- ☑ (*following* I82.7)
    basilic I82.61- ☑
      chronic I82.71- ☑
    brachial I82.62- ☑
      chronic I82.72- ☑
    brachiocephalic (innominate) I82.290
      chronic I82.291
    cephalic I82.61- ☑
      chronic I82.71- ☑
    chronic I82.91
    deep (DVT) I82.40- ☑
      calf I82.4Z- ☑
        chronic I82.5Z- ☑
      lower leg I82.4Z- ☑
        chronic I82.5Z- ☑
      thigh I82.4Y- ☑
        chronic I82.5Y- ☑
      upper leg I82.4Y ☑
        chronic I82.5Y-
    femoral I82.41- ☑
      chronic I82.51- ☑
    iliac (iliofemoral) I82.42- ☑
      chronic I82.52- ☑
    innominate I82.290
      chronic I82.291
    internal jugular I82.C1- ☑ (*following* I82.7)
      chronic I82.C2- ☑ (*following* I82.7)
    lower extremity
      deep I82.40- ☑
        chronic I82.50- ☑
        specified NEC I82.49- ☑
          chronic NEC I82.59- ☑
      distal
        deep I82.4Z- ☑
      proximal
        deep I82.4Y- ☑
          chronic I82.5Y- ☑
      superficial I82.81- ☑
    popliteal I82.43- ☑
      chronic I82.53- ☑
    radial I82.62- ☑
      chronic I82.72- ☑
    renal I82.3
    saphenous (greater) (lesser) I82.81- ☑
    specified NEC I82.890
      chronic NEC I82.891
    subclavian I82.B1- ☑ (*following* I82.7)
      chronic I82.B2- ☑ (*following* I82.7)
    thoracic NEC I82.290
      chronic I82.291
    tibial I82.44- ☑
      chronic I82.54- ☑
    ulnar I82.62- ☑
      chronic I82.72- ☑
    upper extremity I82.60- ☑
      chronic I82.70- ☑
      deep I82.62- ☑
        chronic I82.72- ☑
      superficial I82.61- ☑
        chronic I82.71- ☑
  vena cava
    inferior (acute) I82.220
      chronic I82.221
    superior (acute) I82.210
      chronic I82.211
  venous sinus G08
  vessels of brain — *see* Occlusion, artery, cerebral
Embolus — *see* Embolism

Embryoma — *see also* Neoplasm, uncertain behavior, by site
  benign — *see* Neoplasm, benign, by site
  kidney C64.- ☑
  liver C22.0
  malignant — *see also* Neoplasm, malignant, by site
    kidney C64.- ☑
    liver C22.0
    testis C62.9- ☑
      descended (scrotal) C62.1- ☑
      undescended C62.0- ☑
    testis C62.9- ☑
      descended (scrotal) C62.1- ☑
      undescended C62.0- ☑
Embryonic
  circulation Q28.9
  heart Q28.9
  vas deferens Q55.4
Embryopathia NOS Q89.9
Embryotoxon Q13.4
Emesis — *see* Vomiting
Emotional lability R45.86
Emotionality, pathological F60.3
Emotogenic disease — *see* Disorder, psychogenic
Emphysema (atrophic) (bullous) (chronic) (interlobular) (lung) (obstructive) (pulmonary) (senile) (vesicular) J43.9
  cellular tissue (traumatic) T79.7 ☑
    surgical T81.82 ☑
  centrilobular J43.2
  compensatory J98.3
  congenital (interstitial) P25.0
  conjunctiva H11.89
  connective tissue (traumatic) T79.7 ☑
    surgical T81.82 ☑
  due to chemicals, gases, fumes or vapors J68.4
  eyelid(s) — *see* Disorder, eyelid, specified type NEC
    surgical T81.82 ☑
    traumatic T79.7 ☑
  interstitial J98.2
    congenital P25.0
    perinatal period P25.0
  laminated tissue T79.7 ☑
    surgical T81.82 ☑
  mediastinal J98.2
    newborn P25.2
  orbit, orbital — *see* Disorder, orbit, specified type NEC
  panacinar J43.1
  panlobular J43.1
  specified NEC J43.8
  subcutaneous (traumatic) T79.7 ☑
    nontraumatic J98.2
    postprocedural T81.82 ☑
    surgical T81.82 ☑
  surgical T81.82 ☑
  thymus (gland) (congenital) E32.8
  traumatic (subcutaneous) T79.7 ☑
  unilateral J43.0
Empty nest syndrome Z60.0
Empyema (acute) (chest) (double) (pleura) (supradiaphragmatic) (thorax) J86.9
  with fistula J86.0
  accessory sinus (chronic) — *see* Sinusitis
  antrum (chronic) — *see* Sinusitis, maxillary
  brain (any part) — *see* Abscess, brain
  ethmoidal (chronic) (sinus) — *see* Sinusitis, ethmoidal
  extradural — *see* Abscess, extradural
  frontal (chronic) (sinus) — *see* Sinusitis, frontal
  gallbladder K81.0
  mastoid (process) (acute) — *see* Mastoiditis, acute
  maxilla, maxillary M27.2
    sinus (chronic) — *see* Sinusitis, maxillary
  nasal sinus (chronic) — *see* Sinusitis
  sinus (accessory) (chronic) (nasal) — *see* Sinusitis
  sphenoidal (sinus) (chronic) — *see* Sinusitis, sphenoidal
  subarachnoid — *see* Abscess, extradural
  subdural — *see* Abscess, subdural
  tuberculous A15.6
  ureter — *see* Ureteritis
  ventricular — *see* Abscess, brain
En coup de sabre lesion L94.1
Enamel pearls K00.2
Enameloma K00.2
Enanthema, viral B09
Encephalitis (chronic) (hemorrhagic) (idiopathic) (nonepidemic) (spurious) (subacute) G04.90
  acute — *see also* Encephalitis, viral A86

Encephalitis — *continued*
  acute — *see also* Encephalitis, viral — *continued*
    disseminated G04.00
      infectious G04.01
      noninfectious G04.81
      postimmunization (postvaccination) G04.02
      postinfectious G04.01
    inclusion body A85.8
    necrotizing hemorrhagic G04.30
      postimmunization G04.32
      postinfectious G04.31
      specified NEC G04.39
  arboviral, arbovirus NEC A85.2
  arthropod-borne NEC (viral) A85.2
  Australian A83.4
  California (virus) A83.5
  Central European (tick-borne) A84.1
  Czechoslovakian A84.1
  Dawson's (inclusion body) A81.1
  diffuse sclerosing A81.1
  disseminated, acute G04.00
  due to
    cat scratch disease A28.1
    human immunodeficiency virus (HIV) disease B20 [G05.3]
    malaria — *see* Malaria
    rickettsiosis — *see* Rickettsiosis
    smallpox inoculation G04.02
    typhus — *see* Typhus
  Eastern equine A83.2
  endemic (viral) A86
  epidemic NEC (viral) A86
  equine (acute) (infectious) (viral) A83.9
    Eastern A83.2
    Venezuelan A92.2
    Western A83.1
  Far Eastern (tick-borne) A84.0
  following vaccination or other immunization procedure G04.02
  herpes zoster B02.0
  herpesviral B00.4
    due to herpesvirus 6 B10.01
    due to herpesvirus 7 B10.09
    specified NEC B10.09
  Ilheus (virus) A83.8
  in (due to)
    actinomycosis A42.82
    adenovirus A85.1
    African trypanosomiasis B56.9 [G05.3]
    Chagas' disease (chronic) B57.42
    cytomegalovirus B25.8
    enterovirus A85.0
    herpes (simplex) virus B00.4
      due to herpesvirus 6 B10.01
      due to herpesvirus 7 B10.09
      specified NEC B10.09
    infectious disease NEC B99 ☑ [G05.3]
    influenza — *see* Influenza, with, encephalopathy
    listeriosis A32.12
    measles B05.0
    mumps B26.2
    naegleriasis B60.2
    parasitic disease NEC B89 [G05.3]
    poliovirus A80.9 [G05.3]
    rubella B06.01
    syphilis
      congenital A50.42
      late A52.14
    systemic lupus erythematosus M32.19
    toxoplasmosis (acquired) B58.2
      congenital P37.1
    tuberculosis A17.82
    zoster B02.0
  inclusion body A81.1
  infectious (acute) (virus) NEC A86
  Japanese (B type) A83.0
  La Crosse A83.5
  lead — *see* Poisoning, lead
  lethargica (acute) (infectious) A85.8
  louping ill A84.89
  lupus erythematosus, systemic M32.19
  lymphatica A87.2
  Mengo A85.8
  meningococcal A39.81
  Murray Valley A83.4
  otitic NEC H66.40 [G05.3]
  parasitic NOS B71.9
  periaxial G37.0

☑ **Additional Character Required** — Refer to the Tabular List for Character Selection

⬩ **Subterms under main terms may continue to next column or page**

Encephalitis — *continued*
  periaxialis (concentrica) (diffuse) G37.5
  postchickenpox B01.11
  postexanthematous NEC B09
  postimmunization G04.02
  postinfectious NEC G04.01
  postmeasles B05.0
  postvaccinal G04.02
  postvaricella B01.11
  postviral NEC A86
  Powassan A84.81
  Rasmussen G04.81
  Rio Bravo A85.8
  Russian
    autumnal A83.0
    spring-summer (taiga) A84.0
  saturnine — *see* Poisoning, lead
  specified NEC G04.81
  St. Louis A83.3
  subacute sclerosing A81.1
  summer A83.0
  suppurative G04.81
  tick-borne A84.9
  Torula, torular (cryptococcal) B45.1
  toxic NEC G92
  trichinosis B75 *[G05.3]*
  type
    B A83.0
    C A83.3
  van Bogaert's A81.1
  Venezuelan equine A92.2
  Vienna A85.8
  viral, virus A86
    arthropod-borne NEC A85.2
      mosquito-borne A83.9
        Australian X disease A83.4
        California virus A83.5
        Eastern equine A83.2
        Japanese (B type) A83.0
        Murray Valley A83.4
        specified NEC A83.8
        St. Louis A83.3
        type B A83.0
        type C A83.3
        Western equine A83.1
      tick-borne A84.9
        biundulant A84.1
        central European A84.1
        Czechoslovakian A84.1
        diphasic meningoencephalitis A84.1
        Far Eastern A84.0
        Russian spring-summer (taiga) A84.0
        specified NEC A84.89
      specified type NEC A85.8
      tick-borne, specified NEC A84.89
  Western equine A83.1
Encephalocele Q01.9
  frontal Q01.0
  nasofrontal Q01.1
  occipital Q01.2
  specified NEC Q01.8
Encephalocystocele — *see* Encephalocele
Encephaloduroarteriomyosynangiosis (EDAMS) I67.5
Encephalomalacia (brain) (cerebellar) (cerebral) — *see* Softening, brain
Encephalomeningitis — *see* Meningoencephalitis
Encephalomeningocele — *see* Encephalocele
Encephalomeningomyelitis — *see* Meningoencephalitis
Encephalomyelitis — *see also* Encephalitis G04.90
  acute disseminated G04.00
    infectious G04.01
    noninfectious G04.81
    postimmunization G04.02
    postinfectious G04.01
  acute necrotizing hemorrhagic G04.30
    postimmunization G04.32
    postinfectious G04.31
    specified NEC G04.39
  benign myalgic G93.3
  equine A83.9
    Eastern A83.2
    Venezuelan A92.2
    Western A83.1
  in diseases classified elsewhere G05.3
  myalgic, benign G93.3
  postchickenpox B01.11
  postinfectious NEC G04.01
  postmeasles B05.0

Encephalomyelitis — *continued*
  postvaccinal G04.02
  postvaricella B01.11
  rubella B06.01
  specified NEC G04.81
  Venezuelan equine A92.2
Encephalomyelocele — *see* Encephalocele
Encephalomyelomeningitis — *see* Meningoencephalitis
Encephalomyelopathy G96.9
Encephalomyeloradiculitis (acute) G61.0
Encephalomyeloradiculoneuritis (acute) (Guillain-Barré) G61.0
Encephalomyeloradiculopathy G96.9
Encephalopathia hyperbilirubinemica, newborn P57.9
  due to isoimmunization (conditions in P55) P57.0
Encephalopathy (acute) G93.40
  acute necrotizing hemorrhagic G04.30
    postimmunization G04.32
    postinfectious G04.31
    specified NEC G04.39
  alcoholic G31.2
  anoxic — *see* Damage, brain, anoxic
  arteriosclerotic I67.2
  centrolobar progressive (Schilder) G37.0
  congenital Q07.9
  degenerative, in specified disease NEC G32.89
  demyelinating callosal G37.1
  due to
    drugs — *see also* Table of Drugs and Chemicals G92
  hepatic — *see* Failure, hepatic
  hyperbilirubinemic, newborn P57.9
    due to isoimmunization (conditions in P55) P57.0
  hypertensive I67.4
  hypoglycemic E16.2
  hypoxic — *see* Damage, brain, anoxic
  hypoxic ischemic P91.60
    mild P91.61
    moderate P91.62
    severe P91.63
  in (due to) (with)
    birth injury P11.1
    hyperinsulinism E16.1 *[G94]*
    influenza — *see* Influenza, with, encephalopathy
    lack of vitamin — *see also* Deficiency, vitamin E56.9 *[G32.89]*
    neoplastic disease — *see also* Neoplasm D49.9 *[G13.1]*
    serum — *see also* Reaction, serum T80.69 ☑
    syphilis A52.17
    trauma (postconcussional) F07.81
      current injury — *see* Injury, intracranial
    vaccination G04.02
  lead — *see* Poisoning, lead
  metabolic G93.41
    drug induced G92
    toxic G92
  myoclonic, early, symptomatic — *see* Epilepsy, generalized, specified NEC
  necrotizing, subacute (Leigh) G31.82
  neonatal P91.819
    in diseases classified elsewhere P91.811
  pellagrous E52 *[G32.89]*
  portosystemic — *see* Failure, hepatic
  postcontusional F07.81
    current injury — *see* Injury, intracranial, diffuse
  posthypoglycemic (coma) E16.1 *[G94]*
  postradiation G93.89
  saturnine — *see* Poisoning, lead
  septic G93.41
  specified NEC G93.49
  spongiform, subacute (viral) A81.09
  toxic G92
    metabolic G92
  traumatic (postconcussional) F07.81
    current injury — *see* Injury, intracranial
  vitamin B deficiency NEC E53.9 *[G32.89]*
    vitamin B1 E51.2
  Wernicke's E51.2
Encephalorrhagia — *see* Hemorrhage, intracranial, intracerebral
Encephalosis, posttraumatic F07.81
Enchondroma — *see also* Neoplasm, bone, benign
Enchondromatosis (cartilaginous) (multiple) Q78.4
Encopresis R15.9
  functional F98.1
  nonorganic origin F98.1
  psychogenic F98.1

Encounter (with health service) (for) Z76.89
  adjustment and management (of)
    breast implant Z45.81 ☑
    implanted device NEC Z45.89
    myringotomy device (stent) (tube) Z45.82
    neurostimulator (brain) (gastric) (peripheral nerve) (sacral nerve) (spinal cord) (vagus nerve) Z45.42
  administrative purpose only Z02.9
    examination for
      adoption Z02.82
      armed forces Z02.3
      disability determination Z02.71
      driving license Z02.4
      employment Z02.1
      insurance Z02.6
      medical certificate NEC Z02.79
      paternity testing Z02.81
      residential institution admission Z02.2
      school admission Z02.0
      sports Z02.5
      specified reason NEC Z02.89
  aftercare — *see* Aftercare
  antenatal screening Z36.9
    cervical length Z36.86
    chromosomal anomalies Z36.0
    congenital cardiac abnormalities Z36.83
    elevated maternal serum alphafetoprotein Z36.1
    fetal growth retardation Z36.4
    fetal lung maturity Z36.84
    fetal macrosomia Z36.88
    hydrops fetalis Z36.81
    intrauterine growth restriction (IUGR) /small-for-dates Z36.4
    isoimmunization Z36.5
    large-for-dates Z36.88
    malformations Z36.3
    non-visualized anatomy on a previous scan Z36.2
    nuchal translucency Z36.82
    raised alphafetoprotein level Z36.1
    risk of pre-term labor Z36.86
    specified follow-up NEC Z36.2
    specified genetic defects NEC Z36.8A
    specified type NEC Z36.89
    Streptococcus B Z36.85
    suspected anomaly Z36.3
    uncertain dates Z36.87
  assisted reproductive fertility procedure cycle Z31.83
  blood typing Z01.83
    Rh typing Z01.83
  breast augmentation or reduction Z41.1
  breast implant exchange (different material) (different size) Z45.81 ☑
  breast reconstruction following mastectomy Z42.1
  check-up — *see* Examination
  chemotherapy for neoplasm Z51.11
  colonoscopy, screening Z12.11
  counseling — *see* Counseling
  delivery, full-term, uncomplicated O80
    cesarean, without indication O82
  desensitization to allergens Z51.6
  ear piercing Z41.3
  examination — *see* Examination
  expectant parent(s) (adoptive) pre-birth pediatrician visit Z76.81
  fertility preservation procedure (prior to cancer therapy) (prior to removal of gonads) Z31.84
  fitting (of) — *see* Fitting (and adjustment) (of)
  genetic
    counseling
      nonprocreative Z71.83
      procreative Z31.5
    testing — *see* Test, genetic
  hearing conservation and treatment Z01.12
  immunotherapy for neoplasm Z51.12
  in vitro fertilization cycle Z31.83
  instruction (in)
    child care (postpartal) (prenatal) Z32.3
    childbirth Z32.2
    natural family planning
      procreative Z31.61
      to avoid pregnancy Z30.02
  insulin pump titration Z46.81
  joint prosthesis insertion following prior explantation of joint prosthesis (staged procedure)
    hip Z47.32
    knee Z47.33
    shoulder Z47.31

▽ Subterms under main terms may continue to next column or page   ☑ Additional Character Required — Refer to the Tabular List for Character Selection   **133**

Encephalitis — Encounter

Endocarditis — *continued*
　pulmonary — *continued*
　　congenital Q22.2
　　rheumatic (chronic) (inactive) (with chorea) I09.89
　　　active or acute I01.1
　　　　with chorea (acute) (rheumatic) (Sydenham's) I02.0
　　syphilitic A52.03
　purulent (acute) (any valve) (subacute) I33.0
　Q fever A78 [I39]
　rheumatic (chronic) (inactive) (with chorea) I09.1
　　active or acute (aortic) (mitral) (pulmonary) (tricuspid) I01.1
　　　with chorea (acute) (rheumatic) (Sydenham's) I02.0
　rheumatoid — *see* Rheumatoid, carditis
　septic (acute) (any valve) (subacute) I33.0
　streptococcal (acute) (any valve) (subacute) I33.0
　subacute — *see* Endocarditis, acute
　suppurative (acute) (any valve) (subacute) I33.0
　syphilitic A52.03
　toxic I33.9
　tricuspid (chronic) (heart) (inactive) (rheumatic) (valve) (with chorea) I07.9
　　with
　　　aortic (valve) disease I08.2
　　　　mitral (valve) disease I08.3
　　　mitral (valve) disease I08.1
　　　　aortic (valve) disease I08.3
　　　rheumatic fever (conditions in I00)
　　　　active — *see* Endocarditis, acute, rheumatic
　　　　inactive or quiescent (with chorea) I07.8
　　active or acute I01.1
　　　with chorea (acute) (rheumatic) (Sydenham's) I02.0
　arteriosclerotic I36.8
　nonrheumatic I36.8
　　acute or subacute I33.9
　specified cause, except rheumatic I36.8
　tuberculous — *see* Tuberculosis, endocarditis
　typhoid A01.02
　ulcerative (acute) (any valve) (subacute) I33.0
　vegetative (acute) (any valve) (subacute) I33.0
　verrucous (atypical) (nonbacterial) (nonrheumatic) M32.11
Endocardium, endocardial — *see also* condition
　cushion defect Q21.2
Endocervicitis — *see also* Cervicitis
　due to intrauterine (contraceptive) device T83.69 ☑
　hyperplastic N72
Endocrine — *see* condition
Endocrinopathy, pluriglandular E31.9
Endodontic
　overfill M27.52
　underfill M27.53
Endodontitis K04.01
　irreversible K04.02
　reversible K04.01
Endomastoiditis — *see* Mastoiditis
Endometrioma N80.9
Endometriosis N80.9
　appendix N80.5
　bladder N80.8
　bowel N80.5
　broad ligament N80.3
　cervix N80.0
　colon N80.5
　cul-de-sac (Douglas') N80.3
　exocervix N80.0
　fallopian tube N80.2
　female genital organ NEC N80.8
　gallbladder N80.8
　in scar of skin N80.6
　internal N80.0
　intestine N80.5
　lung N80.8
　myometrium N80.0
　ovary N80.1
　parametrium N80.3
　pelvic peritoneum N80.3
　peritoneal (pelvic) N80.3
　rectovaginal septum N80.4
　rectum N80.5
　round ligament N80.3
　skin (scar) N80.6
　specified site NEC N80.8
　stromal D39.0
　thorax N80.8

Endometriosis — *continued*
　umbilicus N80.8
　uterus (internal) N80.0
　vagina N80.4
　vulva N80.8
Endometritis (decidual) (nonspecific) (purulent) (senile) (atrophic) (suppurative) N71.9
　with ectopic pregnancy O08.0
　acute N71.0
　blenorrhagic (gonococcal) (acute) (chronic) A54.24
　cervix, cervical (with erosion or ectropion) — *see also* Cervicitis
　　hyperplastic N72
　chlamydial A56.11
　chronic N71.1
　following
　　abortion — *see* Abortion by type complicated by genital infection
　　ectopic or molar pregnancy O08.0
　gonococcal, gonorrheal (acute) (chronic) A54.24
　hyperplastic — *see also* Hyperplasia, endometrial N85.00
　　cervix N72
　puerperal, postpartum, childbirth O86.12
　subacute N71.0
　tuberculous A18.17
Endometrium — *see* condition
Endomyocardiopathy, South African I42.3
Endomyocarditis — *see* Endocarditis
Endomyofibrosis I42.3
Endomyometritis — *see* Endometritis
Endopericarditis — *see* Endocarditis
Endoperineuritis — *see* Disorder, nerve
Endophlebitis — *see* Phlebitis
Endophthalmia — *see* Endophthalmitis, purulent
Endophthalmitis (acute) (infective) (metastatic) (subacute) H44.009
　bleb associated — *see also* Bleb, inflamed (infected), postprocedural H59.4 ☑
　gonorrheal A54.39
　in (due to)
　　cysticercosis B69.1
　　onchocerciasis B73.01
　　toxocariasis B83.0
　panuveitis — *see* Panuveitis
　parasitic H44.12- ☑
　purulent H44.00- ☑
　　panophthalmitis — *see* Panophthalmitis
　　vitreous abscess H44.02- ☑
　specified NEC H44.19
　sympathetic — *see* Uveitis, sympathetic
Endosalpingioma D28.2
Endosalpingiosis N94.89
Endosteitis — *see* Osteomyelitis
Endothelioma, bone — *see* Neoplasm, bone, malignant
Endotheliosis (hemorrhagic infectional) D69.8
Endotoxemia — code to condition
Endotrachelitis — *see* Cervicitis
Engelmann (-Camurati) **syndrome** Q78.3
English disease — *see* Rickets
Engman's disease L30.3
Engorgement
　breast N64.59
　　newborn P83.4
　　puerperal, postpartum O92.79
　lung (passive) — *see* Edema, lung
　pulmonary (passive) — *see* Edema, lung
　stomach K31.89
　venous, retina — *see* Occlusion, retina, vein, engorgement
Enlargement, enlarged — *see also* Hypertrophy
　adenoids J35.2
　　with tonsils J35.3
　alveolar ridge K08.89
　　congenital — *see* Anomaly, alveolar
　apertures of diaphragm (congenital) Q79.1
　gingival K06.1
　heart, cardiac — *see* Hypertrophy, cardiac
　labium majus, childhood asymmetric (CALME) N90.61
　lacrimal gland, chronic H04.03- ☑
　liver — *see* Hypertrophy, liver
　lymph gland or node R59.9
　　generalized R59.1
　　localized R59.0
　orbit H05.34- ☑
　organ or site, congenital NEC — *see* Anomaly, by site
　parathyroid (gland) E21.0

Enlargement, enlarged — *continued*
　pituitary fossa R93.0
　prostate N40.0
　　with lower urinary tract symptoms (LUTS) N40.1
　　without lower urinary tract symtpoms (LUTS) N40.0
　sella turcica R93.0
　spleen — *see* Splenomegaly
　thymus (gland) (congenital) E32.0
　thyroid (gland) — *see* Goiter
　tongue K14.8
　tonsils J35.1
　　with adenoids J35.3
　uterus N85.2
　vestibular aqueduct Q16.5
Enophthalmos H05.40- ☑
　due to
　　orbital tissue atrophy H05.41- ☑
　　trauma or surgery H05.42- ☑
Enostosis M27.8
Entamebic, entamebiasis — *see* Amebiasis
Entanglement
　umbilical cord(s) O69.82 ☑
　　with compression O69.2 ☑
　　around neck (with compression) O69.81 ☑
　　　with compression O69.1 ☑
　　　without compression O69.81 ☑
　　of twins in monoamniotic sac O69.2 ☑
　　without compression O69.82 ☑
Enteralgia — *see* Pain, abdominal
Enteric — *see* condition
Enteritis (acute) (diarrheal) (hemorrhagic) (noninfective) K52.9
　adenovirus A08.2
　aertrycke infection A02.0
　allergic K52.29
　　with
　　　eosinophilic gastritis or gastroenteritis K52.81
　　　food protein-induced enterocolitis syndrome K52.21
　　　food protein-induced enteropathy K52.22
　　　FPIES K52.21
　amebic (acute) A06.0
　　with abscess — *see* Abscess, amebic
　　chronic A06.1
　　　with abscess — *see* Abscess, amebic
　　　nondysenteric A06.2
　　nondysenteric A06.2
　astrovirus A08.32
　bacillary NOS A03.9
　bacterial A04.9
　　specified NEC A04.8
　calicivirus A08.31
　candidal B37.82
　Chilomastix A07.8
　choleriformis A00.1
　chronic (noninfectious) K52.9
　　ulcerative — *see* Colitis, ulcerative
　cicatrizing (chronic) — *see* Enteritis, regional, small intestine
　Clostridium
　　botulinum (food poisoning) A05.1
　　difficile
　　　not specified as recurrent A04.72
　　　recurrent A04.71
　coccidial A07.3
　coxsackie virus A08.39
　dietetic — *see also* Enteritis, allergic K52.29
　drug-induced K52.1
　due to
　　astrovirus A08.32
　　calicivirus A08.31
　　coxsackie virus A08.39
　　drugs K52.1
　　echovirus A08.39
　　enterovirus NEC A08.39
　　food hypersensitivity — *see also* Enteritis, allergic K52.29
　　infectious organism (bacterial) (viral) — *see* Enteritis, infectious
　　torovirus A08.39
　　Yersinia enterocolitica A04.6
　echovirus A08.39
　eltor A00.1
　enterovirus NEC A08.39
　eosinophilic K52.81
　epidemic (infectious) A09
　fulminant — *see also* Ischemia, intestine, acute K55.019
　gangrenous — *see* Enteritis, infectious

Enteritis — *continued*
  giardial A07.1
  infectious NOS A09
    due to
      adenovirus A08.2
      Aerobacter aerogenes A04.8
      Arizona (bacillus) A02.0
      bacteria NOS A04.9
        specified NEC A04.8
      Campylobacter A04.5
      Clostridium difficile
        not specified as recurrent A04.72
        recurrent A04.71
      Clostridium perfringens A04.8
      Enterobacter aerogenes A04.8
      enterovirus A08.39
      Escherichia coli A04.4
        enteroaggregative A04.4
        enterohemorrhagic A04.3
        enteroinvasive A04.2
        enteropathogenic A04.0
        enterotoxigenic A04.1
        specified NEC A04.4
      specified
        bacteria NEC A04.8
        virus NEC A08.39
      Staphylococcus A04.8
      virus NEC A08.4
        specified type NEC A08.39
      Yersinia enterocolitica A04.6
    specified organism NEC A08.8
  influenzal — *see* Influenza, with, digestive manifestations
  ischemic K55.9
    acute — *see also* Ischemia, intestine, acute K55.019
    chronic K55.1
  microsporidial A07.8
  mucomembranous, myxomembranous — *see* Syndrome, irritable bowel
  mucous — *see* Syndrome, irritable bowel
  necroticans A05.2
  necrotizing of newborn — *see* Enterocolitis, necrotizing, in newborn
  neurogenic — *see* Syndrome, irritable bowel
  newborn necrotizing — *see* Enterocolitis, necrotizing, in newborn
  noninfectious K52.9
  norovirus A08.11
  parasitic NEC B82.9
  paratyphoid (fever) — *see* Fever, paratyphoid
  protozoal A07.9
    specified NEC A07.8
  radiation K52.0
  regional (of) K50.90
    with
      complication K50.919
        abscess K50.914
        fistula K50.913
        intestinal obstruction K50.912
        rectal bleeding K50.911
        specified complication NEC K50.918
    colon — *see* Enteritis, regional, large intestine
    duodenum — *see* Enteritis, regional, small intestine
    ileum — *see* Enteritis, regional, small intestine
    jejunum — *see* Enteritis, regional, small intestine
    large bowel — *see* Enteritis, regional, large intestine
    large intestine (colon) (rectum) K50.10
      with
        complication K50.119
          abscess K50.114
          fistula K50.113
          intestinal obstruction K50.112
          rectal bleeding K50.111
          small intestine (duodenum) (ileum) (jejunum) involvement K50.80
            with
              complication K50.819
                abscess K50.814
                fistula K50.813
                intestinal obstruction K50.812
                rectal bleeding K50.811
                specified complication NEC K50.818
          specified complication NEC K50.118
    rectum — *see* Enteritis, regional, large intestine
    small intestine (duodenum) (ileum) (jejunum) K50.00

Enteritis — *continued*
  regional — *continued*
    small intestine — *continued*
      with
        complication K50.019
          abscess K50.014
          fistula K50.013
          intestinal obstruction K50.012
          large intestine (colon) (rectum) involvement K50.80
            with
              complication K50.819
                abscess K50.814
                fistula K50.813
                intestinal obstruction K50.812
                rectal bleeding K50.811
                specified complication NEC K50.818
          rectal bleeding K50.011
          specified complication NEC K50.018
  rotaviral A08.0
  Salmonella, salmonellosis (arizonae) (cholerae-suis) (enteritidis) (typhimurium) A02.0
  segmental — *see* Enteritis, regional
  septic A09
  Shigella — *see* Infection, Shigella
  small round structured NEC A08.19
  spasmodic, spastic — *see* Syndrome, irritable bowel
  staphylococcal A04.8
    due to food A05.0
  torovirus A08.39
  toxic NEC K52.1
    due to Clostridium difficile
      not specified as recurrent A04.72
      recurrent A04.71
  trichomonal A07.8
  tuberculous A18.32
  typhosa A01.00
  ulcerative (chronic) — *see* Colitis, ulcerative
  viral A08.4
    adenovirus A08.2
    enterovirus A08.39
    Rotavirus A08.0
    small round structured NEC A08.19
    specified NEC A08.39
    virus specified NEC A08.39

Enterobiasis B80
Enterobius vermicularis (infection) (infestation) B80
Enterocele — *see also* Hernia, abdomen
  pelvic, pelvis (acquired) (congenital) N81.5
  vagina, vaginal (acquired) (congenital) NEC N81.5
Enterocolitis — *see also* Enteritis K52.9
  due to Clostridium difficile
    not specified as recurrent A04.72
    recurrent A04.71
  fulminant ischemic — *see also* Ischemia, intestine, acute K55.059
  granulomatous — *see* Enteritis, regional
  hemorrhagic (acute) — *see also* Ischemia, intestine, acute K55.059
  chronic K55.1
  infectious NEC A09
  ischemic K55.9
  necrotizing K55.30
    with
      perforation K55.33
      pneumatosis K55.32
        and perforation K55.33
    due to Clostridium difficile
      not specified as recurrent A04.72
      recurrent A04.71
    in non-newborn K55.30
      stage 1 (without pneumatosis, without perforation) K55.31
      stage 2 (with pneumatosis, without perforation) K55.32
      stage 3 (with pneumatosis, with perforation) K55.33
    in newborn P77.9
      stage 1 (without pneumatosis, without perforation) P77.1
      stage 2 (with pneumatosis, without perforation) P77.2
      stage 3 (with pneumatosis, with perforation) P77.3
    without pneumatosis or perforation K55.31
  noninfectious K52.9

Enterocolitis — *continued*
  noninfectious — *continued*
    newborn — *see* Enterocolitis, necrotizing, in newborn
    pseudomembranous (newborn)
      not specified as recurrent A04.72
      recurrent A04.71
    radiation K52.0
      newborn — *see* Enterocolitis, necrotizing, in newborn
    ulcerative (chronic) — *see* Pancolitis, ulcerative (chronic)
Enterogastritis — *see* Enteritis
Enteropathy K63.9
  celiac-gluten-sensitive K90.0
    non-celiac K90.41
  food protein-induced K52.22
  hemorrhagic, terminal — *see also* Ischemia, intestine, acute K55.059
  protein-losing K90.49
Enteroperitonitis — *see* Peritonitis
Enteroptosis K63.4
Enterorrhagia K92.2
Enterospasm — *see also* Syndrome, irritable, bowel
  psychogenic F45.8
Enterostenosis — *see also* Obstruction, intestine, specified NEC K56.699
Enterostomy
  complication — *see* Complication, enterostomy
  status Z93.4
Enterovirus, as cause of disease classified elsewhere B97.10
  coxsackievirus B97.11
  echovirus B97.12
  other specified B97.19
Enthesopathy (peripheral) M77.9
  Achilles tendinitis — *see* Tendinitis, Achilles
  ankle and tarsus M77.5- ☑
    specified type NEC — *see* Enthesopathy, foot, specified type NEC
  anterior tibial syndrome M76.81- ☑
  calcaneal spur — *see* Spur, bone, calcaneal
  elbow region M77.8
    lateral epicondylitis — *see* Epicondylitis, lateral
    medial epicondylitis — *see* Epicondylitis, medial
  foot NEC M77.8
    metatarsalgia — *see* Metatarsalgia
    specified type NEC M77.5- ☑
  forearm M77.8
  gluteal tendinitis — *see* Tendinitis, gluteal
  hand M77.8
  hip — *see* Enthesopathy, lower limb, specified type NEC
  iliac crest spur — *see* Spur, bone, iliac crest
  iliotibial band syndrome — *see* Syndrome, iliotibial band
  knee — *see* Enthesopathy, lower limb, lower leg, specified type NEC
  lateral epicondylitis — *see* Epicondylitis, lateral
  lower limb (excluding foot) M76.9
    Achilles tendinitis — *see* Tendinitis, Achilles
    ankle and tarsus M77.5- ☑
      specified type NEC — *see* Enthesopathy, foot, specified type NEC
    anterior tibial syndrome M76.81- ☑
    gluteal tendinitis — *see* Tendinitis, gluteal
    iliac crest spur — *see* Spur, bone, iliac crest
    iliotibial band syndrome — *see* Syndrome, iliotibial band
    patellar tendinitis — *see* Tendinitis, patellar
    pelvic region — *see* Enthesopathy, lower limb, specified type NEC
    peroneal tendinitis — *see* Tendinitis, peroneal
    posterior tibial syndrome M76.82- ☑
    psoas tendinitis — *see* Tendinitis, psoas
    specified type NEC M76.89- ☑
    tibial collateral bursitis — *see* Bursitis, tibial collateral
  medial epicondylitis — *see* Epicondylitis, medial
  metatarsalgia — *see* Metatarsalgia
  multiple sites M77.8
  patellar tendinitis — *see* Tendinitis, patellar
  pelvis M77.8
  periarthritis of wrist — *see* Periarthritis, wrist
  peroneal tendinitis — *see* Tendinitis, peroneal
  posterior tibial syndrome M76.82- ☑
  psoas tendinitis — *see* Tendinitis, psoas

Enthesopathy — *continued*
  shoulder M77.8
  shoulder region — *see* Lesion, shoulder
  specified type NEC M77.8
  spinal M46.00
    cervical region M46.02
    cervicothoracic region M46.03
    lumbar region M46.06
    lumbosacral region M46.07
    multiple sites M46.09
    occipito-atlanto-axial region M46.01
    sacrococcygeal region M46.08
    thoracic region M46.04
    thoracolumbar region M46.05
  tibial collateral bursitis — *see* Bursitis, tibial collateral
  upper arm M77.8
  wrist and carpus NEC M77.8
    calcaneal spur — *see* Spur, bone, calcaneal
    periarthritis of wrist — *see* Periarthritis, wrist
Entomophobia F40.218
Entomophthoromycosis B46.8
Entrance, air into vein — *see* Embolism, air
Entrapment, nerve — *see* Neuropathy, entrapment
Entropion (eyelid) (paralytic) H02.009
  cicatricial H02.019
    left H02.016
      lower H02.015
      upper H02.014
    right H02.013
      lower H02.012
      upper H02.011
  congenital Q10.2
  left H02.006
    lower H02.005
    upper H02.004
  mechanical H02.029
    left H02.026
      lower H02.025
      upper H02.024
    right H02.023
      lower H02.022
      upper H02.021
  right H02.003
    lower H02.002
    upper H02.001
  senile H02.039
    left H02.036
      lower H02.035
      upper H02.034
    right H02.033
      lower H02.032
      upper H02.031
  spastic H02.049
    left H02.046
      lower H02.045
      upper H02.044
    right H02.043
      lower H02.042
      upper H02.041
Enucleated eye (traumatic, current) S05.7- ☑
Enuresis R32
  functional F98.0
  habit disturbance F98.0
  nocturnal N39.44
    psychogenic F98.0
  nonorganic origin F98.0
  psychogenic F98.0
Eosinopenia — *see* Agranulocytosis
Eosinophilia (allergic) (idiopathic) (secondary) D72.10
  with
    angiolymphoid hyperplasia (ALHE) D18.01
  familial D72.19
  hereditary D72.19
  in disease classified elsewhere D72.18
  infiltrative — *see* Eosinophilia, pulmonary
  Löffler's J82.89
  peritoneal — *see* Peritonitis, eosinophilic
  pulmonary NEC J82.89
    acute J82.82
    asthmatic J82.83
    chronic J82.81
  specified NEC D72.19
  tropical (pulmonary) J82.89
Eosinophilia-myalgia syndrome M35.8
Ependymitis (acute) (cerebral) (chronic) (granular) — *see* Encephalomyelitis
Ependymoblastoma
  specified site — *see* Neoplasm, malignant, by site

Ependymoblastoma — *continued*
  unspecified site C71.9
Ependymoma (epithelial) (malignant)
  anaplastic
    specified site — *see* Neoplasm, malignant, by site
    unspecified site C71.9
  benign
    specified site — *see* Neoplasm, benign, by site
    unspecified site D33.2
  myxopapillary D43.2
    specified site — *see* Neoplasm, uncertain behavior, by site
    unspecified site D43.2
  papillary D43.2
    specified site — *see* Neoplasm, uncertain behavior, by site
    unspecified site D43.2
  specified site — *see* Neoplasm, malignant, by site
  unspecified site C71.9
Ependymopathy G93.89
Ephelis, ephelides L81.2
Epiblepharon (congenital) Q10.3
Epicanthus, epicanthic fold (eyelid) (congenital) Q10.3
Epicondylitis (elbow)
  lateral M77.1- ☑
  medial M77.0- ☑
Epicystitis — *see* Cystitis
Epidemic — *see* condition
Epidermidalization, cervix — *see* Dysplasia, cervix
Epidermis, epidermal — *see* condition
Epidermodysplasia verruciformis B07.8
Epidermolysis
  bullosa (congenital) Q81.9
    acquired L12.30
      drug-induced L12.31
      specified cause NEC L12.35
    dystrophica Q81.2
    letalis Q81.1
    simplex Q81.0
    specified NEC Q81.8
  necroticans combustiformis L51.2
    due to drug — *see* Table of Drugs and Chemicals, by drug
Epidermophytid — *see* Dermatophytosis
Epidermophytosis (infected) — *see* Dermatophytosis
Epididymis — *see* condition
Epididymitis (acute) (nonvenereal) (recurrent) (residual) N45.1
  with orchitis N45.3
  blennorrhagic (gonococcal) A54.23
  caseous (tuberculous) A18.15
  chlamydial A56.19
  filarial — *see also* Infestation, filarial B74.9 *[N51]*
  gonococcal A54.23
  syphilitic A52.76
  tuberculous A18.15
Epididymo-orchitis — *see also* Epididymitis N45.3
Epidural — *see* condition
Epigastrium, epigastric — *see* condition
Epigastrocele — *see* Hernia, ventral
Epiglottis — *see* condition
Epiglottitis, epiglottiditis (acute) J05.10
  with obstruction J05.11
  chronic J37.0
Epignathus Q89.4
Epilepsia partialis continua — *see also* Kozhevnikof's epilepsy G40.1- ☑
Epilepsy, epileptic, epilepsia (attack) (cerebral) (convulsion) (fit) (seizure) G40.909

> *Note: the following terms are to be considered equivalent to intractable: pharmacoresistant (pharmacologically resistant), treatment resistant, refractory (medically) and poorly controlled*

  with
    complex partial seizures — *see* Epilepsy, localization-related, symptomatic, with complex partial seizures
    grand mal seizures on awakening — *see* Epilepsy, generalized, specified NEC
    myoclonic absences — *see* Epilepsy, generalized, specified NEC
    myoclonic-astatic seizures — *see* Epilepsy, generalized, specified NEC
    simple partial seizures — *see* Epilepsy, localization-related, symptomatic, with simple partial seizures

Epilepsy, epileptic, epilepsia — *continued*
  akinetic — *see* Epilepsy, generalized, specified NEC
  benign childhood with centrotemporal EEG spikes — *see* Epilepsy, localization-related, idiopathic
  benign myoclonic in infancy G40.80- ☑
  Bravais-jacksonian — *see* Epilepsy, localization-related, symptomatic, with simple partial seizures
  childhood
    with occipital EEG paroxysms — *see* Epilepsy, localization-related, idiopathic
    absence G40.A09 (*following* G40.3)
      intractable G40.A19 (*following* G40.3)
        with status epilepticus G40.A11 (*following* G40.3)
        without status epilepticus G40.A19 (*following* G40.3)
      not intractable G40.A09 (*following* G40.3)
        with status epilepticus G40.A01 (*following* G40.3)
        without status epilepticus G40.A09 (*following* G40.3)
  climacteric — *see* Epilepsy, specified NEC
  cysticercosis B69.0
  deterioration (mental) F06.8
  due to syphilis A52.19
  focal — *see* Epilepsy, localization-related, symptomatic, with simple partial seizures
  generalized
    idiopathic G40.309
      intractable G40.319
        with status epilepticus G40.311
        without status epilepticus G40.319
      not intractable G40.309
        with status epilepticus G40.301
        without status epilepticus G40.309
    specified NEC G40.409
      intractable G40.419
        with status epilepticus G40.411
        without status epilepticus G40.419
      not intractable G40.409
        with status epilepticus G40.401
        without status epilepticus G40.409
  impulsive petit mal — *see* Epilepsy, juvenile myoclonic
  intractable G40.919
    with status epilepticus G40.911
    without status epilepticus G40.919
  juvenile absence G40.A09 (*following* G40.3)
    intractable G40.A19 (*following* G40.3)
      with status epilepticus G40.A11 (*following* G40.3)
      without status epilepticus G40.A19 (*following* G40.3)
    not intractable G40.A09 (*following* G40.3)
      with status epilepticus G40.A01 (*following* G40.3)
      without status epilepticus G40.A09 (*following* G40.3)
  juvenile myoclonic G40.B09 (*following* G40.3)
    intractable G40.B19 (*following* G40.3)
      with status epilepticus G40.B11 (*following* G40.3)
      without status epilepticus G40.B19 (*following* G40.3)
    not intractable G40.B09 (*following* G40.3)
      with status epilepticus G40.B01 (*following* G40.3)
      without status epilepticus G40.B09 (*following* G40.3)
  localization-related (focal) (partial)
    idiopathic G40.009
      with seizures of localized onset G40.009
        intractable G40.019
          with status epilepticus G40.011
          without status epilepticus G40.019
        not intractable G40.009
          with status epilepticus G40.001
          without status epilepticus G40.009
    symptomatic
      with complex partial seizures G40.209
        intractable G40.219
          with status epilepticus G40.211
          without status epilepticus G40.219
        not intractable G40.209
          with status epilepticus G40.201
          without status epilepticus G40.209
      with simple partial seizures G40.109
        intractable G40.119
          with status epilepticus G40.111
          without status epilepticus G40.119
        not intractable G40.109
          with status epilepticus G40.101
          without status epilepticus G40.109

⚫ Subtterms under main terms may continue to next column or page   ☑ Additional Character Required — Refer to the Tabular List for Character Selection   137

Enthesopathy — Epilepsy, epileptic, epilepsia

Epilepsy, epileptic, epilepsia — *continued*
  myoclonus, myoclonic — *see also* Epilepsy, generalized, specified NEC
    progressive — *see* Epilepsy, generalized, idiopathic
    severe, in infancy (SMEI) G40.83- ☑
  not intractable G40.909
    with status epilepticus G40.901
    without status epilepticus G40.909
  on awakening — *see* Epilepsy, generalized, specified NEC
  parasitic NOS B71.9 *[G94]*
  partialis continua — *see also* Kozhevnikof's epilepsy G40.1- ☑
  peripheral — *see* Epilepsy, specified NEC
  polymorphic, in infancy (PMEI) G40.83- ☑
  procursiva — *see* Epilepsy, localization-related, symptomatic, with simple partial seizures
  progressive (familial) myoclonic — *see* Epilepsy, generalized, idiopathic
  reflex — *see* Epilepsy, specified NEC
  related to
    alcohol G40.509
      not intractable G40.509
        with status epilepticus G40.501
        without status epliepticus G40.509
    drugs G40.509
      not intractable G40.509
        with status epilepticus G40.501
        without status epliepticus G40.509
    external causes G40.509
      not intractable G40.509
        with status epilepticus G40.501
        without status epliepticus G40.509
    hormonal changes G40.509
      not intractable G40.509
        with status epilepticus G40.501
        without status epliepticus G40.509
    sleep deprivation G40.509
      not intractable G40.509
        with status epilepticus G40.501
        without status epliepticus G40.509
    stress G40.509
      not intractable G40.509
        with status epilepticus G40.501
        without status epliepticus G40.509
  somatomotor — *see* Epilepsy, localization-related, symptomatic, with simple partial seizures
  somatosensory — *see* Epilepsy, localization-related, symptomatic, with simple partial seizures
  spasms G40.822
    intractable G40.824
      with status epilepticus G40.823
      without status epilepticus G40.824
    not intractable G40.822
      with status epilepticus G40.821
      without status epilepticus G40.822
  specified NEC G40.802
    intractable G40.804
      with status epilepticus G40.803
      without status epilepticus G40.804
    not intractable G40.802
      with status epilepticus G40.801
      without status epilepticus G40.802
  syndromes
    generalized
      idiopathic G40.309
        intractable G40.319
          with status epilepticus G40.311
          without status epilepticus G40.319
        not intractable G40.309
          with status epilepticus G40.301
          without status epilepticus G40.309
      specified NEC G40.409
        intractable G40.419
          with status epilepticus G40.411
          without status epilepticus G40.419
        not intractable G40.409
          with status epilepticus G40.401
          without status epilepticus G40.409
    localization-related (focal) (partial)
      idiopathic G40.009
        with seizures of localized onset G40.009
          intractable G40.019
            with status epilepticus G40.011
            without status epilepticus G40.019
          not intractable G40.009
            with status epilepticus G40.001
            without status epilepticus G40.009

Epilepsy, epileptic, epilepsia — *continued*
  syndromes — *continued*
    localization-related — *continued*
      symptomatic
        with complex partial seizures G40.209
          intractable G40.219
            with status epilepticus G40.211
            without status epilepticus G40.219
          not intractable G40.209
            with status epilepticus G40.201
            without status epilepticus G40.209
        with simple partial seizures G40.109
          intractable G40.119
            with status epilepticus G40.111
            without status epilepticus G40.119
          not intractable G40.109
            with status epilepticus G40.101
            without status epilepticus G40.109
    specified NEC G40.802
      intractable G40.804
        with status epilepticus G40.803
        without status epilepticus G40.804
      not intractable G40.802
        with status epilepticus G40.801
        without status epilepticus G40.802
    tonic (-clonic) — *see* Epilepsy, generalized, specified NEC
    twilight F05
    uncinate (gyrus) — *see* Epilepsy, localization-related, symptomatic, with complex partial seizures
    Unverricht (-Lundborg) (familial myoclonic) — *see* Epilepsy, generalized, idiopathic
    visceral — *see* Epilepsy, specified NEC
    visual — *see* Epilepsy, specified NEC
Epiloia Q85.1
Epimenorrhea N92.0
Epipharyngitis — *see* Nasopharyngitis
Epiphora H04.20- ☑
  due to
    excess lacrimation H04.21- ☑
    insufficient drainage H04.22- ☑
Epiphyseal arrest — *see* Arrest, epiphyseal
Epiphyseolysis, epiphysiolysis — *see* Osteochondropathy
Epiphysitis — *see also* Osteochondropathy
  juvenile M92.9
  syphilitic (congenital) A50.02
Epiplocele — *see* Hernia, abdomen
Epiploitis — *see* Peritonitis
Epiplosarcomphalocele — *see* Hernia, umbilicus
Episcleritis (suppurative) H15.10- ☑
  in (due to)
    syphilis A52.71
    tuberculosis A18.51
  nodular H15.12- ☑
  periodica fugax H15.11- ☑
    angioneurotic — *see* Edema, angioneurotic
  syphilitic (late) A52.71
  tuberculous A18.51
Episode
  affective, mixed F39
  depersonalization (in neurotic state) F48.1
  depressive F32.9
    major F32.9
      mild F32.0
      moderate F32.1
      severe (without psychotic symptoms) F32.2
        with psychotic symptoms F32.3
    recurrent F33.9
      brief F33.8
    specified NEC F32.89
  hypomanic F30.8
  manic F30.9
    with
      psychotic symptoms F30.2
      remission (full) F30.4
        partial F30.3
    other specified F30.8
    recurrent F31.89
    without psychotic symptoms F30.10
      mild F30.11
      moderate F30.12
      severe (without psychotic symptoms) F30.13
        with psychotic symptoms F30.2
  psychotic F23
    organic F06.8
  schizophrenic (acute) NEC, brief F23
Epispadias (female) (male) Q64.0

Episplenitis D73.89
Epistaxis (multiple) R04.0
  hereditary I78.0
  vicarious menstruation N94.89
Epithelioma (malignant) — *see also* Neoplasm, malignant, by site
  adenoides cysticum — *see* Neoplasm, skin, benign
  basal cell — *see* Neoplasm, skin, malignant
  benign — *see* Neoplasm, benign, by site
  Bowen's — *see* Neoplasm, skin, in situ
  calcifying, of Malherbe — *see* Neoplasm, skin, benign
  external site — *see* Neoplasm, skin, malignant
  intraepidermal, Jadassohn — *see* Neoplasm, skin, benign
  squamous cell — *see* Neoplasm, malignant, by site
Epitheliomatosis pigmented Q82.1
Epitheliopathy, multifocal placoid pigment H30.14- ☑
Epithelium, epithelial — *see* condition
Epituberculosis (with atelectasis) (allergic) A15.7
Eponychia Q84.6
Epstein's
  nephrosis or syndrome — *see* Nephrosis
  pearl K09.8
Epulis (gingiva) (fibrous) (giant cell) K06.8
Equinia A24.0
Equinovarus (congenital) (talipes) Q66.0- ☑
  acquired — *see* Deformity, limb, clubfoot
Equivalent
  convulsive (abdominal) — *see* Epilepsy, specified NEC
  epileptic (psychic) — *see* Epilepsy, localization-related, symptomatic, with complex partial seizures
Erb (-Duchenne) **paralysis** (birth injury) (newborn) P14.0
Erb-Goldflam disease or syndrome G70.00
  with exacerbation (acute) G70.01
  in crisis G70.01
Erb's
  disease G71.02
  palsy, paralysis (brachial) (birth) (newborn) P14.0
    spinal (spastic) syphilitic A52.17
  pseudohypertrophic muscular dystrophy G71.02
Erdheim's syndrome (acromegalic macrospondylitis) E22.0
Erection, painful (persistent) — *see* Priapism
Ergosterol deficiency (vitamin D) E55.9
  with
    adult osteomalacia M83.8
    rickets — *see* Rickets
Ergotism — *see also* Poisoning, food, noxious, plant
  from ergot used as drug (migraine therapy) — *see* Table of Drugs and Chemicals
Erosio interdigitalis blastomycetica B37.2
Erosion
  artery I77.2
    without rupture I77.89
  bone — *see* Disorder, bone, density and structure, specified NEC
  bronchus J98.09
  cartilage (joint) — *see* Disorder, cartilage, specified type NEC
  cervix (uteri) (acquired) (chronic) (congenital) N86
    with cervicitis N72
  cornea (nontraumatic) — *see* Ulcer, cornea
    recurrent H18.83- ☑
    traumatic — *see* Abrasion, cornea
  dental (idiopathic) (occupational) (due to diet, drugs or vomiting) K03.2
  duodenum, postpyloric — *see* Ulcer, duodenum
  esophagus K22.10
    with bleeding K22.11
  gastric — *see* Ulcer, stomach
  gastrojejunal — *see* Ulcer, gastrojejunal
  implanted mesh — *see* Complications, prosthetic device or implant, mesh
  intestine K63.3
  lymphatic vessel I89.8
  pylorus, pyloric (ulcer) — *see* Ulcer, stomach
  spine, aneurysmal A52.09
  stomach — *see* Ulcer, stomach
  subcutaneous device pocket
    nervous system prosthetic device, implant, or graft T85.890 ☑
    other internal prosthetic device, implant, or graft T85.898 ☑
  teeth (idiopathic) (occupational) (due to diet, drugs or vomiting) K03.2
  urethra N36.8

Erosion — *continued*
uterus N85.8
Erotomania F52.8
Error
metabolism, inborn — *see* Disorder, metabolism
refractive — *see* Disorder, refraction
Eructation R14.2
nervous or psychogenic F45.8
Eruption
creeping B76.9
drug (generalized) (taken internally) L27.0
fixed L27.1
in contact with skin — *see* Dermatitis, due to drugs
localized L27.1
Hutchinson, summer L56.4
Kaposi's varicelliform B00.0
napkin L22
polymorphous light (sun) L56.4
recalcitrant pustular L13.8
ringed R23.8
skin (nonspecific) R21
creeping (meaning hookworm) B76.9
due to inoculation/vaccination (generalized) — *see
also* Dermatitis, due to, vaccine L27.0
localized L27.1
erysipeloid A26.0
feigned L98.1
Kaposi's varicelliform B00.0
lichenoid L28.0
meaning dermatitis — *see* Dermatitis
toxic NEC L53.0
tooth, teeth, abnormal (incomplete) (late) (premature)
(sequence) K00.6
vesicular R23.8
Erysipelas (gangrenous) (infantile) (newborn) (phlegmonous) (suppurative) A46
external ear A46 *[H62.40]*
puerperal, postpartum O86.89
Erysipeloid A26.9
cutaneous (Rosenbach's) A26.0
disseminated A26.8
sepsis A26.7
specified NEC A26.8
Erythema, erythematous (infectional) (inflammation)
L53.9
ab igne L59.0
annulare (centrifugum) (rheumaticum) L53.1
arthriticum epidemicum A25.1
brucellum — *see* Brucellosis
chronic figurate NEC L53.3
chronicum migrans (Borrelia burgdorferi) A69.20
diaper L22
due to
chemical NEC L53.0
in contact with skin L24.5
drug (internal use) — *see* Dermatitis, due to, drugs
elevatum diutinum L95.1
endemic E52
epidemic, arthritic A25.1
figuratum perstans L53.3
gluteal L22
heat — *code by site under* Burn, first degree
ichthyosiforme congenitum bullous Q80.3
in diseases classified elsewhere L54
induratum (nontuberculous) L52
tuberculous A18.4
infectiosum B08.3
intertrigo L30.4
iris L51.9
marginatum L53.2
in (due to) acute rheumatic fever I00
medicamentosum — *see* Dermatitis, due to, drugs
migrans A26.0
chronicum A69.20
tongue K14.1
multiforme (major) (minor) L51.9
bullous, bullosum L51.1
conjunctiva L51.1
nonbullous L51.0
pemphigoides L12.0
specified NEC L51.8
napkin L22
neonatorum P83.88
toxic P83.1
nodosum L52
tuberculous A18.4
palmar L53.8
pernio T69.1 ☑

Erythema, erythematous — *continued*
rash, newborn P83.88
scarlatiniform (recurrent) (exfoliative) L53.8
solare L55.0
specified NEC L53.8
toxic, toxicum NEC L53.0
newborn P83.1
tuberculous (primary) A18.4
Erythematous, erythematosus — *see* condition
Erythermalgia (primary) I73.81
Erythralgia I73.81
Erythrasma L08.1
Erythredema (polyneuropathy) — *see* Poisoning, mer-
cury
Erythremia (acute) C94.0- ☑
chronic D45
secondary D75.1
Erythroblastopenia — *see also* Aplasia, red cell D60.9
congenital D61.01
Erythroblastophthisis D61.09
Erythroblastosis (fetalis) (newborn) P55.9
due to
ABO (antibodies) (incompatibility) (isoimmunization)
P55.1
Rh (antibodies) (incompatibility) (isoimmunization)
P55.0
Erythrocyanosis (crurum) I73.89
Erythrocythemia — *see* Erythremia
Erythrocytosis (megalosplenic) (secondary) D75.1
familial D75.0
oval, hereditary — *see* Elliptocytosis
secondary D75.1
stress D75.1
Erythroderma (secondary) — *see also* Erythema L53.9
bullous ichthyosiform, congenital Q80.3
desquamativum L21.1
ichthyosiform, congenital (bullous) Q80.3
neonatorum P83.88
psoriaticum L40.8
Erythrodysesthesia, palmar plantar (PPE) L27.1
Erythrogenesis imperfecta D61.09
Erythroleukemia C94.0- ☑
Erythromelalgia I73.81
Erythrophagocytosis D75.89
Erythrophobia F40.298
Erythroplakia, oral epithelium, and tongue K13.29
Erythroplasia (Queyrat) D07.4
specified site — *see* Neoplasm, skin, in situ
unspecified site D07.4
Escherichia coli (E. coli), **as cause of disease classified
elsewhere** B96.20
non-O157 Shiga toxin-producing (with known O group)
B96.22
non-Shiga toxin-producing B96.29
O157 with confirmation of Shiga toxin when H antigen
is unknown, or is not H7 B96.21
O157:H- (nonmotile) with confirmation of Shiga toxin
B96.21
O157:H7 with or without confirmation of Shiga toxin-
production B96.21
Shiga toxin-producing (with unspecified O group)
(STEC) B96.23
O157 B96.21
specified NEC B96.29
Esophagismus K22.4
Esophagitis (acute) (alkaline) (chemical) (chronic) (infectional) (necrotic) (peptic) (postoperative) (without
bleeding) K20.90
with bleeding K20.91
candidal B37.81
due to gastrointestinal reflux disease (without bleeding) K21.00
with bleeding K21.01
eosinophilic K20.0
reflux K21.00
specified NEC (without bleeding) K20.80
with bleeding K20.81
tuberculous A18.83
ulcerative K22.10
with bleeding K22.11
Esophagocele K22.5
Esophagomalacia K22.8
Esophagospasm K22.4
Esophagostenosis K22.2
Esophagostomiasis B81.8
Esophagotracheal — *see* condition
Esophagus — *see* condition
Esophoria H50.51

Esophoria — *continued*
convergence, excess H51.12
divergence, insufficiency H51.8
Esotropia — *see* Strabismus, convergent concomitant
Espundia B55.2
Essential — *see* condition
Esthesioneuroblastoma C30.0
Esthesioneurocytoma C30.0
Esthesioneuroepithelioma C30.0
Esthiomene A55
Estivo-autumnal malaria (fever) B50.9
Estrangement (marital) Z63.5
parent-child NEC Z62.890
Estriasis — *see* Myiasis
Ethanolism — *see* Alcoholism
Etherism — *see* Dependence, drug, inhalant
Ethmoid, ethmoidal — *see* condition
Ethmoiditis (chronic) (nonpurulent) (purulent) — *see
also* Sinusitis, ethmoidal
influenzal — *see* Influenza, with, respiratory manifesta-
tions NEC
Woakes' J33.1
Ethylism — *see* Alcoholism
Eulenburg's disease (congenital paramyotonia) G71.19
Eumycetoma B47.0
Eunuchoidism E29.1
hypogonadotropic E23.0
European blastomycosis — *see* Cryptococcosis
Eustachian — *see* condition
Evaluation (for) (of)
development state
adolescent Z00.3
period of
delayed growth in childhood Z00.70
with abnormal findings Z00.71
rapid growth in childhood Z00.2
puberty Z00.3
growth and developmental state (period of rapid
growth) Z00.2
delayed growth Z00.70
with abnormal findings Z00.71
mental health (status) Z00.8
requested by authority Z04.6
period of
delayed growth in childhood Z00.70
with abnormal findings Z00.71
rapid growth in childhood Z00.2
suspected condition — *see* Observation
Evans syndrome D69.41
Event
apparent life threatening in newborn and infant (ALTE)
R68.13
brief resolved unexplained event (BRUE) R68.13
Eventration — *see also* Hernia, ventral
colon into chest — *see* Hernia, diaphragm
diaphragm (congenital) Q79.1
Eversion
bladder N32.89
cervix (uteri) N86
with cervicitis N72
foot NEC — *see also* Deformity, valgus, ankle
congenital Q66.6
punctum lacrimale (postinfectional) (senile) H04.52- ☑
ureter (meatus) N28.89
urethra (meatus) N36.8
uterus N81.4
Evidence
cytologic
of malignancy on anal smear R85.614
of malignancy on cervical smear R87.614
of malignancy on vaginal smear R87.624
Evisceration
birth injury P15.8
traumatic NEC
eye — *see* Enucleated eye
Evulsion — *see* Avulsion
Ewing's sarcoma or tumor — *see* Neoplasm, bone,
malignant
Examination (for) (following) (general) (of) (routine)
Z00.00
with abnormal findings Z00.01
abuse, physical (alleged), ruled out
adult Z04.71
child Z04.72
adolescent (development state) Z00.3
alleged rape or sexual assault (victim), ruled out
adult Z04.41
child Z04.42

Examination — continued
- allergy Z01.82
- annual (adult) (periodic) (physical) Z00.00
  - with abnormal findings Z00.01
    - gynecological Z01.419
      - with abnormal findings Z01.411
- antibody response Z01.84
- blood — see Examination, laboratory
- blood pressure Z01.30
  - with abnormal findings Z01.31
- cancer staging — see Neoplasm, malignant, by site
- cervical Papanicolaou smear Z12.4
  - as part of routine gynecological examination Z01.419
    - with abnormal findings Z01.411
- child (over 28 days old) Z00.129
  - with abnormal findings Z00.121
  - under 28 days old — see Newborn, examination
- clinical research control or normal comparison (control) (participant) Z00.6
- contraceptive (drug) maintenance (routine) Z30.8
  - device (intrauterine) Z30.431
- dental Z01.20
  - with abnormal findings Z01.21
- developmental — see Examination, child
- donor (potential) Z00.5
- ear Z01.10
  - with abnormal findings NEC Z01.118
- eye Z01.00
  - with abnormal findings Z01.01
  - following failed vision screening Z01.020
    - with abnormal findings Z01.021
- follow-up (routine) (following) Z09
  - chemotherapy NEC Z09
    - malignant neoplasm Z08
  - fracture Z09
  - malignant neoplasm Z08
  - postpartum Z39.2
  - psychotherapy Z09
  - radiotherapy NEC Z09
    - malignant neoplasm Z08
  - surgery NEC Z09
    - malignant neoplasm Z08
- following
  - accident NEC Z04.3
    - transport Z04.1
    - work Z04.2
  - assault, alleged, ruled out
    - adult Z04.71
    - child Z04.72
  - motor vehicle accident Z04.1
  - treatment (for) Z09
    - combined NEC Z09
      - fracture Z09
        - malignant neoplasm Z08
    - malignant neoplasm Z08
    - mental disorder Z09
    - specified condition NEC Z09
- forced sexual exploitation Z04.81
- forced labor exploitation Z04.82
- gynecological Z01.419
  - with abnormal findings Z01.411
  - for contraceptive maintenance Z30.8
- health — see Examination, medical
- hearing Z01.10
  - with abnormal findings NEC Z01.118
  - following failed hearing screening Z01.110
  - infant or child (over 28 days old) Z00.129
    - with abnormal findings Z00.121
- immunity status testing Z01.84
- laboratory (as part of a general medical examination) Z00.00
  - with abnormal findings Z00.01
  - preprocedural Z01.812
- lactating mother Z39.1
- medical (adult) (for) (of) Z00.00
  - with abnormal findings Z00.01
  - administrative purpose only Z02.9
    - specified NEC Z02.89
  - admission to
    - armed forces Z02.3
    - old age home Z02.2
    - prison Z02.89
    - residential institution Z02.2
    - school Z02.0
      - following illness or medical treatment Z02.0
    - summer camp Z02.89
  - adoption Z02.82
  - blood alcohol or drug level Z02.83

Examination — continued
- medical — continued
  - camp (summer) Z02.89
  - clinical research, normal subject (control) (participant) Z00.6
  - control subject in clinical research (normal comparison) (participant) Z00.6
  - donor (potential) Z00.5
  - driving license Z02.4
  - general (adult) Z00.00
    - with abnormal findings Z00.01
  - immigration Z02.89
  - insurance purposes Z02.6
  - marriage Z02.89
  - medicolegal reasons NEC Z04.89
  - naturalization Z02.89
  - participation in sport Z02.5
  - paternity testing Z02.81
  - population survey Z00.8
  - pre-employment Z02.1
  - pre-operative — see Examination, pre-procedural
  - pre-procedural
    - cardiovascular Z01.810
    - respiratory Z01.811
    - specified NEC Z01.818
  - preschool children
    - for admission to school Z02.0
  - prisoners
    - for entrance into prison Z02.89
  - recruitment for armed forces Z02.3
  - specified NEC Z00.8
  - sport competition Z02.5
- medicolegal reason NEC Z04.89
  - following
    - forced sexual exploitation Z04.81
    - forced labor exploitation Z04.82
- newborn — see Newborn, examination
- pelvic (annual) (periodic) Z01.419
  - with abnormal findings Z01.411
- period of rapid growth in childhood Z00.2
- periodic (adult) (annual) (routine) Z00.00
  - with abnormal findings Z00.01
- physical (adult) — see also Examination, medical Z00.00
  - sports Z02.5
- postpartum
  - immediately after delivery Z39.0
  - routine follow-up Z39.2
- pre-chemotherapy (antineoplastic) Z01.818
- prenatal (normal pregnancy) — see also Pregnancy, normal Z34.9- ☑
- pre-procedural (pre-operative)
  - cardiovascular Z01.810
  - laboratory Z01.812
  - respiratory Z01.811
  - specified NEC Z01.818
- prior to chemotherapy (antineoplastic) Z01.818
- psychiatric NEC Z00.8
  - follow-up not needing further care Z09
  - requested by authority Z04.6
- radiological (as part of a general medical examination) Z00.00
  - with abnormal findings Z00.01
- repeat cervical smear to confirm findings of recent normal smear following initial abnormal smear Z01.42
- skin (hypersensitivity) Z01.82
- special — see also Examination, by type Z01.89
  - specified type NEC Z01.89
- specified type or reason NEC Z04.89
- teeth Z01.20
  - with abnormal findings Z01.21
- urine — see Examination, laboratory
- vision Z01.00
  - with abnormal findings Z01.01
  - following failed vision screening Z01.020
    - with abnormal findings Z01.021
  - infant or child (over 28 days old) Z00.129
    - with abnormal findings Z00.121

Exanthem, exanthema — see also Rash
- with enteroviral vesicular stomatitis B08.4
- Boston A88.0
- epidemic with meningitis A88.0 [G02]
- subitum B08.20
  - due to human herpesvirus 6 B08.21
  - due to human herpesvirus 7 B08.22
- viral, virus B09
  - specified type NEC B08.8

Excess, excessive, excessively
- alcohol level in blood R78.0
- androgen (ovarian) E28.1
- attrition, tooth, teeth K03.0
- carotene, carotin (dietary) E67.1
- cold, effects of T69.9 ☑
  - specified effect NEC T69.8 ☑
- convergence H51.12
- crying
  - in child, adolescent, or adult R45.83
  - in infant R68.11
- development, breast N62
- divergence H51.8
- drinking (alcohol) NEC (without dependence) F10.10
  - habitual (continual) (without remission) F10.20
- eating R63.2
- estrogen E28.0
- fat — see also Obesity
  - in heart — see Degeneration, myocardial
  - localized E65
- foreskin N47.8
- gas R14.0
- glucagon E16.3
- heat — see Heat
- intermaxillary vertical dimension of fully erupted teeth M26.37
- interocclusal distance of fully erupted teeth M26.37
- kalium E87.5
- large
  - colon K59.39
    - congenital Q43.8
  - infant P08.0
  - organ or site, congenital NEC — see Anomaly, by site
- long
  - organ or site, congenital NEC — see Anomaly, by site
- menstruation (with regular cycle) N92.0
  - with irregular cycle N92.1
- napping Z72.821
- natrium E87.0
- number of teeth K00.1
- nutrient (dietary) NEC R63.2
- potassium (K) E87.5
- salivation K11.7
- secretion — see also Hypersecretion
  - milk O92.6
  - sputum R09.3
  - sweat R61
- sexual drive F52.8
- short
  - organ or site, congenital NEC — see Anomaly, by site
  - umbilical cord in labor or delivery O69.3 ☑
- skin L98.7
  - and subcutaneous tissue L98.7
  - eyelid (acquired) — see Blepharochalasis
    - congenital Q10.3
- sodium (Na) E87.0
- spacing of fully erupted teeth M26.32
- sputum R09.3
- sweating R61
- thirst R63.1
  - due to deprivation of water T73.1 ☑
- tuberosity of jaw M26.07
- vitamin
  - A (dietary) E67.0
    - administered as drug (prolonged intake) — see Table of Drugs and Chemicals, vitamins, adverse effect
    - overdose or wrong substance given or taken — see Table of Drugs and Chemicals, vitamins, poisoning
  - D (dietary) E67.3
    - administered as drug (prolonged intake) — see Table of Drugs and Chemicals, vitamins, adverse effect
    - overdose or wrong substance given or taken — see Table of Drugs and Chemicals, vitamins, poisoning
- weight
  - gain R63.5
  - loss R63.4

Excitability, abnormal, under minor stress (personality disorder) F60.3

Excitation
- anomalous atrioventricular I45.6
- psychogenic F30.8

Excitation — *continued*
  reactive (from emotional stress, psychological trauma)
      F30.8
Excitement
  hypomanic F30.8
  manic F30.9
  mental, reactive (from emotional stress, psychological
      trauma) F30.8
  state, reactive (from emotional stress, psychological
      trauma) F30.8
Excoriation (traumatic) — *see also* Abrasion
  neurotic L98.1
  skin picking disorder F42.4
Exfoliation
  due to erythematous conditions according to extent
      of body surface involved L49.0
    10-19 percent of body surface L49.1
    20-29 percent of body surface L49.2
    30-39 percent of body surface L49.3
    40-49 percent of body surface L49.4
    50-59 percent of body surface L49.5
    60-69 percent of body surface L49.6
    70-79 percent of body surface L49.7
    80-89 percent of body surface L49.8
    90-99 percent of body surface L49.9
    less than 10 percent of body surface L49.0
  teeth, due to systemic causes K08.0
Exfoliative — *see* condition
Exhaustion, exhaustive (physical NEC) R53.83
  battle F43.0
  cardiac — *see* Failure, heart
  delirium F43.0
  due to
    cold T69.8 ☑
    excessive exertion T73.3 ☑
    exposure T73.2 ☑
    neurasthenia F48.8
  heart — *see* Failure, heart
  heat — *see also* Heat, exhaustion T67.5 ☑
    due to
      salt depletion T67.4 ☑
      water depletion T67.3 ☑
  maternal, complicating delivery O75.81
  mental F48.8
  myocardium, myocardial — *see* Failure, heart
  nervous F48.8
  old age R54
  psychogenic F48.8
  psychosis F43.0
  senile R54
  vital NEC Z73.0
Exhibitionism F65.2
Exocervicitis — *see* Cervicitis
Exomphalos Q79.2
  meaning hernia — *see* Hernia, umbilicus
Exophoria H50.52
  convergence, insufficiency H51.11
  divergence, excess H51.8
Exophthalmos H05.2- ☑
  congenital Q15.8
  constant NEC H05.24- ☑
  displacement, globe — *see* Displacement, globe
  due to thyrotoxicosis (hyperthyroidism) — *see* Hyper-
      thyroidism, with, goiter (diffuse)
  dysthyroid — *see* Hyperthyroidism, with, goiter (dif-
      fuse)
  goiter — *see* Hyperthyroidism, with, goiter (diffuse)
  intermittent NEC H05.25- ☑
  malignant — *see* Hyperthyroidism, with, goiter (diffuse)
  orbital
    edema — *see* Edema, orbit
    hemorrhage — *see* Hemorrhage, orbit
  pulsating NEC H05.26- ☑
  thyrotoxic, thyrotropic — *see* Hyperthyroidism, with,
      goiter (diffuse)
Exostosis — *see also* Disorder, bone
  cartilaginous — *see* Neoplasm, bone, benign
  congenital (multiple) Q78.6
  external ear canal H61.81- ☑
  gonococcal A54.49
  jaw (bone) M27.8
  multiple, congenital Q78.6
  orbit H05.35- ☑
  osteocartilaginous — *see* Neoplasm, bone, benign
  syphilitic A52.77
Exotropia — *see* Strabismus, divergent concomitant

Explanation of
  investigation finding Z71.2
  medication Z71.89
Exposure (to) — *see also* Contact, with T75.89 ☑
  acariasis Z20.7
  AIDS virus Z20.6
  air pollution Z77.110
  algae and algae toxins Z77.121
  algae bloom Z77.121
  anthrax Z20.810
  aromatic amines Z77.020
  aromatic (hazardous) compounds NEC Z77.028
  aromatic dyes NOS Z77.028
  arsenic Z77.010
  asbestos Z77.090
  bacterial disease NEC Z20.818
  benzene Z77.021
  blue-green algae bloom Z77.121
  body fluids (potentially hazardous) Z77.21
  brown tide Z77.121
  chemicals (chiefly nonmedicinal) (hazardous) NEC
      Z77.098
  cholera Z20.09
  chromium compounds Z77.018
  cold, effects of T69.9 ☑
    specified effect NEC T69.8 ☑
  communicable disease Z20.9
    bacterial NEC Z20.818
    specified NEC Z20.89
    viral NEC Z20.828
    Zika virus Z20.821
  cyanobacteria bloom Z77.121
  disaster Z65.5
  discrimination Z60.5
  dyes Z77.098
  effects of T73.9 ☑
  environmental tobacco smoke (acute) (chronic) Z77.22
  Escherichia coli (E. coli) Z20.01
  exhaustion due to T73.2 ☑
  fiberglass — *see* Table of Drugs and Chemicals, fiber-
      glass
  German measles Z20.4
  gonorrhea Z20.2
  hazardous metals NEC Z77.018
  hazardous substances NEC Z77.29
  hazards in the physical environment NEC Z77.128
  hazards to health NEC Z77.9
  human immunodeficiency virus (HIV) Z20.6
  human T-lymphotropic virus type-1 (HTLV-1) Z20.89
  implanted
    mesh — *see* Complications, prosthetic devise or
        implant, mesh
    prosthetic materials NEC — *see* Complications,
        prosthetic materials NEC
  infestation (parasitic) NEC Z20.7
  intestinal infectious disease NEC Z20.09
    Escherichia coli (E. coli) Z20.01
  lead Z77.011
  meningococcus Z20.811
  mold (toxic) Z77.120
  nickel dust Z77.018
  noise Z77.122
  occupational
    air contaminants NEC Z57.39
    dust Z57.2
    environmental tobacco smoke Z57.31
    extreme temperature Z57.6
    noise Z57.0
    radiation Z57.1
    risk factors Z57.9
      specified NEC Z57.8
    toxic agents (gases) (liquids) (solids) (vapors) in
        agriculture Z57.4
    toxic agents (gases) (liquids) (solids) (vapors) in in-
        dustry NEC Z57.5
    vibration Z57.7
  parasitic disease NEC Z20.7
  pediculosis Z20.7
  persecution Z60.5
  pfiesteria piscicida Z77.121
  poliomyelitis Z20.89
  pollution
    air Z77.110
    environmental NEC Z77.118
    soil Z77.112
    water Z77.111
  polycyclic aromatic hydrocarbons Z77.028

Exposure — *continued*
  prenatal (drugs) (toxic chemicals) — *see* Newborn, af-
      fected by, noxious substances transmitted via
      placenta or breast milk
  rabies Z20.3
  radiation, naturally occurring NEC Z77.123
  radon Z77.123
  red tide (Florida) Z77.121
  rubella Z20.4
  second hand tobacco smoke (acute) (chronic) Z77.22
    in the perinatal period P96.81
  sexually-transmitted disease Z20.2
  smallpox (laboratory) Z20.89
  syphilis Z20.2
  terrorism Z65.4
  torture Z65.4
  tuberculosis Z20.1
  uranium Z77.012
  varicella Z20.820
  venereal disease Z20.2
  viral disease NEC Z20.828
  war Z65.5
  water pollution Z77.111
  Zika virus Z20.821
Exsanguination — *see* Hemorrhage
Exstrophy
  abdominal contents Q45.8
  bladder Q64.10
    cloacal Q64.12
    specified type NEC Q64.19
    supravesical fissure Q64.11
Extensive — *see* condition
Extra — *see also* Accessory
  marker chromosomes (normal individual) Q92.61
    in abnormal individual Q92.62
  rib Q76.6
    cervical Q76.5
Extrasystoles (supraventricular) I49.49
  atrial I49.1
  auricular I49.1
  junctional I49.2
  ventricular I49.3
Extrauterine gestation or pregnancy — *see* Pregnancy,
      by site
Extravasation
  blood R58
  chyle into mesentery I89.8
  pelvicalyceal N13.8
  pyelosinus N13.8
  urine (from ureter) R39.0
  vesicant agent
    antineoplastic chemotherapy T80.810 ☑
    other agent NEC T80.818 ☑
Extremity — *see* condition, limb
Extrophy — *see* Exstrophy
Extroversion
  bladder Q64.19
  uterus N81.4
    complicating delivery O71.2
    postpartal (old) N81.4
Extruded tooth (teeth) M26.34
Extrusion
  breast implant (prosthetic) T85.42 ☑
  eye implant (globe) (ball) T85.328 ☑
  intervertebral disc — *see* Displacement, intervertebral
      disc
  ocular lens implant (prosthetic) — *see* Complications,
      intraocular lens
  vitreous — *see* Prolapse, vitreous
Exudate
  pleural — *see* Effusion, pleura
  retina H35.89
Exudative — *see* condition
Eye, eyeball, eyelid — *see* condition
Eyestrain — *see* Disturbance, vision, subjective
Eyeworm disease of Africa B74.3

F

Faber's syndrome (achlorhydric anemia) D50.9
Fabry (-Anderson) **disease** E75.21
Facet syndrome M47.89- ☑
Faciocephalalgia, autonomic — *see also* Neuropathy,
      peripheral, autonomic G90.09
Factor(s)
  psychic, associated with diseases classified elsewhere
      F54

Factor(s) — *continued*
- psychological
  - affecting physical conditions F54
  - or behavioral
    - affecting general medical condition F54
    - associated with disorders or diseases classified elsewhere F54

Fahr disease (of brain) G23.8

Fahr Volhard disease (of kidney) I12.- ☑

Failure, failed
- abortion — *see* Abortion, attempted
- aortic (valve) I35.8
  - rheumatic I06.8
- attempted abortion — *see* Abortion, attempted
- biventricular I50.82
  - due to left heart failure I50.814
- bone marrow — *see* Anemia, aplastic
- cardiac — *see* Failure, heart
- cardiorenal (chronic) — *see also* Failure, renal, and Failure, heart I50.9
  - hypertensive I13.2
- cardiorespiratory — *see also* Failure, heart R09.2
- cardiovascular (chronic) — *see* Failure, heart
- cerebrovascular I67.9
- cervical dilatation in labor O62.0
- circulation, circulatory (peripheral) R57.9
  - newborn P29.89
- compensation — *see* Disease, heart
- compliance with medical treatment or regimen — *see* Noncompliance
- congestive — *see* Failure, heart, congestive
- dental implant (endosseous) M27.69
  - due to
    - failure of dental prosthesis M27.63
    - lack of attached gingiva M27.62
    - occlusal trauma (poor prosthetic design) M27.62
    - parafunctional habits M27.62
    - periodontal infection (peri-implantitis) M27.62
    - poor oral hygiene M27.62
  - osseointegration M27.61
    - due to
      - complications of systemic disease M27.61
      - poor bone quality M27.61
    - iatrogenic M27.61
  - post-osseointegration
    - biological M27.62
    - due to complications of systemic disease M27.62
    - iatrogenic M27.62
    - mechanical M27.63
  - pre-integration M27.61
  - pre-osseointegration M27.61
  - specified NEC M27.69
- descent of head (at term) of pregnancy (mother) O32.4 ☑
- endosseous dental implant — *see* Failure, dental implant
- engagement of head (term of pregnancy) (mother) O32.4 ☑
- erection (penile) — *see also* Dysfunction, sexual, male, erectile N52.9
  - nonorganic F52.21
- examination(s), anxiety concerning Z55.2
- expansion terminal respiratory units (newborn) (primary) P28.0
- forceps NOS (with subsequent cesarean delivery) O66.5
- gain weight (child over 28 days old) R62.51
  - adult R62.7
  - newborn P92.6
- genital response (male) F52.21
  - female F52.22
- heart (acute) (senile) (sudden) I50.9
  - with
    - acute pulmonary edema — *see* Failure, ventricular, left
    - decompensation — *see also* Failure, heart, by type as diastolic or systolic, acute and chronic I50.9
    - dilatation — *see* Disease, heart
    - hypertension — *see* Hypertension, heart
    - normal ejection fraction — *see* Failure, heart, diastolic
    - preserved ejection fraction — *see* Failure, heart, diastolic
    - reduced ejection fraction — *see* Failure, heart, systolic
  - arteriosclerotic I70.90
  - biventricular I50.82
    - due to left heart failure I50.814

Failure, failed — *continued*
- heart — *continued*
  - combined left-right sided I50.82
    - due to left heart failure I50.814
  - compensated — *see also* Failure, heart, by type as diastolic or systolic, chronic I50.9
  - complicating
    - anesthesia (general) (local) or other sedation
      - in labor and delivery O74.2
      - in pregnancy O29.12- ☑
      - postpartum, puerperal O89.1
    - delivery (cesarean) (instrumental) O75.4
  - congestive I50.9
    - with rheumatic fever (conditions in I00)
      - active I01.8
      - inactive or quiescent (with chorea) I09.81
    - newborn P29.0
    - rheumatic (chronic) (inactive) (with chorea) I09.81
      - active or acute I01.8
        - with chorea I02.0
  - decompensated — *see also* Failure, heart, by type as diastolic or systolic, acute and chronic I50.9
  - degenerative — *see* Degeneration, myocardial
  - diastolic (congestive) (left ventricular) I50.30
    - acute (congestive) I50.31
      - and (on) chronic (congestive) I50.33
    - chronic (congestive) I50.32
      - and (on) acute (congestive) I50.33
    - combined with systolic (congestive) I50.40
      - acute (congestive) I50.41
        - and (on) chronic (congestive) I50.43
      - chronic (congestive) I50.42
        - and (on) acute (congestive) I50.43
  - due to presence of cardiac prosthesis I97.13- ☑
  - end stage — *see also* Failure, heart, by type as diastolic or systolic, chronic I50.84
  - following cardiac surgery I97.13- ☑
  - high output NOS I50.83
  - hypertensive — *see* Hypertension, heart
  - left (ventricular) — *see also* Failure, ventricular, left
    - combined diastolic and systolic — *see* Failure, heart, diastolic, combined with systolic
    - diastolic — *see* Failure, heart, diastolic
    - systolic — *see* Failure, heart, systolic
  - low output (syndrome) NOS I50.9
  - newborn P29.0
  - organic — *see* Disease, heart
  - peripartum O90.3
  - postprocedural I97.13- ☑
  - rheumatic (chronic) (inactive) I09.9
  - right (isolated) (ventricular) I50.810
    - acute I50.811
      - and (on) chronic I50.813
    - chronic I50.812
      - and acute I50.813
    - secondary to left heart failure I50.814
  - specified NEC I50.89

Note: heart failure stages A, B, C, and D are based on the American College of Cardiology and American Heart Association stages of heart failure, which complement and should not be confused with the New York Heart Association Classification of Heart Failure, into Class I, Class II, Class III, and Class IV

  - stage A Z91.89
  - stage B — *see also* Failure, heart, by type as diastolic or systolic I50.9
  - stage C — *see also* Failure, heart, by type as diastolic or systolic I50.9
  - stage D — *see also* Failure, heart, by type as diastolic or systolic, chronic I50.84
  - systolic (congestive) (left ventricular) I50.20
    - acute (congestive) I50.21
      - and (on) chronic (congestive) I50.23
    - chronic (congestive) I50.22
      - and (on) acute (congestive) I50.23
    - combined with diastolic (congestive) I50.40
      - acute (congestive) I50.41
        - and (on) chronic (congestive) I50.43
      - chronic (congestive) I50.42
        - and (on) acute (congestive) I50.43
  - thyrotoxic — *see also* Thyrotoxicosis E05.90 *[I43]*
    - with
      - high output — *see also* Thyrotoxicosis I50.83
      - thyroid storm E05.91 *[I43]*
        - high output — *see also* Thyrotoxicosis I50.83

Failure, failed — *continued*
- heart — *continued*
  - valvular — *see* Endocarditis
- hepatic K72.90
  - with coma K72.91
  - acute or subacute K72.00
    - with coma K72.01
    - due to drugs K71.10
      - with coma K71.11
  - alcoholic (acute) (chronic) (subacute) K70.40
    - with coma K70.41
  - chronic K72.10
    - with coma K72.11
    - due to drugs (acute) (subacute) (chronic) K71.10
      - with coma K71.11
  - due to drugs (acute) (subacute) (chronic) K71.10
    - with coma K71.11
  - postprocedural K91.82
- hepatorenal K76.7
- induction (of labor) O61.9
  - abortion — *see* Abortion, attempted
  - by
    - oxytocic drugs O61.0
    - prostaglandins O61.0
  - instrumental O61.1
  - mechanical O61.1
  - medical O61.0
  - specified NEC O61.8
  - surgical O61.1
- intubation during anesthesia T88.4 ☑
  - in pregnancy O29.6- ☑
  - labor and delivery O74.7
  - postpartum, puerperal O89.6
- involution, thymus (gland) E32.0
- kidney — *see also* Disease, kidney, chronic N19
  - acute — *see also* Failure, renal, acute N17.9
- lactation (complete) O92.3
  - partial O92.4
- Leydig's cell, adult E29.1
- liver — *see* Failure, hepatic
- menstruation at puberty N91.0
- mitral I05.8
- myocardial, myocardium — *see also* Failure, heart I50.9
  - chronic — *see also* Failure, heart, congestive I50.9
  - congestive — *see also* Failure, heart, congestive I50.9
- orgasm (female) (psychogenic) F52.31
  - male F52.32
- ovarian (primary) E28.39
  - iatrogenic E89.40
    - asymptomatic E89.40
    - symptomatic E89.41
  - postprocedural (postablative) (postirradiation) (postsurgical) E89.40
    - asymptomatic E89.40
    - symptomatic E89.41
- ovulation causing infertility N97.0
- polyglandular, autoimmune E31.0
- prosthetic joint implant — *see* Complications, joint prosthesis, mechanical, breakdown, by site
- renal N19
  - with
    - tubular necrosis (acute) N17.0
  - acute N17.9
    - with
      - cortical necrosis N17.1
      - medullary necrosis N17.2
      - tubular necrosis N17.0
    - specified NEC N17.8
  - chronic N18.9
    - hypertensive — *see* Hypertension, kidney
  - congenital P96.0
  - end stage (chronic) N18.6
    - due to hypertension I12.0
  - following
    - abortion — *see* Abortion by type complicated by specified condition NEC
    - crushing T79.5 ☑
    - ectopic or molar pregnancy O08.4
    - labor and delivery (acute) O90.4
  - hypertensive — *see* Hypertension, kidney
  - postprocedural N99.0
- respiration, respiratory J96.90
  - with
    - hypercapnia J96.92
    - hypercarbia J96.92
    - hypoxia J96.91
  - acute J96.00

Failure, failed — *continued*
  respiration, respiratory — *continued*
    acute — *continued*
      with
        hypercapnia J96.02
        hypercarbia J96.02
        hypoxia J96.01
      center G93.89
    acute and (on) chronic J96.20
      with
        hypercapnia J96.22
        hypercarbia J96.22
        hypoxia J96.21
    chronic J96.10
      with
        hypercapnia J96.12
        hypercarbia J96.12
        hypoxia J96.11
    newborn P28.5
    postprocedural (acute) J95.821
      acute and chronic J95.822
  rotation
    cecum Q43.3
    colon Q43.3
    intestine Q43.3
    kidney Q63.2
  sedation (conscious) (moderate) during procedure
    T88.52 ☑
    history of Z92.83
  segmentation — *see also* Fusion
    fingers — *see* Syndactylism, complex, fingers
    vertebra Q76.49
      with scoliosis Q76.3
  seminiferous tubule, adult E29.1
  senile (general) R54
  sexual arousal (male) F52.21
    female F52.22
  testicular endocrine function E29.1
  to thrive (child over 28 days old) R62.51
    adult R62.7
    newborn P92.6
  transplant T86.92
    bone T86.831
      marrow T86.02
    cornea T86.841- ☑
    heart T86.22
      with lung(s) T86.32
    intestine T86.851
    kidney T86.12
    liver T86.42
    lung(s) T86.811
      with heart T86.32
    pancreas T86.891
    skin (allograft) (autograft) T86.821
    specified organ or tissue NEC T86.891
    stem cell (peripheral blood) (umbilical cord) T86.5
  trial of labor (with subsequent cesarean delivery)
    O66.40
    following previous cesarean delivery O66.41
  tubal ligation N99.89
  urinary — *see* Disease, kidney, chronic
  vacuum extraction NOS (with subsequent cesarean
    delivery) O66.5
  vasectomy N99.89
  ventouse NOS (with subsequent cesarean delivery)
    O66.5
  ventricular — *see also* Failure, heart I50.9
    left — *see also* Failure, heart, left I50.1
      with rheumatic fever (conditions in I00)
        active I01.8
          with chorea I02.0
        inactive or quiescent (with chorea) I09.81
        rheumatic (chronic) (inactive) (with chorea)
          I09.81
          active or acute I01.8
            with chorea I02.0
    right — *see* Failure, heart, right
  vital centers, newborn P91.88
Fainting (fit) R55
Fallen arches — *see* Deformity, limb, flat foot
Falling, falls (repeated) R29.6
  any organ or part — *see* Prolapse
Fallopian
  insufflation Z31.41
  tube — *see* condition
Fallot's
  pentalogy Q21.8
  tetrad or tetralogy Q21.3

Fallot's — *continued*
  triad or trilogy Q22.3
False — *see also* condition
  croup J38.5
  joint — *see* Nonunion, fracture
  labor (pains) O47.9
    at or after 37 completed weeks of gestation O47.1
    before 37 completed weeks of gestation O47.0- ☑
  passage, urethra (prostatic) N36.5
  pregnancy F45.8
Family, familial — *see also* condition
  disruption Z63.8
    involving divorce or separation Z63.5
  Li-Fraumeni (syndrome) Z15.01
  planning advice Z30.09
  problem Z63.9
    specified NEC Z63.8
  retinoblastoma C69.2- ☑
Famine (effects of) T73.0 ☑
  edema — *see* Malnutrition, severe
Fanconi (-de Toni)(-Debré) **syndrome** E72.09
  with cystinosis E72.04
Fanconi's anemia (congenital pancytopenia) D61.09
Farber's disease or syndrome E75.29
Farcy A24.0
Farmer's
  lung J67.0
  skin L57.8
Farsightedness — *see* Hypermetropia
Fascia — *see* condition
Fasciculation R25.3
Fasciitis M72.9
  diffuse (eosinophilic) M35.4
  infective M72.8
    necrotizing M72.6
  necrotizing M72.6
  nodular M72.4
  perirenal (with ureteral obstruction) N13.5
    with infection N13.6
  plantar M72.2
  specified NEC M72.8
  traumatic (old) M72.8
    current — *code by* site under Sprain
Fascioliasis B66.3
Fasciolopsis, fasciolopsiasis (intestinal) B66.5
Fascioscapulohumeral myopathy G71.02
Fast pulse R00.0
Fat
  embolism — *see* Embolism, fat
  excessive — *see also* Obesity
    in heart — *see* Degeneration, myocardial
  in stool R19.5
  localized (pad) E65
    heart — *see* Degeneration, myocardial
    knee M79.4
    retropatellar M79.4
  necrosis
    breast N64.1
    mesentery K65.4
    omentum K65.4
  pad E65
    knee M79.4
Fatigue R53.83
  auditory deafness — *see* Deafness
  chronic R53.82
  combat F43.0
  general R53.83
    psychogenic F48.8
  heat (transient) T67.6 ☑
  muscle M62.89
  myocardium — *see* Failure, heart
  neoplasm-related R53.0
  nervous, neurosis F48.8
  operational F48.8
  psychogenic (general) F48.8
  senile R54
  voice R49.8
Fatness — *see* Obesity
Fatty — *see also* condition
  apron E65
  degeneration — *see* Degeneration, fatty
  heart (enlarged) — *see* Degeneration, myocardial
  liver NEC K76.0
    alcoholic K70.0
    nonalcoholic K76.0
  necrosis — *see* Degeneration, fatty
Fauces — *see* condition
Fauchard's disease (periodontitis) — *see* Periodontitis

Faucitis J02.9
Favism (anemia) D55.0
Favus — *see* Dermatophytosis
Fazio-Londe disease or syndrome G12.1
Fear complex or reaction F40.9
Fear of — *see* Phobia
Feared complaint unfounded Z71.1
Febris, febrile — *see also* Fever
  flava — *see also* Fever, yellow A95.9
  melitensis A23.0
  pestis — *see* Plague
  recurrens — *see* Fever, relapsing
  rubra A38.9
Fecal
  incontinence R15.9
  smearing R15.1
  soiling R15.1
  urgency R15.2
Fecalith (impaction) K56.41
  appendix K38.1
  congenital P76.8
Fede's disease K14.0
Feeble rapid pulse due to shock following injury
  T79.4 ☑
Feeble-minded F70
Feeding
  difficulties R63.3
  problem R63.3
    newborn P92.9
      specified NEC P92.8
    nonorganic (adult) — *see* Disorder, eating
Feeling (of)
  foreign body in throat R09.89
Feer's disease — *see* Poisoning, mercury
Feet — *see* condition
Feigned illness Z76.5
Feil-Klippel syndrome (brevicollis) Q76.1
Feinmesser's (hidrotic) **ectodermal dysplasia** Q82.4
Felon — *see also* Cellulitis, digit
  with lymphangitis — *see* Lymphangitis, acute, digit
Felty's syndrome M05.00
  ankle M05.07- ☑
  elbow M05.02- ☑
  foot joint M05.07- ☑
  hand joint M05.04- ☑
  hip M05.05- ☑
  knee M05.06- ☑
  multiple site M05.09
  shoulder M05.01- ☑
  vertebra — *see* Spondylitis, ankylosing
  wrist M05.03- ☑
Female genital cutting status — *see* Female genital
  mutilation status (FGM)
Female genital mutilation status (FGM) N90.810
  specified NEC N90.818
  type I (clitorectomy status) N90.811
  type II (clitorectomy with excision of labia minora sta-
    tus) N90.812
  type III (infibulation status) N90.813
  type IV N90.818
Femur, femoral — *see* condition
Fenestration, fenestrated — *see also* Imperfect, closure
  aortico-pulmonary Q21.4
  cusps, heart valve NEC Q24.8
    pulmonary Q22.3
  pulmonic cusps Q22.3
Fernell's disease (aortic aneurysm) I71.9
Fertile eunuch syndrome E23.0
Fetid
  breath R19.6
  sweat L75.0
Fetishism F65.0
  transvestic F65.1
Fetus, fetal — *see also* condition
  alcohol syndrome (dysmorphic) Q86.0
  compressus O31.0- ☑
  hydantoin syndrome Q86.1
  lung tissue P28.0
  papyraceous O31.0- ☑
Fever (inanition) (of unknown origin) (persistent) (with
  chills) (with rigor) R50.9
  abortus A23.1
  Aden (dengue) A90
  African tick bite A77.8
  African tick-borne A68.1

Index

Fever — Fever

☑ Additional Character Required — Refer to the Tabular List for Character Selection   ▼ Subterms under main terms may continue to next column or page

Fever — *continued*
  spotted A77.9
    American A77.0
    Brazilian A77.0
    cerebrospinal meningitis A39.0
    Colombian A77.0
    due to Rickettsia
      africae (African tick bite fever) A77.8
      australis A77.3
      conorii A77.1
      parkeri A77.8
      rickettsii A77.0
      sibirica A77.2
      specified type NEC A77.8
    Ehrlichiosis A77.40
      due to
        E. chafeensis A77.41
        specified organism NEC A77.49
    Rocky Mountain A77.0
  steroid R50.2
  streptobacillary A25.1
  subtertian B50.9
  Sumatran mite A75.3
  sun A90
  swamp A27.9
  swine A02.8
  sylvatic, yellow A95.0
  Tahyna B33.8
  tertian — *see* Malaria, tertian
  Thailand hemorrhagic A91
  thermic T67.01 ☑
  three-day A93.1
  tick
    American mountain A93.2
    Colorado A93.2
    Kemerovo A93.8
    Mediterranean A77.1
    mountain A93.2
    nonexanthematous A93.2
    Quaranfil A93.8
  tick-bite NEC A93.8
  tick-borne (hemorrhagic) NEC A93.8
  trench A79.0
  tsutsugamushi A75.3
  typhogastric A01.00
  typhoid (abortive) (hemorrhagic) (intermittent) (malignant) A01.00
    complicated by
      arthritis A01.04
      heart involvement A01.02
      meningitis A01.01
      osteomyelitis A01.05
      pneumonia A01.03
      specified NEC A01.09
  typhomalarial — *see* Malaria
  typhus — *see* Typhus (fever)
  undulant — *see* Brucellosis
  unknown origin R50.9
  uveoparotid D86.89
  valley B38.0
  Venezuelan equine A92.2
  vesicular stomatitis A93.8
  viral hemorrhagic — *see* Fever, hemorrhagic, by type of virus
  Volhynian A79.0
  Wesselsbron (viral) A92.8
  West
    African B50.8
    Nile (viral) A92.30
      with
        complications NEC A92.39
        cranial nerve disorders A92.32
        encephalitis A92.31
        encephalomyelitis A92.31
        neurologic manifestation NEC A92.32
        optic neuritis A92.32
        polyradiculitis A92.32
  Whitmore's — *see* Melioidosis
  Wolhynian A79.0
  worm B83.9
  yellow A95.9
    jungle A95.0
    sylvatic A95.0
    urban A95.1
  Zika virus A92.5
Fibrillation
  atrial or auricular (established) I48.91
    chronic I48.20

Fibrillation — *continued*
  atrial or auricular — *continued*
    chronic — *continued*
      persistent I48.19
      paroxysmal I48.0
      permanent I48.21
      persistent (chronic) (NOS) (other) I48.19
      longstanding I48.11
  cardiac I49.8
  heart I49.8
  muscular M62.89
  ventricular I49.01
Fibrin
  ball or bodies, pleural (sac) J94.1
  chamber, anterior (eye) (gelatinous exudate) — *see* Iridocyclitis, acute
Fibrinogenolysis — *see* Fibrinolysis
Fibrinogenopenia D68.8
  acquired D65
  congenital D68.2
Fibrinolysis (hemorrhagic) (acquired) D65
  antepartum hemorrhage — *see* Hemorrhage, antepartum, with coagulation defect
  following
    abortion — *see* Abortion by type complicated by hemorrhage
    ectopic or molar pregnancy O08.1
  intrapartum O67.0
  newborn, transient P60
  postpartum O72.3
Fibrinopenia (hereditary) D68.2
  acquired D68.4
Fibrinopurulent — *see* condition
Fibrinous — *see* condition
Fibroadenoma
  cellular intracanalicular D24- ☑
  giant D24- ☑
  intracanalicular
    cellular D24- ☑
    giant D24- ☑
    specified site — *see* Neoplasm, benign, by site
    unspecified site D24- ☑
  juvenile D24- ☑
  pericanalicular
    specified site — *see* Neoplasm, benign, by site
    unspecified site D24- ☑
  phyllodes D24- ☑
  prostate D29.1
  specified site NEC — *see* Neoplasm, benign, by site
  unspecified site D24- ☑
Fibroadenosis, breast (chronic) (cystic) (diffuse) (periodic) (segmental) N60.2- ☑
Fibroangioma — *see also* Neoplasm, benign, by site
  juvenile
    specified site — *see* Neoplasm, benign, by site
    unspecified site D10.6
Fibrochondrosarcoma — *see* Neoplasm, cartilage, malignant
Fibrocystic
  disease — *see also* Fibrosis, cystic
    breast — *see* Mastopathy, cystic
    jaw M27.49
    kidney (congenital) Q61.8
    liver Q44.6
    pancreas E84.9
  kidney (congenital) Q61.8
Fibrodysplasia ossificans progressiva — *see* Myositis, ossificans, progressiva
Fibroelastosis (cordis) (endocardial) (endomyocardial) I42.4
Fibroid (tumor) — *see also* Neoplasm, connective tissue, benign
  disease, lung (chronic) — *see* Fibrosis, lung
  heart (disease) — *see* Myocarditis
  in pregnancy or childbirth O34.1- ☑
    causing obstructed labor O65.5
  induration, lung (chronic) — *see* Fibrosis, lung
  lung — *see* Fibrosis, lung
  pneumonia (chronic) — *see* Fibrosis, lung
  uterus — *see also* Leiomyoma, uterus D25.9
Fibrolipoma — *see* Lipoma
Fibroliposarcoma — *see* Neoplasm, connective tissue, malignant
Fibroma — *see also* Neoplasm, connective tissue, benign
  ameloblastic — *see* Cyst, calcifying odontogenic
  bone (nonossifying) — *see* Disorder, bone, specified type NEC

Fibroma — *continued*
  bone — *see* Disorder, bone, specified type — *continued*
    ossifying — *see* Neoplasm, bone, benign
  cementifying — *see* Neoplasm, bone, benign
  chondromyoid — *see* Neoplasm, bone, benign
  desmoplastic — *see* Neoplasm, connective tissue, uncertain behavior
  durum — *see* Neoplasm, connective tissue, benign
  fascial — *see* Neoplasm, connective tissue, benign
  invasive — *see* Neoplasm, connective tissue, uncertain behavior
  molle — *see* Lipoma
  myxoid — *see* Neoplasm, connective tissue, benign
  nasopharynx, nasopharyngeal (juvenile) D10.6
  nonosteogenic (nonossifying) — *see* Dysplasia, fibrous
  odontogenic (central) — *see* Cyst, calcifying odontogenic
  ossifying — *see* Neoplasm, bone, benign
  periosteal — *see* Neoplasm, bone, benign
  soft — *see* Lipoma
Fibromatosis M72.9
  abdominal — *see* Neoplasm, connective tissue, uncertain behavior
  aggressive — *see* Neoplasm, connective tissue, uncertain behavior
  congenital generalized — *see* Neoplasm, connective tissue, uncertain behavior
  Dupuytren's M72.0
  gingival K06.1
  palmar (fascial) M72.0
  plantar (fascial) M72.2
  pseudosarcomatous (proliferative) (subcutaneous) M72.4
  retroperitoneal D48.3
  specified NEC M72.8
Fibromyalgia M79.7
Fibromyoma — *see also* Neoplasm, connective tissue, benign
  uterus (corpus) — *see also* Leiomyoma, uterus
    in pregnancy or childbirth — *see* Fibroid, in pregnancy or childbirth
    causing obstructed labor O65.5
Fibromyositis M79.7
Fibromyxolipoma D17.9
Fibromyxoma — *see* Neoplasm, connective tissue, benign
Fibromyxosarcoma — *see* Neoplasm, connective tissue, malignant
Fibro-odontoma, ameloblastic — *see* Cyst, calcifying odontogenic
Fibro-osteoma — *see* Neoplasm, bone, benign
Fibroplasia, retrolental H35.17- ☑
Fibropurulent — *see* condition
Fibrosarcoma — *see also* Neoplasm, connective tissue, malignant
  ameloblastic C41.1
    upper jaw (bone) C41.0
  congenital — *see* Neoplasm, connective tissue, malignant
  fascial — *see* Neoplasm, connective tissue, malignant
  infantile — *see* Neoplasm, connective tissue, malignant
  odontogenic C41.1
    upper jaw (bone) C41.0
  periosteal — *see* Neoplasm, bone, malignant
Fibrosclerosis
  breast N60.3- ☑
  multifocal M35.5
  penis (corpora cavernosa) N48.6
Fibrosis, fibrotic
  adrenal (gland) E27.8
  amnion O41.8X- ☑
  anal papillae K62.89
  arteriocapillary — *see* Arteriosclerosis
  bladder N32.89
    interstitial — *see* Cystitis, chronic, interstitial
    localized submucosal — *see* Cystitis, chronic, interstitial
    panmural — *see* Cystitis, chronic, interstitial
  breast — *see* Fibrosclerosis, breast
  capillary — *see also* Arteriosclerosis I70.90
    lung (chronic) — *see* Fibrosis, lung
  cardiac — *see* Myocarditis
  cervix N88.8
  chorion O41.8X- ☑
  corpus cavernosum (sclerosing) N48.6
  cystic (of pancreas) E84.9

Fibrosis, fibrotic — *continued*
  cystic — *continued*
    with
      distal intestinal obstruction syndrome E84.19
      fecal impaction E84.19
      intestinal manifestations NEC E84.19
      pulmonary manifestations E84.0
      specified manifestations NEC E84.8
    due to device, implant or graft — *see also* Complications, by site and type, specified NEC T85.828 ☑
      arterial graft NEC T82.828 ☑
      breast (implant) T85.828 ☑
      catheter NEC T85.828 ☑
        dialysis (renal) T82.828 ☑
          intraperitoneal T85.828 ☑
        infusion NEC T82.828 ☑
          spinal (epidural) (subdural) T85.820 ☑
        urinary (indwelling) T83.82 ☑
      electronic (electrode) (pulse generator) (stimulator)
        bone T84.82 ☑
        cardiac T82.827 ☑
        nervous system (brain) (peripheral nerve) (spinal)
          T85.820 ☑
        urinary T83.82 ☑
      fixation, internal (orthopedic) NEC T84.82 ☑
      gastrointestinal (bile duct) (esophagus) T85.828 ☑
      genital NEC T83.82 ☑
      heart NEC T82.827 ☑
      joint prosthesis T84.82 ☑
      ocular (corneal graft) (orbital implant) NEC
        T85.828 ☑
      orthopedic NEC T84.82 ☑
      specified NEC T85.828 ☑
      urinary NEC T83.82 ☑
      vascular NEC T82.828 ☑
      ventricular intracranial shunt T85.820 ☑
    ejaculatory duct N50.89
    endocardium — *see* Endocarditis
    endomyocardial (tropical) I42.3
    epididymis N50.89
    eye muscle — *see* Strabismus, mechanical
    heart — *see* Myocarditis
    hepatic — *see* Fibrosis, liver
    hepatolienal (portal hypertension) K76.6
    hepatosplenic (portal hypertension) K76.6
    infrapatellar fat pad M79.4
    intrascrotal N50.89
    kidney N26.9
    liver K74.00
      with sclerosis K74.2
      advanced K74.02
      alcoholic K70.2
      early K74.01
      stage
        F1 or F2 K74.01
        F3 K74.02
    lung (atrophic) (chronic) (confluent) (massive) (perialveolar) (peribronchial) J84.10
      with
        anthracosilicosis J60
        anthracosis J60
        asbestosis J61
        bagassosis J67.1
        bauxite J63.1
        berylliosis J63.2
        byssinosis J66.0
        calcicosis J62.8
        chalicosis J62.8
        dust reticulation J64
        farmer's lung J67.0
        ganister disease J62.8
        graphite J63.3
        pneumoconiosis NOS J64
        siderosis J63.4
        silicosis J62.8
      capillary J84.10
      congenital P27.8
      diffuse (idiopathic) J84.10
        chemicals, gases, fumes or vapors (inhalation)
          J68.4
        interstitial J84.10
          acute J84.114
        talc J62.0
      following radiation J70.1
      idiopathic J84.112
      postinflammatory J84.10
      silicotic J62.8
      tuberculous — *see* Tuberculosis, pulmonary

Fibrosis, fibrotic — *continued*
  lymphatic gland I89.8
  median bar — *see* Hyperplasia, prostate
  mediastinum (idiopathic) J98.59
  meninges G96.198
  myocardium, myocardial — *see* Myocarditis
  ovary N83.8
  oviduct N83.8
  pancreas K86.89
  penis NEC N48.6
  pericardium I31.0
  perineum, in pregnancy or childbirth O34.7- ☑
    causing obstructed labor O65.5
  pleura J94.1
  popliteal fat pad M79.4
  prostate (chronic) — *see* Hyperplasia, prostate
  pulmonary — *see also* Fibrosis, lung J84.10
    congenital P27.8
    idiopathic J84.112
  rectal sphincter K62.89
  retroperitoneal, idiopathic (with ureteral obstruction)
    N13.5
    with infection N13.6
  sclerosing mesenteric (idiopathic) K65.4
  scrotum N50.89
  seminal vesicle N50.89
  senile R54
  skin L90.5
  spermatic cord N50.89
  spleen D73.89
    in schistosomiasis (bilharziasis) B65.9 *[D77]*
  subepidermal nodular — *see* Neoplasm, skin, benign
  submucous (oral) (tongue) K13.5
  testis N44.8
    chronic, due to syphilis A52.76
  thymus (gland) E32.8
  tongue, submucous K13.5
  tunica vaginalis N50.89
  uterus (non-neoplastic) N85.8
  vagina N89.8
  valve, heart — *see* Endocarditis
  vas deferens N50.89
  vein I87.8
Fibrositis (periarticular) M79.7
  nodular, chronic (Jaccoud's) (rheumatoid) — *see*
    Arthropathy, postrheumatic, chronic
Fibrothorax J94.1
Fibrotic — *see* Fibrosis
Fibrous — *see* condition
Fibroxanthoma — *see also* Neoplasm, connective tissue,
    benign
  atypical — *see* Neoplasm, connective tissue, uncertain
    behavior
  malignant — *see* Neoplasm, connective tissue, malignant
Fibroxanthosarcoma — *see* Neoplasm, connective tissue, malignant
Fiedler's
  disease (icterohemorrhagic leptospirosis) A27.0
  myocarditis (acute) I40.1
Fifth disease B08.3
  venereal A55
Filaria, filarial, filariasis — *see* Infestation, filarial
Filatov's disease — *see* Mononucleosis, infectious
File-cutter's disease — *see* Poisoning, lead
Filling defect
  biliary tract R93.2
  bladder R93.41
  duodenum R93.3
  gallbladder R93.2
  gastrointestinal tract R93.3
  intestine R93.3
  kidney R93.42- ☑
  stomach R93.3
  ureter R93.41
  urinary organs, specified NEC R93.49
Fimbrial cyst Q50.4
Financial problem affecting care NOS Z59.9
  bankruptcy Z59.8
  foreclosure on loan Z59.8
Findings, abnormal, inconclusive, without diagnosis
    — *see also* Abnormal
  17-ketosteroids, elevated R82.5
  acetonuria R82.4
  alcohol in blood R78.0
  anisocytosis R71.8
  antenatal screening of mother O28.9
    biochemical O28.1

Findings, abnormal, inconclusive, without diagnosis
    — *continued*
  antenatal screening of mother — *continued*
    chromosomal O28.5
    cytological O28.2
    genetic O28.5
    hematological O28.0
    radiological O28.4
    specified NEC O28.8
    ultrasonic O28.3
  antibody titer, elevated R76.0
  anticardiolipin antibody R76.0
  antiphosphatidylglycerol antibody R76.0
  antiphosphatidylinositol antibody R76.0
  antiphosphatidylserine antibody R76.0
  antiphospholipid antibody R76.0
  bacteriuria R82.71
  bicarbonate E87.8
  bile in urine R82.2
  blood sugar R73.09
    high R73.9
    low (transient) E16.2
  body fluid or substance, specified NEC R88.8
  casts, urine R82.998
  catecholamines R82.5
  cells, urine R82.998
  chloride E87.8
  cholesterol E78.9
    high E78.00
      with high triglycerides E78.2
  chyluria R82.0
  cloudy
    dialysis effluent R88.0
    urine R82.90
  creatinine clearance R94.4
  crystals, urine R82.998
  culture
    blood R78.81
    positive — *see* Positive, culture
  echocardiogram R93.1
  electrolyte level, urinary R82.998
  function study NEC R94.8
    bladder R94.8
    endocrine NEC R94.7
      thyroid R94.6
    kidney R94.4
    liver R94.5
    pancreas R94.8
    placenta R94.8
    pulmonary R94.2
    spleen R94.8
  gallbladder, nonvisualization R93.2
  glucose (tolerance test) (non-fasting) R73.09
  glycosuria R81
  heart
    shadow R93.1
    sounds R01.2
  hematinuria R82.3
  hematocrit drop (precipitous) R71.0
  hemoglobinuria R82.3
  human papillomavirus (HPV) DNA test positive
    cervix
      high risk R87.810
      low risk R87.820
    vagina
      high risk R87.811
      low risk R87.821
  in blood (of substance not normally found in blood)
    R78.9
    addictive drug NEC R78.4
    alcohol (excessive level) R78.0
    cocaine R78.2
    hallucinogen R78.3
    heavy metals (abnormal level) R78.79
    lead R78.71
    lithium (abnormal level) R78.89
    opiate drug R78.1
    psychotropic drug R78.5
    specified substance NEC R78.89
    steroid agent R78.6
  indoleacetic acid, elevated R82.5
  ketonuria R82.4
  lactic acid dehydrogenase (LDH) R74.02
  liver function test R79.89
  mammogram NEC R92.8
    calcification (calculus) R92.1
    inconclusive result (due to dense breasts) R92.2
    microcalcification R92.0
  mediastinal shift R93.89

☑ **Additional Character Required** — Refer to the Tabular List for Character Selection

☑ Subterms under main terms may continue to next column or page

Findings, abnormal, inconclusive, without diagnosis
— *continued*
  melanin, urine R82.998
  myoglobinuria R82.1
  neonatal screening P09
  nonvisualization of gallbladder R93.2
  odor of urine NOS R82.90
  Papanicolaou cervix R87.619
    non-atypical endometrial cells R87.618
  pneumoencephalogram R93.0
  poikilocytosis R71.8
  potassium (deficiency) E87.6
    excess E87.5
  PPD R76.11
  radiologic (X-ray) R93.89
    abdomen R93.5
    biliary tract R93.2
    breast R92.8
    gastrointestinal tract R93.3
    genitourinary organs R93.89
    head R93.0
    inconclusive due to excess body fat of patient R93.9
    intrathoracic organs NEC R93.1
    musculoskeletal
      limbs R93.6
      other than limb R93.7
    placenta R93.89
    retroperitoneum R93.5
    skin R93.89
    skull R93.0
    subcutaneous tissue R93.89
    testis R93.81- ☑
  red blood cell (count) (morphology) (sickling) (volume)
      R71.8
  scan NEC R94.8
    bladder R94.8
    bone R94.8
    kidney R94.4
    liver R93.2
    lung R94.2
    pancreas R94.8
    placental R94.8
    spleen R94.8
    thyroid R94.6
  sedimentation rate, elevated R70.0
  SGOT R74.01
  SGPT R74.01
  sodium (deficiency) E87.1
    excess E87.0
  specified body fluid NEC R88.8
  stress test R94.39
  testis R93.81- ☑
  thyroid (function) (metabolic rate) (scan) (uptake) R94.6
  transaminase (level) R74.01
  triglycerides E78.9
    high E78.1
      with high cholesterol E78.2
  tuberculin skin test (without active tuberculosis) R76.11
  urine R82.90
    acetone R82.4
    bacteria R82.71
    bile R82.2
    casts or cells R82.998
    chyle R82.0
    culture positive R82.79
    glucose R81
    hemoglobin R82.3
    ketone R82.4
    sugar R81
  vanillylmandelic acid (VMA), elevated R82.5
  vectorcardiogram (VCG) R94.39
  ventriculogram R93.0
  white blood cell (count) (differential) (morphology)
      D72.9
  xerography R92.8
Finger — *see* condition
Fire, Saint Anthony's — *see* Erysipelas
Fire-setting
  pathological (compulsive) F63.1
Fish hook stomach K31.89
Fishmeal-worker's lung J67.8
Fissure, fissured
  anus, anal K60.2
    acute K60.0
    chronic K60.1
    congenital Q43.8
  ear, lobule, congenital Q17.8
  epiglottis (congenital) Q31.8

Fissure, fissured — *continued*
  larynx J38.7
    congenital Q31.8
  lip K13.0
    congenital — *see* Cleft, lip
  nipple N64.0
    associated with
      lactation O92.13
      pregnancy O92.11- ☑
      puerperium O92.12
  nose Q30.2
  palate (congenital) — *see* Cleft, palate
  skin R23.4
  spine (congenital) — *see also* Spina bifida
    with hydrocephalus — *see* Spina bifida, by site, with
        hydrocephalus
  tongue (acquired) K14.5
    congenital Q38.3
Fistula (cutaneous) L98.8
  abdomen (wall) K63.2
    bladder N32.2
    intestine NEC K63.2
    ureter N28.89
    uterus N82.5
  abdominorectal K63.2
  abdominosigmoidal K63.2
  abdominothoracic J86.0
  abdominouterine N82.5
    congenital Q51.7
  abdominovesical N32.2
  accessory sinuses — *see* Sinusitis
  actinomycotic — *see* Actinomycosis
  alveolar antrum — *see* Sinusitis, maxillary
  alveolar process K04.6
  anorectal K60.5
  antrobuccal — *see* Sinusitis, maxillary
  antrum — *see* Sinusitis, maxillary
  anus, anal (recurrent) (infectional) K60.3
    congenital Q43.6
      with absence, atresia and stenosis Q42.2
    tuberculous A18.32
  aorta-duodenal I77.2
  appendix, appendicular K38.3
  arteriovenous (acquired) (nonruptured) I77.0
    brain I67.1
      congenital Q28.2
        ruptured — *see* Fistula, arteriovenous, brain,
            ruptured
      ruptured I60.8
        intracerebral I61.8
        intraparenchymal I61.8
        intraventricular I61.5
        subarachnoid I60.8
    cerebral — *see* Fistula, arteriovenous, brain
    congenital (peripheral) — *see also* Malformation,
        arteriovenous
      brain Q28.2
        ruptured — *see* Fistula, arteriovenous, brain,
            ruptured
      coronary Q24.5
      pulmonary Q25.72
    coronary I25.41
      congenital Q24.5
    pulmonary I28.0
      congenital Q25.72
    surgically created (for dialysis) Z99.2
      complication — *see* Complication, arteriovenous,
          fistula, surgically created
    traumatic — *see* Injury, blood vessel
  artery I77.2
  aural (mastoid) — *see* Mastoiditis, chronic
  auricle — *see also* Disorder, pinna, specified type NEC
    congenital Q18.1
  Bartholin's gland N82.8
  bile duct (common) (hepatic) K83.3
    with calculus, stones — *see also* Calculus, bile duct
        K83.3
  biliary (tract) — *see* Fistula, bile duct
  bladder (sphincter) NEC — *see also* Fistula, vesico-
      N32.2
    into seminal vesicle N32.2
  bone — *see also* Disorder, bone, specified type NEC
    with osteomyelitis, chronic — *see* Osteomyelitis,
        chronic, with draining sinus
  brain G93.89
    arteriovenous (acquired) — *see also* Fistula, arteri-
        ovenous, brain I67.1
      congenital Q28.2

Fistula — *continued*
  branchial (cleft) Q18.0
  branchiogenous Q18.0
  breast N61.0
    puerperal, postpartum or gestational, due to mastitis
        (purulent) — *see* Mastitis, obstetric, purulent
  bronchial J86.0
  bronchocutaneous, bronchomediastinal, bronchopleu-
      ral, bronchopleuromediastinal (infective) J86.0
    tuberculous NEC A15.5
  bronchoesophageal J86.0
    congenital Q39.2
      with atresia of esophagus Q39.1
  bronchovisceral J86.0
  buccal cavity (infective) K12.2
  cecosigmoidal K63.2
  cecum K63.2
  cerebrospinal (fluid) G96.08
  cervical, lateral Q18.1
  cervicoaural Q18.1
  cervicosigmoidal N82.4
  cervicovesical N82.1
  cervix N82.8
  chest (wall) J86.0
  cholecystenteric — *see* Fistula, gallbladder
  cholecystocolic — *see* Fistula, gallbladder
  cholecystocolonic — *see* Fistula, gallbladder
  cholecystoduodenal — *see* Fistula, gallbladder
  cholecystogastric — *see* Fistula, gallbladder
  cholecystointestinal — *see* Fistula, gallbladder
  choledochoduodenal — *see* Fistula, bile duct
  cholocolic K82.3
  coccyx — *see* Sinus, pilonidal
  colon K63.2
  colostomy K94.09
  colovesical N32.1
  common duct — *see* Fistula, bile duct
  congenital, site not listed — *see* Anomaly, by site
  coronary, arteriovenous I25.41
    congenital Q24.5
  costal region J86.0
  cul-de-sac, Douglas' N82.8
  cystic duct — *see also* Fistula, gallbladder
    congenital Q44.5
  dental K04.6
  diaphragm J86.0
  duodenum K31.6
  ear (external) (canal) — *see* Disorder, ear, external,
      specified type NEC
  enterocolic K63.2
  enterocutaneous K63.2
  enterouterine N82.4
    congenital Q51.7
  enterovaginal N82.4
    congenital Q52.2
    large intestine N82.3
    small intestine N82.2
  enterovesical N32.1
  epididymis N50.89
    tuberculous A18.15
  esophagobronchial J86.0
    congenital Q39.2
      with atresia of esophagus Q39.1
  esophagocutaneous K22.8
  esophagopleural-cutaneous J86.0
  esophagotracheal J86.0
    congenital Q39.2
      with atresia of esophagus Q39.1
  esophagus K22.8
    congenital Q39.2
      with atresia of esophagus Q39.1
  ethmoid — *see* Sinusitis, ethmoidal
  eyeball (cornea) (sclera) — *see* Disorder, globe, hy-
      potony
  eyelid H01.8
  fallopian tube, external N82.5
  fecal K63.2
    congenital Q43.6
  from periapical abscess K04.6
  frontal sinus — *see* Sinusitis, frontal
  gallbladder K82.3
    with calculus, cholelithiasis, stones — *see* Calculus,
        gallbladder
  gastric K31.6
  gastrocolic K31.6
    congenital Q40.2
    tuberculous A18.32
  gastroenterocolic K31.6

Index

Fistula — *continued*
- gastroesophageal K31.6
- gastrojejunal K31.6
- gastrojejunocolic K31.6
- genital tract (female) N82.9
  - specified NEC N82.8
  - to intestine NEC N82.4
  - to skin N82.5
- hepatic artery-portal vein, congenital Q26.6
- hepatopleural J86.0
- hepatopulmonary J86.0
- ileorectal or ileosigmoidal K63.2
- ileovaginal N82.2
- ileovesical N32.1
- ileum K63.2
- in ano K60.3
  - tuberculous A18.32
- inner ear (labyrinth) — *see* subcategory H83.1 ☑
- intestine NEC K63.2
- intestinocolonic (abdominal) K63.2
- intestinoureteral N28.89
- intestinouterine N82.4
- intestinovaginal N82.4
  - large intestine N82.3
  - small intestine N82.2
- intestinovesical N32.1
- ischiorectal (fossa) K61.39
- jejunum K63.2
- joint M25.10
  - ankle M25.17- ☑
  - elbow M25.12- ☑
  - foot joint M25.17- ☑
  - hand joint M25.14- ☑
  - hip M25.15- ☑
  - knee M25.16- ☑
  - shoulder M25.11- ☑
  - specified joint NEC M25.18
  - tuberculous — *see* Tuberculosis, joint
  - vertebrae M25.18
  - wrist M25.13- ☑
- kidney N28.89
- labium (majus) (minus) N82.8
- labyrinth — *see* subcategory H83.1 ☑
- lacrimal (gland) (sac) H04.61- ☑
- lacrimonasal duct — *see* Fistula, lacrimal
- laryngotracheal, congenital Q34.8
- larynx J38.7
- lip K13.0
  - congenital Q38.0
- lumbar, tuberculous A18.01
- lung J86.0
- lymphatic I89.8
- mammary (gland) N61.0
- mastoid (process) (region) — *see* Mastoiditis, chronic
- maxillary J32.0
- medial, face and neck Q18.8
- mediastinal J86.0
- mediastinobronchial J86.0
- mediastinocutaneous J86.0
- middle ear — *see* subcategory H74.8 ☑
- mouth K12.2
- nasal J34.89
  - sinus — *see* Sinusitis
- nasopharynx J39.2
- nipple N64.0
- nose J34.89
- oral (cutaneous) K12.2
  - maxillary J32.0
  - nasal (with cleft palate) — *see* Cleft, palate
- orbit, orbital — *see* Disorder, orbit, specified type NEC
- oroantral J32.0
- oviduct, external N82.5
- palate (hard) M27.8
- pancreatic K86.89
- pancreaticoduodenal K86.89
- parotid (gland) K11.4
  - region K12.2
- penis N48.89
- perianal K60.3
- pericardium (pleura) (sac) — *see* Pericarditis
- pericecal K63.2
- perineorectal K60.4
- perineosigmoidal K63.2
- perineum, perineal (with urethral involvement) NEC N36.0
  - tuberculous A18.13
  - ureter N28.89
- perirectal K60.4

Fistula — *continued*
- perirectal — *continued*
  - tuberculous A18.32
- peritoneum K65.9
- pharyngoesophageal J39.2
- pharynx J39.2
  - branchial cleft (congenital) Q18.0
- pilonidal (infected) (rectum) — *see* Sinus, pilonidal
- pleura, pleural, pleurocutaneous, pleuroperitoneal J86.0
  - tuberculous NEC A15.6
- pleuropericardial I31.8
- portal vein-hepatic artery, congenital Q26.6
- postauricular H70.81- ☑
- postoperative, persistent T81.83 ☑
  - specified site — *see* Fistula, by site
- preauricular (congenital) Q18.1
- prostate N42.89
- pulmonary J86.0
  - arteriovenous I28.0
    - congenital Q25.72
  - tuberculous — *see* Tuberculosis, pulmonary
- pulmonoperitoneal J86.0
- rectolabial N82.4
- rectosigmoid (intercommunicating) K63.2
- rectoureteral N28.89
- rectourethral N36.0
  - congenital Q64.73
- rectouterine N82.4
  - congenital Q51.7
- rectovaginal N82.3
  - congenital Q52.2
  - tuberculous A18.18
- rectovesical N32.1
  - congenital Q64.79
- rectovesicovaginal N82.3
- rectovulval N82.4
  - congenital Q52.79
- rectum (to skin) K60.4
  - congenital Q43.6
    - with absence, atresia and stenosis Q42.0
  - tuberculous A18.32
- renal N28.89
- retroauricular — *see* Fistula, postauricular
- salivary duct or gland (any) K11.4
  - congenital Q38.4
- scrotum (urinary) N50.89
  - tuberculous A18.15
- semicircular canals — *see* subcategory H83.1 ☑
- sigmoid K63.2
  - to bladder N32.1
- sinus — *see* Sinusitis
- skin L98.8
  - to genital tract (female) N82.5
- splenocolic D73.89
- stercoral K63.2
- stomach K31.6
- sublingual gland K11.4
- submandibular gland K11.4
- submaxillary (gland) K11.4
  - region K12.2
- thoracic J86.0
  - duct I89.8
- thoracoabdominal J86.0
- thoracogastric J86.0
- thoracointestinal J86.0
- thorax J86.0
- thyroglossal duct Q89.2
- thyroid E07.89
- trachea, congenital (external) (internal) Q32.1
- tracheoesophageal J86.0
  - congenital Q39.2
    - with atresia of esophagus Q39.1
  - following tracheostomy J95.04
- traumatic arteriovenous — *see* Injury, blood vessel, by site
- tuberculous — *code by* site under Tuberculosis
- typhoid A01.09
- umbilicourinary Q64.8
- urachus, congenital Q64.4
- ureter (persistent) N28.89
- ureteroabdominal N28.89
- ureterorectal N28.89
- ureterosigmoido-abdominal N28.89
- ureterovaginal N82.1
- ureterovesical N32.2
- urethra N36.0
  - congenital Q64.79

Fistula — *continued*
- urethra — *continued*
  - tuberculous A18.13
- urethroperineal N36.0
- urethroperineovesical N32.2
- urethrorectal N36.0
  - congenital Q64.73
- urethroscrotal N50.89
- urethrovaginal N82.1
- urethrovesical N32.2
- urinary (tract) (persistent) (recurrent) N36.0
- uteroabdominal N82.5
  - congenital Q51.7
- uteroenteric, uterointestinal N82.4
  - congenital Q51.7
- uterorectal N82.4
  - congenital Q51.7
- uteroureteric N82.1
- uterourethral Q51.7
- uterovaginal N82.8
- uterovesical N82.1
  - congenital Q51.7
- uterus N82.8
- vagina (postpartal) (wall) N82.8
- vaginocutaneous (postpartal) N82.5
- vaginointestinal NEC N82.4
  - large intestine N82.3
  - small intestine N82.2
- vaginoperineal N82.5
- vasocutaneous, congenital Q55.7
- vesical NEC N32.2
- vesicoabdominal N32.2
- vesicocervicovaginal N82.1
- vesicocolic N32.1
- vesicocutaneous N32.2
- vesicoenteric N32.1
- vesicointestinal N32.1
- vesicometrorectal N82.4
- vesicoperineal N32.2
- vesicorectal N32.1
  - congenital Q64.79
- vesicosigmoidal N32.1
- vesicosigmoidovaginal N82.3
- vesicoureteral N32.2
- vesicoureterovaginal N82.1
- vesicourethral N32.2
- vesicourethrorectal N32.1
- vesicouterine N82.1
  - congenital Q51.7
- vesicovaginal N82.0
- vulvorectal N82.4
  - congenital Q52.79

Fit R56.9
- epileptic — *see* Epilepsy
- fainting R55
- hysterical F44.5
- newborn P90

Fitting (and adjustment) (of)
- artificial
  - arm — *see* Admission, adjustment, artificial, arm
  - breast Z44.3 ☑
  - eye Z44.2 ☑
  - leg — *see* Admission, adjustment, artificial, leg
- automatic implantable cardiac defibrillator (with synchronous cardiac pacemaker) Z45.02
- brain neuropacemaker Z46.2
  - implanted Z45.42
- cardiac defibrillator — *see* Fitting (and adjustment) (of), automatic implantable cardiac defibrillator
- catheter, non-vascular Z46.82
- colostomy belt Z46.89
- contact lenses Z46.0
- CRT-D (resynchronization therapy defibrillator) Z45.0
- CRT-P (cardiac resynchronization therapy pacemaker) Z45.018
  - pulse generator Z45.010
- cystostomy device Z46.6
- defibrillator, cardiac — *see* Fitting (and adjustment) (of), automatic implantable cardiac defibrillator
- dentures Z46.3
- device NOS Z46.9
  - abdominal Z46.89
  - gastrointestinal NEC Z46.59
  - implanted NEC Z45.89
  - nervous system Z46.2
    - implanted — *see* Admission, adjustment, device implanted, nervous system
  - orthodontic Z46.4

☑ **Additional Character Required — Refer to the Tabular List for Character Selection**

🔄 **Subterms under main terms may continue to next column or page**

Fistula — Fitting

Fitting — *continued*
  device — *continued*
    orthoptic Z46.0
    orthotic Z46.89
    prosthetic (external) Z44.9
      breast Z44.3 ☑
      dental Z46.3
      eye Z44.2 ☑
      specified NEC Z44.8
    specified NEC Z46.89
    substitution
      auditory Z46.2
        implanted — *see* Admission, adjustment, device, implanted, hearing device
      nervous system Z46.2
        implanted — *see* Admission, adjustment, device, implanted, nervous system
      visual Z46.2
        implanted Z45.31
    urinary Z46.6
  gastric lap band Z46.51
  gastrointestinal appliance NEC Z46.59
  glasses (reading) Z46.0
  hearing aid Z46.1
  ileostomy device Z46.89
  insulin pump Z46.81
  intestinal appliance NEC Z46.89
  myringotomy device (stent) (tube) Z45.82
  neuropacemaker Z46.2
    implanted Z45.42
  non-vascular catheter Z46.82
  orthodontic device Z46.4
  orthopedic device (brace) (cast) (corset) (shoes) Z46.89
  pacemaker (cardiac) (cardiac resynchronization therapy (CRT-P)) Z45.018
    nervous system (brain) (peripheral nerve) (spinal cord) Z46.2
      implanted Z45.42
    pulse generator Z45.010
  portacath (port-a-cath) Z45.2
  prosthesis (external) Z44.9
    arm — *see* Admission, adjustment, artificial, arm
    breast Z44.3 ☑
    dental Z46.3
    eye Z44.2 ☑
    leg — *see* Admission, adjustment, artificial, leg
    specified NEC Z44.8
  spectacles Z46.0
  wheelchair Z46.89
Fitzhugh-Curtis syndrome
  due to
    Chlamydia trachomatis A74.81
    Neisseria gonorrhorea (gonococcal peritonitis) A54.85
Fitz's syndrome (acute hemorrhagic pancreatitis) — *see also* Pancreatitis, acute K85.80
Fixation
  joint — *see* Ankylosis
  larynx J38.7
  stapes — *see* Ankylosis, ear ossicles
    deafness — *see* Deafness, conductive
  uterus (acquired) — *see* Malposition, uterus
  vocal cord J38.3
Flabby ridge K06.8
Flaccid — *see also* condition
  palate, congenital Q38.5
Flail
  chest S22.5 ☑
    newborn (birth injury) P13.8
  joint (paralytic) M25.20
    ankle M25.27- ☑
    elbow M25.22- ☑
    foot joint M25.27- ☑
    hand joint M25.24- ☑
    hip M25.25- ☑
    knee M25.26- ☑
    shoulder M25.21- ☑
    specified joint NEC M25.28
    wrist M25.23- ☑
Flajani's disease — *see* Hyperthyroidism, with, goiter (diffuse)
Flap, liver K71.3
Flashbacks (residual to hallucinogen use) F16.283
Flat
  chamber (eye) — *see* Disorder, globe, hypotony, flat anterior chamber
  chest, congenital Q67.8

Flat — *continued*
  foot (acquired) (fixed type) (painful) (postural) — *see also* Deformity, limb, flat foot
    congenital (rigid) (spastic (everted)) Q66.5- ☑
    rachitic sequelae (late effect) E64.3
  organ or site, congenital NEC — *see* Anomaly, by site
  pelvis M95.5
    with disproportion (fetopelvic) O33.0
      causing obstructed labor O65.0
    congenital Q74.2
Flatau-Schilder disease G37.0
Flatback syndrome M40.30
  lumbar region M40.36
  lumbosacral region M40.37
  thoracolumbar region M40.35
Flattening
  head, femur M89.8X5
  hip — *see* Coxa, plana
  lip (congenital) Q18.8
  nose (congenital) Q67.4
    acquired M95.0
Flatulence R14.3
  psychogenic F45.8
Flatus R14.3
  vaginalis N89.8
Flax-dresser's disease J66.1
Flea bite — *see* Injury, bite, by site, superficial, insect
Flecks, glaucomatous (subcapsular) — *see* Cataract, complicated
Fleischer (-Kayser) **ring** (cornea) H18.04- ☑
Fleshy mole O02.0
Flexibilitas cerea — *see* Catalepsy
Flexion
  amputation stump (surgical) T87.89
  cervix — *see* Malposition, uterus
  contracture, joint — *see* Contraction, joint
  deformity, joint — *see also* Deformity, limb, flexion M21.20
    hip, congenital Q65.89
  uterus — *see also* Malposition, uterus
    lateral — *see* Lateroversion, uterus
Flexner-Boyd dysentery A03.2
Flexner's dysentery A03.1
Flexure — *see* Flexion
Flint murmur (aortic insufficiency) I35.1
Floater, vitreous — *see* Opacity, vitreous
Floating
  cartilage (joint) — *see also* Loose, body, joint
    knee — *see* Derangement, knee, loose body
  gallbladder, congenital Q44.1
  kidney N28.89
    congenital Q63.8
  spleen D73.89
Flooding N92.0
Floor — *see* condition
Floppy
  baby syndrome (nonspecific) P94.2
  iris syndrome (intraoperative) (IFIS) H21.81
  nonrheumatic mitral valve syndrome I34.1
Flu — *see also* Influenza
  avian — *see also* Influenza, due to, identified novel influenza A virus J09.X2
  bird — *see also* Influenza, due to, identified novel influenza A virus J09.X2
  intestinal NEC A08.4
  swine (viruses that normally cause infections in pigs) — *see also* Influenza, due to, identified novel influenza A virus J09.X2
Fluctuating blood pressure I99.8
Fluid
  abdomen R18.8
  chest J94.8
  heart — *see* Failure, heart, congestive
  joint — *see* Effusion, joint
  loss (acute) E86.9
  lung — *see* Edema, lung
  overload E87.70
    specified NEC E87.79
  peritoneal cavity R18.8
  pleural cavity J94.8
  retention R60.9
Flukes NEC — *see also* Infestation, fluke
  blood NEC — *see* Schistosomiasis
  liver B66.3
Fluor (vaginalis) N89.8
  trichomonal or due to Trichomonas (vaginalis) A59.00

Fluorosis
  dental K00.3
  skeletal M85.10
    ankle M85.17- ☑
    foot M85.17- ☑
    forearm M85.13- ☑
    hand M85.14- ☑
    lower leg M85.16- ☑
    multiple site M85.19
    neck M85.18
    rib M85.18
    shoulder M85.11- ☑
    skull M85.18
    specified site NEC M85.18
    thigh M85.15- ☑
    toe M85.17- ☑
    upper arm M85.12- ☑
    vertebra M85.18
Flush syndrome E34.0
Flushing R23.2
  menopausal N95.1
Flutter
  atrial or auricular I48.92
    atypical I48.4
    type I I48.3
    type II I48.4
    typical I48.3
  heart I49.8
    atrial or auricular I48.92
      atypical I48.4
      type I I48.3
      type II I48.4
      typical I48.3
    ventricular I49.02
  ventricular I49.02
FNHTR (febrile nonhemolytic transfusion reaction) R50.84
Fochier's abscess — *code by* site under Abscess
Focus, Assmann's — *see* Tuberculosis, pulmonary
Fogo selvagem L10.3
Foix-Alajouanine syndrome G95.19
Fold, folds (anomalous) — *see also* Anomaly, by site
  Descemet's membrane — *see* Change, corneal membrane, Descemet's, fold
  epicanthic Q10.3
  heart Q24.8
Folie à deux F24
Follicle
  cervix (nabothian) (ruptured) N88.8
  graafian, ruptured, with hemorrhage N83.0- ☑
  nabothian N88.8
Follicular — *see* condition
Folliculitis (superficial) L73.9
  abscedens et suffodiens L66.3
  cyst N83.0- ☑
  decalvans L66.2
  deep — *see* Furuncle, by site
  gonococcal (acute) (chronic) A54.01
  keloid, keloidalis L73.0
  pustular L01.02
  ulerythematosa reticulata L66.4
Folliculome lipidique
  specified site — *see* Neoplasm, benign, by site
  unspecified site
    female D27.9
    male D29.20
Følling's disease E70.0
Follow-up — *see* Examination, follow-up
Fong's syndrome (hereditary osteo-onychodysplasia) Q87.2
Food
  allergy L27.2
  asphyxia (from aspiration or inhalation) — *see* Foreign body, by site
  choked on — *see* Foreign body, by site
  deprivation T73.0 ☑
    specified kind of food NEC E63.8
  intoxication — *see* Poisoning, food
  lack of T73.0 ☑
  poisoning — *see* Poisoning, food
  rejection NEC — *see* Disorder, eating
  strangulation or suffocation — *see* Foreign body, by site
  toxemia — *see* Poisoning, food
Foot — *see* condition
Foramen ovale (nonclosure) (patent) (persistent) Q21.1
Forbes' glycogen storage disease E74.03
Fordyce-Fox disease L75.2

Fordyce's disease (mouth) Q38.6
Forearm — *see* condition
Foreign body
  with
    laceration — *see* Laceration, by site, with foreign body
    puncture wound — *see* Puncture, by site, with foreign body
  accidentally left following a procedure T81.509 ☑
    aspiration T81.506 ☑
      resulting in
        adhesions T81.516 ☑
        obstruction T81.526 ☑
        perforation T81.536 ☑
        specified complication NEC T81.596 ☑
    cardiac catheterization T81.505 ☑
      resulting in
        acute reaction T81.60 ☑
          aseptic peritonitis T81.61 ☑
          specified NEC T81.69 ☑
        adhesions T81.515 ☑
        obstruction T81.525 ☑
        perforation T81.535 ☑
        specified complication NEC T81.595 ☑
    causing
      acute reaction T81.60 ☑
        aseptic peritonitis T81.61 ☑
        specified complication NEC T81.69 ☑
      adhesions T81.519 ☑
      aseptic peritonitis T81.61 ☑
      obstruction T81.529 ☑
      perforation T81.539 ☑
      specified complication NEC T81.599 ☑
    endoscopy T81.504 ☑
      resulting in
        adhesions T81.514 ☑
        obstruction T81.524 ☑
        perforation T81.534 ☑
        specified complication NEC T81.594 ☑
    immunization T81.503 ☑
      resulting in
        adhesions T81.513 ☑
        obstruction T81.523 ☑
        perforation T81.533 ☑
        specified complication NEC T81.593 ☑
    infusion T81.501 ☑
      resulting in
        adhesions T81.511 ☑
        obstruction T81.521 ☑
        perforation T81.531 ☑
        specified complication NEC T81.591 ☑
    injection T81.503 ☑
      resulting in
        adhesions T81.513 ☑
        obstruction T81.523 ☑
        perforation T81.533 ☑
        specified complication NEC T81.593 ☑
    kidney dialysis T81.502 ☑
      resulting in
        adhesions T81.512 ☑
        obstruction T81.522 ☑
        perforation T81.532 ☑
        specified complication NEC T81.592 ☑
    packing removal T81.507 ☑
      resulting in
        acute reaction T81.60 ☑
          aseptic peritonitis T81.61 ☑
          specified NEC T81.69 ☑
        adhesions T81.517 ☑
        obstruction T81.527 ☑
        perforation T81.537 ☑
        specified complication NEC T81.597 ☑
    puncture T81.506 ☑
      resulting in
        adhesions T81.516 ☑
        obstruction T81.526 ☑
        perforation T81.536 ☑
        specified complication NEC T81.596 ☑
    specified procedure NEC T81.508 ☑
      resulting in
        acute reaction T81.60 ☑
          aseptic peritonitis T81.61 ☑
          specified NEC T81.69 ☑
        adhesions T81.518 ☑
        obstruction T81.528 ☑
        perforation T81.538 ☑

Foreign body — *continued*
  accidentally left following a procedure — *continued*
    specified procedure — *continued*
      resulting in — *continued*
        specified complication NEC T81.598 ☑
    surgical operation T81.500 ☑
      resulting in
        acute reaction T81.60 ☑
          aseptic peritonitis T81.61 ☑
          specified NEC T81.69 ☑
        adhesions T81.510 ☑
        obstruction T81.520 ☑
        perforation T81.530 ☑
        specified complication NEC T81.590 ☑
    transfusion T81.501 ☑
      resulting in
        adhesions T81.511 ☑
        obstruction T81.521 ☑
        perforation T81.531 ☑
        specified complication NEC T81.591 ☑
  alimentary tract T18.9 ☑
    anus T18.5 ☑
    colon T18.4 ☑
    esophagus — *see* Foreign body, esophagus
    mouth T18.0 ☑
    multiple sites T18.8 ☑
    rectosigmoid (junction) T18.5 ☑
    rectum T18.5 ☑
    small intestine T18.3 ☑
    specified site NEC T18.8 ☑
    stomach T18.2 ☑
  anterior chamber (eye) S05.5- ☑
  auditory canal — *see* Foreign body, entering through orifice, ear
  bronchus T17.508 ☑
    causing
      asphyxiation T17.500 ☑
        food (bone) (seed) T17.520 ☑
        gastric contents (vomitus) T17.510 ☑
        specified type NEC T17.590 ☑
      injury NEC T17.508 ☑
        food (bone) (seed) T17.528 ☑
        gastric contents (vomitus) T17.518 ☑
        specified type NEC T17.598 ☑
  canthus — *see* Foreign body, conjunctival sac
  ciliary body (eye) S05.5- ☑
  conjunctival sac T15.1- ☑
  cornea T15.0- ☑
  entering through orifice
    accessory sinus T17.0 ☑
    alimentary canal T18.9 ☑
      multiple parts T18.8 ☑
      specified part NEC T18.8 ☑
    alveolar process T18.0 ☑
    antrum (Highmore's) T17.0 ☑
    anus T18.5 ☑
    appendix T18.4 ☑
    auditory canal — *see* Foreign body, entering through orifice, ear
    auricle — *see* Foreign body, entering through orifice, ear
    bladder T19.1 ☑
    bronchioles — *see* Foreign body, respiratory tract, specified site NEC
    bronchus (main) — *see* Foreign body, bronchus
    buccal cavity T18.0 ☑
    canthus (inner) — *see* Foreign body, conjunctival sac
    cecum T18.4 ☑
    cervix (canal) (uteri) T19.3 ☑
    colon T18.4 ☑
    conjunctival sac — *see* Foreign body, conjunctival sac
    cornea — *see* Foreign body, cornea
    digestive organ or tract NOS T18.9 ☑
      multiple parts T18.8 ☑
      specified part NEC T18.8 ☑
    duodenum T18.3 ☑
    ear (external) T16.- ☑
    esophagus — *see* Foreign body, esophagus
    eye (external) NOS T15.9- ☑
      conjunctival sac — *see* Foreign body, conjunctival sac
      cornea — *see* Foreign body, cornea
      specified part NEC T15.8- ☑

Foreign body — *continued*
  entering through orifice — *continued*
    eyeball — *see also* Foreign body, entering through orifice, eye, specified part NEC
      with penetrating wound — *see* Puncture, eyeball
    eyelid — *see also* Foreign body, conjunctival sac
      with
        laceration — *see* Laceration, eyelid, with foreign body
        puncture — *see* Puncture, eyelid, with foreign body
        superficial injury — *see* Foreign body, superficial, eyelid
    gastrointestinal tract T18.9 ☑
      multiple parts T18.8 ☑
      specified part NEC T18.8 ☑
    genitourinary tract T19.9 ☑
      multiple parts T19.8 ☑
      specified part NEC T19.8 ☑
    globe — *see* Foreign body, entering through orifice, eyeball
    gum T18.0 ☑
    Highmore's antrum T17.0 ☑
    hypopharynx — *see* Foreign body, pharynx
    ileum T18.3 ☑
    intestine (small) T18.3 ☑
      large T18.4 ☑
    lacrimal apparatus (punctum) — *see* Foreign body, entering through orifice, eye, specified part NEC
    large intestine T18.4 ☑
    larynx — *see* Foreign body, larynx
    lung — *see* Foreign body, respiratory tract, specified site NEC
    maxillary sinus T17.0 ☑
    mouth T18.0 ☑
    nasal sinus T17.0 ☑
    nasopharynx — *see* Foreign body, pharynx
    nose (passage) T17.1 ☑
    nostril T17.1 ☑
    oral cavity T18.0 ☑
    palate T18.0 ☑
    penis T19.4 ☑
    pharynx — *see* Foreign body, pharynx
    piriform sinus — *see* Foreign body, pharynx
    rectosigmoid (junction) T18.5 ☑
    rectum T18.5 ☑
    respiratory tract — *see* Foreign body, respiratory tract
    sinus (accessory) (frontal) (maxillary) (nasal) T17.0 ☑
      piriform — *see* Foreign body, pharynx
    small intestine T18.3 ☑
    stomach T18.2 ☑
    suffocation by — *see* Foreign body, by site
    tear ducts or glands — *see* Foreign body, entering through orifice, eye, specified part NEC
    throat — *see* Foreign body, pharynx
    tongue T18.0 ☑
    tonsil, tonsillar (fossa) — *see* Foreign body, pharynx
    trachea — *see* Foreign body, trachea
    ureter T19.8 ☑
    urethra T19.0 ☑
    uterus (any part) T19.3 ☑
    vagina T19.2 ☑
    vulva T19.2 ☑
  esophagus T18.108 ☑
    causing
      injury NEC T18.108 ☑
        food (bone) (seed) T18.128 ☑
        gastric contents (vomitus) T18.118 ☑
        specified type NEC T18.198 ☑
      tracheal compression T18.100 ☑
        food (bone) (seed) T18.120 ☑
        gastric contents (vomitus) T18.110 ☑
        specified type NEC T18.190 ☑
  feeling of, in throat R09.89
  fragment — *see* Retained, foreign body fragments (type of)
  genitourinary tract T19.9 ☑
    bladder T19.1 ☑
    multiple parts T19.8 ☑
    penis T19.4 ☑
    specified site NEC T19.8 ☑
    urethra T19.0 ☑
    uterus T19.3 ☑
      IUD Z97.5

☑ Additional Character Required — Refer to the Tabular List for Character Selection

▽ Subterms under main terms may continue to next column or page

Foreign body — *continued*
  genitourinary tract — *continued*
    vagina T19.2 ☑
      contraceptive device Z97.5
    vulva T19.2 ☑
  granuloma (old) (soft tissue) — *see also* Granuloma,
      foreign body
    skin L92.3
  in
    laceration — *see* Laceration, by site, with foreign
        body
    puncture wound — *see* Puncture, by site, with for-
        eign body
    soft tissue (residual) M79.5
  inadvertently left in operation wound — *see* Foreign
      body, accidentally left during a procedure
  ingestion, ingested NOS T18.9 ☑
  inhalation or inspiration — *see* Foreign body, by site
  internal organ, not entering through a natural orifice
      — code as specific injury with foreign body
  intraocular S05.5- ☑
    old, retained (nonmagnetic) H44.70- ☑
      anterior chamber H44.71- ☑
      ciliary body H44.72- ☑
      iris H44.72- ☑
      lens H44.73- ☑
      magnetic H44.60- ☑
        anterior chamber H44.61- ☑
        ciliary body H44.62- ☑
        iris H44.62- ☑
        lens H44.63- ☑
        posterior wall H44.64- ☑
        specified site NEC H44.69- ☑
        vitreous body H44.65- ☑
      posterior wall H44.74- ☑
      specified site NEC H44.79- ☑
      vitreous body H44.75- ☑
    iris — *see* Foreign body, intraocular
  lacrimal punctum — *see* Foreign body, entering
      through orifice, eye, specified part NEC
  larynx T17.308 ☑
    causing
      asphyxiation T17.300 ☑
        food (bone) (seed) T17.320 ☑
        gastric contents (vomitus) T17.310 ☑
        specified type NEC T17.390 ☑
      injury NEC T17.308 ☑
        food (bone) (seed) T17.328 ☑
        gastric contents (vomitus) T17.318 ☑
        specified type NEC T17.398 ☑
  lens — *see* Foreign body, intraocular
  ocular muscle S05.4- ☑
    old, retained — *see* Foreign body, orbit, old
  old or residual
    soft tissue (residual) M79.5
  operation wound, left accidentally — *see* Foreign body,
      accidentally left during a procedure
  orbit S05.4- ☑
    old, retained H05.5- ☑
  pharynx T17.208 ☑
    causing
      asphyxiation T17.200 ☑
        food (bone) (seed) T17.220 ☑
        gastric contents (vomitus) T17.210 ☑
        specified type NEC T17.290 ☑
      injury NEC T17.208 ☑
        food (bone) (seed) T17.228 ☑
        gastric contents (vomitus) T17.218 ☑
        specified type NEC T17.298 ☑
  respiratory tract T17.908 ☑
    bronchioles — *see* Foreign body, respiratory tract,
        specified site NEC
    bronchus — *see* Foreign body, bronchus
    causing
      asphyxiation T17.900 ☑
        food (bone) (seed) T17.920 ☑
        gastric contents (vomitus) T17.910 ☑
        specified type NEC T17.990 ☑
      injury NEC T17.908 ☑
        food (bone) (seed) T17.928 ☑
        gastric contents (vomitus) T17.918 ☑
        specified type NEC T17.998 ☑
    larynx — *see* Foreign body, larynx
    lung — *see* Foreign body, respiratory tract, specified
        site NEC

Foreign body — *continued*
  respiratory tract — *continued*
    multiple parts — *see* Foreign body, respiratory tract,
        specified site NEC
    nasal sinus T17.0 ☑
    nasopharynx — *see* Foreign body, pharynx
    nose T17.1 ☑
    nostril T17.1 ☑
    pharynx — *see* Foreign body, pharynx
    specified site NEC T17.808 ☑
      causing
        asphyxiation T17.800 ☑
          food (bone) (seed) T17.820 ☑
          gastric contents (vomitus) T17.810 ☑
          specified type NEC T17.890 ☑
        injury NEC T17.808 ☑
          food (bone) (seed) T17.828 ☑
          gastric contents (vomitus) T17.818 ☑
          specified type NEC T17.898 ☑
    throat — *see* Foreign body, pharynx
    trachea — *see* Foreign body, trachea
  retained (old) (nonmagnetic) (in)
    anterior chamber (eye) — *see* Foreign body, intraoc-
        ular, old, retained, anterior chamber
      magnetic — *see* Foreign body, intraocular, old,
          retained, magnetic, anterior chamber
    ciliary body — *see* Foreign body, intraocular, old,
        retained, ciliary body
      magnetic — *see* Foreign body, intraocular, old,
          retained, magnetic, ciliary body
    eyelid H02.819
      left H02.816
        lower H02.815
        upper H02.814
      right H02.813
        lower H02.812
        upper H02.811
    fragments — *see* Retained, foreign body fragments
        (type of)
    globe — *see* Foreign body, intraocular, old, retained
      magnetic — *see* Foreign body, intraocular, old,
          retained, magnetic
    intraocular — *see* Foreign body, intraocular, old,
        retained
      magnetic — *see* Foreign body, intraocular, old,
          retained, magnetic
    iris — *see* Foreign body, intraocular, old, retained,
        iris
      magnetic — *see* Foreign body, intraocular, old,
          retained, magnetic, iris
    lens — *see* Foreign body, intraocular, old, retained,
        lens
      magnetic — *see* Foreign body, intraocular, old,
          retained, magnetic, lens
    muscle — *see* Foreign body, retained, soft tissue
    orbit — *see* Foreign body, orbit, old
    posterior wall of globe — *see* Foreign body, intraoc-
        ular, old, retained, posterior wall
      magnetic — *see* Foreign body, intraocular, old,
          retained, magnetic, posterior wall
    retrobulbar — *see* Foreign body, orbit, old, retrob-
        ulbar
    soft tissue M79.5
    vitreous — *see* Foreign body, intraocular, old, re-
        tained, vitreous body
      magnetic — *see* Foreign body, intraocular, old,
          retained, magnetic, vitreous body
  retina S05.5- ☑
  superficial, without open wound
    abdomen, abdominal (wall) S30.851 ☑
    alveolar process S00.552 ☑
    ankle S90.55- ☑
    antecubital space — *see* Foreign body, superficial,
        forearm
    anus S30.857 ☑
    arm (upper) S40.85- ☑
    auditory canal — *see* Foreign body, superficial, ear
    auricle — *see* Foreign body, superficial, ear
    axilla — *see* Foreign body, superficial, arm
    back, lower S30.850 ☑
    breast S20.15- ☑
    brow S00.85 ☑
    buttock S30.850 ☑
    calf — *see* Foreign body, superficial, leg
    canthus — *see* Foreign body, superficial, eyelid
    cheek S00.85 ☑
      internal S00.552 ☑

Foreign body — *continued*
  superficial, without open wound — *continued*
    chest wall — *see* Foreign body, superficial, thorax
    chin S00.85 ☑
    clitoris S30.854 ☑
    costal region — *see* Foreign body, superficial, thorax
    digit(s)
      foot — *see* Foreign body, superficial, toe
      hand — *see* Foreign body, superficial, finger
    ear S00.45- ☑
    elbow S50.35- ☑
    epididymis S30.853 ☑
    epigastric region S30.851 ☑
    epiglottis S10.15 ☑
    esophagus, cervical S10.15 ☑
    eyebrow — *see* Foreign body, superficial, eyelid
    eyelid S00.25- ☑
    face S00.85 ☑
    finger(s) S60.459 ☑
      index S60.45- ☑
      little S60.45- ☑
      middle S60.45- ☑
      ring S60.45- ☑
    flank S30.851 ☑
    foot (except toe(s) alone) S90.85- ☑
      toe — *see* Foreign body, superficial, toe
    forearm S50.85- ☑
      elbow only — *see* Foreign body, superficial, el-
          bow
    forehead S00.85 ☑
    genital organs, external
      female S30.856 ☑
      male S30.855 ☑
    groin S30.851 ☑
    gum S00.552 ☑
    hand S60.55- ☑
    head S00.95 ☑
      ear — *see* Foreign body, superficial, ear
      eyelid — *see* Foreign body, superficial, eyelid
      lip S00.551 ☑
      nose S00.35 ☑
      oral cavity S00.552 ☑
      scalp S00.05 ☑
      specified site NEC S00.85 ☑
    heel — *see* Foreign body, superficial, foot
    hip S70.25- ☑
    inguinal region S30.851 ☑
    interscapular region S20.459 ☑
    jaw S00.85 ☑
    knee S80.25- ☑
    labium (majus) (minus) S30.854 ☑
    larynx S10.15 ☑
    leg (lower) S80.85- ☑
      knee — *see* Foreign body, superficial, knee
      upper — *see* Foreign body, superficial, thigh
    lip S00.551 ☑
    lower back S30.850 ☑
    lumbar region S30.850 ☑
    malar region S00.85 ☑
    mammary — *see* Foreign body, superficial, breast
    mastoid region S00.85 ☑
    mouth S00.552 ☑
    nail
      finger — *see* Foreign body, superficial, finger
      toe — *see* Foreign body, superficial, toe
    nape S10.85 ☑
    nasal S00.35 ☑
    neck S10.95 ☑
      specified site NEC S10.85 ☑
      throat S10.15 ☑
    nose S00.35 ☑
    occipital region S00.05 ☑
    oral cavity S00.552 ☑
    orbital region — *see* Foreign body, superficial, eyelid
    palate S00.552 ☑
    palm — *see* Foreign body, superficial, hand
    parietal region S00.05 ☑
    pelvis S30.850 ☑
    penis S30.852 ☑
    perineum
      female S30.854 ☑
      male S30.850 ☑
    periocular area — *see* Foreign body, superficial,
        eyelid
    phalanges
      finger — *see* Foreign body, superficial, finger

Fracture, traumatic — *continued*
  ankle — *continued*
    bimalleolar (displaced) S82.84- ☑
      nondisplaced S82.84- ☑
    lateral malleolus only (displaced) S82.6- ☑
      nondisplaced S82.6- ☑
    medial malleolus (displaced) S82.5- ☑
      associated with Maisonneuve's fracture — *see*
        Fracture, Maisonneuve's
      nondisplaced S82.5- ☑
    talus — *see* Fracture, tarsal, talus
    trimalleolar (displaced) S82.85- ☑
      nondisplaced S82.85- ☑
  arm (upper) — *see also* Fracture, humerus, shaft
    humerus — *see* Fracture, humerus
    radius — *see* Fracture, radius
    ulna — *see* Fracture, ulna
  astragalus — *see* Fracture, tarsal, talus
  atlas — *see* Fracture, neck, cervical vertebra, first
  axis — *see* Fracture, neck, cervical vertebra, second
  back — *see* Fracture, vertebra
  Barton's — *see* Barton's fracture
  base of skull — *see* Fracture, skull, base
  basicervical (basal) (femoral) S72.0 ☑
  Bennett's — *see* Bennett's fracture
  bimalleolar — *see* Fracture, ankle, bimalleolar
  blow-out S02.3- ☑
  bone NEC T14.8 ☑
    birth injury P13.9
    following insertion of orthopedic implant, joint
        prosthesis or bone plate — *see* Fracture, fol-
        lowing insertion of orthopedic implant, joint
        prosthesis or bone plate
    in (due to) neoplastic disease NEC — *see* Fracture,
        pathological, due to, neoplastic disease
    pathological (cause unknown) — *see* Fracture,
        pathological
  breast bone — *see* Fracture, sternum
  bucket handle (semilunar cartilage) — *see* Tear,
      meniscus
  buckle — *see* Fracture, by site, torus
  burst — *see* Fracture, traumatic, by site
  calcaneus — *see* Fracture, tarsal, calcaneus
  carpal bone(s) S62.10- ☑
    capitate (displaced) S62.13- ☑
      nondisplaced S62.13- ☑
    cuneiform — *see* Fracture, carpal bone, triquetrum
    hamate (body) (displaced) S62.143 ☑
      hook process (displaced) S62.15- ☑
        nondisplaced S62.15- ☑
      nondisplaced S62.14- ☑
    larger multangular — *see* Fracture, carpal bones,
        trapezium
    lunate (displaced) S62.12- ☑
      nondisplaced S62.12- ☑
    navicular S62.00- ☑
      distal pole (displaced) S62.01- ☑
        nondisplaced S62.01- ☑
      middle third (displaced) S62.02- ☑
        nondisplaced S62.02- ☑
      proximal third (displaced) S62.03- ☑
        nondisplaced S62.03- ☑
      volar tuberosity — *see* Fracture, carpal bones,
          navicular, distal pole
    os magnum — *see* Fracture, carpal bones, capitate
    pisiform (displaced) S62.16- ☑
      nondisplaced S62.16- ☑
    semilunar — *see* Fracture, carpal bones, lunate
    smaller multangular — *see* Fracture, carpal bones,
        trapezoid
    trapezium (displaced) S62.17- ☑
      nondisplaced S62.17- ☑
    trapezoid (displaced) S62.18- ☑
      nondisplaced S62.18- ☑
    triquetrum (displaced) S62.11- ☑
      nondisplaced S62.11- ☑
    unciform — *see* Fracture, carpal bones, hamate
  cervical — *see* Fracture, vertebra, cervical
  clavicle S42.00- ☑
    acromial end (displaced) S42.03- ☑
      nondisplaced S42.03- ☑
    birth injury P13.4
    lateral end — *see* Fracture, clavicle, acromial end
    shaft (displaced) S42.02- ☑
      nondisplaced S42.02- ☑
    sternal end (anterior) (displaced) S42.01- ☑

Fracture, traumatic — *continued*
  clavicle — *continued*
    sternal end — *continued*
      nondisplaced S42.01- ☑
      posterior S42.01- ☑
  coccyx S32.2 ☑
  collapsed — *see* Collapse, vertebra
  collar bone — *see* Fracture, clavicle
  Colles' — *see* Colles' fracture
  coronoid process — *see* Fracture, ulna, upper end,
      coronoid process
  corpus cavernosum penis S39.840 ☑
  costochondral cartilage S23.41 ☑
  costochondral, costosternal junction — *see* Fracture,
      rib
  cranium — *see* Fracture, skull
  cricoid cartilage S12.8 ☑
  cuboid (ankle) — *see* Fracture, tarsal, cuboid
  cuneiform
    foot — *see* Fracture, tarsal, cuneiform
    wrist — *see* Fracture, carpal, triquetrum
  delayed union — *see* Delay, union, fracture
  dental restorative material K08.539
    with loss of material K08.531
    without loss of material K08.530
  due to
    birth injury — *see* Birth, injury, fracture
    osteoporosis — *see* Osteoporosis, with fracture
  Dupuytren's — *see* Fracture, ankle, lateral malleolus
  elbow S42.40- ☑
  ethmoid (bone) (sinus) — *see* Fracture, skull, base
  face bone S02.92 ☑
  fatigue — *see also* Fracture, stress
    vertebra M48.40 ☑
      cervical region M48.42 ☑
      cervicothoracic region M48.43 ☑
      lumbar region M48.46 ☑
      lumbosacral region M48.47 ☑
      occipito-atlanto-axial region M48.41 ☑
      sacrococcygeal region M48.48 ☑
      thoracic region M48.44 ☑
      thoracolumbar region M48.45 ☑
  femur, femoral S72.9- ☑
    basicervical (basal) S72.0 ☑
    birth injury P13.2
    capital epiphyseal S79.01- ☑
    condyles, epicondyles — *see* Fracture, femur, lower
        end
    distal end — *see* Fracture, femur, lower end
    epiphysis
      head — *see* Fracture, femur, upper end, epiphysis
      lower — *see* Fracture, femur, lower end, epiph-
          ysis
      upper — *see* Fracture, femur, upper end, epiph-
          ysis
    following insertion of implant, prosthesis or plate
        M96.66- ☑
    head — *see* Fracture, femur, upper end, head
    intertrochanteric — *see* Fracture, femur,
        trochanteric
    intratrochanteric — *see* Fracture, femur,
        trochanteric
    lower end S72.40- ☑
      condyle (displaced) S72.41- ☑
        lateral (displaced) S72.42- ☑
          nondisplaced S72.42- ☑
        medial (displaced) S72.43- ☑
          nondisplaced S72.43- ☑
        nondisplaced S72.41- ☑
      epiphysis (displaced) S72.44- ☑
        nondisplaced S72.44- ☑
      physeal S79.10- ☑
        Salter-Harris
          Type I S79.11- ☑
          Type II S79.12- ☑
          Type III S79.13- ☑
          Type IV S79.14- ☑
        specified NEC S79.19- ☑
      specified NEC S72.49- ☑
      supracondylar (displaced) S72.45- ☑
        with intracondylar extension (displaced)
            S72.46- ☑
          nondisplaced S72.46- ☑
        nondisplaced S72.45- ☑
      torus S72.47- ☑
    neck — *see* Fracture, femur, upper end, neck

Fracture, traumatic — *continued*
  femur, femoral — *continued*
    pertrochanteric — *see* Fracture, femur, trochanteric
    shaft (lower third) (middle third) (upper third)
        S72.30- ☑
      comminuted (displaced) S72.35- ☑
        nondisplaced S72.35- ☑
      oblique (displaced) S72.33- ☑
        nondisplaced S72.33- ☑
      segmental (displaced) S72.36- ☑
        nondisplaced S72.36- ☑
      specified NEC S72.39- ☑
      spiral (displaced) S72.34- ☑
        nondisplaced S72.34- ☑
      transverse (displaced) S72.32- ☑
        nondisplaced S72.32- ☑
    specified site NEC — *see* subcategory S72.8 ☑
    subcapital (displaced) S72.01- ☑
    subtrochanteric (region) (section) (displaced)
        S72.2- ☑
      nondisplaced S72.2- ☑
    transcervical — *see* Fracture, femur, midcervical
    transtrochanteric — *see* Fracture, femur,
        trochanteric
    trochanteric S72.10- ☑
      apophyseal (displaced) S72.13- ☑
        nondisplaced S72.13- ☑
      greater trochanter (displaced) S72.11- ☑
        nondisplaced S72.11- ☑
      intertrochanteric (displaced) S72.14- ☑
        nondisplaced S72.14- ☑
      lesser trochanter (displaced) S72.12- ☑
        nondisplaced S72.12- ☑
    upper end S72.00- ☑
      apophyseal (displaced) S72.13- ☑
        nondisplaced S72.13- ☑
      cervicotrochanteric — *see* Fracture, femur, upper
          end, neck, base
      epiphysis (displaced) S72.02- ☑
        nondisplaced S72.02- ☑
      head S72.05- ☑
        articular (displaced) S72.06- ☑
          nondisplaced S72.06- ☑
        specified NEC S72.09- ☑
      intertrochanteric (displaced) S72.14- ☑
        nondisplaced S72.14- ☑
      intracapsular S72.01- ☑
      midcervical (displaced) S72.03- ☑
        nondisplaced S72.03- ☑
      neck S72.00- ☑
        base (displaced) S72.04- ☑
          nondisplaced S72.04- ☑
        specified NEC S72.09- ☑
      pertrochanteric — *see* Fracture, femur, upper
          end, trochanteric
      physeal S79.00- ☑
        Salter-Harris type I S79.01- ☑
        specified NEC S79.09- ☑
      subcapital (displaced) S72.01- ☑
      subtrochanteric (displaced) S72.2- ☑
        nondisplaced S72.2- ☑
      transcervical — *see* Fracture, femur, upper end,
          midcervical
      trochanteric S72.10- ☑
        greater (displaced) S72.11- ☑
          nondisplaced S72.11- ☑
        lesser (displaced) S72.12- ☑
          nondisplaced S72.12- ☑
  fibula (shaft) (styloid) S82.40- ☑
    comminuted (displaced) S82.45- ☑
      nondisplaced S82.45- ☑
    following insertion of implant, prosthesis or plate
        M96.67- ☑
    involving ankle or malleolus — *see* Fracture, fibula,
        lateral malleolus
    lateral malleolus (displaced) S82.6- ☑
      nondisplaced S82.6- ☑
    lower end
      physeal S89.30- ☑
        Salter-Harris
          Type I S89.31- ☑
          Type II S89.32- ☑
        specified NEC S89.39- ☑
      specified NEC S82.83- ☑
      torus S82.82- ☑
    oblique (displaced) S82.43- ☑

Fracture, traumatic — *continued*
fibula — *continued*
oblique — *continued*
nondisplaced S82.43- ☑
segmental (displaced) S82.46- ☑
nondisplaced S82.46- ☑
specified NEC S82.49- ☑
spiral (displaced) S82.44- ☑
nondisplaced S82.44- ☑
transverse (displaced) S82.42- ☑
nondisplaced S82.42- ☑
upper end
physeal S89.20- ☑
Salter-Harris
Type I S89.21- ☑
Type II S89.22- ☑
specified NEC S89.29- ☑
specified NEC S82.83- ☑
torus S82.81- ☑
finger (except thumb) S62.60- ☑
distal phalanx (displaced) S62.63- ☑
nondisplaced S62.66- ☑
index S62.60- ☑
distal phalanx (displaced) S62.63- ☑
nondisplaced S62.66- ☑
middle phalanx (displaced) S62.62- ☑
nondisplaced S62.65- ☑
proximal phalanx (displaced) S62.61- ☑
nondisplaced S62.64- ☑
little S62.60- ☑
distal phalanx (displaced) S62.63- ☑
nondisplaced S62.66- ☑
middle phalanx (displaced) S62.62- ☑
nondisplaced S62.65- ☑
proximal phalanx (displaced) S62.61- ☑
nondisplaced S62.64- ☑
middle S62.60- ☑
distal phalanx (displaced) S62.63- ☑
nondisplaced S62.66- ☑
middle phalanx (displaced) S62.62- ☑
nondisplaced S62.65- ☑
proximal phalanx (displaced) S62.61- ☑
nondisplaced S62.64- ☑
middle phalanx (displaced) S62.62- ☑
nondisplaced S62.65- ☑
proximal phalanx (displaced) S62.61- ☑
nondisplaced S62.64- ☑
ring S62.60- ☑
distal phalanx (displaced) S62.63- ☑
nondisplaced S62.66- ☑
middle phalanx (displaced) S62.62- ☑
nondisplaced S62.65- ☑
proximal phalanx (displaced) S62.61- ☑
nondisplaced S62.64- ☑
thumb — *see* Fracture, thumb
following insertion (intraoperative) (postoperative) of
orthopedic implant, joint prosthesis or bone
plate M96.69
femur M96.66- ☑
fibula M96.67- ☑
humerus M96.62- ☑
pelvis M96.65
radius M96.63- ☑
specified bone NEC M96.69
tibia M96.67- ☑
ulna M96.63- ☑
foot S92.90- ☑
astragalus — *see* Fracture, tarsal, talus
calcaneus — *see* Fracture, tarsal, calcaneus
cuboid — *see* Fracture, tarsal, cuboid
cuneiform — *see* Fracture, tarsal, cuneiform
metatarsal — *see* Fracture, metatarsal
navicular — *see* Fracture, tarsal, navicular
sesamoid S92.81- ☑
specified NEC S92.81- ☑
talus — *see* Fracture, tarsal, talus
tarsal — *see* Fracture, tarsal
toe — *see* Fracture, toe
forearm S52.9- ☑
radius — *see* Fracture, radius
ulna — *see* Fracture, ulna
fossa (anterior) (middle) (posterior) S02.19 ☑
fragility — *see* Fracture, pathological, due to osteoporosis
frontal (bone) (skull) S02.0 ☑
sinus S02.19 ☑

Fracture, traumatic — *continued*
glenoid (cavity) (scapula) — *see* Fracture, scapula,
glenoid cavity
greenstick — *see* Fracture, by site
hallux — *see* Fracture, toe, great
hand S62.9- ☑
carpal — *see* Fracture, carpal bone
finger (except thumb) — *see* Fracture, finger
metacarpal — *see* Fracture, metacarpal
navicular (scaphoid) (hand) — *see* Fracture, carpal
bone, navicular
thumb — *see* Fracture, thumb
healed or old
with complications — *code by* Nature of the complication
heel bone — *see* Fracture, tarsal, calcaneus
Hill-Sachs S42.29- ☑
hip — *see* Fracture, femur, neck
humerus S42.30- ☑
anatomical neck — *see* Fracture, humerus, upper
end
articular process — *see* Fracture, humerus, lower
end
capitellum — *see* Fracture, humerus, lower end,
condyle, lateral
distal end — *see* Fracture, humerus, lower end
epiphysis
lower — *see* Fracture, humerus, lower end, physeal
upper — *see* Fracture, humerus, upper end,
physeal
external condyle — *see* Fracture, humerus, lower
end, condyle, lateral
following insertion of implant, prosthesis or plate
M96.62- ☑
great tuberosity — *see* Fracture, humerus, upper
end, greater tuberosity
intercondylar — *see* Fracture, humerus, lower end
internal epicondyle — *see* Fracture, humerus, lower
end, epicondyle, medial
lesser tuberosity — *see* Fracture, humerus, upper
end, lesser tuberosity
lower end S42.40- ☑
condyle
lateral (displaced) S42.45- ☑
nondisplaced S42.45- ☑
medial (displaced) S42.46- ☑
nondisplaced S42.46- ☑
epicondyle
lateral (displaced) S42.43- ☑
nondisplaced S42.43- ☑
medial (displaced) S42.44- ☑
incarcerated S42.44- ☑
nondisplaced S42.44- ☑
physeal S49.10- ☑
Salter-Harris
Type I S49.11- ☑
Type II S49.12- ☑
Type III S49.13- ☑
Type IV S49.14- ☑
specified NEC S49.19- ☑
specified NEC (displaced) S42.49- ☑
nondisplaced S42.49- ☑
supracondylar (simple) (displaced) S42.41- ☑
with intercondylar fracture — *see* Fracture,
humerus, lower end
comminuted (displaced) S42.42- ☑
nondisplaced S42.42- ☑
nondisplaced S42.41- ☑
torus S42.48- ☑
transcondylar (displaced) S42.47- ☑
nondisplaced S42.47- ☑
proximal end — *see* Fracture, humerus, upper end
shaft S42.30- ☑
comminuted (displaced) S42.35- ☑
nondisplaced S42.35- ☑
greenstick S42.31- ☑
oblique (displaced) S42.33- ☑
nondisplaced S42.33- ☑
segmental (displaced) S42.36- ☑
nondisplaced S42.36- ☑
specified NEC S42.39- ☑
spiral (displaced) S42.34- ☑
nondisplaced S42.34- ☑
transverse (displaced) S42.32- ☑
nondisplaced S42.32- ☑

Fracture, traumatic — *continued*
humerus — *continued*
supracondylar — *see* Fracture, humerus, lower en
surgical neck — *see* Fracture, humerus, upper en
surgical neck
trochlea — *see* Fracture, humerus, lower end,
condyle, medial
tuberosity — *see* Fracture, humerus, upper end
upper end S42.20- ☑
anatomical neck — *see* Fracture, humerus, uppe
end, specified NEC
articular head — *see* Fracture, humerus, uppe
end, specified NEC
epiphysis — *see* Fracture, humerus, upper en
physeal
greater tuberosity (displaced) S42.25- ☑
nondisplaced S42.25- ☑
lesser tuberosity (displaced) S42.26- ☑
nondisplaced S42.26- ☑
physeal S49.00- ☑
Salter-Harris
Type I S49.01- ☑
Type II S49.02- ☑
Type III S49.03- ☑
Type IV S49.04- ☑
specified NEC S49.09- ☑
specified NEC (displaced) S42.29- ☑
nondisplaced S42.29- ☑
surgical neck (displaced) S42.21- ☑
four-part S42.24- ☑
nondisplaced S42.21- ☑
three-part S42.23- ☑
two-part (displaced) S42.22- ☑
nondisplaced S42.22- ☑
torus S42.27- ☑
transepiphyseal — *see* Fracture, humerus, uppe
end, physeal
hyoid bone S12.8 ☑
ilium S32.30- ☑
with disruption of pelvic ring — *see* Disruption,
pelvic ring
avulsion (displaced) S32.31- ☑
nondisplaced S32.31- ☑
specified NEC S32.39- ☑
impaction, impacted — *code as* Fracture, by site
innominate bone — *see* Fracture, ilium
instep — *see* Fracture, foot
ischium S32.60- ☑
with disruption of pelvic ring — *see* Disruption,
pelvic ring
avulsion (displaced) S32.61- ☑
nondisplaced S32.61- ☑
specified NEC S32.69- ☑
jaw (bone) (lower) — *see* Fracture, mandible
upper — *see* Fracture, maxilla
joint prosthesis — *see* Complications, joint prosthesi
mechanical, breakdown, by site
periprosthetic — *see* Fracture, traumatic, peripros
thetic
knee cap — *see* Fracture, patella
larynx S12.8 ☑
late effects — *see* Sequelae, fracture
leg (lower) S82.9- ☑
ankle — *see* Fracture, ankle
femur — *see* Fracture, femur
fibula — *see* Fracture, fibula
malleolus — *see* Fracture, ankle
patella — *see* Fracture, patella
specified site NEC S82.89- ☑
tibia — *see* Fracture, tibia
lumbar spine — *see* Fracture, vertebra, lumbar
lumbosacral spine S32.9 ☑
Maisonneuve's (displaced) S82.86- ☑
nondisplaced S82.86- ☑
malar bone — *see also* Fracture, maxilla S02.400 ☑
left side S02.40B ☑
right side S02.40A ☑
malleolus — *see* Fracture, ankle
malunion — *see* Fracture, by site
mandible (lower jaw (bone)) S02.609 ☑
alveolus S02.67- ☑
angle (of jaw) S02.65- ☑
body, unspecified S02.600 ☑
left side S02.602 ☑
right side S02.601 ☑
condylar process S02.61- ☑

☑ **Additional Character Required** — Refer to the Tabular List for Character Selection

▽ **Subterms under main terms may continue to next column or page**

Fracture, traumatic — *continued*
- mandible — *continued*
  - coronoid process S02.63- ☑
  - ramus, unspecified S02.64- ☑
  - specified site NEC S02.69 ☑
  - subcondylar process S02.62- ☑
  - symphysis S02.66 ☑
- manubrium (sterni) S22.21 ☑
  - dissociation from sternum S22.23 ☑
- march — *see* Fracture, traumatic, stress, by site
- maxilla, maxillary (bone) (sinus) (superior) (upper jaw) S02.401 ☑
  - alveolus S02.42 ☑
  - inferior — *see* Fracture, mandible
  - LeFort I S02.411 ☑
  - LeFort II S02.412 ☑
  - LeFort III S02.413 ☑
  - left side S02.40D ☑
  - right side S02.40C ☑
- metacarpal S62.309 ☑
  - base (displaced) S62.319 ☑
    - nondisplaced S62.349 ☑
  - fifth S62.30- ☑
    - base (displaced) S62.31- ☑
      - nondisplaced S62.34- ☑
    - neck (displaced) S62.33- ☑
      - nondisplaced S62.36- ☑
    - shaft (displaced) S62.32- ☑
      - nondisplaced S62.35- ☑
    - specified NEC S62.398 ☑
  - first S62.20- ☑
    - base NEC (displaced) S62.23- ☑
      - nondisplaced S62.23- ☑
    - Bennett's — *see* Bennett's fracture
    - neck (displaced) S62.25- ☑
      - nondisplaced S62.25- ☑
    - shaft (displaced) S62.24- ☑
      - nondisplaced S62.24- ☑
    - specified NEC S62.29- ☑
  - fourth S62.30- ☑
    - base (displaced) S62.31- ☑
      - nondisplaced S62.34- ☑
    - neck (displaced) S62.33- ☑
      - nondisplaced S62.36- ☑
    - shaft (displaced) S62.32- ☑
      - nondisplaced S62.35- ☑
    - specified NEC S62.39- ☑
  - neck (displaced) S62.33- ☑
    - nondisplaced S62.36- ☑
  - Rolando's — *see* Rolando's fracture
  - second S62.30- ☑
    - base (displaced) S62.31- ☑
      - nondisplaced S62.34- ☑
    - neck (displaced) S62.33- ☑
      - nondisplaced S62.36- ☑
    - shaft (displaced) S62.32- ☑
      - nondisplaced S62.35- ☑
    - specified NEC S62.39- ☑
  - shaft (displaced) S62.32- ☑
    - nondisplaced S62.35- ☑
  - specified NEC S62.399 ☑
  - third S62.30- ☑
    - base (displaced) S62.31- ☑
      - nondisplaced S62.34- ☑
    - neck (displaced) S62.33- ☑
      - nondisplaced S62.36- ☑
    - shaft (displaced) S62.32- ☑
      - nondisplaced S62.35- ☑
    - specified NEC S62.39- ☑
- metaphyseal — *see* Fracture, traumatic, by site, shaft
- metastatic — *see* Fracture, pathological, due to, neoplastic disease — *see also* Neoplasm
- metatarsal bone S92.30- ☑
  - fifth (displaced) S92.35- ☑
    - nondisplaced S92.35- ☑
  - first (displaced) S92.31- ☑
    - nondisplaced S92.31- ☑
  - fourth (displaced) S92.34- ☑
    - nondisplaced S92.34- ☑
  - physeal S99.10- ☑
    - Salter-Harris
      - Type I S99.11- ☑
      - Type II S99.12- ☑
      - Type III S99.13- ☑
      - Type IV S99.14- ☑
    - specified NEC S99.19- ☑

Fracture, traumatic — *continued*
- metatarsal bone — *continued*
  - second (displaced) S92.32- ☑
    - nondisplaced S92.32- ☑
  - third (displaced) S92.33- ☑
    - nondisplaced S92.33- ☑
- Montegia's — *see* Montegia's fracture
- multiple
  - hand (and wrist) NEC — *see* Fracture, by site
  - ribs — *see* Fracture, rib, multiple
- nasal (bone(s)) S02.2 ☑
- navicular (scaphoid) (foot) — *see also* Fracture, tarsal, navicular
  - hand — *see* Fracture, carpal, navicular
- neck S12.9 ☑
  - cervical vertebra S12.9 ☑
    - fifth (displaced) S12.400 ☑
      - nondisplaced S12.401 ☑
      - specified type NEC (displaced) S12.490 ☑
        - nondisplaced S12.491 ☑
    - first (displaced) S12.000 ☑
      - burst (stable) S12.01 ☑
        - unstable S12.02 ☑
      - lateral mass (displaced) S12.040 ☑
        - nondisplaced S12.041 ☑
      - nondisplaced S12.001 ☑
      - posterior arch (displaced) S12.030 ☑
        - nondisplaced S12.031 ☑
      - specified type NEC (displaced) S12.090 ☑
        - nondisplaced S12.091 ☑
    - fourth (displaced) S12.300 ☑
      - nondisplaced S12.301 ☑
      - specified type NEC (displaced) S12.390 ☑
        - nondisplaced S12.391 ☑
    - second (displaced) S12.100 ☑
      - dens (anterior) (displaced) (type II) S12.110 ☑
        - nondisplaced S12.112 ☑
        - posterior S12.111 ☑
        - specified type NEC (displaced) S12.120 ☑
          - nondisplaced S12.121 ☑
      - nondisplaced S12.101 ☑
      - specified type NEC (displaced) S12.190 ☑
        - nondisplaced S12.191 ☑
    - seventh (displaced) S12.600 ☑
      - nondisplaced S12.601 ☑
      - specified type NEC (displaced) S12.690 ☑
        - nondisplaced S12.691 ☑
    - sixth (displaced) S12.500 ☑
      - nondisplaced S12.501 ☑
      - specified type NEC (displaced) S12.590 ☑
        - nondisplaced S12.591 ☑
    - third (displaced) S12.200 ☑
      - nondisplaced S12.201 ☑
      - specified type NEC (displaced) S12.290 ☑
        - nondisplaced S12.291 ☑
  - hyoid bone S12.8 ☑
  - larynx S12.8 ☑
  - specified site NEC S12.8 ☑
  - thyroid cartilage S12.8 ☑
  - trachea S12.8 ☑
- neoplastic NEC — *see* Fracture, pathological, due to, neoplastic disease
- neural arch — *see* Fracture, vertebra
- newborn — *see* Birth, injury, fracture
- nontraumatic — *see* Fracture, pathological
- nonunion — *see* Nonunion, fracture
- nose, nasal (bone) (septum) S02.2 ☑
- occiput — *see* Fracture, skull, base, occiput
- odontoid process — *see* Fracture, neck, cervical vertebra, second
- olecranon (process) (ulna) — *see* Fracture, ulna, upper end, olecranon process
- orbit, orbital (bone) (region) S02.85 ☑
  - floor (blow-out) S02.3- ☑
  - roof S02.12- ☑
  - wall S02.85 ☑
    - lateral S02.84- ☑
    - medial S02.83- ☑
- os
  - calcis — *see* Fracture, tarsal, calcaneus
  - magnum — *see* Fracture, carpal, capitate
  - pubis — *see* Fracture, pubis
- palate S02.8- ☑
- parietal bone (skull) S02.0 ☑
- patella S82.00- ☑
  - comminuted (displaced) S82.04- ☑

Fracture, traumatic — *continued*
- patella — *continued*
  - comminuted — *continued*
    - nondisplaced S82.04- ☑
  - longitudinal (displaced) S82.02- ☑
    - nondisplaced S82.02- ☑
  - osteochondral (displaced) S82.01- ☑
    - nondisplaced S82.01- ☑
  - specified NEC S82.09- ☑
  - transverse (displaced) S82.03- ☑
    - nondisplaced S82.03- ☑
- pedicle (of vertebral arch) — *see* Fracture, vertebra
- pelvis, pelvic (bone) S32.9 ☑
  - acetabulum — *see* Fracture, acetabulum
  - circle — *see* Disruption, pelvic ring
  - following insertion of implant, prosthesis or plate M96.65
  - ilium — *see* Fracture, ilium
  - ischium — *see* Fracture, ischium
  - multiple
    - with disruption of pelvic ring (circle) — *see* Disruption, pelvic ring
    - without disruption of pelvic ring (circle) S32.82 ☑
  - pubis — *see* Fracture, pubis
  - sacrum — *see* Fracture, sacrum
  - specified site NEC S32.89 ☑
- periprosthetic, around internal prosthetic joint M97.9 ☑
  - ankle M97.2- ☑
  - elbow M97.4- ☑
  - finger M97.8 ☑
  - hip M97.0- ☑
  - knee M97.1- ☑
  - shoulder M97.3- ☑
  - specified joint NEC M97.8 ☑
  - spine M97.8 ☑
  - toe M97.8 ☑
  - wrist M97.8 ☑
- phalanx
  - foot — *see* Fracture, toe
  - hand — *see* Fracture, finger
- pisiform — *see* Fracture, carpal, pisiform
- pond — *see* Fracture, skull
- prosthetic device, internal — *see* Complications, prosthetic device, by site, mechanical
- pubis S32.50- ☑
  - with disruption of pelvic ring — *see* Disruption, pelvic ring
  - specified site NEC S32.59- ☑
  - superior rim S32.51- ☑
- radius S52.9- ☑
  - distal end — *see* Fracture, radius, lower end
  - following insertion of implant, prosthesis or plate M96.63- ☑
  - head — *see* Fracture, radius, upper end, head
  - lower end S52.50- ☑
    - Barton's — *see* Barton's fracture
    - Colles' — *see* Colles' fracture
    - extraarticular NEC S52.55- ☑
    - intraarticular NEC S52.57- ☑
    - physeal S59.20- ☑
      - Salter-Harris
        - Type I S59.21- ☑
        - Type II S59.22- ☑
        - Type III S59.23- ☑
        - Type IV S59.24- ☑
      - specified NEC S59.29- ☑
    - Smith's — *see* Smith's fracture
    - specified NEC S52.59- ☑
    - styloid process (displaced) S52.51- ☑
      - nondisplaced S52.51- ☑
    - torus S52.52- ☑
  - neck — *see* Fracture, radius, upper end
  - proximal end — *see* Fracture, radius, upper end
  - shaft S52.30- ☑
    - bent bone S52.38- ☑
    - comminuted (displaced) S52.35- ☑
      - nondisplaced S52.35- ☑
    - Galeazzi's — *see* Galeazzi's fracture
    - greenstick S52.31- ☑
    - oblique (displaced) S52.33- ☑
      - nondisplaced S52.33- ☑
    - segmental (displaced) S52.36- ☑
      - nondisplaced S52.36- ☑
    - specified NEC S52.39- ☑

Fracture, traumatic — *continued*
  radius — *continued*
    shaft — *continued*
      spiral (displaced) S52.34- ☑
        nondisplaced S52.34- ☑
      transverse (displaced) S52.32- ☑
        nondisplaced S52.32- ☑
    upper end S52.10- ☑
      head (displaced) S52.12- ☑
        nondisplaced S52.12- ☑
      neck (displaced) S52.13- ☑
        nondisplaced S52.13- ☑
      physeal S59.10- ☑
        Salter-Harris
          Type I S59.11- ☑
          Type II S59.12- ☑
          Type III S59.13- ☑
          Type IV S59.14- ☑
        specified NEC S59.19- ☑
      specified NEC S52.18- ☑
      torus S52.11- ☑
  ramus
    inferior or superior, pubis — *see* Fracture, pubis
    mandible — *see* Fracture, mandible
  restorative material (dental) K08.539
    with loss of material K08.531
    without loss of material K08.530
  rib S22.3- ☑
    with flail chest — *see* Flail, chest
    multiple S22.4- ☑
      with flail chest — *see* Flail, chest
  root, tooth — *see* Fracture, tooth
  sacrum S32.10 ☑
    specified NEC S32.19 ☑
    Type
      1 S32.14 ☑
      2 S32.15 ☑
      3 S32.16 ☑
      4 S32.17 ☑
    Zone
      I S32.119 ☑
        displaced (minimally) S32.111 ☑
          severely S32.112 ☑
        nondisplaced S32.110 ☑
      II S32.129 ☑
        displaced (minimally) S32.121 ☑
          severely S32.122 ☑
        nondisplaced S32.120 ☑
      III S32.139 ☑
        displaced (minimally) S32.131 ☑
          severely S32.132 ☑
        nondisplaced S32.130 ☑
  scaphoid (hand) — *see also* Fracture, carpal, navicular
    foot — *see* Fracture, tarsal, navicular
  scapula S42.10- ☑
    acromial process (displaced) S42.12- ☑
      nondisplaced S42.12- ☑
    body (displaced) S42.11- ☑
      nondisplaced S42.11- ☑
    coracoid process (displaced) S42.13- ☑
      nondisplaced S42.13- ☑
    glenoid cavity (displaced) S42.14- ☑
      nondisplaced S42.14- ☑
    neck (displaced) S42.15- ☑
      nondisplaced S42.15- ☑
    specified NEC S42.19- ☑
  semilunar bone, wrist — *see* Fracture, carpal, lunate
  sequelae — *see* Sequelae, fracture
  sesamoid bone
    foot S92.81- ☑
    hand — *see* Fracture, carpal
    other — *see* Fracture, traumatic, by site
  shepherd's — *see* Fracture, tarsal, talus
  shoulder (girdle) S42.9- ☑
    blade — *see* Fracture, scapula
  sinus (ethmoid) (frontal) S02.19 ☑
  skull S02.91 ☑
    base S02.10- ☑
      occiput S02.119 ☑
        condyle S02.113 ☑
          specified NEC S02.118 ☑
            left side S02.11H ☑
            right side S02.11G ☑
          type I S02.110 ☑
            left side S02.11B ☑
            right side S02.11A ☑

Fracture, traumatic — *continued*
  skull — *continued*
    base — *continued*
      occiput — *continued*
        condyle — *continued*
          type II S02.111 ☑
            left side S02.11D ☑
            right side S02.11C ☑
          type III S02.112 ☑
            left side S02.11F ☑
            right side S02.11E ☑
        specified NEC S02.19 ☑
    birth injury P13.0
    frontal bone S02.0 ☑
    parietal bone S02.0 ☑
    specified site NEC S02.8- ☑
    temporal bone S02.19 ☑
    vault S02.0 ☑
  Smith's — *see* Smith's fracture
  sphenoid (bone) (sinus) S02.19 ☑
  spine — *see* Fracture, vertebra
  spinous process — *see* Fracture, vertebra
  spontaneous (cause unknown) — *see* Fracture, patho-
    logical
  stave (of thumb) — *see* Fracture, metacarpal, first
  sternum S22.20 ☑
    with flail chest — *see* Flail, chest
    body S22.22 ☑
    manubrium S22.21 ☑
    xiphoid (process) S22.24 ☑
  stress M84.30 ☑
    ankle M84.37- ☑
    carpus M84.34- ☑
    clavicle M84.31- ☑
    femoral neck M84.359 ☑
    femur M84.35- ☑
    fibula M84.36- ☑
    finger M84.34- ☑
    hip M84.359 ☑
    humerus M84.32- ☑
    ilium M84.350 ☑
    ischium M84.350 ☑
    metacarpus M84.34- ☑
    metatarsus M84.37- ☑
    neck — *see* Fracture, fatigue, vertebra
    pelvis M84.350 ☑
    radius M84.33- ☑
    rib M84.38 ☑
    scapula M84.31- ☑
    skull M84.38 ☑
    tarsus M84.37- ☑
    tibia M84.36- ☑
    toe M84.37- ☑
    ulna M84.33- ☑
    vertebra — *see* Fracture, fatigue, vertebra
  supracondylar, elbow — *see* Fracture, humerus, lower
    end, supracondylar
  symphysis pubis — *see* Fracture, pubis
  talus (ankle bone) — *see* Fracture, tarsal, talus
  tarsal bone(s) S92.20- ☑
    astragalus — *see* Fracture, tarsal, talus
    calcaneus S92.00- ☑
      anterior process (displaced) S92.02- ☑
        nondisplaced S92.02- ☑
      body (displaced) S92.01- ☑
        nondisplaced S92.01- ☑
      extraarticular NEC (displaced) S92.05- ☑
        nondisplaced S92.05- ☑
      intraarticular (displaced) S92.06- ☑
        nondisplaced S92.06- ☑
      physeal S99.00- ☑
        Salter-Harris
          Type I S99.01- ☑
          Type II S99.02- ☑
          Type III S99.03- ☑
          Type IV S99.04- ☑
        specified NEC S99.09- ☑
      tuberosity (displaced) S92.04- ☑
        avulsion (displaced) S92.03- ☑
          nondisplaced S92.03- ☑
        nondisplaced S92.04- ☑
    cuboid (displaced) S92.21- ☑
      nondisplaced S92.21- ☑
    cuneiform
      intermediate (displaced) S92.23- ☑
        nondisplaced S92.23- ☑

Fracture, traumatic — *continued*
  tarsal bone(s) — *continued*
    cuneiform — *continued*
      lateral (displaced) S92.22- ☑
        nondisplaced S92.22- ☑
      medial (displaced) S92.24- ☑
        nondisplaced S92.24- ☑
    navicular (displaced) S92.25- ☑
      nondisplaced S92.25- ☑
    scaphoid — *see* Fracture, tarsal, navicular
    talus S92.10- ☑
      avulsion (displaced) S92.15- ☑
        nondisplaced S92.15- ☑
      body (displaced) S92.12- ☑
        nondisplaced S92.12- ☑
      dome (displaced) S92.14- ☑
        nondisplaced S92.14- ☑
      head (displaced) S92.12- ☑
        nondisplaced S92.12- ☑
      lateral process (displaced) S92.14- ☑
        nondisplaced S92.14- ☑
      neck (displaced) S92.11- ☑
        nondisplaced S92.11- ☑
      posterior process (displaced) S92.13- ☑
        nondisplaced S92.13- ☑
      specified NEC S92.19- ☑
  temporal bone (styloid) S02.19 ☑
  thorax (bony) S22.9 ☑
    with flail chest — *see* Flail, chest
    rib S22.3- ☑
      multiple S22.4- ☑
        with flail chest — *see* Flail, chest
    sternum S22.20 ☑
      body S22.22 ☑
      manubrium S22.21 ☑
      xiphoid process S22.24 ☑
    vertebra (displaced) S22.009 ☑
      burst (stable) S22.001 ☑
        unstable S22.002 ☑
      eighth S22.069 ☑
        burst (stable) S22.061 ☑
          unstable S22.062 ☑
        specified type NEC S22.068 ☑
        wedge compression S22.060 ☑
      eleventh S22.089 ☑
        burst (stable) S22.081 ☑
          unstable S22.082 ☑
        specified type NEC S22.088 ☑
        wedge compression S22.080 ☑
      fifth S22.059 ☑
        burst (stable) S22.051 ☑
          unstable S22.052 ☑
        specified type NEC S22.058 ☑
        wedge compression S22.050 ☑
      first S22.019 ☑
        burst (stable) S22.011 ☑
          unstable S22.012 ☑
        specified type NEC S22.018 ☑
        wedge compression S22.010 ☑
      fourth S22.049 ☑
        burst (stable) S22.041 ☑
          unstable S22.042 ☑
        specified type NEC S22.048 ☑
        wedge compression S22.040 ☑
      ninth S22.079 ☑
        burst (stable) S22.071 ☑
          unstable S22.072 ☑
        specified type NEC S22.078 ☑
        wedge compression S22.070 ☑
      nondisplaced S22.001 ☑
      second S22.029 ☑
        burst (stable) S22.021 ☑
          unstable S22.022 ☑
        specified type NEC S22.028 ☑
        wedge compression S22.020 ☑
      seventh S22.069 ☑
        burst (stable) S22.061 ☑
          unstable S22.062 ☑
        specified type NEC S22.068 ☑
        wedge compression S22.060 ☑
      sixth S22.059 ☑
        burst (stable) S22.051 ☑
          unstable S22.052 ☑
        specified type NEC S22.058 ☑
        wedge compression S22.050 ☑
      specified type NEC S22.008 ☑

☑ **Additional Character Required** — Refer to the Tabular List for Character Selection   ▽ Subterms under main terms may continue to next column or pag

Fragile, fragility — *continued*
- nails L60.3
- non-sex chromosome site Q95.5
- X chromosome Q99.2

Fragilitas
- crinium L67.8
- ossium (with blue sclerae) (hereditary) Q78.0
- unguium L60.3
  - congenital Q84.6

Fragments, cataract (lens), **following cataract surgery** H59.02- ☑
- retained foreign body — *see* Retained, foreign body fragments (type of)

Frailty (frail) R54
- mental R41.81

Frambesia, frambesial (tropica) — *see also* Yaws
- initial lesion or ulcer A66.0
- primary A66.0

Frambeside
- gummatous A66.4
- of early yaws A66.2

Frambesioma A66.1

Franceschetti-Klein (-Wildervanck) **disease or syndrome** Q75.4

Francis' disease — *see* Tularemia

Franklin disease C88.2

Frank's essential thrombocytopenia D69.3

Fraser's syndrome Q87.0

Freckle(s) L81.2
- malignant melanoma in — *see* Melanoma
- melanotic (Hutchinson's) — *see* Melanoma, in situ
- retinal D49.81

Frederickson's hyperlipoproteinemia, type
- I and V E78.3
- IIA E78.00
- IIB and III E78.2
- IV E78.1

Freeman Sheldon syndrome Q87.0

Freezing — *see also* Effect, adverse, cold T69.9 ☑

Freiberg's disease (infraction of metatarsal head or osteochondrosis) — *see* Osteochondrosis, juvenile, metatarsus

Frei's disease A55

Fremitus, friction, cardiac R01.2

Frenum, frenulum
- external os Q51.828
- tongue (shortening) (congenital) Q38.1

Frequency micturition (nocturnal) R35.0
- psychogenic F45.8

Frey's syndrome
- auriculotemporal G50.8
- hyperhidrosis L74.52

Friction
- burn — *see* Burn, by site
- fremitus, cardiac R01.2
- precordial R01.2
- sounds, chest R09.89

Friderichsen-Waterhouse syndrome or disease A39.1

Friedländer's B (bacillus) **NEC** — *see also* condition A49.8

Friedreich's
- ataxia G11.11
- combined systemic disease G11.11
- facial hemihypertrophy Q67.4
- sclerosis (cerebellum) (spinal cord) G11.11

Frigidity F52.22

Fröhlich's syndrome E23.6

Frontal — *see also* condition
- lobe syndrome F07.0

Frostbite (superficial) T33.90 ☑
- with
  - partial thickness skin loss — *see* Frostbite (superficial), by site
  - tissue necrosis T34.90 ☑
- abdominal wall T33.3 ☑
  - with tissue necrosis T34.3 ☑
- ankle T33.81- ☑
  - with tissue necrosis T34.81- ☑
- arm T33.4- ☑
  - with tissue necrosis T34.4- ☑
  - finger(s) — *see* Frostbite, finger
  - hand — *see* Frostbite, hand
  - wrist — *see* Frostbite, wrist
- ear T33.01- ☑
  - with tissue necrosis T34.01- ☑
- face T33.09 ☑
  - with tissue necrosis T34.09 ☑
- finger T33.53- ☑

Frostbite — *continued*
- finger — *continued*
  - with tissue necrosis T34.53- ☑
- foot T33.82- ☑
  - with tissue necrosis T34.82- ☑
- hand T33.52- ☑
  - with tissue necrosis T34.52- ☑
- head T33.09 ☑
  - with tissue necrosis T34.09 ☑
  - ear — *see* Frostbite, ear
  - nose — *see* Frostbite, nose
- hip (and thigh) T33.6- ☑
  - with tissue necrosis T34.6- ☑
- knee T33.7- ☑
  - with tissue necrosis T34.7- ☑
- leg T33.9- ☑
  - with tissue necrosis T34.9- ☑
  - ankle — *see* Frostbite, ankle
  - foot — *see* Frostbite, foot
  - knee — *see* Frostbite, knee
  - lower T33.7- ☑
    - with tissue necrosis T34.7- ☑
  - thigh — *see* Frostbite, hip
  - toe — *see* Frostbite, toe
- limb
  - lower T33.99 ☑
    - with tissue necrosis T34.99 ☑
  - upper — *see* Frostbite, arm
- neck T33.1 ☑
  - with tissue necrosis T34.1 ☑
- nose T33.02 ☑
  - with tissue necrosis T34.02 ☑
- pelvis T33.3 ☑
  - with tissue necrosis T34.3 ☑
- specified site NEC T33.99 ☑
  - with tissue necrosis T34.99 ☑
- thigh — *see* Frostbite, hip
- thorax T33.2 ☑
  - with tissue necrosis T34.2 ☑
- toes T33.83- ☑
  - with tissue necrosis T34.83- ☑
- trunk T33.99 ☑
  - with tissue necrosis T34.99 ☑
- wrist T33.51- ☑
  - with tissue necrosis T34.51- ☑

Frotteurism F65.81

Frozen — *see also* Effect, adverse, cold T69.9 ☑
- pelvis (female) N94.89
  - male K66.8
- shoulder — *see* Capsulitis, adhesive

Fructokinase deficiency E74.11

Fructose 1,6 diphosphatase deficiency E74.19

Fructosemia (benign) (essential) E74.12

Fructosuria (benign) (essential) E74.11

Fuchs'
- black spot (myopic) — *see also* Myopia, degenerative H44.2- ☑
- dystrophy (corneal endothelium) H18.51- ☑
- heterochromic cyclitis — *see* Cyclitis, Fuchs' heterochromic

Fucosidosis E77.1

Fugue R68.89
- dissociative F44.1
- hysterical (dissociative) F44.1
- postictal in epilepsy — *see* Epilepsy
- reaction to exceptional stress (transient) F43.0

Fulminant, fulminating — *see* condition

Functional — *see also* condition
- bleeding (uterus) N93.8

Functioning, intellectual, borderline R41.83

Fundus — *see* condition

Fungemia NOS B49

Fungus, fungous
- cerebral G93.89
- disease NOS B49
- infection — *see* Infection, fungus

Funiculitis (acute) (chronic) (endemic) N49.1
- gonococcal (acute) (chronic) A54.23
- tuberculous A18.15

Funnel
- breast (acquired) M95.4
  - congenital Q67.6
  - sequelae (late effect) of rickets E64.3
- chest (acquired) M95.4
  - congenital Q67.6
  - sequelae (late effect) of rickets E64.3

Funnel — *continued*
- pelvis (acquired) M95.5
  - with disproportion (fetopelvic) O33.3 ☑
    - causing obstructed labor O65.3
  - congenital Q74.2

FUO (fever of unknown origin) R50.9

Furfur L21.0
- microsporon B36.0

Furrier's lung J67.8

Furrowed K14.5
- nail(s) (transverse) L60.4
  - congenital Q84.6
- tongue K14.5
  - congenital Q38.3

Furuncle L02.92
- abdominal wall L02.221
- ankle — *see* Furuncle, lower limb
- antecubital space — *see* Furuncle, upper limb
- anus K61.0
- arm — *see* Furuncle, upper limb
- auditory canal, external — *see* Abscess, ear, external
- auricle (ear) — *see* Abscess, ear, external
- axilla (region) L02.42- ☑
- back (any part) L02.222
- breast N61.1
- buttock L02.32
- cheek (external) L02.02
- chest wall L02.223
- chin L02.02
- corpus cavernosum N48.21
- ear, external — *see* Abscess, ear, external
- external auditory canal — *see* Abscess, ear, external
- eyelid — *see* Abscess, eyelid
- face L02.02
- femoral (region) — *see* Furuncle, lower limb
- finger — *see* Furuncle, hand
- flank L02.221
- foot L02.62- ☑
- forehead L02.02
- gluteal (region) L02.32
- groin L02.224
- hand L02.52- ☑
- head L02.821
  - face L02.02
- hip — *see* Furuncle, lower limb
- kidney — *see* Abscess, kidney
- knee — *see* Furuncle, lower limb
- labium (majus) (minus) N76.4
- lacrimal
  - gland — *see* Dacryoadenitis
  - passages (duct) (sac) — *see* Inflammation, lacrimal passages, acute
- leg (any part) — *see* Furuncle, lower limb
- lower limb L02.42- ☑
- malignant A22.0
- mouth K12.2
- navel L02.226
- neck L02.12
- nose J34.0
- orbit, orbital — *see* Abscess, orbit
- palmar (space) — *see* Furuncle, hand
- partes posteriores L02.32
- pectoral region L02.223
- penis N48.21
- perineum L02.225
- pinna — *see* Abscess, ear, external
- popliteal — *see* Furuncle, lower limb
- prepatellar — *see* Furuncle, lower limb
- scalp L02.821
- seminal vesicle N49.0
- shoulder — *see* Furuncle, upper limb
- specified site NEC L02.828
- submandibular K12.2
- temple (region) L02.02
- thumb — *see* Furuncle, hand
- toe — *see* Furuncle, foot
- trunk L02.229
  - abdominal wall L02.221
  - back L02.222
  - chest wall L02.223
  - groin L02.224
  - perineum L02.225
  - umbilicus L02.226
- umbilicus L02.226
- upper limb L02.42- ☑
- vulva N76.4

Furunculosis — *see* Furuncle

☑ **Additional Character Required** — **Refer to the Tabular List for Character Selection**

⬇ Subterms under main terms may continue to next column or page

ised — *see* Fusion, fused
usion, fused (congenital)
  astragaloscaphoid Q74.2
  atria Q21.1
  auditory canal Q16.1
  auricles, heart Q21.1
  binocular with defective stereopsis H53.32
  bone Q79.8
  cervical spine M43.22
  choanal Q30.0
  commissure, mitral valve Q23.2
  cusps, heart valve NEC Q24.8
    mitral Q23.2
    pulmonary Q22.1
    tricuspid Q22.4
  ear ossicles Q16.3
  fingers Q70.0 ☑
  hymen Q52.3
  joint (acquired) — *see also* Ankylosis
    congenital Q74.8
  kidneys (incomplete) Q63.1
  labium (majus) (minus) Q52.5
  larynx and trachea Q34.8

Fusion, fused — *continued*
  limb, congenital Q74.8
    lower Q74.2
    upper Q74.0
  lobes, lung Q33.8
  lumbosacral (acquired) M43.27
    arthrodesis status Z98.1
    congenital Q76.49
    postprocedural status Z98.1
  nares, nose, nasal, nostril(s) Q30.0
  organ or site not listed — *see* Anomaly, by site
  ossicles Q79.9
    auditory Q16.3
  pulmonic cusps Q22.1
  ribs Q76.6
  sacroiliac (joint) (acquired) M43.28
    arthrodesis status Z98.1
    congenital Q74.2
    postprocedural status Z98.1
  spine (acquired) NEC M43.20
    arthrodesis status Z98.1
    cervical region M43.22
    cervicothoracic region M43.23

Fusion, fused — *continued*
  spine — *continued*
    congenital Q76.49
    lumbar M43.26
    lumbosacral region M43.27
    occipito-atlanto-axial region M43.21
    postoperative status Z98.1
    sacrococcygeal region M43.28
    thoracic region M43.24
    thoracolumbar region M43.25
  sublingual duct with submaxillary duct at opening in
    mouth Q38.4
  testes Q55.1
  toes Q70.2- ☑
  tooth, teeth K00.2
  trachea and esophagus Q39.8
  twins Q89.4
  vagina Q52.4
  ventricles, heart Q21.0
  vertebra (arch) — *see* Fusion, spine
  vulva Q52.5
Fusospirillosis (mouth) (tongue) (tonsil) A69.1
Fussy baby R68.12

G

Gain in weight (abnormal) (excessive) — *see also* Weight, gain
Gaisböck's disease (polycythemia hypertonica) D75.1
Gait abnormality R26.9
  ataxic R26.0
  falling R29.6
  hysterical (ataxic) (staggering) F44.4
  paralytic R26.1
  spastic R26.1
  specified type NEC R26.89
  staggering R26.0
  unsteadiness R26.81
  walking difficulty NEC R26.2
Galactocele (breast) N64.89
  puerperal, postpartum O92.79
Galactokinase deficiency E74.29
Galactophoritis N61.0
  gestational, puerperal, postpartum O91.2- ☑
Galactorrhea O92.6
  not associated with childbirth N64.3
Galactosemia (classic) (congenital) E74.21
Galactosuria E74.29
Galacturia R82.0
  schistosomiasis (bilharziasis) B65.0
GALD (gestational alloimmune liver disease) P78.84
Galeazzi's fracture S52.37- ☑
Galen's vein — *see* condition
Galeophobia F40.218
Gall duct — *see* condition
Gallbladder — *see also* condition
  acute K81.0
Gallop rhythm R00.8
Gallstone (colic) (cystic duct) (gallbladder) (impacted) (multiple) — *see also* Calculus, gallbladder
  with
    cholecystitis — *see* Calculus, gallbladder, with cholecystitis
  bile duct (common) (hepatic) — *see* Calculus, bile duct
  causing intestinal obstruction K56.3
  specified NEC K80.80
    with obstruction K80.81
Gambling Z72.6
  pathological (compulsive) F63.0
Gammopathy (of undetermined significance [MGUS]) D47.2
  associated with lymphoplasmacytic dyscrasia D47.2
  monoclonal D47.2
  polyclonal D89.0
Gamna's disease (siderotic splenomegaly) D73.1
Gamophobia F40.298
Gampsodactylia (congenital) Q66.7- ☑
Gamstorp's disease (adynamia episodica hereditaria) G72.3
Gandy-Nanta disease (siderotic splenomegaly) D73.1
Gang
  membership offenses Z72.810
Gangliocytoma D36.10
Ganglioglioma — *see* Neoplasm, uncertain behavior, by site
Ganglion (compound) (diffuse) (joint) (tendon (sheath)) M67.40
  ankle M67.47- ☑
  foot M67.47- ☑
  forearm M67.43- ☑
  hand M67.44- ☑
  lower leg M67.46- ☑
  multiple sites M67.49
  of yaws (early) (late) A66.6
  pelvic region M67.45- ☑
  periosteal — *see* Periostitis
  shoulder region M67.41- ☑
  specified site NEC M67.48
  thigh region M67.45- ☑
  tuberculous A18.09
  upper arm M67.42- ☑
  wrist M67.43- ☑
Ganglioneuroblastoma — *see* Neoplasm, nerve, malignant
Ganglioneuroma D36.10
  malignant — *see* Neoplasm, nerve, malignant
Ganglioneuromatosis D36.10
Ganglionitis
  fifth nerve — *see* Neuralgia, trigeminal
  gasserian (postherpetic) (postzoster) B02.21

Ganglionitis — *continued*
  geniculate G51.1
    newborn (birth injury) P11.3
    postherpetic, postzoster B02.21
  herpes zoster B02.21
  postherpetic geniculate B02.21
Gangliosidosis E75.10
  GM1 E75.19
  GM2 E75.00
    other specified E75.09
    Sandhoff disease E75.01
    Tay-Sachs disease E75.02
  GM3 E75.19
  mucolipidosis IV E75.11
Gangosa A66.5
Gangrene, gangrenous (connective tissue) (dropsical) (dry) (moist) (skin) (ulcer) — *see also* Necrosis I96
  with diabetes (mellitus) — *see* Diabetes, gangrene
  abdomen (wall) I96
  alveolar M27.3
  appendix K35.80
    with
      peritonitis, localized — *see also* Appendicitis K35.31
  arteriosclerotic (general) (senile) — *see* Arteriosclerosis, extremities, with, gangrene
  auricle I96
  Bacillus welchii A48.0
  bladder (infectious) — *see* Cystitis, specified type NEC
  bowel, cecum, or colon — *see* Gangrene, intestine
  Clostridium perfringens or welchii A48.0
  cornea H18.89- ☑
  corpora cavernosa N48.29
    noninfective N48.89
  cutaneous, spreading I96
  decubital — *see* Ulcer, pressure, by site
  diabetic (any site) — *see* Diabetes, gangrene
  emphysematous — *see* Gangrene, gas
  epidemic — *see* Poisoning, food, noxious, plant
  epididymis (infectional) N45.1
  erysipelas — *see* Erysipelas
  extremity (lower) (upper) I96
  Fournier N49.3
    female N76.89
  fusospirochetal A69.0
  gallbladder — *see* Cholecystitis, acute
  gas (bacillus) A48.0
    following
      abortion — *see* Abortion by type complicated by infection
      ectopic or molar pregnancy O08.0
  glossitis K14.0
  hernia — *see* Hernia, by site, with gangrene
  intestine, intestinal (hemorrhagic) (massive) — *see also* Infarct, intestine K55.069
    with
      mesenteric embolism — *see also* Infarct, intestine K55.069
      obstruction — *see* Obstruction, intestine
  laryngitis J04.0
  limb (lower) (upper) I96
  lung J85.0
    spirochetal A69.8
  lymphangitis I89.1
  Meleney's (synergistic) — *see* Ulcer, skin
  mesentery — *see also* Infarct, intestine K55.069
    with
      embolism — *see also* Infarct, intestine K55.069
      intestinal obstruction — *see* Obstruction, intestine
  mouth A69.0
  ovary — *see* Oophoritis
  pancreas — *see* Pancreatitis, acute
  penis N48.29
    noninfective N48.89
  perineum I96
  pharynx — *see also* Pharyngitis
    Vincent's A69.1
  presenile I73.1
  progressive synergistic — *see* Ulcer, skin
  pulmonary J85.0
  pulpal (dental) K04.1
  quinsy J36
  Raynaud's (symmetric gangrene) I73.01
  retropharyngeal J39.2
  scrotum N49.3
    noninfective N50.89

Gangrene, gangrenous — *continued*
  senile (atherosclerotic) — *see* Arteriosclerosis, extremities, with, gangrene
  spermatic cord N49.1
    noninfective N50.89
  spine I96
  spirochetal NEC A69.8
  spreading cutaneous I96
  stomatitis A69.0
  symmetrical I73.01
  testis (infectional) N45.2
    noninfective N44.8
  throat — *see also* Pharyngitis
    diphtheritic A36.0
    Vincent's A69.1
  thyroid (gland) E07.89
  tooth (pulp) K04.1
  tuberculous NEC — *see* Tuberculosis
  tunica vaginalis N49.1
    noninfective N50.89
  umbilicus I96
  uterus — *see* Endometritis
  uvulitis K12.2
  vas deferens N49.1
    noninfective N50.89
  vulva N76.89
Ganister disease J62.8
Ganser's syndrome (hysterical) F44.89
Gardner-Diamond syndrome (autoerythrocyte sensitization) D69.2
Gargoylism E76.01
Garré's disease, osteitis (sclerosing), osteomyelitis — *see* Osteomyelitis, specified type NEC
Garrod's pad, knuckle M72.1
Gartner's duct
  cyst Q52.4
  persistent Q50.6
Gas R14.3
  asphyxiation, inhalation, poisoning, suffocation NEC — *see* Table of Drugs and Chemicals
  excessive R14.0
  gangrene A48.0
    following
      abortion — *see* Abortion by type complicated by infection
      ectopic or molar pregnancy O08.0
  on stomach R14.0
  pains R14.1
Gastralgia — *see also* Pain, abdominal
Gastrectasis K31.0
  psychogenic F45.8
Gastric — *see* condition
Gastrinoma
  malignant
    pancreas C25.4
    specified site NEC — *see* Neoplasm, malignant, by site
    unspecified site C25.4
  specified site — *see* Neoplasm, uncertain behavior
  unspecified site D37.9
Gastritis (simple) K29.70
  with bleeding K29.71
  acute (erosive) K29.00
    with bleeding K29.01
  alcoholic K29.20
    with bleeding K29.21
  allergic K29.60
    with bleeding K29.61
  atrophic (chronic) K29.40
    with bleeding K29.41
  chronic (antral) (fundal) K29.50
    with bleeding K29.51
    atrophic K29.40
      with bleeding K29.41
    superficial K29.30
      with bleeding K29.31
  dietary counseling and surveillance Z71.3
  due to diet deficiency E63.9
  eosinophilic K52.81
  giant hypertrophic K29.60
    with bleeding K29.61
  granulomatous K29.60
    with bleeding K29.61
  hypertrophic (mucosa) K29.60
    with bleeding K29.61
  nervous F54
  spastic K29.60
    with bleeding K29.61

☑ **Additional Character Required — Refer to the Tabular List for Character Selection**

▽ **Subterms under main terms may continue to next column or pag**

Gastritis — *continued*
  specified NEC K29.60
    with bleeding K29.61
  superficial chronic K29.30
    with bleeding K29.31
  tuberculous A18.83
  viral NEC A08.4
Gastrocarcinoma — *see* Neoplasm, malignant, stomach
Gastrocolic — *see* condition
Gastrodisciasis, gastrodiscoidiasis B66.8
Gastroduodenitis K29.90
  with bleeding K29.91
  virus, viral A08.4
    specified type NEC A08.39
Gastrodynia — *see* Pain, abdominal
Gastroenteritis (acute) (chronic) (noninfectious) — *see also* Enteritis K52.9
  allergic K52.29
    with
      eosinophilic gastritis or gastroenteritis K52.81
      food protein-induced enterocolitis syndrome K52.21
      food protein-induced enteropathy K52.22
  dietetic — *see also* Gastroenteritis, allergic K52.29
  drug-induced K52.1
  due to
    Cryptosporidium A07.2
    drugs K52.1
    food poisoning — *see* Intoxication, foodborne
    radiation K52.0
  eosinophilic K52.81
  epidemic (infectious) A09
  food hypersensitivity — *see also* Gastroenteritis, allergic K52.29
  infectious — *see* Enteritis, infectious
  influenzal — *see* Influenza, with gastroenteritis
  noninfectious K52.9
    specified NEC K52.89
  rotaviral A08.0
  Salmonella A02.0
  toxic K52.1
  viral NEC A08.4
    acute infectious A08.39
      type Norwalk A08.11
    infantile (acute) A08.39
    Norwalk agent A08.11
    rotaviral A08.0
    severe of infants A08.39
    specified type NEC A08.39
Gastroenteropathy — *see also* Gastroenteritis K52.9
  acute, due to Norovirus A08.11
  acute, due to Norwalk agent A08.11
  infectious A09
Gastroenteroptosis K63.4
Gastroesophageal laceration- hemorrhage syndrome K22.6
Gastrointestinal — *see* condition
Gastrojejunal — *see* condition
Gastrojejunitis — *see also* Enteritis K52.9
Gastrojejunocolic — *see* condition
Gastroliths K31.89
Gastromalacia K31.89
Gastroparalysis K31.84
  diabetic — *see* Diabetes, gastroparalysis
Gastroparesis K31.84
  diabetic — *see* Diabetes, by type, with gastroparesis
Gastropathy K31.9
  congestive portal K31.89
  erythematous K29.70
  exudative K90.89
  portal hypertensive K31.89
Gastroptosis K31.89
Gastrorrhagia K92.2
  psychogenic F45.8
Gastroschisis (congenital) Q79.3
Gastrospasm (neurogenic) (reflex) K31.89
  neurotic F45.8
  psychogenic F45.8
Gastrostaxis — *see* Gastritis, with bleeding
Gastrostenosis K31.89
Gastrostomy
  attention to Z43.1
  status Z93.1
Gastrosuccorrhea (continuous) (intermittent) K31.89
  neurotic F45.8
  psychogenic F45.8
Gatophobia F40.218

Gaucher's disease or splenomegaly (adult) (infantile) E75.22
Gee (-Herter)(-Thaysen) **disease** (nontropical sprue) K90.0
Gélineau's syndrome G47.419
  with cataplexy G47.411
Gemination, tooth, teeth K00.2
Gemistocytoma
  specified site — *see* Neoplasm, malignant, by site
  unspecified site C71.9
General, generalized — *see* condition
Genetic
  carrier (status)
    cystic fibrosis Z14.1
    hemophilia A (asymptomatic) Z14.01
      symptomatic Z14.02
    specified NEC Z14.8
  susceptibility to disease NEC Z15.89
    malignant neoplasm Z15.09
      breast Z15.01
      endometrium Z15.04
      ovary Z15.02
      prostate Z15.03
      specified NEC Z15.09
    multiple endocrine neoplasia Z15.81
Genital — *see* condition
Genito-anorectal syndrome A55
Genitourinary system — *see* condition
Genu
  congenital Q74.1
  extrorsum (acquired) — *see also* Deformity, varus, knee
    congenital Q74.1
    sequelae (late effect) of rickets E64.3
  introrsum (acquired) — *see also* Deformity, valgus, knee
    congenital Q74.1
    sequelae (late effect) of rickets E64.3
  rachitic (old) E64.3
  recurvatum (acquired) — *see also* Deformity, limb, specified type NEC, lower leg
    congenital Q68.2
    sequelae (late effect) of rickets E64.3
  valgum (acquired) (knock-knee) M21.06- ☑
    congenital Q74.1
    sequelae (late effect) of rickets E64.3
  varum (acquired) (bowleg) M21.16- ☑
    congenital Q74.1
    sequelae (late effect) of rickets E64.3
Geographic tongue K14.1
Geophagia — *see* Pica
Geotrichosis B48.3
  stomatitis B48.3
Gephyrophobia F40.242
Gerbode defect Q21.0
GERD (gastroesophageal reflux disease) K21.9
Gerhardt's
  disease (erythromelalgia) I73.81
  syndrome (vocal cord paralysis) J38.00
    bilateral J38.02
    unilateral J38.01
German measles — *see also* Rubella
  exposure to Z20.4
Germinoblastoma (diffuse) C85.9- ☑
  follicular C82.9- ☑
Germinoma — *see* Neoplasm, malignant, by site
Gerontoxon — *see* Degeneration, cornea, senile
Gerstmann's syndrome R48.8
  developmental F81.2
Gerstmann-Sträussler-Scheinker syndrome (GSS) A81.82
Gestation (period) — *see also* Pregnancy
  ectopic — *see* Pregnancy, by site
  multiple O30.9- ☑
    greater than quadruplets — *see* Pregnancy, multiple (gestation), specified NEC
    specified NEC — *see* Pregnancy, multiple (gestation), specified NEC
Gestational
  mammary abscess O91.11- ☑
  purulent mastitis O91.11- ☑
  subareolar abscess O91.11- ☑
Ghon tubercle, primary infection A15.7
Ghost
  teeth K00.4
  vessels (cornea) H16.41- ☑
Ghoul hand A66.3
Gianotti-Crosti disease L44.4

Giant
  cell
    epulis K06.8
    peripheral granuloma K06.8
  esophagus, congenital Q39.5
  kidney, congenital Q63.3
  urticaria T78.3 ☑
    hereditary D84.1
Giardiasis A07.1
Gibert's disease or pityriasis L42
Giddiness R42
  hysterical F44.89
  psychogenic F45.8
Gierke's disease (glycogenosis I) E74.01
Gigantism (cerebral) (hypophyseal) (pituitary) E22.0
  constitutional E34.4
Gilbert's disease or syndrome E80.4
Gilchrist's disease B40.9
Gilford-Hutchinson disease E34.8
Gilles de la Tourette's disease or syndrome (motor-verbal tic) F95.2
Gingivitis K05.10
  acute (catarrhal) K05.00
    necrotizing A69.1
    nonplaque induced K05.01
    plaque induced K05.00
  chronic (desquamative) (hyperplastic) (simple marginal) (pregnancy associated) (ulcerative) K05.10
    nonplaque induced K05.11
    plaque induced K05.10
  expulsiva — *see* Periodontitis
  necrotizing ulcerative (acute) A69.1
  pellagrous E52
    acute necrotizing A69.1
  Vincent's A69.1
Gingivoglossitis K14.0
Gingivopericementitis — *see* Periodontitis
Gingivosis — *see* Gingivitis, chronic
Gingivostomatitis K05.10
  herpesviral B00.2
  necrotizing ulcerative (acute) A69.1
Gland, glandular — *see* condition
Glanders A24.0
Glanzmann (-Naegeli) **disease or thrombasthenia** D69.1
Glasgow coma scale
  total score
    3-8 R40.243 ☑
    9-12 R40.242 ☑
    13-15 R40.241 ☑
Glass-blower's disease (cataract) — *see* Cataract, specified NEC
Glaucoma H40.9
  with
    increased episcleral venous pressure H40.81- ☑
    pseudoexfoliation of lens — *see* Glaucoma, open angle, primary, capsular
  absolute H44.51- ☑
  angle-closure (primary) H40.20- ☑
    acute (attack) (crisis) H40.21- ☑
    chronic H40.22- ☑
    intermittent H40.23- ☑
    residual stage H40.24- ☑
  borderline H40.00- ☑
  capsular (with pseudoexfoliation of lens) — *see* Glaucoma, open angle, primary, capsular
  childhood Q15.0
  closed angle — *see* Glaucoma, angle-closure
  congenital Q15.0
  corticosteroid-induced — *see* Glaucoma, secondary, drugs
  hypersecretion H40.82- ☑
  in (due to)
    amyloidosis E85.4 *[H42]*
    aniridia Q13.1 *[H42]*
    concussion of globe — *see* Glaucoma, secondary, trauma
    dislocation of lens — *see* Glaucoma, secondary
    disorder of lens NEC — *see* Glaucoma, secondary
    drugs — *see* Glaucoma, secondary, drugs
    endocrine disease NOS E34.9 *[H42]*
    eye
      inflammation — *see* Glaucoma, secondary, inflammation
      trauma — *see* Glaucoma, secondary, trauma
    hypermature cataract — *see* Glaucoma, secondary

Glaucoma — *continued*
 in — *continued*
  iridocyclitis — *see* Glaucoma, secondary, inflammation
  lens disorder — *see* Glaucoma, secondary
  Lowe's syndrome E72.03 *[H42]*
  metabolic disease NOS E88.9 *[H42]*
  ocular disorders NEC — *see* Glaucoma, secondary
  onchocerciasis B73.02
  pupillary block — *see* Glaucoma, secondary
  retinal vein occlusion — *see* Glaucoma, secondary
  Rieger's anomaly Q13.81 *[H42]*
  rubeosis of iris — *see* Glaucoma, secondary
  tumor of globe — *see* Glaucoma, secondary
 infantile Q15.0
 low tension — *see* Glaucoma, open angle, primary, low-tension
 malignant H40.83- ☑
 narrow angle — *see* Glaucoma, angle-closure
 newborn Q15.0
 noncongestive (chronic) — *see* Glaucoma, open angle
 nonobstructive — *see* Glaucoma, open angle
 obstructive — *see also* Glaucoma, angle-closure
  due to lens changes — *see* Glaucoma, secondary
 open angle H40.10- ☑
  primary H40.11- ☑
   capsular (with pseudoexfoliation of lens) H40.14- ☑
   low-tension H40.12- ☑
   pigmentary H40.13- ☑
   residual stage H40.15- ☑
 phacolytic — *see* Glaucoma, secondary
 pigmentary — *see* Glaucoma, open angle, primary, pigmentary
 postinfectious — *see* Glaucoma, secondary, inflammation
 secondary (to) H40.5- ☑
  drugs H40.6- ☑
  inflammation H40.4- ☑
  trauma H40.3- ☑
 simple (chronic) H40.11- ☑
 simplex H40.11- ☑
 specified type NEC H40.89
 suspect H40.00- ☑
 syphilitic A52.71
 traumatic — *see also* Glaucoma, secondary, trauma
  newborn (birth injury) P15.3
 tuberculous A18.59
Glaucomatous flecks (subcapsular) — *see* Cataract, complicated
Glazed tongue K14.4
Gleet (gonococcal) A54.01
Glénard's disease K63.4
Glioblastoma (multiforme)
 with sarcomatous component
  specified site — *see* Neoplasm, malignant, by site
  unspecified site C71.9
 giant cell
  specified site — *see* Neoplasm, malignant, by site
  unspecified site C71.9
 specified site — *see* Neoplasm, malignant, by site
 unspecified site C71.9
Glioma (malignant)
 astrocytic
  specified site — *see* Neoplasm, malignant, by site
  unspecified site C71.9
 mixed
  specified site — *see* Neoplasm, malignant, by site
  unspecified site C71.9
 nose Q30.8
 specified site NEC — *see* Neoplasm, malignant, by site
 subependymal D43.2
  specified site — *see* Neoplasm, uncertain behavior, by site
  unspecified site D43.2
 unspecified site C71.9
Gliomatosis cerebri C71.0
Glioneuroma — *see* Neoplasm, uncertain behavior, by site
Gliosarcoma
 specified site — *see* Neoplasm, malignant, by site
 unspecified site C71.9
Gliosis (cerebral) G93.89
 spinal G95.89
Glisson's disease — *see* Rickets
Globinuria R82.3
Globus (hystericus) F45.8

Glomangioma D18.00
 intra-abdominal D18.03
 intracranial D18.02
 skin D18.01
 specified site NEC D18.09
Glomangiomyoma D18.00
 intra-abdominal D18.03
 intracranial D18.02
 skin D18.01
 specified site NEC D18.09
Glomangiosarcoma — *see* Neoplasm, connective tissue, malignant
Glomerular
 disease in syphilis A52.75
 nephritis — *see* Glomerulonephritis
Glomerulitis — *see* Glomerulonephritis
Glomerulonephritis — *see also* Nephritis N05.9
 with
  C3
   glomerulonephritis N05.A
   glomerulopathy N05.A
    with dense deposit disease N05.6
  edema — *see* Nephrosis
  minimal change N05.0
  minor glomerular abnormality N05.0
 acute N00.9
 chronic N03.9
 crescentic (diffuse) NEC — *see also* N00-N07 with fourth character .7 N05.7
 dense deposit — *see also* N00-N07 with fourth character .6 N05.6
 diffuse
  crescentic — *see also* N00-N07 with fourth character .7 N05.7
  endocapillary proliferative — *see also* N00-N07 with fourth character .4 N05.4
  membranous — *see also* N00-N07 with fourth character .2 N05.2
  mesangial proliferative — *see also* N00-N07 with fourth character .3 N05.3
  mesangiocapillary — *see also* N00-N07 with fourth character .5 N05.5
  sclerosing N18.9
 endocapillary proliferative (diffuse) NEC — *see also* N00-N07 with fourth character .4 N05.4
 extracapillary NEC — *see also* N00-N07 with fourth character .7 N05.7
 focal (and segmental) — *see also* N00-N07 with fourth character .1 N05.1
 hypocomplementemic — *see* Glomerulonephritis, membranoproliferative
 IgA — *see* Nephropathy, IgA
 immune complex (circulating) NEC N05.8
 in (due to)
  amyloidosis E85.4 *[N08]*
  bilharziasis B65.9 *[N08]*
  cryoglobulinemia D89.1 *[N08]*
  defibrination syndrome D65 *[N08]*
  diabetes mellitus — *see* Diabetes, glomerulosclerosis
  disseminated intravascular coagulation D65 *[N08]*
  Fabry (-Anderson) disease E75.21 *[N08]*
  Goodpasture's syndrome M31.0
  hemolytic-uremic syndrome D59.3
  Henoch (-Schönlein) purpura D69.0 *[N08]*
  lecithin cholesterol acyltransferase deficiency E78.6 *[N08]*
  microscopic polyangiitis M31.7 *[N08]*
  multiple myeloma C90.0- ☑ *[N08]*
  Plasmodium malariae B52.0
  schistosomiasis B65.9 *[N08]*
  sepsis A41.9 *[N08]*
   streptococcal A40- ☑ *[N08]*
  sickle-cell disorders D57.- ☑ *[N08]*
  strongyloidiasis B78.9 *[N08]*
  subacute bacterial endocarditis I33.0 *[N08]*
  syphilis (late) congenital A50.59 *[N08]*
  systemic lupus erythematosus M32.14
  thrombotic thrombocytopenic purpura M31.1 *[N08]*
  typhoid fever A01.09
  Waldenström macroglobulinemia C88.0 *[N08]*
  Wegener's granulomatosis M31.31
 latent or quiescent N03.9
 lobular, lobulonodular — *see* Glomerulonephritis, membranoproliferative
 membranoproliferative (diffuse)(type 1 or 3) — *see also* N00-N07 with fourth character .5 N05.5

Glomerulonephritis — *continued*
 membranoproliferative — *see also* N00-N07 with fourth character .5 — *continued*
  dense deposit (type 2) NEC — *see also* N00-N07 with fourth character .6 N05.6
 membranous (diffuse) NEC — *see also* N00-N07 with fourth character .2 N05.2
 mesangial
  IgA/IgG — *see* Nephropathy, IgA
  proliferative (diffuse) NEC — *see also* N00-N07 with fourth character .3 N05.3
 mesangiocapillary (diffuse) NEC — *see also* N00-N07 with fourth character .5 N05.5
 necrotic, necrotizing NEC — *see also* N00- N07 with fourth character .8 N05.8
 nodular — *see* Glomerulonephritis, membranoproliferative
 poststreptococcal NEC N05.9
  acute N00.9
  chronic N03.9
  rapidly progressive N01.9
 proliferative NEC — *see also* N00-N07 with fourth character .8 N05.8
  diffuse (lupus) M32.14
 rapidly progressive N01.9
 sclerosing, diffuse N18.9
 specified pathology NEC — *see also* N00- N07 with fourth character .8 N05.8
 subacute N01.9
Glomerulopathy — *see* Glomerulonephritis
Glomerulosclerosis — *see also* Sclerosis, renal
 intercapillary (nodular) (with diabetes) — *see* Diabetes, glomerulosclerosis
 intracapillary — *see* Diabetes, glomerulosclerosis
Glossagra K14.6
Glossalgia K14.6
Glossitis (chronic superficial) (gangrenous) (Moeller's) K14.0
 areata exfoliativa K14.1
 atrophic K14.4
 benign migratory K14.1
 cortical superficial, sclerotic K14.0
 Hunter's D51.0
 interstitial, sclerous K14.0
 median rhomboid K14.2
 pellagrous E52
 superficial, chronic K14.0
Glossocele K14.8
Glossodynia K14.6
 exfoliativa K14.4
Glossoncus K14.8
Glossopathy K14.9
Glossophytia K14.3
Glossoplegia K14.8
Glossoptosis K14.8
Glossopyrosis K14.6
Glossotrichia K14.3
Glossy skin L90.8
Glottis — *see* condition
Glottitis — *see also* Laryngitis J04.0
Glucagonoma
 pancreas
  benign D13.7
  malignant C25.4
  uncertain behavior D37.8
 specified site NEC
  benign — *see* Neoplasm, benign, by site
  malignant — *see* Neoplasm, malignant, by site
  uncertain behavior — *see* Neoplasm, uncertain behavior, by site
 unspecified site
  benign D13.7
  malignant C25.4
  uncertain behavior D37.8
Glucoglycinuria E72.51
Glucose-galactose malabsorption E74.39
Glue
 ear — *see* Otitis, media, nonsuppurative, chronic, mucoid
 sniffing (airplane) — *see* Abuse, drug, inhalant
  dependence — *see* Dependence, drug, inhalant
GLUT1 deficiency syndrome 1, infantile onset E74.81
GLUT1 deficiency syndrome 2, childhood onset E74.810
Glutaric aciduria E72.3
Glycinemia E72.51
Glycinuria (renal) (with ketosis) E72.09

Glycogen
infiltration — *see* Disease, glycogen storage
storage disease — *see* Disease, glycogen storage
Glycogenosis (diffuse) (generalized) — *see also* Disease, glycogen storage
cardiac E74.02 *[I43]*
diabetic, secondary — *see* Diabetes, glycogenosis, secondary
pulmonary interstitial J84.842
Glycopenia E16.2
Glycosuria R81
renal E74.818
Gnathostoma spinigerum (infection) (infestation), **gnathostomiasis** (wandering swelling) B83.1
Goiter (plunging) (substernal) E04.9
with
hyperthyroidism (recurrent) — *see* Hyperthyroidism, with, goiter
thyrotoxicosis — *see* Hyperthyroidism, with, goiter
adenomatous — *see* Goiter, nodular
cancerous C73
congenital (nontoxic) E03.0
diffuse E03.0
parenchymatous E03.0
transitory, with normal functioning P72.0
cystic E04.2
due to iodine-deficiency E01.1
due to
enzyme defect in synthesis of thyroid hormone E07.1
iodine-deficiency (endemic) E01.2
dyshormonogenetic (familial) E07.1
endemic (iodine-deficiency) E01.2
diffuse E01.0
multinodular E01.1
exophthalmic — *see* Hyperthyroidism, with, goiter
iodine-deficiency (endemic) E01.2
diffuse E01.0
multinodular E01.1
nodular E01.1
lingual Q89.2
lymphadenoid E06.3
malignant C73
multinodular (cystic) (nontoxic) E04.2
toxic or with hyperthyroidism E05.20
with thyroid storm E05.21
neonatal NEC P72.0
nodular (nontoxic) (due to) E04.9
with
hyperthyroidism E05.20
with thyroid storm E05.21
thyrotoxicosis E05.20
with thyroid storm E05.21
endemic E01.1
iodine-deficiency E01.1
sporadic E04.9
toxic E05.20
with thyroid storm E05.21
nontoxic E04.9
diffuse (colloid) E04.0
multinodular E04.2
simple E04.0
specified NEC E04.8
uninodular E04.1
simple E04.0
toxic — *see* Hyperthyroidism, with, goiter
uninodular (nontoxic) E04.1
toxic or with hyperthyroidism E05.10
with thyroid storm E05.11
Goiter-deafness syndrome E07.1
Goldberg syndrome Q89.8
Goldberg-Maxwell syndrome E34.51
Goldblatt's hypertension or kidney I70.1
Goldenhar (-Gorlin) **syndrome** Q87.0
Goldflam-Erb disease or syndrome G70.00
with exacerbation (acute) G70.01
in crisis G70.01
Goldscheider's disease Q81.8
Goldstein's disease (familial hemorrhagic telangiectasia) I78.0
Golfer's elbow — *see* Epicondylitis, medial
Gonadoblastoma
specified site — *see* Neoplasm, uncertain behavior, by site
unspecified site
female D39.10
male D40.10
Gonecystitis — *see* Vesiculitis

Gongylonemiasis B83.8
Goniosynechiae — *see* Adhesions, iris, goniosynechiae
Gonococcemia A54.86
Gonococcus, gonococcal (disease) (infection) — *see also* condition A54.9
anus A54.6
bursa, bursitis A54.49
conjunctiva, conjunctivitis (neonatorum) A54.31
endocardium A54.83
eye A54.30
conjunctivitis A54.31
iridocyclitis A54.32
keratitis A54.33
newborn A54.31
other specified A54.39
fallopian tubes (acute) (chronic) A54.24
genitourinary (organ) (system) (tract) (acute)
lower A54.00
with abscess (accessory gland) (periurethral) A54.1
upper — *see also* condition A54.29
heart A54.83
iridocyclitis A54.32
joint A54.42
lymphatic (gland) (node) A54.89
meninges, meningitis A54.81
musculoskeletal A54.40
arthritis A54.42
osteomyelitis A54.43
other specified A54.49
spondylopathy A54.41
pelviperitonitis A54.24
pelvis (acute) (chronic) A54.24
pharynx A54.5
proctitis A54.6
pyosalpinx (acute) (chronic) A54.24
rectum A54.6
skin A54.89
specified site NEC A54.89
tendon sheath A54.49
throat A54.5
urethra (acute) (chronic) A54.01
with abscess (accessory gland) (periurethral) A54.1
vulva (acute) (chronic) A54.02
Gonocytoma
specified site — *see* Neoplasm, uncertain behavior, by site
unspecified site
female D39.10
male D40.10
Gonorrhea (acute) (chronic) A54.9
Bartholin's gland (acute) (chronic) (purulent) A54.02
with abscess (accessory gland) (periurethral) A54.1
bladder A54.01
cervix A54.03
conjunctiva, conjunctivitis (neonatorum) A54.31
contact Z20.2
Cowper's gland (with abscess) A54.1
exposure to Z20.2
fallopian tube (acute) (chronic) A54.24
kidney (acute) (chronic) A54.21
lower genitourinary tract A54.00
with abscess (accessory gland) (periurethral) A54.1
ovary (acute) (chronic) A54.24
pelvis (acute) (chronic) A54.24
female pelvic inflammatory disease A54.24
penis A54.09
prostate (acute) (chronic) A54.22
seminal vesicle (acute) (chronic) A54.23
specified site not listed — *see also* Gonococcus A54.89
spermatic cord (acute) (chronic) A54.23
urethra A54.01
with abscess (accessory gland) (periurethral) A54.1
vagina A54.02
vas deferens (acute) (chronic) A54.23
vulva A54.02
Goodall's disease A08.19
Goodpasture's syndrome M31.0
Gopalan's syndrome (burning feet) E53.0
Gorlin-Chaudry-Moss syndrome Q87.0
Gottron's papules L94.4
Gougerot-Blum syndrome (pigmented purpuric lichenoid dermatitis) L81.7
Gougerot-Carteaud disease or syndrome (confluent reticulate papillomatosis) L83
Gougerot's syndrome (trisymptomatic) L81.7
Gouley's syndrome (constrictive pericarditis) I31.1
Goundou A66.6

Gout, chronic — *see also* Gout, gouty M1A.9 ☑ (*following* M08)
drug-induced M1A.20 ☑ (*following* M08)
ankle M1A.27- ☑ (*following* M08)
elbow M1A.22- ☑ (*following* M08)
foot joint M1A.27- ☑ (*following* M08)
hand joint M1A.24- ☑ (*following* M08)
hip M1A.25- ☑ (*following* M08)
knee M1A.26- ☑ (*following* M08)
multiple site M1A.29- ☑ (*following* M08)
shoulder M1A.21- ☑ (*following* M08)
vertebrae M1A.28 ☑ (*following* M08)
wrist M1A.23- ☑ (*following* M08)
idiopathic M1A.00 ☑ (*following* M08)
ankle M1A.07- ☑ (*following* M08)
elbow M1A.02- ☑ (*following* M08)
foot joint M1A.07- ☑ (*following* M08)
hand joint M1A.04- ☑ (*following* M08)
hip M1A.05- ☑ (*following* M08)
knee M1A.06- ☑ (*following* M08)
multiple site M1A.09 ☑ (*following* M08)
shoulder M1A.01- ☑ (*following* M08)
vertebrae M1A.08 ☑ (*following* M08)
wrist M1A.03- ☑ (*following* M08)
in (due to) renal impairment M1A.30 ☑ (*following* M08)
ankle M1A.37- ☑ (*following* M08)
elbow M1A.32- ☑ (*following* M08)
foot joint M1A.37- ☑ (*following* M08)
hand joint M1A.34- ☑ (*following* M08)
hip M1A.35- ☑ (*following* M08)
knee M1A.36- ☑ (*following* M08)
multiple site M1A.39 ☑ (*following* M08)
shoulder M1A.31- ☑ (*following* M08)
vertebrae M1A.38 ☑ (*following* M08)
wrist M1A.33- ☑ (*following* M08)
lead-induced M1A.10 ☑ (*following* M08)
ankle M1A.17- ☑ (*following* M08)
elbow M1A.12- ☑ (*following* M08)
foot joint M1A.17- ☑ (*following* M08)
hand joint M1A.14- ☑ (*following* M08)
hip M1A.15- ☑ (*following* M08)
knee M1A.16- ☑ (*following* M08)
multiple site M1A.19 ☑ (*following* M08)
shoulder M1A.11- ☑ (*following* M08)
vertebrae M1A.18 ☑ (*following* M08)
wrist M1A.13- ☑ (*following* M08)
primary — *see* Gout, chronic, idiopathic
saturnine — *see* Gout, chronic, lead-induced
secondary NEC M1A.40 ☑ (*following* M08)
ankle M1A.47- ☑ (*following* M08)
elbow M1A.42- ☑ (*following* M08)
foot joint M1A.47- ☑ (*following* M08)
hand joint M1A.44- ☑ (*following* M08)
hip M1A.45- ☑ (*following* M08)
knee M1A.46- ☑ (*following* M08)
multiple site M1A.49 ☑ (*following* M08)
shoulder M1A.41- ☑ (*following* M08)
vertebrae M1A.48 ☑ (*following* M08)
wrist M1A.43- ☑ (*following* M08)
syphilitic — *see also* subcategory M14.8- A52.77
tophi M1A.9 ☑ (*following* M08)
Gout, gouty (acute) (attack) (flare) — *see also* Gout, chronic M10.9
drug-induced M10.20
ankle M10.27- ☑
elbow M10.22- ☑
foot joint M10.27- ☑
hand joint M10.24- ☑
hip M10.25- ☑
knee M10.26- ☑
multiple site M10.29
shoulder M10.21- ☑
vertebrae M10.28
wrist M10.23- ☑
idiopathic M10.00
ankle M10.07- ☑
elbow M10.02- ☑
foot joint M10.07- ☑
hand joint M10.04- ☑
hip M10.05- ☑
knee M10.06- ☑
multiple site M10.09
shoulder M10.01- ☑
vertebrae M10.08
wrist M10.03- ☑
in (due to) renal impairment M10.30

Glycogen — Gout, gouty

Subterms under main terms may continue to next column or page   ☑ Additional Character Required — Refer to the Tabular List for Character Selection   163

Gout, gouty — *continued*
in renal impairment — *continued*
ankle M10.37- ☑
elbow M10.32- ☑
foot joint M10.37- ☑
hand joint M10.34- ☑
hip M10.35- ☑
knee M10.36- ☑
multiple site M10.39
shoulder M10.31- ☑
vertebrae M10.38
wrist M10.33- ☑
lead-induced M10.10
ankle M10.17- ☑
elbow M10.12- ☑
foot joint M10.17- ☑
hand joint M10.14- ☑
hip M10.15- ☑
knee M10.16- ☑
multiple site M10.19
shoulder M10.11- ☑
vertebrae M10.18
wrist M10.13- ☑
primary — *see* Gout, idiopathic
saturnine — *see* Gout, lead-induced
secondary NEC M10.40
ankle M10.47- ☑
elbow M10.42- ☑
foot joint M10.47- ☑
hand joint M10.44- ☑
hip M10.45- ☑
knee M10.46- ☑
multiple site M10.49
shoulder M10.41- ☑
vertebrae M10.48
wrist M10.43- ☑
syphilitic — *see also* subcategory M14.8- A52.77
tophi — *see* Gout, chronic
Gower's
muscular dystrophy G71.01
syndrome (vasovagal attack) R55
Gradenigo's syndrome — *see* Otitis, media, suppurative, acute
Graefe's disease — *see* Strabismus, paralytic, ophthalmoplegia, progressive
Graft-versus-host disease D89.813
acute D89.810
acute on chronic D89.812
chronic D89.811
Grain mite (itch) B88.0
Grainhandler's disease or lung J67.8
Grand mal — *see* Epilepsy, generalized, specified NEC
Grand multipara status only (not pregnant) Z64.1
pregnant — *see* Pregnancy, complicated by, grand multiparity
Granite worker's lung J62.8
Granular — *see also* condition
inflammation, pharynx J31.2
kidney (contracting) — *see* Sclerosis, renal
liver K74.69
Granulation tissue (abnormal) (excessive) L92.9
postmastoidectomy cavity — *see* Complications, postmastoidectomy, granulation
Granulocytopenia (primary) (malignant) — *see* Agranulocytosis
Granuloma L92.9
abdomen K66.8
from residual foreign body L92.3
pyogenicum L98.0
actinic L57.5
annulare (perforating) L92.0
apical K04.5
aural — *see* Otitis, externa, specified NEC
beryllium (skin) L92.3
bone
eosinophilic C96.6
from residual foreign body — *see* Osteomyelitis, specified type NEC
lung C96.6
brain (any site) G06.0
schistosomiasis B65.9 *[G07]*
canaliculus lacrimalis — *see* Granuloma, lacrimal
candidal (cutaneous) B37.2
cerebral (any site) G06.0
coccidioidal (primary) (progressive) B38.7
lung B38.1
meninges B38.4

Granuloma — *continued*
colon K63.89
conjunctiva H11.22- ☑
dental K04.5
ear, middle — *see* Cholesteatoma
eosinophilic C96.6
bone C96.6
lung C96.6
oral mucosa K13.4
skin L92.2
eyelid H01.8
facial (e) L92.2
foreign body (in soft tissue) NEC M60.20
ankle M60.27- ☑
foot M60.27- ☑
forearm M60.23- ☑
hand M60.24- ☑
in operation wound — *see* Foreign body, accidentally left during a procedure
lower leg M60.26- ☑
pelvic region M60.25- ☑
shoulder region M60.21- ☑
skin L92.3
specified site NEC M60.28
subcutaneous tissue L92.3
thigh M60.25- ☑
upper arm M60.22- ☑
gangraenescens M31.2
genito-inguinale A58
giant cell (central) (reparative) (jaw) M27.1
gingiva (peripheral) K06.8
gland (lymph) I88.8
hepatic NEC K75.3
in (due to)
berylliosis J63.2 *[K77]*
sarcoidosis D86.89
Hodgkin C81.9 ☑
ileum K63.89
infectious B99.9
specified NEC B99.8
inguinale (Donovan) (venereal) A58
intestine NEC K63.89
intracranial (any site) G06.0
intraspinal (any part) G06.1
iridocyclitis — *see* Iridocyclitis, chronic
jaw (bone) (central) M27.1
reparative giant cell M27.1
kidney — *see also* Infection, kidney N15.8
lacrimal H04.81- ☑
larynx J38.7
lethal midline (faciale(e)) M31.2
liver NEC — *see* Granuloma, hepatic
lung (infectious) — *see also* Fibrosis, lung
coccidioidal B38.1
eosinophilic C96.6
Majocchi's B35.8
malignant (facial(e)) M31.2
mandible (central) M27.1
midline (lethal) M31.2
monilial (cutaneous) B37.2
nasal sinus — *see* Sinusitis
operation wound T81.89 ☑
foreign body — *see* Foreign body, accidentally left during a procedure
stitch T81.89 ☑
talc — *see* Foreign body, accidentally left during a procedure
oral mucosa K13.4
orbit, orbital H05.11- ☑
paracoccidioidal B41.8
penis, venereal A58
periapical K04.5
peritoneum K66.8
due to ova of helminths NOS — *see also* Helminthiasis B83.9 *[K67]*
postmastoidectomy cavity — *see* Complications, postmastoidectomy, recurrent cholesteatoma
prostate N42.89
pudendi (ulcerating) A58
pulp, internal (tooth) K03.3
pyogenic, pyogenicum (of) (skin) L98.0
gingiva K06.8
maxillary alveolar ridge K04.5
oral mucosa K13.4
rectum K62.89
reticulohistiocytic D76.3
rubrum nasi L74.8
Schistosoma — *see* Schistosomiasis

Granuloma — *continued*
septic (skin) L98.0
silica (skin) L92.3
sinus (accessory) (infective) (nasal) — *see* Sinusitis
skin L92.9
from residual foreign body L92.3
pyogenicum L98.0
spine
syphilitic (epidural) A52.19
tuberculous A18.01
stitch (postoperative) T81.89 ☑
suppurative (skin) L98.0
swimming pool A31.1
talc — *see also* Granuloma, foreign body
in operation wound — *see* Foreign body, accidentally left during a procedure
telangiectaticum (skin) L98.0
tracheostomy J95.09
trichophyticum B35.8
tropicum A66.4
umbilical P83.81
umbilicus P83.81
urethra N36.8
uveitis — *see* Iridocyclitis, chronic
vagina A58
venereum A58
vocal cord J38.3
Granulomatosis L92.9
with polyangiitis M31.3 ☑
eosinophilic, with polyangiitis [EGPA] M30.1
lymphoid C83.8- ☑
miliary (listerial) A32.89
necrotizing, respiratory M31.30
progressive septic D71
specified NEC L92.8
Wegener's M31.30
with renal involvement M31.31
Granulomatous tissue (abnormal) (excessive) L92.9
Granulosis rubra nasi L74.8
Graphite fibrosis (of lung) J63.3
Graphospasm F48.8
organic G25.89
Grating scapula M89.8X1
Gravel (urinary) — *see* Calculus, urinary
Graves' disease — *see* Hyperthyroidism, with, goiter
Gravis — *see* condition
Grawitz tumor C64.- ☑
Gray syndrome (newborn) P93.0
Grayness, hair (premature) L67.1
congenital Q84.2
Green sickness D50.8
Greenfield's disease
meaning
concentric sclerosis (encephalitis periaxialis conce
trica) G37.5
metachromatic leukodystrophy E75.25
Greenstick fracture — *code as* Fracture, by site
Grey syndrome (newborn) P93.0
Grief F43.21
prolonged F43.29
reaction — *see also* Disorder, adjustment F43.20
Griesinger's disease B76.0
Grinder's lung or pneumoconiosis J62.8
Grinding, teeth
psychogenic F45.8
sleep related G47.63
Grip
Dabney's B33.0
devil's B33.0
Grippe, grippal — *see also* Influenza
Balkan A78
summer, of Italy A93.1
Grisel's disease M43.6
Groin — *see* condition
Grooved tongue K14.5
Ground itch B76.9
Grover's disease or syndrome L11.1
Growing pains, children R29.898
Growth (fungoid) (neoplastic) (new) — *see also* Neoplas
adenoid (vegetative) J35.8
benign — *see* Neoplasm, benign, by site
malignant — *see* Neoplasm, malignant, by site
rapid, childhood Z00.2
secondary — *see* Neoplasm, secondary, by site
Gruby's disease B35.0
Gubler-Millard paralysis or syndrome G46.3
Guerin-Stern syndrome Q74.3

uidance, insufficient anterior (occlusal) M26.54
uillain-Barré disease or syndrome G61.0
  sequelae G65.0
uinea worms (infection) (infestation) B72
uinon's disease (motor-verbal tic) F95.2
ull's disease E03.4
um — *see* condition
umboil K04.7
  with sinus K04.6
umma (syphilitic) A52.79
  artery A52.09
    cerebral A52.04
  bone A52.77
    of yaws (late) A66.6
  brain A52.19
  cauda equina A52.19
  central nervous system A52.3
  ciliary body A52.71
  congenital A50.59
  eyelid A52.71
  heart A52.06
  intracranial A52.19
  iris A52.71
  kidney A52.75
  larynx A52.73
  leptomeninges A52.19
  liver A52.74
  meninges A52.19
  myocardium A52.06
  nasopharynx A52.73
  neurosyphilitic A52.3
  nose A52.73
  orbit A52.71
  palate (soft) A52.79
  penis A52.76
  pericardium A52.06
  pharynx A52.73
  pituitary A52.79
  scrofulous (tuberculous) A18.4
  skin A52.79
  specified site NEC A52.79
  spinal cord A52.19
  tongue A52.79
  tonsil A52.73
  trachea A52.73
  tuberculous A18.4
  ulcerative due to yaws A66.4
  ureter A52.75
  yaws A66.4
    bone A66.6
unn's syndrome Q07.8
unshot wound — *see also* Puncture, open
  fracture — *code as* Fracture, by site
  internal organs — *see* Injury, by site
ynandrism Q56.0
ynandroblastoma
  specified site — *see* Neoplasm, uncertain behavior, by
    site
  unspecified site
    female D39.10
    male D40.10
ynecological examination (periodic) (routine) Z01.419
  with abnormal findings Z01.411
ynecomastia N62
ynephobia F40.291
yrate scalp Q82.8

H

(Hartnup's) **disease** E72.02
aas' disease or osteochondrosis (juvenile) (head of
  humerus) — *see* Osteochondrosis, juvenile, humerus
abit, habituation
  bad sleep Z72.821
  chorea F95.8
  disturbance, child F98.9
  drug — *see* Dependence, drug
  irregular sleep Z72.821
  laxative F55.2
  spasm — *see* Tic
  tic — *see* Tic
aemophilus (H.) **influenzae, as cause of disease**
  classified elsewhere B96.3
aff disease — *see* Poisoning, mercury
ageman's factor defect, deficiency or disease D68.2
aglund's disease or osteochondrosis (juvenile) (os
  tibiale externum) — *see* Osteochondrosis, juvenile,
  tarsus

Hailey-Hailey disease Q82.8
Hair — *see also* condition
  plucking F63.3
    in stereotyped movement disorder F98.4
  tourniquet syndrome — *see also* Constriction, external,
    by site
    finger S60.44- ☑
    penis S30.842 ☑
    thumb S60.34- ☑
    toe S90.44- ☑
Hairball in stomach T18.2 ☑
Hair-pulling, pathological (compulsive) F63.3
Hairy black tongue K14.3
Half vertebra Q76.49
Halitosis R19.6
Hallerman-Streiff syndrome Q87.0
Hallervorden-Spatz disease G23.0
Hallopeau's acrodermatitis or disease L40.2
Hallucination R44.3
  auditory R44.0
  gustatory R44.2
  olfactory R44.2
  specified NEC R44.2
  tactile R44.2
  visual R44.1
Hallucinosis (chronic) F28
  alcoholic (acute) F10.951
    in
      abuse F10.151
      dependence F10.251
  drug-induced F19.951
    cannabis F12.951
    cocaine F14.951
    hallucinogen F16.151
    in
      abuse F19.151
        cannabis F12.151
        cocaine F14.151
        hallucinogen F16.151
        inhalant F18.151
        opioid F11.151
        sedative, anxiolytic or hypnotic F13.151
        stimulant NEC F15.151
      dependence F19.251
        cannabis F12.251
        cocaine F14.251
        hallucinogen F16.251
        inhalant F18.251
        opioid F11.251
        sedative, anxiolytic or hypnotic F13.251
        stimulant NEC F15.251
    inhalant F18.951
    opioid F11.951
    sedative, anxiolytic or hypnotic F13.951
    stimulant NEC F15.951
  organic F06.0
Hallux
  deformity (acquired) NEC M20.5X- ☑
  limitus M20.5X- ☑
  malleus (acquired) NEC M20.3- ☑
  rigidus (acquired) M20.2- ☑
    congenital Q74.2
    sequelae (late effect) of rickets E64.3
  valgus (acquired) M20.1- ☑
    congenital Q66.6
  varus (acquired) M20.3- ☑
    congenital Q66.3- ☑
Halo, visual H53.19
Hamartoma, hamartoblastoma Q85.9
  epithelial (gingival), odontogenic, central or peripheral
    — *see* Cyst, calcifying odontogenic
Hamartosis Q85.9
Hamman-Rich syndrome J84.114
Hammer toe (acquired) NEC — *see also* Deformity, toe,
  hammer toe
  congenital Q66.89
  sequelae (late effect) of rickets E64.3
Hand — *see* condition
Hand-foot syndrome L27.1
Handicap, handicapped
  educational Z55.9
    specified NEC Z55.8
Hand-Schüller-Christian disease or syndrome C96.5
Hanging (asphyxia) (strangulation) (suffocation) — *see*
  Asphyxia, traumatic, due to mechanical threat
Hangnail — *see also* Cellulitis, digit
  with lymphangitis — *see* Lymphangitis, acute, digit

Hangover (alcohol) F10.129
Hanhart's syndrome Q87.0
Hanot-Chauffard (-Troisier) **syndrome** E83.19
Hanot's cirrhosis or disease K74.3
Hansen's disease — *see* Leprosy
Hantaan virus disease (Korean hemorrhagic fever) A98.5
Hantavirus disease (with renal manifestations) (Dobrava)
  (Puumala) (Seoul) A98.5
  with pulmonary manifestations (Andes) (Bayou)
    (Bermejo) (Black Creek Canal) (Choclo) (Juquitiba)
    (Laguna negra) (Lechiguanas) (New York) (Oran)
    (Sin nombre) B33.4
Happy puppet syndrome Q93.51
Harada's disease or syndrome H30.81- ☑
Hardening
  artery — *see* Arteriosclerosis
  brain G93.89
Harelip (complete) (incomplete) — *see* Cleft, lip
Harlequin (newborn) Q80.4
Harley's disease D59.6
Harmful use (of)
  alcohol F10.10
  anxiolytics — *see* Abuse, drug, sedative
  cannabinoids — *see* Abuse, drug, cannabis
  cocaine — *see* Abuse, drug, cocaine
  drug — *see* Abuse, drug
  hallucinogens — *see* Abuse, drug, hallucinogen
  hypnotics — *see* Abuse, drug, sedative
  opioids — *see* Abuse, drug, opioid
  PCP (phencyclidine) — *see* Abuse, drug, hallucinogen
  sedatives — *see* Abuse, drug, sedative
  stimulants NEC — *see* Abuse, drug, stimulant
Harris' lines — *see* Arrest, epiphyseal
Hartnup's disease E72.02
Harvester's lung J67.0
Harvesting ovum for in vitro fertilization Z31.83
Hashimoto's disease or thyroiditis E06.3
Hashitoxicosis (transient) E06.3
Hassal-Henle bodies or warts (cornea) H18.49
Haut mal — *see* Epilepsy, generalized, specified NEC
Haverhill fever A25.1
Hay fever — *see also* Fever, hay J30.1
Hayem-Widal syndrome D59.8
Haygarth's nodes M15.8
Haymaker's lung J67.0
Hb (abnormal)
  Bart's disease D56.0
  disease — *see* Disease, hemoglobin
  trait — *see* Trait
Head — *see* condition
Headache R51.9
  with
    orthostatic component NEC R51.0
    positional component NEC R51.0
  allergic NEC G44.89
  associated with sexual activity G44.82
  chronic daily R51.9
  cluster G44.009
    chronic G44.029
      intractable G44.021
      not intractable G44.029
    episodic G44.019
      intractable G44.011
      not intractable G44.019
    intractable G44.001
    not intractable G44.009
  cough (primary) G44.83
  daily chronic R51.9
  drug-induced NEC G44.40
    intractable G44.41
    not intractable G44.40
  exertional (primary) G44.84
  histamine G44.009
    intractable G44.001
    not intractable G44.009
  hypnic G44.81
  lumbar puncture G97.1
  medication overuse G44.40
    intractable G44.41
    not intractable G44.40
  menstrual — *see* Migraine, menstrual
  migraine (type) — *see also* Migraine G43.909
  nasal septum R51.9
  neuralgiform, short lasting unilateral, with conjunctival
    injection and tearing (SUNCT) G44.059
    intractable G44.051
    not intractable G44.059

Headache — continued
  new daily persistent (NDPH) G44.52
  orgasmic G44.82
  periodic syndromes in adults and children G43.C0 (following G43.7)
    with refractory migraine G43.C1 (following G43.7)
    intractable G43.C1 (following G43.7)
    not intractable G43.C0 (following G43.7)
    without refractory migraine G43.C0 (following G43.7)
  postspinal puncture G97.1
  post-traumatic G44.309
    acute G44.319
      intractable G44.311
      not intractable G44.319
    chronic G44.329
      intractable G44.321
      not intractable G44.329
    intractable G44.301
    not intractable G44.309
  pre-menstrual — see Migraine, menstrual
  preorgasmic G44.82
  primary
    cough G44.83
    exertional G44.84
    stabbing G44.85
    thunderclap G44.53
  rebound G44.40
    intractable G44.41
    not intractable G44.40
  short lasting unilateral neuralgiform, with conjunctival injection and tearing (SUNCT) G44.059
    intractable G44.051
    not intractable G44.059
  specified syndrome NEC G44.89
  spinal and epidural anesthesia - induced T88.59 ☑
    in labor and delivery O74.5
    in pregnancy O29.4- ☑
    postpartum, puerperal O89.4
  spinal fluid loss (from puncture) G97.1
  stabbing (primary) G44.85
  tension (-type) G44.209
    chronic G44.229
      intractable G44.221
      not intractable G44.229
    episodic G44.219
      intractable G44.211
      not intractable G44.219
    intractable G44.201
    not intractable G44.209
  thunderclap (primary) G44.53
  vascular NEC G44.1
Healthy
  infant
    accompanying sick mother Z76.3
    receiving care Z76.2
  person accompanying sick person Z76.3
Hearing examination Z01.10
  with abnormal findings NEC Z01.118
  following failed hearing screening Z01.110
  for hearing conservation and treatment Z01.12
  infant or child (over 28 days old) Z00.129
    with abnormal findings Z00.121
Heart — see condition
Heart beat
  abnormality R00.9
    specified NEC R00.8
  awareness R00.2
  rapid R00.0
  slow R00.1
Heartburn R12
  psychogenic F45.8
Heartland virus disease A93.8
Heat (effects) T67.9 ☑
  apoplexy T67.01 ☑
  burn — see also Burn L55.9
  collapse T67.1 ☑
  cramps T67.2 ☑
  dermatitis or eczema L59.0
  edema T67.7 ☑
  erythema — code by site under Burn, first degree
  excessive T67.9 ☑
    specified effect NEC T67.8 ☑
  exhaustion T67.5 ☑
    anhydrotic T67.3 ☑
    due to
      salt (and water) depletion T67.4 ☑
      water depletion T67.3 ☑
        with salt depletion T67.4 ☑

Heat — continued
  fatigue (transient) T67.6 ☑
  fever T67.01 ☑
  hyperpyrexia T67.01 ☑
  prickly L74.0
  prostration — see Heat, exhaustion
  pyrexia T67.01 ☑
  rash L74.0
  specified effect NEC T67.8 ☑
  stroke T67.01 ☑
    exertional T67.02 ☑
    specified NEC T67.09 ☑
  sunburn — see Sunburn
  syncope T67.1 ☑
Heavy-for-dates NEC (infant) (4000g to 4499g) P08.1
  exceptionally (4500g or more) P08.0
Hebephrenia, hebephrenic (schizophrenia) F20.1
Heberden's disease or nodes (with arthropathy) M15.1
Hebra's
  pityriasis L26
  prurigo L28.2
Heel — see condition
Heerfordt's disease D86.89
Hegglin's anomaly or syndrome D72.0
Heilmeyer-Schoner disease D45
Heine-Medin disease A80.9
Heinz body anemia, congenital D58.2
Heliophobia F40.228
Heller's disease or syndrome F84.3
HELLP syndrome (hemolysis, elevated liver enzymes and low platelet count) O14.2- ☑
  complicating
    childbirth O14.24
    puerperium O14.25
Helminthiasis — see also Infestation, helminth
  Ancylostoma B76.0
  intestinal B82.0
    mixed types (types classifiable to more than one of the titles B65.0-B81.3 and B81.8) B81.4
    specified type NEC B81.8
  mixed types (intestinal) (types classifiable to more than one of the titles B65.0-B81.3 and B81.8) B81.4
  Necator (americanus) B76.1
  specified type NEC B83.8
Heloma L84
Hemangioblastoma — see Neoplasm, connective tissue, uncertain behavior
  malignant — see Neoplasm, connective tissue, malignant
Hemangioendothelioma — see also Neoplasm, uncertain behavior, by site
  benign D18.00
    intra-abdominal D18.03
    intracranial D18.02
    skin D18.01
    specified site NEC D18.09
  bone (diffuse) — see Neoplasm, bone, malignant
  epithelioid — see also Neoplasm, uncertain behavior, by site
    malignant — see Neoplasm, malignant, by site
  malignant — see Neoplasm, connective tissue, malignant
Hemangiofibroma — see Neoplasm, benign, by site
Hemangiolipoma — see Lipoma
Hemangioma D18.00
  arteriovenous D18.00
    intra-abdominal D18.03
    intracranial D18.02
    skin D18.01
    specified site NEC D18.09
  capillary I78.1
    intra-abdominal D18.03
    intracranial D18.02
    skin D18.01
    specified site NEC D18.09
  cavernous D18.00
    intra-abdominal D18.03
    intracranial D18.02
    skin D18.01
    specified site NEC D18.09
  epithelioid D18.00
    intra-abdominal D18.03
    intracranial D18.02
    skin D18.01
    specified site NEC D18.09
  histiocytoid D18.00
    intra-abdominal D18.03

Hemangioma — continued
  histiocytoid — continued
    intracranial D18.02
    skin D18.01
    specified site NEC D18.09
  infantile D18.00
    intra-abdominal D18.03
    intracranial D18.02
    skin D18.01
    specified site NEC D18.09
  intra-abdominal D18.03
  intracranial D18.02
  intramuscular D18.00
    intra-abdominal D18.03
    intracranial D18.02
    skin D18.01
    specified site NEC D18.09
  intrathoracic structures D18.09
  juvenile D18.00
  malignant — see Neoplasm, connective tissue, malignant
  plexiform D18.00
    intra-abdominal D18.03
    intracranial D18.02
    skin D18.01
    specified site NEC D18.09
  racemose D18.00
    intra-abdominal D18.03
    intracranial D18.02
    skin D18.01
    specified site NEC D18.09
  sclerosing — see Neoplasm, skin, benign
  simplex D18.00
    intra-abdominal D18.03
    intracranial D18.02
    skin D18.01
    specified site NEC D18.09
  skin D18.01
  specified site NEC D18.09
  venous D18.00
    intra-abdominal D18.03
    intracranial D18.02
    skin D18.01
    specified site NEC D18.09
  verrucous keratotic D18.00
    intra-abdominal D18.03
    intracranial D18.02
    skin D18.01
    specified site NEC D18.09
Hemangiomatosis (systemic) I78.8
  involving single site — see Hemangioma
Hemangiopericytoma — see also Neoplasm, connecti
  tissue, uncertain behavior
  benign — see Neoplasm, connective tissue, benign
  malignant — see Neoplasm, connective tissue, mali
    nant
Hemangiosarcoma — see Neoplasm, connective tissu
  malignant
Hemarthrosis (nontraumatic) M25.00
  ankle M25.07- ☑
  elbow M25.02- ☑
  foot joint M25.07- ☑
  hand joint M25.04- ☑
  hip M25.05- ☑
  in hemophilic arthropathy — see Arthropathy, hemophilic
  knee M25.06- ☑
  shoulder M25.01- ☑
  specified joint NEC M25.08
  traumatic — see Sprain, by site
  vertebrae M25.08
  wrist M25.03- ☑
Hematemesis K92.0
  with ulcer — code by site under Ulcer, with hemorrha
    K27.4
  newborn, neonatal P54.0
    due to swallowed maternal blood P78.2
Hematidrosis L74.8
Hematinuria — see also Hemoglobinuria
  malarial B50.8
Hematobilia K83.8
Hematocele
  female NEC N94.89
    with ectopic pregnancy O00.90
      with intrauterine pregnancy O00.91
    ovary N83.8
  male N50.1
Hematochezia — see also Melena K92.1

Hematochyluria — see also Infestation, filarial
  schistosomiasis (bilharziasis) B65.0
Hematocolpos (with hematometra or hematosalpinx)
  N89.7
Hematocornea — see Pigmentation, cornea, stromal
Hematogenous — see condition
Hematoma (traumatic) (skin surface intact) — see also
  Contusion
  with
    injury of internal organs — see Injury, by site
    open wound — see Wound, open
  amputation stump (surgical) (late) T87.89
  aorta, dissecting I71.00
    abdominal I71.02
    thoracic I71.01
    thoracoabdominal I71.03
  aortic intramural — see Dissection, aorta
  arterial (complicating trauma) — see Injury, blood
    vessel, by site
  auricle — see Contusion, ear
    nontraumatic — see Disorder, pinna, hematoma
  birth injury NEC P15.8
  brain (traumatic)
    with
      cerebral laceration or contusion (diffuse) — see
        Injury, intracranial, diffuse
        focal — see Injury, intracranial, focal
    cerebellar, traumatic S06.37- ☑
    intracerebral, traumatic — see Injury, intracranial,
      intracerebral hemorrhage
    newborn NEC P52.4
      birth injury P10.1
    nontraumatic — see Hemorrhage, intracranial
    subarachnoid, arachnoid, traumatic — see Injury,
      intracranial, subarachnoid hemorrhage
    subdural, traumatic — see Injury, intracranial, sub-
      dural hemorrhage
  breast (nontraumatic) N64.89
  broad ligament (nontraumatic) N83.7
    traumatic S37.892 ☑
  cerebellar, traumatic S06.37- ☑
  cerebral — see Hematoma, brain
  cerebrum S06.36- ☑
    left S06.35- ☑
    right S06.34- ☑
  cesarean delivery wound O90.2
  complicating delivery (perineal) (pelvic) (vagina) (vulva)
    O71.7
  corpus cavernosum (nontraumatic) N48.89
  epididymis (nontraumatic) N50.1
  epidural (traumatic) — see Injury, intracranial, epidural
    hemorrhage
    spinal — see Injury, spinal cord, by region
  episiotomy O90.2
  face, birth injury P15.4
  genital organ NEC (nontraumatic)
    female (nonobstetric) N94.89
      traumatic S30.202 ☑
    male N50.1
      traumatic S30.201 ☑
  internal organs — see Injury, by site
  intracerebral, traumatic — see Injury, intracranial, in-
    tracerebral hemorrhage
  intraoperative — see Complications, intraoperative,
    hemorrhage
  labia (nontraumatic) (nonobstetric) N90.89
  liver (subcapsular) (nontraumatic) K76.89
    birth injury P15.0
  mediastinum — see Injury, intrathoracic
  mesosalpinx (nontraumatic) N83.7
    traumatic S37.898 ☑
  muscle — code by site under Contusion
  nontraumatic
    muscle M79.81
    soft tissue M79.81
  obstetrical surgical wound O90.2
  orbit, orbital (nontraumatic) — see also Hemorrhage,
    orbit
    traumatic — see Contusion, orbit
  pelvis (female) (nontraumatic) (nonobstetric) N94.89
    obstetric O71.7
    traumatic — see Injury, by site
  penis (nontraumatic) N48.89
    birth injury P15.5
  perianal (nontraumatic) K64.5
  perineal S30.23 ☑
    complicating delivery O71.7

Hematoma — continued
  perirenal — see Injury, kidney
  pinna — see Contusion, ear
    nontraumatic — see Disorder, pinna, hematoma
  placenta O43.89- ☑
  postoperative (postprocedural) — see Complication,
    postprocedural, hematoma
  retroperitoneal (nontraumatic) K66.1
    traumatic S36.892 ☑
  scrotum, superficial S30.22 ☑
    birth injury P15.5
  seminal vesicle (nontraumatic) N50.1
    traumatic S37.892 ☑
  spermatic cord (traumatic) S37.892 ☑
    nontraumatic N50.1
  spinal (cord) (meninges) — see also Injury, spinal cord,
    by region
    newborn (birth injury) P11.5
  spleen D73.5
    intraoperative — see Complications, intraoperative,
      hemorrhage, spleen
    postprocedural (postoperative) — see Complica-
      tions, postprocedural, hemorrhage, spleen
  sternocleidomastoid, birth injury P15.2
  sternomastoid, birth injury P15.2
  subarachnoid (traumatic) — see Injury, intracranial,
    subarachnoid hemorrhage
    newborn (nontraumatic) P52.5
      due to birth injury P10.3
    nontraumatic — see Hemorrhage, intracranial,
      subarachnoid
  subdural (traumatic) — see Injury, intracranial, subdural
    hemorrhage
    newborn (localized) P52.8
      birth injury P10.0
    nontraumatic — see Hemorrhage, intracranial,
      subdural
  superficial, newborn P54.5
  testis (nontraumatic) N50.1
    birth injury P15.5
  tunica vaginalis (nontraumatic) N50.1
  umbilical cord, complicating delivery O69.5 ☑
  uterine ligament (broad) (nontraumatic) N83.7
    traumatic S37.892 ☑
  vagina (ruptured) (nontraumatic) N89.8
    complicating delivery O71.7
  vas deferens (nontraumatic) N50.1
    traumatic S37.892 ☑
  vitreous — see Hemorrhage, vitreous
  vulva (nontraumatic) (nonobstetric) N90.89
    complicating delivery O71.7
    newborn (birth injury) P15.5
Hematometra N85.7
  with hematocolpos N89.7
Hematomyelia (central) G95.19
  newborn (birth injury) P11.5
  traumatic T14.8 ☑
Hematomyelitis G04.90
Hematoperitoneum — see Hemoperitoneum
Hematophobia F40.230
Hematopneumothorax (see Hemothorax)
Hematopoiesis, cyclic D70.4
Hematoporphyria — see Porphyria
Hematorachis, hematorrhachis G95.19
  newborn (birth injury) P11.5
Hematosalpinx N83.6
  with
    hematocolpos N89.7
    hematometra N85.7
      with hematocolpos N89.7
    infectional — see Salpingitis
Hematospermia R36.1
Hematothorax (see Hemothorax)
Hematuria R31.9
  benign (familial) (of childhood) — see also Hematuria,
    idiopathic
    essential microscopic R31.1
  due to sulphonamide, sulfonamide — see Table of
    Drugs and Chemicals, by drug
  endemic — see also Schistosomiasis B65.0
  gross R31.0
  idiopathic N02.9
    with glomerular lesion
      C3
        glomerulonephritis N02.A
        glomerulopathy N02.A
          with dense deposit disease N02.6

Hematuria — continued
  idiopathic — continued
    with glomerular lesion — continued
      crescentic (diffuse) glomerulonephritis N02.7
      dense deposit disease N02.6
      endocapillary proliferative glomerulonephritis
        N02.4
      focal and segmental hyalinosis or sclerosis N02.1
      membranoproliferative (diffuse) N02.5
      membranous (diffuse) N02.2
      mesangial proliferative (diffuse) N02.3
      mesangiocapillary (diffuse) N02.5
      minor abnormality N02.0
      proliferative NEC N02.8
      specified pathology NEC N02.8
    intermittent — see Hematuria, idiopathic
  malarial B50.8
  microscopic NEC (with symptoms) R31.29
    asymptomatic R31.21
    benign essential R31.1
  paroxysmal — see also Hematuria, idiopathic
    nocturnal D59.5
  persistent — see Hematuria, idiopathic
  recurrent — see Hematuria, idiopathic
  tropical — see also Schistosomiasis B65.0
  tuberculous A18.13
Hemeralopia (day blindness) H53.11
  vitamin A deficiency E50.5
Hemi-akinesia R41.4
Hemianalgesia R20.0
Hemianencephaly Q00.0
Hemianesthesia R20.0
Hemianopia, hemianopsia (heteronymous) H53.47
  homonymous H53.46- ☑
  syphilitic A52.71
Hemiathetosis R25.8
Hemiatrophy R68.89
  cerebellar G31.9
  face, facial, progressive (Romberg) G51.8
  tongue K14.8
Hemiballism (us) G25.5
Hemicardia Q24.8
Hemicephalus, hemicephaly Q00.0
Hemichorea G25.5
Hemicolitis, left — see Colitis, left sided
Hemicrania
  congenital malformation Q00.0
  continua G44.51
  meaning migraine — see also Migraine G43.909
  paroxysmal G44.039
    chronic G44.049
      intractable G44.041
      not intractable G44.049
    episodic G44.039
      intractable G44.031
      not intractable G44.039
    intractable G44.031
    not intractable G44.039
Hemidystrophy — see Hemiatrophy
Hemiectromelia Q73.8
Hemihypalgesia R20.8
Hemihypesthesia R20.1
Hemi-inattention R41.4
Hemimelia Q73.8
  lower limb — see Defect, reduction, lower limb, speci-
    fied type NEC
  upper limb — see Defect, reduction, upper limb, spec-
    ified type NEC
Hemiparalysis — see Hemiplegia
Hemiparesis — see Hemiplegia
Hemiparesthesia R20.2
Hemiparkinsonism G20
Hemiplegia G81.9- ☑
  alternans facialis G83.89
  ascending NEC G81.90
    spinal G95.89
  congenital (cerebral) G80.8
    spastic G80.2
  embolic (current episode) I63.4- ☑
  flaccid G81.0- ☑
  following
    cerebrovascular disease I69.959
      cerebral infarction I69.35- ☑
      intracerebral hemorrhage I69.15- ☑
      nontraumatic intracranial hemorrhage NEC
        I69.25- ☑
      specified disease NEC I69.85- ☑

Hemiplegia — *continued*
  following — *continued*
    cerebrovascular disease — *continued*
      stroke NOS I69.35- ☑
      subarachnoid hemorrhage I69.05- ☑
  hysterical F44.4
  newborn NEC P91.88
    birth injury P11.9
  spastic G81.1- ☑
    congenital G80.2
  thrombotic (current episode) I63.3- ☑
Hemisection, spinal cord — *see* Injury, spinal cord, by region
Hemispasm (facial) R25.2
Hemisporosis B48.8
Hemitremor R25.1
Hemivertebra Q76.49
  failure of segmentation with scoliosis Q76.3
  fusion with scoliosis Q76.3
Hemochromatosis E83.119
  with refractory anemia D46.1
  due to repeated red blood cell transfusion E83.111
  hereditary (primary) E83.110
  neonatal P78.84
  primary E83.110
  specified NEC E83.118
Hemoglobin — *see also* condition
  abnormal (disease) — *see* Disease, hemoglobin
  AS genotype D57.3
  Constant Spring D58.2
  E-beta thalassemia D56.5
  fetal, hereditary persistence (HPFH) D56.4
  H Constant Spring D56.0
  low NOS D64.9
  S (Hb S), heterozygous D57.3
Hemoglobinemia D59.9
  due to blood transfusion T80.89 ☑
  paroxysmal D59.6
    nocturnal D59.5
Hemoglobinopathy (mixed) D58.2
  with thalassemia D56.8
  sickle-cell D57.1
    with thalassemia D57.40
      with
        acute chest syndrome D57.411
        cerebral vascular involvement D57.413
        crisis (painful) D57.419
          with specified complication NEC D57.418
        splenic sequestration D57.412
        vasoocclusive pain D57.419
      without crisis D57.40
Hemoglobinuria R82.3
  with anemia, hemolytic, acquired (chronic) NEC D59.6
  cold (paroxysmal) (with Raynaud's syndrome) D59.6
    agglutinin D59.12
  due to exertion or hemolysis NEC D59.6
  intermittent D59.6
  malarial B50.8
  march D59.6
  nocturnal (paroxysmal) D59.5
  paroxysmal (cold) D59.6
    nocturnal D59.5
Hemolymphangioma D18.1
Hemolysis
  intravascular
    with
      abortion — *see* Abortion, by type, complicated by, hemorrhage
      ectopic or molar pregnancy O08.1
      hemorrhage
        antepartum — *see* Hemorrhage, antepartum, with coagulation defect
        intrapartum — *see also* Hemorrhage, complicating, delivery O67.0
      postpartum O72.3
  neonatal (excessive) P58.9
    specified NEC P58.8
Hemolytic — *see* condition
Hemopericardium I31.2
  following acute myocardial infarction (current complication) I23.0
  newborn P54.8
  traumatic — *see* Injury, heart, with hemopericardium
Hemoperitoneum K66.1
  infectional K65.9
  traumatic S36.899 ☑
    with open wound — *see* Wound, open, with penetration into peritoneal cavity

Hemophilia (classical) (familial) (hereditary) D66
  A D66
  acquired D68.311
  autoimmune D68.311
  B D67
  C D68.1
  calcipriva — *see also* Defect, coagulation D68.4
  nonfamilial — *see also* Defect, coagulation D68.4
  secondary D68.311
  vascular D68.0
Hemophthalmos H44.81- ☑
Hemopneumothorax — *see also* Hemothorax
  traumatic S27.2 ☑
Hemoptysis R04.2
  newborn P26.9
  tuberculous — *see* Tuberculosis, pulmonary
Hemorrhage, hemorrhagic (concealed) R58
  abdomen R58
  accidental antepartum — *see* Hemorrhage, antepartum
  acute idiopathic pulmonary, in infants R04.81
  adenoid J35.8
  adrenal (capsule) (gland) E27.49
    medulla E27.8
    newborn P54.4
  after delivery — *see* Hemorrhage, postpartum
  alveolar
    lung, newborn P26.8
    process K08.89
  alveolus K08.89
  amputation stump (surgical) T87.89
  anemia (chronic) D50.0
    acute D62
  antepartum (with) O46.90
    with coagulation defect O46.00- ☑
      afibrinogenemia O46.01- ☑
      disseminated intravascular coagulation O46.02- ☑
      hypofibrinogenemia O46.01- ☑
      specified defect NEC O46.09- ☑
    before 20 weeks gestation O20.9
      specified type NEC O20.8
      threatened abortion O20.0
    due to
      abruptio placenta — *see also* Abruptio placentae O45.9- ☑
      leiomyoma, uterus — *see* Hemorrhage, antepartum, specified cause NEC
      placenta previa O44.1- ☑
    specified cause NEC — *see* subcategory O46.8X- ☑
  anus (sphincter) K62.5
  apoplexy (stroke) — *see* Hemorrhage, intracranial, intracerebral
  arachnoid — *see* Hemorrhage, intracranial, subarachnoid
  artery R58
    brain — *see* Hemorrhage, intracranial, intracerebral
  basilar (ganglion) I61.0
  bladder N32.89
  bowel K92.2
    newborn P54.3
  brain (miliary) (nontraumatic) — *see* Hemorrhage, intracranial, intracerebral
    due to
      birth injury P10.1
      syphilis A52.05
    epidural or extradural (traumatic) — *see* Injury, intracranial, epidural hemorrhage
    newborn P52.4
      birth injury P10.1
    subarachnoid — *see* Hemorrhage, intracranial, subarachnoid
    subdural — *see* Hemorrhage, intracranial, subdural
  brainstem (nontraumatic) I61.3
    traumatic S06.38- ☑
  breast N64.59
  bronchial tube — *see* Hemorrhage, lung
  bronchopulmonary — *see* Hemorrhage, lung
  bronchus — *see* Hemorrhage, lung
  bulbar I61.5
  capillary I78.8
    primary D69.8
  cecum K92.2
  cerebellar, cerebellum (nontraumatic) I61.4
    newborn P52.6
    traumatic S06.37- ☑
  cerebral, cerebrum — *see also* Hemorrhage, intracranial, intracerebral
    lobe I61.1

Hemorrhage, hemorrhagic — *continued*
  cerebral, cerebrum — *see also* Hemorrhage, intracranial, intracerebral — *continued*
    newborn (anoxic) P52.4
      birth injury P10.1
  cerebromeningeal I61.8
  cerebrospinal — *see* Hemorrhage, intracranial, intracerebral
  cervix (uteri) (stump) NEC N88.8
  chamber, anterior (eye) — *see* Hyphema
  childbirth — *see* Hemorrhage, complicating, delivery
  choroid H31.30- ☑
    expulsive H31.31- ☑
  ciliary body — *see* Hyphema
  cochlea — *see* subcategory H83.8 ☑
  colon K92.2
  complicating
    abortion — *see* Abortion, by type, complicated by, hemorrhage
    delivery O67.9
      associated with coagulation defect (afibrinogenemia) (DIC) (hyperfibrinolysis) O67.0
      specified cause NEC O67.8
      surgical procedure — *see* Hemorrhage, intraoperative
  conjunctiva H11.3- ☑
    newborn P54.8
  cord, newborn (stump) P51.9
  corpus luteum (ruptured) cyst N83.1- ☑
  cortical (brain) I61.1
  cranial — *see* Hemorrhage, intracranial
  cutaneous R23.3
    due to autosensitivity, erythrocyte D69.2
    newborn P54.5
  delayed
    following ectopic or molar pregnancy O08.1
    postpartum O72.2
  diathesis (familial) D69.9
  disease D69.9
    newborn P53
    specified type NEC D69.8
  due to or associated with
    afibrinogenemia or other coagulation defect (conditions in categories D65- D69)
      antepartum — *see* Hemorrhage, antepartum, with coagulation defect
      intrapartum O67.0
    dental implant M27.61
    device, implant or graft — *see also* Complications, by site and type, specified NEC T85.838 ☑
      arterial graft NEC T82.838 ☑
      breast T85.838 ☑
      catheter NEC T85.838 ☑
        dialysis (renal) T82.838 ☑
          intraperitoneal T85.838 ☑
        infusion NEC T82.838 ☑
          spinal (epidural) (subdural) T85.830 ☑
        urinary (indwelling) T83.83 ☑
      electronic (electrode) (pulse generator) (stimulator)
        bone T84.83 ☑
        cardiac T82.837 ☑
        nervous system (brain) (peripheral nerve) (spinal) T85.830 ☑
        urinary T83.83 ☑
      fixation, internal (orthopedic) NEC T84.83 ☑
      gastrointestinal (bile duct) (esophagus) T85.838 ☑
      genital NEC T83.83 ☑
      heart NEC T82.837 ☑
      joint prosthesis T84.83 ☑
      ocular (corneal graft) (orbital implant) NEC T85.838 ☑
      orthopedic NEC T84.83 ☑
        bone graft T86.838 ☑
      specified NEC T85.838 ☑
      urinary NEC T83.83 ☑
      vascular NEC T82.838 ☑
      ventricular intracranial shunt T85.830 ☑
  duodenum, duodenal K92.2
    ulcer — *see* Ulcer, duodenum, with hemorrhage
  dura mater — *see* Hemorrhage, intracranial, subdural
  endotracheal — *see* Hemorrhage, lung
  epicranial subaponeurotic (massive), birth injury P12.2
  epidural (traumatic) — *see also* Injury, intracranial, epidural hemorrhage
    nontraumatic I62.1

Hemorrhage, hemorrhagic — *continued*
　esophagus K22.8
　　varix I85.01
　　　secondary I85.11
　excessive, following ectopic gestation (subsequent
　　　episode) O08.1
　extradural (traumatic) — *see* Injury, intracranial,
　　　epidural hemorrhage
　　birth injury P10.8
　　newborn (anoxic) (nontraumatic) P52.8
　　nontraumatic I62.1
　eye NEC H57.89
　　fundus — *see* Hemorrhage, retina
　　lid — *see* Disorder, eyelid, specified type NEC
　fallopian tube N83.6
　fibrinogenolysis — *see* Fibrinolysis
　fibrinolytic (acquired) — *see* Fibrinolysis
　from
　　ear (nontraumatic) — *see* Otorrhagia
　　tracheostomy stoma J95.01
　fundus, eye — *see* Hemorrhage, retina
　funis — *see* Hemorrhage, umbilicus, cord
　gastric — *see* Hemorrhage, stomach
　gastroenteric K92.2
　　newborn P54.3
　gastrointestinal (tract) K92.2
　　newborn P54.3
　genital organ, male N50.1
　genitourinary (tract) NOS R31.9
　gingiva K06.8
　globe (eye) — *see* Hemophthalmos
　graafian follicle cyst (ruptured) N83.0- ☑
　gum K06.8
　heart I51.89
　hypopharyngeal (throat) R04.1
　intermenstrual (regular) N92.3
　　irregular N92.1
　internal (organs) NEC R58
　　capsule I61.0
　　ear — *see* subcategory H83.8 ☑
　　newborn P54.8
　intestine K92.2
　　newborn P54.3
　intra-abdominal R58
　intra-alveolar (lung), newborn P26.8
　intracerebral (nontraumatic) — *see* Hemorrhage, in-
　　　tracranial, intracerebral
　intracranial (nontraumatic) I62.9
　　birth injury P10.9
　　epidural, nontraumatic I62.1
　　extradural, nontraumatic I62.1
　　intracerebral (nontraumatic) (in) I61.9
　　　brain stem I61.3
　　　cerebellum I61.4
　　　hemisphere I61.2
　　　　cortical (superficial) I61.1
　　　　subcortical (deep) I61.0
　　　intraoperative
　　　　during a nervous system procedure G97.31
　　　　during other procedure G97.32
　　　intraventricular I61.5
　　　multiple localized I61.6
　　　newborn P52.4
　　　　birth injury P10.1
　　　postprocedural
　　　　following a nervous system procedure G97.51
　　　　following other procedure G97.52
　　　specified NEC I61.8
　　　superficial I61.1
　　　traumatic (diffuse) — *see* Injury, intracranial,
　　　　diffuse
　　　focal — *see* Injury, intracranial, focal
　　newborn P52.9
　　　specified NEC P52.8
　　subarachnoid (nontraumatic) (from) I60.9
　　　intracranial (cerebral) artery I60.7
　　　　anterior communicating I60.2
　　　　basilar I60.4
　　　　carotid siphon and bifurcation I60.0- ☑
　　　　communicating I60.7
　　　　　anterior I60.2
　　　　　posterior I60.3- ☑
　　　　middle cerebral I60.1- ☑
　　　　posterior communicating I60.3- ☑
　　　　specified artery NEC I60.6
　　　　vertebral I60.5- ☑
　　　newborn P52.5
　　　　birth injury P10.3

Hemorrhage, hemorrhagic — *continued*
　intracranial — *continued*
　　subarachnoid — *continued*
　　　specified NEC I60.8
　　　traumatic S06.6X- ☑
　　subdural (nontraumatic) I62.00
　　　acute I62.01
　　　birth injury P10.0
　　　chronic I62.03
　　　newborn (anoxic) (hypoxic) P52.8
　　　　birth injury P10.0
　　　spinal G95.19
　　　subacute I62.02
　　　traumatic — *see* Injury, intracranial, subdural
　　　　hemorrhage
　　　traumatic — *see* Injury, intracranial, focal brain in-
　　　　jury
　intramedullary NEC G95.19
　intraocular — *see* Hemophthalmos
　intraoperative, intraprocedural — *see* Complication,
　　　hemorrhage (hematoma), intraoperative (in-
　　　traprocedural), by site
　intrapartum — *see* Hemorrhage, complicating, delivery
　intrapelvic
　　female N94.89
　　male K66.1
　intraperitoneal K66.1
　intrapontine I61.3
　intraprocedural — *see* Complication, hemorrhage
　　　(hematoma), intraoperative (intraprocedural),
　　　by site
　intrauterine N85.7
　　complicating delivery — *see also* Hemorrhage,
　　　complicating, delivery O67.9
　　postpartum — *see* Hemorrhage, postpartum
　intraventricular I61.5
　　newborn (nontraumatic) — *see also* Newborn, af-
　　　fected by, hemorrhage P52.3
　　　due to birth injury P10.2
　　　grade
　　　　1 P52.0
　　　　2 P52.1
　　　　3 P52.21
　　　　4 P52.22
　intravesical N32.89
　iris (postinfectional) (postinflammatory) (toxic) — *see*
　　　Hyphema
　joint (nontraumatic) — *see* Hemarthrosis
　kidney N28.89
　knee (joint) (nontraumatic) — *see* Hemarthrosis, knee
　labyrinth — *see* subcategory H83.8 ☑
　lenticular striate artery I61.0
　ligature, vessel — *see* Hemorrhage, postoperative
　liver K76.89
　lung R04.89
　　newborn P26.9
　　　massive P26.1
　　　specified NEC P26.8
　　tuberculous — *see* Tuberculosis, pulmonary
　massive umbilical, newborn P51.0
　mediastinum — *see* Hemorrhage, lung
　medulla I61.3
　membrane (brain) I60.8
　　spinal cord — *see* Hemorrhage, spinal cord
　meninges, meningeal (brain) (middle) I60.8
　　spinal cord — *see* Hemorrhage, spinal cord
　mesentery K66.1
　metritis — *see* Endometritis
　mouth K13.79
　mucous membrane NEC R58
　　newborn P54.8
　muscle M62.89
　nail (subungual) L60.8
　nasal turbinate R04.0
　　newborn P54.8
　navel, newborn P51.9
　newborn P54.9
　　specified NEC P54.8
　nipple N64.59
　nose R04.0
　　newborn P54.8
　omentum K66.1
　optic nerve (sheath) H47.02- ☑
　orbit, orbital H05.23- ☑
　ovary NEC N83.8
　oviduct N83.6
　pancreas K86.89
　parathyroid (gland) (spontaneous) E21.4

Hemorrhage, hemorrhagic — *continued*
　parturition — *see* Hemorrhage, complicating, delivery
　penis N48.89
　pericardium, pericarditis I31.2
　peritoneum, peritoneal K66.1
　peritonsillar tissue J35.8
　　due to infection J36
　petechial R23.3
　　due to autosensitivity, erythrocyte D69.2
　pituitary (gland) E23.6
　pleura — *see* Hemorrhage, lung
　polioencephalitis, superior E51.2
　polymyositis — *see* Polymyositis
　pons, pontine I61.3
　posterior fossa (nontraumatic) I61.8
　　newborn P52.6
　postmenopausal N95.0
　postnasal R04.0
　postoperative — *see* Complications, postprocedural,
　　　hemorrhage, by site
　postpartum NEC (following delivery of placenta) O72.1
　　delayed or secondary O72.2
　　retained placenta O72.0
　　third stage O72.0
　pregnancy — *see* Hemorrhage, antepartum
　preretinal — *see* Hemorrhage, retina
　prostate N42.1
　puerperal — *see* Hemorrhage, postpartum
　　delayed or secondary O72.2
　pulmonary R04.89
　　newborn P26.9
　　　massive P26.1
　　　specified NEC P26.8
　　tuberculous — *see* Tuberculosis, pulmonary
　purpura (primary) D69.3
　rectum (sphincter) K62.5
　　newborn P54.2
　recurring, following initial hemorrhage at time of injury
　　　T79.2 ☑
　renal N28.89
　respiratory passage or tract R04.9
　　specified NEC R04.89
　retina, retinal (vessels) H35.6- ☑
　　diabetic — *see* Diabetes, retinal, hemorrhage
　retroperitoneal R58
　scalp R58
　scrotum N50.1
　secondary (nontraumatic) R58
　　following initial hemorrhage at time of injury
　　　T79.2 ☑
　seminal vesicle N50.1
　skin R23.3
　　newborn P54.5
　slipped umbilical ligature P51.8
　spermatic cord N50.1
　spinal (cord) G95.19
　　newborn (birth injury) P11.5
　spleen D73.5
　　intraoperative — *see* Complications, intraoperative,
　　　hemorrhage, spleen
　　postprocedural — *see* Complications, postprocedu-
　　　ral, hemorrhage, spleen
　stomach K92.2
　　newborn P54.3
　　ulcer — *see* Ulcer, stomach, with hemorrhage
　subarachnoid (nontraumatic) — *see* Hemorrhage, in-
　　　tracranial, subarachnoid
　subconjunctival — *see also* Hemorrhage, conjunctiva
　　birth injury P15.3
　subcortical (brain) I61.0
　subcutaneous R23.3
　subdiaphragmatic R58
　subdural (acute) (nontraumatic) — *see* Hemorrhage,
　　　intracranial, subdural
　subependymal
　　newborn P52.0
　　　with intraventricular extension P52.1
　　　　and intracerebral extension P52.22
　subgaleal P12.2
　subhyaloid — *see* Hemorrhage, retina
　subperiosteal — *see* Disorder, bone, specified type NEC
　subretinal — *see* Hemorrhage, retina
　subtentorial — *see* Hemorrhage, intracranial, subdural
　subungual L60.8
　suprarenal (capsule) (gland) E27.49
　　newborn P54.4
　tentorium (traumatic) NEC — *see* Hemorrhage, brain
　　newborn (birth injury) P10.4

Hemorrhage, hemorrhagic — *continued*
testis N50.1
third stage (postpartum) O72.0
thorax — *see* Hemorrhage, lung
throat R04.1
thymus (gland) E32.8
thyroid (cyst) (gland) E07.89
tongue K14.8
tonsil J35.8
trachea — *see* Hemorrhage, lung
tracheobronchial R04.89
newborn P26.0
traumatic — *code to* specific injury
cerebellar — *see* Hemorrhage, brain
intracranial — *see* Hemorrhage, brain
recurring or secondary (following initial hemorrhage
at time of injury) T79.2 ☑
tuberculous NEC — *see also* Tuberculosis, pulmonary
A15.0
tunica vaginalis N50.1
ulcer — *code by* site under Ulcer, with hemorrhage
K27.4
umbilicus, umbilical
cord
after birth, newborn P51.9
complicating delivery O69.5 ☑
newborn P51.9
massive P51.0
slipped ligature P51.8
stump P51.9
urethra (idiopathic) N36.8
uterus, uterine (abnormal) N93.9
climacteric N92.4
complicating delivery — *see* Hemorrhage, complicating, delivery
dysfunctional or functional N93.8
intermenstrual (regular) N92.3
irregular N92.1
postmenopausal N95.0
postpartum — *see* Hemorrhage, postpartum
preclimacteric or premenopausal N92.4
prepubertal N93.8
pubertal N92.2
vagina (abnormal) N93.9
newborn P54.6
vas deferens N50.1
vasa previa O69.4 ☑
ventricular I61.5
vesical N32.89
viscera NEC R58
newborn P54.8
vitreous (humor) (intraocular) H43.1- ☑
vulva N90.89
Hemorrhoids (bleeding) (without mention of degree)
K64.9
1st degree (grade/stage I) (without prolapse outside
of anal canal) K64.0
2nd degree (grade/stage II) (that prolapse with straining but retract spontaneously) K64.1
3rd degree (grade/stage III) (that prolapse with straining and require manual replacement back inside
anal canal) K64.2
4th degree (grade/stage IV) (with prolapsed tissue that
cannot be manually replaced) K64.3
complicating
pregnancy O22.4 ☑
puerperium O87.2
external K64.4
with
thrombosis K64.5
internal (without mention of degree) K64.8
prolapsed K64.8
skin tags
anus K64.4
residual K64.4
specified NEC K64.8
strangulated — *see also* Hemorrhoids, by degree K64.8
thrombosed — *see also* Hemorrhoids, by degree K64.5
ulcerated — *see also* Hemorrhoids, by degree K64.8
Hemosalpinx N83.6
with
hematocolpos N89.7
hematometra N85.7
with hematocolpos N89.7
Hemosiderosis (dietary) E83.19
pulmonary, idiopathic E83.1- ☑ *[J84.03]*
transfusion T80.89 ☑
Hemothorax (bacterial) (nontuberculous) J94.2

Hemothorax — *continued*
newborn P54.8
traumatic S27.1 ☑
with pneumothorax S27.2 ☑
tuberculous NEC A15.6
Henoch (-Schönlein) **disease or syndrome** (purpura)
D69.0
Henpue, henpuye A66.6
Hepar lobatum (syphilitic) A52.74
Hepatalgia K76.89
Hepatitis K75.9
acute B17.9
with coma K72.01
with hepatic failure — *see* Failure, hepatic
alcoholic — *see* Hepatitis, alcoholic
infectious B17.9
non-viral K72.0 ☑
viral B17.9
alcoholic (acute) (chronic) K70.10
with ascites K70.11
amebic — *see* Abscess, liver, amebic
anicteric, (viral) — *see* Hepatitis, viral
antigen-associated (HAA) — *see* Hepatitis, B
Australia-antigen (positive) — *see* Hepatitis, B
autoimmune K75.4
B B19.10
with hepatic coma B19.11
acute B16.9
with
delta-agent (coinfection) (without hepatic
coma) B16.1
with hepatic coma B16.0
hepatic coma (without delta-agent coinfection) B16.2
chronic B18.1
with delta-agent B18.0
bacterial NEC K75.89
C (viral) B19.20
with hepatic coma B19.21
acute B17.10
with hepatic coma B17.11
chronic B18.2
catarrhal (acute) B15.9
with hepatic coma B15.0
cholangiolitic K75.89
cholestatic K75.89
chronic K73.9
active K73.2
lobular NEC K73.1
persistent NEC K73.0
specified NEC K73.8
cytomegaloviral B25.1
due to ethanol (acute) (chronic) — *see* Hepatitis, alcoholic
epidemic B15.9
with hepatic coma B15.0
fulminant NEC (viral) — *see* Hepatitis, viral
granulomatous NEC K75.3
herpesviral B00.81
history of
B Z86.19
C Z86.19
homologous serum — *see* Hepatitis, viral, type B
in (due to)
mumps B26.81
toxoplasmosis (acquired) B58.1
congenital (active) P37.1 *[K77]*
infectious, infective B15.9
acute (subacute) B17.9
chronic B18.9
inoculation — *see* Hepatitis, viral, type B
interstitial (chronic) K74.69
lupoid NEC K75.4
malignant NEC (with hepatic failure) K72.90
with coma K72.91
neonatal (idiopathic) (toxic) P59.29
neonatal giant cell P59.29
newborn P59.29
non-viral K72.0 ☑
postimmunization — *see* Hepatitis, viral, type B
post-transfusion — *see* Hepatitis, viral, type B
reactive, nonspecific K75.2
serum — *see* Hepatitis, viral, type B
specified type NEC
with hepatic failure — *see* Failure, hepatic
syphilitic (late) A52.74
congenital (early) A50.08 *[K77]*
late A50.59 *[K77]*

Hepatitis — *continued*
syphilitic — *continued*
secondary A51.45
toxic — *see also* Disease, liver, toxic K71.6
tuberculous A18.83
viral, virus B19.9
with hepatic coma B19.0
acute B17.9
chronic B18.9
specified NEC B18.8
type
B B18.1
with delta-agent B18.0
C B18.2
congenital P35.3
coxsackie B33.8 *[K77]*
cytomegalic inclusion B25.1
in remission, any type — *code to* Hepatitis, chroni
by type
non-A, non-B B17.8
specified type NEC (with or without coma) B17.8
type
A B15.9
with hepatic coma B15.0
B B19.10
with hepatic coma B19.11
acute B16.9
with
delta-agent (coinfection) (without
hepatic coma) B16.1
with hepatic coma B16.0
hepatic coma (without delta-agent
coinfection) B16.2
chronic B18.1
with delta-agent B18.0
C B19.20
with hepatic coma B19.21
acute B17.10
with hepatic coma B17.11
chronic B18.2
E B17.2
non-A, non-B B17.8
Hepatization lung (acute) — *see* Pneumonia, lobar
Hepatoblastoma C22.2
Hepatocarcinoma C22.0
Hepatocholangiocarcinoma C22.0
Hepatocholangioma, benign D13.4
Hepatocholangitis K75.89
Hepatolenticular degeneration E83.01
Hepatoma (malignant) C22.0
benign D13.4
embryonal C22.0
Hepatomegaly — *see also* Hypertrophy, liver
with splenomegaly R16.2
congenital Q44.7
in mononucleosis
gammaherpesviral B27.09
infectious specified NEC B27.89
Hepatoptosis K76.89
Hepatorenal syndrome following labor and delive
O90.4
Hepatosis K76.89
Hepatosplenomegaly R16.2
hyperlipemic (Bürger-Grütz type) E78.3 *[K77]*
Hereditary — *see* condition
Heredodegeneration, macular — *see* Dystrophy, reti
Heredopathia atactica polyneuritiformis G60.1
Heredosyphilis — *see* Syphilis, congenital
Herlitz' syndrome Q81.1
Hermansky-Pudlak syndrome E70.331
Hermaphrodite, hermaphroditism (true) Q56.0
46,XX with streak gonads Q99.1
46,XX/46,XY Q99.0
46,XY with streak gonads Q99.1
chimera 46,XX/46,XY Q99.0
Hernia, hernial (acquired) (recurrent) K46.9
with
gangrene — *see* Hernia, by site, with, gangrene
incarceration — *see* Hernia, by site, with, obstructic
irreducible — *see* Hernia, by site, with, obstructic
obstruction — *see* Hernia, by site, with, obstructic
strangulation — *see* Hernia, by site, with, obstru
tion
abdomen, abdominal K46.9
with
gangrene (and obstruction) K46.1
obstruction K46.0
femoral — *see* Hernia, femoral

Hernia, hernial — *continued*
  abdomen, abdominal — *continued*
    incisional — *see* Hernia, incisional
    inguinal — *see* Hernia, inguinal
    specified site NEC K45.8
      with
        gangrene (and obstruction) K45.1
        obstruction K45.0
    umbilical — *see* Hernia, umbilical
    wall — *see* Hernia, ventral
  appendix — *see* Hernia, abdomen
  bladder (mucosa) (sphincter)
    congenital (female) (male) Q79.51
    female — *see* Cystocele
    male N32.89
  brain, congenital — *see* Encephalocele
  cartilage, vertebra — *see* Displacement, intervertebral
    disc
  cerebral, congenital — *see also* Encephalocele
    endaural Q01.8
  ciliary body (traumatic) S05.2- ☑
  colon — *see* Hernia, abdomen
  Cooper's — *see* Hernia, abdomen, specified site NEC
  crural — *see* Hernia, femoral
  diaphragm, diaphragmatic K44.9
    with
      gangrene (and obstruction) K44.1
      obstruction K44.0
    congenital Q79.0
  direct (inguinal) — *see* Hernia, inguinal
  diverticulum, intestine — *see* Hernia, abdomen
  double (inguinal) — *see* Hernia, inguinal, bilateral
  due to adhesions (with obstruction) K56.50
  epigastric — *see also* Hernia, ventral K43.9
  esophageal hiatus — *see* Hernia, hiatal
  external (inguinal) — *see* Hernia, inguinal
  fallopian tube N83.4- ☑
  fascia M62.89
  femoral K41.90
    with
      gangrene (and obstruction) K41.40
        not specified as recurrent K41.40
        recurrent K41.41
      obstruction K41.30
        not specified as recurrent K41.30
        recurrent K41.31
    not specified as recurrent K41.90
    recurrent K41.91
    bilateral K41.20
      with
        gangrene (and obstruction) K41.10
          not specified as recurrent K41.10
          recurrent K41.11
        obstruction K41.00
          not specified as recurrent K41.00
          recurrent K41.01
      not specified as recurrent K41.20
      recurrent K41.21
    unilateral K41.90
      with
        gangrene (and obstruction) K41.40
          not specified as recurrent K41.40
          recurrent K41.41
        obstruction K41.30
          not specified as recurrent K41.30
          recurrent K41.31
      not specified as recurrent K41.90
      recurrent K41.91
  foramen magnum G93.5
    congenital Q01.8
  funicular (umbilical) — *see also* Hernia, umbilicus
    spermatic (cord) — *see* Hernia, inguinal
  gastrointestinal tract — *see* Hernia, abdomen
  Hesselbach's — *see* Hernia, femoral, specified site NEC
  hiatal (esophageal) (sliding) K44.9
    with
      gangrene (and obstruction) K44.1
      obstruction K44.0
    congenital Q40.1
  hypogastric — *see* Hernia, ventral
  incarcerated — *see also* Hernia, by site, with obstruction
    with gangrene — *see* Hernia, by site, with gangrene
  incisional K43.2
    with
      gangrene (and obstruction) K43.1
      obstruction K43.0
  indirect (inguinal) — *see* Hernia, inguinal

Hernia, hernial — *continued*
  inguinal (direct) (external) (funicular) (indirect) (internal) (oblique) (scrotal) (sliding) K40.90
    with
      gangrene (and obstruction) K40.40
        not specified as recurrent K40.40
        recurrent K40.41
      obstruction K40.30
        not specified as recurrent K40.30
        recurrent K40.31
    not specified as recurrent K40.90
    recurrent K40.91
    bilateral K40.20
      with
        gangrene (and obstruction) K40.10
          not specified as recurrent K40.10
          recurrent K40.11
        obstruction K40.00
          not specified as recurrent K40.00
          recurrent K40.01
      not specified as recurrent K40.20
      recurrent K40.21
    unilateral K40.90
      with
        gangrene (and obstruction) K40.40
          not specified as recurrent K40.40
          recurrent K40.41
        obstruction K40.30
          not specified as recurrent K40.30
          recurrent K40.31
      not specified as recurrent K40.90
      recurrent K40.91
  internal — *see also* Hernia, abdomen
    inguinal — *see* Hernia, inguinal
  interstitial — *see* Hernia, abdomen
  intervertebral cartilage or disc — *see* Displacement, intervertebral disc
  intestine, intestinal — *see* Hernia, by site
  intra-abdominal — *see* Hernia, abdomen
  iris (traumatic) S05.2- ☑
  irreducible — *see also* Hernia, by site, with obstruction
    with gangrene — *see* Hernia, by site, with gangrene
  ischiatic — *see* Hernia, abdomen, specified site NEC
  ischiorectal — *see* Hernia, abdomen, specified site NEC
  lens (traumatic) S05.2- ☑
  linea (alba) (semilunaris) — *see* Hernia, ventral
  Littre's — *see* Hernia, abdomen
  lumbar — *see* Hernia, abdomen, specified site NEC
  lung (subcutaneous) J98.4
  mediastinum J98.59
  mesenteric (internal) — *see* Hernia, abdomen
  midline — *see* Hernia, ventral
  muscle (sheath) M62.89
  nucleus pulposus — *see* Displacement, intervertebral disc
  oblique (inguinal) — *see* Hernia, inguinal
  obstructive — *see also* Hernia, by site, with obstruction
    with gangrene — *see* Hernia, by site, with gangrene
  obturator — *see* Hernia, abdomen, specified site NEC
  omental — *see* Hernia, abdomen
  ovary N83.4- ☑
  oviduct N83.4- ☑
  paraesophageal — *see also* Hernia, diaphragm
    congenital Q40.1
  parastomal K43.5
    with
      gangrene (and obstruction) K43.4
      obstruction K43.3
  paraumbilical — *see* Hernia, umbilicus
  perineal — *see* Hernia, abdomen, specified site NEC
  Petit's — *see* Hernia, abdomen, specified site NEC
  postoperative — *see* Hernia, incisional
  pregnant uterus — *see* Abnormal, uterus in pregnancy or childbirth
  prevesical N32.89
  properitoneal — *see* Hernia, abdomen, specified site NEC
  pudendal — *see* Hernia, abdomen, specified site NEC
  rectovaginal N81.6
  retroperitoneal — *see* Hernia, abdomen, specified site NEC
  Richter's — *see* Hernia, abdomen, with obstruction
  Rieux's, Riex's — *see* Hernia, abdomen, specified site NEC

Hernia, hernial — *continued*
  sac condition (adhesion) (dropsy) (inflammation) (laceration) (suppuration) — *code by site under* Hernia
  sciatic — *see* Hernia, abdomen, specified site NEC
  scrotum, scrotal — *see* Hernia, inguinal
  sliding (inguinal) — *see also* Hernia, inguinal
    hiatus — *see* Hernia, hiatal
  spigelian — *see* Hernia, ventral
  spinal — *see* Spina bifida
  strangulated — *see also* Hernia, by site, with obstruction
    with gangrene — *see* Hernia, by site, with gangrene
  subxiphoid — *see* Hernia, ventral
  supra-umbilicus — *see* Hernia, ventral
  tendon — *see* Disorder, tendon, specified type NEC
  Treitz's (fossa) — *see* Hernia, abdomen, specified site NEC
  tunica vaginalis Q55.29
  umbilicus, umbilical K42.9
    with
      gangrene (and obstruction) K42.1
      obstruction K42.0
  ureter N28.89
  urethra, congenital Q64.79
  urinary meatus, congenital Q64.79
  uterus N81.4
    pregnant — *see* Abnormal, uterus in pregnancy or childbirth
  vaginal (anterior) (wall) — *see* Cystocele
  Velpeau's — *see* Hernia, femoral
  ventral K43.9
    with
      gangrene (and obstruction) K43.7
      obstruction K43.6
    incisional K43.2
      with
        gangrene (and obstruction) K43.1
        obstruction K43.0
      recurrent — *see* Hernia, incisional
    specified NEC K43.9
      with
        gangrene (and obstruction) K43.7
        obstruction K43.6
  vesical
    congenital (female) (male) Q79.51
    female — *see* Cystocele
    male N32.89
  vitreous (into wound) S05.2- ☑
    into anterior chamber — *see* Prolapse, vitreous
Herniation — *see also* Hernia
  brain (stem) G93.5
  cerebral G93.5
  mediastinum J98.59
  nucleus pulposus — *see* Displacement, intervertebral disc
Herpangina B08.5
Herpes, herpesvirus, herpetic B00.9
  anogenital A60.9
    perianal skin A60.1
    rectum A60.1
    urogenital tract A60.00
      cervix A60.03
      male genital organ NEC A60.02
      penis A60.01
      specified site NEC A60.09
      vagina A60.04
      vulva A60.04
  blepharitis (zoster) B02.39
    simplex B00.59
  circinatus B35.4
    bullosus L12.0
  conjunctivitis (simplex) B00.53
    zoster B02.31
  cornea B02.33
  encephalitis B00.4
    due to herpesvirus 6 B10.01
    due to herpesvirus 7 B10.09
    specified NEC B10.09
  eye (zoster) B02.30
    simplex B00.50
  eyelid (zoster) B02.39
    simplex B00.59
  facialis B00.1
  febrilis B00.1
  geniculate ganglionitis B02.21
  genital, genitalis A60.00
    female A60.09

▸ Subterms under main terms may continue to next column or page   ☑ **Additional Character Required** — Refer to the Tabular List for Character Selection   **171**

Hernia, hernial — Herpes, herpesvirus, herpetic

Herpes, herpesvirus, herpetic — *continued*
  genital, genitalis — *continued*
    male A60.02
  gestational, gestationis O26.4- ☑
  gingivostomatitis B00.2
  human B00.9
    1 — *see* Herpes, simplex
    2 — *see* Herpes, simplex
    3 — *see* Varicella
    4 — *see* Mononucleosis, Epstein-Barr (virus)
    5 — *see* Disease, cytomegalic inclusion (generalized)
    6
        encephalitis B10.01
        specified NEC B10.81
    7
        encephalitis B10.09
        specified NEC B10.82
    8 B10.89
  infection NEC B10.89
    Kaposi's sarcoma associated B10.89
  iridocyclitis (simplex) B00.51
    zoster B02.32
  iris (vesicular erythema multiforme) L51.9
  iritis (simplex) B00.51
  Kaposi's sarcoma associated B10.89
  keratitis (simplex) (dendritic) (disciform) (interstitial) B00.52
    zoster (interstitial) B02.33
  keratoconjunctivitis (simplex) B00.52
    zoster B02.33
  labialis B00.1
  lip B00.1
  meningitis (simplex) B00.3
    zoster B02.1
  ophthalmicus (zoster) NEC B02.30
    simplex B00.50
  penis A60.01
  perianal skin A60.1
  pharyngitis, pharyngotonsillitis B00.2
  rectum A60.1
  scrotum A60.02
  sepsis B00.7
  simplex B00.9
    complicated NEC B00.89
    congenital P35.2
    conjunctivitis B00.53
    external ear B00.1
    eyelid B00.59
    hepatitis B00.81
    keratitis (interstitial) B00.52
    myelitis B00.82
    specified complication NEC B00.89
    visceral B00.89
  stomatitis B00.2
  tonsurans B35.0
  visceral B00.89
  vulva A60.04
  whitlow B00.89
  zoster — *see also* condition B02.9
    auricularis B02.21
    complicated NEC B02.8
    conjunctivitis B02.31
    disseminated B02.7
    encephalitis B02.0
    eye (lid) B02.39
    geniculate ganglionitis B02.21
    keratitis (interstitial) B02.33
    meningitis B02.1
    myelitis B02.24
    neuritis, neuralgia B02.29
    ophthalmicus NEC B02.30
    oticus B02.21
    polyneuropathy B02.23
    specified complication NEC B02.8
    trigeminal neuralgia B02.22
Herpesvirus (human) — *see* Herpes
Herpetophobia F40.218
Herrick's anemia — *see* Disease, sickle-cell
Hers' disease E74.09
Herter-Gee syndrome K90.0
Herxheimer's reaction R68.89
Hesitancy
  of micturition R39.11
  urinary R39.11
Hesselbach's hernia — *see* Hernia, femoral, specified site NEC
Heterochromia (congenital) Q13.2
  cataract — *see* Cataract, complicated

Heterochromia — *continued*
  cyclitis (Fuchs) — *see* Cyclitis, Fuchs' heterochromic
  hair L67.1
  iritis — *see* Cyclitis, Fuchs' heterochromic
  retained metallic foreign body (nonmagnetic) — *see* Foreign body, intraocular, old, retained
    magnetic — *see* Foreign body, intraocular, old, retained, magnetic
  uveitis — *see* Cyclitis, Fuchs' heterochromic
Heterophoria — *see* Strabismus, heterophoria
Heterophyes, heterophyiasis (small intestine) B66.8
Heterotopia, heterotopic — *see also* Malposition, congenital
  cerebralis Q04.8
Heterotropia — *see* Strabismus
Heubner-Herter disease K90.0
Hexadactylism Q69.9
HGSIL (cytology finding) (high grade squamous intraepithelial lesion on cytologic smear) (Pap smear finding)
  anus R85.613
  cervix R87.613
    biopsy (histology) finding — *see* Neoplasia, intraepithelial, cervix, grade II or grade III
  vagina R87.623
    biopsy (histology) finding — *see* Neoplasia, intraepithelial, cervix, grade II or grade III
Hibernoma — *see* Lipoma
Hiccup, hiccough R06.6
  epidemic B33.0
  psychogenic F45.8
Hidden penis (congenital) Q55.64
  acquired N48.83
Hidradenitis (axillaris) (suppurative) L73.2
Hidradenoma (nodular) — *see also* Neoplasm, skin, benign
  clear cell — *see* Neoplasm, skin, benign
  papillary — *see* Neoplasm, skin, benign
Hidrocystoma — *see* Neoplasm, skin, benign
High
  altitude effects T70.20 ☑
    anoxia T70.29 ☑
    on
        ears T70.0 ☑
        sinuses T70.1 ☑
    polycythemia D75.1
  arch
    foot Q66.7- ☑
    palate, congenital Q38.5
  arterial tension — *see* Hypertension
  basal metabolic rate R94.8
  blood pressure — *see also* Hypertension
    borderline R03.0
    reading (incidental) (isolated) (nonspecific), without diagnosis of hypertension R03.0
  cholesterol E78.00
    with high triglycerides E78.2
  diaphragm (congenital) Q79.1
  expressed emotional level within family Z63.8
  head at term O32.4 ☑
  palate, congenital Q38.5
  risk
    infant NEC Z76.2
    sexual behavior (heterosexual) Z72.51
        bisexual Z72.53
        homosexual Z72.52
  scrotal testis, testes
    bilateral Q53.23
    unilateral Q53.13
  temperature (of unknown origin) R50.9
  thoracic rib Q76.6
  triglycerides E78.1
    with high cholesterol E78.2
Hildenbrand's disease A75.0
Hilum — *see* condition
Hip — *see* condition
Hippel's disease Q85.8
Hippophobia F40.218
Hippus H57.09
Hirschsprung's disease or megacolon Q43.1
Hirsutism, hirsuties L68.0
Hirudiniasis
  external B88.3
  internal B83.4
Hiss-Russell dysentery A03.1
Histidinemia, histidinuria E70.41
Histiocytoma — *see also* Neoplasm, skin, benign

Histiocytoma — *continued*
  fibrous — *see also* Neoplasm, skin, benign
    atypical — *see* Neoplasm, connective tissue, uncertain behavior
    malignant — *see* Neoplasm, connective tissue, malignant
Histiocytosis D76.3
  acute differentiated progressive C96.0
  Langerhans' cell NEC C96.6
    multifocal X
        multisystemic (disseminated) C96.0
        unisystemic C96.5
    pulmonary, adult (adult PLCH) J84.82
    unifocal (X) C96.6
  lipid, lipoid D76.3
    essential E75.29
  malignant C96.A (*following* C96.6)
  mononuclear phagocytes NEC D76.1
    Langerhans' cells C96.6
  non-Langerhans cell D76.3
  polyostotic sclerosing D76.3
  sinus, with massive lymphadenopathy D76.3
  syndrome NEC D76.3
  X NEC C96.6
    acute (progressive) C96.0
    chronic C96.6
    multifocal C96.5
    multisystemic C96.0
    unifocal C96.6
Histoplasmosis B39.9
  with pneumonia NEC B39.2
  African B39.5
  American — *see* Histoplasmosis, capsulati
  capsulati B39.4
    disseminated B39.3
    generalized B39.3
    pulmonary B39.2
        acute B39.0
        chronic B39.1
  Darling's B39.4
  duboisii B39.5
  lung NEC B39.2
History
  family (of) — *see also* History, personal (of)
    alcohol abuse Z81.1
    allergy NEC Z84.89
    anemia Z83.2
    arthritis Z82.61
    asthma Z82.5
    blindness Z82.1
    cardiac death (sudden) Z82.41
    carrier of genetic disease Z84.81
    chromosomal anomaly Z82.79
    chronic
        disabling disease NEC Z82.8
        lower respiratory disease Z82.5
    colonic polyps Z83.71
    congenital malformations and deformations Z82.7
        polycystic kidney Z82.71
    consanguinity Z84.3
    deafness Z82.2
    diabetes mellitus Z83.3
    disability NEC Z82.8
    disease or disorder (of)
        allergic NEC Z84.89
        behavioral NEC Z81.8
        blood and blood-forming organs Z83.2
        cardiovascular NEC Z82.49
        chronic disabling NEC Z82.8
        digestive Z83.79
        ear NEC Z83.52
        elevated lipoprotein (a) (Lp(a)) Z83.430
        endocrine NEC Z83.49
        eye NEC Z83.518
            glaucoma Z83.511
        familial hypercholesterolemia Z83.42
        genitourinary NEC Z84.2
        glaucoma Z83.511
        hematological Z83.2
        immune mechanism Z83.2
        infectious NEC Z83.1
        ischemic heart Z82.49
        kidney Z84.1
        lipoprotein metabolism Z83.438
        mental NEC Z81.8
        metabolic Z83.49
        musculoskeletal NEC Z82.69
        neurological NEC Z82.0

☑ **Additional Character Required** — Refer to the Tabular List for Character Selection   ▽ Subterms under main terms may continue to next column or page

History — *continued*
  family — *see also* History, personal — *continued*
    disease or disorder — *continued*
      nutritional Z83.49
      parasitic NEC Z83.1
      psychiatric NEC Z81.8
      respiratory NEC Z83.6
      skin and subcutaneous tissue NEC Z84.0
      specified NEC Z84.89
    drug abuse NEC Z81.3
    elevated lipoprotein (a) (Lp(a)) Z83.430
    epilepsy Z82.0
    familial hypercholesterolemia Z83.42
    genetic disease carrier Z84.81
    glaucoma Z83.511
    hearing loss Z82.2
    human immunodeficiency virus (HIV) infection Z83.0
    Huntington's chorea Z82.0
    hyperlipidemia, familial combined Z83.438
    intellectual disability Z81.0
    leukemia Z80.6
    lipidemia NEC Z83.438
    malignant neoplasm (of) NOS Z80.9
      bladder Z80.52
      breast Z80.3
      bronchus Z80.1
      digestive organ Z80.0
      gastrointestinal tract Z80.0
      genital organ Z80.49
        ovary Z80.41
        prostate Z80.42
        specified organ NEC Z80.49
        testis Z80.43
      hematopoietic NEC Z80.7
      intrathoracic organ NEC Z80.2
      kidney Z80.51
      lung Z80.1
      lymphatic NEC Z80.7
      ovary Z80.41
      prostate Z80.42
      respiratory organ NEC Z80.2
      specified site NEC Z80.8
      testis Z80.43
      trachea Z80.1
      urinary organ or tract Z80.59
        bladder Z80.52
        kidney Z80.51
    mental
      disorder NEC Z81.8
    multiple endocrine neoplasia (MEN) syndrome Z83.41
    osteoporosis Z82.62
    polycystic kidney Z82.71
    polyps (colon) Z83.71
    psychiatric disorder Z81.8
    psychoactive substance abuse NEC Z81.3
    respiratory condition NEC Z83.6
      asthma and other lower respiratory conditions Z82.5
    self-harmful behavior Z81.8
    SIDS (sudden infant death syndrome) Z84.82
    skin condition Z84.0
    specified condition NEC Z84.89
    stroke (cerebrovascular) Z82.3
    substance abuse NEC Z81.4
      alcohol Z81.1
      drug NEC Z81.3
      psychoactive NEC Z81.3
      tobacco Z81.2
    sudden
      cardiac death Z82.41
      infant death syndrome (SIDS) Z84.82
    tobacco abuse Z81.2
    violence, violent behavior Z81.8
    visual loss Z82.1
  personal (of) — *see also* History, family (of)
    abuse
      adult Z91.419
        forced labor or sexual exploitation Z91.42
        physical and sexual Z91.410
        psychological Z91.411
      childhood Z62.819
        forced labor or sexual exploitation in childhood Z62.813
        physical Z62.810
        psychological Z62.811
        sexual Z62.810
    alcohol dependence F10.21
    allergy (to) Z88.9

History — *continued*
  personal — *see also* History, family — *continued*
    allergy — *continued*
      analgesic agent NEC Z88.6
      anesthetic Z88.4
      antibiotic agent NEC Z88.1
      anti-infective agent NEC Z88.3
      contrast media Z91.041
      drugs, medicaments and biological substances Z88.9
        specified NEC Z88.8
      food Z91.018
        additives Z91.02
        eggs Z91.012
        milk products Z91.011
        peanuts Z91.010
        seafood Z91.013
        specified food NEC Z91.018
      insect Z91.038
        bee Z91.030
      latex Z91.040
      medicinal agents Z88.9
        specified NEC Z88.8
      narcotic agent NEC Z88.5
      nonmedicinal agents Z91.048
      penicillin Z88.0
      serum Z88.7
      specified NEC Z91.09
      sulfonamides Z88.2
      vaccine Z88.7
    anaphylactic shock Z87.892
    anaphylaxis Z87.892
    behavioral disorders Z86.59
    benign carcinoid tumor Z86.012
    benign neoplasm Z86.018
      brain Z86.011
      carcinoid Z86.012
      colonic polyps Z86.010
    brain injury (traumatic) Z87.820
    breast implant removal Z98.86
    calculi, renal Z87.442
    cancer — *see* History, personal (of), malignant neoplasm (of)
    cardiac arrest (death), successfully resuscitated Z86.74
    cerebral infarction without residual deficit Z86.73
    cervical dysplasia Z87.410
    chemotherapy for neoplastic condition Z92.21
    childhood abuse — *see* History, personal (of), abuse
    cleft lip (corrected) Z87.730
    cleft palate (corrected) Z87.730
    collapsed vertebra (healed) Z87.311
      due to osteoporosis Z87.310
    combat and operational stress reaction Z86.51
    congenital malformation (corrected) Z87.798
      circulatory system (corrected) Z87.74
      digestive system (corrected) NEC Z87.738
      ear (corrected) Z87.721
      eye (corrected) Z87.720
      face and neck (corrected) Z87.790
      genitourinary system (corrected) NEC Z87.718
      heart (corrected) Z87.74
      integument (corrected) Z87.76
      limb(s) (corrected) Z87.76
      musculoskeletal system (corrected) Z87.76
      neck (corrected) Z87.790
      nervous system (corrected) NEC Z87.728
      respiratory system (corrected) Z87.75
      sense organs (corrected) NEC Z87.728
      specified NEC Z87.798
    contraception Z92.0
    deployment (military) Z91.82
    diabetic foot ulcer Z86.31
    disease or disorder (of) Z87.898
      anaphylaxis Z87.892
      blood and blood-forming organs Z86.2
      circulatory system Z86.79
        specified condition NEC Z86.79
      connective tissue Z87.39
      digestive system Z87.19
        colonic polyp Z86.010
        peptic ulcer disease Z87.11
        specified condition NEC Z87.19
      ear Z86.69
      endocrine Z86.39
        diabetic foot ulcer Z86.31
        gestational diabetes Z86.32
        specified type NEC Z86.39
      eye Z86.69

History — *continued*
  personal — *see also* History, family — *continued*
    disease or disorder — *continued*
      genital (track) system NEC
        female Z87.42
        male Z87.438
      hematological Z86.2
      Hodgkin Z85.71
      immune mechanism Z86.2
      infectious Z86.19
        malaria Z86.13
        Methicillin resistant Staphylococcus aureus (MRSA) Z86.14
        poliomyelitis Z86.12
        specified NEC Z86.19
        tuberculosis Z86.11
      mental NEC Z86.59
      metabolic Z86.39
        diabetic foot ulcer Z86.31
        gestational diabetes Z86.32
        specified type NEC Z86.39
      musculoskeletal NEC Z87.39
      nervous system Z86.69
      nutritional Z86.39
      parasitic Z86.19
      respiratory system NEC Z87.09
      sense organs Z86.69
      skin Z87.2
      specified site or type NEC Z87.898
      subcutaneous tissue Z87.2
      trophoblastic Z87.59
      urinary system NEC Z87.448
    drug dependence — *see* Dependence, drug, by type, in remission
    drug therapy
      antineoplastic chemotherapy Z92.21
      estrogen Z92.23
      immunosupression Z92.25
      inhaled steroids Z92.240
      monoclonal drug Z92.22
      specified NEC Z92.29
      steroid Z92.241
      systemic steroids Z92.241
    dysplasia
      cervical (mild) (moderate) Z87.410
        severe (grade III) Z86.001
      prostatic Z87.430
      vaginal (mild) (moderate) Z87.411
        severe (grade III) Z86.002
      vulvar (mild) (moderate) Z87.412
        severe (grade III) Z86.002
    embolism (venous) Z86.718
      pulmonary Z86.711
    encephalitis Z86.61
    estrogen therapy Z92.23
    extracorporeal membrane oxygenation (ECMO) Z92.81
    failed conscious sedation Z92.83
    failed moderate sedation Z92.83
    fall, falling Z91.81
    forced labor or sexual exploitation Z91.42
      in childhood Z62.813
    fracture (healed)
      fatigue Z87.312
      fragility Z87.310
      osteoporosis Z87.310
      pathological NEC Z87.311
      stress Z87.312
      traumatic Z87.81
    gestational diabetes Z86.32
    hepatitis
      B Z86.19
      C Z86.19
    Hodgkin disease Z85.71
    hyperthermia, malignant Z88.4
    hypospadias (corrected) Z87.710
    hysterectomy Z90.710
    immunosupression therapy Z92.25
    in situ neoplasm
      breast Z86.000
      cervix uteri Z86.001
      digestive organs, specified NEC Z86.004
      esophagus Z86.003
      genital organs, specified NEC Z86.002
      melanoma Z86.006
      middle ear Z86.005
      oral cavity Z86.003
      respiratory system Z86.005
      skin Z86.007

History — *continued*
  personal — *see also* History, family — *continued*
    in situ neoplasm — *continued*
      specified NEC Z86.008
      stomach Z86.003
    in utero procedure during pregnancy Z98.870
    in utero procedure while a fetus Z98.871
    infection NEC Z86.19
      central nervous system Z86.61
      latent tuberculosis Z86.15
      Methicillin resistant Staphylococcus aureus (MRSA) Z86.14
      urinary (recurrent) (tract) Z87.440
    injury NEC Z87.828
    irradiation Z92.3
    kidney stones Z87.442
    latent tuberculosis infection Z86.15
    leukemia Z85.6
    lymphoma (non-Hodgkin) Z85.72
    malignant melanoma (skin) Z85.820
    malignant neoplasm (of) Z85.9
      accessory sinuses Z85.22
      anus NEC Z85.048
        carcinoid Z85.040
      bladder Z85.51
      bone Z85.830
      brain Z85.841
      breast Z85.3
      bronchus NEC Z85.118
        carcinoid Z85.110
      carcinoid — *see* History, personal (of), malignant neoplasm, by site, carcinoid
      cervix Z85.41
      colon NEC Z85.038
        carcinoid Z85.030
      digestive organ Z85.00
        specified NEC Z85.09
      endocrine gland NEC Z85.858
      epididymis Z85.48
      esophagus Z85.01
      eye Z85.840
      gastrointestinal tract — *see* History, malignant neoplasm, digestive organ
      genital organ
        female Z85.40
          specified NEC Z85.44
        male Z85.45
          specified NEC Z85.49
      hematopoietic NEC Z85.79
      intrathoracic organ Z85.20
      kidney NEC Z85.528
        carcinoid Z85.520
      large intestine NEC Z85.038
        carcinoid Z85.030
      larynx Z85.21
      liver Z85.05
      lung NEC Z85.118
        carcinoid Z85.110
      mediastinum Z85.29
      Merkel cell Z85.821
      middle ear Z85.22
      nasal cavities Z85.22
      nervous system NEC Z85.848
      oral cavity Z85.819
        specified site NEC Z85.818
      ovary Z85.43
      pancreas Z85.07
      pelvis Z85.53
      pharynx Z85.819
        specified site NEC Z85.818
      pleura Z85.29
      prostate Z85.46
      rectosigmoid junction NEC Z85.048
        carcinoid Z85.040
      rectum NEC Z85.048
        carcinoid Z85.040
      respiratory organ Z85.20
      sinuses, accessory Z85.22
      skin NEC Z85.828
        melanoma Z85.820
        Merkel cell Z85.821
      small intestine NEC Z85.068
        carcinoid Z85.060
      soft tissue Z85.831
      specified site NEC Z85.89
      stomach NEC Z85.028
        carcinoid Z85.020
      testis Z85.47
      thymus NEC Z85.238

History — *continued*
  personal — *see also* History, family — *continued*
    malignant neoplasm — *continued*
      thymus — *continued*
        carcinoid Z85.230
      thyroid Z85.850
      tongue Z85.810
      trachea Z85.12
      urinary organ or tract Z85.50
        specified NEC Z85.59
      uterus Z85.42
    maltreatment Z91.89
    medical treatment NEC Z92.89
    melanoma Z85.820
      in situ Z86.006
      malignant (skin) Z85.820
    meningitis Z86.61
    mental disorder Z86.59
    Merkel cell carcinoma (skin) Z85.821
    Methicillin resistant Staphylococcus aureus (MRSA) Z86.14
    military deployment Z91.82
    military war, peacekeeping and humanitarian deployment (current or past conflict) Z91.82
    myocardial infarction (old) I25.2
    neglect (in)
      adult Z91.412
      childhood Z62.812
    neoplasia
      anal intraepithelial, III [AIN III] Z86.004
      high-grade prostatic intraepithelial, III [HGPIN III] Z86.002
      vaginal intraepithelial, III [VAIN III] Z86.002
      vulvar intraepithelial, III [VIN III] Z86.002
    neoplasm
      benign Z86.018
        brain Z86.011
        colon polyp Z86.010
      in situ
        breast Z86.000
        cervix uteri Z86.001
        digestive organs, specified NEC Z86.004
        esophagus Z86.003
        genital organs, specified NEC Z86.002
        melanoma Z86.006
        middle ear Z86.005
        oral cavity Z86.003
        respiratory system Z86.005
        skin Z86.007
        specified NEC Z86.008
        stomach Z86.003
      malignant — *see* History of, malignant neoplasm
      uncertain behavior Z86.03
    nephrotic syndrome Z87.441
    nicotine dependence Z87.891
    noncompliance with medical treatment or regimen — *see* Noncompliance
    nutritional deficiency Z86.39
    obstetric complications Z87.59
      childbirth Z87.59
      pregnancy Z87.59
      pre-term labor Z87.51
      puerperium Z87.59
    osteoporosis fractures Z87.31 ☑
    parasuicide (attempt) Z91.5
    physical trauma NEC Z87.828
      self-harm or suicide attempt Z91.5
    pneumonia (recurrent) Z87.01
    poisoning NEC Z91.89
      self-harm or suicide attempt Z91.5
    poor personal hygiene Z91.89
    preterm labor Z87.51
    procedure during pregnancy Z98.870
    procedure while a fetus Z98.871
    prolonged reversible ischemic neurologic deficit (PRIND) Z86.73
    prostatic dysplasia Z87.430
    psychological
      abuse
        adult Z91.411
        child Z62.811
      trauma, specified NEC Z91.49
    radiation therapy Z92.3
    removal
      implant
        breast Z98.86
    renal calculi Z87.442
    respiratory condition NEC Z87.09
    retained foreign body fully removed Z87.821

History — *continued*
  personal — *see also* History, family — *continued*
    risk factors NEC Z91.89
    self-harm Z91.5
    self-poisoning attempt Z91.5
    sex reassignment Z87.890
    sleep-wake cycle problem Z72.821
    specified NEC Z87.898
    steroid therapy (systemic) Z92.241
      inhaled Z92.240
    stroke without residual deficits Z86.73
    substance abuse NEC F10-F19
    sudden cardiac arrest Z86.74
    sudden cardiac death successfully resuscitated Z86.74
    suicide attempt Z91.5
    surgery NEC Z98.890
      with uterine scar Z98.891
      sex reassignment Z87.890
      transplant — *see* Transplant
    thrombophlebitis Z86.72
    thrombosis (venous) Z86.718
      pulmonary Z86.711
    tobacco dependence Z87.891
    transient ischemic attack (TIA) without residual deficits Z86.73
    trauma (physical) NEC Z87.828
      psychological NEC Z91.49
      self-harm Z91.5
    traumatic brain injury Z87.820
    tuberculosis, latent infection Z86.15
    unhealthy sleep-wake cycle Z72.821
    unintended awareness under general anesthesia Z92.84
    urinary calculi Z87.442
    urinary (recurrent) (tract) infection(s) Z87.440
    uterine scar from previous surgery Z98.891
    vaginal dysplasia Z87.411
    venous thrombosis or embolism Z86.718
      pulmonary Z86.711
    vulvar dysplasia Z87.412

His-Werner disease A79.0
HIV — *see also* Human, immunodeficiency virus B20
  laboratory evidence (nonconclusive) R75
  nonconclusive test (in infants) R75
  positive, seropositive Z21
Hives (bold) — *see* Urticaria
Hoarseness R49.0
Hobo Z59.0
Hodgkin disease — *see* Lymphoma, Hodgkin
Hodgson's disease I71.2
  ruptured I71.1
Hoffa-Kastert disease E88.89
Hoffa's disease E88.89
Hoffmann-Bouveret syndrome I47.9
Hoffmann's syndrome E03.9 *[G73.7]*
Hole (round)
  macula H35.34- ☑
  retina (without detachment) — *see* Break, retina, round hole
    with detachment — *see* Detachment, retina, with retinal, break
Holiday relief care Z75.5
Hollenhorst's plaque — *see* Occlusion, artery, retina
Hollow foot (congenital) Q66.7- ☑
  acquired — *see* Deformity, limb, foot, specified NEC
Holoprosencephaly Q04.2
Holt-Oram syndrome Q87.2
Homelessness Z59.0
Homesickness — *see* Disorder, adjustment
Homocystinemia, homocystinuria E72.11
Homogentisate 1,2-dioxygenase deficiency E70.29
Homologous serum hepatitis (prophylactic) (therapeutic) — *see* Hepatitis, viral, type B
Honeycomb lung J98.4
  congenital Q33.0
Hooded
  clitoris Q52.6
  penis Q55.69
Hookworm (disease) (infection) (infestation) B76.9
  with anemia B76.9 *[D63.8]*
  specified NEC B76.8
Hordeolum (eyelid) (externum) (recurrent) H00.019
  internum H00.029
    left H00.026
      lower H00.025
      upper H00.024
    right H00.023

Hordeolum — *continued*
  internum — *continued*
    right — *continued*
      lower H00.022
      upper H00.021
    left H00.016
      lower H00.015
      upper H00.014
    right H00.013
      lower H00.012
      upper H00.011
Horn
  cutaneous L85.8
  nail L60.2
    congenital Q84.6
Horner (-Claude Bernard) **syndrome** G90.2
  traumatic — *see* Injury, nerve, cervical sympathetic
Horseshoe kidney (congenital) Q63.1
Horton's headache or neuralgia G44.099
  intractable G44.091
  not intractable G44.099
Hospital hopper syndrome — *see* Disorder, factitious
Hospitalism in children — *see* Disorder, adjustment
Hostility R45.5
  towards child Z62.3
Hot flashes
  menopausal N95.1
Hourglass (contracture) — *see also* Contraction, hour-
    glass
  stomach K31.89
    congenital Q40.2
    stricture K31.2
Household, housing circumstance affecting care
    Z59.9
  specified NEC Z59.8
Housemaid's knee — *see* Bursitis, prepatellar
Hudson (-Stähli) **line** (cornea) — *see* Pigmentation,
    cornea, anterior
Human
  bite (open wound) — *see also* Bite
    intact skin surface — *see* Bite, superficial
  herpesvirus — *see* Herpes
  immunodeficiency virus (HIV) disease (infection) B20
    asymptomatic status Z21
    contact Z20.6
    counseling Z71.7
    dementia B20 *[F02.80]*
      with behavioral disturbance B20 *[F02.81]*
    exposure to Z20.6
    laboratory evidence R75
    type-2 (HIV 2) as cause of disease classified else-
      where B97.35
  papillomavirus (HPV)
    DNA test positive
      high risk
        cervix R87.810
        vagina R87.811
      low risk
        cervix R87.820
        vagina R87.821
    screening for Z11.51
  T-cell lymphotropic virus
    type-1 (HTLV-I) infection B33.3
      as cause of disease classified elsewhere B97.33
      carrier Z22.6
    type-2 (HTLV-II) as cause of disease classified else-
      where B97.34
Humidifier lung or pneumonitis J67.7
Humiliation (experience) **in childhood** Z62.898
Humpback (acquired) — *see* Kyphosis
Hunchback (acquired) — *see* Kyphosis
Hunger T73.0 ☑
  air, psychogenic F45.8
Hungry bone syndrome E83.81
Hunner's ulcer — *see* Cystitis, chronic, interstitial
Hunter's
  glossitis D51.0
  syndrome E76.1
Huntington's disease or chorea G10
  with dementia G10 *[F02.80]*
    with behavioral disturbance G10 *[F02.81]*
Hunt's
  disease or syndrome (herpetic geniculate ganglionitis)
    B02.21
    dyssynergia cerebellaris myoclonica G11.19
  neuralgia B02.21
Hurler (-Scheie) **disease or syndrome** E76.02
Hurst's disease G36.1

Hurthle cell
  adenocarcinoma C73
  adenoma D34
  carcinoma C73
  tumor D34
Hutchinson-Boeck disease or syndrome — *see* Sar-
    coidosis
Hutchinson-Gilford disease or syndrome E34.8
Hutchinson's
  disease, meaning
    angioma serpiginosum L81.7
    pompholyx (cheiropompholyx) L30.1
    prurigo estivalis L56.4
    summer eruption or summer prurigo L56.4
  melanotic freckle — *see* Melanoma, in situ
    malignant melanoma in — *see* Melanoma
  teeth or incisors (congenital syphilis) A50.52
  triad (congenital syphilis) A50.53
Hyalin plaque, sclera, senile H15.89
Hyaline membrane (disease) (lung) (pulmonary) (new-
    born) P22.0
Hyalinosis
  cutis (et mucosae) E78.89
  focal and segmental (glomerular) — *see also* N00-N07
    with fourth character .1 N05.1
Hyalitis, hyalosis, asteroid — *see also* Deposit, crys-
    talline
  syphilitic (late) A52.71
Hydatid
  cyst or tumor — *see* Echinococcus
  mole — *see* Hydatidiform mole
  Morgagni
    female Q50.5
    male (epididymal) Q55.4
      testicular Q55.29
Hydatidiform mole (benign) (complicating pregnancy)
    (delivered) (undelivered) O01.9
  classical O01.0
  complete O01.0
  incomplete O01.1
  invasive D39.2
  malignant D39.2
  partial O01.1
Hydatidosis — *see* Echinococcus
Hydradenitis (axillaris) (suppurative) L73.2
Hydradenoma — *see* Hidradenoma
Hydramnios O40.- ☑
Hydrancephaly, hydranencephaly Q04.3
  with spina bifida — *see* Spina bifida, with hydro-
    cephalus
Hydrargyrism NEC — *see* Poisoning, mercury
Hydrarthrosis — *see also* Effusion, joint
  gonococcal A54.42
  intermittent M12.40
    ankle M12.47- ☑
    elbow M12.42- ☑
    foot joint M12.47- ☑
    hand joint M12.44- ☑
    hip M12.45- ☑
    knee M12.46- ☑
    multiple site M12.49
    shoulder M12.41- ☑
    specified joint NEC M12.48
    wrist M12.43- ☑
  of yaws (early) (late) — *see also* subcategory M14.8-
    A66.6
  syphilitic (late) A52.77
    congenital A50.55 *[M12.80]*
Hydremia D64.89
Hydrencephalocele (congenital) — *see* Encephalocele
Hydrencephalomeningocele (congenital) — *see* En-
    cephalocele
Hydroa R23.8
  aestivale L56.4
  vacciniforme L56.4
Hydroadenitis (axillaris) (suppurative) L73.2
Hydrocalycosis — *see* Hydronephrosis
Hydrocele (spermatic cord) (testis) (tunica vaginalis)
    N43.3
  canal of Nuck N94.89
  communicating N43.2
    congenital P83.5
  congenital P83.5
  encysted N43.0
  female NEC N94.89
  infected N43.1
  newborn P83.5

Hydrocele — *continued*
  round ligament N94.89
  specified NEC N43.2
  spinalis — *see* Spina bifida
  vulva N90.89
Hydrocephalus (acquired) (external) (internal) (malig-
    nant) (recurrent) G91.9
  aqueduct Sylvius stricture Q03.0
  causing disproportion O33.6 ☑
    with obstructed labor O66.3
  communicating G91.0
  congenital (external) (internal) Q03.9
    with spina bifida Q05.4
      cervical Q05.0
      dorsal Q05.1
      lumbar Q05.2
      lumbosacral Q05.2
      sacral Q05.3
      thoracic Q05.1
      thoracolumbar Q05.1
    specified NEC Q03.8
  due to toxoplasmosis (congenital) P37.1
  foramen Magendie block (acquired) G91.1
    congenital — *see also* Hydrocephalus, congenital
      Q03.1
  in (due to)
    infectious disease NEC B89 *[G91.4]*
    neoplastic disease NEC — *see also* Neoplasm G91.4
    parasitic disease B89 *[G91.4]*
  newborn Q03.9
    with spina bifida — *see* Spina bifida, with hydro-
      cephalus
  noncommunicating G91.1
  normal pressure G91.2
    secondary G91.0
  obstructive G91.1
  otitic G93.2
  post-traumatic NEC G91.3
  secondary G91.4
    post-traumatic G91.3
  specified NEC G91.8
  syphilitic, congenital A50.49
Hydrocolpos (congenital) N89.8
Hydrocystoma — *see* Neoplasm, skin, benign
Hydroencephalocele (congenital) — *see* Encephalocele
Hydroencephalomeningocele (congenital) — *see* En-
    cephalocele
Hydrohematopneumothorax — *see* Hemothorax
Hydromeningitis — *see* Meningitis
Hydromeningocele (spinal) — *see also* Spina bifida
  cranial — *see* Encephalocele
Hydrometra N85.8
Hydrometrocolpos N89.8
Hydromicrocephaly Q02
Hydromphalos (since birth) Q45.8
Hydromyelia Q06.4
Hydromyelocele — *see* Spina bifida
Hydronephrosis (atrophic) (early) (functionless) (inter-
    mittent) (primary) (secondary) NEC N13.30
  with
    infection N13.6
    obstruction (by) (of)
      renal calculus N13.2
        with infection N13.6
      ureteral NEC N13.1
        with infection N13.6
        calculus N13.2
          with infection N13.6
      ureteropelvic junction (congenital) Q62.11
        acquired N13.0
          with infection N13.6
      ureteral stricture NEC N13.1
        with infection N13.6
  congenital Q62.0
  due to acquired occlusion of ureteropelvic junction
    N13.0
  specified type NEC N13.39
  tuberculous A18.11
Hydropericarditis — *see* Pericarditis
Hydropericardium — *see* Pericarditis
Hydroperitoneum R18.8
Hydrophobia — *see* Rabies
Hydrophthalmos Q15.0
Hydropneumohemothorax — *see* Hemothorax
Hydropneumopericarditis — *see* Pericarditis
Hydropneumopericardium — *see* Pericarditis
Hydropneumothorax J94.8
  traumatic — *see* Injury, intrathoracic, lung

Hydropneumothorax — *continued*
  tuberculous NEC A15.6
Hydrops R60.9
  abdominis R18.8
  articulorum intermittens — *see* Hydrarthrosis, intermittent
  cardiac — *see* Failure, heart, congestive
  causing obstructed labor (mother) O66.3
  endolymphatic H81.0- ☑
  fetal — *see* Pregnancy, complicated by, hydrops, fetalis
  fetalis P83.2
    due to
      ABO isoimmunization P56.0
      alpha thalassemia D56.0
      hemolytic disease P56.90
        specified NEC P56.99
      isoimmunization (ABO) (Rh) P56.0
      other specified nonhemolytic disease NEC P83.2
      Rh incompatibility P56.0
    during pregnancy — *see* Pregnancy, complicated by, hydrops, fetalis
  gallbladder K82.1
  joint — *see* Effusion, joint
  labyrinth H81.0- ☑
  newborn (idiopathic) P83.2
    due to
      ABO isoimmunization P56.0
      alpha thalassemia D56.0
      hemolytic disease P56.90
        specified NEC P56.99
      isoimmunization (ABO) (Rh) P56.0
      Rh incompatibility P56.0
  nutritional — *see* Malnutrition, severe
  pericardium — *see* Pericarditis
  pleura — *see* Hydrothorax
  spermatic cord — *see* Hydrocele
Hydropyonephrosis N13.6
Hydrorachis Q06.4
Hydrorrhea (nasal) J34.89
  pregnancy — *see* Rupture, membranes, premature
Hydrosadenitis (axillaris) (suppurative) L73.2
Hydrosalpinx (fallopian tube) (follicularis) N70.11
Hydrothorax (double) (pleura) J94.8
  chylous (nonfilarial) I89.8
    filarial — *see also* Infestation, filarial B74.9 [*J91.8*]
  traumatic — *see* Injury, intrathoracic
  tuberculous NEC (non primary) A15.6
Hydroureter — *see also* Hydronephrosis N13.4
  with infection N13.6
  congenital Q62.39
Hydroureteronephrosis — *see* Hydronephrosis
Hydrourethra N36.8
Hydroxykynureninuria E70.89
Hydroxylysinemia E72.3
Hydroxyprolinemia E72.59
Hygiene, sleep
  abuse Z72.821
  inadequate Z72.821
  poor Z72.821
Hygroma (congenital) (cystic) D18.1
  praepatellare, prepatellar — *see* Bursitis, prepatellar
Hymen — *see* condition
Hymenolepis, hymenolepiasis (diminuta) (infection) (infestation) (nana) B71.0
Hypalgesia R20.8
Hyperacidity (gastric) K31.89
  psychogenic F45.8
Hyperactive, hyperactivity F90.9
  basal cell, uterine cervix — *see* Dysplasia, cervix
  bowel sounds R19.12
  cervix epithelial (basal) — *see* Dysplasia, cervix
  child F90.9
    attention deficit — *see* Disorder, attention-deficit hyperactivity
  detrusor muscle N32.81
  gastrointestinal K31.89
    psychogenic F45.8
  nasal mucous membrane J34.3
  stomach K31.89
  thyroid (gland) — *see* Hyperthyroidism
Hyperacusis H93.23- ☑
Hyperadrenalism E27.5
Hyperadrenocorticism E24.9
  congenital E25.0
  iatrogenic E24.2

Hyperadrenocorticism — *continued*
  iatrogenic — *continued*
    correct substance properly administered — *see* Table of Drugs and Chemicals, by drug, adverse effect
    overdose or wrong substance given or taken — *see* Table of Drugs and Chemicals, by drug, poisoning
  not associated with Cushing's syndrome E27.0
  pituitary-dependent E24.0
Hyperaldosteronism E26.9
  familial (type I) E26.02
  glucocorticoid-remediable E26.02
  primary (due to (bilateral) adrenal hyperplasia) E26.09
  primary NEC E26.09
  secondary E26.1
  specified NEC E26.89
Hyperalgesia R20.8
Hyperalimentation R63.2
  carotene, carotin E67.1
  specified NEC E67.8
  vitamin
    A E67.0
    D E67.3
Hyperaminoaciduria
  arginine E72.21
  cystine E72.01
  lysine E72.3
  ornithine E72.4
Hyperammonemia (congenital) E72.20
Hyperazotemia — *see* Uremia
Hyperbetalipoproteinemia (familial) E78.00
  with prebetalipoproteinemia E78.2
Hyperbicarbonatemia P74.41
Hyperbilirubinemia
  constitutional E80.6
  familial conjugated E80.6
  neonatal (transient) — *see* Jaundice, newborn
Hypercalcemia, hypocalciuric, familial E83.52
Hypercalciuria, idiopathic R82.994
Hypercapnia R06.89
  newborn P84
Hypercarotenemia (dietary) E67.1
Hypercementosis K03.4
Hyperchloremia E87.8
Hyperchlorhydria K31.89
  neurotic F45.8
  psychogenic F45.8
Hypercholesterinemia — *see* Hypercholesterolemia
Hypercholesterolemia (essential) (primary) (pure) E78.00
  with hyperglyceridemia, endogenous E78.2
  dietary counseling and surveillance Z71.3
  familial E78.01
  hereditary E78.01
Hyperchylia gastrica, psychogenic F45.8
Hyperchylomicronemia (familial) (primary) E78.3
  with hyperbetalipoproteinemia E78.3
Hypercoagulable (state) D68.59
  activated protein C resistance D68.51
  antithrombin (III) deficiency D68.59
  factor V Leiden mutation D68.51
  primary NEC D68.59
  protein C deficiency D68.59
  protein S deficiency D68.59
  prothrombin gene mutation D68.52
  secondary D68.69
  specified NEC D68.69
Hypercoagulation (state) D68.59
Hypercorticalism, pituitary-dependent E24.0
Hypercorticosolism — *see* Cushing's, syndrome
Hypercorticosteronism E24.2
  correct substance properly administered — *see* Table of Drugs and Chemicals, by drug, adverse effect
  overdose or wrong substance given or taken — *see* Table of Drugs and Chemicals, by drug, poisoning
Hypercortisonism E24.2
  correct substance properly administered — *see* Table of Drugs and Chemicals, by drug, adverse effect
  overdose or wrong substance given or taken — *see* Table of Drugs and Chemicals, by drug, poisoning
Hyperekplexia Q89.8
Hyperelectrolytemia E87.8
Hyperemesis R11.10
  with nausea R11.2
  gravidarum (mild) O21.0
    with
      carbohydrate depletion O21.1
      dehydration O21.1

Hyperemesis — *continued*
  gravidarum — *continued*
    with — *continued*
      electrolyte imbalance O21.1
      metabolic disturbance O21.1
    severe (with metabolic disturbance) O21.1
  projectile R11.12
  psychogenic F45.8
Hyperemia (acute) (passive) R68.89
  anal mucosa K62.89
  bladder N32.89
  cerebral I67.89
  conjunctiva H11.43- ☑
  ear internal, acute — *see* subcategory H83.0 ☑
  enteric K59.89
  eye — *see* Hyperemia, conjunctiva
  eyelid (active) (passive) — *see* Disorder, eyelid, specified type NEC
  intestine K59.89
  iris — *see* Disorder, iris, vascular
  kidney N28.89
  labyrinth — *see* subcategory H83.0 ☑
  liver (active) K76.89
  lung (passive) — *see* Edema, lung
  pulmonary (passive) — *see* Edema, lung
  renal N28.89
  retina H35.89
  stomach K31.89
Hyperesthesia (body surface) R20.3
  larynx (reflex) J38.7
    hysterical F44.89
  pharynx (reflex) J39.2
    hysterical F44.89
Hyperestrogenism (drug-induced) (iatrogenic) E28.0
Hyperexplexia Q89.8
Hyperfibrinolysis — *see* Fibrinolysis
Hyperfructosemia E74.19
Hyperfunction
  adrenal cortex, not associated with Cushing's syndrome E27.0
  medulla E27.5
    adrenomedullary E27.5
  virilism E25.9
    congenital E25.0
  ovarian E28.8
  pancreas K86.89
  parathyroid (gland) E21.3
  pituitary (gland) (anterior) E22.9
    specified NEC E22.8
  polyglandular E31.1
  testicular E29.0
Hypergammaglobulinemia D89.2
  polyclonal D89.0
  Waldenström D89.0
Hypergastrinemia E16.4
Hyperglobulinemia R77.1
Hyperglycemia, hyperglycemic (transient) R73.9
  coma — *see* Diabetes, by type, with coma
  postpancreatectomy E89.1
Hyperglyceridemia (endogenous) (essential) (familial) (hereditary) (pure) E78.1
  mixed E78.3
Hyperglycinemia (non-ketotic) E72.51
Hypergonadism
  ovarian E28.8
  testicular (primary) (infantile) E29.0
Hyperheparinemia D68.32
Hyperhidrosis, hyperidrosis R61
  focal
    primary L74.519
      axilla L74.510
      face L74.511
      palms L74.512
      soles L74.513
    secondary L74.52
  generalized R61
  localized
    primary L74.519
      axilla L74.510
      face L74.511
      palms L74.512
      soles L74.513
    secondary L74.52
  psychogenic F45.8
  secondary R61
    focal L74.52
Hyperhistidinemia E70.41
Hyperhomocysteinemia E72.11

☑ **Additional Character Required** — **Refer to the Tabular List for Character Selection**   ▽ **Subterms under main terms may continue to next column or page**

Hyperhydroxyprolinemia E72.59
Hyperinsulinism (functional) E16.1
  with
    coma (hypoglycemic) E15
    encephalopathy E16.1 *[G94]*
  ectopic E16.1
  therapeutic misadventure (from administration of insulin) — *see* subcategory T38.3 ☑
Hyperkalemia E87.5
Hyperkeratosis — *see also* Keratosis L85.9
  cervix N88.0
  due to yaws (early) (late) (palmar or plantar) A66.3
  follicularis Q82.8
    penetrans (in cutem) L87.0
  palmoplantaris climacterica L85.1
  pinta A67.1
  senile (with pruritus) L57.0
  universalis congenita Q80.8
  vocal cord J38.3
  vulva N90.4
Hyperkinesia, hyperkinetic (disease) (reaction) (syndrome) (childhood) (adolescence) — *see also* Disorder, attention-deficit hyperactivity
  heart I51.89
Hyperleucine-isoleucinemia E71.19
Hyperlipemia, hyperlipidemia E78.5
  combined E78.2
    familial E78.49
  group
    A E78.00
    B E78.1
    C E78.2
    D E78.3
  mixed E78.2
  specified NEC E78.49
Hyperlipidosis E75.6
  hereditary NEC E75.5
Hyperlipoproteinemia E78.5
  Fredrickson's type
    I E78.3
    IIa E78.00
    IIb E78.2
    III E78.2
    IV E78.1
    V E78.3
  low-density-lipoprotein-type (LDL) E78.00
  very-low-density-lipoprotein-type (VLDL) E78.1
Hyperlucent lung, unilateral J43.0
Hyperlysinemia E72.3
Hypermagnesemia E83.41
  neonatal P71.8
Hypermenorrhea N92.0
Hypermethioninemia E72.19
Hypermetropia (congenital) H52.0- ☑
Hypermobility, hypermotility
  cecum — *see* Syndrome, irritable bowel
  coccyx — *see* subcategory M53.2 ☑
  colon — *see* Syndrome, irritable bowel
    psychogenic F45.8
  ileum K58.9
  intestine — *see also* Syndrome, irritable bowel K58.9
    psychogenic F45.8
  meniscus (knee) — *see* Derangement, knee, meniscus
  scapula — *see* Instability, joint, shoulder
  stomach K31.89
    psychogenic F45.8
  syndrome M35.7
  urethra N36.41
    with intrinsic sphincter deficiency N36.43
Hypernasality R49.21
Hypernatremia E87.0
Hypernephroma C64.- ☑
Hyperopia — *see* Hypermetropia
Hyperorexia nervosa F50.2
Hyperornithinemia E72.4
Hyperosmia R43.1
Hyperosmolality E87.0
Hyperostosis (monomelic) — *see also* Disorder, bone, density and structure, specified NEC
  ankylosing (spine) M48.10
    cervical region M48.12
    cervicothoracic region M48.13
    lumbar region M48.16
    lumbosacral region M48.17
    multiple sites M48.19
    occipito-atlanto-axial region M48.11
    sacrococcygeal region M48.18
    thoracic region M48.14

Hyperostosis — *continued*
  ankylosing — *continued*
    thoracolumbar region M48.15
  cortical (skull) M85.2
    infantile M89.8X- ☑
  frontal, internal of skull M85.2
  interna frontalis M85.2
  skeletal, diffuse idiopathic — *see* Hyperostosis, ankylosing
  skull M85.2
    congenital Q75.8
  vertebral, ankylosing — *see* Hyperostosis, ankylosing
Hyperovarism E28.8
Hyperoxaluria R82.992
  primary E72.53
Hyperparathyroidism E21.3
  primary E21.0
  secondary (renal) N25.81
    non-renal E21.1
  specified NEC E21.2
  tertiary E21.2
Hyperpathia R20.8
Hyperperistalsis R19.2
  psychogenic F45.8
Hyperpermeability, capillary I78.8
Hyperphagia R63.2
Hyperphenylalaninemia NEC E70.1
Hyperphoria (alternating) H50.53
Hyperphosphatemia E83.39
Hyperpiesis, hyperpiesia — *see* Hypertension
Hyperpigmentation — *see also* Pigmentation
  melanin NEC L81.4
  postinflammatory L81.0
Hyperpinealism E34.8
Hyperpituitarism E22.9
Hyperplasia, hyperplastic
  adenoids J35.2
  adrenal (capsule) (cortex) (gland) E27.8
    with
      sexual precocity (male) E25.9
        congenital E25.0
      virilism, adrenal E25.9
        congenital E25.0
      virilization (female) E25.9
        congenital E25.0
    congenital E25.0
    salt-losing E25.0
  adrenomedullary E27.5
  angiolymphoid, eosinophilia (ALHE) D18.01
  appendix (lymphoid) K38.0
  artery, fibromuscular I77.3
  bone — *see also* Hypertrophy, bone
    marrow D75.89
  breast — *see also* Hypertrophy, breast
    atypical, atypia N60.9- ☑
      ductal N60.9- ☑
      lobular N60.9- ☑
  C-cell, thyroid E07.0
  cementation (tooth) (teeth) K03.4
  cervical gland R59.0
  cervix (uteri) (basal cell) (endometrium) (polypoid) — *see also* Dysplasia, cervix
    congenital Q51.828
  clitoris, congenital Q52.6
  denture K06.2
  endocervicitis N72
  endometrium, endometrial (adenomatous) (cystic) (glandular) (glandular-cystic) (polypoid) N85.00
    with atypia N85.02
    benign N85.01
    cervix — *see* Dysplasia, cervix
    complex (without atypia) N85.01
    simple (without atypia) N85.01
  epithelial L85.9
    focal, oral, including tongue K13.29
    nipple N62
    skin L85.9
    tongue K13.29
    vaginal wall N89.3
  erythroid D75.89
  fibromuscular of artery (carotid) (renal) I77.3
  genital
    female NEC N94.89
    male N50.89
  gingiva K06.1
  glandularis cystica uteri (interstitialis) — *see also* Hyperplasia, endometrial N85.00
  gum K06.1

Hyperplasia, hyperplastic — *continued*
  hymen, congenital Q52.4
  irritative, edentulous (alveolar) K06.2
  jaw M26.09
    alveolar M26.79
      lower M26.03
        alveolar M26.72
      upper M26.01
        alveolar M26.71
  kidney (congenital) Q63.3
  labia N90.69
    epithelial N90.3
  liver (congenital) Q44.7
    nodular, focal K76.89
  lymph gland or node R59.9
  mandible, mandibular M26.03
    alveolar M26.72
    unilateral condylar M27.8
  maxilla, maxillary M26.01
    alveolar M26.71
  myometrium, myometrial N85.2
  neuroendocrine cell, of infancy J84.841
  nose
    lymphoid J34.89
    polypoid J33.9
  oral mucosa (irritative) K13.6
  organ or site, congenital NEC — *see* Anomaly, by site
  ovary N83.8
  palate, papillary (irritative) K13.6
  pancreatic islet cells E16.9
    alpha E16.8
      with excess
        gastrin E16.4
        glucagon E16.3
    beta E16.1
  parathyroid (gland) E21.0
  pharynx (lymphoid) J39.2
  prostate (adenofibromatous) (nodular) N40.0
    with lower urinary tract symptoms (LUTS) N40.1
    without lower urinary tract symtpoms (LUTS) N40.0
  renal artery I77.89
  reticulo-endothelial (cell) D75.89
  salivary gland (any) K11.1
  Schimmelbusch's — *see* Mastopathy, cystic
  suprarenal capsule (gland) E27.8
  thymus (gland) (persistent) E32.0
  thyroid (gland) — *see* Goiter
  tonsils (faucial) (infective) (lingual) (lymphoid) J35.1
    with adenoids J35.3
  unilateral condylar M27.8
  uterus, uterine N85.2
    endometrium (glandular) — *see also* Hyperplasia, endometrial N85.00
  vulva N90.69
    epithelial N90.3
Hyperpnea — *see* Hyperventilation
Hyperpotassemia E87.5
Hyperprebetalipoproteinemia (familial) E78.1
Hyperprolactinemia E22.1
Hyperprolinemia (type I) (type II) E72.59
Hyperproteinemia E88.09
Hyperprothrombinemia, causing coagulation factor deficiency D68.4
Hyperpyrexia R50.9
  heat (effects) T67.01 ☑
  malignant, due to anesthetic T88.3 ☑
  rheumatic — *see* Fever, rheumatic
  unknown origin R50.9
Hyper-reflexia R29.2
Hypersalivation K11.7
Hypersecretion
  ACTH (not associated with Cushing's syndrome) E27.0
    pituitary E24.0
  adrenaline E27.5
  adrenomedullary E27.5
  androgen (testicular) E29.0
    ovarian (drug-induced) (iatrogenic) E28.1
  calcitonin E07.0
  catecholamine E27.5
  corticoadrenal E24.9
  cortisol E24.9
  epinephrine E27.5
  estrogen E28.0
  gastric K31.89
    psychogenic F45.8
  gastrin E16.4
  glucagon E16.3

Hypersecretion — *continued*
  hormone(s)
    ACTH (not associated with Cushing's syndrome)
        E27.0
      pituitary E24.0
    antidiuretic E22.2
    growth E22.0
    intestinal NEC E34.1
    ovarian androgen E28.1
    pituitary E22.9
    testicular E29.0
    thyroid stimulating E05.80
      with thyroid storm E05.81
  insulin — *see* Hyperinsulinism
  lacrimal glands — *see* Epiphora
  medulloadrenal E27.5
  milk O92.6
  ovarian androgens E28.1
  salivary gland (any) K11.7
  thyrocalcitonin E07.0
  upper respiratory J39.8
Hypersegmentation, leukocytic, hereditary D72.0
Hypersensitive, hypersensitiveness, hypersensitivity
    — *see also* Allergy
  carotid sinus G90.01
  colon — *see* Irritable, colon
  drug T88.7 ☑
  gastrointestinal K52.29
    immediate K52.29
    psychogenic F45.8
  labyrinth — *see* subcategory H83.2 ☑
  pain R20.8
  pneumonitis — *see* Pneumonitis, allergic
  reaction T78.40 ☑
  upper respiratory tract NEC J39.3
Hypersomnia (organic) G47.10
  due to
    alcohol
      abuse F10.182
      dependence F10.282
      use F10.982
    amphetamines
      abuse F15.182
      dependence F15.282
      use F15.982
    caffeine
      abuse F15.182
      dependence F15.282
      use F15.982
    cocaine
      abuse F14.182
      dependence F14.282
      use F14.982
    drug NEC
      abuse F19.182
      dependence F19.282
      use F19.982
    medical condition G47.14
    mental disorder F51.13
    opioid
      abuse F11.182
      dependence F11.282
      use F11.982
    psychoactive substance NEC
      abuse F19.182
      dependence F19.282
      use F19.982
    sedative, hypnotic, or anxiolytic
      abuse F13.182
      dependence F13.282
      use F13.982
    stimulant NEC
      abuse F15.182
      dependence F15.282
      use F15.982
  idiopathic G47.11
    with long sleep time G47.11
    without long sleep time G47.12
  menstrual related G47.13
  nonorganic origin F51.11
    specified NEC F51.19
  not due to a substance or known physiological condition F51.11
    specified NEC F51.19
  primary F51.11
  recurrent G47.13
  specified NEC G47.19
Hypersplenia, hypersplenism D73.1

Hyperstimulation, ovaries (associated with induced ovulation) N98.1
Hypersusceptibility — *see* Allergy
Hypertelorism (ocular) (orbital) Q75.2
Hypertension, hypertensive (accelerated) (benign) (essential) (idiopathic) (malignant) (systemic) I10
  with
    heart failure (congestive) I11.0
    heart involvement (conditions in I50.- or I51.4-I51.7, I51.89, I51.9, due to hypertension) — *see* Hypertension, heart
    kidney involvement — *see* Hypertension, kidney
  benign, intracranial G93.2
  borderline R03.0
  cardiorenal (disease) I13.10
    with heart failure I13.0
      with stage 1 through stage 4 chronic kidney disease I13.0
      with stage 5 or end stage renal disease I13.2
    without heart failure I13.10
      with stage 1 through stage 4 chronic kidney disease I13.10
      with stage 5 or end stage renal disease I13.11
  cardiovascular
    disease (arteriosclerotic) (sclerotic) — *see* Hypertension, heart
    renal (disease) — *see* Hypertension, cardiorenal
  chronic venous — *see* Hypertension, venous (chronic)
  complicating
    childbirth (labor) O16.4
    pre-existing O10.92
      with
        heart disease O10.12
          with renal disease O10.32
        pre-eclampsia O11.4
        renal disease O10.22
          with heart disease O10.32
      essential O10.02
    secondary O10.42
  pregnancy O16.- ☑
    with edema — *see also* Pre-eclampsia O14.9- ☑
    gestational (pregnancy induced) (without proteinuria) O13.- ☑
      with proteinuria O14.9- ☑
        mild pre-eclampsia O14.0- ☑
        moderate pre-eclampsia O14.0- ☑
        severe pre-eclampsia O14.1- ☑
          with hemolysis, elevated liver enzymes and low platelet count (HELLP) O14.2- ☑
    pre-existing O10.91- ☑
      with
        heart disease O10.11- ☑
          with renal disease O10.31- ☑
        pre-eclampsia — *see* category O11
        renal disease O10.21- ☑
          with heart disease O10.31- ☑
      essential O10.01- ☑
      secondary O10.41- ☑
    transient O13- ☑
  puerperium, pre-existing O16.5
    pre-existing
      with
        heart disease O10.13
          with renal disease O10.33
        pre-eclampsia O11.5
        renal disease O10.23
          with heart disease O10.33
      essential O10.03
    pregnancy-induced O13.9
    secondary O10.43
  crisis I16.9
  due to
    endocrine disorders I15.2
    pheochromocytoma I15.2
    renal disorders NEC I15.1
      arterial I15.0
    renovascular disorders I15.0
    specified disease NEC I15.8
  emergency I16.1
  encephalopathy I67.4
  gestational (without significant proteinuria) (pregnancy-induced) (transient) O13.- ☑
    with significant proteinuria — *see* Pre-eclampsia
  complicating
    delivery O13.4
    puerperium O13.5
  Goldblatt's I70.1

Hypertension, hypertensive — *continued*
  heart (disease) (conditions in I51.4-I51.9 due to hypertension) I11.9
    with
      heart failure (congestive) I11.0
      kidney disease (chronic) — *see* Hypertension, cardiorenal
  intracranial, benign G93.2
  kidney I12.9
    with
      heart disease — *see* Hypertension, cardiorenal
      stage 1 through stage 4 chronic kidney disease I12.9
      stage 5 chronic kidney disease (CKD) or end stage renal disease (ESRD) I12.0
  lesser circulation I27.0
  maternal O16- ☑
  newborn P29.2
    pulmonary (persistent) P29.30
  ocular H40.05- ☑
  pancreatic duct — *code to* underlying condition
    with chronic pancreatitis K86.1
  portal (due to chronic liver disease) (idiopathic) K76.6
    gastropathy K31.89
    in (due to) schistosomiasis (bilharziasis) B65.9 *[K77]*
  postoperative I97.3
  psychogenic F45.8
  pulmonary I27.20
    with
      cor pulmonale (chronic) I27.29
        acute I26.09
      right heart ventricular strain/failure I27.29
        acute I26.09
      right to left shunt related to congenital heart disease I27.83
      unclear multifactorial mechanisms I27.29
    arterial (associated) (drug-induced) (toxin-induced) I27.21
    chronic thromboembolic I27.24
    due to
      hematologic disorders I27.29
      left heart disease I27.22
      lung diseases and hypoxia I27.23
      metabolic disorders I27.29
      specified systemic disorders I27.29
    group 1 (associated) (drug-induced) (toxin-induced) I27.21
    group 2 I27.22
    group 3 I27.23
    group 4 I27.24
    group 5 I27.29
    of newborn (persistent) P29.30
    primary (idiopathic) I27.0
    secondary
      arterial I27.21
      specified NEC I27.29
  renal — *see* Hypertension, kidney
  renovascular I15.0
  secondary NEC I15.9
    due to
      endocrine disorders I15.2
      pheochromocytoma I15.2
      renal disorders NEC I15.1
        arterial I15.0
      renovascular disorders I15.0
    specified NEC I15.8
  transient R03.0
    of pregnancy O13.- ☑
  urgency I16.0
  venous (chronic)
    due to
      deep vein thrombosis — *see* Syndrome, post-thrombotic
    idiopathic I87.309
      with
        inflammation I87.32- ☑
          with ulcer I87.33- ☑
        specified complication NEC I87.39- ☑
        ulcer I87.31- ☑
          with inflammation I87.33- ☑
      asymptomatic I87.30- ☑
Hypertensive urgency — *see* Hypertension
Hyperthecosis ovary E28.8
Hyperthermia (of unknown origin) — *see also* Hyperpyrexia
  malignant, due to anesthesia T88.3 ☑
  newborn P81.9
    environmental P81.0

☑ **Additional Character Required** — Refer to the Tabular List for Character Selection   ▽ Subterms under main terms may continue to next column or page

Hyperthyroid (recurrent) — see Hyperthyroidism
Hyperthyroidism (latent) (pre-adult) (recurrent) E05.90
  with
    goiter (diffuse) E05.00
      with thyroid storm E05.01
      nodular (multinodular) E05.20
        with thyroid storm E05.21
        uninodular E05.10
          with thyroid storm E05.11
    storm E05.91
  due to ectopic thyroid tissue E05.30
    with thyroid storm E05.31
  neonatal, transitory P72.1
  specified NEC E05.80
    with thyroid storm E05.81
Hypertony, hypertonia, hypertonicity
  bladder N31.8
  congenital P94.1
  stomach K31.89
    psychogenic F45.8
  uterus, uterine (contractions) (complicating delivery) O62.4
Hypertrichosis L68.9
  congenital Q84.2
  eyelid H02.869
    left H02.866
      lower H02.865
      upper H02.864
    right H02.863
      lower H02.862
      upper H02.861
  lanuginosa Q84.2
    acquired L68.1
  localized L68.2
  specified NEC L68.8
Hypertriglyceridemia, essential E78.1
Hypertrophy, hypertrophic
  adenofibromatous, prostate — see Enlargement, enlarged, prostate
  adenoids (infective) J35.2
    with tonsils J35.3
  adrenal cortex E27.8
  alveolar process or ridge — see Anomaly, alveolar
  anal papillae K62.89
  artery I77.89
    congenital NEC Q27.8
      digestive system Q27.8
      lower limb Q27.8
      specified site NEC Q27.8
      upper limb Q27.8
  auricular — see Hypertrophy, cardiac
  Bartholin's gland N75.8
  bile duct (common) (hepatic) K83.8
  bladder (sphincter) (trigone) N32.89
  bone M89.30
    carpus M89.34- ☑
    clavicle M89.31- ☑
    femur M89.35- ☑
    fibula M89.36- ☑
    finger M89.34- ☑
    humerus M89.32- ☑
    ilium M89.359
    ischium M89.359
    metacarpus M89.34- ☑
    metatarsus M89.37- ☑
    multiple sites M89.39
    neck M89.38
    radius M89.33- ☑
    rib M89.38
    scapula M89.31- ☑
    skull M89.38
    tarsus M89.37- ☑
    tibia M89.36- ☑
    toe M89.37- ☑
    ulna M89.33- ☑
    vertebra M89.38
  brain G93.89
  breast N62
    cystic — see Mastopathy, cystic
    newborn P83.4
    pubertal, massive N62
    puerperal, postpartum — see Disorder, breast, specified type NEC
    senile (parenchymatous) N62
  cardiac (chronic) (idiopathic) I51.7
    with rheumatic fever (conditions in I00)
      active I01.8
      inactive or quiescent (with chorea) I09.89

Hypertrophy, hypertrophic — continued
  cardiac — continued
    congenital NEC Q24.8
    fatty — see Degeneration, myocardial
    hypertensive — see Hypertension, heart
    rheumatic (with chorea) I09.89
      active or acute I01.8
        with chorea I02.0
    valve — see Endocarditis
  cartilage — see Disorder, cartilage, specified type NEC
  cecum — see Megacolon
  cervix (uteri) N88.8
    congenital Q51.828
    elongation N88.4
  clitoris (cirrhotic) N90.89
    congenital Q52.6
  colon — see also Megacolon
    congenital Q43.2
  conjunctiva, lymphoid H11.89
  corpora cavernosa N48.89
  cystic duct K82.8
  duodenum K31.89
  endometrium (glandular) — see also Hyperplasia, endometrial N85.00
    cervix N88.8
  epididymis N50.89
  esophageal hiatus (congenital) Q79.1
    with hernia — see Hernia, hiatal
  eyelid — see Disorder, eyelid, specified type NEC
  fat pad E65
    knee (infrapatellar) (popliteal) (prepatellar) (retropatellar) M79.4
  foot (congenital) Q74.2
  frenulum, frenum (tongue) K14.8
    lip K13.0
  gallbladder K82.8
  gastric mucosa K29.60
    with bleeding K29.61
  gland, glandular R59.9
    generalized R59.1
    localized R59.0
  gum (mucous membrane) K06.1
  heart (idiopathic) — see also Hypertrophy, cardiac
    valve — see also Endocarditis I38
  hemifacial Q67.4
  hepatic — see Hypertrophy, liver
  hiatus (esophageal) Q79.1
  hilus gland R59.0
  hymen, congenital Q52.4
  ileum K63.89
  intestine NEC K63.89
  jejunum K63.89
  kidney (compensatory) N28.81
    congenital Q63.3
  labium (majus) (minus) N90.60
  ligament — see Disorder, ligament
  lingual tonsil (infective) J35.1
    with adenoids J35.3
  lip K13.0
    congenital Q18.6
  liver R16.0
    acute K76.89
    cirrhotic — see Cirrhosis, liver
    congenital Q44.7
    fatty — see Fatty, liver
  lymph, lymphatic gland R59.9
    generalized R59.1
    localized R59.0
    tuberculous — see Tuberculosis, lymph gland
  mammary gland — see Hypertrophy, breast
  Meckel's diverticulum (congenital) Q43.0
    malignant — see Table of Neoplasms, small intestine, malignant
  median bar — see Hyperplasia, prostate
  meibomian gland — see Chalazion
  meniscus, knee, congenital Q74.1
  metatarsal head — see Hypertrophy, bone, metatarsus
  metatarsus — see Hypertrophy, bone, metatarsus
  mucous membrane
    alveolar ridge K06.2
    gum K06.1
    nose (turbinate) J34.3
  muscle M62.89
  muscular coat, artery I77.89
  myocardium — see also Hypertrophy, cardiac
    idiopathic I42.2
  myometrium N85.2
  nail L60.2

Hypertrophy, hypertrophic — continued
  nail — continued
    congenital Q84.5
  nasal J34.89
    alae J34.89
    bone J34.89
    cartilage J34.89
    mucous membrane (septum) J34.3
    sinus J34.89
    turbinate J34.3
  nasopharynx, lymphoid (infectional) (tissue) (wall) J35.2
  nipple N62
  organ or site, congenital NEC — see Anomaly, by site
  ovary N83.8
  palate (hard) M27.8
    soft K13.79
  pancreas, congenital Q45.3
  parathyroid (gland) E21.0
  parotid gland K11.1
  penis N48.89
  pharyngeal tonsil J35.2
  pharynx J39.2
    lymphoid (infectional) (tissue) (wall) J35.2
  pituitary (anterior) (fossa) (gland) E23.6
  prepuce (congenital) N47.8
    female N90.89
  prostate — see Enlargement, enlarged, prostate
    congenital Q55.4
  pseudomuscular G71.09
  pylorus (adult) (muscle) (sphincter) K31.1
    congenital or infantile Q40.0
  rectal, rectum (sphincter) K62.89
  rhinitis (turbinate) J31.0
  salivary gland (any) K11.1
    congenital Q38.4
  scaphoid (tarsal) — see Hypertrophy, bone, tarsus
  scar L91.0
  scrotum N50.89
  seminal vesicle N50.89
  sigmoid — see Megacolon
  skin L91.9
    specified NEC L91.8
  spermatic cord N50.89
  spleen — see Splenomegaly
  spondylitis — see Spondylosis
  stomach K31.89
  sublingual gland K11.1
  submandibular gland K11.1
  suprarenal cortex (gland) E27.8
  synovial NEC M67.20
    acromioclavicular M67.21- ☑
    ankle M67.27- ☑
    elbow M67.22- ☑
    foot M67.27- ☑
    hand M67.24- ☑
    hip M67.25- ☑
    knee M67.26- ☑
    multiple sites M67.29
    specified site NEC M67.28
    wrist M67.23- ☑
  tendon — see Disorder, tendon, specified type NEC
  testis N44.8
    congenital Q55.29
  thymic, thymus (gland) (congenital) E32.0
  thyroid (gland) — see Goiter
  toe (congenital) Q74.2
    acquired — see also Deformity, toe, specified NEC
  tongue K14.8
    congenital Q38.2
    papillae (foliate) K14.3
  tonsils (faucial) (infective) (lingual) (lymphoid) J35.1
    with adenoids J35.3
  tunica vaginalis N50.89
  ureter N28.89
  urethra N36.8
  uterus N85.2
    neck (with elongation) N88.4
    puerperal O90.89
  uvula K13.79
  vagina N89.8
  vas deferens N50.89
  vein I87.8
  ventricle, ventricular (heart) — see also Hypertrophy, cardiac
    congenital Q24.8
    in tetralogy of Fallot Q21.3
  verumontanum N36.8
  vocal cord J38.3

Hypertrophy, hypertrophic — *continued*
  vulva N90.60
    stasis (nonfilarial) N90.69
Hypertropia H50.2- ☑
Hypertyrosinemia E70.21
Hyperuricemia (asymptomatic) E79.0
Hyperuricosuria R82.993
Hypervalinemia E71.19
Hyperventilation (tetany) R06.4
  hysterical F45.8
  psychogenic F45.8
  syndrome F45.8
Hypervitaminosis (dietary) NEC E67.8
  A E67.0
    administered as drug (prolonged intake) — *see* Table of Drugs and Chemicals, vitamins, adverse effect
    overdose or wrong substance given or taken — *see* Table of Drugs and Chemicals, vitamins, poisoning
  B6 E67.2
  D E67.3
    administered as drug (prolonged intake) — *see* Table of Drugs and Chemicals, vitamins, adverse effect
    overdose or wrong substance given or taken — *see* Table of Drugs and Chemicals, vitamins, poisoning
  K E67.8
    administered as drug (prolonged intake) — *see* Table of Drugs and Chemicals, vitamins, adverse effect
    overdose or wrong substance given or taken — *see* Table of Drugs and Chemicals, vitamins, poisoning
Hypervolemia E87.70
  specified NEC E87.79
Hypesthesia R20.1
  cornea — *see* Anesthesia, cornea
Hyphema H21.0- ☑
  traumatic S05.1- ☑
Hypoacidity, gastric K31.89
  psychogenic F45.8
Hypoadrenalism, hypoadrenia E27.40
  primary E27.1
  tuberculous A18.7
Hypoadrenocorticism E27.40
  pituitary E23.0
  primary E27.1
Hypoalbuminemia E88.09
Hypoaldosteronism E27.40
Hypoalphalipoproteinemia E78.6
Hypobarism T70.29 ☑
Hypobaropathy T70.29 ☑
Hypobetalipoproteinemia (familial) E78.6
Hypocalcemia E83.51
  dietary E58
  neonatal P71.1
    due to cow's milk P71.0
  phosphate-loading (newborn) P71.1
Hypochloremia E87.8
Hypochlorhydria K31.89
  neurotic F45.8
  psychogenic F45.8
Hypochondria, hypochondriac, hypochondriasis (reaction) F45.21
  sleep F51.03
Hypochondrogenesis Q77.0
Hypochondroplasia Q77.4
Hypochromasia, blood cells D50.8
Hypocitraturia R82.991
Hypodontia — *see* Anodontia
Hypoeosinophilia D72.89
Hypoesthesia R20.1
Hypofibrinogenemia D68.8
  acquired D65
  congenital (hereditary) D68.2
Hypofunction
  adrenocortical E27.40
    drug-induced E27.3
    postprocedural E89.6
    primary E27.1
  adrenomedullary, postprocedural E89.6
  cerebral R29.818
  corticoadrenal NEC E27.40
  intestinal K59.89
  labyrinth — *see* subcategory H83.2 ☑

Hypofunction — *continued*
  ovary E28.39
  pituitary (gland) (anterior) E23.0
  testicular E29.1
    postprocedural (postsurgical) (postirradiation) (iatrogenic) E89.5
Hypogalactia O92.4
Hypogammaglobulinemia — *see also* Agammaglobulinemia D80.1
  hereditary D80.0
  nonfamilial D80.1
  transient, of infancy D80.7
Hypogenitalism (congenital) — *see* Hypogonadism
Hypoglossia Q38.3
Hypoglycemia (spontaneous) E16.2
  coma E15
    diabetic — *see* Diabetes, by type, with hypoglycemia, with coma
  diabetic — *see* Diabetes, hypoglycemia
  dietary counseling and surveillance Z71.3
  drug-induced E16.0
    with coma (nondiabetic) E15
  due to insulin E16.0
    with coma (nondiabetic) E15
    therapeutic misadventure — *see* subcategory T38.3 ☑
  functional, nonhyperinsulinemic E16.1
  iatrogenic E16.0
    with coma (nondiabetic) E15
  in infant of diabetic mother P70.1
    gestational diabetes P70.0
  infantile E16.1
  leucine-induced E71.19
  neonatal (transitory) P70.4
    iatrogenic P70.3
  reactive (not drug-induced) E16.1
  transitory neonatal P70.4
Hypogonadism
  female E28.39
  hypogonadotropic E23.0
  male E29.1
  ovarian (primary) E28.39
  pituitary E23.0
  testicular (primary) E29.1
Hypohidrosis, hypoidrosis L74.4
Hypoinsulinemia, postprocedural E89.1
Hypokalemia E87.6
Hypoleukocytosis — *see* Agranulocytosis
Hypolipoproteinemia (alpha) (beta) E78.6
Hypomagnesemia E83.42
  neonatal P71.2
Hypomania, hypomanic reaction F30.8
Hypomenorrhea — *see* Oligomenorrhea
Hypometabolism R63.8
Hypomotility
  gastrointestinal (tract) K31.89
    psychogenic F45.8
  intestine K59.89
    psychogenic F45.8
  stomach K31.89
    psychogenic F45.8
Hyponasality R49.22
Hyponatremia E87.1
Hypo-osmolality E87.1
Hypo-ovarianism, hypo-ovarism E28.39
Hypoparathyroidism E20.9
  familial E20.8
  idiopathic E20.0
  neonatal, transitory P71.4
  postprocedural E89.2
  specified NEC E20.8
Hypoperfusion (in)
  newborn P96.89
Hypopharyngitis — *see* Laryngopharyngitis
Hypophoria H50.53
Hypophosphatemia, hypophosphatasia (acquired) (congenital) (renal) E83.39
  familial E83.31
Hypophyseal, hypophysis — *see also* condition
  dwarfism E23.0
  gigantism E22.0
Hypopiesis — *see* Hypotension
Hypopinealism E34.8
Hypopituitarism (juvenile) E23.0
  drug-induced E23.1
  due to
    hypophysectomy E89.3
    radiotherapy E89.3

Hypopituitarism — *continued*
  iatrogenic NEC E23.1
  postirradiation E89.3
  postpartum O99.285
  postprocedural E89.3
Hypoplasia, hypoplastic
  adrenal (gland), congenital Q89.1
  alimentary tract, congenital Q45.8
    upper Q40.8
  anus, anal (canal) Q42.3
    with fistula Q42.2
  aorta, aortic Q25.42
    ascending, in hypoplastic left heart syndrome Q23.4
    valve Q23.1
      in hypoplastic left heart syndrome Q23.4
  areola, congenital Q83.8
  arm (congenital) — *see* Defect, reduction, upper limb
  artery (peripheral) Q27.8
    brain (congenital) Q28.3
    coronary Q24.5
    digestive system Q27.8
    lower limb Q27.8
    pulmonary Q25.79
      functional, unilateral J43.0
    retinal (congenital) Q14.1
    specified site NEC Q27.8
    umbilical Q27.0
    upper limb Q27.8
  auditory canal Q17.8
    causing impairment of hearing Q16.9
  biliary duct or passage Q44.5
  bone NOS Q79.9
    face Q75.8
    marrow D61.9
      megakaryocytic D69.49
    skull — *see* Hypoplasia, skull
  brain Q02
    gyri Q04.3
    part of Q04.3
  breast (areola) N64.82
  bronchus Q32.4
  cardiac Q24.8
  carpus — *see* Defect, reduction, upper limb, specified type NEC
  cartilage hair Q78.8
  cecum Q42.8
  cementum K00.4
  cephalic Q02
  cerebellum Q04.3
  cervix (uteri), congenital Q51.821
  clavicle (congenital) Q74.0
  coccyx Q76.49
  colon Q42.9
    specified NEC Q42.8
  corpus callosum Q04.0
  cricoid cartilage Q31.2
  digestive organ(s) or tract NEC Q45.8
    upper (congenital) Q40.8
  ear (auricle) (lobe) Q17.2
    middle Q16.4
  enamel of teeth (neonatal) (postnatal) (prenatal) K00.40
  endocrine (gland) NEC Q89.2
  endometrium N85.8
  epididymis (congenital) Q55.4
  epiglottis Q31.2
  erythroid, congenital D61.01
  esophagus (congenital) Q39.8
  eustachian tube Q17.8
  eye Q11.2
  eyelid (congenital) Q10.3
  face Q18.8
    bone(s) Q75.8
  femur (congenital) — *see* Defect, reduction, lower limb, specified type NEC
  fibula (congenital) — *see* Defect, reduction, lower limb, specified type NEC
  finger (congenital) — *see* Defect, reduction, upper limb, specified type NEC
  focal dermal Q82.8
  foot — *see* Defect, reduction, lower limb, specified type NEC
  gallbladder Q44.0
  genitalia, genital organ(s)
    female, congenital Q52.8
      external Q52.79
      internal NEC Q52.8
    in adiposogenital dystrophy E23.6
  glottis Q31.2

☑ **Additional Character Required** — Refer to the Tabular List for Character Selection   ▽ **Subterms under main terms may continue to next column or page**

Hypoplasia, hypoplastic — *continued*
  hair Q84.2
  hand (congenital) — *see* Defect, reduction, upper limb, specified type NEC
  heart Q24.8
  humerus (congenital) — *see* Defect, reduction, upper limb, specified type NEC
  intestine (small) Q41.9
    large Q42.9
      specified NEC Q42.8
  jaw M26.09
    alveolar M26.79
    lower M26.04
      alveolar M26.74
    upper M26.02
      alveolar M26.73
  kidney(s) Q60.5
    bilateral Q60.4
    unilateral Q60.3
  labium (majus) (minus), congenital Q52.79
  larynx Q31.2
  left heart syndrome Q23.4
  leg (congenital) — *see* Defect, reduction, lower limb
  limb Q73.8
    lower (congenital) — *see* Defect, reduction, lower limb
    upper (congenital) — *see* Defect, reduction, upper limb
  liver Q44.7
  lung (lobe) (not associated with short gestation) Q33.6
    associated with immaturity, low birth weight, prematurity, or short gestation P28.0
  mammary (areola), congenital Q83.8
  mandible, mandibular M26.04
    alveolar M26.74
    unilateral condylar M27.8
  maxillary M26.02
    alveolar M26.73
  medullary D61.9
  megakaryocytic D69.49
  metacarpus — *see* Defect, reduction, upper limb, specified type NEC
  metatarsus — *see* Defect, reduction, lower limb, specified type NEC
  muscle Q79.8
  nail(s) Q84.6
  nose, nasal Q30.1
  optic nerve H47.03- ☑
  osseous meatus (ear) Q17.8
  ovary, congenital Q50.39
  pancreas Q45.0
  parathyroid (gland) Q89.2
  parotid gland Q38.4
  patella Q74.1
  pelvis, pelvic girdle Q74.2
  penis (congenital) Q55.62
  peripheral vascular system Q27.8
    digestive system Q27.8
    lower limb Q27.8
    specified site NEC Q27.8
    upper limb Q27.8
  pituitary (gland) (congenital) Q89.2
  pulmonary (not associated with short gestation) Q33.6
    artery, functional J43.0
    associated with short gestation P28.0
  radioulnar — *see* Defect, reduction, upper limb, specified type NEC
  radius — *see* Defect, reduction, upper limb
  rectum Q42.1
    with fistula Q42.0
  respiratory system NEC Q34.8
  rib Q76.6
  right heart syndrome Q22.6
  sacrum Q76.49
  scapula Q74.0
  scrotum Q55.1
  shoulder girdle Q74.0
  skin Q82.8
  skull (bone) Q75.8
    with
      anencephaly Q00.0
      encephalocele — *see* Encephalocele
      hydrocephalus Q03.9
        with spina bifida — *see* Spina bifida, by site, with hydrocephalus
      microcephaly Q02
  spinal (cord) (ventral horn cell) Q06.1
  spine Q76.49

Hypoplasia, hypoplastic — *continued*
  sternum Q76.7
  tarsus — *see* Defect, reduction, lower limb, specified type NEC
  testis Q55.1
  thymic, with immunodeficiency D82.1
  thymus (gland) Q89.2
    with immunodeficiency D82.1
  thyroid (gland) E03.1
    cartilage Q31.2
  tibiofibular (congenital) — *see* Defect, reduction, lower limb, specified type NEC
  toe — *see* Defect, reduction, lower limb, specified type NEC
  tongue Q38.3
  Turner's K00.4
  ulna (congenital) — *see* Defect, reduction, upper limb
  umbilical artery Q27.0
  unilateral condylar M27.8
  ureter Q62.8
  uterus, congenital Q51.811
  vagina Q52.4
  vascular NEC peripheral Q27.8
    brain Q28.3
    digestive system Q27.8
    lower limb Q27.8
    specified site NEC Q27.8
    upper limb Q27.8
  vein(s) (peripheral) Q27.8
    brain Q28.3
    digestive system Q27.8
    great Q26.8
    lower limb Q27.8
    specified site NEC Q27.8
    upper limb Q27.8
  vena cava (inferior) (superior) Q26.8
  vertebra Q76.49
  vulva, congenital Q52.79
  zonule (ciliary) Q12.8
Hypoplasminogenemia E88.02
Hypopnea, obstructive sleep apnea G47.33
Hypopotassemia E87.6
Hypoproconvertinemia, congenital (hereditary) D68.2
Hypoproteinemia E77.8
Hypoprothrombinemia (congenital) (hereditary) (idiopathic) D68.2
  acquired D68.4
  newborn, transient P61.6
Hypoptyalism K11.7
Hypopyon (eye) (anterior chamber) — *see* Iridocyclitis, acute, hypopyon
Hypopyrexia R68.0
Hyporeflexia R29.2
Hyposecretion
  ACTH E23.0
  antidiuretic hormone E23.2
  ovary E28.39
  salivary gland (any) K11.7
  vasopressin E23.2
Hyposegmentation, leukocytic, hereditary D72.0
Hyposiderinemia D50.9
Hypospadias Q54.9
  balanic Q54.0
  coronal Q54.0
  glandular Q54.0
  penile Q54.1
  penoscrotal Q54.2
  perineal Q54.3
  specified NEC Q54.8
Hypospermatogenesis — *see* Oligospermia
Hyposplenism D73.0
Hypostasis pulmonary, passive — *see* Edema, lung
Hypostatic — *see* condition
Hyposthenuria N28.89
Hypotension (arterial) (constitutional) I95.9
  chronic I95.89
  due to (of) hemodialysis I95.3
  drug-induced I95.2
  iatrogenic I95.89
  idiopathic (permanent) I95.0
  intracranial G96.810
    following
      lumbar cerebrospinal fluid shunting G97.83
      specified procedure NEC G97.84
      ventricular shunting (ventriculostomy) G97.2
    specified NEC G96.819
    spontaneous G96.811
  intra-dialytic I95.3

Hypotension — *continued*
  maternal, syndrome (following labor and delivery) O26.5- ☑
  neurogenic, orthostatic G90.3
  orthostatic (chronic) I95.1
    due to drugs I95.2
    neurogenic G90.3
  postoperative I95.81
  postural I95.1
  specified NEC I95.89
Hypothermia (accidental) T68 ☑
  due to anesthesia, anesthetic T88.51 ☑
  low environmental temperature T68 ☑
  neonatal P80.9
    environmental (mild) NEC P80.8
    mild P80.8
    severe (chronic) (cold injury syndrome) P80.0
    specified NEC P80.8
  not associated with low environmental temperature R68.0
Hypothyroidism (acquired) E03.9
  autoimmune — *see* Thyroiditis, autoimmune
  congenital (without goiter) E03.1
    with goiter (diffuse) E03.0
  due to
    exogenous substance NEC E03.2
    iodine-deficiency, acquired E01.8
      subclinical E02
    irradiation therapy E89.0
    medicament NEC E03.2
    P-aminosalicylic acid (PAS) E03.2
    phenylbutazone E03.2
    resorcinol E03.2
    sulfonamide E03.2
    surgery E89.0
    thiourea group drugs E03.2
  iatrogenic NEC E03.2
  iodine-deficiency (acquired) E01.8
    congenital — *see* Syndrome, iodine- deficiency, congenital
    subclinical E02
  neonatal, transitory P72.2
  postinfectious E03.3
  postirradiation E89.0
  postprocedural E89.0
  postsurgical E89.0
  specified NEC E03.8
  subclinical, iodine-deficiency related E02
Hypotonia, hypotonicity, hypotony
  bladder N31.2
  congenital (benign) P94.2
  eye — *see* Disorder, globe, hypotony
Hypotrichosis — *see* Alopecia
Hypotropia H50.2- ☑
Hypoventilation R06.89
  congenital central alveolar G47.35
  sleep related
    idiopathic nonobstructive alveolar G47.34
    in conditions classified elsewhere G47.36
Hypovitaminosis — *see* Deficiency, vitamin
Hypovolemia E86.1
  surgical shock T81.19 ☑
  traumatic (shock) T79.4 ☑
Hypoxemia R09.02
  newborn P84
  sleep related, in conditions classified elsewhere G47.36
Hypoxia — *see also* Anoxia R09.02
  cerebral, during a procedure NEC G97.81
    postprocedural NEC G97.82
  intrauterine P84
  myocardial — *see* Insufficiency, coronary
  newborn P84
  sleep-related G47.34
Hypsarrhythmia — *see* Epilepsy, generalized, specified NEC
Hysteralgia, pregnant uterus O26.89- ☑
Hysteria, hysterical (conversion) (dissociative state) F44.9
  anxiety F41.8
  convulsions F44.5
  psychosis, acute F44.9
Hysteroepilepsy F44.5

I

IBDU (colonic inflammatory bowel dissease unclassified) K52.3
Ichthyoparasitism due to Vandellia cirrhosa B88.8

Ichthyosis (congenital) Q80.9
    acquired L85.0
    fetalis Q80.4
    hystrix Q80.8
    lamellar Q80.2
    lingual K13.29
    palmaris and plantaris Q82.8
    simplex Q80.0
    vera Q80.8
    vulgaris Q80.0
    X-linked Q80.1
Ichthyotoxism — see Poisoning, fish
    bacterial — see Intoxication, foodborne
Icteroanemia, hemolytic (acquired) D59.9
    congenital — see Spherocytosis
Icterus — see also Jaundice
    conjunctiva R17
    gravis, newborn P55.0
    hematogenous (acquired) D59.9
    hemolytic (acquired) D59.9
        congenital — see Spherocytosis
    hemorrhagic (acute) (leptospiral) (spirochetal) A27.0
        newborn P53
    infectious B15.9
        with hepatic coma B15.0
        leptospiral A27.0
        spirochetal A27.0
    neonatorum — see Jaundice, newborn
    newborn P59.9
    spirochetal A27.0
Ictus solaris, solis T67.01 ☑
Id reaction (due to bacteria) L30.2
Ideation
    homicidal R45.850
    suicidal R45.851
Identity disorder (child) F64.9
    gender role F64.2
    psychosexual F64.2
Idioglossia F80.0
Idiopathic — see condition
Idiot, idiocy (congenital) F73
    amaurotic (Bielschowsky(-Jansky)) (family) (infantile
        (late)) (juvenile (late)) (Vogt-Spielmeyer) E75.4
    microcephalic Q02
IgE asthma J45.909
IIAC (idiopathic infantile arterial calcification) Q28.8
Ileitis (chronic) (noninfectious) — see also Enteritis K52.9
    backwash — see Pancolitis, ulcerative (chronic)
    infectious A09
    regional (ulcerative) — see Enteritis, regional, small
        intestine
    segmental — see Enteritis, regional
    terminal (ulcerative) — see Enteritis, regional, small
        intestine
Ileocolitis — see also Enteritis K52.9
    infectious A09
    regional — see Enteritis, regional
    ulcerative K51.0- ☑
Ileostomy
    attention to Z43.2
    malfunctioning K94.13
    status Z93.2
        with complication — see Complications, enterosto-
            my
Ileotyphus — see Typhoid
Ileum — see condition
Ileus (bowel) (colon) (inhibitory) (intestine) K56.7
    adynamic K56.0
    due to gallstone (in intestine) K56.3
    duodenal (chronic) K31.5
    gallstone K56.3
    mechanical NEC — see also Obstruction, intestine,
        specified NEC K56.699
    meconium P76.0
        in cystic fibrosis E84.11
        meaning meconium plug (without cystic fibrosis)
            P76.0
    myxedema K59.89
    neurogenic K56.0
        Hirschsprung's disease or megacolon Q43.1
    newborn
        due to meconium P76.0
            in cystic fibrosis E84.11
            meaning meconium plug (without cystic fibrosis)
                P76.0
        transitory P76.1
    obstructive — see also Obstruction, intestine, specified
        NEC K56.699

Ileus — continued
    paralytic K56.0
    postoperative K91.89
Iliac — see condition
Iliotibial band syndrome M76.3- ☑
Illiteracy Z55.0
Illness — see also Disease R69
    manic-depressive — see Disorder, bipolar
Imbalance R26.89
    autonomic G90.8
    constituents of food intake E63.1
    electrolyte E87.8
        with
            abortion — see Abortion by type, complicated
                by, electrolyte imbalance
            molar pregnancy O08.5
        due to hyperemesis gravidarum O21.1
        following ectopic or molar pregnancy O08.5
        neonatal, transitory NEC P74.49
            potassium
                hyperkalemia P74.31
                hypokalemia P74.32
            sodium
                hypernatremia P74.21
                hyponatremia P74.22
    endocrine E34.9
    eye muscle NOS H50.9
    hormone E34.9
    hysterical F44.4
    labyrinth — see subcategory H83.2 ☑
    posture R29.3
    protein-energy — see Malnutrition
    sympathetic G90.8
Imbecile, imbecility (I.Q. 35-49) F71
Imbedding, intrauterine device T83.39 ☑
Imbibition, cholesterol (gallbladder) K82.4
Imbrication, teeth,, fully erupted M26.30
Imerslund (-Gräsbeck) **syndrome** D51.1
Immature — see also Immaturity
    birth (less than 37 completed weeks) — see Preterm,
        newborn
        extremely (less than 28 completed weeks) — see
            Immaturity, extreme
    personality F60.89
Immaturity (less than 37 completed weeks) — see also
    Preterm, newborn
    extreme of newborn (less than 28 completed weeks of
        gestation) (less than 196 completed days of
        gestation) (unspecified weeks of gestation)
        P07.20
        gestational age
            23 completed weeks (23 weeks, 0 days through
                23 weeks, 6 days) P07.22
            24 completed weeks (24 weeks, 0 days through
                24 weeks, 6 days) P07.23
            25 completed weeks (25 weeks, 0 days through
                25 weeks, 6 days) P07.24
            26 completed weeks (26 weeks, 0 days through
                26 weeks, 6 days) P07.25
            27 completed weeks (27 weeks, 0 days through
                27 weeks, 6 days) P07.26
            less than 23 completed weeks P07.21
    fetus or infant light-for-dates — see Light-for-dates
    lung, newborn P28.0
    organ or site NEC — see Hypoplasia
    pulmonary, newborn P28.0
    reaction F60.89
    sexual (female) (male), after puberty E30.0
Immersion T75.1 ☑
    foot T69.02- ☑
    hand T69.01- ☑
Immobile, immobility
    complete, due to severe physical disability or frailty
        R53.2
    intestine K59.89
    syndrome (paraplegic) M62.3
Immune reconstitution (inflammatory) syndrome [IRIS]
    D89.3
Immunization — see also Vaccination
    ABO — see Incompatibility, ABO
        in newborn P55.1
    appropriate for age
        child (over 28 days old) Z00.129
            with abnormal findings Z00.121
    complication — see Complications, vaccination
    encounter for Z23
    not done (not carried out) Z28.9
        because (of)

Immunization — continued
    not done — continued
        because — continued
            acute illness of patient Z28.01
            allergy to vaccine (or component) Z28.04
            caregiver refusal Z28.82
            chronic illness of patient Z28.02
            contraindication NEC Z28.09
            delay in delivery of vaccine Z28.83
            group pressure Z28.1
            guardian refusal Z28.82
            immune compromised state of patient Z28.03
            lack of availability of vaccine Z28.83
            manufacturer delay of vaccine Z28.83
            parent refusal Z28.82
            patient had disease being vaccinated against
                Z28.81
            patient refusal Z28.21
            patient's belief Z28.1
            religious beliefs of patient Z28.1
            specified reason NEC Z28.89
                of patient Z28.29
            unavailability of vaccine Z28.83
            unspecified patient reason Z28.20
    Rh factor
        affecting management of pregnancy NEC O36.09- ☑
            anti-D antibody O36.01- ☑
        from transfusion — see Complication(s), transfusion,
            incompatibility reaction, Rh (factor)
Immunocompromised NOS D84.9
Immunocytoma C83.0- ☑
Immunodeficiency D84.9
    with
        adenosine-deaminase deficiency — see also Defi-
            ciency, adenosine deaminase D81.30
        antibody defects D80.9
            specified type NEC D80.8
        hyperimmunoglobulinemia D80.6
        increased immunoglobulin M (IgM) D80.5
        major defect D82.9
            specified type NEC D82.8
        partial albinism D82.8
        short-limbed stature D82.2
        thrombocytopenia and eczema D82.0
    antibody with
        hyperimmunoglobulinemia D80.6
        near-normal immunoglobulins D80.6
    autosomal recessive, Swiss type D80.0
    combined D81.9
        biotin-dependent carboxylase D81.819
            biotinidase D81.810
            holocarboxylase synthetase D81.818
            specified type NEC D81.818
        severe (SCID) D81.9
            with
                low or normal B-cell numbers D81.2
                low T- and B-cell numbers D81.1
                reticular dysgenesis D81.0
        specified type NEC D81.89
    common variable D83.9
        with
            abnormalities of B-cell numbers and function
                D83.0
            autoantibodies to B- or T-cells D83.2
            immunoregulatory T-cell disorders D83.1
        specified type NEC D83.8
    due to
        conditions classified elsewhere D84.81
        drugs D84.821
        external causes D84.822
        medication (current or past) D84.821
    following hereditary defective response to Epstein-Barr
        virus (EBV) D82.3
    selective, immunoglobulin
        A (IgA) D80.2
        G (IgG) (subclasses) D80.3
        M (IgM) D80.4
    severe combined (SCID) D81.9
        due to adenosine deaminase deficiency D81.31
    specified type NEC D84.89
    X-linked, with increased IgM D80.5
Immunodeficient NOS D84.9
Immunosuppressed NOS D84.9
Immunotherapy (encounter for)
    antineoplastic Z51.12
Impaction, impacted
    bowel, colon, rectum — see also Impaction, fecal
        K56.49

182

☑ Additional Character Required — Refer to the Tabular List for Character Selection   ▽ Subterms under main terms may continue to next column or page

Impaction, impacted — *continued*
  bowel, colon, rectum — *see also* Impaction, fecal — *continued*
    by gallstone K56.3
  calculus — *see* Calculus
  cerumen (ear) (external) H61.2- ☑
  cuspid — *see* Impaction, tooth
  dental (same or adjacent tooth) K01.1
  fecal, feces K56.41
  fracture — *see* Fracture, by site
  gallbladder — *see* Calculus, gallbladder
  gallstone(s) — *see* Calculus, gallbladder
    bile duct (common) (hepatic) — *see* Calculus, bile duct
    cystic duct — *see* Calculus, gallbladder
    in intestine, with obstruction (any part) K56.3
  intestine (calculous) NEC — *see also* Impaction, fecal K56.49
    gallstone, with ileus K56.3
  intrauterine device (IUD) T83.39 ☑
  molar — *see* Impaction, tooth
  shoulder, causing obstructed labor O66.0
  tooth, teeth K01.1
  turbinate J34.89
Impaired, impairment (function)
  auditory discrimination — *see* Abnormal, auditory perception
  cognitive, mild, so stated G31.84
  dual sensory Z73.82
  fasting glucose R73.01
  glucose tolerance (oral) R73.02
  hearing — *see* Deafness
  heart — *see* Disease, heart
  kidney N28.9
    disorder resulting from N25.9
      specified NEC N25.89
  liver K72.90
    with coma K72.91
  mastication K08.89
  mild cognitive, so stated G31.84
  mobility
    ear ossicles — *see* Ankylosis, ear ossicles
    requiring care provider Z74.09
  myocardium, myocardial — *see* Insufficiency, myocardial
  rectal sphincter R19.8
  renal (acute) (chronic) N28.9
    disorder resulting from N25.9
      specified NEC N25.89
  vision NEC H54.7
    both eyes H54.3
Impediment, speech — *see also* Disorder, speech R47.9
  psychogenic (childhood) F98.8
  slurring R47.81
  specified NEC R47.89
Impending
  coronary syndrome I20.0
  delirium tremens F10.239
  myocardial infarction I20.0
Imperception auditory (acquired) — *see also* Deafness
  congenital H93.25
Imperfect
  aeration, lung (newborn) NEC — *see* Atelectasis
  closure (congenital)
    alimentary tract NEC Q45.8
      lower Q43.8
      upper Q40.8
    atrioventricular ostium Q21.2
    atrium (secundum) Q21.1
    branchial cleft NOS Q18.2
      cyst Q18.0
      fistula Q18.0
      sinus Q18.0
    choroid Q14.3
    cricoid cartilage Q31.8
    cusps, heart valve NEC Q24.8
      pulmonary Q22.3
    ductus
      arteriosus Q25.0
      Botalli Q25.0
    ear drum (causing impairment of hearing) Q16.4
    esophagus with communication to bronchus or trachea Q39.1
    eyelid Q10.3
    foramen
      botalli Q21.1
      ovale Q21.1

Imperfect — *continued*
  closure — *continued*
    genitalia, genital organ(s) or system
      female Q52.8
        external Q52.79
        internal NEC Q52.8
      male Q55.8
    glottis Q31.8
    interatrial ostium or septum Q21.1
    interauricular ostium or septum Q21.1
    interventricular ostium or septum Q21.0
    larynx Q31.8
    lip — *see* Cleft, lip
    nasal septum Q30.3
    nose Q30.2
    omphalomesenteric duct Q43.0
    optic nerve entry Q14.2
    organ or site not listed — *see* Anomaly, by site
    ostium
      interatrial Q21.1
      interauricular Q21.1
      interventricular Q21.0
    palate — *see* Cleft, palate
    preauricular sinus Q18.1
    retina Q14.1
    roof of orbit Q75.8
    sclera Q13.5
    septum
      aorticopulmonary Q21.4
      atrial (secundum) Q21.1
      between aorta and pulmonary artery Q21.4
      heart Q21.9
      interatrial (secundum) Q21.1
      interauricular (secundum) Q21.1
      interventricular Q21.0
        in tetralogy of Fallot Q21.3
      nasal Q30.3
      ventricular Q21.0
        with pulmonary stenosis or atresia, dextraposition of aorta, and hypertrophy of right ventricle Q21.3
        in tetralogy of Fallot Q21.3
    skull Q75.0
      with
        anencephaly Q00.0
        encephalocele — *see* Encephalocele
        hydrocephalus Q03.9
          with spina bifida — *see* Spina bifida, by site, with hydrocephalus
        microcephaly Q02
    spine (with meningocele) — *see* Spina bifida
    trachea Q32.1
    tympanic membrane (causing impairment of hearing) Q16.4
    uterus Q51.818
    vitelline duct Q43.0
  erection — *see* Dysfunction, sexual, male, erectile
  fusion — *see* Imperfect, closure
  inflation, lung (newborn) — *see* Atelectasis
  posture R29.3
  rotation, intestine Q43.3
  septum, ventricular Q21.0
Imperfectly descended testis — *see* Cryptorchid
Imperforate (congenital) — *see also* Atresia
  anus Q42.3
    with fistula Q42.2
  cervix (uteri) Q51.828
  esophagus Q39.0
    with tracheoesophageal fistula Q39.1
  hymen Q52.3
  jejunum Q41.1
  pharynx Q38.8
  rectum Q42.1
    with fistula Q42.0
  urethra Q64.39
  vagina Q52.4
Impervious (congenital) — *see also* Atresia
  anus Q42.3
    with fistula Q42.2
  bile duct Q44.2
  esophagus Q39.0
    with tracheoesophageal fistula Q39.1
  intestine (small) Q41.9
    large Q42.9
      specified NEC Q42.8
  rectum Q42.1
    with fistula Q42.0
  ureter — *see* Atresia, ureter

Impervious — *continued*
  urethra Q64.39
Impetiginization of dermatoses L01.1
Impetigo (any organism) (any site) (circinate) (contagiosa) (simplex) (vulgaris) L01.00
  Bockhart's L01.02
  bullous, bullosa L01.03
  external ear L01.00 *[H62.40]*
  follicularis L01.02
  furfuracea L30.5
  herpetiformis L40.1
    nonobstetrical L40.1
  neonatorum L01.03
  nonbullous L01.01
  specified type NEC L01.09
  ulcerative L01.09
Impingement (on teeth)
  joint — *see* Disorder, joint, specified type NEC
  soft tissue
    anterior M26.81
    posterior M26.82
Implant, endometrial N80.9
Implantation
  anomalous — *see* Anomaly, by site
    ureter Q62.63
  cyst
    external area or site (skin) NEC L72.0
    iris — *see* Cyst, iris, implantation
    vagina N89.8
    vulva N90.7
  dermoid (cyst) — *see* Implantation, cyst
Impotence (sexual) N52.9
  counseling Z70.1
  organic origin — *see also* Dysfunction, sexual, male, erectile N52.9
  psychogenic F52.21
Impression, basilar Q75.8
Imprisonment, anxiety concerning Z65.1
Improper care (child) (newborn) — *see* Maltreatment
Improperly tied umbilical cord (causing hemorrhage) P51.8
Impulsiveness (impulsive) R45.87
Inability to swallow — *see* Aphagia
Inaccessible, inaccessibility
  health care NEC Z75.3
    due to
      waiting period Z75.2
        for admission to facility elsewhere Z75.1
      other helping agencies Z75.4
Inactive — *see* condition
Inadequate, inadequacy
  aesthetics of dental restoration K08.56
  biologic, constitutional, functional, or social F60.7
  development
    child R62.50
    genitalia
      after puberty NEC E30.0
      congenital
        female Q52.8
          external Q52.79
          internal Q52.8
        male Q55.8
    lungs Q33.6
      associated with short gestation P28.0
    organ or site not listed — *see* Anomaly, by site
  diet (causing nutritional deficiency) E63.9
  eating habits Z72.4
  environment, household Z59.1
  family support Z63.8
  food (supply) NEC Z59.4
    hunger effects T73.0 ☑
  functional F60.7
  household care, due to
    family member
      handicapped or ill Z74.2
      on vacation Z75.5
      temporarily away from home Z74.2
    technical defects in home Z59.1
    temporary absence from home of person rendering care Z74.2
  housing (heating) (space) Z59.1
  income (financial) Z59.6
  intrafamilial communication Z63.8
  material resources Z59.9
  mental — *see* Disability, intellectual
  parental supervision or control of child Z62.0
  personality F60.7

Inadequate, inadequacy — continued
pulmonary
function R06.89
newborn P28.5
ventilation, newborn P28.5
sample of cytologic smear
anus R85.615
cervix R87.615
vagina R87.625
social F60.7
insurance Z59.7
skills NEC Z73.4
supervision of child by parent Z62.0
teaching affecting education Z55.8
welfare support Z59.7
Inanition R64
with edema — see Malnutrition, severe
due to
deprivation of food T73.0 ☑
malnutrition — see Malnutrition
fever R50.9
Inappropriate
change in quantitative human chorionic gonadotropin (hCG) in early pregnancy O02.81
diet or eating habits Z72.4
level of quantitative human chorionic gonadotropin (hCG) for gestational age in early pregnancy O02.81
secretion
antidiuretic hormone (ADH) (excessive) E22.2
deficiency E23.2
pituitary (posterior) E22.2
Inattention at or after birth — see Neglect
Incarceration, incarcerated
enterocele K46.0
gangrenous K46.1
epiplocele K46.0
gangrenous K46.1
exomphalos K42.0
gangrenous K42.1
hernia — see also Hernia, by site, with obstruction
with gangrene — see Hernia, by site, with gangrene
iris, in wound — see Injury, eye, laceration, with prolapse
lens, in wound — see Injury, eye, laceration, with prolapse
omphalocele K42.0
prison, anxiety concerning Z65.1
rupture — see Hernia, by site
sarcoepiplocele K46.0
gangrenous K46.1
sarcoepiplomphalocele K42.0
with gangrene K42.1
uterus N85.8
gravid O34.51- ☑
causing obstructed labor O65.5
Incised wound
external — see Laceration
internal organs — see Injury, by site
Incision, incisional
hernia K43.2
with
gangrene (and obstruction) K43.1
obstruction K43.0
surgical, complication — see Complications, surgical procedure
traumatic
external — see Laceration
internal organs — see Injury, by site
Inclusion
azurophilic leukocytic D72.0
blennorrhea (neonatal) (newborn) P39.1
gallbladder in liver (congenital) Q44.1
Incompatibility
ABO
affecting management of pregnancy O36.11- ☑
anti-A sensitization O36.11- ☑
anti-B sensitization O36.19- ☑
specified NEC O36.19- ☑
infusion or transfusion reaction — see Complication(s), transfusion, incompatibility reaction, ABO
newborn P55.1
blood (group) (Duffy) (K) (Kell) (Kidd) (Lewis) (M) (S) NEC
affecting management of pregnancy O36.11- ☑
anti-A sensitization O36.11- ☑
anti-B sensitization O36.19- ☑

Incompatibility — continued
blood (S) — continued
infusion or transfusion reaction T80.89 ☑
newborn P55.8
divorce or estrangement Z63.5
Rh (blood group) (factor) Z31.82
affecting management of pregnancy NEC O36.09- ☑
anti-D antibody O36.01- ☑
infusion or transfusion reaction — see Complication(s), transfusion, incompatibility reaction, Rh (factor)
newborn P55.0
rhesus — see Incompatibility, Rh
Incompetency, incompetent, incompetence
annular
aortic (valve) — see Insufficiency, aortic
mitral (valve) I34.0
pulmonary valve (heart) I37.1
aortic (valve) — see Insufficiency, aortic
cardiac valve — see Endocarditis
cervix, cervical (os) N88.3
in pregnancy O34.3- ☑
chronotropic I45.89
with
autonomic dysfunction G90.8
ischemic heart disease I25.89
left ventricular dysfunction I51.89
sinus node dysfunction I49.8
esophagogastric (junction) (sphincter) K22.0
mitral (valve) — see Insufficiency, mitral
pelvic fundus N81.89
pubocervical tissue N81.82
pulmonary valve (heart) I37.1
congenital Q22.3
rectovaginal tissue N81.83
tricuspid (annular) (valve) — see Insufficiency, tricuspid
valvular — see Endocarditis
congenital Q24.8
vein, venous (saphenous) (varicose) — see Varix, leg
Incomplete — see also condition
bladder, emptying R33.9
defecation R15.0
expansion lungs (newborn) NEC — see Atelectasis
rotation, intestine Q43.3
Inconclusive
diagnostic imaging due to excess body fat of patient R93.9
findings on diagnostic imaging of breast NEC R92.8
mammogram (due to dense breasts) R92.2
Incontinence R32
anal sphincter R15.9
coital N39.491
feces R15.9
nonorganic origin F98.1
insensible (urinary) N39.42
overflow N39.490
postural (urinary) N39.492
psychogenic F45.8
rectal R15.9
reflex N39.498
stress (female) (male) N39.3
and urge N39.46
urethral sphincter R32
urge N39.41
and stress (female) (male) N39.46
urine (urinary) R32
continuous N39.45
due to cognitive impairment, or severe physical disability or immobility R39.81
functional R39.81
insensible N39.42
mixed (stress and urge) N39.46
nocturnal N39.44
nonorganic origin F98.0
overflow N39.490
post dribbling N39.43
postural N39.492
reflex N39.498
specified NEC N39.498
stress (female) (male) N39.3
and urge N39.46
total N39.498
unaware N39.42
urge N39.41
and stress (female) (male) N39.46
Incontinentia pigmenti Q82.3
Incoordinate, incoordination
esophageal-pharyngeal (newborn) — see Dysphagia

Incoordinate, incoordination — continued
muscular R27.8
uterus (action) (contractions) (complicating delivery) O62.4
Increase, increased
abnormal, in development R63.8
androgens (ovarian) E28.1
anticoagulants (antithrombin) (anti-VIIIa) (anti-IXa) (anti-Xa) (anti-XIa) — see Circulating anticoagulants
cold sense R20.8
estrogen E28.0
function
adrenal
cortex — see Cushing's, syndrome
medulla E27.5
pituitary (gland) (anterior) (lobe) E22.9
posterior E22.2
heat sense R20.8
intracranial pressure (benign) G93.2
permeability, capillaries I78.8
pressure, intracranial G93.2
secretion
gastrin E16.4
glucagon E16.3
pancreas, endocrine E16.9
growth hormone-releasing hormone E16.8
pancreatic polypeptide E16.8
somatostatin E16.8
vasoactive-intestinal polypeptide E16.8
sphericity, lens Q12.4
splenic activity D73.1
venous pressure I87.8
portal K76.6
Increta placenta O43.22- ☑
Incrustation, cornea, foreign body (lead)(zinc) — see Foreign body, cornea
Incyclophoria H50.54
Incyclotropia — see Cyclotropia
Indeterminate sex Q56.4
India rubber skin Q82.8
Indigestion (acid) (bilious) (functional) K30
catarrhal K31.89
due to decomposed food NOS A05.9
nervous F45.8
psychogenic F45.8
Indirect — see condition
Induratio penis plastica N48.6
Induration, indurated
brain G93.89
breast (fibrous) N64.51
puerperal, postpartum O92.29
broad ligament N83.8
chancre
anus A51.1
congenital A50.07
extragenital NEC A51.2
corpora cavernosa (penis) (plastic) N48.6
liver (chronic) K76.89
lung (black) (chronic) (fibroid) — see also Fibrosis, lung J84.10
essential brown J84.03
penile (plastic) N48.6
phlebitic — see Phlebitis
skin R23.4
Inebriety (without dependence) — see Alcohol, intoxication
Inefficiency, kidney N28.9
Inelasticity, skin R23.4
Inequality, leg (length) (acquired) — see also Deformity, limb, unequal length
congenital — see Defect, reduction, lower limb
lower leg — see Deformity, limb, unequal length
Inertia
bladder (neurogenic) N31.2
stomach K31.89
psychogenic F45.8
uterus, uterine during labor O62.2
during latent phase of labor O62.0
primary O62.0
secondary O62.1
vesical (neurogenic) N31.2
Infancy, infantile, infantilism — see also condition
celiac K90.0
genitalia, genitals (after puberty) E30.0
Herter's (nontropical sprue) K90.0
intestinal K90.0
Lorain E23.0

☑ Additional Character Required — Refer to the Tabular List for Character Selection

▽ Subterms under main terms may continue to next column or page

Infancy, infantile, infantilism — *continued*
  pancreatic K86.89
  pelvis M95.5
    with disproportion (fetopelvic) O33.1
      causing obstructed labor O65.1
  pituitary E23.0
  renal N25.0
  uterus — *see* Infantile, genitalia
Infant(s) — *see also* Infancy
  excessive crying R68.11
  irritable child R68.12
  lack of care — *see* Neglect
  liveborn (singleton) Z38.2
    born in hospital Z38.00
      by cesarean Z38.01
    born outside hospital Z38.1
    multiple NEC Z38.8
      born in hospital Z38.68
        by cesarean Z38.69
      born outside hospital Z38.7
    quadruplet Z38.8
      born in hospital Z38.63
        by cesarean Z38.64
      born outside hospital Z38.7
    quintuplet Z38.8
      born in hospital Z38.65
        by cesarean Z38.66
      born outside hospital Z38.7
    triplet Z38.8
      born in hospital Z38.61
        by cesarean Z38.62
      born outside hospital Z38.7
    twin Z38.5
      born in hospital Z38.30
        by cesarean Z38.31
      born outside hospital Z38.4
  of diabetic mother (syndrome of) P70.1
    gestational diabetes P70.0
Infantile — *see also* condition
  genitalia, genitals E30.0
  os, uterine E30.0
  penis E30.0
  testis E29.1
  uterus E30.0
Infantilism — *see* Infancy
Infarct, infarction
  adrenal (capsule) (gland) E27.49
  appendices epiploicae — *see also* Infarct, intestine
    K55.069
  bowel — *see also* Infarct, intestine K55.069
  brain (stem) — *see* Infarct, cerebral
  breast N64.89
  brewer's (kidney) N28.0
  cardiac — *see* Infarct, myocardium
  cerebellar — *see* Infarct, cerebral
  cerebral (acute) (chronic) — *see also* Occlusion, artery
    cerebral or precerebral, with infarction I63.9-
    aborted I63.9
    cortical I63.9
    due to
      cerebral venous thrombosis, nonpyogenic I63.6
      embolism
        cerebral arteries I63.4- ☑
        precerebral arteries I63.1- ☑
      occlusion NEC
        cerebral arteries I63.5- ☑
        precerebral arteries I63.2- ☑
        small artery I63.81
      stenosis NEC
        cerebral arteries I63.5- ☑
        precerebral arteries I63.2- ☑
        small artery I63.81
      thrombosis
        cerebral artery I63.3- ☑
        precerebral artery I63.0- ☑
    intraoperative
      during cardiac surgery I97.810
      during other surgery I97.811
    neonatal P91.82- ☑
    perinatal (arterial ischemic) P91.82- ☑
    postprocedural
      following cardiac surgery I97.820
      following other surgery I97.821
    specified NEC I63.89
  colon (acute) (agnogenic) (embolic) (hemorrhagic)
    (nonocclusive) (nonthrombotic) (occlusive)
    (segmental) (thrombotic) (with gangrene) — *see*
    also Infarct, intestine K55.049

Infarct, infarction — *continued*
  coronary artery — *see* Infarct, myocardium
  embolic — *see* Embolism
  fallopian tube N83.8
  gallbladder K82.8
  heart — *see* Infarct, myocardium
  hepatic K76.3
  hypophysis (anterior lobe) E23.6
  impending (myocardium) I20.0
  intestine (acute) (agnogenic) (embolic) (hemorrhagic)
    (nonocclusive) (nonthrombotic) (occlusive)
    (thrombotic) (with gangrene) K55.069
    diffuse K55.062
    focal K55.061
    large K55.049
      diffuse K55.042
      focal K55.041
    small K55.029
      diffuse K55.022
      focal K55.021
  kidney N28.0
  lacunar I63.81
  liver K76.3
  lung (embolic) (thrombotic) — *see* Embolism, pul-
    monary
  lymph node I89.8
  mesentery, mesenteric (embolic) (thrombotic) (with
    gangrene) — *see also* Infarct, intestine K55.069
  muscle (ischemic) M62.20
    ankle M62.27- ☑
    foot M62.27- ☑
    forearm M62.23- ☑
    hand M62.24- ☑
    lower leg M62.26- ☑
    pelvic region M62.25- ☑
    shoulder region M62.21- ☑
    specified site NEC M62.28
    thigh M62.25- ☑
    upper arm M62.22- ☑
  myocardium, myocardial (acute) (with stated duration
    of 4 weeks or less) I21.9
    associated with revascularization procedure I21.A9
    diagnosed on ECG, but presenting no symptoms
      I25.2
    due to
      demand ischemia I21.A1
      ischemic imbalance I21.A1
    healed or old I25.2
    intraoperative — *see also* Infarct, myocardium, as-
      sociated with revascularization procedure
      during cardiac surgery I97.790
      during other surgery I97.791
    non-Q wave I21.4
    non-ST elevation (NSTEMI) I21.4
      subsequent I22.2
    nontransmural I21.4
    past (diagnosed on ECG or other investigation, but
      currently presenting no symptoms) I25.2
    postprocedural — *see also* Infarct, myocardium,
      associated with revascularization procedure
      following cardiac surgery — *see also* Infarct,
        myocardium, type 4 or type 5 I97.190
      following other surgery I97.191
    Q wave (*see also* Infarct, myocardium, by site) I21.3
    secondary to
      demand ischemia I21.A1
      ischemic imbalance I21.A1
    ST elevation (STEMI) I21.3
      anterior (anteroapical) (anterolateral) (anterosep-
        tal) (Q wave) (wall) I21.09
        subsequent I22.0
      inferior (diaphragmatic) (inferolateral) (inferopos-
        terior) (wall) NEC I21.19
        subsequent I22.1
      inferoposterior transmural (Q wave) I21.11
      involving
        coronary artery of anterior wall NEC I21.09
        coronary artery of inferior wall NEC I21.19
        diagonal coronary artery I21.02
        left anterior descending coronary artery I21.02
        left circumflex coronary artery I21.21
        left main coronary artery I21.01
        oblique marginal coronary artery I21.21
        right coronary artery I21.11
      lateral (apical-lateral) (basal-lateral) (high) I21.29
        subsequent I22.8
      posterior (posterobasal) (posterolateral) (pos-
        teroseptal) (true) I21.29

Infarct, infarction — *continued*
  myocardium, myocardial — *continued*
    ST elevation — *continued*
      posterior — *continued*
        subsequent I22.8
      septal I21.29
        subsequent I22.8
      specified NEC I21.29
        subsequent I22.8
      subsequent I22.9
    subsequent (recurrent) (reinfarction) I22.9
      anterior (anteroapical) (anterolateral) (anterosep-
        tal) (wall) I22.0
      diaphragmatic (wall) I22.1
      inferior (diaphragmatic) (inferolateral) (inferopos-
        terior) (wall) I22.1
      lateral (apical-lateral) (basal-lateral) (high) I22.8
      non-ST elevation (NSTEMI) I22.2
      posterior (posterobasal) (posterolateral) (pos-
        teroseptal) (true) I22.8
      septal I22.8
      specified NEC I22.8
      ST elevation I22.9
        anterior (anteroapical) (anterolateral) (an-
          teroseptal) (wall) I22.0
        inferior (diaphragmatic) (inferolateral) (infer-
          oposterior) (wall) I22.1
        specified NEC I22.8
      subendocardial I22.2
      transmural I21.3
        anterior (anteroapical) (anterolateral) (an-
          teroseptal) (wall) I22.0
        diaphragmatic (wall) I22.1
        inferior (diaphragmatic) (inferolateral) (infer-
          oposterior) (wall) I22.1
        lateral (apical-lateral) (basal-lateral) (high)
          I22.8
        posterior (posterobasal) (posterolateral)
          (posteroseptal) (true) I22.8
        specified NEC I22.8
    type 1 — *see also* Infarction, myocardial, subse-
      quent, by site, or by ST elevation or non-
      ST elevation I22.9
    type 2 I21.A1
    type 3 I21.A9
    type 4 I21.A9
    type 5 I21.A9
  syphilitic A52.06
  transmural I21.9
    anterior (anteroapical) (anterolateral) (anterosep-
      tal) (Q wave) (wall) NEC I21.09
    inferior (diaphragmatic) (inferolateral) (inferopos-
      terior) (Q wave) (wall) NEC I21.19
    inferoposterior (Q wave) I21.11
    lateral (apical-lateral) (basal-lateral) (high) NEC
      I21.29
    posterior (posterobasal) (posterolateral) (pos-
      teroseptal) (true) NEC I21.29
    septal NEC I21.29
    specified NEC I21.29
    type 1 — *see also* Infarction, myocardial, by site, or
      by ST elevation or non-ST elevation I21.9
    type 2 I21.A1
    type 3 I21.A9
    type 4 (a) (b) (c) I21.A9
    type 5 I21.A9
  nontransmural I21.4
  omentum — *see also* Infarct, intestine K55.069
  ovary N83.8
  pancreas K86.89
  papillary muscle — *see* Infarct, myocardium
  parathyroid gland E21.4
  pituitary (gland) E23.6
  placenta O43.81- ☑
  prostate N42.89
  pulmonary (artery) (vein) (hemorrhagic) — *see* Em-
    bolism, pulmonary
  renal (embolic) (thrombotic) N28.0
  retina, retinal (artery) — *see* Occlusion, artery, retina
  spinal (cord) (acute) (embolic) (nonembolic) G95.11
  spleen D73.5
    embolic or thrombotic I74.8
  subendocardial (acute) (nontransmural) I21.4
  suprarenal (capsule) (gland) E27.49
  testis N50.1
  thrombotic — *see also* Thrombosis
    artery, arterial — *see* Embolism
  thyroid (gland) E07.89

Infarct, infarction — *continued*
  ventricle (heart) — *see* Infarct, myocardium
Infecting — *see* condition
Infection, infected, infective (opportunistic) B99.9
  with
    drug resistant organism — *see* Resistance (to), drug
        — *see also* specific organism
    lymphangitis — *see* Lymphangitis
    organ dysfunction (acute) R65.20
      with septic shock R65.21
  abscess (skin) — *code by* site under Abscess
  Absidia — *see* Mucormycosis
  Acanthamoeba — *see* Acanthamebiasis
  Acanthocheilonema (perstans) (streptocerca) B74.4
  accessory sinus (chronic) — *see* Sinusitis
  achorion — *see* Dermatophytosis
  Acremonium falciforme B47.0
  acromioclavicular M00.9
  Actinobacillus (actinomycetem-comitans) A28.8
    mallei A24.0
    muris A25.1
  Actinomadura B47.1
  Actinomyces (israelii) — *see also* Actinomycosis A42.9
  Actinomycetales — *see* Actinomycosis
  actinomycotic NOS — *see* Actinomycosis
  adenoid (and tonsil) J03.90
    chronic J35.02
  adenovirus NEC
    as cause of disease classified elsewhere B97.0
    unspecified nature or site B34.0
  aerogenes capsulatus A48.0
  aertrycke — *see* Infection, salmonella
  alimentary canal NOS — *see* Enteritis, infectious
  Allescheria boydii B48.2
  Alternaria B48.8
  alveolus, alveolar (process) K04.7
  Ameba, amebic (histolytica) — *see* Amebiasis
  amniotic fluid, sac or cavity O41.10- ☑
    chorioamnionitis O41.12- ☑
    placentitis O41.14- ☑
  amputation stump (surgical) — *see* Complication,
      amputation stump, infection
  Ancylostoma (duodenalis) B76.0
  Anisakiasis, Anisakis larvae B81.0
  anthrax — *see* Anthrax
  antrum (chronic) — *see* Sinusitis, maxillary
  anus, anal (papillae) (sphincter) K62.89
  arbovirus (arbor virus) A94
    specified type NEC A93.8
  artificial insemination N98.0
  Ascaris lumbricoides — *see* Ascariasis
  Ascomycetes B47.0
  Aspergillus (flavus) (fumigatus) (terreus) — *see* As-
      pergillosis
  atypical
    acid-fast (bacilli) — *see* Mycobacterium, atypical
    mycobacteria — *see* Mycobacterium, atypical
    virus A81.9
      specified type NEC A81.89
  auditory meatus (external) — *see* Otitis, externa, infec-
      tive
  auricle (ear) — *see* Otitis, externa, infective
  axillary gland (lymph) L04.2
  Bacillus A49.9
    abortus A23.1
    anthracis — *see* Anthrax
    Ducrey's (any location) A57
    Flexner's A03.1
    Friedländer's NEC A49.8
    gas (gangrene) A48.0
    mallei A24.0
    melitensis A23.0
    paratyphoid, paratyphosus A01.4
      A A01.1
      B A01.2
      C A01.3
    Shiga (-Kruse) A03.0
    suipestifer — *see* Infection, salmonella
    swimming pool A31.1
    typhosa A01.00
    welchii — *see* Gangrene, gas
  bacterial NOS A49.9
    as cause of disease classified elsewhere B96.89
      Bacteroides fragilis [B. fragilis] B96.6
      Clostridium perfringens [C. perfringens] B96.7
      Enterobacter sakazakii B96.89
      Enterococcus B95.2

Infection, infected, infective — *continued*
  bacterial — *continued*
    as cause of disease classified elsewhere — *contin-
        ued*
      Escherichia coli [E. coli] — *see also* Escherichia
          coli B96.20
      Helicobacter pylori [H.pylori] B96.81
      Hemophilus influenzae [H. influenzae] B96.3
      Klebsiella pneumoniae [K. pneumoniae] B96.1
      Mycoplasma pneumoniae [M. pneumoniae]
          B96.0
      Proteus (mirabilis) (morganii) B96.4
      Pseudomonas (aeruginosa) (mallei) (pseudoma-
          llei) B96.5
      Staphylococcus B95.8
        aureus (methicillin susceptible) (MSSA) B95.61
          methicillin resistant (MRSA) B95.62
        specified NEC B95.7
      Streptococcus B95.5
        group A B95.0
        group B B95.1
        pneumoniae B95.3
        specified NEC B95.4
      Vibrio vulnificus B96.82
    specified NEC A48.8
  Bacterium
    paratyphosum A01.4
      A A01.1
      B A01.2
      C A01.3
    typhosum A01.00
  Bacteroides NEC A49.8
    fragilis, as cause of disease classified elsewhere
        B96.6
  Balantidium coli A07.0
  Bartholin's gland N75.8
  Basidiobolus B46.8
  bile duct (common) (hepatic) — *see* Cholangitis
  bladder — *see* Cystitis
  Blastomyces, blastomycotic — *see also* Blastomycosis
    brasiliensis — *see* Paracoccidioidomycosis
    dermatitidis — *see* Blastomycosis
    European — *see* Cryptococcosis
    Loboi B48.0
    North American B40.9
    South American — *see* Paracoccidioidomycosis
  bleb, postprocedure — *see* Blebitis
  bone — *see* Osteomyelitis
  Bordetella — *see* Whooping cough
  Borrelia bergdorfi A69.20
  brain — *see also* Encephalitis G04.90
    membranes — *see* Meningitis
    septic G06.0
      meninges — *see* Meningitis, bacterial
  branchial cyst Q18.0
  breast — *see* Mastitis
  bronchus — *see* Bronchitis
  Brucella A23.9
    abortus A23.1
    canis A23.3
    melitensis A23.0
    mixed A23.8
    specified NEC A23.8
    suis A23.2
  Brugia (malayi) B74.1
    timori B74.2
  bursa — *see* Bursitis, infective
  buttocks (skin) L08.9
  Campylobacter, intestinal A04.5
    as cause of disease classified elsewhere B96.81
  Candida (albicans) (tropicalis) — *see* Candidiasis
  candiru B88.8
  Capillaria (intestinal) B81.1
    hepatica B83.8
    philippinensis B81.1
  cartilage — *see* Disorder, cartilage, specified type NEC
  cat liver fluke B66.0
  catheter-related bloodstream (CRBSI) T80.211 ☑
  cellulitis — *code by* site under Cellulitis
  central line-associated T80.219 ☑
    bloodstream (CLABSI) T80.211 ☑
    specified NEC T80.218 ☑
  Cephalosporium falciforme B47.0
  cerebrospinal — *see* Meningitis
  cervical gland (lymph) L04.0
  cervix — *see* Cervicitis
  cesarean delivery wound (puerperal) O86.00
  cestodes — *see* Infestation, cestodes

Infection, infected, infective — *continued*
  chest J22
  Chilomastix (intestinal) A07.8
  Chlamydia, chlamydial A74.9
    anus A56.3
    genitourinary tract A56.2
      lower A56.00
      specified NEC A56.19
    lymphogranuloma A55
    pharynx A56.4
    psittaci A70
    rectum A56.3
    sexually transmitted NEC A56.8
  cholera — *see* Cholera
  Cladosporium
    bantianum (brain abscess) B43.1
    carrionii B43.0
    castellanii B36.1
    trichoides (brain abscess) B43.1
    werneckii B36.1
  Clonorchis (sinensis) (liver) B66.1
  Clostridium NEC
    bifermentans A48.0
    botulinum (food poisoning) A05.1
      infant A48.51
      wound A48.52
    difficile
      as cause of disease classified elsewhere B96.89
      foodborne (disease)
        not specified as recurrent A04.72
        recurrent A04.71
      gas gangrene A48.0
      necrotizing enterocolitis
        not specified as recurrent A04.72
        recurrent A04.71
      sepsis A41.4
    gas-forming NEC A48.0
    histolyticum A48.0
    novyi, causing gas gangrene A48.0
    oedematiens A48.0
    perfringens
      as cause of disease classified elsewhere B96.7
      due to food A05.2
      foodborne (disease) A05.2
      gas gangrene A48.0
      sepsis A41.4
    septicum, causing gas gangrene A48.0
    sordellii, causing gas gangrene A48.0
    welchii
      as cause of disease classified elsewhere B96.7
      foodborne (disease) A05.2
      gas gangrene A48.0
      necrotizing enteritis A05.2
      sepsis A41.4
  Coccidioides (immitis) — *see* Coccidioidomycosis
  colon — *see* Enteritis, infectious
  colostomy K94.02
  common duct — *see* Cholangitis
  congenital P39.9
    Candida (albicans) P37.5
    cytomegalovirus P35.1
    hepatitis, viral P35.3
    herpes simplex P35.2
    infectious or parasitic disease P37.9
      specified NEC P37.8
    listeriosis (disseminated) P37.2
    malaria NEC P37.4
      falciparum P37.3
    Plasmodium falciparum P37.3
    poliomyelitis P35.8
    rubella P35.0
    skin P39.4
    toxoplasmosis (acute) (subacute) (chronic) P37.1
    tuberculosis P37.0
    urinary (tract) P39.3
    vaccinia P35.8
    virus P35.9
      specified type NEC P35.8
  Conidiobolus B46.8
  coronavirus-2019 U07.1
  coronavirus NEC B34.2
    as cause of disease classified elsewhere B97.29
    severe acute respiratory syndrome (SARS associate*
        B97.21
  corpus luteum — *see* Salpingo-oophoritis
  Corynebacterium diphtheriae — *see* Diphtheria
  cotia virus B08.8
  COVID-19 U07.1
  Coxiella burnetii A78

☑ **Additional Character Required** — Refer to the Tabular List for Character Selection   ▽ **Subterms under main terms may continue to next column or pag**

Infection, infected, infective — *continued*
- coxsackie — *see* Coxsackie
- Cryptococcus neoformans — *see* Cryptococcosis
- Cryptosporidium A07.2
- Cunninghamella — *see* Mucormycosis
- cyst — *see* Cyst
- cystic duct — *see also* Cholecystitis K81.9
- Cysticercus cellulosae — *see* Cysticercosis
- cytomegalovirus, cytomegaloviral B25.9
  - congenital P35.1
  - maternal, maternal care for (suspected) damage to fetus O35.3 ☑
  - mononucleosis B27.10
    - with
      - complication NEC B27.19
      - meningitis B27.12
      - polyneuropathy B27.11
- delta-agent (acute), in hepatitis B carrier B17.0
- dental (pulpal origin) K04.7
- Deuteromycetes B47.0
- Dicrocoelium dendriticum B66.2
- Dipetalonema (perstans) (streptocerca) B74.4
- diphtherial — *see* Diphtheria
- Diphyllobothrium (adult) (latum) (pacificum) B70.0
  - larval B70.1
- Diplogonoporus (grandis) B71.8
- Dipylidium caninum B67.4
- Dirofilaria B74.8
- Dracunculus medinensis B72
- Drechslera (hawaiiensis) B43.8
- Ducrey Haemophilus (any location) A57
- due to or resulting from
  - artificial insemination N98.0
  - Babesia
    - divergens (-like) strain B60.03
    - duncani (-type) species B60.02
    - microti B60.01
    - species
      - specified NEC B60.09
  - central venous catheter T80.219 ☑
    - bloodstream T80.211 ☑
    - exit or insertion site T80.212 ☑
    - localized T80.212 ☑
    - port or reservoir T80.212 ☑
    - specified NEC T80.218 ☑
    - tunnel T80.212 ☑
  - device, implant or graft — *see also* Complications, by site and type, infection or inflammation T85.79 ☑
    - arterial graft NEC T82.7 ☑
    - breast (implant) T85.79 ☑
    - catheter NEC T85.79 ☑
      - dialysis (renal) T82.7 ☑
        - central line T80.211 ☑
        - intraperitoneal T85.71 ☑
      - infusion NEC T82.7 ☑
        - cranial T85.735 ☑
        - intrathecal T85.735 ☑
        - spinal (epidural) (subdural) T85.735 ☑
        - subarachnoid T85.735 ☑
      - urinary T83.518 ☑
        - cystostomy T83.510 ☑
        - Hopkins T83.518 ☑
        - ileostomy T83.518 ☑
        - nephrostomy T83.512 ☑
        - specified NEC T83.518 ☑
        - urethral indwelling T83.511 ☑
        - urostomy T83.518 ☑
    - electronic (electrode) (pulse generator) (stimulator)
      - bone T84.7 ☑
      - cardiac T82.7 ☑
      - nervous system T85.738 ☑
        - brain T85.731 ☑
        - cranial nerve T85.732 ☑
        - gastric nerve T85.732 ☑
        - generator pocket T85.734 ☑
        - neurostimulator generator T85.734 ☑
        - peripheral nerve T85.732 ☑
        - sacral nerve T85.732 ☑
        - spinal cord T85.733 ☑
        - vagal nerve T85.732 ☑
      - urinary (indwelling) T83.51 ☑
    - fixation, internal (orthopedic) NEC — *see* Complication, fixation device, infection
    - gastrointestinal (bile duct) (esophagus) T85.79 ☑
      - neurostimulator electrode (lead) T85.732 ☑

Infection, infected, infective — *continued*
- due to or resulting from — *continued*
  - device, implant or graft — *see also* Complications, by site and type, infection or inflammation — *continued*
    - genital NEC T83.69 ☑
    - heart NEC T82.7 ☑
      - valve (prosthesis) T82.6 ☑
        - graft T82.7 ☑
    - joint prosthesis — *see* Complication, joint prosthesis, infection
    - ocular (corneal graft) (orbital implant) NEC T85.79 ☑
    - orthopedic NEC T84.7 ☑
    - penile (cylinder) (pump) (resevoir) T83.61 ☑
    - specified NEC T85.79 ☑
    - testicular T83.62 ☑
    - urinary NEC T83.598 ☑
      - ileal conduit stent T83.593 ☑
      - implanted neurostimulation T83.590 ☑
      - implanted sphincter T83.591 ☑
      - indwelling ureteral stent T83.592 ☑
      - nephroureteral stent T83.593 ☑
      - specified stent NEC T83.593 ☑
    - vascular NEC T82.7 ☑
    - ventricular intracranial (communicating) shunt T85.730 ☑
  - Hickman catheter T80.219 ☑
    - bloodstream T80.211 ☑
    - localized T80.212 ☑
    - specified NEC T80.218 ☑
  - immunization or vaccination T88.0 ☑
  - infusion, injection or transfusion NEC T80.29 ☑
  - injury NEC — *code by* site under Wound, open
  - peripherally inserted central catheter (PICC) T80.219 ☑
    - bloodstream T80.211 ☑
    - localized T80.212 ☑
    - specified NEC T80.218 ☑
  - portacath (port-a-cath) T80.219 ☑
    - bloodstream T80.211 ☑
    - localized T80.212 ☑
    - specified NEC T80.218 ☑
  - protozoa of the order Piroplasmida NEC B60.09
  - pulmonary artery catheter — *see* Infection, due to or resulting from, central venous catheter
  - surgery T81.40 ☑
  - Swan Ganz catheter — *see* Infection, due to or resulting from, central venous catheter
  - triple lumen catheter T80.219 ☑
    - bloodstream T80.211 ☑
    - localized T80.212 ☑
    - specified NEC T80.218 ☑
  - umbilical venous catheter T80.219 ☑
    - bloodstream T80.211 ☑
    - localized T80.212 ☑
    - specified NEC T80.218 ☑
- during labor NEC O75.3
- ear (middle) — *see also* Otitis media
  - external — *see* Otitis, externa, infective
  - inner — *see* subcategory H83.0 ☑
- Eberthella typhosa A01.00
- Echinococcus — *see* Echinococcus
- echovirus
  - as cause of disease classified elsewhere B97.12
  - unspecified nature or site B34.1
- endocardium I33.0
- endocervix — *see* Cervicitis
- Entamoeba — *see* Amebiasis
- enteric — *see* Enteritis, infectious
- Enterobacter sakazakii B96.89
- Enterobius vermicularis B80
- enterostomy K94.12
- enterovirus B34.1
  - as cause of disease classified elsewhere B97.10
    - coxsackievirus B97.11
    - echovirus B97.12
    - specified NEC B97.19
- Entomophthora B46.8
- Epidermophyton — *see* Dermatophytosis
- epididymis — *see* Epididymitis
- episiotomy (puerperal) O86.09
- Erysipelothrix (insidiosa) (rhusiopathiae) — *see* Erysipeloid
- erythema infectiosum B08.3
- Escherichia (E.) coli NEC A49.8

Infection, infected, infective — *continued*
- Escherichia coli — *continued*
  - as cause of disease classified elsewhere — *see also* Escherichia coli B96.20
  - congenital P39.8
    - sepsis P36.4
  - generalized A41.51
  - intestinal — *see* Enteritis, infectious, due to, Escherichia coli
- ethmoidal (chronic) (sinus) — *see* Sinusitis, ethmoidal
- eustachian tube (ear) — *see* Salpingitis, eustachian
- external auditory canal (meatus) NEC — *see* Otitis, externa, infective
- eye (purulent) — *see* Endophthalmitis, purulent
- eyelid — *see* Inflammation, eyelid
- fallopian tube — *see* Salpingo-oophoritis
- Fasciola (gigantica) (hepatica) (indica) B66.3
- Fasciolopsis (buski) B66.5
- filarial — *see* Infestation, filarial
- finger (skin) L08.9
  - nail L03.01- ☑
    - fungus B35.1
- fish tapeworm B70.0
  - larval B70.1
- flagellate, intestinal A07.9
- fluke — *see* Infestation, fluke
- focal
  - teeth (pulpal origin) K04.7
  - tonsils J35.01
- Fonsecaea (compactum) (pedrosoi) B43.0
- food — *see* Intoxication, foodborne
- foot (skin) L08.9
  - dermatophytic fungus B35.3
- Francisella tularensis — *see* Tularemia
- frontal (sinus) (chronic) — *see* Sinusitis, frontal
- fungus NOS B49
  - beard B35.0
  - dermatophytic — *see* Dermatophytosis
  - foot B35.3
  - groin B35.6
  - hand B35.2
  - nail B35.1
  - pathogenic to compromised host only B48.8
  - perianal (area) B35.6
  - scalp B35.0
  - skin B36.9
    - foot B35.3
    - hand B35.2
    - toenails B35.1
- Fusarium B48.8
- gallbladder — *see* Cholecystitis
- gas bacillus — *see* Gangrene, gas
- gastrointestinal — *see* Enteritis, infectious
- generalized NEC — *see* Sepsis
- generator pocket, implanted electronic neurostimulator T85.734 ☑
- genital organ or tract
  - female — *see* Disease, pelvis, inflammatory
  - male N49.9
    - multiple sites N49.8
    - specified NEC N49.8
- Ghon tubercle, primary A15.7
- Giardia lamblia A07.1
- gingiva (chronic) K05.10
  - acute K05.00
    - nonplaque induced K05.01
    - plaque induced K05.00
  - nonplaque induced K05.11
  - plaque induced K05.10
- glanders A24.0
- glenosporopsis B48.0
- Gnathostoma (spinigerum) B83.1
- Gongylonema B83.8
- gonococcal — *see* Gonococcus
- gram-negative bacilli NOS A49.9
- guinea worm B72
- gum (chronic) K05.10
  - acute K05.00
    - nonplaque induced K05.01
    - plaque induced K05.00
  - nonplaque induced K05.11
  - plaque induced K05.10
- Haemophilus — *see* Infection, Hemophilus
- heart — *see* Carditis
- Helicobacter pylori A04.8
  - as cause of disease classified elsewhere B96.81
- helminths B83.9
  - intestinal B82.0

▼ Subterms under main terms may continue to next column or page   ☑ Additional Character Required — Refer to the Tabular List for Character Selection   187

Infection, infected, infective — Infection, infected, infective

Infection, infected, infective — *continued*
  helminths — *continued*
    intestinal — *continued*
      mixed (types classifiable to more than one of the titles B65.Ø-B81.3 and B81.8) B81.4
      specified type NEC B81.8
    specified type NEC B83.8
  Hemophilus
    aegyptius, systemic A48.4
    ducrey (any location) A57
    generalized A41.3
    influenzae NEC A49.2
      as cause of disease classified elsewhere B96.3
  herpes (simplex) — *see also* Herpes
    congenital P35.2
    disseminated BØØ.7
    zoster BØ2.9
  herpesvirus, herpesviral — *see* Herpes
  Heterophyes (heterophyes) B66.8
  hip (joint) NEC MØØ.9
    due to internal joint prosthesis
      left T84.52 ☑
      right T84.51 ☑
    skin NEC LØ8.9
  Histoplasma — *see* Histoplasmosis
    American B39.4
    capsulatum B39.4
  hookworm B76.9
  human
    papilloma virus A63.Ø
    T-cell lymphotropic virus type-1 (HTLV-1) B33.3
  hydrocele N43.Ø
  Hymenolepis B71.Ø
  hypopharynx — *see* Pharyngitis
  inguinal (lymph) glands LØ4.1
    due to soft chancre A57
  intervertebral disc, pyogenic M46.3Ø
    cervical region M46.32
    cervicothoracic region M46.33
    lumbar region M46.36
    lumbosacral region M46.37
    multiple sites M46.39
    occipito-atlanto-axial region M46.31
    sacrococcygeal region M46.38
    thoracic region M46.34
    thoracolumbar region M46.35
  intestine, intestinal — *see* Enteritis, infectious
    specified NEC AØ8.8
  intra-amniotic affecting newborn NEC P39.2
  intrauterine inflammation O41.12- ☑
  Isospora belli or hominis AØ7.3
  Japanese B encephalitis A83.Ø
  jaw (bone) (lower) (upper) M27.2
  joint NEC MØØ.9
    due to internal joint prosthesis T84.5Ø ☑
  kidney (cortex) (hematogenous) N15.9
    with calculus N20.Ø
      with hydronephrosis N13.6
    following ectopic gestation OØ8.83
    pelvis and ureter (cystic) N28.85
    puerperal (postpartum) Oage86.21
    specified NEC N15.8
  Klebsiella (K.) pneumoniae NEC A49.8
    as cause of disease classified elsewhere B96.1
  knee (joint) NEC MØØ.9
    joint MØØ.9
    due to internal joint prosthesis
      left T84.54 ☑
      right T84.53 ☑
    skin LØ8.9
  Koch's — *see* Tuberculosis
  labia (majora) (minora) (acute) — *see* Vulvitis
  lacrimal
    gland — *see* Dacryoadenitis
    passages (duct) (sac) — *see* Inflammation, lacrimal, passages
  lancet fluke B66.2
  larynx NEC J38.7
  leg (skin) NOS LØ8.9
  Legionella pneumophila A48.1
    nonpneumonic A48.2
  Leishmania — *see also* Leishmaniasis
    aethiopica B55.1
    braziliensis B55.2
    chagasi B55.Ø
    donovani B55.Ø
    infantum B55.Ø
    major B55.1

Infection, infected, infective — *continued*
  Leishmania — *see also* Leishmaniasis — *continued*
    mexicana B55.1
    tropica B55.1
  lentivirus, as cause of disease classified elsewhere B97.31
  Leptosphaeria senegalensis B47.Ø
  Leptospira interrogans A27.9
    autumnalis A27.89
    canicola A27.89
    hebdomadis A27.89
    icterohaemorrhagiae A27.Ø
    pomona A27.89
    specified type NEC A27.89
  leptospirochetal NEC — *see* Leptospirosis
  Listeria monocytogenes — *see also* Listeriosis
    congenital P37.2
  Loa loa B74.3
    with conjunctival infestation B74.3
    eyelid B74.3
  Loboa loboi B48.Ø
  local, skin (staphylococcal) (streptococcal) LØ8.9
    abscess — *code by* site under Abscess
    cellulitis — *code by* site under Cellulitis
    specified NEC LØ8.89
    ulcer — *see* Ulcer, skin
  Loefflerella mallei A24.Ø
  lung — *see also* Pneumonia J18.9
    atypical Mycobacterium A31.Ø
    spirochetal A69.8
    tuberculous — *see* Tuberculosis, pulmonary
    virus — *see* Pneumonia, viral
  lymph gland — *see also* Lymphadenitis, acute
    mesenteric I88.Ø
  lymphoid tissue, base of tongue or posterior pharynx, NEC (chronic) J35.Ø3
  Madurella (grisea) (mycetomii) B47.Ø
  major
    following ectopic or molar pregnancy OØ8.Ø
    puerperal, postpartum, childbirth O85
  Malassezia furfur B36.Ø
  Malleomyces
    mallei A24.Ø
    pseudomallei (whitmori) — *see* Melioidosis
  mammary gland N61.Ø
  Mansonella (ozzardi) (perstans) (streptocerca) B74.4
  mastoid — *see* Mastoiditis
  maxilla, maxillary M27.2
    sinus (chronic) — *see* Sinusitis, maxillary
  mediastinum J98.51
  Medina (worm) B72
  meibomian cyst or gland — *see* Hordeolum
  meninges — *see* Meningitis, bacterial
  meningococcal — *see also* condition A39.9
    adrenals A39.1
    brain A39.81
    cerebrospinal A39.Ø
    conjunctiva A39.89
    endocardium A39.51
    heart A39.5Ø
      endocardium A39.51
      myocardium A39.52
      pericardium A39.53
    joint A39.83
    meninges A39.Ø
    meningococcemia A39.4
      acute A39.2
      chronic A39.3
    myocardium A39.52
    pericardium A39.53
    retrobulbar neuritis A39.82
    specified site NEC A39.89
  mesenteric lymph nodes or glands NEC I88.Ø
  Metagonimus B66.8
  metatarsophalangeal MØØ.9
  methicillin
    resistant Staphylococcus aureus (MRSA) A49.Ø2
    susceptible Staphylococcus aureus (MSSA) A49.Ø1
  Microsporum, microsporic — *see* Dermatophytosis
  mixed flora (bacterial) NEC A49.8
  Monilia — *see* Candidiasis
  Monosporium apiospermum B48.2
  mouth, parasitic B37.Ø
  Mucor — *see* Mucormycosis
  muscle NEC — *see* Myositis, infective
  mycelium NOS B49
  mycetoma B47.9
    actinomycotic NEC B47.1

Infection, infected, infective — *continued*
  mycetoma — *continued*
    mycotic NEC B47.Ø
  Mycobacterium, mycobacterial — *see* Mycobacterium
  Mycoplasma NEC A49.3
    pneumoniae, as cause of disease classified elsewhere B96.Ø
  mycotic NOS B49
    pathogenic to compromised host only B48.8
    skin NOS B36.9
  myocardium NEC I4Ø.Ø
  nail (chronic)
    with lymphangitis — *see* Lymphangitis, acute, digit
    finger LØ3.Ø1- ☑
      fungus B35.1
    ingrowing L6Ø.Ø
    toe LØ3.Ø3- ☑
      fungus B35.1
  nasal sinus (chronic) — *see* Sinusitis
  nasopharynx — *see* Nasopharyngitis
  navel LØ8.82
  Necator americanus B76.1
  Neisseria — *see* Gonococcus
  Neotestudina rosatii B47.Ø
  newborn P39.9
    intra-amniotic NEC P39.2
    skin P39.4
    specified type NEC P39.8
  nipple N61.Ø
    associated with
      lactation O91.Ø3
      pregnancy O91.Ø1- ☑
      puerperium O91.Ø2
  Nocardia — *see* Nocardiosis
  obstetrical surgical wound (puerperal) O86.ØØ
    incisional site
      deep O86.Ø2
      superficial O86.Ø1
    organ and space site O86.Ø3
    surgical site specified NEC O86.Ø9
  Oesophagostomum (apiostomum) B81.8
  Oestrus ovis — *see* Myiasis
  Oidium albicans B37.9
  Onchocerca (volvulus) — *see* Onchocerciasis
  oncovirus, as cause of disease classified elsewhere B97.32
  operation wound T81.49 ☑
  Opisthorchis (felineus) (viverrini) B66.Ø
  orbit, orbital — *see* Inflammation, orbit
  orthopoxvirus NEC BØ8.Ø9
  ovary — *see* Salpingo-oophoritis
  Oxyuris vermicularis B8Ø
  pancreas (acute) — *see* Pancreatitis, acute
    abscess — *see* Pancreatitis, acute
    specified NEC — *see also* Pancreatitis, acute K85.8Ø
  papillomavirus, as cause of disease classified elsewhere B97.7
  papovavirus NEC B34.4
  Paracoccidioides brasiliensis — *see* Paracoccidioidomycosis
  Paragonimus (westermani) B66.4
  parainfluenza virus B34.8
  parameningococcus NOS A39.9
  parapoxvirus BØ8.6Ø
    specified NEC BØ8.69
  parasitic B89
  Parastrongylus
    cantonensis B83.2
    costaricensis B81.3
    paratyphoid AØ1.4
      Type A AØ1.1
      Type B AØ1.2
      Type C AØ1.3
  paraurethral ducts N34.2
  parotid gland — *see* Sialoadenitis
  parvovirus NEC B34.3
    as cause of disease classified elsewhere B97.6
  Pasteurella NEC A28.9
    multocida A28.Ø
    pestis — *see* Plague
    pseudotuberculosis A28.2
    septica (cat bite) (dog bite) A28.Ø
    tularensis — *see* Tularemia
  pelvic, female — *see* Disease, pelvis, inflammatory
  Penicillium (marneffei) B48.4
  penis (glans) (retention) NEC N48.29
  periapical KØ4.5
  peridental, periodontal KØ5.2Ø

☑ **Additional Character Required — Refer to the Tabular List for Character Selection**   ▽ Subterms under main terms may continue to next column or page

Infection, infected, infective — *continued*
 peridental, periodontal — *continued*
  generalized — *see* Periodontitis, aggressive, generalized
  localized — *see* Periodontitis, aggressive, localized
 perinatal period P39.9
  specified type NEC P39.8
 perineal repair (puerperal) O86.09
 periorbital — *see* Inflammation, orbit
 perirectal K62.89
 perirenal — *see* Infection, kidney
 peritoneal — *see* Peritonitis
 periureteral N28.89
 Petriellidium boydii B48.2
 pharynx — *see also* Pharyngitis
  coxsackievirus B08.5
  posterior, lymphoid (chronic) J35.03
 Phialophora
  gougerotii (subcutaneous abscess or cyst) B43.2
  jeanselmei (subcutaneous abscess or cyst) B43.2
  verrucosa (skin) B43.0
 Piedraia hortae B36.3
 pinta A67.9
  intermediate A67.1
  late A67.2
  mixed A67.3
  primary A67.0
 pinworm B80
 pityrosporum furfur B36.0
 pleuro-pneumonia-like organism (PPLO) NEC A49.3
  as cause of disease classified elsewhere B96.0
 pneumococcus, pneumococcal NEC A49.1
  as cause of disease classified elsewhere B95.3
  generalized (purulent) A40.3
   with pneumonia J13
 Pneumocystis carinii (pneumonia) B59
 Pneumocystis jiroveci (pneumonia) B59
 port or reservoir T80.212 ☑
 postoperative T81.40 ☑
 postoperative wound T81.49 ☑
  surgical site
   deep incisional T81.42 ☑
   organ and space T81.43 ☑
   specified NEC T81.49 ☑
   superficial incisional T81.41 ☑
 postprocedural T81.40 ☑
 postvaccinal T88.0 ☑
 prepuce NEC N47.7
  with penile inflammation N47.6
 prion — *see* Disease, prion, central nervous system
 prostate (capsule) — *see* Prostatitis
 Proteus (mirabilis) (morganii) (vulgaris) NEC A49.8
  as cause of disease classified elsewhere B96.4
 protozoal NEC B64
  intestinal A07.9
   specified NEC A07.8
  specified NEC B60.8
 Pseudoallescheria boydii B48.2
 Pseudomonas NEC A49.8
  as cause of disease classified elsewhere B96.5
  mallei A24.0
  pneumonia J15.1
  pseudomallei — *see* Melioidosis
 puerperal O86.4
  genitourinary tract NEC O86.89
  major or generalized O85
  minor O86.4
  specified NEC O86.89
 pulmonary — *see* Infection, lung
 purulent — *see* Abscess
 Pyrenochaeta romeroi B47.0
 Q fever A78
 rectum (sphincter) K62.89
 renal — *see also* Infection, kidney
  pelvis and ureter (cystic) N28.85
 reovirus, as cause of disease classified elsewhere B97.5
 respiratory (tract) NEC J98.8
  acute J22
  chronic J98.8
  influenzal (upper) (acute) — *see* Influenza, with, respiratory manifestations NEC
  lower (acute) J22
   chronic — *see* Bronchitis, chronic
  rhinovirus J00
  syncytial virus (RSV) — *see* Infection, virus, respiratory syncytial (RSV)
  upper (acute) NOS J06.9
   chronic J39.8

Infection, infected, infective — *continued*
 respiratory — *continued*
  upper — *continued*
   streptococcal J06.9
   viral NOS J06.9
    due to respiratory syncytial virus (RSV) J06.9 [B97.4]
 resulting from
  presence of internal prosthesis, implant, graft — *see* Complications, by site and type, infection
 retortamoniasis A07.8
 retroperitoneal NEC K68.9
 retrovirus B33.3
  as cause of disease classified elsewhere B97.30
   human
    immunodeficiency, type 2 (HIV 2) B97.35
    T-cell lymphotropic
     type I (HTLV-I) B97.33
     type II (HTLV-II) B97.34
   lentivirus B97.31
   oncovirus B97.32
   specified NEC B97.39
 Rhinosporidium (seeberi) B48.1
 rhinovirus
  as cause of disease classified elsewhere B97.89
  unspecified nature or site B34.8
 Rhizopus — *see* Mucormycosis
 rickettsial NOS A79.9
 roundworm (large) NEC B82.0
  Ascariasis — *see also* Ascariasis B77.9
 rubella — *see* Rubella
 Saccharomyces — *see* Candidiasis
 salivary duct or gland (any) — *see* Sialoadenitis
 Salmonella (aertrycke) (arizonae) (callinarum) (cholerae-suis) (enteritidis) (suipestifer) (typhimurium) A02.9
  with
   (gastro)enteritis A02.0
   sepsis A02.1
   specified manifestation NEC A02.8
  due to food (poisoning) A02.9
  hirschfeldii A01.3
  localized A02.20
   arthritis A02.23
   meningitis A02.21
   osteomyelitis A02.24
   pneumonia A02.22
   pyelonephritis A02.25
   specified NEC A02.29
  paratyphi A01.4
   A A01.1
   B A01.2
   C A01.3
  schottmuelleri A01.2
  typhi, typhosa — *see* Typhoid
 Sarcocystis A07.8
 scabies B86
 Schistosoma — *see* Infestation, Schistosoma
 scrotum (acute) NEC N49.2
 seminal vesicle — *see* Vesiculitis
 septic
  localized, skin — *see* Abscess
 sheep liver fluke B66.3
 Shigella A03.9
  boydii A03.2
  dysenteriae A03.0
  flexneri A03.1
  group
   A A03.0
   B A03.1
   C A03.2
   D A03.3
  Schmitz (-Stutzer) A03.0
  schmitzii A03.0
  shigae A03.0
  sonnei A03.3
  specified NEC A03.8
 shoulder (joint) NEC M00.9
  due to internal joint prosthesis T84.59 ☑
  skin NEC L08.9
 sinus (accessory) (chronic) (nasal) — *see also* Sinusitis
  pilonidal — *see* Sinus, pilonidal
  skin NEC L08.89
 Skene's duct or gland — *see* Urethritis
 skin (local) (staphylococcal) (streptococcal) L08.9
  abscess — *code by* site under Abscess
  cellulitis — *code by* site under Cellulitis
  due to fungus B36.9

Infection, infected, infective — *continued*
 skin — *continued*
  due to fungus — *continued*
   specified type NEC B36.8
  mycotic B36.9
   specified type NEC B36.8
  newborn P39.4
  ulcer — *see* Ulcer, skin
 slow virus A81.9
  specified NEC A81.89
 Sparganum (mansoni) (proliferum) (baxteri) B70.1
 specific — *see also* Syphilis
  to perinatal period — *see* Infection, congenital
 specified NEC B99.8
 spermatic cord NEC N49.1
 sphenoidal (sinus) — *see* Sinusitis, sphenoidal
 spinal cord NOS — *see also* Myelitis G04.91
  abscess G06.1
  meninges — *see* Meningitis
  streptococcal G04.89
 Spirillum A25.0
 spirochetal NOS A69.9
  lung A69.8
  specified NEC A69.8
 Spirometra larvae B70.1
 spleen D73.89
 Sporotrichum, Sporothrix (schenckii) — *see* Sporotrichosis
 staphylococcal, unspecified site
  as cause of disease classified elsewhere B95.8
   aureus (methicillin susceptible) (MSSA) B95.61
    methicillin resistant (MRSA) B95.62
   specified NEC B95.7
  aureus (methicillin susceptible) (MSSA) A49.01
   methicillin resistant (MRSA) A49.02
  food poisoning A05.0
  generalized (purulent) A41.2
  pneumonia — *see* Pneumonia, staphylococcal
 Stellantchasmus falcatus B66.8
 streptobacillus moniliformis A25.1
 streptococcal NEC A49.1
  as cause of disease classified elsewhere B95.5
  B genitourinary complicating
   childbirth O98.82
   pregnancy O98.81- ☑
   puerperium O98.83
  congenital
   sepsis P36.10
    group B P36.0
    specified NEC P36.19
  generalized (purulent) A40.9
 Streptomyces B47.1
 Strongyloides (stercoralis) — *see* Strongyloidiasis
 stump (amputation) (surgical) — *see* Complication, amputation stump, infection
 subcutaneous tissue, local L08.9
 suipestifer — *see* Infection, salmonella
 swimming pool bacillus A31.1
 Taenia — *see* Infestation, Taenia
 Taeniarhynchus saginatus B68.1
 tapeworm — *see* Infestation, tapeworm
 tendon (sheath) — *see* Tenosynovitis, infective NEC
 Ternidens diminutus B81.8
 testis — *see* Orchitis
 threadworm B80
 throat — *see* Pharyngitis
 thyroglossal duct K14.8
 toe (skin) L08.9
  cellulitis L03.03- ☑
   fungus B35.1
  nail L03.03- ☑
   fungus B35.1
 tongue NEC K14.0
  parasitic B37.0
 tonsil (and adenoid) (faucial) (lingual) (pharyngeal) — *see* Tonsillitis
 tooth, teeth K04.7
  periapical K04.7
  peridental, periodontal K05.20
   generalized — *see* Periodontitis, aggressive, generalized
   localized — *see* Periodontitis, aggressive, localized
  pulp K04.01
   irreversible K04.02
   reversible K04.01
  socket M27.3
 TORCH — *see* Infection, congenital

Infection, infected, infective — *continued*
TORCH — *see* Infection, congenital — *continued*
without active infection P00.2
Torula histolytica — *see* Cryptococcosis
Toxocara (canis) (cati) (felis) B83.0
Toxoplasma gondii — *see* Toxoplasma
trachea, chronic J42
trematode NEC — *see* Infestation, fluke
trench fever A79.0
Treponema pallidum — *see* Syphilis
Trichinella (spiralis) B75
Trichomonas A59.9
cervix A59.09
intestine A07.8
prostate A59.02
specified site NEC A59.8
urethra A59.03
urogenitalis A59.00
vagina A59.01
vulva A59.01
Trichophyton, trichophytic — *see* Dermatophytosis
Trichosporon (beigelii) cutaneum B36.2
Trichostrongylus B81.2
Trichuris (trichiura) B79
Trombicula (irritans) B88.0
Trypanosoma
brucei
gambiense B56.0
rhodesiense B56.1
cruzi — *see* Chagas' disease
tubal — *see* Salpingo-oophoritis
tuberculous
latent (LTBI) Z22.7
NEC — *see* Tuberculosis
tubo-ovarian — *see* Salpingo-oophoritis
tunica vaginalis N49.1
tunnel T80.212 ☑
tympanic membrane NEC — *see* Myringitis
typhoid (abortive) (ambulant) (bacillus) — *see* Typhoid
typhus A75.9
flea-borne A75.2
mite-borne A75.3
recrudescent A75.1
tick-borne A77.9
African A77.1
North Asian A77.2
umbilicus L08.82
ureter — *see* Ureteritis
urethra — *see* Urethritis
urinary (tract) N39.0
bladder — *see* Cystitis
complicating
pregnancy O23.4- ☑
specified type NEC O23.3- ☑
kidney — *see* Infection, kidney
newborn P39.3
puerperal (postpartum) O86.20
tuberculous A18.13
urethra — *see* Urethritis
uterus, uterine — *see* Endometritis
vaccination T88.0 ☑
vaccinia not from vaccination B08.011
vagina (acute) — *see* Vaginitis
varicella B01.9
varicose veins — *see* Varix
vas deferens NEC N49.1
vesical — *see* Cystitis
Vibrio
cholerae A00.0
El Tor A00.1
parahaemolyticus (food poisoning) A05.3
vulnificus
as cause of disease classified elsewhere B96.82
foodborne intoxication A05.5
Vincent's (gum) (mouth) (tonsil) A69.1
virus, viral NOS B34.9
adenovirus
as cause of disease classified elsewhere B97.0
unspecified nature or site B34.0
arborvirus, arbovirus arthropod-borne A94
as cause of disease classified elsewhere B97.89
adenovirus B97.0
coronavirus B97.29
SARS-associated B97.21
coxsackievirus B97.11
echovirus B97.12
enterovirus B97.10
coxsackievirus B97.11

Infection, infected, infective — *continued*
virus, viral — *continued*
as cause of disease classified elsewhere — *continued*
enterovirus — *continued*
echovirus B97.12
specified NEC B97.19
human
immunodeficiency, type 2 (HIV 2) B97.35
metapneumovirus B97.81
T-cell lymphotropic,
type I (HTLV-I) B97.33
type II (HTLV-II) B97.34
papillomavirus B97.7
parvovirus B97.6
reovirus B97.5
respiratory syncytial (RSV) — *see* Infection, virus, respiratory syncytial (RSV)
retrovirus B97.30
human
immunodeficiency, type 2 (HIV 2) B97.35
T-cell lymphotropic,
type I (HTLV-I) B97.33
type II (HTLV-II) B97.34
lentivirus B97.31
oncovirus B97.32
specified NEC B97.39
specified NEC B97.89
central nervous system A89
atypical A81.9
specified NEC A81.89
enterovirus NEC A88.8
meningitis A87.0
slow virus A81.9
specified NEC A81.89
specified NEC A88.8
chest J98.8
cotia B08.8
COVID-19 U07.1
coxsackie — *see also* Infection, coxsackie B34.1
as cause of disease classified elsewhere B97.11
ECHO
as cause of disease classified elsewhere B97.12
unspecified nature or site B34.1
encephalitis, tick-borne A84.9
enterovirus, as cause of disease classified elsewhere B97.10
coxsackievirus B97.11
echovirus B97.12
specified NEC B97.19
exanthem NOS B09
human metapneumovirus as cause of disease classified elsewhere B97.81
human papilloma as cause of disease classified elsewhere B97.7
intestine — *see* Enteritis, viral
respiratory syncytial (RSV)
as cause of disease classified elsewhere B97.4
bronchiolitis J21.0
bronchitis J20.5
bronchopneumonia J12.1
otitis media H65- ☑ *[B97.4]*
pneumonia J12.1
upper respiratory infection J06.9 *[B97.4]*
rhinovirus
as cause of disease classified elsewhere B97.89
unspecified nature or site B34.8
slow A81.9
specified NEC A81.89
specified type NEC B33.8
as cause of disease classified elsewhere B97.89
unspecified nature or site B34.8
unspecified nature or site B34.9
West Nile — *see* Virus, West Nile
vulva (acute) — *see* Vulvitis
West Nile — *see* Virus, West Nile
whipworm B79
worms B83.9
specified type NEC B83.8
Wuchereria (bancrofti) B74.0
malayi B74.1
yatapoxvirus B08.70
specified NEC B08.79
yeast — *see also* Candidiasis B37.9
yellow fever — *see* Fever, yellow
Yersinia
enterocolitica (intestinal) A04.6
pestis — *see* Plague

Infection, infected, infective — *continued*
Yersinia — *continued*
pseudotuberculosis A28.2
Zeis' gland — *see* Hordeolum
Zika virus A92.5
congenital P35.4
zoonotic bacterial NOS A28.9
Zopfia senegalensis B47.0
Infective, infectious — *see* condition
Infertility
female N97.9
age-related N97.8
associated with
anovulation N97.0
cervical (mucus) disease or anomaly N88.3
congenital anomaly
cervix N88.3
fallopian tube N97.1
uterus N97.2
vagina N97.8
dysmucorrhea N88.3
fallopian tube disease or anomaly N97.1
pituitary-hypothalamic origin E23.0
specified origin NEC N97.8
Stein-Leventhal syndrome E28.2
uterine disease or anomaly N97.2
vaginal disease or anomaly N97.8
due to
cervical anomaly N88.3
fallopian tube anomaly N97.1
ovarian failure E28.39
Stein-Leventhal syndrome E28.2
uterine anomaly N97.2
vaginal anomaly N97.8
nonimplantation N97.2
origin
cervical N88.3
tubal (block) (occlusion) (stenosis) N97.1
uterine N97.2
vaginal N97.8
male N46.9
azoospermia N46.01
extratesticular cause N46.029
drug therapy N46.021
efferent duct obstruction N46.023
infection N46.022
radiation N46.024
specified cause NEC N46.029
systemic disease N46.025
oligospermia N46.11
extratesticular cause N46.129
drug therapy N46.121
efferent duct obstruction N46.123
infection N46.122
radiation N46.124
specified cause NEC N46.129
systemic disease N46.125
specified type NEC N46.8
Infestation B88.9
Acanthocheilonema (perstans) (streptocerca) B74.4
Acariasis B88.0
demodex folliculorum B88.0
sarcoptes scabiei B86
trombiculae B88.0
Agamofilaria streptocerca B74.4
Ancylostoma, ankylostoma (braziliense) (caninum) (ceylanicum) (duodenale) B76.0
americanum B76.1
new world B76.1
Anisakis larvae, anisakiasis B81.0
arthropod NEC B88.2
Ascaris lumbricoides — *see* Ascariasis
Balantidium coli A07.0
beef tapeworm B68.1
Bothriocephalus (latus) B70.0
larval B70.1
broad tapeworm B70.0
larval B70.1
Brugia (malayi) B74.1
timori B74.2
candiru B88.8
Capillaria
hepatica B83.8
philippinensis B81.1
cat liver fluke B66.0
cestodes B71.9
diphyllobothrium — *see* Infestation, diphyllobothrium
dipylidiasis B71.1

☑ Additional Character Required — Refer to the Tabular List for Character Selection   ▽ Subterms under main terms may continue to next column or page

◤ Subterms under main terms may continue to next column or page   ☑ Additional Character Required — Refer to the Tabular List for Character Selection   191

Infestation — Infiltrate, infiltration

Infiltrate, infiltration — *continued*
  cardiac — *continued*
    glycogenic E74.02 *[I43]*
  corneal — *see* Edema, cornea
  eyelid — *see* Inflammation, eyelid
  glycogen, glycogenic — *see* Disease, glycogen storage
  heart, cardiac
    fatty — *see* Degeneration, myocardial
    glycogenic E74.02 *[I43]*
    inflammatory in vitreous H43.89
  kidney N28.89
  leukemic — *see* Leukemia
  liver K76.89
    fatty — *see* Fatty, liver NEC
    glycogen — *see also* Disease, glycogen storage
      E74.03 *[K77]*
  lung R91.8
    eosinophilic — *see* Eosinophilia, pulmonary
  lymphatic — *see also* Leukemia, lymphatic C91.9-
    gland I88.9
  muscle, fatty M62.89
  myocardium, myocardial
    fatty — *see* Degeneration, myocardial
    glycogenic E74.02 *[I43]*
  on chest x-ray R91.8
  pulmonary R91.8
    with eosinophilia — *see* Eosinophilia, pulmonary
  skin (lymphocytic) L98.6
  thymus (gland) (fatty) E32.8
  urine R39.0
  vesicant agent
    antineoplastic chemotherapy T80.810 ☑
    other agent NEC T80.818 ☑
  vitreous body H43.89

Infirmity R68.89
  senile R54

Inflammation, inflamed, inflammatory (with exudation)
  abducent (nerve) — *see* Strabismus, paralytic, sixth
    nerve
  accessory sinus (chronic) — *see* Sinusitis
  adrenal (gland) E27.8
  alveoli, teeth M27.3
    scorbutic E54
  anal canal, anus K62.89
  antrum (chronic) — *see* Sinusitis, maxillary
  appendix — *see* Appendicitis
  arachnoid — *see* Meningitis
  areola N61.0
    puerperal, postpartum or gestational — *see* Infection, nipple
  areolar tissue NOS L08.9
  artery — *see* Arteritis
  auditory meatus (external) — *see* Otitis, externa
  Bartholin's gland N75.8
  bile duct (common) (hepatic) or passage — *see*
    Cholangitis
  bladder — *see* Cystitis
  bone — *see* Osteomyelitis
  brain — *see also* Encephalitis
    membrane — *see* Meningitis
  breast N61.0
    puerperal, postpartum, gestational — *see* Mastitis,
      obstetric
  broad ligament — *see* Disease, pelvis, inflammatory
  bronchi — *see* Bronchitis
  catarrhal J00
  cecum — *see* Appendicitis
  cerebral — *see also* Encephalitis
    membrane — *see* Meningitis
  cerebrospinal
    meningococcal A39.0
  cervix (uteri) — *see* Cervicitis
  chest J98.8
  chorioretinal H30.9- ☑
    cyclitis — *see* Cyclitis
    disseminated H30.10- ☑
      generalized H30.13- ☑
      peripheral H30.12- ☑
      posterior pole H30.11- ☑
    epitheliopathy — *see* Epitheliopathy
    focal H30.00- ☑
      juxtapapillary H30.01- ☑
      macular H30.04- ☑
      paramacular — *see* Inflammation, chorioretinal,
        focal, macular
      peripheral H30.03- ☑

Inflammation, inflamed, inflammatory —
    continued
  chorioretinal — *continued*
    focal — *continued*
      posterior pole H30.02- ☑
    specified type NEC H30.89- ☑
  choroid — *see* Inflammation, chorioretinal
  chronic, postmastoidectomy cavity — *see* Complications, postmastoidectomy, inflammation
  colon — *see* Enteritis
  connective tissue (diffuse) NEC — *see* Disorder, soft
    tissue, specified type NEC
  cornea — *see* Keratitis
  corpora cavernosa N48.29
  cranial nerve — *see* Disorder, nerve, cranial
  Douglas' cul-de-sac or pouch (chronic) N73.0
  due to device, implant or graft — *see also* Complications, by site and type, infection or inflammation
    arterial graft T82.7 ☑
    breast (implant) T85.79 ☑
    catheter T85.79 ☑
      dialysis (renal) T82.7 ☑
        intraperitoneal T85.71 ☑
      infusion T82.7 ☑
        cranial T85.735 ☑
        intrathecal T85.735 ☑
        spinal (epidural) (subdural) T85.735 ☑
        subarachnoid T85.735 ☑
      urinary T83.518 ☑
        cystostomy T83.510 ☑
        Hopkins T83.518 ☑
        ileostomy T83.518 ☑
        nephrostomy T83.512 ☑
        specified NEC T83.518 ☑
        urethral indwelling T83.511 ☑
        urostomy T83.518 ☑
    electronic (electrode) (pulse generator) (stimulator)
      bone T84.7 ☑
      cardiac T82.7 ☑
      nervous system T85.738 ☑
        brain T85.731 ☑
        cranial nerve T85.732 ☑
        gastric nerve T85.732 ☑
        neurostimulator generator T85.734 ☑
        peripheral nerve T85.732 ☑
        sacral nerve T85.732 ☑
        spinal cord T85.733 ☑
        vagal nerve T85.732 ☑
      urinary T83.590 ☑
    fixation, internal (orthopedic) NEC — *see* Complication, fixation device, infection
    gastrointestinal (bile duct) (esophagus) T85.79 ☑
      neurostimulator electrode (lead) T85.732 ☑
    genital NEC T83.69 ☑
    heart NEC T82.7 ☑
      valve (prosthesis) T82.6 ☑
        graft T82.7 ☑
    joint prosthesis — *see* Complication, joint prosthesis, infection
    ocular (corneal graft) (orbital implant) NEC T85.79 ☑
    orthopedic NEC T84.7 ☑
    penile (cylinder) (pump) (resevoir) T83.61 ☑
    specified NEC T85.79 ☑
    testicular T83.62 ☑
    urinary NEC T83.598 ☑
      ileal conduit stent T83.593 ☑
      implanted neurostimulation T83.590 ☑
      implanted sphincter T83.591 ☑
      indwelling ureteral stent T83.592 ☑
      nephroureteral stent T83.593 ☑
      specified stent NEC T83.593 ☑
    vascular NEC T82.7 ☑
    ventricular intracranial (communicating) shunt
      T85.730 ☑
  duodenum K29.80
    with bleeding K29.81
  dura mater — *see* Meningitis
  ear (middle) — *see also* Otitis, media
    external — *see* Otitis, externa
    inner — *see subcategory* H83.0 ☑
  epididymis — *see* Epididymitis
  esophagus — *see* Esophagitis
  ethmoidal (sinus) (chronic) — *see* Sinusitis, ethmoidal
  eustachian tube (catarrhal) — *see* Salpingitis, eustachian
  eyelid H01.9

Inflammation, inflamed, inflammatory —
    continued
  eyelid — *continued*
    abscess — *see* Abscess, eyelid
    blepharitis — *see* Blepharitis
    chalazion — *see* Chalazion
    dermatosis (noninfectious) — *see* Dermatosis, eye
    hordeolum — *see* Hordeolum
    specified NEC H01.8
  fallopian tube — *see* Salpingo-oophoritis
  fascia — *see* Myositis
  follicular, pharynx J31.2
  frontal (sinus) (chronic) — *see* Sinusitis, frontal
  gallbladder — *see* Cholecystitis
  gastric — *see* Gastritis
  gastrointestinal — *see* Enteritis
  genital organ (internal) (diffuse)
    female — *see* Disease, pelvis, inflammatory
    male N49.9
      multiple sites N49.8
      specified NEC N49.8
  gland (lymph) — *see* Lymphadenitis
  glottis — *see* Laryngitis
  granular, pharynx J31.2
  gum K05.10
    nonplaque induced K05.11
    plaque induced K05.10
  heart — *see* Carditis
  hepatic duct — *see* Cholangitis
  ileoanal (internal) pouch K91.850
  ileum — *see also* Enteritis
    regional or terminal — *see* Enteritis, regional
  intestinal pouch K91.850
  intestine (any part) — *see* Enteritis
  jaw (acute) (bone) (chronic) (lower) (suppurative) (upper) M27.2
  joint NEC — *see* Arthritis
    sacroiliac M46.1
  kidney — *see* Nephritis
  knee (joint) M13.169
    tuberculous A18.02
  labium (majus) (minus) — *see* Vulvitis
  lacrimal
    gland — *see* Dacryoadenitis
    passages (duct) (sac) — *see also* Dacryocystitis
      canaliculitis — *see* Canaliculitis, lacrimal
  larynx — *see* Laryngitis
  leg NOS L08.9
  lip K13.0
  liver (capsule) — *see also* Hepatitis
    chronic K73.9
    suppurative K75.0
  lung (acute) — *see also* Pneumonia
    chronic J98.4
  lymph gland or node — *see* Lymphadenitis
  lymphatic vessel — *see* Lymphangitis
  maxilla, maxillary M27.2
    sinus (chronic) — *see* Sinusitis, maxillary
  membranes of brain or spinal cord — *see* Meningitis
  meninges — *see* Meningitis
  mouth K12.1
  muscle — *see* Myositis
  myocardium — *see* Myocarditis
  nasal sinus (chronic) — *see* Sinusitis
  nasopharynx — *see* Nasopharyngitis
  navel L08.82
  nerve NEC — *see* Neuralgia
  nipple N61.0
    puerperal, postpartum or gestational — *see* Infection, nipple
  nose — *see* Rhinitis
  oculomotor (nerve) — *see* Strabismus, paralytic, third
    nerve
  optic nerve — *see* Neuritis, optic
  orbit (chronic) H05.10
    acute H05.00
      abscess — *see* Abscess, orbit
      cellulitis — *see* Cellulitis, orbit
      osteomyelitis — *see* Osteomyelitis, orbit
      periostitis — *see* Periostitis, orbital
      tenonitis — *see* Tenonitis, eye
    granuloma — *see* Granuloma, orbit
    myositis — *see* Myositis, orbital
  ovary — *see* Salpingo-oophoritis
  oviduct — *see* Salpingo-oophoritis
  pancreas (acute) — *see* Pancreatitis
  parametrium N73.0

☑ **Additional Character Required — Refer to the Tabular List for Character Selection**   ▽ Subterms under main terms may continue to next column or pag

Injury — *continued*
  aorta — *continued*
    abdominal S35.00 ☑
      laceration (minor) (superficial) S35.01 ☑
        major S35.02 ☑
      specified type NEC S35.09 ☑
    laceration (minor) (superficial) S25.01 ☑
      major S25.02 ☑
    specified type NEC S25.09 ☑
  arm (upper) S49.9- ☑
    blood vessel — *see* Injury, blood vessel, arm
    contusion — *see* Contusion, arm, upper
    fracture — *see* Fracture, humerus
    lower — *see* Injury, forearm
    muscle — *see* Injury, muscle, shoulder
    nerve — *see* Injury, nerve, arm
    open — *see* Wound, open, arm
    specified type NEC S49.8- ☑
    superficial — *see* Injury, superficial, arm
  artery (complicating trauma) — *see also* Injury, blood vessel, by site
    cerebral or meningeal — *see* Injury, intracranial
  auditory canal (external) (meatus) S09.91 ☑
  auricle, auris, ear S09.91 ☑
  axilla — *see* Injury, shoulder
  back — *see* Injury, back, lower
  bile duct S36.13 ☑
  birth — *see also* Birth, injury P15.9
  bladder (sphincter) S37.20 ☑
    at delivery O71.5
    contusion S37.22 ☑
    laceration S37.23 ☑
    obstetrical trauma O71.5
    specified type NEC S37.29 ☑
  blast (air) (hydraulic) (immersion) (underwater) NEC T14.8 ☑
    acoustic nerve trauma — *see* Injury, nerve, acoustic
    bladder — *see* Injury, bladder
    brain — *see* Concussion
    colon — *see* Injury, intestine, large
    ear (primary) S09.31- ☑
      secondary S09.39- ☑
    generalized T70.8 ☑
    lung — *see* Injury, intrathoracic, lung
    multiple body organs T70.8 ☑
    peritoneum S36.81 ☑
    rectum S36.61 ☑
    retroperitoneum S36.898 ☑
    small intestine S36.419 ☑
      duodenum S36.410 ☑
      specified site NEC S36.418 ☑
    specified
      intra-abdominal organ NEC S36.898 ☑
      pelvic organ NEC S37.899 ☑
  blood vessel NEC T14.8 ☑
    abdomen S35.9 ☑
      aorta — *see* Injury, aorta, abdominal
      celiac artery — *see* Injury, blood vessel, celiac artery
      iliac vessel — *see* Injury, blood vessel, iliac
      laceration S35.91 ☑
      mesenteric vessel — *see* Injury, mesenteric
      portal vein — *see* Injury, blood vessel, portal vein
      renal vessel — *see* Injury, blood vessel, renal
      specified vessel NEC S35.8X- ☑
      splenic vessel — *see* Injury, blood vessel, splenic
      vena cava — *see* Injury, vena cava, inferior
    ankle — *see* Injury, blood vessel, foot
    aorta (abdominal) (thoracic) — *see* Injury, aorta
    arm (upper) NEC S45.90- ☑
      forearm — *see* Injury, blood vessel, forearm
      laceration S45.91- ☑
      specified
        site NEC S45.80- ☑
          laceration S45.81- ☑
          specified type NEC S45.89- ☑
        type NEC S45.99- ☑
      superficial vein S45.30- ☑
        laceration S45.31- ☑
        specified type NEC S45.39- ☑
    axillary
      artery S45.00- ☑
        laceration S45.01- ☑
        specified type NEC S45.09- ☑
      vein S45.20- ☑
        laceration S45.21- ☑

Injury — *continued*
  blood vessel — *continued*
    axillary — *continued*
      vein — *continued*
        specified type NEC S45.29- ☑
    azygos vein — *see* Injury, blood vessel, thoracic, specified site NEC
    brachial
      artery S45.10- ☑
        laceration S45.11- ☑
        specified type NEC S45.19- ☑
      vein S45.20- ☑
        laceration S45.219 ☑
        specified type NEC S45.29- ☑
    carotid artery (common) (external) (internal, extracranial) S15.00- ☑
      internal, intracranial S06.8- ☑
      laceration (minor) (superficial) S15.01- ☑
        major S15.02- ☑
      specified type NEC S15.09- ☑
    celiac artery S35.219 ☑
      branch S35.299 ☑
        laceration (minor) (superficial) S35.291 ☑
          major S35.292 ☑
        specified NEC S35.298 ☑
      laceration (minor) (superficial) S35.211 ☑
        major S35.212 ☑
      specified type NEC S35.218 ☑
    cerebral — *see* Injury, intracranial
    deep plantar — *see* Injury, blood vessel, plantar artery
    digital (hand) — *see* Injury, blood vessel, finger
    dorsal
      artery (foot) S95.00- ☑
        laceration S95.01- ☑
        specified type NEC S95.09- ☑
      vein (foot) S95.20- ☑
        laceration S95.21- ☑
        specified type NEC S95.29- ☑
    due to accidental laceration during procedure — *see* Laceration, accidental complicating surgery
    extremity — *see* Injury, blood vessel, limb
    femoral
      artery (common) (superficial) S75.00- ☑
        laceration (minor) (superficial) S75.01- ☑
          major S75.02- ☑
        specified type NEC S75.09- ☑
      vein (hip level) (thigh level) S75.10- ☑
        laceration (minor) (superficial) S75.11- ☑
          major S75.12- ☑
        specified type NEC S75.19- ☑
    finger S65.50- ☑
      index S65.50- ☑
        laceration S65.51- ☑
        specified type NEC S65.59- ☑
      laceration S65.51- ☑
      little S65.50- ☑
        laceration S65.51- ☑
        specified type NEC S65.59- ☑
      middle S65.50- ☑
        laceration S65.51- ☑
        specified type NEC S65.59- ☑
      specified type NEC S65.59- ☑
      thumb — *see* Injury, blood vessel, thumb
    foot S95.90- ☑
      dorsal
        artery — *see* Injury, blood vessel, dorsal, artery
        vein — *see* Injury, blood vessel, dorsal, vein
      laceration S95.91- ☑
      plantar artery — *see* Injury, blood vessel, plantar artery
      specified
        site NEC S95.80- ☑
          laceration S95.81- ☑
          specified type NEC S95.89- ☑
        specified type NEC S95.99- ☑
    forearm S55.90- ☑
      laceration S55.91- ☑
      radial artery — *see* Injury, blood vessel, radial artery
      specified
        site NEC S55.80- ☑
          laceration S55.81- ☑
          specified type NEC S55.89- ☑

Injury — *continued*
  blood vessel — *continued*
    forearm — *continued*
      specified — *continued*
        type NEC S55.99- ☑
      ulnar artery — *see* Injury, blood vessel, ulnar artery
      vein S55.20- ☑
        laceration S55.21- ☑
        specified type NEC S55.29- ☑
    gastric
      artery — *see* Injury, mesenteric, artery, branch
      vein — *see* Injury, blood vessel, abdomen
    gastroduodenal artery — *see* Injury, mesenteric, artery, branch
    greater saphenous vein (lower leg level) S85.30- ☑
      hip (and thigh) level S75.20- ☑
        laceration (minor) (superficial) S75.21- ☑
          major S75.22- ☑
        specified type NEC S75.29- ☑
      laceration S85.31- ☑
      specified type NEC S85.39- ☑
    hand (level) S65.90- ☑
      finger — *see* Injury, blood vessel, finger
      laceration S65.91- ☑
      palmar arch — *see* Injury, blood vessel, palmar arch
      radial artery — *see* Injury, blood vessel, radial artery, hand
      specified
        site NEC S65.80- ☑
          laceration S65.81- ☑
          specified type NEC S65.89- ☑
        type NEC S65.99- ☑
      thumb — *see* Injury, blood vessel, thumb
      ulnar artery — *see* Injury, blood vessel, ulnar artery, hand
    head S09.0 ☑
      intracranial — *see* Injury, intracranial
      multiple S09.0 ☑
    hepatic
      artery — *see* Injury, mesenteric, artery
      vein — *see* Injury, vena cava, inferior
    hip S75.90- ☑
      femoral artery — *see* Injury, blood vessel, femoral, artery
      femoral vein — *see* Injury, blood vessel, femoral vein
      greater saphenous vein — *see* Injury, blood vessel, greater saphenous, hip level
      laceration S75.91- ☑
      specified
        site NEC S75.80- ☑
          laceration S75.81- ☑
          specified type NEC S75.89- ☑
        type NEC S75.99- ☑
    hypogastric (artery) (vein) — *see* Injury, blood vessel, iliac
    iliac S35.5- ☑
      artery S35.51- ☑
      specified vessel NEC S35.5- ☑
      uterine vessel — *see* Injury, blood vessel, uterine
      vein S35.51- ☑
    innominate — *see* Injury, blood vessel, thoracic, innominate
    intercostal (artery) (vein) — *see* Injury, blood vessel, thoracic, intercostal
    jugular vein (external) S15.20- ☑
      internal S15.30- ☑
        laceration (minor) (superficial) S15.31- ☑
          major S15.32- ☑
        specified type NEC S15.39- ☑
      laceration (minor) (superficial) S15.21- ☑
        major S15.22- ☑
      specified type NEC S15.29- ☑
    leg (level) (lower) S85.90- ☑
      greater saphenous — *see* Injury, blood vessel, greater saphenous
      laceration S85.91- ☑
      lesser saphenous — *see* Injury, blood vessel, lesser saphenous
      peroneal artery — *see* Injury, blood vessel, peroneal artery
      popliteal
        artery — *see* Injury, blood vessel, popliteal, artery

Index

Injury — Injury

Injury — continued
- esophagus — see also Injury, intrathoracic, esophagus
  - — continued
    - cervical NEC S19.85 ☑
  - eustachian tube S09.30 ☑
  - eye S05.9- ☑
    - avulsion S05.7- ☑
    - ball — see Injury, eyeball
    - conjunctiva S05.0- ☑
    - cornea
      - abrasion S05.0- ☑
      - laceration S05.3- ☑
        - with prolapse S05.2- ☑
    - lacrimal apparatus S05.8X- ☑
    - orbit penetration S05.4- ☑
    - specified site NEC S05.8X- ☑
  - eyeball S05.8X- ☑
    - contusion S05.1- ☑
    - penetrating S05.6- ☑
      - with
        - foreign body S05.5- ☑
        - prolapse or loss of intraocular tissue S05.2- ☑
        - without prolapse or loss of intraocular tissue S05.3- ☑
    - specified type NEC S05.8- ☑
  - eyebrow S09.93 ☑
  - eyelid S09.93 ☑
    - abrasion — see Abrasion, eyelid
    - contusion — see Contusion, eyelid
    - open — see Wound, open, eyelid
  - face S09.93 ☑
  - fallopian tube S37.509 ☑
    - bilateral S37.502 ☑
      - blast injury S37.512 ☑
      - contusion S37.522 ☑
      - laceration S37.532 ☑
      - specified type NEC S37.592 ☑
    - blast injury (primary) S37.519 ☑
      - bilateral S37.512 ☑
      - secondary — see Injury, fallopian tube, specified type NEC
      - unilateral S37.511 ☑
    - contusion S37.529 ☑
      - bilateral S37.522 ☑
      - unilateral S37.521 ☑
    - laceration S37.539 ☑
      - bilateral S37.532 ☑
      - unilateral S37.531 ☑
    - specified type NEC S37.599 ☑
      - bilateral S37.592 ☑
      - unilateral S37.591 ☑
    - unilateral S37.501 ☑
      - blast injury S37.511 ☑
      - contusion S37.521 ☑
      - laceration S37.531 ☑
      - specified type NEC S37.591 ☑
  - fascia — see Injury, muscle
  - fifth cranial nerve (trigeminal) — see Injury, nerve, trigeminal
  - finger (nail) S69.9- ☑
    - blood vessel — see Injury, blood vessel, finger
    - contusion — see Contusion, finger
    - dislocation — see Dislocation, finger
    - fracture — see Fracture, finger
    - muscle — see Injury, muscle, finger
    - nerve — see Injury, nerve, digital, finger
    - open — see Wound, open, finger
    - specified NEC S69.8- ☑
    - sprain — see Sprain, finger
    - superficial — see Injury, superficial, finger
  - first cranial nerve (olfactory) — see Injury, nerve, olfactory
  - flank — see Injury, abdomen
  - foot S99.92- ☑
    - blood vessel — see Injury, blood vessel, foot
    - contusion — see Contusion, foot
    - dislocation — see Dislocation, foot
    - fracture — see Fracture, foot
    - muscle — see Injury, muscle, foot
    - open — see Wound, open, foot
    - specified type NEC S99.82- ☑
    - sprain — see Sprain, foot
    - superficial — see Injury, superficial, foot
  - forceps NOS P15.9
  - forearm S59.91- ☑
    - blood vessel — see Injury, blood vessel, forearm

Injury — continued
- forearm — continued
  - contusion — see Contusion, forearm
  - fracture — see Fracture, forearm
  - muscle — see Injury, muscle, forearm
  - nerve — see Injury, nerve, forearm
  - open — see Wound, open, forearm
  - specified NEC S59.81- ☑
  - superficial — see Injury, superficial, forearm
- forehead S09.90 ☑
- fourth cranial nerve (trochlear) — see Injury, nerve, trochlear
- gallbladder S36.129 ☑
  - contusion S36.122 ☑
  - laceration S36.123 ☑
  - specified NEC S36.128 ☑
- ganglion
  - celiac, coeliac — see Injury, nerve, lumbosacral, sympathetic
  - gasserian — see Injury, nerve, trigeminal
  - stellate — see Injury, nerve, thorax, sympathetic
  - thoracic sympathetic — see Injury, nerve, thorax, sympathetic
- gasserian ganglion — see Injury, nerve, trigeminal
- gastric artery — see Injury, blood vessel, celiac artery, branch
- gastroduodenal artery — see Injury, blood vessel, celiac artery, branch
- gastrointestinal tract — see Injury, intra-abdominal
  - with open wound into abdominal cavity — see Wound, open, with penetration into peritoneal cavity
  - colon — see Injury, intestine, large
  - rectum — see Injury, intestine, large, rectum
    - with open wound into abdominal cavity S36.61 ☑
  - small intestine — see Injury, intestine, small
  - specified site NEC — see Injury, intra-abdominal, specified, site NEC
  - stomach — see Injury, stomach
- genital organ(s)
  - external S39.94 ☑
    - specified NEC S39.848 ☑
  - internal S37.90 ☑
    - fallopian tube — see Injury, fallopian tube
    - ovary — see Injury, ovary
    - prostate — see Injury, prostate
    - seminal vesicle — see Injury, pelvis, organ, specified site NEC
    - uterus — see Injury, uterus
    - vas deferens — see Injury, pelvis, organ, specified site NEC
  - obstetrical trauma O71.9
- gland
  - lacrimal laceration — see Injury, eye, specified site NEC
  - salivary S09.93 ☑
  - thyroid NEC S19.84 ☑
- globe (eye) S05.90 ☑
  - specified NEC S05.8X- ☑
- groin — see Injury, abdomen
- gum S09.90 ☑
- hand S69.9- ☑
  - blood vessel — see Injury, blood vessel, hand
  - contusion — see Contusion, hand
  - fracture — see Fracture, hand
  - muscle — see Injury, muscle, hand
  - nerve — see Injury, nerve, hand
  - open — see Wound, open, hand
  - specified NEC S69.8- ☑
  - sprain — see Sprain, hand
  - superficial — see Injury, superficial, hand
- head S09.90 ☑
  - with loss of consciousness S06.9- ☑
  - specified NEC S09.8 ☑
- heart S26.90 ☑
  - with hemopericardium S26.00 ☑
    - contusion S26.01 ☑
    - laceration (mild) S26.020 ☑
      - major S26.022 ☑
      - moderate S26.021 ☑
    - specified type NEC S26.09 ☑
  - contusion S26.91 ☑
  - laceration S26.92 ☑
  - specified type NEC S26.99 ☑
  - without hemopericardium S26.10 ☑

Injury — continued
- heart — continued
  - without hemopericardium — continued
    - contusion S26.11 ☑
    - laceration S26.12 ☑
    - specified type NEC S26.19 ☑
  - heel — see Injury, foot
  - hepatic
    - artery — see Injury, blood vessel, celiac artery, branch
    - duct — see Injury, liver
    - vein — see Injury, vena cava, inferior
  - hip S79.91- ☑
    - blood vessel — see Injury, blood vessel, hip
    - contusion — see Contusion, hip
    - dislocation — see Dislocation, hip
    - fracture — see Fracture, femur, neck
    - muscle — see Injury, muscle, hip
    - nerve — see Injury, nerve, hip
    - open — see Wound, open, hip
    - specified NEC S79.81- ☑
    - sprain — see Sprain, hip
    - superficial — see Injury, superficial, hip
  - hymen S39.94 ☑
  - hypogastric
    - blood vessel — see Injury, blood vessel, iliac
    - plexus — see Injury, nerve, lumbosacral, sympathetic
  - ileum — see Injury, intestine, small
  - iliac region S39.91 ☑
  - instrumental (during surgery) — see Laceration, accidental complicating surgery
    - birth injury — see Birth, injury
    - nonsurgical — see Injury, by site
    - obstetrical O71.9
      - bladder O71.5
      - cervix O71.3
      - high vaginal O71.4
      - perineal NOS O70.9
      - urethra O71.5
      - uterus O71.5
        - with rupture or perforation O71.1
  - internal T14.8 ☑
    - aorta — see Injury, aorta
    - bladder (sphincter) — see Injury, bladder
      - with
        - ectopic or molar pregnancy O08.6
        - following ectopic or molar pregnancy O08.6
        - obstetrical trauma O71.5
    - bronchus, bronchi — see Injury, intrathoracic, bronchus
    - cecum — see Injury, intestine, large
    - cervix (uteri) — see also Injury, uterus
      - with ectopic or molar pregnancy O08.6
      - following ectopic or molar pregnancy O08.6
      - obstetrical trauma O71.3
    - chest — see Injury, intrathoracic
    - gastrointestinal tract — see Injury, intra-abdominal
    - heart — see Injury, heart
    - intestine NEC — see Injury, intestine
    - intrauterine — see Injury, uterus
    - mesentery — see Injury, intra-abdominal, specified, site NEC
    - pelvis, pelvic (organ) S37.90 ☑
      - following ectopic or molar pregnancy (subsequent episode) O08.6
      - obstetrical trauma NEC O71.5
        - rupture or perforation O71.1
      - specified NEC S39.83 ☑
    - rectum — see Injury, intestine, large, rectum
    - stomach — see Injury, stomach
    - ureter — see Injury, ureter
    - urethra (sphincter) following ectopic or molar pregnancy O08.6
    - uterus — see Injury, uterus
  - interscapular area — see Injury, thorax
  - intestine
    - large S36.509 ☑
      - ascending (right) S36.500 ☑
        - blast injury (primary) S36.510 ☑
          - secondary S36.590 ☑
        - contusion S36.520 ☑
        - laceration S36.530 ☑
        - specified type NEC S36.590 ☑
      - blast injury (primary) S36.519 ☑
        - ascending (right) S36.510 ☑
        - descending (left) S36.512 ☑

☑ **Additional Character Required** — Refer to the Tabular List for Character Selection   ▽ Subterms under main terms may continue to next column or page

Injury — *continued*
  intestine — *continued*
    large — *continued*
      blast injury — *continued*
        rectum S36.61 ☑
        sigmoid S36.513 ☑
        specified site NEC S36.518 ☑
        transverse S36.511 ☑
      contusion S36.529 ☑
        ascending (right) S36.520 ☑
        descending (left) S36.522 ☑
        rectum S36.62 ☑
        sigmoid S36.523 ☑
        specified site NEC S36.528 ☑
        transverse S36.521 ☑
      descending (left) S36.502 ☑
        blast injury (primary) S36.512 ☑
          secondary S36.592 ☑
        contusion S36.522 ☑
        laceration S36.532 ☑
        specified type NEC S36.592 ☑
      laceration S36.539 ☑
        ascending (right) S36.530 ☑
        descending (left) S36.532 ☑
        rectum S36.63 ☑
        sigmoid S36.533 ☑
        specified site NEC S36.538 ☑
        transverse S36.531 ☑
      rectum S36.60 ☑
        blast injury (primary) S36.61 ☑
          secondary S36.69 ☑
        contusion S36.62 ☑
        laceration S36.63 ☑
        specified type NEC S36.69 ☑
      sigmoid S36.503 ☑
        blast injury (primary) S36.513 ☑
          secondary S36.593 ☑
        contusion S36.523 ☑
        laceration S36.533 ☑
        specified type NEC S36.593 ☑
      specified
        site NEC S36.508 ☑
          blast injury (primary) S36.518 ☑
            secondary S36.598 ☑
          contusion S36.528 ☑
          laceration S36.538 ☑
          specified type NEC S36.598 ☑
        type NEC S36.599 ☑
          ascending (right) S36.590 ☑
          descending (left) S36.592 ☑
          rectum S36.69 ☑
          sigmoid S36.593 ☑
          specified site NEC S36.598 ☑
          transverse S36.591 ☑
      transverse S36.501 ☑
        blast injury (primary) S36.511 ☑
          secondary S36.591 ☑
        contusion S36.521 ☑
        laceration S36.531 ☑
        specified type NEC S36.591 ☑
    small S36.409 ☑
      blast injury (primary) S36.419 ☑
        duodenum S36.410 ☑
        secondary S36.499 ☑
          duodenum S36.490 ☑
          specified site NEC S36.498 ☑
        specified site NEC S36.418 ☑
      contusion S36.429 ☑
        duodenum S36.420 ☑
        specified site NEC S36.428 ☑
      duodenum S36.400 ☑
        blast injury (primary) S36.410 ☑
          secondary S36.490 ☑
        contusion S36.420 ☑
        laceration S36.430 ☑
        specified NEC S36.490 ☑
      laceration S36.439 ☑
        duodenum S36.430 ☑
        specified site NEC S36.438 ☑
      specified
        site NEC S36.408 ☑
        type NEC S36.499 ☑
          duodenum S36.490 ☑
          specified site NEC S36.498 ☑
  intra-abdominal S36.90 ☑
    adrenal gland — *see* Injury, adrenal gland

Injury — *continued*
  intra-abdominal — *continued*
    bladder — *see* Injury, bladder
    colon — *see* Injury, intestine, large
    contusion S36.92 ☑
    fallopian tube — *see* Injury, fallopian tube
    gallbladder — *see* Injury, gallbladder
    intestine — *see* Injury, intestine
    kidney — *see* Injury, kidney
    laceration S36.93 ☑
    liver — *see* Injury, liver
    ovary — *see* Injury, ovary
    pancreas — *see* Injury, pancreas
    pelvic NOS S37.90 ☑
    peritoneum — *see* Injury, intra-abdominal, specified, site NEC
    prostate — *see* Injury, prostate
    rectum — *see* Injury, intestine, large, rectum
    retroperitoneum — *see* Injury, intra-abdominal, specified, site NEC
    seminal vesicle — *see* Injury, pelvis, organ, specified site NEC
    small intestine — *see* Injury, intestine, small
    specified
      pelvic S37.90 ☑
        specified
          site NEC S37.899 ☑
            specified type NEC S37.898 ☑
          type NEC S37.99 ☑
      site NEC S36.899 ☑
        contusion S36.892 ☑
        laceration S36.893 ☑
        specified type NEC S36.898 ☑
      type NEC S36.99 ☑
    spleen — *see* Injury, spleen
    stomach — *see* Injury, stomach
    ureter — *see* Injury, ureter
    urethra — *see* Injury, urethra
    uterus — *see* Injury, uterus
    vas deferens — *see* Injury, pelvis, organ, specified site NEC
  intracranial (traumatic) S06.9- ☑
    cerebellar hemorrhage, traumatic — *see* Injury, intracranial, focal
    cerebral edema, traumatic S06.1X- ☑
      diffuse S06.1X- ☑
      focal S06.1X- ☑
    diffuse (axonal) S06.2X- ☑
    epidural hemorrhage (traumatic) S06.4X- ☑
    focal brain injury S06.30- ☑
      contusion — *see* Contusion, cerebral
      laceration — *see* Laceration, cerebral
    intracerebral hemorrhage, traumatic S06.36- ☑
      left side S06.35- ☑
      right side S06.34- ☑
    subarachnoid hemorrhage, traumatic S06.6X- ☑
    subdural hemorrhage, traumatic S06.5X- ☑
  intraocular — *see* Injury, eyeball, penetrating
  intrathoracic S27.9 ☑
    bronchus S27.409 ☑
      bilateral S27.402 ☑
      blast injury (primary) S27.419 ☑
        bilateral S27.412 ☑
        secondary — *see* Injury, intrathoracic, bronchus, specified type NEC
        unilateral S27.411 ☑
      contusion S27.429 ☑
        bilateral S27.422 ☑
        unilateral S27.421 ☑
      laceration S27.439 ☑
        bilateral S27.432 ☑
        unilateral S27.431 ☑
      specified type NEC S27.499 ☑
        bilateral S27.492 ☑
        unilateral S27.491 ☑
      unilateral S27.401 ☑
    diaphragm S27.809 ☑
      contusion S27.802 ☑
      laceration S27.803 ☑
      specified type NEC S27.808 ☑
    esophagus (thoracic) S27.819 ☑
      contusion S27.812 ☑
      laceration S27.813 ☑
      specified type NEC S27.818 ☑
    heart — *see* Injury, heart
    hemopneumothorax S27.2 ☑

Injury — *continued*
  intrathoracic — *continued*
    hemothorax S27.1 ☑
    lung S27.309 ☑
      aspiration J69.0
      bilateral S27.302 ☑
      blast injury (primary) S27.319 ☑
        bilateral S27.312 ☑
        secondary — *see* Injury, intrathoracic, lung, specified type NEC
        unilateral S27.311 ☑
      contusion S27.329 ☑
        bilateral S27.322 ☑
        unilateral S27.321 ☑
      laceration S27.339 ☑
        bilateral S27.332 ☑
        unilateral S27.331 ☑
      specified type NEC S27.399 ☑
        bilateral S27.392 ☑
        unilateral S27.391 ☑
      unilateral S27.301 ☑
    pleura S27.60 ☑
      laceration S27.63 ☑
      specified type NEC S27.69 ☑
    pneumothorax S27.0 ☑
    specified organ NEC S27.899 ☑
      contusion S27.892 ☑
      laceration S27.893 ☑
      specified type NEC S27.898 ☑
    thoracic duct — *see* Injury, intrathoracic, specified organ NEC
    thymus gland — *see* Injury, intrathoracic, specified organ NEC
    trachea, thoracic S27.50 ☑
      blast (primary) S27.51 ☑
      contusion S27.52 ☑
      laceration S27.53 ☑
      specified type NEC S27.59 ☑
  iris — *see* Injury, eye, specified site NEC
    penetrating — *see* Injury, eyeball, penetrating
  jaw S09.93 ☑
  jejunum — *see* Injury, intestine, small
  joint NOS T14.8 ☑
    old or residual — *see* Disorder, joint, specified type NEC
  kidney S37.00- ☑
    acute (nontraumatic) N17.9
    contusion — *see* Contusion, kidney
    laceration — *see* Laceration, kidney
    specified NEC S37.09- ☑
  knee S89.9- ☑
    contusion — *see* Contusion, knee
    dislocation — *see* Dislocation, knee
    meniscus (lateral) (medial) — *see* Sprain, knee, specified site NEC
      old injury or tear — *see* Derangement, knee, meniscus, due to old injury
    open — *see* Wound, open, knee
    specified NEC S89.8- ☑
    sprain — *see* Sprain, knee
    superficial — *see* Injury, superficial, knee
  labium (majus) (minus) S39.94 ☑
  labyrinth, ear S09.30- ☑
  lacrimal apparatus, duct, gland, or sac — *see* Injury, eye, specified site NEC
  larynx NEC S19.81 ☑
  leg (lower) S89.9- ☑
    blood vessel — *see* Injury, blood vessel, leg
    contusion — *see* Contusion, leg
    fracture — *see* Fracture, leg
    muscle — *see* Injury, muscle, leg
    nerve — *see* Injury, nerve, leg
    open — *see* Wound, open, leg
    specified NEC S89.8- ☑
    superficial — *see* Injury, superficial, leg
  lens, eye — *see* Injury, eye, specified site NEC
    penetrating — *see* Injury, eyeball, penetrating
  limb NEC T14.8 ☑
  lip S09.93 ☑
  liver S36.119 ☑
    contusion S36.112 ☑
    laceration S36.113 ☑
      major (stellate) S36.116 ☑
      minor S36.114 ☑
      moderate S36.115 ☑
    specified NEC S36.118 ☑

Injury — *continued*
  lower back S39.92 ☑
    specified NEC S39.82 ☑
  lumbar, lumbosacral (region) S39.92 ☑
    plexus — *see* Injury, lumbosacral plexus
  lumbosacral plexus S34.4 ☑
  lung — *see also* Injury, intrathoracic, lung
    aspiration J69.0
    dabbing (related) U07.0
    electronic cigarette (related) U07.0
    EVALI - [e-cigarette, or vaping, product use associat-
      ed] U07.0
    transfusion-related (TRALI) J95.84
    vaping (associated) (device) (product) (use) U07.0
  lymphatic thoracic duct — *see* Injury, intrathoracic,
    specified organ NEC
  malar region S09.93 ☑
  mastoid region S09.90 ☑
  maxilla S09.93 ☑
  mediastinum — *see* Injury, intrathoracic, specified or-
    gan NEC
  membrane, brain — *see* Injury, intracranial
  meningeal artery — *see* Injury, intracranial, subdural
    hemorrhage
  meninges (cerebral) — *see* Injury, intracranial
  mesenteric
    artery
      branch S35.299 ☑
        laceration (minor) (superficial) S35.291 ☑
          major S35.292 ☑
        specified NEC S35.298 ☑
      inferior S35.239 ☑
        laceration (minor) (superficial) S35.231 ☑
          major S35.232 ☑
        specified NEC S35.238 ☑
      superior S35.229 ☑
        laceration (minor) (superficial) S35.221 ☑
          major S35.222 ☑
        specified NEC S35.228 ☑
    plexus (inferior) (superior) — *see* Injury, nerve,
      lumbosacral, sympathetic
    vein
      inferior S35.349 ☑
        laceration S35.341 ☑
        specified NEC S35.348 ☑
      superior S35.339 ☑
        laceration S35.331 ☑
        specified NEC S35.338 ☑
  mesentery — *see* Injury, intra-abdominal, specified site
    NEC
  mesosalpinx — *see* Injury, pelvic organ, specified site
    NEC
  middle ear S09.30- ☑
  midthoracic region NOS S29.9 ☑
  mouth S09.93 ☑
  multiple NOS T07 ☑
  muscle (and fascia) (and tendon)
    abdomen S39.001 ☑
      laceration S39.021 ☑
      specified type NEC S39.091 ☑
      strain S39.011 ☑
    abductor
      thumb, forearm level — *see* Injury, muscle,
        thumb, abductor
    adductor
      thigh S76.20- ☑
        laceration S76.22- ☑
        specified type NEC S76.29- ☑
        strain S76.21- ☑
    ankle — *see* Injury, muscle, foot
    anterior muscle group, at leg level (lower) S86.20- ☑
      laceration S86.22- ☑
      specified type NEC S86.29- ☑
      strain S86.21- ☑
    arm (upper) — *see* Injury, muscle, shoulder
    biceps (parts NEC) S46.20- ☑
      laceration S46.22- ☑
      long head S46.10- ☑
        laceration S46.12- ☑
        specified type NEC S46.19- ☑
        strain S46.11- ☑
      specified type NEC S46.29- ☑
      strain S46.21- ☑
    extensor
      finger(s) (other than thumb) — *see* Injury, mus-
        cle, finger by site, extensor

Injury — *continued*
  muscle — *continued*
    extensor — *continued*
      forearm level, specified NEC — *see* Injury, muscle,
        forearm, extensor
      thumb — *see* Injury, muscle, thumb, extensor
      toe (large) (ankle level) (foot level) — *see* Injury,
        muscle, toe, extensor
    finger
      extensor (forearm level) S56.40- ☑
        hand level S66.309 ☑
          laceration S66.329 ☑
          specified type NEC S66.399 ☑
          strain S66.319 ☑
        laceration S56.429 ☑
        specified type NEC S56.499 ☑
        strain S56.419 ☑
      flexor (forearm level) S56.10- ☑
        hand level S66.109 ☑
          laceration S66.129 ☑
          specified type NEC S66.199 ☑
          strain S66.119 ☑
        laceration S56.129 ☑
        specified type NEC S56.199 ☑
        strain S56.119 ☑
      index
        extensor (forearm level)
          hand level S66.308 ☑
            laceration S66.32- ☑
            specified type NEC S66.39- ☑
            strain S66.31- ☑
          specified type NEC S56.492- ☑
        flexor (forearm level)
          hand level S66.108 ☑
            laceration S66.12- ☑
            specified type NEC S66.19- ☑
            strain S66.11- ☑
          specified type NEC S56.19- ☑
          strain S56.11- ☑
        intrinsic S66.50- ☑
          laceration S66.52- ☑
          specified type NEC S66.59- ☑
          strain S66.51- ☑
      intrinsic S66.509 ☑
        laceration S66.529 ☑
        specified type NEC S66.599 ☑
        strain S66.519 ☑
      little
        extensor (forearm level)
          hand level S66.30- ☑
            laceration S66.32- ☑
            specified type NEC S66.39- ☑
            strain S66.31- ☑
          laceration S56.42- ☑
          specified type NEC S56.49- ☑
          strain S56.41- ☑
        flexor (forearm level)
          hand level S66.10- ☑
            laceration S66.12- ☑
            specified type NEC S66.19- ☑
            strain S66.11- ☑
          laceration S56.12- ☑
          specified type NEC S56.19- ☑
          strain S56.11- ☑
        intrinsic S66.50- ☑
          laceration S66.52- ☑
          specified type NEC S66.59- ☑
          strain S66.51- ☑
      middle
        extensor (forearm level)
          hand level S66.30- ☑
            laceration S66.32- ☑
            specified type NEC S66.39- ☑
            strain S66.31- ☑
          laceration S56.42- ☑
          specified type NEC S56.49- ☑
          strain S56.41- ☑
        flexor (forearm level)
          hand level S66.10- ☑
            laceration S66.12- ☑
            specified type NEC S66.19- ☑
            strain S66.11- ☑
          laceration S56.12- ☑
          specified type NEC S56.19- ☑
          strain S56.11- ☑
        intrinsic S66.50- ☑

Injury — *continued*
  muscle — *continued*
    finger — *continued*
      middle — *continued*
        intrinsic — *continued*
          laceration S66.52- ☑
          specified type NEC S66.59- ☑
          strain S66.51- ☑
      ring
        extensor (forearm level)
          hand level S66.30- ☑
            laceration S66.32- ☑
            specified type NEC S66.39- ☑
            strain S66.31- ☑
          laceration S56.42- ☑
          specified type NEC S56.49- ☑
          strain S56.41- ☑
        flexor (forearm level)
          hand level S66.10- ☑
            laceration S66.12- ☑
            specified type NEC S66.19- ☑
            strain S66.11- ☑
          laceration S56.12- ☑
          specified type NEC S56.19- ☑
          strain S56.11- ☑
        intrinsic S66.50- ☑
          laceration S66.52- ☑
          specified type NEC S66.59- ☑
          strain S66.51- ☑
    flexor
      finger(s) (other than thumb) — *see* Injury, mu
        cle, finger
      forearm level, specified NEC — *see* Injury, musc
        forearm, flexor
      thumb — *see* Injury, muscle, thumb, flexor
      toe (long) (ankle level) (foot level) — *see* Inju
        muscle, toe, flexor
    foot S96.90- ☑
      intrinsic S96.20- ☑
        laceration S96.22- ☑
        specified type NEC S96.29- ☑
        strain S96.21- ☑
      laceration S96.92- ☑
      long extensor, toe — *see* Injury, muscle, toe, e
        tensor
      long flexor, toe — *see* Injury, muscle, toe, flex
      specified
        site NEC S96.80- ☑
          laceration S96.82- ☑
          specified type NEC S96.89- ☑
          strain S96.81- ☑
        type S96.99- ☑
      strain S96.91- ☑
    forearm (level) S56.90- ☑
      extensor S56.50- ☑
        laceration S56.52- ☑
        specified type NEC S56.59- ☑
        strain S56.51- ☑
      flexor S56.20- ☑
        laceration S56.22- ☑
        specified type NEC S56.29- ☑
        strain S56.21- ☑
      laceration S56.92- ☑
      specified S56.99- ☑
        site NEC S56.80- ☑
          laceration S56.82- ☑
          strain S56.81- ☑
          type NEC S56.89- ☑
      strain S56.91- ☑
    hand (level) S66.90- ☑
      laceration S66.92- ☑
      specified
        site NEC S66.80- ☑
          laceration S66.82- ☑
          specified type NEC S66.89- ☑
          strain S66.81- ☑
        type NEC S66.99- ☑
      strain S66.91- ☑
    head S09.10 ☑
      laceration S09.12 ☑
      specified type NEC S09.19 ☑
      strain S09.11 ☑
    hip NEC S76.00- ☑
      laceration S76.02- ☑
      specified type NEC S76.09- ☑
      strain S76.01- ☑

☑ **Additional Character Required — Refer to the Tabular List for Character Selection**   ▽ Subterms under main terms may continue to next column or pa

Injury — *continued*
  muscle — *continued*
    intrinsic
      ankle and foot level — *see* Injury, muscle, foot, intrinsic
      finger (other than thumb) — *see* Injury, muscle, finger by site, intrinsic
      foot (level) — *see* Injury, muscle, foot, intrinsic
      thumb — *see* Injury, muscle, thumb, intrinsic
    leg (level) (lower) S86.90- ☑
      Achilles tendon — *see* Injury, Achilles tendon
      anterior muscle group — *see* Injury, muscle, anterior muscle group
      laceration S86.92- ☑
      peroneal muscle group — *see* Injury, muscle, peroneal muscle group
      posterior muscle group — *see* Injury, muscle, posterior muscle group, leg level
      specified
        site NEC S86.80- ☑
          laceration S86.82- ☑
          specified type NEC S86.89- ☑
          strain S86.81- ☑
        type NEC S86.99- ☑
      strain S86.91- ☑
    long
      extensor toe, at ankle and foot level — *see* Injury, muscle, toe, extensor
      flexor, toe, at ankle and foot level — *see* Injury, muscle, toe, flexor
      head, biceps — *see* Injury, muscle, biceps, long head
    lower back S39.002 ☑
      laceration S39.022 ☑
      specified type NEC S39.092 ☑
      strain S39.012 ☑
    neck (level) S16.9 ☑
      laceration S16.2 ☑
      specified type NEC S16.8 ☑
      strain S16.1 ☑
    pelvis S39.003 ☑
      laceration S39.023 ☑
      specified type NEC S39.093 ☑
      strain S39.013 ☑
    peroneal muscle group, at leg level (lower) S86.30- ☑
      laceration S86.32- ☑
      specified type NEC S86.39- ☑
      strain S86.31- ☑
    posterior muscle (group)
      leg level (lower) S86.10- ☑
        laceration S86.12- ☑
        specified type NEC S86.19- ☑
        strain S86.11- ☑
      thigh level S76.30- ☑
        laceration S76.32- ☑
        specified type NEC S76.39- ☑
        strain S76.31- ☑
    quadriceps (thigh) S76.10- ☑
      laceration S76.12- ☑
      specified type NEC S76.19- ☑
      strain S76.11- ☑
    shoulder S46.90- ☑
      laceration S46.92- ☑
      rotator cuff — *see* Injury, rotator cuff
      specified site NEC S46.80- ☑
        laceration S46.82- ☑
        specified type NEC S46.89- ☑
        strain S46.81- ☑
      specified type NEC S46.99- ☑
      strain S46.91- ☑
    thigh NEC (level) S76.90- ☑
      adductor — *see* Injury, muscle, adductor, thigh
      laceration S76.92- ☑
      posterior muscle (group) — *see* Injury, muscle, posterior muscle, thigh level
      quadriceps — *see* Injury, muscle, quadriceps
      specified
        site NEC S76.80- ☑
          laceration S76.82- ☑
          specified type NEC S76.89- ☑
          strain S76.81- ☑
        type NEC S76.99- ☑
      strain S76.91- ☑
    thorax (level) S29.009 ☑
      back wall S29.002 ☑

Injury — *continued*
  muscle — *continued*
    thorax — *continued*
      front wall S29.001 ☑
      laceration S29.029 ☑
        back wall S29.022 ☑
        front wall S29.021 ☑
      specified type NEC S29.099 ☑
        back wall S29.092 ☑
        front wall S29.091 ☑
      strain S29.019 ☑
        back wall S29.012 ☑
        front wall S29.011 ☑
    thumb
      abductor (forearm level) S56.30- ☑
        laceration S56.32- ☑
        specified type NEC S56.39- ☑
        strain S56.31- ☑
      extensor (forearm level) S56.30- ☑
        hand level S66.20- ☑
          laceration S66.22- ☑
          specified type NEC S66.29- ☑
          strain S66.21- ☑
        laceration S56.32- ☑
        specified type NEC S56.39- ☑
        strain S56.31- ☑
      flexor (forearm level) S56.00- ☑
        hand level S66.00- ☑
          laceration S66.02- ☑
          specified type NEC S66.09- ☑
          strain S66.01- ☑
        laceration S56.02- ☑
        specified type NEC S56.09- ☑
        strain S56.01- ☑
        wrist level — *see* Injury, muscle, thumb, flexor, hand level
      intrinsic S66.40- ☑
        laceration S66.42- ☑
        specified type NEC S66.49- ☑
        strain S66.41- ☑
    toe — *see also* Injury, muscle, foot
      extensor, long S96.10- ☑
        laceration S96.12- ☑
        specified type NEC S96.19- ☑
        strain S96.11- ☑
      flexor, long S96.00- ☑
        laceration S96.02- ☑
        specified type NEC S96.09- ☑
        strain S96.01- ☑
    triceps S46.30- ☑
      laceration S46.32- ☑
      specified type NEC S46.39- ☑
      strain S46.31- ☑
    wrist (and hand) level — *see* Injury, muscle, hand
  musculocutaneous nerve — *see* Injury, nerve, musculocutaneous
  myocardium — *see* Injury, heart
  nape — *see* Injury, neck
  nasal (septum) (sinus) S09.92 ☑
  nasopharynx S09.92 ☑
  neck S19.9 ☑
    specified NEC S19.80 ☑
      specified site NEC S19.89 ☑
  nerve NEC T14.8 ☑
    abdomen S34.9 ☑
      peripheral S34.6 ☑
      specified site NEC S34.8 ☑
    abducens S04.4- ☑
      contusion S04.4- ☑
      laceration S04.4- ☑
      specified type NEC S04.4- ☑
    abducent — *see* Injury, nerve, abducens
    accessory S04.7- ☑
      contusion S04.7- ☑
      laceration S04.7- ☑
      specified type NEC S04.7- ☑
    acoustic S04.6- ☑
      contusion S04.6- ☑
      laceration S04.6- ☑
      specified type NEC S04.6- ☑
    ankle S94.9- ☑
      cutaneous sensory S94.3- ☑
      specified site NEC — *see* subcategory S94.8 ☑
    anterior crural, femoral — *see* Injury, nerve, femoral
    arm (upper) S44.9- ☑
      axillary — *see* Injury, nerve, axillary

Injury — *continued*
  nerve — *continued*
    arm — *continued*
      cutaneous — *see* Injury, nerve, cutaneous, arm
      median — *see* Injury, nerve, median, upper arm
      musculocutaneous — *see* Injury, nerve, musculocutaneous
      radial — *see* Injury, nerve, radial, upper arm
      specified site NEC — *see* subcategory S44.8 ☑
      ulnar — *see* Injury, nerve, ulnar, arm
    auditory — *see* Injury, nerve, acoustic
    axillary S44.3- ☑
    brachial plexus — *see* Injury, brachial plexus
    cervical sympathetic S14.5 ☑
    cranial S04.9 ☑
      contusion S04.9 ☑
      eighth (acoustic or auditory) — *see* Injury, nerve, acoustic
      eleventh (accessory) — *see* Injury, nerve, accessory
      fifth (trigeminal) — *see* Injury, nerve, trigeminal
      first (olfactory) — *see* Injury, nerve, olfactory
      fourth (trochlear) — *see* Injury, nerve, trochlear
      laceration S04.9 ☑
      ninth (glossopharyngeal) — *see* Injury, nerve, glossopharyngeal
      second (optic) — *see* Injury, nerve, optic
      seventh (facial) — *see* Injury, nerve, facial
      sixth (abducent) — *see* Injury, nerve, abducens
      specified
        nerve NEC S04.89- ☑
          contusion S04.89- ☑
          laceration S04.89- ☑
          specified type NEC S04.89- ☑
        type NEC S04.9 ☑
      tenth (pneumogastric or vagus) — *see* Injury, nerve, vagus
      third (oculomotor) — *see* Injury, nerve, oculomotor
      twelfth (hypoglossal) — *see* Injury, nerve, hypoglossal
    cutaneous sensory
      ankle (level) S94.3- ☑
      arm (upper) (level) S44.5- ☑
      foot (level) — *see* Injury, nerve, cutaneous sensory, ankle
      forearm (level) S54.3- ☑
      hip (level) S74.2- ☑
      leg (lower level) S84.2- ☑
      shoulder (level) — *see* Injury, nerve, cutaneous sensory, arm
      thigh (level) — *see* Injury, nerve, cutaneous sensory, hip
    deep peroneal — *see* Injury, nerve, peroneal, foot
    digital
      finger S64.4- ☑
        index S64.49- ☑
        little S64.49- ☑
        middle S64.49- ☑
        ring S64.49- ☑
      thumb S64.3- ☑
      toe — *see* Injury, nerve, ankle, specified site NEC
    eighth cranial (acoustic or auditory) — *see* Injury, nerve, acoustic
    eleventh cranial (accessory) — *see* Injury, nerve, accessory
    facial S04.5- ☑
      contusion S04.5- ☑
      laceration S04.5- ☑
      newborn P11.3
      specified type NEC S04.5- ☑
    femoral (hip level) (thigh level) S74.1- ☑
    fifth cranial (trigeminal) — *see* Injury, nerve, trigeminal
    finger (digital) — *see* Injury, nerve, digital, finger
    first cranial (olfactory) — *see* Injury, nerve, olfactory
    foot S94.9- ☑
      cutaneous sensory S94.3- ☑
      deep peroneal S94.2- ☑
      lateral plantar S94.0- ☑
      medial plantar S94.1- ☑
      specified site NEC — *see* subcategory S94.8 ☑
    forearm (level) S54.9- ☑
      cutaneous sensory — *see* Injury, nerve, cutaneous sensory, forearm
      median — *see* Injury, nerve, median

Index

Injury — *continued*
  nerve — *continued*
    forearm — *continued*
      radial — *see* Injury, nerve, radial
      specified NEC — *see* subcategory S54.8 ☑
      ulnar — *see* Injury, nerve, ulnar
    fourth cranial (trochlear) — *see* Injury, nerve, trochlear
    glossopharyngeal S04.89- ☑
      specified type NEC S04.89- ☑
    hand S64.9- ☑
      median — *see* Injury, nerve, median, hand
      radial — *see* Injury, nerve, radial, hand
      specified NEC — *see* subcategory S64.8 ☑
      ulnar — *see* Injury, nerve, ulnar, hand
    hip (level) S74.9- ☑
      cutaneous sensory — *see* Injury, nerve, cutaneous sensory, hip
      femoral — *see* Injury, nerve, femoral
      sciatic — *see* Injury, nerve, sciatic
      specified site NEC — *see* subcategory S74.8 ☑
    hypoglossal S04.89- ☑
      specified type NEC S04.89- ☑
    lateral plantar S94.0- ☑
    leg (lower) S84.9- ☑
      cutaneous sensory — *see* Injury, nerve, cutaneous sensory, leg
      peroneal — *see* Injury, nerve, peroneal
      specified site NEC — *see* subcategory S84.8 ☑
      tibial — *see* Injury, nerve, tibial
      upper — *see* Injury, nerve, thigh
    lower
      back — *see* Injury, nerve, abdomen, specified site NEC
        peripheral — *see* Injury, nerve, abdomen, peripheral
      limb — *see* Injury, nerve, leg
    lumbar plexus — *see* Injury, nerve, lumbosacral, sympathetic
    lumbar spinal — *see* Injury, nerve, spinal, lumbar
    lumbosacral
      plexus — *see* Injury, nerve, lumbosacral, sympathetic
      sympathetic S34.5 ☑
    medial plantar S94.1- ☑
    median (forearm level) S54.1- ☑
      hand (level) S64.1- ☑
      upper arm (level) S44.1- ☑
      wrist (level) — *see* Injury, nerve, median, hand
    musculocutaneous S44.4- ☑
    musculospiral (upper arm level) — *see* Injury, nerve, radial, upper arm
    neck S14.9 ☑
      peripheral S14.4 ☑
      specified site NEC S14.8 ☑
      sympathetic S14.5 ☑
    ninth cranial (glossopharyngeal) — *see* Injury, nerve, glossopharyngeal
    oculomotor S04.1- ☑
      contusion S04.1- ☑
      laceration S04.1- ☑
      specified type NEC S04.1- ☑
    olfactory S04.81- ☑
      specified type NEC S04.81- ☑
    optic S04.01- ☑
      contusion S04.01- ☑
      laceration S04.01- ☑
      specified type NEC S04.01- ☑
    pelvic girdle — *see* Injury, nerve, hip
    pelvis — *see* Injury, nerve, abdomen, specified site NEC
      peripheral — *see* Injury, nerve, abdomen, peripheral
    peripheral NEC T14.8 ☑
      abdomen — *see* Injury, nerve, abdomen, peripheral
      lower back — *see* Injury, nerve, abdomen, peripheral
      neck — *see* Injury, nerve, neck, peripheral
      pelvis — *see* Injury, nerve, abdomen, peripheral
      specified NEC T14.8 ☑
    peroneal (lower leg level) S84.1- ☑
      foot S94.2- ☑
    plexus
      brachial — *see* Injury, brachial plexus

Injury — *continued*
  nerve — *continued*
    plexus — *continued*
      celiac, coeliac — *see* Injury, nerve, lumbosacral, sympathetic
      mesenteric, inferior — *see* Injury, nerve, lumbosacral, sympathetic
      sacral — *see* Injury, lumbosacral plexus
      spinal
        brachial — *see* Injury, brachial plexus
        lumbosacral — *see* Injury, lumbosacral plexus
    pneumogastric — *see* Injury, nerve, vagus
    radial (forearm level) S54.2- ☑
      hand (level) S64.2- ☑
      upper arm (level) S44.2- ☑
      wrist (level) — *see* Injury, nerve, radial, hand
    root — *see* Injury, nerve, spinal, root
    sacral plexus — *see* Injury, lumbosacral plexus
    sacral spinal — *see* Injury, nerve, spinal, sacral
    sciatic (hip level) (thigh level) S74.0- ☑
    second cranial (optic) — *see* Injury, nerve, optic
    seventh cranial (facial) — *see* Injury, nerve, facial
    shoulder — *see* Injury, nerve, arm
    sixth cranial (abducent) — *see* Injury, nerve, abducens
    spinal
      plexus — *see* Injury, nerve, plexus, spinal
      root
        cervical S14.2 ☑
        dorsal S24.2 ☑
        lumbar S34.21 ☑
        sacral S34.22 ☑
        thoracic — *see* Injury, nerve, spinal, root, dorsal
    splanchnic — *see* Injury, nerve, lumbosacral, sympathetic
    sympathetic NEC — *see* Injury, nerve, lumbosacral, sympathetic
      cervical — *see* Injury, nerve, cervical sympathetic
    tenth cranial (pneumogastric or vagus) — *see* Injury, nerve, vagus
    thigh (level) — *see* Injury, nerve, hip
      cutaneous sensory — *see* Injury, nerve, cutaneous sensory, hip
      femoral — *see* Injury, nerve, femoral
      sciatic — *see* Injury, nerve, sciatic
      specified NEC — *see* Injury, nerve, hip
    third cranial (oculomotor) — *see* Injury, nerve, oculomotor
    thorax S24.9 ☑
      peripheral S24.3 ☑
      specified site NEC S24.8 ☑
      sympathetic S24.4 ☑
    thumb, digital — *see* Injury, nerve, digital, thumb
    tibial (lower leg level) (posterior) S84.0- ☑
    toe — *see* Injury, nerve, ankle
    trigeminal S04.3- ☑
      contusion S04.3- ☑
      laceration S04.3- ☑
      specified type NEC S04.3- ☑
    trochlear S04.2- ☑
      contusion S04.2- ☑
      laceration S04.2- ☑
      specified type NEC S04.2- ☑
    twelfth cranial (hypoglossal) — *see* Injury, nerve, hypoglossal
    ulnar (forearm level) S54.0- ☑
      arm (upper) (level) S44.0- ☑
      hand (level) S64.0- ☑
      wrist (level) — *see* Injury, nerve, ulnar, hand
    vagus S04.89- ☑
      specified type NEC S04.89- ☑
    wrist (level) — *see* Injury, nerve, hand
    ninth cranial nerve (glossopharyngeal) — *see* Injury, nerve, glossopharyngeal
  nose (septum) S09.92 ☑
  obstetrical O71.9
    specified NEC O71.89
  occipital (region) (scalp) S09.90 ☑
    lobe — *see* Injury, intracranial
  optic chiasm S04.02 ☑
  optic radiation S04.03- ☑
  optic tract and pathways S04.03- ☑
  orbit, orbital (region) — *see* Injury, eye
    penetrating (with foreign body) — *see* Injury, eye, orbit, penetrating

Injury — *continued*
  orbit, orbital — *see* Injury, eye — *continued*
    specified NEC — *see* Injury, eye, specified site NEC
  ovary, ovarian S37.409 ☑
    bilateral S37.402 ☑
      contusion S37.422 ☑
      laceration S37.432 ☑
      specified type NEC S37.492 ☑
    blood vessel — *see* Injury, blood vessel, ovarian
    contusion S37.429 ☑
      bilateral S37.422 ☑
      unilateral S37.421 ☑
    laceration S37.439 ☑
      bilateral S37.432 ☑
      unilateral S37.431 ☑
    specified type NEC S37.499 ☑
      bilateral S37.492 ☑
      unilateral S37.491 ☑
    unilateral S37.401 ☑
      contusion S37.421 ☑
      laceration S37.431 ☑
      specified type NEC S37.491 ☑
  palate (hard) (soft) S09.93 ☑
  pancreas S36.209 ☑
    body S36.201 ☑
      contusion S36.221 ☑
      laceration S36.231 ☑
        major S36.261 ☑
        minor S36.241 ☑
        moderate S36.251 ☑
      specified type NEC S36.291 ☑
    contusion S36.229 ☑
    head S36.200 ☑
      contusion S36.220 ☑
      laceration S36.230 ☑
        major S36.260 ☑
        minor S36.240 ☑
        moderate S36.250 ☑
      specified type NEC S36.290 ☑
    laceration S36.239 ☑
      major S36.269 ☑
      minor S36.249 ☑
      moderate S36.259 ☑
    specified type NEC S36.299 ☑
    tail S36.202 ☑
      contusion S36.222 ☑
      laceration S36.232 ☑
        major S36.262 ☑
        minor S36.242 ☑
        moderate S36.252 ☑
      specified type NEC S36.292 ☑
  parietal (region) (scalp) S09.90 ☑
    lobe — *see* Injury, intracranial
  patellar ligament (tendon) S76.10- ☑
    laceration S76.12- ☑
    specified NEC S76.19- ☑
    strain S76.11- ☑
  pelvis, pelvic (floor) S39.93 ☑
    complicating delivery O70.1
    joint or ligament, complicating delivery O71.6
    organ S37.90 ☑
      with ectopic or molar pregnancy O08.6
      complication of abortion — *see* Abortion
      contusion S37.92 ☑
      following ectopic or molar pregnancy O08.6
      laceration S37.93 ☑
      obstetrical trauma NEC O71.5
      specified
        site NEC S37.899 ☑
          contusion S37.892 ☑
          laceration S37.893 ☑
          specified type NEC S37.898 ☑
        type NEC S37.99 ☑
    specified NEC S39.83 ☑
  penis S39.94 ☑
  perineum S39.94 ☑
  peritoneum S36.81 ☑
    laceration S36.893 ☑
  periurethral tissue — *see* Injury, urethra
    complicating delivery O71.82
  phalanges
    foot — *see* Injury, foot
    hand — *see* Injury, hand
  pharynx NEC S19.85 ☑
  pleura — *see* Injury, intrathoracic, pleura

Injury — Injury

njury — *continued*
  plexus
    brachial — *see* Injury, brachial plexus
    cardiac — *see* Injury, nerve, thorax, sympathetic
    celiac, coeliac — *see* Injury, nerve, lumbosacral, sympathetic
    esophageal — *see* Injury, nerve, thorax, sympathetic
    hypogastric — *see* Injury, nerve, lumbosacral, sympathetic
    lumbar, lumbosacral — *see* Injury, lumbosacral plexus
    mesenteric — *see* Injury, nerve, lumbosacral, sympathetic
    pulmonary — *see* Injury, nerve, thorax, sympathetic
  postcardiac surgery (syndrome) I97.0
  prepuce S39.94 ☑
  pressure
    injury — *see* Ulcer, pressure, by site
  prostate S37.829 ☑
    contusion S37.822 ☑
    laceration S37.823 ☑
    specified type NEC S37.828 ☑
  pubic region S39.94 ☑
  pudendum S39.94 ☑
  pulmonary plexus — *see* Injury, nerve, thorax, sympathetic
  rectovaginal septum NEC S39.83 ☑
  rectum — *see* Injury, intestine, large, rectum
  retina — *see* Injury, eye, specified site NEC
    penetrating — *see* Injury, eyeball, penetrating
  retroperitoneal — *see* Injury, intra-abdominal, specified site NEC
  rotator cuff (muscle(s)) (tendon(s)) S46.00- ☑
    laceration S46.02- ☑
    specified type NEC S46.09- ☑
    strain S46.01- ☑
  round ligament — *see* Injury, pelvic organ, specified site NEC
  sacral plexus — *see* Injury, lumbosacral plexus
  salivary duct or gland S09.93 ☑
  scalp S09.90 ☑
    newborn (birth injury) P12.9
      due to monitoring (electrode) (sampling incision) P12.4
      specified NEC P12.89
        caput succedaneum P12.81
  scapular region — *see* Injury, shoulder
  sclera — *see* Injury, eye, specified site NEC
    penetrating — *see* Injury, eyeball, penetrating
  scrotum S39.94 ☑
  second cranial nerve (optic) — *see* Injury, nerve, optic
  seminal vesicle — *see* Injury, pelvic organ, specified site NEC
  seventh cranial nerve (facial) — *see* Injury, nerve, facial
  shoulder S49.9- ☑
    blood vessel — *see* Injury, blood vessel, arm
    contusion — *see* Contusion, shoulder
    dislocation — *see* Dislocation, shoulder
    fracture — *see* Fracture, shoulder
    muscle — *see* Injury, muscle, shoulder
    nerve — *see* Injury, nerve, shoulder
    open — *see* Wound, open, shoulder
    specified type NEC S49.8- ☑
    sprain — *see* Sprain, shoulder girdle
    superficial — *see* Injury, superficial, shoulder
  sinus
    cavernous — *see* Injury, intracranial
    nasal S09.92 ☑
  sixth cranial nerve (abducent) — *see* Injury, nerve, abducens
  skeleton, birth injury P13.9
    specified part NEC P13.8
  skin NEC T14.8 ☑
    surface intact — *see* Injury, superficial
  skull NEC S09.90 ☑
  specified NEC T14.8 ☑
  spermatic cord (pelvic region) S37.898 ☑
    scrotal region S39.848 ☑
  spinal (cord)
    cervical (neck) S14.109 ☑
      anterior cord syndrome S14.139 ☑
        C1 level S14.131 ☑
        C2 level S14.132 ☑
        C3 level S14.133 ☑
        C4 level S14.134 ☑
        C5 level S14.135 ☑

Injury — *continued*
  spinal — *continued*
    cervical — *continued*
      anterior cord syndrome — *continued*
        C6 level S14.136 ☑
        C7 level S14.137 ☑
        C8 level S14.138 ☑
      Brown-Séquard syndrome S14.149 ☑
        C1 level S14.141 ☑
        C2 level S14.142 ☑
        C3 level S14.143 ☑
        C4 level S14.144 ☑
        C5 level S14.145 ☑
        C6 level S14.146 ☑
        C7 level S14.147 ☑
        C8 level S14.148 ☑
      C1 level S14.101 ☑
      C2 level S14.102 ☑
      C3 level S14.103 ☑
      C4 level S14.104 ☑
      C5 level S14.105 ☑
      C6 level S14.106 ☑
      C7 level S14.107 ☑
      C8 level S14.108 ☑
      central cord syndrome S14.129 ☑
        C1 level S14.121 ☑
        C2 level S14.122 ☑
        C3 level S14.123 ☑
        C4 level S14.124 ☑
        C5 level S14.125 ☑
        C6 level S14.126 ☑
        C7 level S14.127 ☑
        C8 level S14.128 ☑
      complete lesion S14.119 ☑
        C1 level S14.111 ☑
        C2 level S14.112 ☑
        C3 level S14.113 ☑
        C4 level S14.114 ☑
        C5 level S14.115 ☑
        C6 level S14.116 ☑
        C7 level S14.117 ☑
        C8 level S14.118 ☑
      concussion S14.0 ☑
      edema S14.0 ☑
      incomplete lesion specified NEC S14.159 ☑
        C1 level S14.151 ☑
        C2 level S14.152 ☑
        C3 level S14.153 ☑
        C4 level S14.154 ☑
        C5 level S14.155 ☑
        C6 level S14.156 ☑
        C7 level S14.157 ☑
        C8 level S14.158 ☑
      posterior cord syndrome S14.159 ☑
        C1 level S14.151 ☑
        C2 level S14.152 ☑
        C3 level S14.153 ☑
        C4 level S14.154 ☑
        C5 level S14.155 ☑
        C6 level S14.156 ☑
        C7 level S14.157 ☑
        C8 level S14.158 ☑
    dorsal — *see* Injury, spinal, thoracic
    lumbar S34.109 ☑
      complete lesion S34.119 ☑
        L1 level S34.111 ☑
        L2 level S34.112 ☑
        L3 level S34.113 ☑
        L4 level S34.114 ☑
        L5 level S34.115 ☑
      concussion S34.01 ☑
      edema S34.01 ☑
      incomplete lesion S34.129 ☑
        L1 level S34.121 ☑
        L2 level S34.122 ☑
        L3 level S34.123 ☑
        L4 level S34.124 ☑
        L5 level S34.125 ☑
      L1 level S34.101 ☑
      L2 level S34.102 ☑
      L3 level S34.103 ☑
      L4 level S34.104 ☑
      L5 level S34.105 ☑
    nerve root NEC
      cervical — *see* Injury, nerve, spinal, root, cervical
      dorsal — *see* Injury, nerve, spinal, root, dorsal

Injury — *continued*
  spinal — *continued*
    nerve root — *continued*
      lumbar S34.21 ☑
      sacral S34.22 ☑
      thoracic — *see* Injury, nerve, spinal, root, dorsal
    plexus
      brachial — *see* Injury, brachial plexus
      lumbosacral — *see* Injury, lumbosacral plexus
    sacral S34.139 ☑
      complete lesion S34.131 ☑
      incomplete lesion S34.132 ☑
    thoracic S24.109 ☑
      anterior cord syndrome S24.139 ☑
        T1 level S24.131 ☑
        T2-T6 level S24.132 ☑
        T7-T10 level S24.133 ☑
        T11-T12 level S24.134 ☑
      Brown-Séquard syndrome S24.149 ☑
        T1 level S24.141 ☑
        T2-T6 level S24.142 ☑
        T7-T10 level S24.143 ☑
        T11-T12 level S24.144 ☑
      complete lesion S24.119 ☑
        T1 level S24.111 ☑
        T2-T6 level S24.112 ☑
        T7-T10 level S24.113 ☑
        T11-T12 level S24.114 ☑
      concussion S24.0 ☑
      edema S24.0 ☑
      incomplete lesion specified NEC S24.159 ☑
        T1 level S24.151 ☑
        T2-T6 level S24.152 ☑
        T7-T10 level S24.153 ☑
        T11-T12 level S24.154 ☑
      posterior cord syndrome S24.159 ☑
        T1 level S24.151 ☑
        T2-T6 level S24.152 ☑
        T7-T10 level S24.153 ☑
        T11-T12 level S24.154 ☑
      T1 level S24.101 ☑
      T2-T6 level S24.102 ☑
      T7-T10 level S24.103 ☑
      T11-T12 level S24.104 ☑
  splanchnic nerve — *see* Injury, nerve, lumbosacral, sympathetic
  spleen S36.00 ☑
    contusion S36.029 ☑
      major S36.021 ☑
      minor S36.020 ☑
    laceration S36.039 ☑
      major (massive) (stellate) S36.032 ☑
      moderate S36.031 ☑
      superficial (capsular) (minor) S36.030 ☑
    specified type NEC S36.09 ☑
  splenic artery — *see* Injury, blood vessel, celiac artery, branch
  stellate ganglion — *see* Injury, nerve, thorax, sympathetic
  sternal region S29.9 ☑
  stomach S36.30 ☑
    contusion S36.32 ☑
    laceration S36.33 ☑
    specified type NEC S36.39 ☑
  subconjunctival — *see* Injury, eye, conjunctiva
  subcutaneous NEC T14.8 ☑
  submaxillary region S09.93 ☑
  submental region S09.93 ☑
  subungual
    fingers — *see* Injury, hand
    toes — *see* Injury, foot
  superficial NEC T14.8 ☑
    abdomen, abdominal (wall) S30.92 ☑
      abrasion S30.811 ☑
      bite S30.871 ☑
        insect S30.861 ☑
      contusion S30.1 ☑
      external constriction S30.841 ☑
      foreign body S30.851 ☑
    abrasion — *see* Abrasion, by site
    adnexa, eye NEC — *see* Injury, eye, specified site NEC
    alveolar process — *see* Injury, superficial, oral cavity
  ankle S90.91- ☑
    abrasion — *see* Abrasion, ankle
    bite — *see* Bite, ankle

▽ **Subterms under main terms may continue to next column or page**   ☑ **Additional Character Required — Refer to the Tabular List for Character Selection**   **201**

Injury — Injury

☑ Additional Character Required — Refer to the Tabular List for Character Selection   ▽ Subterms under main terms may continue to next column or page

Inoculation — *continued*
complication or reaction — *see* Complications, vaccination

Insanity, insane — *see also* Psychosis
adolescent — *see* Schizophrenia
confusional F28
acute or subacute F05
delusional F22
senile F03 ☑

Insect
bite — *see* Bite, by site, superficial, insect
venomous, poisoning NEC (by) — *see* Venom, arthropod

Insensitivity
adrenocorticotropin hormone (ACTH) E27.49
androgen E34.50
complete E34.51
partial E34.52

Insertion
cord (umbilical) lateral or velamentous O43.12- ☑
intrauterine contraceptive device (encounter for) — *see* Intrauterine contraceptive device

Insolation (sunstroke) T67.01 ☑

Insomnia (organic) G47.00
adjustment F51.02
adjustment disorder F51.02
behavioral, of childhood Z73.819
combined type Z73.812
limit setting type Z73.811
sleep-onset association type Z73.810
childhood Z73.819
chronic F51.04
somatized tension F51.04
conditioned F51.04
due to
alcohol
abuse F10.182
dependence F10.282
use F10.982
amphetamines
abuse F15.182
dependence F15.282
use F15.982
anxiety disorder F51.05
caffeine
abuse F15.182
dependence F15.282
use F15.982
cocaine
abuse F14.182
dependence F14.282
use F14.982
depression F51.05
drug NEC
abuse F19.182
dependence F19.282
use F19.982
medical condition G47.01
mental disorder NEC F51.05
opioid
abuse F11.182
dependence F11.282
use F11.982
psychoactive substance NEC
abuse F19.182
dependence F19.182
use F19.982
sedative, hypnotic, or anxiolytic
abuse F13.182
dependence F13.282
use F13.982
stimulant NEC
abuse F15.182
dependence F15.282
use F15.982
fatal familial (FFI) A81.83
idiopathic F51.01
learned F51.3
nonorganic origin F51.01
not due to a substance or known physiological condition F51.01
specified NEC F51.09
paradoxical F51.03
primary F51.01
psychiatric F51.05
psychophysiologic F51.04
related to psychopathology F51.05
short-term F51.02

Insomnia — *continued*
specified NEC G47.09
stress-related F51.02
transient F51.02
without objective findings F51.02

Inspiration
food or foreign body — *see* Foreign body, by site
mucus — *see* Asphyxia, mucus

Inspissated bile syndrome (newborn) P59.1

Instability
emotional (excessive) F60.3
joint (post-traumatic) M25.30
ankle M25.37- ☑
due to old ligament injury — *see* Disorder, ligament
elbow M25.32- ☑
flail — *see* Flail, joint
foot M25.37- ☑
hand M25.34- ☑
hip M25.35- ☑
knee M25.36- ☑
lumbosacral — *see* subcategory M53.2 ☑
prosthesis — *see* Complications, joint prosthesis, mechanical, displacement, by site
sacroiliac — *see* subcategory M53.2 ☑
secondary to
old ligament injury — *see* Disorder, ligament
removal of joint prosthesis M96.89
shoulder (region) M25.31- ☑
specified site NEC M25.39
spine — *see* subcategory M53.2 ☑
wrist M25.33- ☑
knee (chronic) M23.5- ☑
lumbosacral — *see* subcategory M53.2 ☑
nervous F48.8
personality (emotional) F60.3
spine — *see* Instability, joint, spine
vasomotor R55

Institutional syndrome (childhood) F94.2
Institutionalization, affecting child Z62.22
disinhibited attachment F94.2

Insufficiency, insufficient
accommodation, old age H52.4
adrenal (gland) E27.40
primary E27.1
adrenocortical E27.40
drug-induced E27.3
iatrogenic E27.3
primary E27.1
anatomic crown height K08.89
anterior (occlusal) guidance M26.54
anus K62.89
aortic (valve) I35.1
with
mitral (valve) disease I08.0
with tricuspid (valve) disease I08.3
stenosis I35.2
tricuspid (valve) disease I08.2
with mitral (valve) disease I08.3
congenital Q23.1
rheumatic I06.1
with
mitral (valve) disease I08.0
with tricuspid (valve) disease I08.3
stenosis I06.2
with mitral (valve) disease I08.0
with tricuspid (valve) disease I08.3
tricuspid (valve) disease I08.2
with mitral (valve) disease I08.3
specified cause NEC I35.1
syphilitic A52.03
arterial I77.1
basilar G45.0
carotid (hemispheric) G45.1
cerebral I67.81
coronary (acute or subacute) I24.8
mesenteric K55.1
peripheral I73.9
precerebral (multiple) (bilateral) G45.2
vertebral G45.0
arteriovenous I99.8
biliary K83.8
cardiac — *see also* Insufficiency, myocardial
due to presence of (cardiac) prosthesis I97.11- ☑
postprocedural I97.11- ☑
cardiorenal, hypertensive I13.2
cardiovascular — *see* Disease, cardiovascular
cerebrovascular (acute) I67.81

Insufficiency, insufficient — *continued*
cerebrovascular — *continued*
with transient focal neurological signs and symptoms G45.8
circulatory NEC I99.8
newborn P29.89
clinical crown length K08.89
convergence H51.11
coronary (acute or subacute) I24.8
chronic or with a stated duration of over 4 weeks I25.89
corticoadrenal E27.40
primary E27.1
dietary E63.9
divergence H51.8
food T73.0 ☑
gastroesophageal K22.8
gonadal
ovary E28.39
testis E29.1
heart — *see also* Insufficiency, myocardial
newborn P29.0
valve — *see* Endocarditis
hepatic — *see* Failure, hepatic
idiopathic autonomic G90.09
interocclusal distance of fully erupted teeth (ridge) M26.36
kidney N28.9
acute N28.9
chronic N18.9
lacrimal (secretion) H04.12- ☑
passages — *see* Stenosis, lacrimal
liver — *see* Failure, hepatic
lung — *see* Insufficiency, pulmonary
mental (congenital) — *see* Disability, intellectual
mesenteric K55.1
mitral (valve) I34.0
with
aortic valve disease I08.0
with tricuspid (valve) disease I08.3
obstruction or stenosis I05.2
with aortic valve disease I08.0
tricuspid (valve) disease I08.1
with aortic (valve) disease I08.3
congenital Q23.3
rheumatic I05.1
with
aortic valve disease I08.0
with tricuspid (valve) disease I08.3
obstruction or stenosis I05.2
with aortic valve disease I08.0
with tricuspid (valve) disease I08.3
tricuspid (valve) disease I08.1
with aortic (valve) disease I08.3
active or acute I01.1
with chorea, rheumatic (Sydenham's) I02.0
specified cause, except rheumatic I34.0
muscle — *see also* Disease, muscle
heart — *see* Insufficiency, myocardial
ocular NEC H50.9
myocardial, myocardium (with arteriosclerosis) — *see also* Failure, heart I50.9
with
rheumatic fever (conditions in I00) I09.0
active, acute or subacute I01.2
with chorea I02.0
inactive or quiescent (with chorea) I09.0
congenital Q24.8
hypertensive — *see* Hypertension, heart
newborn P29.0
rheumatic I09.0
active, acute, or subacute I01.2
syphilitic A52.06
nourishment T73.0 ☑
pancreatic K86.89
exocrine K86.81
parathyroid (gland) E20.9
peripheral vascular (arterial) I73.9
pituitary E23.0
placental (mother) O36.51- ☑
platelets D69.6
prenatal care affecting management of pregnancy O09.3- ☑
progressive pluriglandular E31.0
pulmonary J98.4
acute, following surgery (nonthoracic) J95.2
thoracic J95.1
chronic, following surgery J95.3

Insufficiency, insufficient — *continued*
  pulmonary — *continued*
    following
      shock J98.4
      trauma J98.4
    newborn P28.89
    valve I37.1
      with stenosis I37.2
      congenital Q22.2
      rheumatic I09.89
        with aortic, mitral or tricuspid (valve) disease
          I08.8
  pyloric K31.89
  renal (acute) N28.9
    chronic N18.9
  respiratory R06.89
    newborn P28.5
  rotation — *see* Malrotation
  sleep syndrome F51.12
  social insurance Z59.7
  suprarenal E27.40
    primary E27.1
  tarso-orbital fascia, congenital Q10.3
  testis E29.1
  thyroid (gland) (acquired) E03.9
    congenital E03.1
  tricuspid (valve) (rheumatic) I07.1
    with
      aortic (valve) disease I08.2
        with mitral (valve) disease I08.3
      mitral (valve) disease I08.1
        with aortic (valve) disease I08.3
      obstruction or stenosis I07.2
        with aortic (valve) disease I08.2
          with mitral (valve) disease I08.3
    congenital Q22.8
    nonrheumatic I36.1
      with stenosis I36.2
  urethral sphincter R32
  valve, valvular (heart) I38
    aortic — *see* Insufficiency, aortic (valve)
    congenital Q24.8
    mitral — *see* Insufficiency, mitral (valve)
    pulmonary — *see* Insufficiency, pulmonary, valve
    tricuspid — *see* Insufficiency, tricuspid (valve)
  vascular I99.8
    intestine K55.9
      acute — *see also* Ischemia, intestine, acute
        K55.059
    mesenteric K55.1
    peripheral I73.9
    renal — *see* Hypertension, kidney
  velopharyngeal
    acquired K13.79
    congenital Q38.8
  venous (chronic) (peripheral) I87.2
  ventricular — *see* Insufficiency, myocardial
  welfare support Z59.7
Insufflation, fallopian Z31.41
Insular — *see* condition
Insuloma
  pancreas
    benign D13.7
    malignant C25.4
    uncertain behavior D37.8
  specified site
    benign — *see* Neoplasm, by site, benign
    malignant — *see* Neoplasm, by site, malignant
    uncertain behavior — *see* Neoplasm, by site, uncer-
      tain behavior
  unspecified site
    benign D13.7
    malignant C25.4
    uncertain behavior D37.8
Insuloma — *see* Insulinoma
Interference
  balancing side M26.56
  non-working side M26.56
Intermenstrual — *see* condition
Intermittent — *see* condition
Internal — *see* condition
Interrogation
  cardiac defibrillator (automatic) (implantable) Z45.02
  cardiac pacemaker Z45.018
  cardiac (event) (loop) recorder Z45.09
  infusion pump (implanted) (intrathecal) Z45.1
  neurostimulator Z46.2

Interruption
  aortic arch Q25.21
  bundle of His I44.30
  phase-shift, sleep cycle — *see* Disorder, sleep, circadian
    rhythm
  sleep phase-shift, or 24 hour sleep-wake cycle — *see*
    Disorder, sleep, circadian rhythm
Interstitial — *see* condition
Intertrigo L30.4
  labialis K13.0
Intervertebral disc — *see* condition
Intestine, intestinal — *see* condition
Intolerance
  carbohydrate K90.49
  disaccharide, hereditary E73.0
  fat NEC K90.49
    pancreatic K90.3
  food K90.49
    dietary counseling and surveillance Z71.3
  fructose E74.10
    hereditary E74.12
  glucose (-galactose) E74.39
  gluten K90.41
  lactose E73.9
    specified NEC E73.8
  lysine E72.3
  milk NEC K90.49
    lactose E73.9
  protein K90.49
  starch NEC K90.49
  sucrose (-isomaltose) E74.31
Intoxicated NEC (without dependence) — *see* Alcohol,
  intoxication
Intoxication
  acid E87.2
  alcoholic (acute) (without dependence) — *see* Alcohol,
    intoxication
  alimentary canal K52.1
  amphetamine (without dependence) — *see also* Abuse,
    drug, stimulant, with intoxication
    with dependence — *see* Dependence, drug, stimu-
      lant, with intoxication
    stimulant NEC F15.10
      with
        anxiety disorder F15.180
        intoxication F15.129
          with
            delirium F15.121
            perceptual disturbance F15.122
  anxiolytic (acute) (without dependence) — *see* Abuse,
    drug, sedative, with intoxication
    with dependence — *see* Dependence, drug, seda-
      tive, with intoxication
  caffeine F15.929
    with dependence — *see* Dependence, drug, stimu-
      lant, with intoxication
  cannabinoids (acute) (without dependence) — *see*
    Use, cannabis, with intoxication
    with
      abuse — *see* Abuse, drug, cannabis, with intoxi-
        cation
      dependence — *see* Dependence, drug, cannabis,
        with intoxication
  chemical — *see* Table of Drugs and Chemicals
    via placenta or breast milk — *see* - Absorption,
      chemical, through placenta
  cocaine (acute) (without dependence) — *see* Abuse,
    drug, cocaine, with intoxication
    with dependence — *see* Dependence, drug, cocaine,
      with intoxication
  drug
    acute (without dependence) — *see* Abuse, drug, by
      type with intoxication
    with dependence — *see* Dependence, drug, by
      type with intoxication
    addictive
      via placenta or breast milk — *see* Absorption,
        drug, addictive, through placenta
    newborn P93.8
      gray baby syndrome P93.0
    overdose or wrong substance given or taken — *see*
      Table of Drugs and Chemicals, by drug, poi-
      soning
  enteric K52.1
  foodborne A05.9
    bacterial A05.9
    classical (Clostridium botulinum) A05.1

Intoxication — *continued*
  foodborne — *continued*
    due to
      Bacillus cereus A05.4
      bacterium A05.9
        specified NEC A05.8
      Clostridium
        botulinum A05.1
        perfringens A05.2
        welchii A05.2
      Salmonella A02.9
        with
          (gastro)enteritis A02.0
          localized infection(s) A02.20
            arthritis A02.23
            meningitis A02.21
            osteomyelitis A02.24
            pneumonia A02.22
            pyelonephritis A02.25
            specified NEC A02.29
          sepsis A02.1
          specified manifestation NEC A02.8
      Staphylococcus A05.0
      Vibrio
        parahaemolyticus A05.3
        vulnificus A05.5
    enterotoxin, staphylococcal A05.0
    noxious — *see* Poisoning, food, noxious
  gastrointestinal K52.1
  hallucinogenic (without dependence) — *see* Abuse,
    drug, hallucinogen, with intoxication
    with dependence — *see* Dependence, drug, hallu-
      cinogen, with intoxication
  hypnotic (acute) (without dependence) — *see* Abuse,
    drug, sedative, with intoxication
    with dependence — *see* Dependence, drug, seda-
      tive, with intoxication
  inhalant (acute) (without dependence) — *see* Abuse,
    drug, inhalant, with intoxication
    with dependence — *see* Dependence, drug, in-
      halant, with intoxication
  meaning
    inebriation — *see* category F10 ☑
    poisoning — *see* Table of Drugs and Chemicals
  methyl alcohol (acute) (without dependence) — *see*
    Alcohol, intoxication
  opioid (acute) (without dependence) — *see* Abuse,
    drug, opioid, with intoxication
    with dependence — *see* Dependence, drug, opioid,
      with intoxication
  pathologic NEC (without dependence) — *see* Alcohol,
    intoxication
  phencyclidine (without dependence) — *see* Abuse,
    drug, hallucinogen, with intoxication
    with dependence — *see* Dependence, drug, hallu-
      cinogen, with intoxication
  potassium (K) E87.5
  psychoactive substance NEC (without dependence) —
    see Abuse, drug, psychoactive NEC, with intoxi-
    cation
    with dependence — *see* Dependence, drug, psy-
      choactive NEC, with intoxication
  sedative (acute) (without dependence) — *see* Abuse,
    drug, sedative, with intoxication
    with dependence — *see* Dependence, drug, seda-
      tive, with intoxication
  serum — *see also* Reaction, serum T80.69 ☑
  uremic — *see* Uremia
  volatile solvents (acute) (without dependence) — *see*
    Abuse, drug, inhalant, with intoxication
    with dependence — *see* Dependence, drug, in-
      halant, with intoxication
  water E87.79
Intraabdominal testis, testes
  bilateral Q53.211
  unilateral Q53.111
Intracranial — *see* condition
Intrahepatic gallbladder Q44.1
Intraligamentous — *see* condition
Intrathoracic — *see also* condition
  kidney Q63.2
Intrauterine contraceptive device
  checking Z30.431
  in situ Z97.5
  insertion Z30.430
    immediately following removal Z30.433
  management Z30.431
  reinsertion Z30.433

Intrauterine contraceptive device — *continued*
  removal Z30.432
  replacement Z30.433
  retention in pregnancy O26.3- ☑
Intraventricular — *see* condition
Intrinsic deformity — *see* Deformity
Intubation, difficult or failed T88.4 ☑
Intumescence, lens (eye) (cataract) — *see* Cataract
Intussusception (bowel) (colon) (enteric) (ileocecal)
  (ileocolic) (intestine) (rectum) K56.1
  appendix K38.8
  congenital Q43.8
  ureter (with obstruction) N13.5
Invagination (bowel, colon, intestine or rectum) K56.1
Inversion
  albumin-globulin (A-G) ratio E88.09
  bladder N32.89
  cecum — *see* Intussusception
  cervix N88.8
  chromosome in normal individual Q95.1
  circadian rhythm — *see* Disorder, sleep, circadian
    rhythm
  nipple N64.59
    congenital Q83.8
    gestational — *see* Retraction, nipple
    puerperal, postpartum — *see* Retraction, nipple
  nyctohemeral rhythm — *see* Disorder, sleep, circadian
    rhythm
  optic papilla Q14.2
  organ or site, congenital NEC — *see* Anomaly, by site
  sleep rhythm — *see* Disorder, sleep, circadian rhythm
  testis (congenital) Q55.29
  uterus (chronic) (postinfectional) (postpartal, old) N85.5
    postpartum O71.2
  vagina (posthysterectomy) N99.3
  ventricular Q20.5
Investigation — *see also* Examination Z04.9
  clinical research subject (control) (normal comparison)
    (participant) Z00.6
Involuntary movement, abnormal R25.9
Involution, involutional — *see also* condition
  breast, cystic — *see* Dysplasia, mammary, specified
    type NEC
  depression (single episode) F32.89
    recurrent episode F33.9
  melancholia (single episode) F32.89
    recurrent episode F33.8
  ovary, senile — *see* Atrophy, ovary
  thymus failure E32.8
I.Q.
  20-34 F72
  35-49 F71
  50-69 F70
  under 20 F73
IRDS (type I) P22.0
  type II P22.1
Irideremia Q13.1
Iridis rubeosis — *see* Disorder, iris, vascular
Iridochoroiditis (panuveitis) — *see* Panuveitis
Iridocyclitis H20.9
  acute H20.0- ☑
    hypopyon H20.05- ☑
    primary H20.01- ☑
    recurrent H20.02- ☑
    secondary (noninfectious) H20.04- ☑
      infectious H20.03- ☑
  chronic H20.1- ☑
  due to allergy — *see* Iridocyclitis, acute, secondary
  endogenous — *see* Iridocyclitis, acute, primary
  Fuchs' — *see* Cyclitis, Fuchs' heterochromic
  gonococcal A54.32
  granulomatous — *see* Iridocyclitis, chronic
  herpes, herpetic (simplex) B00.51
    zoster B02.32
  hypopyon — *see* Iridocyclitis, acute, hypopyon
  in (due to)
    ankylosing spondylitis M45.9
    gonococcal infection A54.32
    herpes (simplex) virus B00.51
      zoster B02.32
    infectious disease NOS B99 ☑
    parasitic disease NOS B89 *[H22]*
    sarcoidosis D86.83
    syphilis A51.43
    tuberculosis A18.54
    zoster B02.32
  lens-induced H20.2- ☑

Iridocyclitis — *continued*
  nongranulomatous — *see* Iridocyclitis, acute
  recurrent — *see* Iridocyclitis, acute, recurrent
  rheumatic — *see* Iridocyclitis, chronic
  subacute — *see* Iridocyclitis, acute
  sympathetic — *see* Uveitis, sympathetic
  syphilitic (secondary) A51.43
  tuberculous (chronic) A18.54
  Vogt-Koyanagi H20.82- ☑
Iridocyclochoroiditis (panuveitis) — *see* Panuveitis
Iridodialysis H21.53- ☑
Iridodonesis H21.89
Iridoplegia (complete) (partial) (reflex) H57.09
Iridoschisis H21.25- ☑
Iris — *see also* condition
  bombé — *see* Membrane, pupillary
Iritis — *see also* Iridocyclitis
  chronic — *see* Iridocyclitis, chronic
  diabetic — *see* E08-E13 with .39
  due to
    herpes simplex B00.51
    leprosy A30.9 *[H22]*
  gonococcal A54.32
  gouty — *see also* Gout, by type M10.9 *[H22]*
  granulomatous — *see* Iridocyclitis, chronic
  lens induced — *see* Iridocyclitis, lens-induced
  papulosa (syphilitic) A52.71
  rheumatic — *see* Iridocyclitis, chronic
  syphilitic (secondary) A51.43
    congenital (early) A50.01
    late A52.71
  tuberculous A18.54
Iron — *see* condition
Iron-miner's lung J63.4
Irradiated enamel (tooth, teeth) K03.89
Irradiation effects, adverse T66 ☑
Irreducible, irreducibility — *see* condition
Irregular, irregularity
  action, heart I49.9
  alveolar process K08.89
  bleeding N92.6
  breathing R06.89
  contour of cornea (acquired) — *see* Deformity, cornea
    congenital Q13.4
  contour, reconstructed breast N65.0
  dentin (in pulp) K04.3
  eye movements H55.89
    deficient
      saccadic H55.81
      smooth H55.82
    nystagmus — *see* Nystagmus
  labor O62.2
  menstruation (cause unknown) N92.6
  periods N92.6
  prostate N42.9
  pupil — *see* Abnormality, pupillary
  reconstructed breast N65.0
  respiratory R06.89
  septum (nasal) J34.2
  shape, organ or site, congenital NEC — *see* Distortion
  sleep-wake pattern (rhythm) G47.23
Irritable, irritability R45.4
  bladder N32.89
  bowel (syndrome) K58.9
    with
      constipation K58.1
      diarrhea K58.0
    mixed K58.2
    psychogenic F45.8
    specified NEC K58.8
  bronchial — *see* Bronchitis
  cerebral, in newborn P91.3
  colon — *see also* Irritable, bowel K58.9
    with diarrhea K58.0
    psychogenic F45.8
  duodenum K59.89
  heart (psychogenic) F45.8
  hip — *see* Derangement, joint, specified type NEC, hip
  ileum K59.89
  infant R68.12
  jejunum K59.89
  rectum K59.89
  stomach K31.89
    psychogenic F45.8
  sympathetic G90.8
  urethra N36.8
Irritation
  anus K62.89

Irritation — *continued*
  axillary nerve G54.0
  bladder N32.89
  brachial plexus G54.0
  bronchial — *see* Bronchitis
  cervical plexus G54.2
  cervix — *see* Cervicitis
  choroid, sympathetic — *see* Endophthalmitis
  cranial nerve — *see* Disorder, nerve, cranial
  gastric K31.89
    psychogenic F45.8
  globe, sympathetic — *see* Uveitis, sympathetic
  labyrinth — *see* subcategory H83.2 ☑
  lumbosacral plexus G54.1
  meninges (traumatic) — *see* Injury, intracranial
    nontraumatic — *see* Meningismus
  nerve — *see* Disorder, nerve
  nervous R45.0
  penis N48.89
  perineum NEC L29.3
  peripheral autonomic nervous system G90.8
  peritoneum — *see* Peritonitis
  pharynx J39.2
  plantar nerve — *see* Lesion, nerve, plantar
  spinal (cord) (traumatic) — *see also* Injury, spinal cord
    by region
    nerve G58.9
      root NEC — *see* Radiculopathy
    nontraumatic — *see* Myelopathy
  stomach K31.89
    psychogenic F45.8
  sympathetic nerve NEC G90.8
  ulnar nerve — *see* Lesion, nerve, ulnar
  vagina N89.8
Ischemia, ischemic I99.8
  bowel (transient)
    acute — *see also* Ischemia, intestine, acute K55.05
    chronic K55.1
    due to mesenteric artery insufficiency K55.1
  brain — *see* Ischemia, cerebral
  cardiac (see Disease, heart, ischemic)
  cardiomyopathy I25.5
  cerebral (chronic) (generalized) I67.82
    arteriosclerotic I67.2
    intermittent G45.9
    newborn P91.0
    recurrent focal G45.8
    transient G45.9
  colon chronic (due to mesenteric artery insufficiency)
    K55.1
  coronary — *see* Disease, heart, ischemic
  demand (coronary) — *see also* Angina I24.8
    with myocardial infarction I21.A1
    resulting in myocardial infarction I21.A1
  heart (chronic or with a stated duration of over 4 weeks)
    I25.9
    acute or with a stated duration of 4 weeks or less
      I24.9
    subacute I24.9
  infarction, muscle — *see* Infarct, muscle
  intestine (large) (small) (transient) K55.9
    acute K55.059
      diffuse K55.052
      focal K55.051
      large K55.039
        diffuse K55.032
        focal K55.031
      small K55.019
        diffuse K55.012
        focal K55.011
    chronic K55.1
    due to mesenteric artery insufficiency K55.1
  kidney N28.0
  limb, critical — *see* Arteriosclerosis, with critical limb
    ischemia
  limb-threatening, chronic — *see* Arteriosclerosis, with
    critical limb ischemia
  mesenteric, acute — *see also* Ischemia, intestine, acute
    K55.059
  muscle, traumatic T79.6 ☑
  myocardium, myocardial (chronic or with a stated du-
    ration of over 4 weeks) I25.9
    acute, without myocardial infarction I51.3
    silent (asymptomatic) I25.6
    transient of newborn P29.4
  renal N28.0
  retina, retinal — *see* Occlusion, artery, retina

Ischemia, ischemic — *continued*
  small bowel
    acute K55.019
      diffuse K55.012
      focal K55.011
    chronic K55.1
    due to mesenteric artery insufficiency K55.1
  spinal cord G95.11
  subendocardial — *see* Insufficiency, coronary
  supply (coronary) — *see also* Angina I25.9
    due to vasospasm I20.1
Ischial spine — *see* condition
Ischialgia — *see* Sciatica
Ischiopagus Q89.4
Ischium, ischial — *see* condition
Ischuria R34
Iselin's disease or osteochondrosis — *see* Osteochondrosis, juvenile, metatarsus
Islands of
  parotid tissue in
    lymph nodes Q38.6
    neck structures Q38.6
  submaxillary glands in
    fascia Q38.6
    lymph nodes Q38.6
    neck muscles Q38.6
Islet cell tumor, pancreas D13.7
Isoimmunization NEC — *see also* Incompatibility
  affecting management of pregnancy (ABO) (with hydrops fetalis) O36.11- ☑
    anti-A sensitization O36.11- ☑
    anti-B sensitization O36.19- ☑
    anti-c sensitization O36.09- ☑
    anti-C sensitization O36.09- ☑
    anti-e sensitization O36.09- ☑
    anti-E sensitization O36.09- ☑
    Rh NEC O36.09- ☑
      anti-D antibody O36.01- ☑
    specified NEC O36.19- ☑
  newborn P55.9
    with
      hydrops fetalis P56.0
      kernicterus P57.0
    ABO (blood groups) P55.1
    Rhesus (Rh) factor P55.0
    specified type NEC P55.8
Isolation, isolated
  dwelling Z59.8
  family Z63.79
  social Z60.4
Isoleucinosis E71.19
Isomerism atrial appendages (with asplenia or polysplenia) Q20.6
Isosporiasis, isosporosis A07.3
Isovaleric acidemia E71.110
Issue of
  medical certificate Z02.79
    for disability determination Z02.71
  repeat prescription (appliance) (glasses) (medicinal substance, medicament, medicine) Z76.0
    contraception — *see* Contraception
Itch, itching — *see also* Pruritus
  baker's L23.6
  barber's B35.0
  bricklayer's L24.5
  cheese B88.0
  clam digger's B65.3
  coolie B76.9
  copra B88.0
  dew B76.9
  dhobi B35.6
  filarial — *see* Infestation, filarial
  grain B88.0
  grocer's B88.0
  ground B76.9
  harvest B88.0
  jock B35.6
  Malabar B35.5
    beard B35.0
    foot B35.3
    scalp B35.0
  meaning scabies B86
  Norwegian B86
  perianal L29.0
  poultrymen's B88.0
  sarcoptic B86
  scabies B86
  scrub B88.0

Itch, itching — *continued*
  straw B88.0
  swimmer's B65.3
  water B76.9
  winter L29.8
Ivemark's syndrome (asplenia with congenital heart disease) Q89.01
Ivory bones Q78.2
Ixodiasis NEC B88.8

J

Jaccoud's syndrome — *see* Arthropathy, postrheumatic, chronic
Jackson's
  membrane Q43.3
  paralysis or syndrome G83.89
  veil Q43.3
Jacquet's dermatitis (diaper dermatitis) L22
Jadassohn-Pellizari's disease or anetoderma L90.2
Jadassohn's
  blue nevus — *see* Nevus
  intraepidermal epithelioma — *see* Neoplasm, skin, benign
Jaffe-Lichtenstein (-Uehlinger) **syndrome** — *see* Dysplasia, fibrous, bone NEC
Jakob-Creutzfeldt disease or syndrome — *see* Creutzfeldt-Jakob disease or syndrome
Jaksch-Luzet disease D64.89
Jamaican
  neuropathy G92
  paraplegic tropical ataxic-spastic syndrome G92
Janet's disease F48.8
Janiceps Q89.4
Jansky-Bielschowsky amaurotic idiocy E75.4
Japanese
  B-type encephalitis A83.0
  river fever A75.3
Jaundice (yellow) R17
  acholuric (familial) (splenomegalic) — *see also* Spherocytosis
    acquired D59.8
  breast-milk (inhibitor) P59.3
  catarrhal (acute) B15.9
    with hepatic coma B15.0
  cholestatic (benign) R17
  due to or associated with
    delayed conjugation P59.8
      associated with (due to) preterm delivery P59.0
    preterm delivery P59.0
  epidemic (catarrhal) B15.9
    with hepatic coma B15.0
    leptospiral A27.0
    spirochetal A27.0
  familial nonhemolytic (congenital) (Gilbert) E80.4
    Crigler-Najjar E80.5
  febrile (acute) B15.9
    with hepatic coma B15.0
    leptospiral A27.0
    spirochetal A27.0
  hematogenous D59.9
  hemolytic (acquired) D59.9
    congenital — *see* Spherocytosis
  hemorrhagic (acute) (leptospiral) (spirochetal) A27.0
  infectious (acute) (subacute) B15.9
    with hepatic coma B15.0
    leptospiral A27.0
    spirochetal A27.0
  leptospiral (hemorrhagic) A27.0
  malignant (without coma) K72.90
    with coma K72.91
  neonatal — *see* Jaundice, newborn
  newborn P59.9
    due to or associated with
      ABO
        antibodies P55.1
        incompatibility, maternal/fetal P55.1
        isoimmunization P55.1
      absence or deficiency of enzyme system for bilirubin conjugation (congenital) P59.8
      bleeding P58.1
      breast milk inhibitors to conjugation P59.3
        associated with preterm delivery P59.0
      bruising P58.0
      Crigler-Najjar syndrome E80.5
      delayed conjugation P59.8
        associated with preterm delivery P59.0

Jaundice — *continued*
  newborn — *continued*
    due to or associated with — *continued*
      drugs or toxins
        given to newborn P58.42
        transmitted from mother P58.41
      excessive hemolysis P58.9
        due to
          bleeding P58.1
          bruising P58.0
          drugs or toxins
            given to newborn P58.42
            transmitted from mother P58.41
          infection P58.2
          polycythemia P58.3
          swallowed maternal blood P58.5
        specified type NEC P58.8
      galactosemia E74.21
      Gilbert syndrome E80.4
      hemolytic disease P55.9
        ABO isoimmunization P55.1
        Rh isoimmunization P55.0
        specified NEC P55.8
      hepatocellular damage P59.20
        specified NEC P59.29
      hereditary hemolytic anemia P58.8
      hypothyroidism, congenital E03.1
      incompatibility, maternal/fetal NOS P55.9
      infection P58.2
      inspissated bile syndrome P59.1
      isoimmunization NOS P55.9
      mucoviscidosis E84.9
      polycythemia P58.3
      preterm delivery P59.0
      Rh
        antibodies P55.0
        incompatibility, maternal/fetal P55.0
        isoimmunization P55.0
      specified cause NEC P59.8
      swallowed maternal blood P58.5
      spherocytosis (congenital) D58.0
  nonhemolytic congenital familial (Gilbert) E80.4
  nuclear, newborn — *see also* Kernicterus of newborn P57.9
  obstructive — *see also* Obstruction, bile duct K83.1
  post-immunization — *see* Hepatitis, viral, type, B
  post-transfusion — *see* Hepatitis, viral, type, B
  regurgitation — *see also* Obstruction, bile duct K83.1
  serum (homologous) (prophylactic) (therapeutic) — *see* Hepatitis, viral, type, B
  spirochetal (hemorrhagic) A27.0
  symptomatic R17
    newborn P59.9
Jaw — *see* condition
Jaw-winking phenomenon or syndrome Q07.8
Jealousy
  alcoholic F10.988
  childhood F93.8
  sibling F93.8
Jejunitis — *see* Enteritis
Jejunostomy status Z93.4
Jejunum, jejunal — *see* condition
Jensen's disease — *see* Inflammation, chorioretinal, focal, juxtapapillary
Jerks, myoclonic G25.3
Jervell-Lange-Nielsen syndrome I45.81
Jeune's disease Q77.2
Jigger disease B88.1
Job's syndrome (chronic granulomatous disease) D71
Joint — *see also* condition
  mice — *see* Loose, body, joint
    knee M23.4- ☑
Jordan's anomaly or syndrome D72.0
Joseph-Diamond-Blackfan anemia (congenital hypoplastic) D61.01
Jungle yellow fever A95.0
Jüngling's disease — *see* Sarcoidosis
Juvenile — *see* condition

K

Kahler's disease C90.0- ☑
Kakke E51.11
Kala-azar B55.0
Kallmann's syndrome E23.0
Kanner's syndrome (autism) — *see* Psychosis, childhood

▽ Subterms under main terms may continue to next column or page   ☑ Additional Character Required — Refer to the Tabular List for Character Selection   **207**

Ischemia, ischemic — Kanner's syndrome

Index

Kaposi's — Kissing spine

Kaposi's
  dermatosis (xeroderma pigmentosum) Q82.1
  lichen ruber L44.0
    acuminatus L44.0
  sarcoma
    colon C46.4
    connective tissue C46.1
    gastrointestinal organ C46.4
    lung C46.5- ☑
    lymph node (multiple) C46.3
    palate (hard) (soft) C46.2
    rectum C46.4
    skin (multiple sites) C46.0
    specified site NEC C46.7
    stomach C46.4
    unspecified site C46.9
  varicelliform eruption B00.0
    vaccinia T88.1 ☑
Kartagener's syndrome or triad (sinusitis, bronchiecta-
    sis, situs inversus) Q89.3
Karyotype
  with abnormality except iso (Xq) Q96.2
  45,X Q96.0
  46,X
    iso (Xq) Q96.1
  46,XX Q98.3
    with streak gonads Q50.32
    hermaphrodite (true) Q99.1
    male Q98.3
  46,XY
    with streak gonads Q56.1
    female Q97.3
    hermaphrodite (true) Q99.1
  47,XXX Q97.0
  47,XXY Q98.0
  47,XYY Q98.5
Kaschin-Beck disease — see Disease, Kaschin-Beck
Katayama's disease or fever B65.2
Kawasaki's syndrome M30.3
Kayser-Fleischer ring (cornea) (pseudosclerosis)
    H18.04- ☑
Kaznelson's syndrome (congenital hypoplastic anemia)
    D61.01
Kearns-Sayre syndrome H49.81- ☑
Kedani fever A75.3
Kelis L91.0
Kelly (-Patterson) **syndrome** (sideropenic dysphagia)
    D50.1
Keloid, cheloid L91.0
  acne L73.0
  Addison's L94.0
  cornea — see Opacity, cornea
  Hawkin's L91.0
  scar L91.0
Keloma L91.0
Kenya fever A77.1
Keratectasia — see also Ectasia, cornea
  congenital Q13.4
Keratinization of alveolar ridge mucosa
  excessive K13.23
  minimal K13.22
Keratinized residual ridge mucosa
  excessive K13.23
  minimal K13.22
Keratitis (nodular) (nonulcerative) (simple) (zonular)
    H16.9
  with ulceration (central) (marginal) (perforated) (ring)
    — see Ulcer, cornea
  actinic — see Photokeratitis
  arborescens (herpes simplex) B00.52
  areolar H16.11- ☑
  bullosa H16.8
  deep H16.309
    specified type NEC H16.399
  dendritic (a) (herpes simplex) B00.52
  disciform (is) (herpes simplex) B00.52
    varicella B01.81
  filamentary H16.12- ☑
  gonococcal (congenital or prenatal) A54.33
  herpes, herpetic (simplex) B00.52
    zoster B02.33
  in (due to)
    acanthamebiasis B60.13
    adenovirus B30.0
    exanthema — see also Exanthem B09
    herpes (simplex) virus B00.52
    measles B05.81
    syphilis A50.31

Keratitis — continued
  in — continued
    tuberculosis A18.52
    zoster B02.33
  interstitial (nonsyphilitic) H16.30- ☑
    diffuse H16.32- ☑
    herpes, herpetic (simplex) B00.52
      zoster B02.33
    sclerosing H16.33- ☑
    specified type NEC H16.39- ☑
    syphilitic (congenital) (late) A50.31
    tuberculous A18.52
  macular H16.11- ☑
  nummular H16.11- ☑
  oyster shuckers' H16.8
  parenchymatous — see Keratitis, interstitial
  petrificans H16.8
  postmeasles B05.81
  punctata
    leprosa A30.9 [H16.14-] ☑
    syphilitic (profunda) A50.31
  punctate H16.14- ☑
  purulent H16.8
  rosacea L71.8
  sclerosing H16.33- ☑
  specified type NEC H16.8
  stellate H16.11- ☑
  striate H16.11- ☑
  superficial H16.10- ☑
    with conjunctivitis — see Keratoconjunctivitis
    due to light — see Photokeratitis
  suppurative H16.8
  syphilitic (congenital) (prenatal) A50.31
  trachomatous A71.1
    sequelae B94.0
  tuberculous A18.52
  vesicular H16.8
  xerotic — see also Keratomalacia H16.8
    vitamin A deficiency E50.4
Keratoacanthoma L85.8
Keratocele — see Descemetocele
Keratoconjunctivitis H16.20- ☑
  Acanthamoeba B60.13
  adenoviral B30.0
  epidemic B30.0
  exposure H16.21- ☑
  herpes, herpetic (simplex) B00.52
    zoster B02.33
  in exanthema — see also Exanthem B09
  infectious B30.0
  lagophthalmic — see Keratoconjunctivitis, specified
      type NEC
  neurotrophic H16.23- ☑
  phlyctenular H16.25- ☑
  postmeasles B05.81
  shipyard B30.0
  sicca (Sjogren's) M35.0- ☑
    not Sjogren's H16.22- ☑
  specified type NEC H16.29- ☑
  tuberculous (phlyctenular) A18.52
  vernal H16.26- ☑
Keratoconus H18.60- ☑
  congenital Q13.4
  stable H18.61- ☑
  unstable H18.62- ☑
Keratocyst (dental) (odontogenic) — see Cyst, calcifying
    odontogenic
Keratoderma, keratodermia (congenital) (palmaris et
    plantaris) (symmetrical) Q82.8
  acquired L85.1
    in diseases classified elsewhere L86
  climactericum L85.1
  gonococcal A54.89
  gonorrheal A54.89
  punctata L85.2
  Reiter's — see Reiter's disease
Keratodermatocele — see Descemetocele
Keratoglobus H18.79 ☑
  congenital Q15.8
    with glaucoma Q15.0
Keratohemia — see Pigmentation, cornea, stromal
Keratoiritis — see also Iridocyclitis
  syphilitic A50.39
  tuberculous A18.54
Keratoma L57.0
  palmaris and plantaris hereditarium Q82.8
  senile L57.0

Keratomalacia H18.44- ☑
  vitamin A deficiency E50.4
Keratomegaly Q13.4
Keratomycosis B49
  nigrans, nigricans (palmaris) B36.1
Keratopathy H18.9
  band H18.42- ☑
  bullous (aphakic), following cataract surgery H59.01- ☑
  bullous H18.1- ☑
Keratoscleritis, tuberculous A18.52
Keratosis L57.0
  actinic L57.0
  arsenical L85.8
  congenital, specified NEC Q80.8
  female genital NEC N94.89
  follicularis Q82.8
    acquired L11.0
    congenita Q82.8
    et parafollicularis in cutem penetrans L87.0
    spinulosa (decalvans) Q82.8
    vitamin A deficiency E50.8
  gonococcal A54.89
  male genital (external) N50.89
  nigricans L83
  obturans, external ear (canal) — see Cholesteatoma,
      external ear
  palmaris et plantaris (inherited) (symmetrical) Q82.8
    acquired L85.1
  penile N48.89
  pharynx J39.2
  pilaris, acquired L85.8
  punctata (palmaris et plantaris) L85.2
  scrotal N50.89
  seborrheic L82.1
    inflamed L82.0
  senile L57.0
  solar L57.0
  tonsillaris J35.8
  vagina N89.4
  vegetans Q82.8
  vitamin A deficiency E50.8
  vocal cord J38.3
Kerato-uveitis — see Iridocyclitis
Kerion (celsi) B35.0
Kernicterus of newborn (not due to isoimmunization)
    P57.9
  due to isoimmunization (conditions in P55.0-P55.9)
    P57.0
  specified type NEC P57.8
Kerunoparalysis T75.09 ☑
Keshan disease E59
Ketoacidosis E87.2
  diabetic — see Diabetes, by type, with ketoacidosis
Ketonuria R82.4
Ketosis NEC E88.89
  diabetic — see Diabetes, by type, with ketoacidosis
Kew Garden fever A79.1
Kidney — see condition
Kienböck's disease — see also Osteochondrosis, juvenile
    hand, carpal lunate
  adult M93.1
Kimmelstiel (-Wilson) **disease** — see Diabetes, Kimmel-
    stiel (-Wilson) disease
Kink, kinking
  artery I77.1
  hair (acquired) L67.8
  ileum or intestine — see Obstruction, intestine
  Lane's — see Obstruction, intestine
  organ or site, congenital NEC — see Anomaly, by site
  ureter (pelvic junction) N13.5
    with
      hydronephrosis N13.1
        with infection N13.6
      pyelonephritis (chronic) N11.1
    congenital Q62.39
  vein(s) I87.8
    caval I87.1
    peripheral I87.1
Kinnier Wilson's disease (hepatolenticular degenera-
    tion) E83.01
Kissing spine M48.20
  cervical region M48.22
  cervicothoracic region M48.23
  lumbar region M48.26
  lumbosacral region M48.27
  occipito-atlanto-axial region M48.21
  thoracic region M48.24
  thoracolumbar region M48.25

Klatskin's tumor C22.1
Klauder's disease A26.8
Klebs' disease — *see also* Glomerulonephritis N05- ☑
Klebsiella (K.) pneumoniae, as cause of disease classified elsewhere B96.1
Klein (e)-Levin syndrome G47.13
Kleptomania F63.2
Klinefelter's syndrome Q98.4
  karyotype 47,XXY Q98.0
  male with more than two X chromosomes Q98.1
Klippel-Feil deficiency, disease, or syndrome (brevicollis) Q76.1
Klippel's disease I67.2
Klippel-Trenaunay (-Weber) **syndrome** Q87.2
Klumpke (-Déjerine) **palsy, paralysis** (birth) (newborn) P14.1
Knee — *see* condition
Knock knee (acquired) M21.06- ☑
  congenital Q74.1
Knot(s)
  intestinal, syndrome (volvulus) K56.2
  surfer S89.8- ☑
  umbilical cord (true) O69.2 ☑
Knotting (of)
  hair L67.8
  intestine K56.2
Knuckle pad (Garrod's) M72.1
Koch's
  infection — *see* Tuberculosis
  relapsing fever A68.9
Koch-Weeks' conjunctivitis — *see* Conjunctivitis, acute, mucopurulent
Koebner's syndrome Q81.8
Koenig's disease (osteochondritis dissecans) — *see* Osteochondritis, dissecans
Köhler-Pellegrini-Steida disease or syndrome (calcification, knee joint) — *see* Bursitis, tibial collateral
Köhler's disease
  patellar — *see* Osteochondrosis, juvenile, patella
  tarsal navicular — *see* Osteochondrosis, juvenile, tarsus
Koilonychia L60.3
  congenital Q84.6
Kojevnikov's, epilepsy — *see* Kozhevnikof's epilepsy
Koplik's spots B05.9
Kopp's asthma E32.8
Korsakoff's (Wernicke) **disease, psychosis or syndrome** (alcoholic) F10.96
  with dependence F10.26
  drug-induced
    due to drug abuse — *see* Abuse, drug, by type, with amnestic disorder
    due to drug dependence — *see* Dependence, drug, by type, with amnestic disorder
  nonalcoholic F04
Korsakov's disease, psychosis or syndrome — *see* Korsakoff's disease
Korsakow's disease, psychosis or syndrome — *see* Korsakoff's disease
Kostmann's disease or syndrome (infantile genetic agranulocytosis) — *see* Agranulocytosis
Kozhevnikof's epilepsy G40.109
  intractable G40.119
    with status epilepticus G40.111
    without status epilepticus G40.119
  not intractable G40.109
    with status epilepticus G40.101
    without status epilepticus G40.109
Krabbe's
  disease E75.23
  syndrome, congenital muscle hypoplasia Q79.8
Kraepelin-Morel disease — *see* Schizophrenia
Kraft-Weber-Dimitri disease Q85.8
Kraurosis
  ani K62.89
  penis N48.0
  vagina N89.8
  vulva N90.4
Kreotoxism A05.9
Krukenberg's
  spindle — *see* Pigmentation, cornea, posterior
  tumor C79.6- ☑
Kufs' disease E75.4
Kugelberg-Welander disease G12.1
Kuhnt-Junius degeneration — *see also* Degeneration, macula H35.32- ☑
Kümmell's disease or spondylitis — *see* Spondylopathy, traumatic

Kupffer cell sarcoma C22.3
Kuru A81.81
Kussmaul's
  disease M30.0
  respiration E87.2
    in diabetic acidosis — *see* Diabetes, by type, with ketoacidosis
Kwashiorkor E40
  marasmus, marasmus type E42
Kyasanur Forest disease A98.2
Kyphoscoliosis, kyphoscoliotic (acquired) — *see also* Scoliosis M41.9
  congenital Q67.5
  heart (disease) I27.1
  sequelae of rickets E64.3
  tuberculous A18.01
Kyphosis, kyphotic (acquired) M40.209
  cervical region M40.202
  cervicothoracic region M40.203
  congenital Q76.419
    cervical region Q76.412
    cervicothoracic region Q76.413
    occipito-atlanto-axial region Q76.411
    thoracic region Q76.414
    thoracolumbar region Q76.415
  Morquio-Brailsford type (spinal) — *see also* subcategory M49.8 E76.219
  postlaminectomy M96.3
  postradiation therapy M96.2
  postural (adolescent) M40.00
    cervicothoracic region M40.03
    thoracic region M40.04
    thoracolumbar region M40.05
  secondary NEC M40.10
    cervical region M40.12
    cervicothoracic region M40.13
    thoracic region M40.14
    thoracolumbar region M40.15
  sequelae of rickets E64.3
  specified type NEC M40.299
    cervical region M40.292
    cervicothoracic region M40.293
    thoracic region M40.294
    thoracolumbar region M40.295
  syphilitic, congenital A50.56
  thoracic region M40.204
  thoracolumbar region M40.205
  tuberculous A18.01
Kyrle disease L87.0

L

Labia, labium — *see* condition
Labile
  blood pressure R09.89
  vasomotor system I73.9
Labioglossal paralysis G12.29
Labium leporinum — *see* Cleft, lip
Labor — *see* Delivery
Labored breathing — *see* Hyperventilation
Labyrinthitis (circumscribed) (destructive) (diffuse) (inner ear) (latent) (purulent) (suppurative) — *see also* subcategory H83.0 ☑
  syphilitic A52.79
Laceration
  with abortion — *see* Abortion, by type, complicated by laceration of pelvic organs
  abdomen, abdominal
    wall S31.119 ☑
      with
        foreign body S31.129 ☑
        penetration into peritoneal cavity S31.619 ☑
          with foreign body S31.629 ☑
      epigastric region S31.112 ☑
        with
          foreign body S31.122 ☑
          penetration into peritoneal cavity S31.612 ☑
            with foreign body S31.622 ☑
      left
        lower quadrant S31.114 ☑
          with
            foreign body S31.124 ☑
            penetration into peritoneal cavity S31.614 ☑
              with foreign body S31.624 ☑
        upper quadrant S31.111 ☑

Laceration — *continued*
  abdomen, abdominal — *continued*
    wall — *continued*
      left — *continued*
        upper quadrant — *continued*
          with
            foreign body S31.121 ☑
            penetration into peritoneal cavity S31.611 ☑
              with foreign body S31.621 ☑
      periumbilic region S31.115 ☑
        with
          foreign body S31.125 ☑
          penetration into peritoneal cavity S31.615 ☑
            with foreign body S31.625 ☑
      right
        lower quadrant S31.113 ☑
          with
            foreign body S31.123 ☑
            penetration into peritoneal cavity S31.613 ☑
              with foreign body S31.623 ☑
        upper quadrant S31.110 ☑
          with
            foreign body S31.120 ☑
            penetration into peritoneal cavity S31.610 ☑
              with foreign body S31.620 ☑
  accidental, complicating surgery — *see* Complications, surgical, accidental puncture or laceration
  Achilles tendon S86.02- ☑
  adrenal gland S37.813 ☑
  alveolar (process) — *see* Laceration, oral cavity
  ankle S91.01- ☑
    with
      foreign body S91.02- ☑
  antecubital space — *see* Laceration, elbow
  anus (sphincter) S31.831 ☑
    with
      ectopic or molar pregnancy O08.6
      foreign body S31.832 ☑
    complicating delivery — *see* Delivery, complicated, by, laceration, anus (sphincter)
    following ectopic or molar pregnancy O08.6
    nontraumatic, nonpuerperal — *see* Fissure, anus
  arm (upper) S41.11- ☑
    with foreign body S41.12- ☑
    lower — *see* Laceration, forearm
  auditory canal (external) (meatus) — *see* Laceration, ear
  auricle, ear — *see* Laceration, ear
  axilla — *see* Laceration, arm
  back — *see also* Laceration, thorax, back
    lower S31.010 ☑
      with
        foreign body S31.020 ☑
          with penetration into retroperitoneal space S31.021 ☑
        penetration into retroperitoneal space S31.011 ☑
  bile duct S36.13 ☑
  bladder S37.23 ☑
    with ectopic or molar pregnancy O08.6
    following ectopic or molar pregnancy O08.6
    obstetrical trauma O71.5
  blood vessel — *see* Injury, blood vessel
  bowel — *see also* Laceration, intestine
    with ectopic or molar pregnancy O08.6
    complicating abortion — *see* Abortion, by type, complicated by, specified condition NEC
    following ectopic or molar pregnancy O08.6
    obstetrical trauma O71.5
  brain (any part) (cortex) (diffuse) (membrane) — *see also* Injury, intracranial, diffuse
    during birth P10.8
      with hemorrhage P10.1
    focal — *see* Injury, intracranial, focal brain injury
  brainstem S06.38- ☑
  breast S21.01- ☑
    with foreign body S21.02- ☑
  broad ligament S37.893 ☑
    with ectopic or molar pregnancy O08.6
    following ectopic or molar pregnancy O08.6
    laceration syndrome N83.8
    obstetrical trauma O71.6
    syndrome (laceration) N83.8

▽ **Subterms under main terms may continue to next column or page**   ☑ **Additional Character Required — Refer to the Tabular List for Character Selection**   **209**

Klatskin's tumor — Laceration

Laceration — continued
- buttock S31.801 ☑
  - with foreign body S31.802 ☑
  - left S31.821 ☑
    - with foreign body S31.822 ☑
  - right S31.811 ☑
    - with foreign body S31.812 ☑
- calf — see Laceration, leg
- canaliculus lacrimalis — see Laceration, eyelid
- canthus, eye — see Laceration, eyelid
- capsule, joint — see Sprain
- causing eversion of cervix uteri (old) N86
- central (perineal), complicating delivery O70.9
- cerebellum, traumatic S06.37- ☑
- cerebral S06.33- ☑
  - during birth P10.8
    - with hemorrhage P10.1
  - left side S06.32- ☑
  - right side S06.31- ☑
- cervix (uteri)
  - with ectopic or molar pregnancy O08.6
  - following ectopic or molar pregnancy O08.6
  - nonpuerperal, nontraumatic N88.1
  - obstetrical trauma (current) O71.3
  - old (postpartal) N88.1
  - traumatic S37.63 ☑
- cheek (external) S01.41- ☑
  - with foreign body S01.42- ☑
  - internal — see Laceration, oral cavity
- chest wall — see Laceration, thorax
- chin — see Laceration, head, specified site NEC
- chordae tendinae NEC I51.1
  - concurrent with acute myocardial infarction — see Infarct, myocardium
  - following acute myocardial infarction (current complication) I23.4
- clitoris — see Laceration, vulva
- colon — see Laceration, intestine, large, colon
- common bile duct S36.13 ☑
- cortex (cerebral) — see Injury, intracranial, diffuse
- costal region — see Laceration, thorax
- cystic duct S36.13 ☑
- diaphragm S27.803 ☑
- digit(s)
  - foot — see Laceration, toe
  - hand — see Laceration, finger
- duodenum S36.430 ☑
- ear (canal) (external) S01.31- ☑
  - with foreign body S01.32- ☑
  - drum S09.2- ☑
- elbow S51.01- ☑
  - with
    - foreign body S51.02- ☑
- epididymis — see Laceration, testis
- epigastric region — see Laceration, abdomen, wall, epigastric region
- esophagus K22.8
  - traumatic
    - cervical S11.21 ☑
      - with foreign body S11.22 ☑
    - thoracic S27.813 ☑
- eye (ball) S05.3- ☑
  - with prolapse or loss of intraocular tissue S05.2- ☑
  - penetrating S05.6- ☑
- eyebrow — see Laceration, eyelid
- eyelid S01.11- ☑
  - with foreign body S01.12- ☑
- face NEC — see Laceration, head, specified site NEC
- fallopian tube S37.539 ☑
  - bilateral S37.532 ☑
  - unilateral S37.531 ☑
- finger(s) S61.219 ☑
  - with
    - damage to nail S61.319 ☑
      - with
        - foreign body S61.329 ☑
    - foreign body S61.229 ☑
  - index S61.218 ☑
    - with
      - damage to nail S61.318 ☑
        - with
          - foreign body S61.328 ☑
      - foreign body S61.228 ☑
    - left S61.211 ☑
      - with
        - damage to nail S61.311 ☑

Laceration — continued
- finger(s) — continued
  - index — continued
    - left — continued
      - with — continued
        - damage to nail — continued
          - with
            - foreign body S61.321 ☑
          - foreign body S61.221 ☑
    - right S61.210 ☑
      - with
        - damage to nail S61.310 ☑
          - with
            - foreign body S61.320 ☑
        - foreign body S61.220 ☑
  - little S61.218 ☑
    - with
      - damage to nail S61.318 ☑
        - with
          - foreign body S61.328 ☑
      - foreign body S61.228 ☑
    - left S61.217 ☑
      - with
        - damage to nail S61.317 ☑
          - with
            - foreign body S61.327 ☑
        - foreign body S61.227 ☑
    - right S61.216 ☑
      - with
        - damage to nail S61.316 ☑
          - with
            - foreign body S61.326 ☑
        - foreign body S61.226 ☑
  - middle S61.218 ☑
    - with
      - damage to nail S61.318 ☑
        - with
          - foreign body S61.328 ☑
      - foreign body S61.228 ☑
    - left S61.213 ☑
      - with
        - damage to nail S61.313 ☑
          - with
            - foreign body S61.323 ☑
        - foreign body S61.223 ☑
    - right S61.212 ☑
      - with
        - damage to nail S61.312 ☑
          - with
            - foreign body S61.322 ☑
        - foreign body S61.222 ☑
  - ring S61.218 ☑
    - with
      - damage to nail S61.318 ☑
        - with
          - foreign body S61.328 ☑
      - foreign body S61.228 ☑
    - left S61.215 ☑
      - with
        - damage to nail S61.315 ☑
          - with
            - foreign body S61.325 ☑
        - foreign body S61.225 ☑
    - right S61.214 ☑
      - with
        - damage to nail S61.314 ☑
          - with
            - foreign body S61.324 ☑
        - foreign body S61.224 ☑
- flank S31.119 ☑
  - with foreign body S31.129 ☑
- foot (except toe(s) alone) S91.319 ☑
  - with foreign body S91.329 ☑
  - left S91.312 ☑
    - with foreign body S91.322 ☑
  - right S91.311 ☑
    - with foreign body S91.321 ☑
  - toe — see Laceration, toe
- forearm S51.819 ☑
  - with
    - foreign body S51.829 ☑
  - elbow only — see Laceration, elbow
  - left S51.812 ☑
    - with
      - foreign body S51.822 ☑
  - right S51.811 ☑

Laceration — continued
- forearm — continued
  - right — continued
    - with
      - foreign body S51.821 ☑
- forehead S01.81 ☑
  - with foreign body S01.82 ☑
- fourchette O70.0
  - with ectopic or molar pregnancy O08.6
  - complicating delivery O70.0
  - following ectopic or molar pregnancy O08.6
- gallbladder S36.123 ☑
- genital organs, external
  - female S31.512 ☑
    - with foreign body S31.522 ☑
    - vagina — see Laceration, vagina
    - vulva — see Laceration, vulva
  - male S31.511 ☑
    - with foreign body S31.521 ☑
    - penis — see Laceration, penis
    - scrotum — see Laceration, scrotum
    - testis — see Laceration, testis
- groin — see Laceration, abdomen, wall
- gum — see Laceration, oral cavity
- hand S61.419 ☑
  - with
    - foreign body S61.429 ☑
  - finger — see Laceration, finger
  - left S61.412 ☑
    - with
      - foreign body S61.422 ☑
  - right S61.411 ☑
    - with
      - foreign body S61.421 ☑
  - thumb — see Laceration, thumb
- head S01.91 ☑
  - with foreign body S01.92 ☑
  - cheek — see Laceration, cheek
  - ear — see Laceration, ear
  - eyelid — see Laceration, eyelid
  - lip — see Laceration, lip
  - nose — see Laceration, nose
  - oral cavity — see Laceration, oral cavity
  - scalp S01.01 ☑
    - with foreign body S01.02 ☑
  - specified site NEC S01.81 ☑
    - with foreign body S01.82 ☑
  - temporomandibular area — see Laceration, cheek
- heart — see Injury, heart, laceration
- heel — see Laceration, foot
- hepatic duct S36.13 ☑
- hip S71.019 ☑
  - with foreign body S71.029 ☑
  - left S71.012 ☑
    - with foreign body S71.022 ☑
  - right S71.011 ☑
    - with foreign body S71.021 ☑
- hymen — see Laceration, vagina
- hypochondrium — see Laceration, abdomen, wall
- hypogastric region — see Laceration, abdomen, wall
- ileum S36.438 ☑
- inguinal region — see Laceration, abdomen, wall
- instep — see Laceration, foot
- internal organ — see Injury, by site
- interscapular region — see Laceration, thorax, back
- intestine
  - large
    - colon S36.539 ☑
      - ascending S36.530 ☑
      - descending S36.532 ☑
      - sigmoid S36.533 ☑
      - specified site NEC S36.538 ☑
    - rectum S36.63 ☑
      - transverse S36.531 ☑
    - small S36.439 ☑
      - duodenum S36.430 ☑
      - specified site NEC S36.438 ☑
- intra-abdominal organ S36.93 ☑
  - intestine — see Laceration, intestine
  - liver — see Laceration, liver
  - pancreas — see Laceration, pancreas
  - peritoneum S36.81 ☑
  - specified site NEC S36.893 ☑
  - spleen — see Laceration, spleen
  - stomach — see Laceration, stomach
- intracranial NEC — see also Injury, intracranial, diffus

Laceration — Laceration

210

☑ Additional Character Required — Refer to the Tabular List for Character Selection   ▽ Subterms under main terms may continue to next column or page

Laceration — *continued*
  intracranial — *see also* Injury, intracranial, diffuse —
    continued
    birth injury P10.9
  jaw — *see* Laceration, head, specified site NEC
  jejunum S36.438 ☑
  joint capsule — *see* Sprain, by site
  kidney S37.03-
    major (greater than 3 cm) (massive) (stellate)
      S37.06-
    minor (less than 1 cm) S37.04- ☑
    moderate (1 to 3 cm) S37.05- ☑
      multiple S37.06- ☑
  knee S81.01- ☑
    with foreign body S81.02- ☑
  labium (majus) (minus) — *see* Laceration, vulva
  lacrimal duct — *see* Laceration, eyelid
  large intestine — *see* Laceration, intestine, large
  larynx S11.011 ☑
    with foreign body S11.012 ☑
  leg (lower) S81.819 ☑
    with foreign body S81.829 ☑
    foot — *see* Laceration, foot
    knee — *see* Laceration, knee
    left S81.812 ☑
      with foreign body S81.822 ☑
    right S81.811 ☑
      with foreign body S81.821 ☑
    upper — *see* Laceration, thigh
  ligament — *see* Sprain
  lip S01.511 ☑
    with foreign body S01.521 ☑
  liver S36.113 ☑
    major (stellate) S36.116 ☑
    minor S36.114 ☑
    moderate S36.115 ☑
  loin — *see* Laceration, abdomen, wall
  lower back — *see* Laceration, back, lower
  lumbar region — *see* Laceration, back, lower
  lung S27.339 ☑
    bilateral S27.332 ☑
    unilateral S27.331 ☑
  malar region — *see* Laceration, head, specified site NEC
  mammary — *see* Laceration, breast
  mastoid region — *see* Laceration, head, specified site
    NEC
  meninges — *see* Injury, intracranial, diffuse
  meniscus — *see* Tear, meniscus
  mesentery S36.893 ☑
  mesosalpinx S37.893 ☑
  mouth — *see* Laceration, oral cavity
  muscle — *see* Injury, muscle, by site, laceration
  nail
    finger — *see* Laceration, finger, with damage to nail
    toe — *see* Laceration, toe, with damage to nail
  nasal (septum) (sinus) — *see* Laceration, nose
  nasopharynx — *see* Laceration, head, specified site
    NEC
  neck S11.91 ☑
    with foreign body S11.92 ☑
    involving
      cervical esophagus S11.21 ☑
        with foreign body S11.22 ☑
      larynx — *see* Laceration, larynx
      pharynx — *see* Laceration, pharynx
      thyroid gland — *see* Laceration, thyroid gland
      trachea — *see* Laceration, trachea
    specified site NEC S11.81 ☑
      with foreign body S11.82 ☑
  nerve — *see* Injury, nerve
  nose (septum) (sinus) S01.21 ☑
    with foreign body S01.22 ☑
  ocular NOS S05.3-
    adnexa NOS S01.11- ☑
  oral cavity S01.512 ☑
    with foreign body S01.522 ☑
  orbit (eye) — *see* Wound, open, ocular, orbit
  ovary S37.439 ☑
    bilateral S37.432 ☑
    unilateral S37.431 ☑
  palate — *see* Laceration, oral cavity
  palm — *see* Laceration, hand
  pancreas S36.239 ☑
  pelvic S31.010 ☑
    with
      foreign body S31.020 ☑

Laceration — *continued*
  pelvic — *continued*
    with — *continued*
      foreign body — *continued*
        penetration into retroperitoneal cavity
          S31.021 ☑
      penetration into retroperitoneal cavity
        S31.011 ☑
    floor — *see also* Laceration, back, lower
      with ectopic or molar pregnancy O08.6
      complicating delivery O70.1
      following ectopic or molar pregnancy O08.6
      old (postpartal) N81.89
    organ S37.93 ☑
  penis S31.21 ☑
    with foreign body S31.22 ☑
  perineum
    female S31.41 ☑
      with
        ectopic or molar pregnancy O08.6
        foreign body S31.42 ☑
      during delivery O70.9
        first degree O70.0
        fourth degree O70.3
        second degree O70.1
        third degree — *see also* Delivery, complicat-
          ed, by, laceration, perineum, third de-
          gree O70.20
      old (postpartal) N81.89
      postpartal N81.89
      secondary (postpartal) O90.1
    male S31.119 ☑
      with foreign body S31.129 ☑
  periocular area (with or without lacrimal passages) —
    see Laceration, eyelid
  peritoneum S36.893 ☑
  periumbilic region — *see* Laceration, abdomen, wall,
    periumbilic
  periurethral tissue — *see* Laceration, urethra
  phalanges
    finger — *see* Laceration, finger
    toe — *see* Laceration, toe
  pharynx S11.21 ☑
    with foreign body S11.22 ☑
  pinna — *see* Laceration, ear
  popliteal space — *see* Laceration, knee
  prepuce — *see* Laceration, penis
  prostate S37.823 ☑
  pubic region S31.119 ☑
    with foreign body S31.129 ☑
  pudendum — *see* Laceration, genital organs, external
  rectovaginal septum — *see* Laceration, vagina
  rectum S36.63 ☑
  retroperitoneum S36.893 ☑
  round ligament S37.893 ☑
  sacral region — *see* Laceration, back, lower
  sacroiliac region — *see* Laceration, back, lower
  salivary gland — *see* Laceration, oral cavity
  scalp S01.01 ☑
    with foreign body S01.02 ☑
  scapular region — *see* Laceration, shoulder
  scrotum S31.31 ☑
    with foreign body S31.32 ☑
  seminal vesicle S37.893 ☑
  shin — *see* Laceration, leg
  shoulder S41.019 ☑
    with foreign body S41.029 ☑
    left S41.012 ☑
      with foreign body S41.022 ☑
    right S41.011 ☑
      with foreign body S41.021 ☑
  small intestine — *see* Laceration, intestine, small
  spermatic cord — *see* Laceration, testis
  spinal cord (meninges) — *see also* Injury, spinal cord,
    by region
    due to injury at birth P11.5
    newborn (birth injury) P11.5
  spleen S36.039 ☑
    major (massive) (stellate) S36.032 ☑
    moderate S36.031 ☑
    superficial (minor) S36.030 ☑
  sternal region — *see* Laceration, thorax, front
  stomach S36.33 ☑
  submaxillary region — *see* Laceration, head, specified
    site NEC
  submental region — *see* Laceration, head, specified
    site NEC

Laceration — *continued*
  subungual
    finger(s) — *see* Laceration, finger, with damage to
      nail
    toe(s) — *see* Laceration, toe, with damage to nail
  suprarenal gland — *see* Laceration, adrenal gland
  temple, temporal region — *see* Laceration, head,
    specified site NEC
  temporomandibular area — *see* Laceration, cheek
  tendon — *see* Injury, muscle, by site, laceration
    Achilles S86.02- ☑
  tentorium cerebelli — *see* Injury, intracranial, diffuse
  testis S31.31 ☑
    with foreign body S31.32 ☑
  thigh S71.11- ☑
    with foreign body S71.12- ☑
  thorax, thoracic (wall) S21.91 ☑
    with foreign body S21.92 ☑
    back S21.22- ☑
      with penetration into thoracic cavity
        S21.42- ☑
    front S21.12- ☑
      with penetration into thoracic cavity
        S21.32- ☑
    back S21.21- ☑
      with
        foreign body S21.22- ☑
          with penetration into thoracic cavity
            S21.42- ☑
        penetration into thoracic cavity S21.41- ☑
    breast — *see* Laceration, breast
    front S21.11- ☑
      with
        foreign body S21.12- ☑
          with penetration into thoracic cavity
            S21.32- ☑
        penetration into thoracic cavity S21.31- ☑
  thumb S61.019 ☑
    with
      damage to nail S61.119 ☑
        with
          foreign body S61.129 ☑
      foreign body S61.029 ☑
    left S61.012 ☑
      with
        damage to nail S61.112 ☑
          with
            foreign body S61.122 ☑
        foreign body S61.022 ☑
    right S61.011 ☑
      with
        damage to nail S61.111 ☑
          with
            foreign body S61.121 ☑
        foreign body S61.021 ☑
  thyroid gland S11.11 ☑
    with foreign body S11.12 ☑
  toe(s) S91.119 ☑
    with
      damage to nail S91.219 ☑
        with
          foreign body S91.229 ☑
      foreign body S91.129 ☑
    great S91.113 ☑
      with
        damage to nail S91.213 ☑
          with
            foreign body S91.223 ☑
        foreign body S91.123 ☑
      left S91.112 ☑
        with
          damage to nail S91.212 ☑
            with
              foreign body S91.222 ☑
          foreign body S91.122 ☑
      right S91.111 ☑
        with
          damage to nail S91.211 ☑
            with
              foreign body S91.221 ☑
          foreign body S91.121 ☑
    lesser S91.116 ☑
      with
        damage to nail S91.216 ☑
          with
            foreign body S91.226 ☑

Laceration — *continued*
toe(s) — *continued*
lesser — *continued*
with — *continued*
foreign body S91.126 ☑
left S91.115 ☑
with
damage to nail S91.215 ☑
with
foreign body S91.225 ☑
foreign body S91.125 ☑
right S91.114 ☑
with
damage to nail S91.214 ☑
with
foreign body S91.224 ☑
foreign body S91.124 ☑
tongue — *see* Laceration, oral cavity
trachea S11.021 ☑
with foreign body S11.022 ☑
tunica vaginalis — *see* Laceration, testis
tympanum, tympanic membrane — *see* Laceration, ear, drum
umbilical region S31.115 ☑
with foreign body S31.125 ☑
ureter S37.13 ☑
urethra S37.33 ☑
with or following ectopic or molar pregnancy O08.6
obstetrical trauma O71.5
urinary organ NEC S37.893 ☑
uterus S37.63 ☑
with ectopic or molar pregnancy O08.6
following ectopic or molar pregnancy O08.6
nonpuerperal, nontraumatic N85.8
obstetrical trauma NEC O71.81
old (postpartal) N85.8
uvula — *see* Laceration, oral cavity
vagina S31.41 ☑
with
ectopic or molar pregnancy O08.6
foreign body S31.42 ☑
during delivery O71.4
with perineal laceration — *see* Laceration, perineum, female, during delivery
following ectopic or molar pregnancy O08.6
nonpuerperal, nontraumatic N89.8
old (postpartal) N89.8
vas deferens S37.893 ☑
vesical — *see* Laceration, bladder
vocal cords S11.031 ☑
with foreign body S11.032 ☑
vulva S31.41 ☑
with
ectopic or molar pregnancy O08.6
foreign body S31.42 ☑
complicating delivery O70.0
following ectopic or molar pregnancy O08.6
nonpuerperal, nontraumatic N90.89
old (postpartal) N90.89
wrist S61.519 ☑
with
foreign body S61.529 ☑
left S61.512 ☑
with
foreign body S61.522 ☑
right S61.511 ☑
with
foreign body S61.521 ☑
Lack of
achievement in school Z55.3
adequate
food Z59.4
intermaxillary vertical dimension of fully erupted teeth M26.36
sleep Z72.820
appetite (see Anorexia) R63.0
awareness R41.9
care
in home Z74.2
of infant (at or after birth) T76.02 ☑
confirmed T74.02 ☑
cognitive functions R41.9
coordination R27.9
ataxia R27.0
specified type NEC R27.8
development (physiological) R62.50
failure to thrive (child over 28 days old) R62.51

Lack of — *continued*
development — *continued*
failure to thrive — *continued*
adult R62.7
newborn P92.6
short stature R62.52
specified type NEC R62.59
energy R53.83
financial resources Z59.6
food T73.0 ☑
growth R62.52
heating Z59.1
housing (permanent) (temporary) Z59.0
adequate Z59.1
learning experiences in childhood Z62.898
leisure time (affecting life-style) Z73.2
material resources Z59.9
memory — *see also* Amnesia
mild, following organic brain damage F06.8
ovulation N97.0
parental supervision or control of child Z62.0
person able to render necessary care Z74.2
physical exercise Z72.3
play experience in childhood Z62.898
posterior occlusal support M26.57
relaxation (affecting life-style) Z73.2
sexual
desire F52.0
enjoyment F52.1
shelter Z59.0
sleep (adequate) Z72.820
supervision of child by parent Z62.0
support, posterior occlusal M26.57
water T73.1 ☑
Lacrimal — *see* condition
Lacrimation, abnormal — *see* Epiphora
Lacrimonasal duct — *see* condition
Lactation, lactating (breast) (puerperal, postpartum)
associated
cracked nipple O92.13
retracted nipple O92.03
defective O92.4
disorder NEC O92.79
excessive O92.6
failed (complete) O92.3
partial O92.4
mastitis NEC — *see* Mastitis, obstetric
mother (care and/or examination) Z39.1
nonpuerperal N64.3
Lacticemia, excessive E87.2
Lacunar skull Q75.8
Laennec's cirrhosis K70.30
with ascites K70.31
nonalcoholic K74.69
Lafora's disease — *see* Epilepsy, generalized, idiopathic
Lag, lid (nervous) — *see* Retraction, lid
Lagophthalmos (eyelid) (nervous) H02.209
bilateral, upper and lower eyelids H02.20C
cicatricial H02.219
bilateral, upper and lower eyelids H02.21C
left H02.216
lower H02.215
upper H02.214
upper and lower eyelids H02.21B
right H02.213
lower H02.212
upper H02.211
upper and lower eyelids H02.21A
keratoconjunctivitis — *see* Keratoconjunctivitis
left H02.206
lower H02.205
upper H02.204
upper and lower eyelids H02.20B
mechanical H02.229
bilateral, upper and lower eyelids H02.22C
left H02.226
lower H02.225
upper H02.224
upper and lower eyelids H02.22B
right H02.223
lower H02.222
upper H02.221
upper and lower eyelids H02.22A
paralytic H02.239
bilateral, upper and lower eyelids H02.23C
left H02.236
lower H02.235
upper H02.234

Lagophthalmos — *continued*
paralytic — *continued*
left — *continued*
upper and lower eyelids H02.23B
right H02.233
lower H02.232
upper H02.231
upper and lower eyelids H02.23A
right H02.203
lower H02.202
upper H02.201
upper and lower eyelids H02.20A
Laki-Lorand factor deficiency — *see* Defect, coagulation, specified type NEC
Lalling F80.0
Lambert-Eaton syndrome — *see* Syndrome, Lambert-Eaton
Lambliasis, lambliosis A07.1
Landau-Kleffner syndrome — *see* Epilepsy, specified NEC
Landouzy-Déjérine dystrophy or facioscapulohumeral atrophy G71.02
Landouzy's disease (icterohemorrhagic leptospirosis) A27.0
Landry-Guillain-Barré, syndrome or paralysis G61.0
Landry's disease or paralysis G61.0
Lane's
band Q43.3
kink — *see* Obstruction, intestine
syndrome K90.2
Langdon Down syndrome — *see* Trisomy, 21
Lapsed immunization schedule status Z28.3
Large
baby (regardless of gestational age) (4000g to 4499g) P08.1
ear, congenital Q17.1
physiological cup Q14.2
stature R68.89
Large-for-dates NEC (infant) (4000g to 4499g) P08.1
affecting management of pregnancy O36.6- ☑
exceptionally (4500g or more) P08.0
Larsen-Johansson disease orosteochondrosis — *see* Osteochondrosis, juvenile, patella
Larsen's syndrome (flattened facies and multiple congenital dislocations) Q74.8
Larva migrans
cutaneous B76.9
Ancylostoma B76.0
visceral B83.0
Laryngeal — *see* condition
Laryngismus (stridulus) J38.5
congenital P28.89
diphtheritic A36.2
Laryngitis (acute) (edematous) (fibrinous) (infective) (infiltrative) (malignant) (membranous) (phlegmonous) (pneumococcal) (pseudomembranous) (septic) (subglottic) (suppurative) (ulcerative) J04.0
with
influenza, flu, or grippe — *see* Influenza, with, laryngitis
tracheitis (acute) — *see* Laryngotracheitis
atrophic J37.0
catarrhal J37.0
chronic J37.0
with tracheitis (chronic) J37.1
diphtheritic A36.2
due to external agent — *see* Inflammation, respiratory, upper, due to
H. influenzae J04.0
Hemophilus influenzae J04.0
hypertrophic J37.0
influenzal — *see* Influenza, with, respiratory manifestations NEC
obstructive J05.0
sicca J37.0
spasmodic J05.0
acute J04.0
streptococcal J04.0
stridulous J05.0
syphilitic (late) A52.73
congenital A50.59 *[J99]*
early A50.03 *[J99]*
tuberculous A15.5
Vincent's A69.1
Laryngocele (congenital) (ventricular) Q31.3
Laryngofissure J38.7
congenital Q31.8
Laryngomalacia (congenital) Q31.5

212

☑ **Additional Character Required** — Refer to the Tabular List for Character Selection   ⬙ **Subterms under main terms may continue to next column or page**

Laryngopharyngitis (acute) J06.0
  chronic J37.0
  due to external agent — *see* Inflammation, respiratory, upper, due to
Laryngoplegia J38.00
  bilateral J38.02
  unilateral J38.01
Laryngoptosis J38.7
Laryngospasm J38.5
Laryngostenosis J38.6
Laryngotracheitis (acute) (Infectional) (infective) (viral) J04.2
  atrophic J37.1
  catarrhal J37.1
  chronic J37.1
  diphtheritic A36.2
  due to external agent — *see* Inflammation, respiratory, upper, due to
  Hemophilus influenzae J04.2
  hypertrophic J37.1
  influenzal — *see* Influenza, with, respiratory manifestations NEC
  pachydermic J38.7
  sicca J37.1
  spasmodic J38.5
    acute J05.0
  streptococcal J04.2
  stridulous J38.5
  syphilitic (late) A52.73
    congenital A50.59 *[J99]*
    early A50.03 *[J99]*
  tuberculous A15.5
  Vincent's A69.1
Laryngotracheobronchitis — *see* Bronchitis
Larynx, laryngeal — *see* condition
Lassa fever A96.2
Lassitude — *see* Weakness
Late
  talker R62.0
  walker R62.0
Late effect(s) — *see* Sequelae
Latent — *see* condition
Laterocession — *see* Lateroversion
Lateroflexion — *see* Lateroversion
Lateroversion
  cervix — *see* Lateroversion, uterus
  uterus, uterine (cervix) (postinfectional) (postpartal, old) N85.4
    congenital Q51.818
    in pregnancy or childbirth O34.59- ☑
Lathyrism — *see* Poisoning, food, noxious, plant
Launois' syndrome (pituitary gigantism) E22.0
Launois-Bensaude adenolipomatosis E88.89
Laurence-Moon (-Bardet)-**Biedl syndrome** Q87.89
Lax, laxity — *see also* Relaxation
  ligament (ous) — *see also* Disorder, ligament
    familial M35.7
    knee — *see* Derangement, knee
  skin (acquired) L57.4
    congenital Q82.8
Laxative habit F55.2
Lazy leukocyte syndrome D70.8
Lead miner's lung J63.6
Leak, leakage
  air NEC J93.82
    postprocedural J95.812
  amniotic fluid — *see* Rupture, membranes, premature
  blood (microscopic), fetal, into maternal circulation
    affecting management of pregnancy — *see* Pregnancy, complicated by
  cerebrospinal fluid G96.00
    cranial
      postoperative G96.08
      specified NEC G96.08
      spontaneous G96.01
      traumatic G96.08
    from spinal (lumbar) puncture G97.0
    spinal
      postoperative G96.09
      post-traumatic G96.09
      specified NEC G96.09
      spontaneous G96.02
    spontaneous
      from
        skull base G96.01
        spine G96.02
    CSF — *see* Leak, cerebrospinal fluid

Leak, leakage — *continued*
  device, implant or graft — *see also* Complications, by site and type, mechanical
    arterial graft NEC — *see* Complication, cardiovascular device, mechanical, vascular
    breast (implant) T85.43 ☑
    catheter NEC T85.638 ☑
      dialysis (renal) T82.43 ☑
        intraperitoneal T85.631 ☑
      infusion NEC T82.534 ☑
        spinal (epidural) (subdural) T85.630 ☑
      urinary T83.038 ☑
        cystostomy T83.030 ☑
        Hopkins T83.038 ☑
        ileostomy T83.038 ☑
        indwelling T83.031 ☑
        nephrostomy T83.032 ☑
        specified T83.038 ☑
        urostomy T83.038 ☑
    gastrointestinal — *see* Complications, prosthetic device, mechanical, gastrointestinal device
    genital NEC T83.498 ☑
      penile prosthesis (cylinder) (implanted) (pump) (reservoir) T83.490 ☑
      testicular prosthesis T83.491 ☑
    heart NEC — *see* Complication, cardiovascular device, mechanical
    joint prosthesis — *see* Complications, joint prosthesis, mechanical, specified NEC, by site
    ocular NEC — *see* Complications, prosthetic device, mechanical, ocular device
    orthopedic NEC — *see* Complication, orthopedic, device, mechanical
    persistent air J93.82
    specified NEC T85.638 ☑
    urinary NEC — *see also* Complication, genitourinary, device, urinary, mechanical
      graft T83.23 ☑
    vascular NEC — *see* Complication, cardiovascular device, mechanical
    ventricular intracranial shunt T85.03 ☑
  urine — *see* Incontinence
Leaky heart — *see* Endocarditis
Learning defect (specific) F81.9
Leather bottle stomach C16.9
Leber's
  congenital amaurosis H35.50
  optic atrophy (hereditary) H47.22
Lederer's anemia D59.19
Leeches (external) — *see* Hirudiniasis
Leg — *see* condition
Legg (-Calvé)-**Perthes disease, syndrome or osteochondrosis** M91.1- ☑
Legionellosis A48.1
  nonpneumonic A48.2
Legionnaires'
  disease A48.1
    nonpneumonic A48.2
  pneumonia A48.1
Leigh's disease G31.82
Leiner's disease L21.1
Leiofibromyoma — *see* Leiomyoma
Leiomyoblastoma — *see* Neoplasm, connective tissue, benign
Leiomyofibroma — *see also* Neoplasm, connective tissue, benign
  uterus (cervix) (corpus) D25.9
Leiomyoma — *see also* Neoplasm, connective tissue, benign
  bizarre — *see* Neoplasm, connective tissue, benign
  cellular — *see* Neoplasm, connective tissue, benign
  epithelioid — *see* Neoplasm, connective tissue, benign
  uterus (cervix) (corpus) D25.9
    intramural D25.1
    submucous D25.0
    subserosal D25.2
  vascular — *see* Neoplasm, connective tissue, benign
Leiomyoma, leiomyomatosis (intravascular) — *see* Neoplasm, connective tissue, uncertain behavior
Leiomyosarcoma — *see also* Neoplasm, connective tissue, malignant
  epithelioid — *see* Neoplasm, connective tissue, malignant
  myxoid — *see* Neoplasm, connective tissue, malignant
Leishmaniasis B55.9
  American (mucocutaneous) B55.2
  cutaneous B55.1

Leishmaniasis — *continued*
  Asian Desert B55.1
  Brazilian B55.2
  cutaneous (any type) B55.1
  dermal — *see also* Leishmaniasis, cutaneous
    post-kala-azar B55.0
  eyelid B55.1
  infantile B55.0
  Mediterranean B55.0
  mucocutaneous (American) (New World) B55.2
  naso-oral B55.2
  nasopharyngeal B55.2
  old world B55.1
  tegumentaria diffusa B55.1
  visceral B55.0
Leishmanoid, dermal — *see also* Leishmaniasis, cutaneous
  post-kala-azar B55.0
Lenegre's disease I44.2
Lengthening, leg — *see* Deformity, limb, unequal length
Lennert's lymphoma — *see* Lymphoma, Lennert's
Lennox-Gastaut syndrome G40.812
  intractable G40.814
    with status epilepticus G40.813
    without status epilepticus G40.814
  not intractable G40.812
    with status epilepticus G40.811
    without status epilepticus G40.812
Lens — *see* condition
Lenticonus (anterior) (posterior) (congenital) Q12.8
Lenticular degeneration, progressive E83.01
Lentiglobus (posterior) (congenital) Q12.8
Lentigo (congenital) L81.4
  maligna — *see also* Melanoma, in situ
    melanoma — *see* Melanoma
Lentivirus, as cause of disease classified elsewhere B97.31
Leontiasis
  ossium M85.2
  syphilitic (late) A52.78
    congenital A50.59
Lepothrix A48.8
Lepra — *see* Leprosy
Leprechaunism E34.8
Leprosy A30.- ☑
  with muscle disorder A30.9 *[M63.80]*
    ankle A30.9 *[M63.87-]* ☑
    foot A30.9 *[M63.87-]* ☑
    forearm A30.9 *[M63.83-]* ☑
    hand A30.9 *[M63.84-]* ☑
    lower leg A30.9 *[M63.86-]* ☑
    multiple sites A30.9 *[M63.89]*
    pelvic region A30.9 *[M63.85-]* ☑
    shoulder region A30.9 *[M63.81-]* ☑
    specified site NEC A30.9 *[M63.88]*
    thigh A30.9 *[M63.85-]* ☑
    upper arm A30.9 *[M63.82-]* ☑
  anesthetic A30.9
  BB A30.3
  BL A30.4
  borderline (infiltrated) (neuritic) A30.3
    lepromatous A30.4
    tuberculoid A30.2
  BT A30.2
  dimorphous (infiltrated) (neuritic) A30.3
  I A30.0
  indeterminate (macular) (neuritic) A30.0
  lepromatous (diffuse) (infiltrated) (macular) (neuritic) (nodular) A30.5
  LL A30.5
  macular (early) (neuritic) (simple) A30.9
  maculoanesthetic A30.9
  mixed A30.3
  neural A30.9
  nodular A30.5
  primary neuritic A30.3
  specified type NEC A30.8
  TT A30.1
  tuberculoid (major) (minor) A30.1
Leptocytosis, hereditary D56.9
Leptomeningitis (chronic) (circumscribed) (hemorrhagic) (nonsuppurative) — *see* Meningitis
Leptomeningopathy G96.198
Leptospiral — *see* condition
Leptospirochetal — *see* condition
Leptospirosis A27.9
  canicola A27.89

Leptospirosis — continued
 due to Leptospira interrogans serovar icterohaemorrhagiae A27.0
 icterohemorrhagica A27.0
 pomona A27.89
 Weil's disease A27.0
Leptus dermatitis B88.0
Leriche's syndrome (aortic bifurcation occlusion) I74.09
Leri's pleonosteosis Q78.8
Leri-Weill syndrome Q77.8
Lermoyez' syndrome — see Vertigo, peripheral NEC
Lesch-Nyhan syndrome E79.1
Leser-Trélat disease L82.1
 inflamed L82.0
Lesion(s) (nontraumatic)
 abducens nerve — see Strabismus, paralytic, sixth nerve
 alveolar process K08.9
 angiocentric immunoproliferative D47.Z9 (following D47.4)
 anorectal K62.9
 aortic (valve) I35.9
 auditory nerve — see subcategory H93.3 ☑
 basal ganglion G25.9
 bile duct — see Disease, bile duct
 biomechanical M99.9
  specified type NEC M99.89
   abdomen M99.89
   acromioclavicular M99.87
   cervical region M99.81
   cervicothoracic M99.81
   costochondral M99.88
   costovertebral M99.88
   head region M99.80
   hip M99.85
   lower extremity M99.86
   lumbar region M99.83
   lumbosacral M99.83
   occipitocervical M99.80
   pelvic region M99.85
   pubic M99.85
   rib cage M99.88
   sacral region M99.84
   sacrococcygeal M99.84
   sacroiliac M99.84
   specified NEC M99.89
   sternochondral M99.88
   sternoclavicular M99.87
   thoracic region M99.82
   thoracolumbar M99.82
   upper extremity M99.87
 bladder N32.9
 bone — see Disorder, bone
 brachial plexus G54.0
 brain G93.9
  congenital Q04.9
  vascular I67.9
   degenerative I67.9
   hypertensive I67.4
 buccal cavity K13.79
 calcified — see Calcification
 canthus — see Disorder, eyelid
 carate — see Pinta, lesions
 cardia K31.9
 cardiac — see also Disease, heart I51.9
  congenital Q24.9
  valvular — see Endocarditis
 cauda equina G83.4
 cecum K63.9
 cerebral — see Lesion, brain
 cerebrovascular I67.9
  degenerative I67.9
  hypertensive I67.4
 cervical (nerve) root NEC G54.2
 chiasmal — see Disorder, optic, chiasm
 chorda tympani G51.8
 coin, lung R91.1
 colon K63.9
 combined periodontic - endodontic K05.5
 congenital — see Anomaly, by site
 conjunctiva H11.9
 conus medullaris — see Injury, conus medullaris
 coronary artery — see Ischemia, heart
 cranial nerve G52.9
  eighth — see Disorder, ear
  eleventh G52.9
  fifth G50.9
  first G52.0
  fourth — see Strabismus, paralytic, fourth nerve

Lesion(s) — continued
 cranial nerve — continued
  seventh G51.9
  sixth — see Strabismus, paralytic, sixth nerve
  tenth G52.2
  twelfth G52.3
 cystic — see Cyst
 degenerative — see Degeneration
 duodenum K31.9
 edentulous (alveolar) ridge, associated with trauma, due to traumatic occlusion K06.2
 en coup de sabre L94.1
 eyelid — see Disorder, eyelid
 gasserian ganglion G50.8
 gastric K31.9
 gastroduodenal K31.9
 gastrointestinal K63.9
 gingiva, associated with trauma K06.2
 glomerular
  focal and segmental — see also N00-N07 with fourth character .1 N05.1
  minimal change — see also N00-N07 with fourth character .0 N05.0
 heart (organic) — see Disease, heart
 hyperchromic, due to pinta (carate) A67.1
 hyperkeratotic — see Hyperkeratosis
 hypothalamic E23.7
 ileocecal K63.9
 ileum K63.9
 iliohypogastric nerve G57.8- ☑
 inflammatory — see Inflammation
 intestine K63.9
 intracerebral — see Lesion, brain
 intrachiasmal (optic) — see Disorder, optic, chiasm
 intracranial, space-occupying R90.0
 joint — see Disorder, joint
  sacroiliac (old) M53.3
 keratotic — see Keratosis
 kidney — see Disease, renal
 laryngeal nerve (recurrent) G52.2
 lip K13.0
 liver K76.9
 lumbosacral
  plexus G54.1
  root (nerve) NEC G54.4
 lung (coin) R91.1
 maxillary sinus J32.0
 mitral I05.9
 Morel-Lavallée — see Hematoma, by site
 motor cortex NEC G93.89
 mouth K13.79
 nerve G58.9
  femoral G57.2- ☑
  median G56.1- ☑
   carpal tunnel syndrome — see Syndrome, carpal tunnel
  plantar G57.6- ☑
  popliteal (lateral) G57.3- ☑
   medial G57.4- ☑
  radial G56.3- ☑
  sciatic G57.0- ☑
  spinal — see Injury, nerve, spinal
  ulnar G56.2- ☑
 nervous system, congenital Q07.9
 nonallopathic — see Lesion, biomechanical
 nose (internal) J34.89
 obstructive — see Obstruction
 obturator nerve G57.8- ☑
 oral mucosa K13.70
 organ or site NEC — see Disease, by site
 osteolytic — see Osteolysis
 peptic K27.9
 periodontal, due to traumatic occlusion K05.5
 pharynx J39.2
 pigment, pigmented (skin) L81.9
 pinta — see Pinta, lesions
 polypoid — see Polyp
 prechiasmal (optic) — see Disorder, optic, chiasm
 primary — see also Syphilis, primary A51.0
  carate A67.0
  pinta A67.0
  yaws A66.0
 pulmonary J98.4
  valve I37.9
 pylorus K31.9
 rectosigmoid K63.9
 retina, retinal H35.9
 sacroiliac (joint) (old) M53.3

Lesion(s) — continued
 salivary gland K11.9
  benign lymphoepithelial K11.8
 saphenous nerve G57.8- ☑
 sciatic nerve G57.0- ☑
 secondary — see Syphilis, secondary
 shoulder (region) M75.9- ☑
  specified NEC M75.8- ☑
 sigmoid K63.9
 sinus (accessory) (nasal) J34.89
 skin L98.9
  suppurative L08.0
 SLAP S43.43- ☑
 spinal cord G95.9
  congenital Q06.9
 spleen D73.89
 stomach K31.9
 superior glenoid labrum S43.43- ☑
 syphilitic — see Syphilis
 tertiary — see Syphilis, tertiary
 thoracic root (nerve) NEC G54.3
 tonsillar fossa J35.9
 tooth, teeth K08.9
  white spot
   chewing surface K02.51
   pit and fissure surface K02.51
   smooth surface K02.61
 traumatic — see specific type of injury by site
 tricuspid (valve) I07.9
  nonrheumatic I36.9
 trigeminal nerve G50.9
 ulcerated or ulcerative — see Ulcer, skin
 uterus N85.9
 vagina N89.8
 vagus nerve G52.2
 valvular — see Endocarditis
 vascular I99.9
  affecting central nervous system I67.9
  following trauma NEC T14.8 ☑
  umbilical cord, complicating delivery O69.5 ☑
 vulva N90.89
 warty — see Verruca
 white spot (tooth)
  chewing surface K02.51
  pit and fissure surface K02.51
  smooth surface K02.61
Lethargic — see condition
Lethargy R53.83
Letterer-Siwe's disease C96.0
Leukemia, leukemic C95.9- ☑
 acute basophilic C94.8- ☑
 acute bilineal C95.0- ☑
 acute erythroid C94.0- ☑
 acute lymphoblastic C91.0- ☑
 acute megakaryoblastic C94.2- ☑
 acute megakaryocytic C94.2- ☑
 acute mixed lineage C95.0- ☑
 acute monoblastic (monoblastic/monocytic) C93.0- ☑
 acute monocytic (monoblastic/monocytic) C93.0- ☑
 acute myeloblastic (minimal differentiation) (with maturation) C92.0- ☑
 acute myeloid, NOS C92.0- ☑
  with
   11q23-abnormality C92.6- ☑
   dysplasia of remaining hematopoesis and/or myelodysplastic disease in its history C92.A- ☑ (following C92.6)
   multilineage dysplasia C92.A- ☑ (following C92.6)
   variation of MLL-gene C92.6- ☑
  M6 (a)(b) C94.0- ☑
  M7 C94.2- ☑
 acute myelomonocytic C92.5- ☑
 acute promyelocytic C92.4- ☑
 adult T-cell (HTLV-1-associated) (acute variant) (chronic variant) (lymphomatoid variant) (smouldering variant) C91.5- ☑
 aggressive NK-cell C94.8- ☑
 AML (1/ETO) (M0) (M1) (M2) (without a FAB classification) C92.0- ☑
 AML M3 C92.4- ☑
 AML M4 (Eo with inv(16) or t(16;16)) C92.5- ☑
 AML M5 C93.0- ☑
 AML M5a C93.0- ☑
 AML M5b C93.0- ☑
 AML Me with t (15;17) and variants C92.4- ☑
 atypical chronic myeloid, BCR/ABL-negative C92.2- ☑

☑ Additional Character Required — Refer to the Tabular List for Character Selection
▼ Subterms under main terms may continue to next column or page

Leukemia, leukemic — continued
- biphenotypic acute C95.0- ☑
- blast cell C95.0- ☑
- Burkitt-type, mature B-cell C91.A- ☑ (following C91.6)
- chronic eosinophilic — see Syndrome, hypereosinophilic, myeloid C94.8- ☑
- chronic lymphocytic, of B-cell type C91.1- ☑
- chronic monocytic C93.1- ☑
- chronic myelogenous (Philadelphia chromosome (Ph1) positive) (t(9;22)) (q34;q11) (with crisis of blast cells) C92.1- ☑
- chronic myeloid, BCR/ABL-positive C92.1- ☑
  - atypical, BCR/ABL-negative C92.2- ☑
- chronic myelomonocytic C93.1- ☑
- chronic neutrophilic D47.1
- CMML (-1) (-2) (with eosinophilia) C93.1- ☑
- granulocytic — see also Category C92 C92.9- ☑
- hairy cell C91.4- ☑
- juvenile myelomonocytic C93.3- ☑
- lymphoid C91.9- ☑
  - specified NEC C91.Z- ☑ (following C91.6)
- mast cell C94.3- ☑
- mature B-cell, Burkitt-type C91.A- ☑ (following C91.6)
- monocytic (subacute) C93.9- ☑
  - specified NEC C93.Z- ☑ (following C93.3)
- myelogenous — see also Category C92 C92.9- ☑
- myeloid C92.9- ☑
  - specified NEC C92.Z- ☑ (following C92.6)
- plasma cell C90.1- ☑
- plasmacytic C90.1- ☑
- prolymphocytic
  - of B-cell type C91.3- ☑
  - of T-cell type C91.6- ☑
- specified NEC C94.8- ☑
- stem cell, of unclear lineage C95.0- ☑
- subacute lymphocytic C91.9- ☑
- T-cell large granular lymphocytic C91.Z- ☑ (following C91.6)
- unspecified cell type C95.9- ☑
  - acute C95.0- ☑
  - chronic C95.1- ☑

Leukemoid reaction — see also Reaction, leukemoid D72.823

Leukoaraiosis (hypertensive) I67.81

Leukoariosis — see Leukoaraiosis

Leukocoria — see Disorder, globe, degenerated condition, leucocoria

Leukocytopenia D72.819

Leukocytosis D72.829
- eosinophilic D72.19

Leukoderma, leukodermia NEC L81.5
- syphilitic A51.39
  - late A52.79

Leukodystrophy E75.29

Leukoedema, oral epithelium K13.29

Leukoencephalitis G04.81
- acute (subacute) hemorrhagic G36.1
  - postimmunization or postvaccinal G04.02
- postinfectious G04.01
- subacute sclerosing A81.1
- van Bogaert's (sclerosing) A81.1

Leukoencephalopathy — see also Encephalopathy G93.49
- Binswanger's I67.3
- heroin vapor G92
- metachromatic E75.25
- multifocal (progressive) A81.2
- postimmunization and postvaccinal G04.02
- progressive multifocal A81.2
- reversible, posterior G93.6
- van Bogaert's (sclerosing) A81.1
- vascular, progressive I67.3

Leukoerythroblastosis D75.9

Leukokeratosis — see also Leukoplakia
- mouth K13.21
- nicotina palati K13.24
- oral mucosa K13.21
- tongue K13.21
- vocal cord J38.3

Leukokraurosis vulva (e) N90.4

Leukoma (cornea) — see also Opacity, cornea
- adherent H17.0- ☑
- interfering with central vision — see Opacity, cornea, central

Leukomalacia, cerebral, newborn P91.2
- periventricular P91.2

Leukomelanopathy, hereditary D72.0

Leukonychia (punctata) (striata) L60.8
- congenital Q84.4

Leukopathia unguium L60.8
- congenital Q84.4

Leukopenia D72.819
- basophilic D72.818
- chemotherapy (cancer) induced D70.1
- congenital D70.0
- cyclic D70.0
- drug induced NEC D70.2
  - due to cytoreductive cancer chemotherapy D70.1
- eosinophilic D72.818
- familial D70.0
- infantile genetic D70.0
- malignant D70.9
- periodic D70.0
- transitory neonatal P61.5

Leukopenic — see condition

Leukoplakia
- anus K62.89
- bladder (postinfectional) N32.89
- buccal K13.21
- cervix (uteri) N88.0
- esophagus K22.8
- gingiva K13.21
- hairy (oral mucosa) (tongue) K13.3
- kidney (pelvis) N28.89
- larynx J38.7
- lip K13.21
- mouth K13.21
- oral epithelium, including tongue (mucosa) K13.21
- palate K13.21
- pelvis (kidney) N28.89
- penis (infectional) N48.0
- rectum K62.89
- syphilitic (late) A52.79
- tongue K13.21
- ureter (postinfectional) N28.89
- urethra (postinfectional) N36.8
- uterus N85.8
- vagina N89.4
- vocal cord J38.3
- vulva N90.4

Leukorrhea N89.8
- due to Trichomonas (vaginalis) A59.00
- trichomonal A59.00

Leukosarcoma C85.9- ☑

Levocardia (isolated) Q24.1
- with situs inversus Q89.3

Levotransposition Q20.5

Lev's disease or syndrome (acquired complete heart block) I44.2

Levulosuria — see Fructosuria

Levurid L30.2

Lewy body (ies) (dementia) (disease) G31.83

Leyden-Moebius dystrophy G71.09

Leydig cell
- carcinoma
  - specified site — see Neoplasm, malignant, by site
  - unspecified site
    - female C56.9
    - male C62.9- ☑
- tumor
  - benign
    - specified site — see Neoplasm, benign, by site
    - unspecified site
      - female D27.- ☑
      - male D29.2- ☑
  - malignant
    - specified site — see Neoplasm, malignant, by site
    - unspecified site
      - female C56.- ☑
      - male C62.9- ☑
  - specified site — see Neoplasm, uncertain behavior, by site
  - unspecified site
    - female D39.1- ☑
    - male D40.1- ☑

Leydig-Sertoli cell tumor
- specified site — see Neoplasm, benign, by site
- unspecified site
  - female D27.- ☑
  - male D29.2- ☑

LGSIL (Low grade squamous intraepithelial lesion on cytologic smear of)
- anus R85.612
- cervix R87.612

LGSIL — continued
- vagina R87.622

Liar, pathologic F60.2

Libido
- decreased R68.82

Libman-Sacks disease M32.11

Lice (infestation) B85.2
- body (Pediculus corporis) B85.1
- crab B85.3
- head (Pediculus capitis) B85.0
- mixed (classifiable to more than one of the titles B85.0-B85.3) B85.4
- pubic (Phthirus pubis) B85.3

Lichen L28.0
- albus L90.0
  - penis N48.0
  - vulva N90.4
- amyloidosis E85.4 [L99]
- atrophicus L90.0
  - penis N48.0
  - vulva N90.4
- congenital Q82.8
- myxedematosus L98.5
- nitidus L44.1
- pilaris Q82.8
  - acquired L85.8
- planopilaris L66.1
- planus (chronicus) L43.9
  - annularis L43.8
  - bullous L43.1
  - follicular L66.1
  - hypertrophic L43.0
  - moniliformis L44.3
  - of Wilson L43.9
  - specified NEC L43.8
  - subacute (active) L43.3
  - tropicus L43.3
- ruber
  - acuminatus L44.0
  - moniliformis L44.3
  - planus L43.9
- sclerosus (et atrophicus) L90.0
  - penis N48.0
  - vulva N90.4
- scrofulosus (primary) (tuberculous) A18.4
- simplex (chronicus) (circumscriptus) L28.0
- striatus L44.2
- urticatus L28.2

Lichenification L28.0

Lichenoides tuberculosis (primary) A18.4

Lichtheim's disease or syndrome D51.0

Lien migrans D73.89

Ligament — see condition

Light
- for gestational age — see Light for dates
- headedness R42

Light-for-dates (infant) P05.00
- with weight of
  - 499 grams or less P05.01
  - 500-749 grams P05.02
  - 750-999 grams P05.03
  - 1000-1249 grams P05.04
  - 1250-1499 grams P05.05
  - 1500-1749 grams P05.06
  - 1750-1999 grams P05.07
  - 2000-2499 grams P05.08
  - 2500 grams and over P05.09
- affecting management of pregnancy O36.59- ☑
- and small-for-dates — see Small for dates
- specified NEC P05.09

Lightning (effects) (stroke) (struck by) T75.00 ☑
- burn — see Burn
- foot E53.8
- shock T75.01 ☑
- specified effect NEC T75.09 ☑

Lightwood-Albright syndrome N25.89

Lightwood's disease or syndrome (renal tubular acidosis) N25.89

Lignac (-de Toni) (-Fanconi) (-Debré) disease or syndrome E72.09
- with cystinosis E72.04

Ligneous thyroiditis E06.5

Likoff's syndrome I20.8

Limb — see condition

Limbic epilepsy personality syndrome F07.0

Limitation, limited
- activities due to disability Z73.6
- cardiac reserve — see Disease, heart

Limitation, limited — *continued*
  eye muscle duction, traumatic — *see* Strabismus, mechanical
  mandibular range of motion M26.52
Lindau (-von Hippel) **disease** Q85.8
Line(s)
  Beau's L60.4
  Harris' — *see* Arrest, epiphyseal
  Hudson's (cornea) — *see* Pigmentation, cornea, anterior
  Stähli's (cornea) — *see* Pigmentation, cornea, anterior
Linea corneae senilis — *see* Change, cornea, senile
Lingua
  geographica K14.1
  nigra (villosa) K14.3
  plicata K14.5
  tylosis K13.29
Lingual — *see* condition
Linguatulosis B88.8
Linitis (gastric) **plastica** C16.9
Lip — *see* condition
Lipedema — *see* Edema
Lipemia — *see also* Hyperlipidemia
  retina, retinalis E78.3
Lipidosis E75.6
  cerebral (infantile) (juvenile) (late) E75.4
  cerebroretinal E75.4
  cerebroside E75.22
  cholesterol (cerebral) E75.5
  glycolipid E75.21
  hepatosplenomegalic E78.3
  sphingomyelin — *see* Niemann-Pick disease or syndrome
  sulfatide E75.29
Lipoadenoma — *see* Neoplasm, benign, by site
Lipoblastoma — *see* Lipoma
Lipoblastomatosis — *see* Lipoma
Lipochondrodystrophy E76.01
Lipochrome histiocytosis (familial) D71
Lipodermatosclerosis — *see* Varix, leg, with, inflammation
  ulcerated — *see* Varix, leg, with, ulcer, with inflammation by site
Lipodystrophia progressiva E88.1
Lipodystrophy (progressive) E88.1
  insulin E88.1
  intestinal K90.81
  mesenteric K65.4
Lipofibroma — *see* Lipoma
Lipofuscinosis, neuronal (with ceroidosis) E75.4
Lipogranuloma, sclerosing L92.8
Lipogranulomatosis E78.89
Lipoid — *see also* condition
  histiocytosis D76.3
    essential E75.29
  nephrosis N04.9
  proteinosis of Urbach E78.89
Lipoidemia — *see* Hyperlipidemia
Lipoidosis — *see* Lipidosis
Lipoma D17.9
  fetal D17.9
    fat cell D17.9
  infiltrating D17.9
  intramuscular D17.9
  pleomorphic D17.9
  site classification
    arms (skin) (subcutaneous) D17.2- ☑
    connective tissue D17.30
      intra-abdominal D17.5
      intrathoracic D17.4
      peritoneum D17.79
      retroperitoneum D17.79
      specified site NEC D17.39
      spermatic cord D17.6
    face (skin) (subcutaneous) D17.0
    genitourinary organ NEC D17.72
    head (skin) (subcutaneous) D17.0
    intra-abdominal D17.5
    intrathoracic D17.4
    kidney D17.71
    legs (skin) (subcutaneous) D17.2- ☑
    neck (skin) (subcutaneous) D17.0
    peritoneum D17.79
    retroperitoneum D17.79
    skin D17.30
      specified site NEC D17.39
    specified site NEC D17.79
    spermatic cord D17.6
    subcutaneous D17.30

Lipoma — *continued*
  site classification — *continued*
    subcutaneous — *continued*
      specified site NEC D17.39
      trunk (skin) (subcutaneous) D17.1
      unspecified D17.9
  spindle cell D17.9
Lipomatosis E88.2
  dolorosa (Dercum) E88.2
  fetal — *see* Lipoma
  Launois-Bensaude E88.89
Lipomyoma — *see* Lipoma
Lipomyxoma — *see* Lipoma
Lipomyxosarcoma — *see* Neoplasm, connective tissue, malignant
Lipoprotein metabolism disorder E78.9
Lipoproteinemia E78.5
  broad-beta E78.2
  floating-beta E78.2
  hyper-pre-beta E78.1
Liposarcoma — *see also* Neoplasm, connective tissue, malignant
  dedifferentiated — *see* Neoplasm, connective tissue, malignant
  differentiated type — *see* Neoplasm, connective tissue, malignant
  embryonal — *see* Neoplasm, connective tissue, malignant
  mixed type — *see* Neoplasm, connective tissue, malignant
  myxoid — *see* Neoplasm, connective tissue, malignant
  pleomorphic — *see* Neoplasm, connective tissue, malignant
  round cell — *see* Neoplasm, connective tissue, malignant
  well differentiated type — *see* Neoplasm, connective tissue, malignant
Liposynovitis prepatellaris E88.89
Lipping, cervix N86
Lipschütz disease or ulcer N76.6
Lipuria R82.0
  schistosomiasis (bilharziasis) B65.0
Lisping F80.0
Lissauer's paralysis A52.17
Lissencephalia, lissencephaly Q04.3
Listeriosis, listerellosis A32.9
  congenital (disseminated) P37.2
  cutaneous A32.0
  neonatal, newborn (disseminated) P37.2
  oculoglandular A32.81
  specified NEC A32.89
Lithemia E79.0
Lithiasis — *see* Calculus
Lithosis J62.8
Lithuria R82.998
Litigation, anxiety concerning Z65.3
Little leaguer's elbow — *see* Epicondylitis, medial
Little's disease G80.9
Littre's
  gland — *see* condition
  hernia — *see* Hernia, abdomen
Littritis — *see* Urethritis
Livedo (annularis) (racemosa) (reticularis) R23.1
Liver — *see* condition
Living alone (problems with) Z60.2
  with handicapped person Z74.2
Lloyd's syndrome — *see* Adenomatosis, endocrine
Loa loa, loaiasis, loasis B74.3
Lobar — *see* condition
Lobomycosis B48.0
Lobo's disease B48.0
Lobotomy syndrome F07.0
Lobstein (-Ekman) **disease or syndrome** Q78.0
Lobster-claw hand Q71.6- ☑
Lobulation (congenital) — *see also* Anomaly, by site
  kidney, Q63.1
  liver, abnormal Q44.7
  spleen Q89.09
Lobule, lobular — *see* condition
Local, localized — *see* condition
Locked twins causing obstructed labor O66.1
Locked-in state G83.5
Locking
  joint — *see* Derangement, joint, specified type NEC
  knee — *see* Derangement, knee
Lockjaw — *see* Tetanus

Löffler's
  endocarditis I42.3
  eosinophilia J82.89
  pneumonia J82.89
  syndrome (eosinophilic pneumonitis) J82.89
Loiasis (with conjunctival infestation) (eyelid) B74.3
Lone Star fever A77.0
Long
  labor O63.9
    first stage O63.0
    second stage O63.1
  QT syndrome I45.81
Longitudinal stripes or grooves, nails L60.8
  congenital Q84.6
Long-term (current) (prophylactic) **drug therapy** (use of)
  agents affecting estrogen receptors and estrogen levels NEC Z79.818
  anastrozole (Arimidex) Z79.811
  antibiotics Z79.2
    short-term use — *omit code*
  anticoagulants Z79.01
  anti-inflammatory, non-steroidal (NSAID) Z79.1
  antiplatelet Z79.02
  antithrombotics Z79.02
  aromatase inhibitors Z79.811
  aspirin Z79.82
  birth control pill or patch Z79.3
  bisphosphonates Z79.83
  contraceptive, oral Z79.3
  drug, specified NEC Z79.899
  estrogen receptor downregulators Z79.818
  Evista Z79.810
  exemestane (Aromasin) Z79.811
  Fareston Z79.810
  fulvestrant (Faslodex) Z79.818
  gonadotropin-releasing hormone (GnRH) agonist Z79.818
  goserelin acetate (Zoladex) Z79.818
  hormone replacement Z79.890
  insulin Z79.4
  letrozole (Femara) Z79.811
  leuprolide acetate (leuprorelin) (Lupron) Z79.818
  megestrol acetate (Megace) Z79.818
  methadone for pain management Z79.891
  Nolvadex Z79.810
  non-steroidal anti-inflammatories (NSAID) Z79.1
  opiate analgesic Z79.891
  oral
    antidiabetic Z79.84
    contraceptive Z79.3
    hypoglycemic Z79.84
  raloxifene (Evista) Z79.810
  selective estrogen receptor modulators (SERMs) Z79.810
  steroids
    inhaled Z79.51
    systemic Z79.52
  tamoxifen (Nolvadex) Z79.810
  toremifene (Fareston) Z79.810
Loop
  intestine — *see* Volvulus
  vascular on papilla (optic) Q14.2
Loose — *see also* condition
  body
    joint M24.00
      ankle M24.07- ☑
      elbow M24.02- ☑
      hand M24.04- ☑
      hip M24.05- ☑
      knee M23.4- ☑
      shoulder (region) M24.01- ☑
      specified site NEC M24.08
      toe M24.07- ☑
      vertebra M24.08
      wrist M24.03- ☑
    knee M23.4- ☑
    sheath, tendon — *see* Disorder, tendon, specified type NEC
  cartilage — *see* Loose, body, joint
  skin and subcutaneous tissue (following bariatric surgery weight loss) (following dietary weight loss) L98.7
  tooth, teeth K08.89
Loosening
  aseptic
    joint prosthesis — *see* Complications, joint prosthesis, mechanical, loosening, by site

Loosening — continued
  epiphysis — see Osteochondropathy
  mechanical
    joint prosthesis — see Complications, joint prosthesis, mechanical, loosening, by site
Looser-Milkman (-Debray) **syndrome** M83.8
Lop ear (deformity) Q17.3
Lorain (-Levi) **short stature syndrome** E23.0
Lordosis M40.50
  acquired — see Lordosis, specified type NEC
  congenital Q76.429
    lumbar region Q76.426
    lumbosacral region Q76.427
    sacral region Q76.428
    sacrococcygeal region Q76.428
    thoracolumbar region Q76.425
  lumbar region M40.56
  lumbosacral region M40.57
  postsurgical M96.4
  postural — see Lordosis, specified type NEC
  rachitic (late effect) (sequelae) E64.3
  sequelae of rickets E64.3
  specified type NEC M40.40
    lumbar region M40.46
    lumbosacral region M40.47
    thoracolumbar region M40.45
  thoracolumbar region M40.55
  tuberculous A18.01
Loss (of)
  appetite — see also Anorexia R63.0
    hysterical F50.89
    nonorganic origin F50.89
    psychogenic F50.89
  blood — see Hemorrhage
  bone — see Loss, substance of, bone
  consciousness, transient R55
    traumatic — see Injury, intracranial
  control, sphincter, rectum R15.9
    nonorganic origin F98.1
  elasticity, skin R23.4
  family (member) in childhood Z62.898
  fluid (acute) E86.9
  function of labyrinth — see subcategory H83.2 ☑
  hair, nonscarring — see Alopecia
  hearing — see also Deafness
    central NOS H90.5
    conductive H90.2
      bilateral H90.0
      unilateral
        with
          restricted hearing on the contralateral side H90.A1- ☑
          unrestricted hearing on the contralateral side H90.1- ☑
    mixed conductive and sensorineural hearing loss H90.8
      bilateral H90.6
      unilateral
        with
          restricted hearing on the contralateral side H90.A3- ☑
          unrestricted hearing on the contralateral side H90.7- ☑
    neural NOS H90.5
    perceptive NOS H90.5
    sensorineural NOS H90.5
      bilateral H90.3
      unilateral
        with
          restricted hearing onthe contralateral side H90.A2- ☑
          unrestricted hearing on the contralateral side H90.4- ☑
    sensory NOS H90.5
  height R29.890
  limb or member, traumatic, current — see Amputation, traumatic
  love relationship in childhood Z62.898
  memory — see also Amnesia
    mild, following organic brain damage F06.8
  mind — see Psychosis
  occlusal vertical dimension of fully erupted teeth M26.37
  organ or part — see Absence, by site, acquired
  ossicles, ear (partial) H74.32- ☑
  parent in childhood Z63.4
  pregnancy, recurrent N96
    care in current pregnancy O26.2- ☑

Loss — continued
  pregnancy, recurrent — continued
    without current pregnancy N96
  recurrent pregnancy — see Loss, pregnancy, recurrent
  self-esteem, in childhood Z62.898
  sense of
    smell — see Disturbance, sensation, smell
    taste — see Disturbance, sensation, taste
    touch R20.8
  sensory R44.9
    dissociative F44.6
  sexual desire F52.0
  sight (acquired) (complete) (congenital) — see Blindness
  substance of
    bone — see Disorder, bone, density and structure, specified NEC
      horizontal alveolar K06.3
    cartilage — see Disorder, cartilage, specified type NEC
      auricle (ear) — see Disorder, pinna, specified type NEC
    vitreous (humor) H15.89
  tooth, teeth — see Absence, teeth, acquired
  vision, visual H54.7
    both eyes H54.3
    one eye H54.60
      left (normal vision on right) H54.62
      right (normal vision on left) H54.61
    specified as blindness — see Blindness
    subjective
      sudden H53.13- ☑
      transient H53.12- ☑
  vitreous — see Prolapse, vitreous
  voice — see Aphonia
  weight (abnormal) (cause unknown) R63.4
Louis-Bar syndrome (ataxia-telangiectasia) G11.3
Louping ill (encephalitis) A84.89
Louse, lousiness — see Lice
Low
  achiever, school Z55.3
  back syndrome M54.5
  basal metabolic rate R94.8
  birthweight (2499 grams or less) P07.10
    with weight of
      1000-1249 grams P07.14
      1250-1499 grams P07.15
      1500-1749 grams P07.16
      1750-1999 grams P07.17
      2000-2499 grams P07.18
    extreme (999 grams or less) P07.00
      with weight of
        499 grams or less P07.01
        500-749 grams P07.02
        750-999 grams P07.03
    for gestational age — see Light for dates
  blood pressure — see also Hypotension
    reading (incidental) (isolated) (nonspecific) R03.1
  cardiac reserve — see Disease, heart
  function — see also Hypofunction
    kidney N28.9
  hematocrit D64.9
  hemoglobin D64.9
  income Z59.6
  level of literacy Z55.0
  lying
    kidney N28.89
    organ or site, congenital — see Malposition, congenital
  output syndrome (cardiac) — see Failure, heart
  platelets (blood) — see Thrombocytopenia
  reserve, kidney N28.89
  salt syndrome E87.1
  self esteem R45.81
  set ears Q17.4
  vision H54.2X- ☑
    one eye (other eye normal) H54.50
      left (normal vision on right) H54.52A- ☑
      other eye blind — see Blindness
      right (normal vision on left) H54.511- ☑
Low-density-lipoprotein-type (LDL) **hyperlipoproteinemia** E78.00
Lowe's syndrome E72.03
Lown-Ganong-Levine syndrome I45.6
LSD reaction (acute) (without dependence) F16.90
  with dependence F16.20
L-shaped kidney Q63.8
LTBI (latent tuberculosis infection) Z22.7

Ludwig's angina or disease K12.2
Lues (venerea), **luetic** — see Syphilis
Luetscher's syndrome (dehydration) E86.0
Lumbago, lumbalgia M54.5
  with sciatica M54.4- ☑
    due to intervertebral disc disorder M51.17
  due to displacement, intervertebral disc M51.27
    with sciatica M51.17
Lumbar — see condition
Lumbarization, vertebra, congenital Q76.49
Lumbermen's itch B88.0
Lump — see also Mass
  breast N63.0
    axillary tail
      left N63.32
      right N63.31
    left
      lower inner quadrant N63.24
      lower outer quadrant N63.23
      overlapping quadrants N63.25
      unspecified quadrant N63.20
      upper inner quadrant N63.22
      upper outer quadrant N63.21
    right
      lower inner quadrant N63.14
      lower outer quadrant N63.13
      overlapping quadrants N63.15
      unspecified quadrant N63.10
      upper inner quadrant N63.12
      upper outer quadrant N63.11
    subareolar
      left N63.42
      right N63.41
Lunacy — see Psychosis
Lung — see condition
Lupoid (miliary) **of Boeck** D86.3
Lupus
  anticoagulant D68.62
    with
      hemorrhagic disorder D68.312
      hypercoagulable state D68.62
    finding without diagnosis R76.0
  discoid (local) L93.0
  erythematosus (discoid) (local) L93.0
    disseminated — see Lupus, erythematosus, systemic
    eyelid H01.129
      left H01.126
        lower H01.125
        upper H01.124
      right H01.123
        lower H01.122
        upper H01.121
    profundus L93.2
    specified NEC L93.2
    subacute cutaneous L93.1
    systemic M32.9
      with organ or system involvement M32.10
        endocarditis M32.11
        lung M32.13
        pericarditis M32.12
        renal (glomerular) M32.14
          tubulo-interstitial M32.15
        specified organ or system NEC M32.19
      drug-induced M32.0
      inhibitor (presence of) D68.62
        with
          hemorrhagic disorder D68.312
          hypercoagulable state D68.62
        finding without diagnosis R76.0
      specified NEC M32.8
  exedens A18.4
  hydralazine M32.0
    correct substance properly administered — see Table of Drugs and Chemicals, by drug, adverse effect
    overdose or wrong substance given or taken — see Table of Drugs and Chemicals, by drug, poisoning
  nephritis (chronic) M32.14
  nontuberculous, not disseminated L93.0
  panniculitis L93.2
  pernio (Besnier) D86.3
  systemic — see Lupus, erythematosus, systemic
  tuberculous A18.4
    eyelid A18.4
  vulgaris A18.4
    eyelid A18.4
Luteinoma D27.- ☑

☑ Subterms under main terms may continue to next column or page   ☑ Additional Character Required — Refer to the Tabular List for Character Selection   217

Loosening — Luteinoma

Lutembacher's disease or syndrome (atrial septal defect with mitral stenosis) Q21.1
Luteoma D27.- ☑
Lutz (-Splendore-de Almeida) **disease** — see Paracoccidioidomycosis
Luxation — see also Dislocation
    eyeball (nontraumatic) — see Luxation, globe
        birth injury P15.3
    globe, nontraumatic H44.82- ☑
    lacrimal gland — see Dislocation, lacrimal gland
    lens (old) (partial) (spontaneous)
        congenital Q12.1
        syphilitic A50.39
Lycanthropy F22
Lyell's syndrome L51.2
    due to drug L51.2
        correct substance properly administered — see Table of Drugs and Chemicals, by drug, adverse effect
        overdose or wrong substance given or taken — see Table of Drugs and Chemicals, by drug, poisoning
Lyme disease A69.20
Lymph
    gland or node — see condition
    scrotum — see Infestation, filarial
Lymphadenitis I88.9
    with ectopic or molar pregnancy O08.0
    acute L04.9
        axilla L04.2
        face L04.0
        head L04.0
        hip L04.3
        limb
            lower L04.3
            upper L04.2
        neck L04.0
        shoulder L04.2
        specified site NEC L04.8
        trunk L04.1
    anthracosis (occupational) J60
    any site, except mesenteric I88.9
        chronic I88.1
        subacute I88.1
    breast
        gestational — see Mastitis, obstetric
        puerperal, postpartum (nonpurulent) O91.22
    chancroidal (congenital) A57
    chronic I88.1
        mesenteric I88.0
    due to
        Brugia (malayi) B74.1
            timori B74.2
        chlamydial lymphogranuloma A55
        diphtheria (toxin) A36.89
        lymphogranuloma venereum A55
        Wuchereria bancrofti B74.0
    following ectopic or molar pregnancy O08.0
    gonorrheal A54.89
    infective — see Lymphadenitis, acute
    mesenteric (acute) (chronic) (nonspecific) (subacute) I88.0
        due to Salmonella typhi A01.09
        tuberculous A18.39
    mycobacterial A31.8
    purulent — see Lymphadenitis, acute
    pyogenic — see Lymphadenitis, acute
    regional, nonbacterial I88.8
    septic — see Lymphadenitis, acute
    subacute, unspecified site I88.1
    suppurative — see Lymphadenitis, acute
    syphilitic (early) (secondary) A51.49
        late A52.79
    tuberculous — see Tuberculosis, lymph gland
    venereal (chlamydial) A55
Lymphadenoid goiter E06.3
Lymphadenopathy (generalized) R59.1
    angioimmunoblastic, with dysproteinemia (AILD) C86.5
    due to toxoplasmosis (acquired) B58.89
        congenital (acute) (subacute) (chronic) P37.1
    localized R59.0
    syphilitic (early) (secondary) A51.49
Lymphadenosis R59.1
Lymphangiectasis I89.0
    conjunctiva H11.89
    postinfectional I89.0
    scrotum I89.0
Lymphangiectatic elephantiasis, nonfilarial I89.0

Lymphangioendothelioma D18.1
    malignant — see Neoplasm, connective tissue, malignant
Lymphangioleiomyomatosis J84.81
Lymphangioma D18.1
    capillary D18.1
    cavernous D18.1
    cystic D18.1
    malignant — see Neoplasm, connective tissue, malignant
Lymphangiomyoma D18.1
Lymphangiomyomatosis J84.81
Lymphangiosarcoma — see Neoplasm, connective tissue, malignant
Lymphangitis I89.1
    with
        abscess — code by site under Abscess
        cellulitis — code by site under Cellulitis
        ectopic or molar pregnancy O08.0
    acute L03.91
        abdominal wall L03.321
        ankle — see Lymphangitis, acute, lower limb
        arm — see Lymphangitis, acute, upper limb
        auricle (ear) — see Lymphangitis, acute, ear
        axilla L03.12- ☑
        back (any part) L03.322
        buttock L03.327
        cervical (meaning neck) L03.222
        cheek (external) L03.212
        chest wall L03.323
        digit
            finger — see Lymphangitis, acute, finger
            toe — see Lymphangitis, acute, toe
        ear (external) H60.1- ☑
        external auditory canal — see Lymphangitis, acute, ear
        eyelid — see Abscess, eyelid
        face NEC L03.212
        finger (intrathecal) (periosteal) (subcutaneous) (subcuticular) L03.02- ☑
        foot — see Lymphangitis, acute, lower limb
        gluteal (region) L03.327
        groin L03.324
        hand — see Lymphangitis, acute, upper limb
        head NEC L03.891
            face (any part, except ear, eye and nose) L03.212
        heel — see Lymphangitis, acute, lower limb
        hip — see Lymphangitis, acute, lower limb
        jaw (region) L03.212
        knee — see Lymphangitis, acute, lower limb
        leg — see Lymphangitis, acute, lower limb
        lower limb L03.12- ☑
            toe — see Lymphangitis, acute, toe
        navel L03.326
        neck (region) L03.222
        orbit, orbital — see Cellulitis, orbit
        pectoral (region) L03.323
        perineal, perineum L03.325
        scalp (any part) L03.891
        shoulder — see Lymphangitis, acute, upper limb
        specified site NEC L03.898
        thigh — see Lymphangitis, acute, lower limb
        thumb (intrathecal) (periosteal) (subcutaneous) (subcuticular) — see Lymphangitis, acute, finger
        toe (intrathecal) (periosteal) (subcutaneous) (subcuticular) L03.04- ☑
        trunk L03.329
            abdominal wall L03.321
            back (any part) L03.322
            buttock L03.327
            chest wall L03.323
            groin L03.324
            perineal, perineum L03.325
            umbilicus L03.326
        umbilicus L03.326
        upper limb L03.12- ☑
            axilla — see Lymphangitis, acute, axilla
            finger — see Lymphangitis, acute, finger
            thumb — see Lymphangitis, acute, finger
        wrist — see Lymphangitis, acute, upper limb
    breast
        gestational — see Mastitis, obstetric
    chancroidal A57
    chronic (any site) I89.1
    due to
        Brugia (malayi) B74.1

Lymphangitis — continued
    due to — continued
        Brugia — continued
            timori B74.2
        Wuchereria bancrofti B74.0
    following ectopic or molar pregnancy O08.89
    penis
        acute N48.29
        gonococcal (acute) (chronic) A54.09
    puerperal, postpartum, childbirth O86.89
    strumous, tuberculous A18.2
    subacute (any site) I89.1
    tuberculous — see Tuberculosis, lymph gland
Lymphatic (vessel) — see condition
Lymphatism E32.8
Lymphectasia I89.0
Lymphedema (acquired) — see also Elephantiasis
    congenital Q82.0
    hereditary (chronic) (idiopathic) Q82.0
    postmastectomy I97.2
    praecox I89.0
    secondary I89.0
    surgical NEC I97.89
        postmastectomy (syndrome) I97.2
Lymphoblastic — see condition
Lymphoblastoma (diffuse) — see Lymphoma, lymphoblastic (diffuse)
    giant follicular — see Lymphoma, lymphoblastic (diffuse)
    macrofollicular — see Lymphoma, lymphoblastic (diffuse)
Lymphocele I89.8
Lymphocytic
    chorioencephalitis (acute) (serous) A87.2
    choriomeningitis (acute) (serous) A87.2
    meningoencephalitis A87.2
Lymphocytoma, benign cutis L98.8
Lymphocytopenia D72.810
Lymphocytosis (symptomatic) D72.820
    infectious (acute) B33.8
Lymphoepithelioma — see Neoplasm, malignant, by site
Lymphogranuloma (malignant) — see also Lymphoma, Hodgkin
    chlamydial A55
    inguinale A55
    venereum (any site) (chlamydial) (with stricture of rectum) A55
Lymphogranulomatosis (malignant) — see also Lymphoma, Hodgkin
    benign (Boeck's sarcoid) (Schaumann's) D86.1
Lymphohistiocytosis, hemophagocytic (familial) D76.1
Lymphoid — see condition
Lymphoma (of) (malignant) C85.90
    adult T-cell (HTLV-1-associated) (acute variant) (chronic variant) (lymphomatoid variant) (smoldering variant) C91.5- ☑
    anaplastic large cell
        ALK-negative C84.7- ☑
        ALK-positive C84.6- ☑
        CD30-positive C84.6- ☑
        primary cutaneous C86.6
    angioimmunoblastic T-cell C86.5
    BALT C88.4
    B-cell C85.1- ☑
    blastic NK-cell C86.4
    blastic plasmacytoid dendritic cell neoplasm (BPDCN) C86.4
    B-precursor C83.5- ☑
    bronchial-associated lymphoid tissue [BALT-lymphoma] C88.4
    Burkitt (atypical) C83.7- ☑
    Burkitt-like C83.7- ☑
    centrocytic C83.1- ☑
    cutaneous follicle center C82.6- ☑
    cutaneous T-cell C84.A- ☑ (following C84.7)
    diffuse follicle center C82.5- ☑
    diffuse large cell C83.3- ☑
        anaplastic C83.3- ☑
        B-cell C83.3- ☑
        CD30-positive C83.3- ☑
        centroblastic C83.3- ☑
        immunoblastic C83.3- ☑
        plasmablastic C83.3- ☑
        subtype not specified C83.3- ☑
        T-cell rich C83.3- ☑
    enteropathy-type (associated) (intestinal) T-cell C86.2

Index

Lymphoma — Malaria, malarial

Malaria, malarial — *continued*
 recurrent B54
 remittent B54
 specified type NEC (parasitologically confirmed) B53.8
 spleen B54
 subtertian (fever) — *see* Malaria, falciparum
 tertian (benign) — *see also* Malaria, vivax
  malignant B50.9
 tropical B50.9
 typhoid B54
 vivax B51.9
  with
   complications NEC B51.8
   ruptured spleen B51.0
Malassez's disease (cystic) N50.89
Malassimilation K90.9
Maldescent, testis Q53.9
 bilateral Q53.20
  abdominal Q53.211
  perineal Q53.22
 unilateral Q53.10
  abdominal Q53.111
  perineal Q53.12
Maldevelopment — *see also* Anomaly
 brain Q07.9
 colon Q43.9
 hip Q74.2
  congenital dislocation Q65.2
   bilateral Q65.1
   unilateral Q65.0- ☑
 mastoid process Q75.8
 middle ear Q16.4
  except ossicles Q16.4
  ossicles Q16.3
 ossicles Q16.3
 spine Q76.49
 toe Q74.2
Male type pelvis Q74.2
 with disproportion (fetopelvic) O33.3 ☑
  causing obstructed labor O65.3
Malformation (congenital) — *see also* Anomaly
 adrenal gland Q89.1
 affecting multiple systems with skeletal changes NEC Q87.5
 alimentary tract Q45.9
  specified type NEC Q45.8
  upper Q40.9
   specified type NEC Q40.8
 aorta Q25.40
  absence Q25.41
  aneurysm, congenital Q25.43
  aplasia Q25.41
  atresia Q25.29
   aortic arch Q25.21
  coarctation (preductal) (postductal) Q25.1
  dilatation, congenital Q25.44
  hypoplasia Q25.42
  patent ductus arteriosus Q25.0
  specified type NEC Q25.49
  stenosis Q25.1
   supravalvular Q25.3
 aortic valve Q23.9
  specified NEC Q23.8
 arteriovenous, aneurysmatic (congenital) Q27.30
  brain Q28.2
   ruptured I60.8
    intracerebral I61.8
    intraparenchymal I61.8
    intraventricular I61.5
    subarachnoid I60.8
  cerebral — *see also* Malformation, arteriovenous, brain Q28.2
  peripheral Q27.30
   digestive system — *see* Angiodysplasia
    congenital Q27.33
   lower limb Q27.32
   other specified site Q27.39
   renal vessel Q27.34
   upper limb Q27.31
  precerebral vessels (nonruptured) Q28.0
 auricle
  ear (congenital) Q17.3
   acquired H61.119
    left H61.112
     with right H61.113
    right H61.111
     with left H61.113
  bile duct Q44.5

Malformation — *continued*
 bladder Q64.79
  aplasia Q64.5
  diverticulum Q64.6
  exstrophy — *see* Exstrophy, bladder
  neck obstruction Q64.31
 bone Q79.9
  face Q75.9
   specified type NEC Q75.8
  skull Q75.9
   specified type NEC Q75.8
 brain (multiple) Q04.9
  arteriovenous Q28.2
  specified type NEC Q04.8
 branchial cleft Q18.2
 breast Q83.9
  specified type NEC Q83.8
 broad ligament Q50.6
 bronchus Q32.4
 bursa Q79.9
 cardiac
  chambers Q20.9
   specified type NEC Q20.8
  septum Q21.9
   specified type NEC Q21.8
 cerebral Q04.9
  vessels Q28.3
 cervix uteri Q51.9
  specified type NEC Q51.828
 Chiari
  Type I G93.5
  Type II Q07.01
 choroid (congenital) Q14.3
  plexus Q07.8
 circulatory system Q28.9
 cochlea Q16.5
 cornea Q13.4
 coronary vessels Q24.5
 corpus callosum (congenital) Q04.0
 diaphragm Q79.1
 digestive system NEC, specified type NEC Q45.8
 dura Q07.9
  brain Q04.9
  spinal Q06.9
 ear Q17.9
  causing impairment of hearing Q16.9
  external Q17.9
   accessory auricle Q17.0
   causing impairment of hearing Q16.9
    absence of
     auditory canal Q16.1
     auricle Q16.0
   macrotia Q17.1
   microtia Q17.2
   misplacement Q17.4
   misshapen NEC Q17.3
   prominence Q17.5
   specified type NEC Q17.8
  inner Q16.5
  middle Q16.4
   absence of eustachian tube Q16.2
   ossicles (fusion) Q16.3
  ossicles Q16.3
  specified type NEC Q17.8
 epididymis Q55.4
 esophagus Q39.9
  specified type NEC Q39.8
 eye Q15.9
  lid Q10.3
  specified NEC Q15.8
 fallopian tube Q50.6
 genital organ — *see* Anomaly, genitalia
 great
  artery Q25.9
   aorta — *see* Malformation, aorta
   pulmonary artery — *see* Malformation, pulmonary, artery
   specified type NEC Q25.8
  vein Q26.9
   anomalous
    portal venous connection Q26.5
    pulmonary venous connection Q26.4
     partial Q26.3
     total Q26.2
   persistent left superior vena cava Q26.1
   portal vein-hepatic artery fistula Q26.6
   specified type NEC Q26.8
   vena cava stenosis, congenital Q26.0
 gum Q38.6

Malformation — *continued*
 hair Q84.2
 heart Q24.9
  specified type NEC Q24.8
 integument Q84.9
  specified type NEC Q84.8
 internal ear Q16.5
 intestine Q43.9
  specified type NEC Q43.8
 iris Q13.2
 joint Q74.9
  ankle Q74.2
  lumbosacral Q76.49
  sacroiliac Q74.2
  specified type NEC Q74.8
 kidney Q63.9
  accessory Q63.0
  giant Q63.3
  horseshoe Q63.1
  hydronephrosis Q62.0
  malposition Q63.2
  specified type NEC Q63.8
 lacrimal apparatus Q10.6
 lingual Q38.3
 lip Q38.0
 liver Q44.7
 lung Q33.9
 meninges or membrane (congenital) Q07.9
  cerebral Q04.8
  spinal (cord) Q06.9
 middle ear Q16.4
  ossicles Q16.3
 mitral valve Q23.9
  specified NEC Q23.8
 Mondini's (congenital) (malformation, cochlea) Q16.5
 mouth (congenital) Q38.6
 multiple types NEC Q89.7
 musculoskeletal system Q79.9
 myocardium Q24.8
 nail Q84.6
 nervous system (central) Q07.9
 nose Q30.9
  specified type NEC Q30.8
 optic disc Q14.2
 orbit Q10.7
 ovary Q50.39
 palate Q38.5
 parathyroid gland Q89.2
 pelvic organs or tissues NEC
  in pregnancy or childbirth O34.8- ☑
   causing obstructed labor O65.5
 penis Q55.69
  aplasia Q55.5
  curvature (lateral) Q55.61
  hypoplasia Q55.62
 pericardium Q24.8
 peripheral vascular system Q27.9
  specified type NEC Q27.8
 pharynx Q38.8
 precerebral vessels Q28.1
 prostate Q55.4
 pulmonary
  arteriovenous Q25.72
  artery Q25.9
   atresia Q25.5
   specified type NEC Q25.79
   stenosis Q25.6
  valve Q22.3
 renal artery Q27.2
 respiratory system Q34.9
 retina Q14.1
 scrotum — *see* Malformation, testis and scrotum
 seminal vesicles Q55.4
 sense organs NEC Q07.9
 skin Q82.9
 specified NEC Q89.8
 spinal
  cord Q06.9
  nerve root Q07.8
 spine Q76.49
  kyphosis — *see* Kyphosis, congenital
  lordosis — *see* Lordosis, congenital
 spleen Q89.09
 stomach Q40.3
  specified type NEC Q40.2
 teeth, tooth K00.9
 tendon Q79.9
 testis and scrotum Q55.20
  aplasia Q55.0

☑ **Additional Character Required — Refer to the Tabular List for Character Selection**   ▽ Subterms under main terms may continue to next column or page

Malformation — continued
 testis and scrotum — continued
  hypoplasia Q55.1
  polyorchism Q55.21
  retractile testis Q55.22
  scrotal transposition Q55.23
  specified NEC Q55.29
 thorax, bony Q76.9
 throat Q38.8
 thyroid gland Q89.2
 tongue (congenital) Q38.3
  hypertrophy Q38.2
  tie Q38.1
 trachea Q32.1
 tricuspid valve Q22.9
  specified type NEC Q22.8
 umbilical cord NEC (complicating delivery) O69.89 ☑
 umbilicus Q89.9
 ureter Q62.8
  agenesis Q62.4
  duplication Q62.5
  malposition — see Malposition, congenital, ureter
  obstructive defect — see Defect, obstructive, ureter
  vesico-uretero-renal reflux Q62.7
 urethra Q64.79
  aplasia Q64.5
  duplication Q64.74
  posterior valves Q64.2
  prolapse Q64.71
  stricture Q64.32
 urinary system Q64.9
 uterus Q51.9
  specified type NEC Q51.818
 vagina Q52.4
 vas deferens Q55.4
  atresia Q55.3
 vascular system, peripheral Q27.9
 venous — see Anomaly, vein(s)
 vulva Q52.70
Malfunction — see also Dysfunction
 cardiac electronic device T82.119 ☑
  electrode T82.110 ☑
  pulse generator T82.111 ☑
  specified type NEC T82.118 ☑
 catheter device NEC T85.618 ☑
  cystostomy T83.010 ☑
  dialysis (renal) (vascular) T82.41 ☑
   intraperitoneal T85.611 ☑
  infusion NEC T82.514 ☑
   cranial T85.610 ☑
   epidural T85.610 ☑
   intrathecal T85.610 ☑
   spinal T85.610 ☑
   subarachnoid T85.610 ☑
   subdural T85.610 ☑
  urinary — see also Breakdown, device, catheter
    T83.018 ☑
 colostomy K94.03
  valve K94.03
 cystostomy (stoma) N99.512
  catheter T83.010 ☑
 enteric stoma K94.13
 enterostomy K94.13
 esophagostomy K94.33
 gastroenteric K31.89
 gastrostomy K94.23
 ileostomy K94.13
  valve K94.13
 intrathecal infusion pump T85.615 ☑
 jejunostomy K94.13
 nervous system device, implant or graft, specified NEC
    T85.615 ☑
 pacemaker — see Malfunction, cardiac electronic de-
    vice
 prosthetic device, internal — see Complications, pros-
    thetic device, by site, mechanical
 tracheostomy J95.03
 urinary device NEC — see Complication, genitourinary,
    device, urinary, mechanical
 valve
  colostomy K94.03
  heart T82.09 ☑
  ileostomy K94.13
 vascular graft or shunt NEC — see Complication, car-
    diovascular device, mechanical, vascular
 ventricular (communicating shunt) T85.01 ☑
Malherbe's tumor — see Neoplasm, skin, benign
Malibu disease L98.8

Malignancy — see also Neoplasm, malignant, by site
 unspecified site (primary) C80.1
Malignant — see condition
Malingerer, malingering Z76.5
Mallet finger (acquired) — see Deformity, finger, mallet
  finger
  congenital Q74.0
  sequelae of rickets E64.3
Malleus A24.0
Mallory's bodies R89.7
Mallory-Weiss syndrome K22.6
Malnutrition E46
 degree
  first E44.1
  mild (protein) E44.1
  moderate (protein) E44.0
  second E44.0
  severe (protein-energy) E43
   intermediate form E42
    with
     kwashiorkor (and marasmus) E42
     marasmus E41
  third E43
 following gastrointestinal surgery K91.2
 intrauterine
  light-for-dates — see Light for dates
  small-for-dates — see Small for dates
 lack of care, or neglect (child) (infant) T76.02 ☑
  confirmed T74.02 ☑
 malignant E40
 protein E46
  calorie E46
   mild E44.1
   moderate E44.0
   severe E43
    intermediate form E42
     with
      kwashiorkor (and marasmus) E42
      marasmus E41
  energy E46
   mild E44.1
   moderate E44.0
   severe E43
    intermediate form E42
     with
      kwashiorkor (and marasmus) E42
      marasmus E41
 severe (protein-energy) E43
  with
   kwashiorkor (and marasmus) E42
   marasmus E41
Malocclusion (teeth) M26.4
 Angle's M26.219
  class I M26.211
  class II M26.212
  class III M26.213
 due to
  abnormal swallowing M26.59
  mouth breathing M26.59
  tongue, lip or finger habits M26.59
 temporomandibular (joint) M26.69
Malposition
 cervix — see Malposition, uterus
 congenital
  adrenal (gland) Q89.1
  alimentary tract Q45.8
   lower Q43.8
   upper Q40.8
  aorta Q25.49
  appendix Q43.8
  arterial trunk Q20.0
  artery (peripheral) Q27.8
   coronary Q24.5
   digestive system Q27.8
   lower limb Q27.8
   pulmonary Q25.79
   specified site NEC Q27.8
   upper limb Q27.8
  auditory canal Q17.8
   causing impairment of hearing Q16.9
  auricle (ear) Q17.4
   causing impairment of hearing Q16.9
   cervical Q18.2
  biliary duct or passage Q44.5
  bladder (mucosa) — see Exstrophy, bladder
  brachial plexus Q07.8
  brain tissue Q04.8
  breast Q83.8

Malposition — continued
 congenital — continued
  bronchus Q32.4
  cecum Q43.8
  clavicle Q74.0
  colon Q43.8
  digestive organ or tract NEC Q45.8
   lower Q43.8
   upper Q40.8
  ear (auricle) (external) Q17.4
   ossicles Q16.3
  endocrine (gland) NEC Q89.2
  epiglottis Q31.8
  eustachian tube Q17.8
  eye Q15.8
  facial features Q18.8
  fallopian tube Q50.6
  finger(s) Q68.1
   supernumerary Q69.0
  foot Q66.9- ☑
  gallbladder Q44.1
  gastrointestinal tract Q45.8
  genitalia, genital organ(s) or tract
   female Q52.8
    external Q52.79
    internal NEC Q52.8
   male Q55.8
  glottis Q31.8
  hand Q68.1
  heart Q24.8
   dextrocardia Q24.0
    with complete transposition of viscera Q89.3
  hepatic duct Q44.5
  hip (joint) Q65.89
  intestine (large) (small) Q43.8
   with anomalous adhesions, fixation or malrota-
     tion Q43.3
  joint NEC Q68.8
  kidney Q63.2
  larynx Q31.8
  limb Q68.8
   lower Q68.8
   upper Q68.8
  liver Q44.7
  lung (lobe) Q33.8
  nail(s) Q84.6
  nerve Q07.8
  nervous system NEC Q07.8
  nose, nasal (septum) Q30.8
  organ or site not listed — see Anomaly, by site
  ovary Q50.39
  pancreas Q45.3
  parathyroid (gland) Q89.2
  patella Q74.1
  peripheral vascular system Q27.8
  pituitary (gland) Q89.2
  respiratory organ or system NEC Q34.8
  rib (cage) Q76.6
   supernumerary in cervical region Q76.5
  scapula Q74.0
  shoulder Q74.0
  spinal cord Q06.8
  spleen Q89.09
  sternum NEC Q76.7
  stomach Q40.2
  symphysis pubis Q74.2
  thymus (gland) Q89.2
  thyroid (gland) (tissue) Q89.2
   cartilage Q31.8
  toe(s) Q66.9- ☑
   supernumerary Q69.2
  tongue Q38.3
  trachea Q32.1
  ureter Q62.60
   deviation Q62.61
   displacement Q62.62
   ectopia Q62.63
   specified type NEC Q62.69
  uterus Q51.818
  vein(s) (peripheral) Q27.8
   great Q26.8
  vena cava (inferior) (superior) Q26.8
 device, implant or graft — see also Complications, by
   site and type, mechanical T85.628 ☑
  arterial graft NEC — see Complication, cardiovascu-
    lar device, mechanical, vascular
  breast (implant) T85.42 ☑
  catheter NEC T85.628 ☑

Malposition — *continued*
  device, implant or graft — *see also* Complications, by
      site and type, mechanical — *continued*
    catheter — *continued*
      cystostomy T83.020 ☑
      dialysis (renal) T82.42 ☑
        intraperitoneal T85.621 ☑
      infusion NEC T82.524 ☑
        spinal (epidural) (subdural) T85.620 ☑
      urinary — *see also* Displacement, device,
          catheter, urinary T83.028 ☑
    electronic (electrode) (pulse generator) (stimulator)
      bone T84.320 ☑
      cardiac T82.129 ☑
        electrode T82.120 ☑
        pulse generator T82.121 ☑
        specified type NEC T82.128 ☑
      nervous system — *see* Complication, prosthetic
          device, mechanical, electronic nervous
          system stimulator
      urinary — *see* Complication, genitourinary, de-
          vice, urinary, mechanical
    fixation, internal (orthopedic) NEC — *see* Complica-
        tion, fixation device, mechanical
    gastrointestinal — *see* Complications, prosthetic
        device, mechanical, gastrointestinal device
    genital NEC T83.428 ☑
      intrauterine contraceptive device (string)
          T83.32 ☑
      penile prosthesis (cylinder) (implanted) (pump)
          (reservoir) T83.420 ☑
      testicular prosthesis T83.421 ☑
    heart NEC — *see* Complication, cardiovascular de-
        vice, mechanical
    joint prosthesis — *see* Complication, joint prosthe-
        sis, mechanical
    ocular NEC — *see* Complications, prosthetic device,
        mechanical, ocular device
    orthopedic NEC — *see* Complication, orthopedic,
        device, mechanical
    specified NEC T85.628 ☑
    urinary NEC — *see also* Complication, genitourinary,
        device, urinary, mechanical
      graft T83.22 ☑
    vascular NEC — *see* Complication, cardiovascular
        device, mechanical
    ventricular intracranial shunt T85.02 ☑
  fetus — *see* Pregnancy, complicated by (management
      affected by), presentation, fetal
  gallbladder K82.8
  gastrointestinal tract, congenital Q45.8
  heart, congenital NEC Q24.8
  joint prosthesis — *see* Complications, joint prosthesis,
      mechanical, displacement, by site
  stomach K31.89
    congenital Q40.2
  tooth, teeth, fully erupted M26.30
  uterus (acute) (acquired) (adherent) (asymptomatic)
      (postinfectional) (postpartal, old) N85.4
    anteflexion or anteversion N85.4
      congenital Q51.818
    flexion N85.4
      lateral — *see* Lateroversion, uterus
    inversion N85.5
    lateral (flexion) (version) — *see* Lateroversion, uterus
      in pregnancy or childbirth — *see* subcategory
          O34.5 ☑
    retroflexion or retroversion — *see* Retroversion,
        uterus
Malposture R29.3
Malrotation
  cecum Q43.3
  colon Q43.3
  intestine Q43.3
  kidney Q63.2
Malta fever — *see* Brucellosis
Maltreatment
  adult
    abandonment
      confirmed T74.01 ☑
      suspected T76.01 ☑
    bullying
      confirmed T74.31 ☑
      suspected T76.31 ☑
    confirmed T74.91 ☑
    history of Z91.419

Maltreatment — *continued*
  adult — *continued*
    intimidation (through social media)
      confirmed T74.31 ☑
      suspected T76.31 ☑
    neglect
      confirmed T74.01 ☑
      suspected T76.01 ☑
    physical abuse
      confirmed T74.11 ☑
      suspected T76.11 ☑
    psychological abuse
      confirmed T74.31 ☑
      history of Z91.411
      suspected T76.31 ☑
    sexual abuse
      confirmed T74.21 ☑
      suspected T76.21 ☑
    suspected T76.91 ☑
  child
    abandonment
      confirmed T74.02 ☑
      suspected T76.02 ☑
    bullying
      confirmed T74.32 ☑
      suspected T76.32 ☑
    confirmed T74.92 ☑
    history of — *see* History, personal (of), abuse
    intimidation (through social media)
      confirmed T74.32 ☑
      suspected T76.32 ☑
    neglect
      confirmed T74.02 ☑
      history of — *see* History, personal (of), abuse
      suspected T76.02 ☑
    physical abuse
      confirmed T74.12 ☑
      history of — *see* History, personal (of), abuse
      suspected T76.12 ☑
    psychological abuse
      confirmed T74.32 ☑
      history of — *see* History, personal (of), abuse
      suspected T76.32 ☑
    sexual abuse
      confirmed T74.22 ☑
      history of — *see* History, personal (of), abuse
      suspected T76.22 ☑
    suspected T76.92 ☑
  personal history of Z91.89
Maltworker's lung J67.4
Malunion, fracture — *see* Fracture, by site
Mammillitis N61.0
  puerperal, postpartum O91.02
Mammitis — *see* Mastitis
Mammogram (examination) Z12.39
  routine Z12.31
Mammoplasia N62
Management (of)
  bone conduction hearing device (implanted) Z45.320
  cardiac pacemaker NEC Z45.018
  cerebrospinal fluid drainage device Z45.41
  cochlear device (implanted) Z45.321
  contraceptive Z30.9
    specified NEC Z30.8
  implanted device Z45.9
    specified NEC Z45.89
  infusion pump Z45.1
  procreative Z31.9
    male factor infertility in female Z31.81
    specified NEC Z31.89
  prosthesis (external) — *see also* Fitting Z44.9
    implanted Z45.9
      specified NEC Z45.89
  renal dialysis catheter Z49.01
  vascular access device Z45.2
Mangled — *see* specified injury by site
Mania (monopolar) — *see also* Disorder, mood, manic
    episode
  with psychotic symptoms F30.2
  without psychotic symptoms F30.10
    mild F30.11
    moderate F30.12
    severe F30.13
  Bell's F30.8
  chronic (recurrent) F31.89
  hysterical F44.89
  puerperal F30.8

Mania — *continued*
  recurrent F31.89
Manic depression F31.9
Manic-depressive insanity, psychosis, or syndrome
    — *see* Disorder, bipolar
Mannosidosis E77.1
Mansonelliasis, mansonellosis B74.4
Manson's
  disease B65.1
  schistosomiasis B65.1
Manual — *see* condition
Maple-bark-stripper's lung (disease) J67.6
Maple-syrup-urine disease E71.0
Marable's syndrome (celiac artery compression) I77.4
Marasmus E41
  due to malnutrition E41
  intestinal E41
  nutritional E41
  senile R54
  tuberculous NEC — *see* Tuberculosis
Marble
  bones Q78.2
  skin R23.8
Marburg virus disease A98.3
March
  fracture — *see* Fracture, traumatic, stress, by site
  hemoglobinuria D59.6
Marchesani (-Weill) **syndrome** Q87.0
Marchiafava (-Bignami) **syndrome or disease** G37.1
Marchiafava-Micheli syndrome D59.5
Marcus Gunn's syndrome Q07.8
Marfan's syndrome — *see* Syndrome, Marfan's
Marie-Bamberger disease — *see* Osteoarthropathy,
    hypertrophic, specified NEC
Marie-Charcot-Tooth neuropathic muscular atrophy
    G60.0
Marie's
  cerebellar ataxia (late-onset) G11.2
  disease or syndrome (acromegaly) E22.0
Marie-Strümpell arthritis, disease or spondylitis —
    see Spondylitis, ankylosing
Marion's disease (bladder neck obstruction) N32.0
Marital conflict Z63.0
Mark
  port wine Q82.5
  raspberry Q82.5
  strawberry Q82.5
  stretch L90.6
  tattoo L81.8
Marker heterochromatin — *see* Extra, marker chromo-
    somes
Maroteaux-Lamy syndrome (mild) (severe) E76.29
Marrow (bone)
  arrest D61.9
  poor function D75.89
Marseilles fever A77.1
Marsh fever — *see* Malaria
Marshall's (hidrotic) **ectodermal dysplasia** Q82.4
Marsh's disease (exophthalmic goiter) E05.00
  with storm E05.01
Masculinization (female) **with adrenal hyperplasia**
    E25.9
  congenital E25.0
Masculinovoblastoma D27.- ☑
Masochism (sexual) F65.51
Mason's lung J62.8
Mass
  abdominal R19.00
    epigastric R19.06
    generalized R19.07
    left lower quadrant R19.04
    left upper quadrant R19.02
    periumbilic R19.05
    right lower quadrant R19.03
    right upper quadrant R19.01
    specified site NEC R19.09
  breast — *see also* Lump, breast N63.0
  chest R22.2
  cystic — *see* Cyst
  ear H93.8- ☑
  head R22.0
  intra-abdominal (diffuse) (generalized) — *see* Mass,
    abdominal
  kidney N28.89
  liver R16.0
  localized (skin) R22.9
    chest R22.2

Mass — *continued*
  localized — *continued*
    head R22.0
    limb
      lower R22.4- ☑
      upper R22.3- ☑
    neck R22.1
    trunk R22.2
  lung R91.8
  malignant — *see* Neoplasm, malignant, by site
  neck R22.1
  pelvic (diffuse) (generalized) — *see* Mass, abdominal
  specified organ NEC — *see* Disease, by site
  splenic R16.1
  substernal thyroid — *see* Goiter
  superficial (localized) R22.9
  umbilical (diffuse) (generalized) R19.09
Massive — *see* condition
Mast cell
  disease, systemic tissue D47.02
  leukemia C94.3- ☑
  neoplasm
    malignant C96.20
      specified type NEC C96.29
    of uncertain behavior NEC D47.09
  sarcoma C96.22
  tumor D47.09
Mastalgia N64.4
Masters-Allen syndrome N83.8
Mastitis (acute) (diffuse) (nonpuerperal) (subacute) N61.0
  with abscess N61.1
  chronic (cystic) — *see* Mastopathy, cystic
  cystic (Schimmelbusch's type) — *see* Mastopathy, cystic
  fibrocystic — *see* Mastopathy, cystic
  granulomatous N61.2- ☑
  infective N61.0
    newborn P39.0
  interstitial, gestational or puerperal — *see* Mastitis, obstetric
  neonatal (noninfective) P83.4
    infective P39.0
  obstetric (interstitial) (nonpurulent)
    associated with
      lactation O91.23
      pregnancy O91.21- ☑
      puerperium O91.22
    purulent
      associated with
        lactation O91.13
        pregnancy O91.11- ☑
        puerperium O91.12
  periductal — *see* Ectasia, mammary duct
  phlegmonous — *see* Mastopathy, cystic
  plasma cell — *see* Ectasia, mammary duct
  without abscess N61.0
Mastocytoma (extracutaneous) D47.09
  malignant C96.29
  solitary D47.01
Mastocytosis D47.09
  aggressive systemic C96.21
  cutaneous (diffuse) (maculopapular) D47.01
    congenital Q82.2
    of neonatal onset Q82.2
    of newborn onset Q82.2
  indolent systemic D47.02
  isolated bone marrow D47.02
  malignant C96.29
  systemic (indolent) (smoldering)
    with an associated hematological non-mast cell lineage disease (SM-AHNMD) D47.02
Mastodynia N64.4
Mastoid — *see* condition
Mastoidalgia — *see* subcategory H92.0 ☑
Mastoiditis (coalescent) (hemorrhagic) (suppurative) H70.9- ☑
  acute, subacute H70.00- ☑
    complicated NEC H70.09- ☑
    subperiosteal H70.01- ☑
  chronic (necrotic) (recurrent) H70.1- ☑
  in (due to)
    infectious disease NEC B99 ☑ *[H75.0-]* ☑
    parasitic disease NEC B89 *[H75.0-]* ☑
    tuberculosis A18.03
  petrositis — *see* Petrositis
  postauricular fistula — *see* Fistula, postauricular
  specified NEC H70.89- ☑
  tuberculous A18.03

Mastopathy, mastopathia N64.9
  chronica cystica — *see* Mastopathy, cystic
  cystic (chronic) (diffuse) N60.1- ☑
    with epithelial proliferation N60.3- ☑
  diffuse cystic — *see* Mastopathy, cystic
  estrogenic, oestrogenica N64.89
  ovarian origin N64.89
Mastoplasia, mastoplastia N62
Masturbation (excessive) F98.8
Maternal care (for) — *see* Pregnancy (complicated by) (management affected by)
Matheiu's disease (leptospiral jaundice) A27.0
Mauclaire's disease or osteochondrosis — *see* Osteochondrosis, juvenile, hand, metacarpal
Maxcy's disease A75.2
Maxilla, maxillary — *see* condition
May (-Hegglin) **anomaly or syndrome** D72.0
McArdle (-Schmid)(-Pearson) **disease** (glycogen storage) E74.04
McCune-Albright syndrome Q78.1
McQuarrie's syndrome (idiopathic familial hypoglycemia) E16.2
Meadow's syndrome Q86.1
Measles (black) (hemorrhagic) (suppressed) B05.9
  with
    complications NEC B05.89
    encephalitis B05.0
    intestinal complications B05.4
    keratitis (keratoconjunctivitis) B05.81
    meningitis B05.1
    otitis media B05.3
    pneumonia B05.2
  French — *see* Rubella
  German — *see* Rubella
  Liberty — *see* Rubella
Meatitis, urethral — *see* Urethritis
Meatus, meatal — *see* condition
Meat-wrappers' asthma J68.9
Meckel-Gruber syndrome Q61.9
Meckel's diverticulitis, diverticulum (displaced) (hypertrophic) Q43.0
  malignant — *see* Table of Neoplasms, small intestine, malignant
Meconium
  ileus, newborn P76.0
    in cystic fibrosis E84.11
    meaning meconium plug (without cystic fibrosis) P76.0
  obstruction, newborn P76.0
    due to fecaliths P76.0
    in mucoviscidosis E84.11
  peritonitis P78.0
  plug syndrome (newborn) NEC P76.0
Median — *see also* condition
  arcuate ligament syndrome I77.4
  bar (prostate) (vesical orifice) — *see* Hyperplasia, prostate
  rhomboid glossitis K14.2
Mediastinal shift R93.89
Mediastinitis (acute) (chronic) J98.51
  syphilitic A52.73
  tuberculous A15.8
Mediastinopericarditis — *see also* Pericarditis
  acute I30.9
  adhesive I31.0
  chronic I31.8
    rheumatic I09.2
Mediastinum, mediastinal — *see* condition
Medicine poisoning — *see* Table of Drugs and Chemicals, by drug, poisoning
Mediterranean
  fever — *see* Brucellosis
    familial M04.1
    tick A77.1
  kala-azar B55.0
  leishmaniasis B55.0
  tick fever A77.1
Medulla — *see* condition
Medullary cystic kidney Q61.5
Medullated fibers
  optic (nerve) Q14.8
  retina Q14.1
Medulloblastoma
  desmoplastic C71.6
  specified site — *see* Neoplasm, malignant, by site
  unspecified site C71.6

Medulloepithelioma — *see also* Neoplasm, malignant, by site
  teratoid — *see* Neoplasm, malignant, by site
Medullomyoblastoma
  specified site — *see* Neoplasm, malignant, by site
  unspecified site C71.6
Meekeren-Ehlers-Danlos syndrome — *see also* Syndrome, Ehlers-Danlos Q79.69
Megacolon (acquired) (functional) (not Hirschsprung's disease) (in) K59.39
  Chagas' disease B57.32
  congenital, congenitum (aganglionic) Q43.1
  Hirschsprung's (disease) Q43.1
  toxic NEC K59.31
    due to Clostridium difficile
      not specified as recurrent A04.72
      recurrent A04.71
Megaesophagus (functional) K22.0
  congenital Q39.5
  in (due to) Chagas' disease B57.31
Megalencephaly Q04.5
Megalerythema (epidemic) B08.3
Megaloappendix Q43.8
Megalocephalus, megalocephaly NEC Q75.3
Megalocornea Q15.8
  with glaucoma Q15.0
Megalocytic anemia D53.1
Megalodactylia (fingers) (thumbs) (congenital) Q74.0
  toes Q74.2
Megaloduodenum Q43.8
Megaloesophagus (functional) K22.0
  congenital Q39.5
Megalogastria (acquired) K31.89
  congenital Q40.2
Megalophthalmos Q11.3
Megalopsia H53.15
Megalosplenia — *see* Splenomegaly
Megaloureter N28.82
  congenital Q62.2
Megarectum K62.89
Megasigmoid K59.39
  congenital Q43.2
Megaureter N28.82
  congenital Q62.2
Megavitamin-B6 syndrome E67.2
Megrim — *see* Migraine
Meibomian
  cyst, infected — *see* Hordeolum
  gland — *see* condition
  sty, stye — *see* Hordeolum
Meibomitis — *see* Hordeolum
Meige-Milroy disease (chronic hereditary edema) Q82.0
Meige's syndrome Q82.0
Melalgia, nutritional E53.8
Melancholia F32.9
  climacteric (single episode) F32.89
    recurrent episode F33.8
  hypochondriac F45.29
  intermittent (single episode) F32.89
    recurrent episode F33.8
  involutional (single episode) F32.89
    recurrent episode F33.8
  menopausal (single episode) F32.89
    recurrent episode F33.8
  puerperal F32.89
  reactive (emotional stress or trauma) F32.3
  recurrent F33.9
  senile F03 ☑
  stuporous (single episode) F32.89
    recurrent episode F33.8
Melanemia R79.89
Melanoameloblastoma — *see* Neoplasm, bone, benign
Melanoblastoma — *see* Melanoma
Melanocarcinoma — *see* Melanoma
Melanocytoma, eyeball D31.9- ☑
Melanocytosis, neurocutaneous Q82.8
Melanoderma, melanodermia L81.4
Melanodontia, infantile K03.89
Melanodontoclasia K03.89
Melanoepithelioma — *see* Melanoma
Melanoma (malignant) C43.9
  acral lentiginous, malignant — *see* Melanoma, skin, by site
  amelanotic — *see* Melanoma, skin, by site
  balloon cell — *see* Melanoma, skin, by site
  benign — *see* Nevus

Melanoma — continued
- desmoplastic, malignant — see Melanoma, skin, by site
- epithelioid cell — see Melanoma, skin, by site
  - with spindle cell, mixed — see Melanoma, skin, by site
- in
  - giant pigmented nevus — see Melanoma, skin, by site
  - Hutchinson's melanotic freckle — see Melanoma, skin, by site
  - junctional nevus — see Melanoma, skin, by site
  - precancerous melanosis — see Melanoma, skin, by site
- in situ D03.9
  - abdominal wall D03.59
  - ala nasi D03.39
  - ankle D03.7- ☑
  - anus, anal (margin) (skin) D03.51
  - arm D03.6- ☑
  - auditory canal D03.2- ☑
  - auricle (ear) D03.2- ☑
  - auricular canal (external) D03.2- ☑
  - axilla, axillary fold D03.59
  - back D03.59
  - breast D03.52
  - brow D03.39
  - buttock D03.59
  - canthus (eye) D03.1- ☑
  - cheek (external) D03.39
  - chest wall D03.59
  - chin D03.39
  - choroid D03.8
  - conjunctiva D03.8
  - ear (external) D03.2- ☑
  - external meatus (ear) D03.2- ☑
  - eye D03.8
  - eyebrow D03.39
  - eyelid (lower) (upper) D03.1- ☑
  - face D03.30
    - specified NEC D03.39
  - female genital organ (external) NEC D03.8
  - finger D03.6- ☑
  - flank D03.59
  - foot D03.7- ☑
  - forearm D03.6- ☑
  - forehead D03.39
  - foreskin D03.8
  - gluteal region D03.59
  - groin D03.59
  - hand D03.6- ☑
  - heel D03.7- ☑
  - helix D03.2- ☑
  - hip D03.7- ☑
  - interscapular region D03.59
  - iris D03.8
  - jaw D03.39
  - knee D03.7- ☑
  - labium (majus) (minus) D03.8
  - lacrimal gland D03.8
  - leg D03.7- ☑
  - lip (lower) (upper) D03.0
  - lower limb NEC D03.7- ☑
  - male genital organ (external) NEC D03.8
  - nail D03.9
    - finger D03.6- ☑
    - toe D03.7- ☑
  - neck D03.4
  - nose (external) D03.39
  - orbit D03.8
  - penis D03.8
  - perianal skin D03.51
  - perineum D03.51
  - pinna D03.2- ☑
  - popliteal fossa or space D03.7- ☑
  - prepuce D03.8
  - pudendum D03.8
  - retina D03.8
  - retrobulbar D03.8
  - scalp D03.4
  - scrotum D03.8
  - shoulder D03.6- ☑
  - specified site NEC D03.8
  - submammary fold D03.52
  - temple D03.39
  - thigh D03.7- ☑
  - toe D03.7- ☑

Melanoma — continued
- in situ — continued
  - trunk NEC D03.59
  - umbilicus D03.59
  - upper limb NEC D03.6- ☑
  - vulva D03.8
- juvenile — see Nevus
- malignant, of soft parts except skin — see Neoplasm, connective tissue, malignant
- metastatic
  - breast C79.81
  - genital organ C79.82
  - specified site NEC C79.89
- neurotropic, malignant — see Melanoma, skin, by site
- nodular — see Melanoma, skin, by site
- regressing, malignant — see Melanoma, skin, by site
- skin C43.9
  - abdominal wall C43.59
  - ala nasi C43.31
  - ankle C43.7- ☑
  - anus, anal (skin) C43.51
  - arm C43.6- ☑
  - auditory canal (external) C43.2- ☑
  - auricle (ear) C43.2- ☑
  - auricular canal (external) C43.2- ☑
  - axilla, axillary fold C43.59
  - back C43.59
  - breast (female) (male) C43.52
  - brow C43.39
  - buttock C43.59
  - canthus (eye) C43.1- ☑
  - cheek (external) C43.39
  - chest wall C43.59
  - chin C43.39
  - ear (external) C43.2- ☑
  - elbow C43.6- ☑
  - external meatus (ear) C43.2- ☑
  - eyebrow C43.39
  - eyelid (lower) (upper) C43.1- ☑
  - face C43.39
    - specified NEC C43.39
  - female genital organ (external) NEC C51.9
  - finger C43.6- ☑
  - flank C43.59
  - foot C43.7- ☑
  - forearm C43.6- ☑
  - forehead C43.39
  - foreskin C60.0
  - glabella C43.39
  - gluteal region C43.59
  - groin C43.59
  - hand C43.6- ☑
  - heel C43.7- ☑
  - helix C43.2- ☑
  - hip C43.7- ☑
  - interscapular region C43.59
  - jaw (external) C43.39
  - knee C43.7- ☑
  - labium C51.9
    - majus C51.0
    - minus C51.1
  - leg C43.7- ☑
  - lip (lower) (upper) C43.0
  - lower limb NEC C43.7- ☑
  - male genital organ (external) NEC C63.9
  - nail
    - finger C43.6- ☑
    - toe C43.7- ☑
  - nasolabial groove C43.39
  - nates C43.59
  - neck C43.4
  - nose (external) C43.31
  - overlapping site C43.8
  - palpebra C43.1- ☑
  - penis C60.9
  - perianal skin C43.51
  - perineum C43.51
  - pinna C43.2- ☑
  - popliteal fossa or space C43.7- ☑
  - prepuce C60.0
  - pudendum C51.9
  - scalp C43.4
  - scrotum C63.2
  - shoulder C43.6- ☑
  - skin NEC C43.9
  - submammary fold C43.52
  - temple C43.39

Melanoma — continued
- skin — continued
  - thigh C43.7- ☑
  - toe C43.7- ☑
  - trunk NEC C43.59
  - umbilicus C43.59
  - upper limb NEC C43.6- ☑
  - vulva C51.9
    - overlapping sites C51.8
- spindle cell
  - with epithelioid, mixed — see Melanoma, skin, by site
  - type A C69.4- ☑
  - type B C69.4- ☑
- superficial spreading — see Melanoma, skin, by site

Melanosarcoma — see also Melanoma
- epithelioid cell — see Melanoma

Melanosis L81.4
- addisonian E27.1
  - tuberculous A18.7
- adrenal E27.1
- colon K63.89
- conjunctiva — see Pigmentation, conjunctiva
  - congenital Q13.89
- cornea (presenile) (senile) — see also Pigmentation, cornea
  - congenital Q13.4
- eye NEC H57.89
  - congenital Q15.8
- lenticularis progressiva Q82.1
- liver K76.89
- precancerous — see also Melanoma, in situ
  - malignant melanoma in — see Melanoma
- Riehl's L81.4
- sclera H15.89
  - congenital Q13.89
- suprarenal E27.1
- tar L81.4
- toxic L81.4

Melanuria R82.998

MELAS syndrome E88.41

Melasma L81.1
- adrenal (gland) E27.1
- suprarenal (gland) E27.1

Melena K92.1
- with ulcer — code by site under Ulcer, with hemorrhage K27.4
- due to swallowed maternal blood P78.2
- newborn, neonatal P54.1
  - due to swallowed maternal blood P78.2

Meleney's
- gangrene (cutaneous) — see Ulcer, skin
- ulcer (chronic undermining) — see Ulcer, skin

Melioidosis A24.9
- acute A24.1
- chronic A24.2
- fulminating A24.1
- pneumonia A24.1
- pulmonary (chronic) A24.2
  - acute A24.1
  - subacute A24.2
- sepsis A24.1
- specified NEC A24.3
- subacute A24.2

Melitensis, febris A23.0

Melkersson (-Rosenthal) **syndrome** G51.2

Mellitus, diabetes — see Diabetes

Melorheostosis (bone) — see Disorder, bone, density and structure, specified NEC

Meloschisis Q18.4

Melotia Q17.4

Membrana
- capsularis lentis posterior Q13.89
- epipapillaris Q14.2

Membranacea placenta O43.19- ☑

Membranaceous uterus N85.8

Membrane(s), membranous — see also condition
- cyclitic — see Membrane, pupillary
- folds, congenital — see Web
- Jackson's Q43.3
- over face of newborn P28.9
- premature rupture — see Rupture, membranes, premature
- pupillary H21.4- ☑
  - persistent Q13.89
- retained (with hemorrhage) (complicating delivery) O72.2

Membrane(s), membranous — *continued*
  retained — *continued*
    without hemorrhage O73.1
  secondary cataract, secondary
    secondary cataract — *see* Cataract, secondary
  unruptured (causing asphyxia) — *see* Asphyxia, new-
    born
  vitreous — *see* Opacity, vitreous, membranes and
    strands
Membranitis — *see* Chorioamnionitis
Memory disturbance, lack or loss — *see also* Amnesia
  mild, following organic brain damage F06.8
Menadione deficiency E56.1
Menarche
  delayed E30.0
  precocious E30.1
Mendacity, pathologic F60.2
Mendelson's syndrome (due to anesthesia) J95.4
  in labor and delivery O74.0
  in pregnancy O29.01- ☑
  obstetric O74.0
  postpartum, puerperal O89.01
Ménétrier's disease or syndrome K29.60
  with bleeding K29.61
Ménière's disease, syndrome or vertigo H81.0- ☑
Meninges, meningeal — *see* condition
Meningioma — *see also* Neoplasm, meninges, benign
  angioblastic — *see* Neoplasm, meninges, benign
  angiomatous — *see* Neoplasm, meninges, benign
  atypical — *see* Neoplasm, meninges, uncertain behav-
    ior
  endotheliomatous — *see* Neoplasm, meninges, benign
  fibroblastic — *see* Neoplasm, meninges, benign
  fibrous — *see* Neoplasm, meninges, benign
  hemangioblastic — *see* Neoplasm, meninges, benign
  hemangiopericytic — *see* Neoplasm, meninges, benign
  malignant — *see* Neoplasm, meninges, malignant
  meningiothelial — *see* Neoplasm, meninges, benign
  meningotheliomatous — *see* Neoplasm, meninges,
    benign
  mixed — *see* Neoplasm, meninges, benign
  multiple — *see* Neoplasm, meninges, uncertain behav-
    ior
  papillary — *see* Neoplasm, meninges, uncertain behav-
    ior
  psammomatous — *see* Neoplasm, meninges, benign
  syncytial — *see* Neoplasm, meninges, benign
  transitional — *see* Neoplasm, meninges, benign
Meningiomatosis (diffuse) — *see* Neoplasm, meninges,
  uncertain behavior
Meningism — *see* Meningismus
Meningismus (infectional) (pneumococcal) R29.1
  due to serum or vaccine R29.1
  influenzal — *see* Influenza, with, manifestations NEC
Meningitis (basal) (basic) (brain) (cerebral) (cervical)
  (congestive) (diffuse) (hemorrhagic) (infantile)
  (membranous) (metastatic) (nonspecific) (pontine)
  (progressive) (simple) (spinal) (subacute) (sympathetic) (toxic) G03.9
  abacterial G03.0
  actinomycotic A42.81
  adenoviral A87.1
  arbovirus A87.8
  aseptic (acute) G03.0
  bacterial G00.9
    Escherichia coli (E. coli) G00.8
    Friedländer (bacillus) G00.8
    gram-negative G00.9
    H. influenzae G00.0
    Klebsiella G00.8
    pneumococcal G00.1
    specified organism NEC G00.8
    staphylococcal G00.3
    streptococcal (acute) G00.2
  benign recurrent (Mollaret) G03.2
  candidal B37.5
  caseous (tuberculous) A17.0
  cerebrospinal A39.0
  chronic NEC G03.1
  clear cerebrospinal fluid NEC G03.0
  coxsackievirus A87.0
  cryptococcal B45.1
  diplococcal (gram positive) A39.0
  echovirus A87.0
  enteroviral A87.0
  eosinophilic B83.2
  epidemic NEC A39.0
  Escherichia coli (E. coli) G00.8
  fibrinopurulent G00.9

Meningitis — *continued*
  fibrinopurulent — *continued*
    specified organism NEC G00.8
  Friedländer (bacillus) G00.8
  gonococcal A54.81
  gram-negative cocci G00.9
  gram-positive cocci G00.9
  H. influenzae G00.0
  Haemophilus (influenzae) G00.0
  in (due to)
    adenovirus A87.1
    African trypanosomiasis B56.9 *[G02]*
    anthrax A22.8
    bacterial disease NEC A48.8 *[G01]*
    Chagas' disease (chronic) B57.41
    chickenpox B01.0
    coccidioidomycosis B38.4
    Diplococcus pneumoniae G00.1
    enterovirus A87.0
    herpes (simplex) virus B00.3
      zoster B02.1
    infectious mononucleosis B27.92
    leptospirosis A27.81
    Listeria monocytogenes A32.11
    Lyme disease A69.21
    measles B05.1
    mumps (virus) B26.1
    neurosyphilis (late) A52.13
    parasitic disease NEC B89 *[G02]*
    poliovirus A80.9 *[G02]*
    preventive immunization, inoculation or vaccination
      G03.8
    rubella B06.02
    Salmonella infection A02.21
    specified cause NEC G03.8
    Streptococcal pneumoniae G00.1
    typhoid fever A01.01
    varicella B01.0
    viral disease NEC A87.8
    whooping cough A37.90
    zoster B02.1
  infectious G00.9
  influenzal (H. influenzae) G00.0
  Klebsiella G00.8
  leptospiral (aseptic) A27.81
  lymphocytic (acute) (benign) (serous) A87.2
  meningococcal A39.0
  Mima polymorpha G00.8
  Mollaret (benign recurrent) G03.2
  monilial B37.5
  mycotic NEC B49 *[G02]*
  Neisseria A39.0
  nonbacterial G03.0
  nonpyogenic NEC G03.0
  ossificans G96.198
  pneumococcal streptococcus pneumoniae G00.1
  poliovirus A80.9 *[G02]*
  postmeasles B05.1
  purulent G00.9
    specified organism NEC G00.8
  pyogenic G00.9
    specified organism NEC G00.8
  Salmonella (arizonae) (Cholerae-Suis) (enteritidis) (ty-
    phimurium) A02.21
  septic G00.9
    specified organism NEC G00.8
  serosa circumscripta NEC G03.0
  serous NEC G93.2
  specified organism NEC G00.8
  sporotrichosis B42.81
  staphylococcal G00.3
  sterile G03.0
  Streptococcal (acute) G00.2
    pneumoniae G00.1
  suppurative G00.9
    specified organism NEC G00.8
  syphilitic (late) (tertiary) A52.13
    acute A51.41
    congenital A50.41
    secondary A51.41
  Torula histolytica (cryptococcal) B45.1
  traumatic (complication of injury) T79.8 ☑
  tuberculous A17.0
  typhoid A01.01
  viral NEC A87.9
  Yersinia pestis A20.3
Meningocele (spinal) — *see also* Spina bifida

Meningocele — *continued*
  with hydrocephalus — *see* Spina bifida, by site, with
    hydrocephalus
  acquired (traumatic) G96.198
  cerebral — *see* Encephalocele
Meningocerebritis — *see* Meningoencephalitis
Meningococcemia A39.4
  acute A39.2
  chronic A39.3
Meningococcus, meningococcal — *see also* condition
  A39.9
  adrenalitis, hemorrhagic A39.1
  carrier (suspected) of Z22.31
  meningitis (cerebrospinal) A39.0
Meningoencephalitis — *see also* Encephalitis G04.90
  acute NEC — *see also* Encephalitis, viral A86
  bacterial NEC G04.2
  California A83.5
  diphasic A84.1
  eosinophilic B83.2
  epidemic A39.81
  herpesviral, herpetic B00.4
    due to herpesvirus 6 B10.01
    due to herpesvirus 7 B10.09
    specified NEC B10.09
  in (due to)
    blastomycosis NEC B40.81
    diseases classified elsewhere G05.3
    free-living amebae B60.2
    H. influenzae G00.0
    Hemophilus influenzae (H .influenzae) G00.0
    herpes B00.4
      due to herpesvirus 6 B10.01
      due to herpesvirus 7 B10.09
      specified NEC B10.09
    Lyme disease A69.22
    mercury — *see* subcategory T56.1 ☑
    mumps B26.2
    Naegleria (amebae) (organisms) (fowleri) B60.2
    Parastrongylus cantonensis B83.2
    toxoplasmosis (acquired) B58.2
      congenital P37.1
  infectious (acute) (viral) A86
  influenzal (H. influenzae) G00.0
  Listeria monocytogenes A32.12
  lymphocytic (serous) A87.2
  mumps B26.2
  parasitic NEC B89 *[G05.3]*
  pneumococcal G04.2
  primary ambic B60.2
  specific (syphilitic) A52.14
  specified organism NEC G04.81
  staphylococcal G04.2
  streptococcal G04.2
  syphilitic A52.14
  toxic NEC G92
    due to mercury — *see* subcategory T56.1 ☑
  tuberculous A17.82
  virus NEC A86
Meningoencephalocele — *see also* Encephalocele
  syphilitic A52.19
    congenital A50.49
Meningoencephalomyelitis — *see also* Meningoencephalitis
  acute NEC (viral) A86
    disseminated G04.00
      postimmunization or postvaccination G04.02
      postinfectious G04.01
  due to
    actinomycosis A42.82
    Torula B45.1
    Toxoplasma or toxoplasmosis (acquired) B58.2
      congenital P37.1
  postimmunization or postvaccination G04.02
Meningoencephalomyelopathy G96.9
Meningoencephalopathy G96.9
Meningomyelitis — *see also* Meningoencephalitis
  bacterial NEC G04.2
  blastomycotic NEC B40.81
  cryptococcal B45.1
  in diseases classified elsewhere G05.4
  meningococcal A39.81
  syphilitic A52.14
  tuberculous A17.82
Meningomyelocele — *see also* Spina bifida
  syphilitic A52.19
Meningomyeloneuritis — *see* Meningoencephalitis
Meningoradiculitis — *see* Meningitis

Meningovascular — see condition
Menkes' disease or syndrome E83.09
  meaning maple-syrup-urine disease E71.0
Menometrorrhagia N92.1
Menopause, menopausal (asymptomatic) (state) Z78.0
  arthritis (any site) NEC — see Arthritis, specified form NEC
  bleeding N92.4
  depression (single episode) F32.89
    agitated (single episode) F32.2
      recurrent episode F33.9
    psychotic (single episode) F32.89
      recurrent episode F33.9
    recurrent episode F33.8
    melancholia (single episode) F32.89
      recurrent episode F33.8
  paranoid state F22
  premature E28.319
    asymptomatic E28.319
      postirradiation E89.40
      postsurgical E89.40
    symptomatic E28.310
      postirradiation E89.41
      postsurgical E89.41
  psychosis NEC F28
  symptomatic N95.1
  toxic polyarthritis NEC — see Arthritis, specified form NEC
Menorrhagia (primary) N92.0
  climacteric N92.4
    menopausal N92.4
  menopausal N92.4
  perimenopausal N92.4
  postclimacteric N95.0
  postmenopausal N95.0
  preclimacteric or premenopausal N92.4
  pubertal (menses retained) N92.2
Menostaxis N92.0
Menses, retention N94.89
Menstrual — see Menstruation
Menstruation
  absent — see Amenorrhea
  anovulatory N97.0
  cycle, irregular N92.6
  delayed N91.0
  disorder N93.9
    psychogenic F45.8
  during pregnancy O20.8
  excessive (with regular cycle) N92.0
    with irregular cycle N92.1
    at puberty N92.2
  frequent N92.0
  infrequent — see Oligomenorrhea
  irregular N92.6
    specified NEC N92.5
  latent N92.5
  membranous N92.5
  painful — see also Dysmenorrhea N94.6
    primary N94.4
    psychogenic F45.8
    secondary N94.5
  passage of clots N92.0
  precocious E30.1
  protracted N92.5
  rare — see Oligomenorrhea
  retained N94.89
  retrograde N92.5
  scanty — see Oligomenorrhea
  suppression N94.89
  vicarious (nasal) N94.89
Mental — see also condition
  deficiency — see Disability, intellectual
  deterioration — see Psychosis
  disorder — see Disorder, mental
  exhaustion F48.8
  insufficiency (congenital) — see Disability, intellectual
  observation without need for further medical care Z03.89
  retardation — see Disability, intellectual
  subnormality — see Disability, intellectuall
  upset — see Disorder, mental
Meralgia paresthetica G57.1- ☑
Mercurial — see condition
Mercurialism — see subcategory T56.1 ☑
Merkel cell tumor — see Carcinoma, Merkel cell
Merocele — see Hernia, femoral
Meromelia
  lower limb — see Defect, reduction, lower limb

Meromelia — continued
  lower limb — see Defect, reduction, lower limb — continued
    intercalary
      femur — see Defect, reduction, lower limb, specified type NEC
        tibiofibular (complete) (incomplete) — see Defect, reduction, lower limb
  upper limb — see Defect, reduction, upper limb
    intercalary, humeral, radioulnar — see Agenesis, arm, with hand present
MERRF syndrome (myoclonic epilepsy associated with ragged-red fiber) E88.42
Merzbacher-Pelizaeus disease E75.29
Mesaortitis — see Aortitis
Mesarteritis — see Arteritis
Mesencephalitis — see Encephalitis
Mesenchymoma — see also Neoplasm, connective tissue, uncertain behavior
  benign — see Neoplasm, connective tissue, benign
  malignant — see Neoplasm, connective tissue, malignant
Mesenteritis
  retractile K65.4
  sclerosing K65.4
Mesentery, mesenteric — see condition
Mesiodens, mesiodentes K00.1
Mesio-occlusion M26.213
Mesocolon — see condition
Mesonephroma (malignant) — see Neoplasm, malignant, by site
  benign — see Neoplasm, benign, by site
Mesophlebitis — see Phlebitis
Mesostromal dysgenesia Q13.89
Mesothelioma (malignant) C45.9
  benign
    mesentery D19.1
    mesocolon D19.1
    omentum D19.1
    peritoneum D19.1
    pleura D19.0
    specified site NEC D19.7
    unspecified site D19.9
  biphasic C45.9
    benign
      mesentery D19.1
      mesocolon D19.1
      omentum D19.1
      peritoneum D19.1
      pleura D19.0
      specified site NEC D19.7
      unspecified site D19.9
  cystic D48.4
  epithelioid C45.9
    benign
      mesentery D19.1
      mesocolon D19.1
      omentum D19.1
      peritoneum D19.1
      pleura D19.0
      specified site NEC D19.7
      unspecified site D19.9
  fibrous C45.9
    benign
      mesentery D19.1
      mesocolon D19.1
      omentum D19.1
      peritoneum D19.1
      pleura D19.0
      specified site NEC D19.7
      unspecified site D19.9
  site classification
    liver C45.7
    lung C45.7
    mediastinum C45.7
    mesentery C45.1
    mesocolon C45.1
    omentum C45.1
    pericardium C45.2
    peritoneum C45.1
    pleura C45.0
      parietal C45.0
    retroperitoneum C45.7
    specified site NEC C45.7
    unspecified C45.9
Metabolic syndrome E88.81
Metagonimiasis B66.8
Metagonimus infestation (intestine) B66.8

Metal
  pigmentation L81.8
  polisher's disease J62.8
Metamorphopsia H53.15
Metaplasia
  apocrine (breast) — see Dysplasia, mammary, specified type NEC
  cervix (squamous) — see Dysplasia, cervix
  endometrium (squamous) (uterus) N85.8
  esophagus K22.7- ☑
  kidney (pelvis) (squamous) N28.89
  myelogenous D73.1
  myeloid (agnogenic) (megakaryocytic) D73.1
  spleen D73.1
  squamous cell, bladder N32.89
Metastasis, metastatic
  abscess — see Abscess
  calcification E83.59
  cancer
    from specified site — see Neoplasm, malignant, by site
    to specified site — see Neoplasm, secondary, by site
  deposits (in) — see Neoplasm, secondary, by site
  disease — see also Neoplasm, secondary, by site C79.9
  spread (to) — see Neoplasm, secondary, by site
Metastrongyliasis B83.8
Metatarsalgia M77.4- ☑
  anterior G57.6- ☑
  Morton's G57.6- ☑
Metatarsus, metatarsal — see also condition
  adductus, congenital Q66.22- ☑
  valgus (abductus), congenital Q66.6
  varus (congenital) Q66.22- ☑
    primus Q66.21- ☑
Methadone use — see Use, opioid
Methemoglobinemia D74.9
  acquired (with sulfhemoglobinemia) D74.8
  congenital D74.0
  enzymatic (congenital) D74.0
  Hb M disease D74.0
  hereditary D74.0
  toxic D74.8
Methemoglobinuria — see Hemoglobinuria
Methioninemia E72.19
Methylmalonic acidemia E71.120
Metritis (catarrhal) (hemorrhagic) (septic) (suppurative) — see also Endometritis
  cervical — see Cervicitis
Metropathia hemorrhagica N93.8
Metroperitonitis — see Peritonitis, pelvic, female
Metrorrhagia N92.1
  climacteric N92.4
  menopausal N92.4
  perimenopausal N92.4
  postpartum NEC (atonic) (following delivery of placenta) O72.1
    delayed or secondary O72.2
  preclimacteric or premenopausal N92.4
  psychogenic F45.8
Metrorrhexis — see Rupture, uterus
Metrosalpingitis N70.91
Metrostaxis N93.8
Metrovaginitis — see Endometritis
Meyer-Schwickerath and Weyers syndrome Q87.0
Meynert's amentia (nonalcoholic) F04
  alcoholic F10.96
    with dependence F10.26
Mibelli's disease (porokeratosis) Q82.8
Mice, joint — see Loose, body, joint
  knee M23.4- ☑
Micrencephalon, micrencephaly Q02
Microalbuminuria R80.9
Microaneurysm, retinal — see also Disorder, retina, microaneurysms
  diabetic — see E08-E13 with .31
Microangiopathy (peripheral) I73.9
  thrombotic M31.1
Microcalcifications, breast R92.0
Microcephalus, microcephalic, microcephaly Q02
  due to toxoplasmosis (congenital) P37.1
Microcheilia Q18.7
Microcolon (congenital) Q43.8
Microcornea (congenital) Q13.4
Microcytic — see condition
Microdeletions NEC Q93.88
Microdontia K00.2
Microdrepanocytosis D57.40

☑ Additional Character Required — Refer to the Tabular List for Character Selection   ▽ Subterms under main terms may continue to next column or page

Microdrepanocytosis — *continued*
  with
    acute chest syndrome D57.411
    cerebral vascular involvement D57.413
    crisis (painful) D57.419
      with specified complication NEC D57.418
    splenic sequestration D57.412
    vasoocclusive pain D57.419
Microembolism
  atherothrombotic — *see* Atheroembolism
  retinal — *see* Occlusion, artery, retina
Microencephalon Q02
Microfilaria streptocerca infestation — *see* Onchocerciasis
Microgastria (congenital) Q40.2
Microgenia M26.06
Microgenitalia, congenital
  female Q52.8
  male Q55.8
Microglioma — *see* Lymphoma, non-Hodgkin, specified NEC
Microglossia (congenital) Q38.3
Micrognathia, micrognathism (congenital) (mandibular) (maxillary) M26.09
Microgyria (congenital) Q04.3
Microinfarct of heart — *see* Insufficiency, coronary
Microlentia (congenital) Q12.8
Microlithiasis, alveolar, pulmonary J84.02
Micromastia N64.82
Micromyelia (congenital) Q06.8
Micropenis Q55.62
Microphakia (congenital) Q12.8
Microphthalmos, microphthalmia (congenital) Q11.2
  due to toxoplasmosis P37.1
Micropsia H53.15
Microscopic polyangiitis (polyarteritis) M31.7
Microsporidiosis B60.8
  intestinal A07.8
Microsporon furfur infestation B36.0
Microsporosis — *see also* Dermatophytosis
  nigra B36.1
Microstomia (congenital) Q18.5
Microtia (congenital) (external ear) Q17.2
Microtropia H50.40
Microvillus inclusion disease (MVD) (MVID) Q43.8
Micturition
  disorder NEC — *see also* Difficulty, micturition R39.198
    psychogenic F45.8
  frequency R35.0
    psychogenic F45.8
  hesitancy R39.11
  incomplete emptying R39.14
  nocturnal R35.1
  painful R30.9
    dysuria R30.0
    psychogenic F45.8
    tenesmus R30.1
  poor stream R39.12
  position dependent R39.192
  split stream R39.13
  straining R39.16
  urgency R39.15
Mid plane — *see* condition
Middle
  ear — *see* condition
  lobe (right) syndrome J98.19
Miescher's elastoma L87.2
Mietens' syndrome Q87.2
Migraine (idiopathic) G43.909
  with refractory migraine G43.919
    with status migrainosus G43.911
    without status migrainosus G43.919
  with aura (acute-onset) (prolonged) (typical) (without headache) G43.109
    with refractory migraine G43.119
      with status migrainosus G43.111
      without status migrainosus G43.119
    intractable G43.119
      with status migrainosus G43.111
      without status migrainosus G43.119
    not intractable G43.109
      with status migrainosus G43.101
      without status migrainosus G43.109
    persistent G43.509
      with cerebral infarction G43.609
        with refractory migraine G43.619
          with status migrainosus G43.611
          without status migrainosus G43.619

Migraine — *continued*
  with aura — *continued*
    persistent — *continued*
      with cerebral infarction — *continued*
        intractable G43.619
          with status migrainosus G43.611
          without status migrainosus G43.619
        not intractable G43.609
          with status migrainosus G43.601
          without status migrainosus G43.609
        without refractory migraine G43.609
          with status migrainosus G43.601
          without status migrainosus G43.609
      without cerebral infarction G43.509
        with refractory migraine G43.519
          with status migrainosus G43.511
          without status migrainosus G43.519
        intractable G43.519
          with status migrainosus G43.511
          without status migrainosus G43.519
        not intractable G43.509
          with status migrainosus G43.501
          without status migrainosus G43.509
        without refractory migraine G43.509
          with status migrainosus G43.501
          without status migrainosus G43.509
    without mention of refractory migraine G43.109
      with status migrainosus G43.101
      without status migrainosus G43.109
  abdominal G43.D0 (*following* G43.7)
    with refractory migraine G43.D1 (*following* G43.7)
    intractable G43.D1 (*following* G43.7)
    not intractable G43.D0 (*following* G43.7)
    without refractory migraine G43.D0 (*following* G43.7)
  basilar — *see* Migraine, with aura
  classical — *see* Migraine, with aura
  common — *see* Migraine, without aura
  complicated G43.109
  equivalents — *see* Migraine, with aura
  familiar — *see* Migraine, hemiplegic
  hemiplegic G43.409
    with refractory migraine G43.419
      with status migrainosus G43.411
      without status migrainosus G43.419
    intractable G43.419
      with status migrainosus G43.411
      without status migrainosus G43.419
    not intractable G43.409
      with status migrainosus G43.401
      without status migrainosus G43.409
    without refractory migraine G43.409
      with status migrainosus G43.401
      without status migrainosus G43.409
  intractable G43.919
    with status migrainosus G43.911
    without status migrainosus G43.919
  menstrual G43.829
    with refractory migraine G43.839
      with status migrainosus G43.831
      without status migrainosus G43.839
    intractable G43.839
      with status migrainosus G43.831
      without status migrainosus G43.839
    not intractable 4G43.829
      with status migrainosus G43.821
      without status migrainosus G43.829
    without refractory migraine G43.829
      with status migrainosus G43.821
      without status migrainosus G43.829
  menstrually related — *see* Migraine, menstrual
  not intractable G43.909
    with status migrainosus G43.901
    without status migrainosus G43.919
  ophthalmoplegic G43.B0 (*following* G43.7)
    with refractory migraine G43.B1 (*following* G43.7)
    intractable G43.B1 (*following* G43.7)
    not intractable G43.B0 (*following* G43.7)
    without refractory migraine G43.B0 (*following* G43.7)
  persistent aura (with, without) cerebral infarction — *see* Migraine, with aura, persistent
  preceded or accompanied by transient focal neurological phenomena — *see* Migraine, with aura
  pre-menstrual — *see* Migraine, menstrual
  pure menstrual — *see* Migraine, menstrual
  retinal — *see* Migraine, with aura
  specified NEC G43.809
    intractable G43.819
      with status migrainosus G43.811

Migraine — *continued*
  specified — *continued*
    intractable — *continued*
      without status migrainosus G43.819
    not intractable G43.809
      with status migrainosus G43.801
      without status migrainosus G43.809
  sporadic — *see* Migraine, hemiplegic
  transformed — *see* Migraine, without aura, chronic
  triggered seizures — *see* Migraine, with aura
  without aura G43.009
    with refractory migraine G43.019
      with status migrainosus G43.011
      without status migrainosus G43.019
    chronic G43.709
      with refractory migraine G43.719
        with status migrainosus G43.711
        without status migrainosus G43.719
      intractable
        with status migrainosus G43.711
        without status migrainosus G43.719
      not intractable
        with status migrainosus G43.701
        without status migrainosus G43.709
      without refractory migraine G43.709
        with status migrainosus G43.701
        without status migrainosus G43.709
    intractable
      with status migrainosus G43.011
      without status migrainosus G43.019
    not intractable
      with status migrainosus G43.001
      without status migrainosus G43.009
    without mention of refractory migraine G43.009
      with status migrainosus G43.001
      without status migrainosus G43.009
    without refractory migraine G43.909
      with status migrainosus G43.901
      without status migrainosus G43.919
Migrant, social Z59.0
Migration, anxiety concerning Z60.3
Migratory, migrating — *see also* condition
  person Z59.0
  testis Q55.29
Mikity-Wilson disease or syndrome P27.0
Mikulicz' disease or syndrome K11.8
Miliaria L74.3
  alba L74.1
  apocrine L75.2
  crystallina L74.1
  profunda L74.2
  rubra L74.0
  tropicalis L74.2
Miliary — *see* condition
Milium L72.0
  colloid L57.8
Milk
  crust L21.0
  excessive secretion O92.6
  poisoning — *see* Poisoning, food, noxious
  retention O92.79
  sickness — *see* Poisoning, food, noxious
  spots I31.0
Milk-alkali disease or syndrome E83.52
Milk-leg (deep vessels) (nonpuerperal) — *see* Embolism, vein, lower extremity
  complicating pregnancy O22.3- ☑
  puerperal, postpartum, childbirth O87.1
Milkman's disease or syndrome M83.8
Milky urine — *see* Chyluria
Millard-Gubler (-Foville) **paralysis or syndrome** G46.3
Millar's asthma J38.5
Miller Fisher syndrome G61.0
Mills' disease — *see* Hemiplegia
Millstone maker's pneumoconiosis J62.8
Milroy's disease (chronic hereditary edema) Q82.0
Minamata disease T56.1 ☑
Miners' asthma or lung J60
Minkowski-Chauffard syndrome — *see* Spherocytosis
Minor — *see* condition
Minor's disease (hematomyelia) G95.19
Minot's disease (hemorrhagic disease), newborn P53
Minot-von Willebrand-Jurgens disease or syndrome (angiohemophilia) D68.0
Minus (and plus) **hand** (intrinsic) — *see* Deformity, limb, specified type NEC, forearm
Miosis (pupil) H57.03
Mirizzi's syndrome (hepatic duct stenosis) K83.1

Mirror writing F81.0
Misadventure (of) (prophylactic) (therapeutic) — *see also* Complications T88.9 ☑
   administration of insulin (by accident) — *see* subcategory T38.3 ☑
   infusion — *see* Complications, infusion
   local applications (of fomentations, plasters, etc.) T88.9 ☑
     burn or scald — *see* Burn
     specified NEC T88.8 ☑
   medical care (early) (late) T88.9 ☑
     adverse effect of drugs or chemicals — *see* Table of Drugs and Chemicals
     burn or scald — *see* Burn
     specified NEC T88.8 ☑
   specified NEC T88.8 ☑
   surgical procedure (early) (late) — *see* Complications, surgical procedure
   transfusion — *see* Complications, transfusion
   vaccination or other immunological procedure — *see* Complications, vaccination
Miscarriage O03.9
Misdirection, aqueous H40.83- ☑
Misperception, sleep state F51.02
Misplaced, misplacement
   ear Q17.4
   kidney (acquired) N28.89
     congenital Q63.2
   organ or site, congenital NEC — *see* Malposition, congenital
Missed
   abortion O02.1
   delivery O36.4 ☑
Missing — *see also* Absence
   string of intrauterine contraceptive device T83.32- ☑
Misuse of drugs F19.99
Mitchell's disease (erythromelalgia) I73.81
Mite(s) (infestation) B88.9
   diarrhea B88.0
   grain (itch) B88.0
   hair follicle (itch) B88.0
   in sputum B88.0
Mitral — *see* condition
Mittelschmerz N94.0
Mixed — *see* condition
MMN (multifocal motor neuropathy) G61.82
MNGIE (Mitochondrial Neurogastrointestinal Encephalopathy) **syndrome** E88.49
Mobile, mobility
   cecum Q43.3
   excessive — *see* Hypermobility
   gallbladder, congenital Q44.1
   kidney N28.89
   organ or site, congenital NEC — *see* Malposition, congenital
Mobitz heart block (atrioventricular) I44.1
Moebius, Möbius
   disease (ophthalmoplegic migraine) — *see* Migraine, ophthalmoplegic
   syndrome Q87.0
     congenital oculofacial paralysis (with other anomalies) Q87.0
     ophthalmoplegic migraine — *see* Migraine, ophthalmoplegic
Moeller's glossitis K14.0
Mohr's syndrome (Types I and II) Q87.0
Mola destruens D39.2
Molar pregnancy O02.0
Molarization of premolars K00.2
Molding, head (during birth) — *omit code*
Mole (pigmented) — *see also* Nevus
   blood O02.0
   Breus' O02.0
   cancerous — *see* Melanoma
   carneous O02.0
   destructive D39.2
   fleshy O02.0
   hydatid, hydatidiform (benign) (complicating pregnancy) (delivered) (undelivered) O01.9
     classical O01.0
     complete O01.0
     incomplete O01.1
     invasive D39.2
     malignant D39.2
     partial O01.1
   intrauterine O02.0
   invasive (hydatidiform) D39.2

Mole — *continued*
   malignant
     meaning
       malignant hydatidiform mole D39.2
       melanoma — *see* Melanoma
   nonhydatidiform O02.0
   nonpigmented — *see* Nevus
   pregnancy NEC O02.0
   skin — *see* Nevus
   tubal O00.10- ☑
     with intrauterine pregnancy O00.11- ☑
   vesicular — *see* Mole, hydatidiform
Molimen, molimina (menstrual) N94.3
Molluscum contagiosum (epitheliale) B08.1
Mönckeberg's arteriosclerosis, disease, or sclerosis — *see* Arteriosclerosis, extremities
Mondini's malformation (cochlea) Q16.5
Mondor's disease I80.8
Monge's disease T70.29 ☑
Monilethrix (congenital) Q84.1
Moniliasis — *see also* Candidiasis B37.9
   neonatal P37.5
Monitoring (encounter for)
   therapeutic drug level Z51.81
Monkey malaria B53.1
Monkeypox B04
Monoarthritis M13.10
   ankle M13.17- ☑
   elbow M13.12- ☑
   foot joint M13.17- ☑
   hand joint M13.14- ☑
   hip M13.15- ☑
   knee M13.16- ☑
   shoulder M13.11- ☑
   wrist M13.13- ☑
Monoblastic — *see* condition
Monochromat (ism), monochromatopsia (acquired) (congenital) H53.51
Monocytic — *see* condition
Monocytopenia D72.818
Monocytosis (symptomatic) D72.821
Monomania — *see* Psychosis
Mononeuritis G58.9
   cranial nerve — *see* Disorder, nerve, cranial
   femoral nerve G57.2- ☑
   lateral
     cutaneous nerve of thigh G57.1- ☑
     popliteal nerve G57.3- ☑
   lower limb G57.9- ☑
     specified nerve NEC G57.8- ☑
   medial popliteal nerve G57.4- ☑
   median nerve G56.1- ☑
   multiplex G58.7
   plantar nerve G57.6- ☑
   posterior tibial nerve G57.5- ☑
   radial nerve G56.3- ☑
   sciatic nerve G57.0- ☑
   specified NEC G58.8
   tibial nerve G57.4- ☑
   ulnar nerve G56.2- ☑
   upper limb G56.9- ☑
     specified nerve NEC G56.8- ☑
   vestibular — *see* subcategory H93.3 ☑
Mononeuropathy G58.9
   carpal tunnel syndrome — *see* Syndrome, carpal tunnel
   diabetic NEC — *see* E08-E13 with .41
   femoral nerve — *see* Lesion, nerve, femoral
   ilioinguinal nerve G57.8- ☑
   in diseases classified elsewhere — *see* category G59
   intercostal G58.0
   lower limb G57.9- ☑
     causalgia — *see* Causalgia, lower limb
     femoral nerve — *see* Lesion, nerve, femoral
     meralgia paresthetica G57.1- ☑
     plantar nerve — *see* Lesion, nerve, plantar
     popliteal nerve — *see* Lesion, nerve, popliteal
     sciatic nerve — *see* Lesion, nerve, sciatic
     specified NEC G57.8- ☑
     tarsal tunnel syndrome — *see* Syndrome, tarsal tunnel
   median nerve — *see* Lesion, nerve, median
   multiplex G58.7
   obturator nerve G57.8- ☑
   popliteal nerve — *see* Lesion, nerve, popliteal
   radial nerve — *see* Lesion, nerve, radial
   saphenous nerve G57.8- ☑

Mononeuropathy — *continued*
   specified NEC G58.8
   tarsal tunnel syndrome — *see* Syndrome, tarsal tunnel
   tuberculous A17.83
   ulnar nerve — *see* Lesion, nerve, ulnar
   upper limb G56.9- ☑
     carpal tunnel syndrome — *see* Syndrome, carpal tunnel
     causalgia — *see* Causalgia
     median nerve — *see* Lesion, nerve, median
     radial nerve — *see* Lesion, nerve, radial
     specified site NEC G56.8- ☑
     ulnar nerve — *see* Lesion, nerve, ulnar
Mononucleosis, infectious B27.90
   with
     complication NEC B27.99
     meningitis B27.92
     polyneuropathy B27.91
   cytomegaloviral B27.10
     with
       complication NEC B27.19
       meningitis B27.12
       polyneuropathy B27.11
   Epstein-Barr (virus) B27.00
     with
       complication NEC B27.09
       meningitis B27.02
       polyneuropathy B27.01
   gammaherpesviral B27.00
     with
       complication NEC B27.09
       meningitis B27.02
       polyneuropathy B27.01
   specified NEC B27.80
     with
       complication NEC B27.89
       meningitis B27.82
       polyneuropathy B27.81
Monoplegia G83.3- ☑
   congenital (cerebral) G80.8
     spastic G80.1
   embolic (current episode) I63.4- ☑
   following
     cerebrovascular disease
       cerebral infarction
         lower limb I69.34- ☑
         upper limb I69.33- ☑
       intracerebral hemorrhage
         lower limb I69.14- ☑
         upper limb I69.13- ☑
       lower limb I69.94- ☑
       nontraumatic intracranial hemorrhage NEC
         lower limb I69.24- ☑
         upper limb I69.23- ☑
       specified disease NEC
         lower limb I69.84- ☑
         upper limb I69.83- ☑
       stroke NOS
         lower limb I69.34- ☑
         upper limb I69.33- ☑
       subarachnoid hemorrhage
         lower limb I69.04- ☑
         upper limb I69.03- ☑
       upper limb I69.93- ☑
   hysterical (transient) F44.4
   lower limb G83.1- ☑
   psychogenic (conversion reaction) F44.4
   thrombotic (current episode) I63.3- ☑
   transient R29.818
   upper limb G83.2- ☑
Monorchism, monorchidism Q55.0
Monosomy — *see also* Deletion, chromosome Q93.9
   specified NEC Q93.89
   whole chromosome
     meiotic nondisjunction Q93.0
     mitotic nondisjunction Q93.1
     mosaicism Q93.1
   X Q96.9
Monster, monstrosity (single) Q89.7
   acephalic Q00.0
   twin Q89.4
Monteggia's fracture (-dislocation) S52.27- ☑
Mooren's ulcer (cornea) — *see* Ulcer, cornea, Mooren's
Moore's syndrome — *see* Epilepsy, specified NEC
Mooser-Neill reaction A75.2
Mooser's bodies A75.2
Morbidity not stated or unknown R69

☑ Additional Character Required — Refer to the Tabular List for Character Selection
▽ Subterms under main terms may continue to next column or page

Morbilli — *see* Measles
Morbus — *see also* Disease
  angelicus, anglorum E55.0
  Beigel B36.2
  caducus — *see* Epilepsy
  celiacus K90.0
  comitialis — *see* Epilepsy
  cordis — *see also* Disease, heart I51.9
    valvulorum — *see* Endocarditis
  coxae senilis M16.9
    tuberculous A18.02
  hemorrhagicus neonatorum P53
  maculosus neonatorum P54.5
Morel (-Stewart)(-Morgagni) **syndrome** M85.2
Morel-Kraepelin disease — *see* Schizophrenia
Morel-Moore syndrome M85.2
Morgagni's
  cyst, organ, hydatid, or appendage
    female Q50.5
    male (epididymal) Q55.4
      testicular Q55.29
  syndrome M85.2
Morgagni-Stewart-Morel syndrome M85.2
Morgagni-Stokes-Adams syndrome I45.9
Morgagni-Turner (-Albright) **syndrome** Q96.9
Moria F07.0
Moron (I.Q. 50-69) F70
Morphea L94.0
Morphinism (without remission) F11.20
  with remission F11.21
Morphinomania (without remission) F11.20
  with remission F11.21
Morquio (-Ullrich)(-Brailsford) **disease or syndrome** —
  see Mucopolysaccharidosis
Mortification (dry) (moist) — *see* Gangrene
Morton's metatarsalgia (neuralgia)(neuroma) (syndrome) G57.6- ☑
Morvan's disease or syndrome G60.8
Mosaicism, mosaic (autosomal) (chromosomal)
  45,X/46,XX Q96.3
  45,X/other cell lines NEC with abnormal sex chromosome Q96.4
  sex chromosome
    female Q97.8
    lines with various numbers of X chromosomes Q97.2
    male Q98.7
    XY Q96.3
Moschowitz' disease M31.1
Mother yaw A66.0
Motion sickness (from travel, any vehicle) (from roundabouts or swings) T75.3 ☑
Mottled, mottling, teeth (enamel) (endemic) (nonendemic) K00.3
Mounier-Kuhn syndrome Q32.4
  with bronchiectasis J47.9
    exacerbation (acute) J47.1
    lower respiratory infection J47.0
  acquired J98.09
    with bronchiectasis J47.9
      with
        exacerbation (acute) J47.1
        lower respiratory infection J47.0
Mountain
  sickness T70.29 ☑
    with polycythemia , acquired (acute) D75.1
  tick fever A93.2
Mouse, joint — *see* Loose, body, joint
  knee M23.4- ☑
Mouth — *see* condition
Movable
  coccyx — *see* subcategory M53.2 ☑
  kidney N28.89
    congenital Q63.8
  spleen D73.89
Movements, dystonic R25.8
Moyamoya disease I67.5
MRSA (Methicillin resistant Staphylococcus aureus)
  infection A49.02
    as the cause of diseases classified elsewhere B95.62
  sepsis A41.02
MSD (multiple sulfatase deficiency) E75.26
MSSA (Methicillin susceptible Staphylococcus aureus)
  infection A49.01
    as the cause of diseases classified elsewhere B95.61
  sepsis A41.01
Mucha-Habermann disease L41.0
Mucinosis (cutaneous) (focal) (papular) (skin) L98.5

Mucinosis — *continued*
  oral K13.79
Mucocele
  appendix K38.8
  buccal cavity K13.79
  gallbladder K82.1
  lacrimal sac, chronic H04.43- ☑
  nasal sinus J34.1
  nose J34.1
  salivary gland (any) K11.6
  sinus (accessory) (nasal) J34.1
  turbinate (bone) (middle) (nasal) J34.1
  uterus N85.8
Mucolipidosis
  I E77.1
  II, III E77.0
  IV E75.11
Mucopolysaccharidosis E76.3
  beta-gluduronidase deficiency E76.29
  cardiopathy E76.3 *[I52]*
  Hunter's syndrome E76.1
  Hurler's syndrome E76.01
  Hurler-Scheie syndrome E76.02
  Maroteaux-Lamy syndrome E76.29
  Morquio syndrome E76.219
    A E76.210
    B E76.211
    classic E76.210
  Sanfilippo syndrome E76.22
  Scheie's syndrome E76.03
  specified NEC E76.29
  type
    I
      Hurler's syndrome E76.01
      Hurler-Scheie syndrome E76.02
      Scheie's syndrome E76.03
    II E76.1
    III E76.22
    IV E76.219
    IVA E76.210
    IVB E76.211
    VI E76.29
    VII E76.29
Mucormycosis B46.5
  cutaneous B46.3
  disseminated B46.4
  gastrointestinal B46.2
  generalized B46.4
  pulmonary B46.0
  rhinocerebral B46.1
  skin B46.3
  subcutaneous B46.3
Mucositis (ulcerative) K12.30
  due to drugs NEC K12.32
  gastrointestinal K92.81
  mouth (oral) (oropharyngeal) K12.30
    due to antineoplastic therapy K12.31
    due to drugs NEC K12.32
    due to radiation K12.33
    specified NEC K12.39
    viral K12.39
  nasal J34.81
  oral cavity — *see* Mucositis, mouth
  oral soft tissues — *see* Mucositis, mouth
  vagina and vulva N76.81
Mucositis necroticans agranulocytica — *see* Agranulocytosis
Mucous — *see also* condition
  patches (syphilitic) A51.39
    congenital A50.07
Mucoviscidosis E84.9
  with meconium obstruction E84.11
Mucus
  asphyxia or suffocation — *see* Asphyxia, mucus
  in stool R19.5
  plug — *see* Asphyxia, mucus
Muguet B37.0
Mulberry molars (congenital syphilis) A50.52
Müllerian mixed tumor
  specified site — *see* Neoplasm, malignant, by site
  unspecified site C54.9
Multicystic kidney (development) Q61.4
Multiparity (grand) Z64.1
  affecting management of pregnancy, labor and delivery (supervision only) O09.4- ☑
  requiring contraceptive management — *see* Contraception
Multipartita placenta O43.19- ☑

Multiple, multiplex — *see also* condition
  digits (congenital) Q69.9
  endocrine neoplasia — *see* Neoplasia, endocrine, multiple (MEN)
  personality F44.81
Mumps B26.9
  arthritis B26.85
  complication NEC B26.89
  encephalitis B26.2
  hepatitis B26.81
  meningitis (aseptic) B26.1
  meningoencephalitis B26.2
  myocarditis B26.82
  oophoritis B26.89
  orchitis B26.0
  pancreatitis B26.3
  polyneuropathy B26.84
Mumu — *see also* Infestation, filarial B74.9 *[N51]*
Münchhausen's syndrome — *see* Disorder, factitious
Münchmeyer's syndrome — *see* Myositis, ossificans, progressiva
Mural — *see* condition
Murmur (cardiac) (heart) (organic) R01.1
  abdominal R19.15
  aortic (valve) — *see* Endocarditis, aortic
  benign R01.0
  diastolic — *see* Endocarditis
  Flint I35.1
  functional R01.0
  Graham Steell I37.1
  innocent R01.0
  mitral (valve) — *see* Insufficiency, mitral
  nonorganic R01.0
  presystolic, mitral — *see* Insufficiency, mitral
  pulmonic (valve) I37.8
  systolic R01.1
  tricuspid (valve) I07.9
  valvular — *see* Endocarditis
Murri's disease (intermittent hemoglobinuria) D59.6
Muscle, muscular — *see also* condition
  carnitine (palmityltransferase) deficiency E71.314
Musculoneuralgia — *see* Neuralgia
Mushrooming hip — *see* Derangement, joint, specified NEC, hip
Mushroom-workers' (pickers') **disease or lung** J67.5
Mutation(s)
  factor V Leiden D68.51
  prothrombin gene D68.52
  surfactant, of lung J84.83
Mutism — *see also* Aphasia
  deaf (acquired) (congenital) NEC H91.3
  elective (adjustment reaction) (childhood) F94.0
  hysterical F44.4
  selective (childhood) F94.0
MVD (microvillus inclusion disease) Q43.8
MVID (microvillus inclusion disease) Q43.8
Myalgia M79.10
  auxiliary muscles, head and neck M79.12
  epidemic (cervical) B33.0
  mastication muscle M79.11
  site specified NEC M79.18
  traumatic NEC T14.8 ☑
Myasthenia G70.9
  congenital G70.2
  cordis — *see* Failure, heart
  developmental G70.2
  gravis G70.00
    with exacerbation (acute) G70.01
    in crisis G70.01
    neonatal, transient P94.0
    pseudoparalytica G70.00
      with exacerbation (acute) G70.01
      in crisis G70.01
  stomach, psychogenic F45.8
  syndrome
    in
      diabetes mellitus — *see* E08-E13 with .44
      neoplastic disease — *see also* Neoplasm D49.9 *[G73.3]*
      pernicious anemia D51.0 *[G73.3]*
      thyrotoxicosis E05.90 *[G73.3]*
        with thyroid storm E05.91 *[G73.3]*
Myasthenic M62.81
Mycelium infection B49
Mycetismus — *see* Poisoning, food, noxious, mushroom
Mycetoma B47.9
  actinomycotic B47.1
  bone (mycotic) B47.9 *[M90.80]*

Mycetoma — *continued*
eumycotic B47.0
foot B47.9
actinomycotic B47.1
mycotic B47.0
madurae NEC B47.9
mycotic B47.0
maduromycotic B47.0
mycotic B47.0
nocardial B47.1
Mycobacteriosis — *see* Mycobacterium
Mycobacterium, mycobacterial (infection) A31.9
anonymous A31.9
atypical A31.9
cutaneous A31.1
pulmonary A31.0
tuberculous — *see* Tuberculosis, pulmonary
specified site NEC A31.8
avium (intracellulare complex) A31.0
balnei A31.1
Battey A31.0
chelonei A31.8
cutaneous A31.1
extrapulmonary systemic A31.8
fortuitum A31.8
intracellulare (Battey bacillus) A31.0
kakaferifu A31.8
kansasii (yellow bacillus) A31.0
kasongo A31.8
leprae — *see also* Leprosy A30.9
luciflavum A31.1
marinum (M. balnei) A31.1
nonspecific — *see* Mycobacterium, atypical
pulmonary (atypical) A31.0
tuberculous — *see* Tuberculosis, pulmonary
scrofulaceum A31.8
simiae A31.8
systemic, extrapulmonary A31.8
szulgai A31.8
terrae A31.8
triviale A31.8
tuberculosis (human, bovine) — *see* Tuberculosis
ulcerans A31.1
xenopi A31.8
Mycoplasma (M.) **pneumoniae, as cause of disease classified elsewhere** B96.0
Mycosis, mycotic B49
cutaneous NEC B36.9
ear B36.9
in
aspergillosis B44.89
candidiasis B37.84
moniliasis B37.84
fungoides (extranodal) (solid organ) C84.0- ☑
mouth B37.0
nails B35.1
opportunistic B48.8
skin NEC B36.9
specified NEC B48.8
stomatitis B37.0
vagina, vaginitis (candidal) B37.3
Mydriasis (pupil) H57.04
Myelatelia Q06.1
Myelinolysis, pontine, central G37.2
Myelitis (acute) (ascending) (childhood) (chronic) (descending) (diffuse) (disseminated) (idiopathic) (pressure) (progressive) (spinal cord) (subacute) — *see also* Encephalitis G04.91
flaccid G04.89
herpes simplex B00.82
herpes zoster B02.24
in diseases classified elsewhere G05.4
necrotizing, subacute G37.4
optic neuritis in G36.0
postchickenpox B01.12
postherpetic B02.24
postimmunization G04.02
postinfectious NEC G04.89
postvaccinal G04.02
specified NEC G04.89
syphilitic (transverse) A52.14
toxic G92
transverse (in demyelinating diseases of central nervous system) G37.3
tuberculous A17.82
varicella B01.12
Myeloblastic — *see* condition

Myeloblastoma
granular cell — *see also* Neoplasm, connective tissue
malignant — *see* Neoplasm, connective tissue, malignant
tongue D10.1
Myelocele — *see* Spina bifida
Myelocystocele — *see* Spina bifida
Myelocytic — *see* condition
Myelodysplasia D46.9
specified NEC D46.Z (*following* D46.4)
spinal cord (congenital) Q06.1
Myelodysplastic syndrome — *see also* Syndrome, myelodysplastic D46.9
with
5q deletion D46.C (*following* D46.2)
isolated del (5q) chromosomal abnormality D46.C (*following* D46.2)
specified NEC D46.Z (*following* D46.4)
Myeloencephalitis — *see* Encephalitis
Myelofibrosis D75.81
with myeloid metaplasia D47.4
acute C94.4- ☑
idiopathic (chronic) D47.4
primary D47.1
secondary D75.81
in myeloproliferative disease D47.4
Myelogenous — *see* condition
Myeloid — *see* condition
Myelokathexis D70.9
Myeloleukodystrophy E75.29
Myelolipoma — *see* Lipoma
Myeloma (multiple) C90.0- ☑
monostotic C90.3 ☑
plasma cell C90.0- ☑
plasma cell C90.0- ☑
solitary — *see also* Plasmacytoma, solitary C90.3- ☑
Myelomalacia G95.89
Myelomatosis C90.0- ☑
Myelomeningitis — *see* Meningoencephalitis
Myelomeningocele (spinal cord) — *see* Spina bifida
Myelo-osteo-musculodysplasia hereditaria Q79.8
Myelopathic
anemia D64.89
muscle atrophy — *see* Atrophy, muscle, spinal
pain syndrome G89.0
Myelopathy (spinal cord) G95.9
drug-induced G95.89
in (due to)
degeneration or displacement, intervertebral disc NEC — *see* Disorder, disc, with, myelopathy
infection — *see* Encephalitis
intervertebral disc disorder — *see also* Disorder, disc, with, myelopathy
mercury — *see* subcategory T56.1 ☑
neoplastic disease — *see also* Neoplasm D49.9 [G99.2]
pernicious anemia D51.0 [G99.2]
spondylosis — *see* Spondylosis, with myelopathy NEC
necrotic (subacute) (vascular) G95.19
radiation-induced G95.89
spondylogenic NEC — *see* Spondylosis, with myelopathy NEC
toxic G95.89
transverse, acute G37.3
vascular G95.19
vitamin B12 E53.8 [G32.0]
Myelophthisis D61.82
Myeloradiculitis G04.91
Myeloradiculodysplasia (spinal) Q06.1
Myelosarcoma C92.3- ☑
Myelosclerosis D75.89
with myeloid metaplasia D47.4
disseminated, of nervous system G35
megakaryocytic D47.4
with myeloid metaplasia D47.4
Myelosis
acute C92.0- ☑
aleukemic C92.9- ☑
chronic D47.1
erythremic (acute) C94.0- ☑
megakaryocytic C94.2- ☑
nonleukemic D72.828
subacute C92.9- ☑
Myiasis (cavernous) B87.9
aural B87.4
creeping B87.0

Myiasis — *continued*
cutaneous B87.0
dermal B87.0
ear (external) (middle) B87.4
eye B87.2
genitourinary B87.81
intestinal B87.82
laryngeal B87.3
nasopharyngeal B87.3
ocular B87.2
orbit B87.2
skin B87.0
specified site NEC B87.89
traumatic B87.1
wound B87.1
Myoadenoma, prostate — *see* Hyperplasia, prostate
Myoblastoma
granular cell — *see also* Neoplasm, connective tissue, benign
malignant — *see* Neoplasm, connective tissue, malignant
tongue D10.1
Myocardial — *see* condition
Myocardiopathy (congestive) (constrictive) (familial) (hypertrophic nonobstructive) (idiopathic) (infiltrative) (obstructive) (primary) (restrictive) (sporadic) — *see also* Cardiomyopathy I42.9
alcoholic I42.6
cobalt-beer I42.6
glycogen storage E74.02 [I43]
hypertrophic obstructive I42.1
in (due to)
beriberi E51.12
cardiac glycogenosis E74.02 [I43]
Friedreich's ataxia G11.11 [I43]
myotonia atrophica G71.11 [I43]
progressive muscular dystrophy G71.09 [I43]
obscure (African) I42.8
secondary I42.9
thyrotoxic E05.90 [I43]
with storm E05.91 [I43]
toxic NEC I42.7
Myocarditis (with arteriosclerosis)(chronic)(fibroid) (interstitial) (old) (progressive) (senile) I51.4
with
rheumatic fever (conditions in I00) I09.0
active — *see* Myocarditis, acute, rheumatic
inactive or quiescent (with chorea) I09.0
active I40.9
rheumatic I01.2
with chorea (acute) (rheumatic) (Sydenham's) I02.0
acute or subacute (interstitial) I40.9
due to
streptococcus (beta-hemolytic) I01.2
idiopathic I40.1
rheumatic I01.2
with chorea (acute) (rheumatic) (Sydenham's) I02.0
specified NEC I40.8
aseptic of newborn B33.22
bacterial (acute) I40.0
Coxsackie (virus) B33.22
diphtheritic A36.81
eosinophilic I40.1
epidemic of newborn (Coxsackie) B33.22
Fiedler's (acute) (isolated) I40.1
giant cell (acute) (subacute) I40.1
gonococcal A54.83
granulomatous (idiopathic) (isolated) (nonspecific) I40.1
hypertensive — *see* Hypertension, heart
idiopathic (granulomatous) I40.1
in (due to)
diphtheria A36.81
epidemic louse-borne typhus A75.0 [I41]
Lyme disease A69.29
sarcoidosis D86.85
scarlet fever A38.1
toxoplasmosis (acquired) B58.81
typhoid A01.02
typhus NEC A75.9 [I41]
infective I40.0
influenzal — *see* Influenza, with, myocarditis
isolated (acute) I40.1
meningococcal A39.52
mumps B26.82
nonrheumatic, active I40.9
parenchymatous I40.9

☑ **Additional Character Required** — Refer to the Tabular List for Character Selection

▽ **Subterms under main terms may continue to next column or page**

Myocarditis — *continued*
  pneumococcal I40.0
  rheumatic (chronic) (inactive) (with chorea) I09.0
    active or acute I01.2
      with chorea (acute) (rheumatic) (Sydenham's)
        I02.0
  rheumatoid — *see* Rheumatoid, carditis
  septic I40.0
  staphylococcal I40.0
  suppurative I40.0
  syphilitic (chronic) A52.06
  toxic I40.8
    rheumatic — *see* Myocarditis, acute, rheumatic
  tuberculous A18.84
  typhoid A01.02
  valvular — *see* Endocarditis
  virus, viral I40.0
    of newborn (Coxsackie) B33.22
Myocardium, myocardial — *see* condition
Myocardosis — *see* Cardiomyopathy
Myoclonus, myoclonic, myoclonia (familial) (essential)
    (multifocal) (simplex) G25.3
  drug-induced G25.3
  epilepsy — *see also* Epilepsy, generalized, specified
    NEC G40.4- ☑
    familial (progressive) G25.3
  epileptica G40.409
    with status epilepticus G40.401
  facial G51.3- ☑
  familial progressive G25.3
  Friedreich's G25.3
  jerks G25.3
  massive G25.3
  palatal G25.3
  pharyngeal G25.3
Myocytolysis I51.5
Myodiastasis — *see* Diastasis, muscle
Myoendocarditis — *see* Endocarditis
Myoepithelioma — *see* Neoplasm, benign, by site
Myofasciitis (acute) — *see* Myositis
Myofibroma — *see also* Neoplasm, connective tissue,
    benign
  uterus (cervix) (corpus) — *see* Leiomyoma
Myofibromatosis D48.1
  infantile Q89.8
Myofibrosis M62.89
  heart — *see* Myocarditis
  scapulohumeral — *see* Lesion, shoulder, specified NEC
Myofibrositis M79.7
  scapulohumeral — *see* Lesion, shoulder, specified NEC
Myoglobulinuria, myoglobinuria (primary) R82.1
Myokymia, facial G51.4
Myolipoma — *see* Lipoma
Myoma — *see also* Neoplasm, connective tissue, benign
  malignant — *see* Neoplasm, connective tissue, malig-
    nant
  prostate D29.1
  uterus (cervix) (corpus) — *see* Leiomyoma
Myomalacia M62.89
Myometritis — *see* Endometritis
Myometrium — *see* condition
Myonecrosis, clostridial A48.0
Myopathy G72.9
  acute
    necrotizing G72.81
    quadriplegic G72.81
  alcoholic G72.1
  benign congenital G71.20
  central core G71.29
  centronuclear G71.228
    autosomal (dominant) (recessive) G71.228
    other specified NEC G71.228
  congenital (benign) G71.20
  critical illness G72.81
  distal G71.09
  drug-induced G72.0
  endocrine NEC E34.9 *[G73.7]*
  extraocular muscles H05.82- ☑
  facioscapulohumeral G71.02
  hereditary G71.9
    specified NEC G71.8
  hyaline body G71.29
  immune NEC G72.49
  in (due to)
    Addison's disease E27.1 *[G73.7]*
    alcohol G72.1
    amyloidosis E85.0 *[G73.7]*

Myopathy — *continued*
  in — *continued*
    cretinism E00.9 *[G73.7]*
    Cushing's syndrome E24.9 *[G73.7]*
    drugs G72.0
    endocrine disease NEC E34.9 *[G73.7]*
    giant cell arteritis M31.6 *[G73.7]*
    glycogen storage disease E74.00 *[G73.7]*
    hyperadrenocorticism E24.9 *[G73.7]*
    hyperparathyroidism NEC E21.3 *[G73.7]*
    hypoparathyroidism E20.9 *[G73.7]*
    hypopituitarism E23.0 *[G73.7]*
    hypothyroidism E03.9 *[G73.7]*
    infectious disease NEC B99 ☑ *[G73.7]*
    lipid storage disease E75.6 *[G73.7]*
    metabolic disease NEC E88.9 *[G73.7]*
    myxedema E03.9 *[G73.7]*
    parasitic disease NEC B89 *[G73.7]*
    polyarteritis nodosa M30.0 *[G73.7]*
    rheumatoid arthritis — *see* Rheumatoid, myopathy
    sarcoidosis D86.87
    scleroderma M34.82
    sicca syndrome M35.03
    Sjögren's syndrome M35.03
    systemic lupus erythematosus M32.19
    thyrotoxicosis (hyperthyroidism) E05.90 *[G73.7]*
      with thyroid storm E05.91 *[G73.7]*
    toxic agent NEC G72.2
  inflammatory NEC G72.49
  intensive care (ICU) G72.81
  limb-girdle G71.09
  mitochondrial NEC G71.3
  myosin storage G71.29
  myotubular (centronuclear) G71.220
    X-linked G71.220
  mytonic, proximal (PROMM) G71.11
  nemaline G71.21
  ocular G71.09
  oculopharyngeal G71.09
  of critical illness G72.81
  primary G71.9
    specified NEC G71.8
  progressive NEC G72.89
  proximal myotonic (PROMM) G71.11
  rod (body) G71.21
  scapulohumeral G71.02
  specified NEC G72.89
  toxic G72.2
Myopericarditis — *see also* Pericarditis
  chronic rheumatic I09.2
Myopia (axial) (congenital) H52.1- ☑
  degenerative (malignant) H44.20
    with
      choroidal neovascularization H44.2A- ☑
      foveoschisis H44.2D- ☑
      macular hole H44.2B- ☑
      retinal detachment H44.2C- ☑
      specified maculopathy NEC H44.2E- ☑
    bilateral H44.23
    left eye H44.22
    right eye H44.21
  malignant — *see also* Myopia, degenerative H44.2- ☑
  pernicious — *see also* Myopia, degenerative H44.2- ☑
  progressive high (degenerative) — *see also* Myopia,
    degenerative H44.2- ☑
Myosarcoma — *see* Neoplasm, connective tissue, malig-
    nant
Myosis (pupil) H57.03
  stromal (endolymphatic) D39.0
Myositis M60.9
  clostridial A48.0
  due to posture — *see* Myositis, specified type NEC
  epidemic B33.0
  fibrosa or fibrous (chronic), Volkmann's T79.6 ☑
  foreign body granuloma — *see* Granuloma, foreign
    body
  in (due to)
    bilharziasis B65.9 *[M63.8-]* ☑
    cysticercosis B69.81
    leprosy A30.9 *[M63.8-]* ☑
    mycosis B49 *[M63.8-]* ☑
    sarcoidosis D86.87
    schistosomiasis B65.9 *[M63.8-]* ☑
    syphilis
      late A52.78
      secondary A51.49
    toxoplasmosis (acquired) B58.82

Myositis — *continued*
  in — *continued*
    trichinellosis B75 *[M63.8-]* ☑
    tuberculosis A18.09
  inclusion body [IBM] G72.41
  infective M60.009
    arm M60.002
      left M60.001
      right M60.000
    leg M60.005
      left M60.004
      right M60.003
    lower limb M60.005
      ankle M60.07- ☑
      foot M60.07- ☑
      lower leg M60.06- ☑
      thigh M60.05- ☑
      toe M60.07- ☑
    multiple sites M60.09
    specified site NEC M60.08
    upper limb M60.002
      finger M60.04- ☑
      forearm M60.03- ☑
      hand M60.04- ☑
      shoulder region M60.01- ☑
      upper arm M60.02- ☑
  interstitial M60.10
    ankle M60.17- ☑
    foot M60.17- ☑
    forearm M60.13- ☑
    hand M60.14- ☑
    lower leg M60.16- ☑
    multiple sites M60.19
    shoulder region M60.11- ☑
    specified site NEC M60.18
    thigh M60.15- ☑
    upper arm M60.12- ☑
  mycotic B49 *[M63.8-]* ☑
  orbital, chronic H05.12- ☑
  ossificans or ossifying (circumscripta) — *see also* Ossi-
    fication, muscle, specified NEC
    in (due to)
      burns M61.30
        ankle M61.37- ☑
        foot M61.37- ☑
        forearm M61.33- ☑
        hand M61.34- ☑
        lower leg M61.36- ☑
        multiple sites M61.39
        pelvic region M61.35- ☑
        shoulder region M61.31- ☑
        specified site NEC M61.38
        thigh M61.35- ☑
        upper arm M61.32- ☑
      quadriplegia or paraplegia M61.20
        ankle M61.27- ☑
        foot M61.27- ☑
        forearm M61.23- ☑
        hand M61.24- ☑
        lower leg M61.26- ☑
        multiple sites M61.29
        pelvic region M61.25- ☑
        shoulder region M61.21- ☑
        specified site NEC M61.28
        thigh M61.25- ☑
        upper arm M61.22- ☑
    progressiva M61.10
      ankle M61.17- ☑
      finger M61.14- ☑
      foot M61.17- ☑
      forearm M61.13- ☑
      hand M61.14- ☑
      lower leg M61.16- ☑
      multiple sites M61.19
      pelvic region M61.15- ☑
      shoulder region M61.11- ☑
      specified site NEC M61.18
      thigh M61.15- ☑
      toe M61.17- ☑
      upper arm M61.12- ☑
    traumatica M61.00
      ankle M61.07- ☑
      foot M61.07- ☑
      forearm M61.03- ☑
      hand M61.04- ☑
      lower leg M61.06- ☑
      multiple sites M61.09

Myositis — *continued*
  ossificans or ossifying — *see also* Ossification, muscle,
      specified — *continued*
    traumatica — *continued*
      pelvic region M61.05- ☑
      shoulder region M61.01- ☑
      specified site NEC M61.08
      thigh M61.05- ☑
      upper arm M61.02- ☑
  purulent — *see* Myositis, infective
  specified type NEC M60.80
    ankle M60.87- ☑
    foot M60.87- ☑
    forearm M60.83- ☑
    hand M60.84- ☑
    lower leg M60.86- ☑
    multiple sites M60.89
    pelvic region M60.85- ☑
    shoulder region M60.81- ☑
    specified site NEC M60.88
    thigh M60.85- ☑
    upper arm M60.82- ☑
  suppurative — *see* Myositis, infective
  traumatic (old) — *see* Myositis, specified type NEC

Myospasia impulsiva F95.2
Myotonia (acquisita) (intermittens) M62.89
  atrophica G71.11
  chondrodystrophic G71.13
  congenita (acetazolamide responsive) (dominant) (recessive) G71.12
  drug-induced G71.14
  dystrophica G71.11
  fluctuans G71.19
  levior G71.12
  permanens G71.19
  symptomatic G71.19
Myotonic pupil — *see* Anomaly, pupil, function, tonic pupil
Myriapodiasis B88.2
Myringitis H73.2- ☑
  with otitis media — *see* Otitis, media
  acute H73.00- ☑
    bullous H73.01- ☑
    specified NEC H73.09- ☑
  bullous — *see* Myringitis, acute, bullous
  chronic H73.1- ☑
Mysophobia F40.228
Mytilotoxism — *see* Poisoning, fish
Myxadenitis labialis K13.0

Myxedema (adult) (idiocy) (infantile) (juvenile) — *see also* Hypothyroidism E03.9
  circumscribed E05.90
    with storm E05.91
  coma E03.5
  congenital E00.1
  cutis L98.5
  localized (pretibial) E05.90
    with storm E05.91
  papular L98.5
Myxochondrosarcoma — *see* Neoplasm, cartilage, malignant
Myxofibroma — *see* Neoplasm, connective tissue, benign
  odontogenic — *see* Cyst, calcifying odontogenic
Myxofibrosarcoma — *see* Neoplasm, connective tissue, malignant
Myxolipoma D17.9
Myxoliposarcoma — *see* Neoplasm, connective tissue, malignant
Myxoma — *see also* Neoplasm, connective tissue, benign
  nerve sheath — *see* Neoplasm, nerve, benign
  odontogenic — *see* Cyst, calcifying odontogenic
Myxosarcoma — *see* Neoplasm, connective tissue, malignant

N

Naegeli's
  disease Q82.8
  leukemia, monocytic C93.1- ☑
Naegleriasis (with meningoencephalitis) B60.2
Naffziger's syndrome G54.0
Naga sore — *see* Ulcer, skin
Nägele's pelvis M95.5
  with disproportion (fetopelvic) O33.0
    causing obstructed labor O65.0
Nail — *see also* condition
  biting F98.8
  patella syndrome Q87.2
Nanism, nanosomia — *see* Dwarfism
Nanophyetiasis B66.8
Nanukayami A27.89
Napkin rash L22
Narcolepsy G47.419
  with cataplexy G47.411
  in conditions classified elsewhere G47.429
    with cataplexy G47.421
Narcosis R06.89
Narcotism — *see* Dependence
NARP (Neuropathy, Ataxia and Retinitis pigmentosa)
  syndrome E88.49
Narrow
  anterior chamber angle H40.03- ☑
  gingival width (of periodontal soft tissue) K05.5
  pelvis — *see* Contraction, pelvis
Narrowing — *see also* Stenosis
  artery I77.1
    auditory, internal I65.8
    basilar — *see* Occlusion, artery, basilar
    carotid — *see* Occlusion, artery, carotid
    cerebellar — *see* Occlusion, artery, cerebellar
    cerebral — *see* Occlusion artery, cerebral
    choroidal — *see* Occlusion, artery, precerebral,
      specified NEC
    communicating posterior — *see* Occlusion, artery,
      precerebral, specified NEC
    coronary — *see also* Disease, heart, ischemic,
      atherosclerotic
      congenital Q24.5
        syphilitic A50.54 [I52]
      due to syphilis NEC A52.06
    hypophyseal — *see* Occlusion, artery, precerebral,
      specified NEC
    pontine — *see* Occlusion, artery, precerebral, spec-
      ified NEC
    precerebral — *see* Occlusion, artery, precerebral
    vertebral — *see* Occlusion, artery, vertebral
  auditory canal (external) — *see* Stenosis, external ear
    canal
  eustachian tube — *see* Obstruction, eustachian tube
  eyelid — *see* Disorder, eyelid function
  larynx J38.6
  mesenteric artery — *see also* Ischemia, intestine, acute
    K55.059
  palate M26.89
  palpebral fissure — *see* Disorder, eyelid function
  ureter N13.5
    with infection N13.6
  urethra — *see* Stricture, urethra
Narrowness, abnormal, eyelid Q10.3
Nasal — *see* condition
Nasolachrymal, nasolacrimal — *see* condition
Nasopharyngeal — *see also* condition
  pituitary gland Q89.2
  torticollis M43.6
Nasopharyngitis (acute) (infective) (streptococcal)
  (subacute) J00
  chronic (suppurative) (ulcerative) J31.1
Nasopharynx, nasopharyngeal — *see* condition
Natal tooth, teeth K00.6
Nausea (without vomiting) R11.0
  with vomiting R11.2
  gravidarum — *see* Hyperemesis, gravidarum
  marina T75.3 ☑
  navalis T75.3 ☑
Navel — *see* condition
Neapolitan fever — *see* Brucellosis
Near drowning T75.1 ☑
Nearsightedness — *see* Myopia
Near-syncope R55
Nebula, cornea — *see* Opacity, cornea

Necator americanus infestation B76.1
Necatoriasis B76.1
Neck — *see* condition
Necrobiosis R68.89
  lipoidica NEC L92.1
    with diabetes — *see* E08-E13 with .620
Necrolysis, toxic epidermal L51.2
  due to drug
    correct substance properly administered — *see* Ta-
      ble of Drugs and Chemicals, by drug, adverse
      effect
    overdose or wrong substance given or taken — *see*
      Table of Drugs and Chemicals, by drug, poi-
      soning
Necrophilia F65.89
Necrosis, necrotic (ischemic) — *see also* Gangrene
  adrenal (capsule) (gland) E27.49
  amputation stump (surgical) (late) T87.50
    arm T87.5- ☑
    leg T87.5- ☑
  antrum J32.0
  aorta (hyaline) — *see also* Aneurysm, aorta
    cystic medial — *see* Dissection, aorta
  artery I77.5
  bladder (aseptic) (sphincter) N32.89
  bone — *see also* Osteonecrosis M87.9
    aseptic or avascular — *see* Osteonecrosis
      idiopathic M87.00
    ethmoid J32.2
    jaw M27.2
    tuberculous — *see* Tuberculosis, bone
  brain I67.89
  breast (aseptic) (fat) (segmental) N64.1
  bronchus J98.09
  central nervous system NEC I67.89
  cerebellar I67.89
  cerebral I67.89
  colon — *see also* Infarct, intestine K55.049
  cornea H18.89- ☑
  cortical (acute) (renal) N17.1
  cystic medial (aorta) — *see* Dissection, aorta
  dental pulp K04.1
  esophagus K22.8
  ethmoid (bone) J32.2
  eyelid — *see* Disorder, eyelid, degenerative
  fat, fatty (generalized) — *see also* Disorder, soft tissue,
    specified type NEC)
    abdominal wall K65.4
    breast (aseptic) (segmental) N64.1
    localized — *see* Degeneration, by site, fatty
    mesentery K65.4
    omentum K65.4
    pancreas K86.89
    peritoneum K65.4
    skin (subcutaneous), newborn P83.0
    subcutaneous, due to birth injury P15.6
  gallbladder — *see* Cholecystitis, acute
  heart — *see* Infarct, myocardium
  hip, aseptic or avascular — *see* Osteonecrosis, by type,
    femur
  intestine (acute) (hemorrhagic) (massive) — *see also*
    Infarct, intestine K55.069
  jaw M27.2
  kidney (bilateral) N28.0
    acute N17.9
    cortical (acute) (bilateral) N17.1
      with ectopic or molar pregnancy O08.4
    medullary (bilateral) (in acute renal failure) (papil-
      lary) N17.2
    papillary (bilateral) (in acute renal failure) N17.2
    tubular N17.0
      with ectopic or molar pregnancy O08.4
      complicating
        abortion — *see* Abortion, by type, complicat-
          ed by, tubular necrosis
        ectopic or molar pregnancy O08.4
        pregnancy — *see* Pregnancy, complicated by,
          diseases of, specified type or system
          NEC
      following ectopic or molar pregnancy O08.4
      traumatic T79.5 ☑
  larynx J38.7
  liver (with hepatic failure) (cell) — *see* Failure, hepatic
    hemorrhagic, central K76.2
  lung J85.0
  lymphatic gland — *see* Lymphadenitis, acute
  mammary gland (fat) (segmental) N64.1
  mastoid (chronic) — *see* Mastoiditis, chronic

Necrosis, necrotic — *continued*
  medullary (acute) (renal) N17.2
  mesentery — *see also* Infarct, intestine K55.069
    fat K65.4
  mitral valve — *see* Insufficiency, mitral
  myocardium, myocardial — *see* Infarct, myocardium
  nose J34.0
  omentum (with mesenteric infarction) — *see also* In-
    farct, intestine K55.069
    fat K65.4
  orbit, orbital — *see* Osteomyelitis, orbit
  ossicles, ear — *see* Abnormal, ear ossicles
  ovary N70.92
  pancreas (aseptic) (duct) (fat) K86.89
    acute (infective) — *see* Pancreatitis, acute
    infective — *see* Pancreatitis, acute
  papillary (acute) (renal) N17.2
  perineum N90.89
  peritoneum (with mesenteric infarction) — *see also*
    Infarct, intestine K55.069
    fat K65.4
  pharynx J02.9
    in granulocytopenia — *see* Neutropenia
    Vincent's A69.1
  phosphorus — *see* subcategory T54.2 ☑
  pituitary (gland) E23.0
    postpartum O99.285
    Sheehan O99.285
  pressure — *see* Ulcer, pressure, by site
  pulmonary J85.0
  pulp (dental) K04.1
  radiation — *see* Necrosis, by site
  radium — *see* Necrosis, by site
  renal — *see* Necrosis, kidney
  sclera H15.89
  scrotum N50.89
  skin or subcutaneous tissue NEC I96
  spine, spinal (column) — *see also* Osteonecrosis, by
    type, vertebra
    cord G95.19
  spleen D73.5
  stomach K31.89
  stomatitis (ulcerative) A69.0
  subcutaneous fat, newborn P83.88
  subendocardial (acute) I21.4
    chronic I25.89
  suprarenal (capsule) (gland) E27.49
  testis N50.89
  thymus (gland) E32.8
  tonsil J35.8
  trachea J39.8
  tuberculous NEC — *see* Tuberculosis
  tubular (acute) (anoxic) (renal) (toxic) N17.0
    postprocedural N99.0
  vagina N89.8
  vertebra — *see also* Osteonecrosis, by type, vertebra
    tuberculous A18.01
  vulva N90.89
  X-ray — *see* Necrosis, by site
Necrospermia — *see* Infertility, male
Need (for)
  care provider because (of)
    assistance with personal care Z74.1
    continuous supervision required Z74.3
    impaired mobility Z74.09
    no other household member able to render care
      Z74.2
    specified reason NEC Z74.8
  immunization — *see* Vaccination
  vaccination — *see* Vaccination
Neglect
  adult
    confirmed T74.01 ☑
    history of Z91.412
    suspected T76.01 ☑
  child (childhood)
    confirmed T74.02 ☑
    history of Z62.812
    suspected T76.02 ☑
  emotional, in childhood Z62.898
  hemispatial R41.4
  left-sided R41.4
  sensory R41.4
  visuospatial R41.4
Neisserian infection NEC — *see* Gonococcus
Nelaton's syndrome G60.8
Nelson's syndrome E24.1
Nematodiasis (intestinal) B82.0

Nematodiasis — *continued*
Ancylostoma B76.0
Neonatal — *see also* Newborn
acne L70.4
bradycardia P29.12
screening, abnormal findings on P09
tachycardia P29.11
tooth, teeth K00.6
Neonatorum — *see* condition
Neoplasia
endocrine, multiple (MEN) E31.20
type I E31.21
type IIA E31.22
type IIB E31.23
intraepithelial (histologically confirmed)
anal (AIN) (histologically confirmed) K62.82
grade I K62.82
grade II K62.82
severe D01.3
cervical glandular (histologically confirmed) D06.9
cervix (uteri) (CIN) (histologically confirmed) N87.9
glandular D06.9
grade I N87.0
grade II N87.1
grade III (severe dysplasia) — *see also* Carcinoma, cervix uteri, in situ D06.9
prostate (histologically confirmed) (PIN) N42.31
grade I N42.31
grade II N42.31
grade III (severe dysplasia) D07.5
vagina (histologically confirmed) (VAIN) N89.3
grade I N89.0
grade II N89.1
grade III (severe dysplasia) D07.2
vulva (histologically confirmed) (VIN) N90.3
grade I N90.0
grade II N90.1
grade III (severe dysplasia) D07.1
Neoplasm, neoplastic — *see also* Table of Neoplasms
lipomatous, benign — *see* Lipoma
malignant mast cell C96.20
specified type NEC C96.29
mast cell, of uncertain behavior NEC D47.09
Neovascularization
ciliary body — *see* Disorder, iris, vascular
cornea H16.40- ☑
deep H16.44- ☑
ghost vessels — *see* Ghost, vessels
localized H16.43- ☑
pannus — *see* Pannus
iris — *see* Disorder, iris, vascular
retina H35.05- ☑
Nephralgia N23
Nephritis, nephritic (albuminuric) (azotemic) (congenital) (disseminated) (epithelial) (familial) (focal) (granulomatous) (hemorrhagic) (infantile) (nonsuppurative, excretory) (uremic) N05.9
with
C3
glomerulonephritis N05.A
glomerulopathy N05.A
with dense deposit disease N05.6
dense deposit disease N05.6
diffuse
crescentic glomerulonephritis N05.7
endocapillary proliferative glomerulonephritis N05.4
membranous glomerulonephritis N05.2
mesangial proliferative glomerulonephritis N05.3
mesangiocapillary glomerulonephritis N05.5
edema — *see* Nephrosis
focal and segmental glomerular lesions N05.1
foot process disease N04.9
glomerular lesion
diffuse sclerosing N05.8
hypocomplementemic — *see* Nephritis, membranoproliferative
IgA — *see* Nephropathy, IgA
lobular, lobulonodular — *see* Nephritis, membranoproliferative
nodular — *see* Nephritis, membranoproliferative
lesion of
glomerulonephritis, proliferative N05.8
renal necrosis N05.9
minor glomerular abnormality N05.0
specified morphological changes NEC N05.8
acute N00.9

Nephritis, nephritic — *continued*
acute — *continued*
with
C3
glomerulonephritis N00.A
glomerulopathy N00.A
with dense deposit disease N00.6
dense deposit disease N00.6
diffuse
crescentic glomerulonephritis N00.7
endocapillary proliferative glomerulonephritis N00.4
membranous glomerulonephritis N00.2
mesangial proliferative glomerulonephritis N00.3
mesangiocapillary glomerulonephritis N00.5
focal and segmental glomerular lesions N00.1
minor glomerular abnormality N00.0
specified morphological changes NEC N00.8
amyloid E85.4 *[N08]*
antiglomerular basement membrane (anti-GBM) antibody NEC
in Goodpasture's syndrome M31.0
antitubular basement membrane (tubulo-interstitial) NEC N12
toxic — *see* Nephropathy, toxic
arteriolar — *see* Hypertension, kidney
arteriosclerotic — *see* Hypertension, kidney
ascending — *see* Nephritis, tubulo-interstitial
atrophic N03.9
Balkan (endemic) N15.0
calculous, calculus — *see* Calculus, kidney
cardiac — *see* Hypertension, kidney
cardiovascular — *see* Hypertension, kidney
chronic N03.9
with
C3
glomerulonephritis N03.A
glomerulopathy N03.A
with dense deposit disease N03.6
dense deposit disease N03.6
diffuse
crescentic glomerulonephritis N03.7
endocapillary proliferative glomerulonephritis N03.4
membranous glomerulonephritis N03.2
mesangial proliferative glomerulonephritis N03.3
mesangiocapillary glomerulonephritis N03.5
focal and segmental glomerular lesions N03.1
minor glomerular abnormality N03.0
specified morphological changes NEC N03.8
arteriosclerotic — *see* Hypertension, kidney
cirrhotic N26.9
complicating pregnancy O26.83- ☑
croupous N00.9
degenerative — *see* Nephrosis
diffuse sclerosing N05.8
due to
diabetes mellitus — *see* E08-E13 with .21
subacute bacterial endocarditis I33.0
systemic lupus erythematosus (chronic) M32.14
typhoid fever A01.09
gonococcal (acute) (chronic) A54.21
hypocomplementemic — *see* Nephritis, membranoproliferative
IgA — *see* Nephropathy, IgA
immune complex (circulating) NEC N05.8
infective — *see* Nephritis, tubulo-interstitial
interstitial — *see* Nephritis, tubulo-interstitial
lead N14.3
membranoproliferative (diffuse) (type 1 or 3) — *see also* N00-N07 with fourth character .5 N05.5
type 2 — *see also* N00-N07 with fourth character .6 N05.6
minimal change N05.0
necrotic, necrotizing NEC — *see also* N00-N07 with fourth character .8 N05.8
nephrotic — *see* Nephrosis
nodular — *see* Nephritis, membranoproliferative
polycystic Q61.3
adult type Q61.2
autosomal
dominant Q61.2
recessive NEC Q61.19
childhood type NEC Q61.19
infantile type NEC Q61.19
poststreptococcal N05.9

Nephritis, nephritic — *continued*
poststreptococcal — *continued*
acute N00.9
chronic N03.9
rapidly progressive N01.9
proliferative NEC — *see also* N00-N07 with fourth character .8 N05.8
purulent — *see* Nephritis, tubulo-interstitial
rapidly progressive N01.9
with
C3
glomerulonephritis N01.A
glomerulopathy N01.A
with dense deposit disease N01.6
dense deposit disease N01.6
diffuse
crescentic glomerulonephritis N01.7
endocapillary proliferative glomerulonephritis N01.4
membranous glomerulonephritis N01.2
mesangial proliferative glomerulonephritis N01.3
mesangiocapillary glomerulonephritis N01.5
focal and segmental glomerular lesions N01.1
minor glomerular abnormality N01.0
specified morphological changes NEC N01.8
salt losing or wasting NEC N28.89
saturnine N14.3
sclerosing, diffuse N05.8
septic — *see* Nephritis, tubulo-interstitial
specified pathology NEC — *see also* N00-N07 with fourth character .8 N05.8
subacute N01.9
suppurative — *see* Nephritis, tubulo-interstitial
syphilitic (late) A52.75
congenital A50.59 *[N08]*
early (secondary) A51.44
toxic — *see* Nephropathy, toxic
tubal, tubular — *see* Nephritis, tubulo-interstitial
tuberculous A18.11
tubulo-interstitial (in) N12
acute (infectious) N10
chronic (infectious) N11.9
nonobstructive N11.8
reflux-associated N11.0
obstructive N11.1
specified NEC N11.8
due to
brucellosis A23.9 *[N16]*
cryoglobulinemia D89.1 *[N16]*
glycogen storage disease E74.00 *[N16]*
Sjögren's syndrome M35.04
vascular — *see* Hypertension, kidney
war N00.9
Nephroblastoma (epithelial) (mesenchymal) C64- ☑
Nephrocalcinosis E83.59 *[N29]*
Nephrocystitis, pustular — *see* Nephritis, tubulo-interstitial
Nephrolithiasis (congenital) (pelvis) (recurrent) — *see also* Calculus, kidney
Nephroma C64- ☑
mesoblastic D41.0- ☑
Nephronephritis — *see* Nephrosis
Nephronophthisis Q61.5
Nephropathia epidemica A98.5
Nephropathy — *see also* Nephritis N28.9
with
edema — *see* Nephrosis
glomerular lesion — *see* Glomerulonephritis
amyloid, hereditary E85.0
analgesic N14.0
with medullary necrosis, acute N17.2
Balkan (endemic) N15.0
chemical — *see* Nephropathy, toxic
diabetic — *see* E08-E13 with .21
drug-induced N14.2
specified NEC N14.1
focal and segmental hyalinosis or sclerosis N02.1
heavy metal-induced N14.3
hereditary NEC N07.9
with
C3
glomerulonephritis N07.A
glomerulopathy N07.A
with dense deposit disease N07.6
dense deposit disease N07.6
diffuse
crescentic glomerulonephritis N07.7

☑ Additional Character Required — Refer to the Tabular List for Character Selection

☒ Subterms under main terms may continue to next column or page

Nephropathy — *continued*
  hereditary — *continued*
    with — *continued*
      diffuse — *continued*
        endocapillary proliferative glomerulonephritis N07.4
        membranous glomerulonephritis N07.2
        mesangial proliferative glomerulonephritis N07.3
        mesangiocapillary glomerulonephritis N07.5
        focal and segmental glomerular lesions N07.1
        minor glomerular abnormality N07.0
        specified morphological changes NEC N07.8
  hypercalcemic N25.89
  hypertensive — *see* Hypertension, kidney
  hypokalemic (vacuolar) N25.89
  IgA N02.8
    with glomerular lesion N02.9
      focal and segmental hyalinosis or sclerosis N02.1
      membranoproliferative (diffuse) N02.5
      membranous (diffuse) N02.2
      mesangial proliferative (diffuse) N02.3
      mesangiocapillary (diffuse) N02.5
      proliferative NEC N02.8
      specified pathology NEC N02.8
  lead N14.3
  membranoproliferative (diffuse) N02.5
  membranous (diffuse) N02.2
  mesangial (IgA/IgG) — *see* Nephropathy, IgA
    proliferative (diffuse) N02.3
  mesangiocapillary (diffuse) N02.5
  obstructive N13.8
  phenacetin N17.2
  phosphate-losing N25.0
  potassium depletion N25.89
  pregnancy-related O26.83- ☑
  proliferative NEC — *see also* N00-N07 with fourth character .8 N05.8
  protein-losing N25.89
  saturnine N14.3
  sickle-cell D57.- ☑ *[N08]*
  toxic NEC N14.4
    due to
      drugs N14.2
        analgesic N14.0
        specified NEC N14.1
      heavy metals N14.3
  vasomotor N17.0
  water-losing N25.89
Nephroptosis N28.83
Nephropyosis — *see* Abscess, kidney
Nephrorrhagia N28.89
Nephrosclerosis (arteriolar)(arteriosclerotic) (chronic) (hyaline) — *see also* Hypertension, kidney
  hyperplastic — *see* Hypertension, kidney
  senile N26.9
Nephrosis, nephrotic (Epstein's) (syndrome) (congenital) N04.9
  with
    foot process disease N04.9
    glomerular lesion N04.1
    hypocomplementemic N04.5
  acute N04.9
  anoxic — *see* Nephrosis, tubular
  chemical — *see* Nephrosis, tubular
  cholemic K76.7
  diabetic — *see* E08-E13 with .21
  Finnish type (congenital) Q89.8
  hemoglobin N10
  hemoglobinuric — *see* Nephrosis, tubular
  in
    amyloidosis E85.4 *[N08]*
    diabetes mellitus — *see* E08-E13 with .21
    epidemic hemorrhagic fever A98.5
    malaria (malariae) B52.0
  ischemic — *see* Nephrosis, tubular
  lipoid N04.9
  lower nephron — *see* Nephrosis, tubular
  malarial (malariae) B52.0
  minimal change N04.0
  myoglobin N10
  necrotizing — *see* Nephrosis, tubular
  osmotic (sucrose) N25.89
  radiation N04.9
  syphilitic (late) A52.75
  toxic — *see* Nephrosis, tubular
  tubular (acute) N17.0
    postprocedural N99.0

Nephrosis, nephrotic — *continued*
  tubular — *continued*
    radiation N04.9
Nephrosonephritis, hemorrhagic (endemic) A98.5
Nephrostomy
  attention to Z43.6
  status Z93.6
Nerve — *see also* condition
  injury — *see* Injury, nerve, by body site
Nerves R45.0
Nervous — *see also* condition R45.0
  heart F45.8
  stomach F45.8
  tension R45.0
Nervousness R45.0
Nesidioblastoma
  pancreas D13.7
  specified site NEC — *see* Neoplasm, benign, by site
  unspecified site D13.7
Nettleship's syndrome — *see* Urticaria pigmentosa
Neumann's disease or syndrome L10.1
Neuralgia, neuralgic (acute) M79.2
  accessory (nerve) G52.8
  acoustic (nerve) — *see* subcategory H93.3 ☑
  auditory (nerve) — *see* subcategory H93.3 ☑
  ciliary G44.009
    intractable G44.001
    not intractable G44.009
  cranial
    nerve — *see also* Disorder, nerve, cranial
      fifth or trigeminal — *see* Neuralgia, trigeminal
      postherpetic, postzoster B02.29
  ear — *see* subcategory H92.0 ☑
  facialis vera G51.1
  Fothergill's — *see* Neuralgia, trigeminal
  glossopharyngeal (nerve) G52.1
  Horton's G44.099
    intractable G44.091
    not intractable G44.099
  Hunt's B02.21
  hypoglossal (nerve) G52.3
  infraorbital — *see* Neuralgia, trigeminal
  malarial — *see* Malaria
  migrainous G44.009
    intractable G44.001
    not intractable G44.009
  Morton's G57.6- ☑
  nerve, cranial — *see* Disorder, nerve, cranial
  nose G52.0
  occipital M54.81
  olfactory G52.0
  penis N48.9
  perineum R10.2
  postherpetic NEC B02.29
    trigeminal B02.22
  pubic region R10.2
  scrotum R10.2
  Sluder's G44.89
  specified nerve NEC G58.8
  spermatic cord R10.2
  sphenopalatine (ganglion) G90.09
  trifacial — *see* Neuralgia, trigeminal
  trigeminal G50.0
    postherpetic, postzoster B02.22
  vagus (nerve) G52.2
  writer's F48.8
    organic G25.89
Neurapraxia — *see* Injury, nerve
Neurasthenia F48.8
  cardiac F45.8
  gastric F45.8
  heart F45.8
Neurilemmoma — *see also* Neoplasm, nerve, benign
  acoustic (nerve) D33.3
  malignant — *see also* Neoplasm, nerve, malignant
    acoustic (nerve) C72.4- ☑
Neurilemmosarcoma — *see* Neoplasm, nerve, malignant
Neurinoma — *see* Neoplasm, nerve, benign
Neurinomatosis — *see* Neoplasm, nerve, uncertain behavior
Neuritis (rheumatoid) M79.2
  abducens (nerve) — *see* Strabismus, paralytic, sixth nerve
  accessory (nerve) G52.8
  acoustic (nerve) — *see also* subcategory H93.3 ☑
    in (due to)
      infectious disease NEC B99 ☑ *[H94.0-]* ☑

Neuritis — *continued*
  acoustic — *see also* subcategory — *continued*
    in — *continued*
      parasitic disease NEC B89 *[H94.0-]* ☑
      syphilitic A52.15
  alcoholic G62.1
    with psychosis — *see* Psychosis, alcoholic
  amyloid, any site E85.4 *[G63]*
  auditory (nerve) — *see* subcategory H93.3 ☑
  brachial — *see* Radiculopathy
    due to displacement, intervertebral disc — *see* Disorder, disc, cervical, with neuritis
  cranial nerve
    due to Lyme disease A69.22
    eighth or acoustic or auditory — *see* subcategory H93.3 ☑
    eleventh or accessory G52.8
    fifth or trigeminal G51.0
    first or olfactory G52.0
    fourth or trochlear — *see* Strabismus, paralytic, fourth nerve
    second or optic — *see* Neuritis, optic
    seventh or facial G51.8
      newborn (birth injury) P11.3
    sixth or abducent — *see* Strabismus, paralytic, sixth nerve
    tenth or vagus G52.2
    third or oculomotor — *see* Strabismus, paralytic, third nerve
    twelfth or hypoglossal G52.3
  Déjérine-Sottas G60.0
  diabetic (mononeuropathy) — *see* E08-E13 with .41
    polyneuropathy — *see* E08-E13 with .42
  due to
    beriberi E51.11
    displacement, prolapse or rupture, intervertebral disc — *see* Disorder, disc, with, radiculopathy
    herniation, nucleus pulposus M51.9 *[G55]*
  endemic E51.11
  facial G51.8
    newborn (birth injury) P11.3
  general — *see* Polyneuropathy
  geniculate ganglion G51.1
    due to herpes (zoster) B02.21
  gouty — *see also* Gout, by type M10.9 *[G63]*
  hypoglossal (nerve) G52.3
  ilioinguinal (nerve) G57.9- ☑
  infectious (multiple) NEC G61.0
  interstitial hypertrophic progressive G60.0
  lumbar M54.16
  lumbosacral M54.17
  multiple — *see also* Polyneuropathy
    endemic E51.11
    infective, acute G61.0
  multiplex endemica E51.11
  nerve root — *see* Radiculopathy
  oculomotor (nerve) — *see* Strabismus, paralytic, third nerve
  olfactory nerve G52.0
  optic (nerve) (hereditary) (sympathetic) H46.9
    with demyelination G36.0
    in myelitis G36.0
    nutritional H46.2
    papillitis — *see* Papillitis, optic
    retrobulbar H46.1- ☑
    specified type NEC H46.8
    toxic H46.3
  peripheral (nerve) G62.9
    multiple — *see* Polyneuropathy
    single — *see* Mononeuritis
  pneumogastric (nerve) G52.2
  postherpetic, postzoster B02.29
  progressive hypertrophic interstitial G60.0
  retrobulbar — *see also* Neuritis, optic, retrobulbar
    in (due to)
      late syphilis A52.15
      meningococcal infection A39.82
    meningococcal A39.82
    syphilitic A52.15
  sciatic (nerve) — *see also* Sciatica
    due to displacement of intervertebral disc — *see* Disorder, disc, with, radiculopathy
  serum — *see also* Reaction, serum T80.69 ☑
  shoulder-girdle G54.5
  specified nerve NEC G58.8
  spinal (nerve) root — *see* Radiculopathy
  syphilitic A52.15
  thenar (median) G56.1- ☑

Neuritis — *continued*
  thoracic M54.14
  toxic NEC G62.2
  trochlear (nerve) — *see* Strabismus, paralytic, fourth
    nerve
  vagus (nerve) G52.2
Neuroastrocytoma — *see* Neoplasm, uncertain behavior,
    by site
Neuroavitaminosis E56.9 *[G99.8]*
Neuroblastoma
  olfactory C30.0
  specified site — *see* Neoplasm, malignant, by site
  unspecified site C74.90
Neurochorioretinitis — *see* Chorioretinitis
Neurocirculatory asthenia F45.8
Neurocysticercosis B69.0
Neurocytoma — *see* Neoplasm, benign, by site
Neurodermatitis (circumscribed) (circumscripta) (local)
    L28.0
  atopic L20.81
  diffuse (Brocq) L20.81
  disseminated L20.81
Neuroencephalomyelopathy, optic G36.0
Neuroepithelioma — *see also* Neoplasm, malignant, by
    site
  olfactory C30.0
Neurofibroma — *see also* Neoplasm, nerve, benign
  melanotic — *see* Neoplasm, nerve, benign
  multiple — *see* Neurofibromatosis
  plexiform — *see* Neoplasm, nerve, benign
Neurofibromatosis (multiple) (nonmalignant) Q85.00
  acoustic Q85.02
  malignant — *see* Neoplasm, nerve, malignant
  specified NEC Q85.09
  type 1 (von Recklinghausen) Q85.01
  type 2 Q85.02
Neurofibrosarcoma — *see* Neoplasm, nerve, malignant
Neurogenic — *see also* condition
  bladder — *see also* Dysfunction, bladder, neuromuscu-
    lar N31.9
    cauda equina syndrome G83.4
  bowel NEC K59.2
  heart F45.8
Neuroglioma — *see* Neoplasm, uncertain behavior, by
    site
Neurolabyrinthitis (of Dix and Hallpike) — *see* Neuroni-
    tis, vestibular
Neurolathyrism — *see* Poisoning, food, noxious, plant
Neuroleprosy A30.9
Neuroma — *see also* Neoplasm, nerve, benign
  acoustic (nerve) D33.3
  amputation (stump) (traumatic) (surgical complication)
      (late) T87.3- ☑
    arm T87.3- ☑
    leg T87.3- ☑
  digital (toe) G57.6- ☑
  interdigital G58.8
    lower limb (toe) G57.8- ☑
    upper limb G56.8- ☑
  intermetatarsal G57.8- ☑
  Morton's G57.6- ☑
  nonneoplastic
    arm G56.9- ☑
    leg G57.9- ☑
    lower extremity G57.9- ☑
    upper extremity G56.9- ☑
  optic (nerve) D33.3
  plantar G57.6- ☑
  plexiform — *see* Neoplasm, nerve, benign
  surgical (nonneoplastic)
    arm G56.9- ☑
    leg G57.9- ☑
    lower extremity G57.9- ☑
    upper extremity G56.9- ☑
Neuromyalgia — *see* Neuralgia
Neuromyasthenia (epidemic) (postinfectious) G93.3
Neuromyelitis G36.9
  ascending G61.0
  optica G36.0
Neuromyopathy G70.9
  paraneoplastic D49.9 *[G13.0]*
Neuromyotonia (Isaacs) G71.19
Neuronevus — *see* Nevus
Neuronitis G58.9
  ascending (acute) G57.2- ☑
  vestibular H81.2- ☑
Neuroparalytic — *see* condition

Neuropathy, neuropathic G62.9
  acute motor G62.81
  alcoholic G62.1
    with psychosis — *see* Psychosis, alcoholic
  arm G56.9- ☑
  autonomic, peripheral — *see* Neuropathy, peripheral,
    autonomic
  axillary G56.9- ☑
  bladder N31.9
    atonic (motor) (sensory) N31.2
    autonomous N31.2
    flaccid N31.2
    nonreflex N31.2
    reflex N31.1
    uninhibited N31.0
  brachial plexus G54.0
  cervical plexus G54.2
  chronic
    progressive segmentally demyelinating G62.89
    relapsing demyelinating G62.89
  Déjérine-Sottas G60.0
  diabetic — *see* E08-E13 with .40
    mononeuropathy — *see* E08-E13 with .41
    polyneuropathy — *see* E08-E13 with .42
  entrapment G58.9
    iliohypogastric nerve G57.8- ☑
    ilioinguinal nerve G57.8- ☑
    lateral cutaneous nerve of thigh G57.1- ☑
    median nerve G56.0- ☑
    obturator nerve G57.8- ☑
    peroneal nerve G57.3- ☑
    posterior tibial nerve G57.5- ☑
    saphenous nerve G57.8- ☑
    ulnar nerve G56.2- ☑
  facial nerve G51.9
  hereditary G60.9
    motor and sensory (types I-IV) G60.0
    sensory G60.8
    specified NEC G60.8
  hypertrophic G60.0
    Charcot-Marie-Tooth G60.0
    Déjérine-Sottas G60.0
    interstitial progressive G60.0
    of infancy G60.0
    Refsum G60.1
  idiopathic G60.9
    progressive G60.3
    specified NEC G60.8
  in association with hereditary ataxia G60.2
  intercostal G58.0
  ischemic — *see* Disorder, nerve
  Jamaica (ginger) G62.2
  leg NEC G57.9- ☑
  lower extremity G57.9- ☑
  lumbar plexus G54.1
  median nerve G56.1- ☑
  motor and sensory — *see also* Polyneuropathy
    hereditary (types I-IV) G60.0
  multifocal motor (MMN) G61.82
  multiple (acute) (chronic) — *see* Polyneuropathy
  optic (nerve) — *see also* Neuritis, optic
    ischemic H47.01- ☑
  paraneoplastic (sensorial) (Denny Brown) D49.9 *[G13.0]*
  peripheral (nerve) — *see also* Polyneuropathy G62.9
    autonomic G90.9
      idiopathic G90.09
      in (due to)
        amyloidosis E85.4 *[G99.0]*
        diabetes mellitus — *see* E08-E13 with .43
        endocrine disease NEC E34.9 *[G99.0]*
        gout M10.00 *[G99.0]*
        hyperthyroidism E05.90 *[G99.0]*
          with thyroid storm E05.91 *[G99.0]*
        metabolic disease NEC E88.9 *[G99.0]*
    idiopathic G60.9
      progressive G60.3
    in (due to)
      antitetanus serum G62.0
      arsenic G62.2
      drugs NEC G62.0
      lead G62.2
      organophosphate compounds G62.2
      toxic agent NEC G62.2
  plantar nerves G57.6- ☑
  progressive
    hypertrophic interstitial G60.0
    inflammatory G62.81

Neuropathy, neuropathic — *continued*
  radicular NEC — *see* Radiculopathy
  sacral plexus G54.1
  sciatic G57.0- ☑
  serum G61.1
  toxic NEC G62.2
  trigeminal sensory G50.8
  ulnar nerve G56.2- ☑
  uremic N18.9 *[G63]*
  vitamin B12 E53.8 *[G63]*
    with anemia (pernicious) D51.0 *[G63]*
      due to dietary deficiency D51.3 *[G63]*
Neurophthisis — *see also* Disorder, nerve
  peripheral, diabetic — *see* E08-E13 with .42
Neuroretinitis — *see* Chorioretinitis
Neuroretinopathy, hereditary optic H47.22
Neurosarcoma — *see* Neoplasm, nerve, malignant
Neurosclerosis — *see* Disorder, nerve
Neurosis, neurotic F48.9
  anankastic F42.8
  anxiety (state) F41.1
    panic type F41.0
  asthenic F48.8
  bladder F45.8
  cardiac (reflex) F45.8
  cardiovascular F45.8
  character F60.9
  colon F45.8
  compensation F68.10
  compulsive, compulsion F42.8
  conversion F44.9
  craft F48.8
  cutaneous F45.8
  depersonalization F48.1
  depressive (reaction) (type) F34.1
  environmental F48.8
  excoriation L98.1
  fatigue F48.8
  functional — *see* Disorder, somatoform
  gastric F45.8
  gastrointestinal F45.8
  heart F45.8
  hypochondriacal F45.21
  hysterical F44.9
  incoordination F45.8
    larynx F45.8
    vocal cord F45.8
  intestine F45.8
  larynx (sensory) F45.8
    hysterical F44.4
  mixed NEC F48.8
  musculoskeletal F45.8
  obsessional F42.8
  obsessive-compulsive F42.8
  occupational F48.8
  ocular NEC F45.8
  organ — *see* Disorder, somatoform
  pharynx F45.8
  phobic F40.9
  posttraumatic (situational) F43.10
    acute F43.11
    chronic F43.12
  psychasthenic (type) F48.8
  railroad F48.8
  rectum F45.8
  respiratory F45.8
  rumination F45.8
  sexual F65.9
  situational F48.8
  social F40.10
    generalized F40.11
  specified type NEC F48.8
  state F48.9
    with depersonalization episode F48.1
  stomach F45.8
  traumatic F43.10
    acute F43.11
    chronic F43.12
  vasomotor F45.8
  visceral F45.8
  war F48.8
Neurospongioblastosis diffusa Q85.1
Neurosyphilis (arrested) (early) (gumma) (late) (latent)▼
    (recurrent) (relapse) A52.3
  with ataxia (cerebellar) (locomotor) (spastic) (spinal)
    A52.19
  aneurysm (cerebral) A52.05
  arachnoid (adhesive) A52.13

☑ Additional Character Required — Refer to the Tabular List for Character Selection   ▼ Subterms under main terms may continue to next column or page

Neurosyphilis — *continued*
- arteritis (any artery) (cerebral) A52.04
- asymptomatic A52.2
- congenital A50.40
- dura (mater) A52.13
- general paresis A52.17
- hemorrhagic A52.05
- juvenile (asymptomatic) (meningeal) A50.40
- leptomeninges (aseptic) A52.13
- meningeal, meninges (adhesive) A52.13
- meningitis A52.13
- meningovascular (diffuse) A52.13
- optic atrophy A52.15
- parenchymatous (degenerative) A52.19
- paresis, paretic A52.17
  - juvenile A50.45
- remission in (sustained) A52.3
- serological (without symptoms) A52.2
- specified nature or site NEC A52.19
- tabes, tabetic (dorsalis) A52.11
  - juvenile A50.45
- taboparesis A52.17
  - juvenile A50.45
- thrombosis (cerebral) A52.05
- vascular (cerebral) NEC A52.05

Neurothekeoma — *see* Neoplasm, nerve, benign

Neurotic — *see* Neurosis

Neurotoxemia — *see* Toxemia

Neutroclusion M26.211

Neutropenia, neutropenic (chronic) (genetic) (idiopathic) (immune) (infantile) (malignant) (pernicious) (splenic) D70.9
- congenital (primary) D70.0
- cyclic D70.4
- cytoreductive cancer chemotherapy sequela D70.1
- drug-induced D70.2
  - due to cytoreductive cancer chemotherapy D70.1
- due to infection D70.3
- fever D70.9
- neonatal, transitory (isoimmune) (maternal transfer) P61.5
- periodic D70.4
- secondary (cyclic) (periodic) (splenic) D70.4
  - drug-induced D70.2
    - due to cytoreductive cancer chemotherapy D70.1
- toxic D70.8

Neutrophilia, hereditary giant D72.0

Nevocarcinoma — *see* Melanoma

Nevus D22.9
- achromic — *see* Neoplasm, skin, benign
- amelanotic — *see* Neoplasm, skin, benign
- angiomatous D18.00
  - intra-abdominal D18.03
  - intracranial D18.02
  - skin D18.01
  - specified site NEC D18.09
- araneus I78.1
- balloon cell — *see* Neoplasm, skin, benign
- bathing trunk D48.5
- blue — *see* Neoplasm, skin, benign
  - cellular — *see* Neoplasm, skin, benign
  - giant — *see* Neoplasm, skin, benign
  - Jadassohn's — *see* Neoplasm, skin, benign
  - malignant — *see* Melanoma
- capillary D18.00
  - intra-abdominal D18.03
  - intracranial D18.02
  - skin D18.01
  - specified site NEC D18.09
- cavernous D18.00
  - intra-abdominal D18.03
  - intracranial D18.02
  - skin D18.01
  - specified site NEC D18.09
- cellular — *see* Neoplasm, skin, benign
  - blue — *see* Neoplasm, skin, benign
- choroid D31.3- ☑
- comedonicus Q82.5
- conjunctiva D31.0- ☑
- dermal — *see* Neoplasm, skin, benign
  - with epidermal nevus — *see* Neoplasm, skin, benign
- dysplastic — *see* Neoplasm, skin, benign
- eye D31.9- ☑
- flammeus Q82.5
- hemangiomatous D18.00
  - intra-abdominal D18.03
  - intracranial D18.02
  - skin D18.01

Nevus — *continued*
- hemangiomatous — *continued*
  - specified site NEC D18.09
- iris D31.4- ☑
- lacrimal gland D31.5- ☑
- lymphatic D18.1
- magnocellular
  - specified site — *see* Neoplasm, benign, by site
  - unspecified site D31.40
- malignant — *see* Melanoma
- meaning hemangioma D18.00
  - intra-abdominal D18.03
  - intracranial D18.02
  - skin D18.01
  - specified site NEC D18.09
- mouth (mucosa) D10.30
  - specified site NEC D10.39
  - white sponge Q38.6
- multiplex Q85.1
- non-neoplastic I78.1
- oral mucosa D10.30
  - specified site NEC D10.39
  - white sponge Q38.6
- orbit D31.6- ☑
- pigmented
  - giant — *see also* Neoplasm, skin, uncertain behavior D48.5
    - malignant melanoma in — *see* Melanoma
- portwine Q82.5
- retina D31.2- ☑
- retrobulbar D31.6- ☑
- sanguineous Q82.5
- senile I78.1
- skin D22.9
  - abdominal wall D22.5
  - ala nasi D22.39
  - ankle D22.7- ☑
  - anus, anal D22.5
  - arm D22.6- ☑
  - auditory canal (external) D22.2- ☑
  - auricle (ear) D22.2- ☑
  - auricular canal (external) D22.2- ☑
  - axilla, axillary fold D22.5
  - back D22.5
  - breast D22.5
  - brow D22.39
  - buttock D22.5
  - canthus (eye) D22.1- ☑
  - cheek (external) D22.39
  - chest wall D22.5
  - chin D22.39
  - ear (external) D22.2- ☑
  - external meatus (ear) D22.2- ☑
  - eyebrow D22.39
  - eyelid (lower) (upper) D22.1- ☑
  - face D22.30
    - specified NEC D22.39
  - female genital organ (external) NEC D28.0
  - finger D22.6- ☑
  - flank D22.5
  - foot D22.7- ☑
  - forearm D22.6- ☑
  - forehead D22.39
  - foreskin D29.0
  - genital organ (external) NEC
    - female D28.0
    - male D29.9
  - gluteal region D22.5
  - groin D22.5
  - hand D22.6- ☑
  - heel D22.7- ☑
  - helix D22.2- ☑
  - hip D22.7- ☑
  - interscapular region D22.5
  - jaw D22.39
  - knee D22.7- ☑
  - labium (majus) (minus) D28.0
  - leg D22.7- ☑
  - lip (lower) (upper) D22.0
  - lower limb D22.7- ☑
  - male genital organ (external) D29.9
  - nail D22.9
    - finger D22.6- ☑
    - toe D22.7- ☑
  - nasolabial groove D22.39
  - nates D22.5
  - neck D22.4
  - nose (external) D22.39

Nevus — *continued*
- skin — *continued*
  - palpebra D22.1- ☑
  - penis D29.0
  - perianal skin D22.5
  - perineum D22.5
  - pinna D22.2- ☑
  - popliteal fossa or space D22.7- ☑
  - prepuce D29.0
  - pudendum D28.0
  - scalp D22.4
  - scrotum D29.4
  - shoulder D22.6- ☑
  - submammary fold D22.5
  - temple D22.39
  - thigh D22.7- ☑
  - toe D22.7- ☑
  - trunk NEC D22.5
  - umbilicus D22.5
  - upper limb D22.6- ☑
  - vulva D28.0
- specified site NEC — *see* Neoplasm, by site, benign
- spider I78.1
- stellar I78.1
- strawberry Q82.5
- Sutton's benign D22.9
- unius lateris Q82.5
- Unna's Q82.5
- vascular Q82.5
- verrucous Q82.5

Newborn (infant) (liveborn) (singleton) Z38.2
- abstinence syndrome P96.1
- acne L70.4
- affected by
  - abnormalities of membranes P02.9
    - specified NEC P02.8
  - abruptio placenta P02.1
  - amino-acid metabolic disorder, transitory P74.8
  - amniocentesis (while in utero) P00.6
  - amnionitis P02.78
  - apparent life threatening event (ALTE) R68.13
  - bleeding (into)
    - cerebral cortex P52.22
    - germinal matrix P52.0
    - ventricles P52.1
  - breech delivery P03.0
  - cardiac arrest P29.81
  - cardiomyopathy I42.8
    - congenital I42.4
  - cerebral ischemia P91.0
  - Cesarean delivery P03.4
  - chemotherapy agents P04.11
  - chorioamnionitis P02.78
  - cocaine (crack) P04.41
  - complications of labor and delivery P03.9
    - specified NEC P03.89
  - compression of umbilical cord NEC P02.5
  - contracted pelvis P03.1
  - cyanosis P28.2
  - delivery P03.9
    - Cesarean P03.4
    - forceps P03.2
    - vacuum extractor P03.3
  - drugs of addiction P04.40
    - cocaine P04.41
    - hallucinogens P04.42
    - specified drug NEC P04.49
  - entanglement (knot) in umbilical cord P02.5
  - environmental chemicals P04.6
  - fetal (intrauterine)
    - growth retardation P05.9
    - inflammatory response syndrome (FIRS) P02.70
    - malnutrition not light or small for gestational age P05.2
  - FIRS (fetal inflammatory response syndrome) P02.70
  - forceps delivery P03.2
  - heart rate abnormalities
    - bradycardia P29.12
    - intrauterine P03.819
      - before onset of labor P03.810
      - during labor P03.811
    - tachycardia P29.11
  - hemorrhage (antepartum) P02.1
    - cerebellar (nontraumatic) P52.6
    - intracerebral (nontraumatic) P52.4
    - intracranial (nontraumatic) P52.9
      - specified NEC P52.8
    - intraventricular (nontraumatic) P52.3

238
☑ Additional Character Required — Refer to the Tabular List for Character Selection
🖝 Subterms under main terms may continue to next column or pag

Newborn — Nodule

Index

Nodule(s), **nodular** — *continued*
  Haygarth's M15.8
  inflammatory — *see* Inflammation
  juxta-articular
    syphilitic A52.77
    yaws A66.7
  larynx J38.7
  lung, solitary (subsegmental branch of the bronchial tree) R91.1
    multiple R91.8
  milker's B08.03
  prostate N40.2
    with lower urinary tract symptoms (LUTS) N40.3
    without lower urinary tract symptoms (LUTS) N40.2
  pulmonary, solitary (subsegmental branch of the bronchial tree) R91.1
  retrocardiac R09.89
  rheumatoid M06.30
    ankle M06.37- ☑
    elbow M06.32- ☑
    foot joint M06.37- ☑
    hand joint M06.34- ☑
    hip M06.35- ☑
    knee M06.36- ☑
    multiple site M06.39
    shoulder M06.31- ☑
    vertebra M06.38
    wrist M06.33- ☑
  scrotum (inflammatory) N49.2
  singer's J38.2
  solitary, lung (subsegmental branch of the bronchial tree) R91.1
    multiple R91.8
  subcutaneous — *see* Swelling, localized
  teacher's J38.2
  thyroid (cold) (gland) (nontoxic) E04.1
    with thyrotoxicosis E05.20
      with thyroid storm E05.21
    toxic or with hyperthyroidism E05.20
      with thyroid storm E05.21
  vocal cord J38.2
Noma (gangrenous) (hospital) (infective) A69.0
  auricle I96
  mouth A69.0
  pudendi N76.89
  vulvae N76.89
Nomad, nomadism Z59.0
NOMID (neonatal onset multisystemic inflammatory disorder) M04.2
Nonadherence to medical treatment Z91.19
Nonautoimmune hemolytic anemia D59.4
  drug-induced D59.2
Nonclosure — *see also* Imperfect, closure
  ductus arteriosus (Botallo's) Q25.0
  foramen
    botalli Q21.1
    ovale Q21.1
Noncompliance Z91.19
  with
    dialysis Z91.15
    dietary regimen Z91.11
    medical treatment Z91.19
    medication regimen NEC Z91.14
      underdosing — *see also* Table of Drugs and Chemicals, categories T36-T50, with final character 6 Z91.14
        intentional NEC Z91.128
          due to financial hardship of patient Z91.120
        unintentional NEC Z91.138
          due to patient's age related debility Z91.130
    renal dialysis Z91.15
Nondescent (congenital) — *see also* Malposition, congenital
  cecum Q43.3
  colon Q43.3
  testicle Q53.9
    bilateral Q53.20
      abdominal Q53.211
      perineal Q53.22
    unilateral Q53.10
      abdominal Q53.111
      perineal Q53.12
Nondevelopment
  brain Q02
    part of Q04.3
  heart Q24.8

Nondevelopment — *continued*
  organ or site, congenital NEC — *see* Hypoplasia
Nonengagement
  head NEC O32.4 ☑
    in labor, causing obstructed labor O64.8 ☑
Nonexanthematous tick fever A93.2
Nonexpansion, lung (newborn) P28.0
Nonfunctioning
  cystic duct — *see also* Disease, gallbladder K82.8
  gallbladder — *see also* Disease, gallbladder K82.8
  kidney N28.9
  labyrinth — *see* subcategory H83.2 ☑
Non-Hodgkin lymphoma NEC — *see* Lymphoma, non-Hodgkin
Nonimplantation, ovum N97.2
Noninsufflation, fallopian tube N97.1
Non-ketotic hyperglycinemia E72.51
Nonne-Milroy syndrome Q82.0
Nonovulation N97.0
Non-palpable testicle(s)
  bilateral R39.84
  unilateral R39.83
Nonpatent fallopian tube N97.1
Nonpneumatization, lung NEC P28.0
Nonrotation — *see* Malrotation
Nonsecretion, urine — *see* Anuria
Nonunion
  fracture — *see* Fracture, by site
  joint, following fusion or arthrodesis M96.0
  organ or site, congenital NEC — *see* Imperfect, closure
  symphysis pubis, congenital Q74.2
Nonvisualization, gallbladder R93.2
Nonvital, nonvitalized tooth K04.99
Non-working side interference M26.56
Noonan's syndrome Q87.19
Normocytic anemia (infectional) due to blood loss (chronic) D50.0
  acute D62
Norrie's disease (congenital) Q15.8
North American blastomycosis B40.9
Norwegian itch B86
Nose, nasal — *see* condition
Nosebleed R04.0
Nose-picking F98.8
Nosomania F45.21
Nosophobia F45.22
Nostalgia F43.20
Notch of iris Q13.2
Notching nose, congenital (tip) Q30.2
Nothnagel's
  syndrome — *see* Strabismus, paralytic, third nerve
  vasomotor acroparesthesia I73.89
Novy's relapsing fever A68.9
  louse-borne A68.0
  tick-borne A68.1
Noxious
  foodstuffs, poisoning by — *see* Poisoning, food, noxious, plant
  substances transmitted through placenta or breast milk P04.9
Nucleus pulposus — *see* condition
Numbness R20.0
Nuns' knee — *see* Bursitis, prepatellar
Nursemaid's elbow S53.03- ☑
Nutcracker esophagus K22.4
Nutmeg liver K76.1
Nutrient element deficiency E61.9
  specified NEC E61.8
Nutrition deficient or insufficient — *see also* Malnutrition E46
  due to
    insufficient food T73.0 ☑
    lack of
      care (child) T76.02 ☑
        adult T76.01 ☑
      food T73.0 ☑
Nutritional stunting E45
Nyctalopia (night blindness) — *see* Blindness, night
Nycturia R35.1
  psychogenic F45.8
Nymphomania F52.8
Nystagmus H55.00
  benign paroxysmal — *see* Vertigo, benign paroxysmal
  central positional H81.4
  congenital H55.01
  dissociated H55.04
  latent H55.02

Nystagmus — *continued*
  miners' H55.09
  positional
    benign paroxysmal H81.4
    central H81.4
  specified form NEC H55.09
  visual deprivation H55.03

O

Obermeyer's relapsing fever (European) A68.0
Obesity E66.9
  with alveolar hypoventilation E66.2
  adrenal E27.8
  complicating
    childbirth O99.214
    pregnancy O99.21- ☑
    puerperium O99.215
  constitutional E66.8
  dietary counseling and surveillance Z71.3
  drug-induced E66.1
  due to
    drug E66.1
    excess calories E66.09
      morbid E66.01
      severe E66.01
  endocrine E66.8
  endogenous E66.8
  exogenous E66.09
  familial E66.8
  glandular E66.8
  hypothyroid — *see* Hypothyroidism
  hypoventilation syndrome (OHS) E66.2
  morbid E66.01
    with
      alveolar hypoventilation E66.2
      obesity hypoventilation syndrome (OHS) E66.2
    due to excess calories E66.01
  nutritional E66.09
  pituitary E23.6
  severe E66.01
  specified type NEC E66.8
Oblique — *see* condition
Obliteration
  appendix (lumen) K38.8
  artery I77.1
  bile duct (noncalculous) K83.1
  common duct (noncalculous) K83.1
  cystic duct — *see* Obstruction, gallbladder
  disease, arteriolar I77.1
  endometrium N85.8
  eye, anterior chamber — *see* Disorder, globe, hypotony
  fallopian tube N97.1
  lymphatic vessel I89.0
    due to mastectomy I97.2
  organ or site, congenital NEC — *see* Atresia, by site
  ureter N13.5
    with infection N13.6
  urethra — *see* Stricture, urethra
  vein I87.8
  vestibule (oral) K08.89
Observation (following) (for) (without need for further medical care) Z04.9
  accident NEC Z04.3
    at work Z04.2
    transport Z04.1
  adverse effect of drug Z03.6
  alleged rape or sexual assault (victim), ruled out
    adult Z04.41
    child Z04.42
  criminal assault Z04.89
  development state
    adolescent Z00.3
    period of rapid growth in childhood Z00.2
    puberty Z00.3
  disease, specified NEC Z03.89
  following work accident Z04.2
  forced sexual exploitation Z04.81
  forced labor exploitation Z04.82
  growth and development state — *see* Observation, development state
  injuries (accidental) NEC — *see also* Observation, accident
  newborn (for)
    suspected condition, related to exposure from the mother or birth process — *see* Newborn, affected by, maternal
    ruled out Z05.9

Observation — *continued*
  newborn — *continued*
    suspected condition, related to exposure from the mother or birth process — *see* Newborn, affected by, maternal — *continued*
      ruled out — *continued*
        cardiac Z05.0
        connective tissue Z05.73
        gastrointestinal Z05.5
        genetic Z05.41
        genitourinary Z05.6
        immunologic Z05.43
        infectious Z05.1
        metabolic Z05.42
        musculoskeletal Z05.72
        neurological Z05.2
        respiratory Z05.3
        skin and subcutaneous tissue Z05.71
        specified condition NEC Z05.8
  postpartum
    immediately after delivery Z39.0
    routine follow-up Z39.2
  pregnancy (normal) (without complication) Z34.9- ☑
    high risk O09.9- ☑
  suicide attempt, alleged NEC Z03.89
    self-poisoning Z03.6
  suspected, ruled out — *see also* Suspected condition, ruled out
    abuse, physical
      adult Z04.71
      child Z04.72
    accident at work Z04.2
    adult battering victim Z04.71
    child battering victim Z04.72
    condition NEC Z03.89
      newborn — *see also* Observation, newborn (for), suspected condition, ruled out Z05.9
    drug poisoning or adverse effect Z03.6
    exposure (to)
      anthrax Z03.810
      biological agent NEC Z03.818
    foreign body
      aspirated (inhaled) Z03.822
      ingested Z03.821
      inserted (injected), in (eye) (orifice) (skin) Z03.823
    inflicted injury NEC Z04.89
    suicide attempt, alleged Z03.89
      self-poisoning Z03.6
    toxic effects from ingested substance (drug) (poison) Z03.6
  toxic effects from ingested substance (drug) (poison) Z03.6

Obsession, obsessional state F42.8
  mixed thoughts and acts F42.2
Obsessive-compulsive neurosis or reaction F42.8
Obstetric embolism, septic — *see* Embolism, obstetric, septic
Obstetrical trauma (complicating delivery) O71.9
  with or following ectopic or molar pregnancy O08.6
  specified type NEC O71.89
Obstipation — *see* Constipation
Obstruction, obstructed, obstructive
  airway J98.8
    with
      allergic alveolitis J67.9
      asthma J45.909
        with
          exacerbation (acute) J45.901
          status asthmaticus J45.902
      bronchiectasis J47.9
        with
          exacerbation (acute) J47.1
          lower respiratory infection J47.0
      bronchitis (chronic) J44.9
      emphysema J43.9
    chronic J44.9
      with
        allergic alveolitis — *see* Pneumonitis, hypersensitivity
        bronchiectasis J47.9
          with
            exacerbation (acute) J47.1
            lower respiratory infection J47.0
    due to
      foreign body — *see* Foreign body, by site, causing asphyxia
      inhalation of fumes or vapors J68.9
      laryngospasm J38.5

Obstruction, obstructed, obstructive — *continued*
  ampulla of Vater K83.1
  aortic (heart) (valve) — *see* Stenosis, aortic
  aortoiliac I74.09
  aqueduct of Sylvius G91.1
    congenital Q03.0
      with spina bifida — *see* Spina bifida, by site, with hydrocephalus
  Arnold-Chiari — *see* Arnold-Chiari disease
  artery — *see also* Atherosclerosis, artery I70.9 ☑
    basilar (complete) (partial) — *see* Occlusion, artery, basilar
    carotid (complete) (partial) — *see* Occlusion, artery, carotid
    cerebellar — *see* Occlusion, artery, cerebellar
    cerebral (anterior) (middle) (posterior) — *see* Occlusion, artery, cerebral
    precerebral — *see* Occlusion, artery, precerebral
    renal N28.0
    retinal NEC — *see* Occlusion, artery, retina
    stent — *see* Restenosis, stent
    vertebral (complete) (partial) — *see* Occlusion, artery, vertebral
  band (intestinal) — *see also* Obstruction, intestine, specified NEC K56.699
  bile duct or passage (common) (hepatic) (noncalculous) K83.1
    with calculus K80.51
    congenital (causing jaundice) Q44.3
  biliary (duct) (tract) K83.1
    gallbladder K82.0
  bladder-neck (acquired) N32.0
    congenital Q64.31
    due to hyperplasia (hypertrophy) of prostate — *see* Hyperplasia, prostate
  bowel — *see* Obstruction, intestine
  bronchus J98.09
  canal, ear — *see* Stenosis, external ear canal
  cardia K22.2
  caval veins (inferior) (superior) I87.1
  cecum — *see* Obstruction, intestine
  circulatory I99.8
  colon — *see* Obstruction, intestine
  common duct (noncalculous) K83.1
  coronary (artery) — *see* Occlusion, coronary
  cystic duct — *see also* Obstruction, gallbladder
    with calculus K80.21
  device, implant or graft — *see also* Complications, by site and type, mechanical T85.698 ☑
    arterial graft NEC — *see* Complication, cardiovascular device, mechanical, vascular
    catheter NEC T85.628 ☑
      cystostomy T83.090 ☑
      dialysis (renal) T82.49 ☑
        intraperitoneal T85.691 ☑
      Hopkins T83.098 ☑
      ileostomy T83.098 ☑
      infusion NEC T82.594 ☑
        spinal (epidural) (subdural) T85.690 ☑
      nephrostomy T83.092 ☑
      urethral indwelling T83.091 ☑
      urinary T83.098 ☑
      urostomy T83.098 ☑
    due to infection T85.79 ☑
    gastrointestinal — *see* Complications, prosthetic device, mechanical, gastrointestinal device
    genital NEC T83.498 ☑
      intrauterine contraceptive device T83.39 ☑
      penile prosthesis (cylinder) (implanted) (pump) (resevoir) T83.490 ☑
      testicular prosthesis T83.491 ☑
    heart NEC — *see* Complication, cardiovascular device, mechanical
    joint prosthesis — *see* Complications, joint prosthesis, mechanical, specified NEC, by site
    orthopedic NEC — *see* Complication, orthopedic, device, mechanical
    specified NEC T85.628 ☑
    urinary NEC — *see also* Complication, genitourinary, device, urinary, mechanical
      graft T83.29 ☑
    vascular NEC — *see* Complication, cardiovascular device, mechanical
    ventricular intracranial shunt T85.09 ☑
  due to foreign body accidentally left in operative wound T81.529 ☑
  duodenum K31.5

Obstruction, obstructed, obstructive — *continued*
  ejaculatory duct N50.89
  esophagus K22.2
  eustachian tube (complete) (partial) H68.10- ☑
    cartilagenous (extrinsic) H68.13- ☑
      intrinsic H68.12- ☑
    osseous H68.11- ☑
  fallopian tube (bilateral) N97.1
  fecal K56.41
    with hernia — *see* Hernia, by site, with obstruction
  foramen of Monro (congenital) Q03.8
    with spina bifida — *see* Spina bifida, by site, with hydrocephalus
  foreign body — *see* Foreign body
  gallbladder K82.0
    with calculus, stones K80.21
    congenital Q44.1
  gastric outlet K31.1
  gastrointestinal — *see* Obstruction, intestine
  hepatic K76.89
    duct (noncalculous) K83.1
  ileum — *see* Obstruction, intestine
  iliofemoral (artery) I74.5
  intestine K56.609
    with
      adhesions (intestinal) (peritoneal) K56.50
        complete K56.52
        incomplete K56.51
        partial K56.51
    adynamic K56.0
    by gallstone K56.3
    complete K56.601
    congenital (small) Q41.9
      large Q42.9
      specified part NEC Q42.8
    incomplete K56.600
    neurogenic K56.0
      Hirschsprung's disease or megacolon Q43.1
    newborn P76.9
      due to
        fecaliths P76.8
        inspissated milk P76.2
        meconium (plug) P76.0
          in mucoviscidosis E84.11
      specified NEC P76.8
    partial K56.600
    postoperative K91.30
      complete K91.32
      incomplete K91.31
      partial K91.31
    reflex K56.0
    specified NEC K56.699
      complete K56.691
      incomplete K56.690
      partial K56.690
    volvulus K56.2
  intracardiac ball valve prosthesis T82.09 ☑
  jejunum — *see* Obstruction, intestine
  joint prosthesis — *see* Complications, joint prosthesis, mechanical, specified NEC, by site
  kidney (calices) N28.89
  labor — *see* Delivery
  lacrimal (passages) (duct)
    by
      dacryolith — *see* Dacryolith
      stenosis — *see* Stenosis, lacrimal
    congenital Q10.5
    neonatal H04.53- ☑
  lacrimonasal duct — *see* Obstruction, lacrimal
  lacteal, with steatorrhea K90.2
  laryngitis — *see* Laryngitis
  larynx NEC J38.6
    congenital Q31.8
  lung J98.4
    disease, chronic J44.9
  lymphatic I89.0
  meconium (plug)
    newborn P76.0
      due to fecaliths P76.0
      in mucoviscidosis E84.11
  mitral — *see* Stenosis, mitral
  nasal J34.89
  nasolacrimal duct — *see also* Obstruction, lacrimal
    congenital Q10.5
  nasopharynx J39.2
  nose J34.89
  organ or site, congenital NEC — *see* Atresia, by site
  pancreatic duct K86.89

Obstruction, obstructed, obstructive — *continued*
 parotid duct or gland K11.8
 pelviureteral junction N13.5
  with hydronephrosis N13.0
  congenital Q62.39
 pharynx J39.2
 portal (circulation) (vein) I81
 prostate — *see also* Hyperplasia, prostate
  valve (urinary) N32.0
 pulmonary valve (heart) I37.0
 pyelonephritis (chronic) N11.1
 pylorus
  adult K31.1
  congenital or infantile Q40.0
 rectosigmoid — *see* Obstruction, intestine
 rectum K62.4
 renal N28.89
  outflow N13.8
  pelvis, congenital Q62.39
 respiratory J98.8
  chronic J44.9
 retinal (vessels) H34.9
 salivary duct (any) K11.8
  with calculus K11.5
 sigmoid — *see* Obstruction, intestine
 sinus (accessory) (nasal) J34.89
 Stensen's duct K11.8
 stomach NEC K31.89
  acute K31.0
  congenital Q40.2
  due to pylorospasm K31.3
 submandibular duct K11.8
 submaxillary gland K11.8
  with calculus K11.5
 thoracic duct I89.0
 thrombotic — *see* Thrombosis
 trachea J39.8
 tracheostomy airway J95.03
 tricuspid (valve) — *see* Stenosis, tricuspid
 upper respiratory, congenital Q34.8
 ureter (functional) (pelvic junction) NEC N13.5
  with
    hydronephrosis N13.1
      with infection N13.6
    pyelonephritis (chronic) N11.1
  congenital Q62.39
  due to calculus — *see* Calculus, ureter
 urethra NEC N36.8
  congenital Q64.39
 urinary (moderate) N13.9
  due to hyperplasia (hypertrophy) of prostate — *see*
    Hyperplasia, prostate
  organ or tract (lower) N13.9
  prostatic valve N32.0
  specified NEC N13.8
 uropathy N13.9
 uterus N85.8
 vagina N89.5
 valvular — *see* Endocarditis
 vein, venous I87.1
  caval (inferior) (superior) I87.1
  thrombotic — *see* Thrombosis
 vena cava (inferior) (superior) I87.1
 vesical NEC N32.0
 vesicourethral orifice N32.0
  congenital Q64.31
 vessel NEC I99.8
  stent — *see* Restenosis, stent

Obturator — *see* condition
Occlusal wear, teeth K03.0
Occlusio pupillae — *see* Membrane, pupillary
Occlusion, occluded
 anus K62.4
  congenital Q42.3
    with fistula Q42.2
 aortoiliac (chronic) I74.09
 aqueduct of Sylvius G91.1
  congenital Q03.0
    with spina bifida — *see* Spina bifida, by site, with
      hydrocephalus
 artery — *see also* Atherosclerosis, artery I70.9 ☑
  auditory, internal I65.8
  basilar I65.1
    with
      infarction I63.22
        due to
          embolism I63.12
          thrombosis I63.02

Occlusion, occluded — *continued*
 artery — *see also* Atherosclerosis, artery — *continued*
  brain or cerebral I66.9
    with infarction (due to) I63.5- ☑
      embolism I63.4- ☑
      thrombosis I63.3- ☑
  carotid I65.2- ☑
    with
      infarction I63.23- ☑
        due to
          embolism I63.13- ☑
          thrombosis I63.03- ☑
  cerebellar (anterior inferior) (posterior inferior) (superior) I66.3
    with infarction I63.54- ☑
      due to
        embolism I63.44- ☑
        thrombosis I63.34- ☑
  cerebral I66.9
    with infarction I63.50
      due to
        embolism I63.40
          specified NEC I63.49
        thrombosis I63.30
          specified NEC I63.39
    anterior I66.1- ☑
      with infarction I63.52- ☑
        due to
          embolism I63.42- ☑
          thrombosis I63.32- ☑
    middle I66.0- ☑
      with infarction I63.51- ☑
        due to
          embolism I63.41- ☑
          thrombosis I63.31- ☑
    posterior I66.2- ☑
      with infarction I63.53- ☑
        due to
          embolism I63.43- ☑
          thrombosis I63.33- ☑
    specified NEC I66.8
      with infarction I63.59
        due to
          embolism I63.4- ☑
          thrombosis I63.3- ☑
  choroidal (anterior) — *see* Occlusion, artery, precerebral, specified NEC
  communicating posterior — *see* Occlusion, artery, precerebral, specified NEC
  complete
    coronary I25.82
    extremities I70.92
  coronary (acute) (thrombotic) (without myocardial infarction) I24.0
    with myocardial infarction — *see* Infarction, myocardium
    chronic total I25.82
    complete I25.82
    healed or old I25.2
    total (chronic) I25.82
  hypophyseal — *see* Occlusion, artery, precerebral, specified NEC
  iliac I74.5
  lower extremities due to stenosis or stricture I77.1
  mesenteric (embolic) (thrombotic) — *see also* Infarct, intestine K55.069
  perforating — *see* Occlusion, artery, cerebral, specified NEC
  peripheral I77.9
    thrombotic or embolic I74.4
  pontine — *see* Occlusion, artery, precerebral, specified NEC
  precerebral I65.9
    with infarction I63.20
      specified NEC I63.29
      due to
        embolism I63.10
          specified NEC I63.19
        thrombosis I63.00
          specified NEC I63.09
    basilar — *see* Occlusion, artery, basilar
    carotid — *see* Occlusion, artery, carotid
    puerperal O88.23
    specified NEC I65.8
      with infarction I63.29

Occlusion, occluded — *continued*
 artery — *see also* Atherosclerosis, artery — *continued*
  precerebral — *continued*
    specified — *continued*
      with infarction — *continued*
        due to
          embolism I63.19
          thrombosis I63.09
      vertebral — *see* Occlusion, artery, vertebral
  renal N28.0
  retinal
    branch H34.23- ☑
    central H34.1- ☑
    partial H34.21- ☑
    transient H34.0- ☑
  spinal — *see* Occlusion, artery, precerebral, vertebral
  total (chronic)
    coronary I25.82
    extremities I70.92
  vertebral I65.0- ☑
    with
      infarction I63.21- ☑
        due to
          embolism I63.11- ☑
          thrombosis I63.01- ☑
 basilar artery — *see* Occlusion, artery, basilar
 bile duct (common) (hepatic) (noncalculous) K83.1
 bowel — *see* Obstruction, intestine
 carotid (artery) (common) (internal) — *see* Occlusion, artery, carotid
 centric (of teeth) M26.59
  maximum intercuspation discrepancy M26.55
 cerebellar (artery) — *see* Occlusion, artery, cerebellar
 cerebral (artery) — *see* Occlusion, artery, cerebral
 cerebrovascular — *see also* Occlusion, artery, cerebral
  with infarction I63.5- ☑
 cervical canal — *see* Stricture, cervix
 cervix (uteri) — *see* Stricture, cervix
 choanal Q30.0
 choroidal (artery) — *see* Occlusion, artery, precerebral, specified NEC
 colon — *see* Obstruction, intestine
 communicating posterior artery — *see* Occlusion, artery, precerebral, specified NEC
 coronary (artery) (vein) (thrombotic) — *see also* Infarct, myocardium
  chronic total I25.82
  healed or old I25.2
  not resulting in infarction I24.0
  total (chronic) I25.82
 cystic duct — *see* Obstruction, gallbladder
 embolic — *see* Embolism
 fallopian tube N97.1
  congenital Q50.6
 gallbladder — *see also* Obstruction, gallbladder
  congenital (causing jaundice) Q44.1
 gingiva, traumatic K06.2
 hymen N89.6
  congenital Q52.3
 hypophyseal (artery) — *see* Occlusion, artery, precerebral, specified NEC
 iliac artery I74.5
 intestine — *see* Obstruction, intestine
 lacrimal passages — *see* Obstruction, lacrimal
 lung J98.4
 lymph or lymphatic channel I89.0
 mammary duct N64.89
 mesenteric artery (embolic) (thrombotic) — *see also*
  Infarct, intestine K55.069
 nose J34.89
  congenital Q30.0
 organ or site, congenital NEC — *see* Atresia, by site
 oviduct N97.1
  congenital Q50.6
 peripheral arteries
  due to stricture or stenosis I77.1
  upper extremity I74.2
 pontine (artery) — *see* Occlusion, artery, precerebral, specified NEC
 posterior lingual, of mandibular teeth M26.29
 precerebral artery — *see* Occlusion, artery, precerebral
 punctum lacrimale — *see* Obstruction, lacrimal
 pupil — *see* Membrane, pupillary
 pylorus, adult — *see also* Stricture, pylorus K31.1
 renal artery N28.0

Occlusion, occluded — *continued*
  retina, retinal
    artery — *see* Occlusion, artery, retinal
    vein (central) H34.81- ☑
      engorgement H34.82- ☑
      tributary H34.83- ☑
    vessels H34.9
  spinal artery — *see* Occlusion, artery, precerebral, vertebral
  teeth (mandibular) (posterior lingual) M26.29
  thoracic duct I89.0
  thrombotic — *see* Thrombosis, artery
  traumatic
    edentulous (alveolar) ridge K06.2
    gingiva K06.2
    periodontal K05.5
  tubal N97.1
  ureter (complete) (partial) N13.5
    congenital Q62.10
  ureteropelvic junction N13.5
    congenital Q62.11
  ureterovesical orifice N13.5
    congenital Q62.12
  urethra — *see* Stricture, urethra
  uterus N85.8
  vagina N89.5
  vascular NEC I99.8
  vein — *see* Thrombosis
    retinal — *see* Occlusion, retinal, vein
  vena cava (inferior) (superior) — *see* Embolism, vena cava
  ventricle (brain) NEC G91.1
  vertebral (artery) — *see* Occlusion, artery, vertebral
  vessel (blood) I99.8
  vulva N90.5
Occult
  blood in feces (stools) R19.5
Occupational
  problems NEC Z56.89
Ochlophobia — *see* Agoraphobia
Ochronosis (endogenous) E70.29
Ocular muscle — *see* condition
Oculogyric crisis or disturbance H51.8
  psychogenic F45.8
Oculomotor syndrome H51.9
Oculopathy
  syphilitic NEC A52.71
    congenital
      early A50.01
      late A50.30
    early (secondary) A51.43
    late A52.71
Oddi's sphincter spasm K83.4
Odontalgia K08.89
Odontoameloblastoma — *see* Cyst, calcifying odontogenic
Odontoclasia K03.89
Odontodysplasia, regional K00.4
Odontogenesis imperfecta K00.5
Odontoma (ameloblastic) (complex) (compound) (fibroameloblastic) — *see* Cyst, calcifying odontogenic
Odontomyelitis (closed) (open) K04.01
  irreversible K04.02
  reversible K04.01
Odontorrhagia K08.89
Odontosarcoma, ameloblastic C41.1
  upper jaw (bone) C41.0
Oestriasis — *see* Myiasis
Oguchi's disease H53.63
Ohara's disease — *see* Tularemia
OHS (obesity hypoventilation syndrome) E66.2
Oidiomycosis — *see* Candidiasis
Oidium albicans infection — *see* Candidiasis
Old age (without mention of debility) R54
  dementia F03 ☑
Old (previous) **myocardial infarction** I25.2
Olfactory — *see* condition
Oligemia — *see* Anemia
Oligoastrocytoma
  specified site — *see* Neoplasm, malignant, by site
  unspecified site C71.9
Oligocythemia D64.9
Oligodendroblastoma
  specified site — *see* Neoplasm, malignant
  unspecified site C71.9

Oligodendroglioma
  anaplastic type
    specified site — *see* Neoplasm, malignant, by site
    unspecified site C71.9
  specified site — *see* Neoplasm, malignant, by site
  unspecified site C71.9
Oligodontia — *see* Anodontia
Oligoencephalon Q02
Oligohidrosis L74.4
Oligohydramnios O41.0- ☑
Oligohydrosis L74.4
Oligomenorrhea N91.5
  primary N91.3
  secondary N91.4
Oligophrenia — *see also* Disability, intellectual
  phenylpyruvic E70.0
Oligospermia N46.11
  due to
    drug therapy N46.121
    efferent duct obstruction N46.123
    infection N46.122
    radiation N46.124
    specified cause NEC N46.129
    systemic disease N46.125
Oligotrichia — *see* Alopecia
Oliguria R34
  with, complicating or following ectopic or molar pregnancy O08.4
  postprocedural N99.0
Ollier's disease Q78.4
Omenotocele — *see* Hernia, abdomen, specified site NEC
Omentitis — *see* Peritonitis
Omentum, omental — *see* condition
Omphalitis (congenital) (newborn) P38.9
  with mild hemorrhage P38.1
  without hemorrhage P38.9
  not of newborn L08.82
  tetanus A33
Omphalocele Q79.2
Omphalomesenteric duct, persistent Q43.0
Omphalorrhagia, newborn P51.9
Omsk hemorrhagic fever A98.1
Onanism (excessive) F98.8
Onchocerciasis, onchocercosis B73.1
  with
    eye disease B73.00
      endophthalmitis B73.01
      eyelid B73.09
      glaucoma B73.02
      specified NEC B73.09
    eyelid B73.09
    eye NEC B73.00
Oncocytoma — *see* Neoplasm, benign, by site
Oncovirus, as cause of disease classified elsewhere B97.32
Ondine's curse — *see* Apnea, sleep
Oneirophrenia F23
Onychauxis L60.2
  congenital Q84.5
Onychia — *see also* Cellulitis, digit
  with lymphangitis — *see* Lymphangitis, acute, digit
  candidal B37.2
  dermatophytic B35.1
Onychitis — *see also* Cellulitis, digit
  with lymphangitis — *see* Lymphangitis, acute, digit
Onychocryptosis L60.0
Onychodystrophy L60.3
  congenital Q84.6
Onychogryphosis, onychogryposis L60.2
Onycholysis L60.1
Onychomadesis L60.8
Onychomalacia L60.3
Onychomycosis (finger) (toe) B35.1
Onycho-osteodysplasia Q87.2
Onychophagia F98.8
Onychophosis L60.8
Onychoptosis L60.8
Onychorrhexis L60.3
  congenital Q84.6
Onychoschizia L60.3
Onyxis (finger) (toe) L60.0
Onyxitis — *see also* Cellulitis, digit
  with lymphangitis — *see* Lymphangitis, acute, digit
Oophoritis (cystic) (infectional) (interstitial) N70.92
  with salpingitis N70.93
  acute N70.02
    with salpingitis N70.03

Oophoritis — *continued*
  chronic N70.12
    with salpingitis N70.13
  complicating abortion — *see* Abortion, by type, complicated by, oophoritis
Oophorocele N83.4- ☑
Opacity, opacities
  cornea H17.- ☑
    central H17.1- ☑
    congenital Q13.3
    degenerative — *see* Degeneration, cornea
    hereditary — *see* Dystrophy, cornea
    inflammatory — *see* Keratitis
    minor H17.81- ☑
    peripheral H17.82- ☑
    sequelae of trachoma (healed) B94.0
    specified NEC H17.89
  enamel (teeth) (fluoride) (nonfluoride) K00.3
  lens — *see* Cataract
  snowball — *see* Deposit, crystalline
  vitreous (humor) NEC H43.39- ☑
    congenital Q14.0
    membranes and strands H43.31- ☑
Opalescent dentin (hereditary) K00.5
Open, opening
  abnormal, organ or site, congenital — *see* Imperfect, closure
  angle with
    borderline
      findings
        high risk H40.02- ☑
        low risk H40.01- ☑
      intraocular pressure H40.00- ☑
    cupping of discs H40.01- ☑
    glaucoma (primary) — *see* Glaucoma, open angle
  bite
    anterior M26.220
    posterior M26.221
  false — *see* Imperfect, closure
  margin on tooth restoration K08.51
  restoration margins of tooth K08.51
  wound — *see* Wound, open
Operational fatigue F48.8
Operative — *see* condition
Operculitis — *see* Periodontitis
Operculum — *see* Break, retina
Ophiasis L63.2
Ophthalmia — *see also* Conjunctivitis H10.9
  actinic rays — *see* Photokeratitis
  allergic (acute) — *see* Conjunctivitis, acute, atopic
  blennorrhagic (gonococcal) (neonatorum) A54.31
  diphtheritic A36.86
  Egyptian A71.1
  electrica — *see* Photokeratitis
  gonococcal (neonatorum) A54.31
  metastatic — *see* Endophthalmitis, purulent
  migraine — *see* Migraine, ophthalmoplegic
  neonatorum, newborn P39.1
    gonococcal A54.31
  nodosa H16.24- ☑
  purulent — *see* Conjunctivitis, acute, mucopurulent
  spring — *see* Conjunctivitis, acute, atopic
  sympathetic — *see* Uveitis, sympathetic
Ophthalmitis — *see* Ophthalmia
Ophthalmocele (congenital) Q15.8
Ophthalmoneuromyelitis G36.0
Ophthalmoplegia — *see also* Strabismus, paralytic
  anterior internuclear — *see* Ophthalmoplegia, internuclear
  ataxia-areflexia G61.0
  diabetic — *see* E08-E13 with .39
  exophthalmic E05.00
    with thyroid storm E05.01
  external H49.88- ☑
    progressive H49.4- ☑
      with pigmentary retinopathy — *see* Kearns-Sayre syndrome
    total H49.3- ☑
  internal (complete) (total) H52.51- ☑
  internuclear H51.2- ☑
  migraine — *see* Migraine, ophthalmoplegic
  Parinaud's H49.88- ☑
  progressive external — *see* Ophthalmoplegia, external, progressive
  supranuclear, progressive G23.1
  total (external) — *see* Ophthalmoplegia, external, total

pioid(s)
abuse — see Abuse, drug, opioids
dependence — see Dependence, drug, opioids
induced, without use disorder
  anxiety disorder F11.988
  delirium F11.921
  depressive disorder F11.94
  sexual dysfunction F11.981
  sleep disorder F11.982
pisthognathism M26.09
pisthorchiasis (felineus) (viverrini) B66.0
pitz' disease D73.2
piumism — see Dependence, drug, opioid
ppenheim's disease G70.2
ppenheim-Urbach disease (necrobiosis lipoidica dia-
  beticorum) — see E08-E13 with .620
ptic nerve — see condition
rbit — see condition
rchioblastoma C62.9- ☑
rchitis (gangrenous) (nonspecific) (septic) (suppurative)
  N45.2
blennorrhagic (gonococcal) (acute) (chronic) A54.23
chlamydial A56.19
filarial — see also Infestation, filarial B74.9 [N51]
gonococcal (acute) (chronic) A54.23
mumps B26.0
syphilitic A52.76
tuberculous A18.15
rf (virus disease) B08.02
rganic — see also condition
brain syndrome F09
heart — see Disease, heart
mental disorder F09
psychosis F09
rgasm
anejaculatory N53.13
riental
bilharziasis B65.2
schistosomiasis B65.2
rifice — see condition
rigin of both great vessels from right ventricle
  Q20.1
rmond's disease (with ureteral obstruction) N13.5
with infection N13.6
rnithine metabolism disorder E72.4
rnithinemia (Type I) (Type II) E72.4
rnithosis A70
rotaciduria, oroticaciduria (congenital) (hereditary)
  (pyrimidine deficiency) E79.8
anemia D53.0
rthodontics
adjustment Z46.4
fitting Z46.4
rthopnea R06.01
rthopoxvirus B08.09
s, uterus — see condition
sgood-Schlatter disease or osteochondrosis
  M92.52- ☑
sler (-Weber)-**Rendu disease** I78.0
sler's nodes I33.0
smidrosis L75.0
sseous — see condition
ssification
artery — see Arteriosclerosis
auricle (ear) — see Disorder, pinna, specified type NEC
bronchial J98.09
cardiac — see Degeneration, myocardial
cartilage (senile) — see Disorder, cartilage, specified
  type NEC
coronary (artery) — see Disease, heart, ischemic,
  atherosclerotic
diaphragm J98.6
ear, middle — see Otosclerosis
falx cerebri G96.198
fontanel, premature Q75.0
heart — see also Degeneration, myocardial
  valve — see Endocarditis
larynx J38.7
ligament — see Disorder, tendon, specified type NEC
  posterior longitudinal — see Spondylopathy, specified NEC
meninges (cerebral) (spinal) G96.198
multiple, eccentric centers — see Disorder, bone, development or growth
muscle — see also Calcification, muscle
  due to burns — see Myositis, ossificans, in, burns
  paralytic — see Myositis, ossificans, in, quadriplegia

Ossification — continued
muscle — see also Calcification, muscle — continued
  progressive — see Myositis, ossificans, progressiva
  specified NEC M61.50
   ankle M61.57- ☑
   foot M61.57- ☑
   forearm M61.53- ☑
   hand M61.54- ☑
   lower leg M61.56- ☑
   multiple sites M61.59
   pelvic region M61.55- ☑
   shoulder region M61.51- ☑
   specified site NEC M61.58
   thigh M61.55- ☑
   upper arm M61.52- ☑
  traumatic — see Myositis, ossificans, traumatica
myocardium, myocardial — see Degeneration, myocardial
penis N48.89
periarticular — see Disorder, joint, specified type NEC
pinna — see Disorder, pinna, specified type NEC
rider's bone — see Ossification, muscle, specified NEC
sclera H15.89
subperiosteal, post-traumatic M89.8X- ☑
tendon — see Disorder, tendon, specified type NEC
trachea J39.8
tympanic membrane — see Disorder, tympanic membrane, specified NEC
vitreous (humor) — see Deposit, crystalline
Osteitis — see also Osteomyelitis
alveolar M27.3
condensans M85.30
  ankle M85.37- ☑
  foot M85.37- ☑
  forearm M85.33- ☑
  hand M85.34- ☑
  lower leg M85.36- ☑
  multiple site M85.39
  neck M85.38
  rib M85.38
  shoulder M85.31- ☑
  skull M85.38
  specified site NEC M85.38
  thigh M85.35- ☑
  toe M85.37- ☑
  upper arm M85.32- ☑
  vertebra M85.38
deformans M88.9
  in (due to)
   malignant neoplasm of bone C41.9 [M90.60]
   neoplastic disease — see also Neoplasm
    D49.9 [M90.60]
    carpus D49.9 [M90.64-] ☑
    clavicle D49.9 [M90.61-] ☑
    femur D49.9 [M90.65-] ☑
    fibula D49.9 [M90.66-] ☑
    finger D49.9 [M90.64-] ☑
    humerus D49.9 [M90.62-] ☑
    ilium D49.9 [M90.65-] ☑
    ischium D49.9 [M90.65-] ☑
    metacarpus D49.9 [M90.64-] ☑
    metatarsus D49.9 [M90.67-] ☑
    multiple sites D49.9 [M90.69]
    neck D49.9 [M90.68]
    radius D49.9 [M90.63-] ☑
    rib D49.9 [M90.68]
    scapula D49.9 [M90.61-] ☑
    skull D49.9 [M90.68]
    tarsus D49.9 [M90.67-] ☑
    tibia D49.9 [M90.66-] ☑
    toe D49.9 [M90.67-] ☑
    ulna D49.9 [M90.63-] ☑
    vertebra D49.9 [M90.68]
  skull M88.0
  specified NEC — see Paget's disease, bone, by site
  vertebra M88.1
due to yaws A66.6
fibrosa NEC — see Cyst, bone, by site
  circumscripta — see Dysplasia, fibrous, bone NEC
  cystica (generalisata) E21.0
  disseminata Q78.1
  osteoplastica E21.0
fragilitans Q78.0
Garr's (sclerosing) — see Osteomyelitis, specified type
  NEC

Osteitis — continued
jaw (acute) (chronic) (lower) (suppurative) (upper)
  M27.2
parathyroid E21.0
petrous bone (acute) (chronic) — see Petrositis
sclerotic, nonsuppurative — see Osteomyelitis, specified type NEC
tuberculosa A18.09
  cystica D86.89
  multiplex cystoides D86.89
Osteoarthritis M19.90
ankle M19.07- ☑
elbow M19.02- ☑
foot joint M19.07- ☑
generalized M15.9
  erosive M15.4
  primary M15.0
  specified NEC M15.8
hand joint M19.04- ☑
  first carpometacarpal joint M18.9
hip M16.1- ☑
  bilateral M16.0
  due to hip dysplasia (unilateral) M16.3- ☑
   bilateral M16.2
interphalangeal
  distal (Heberden) M15.1
  proximal (Bouchard) M15.2
knee M17.1- ☑
  bilateral M17.0
post-traumatic NEC M19.92
  ankle M19.17- ☑
  elbow M19.12- ☑
  foot joint M19.17- ☑
  hand joint M19.14- ☑
   first carpometacarpal joint M18.3- ☑
    bilateral M18.2
  hip M16.5- ☑
   bilateral M16.4
  knee M17.3- ☑
   bilateral M17.2
  shoulder M19.11- ☑
  specified site NEC M19.19
  wrist M19.13- ☑
primary M19.91
  ankle M19.07- ☑
  elbow M19.02- ☑
  foot joint M19.07- ☑
  hand joint M19.04- ☑
   first carpometacarpal joint M18.1- ☑
    bilateral M18.0
  hip M16.1- ☑
   bilateral M16.0
  knee M17.1- ☑
   bilateral M17.0
  multiple sites M89.49
  shoulder M19.01- ☑
  spine — see Spondylosis
  wrist M19.03- ☑
secondary M19.93
  ankle M19.27- ☑
  elbow M19.22- ☑
  foot joint M19.27- ☑
  hand joint M19.24- ☑
   first carpometacarpal joint M18.5- ☑
    bilateral M18.4
  hip M16.7
   bilateral M16.6
  knee M17.5
   bilateral M17.4
  multiple M15.3
  shoulder M19.21- ☑
  specified site NEC M19.29
  spine — see Spondylosis
  wrist M19.23- ☑
shoulder M19.01- ☑
specified site NEC M19.09
spine — see Spondylosis
wrist M19.03- ☑
Osteoarthropathy (hypertrophic) M19.90
ankle — see Osteoarthritis, primary, ankle
elbow — see Osteoarthritis, primary, elbow
foot joint — see Osteoarthritis, primary, foot
hand joint — see Osteoarthritis, primary, hand joint
knee joint — see Osteoarthritis, primary, knee
multiple site — see Osteoarthritis, primary, multiple
  joint

Osteoarthropathy — *continued*
- pulmonary — *see also* Osteoarthropathy, specified type NEC
  - hypertrophic — *see* Osteoarthropathy, hypertrophic, specified type NEC
- secondary — *see* Osteoarthropathy, specified type NEC
- secondary hypertrophic — *see* Osteoarthropathy, specified type NEC
- shoulder — *see* Osteoarthritis, primary, shoulder
- specified joint NEC — *see* Osteoarthritis, primary, specified joint NEC
- specified type NEC M89.40
  - carpus M89.44- ☑
  - clavicle M89.41- ☑
  - femur M89.45- ☑
  - fibula M89.46- ☑
  - finger M89.44- ☑
  - humerus M89.42- ☑
  - ilium M89.459
  - ischium M89.459
  - metacarpus M89.44- ☑
  - metatarsus M89.47- ☑
  - multiple sites M89.49
  - neck M89.48
  - radius M89.43- ☑
  - rib M89.48
  - scapula M89.41- ☑
  - skull M89.48
  - tarsus M89.47- ☑
  - tibia M89.46- ☑
  - toe M89.47- ☑
  - ulna M89.43- ☑
  - vertebra M89.48
- spine — *see* Spondylosis
- wrist — *see* Osteoarthritis, primary, wrist

Osteoarthrosis (degenerative) (hypertrophic) (joint) — *see also* Osteoarthritis
- deformans alkaptonurica E70.29 *[M36.8]*
- erosive M15.4
- generalized M15.9
  - primary M15.0
- polyarticular M15.9
- spine — *see* Spondylosis

Osteoblastoma — *see* Neoplasm, bone, benign
- aggressive — *see* Neoplasm, bone, uncertain behavior

Osteochondritis — *see also* Osteochondropathy, by site
- Brailsford's — *see* Osteochondrosis, juvenile, radius
- dissecans M93.20
  - ankle M93.27- ☑
  - elbow M93.22- ☑
  - foot M93.27- ☑
  - hand M93.24- ☑
  - hip M93.25- ☑
  - knee M93.26- ☑
  - multiple sites M93.29
  - shoulder joint M93.21- ☑
  - specified site NEC M93.28
  - wrist M93.23- ☑
- juvenile M92.9
  - patellar — *see* Osteochondrosis, juvenile, patella
- syphilitic (congenital) (early) A50.02 *[M90.80]*
  - ankle A50.02 *[M90.87-]* ☑
  - elbow A50.02 *[M90.82-]* ☑
  - foot A50.02 *[M90.87-]* ☑
  - forearm A50.02 *[M90.83-]* ☑
  - hand A50.02 *[M90.84-]* ☑
  - hip A50.02 *[M90.85-]* ☑
  - knee A50.02 *[M90.86-]* ☑
  - multiple sites A50.02 *[M90.89]*
  - shoulder joint A50.02 *[M90.81-]* ☑
  - specified site NEC A50.02 *[M90.88]*

Osteochondroarthrosis deformans endemica — *see* Disease, Kaschin-Beck

Osteochondrodysplasia Q78.9
- with defects of growth of tubular bones and spine Q77.9
  - specified NEC Q77.8
- specified NEC Q78.8

Osteochondrodystrophy E78.9

Osteochondrolysis — *see* Osteochondritis, dissecans

Osteochondroma — *see* Neoplasm, bone, benign

Osteochondromatosis D48.0
- syndrome Q78.4

Osteochondromyxosarcoma — *see* Neoplasm, bone, malignant

Osteochondropathy M93.90
- ankle M93.97- ☑

Osteochondropathy — *continued*
- elbow M93.92- ☑
- foot M93.97- ☑
- hand M93.94- ☑
- hip M93.95- ☑
- Kienböck's disease of adults M93.1
- knee M93.96- ☑
- multiple joints M93.99
- osteochondritis dissecans — *see* Osteochondritis, dissecans
- osteochondrosis — *see* Osteochondrosis
- shoulder region M93.91- ☑
- slipped upper femoral epiphysis — *see* Slipped, epiphysis, upper femoral
- specified joint NEC M93.98
- specified type NEC M93.80
  - ankle M93.87- ☑
  - elbow M93.82- ☑
  - foot M93.87- ☑
  - hand M93.84- ☑
  - hip M93.85- ☑
  - knee M93.86- ☑
  - multiple joints M93.89
  - shoulder region M93.81- ☑
  - specified joint NEC M93.88
  - wrist M93.83- ☑
- syphilitic, congenital
  - early A50.02 *[M90.80]*
  - late A50.56 *[M90.80]*
- wrist M93.93- ☑

Osteochondrosarcoma — *see* Neoplasm, bone, malignant

Osteochondrosis — *see also* Osteochondropathy, by site
- acetabulum (juvenile) M91.0
- adult — *see* Osteochondropathy, specified type NEC, by site
- astragalus (juvenile) — *see* Osteochondrosis, juvenile, tarsus
- Blount M92.51- ☑
- Buchanan's M91.0
- Burns' — *see* Osteochondrosis, juvenile, ulna
- calcaneus (juvenile) — *see* Osteochondrosis, juvenile, tarsus
- capitular epiphysis (femur) (juvenile) — *see* Legg-Calvé-Perthes disease
- carpal (juvenile) (lunate) (scaphoid) — *see* Osteochondrosis, juvenile, hand, carpal lunate
  - adult M93.1
- coxae juvenilis — *see* Legg-Calvé-Perthes disease
- deformans juvenilis, coxae — *see* Legg-Calvé-Perthes disease
- Diaz's — *see* Osteochondrosis, juvenile, tarsus
- dissecans (knee) (shoulder) — *see* Osteochondritis, dissecans
- femoral capital epiphysis (juvenile) — *see* Legg-Calvé-Perthes disease
- femur (head), juvenile — *see* Legg-Calvé-Perthes disease
- fibula (juvenile) — *see* Osteochondrosis, juvenile, fibula
- foot NEC (juvenile) M92.8
- Freiberg's — *see* Osteochondrosis, juvenile, metatarsus
- Haas' (juvenile) — *see* Osteochondrosis, juvenile, humerus
- Haglund's — *see* Osteochondrosis, juvenile, tarsus
- hip (juvenile) — *see* Legg-Calvé-Perthes disease
- humerus (capitulum) (head) (juvenile) — *see* Osteochondrosis, juvenile, humerus
- ilium, iliac crest (juvenile) M91.0
- ischiopubic synchondrosis M91.0
- Iselin's — *see* Osteochondrosis, juvenile, metatarsus
- juvenile, juvenilis M92.9
  - after congenital dislocation of hip reduction — *see* Osteochondrosis, juvenile, hip, specified NEC
  - arm — *see* Osteochondrosis, juvenile, upper limb NEC
  - capitular epiphysis (femur) — *see* Legg-Calvé-Perthes disease
  - clavicle, sternal epiphysis — *see* Osteochondrosis, juvenile, upper limb NEC
  - coxae — *see* Legg-Calvé-Perthes disease
  - deformans M92.9
  - fibula M92.50- ☑
  - foot NEC M92.8
  - hand M92.20- ☑
    - carpal lunate M92.21- ☑

Osteochondrosis — *continued*
- juvenile, juvenilis — *continued*
  - hand — *continued*
    - metacarpal head M92.22- ☑
    - specified site NEC M92.29- ☑
  - head of femur — *see* Legg-Calvé-Perthes disease
  - hip and pelvis M91.9- ☑
    - coxa plana — *see* Coxa, plana
    - femoral head — *see* Legg-Calvé-Perthes disease
    - pelvis M91.0
    - pseudocoxalgia — *see* Pseudocoxalgia
    - specified NEC M91.8- ☑
  - humerus M92.0- ☑
  - limb
    - lower NEC M92.8
    - upper NEC — *see* Osteochondrosis, juvenile, upper limb NEC
  - medial cuneiform bone — *see* Osteochondrosis, juvenile, tarsus
  - metatarsus M92.7- ☑
  - patella M92.4- ☑
  - radius M92.1- ☑
  - specified
    - site NEC M92.8
    - type NEC M92.8
      - tibia and fibula M92.59- ☑
  - spine M42.00
    - cervical region M42.02
    - cervicothoracic region M42.03
    - lumbar region M42.06
    - lumbosacral region M42.07
    - multiple sites M42.09
    - occipito-atlanto-axial region M42.01
    - sacrococcygeal region M42.08
    - thoracic region M42.04
    - thoracolumbar region M42.05
  - tarsus M92.6- ☑
  - tibia M92.50- ☑
    - proximal M92.51- ☑
    - tubercle M92.52- ☑
  - ulna M92.1- ☑
  - upper limb NEC M92.3- ☑
  - vertebra (body) (epiphyseal plates) (Calvé's) (Scheuermann's) — *see* Osteochondrosis, j venile, spine
- Kienböck's — *see* Osteochondrosis, juvenile, hand, carpal lunate
  - adult M93.1
- Köhler's
  - patellar — *see* Osteochondrosis, juvenile, patella
  - tarsal navicular — *see* Osteochondrosis, juvenile tarsus
- Legg-Perthes (-Calvé)(-Waldenström) — *see* Legg-Calvé-Perthes disease
- limb
  - lower NEC (juvenile) M92.8
    - tibia and fibula M92.59- ☑
    - upper NEC (juvenile) — *see* Osteochondrosis, juv nile, upper limb NEC
- lunate bone (carpal) (juvenile) — *see also* Osteocho drosis, juvenile, hand, carpal lunate
  - adult M93.1
- Mauclaire's — *see* Osteochondrosis, juvenile, hand, metacarpal
- metacarpal (head) (juvenile) — *see* Osteochondrosi juvenile, hand, metacarpal
- metatarsus (fifth) (head) (juvenile) (second) — *see* O teochondrosis, juvenile, metatarsus
- navicular (juvenile) — *see* Osteochondrosis, juvenil tarsus
- os
  - calcis (juvenile) — *see* Osteochondrosis, juvenile tarsus
  - tibiale externum (juvenile) — *see* Osteochondros juvenile, tarsus
- Osgood-Schlatter M92.52- ☑
- Panner's — *see* Osteochondrosis, juvenile, humerus
- patellar center (juvenile) (primary) (secondary) — s Osteochondrosis, juvenile, patella
- pelvis (juvenile) M91.0
- Pierson's M91.0
- radius (head) (juvenile) — *see* Osteochondrosis, juv nile, radius
- Scheuermann's — *see* Osteochondrosis, juvenile, spi
- Sever's — *see* Osteochondrosis, juvenile, tarsus
- Sinding-Larsen — *see* Osteochondrosis, juvenile, patella

☑ **Additional Character Required** — **Refer to the Tabular List for Character Selection**　　　▽ **Subterms under main terms may continue to next column or pag**

Osteochondrosis — continued
  spine M42.9
    adult M42.10
      cervical region M42.12
      cervicothoracic region M42.13
      lumbar region M42.16
      lumbosacral region M42.17
      multiple sites M42.19
      occipito-atlanto-axial region M42.11
      sacrococcygeal region M42.18
      thoracic region M42.14
      thoracolumbar region M42.15
    juvenile — see Osteochondrosis, juvenile, spine
  symphysis pubis (juvenile) M91.0
  syphilitic (congenital) A50.02
  talus (juvenile) — see Osteochondrosis, juvenile, tarsus
  tarsus (navicular) (juvenile) — see Osteochondrosis, juvenile, tarsus
  tibia (proximal) (tubercle) (juvenile) — see Osteochondrosis, juvenile, tibia
  tuberculous — see Tuberculosis, bone
  ulna (lower) (juvenile) — see Osteochondrosis, juvenile, ulna
  van Neck's M91.0
  vertebral — see Osteochondrosis, spine
Osteoclastoma D48.0
  malignant — see Neoplasm, bone, malignant
Osteodynia — see Disorder, bone, specified type NEC
Osteodystrophy Q78.9
  azotemic N25.0
  congenital Q78.9
  parathyroid, secondary E21.1
  renal N25.0
Osteofibroma — see Neoplasm, bone, benign
Osteofibrosarcoma — see Neoplasm, bone, malignant
Osteogenesis imperfecta Q78.0
Osteogenic — see condition
Osteolysis M89.50
  carpus M89.54- ☑
  clavicle M89.51- ☑
  femur M89.55- ☑
  fibula M89.56- ☑
  finger M89.54- ☑
  humerus M89.52- ☑
  ilium M89.559
  ischium M89.559
  joint prosthesis (periprosthetic) — see Complications, joint prosthesis, mechanical, periprosthetic, osteolysis, by site
  metacarpus M89.54- ☑
  metatarsus M89.57- ☑
  multiple sites M89.59
  neck M89.58
  periprosthetic — see Complications, joint prosthesis, mechanical, periprosthetic, osteolysis, by site
  radius M89.53- ☑
  rib M89.58
  scapula M89.51- ☑
  skull M89.58
  tarsus M89.57- ☑
  tibia M89.56- ☑
  toe M89.57- ☑
  ulna M89.53- ☑
  vertebra M89.58
Osteoma — see also Neoplasm, bone, benign
  osteoid — see also Neoplasm, bone, benign
    giant — see Neoplasm, bone, benign
Osteomalacia M83.9
  adult M83.9
    drug-induced NEC M83.5
    due to
      malabsorption (postsurgical) M83.2
      malnutrition M83.3
    specified NEC M83.8
  aluminium-induced M83.4
  infantile — see Rickets
  juvenile — see Rickets
  oncogenic E83.89
  pelvis M83.8
  puerperal M83.0
  senile M83.1
  vitamin-D-resistant in adults E83.31 [M90.8-] ☑
    carpus E83.31 [M90.84-] ☑
    clavicle E83.31 [M90.81-] ☑
    femur E83.31 [M90.85-] ☑
    fibula E83.31 [M90.86-] ☑
    finger E83.31 [M90.84-] ☑

Osteomalacia — continued
  vitamin-D-resistant in adults — continued
    humerus E83.31 [M90.82-] ☑
    ilium E83.31 [M90.859]
    ischium E83.31 [M90.859]
    metacarpus E83.31 [M90.84-] ☑
    metatarsus E83.31 [M90.87-] ☑
    multiple sites E83.31 [M90.89]
    neck E83.31 [M90.88]
    radius E83.31 [M90.83-] ☑
    rib E83.31 [M90.88]
    scapula E83.31 [M90.819]
    skull E83.31 [M90.88]
    tarsus E83.31 [M90.879]
    tibia E83.31 [M90.869]
    toe E83.31 [M90.879]
    ulna E83.31 [M90.839]
    vertebra E83.31 [M90.88]
Osteomyelitis (general) (infective) (localized) (neonatal) (purulent) (septic) (staphylococcal) (streptococcal) (suppurative) (with periostitis) M86.9
  acute M86.10
    carpus M86.14- ☑
    clavicle M86.11- ☑
    femur M86.15- ☑
    fibula M86.16- ☑
    finger M86.14- ☑
    hematogenous M86.00
      carpus M86.04- ☑
      clavicle M86.01- ☑
      femur M86.05- ☑
      fibula M86.06- ☑
      finger M86.04- ☑
      humerus M86.02- ☑
      ilium M86.059
      ischium M86.059
      mandible M27.2
      metacarpus M86.04- ☑
      metatarsus M86.07- ☑
      multiple sites M86.09
      neck M86.08
      orbit H05.02- ☑
      petrous bone — see Petrositis
      radius M86.03- ☑
      rib M86.08
      scapula M86.01- ☑
      skull M86.08
      tarsus M86.07- ☑
      tibia M86.06- ☑
      toe M86.07- ☑
      ulna M86.03- ☑
      vertebra — see Osteomyelitis, vertebra
    humerus M86.12- ☑
    ilium M86.18
    ischium M86.18
    mandible M27.2
    metacarpus M86.14- ☑
    metatarsus M86.17- ☑
    multiple sites M86.19
    neck M86.18
    orbit H05.02- ☑
    petrous bone — see Petrositis
    radius M86.13- ☑
    rib M86.18
    scapula M86.11- ☑
    skull M86.18
    tarsus M86.17- ☑
    tibia M86.16- ☑
    toe M86.17- ☑
    ulna M86.13- ☑
    vertebra — see Osteomyelitis, vertebra
  chronic (or old) M86.60
    with draining sinus M86.40
      carpus M86.44- ☑
      clavicle M86.41- ☑
      femur M86.45- ☑
      fibula M86.46- ☑
      finger M86.44- ☑
      humerus M86.42- ☑
      ilium M86.459
      ischium M86.459
      mandible M27.2
      metacarpus M86.44- ☑
      metatarsus M86.47- ☑
      multiple sites M86.49
      neck M86.48

Osteomyelitis — continued
  chronic — continued
    with draining sinus — continued
      orbit H05.02- ☑
      petrous bone — see Petrositis
      radius M86.43- ☑
      rib M86.48
      scapula M86.41- ☑
      skull M86.48
      tarsus M86.47- ☑
      tibia M86.46- ☑
      toe M86.47- ☑
      ulna M86.43- ☑
      vertebra — see Osteomyelitis, vertebra
    carpus M86.64- ☑
    clavicle M86.61- ☑
    femur M86.65- ☑
    fibula M86.66- ☑
    finger M86.64- ☑
    hematogenous NEC M86.50
      carpus M86.54- ☑
      clavicle M86.51- ☑
      femur M86.55- ☑
      fibula M86.56- ☑
      finger M86.54- ☑
      humerus M86.52- ☑
      ilium M86.559
      ischium M86.559
      mandible M27.2
      metacarpus M86.54- ☑
      metatarsus M86.57- ☑
      multifocal M86.30
        carpus M86.34- ☑
        clavicle M86.31- ☑
        femur M86.35- ☑
        fibula M86.36- ☑
        finger M86.34- ☑
        humerus M86.32- ☑
        ilium M86.359
        ischium M86.359
        metacarpus M86.34- ☑
        metatarsus M86.37- ☑
        multiple sites M86.39
        neck M86.38
        radius M86.33- ☑
        rib M86.38
        scapula M86.31- ☑
        skull M86.38
        tarsus M86.37- ☑
        tibia M86.36- ☑
        toe M86.37- ☑
        ulna M86.33- ☑
        vertebra — see Osteomyelitis, vertebra
      multiple sites M86.59
      neck M86.58
      orbit H05.02- ☑
      petrous bone — see Petrositis
      radius M86.53- ☑
      rib M86.58
      scapula M86.51- ☑
      skull M86.58
      tarsus M86.57- ☑
      tibia M86.56- ☑
      toe M86.57- ☑
      ulna M86.53- ☑
      vertebra — see Osteomyelitis, vertebra
    humerus M86.62- ☑
    ilium M86.659
    ischium M86.659
    mandible M27.2
    metacarpus M86.64- ☑
    metatarsus M86.67- ☑
    multifocal — see Osteomyelitis, chronic, hematogenous, multifocal
    multiple sites M86.69
    neck M86.68
    orbit H05.02- ☑
    petrous bone — see Petrositis
    radius M86.63- ☑
    rib M86.68
    scapula M86.61- ☑
    skull M86.68
    tarsus M86.67- ☑
    tibia M86.66- ☑
    toe M86.67- ☑
    ulna M86.63- ☑

Osteomyelitis — continued
  chronic — continued
    vertebra — see Osteomyelitis, vertebra
  echinococcal B67.2
  Garr's — see Osteomyelitis, specified type NEC
  in diabetes mellitus — see E08-E13 with .69
  jaw (acute) (chronic) (lower) (neonatal) (suppurative)
    (upper) M27.2
  nonsuppurating — see Osteomyelitis, specified type
    NEC
  orbit H05.02- ☑
  petrous bone — see Petrositis
  Salmonella (arizonae) (cholerae-suis) (enteritidis) (ty-
    phimurium) A02.24
  sclerosing, nonsuppurative — see Osteomyelitis,
    specified type NEC
  specified type NEC — see also subcategory M86.8X- ☑
    mandible M27.2
    orbit H05.02- ☑
    petrous bone — see Petrositis
    vertebra — see Osteomyelitis, vertebra
  subacute M86.20
    carpus M86.24- ☑
    clavicle M86.21- ☑
    femur M86.25- ☑
    fibula M86.26- ☑
    finger M86.24- ☑
    humerus M86.22- ☑
    mandible M27.2
    metacarpus M86.24- ☑
    metatarsus M86.27- ☑
    multiple sites M86.29
    neck M86.28
    orbit H05.02- ☑
    petrous bone — see Petrositis
    radius M86.23- ☑
    rib M86.28
    scapula M86.21- ☑
    skull M86.28
    tarsus M86.27- ☑
    tibia M86.26- ☑
    toe M86.27- ☑
    ulna M86.23- ☑
    vertebra — see Osteomyelitis, vertebra
  syphilitic A52.77
    congenital (early) A50.02 [M90.80]
  tuberculous — see Tuberculosis, bone
  typhoid A01.05
  vertebra M46.20
    cervical region M46.22
    cervicothoracic region M46.23
    lumbar region M46.26
    lumbosacral region M46.27
    occipito-atlanto-axial region M46.21
    sacrococcygeal region M46.28
    thoracic region M46.24
    thoracolumbar region M46.25
Osteomyelofibrosis D47.4
Osteomyelosclerosis D75.89
Osteonecrosis M87.9
  due to
    drugs — see Osteonecrosis, secondary, due to, drugs
    trauma — see Osteonecrosis, secondary, due to,
      trauma
  idiopathic aseptic M87.00
    ankle M87.07- ☑
    carpus M87.03- ☑
    clavicle M87.01- ☑
    femur M87.05- ☑
    fibula M87.06- ☑
    finger M87.04- ☑
    humerus M87.02- ☑
    ilium M87.050
    ischium M87.050
    metacarpus M87.04- ☑
    metatarsus M87.07- ☑
    multiple sites M87.09
    neck M87.08
    pelvis M87.050
    radius M87.03- ☑
    rib M87.08
    scapula M87.01- ☑
    skull M87.08
    tarsus M87.07- ☑
    tibia M87.06- ☑
    toe M87.07- ☑
    ulna M87.03- ☑

Osteonecrosis — continued
  idiopathic aseptic — continued
    vertebra M87.08
  secondary NEC M87.30
    carpus M87.33- ☑
    clavicle M87.31- ☑
    due to
      drugs M87.10
        carpus M87.13- ☑
        clavicle M87.11- ☑
        femur M87.15- ☑
        fibula M87.16- ☑
        finger M87.14- ☑
        humerus M87.12- ☑
        ilium M87.159
        ischium M87.159
        jaw M87.180
        metacarpus M87.14- ☑
        metatarsus M87.17- ☑
        multiple sites M87.19
        neck M87.18
        radius M87.13- ☑
        rib M87.18
        scapula M87.11- ☑
        skull M87.18
        tarsus M87.17- ☑
        tibia M87.16- ☑
        toe M87.17- ☑
        ulna M87.13- ☑
        vertebra M87.18
      hemoglobinopathy NEC D58.2 [M90.50]
        carpus D58.2 [M90.54-] ☑
        clavicle D58.2 [M90.51-] ☑
        femur D58.2 [M90.55-] ☑
        fibula D58.2 [M90.56-] ☑
        finger D58.2 [M90.54-] ☑
        humerus D58.2 [M90.52-] ☑
        ilium D58.2 [M90.55-] ☑
        ischium D58.2 [M90.55-] ☑
        metacarpus D58.2 [M90.54-] ☑
        metatarsus D58.2 [M90.57-] ☑
        multiple sites D58.2 [M90.58]
        neck D58.2 [M90.58]
        radius D58.2 [M90.53-] ☑
        rib D58.2 [M90.58]
        scapula D58.2 [M90.51-] ☑
        skull D58.2 [M90.58]
        tarsus D58.2 [M90.57-] ☑
        tibia D58.2 [M90.56-] ☑
        toe D58.2 [M90.57-] ☑
        ulna D58.2 [M90.53-] ☑
        vertebra D58.2 [M90.58]
      trauma (previous) M87.20
        carpus M87.23- ☑
        clavicle M87.21- ☑
        femur M87.25- ☑
        fibula M87.26- ☑
        finger M87.24- ☑
        humerus M87.22- ☑
        ilium M87.25- ☑
        ischium M87.25- ☑
        metacarpus M87.24- ☑
        metatarsus M87.27- ☑
        multiple sites M87.29
        neck M87.28
        radius M87.23- ☑
        rib M87.28
        scapula M87.21- ☑
        skull M87.28
        tarsus M87.27- ☑
        tibia M87.26- ☑
        toe M87.27- ☑
        ulna M87.23- ☑
        vertebra M87.28
    femur M87.35- ☑
    fibula M87.36- ☑
    finger M87.34- ☑
    humerus M87.32- ☑
    ilium M87.350
    in
      caisson disease T70.3 ☑ [M90.50]
        carpus T70.3 ☑ [M90.54-] ☑
        clavicle T70.3 ☑ [M90.51-] ☑
        femur T70.3 ☑ [M90.55-] ☑
        fibula T70.3 ☑ [M90.56-] ☑
        finger T70.3 ☑ [M90.54-] ☑

Osteonecrosis — continued
  secondary — continued
    in — continued
      caisson disease — continued
        humerus T70.3 ☑ [M90.52-] ☑
        ilium T70.3 ☑ [M90.55-] ☑
        ischium T70.3 ☑ [M90.55-] ☑
        metacarpus T70.3 ☑ [M90.54-] ☑
        metatarsus T70.3 ☑ [M90.57-] ☑
        multiple sites T70.3 ☑ [M90.59]
        neck T70.3 ☑ [M90.58]
        radius T70.3 ☑ [M90.53-] ☑
        rib T70.3 ☑ [M90.58]
        scapula T70.3 ☑ [M90.51-] ☑
        skull T70.3 ☑ [M90.58]
        tarsus T70.3 ☑ [M90.57-] ☑
        tibia T70.3 ☑ [M90.56-] ☑
        toe T70.3 ☑ [M90.57-] ☑
        ulna T70.3 ☑ [M90.53-] ☑
        vertebra T70.3 ☑ [M90.58]
    ischium M87.350
    metacarpus M87.34- ☑
    metatarsus M87.37- ☑
    multiple site M87.39
    neck M87.38
    radius M87.33- ☑
    rib M87.38
    scapula M87.319
    skull M87.38
    tarsus M87.379
    tibia M87.366
    toe M87.379
    ulna M87.33- ☑
    vertebra M87.38
  specified type NEC M87.80
    carpus M87.83- ☑
    clavicle M87.81- ☑
    femur M87.85- ☑
    fibula M87.86- ☑
    finger M87.84- ☑
    humerus M87.82- ☑
    ilium M87.85- ☑
    ischium M87.85- ☑
    metacarpus M87.84- ☑
    metatarsus M87.87- ☑
    multiple sites M87.89
    neck M87.88
    radius M87.83- ☑
    rib M87.88
    scapula M87.81- ☑
    skull M87.88
    tarsus M87.87- ☑
    tibia M87.86- ☑
    toe M87.87- ☑
    ulna M87.83- ☑
    vertebra M87.88
Osteo-onycho-arthro-dysplasia Q87.2
Osteo-onychodysplasia, hereditary Q87.2
Osteopathia condensans disseminata Q78.8
Osteopathy — see also Osteomyelitis, Osteonecrosis,
  Osteoporosis
  after poliomyelitis M89.60
    carpus M89.64- ☑
    clavicle M89.61- ☑
    femur M89.65- ☑
    fibula M89.66- ☑
    finger M89.64- ☑
    humerus M89.62- ☑
    ilium M89.659
    ischium M89.659
    metacarpus M89.64- ☑
    metatarsus M89.67- ☑
    multiple sites M89.69
    neck M89.68
    radius M89.63- ☑
    rib M89.68
    scapula M89.61- ☑
    skull M89.68
    tarsus M89.67- ☑
    tibia M89.66- ☑
    toe M89.67- ☑
    ulna M89.63- ☑
    vertebra M89.68
  in (due to)
    renal osteodystrophy N25.0

Osteopathy — *continued*
  in — *continued*
    specified diseases classified elsewhere — *see* sub-
      category M90.8 ☑
Osteopenia M85.8-
  borderline M85.8- ☑
Osteoperiostitis — *see* Osteomyelitis, specified type
  NEC
Osteopetrosis (familial) Q78.2
Osteophyte M25.70
  ankle M25.77- ☑
  elbow M25.72- ☑
  foot joint M25.77- ☑
  hand joint M25.74- ☑
  hip M25.75- ☑
  knee M25.76- ☑
  shoulder M25.71- ☑
  spine M25.78
  vertebrae M25.78
  wrist M25.73- ☑
Osteopoikilosis Q78.8
Osteoporosis (female) (male) M81.0
  with current pathological fracture M80.00 ☑
  age-related M81.0
    with current pathologic fracture M80.00 ☑
      carpus M80.04- ☑
      clavicle M80.01- ☑
      fibula M80.06- ☑
      finger M80.04- ☑
      humerus M80.02- ☑
      ilium M80.05- ☑
      ischium M80.05- ☑
      metacarpus M80.04- ☑
      metatarsus M80.07- ☑
      pelvis M80.05- ☑
      radius M80.03- ☑
      scapula M80.01- ☑
      site specified NEC M80.0A ☑
      tarsus M80.07- ☑
      tibia M80.06- ☑
      toe M80.07- ☑
      ulna M80.03- ☑
      vertebra M80.08 ☑
  disuse M81.8
    with current pathological fracture M80.80 ☑
      carpus M80.84- ☑
      clavicle M80.81- ☑
      fibula M80.86- ☑
      finger M80.84- ☑
      humerus M80.82- ☑
      ilium M80.85- ☑
      ischium M80.85- ☑
      metacarpus M80.84- ☑
      metatarsus M80.87- ☑
      pelvis M80.85- ☑
      radius M80.83- ☑
      scapula M80.81- ☑
      site specified NEC M80.8A ☑
      tarsus M80.87- ☑
      tibia M80.86- ☑
      toe M80.87- ☑
      ulna M80.83- ☑
      vertebra M80.88 ☑
  drug-induced — *see* Osteoporosis, specified type NEC
  idiopathic — *see* Osteoporosis, specified type NEC
  involutional — *see* Osteoporosis, age-related
  Lequesne M81.6
  localized M81.6
  postmenopausal M81.0
    with pathological fracture M80.00 ☑
      carpus M80.04- ☑
      clavicle M80.01- ☑
      fibula M80.06- ☑
      finger M80.04- ☑
      humerus M80.02- ☑
      ilium M80.05- ☑
      ischium M80.05- ☑
      metacarpus M80.04- ☑
      metatarsus M80.07- ☑
      pelvis M80.05- ☑
      radius M80.03- ☑
      scapula M80.01- ☑
      site specified NEC M80.0A ☑
      tarsus M80.07- ☑
      tibia M80.06- ☑
      toe M80.07- ☑

Osteoporosis — *continued*
  postmenopausal — *continued*
    with pathological fracture — *continued*
      ulna M80.03- ☑
      vertebra M80.08 ☑
  postoophorectomy — *see* Osteoporosis, specified type
    NEC
  postsurgical malabsorption — *see* Osteoporosis,
    specified type NEC
  post-traumatic — *see* Osteoporosis, specified type NEC
  senile — *see* Osteoporosis, age-related
  specified type NEC M81.8
    with pathological fracture M80.80 ☑
      carpus M80.84- ☑
      clavicle M80.81- ☑
      fibula M80.86- ☑
      finger M80.84- ☑
      humerus M80.82- ☑
      ilium M80.85- ☑
      ischium M80.85- ☑
      metacarpus M80.84- ☑
      metatarsus M80.87- ☑
      pelvis M80.85- ☑
      radius M80.83- ☑
      scapula M80.81- ☑
      site specified NEC M80.8A ☑
      tarsus M80.87- ☑
      tibia M80.86- ☑
      toe M80.87- ☑
      ulna M80.83- ☑
      vertebra M80.88 ☑
Osteopsathyrosis (idiopathica) Q78.0
Osteoradionecrosis, jaw (acute) (chronic) (lower) (suppurative) (upper) M27.2
Osteosarcoma (any form) — *see* Neoplasm, bone, malignant
Osteosclerosis Q78.2
  acquired M85.8- ☑
  congenita Q77.4
  fragilitas (generalisata) Q78.2
  myelofibrosis D75.81
Osteosclerotic anemia D64.89
Osteosis
  cutis L94.2
  renal fibrocystic N25.0
Österreicher-Turner syndrome Q87.2
Ostium
  atrioventriculare commune Q21.2
  primum (arteriosum) (defect) (persistent) Q21.2
  secundum (arteriosum) (defect) (patent) (persistent)
    Q21.1
Ostrum-Furst syndrome Q75.8
Otalgia H92.0 ☑
Otitis (acute) H66.90
  with effusion — *see also* Otitis, media, nonsuppurative
    purulent — *see* Otitis, media, suppurative
  adhesive — *see* subcategory H74.1 ☑
  chronic — *see also* Otitis, media, chronic
    with effusion — *see also* Otitis, media, nonsuppura-
      tive, chronic
  externa H60.9- ☑
    abscess — *see* Abscess, ear, external
    acute (noninfective) H60.50- ☑
      actinic H60.51- ☑
      chemical H60.52- ☑
      contact H60.53- ☑
      eczematoid H60.54- ☑
      infective — *see* Otitis, externa, infective
      reactive H60.55- ☑
      specified NEC H60.59- ☑
    cellulitis — *see* Cellulitis, ear
    chronic H60.6- ☑
    diffuse — *see* Otitis, externa, infective, diffuse
    hemorrhagic — *see* Otitis, externa, infective, hem-
      orrhagic
    in (due to)
      aspergillosis B44.89
      candidiasis B37.84
      erysipelas A46 [H62.40]
      herpes (simplex) virus infection B00.1
        zoster B02.8
      impetigo L01.00 [H62.40]
      infectious disease NEC B99 ☑ [H62.4-] ☑
      mycosis NEC B36.9 [H62.40]
      parasitic disease NEC B89 [H62.40]
      viral disease NEC B34.9 [H62.40]

Otitis — *continued*
  externa — *continued*
    in — *continued*
      zoster B02.8
    infective NEC H60.39- ☑
      abscess — *see* Abscess, ear, external
      cellulitis — *see* Cellulitis, ear
      diffuse H60.31- ☑
      hemorrhagic H60.32- ☑
      swimmer's ear — *see* Swimmer's, ear
    malignant H60.2- ☑
    mycotic NEC B36.9 [H62.40]
      in
        aspergillosis B44.89
        candidiasis B37.84
        moniliasis B37.84
    necrotizing — *see* Otitis, externa, malignant
    Pseudomonas aeruginosa — *see* Otitis, externa,
      malignant
    reactive — *see* Otitis, externa, acute, reactive
    specified NEC — *see* subcategory H60.8 ☑
    tropical NEC B36.9 [H62.40]
      in
        aspergillosis B44.89
        candidiasis B37.84
        moniliasis B37.84
  insidiosa — *see* Otosclerosis
  interna H83.0 ☑
  media (hemorrhagic) (staphylococcal) (streptococcal)
    H66.9- ☑
    with effusion (nonpurulent) — *see* Otitis, media,
      nonsuppurative
    acute, subacute H66.90
      allergic — *see* Otitis, media, nonsuppurative,
        acute, allergic
      exudative — *see* Otitis, media, suppurative, acute
      mucoid — *see* Otitis, media, nonsuppurative,
        acute
      necrotizing — *see also* Otitis, media, suppurative,
        acute
        in
          measles B05.3
          scarlet fever A38.0
      nonsuppurative NEC — *see* Otitis, media, non-
        suppurative, acute
      purulent — *see* Otitis, media, suppurative, acute
      sanguinous — *see* Otitis, media, nonsuppurative,
        acute
      secretory — *see* Otitis, media, nonsuppurative,
        acute, serous
      seromucinous — *see* Otitis, media, nonsuppura-
        tive, acute
      serous — *see* Otitis, media, nonsuppurative,
        acute, serous
      suppurative — *see* Otitis, media, suppurative,
        acute
    allergic — *see* Otitis, media, nonsuppurative
    catarrhal — *see* Otitis, media, nonsuppurative
    chronic H66.90
      with effusion (nonpurulent) — *see* Otitis, media,
        nonsuppurative, chronic
      allergic — *see* Otitis, media, nonsuppurative,
        chronic, allergic
      benign suppurative — *see* Otitis, media, suppu-
        rative, chronic, tubotympanic
      catarrhal — *see* Otitis, media, nonsuppurative,
        chronic, serous
      exudative — *see* Otitis, media, nonsuppurative,
        chronic
      mucinous — *see* Otitis, media, nonsuppurative,
        chronic, mucoid
      mucoid — *see* Otitis, media, nonsuppurative,
        chronic, mucoid
      nonsuppurative NEC — *see* Otitis, media, non-
        suppurative, chronic
      purulent — *see* Otitis, media, suppurative,
        chronic
      secretory — *see* Otitis, media, nonsuppurative,
        chronic, mucoid
      seromucinous — *see* Otitis, media, nonsuppura-
        tive, chronic
      serous — *see* Otitis, media, nonsuppurative,
        chronic, serous
      suppurative — *see* Otitis, media, suppurative,
        chronic
      transudative — *see* Otitis, media, nonsuppura-
        tive, chronic, mucoid

Otitis — *continued*
  media — *continued*
    exudative — *see* Otitis, media, suppurative
    in (due to) (with)
      influenza — *see* Influenza, with, otitis media
      measles B05.3
      scarlet fever A38.0
      tuberculosis A18.6
      viral disease NEC B34.- ☑ *[H67.-]* ☑
    mucoid — *see* Otitis, media, nonsuppurative
    nonsuppurative H65.9- ☑
      acute or subacute NEC H65.19- ☑
        allergic H65.11- ☑
          recurrent H65.11- ☑
        recurrent H65.19- ☑
        secretory — *see* Otitis, media, nonsuppura-
          tive, serous
        serous H65.0- ☑
          recurrent H65.0- ☑
      chronic H65.49- ☑
        allergic H65.41- ☑
        mucoid H65.3- ☑
        serous H65.2- ☑
      postmeasles B05.3
    purulent — *see* Otitis, media, suppurative
    secretory — *see* Otitis, media, nonsuppurative
    seromucinous — *see* Otitis, media, nonsuppurative
    serous — *see* Otitis, media, nonsuppurative
    suppurative H66.4- ☑
      acute H66.00- ☑
        with rupture of ear drum H66.01- ☑
        recurrent H66.00- ☑
          with rupture of ear drum H66.01- ☑
      chronic — *see also* subcategory H66.3 ☑
        atticoantral H66.2- ☑
        benign — *see* Otitis, media, suppurative,
          chronic, tubotympanic
        tubotympanic H66.1- ☑
    transudative — *see* Otitis, media, nonsuppurative
    tuberculous A18.6
Otocephaly Q18.2
Otolith syndrome — *see* subcategory H81.8 ☑
Otomycosis (diffuse) **NEC** B36.9 *[H62.40]*
  in
    aspergillosis B44.89
    candidiasis B37.84
    moniliasis B37.84
Otoporosis — *see* Otosclerosis
Otorrhagia (nontraumatic) H92.2- ☑
  traumatic — *code by* Type of injury
Otorrhea H92.1- ☑
  cerebrospinal (fluid) G96.01
    postoperative G96.08
    specified NEC G96.08
    spontaneous G96.01
    traumatic G96.08
Otosclerosis (general) H80.9- ☑
  cochlear (endosteal) H80.2- ☑
  involving
    otic capsule — *see* Otosclerosis, cochlear
    oval window
      nonobliterative H80.0- ☑
      obliterative H80.1- ☑
    round window — *see* Otosclerosis, cochlear
  nonobliterative — *see* Otosclerosis, involving, oval
    window, nonobliterative
  obliterative — *see* Otosclerosis, involving, oval window,
    obliterative
  specified NEC H80.8- ☑
Otospongiosis — *see* Otosclerosis
Otto's disease or pelvis M24.7
Outcome of delivery Z37.9
  multiple births Z37.9
    all liveborn Z37.50
      quadruplets Z37.52
      quintuplets Z37.53
      sextuplets Z37.54
      specified number NEC Z37.59
      triplets Z37.51
    all stillborn Z37.7
    some liveborn Z37.60
      quadruplets Z37.62
      quintuplets Z37.63
      sextuplets Z37.64
      specified number NEC Z37.69
      triplets Z37.61
  single NEC Z37.9

Outcome of delivery — *continued*
  single — *continued*
    liveborn Z37.0
    stillborn Z37.1
  twins NEC Z37.9
    both liveborn Z37.2
    both stillborn Z37.4
    one liveborn, one stillborn Z37.3
Outlet — *see* condition
Ovalocytosis (congenital) (hereditary) — *see* Elliptocytosis
Ovarian — *see* Condition
Ovariocele N83.4- ☑
Ovaritis (cystic) — *see* Oophoritis
Ovary, ovarian — *see also* condition
  resistant syndrome E28.39
  vein syndrome N13.8
Overactive — *see also* Hyperfunction
  adrenal cortex NEC E27.0
  bladder N32.81
  hypothalamus E23.3
  thyroid — *see* Hyperthyroidism
Overactivity R46.3
  child — *see* Disorder, attention-deficit hyperactivity
Overbite (deep) (excessive) (horizontal) (vertical) M26.29
Overbreathing — *see* Hyperventilation
Overconscientious personality F60.5
Overdevelopment — *see* Hypertrophy
Overdistension — *see* Distension
Overdose, overdosage (drug) — *see* Table of Drugs and
  Chemicals, by drug, poisoning
Overeating R63.2
  nonorganic origin F50.89
  psychogenic F50.89
Overexertion (effects) (exhaustion) T73.3 ☑
Overexposure (effects) T73.9 ☑
  exhaustion T73.2 ☑
Overfeeding — *see* Overeating
  newborn P92.4
Overfill, endodontic M27.52
Overgrowth, bone — *see* Hypertrophy, bone
Overhanging of dental restorative material (unre-
  pairable) K08.52
Overheated (places) (effects) — *see* Heat
Overjet (excessive horizontal) M26.23
Overlaid, overlying (suffocation) — *see* Asphyxia, trau-
  matic, due to mechanical threat
Overlap, excessive horizontal (teeth) M26.23
Overlapping toe (acquired) — *see also* Deformity, toe,
  specified NEC
  congenital (fifth toe) Q66.89
Overload
  circulatory, due to transfusion (blood) (blood compo-
    nents) (TACO) E87.71
  fluid E87.70
    due to transfusion (blood) (blood components)
      E87.71
    specified NEC E87.79
  iron, due to repeated red blood cell transfusions
    E83.111
  potassium (K) E87.5
  sodium (Na) E87.0
Overnutrition — *see* Hyperalimentation
Overproduction — *see also* Hypersecretion
  ACTH E27.0
  catecholamine E27.5
  growth hormone E22.0
Overprotection, child by parent Z62.1
Overriding
  aorta Q25.49
  finger (acquired) — *see* Deformity, finger
    congenital Q68.1
  toe (acquired) — *see also* Deformity, toe, specified NEC
    congenital Q66.89
Overstrained R53.83
  heart — *see* Hypertrophy, cardiac
Overuse, muscle NEC M70.8- ☑
Overweight E66.3
Overworked R53.83
Oviduct — *see* condition
Ovotestis Q56.0
Ovulation (cycle)
  failure or lack of N97.0
  pain N94.0
Ovum — *see* condition
Owren's disease or syndrome (parahemophilia) D68.2
Ox heart — *see* Hypertrophy, cardiac

Oxalosis E72.53
Oxaluria E72.53
Oxycephaly, oxycephalic Q75.0
  syphilitic, congenital A50.02
Oxyuriasis B80
Oxyuris vermicularis (infestation) B80
Ozena J31.0

P

Pachyderma, pachydermia L85.9
  larynx (verrucosa) J38.7
Pachydermatocele (congenital) Q82.8
Pachydermoperiostosis — *see also* Osteoarthropathy
  hypertrophic, specified type NEC
  clubbed nail M89.40 *[L62]*
Pachygyria Q04.3
Pachymeningitis (adhesive) (basal) (brain) (cervical)
  (chronic)(circumscribed) (external) (fibrous) (hemor
  rhagic) (hypertrophic) (internal) (purulent) (spina
  (suppurative) — *see* Meningitis
Pachyonychia (congenital) Q84.5
Pacinian tumor — *see* Neoplasm, skin, benign
Pad, knuckle or Garrod's M72.1
Paget's disease
  with infiltrating duct carcinoma — *see* Neoplasm,
    breast, malignant
  bone M88.9
    carpus M88.84- ☑
    clavicle M88.81- ☑
    femur M88.85- ☑
    fibula M88.86- ☑
    finger M88.84- ☑
    humerus M88.82- ☑
    ilium M88.85- ☑
    in neoplastic disease — *see* Osteitis, deformans, i
      neoplastic disease
    ischium M88.85- ☑
    metacarpus M88.84- ☑
    metatarsus M88.87- ☑
    multiple sites M88.89
    neck M88.88
    radius M88.83- ☑
    rib M88.88
    scapula M88.81- ☑
    skull M88.0
    specified NEC M88.88
    tarsus M88.87- ☑
    tibia M88.86- ☑
    toe M88.87- ☑
    ulna M88.83- ☑
    vertebra M88.1
  breast (female) C50.01- ☑
    male C50.02- ☑
  extramammary — *see also* Neoplasm, skin, malignan
    anus C21.0
      margin C44.590
      skin C44.590
  intraductal carcinoma — *see* Neoplasm, breast, malig
    nant
  malignant — *see* Neoplasm, skin, malignant
    breast (female) C50.01- ☑
      male C50.02- ☑
    unspecified site (female) C50.01- ☑
      male C50.02- ☑
  mammary — *see* Paget's disease, breast
  nipple — *see* Paget's disease, breast
  osteitis deformans — *see* Paget's disease, bone
Paget-Schroetter syndrome I82.890
Pain(s) — *see also* Painful R52
  abdominal R10.9
    colic R10.83
    generalized R10.84
      with acute abdomen R10.0
    lower R10.30
      left quadrant R10.32
      pelvic or perineal R10.2
      periumbilical R10.33
      right quadrant R10.31
    rebound — *see* Tenderness, abdominal, rebound
    severe with abdominal rigidity R10.0
    tenderness — *see* Tenderness, abdominal
    upper R10.10
      epigastric R10.13
      left quadrant R10.12
      right quadrant R10.11
  acute R52

248

☑ **Additional Character Required — Refer to the Tabular List for Character Selection**
    Ⓥ **Subterms under main terms may continue to next column or page**

Otitis — Pain

Pain(s) — *continued*
  acute — *continued*
    due to trauma G89.11
    neoplasm related G89.3
    postprocedural NEC G89.18
    post-thoracotomy G89.12
    specified by site — *code to* Pain, by site
  adnexa (uteri) R10.2
  anginoid — *see* Pain, precordial
  anus K62.89
  arm — *see* Pain, limb, upper
  axillary (axilla) M79.62- ☑
  back (postural) M54.9
  bladder R39.89
    associated with micturition — *see* Micturition,
        painful
    chronic R39.82
  bone — *see* Disorder, bone, specified type NEC
  breast N64.4
  broad ligament R10.2
  cancer associated (acute) (chronic) G89.3
  cecum — *see* Pain, abdominal
  cervicobrachial M53.1
  chest (central) R07.9
    anterior wall R07.89
    atypical R07.89
    ischemic I20.9
    musculoskeletal R07.89
    non-cardiac R07.89
    on breathing R07.1
    pleurodynia R07.81
    precordial R07.2
    wall (anterior) R07.89
  chronic G89.29
    associated with significant psychosocial dysfunction
        G89.4
    due to trauma G89.21
    neoplasm related G89.3
    postoperative NEC G89.28
    postprocedural NEC G89.28
    post-thoracotomy G89.22
    specified NEC G89.29
  coccyx M53.3
  colon — *see* Pain, abdominal
  coronary — *see* Angina
  costochondral R07.1
  diaphragm R07.1
  due to cancer G89.3
  due to device, implant or graft — *see also* Complica-
        tions, by site and type, specified NEC T85.848 ☑
    arterial graft NEC T82.848 ☑
    breast (implant) T85.848 ☑
    catheter NEC T85.848 ☑
      dialysis (renal) T82.848 ☑
        intraperitoneal T85.848 ☑
      infusion NEC T82.848 ☑
        spinal (epidural) (subdural) T85.840 ☑
      urinary (indwelling) T83.84 ☑
    electronic (electrode) (pulse generator) (stimulator)
      bone T85.840 ☑
      cardiac T82.847 ☑
      nervous system (brain) (peripheral nerve) (spinal)
          T85.84 ☑
      urinary T83.84 ☑
    fixation, internal (orthopedic) NEC T84.84 ☑
    gastrointestinal (bile duct) (esophagus) T85.848 ☑
    genital NEC T83.84 ☑
    heart NEC T82.847 ☑
    infusion NEC T85.848 ☑
    joint prosthesis T84.84 ☑
    ocular (corneal graft) (orbital implant) NEC
        T85.848 ☑
    orthopedic NEC T84.84 ☑
    specified NEC T85.848 ☑
    urinary NEC T83.84 ☑
    vascular NEC T82.848 ☑
    ventricular intracranial shunt T85.840 ☑
  due to malignancy (primary) (secondary) G89.3
  ear — *see subcategory* H92.0 ☑
  epigastric, epigastrium R10.13
  eye — *see* Pain, ocular
  face, facial R51.9
    atypical G50.1
  female genital organs NEC N94.89
  finger — *see* Pain, limb, upper
  flank — *see* Pain, abdominal
  foot — *see* Pain, limb, lower

Pain(s) — *continued*
  gallbladder K82.9
  gas (intestinal) R14.1
  gastric — *see* Pain, abdominal
  generalized NOS R52
  genital organ
    female N94.89
    male N50.89
  groin — *see* Pain, abdominal, lower
  hand — *see* Pain, limb, upper
  head — *see* Headache
  heart — *see* Pain, precordial
  infra-orbital — *see* Neuralgia, trigeminal
  intercostal R07.82
  intermenstrual N94.0
  jaw R68.84
  joint M25.50
    ankle M25.57- ☑
    elbow M25.52- ☑
    finger M25.54- ☑
    foot M25.57- ☑
    hand M25.54- ☑
    hip M25.55- ☑
    knee M25.56- ☑
    shoulder M25.51- ☑
    specified site NEC M25.59
    toe M25.57- ☑
    wrist M25.53- ☑
  kidney N23
  laryngeal R07.0
  leg — *see* Pain, limb, lower
  limb M79.609
    lower M79.60- ☑
      foot M79.67- ☑
      lower leg M79.66- ☑
      thigh M79.65- ☑
      toe M79.67- ☑
    upper M79.60- ☑
      axilla M79.62- ☑
      finger M79.64- ☑
      forearm M79.63- ☑
      hand M79.64- ☑
      upper arm M79.62- ☑
  loin M54.5
  low back M54.5
  lumbar region M54.5
  mandibular R68.84
  mastoid — *see subcategory* H92.0 ☑
  maxilla R68.84
  menstrual — *see also* Dysmenorrhea N94.6
  metacarpophalangeal (joint) — *see* Pain, joint, hand
  metatarsophalangeal (joint) — *see* Pain, joint, foot
  mouth K13.79
  muscle — *see* Myalgia
  musculoskeletal — *see also* Pain, by site M79.18
  myofascial M79.18
  nasal J34.89
  nasopharynx J39.2
  neck NEC M54.2
  nerve NEC — *see* Neuralgia
  neuromuscular — *see* Neuralgia
  nose J34.89
  ocular H57.1- ☑
  ophthalmic — *see* Pain, ocular
  orbital region — *see* Pain, ocular
  ovary N94.89
  over heart — *see* Pain, precordial
  ovulation N94.0
  pelvic (female) R10.2
  penis N48.89
  pericardial — *see* Pain, precordial
  perineal, perineum R10.2
  pharynx J39.2
  pleura, pleural, pleuritic R07.81
  postoperative NOS G89.18
  postprocedural NOS G89.18
  post-thoracotomy G89.12
  precordial (region) R07.2
  premenstrual N94.3
  psychogenic (persistent) (any site) F45.41
  radicular (spinal) — *see* Radiculopathy
  rectum K62.89
  respiration R07.1
  retrosternal R07.2
  rheumatoid, muscular — *see* Myalgia
  rib R07.81
  root (spinal) — *see* Radiculopathy

Pain(s) — *continued*
  round ligament (stretch) R10.2
  sacroiliac M53.3
  sciatic — *see* Sciatica
  scrotum N50.82
  seminal vesicle N50.89
  shoulder M25.51- ☑
  spermatic cord N50.89
  spinal root — *see* Radiculopathy
  spine M54.9
    cervical M54.2
    low back M54.5
      with sciatica M54.4- ☑
    thoracic M54.6
  stomach — *see* Pain, abdominal
  substernal R07.2
  temporomandibular (joint) M26.62- ☑
  testis N50.81- ☑
  thoracic spine M54.6
    with radicular and visceral pain M54.14
  throat R07.0
  tibia — *see* Pain, limb, lower
  toe — *see* Pain, limb, lower
  tongue K14.6
  tooth K08.89
  trigeminal — *see* Neuralgia, trigeminal
  tumor associated G89.3
  ureter N23
  urinary (organ) (system) N23
  uterus NEC N94.89
  vagina R10.2
  vertebrogenic (syndrome) M54.89
  vesical R39.89
    associated with micturition — *see* Micturition,
        painful
  vulva R10.2
Painful — *see also* Pain
  coitus
    female N94.10
    male N53.12
    psychogenic F52.6
  ejaculation (semen) N53.12
    psychogenic F52.6
  erection — *see* Priapism
  feet syndrome E53.8
  joint replacement (hip) (knee) T84.84 ☑
  menstruation — *see* Dysmenorrhea
    psychogenic F45.8
  micturition — *see* Micturition, painful
  respiration R07.1
  scar NEC L90.5
  wire sutures T81.89 ☑
Painter's colic — *see subcategory* T56.0 ☑
Palate — *see* condition
Palatoplegia K13.79
Palatoschisis — *see* Cleft, palate
Palilalia R48.8
Palliative care Z51.5
Pallor R23.1
  optic disc, temporal — *see* Atrophy, optic
Palmar — *see also* condition
  fascia — *see* condition
Palpable
  cecum K63.89
  kidney N28.89
  ovary N83.8
  prostate N42.9
  spleen — *see* Splenomegaly
Palpitations (heart) R00.2
  psychogenic F45.8
Palsy — *see also* Paralysis G83.9
  atrophic diffuse (progressive) G12.22
  Bell's — *see also* Palsy, facial
    newborn P11.3
  brachial plexus NEC G54.0
    newborn (birth injury) P14.3
  brain — *see* Palsy, cerebral
  bulbar (progressive) (chronic) G12.22
    of childhood (Fazio-Londe) G12.1
    pseudo NEC G12.29
    supranuclear (progressive) G23.1
  cerebral (congenital) G80.9
    ataxic G80.4
    athetoid G80.3
    choreathetoid G80.3
    diplegic G80.8
      spastic G80.1
    dyskinetic G80.3

Palsy — continued
  cerebral — continued
    dyskinetic — continued
      athetoid G80.3
      choreathetoid G80.3
      distonic G80.3
    dystonic G80.3
    hemiplegic G80.8
      spastic G80.2
    mixed G80.8
    monoplegic G80.8
      spastic G80.1
    paraplegic G80.8
      spastic G80.1
    quadriplegic G80.8
      spastic G80.0
    spastic G80.1
      diplegic G80.1
      hemiplegic G80.2
      monoplegic G80.1
      quadriplegic G80.0
      specified NEC G80.1
      tetrapelgic G80.0
    specified NEC G80.8
    syphilitic A52.12
      congenital A50.49
    tetraplegic G80.8
      spastic G80.0
  cranial nerve — see also Disorder, nerve, cranial
    multiple G52.7
      in
          infectious disease B99 ☑ [G53]
          neoplastic disease — see also Neoplasm
            D49.9 [G53]
          parasitic disease B89 [G53]
          sarcoidosis D86.82
  creeping G12.22
  diver's T70.3 ☑
  Erb's P14.0
  facial G51.0
    newborn (birth injury) P11.3
  glossopharyngeal G52.1
  Klumpke (-Déjérine) P14.1
  lead — see subcategory T56.0 ☑
  median nerve (tardy) G56.1- ☑
  nerve G58.9
    specified NEC G58.8
  peroneal nerve (acute) (tardy) G57.3- ☑
  progressive supranuclear G23.1
  pseudobulbar NEC G12.29
  radial nerve (acute) G56.3- ☑
  seventh nerve — see also Palsy, facial
    newborn P11.3
  shaking — see Parkinsonism
  spastic (cerebral) (spinal) G80.1
  ulnar nerve (tardy) G56.2- ☑
  wasting G12.29
Paludism — see Malaria
Panangiitis M30.0
Panaris, panaritium — see also Cellulitis, digit
  with lymphangitis — see Lymphangitis, acute, digit
Panarteritis nodosa M30.0
  brain or cerebral I67.7
Pancake heart R93.1
  with cor pulmonale (chronic) I27.81
Pancarditis (acute) (chronic) I51.89
  rheumatic I09.89
    active or acute I01.8
Pancoast's syndrome or tumor C34.1- ☑
Pancolitis, ulcerative (chronic) K51.00
  with
    abscess K51.014
    complication K51.019
    fistula K51.013
    obstruction K51.012
    rectal bleeding K51.011
    specified complication NEC K51.018
Pancreas, pancreatic — see condition
Pancreatitis (annular) (apoplectic) (calcareous) (edematous) (hemorrhagic) (malignant) (subacute) (suppurative) K85.90
  with necrosis (uninfected) K85.91
    infected K85.92
  acute (without necrosis or infection) K85.90
    with necrosis (uninfected) K85.91
      infected K85.92
    alcohol induced (without necrosis or infection)
      K85.20

Pancreatitis — continued
  acute — continued
    alcohol induced — continued
      with necrosis (uninfected) K85.21
        infected K85.22
      biliary (without necrosis or infection) K85.10
        with necrosis (uninfected) K85.11
          infected K85.12
      drug induced (without necrosis or infection) K85.30
        with necrosis (uninfected) K85.31
          infected K85.32
      gallstone (without necrosis or infection) K85.10
        with necrosis (uninfected) K85.11
          infected K85.12
      idiopathic (without necrosis or infection) K85.00
        with necrosis (uninfected) K85.01
          infected K85.02
      specified NEC (without necrosis or infection) K85.80
        with necrosis (uninfected) K85.81
          infected K85.82
  chronic (infectious) K86.1
    alcohol-induced K86.0
    recurrent K86.1
    relapsing K86.1
  cystic (chronic) K86.1
  cytomegaloviral B25.2
  fibrous (chronic) K86.1
  gallstone (without necrosis or infection) K85.10
    with necrosis (uninfected) K85.11
      infected K85.12
  gangrenous — see Pancreatitis, acute
  interstitial (chronic) K86.1
    acute — see also Pancreatitis, acute K85.80
  mumps B26.3
  recurrent
    acute K85.- ☑
    chronic K86.1
  relapsing, chronic K86.1
  syphilitic A52.74
Pancreatoblastoma — see Neoplasm, pancreas, malignant
Pancreolithiasis K86.89
Pancytolysis D75.89
Pancytopenia (acquired) D61.818
  with
    malformations D61.09
    myelodysplastic syndrome — see Syndrome,
      myelodysplastic
  antineoplastic chemotherapy induced D61.810
  congenital D61.09
  drug-induced NEC D61.811
PANDAS (pediatric autoimmune neuropsychiatric disorders associated with streptococcal infections syndrome) D89.89
Panencephalitis, subacute, sclerosing A81.1
Panhematopenia D61.9
  congenital D61.09
  constitutional D61.09
  splenic, primary D73.1
Panhemocytopenia D61.9
  congenital D61.09
  constitutional D61.09
Panhypogonadism E29.1
Panhypopituitarism E23.0
  prepubertal E23.0
Panic (attack) (state) F41.0
  reaction to exceptional stress (transient) F43.0
Panmyelopathy, familial, constitutional D61.09
Panmyelophthisis D61.82
  congenital D61.09
Panmyelosis (acute) (with myelofibrosis) C94.4- ☑
Panner's disease — see Osteochondrosis, juvenile,
  humerus
Panneuritis endemica E51.11
Panniculitis (nodular) (nonsuppurative) M79.3
  back M54.00
    cervical region M54.02
    cervicothoracic region M54.03
    lumbar region M54.06
    lumbosacral region M54.07
    multiple sites M54.09
    occipito-atlanto-axial region M54.01
    sacrococcygeal region M54.08
    thoracic region M54.04
    thoracolumbar region M54.05
  lupus L93.2
  mesenteric K65.4
  neck M54.02

Panniculitis — continued
  neck — continued
    cervicothoracic region M54.03
    occipito-atlanto-axial region M54.01
  relapsing M35.6
Panniculus adiposus (abdominal) E65
Pannus (allergic) (cornea) (degenerativus) (keratic)
  H16.42- ☑
  abdominal (symptomatic) E65
  trachomatosus, trachomatous (active) A71.1
Panophthalmitis H44.01- ☑
Pansinusitis (chronic) (hyperplastic) (nonpurulent) (purulent) J32.4
  acute J01.40
    recurrent J01.41
  tuberculous A15.8
Panuveitis (sympathetic) H44.11- ☑
Panvalvular disease I08.9
  specified NEC I08.8
PAPA (pyogenic arthritis, pyoderma gangrenosum, an
  acne syndrome) M04.8
Papanicolaou smear, cervix Z12.4
  as part of routine gynecological examination Z01.41☑
    with abnormal findings Z01.411
  for suspected neoplasm Z12.4
  nonspecific abnormal finding R87.619
  routine Z01.419
    with abnormal findings Z01.411
Papilledema (choked disc) H47.10
  associated with
    decreased ocular pressure H47.12
    increased intracranial pressure H47.11
    retinal disorder H47.13
  Foster-Kennedy syndrome H47.14- ☑
Papillitis H46.00
  anus K62.89
  chronic lingual K14.4
  necrotizing, kidney N17.2
  optic H46.0- ☑
  rectum K62.89
  renal, necrotizing N17.2
  tongue K14.0
Papilloma — see also Neoplasm, benign, by site
  acuminatum (female) (male) (anogenital) A63.0
  basal cell L82.1
    inflamed L82.0
  benign pinta (primary) A67.0
  bladder (urinary) (transitional cell) D41.4
  choroid plexus (lateral ventricle) (third ventricle) D33☑
    anaplastic C71.5
    fourth ventricle D33.1
    malignant C71.5
  renal pelvis (transitional cell) D41.1- ☑
    benign D30.1- ☑
  Schneiderian
    specified site — see Neoplasm, benign, by site
    unspecified site D14.0
  serous surface
    borderline malignancy
      specified site — see Neoplasm, uncertain behavior, by site
      unspecified site D39.10
    specified site — see Neoplasm, benign, by site
    unspecified site D27.9
  transitional (cell)
    bladder (urinary) D41.4
    inverted type — see Neoplasm, uncertain behavior,
      by site
    renal pelvis D41.1- ☑
    ureter D41.2- ☑
  ureter (transitional cell) D41.2- ☑
    benign D30.2- ☑
  urothelial — see Neoplasm, uncertain behavior, by site
  villous — see Neoplasm, uncertain behavior, by site
    adenocarcinoma in — see Neoplasm, malignant, ☑
      site
    in situ — see Neoplasm, in situ
  yaws, plantar or palmar A66.1
Papillomata, multiple, of yaws A66.1
Papillomatosis — see also Neoplasm, benign, by site
  confluent and reticulated L83
  cystic, breast — see Mastopathy, cystic
  ductal, breast — see Mastopathy, cystic
  intraductal (diffuse) — see Neoplasm, benign, by site
  subareolar duct D24- ☑
Papillomavirus, as cause of disease classified elsewhere B97.7

Papillon-Léage and Psaume syndrome Q87.0
Papule(s) R23.8
  carate (primary) A67.0
  fibrous, of nose D22.39
  Gottron's L94.4
  pinta (primary) A67.0
Papulosis
  lymphomatoid C86.6
  malignant I77.89
Papyraceous fetus O31.0- ☑
Para-albuminemia E88.09
Paracephalus Q89.7
Parachute mitral valve Q23.2
Paracoccidioidomycosis B41.9
  disseminated B41.7
  generalized B41.7
  mucocutaneous-lymphangitic B41.8
  pulmonary B41.0
  specified NEC B41.8
  visceral B41.8
Paradentosis K05.4
Paraffinoma T88.8 ☑
Paraganglioma D44.7
  adrenal D35.0- ☑
    malignant C74.1- ☑
  aortic body D44.7
    malignant C75.5
  carotid body D44.6
    malignant C75.4
  chromaffin — see also Neoplasm, benign, by site
    malignant — see Neoplasm, malignant, by site
  extra-adrenal D44.7
    malignant C75.5
      specified site — see Neoplasm, malignant, by
        site
      unspecified site C75.5
    specified site — see Neoplasm, uncertain behavior,
      by site
    unspecified site D44.7
  gangliocytic D13.2
    specified site — see Neoplasm, benign, by site
    unspecified site D13.2
  glomus jugulare D44.7
    malignant C75.5
  jugular D44.7
  malignant C75.5
    specified site — see Neoplasm, malignant, by site
    unspecified site C75.5
  nonchromaffin D44.7
    malignant C75.5
      specified site — see Neoplasm, malignant, by
        site
      unspecified site C75.5
    specified site — see Neoplasm, uncertain behavior,
      by site
    unspecified site D44.7
  parasympathetic D44.7
    specified site — see Neoplasm, uncertain behavior,
      by site
    unspecified site D44.7
  specified site — see Neoplasm, uncertain behavior, by
    site
  sympathetic D44.7
    specified site — see Neoplasm, uncertain behavior,
      by site
    unspecified site D44.7
  unspecified site D44.7
Parageusia R43.2
  psychogenic F45.8
Paragonimiasis B66.4
Paragranuloma, Hodgkin — see Lymphoma, Hodgkin,
  specified NEC
Parahemophilia — see also Defect, coagulation D68.2
Parakeratosis R23.4
  variegata L41.0
Paralysis, paralytic (complete) (incomplete) G83.9
  with
    syphilis A52.17
  abducens, abducent (nerve) — see Strabismus, paralyt-
    ic, sixth nerve
  abductor, lower extremity G57.9- ☑
  accessory nerve G52.8
  accommodation — see also Paresis, of accommodation
    hysterical F44.89
  acoustic nerve (except Deafness) H93.3 ☑
  agitans — see also Parkinsonism G20
    arteriosclerotic G21.4
  alternating (oculomotor) G83.89

Paralysis, paralytic — continued
  amyotrophic G12.21
  ankle G57.9- ☑
  anus (sphincter) K62.89
  arm — see Monoplegia, upper limb
  ascending (spinal), acute G61.0
  association G12.29
  asthenic bulbar G70.00
    with exacerbation (acute) G70.01
    in crisis G70.01
  ataxic (hereditary) G11.9
    general (syphilitic) A52.17
  atrophic G58.9
    infantile, acute — see Poliomyelitis, paralytic
    progressive G12.22
    spinal (acute) — see Poliomyelitis, paralytic
  axillary G54.0
  Babinski-Nageotte's G83.89
  Bell's G51.0
    newborn P11.3
  Benedikt's G46.3
  birth injury P14.9
    spinal cord P11.5
  bladder (neurogenic) (sphincter) N31.2
  bowel, colon or intestine K56.0
  brachial plexus G54.0
    birth injury P14.3
    newborn (birth injury) P14.3
  brain G83.9
    diplegia G83.0
    triplegia G83.89
  bronchial J98.09
  Brown-Séquard G83.81
  bulbar (chronic) (progressive) G12.22
    infantile — see Poliomyelitis, paralytic
    poliomyelitic — see Poliomyelitis, paralytic
    pseudo G12.29
  bulbospinal G70.00
    with exacerbation (acute) G70.01
    in crisis G70.01
  cardiac — see also Failure, heart I50.9
  cerebrocerebellar, diplegic G80.1
  cervical
    plexus G54.2
    sympathetic G90.09
  Céstan-Chenais G46.3
  Charcot-Marie-Tooth type G60.0
  Clark's G80.9
  colon K56.0
  compressed air T70.3 ☑
  compression
    arm G56.9- ☑
    leg G57.9- ☑
    lower extremity G57.9- ☑
    upper extremity G56.9- ☑
  congenital (cerebral) — see Palsy, cerebral
  conjugate movement (gaze) (of eye) H51.0
    cortical (nuclear) (supranuclear) H51.0
  cordis — see Failure, heart
  cranial or cerebral nerve G52.9
  creeping G12.22
  crossed leg G83.89
  crutch — see Injury, brachial plexus
  deglutition R13.0
    hysterical F44.4
  dementia A52.17
  descending (spinal) NEC G12.29
  diaphragm (flaccid) J98.6
    due to accidental dissection of phrenic nerve during
      procedure — see Puncture, accidental compli-
      cating surgery
  digestive organs NEC K59.89
  diplegic — see Diplegia
  divergence (nuclear) H51.8
  diver's T70.3 ☑
  Duchenne's
    birth injury P14.0
    due to or associated with
      motor neuron disease G12.22
      muscular dystrophy G71.01
  due to intracranial or spinal birth injury — see Palsy,
    cerebral
  embolic (current episode) I63.4- ☑
  Erb (-Duchenne) (birth) (newborn) P14.0
  Erb's syphilitic spastic spinal A52.17
  esophagus K22.8
  eye muscle (extrinsic) H49.9
    intrinsic — see also Paresis, of accommodation

Paralysis, paralytic — continued
  facial (nerve) G51.0
    birth injury P11.3
    congenital P11.3
    following operation NEC — see Puncture, accidental
      complicating surgery
    newborn (birth injury) P11.3
  familial (recurrent) (periodic) G72.3
    spastic G11.4
  fauces J39.2
  finger G56.9- ☑
  gait R26.1
  gastric nerve (nondiabetic) G52.2
  gaze, conjugate H51.0
  general (progressive) (syphilitic) A52.17
    juvenile A50.45
  glottis J38.00
    bilateral J38.02
    unilateral J38.01
  gluteal G54.1
  Gubler (-Millard) G46.3
  hand — see Monoplegia, upper limb
  heart — see Arrest, cardiac
  hemiplegic — see Hemiplegia
  hyperkalemic periodic (familial) G72.3
  hypoglossal (nerve) G52.3
  hypokalemic periodic G72.3
  hysterical F44.4
  ileus K56.0
  infantile — see also Poliomyelitis, paralytic A80.30
    bulbar — see Poliomyelitis, paralytic
    cerebral — see Palsy, cerebral
    spastic — see Palsy, cerebral, spastic
  infective — see Poliomyelitis, paralytic
  inferior nuclear G83.9
  internuclear — see Ophthalmoplegia, internuclear
  intestine K56.0
  iris H57.09
    due to diphtheria (toxin) A36.89
  ischemic, Volkmann's (complicating trauma) T79.6 ☑
  Jackson's G83.89
  jake — see Poisoning, food, noxious, plant
  Jamaica ginger (jake) G62.2
  juvenile general A50.45
  Klumpke (-Déjérine) (birth) (newborn) P14.1
  labioglossal (laryngeal) (pharyngeal) G12.29
  Landry's G61.0
  laryngeal nerve (recurrent) (superior) (unilateral) J38.00
    bilateral J38.02
    unilateral J38.01
  larynx J38.00
    bilateral J38.02
    due to diphtheria (toxin) A36.2
    unilateral J38.01
  lateral G12.23
  lead T56.0 ☑
  left side — see Hemiplegia
  leg G83.1- ☑
    both — see Paraplegia
    crossed G83.89
    hysterical F44.4
    psychogenic F44.4
    transient or transitory R29.818
      traumatic NEC — see Injury, nerve, leg
  levator palpebrae superioris — see Blepharoptosis,
    paralytic
  limb — see Monoplegia
  lip K13.0
  Lissauer's A52.17
  lower limb — see Monoplegia, lower limb
    both — see Paraplegia
  lung J98.4
  median nerve G56.1- ☑
  medullary (tegmental) G83.89
  mesencephalic NEC G83.89
    tegmental G83.89
  middle alternating G83.89
  Millard-Gubler-Foville G46.3
  monoplegic — see Monoplegia
  motor G83.9
  muscle, muscular NEC G72.89
    due to nerve lesion G58.9
    eye (extrinsic) H49.9
      intrinsic — see Paresis, of accommodation
      oblique — see Strabismus, paralytic, fourth nerve
    iris sphincter H21.9
    ischemic (Volkmann's) (complicating trauma)
      T79.6 ☑

Paralysis, paralytic — *continued*
  muscle, muscular — *continued*
    progressive G12.21
    progressive, spinal G12.25
    pseudohypertrophic G71.02
    spinal progressive G12.25
  musculocutaneous nerve G56.9- ☑
  musculospiral G56.9- ☑
  nerve — *see also* Disorder, nerve
    abducent — *see* Strabismus, paralytic, sixth nerve
    accessory G52.8
    auditory (except Deafness) H93.3 ☑
    birth injury P14.9
    cranial or cerebral G52.9
    facial G51.0
      birth injury P11.3
      congenital P11.3
      newborn (birth injury) P11.3
    fourth or trochlear — *see* Strabismus, paralytic, fourth nerve
    newborn (birth injury) P14.9
    oculomotor — *see* Strabismus, paralytic, third nerve
    phrenic (birth injury) P14.2
    radial G56.3- ☑
    seventh or facial G51.0
      newborn (birth injury) P11.3
    sixth or abducent — *see* Strabismus, paralytic, sixth nerve
    syphilitic A52.15
    third or oculomotor — *see* Strabismus, paralytic, third nerve
    trigeminal G50.9
    trochlear — *see* Strabismus, paralytic, fourth nerve
    ulnar G56.2- ☑
  normokalemic periodic G72.3
  ocular H49.9
    alternating G83.89
  oculofacial, congenital (Moebius) Q87.0
  oculomotor (external bilateral) (nerve) — *see* Strabismus, paralytic, third nerve
  palate (soft) K13.79
  paratrigeminal G50.9
  periodic (familial) (hyperkalemic) (hypokalemic) (myotonic) (normokalemic) (potassium sensitive) (secondary) G72.3
  peripheral autonomic nervous system — *see* Neuropathy, peripheral, autonomic
  peroneal (nerve) G57.3- ☑
  pharynx J39.2
  phrenic nerve G56.8- ☑
  plantar nerve(s) G57.6- ☑
  pneumogastric nerve G52.2
  poliomyelitis (current) — *see* Poliomyelitis, paralytic
  popliteal nerve G57.3- ☑
  postepileptic transitory G83.84
  progressive (atrophic) (bulbar) (spinal) G12.22
    general A52.17
    infantile acute — *see* Poliomyelitis, paralytic
    supranuclear G23.1
  pseudobulbar G12.29
  pseudohypertrophic (muscle) G71.09
  psychogenic F44.4
  quadriceps G57.9- ☑
  quadriplegic — *see* Tetraplegia
  radial nerve G56.3- ☑
  rectus muscle (eye) H49.9
  recurrent isolated sleep G47.53
  respiratory (muscle) (system) (tract) R06.81
    center NEC G93.89
    congenital P28.89
    newborn P28.89
  right side — *see* Hemiplegia
  saturnine T56.0 ☑
  sciatic nerve G57.0- ☑
  senile G83.9
  shaking — *see* Parkinsonism
  shoulder G56.9- ☑
  sleep, recurrent isolated G47.53
  spastic G83.9
    cerebral — *see* Palsy, cerebral, spastic
    congenital (cerebral) — *see* Palsy, cerebral, spastic
    familial G11.4
    hereditary G11.4
    quadriplegic G80.0
    syphilitic (spinal) A52.17
  sphincter, bladder — *see* Paralysis, bladder
  spinal (cord) G83.9
    accessory nerve G52.8

Paralysis, paralytic — *continued*
  spinal — *continued*
    acute — *see* Poliomyelitis, paralytic
    ascending acute G61.0
    atrophic (acute) — *see also* Poliomyelitis, paralytic
      spastic, syphilitic A52.17
    congenital NEC — *see* Palsy, cerebral
    hereditary G95.89
    infantile — *see* Poliomyelitis, paralytic
    progressive G12.21
      muscle G12.25
    sequelae NEC G83.89
  sternomastoid G52.8
  stomach K31.84
    diabetic — *see* Diabetes, by type, with gastroparesis
    nerve G52.2
      diabetic — *see* Diabetes, by type, with gastroparesis
  stroke — *see* Infarct, brain
  subcapsularis G56.8- ☑
  supranuclear (progressive) G23.1
  sympathetic G90.8
    cervical G90.09
    nervous system — *see* Neuropathy, peripheral, autonomic
  syndrome G83.9
    specified NEC G83.89
  syphilitic spastic spinal (Erb's) A52.17
  thigh G57.9- ☑
  throat J39.2
    diphtheritic A36.0
    muscle J39.2
  thrombotic (current episode) I63.3- ☑
  thumb G56.9- ☑
  tick — *see* Toxicity, venom, arthropod, specified NEC
  Todd's (postepileptic transitory paralysis) G83.84
  toe G57.6- ☑
  tongue K14.8
  transient R29.5
    arm or leg NEC R29.818
    traumatic NEC — *see* Injury, nerve
  trapezius G52.8
  traumatic, transient NEC — *see* Injury, nerve
  trembling — *see* Parkinsonism
  triceps brachii G56.9- ☑
  trigeminal nerve G50.9
  trochlear (nerve) — *see* Strabismus, paralytic, fourth nerve
  ulnar nerve G56.2- ☑
  upper limb — *see* Monoplegia, upper limb
  uremic N18.9 *[G99.8]*
  uveoparotitic D86.89
  uvula K13.79
    postdiphtheritic A36.0
  vagus nerve G52.2
  vasomotor NEC G90.8
  velum palati K13.79
  vesical — *see* Paralysis, bladder
  vestibular nerve (except Vertigo) H93.3 ☑
  vocal cords J38.00
    bilateral J38.02
    unilateral J38.01
  Volkmann's (complicating trauma) T79.6 ☑
  wasting G12.29
  Weber's G46.3
  wrist G56.9- ☑
Paramedial urethrovesical orifice Q64.79
Paramenia N92.6
Parametritis — *see also* Disease, pelvis, inflammatory N73.2
  acute N73.0
  complicating abortion — *see* Abortion, by type, complicated by, parametritis
Parametrium, parametric — *see* condition
Paramnesia — *see* Amnesia
Paramolar K00.1
Paramyloidosis E85.89
Paramyoclonus multiplex G25.3
Paramyotonia (congenita) G71.19
Parangi — *see* Yaws
Paranoia (querulans) F22
  senile F03 ☑
Paranoid
  dementia (senile) F03 ☑
    praecox — *see* Schizophrenia
  personality F60.0
  psychosis (climacteric) (involutional) (menopausal) F22

Paranoid — *continued*
  psychosis — *continued*
    psychogenic (acute) F23
    senile F03 ☑
  reaction (acute) F23
    chronic F22
  schizophrenia F20.0
  state (climacteric) (involutional) (menopausal) (simple) F22
    senile F03 ☑
  tendencies F60.0
  traits F60.0
  trends F60.0
  type, psychopathic personality F60.0
Paraparesis — *see* Paraplegia
Paraphasia R47.02
Paraphilia F65.9
Paraphimosis (congenital) N47.2
  chancroidal A57
Paraphrenia, paraphrenic (late) F22
  schizophrenia F20.0
Paraplegia (lower) G82.20
  ataxic — *see* Degeneration, combined, spinal cord
  complete G82.21
  congenital (cerebral) G80.8
    spastic G80.1
  familial spastic G11.4
  functional (hysterical) F44.4
  hereditary, spastic G11.4
  hysterical F44.4
  incomplete G82.22
  Pott's A18.01
  psychogenic F44.4
  spastic
    Erb's spinal, syphilitic A52.17
    hereditary G11.4
    tropical G04.1
  syphilitic (spastic) A52.17
  traumatic
    current injury — code to injury with seventh character A
      sequela of previous injury — code to injury with seventh character S
  tropical spastic G04.1
Parapoxvirus B08.60
  specified NEC B08.69
Paraproteinemia D89.2
  benign (familial) D89.2
  monoclonal D47.2
  secondary to malignant disease D47.2
Parapsoriasis L41.9
  en plaques L41.4
  guttata L41.1
  large plaque L41.4
  retiform, retiformis L41.5
  small plaque L41.3
  specified NEC L41.8
  varioliformis (acuta) L41.0
Parasitic — *see also* condition
  disease NEC B89
  stomatitis B37.0
  sycosis (beard) (scalp) B35.0
  twin Q89.4
Parasitism B89
  intestinal B82.9
  skin B88.9
  specified — *see* Infestation
Parasitophobia F40.218
Parasomnia G47.50
  due to
    alcohol
      abuse F10.182
      dependence F10.282
      use F10.982
    amphetamines
      abuse F15.182
      dependence F15.282
      use F15.982
    caffeine
      abuse F15.182
      dependence F15.282
      use F15.982
    cocaine
      abuse F14.182
      dependence F14.282
      use F14.982
    drug NEC
      abuse F19.182

☑ **Additional Character Required** — Refer to the Tabular List for Character Selection   ▽ Subterms under main terms may continue to next column or page

Parasomnia — *continued*
  due to — *continued*
    drug — *continued*
      dependence F19.282
      use F19.982
    opioid
      abuse F11.182
      dependence F11.282
      use F11.982
    psychoactive substance NEC
      abuse F19.182
      dependence F19.282
      use F19.982
    sedative, hypnotic, or anxiolytic
      abuse F13.182
      dependence F13.282
      use F13.982
    stimulant NEC
      abuse F15.182
      dependence F15.282
      use F15.982
  in conditions classified elsewhere G47.54
  nonorganic origin F51.8
  organic G47.50
  specified NEC G47.59
Paraspadias Q54.9
Paraspasmus facialis G51.8
Parasuicide (attempt)
  history of (personal) Z91.5
    in family Z81.8
Parathyroid gland — *see* condition
Parathyroid tetany E20.9
Paratrachoma A74.0
Paratyphilitis — *see* Appendicitis
Paratyphoid (fever) — *see* Fever, paratyphoid
Paratyphus — *see* Fever, paratyphoid
Paraurethral duct Q64.79
Paraurethritis — *see also* Urethritis
  gonococcal (acute) (chronic) (with abscess) A54.1
Paravaccinia NEC B08.04
Paravaginitis — *see* Vaginitis
Parencephalitis — *see also* Encephalitis
  sequelae G09
Parent-child conflict — *see* Conflict, parent-child
  estrangement NEC Z62.890
Paresis — *see also* Paralysis
  accommodation — *see* Paresis, of accommodation
  Bernhardt's G57.1- ☑
  bladder (sphincter) — *see also* Paralysis, bladder
    tabetic A52.17
  bowel, colon or intestine K56.0
  extrinsic muscle, eye H49.9
  general (progressive) (syphilitic) A52.17
    juvenile A50.45
  heart — *see* Failure, heart
  insane (syphilitic) A52.17
  juvenile (general) A50.45
  of accommodation H52.52- ☑
  peripheral progressive (idiopathic) G60.3
  pseudohypertrophic G71.09
  senile G83.9
  syphilitic (general) A52.17
    congenital A50.45
  vesical NEC N31.2
Paresthesia — *see also* Disturbance, sensation, skin R20.2
  Bernhardt G57.1- ☑
Paretic — *see* condition
Parinaud's
  conjunctivitis H10.89
  oculoglandular syndrome H10.89
  ophthalmoplegia H49.88- ☑
Parkinsonism (idiopathic) (primary) G20
  with neurogenic orthostatic hypotension (symptomatic) G90.3
  arteriosclerotic G21.4
  dementia G31.83 *[F02.80]*
    with behavioral disturbance G31.83 *[F02.81]*
  due to
    drugs NEC G21.19
      neuroleptic G21.11
  medication-induced NEC G21.19
  neuroleptic induced G21.11
  postencephalitic G21.3
  secondary G21.9
    due to
      arteriosclerosis G21.4
      drugs NEC G21.19
        neuroleptic G21.11

Parkinsonism — *continued*
  secondary — *continued*
    due to — *continued*
      encephalitis G21.3
      external agents NEC G21.2
      syphilis A52.19
    specified NEC G21.8
  syphilitic A52.19
  treatment-induced NEC G21.19
  vascular G21.4
Parkinson's disease, syndrome or tremor — *see* Parkinsonism
Parodontitis — *see* Periodontitis
Parodontosis K05.4
Paronychia — *see also* Cellulitis, digit
  with lymphangitis — *see* Lymphangitis, acute, digit
  candidal (chronic) B37.2
  tuberculous (primary) A18.4
Parorexia (psychogenic) F50.89
Parosmia R43.1
  psychogenic F45.8
Parotid gland — *see* condition
Parotitis, parotiditis (allergic)(nonspecific toxic) (purulent) (septic) (suppurative) — *see also* Sialoadenitis
  epidemic — *see* Mumps
  infectious — *see* Mumps
  postoperative K91.89
  surgical K91.89
Parrot fever A70
Parrot's disease (early congenital syphilitic pseudoparalysis) A50.02
Parry-Romberg syndrome G51.8
Parry's disease or syndrome E05.00
  with thyroid storm E05.01
Pars planitis — *see* Cyclitis
Parsonage (-Aldren)-**Turner syndrome** G54.5
Parson's disease (exophthalmic goiter) E05.00
  with thyroid storm E05.01
Particolored infant Q82.8
Parturition — *see* Delivery
Parulis K04.7
  with sinus K04.6
Parvovirus, as cause of disease classified elsewhere B97.6
Pasini and Pierini's atrophoderma L90.3
Passage
  false, urethra N36.5
  meconium (newborn) during delivery P03.82
  of sounds or bougies — *see* Attention to, artificial, opening
Passive — *see* condition
  smoking Z77.22
Pasteurella septica A28.0
Pasteurellosis — *see* Infection, Pasteurella
PAT (paroxysmal atrial tachycardia) I47.1
Patau's syndrome — *see* Trisomy, 13
Patches
  mucous (syphilitic) A51.39
    congenital A50.07
  smokers' (mouth) K13.24
Patellar — *see* condition
Patent — *see also* Imperfect, closure
  canal of Nuck Q52.4
  cervix N88.3
  ductus arteriosus or Botallo's Q25.0
  foramen
    botalli Q21.1
    ovale Q21.1
  interauricular septum Q21.1
  interventricular septum Q21.0
  omphalomesenteric duct Q43.0
  os (uteri) — *see* Patent, cervix
  ostium secundum Q21.1
  urachus Q64.4
  vitelline duct Q43.0
Paterson (-Brown)(-Kelly) **syndrome or web** D50.1
Pathologic, pathological — *see also* condition
  asphyxia R09.01
  fire-setting F63.1
  gambling F63.0
  ovum O02.0
  resorption, tooth K03.3
  stealing F63.2
Pathology (of) — *see* Disease
  periradicular, associated with previous endodontic treatment NEC M27.59
Pattern, sleep-wake, irregular G47.23

Patulous — *see also* Imperfect, closure (congenital)
  alimentary tract Q45.8
    lower Q43.8
    upper Q40.8
  eustachian tube H69.0- ☑
Pause, sinoatrial I49.5
Paxton's disease B36.2
Pearl(s)
  enamel K00.2
  Epstein's K09.8
Pearl-worker's disease — *see* Osteomyelitis, specified type NEC
Pectenosis K62.4
Pectoral — *see* condition
Pectus
  carinatum (congenital) Q67.7
    acquired M95.4
    rachitic sequelae (late effect) E64.3
  excavatum (congenital) Q67.6
    acquired M95.4
    rachitic sequelae (late effect) E64.3
  recurvatum (congenital) Q67.6
Pedatrophia E41
Pederosis F65.4
Pediculosis (infestation) B85.2
  capitis (head-louse) (any site) B85.0
  corporis (body-louse) (any site) B85.1
  eyelid B85.0
  mixed (classifiable to more than one of the titles B85.0-B85.3) B85.4
  pubis (pubic louse) (any site) B85.3
  vestimenti B85.1
  vulvae B85.3
Pediculus (infestation) — *see* Pediculosis
Pedophilia F65.4
Peg-shaped teeth K00.2
Pelade — *see* Alopecia, areata
Pelger-Huët anomaly or syndrome D72.0
Peliosis (rheumatica) D69.0
  hepatis K76.4
    with toxic liver disease K71.8
Pelizaeus-Merzbacher disease E75.29
Pellagra (alcoholic) (with polyneuropathy) E52
Pellagra-cerebellar-ataxia-renal aminoaciduria syndrome E72.02
Pellegrini (-Stieda) **disease or syndrome** — *see* Bursitis, tibial collateral
Pellizzi's syndrome E34.8
Pel's crisis A52.11
Pelvic — *see also* condition
  examination (periodic) (routine) Z01.419
    with abnormal findings Z01.411
  kidney, congenital Q63.2
Pelviolithiasis — *see* Calculus, kidney
Pelviperitonitis — *see also* Peritonitis, pelvic
  gonococcal A54.24
  puerperal O85
Pelvis — *see* condition or type
Pemphigoid L12.9
  benign, mucous membrane L12.1
  bullous L12.0
  cicatricial L12.1
  juvenile L12.2
  ocular L12.1
  specified NEC L12.8
Pemphigus L10.9
  benign familial (chronic) Q82.8
  Brazilian L10.3
  circinatus L13.0
  conjunctiva L12.1
  drug-induced L10.5
  erythematosus L10.4
  foliaceus L10.2
  gangrenous — *see* Gangrene
  neonatorum L01.03
  ocular L12.1
  paraneoplastic L10.81
  specified NEC L10.89
  syphilitic (congenital) A50.06
  vegetans L10.1
  vulgaris L10.0
  wildfire L10.3
Pendred's syndrome E07.1
Pendulous
  abdomen, in pregnancy — *see* Pregnancy, complicated by, abnormal, pelvic organs or tissues NEC
  breast N64.89
Penetrating wound — *see also* Puncture

▽ **Subterms under main terms may continue to next column or page**   ☑ **Additional Character Required — Refer to the Tabular List for Character Selection**

Penetrating wound — *continued*
  with internal injury — *see* Injury, by site
  eyeball — *see* Puncture, eyeball
  orbit (with or without foreign body) — *see* Puncture, orbit
  uterus by instrument with or following ectopic or molar pregnancy O08.6
Penicillosis B48.4
Penis — *see* condition
Penitis N48.29
Pentalogy of Fallot Q21.8
Pentasomy X syndrome Q97.1
Pentosuria (essential) E74.89
Percreta placenta - O43.23
Peregrinating patient — *see* Disorder, factitious
Perforation, perforated (nontraumatic) (of)
  accidental during procedure (blood vessel) (nerve) (organ) — *see* Complication, accidental puncture or laceration
  antrum — *see* Sinusitis, maxillary
  appendix K35.32
    with localized peritonitis K35.32
  atrial septum, multiple Q21.1
  attic, ear — *see* Perforation, tympanum, attic
  bile duct (common) (hepatic) K83.2
    cystic K82.2
  bladder (urinary)
    with or following ectopic or molar pregnancy O08.6
    obstetrical trauma O71.5
    traumatic S37.29 ☑
      at delivery O71.5
  bowel K63.1
    with or following ectopic or molar pregnancy O08.6
    newborn P78.0
    obstetrical trauma O71.5
    traumatic — *see* Laceration, intestine
  broad ligament N83.8
    with or following ectopic or molar pregnancy O08.6
    obstetrical trauma O71.6
  by
    device, implant or graft — *see also* Complications, by site and type, mechanical T85.628 ☑
      arterial graft NEC — *see* Complication, cardiovascular device, mechanical, vascular
      breast (implant) T85.49 ☑
      catheter NEC T85.698 ☑
        cystostomy T83.090 ☑
        dialysis (renal) T82.49 ☑
          intraperitoneal T85.691 ☑
        infusion NEC T82.594 ☑
          spinal (epidural) (subdural) T85.690 ☑
        urinary — *see also* Complications, catheter, urinary T83.098 ☑
      electronic (electrode) (pulse generator) (stimulator)
        bone T84.390 ☑
        cardiac T82.199 ☑
          electrode T82.190 ☑
          pulse generator T82.191 ☑
          specified type NEC T82.198 ☑
        nervous system — *see* Complication, prosthetic device, mechanical, electronic nervous system stimulator
        urinary — *see* Complication, genitourinary, device, urinary, mechanical
      fixation, internal (orthopedic) NEC — *see* Complication, fixation device, mechanical
      gastrointestinal — *see* Complications, prosthetic device, mechanical, gastrointestinal device
      genital NEC T83.498 ☑
        intrauterine contraceptive device T83.39 ☑
        penile prosthesis T83.490 ☑
      heart NEC — *see* Complication, cardiovascular device, mechanical
      joint prosthesis — *see* Complications, joint prosthesis, mechanical, specified NEC, by site
      ocular NEC — *see* Complications, prosthetic device, mechanical, ocular device
      orthopedic NEC — *see* Complication, orthopedic, device, mechanical
      specified NEC T85.628 ☑
      urinary NEC — *see also* Complication, genitourinary, device, urinary, mechanical
        graft T83.29 ☑
      vascular NEC — *see* Complication, cardiovascular device, mechanical

Perforation, perforated — *continued*
  by — *continued*
    device, implant or graft — *see also* Complications, by site and type, mechanical — *continued*
      ventricular intracranial shunt T85.09 ☑
    foreign body left accidentally in operative wound T81.539 ☑
    instrument (any) during a procedure, accidental — *see* Puncture, accidental complicating surgery
  cecum K35.32
    with localized peritonitis K35.32
  cervix (uteri) N88.8
    with or following ectopic or molar pregnancy O08.6
    obstetrical trauma O71.3
  colon K63.1
    newborn P78.0
    obstetrical trauma O71.5
    traumatic — *see* Laceration, intestine, large
  common duct (bile) K83.2
  cornea (due to ulceration) — *see* Ulcer, cornea, perforated
  cystic duct K82.2
  diverticulum (intestine) K57.80
    with bleeding K57.81
    large intestine K57.20
      with
        bleeding K57.21
        small intestine K57.40
          with bleeding K57.41
      small intestine K57.00
        with
          bleeding K57.01
          large intestine K57.40
            with bleeding K57.41
  ear drum — *see* Perforation, tympanum
  esophagus K22.3
  ethmoidal sinus — *see* Sinusitis, ethmoidal
  frontal sinus — *see* Sinusitis, frontal
  gallbladder K82.2
  heart valve — *see* Endocarditis
  ileum K63.1
    newborn P78.0
    obstetrical trauma O71.5
    traumatic — *see* Laceration, intestine, small
  instrumental, surgical (accidental) (blood vessel) (nerve) (organ) — *see* Puncture, accidental complicating surgery
  intestine NEC K63.1
    with ectopic or molar pregnancy O08.6
    newborn P78.0
    obstetrical trauma O71.5
    traumatic — *see* Laceration, intestine
    ulcerative NEC K63.1
      newborn P78.0
  jejunum, jejunal K63.1
    obstetrical trauma O71.5
    traumatic — *see* Laceration, intestine, small
    ulcer — *see* Ulcer, gastrojejunal, with perforation
  joint prosthesis — *see* Complications, joint prosthesis, mechanical, specified NEC, by site
  mastoid (antrum) (cell) — *see* Disorder, mastoid, specified NEC
  maxillary sinus — *see* Sinusitis, maxillary
  membrana tympani — *see* Perforation, tympanum
  nasal
    septum J34.89
      congenital Q30.3
      syphilitic A52.73
    sinus J34.89
      congenital Q30.8
      due to sinusitis — *see* Sinusitis
  palate — *see also* Cleft, palate Q35.9
    syphilitic A52.79
  palatine vault — *see also* Cleft, palate, hard Q35.1
    syphilitic A52.79
    congenital A50.59
  pars flaccida (ear drum) — *see* Perforation, tympanum, attic
  pelvic
    floor S31.030 ☑
      with
        ectopic or molar pregnancy O08.6
        penetration into retroperitoneal space S31.031 ☑
        retained foreign body S31.040 ☑
          with penetration into retroperitoneal space S31.041 ☑
      following ectopic or molar pregnancy O08.6

Perforation, perforated — *continued*
  pelvic — *continued*
    floor — *continued*
      obstetrical trauma O70.1
    organ S37.99 ☑
      adrenal gland S37.818 ☑
      bladder — *see* Perforation, bladder
      fallopian tube S37.599 ☑
        bilateral S37.592 ☑
        unilateral S37.591 ☑
      kidney S37.09- ☑
      obstetrical trauma O71.5
      ovary S37.499 ☑
        bilateral S37.492 ☑
        unilateral S37.491 ☑
      prostate S37.828 ☑
      specified organ NEC S37.898 ☑
      ureter — *see* Perforation, ureter
      urethra — *see* Perforation, urethra
      uterus — *see* Perforation, uterus
  perineum — *see* Laceration, perineum
  pharynx J39.2
  rectum K63.1
    newborn P78.0
    obstetrical trauma O71.5
    traumatic S36.63 ☑
  root canal space due to endodontic treatment M27.5
  sigmoid K63.1
    newborn P78.0
    obstetrical trauma O71.5
    traumatic S36.533 ☑
  sinus (accessory) (chronic) (nasal) J34.89
  sphenoidal sinus — *see* Sinusitis, sphenoidal
  surgical (accidental) (by instrument) (blood vessel) (nerve) (organ) — *see* Puncture, accidental complicating surgery
  traumatic
    external — *see* Puncture
    eye — *see* Puncture, eyeball
    internal organ — *see* Injury, by site
  tympanum, tympanic (membrane) (persistent post-traumatic) (postinflammatory) H72.9- ☑
    attic H72.1- ☑
      multiple — *see* Perforation, tympanum, multipl
      total — *see* Perforation, tympanum, total
    central H72.0- ☑
      multiple — *see* Perforation, tympanum, multipl
      total — *see* Perforation, tympanum, total
    marginal NEC — *see* subcategory H72.2 ☑
    multiple H72.81- ☑
    pars flaccida — *see* Perforation, tympanum, attic
    total H72.82- ☑
    traumatic, current episode S09.2- ☑
  typhoid, gastrointestinal — *see* Typhoid
  ulcer — *see* Ulcer, by site, with perforation
  ureter N28.89
    traumatic S37.19 ☑
  urethra N36.8
    with ectopic or molar pregnancy O08.6
    following ectopic or molar pregnancy O08.6
    obstetrical trauma O71.5
    traumatic S37.39 ☑
      at delivery O71.5
  uterus
    with ectopic or molar pregnancy O08.6
    by intrauterine contraceptive device T83.39 ☑
    following ectopic or molar pregnancy O08.6
    obstetrical trauma O71.1
    traumatic S37.69 ☑
      obstetric O71.1
  uvula K13.79
    syphilitic A52.79
  vagina O71.4
    obstetrical trauma O71.4
    other trauma — *see* Puncture, vagina
Periadenitis mucosa necrotica recurrens K12.0
Periappendicitis (acute) — *see* Appendicitis
Periarteritis nodosa (disseminated) (infectious) (necro tizing) M30.0
Periarthritis (joint) — *see also* Enthesopathy
  Duplay's M75.0- ☑
  gonococcal A54.42
  humeroscapularis — *see* Capsulitis, adhesive
  scapulohumeral — *see* Capsulitis, adhesive
  shoulder — *see* Capsulitis, adhesive
  wrist M77.2- ☑
Periarthrosis (angioneural) — *see* Enthesopathy

ericapsulitis, adhesive (shoulder) — *see* Capsulitis, adhesive
ericarditis (with decompensation) (with effusion) I31.9
with rheumatic fever (conditions in I00)
active — *see* Pericarditis, rheumatic
inactive or quiescent I09.2
acute (hemorrhagic) (nonrheumatic) (Sicca) I30.9
with chorea (acute) (rheumatic) (Sydenham's) I02.0
benign I30.8
nonspecific I30.0
rheumatic I01.0
with chorea (acute) (Sydenham's) I02.0
adhesive or adherent (chronic) (external) (internal) I31.0
acute — *see* Pericarditis, acute
rheumatic I09.2
bacterial (acute) (subacute) (with serous or seropurulent effusion) I30.1
calcareous I31.1
cholesterol (chronic) I31.8
acute I30.9
chronic (nonrheumatic) I31.9
rheumatic I09.2
constrictive (chronic) I31.1
coxsackie B33.23
fibrinocaseous (tuberculous) A18.84
fibrinopurulent I30.1
fibrinous I30.8
fibrous I31.0
gonococcal A54.83
idiopathic I30.0
in systemic lupus erythematosus M32.12
infective I30.1
meningococcal A39.53
neoplastic (chronic) I31.8
acute I30.9
obliterans, obliterating I31.0
plastic I31.0
pneumococcal I30.1
postinfarction I24.1
purulent I30.1
rheumatic (active) (acute) (with effusion) (with pneumonia) I01.0
with chorea (acute) (rheumatic) (Sydenham's) I02.0
chronic or inactive (with chorea) I09.2
rheumatoid — *see* Rheumatoid, carditis
septic I30.1
serofibrinous I30.8
staphylococcal I30.1
streptococcal I30.1
suppurative I30.1
syphilitic A52.06
tuberculous A18.84
uremic N18.9 *[I32]*
viral I30.1
ericardium, pericardial — *see* condition
ericellulitis — *see* Cellulitis
ericementitis (chronic) (suppurative) — *see also* Periodontitis
acute K05.20
generalized — *see* Periodontitis, aggressive, generalized
localized — *see* Periodontitis, aggressive, localized
erichondritis
auricle — *see* Perichondritis, ear
bronchus J98.09
ear (external) H61.00- ☑
acute H61.01- ☑
chronic H61.02- ☑
external auditory canal — *see* Perichondritis, ear
larynx J38.7
syphilitic A52.73
typhoid A01.09
nose J34.89
pinna — *see* Perichondritis, ear
trachea J39.8
ericlasia K05.4
ericoronitis — *see* Periodontitis
ericystitis N30.90
with hematuria N30.91
eridiverticulitis (intestine) K57.92
cecum — *see* Diverticulitis, intestine, large
colon — *see* Diverticulitis, intestine, large
duodenum — *see* Diverticulitis, intestine, small
intestine — *see* Diverticulitis, intestine
jejunum — *see* Diverticulitis, intestine, small
rectosigmoid — *see* Diverticulitis, intestine, large
rectum — *see* Diverticulitis, intestine, large
sigmoid — *see* Diverticulitis, intestine, large

Periendocarditis — *see* Endocarditis
Periepididymitis N45.1
Perifolliculitis L01.02
abscedens, caput, scalp L66.3
capitis, abscedens (et suffodiens) L66.3
superficial pustular L01.02
Perihepatitis K65.8
Perilabyrinthitis (acute) — *see* subcategory H83.0 ☑
Perimeningitis — *see* Meningitis
Perimetritis — *see* Endometritis
Perimetrosalpingitis — *see* Salpingo-oophoritis
Perineocele N81.81
Perinephric, perinephritic — *see* condition
Perinephritis — *see also* Infection, kidney
purulent — *see* Abscess, kidney
Perineum, perineal — *see* condition
Perineuritis NEC — *see* Neuralgia
Periodic — *see* condition
Periodontitis (chronic) (complex) (compound) (local)
(simplex) K05.30
acute K05.20
generalized K05.229
moderate K05.222
severe K05.223
slight K05.221
localized K05.219
moderate K05.212
severe K05.213
slight K05.211
apical K04.5
acute (pulpal origin) K04.4
generalized K05.329
moderate K05.322
severe K05.323
slight K05.321
localized K05.319
moderate K05.312
severe K05.313
slight K05.311
Periodontoclasia K05.4
Periodontosis (juvenile) K05.4
Periods — *see also* Menstruation
heavy N92.0
irregular N92.6
shortened intervals (irregular) N92.1
Perionychia — *see also* Cellulitis, digit
with lymphangitis — *see* Lymphangitis, acute, digit
Perioophoritis — *see* Salpingo-oophoritis
Periorchitis N45.2
Periosteum, periosteal — *see* condition
Periostitis (albuminosa) (circumscribed) (diffuse) (infective) (monomelic) — *see also* Osteomyelitis
alveolar M27.3
alveolodental M27.3
dental M27.3
gonorrheal A54.43
jaw (lower) (upper) M27.2
orbit H05.03- ☑
syphilitic A52.77
congenital (early) A50.02 *[M90.80]*
secondary A51.46
tuberculous — *see* Tuberculosis, bone
yaws (hypertrophic) (early) (late) A66.6 *[M90.80]*
Periostosis (hyperplastic) — *see also* Disorder, bone,
specified type NEC
with osteomyelitis — *see* Osteomyelitis, specified type
NEC
Peripartum
cardiomyopathy O90.3
Periphlebitis — *see* Phlebitis
Periproctitis K62.89
Periprostatitis — *see* Prostatitis
Perirectal — *see* condition
Perirenal — *see* condition
Perisalpingitis — *see* Salpingo-oophoritis
Perisplenitis (infectional) D73.89
Peristalsis, visible or reversed R19.2
Peritendinitis — *see* Enthesopathy
Peritoneum, peritoneal — *see* condition
Peritonitis (adhesive) (bacterial) (fibrinous) (hemorrhagic)
(idiopathic) (localized) (perforative) (primary) (with
adhesions) (with effusion) K65.9
with or following
abscess K65.1
appendicitis
with perforation or rupture K35.32
generalized — *see also* Appendicitis K35.20

Peritonitis — *continued*
with or following — *continued*
appendicitis — *continued*
localized — *see also* Appendicitis K35.30
diverticular disease (intestine) K57.80
with bleeding K57.81
ectopic or molar pregnancy O08.0
large intestine K57.20
with
bleeding K57.21
small intestine K57.40
with bleeding K57.41
small intestine K57.00
with
bleeding K57.01
large intestine K57.40
with bleeding K57.41
acute (generalized) K65.0
aseptic T81.61 ☑
bile, biliary K65.3
chemical T81.61 ☑
chlamydial A74.81
chronic proliferative K65.8
complicating abortion — *see* Abortion, by type, complicated by, pelvic peritonitis
congenital P78.1
diaphragmatic K65.0
diffuse K65.0
diphtheritic A36.89
disseminated K65.0
due to
bile K65.3
foreign
body or object accidentally left during a procedure (instrument) (sponge) (swab)
T81.599 ☑
substance accidentally left during a procedure
(chemical) (powder) (talc) T81.61 ☑
talc T81.61 ☑
urine K65.8
eosinophilic K65.8
acute K65.0
fibrocaseous (tuberculous) A18.31
fibropurulent K65.0
following ectopic or molar pregnancy O08.0
general (ized) K65.0
gonococcal A54.85
meconium (newborn) P78.0
neonatal P78.1
meconium P78.0
pancreatic K65.0
paroxysmal, familial E85.0
benign E85.0
pelvic
female N73.5
acute N73.3
chronic N73.4
with adhesions N73.6
male K65.0
periodic, familial E85.0
proliferative, chronic K65.8
puerperal, postpartum, childbirth O85
purulent K65.0
septic K65.0
specified NEC K65.8
spontaneous bacterial K65.2
subdiaphragmatic K65.0
subphrenic K65.0
suppurative K65.0
syphilitic A52.74
congenital (early) A50.08 *[K67]*
talc T81.61 ☑
tuberculous A18.31
urine K65.8
Peritonsillar — *see* condition
Peritonsillitis J36
Perityphlitis K37
Periureteritis N28.89
Periurethral — *see* condition
Periurethritis (gangrenous) — *see* Urethritis
Periuterine — *see* condition
Perivaginitis — *see* Vaginitis
Perivasculitis, retinal H35.06- ☑
Perivasitis (chronic) N49.1
Perivesiculitis (seminal) — *see* Vesiculitis
Perlèche NEC K13.0
due to
candidiasis B37.83

Perlèche — continued
  due to — continued
    moniliasis B37.83
    riboflavin deficiency E53.0
    vitamin B2 (riboflavin) deficiency E53.0
Pernicious — see condition
Pernio, perniosis T69.1 ☑
Perpetrator (of abuse) — see Index to External Causes
  of Injury, Perpetrator
Persecution
  delusion F22
  social Z60.5
Perseveration (tonic) R48.8
Persistence, persistent (congenital)
  anal membrane Q42.3
    with fistula Q42.2
  arteria stapedia Q16.3
  atrioventricular canal Q21.2
  branchial cleft NOS Q18.2
    cyst Q18.0
    fistula Q18.0
    sinus Q18.0
  bulbus cordis in left ventricle Q21.8
  canal of Cloquet Q14.0
  capsule (opaque) Q12.8
  cilioretinal artery or vein Q14.8
  cloaca Q43.7
  communication — see Fistula, congenital
  convolutions
    aortic arch Q25.46
    fallopian tube Q50.6
    oviduct Q50.6
    uterine tube Q50.6
  double aortic arch Q25.45
  ductus arteriosus (Botalli) Q25.0
  fetal
    circulation P29.38
    form of cervix (uteri) Q51.828
    hemoglobin, hereditary (HPFH) D56.4
  foramen
    Botalli Q21.1
    ovale Q21.1
  Gartner's duct Q52.4
  hemoglobin, fetal (hereditary) (HPFH) D56.4
  hyaloid
    artery (generally incomplete) Q14.0
    system Q14.8
  hymen, in pregnancy or childbirth — see Pregnancy,
    complicated by, abnormal, vulva
  lanugo Q84.2
  left
    posterior cardinal vein Q26.8
    root with right arch of aorta Q25.49
    superior vena cava Q26.1
  Meckel's diverticulum Q43.0
    malignant — see Table of Neoplasms, small intes-
     tine, malignant
  mucosal disease (middle ear) — see Otitis, media,
    suppurative, chronic, tubotympanic
  nail(s), anomalous Q84.6
  omphalomesenteric duct Q43.0
  organ or site not listed — see Anomaly, by site
  ostium
    atrioventriculare commune Q21.2
    primum Q21.2
    secundum Q21.1
  ovarian rests in fallopian tube Q50.6
  pancreatic tissue in intestinal tract Q43.8
  primary (deciduous)
    teeth K00.6
    vitreous hyperplasia Q14.0
  pupillary membrane Q13.89
  rhesus (Rh) titer — see Complication(s), transfusion,
    incompatibility reaction, Rh (factor)
  right aortic arch Q25.47
  sinus
    urogenitalis
     female Q52.8
     male Q55.8
    venosus with imperfect incorporation in right auricle
     Q26.8
  thymus (gland) (hyperplasia) E32.0
  thyroglossal duct Q89.2
  thyrolingual duct Q89.2
  truncus arteriosus or communis Q20.0
  tunica vasculosa lentis Q12.2
  umbilical sinus Q64.4
  urachus Q64.4

Persistence, persistent — continued
  vitelline duct Q43.0
Person (with)
  admitted for clinical research, as a control subject
    (normal comparison) (participant) Z00.6
  awaiting admission to adequate facility elsewhere
    Z75.1
  concern (normal) about sick person in family Z63.6
  consulting on behalf of another Z71.0
  feigning illness Z76.5
  living (in)
    alone Z60.2
    boarding school Z59.3
    residential institution Z59.3
    without
     adequate housing (heating) (space) Z59.1
     housing (permanent) (temporary) Z59.0
     person able to render necessary care Z74.2
     shelter Z59.0
  on waiting list Z75.1
  sick or handicapped in family Z63.6
Personality (disorder) F60.9
  accentuation of traits (type A pattern) Z73.1
  affective F34.0
  aggressive F60.3
  amoral F60.2
  anacastic, anankastic F60.5
  antisocial F60.2
  anxious F60.6
  asocial F60.2
  asthenic F60.7
  avoidant F60.6
  borderline F60.3
  change due to organic condition (enduring) F07.0
  compulsive F60.5
  cycloid F34.0
  cyclothymic F34.0
  dependent F60.7
  depressive F34.1
  dissocial F60.2
  dual F44.81
  eccentric F60.89
  emotionally unstable F60.3
  expansive paranoid F60.0
  explosive F60.3
  fanatic F60.0
  haltose type F60.89
  histrionic F60.4
  hyperthymic F34.0
  hypothymic F34.1
  hysterical F60.4
  immature F60.89
  inadequate F60.7
  labile (emotional) F60.3
  mixed (nonspecific) F60.89
  morally defective F60.2
  multiple F44.81
  narcissistic F60.81
  obsessional F60.5
  obsessive (-compulsive) F60.5
  organic F07.0
  overconscientious F60.5
  paranoid F60.0
  passive (-dependent) F60.7
  passive-aggressive F60.89
  pathologic F60.9
  pattern defect or disturbance F60.9
  pseudopsychopathic (organic) F07.0
  pseudoretarded (organic) F07.0
  psychoinfantile F60.4
  psychoneurotic NEC F60.89
  psychopathic F60.2
  querulant F60.0
  sadistic F60.89
  schizoid F60.1
  self-defeating F60.89
  sensitive paranoid F60.0
  sociopathic (amoral) (antisocial) (asocial) (dissocial)
    F60.2
  specified NEC F60.89
  type A Z73.1
  unstable (emotional) F60.3
Perthes' disease — see Legg-Calvé-Perthes disease
Pertussis — see also Whooping cough A37.90
Perversion, perverted
  appetite F50.89
    psychogenic F50.89
  function
    pituitary gland E23.2

Perversion, perverted — continued
  function — continued
    pituitary gland — continued
     posterior lobe E22.2
  sense of smell and taste R43.8
    psychogenic F45.8
  sexual — see Deviation, sexual
Pervious, congenital — see also Imperfect, closure
  ductus arteriosus Q25.0
Pes (congenital) — see also Talipes
  acquired — see also Deformity, limb, foot, specified
    NEC
    planus — see Deformity, limb, flat foot
  adductus Q66.89
  cavus Q66.7- ☑
  deformity NEC, acquired — see Deformity, limb, foot,
    specified NEC
  planus (acquired) (any degree) — see also Deformity,
    limb, flat foot
    rachitic sequelae (late effect) E64.3
  valgus Q66.6
Pest, pestis — see Plague
Petechia, petechiae R23.3
  newborn P54.5
Petechial typhus A75.9
Peter's anomaly Q13.4
Petit mal seizure — see Epilepsy, childhood, absence
Petit's hernia — see Hernia, abdomen, specified site NE
Petrellidosis B48.2
Petrositis H70.20- ☑
  acute H70.21- ☑
  chronic H70.22- ☑
Peutz-Jeghers disease or syndrome Q85.8
Peyronie's disease N48.6
PFAPA (periodic fever, aphthous stomatitis, pharyngiti
  and adenopathy syndrome) M04.8
Pfeiffer's disease — see Mononucleosis, infectious
Phagedena (dry) (moist) (sloughing) — see also Gan-
  grene
  geometric L88
  penis N48.29
  tropical — see Ulcer, skin
  vulva N76.6
Phagedenic — see condition
Phakoma H35.89
Phakomatosis — see also specific eponymous syndrome
  Q85.9
  Bourneville's Q85.1
  specified NEC Q85.8
Phantom limb syndrome (without pain) G54.7
  with pain G54.6
Pharyngeal pouch syndrome D82.1
Pharyngitis (acute) (catarrhal)(gangrenous) (infective)
  (malignant) (membranous) (phlegmonous) (pseudomembranous) (simple) (subacute) (suppurative)
  (ulcerative) (viral) J02.9
  with influenza, flu, or grippe — see Influenza, with,
    pharyngitis
  aphthous B08.5
  atrophic J31.2
  chlamydial A56.4
  chronic (atrophic) (granular) (hypertrophic) J31.2
  coxsackievirus B08.5
  diphtheritic A36.0
  enteroviral vesicular B08.5
  follicular (chronic) J31.2
  fusospirochetal A69.1
  gonococcal A54.5
  granular (chronic) J31.2
  herpesviral B00.2
  hypertrophic J31.2
  infectional, chronic J31.2
  influenzal — see Influenza, with, respiratory manifesta
    tions NEC
  lymphonodular, acute (enteroviral) B08.8
  pneumococcal J02.8
  purulent J02.9
  putrid J02.9
  septic J02.0
  sicca J31.2
  specified organism NEC J02.8
  staphylococcal J02.8
  streptococcal J02.0
  syphilitic, congenital (early) A50.03
  tuberculous A15.8
  vesicular, enteroviral B08.5
  viral NEC J02.8
Pharyngoconjunctivitis, viral B30.2

Pharyngolaryngitis (acute) J06.0
  chronic J37.0
Pharyngoplegia J39.2
Pharyngotonsillitis, herpesviral B00.2
Pharyngotracheitis, chronic J42
Pharynx, pharyngeal — see condition
Phencyclidine-induced
  anxiety disorder F16.980
  bipolar and related disorder F16.94
  depressive disorder F16.94
  psychotic disorder F16.959
Phenomenon
  Arthus' — see Arthus' phenomenon
  jaw-winking Q07.8
  lupus erythematosus (LE) cell M32.9
  Raynaud's (secondary) I73.00
    with gangrene I73.01
  vasomotor R55
  vasospastic I73.9
  vasovagal R55
  Wenckebach's I44.1
Phenylketonuria E70.1
  classical E70.0
  maternal E70.1
Pheochromoblastoma
  specified site — see Neoplasm, malignant, by site
  unspecified site C74.10
Pheochromocytoma
  malignant
    specified site — see Neoplasm, malignant, by site
    unspecified site C74.10
  specified site — see Neoplasm, benign, by site
  unspecified site D35.00
Pheohyphomycosis — see Chromomycosis
Pheomycosis — see Chromomycosis
Phimosis (congenital) (due to infection) N47.1
  chancroidal A57
Phlebectasia — see also Varix
  congenital Q27.4
Phlebitis (infective) (pyemic) (septic) (suppurative) I80.9
  antepartum — see Thrombophlebitis, antepartum
  blue — see Phlebitis, leg, deep
  breast, superficial I80.8
  calf muscular vein (NOS) I80.25- ☑
  cavernous (venous) sinus — see Phlebitis, intracranial (venous) sinus
  cerebral (venous) sinus — see Phlebitis, intracranial (venous) sinus
  chest wall, superficial I80.8
  cranial (venous) sinus — see Phlebitis, intracranial (venous) sinus
  deep (vessels) — see Phlebitis, leg, deep
  due to implanted device — see Complications, by site and type, specified NEC
  during or resulting from a procedure T81.72 ☑
  femoral vein (superficial) I80.1- ☑
  femoropopliteal vein I80.0- ☑
  gastrocnemial vein I80.25- ☑
  gestational — see Phlebopathy, gestational
  hepatic veins I80.8
  iliac vein (common) (external) (internal) I80.21- ☑
  iliofemoral — see Phlebitis, femoral vein
  intracranial (venous) sinus (any) G08
    nonpyogenic I67.6
  intraspinal venous sinuses and veins G08
    nonpyogenic G95.19
  lateral (venous) sinus — see Phlebitis, intracranial (venous) sinus
  leg I80.3
    antepartum — see Thrombophlebitis, antepartum
    deep (vessels) NEC I80.20- ☑
      iliac I80.21- ☑
      popliteal vein I80.22- ☑
      specified vessel NEC I80.29- ☑
      tibial vein (anterior) (posterior) I80.23- ☑
    femoral vein (superficial) I80.1- ☑
    superficial (vessels) I80.0- ☑
  longitudinal sinus — see Phlebitis, intracranial (venous) sinus
  lower limb — see Phlebitis, leg
  migrans, migrating (superficial) I82.1
  pelvic
    with ectopic or molar pregnancy O08.0
    following ectopic or molar pregnancy O08.0
    puerperal, postpartum O87.1
  peroneal vein I80.24- ☑
  popliteal vein — see Phlebitis, leg, deep, popliteal

Phlebitis — continued
  portal (vein) K75.1
  postoperative T81.72 ☑
  pregnancy — see Thrombophlebitis, antepartum
  puerperal, postpartum, childbirth O87.0
    deep O87.1
    pelvic O87.1
    superficial O87.0
  retina — see Vasculitis, retina
  saphenous (accessory) (great) (long) (small) — see Phlebitis, leg, superficial
  sinus (meninges) — see Phlebitis, intracranial (venous) sinus
  soleal vein I80.25- ☑
  specified site NEC I80.8
  syphilitic A52.09
  tibial vein — see Phlebitis, leg, deep, tibial
  ulcerative I80.9
    leg — see Phlebitis, leg
  umbilicus I80.8
  uterus (septic) — see Endometritis
  varicose (leg) (lower limb) — see Varix, leg, with, inflammation
Phlebofibrosis I87.8
Phleboliths I87.8
Phlebopathy,
  gestational O22.9- ☑
  puerperal O87.9
Phlebosclerosis I87.8
Phlebothrombosis — see also Thrombosis
  antepartum — see Thrombophlebitis, antepartum
  pregnancy — see Thrombophlebitis, antepartum
  puerperal — see Thrombophlebitis, puerperal
Phlebotomus fever A93.1
Phlegmasia
  alba dolens O87.1
    nonpuerperal — see Phlebitis, femoral vein
  cerulea dolens — see Phlebitis, leg, deep
Phlegmon — see Abscess
Phlegmonous — see condition
Phlyctenulosis (allergic) (keratoconjunctivitis) (nontuberculous) — see also Keratoconjunctivitis
  cornea — see Keratoconjunctivitis
  tuberculous A18.52
Phobia, phobic F40.9
  animal F40.218
    spiders F40.210
  examination F40.298
  reaction F40.9
  simple F40.298
  social F40.10
    generalized F40.11
  specific (isolated) F40.298
    animal F40.218
      spiders F40.210
    blood F40.230
    injection F40.231
    injury F40.233
    men F40.290
    natural environment F40.228
      thunderstorms F40.220
    situational F40.248
      bridges F40.242
      closed in spaces F40.240
      flying F40.243
      heights F40.241
    specified focus NEC F40.298
    transfusion F40.231
    women F40.291
  specified NEC F40.8
    medical care NEC F40.232
  state F40.9
Phocas' disease — see Mastopathy, cystic
Phocomelia Q73.1
  lower limb — see Agenesis, leg, with foot present
  upper limb — see Agenesis, arm, with hand present
Phoria H50.50
Phosphate-losing tubular disorder N25.0
Phosphatemia E83.39
Phosphaturia E83.39
Photodermatitis (sun) L56.8
  chronic L57.8
  due to drug L56.8
  light other than sun L59.8
Photokeratitis H16.13- ☑
Photophobia H53.14- ☑
Photophthalmia — see Photokeratitis

Photopsia H53.19
Photoretinitis — see Retinopathy, solar
Photosensitivity, photosensitization (sun) skin L56.8
  light other than sun L59.8
Phrenitis — see Encephalitis
Phrynoderma (vitamin A deficiency) E50.8
Phthiriasis (pubis) B85.3
  with any infestation classifiable to B85.0-B85.2 B85.4
Phthirus infestation — see Phthiriasis
Phthisis — see also Tuberculosis
  bulbi (infectional) — see Disorder, globe, degenerated condition, atrophy
  eyeball (due to infection) — see Disorder, globe, degenerated condition, atrophy
Phycomycosis — see Zygomycosis
Physalopteriasis B81.8
Physical restraint status Z78.1
Phytobezoar T18.9 ☑
  intestine T18.3 ☑
  stomach T18.2 ☑
Pian — see Yaws
Pianoma A66.1
Pica F50.89
  in adults F50.89
  infant or child F98.3
Picking, nose F98.8
Pick-Niemann disease — see Niemann-Pick disease or syndrome
Pick's
  cerebral atrophy G31.01 [F02.80]
    with behavioral disturbance G31.01 [F02.81]
  disease or syndrome (brain) G31.01 [F02.80]
    with behavioral disturbance G31.01 [F02.81]
    brain G31.01 [F02.80]
      with behavioral disturbance G31.01 [F02.81]
    pericardium (pericardial pseudocirrhosis of liver) I31.1
  syndrome
    brain G31.01 [F02.80]
      with behavioral disturbance G31.01 [F02.81]
    of heart (pericardial pseudocirrhosis of liver) I31.1
Pickwickian syndrome E66.2
Piebaldism E70.39
Piedra (beard) (scalp) B36.8
  black B36.3
  white B36.2
Pierre Robin deformity or syndrome Q87.0
Pierson's disease or osteochondrosis M91.0
Pig-bel A05.2
Pigeon
  breast or chest (acquired) M95.4
    congenital Q67.7
    rachitic sequelae (late effect) E64.3
  breeder's disease or lung J67.2
  fancier's disease or lung J67.2
  toe — see Deformity, toe, specified NEC
Pigmentation (abnormal) (anomaly) L81.9
  conjunctiva H11.13- ☑
  cornea (anterior) H18.01- ☑
    posterior H18.05- ☑
    stromal H18.06- ☑
  diminished melanin formation NEC L81.6
  iron L81.8
  lids, congenital Q82.8
  limbus corneae — see Pigmentation, cornea
  metals L81.8
  optic papilla, congenital Q14.2
  retina, congenital (grouped) (nevoid) Q14.1
  scrotum, congenital Q82.8
  tattoo L81.8
Piles — see also Hemorrhoids K64.9
Pili
  annulati or torti (congenital) Q84.1
  incarnati L73.1
Pill roller hand (intrinsic) — see Parkinsonism
Pilomatrixoma — see Neoplasm, skin, benign
  malignant — see Neoplasm, skin, malignant
Pilonidal — see condition
Pimple R23.8
PIN — see Neoplasia, intraepithelial, prostate
Pinched nerve — see Neuropathy, entrapment
Pindborg tumor — see Cyst, calcifying odontogenic
Pineal body or gland — see condition
Pinealoblastoma C75.3
Pinealoma D44.5
  malignant C75.3
Pineoblastoma C75.3

Pineocytoma D44.5
Pinguecula H11.15- ☑
Pingueculitis H10.81- ☑
Pinhole meatus — *see also* Stricture, urethra N35.919
Pink
  disease — *see* subcategory T56.1 ☑
  eye — *see* Conjunctivitis, acute, mucopurulent
Pinkus' disease (lichen nitidus) L44.1
Pinpoint
  meatus — *see* Stricture, urethra
  os (uteri) — *see* Stricture, cervix
Pins and needles R20.2
Pinta A67.9
  cardiovascular lesions A67.2
  chancre (primary) A67.0
  erythematous plaques A67.1
  hyperchromic lesions A67.1
  hyperkeratosis A67.1
  lesions A67.9
    cardiovascular A67.2
    hyperchromic A67.1
    intermediate A67.1
    late A67.2
    mixed A67.3
    primary A67.0
    skin (achromic) (cicatricial) (dyschromic) A67.2
      hyperchromic A67.1
      mixed (achromic and hyperchromic) A67.3
  papule (primary) A67.0
  skin lesions (achromic) (cicatricial) (dyschromic) A67.2
    hyperchromic A67.1
    mixed (achromic and hyperchromic) A67.3
  vitiligo A67.2
Pintids A67.1
Pinworm (disease) (infection) (infestation) B80
Piroplasmosis — *see also* Babesiosis B60.00
  specified NEC B60.09
Pistol wound — *see* Gunshot wound
Pitchers' elbow — *see* Derangement, joint, specified
    type NEC, elbow
Pithecoid pelvis Q74.2
  with disproportion (fetopelvic) O33.0
    causing obstructed labor O65.0
Pithiatism F48.8
Pitted — *see* Pitting
Pitting — *see also* Edema R60.9
  lip R60.0
  nail L60.8
  teeth K00.4
Pituitary gland — *see* condition
Pituitary-snuff-taker's disease J67.8
Pityriasis (capitis) L21.0
  alba L30.5
  circinata (et maculata) L42
  furfuracea L21.0
  Hebra's L26
  lichenoides L41.0
    chronica L41.1
    et varioliformis (acuta) L41.0
  maculata (et circinata) L30.5
  nigra B36.1
  pilaris, Hebra's L44.0
  rosea L42
  rotunda L44.8
  rubra (Hebra) pilaris L44.0
  simplex L30.5
  specified type NEC L30.5
  streptogenes L30.5
  versicolor (scrotal) B36.0
Placenta, placental — *see* Pregnancy, complicated by
    (care of) (management affected by), specified con-
    dition
Placentitis O41.14- ☑
Plagiocephaly Q67.3
Plague A20.9
  abortive A20.8
  ambulatory A20.8
  asymptomatic A20.8
  bubonic A20.0
  cellulocutaneous A20.1
  cutaneobubonic A20.1
  lymphatic gland A20.0
  meningitis A20.3
  pharyngeal A20.8
  pneumonic (primary) (secondary) A20.2
  pulmonary, pulmonic A20.2
  septicemic A20.7
  tonsillar A20.8

Plague — *continued*
  tonsillar — *continued*
    septicemic A20.7
Planning, family
  contraception Z30.9
  procreation Z31.69
Plaque(s)
  artery, arterial — *see* Arteriosclerosis
  calcareous — *see* Calcification
  coronary, lipid rich I25.83
  epicardial I31.8
  erythematous, of pinta A67.1
  Hollenhorst's — *see* Occlusion, artery, retina
  lipid rich, coronary I25.83
  pleural (without asbestos) J92.9
    with asbestos J92.0
  tongue K13.29
Plasmacytoma C90.3- ☑
  extramedullary C90.2- ☑
  medullary C90.0- ☑
  solitary C90.3- ☑
Plasmacytopenia D72.818
Plasmacytosis D72.822
Plaster ulcer — *see* Ulcer, pressure, by site
Plateau iris syndrome (post-iridectomy) (postprocedu-
    ral) (without glaucoma) H21.82
  with glaucoma H40.22- ☑
Platybasia Q75.8
Platyonychia (congenital) Q84.6
  acquired L60.8
Platypelloid pelvis M95.5
  with disproportion (fetopelvic) O33.0
    causing obstructed labor O65.0
  congenital Q74.2
Platyspondylisis Q76.49
Plaut (-Vincent) **disease** — *see also* Vincent's A69.1
Plethora R23.2
  newborn P61.1
Pleura, pleural — *see* condition
Pleuralgia R07.81
Pleurisy (acute) (adhesive) (chronic) (costal) (diaphrag-
    matic) (double) (dry) (fibrinous) (fibrous) (interlobar)
    (latent) (plastic) (primary) (residual) (sicca) (sterile)
    (subacute) (unresolved) R09.1
  with
    adherent pleura J86.0
    effusion J90
      chylous, chyliform J94.0
      tuberculous (non primary) A15.6
        primary (progressive) A15.7
      tuberculosis — *see* Pleurisy, tuberculous (non pri-
        mary)
  encysted — *see* Pleurisy, with effusion
  exudative — *see* Pleurisy, with effusion
  fibrinopurulent, fibropurulent — *see* Pyothorax
  hemorrhagic — *see* Hemothorax
  pneumococcal J90
  purulent — *see* Pyothorax
  septic — *see* Pyothorax
  serofibrinous — *see* Pleurisy, with effusion
  seropurulent — *see* Pyothorax
  serous — *see* Pleurisy, with effusion
  staphylococcal J86.9
  streptococcal J90
  suppurative — *see* Pyothorax
  traumatic (post) (current) — *see* Injury, intrathoracic,
    pleura
  tuberculous (with effusion) (non primary) A15.6
    primary (progressive) A15.7
Pleuritis sicca — *see* Pleurisy
Pleurobronchopneumonia — *see* Pneumonia, broncho-
Pleurodynia R07.81
  epidemic B33.0
  viral B33.0
Pleuropericarditis — *see also* Pericarditis
  acute I30.9
Pleuropneumonia (acute) (bilateral) (double) (septic)
    — *see also* Pneumonia J18.8
  chronic — *see* Fibrosis, lung
Pleuro-pneumonia-like-organism (PPLO), as cause of
    disease classified elsewhere B96.0
Pleurorrhea — *see* Pleurisy, with effusion
Plexitis, brachial G54.0
Plica
  polonica B85.0
  syndrome, knee M67.5- ☑
  tonsil J35.8

Plicated tongue K14.5
Plug
  bronchus NEC J98.09
  meconium (newborn) NEC syndrome P76.0
  mucus — *see* Asphyxia, mucus
Plumbism — *see* subcategory T56.0 ☑
Plummer's disease E05.20
  with thyroid storm E05.21
Plummer-Vinson syndrome D50.1
Pluricarential syndrome of infancy E40
Plus (and minus) **hand** (intrinsic) — *see* Deformity, limb,
    specified type NEC, forearm
PMEI (polymorphic epilepsy in infancy) G40.83- ☑
Pneumathemia — *see* Air, embolism
Pneumatic hammer (drill) syndrome T75.21 ☑
Pneumatocele (lung) J98.4
  intracranial G93.89
  tension J44.9
Pneumatosis
  cystoides intestinalis K63.89
  intestinalis K63.89
  peritonei K66.8
Pneumaturia R39.89
Pneumoblastoma — *see* Neoplasm, lung, malignant
Pneumocephalus G93.89
Pneumococcemia A40.3
Pneumococcus, pneumococcal — *see* condition
Pneumoconiosis (due to) (inhalation of) J64
  with tuberculosis (any type in A15) J65
  aluminum J63.0
  asbestos J61
  bagasse, bagassosis J67.1
  bauxite J63.1
  beryllium J63.2
  coal miners' (simple) J60
  coalworkers' (simple) J60
  collier's J60
  cotton dust J66.0
  diatomite (diatomaceous earth) J62.8
  dust
    inorganic NEC J63.6
    lime J62.8
    marble J62.8
    organic NEC J66.8
  fumes or vapors (from silo) J68.9
  graphite J63.3
  grinder's J62.8
  kaolin J62.8
  mica J62.8
  millstone maker's J62.8
  mineral fibers NEC J61
  miner's J60
  moldy hay J67.0
  potter's J62.8
  rheumatoid — *see* Rheumatoid, lung
  sandblaster's J62.8
  silica, silicate NEC J62.8
    with carbon J60
  stonemason's J62.8
  talc (dust) J62.0
Pneumocystis carinii pneumonia B59
Pneumocystis jiroveci (pneumonia) B59
Pneumocystosis (with pneumonia) B59
Pneumohemopericardium I31.2
Pneumohemothorax J94.2
  traumatic S27.2 ☑
Pneumohydropericardium — *see* Pericarditis
Pneumohydrothorax — *see* Hydrothorax
Pneumomediastinum J98.2
  congenital or perinatal P25.2
Pneumomycosis B49 *[J99]*
Pneumonia (acute) (double) (migratory) (purulent)
    (septic) (unresolved) J18.9
  with
    influenza — *see* Influenza, with, pneumonia
    lung abscess J85.1
      due to specified organism — *see* Pneumonia, i◼
        (due to)
  adenoviral J12.0
  adynamic J18.2
  alba A50.04
  allergic — *see also* Pneumonitis, hypersensitivity J82.8◼
  alveolar — *see* Pneumonia, lobar
  anaerobes J15.8
  anthrax A22.1
  apex, apical — *see* Pneumonia, lobar
  Ascaris B77.81
  aspiration J69.0

☑ **Additional Character Required** — Refer to the Tabular List for Character Selection   ▽ **Subterms under main terms may continue to next column or page**

Pneumonia — *continued*
  aspiration — *continued*
    due to
      aspiration of microorganisms
        bacterial J15.9
        viral J12.9
      food (regurgitated) J69.0
      gastric secretions J69.0
      milk (regurgitated) J69.0
      oils, essences J69.1
      solids, liquids NEC J69.8
      vomitus J69.0
    newborn P24.81
      amniotic fluid (clear) P24.11
      blood P24.21
      food (regurgitated) P24.31
      liquor (amnii) P24.11
      meconium P24.01
      milk P24.31
      mucus P24.11
      specified NEC P24.81
      stomach contents P24.31
    postprocedural J95.4
  atypical NEC J18.9
  bacillus J15.9
    specified NEC J15.8
  bacterial J15.9
    specified NEC J15.8
  Bacteroides (fragilis) (oralis) (melaninogenicus) J15.8
  basal, basic, basilar — *see* Pneumonia, by type
  bronchiolitis obliterans organized (BOOP) J84.89
  broncho-, bronchial (confluent) (croupous) (diffuse)
    (disseminated) (hemorrhagic) (involving lobes)
    (lobar) (terminal) J18.0
    allergic — *see also* Pneumonitis, hypersensitivity
      J82.89
    aspiration — *see* Pneumonia, aspiration
    bacterial J15.9
      specified NEC J15.8
    chronic — *see* Fibrosis, lung
    diplococcal J13
    Eaton's agent J15.7
    Escherichia coli (E. coli) J15.5
    Friedländer's bacillus J15.0
    Hemophilus influenzae J14
    hypostatic J18.2
    inhalation — *see also* Pneumonia, aspiration
      due to fumes or vapors (chemical) J68.0
      of oils or essences J69.1
    Klebsiella (pneumoniae) J15.0
    lipid, lipoid J69.1
      endogenous J84.89
    Mycoplasma (pneumoniae) J15.7
    pleuro-pneumonia-like-organisms (PPLO) J15.7
    pneumococcal J13
    Proteus J15.6
    Pseudomonas J15.1
    Serratia marcescens J15.6
    specified organism NEC J16.8
    staphylococcal — *see* Pneumonia, staphylococcal
    streptococcal NEC J15.4
      group B J15.3
      pneumoniae J13
    viral, virus — *see* Pneumonia, viral
  Butyrivibrio (fibriosolvens) J15.8
  Candida B37.1
  caseous — *see* Tuberculosis, pulmonary
  catarrhal — *see* Pneumonia, broncho
  chlamydial J16.0
    congenital P23.1
  cholesterol J84.89
  cirrhotic (chronic) — *see* Fibrosis, lung
  Clostridium (haemolyticum) (novyi) J15.8
  confluent — *see* Pneumonia, broncho
  congenital (infective) P23.9
    due to
      bacterium NEC P23.6
      Chlamydia P23.1
      Escherichia coli P23.4
      Haemophilus influenzae P23.6
      infective organism NEC P23.8
      Klebsiella pneumoniae P23.6
      Mycoplasma P23.6
      Pseudomonas P23.5
      Staphylococcus P23.2
      Streptococcus (except group B) P23.6
        group B P23.3
      viral agent P23.0

Pneumonia — *continued*
  congenital — *continued*
    specified NEC P23.8
  croupous — *see* Pneumonia, lobar
  cryptogenic organizing J84.116
  cytomegalic inclusion B25.0
  cytomegaloviral B25.0
  deglutition — *see* Pneumonia, aspiration
  desquamative interstitial J84.117
  diffuse — *see* Pneumonia, broncho
  diplococcal, diplococcus (broncho-) (lobar) J13
  disseminated (focal) — *see* Pneumonia, broncho
  Eaton's agent J15.7
  embolic, embolism — *see* Embolism, pulmonary
  Enterobacter J15.6
  eosinophilic J82.81
    acute J82.82
    chronic J82.81
  Escherichia coli (E. coli) J15.5
  Eubacterium J15.8
  fibrinous — *see* Pneumonia, lobar
  fibroid, fibrous (chronic) — *see* Fibrosis, lung
  Friedländer's bacillus J15.0
  Fusobacterium (nucleatum) J15.8
  gangrenous J85.0
  giant cell (measles) B05.2
  gonococcal A54.84
  gram-negative bacteria NEC J15.6
    anaerobic J15.8
  Hemophilus influenzae (broncho) (lobar) J14
  human metapneumovirus J12.3
  hypostatic (broncho) (lobar) J18.2
  in (due to)
    actinomycosis A42.0
    adenovirus J12.0
    anthrax A22.1
    ascariasis B77.81
    aspergillosis B44.9
    Bacillus anthracis A22.1
    Bacterium anitratum J15.6
    candidiasis B37.1
    chickenpox B01.2
    Chlamydia J16.0
      neonatal P23.1
    coccidioidomycosis B38.2
      acute B38.0
      chronic B38.1
    cytomegalovirus disease B25.0
    Diplococcus (pneumoniae) J13
    Eaton's agent J15.7
    Enterobacter J15.6
    Escherichia coli (E. coli) J15.5
    Friedländer's bacillus J15.0
    fumes and vapors (chemical) (inhalation) J68.0
    gonorrhea A54.84
    Hemophilus influenzae (H. influenzae) J14
    Herellea J15.6
    histoplasmosis B39.2
      acute B39.0
      chronic B39.1
    human metapneumovirus J12.3
    Klebsiella (pneumoniae) J15.0
    measles B05.2
    Mycoplasma (pneumoniae) J15.7
    nocardiosis, nocardiasis A43.0
    ornithosis A70
    parainfluenza virus J12.2
    pleuro-pneumonia-like-organism (PPLO) J15.7
    pneumococcus J13
    pneumocystosis (Pneumocystis carinii) (Pneumocys-
      tis jiroveci) B59
    Proteus J15.6
    Pseudomonas NEC J15.1
      pseudomallei A24.1
    psittacosis A70
    Q fever A78
    respiratory syncytial virus (RSV) J12.1
    rheumatic fever I00 *[J17]*
    rubella B06.81
    Salmonella (infection) A02.22
      typhi A01.03
    schistosomiasis B65.9 *[J17]*
    Serratia marcescens J15.6
    specified
      bacterium NEC J15.8
      organism NEC J16.8
    spirochetal NEC A69.8
    Staphylococcus J15.20

Pneumonia — *continued*
  in — *continued*
    Staphylococcus — *continued*
      aureus (methicillin susceptible) (MSSA) J15.211
        methicillin resistant (MRSA) J15.212
      specified NEC J15.29
    Streptococcus J15.4
      group B J15.3
      pneumoniae J13
      specified NEC J15.4
    toxoplasmosis B58.3
    tularemia A21.2
    typhoid (fever) A01.03
    varicella B01.2
    virus — *see* Pneumonia, viral
    whooping cough A37.91
      due to
        Bordetella parapertussis A37.11
        Bordetella pertussis A37.01
        specified NEC A37.81
    Yersinia pestis A20.2
  inhalation of food or vomit — *see* Pneumonia, aspira-
    tion
  interstitial J84.9
    chronic J84.111
    desquamative J84.117
    due to
      collagen vascular disease J84.178
      known underlying cause J84.178
    idiopathic NOS J84.111
    in disease classified elsewhere J84.178
    lymphocytic (due to collagen vascular disease) (in
      diseases classified elsewhere) J84.178
    lymphoid J84.2
    non-specific J84.89
      due to
        collagen vascular disease J84.178
        known underlying cause J84.178
      idiopathic J84.113
      in diseases classified elsewhere J84.178
    plasma cell B59
    pseudomonas J15.1
    usual J84.112
      due to collagen vascular disease J84.178
      idiopathic J84.112
      in diseases classified elsewhere J84.178
  Klebsiella (pneumoniae) J15.0
  lipid, lipoid (exogenous) J69.1
    endogenous J84.89
  lobar (disseminated) (double) (interstitial) J18.1
    bacterial J15.9
      specified NEC J15.8
    chronic — *see* Fibrosis, lung
    Escherichia coli (E. coli) J15.5
    Friedländer's bacillus J15.0
    Hemophilus influenzae J14
    hypostatic J18.2
    Klebsiella (pneumoniae) J15.0
    pneumococcal J13
    Proteus J15.6
    Pseudomonas J15.1
    specified organism NEC J16.8
    staphylococcal — *see* Pneumonia, staphylococcal
    streptococcal NEC J15.4
    Streptococcus pneumoniae J13
    viral, virus — *see* Pneumonia, viral
  lobular — *see* Pneumonia, broncho
  Löffler's J82.89
  lymphoid interstitial J84.2
  massive — *see* Pneumonia, lobar
  meconium P24.01
  MRSA (methicillin resistant Staphylococcus aureus)
    J15.212
  MSSA (methicillin susceptible Staphylococcus aureus)
    J15.211
  multilobar — *see* Pneumonia, by type
  Mycoplasma (pneumoniae) J15.7
  necrotic J85.0
  neonatal P23.9
    aspiration — *see* Aspiration, by substance, with
      pneumonia
  nitrogen dioxide J68.0
  organizing J84.89
    due to
      collagen vascular disease J84.178
      known underlying cause J84.178
    in diseases classified elsewhere J84.178
  orthostatic J18.2

Pneumonia — *continued*
parainfluenza virus J12.2
parenchymatous — *see* Fibrosis, lung
passive J18.2
patchy — *see* Pneumonia, broncho
Peptococcus J15.8
Peptostreptococcus J15.8
plasma cell (of infants) B59
pleurolobar — *see* Pneumonia, lobar
pleuro-pneumonia-like organism (PPLO) J15.7
pneumococcal (broncho) (lobar) J13
Pneumocystis (carinii) (jiroveci) B59
postinfectional NEC B99 ☑ *[J17]*
postmeasles B05.2
Proteus J15.6
Pseudomonas J15.1
psittacosis A70
radiation J70.0
respiratory syncytial virus (RSV) J12.1
resulting from a procedure J95.89
rheumatic I00 *[J17]*
Salmonella (arizonae) (cholerae-suis) (enteritidis) (typhimurium) A02.22
typhi A01.03
typhoid fever A01.03
SARS-associated coronavirus J12.81
segmented, segmental — *see* Pneumonia, broncho-
Serratia marcescens J15.6
specified NEC J18.8
bacterium NEC J15.8
organism NEC J16.8
virus NEC J12.89
spirochetal NEC A69.8
staphylococcal (broncho) (lobar) J15.20
aureus (methicillin susceptible) (MSSA) J15.211
methicillin resistant (MRSA) J15.212
specified NEC J15.29
static, stasis J18.2
streptococcal NEC (broncho) (lobar) J15.4
group
A J15.4
B J15.3
specified NEC J15.4
Streptococcus pneumoniae J13
syphilitic, congenital (early) A50.04
traumatic (complication) (early) (secondary) T79.8 ☑
tuberculous (any) — *see* Tuberculosis, pulmonary
tularemic A21.2
varicella B01.2
Veillonella J15.8
ventilator associated J95.851
viral, virus (broncho) (interstitial) (lobar) J12.9
adenoviral J12.0
congenital P23.0
human metapneumovirus J12.3
parainfluenza J12.2
respiratory syncytial (RSV) J12.1
SARS-associated coronavirus J12.81
specified NEC J12.89
white (congenital) A50.04
Pneumonic — *see* condition
Pneumonitis (acute) (primary) — *see also* Pneumonia
air-conditioner J67.7
allergic (due to) J67.9
organic dust NEC J67.8
red cedar dust J67.8
sequoiosis J67.8
wood dust J67.8
aspiration J69.0
due to
anesthesia J95.4
during
labor and delivery O74.0
pregnancy O29.01- ☑
puerperium O89.01
fumes or gases J68.0
obstetric O74.0
chemical (due to gases, fumes or vapors) (inhalation)
J68.0
due to anesthesia J95.4
cholesterol J84.89
chronic — *see* Fibrosis, lung
congenital rubella P35.0
crack (cocaine) J68.0
due to
beryllium J68.0
cadmium J68.0
crack (cocaine) J68.0

Pneumonitis — *continued*
due to — *continued*
detergent J69.8
fluorocarbon-polymer J68.0
food, vomit (aspiration) J69.0
fumes or vapors J68.0
gases, fumes or vapors (inhalation) J68.0
inhalation
blood J69.8
essences J69.1
food (regurgitated), milk, vomit J69.0
oils, essences J69.1
saliva J69.0
solids, liquids NEC J69.8
manganese J68.0
nitrogen dioxide J68.0
oils, essences J69.1
solids, liquids NEC J69.8
toxoplasmosis (acquired) B58.3
congenital P37.1
vanadium J68.0
ventilator J95.851
eosinophilic J82.81
acute J82.82
chronic J82.81
hypersensitivity J67.9
air conditioner lung J67.7
bagassosis J67.1
bird fancier's lung J67.2
farmer's lung J67.0
maltworker's lung J67.4
maple bark-stripper's lung J67.6
mushroom worker's lung J67.5
specified organic dust NEC J67.8
suberosis J67.3
interstitial (chronic) J84.89
acute J84.114
lymphoid J84.2
non-specific J84.89
idiopathic J84.113
lymphoid, interstitial J84.2
meconium P24.01
postanesthetic J95.4
correct substance properly administered — *see* Table of Drugs and Chemicals, by drug, adverse
effect
in labor and delivery O74.0
in pregnancy O29.01- ☑
obstetric O74.0
overdose or wrong substance given or taken (by
accident) — *see* Table of Drugs and Chemicals, by drug, poisoning
postpartum, puerperal O89.01
postoperative J95.4
obstetric O74.0
radiation J70.0
rubella, congenital P35.0
ventilation (air-conditioning) J67.7
ventilator associated J95.851
wood-dust J67.8
Pneumonoconiosis — *see* Pneumoconiosis
Pneumoparotid K11.8
Pneumopathy NEC J98.4
alveolar J84.09
due to organic dust NEC J66.8
parietoalveolar J84.09
Pneumopericarditis — *see also* Pericarditis
acute I30.9
Pneumopericardium — *see also* Pericarditis
congenital P25.3
newborn P25.3
traumatic (post) — *see* Injury, heart
Pneumophagia (psychogenic) F45.8
Pneumopleurisy, pneumopleuritis — *see also* Pneumonia J18.8
Pneumopyopericardium I30.1
Pneumopyothorax — *see* Pyopneumothorax
with fistula J86.0
Pneumorrhagia — *see also* Hemorrhage, lung
tuberculous — *see* Tuberculosis, pulmonary
Pneumothorax NOS J93.9
acute J93.83
chronic J93.81
congenital P25.1
perinatal period P25.1
postprocedural J95.811
specified NEC J93.83
spontaneous NOS J93.83

Pneumothorax — *continued*
spontaneous — *continued*
newborn P25.1
primary J93.11
secondary J93.12
tension J93.0
tense valvular, infectional J93.0
tension (spontaneous) J93.0
traumatic S27.0 ☑
with hemothorax S27.2 ☑
tuberculous — *see* Tuberculosis, pulmonary
Podagra — *see also* Gout M10.9
Podencephalus Q01.9
Poikilocytosis R71.8
Poikiloderma L81.6
Civatte's L57.3
congenital Q82.8
vasculare atrophicans L94.5
Poikilodermatomyositis M33.10
with
myopathy M33.12
respiratory involvement M33.11
specified organ involvement NEC M33.19
Pointed ear (congenital) Q17.3
Poison ivy, oak, sumac or other plant dermatitis (allergic) (contact) L23.7
Poisoning (acute) — *see also* Table of Drugs and Chemicals
algae and toxins T65.82- ☑
Bacillus B (aertrycke) (cholerae (suis)) (paratyphosus)
(suipestifer) A02.9
botulinus A05.1
bacterial toxins A05.9
berries, noxious — *see* Poisoning, food, noxious, berrie
botulism A05.1
ciguatera fish T61.0- ☑
Clostridium botulinum A05.1
death-cap (Amanita phalloides) (Amanita verna) —
see Poisoning, food, noxious, mushrooms
drug — *see* Table of Drugs and Chemicals, by drug,
poisoning
epidemic, fish (noxious) — *see* Poisoning, seafood
bacterial A05.9
fava bean D55.0
fish (noxious) T61.9- ☑
bacterial — *see* Intoxication, foodborne, by agent
ciguatera fish — *see* Poisoning, ciguatera fish
scombroid fish — *see* Poisoning, scombroid fish
specified type NEC T61.77- ☑
food NEC A05.9
bacterial — *see* Intoxication, foodborne, by agent
due to
Bacillus (aertrycke) (choleraesuis) (paratyphosus
(suipestifer) A02.9
botulinus A05.1
Clostridium (perfringens) (Welchii) A05.2
salmonella (aertrycke) (callinarum) (choleraesuis
(enteritidis) (paratyphi) (suipestifer) A02.
with
gastroenteritis A02.0
sepsis A02.1
staphylococcus A05.0
Vibrio
parahaemolyticus A05.3
vulnificus A05.5
noxious or naturally toxic T62.9- ☑
berries — *see* subcategory T62.1 ☑
fish — *see* Poisoning, seafood
mushrooms — *see* subcategory T62.0X ☑
plants NEC — *see* subcategory T62.2X ☑
seafood — *see* Poisoning, seafood
specified NEC — *see* subcategory T62.8X ☑
ichthyotoxism — *see* Poisoning, seafood
kreotoxism, food A05.9
latex T65.81- ☑
lead T56.0- ☑
mushroom — *see* Poisoning, food, noxious, mushroom
mussels — *see also* Poisoning, shellfish
bacterial — *see* Intoxication, foodborne, by agent
nicotine (tobacco) T65.2- ☑
noxious foodstuffs — *see* Poisoning, food, noxious
plants, noxious — *see* Poisoning, food, noxious, plant
NEC
ptomaine — *see* Poisoning, food
radiation J70.0
Salmonella (arizonae) (cholerae-suis) (enteritidis) (typhimurium) A02.9

Poisoning — continued
  scombroid fish T61.1- ☑
  seafood (noxious) T61.9- ☑
    bacterial — see Intoxication, foodborne, by agent
    fish — see Poisoning, fish
    shellfish — see Poisoning, shellfish
    specified NEC — see subcategory T61.8X ☑
  shellfish (amnesic) (azaspiracid) (diarrheic) (neurotoxic)
    (noxious) (paralytic) T61.78- ☑
    bacterial — see Intoxication, foodborne, by agent
    ciguatera mollusk — see Poisoning, ciguatera fish
  specified substance NEC T65.891 ☑
  Staphylococcus, food A05.0
  tobacco (nicotine) T65.2- ☑
  water E87.79
Poker spine — see Spondylitis, ankylosing
Poland syndrome Q79.8
Polioencephalitis (acute) (bulbar) A80.9
  inferior G12.22
  influenzal — see Influenza, with, encephalopathy
  superior hemorrhagic (acute) (Wernicke's) E51.2
  Wernicke's E51.2
Polioencephalomyelitis (acute) (anterior) A80.9
  with beriberi E51.2
Polioencephalopathy, superior hemorrhagic E51.2
  with
    beriberi E51.11
    pellagra E52
Poliomeningoencephalitis — see Meningoencephalitis
Poliomyelitis (acute) (anterior) (epidemic) A80.9
  with paralysis (bulbar) — see Poliomyelitis, paralytic
  abortive A80.4
  ascending (progressive) — see Poliomyelitis, paralytic
  bulbar (paralytic) — see Poliomyelitis, paralytic
  congenital P35.8
  nonepidemic A80.9
  nonparalytic A80.4
  paralytic A80.30
    specified NEC A80.39
    vaccine-associated A80.0
    wild virus
      imported A80.1
      indigenous A80.2
  spinal, acute A80.9
Poliosis (eyebrow) (eyelashes) L67.1
  circumscripta, acquired L67.1
Pollakiuria R35.0
  psychogenic F45.8
Pollinosis J30.1
Pollitzer's disease L73.2
Polyadenitis — see also Lymphadenitis
  malignant A20.0
Polyalgia M79.89
Polyangiitis M30.0
  microscopic M31.7
  overlap syndrome M30.8
Polyarteritis
  microscopic M31.7
  nodosa M30.0
    with lung involvement M30.1
    juvenile M30.2
    related condition NEC M30.8
Polyarthralgia — see Pain, joint
Polyarthritis, polyarthropathy — see also Arthritis
  M13.0
  due to or associated with other specified conditions
    — see Arthritis
  epidemic (Australian) (with exanthema) B33.1
  infective — see Arthritis, pyogenic or pyemic
  inflammatory M06.4
  juvenile (chronic) (seronegative) M08.3
  migratory M13.8- ☑
  rheumatic, acute — see Fever, rheumatic
Polyarthrosis M15.9
  post-traumatic M15.3
  primary M15.0
  specified NEC M15.8
Polycarential syndrome of infancy E40
Polychondritis (atrophic) (chronic) — see also Disorder,
  cartilage, specified type NEC
  relapsing M94.1
Polycoria Q13.2
Polycystic (disease)
  degeneration, kidney Q61.3
    autosomal dominant (adult type) Q61.2
    autosomal recessive (infantile type) NEC Q61.19
  kidney Q61.3

Polycystic — continued
  kidney — continued
    autosomal
      dominant Q61.2
      recessive NEC Q61.19
    autosomal dominant (adult type) Q61.2
    autosomal recessive (childhood type) NEC Q61.19
    infantile type NEC Q61.19
  liver Q44.6
  lung J98.4
    congenital Q33.0
  ovary, ovaries E28.2
  spleen Q89.09
Polycythemia (secondary) D75.1
  acquired D75.1
  benign (familial) D75.0
  due to
    donor twin P61.1
    erythropoietin D75.1
    fall in plasma volume D75.1
    high altitude D75.1
    maternal-fetal transfusion P61.1
    stress D75.1
  emotional D75.1
  erythropoietin D75.1
  familial (benign) D75.0
  Gaisböck's (hypertonica) D75.1
  high altitude D75.1
  hypertonica D75.1
  hypoxemic D75.1
  neonatorum P61.1
  nephrogenous D75.1
  relative D75.1
  secondary D75.1
  spurious D75.1
  stress D75.1
  vera D45
Polycytosis cryptogenica D75.1
Polydactylism, polydactyly Q69.9
  toes Q69.2
Polydipsia R63.1
Polydystrophy, pseudo-Hurler E77.0
Polyembryoma — see Neoplasm, malignant, by site
Polyglandular
  deficiency E31.0
  dyscrasia E31.9
  dysfunction E31.9
  syndrome E31.8
Polyhydramnios O40.- ☑
Polymastia Q83.1
Polymenorrhea N92.0
Polymyalgia M35.3
  arteritica, giant cell M31.5
  rheumatica M35.3
    with giant cell arteritis M31.5
Polymyositis (acute) (chronic) (hemorrhagic) M33.20
  with
    myopathy M33.22
    respiratory involvement M33.21
    skin involvement — see Dermatopolymyositis
    specified organ involvement NEC M33.29
  ossificans (generalisata) (progressiva) — see Myositis,
    ossificans, progressiva
Polyneuritis, polyneuritic — see also Polyneuropathy
  acute (post-)infective G61.0
  alcoholic G62.1
  cranialis G52.7
  demyelinating, chronic inflammatory (CIDP) G61.81
  diabetic — see Diabetes, polyneuropathy
  diphtheritic A36.83
  due to lack of vitamin NEC E56.9 [G63]
  endemic E51.11
  erythredema — see subcategory T56.1 ☑
  febrile, acute G61.0
  hereditary ataxic G60.1
  idiopathic, acute G61.0
  infective (acute) G61.0
  inflammatory, chronic demyelinating (CIDP) G61.81
  nutritional E63.9 [G63]
  postinfective (acute) G61.0
  specified NEC G62.89
Polyneuropathy (peripheral) G62.9
  alcoholic G62.1
  amyloid (Portuguese) E85.1 [G63]
    transthyretin-related (ATTR) familial E85.1 [G63]
  arsenical G62.2
  critical illness G62.81
  demyelinating, chronic inflammatory (CIDP) G61.81

Polyneuropathy — continued
  diabetic — see Diabetes, polyneuropathy
  drug-induced G62.0
  hereditary G60.9
    specified NEC G60.8
  idiopathic G60.9
    progressive G60.3
  in (due to)
    alcohol G62.1
      sequelae G65.2
    amyloidosis, familial (Portuguese) E85.1 [G63]
    antitetanus serum G61.1
    arsenic G62.2
      sequelae G65.2
    avitaminosis NEC E56.9 [G63]
    beriberi E51.11
    collagen vascular disease NEC M35.9 [G63]
    deficiency (of)
      B (-complex) vitamins E53.9 [G63]
      vitamin B6 E53.1 [G63]
    diabetes — see Diabetes, polyneuropathy
    diphtheria A36.83
    drug or medicament G62.0
      correct substance properly administered — see
        Table of Drugs and Chemicals, by drug,
        adverse effect
      overdose or wrong substance given or taken —
        see Table of Drugs and Chemicals, by drug,
        poisoning
    endocrine disease NEC E34.9 [G63]
    herpes zoster B02.23
    hypoglycemia E16.2 [G63]
    infectious
      disease NEC B99 ☑ [G63]
      mononucleosis B27.91
    lack of vitamin NEC E56.9 [G63]
    lead G62.2
      sequelae G65.2
    leprosy A30.9 [G63]
    Lyme disease A69.22
    metabolic disease NEC E88.9 [G63]
    microscopic polyangiitis M31.7 [G63]
    mumps B26.84
    neoplastic disease — see also Neoplasm D49.9 [G63]
    nutritional deficiency NEC E63.9 [G63]
    organophosphate compounds G62.2
      sequelae G65.2
    parasitic disease NEC B89 [G63]
    pellagra E52 [G63]
    polyarteritis nodosa M30.0
    porphyria E80.20 [G63]
    radiation G62.82
    rheumatoid arthritis — see Rheumatoid, polyneu-
      ropathy
    sarcoidosis D86.89
    serum G61.1
    syphilis (late) A52.15
      congenital A50.43
    systemic
      connective tissue disorder M35.9 [G63]
      lupus erythematosus M32.19
    toxic agent NEC G62.2
      sequelae G65.2
  inflammatory G61.9
    chronic demyelinating (CIDP) G61.81
    sequelae G65.1
    specified NEC G61.89
  lead G62.2
    sequelae G65.2
  nutritional NEC E63.9 [G63]
  postherpetic (zoster) B02.23
  progressive G60.3
  radiation-induced G62.82
  sensory (hereditary) (idiopathic) G60.8
  specified NEC G62.89
  syphilitic (late) A52.15
    congenital A50.43
  transthyretin-related (ATTR) familial amyloid E85.1
    triorthocresyl phosphate G62.2
      sequelae G65.2
    tuberculosis A17.89
    uremia N18.9 [G63]
    vitamin B12 deficiency E53.8 [G63]
      with anemia (pernicious) D51.0 [G63]
        due to dietary deficiency D51.3 [G63]
    zoster B02.23
Polyopia H53.8
Polyorchism, polyorchidism Q55.21

Polyosteoarthritis — *see also* Osteoarthritis, generalized
    M15.9
  post-traumatic M15.3
  specified NEC M15.8
Polyostotic fibrous dysplasia Q78.1
Polyotia Q17.0
Polyp, polypus
  accessory sinus J33.8
  adenocarcinoma in — *see* Neoplasm, malignant, by
      site
  adenocarcinoma in situ — *see* Neoplasm, in situ, by
      site
  adenoid tissue J33.0
  adenomatous — *see also* Neoplasm, benign, by site
    adenocarcinoma in — *see* Neoplasm, malignant, by
        site
    adenocarcinoma in situ in — *see* Neoplasm, in situ,
        by site
    carcinoma in — *see* Neoplasm, malignant, by site
    carcinoma in situ in — *see* Neoplasm, in situ, by site
    multiple — *see* Neoplasm, benign
      adenocarcinoma in — *see* Neoplasm, malignant,
          by site
      adenocarcinoma in situ in — *see* Neoplasm, in
          situ, by site
  antrum J33.8
  anus, anal (canal) K62.0
  Bartholin's gland N84.3
  bladder D41.4
  carcinoma in — *see* Neoplasm, malignant, by site
  carcinoma in situ in — *see* Neoplasm, in situ, by site
  cecum D12.0
  cervix (uteri) N84.1
    in pregnancy or childbirth — *see* Pregnancy, com-
        plicated by, abnormal, cervix
    mucous N84.1
    nonneoplastic N84.1
  choanal J33.0
  cholesterol K82.4
  clitoris N84.3
  colon K63.5
    adenomatous D12.6
      ascending D12.2
      cecum D12.0
      descending D12.4
    hyperplastic, (any site) K63.5
    inflammatory K51.40
      with
        abscess K51.414
        complication K51.419
          specified NEC K51.418
        fistula K51.413
        intestinal obstruction K51.412
        rectal bleeding K51.411
    sigmoid D12.5
    transverse D12.3
  corpus uteri N84.0
  dental K04.01
    irreversible K04.02
    reversible K04.01
  duodenum K31.7
  ear (middle) H74.4- ☑
  endometrium N84.0
  ethmoidal (sinus) J33.8
  fallopian tube N84.8
  female genital tract N84.9
    specified NEC N84.8
  frontal (sinus) J33.8
  gallbladder K82.4
  gingiva, gum K06.8
  labia, labium (majus) (minus) N84.3
  larynx (mucous) J38.1
    adenomatous D14.1
  malignant — *see* Neoplasm, malignant, by site
  maxillary (sinus) J33.8
  middle ear — *see* Polyp, ear (middle)
  myometrium N84.0
  nares
    anterior J33.9
    posterior J33.0
  nasal (mucous) J33.9
    cavity J33.0
    septum J33.0
  nasopharyngeal J33.0
  nose (mucous) J33.9
  oviduct N84.8
  pharynx J39.2
  placenta O90.89

Polyp, polypus — *continued*
  prostate — *see* Enlargement, enlarged, prostate
  pudenda, pudendum N84.3
  pulpal (dental) K04.01
    irreversible K04.02
    reversible K04.01
  rectum (nonadenomatous) K62.1
    adenomatous — *see* Polyp, adenomatous
  septum (nasal) J33.0
  sinus (accessory) (ethmoidal) (frontal) (maxillary)
      (sphenoidal) J33.8
  sphenoidal (sinus) J33.8
  stomach K31.7
    adenomatous D13.1
  tube, fallopian N84.8
  turbinate, mucous membrane J33.8
  umbilical, newborn P83.6
  ureter N28.89
  urethra N36.2
  uterus (body) (corpus) (mucous) N84.0
    cervix N84.1
    in pregnancy or childbirth — *see* Pregnancy, com-
        plicated by, tumor, uterus
  vagina N84.2
  vocal cord (mucous) J38.1
  vulva N84.3
Polyphagia R63.2
Polyploidy Q92.7
Polypoid — *see* condition
Polyposis — *see also* Polyp
  coli (adenomatous) D12.6
    adenocarcinoma in C18.9
    adenocarcinoma in situ in — *see* Neoplasm, in situ,
        by site
    carcinoma in C18.9
  colon (adenomatous) D12.6
  familial D12.6
    adenocarcinoma in situ in — *see* Neoplasm, in situ,
        by site
  intestinal (adenomatous) D12.6
  malignant lymphomatous C83.1- ☑
  multiple, adenomatous — *see also* Neoplasm, benign
      D36.9
Polyradiculitis — *see* Polyneuropathy
Polyradiculoneuropathy (acute) (postinfective) (seg-
    mentally demyelinating) G61.0
Polyserositis
  due to pericarditis I31.1
  pericardial I31.1
  periodic, familial E85.0
  tuberculous A19.9
    acute A19.1
    chronic A19.8
Polysplenia syndrome Q89.09
Polysyndactyly — *see also* Syndactylism, syndactyly
    Q70.4
Polytrichia L68.3
Polyunguia Q84.6
Polyuria R35.8
  nocturnal R35.1
  psychogenic F45.8
Pompe's disease (glycogen storage) E74.02
Pompholyx L30.1
Poncet's disease (tuberculous rheumatism) A18.09
Pond fracture — *see* Fracture, skull
Ponos B55.0
Pons, pontine — *see* condition
Poor
  aesthetic of existing restoration of tooth K08.56
  contractions, labor O62.2
  gingival margin to tooth restoration K08.51
  personal hygiene R46.0
  prenatal care, affecting management of pregnancy —
      see Pregnancy, complicated by, insufficient,
      prenatal care
  sucking reflex (newborn) R29.2
  urinary stream R39.12
  vision NEC H54.7
Poradenitis, nostras inguinalis or venerea A55
Porencephaly (congenital) (developmental) (true) Q04.6
  acquired G93.0
  nondevelopmental G93.0
  traumatic (post) F07.89
Porocephaliasis B88.8
Porokeratosis Q82.8
Poroma, eccrine — *see* Neoplasm, skin, benign
Porphyria (South African) E80.20
  acquired E80.20

Porphyria — *continued*
  acute intermittent (hepatic) (Swedish) E80.21
  cutanea tarda (hereditary) (symptomatic) E80.1
  due to drugs E80.20
    correct substance properly administered — *see* Ta-
        ble of Drugs and Chemicals, by drug, adverse
        effect
    overdose or wrong substance given or taken — *see*
        Table of Drugs and Chemicals, by drug, poi-
        soning
  erythropoietic (congenital) (hereditary) E80.0
  hepatocutaneous type E80.1
  secondary E80.20
  toxic NEC E80.20
  variegata E80.20
Porphyrinuria — *see* Porphyria
Porphyruria — *see* Porphyria
Port wine nevus, mark, or stain Q82.5
Portal — *see* condition
Posadas-Wernicke disease B38.9
Positive
  culture (nonspecific)
    blood R78.81
    bronchial washings R84.5
    cerebrospinal fluid R83.5
    cervix uteri R87.5
    nasal secretions R84.5
    nipple discharge R89.5
    nose R84.5
      staphylococcus (Methicillin susceptible) Z22.321
        Methicillin resistant Z22.322
    peritoneal fluid R85.5
    pleural fluid R84.5
    prostatic secretions R86.5
    saliva R85.5
    seminal fluid R86.5
    sputum R84.5
    synovial fluid R89.5
    throat scrapings R84.5
    urine R82.79
    vagina R87.5
    vulva R87.5
    wound secretions R89.5
  PPD (skin test) R76.11
  serology for syphilis A53.0
    false R76.8
    with signs or symptoms — *code as* Syphilis, by site
        and stage
  skin test, tuberculin (without active tuberculosis) R76.11
  test, human immunodeficiency virus (HIV) R75
  VDRL A53.0
    with signs or symptoms — *code by* site and stage
        under Syphilis A53.9
  Wassermann reaction A53.0
Postcardiotomy syndrome I97.0
Postcaval ureter Q62.62
Postcholecystectomy syndrome K91.5
Postclimacteric bleeding N95.0
Postcommissurotomy syndrome I97.0
Postconcussional syndrome F07.81
Postcontusional syndrome F07.81
Postcricoid region — *see* condition
Post-dates (40-42 weeks) (pregnancy) (mother) O48.0
  more than 42 weeks gestation O48.1
Postencephalitic syndrome F07.89
Posterior — *see* condition
Posterolateral sclerosis (spinal cord) — *see* Degenera-
    tion, combined
Postexanthematous — *see* condition
Postfebrile — *see* condition
Postgastrectomy dumping syndrome K91.1
Posthemiplegic chorea — *see* Monoplegia
Posthemorrhagic anemia (chronic) D50.0
  acute D62
  newborn P61.3
Postherpetic neuralgia (zoster) B02.29
  trigeminal B02.22
Posthitis N47.7
Postimmunization complication or reaction — *see*
    Complications, vaccination
Postinfectious — *see* condition
Postlaminectomy syndrome NEC M96.1
Postleukotomy syndrome F07.0
Postmastectomy lymphedema (syndrome) I97.2
Postmaturity, postmature (over 42 weeks)
  maternal (over 42 weeks gestation) O48.1
  newborn P08.22

Polyosteoarthritis — Postmaturity, postmature

262   ☑ **Additional Character Required — Refer to the Tabular List for Character Selection**   ▼ **Subterms under main terms may continue to next column or page**

Postmeasles complication NEC — *see also* condition
  B05.89
Postmenopausal
  endometrium (atrophic) N95.8
    suppurative — *see also* Endometritis N71.9
  osteoporosis — *see* Osteoporosis, postmenopausal
Postnasal drip R09.82
  due to
    allergic rhinitis — *see* Rhinitis, allergic
    common cold J00
    gastroesophageal reflux — *see* Reflux, gastroe-
      sophageal
    nasopharyngitis — *see* Nasopharyngitis
    other known condition — *code to* condition
    sinusitis — *see* Sinusitis
Postnatal — *see* condition
Postoperative (postprocedural) — *see* Complication,
  postoperative
  pneumothorax, therapeutic Z98.3
  state NEC Z98.890
Postpancreatectomy hyperglycemia E89.1
Postpartum — *see* Puerperal
Postphlebitic syndrome — *see* Syndrome, postthrom-
  botic
Postpolio (myelitic) **syndrome** G14
Postpoliomyelitic — *see also* condition
  osteopathy — *see* Osteopathy, after poliomyelitis
Postprocedural — *see also* Postoperative
  hypoinsulinemia E89.1
Postschizophrenic depression F32.89
Postsurgery status — *see also* Status (post)
  pneumothorax, therapeutic Z98.3
Post-term (40-42 weeks) (pregnancy) (mother) O48.0
  infant P08.21
  more than 42 weeks gestation (mother) O48.1
Post-traumatic brain syndrome, nonpsychotic F07.81
Post-typhoid abscess A01.09
Postures, hysterical F44.2
Postvaccinal reaction or complication — *see* Complications, vaccination
Postvalvulotomy syndrome I97.0
Potain's
  disease (pulmonary edema) — *see* Edema, lung
  syndrome (gastrectasis with dyspepsia) K31.0
Potter's
  asthma J62.8
  facies Q60.6
  lung J62.8
  syndrome (with renal agenesis) Q60.6
Pott's
  curvature (spinal) A18.01
  disease or paraplegia A18.01
  spinal curvature A18.01
  tumor, puffy — *see* Osteomyelitis, specified type NEC
Pouch
  bronchus Q32.4
  Douglas' — *see* condition
  esophagus, esophageal, congenital Q39.6
    acquired K22.5
  gastric K31.4
  Hartmann's K82.8
  pharynx, pharyngeal (congenital) Q38.7
Pouchitis K91.850
Poultrymen's itch B88.0
Poverty NEC Z59.6
  extreme Z59.5
Poxvirus NEC B08.8
Prader-Willi syndrome Q87.11
Prader-Willi-like syndrome Q87.19
Preauricular appendage or tag Q17.0
Prebetalipoproteinemia (acquired) (essential) (familial)
  (hereditary) (primary) (secondary) E78.1
  with chylomicronemia E78.3
Precipitate labor or delivery O62.3
Preclimacteric bleeding (menorrhagia) N92.4
Precocious
  adrenarche E30.1
  menarche E30.1
  menstruation E30.1
  pubarche E30.1
  puberty E30.1
    central E22.8
  sexual development NEC E30.1
  thelarche E30.8
Precocity, sexual (constitutional) (cryptogenic) (female)
  (idiopathic) (male) E30.1
  with adrenal hyperplasia E25.9

Precocity, sexual — *continued*
  with adrenal hyperplasia — *continued*
    congenital E25.0
Precordial pain R07.2
Predeciduous teeth K00.2
Prediabetes, prediabetic R73.03
  complicating
    pregnancy — *see* Pregnancy, complicated by, dis-
      eases of, specified type or system NEC
    puerperium O99.893
Predislocation status of hip at birth Q65.6
Pre-eclampsia O14.9- ☑
  with pre-existing hypertension — *see* Hypertension,
    complicating pregnancy, pre-existing, with, pre-
    eclampsia
  complicating
    childbirth O14.94
    puerperium O14.95
  mild O14.0- ☑
    complicating
      childbirth O14.04
      puerperium O14.05
  moderate O14.0- ☑
    complicating
      childbirth O14.04
      puerperium O14.05
  severe O14.1- ☑
    with hemolysis, elevated liver enzymes and low
      platelet count (HELLP) O14.2- ☑
      complicating
        childbirth O14.24
        puerperium O14.25
    complicating
      childbirth O14.14
      puerperium O14.15
Pre-eruptive color change, teeth, tooth K00.8
Pre-excitation atrioventricular conduction I45.6
Preglaucoma H40.00- ☑
Pregnancy (single) (uterine) — *see also* Delivery and
  Puerperal Z33.1

  Note: The Tabular must be reviewed for assign-
  ment of appropriate seventh character for mul-
  tiple gestation codes in Chapter 15

  Note: The Tabular must be reviewed for assign-
  ment of the appropriate character indicating the
  trimester of the pregnancy

  abdominal (ectopic) O00.00
    with intrauterine pregnancy O00.01
      with viable fetus O36.7- ☑
  ampullar O00.10- ☑
    with intrauterine pregnancy O00.11- ☑
  biochemical O02.81
  broad ligament O00.80
    with intrauterine pregnancy O00.81
  cervical O00.8
    with intrauterine pregnancy O00.81
  chemical O02.81
  complicated by (care of) (management affected by)
    abnormal, abnormality
      cervix O34.4- ☑
        causing obstructed labor O65.5
      cord (umbilical) O69.9 ☑
      fetal heart rate or rhythm O36.83- ☑
      findings on antenatal screening of mother O28.9
        biochemical O28.1
        chromosomal O28.5
        cytological O28.2
        genetic O28.5
        hematological O28.0
        radiological O28.4
        specified NEC O28.8
        ultrasonic O28.3
      glucose (tolerance) NEC O99.810
      pelvic organs O34.9- ☑
        specified NEC O34.8- ☑
          causing obstructed labor O65.5
      pelvis (bony) (major) NEC O33.0
      perineum O34.7- ☑
      position
        placenta O44.0- ☑
          with hemorrhage O44.1- ☑
        uterus O34.59- ☑
      uterus O34.59- ☑
        causing obstructed labor O65.5
        congenital O34.0- ☑

Pregnancy — *continued*
  complicated by — *continued*
    abnormal, abnormality — *continued*
      vagina O34.6- ☑
        causing obstructed labor O65.5
      vulva O34.7- ☑
        causing obstructed labor O65.5
    abruptio placentae — *see* Abruptio placentae
    abscess or cellulitis
      bladder O23.1- ☑
      breast O91.11- ☑
      genital organ or tract O23.9- ☑
    abuse
      physical O9A.31 ☑ (*following* O99)
      psychological O9A.51 ☑ (*following* O99)
      sexual O9A.41 ☑ (*following* O99)
    adverse effect anesthesia O29.9- ☑
      aspiration pneumonitis O29.01- ☑
      cardiac arrest O29.11- ☑
      cardiac complication NEC O29.19- ☑
      cardiac failure O29.12- ☑
      central nervous system complication NEC
        O29.29- ☑
      cerebral anoxia O29.21- ☑
      failed or difficult intubation O29.6- ☑
      inhalation of stomach contents or secretions NOS
        O29.01- ☑
      local, toxic reaction O29.3X ☑
      Mendelson's syndrome O29.01- ☑
      pressure collapse of lung O29.02- ☑
      pulmonary complications NEC O29.09- ☑
      specified NEC O29.8X- ☑
      spinal and epidural type NEC O29.5X ☑
        induced headache O29.4- ☑
    albuminuria — *see also* Proteinuria, gestational
      O12.1- ☑
    alcohol use O99.31- ☑
    amnionitis O41.12- ☑
    anaphylactoid syndrome of pregnancy O88.01- ☑
    anemia (conditions in D50-D64) (pre-existing)
      O99.01- ☑
      complicating the puerperium O99.03
    antepartum hemorrhage O46.9- ☑
      with coagulation defect — *see* Hemorrhage,
        antepartum, with coagulation defect
      specified NEC O46.8X- ☑
    appendicitis O99.61- ☑
    atrophy (yellow) (acute) liver (subacute) O26.61- ☑
    bariatric surgery status O99.84- ☑
    bicornis or bicornuate uterus O34.0- ☑
    biliary tract problems O26.61- ☑
    breech presentation O32.1 ☑
    cardiovascular diseases (conditions in I00-I09, I20-
      I52, I70-I99) O99.41- ☑
    cerebrovascular disorders (conditions in I60-I69)
      O99.41- ☑
    cervical shortening O26.87- ☑
    cervicitis O23.51- ☑
    cesarean scar defect (isthmocele) O34.22
    chloasma (gravidarum) O26.89- ☑
    cholecystitis O99.61- ☑
    cholestasis (intrahepatic) O26.61- ☑
    chorioamnionitis O41.12- ☑
    circulatory system disorder (conditions in I00-I09,
      I20-I99, O99.41-)
    compound presentation O32.6 ☑
    conjoined twins O30.02- ☑
    connective system disorders (conditions in M00-
      M99) O99.891
    contracted pelvis (general) O33.1
      inlet O33.2
      outlet O33.3 ☑
    convulsions (eclamptic) (uremic) — *see also*
      Eclampsia O15.9
    cracked nipple O92.11- ☑
    cystitis O23.1- ☑
    cystocele O34.8- ☑
    death of fetus (near term) O36.4 ☑
      early pregnancy O02.1
      of one fetus or more in multiple gestation
        O31.2- ☑
    deciduitis O41.14- ☑
    decreased fetal movement O36.81- ☑
    dental problems O99.61- ☑
    diabetes (mellitus) O24.91- ☑

Pregnancy — *continued*
  complicated by — *continued*
    diabetes — *continued*
      gestational (pregnancy induced) — *see* Diabetes, gestational
      pre-existing O24.31- ☑
        specified NEC O24.81- ☑
        type 1 O24.01- ☑
        type 2 O24.11- ☑
    digestive system disorders (conditions in K00-K93) O99.61- ☑
    diseases of — *see* Pregnancy, complicated by, specified body system disease
      biliary tract O26.61- ☑
      blood NEC (conditions in D65-D77) O99.11- ☑
      liver O26.61- ☑
      specified NEC O99.891
    disorders of — *see* Pregnancy, complicated by, specified body system disorder
      amniotic fluid and membranes O41.9- ☑
        specified NEC O41.8X- ☑
      biliary tract O26.61- ☑
      ear and mastoid process (conditions in H60-H95) O99.891
      eye and adnexa (conditions in H00-H59) O99.891
      liver O26.61- ☑
      skin (conditions in L00-L99) O99.71- ☑
      specified NEC O99.891
    displacement, uterus NEC O34.59- ☑
      causing obstructed labor O65.5
    disproportion (due to) O33.9
      fetal (ascites) (hydrops) (meningomyelocele) (sacral teratoma) (tumor) deformities NEC O33.7 ☑
      generally contracted pelvis O33.1
      hydrocephalic fetus O33.6 ☑
      inlet contraction of pelvis O33.2
      mixed maternal and fetal origin O33.4 ☑
      specified NEC O33.8
    double uterus O34.0- ☑
      causing obstructed labor O65.5
    drug use (conditions in F11-F19) O99.32- ☑
    eclampsia, eclamptic (coma) (convulsions) (delirium) (nephritis) (uremia) — *see also* Eclampsia O15.- ☑
    ectopic pregnancy — *see* Pregnancy, ectopic
    edema O12.0- ☑
      with
        gestational hypertension, mild — *see also* Pre-eclampsia O14.0- ☑
        proteinuria O12.2- ☑
    effusion, amniotic fluid — *see* Pregnancy, complicated by, premature rupture of membranes
    elderly
      multigravida O09.52- ☑
      primigravida O09.51- ☑
    embolism — *see also* Embolism, obstetric, pregnancy O88.- ☑
    endocrine diseases NEC O99.28- ☑
    endometritis O86.12
    excessive weight gain O26.0- ☑
    exhaustion O26.81- ☑
      during labor and delivery O75.81
    face presentation O32.3 ☑
    failed induction of labor O61.9
      instrumental O61.1
      mechanical O61.1
      medical O61.0
      specified NEC O61.8
      surgical O61.1
    failed or difficult intubation for anesthesia O29.6- ☑
    false labor (pains) O47.9
      at or after 37 completed weeks of pregnancy O47.1
      before 37 completed weeks of pregnancy O47.0- ☑
    fatigue O26.81- ☑
      during labor and delivery O75.81
    fatty metamorphosis of liver O26.61- ☑
    female genital mutilation O34.8- ☑ *[N90.81-]*
    fetal (maternal care for)
      abnormality or damage O35.9 ☑
        acid-base balance O68
        specified type NEC O35.8 ☑
      acidemia O68
      acidosis O68
      alkalosis O68

Pregnancy — *continued*
  complicated by — *continued*
    fetal — *continued*
      anemia and thrombocytopenia O36.82- ☑
      anencephaly O35.0 ☑
      bradycardia O36.83- ☑
      chromosomal abnormality (conditions in Q90-Q99) O35.1 ☑
      conjoined twins O30.02- ☑
      damage from
        amniocentesis O35.7 ☑
        biopsy procedures O35.7 ☑
        drug addiction O35.5 ☑
        hematological investigation O35.7 ☑
        intrauterine contraceptive device O35.7 ☑
        maternal
          alcohol addiction O35.4 ☑
          cytomegalovirus infection O35.3 ☑
          disease NEC O35.8 ☑
          drug addiction O35.5 ☑
          listeriosis O35.8 ☑
          rubella O35.3 ☑
          toxoplasmosis O35.8 ☑
          viral infection O35.3 ☑
        medical procedure NEC O35.7 ☑
        radiation O35.6 ☑
      death (near term) O36.4 ☑
        early pregnancy O02.1
      decreased movement O36.81- ☑
      depressed heart rate tones O36.83- ☑
      disproportion due to deformity (fetal) O33.7 ☑
      excessive growth (large for dates) O36.6- ☑
      growth retardation O36.59- ☑
        light for dates O36.59- ☑
        small for dates O36.59- ☑
      heart rate irregularity (abnormal variability) (bradycardia) (decelerations) (tachycardia) O36.83- ☑
      hereditary disease O35.2 ☑
      hydrocephalus O35.0 ☑
      intrauterine death O36.4 ☑
      non-reassuring heart rate or rhythm O36.83- ☑
      poor growth O36.59- ☑
        light for dates O36.59- ☑
        small for dates O36.59- ☑
      problem O36.9- ☑
        specified NEC O36.89- ☑
      reduction (elective) O31.3- ☑
      selective termination O31.3- ☑
      spina bifida O35.0 ☑
      thrombocytopenia O36.82- ☑
    fibroid (tumor) (uterus) O34.1- ☑
    fissure of nipple O92.11- ☑
    gallstones O99.61- ☑
    gastric banding status O99.84- ☑
    gastric bypass status O99.84- ☑
    genital herpes (asymptomatic) (history of) (inactive) O98.3- ☑
    genital tract infection O23.9- ☑
    glomerular diseases (conditions in N00-N07) O26.83- ☑
      with hypertension, pre-existing — *see* Hypertension, complicating, pregnancy, pre-existing, with, renal disease
    gonorrhea O98.21- ☑
    grand multiparity O09.4 ☑
    habitual aborter — *see* Pregnancy, complicated by, recurrent pregnancy loss
    HELLP syndrome (hemolysis, elevated liver enzymes and low platelet count) O14.2- ☑
    hemorrhage
      antepartum — *see* Hemorrhage, antepartum
      before 20 completed weeks gestation O20.9
        specified NEC O20.8
      due to premature separation, placenta — *see also* Abruptio placentae O45.9- ☑
      early O20.9
        specified NEC O20.8
      threatened abortion O20.0
    hemorrhoids O22.4- ☑
    hepatitis (viral) O98.41- ☑
    herniation of uterus O34.59- ☑
    high
      head at term O32.4 ☑
      risk — *see* Supervision (of) (for), high-risk

Pregnancy — *continued*
  complicated by — *continued*
    history of in utero procedure during previous pregnancy O09.82- ☑
    HIV O98.71- ☑
    human immunodeficiency virus (HIV) disease O98.71- ☑
    hydatidiform mole — *see also* Mole, hydatidiform O01.9
    hydramnios O40.- ☑
    hydrocephalic fetus (disproportion) O33.6 ☑
    hydrops
      amnii O40.- ☑
      fetalis O36.2- ☑
        associated with isoimmunization — *see also* Pregnancy, complicated by, isoimmunization O36.11- ☑
    hydrorrhea O42.90
    hyperemesis (gravidarum) (mild) — *see also* Hyperemesis, gravidarum O21.0
    hypertension — *see* Hypertension, complicating pregnancy
    hypertensive
      heart and renal disease, pre-existing — *see* Hypertension, complicating, pregnancy, pre-existing, with, heart disease, with renal disease
      heart disease, pre-existing — *see* Hypertension, complicating, pregnancy, pre-existing, with, heart disease
      renal disease, pre-existing — *see* Hypertension, complicating, pregnancy, pre-existing, with, renal disease
    hypotension O26.5- ☑
    immune disorders NEC (conditions in D80-D89) O99.11- ☑
    incarceration, uterus O34.51- ☑
    incompetent cervix O34.3- ☑
    inconclusive fetal viability O36.80 ☑
    infection(s) O98.91- ☑
      amniotic fluid or sac O41.10- ☑
      bladder O23.1- ☑
      carrier state NEC O99.830
        streptococcus B O99.820
      genital organ or tract O23.9- ☑
        specified NEC O23.59- ☑
      genitourinary tract O23.9- ☑
      gonorrhea O98.21- ☑
      hepatitis (viral) O98.41- ☑
      HIV O98.71- ☑
      human immunodeficiency virus (HIV) O98.71- ☑
      kidney O23.0- ☑
      nipple O91.01- ☑
      parasitic disease O98.91- ☑
        specified NEC O98.81- ☑
      protozoal disease O98.61- ☑
      sexually transmitted NEC O98.31- ☑
      specified type NEC O98.81- ☑
      syphilis O98.11- ☑
      tuberculosis O98.01- ☑
      urethra O23.2- ☑
      urinary (tract) O23.4- ☑
        specified NEC O23.3- ☑
      viral disease O98.51- ☑
    injury or poisoning (conditions in S00-T88) O9A.21- ☑ (*following* O99)
      due to abuse
        physical O9A.31- ☑ (*following* O99)
        psychological O9A.51- ☑ (*following* O99)
        sexual O9A.41- ☑ (*following* O99)
    insufficient
      prenatal care O09.3- ☑
      weight gain O26.1- ☑
    insulin resistance O26.89 ☑
    intrauterine fetal death (near term) O36.4 ☑
      early pregnancy O02.1
      multiple gestation (one fetus or more) O31.2- ☑
    isoimmunization O36.11- ☑
      anti-A sensitization O36.11- ☑
      anti-B sensitization O36.19- ☑
      Rh O36.09- ☑
        anti-D antibody O36.01- ☑
      specified NEC O36.19- ☑
    laceration of uterus NEC O71.81
    malformation
      placenta, placental (vessel) O43.10- ☑

☑ **Additional Character Required** — Refer to the Tabular List for Character Selection   Ⓥ **Subterms under main terms may continue to next column or page**

Pregnancy — *continued*
  cornual — *continued*
    with intrauterine pregnancy O00.81
  ectopic (ruptured) O00.90
    with intrauterine pregnancy O00.91
    abdominal O00.00
      with
        intrauterine pregnancy O00.01
          viable fetus O36.7- ☑
    cervical O00.80
      with intrauterine pregnancy O00.81
    complicated (by) O08.9
      afibrinogenemia O08.1
      cardiac arrest O08.81
      chemical damage of pelvic organ(s) O08.6
      circulatory collapse O08.3
      defibrination syndrome O08.1
      electrolyte imbalance O08.5
      embolism (amniotic fluid) (blood clot) (pulmonary) (septic) O08.2
      endometritis O08.0
      genital tract and pelvic infection O08.0
      hemorrhage (delayed) (excessive) O08.1
      infection
        genital tract or pelvic O08.0
        kidney O08.83
        urinary tract O08.3
      intravascular coagulation O08.1
      laceration of pelvic organ(s) O08.6
      metabolic disorder O08.5
      oliguria O08.4
      oophoritis O08.0
      parametritis O08.0
      pelvic peritonitis O08.0
      perforation of pelvic organ(s) O08.6
      renal failure or shutdown O08.4
      salpingitis or salpingo-oophoritis O08.0
      sepsis O08.82
      shock O08.83
        septic O08.82
      specified condition NEC O08.89
      tubular necrosis (renal) O08.4
      uremia O08.4
      urinary infection O08.83
      venous complication NEC O08.7
        embolism O08.2
    cornual O00.80
      with intrauterine pregnancy O00.81
    intraligamentous O00.80
      with intrauterine pregnancy O00.81
    mural O00.80
      with intrauterine pregnancy O00.81
    ovarian O00.20- ☑
      with intrauterine pregnancy O00.21- ☑
    specified site NEC O00.80
      with intrauterine pregnancy O00.81
    tubal (ruptured) O00.10- ☑
      with intrauterine pregnancy O00.11- ☑
  examination (normal) Z34.9- ☑
    first Z34.0- ☑
    high-risk — *see* Pregnancy, supervision of, high-risk
    specified Z34.8- ☑
  extrauterine — *see* Pregnancy, ectopic
  fallopian O00.10- ☑
    with intrauterine pregnancy O00.11- ☑
  false F45.8
  gestational carrier Z33.3
  heptachorionic, hepta-amniotic (septuplets) O30.83- ☑
  hexachorionic, hexa-amniotic (sextuplets) O30.83- ☑
  hidden O09.3- ☑
  high-risk — *see* Pregnancy, supervision of, high-risk
  incidental finding Z33.1
  interstitial O00.80
    with intrauterine pregnancy O00.81
  intraligamentous O00.80
    with intrauterine pregnancy O00.81
  intramural O00.80
    with intrauterine pregnancy O00.81
  intraperitoneal O00.00
    with intrauterine pregnancy O00.01
  isthmian O00.10- ☑
    with intrauterine pregnancy O00.11- ☑
  mesometric (mural) O00.80
    with intrauterine pregnancy O00.81
  molar NEC O02.0
    complicated (by) O08.9
      afibrinogenemia O08.1
      cardiac arrest O08.81

Pregnancy — *continued*
  molar — *continued*
    complicated — *continued*
      chemical damage of pelvic organ(s) O08.6
      circulatory collapse O08.3
      defibrination syndrome O08.1
      electrolyte imbalance O08.5
      embolism (amniotic fluid) (blood clot) (pulmonary) (septic) O08.2
      endometritis O08.0
      genital tract and pelvic infection O08.0
      hemorrhage (delayed) (excessive) O08.1
      infection
        genital tract or pelvic O08.0
        kidney O08.83
        urinary tract O08.83
      intravascular coagulation O08.1
      laceration of pelvic organ(s) O08.6
      metabolic disorder O08.5
      oliguria O08.4
      oophoritis O08.0
      parametritis O08.0
      pelvic peritonitis O08.0
      perforation of pelvic organ(s) O08.6
      renal failure or shutdown O08.4
      salpingitis or salpingo-oophoritis O08.0
      sepsis O08.82
      shock O08.3
        septic O08.82
      specified condition NEC O08.89
      tubular necrosis (renal) O08.4
      uremia O08.4
      urinary infection O08.83
      venous complication NEC O08.7
        embolism O08.2
    hydatidiform — *see also* Mole, hydatidiform O01.9
  multiple (gestation) O30.9- ☑
    greater than quadruplets — *see* Pregnancy, multiple (gestation), specified NEC
    specified NEC O30.80- ☑
      with
        two or more monoamniotic fetuses O30.82- ☑
        two or more monochorionic fetuses O30.81- ☑
        number of chorions and amnions are both equal to the number of fetuses O30.83- ☑
      two or more monoamniotic fetuses O30.82- ☑
      two or more monochorionic fetuses O30.81- ☑
      unable to determine number of placenta and number of amniotic sacs O30.89- ☑
      unspecified number of placenta and unspecified number of amniotic sacs O30.80- ☑
  mural O00.80
    with intrauterine pregnancy O00.81
  normal (supervision of) Z34.9- ☑
    first Z34.0- ☑
    high-risk — *see* Pregnancy, supervision of, high-risk
    specified Z34.8- ☑
  ovarian O00.20- ☑
    with intrauterine pregnancy O00.21- ☑
  pentachorionic, penta-amniotic (quintuplets) O30.83- ☑
  postmature (40 to 42 weeks) O48.0
    more than 42 weeks gestation O48.1
  post-term (40 to 42 weeks) O48.0
  prenatal care only Z34.9- ☑
    first Z34.0- ☑
    high-risk — *see* Pregnancy, supervision of, high-risk
    specified Z34.8- ☑
  prolonged (more than 42 weeks gestation) O48.1
  quadruplet O30.20- ☑
    with
      two or more monoamniotic fetuses O30.22- ☑
      two or more monochorionic fetuses O30.21- ☑
      quadrachorionic/quadra-amniotic O30.23- ☑
    two or more monoamniotic fetuses O30.22- ☑
    two or more monochorionic fetuses O30.21- ☑
    unable to determine number of placenta and number of amniotic sacs O30.29- ☑
    unspecified number of placenta and unspecified number of amniotic sacs O30.20- ☑
  quintuplet — *see* Pregnancy, multiple (gestation), specified NEC
  sextuplet — *see* Pregnancy, multiple (gestation), specified NEC

Pregnancy — *continued*
  supervision of
    concealed pregnancy O09.3- ☑
    elderly mother
      multigravida O09.52- ☑
      primigravida O09.51- ☑
    hidden pregnancy O09.3- ☑
    high-risk O09.9- ☑
      due to (history of)
        ectopic pregnancy O09.1- ☑
        elderly — *see* Pregnancy, supervision, elderl? mother
        grand multiparity O09.4 ☑
        in utero procedure during previous pregnancy O09.82- ☑
        in vitro fertilization O09.81- ☑
        infertility O09.0- ☑
        insufficient prenatal care O09.3- ☑
        molar pregnancy O09.A- ☑
        multiple previous pregnancies O09.4- ☑
        older mother — *see* Pregnancy, supervision of, elderly mother
        poor reproductive or obstetric history NEC O09.29- ☑
        pre-term labor O09.21- ☑
        previous
          neonatal death O09.29- ☑
        social problems O09.7- ☑
        specified NEC O09.89- ☑
        very young mother — *see* Pregnancy, supervision, young mother
      resulting from in vitro fertilization O09.81- ☑
    normal Z34.9- ☑
      first Z34.0- ☑
      specified NEC Z34.8- ☑
    young mother
      multigravida O09.62- ☑
      primigravida O09.61- ☑
  triplet O30.10- ☑
    with
      two or more monoamniotic fetuses O30.12- ☑
      two or more monochorionic fetuses O30.11- ☑
    trichorionic/triamniotic O30.13- ☑
    two or more monoamniotic fetuses O30.12- ☑
    two or more monochorionic fetuses O30.11- ☑
    unable to determine number of placenta and number of amniotic sacs O30.19- ☑
    unspecified number of placenta and unspecified number of amniotic sacs O30.10- ☑
  tubal (with abortion) (with rupture) O00.10- ☑
    with intrauterine pregnancy O00.11- ☑
  twin O30.00- ☑
    conjoined O30.02- ☑
    dichorionic/diamniotic (two placenta, two amnioti? sacs) O30.04- ☑
    monochorionic/diamniotic (one placenta, two amniotic sacs) O30.03- ☑
    monochorionic/monoamniotic (one placenta, one amniotic sac) O30.01- ☑
    unable to determine number of placenta and number of amniotic sacs O30.09- ☑
    unspecified number of placenta and unspecified number of amniotic sacs O30.00- ☑
  unwanted Z64.0
  weeks of gestation
    8 weeks Z3A.08 (*following* Z36)
    9 weeks Z3A.09 (*following* Z36)
    10 weeks Z3A.10 (*following* Z36)
    11 weeks Z3A.11 (*following* Z36)
    12 weeks Z3A.12 (*following* Z36)
    13 weeks Z3A.13 (*following* Z36)
    14 weeks Z3A.14 (*following* Z36)
    15 weeks Z3A.15 (*following* Z36)
    16 weeks Z3A.16 (*following* Z36)
    17 weeks Z3A.17 (*following* Z36)
    18 weeks Z3A.18 (*following* Z36)
    19 weeks Z3A.19 (*following* Z36)
    20 weeks Z3A.20 (*following* Z36)
    21 weeks Z3A.21 (*following* Z36)
    22 weeks Z3A.22 (*following* Z36)
    23 weeks Z3A.23 (*following* Z36)
    24 weeks Z3A.24 (*following* Z36)
    25 weeks Z3A.25 (*following* Z36)
    26 weeks Z3A.26 (*following* Z36)
    27 weeks Z3A.27 (*following* Z36)
    28 weeks Z3A.28 (*following* Z36)
    29 weeks Z3A.29 (*following* Z36)

☑ Additional Character Required — Refer to the Tabular List for Character Selection   ▽ Subterms under main terms may continue to next column or page

Pregnancy — continued
  weeks of gestation — continued
    30 weeks Z3A.30 (following Z36)
    31 weeks Z3A.31 (following Z36)
    32 weeks Z3A.32 (following Z36)
    33 weeks Z3A.33 (following Z36)
    34 weeks Z3A.34 (following Z36)
    35 weeks Z3A.35 (following Z36)
    36 weeks Z3A.36 (following Z36)
    37 weeks Z3A.37 (following Z36)
    38 weeks Z3A.38 (following Z36)
    39 weeks Z3A.39 (following Z36)
    40 weeks Z3A.40 (following Z36)
    41 weeks Z3A.41 (following Z36)
    42 weeks Z3A.42 (following Z36)
    greater than 42 weeks Z3A.49 (following Z36)
    less than 8 weeks Z3A.01 (following Z36)
    not specified Z3A.00 (following Z36)
Preiser's disease — see Osteonecrosis, secondary, due to, trauma, metacarpus
Pre-kwashiorkor — see Malnutrition, severe
Preleukemia (syndrome) D46.9
Preluxation, hip, congenital Q65.6
Premature — see also condition
  adrenarche E27.0
  aging E34.8
  beats I49.40
    atrial I49.1
    auricular I49.1
    supraventricular I49.1
  birth NEC — see Preterm, newborn
  closure, foramen ovale Q21.8
  contraction
    atrial I49.1
    atrioventricular I49.2
    auricular I49.1
    auriculoventricular I49.49
    heart (extrasystole) I49.49
    junctional I49.2
    ventricular I49.3
  delivery — see also Pregnancy, complicated by, preterm labor O60.10 ☑
  ejaculation F52.4
  infant NEC — see Preterm, newborn
    light-for-dates — see Light for dates
  labor — see Pregnancy, complicated by, preterm labor
  lungs P28.0
  menopause E28.319
    asymptomatic E28.319
    symptomatic E28.310
  newborn
    extreme (less than 28 completed weeks) — see Immaturity, extreme
    less than 37 completed weeks — see Preterm, newborn
  puberty E30.1
  rupture membranes or amnion — see Pregnancy, complicated by, premature rupture of membranes
  senility E34.8
  thelarche E30.8
  ventricular systole I49.3
Prematurity NEC (less than 37 completed weeks) — see Preterm, newborn
  extreme (less than 28 completed weeks) — see Immaturity, extreme
Premenstrual
  dysphoric disorder (PMDD) F32.81
  tension (syndrome) N94.3
Premolarization, cuspids K00.2
Prenatal
  care, normal pregnancy — see Pregnancy, normal
  screening of mother — see also Encounter, antenatal screening Z36.9
  teeth K00.6
Preparatory care for subsequent treatment NEC
  for dialysis Z49.01
    peritoneal Z49.02
Prepartum — see condition
Preponderance, left or right ventricular I51.7
Prepuce — see condition
PRES (posterior reversible encephalopathy syndrome) I67.83
Presbycardia R54
Presbycusis, presbyacusia H91.1- ☑
Presbyesophagus K22.8
Presbyophrenia F03 ☑
Presbyopia H52.4

Prescription of contraceptives (initial) Z30.019
  barrier Z30.018
  diaphragm Z30.018
  emergency (postcoital) Z30.012
  implantable subdermal Z30.017
  injectable Z30.013
  intrauterine contraceptive device Z30.014
  pills Z30.011
  postcoital (emergency) Z30.012
  repeat Z30.40
    barrier Z30.49
    diaphragm Z30.49
    implantable subdermal Z30.46
    injectable Z30.42
    pills Z30.41
    specified type NEC Z30.49
    transdermal patch hormonal Z30.45
    vaginal ring hormonal Z30.44
  specified type NEC Z30.018
    transdermal patch hormonal Z30.016
    vaginal ring hormonal Z30.015
Presence (of)
  ankle-joint implant (functional) (prosthesis) Z96.66- ☑
  aortocoronary (bypass) graft Z95.1
  arterial-venous shunt (dialysis) Z99.2
  artificial
    eye (globe) Z97.0
    heart (fully implantable) (mechanical) Z95.812
      valve Z95.2
    larynx Z96.3
    lens (intraocular) Z96.1
    limb (complete) (partial) Z97.1- ☑
      arm Z97.1- ☑
        bilateral Z97.15
      leg Z97.1- ☑
        bilateral Z97.16
  audiological implant (functional) Z96.29
  bladder implant (functional) Z96.0
  bone
    conduction hearing device Z96.29
    implant (functional) NEC Z96.7
    joint (prosthesis) — see Presence, joint implant
  cardiac
    defibrillator (functional) (with synchronous cardiac pacemaker) Z95.810
    implant or graft Z95.9
      specified type NEC Z95.818
    pacemaker Z95.0
    resynchronization therapy
      defibrillator Z95.810
      pacemaker Z95.0
  cardioverter-defibrillator (ICD) Z95.810
  cerebrospinal fluid drainage device Z98.2
  cochlear implant (functional) Z96.21
  contact lens (es) Z97.3
  coronary artery graft or prosthesis Z95.5
  CRT-D (cardiac resynchronization therapy defibrillator) Z95.810
  CRT-P (cardiac resynchronization therapy pacemaker) Z95.0
  CSF shunt Z98.2
  dental prosthesis device Z97.2
  dentures Z97.2
  device (external) NEC Z97.8
    cardiac NEC Z95.818
    heart assist Z95.811
    implanted (functional) Z96.9
      specified NEC Z96.89
    prosthetic Z97.8
  ear implant Z96.20
    cochlear implant Z96.21
    myringotomy tube Z96.22
    specified type NEC Z96.29
  elbow-joint implant (functional) (prosthesis) Z96.62- ☑
  endocrine implant (functional) NEC Z96.49
  eustachian tube stent or device (functional) Z96.29
  external hearing-aid or device Z97.4
  finger-joint implant (functional) (prosthetic) Z96.69- ☑
  functional implant Z96.9
    specified NEC Z96.89
  graft
    cardiac NEC Z95.818
    vascular NEC Z95.828
  hearing-aid or device (external) Z97.4
    implant (bone) (cochlear) (functional) Z96.21
  heart assist device Z95.811
  heart valve implant (functional) Z95.2
    prosthetic Z95.2

Presence — continued
  heart valve implant — continued
    specified type NEC Z95.4
    xenogenic Z95.3
  hip-joint implant (functional) (prosthesis) Z96.64- ☑
  ICD (cardioverter-defibrillator) Z95.810
  implanted device (artificial) (functional) (prosthetic) Z96.9
    automatic cardiac defibrillator (with synchronous cardiac pacemaker) Z95.810
    cardiac pacemaker Z95.0
    cochlear Z96.21
    dental Z96.5
    heart Z95.812
    heart valve Z95.2
      prosthetic Z95.2
      specified NEC Z95.4
      xenogenic Z95.3
    insulin pump Z96.41
    intraocular lens Z96.1
    joint Z96.60
      ankle Z96.66- ☑
      elbow Z96.62- ☑
      finger Z96.69- ☑
      hip Z96.64- ☑
      knee Z96.65- ☑
      shoulder Z96.61- ☑
      specified NEC Z96.698
      wrist Z96.63- ☑
    larynx Z96.3
    myringotomy tube Z96.22
    otological Z96.20
      cochlear Z96.21
      eustachian stent Z96.29
      myringotomy Z96.22
      specified NEC Z96.29
      stapes Z96.29
    skin Z96.81
    skull plate Z96.7
    specified NEC Z96.89
    urogenital Z96.0
  insulin pump (functional) Z96.41
  intestinal bypass or anastomosis Z98.0
  intraocular lens (functional) Z96.1
  intrauterine contraceptive device (IUD) Z97.5
  intravascular implant (functional) (prosthetic) NEC Z95.9
    coronary artery Z95.5
    defibrillator (with synchronous cardiac pacemaker) Z95.810
    peripheral vessel (with angioplasty) Z95.820
  joint implant (prosthetic) (any) Z96.60
    ankle — see Presence, ankle joint implant
    elbow — see Presence, elbow joint implant
    finger — see Presence, finger joint implant
    hip — see Presence, hip joint implant
    knee — see Presence, knee joint implant
    shoulder — see Presence, shoulder joint implant
    specified joint NEC Z96.698
    wrist — see Presence, wrist joint implant
  knee-joint implant (functional) (prosthesis) Z96.65- ☑
  laryngeal implant (functional) Z96.3
  mandibular implant (dental) Z96.5
  myringotomy tube(s) Z96.22
  neurostimulator (brain) (gastric) (peripheral nerve) (sacral nerve) (spinal cord) (vagus nerve) Z96.82
  orthopedic-joint implant (prosthetic) (any) — see Presence, joint implant
  otological implant (functional) Z96.29
  shoulder-joint implant (functional) (prosthesis) Z96.61- ☑
  skull-plate implant Z96.7
  spectacles Z97.3
  stapes implant (functional) Z96.29
  systemic lupus erythematosus [SLE] inhibitor D68.62
  tendon implant (functional) (graft) Z96.7
  tooth root(s) implant Z96.5
  ureteral stent Z96.0
  urethral stent Z96.0
  urogenital implant (functional) Z96.0
  vascular implant or device Z95.9
    access port device Z95.828
    specified type NEC Z95.828
  wrist-joint implant (functional) (prosthesis) Z96.63- ☑
Presenile — see also condition
  dementia F03 ☑
  premature aging E34.8

Presentation, fetal — see Delivery, complicated by,
malposition
Prespondylolisthesis (congenital) Q76.2
Pressure
  area, skin — see Ulcer, pressure, by site
  brachial plexus G54.0
  brain G93.5
    injury at birth NEC P11.1
  cerebral — see Pressure, brain
  chest R07.89
  cone, tentorial G93.5
  hyposystolic — see also Hypotension
    incidental reading, without diagnosis of hypoten-
sion R03.1
  increased
    intracranial benign G93.2
      injury at birth P11.0
    intraocular H40.05- ☑
  injury — see Ulcer, pressure, by site
  lumbosacral plexus G54.1
  mediastinum J98.59
  necrosis (chronic) — see Ulcer, pressure, by site
  parental, inappropriate (excessive) Z62.6
  sore (chronic) — see Ulcer, pressure, by site
  spinal cord G95.20
  ulcer (chronic) — see Ulcer, pressure, by site
  venous, increased I87.8
Pre-syncope R55
Preterm
  delivery — see also Pregnancy, complicated by,
preterm labor O60.10 ☑
  labor — see Pregnancy, complicated by, preterm labor
  newborn (infant) P07.30
    gestational age
      28 completed weeks (28 weeks, 0 days through
28 weeks, 6 days) P07.31
      29 completed weeks (29 weeks, 0 days through
29 weeks, 6 days) P07.32
      30 completed weeks (30 weeks, 0 days through
30 weeks, 6 days) P07.33
      31 completed weeks (31 weeks, 0 days through
31 weeks, 6 days) P07.34
      32 completed weeks (32 weeks, 0 days through
32 weeks, 6 days) P07.35
      33 completed weeks (33 weeks, 0 days through
33 weeks, 6 days) P07.36
      34 completed weeks (34 weeks, 0 days through
34 weeks, 6 days) P07.37
      35 completed weeks (35 weeks, 0 days through
35 weeks, 6 days) P07.38
      36 completed weeks (36 weeks, 0 days through
36 weeks, 6 days) P07.39
Previa
  placenta (total) (without hemorrhage) O44.0- ☑
    with hemorrhage O44.1- ☑
    complete O44.0- ☑
      with hemorrhage O44.1- ☑
    low — see also Delivery, complicated, by, placenta,
low O44.4- ☑
      with hemorrhage O44.5- ☑
    marginal O44.2- ☑
      with hemorrhage O44.3- ☑
    partial O44.2- ☑
      with hemorrhage O44.3- ☑
  vasa O69.4 ☑
Priapism N48.30
  due to
    disease classified elsewhere N48.32
    drug N48.33
    specified cause NEC N48.39
    trauma N48.31
Prickling sensation (skin) R20.2
Prickly heat L74.0
Primary — see condition
Primigravida
  elderly, affecting management of pregnancy, labor and
delivery (supervision only) — see Pregnancy,
complicated by, elderly, primigravida
  older, affecting management of pregnancy, labor and
delivery (supervision only) — see Pregnancy,
complicated by, elderly, primigravida
  very young, affecting management of pregnancy, labor
and delivery (supervision only) — see Pregnancy,
complicated by, young mother, primigravida

Primipara
  elderly, affecting management of pregnancy, labor and
delivery (supervision only) — see Pregnancy,
complicated by, elderly, primigravida
  older, affecting management of pregnancy, labor and
delivery (supervision only) — see Pregnancy,
complicated by, elderly, primigravida
  very young, affecting management of pregnancy, labor
and delivery (supervision only) — see Pregnancy,
complicated by, young mother, primigravida
Primus varus Q66.21- ☑
PRIND (Prolonged reversible ischemic neurologic deficit)
  I63.9
Pringle's disease (tuberous sclerosis) Q85.1
Prinzmetal angina I20.1
Prizefighter ear — see Cauliflower ear
Problem (with) (related to)
  academic Z55.8
  acculturation Z60.3
  adjustment (to)
    change of job Z56.1
    life-cycle transition Z60.0
    pension Z60.0
    retirement Z60.0
  adopted child Z62.821
  alcoholism in family Z63.72
  atypical parenting situation Z62.9
  bankruptcy Z59.8
  behavioral (adult) F69
    drug seeking Z76.5
  birth of sibling affecting child Z62.898
  care (of)
    provider dependency Z74.9
      specified NEC Z74.8
    sick or handicapped person in family or household
Z63.6
  child
    abuse (affecting the child) — see Maltreatment,
child
    custody or support proceedings Z65.3
    in care of non-parental family member Z62.21
    in foster care Z62.21
    in welfare custody Z62.21
    living in orphanage or group home Z62.22
  child-rearing Z62.9
    specified NEC Z62.898
  communication (developmental) F80.9
  conflict or discord (with)
    boss Z56.4
    classmates Z55.4
    counselor Z64.4
    employer Z56.4
    family Z63.9
      specified NEC Z63.8
    probation officer Z64.4
    social worker Z64.4
    teachers Z55.4
    workmates Z56.4
  conviction in legal proceedings Z65.0
    with imprisonment Z65.1
  counselor Z64.4
  creditors Z59.8
  digestive K92.9
  drug addict in family Z63.72
  ear — see Disorder, ear
  economic Z59.9
    affecting care Z59.9
    specified NEC Z59.8
  education Z55.9
    specified NEC Z55.8
  employment Z56.9
    change of job Z56.1
    discord Z56.4
    environment Z56.5
    sexual harassment Z56.81
    specified NEC Z56.89
    stressful schedule Z56.3
    stress NEC Z56.6
    threat of job loss Z56.2
    unemployment Z56.0
  enuresis, child F98.0
  eye H57.9
  failed examinations (school) Z55.2
  falling Z91.81
  family — see also Disruption, family Z63.9
    specified NEC Z63.8
  feeding (elderly) (infant) R63.3
    newborn P92.9

Problem — continued
  feeding — continued
    newborn — continued
      breast P92.5
      overfeeding P92.4
      slow P92.2
      specified NEC P92.8
      underfeeding P92.3
    nonorganic F50.89
  finance Z59.9
    specified NEC Z59.8
  foreclosure on loan Z59.8
  foster child Z62.822
  frightening experience(s) in childhood Z62.898
  genital NEC
    female N94.9
    male N50.9
  health care Z75.9
    specified NEC Z75.8
  hearing — see Deafness
  homelessness Z59.0
  housing Z59.9
    inadequate Z59.1
    isolated Z59.8
    specified NEC Z59.8
  identity (of childhood) F93.8
  illegitimate pregnancy (unwanted) Z64.0
  illiteracy Z55.0
  impaired mobility Z74.09
  imprisonment or incarceration Z65.1
  inadequate teaching affecting education Z55.8
  inappropriate (excessive) parental pressure Z62.6
  influencing health status NEC Z78.9
  in-law Z63.1
  institutionalization, affecting child Z62.22
  intrafamilial communication Z63.8
  jealousy, child F93.8
  landlord Z59.2
  language (developmental) F80.9
  learning (developmental) F81.9
  legal Z65.3
    conviction without imprisonment Z65.0
    imprisonment Z65.1
    release from prison Z65.2
  life-management Z73.9
    specified NEC Z73.89
  life-style Z72.9
    gambling Z72.6
    high-risk sexual behavior (heterosexual) Z72.51
      bisexual Z72.53
      homosexual Z72.52
    inappropriate eating habits Z72.4
    self-damaging behavior NEC Z72.89
    specified NEC Z72.89
    tobacco use Z72.0
  literacy Z55.9
    low level Z55.0
    specified NEC Z55.8
  living alone Z60.2
  lodgers Z59.2
  loss of love relationship in childhood Z62.898
  marital Z63.0
    involving
      divorce Z63.5
      estrangement Z63.5
      gender identity F66
  mastication K08.89
  medical
    care, within family Z63.6
    facilities Z75.9
      specified NEC Z75.8
  mental F48.9
  multiparity Z64.1
  negative life events in childhood Z62.9
    altered pattern of family relationships Z62.898
    frightening experience Z62.898
    loss of
      love relationship Z62.898
      self-esteem Z62.898
    physical abuse (alleged) — see Maltreatment, child
    removal from home Z62.29
    specified event NEC Z62.898
  neighbor Z59.2
  neurological NEC R29.818
  new step-parent affecting child Z62.898
  none (feared complaint unfounded) Z71.1
  occupational NEC Z56.89
  parent-child — see Conflict, parent-child
  personal hygiene Z91.89

Problem — *continued*
personality F69
phase-of-life transition, adjustment Z60.0
presence of sick or disabled person in family or household Z63.79
needing care Z63.6
primary support group (family) Z63.9
specified NEC Z63.8
probation officer Z64.4
psychiatric F99
psychosexual (development) F66
psychosocial Z65.9
religious or spiritual Z65.8
specified NEC Z65.8
relationship Z63.9
childhood F93.8
release from prison Z65.2
religious or spiritual Z65.8
removal from home affecting child Z62.29
seeking and accepting known hazardous and harmful behavioral or psychological interventions Z65.8
chemical, nutritional or physical interventions Z65.8
sexual function (nonorganic) F52.9
sight H54.7
sleep disorder, child F51.9
smell — *see* Disturbance, sensation, smell
social
environment Z60.9
specified NEC Z60.8
exclusion and rejection Z60.4
worker Z64.4
speech R47.9
developmental F80.9
specified NEC R47.89
swallowing — *see* Dysphagia
taste — *see* Disturbance, sensation, taste
tic, child F95.0
underachievement in school Z55.3
unemployment Z56.0
threatened Z56.2
unwanted pregnancy Z64.0
upbringing Z62.9
specified NEC Z62.898
urinary N39.9
voice production R47.89
work schedule (stressful) Z56.3
Procedure (surgical)
converted
arthroscopic to open Z53.33
laparoscopic to open Z53.31
specified procedure NEC to open Z53.39
thoracoscopic to open Z53.32
for purpose other than remedying health state Z41.9
specified NEC Z41.8
not done Z53.9
because of
administrative reasons Z53.8
contraindication Z53.09
smoking Z53.01
patient's decision Z53.20
for reasons of belief or group pressure Z53.1
left against medical advice (AMA) Z53.21
specified reason NEC Z53.29
specified reason NEC Z53.8
Procidentia (uteri) N81.3
Proctalgia K62.89
fugax K59.4
spasmodic K59.4
Proctitis K62.89
amebic (acute) A06.0
chlamydial A56.3
gonococcal A54.6
granulomatous — *see* Enteritis, regional, large intestine
herpetic A60.1
radiation K62.7
tuberculous A18.32
ulcerative (chronic) K51.20
with
complication K51.219
abscess K51.214
fistula K51.213
obstruction K51.212
rectal bleeding K51.211
specified NEC K51.218
Proctocele
female (without uterine prolapse) N81.6
with uterine prolapse N81.2
complete N81.3

Proctocele — *continued*
male K62.3
Proctocolitis
food protein-induced K52.82
food-induced eosinophilic K52.82
milk protein-induced K52.82
mucosal — *see* Rectosigmoiditis, ulcerative
Proctoptosis K62.3
Proctorrhagia K62.5
Proctosigmoiditis K63.89
ulcerative (chronic) — *see* Rectosigmoiditis, ulcerative
Proctospasm K59.4
psychogenic F45.8
Profichet's disease — *see* Disorder, soft tissue, specified type NEC
Progeria E34.8
Prognathism (mandibular) (maxillary) M26.19
Progonoma (melanotic) — *see* Neoplasm, benign, by site
Progressive — *see* condition
Prolactinoma
specified site — *see* Neoplasm, benign, by site
unspecified site D35.2
Prolapse, prolapsed
anus, anal (canal) (sphincter) K62.2
arm or hand O32.2 ☑
causing obstructed labor O64.4 ☑
bladder (mucosa) (sphincter) (acquired)
congenital Q79.4
female — *see* Cystocele
male N32.89
breast implant (prosthetic) T85.49 ☑
cecostomy K94.09
cecum K63.4
cervix, cervical (hypertrophied) N81.2
anterior lip, obstructing labor O65.5
congenital Q51.828
postpartal, old N81.2
stump N81.85
ciliary body (traumatic) — *see* Laceration, eye(ball), with prolapse or loss of interocular tissue
colon (pedunculated) K63.4
colostomy K94.09
disc (intervertebral) — *see* Displacement, intervertebral disc
eye implant (orbital) T85.398 ☑
lens (ocular) — *see* Complications, intraocular lens
fallopian tube N83.4- ☑
gastric (mucosa) K31.89
genital, female N81.9
specified NEC N81.89
globe, nontraumatic — *see* Luxation, globe
ileostomy bud K94.19
intervertebral disc — *see* Displacement, intervertebral disc
intestine (small) K63.4
iris (traumatic) — *see* Laceration, eye(ball), with prolapse or loss of interocular tissue
nontraumatic H21.89
kidney N28.83
congenital Q63.2
laryngeal muscles or ventricle J38.7
liver K76.89
meatus urinarius N36.8
mitral (valve) I34.1
ocular lens implant — *see* Complications, intraocular lens
organ or site, congenital NEC — *see* Malposition, congenital
ovary N83.4- ☑
pelvic floor, female N81.89
perineum, female N81.89
rectum (mucosa) (sphincter) K62.3
due to trichuris trichuria B79
spleen D73.89
stomach K31.89
umbilical cord
complicating delivery O69.0 ☑
urachus, congenital Q64.4
ureter N28.89
with obstruction N13.5
with infection N13.6
ureterovesical orifice N28.89
urethra (acquired) (infected) (mucosa) N36.8
congenital Q64.71
urinary meatus N36.8
congenital Q64.72
uterovaginal N81.4

Prolapse, prolapsed — *continued*
uterovaginal — *continued*
complete N81.3
incomplete N81.2
uterus (with prolapse of vagina) N81.4
complete N81.3
congenital Q51.818
first degree N81.2
in pregnancy or childbirth — *see* Pregnancy, complicated by, abnormal, uterus
incomplete N81.2
postpartal (old) N81.4
second degree N81.2
third degree N81.3
uveal (traumatic) — *see* Laceration, eye(ball), with prolapse or loss of interocular tissue
vagina (anterior) (wall) — *see* Cystocele
with prolapse of uterus N81.4
complete N81.3
incomplete N81.2
posterior wall N81.6
posthysterectomy N99.3
vitreous (humor) H43.0- ☑
in wound — *see* Laceration, eye(ball), with prolapse or loss of interocular tissue
womb — *see* Prolapse, uterus
Prolapsus, female N81.9
specified NEC N81.89
Proliferation(s)
primary cutaneous CD30-positive large T-cell C86.6
prostate, atypical small acinar N42.32
Proliferative — *see* condition
Prolonged, prolongation (of)
bleeding (time) (idiopathic) R79.1
coagulation (time) R79.1
gestation (over 42 completed weeks)
mother O48.1
newborn P08.22
interval I44.0
labor O63.9
first stage O63.0
second stage O63.1
partial thromboplastin time (PTT) R79.1
pregnancy (more than 42 weeks gestation) O48.1
prothrombin time R79.1
QT interval R94.31
uterine contractions in labor O62.4
Prominence, prominent
auricle (congenital) (ear) Q17.5
ischial spine or sacral promontory with disproportion (fetopelvic) O33.0
causing obstructed labor O65.0
nose (congenital) acquired M95.0
Promiscuity — *see* High, risk, sexual behavior
Pronation
ankle — *see* Deformity, limb, foot, specified NEC
foot — *see also* Deformity, limb, foot, specified NEC
congenital Q74.2
Prophylactic
administration of
antibiotics, long-term Z79.2
short-term use — *omit code*
drug — *see also* Long-term (current) drug therapy (use of) Z79.899
medication Z79.899
organ removal (for neoplasia management) Z40.00
breast Z40.01
fallopian tube(s) Z40.03
with ovary(s) Z40.02
ovary(s) Z40.02
specified site NEC Z40.09
surgery Z40.9
for risk factors related to malignant neoplasm — *see* Prophylactic, organ removal
specified NEC Z40.8
vaccination Z23
Propionic acidemia E71.121
Proptosis (ocular) — *see also* Exophthalmos
thyroid — *see* Hyperthyroidism, with goiter
Prosecution, anxiety concerning Z65.3
Prosopagnosia R48.3
Prostadynia N42.81
Prostate, prostatic — *see* condition
Prostatism — *see* Hyperplasia, prostate
Prostatitis (congestive) (suppurative) (with cystitis) N41.9
acute N41.0
cavitary N41.8
chronic N41.1

Prostatitis — continued
  diverticular N41.8
  due to Trichomonas (vaginalis) A59.02
  fibrous N41.1
  gonococcal (acute) (chronic) A54.22
  granulomatous N41.4
  hypertrophic N41.1
  subacute N41.1
  trichomonal A59.02
  tuberculous A18.14
Prostatocystitis N41.3
Prostatorrhea N42.89
Prostatosis N42.82
Prostration R53.83
  heat — see also Heat, exhaustion
    anhydrotic T67.3 ☑
    due to
      salt (and water) depletion T67.4 ☑
      water depletion T67.3 ☑
  nervous F48.8
  senile R54
Protanomaly (anomalous trichromat) H53.54
Protanopia (complete) (incomplete) H53.54
Protection (against) (from) — see Prophylactic
Protein
  deficiency NEC — see Malnutrition
  malnutrition — see Malnutrition
  sickness — see also Reaction, serum T80.69 ☑
Proteinemia R77.9
Proteinosis
  alveolar (pulmonary) J84.01
  lipid or lipoid (of Urbach) E78.89
Proteinuria R80.9
  Bence Jones R80.3
  complicating pregnancy — see Proteinuria, gestational
  gestational
    complicating
      childbirth O12.14
      pregnancy O12.1- ☑
        with edema O12.2- ☑
      puerperium O12.15
  idiopathic R80.0
  isolated R80.0
    with glomerular lesion N06.9
      C3
        glomerulonephritis N06.A
        glomerulopathy N06.A
          with dense deposit disease N06.6
        dense deposit disease N06.6
        diffuse
          crescentic glomerulonephritis N06.7
          endocapillary proliferative glomerulonephritis N06.4
          mesangiocapillary glomerulonephritis N06.5
        focal and segmental hyalinosis or sclerosis N06.1
        membranous (diffuse) N06.2
        mesangial proliferative (diffuse) N06.3
        minimal change N06.0
        specified pathology NEC N06.8
  orthostatic R80.2
    with glomerular lesion — see Proteinuria, isolated, with glomerular lesion
  persistent R80.1
    with glomerular lesion — see Proteinuria, isolated, with glomerular lesion
  postural R80.2
    with glomerular lesion — see Proteinuria, isolated, with glomerular lesion
  pre-eclamptic — see Pre-eclampsia
  puerperal O12.15
  specified type NEC R80.8
Proteolysis, pathologic D65
Proteus (mirabilis) (morganii), as cause of disease classified elsewhere B96.4
Prothrombin gene mutation D68.52
Protoporphyria, erythropoietic E80.0
Protozoal — see also condition
  disease B64
  specified NEC B60.8
Protrusion, protrusio
  acetabuli M24.7
  acetabulum (into pelvis) M24.7
  device, implant or graft — see also Complications, by site and type, mechanical T85.698 ☑
    arterial graft NEC — see Complication, cardiovascular device, mechanical, vascular
    breast (implant) T85.49 ☑

Protrusion, protrusio — continued
  device, implant or graft — see also Complications, by site and type, mechanical — continued
    catheter NEC T85.698 ☑
      cystostomy T83.090 ☑
      dialysis (renal) T82.49 ☑
        intraperitoneal T85.691 ☑
      infusion NEC T82.594 ☑
        spinal (epidural) (subdural) T85.690 ☑
      urinary — see also Complications, catheter, urinary T83.098 ☑
    electronic (electrode) (pulse generator) (stimulator)
      bone T84.390 ☑
      nervous system — see Complication, prosthetic device, mechanical, electronic nervous system stimulator
    fixation, internal (orthopedic) NEC — see Complication, fixation device, mechanical
    gastrointestinal — see Complications, prosthetic device, mechanical, gastrointestinal device
    genital NEC T83.498 ☑
      intrauterine contraceptive device T83.39 ☑
      penile prosthesis (cylinder) (implanted) (pump) (resevoir) T83.490 ☑
      testicular prosthesis T83.491 ☑
    heart NEC — see Complication, cardiovascular device, mechanical
    joint prosthesis — see Complications, joint prosthesis, mechanical, specified NEC, by site
    ocular NEC — see Complications, prosthetic device, mechanical, ocular device
    orthopedic NEC — see Complication, orthopedic, device, mechanical
    specified NEC T85.628 ☑
    urinary NEC — see also Complication, genitourinary, device, urinary, mechanical
      graft T83.29 ☑
    vascular NEC — see Complication, cardiovascular device, mechanical
    ventricular intracranial shunt T85.09 ☑
  intervertebral disc — see Displacement, intervertebral disc
  joint prosthesis — see Complications, joint prosthesis, mechanical, specified NEC, by site
  nucleus pulposus — see Displacement, intervertebral disc
Prune belly (syndrome) Q79.4
Prurigo (ferox) (gravis) (Hebrae) (Hebra's) (mitis) (simplex) L28.2
  Besnier's L20.0
  estivalis L56.4
  nodularis L28.1
  psychogenic F45.8
Pruritus, pruritic (essential) L29.9
  ani, anus L29.0
    psychogenic F45.8
  anogenital L29.3
    psychogenic F45.8
  due to onchocerca volvulus B73.1
  gravidarum — see Pregnancy, complicated by, specified pregnancy-related condition NEC
  hiemalis L29.8
  neurogenic (any site) F45.8
  perianal L29.0
  psychogenic (any site) F45.8
  scroti, scrotum L29.1
    psychogenic F45.8
  senile, senilis L29.8
  specified NEC L29.8
    psychogenic F45.8
  Trichomonas A59.9
  vulva, vulvae L29.2
    psychogenic F45.8
Pseudarthrosis, pseudoarthrosis (bone) — see Nonunion, fracture
  clavicle, congenital Q74.0
  joint, following fusion or arthrodesis M96.0
Pseudoaneurysm — see Aneurysm
Pseudoangina (pectoris) — see Angina
Pseudoangioma I81
Pseudoarteriosus Q28.8
Pseudoarthrosis — see Pseudarthrosis
Pseudobulbar affect (PBA) F48.2
Pseudochromhidrosis L67.8
Pseudocirrhosis, liver, pericardial I31.1
Pseudocowpox B08.03
Pseudocoxalgia M91.3- ☑

Pseudocroup J38.5
Pseudo-Cushing's syndrome, alcohol-induced E24.4
Pseudocyesis F45.8
Pseudocyst
  lung J98.4
  pancreas K86.3
  retina — see Cyst, retina
Pseudoelephantiasis neuroarthritica Q82.0
Pseudoexfoliation, capsule (lens) — see Cataract, specified NEC
Pseudofolliculitis barbae L73.1
Pseudoglioma H44.89
Pseudohemophilia (Bernuth's) (hereditary) (type B) D68.6
  Type A D69.8
  vascular D69.8
Pseudohermaphroditism Q56.3
  adrenal E25.8
  female Q56.2
    with adrenocortical disorder E25.8
    without adrenocortical disorder Q56.2
    adrenal (congenital) E25.0
    unspecified E25.9
  male Q56.1
    with
      5-alpha-reductase deficiency E29.1
      adrenocortical disorder E25.8
      androgen resistance E34.51
      cleft scrotum Q56.1
      feminizing testis E34.51
    without gonadal disorder Q56.1
    adrenal E25.8
    unspecified E25.9
Pseudo-Hurler's polydystrophy E77.0
Pseudohydrocephalus G93.2
Pseudohypertrophic muscular dystrophy (Erb's) G71.02
Pseudohypertrophy, muscle G71.09
Pseudohypoparathyroidism E20.1
Pseudoinsomnia F51.03
Pseudoleukemia, infantile D64.89
Pseudomembranous — see condition
Pseudomeningocele (cerebral) (infective) (post-traumatic) G96.198
  postprocedural (spinal) G97.82
Pseudomenses (newborn) P54.6
Pseudomenstruation (newborn) P54.6
Pseudomonas
  aeruginosa, as cause of disease classified elsewhere B96.5
  mallei infection A24.0
    as cause of disease classified elsewhere B96.5
  pseudomallei, as cause of disease classified elsewhere B96.5
Pseudomyotonia G71.19
Pseudomyxoma peritonei C78.6
Pseudoneuritis, optic (nerve) (disc) (papilla), **congenital** Q14.2
Pseudo-obstruction intestine (acute) (chronic) (idiopathic) (intermittent secondary) (primary) K59.89
  colonic K59.81
Pseudopapilledema H47.33- ☑
  congenital Q14.2
Pseudoparalysis
  arm or leg R29.818
  atonic, congenital P94.2
Pseudopelade L66.0
Pseudophakia Z96.1
Pseudopolyarthritis, rhizomelic M35.3
Pseudopolycythemia D75.1
Pseudopseudohypoparathyroidism E20.1
Pseudopterygium H11.81- ☑
Pseudoptosis (eyelid) — see Blepharochalasis
Pseudopuberty, precocious
  female heterosexual E25.8
  male isosexual E25.8
Pseudorickets (renal) N25.0
Pseudorubella B08.20
Pseudosclerema, newborn P83.88
Pseudosclerosis (brain)
  Jakob's — see Creutzfeldt-Jakob disease or syndrome
  of Westphal (Strümpell) E83.01
  spastic — see Creutzfeldt-Jakob disease or syndrome
Pseudotetanus — see Convulsions
Pseudotetany R29.0
  hysterical F44.5
Pseudotruncus arteriosus Q25.49

☑ Additional Character Required — Refer to the Tabular List for Character Selection   ▽ Subterms under main terms may continue to next column or page

Pseudotuberculosis A28.2
    enterocolitis A04.8
    pasteurella (infection) A28.0
Pseudotumor G93.2
    cerebri G93.2
    orbital H05.11 ☑
Pseudoxanthoma elasticum Q82.8
Psilosis (sprue) (tropical) K90.1
    nontropical K90.0
Psittacosis A70
Psoitis M60.88
Psoriasis L40.9
    arthropathic L40.50
        arthritis mutilans L40.52
        distal interphalangeal L40.51
        juvenile L40.54
        other specified L40.59
        spondylitis L40.53
    buccal K13.29
    flexural L40.8
    guttate L40.4
    mouth K13.29
    nummular L40.0
    plaque L40.0
    psychogenic F54
    pustular (generalized) L40.1
        palmaris et plantaris L40.3
    specified NEC L40.8
    vulgaris L40.0
Psychasthenia F48.8
Psychiatric disorder or problem F99
Psychogenic — *see also* condition
    factors associated with physical conditions F54
Psychological and behavioral factors affecting
        medical condition F59
Psychoneurosis, psychoneurotic — *see also* Neurosis
    anxiety (state) F41.1
    depersonalization F48.1
    hypochondriacal F45.21
    hysteria F44.9
    neurasthenic F48.8
    personality NEC F60.89
Psychopathy, psychopathic
    affectionless F94.2
    autistic F84.5
    constitution, post-traumatic F07.81
    personality — *see* Disorder, personality
    sexual — *see* Deviation, sexual
    state F60.2
Psychosexual identity disorder of childhood F64.2
Psychosis, psychotic F29
    acute (transient) F23
        hysterical F44.9
    affective — *see* Disorder, mood
    alcoholic F10.959
        with
            abuse F10.159
            anxiety disorder F10.980
                with
                    abuse F10.180
                    dependence F10.280
            delirium tremens F10.231
            delusions F10.950
                with
                    abuse F10.150
                    dependence F10.250
            dementia F10.97
                with dependence F10.27
            dependence F10.259
            hallucinosis F10.951
                with
                    abuse F10.151
                    dependence F10.251
            mood disorder F10.94
                with
                    abuse F10.14
                    dependence F10.24
            paranoia F10.950
                with
                    abuse F10.150
                    dependence F10.250
            persisting amnesia F10.96
                with dependence F10.26
        amnestic confabulatory F10.96
            with dependence F10.26
        delirium tremens F10.231
        Korsakoff's, Korsakov's, Korsakow's F10.26
        paranoid type F10.950

Psychosis, psychotic — *continued*
    alcoholic — *continued*
        paranoid type — *continued*
            with
                abuse F10.150
                dependence F10.250
    anergastic — *see* Psychosis, organic
    arteriosclerotic (simple type) (uncomplicated) F01.50
        with behavioral disturbance F01.51
    childhood F84.0
        atypical F84.8
    climacteric — *see* Psychosis, involutional
    confusional F29
        acute or subacute F05
        reactive F23
    cycloid F23
    depressive — *see* Disorder, depressive
    disintegrative (childhood) F84.3
    drug-induced — *see* F11-F19 with .X59
        paranoid and hallucinatory states — *see* F11-F19
            with .X50 or .X51
    due to or associated with
        addiction, drug — *see* F11-F19 with .X59
        dependence
            alcohol F10.259
            drug — *see* F11-F19 with .X59
        epilepsy F06.8
        Huntington's chorea F06.8
        ischemia, cerebrovascular (generalized) F06.8
        multiple sclerosis F06.8
        physical disease F06.8
        presenile dementia F03 ☑
        senile dementia F03 ☑
        vascular disease (arteriosclerotic) (cerebral) F01.50
            with behavioral disturbance F01.51
    epileptic F06.8
    episode F23
        due to or associated with physical condition F06.8
    exhaustive F43.0
    hallucinatory, chronic F28
    hypomanic F30.8
    hysterical (acute) F44.9
    induced F24
    infantile F84.0
        atypical F84.8
    infective (acute) (subacute) F05
    involutional F28
        depressive — *see* Disorder, depressive
        melancholic — *see* Disorder, depressive
        paranoid (state) F22
    Korsakoff's, Korsakov's, Korsakow's (nonalcoholic) F04
        alcoholic F10.96
            in dependence F10.26
        induced by other psychoactive substance — *see*
            categories F11-F19 with .X5X
    mania, manic (single episode) F30.2
        recurrent type F31.89
    manic-depressive — *see* Disorder, bipolar
    menopausal — *see* Psychosis, involutional
    mixed schizophrenic and affective F25.8
    multi-infarct (cerebrovascular) F01.50
        with behavioral disturbance F01.51
    nonorganic F29
        specified NEC F28
    organic F09
        due to or associated with
            arteriosclerosis (cerebral) — *see* Psychosis, arte-
                riosclerotic
            cerebrovascular disease, arteriosclerotic — *see*
                Psychosis, arteriosclerotic
            childbirth — *see* Psychosis, puerperal
            Creutzfeldt-Jakob disease or syndrome — *see*
                Creutzfeldt-Jakob disease or syndrome
            dependence, alcohol F10.259
            disease
                alcoholic liver F10.259
                brain, arteriosclerotic — *see* Psychosis, arte-
                    riosclerotic
                cerebrovascular F01.50
                    with behavioral disturbance F01.51
                Creutzfeldt-Jakob — *see* Creutzfeldt-Jakob
                    disease or syndrome
                endocrine or metabolic F06.8
                    acute or subacute F05
                liver, alcoholic F10.259
            epilepsy transient (acute) F05
            infection
                brain (intracranial) F06.8

Psychosis, psychotic — *continued*
    organic — *continued*
        due to or associated with — *continued*
            infection — *continued*
                brain — *continued*
                    acute or subacute F05
                intoxication
                    alcoholic (acute) F10.259
                    drug F11-F19 with .x59
                ischemia, cerebrovascular (generalized) — *see*
                    Psychosis, arteriosclerotic
                puerperium — *see* Psychosis, puerperal
                trauma, brain (birth) (from electric current) (sur-
                    gical) F06.8
                    acute or subacute F05
            infective F06.8
                acute or subacute F05
            post-traumatic F06.8
                acute or subacute F05
    paranoiac F22
    paranoid (climacteric) (involutional) (menopausal) F22
        psychogenic (acute) F23
        schizophrenic F20.0
        senile F03 ☑
    postpartum (NOS) F53.1
    presbyophrenic (type) F03 ☑
    presenile F03 ☑
    psychogenic (paranoid) F23
        depressive F32.3
    puerperal (NOS) F53.1
        specified type — *see* Psychosis, by type
    reactive (brief) (transient) (emotional stress) (psycho-
        logical trauma) F23
        depressive F32.3
            recurrent F33.3
        excitative type F30.8
    schizoaffective F25.9
        depressive type F25.1
        manic type F25.0
    schizophrenia, schizophrenic — *see* Schizophrenia
    schizophrenia-like, in epilepsy F06.2
    schizophreniform F20.81
        affective type F25.9
        brief F23
        confusional type F23
        mixed type F25.0
    senile NEC F03 ☑
        depressed or paranoid type F03 ☑
        simple deterioration F03 ☑
        specified type — *code to* condition
    shared F24
    situational (reactive) F23
    symbiotic (childhood) F84.3
    symptomatic F09
Psychosomatic — *see* Disorder, psychosomatic
Psychosyndrome, organic F07.9
Psychotic episode due to or associated with physical
    condition F06.8
Pterygium (eye) H11.00- ☑
    amyloid H11.01- ☑
    central H11.02- ☑
    colli Q18.3
    double H11.03- ☑
    peripheral
        progressive H11.05- ☑
        stationary H11.04- ☑
    recurrent H11.06- ☑
Ptilosis (eyelid) — *see* Madarosis
Ptomaine (poisoning) — *see* Poisoning, food
Ptosis — *see also* Blepharoptosis
    adiposa (false) — *see* Blepharoptosis
    breast N64.81-
    brow H57.81- ☑
    cecum K63.4
    colon K63.4
    congenital (eyelid) Q10.0
        specified site NEC — *see* Anomaly, by site
    eyebrow H57.81- ☑
    eyelid — *see* Blepharoptosis
        congenital Q10.0
    gastric K31.89
    intestine K63.4
    kidney N28.83
    liver K76.89
    renal N28.83
    splanchnic K63.4
    spleen D73.89
    stomach K31.89

Ptosis — *continued*
  viscera K63.4
PTP D69.51
Ptyalism (periodic) K11.7
  hysterical F45.8
  pregnancy — *see* Pregnancy, complicated by, specified
      pregnancy-related condition NEC
  psychogenic F45.8
Ptyalolithiasis K11.5
Pubarche, precocious E30.1
Pubertas praecox E30.1
Puberty (development state) Z00.3
  bleeding (excessive) N92.2
  delayed E30.0
  precocious (constitutional) (cryptogenic) (idiopathic)
      E30.1
    central E22.8
    due to
      ovarian hyperfunction E28.1
        estrogen E28.0
      testicular hyperfunction E29.0
  premature E30.1
    due to
      adrenal cortical hyperfunction E25.8
      pineal tumor E34.8
      pituitary (anterior) hyperfunction E22.8
Puckering, macula — *see* Degeneration, macula, puckering
Pudenda, pudendum — *see* condition
Puente's disease (simple glandular cheilitis) K13.0
Puerperal, puerperium (complicated by, complications)
  abnormal glucose (tolerance test) O99.815
  abscess
    areola O91.02
      associated with lactation O91.03
    Bartholin's gland O86.19
    breast O91.12
      associated with lactation O91.13
    cervix (uteri) O86.11
    genital organ NEC O86.19
    kidney O86.21
    mammary O91.12
      associated with lactation O91.13
    nipple O91.02
      associated with lactation O91.03
    peritoneum O85
    subareolar O91.12
      associated with lactation O91.13
    urinary tract — *see* Puerperal, infection, urinary
    uterus O86.12
    vagina (wall) O86.13
    vaginorectal O86.13
    vulvovaginal gland O86.13
  adnexitis O86.19
  afibrinogenemia, or other coagulation defect O72.3
  albuminuria (acute) (subacute) — *see* Proteinuria,
    gestational
  alcohol use O99.315
  anemia O90.81
    pre-existing (pre-pregnancy) O99.03
  anesthetic death O89.8
  apoplexy O99.43
  bariatric surgery status O99.845
  blood disorder NEC O99.13
  blood dyscrasia O72.3
  cardiomyopathy O90.3
  cerebrovascular disorder (conditions in I60-I69) O99.43
  cervicitis O86.11
  circulatory system disorder O99.43
  coagulopathy (any) O99.13
    with hemorrhage O72.3
  complications O90.9
    specified NEC O90.89
  convulsions — *see* Eclampsia
  cystitis O86.22
  cystopyelitis O86.29
  delirium NEC F05
  diabetes O24.93
    gestational — *see* Puerperal, gestational diabetes
    pre-existing O24.33
      specified NEC O24.83
      type 1 O24.03
      type 2 O24.13
  digestive system disorder O99.63
  disease O90.9
    breast NEC O92.29
    cerebrovascular (acute) O99.43
    nonobstetric NEC O99.893

Puerperal, puerperium — *continued*
  disease — *continued*
    tubo-ovarian O86.19
    Valsuani's O99.03
  disorder O90.9
    biliary tract O26.63
    lactation O92.70
    liver O26.63
    nonobstetric NEC O99.893
  disruption
    cesarean wound O90.0
    episiotomy wound O90.1
    perineal laceration wound O90.1
  drug use O99.325
  eclampsia (with pre-existing hypertension) O15.2
  embolism (pulmonary) (blood clot) — *see* Embolism,
    obstetric, puerperal
  endocrine, nutritional or metabolic disease NEC
    O99.285
  endophlebitis — *see* Puerperal, phlebitis
  endotrachelitis O86.11
  failure
    lactation (complete) O92.3
      partial O92.4
    renal, acute O90.4
  fever (of unknown origin) O86.4
    septic O85
  fissure, nipple O92.12
    associated with lactation O92.13
  fistula
    breast (due to mastitis) O91.12
      associated with lactation O91.13
    nipple O91.02
      associated with lactation O91.03
  galactophoritis O91.22
    associated with lactation O91.23
  galactorrhea O92.6
  gastric banding status O99.845
  gastric bypass status O99.845
  gastrointestinal disease NEC O99.63
  gestational
    diabetes O24.439
      diet controlled O24.430
      insulin (and diet) controlled O24.434
      oral drug controlled (antidiabetic) (hypo-
        glycemic) O24.435
    edema O12.05
      with proteinuria O12.25
    proteinuria O12.15
  gonorrhea O98.23
  hematoma, subdural O99.43
  hemiplegia, cerebral O99.355
    due to cerbrovascular disorder O99.43
  hemorrhage O72.1
    brain O99.43
    bulbar O99.43
    cerebellar O99.43
    cerebral O99.43
    cortical O99.43
    delayed or secondary O72.2
    extradural O99.43
    internal capsule O99.43
    intracranial O99.43
    intrapontine O99.43
    meningeal O99.43
    pontine O99.43
    retained placenta O72.0
    subarachnoid O99.43
    subcortical O99.43
    subdural O99.43
    third stage O72.0
    uterine, delayed O72.2
    ventricular O99.43
  hemorrhoids O87.2
  hepatorenal syndrome O90.4
  hypertension — *see* Hypertension, complicating,
    puerperium
  hypertrophy, breast O92.29
  induration breast (fibrous) O92.29
  infection O86.4
    cervix O86.11
    generalized O85
    genital tract NEC O86.19
      obstetric surgical wound O86.09
    kidney (bacillus coli) O86.21
    maternal O98.93
      carrier state NEC O99.835
      gonorrhea O98.23
      human immunodeficiency virus (HIV) O98.73

Puerperal, puerperium — *continued*
  infection — *continued*
    maternal — *continued*
      protozoal O98.63
      sexually transmitted NEC O98.33
      specified NEC O98.83
      streptococcus group B (GBS) carrier state O99.825
      syphilis O98.13
      tuberculosis O98.03
      viral hepatitis O98.43
      viral NEC O98.53
    nipple O91.02
      associated with lactation O91.03
    peritoneum O85
    renal O86.21
    specified NEC O86.89
    urinary (asymptomatic) (tract) NEC O86.20
      bladder O86.22
      kidney O86.21
      specified site NEC O86.29
      urethra O86.22
    vagina O86.13
    vein — *see* Puerperal, phlebitis
  ischemia, cerebral O99.43
  lymphangitis O86.89
    breast O91.22
      associated with lactation O91.23
  malignancy O9A.13 (*following* O99)
  malnutrition O25.3
  mammillitis O91.02
    associated with lactation O91.03
  mammitis O91.22
    associated with lactation O91.23
  mania F30.8
  mastitis O91.22
    associated with lactation O91.23
    purulent O91.12
      associated with lactation O91.13
  melancholia — *see* Disorder, depressive
  mental disorder NEC O99.345
  metroperitonitis O85
  metrorrhagia — *see* Hemorrhage, postpartum
  metrosalpingitis O86.19
  metrovaginitis O86.13
  milk leg O87.1
  monoplegia, cerebral O99.43
  mood disturbance O90.6
  necrosis, liver (acute) (subacute) (conditions in subcat
    egory K72.0) O26.63
    with renal failure O90.4
  nervous system disorder O99.355
  obesity (pre-existing prior to pregnancy) O99.215
  obesity surgery status O99.845
  occlusion, precerebral artery O99.43
  paralysis
    bladder (sphincter) O90.89
    cerebral O99.43
  paralytic stroke O99.43
  parametritis O85
  paravaginitis O86.13
  pelviperitonitis O85
  perimetritis O86.12
  perimetrosalpingitis O86.19
  perinephritis O86.21
  periphlebitis — *see* Puerperal phlebitis
  peritoneal infection O85
  peritonitis (pelvic) O85
  perivaginitis O86.13
  phlebitis O87.0
    deep O87.1
    pelvic O87.1
    superficial O87.0
  phlebothrombosis, deep O87.1
  phlegmasia alba dolens O87.1
  placental polyp O90.89
  pneumonia, embolic — *see* Embolism, obstetric,
    puerperal
  pre-eclampsia — *see* Pre-eclampsia
  psychosis (NOS) F53.1
  pyelitis O86.21
  pyelocystitis O86.29
  pyelonephritis O86.21
  pyelonephrosis O86.21
  pyemia O85
  pyocystitis O86.29
  pyohemia O85
  pyometra O86.12
  pyonephritis O86.21
  pyosalpingitis O86.19

Puerperal, puerperium — *continued*
  pyrexia (of unknown origin) O86.4
  renal
    disease NEC O90.89
    failure O90.4
  respiratory disease NEC O99.53
  retention
    decidua — *see* Retention, decidua
    placenta O72.0
    secundines — *see* Retention, secundines
  retrated nipple O92.02
  salpingo-ovaritis O86.19
  salpingoperitonitis O85
  secondary perineal tear O90.1
  sepsis (pelvic) O85
  sepsis O85
  septic thrombophlebitis O86.81
  skin disorder NEC O99.73
  specified condition NEC O99.893
  stroke O99.43
  subinvolution (uterus) O90.89
  subluxation of symphysis (pubis) O26.73
  suppuration — *see* Puerperal, abscess
  tetanus A34
  thelitis O91.02
    associated with lactation O91.03
  thrombocytopenia O72.3
  thrombophlebitis (superficial) O87.0
    deep O87.1
    pelvic O87.1
    septic O86.81
  thrombosis (venous) — *see* Thrombosis, puerperal
  thyroiditis O90.5
  toxemia (eclamptic) (pre-eclamptic) (with convulsions) O15.2
  trauma, non-obstetric O9A.23 (*following* O99)
    caused by abuse (physical) (suspected) O9A.33 (*following* O99)
      confirmed O9A.33 (*following* O99)
      psychological (suspected) O9A.53 (*following* O99)
        confirmed O9A.53 (*following* O99)
      sexual (suspected) O9A.43 (*following* O99)
        confirmed O9A.43 (*following* O99)
  uremia (due to renal failure) O90.4
  urethritis O86.22
  vaginitis O86.13
  varicose veins (legs) O87.4
    vulva or perineum O87.8
  venous O87.9
  vulvitis O86.19
  vulvovaginitis O86.13
  white leg O87.1
Puerperium — *see* Puerperal
Pulmolithiasis J98.4
Pulmonary — *see* condition
Pulpitis (acute) (anachoretic) (chronic) (hyperplastic) (putrescent) (suppurative) (ulcerative) K04.01
  irreversible K04.02
  reversible K04.01
Pulpless tooth K04.99
Pulse
  alternating R00.8
  bigeminal R00.8
  fast R00.0
  feeble, rapid due to shock following injury T79.4 ☑
  rapid R00.0
  weak R09.89
Pulsus alternans or trigeminus R00.8
Punch drunk F07.81
Punctum lacrimale occlusion — *see* Obstruction, lacrimal
Puncture
  abdomen, abdominal
    wall S31.139 ☑
      with
        foreign body S31.149 ☑
        penetration into peritoneal cavity S31.639 ☑
          with foreign body S31.649 ☑
      epigastric region S31.132 ☑
        with
          foreign body S31.142 ☑
          penetration into peritoneal cavity S31.632 ☑
            with foreign body S31.642 ☑
      left
        lower quadrant S31.134 ☑
          with
            foreign body S31.144 ☑

Puncture — *continued*
  abdomen, abdominal — *continued*
    wall — *continued*
      left — *continued*
        lower quadrant — *continued*
          with — *continued*
            penetration into peritoneal cavity S31.634 ☑
              with foreign body S31.644 ☑
        upper quadrant S31.131 ☑
          with
            foreign body S31.141 ☑
            penetration into peritoneal cavity S31.631 ☑
              with foreign body S31.641 ☑
      periumbilic region S31.135 ☑
        with
          foreign body S31.145 ☑
          penetration into peritoneal cavity S31.635 ☑
            with foreign body S31.645 ☑
      right
        lower quadrant S31.133 ☑
          with
            foreign body S31.143 ☑
            penetration into peritoneal cavity S31.633 ☑
              with foreign body S31.643 ☑
        upper quadrant S31.130 ☑
          with
            foreign body S31.140 ☑
            penetration into peritoneal cavity S31.630 ☑
              with foreign body S31.640 ☑
    accidental, complicating surgery — *see* Complication, accidental puncture or laceration
    alveolar (process) — *see* Puncture, oral cavity
    ankle S91.039 ☑
      with
        foreign body S91.049 ☑
      left S91.032 ☑
        with
          foreign body S91.042 ☑
      right S91.031 ☑
        with
          foreign body S91.041 ☑
    anus S31.833 ☑
      with foreign body S31.834 ☑
    arm (upper) S41.139 ☑
      with foreign body S41.149 ☑
      left S41.132 ☑
        with foreign body S41.142 ☑
      lower — *see* Puncture, forearm
      right S41.131 ☑
        with foreign body S41.141 ☑
    auditory canal (external) (meatus) — *see* Puncture, ear
    auricle, ear — *see* Puncture, ear
    axilla — *see* Puncture, arm
    back — *see also* Puncture, thorax, back
      lower S31.030 ☑
        with
          foreign body S31.040 ☑
            with penetration into retroperitoneal space S31.041 ☑
          penetration into retroperitoneal space S31.031 ☑
    bladder (traumatic) S37.29 ☑
      nontraumatic N32.89
    breast S21.039 ☑
      with foreign body S21.049 ☑
      left S21.032 ☑
        with foreign body S21.042 ☑
      right S21.031 ☑
        with foreign body S21.041 ☑
    buttock S31.803 ☑
      with foreign body S31.804 ☑
      left S31.823 ☑
        with foreign body S31.824 ☑
      right S31.813 ☑
        with foreign body S31.814 ☑
    by
      device, implant or graft — *see* Complications, by site and type, mechanical
      foreign body left accidentally in operative wound T81.539 ☑

Puncture — *continued*
  by — *continued*
    instrument (any) during a procedure, accidental — *see* Puncture, accidental complicating surgery
  calf — *see* Puncture, leg
  canaliculus lacrimalis — *see* Puncture, eyelid
  canthus, eye — *see* Puncture, eyelid
  cervical esophagus S11.23 ☑
    with foreign body S11.24 ☑
  cheek (external) S01.439 ☑
    with foreign body S01.449 ☑
    internal — *see* Puncture, oral cavity
    left S01.432 ☑
      with foreign body S01.442 ☑
    right S01.431 ☑
      with foreign body S01.441 ☑
  chest wall — *see* Puncture, thorax
  chin — *see* Puncture, head, specified site NEC
  clitoris — *see* Puncture, vulva
  costal region — *see* Puncture, thorax
  digit(s)
    foot — *see* Puncture, toe
    hand — *see* Puncture, finger
  ear (canal) (external) S01.339 ☑
    with foreign body S01.349 ☑
    drum S09.2- ☑
    left S01.332 ☑
      with foreign body S01.342 ☑
    right S01.331 ☑
      with foreign body S01.341 ☑
  elbow S51.039 ☑
    with
      foreign body S51.049 ☑
    left S51.032 ☑
      with
        foreign body S51.042 ☑
    right S51.031 ☑
      with
        foreign body S51.041 ☑
  epididymis — *see* Puncture, testis
  epigastric region — *see* Puncture, abdomen, wall, epigastric
  epiglottis S11.83 ☑
    with foreign body S11.84 ☑
  esophagus
    cervical S11.23 ☑
      with foreign body S11.24 ☑
    thoracic S27.818 ☑
  eyeball S05.6- ☑
    with foreign body S05.5- ☑
  eyebrow — *see* Puncture, eyelid
  eyelid S01.13- ☑
    with foreign body S01.14- ☑
    left S01.132 ☑
      with foreign body S01.142 ☑
    right S01.131 ☑
      with foreign body S01.141 ☑
  face NEC — *see* Puncture, head, specified site NEC
  finger(s) S61.239 ☑
    with
      damage to nail S61.339 ☑
        with
          foreign body S61.349 ☑
      foreign body S61.249 ☑
    index S61.238 ☑
      with
        damage to nail S61.338 ☑
          with
            foreign body S61.348 ☑
        foreign body S61.248 ☑
      left S61.231 ☑
        with
          damage to nail S61.331 ☑
            with
              foreign body S61.341 ☑
          foreign body S61.241 ☑
      right S61.230 ☑
        with
          damage to nail S61.330 ☑
            with
              foreign body S61.340 ☑
          foreign body S61.240 ☑
    little S61.238 ☑
      with
        damage to nail S61.338 ☑

Puncture — *continued*
  finger(s) — *continued*
    little — *continued*
      with — *continued*
        damage to nail — *continued*
          with
            foreign body S61.348 ☑
          foreign body S61.248 ☑
        left S61.237 ☑
          with
            damage to nail S61.337 ☑
              with
                foreign body S61.347 ☑
              foreign body S61.247 ☑
        right S61.236 ☑
          with
            damage to nail S61.336 ☑
              with
                foreign body S61.346 ☑
              foreign body S61.246 ☑
    middle S61.238 ☑
      with
        damage to nail S61.338 ☑
          with
            foreign body S61.348 ☑
        foreign body S61.248 ☑
      left S61.233 ☑
        with
          damage to nail S61.333 ☑
            with
              foreign body S61.343 ☑
          foreign body S61.243 ☑
      right S61.232 ☑
        with
          damage to nail S61.332 ☑
            with
              foreign body S61.342 ☑
          foreign body S61.242 ☑
    ring S61.238 ☑
      with
        damage to nail S61.338 ☑
          with
            foreign body S61.348 ☑
        foreign body S61.248 ☑
      left S61.235 ☑
        with
          damage to nail S61.335 ☑
            with
              foreign body S61.345 ☑
          foreign body S61.245 ☑
      right S61.234 ☑
        with
          damage to nail S61.334 ☑
            with
              foreign body S61.344 ☑
          foreign body S61.244 ☑
  flank S31.139 ☑
    with foreign body S31.149 ☑
  foot (except toe(s) alone) S91.339 ☑
    with foreign body S91.349 ☑
    left S91.332 ☑
      with foreign body S91.342 ☑
    right S91.331 ☑
      with foreign body S91.341 ☑
    toe — *see* Puncture, toe
  forearm S51.839 ☑
    with
      foreign body S51.849 ☑
    elbow only — *see* Puncture, elbow
    left S51.832 ☑
      with
        foreign body S51.842 ☑
    right S51.831 ☑
      with
        foreign body S51.841 ☑
  forehead — *see* Puncture, head, specified site NEC
  genital organs, external
    female S31.532 ☑
      with foreign body S31.542 ☑
      vagina — *see* Puncture, vagina
      vulva — *see* Puncture, vulva
    male S31.531 ☑
      with foreign body S31.541 ☑
      penis — *see* Puncture, penis
      scrotum — *see* Puncture, scrotum
      testis — *see* Puncture, testis

Puncture — *continued*
  groin — *see* Puncture, abdomen, wall
  gum — *see* Puncture, oral cavity
  hand S61.439 ☑
    with
      foreign body S61.449 ☑
    finger — *see* Puncture, finger
    left S61.432 ☑
      with
        foreign body S61.442 ☑
    right S61.431 ☑
      with
        foreign body S61.441 ☑
    thumb — *see* Puncture, thumb
  head S01.93 ☑
    with foreign body S01.94 ☑
    cheek — *see* Puncture, cheek
    ear — *see* Puncture, ear
    eyelid — *see* Puncture, eyelid
    lip — *see* Puncture, oral cavity
    nose — *see* Puncture, nose
    oral cavity — *see* Puncture, oral cavity
    scalp S01.03 ☑
      with foreign body S01.04 ☑
    specified site NEC S01.83 ☑
      with foreign body S01.84 ☑
    temporomandibular area — *see* Puncture, cheek
  heart S26.99 ☑
    with hemopericardium S26.09 ☑
    without hemopericardium S26.19 ☑
  heel — *see* Puncture, foot
  hip S71.039 ☑
    with foreign body S71.049 ☑
    left S71.032 ☑
      with foreign body S71.042 ☑
    right S71.031 ☑
      with foreign body S71.041 ☑
  hymen — *see* Puncture, vagina
  hypochondrium — *see* Puncture, abdomen, wall
  hypogastric region — *see* Puncture, abdomen, wall
  inguinal region — *see* Puncture, abdomen, wall
  instep — *see* Puncture, foot
  internal organs — *see* Injury, by site
  interscapular region — *see* Puncture, thorax, back
  intestine
    large
      colon S36.599 ☑
        ascending S36.590 ☑
        descending S36.592 ☑
        sigmoid S36.593 ☑
        specified site NEC S36.598 ☑
        transverse S36.591 ☑
      rectum S36.69 ☑
    small S36.499 ☑
      duodenum S36.490 ☑
      specified site NEC S36.498 ☑
  intra-abdominal organ S36.99 ☑
    gallbladder S36.128 ☑
    intestine — *see* Puncture, intestine
    liver S36.118 ☑
    pancreas — *see* Puncture, pancreas
    peritoneum S36.81 ☑
    specified site NEC S36.898 ☑
    spleen S36.09 ☑
    stomach S36.39 ☑
  jaw — *see* Puncture, head, specified site NEC
  knee S81.039 ☑
    with foreign body S81.049 ☑
    left S81.032 ☑
      with foreign body S81.042 ☑
    right S81.031 ☑
      with foreign body S81.041 ☑
  labium (majus) (minus) — *see* Puncture, vulva
  lacrimal duct — *see* Puncture, eyelid
  larynx S11.013 ☑
    with foreign body S11.014 ☑
  leg (lower) S81.839 ☑
    with foreign body S81.849 ☑
    foot — *see* Puncture, foot
    knee — *see* Puncture, knee
    left S81.832 ☑
      with foreign body S81.842 ☑
    right S81.831 ☑
      with foreign body S81.841 ☑
    upper — *see* Puncture, thigh
  lip S01.531 ☑

Puncture — *continued*
  lip — *continued*
    with foreign body S01.541 ☑
  loin — *see* Puncture, abdomen, wall
  lower back — *see* Puncture, back, lower
  lumbar region — *see* Puncture, back, lower
  malar region — *see* Puncture, head, specified site NEC
  mammary — *see* Puncture, breast
  mastoid region — *see* Puncture, head, specified site NEC
  mouth — *see* Puncture, oral cavity
  nail
    finger — *see* Puncture, finger, with damage to nail
    toe — *see* Puncture, toe, with damage to nail
  nasal (septum) (sinus) — *see* Puncture, nose
  nasopharynx — *see* Puncture, head, specified site NEC
  neck S11.93 ☑
    with foreign body S11.94 ☑
    involving
      cervical esophagus — *see* Puncture, cervical esophagus
      larynx — *see* Puncture, larynx
      pharynx — *see* Puncture, pharynx
      thyroid gland — *see* Puncture, thyroid gland
      trachea — *see* Puncture, trachea
    specified site NEC S11.83 ☑
      with foreign body S11.84 ☑
  nose (septum) (sinus) S01.23 ☑
    with foreign body S01.24 ☑
  ocular — *see* Puncture, eyeball
  oral cavity S01.532 ☑
    with foreign body S01.542 ☑
  orbit S05.4- ☑
  palate — *see* Puncture, oral cavity
  palm — *see* Puncture, hand
  pancreas S36.299 ☑
    body S36.291 ☑
    head S36.290 ☑
    tail S36.292 ☑
  pelvis — *see* Puncture, back, lower
  penis S31.23 ☑
    with foreign body S31.24 ☑
  perineum
    female S31.43 ☑
      with foreign body S31.44 ☑
    male S31.139 ☑
      with foreign body S31.149 ☑
  periocular area (with or without lacrimal passages) — *see* Puncture, eyelid
  phalanges
    finger — *see* Puncture, finger
    toe — *see* Puncture, toe
  pharynx S11.23 ☑
    with foreign body S11.24 ☑
  pinna — *see* Puncture, ear
  popliteal space — *see* Puncture, knee
  prepuce — *see* Puncture, penis
  pubic region S31.139 ☑
    with foreign body S31.149 ☑
  pudendum — *see* Puncture, genital organs, external
  rectovaginal septum — *see* Puncture, vagina
  sacral region — *see* Puncture, back, lower
  sacroiliac region — *see* Puncture, back, lower
  salivary gland — *see* Puncture, oral cavity
  scalp S01.03 ☑
    with foreign body S01.04 ☑
  scapular region — *see* Puncture, shoulder
  scrotum S31.33 ☑
    with foreign body S31.34 ☑
  shin — *see* Puncture, leg
  shoulder S41.039 ☑
    with foreign body S41.049 ☑
    left S41.032 ☑
      with foreign body S41.042 ☑
    right S41.031 ☑
      with foreign body S41.041 ☑
  spermatic cord — *see* Puncture, testis
  sternal region — *see* Puncture, thorax, front
  submaxillary region — *see* Puncture, head, specified site NEC
  submental region — *see* Puncture, head, specified site NEC
  subungual
    finger(s) — *see* Puncture, finger, with damage to nail
    toe — *see* Puncture, toe, with damage to nail

Puncture — *continued*
  supraclavicular fossa — *see* Puncture, neck, specified site NEC
  temple, temporal region — *see* Puncture, head, specified site NEC
  temporomandibular area — *see* Puncture, cheek
  testis S31.33 ☑
    with foreign body S31.34 ☑
  thigh S71.139 ☑
    with foreign body S71.149 ☑
    left S71.132 ☑
      with foreign body S71.142 ☑
    right S71.131 ☑
      with foreign body S71.141 ☑
  thorax, thoracic (wall) S21.93 ☑
    with foreign body S21.94 ☑
    back S21.23- ☑
      with
        foreign body S21.24- ☑
          with penetration S21.44 ☑
        penetration S21.43 ☑
    breast — *see* Puncture, breast
    front S21.13- ☑
      with
        foreign body S21.14- ☑
          with penetration S21.34 ☑
        penetration S21.33 ☑
  throat — *see* Puncture, neck
  thumb S61.039 ☑
    with
      damage to nail S61.139 ☑
        with
          foreign body S61.149 ☑
      foreign body S61.049 ☑
    left S61.032 ☑
      with
        damage to nail S61.132 ☑
          with
            foreign body S61.142 ☑
        foreign body S61.042 ☑
    right S61.031 ☑
      with
        damage to nail S61.131 ☑
          with
            foreign body S61.141 ☑
        foreign body S61.041 ☑
  thyroid gland S11.13 ☑
    with foreign body S11.14 ☑
  toe(s) S91.139 ☑
    with
      damage to nail S91.239 ☑
        with
          foreign body S91.249 ☑
      foreign body S91.149 ☑
    great S91.133 ☑
      with
        damage to nail S91.233 ☑
          with
            foreign body S91.243 ☑
        foreign body S91.143 ☑
      left S91.132 ☑
        with
          damage to nail S91.232 ☑
            with
              foreign body S91.242 ☑
          foreign body S91.142 ☑
      right S91.131 ☑
        with
          damage to nail S91.231 ☑
            with
              foreign body S91.241 ☑
          foreign body S91.141 ☑
    lesser S91.136 ☑
      with
        damage to nail S91.236 ☑
          with
            foreign body S91.246 ☑
        foreign body S91.146 ☑
      left S91.135 ☑
        with
          damage to nail S91.235 ☑
            with
              foreign body S91.245 ☑
          foreign body S91.145 ☑
      right S91.134 ☑

Puncture — *continued*
  toe(s) — *continued*
    lesser — *continued*
      right — *continued*
        with
          damage to nail S91.234 ☑
            with
              foreign body S91.244 ☑
          foreign body S91.144 ☑
  tongue — *see* Puncture, oral cavity
  trachea S11.023 ☑
    with foreign body S11.024 ☑
  tunica vaginalis — *see* Puncture, testis
  tympanum, tympanic membrane S09.2- ☑
  umbilical region S31.135 ☑
    with foreign body S31.145 ☑
  uvula — *see* Puncture, oral cavity
  vagina S31.43 ☑
    with foreign body S31.44 ☑
  vocal cords S11.033 ☑
    with foreign body S11.034 ☑
  vulva S31.43 ☑
    with foreign body S31.44 ☑
  wrist S61.539 ☑
    with
      foreign body S61.549 ☑
    left S61.532 ☑
      with
        foreign body S61.542 ☑
    right S61.531 ☑
      with
        foreign body S61.541 ☑
PUO (pyrexia of unknown origin) R50.9
Pupillary membrane (persistent) Q13.89
Pupillotonia — *see* Anomaly, pupil, function, tonic pupil
Purpura D69.2
  abdominal D69.0
  allergic D69.0
  anaphylactoid D69.0
  annularis telangiectodes L81.7
  arthritic D69.0
  autoerythrocyte sensitization D69.2
  autoimmune D69.0
  bacterial D69.0
  Bateman's (senile) D69.2
  capillary fragility (hereditary) (idiopathic) D69.8
  cryoglobulinemic D89.1
  Devil's pinches D69.2
  fibrinolytic — *see* Fibrinolysis
  fulminans, fulminous D65
  gangrenous D65
  hemorrhagic, hemorrhagica D69.3
    not due to thrombocytopenia D69.0
  Henoch (-Schönlein) (allergic) D69.0
  hypergammaglobulinemic (benign) (Waldenström) D89.0
  idiopathic (thrombocytopenic) D69.3
    nonthrombocytopenic D69.0
  immune thrombocytopenic D69.3
  infectious D69.0
  malignant D69.0
  neonatorum P54.5
  nervosa D69.0
  newborn P54.5
  nonthrombocytopenic D69.2
    hemorrhagic D69.0
    idiopathic D69.0
  nonthrombopenic D69.2
  peliosis rheumatica D69.0
  posttransfusion (post-transfusion) (from (fresh) whole blood or blood products) D69.51
  primary D69.49
  red cell membrane sensitivity D69.2
  rheumatica D69.0
  Schönlein (-Henoch) (allergic) D69.0
  scorbutic E54 [D77]
  senile D69.2
  simplex D69.2
  symptomatica D69.0
  telangiectasia annularis L81.7
  thrombocytopenic D69.49
    congenital D69.42
    hemorrhagic D69.3
    hereditary D69.42
    idiopathic D69.3
    immune D69.3
    neonatal, transitory P61.0
    thrombotic M31.1

Purpura — *continued*
  thrombohemolytic — *see* Fibrinolysis
  thrombolytic — *see* Fibrinolysis
  thrombopenic D69.49
  thrombotic, thrombocytopenic M31.1
  toxic D69.0
  vascular D69.0
  visceral symptoms D69.0
Purpuric spots R23.3
Purulent — *see* condition
Pus
  in
    stool R19.5
    urine N39.0
  tube (rupture) — *see* Salpingo-oophoritis
Pustular rash L08.0
Pustule (nonmalignant) L08.9
  malignant A22.0
Pustulosis palmaris et plantaris L40.3
Putnam (-Dana) **disease or syndrome** — *see* Degeneration, combined
Putrescent pulp (dental) K04.1
Pyarthritis, pyarthrosis — *see* Arthritis, pyogenic or pyemic
  tuberculous — *see* Tuberculosis, joint
Pyelectasis — *see* Hydronephrosis
Pyelitis (congenital) (uremic) — *see also* Pyelonephritis
  with
    calculus — *see* category N20 ☑
      with hydronephrosis N13.6
    contracted kidney N11.9
  acute N10
  chronic N11.9
    with calculus — *see* category N20 ☑
      with hydronephrosis N13.6
  cystica N28.84
  puerperal (postpartum) O86.21
  tuberculous A18.11
Pyelocystitis — *see* Pyelonephritis
Pyelonephritis — *see also* Nephritis, tubulo-interstitial
  with
    calculus — *see* category N20 ☑
      with hydronephrosis N13.6
    contracted kidney N11.9
  acute N10
  calculous — *see* category N20 ☑
    with hydronephrosis N13.6
  chronic N11.9
    with calculus — *see* category N20 ☑
      with hydronephrosis N13.6
    associated with ureteral obstruction or stricture N11.1
    nonobstructive N11.8
      with reflux (vesicoureteral) N11.0
    obstructive N11.1
    specified NEC N11.8
  in (due to)
    brucellosis A23.9 [N16]
    cryoglobulinemia (mixed) D89.1 [N16]
    cystinosis E72.04
    diphtheria A36.84
    glycogen storage disease E74.09 [N16]
    leukemia NEC C95.9- ☑ [N16]
    lymphoma NEC C85.90 [N16]
    multiple myeloma C90.0- ☑ [N16]
    obstruction N11.1
    Salmonella infection A02.25
    sarcoidosis D86.84
    sepsis A41.9 [N16]
    Sjögren's disease M35.04
    toxoplasmosis B58.83
    transplant rejection T86.91 [N16]
    Wilson's disease E83.01 [N16]
    nonobstructive N12
      with reflux (vesicoureteral) N11.0
      chronic N11.8
  syphilitic A52.75
Pyelonephrosis (obstructive) N11.1
  chronic N11.9
Pyelophlebitis I80.8
Pyeloureteritis cystica N28.85
Pyemia, pyemic (fever) (infection) (purulent) — *see also* Sepsis
  joint — *see* Arthritis, pyogenic or pyemic
  liver K75.1
  pneumococcal A40.3
  portal K75.1

🐢 Subterms under main terms may continue to next column or page   ☑ Additional Character Required — Refer to the Tabular List for Character Selection   275

Puncture — Pyemia, pyemic

Pyemia, pyemic — continued
  postvaccinal T88.0 ☑
  puerperal, postpartum, childbirth O85
  specified organism NEC A41.89
  tuberculous — see Tuberculosis, miliary
Pygopagus Q89.4
Pyknoepilepsy (idiopathic) — see Pyknolepsy
Pyknolepsy G40.A09 (following G40.3)
  intractable G40.A19 (following G40.3)
    with status epilepticus G40.A11 (following G40.3)
    without status epilepticus G40.A19 (following G40.3)
  not intractable G40.A09 (following G40.3)
    with status epilepticus G40.A01 (following G40.3)
    without status epilepticus G40.A09 (following G40.3)
Pylephlebitis K75.1
Pyle's syndrome Q78.5
Pylethrombophlebitis K75.1
Pylethrombosis K75.1
Pyloritis K29.90
  with bleeding K29.91
Pylorospasm (reflex) **NEC** K31.3
  congenital or infantile Q40.0
  neurotic F45.8
  newborn Q40.0
  psychogenic F45.8
Pylorus, pyloric — see condition
Pyoarthrosis — see Arthritis, pyogenic or pyemic
Pyocele
  mastoid — see Mastoiditis, acute
  sinus (accessory) — see Sinusitis
  turbinate (bone) J32.9
  urethra — see also Urethritis N34.0
Pyocolpos — see Vaginitis
Pyocystitis N30.80
  with hematuria N30.81
Pyoderma, pyodermia L08.0
  gangrenosum L88
  newborn P39.4
  phagedenic L88
  vegetans L08.81
Pyodermatitis L08.0
  vegetans L08.81
Pyogenic — see condition
Pyohydronephrosis N13.6
Pyometra, pyometrium, pyometritis — see Endometritis
Pyomyositis (tropical) — see Myositis, infective
Pyonephritis N12
Pyonephrosis N13.6
  tuberculous A18.11
Pyo-oophoritis — see Salpingo-oophoritis
Pyo-ovarium — see Salpingo-oophoritis
Pyopericarditis, pyopericardium I30.1
Pyophlebitis — see Phlebitis
Pyopneumopericardium I30.1
Pyopneumothorax (infective) J86.9
  with fistula J86.0
  tuberculous NEC A15.6
Pyosalpinx, pyosalpingitis — see also Salpingo-
    oophoritis
Pyothorax J86.9
  with fistula J86.0
  tuberculous NEC A15.6
Pyoureter N28.89
  tuberculous A18.11
Pyramidopallidonigral syndrome G20
Pyrexia (of unknown origin) R50.9
  atmospheric T67.01 ☑
  during labor NEC O75.2
  heat T67.01 ☑
  newborn P81.9
    environmentally-induced P81.0
  persistent R50.9
  puerperal O86.4
Pyroglobulinemia NEC E88.09
Pyromania F63.1
Pyrosis R12
Pyuria (bacterial) (sterile) R82.81

Q

Q fever A78
  with pneumonia A78
Quadricuspid aortic valve Q23.8
Quadrilateral fever A78
Quadriparesis — see Quadriplegia
  meaning muscle weakness M62.81

Quadriplegia G82.50
  complete
    C1-C4 level G82.51
    C5-C7 level G82.53
  congenital (cerebral) (spinal) G80.8
    spastic G80.0
  embolic (current episode) I63.4- ☑
  functional R53.2
  incomplete
    C1-C4 level G82.52
    C5-C7 level G82.54
  thrombotic (current episode) I63.3- ☑
  traumatic — code to injury with seventh character S
    current episode — see Injury, spinal (cord), cervical
Quadruplet, pregnancy — see Pregnancy, quadruplet
Quarrelsomeness F60.3
Queensland fever A77.3
Quervain's disease M65.4
  thyroid E06.1
Queyrat's erythroplasia D07.4
  penis D07.4
  specified site — see Neoplasm, skin, in situ
  unspecified site D07.4
Quincke's disease or edema T78.3 ☑
  hereditary D84.1
Quinsy (gangrenous) J36
Quintan fever A79.0
Quintuplet, pregnancy — see Pregnancy, quintuplet

R

Rabbit fever — see Tularemia
Rabies A82.9
  contact Z20.3
  exposure to Z20.3
  inoculation reaction — see Complications, vaccination
  sylvatic A82.0
  urban A82.1
Rachischisis — see Spina bifida
Rachitic — see also condition
  deformities of spine (late effect) (sequelae) E64.3
  pelvis (late effect) (sequelae) E64.3
    with disproportion (fetopelvic) O33.0
      causing obstructed labor O65.0
Rachitis, rachitism (acute) (tarda) — see also Rickets
  renalis N25.0
  sequelae E64.3
Radial nerve — see condition
Radiation
  burn — see Burn
  effects NOS T66 ☑
  sickness NOS T66 ☑
  therapy, encounter for Z51.0
Radiculitis (pressure) (vertebrogenic) — see Radiculopathy
Radiculomyelitis — see also Encephalitis
  toxic, due to
    Clostridium tetani A35
    Corynebacterium diphtheriae A36.82
Radiculopathy M54.10
  cervical region M54.12
  cervicothoracic region M54.13
  due to
    disc disorder
      C3 M50.11
      C4 M50.11
      C5 M50.121
      C6 M50.122
      C7 M50.123
    displacement of intervertebral disc — see Disorder,
      disc, with, radiculopathy
  leg M54.1- ☑
  lumbar region M54.16
  lumbosacral region M54.17
  occipito-atlanto-axial region M54.11
  postherpetic B02.29
  sacrococcygeal region M54.18
  syphilitic A52.11
  thoracic region (with visceral pain) M54.14
  thoracolumbar region M54.15
Radiodermal burns (acute, chronic, or occupational) —
    see Burn
Radiodermatitis L58.9
  acute L58.0
  chronic L58.1
Radiotherapy session Z51.0
RAEB (refractory anemia with excess blasts) D46.2- ☑

Rage, meaning rabies — see Rabies
Ragpicker's disease A22.1
Ragsorter's disease A22.1
Raillietiniasis B71.8
Railroad neurosis F48.8
Railway spine F48.8
Raised — see also Elevated
  antibody titer R76.0
Rake teeth, tooth M26.39
Rales R09.89
Ramifying renal pelvis Q63.8
Ramsay-Hunt disease or syndrome — see also Hunt's
    disease B02.21
  meaning dyssynergia cerebellaris myoclonica G11.19
Ranula K11.6
  congenital Q38.4
Rape
  adult
    confirmed T74.21 ☑
    suspected T76.21 ☑
  alleged, observation or examination, ruled out
    adult Z04.41
    child Z04.42
  child
    confirmed T74.22 ☑
    suspected T76.22 ☑
Rapid
  feeble pulse, due to shock, following injury T79.4 ☑
  heart (beat) R00.0
    psychogenic F45.8
  second stage (delivery) O62.3
  time-zone change syndrome G47.25
Rarefaction, bone — see Disorder, bone, density and
    structure, specified NEC
Rash (toxic) R21
  canker A38.9
  diaper L22
  drug (internal use) L27.0
    contact — see also Dermatitis, due to, drugs, exter-
      nal L25.1
  following immunization T88.1 ☑
  food — see Dermatitis, due to, food
  heat L74.0
  napkin (psoriasiform) L22
  nettle — see Urticaria
  pustular L08.0
  rose R21
    epidemic B06.9
  scarlet A38.9
  serum — see also Reaction, serum T80.69 ☑
  wandering tongue K14.1
Rasmussen aneurysm — see Tuberculosis, pulmonary
Rasmussen encephalitis G04.81
Rat-bite fever A25.9
  due to Streptobacillus moniliformis A25.1
  spirochetal (morsus muris) A25.0
Rathke's pouch tumor D44.3
Raymond (-Céstan) **syndrome** I65.8
Raynaud's disease, phenomenon or syndrome (sec-
    ondary) I73.00
  with gangrene (symmetric) I73.01
RDS (newborn) (type I) P22.0
  type II P22.1
Reaction — see also Disorder
  withdrawing, child or adolescent F93.8
  adaptation — see Disorder, adjustment
  adjustment (anxiety) (conduct disorder) (depressive-
    ness) (distress) — see Disorder, adjustment
    with
      mutism, elective (child) (adolescent) F94.0
  adverse
    food (any) (ingested) NEC T78.1 ☑
      anaphylactic — see Shock, anaphylactic, due to
        food
  affective — see Disorder, mood
  allergic — see Allergy
  anaphylactic — see Shock, anaphylactic
  anaphylactoid — see Shock, anaphylactic
  anesthesia — see Anesthesia, complication
  antitoxin (prophylactic) (therapeutic) — see Complica-
    tions, vaccination
  anxiety F41.1
  Arthus — see Arthus' phenomenon
  asthenic F48.8
  combat and operational stress F43.0
  compulsive F42.8
  conversion F44.9

Reaction — *continued*
- crisis, acute F43.0
- deoxyribonuclease (DNA) (DNase) hypersensitivity D69.2
- depressive (single episode) F32.9
  - affective (single episode) F31.4
    - recurrent episode F33.9
  - neurotic F34.1
  - psychoneurotic F34.1
  - psychotic F32.3
  - recurrent — *see* Disorder, depressive, recurrent
- dissociative F44.9
- drug NEC T88.7 ☑
  - addictive — *see* Dependence, drug
    - transmitted via placenta or breast milk — *see* Absorption, drug, addictive, through placenta
  - allergic — *see* Allergy, drug
  - lichenoid L43.2
  - newborn P93.8
    - gray baby syndrome P93.0
  - overdose or poisoning (by accident) — *see* Table of Drugs and Chemicals, by drug, poisoning
  - photoallergic L56.1
  - phototoxic L56.0
  - withdrawal — *see* Dependence, by drug, with, withdrawal
    - infant of dependent mother P96.1
    - newborn P96.1
  - wrong substance given or taken (by accident) — *see* Table of Drugs and Chemicals, by drug, poisoning
- fear F40.9
  - child (abnormal) F93.8
- febrile nonhemolytic transfusion (FNHTR) R50.84
- fluid loss, cerebrospinal G97.1
- foreign
  - body NEC — *see* Granuloma, foreign body
    - in operative wound (inadvertently left) — *see* Foreign body, accidentally left during a procedure
  - substance accidentally left during a procedure (chemical) (powder) (talc) T81.60 ☑
    - aseptic peritonitis T81.61 ☑
    - body or object (instrument) (sponge) (swab) — *see* Foreign body, accidentally left during a procedure
    - specified reaction NEC T81.69 ☑
- grief — *see* Disorder, adjustment
- Herxheimer's R68.89
- hyperkinetic — *see* Hyperkinesia
- hypochondriacal F45.20
- hypoglycemic, due to insulin E16.0
  - with coma (diabetic) — *see* Diabetes, coma
    - nondiabetic E15
  - therapeutic misadventure — *see* subcategory T38.3 ☑
- hypomanic F30.8
- hysterical F44.9
- immunization — *see* Complications, vaccination
- incompatibility
  - ABO blood group (infusion) (transfusion) — *see* Complication(s), transfusion, incompatibility reaction, ABO
    - delayed serologic T80.39 ☑
  - minor blood group (Duffy) (E) (K) (Kell) (Kidd) (Lewis) (M) (N) (P) (S) T80.89 ☑
  - Rh (factor) (infusion) (transfusion) — *see* Complication(s), transfusion, incompatibility reaction, Rh (factor)
- inflammatory — *see* Infection
- infusion — *see* Complications, infusion
- inoculation (immune serum) — *see* Complications, vaccination
- insulin T38.3- ☑
- involutional psychotic — *see* Disorder, depressive
- leukemoid D72.823
  - basophilic D72.823
  - lymphocytic D72.823
  - monocytic D72.823
  - myelocytic D72.823
  - neutrophilic D72.823
- LSD (acute)
  - due to drug abuse — *see* Abuse, drug, hallucinogen
  - due to drug dependence — *see* Dependence, drug, hallucinogen
- lumbar puncture G97.1
- manic-depressive — *see* Disorder, bipolar

Reaction — *continued*
- neurasthenic F48.8
- neurogenic — *see* Neurosis
- neurotic F48.9
- neurotic-depressive F34.1
- nitritoid — *see* Crisis, nitritoid
- nonspecific
  - to
    - cell mediated immunity measurement of gamma interferon antigen response without active tuberculosis R76.12
    - QuantiFERON-TB test (QFT) without active tuberculosis R76.12
    - tuberculin test — *see also* Reaction, tuberculin skin test R76.11
- obsessive-compulsive F42.8
- organic, acute or subacute — *see* Delirium
- paranoid (acute) F23
  - chronic F22
  - senile F03 ☑
- passive dependency F60.7
- phobic F40.9
- post-traumatic stress, uncomplicated Z73.3
- psychogenic F99
- psychoneurotic — *see also* Neurosis
  - compulsive F42.8
  - depersonalization F48.1
  - depressive F34.1
  - hypochondriacal F45.20
  - neurasthenic F48.8
  - obsessive F42.8
- psychophysiologic — *see* Disorder, somatoform
- psychosomatic — *see* Disorder, somatoform
- psychotic — *see* Psychosis
- scarlet fever toxin — *see* Complications, vaccination
- schizophrenic F23
  - acute (brief) (undifferentiated) F23
  - latent F21
  - undifferentiated (acute) (brief) F23
- serological for syphilis — *see* Serology for syphilis
- serum T80.69 ☑
  - anaphylactic (immediate) — *see also* Shock, anaphylactic T80.59 ☑
  - specified reaction NEC
    - due to
      - administration of blood and blood products T80.61 ☑
      - immunization T80.62 ☑
      - serum specified NEC T80.69 ☑
      - vaccination T80.62 ☑
- situational — *see* Disorder, adjustment
- somatization — *see* Disorder, somatoform
- spinal puncture G97.1
  - dural G97.1
- stress (severe) F43.9
  - acute (agitation) ("daze") (disorientation) (disturbance of consciousness) (flight reaction) (fugue) F43.0
  - specified NEC F43.8
- surgical procedure — *see* Complications, surgical procedure
- tetanus antitoxin — *see* Complications, vaccination
- toxic, to local anesthesia T88.59 ☑
  - in labor and delivery O74.4
  - in pregnancy O29.3X- ☑
  - postpartum, puerperal O89.3
- toxin-antitoxin — *see* Complications, vaccination
- transfusion (blood) (bone marrow) (lymphocytes) (allergic) — *see* Complications, transfusion
- tuberculin skin test, abnormal R76.11
- vaccination (any) — *see* Complications, vaccination

Reactive airway disease — *see* Asthma
Reactive depression — *see* Reaction, depressive
Rearrangement
- chromosomal
  - balanced (in) Q95.9
    - abnormal individual (autosomal) Q95.2
    - non-sex (autosomal) chromosomes Q95.2
    - sex/non-sex chromosomes Q95.3
    - specified NEC Q95.8

Recalcitrant patient — *see* Noncompliance
Recanalization, thrombus — *see* Thrombosis
Recession, receding
- chamber angle (eye) H21.55- ☑
- chin M26.09
- gingival (postinfective) (postoperative)
  - generalized K06.020
    - minimal K06.021

Recession, receding — *continued*
- gingival — *continued*
  - generalized — *continued*
    - moderate K06.022
    - severe K06.023
  - localized K06.010
    - minimal K06.011
    - moderate K06.012
    - severe K06.013

Recklinghausen disease Q85.01
- bones E21.0
Reclus' disease (cystic) — *see* Mastopathy, cystic
Recrudescent typhus (fever) A75.1
Recruitment, auditory H93.21- ☑
Rectalgia K62.89
Rectitis K62.89
Rectocele
- female (without uterine prolapse) N81.6
  - with uterine prolapse N81.4
    - incomplete N81.2
- in pregnancy — *see* Pregnancy, complicated by, abnormal, pelvic organs or tissues NEC
- male K62.3
Rectosigmoid junction — *see* condition
Rectosigmoiditis K63.89
- ulcerative (chronic) K51.30
  - with
    - complication K51.319
      - abscess K51.314
      - fistula K51.313
      - obstruction K51.312
      - rectal bleeding K51.311
      - specified NEC K51.318
Rectourethral — *see* condition
Rectovaginal — *see* condition
Rectovesical — *see* condition
Rectum, rectal — *see* condition
Recurrent — *see* condition
- pregnancy loss — *see* Loss (of), pregnancy, recurrent
Red bugs B88.0
Red tide — *see also* Table of Drugs and Chemicals T65.82- ☑
Red-cedar lung or pneumonitis J67.8
Reduced
- mobility Z74.09
- ventilatory or vital capacity R94.2
Redundant, redundancy
- anus (congenital) Q43.8
- clitoris N90.89
- colon (congenital) Q43.8
- foreskin (congenital) N47.8
- intestine (congenital) Q43.8
- labia N90.69
- organ or site, congenital NEC — *see* Accessory
- panniculus (abdominal) E65
- prepuce (congenital) N47.8
- pylorus K31.89
- rectum (congenital) Q43.8
- scrotum N50.89
- sigmoid (congenital) Q43.8
- skin L98.7
  - and subcutaneous tissue L98.7
  - of face L57.4
    - eyelids — *see* Blepharochalasis
- stomach K31.89
Reduplication — *see* Duplication
Reflex R29.2
- hyperactive gag J39.2
- pupillary, abnormal — *see* Anomaly, pupil, function
- vasoconstriction I73.9
- vasovagal R55
Reflux K21.9
- acid K21.9
- esophageal K21.9
  - with esophagitis (without bleeding) K21.00
    - with bleeding K21.01
  - newborn P78.83
- gastroesophageal K21.9
  - with esophagitis (without bleeding) K21.00
    - with bleeding K21.01
- mitral — *see* Insufficiency, mitral
- ureteral — *see* Reflux, vesicoureteral
- vesicoureteral (with scarring) N13.70
  - with
    - nephropathy N13.729
      - with hydroureter N13.739
        - bilateral N13.732
        - unilateral N13.731

Reflux — *continued*
    vesicoureteral — *continued*
        with — *continued*
            nephropathy — *continued*
                bilateral N13.722
                unilateral N13.721
                    without hydroureter N13.729
                        bilateral N13.722
                        unilateral N13.721
                pyelonephritis (chronic) N11.0
            congenital Q62.7
            without nephropathy N13.71
Reforming, artificial openings — *see* Attention to, artificial, opening
Refractive error — *see* Disorder, refraction
Refsum's disease or syndrome G60.1
Refusal of
    food, psychogenic F50.89
    treatment (because of) Z53.20
        left against medical advice (AMA) Z53.21
        patient's decision NEC Z53.29
        reasons of belief or group pressure Z53.1
Regional — *see* condition
Regurgitation R11.10
    aortic (valve) — *see* Insufficiency, aortic
    food — *see also* Vomiting
        with reswallowing — *see* Rumination
        newborn P92.1
    gastric contents — *see* Vomiting
    heart — *see* Endocarditis
    mitral (valve) — *see* Insufficiency, mitral
        congenital Q23.3
    myocardial — *see* Endocarditis
    pulmonary (valve) (heart) I37.1
        congenital Q22.2
        syphilitic A52.03
    tricuspid — *see* Insufficiency, tricuspid
    valve, valvular — *see* Endocarditis
        congenital Q24.8
    vesicoureteral — *see* Reflux, vesicoureteral
Reichmann's disease or syndrome K31.89
Reifenstein syndrome E34.52
Reinsertion
    implantable subdermal contraceptive Z30.46
    intrauterine contraceptive device Z30.433
Reiter's disease, syndrome, or urethritis M02.30
    ankle M02.37- ☑
    elbow M02.32- ☑
    foot joint M02.37- ☑
    hand joint M02.34- ☑
    hip M02.35- ☑
    knee M02.36- ☑
    multiple site M02.39
    shoulder M02.31- ☑
    vertebra M02.38
    wrist M02.33- ☑
Rejection
    food, psychogenic F50.89
    transplant T86.91
        bone T86.830
            marrow T86.01
        cornea T86.840- ☑
        heart T86.21
            with lung(s) T86.31
        intestine T86.850
        kidney T86.11
        liver T86.41
        lung(s) T86.810
            with heart T86.31
        organ (immune or nonimmune cause) T86.91
        pancreas T86.890
        skin (allograft) (autograft) T86.820
        specified NEC T86.890
        stem cell (peripheral blood) (umbilical cord) T86.5
Relapsing fever A68.9
    Carter's (Asiatic) A68.1
    Dutton's (West African) A68.1
    Koch's A68.9
    louse-borne (epidemic) A68.0
    Novy's (American) A68.1
    Obermeyers's (European) A68.0
    Spirillum A68.9
    tick-borne (endemic) A68.1
Relationship
    occlusal
        open anterior M26.220
        open posterior M26.221

Relaxation
    anus (sphincter) K62.89
        psychogenic F45.8
    arch (foot) — *see also* Deformity, limb, flat foot
    back ligaments — *see* Instability, joint, spine
    bladder (sphincter) N31.2
    cardioesophageal K21.9
    cervix — *see* Incompetency, cervix
    diaphragm J98.6
    joint (capsule) (ligament) (paralytic) — *see* Flail, joint
        congenital NEC Q74.8
    lumbosacral (joint) — *see* subcategory M53.2 ☑
    pelvic floor N81.89
    perineum N81.89
    posture R29.3
    rectum (sphincter) K62.89
    sacroiliac (joint) — *see* subcategory M53.2 ☑
    scrotum N50.89
    urethra (sphincter) N36.44
    vesical N31.2
Release from prison, anxiety concerning Z65.2
Remains
    canal of Cloquet Q14.0
    capsule (opaque) Q14.8
Remittent fever (malarial) B54
Remnant
    canal of Cloquet Q14.0
    capsule (opaque) Q14.8
    cervix, cervical stump (acquired) (postoperative) N88.8
    cystic duct, postcholecystectomy K91.5
    fingernail L60.8
        congenital Q84.6
    meniscus, knee — *see* Derangement, knee, meniscus, specified NEC
    thyroglossal duct Q89.2
    tonsil J35.8
        infected (chronic) J35.01
    urachus Q64.4
Removal (from) (of)
    artificial
        arm Z44.00- ☑
            complete Z44.01- ☑
            partial Z44.02- ☑
        eye Z44.2- ☑
        leg Z44.10- ☑
            complete Z44.11- ☑
            partial Z44.12- ☑
    breast implant Z45.81 ☑
    cardiac pulse generator (battery) (end-of-life) Z45.010
    catheter (urinary) (indwelling) Z46.6
        from artificial opening — *see* Attention to, artificial, opening
        non-vascular Z46.82
        vascular NEC Z45.2
    device Z46.9
        contraceptive Z30.432
            implantable subdermal Z30.46
        implanted NEC Z45.89
        specified NEC Z46.89
    drains Z48.03
    dressing (nonsurgical) Z48.00
        surgical Z48.01
    external
        fixation device — *code to* fracture with seventh character D
        prosthesis, prosthetic device Z44.9
            breast Z44.3- ☑
            specified NEC Z44.8
    home in childhood (to foster home or institution) Z62.29
    ileostomy Z43.2
    insulin pump Z46.81
    myringotomy device (stent) (tube) Z45.82
    nervous system device NEC Z46.2
        brain neuropacemaker Z46.2
        visual substitution device Z46.2
            implanted Z45.31
    non-vascular catheter Z46.82
    organ, prophylactic (for neoplasia management) — *see* Prophylactic, organ removal
    orthodontic device Z46.4
    staples Z48.02
    stent
        ureteral Z46.6
    suture Z48.02
    urinary device Z46.6
    vascular access device or catheter Z45.2

Ren
    arcuatus Q63.1
    mobile, mobilis N28.89
        congenital Q63.8
    unguliformis Q63.1
Renal — *see* condition
Rendu-Osler-Weber disease or syndrome I78.0
Reninoma D41.0- ☑
Renon-Delille syndrome E23.3
Reovirus, as cause of disease classified elsewhere B97.5
Repeated falls NEC R29.6
Replaced chromosome by dicentric ring Q93.2
Replacement by artificial or mechanical device or prosthesis of
    bladder Z96.0
    blood vessel NEC Z95.828
    bone NEC Z96.7
    cochlea Z96.21
    coronary artery Z95.5
    eustachian tube Z96.29
    eye globe Z97.0
    heart Z95.812
        valve Z95.2
            prosthetic Z95.2
            specified NEC Z95.4
            xenogenic Z95.3
    intestine Z96.89
    joint Z96.60
        hip — *see* Presence, hip joint implant
        knee — *see* Presence, knee joint implant
        specified site NEC Z96.698
    larynx Z96.3
    lens Z96.1
    limb(s) — *see* Presence, artificial, limb
    mandible NEC (for tooth root implant(s)) Z96.5
    organ NEC Z96.89
    peripheral vessel NEC Z95.828
    stapes Z96.29
    teeth Z97.2
    tendon Z96.7
    tissue NEC Z96.89
    tooth root(s) Z96.5
    vessel NEC Z95.828
        coronary (artery) Z95.5
Request for expert evidence Z04.89
Reserve, decreased or low
    cardiac — *see* Disease, heart
    kidney N28.89
Residual — *see also* condition
    ovary syndrome N99.83
    state, schizophrenic F20.5
    urine R39.198
Resistance, resistant (to)
    activated protein C D68.51
    complicating pregnancy O26.89 ☑
    insulin E88.81
    organism(s)
        to
            drug Z16.30
                aminoglycosides Z16.29
                amoxicillin Z16.11
                ampicillin Z16.11
                antibiotic(s) Z16.20
                    multiple Z16.24
                    specified NEC Z16.29
                antifungal Z16.32
                antimicrobial (single) Z16.30
                    multiple Z16.35
                    specified NEC Z16.39
                antimycobacterial (single) Z16.341
                    multiple Z16.342
                antiparasitic Z16.31
                antiviral Z16.33
                beta lactam antibiotics Z16.10
                    specified NEC Z16.19
                cephalosporins Z16.19
                extended beta lactamase (ESBL) Z16.12
                fluoroquinolones Z16.23
                macrolides Z16.29
                methicillin — *see* MRSA
                multiple drugs (MDRO)
                    antibiotics Z16.24
                    antimicrobial Z16.35
                    antimycobacterials Z16.342
                penicillins Z16.11
                quinine (and related compounds) Z16.31
                quinolones Z16.23

Resistance, resistant — *continued*
  organism(s) — *continued*
    to — *continued*
      drug — *continued*
        sulfonamides Z16.29
        tetracyclines Z16.29
        tuberculostatics (single) Z16.341
          multiple Z16.342
        vancomycin Z16.21
          related antibiotics Z16.22
  thyroid hormone E07.89
Resorption
  dental (roots) K03.3
    alveoli M26.79
  teeth (external) (internal) (pathological) (roots) K03.3
Respiration
  Cheyne-Stokes R06.3
  decreased due to shock, following injury T79.4 ☑
  disorder of, psychogenic F45.8
  insufficient, or poor R06.89
    newborn P28.5
  painful R07.1
  sighing, psychogenic F45.8
Respiratory — *see also* condition
  distress syndrome (newborn) (type I) P22.0
    type II P22.1
  syncytial virus, as cause of disease classified elsewhere
    — *see also* Virus, respiratory syncytial (RSV) B97.4
Respite care Z75.5
Response (drug)
  photoallergic L56.1
  phototoxic L56.0
Restenosis
  stent
    vascular
      end stent
        adjacent to stent — *see* Arteriosclerosis
        within the stent
          coronary T82.855 ☑
          peripheral T82.856 ☑
      in stent
        coronary vessel T82.855 ☑
        peripheral vessel T82.856 ☑
Restless legs (syndrome) G25.81
Restlessness R45.1
Restoration (of)
  dental
    aesthetically inadequate or displeasing K08.56
    defective K08.50
      specified NEC K08.59
    failure of marginal integrity K08.51
    failure of periodontal anatomical intergrity K08.54
  organ continuity from previous sterilization (tuboplas-
    ty) (vasoplasty) Z31.0
    aftercare Z31.42
  tooth (existing)
    contours biologically incompatible with oral health
      K08.54
    open margins K08.51
    overhanging K08.52
    poor aesthetic K08.56
    poor gingival margins K08.51
  unsatisfactory, of tooth K08.50
    specified NEC K08.59
Restorative material (dental)
  allergy to K08.55
  fractured K08.539
    with loss of material K08.531
    without loss of material K08.530
  unrepairable overhanging of K08.52
Restriction of housing space Z59.1
Rests, ovarian, in fallopian tube Q50.6
Restzustand (schizophrenic) F20.5
Retained — *see also* Retention
  cholelithiasis following cholecystectomy K91.86
  foreign body fragments (type of) Z18.9
    acrylics Z18.2
    animal quill(s) or spines Z18.31
    cement Z18.83
    concrete Z18.83
    crystalline Z18.83
    depleted isotope Z18.09
    depleted uranium Z18.01
    diethylhexyl phthalates Z18.2
    glass Z18.81
    isocyanate Z18.2
    magnetic metal Z18.11
    metal Z18.10

Retained — *continued*
  foreign body fragments — *continued*
    nonmagnetic metal Z18.12
    nontherapeutic radioactive Z18.09
    organic NEC Z18.39
    plastic Z18.2
    quill(s) (animal) Z18.31
    radioactive (nontherapeutic) NEC Z18.09
    specified NEC Z18.89
    spine(s) (animal) Z18.31
    stone Z18.83
    tooth (teeth) Z18.32
    wood Z18.33
  fragments (type of) Z18.9
    acrylics Z18.2
    animal quill(s) or spines Z18.31
    cement Z18.83
    concrete Z18.83
    crystalline Z18.83
    depleted isotope Z18.09
    depleted uranium Z18.01
    diethylhexyl phthalates Z18.2
    glass Z18.81
    isocyanate Z18.2
    magnetic metal Z18.11
    metal Z18.10
    nonmagnetic metal Z18.12
    nontherapeutic radioactive Z18.09
    organic NEC Z18.39
    plastic Z18.2
    quill(s) (animal) Z18.31
    radioactive (nontherapeutic) NEC Z18.09
    specified NEC Z18.89
    spine(s) (animal) Z18.31
    stone Z18.83
    tooth (teeth) Z18.32
    wood Z18.33
  gallstones, following cholecystectomy K91.86
Retardation
  development, developmental, specific — *see* Disorder,
    developmental
  endochondral bone growth — *see* Disorder, bone, de-
    velopment or growth
  growth R62.50
    due to malnutrition E45
  mental — *see* Disability, intellectual
  motor function, specific F82
  physical (child) R62.52
    due to malnutrition E45
  reading (specific) F81.0
  spelling (specific) (without reading disorder) F81.81
Retching — *see* Vomiting
Retention — *see also* Retained
  bladder — *see* Retention, urine
  carbon dioxide E87.2
  cholelithiasis following cholecystectomy K91.86
  cyst — *see* Cyst
  dead
    fetus (at or near term) (mother) O36.4 ☑
      early fetal death O02.1
    ovum O02.0
  decidua (fragments) (following delivery) (with hemor-
    rhage) O72.2
    without hemorrhage O73.1
  deciduous tooth K00.6
  dental root K08.3
  fecal — *see* Constipation
  fetus
    dead O36.4 ☑
    early O02.1
  fluid R60.9
  foreign body — *see also* Foreign body, retained
    current trauma — *code as* Foreign body, by site or
      type
  gallstones, following cholecystectomy K91.86
  gastric K31.89
  intrauterine contraceptive device, in pregnancy — *see*
    Pregnancy, complicated by, retention, intrauter-
    ine device
  membranes (complicating delivery) (with hemorrhage)
    O72.2
    with abortion — *see* Abortion, by type
    without hemorrhage O73.1
  meniscus — *see* Derangement, meniscus
  menses N94.89
  milk (puerperal, postpartum) O92.79
  nitrogen, extrarenal R39.2
  ovary syndrome N99.83

Retention — *continued*
  placenta (total) (with hemorrhage) O72.0
    without hemorrhage O73.0
    portions or fragments (with hemorrhage) O72.2
      without hemorrhage O73.1
  products of conception
    early pregnancy (dead fetus) O02.1
    following
      delivery (with hemorrhage) O72.2
        without hemorrhage O73.1
  secundines (following delivery) (with hemorrhage)
    O72.0
    without hemorrhage O73.0
    complicating puerperium (delayed hemorrhage)
      O72.2
    partial O72.2
      without hemorrhage O73.1
  smegma, clitoris N90.89
  urine R33.9
    due to hyperplasia (hypertrophy) of prostate — *see*
      Hyperplasia, prostate
    drug-induced R33.0
    organic R33.8
      drug-induced R33.0
    psychogenic F45.8
    specified NEC R33.8
  water (in tissues) — *see* Edema
Reticulation, dust — *see* Pneumoconiosis
Reticulocytosis R70.1
Reticuloendotheliosis
  acute infantile C96.0
  leukemic C91.4- ☑
  nonlipid C96.0
Reticulohistiocytoma (giant-cell) D76.3
Reticuloid, actinic L57.1
Reticulosis (skin)
  acute of infancy C96.0
  hemophagocytic, familial D76.1
  histiocytic medullary C96.A (*following* C96.6)
  lipomelanotic I89.8
  malignant (midline) C86.0
  polymorphic C83.8- ☑
  Sézary — *see* Sézary disease
Retina, retinal — *see also* condition
  dark area D49.81
Retinitis — *see also* Inflammation, chorioretinal
  albuminurica N18.9 *[H32]*
  diabetic — *see* Diabetes, retinitis
  disciformis — *see* Degeneration, macula
  focal — *see* Inflammation, chorioretinal, focal
  gravidarum — *see* Pregnancy, complicated by, speci-
    fied pregnancy-related condition NEC
  juxtapapillaris — *see* Inflammation, chorioretinal, focal,
    juxtapapillary
  luetic — *see* Retinitis, syphilitic
  pigmentosa H35.52
  proliferans — *see* Disorder, globe, degenerative, spec-
    ified type NEC
  proliferating — *see* Disorder, globe, degenerative,
    specified type NEC
  renal N18.9 *[H32]*
  syphilitic (early) (secondary) A51.43
    central, recurrent A52.71
    congenital (early) A50.01 *[H32]*
    late A52.71
  tuberculous A18.53
Retinoblastoma C69.2- ☑
  differentiated C69.2- ☑
  undifferentiated C69.2- ☑
Retinochoroiditis — *see also* Inflammation, chorioretinal
  disseminated — *see* Inflammation, chorioretinal, dis-
    seminated
    syphilitic A52.71
  focal — *see* Inflammation, chorioretinal
  juxtapapillaris — *see* Inflammation, chorioretinal, focal,
    juxtapapillary
Retinopathy (background) H35.00
  arteriosclerotic I70.8 *[H35.0-]* ☑
  atherosclerotic I70.8 *[H35.0-]* ☑
  central serous — *see* Chorioretinopathy, central serous
  Coats H35.02- ☑
  diabetic — *see* Diabetes, retinopathy
  exudative H35.02- ☑
  hypertensive H35.03- ☑
  in (due to)
    diabetes — *see* Diabetes, retinopathy
    sickle-cell disorders D57.- ☑ *[H36]*

Retinopathy — *continued*
  of prematurity H35.10- ☑
    stage 0 H35.11- ☑
    stage 1 H35.12- ☑
    stage 2 H35.13- ☑
    stage 3 H35.14- ☑
    stage 4 H35.15- ☑
    stage 5 H35.16- ☑
  pigmentary, congenital — *see* Dystrophy, retina
  proliferative NEC H35.2- ☑
    diabetic — *see* Diabetes, retinopathy, proliferative
    sickle-cell D57.- ☑ *[H36]*
  solar H31.02- ☑
Retinoschisis H33.10- ☑
  congenital Q14.1
  specified type NEC H33.19- ☑
Retortamoniasis A07.8
Retractile testis Q55.22
Retraction
  cervix — *see* Retroversion, uterus
  drum (membrane) — *see* Disorder, tympanic membrane, specified NEC
  finger — *see* Deformity, finger
  lid H02.539
    left H02.536
      lower H02.535
      upper H02.534
    right H02.533
      lower H02.532
      upper H02.531
  lung J98.4
  mediastinum J98.59
  nipple N64.53
    associated with
      lactation O92.03
      pregnancy O92.01- ☑
      puerperium O92.02
    congenital Q83.8
  palmar fascia M72.0
  pleura — *see* Pleurisy
  ring, uterus (Bandl's) (pathological) O62.4
  sternum (congenital) Q76.7
    acquired M95.4
  uterus — *see* Retroversion, uterus
  valve (heart) — *see* Endocarditis
Retrobulbar — *see* condition
Retrocecal — *see* condition
Retrocession — *see* Retroversion
Retrodisplacement — *see* Retroversion
Retroflection, retroflexion — *see* Retroversion
Retrognathia, retrognathism (mandibular) (maxillary) M26.19
Retrograde menstruation N92.5
Retroperineal — *see* condition
Retroperitoneal — *see* condition
Retroperitonitis K68.9
Retropharyngeal — *see* condition
Retroplacental — *see* condition
Retroposition — *see* Retroversion
Retroprosthetic membrane T85.398 ☑
Retrosternal thyroid (congenital) Q89.2
Retroversion, retroverted
  cervix — *see* Retroversion, uterus
  female NEC — *see* Retroversion, uterus
  iris H21.89
  testis (congenital) Q55.29
  uterus (acquired) (acute) (any degree) (asymptomatic) (cervix) (postinfectional) (postpartal, old) N85.4
    congenital Q51.818
    in pregnancy O34.53- ☑
Retrovirus, as cause of disease classified elsewhere B97.30
  human
    immunodeficiency, type 2 (HIV 2) B97.35
    T-cell lymphotropic
      type I (HTLV-I) B97.33
      type II (HTLV-II) B97.34
  lentivirus B97.31
  oncovirus B97.32
  specified NEC B97.39
Retrusion, premaxilla (developmental) M26.09
Rett's disease or syndrome F84.2
Reverse peristalsis R19.2
Reye's syndrome G93.7
Rh (factor)
  hemolytic disease (newborn) P55.0

Rh — *continued*
  incompatibility, immunization or sensitization
    affecting management of pregnancy NEC O36.09- ☑
      anti-D antibody O36.01- ☑
    newborn P55.0
    transfusion reaction — *see* Complication(s), transfusion, incompatibility reaction, Rh (factor)
  negative mother affecting newborn P55.0
  titer elevated — *see* Complication(s), transfusion, incompatibility reaction, Rh (factor)
  transfusion reaction — *see* Complication(s), transfusion, incompatibility reaction, Rh (factor)
Rhabdomyolysis (idiopathic) NEC M62.82
  traumatic T79.6
Rhabdomyoma — *see also* Neoplasm, connective tissue, benign
  adult — *see* Neoplasm, connective tissue, benign
  fetal — *see* Neoplasm, connective tissue, benign
  glycogenic — *see* Neoplasm, connective tissue, benign
Rhabdomyosarcoma (any type) — *see* Neoplasm, connective tissue, malignant
Rhabdosarcoma — *see* Rhabdomyosarcoma
Rhesus (factor) **incompatibility** — *see* Rh, incompatibility
Rheumatic (acute) (subacute)
  adherent pericardium I09.2
  chronic I09.89
  coronary arteritis I01.8
  degeneration, myocardium I09.0
  fever (acute) — *see* Fever, rheumatic
  heart — *see* Disease, heart, rheumatic
  myocardial degeneration — *see* Degeneration, myocardium
  myocarditis (chronic) (inactive) (with chorea) I09.0
    active or acute I01.2
      with chorea (acute) (rheumatic) (Sydenham's) I02.0
  pancarditis, acute I01.8
    with chorea (acute (rheumatic) Sydenham's) I02.0
  pericarditis (active) (acute) (with effusion) (with pneumonia) I01.0
    with chorea (acute) (rheumatic) (Sydenham's) I02.0
    chronic or inactive I09.2
  pneumonia I00 *[J17]*
  torticollis M43.6
  typhoid fever A01.09
Rheumatism (articular) (neuralgic) (nonarticular) M79.0
  gout — *see* Arthritis, rheumatoid
  intercostal, meaning Tietze's disease M94.0
  palindromic (any site) M12.30
    ankle M12.37- ☑
    elbow M12.32- ☑
    foot joint M12.37- ☑
    hand joint M12.34- ☑
    hip M12.35- ☑
    knee M12.36- ☑
    multiple site M12.39
    shoulder M12.31- ☑
    specified joint NEC M12.38
    vertebrae M12.38
    wrist M12.33- ☑
  sciatic M54.4- ☑
Rheumatoid — *see also* condition
  arthritis — *see also* Arthritis, rheumatoid
    with involvement of organs NEC M05.60
      ankle M05.67- ☑
      elbow M05.62- ☑
      foot joint M05.67- ☑
      hand joint M05.64- ☑
      hip M05.65- ☑
      knee M05.66- ☑
      multiple site M05.69
      shoulder M05.61- ☑
      vertebra — *see* Spondylitis, ankylosing
      wrist M05.63- ☑
    seronegative — *see* Arthritis, rheumatoid, seronegative
    seropositive — *see* Arthritis, rheumatoid, seropositive
  carditis M05.30
    ankle M05.37- ☑
    elbow M05.32- ☑
    foot joint M05.37- ☑
    hand joint M05.34- ☑
    hip M05.35- ☑
    knee M05.36- ☑
    multiple site M05.39
    shoulder M05.31- ☑

Rheumatoid — *continued*
  carditis — *continued*
    vertebra — *see* Spondylitis, ankylosing
    wrist M05.33- ☑
  endocarditis — *see* Rheumatoid, carditis
  lung (disease) M05.10
    ankle M05.17- ☑
    elbow M05.12- ☑
    foot joint M05.17- ☑
    hand joint M05.14- ☑
    hip M05.15- ☑
    knee M05.16- ☑
    multiple site M05.19
    shoulder M05.11- ☑
    vertebra — *see* Spondylitis, ankylosing
    wrist M05.13- ☑
  myocarditis — *see* Rheumatoid, carditis
  myopathy M05.40
    ankle M05.47- ☑
    elbow M05.42- ☑
    foot joint M05.47- ☑
    hand joint M05.44- ☑
    hip M05.45- ☑
    knee M05.46- ☑
    multiple site M05.49
    shoulder M05.41- ☑
    vertebra — *see* Spondylitis, ankylosing
    wrist M05.43- ☑
  pericarditis — *see* Rheumatoid, carditis
  polyarthritis — *see* Arthritis, rheumatoid
  polyneuropathy M05.50
    ankle M05.57- ☑
    elbow M05.52- ☑
    foot joint M05.57- ☑
    hand joint M05.54- ☑
    hip M05.55- ☑
    knee M05.56- ☑
    multiple site M05.59
    shoulder M05.51- ☑
    vertebra — *see* Spondylitis, ankylosing
    wrist M05.53- ☑
  vasculitis M05.20
    ankle M05.27- ☑
    elbow M05.22- ☑
    foot joint M05.27- ☑
    hand joint M05.24- ☑
    hip M05.25- ☑
    knee M05.26- ☑
    multiple site M05.29
    shoulder M05.21- ☑
    vertebra — *see* Spondylitis, ankylosing
    wrist M05.23- ☑
Rhinitis (atrophic) (catarrhal) (chronic) (croupous) (fibrinous) (granulomatous) (hyperplastic) (hypertrophic) (membranous) (obstructive) (purulent) (suppurative) (ulcerative) J31.0
  with
    sore throat — *see* Nasopharyngitis
  acute J00
  allergic J30.9
    with asthma J45.909
      with
        exacerbation (acute) J45.901
        status asthmaticus J45.902
    due to
      food J30.5
      pollen J30.1
    nonseasonal J30.89
    perennial J30.89
    seasonal NEC J30.2
    specified NEC J30.89
  infective J00
  pneumococcal J00
  syphilitic A52.73
    congenital A50.05 *[J99]*
  tuberculous A15.8
  vasomotor J30.0
Rhinoantritis (chronic) — *see* Sinusitis, maxillary
Rhinodacryolith — *see* Dacryolith
Rhinolith (nasal sinus) J34.89
Rhinomegaly J34.89
Rhinopharyngitis (acute) (subacute) — *see also* Nasopharyngitis
  chronic J31.1
  destructive ulcerating A66.5
  mutilans A66.5
Rhinophyma L71.1

☑ Additional Character Required — Refer to the Tabular List for Character Selection   ▽ Subterms under main terms may continue to next column or page

Rhinorrhea J34.89
  cerebrospinal (fluid) G96.01
    postoperative G96.08
    specified NEC G96.08
    spontaneous G96.01
    traumatic G96.08
  paroxysmal — *see* Rhinitis, allergic
  spasmodic — *see* Rhinitis, allergic
Rhinosalpingitis — *see* Salpingitis, eustachian
Rhinoscleroma A48.8
Rhinosporidiosis B48.1
Rhinovirus infection NEC B34.8
Rhizomelic chondrodysplasia punctata E71.540
Rhythm
  atrioventricular nodal I49.8
  disorder I49.9
    coronary sinus I49.8
    ectopic I49.8
    nodal I49.8
  escape I49.9
  heart, abnormal I49.9
  idioventricular I44.2
  nodal I49.8
  sleep, inversion G47.2- ☑
    nonorganic origin — *see* Disorder, sleep, circadian rhythm, psychogenic
Rhytidosis facialis L98.8
Rib — *see also* condition
  cervical Q76.5
Riboflavin deficiency E53.0
Rice bodies — *see also* Loose, body, joint
  knee M23.4- ☑
Richter syndrome — *see* Leukemia, chronic lymphocytic, B-cell type
Richter's hernia — *see* Hernia, abdomen, with obstruction
Ricinism — *see* Poisoning, food, noxious, plant
Rickets (active) (acute) (adolescent) (chest wall) (congenital) (current) (infantile) (intestinal) E55.0
  adult — *see* Osteomalacia
  celiac K90.0
  hypophosphatemic with nephrotic-glycosuric dwarfism E72.09
  inactive E64.3
  kidney N25.0
  renal N25.0
  sequelae, any E64.3
  vitamin-D-resistant E83.31 *[M90.80]*
Rickettsia 364D/R. philipii (Pacific Coast tick fever) A77.8
Rickettsial disease A79.9
  specified type NEC A79.89
Rickettsialpox (Rickettsia akari) A79.1
Rickettsiosis A79.9
  due to
    Ehrlichia sennetsu A79.81
    Neorickettsia sennetsu A79.81
    Rickettsia akari (rickettsialpox) A79.1
  specified type NEC A79.89
  tick-borne A77.9
  vesicular A79.1
Rider's bone — *see* Ossification, muscle, specified NEC
Ridge, alveolus — *see also* condition
  flabby K06.8
Ridged ear, congenital Q17.3
Riedel's
  lobe, liver Q44.7
  struma, thyroiditis or disease E06.5
Rieger's anomaly or syndrome Q13.81
Riehl's melanosis L81.4
Rietti-Greppi-Micheli anemia D56.9
Rieux's hernia — *see* Hernia, abdomen, specified site NEC
Riga (-Fede) **disease** K14.0
Riggs' disease — *see* Periodontitis
Right aortic arch Q25.47
Right middle lobe syndrome J98.11
Rigid, rigidity — *see also* condition
  abdominal R19.30
    with severe abdominal pain R10.0
    epigastric R19.36
    generalized R19.37
    left lower quadrant R19.34
    left upper quadrant R19.32
    periumbilic R19.35
    right lower quadrant R19.33
    right upper quadrant R19.31

Rigid, rigidity — *continued*
  articular, multiple, congenital Q68.8
  cervix (uteri) in pregnancy — *see* Pregnancy, complicated by, abnormal, cervix
  hymen (acquired) (congenital) N89.6
  nuchal R29.1
  pelvic floor in pregnancy — *see* Pregnancy, complicated by, abnormal, pelvic organs or tissues NEC
  perineum or vulva in pregnancy — *see* Pregnancy, complicated by, abnormal, vulva
  spine — *see* Dorsopathy, specified NEC
  vagina in pregnancy — *see* Pregnancy, complicated by, abnormal, vagina
Rigors R68.89
  with fever R50.9
Riley-Day syndrome G90.1
RIND (reversible ischemic neurologic deficit) I63.9
Ring(s)
  aorta (vascular) Q25.45
  Bandl's O62.4
  contraction, complicating delivery O62.4
  esophageal, lower (muscular) K22.2
  Fleischer's (cornea) H18.04- ☑
  hymenal, tight (acquired) (congenital) N89.6
  Kayser-Fleischer (cornea) H18.04- ☑
  retraction, uterus, pathological O62.4
  Schatzki's (esophagus) (lower) K22.2
    congenital Q39.3
  Soemmerring's — *see* Cataract, secondary
  vascular (congenital) Q25.8
    aorta Q25.45
Ringed hair (congenital) Q84.1
Ringworm B35.9
  beard B35.0
  black dot B35.0
  body B35.4
  Burmese B35.5
  corporeal B35.4
  foot B35.3
  groin B35.6
  hand B35.2
  honeycomb B35.0
  nails B35.1
  perianal (area) B35.6
  scalp B35.0
  specified NEC B35.8
  Tokelau B35.5
Rise, venous pressure I87.8
Rising, PSA following treatment for malignant neoplasm of prostate R97.21
Risk
  for
    dental caries Z91.849
      high Z91.843
      low Z91.841
      moderate Z91.842
  suicidal
    meaning personal history of attempted suicide Z91.5
    meaning suicidal ideation — *see* Ideation, suicidal
Ritter's disease L00
Rivalry, sibling Z62.891
Rivalta's disease A42.2
River blindness B73.01
Robert's pelvis Q74.2
  with disproportion (fetopelvic) O33.0
    causing obstructed labor O65.0
Robin (-Pierre) **syndrome** Q87.0
Robinow-Silverman-Smith syndrome Q87.19
Robinson's (hidrotic) **ectodermal dysplasia or syndrome** Q82.4
Robles' disease B73.01
Rocky Mountain (spotted) **fever** A77.0
Roetheln — *see* Rubella
Roger's disease Q21.0
Rokitansky-Aschoff sinuses (gallbladder) K82.8
Rolando's fracture (displaced) S62.22- ☑
  nondisplaced S62.22- ☑
Romano-Ward (prolonged QT interval) **syndrome** I45.81
Romberg's disease or syndrome G51.8
Roof, mouth — *see* condition
Rosacea L71.9
  acne L71.9
  keratitis L71.8
  specified NEC L71.8
Rosary, rachitic E55.0
Rose
  cold J30.1

Rose — *continued*
  fever J30.1
  rash R21
    epidemic B06.9
Rosenbach's erysipeloid A26.0
Rosenthal's disease or syndrome D68.1
Roseola B09
  infantum B08.20
    due to human herpesvirus 6 B08.21
    due to human herpesvirus 7 B08.22
Ross River disease or fever B33.1
Rossbach's disease K31.89
  psychogenic F45.8
Rostan's asthma (cardiac) — *see* Failure, ventricular, left
Rotation
  anomalous, incomplete or insufficient, intestine Q43.3
  cecum (congenital) Q43.3
  colon (congenital) Q43.3
  spine, incomplete or insufficient — *see* Dorsopathy, deforming, specified NEC
  tooth, teeth, fully erupted M26.35
  vertebra, incomplete or insufficient — *see* Dorsopathy, deforming, specified NEC
Rotes Quérol disease or syndrome — *see* Hyperostosis, ankylosing
Roth (-Bernhardt) **disease or syndrome** — *see* Meralgia paraesthetica
Rothmund (-Thomson) **syndrome** Q82.8
Rotor's disease or syndrome E80.6
Round
  back (with wedging of vertebrae) — *see* Kyphosis
    sequelae (late effect) of rickets E64.3
  worms (large) (infestation) NEC B82.0
    Ascariasis — *see also* Ascariasis B77.9
Roussy-Lévy syndrome G60.0
Rubella (German measles) B06.9
  complication NEC B06.09
    neurological B06.00
  congenital P35.0
  contact Z20.4
  exposure to Z20.4
  maternal
    care for (suspected) damage to fetus O35.3 ☑
    manifest rubella in infant P35.0
    suspected damage to fetus affecting management of pregnancy O35.3 ☑
  specified complications NEC B06.89
Rubeola (meaning measles) — *see* Measles
  meaning rubella — *see* Rubella
Rubeosis, iris — *see* Disorder, iris, vascular
Rubinstein-Taybi syndrome Q87.2
Rudimentary (congenital) — *see also* Agenesis
  arm — *see* Defect, reduction, upper limb
  bone Q79.9
  cervix uteri Q51.828
  eye Q11.2
  lobule of ear Q17.3
  patella Q74.1
  respiratory organs in thoracopagus Q89.4
  tracheal bronchus Q32.4
  uterus Q51.818
    in male Q56.1
  vagina Q52.0
Ruled out condition — *see* Observation, suspected
Rumination R11.10
  with nausea R11.2
  disorder of infancy F98.21
  neurotic F42.8
  newborn P92.1
  obsessional F42.8
  psychogenic F42.8
Runeberg's disease D51.0
Runny nose R09.89
Rupia (syphilitic) A51.39
  congenital A50.06
  tertiary A52.79
Rupture, ruptured
  abscess (spontaneous) — *code by* site under Abscess
  aneurysm — *see* Aneurysm
  anus (sphincter) — *see* Laceration, anus
  aorta, aortic I71.8
    abdominal I71.3
    arch I71.1
    ascending I71.1
    descending I71.8
      abdominal I71.3
      thoracic I71.1
    syphilitic A52.01

Rupture, ruptured — continued
  aorta, aortic — continued
    thoracoabdominal I71.5
    thorax, thoracic I71.1
    transverse I71.1
    traumatic — see Injury, aorta, laceration, major
    valve or cusp — see also Endocarditis, aortic I35.8
  appendix (with peritonitis) — see also Appendicitis K35.32
    with localized peritonitis — see also Appendicitis K35.32
  arteriovenous fistula, brain — see Fistula, arteriovenous, brain, ruptured
  artery I77.2
    brain — see Hemorrhage, intracranial, intracerebral
    coronary — see Infarct, myocardium
    heart — see Infarct, myocardium
    pulmonary I28.8
    traumatic (complication) — see Injury, blood vessel
  bile duct (common) (hepatic) K83.2
    cystic K82.2
  bladder (sphincter) (nontraumatic) (spontaneous) N32.89
    following ectopic or molar pregnancy O08.6
    obstetrical trauma O71.5
    traumatic S37.29 ☑
  blood vessel — see also Hemorrhage
    brain — see Hemorrhage, intracranial, intracerebral
    heart — see Infarct, myocardium
    traumatic (complication) — see Injury, blood vessel, laceration, major, by site
  bone — see Fracture
  bowel (nontraumatic) K63.1
  brain
    aneurysm (congenital) — see also Hemorrhage, intracranial, subarachnoid
      syphilitic A52.05
    hemorrhagic — see Hemorrhage, intracranial, intracerebral
  capillaries I78.8
  cardiac (auricle) (ventricle) (wall) I23.3
    with hemopericardium I23.0
    infectional I40.9
    traumatic — see Injury, heart
  cartilage (articular) (current) — see also Sprain
    knee S83.3- ☑
    semilunar — see Tear, meniscus
  cecum (with peritonitis) K65.0
    with peritoneal abscess K35.33
    traumatic S36.598 ☑
  celiac artery, traumatic — see Injury, blood vessel, celiac artery, laceration, major
  cerebral aneurysm (congenital) (see Hemorrhage, intracranial, subarachnoid)
  cervix (uteri)
    with ectopic or molar pregnancy O08.6
    following ectopic or molar pregnancy O08.6
    obstetrical trauma O71.3
    traumatic S37.69 ☑
  chordae tendineae NEC I51.1
    concurrent with acute myocardial infarction — see Infarct, myocardium
    following acute myocardial infarction (current complication) I23.4
  choroid (direct) (indirect) (traumatic) H31.32- ☑
  circle of Willis I60.6
  colon (nontraumatic) K63.1
    traumatic — see Injury, intestine, large
  cornea (traumatic) — see Injury, eye, laceration
  coronary (artery) (thrombotic) — see Infarct, myocardium
  corpus luteum (infected) (ovary) N83.1- ☑
  cyst — see Cyst
  cystic duct K82.2
  Descemet's membrane — see Change, corneal membrane, Descemet's, rupture
    traumatic — see Injury, eye, laceration
  diaphragm, traumatic — see Injury, intrathoracic, diaphragm
  disc — see Rupture, intervertebral disc
  diverticulum (intestine) K57.80
    with bleeding K57.81
    bladder N32.3
    large intestine K57.20
      with
        bleeding K57.21
        small intestine K57.40
          with bleeding K57.41

Rupture, ruptured — continued
  diverticulum — continued
    small intestine K57.00
      with
        bleeding K57.01
        large intestine K57.40
          with bleeding K57.41
  duodenal stump K31.89
  ear drum (nontraumatic) — see also Perforation, tympanum
    traumatic S09.2- ☑
      due to blast injury — see Injury, blast, ear
  esophagus K22.3
  eye (without prolapse or loss of intraocular tissue) — see Injury, eye, laceration
  fallopian tube NEC (nonobstetric) (nontraumatic) N83.8
    due to pregnancy O00.10- ☑
      with intrauterine pregnancy O00.11- ☑
  fontanel P13.1
  gallbladder K82.2
    traumatic S36.128 ☑
  gastric — see also Rupture, stomach
    vessel K92.2
  globe (eye) (traumatic) — see Injury, eye, laceration
  graafian follicle (hematoma) N83.0- ☑
  heart — see Rupture, cardiac
  hymen (nontraumatic) (nonintentional) N89.8
  internal organ, traumatic — see Injury, by site
  intervertebral disc — see Displacement, intervertebral disc
    traumatic — see Rupture, traumatic, intervertebral disc
  intestine NEC (nontraumatic) K63.1
    traumatic — see Injury, intestine
  iris — see also Abnormality, pupillary
    traumatic — see Injury, eye, laceration
  joint capsule, traumatic — see Sprain
  kidney (traumatic) S37.06- ☑
    birth injury P15.8
    nontraumatic N28.89
  lacrimal duct (traumatic) — see Injury, eye, specified site NEC
  lens (cataract) (traumatic) — see Cataract, traumatic
  ligament, traumatic — see Rupture, traumatic, ligament, by site
  liver S36.116 ☑
    birth injury P15.0
  lymphatic vessel I89.8
  marginal sinus (placental) (with hemorrhage) — see Hemorrhage, antepartum, specified cause NEC
  membrana tympani (nontraumatic) — see Perforation, tympanum
  membranes (spontaneous)
    artificial
      delayed delivery following O75.5
    delayed delivery following — see Pregnancy, complicated by, premature rupture of membranes
  meningeal artery I60.8
  meniscus (knee) — see also Tear, meniscus
    old — see Derangement, meniscus
    site other than knee — code as Sprain
  mesenteric artery, traumatic — see Injury, mesenteric, artery, laceration, major
  mesentery (nontraumatic) K66.8
    traumatic — see Injury, intra-abdominal, specified, site NEC
  mitral (valve) I34.8
  muscle (traumatic) — see also Strain
    diastasis — see Diastasis, muscle
    nontraumatic M62.10
      ankle M62.17- ☑
      foot M62.17- ☑
      forearm M62.13- ☑
      hand M62.14- ☑
      lower leg M62.16- ☑
      pelvic region M62.15- ☑
      shoulder region M62.11- ☑
      specified site NEC M62.18
      thigh M62.15- ☑
      upper arm M62.12- ☑
    traumatic — see Strain, by site
  musculotendinous junction NEC, nontraumatic — see Rupture, tendon, spontaneous
  mycotic aneurysm causing cerebral hemorrhage — see Hemorrhage, intracranial, subarachnoid
  myocardium, myocardial — see Rupture, cardiac
    traumatic — see Injury, heart

Rupture, ruptured — continued
  nontraumatic, meaning hernia — see Hernia
  obstructed — see Hernia, by site, obstructed
  operation wound — see Disruption, wound, operation
  ovary, ovarian N83.8
    corpus luteum cyst N83.1- ☑
    follicle (graafian) N83.0- ☑
  oviduct (nonobstetric) (nontraumatic) N83.8
    due to pregnancy O00.10- ☑
      with intrauterine pregnancy O00.11- ☑
  pancreas (nontraumatic) K86.89
    traumatic S36.299 ☑
  papillary muscle NEC I51.2
    following acute myocardial infarction (current complication) I23.5
  pelvic
    floor, complicating delivery O70.1
    organ NEC, obstetrical trauma O71.5
  perineum (nonobstetric) (nontraumatic) N90.89
    complicating delivery — see Delivery, complicated by, laceration, anus (sphincter)
  postoperative wound — see Disruption, wound, operation
  prostate (traumatic) S37.828 ☑
  pulmonary
    artery I28.8
    valve (heart) I37.8
    vein I28.8
    vessel I28.8
  pus tube — see Salpingitis
  pyosalpinx — see Salpingitis
  rectum (nontraumatic) K63.1
    traumatic S36.69 ☑
  retina, retinal (traumatic) (without detachment) — see also Break, retina
    with detachment — see Detachment, retina, with retinal, break
  rotator cuff (nontraumatic) M75.10- ☑
    complete M75.12- ☑
    incomplete M75.11- ☑
  sclera — see Injury, eye, laceration
  sigmoid (nontraumatic) K63.1
    traumatic S36.593 ☑
  spinal cord — see also Injury, spinal cord, by region
    due to injury at birth P11.5
    newborn (birth injury) P11.5
  spleen (traumatic) S36.09 ☑
    birth injury P15.1
    congenital (birth injury) P15.1
    due to P. vivax malaria B51.0
    nontraumatic D73.5
    spontaneous D73.5
  splenic vein R58
    traumatic — see Injury, blood vessel, splenic vein
  stomach (nontraumatic) (spontaneous) K31.89
    traumatic S36.39 ☑
  supraspinatus (complete) (incomplete) (nontraumatic) — see Tear, rotator cuff
  symphysis pubis
    obstetric O71.6
    traumatic S33.4 ☑
  synovium (cyst) M66.10
    ankle M66.17- ☑
    elbow M66.12- ☑
    finger M66.14- ☑
    foot M66.17- ☑
    forearm M66.13- ☑
    hand M66.14- ☑
    pelvic region M66.15- ☑
    shoulder region M66.11- ☑
    specified site NEC M66.18
    thigh M66.15- ☑
    toe M66.17- ☑
    upper arm M66.12- ☑
    wrist M66.13- ☑
  tendon (traumatic) — see Strain
    nontraumatic (spontaneous) M66.9
      ankle M66.87- ☑
      extensor M66.20
        ankle M66.27- ☑
        foot M66.27- ☑
        forearm M66.23- ☑
        hand M66.24- ☑
        lower leg M66.26- ☑
        multiple sites M66.29
        pelvic region M66.25- ☑
        shoulder region M66.21- ☑

☑ Additional Character Required — Refer to the Tabular List for Character Selection   ▽ Subterms under main terms may continue to next column or page

Rupture, ruptured — *continued*
  tendon — *see* Strain — *continued*
    nontraumatic — *continued*
      extensor — *continued*
        specified site NEC M66.28
        thigh M66.25- ☑
        upper arm M66.22- ☑
      flexor M66.30
        ankle M66.37- ☑
        foot M66.37- ☑
        forearm M66.33- ☑
        hand M66.34- ☑
        lower leg M66.36- ☑
        multiple sites M66.39
        pelvic region M66.35- ☑
        shoulder region M66.31- ☑
        specified site NEC M66.38
        thigh M66.35- ☑
        upper arm M66.32- ☑
      foot M66.87- ☑
      forearm M66.83- ☑
      hand M66.84- ☑
      lower leg M66.86- ☑
      multiple sites M66.89
      pelvic region M66.85- ☑
      shoulder region M66.81- ☑
      specified
        site NEC M66.88
        tendon M66.80
      thigh M66.85- ☑
      upper arm M66.82- ☑
  thoracic duct I89.8
  tonsil J35.8
  traumatic
    aorta — *see* Injury, aorta, laceration, major
    diaphragm — *see* Injury, intrathoracic, diaphragm
    external site — *see* Wound, open, by site
    eye — *see* Injury, eye, laceration
    internal organ — *see* Injury, by site
    intervertebral disc
      cervical S13.0 ☑
      lumbar S33.0 ☑
      thoracic S23.0 ☑
    kidney S37.06- ☑
    ligament — *see also* Sprain
      ankle — *see* Sprain, ankle
      carpus — *see* Rupture, traumatic, ligament, wrist
      collateral (hand) — *see* Rupture, traumatic, liga-
        ment, finger, collateral
      finger (metacarpophalangeal) (interphalangeal)
        S63.40- ☑
        collateral S63.41- ☑
          index S63.41- ☑
          little S63.41- ☑
          middle S63.41- ☑
          ring S63.41- ☑
        index S63.40- ☑
        little S63.40- ☑
        middle S63.40- ☑
        palmar S63.42- ☑
          index S63.42- ☑
          little S63.42- ☑
          middle S63.42- ☑
          ring S63.42- ☑
        ring S63.40- ☑
        specified site NEC S63.499 ☑
          index S63.49- ☑
          little S63.49- ☑
          middle S63.49- ☑
          ring S63.49- ☑
        volar plate S63.43- ☑
          index S63.43- ☑
          little S63.43- ☑
          middle S63.43- ☑
          ring S63.43- ☑
      foot — *see* Sprain, foot
      radial collateral S53.2- ☑
      radiocarpal — *see* Rupture, traumatic, ligament,
        wrist, radiocarpal
      ulnar collateral S53.3- ☑
      ulnocarpal — *see* Rupture, traumatic, ligament,
        wrist, ulnocarpal
      wrist S63.30- ☑
        collateral S63.31- ☑
        radiocarpal S63.32- ☑
        specified site NEC S63.39- ☑

Rupture, ruptured — *continued*
  traumatic — *continued*
    ligament — *see also* Sprain — *continued*
      wrist — *continued*
        ulnocarpal (palmar) S63.33- ☑
    liver S36.116 ☑
    membrana tympani — *see* Rupture, ear drum,
      traumatic
    muscle or tendon — *see* Strain
    myocardium — *see* Injury, heart
    pancreas S36.299 ☑
    rectum S36.69 ☑
    sigmoid S36.593 ☑
    spleen S36.09 ☑
    stomach S36.39 ☑
    symphysis pubis S33.4 ☑
    tympanum, tympanic (membrane) — *see* Rupture,
      ear drum, traumatic
    ureter S37.19 ☑
    uterus S37.69 ☑
    vagina — *see* Injury, vagina
    vena cava — *see* Injury, vena cava, laceration, major
  tricuspid (heart) (valve) I07.8
  tube, tubal (nonobstetric) (nontraumatic) N83.8
    abscess — *see* Salpingitis
    due to pregnancy O00.10- ☑
      with intrauterine pregnancy O00.11- ☑
  tympanum, tympanic (membrane) (nontraumatic) —
    see also Perforation, tympanic membrane
    H72.9- ☑
    traumatic — *see* Rupture, ear drum, traumatic
  umbilical cord, complicating delivery O69.89 ☑
  ureter (traumatic) S37.19 ☑
    nontraumatic N28.89
  urethra (nontraumatic) N36.8
    with ectopic or molar pregnancy O08.6
    following ectopic or molar pregnancy O08.6
    obstetrical trauma O71.5
    traumatic S37.39 ☑
  uterosacral ligament (nonobstetric) (nontraumatic)
    N83.8
  uterus (traumatic) S37.69 ☑
    before labor O71.0- ☑
    during or after labor O71.1
    nonpuerperal, nontraumatic N85.8
    pregnant (during labor) O71.1
      before labor O71.0- ☑
  vagina — *see* Injury, vagina
  valve, valvular (heart) — *see* Endocarditis
  varicose vein — *see* Varix
  varix — *see* Varix
  vena cava R58
    traumatic — *see* Injury, vena cava, laceration, major
  vesical (urinary) N32.89
  vessel (blood) R58
    pulmonary I28.8
    traumatic — *see* Injury, blood vessel
  viscus R19.8
  vulva complicating delivery O70.0
Russell-Silver syndrome Q87.19
Russian spring-summer type encephalitis A84.0
Rust's disease (tuberculous cervical spondylitis) A18.01
Ruvalcaba-Myhre-Smith syndrome E71.440
Rytand-Lipsitch syndrome I44.2

S

Saber, sabre shin or tibia (syphilitic) A50.56 *[M90.8-]* ☑
Sac lacrimal — *see* condition
Saccharomyces infection B37.9
Saccharopinuria E72.3
Saccular — *see* condition
Sacculation
  aorta (nonsyphilitic) — *see* Aneurysm, aorta
  bladder N32.3
  intralaryngeal (congenital) (ventricular) Q31.3
  larynx (congenital) (ventricular) Q31.3
  organ or site, congenital — *see* Distortion
  pregnant uterus — *see* Pregnancy, complicated by,
    abnormal, uterus
  ureter N28.89
  urethra N36.1
  vesical N32.3
Sachs' amaurotic familial idiocy or disease E75.02
Sachs-Tay disease E75.02
Sacks-Libman disease M32.11
Sacralgia M53.3

Sacralization Q76.49
Sacrodynia M53.3
Sacroiliac joint — *see* condition
Sacroiliitis NEC M46.1
Sacrum — *see* condition
Saddle
  back — *see* Lordosis
  embolus
    abdominal aorta I74.01
    pulmonary artery I26.92
      with acute cor pulmonale I26.02
  injury — *code to* condition
  nose M95.0
    due to syphilis A50.57
Sadism (sexual) F65.52
Sadness, postpartal O90.6
Sadomasochism F65.50
Saemisch's ulcer (cornea) — *see* Ulcer, cornea, central
Sagging
  skin and subcutaneous tissue (following bariatric
    surgery weight loss) (following dietary weight
    loss) L98.7
Sahib disease B55.0
Sailors' skin L57.8
Saint
  Anthony's fire — *see* Erysipelas
  triad — *see* Hernia, diaphragm
  Vitus' dance — *see* Chorea, Sydenham's
Salaam
  attack(s) — *see* Epilepsy, spasms
  tic R25.8
Salicylism
  abuse F55.8
  overdose or wrong substance given — *see* Table of
    Drugs and Chemicals, by drug, poisoning
Salivary duct or gland — *see* condition
Salivation, excessive K11.7
Salmonella — *see* Infection, Salmonella
Salmonellosis A02.0
Salpingitis (catarrhal) (fallopian tube) (nodular) (pseud-
  ofollicular) (purulent) (septic) N70.91
  with oophoritis N70.93
  acute N70.01
    with oophoritis N70.03
  chlamydial A56.11
  chronic N70.11
    with oophoritis N70.13
  complicating abortion — *see* Abortion, by type, com-
    plicated by, salpingitis
  ear — *see* Salpingitis, eustachian
  eustachian (tube) H68.00- ☑
    acute H68.01- ☑
    chronic H68.02- ☑
  follicularis N70.11
    with oophoritis N70.13
  gonococcal (acute) (chronic) A54.24
  interstitial, chronic N70.11
    with oophoritis N70.13
  isthmica nodosa N70.11
    with oophoritis N70.13
  specific (gonococcal) (acute) (chronic) A54.24
  tuberculous (acute) (chronic) A18.17
  venereal (gonococcal) (acute) (chronic) A54.24
Salpingocele N83.4- ☑
Salpingo-oophoritis (catarrhal) (purulent) (ruptured)
  (septic) (suppurative) N70.93
  acute N70.03
    with ectopic or molar pregnancy O08.0
    following ectopic or molar pregnancy O08.0
    gonococcal A54.24
  chronic N70.13
  following ectopic or molar pregnancy O08.0
  gonococcal (acute) (chronic) A54.24
  puerperal O86.19
  specific (gonococcal) (acute) (chronic) A54.24
  subacute N70.03
  tuberculous (acute) (chronic) A18.17
  venereal (gonococcal) (acute) (chronic) A54.24
Salpingo-ovaritis — *see* Salpingo-oophoritis
Salpingoperitonitis — *see* Salpingo-oophoritis
Salzmann's nodular dystrophy — *see* Degeneration,
  cornea, nodular
Sampson's cyst or tumor N80.1
San Joaquin (Valley) **fever** B38.0
Sandblaster's asthma, lung or pneumoconiosis J62.8
Sander's disease (paranoia) F22
Sandfly fever A93.1

Sandhoff's disease E75.01
Sanfilippo (Type B) (Type C) (Type D) **syndrome** E76.22
Sanger-Brown ataxia G11.2
Sao Paulo fever or typhus A77.0
Saponification, mesenteric K65.8
Sarcocele (benign)
  syphilitic A52.76
    congenital A50.59
Sarcocystosis A07.8
Sarcoepiplocele — *see* Hernia
Sarcoepiplomphalocele Q79.2
Sarcoid — *see also* Sarcoidosis
  arthropathy D86.86
  Boeck's D86.9
  Darier-Roussy D86.3
  iridocyclitis D86.83
  meningitis D86.81
  myocarditis D86.85
  myositis D86.87
  pyelonephritis D86.84
  Spiegler-Fendt L08.89
Sarcoidosis D86.9
  with
    cranial nerve palsies D86.82
    hepatic granuloma D86.89
    polyarthritis D86.86
    tubulo-interstitial nephropathy D86.84
  combined sites NEC D86.89
  lung D86.0
    and lymph nodes D86.2
  lymph nodes D86.1
    and lung D86.2
  meninges D86.81
  skin D86.3
  specified type NEC D86.89
Sarcoma (of) — *see also* Neoplasm, connective tissue, malignant
  alveolar soft part — *see* Neoplasm, connective tissue, malignant
  ameloblastic C41.1
    upper jaw (bone) C41.0
  botryoid — *see* Neoplasm, connective tissue, malignant
  botryoides — *see* Neoplasm, connective tissue, malignant
  cerebellar C71.6
    circumscribed (arachnoidal) C71.6
  circumscribed (arachnoidal) cerebellar C71.6
  clear cell — *see also* Neoplasm, connective tissue, malignant
    kidney C64.- ☑
  dendritic cells (accessory cells) C96.4
  embryonal — *see* Neoplasm, connective tissue, malignant
  endometrial (stromal) C54.1
    isthmus C54.0
  epithelioid (cell) — *see* Neoplasm, connective tissue, malignant
  Ewing's — *see* Neoplasm, bone, malignant
  follicular dendritic cell C96.4
  germinoblastic (diffuse) — *see* Lymphoma, diffuse large cell
    follicular — *see* Lymphoma, follicular, specified NEC
  giant cell (except of bone) — *see also* Neoplasm, connective tissue, malignant
    bone — *see* Neoplasm, bone, malignant
  glomoid — *see* Neoplasm, connective tissue, malignant
  granulocytic C92.3- ☑
  hemangioendothelial — *see* Neoplasm, connective tissue, malignant
  hemorrhagic, multiple — *see* Sarcoma, Kaposi's
  histiocytic C96.A (following C96.6)
  Hodgkin — *see* Lymphoma, Hodgkin
  immunoblastic (diffuse) — *see* Lymphoma, diffuse large cell
  interdigitating dendritic cell C96.4
  Kaposi's
    colon C46.4
    connective tissue C46.1
    gastrointestinal organ C46.4
    lung C46.5- ☑
    lymph node(s) C46.3
    palate (hard) (soft) C46.2
    rectum C46.4
    skin C46.0
    specified site NEC C46.7
    stomach C46.4
    unspecified site C46.9
  Kupffer cell C22.3

Sarcoma — *continued*
  Langerhans cell C96.4
  leptomeningeal — *see* Neoplasm, meninges, malignant
  liver NEC C22.4
  lymphangioendothelial — *see* Neoplasm, connective tissue, malignant
  lymphoblastic — *see* Lymphoma, lymphoblastic (diffuse)
  lymphocytic — *see* Lymphoma, small cell B-cell
  mast cell C96.22
  melanotic — *see* Melanoma
  meningeal — *see* Neoplasm, meninges, malignant
  meningothelial — *see* Neoplasm, meninges, malignant
  mesenchymal — *see also* Neoplasm, connective tissue, malignant
    mixed — *see* Neoplasm, connective tissue, malignant
  mesothelial — *See* Mesothelioma
  monstrocellular
    specified site — *see* Neoplasm, malignant, by site
    unspecified site C71.9
  myeloid C92.3- ☑
  neurogenic — *see* Neoplasm, nerve, malignant
  odontogenic C41.1
    upper jaw (bone) C41.0
  osteoblastic — *see* Neoplasm, bone, malignant
  osteogenic — *see also* Neoplasm, bone, malignant
    juxtacortical — *see* Neoplasm, bone, malignant
    periosteal — *see* Neoplasm, bone, malignant
  periosteal — *see also* Neoplasm, bone, malignant
    osteogenic — *see* Neoplasm, bone, malignant
  pleomorphic cell — *see* Neoplasm, connective tissue, malignant
  reticulum cell (diffuse) — *see* Lymphoma, diffuse large cell
    nodular — *see* Lymphoma, follicular
    pleomorphic cell type — *see* Lymphoma, diffuse large cell
  rhabdoid — *see* Neoplasm, malignant, by site
  round cell — *see* Neoplasm, connective tissue, malignant
  small cell — *see* Neoplasm, connective tissue, malignant
  soft tissue — *see* Neoplasm, connective tissue, malignant
  spindle cell — *see* Neoplasm, connective tissue, malignant
  stromal (endometrial) C54.1
    isthmus C54.0
  synovial — *see also* Neoplasm, connective tissue, malignant
    biphasic — *see* Neoplasm, connective tissue, malignant
    epithelioid cell — *see* Neoplasm, connective tissue, malignant
    spindle cell — *see* Neoplasm, connective tissue, malignant
Sarcomatosis
  meningeal — *see* Neoplasm, meninges, malignant
  specified site NEC — *see* Neoplasm, connective tissue, malignant
  unspecified site C80.1
Sarcopenia (age-related) M62.84
Sarcosinemia E72.59
Sarcosporidiosis (intestinal) A07.8
Satiety, early R68.81
Saturnine — *see* condition
Saturnism
  overdose or wrong substance given or taken — *see* Table of Drugs and Chemicals, by drug, poisoning
Satyriasis F52.8
Sauriasis — *see* Ichthyosis
SBE (subacute bacterial endocarditis) I33.0
Scabies (any site) B86
Scabs R23.4
Scaglietti-Dagnini syndrome E22.0
Scald — *see* Burn
Scalenus anticus (anterior) **syndrome** G54.0
Scales R23.4
Scaling, skin R23.4
Scalp — *see* condition
Scapegoating affecting child Z62.3
Scaphocephaly Q75.0
Scapulalgia M89.8X1
Scapulohumeral myopathy G71.02
Scar, scarring — *see also* Cicatrix L90.5
  adherent L90.5

Scar, scarring — *continued*
  atrophic L90.5
  cervix
    in pregnancy or childbirth — *see* Pregnancy, complicated by, abnormal cervix
  cheloid L91.0
  chorioretinal H31.00- ☑
    posterior pole macula H31.01- ☑
    postsurgical H59.81- ☑
    solar retinopathy H31.02- ☑
    specified type NEC H31.09- ☑
  choroid — *see* Scar, chorioretinal
  conjunctiva H11.24- ☑
  cornea H17.9
    xerophthalmic — *see also* Opacity, cornea
      vitamin A deficiency E50.6
  defect (isthmocele) O34.22
  duodenum, obstructive K31.5
  hypertrophic L91.0
  keloid L91.0
  labia N90.89
  lung (base) J98.4
  macula — *see* Scar, chorioretinal, posterior pole
  muscle M62.89
  myocardium, myocardial I25.2
  painful L90.5
  posterior pole (eye) — *see* Scar, chorioretinal, posterior pole
  retina — *see* Scar, chorioretinal
  trachea J39.8
  transmural uterine, in pregnancy O34.29
  uterus N85.8
    in pregnancy O34.29
  vagina N89.8
    postoperative N99.2
  vulva N90.89
Scarabiasis B88.2
Scarlatina (anginosa) (maligna) A38.9
  myocarditis (acute) A38.1
    old — *see* Myocarditis
  otitis media A38.0
  ulcerosa A38.8
Scarlet fever (albuminuria) (angina) A38.9
Schamberg's disease (progressive pigmentary dermatosis) L81.7
Schatzki's ring (acquired) (esophagus) (lower) K22.2
  congenital Q39.3
Schaufenster krankheit I20.8
Schaumann's
  benign lymphogranulomatosis D86.1
  disease or syndrome — *see* Sarcoidosis
Scheie's syndrome E76.03
Schenck's disease B42.1
Scheuermann's disease or osteochondrosis — *see* Osteochondrosis, juvenile, spine
Schilder (-Flatau) **disease** G37.0
Schilling-type monocytic leukemia C93.0- ☑
Schimmelbusch's disease, cystic mastitis, or hyperplasia — *see* Mastopathy, cystic
Schistosoma infestation — *see* Infestation, Schistosoma
Schistosomiasis B65.9
  with muscle disorder B65.9 *[M63.80]*
    ankle B65.9 *[M63.87-]* ☑
    foot B65.9 *[M63.87-]* ☑
    forearm B65.9 *[M63.83-]* ☑
    hand B65.9 *[M63.84-]* ☑
    lower leg B65.9 *[M63.86-]* ☑
    multiple sites B65.9 *[M63.89]*
    pelvic region B65.9 *[M63.85-]* ☑
    shoulder region B65.9 *[M63.81-]* ☑
    specified site NEC B65.9 *[M63.88]*
    thigh B65.9 *[M63.85-]* ☑
    upper arm B65.9 *[M63.82-]* ☑
  Asiatic B65.2
  bladder B65.0
  chestermani B65.8
  colon B65.1
  cutaneous B65.3
  due to
    S. haematobium B65.0
    S. japonicum B65.2
    S. mansoni B65.1
    S. mattheii B65.8
  Eastern B65.2
  genitourinary tract B65.0
  intestinal B65.1
  lung NEC B65.9 *[J99]*

▼ Subterms under main terms may continue to next column or page   ☑ **Additional Character Required** — Refer to the Tabular List for Character Selection   **285**

Sclerosis, sclerotic — *continued*
  spinal — *continued*
    dorsolateral — *see* Degeneration, combined
    hereditary (Friedreich's) (mixed form) G11.11
    lateral (amyotrophic) G12.21
      progressive G12.23
    multiple G35
    posterior (syphilitic) A52.11
  stomach K31.89
  subendocardial, congenital I42.4
  systemic M34.9
    with
      lung involvement M34.81
      myopathy M34.82
      polyneuropathy M34.83
    drug-induced M34.2
    due to chemicals NEC M34.2
    progressive M34.0
    specified NEC M34.89
  temporal (mesial) G93.81
  tricuspid (heart) (valve) I07.8
  tuberous (brain) Q85.1
  tympanic membrane — *see* Disorder, tympanic membrane, specified NEC
  valve, valvular (heart) — *see* Endocarditis
  vascular — *see* Arteriosclerosis
  vein I87.8
Scoliosis (acquired) (postural) M41.9
  adolescent (idiopathic) — *see* Scoliosis, idiopathic, adolescent
  congenital Q67.5
    due to.bony malformation Q76.3
    failure of segmentation (hemivertebra) Q76.3
    hemivertebra fusion Q76.3
    postural Q67.5
  degenerative M41.8- ☑
  idiopathic M41.20
    adolescent M41.129
      cervical region M41.122
      cervicothoracic region M41.123
      lumbar region M41.126
      lumbosacral region M41.127
      thoracic region M41.124
      thoracolumbar region M41.125
    cervical region M41.22
    cervicothoracic region M41.23
    infantile M41.00
      cervical region M41.02
      cervicothoracic region M41.03
      lumbar region M41.06
      lumbosacral region M41.07
      sacrococcygeal region M41.08
      thoracic region M41.04
      thoracolumbar region M41.05
    juvenile M41.119
      cervical region M41.112
      cervicothoracic region M41.113
      lumbar region M41.116
      lumbosacral region M41.117
      thoracic region M41.114
      thoracolumbar region M41.115
    lumbar region M41.26
    lumbosacral region M41.27
    thoracic region M41.24
    thoracolumbar region M41.25
  infantile — *see* Scoliosis, idiopathic, infantile
  neuromuscular M41.40
    cervical region M41.42
    cervicothoracic region M41.43
    lumbar region M41.46
    lumbosacral region M41.47
    occipito-atlanto-axial region M41.41
    thoracic region M41.44
    thoracolumbar region M41.45
  paralytic — *see* Scoliosis, neuromuscular
  postradiation therapy M96.5
  rachitic (late effect or sequelae) E64.3 *[M49.80]*
    cervical region E64.3 *[M49.82]*
    cervicothoracic region E64.3 *[M49.83]*
    lumbar region E64.3 *[M49.86]*
    lumbosacral region E64.3 *[M49.87]*
    multiple sites E64.3 *[M49.89]*
    occipito-atlanto-axial region E64.3 *[M49.81]*
    sacrococcygeal region E64.3 *[M49.88]*
    thoracic region E64.3 *[M49.84]*
    thoracolumbar region E64.3 *[M49.85]*
  sciatic M54.4- ☑
  secondary (to) NEC M41.50

Scoliosis — *continued*
  secondary — *continued*
    cerebral palsy, Friedreich's ataxia, poliomyelitis, neuromuscular disorders — *see* Scoliosis, neuromuscular
    cervical region M41.52
    cervicothoracic region M41.53
    lumbar region M41.56
    lumbosacral region M41.57
    thoracic region M41.54
    thoracolumbar region M41.55
  specified form NEC M41.80
    cervical region M41.82
    cervicothoracic region M41.83
    lumbar region M41.86
    lumbosacral region M41.87
    thoracic region M41.84
    thoracolumbar region M41.85
  thoracogenic M41.30
    thoracic region M41.34
    thoracolumbar region M41.35
  tuberculous A18.01
Scoliotic pelvis
  with disproportion (fetopelvic) O33.0
    causing obstructed labor O65.0
Scorbutus, scorbutic — *see also* Scurvy
  anemia D53.2
Score, NIHSS (National Institutes of Health Stroke Scale) R29.7- ☑
Scotoma (arcuate) (Bjerrum) (central) (ring) — *see also* Defect, visual field, localized, scotoma
  scintillating H53.19
Scratch — *see* Abrasion
Scratchy throat R09.89
Screening (for) Z13.9
  alcoholism Z13.39
  anemia Z13.0
  anomaly, congenital Z13.89
  antenatal, of mother — *see also* Encounter, antenatal screening Z36.9
  arterial hypertension Z13.6
  arthropod-borne viral disease NEC Z11.59
  autism Z13.41
  bacteriuria, asymptomatic Z13.89
  behavioral disorder Z13.30
    specified NEC Z13.39
  brain injury, traumatic Z13.850
  bronchitis, chronic Z13.83
  brucellosis Z11.2
  cardiovascular disorder Z13.6
  cataract Z13.5
  chlamydial diseases Z11.8
  cholera Z11.0
  chromosomal abnormalities (nonprocreative) NEC Z13.79
  colonoscopy Z12.11
  congenital
    dislocation of hip Z13.89
    eye disorder Z13.5
    malformation or deformation Z13.89
  contamination NEC Z13.88
  cystic fibrosis Z13.228
  dengue fever Z11.59
  dental disorder Z13.84
  depression (adult) (adolescent) (child) Z13.31
    maternal Z13.32
    perinatal Z13.32
  developmental
    delays Z13.40
      global (milestones) Z13.42
      specified NEC Z13.49
    handicap Z13.42
      in early childhood Z13.42
  diabetes mellitus Z13.1
  diphtheria Z11.2
  disability, intellectual Z13.39
  disease or disorder Z13.9
    bacterial NEC Z11.2
      intestinal infectious Z11.0
      respiratory tuberculosis Z11.1
    behavioral Z13.30
      specified NEC Z13.39
    blood or blood-forming organ Z13.0
    cardiovascular Z13.6
    Chagas' Z11.6
    chlamydial Z11.8
    dental Z13.89
    developmental delays Z13.40

Screening — *continued*
  disease or disorder — *continued*
    developmental delays — *continued*
      global (milestones) Z13.42
      specified NEC Z13.49
    digestive tract NEC Z13.818
      lower GI Z13.811
      upper GI Z13.810
    ear Z13.5
    endocrine Z13.29
    eye Z13.5
    genitourinary Z13.89
    heart Z13.6
    human immunodeficiency virus (HIV) infection Z11.4
    immunity Z13.0
    infection
      intestinal Z11.0
        specified NEC Z11.6
    infectious Z11.9
    mental health and behavioral Z13.30
      specified NEC Z13.39
    metabolic Z13.228
    neurological Z13.89
    nutritional Z13.21
      metabolic Z13.228
        lipoid disorders Z13.220
    protozoal Z11.6
      intestinal Z11.0
    respiratory Z13.83
    rheumatic Z13.828
    rickettsial Z11.8
    sexually-transmitted NEC Z11.3
      human immunodeficiency virus (HIV) Z11.4
    sickle-cell (trait) Z13.0
    skin Z13.89
    specified NEC Z13.89
    spirochetal Z11.8
    thyroid Z13.29
    vascular Z13.6
    venereal Z11.3
    viral NEC Z11.59
      human immunodeficiency virus (HIV) Z11.4
      intestinal Z11.0
  elevated titer Z13.89
  emphysema Z13.83
  encephalitis, viral (mosquito- or tick-borne) Z11.59
  exposure to contaminants (toxic) Z13.88
  fever
    dengue Z11.59
    hemorrhagic Z11.59
    yellow Z11.59
  filariasis Z11.6
  galactosemia Z13.228
  gastrointestinal condition Z13.818
  genetic (nonprocreative) - for procreative management — *see* Testing, genetic, for procreative management
    disease carrier status (nonprocreative) Z13.71
    specified NEC (nonprocreative) Z13.79
  genitourinary condition Z13.89
  glaucoma Z13.5
  gonorrhea Z11.3
  gout Z13.89
  helminthiasis (intestinal) Z11.6
  hematopoietic malignancy Z12.89
  hemoglobinopathies NEC Z13.0
  hemorrhagic fever Z11.59
  Hodgkin disease Z12.89
  human immunodeficiency virus (HIV) Z11.4
  human papillomavirus Z11.51
  hypertension Z13.6
  immunity disorders Z13.0
  infant or child (over 28 days old) Z00.129
    with abnormal findings Z00.121
  infection
    mycotic Z11.8
    parasitic Z11.8
  ingestion of radioactive substance Z13.88
  intellectual disability Z13.39
  intestinal
    helminthiasis Z11.6
    infectious disease Z11.0
  leishmaniasis Z11.6
  leprosy Z11.2
  leptospirosis Z11.8
  leukemia Z12.89
  lymphoma Z12.89
  malaria Z11.6
  malnutrition Z13.29

Screening — *continued*
  malnutrition — *continued*
    metabolic Z13.228
    nutritional Z13.21
  measles Z11.59
  mental health disorder Z13.30
    specified NEC Z13.39
  metabolic errors, inborn Z13.228
  multiphasic Z13.89
  musculoskeletal disorder Z13.828
    osteoporosis Z13.820
  mycoses B08.62
  myocardial infarction (acute) Z13.6
  neoplasm (malignant) (of) Z12.9
    bladder Z12.6
    blood Z12.89
    breast Z12.39
      routine mammogram Z12.31
    cervix Z12.4
    colon Z12.11
    genitourinary organs NEC Z12.79
      bladder Z12.6
      cervix Z12.4
      ovary Z12.73
      prostate Z12.5
      testis Z12.71
      vagina Z12.72
    hematopoietic system Z12.89
    intestinal tract Z12.10
      colon Z12.11
      rectum Z12.12
      small intestine Z12.13
    lung Z12.2
    lymph (glands) Z12.89
    nervous system Z12.82
    oral cavity Z12.81
    prostate Z12.5
    rectum Z12.12
    respiratory organs Z12.2
    skin Z12.83
    small intestine Z12.13
    specified site NEC Z12.89
    stomach Z12.0
  nephropathy Z13.89
  nervous system disorders NEC Z13.858
  neurological condition Z13.89
  osteoporosis Z13.820
  parasitic infestation Z11.9
    specified NEC Z11.8
  phenylketonuria Z13.228
  plague Z11.2
  poisoning (chemical) (heavy metal) Z13.88
  poliomyelitis Z11.59
  postnatal, chromosomal abnormalities Z13.89
  prenatal, of mother — *see also* Encounter, antenatal
    screening Z36.9
  protozoal disease Z11.6
    intestinal Z11.0
  pulmonary tuberculosis Z11.1
  radiation exposure Z13.88
  respiratory condition Z13.83
  respiratory tuberculosis Z11.1
  rheumatoid arthritis Z13.828
  rubella Z11.59
  schistosomiasis Z11.6
  sexually-transmitted disease NEC Z11.3
    human immunodeficiency virus (HIV) Z11.4
  sickle-cell disease or trait Z13.0
  skin condition Z13.89
  sleeping sickness Z11.6
  special Z13.9
    specified NEC Z13.89
  syphilis Z11.3
  tetanus Z11.2
  trachoma Z11.8
  traumatic brain injury Z13.850
  trypanosomiasis Z11.6
  tuberculosis, respiratory Z11.1
    active Z11.1
    latent Z11.7
  venereal disease Z11.3
  viral encephalitis (mosquito- or tick-borne) Z11.59
  whooping cough Z11.2
  worms, intestinal Z11.6
  yaws Z11.8
  yellow fever Z11.59
Scrofula, scrofulosis (tuberculosis of cervical lymph glands) A18.2
Scrofulide (primary) (tuberculous) A18.4

Scrofuloderma, scrofulodermia (any site) (primary) A18.4
Scrofulosus lichen (primary) (tuberculous) A18.4
Scrofulous — *see* condition
Scrotal tongue K14.5
Scrotum — *see* condition
Scurvy, scorbutic E54
  anemia D53.2
  gum E54
  infantile E54
  rickets E55.0 *[M90.80]*
Sealpox B08.62
Seasickness T75.3 ☑
Seatworm (infection) (infestation) B80
Sebaceous — *see also* condition
  cyst — *see* Cyst, sebaceous
Seborrhea, seborrheic L21.9
  capillitii R23.8
  capitis L21.0
  dermatitis L21.9
    infantile L21.1
  eczema L21.9
    infantile L21.1
  sicca L21.0
Seckel's syndrome Q87.19
Seclusion, pupil — *see* Membrane, pupillary
Second hand tobacco smoke exposure (acute) (chronic) Z77.22
  in the perinatal period P96.81
Secondary
  dentin (in pulp) K04.3
  neoplasm, secondaries — *see* Table of Neoplasms, secondary
Secretion
  antidiuretic hormone, inappropriate E22.2
  catecholamine, by pheochromocytoma E27.5
  hormone
    antidiuretic, inappropriate (syndrome) E22.2
    by
      carcinoid tumor E34.0
      pheochromocytoma E27.5
    ectopic NEC E34.2
  urinary
    excessive R35.8
    suppression R34
Section
  nerve, traumatic — *see* Injury, nerve
Sedative, hypnotic, or anxiolytic-induced
  anxiety disorder F13.980
  bipolar and related disorder F13.94
  delirium F13.921
  depressive disorder F13.94
  major neurocognitive disorder F13.97
  mild neurocognitive disorder F13.988
  psychotic disorder F13.959
  sexual dysfunction F13.981
  sleep disorder F13.982
Segmentation, incomplete (congenital) — *see also* Fusion
  bone NEC Q78.8
  lumbosacral (joint) (vertebra) Q76.49
Seitelberger's syndrome (infantile neuraxonal dystrophy) G31.89
Seizure(s) — *see also* Convulsions R56.9
  absence G40.A- ☑ *(following G40.3)*
  akinetic — *see* Epilepsy, generalized, specified NEC
  atonic — *see* Epilepsy, generalized, specified NEC
  autonomic (hysterical) F44.5
  convulsive — *see* Convulsions
  cortical (focal) (motor) — *see* Epilepsy, localization-related, symptomatic, with simple partial seizures
  disorder — *see also* Epilepsy G40.909
  due to stroke — *see* Sequelae (of), disease, cerebrovascular, by type, specified NEC
  epileptic — *see* Epilepsy
  febrile (simple) R56.00
    with status epilepticus G40.901
    complex (atypical) (complicated) R56.01
      with status epilepticus G40.901
  grand mal G40.409
    intractable G40.419
      with status epilepticus G40.411
      without status epilepticus G40.419
    not intractable G40.409
      with status epilepticus G40.401
      without status epilepticus G40.409
  heart — *see* Disease, heart
  hysterical F44.5

Seizure(s) — *continued*
  intractable G40.919
    with status epilepticus G40.911
  Jacksonian (focal) (motor type) (sensory type) — *see* Epilepsy, localization-related, symptomatic, with simple partial seizures
  newborn P90
  nonspecific epileptic
    atonic — *see* Epilepsy, generalized, specified NEC
    clonic — *see* Epilepsy, generalized, specified NEC
    myoclonic — *see* Epilepsy, generalized, specified NEC
    tonic — *see* Epilepsy, generalized, specified NEC
    tonic-clonic — *see* Epilepsy, generalized, specified NEC
  partial, developing into secondarily generalized seizures
    complex — *see* Epilepsy, localization-related, symptomatic, with complex partial seizures
    simple — *see* Epilepsy, localization-related, symptomatic, with simple partial seizures
  petit mal G40.A- ☑ *(following G40.3)*
    intractable G40.419
      with status epilepticus G40.411
      without status epilepticus G40.419
    not intractable G40.409
      with status epilepticus G40.401
      without status epilepticus G40.409
  post traumatic R56.1
  recurrent G40.909
  specified NEC G40.89
  uncinate — *see* Epilepsy, localization-related, symptomatic, with complex partial seizures
Selenium deficiency, dietary E59
Self-damaging behavior (life-style) Z72.89
Self-harm (attempted)
  history (personal) Z91.5
    in family Z81.8
Self-mutilation (attempted)
  history (personal) Z91.5
    in family Z81.8
Self-poisoning
  history (personal) Z91.5
    in family Z81.8
  observation following (alleged) attempt Z03.6
Semicoma R40.1
Seminal vesiculitis N49.0
Seminoma C62.9- ☑
  specified site — *see* Neoplasm, malignant, by site
Senear-Usher disease or syndrome L10.4
Senectus R54
Senescence (without mention of psychosis) R54
Senile, senility — *see also* condition R41.81
  with
    acute confusional state F05
    mental changes NOS F03 ☑
    psychosis NEC — *see* Psychosis, senile
  asthenia R54
  cervix (atrophic) N88.8
  debility R54
  endometrium (atrophic) N85.8
  fallopian tube (atrophic) — *see* Atrophy, fallopian tube
  heart (failure) R54
  ovary (atrophic) — *see* Atrophy, ovary
  premature E34.8
  vagina, vaginitis (atrophic) N95.2
  wart L82.1
Sensation
  burning (skin) R20.8
    tongue K14.6
  loss of R20.8
  prickling (skin) R20.2
  tingling (skin) R20.2
Sense loss
  smell — *see* Disturbance, sensation, smell
  taste — *see* Disturbance, sensation, taste
  touch R20.8
Sensibility disturbance (cortical) (deep) (vibratory) R20.9
Sensitive, sensitivity — *see also* Allergy
  carotid sinus G90.01
  child (excessive) F93.8
  cold, autoimmune D59.12
  dentin K03.89
  gluten (non-celiac) K90.41
  latex Z91.040
  methemoglobin D74.8
  tuberculin, without clinical or radiological symptoms R76.11

⚕ Subterms under main terms may continue to next column or page   ☑ **Additional Character Required — Refer to the Tabular List for Character Selection**   **287**

Screening — Sensitive, sensitivity

Sensitive, sensitivity — continued
 visual
  glare H53.71
  impaired contrast H53.72
Sensitiver Beziehungswahn F22
Sensitization, auto-erythrocytic D69.2
Separation
 anxiety, abnormal (of childhood) F93.0
 apophysis, traumatic — code as Fracture, by site
 choroid — see Detachment, choroid
 epiphysis, epiphyseal
  nontraumatic — see also Osteochondropathy,
    specified type NEC
   upper femoral — see Slipped, epiphysis, upper
    femoral
  traumatic — code as Fracture, by site
 fracture — see Fracture
 infundibulum cardiac from right ventricle by a partition
   Q24.3
 joint (traumatic) (current) — code by site under Dislocation
 muscle (nontraumatic) — see Diastasis, muscle
 pubic bone, obstetrical trauma O71.6
 retina, retinal — see Detachment, retina
 symphysis pubis, obstetrical trauma O71.6
 tracheal ring, incomplete, congenital Q32.1
Sepsis (generalized) (unspecified organism) A41.9
 with
  organ dysfunction (acute) (multiple) R65.20
   with septic shock R65.21
 actinomycotic A42.7
 adrenal hemorrhage syndrome (meningococcal) A39.1
 anaerobic A41.4
 Bacillus anthracis A22.7
 Brucella — see also Brucellosis A23.9
 candidal B37.7
 cryptogenic A41.9
 due to device, implant or graft T85.79 ☑
  arterial graft NEC T82.7 ☑
  breast (implant) T85.79 ☑
  catheter NEC T85.79 ☑
   dialysis (renal) T82.7 ☑
    intraperitoneal T85.71 ☑
   infusion NEC T82.7 ☑
    spinal (cranial) (epidural) (intrathecal) (spinal)
      (subarachnoid) (subdural) T85.735 ☑
   urethral indwelling T83.511 ☑
   urinary T83.518 ☑
  ectopic or molar pregnancy O08.82
  electronic (electrode) (pulse generator) (stimulator)
   bone T84.7 ☑
   cardiac T82.7 ☑
   nervous system T85.738 ☑
    brain T85.731 ☑
    neurostimulator generator T85.734 ☑
    peripheral nerve T85.732 ☑
    spinal cord T85.733 ☑
   urinary T83.590 ☑
  fixation, internal (orthopedic) — see Complication,
    fixation device, infection
  gastrointestinal (bile duct) (esophagus) T85.79 ☑
   neurostimulator electrode (lead) T85.732 ☑
  genital T83.69 ☑
  heart NEC T82.7 ☑
   valve (prosthesis) T82.6 ☑
    graft T82.7 ☑
  joint prosthesis — see Complication, joint prosthe-
    sis, infection
  ocular (corneal graft) (orbital implant) T85.79 ☑
  orthopedic NEC T84.7 ☑
   fixation device, internal — see Complication,
    fixation device, infection
  specified NEC T85.79 ☑
  vascular T82.7 ☑
  ventricular intracranial (communicating) shunt
    T85.730 ☑
 during labor O75.3
 Enterococcus A41.81
 Erysipelothrix (rhusiopathiae) (erysipeloid) A26.7
 Escherichia coli (E. coli) A41.5 ☑
 extraintestinal yersiniosis A28.2
 following
  abortion (subsequent episode) O08.0
   current episode — see Abortion
  ectopic or molar pregnancy O08.82
  immunization T88.0 ☑

Sepsis — continued
 following — continued
  infusion, therapeutic injection or transfusion NEC
    T80.29 ☑
  obstetrical procedure O86.04
 gangrenous A41.9
 gonococcal A54.86
 Gram-negative (organism) A41.5 ☑
  anaerobic A41.4
 Haemophilus influenzae A41.3
 herpesviral B00.7
 intra-abdominal K65.1
 intraocular — see Endophthalmitis, purulent
 Listeria monocytogenes A32.7
 localized — code to specific localized infection
  in operation wound T81.49 ☑
  skin — see Abscess
 malleus A24.0
 melioidosis A24.1
 meningeal — see Meningitis
 meningococcal A39.4
  acute A39.2
  chronic A39.3
 MSSA (Methicillin susceptible Staphylococcus aureus)
   A41.01
 newborn P36.9
  due to
   anaerobes NEC P36.5
   Escherichia coli P36.4
   Staphylococcus P36.30
    aureus P36.2
    specified NEC P36.39
   Streptococcus P36.10
    group B P36.0
    specified NEC P36.19
  specified NEC P36.8
 Pasteurella multocida A28.0
 pelvic, puerperal, postpartum, childbirth O85
 pneumococcal A40.3
 postprocedural T81.44 ☑
 puerperal, postpartum, childbirth (pelvic) O85
 Salmonella (arizonae) (cholerae-suis) (enteritidis) (typhimurium) A02.1
 severe R65.20
  with septic shock R65.21
 Shigella — see also Dysentery, bacillary A03.9
 skin, localized — see Abscess
 specified organism NEC A41.89
 Staphylococcus, staphylococcal A41.2
  aureus (methicillin susceptible) (MSSA) A41.01
   methicillin resistant (MRSA) A41.02
  coagulase-negative A41.1
  specified NEC A41.1
 Streptococcus, streptococcal A40.9
  agalactiae A40.1
  group
   A A40.0
   B A40.1
   D A41.81
  neonatal P36.10
   group B P36.0
   specified NEC P36.19
  pneumoniae A40.3
  pyogenes A40.0
  specified NEC A40.8
 tracheostomy stoma J95.02
 tularemic A21.7
 umbilical, umbilical cord (newborn) — see Sepsis,
   newborn
 Yersinia pestis A20.7
Septate — see Septum
Septic — see condition
 arm — see Cellulitis, upper limb
  with lymphangitis — see Lymphangitis, acute, upper
    limb
 embolus — see Embolism
 finger — see Cellulitis, digit
  with lymphangitis — see Lymphangitis, acute, digit
 foot — see Cellulitis, lower limb
  with lymphangitis — see Lymphangitis, acute,
    lower limb
 gallbladder (acute) K81.0
 hand — see Cellulitis, upper limb
  with lymphangitis — see Lymphangitis, acute, upper
    limb
 joint — see Arthritis, pyogenic or pyemic
 leg — see Cellulitis, lower limb

Septic — continued
 leg — see Cellulitis, lower limb — continued
  with lymphangitis — see Lymphangitis, acute,
    lower limb
 nail — see also Cellulitis, digit
  with lymphangitis — see Lymphangitis, acute, digit
 sore — see also Abscess
  throat J02.0
   streptococcal J02.0
 spleen (acute) D73.89
 teeth, tooth (pulpal origin) K04.4
 throat — see Pharyngitis
 thrombus — see Thrombosis
 toe — see Cellulitis, digit
  with lymphangitis — see Lymphangitis, acute, digit
 tonsils, chronic J35.01
  with adenoiditis J35.03
 uterus — see Endometritis
Septicemia A41.9
 meaning sepsis — see Sepsis
Septum, septate (congenital) — see also Anomaly, by
   site
 anal Q42.3
  with fistula Q42.2
 aqueduct of Sylvius Q03.0
  with spina bifida — see Spina bifida, by site, with
    hydrocephalus
 uterus Q51.28
  complete Q51.21
  partial Q51.22
  specified NEC Q51.28
 vagina Q52.10
  in pregnancy — see Pregnancy, complicated by,
    abnormal vagina
  causing obstructed labor O65.5
  longitudinal Q52.129
   microperforate
    left side Q52.124
    right side Q52.123
   nonobstruction Q52.120
   obstructing Q52.129
    left side Q52.122
    right side Q52.121
  transverse Q52.11
Sequelae (of) — see also condition
 abscess, intracranial or intraspinal (conditions in G06,
   G09
 amputation — code to injury with seventh character
   S
 burn and corrosion — code to injury with seventh
   character S
 calcium deficiency E64.8
 cerebrovascular disease — see Sequelae, disease,
   cerebrovascular
 childbirth O94
 contusion — code to injury with seventh character S
 corrosion — see Sequelae, burn and corrosion
 crushing injury — code to injury with seventh character
   S
 disease
  cerebrovascular I69.90
   alteration of sensation I69.998
   aphasia I69.920
   apraxia I69.990
   ataxia I69.993
   cognitive deficits I69.91 ☑
   disturbance of vision I69.998
   dysarthria I69.922
   dysphagia I69.991
   dysphasia I69.921
   facial droop I69.992
   facial weakness I69.992
   fluency disorder I69.923
   hemiplegia I69.95- ☑
   hemorrhage
    intracerebral — see Sequelae, hemorrhage,
      intracerebral
    intracranial, nontraumatic NEC — see Seque-
      lae, hemorrhage, intracranial, nontrau-
      matic
    subarachnoid — see Sequelae, hemorrhage,
      subarachnoid
   language deficit I69.928
   monoplegia
    lower limb I69.94- ☑
    upper limb I69.93- ☑
   paralytic syndrome I69.96- ☑
   specified effect NEC I69.998

☑ Additional Character Required — Refer to the Tabular List for Character Selection

🔺 Subterms under main terms may continue to next column or page

Sequelae — continued
  disease — continued
    cerebrovascular — continued
      specified type NEC I69.80
        alteration of sensation I69.898
        aphasia I69.820
        apraxia I69.890
        ataxia I69.893
        cognitive deficits I69.81 ☑
        disturbance of vision I69.898
        dysarthria I69.822
        dysphagia I69.891
        dysphasia I69.821
        facial droop I69.892
        facial weakness I69.892
        fluency disorder I69.823
        hemiplegia I69.85- ☑
        language deficit I69.828
        monoplegia
          lower limb I69.84- ☑
          upper limb I69.83- ☑
        paralytic syndrome I69.86- ☑
        specified effect NEC I69.898
      speech deficit I69.928
      speech deficit I69.828
      stroke NOS — see Sequelae, stroke NOS
  dislocation — code to injury with seventh character S
  encephalitis or encephalomyelitis (conditions in G04) G09
    in infectious disease NEC B94.8
    viral B94.1
  external cause — code to injury with seventh character S
  foreign body entering natural orifice — code to injury with seventh character S
  fracture — code to injury with seventh character S
  frostbite — code to injury with seventh character S
  Hansen's disease B92
  hemorrhage
    intracerebral I69.10
      alteration of sensation I69.198
      aphasia I69.120
      apraxia I69.190
      ataxia I69.193
      cognitive deficits I69.11 ☑
      disturbance of vision I69.198
      dysarthria I69.122
      dysphagia I69.191
      dysphasia I69.121
      facial droop I69.192
      facial weakness I69.192
      fluency disorder I69.123
      hemiplegia I69.15- ☑
      language deficit NEC I69.128
      monoplegia
        lower limb I69.14- ☑
        upper limb I69.13- ☑
      paralytic syndrome I69.16- ☑
      specified effect NEC I69.198
      speech deficit NEC I69.128
    intracranial, nontraumatic NEC I69.20
      alteration of sensation I69.298
      aphasia I69.220
      apraxia I69.290
      ataxia I69.293
      cognitive deficits I69.21 ☑
      disturbance of vision I69.298
      dysarthria I69.222
      dysphagia I69.291
      dysphasia I69.221
      facial droop I69.292
      facial weakness I69.292
      fluency disorder I69.223
      hemiplegia I69.25- ☑
      language deficit NEC I69.228
      monoplegia
        lower limb I69.24- ☑
        upper limb I69.23- ☑
      paralytic syndrome I69.26- ☑
      specified effect NEC I69.298
      speech deficit NEC I69.228
    subarachnoid I69.00
      alteration of sensation I69.098
      aphasia I69.020
      apraxia I69.090
      ataxia I69.093
      cognitive deficits — see subcategory I69.01- ☑
      disturbance of vision I69.098

Sequelae — continued
  hemorrhage — continued
    subarachnoid — continued
      dysarthria I69.022
      dysphagia I69.091
      dysphasia I69.021
      facial droop I69.092
      facial weakness I69.092
      fluency disorder I69.023
      hemiplegia I69.05- ☑
      language deficit NEC I69.028
      monoplegia
        lower limb I69.04- ☑
        upper limb I69.03- ☑
      paralytic syndrome I69.06- ☑
      specified effect NEC I69.098
      speech deficit NEC I69.028
  hepatitis, viral B94.2
  hyperalimentation E68
  infarction
    cerebral I69.30
      alteration of sensation I69.398
      aphasia I69.320
      apraxia I69.390
      ataxia I69.393
      cognitive deficits I69.31 ☑
      disturbance of vision I69.398
      dysarthria I69.322
      dysphagia I69.391
      dysphasia I69.321
      facial droop I69.392
      facial weakness I69.392
      fluency disorder I69.323
      hemiplegia I69.35- ☑
      language deficit NEC I69.328
      monoplegia
        lower limb I69.34- ☑
        upper limb I69.33- ☑
      paralytic syndrome I69.36- ☑
      specified effect NEC I69.398
      speech deficit NEC I69.328
  infection, pyogenic, intracranial or intraspinal G09
  infectious disease B94.9
    specified NEC B94.8
  injury — code to injury with seventh character S
  leprosy B92
  meningitis
    bacterial (conditions in G00) G09
    other or unspecified cause (conditions in G03) G09
  muscle (and tendon) injury — code to injury with seventh character S
  myelitis — see Sequelae, encephalitis
  niacin deficiency E64.8
  nutritional deficiency E64.9
    specified NEC E64.8
  obstetrical condition O94
  parasitic disease B94.9
  phlebitis or thrombophlebitis of intracranial or intraspinal venous sinuses and veins (conditions in G08) G09
  poisoning — code to poisoning with seventh character S
    nonmedicinal substance — see Sequelae, toxic effect, nonmedicinal substance
  poliomyelitis (acute) B91
  pregnancy O94
  protein-energy malnutrition E64.0
  puerperium O94
  rickets E64.3
  selenium deficiency E64.8
  sprain and strain — code to injury with seventh character S
  stroke NOS I69.30
    alteration in sensation I69.398
    aphasia I69.320
    apraxia I69.390
    ataxia I69.393
    cognitive deficits I69.31 ☑
    disturbance of vision I69.398
    dysarthria I69.322
    dysphagia I69.391
    dysphasia I69.321
    facial droop I69.392
    facial weakness I69.392
    hemiplegia I69.35- ☑
    language deficit NEC I69.328
    monoplegia
      lower limb I69.34- ☑

Sequelae — continued
  stroke — continued
    monoplegia — continued
      upper limb I69.33- ☑
    paralytic syndrome I69.36- ☑
    specified effect NEC I69.398
    speech deficit NEC I69.328
  tendon and muscle injury — code to injury with seventh character S
  thiamine deficiency E64.8
  trachoma B94.0
  tuberculosis B90.9
    bones and joints B90.2
    central nervous system B90.0
    genitourinary B90.1
    pulmonary (respiratory) B90.9
    specified organs NEC B90.8
  viral
    encephalitis B94.1
    hepatitis B94.2
  vitamin deficiency NEC E64.8
    A E64.1
    B E64.8
    C E64.2
  wound, open — code to injury with seventh character S

Sequestration — see also Sequestrum
  disc — see Displacement, intervertebral disc
  lung, congenital Q33.2

Sequestrum
  bone — see Osteomyelitis, chronic
  dental M27.2
  jaw bone M27.2
  orbit — see Osteomyelitis, orbit
  sinus (accessory) (nasal) — see Sinusitis

Sequoiosis lung or pneumonitis J67.8

Serology for syphilis
  doubtful
    with signs or symptoms — code by site and stage under Syphilis
    follow-up of latent syphilis — see Syphilis, latent
  negative, with signs or symptoms — code by site and stage under Syphilis
  positive A53.0
    with signs or symptoms — code by site and stage under Syphilis
  reactivated A53.0

Seroma — see also Hematoma
  postprocedural — see Complication, postprocedural, seroma
  traumatic, secondary and recurrent T79.2 ☑

Seropurulent — see condition

Serositis, multiple K65.8
  pericardial I31.1
  peritoneal K65.8

Serous — see condition

Sertoli cell
  adenoma
    specified site — see Neoplasm, benign, by site
    unspecified site
      female D27.9
      male D29.20
  carcinoma
    specified site — see Neoplasm, malignant, by site
    unspecified site (male) C62.9- ☑
      female C56.9
  tumor
    with lipid storage
      specified site — see Neoplasm, benign, by site
      unspecified site
        female D27.9
        male D29.20
    specified site — see Neoplasm, benign, by site
    unspecified site
      female D27.9
      male D29.20

Sertoli-Leydig cell tumor — see Neoplasm, benign, by site
  specified site — see Neoplasm, benign, by site
  unspecified site
    female D27.9
    male D29.20

Serum
  allergy, allergic reaction — see also Reaction, serum T80.69 ☑
    shock — see also Shock, anaphylactic T80.59 ☑
  arthritis — see also Reaction, serum T80.69 ☑

Index

Serum — Sialidosis

Serum — *continued*
    complication or reaction NEC — *see also* Reaction,
        serum T80.69 ☑
    disease NEC — *see also* Reaction, serum T80.69 ☑
    hepatitis — *see also* Hepatitis, viral, type B
        carrier (suspected) of B18.1
    intoxication — *see also* Reaction, serum T80.69 ☑
    neuritis — *see also* Reaction, serum T80.69 ☑
    neuropathy G61.1
    poisoning NEC — *see also* Reaction, serum T80.69 ☑
    rash NEC — *see also* Reaction, serum T80.69 ☑
    reaction NEC — *see also* Reaction, serum T80.69 ☑
    sickness NEC — *see also* Reaction, serum T80.69 ☑
    urticaria — *see also* Reaction, serum T80.69 ☑
Sesamoiditis M25.8- ☑
Severe sepsis R65.20
    with septic shock R65.21
Sever's disease or osteochondrosis — *see* Osteochon-
    drosis, juvenile, tarsus
Sex
    chromosome mosaics Q97.8
        lines with various numbers of X chromosomes Q97.2
    education Z70.8
    reassignment surgery status Z87.890
Sextuplet pregnancy — *see* Pregnancy, sextuplet
Sexual
    function, disorder of (psychogenic) F52.9
    immaturity (female) (male) E30.0
    impotence (psychogenic) organic origin NEC — *see*
        Dysfunction, sexual, male
    precocity (constitutional) (cryptogenic)(female) (idio-
        pathic) (male) E30.1
Sexuality, pathologic — *see* Deviation, sexual
Sézary disease C84.1- ☑
Shadow, lung R91.8
Shaking palsy or paralysis — *see* Parkinsonism
Shallowness, acetabulum — *see* Derangement, joint,
    specified type NEC, hip
Shaver's disease J63.1
Sheath (tendon) — *see* condition
Sheathing, retinal vessels H35.01- ☑
Shedding
    nail L60.8
    premature, primary (deciduous) teeth K00.6
Sheehan's disease or syndrome E23.0
Shelf, rectal K62.89
Shell teeth K00.5
Shellshock (current) F43.0
    lasting state — *see* Disorder, post-traumatic stress
Shield kidney Q63.1
Shift
    auditory threshold (temporary) H93.24- ☑
    mediastinal R93.89
Shifting sleep-work schedule (affecting sleep) G47.26
Shiga (-Kruse) **dysentery** A03.0
Shiga's bacillus A03.0
Shigella (dysentery) — *see* Dysentery, bacillary
Shigellosis A03.9
    Group A A03.0
    Group B A03.1
    Group C A03.2
    Group D A03.3
Shin splints S86.89- ☑
Shingles — *see* Herpes, zoster
Shipyard disease or eye B30.0
Shirodkar suture, in pregnancy — *see* Pregnancy,
    complicated by, incompetent cervix
Shock R57.9
    with ectopic or molar pregnancy O08.3
    adrenal (cortical) (Addisonian) E27.2
    adverse food reaction (anaphylactic) — *see* Shock,
        anaphylactic, due to food
    allergic — *see* Shock, anaphylactic
    anaphylactic T78.2 ☑
        chemical — *see* Table of Drugs and Chemicals
        due to drug or medicinal substance
            correct substance properly administered T88.6 ☑
            overdose or wrong substance given or taken (by
                accident) — *see* Table of Drugs and
                Chemicals, by drug, poisoning
        due to food (nonpoisonous) T78.00 ☑
            additives T78.06 ☑
            dairy products T78.07 ☑
            eggs T78.08 ☑
            fish T78.03 ☑
                shellfish T78.02 ☑
            fruit T78.04 ☑

Shock — *continued*
    anaphylactic — *continued*
        due to food — *continued*
            milk T78.07 ☑
            nuts T78.05 ☑
                multiple types T78.05 ☑
                peanuts T78.01 ☑
            peanuts T78.01 ☑
            seeds T78.05 ☑
            specified type NEC T78.09 ☑
            vegetable T78.04 ☑
        following sting(s) — *see* Venom
        immunization T80.52 ☑
        serum T80.59 ☑
            blood and blood products T80.51 ☑
            immunization T80.52 ☑
            specified NEC T80.59 ☑
            vaccination T80.52 ☑
    anaphylactoid — *see* Shock, anaphylactic
    anesthetic
        correct substance properly administered T88.2 ☑
        overdose or wrong substance given or taken — *see*
            Table of Drugs and Chemicals, by drug, poi-
            soning
        specified anesthetic — *see* Table of Drugs and
            Chemicals, by drug, poisoning
    cardiogenic R57.0
    chemical substance — *see* Table of Drugs and Chemi-
        cals
    complicating ectopic or molar pregnancy O08.3
    culture — *see* Disorder, adjustment
    drug
        due to correct substance properly administered
            T88.6 ☑
        overdose or wrong substance given or taken (by
            accident) — *see* Table of Drugs and Chemi-
            cals, by drug, poisoning
    during or after labor and delivery O75.1
    electric T75.4 ☑
        (taser) T75.4 ☑
    endotoxic R65.21
        postprocedural (resulting from a procedure, not
            elsewhere classified) T81.12 ☑
    following
        ectopic or molar pregnancy O08.3
        injury (immediate) (delayed) T79.4 ☑
        labor and delivery O75.1
    food (anaphylactic) — *see* Shock, anaphylactic, due to
        food
    from electroshock gun (taser) T75.4 ☑
    gram-negative R65.21
        postprocedural (resulting from a procedure, not
            elsewhere classified) T81.12 ☑
    hematologic R57.8
    hemorrhagic R57.8
        surgery (intraoperative) (postoperative) T81.19 ☑
        trauma T79.4 ☑
    hypovolemic R57.1
        surgical T81.19 ☑
        traumatic T79.4 ☑
    insulin E15
        therapeutic misadventure — *see* subcategory
            T38.3 ☑
    kidney N17.0
        traumatic (following crushing) T79.5 ☑
    lightning T75.01 ☑
    liver K72.00
    lung J80
    obstetric O75.1
        with ectopic or molar pregnancy O08.3
        following ectopic or molar pregnancy O08.3
    pleural (surgical) T81.19 ☑
        due to trauma T79.4 ☑
    postprocedural (postoperative) T81.10 ☑
        with ectopic or molar pregnancy O08.3
        cardiogenic T81.11 ☑
        endotoxic T81.12 ☑
        following ectopic or molar pregnancy O08.3
        gram-negative T81.12 ☑
        hypovolemic T81.19 ☑
        septic T81.12 ☑
        specified type NEC T81.19 ☑
    psychic F43.0
    septic (due to severe sepsis) R65.21
    specified NEC R57.8
    surgical T81.10 ☑
    taser gun (taser) T75.4 ☑

Shock — *continued*
    therapeutic misadventure NEC T81.10 ☑
    thyroxin
        overdose or wrong substance given or taken — *see*
            Table of Drugs and Chemicals, by drug, poi-
            soning
    toxic, syndrome A48.3
    transfusion — *see* Complications, transfusion
    traumatic (immediate) (delayed) T79.4 ☑
Shoemaker's chest M95.4
Short, shortening, shortness
    arm (acquired) — *see also* Deformity, limb, unequal
        length
        congenital Q71.81- ☑
        forearm — *see* Deformity, limb, unequal length
    bowel syndrome K91.2
    breath R06.02
    cervical (complicating pregnancy) O26.87- ☑
        non-gravid uterus N88.3
    common bile duct, congenital Q44.5
    cord (umbilical), complicating delivery O69.3 ☑
    cystic duct, congenital Q44.5
    esophagus (congenital) Q39.8
    femur (acquired) — *see* Deformity, limb, unequal
        length, femur
        congenital — *see* Defect, reduction, lower limb,
            longitudinal, femur
    frenum, frenulum, linguae (congenital) Q38.1
    hip (acquired) — *see also* Deformity, limb, unequal
        length
        congenital Q65.89
    leg (acquired) — *see also* Deformity, limb, unequal
        length
        congenital Q72.81- ☑
        lower leg — *see also* Deformity, limb, unequal
            length
    limbed stature, with immunodeficiency D82.2
    lower limb (acquired) — *see also* Deformity, limb, un-
        equal length
        congenital Q72.81- ☑
    organ or site, congenital NEC — *see* Distortion
    palate, congenital Q38.5
    radius (acquired) — *see also* Deformity, limb, unequal
        length
        congenital — *see* Defect, reduction, upper limb,
            longitudinal, radius
    rib syndrome Q77.2
    stature (child) (hereditary) (idiopathic) NEC R62.52
        constitutional E34.3
        due to endocrine disorder E34.3
        Laron-type E34.3
    tendon — *see also* Contraction, tendon
        with contracture of joint — *see* Contraction, joint
        Achilles (acquired) M67.0- ☑
            congenital Q66.89
        congenital Q79.8
    thigh (acquired) — *see also* Deformity, limb, unequal
        length, femur
        congenital — *see* Defect, reduction, lower limb,
            longitudinal, femur
    tibialis anterior (tendon) — *see* Contraction, tendon
    umbilical cord
        complicating delivery O69.3 ☑
    upper limb, congenital — *see* Defect, reduction, upper
        limb, specified type NEC
    urethra N36.8
    uvula, congenital Q38.5
    vagina (congenital) Q52.4
Shortsightedness — *see* Myopia
Shoshin (acute fulminating beriberi) E51.11
Shoulder — *see* condition
Shovel-shaped incisors K00.2
Shower, thromboembolic — *see* Embolism
Shunt
    arterial-venous (dialysis) Z99.2
    arteriovenous, pulmonary (acquired) I28.0
        congenital Q25.72
    cerebral ventricle (communicating) in situ Z98.2
    surgical, prosthetic, with complications — *see* Compli-
        cations, cardiovascular, device or implant
Shutdown, renal N28.9
Shy-Drager syndrome G90.3
Sialadenitis, sialadenosis (any gland) (chronic) (period-
    ic) (suppurative) — *see* Sialoadenitis
Sialectasia K11.8
Sialidosis E77.1

☑ **Additional Character Required** — Refer to the Tabular List for Character Selection

▽ **Subterms under main terms may continue to next column or page**

ialitis, silitis (any gland) (chronic) (suppurative) — *see* Sialoadenitis

ialoadenitis (any gland) (periodic) (suppurative) K11.20
  acute K11.21
    recurrent K11.22
  chronic K11.23

ialoadenopathy K11.9

ialoangitis — *see* Sialoadenitis

ialodochitis (fibrinosa) — *see* Sialoadenitis

ialodocholithiasis K11.5

ialolithiasis K11.5

ialometaplasia, necrotizing K11.8

ialorrhea — *see also* Ptyalism
  periodic — *see* Sialoadenitis

ialosis K11.7

iamese twin Q89.4

ibling rivalry Z62.891

icard's syndrome G52.7

icca syndrome M35.00
  with
    keratoconjunctivitis M35.01
    lung involvement M35.02
    myopathy M35.03
    renal tubulo-interstitial disorders M35.04
  specified organ involvement NEC M35.09

ick R69
  or handicapped person in family Z63.79
    needing care at home Z63.6
  sinus (syndrome) I49.5

ick-euthyroid syndrome E07.81

ickle-cell
  anemia — *see* Disease, sickle-cell
  beta plus — *see* Disease, sickle-cell, thalassemia, beta
    plus
  beta zero — *see* Disease, sickle-cell, thalassemia, beta
    zero
  trait D57.3

icklemia — *see also* Disease, sickle-cell
  trait D57.3

ickness
  air (travel) T75.3 ☑
  airplane T75.3 ☑
  alpine T70.29 ☑
  altitude T70.20 ☑
  Andes T70.29 ☑
  aviator's T70.29 ☑
  balloon T70.29 ☑
  car T75.3 ☑
  compressed air T70.3 ☑
  decompression T70.3 ☑
  green D50.8
  milk — *see* Poisoning, food, noxious
  motion T75.3 ☑
  mountain T70.29 ☑
    acute D75.1
  protein — *see also* Reaction, serum T80.69 ☑
  radiation T66 ☑
  roundabout (motion) T75.3 ☑
  sea T75.3 ☑
  serum NEC — *see also* Reaction, serum T80.69 ☑
  sleeping (African) B56.9
    by Trypanosoma B56.9
      brucei
        gambiense B56.0
        rhodesiense B56.1
      East African B56.1
      Gambian B56.0
      Rhodesian B56.1
      West African B56.0
  swing (motion) T75.3 ☑
  train (railway) (travel) T75.3 ☑
  travel (any vehicle) T75.3 ☑

ideropenia — *see* Anemia, iron deficiency

iderosilicosis J62.8

iderosis (lung) J63.4
  brain G93.89
  eye (globe) — *see* Disorder, globe, degenerative,
    siderosis

iemens' syndrome (ectodermal dysplasia) Q82.8

ighing R06.89
  psychogenic F45.8

igmoid — *see also* condition
  flexure — *see* condition
  kidney Q63.1

igmoiditis — *see also* Enteritis K52.9
  infectious A09
  noninfectious K52.9

Silfversköld's syndrome Q78.9

Silicosiderosis J62.8

Silicosis, silicotic (simple) (complicated) J62.8
  with tuberculosis J65

Silicotuberculosis J65

Silo-fillers' disease J68.8
  bronchitis J68.0
  pneumonitis J68.0
  pulmonary edema J68.1

Silver's syndrome Q87.19

Simian malaria B53.1

Simmonds' cachexia or disease E23.0

Simons' disease or syndrome (progressive lipodystrophy) E88.1

Simple, simplex — *see* condition

Simulation, conscious (of illness) Z76.5

Simultanagnosia (asimultagnosia) R48.3

Sin Nombre virus disease (Hantavirus) (cardio)-pul-
  monary syndrome) B33.4

Sinding-Larsen disease or osteochondrosis — *see*
  Osteochondrosis, juvenile, patella

Singapore hemorrhagic fever A91

Singer's node or nodule J38.2

Single
  atrium Q21.2
  coronary artery Q24.5
  umbilical artery Q27.0
  ventricle Q20.4

Singultus R06.6
  epidemicus B33.0

Sinus — *see also* Fistula
  abdominal K63.89
  arrest I45.5
  arrhythmia I49.8
  bradycardia R00.1
  branchial cleft (internal) (external) Q18.0
  coccygeal — *see* Sinus, pilonidal
  dental K04.6
  dermal (congenital) Q06.8
    with abscess Q06.8
    coccygeal, pilonidal — *see* Sinus, coccygeal
  infected, skin NEC L08.89
  marginal, ruptured or bleeding — *see* Hemorrhage,
    antepartum, specified cause NEC
  medial, face and neck Q18.8
  pause I45.5
  pericranii Q01.9
  pilonidal (infected) (rectum) L05.92
    with abscess L05.02
  preauricular Q18.1
  rectovaginal N82.3
  Rokitansky-Aschoff (gallbladder) K82.8
  sacrococcygeal (dermoid) (infected) — *see* Sinus, pi-
    lonidal
  tachycardia R00.0
    paroxysmal I47.1
  tarsi syndrome M25.57- ☑
  testis N50.89
  tract (postinfective) — *see* Fistula
  urachus Q64.4

Sinusitis (accessory) (chronic) (hyperplastic) (nasal)
  (nonpurulent) (purulent) J32.9
  acute J01.90
    ethmoidal J01.20
      recurrent J01.21
    frontal J01.10
      recurrent J01.11
    involving more than one sinus, other than pansinusi-
      tis J01.80
      recurrent J01.81
    maxillary J01.00
      recurrent J01.01
    pansinusitis J01.40
      recurrent J01.41
    recurrent J01.91
    specified NEC J01.80
      recurrent J01.81
    sphenoidal J01.30
      recurrent J01.31
  allergic — *see* Rhinitis, allergic
  due to high altitude T70.1 ☑
  ethmoidal J32.2
    acute J01.20
      recurrent J01.21
  frontal J32.1
    acute J01.10
      recurrent J01.11

Sinusitis — *continued*
  influenzal — *see* Influenza, with, respiratory manifesta-
    tions NEC
  involving more than one sinus but not pansinusitis
    J32.8
    acute J01.80
      recurrent J01.81
  maxillary J32.0
    acute J01.00
      recurrent J01.01
  sphenoidal J32.3
    acute J01.30
      recurrent J01.31
  tuberculous, any sinus A15.8

Sinusitis-bronchiectasis-situs inversus (syndrome)
  (triad) Q89.3

Sipple's syndrome E31.22

Sirenomelia (syndrome) Q87.2

Siriasis T67.01 ☑

Sirkari's disease B55.0

Siti A65

Situation, psychiatric F99

Situational
  disturbance (transient) — *see* Disorder, adjustment
    acute F43.0
  maladjustment — *see* Disorder, adjustment
  reaction — *see* Disorder, adjustment
    acute F43.0

Situs inversus or transversus (abdominalis) (thoracis)
  Q89.3

Sixth disease B08.20
  due to human herpesvirus 6 B08.21
  due to human herpesvirus 7 B08.22

Sjögren-Larsson syndrome Q87.19

Sjögren's syndrome or disease — *see* Sicca syndrome

Skeletal — *see* condition

Skene's gland — *see* condition

Skenitis — *see* Urethritis

Skerljevo A65

Skevas-Zerfus disease — *see* Toxicity, venom, marine
  animal, sea anemone

Skin — *see also* condition
  clammy R23.1
  donor — *see* Donor, skin
  hidebound M35.9

Slate-dressers' or slate-miners' lung J62.8

Sleep
  apnea — *see* Apnea, sleep
  deprivation Z72.820
  disorder or disturbance G47.9
    child F51.9
    nonorganic origin F51.9
    specified NEC G47.8
  disturbance G47.9
    nonorganic origin F51.9
  drunkenness F51.9
  rhythm inversion G47.2- ☑
  terrors F51.4
  walking F51.3
    hysterical F44.89

Sleep hygiene
  abuse Z72.821
  inadequate Z72.821
  poor Z72.821

Sleeping sickness — *see* Sickness, sleeping

Sleeplessness — *see* Insomnia
  menopausal N95.1

Sleep-wake schedule disorder G47.20

Slim disease (in HIV infection) B20

Slipped, slipping
  epiphysis (traumatic) — *see also* Osteochondropathy,
    specified type NEC
    capital femoral (traumatic)
      acute (on chronic) S79.01- ☑
    current traumatic — *code as* Fracture, by site
    upper femoral (nontraumatic) M93.00- ☑
      acute M93.01- ☑
        on chronic M93.03- ☑
      chronic M93.02- ☑
  intervertebral disc — *see* Displacement, intervertebral
    disc
  ligature, umbilical P51.8
  patella — *see* Disorder, patella, derangement NEC
  rib M89.8X8
  sacroiliac joint — *see* subcategory M53.2 ☑
  tendon — *see* Disorder, tendon
  ulnar nerve, nontraumatic — *see* Lesion, nerve, ulnar

🦉 **Subterms under main terms may continue to next column or page**   ☑ **Additional Character Required — Refer to the Tabular List for Character Selection**   **291**

Sialitis, silitis — Slipped, slipping

☑ **Additional Character Required** — Refer to the Tabular List for Character Selection   ▽ **Subterms under main terms may continue to next column or page**

Spasm(s), spastic, spasticity — *continued*
- throat J39.2
  - hysterical F45.8
  - psychogenic F45.8
- tic F95.9
  - chronic F95.1
  - transient of childhood F95.0
- tongue K14.8
- torsion (progressive) G24.1
- trigeminal nerve — *see* Neuralgia, trigeminal
- ureter N13.5
- urethra (sphincter) N35.919
- uterus N85.8
  - complicating labor O62.4
- vagina N94.2
  - psychogenic F52.5
- vascular I73.9
- vasomotor I73.9
- vein NEC I87.8
- viscera — *see* Pain, abdominal

Spasmodic — *see* condition
Spasmophilia — *see* Tetany
Spasmus nutans F98.4
Spastic, spasticity — *see also* Spasm
- child (cerebral) (congenital) (paralysis) G80.1
Speaker's throat R49.8
Specific, specified — *see* condition
Speech
- defect, disorder, disturbance, impediment — *see* Disorder, speech R47.9
- psychogenic, in childhood and adolescence F98.8
- slurring R47.81
- specified NEC R47.89
Spencer's disease A08.19
Spens' syndrome (syncope with heart block) I45.9
Sperm counts (fertility testing) Z31.41
- postvasectomy Z30.8
- reversal Z31.42
Spermatic cord — *see* condition
Spermatocele N43.40
- congenital Q55.4
- multiple N43.42
- single N43.41
Spermatocystitis N49.0
Spermatocytoma C62.9- ☑
- specified site — *see* Neoplasm, malignant, by site
Spermatorrhea N50.89
Sphacelus — *see* Gangrene
Sphenoidal — *see* condition
Sphenoiditis (chronic) — *see* Sinusitis, sphenoidal
Sphenopalatine ganglion neuralgia G90.09
Sphericity, increased, lens (congenital) Q12.4
Spherocytosis (congenital) (familial) (hereditary) D58.0
- hemoglobin disease D58.0
- sickle-cell (disease) D57.8- ☑
Spherophakia Q12.4
Sphincter — *see* condition
Sphincteritis, sphincter of Oddi — *see* Cholangitis
Sphingolipidosis E75.3
- specified NEC E75.29
Sphingomyelinosis E75.3
Spicule tooth K00.2
Spider
- bite — *see* Toxicity, venom, spider
  - nonvenomous — *see* Bite, by site, superficial, insect
- fingers — *see* Syndrome, Marfan's
- nevus I78.1
- toes — *see* Syndrome, Marfan's
- vascular I78.1
Spiegler-Fendt
- benign lymphocytoma L98.8
- sarcoid L08.89
Spielmeyer-Vogt disease E75.4
Spina bifida (aperta) Q05.9
- with hydrocephalus NEC Q05.4
- cervical Q05.5
  - with hydrocephalus Q05.0
- dorsal Q05.6
  - with hydrocephalus Q05.1
- lumbar Q05.7
  - with hydrocephalus Q05.2
- lumbosacral Q05.7
  - with hydrocephalus Q05.2
- occulta Q76.0
- sacral Q05.8
  - with hydrocephalus Q05.3
- thoracic Q05.6

Spina bifida — *continued*
- thoracic — *continued*
  - with hydrocephalus Q05.1
  - thoracolumbar Q05.6
    - with hydrocephalus Q05.1
Spindle, Krukenberg's — *see* Pigmentation, cornea, posterior
Spine, spinal — *see* condition
Spiradenoma (eccrine) — *see* Neoplasm, skin, benign
Spirillosis A25.0
Spirillum
- minus A25.0
- obermeieri infection A68.0
Spirochetal — *see* condition
Spirochetosis A69.9
- arthritic, arthritica A69.9
- bronchopulmonary A69.8
- icterohemorrhagic A27.0
- lung A69.8
Spirometrosis B70.1
Spitting blood — *see* Hemoptysis
Splanchnoptosis K63.4
Spleen, splenic — *see* condition
Splenectasis — *see* Splenomegaly
Splenitis (interstitial) (malignant) (nonspecific) D73.89
- malarial — *see also* Malaria B54 *[D77]*
- tuberculous A18.85
Splenocele D73.89
Splenomegaly, splenomegalia (Bengal) (cryptogenic) (idiopathic) (tropical) R16.1
- with hepatomegaly R16.2
- cirrhotic D73.2
- congenital Q89.09
- congestive, chronic D73.2
- Egyptian B65.1
- Gaucher's E75.22
- malarial — *see also* Malaria B54 *[D77]*
- neutropenic D73.81
- Niemann-Pick — *see* Niemann-Pick disease or syndrome
- siderotic D73.2
- syphilitic A52.79
  - congenital (early) A50.08 *[D77]*
Splenopathy D73.9
Splenoptosis D73.89
Splenosis D73.89
Splinter — *see* Foreign body, superficial, by site
Split, splitting
- foot Q72.7- ☑
- hand Q71.6 ☑
- heart sounds R01.2
- lip, congenital — *see* Cleft, lip
- nails L60.3
- urinary stream R39.13
Spondylarthrosis — *see* Spondylosis
Spondylitis (chronic) — *see also* Spondylopathy, inflammatory
- ankylopoietica — *see* Spondylitis, ankylosing
- ankylosing (chronic) M45.9
  - with lung involvement M45.9 *[J99]*
  - cervical region M45.2
  - cervicothoracic region M45.3
  - juvenile M08.1
  - lumbar region M45.6
  - lumbosacral region M45.7
  - multiple sites M45.0
  - occipito-atlanto-axial region M45.1
  - sacrococcygeal region M45.8
  - thoracic region M45.4
  - thoracolumbar region M45.5
- atrophic (ligamentous) — *see* Spondylitis, ankylosing
- deformans (chronic) — *see* Spondylosis
- gonococcal A54.41
- gouty — *see also* Gout, by type, vertebrae M10.08
- in (due to)
  - brucellosis A23.9 *[M49.80]*
    - cervical region A23.9 *[M49.82]*
    - cervicothoracic region A23.9 *[M49.83]*
    - lumbar region A23.9 *[M49.86]*
    - lumbosacral region A23.9 *[M49.87]*
    - multiple sites A23.9 *[M49.89]*
    - occipito-atlanto-axial region A23.9 *[M49.81]*
    - sacrococcygeal region A23.9 *[M49.88]*
    - thoracic region A23.9 *[M49.84]*
    - thoracolumbar region A23.9 *[M49.85]*
  - enterobacteria — *see also* subcategory M49.8 A04.9
  - tuberculosis A18.01

Spondylitis — *continued*
- infectious NEC — *see* Spondylopathy, infective
- juvenile ankylosing (chronic) M08.1
- Kümmell's — *see* Spondylopathy, traumatic
- Marie-Strümpell — *see* Spondylitis, ankylosing
- muscularis — *see* Spondylopathy, specified NEC
- psoriatic L40.53
- rheumatoid — *see* Spondylitis, ankylosing
- rhizomelica — *see* Spondylitis, ankylosing
- sacroiliac NEC M46.1
- senescent, senile — *see* Spondylosis
- traumatic (chronic) or post-traumatic — *see* Spondylopathy, traumatic
- tuberculous A18.01
- typhosa A01.05
Spondyloarthritis
- axial — *see also* Spondlyitis, ankylosing
  - non-radiographic M46.80
    - cervical M46.82
    - cervicothoracic M46.83
    - lumbar M46.84
    - lumbosacral M46.87
    - multiple sites M46.89
    - occipito-atlanto-axial region M46.81
    - sacral and sacrococcygeal M46.88
    - thoracic M46.84
    - thoracolumbar M46.85
Spondylolisthesis (acquired) (degenerative) M43.10
- with disproportion (fetopelvic) O33.0
  - causing obstructed labor O65.0
- cervical region M43.12
- cervicothoracic region M43.13
- congenital Q76.2
- lumbar region M43.16
- lumbosacral region M43.17
- multiple sites M43.19
- occipito-atlanto-axial region M43.11
- sacrococcygeal region M43.18
- thoracic region M43.14
- thoracolumbar region M43.15
- traumatic (old) M43.10
  - acute
    - fifth cervical (displaced) S12.430 ☑
      - nondisplaced S12.431 ☑
      - specified type NEC (displaced) S12.450 ☑
        - nondisplaced S12.451 ☑
      - type III S12.44 ☑
    - fourth cervical (displaced) S12.330 ☑
      - nondisplaced S12.331 ☑
      - specified type NEC (displaced) S12.350 ☑
        - nondisplaced S12.351 ☑
      - type III S12.34 ☑
    - second cervical (displaced) S12.130 ☑
      - nondisplaced S12.131 ☑
      - specified type NEC (displaced) S12.150 ☑
        - nondisplaced S12.151 ☑
      - type III S12.14 ☑
    - seventh cervical (displaced) S12.630 ☑
      - nondisplaced S12.631 ☑
      - specified type NEC (displaced) S12.650 ☑
        - nondisplaced S12.651 ☑
      - type III S12.64 ☑
    - sixth cervical (displaced) S12.530 ☑
      - nondisplaced S12.531 ☑
      - specified type NEC (displaced) S12.550 ☑
        - nondisplaced S12.551 ☑
      - type III S12.54 ☑
    - third cervical (displaced) S12.230 ☑
      - nondisplaced S12.231 ☑
      - specified type NEC (displaced) S12.250 ☑
        - nondisplaced S12.251 ☑
      - type III S12.24 ☑
Spondylolysis (acquired) M43.00
- cervical region M43.02
- cervicothoracic region M43.03
- congenital Q76.2
- lumbar region M43.06
- lumbosacral region M43.07
  - with disproportion (fetopelvic) O33.0
    - causing obstructed labor O65.8
- multiple sites M43.09
- occipito-atlanto-axial region M43.01
- sacrococcygeal region M43.08
- thoracic region M43.04
- thoracolumbar region M43.05
Spondylopathy M48.9
- infective NEC M46.50

▽ Subterms under main terms may continue to next column or page   ☑ Additional Character Required — Refer to the Tabular List for Character Selection

Spondylopathy — *continued*
  infective — *continued*
    cervical region M46.52
    cervicothoracic region M46.53
    lumbar region M46.56
    lumbosacral region M46.57
    multiple sites M46.59
    occipito-atlanto-axial region M46.51
    sacrococcygeal region M46.58
    thoracic region M46.54
    thoracolumbar region M46.55
  inflammatory M46.90
    cervical region M46.92
    cervicothoracic region M46.93
    lumbar region M46.96
    lumbosacral region M46.97
    multiple sites M46.99
    occipito-atlanto-axial region M46.91
    sacrococcygeal region M46.98
    specified type NEC M46.80
      cervical region M46.82
      cervicothoracic region M46.83
      lumbar region M46.86
      lumbosacral region M46.87
      multiple sites M46.89
      occipito-atlanto-axial region M46.81
      sacrococcygeal region M46.88
      thoracic region M46.84
      thoracolumbar region M46.85
    thoracic region M46.94
    thoracolumbar region M46.95
  neuropathic, in
    syringomyelia and syringobulbia G95.0
    tabes dorsalis A52.11
  specified NEC — *see* subcategory M48.8 ☑
  traumatic M48.30
    cervical region M48.32
    cervicothoracic region M48.33
    lumbar region M48.36
    lumbosacral region M48.37
    occipito-atlanto-axial region M48.31
    sacrococcygeal region M48.38
    thoracic region M48.34
    thoracolumbar region M48.35
Spondylosis M47.9
  with
    disproportion (fetopelvic) O33.0
      causing obstructed labor O65.0
    myelopathy NEC M47.10
      cervical region M47.12
      cervicothoracic region M47.13
      lumbar region M47.16
      occipito-atlanto-axial region M47.11
      thoracic region M47.14
      thoracolumbar region M47.15
    radiculopathy M47.20
      cervical region M47.22
      cervicothoracic region M47.23
      lumbar region M47.26
      lumbosacral region M47.27
      occipito-atlanto-axial region M47.21
      sacrococcygeal region M47.28
      thoracic region M47.24
      thoracolumbar region M47.25
  specified NEC M47.899
    cervical region M47.892
    cervicothoracic region M47.893
    lumbar region M47.896
    lumbosacral region M47.897
    occipito-atlanto-axial region M47.891
    sacrococcygeal region M47.898
    thoracic region M47.894
    thoracolumbar region M47.895
  traumatic — *see* Spondylopathy, traumatic
  without myelopathy or radiculopathy M47.819
    cervical region M47.812
    cervicothoracic region M47.813
    lumbar region M47.816
    lumbosacral region M47.817
    occipito-atlanto-axial region M47.811
    sacrococcygeal region M47.818
    thoracic region M47.814
    thoracolumbar region M47.815
Sponge
  inadvertently left in operation wound — *see* Foreign body, accidentally left during a procedure
  kidney (medullary) Q61.5

Sponge-diver's disease — *see* Toxicity, venom, marine animal, sea anemone
Spongioblastoma (any type) — *see* Neoplasm, malignant, by site
  specified site — *see* Neoplasm, malignant, by site
  unspecified site C71.9
Spongioneuroblastoma — *see* Neoplasm, malignant, by site
Spontaneous — *see also* condition
  fracture (cause unknown) — *see* Fracture, pathological
Spoon nail L60.3
  congenital Q84.6
Sporadic — *see* condition
Sporothrix schenckii infection — *see* Sporotrichosis
Sporotrichosis B42.9
  arthritis B42.82
  disseminated B42.7
  generalized B42.7
  lymphocutaneous (fixed) (progressive) B42.1
  pulmonary B42.0
  specified NEC B42.89
Spots, spotting (in) (of)
  Bitot's — *see also* Pigmentation, conjunctiva
    in the young child E50.1
      vitamin A deficiency E50.1
  café, au lait L81.3
  Cayenne pepper I78.1
  cotton wool, retina — *see* Occlusion, artery, retina
  de Morgan's (senile angiomas) I78.1
  Fuchs' black (myopic) — *see also* Myopia, degenerative H44.2- ☑
  intermenstrual (regular) N92.0
    irregular N92.1
  Koplik's B05.9
  liver L81.4
  pregnancy O26.85- ☑
  purpuric R23.3
  ruby I78.1
Spotted fever — *see* Fever, spotted A77.9
Sprain (joint) (ligament)
  acromioclavicular joint or ligament S43.5- ☑
  ankle S93.40- ☑
    calcaneofibular ligament S93.41- ☑
    deltoid ligament S93.42- ☑
    internal collateral ligament — *see* Sprain, ankle, specified ligament NEC
    specified ligament NEC S93.49- ☑
    talofibular ligament — *see* Sprain, ankle, specified ligament NEC
    tibiofibular ligament S93.43- ☑
  anterior longitudinal, cervical S13.4 ☑
  atlas, atlanto-axial, atlanto-occipital S13.4 ☑
  breast bone — *see* Sprain, sternum
  calcaneofibular — *see* Sprain, ankle
  carpal — *see* Sprain, wrist
  carpometacarpal — *see* Sprain, hand, specified site NEC
  cartilage
    costal S23.41 ☑
    semilunar (knee) — *see* Sprain, knee, specified site NEC
      with current tear — *see* Tear, meniscus
    thyroid region S13.5 ☑
    xiphoid — *see* Sprain, sternum
  cervical, cervicodorsal, cervicothoracic S13.4 ☑
  chondrosternal S23.421 ☑
  coracoclavicular S43.8- ☑
  coracohumeral S43.41- ☑
  coronary, knee — *see* Sprain, knee, specified site NEC
  costal cartilage S23.41 ☑
  cricoarytenoid articulation or ligament S13.5 ☑
  cricothyroid articulation S13.5 ☑
  cruciate, knee — *see* Sprain, knee, cruciate
  deltoid, ankle — *see* Sprain, ankle
  dorsal (spine) S23.3 ☑
  elbow S53.40- ☑
    radial collateral ligament S53.43- ☑
    radiohumeral S53.41- ☑
    rupture
      radial collateral ligament — *see* Rupture, traumatic, ligament, radial collateral
      ulnar collateral ligament — *see* Rupture, traumatic, ligament, ulnar collateral
    specified type NEC S53.49- ☑
    ulnar collateral ligament S53.44- ☑
    ulnohumeral S53.42- ☑
  femur, head — *see* Sprain, hip

Sprain — *continued*
  fibular collateral, knee — *see* Sprain, knee, collateral
  fibulocalcaneal — *see* Sprain, ankle
  finger(s) S63.61- ☑
    index S63.61- ☑
    interphalangeal (joint) S63.63- ☑
      index S63.63- ☑
      little S63.63- ☑
      middle S63.63- ☑
      ring S63.63- ☑
    little S63.61- ☑
    metacarpophalangeal (joint) S63.65- ☑
    middle S63.61- ☑
    ring S63.61- ☑
    specified site NEC S63.69- ☑
      index S63.69- ☑
      little S63.69- ☑
      middle S63.69- ☑
      ring S63.69- ☑
  foot S93.60- ☑
    specified ligament NEC S93.69- ☑
    tarsal ligament S93.61- ☑
    tarsometatarsal ligament S93.62- ☑
    toe — *see* Sprain, toe
  hand S63.9- ☑
    finger — *see* Sprain, finger
    specified site NEC — *see* subcategory S63.8 ☑
    thumb — *see* Sprain, thumb
  head S03.9 ☑
  hip S73.10- ☑
    iliofemoral ligament S73.11- ☑
    ischiocapsular (ligament) S73.12- ☑
    specified NEC S73.19- ☑
  iliofemoral — *see* Sprain, hip
  innominate
    acetabulum — *see* Sprain, hip
    sacral junction S33.6 ☑
  internal
    collateral, ankle — *see* Sprain, ankle
    semilunar cartilage — *see* Sprain, knee, specified site NEC
  interphalangeal
    finger — *see* Sprain, finger, interphalangeal (joint)
    toe — *see* Sprain, toe, interphalangeal joint
  ischiocapsular — *see* Sprain, hip
  ischiofemoral — *see* Sprain, hip
  jaw (articular disc) (cartilage) (meniscus) S03.4- ☑
    old M26.69
  knee S83.9- ☑
    collateral ligament S83.40- ☑
      lateral (fibular) S83.42- ☑
      medial (tibial) S83.41- ☑
    cruciate ligament S83.50- ☑
      anterior S83.51- ☑
      posterior S83.52- ☑
    lateral (fibular) collateral ligament S83.42- ☑
    medial (tibial) collateral ligament S83.41- ☑
    patellar ligament S76.11- ☑
    specified site NEC S83.8X- ☑
    superior tibiofibular joint (ligament) S83.6- ☑
  lateral collateral, knee — *see* Sprain, knee, collateral
  lumbar (spine) S33.5 ☑
  lumbosacral S33.9 ☑
  mandible (articular disc) S03.4- ☑
    old M26.69
  medial collateral, knee — *see* Sprain, knee, collateral
  meniscus
    jaw S03.4- ☑
      old M26.69
    knee — *see* Sprain, knee, specified site NEC
      with current tear — *see* Tear, meniscus
        old — *see* Derangement, knee, meniscus, due to old tear
    mandible S03.4- ☑
      old M26.69
  metacarpal (distal) (proximal) — *see* Sprain, hand, specified site NEC
  metacarpophalangeal — *see* Sprain, finger, metacarpophalangeal (joint)
  metatarsophalangeal — *see* Sprain, toe, metatarsophalangeal joint
  midcarpal — *see* Sprain, hand, specified site NEC
  midtarsal — *see* Sprain, foot, specified site NEC
  neck S13.9 ☑
    anterior longitudinal cervical ligament S13.4 ☑
    atlanto-axial joint S13.4 ☑

☑ **Additional Character Required** — Refer to the Tabular List for Character Selection   🐦 **Subterms under main terms may continue to next column or page**

Sprain — *continued*
　neck — *continued*
　　atlanto-occipital joint S13.4 ☑
　　cervical spine S13.4 ☑
　　cricoarytenoid ligament S13.5 ☑
　　cricothyroid ligament S13.5 ☑
　　specified site NEC S13.8 ☑
　　thyroid region (cartilage) S13.5 ☑
　nose S03.8 ☑
　orbicular, hip — *see* Sprain, hip
　patella — *see* Sprain, knee, specified site NEC
　patellar ligament S76.11- ☑
　pelvis NEC S33.8 ☑
　phalanx
　　finger — *see* Sprain, finger
　　toe — *see* Sprain, toe
　pubofemoral — *see* Sprain, hip
　radiocarpal — *see* Sprain, wrist
　radiohumeral — *see* Sprain, elbow
　radius, collateral — *see* Rupture, traumatic, ligament,
　　　radial collateral
　rib (cage) S23.41
　rotator cuff (capsule) S43.42- ☑
　sacroiliac (region)
　　chronic or old — *see* subcategory M53.2 ☑
　　joint S33.6 ☑
　scaphoid (hand) — *see* Sprain, hand, specified site NEC
　scapula (r) — *see* Sprain, shoulder girdle, specified site
　　　NEC
　semilunar cartilage (knee) — *see* Sprain, knee, specified
　　　site NEC
　　with current tear — *see* Tear, meniscus
　　　old — *see* Derangement, knee, meniscus, due to
　　　　old tear
　shoulder joint S43.40- ☑
　　acromioclavicular joint (ligament) — *see* Sprain,
　　　　acromioclavicular joint
　　blade — *see* Sprain, shoulder, girdle, specified site
　　　　NEC
　　coracoclavicular joint (ligament) — *see* Sprain,
　　　　coracoclavicular joint
　　coracohumeral ligament — *see* Sprain, coracohumer-
　　　　al joint
　　girdle S43.9- ☑
　　　specified site NEC S43.8- ☑
　　rotator cuff — *see* Sprain, rotator cuff
　　specified site NEC S43.49- ☑
　　sternoclavicular joint (ligament) — *see* Sprain,
　　　　sternoclavicular joint
　spine
　　cervical S13.4 ☑
　　lumbar S33.5 ☑
　　thoracic S23.3 ☑
　sternoclavicular joint S43.6- ☑
　sternum S23.429 ☑
　　chondrosternal joint S23.421 ☑
　　specified site NEC S23.428 ☑
　　sternoclavicular (joint) (ligament) S23.420 ☑
　symphysis
　　jaw S03.4- ☑
　　　old M26.69
　　mandibular S03.4- ☑
　　　old M26.69
　talofibular — *see* Sprain, ankle
　tarsal — *see* Sprain, foot, specified site NEC
　tarsometatarsal — *see* Sprain, foot, specified site NEC
　temporomandibular S03.4- ☑
　　old M26.69
　thorax S23.9 ☑
　　ribs S23.41 ☑
　　specified site NEC S23.8 ☑
　　spine S23.3 ☑
　　sternum — *see* Sprain, sternum
　thumb S63.60- ☑
　　interphalangeal (joint) S63.62- ☑
　　metacarpophalangeal (joint) S63.64- ☑
　　specified site NEC S63.68- ☑
　thyroid cartilage or region S13.5 ☑
　tibia (proximal end) — *see* Sprain, knee, specified site
　　　NEC
　tibial collateral, knee — *see* Sprain, knee, collateral
　tibiofibular
　　distal — *see* Sprain, ankle
　　superior — *see* Sprain, knee, specified site NEC
　toe(s) S93.50- ☑
　　great S93.50- ☑

Sprain — *continued*
　toe(s) — *continued*
　　interphalangeal joint S93.51- ☑
　　　great S93.51- ☑
　　　lesser S93.51- ☑
　　lesser S93.50- ☑
　　metatarsophalangeal joint S93.52- ☑
　　　great S93.52- ☑
　　　lesser S93.52- ☑
　ulna, collateral — *see* Rupture, traumatic, ligament,
　　　ulnar collateral
　ulnohumeral — *see* Sprain, elbow
　wrist S63.50- ☑
　　carpal S63.51- ☑
　　radiocarpal S63.52- ☑
　　specified site NEC S63.59- ☑
　xiphoid cartilage — *see* Sprain, sternum
Sprengel's deformity (congenital) Q74.0
Sprue (tropical) K90.1
　celiac K90.0
　idiopathic K90.49
　meaning thrush B37.0
　nontropical K90.0
Spur, bone — *see also* Enthesopathy
　calcaneal M77.3- ☑
　iliac crest M76.2- ☑
　nose (septum) J34.89
Spurway's syndrome Q78.0
Sputum
　abnormal (amount) (color) (odor) (purulent) R09.3
　blood-stained R04.2
　excessive (cause unknown) R09.3
Squamous — *see also* condition
　epithelium in
　　cervical canal (congenital) Q51.828
　　uterine mucosa (congenital) Q51.818
Squashed nose M95.0
　congenital Q67.4
Squeeze, diver's T70.3 ☑
Squint — *see also* Strabismus
　accommodative — *see* Strabismus, convergent con-
　　　comitant
SSADHD (succinic semialdehyde dehydrogenase deficien-
　　cy) E72.81
St. Hubert's disease A82.9
Stab — *see also* Laceration
　internal organs — *see* Injury, by site
Stafne's cyst or cavity M27.0
Staggering gait R26.0
　hysterical F44.4
Staghorn calculus — *see* Calculus, kidney
Stähli's line (cornea) (pigment) — *see* Pigmentation,
　　cornea, anterior
Stain, staining
　meconium (newborn) P96.83
　port wine Q82.5
　tooth, teeth (hard tissues) (extrinsic) K03.6
　　due to
　　　accretions K03.6
　　　deposits (betel) (black) (green) (materia alba)
　　　　(orange) (soft) (tobacco) K03.6
　　　metals (copper) (silver) K03.7
　　　nicotine K03.6
　　　pulpal bleeding K03.7
　　　tobacco K03.6
　　intrinsic K00.8
Stammering — *see also* Disorder, fluency F80.81
Standstill
　auricular I45.5
　cardiac — *see* Arrest, cardiac
　sinoatrial I45.5
　ventricular — *see* Arrest, cardiac
Stannosis J63.5
Stanton's disease — *see* Melioidosis
Staphylitis (acute) (catarrhal) (chronic) (gangrenous)
　　(membranous) (suppurative) (ulcerative) K12.2
Staphylococcal scalded skin syndrome L00
Staphylococcemia A41.2
Staphylococcus, staphylococcal — *see also* condition
　as cause of disease classified elsewhere B95.8
　　aureus (methicillin susceptible) (MSSA) B95.61
　　　methicillin resistant (MRSA) B95.62
　　specified NEC, as cause of disease classified elsewhere
　　　B95.7
Staphyloma (sclera)
　cornea H18.72- ☑
　equatorial H15.81- ☑

Staphyloma — *continued*
　localized (anterior) H15.82- ☑
　posticum H15.83- ☑
　ring H15.85- ☑
Stargardt's disease — *see* Dystrophy, retina
Starvation (inanition) (due to lack of food) T73.0 ☑
　edema — *see* Malnutrition, severe
Stasis
　bile (noncalculous) K83.1
　bronchus J98.09
　　with infection — *see* Bronchitis
　cardiac — *see* Failure, heart, congestive
　cecum K59.89
　colon K59.89
　dermatitis I87.2
　　with
　　　varicose ulcer — *see* Varix, leg, with ulcer, with
　　　　inflammation
　　　varicose veins — *see* Varix, leg, with, inflamma-
　　　　tion
　　due to postthrombotic syndrome — *see* Syndrome,
　　　postthrombotic
　duodenal K31.5
　eczema — *see* Varix, leg, with, inflammation
　edema — *see* Hypertension, venous (chronic), idiopath-
　　　ic
　foot T69.0- ☑
　ileocecal coil K59.89
　ileum K59.89
　intestinal K59.89
　jejunum K59.89
　kidney N19
　liver (cirrhotic) K76.1
　lymphatic I89.8
　pneumonia J18.2
　pulmonary — *see* Edema, lung
　rectal K59.89
　renal N19
　　tubular N17.0
　ulcer — *see* Varix, leg, with, ulcer
　　without varicose veins I87.2
　urine — *see* Retention, urine
　venous I87.8
State (of)
　affective and paranoid, mixed, organic psychotic F06.8
　agitated R45.1
　　acute reaction to stress F43.0
　anxiety (neurotic) F41.1
　apprehension F41.1
　burn-out Z73.0
　climacteric, female Z78.0
　　symptomatic N95.1
　compulsive F42.8
　　mixed with obsessional thoughts F42.2
　confusional (psychogenic) F44.89
　　acute — *see also* Delirium
　　　with
　　　　arteriosclerotic dementia F01.50
　　　　　with behavioral disturbance F01.51
　　　　senility or dementia F05
　　　alcoholic F10.231
　　　epileptic F05
　　　reactive (from emotional stress, psychological trau-
　　　　ma) F44.89
　　subacute — *see* Delirium
　convulsive — *see* Convulsions
　crisis F43.0
　depressive F32.9
　　neurotic F34.1
　dissociative F44.9
　emotional shock (stress) R45.7
　hypercoagulation — *see* Hypercoagulable
　locked-in G83.5
　menopausal Z78.0
　　symptomatic N95.1
　neurotic F48.9
　　with depersonalization F48.1
　obsessional F42.8
　oneiroid (schizophrenia-like) F23
　organic
　　hallucinatory (nonalcoholic) F06.0
　　paranoid (-hallucinatory) F06.2
　panic F41.0
　paranoid F22
　　climacteric F22
　　involutional F22
　　menopausal F22
　　organic F06.2

State — *continued*
  paranoid — *continued*
    senile F03 ☑
    simple F22
  persistent vegetative R40.3
  phobic F40.9
  postleukotomy F07.0
  pregnant
    gestational carrier Z33.3
    incidental Z33.1
  psychogenic, twilight F44.89
  psychopathic (constitutional) F60.2
  psychotic, organic — *see also* Psychosis, organic
    mixed paranoid and affective F06.8
    senile or presenile F03 ☑
    transient NEC F06.8
      with
        depression F06.31
        hallucinations F06.0
  residual schizophrenic F20.5
  restlessness R45.1
  stress (emotional) R45.7
  tension (mental) F48.9
    specified NEC F48.8
  transient organic psychotic NEC F06.8
    depressive type F06.31
    hallucinatory type F06.0
  twilight
    epileptic F05
    psychogenic F44.89
  vegetative, persistent R40.3
  vital exhaustion Z73.0
  withdrawal, — *see* Withdrawal, state
Status (post) — *see also* Presence (of)
  absence, epileptic — *see* Epilepsy, by type, with status
      epilepticus
  administration of tPA (rtPA) in a different facility within
      the last 24 hours prior to admission to current
      facility Z92.82
  adrenalectomy (unilateral) (bilateral) E89.6
  anastomosis Z98.0
  anginosus I20.9
  angioplasty (peripheral) Z98.62
    with implant Z95.820
    coronary artery Z98.61
      with implant Z95.5
  aortocoronary bypass Z95.1
  arthrodesis Z98.1
  artificial opening (of) Z93.9
    gastrointestinal tract Z93.4
    specified NEC Z93.8
    urinary tract Z93.6
    vagina Z93.8
  asthmaticus — *see* Asthma, by type, with status asth-
      maticus
  awaiting organ transplant Z76.82
  bariatric surgery Z98.84
  bed confinement Z74.01
  bleb, filtering (vitreous), after glaucoma surgery Z98.83
  breast implant Z98.82
    removal Z98.86
  cataract extraction Z98.4- ☑
  cholecystectomy Z90.49
  clitorectomy N90.811
    with excision of labia minora N90.812
  colectomy (complete) (partial) Z90.49
  colonization — *see* Carrier (suspected) of
  colostomy Z93.3
  convulsivus idiopathicus — *see* Epilepsy, by type, with
      status epilepticus
  coronary artery angioplasty — *see* Status, angioplasty,
      coronary artery
  coronary artery bypass graft Z95.1
  cystectomy (urinary bladder) Z90.6
  cystostomy Z93.50
    appendico-vesicostomy Z93.52
    cutaneous Z93.51
    specified NEC Z93.59
  delinquent immunization Z28.3
  dental Z98.818
    crown Z98.811
    fillings Z98.811
    restoration Z98.811
    sealant Z98.810
    specified NEC Z98.818
  deployment (current) (military) Z56.82
  dialysis (hemodialysis) (peritoneal) Z99.2
  do not resuscitate (DNR) Z66

Status — *continued*
  donor — *see* Donor
  embedded fragments — *see* Retained, foreign body
      fragments (type of)
  embedded splinter — *see* Retained, foreign body
      fragments (type of)
  enterostomy Z93.4
  epileptic, epilepticus — *see also* Epilepsy, by type, with
      status epilepticus G40.901
  estrogen receptor
    negative Z17.1
    positive Z17.0
  female genital cutting — *see* Female genital mutilation
      status
  female genital mutilation — *see* Female genital muti-
      lation status
  filtering (vitreous) bleb after glaucoma surgery Z98.83
  gastrectomy (complete) (partial) Z90.3
  gastric banding Z98.84
  gastric bypass for obesity Z98.84
  gastrostomy Z93.1
  human immunodeficiency virus (HIV) infection,
      asymptomatic Z21
  hysterectomy (complete) (total) Z90.710
    partial (with remaining cervial stump) Z90.711
  ileostomy Z93.2
  implant
    breast Z98.82
  infibulation N90.813
  intestinal bypass Z98.0
  jejunostomy Z93.4
  lapsed immunization schedule Z28.3
  laryngectomy Z90.02
  lymphaticus E32.8
  malignancy
    castrate resistant prostate Z19.2
    hormone resistant Z19.2
    hormone sensitive Z19.1
  marmoratus G80.3
  mastectomy (unilateral) (bilateral) Z90.1- ☑
  military deployment status (current) Z56.82
    in theater or in support of military war, peacekeep-
        ing and humanitarian operations Z56.82
  nephrectomy (unilateral) (bilateral) Z90.5
  nephrostomy Z93.6
  obesity surgery Z98.84
  oophorectomy
    bilateral Z90.722
    unilateral Z90.721
  organ replacement
    by artificial or mechanical device or prosthesis of
      artery Z95.828
      bladder Z96.0
      blood vessel Z95.828
      breast Z97.8
      eye globe Z97.0
      heart Z95.812
        valve Z95.2
      intestine Z97.8
      joint Z96.60
        hip — *see* Presence, hip joint implant
        knee — *see* Presence, knee joint implant
        specified site NEC Z96.698
      kidney Z97.8
      larynx Z96.3
      lens Z96.1
      limbs — *see* Presence, artificial, limb
      liver Z97.8
      lung Z97.8
      pancreas Z97.8
    by organ transplant (heterologous)(homologous)
        — *see* Transplant
  pacemaker
    brain Z96.89
    cardiac Z95.0
    specified NEC Z96.89
  pancreatectomy Z90.410
    complete Z90.410
    partial Z90.411
    total Z90.410
  physical restraint Z78.1
  pneumonectomy (complete) (partial) Z90.2
  pneumothorax, therapeutic Z98.3
  postcommotio cerebri F07.81
  postoperative (postprocedural) NEC Z98.890
    breast implant Z98.82
    dental Z98.818
      crown Z98.811

Status — *continued*
  postoperative — *continued*
    dental — *continued*
      fillings Z98.811
      restoration Z98.811
      sealant Z98.810
      specified NEC Z98.818
    pneumothorax, therapeutic Z98.3
    uterine scar Z98.891
  postpartum (routine follow-up) Z39.2
    care immediately after delivery Z39.0
  postsurgical (postprocedural) NEC Z98.890
    pneumothorax, therapeutic Z98.3
  pregnancy, incidental Z33.1
  prosthesis coronary angioplasty Z95.5
  pseudophakia Z96.1
  renal dialysis (hemodialysis) (peritoneal) Z99.2
  retained foreign body — *see* Retained, foreign body
      fragments (type of)
  reversed jejunal transposition (for bypass) Z98.0
  salpingo-oophorectomy
    bilateral Z90.722
    unilateral Z90.721
  sex reassignment surgery status Z87.890
  shunt
    arteriovenous (for dialysis) Z99.2
    cerebrospinal fluid Z98.2
    ventricular (communicating) (for drainage) Z98.2
  splenectomy Z90.81
  thymicolymphaticus E32.8
  thymicus E32.8
  thymolymphaticus E32.8
  thyroidectomy (hypothyroidism) E89.0
  tooth (teeth) extraction — *see also* Absence, teeth,
      acquired K08.409
  tPA (rtPA) administration in a different facility within
      the last 24 hours prior to admission to current
      facility Z92.82
  tracheostomy Z93.0
  transplant — *see* Transplant
    organ removed Z98.85
  tubal ligation Z98.51
  underimmunization Z28.3
  ureterostomy Z93.6
  urethrostomy Z93.6
  vagina, artificial Z93.8
  vasectomy Z98.52
  wheelchair confinement Z99.3
Stealing
  child problem F91.8
    in company with others Z72.810
  pathological (compulsive) F63.2
Steam burn — *see* Burn
Steatocystoma multiplex L72.2
Steatohepatitis (nonalcoholic) (NASH) K75.81
Steatoma L72.3
  eyelid (cystic) — *see* Dermatosis, eyelid
    infected — *see* Hordeolum
Steatorrhea (chronic) K90.9
  with lacteal obstruction K90.2
  idiopathic (adult) (infantile) K90.9
  pancreatic K90.3
  primary K90.0
  tropical K90.1
Steatosis E88.89
  heart — *see* Degeneration, myocardial
  kidney N28.89
  liver NEC K76.0
Steele-Richardson-Olszewski disease or syndrome
  G23.1
Steinbrocker's syndrome G90.8
Steinert's disease G71.11
Stein-Leventhal syndrome E28.2
Stein's syndrome E28.2
STEMI — *see also* Infarct, myocardium, ST elevation I21.
Stenocardia I20.8
Stenocephaly Q75.8
Stenosis, stenotic (cicatricial) — *see also* Stricture
  ampulla of Vater K83.1
  anus, anal (canal) (sphincter) K62.4
    and rectum K62.4
    congenital Q42.3
      with fistula Q42.2
  aorta (ascending) (supraventricular) (congenital) Q25.
    arteriosclerotic I70.0
    calcified I70.0
    supravalvular Q25.3
  aortic (valve) I35.0

☑ **Additional Character Required** — Refer to the Tabular List for Character Selection   Subterms under main terms may continue to next column or page

Stenosis, stenotic — *continued*
  aortic — *continued*
    .with insufficiency I35.2
    congenital Q23.0
    rheumatic I06.0
      with
        incompetency, insufficiency or regurgitation
          I06.2
          with mitral (valve) disease I08.0
            with tricuspid (valve) disease I08.3
        mitral (valve) disease I08.0
          with tricuspid (valve) disease I08.3
        tricuspid (valve) disease I08.2
          with mitral (valve) disease I08.3
    specified cause NEC I35.0
    syphilitic A52.03
  aqueduct of Sylvius (congenital) Q03.0
    with spina bifida — *see* Spina bifida, by site, with
      hydrocephalus
    acquired G91.1
  artery NEC — *see also* Arteriosclerosis I77.1
    celiac I77.4
    cerebral — *see* Occlusion, artery, cerebral
    extremities — *see* Arteriosclerosis, extremities
    precerebral — *see* Occlusion, artery, precerebral
    pulmonary (congenital) Q25.6
      acquired I28.8
    renal I70.1
    stent
      coronary T82.855 ☑
      peripheral T82.856 ☑
  bile duct (common) (hepatic) K83.1
    congenital Q44.3
  bladder-neck (acquired) N32.0
    congenital Q64.31
  brain G93.89
  bronchus J98.09
    congenital Q32.3
    syphilitic A52.72
  cardia (stomach) K22.2
    congenital Q39.3
  cardiovascular — *see* Disease, cardiovascular
  caudal M48.08
  cervix, cervical (canal) N88.2
    congenital Q51.828
    in pregnancy or childbirth — *see* Pregnancy, com-
      plicated by, abnormal cervix
  colon — *see also* Obstruction, intestine
    congenital Q42.9
      specified NEC Q42.8
  colostomy K94.03
  common (bile) duct K83.1
    congenital Q44.3
  coronary (artery) — *see* Disease, heart, ischemic,
    atherosclerotic
  cystic duct — *see* Obstruction, gallbladder
  due to presence of device, implant or graft — *see also*
    Complications, by site and type, specified NEC
    T85.858 ☑
    arterial graft NEC T82.858 ☑
    breast (implant) T85.858 ☑
    catheter T85.858 ☑
      dialysis (renal) T82.858 ☑
        intraperitoneal T85.858 ☑
      infusion NEC T82.858 ☑
        spinal (epidural) (subdural) T85.850 ☑
      urinary (indwelling) T83.85 ☑
    fixation, internal (orthopedic) NEC T84.85 ☑
    gastrointestinal (bile duct) (esophagus) T85.858 ☑
    genital NEC T83.85 ☑
    heart NEC T82.857 ☑
    joint prosthesis T84.85 ☑
    ocular (corneal graft) (orbital implant) NEC
      T85.858 ☑
    orthopedic NEC T84.85 ☑
    specified NEC T85.858 ☑
    urinary NEC T83.85 ☑
    vascular NEC T82.858 ☑
    ventricular intracranial shunt T85.850 ☑
  duodenum K31.5
    congenital Q41.0
  ejaculatory duct NEC N50.89
    stent
      vascular
        end stent
          adjacent to stent — *see* Arteriosclerosis

Stenosis, stenotic — *continued*
  ejaculatory duct — *continued*
    stent — *continued*
      vascular — *continued*
        end stent — *continued*
          within the stent
            coronary T82.855 ☑
            peripheral T82.856 ☑
        in stent
          coronary vessel T82.855 ☑
          peripheral vessel T82.856 ☑
  endocervical os — *see* Stenosis, cervix
  enterostomy K94.13
  esophagus K22.2
    congenital Q39.3
    syphilitic A52.79
      congenital A50.59 *[K23]*
  eustachian tube — *see* Obstruction, eustachian tube
  external ear canal (acquired) H61.30- ☑
    congenital Q16.1
    due to
      inflammation H61.32- ☑
      trauma H61.31- ☑
    postprocedural H95.81- ☑
    specified cause NEC H61.39- ☑
  gallbladder — *see* Obstruction, gallbladder
  glottis J38.6
  heart valve (congenital) Q24.8
    aortic Q23.0
    mitral Q23.2
    pulmonary Q22.1
    tricuspid Q22.4
  hepatic duct K83.1
  hymen N89.6
  hypertrophic subaortic (idiopathic) I42.1
  ileum — *see also* Obstruction, intestine, specified NEC
    K56.699
    congenital Q41.2
  infundibulum cardia Q24.3
  intervertebral foramina — *see also* Lesion, biomechan-
    ical, specified NEC
    connective tissue M99.79
      abdomen M99.79
      cervical region M99.71
      cervicothoracic M99.71
      head region M99.70
      lumbar region M99.73
      lumbosacral M99.73
      occipitocervical M99.70
      sacral region M99.74
      sacrococcygeal M99.74
      sacroiliac M99.74
      specified NEC M99.79
      thoracic region M99.72
      thoracolumbar M99.72
    disc M99.79
      abdomen M99.79
      cervical region M99.71
      cervicothoracic M99.71
      head region M99.70
      lower extremity M99.76
      lumbar region M99.73
      lumbosacral M99.73
      occipitocervical M99.70
      pelvic M99.75
      rib cage M99.78
      sacral region M99.74
      sacrococcygeal M99.74
      sacroiliac M99.74
      specified NEC M99.79
      thoracic region M99.72
      thoracolumbar M99.72
      upper extremity M99.77
    osseous M99.69
      abdomen M99.69
      cervical region M99.61
      cervicothoracic M99.61
      head region M99.60
      lower extremity M99.66
      lumbar region M99.63
      lumbosacral M99.63
      occipitocervical M99.60
      pelvic M99.65
      rib cage M99.68
      sacral region M99.64
      sacrococcygeal M99.64
      sacroiliac M99.64
      specified NEC M99.69

Stenosis, stenotic — *continued*
  intervertebral foramina — *see also* Lesion, biomechan-
    ical, specified — *continued*
    osseous — *continued*
      thoracic region M99.62
      thoracolumbar M99.62
      upper extremity M99.67
    subluxation — *see* Stenosis, intervertebral foramina,
      osseous
  intestine — *see also* Obstruction, intestine
    congenital (small) Q41.9
      large Q42.9
        specified NEC Q42.8
      specified NEC Q41.8
  jejunum — *see also* Obstruction, intestine, specified
    NEC K56.699
    congenital Q41.1
  lacrimal (passage)
    canaliculi H04.54- ☑
    congenital Q10.5
    duct H04.55- ☑
    punctum H04.56- ☑
    sac H04.57- ☑
  lacrimonasal duct — *see* Stenosis, lacrimal, duct
    congenital Q10.5
  larynx J38.6
    congenital NEC Q31.8
      subglottic Q31.1
    syphilitic A52.73
      congenital A50.59 *[J99]*
  mitral (chronic) (inactive) (valve) I05.0
    with
      aortic valve disease I08.0
      incompetency, insufficiency or regurgitation
        I05.2
    active or acute I01.1
      with rheumatic or Sydenham's chorea I02.0
    congenital Q23.2
    specified cause, except rheumatic I34.2
    syphilitic A52.03
  myocardium, myocardial — *see also* Degeneration,
    myocardial
    hypertrophic subaortic (idiopathic) I42.1
  nares (anterior) (posterior) J34.89
    congenital Q30.0
  nasal duct — *see also* Stenosis, lacrimal, duct
    congenital Q10.5
  nasolacrimal duct — *see also* Stenosis, lacrimal, duct
    congenital Q10.5
  neural canal — *see also* Lesion, biomechanical, speci-
    fied NEC
    connective tissue M99.49
      abdomen M99.49
      cervical region M99.41
      cervicothoracic M99.41
      head region M99.40
      lower extremity M99.46
      lumbar region M99.43
      lumbosacral M99.43
      occipitocervical M99.40
      pelvic M99.45
      rib cage M99.48
      sacral region M99.44
      sacrococcygeal M99.44
      sacroiliac M99.44
      specified NEC M99.49
      thoracic region M99.42
      thoracolumbar M99.42
      upper extremity M99.47
    intervertebral disc M99.59
      abdomen M99.59
      cervical region M99.51
      cervicothoracic M99.51
      head region M99.50
      lower extremity M99.56
      lumbar region M99.53
      lumbosacral M99.53
      occipitocervical M99.50
      pelvic M99.55
      rib cage M99.58
      sacral region M99.54
      sacrococcygeal M99.54
      sacroiliac M99.54
      specified NEC M99.59
      thoracic region M99.52
      thoracolumbar M99.52
      upper extremity M99.57
    osseous M99.39

Stenosis, stenotic — *continued*
  neural canal — *see also* Lesion, biomechanical, specified — *continued*
    osseous — *continued*
      abdomen M99.39
      cervical region M99.31
      cervicothoracic M99.31
      head region M99.30
      lower extremity M99.36
      lumbar region M99.33
      lumbosacral M99.33
      occipitocervical M99.30
      pelvic M99.35
      rib cage M99.38
      sacral region M99.34
      sacrococcygeal M99.34
      sacroiliac M99.34
      specified NEC M99.39
      thoracic region M99.32
      thoracolumbar M99.32
      upper extremity M99.37
    subluxation M99.29
      cervical region M99.21
      cervicothoracic M99.21
      head region M99.20
      lower extremity M99.26
      lumbar region M99.23
      lumbosacral M99.23
      occipitocervical M99.20
      pelvic M99.25
      rib cage M99.28
      sacral region M99.24
      sacrococcygeal M99.24
      sacroiliac M99.24
      specified NEC M99.29
      thoracic region M99.22
      thoracolumbar M99.22
      upper extremity M99.27
  organ or site, congenital NEC — *see* Atresia, by site
  papilla of Vater K83.1
  pulmonary (artery) (congenital) Q25.6
    with ventricular septal defect, transposition of aorta, and hypertrophy of right ventricle Q21.3
    acquired I28.8
    in tetralogy of Fallot Q21.3
    infundibular Q24.3
    subvalvular Q24.3
    supravalvular Q25.6
    valve I37.0
      with insufficiency I37.2
      congenital Q22.1
      rheumatic I09.89
        with aortic, mitral or tricuspid (valve) disease I08.8
    vein, acquired I28.8
    vessel NEC I28.8
  pulmonic (congenital) Q22.1
    infundibular Q24.3
    subvalvular Q24.3
  pylorus (hypertrophic) (acquired) K31.1
    adult K31.1
    congenital Q40.0
    infantile Q40.0
  rectum (sphincter) — *see* Stricture, rectum
  renal artery I70.1
    congenital Q27.1
  salivary duct (any) K11.8
  sphincter of Oddi K83.1
  spinal M48.00
    cervical region M48.02
    cervicothoracic region M48.03
    lumbar region (NOS) (without neurogenic claudication) M48.061
      with neurogenic claudication M48.062
    lumbosacral region M48.07
    occipito-atlanto-axial region M48.01
    sacrococcygeal region M48.08
    thoracic region M48.04
    thoracolumbar region M48.05
  stomach, hourglass K31.2
  subaortic (congenital) Q24.4
    hypertrophic (idiopathic) I42.1
  subglottic J38.6
    congenital Q31.1
    postprocedural J95.5
  trachea J39.8
    congenital Q32.1
    syphilitic A52.73
    tuberculous NEC A15.5

Stenosis, stenotic — *continued*
  tracheostomy J95.03
  tricuspid (valve) I07.0
    with
      aortic (valve) disease I08.2
      incompetency, insufficiency or regurgitation I07.2
        with aortic (valve) disease I08.2
          with mitral (valve) disease I08.3
      mitral (valve) disease I08.1
        with aortic (valve) disease I08.3
    congenital Q22.4
    nonrheumatic I36.0
      with insufficiency I36.2
  tubal N97.1
  ureter — *see* Atresia, ureter
  ureteropelvic junction, congenital Q62.11
  ureterovesical orifice, congenital Q62.12
  urethra (valve) *see also* Stricture, urethra
    congenital Q64.32
  urinary meatus, congenital Q64.33
  vagina N89.5
    congenital Q52.4
    in pregnancy — *see* Pregnancy, complicated by, abnormal vagina
      causing obstructed labor O65.5
  valve (cardiac) (heart) — *see also* Endocarditis I38
    congenital Q24.8
      aortic Q23.0
      mitral Q23.2
      pulmonary Q22.1
      tricuspid Q22.4
  vena cava (inferior) (superior) I87.1
    congenital Q26.0
  vesicourethral orifice Q64.31
  vulva N90.5
Stent jail T82.897 ☑
Stercolith (impaction) K56.41
  appendix K38.1
Stercoraceous, stercoral ulcer K63.3
  anus or rectum K62.6
Stereotypies NEC F98.4
Sterility — *see* Infertility
Sterilization — *see* Encounter (for), sterilization
Sternalgia — *see* Angina
Sternopagus Q89.4
Sternum bifidum Q76.7
Steroid
  effects (adverse) (adrenocortical) (iatrogenic)
    cushingoid E24.2
      correct substance properly administered — *see* Table of Drugs and Chemicals, by drug, adverse effect
      overdose or wrong substance given or taken — *see* Table of Drugs and Chemicals, by drug, poisoning
    diabetes — *see* subcategory E09 ☑
      correct substance properly administered — *see* Table of Drugs and Chemicals, by drug, adverse effect
      overdose or wrong substance given or taken — *see* Table of Drugs and Chemicals, by drug, poisoning
    fever R50.2
    insufficiency E27.3
      correct substance properly administered — *see* Table of Drugs and Chemicals, by drug, adverse effect
      overdose or wrong substance given or taken — *see* Table of Drugs and Chemicals, by drug, poisoning
    responder H40.04- ☑
Stevens-Johnson disease or syndrome L51.1
  toxic epidermal necrolysis overlap L51.3
Stewart-Morel syndrome M85.2
Sticker's disease B08.3
Sticky eye — *see* Conjunctivitis, acute, mucopurulent
Stieda's disease — *see* Bursitis, tibial collateral
Stiff neck — *see* Torticollis
Stiff-man syndrome G25.82
Stiffness, joint NEC M25.60
  ankle M25.67- ☑
  ankylosis — *see* Ankylosis, joint
  contracture — *see* Contraction, joint
  elbow M25.62- ☑
  foot M25.67- ☑
  hand M25.64- ☑

Stiffness, joint — *continued*
  hip M25.65- ☑
  knee M25.66- ☑
  shoulder M25.61- ☑
  specified site NEC M25.69
  wrist M25.63- ☑
Stigmata congenital syphilis A50.59
Stillbirth P95
Still-Felty syndrome — *see* Felty's syndrome
Still's disease or syndrome (juvenile) M08.20
  adult-onset M06.1
  ankle M08.27- ☑
  elbow M08.22- ☑
  foot joint M08.27- ☑
  hand joint M08.24- ☑
  hip M08.25- ☑
  knee M08.26- ☑
  multiple site M08.29
  shoulder M08.21- ☑
  specified site NEC M08.2A
  vertebra M08.28
  wrist M08.23- ☑
Stimulation, ovary E28.1
Sting (venomous) (with allergic or anaphylactic shock) — *see* Table of Drugs and Chemicals, by animal or substance, poisoning
Stippled epiphyses Q78.8
Stitch
  abscess T81.41 ☑
  burst (in operation wound) — *see* Disruption, wound, operation
Stokes' disease E05.00
  with thyroid storm E05.01
Stokes-Adams disease or syndrome I45.9
Stokvis (-Talma) **disease** D74.8
Stoma malfunction
  colostomy K94.03
  enterostomy K94.13
  gastrostomy K94.23
  ileostomy K94.13
  tracheostomy J95.03
Stomach — *see* condition
Stomatitis (denture) (ulcerative) K12.1
  angular K13.0
    due to dietary or vitamin deficiency E53.0
  aphthous K12.0
  bovine B08.61
  candidal B37.0
  catarrhal K12.1
  diphtheritic A36.89
  due to
    dietary deficiency E53.0
    thrush B37.0
    vitamin deficiency
      B group NEC E53.9
      B2 (riboflavin) E53.0
  epidemic B08.8
  epizootic B08.8
  follicular K12.1
  gangrenous A69.0
  Geotrichum B48.3
  herpesviral, herpetic B00.2
  herpetiformis K12.0
  malignant K12.1
  membranous acute K12.1
  monilial B37.0
  mycotic B37.0
  necrotizing ulcerative A69.0
  parasitic B37.0
  septic K12.1
  spirochetal A69.1
  suppurative (acute) K12.2
  ulceromembranous A69.1
  vesicular K12.1
    with exanthem (enteroviral) B08.4
    virus disease A93.8
  Vincent's A69.1
Stomatocytosis D58.8
Stomatomycosis B37.0
Stomatorrhagia K13.79
Stone(s) — *see also* Calculus
  bladder (diverticulum) N21.0
  cystine E72.09
  heart syndrome I50.1
  kidney N20.0
  prostate N42.0
  pulpal (dental) K04.2
  renal N20.0

☑ **Additional Character Required** — Refer to the Tabular List for Character Selection   Subterms under main terms may continue to next column or page

Stone(s) — *continued*
  salivary gland or duct (any) K11.5
  urethra (impacted) N21.1
  urinary (duct) (impacted) (passage) N20.9
    bladder (diverticulum) N21.0
    lower tract N21.9
    specified NEC N21.8
  xanthine E79.8 *[N22]*
Stonecutter's lung J62.8
Stonemason's asthma, disease, lung or pneumoconiosis J62.8
Stoppage
  heart — *see* Arrest, cardiac
  urine — *see* Retention, urine
Storm, thyroid — *see* Thyrotoxicosis
Strabismus (congenital) (nonparalytic) H50.9
  concomitant H50.40
    convergent — *see* Strabismus, convergent concomitant
    divergent — *see* Strabismus, divergent concomitant
  convergent concomitant H50.00
    accommodative component H50.43
    alternating H50.05
      with
        A pattern H50.06
        specified nonconcomitances NEC H50.08
        V pattern H50.07
    monocular H50.01- ☑
      with
        A pattern H50.02- ☑
        specified nonconcomitances NEC H50.04- ☑
        V pattern H50.03- ☑
    intermittent H50.31- ☑
      alternating H50.32
  cyclotropia H50.41 ☑
  divergent concomitant H50.10
    alternating H50.15
      with
        A pattern H50.16
        specified noncomitances NEC H50.18
        V pattern H50.17
    monocular H50.11- ☑
      with
        A pattern H50.12- ☑
        specified noncomitances NEC H50.14- ☑
        V pattern H50.13- ☑
    intermittent H50.33 ☑
      alternating H50.34
  Duane's syndrome H50.81- ☑
  due to adhesions, scars H50.69
  heterophoria H50.50
    alternating H50.55
    cyclophoria H50.54
    esophoria H50.51
    exophoria H50.52
    vertical H50.53
  heterotropia H50.40
    intermittent H50.30
  hypertropia H50.2- ☑
  hypotropia — *see* Hypertropia
  latent H50.50
  mechanical H50.60
    Brown's sheath syndrome H50.61- ☑
    specified type NEC H50.69
  monofixation syndrome H50.42
  paralytic H49.9
    abducens nerve H49.2- ☑
    fourth nerve H49.1- ☑
    Kearns-Sayre syndrome H49.81- ☑
    ophthalmoplegia (external)
      progressive H49.4- ☑
        with pigmentary retinopathy H49.81- ☑
      total H49.3- ☑
    sixth nerve H49.2- ☑
    specified type NEC H49.88- ☑
    third nerve H49.0- ☑
    trochlear nerve H49.1- ☑
  specified type NEC H50.89
  vertical H50.2- ☑
Strain
  back S39.012 ☑
  cervical S16.1 ☑
  eye NEC — *see* Disturbance, vision, subjective
  heart — *see* Disease, heart
  low back S39.012 ☑
  mental NOS Z73.3
    work-related Z56.6

Strain — *continued*
  muscle (tendon) — *see* Injury, muscle, by site, strain
  neck S16.1 ☑
  physical NOS Z73.3
    work-related Z56.6
  postural — *see also* Disorder, soft tissue, due to use
  psychological NEC Z73.3
  tendon — *see* Injury, muscle, by site, strain
Straining, on urination R39.16
Strand, vitreous — *see* Opacity, vitreous, membranes and strands
Strangulation, strangulated — *see also* Asphyxia, traumatic
  appendix K38.8
  bladder-neck N32.0
  bowel or colon K56.2
  food or foreign body — *see* Foreign body, by site
  hemorrhoids — *see* Hemorrhoids, with complication
  hernia — *see also* Hernia, by site, with obstruction
    with gangrene — *see* Hernia, by site, with gangrene
  intestine (large) (small) K56.2
    with hernia — *see also* Hernia, by site, with obstruction
      with gangrene — *see* Hernia, by site, with gangrene
  mesentery K56.2
  mucus — *see* Asphyxia, mucus
  omentum K56.2
  organ or site, congenital NEC — *see* Atresia, by site
  ovary — *see* Torsion, ovary
  penis N48.89
    foreign body T19.4 ☑
  rupture — *see* Hernia, by site, with obstruction
  stomach due to hernia — *see also* Hernia, by site, with obstruction
    with gangrene — *see* Hernia, by site, with gangrene
  vesicourethral orifice N32.0
Strangury R30.0
Straw itch B88.0
Strawberry
  gallbladder K82.4
  mark Q82.5
  tongue (red) (white) K14.3
Streak(s)
  macula, angioid H35.33
  ovarian Q50.32
Strephosymbolia F81.0
  secondary to organic lesion R48.8
Streptobacillary fever A25.1
Streptobacillosis A25.1
Streptobacillus moniliformis A25.1
Streptococcus, streptococcal — *see also* condition
  as cause of disease classified elsewhere B95.5
  group
    A, as cause of disease classified elsewhere B95.0
    B, as cause of disease classified elsewhere B95.1
    D, as cause of disease classified elsewhere B95.2
  pneumoniae, as cause of disease classified elsewhere B95.3
  specified NEC, as cause of disease classified elsewhere B95.4
Streptomycosis B47.1
Streptotrichosis A48.8
Stress F43.9
  family — *see* Disruption, family
  fetal P84
    complicating pregnancy O77.9
      due to drug administration O77.1
  mental NEC Z73.3
    work-related Z56.6
  physical NEC Z73.3
    work-related Z56.6
  polycythemia D75.1
  reaction — *see also* Reaction, stress F43.9
  work schedule Z56.3
Stretching, nerve — *see* Injury, nerve
Striae albicantes, atrophicae or distensae (cutis) L90.6
Stricture — *see also* Stenosis
  ampulla of Vater K83.1
  anus (sphincter) K62.4
    congenital Q42.3
      with fistula Q42.2
    infantile Q42.3
      with fistula Q42.2
  aorta (ascending) (congenital) Q25.1
    arteriosclerotic I70.0
    calcified I70.0
    supravalvular, congenital Q25.3

Stricture — *continued*
  aortic (valve) — *see* Stenosis, aortic
  aqueduct of Sylvius (congenital) Q03.0
    with spina bifida — *see* Spina bifida, by site, with hydrocephalus
    acquired G91.1
  artery I77.1
    basilar — *see* Occlusion, artery, basilar
    carotid — *see* Occlusion, artery, carotid
    celiac I77.4
    congenital (peripheral) Q27.8
      cerebral Q28.3
      coronary Q24.5
      digestive system Q27.8
      lower limb Q27.8
      retinal Q14.1
      specified site NEC Q27.8
      umbilical Q27.0
      upper limb Q27.8
    coronary — *see* Disease, heart, ischemic, atherosclerotic
      congenital Q24.5
    precerebral — *see* Occlusion, artery, precerebral
    pulmonary (congenital) Q25.6
      acquired I28.8
    renal I70.1
    vertebral — *see* Occlusion, artery, vertebral
  auditory canal (external) (congenital)
    acquired — *see* Stenosis, external ear canal
  bile duct (common) (hepatic) K83.1
    congenital Q44.3
    postoperative K91.89
  bladder N32.89
    neck N32.0
  bowel — *see* Obstruction, intestine
  brain G93.89
  bronchus J98.09
    congenital Q32.3
    syphilitic A52.72
  cardia (stomach) K22.2
    congenital Q39.3
  cardiac — *see also* Disease, heart
    orifice (stomach) K22.2
  cecum — *see* Obstruction, intestine
  cervix, cervical (canal) N88.2
    congenital Q51.828
    in pregnancy — *see* Pregnancy, complicated by, abnormal cervix
      causing obstructed labor O65.5
  colon — *see also* Obstruction, intestine
    congenital Q42.9
      specified NEC Q42.8
  colostomy K94.03
  common (bile) duct K83.1
  coronary (artery) — *see* Disease, heart, ischemic, atherosclerotic
  cystic duct — *see* Obstruction, gallbladder
  digestive organs NEC, congenital Q45.8
  duodenum K31.5
    congenital Q41.0
  ear canal (external) (congenital) Q16.1
    acquired — *see* Stricture, auditory canal, acquired
  ejaculatory duct N50.89
  enterostomy K94.13
  esophagus K22.2
    congenital Q39.3
    syphilitic A52.79
      congenital A50.59 *[K23]*
  eustachian tube — *see also* Obstruction, eustachian tube
    congenital Q17.8
  fallopian tube N97.1
    gonococcal A54.24
    tuberculous A18.17
  gallbladder — *see* Obstruction, gallbladder
  glottis J38.6
  heart — *see also* Disease, heart
    valve — *see also* Endocarditis I38
      aortic Q23.0
      mitral Q23.2
      pulmonary Q22.1
      tricuspid Q22.4
  hepatic duct K83.1
  hourglass, of stomach K31.2
  hymen N89.6
  hypopharynx J39.2
  ileum — *see also* Obstruction, intestine, specified NEC K56.699

▽ Subterms under main terms may continue to next column or page   ☑ Additional Character Required — Refer to the Tabular List for Character Selection   **299**

Stone(s) — Stricture

Stricture — *continued*
  ileum — *see also* Obstruction, intestine, specified — *continued*
    congenital Q41.2
  intestine — *see also* Obstruction, intestine
    congenital (small) Q41.9
      large Q42.9
        specified NEC Q42.8
      specified NEC Q41.8
    ischemic K55.1
  jejunum — *see also* Obstruction, intestine, specified NEC K56.699
    congenital Q41.1
  lacrimal passages — *see also* Stenosis, lacrimal
    congenital Q10.5
  larynx J38.6
    congenital NEC Q31.8
      subglottic Q31.1
    syphilitic A52.73
      congenital A50.59 *[J99]*
  meatus
    ear (congenital) Q16.1
      acquired — *see* Stricture, auditory canal, acquired
    osseous (ear) (congenital) Q16.1
      acquired — *see* Stricture, auditory canal, acquired
    urinarius — *see also* Stricture, urethra
      congenital Q64.33
  mitral (valve) — *see* Stenosis, mitral
  myocardium, myocardial I51.5
    hypertrophic subaortic (idiopathic) I42.1
  nares (anterior) (posterior) J34.89
    congenital Q30.0
  nasal duct — *see also* Stenosis, lacrimal, duct
    congenital Q10.5
  nasolacrimal duct — *see also* Stenosis, lacrimal, duct
    congenital Q10.5
  nasopharynx J39.2
    syphilitic A52.73
  nose J34.89
    congenital Q30.0
  nostril (anterior) (posterior) J34.89
    congenital Q30.0
    syphilitic A52.73
      congenital A50.59 *[J99]*
  organ or site, congenital NEC — *see* Atresia, by site
  os uteri — *see* Stricture, cervix
  osseous meatus (ear) (congenital) Q16.1
    acquired — *see* Stricture, auditory canal, acquired
  oviduct — *see* Stricture, fallopian tube
  pelviureteric junction (congenital) Q62.11
    acquired, with hydronephrosis N13.0
  penis, by foreign body T19.4 ☑
  pharynx J39.2
  prostate N42.89
  pulmonary, pulmonic
    artery (congenital) Q25.6
      acquired I28.8
      noncongenital I28.8
    infundibulum (congenital) Q24.3
    valve I37.0
      congenital Q22.1
    vein, acquired I28.8
    vessel NEC I28.8
  punctum lacrimale — *see also* Stenosis, lacrimal, punctum
    congenital Q10.5
  pylorus (hypertrophic) K31.1
    adult K31.1
    congenital Q40.0
    infantile Q40.0
  rectosigmoid — *see also* Obstruction, intestine, specified NEC K56.699
  rectum (sphincter) K62.4
    congenital Q42.1
      with fistula Q42.0
    due to
      chlamydial lymphogranuloma A55
      irradiation K91.89
      lymphogranuloma venereum A55
    gonococcal A54.6
    inflammatory (chlamydial) A55
    syphilitic A52.74
    tuberculous A18.32
  renal artery I70.1
    congenital Q27.1
  salivary duct or gland (any) K11.8

Stricture — *continued*
  sigmoid (flexure) — *see* Obstruction, intestine
  spermatic cord N50.89
  stoma (following) (of)
    colostomy K94.03
    enterostomy K94.13
    gastrostomy K94.23
    ileostomy K94.13
    tracheostomy J95.03
  stomach K31.89
    congenital Q40.2
    hourglass K31.2
  subaortic Q24.4
    hypertrophic (acquired) (idiopathic) I42.1
  subglottic J38.6
  syphilitic NEC A52.79
  trachea J39.8
    congenital Q32.1
    syphilitic A52.73
    tuberculous NEC A15.5
  tracheostomy J95.03
  tricuspid (valve) — *see* Stenosis, tricuspid
  tunica vaginalis N50.89
  ureter (postoperative) N13.5
    with
      hydronephrosis N13.1
        with infection N13.6
      pyelonephritis (chronic) N11.1
    congenital — *see* Atresia, ureter
    tuberculous A18.11
  ureteropelvic junction (congenital) Q62.11
    acquired, with hydronephrosis N13.0
  ureterovesical orifice N13.5
    with infection N13.6
  urethra (organic) (spasmodic) — *see also* Stricture, urethra, male N35.919
    associated with schistosomiasis B65.0 *[N37]*
    congenital Q64.39
      valvular (posterior) Q64.2
    due to
      infection — *see* Stricture, urethra, postinfective
      trauma — *see* Stricture, urethra, post-traumatic
    female N35.92
    gonococcal, gonorrheal A54.01
    infective NEC — *see* Stricture, urethra, postinfective
    late effect (sequelae) of injury — *see* Stricture, urethra, post-traumatic
    male N35.919
      anterior urethra N35.914
      bulbous urethra N35.912
      meatal N35.911
      membranous urethra N35.913
      overlapping sites N35.916
    postcatheterization — *see* Stricture, urethra, postprocedural
    postinfective NEC
      female N35.12
      male N35.119
        anterior urethra N35.114
        bulbous urethra N35.112
        meatal N35.111
        membranous urethra N35.113
        overlapping sites N35.116
    postobstetric N35.021
    postoperative — *see* Stricture, urethra, postprocedural
    postprocedural
      female N99.12
      male N99.114
        anterior bulbous urethra N99.113
        bulbous urethra N99.111
        fossa navicularis N99.115
        meatal N99.110
        membranous urethra N99.112
        overlapping sites N99.116
    post-traumatic
      female N35.028
        due to childbirth N35.021
      male N35.014
        anterior urethra N35.013
        bulbous urethra N35.011
        meatal N35.010
        membranous urethra N35.012
        overlapping sites N35.016
    sequela (late effect) of
      childbirth N35.021
      injury — *see* Stricture, urethra, post-traumatic
    specified cause NEC

Stricture — *continued*
  urethra — *see also* Stricture, urethra, male — *continued*
    specified cause — *continued*
      female N35.82
      male N35.819
        anterior urethra N35.814
        bulbous urethra N35.812
        meatal N35.811
        membranous urethra N35.813
        overlapping sites N35.816
    syphilitic A52.76
    traumatic — *see* Stricture, urethra, post-traumatic
    valvular (posterior), congenital Q64.2
  urinary meatus — *see* Stricture, urethra
  uterus, uterine (synechiae) N85.6
    os (external) (internal) — *see* Stricture, cervix
  vagina (outlet) — *see* Stenosis, vagina
  valve (cardiac) (heart) — *see also* Endocarditis
    congenital
      aortic Q23.0
      mitral Q23.2
      pulmonary Q22.1
      tricuspid Q22.4
  vas deferens N50.89
    congenital Q55.4
  vein I87.1
  vena cava (inferior) (superior) NEC I87.1
    congenital Q26.0
  vesicourethral orifice N32.0
    congenital Q64.31
  vulva (acquired) N90.5

Stridor R06.1
  congenital (larynx) P28.89
Stridulous — *see* condition
Stroke (apoplectic) (brain) (embolic) (ischemic) (paralytic) (thrombotic) I63.9
  cerebral, perinatal P91.82- ☑
  cryptogenic — *see also* infarction, cerebral I63.9
  epileptic — *see* Epilepsy
  heat T67.01 ☑
    exertional T67.02 ☑
    specified NEC T67.09 ☑
  in evolution I63.9
  intraoperative
    during cardiac surgery I97.810
    during other surgery I97.811
  ischemic, perinatal arterial P91.82- ☑
  lightning — *see* Lightning
  meaning
    cerebral hemorrhage — *code to* Hemorrhage, intracranial
    cerebral infarction — *code to* Infarction, cerebral
  neonatal P91.82- ☑
  postprocedural
    following cardiac surgery I97.820
    following other surgery I97.821
  sun T67.01 ☑
    specified NEC T67.09 ☑
  unspecified (NOS) I63.9
Stromatosis, endometrial D39.0
Strongyloidiasis, strongyloidosis B78.9
  cutaneous B78.1
  disseminated B78.7
  intestinal B78.0
Strophulus pruriginosus L28.2
Struck by lightning — *see* Lightning
Struma — *see also* Goiter
  Hashimoto E06.3
  lymphomatosa E06.3
  nodosa (simplex) E04.9
    endemic E01.2
      multinodular E01.1
    multinodular E04.2
      iodine-deficiency related E01.1
    toxic or with hyperthyroidism E05.20
      with thyroid storm E05.21
      multinodular E05.20
        with thyroid storm E05.21
      uninodular E05.10
        with thyroid storm E05.11
    toxicosa E05.20
      with thyroid storm E05.21
      multinodular E05.20
        with thyroid storm E05.21
      uninodular E05.10
        with thyroid storm E05.11
    uninodular E04.1

truma — *continued*
　ovarii D27.- ☑
　Riedel's E06.5
trumipriva cachexia E03.4
trümpell-Marie spine — *see* Spondylitis, ankylosing
trümpell-Westphal pseudosclerosis E83.01
tuart deficiency disease (factor X) D68.2
tuart-Prower factor deficiency (factor X) D68.2
tudent's elbow — *see* Bursitis, elbow, olecranon
tump — *see* Amputation
tunting, nutritional E45
tupor (catatonic) R40.1
　depressive (single episode) F32.89
　　recurrent episode F33.8
　dissociative F44.2
　manic F30.2
　manic-depressive F31.89
　psychogenic (anergic) F44.2
　reaction to exceptional stress (transient) F43.0
turge (-Weber) (-Dimitri) (-Kalischer) **disease or syndrome** Q85.8
tuttering F80.81
　adult onset F98.5
　childhood onset F80.81
　following cerebrovascular disease — *see* Disorder, fluency. following cerebrovascular disease
　in conditions classified elsewhere R47.82
ty, stye (external) (internal) (meibomian) (zeisian) — *see* Hordeolum
ubacidity, gastric K31.89
　psychogenic F45.8
ubacute — *see* condition
ubarachnoid — *see* condition
ubcortical — *see* condition
ubcostal syndrome, nerve compression — *see* Mononeuropathy, upper limb, specified site NEC
ubcutaneous, subcuticular — *see* condition
ubdural — *see* condition
ubendocardium — *see* condition
ubependymoma
　specified site — *see* Neoplasm, uncertain behavior, by site
　unspecified site D43.2
uberosis J67.3
ubglossitis — *see* Glossitis
ubhemophilia D66
ubinvolution
　breast (postlactational) (postpuerperal) N64.89
　puerperal O90.89
　uterus (chronic) (nonpuerperal) N85.3
　　puerperal O90.89
ublingual — *see* condition
ublinguitis — *see* Sialoadenitis
ubluxatable hip Q65.6
ubluxation — *see also* Dislocation
　acromioclavicular S43.11- ☑
　ankle S93.0- ☑
　atlantoaxial, recurrent M43.4
　　with myelopathy M43.3
　carpometacarpal (joint) NEC S63.05- ☑
　　thumb S63.04- ☑
　complex, vertebral — *see* Complex, subluxation
　congenital — *see also* Malposition, congenital
　　hip — *see* Dislocation, hip, congenital, partial
　　joint (excluding hip)
　　　lower limb Q68.8
　　　shoulder Q68.8
　　　upper limb Q68.8
　elbow (traumatic) S53.10- ☑
　　anterior S53.11- ☑
　　lateral S53.14- ☑
　　medial S53.13- ☑
　　posterior S53.12- ☑
　　specified type NEC S53.19- ☑
　finger S63.20- ☑
　　index S63.20- ☑
　　interphalangeal S63.22- ☑
　　　distal S63.24- ☑
　　　　index S63.24- ☑
　　　　little S63.24- ☑
　　　　middle S63.24- ☑
　　　　ring S63.24- ☑
　　　index S63.22- ☑
　　　little S63.22- ☑
　　　middle S63.22- ☑
　　　proximal S63.23- ☑
　　　　index S63.23- ☑

Subluxation — *continued*
　finger — *continued*
　　interphalangeal — *continued*
　　　proximal — *continued*
　　　　little S63.23- ☑
　　　　middle S63.23- ☑
　　　　ring S63.23- ☑
　　　ring S63.22- ☑
　　little S63.20- ☑
　　metacarpophalangeal S63.21- ☑
　　　index S63.21- ☑
　　　little S63.21- ☑
　　　middle S63.21- ☑
　　　ring S63.21- ☑
　　middle S63.20- ☑
　　ring S63.20- ☑
　foot S93.30- ☑
　　specified site NEC S93.33- ☑
　　tarsal joint S93.31- ☑
　　tarsometatarsal joint S93.32- ☑
　　toe — *see* Subluxation, toe
　hip S73.00- ☑
　　anterior S73.03- ☑
　　　obturator S73.02- ☑
　　central S73.04- ☑
　　posterior S73.01- ☑
　interphalangeal (joint)
　　finger S63.22- ☑
　　　distal joint S63.24- ☑
　　　　index S63.24- ☑
　　　　little S63.24- ☑
　　　　middle S63.24- ☑
　　　　ring S63.24- ☑
　　　index S63.22- ☑
　　　little S63.22- ☑
　　　middle S63.22- ☑
　　　proximal joint S63.23- ☑
　　　　index S63.23- ☑
　　　　little S63.23- ☑
　　　　middle S63.23- ☑
　　　　ring S63.23- ☑
　　thumb S63.12- ☑
　　toe S93.13- ☑
　　　great S93.13- ☑
　　　lesser S93.13- ☑
　joint prosthesis — *see* Complications, joint prosthesis, mechanical, displacement, by site
　knee S83.10- ☑
　　cap — *see* Subluxation, patella
　　patella — *see* Subluxation, patella
　　proximal tibia
　　　anteriorly S83.11- ☑
　　　laterally S83.14- ☑
　　　medially S83.13- ☑
　　　posteriorly S83.12- ☑
　　specified type NEC S83.19- ☑
　lens — *see* Dislocation, lens, partial
　ligament, traumatic — *see* Sprain, by site
　metacarpal (bone)
　　proximal end S63.06- ☑
　metacarpophalangeal (joint)
　　finger S63.21- ☑
　　　index S63.21- ☑
　　　little S63.21- ☑
　　　middle S63.21- ☑
　　　ring S63.21- ☑
　　thumb S63.11- ☑
　metatarsophalangeal joint S93.14- ☑
　　great toe S93.14- ☑
　　lesser toe S93.14- ☑
　midcarpal (joint) S63.03- ☑
　patella S83.00- ☑
　　lateral S83.01- ☑
　　recurrent (nontraumatic) — *see* Dislocation, patella, recurrent, incomplete
　　specified type NEC S83.09- ☑
　pathological — *see* Dislocation, pathological
　radial head S53.00- ☑
　　anterior S53.01- ☑
　　nursemaid's elbow S53.03- ☑
　　posterior S53.02- ☑
　　specified type NEC S53.09- ☑
　radiocarpal (joint) S63.02- ☑
　radioulnar (joint)
　　distal S63.01- ☑

Subluxation — *continued*
　radioulnar — *continued*
　　proximal — *see* Subluxation, elbow
　shoulder
　　congenital Q68.8
　　girdle S43.30- ☑
　　　scapula S43.31- ☑
　　　specified site NEC S43.39- ☑
　　traumatic S43.00- ☑
　　　anterior S43.01- ☑
　　　inferior S43.03- ☑
　　　posterior S43.02- ☑
　　　specified type NEC S43.08- ☑
　sternoclavicular (joint) S43.20- ☑
　　anterior S43.21- ☑
　　posterior S43.22- ☑
　symphysis (pubis)
　thumb S63.103
　　interphalangeal joint — *see* Subluxation, interphalangeal (joint), thumb
　　metacarpophalangeal joint — *see* Subluxation, metacarpophalangeal (joint), thumb
　toe(s) S93.10- ☑
　　great S93.10- ☑
　　　interphalangeal joint S93.13- ☑
　　　metatarsophalangeal joint S93.14- ☑
　　interphalangeal joint S93.13- ☑
　　lesser S93.10- ☑
　　　interphalangeal joint S93.13- ☑
　　　metatarsophalangeal joint S93.14- ☑
　　metatarsophalangeal joint S93.149
　ulna
　　distal end S63.07- ☑
　　proximal end — *see* Subluxation, elbow
　ulnohumeral joint — *see* Subluxation, elbow
　vertebral
　　recurrent NEC — *see* subcategory M43.5 ☑
　　traumatic
　　　cervical S13.100 ☑
　　　　atlantoaxial joint S13.120 ☑
　　　　atlantooccipital joint S13.110 ☑
　　　　atloidooccipital joint S13.110 ☑
　　　　joint between
　　　　　C0 and C1 S13.110 ☑
　　　　　C1 and C2 S13.120 ☑
　　　　　C2 and C3 S13.130 ☑
　　　　　C3 and C4 S13.140 ☑
　　　　　C4 and C5 S13.150 ☑
　　　　　C5 and C6 S13.160 ☑
　　　　　C6 and C7 S13.170 ☑
　　　　　C7 and T1 S13.180 ☑
　　　　occipitoatloid joint S13.110 ☑
　　　lumbar S33.100 ☑
　　　　joint between
　　　　　L1 and L2 S33.110 ☑
　　　　　L2 and L3 S33.120 ☑
　　　　　L3 and L4 S33.130 ☑
　　　　　L4 and L5 S33.140 ☑
　　　thoracic S23.100 ☑
　　　　joint between
　　　　　T1 and T2 S23.110 ☑
　　　　　T2 and T3 S23.120 ☑
　　　　　T3 and T4 S23.122 ☑
　　　　　T4 and T5 S23.130 ☑
　　　　　T5 and T6 S23.132 ☑
　　　　　T6 and T7 S23.140 ☑
　　　　　T7 and T8 S23.142 ☑
　　　　　T8 and T9 S23.150 ☑
　　　　　T9 and T10 S23.152 ☑
　　　　　T10 and T11 S23.160 ☑
　　　　　T11 and T12 S23.162 ☑
　　　　　T12 and L1 S23.170 ☑
　wrist (carpal bone) S63.00- ☑
　　carpometacarpal joint — *see* Subluxation, carpometacarpal (joint)
　　distal radioulnar joint — *see* Subluxation, radioulnar (joint), distal
　　metacarpal bone, proximal — *see* Subluxation, metacarpal (bone), proximal end
　　midcarpal — *see* Subluxation, midcarpal (joint)
　　radiocarpal joint — *see* Subluxation, radiocarpal (joint)
　　recurrent — *see* Dislocation, recurrent, wrist
　　specified site NEC S63.09- ☑
　　ulna — *see* Subluxation, ulna, distal end
Submaxillary — *see* condition

Submersion (fatal) (nonfatal) T75.1 ☑
Submucous — see condition
Subnormal, subnormality
  accommodation (old age) H52.4
  mental — see Disability, intellectual
  temperature (accidental) T68 ☑
Subphrenic — see condition
Subscapular nerve — see condition
Subseptus uterus Q51.28
Subsiding appendicitis K36
Substance (other psychoactive) **-induced**
  anxiety disorder F19.980
  bipolar and related disorder F19.94
  delirium F19.921
  depressive disorder F19.94
  major neurocognitive disorder F19.97
  mild neurocognitive disorder F19.988
  obsessive-compulsive and related disorder F19.988
  psychotic disorder F19.959
  sexual dysfunction F19.981
  sleep disorder F19.982
Substernal thyroid E04.9
  congenital Q89.2
Substitution disorder F44.9
Subtentorial — see condition
Subthyroidism (acquired) — see also Hypothyroidism
  congenital E03.1
Succenturiate placenta O43.19- ☑
Sucking thumb, child (excessive) F98.8
Sudamen, sudamina L74.1
Sudanese kala-azar B55.0
Sudden
  hearing loss — see Deafness, sudden
  heart failure — see Failure, heart
Sudeck's atrophy, disease, or syndrome — see Algoneurodystrophy
Suffocation — see Asphyxia, traumatic
Sugar
  blood
    high (transient) R73.9
    low (transient) E16.2
  in urine R81
Suicide, suicidal (attempted) T14.91 ☑
  by poisoning — see Table of Drugs and Chemicals
  history of (personal) Z91.5
    in family Z81.8
  ideation — see Ideation, suicidal
  risk
    meaning personal history of attempted suicide Z91.5
    meaning suicidal ideation — see Ideation, suicidal
  tendencies
    meaning personal history of attempted suicide Z91.5
    meaning suicidal ideation — see Ideation, suicidal
  trauma — see nature of injury by site
Suipestifer infection — see Infection, salmonella
Sulfhemoglobinemia, sulphemoglobinemia (acquired) (with methemoglobinemia) D74.8
Sumatran mite fever A75.3
Summer — see condition
Sunburn L55.9
  due to
    tanning bed (acute) L56.8
      chronic L57.8
    ultraviolet radiation (acute) L56.8
      chronic L57.8
  first degree L55.0
  second degree L55.1
  third degree L55.2
SUNCT (short lasting unilateral neuralgiform headache with conjunctival injection and tearing) G44.059
  intractable G44.051
  not intractable G44.059
Sundowning F05
Sunken acetabulum — see Derangement, joint, specified type NEC, hip
Sunstroke T67.01 ☑
  specified NEC T67.09 ☑
Superfecundation — see Pregnancy, multiple
Superfetation — see Pregnancy, multiple
Superinvolution (uterus) N85.8
Supernumerary (congenital)
  aortic cusps Q23.8
  auditory ossicles Q16.3
  bone Q79.8
  breast Q83.1
  carpal bones Q74.0
  cusps, heart valve NEC Q24.8

Supernumerary — continued
  cusps, heart valve — continued
    aortic Q23.8
    mitral Q23.2
    pulmonary Q22.3
  digit(s) Q69.9
  ear (lobule) Q17.0
  fallopian tube Q50.6
  finger Q69.0
  hymen Q52.4
  kidney Q63.0
  lacrimonasal duct Q10.6
  lobule (ear) Q17.0
  mitral cusps Q23.2
  muscle Q79.8
  nipple(s) Q83.3
  organ or site not listed — see Accessory
  ossicles, auditory Q16.3
  ovary Q50.31
  oviduct Q50.6
  pulmonary, pulmonic cusps Q22.3
  rib Q76.6
    cervical or first (syndrome) Q76.5
  roots (of teeth) K00.2
  spleen Q89.09
  tarsal bones Q74.2
  teeth K00.1
  testis Q55.29
  thumb Q69.1
  toe Q69.2
  uterus Q51.28
  vagina Q52.1 ☑
  vertebra Q76.49
Supervision (of)
  contraceptive — see Prescription, contraceptives
  dietary (for) Z71.3
    allergy (food) Z71.3
    colitis Z71.3
    diabetes mellitus Z71.3
    food allergy or intolerance Z71.3
    gastritis Z71.3
    hypercholesterolemia Z71.3
    hypoglycemia Z71.3
    intolerance (food) Z71.3
    obesity Z71.3
    specified NEC Z71.3
  healthy infant or child Z76.2
    foundling Z76.1
  high-risk pregnancy — see Pregnancy, complicated by, high, risk
  lactation Z39.1
  pregnancy — see Pregnancy, supervision of
Supplemental teeth K00.1
Suppression
  binocular vision H53.34
  lactation O92.5
  menstruation N94.89
  ovarian secretion E28.39
  renal N28.9
  urine, urinary secretion R34
Suppuration, suppurative — see also condition
  accessory sinus (chronic) — see Sinusitis
  adrenal gland
  antrum (chronic) — see Sinusitis, maxillary
  bladder — see Cystitis
  brain G06.0
    sequelae G09
  breast N61.1
    puerperal, postpartum or gestational — see Mastitis, obstetric, purulent
  dental periosteum M27.3
  ear (middle) — see also Otitis, media
    external NEC — see Otitis, externa, infective
    internal — see subcategory H83.0 ☑
  ethmoidal (chronic) (sinus) — see Sinusitis, ethmoidal
  fallopian tube — see Salpingo-oophoritis
  frontal (chronic) (sinus) — see Sinusitis, frontal
  gallbladder (acute) K81.0
  gum K05.20
    generalized — see Periodontitis, aggressive, generalized
    localized — see Periodontitis, aggressive, localized
  intracranial G06.0
  joint — see Arthritis, pyogenic or pyemic
  labyrinthine — see subcategory H83.0 ☑
  lung — see Abscess, lung
  mammary gland N61.1
    puerperal, postpartum O91.12

Suppuration, suppurative — continued
  mammary gland — continued
    puerperal, postpartum — continued
      associated with lactation O91.13
  maxilla, maxillary M27.2
    sinus (chronic) — see Sinusitis, maxillary
  muscle — see Myositis, infective
  nasal sinus (chronic) — see Sinusitis
  pancreas, acute — see also Pancreatitis, acute K85.8
  parotid gland — see Sialoadenitis
  pelvis, pelvic
    female — see Disease, pelvis, inflammatory
    male K65.0
  pericranial — see Osteomyelitis
  salivary duct or gland (any) — see Sialoadenitis
  sinus (accessory) (chronic) (nasal) — see Sinusitis
  sphenoidal sinus (chronic) — see Sinusitis, sphenoidal
  thymus (gland) E32.1
  thyroid (gland) E06.0
  tonsil — see Tonsillitis
  uterus — see Endometritis
Supraeruption of tooth (teeth) M26.34
Supraglottitis J04.30
  with obstruction J04.31
Suprarenal (gland) — see condition
Suprascapular nerve — see condition
Suprasellar — see condition
Surfer's knots or nodules S89.8- ☑
Surgical
  emphysema T81.82 ☑
  procedures, complication or misadventure — see Complications, surgical procedures
  shock T81.10 ☑
Surveillance (of) (for) — see also Observation
  alcohol abuse Z71.41
  contraceptive — see Prescription, contraceptives
  dietary Z71.3
  drug abuse Z71.51
Susceptibility to disease, genetic Z15.89
  malignant neoplasm Z15.09
    breast Z15.01
    endometrium Z15.04
    ovary Z15.02
    prostate Z15.03
    specified NEC Z15.09
  multiple endocrine neoplasia Z15.81
Suspected condition, ruled out — see also Observation, suspected
  amniotic cavity and membrane Z03.71
  cervical shortening Z03.75
  fetal anomaly Z03.73
  fetal growth Z03.74
  maternal and fetal conditions NEC Z03.79
  newborn — see also Observation, newborn, suspected condition ruled out Z05.9
  oligohydramnios Z03.71
  placental problem Z03.72
  polyhydramnios Z03.71
Suspended uterus
  in pregnancy or childbirth — see Pregnancy, complicated by, abnormal uterus
Sutton's nevus D22.9
Suture
  burst (in operation wound) T81.31 ☑
    external operation wound T81.31 ☑
    internal operation wound T81.32 ☑
  inadvertently left in operation wound — see Foreign body, accidentally left during a procedure
  removal Z48.02
Swab inadvertently left in operation wound — see Foreign body, accidentally left during a procedure
Swallowed, swallowing
  difficulty — see Dysphagia
  foreign body — see Foreign body, alimentary tract
Swan-neck deformity (finger) — see Deformity, finger, swan-neck
Swearing, compulsive F42.8
  in Gilles de la Tourette's syndrome F95.2
Sweat, sweats
  fetid L75.0
  night R61
Sweating, excessive R61
Sweeley-Klionsky disease E75.21
Sweet's disease or dermatosis L98.2
Swelling (of) R60.9
  abdomen, abdominal (not referable to any particular organ) — see Mass, abdominal

☑ **Additional Character Required — Refer to the Tabular List for Character Selection**   ▽ Subterms under main terms may continue to next column or page

Swelling — *continued*
- ankle — *see* Effusion, joint, ankle
- arm M79.89
    - forearm M79.89
- breast — *see also* Lump, breast N63.0
- Calabar B74.3
- cervical gland R59.0
- chest, localized R22.2
- ear H93.8- ☑
- extremity (lower) (upper) — *see* Disorder, soft tissue, specified type NEC
- finger M79.89
- foot M79.89
- glands R59.9
    - generalized R59.1
    - localized R59.0
- hand M79.89
- head (localized) R22.0
- inflammatory — *see* Inflammation
- intra-abdominal — *see* Mass, abdominal
- joint — *see* Effusion, joint
- leg M79.89
    - lower M79.89
- limb — *see* Disorder, soft tissue, specified type NEC
- localized (skin) R22.9
    - chest R22.2
    - head R22.0
    - limb
        - lower — *see* Mass, localized, limb, lower
        - upper — *see* Mass, localized, limb, upper
    - neck R22.1
    - trunk R22.2
- neck (localized) R22.1
- pelvic — *see* Mass, abdominal
- scrotum N50.89
- splenic — *see* Splenomegaly
- testis N50.89
- toe M79.89
- umbilical R19.09
- wandering, due to Gnathostoma (spinigerum) B83.1
- white — *see* Tuberculosis, arthritis

Swift (-Feer) disease
- overdose or wrong substance given or taken — *see* Table of Drugs and Chemicals, by drug, poisoning

Swimmer's
- cramp T75.1 ☑
- ear H60.33- ☑
- itch B65.3

Swimming in the head R42

Swollen — *see* Swelling

Swyer syndrome Q99.1

Sycosis L73.8
- barbae (not parasitic) L73.8
- contagiosa (mycotic) B35.0
- lupoides L73.8
- mycotic B35.0
- parasitic B35.0
- vulgaris L73.8

Sydenham's chorea — *see* Chorea, Sydenham's

Sylvatic yellow fever A95.0

Sylvest's disease B33.0

Symblepharon H11.23- ☑
- congenital Q10.3

Symond's syndrome G93.2

Sympathetic — *see* condition

Sympatheticotonia G90.8

Sympathicoblastoma
- specified site — *see* Neoplasm, malignant, by site
- unspecified site C74.90

Sympathogonioma — *see* Sympathicoblastoma

Symphalangy (fingers) (toes) Q70.9

Symptoms NEC R68.89
- breast NEC N64.59
- cold J00
- development NEC R63.8
- factitious, self-induced — *see* Disorder, factitious
- genital organs, female R10.2
- involving
    - abdomen NEC R19.8
    - appearance NEC R46.89
    - awareness R41.9
        - altered mental status R41.82
        - amnesia — *see* Amnesia
        - borderline intellectual functioning R41.83
        - coma — *see* Coma
        - disorientation R41.0
        - neurologic neglect syndrome R41.4
        - senile cognitive decline R41.81

Symptoms — *continued*
- involving — *continued*
    - awareness — *continued*
        - specified symptom NEC R41.89
    - behavior NEC R46.89
    - cardiovascular system NEC R09.89
    - chest NEC R09.89
    - circulatory system NEC R09.89
    - cognitive functions R41.9
        - altered mental status R41.82
        - amnesia — *see* Amnesia
        - borderline intellectual functioning R41.83
        - coma — *see* Coma
        - disorientation R41.0
        - neurologic neglect syndrome R41.4
        - senile cognitive decline R41.81
        - specified symptom NEC R41.89
    - development NEC R62.50
    - digestive system NEC R19.8
    - emotional state NEC R45.89
        - emotional lability R45.86
    - food and fluid intake R63.8
    - general perceptions and sensations R44.9
        - specified NEC R44.8
    - musculoskeletal system R29.91
        - specified NEC R29.898
    - nervous system R29.90
        - specified NEC R29.818
    - pelvis NEC R19.8
    - respiratory system NEC R09.89
    - skin and integument R23.9
    - urinary system R39.9
- menopausal N95.1
- metabolism NEC R63.8
- neurotic F48.8
- of infancy R68.19
- pelvis NEC, female R10.2
- skin and integument NEC R23.9
- subcutaneous tissue NEC R23.9
- viral cold J00

Sympus Q74.2

Syncephalus Q89.4

Synchondrosis
- abnormal (congenital) Q78.8
- ischiopubic M91.0

Synchysis (scintillans) (senile) (vitreous body) H43.89

Syncope (near) (pre-) R55
- anginosa I20.8
- bradycardia R00.1
- cardiac R55
- carotid sinus G90.01
- due to spinal (lumbar) puncture G97.1
- heart R55
- heat T67.1 ☑
- laryngeal R05
- psychogenic F48.8
- tussive R05
- vasoconstriction R55
- vasodepressor R55
- vasomotor R55
- vasovagal R55

Syndactylism, syndactyly Q70.9
- complex (with synostosis)
    - fingers Q70.0- ☑
    - toes Q70.2- ☑
- simple (without synostosis)
    - fingers Q70.1- ☑
    - toes Q70.3- ☑

Syndrome — *see also* Disease
- 5q minus NOS D46.C (*following* D46.2)
- 48,XXXX Q97.1
- 49,XXXXX Q97.1
- abdominal
    - acute R10.0
    - muscle deficiency Q79.4
- abnormal innervation H02.519
    - left H02.516
        - lower H02.515
        - upper H02.514
    - right H02.513
        - lower H02.512
        - upper H02.511
- abstinence, neonatal P96.1
- acid pulmonary aspiration, obstetric O74.0
- acquired immunodeficiency — *see* Human, immunodeficiency virus (HIV) disease
- acute abdominal R10.0
- acute respiratory distress (adult) (child) J80

Syndrome — *continued*
- acute respiratory distress — *continued*
    - idiopathic J84.114
- Adair-Dighton Q78.0
- Adams-Stokes (-Morgagni) I45.9
- adiposogenital E23.6
- adrenal
    - hemorrhage (meningococcal) A39.1
        - meningococcic A39.1
- adrenocortical — *see* Cushing's, syndrome
- adrenogenital E25.9
    - congenital, associated with enzyme deficiency E25.0
- afferent loop NEC K91.89
- Alagille's Q44.7
- alcohol withdrawal (without convulsions) — *see* Dependence, alcohol, with, withdrawal
- Alder's D72.0
- Aldrich (-Wiskott) D82.0
- alien hand R41.4
- Alport Q87.81
- alveolar hypoventilation E66.2
- alveolocapillary block J84.10
- amnesic, amnestic (confabulatory) (due to) — *see* Disorder, amnesic
- amyostatic (Wilson's disease) E83.01
- androgen insensitivity E34.50
    - complete E34.51
    - partial E34.52
- androgen resistance — *see also* Syndrome, androgen insensitivity E34.50
- Angelman Q93.51
- anginal — *see* Angina
- ankyloglossia superior Q38.1
- anterior
    - chest wall R07.89
    - cord G83.82
    - spinal artery G95.19
        - compression M47.019
            - cervical region M47.012
            - cervicothoracic region M47.013
            - lumbar region M47.016
            - occipito-atlanto-axial region M47.011
            - thoracic region M47.014
            - thoracolumbar region M47.015
    - tibial M76.81- ☑
- antibody deficiency D80.9
    - agammaglobulinemic D80.1
        - hereditary D80.0
    - congenital D80.0
    - hypogammaglobulinemic D80.1
        - hereditary D80.0
- anticardiolipin (-antibody) D68.61
- antidepressant discontinuation T43.205 ☑
- antiphospholipid (-antibody) D68.61
- aortic
    - arch M31.4
    - bifurcation I74.09
- aortomesenteric duodenum occlusion K31.5
- apical ballooning (transient left ventricular) I51.81
- arcuate ligament I77.4
- argentaffin, argintaffinoma E34.0
- Arnold-Chiari — *see* Arnold-Chiari disease
- Arrillaga-Ayerza I27.0
- arterial tortuosity Q87.82
- arteriovenous steal T82.898- ☑
- Asherman's N85.6
- aspiration, of newborn — *see* Aspiration, by substance, with pneumonia
    - meconium P24.01
- ataxia-telangiectasia G11.3
- auriculotemporal G50.8
- autoerythrocyte sensitization (Gardner-Diamond) D69.2
- autoimmune lymphoproliferative [ALPS] D89.82
- autoimmune polyglandular E31.0
- autoinflammatory M04.9
    - specified type NEC M04.8
- autosomal — *see* Abnormal, autosomes
- Avellis' G46.8
- Ayerza (-Arrillaga) I27.0
- Babinski-Nageotte G83.89
- Bakwin-Krida Q78.5
- bare lymphocyte D81.6
- Barré-Guillain G61.0
- Barré-Liéou M53.0
- Barrett's — *see* Barrett's, esophagus
- Barsony-Polgar K22.4
- Bársony-Teschendorf K22.4
- Barth E78.71

▽ Subterms under main terms may continue to next column or page   ☑ Additional Character Required — Refer to the Tabular List for Character Selection   303

Swelling — Syndrome

Syndrome — *continued*
Bartter's E26.81
basal cell nevus Q87.89
Basedow's E05.00
   with thyroid storm E05.01
basilar artery G45.0
Batten-Steinert G71.11
battered
   baby or child — *see* Maltreatment, child, physical abuse
   spouse — *see* Maltreatment, adult, physical abuse
Beals Q87.40
Beau's I51.5
Beck's I65.8
Benedikt's G46.3
Béquez César (-Steinbrinck-Chédiak-Higashi) E70.330
Bernhardt-Roth — *see* Meralgia paresthetica
Bernheim's — *see* Failure, heart, right
big spleen D73.1
bilateral polycystic ovarian E28.2
Bing-Horton's — *see* Horton's headache
Birt-Hogg-Dube syndrome Q87.89
Björck (-Thorsen) E34.0
black
   lung J60
   widow spider bite — *see* Toxicity, venom, spider, black widow
Blackfan-Diamond D61.01
Blau M04.8
blind loop K90.2
   congenital Q43.8
   postsurgical K91.2
blue sclera Q78.0
blue toe I75.02- ☑
Boder-Sedgewick G11.3
Boerhaave's K22.3
Borjeson Forssman Lehmann Q89.8
Bouillaud's I01.9
Bourneville (-Pringle) Q85.1
Bouveret (-Hoffman) I47.9
brachial plexus G54.0
bradycardia-tachycardia I49.5
brain (nonpsychotic) F09
   with psychosis, psychotic reaction F09
   acute or subacute — *see* Delirium
   congenital — *see* Disability, intellectual
   organic F09
      post-traumatic (nonpsychotic) F07.81
         psychotic F09
      personality change F07.0
   postcontusional F07.81
   post-traumatic, nonpsychotic F07.81
   psycho-organic F09
   psychotic F06.8
brain stem stroke G46.3
Brandt's (acrodermatitis enteropathica) E83.2
broad ligament laceration N83.8
Brock's J98.11
bronze baby P83.88
Brown-Sequard G83.81
Brugada I49.8
bubbly lung P27.0
Buchem's M85.2
Budd-Chiari I82.0
bulbar (progressive) G12.22
Bürger-Grütz E78.3
Burke's K86.89
Burnett's (milk-alkali) E83.52
burning feet E53.9
Bywaters' T79.5 ☑
Call-Fleming I67.841
carbohydrate-deficient glycoprotein (CDGS) E77.8
carcinogenic thrombophlebitis I82.1
carcinoid E34.0
cardiac asthma I50.1
cardiacos negros I27.0
cardiofaciocutaneous Q87.89
cardiopulmonary-obesity E66.2
cardiorenal — *see* Hypertension, cardiorenal
cardiorespiratory distress (idiopathic), newborn P22.0
cardiovascular renal — *see* Hypertension, cardiorenal
carotid
   artery (hemispheric) (internal) G45.1
      body G90.01
      sinus G90.01
carpal tunnel G56.0- ☑
Cassidy (-Scholte) E34.0
cat cry Q93.4

Syndrome — *continued*
cat eye Q92.8
cauda equina G83.4
causalgia — *see* Causalgia
celiac K90.0
   artery compression I77.4
   axis I77.4
central pain G89.0
cerebellar
   hereditary G11.9
   stroke G46.4
cerebellomedullary malformation — *see* Spina bifida
cerebral
   artery
      anterior G46.1
      middle G46.0
      posterior G46.2
   gigantism E22.0
cervical (root) M53.1
   disc — *see* Disorder, disc, cervical, with neuritis
   fusion Q76.1
   posterior, sympathicus M53.0
   rib Q76.5
   sympathetic paralysis G90.2
cervicobrachial (diffuse) M53.1
cervicocranial M53.0
cervicodorsal outlet G54.2
cervicothoracic outlet G54.0
Céstan (-Raymond) I65.8
Charcot's (angina cruris) (intermittent claudication) I73.9
Charcot-Weiss-Baker G90.09
CHARGE Q89.8
Chédiak-Higashi (-Steinbrinck) E70.330
chest wall R07.1
Chiari's (hepatic vein thrombosis) I82.0
Chilaiditi's Q43.3
child maltreatment — *see* Maltreatment, child
chondrocostal junction M94.0
chondroectodermal dysplasia Q77.6
chromosome 4 short arm deletion Q93.3
chromosome 5 short arm deletion Q93.4
chronic
   infantile neurological, cutaneous and articular (CINCA) M04.2
   pain G89.4
      personality F68.8
Churg-Strauss M30.1
Clarke-Hadfield K86.89
Clerambault's automatism G93.89
Clouston's (hidrotic ectodermal dysplasia) Q82.4
clumsiness, clumsy child F82
cluster headache G44.009
   intractable G44.001
   not intractable G44.009
Coffin-Lowry Q89.8
cold injury (newborn) P80.0
combined immunity deficiency D81.9
compartment (deep) (posterior) (traumatic) T79.A0 ☑ (*following* T79.7)
   abdomen T79.A3 ☑ (*following* T79.7)
   lower extremity (hip, buttock, thigh, leg, foot, toes) T79.A2 ☑ (*following* T79.7)
   nontraumatic
      abdomen M79.A3 (*following* M79.7)
      lower extremity (hip, buttock, thigh, leg, foot, toes) M79.A2- ☑ (*following* M79.7)
      specified site NEC M79.A9 (*following* M79.7)
      upper extremity (shoulder, arm, forearm, wrist, hand, fingers) M79.A1- ☑ (*following* M79.7)
   postprocedural — *see* Syndrome, compartment, nontraumatic
   specified site NEC T79.A9 ☑ (*following* T79.7)
   upper extremity (shoulder, arm, forearm, wrist, hand, fingers) T79.A1 ☑ (*following* T79.7)
complex regional pain — *see* Syndrome, pain, complex regional
compression T79.5 ☑
   anterior spinal — *see* Syndrome, anterior, spinal artery, compression
   cauda equina G83.4
   celiac artery I77.4
   vertebral artery M47.029
      cervical region M47.022
      occipito-atlanto-axial region M47.021
concussion F07.81

Syndrome — *continued*
congenital
   affecting multiple systems NEC Q87.89
   central alveolar hypoventilation G47.35
   facial diplegia Q87.0
   muscular hypertrophy-cerebral Q87.89
   oculo-auriculovertebral Q87.0
   oculofacial diplegia (Moebius) Q87.0
   rubella (manifest) P35.0
congestion-fibrosis (pelvic), female N94.89
congestive dysmenorrhea N94.6
connective tissue M35.9
   overlap NEC M35.1
Conn's E26.01
conus medullaris G95.81
cord
   anterior G83.82
   posterior G83.83
coronary
   acute NEC I24.9
   insufficiency or intermediate I20.0
   slow flow I20.8
Costen's (complex) M26.69
costochondral junction M94.0
costoclavicular G54.0
costovertebral E22.0
Cowden Q85.8
craniovertebral M53.0
Creutzfeldt-Jakob — *see* Creutzfeldt-Jakob disease or syndrome
crib death R99
cricopharyngeal — *see* Dysphagia
cri-du-chat Q93.4
croup J05.0
CRPS I — *see* Syndrome, pain, complex regional I
crush T79.5 ☑
cryopyrin-associated periodic M04.2
cryptophthalmos Q87.0
cubital tunnel — *see* Lesion, nerve, ulnar
Curschmann (-Batten) (-Steinert) G71.11
Cushing's E24.9
   alcohol-induced E24.4
   due to
      alcohol
         drugs E24.2
      ectopic ACTH E24.3
      overproduction of pituitary ACTH E24.0
   drug-induced E24.2
   overdose or wrong substance given or taken — *see* Table of Drugs and Chemicals, by drug, poisoning
   pituitary-dependent E24.0
   specified type NEC E24.8
cystic duct stump K91.5
cytokine release D89.839
   grade 1 D89.831
   grade 2 D89.832
   grade 3 D89.833
   grade 4 D89.834
   grade 5 D89.835
Dana-Putnam D51.0
Danbolt (-Cross) (acrodermatitis enteropathica) E83.2
Dandy-Walker Q03.1
   with spina bifida Q07.01
Danlos' — *see also* Syndrome, Ehlers-Danlos Q79.60
De Quervain E34.51
de Toni-Fanconi (-Debré) E72.09
   with cystinosis E72.04
de Vivo syndrome E74.810
defibrination — *see also* Fibrinolysis
   with
      antepartum hemorrhage — *see* Hemorrhage, antepartum, with coagulation defect
      intrapartum hemorrhage — *see* Hemorrhage, complicating, delivery
   newborn P60
   postpartum O72.3
Degos' I77.89
Déjérine-Roussy G89.0
delayed sleep phase G47.21
demyelinating G37.9
dependence — *see* F10-F19 with fourth character .2
depersonalization (-derealization) F48.1
di George's D82.1
diabetes mellitus in newborn infant P70.2
diabetes mellitus-hypertension-nephrosis — *see* Diabetes, nephrosis
diabetes-nephrosis — *see* Diabetes, nephrosis

Syndrome — *continued*
  diabetic amyotrophy — *see* Diabetes, amyotrophy
  dialysis associated steal T82.898- ☑
  Diamond-Blackfan D61.01
  Diamond-Gardener D69.2
  DIC (diffuse or disseminated intravascular coagulopathy) D65
  Dighton's Q78.0
  disequilibrium E87.8
  Döhle body-panmyelopathic D72.0
  dorsolateral medullary G46.4
  double athetosis G80.3
  Down — *see also* Down syndrome Q90.9
  Dravet (intractable) G40.834
    with status epilepticus G40.833
    without status epilepticus G40.834
  Dresbach's (elliptocytosis) D58.1
  DRESS (drug rash with eosinophilia and systemic symptoms) D72.12
  Dressler's (postmyocardial infarction) I24.1
    postcardiotomy I97.0
  drug rash with eosinophilia and systemic symptoms (DRESS) D72.12
  drug withdrawal, infant of dependent mother P96.1
  dry eye H04.12- ☑
  due to abnormality
    chromosomal Q99.9
      sex
        female phenotype Q97.9
        male phenotype Q98.9
      specified NEC Q99.8
  dumping (postgastrectomy) K91.1
    nonsurgical K31.89
  Dupré's (meningism) R29.1
  dysmetabolic X E88.81
  dyspraxia, developmental F82
  Eagle-Barrett Q79.4
  Eaton-Lambert — *see* Syndrome, Lambert-Eaton
  Ebstein's Q22.5
  ectopic ACTH E24.3
  eczema-thrombocytopenia D82.0
  Eddowes' Q78.8
  effort (psychogenic) F45.8
  Ehlers-Danlos Q79.60
    classical (cEDS) (classical EDS) Q79.61
    hypermobile (hEDS) (hypermobile EDS) Q79.62
    specified NEC Q79.69
    vascular (vascular EDS) (vEDS) Q79.63
  Eisenmenger's I27.83
  Ekman's Q78.0
  electric feet E53.8
  Ellis-van Creveld Q77.6
  empty nest Z60.0
  endocrine-hypertensive E27.0
  entrapment — *see* Neuropathy, entrapment
  eosinophilia-myalgia M35.8
  epileptic — *see also* Epilepsy, by type
    absence G40.A09 (*following* G40.3)
      intractable G40.A19 (*following* G40.3)
        with status epilepticus G40.A11 (*following* G40.3)
        without status epilepticus G40.A19 (*following* G40.3)
      not intractable G40.A09 (*following* G40.3)
        with status epilepticus G40.A01 (*following* G40.3)
        without status epilepticus G40.A09 (*following* G40.3)
  Erdheim-Chester (ECD) E88.89
  Erdheim's E22.0
  erythrocyte fragmentation D59.4
  Evans D69.41
  exhaustion F48.8
  extrapyramidal G25.9
    specified NEC G25.89
  eye retraction — *see* Strabismus
  eyelid-malar-mandible Q87.0
  Faber's D50.9
  facet M47.89- ☑
  facial pain, paroxysmal G50.0
  Fallot's Q21.3
  familial cold autoinflammatory M04.2
  familial eczema-thrombocytopenia (Wiskott-Aldrich) D82.0
  Fanconi (-de Toni) (-Debré) E72.09
    with cystinosis E72.04
  Fanconi's (anemia) (congenital pancytopenia) D61.09

Syndrome — *continued*
  fatigue
    chronic R53.82
    psychogenic F48.8
  faulty bowel habit K59.39
  Feil-Klippel (brevicollis) Q76.1
  Felty's — *see* Felty's syndrome
  fertile eunuch E23.0
  fetal
    alcohol (dysmorphic) Q86.0
    hydantoin Q86.1
  Fiedler's I40.1
  first arch Q87.0
  fish odor E72.89
  Fisher's G61.0
  Fitzhugh-Curtis
    due to
      Chlamydia trachomatis A74.81
      Neisseria gonorrhoea (gonococcal peritonitis) A54.85
  Fitz's — *see also* Pancreatitis, acute K85.80
  Flajani (-Basedow) E05.00
    with thyroid storm E05.01
  flatback — *see* Flatback syndrome
  floppy
    baby P94.2
    iris (intraoperative) (IFIS) H21.81
    mitral valve I34.1
  flush E34.0
  Foix-Alajouanine G95.19
  Fong's Q87.2
  food protein-induced enterocolitis (FPIES) K52.21
  foramen magnum G93.5
  Foster-Kennedy H47.14- ☑
  Foville's (peduncular) G46.3
  fragile X Q99.2
  Franceschetti Q75.4
  Frey's
    auriculotemporal G50.8
    hyperhidrosis L74.52
  Friderichsen-Waterhouse A39.1
  Froin's G95.89
  frontal lobe F07.0
  Fukuhara E88.49
  functional
    bowel K59.9
    prepubertal castrate E29.1
  Gaisböck's D75.1
  ganglion (basal ganglia brain) G25.9
    geniculi G51.1
  Gardner-Diamond D69.2
  gastroesophageal
    junction K22.0
    laceration-hemorrhage K22.6
  gastrojejunal loop obstruction K91.89
  Gee-Herter-Heubner K90.0
  Gelineau's G47.419
    with cataplexy G47.411
  genito-anorectal A55
  Gerstmann-Sträussler-Scheinker (GSS) A81.82
  Gianotti-Crosti L44.4
  giant platelet (Bernard-Soulier) D69.1
  Gilles de la Tourette's F95.2
  Glass Q87.89
  Gleich's D72.118
  goiter-deafness E07.1
  Goldberg Q89.8
  Goldberg-Maxwell E34.51
  Good's D83.8
  Gopalan' (burning feet) E53.8
  Gorlin's Q87.89
  Gougerot-Blum L81.7
  Gouley's I31.1
  Gower's R55
  gray or grey (newborn) P93.0
    platelet D69.1
  Gubler-Millard G46.3
  Guillain-Barré (-Strohl) G61.0
  gustatory sweating G50.8
  Hadfield-Clarke K86.89
  hair tourniquet — *see* Constriction, external, by site
  Hamman's J98.19
  hand-foot L27.1
  hand-shoulder G90.8
  hantavirus (cardio)-pulmonary (HPS) (HCPS) B33.4
  happy puppet Q93.51
  Harada's H30.81- ☑
  Hayem-Faber D50.9
  headache NEC G44.89

Syndrome — *continued*
  headache — *continued*
    complicated NEC G44.59
  Heberden's I20.8
  Hedinger's E34.0
  Hegglin's D72.0
  HELLP (hemolysis, elevated liver enzymes and low platelet count) O14.2- ☑
    complicating
      childbirth O14.24
      puerperium O14.25
  hemolytic-uremic D59.3
  hemophagocytic, infection-associated D76.2
  Henoch-Schönlein D69.0
  hepatic flexure K59.89
  hepatopulmonary K76.81
  hepatorenal K76.7
    following delivery O90.4
    postoperative or postprocedural K91.83
    postpartum, puerperal O90.4
  hepatourologic K76.7
  Herter (-Gee) (nontropical sprue) K90.0
  Heubner-Herter K90.0
  Heyd's K76.7
  Hilger's G90.09
  histamine-like (fish poisoning) — *see* Poisoning, fish
  histiocytic D76.3
  histiocytosis NEC D76.3
  HIV infection, acute B20
  Hoffmann-Werdnig G12.0
  Hollander-Simons E88.1
  Hoppe-Goldflam G70.00
    with exacerbation (acute) G70.01
    in crisis G70.01
  Horner's G90.2
  hungry bone E83.81
  hunterian glossitis D51.0
  Hutchinson's triad A50.53
  hyperabduction G54.0
  hyperammonemia-hyperornithinemia-homocitrullinemia E72.4
  hypereosinophilic (HES) D72.119
    idiopathic (IHES) D72.110
    lymphocytic variant (LHES) D72.111
    specified NEC D72.118
  hyperimmunoglobulin D M04.1
  hyperimmunoglobulin E (IgE) D82.4
  hyperkalemic E87.5
  hyperkinetic — *see* Hyperkinesia
  hypermobility M35.7
  hypernatremia E87.0
  hyperosmolarity E87.0
  hyperperfusion G97.82
  hypersplenic D73.1
  hypertransfusion, newborn P61.1
  hyperventilation F45.8
  hyperviscosity (of serum)
    polycythemic D75.1
    sclerothymic D58.8
  hypoglycemic (familial) (neonatal) E16.2
  hypokalemic E87.6
  hyponatremic E87.1
  hypopituitarism E23.0
  hypoplastic left-heart Q23.4
  hypopotassemia E87.6
  hyposmolality E87.1
  hypotension, maternal O26.5- ☑
  hypothenar hammer I73.89
  hypoventilation, obesity (OHS) E66.2
  ICF (intravascular coagulation-fibrinolysis) D65
  idiopathic
    cardiorespiratory distress, newborn P22.0
    nephrotic (infantile) N04.9
  iliotibial band M76.3- ☑
  immobility, immobilization (paraplegic) M62.3
  immune reconstitution D89.3
  immune reconstitution inflammatory [IRIS] D89.3
  immunity deficiency, combined D81.9
  immunodeficiency
    acquired — *see* Human, immunodeficiency virus (HIV) disease
    combined D81.9
  impending coronary I20.0
  impingement, shoulder M75.4- ☑
  inappropriate secretion of antidiuretic hormone E22.2
  infant
    gestational diabetes P70.0
    of diabetic mother P70.1

Syndrome — *continued*
infantilism (pituitary) E23.0
inferior vena cava I87.1
inspissated bile (newborn) P59.1
institutional (childhood) F94.2
insufficient sleep F51.12
intermediate coronary (artery) I20.0
interspinous ligament — *see* Spondylopathy, specified NEC
intestinal
 carcinoid E34.0
 knot K56.2
intravascular coagulation-fibrinolysis (ICF) D65
iodine-deficiency, congenital E00.9
 type
 mixed E00.2
 myxedematous E00.1
 neurological E00.0
IRDS (idiopathic respiratory distress, newborn) P22.0
irritable
 bowel K58.9
 with
 constipation K58.1
 diarrhea K58.0
 mixed K58.2
 psychogenic F45.8
 specified NEC K58.8
 heart (psychogenic) F45.8
 weakness F48.8
ischemic
 bowel (transient) K55.9
 chronic K55.1
 due to mesenteric artery insufficiency K55.1
 steal T82.898 ☑
IVC (intravascular coagulopathy) D65
Ivemark's Q89.01
Jaccoud's — *see* Arthropathy, postrheumatic, chronic
Jackson's G83.89
Jakob-Creutzfeldt — *see* Creutzfeldt-Jakob disease or syndrome
jaw-winking Q07.8
Jervell-Lange-Nielsen I45.81
jet lag G47.25
Job's D71
Joseph-Diamond-Blackfan D61.01
jugular foramen G52.7
Kabuki Q89.8
Kanner's (autism) F84.0
Kartagener's Q89.3
Kelly's D50.1
Kimmelstiel-Wilson — *see* Diabetes, specified type, with Kimmelstiel-Wilson disease
Klein (e)-Levine G47.13
Klippel-Feil (brevicollis) Q76.1
Köhler-Pellegrini-Steida — *see* Bursitis, tibial collateral
König's K59.89
Korsakoff (-Wernicke) (nonalcoholic) F04
 alcoholic F10.26
Kostmann's D70.0
Krabbe's congenital muscle hypoplasia Q79.8
labyrinthine — *see* subcategory H83.2 ☑
lacunar NEC G46.7
Lambert-Eaton G70.80
 in
 neoplastic disease G73.1
 specified disease NEC G70.81
Landau-Kleffner — *see* Epilepsy, specified NEC
Larsen's Q74.8
lateral
 cutaneous nerve of thigh G57.1- ☑
 medullary G46.4
Launois' E22.0
lazy
 leukocyte D70.8
 posture M62.3
Lemiere I80.8
Lennox-Gastaut G40.812
 intractable G40.814
 with status epilepticus G40.813
 without status epilepticus G40.814
 not intractable G40.812
 with status epilepticus G40.811
 without status epilepticus G40.812
lenticular, progressive E83.01
Leopold-Levi's E05.90
Lev's I44.2
Lichtheim's D51.0
Li-Fraumeni Z15.01

Syndrome — *continued*
Lightwood's N25.89
Lignac (de Toni) (-Fanconi) (-Debré) E72.09
 with cystinosis E72.04
Likoff's I20.8
limbic epilepsy personality F07.0
liver-kidney K76.7
lobotomy F07.0
Löffler's J82.89
long arm 18 or 21 deletion Q93.89
long QT I45.81
Louis-Barré G11.3
low
 atmospheric pressure T70.29 ☑
 back M54.5
 output (cardiac) I50.9
lower radicular, newborn (birth injury) P14.8
Luetscher's (dehydration) E86.0
Lupus anticoagulant D68.62
Lutembacher's Q21.1
macrophage activation D76.1
 due to infection D76.2
magnesium-deficiency R29.3
Majeed M04.8
Mal de Debarquement R42
malabsorption K90.9
 postsurgical K91.2
malformation, congenital, due to
 alcohol Q86.0
 exogenous cause NEC Q86.8
 hydantoin Q86.1
 warfarin Q86.2
malignant
 carcinoid E34.0
 neuroleptic G21.0
Mallory-Weiss K22.6
mandibulofacial dysostosis Q75.4
manic-depressive — *see* Disorder, bipolar
maple-syrup-urine E71.0
Marable's I77.4
Marfan's Q87.40
 with
 cardiovascular manifestations Q87.418
 aortic dilation Q87.410
 ocular manifestations Q87.42
 skeletal manifestations Q87.43
Marie's (acromegaly) E22.0
mast cell activation — *see* Activation, mast cell
maternal hypotension — *see* Syndrome, hypotension, maternal
May (-Hegglin) D72.0
McArdle (-Schmidt) (-Pearson) E74.04
McQuarrie's E16.2
meconium plug (newborn) P76.0
median arcuate ligament I77.4
Meekeren-Ehlers-Danlos Q79.6 ☑
megavitamin-B6 E67.2
Meige G24.4
MELAS E88.41
Mendelson's O74.0
MERRF (myoclonic epilepsy associated with ragged-red fibers) E88.42
mesenteric
 artery (superior) K55.1
 vascular insufficiency K55.1
metabolic E88.81
metastatic carcinoid E34.0
micrognathia-glossoptosis Q87.0
midbrain NEC G93.89
middle lobe (lung) J98.19
middle radicular G54.0
migraine — *see also* Migraine G43.909
Mikulicz' K11.8
milk-alkali E83.52
Millard-Gubler G46.3
Miller-Dieker Q93.88
Miller-Fisher G61.0
Minkowski-Chauffard D58.0
Mirizzi's K83.1
MNGIE (Mitochondrial Neurogastrointestinal En-cephalopathy) E88.49
Möbius, ophthalmoplegic migraine — *see* Migraine, ophthalmoplegic
monofixation H50.42
Morel-Moore M85.2
Morel-Morgagni M85.2
Morgagni (-Morel) (-Stewart) M85.2
Morgagni-Adams-Stokes I45.9

Syndrome — *continued*
Mounier-Kuhn Q32.4
 with bronchiectasis J47.9
 with
 exacerbation (acute) J47.1
 lower respiratory infection J47.0
 acquired J98.09
 with bronchiectasis J47.9
 with
 exacerbation (acute) J47.1
 lower respiratory infection J47.0
Muckle-Wells M04.2
mucocutaneous lymph node (acute febrile) (MCLS) M30.3
multiple endocrine neoplasia (MEN) — *see* Neoplasia, endocrine, multiple (MEN)
multiple operations — *see* Disorder, factitious
myasthenic G70.9
 in
 diabetes mellitus — *see* Diabetes, amyotrophy
 endocrine disease NEC E34.9 *[G73.3]*
 neoplastic disease — *see also* Neoplasm D49.9 *[G73.3]*
 thyrotoxicosis (hyperthyroidism) E05.90 *[G73.3]*
 with thyroid storm E05.91 *[G73.3]*
myelodysplastic D46.9
 with
 5q deletion D46.C (*following* D46.2)
 isolated del (5q) chromosomal abnormality D46.C (*following* D46.2)
 multilineage dysplasia D46.A (*following* D46.2)
 with ringed sideroblasts D46.B (*following* D46.2)
 lesions, low grade D46.20
 specified NEC D46.Z (*following* D46.4)
myeloid hypereosinophilic D72.118
myelopathic pain G89.0
myeloproliferative (chronic) D47.1
myofascial pain M79.18
Naffziger's G54.0
nail patella Q87.2
NARP (Neuropathy, Ataxia and Retinitis pigmentosa) E88.49
neonatal abstinence P96.1
nephritic — *see also* Nephritis
 with edema — *see* Nephrosis
 acute N00.9
 chronic N03.9
 rapidly progressive N01.9
nephrotic (congenital) — *see also* Nephrosis N04.9
 with
 C3
 glomerulonephritis N04.A
 glomerulopathy N04.A
 with dense deposit disease N04.6
 dense deposit disease N04.6
 diffuse
 crescentic glomerulonephritis N04.7
 endocapillary proliferative glomerulonephritis N04.4
 membranous glomerulonephritis N04.2
 mesangial proliferative glomerulonephritis N04.3
 mesangiocapillary glomerulonephritis N04.5
 focal and segmental glomerular lesions N04.1
 minor glomerular abnormality N04.0
 specified morphological changes NEC N04.8
 diabetic — *see* Diabetes, nephrosis
neurologic neglect R41.4
Nezelof's D81.4
Nonne-Milroy-Meige Q82.0
Nothnagel's vasomotor acroparesthesia I73.89
obesity hypoventilation (OHS) E66.2
oculomotor H51.9
Ogilvie K59.81
ophthalmoplegia-cerebellar ataxia — *see* Strabismus, paralytic, third nerve
oral allergy T78.1 ☑
oral-facial-digital Q87.0
organic
 affective F06.30
 amnesic (not alcohol- or drug-induced) F04
 brain F09
 depressive F06.31
 hallucinosis F06.0
 personality F07.0
Ormond's N13.5
oro-facial-digital Q87.0

Syndrome — continued
- os trigonum Q68.8
- Osler-Weber-Rendu I78.0
- osteoporosis-osteomalacia M83.8
- Osterreicher-Turner Q87.2
- otolith — see subcategory H81.8 ☑
- oto-palatal-digital Q87.0
- outlet (thoracic) G54.0
- ovary
  - polycystic E28.2
  - resistant E28.39
  - sclerocystic E28.2
- Owren's D68.2
- Paget-Schroetter I82.890
- pain — see also Pain
  - complex regional I G90.50
    - lower limb G90.52- ☑
    - specified site NEC G90.59
    - upper limb G90.51- ☑
  - complex regional II — see Causalgia
- painful
  - bruising D69.2
  - feet E53.8
  - prostate N42.81
- paralysis agitans — see Parkinsonism
- paralytic G83.9
  - specified NEC G83.89
- Parinaud's H51.0
- parkinsonian — see Parkinsonism
- Parkinson's — see Parkinsonism
- paroxysmal facial pain G50.0
- Parry's E05.00
  - with thyroid storm E05.01
- Parsonage (-Aldren)-Turner G54.5
- patella clunk M25.86- ☑
- Paterson (-Brown) (-Kelly) D50.1
- pectoral girdle I77.89
- pectoralis minor I77.89
- pediatric autoimmune neuropsychiatric disorders associated with streptococcal infections (PANDAS) D89.89
- Pelger-Huet D72.0
- pellagra-cerebellar ataxia-renal aminoaciduria E72.02
- pellagroid E52
- Pellegrini-Stieda — see Bursitis, tibial collateral
- pelvic congestion-fibrosis, female N94.89
- penta X Q97.1
- peptic ulcer — see Ulcer, peptic
- perabduction I77.89
- periodic fever M04.1
- periodic fever, aphthous stomatitis, pharyngitis, and adenopathy [PFAPA] M04.8
- periodic headache, in adults and children — see Headache, periodic syndromes in adults and children
- periurethral fibrosis N13.5
- phantom limb (without pain) G54.7
  - with pain G54.6
- pharyngeal pouch D82.1
- Pick's — see Disease, Pick's
- Pickwickian E66.2
- PIE (pulmonary infiltration with eosinophilia) — see also Eosinophilia, pulmonary J82.89
- pigmentary pallidal degeneration (progressive) G23.0
- pineal E34.8
- pituitary E22.0
- placental transfusion — see Pregnancy, complicated by, placental transfusion syndromes
- plantar fascia M72.2
- plateau iris (post-iridectomy) (postprocedural) H21.82
- Plummer-Vinson D50.1
- pluricarential of infancy E40
- plurideficiency E40
- pluriglandular (compensatory) E31.8
  - autoimmune E31.0
- pneumatic hammer T75.21 ☑
- polyangiitis overlap M30.8
- polycarential of infancy E40
- polyglandular E31.8
  - autoimmune E31.0
- polysplenia Q89.09
- pontine NEC G93.89
- popliteal
  - artery entrapment I77.89
  - web Q87.89
- post chemoembolization — code to associated conditions
- post endometrial ablation N99.85

Syndrome — continued
- postcardiac injury
  - postcardiotomy I97.0
  - postmyocardial infarction I24.1
- postcardiotomy I97.0
- postcholecystectomy K91.5
- postcommissurotomy I97.0
- postconcussional F07.81
- postcontusional F07.81
- postencephalitic F07.89
- posterior
  - cervical sympathetic M53.0
  - cord G83.83
  - fossa compression G93.5
  - reversible encephalopathy (PRES) I67.83
- postgastrectomy (dumping) K91.1
- postgastric surgery K91.1
- postinfarction I24.1
- postlaminectomy NEC M96.1
- postleukotomy F07.0
- postmastectomy lymphedema I97.2
- postmyocardial infarction I24.1
- postoperative NEC T81.9 ☑
  - blind loop K90.2
- postpartum panhypopituitary (Sheehan) E23.0
- postpolio (myelitic) G14
- postthrombotic I87.009
  - with
    - inflammation I87.02- ☑
      - with ulcer I87.03- ☑
    - specified complication NEC I87.09- ☑
    - ulcer I87.01- ☑
      - with inflammation I87.03- ☑
  - asymptomatic I87.00- ☑
- postvagotomy K91.1
- postvalvulotomy I97.0
- postviral NEC G93.3
  - fatigue G93.3
- Potain's K31.0
- potassium intoxication E87.5
- Prader-Willi Q87.11
- Prader-Willi-like Q87.19
- precerebral artery (multiple) (bilateral) G45.2
- preinfarction I20.0
- preleukemic D46.9
- premature senility E34.8
- premenstrual dysphoric F32.81
- premenstrual tension N94.3
- Prinzmetal-Massumi R07.1
- prune belly Q79.4
- pseudo -Turner's Q87.19
- pseudocarpal tunnel (sublimis) — see Syndrome, carpal tunnel
- pseudoparalytica G70.00
  - with exacerbation (acute) G70.01
  - in crisis G70.01
- psycho-organic (nonpsychotic severity) F07.9
  - acute or subacute F05
  - depressive type F06.31
  - hallucinatory type F06.0
  - nonpsychotic severity F07.0
  - specified NEC F07.89
- pulmonary
  - arteriosclerosis I27.0
  - dysmaturity (Wilson-Mikity) P27.0
  - hypoperfusion (idiopathic) P22.0
  - renal (hemorrhagic) (Goodpasture's) M31.0
- pure
  - motor lacunar G46.5
  - sensory lacunar G46.6
- Putnam-Dana D51.0
- pyogenic arthritis, pyoderma gangrenosum, and acne [PAPA] M04.8
- pyramidopallidonigral G20
- pyriformis — see Lesion, nerve, sciatic
- QT interval prolongation I45.81
- radicular NEC — see Radiculopathy
  - upper limbs, newborn (birth injury) P14.3
- rapid time-zone change G47.25
- Rasmussen G04.81
- Raymond (-Céstan) I65.8
- Raynaud's I73.00
  - with gangrene I73.01
- RDS (respiratory distress syndrome, newborn) P22.0
- reactive airways dysfunction J68.3
- Refsum's G60.1
- Reifenstein E34.52

Syndrome — continued
- renal glomerulohyalinosis-diabetic — see Diabetes, nephrosis
- Rendu-Osler-Weber I78.0
- residual ovary N99.83
- resistant ovary E28.39
- respiratory
  - distress
    - acute J80
      - adult J80
      - child J80
      - idiopathic J84.114
    - newborn (idiopathic) (type I) P22.0
      - type II P22.1
- restless legs G25.81
- retinoblastoma (familial) C69.2 ☑
- retroperitoneal fibrosis N13.5
- retroviral seroconversion (acute) Z21
- Reye's G93.7
- Richter — see Leukemia, chronic lymphocytic, B-cell type
- Ridley's I50.1
- right
  - heart, hypoplastic Q22.6
  - ventricular obstruction — see Failure, heart, right
- Romano-Ward (prolonged QT interval) I45.81
- rotator cuff, shoulder — see also Tear, rotator cuff M75.10- ☑
- Rotes Quérol — see Hyperostosis, ankylosing
- Roth — see Meralgia paresthetica
- rubella (congenital) P35.0
- Ruvalcaba-Myhre-Smith E71.440
- Rytand-Lipsitch I44.2
- salt
  - depletion E87.1
    - due to heat NEC T67.8 ☑
      - causing heat exhaustion or prostration T67.4 ☑
  - low E87.1
- salt-losing N28.89
- SATB2-associated Q87.89
- Scaglietti-Dagnini E22.0
- scalenus anticus (anterior) G54.0
- scapulocostal — see Mononeuropathy, upper limb, specified site NEC
- scapuloperoneal G71.09
- schizophrenic, of childhood NEC F84.5
- Schnitzler D47.2
- Scholte's E34.0
- Schroeder's E27.0
- Schüller-Christian C96.5
- Schwachman's — see Syndrome, Shwachman's
- Schwartz (-Jampel) G71.13
- Schwartz-Bartter E22.2
- scimitar Q26.8
- sclerocystic ovary E28.2
- Seitelberger's G31.89
- septicemic adrenal hemorrhage A39.1
- seroconversion, retroviral (acute) Z21
- serous meningitis G93.2
- severe acute respiratory (SARS) J12.81
- shaken infant T74.4 ☑
- shock (traumatic) T79.4 ☑
  - kidney N17.0
    - following crush injury T79.5 ☑
  - toxic A48.3
- shock-lung J80
- Shone's — code to specific anomalies
- short
  - bowel K91.2
  - rib Q77.2
- shoulder-hand — see Algoneurodystrophy
- Shwachman's D70.4
- sicca — see Sicca syndrome
- sick
  - cell E87.1
  - sinus I49.5
- sick-euthyroid E07.81
- sideropenic D50.1
- Siemens' ectodermal dysplasia Q82.4
- Silfversköld's Q78.9
- Simons' E88.1
- sinus tarsi M25.57- ☑
- sinusitis-bronchiectasis-situs inversus Q89.3
- Sipple's E31.22
- sirenomelia Q87.2
- Slocumb's E27.0
- slow flow, coronary I20.8

Syndrome — Syndrome

Syndrome — *continued*
Sluder's G44.89
Smith-Magenis Q93.88
Sneddon-Wilkinson L13.1
Sotos' Q87.3
South African cardiomyopathy I42.8
spasmodic
upward movement, eyes H51.8
winking F95.8
Spen's I45.9
splenic
agenesis Q89.01
flexure K59.89
neutropenia D73.81
Spurway's Q78.0
staphylococcal scalded skin L00
steal
arteriovenous T82.898- ☑
ischemic T82.898- ☑
subclavian G45.8
Stein-Leventhal E28.2
Stein's E28.2
Stevens-Johnson syndrome L51.1
toxic epidermal necrolysis overlap L51.3
Stewart-Morel M85.2
Stickler Q89.8
stiff baby Q89.8
stiff man G25.82
Still-Felty — *see* Felty's syndrome
Stokes (-Adams) I45.9
stone heart I50.1
straight back, congenital Q76.49
subclavian steal G45.8
subcoracoid-pectoralis minor G54.0
subcostal nerve compression I77.89
subphrenic interposition Q43.3
superior
cerebellar artery I63.89
mesenteric artery K55.1
semi-circular canal dehiscence H83.8X- ☑
vena cava I87.1
supine hypotensive (maternal) — *see* Syndrome, hypotension, maternal
suprarenal cortical E27.0
supraspinatus — *see also* Tear, rotator cuff M75.10- ☑
Susac G93.49
swallowed blood P78.2
sweat retention L74.0
Swyer Q99.1
Symond's G93.2
sympathetic
cervical paralysis G90.2
pelvic, female N94.89
systemic inflammatory response (SIRS), of non-infectious origin (without organ dysfunction) R65.10
with acute organ dysfunction R65.11
tachycardia-bradycardia I49.5
takotsubo I51.81
TAR (thrombocytopenia with absent radius) Q87.2
tarsal tunnel G57.5- ☑
teething K00.7
tegmental G93.89
telangiectasic-pigmentation-cataract Q82.8
temporal pyramidal apex — *see* Otitis, media, suppurative, acute
temporomandibular joint-pain-dysfunction M26.62- ☑
Terry's — *see also* Myopia, degenerative H44.2- ☑
testicular feminization — *see also* Syndrome, androgen
insensitivity E34.51
thalamic pain (hyperesthetic) G89.0
thoracic outlet (compression) G54.0
Thorson-Björck E34.0
thrombocytopenia with absent radius (TAR) Q87.2
thyroid-adrenocortical insufficiency E31.0
tibial
anterior M76.81- ☑
posterior M76.82- ☑
Tietze's M94.0
time-zone (rapid) G47.25
Toni-Fanconi E72.09
with cystinosis E72.04
Touraine's Q79.8
tourniquet — *see* Constriction, external, by site
toxic shock A48.3
transient left ventricular apical ballooning I51.81
traumatic vasospastic T75.22 ☑
Treacher Collins Q75.4
triple X, female Q97.0

Syndrome — *continued*
trisomy Q92.9
13 Q91.7
meiotic nondisjunction Q91.4
mitotic nondisjunction Q91.5
mosaicism Q91.5
translocation Q91.6
18 Q91.3
meiotic nondisjunction Q91.0
mitotic nondisjunction Q91.1
mosaicism Q91.1
translocation Q91.2
20 (q)(p) Q92.8
21 Q90.9
meiotic nondisjunction Q90.0
mitotic nondisjunction Q90.1
mosaicism Q90.1
translocation Q90.2
22 Q92.8
tropical wet feet T69.0- ☑
Trousseau's I82.1
tumor lysis (following antineoplastic chemotherapy)
(spontaneous) NEC E88.3
tumor necrosis factor receptor associated periodic
(TRAPS) M04.1
Twiddler's (due to)
automatic implantable defibrillator T82.198 ☑
cardiac pacemaker T82.198 ☑
Unverricht (-Lundborg) — *see* Epilepsy, generalized,
idiopathic
upward gaze H51.8
uremia, chronic — *see also* Disease, kidney, chronic
N18.9
urethral N34.3
urethro-oculo-articular — *see* Reiter's disease
urohepatic K76.7
vago-hypoglossal G52.7
van Buchem's M85.2
van der Hoeve's Q78.0
vascular NEC in cerebrovascular disease G46.8
vasoconstriction, reversible cerebrovascular I67.841
vasomotor I73.9
vasospastic (traumatic) T75.22 ☑
vasovagal R55
VATER Q87.2
velo-cardio-facial Q93.81
vena cava (inferior) (superior) (obstruction) I87.1
vertebral
artery G45.0
compression — *see* Syndrome, anterior, spinal
artery, compression
steal G45.0
vertebro-basilar artery G45.0
vertebrogenic (pain) M54.89
vertiginous — *see* Disorder, vestibular function
Vinson-Plummer D50.1
virus B34.9
visceral larva migrans B83.0
visual disorientation H53.8
vitamin B6 deficiency E53.1
vitreal corneal H59.01- ☑
vitreous (touch) H59.01- ☑
Vogt-Koyanagi H20.82- ☑
Volkmann's T79.6
von Schroetter's I82.890
von Willebrand (-Jürgen) D68.0
Waldenström-Kjellberg D50.1
Wallenberg's G46.3
water retention E87.79
Waterhouse (-Friderichsen) A39.1
Weber-Gubler G46.3
Weber-Leyden G46.3
Weber's G46.3
Wegener's M31.30
with
kidney involvement M31.31
lung involvement M31.30
with kidney involvement M31.31
Weingarten's (tropical eosinophilia) J82.89
Weiss-Baker G90.09
Werdnig-Hoffman G12.0
Wermer's E31.21
Werner's E34.8
Wernicke-Korsakoff (nonalcoholic) F04
alcoholic F10.26
Westphal-Strümpell E83.01
West's — *see* Epilepsy, spasms

Syndrome — *continued*
wet
feet (maceration) (tropical) T69.0- ☑
lung, newborn P22.1
whiplash S13.4 ☑
whistling face Q87.0
Wilkie's K55.1
Wilkinson-Sneddon L13.1
Willebrand (-Jürgens) D68.0
Williams Q93.82
Wilson's (hepatolenticular degeneration) E83.01
Wiskott-Aldrich D82.0
withdrawal — *see* Withdrawal, state
drug
infant of dependent mother P96.1
therapeutic use, newborn P96.2
Woakes' (ethmoiditis) J33.1
Wright's (hyperabduction) G54.0
X I20.9
XXXX Q97.1
XXXXX Q97.1
XXXXY Q98.1
XXY Q98.0
Yao M04.8
yellow nail L60.5
Zahorsky's B08.5
Zellweger syndrome E71.510
Zellweger-like syndrome E71.541
Synechia (anterior) (iris) (posterior) (pupil) — *see also*
Adhesions, iris
intra-uterine (traumatic) N85.6
Synesthesia R20.8
Syngamiasis, syngamosis B83.3
Synodontia K00.2
Synorchidism, synorchism Q55.1
Synostosis (congenital) Q78.8
astragalo-scaphoid Q74.2
radioulnar Q74.0
Synovial sarcoma — *see* Neoplasm, connective tissue,
malignant
Synovioma (malignant) — *see also* Neoplasm, connectiv
tissue, malignant
benign — *see* Neoplasm, connective tissue, benign
Synoviosarcoma — *see* Neoplasm, connective tissue,
malignant
Synovitis — *see also* Tenosynovitis M65.9
crepitant
hand M70.0- ☑
wrist M70.03- ☑
gonococcal A54.49
gouty — *see* Gout
in (due to)
crystals M65.8- ☑
gonorrhea A54.49
syphilis (late) A52.78
use, overuse, pressure — *see* Disorder, soft tissue,
due to use
infective NEC — *see* Tenosynovitis, infective NEC
specified NEC — *see* Tenosynovitis, specified type NE
syphilitic A52.78
congenital (early) A50.02
toxic — *see* Synovitis, transient
transient M67.3- ☑
ankle M67.37- ☑
elbow M67.32- ☑
foot joint M67.37- ☑
hand joint M67.34- ☑
hip M67.35- ☑
knee M67.36- ☑
multiple site M67.39
pelvic region M67.35- ☑
shoulder M67.31- ☑
specified joint NEC M67.38
wrist M67.33- ☑
traumatic, current — *see* Sprain
tuberculous — *see* Tuberculosis, synovitis
villonodular (pigmented) M12.2- ☑
ankle M12.27- ☑
elbow M12.22- ☑
foot joint M12.27- ☑
hand joint M12.24- ☑
hip M12.25- ☑
knee M12.26- ☑
multiple site M12.29
pelvic region M12.25- ☑
shoulder M12.21- ☑
specified joint NEC M12.28

Synovitis — *continued*
  villonodular — *continued*
    vertebrae M12.28
    wrist M12.23- ☑
Syphilid A51.39
  congenital A50.06
    newborn A50.06
  tubercular (late) A52.79
Syphilis, syphilitic (acquired) A53.9
  abdomen (late) A52.79
  acoustic nerve A52.15
  adenopathy (secondary) A51.49
  adrenal (gland) (with cortical hypofunction) A52.79
  age under 2 years NOS — *see also* Syphilis, congenital,
      early
    acquired A51.9
  alopecia (secondary) A51.32
  anemia (late) A52.79 [D63.8]
  aneurysm (aorta) (ruptured) A52.01
    central nervous system A52.05
    congenital A50.54 [I79.0]
  anus (late) A52.74
    primary A51.1
    secondary A51.39
  aorta (arch) (abdominal) (thoracic) A52.02
    aneurysm A52.01
  aortic (insufficiency) (regurgitation) (stenosis) A52.03
    aneurysm A52.01
  arachnoid (adhesive) (cerebral) (spinal) A52.13
  asymptomatic — *see* Syphilis, latent
  ataxia (locomotor) A52.11
  atrophoderma maculatum A51.39
  auricular fibrillation A52.06
  bladder (late) A52.76
  bone A52.77
    secondary A51.46
  brain A52.17
  breast (late) A52.79
  bronchus (late) A52.72
  bubo (primary) A51.0
  bulbar palsy A52.19
  bursa (late) A52.78
  cardiac decompensation A52.06
  cardiovascular A52.00
  central nervous system (late) (recurrent) (relapse) (ter-
      tiary) A52.3
    with
      ataxia A52.11
      general paralysis A52.17
        juvenile A50.45
      paresis (general) A52.17
        juvenile A50.45
      tabes (dorsalis) A52.11
        juvenile A50.45
      taboparesis A52.17
        juvenile A50.45
    aneurysm A52.05
    congenital A50.40
    juvenile A50.40
    remission in (sustained) A52.3
    serology doubtful, negative, or positive A52.3
    specified nature or site NEC A52.19
    vascular A52.05
  cerebral A52.17
    meningovascular A52.13
    nerves (multiple palsies) A52.15
    sclerosis A52.17
    thrombosis A52.05
  cerebrospinal (tabetic type) A52.12
  cerebrovascular A52.05
  cervix (late) A52.76
  chancre (multiple) A51.0
    extragenital A51.2
    Rollet's A51.0
  Charcot's joint A52.16
  chorioretinitis A51.43
    congenital A50.01
    late A52.71
    prenatal A50.01
  choroiditis — *see* Syphilitic chorioretinitis
  choroidoretinitis — *see* Syphilitic chorioretinitis
  ciliary body (secondary) A51.43
    late A52.71
  colon (late) A52.74
  combined spinal sclerosis A52.11
  condyloma (latum) A51.31
  congenital A50.9

Syphilis, syphilitic — *continued*
  congenital — *continued*
    with
      paresis (general) A50.45
      tabes (dorsalis) A50.45
      taboparesis A50.45
    chorioretinitis, choroiditis A50.01 [H32]
    early, or less than 2 years after birth NEC A50.2
      with manifestations — *see* Syphilis, congenital,
          early, symptomatic
      latent (without manifestations) A50.1
        negative spinal fluid test A50.1
        serology positive A50.1
      symptomatic A50.09
        cutaneous A50.06
        mucocutaneous A50.07
        oculopathy A50.01
        osteochondropathy A50.02
        pharyngitis A50.03
        pneumonia A50.04
        rhinitis A50.05
        visceral A50.08
    interstitial keratitis A50.31
    juvenile neurosyphilis A50.45
    late, or 2 years or more after birth NEC A50.7
      chorioretinitis, choroiditis A50.32
      interstitial keratitis A50.31
      juvenile neurosyphilis A50.45
      latent (without manifestations) A50.6
        negative spinal fluid test A50.6
        serology positive A50.6
      symptomatic or with manifestations NEC A50.59
        arthropathy A50.55
        cardiovascular A50.54
        Clutton's joints A50.51
        Hutchinson's teeth A50.52
        Hutchinson's triad A50.53
        osteochondropathy A50.56
        saddle nose A50.57
  conjugal A53.9
    tabes A52.11
  conjunctiva (late) A52.71
  contact Z20.2
  cord bladder A52.19
  cornea, late A52.71
  coronary (artery) (sclerosis) A52.06
  coryza, congenital A50.05
  cranial nerve A52.15
    multiple palsies A52.15
  cutaneous — *see* Syphilis, skin
  dacryocystitis (late) A52.71
  degeneration, spinal cord A52.12
  dementia paralytica A52.17
    juvenilis A50.45
  destruction of bone A52.77
  dilatation, aorta A52.01
  due to blood transfusion A53.9
  dura mater A52.13
  ear A52.79
    inner A52.79
      nerve (eighth) A52.15
      neurorecurrence A52.15
  early A51.9
    cardiovascular A52.00
    central nervous system A52.3
    latent (without manifestations) (less than 2 years
        after infection) A51.5
      negative spinal fluid test A51.5
      serological relapse after treatment A51.5
      serology positive A51.5
    relapse (treated, untreated) A51.9
    skin A51.39
    symptomatic A51.9
      extragenital chancre A51.2
      primary, except extragenital chancre A51.0
      secondary — *see also* Syphilis, secondary A51.39
        relapse (treated, untreated) A51.49
    ulcer A51.39
  eighth nerve (neuritis) A52.15
  endemic A65
  endocarditis A52.03
    aortic A52.03
    pulmonary A52.03
  epididymis (late) A52.76
  epiglottis (late) A52.73
  epiphysitis (congenital) (early) A50.02
  episcleritis (late) A52.71
  esophagus A52.79
  eustachian tube A52.73

Syphilis, syphilitic — *continued*
  exposure to Z20.2
  eye A52.71
  eyelid (late) (with gumma) A52.71
  fallopian tube (late) A52.76
  fracture A52.77
  gallbladder (late) A52.74
  gastric (polyposis) (late) A52.74
  general A53.9
    paralysis A52.17
      juvenile A50.45
  genital (primary) A51.0
  glaucoma A52.71
  gumma NEC A52.79
    cardiovascular system A52.00
    central nervous system A52.3
    congenital A50.59
  heart (block) (decompensation) (disease) (failure)
      A52.06 [I52]
    valve NEC A52.03
  hemianesthesia A52.19
  hemianopsia A52.71
  hemiparesis A52.17
  hemiplegia A52.17
  hepatic artery A52.09
  hepatis A52.74
  hepatomegaly, congenital A50.08
  hereditaria tarda — *see* Syphilis, congenital, late
  hereditary — *see* Syphilis, congenital
  Hutchinson's teeth A50.52
  hyalitis A52.71
  inactive — *see* Syphilis, latent
  infantum — *see* Syphilis, congenital
  inherited — *see* Syphilis, congenital
  internal ear A52.79
  intestine (late) A52.74
  iris, iritis (secondary) A51.43
    late A52.71
  joint (late) A52.77
  keratitis (congenital) (interstitial) (late) A50.31
  kidney (late) A52.75
  lacrimal passages (late) A52.71
  larynx (late) A52.73
  late A52.9
    cardiovascular A52.00
    central nervous system A52.3
    kidney A52.75
    latent or 2 years or more after infection (without
        manifestations) A52.8
      negative spinal fluid test A52.8
      serology positive A52.8
    paresis A52.17
    specified site NEC A52.79
    symptomatic or with manifestations A52.79
    tabes A52.11
  latent A53.0
    with signs or symptoms — *code by* site and stage
        under Syphilis
    central nervous system A52.2
    date of infection unspecified A53.0
    early, or less than 2 years after infection A51.5
    follow-up of latent syphilis A53.0
      date of infection unspecified A53.0
      late, or 2 years or more after infection A52.8
    late, or 2 years or more after infection A52.8
    positive serology (only finding) A53.0
      date of infection unspecified A53.0
      early, or less than 2 years after infection A51.5
      late, or 2 years or more after infection A52.8
  lens (late) A52.71
  leukoderma A51.39
    late A52.79
  lienitis A52.79
  lip A51.39
    chancre (primary) A51.2
    late A52.79
  Lissauer's paralysis A52.17
  liver A52.74
  locomotor ataxia A52.11
  lung A52.72
  lymph gland (early) (secondary) A51.49
    late A52.79
  lymphadenitis (secondary) A51.49
  macular atrophy of skin A51.39
    striated A52.79
  mediastinum (late) A52.73
  meninges (adhesive) (brain) (spinal cord) A52.13
  meningitis A52.13

Syphilis, syphilitic — *continued*
  meningitis — *continued*
    acute (secondary) A51.41
    congenital A50.41
  meningoencephalitis A52.14
  meningovascular A52.13
    congenital A50.41
  mesarteritis A52.09
    brain A52.04
  middle ear A52.77
  mitral stenosis A52.03
  monoplegia A52.17
  mouth (secondary) A51.39
    late A52.79
  mucocutaneous (secondary) A51.39
    late A52.79
  mucous
    membrane (secondary) A51.39
      late A52.79
    patches A51.39
      congenital A50.07
  mulberry molars A50.52
  muscle A52.78
  myocardium A52.06
  nasal sinus (late) A52.73
  neonatorum — *see* Syphilis, congenital
  nephrotic syndrome (secondary) A51.44
  nerve palsy (any cranial nerve) A52.15
    multiple A52.15
  nervous system, central A52.3
  neuritis A52.15
    acoustic A52.15
  neurorecidive of retina A52.19
  neuroretinitis A52.19
  newborn — *see* Syphilis, congenital
  nodular superficial (late) A52.79
  nonvenereal A65
  nose (late) A52.73
    saddle back deformity A50.57
  occlusive arterial disease A52.09
  oculopathy A52.71
  ophthalmic (late) A52.71
  optic nerve (atrophy) (neuritis) (papilla) A52.15
  orbit (late) A52.71
  organic A53.9
  osseous (late) A52.77
  osteochondritis (congenital) (early) A50.02 *[M90.80]*
  osteoporosis A52.77
  ovary (late) A52.76
  oviduct (late) A52.76
  palate (late) A52.79
  pancreas (late) A52.74
  paralysis A52.17
    general A52.17
      juvenile A50.45
  paresis (general) A52.17
    juvenile A50.45
  paresthesia A52.19
  Parkinson's disease or syndrome A52.19
  paroxysmal tachycardia A52.06
  pemphigus (congenital) A50.06
  penis (chancre) A51.0
    late A52.76
  pericardium A52.06
  perichondritis, larynx (late) A52.73
  periosteum (late) A52.77
    congenital (early) A50.02 *[M90.80]*
    early (secondary) A51.46
  peripheral nerve A52.79
  petrous bone (late) A52.77
  pharynx (late) A52.73
    secondary A51.39
  pituitary (gland) A52.79
  pleura (late) A52.73
  pneumonia, white A50.04
  pontine lesion A52.17

Syphilis, syphilitic — *continued*
  portal vein A52.09
  primary A51.0
    anal A51.1
    and secondary — *see* Syphilis, secondary
    central nervous system A52.3
    extragenital chancre NEC A51.2
    fingers A51.2
    genital A51.0
    lip A51.2
    specified site NEC A51.2
    tonsils A51.2
  prostate (late) A52.76
  ptosis (eyelid) A52.71
  pulmonary (late) A52.72
    artery A52.09
  pyelonephritis (late) A52.75
  recently acquired, symptomatic A51.9
  rectum (late) A52.74
  respiratory tract (late) A52.73
  retina, late A52.71
  retrobulbar neuritis A52.15
  salpingitis A52.76
  sclera (late) A52.71
  sclerosis
    cerebral A52.17
    coronary A52.06
    multiple A52.11
  scotoma (central) A52.71
  scrotum (late) A52.76
  secondary (and primary) A51.49
    adenopathy A51.49
    anus A51.39
    bone A51.46
    chorioretinitis, choroiditis A51.43
    hepatitis A51.45
    liver A51.45
    lymphadenitis A51.49
    meningitis (acute) A51.41
    mouth A51.39
    mucous membranes A51.39
    periosteum, periostitis A51.46
    pharynx A51.39
    relapse (treated, untreated) A51.49
    skin A51.39
    specified form NEC A51.49
    tonsil A51.39
    ulcer A51.39
    viscera NEC A51.49
    vulva A51.39
  seminal vesicle (late) A52.76
  seronegative with signs or symptoms — *code by* site and stage under Syphilis
  seropositive
    with signs or symptoms — *code by* site and stage under Syphilis
    follow-up of latent syphilis — *see* Syphilis, latent
    only finding — *see* Syphilis, latent
  seventh nerve (paralysis) A52.15
  sinus, sinusitis (late) A52.73
  skeletal system A52.77
  skin (with ulceration) (early) (secondary) A51.39
    late or tertiary A52.79
  small intestine A52.74
  spastic spinal paralysis A52.17
  spermatic cord (late) A52.76
  spinal (cord) A52.12
  spleen A52.79
  splenomegaly A52.79
  spondylitis A52.77
  staphyloma A52.71
  stigmata (congenital) A50.59
  stomach A52.74
  synovium A52.78
  tabes dorsalis (late) A52.11
    juvenile A50.45

Syphilis, syphilitic — *continued*
  tabetic type A52.11
    juvenile A50.45
  taboparesis A52.17
    juvenile A50.45
  tachycardia A52.06
  tendon (late) A52.78
  tertiary A52.9
    with symptoms NEC A52.79
    cardiovascular A52.00
    central nervous system A52.3
    multiple NEC A52.79
    specified site NEC A52.79
  testis A52.76
  thorax A52.73
  throat A52.73
  thymus (gland) (late) A52.79
  thyroid (late) A52.79
  tongue (late) A52.79
  tonsil (lingual) (late) A52.73
    primary A51.2
    secondary A51.39
  trachea (late) A52.73
  tunica vaginalis (late) A52.76
  ulcer (any site) (early) (secondary) A51.39
    late A52.79
    perforating A52.79
      foot A52.11
  urethra (late) A52.76
  urogenital (late) A52.76
  uterus (late) A52.76
  uveal tract (secondary) A51.43
    late A52.71
  uveitis (secondary) A51.43
    late A52.71
  uvula (late) (perforated) A52.79
  vagina A51.0
    late A52.76
  valvulitis NEC A52.03
  vascular A52.00
    brain (cerebral) A52.05
  ventriculi A52.74
  vesicae urinariae (late) A52.76
  viscera (abdominal) (late) A52.74
    secondary A51.49
  vitreous (opacities) (late) A52.71
    hemorrhage A52.71
  vulva A51.0
    late A52.76
    secondary A51.39
Syphiloma A52.79
  cardiovascular system A52.00
  central nervous system A52.3
  circulatory system A52.00
  congenital A50.59
Syphilophobia F45.29
Syringadenoma — *see also* Neoplasm, skin, benign
  papillary — *see* Neoplasm, skin, benign
Syringobulbia G95.0
Syringocystadenoma — *see* Neoplasm, skin, benign
  papillary — *see* Neoplasm, skin, benign
Syringoma — *see also* Neoplasm, skin, benign
  chondroid — *see* Neoplasm, skin, benign
Syringomyelia G95.0
Syringomyelitis — *see* Encephalitis
Syringomyelocele — *see* Spina bifida
Syringopontia G95.0
System, systemic — *see also* condition
  disease, combined — *see* Degeneration, combined
  inflammatory response syndrome (SIRS) of non-infectious origin (without organ dysfunction) R65.10
    with acute organ dysfunction R65.11
  lupus erythematosus M32.9
    inhibitor present D68.62

T

Tabacism, tabacosis, tabagism — *see also* Poisoning, tobacco
  meaning dependence (without remission) F17.200
    with
      disorder F17.299
        in remission F17.211
        specified disorder NEC F17.298
        withdrawal F17.203
Tabardillo A75.9
  flea-borne A75.2
  louse-borne A75.0
Tabes, tabetic A52.10
  with
    central nervous system syphilis A52.10
    Charcot's joint A52.16
    cord bladder A52.19
    crisis, viscera (any) A52.19
    paralysis, general A52.17
    paresis (general) A52.17
    perforating ulcer (foot) A52.19
  arthropathy (Charcot) A52.16
  bladder A52.19
  bone A52.11
  cerebrospinal A52.12
  congenital A50.45
  conjugal A52.10
  dorsalis A52.11
    juvenile A50.49
  juvenile A50.49
  latent A52.19
  mesenterica A18.39
  paralysis, insane, general A52.17
  spasmodic A52.17
  syphilis (cerebrospinal) A52.12
Taboparalysis A52.17
Taboparesis (remission) A52.17
  juvenile A50.45
TAC (trigeminal autonomic cephalgia) **NEC** G44.099
  intractable G44.091
  not intractable G44.099
Tache noir S60.22- ☑
Tachyalimentation K91.2
Tachyarrhythmia, tachyrhythmia — *see* Tachycardia
Tachycardia R00.0
  atrial (paroxysmal) I47.1
  auricular I47.1
  AV nodal re-entry (re-entrant) I47.1
  junctional (paroxysmal) I47.1
  newborn P29.11
  nodal (paroxysmal) I47.1
  non-paroxysmal AV nodal I45.89
  paroxysmal (sustained) (nonsustained) I47.9
    with sinus bradycardia I49.5
    atrial (PAT) I47.1
    atrioventricular (AV) (re-entrant) I47.1
      psychogenic F54
    junctional I47.1
      ectopic I47.1
    nodal I47.1
    psychogenic (atrial) (supraventricular) (ventricular) F54
    supraventricular (sustained) I47.1
      psychogenic F54
    ventricular I47.2
      psychogenic F54
  psychogenic F45.8
  sick sinus I49.5
  sinoauricular NOS R00.0
    paroxysmal I47.1
  sinus [sinusal] NOS R00.0
    paroxysmal I47.1
  supraventricular I47.1
  ventricular (paroxysmal) (sustained) I47.2
    psychogenic F54
Tachygastria K31.89
Tachypnea R06.82
  hysterical F45.8
  newborn (idiopathic) (transitory) P22.1
  psychogenic F45.8
  transitory, of newborn P22.1
TACO (transfusion associated circulatory overload) E87.71
Taenia (infection) (infestation) B68.9
  diminuta B71.0
  echinococcal infestation B67.90
  mediocanellata B68.1

Taenia — *continued*
  nana B71.0
  saginata B68.1
  solium (intestinal form) B68.0
    larval form — *see* Cysticercosis
Taeniasis (intestine) — *see* Taenia
Tag (hypertrophied skin) (infected) L91.8
  adenoid J35.8
  anus K64.4
  hemorrhoidal K64.4
  hymen N89.8
  perineal N90.89
  preauricular Q17.0
  sentinel K64.4
  skin L91.8
    accessory (congenital) Q82.8
    anus K64.4
    congenital Q82.8
    preauricular Q17.0
  tonsil J35.8
  urethra, urethral N36.8
  vulva N90.89
Tahyna fever B33.8
Takahara's disease E80.3
Takayasu's disease or syndrome M31.4
Talaromycosis B48.4
Talcosis (pulmonary) J62.0
Talipes (congenital) Q66.89
  acquired, planus — *see* Deformity, limb, flat foot
  asymmetric Q66.89
  calcaneovalgus Q66.4- ☑
  calcaneovarus Q66.1- ☑
  calcaneus Q66.89
  cavus Q66.7- ☑
  equinovalgus Q66.6
  equinovarus Q66.0- ☑
  equinus Q66.89
  percavus Q66.7- ☑
  planovalgus Q66.6
  planus (acquired) (any degree) — *see also* Deformity, limb, flat foot
    congenital Q66.5- ☑
    due to rickets (sequelae) E64.3
  valgus Q66.6
  varus Q66.3- ☑
Tall stature, constitutional E34.4
Talma's disease M62.89
Talon noir S90.3- ☑
  hand S60.22- ☑
  heel S90.3- ☑
  toe S90.1- ☑
Tamponade, heart I31.4
Tanapox (virus disease) B08.71
Tangier disease E78.6
Tantrum, child problem F91.8
Tapeworm (infection) (infestation) — *see* Infestation, tapeworm
Tapia's syndrome G52.7
TAR (thrombocytopenia with absent radius) **syndrome** Q87.2
Tarral-Besnier disease L44.0
Tarsal tunnel syndrome — *see* Syndrome, tarsal tunnel
Tarsalgia — *see* Pain, limb, lower
Tarsitis (eyelid) H01.8
  syphilitic A52.71
  tuberculous A18.4
Tartar (teeth) (dental calculus) K03.6
Tattoo (mark) L81.8
Tauri's disease E74.09
Taurodontism K00.2
Taussig-Bing syndrome Q20.1
Taybi's syndrome Q87.2
Tay-Sachs amaurotic familial idiocy or disease E75.02
TBI (traumatic brain injury) S06.9 ☑
Teacher's node or nodule J38.2
Tear, torn (traumatic) — *see also* Laceration
  with abortion — *see* Abortion
  annular fibrosis M51.35
  anus, anal (sphincter) S31.831 ☑
    complicating delivery
      with third degree perineal laceration — *see also* Delivery, complicated, by, laceration, perineum, third degree O70.20
        with mucosa O70.3
      without third degree perineal laceration O70.4
    nontraumatic (healed) (old) K62.81

Tear, torn — *continued*
  articular cartilage, old — *see* Derangement, joint, articular cartilage, by site
  bladder
    with ectopic or molar pregnancy O08.6
    following ectopic or molar pregnancy O08.6
    obstetrical O71.5
    traumatic — *see* Injury, bladder
  bowel
    with ectopic or molar pregnancy O08.6
    following ectopic or molar pregnancy O08.6
    obstetrical trauma O71.5
  broad ligament
    with ectopic or molar pregnancy O08.6
    following ectopic or molar pregnancy O08.6
    obstetrical trauma O71.6
  bucket handle (knee) (meniscus) — *see* Tear, meniscus
  capsule, joint — *see* Sprain
  cartilage — *see also* Sprain
    articular, old — *see* Derangement, joint, articular cartilage, by site
  cervix
    with ectopic or molar pregnancy O08.6
    following ectopic or molar pregnancy O08.6
    obstetrical trauma (current) O71.3
    old N88.1
    traumatic — *see* Injury, uterus
  dural G97.41
    nontraumatic G96.11
  internal organ — *see* Injury, by site
  knee cartilage
    articular (current) S83.3- ☑
    old — *see* Derangement, knee, meniscus, due to old tear
  ligament — *see* Sprain
  meniscus (knee) (current injury) S83.209 ☑
    bucket-handle S83.20- ☑
    lateral
      bucket-handle S83.25- ☑
      complex S83.27- ☑
      peripheral S83.26- ☑
      specified type NEC S83.28- ☑
    medial
      bucket-handle S83.21- ☑
      complex S83.23- ☑
      peripheral S83.22- ☑
      specified type NEC S83.24- ☑
    old — *see* Derangement, knee, meniscus, due to old tear
    site other than knee — *code as* Sprain
    specified type NEC S83.20- ☑
  muscle — *see* Strain
  pelvic
    floor, complicating delivery O70.1
    organ NEC, obstetrical trauma O71.5
      with ectopic or molar pregnancy O08.6
      following ectopic or molar pregnancy O08.6
  perineal, secondary O90.1
  periurethral tissue, obstetrical trauma O71.82
    with ectopic or molar pregnancy O08.6
    following ectopic or molar pregnancy O08.6
  rectovaginal septum — *see* Laceration, vagina
  retina, retinal (without detachment) (horseshoe) — *see also* Break, retina, horseshoe
    with detachment — *see* Detachment, retina, with retinal, break
  rotator cuff (nontraumatic) M75.10- ☑
    complete M75.12- ☑
    incomplete M75.11- ☑
    traumatic S46.01- ☑
      capsule S43.42- ☑
  semilunar cartilage, knee — *see* Tear, meniscus
  supraspinatus (complete) (incomplete) (nontraumatic) — *see also* Tear, rotator cuff M75.10- ☑
  tendon — *see* Strain
  tentorial, at birth P10.4
  umbilical cord
    complicating delivery O69.89 ☑
  urethra
    with ectopic or molar pregnancy O08.6
    following ectopic or molar pregnancy O08.6
    obstetrical trauma O71.5
  uterus — *see* Injury, uterus
  vagina — *see* Laceration, vagina
  vessel, from catheter — *see* Puncture, accidental complicating surgery
  vulva, complicating delivery O70.0

Tear-stone — see Dacryolith
Teeth — see also condition
  grinding
    psychogenic F45.8
    sleep related G47.63
Teething (syndrome) K00.7
Telangiectasia, telangiectasis (verrucous) I78.1
  ataxic (cerebellar) (Louis-Bar) G11.3
  familial I78.0
  hemorrhagic, hereditary (congenital) (senile) I78.0
  hereditary, hemorrhagic (congenital) (senile) I78.0
  juxtafoveal H35.07- ☑
  macular H35.07- ☑
  macularis eruptiva perstans D47.01
  parafoveal H35.07- ☑
  retinal (idiopathic) (juxtafoveal) (macular) (parafoveal) H35.07- ☑
  spider I78.1
Telephone scatologia F65.89
Telescoped bowel or intestine K56.1
  congenital Q43.8
Temperature
  body, high (of unknown origin) R50.9
  cold, trauma from T69.9 ☑
    newborn P80.0
    specified effect NEC T69.8 ☑
Temple — see condition
Temporal — see condition
Temporomandibular joint pain-dysfunction syndrome M26.62- ☑
Temporosphenoidal — see condition
Tendency
  bleeding — see Defect, coagulation
  suicide
    meaning personal history of attempted suicide Z91.5
    meaning suicidal ideation — see Ideation, suicidal
  to fall R29.6
Tenderness, abdominal R10.819
  epigastric R10.816
  generalized R10.817
  left lower quadrant R10.814
  left upper quadrant R10.812
  periumbilic R10.815
  rebound R10.829
    epigastric R10.826
    generalized R10.827
    left lower quadrant R10.824
    left upper quadrant R10.822
    periumbilic R10.825
    right lower quadrant R10.823
    right upper quadrant R10.821
  right lower quadrant R10.813
  right upper quadrant R10.811
Tendinitis, tendonitis — see also Enthesopathy
  Achilles M76.6- ☑
  adhesive — see Tenosynovitis, specified type NEC
    shoulder — see Capsulitis, adhesive
  bicipital M75.2- ☑
  calcific M65.2- ☑
    ankle M65.27- ☑
    foot M65.27- ☑
    forearm M65.23- ☑
    hand M65.24- ☑
    lower leg M65.26- ☑
    multiple sites M65.29
    pelvic region M65.25- ☑
    shoulder M75.3- ☑
    specified site NEC M65.28
    thigh M65.25- ☑
    upper arm M65.22- ☑
  due to use, overuse, pressure — see also Disorder, soft tissue, due to use
    specified NEC — see Disorder, soft tissue, due to use, specified NEC
  gluteal M76.0- ☑
  patellar M76.5- ☑
  peroneal M76.7- ☑
  psoas M76.1- ☑
  tibial (posterior) M76.82- ☑
    anterior M76.81- ☑
  trochanteric — see Bursitis, hip, trochanteric
Tendon — see condition
Tendosynovitis — see Tenosynovitis
Tenesmus (rectal) R19.8
  vesical R30.1
Tennis elbow — see Epicondylitis, lateral
Tenonitis — see also Tenosynovitis

Tenonitis — continued
  eye (capsule) H05.04- ☑
Tenontosynovitis — see Tenosynovitis
Tenontothecitis — see Tenosynovitis
Tenophyte — see Disorder, synovium, specified type NEC
Tenosynovitis — see also Synovitis M65.9
  adhesive — see Tenosynovitis, specified type NEC
    shoulder — see Capsulitis, adhesive
  bicipital (calcifying) — see Tendinitis, bicipital
  gonococcal A54.49
  in (due to)
    crystals M65.8- ☑
    gonorrhea A54.49
    syphilis (late) A52.78
    use, overuse, pressure — see also Disorder, soft tissue, due to use
      specified NEC — see Disorder, soft tissue, due to use, specified NEC
  infective NEC M65.1- ☑
    ankle M65.17- ☑
    foot M65.17- ☑
    forearm M65.13- ☑
    hand M65.14- ☑
    lower leg M65.16- ☑
    multiple sites M65.19
    pelvic region M65.15- ☑
    shoulder region M65.11- ☑
    specified site NEC M65.18
    thigh M65.15- ☑
    upper arm M65.12- ☑
  radial styloid M65.4
  shoulder region M65.81- ☑
    adhesive — see Capsulitis, adhesive
  specified type NEC M65.88
    ankle M65.87- ☑
    foot M65.87- ☑
    forearm M65.83- ☑
    hand M65.84- ☑
    lower leg M65.86- ☑
    multiple sites M65.89
    pelvic region M65.85- ☑
    shoulder region M65.81- ☑
    specified site NEC M65.88
    thigh M65.85- ☑
    upper arm M65.82- ☑
  tuberculous — see Tuberculosis, tenosynovitis
Tenovaginitis — see Tenosynovitis
Tension
  arterial, high — see also Hypertension
    without diagnosis of hypertension R03.0
  headache G44.209
    intractable G44.201
    not intractable G44.209
  nervous R45.0
  pneumothorax J93.0
  premenstrual N94.3
  state (mental) F48.9
Tentorium — see condition
Teratencephalus Q89.8
Teratism Q89.7
Teratoblastoma (malignant) — see Neoplasm, malignant, by site
Teratocarcinoma — see also Neoplasm, malignant, by site
  liver C22.7
Teratoma (solid) — see also Neoplasm, uncertain behavior, by site
  with embryonal carcinoma, mixed — see Neoplasm, malignant, by site
  with malignant transformation — see Neoplasm, malignant, by site
  adult (cystic) — see Neoplasm, benign, by site
  benign — see Neoplasm, benign, by site
  combined with choriocarcinoma — see Neoplasm, malignant, by site
  cystic (adult) — see Neoplasm, benign, by site
  differentiated — see Neoplasm, benign, by site
  embryonal — see also Neoplasm, malignant, by site
    liver C22.7
  immature — see Neoplasm, malignant, by site
  liver C22.7
    adult, benign, cystic, differentiated type or mature D13.4
  malignant — see also Neoplasm, malignant, by site
    anaplastic — see Neoplasm, malignant, by site
    intermediate — see Neoplasm, malignant, by site

Teratoma — continued
  malignant — see also Neoplasm, malignant, by site — continued
    intermediate — see Neoplasm, malignant, by site — continued
      specified site — see Neoplasm, malignant, by site
      unspecified site C62.90
    undifferentiated — see Neoplasm, malignant, by site
  mature — see Neoplasm, uncertain behavior, by site
    malignant — see Neoplasm, by site, malignant, by site
  ovary D27.- ☑
    embryonal, immature or malignant C56- ☑
  solid — see Neoplasm, uncertain behavior, by site
  testis C62.9- ☑
    adult, benign, cystic, differentiated type or mature D29.2- ☑
    scrotal C62.1- ☑
    undescended C62.0- ☑
Termination
  anomalous — see also Malposition, congenital
    right pulmonary vein Q26.3
  pregnancy, elective Z33.2
Ternidens diminutus infestation B81.8
Ternidensiasis B81.8
Terror(s) night (child) F51.4
Terrorism, victim of Z65.4
Terry's syndrome — see also Myopia, degenerative H44.2- ☑
Tertiary — see condition
Test, tests, testing (for)
  adequacy (for dialysis)
    hemodialysis Z49.31
    peritoneal Z49.32
  blood pressure Z01.30
    abnormal reading — see Blood, pressure
  blood typing Z01.83
    Rh typing Z01.83
  blood-alcohol Z04.89
    positive — see Findings, abnormal, in blood
  blood-drug Z04.89
    positive — see Findings, abnormal, in blood
  cardiac pulse generator (battery) Z45.010
  fertility Z31.41
  genetic
    disease carrier status for procreative management
      female Z31.430
      male Z31.440
    male partner of patient with recurrent pregnancy loss Z31.441
    procreative management NEC
      female Z31.438
      male Z31.448
  hearing Z01.10
    with abnormal findings NEC Z01.118
    infant or child (over 28 days old) Z00.129
      with abnormal findings Z00.121
  HIV (human immunodeficiency virus)
    nonconclusive (in infants) R75
    positive Z21
    seropositive Z21
  immunity status Z01.84
  intelligence NEC Z01.89
  laboratory (as part of a general medical examination) Z00.00
    with abnormal finding Z00.01
    for medicolegal reason NEC Z04.89
  male partner of patient with recurrent pregnancy loss Z31.441
  Mantoux (for tuberculosis) Z11.1
    abnormal result R76.11
  pregnancy, positive first pregnancy — see Pregnancy, normal, first
  procreative Z31.49
    fertility Z31.41
  skin, diagnostic
    allergy Z01.82
      special screening examination — see Screening, by name of disease
    Mantoux Z11.1
    tuberculin Z11.1
  specified NEC Z01.89
  tuberculin Z11.1
    abnormal result R76.11
  vision Z01.00
    with abnormal findings Z01.01

est, tests, testing — *continued*
  vision — *continued*
    following failed vision screening Z01.020
      with abnormal findings Z01.021
    infant or child (over 28 days old) Z00.129
      with abnormal findings Z00.121
  Wassermann Z11.3
    positive — *see* Serology for syphilis, positive
esticle, testicular, testis — *see also* condition
  feminization syndrome — *see also* Syndrome, androgen insensitivity E34.51
  migrans Q55.29
etanus, tetanic (cephalic) (convulsions) A35
  with
    abortion A34
    ectopic or molar pregnancy O08.0
  following ectopic or molar pregnancy O08.0
  inoculation reaction (due to serum) — *see* Complications, vaccination
  neonatorum A33
  obstetrical A34
  puerperal, postpartum, childbirth A34
etany (due to) R29.0
  alkalosis E87.3
  associated with rickets E55.0
  convulsions R29.0
    hysterical F44.5
  functional (hysterical) F44.5
  hyperkinetic R29.0
    hysterical F44.5
  hyperpnea R06.4
    hysterical F44.5
    psychogenic F45.8
  hyperventilation — *see also* Hyperventilation R06.4
    hysterical F44.5
  neonatal (without calcium or magnesium deficiency) P71.3
  parathyroid (gland) E20.9
  parathyroprival E89.2
  post- (para)thyroidectomy E89.2
  postoperative E89.2
  pseudotetany R29.0
  psychogenic (conversion reaction) F44.5
etralogy of Fallot Q21.3
etraplegia (chronic) — *see also* Quadriplegia G82.50
hailand hemorrhagic fever A91
halassanemia — *see* Thalassemia
halassemia (anemia) (disease) D56.9
  with other hemoglobinopathy D56.8
  alpha (major) (severe) (triple gene defect) D56.0
    minor D56.3
    silent carrier D56.3
    trait D56.3
  beta (severe) D56.1
    homozygous D56.1
    major D56.1
    minor D56.3
    trait D56.3
  delta-beta (homozygous) D56.2
    minor D56.3
    trait D56.3
  dominant D56.8
  hemoglobin
    C D56.8
    E-beta D56.5
  intermedia D56.1
  major D56.1
  minor D56.3
  mixed D56.8
  sickle-cell — *see* Disease, sickle-cell, thalassemia
  specified type NEC D56.8
  trait D56.3
  variants D56.8
hanatophoric dwarfism or short stature Q77.1
haysen-Gee disease (nontropical sprue) K90.0
haysen's disease K90.0
hecoma D27- ☑
  luteinized D27- ☑
  malignant C56- ☑
helarche, premature E30.8
helaziasis B83.8
helitis N61.0
  puerperal, postpartum or gestational — *see* Infection, nipple
herapeutic — *see* condition

Therapy
  drug, long-term (current) (prophylactic)
    agents affecting estrogen receptors and estrogen levels NEC Z79.818
    anastrozole (Arimidex) Z79.811
    antibiotics Z79.2
      short-term use — *omit code*
    anticoagulants Z79.01
    anti-inflammatory Z79.1
    antiplatelet Z79.02
    antithrombotics Z79.02
    aromatase inhibitors Z79.811
    aspirin Z79.82
    birth control pill or patch Z79.3
    bisphosphonates Z79.83
    contraceptive, oral Z79.3
    drug, specified NEC Z79.899
    estrogen receptor downregulators Z79.818
    Evista Z79.810
    exemestane (Aromasin) Z79.811
    Fareston Z79.810
    fulvestrant (Faslodex) Z79.818
    gonadotropin-releasing hormone (GnRH) agonist Z79.818
    goserelin acetate (Zoladex) Z79.818
    hormone replacement Z79.890
    insulin Z79.4
    letrozole (Femara) Z79.811
    leuprolide acetate (leuprorelin) (Lupron) Z79.818
    megestrol acetate (Megace) Z79.818
    methadone
      for pain management Z79.891
      maintenance therapy F11.20
    Nolvadex Z79.810
    opiate analgesic Z79.891
    oral contraceptive Z79.3
    raloxifene (Evista) Z79.810
    selective estrogen receptor modulators (SERMs) Z79.810
    short term — *omit code*
    steroids
      inhaled Z79.51
      systemic Z79.52
    tamoxifen (Nolvadex) Z79.810
    toremifene (Fareston) Z79.810
Thermic — *see* condition
Thermography (abnormal) — *see also* Abnormal, diagnostic imaging R93.89
  breast R92.8
Thermoplegia T67.01 ☑
Thesaurismosis, glycogen — *see* Disease, glycogen storage
Thiamin deficiency E51.9
  specified NEC E51.8
Thiaminic deficiency with beriberi E51.11
Thibierge-Weissenbach syndrome — *see* Sclerosis, systemic
Thickening
  bone — *see* Hypertrophy, bone
  breast N64.59
  endometrium R93.89
  epidermal L85.9
    specified NEC L85.8
  hymen N89.6
  larynx J38.7
  nail L60.2
    congenital Q84.5
  periosteal — *see* Hypertrophy, bone
  pleura J92.9
    with asbestos J92.0
  skin R23.4
  subepiglottic J38.7
  tongue K14.8
  valve, heart — *see* Endocarditis
Thigh — *see* condition
Thinning vertebra — *see* Spondylopathy, specified NEC
Thirst, excessive R63.1
  due to deprivation of water T73.1 ☑
Thomsen disease G71.12
Thoracic — *see also* condition
  kidney Q63.2
  outlet syndrome G54.0
Thoracogastroschisis (congenital) Q79.8
Thoracopagus Q89.4
Thorax — *see* condition
Thorn's syndrome N28.89
Thorson-Björck syndrome E34.0
Threadworm (infection) (infestation) B80

Threatened
  abortion O20.0
    with subsequent abortion O03.9
  job loss, anxiety concerning Z56.2
  labor (without delivery) O47.9
    at or after 37 completed weeks of gestation O47.1
    before 37 completed weeks of gestation O47.0- ☑
  loss of job, anxiety concerning Z56.2
  miscarriage O20.0
  unemployment, anxiety concerning Z56.2
Three-day fever A93.1
Threshers' lung J67.0
Thrix annulata (congenital) Q84.1
Throat — *see* condition
Thrombasthenia (Glanzmann) (hemorrhagic) (hereditary) D69.1
Thromboangiitis I73.1
  obliterans (general) I73.1
    cerebral I67.89
    vessels
      brain I67.89
      spinal cord I67.89
Thromboarteritis — *see* Arteritis
Thromboasthenia (Glanzmann) (hemorrhagic) (hereditary) D69.1
Thrombocytasthenia (Glanzmann) D69.1
Thrombocythemia (essential) (hemorrhagic) (idiopathic) (primary) D47.3
Thrombocytopathy (dystrophic) (granulopenic) D69.1
Thrombocytopenia, thrombocytopenic D69.6
  with absent radius (TAR) Q87.2
  congenital D69.42
  dilutional D69.59
  due to
    (massive) blood transfusion D69.59
    drugs D69.59
    extracorporeal circulation of blood D69.59
    platelet alloimmunization D69.59
  essential D69.3
  heparin induced (HIT) D75.82
  hereditary D69.42
  idiopathic D69.3
  neonatal, transitory P61.0
    due to
      exchange transfusion P61.0
      idiopathic maternal thrombocytopenia P61.0
      isoimmunization P61.0
  primary NEC D69.49
    idiopathic D69.3
  puerperal, postpartum O72.3
  secondary D69.59
  transient neonatal P61.0
Thrombocytosis, essential D47.3
  primary D47.3
Thromboembolism — *see* Embolism
Thrombopathy (Bernard-Soulier) D69.1
  constitutional D68.0
  Willebrand-Jurgens D68.0
Thrombopenia — *see* Thrombocytopenia
Thrombophilia D68.59
  primary NEC D68.59
  secondary NEC D68.69
  specified NEC D68.69
Thrombophlebitis I80.9
  antepartum O22.2- ☑
    deep O22.3- ☑
    superficial O22.2- ☑
  calf muscular vein (NOS) I80.25- ☑
  cavernous (venous) sinus G08
    complicating pregnancy O22.5- ☑
    nonpyogenic I67.6
  cerebral (sinus) (vein) G08
    nonpyogenic I67.6
    sequelae G09
  due to implanted device — *see* Complications, by site and type, specified NEC
  during or resulting from a procedure NEC T81.72 ☑
  femoral vein (superficial) I80.1- ☑
  femoropopliteal vein I80.0- ☑
  gastrocnemial vein I80.25- ☑
  hepatic (vein) I80.8
  idiopathic, recurrent I82.1
  iliac vein (common) (external) (internal) I80.21- ☑
  iliofemoral I80.1- ☑
  intracranial venous sinus (any) G08
    nonpyogenic I67.6
    sequelae G09
  intraspinal venous sinuses and veins G08

▽ Subterms under main terms may continue to next column or page   ☑ Additional Character Required — Refer to the Tabular List for Character Selection   **313**

Test, tests, testing — Thrombophlebitis

Thrombophlebitis — *continued*
  intraspinal venous sinuses and veins — *continued*
    nonpyogenic G95.19
  lateral (venous) sinus G08
    nonpyogenic I67.6
  leg I80.3
    superficial I80.0- ☑
  longitudinal (venous) sinus G08
    nonpyogenic I67.6
  lower extremity I80.299
  migrans, migrating I82.1
  pelvic
    with ectopic or molar pregnancy O08.0
    following ectopic or molar pregnancy O08.0
    puerperal O87.1
  peroneal vein I80.24- ☑
  popliteal vein — *see* Phlebitis, leg, deep, popliteal
  portal (vein) K75.1
  postoperative T81.72 ☑
  pregnancy — *see* Thrombophlebitis, antepartum
  puerperal, postpartum, childbirth O87.0
    deep O87.1
    pelvic O87.1
    septic O86.81
    superficial O87.0
  saphenous (greater) (lesser) I80.0- ☑
  sinus (intracranial) G08
    nonpyogenic I67.6
  soleal vein I80.25- ☑
  specified site NEC I80.8
  tibial vein (anterior) (posterior) I80.23- ☑

Thrombosis, thrombotic (bland) (multiple) (progressive) (silent) (vessel) I82.90
  anal K64.5
  antepartum — *see* Thrombophlebitis, antepartum
  aorta, aortic I74.10
    abdominal I74.09
      saddle I74.01
    bifurcation I74.09
    saddle I74.01
    specified site NEC I74.19
    terminal I74.09
    thoracic I74.11
    valve — *see* Endocarditis, aortic
  apoplexy I63.3- ☑
  artery, arteries (postinfectional) I74.9
    auditory, internal — *see* Occlusion, artery, precerebral, specified NEC
    basilar — *see* Occlusion, artery, basilar
    carotid (common) (internal) — *see* Occlusion, artery, carotid
    cerebellar (anterior inferior) (posterior inferior) (superior) — *see* Occlusion, artery, cerebellar
    cerebral — *see* Occlusion, artery, cerebral
    choroidal (anterior) — *see* Occlusion, artery, precerebral, specified NEC
    communicating, posterior — *see* Occlusion, artery, precerebral, specified NEC
    coronary — *see also* Infarct, myocardium
      not resulting in infarction I24.0
    hepatic I74.8
    hypophyseal — *see* Occlusion, artery, precerebral, specified NEC
    iliac I74.5
    limb I74.4
      lower I74.3
      upper I74.2
    meningeal, anterior or posterior — *see* Occlusion, artery, cerebral, specified NEC
    mesenteric (with gangrene) — *see also* Infarct, intestine K55.069
    ophthalmic — *see* Occlusion, artery, retina
    pontine — *see* Occlusion, artery, precerebral, specified NEC
    precerebral — *see* Occlusion, artery, precerebral
    pulmonary (iatrogenic) — *see* Embolism, pulmonary
    renal N28.0
    retinal — *see* Occlusion, artery, retina
    spinal, anterior or posterior G95.11
    traumatic NEC T14.8 ☑
    vertebral — *see* Occlusion, artery, vertebral
  atrium, auricular — *see also* Infarct, myocardium
    following acute myocardial infarction (current complication) I23.6
    not resulting in infarction I51.3
    old I51.3
  basilar (artery) — *see* Occlusion, artery, basilar

Thrombosis, thrombotic — *continued*
  brain (artery) (stem) — *see also* Occlusion, artery, cerebral
    due to syphilis A52.05
    puerperal O99.43
    sinus — *see* Thrombosis, intracranial venous sinus
  capillary I78.8
  cardiac — *see also* Infarct, myocardium
    not resulting in infarction I51.3
    old I51.3
    valve — *see* Endocarditis
  carotid (artery) (common) (internal) — *see* Occlusion, artery, carotid
  cavernous (venous) sinus — *see* Thrombosis, intracranial venous sinus
  cerebellar artery (anterior inferior) (posterior inferior) (superior) I66.3
  cerebral (artery) — *see* Occlusion, artery, cerebral
  cerebrovenous sinus — *see also* Thrombosis, intracranial venous sinus
    puerperium O87.3
  chronic I82.91
  coronary (artery) (vein) — *see also* Infarct, myocardium
    not resulting in infarction I24.0
  corpus cavernosum N48.89
  cortical I66.9
  deep — *see* Embolism, vein, lower extremity
  due to device, implant or graft — *see also* Complications, by site and type, specified NEC T85.868 ☑
    arterial graft NEC T82.868 ☑
    breast (implant) T85.868 ☑
    catheter NEC T85.868 ☑
      dialysis (renal) T82.868 ☑
        intraperitoneal T85.868 ☑
      infusion NEC T82.868 ☑
        spinal (epidural) (subdural) T85.860 ☑
      urinary (indwelling) T83.86 ☑
    electronic (electrode) (pulse generator) (stimulator)
      bone T84.86 ☑
      cardiac T82.867 ☑
      nervous system (brain) (peripheral nerve) (spinal) T85.860 ☑
      urinary T83.86 ☑
    fixation, internal (orthopedic) NEC T84.86 ☑
    gastrointestinal (bile duct) (esophagus) T85.868 ☑
    genital NEC T83.86 ☑
    heart T82.867 ☑
    joint prosthesis T84.86 ☑
    ocular (corneal graft) (orbital implant) NEC T85.868 ☑
    orthopedic NEC T84.86 ☑
    specified NEC T85.868 ☑
    urinary NEC T83.86 ☑
    vascular NEC T82.868 ☑
    ventricular intracranial shunt T85.860 ☑
  during the puerperium — *see* Thrombosis, puerperal
  endocardial — *see also* Infarct, myocardium
    not resulting in infarction I51.3
  eye — *see* Occlusion, retina
  genital organ
    female NEC N94.89
      pregnancy — *see* Thrombophlebitis, antepartum
    male N50.1
  gestational — *see* Phlebopathy, gestational
  heart (chamber) — *see also* Infarct, myocardium
    not resulting in infarction I51.3
    old I51.3
  hepatic (vein) I82.0
    artery I74.8
  history (of) Z86.718
  intestine (with gangrene) — *see also* Infarct, intestine K55.069
  intracardiac NEC (apical) (atrial) (auricular) (ventricular) (old) I51.3
  intracranial (arterial) I66.9
    venous sinus (any) G08
      nonpyogenic origin I67.6
      puerperium O87.3
  intramural — *see also* Infarct, myocardium
    not resulting in infarction I51.3
    old I51.3
  intraspinal venous sinuses and veins G08
    nonpyogenic G95.19
  kidney (artery) N28.0
  lateral (venous) sinus — *see* Thrombosis, intracranial venous sinus
  leg — *see* Thrombosis, vein, lower extremity

Thrombosis, thrombotic — *continued*
  leg — *see* Thrombosis, vein, lower extremity — *continued*
    arterial I74.3
  liver (venous) I82.0
    artery I74.8
    portal vein I81
  longitudinal (venous) sinus — *see* Thrombosis, intracranial venous sinus
  lower limb — *see* Thrombosis, vein, lower extremity
  lung (iatrogenic) (postoperative) — *see* Embolism, pulmonary
  meninges (brain) (arterial) I66.8
  mesenteric (artery) (with gangrene) — *see also* Infarct, intestine K55.069
    vein (inferior) (superior) K55.0- ☑
  mitral I34.8
  mural — *see also* Infarct, myocardium
    due to syphilis A52.06
    not resulting in infarction I51.3
    old I51.3
  omentum (with gangrene) — *see also* Infarct, intestine K55.069
  ophthalmic — *see* Occlusion, retina
  pampiniform plexus (male) N50.1
  parietal — *see also* Infarct, myocardium
    not resulting in infarction I24.0
  penis, superficial vein N48.81
  perianal venous K64.5
  peripheral arteries I74.4
    upper I74.2
  personal history (of) Z86.718
  portal I81
    due to syphilis A52.09
  precerebral artery — *see* Occlusion, artery, precerebral
  puerperal, postpartum O87.0
    brain (artery) O99.43
      venous (sinus) O87.3
    cardiac O99.43
    cerebral (artery) O99.43
      venous (sinus) O87.3
    superficial O87.0
  pulmonary (artery) (iatrogenic) (postoperative) (vein) — *see* Embolism, pulmonary
  renal (artery) N28.0
    vein I82.3
  resulting from presence of device, implant or graft — *see* Complications, by site and type, specified NEC
  retina, retinal — *see* Occlusion, retina
  scrotum N50.1
  seminal vesicle N50.1
  sigmoid (venous) sinus — *see* Thrombosis, intracranial venous sinus
  sinus, intracranial (any) — *see* Thrombosis, intracranial venous sinus
  specified site NEC I82.890
    chronic I82.891
  spermatic cord N50.1
  spinal cord (arterial) G95.11
    due to syphilis A52.09
    pyogenic origin G06.1
  spleen, splenic D73.5
    artery I74.8
  testis N50.1
  traumatic NEC T14.8 ☑
  tricuspid I07.8
  tumor — *see* Neoplasm, unspecified behavior, by site
  tunica vaginalis N50.1
  umbilical cord (vessels), complicating delivery O69.5 ☑
  vas deferens N50.1
  vein (acute) I82.90
    antecubital I82.61- ☑
      chronic I82.71- ☑
    axillary I82.A1- ☑ (*following* I82.7)
      chronic I82.A2- ☑ (*following* I82.7)
    basilic I82.61- ☑
      chronic I82.71- ☑
    brachial I82.62- ☑
      chronic I82.72- ☑
    brachiocephalic (innominate) I82.290
      chronic I82.291
    cephalic I82.61- ☑
      chronic I82.71- ☑
    cerebral, nonpyogenic I67.6
    chronic I82.91
    deep (DVT) I82.40- ☑
      calf I82.4Z- ☑

☑ **Additional Character Required** — Refer to the Tabular List for Character Selection

▽ **Subterms under main terms may continue to next column or page**

Thrombosis, thrombotic — *continued*
  vein — *continued*
    deep — *continued*
      calf — *continued*
        chronic I82.5Z- ☑
        lower leg I82.4Z- ☑
          chronic I82.5Z- ☑
        thigh I82.4Y- ☑
          chronic I82.5Y- ☑
        upper leg I82.4Y ☑
          chronic I82.5Y- ☑
      femoral I82.41- ☑
        chronic I82.51- ☑
      iliac (iliofemoral) I82.42- ☑
        chronic I82.52- ☑
      innominate I82.290
        chronic I82.291
      internal jugular I82.C1- ☑ (*following* I82.7)
        chronic I82.C2- ☑ (*following* I82.7)
      lower extremity
        deep I82.40- ☑
          chronic I82.50- ☑
          specified NEC I82.49- ☑
            chronic NEC I82.59- ☑
        distal
          deep I82.4Z- ☑
        proximal
          deep I82.4Y- ☑
            chronic I82.5Y- ☑
        superficial I82.81- ☑
      perianal K64.5
      popliteal I82.43- ☑
        chronic I82.53- ☑
      radial I82.62- ☑
        chronic I82.72- ☑
      renal I82.3
      saphenous (greater) (lesser) I82.81- ☑
      specified NEC I82.890
        chronic NEC I82.891
      subclavian I82.B1- ☑ (*following* I82.7)
        chronic I82.B2- ☑ (*following* I82.7)
      thoracic NEC I82.290
        chronic I82.291
      tibial I82.44- ☑
        chronic I82.54- ☑
      ulnar I82.62- ☑
        chronic I82.72- ☑
      upper extremity I82.60- ☑
        chronic I82.70- ☑
        deep I82.62- ☑
          chronic I82.72- ☑
        superficial I82.61- ☑
          chronic I82.71- ☑
    vena cava
      inferior I82.220
        chronic I82.221
      superior I82.210
        chronic I82.211
    venous, perianal K64.5
    ventricle — *see also* Infarct, myocardium
      following acute myocardial infarction (current complication) I23.6
      not resulting in infarction I24.0
      old I51.3
Thrombus — *see* Thrombosis
Thrush — *see also* Candidiasis
  newborn P37.5
  oral B37.0
  vaginal B37.3
Thumb — *see also* condition
  sucking (child problem) F98.8
Thymitis E32.8
Thymoma — *see also* Neoplasm, thymus, by type
  malignant C37
  metaplastic C37
  microscopic D15.0
  sclerosing C37
  type A C37
  type AB C37
  type B1 C37
  type B2 C37
  type B3 C37
Thymus, thymic (gland) — *see* condition
Thyrocele — *see* Goiter
Thyroglossal — *see also* condition
  cyst Q89.2
  duct, persistent Q89.2

Thyroid (gland) (body) — *see also* condition
  hormone resistance E07.89
  lingual Q89.2
  nodule (cystic) (nontoxic) (single) E04.1
Thyroiditis E06.9
  acute (nonsuppurative) (pyogenic) (suppurative) E06.0
  autoimmune E06.3
  chronic (nonspecific) (sclerosing) E06.5
    with thyrotoxicosis, transient E06.2
    fibrous E06.5
    lymphadenoid E06.3
    lymphocytic E06.3
    lymphoid E06.3
  de Quervain's E06.1
  drug-induced E06.4
  fibrous (chronic) E06.5
  giant-cell (follicular) E06.1
  granulomatous (de Quervain) (subacute) E06.1
  Hashimoto's (struma lymphomatosa) E06.3
  iatrogenic E06.4
  ligneous E06.5
  lymphocytic (chronic) E06.3
  lymphoid E06.3
  lymphomatous E06.3
  nonsuppurative E06.1
  postpartum, puerperal O90.5
  pseudotuberculous E06.1
  pyogenic E06.0
  radiation E06.4
  Riedel's E06.5
  subacute (granulomatous) E06.1
  suppurative E06.0
  tuberculous A18.81
  viral E06.1
  woody E06.5
Thyrolingual duct, persistent Q89.2
Thyromegaly E01.0
Thyrotoxic
  crisis — *see* Thyrotoxicosis
  heart disease or failure — *see also* Thyrotoxicosis E05.90 [I43]
    with thyroid storm E05.91 [I43]
  storm — *see* Thyrotoxicosis
Thyrotoxicosis (recurrent) E05.90
  with
    goiter (diffuse) E05.00
      with thyroid storm E05.01
      adenomatous uninodular E05.10
        with thyroid storm E05.11
      multinodular E05.20
        with thyroid storm E05.21
      nodular E05.20
        with thyroid storm E05.21
      uninodular E05.10
        with thyroid storm E05.11
    infiltrative
      dermopathy E05.00
        with thyroid storm E05.01
      ophthalmopathy E05.00
        with thyroid storm E05.01
    single thyroid nodule E05.10
      with thyroid storm E05.11
    thyroid storm E05.91
  due to
    ectopic thyroid nodule or tissue E05.30
      with thyroid storm E05.31
    ingestion of (excessive) thyroid material E05.40
      with thyroid storm E05.41
    overproduction of thyroid-stimulating hormone E05.80
      with thyroid storm E05.81
    specified cause NEC E05.80
      with thyroid storm E05.81
  factitia E05.40
    with thyroid storm E05.41
  heart — *see also* Failure, heart, high-output E05.90 [I43]
    with thyroid storm — *see also* Failure, heart, high-output E05.91 [I43]
    failure — *see also* Failure, heart, high-output E05.90 [I43]
  neonatal (transient) P72.1
  transient with chronic thyroiditis E06.2
Tibia vara M92.51- ☑
Tic (disorder) F95.9
  breathing F95.8
  child problem F95.0
  compulsive F95.1
  de la Tourette F95.2

Tic — *continued*
  degenerative (generalized) (localized) G25.69
    facial G25.69
  disorder
    chronic
      motor F95.1
      vocal F95.1
    combined vocal and multiple motor F95.2
    transient F95.0
  douloureux G50.0
    atypical G50.1
    postherpetic, postzoster B02.22
  drug-induced G25.61
  eyelid F95.8
  habit F95.9
    chronic F95.1
    transient of childhood F95.0
  lid, transient of childhood F95.0
  motor-verbal F95.2
  occupational F48.8
  orbicularis F95.8
    transient of childhood F95.0
  organic origin G25.69
  postchoreic G25.69
  provisional F95.0
  psychogenic, compulsive F95.1
  salaam R25.8
  spasm (motor or vocal) F95.9
    chronic F95.1
    transient of childhood F95.0
  specified NEC F95.8
Tick-borne — *see* condition
Tietze's disease or syndrome M94.0
Tight, tightness
  anus K62.89
  chest R07.89
  fascia (lata) M62.89
  foreskin (congenital) N47.1
  hymen, hymenal ring N89.6
  introitus (acquired) (congenital) N89.6
  rectal sphincter K62.89
  tendon — *see* Short, tendon
  urethral sphincter N35.919
Tilting vertebra — *see* Dorsopathy, deforming, specified NEC
Timidity, child F93.8
Tinea (intersecta) (tarsi) B35.9
  amiantacea L44.8
  asbestina B35.0
  barbae B35.0
  beard B35.0
  black dot B35.0
  blanca B36.2
  capitis B35.0
  corporis B35.4
  cruris B35.6
  flava B36.0
  foot B35.3
  furfuracea B36.0
  imbricata (Tokelau) B35.5
  kerion B35.0
  manuum B35.2
  microsporic — *see* Dermatophytosis
  nigra B36.1
  nodosa — *see* Piedra
  pedis B35.3
  scalp B35.0
  specified NEC B35.8
  sycosis B35.0
  tonsurans B35.0
  trichophytic — *see* Dermatophytosis
  unguium B35.1
  versicolor B36.0
Tingling sensation (skin) R20.2
Tin-miner's lung J63.5
Tinnitus NOS H93.1- ☑
  audible H93.1- ☑
  aurium H93.1- ☑
  pulsatile H93.A- ☑
  subjective H93.1- ☑
Tipped tooth (teeth) M26.33
Tipping
  pelvis M95.5
    with disproportion (fetopelvic) O33.0
      causing obstructed labor O65.0
  tooth (teeth), fully erupted M26.33
Tiredness R53.83
Tissue — *see* condition

Tobacco (nicotine)
  abuse — *see* Tobacco, use
  dependence — *see* Dependence, drug, nicotine
  harmful use Z72.0
  heart — *see* Tobacco, toxic effect
  maternal use, affecting newborn P04.2
  toxic effect — *see* Table of Drugs and Chemicals, by
    substance, poisoning
    chewing tobacco — *see* Table of Drugs and Chemi-
      cals, by substance, poisoning
    cigarettes — *see* Table of Drugs and Chemicals, by
      substance, poisoning
  use Z72.0
    complicating
      childbirth O99.334
      pregnancy O99.33- ☑
      puerperium O99.335
    counseling and surveillance Z71.6
    history Z87.891
  withdrawal state — *see also* Dependence, drug, nico-
    tine F17.203
Tocopherol deficiency E56.0
Todd's
  cirrhosis K74.3
  paralysis (postepileptic) (transitory) G83.84
Toe — *see* condition
Toilet, artificial opening — *see* Attention to, artificial,
  opening
Tokelau (ringworm) B35.5
Tollwut — *see* Rabies
Tommaselli's disease R31.9
  correct substance properly administered — *see* Table
    of Drugs and Chemicals, by drug, adverse effect
  overdose or wrong substance given or taken — *see*
    Table of Drugs and Chemicals, by drug, poisoning
Tongue — *see also* condition
  tie Q38.1
Tonic pupil — *see* Anomaly, pupil, function, tonic pupil
Toni-Fanconi syndrome (cystinosis) E72.09
  with cystinosis E72.04
Tonsil — *see* condition
Tonsillitis (acute) (catarrhal) (croupous) (follicular) (gangrenous) (infective) (lacunar) (lingual) (malignant)
  (membranous) (parenchymatous) (phlegmonous)
  (pseudomembranous) (purulent) (septic) (subacute)
  (suppurative) (toxic) (ulcerative) (vesicular) (viral)
  J03.90
  chronic J35.01
    with adenoiditis J35.03
  diphtheritic A36.0
  hypertrophic J35.01
    with adenoiditis J35.03
  recurrent J03.91
  specified organism NEC J03.80
    recurrent J03.81
  staphylococcal J03.80
    recurrent J03.81
  streptococcal J03.00
    recurrent J03.01
  tuberculous A15.8
  Vincent's A69.1
Tooth, teeth — *see* condition
Toothache K08.89
Topagnosis R20.8
Tophi — *see* Gout, chronic
TORCH infection — *see* Infection, congenital
  without active infection P00.2
Torn — *see* Tear
Tornwaldt's cyst or disease J39.2
Torsion
  accessory tube — *see* Torsion, fallopian tube
  adnexa (female) — *see* Torsion, fallopian tube
  aorta, acquired I77.1
  appendix epididymis N44.04
  appendix testis N44.03
  bile duct (common) (hepatic) K83.8
    congenital Q44.5
  bowel, colon or intestine K56.2
  cervix — *see* Malposition, uterus
  cystic duct K82.8
  dystonia — *see* Dystonia, torsion
  epididymis (appendix) N44.04
  fallopian tube N83.52- ☑
    with ovary N83.53
  gallbladder K82.8
    congenital Q44.1
  hydatid of Morgagni
    female N83.52- ☑

Torsion — *continued*
  hydatid of Morgagni — *continued*
    male N44.03
  kidney (pedicle) (leading to infarction) N28.0
  Meckel's diverticulum (congenital) Q43.0
    malignant — *see* Table of Neoplasms, small intes-
      tine, malignant
  mesentery K56.2
  omentum K56.2
  organ or site, congenital NEC — *see* Anomaly, by site
  ovary (pedicle) N83.51- ☑
    with fallopian tube N83.53
    congenital Q50.2
  oviduct — *see* Torsion, fallopian tube
  penis (acquired) N48.82
    congenital Q55.63
  spasm — *see* Dystonia, torsion
  spermatic cord N44.02
    extravaginal N44.01
    intravaginal N44.02
  spleen D73.5
  testis, testicle N44.00
    appendix N44.03
  tibia — *see* Deformity, limb, specified type NEC, lower
    leg
  uterus — *see* Malposition, uterus
Torticollis (intermittent) (spastic) M43.6
  congenital (sternomastoid) Q68.0
  due to birth injury P15.8
  hysterical F44.4
  ocular R29.891
  psychogenic F45.8
    conversion reaction F44.4
  rheumatic M43.6
  rheumatoid M06.88
  spasmodic G24.3
  traumatic, current S13.4 ☑
Tortipelvis G24.1
Tortuous
  aortic arch Q25.46
  artery I77.1
  organ or site, congenital NEC — *see* Distortion
  retinal vessel, congenital Q14.1
  ureter N13.8
  urethra N36.8
  vein — *see* Varix
Torture, victim of Z65.4
Torula, torular (histolytica) (infection) — *see* Cryptococcosis
Torulosis — *see* Cryptococcosis
Torus (mandibularis) (palatinus) M27.0
  fracture — *see* Fracture, by site, torus
Touraine's syndrome Q79.8
Tourette's syndrome F95.2
Tourniquet syndrome — *see* Constriction, external, by
  site
Tower skull Q75.0
  with exophthalmos Q87.0
Toxemia R68.89
  bacterial — *see* Sepsis
  burn — *see* Burn
  eclamptic (with pre-existing hypertension) — *see*
    Eclampsia
  erysipelatous — *see* Erysipelas
  fatigue R68.89
  food — *see* Poisoning, food
  gastrointestinal K52.1
  intestinal K52.1
  kidney — *see* Uremia
  malarial — *see* Malaria
  myocardial — *see* Myocarditis, toxic
  of pregnancy — *see* Pre-eclampsia
  pre-eclamptic — *see* Pre-eclampsia
  small intestine K52.1
  staphylococcal, due to food A05.0
  stasis R68.89
  uremic — *see* Uremia
  urinary — *see* Uremia
Toxemica cerebropathia psychica (nonalcoholic) F04
  alcoholic — *see* Alcohol, amnestic disorder
Toxic (poisoning) — *see also* condition T65.91 ☑
  effect — *see* Table of Drugs and Chemicals, by sub-
    stance, poisoning
  shock syndrome A48.3
  thyroid (gland) — *see* Thyrotoxicosis
Toxicemia — *see* Toxemia

Toxicity — *see* Table of Drugs and Chemicals, by substance, poisoning
  fava bean D55.0
  food, noxious — *see* Poisoning, food
  from drug or nonmedicinal substance — *see* Table of
    Drugs and Chemicals, by drug
Toxicosis — *see also* Toxemia
  capillary, hemorrhagic D69.0
Toxinfection, gastrointestinal K52.1
Toxocariasis B83.0
Toxoplasma, toxoplasmosis (acquired) B58.9
  with
    hepatitis B58.1
    meningoencephalitis B58.2
    ocular involvement B58.00
    other organ involvement B58.89
    pneumonia, pneumonitis B58.3
  congenital (acute) (subacute) (chronic) P37.1
  maternal, manifest toxoplasmosis in infant (acute)
    (subacute) (chronic) P37.1
tPA (rtPA) **administation in a different facility within**
  the last 24 hours prior to admission to current
  facility Z92.82
Trabeculation, bladder N32.89
Trachea — *see* condition
Tracheitis (catarrhal) (infantile) (membranous) (plastic)
  (septal) (suppurative) (viral) J04.10
  with
    bronchitis (15 years of age and above) J40
      acute or subacute — *see* Bronchitis, acute
      chronic J42
      tuberculous NEC A15.5
      under 15 years of age J20.9
    laryngitis (acute) J04.2
      chronic J37.1
      tuberculous NEC A15.5
  acute J04.10
    with obstruction J04.11
  chronic J42
    with
      bronchitis (chronic) J42
      laryngitis (chronic) J37.1
  diphtheritic (membranous) A36.89
  due to external agent — *see* Inflammation, respiratory,
    upper, due to
  syphilitic A52.73
  tuberculous A15.5
Trachelitis (nonvenereal) — *see* Cervicitis
Tracheobronchial — *see* condition
Tracheobronchitis (15 years of age and above) — *see*
  also Bronchitis
  due to
    Bordetella bronchiseptica A37.80
      with pneumonia A37.81
    Francisella tularensis A21.8
Tracheobronchomegaly Q32.4
  with bronchiectasis J47.9
    with
      exacerbation (acute) J47.1
      lower respiratory infection J47.0
  acquired J98.09
    with bronchiectasis J47.9
      with
        exacerbation (acute) J47.1
        lower respiratory infection J47.0
Tracheobronchopneumonitis — *see* Pneumonia,
  broncho-
Tracheocele (external) (internal) J39.8
  congenital Q32.1
Tracheomalacia J39.8
  congenital Q32.0
Tracheopharyngitis (acute) J06.9
  chronic J42
  due to external agent — *see* Inflammation, respiratory,
    upper, due to
Tracheostenosis J39.8
Tracheostomy
  complication — *see* Complication, tracheostomy
  status Z93.0
    attention to Z43.0
    malfunctioning J95.03
Trachoma, trachomatous A71.9
  active (stage) A71.1
  contraction of conjunctiva A71.1
  dubium A71.0
  healed or sequelae B94.0
  initial (stage) A71.0
  pannus A71.1

316

☑ **Additional Character Required** — Refer to the Tabular List for Character Selection
▽ Subterms under main terms may continue to next column or page

Trachoma, trachomatous — *continued*
  Türck's J37.0
Traction, vitreomacular H43.82- ☑
Train sickness T75.3 ☑
Trait(s)
  Hb-S D57.3
  hemoglobin
    abnormal NEC D58.2
      with thalassemia D56.3
    C — *see* Disease, hemoglobin C
    S (Hb-S) D57.3
  Lepore D56.3
  personality, accentuated Z73.1
  sickle-cell D57.3
    with elliptocytosis or spherocytosis D57.3
  type A personality Z73.1
Tramp Z59.0
Trance R41.89
  hysterical F44.89
Transaminasemia R74.01
Transection
  abdomen (partial) S38.3 ☑
  aorta (incomplete) — *see also* Injury, aorta
    complete — *see* Injury, aorta, laceration, major
  carotid artery (incomplete) — *see also* Injury, blood
    vessel, carotid, laceration
    complete — *see* Injury, blood vessel, carotid, lacer-
      ation, major
  celiac artery (incomplete) S35.211 ☑
    branch (incomplete) S35.291 ☑
      complete S35.292 ☑
    complete S35.212 ☑
  innominate
    artery (incomplete) — *see also* Injury, blood vessel,
      thoracic, innominate, artery, laceration
      complete — *see* Injury, blood vessel, thoracic,
        innominate, artery, laceration, major
    vein (incomplete) — *see also* Injury, blood vessel,
      thoracic, innominate, vein, laceration
      complete — *see* Injury, blood vessel, thoracic,
        innominate, vein, laceration, major
  jugular vein (external) (incomplete) — *see also* Injury,
    blood vessel, jugular vein, laceration
    complete — *see* Injury, blood vessel, jugular vein,
      laceration, major
    internal (incomplete) — *see also* Injury, blood vessel,
      jugular vein, internal, laceration
      complete — *see* Injury, blood vessel, jugular vein,
        internal, laceration, major
  mesenteric artery (incomplete) — *see also* Injury,
    mesenteric, artery, laceration
    complete — *see* Injury, mesenteric artery, laceration,
      major
  pulmonary vessel (incomplete) — *see also* Injury, blood
    vessel, thoracic, pulmonary, laceration
    complete — *see* Injury, blood vessel, thoracic, pul-
      monary, laceration, major
  subclavian — *see* Transection, innominate
  vena cava (incomplete) — *see also* Injury, vena cava
    complete — *see* Injury, vena cava, laceration, major
  vertebral artery (incomplete) — *see also* Injury, blood
    vessel, vertebral, laceration
    complete — *see* Injury, blood vessel, vertebral, lac-
      eration, major
Transfusion
  associated (red blood cell) hemochromatosis E83.111
  blood
    ABO incompatible — *see* Complication(s), transfu-
      sion, incompatibility reaction, ABO
    minor blood group (Duffy) (E) (K) (Kell) (Kidd) (Lewis)
      (M) (N) (P) (S) T80.89 ☑
    reaction or complication — *see* Complications,
      transfusion
  fetomaternal (mother) — *see* Pregnancy, complicated
    by, placenta, transfusion syndrome
  maternofetal (mother) — *see* Pregnancy, complicated
    by, placenta, transfusion syndrome
  placental (syndrome) (mother) — *see* Pregnancy,
    complicated by, placenta, transfusion syndrome
  reaction (adverse) — *see* Complications, transfusion
  related acute lung injury (TRALI) J95.84
  twin-to-twin — *see* Pregnancy, complicated by, placen-
    ta, transfusion syndrome, fetus to fetus
Transient (meaning homeless) — *see also* condition Z59.0
Translocation
  balanced autosomal Q95.9
    in normal individual Q95.0

Translocation — *continued*
  chromosomes NEC Q99.8
    balanced and insertion in normal individual Q95.0
  Down syndrome Q90.2
  trisomy
    13 Q91.6
    18 Q91.2
    21 Q90.2
Translucency, iris — *see* Degeneration, iris
Transmission of chemical substances through the
  placenta — *see* Absorption, chemical, through
  placenta
Transparency, lung, unilateral J43.0
Transplant (ed) (status) Z94.9
  awaiting organ Z76.82
  bone Z94.6
    marrow Z94.81
  candidate Z76.82
  complication — *see* Complication, transplant
  cornea Z94.7
  heart Z94.1
    and lung(s) Z94.3
    valve Z95.2
      prosthetic Z95.2
      specified NEC Z95.4
      xenogenic Z95.3
  intestine Z94.82
  kidney Z94.0
  liver Z94.4
  lung(s) Z94.2
    and heart Z94.3
  organ (failure) (infection) (rejection) Z94.9
    removal status Z98.85
  pancreas Z94.83
  skin Z94.5
  social Z60.3
  specified organ or tissue NEC Z94.89
  stem cells Z94.84
  tissue Z94.9
Transplants, ovarian, endometrial N80.1
Transposed — *see* Transposition
Transposition (congenital) — *see also* Malposition,
  congenital
  abdominal viscera Q89.3
  aorta (dextra) Q20.3
  appendix Q43.8
  colon Q43.8
  corrected Q20.5
  great vessels (complete) (partial) Q20.3
  heart Q24.0
    with complete transposition of viscera Q89.3
  intestine (large) (small) Q43.8
  reversed jejunal (for bypass) (status) Z98.0
  scrotum Q55.23
  stomach Q40.2
    with general transposition of viscera Q89.3
  tooth, teeth, fully erupted M26.30
  vessels, great (complete) (partial) Q20.3
  viscera (abdominal) (thoracic) Q89.3
Transsexualism F64.0
Transverse — *see also* condition
  arrest (deep), in labor O64.0 ☑
  lie (mother) O32.2 ☑
    causing obstructed labor O64.8 ☑
Transvestism, transvestitism (dual-role) F64.1
  fetishistic F65.1
Trapped placenta (with hemorrhage) O72.0
  without hemorrhage O73.0
TRAPS (tumor necrosis factor receptor associated periodic
  syndrome) M04.1
Trauma, traumatism — *see also* Injury
  acoustic — *see* subcategory H83.3 ☑
  birth — *see* Birth, injury
  complicating ectopic or molar pregnancy O08.6
  during delivery O71.9
  following ectopic or molar pregnancy O08.6
  obstetric O71.9
    specified NEC O71.89
  occusal
    primary K08.81
    secondary K08.82
Traumatic — *see also* condition
  brain injury S06.9 ☑
Treacher Collins syndrome Q75.4
Treitz's hernia — *see* Hernia, abdomen, specified site
  NEC
Trematode infestation — *see* Infestation, fluke
Trematodiasis — *see* Infestation, fluke

Trembling paralysis — *see* Parkinsonism
Tremor(s) R25.1
  drug induced G25.1
  essential (benign) G25.0
  familial G25.0
  hereditary G25.0
  hysterical F44.4
  intention G25.2
  medication induced postural G25.1
  mercurial — *see* subcategory T56.1 ☑
  Parkinson's — *see* Parkinsonism
  psychogenic (conversion reaction) F44.4
  senilis R54
  specified type NEC G25.2
Trench
  fever A79.0
  foot — *see* Immersion, foot
  mouth A69.1
Treponema pallidum infection — *see* Syphilis
Treponematosis
  due to
    T. pallidum — *see* Syphilis
    T. pertenue — *see* Yaws
Triad
  Hutchinson's (congenital syphilis) A50.53
  Kartagener's Q89.3
  Saint's — *see* Hernia, diaphragm
Trichiasis (eyelid) H02.059
  with entropion — *see* Entropion
  left H02.056
    lower H02.055
    upper H02.054
  right H02.053
    lower H02.052
    upper H02.051
Trichinella spiralis (infection) (infestation) B75
Trichinellosis, trichiniasis, trichinelliasis, trichinosis
  B75
  with muscle disorder B75 *[M63.80]*
    ankle B75 *[M63.87-]* ☑
    foot B75 *[M63.87-]* ☑
    forearm B75 *[M63.83-]* ☑
    hand B75 *[M63.84-]* ☑
    lower leg B75 *[M63.86-]* ☑
    multiple sites B75 *[M63.89]*
    pelvic region B75 *[M63.85-]* ☑
    shoulder region B75 *[M63.81-]* ☑
    specified site NEC B75 *[M63.88]*
    thigh B75 *[M63.85-]* ☑
    upper arm B75 *[M63.82-]* ☑
Trichobezoar T18.9 ☑
  intestine T18.3 ☑
  stomach T18.2 ☑
Trichocephaliasis, trichocephalosis B79
Trichocephalus infestation B79
Trichoclasis L67.8
Trichoepithelioma — *see also* Neoplasm, skin, benign
  malignant — *see* Neoplasm, skin, malignant
Trichofolliculoma — *see* Neoplasm, skin, benign
Tricholemmoma — *see* Neoplasm, skin, benign
Trichomoniasis A59.9
  bladder A59.03
  cervix A59.09
  intestinal A07.8
  prostate A59.02
  seminal vesicles A59.09
  specified site NEC A59.8
  urethra A59.03
  urogenitalis A59.00
  vagina A59.01
  vulva A59.01
Trichomycosis
  axillaris A48.8
  nodosa, nodularis B36.8
Trichonodosis L67.8
Trichophytid, trichophyton infection — *see* Dermatophytosis
Trichophytobezoar T18.9 ☑
  intestine T18.3 ☑
  stomach T18.2 ☑
Trichophytosis — *see* Dermatophytosis
Trichoptilosis L67.8
Trichorrhexis (nodosa) (invaginata) L67.0
Trichosis axillaris A48.8
Trichosporosis nodosa B36.2
Trichostasis spinulosa (congenital) Q84.1

Trichostrongyliasis, trichostrongylosis (small intestine) B81.2
Trichostrongylus infection B81.2
Trichotillomania F63.3
Trichromat, trichromatopsia, anomalous (congenital) H53.55
Trichuriasis B79
Trichuris trichiura (infection) (infestation) (any site) B79
Tricuspid (valve) — see condition
Trifid — see also Accessory
  kidney (pelvis) Q63.8
  tongue Q38.3
Trigeminal neuralgia — see Neuralgia, trigeminal
Trigeminy R00.8
Trigger finger (acquired) M65.30
  congenital Q74.0
  index finger M65.32- ☑
  little finger M65.35- ☑
  middle finger M65.33- ☑
  ring finger M65.34- ☑
  thumb M65.31- ☑
Trigonitis (bladder) (chronic) (pseudomembranous) N30.30
  with hematuria N30.31
Trigonocephaly Q75.0
Trilocular heart — see Cor triloculare
Trimethylaminuria E72.52
Tripartite placenta O43.19- ☑
Triphalangeal thumb Q74.0
Triple — see also Accessory
  kidneys Q63.0
  uteri Q51.818
  X, female Q97.0
Triple I O41.12- ☑
Triplegia G83.89
  congenital G80.8
Triplet (newborn) — see also Newborn, triplet
  complicating pregnancy — see Pregnancy, triplet
Triplication — see Accessory
Triploidy Q92.7
Trismus R25.2
  neonatorum A33
  newborn A33
Trisomy (syndrome) Q92.9
  13 (partial) Q91.7
    meiotic nondisjunction Q91.4
    mitotic nondisjunction Q91.5
    mosaicism Q91.5
    translocation Q91.6
  18 (partial) Q91.3
    meiotic nondisjunction Q91.0
    mitotic nondisjunction Q91.1
    mosaicism Q91.1
    translocation Q91.2
  20 Q92.8
  21 (partial) Q90.9
    meiotic nondisjunction Q90.0
    mitotic nondisjunction Q90.1
    mosaicism Q90.1
    translocation Q90.2
  22 Q92.8
  autosomes Q92.9
  chromosome specified NEC Q92.8
    partial Q92.2
      due to unbalanced translocation Q92.5
    specified NEC Q92.8
    whole (nonsex chromosome)
      meiotic nondisjunction Q92.0
      mitotic nondisjunction Q92.1
      mosaicism Q92.1
  due to
    dicentrics — see Extra, marker chromosomes
    extra rings — see Extra, marker chromosomes
    isochromosomes — see Extra, marker chromosomes
  specified NEC Q92.8
  whole chromosome Q92.9
    meiotic nondisjunction Q92.0
    mitotic nondisjunction Q92.1
    mosaicism Q92.1
    partial Q92.9
    specified NEC Q92.8
Tritanomaly, tritanopia H53.55
Trombiculosis, trombiculiasis, trombidiosis B88.0
Trophedema (congenital) (hereditary) Q82.0
Trophoblastic disease — see also Mole, hydatidiform O01.9
Tropholymphedema Q82.0

Trophoneurosis NEC G96.89
  disseminated M34.9
Tropical — see condition
Trouble — see also Disease
  heart — see Disease, heart
  kidney — see Disease, renal
  nervous R45.0
  sinus — see Sinusitis
Trousseau's syndrome (thrombophlebitis migrans) I82.1
Truancy, childhood
  from school Z72.810
Truncus
  arteriosus (persistent) Q20.0
  communis Q20.0
Trunk — see condition
Trypanosomiasis
  African B56.9
    by Trypanosoma brucei
      gambiense B56.0
      rhodesiense B56.1
  American — see Chagas' disease
  Brazilian — see Chagas' disease
  by Trypanosoma
    brucei gambiense B56.0
    brucei rhodesiense B56.1
    cruzi — see Chagas' disease
  gambiense, Gambian B56.0
  rhodesiensis, Rhodesian B56.1
  South American — see Chagas' disease
  where
    African trypanosomiasis is prevalent B56.9
    Chagas' disease is prevalent B57.2
T-shaped incisors K00.2
Tsutsugamushi (disease) (fever) A75.3
Tube, tubal, tubular — see condition
Tubercle — see also Tuberculosis
  brain, solitary A17.81
  Darwin's Q17.8
  Ghon, primary infection A15.7
Tuberculid, tuberculide (indurating, subcutaneous) (lichenoid) (miliary) (papulonecrotic) (primary) (skin) A18.4
Tuberculoma — see also Tuberculosis
  brain A17.81
  meninges (cerebral) (spinal) A17.1
  spinal cord A17.81
Tuberculosis, tubercular, tuberculous (calcification) (calcified) (caseous) (chromogenic acid-fast bacilli) (degeneration) (fibrocaseous) (fistula) (interstitial) (isolated circumscribed lesions) (necrosis) (parenchymatous) (ulcerative) A15.9
  with pneumoconiosis (any condition in J60-J64) J65
  abdomen (lymph gland) A18.39
  abscess (respiratory) A15.9
    bone A18.03
      hip A18.02
      knee A18.02
      sacrum A18.01
      specified site NEC A18.03
      spinal A18.01
      vertebra A18.01
    brain A17.81
    breast A18.89
    Cowper's gland A18.15
    dura (mater) (cerebral) (spinal) A17.81
    epidural (cerebral) (spinal) A17.81
    female pelvis A18.17
    frontal sinus A15.8
    genital organs NEC A18.10
    genitourinary A18.10
    gland (lymphatic) — see Tuberculosis, lymph gland
    hip A18.02
    intestine A18.32
    ischiorectal A18.32
    joint NEC A18.02
      hip A18.02
      knee A18.02
      specified NEC A18.02
      vertebral A18.01
    kidney A18.11
    knee A18.02
    latent Z22.7
    lumbar (spine) A18.01
    lung — see Tuberculosis, pulmonary
    meninges (cerebral) (spinal) A17.0
    muscle A18.09
    perianal (fistula) A18.32
    perinephritic A18.11

Tuberculosis, tubercular, tuberculous — continued
  abscess — continued
    perirectal A18.32
    rectum A18.32
    retropharyngeal A15.8
    sacrum A18.01
    scrofulous A18.2
    scrotum A18.15
    skin (primary) A18.4
    spinal cord A17.81
    spine or vertebra (column) A18.01
    subdiaphragmatic A18.31
    testis A18.15
    urinary A18.13
    uterus A18.17
  accessory sinus — see Tuberculosis, sinus
  Addison's disease A18.7
  adenitis — see Tuberculosis, lymph gland
  adenoids A15.8
  adenopathy — see Tuberculosis, lymph gland
  adherent pericardium A18.84
  adnexa (uteri) A18.17
  adrenal (capsule) (gland) A18.7
  alimentary canal A18.32
  anemia A18.89
  ankle (joint) (bone) A18.02
  anus A18.32
  apex, apical — see Tuberculosis, pulmonary
  appendicitis, appendix A18.32
  arachnoid A17.0
  artery, arteritis A18.89
    cerebral A18.89
  arthritis (chronic) (synovial) A18.02
    spine or vertebra (column) A18.01
  articular — see Tuberculosis, joint
  ascites A18.31
  asthma — see Tuberculosis, pulmonary
  axilla, axillary (gland) A18.2
  bladder A18.12
  bone A18.03
    hip A18.02
    knee A18.02
    limb NEC A18.03
    sacrum A18.01
    spine or vertebral column A18.01
  bowel (miliary) A18.32
  brain A17.81
  breast A18.89
  broad ligament A18.17
  bronchi, bronchial, bronchus A15.5
    ectasia, ectasis (bronchiectasis) — see Tuberculosis, pulmonary
    fistula A15.5
      primary (progressive) A15.7
    gland or node A15.4
      primary (progressive) A15.7
    lymph gland or node A15.4
      primary (progressive) A15.7
  bronchiectasis — see Tuberculosis, pulmonary
  bronchitis A15.5
  bronchopleural A15.6
  bronchopneumonia, bronchopneumonic — see Tuberculosis, pulmonary
  bronchorrhagia A15.5
  bronchotracheal A15.5
  bronze disease A18.7
  buccal cavity A18.83
  bulbourethral gland A18.15
  bursa A18.09
  cachexia A15.9
  cardiomyopathy A18.84
  caries — see Tuberculosis, bone
  cartilage A18.02
    intervertebral A18.01
  catarrhal — see Tuberculosis, respiratory
  cecum A18.32
  cellulitis (primary) A18.4
  cerebellum A17.81
  cerebral, cerebrum A17.81
  cerebrospinal A17.81
    meninges A17.0
  cervical (lymph gland or node) A18.2
  cervicitis, cervix (uteri) A18.16
  chest — see Tuberculosis, respiratory
  chorioretinitis A18.53
  choroid, choroiditis A18.53
  ciliary body A18.54
  colitis A18.32

☑ **Additional Character Required — Refer to the Tabular List for Character Selection**
🔺 **Subterms under main terms may continue to next column or page**

Tuberculosis, tubercular, tuberculous — *continued*
　　collier's J65
　　colliquativa (primary) A18.4
　　colon A18.32
　　complex, primary A15.7
　　congenital P37.0
　　conjunctiva A18.59
　　connective tissue (systemic) A18.89
　　contact Z20.1
　　cornea (ulcer) A18.52
　　Cowper's gland A18.15
　　coxae A18.02
　　coxalgia A18.02
　　cul-de-sac of Douglas A18.17
　　curvature, spine A18.01
　　cutis (colliquativa) (primary) A18.4
　　cyst, ovary A18.18
　　cystitis A18.12
　　dactylitis A18.03
　　diarrhea A18.32
　　diffuse — *see* Tuberculosis, miliary
　　digestive tract A18.32
　　disseminated — *see* Tuberculosis, miliary
　　duodenum A18.32
　　dura (mater) (cerebral) (spinal) A17.0
　　　　abscess (cerebral) (spinal) A17.81
　　dysentery A18.32
　　ear (inner) (middle) A18.6
　　　　bone A18.03
　　　　external (primary) A18.4
　　　　skin (primary) A18.4
　　elbow A18.02
　　emphysema — *see* Tuberculosis, pulmonary
　　empyema A15.6
　　encephalitis A17.82
　　endarteritis A18.89
　　endocarditis A18.84
　　　　aortic A18.84
　　　　mitral A18.84
　　　　pulmonary A18.84
　　　　tricuspid A18.84
　　endocrine glands NEC A18.82
　　endometrium A18.17
　　enteric, enterica, enteritis A18.32
　　enterocolitis A18.32
　　epididymis, epididymitis A18.15
　　epidural abscess (cerebral) (spinal) A17.81
　　epiglottis A15.5
　　episcleritis A18.51
　　erythema (induratum) (nodosum) (primary) A18.4
　　esophagus A18.83
　　eustachian tube A18.6
　　exposure (to) Z20.1
　　exudative — *see* Tuberculosis, pulmonary
　　eye A18.50
　　eyelid (primary) (lupus) A18.4
　　fallopian tube (acute) (chronic) A18.17
　　fascia A18.09
　　fauces A15.8
　　female pelvic inflammatory disease A18.17
　　finger A18.03
　　first infection A15.7
　　gallbladder A18.83
　　ganglion A18.09
　　gastritis A18.83
　　gastrocolic fistula A18.32
　　gastroenteritis A18.32
　　gastrointestinal tract A18.32
　　general, generalized — *see* Tuberculosis, miliary
　　genital organs A18.10
　　genitourinary A18.10
　　genu A18.02
　　glandula suprarenalis A18.7
　　glandular, general A18.2
　　glottis A15.5
　　grinder's J65
　　gum A18.83
　　hand A18.03
　　heart A18.84
　　hematogenous — *see* Tuberculosis, miliary
　　hemoptysis — *see* Tuberculosis, pulmonary
　　hemorrhage NEC — *see* Tuberculosis, pulmonary
　　hemothorax A15.6
　　hepatitis A18.83
　　hilar lymph nodes A15.4
　　　　primary (progressive) A15.7
　　hip (joint) (disease) (bone) A18.02
　　hydropneumothorax A15.6

Tuberculosis, tubercular, tuberculous — *continued*
　　hydrothorax A15.6
　　hypoadrenalism A18.7
　　hypopharynx A15.8
　　ileocecal (hyperplastic) A18.32
　　ileocolitis A18.32
　　ileum A18.32
　　iliac spine (superior) A18.03
　　immunological findings only A15.7
　　indurativa (primary) A18.4
　　infantile A15.7
　　infection A15.9
　　　　without clinical manifestations A15.7
　　infraclavicular gland A18.2
　　inguinal gland A18.2
　　inguinalis A18.2
　　intestine (any part) A18.32
　　iridocyclitis A18.54
　　iris, iritis A18.54
　　ischiorectal A18.32
　　jaw A18.03
　　jejunum A18.32
　　joint A18.02
　　　　vertebral A18.01
　　keratitis (interstitial) A18.52
　　keratoconjunctivitis A18.52
　　kidney A18.11
　　knee (joint) A18.02
　　kyphosis, kyphoscoliosis A18.01
　　laryngitis A15.5
　　larynx A15.5
　　latent Z22.7
　　leptomeninges, leptomeningitis (cerebral) (spinal)
　　　　A17.0
　　lichenoides (primary) A18.4
　　linguae A18.83
　　lip A18.83
　　liver A18.83
　　lordosis A18.01
　　lung — *see* Tuberculosis, pulmonary
　　lupus vulgaris A18.4
　　lymph gland or node (peripheral) A18.2
　　　　abdomen A18.39
　　　　bronchial A15.4
　　　　　　primary (progressive) A15.7
　　　　cervical A18.2
　　　　hilar A15.4
　　　　　　primary (progressive) A15.7
　　　　intrathoracic A15.4
　　　　　　primary (progressive) A15.7
　　　　mediastinal A15.4
　　　　　　primary (progressive) A15.7
　　　　mesenteric A18.39
　　　　retroperitoneal A18.39
　　　　tracheobronchial A15.4
　　　　　　primary (progressive) A15.7
　　lymphadenitis — *see* Tuberculosis, lymph gland
　　lymphangitis — *see* Tuberculosis, lymph gland
　　lymphatic (gland) (vessel) — *see* Tuberculosis, lymph
　　　　gland
　　mammary gland A18.89
　　marasmus A15.9
　　mastoiditis A18.03
　　mediastinal lymph gland or node A15.4
　　　　primary (progressive) A15.7
　　mediastinitis A15.8
　　　　primary (progressive) A15.7
　　mediastinum A15.8
　　　　primary (progressive) A15.7
　　medulla A17.81
　　melanosis, Addisonian A18.7
　　meninges, meningitis (basilar) (cerebral) (cerebrospinal)
　　　　(spinal) A17.0
　　meningoencephalitis A17.82
　　mesentery, mesenteric (gland or node) A18.39
　　miliary A19.9
　　　　acute A19.2
　　　　　　multiple sites A19.1
　　　　　　single specified site A19.0
　　　　chronic A19.8
　　　　specified NEC A19.8
　　millstone makers' J65
　　miner's J65
　　molder's J65
　　mouth A18.83
　　multiple A19.9
　　　　acute A19.1
　　　　chronic A19.8
　　muscle A18.09

Tuberculosis, tubercular, tuberculous — *continued*
　　myelitis A17.82
　　myocardium, myocarditis A18.84
　　nasal (passage) (sinus) A15.8
　　nasopharynx A15.8
　　neck gland A18.2
　　nephritis A18.11
　　nerve (mononeuropathy) A17.83
　　nervous system A17.9
　　nose (septum) A15.8
　　ocular A18.50
　　omentum A18.31
　　oophoritis (acute) (chronic) A18.17
　　optic (nerve trunk) (papilla) A18.59
　　orbit A18.59
　　orchitis A18.15
　　organ, specified NEC A18.89
　　osseous — *see* Tuberculosis, bone
　　osteitis — *see* Tuberculosis, bone
　　osteomyelitis — *see* Tuberculosis, bone
　　otitis media A18.6
　　ovary, ovaritis (acute) (chronic) A18.17
　　oviduct (acute) (chronic) A18.17
　　pachymeningitis A17.0
　　palate (soft) A18.83
　　pancreas A18.83
　　papulonecrotic (a) (primary) A18.4
　　parathyroid glands A18.82
　　paronychia (primary) A18.4
　　parotid gland or region A18.83
　　pelvis (bony) A18.03
　　penis A18.15
　　peribronchitis A15.5
　　pericardium, pericarditis A18.84
　　perichondritis, larynx A15.5
　　periostitis — *see* Tuberculosis, bone
　　perirectal fistula A18.32
　　peritoneum NEC A18.31
　　peritonitis A18.31
　　pharynx, pharyngitis A15.8
　　phlyctenulosis (keratoconjunctivitis) A18.52
　　phthisis NEC — *see* Tuberculosis, pulmonary
　　pituitary gland A18.82
　　pleura, pleural, pleurisy, pleuritis (fibrinous) (oblitera-
　　　　tive) (purulent) (simple plastic) (with effusion)
　　　　A15.6
　　　　primary (progressive) A15.7
　　pneumonia, pneumonic — *see* Tuberculosis, pul-
　　　　monary
　　pneumothorax (spontaneous) (tense valvular) — *see*
　　　　Tuberculosis, pulmonary
　　polyneuropathy A17.89
　　polyserositis A19.9
　　　　acute A19.1
　　　　chronic A19.8
　　potter's J65
　　prepuce A18.15
　　primary (complex) A15.7
　　proctitis A18.32
　　prostate, prostatitis A18.14
　　pulmonalis — *see* Tuberculosis, pulmonary
　　pulmonary (cavitated) (fibrotic) (infiltrative) (nodular)
　　　　A15.0
　　　　childhood type or first infection A15.7
　　　　primary (complex) A15.7
　　pyelitis A18.11
　　pyelonephritis A18.11
　　pyemia — *see* Tuberculosis, miliary
　　pyonephrosis A18.11
　　pyopneumothorax A15.6
　　pyothorax A15.6
　　rectum (fistula) (with abscess) A18.32
　　reinfection stage — *see* Tuberculosis, pulmonary
　　renal A18.11
　　renis A18.11
　　respiratory A15.9
　　　　primary A15.7
　　　　specified site NEC A15.8
　　retina, retinitis A18.53
　　retroperitoneal (lymph gland or node) A18.39
　　rheumatism NEC A18.09
　　rhinitis A15.8
　　sacroiliac (joint) A18.01
　　sacrum A18.01
　　salivary gland A18.83
　　salpingitis (acute) (chronic) A18.17
　　sandblaster's J65
　　sclera A18.51

Tuberculosis, tubercular, tuberculous — *continued*
scoliosis A18.01
scrofulous A18.2
scrotum A18.15
seminal tract or vesicle A18.15
senile A15.9
septic — *see* Tuberculosis, miliary
shoulder (joint) A18.02
blade A18.03
sigmoid A18.32
sinus (any nasal) A15.8
bone A18.03
epididymis A18.15
skeletal NEC A18.03
skin (any site) (primary) A18.4
small intestine A18.32
soft palate A18.83
spermatic cord A18.15
spine, spinal (column) A18.01
cord A17.81
medulla A17.81
membrane A17.0
meninges A17.0
spleen, splenitis A18.85
spondylitis A18.01
sternoclavicular joint A18.02
stomach A18.83
stonemason's J65
subcutaneous tissue (cellular) (primary) A18.4
subcutis (primary) A18.4
subdeltoid bursa A18.83
submaxillary (region) A18.83
supraclavicular gland A18.2
suprarenal (capsule) (gland) A18.7
swelling, joint (*see also* category M01) — *see also* Tuberculosis, joint A18.02
symphysis pubis A18.02
synovitis A18.09
articular A18.02
spine or vertebra A18.01
systemic — *see* Tuberculosis, miliary
tarsitis A18.4
tendon (sheath) — *see* Tuberculosis, tenosynovitis
tenosynovitis A18.09
spine or vertebra A18.01
testis A18.15
throat A15.8
thymus gland A18.82
thyroid gland A18.81
tongue A18.83
tonsil, tonsillitis A15.8
trachea, tracheal A15.5
lymph gland or node A15.4
primary (progressive) A15.7
tracheobronchial A15.5
lymph gland or node A15.4
primary (progressive) A15.7
tubal (acute) (chronic) A18.17
tunica vaginalis A18.15
ulcer (skin) (primary) A18.4
bowel or intestine A18.32
specified NEC — *see* Tuberculosis, by site
unspecified site A15.9
ureter A18.11
urethra, urethral (gland) A18.13
urinary organ or tract A18.13
uterus A18.17
uveal tract A18.54
uvula A18.83
vagina A18.18
vas deferens A18.15
verruca, verrucosa (cutis) (primary) A18.4
vertebra (column) A18.01
vesiculitis A18.15
vulva A18.18
wrist (joint) A18.02
Tuberculum
Carabelli — *see* Excludes Note at K00.2
occlusal — *see* Excludes Note at K00.2
paramolare K00.2
Tuberosity, enitre maxillary M26.07
Tuberous sclerosis (brain) Q85.1
Tubo-ovarian — *see* condition
Tuboplasty, after previous sterilization Z31.0
aftercare Z31.42
Tubotympanitis, catarrhal (chronic) — *see* Otitis, media,
nonsuppurative, chronic, serous
Tularemia A21.9

Tularemia — *continued*
with
conjunctivitis A21.1
pneumonia A21.2
abdominal A21.3
bronchopneumonic A21.2
conjunctivitis A21.1
cryptogenic A21.3
enteric A21.3
gastrointestinal A21.3
generalized A21.7
ingestion A21.3
intestinal A21.3
oculoglandular A21.1
ophthalmic A21.1
pneumonia (any), pneumonic A21.2
pulmonary A21.2
sepsis A21.7
specified NEC A21.8
typhoidal A21.7
ulceroglandular A21.0
Tularensis conjunctivitis A21.1
Tumefaction — *see also* Swelling
liver — *see* Hypertrophy, liver
Tumor — *see also* Neoplasm, unspecified behavior, by
site
acinar cell — *see* Neoplasm, uncertain behavior, by site
acinic cell — *see* Neoplasm, uncertain behavior, by site
adenocarcinoid — *see* Neoplasm, malignant, by site
adenomatoid — *see also* Neoplasm, benign, by site
odontogenic — *see* Cyst, calcifying odontogenic
adnexal (skin) — *see* Neoplasm, skin, benign, by site
adrenal
cortical (benign) D35.0- ☑
malignant C74.0- ☑
rest — *see* Neoplasm, benign, by site
alpha-cell
malignant
pancreas C25.4
specified site NEC — *see* Neoplasm, malignant,
by site
unspecified site C25.4
pancreas D13.7
specified site NEC — *see* Neoplasm, benign, by site
unspecified site D13.7
aneurysmal — *see* Aneurysm
aortic body D44.7
malignant C75.5
Askin's — *see* Neoplasm, connective tissue, malignant
basal cell — *see also* Neoplasm, skin, uncertain behavior D48.5
Bednar — *see* Neoplasm, skin, malignant
benign (unclassified) — *see* Neoplasm, benign, by site
beta-cell
malignant
pancreas C25.4
specified site NEC — *see* Neoplasm, malignant,
by site
unspecified site C25.4
pancreas D13.7
specified site NEC — *see* Neoplasm, benign, by site
unspecified site D13.7
Brenner D27.9
borderline malignancy D39.1- ☑
malignant C56- ☑
proliferating D39.1- ☑
bronchial alveolar, intravascular D38.1
Brooke's — *see* Neoplasm, skin, benign
brown fat — *see* Lipoma
Burkitt — *see* Lymphoma, Burkitt
calcifying epithelial odontogenic — *see* Cyst, calcifying
odontogenic
carcinoid D3A.00 (*following* D36)
benign D3A.00 (*following* D36)
appendix D3A.020 (*following* D36)
ascending colon D3A.022 (*following* D36)
bronchus (lung) D3A.090 (*following* D36)
cecum D3A.021 (*following* D36)
colon D3A.029 (*following* D36)
descending colon D3A.024 (*following* D36)
duodenum D3A.010 (*following* D36)
foregut NOS D3A.094 (*following* D36)
hindgut NOS D3A.096 (*following* D36)
ileum D3A.012 (*following* D36)
jejunum D3A.011 (*following* D36)
kidney D3A.093 (*following* D36)
large intestine D3A.029 (*following* D36)
lung (bronchus) D3A.090 (*following* D36)

Tumor — *continued*
carcinoid — *continued*
benign — *continued*
midgut NOS D3A.095 (*following* D36)
rectum D3A.026 (*following* D36)
sigmoid colon D3A.025 (*following* D36)
small intestine D3A.019 (*following* D36)
specified NEC D3A.098 (*following* D36)
stomach D3A.092 (*following* D36)
thymus D3A.091 (*following* D36)
transverse colon D3A.023 (*following* D36)
malignant C7A.00 (*following* C75)
appendix C7A.020 (*following* C75)
ascending colon C7A.022 (*following* C75)
bronchus (lung) C7A.090 (*following* C75)
cecum C7A.021 (*following* C75)
colon C7A.029 (*following* C75)
descending colon C7A.024 (*following* C75)
duodenum C7A.010 (*following* C75)
foregut NOS C7A.094 (*following* C75)
hindgut NOS C7A.096 (*following* C75)
ileum C7A.012 (*following* C75)
jejunum C7A.011 (*following* C75)
kidney C7A.093 (*following* C75)
large intestine C7A.029 (*following* C75)
lung (bronchus) C7A.090 (*following* C75)
midgut NOS C7A.095 (*following* C75)
rectum C7A.026 (*following* C75)
sigmoid colon C7A.025 (*following* C75)
small intestine C7A.019 (*following* C75)
specified NEC C7A.098 (*following* C75)
stomach C7A.092 (*following* C75)
thymus C7A.091 (*following* C75)
transverse colon C7A.023 (*following* C75)
mesentery metastasis C7B.04 (*following* C75)
secondary C7B.00 (*following* C75)
bone C7B.03 (*following* C75)
distant lymph nodes C7B.01 (*following* C75)
liver C7B.02 (*following* C75)
peritoneum C7B.04 (*following* C75)
specified NEC C7B.09 (*following* C75)
carotid body D44.6
malignant C75.4
cells — *see also* Neoplasm, unspecified behavior, by
site
benign — *see* Neoplasm, benign, by site
malignant — *see* Neoplasm, malignant, by site
uncertain whether benign or malignant — *see*
Neoplasm, uncertain behavior, by site
cervix, in pregnancy or childbirth — *see* Pregnancy,
complicated by, tumor, cervix
chondromatous giant cell — *see* Neoplasm, bone, benign
chromaffin — *see also* Neoplasm, benign, by site
malignant — *see* Neoplasm, malignant, by site
Cock's peculiar L72.3
Codman's — *see* Neoplasm, bone, benign
dentigerous, mixed — *see* Cyst, calcifying odontogenic
dermoid — *see* Neoplasm, benign, by site
with malignant transformation C56- ☑
desmoid (extra-abdominal) — *see also* Neoplasm,
connective tissue, uncertain behavior
abdominal — *see* Neoplasm, connective tissue, uncertain behavior
embolus — *see* Neoplasm, secondary, by site
embryonal (mixed) — *see also* Neoplasm, uncertain
behavior, by site
liver C22.7
endodermal sinus
specified site — *see* Neoplasm, malignant, by site
unspecified site
female C56.- ☑
male C62.90
epithelial
benign — *see* Neoplasm, benign, by site
malignant — *see* Neoplasm, malignant, by site
Ewing's — *see* Neoplasm, bone, malignant, by site
fatty — *see* Lipoma
fibroid — *see* Leiomyoma
G cell
malignant
pancreas C25.4
specified site NEC — *see* Neoplasm, malignant
by site
unspecified site C25.4
specified site — *see* Neoplasm, uncertain behavio
by site
unspecified site D37.8

Tumor — *continued*
  germ cell — *see also* Neoplasm, malignant, by site
    mixed — *see* Neoplasm, malignant, by site
  ghost cell, odontogenic — *see* Cyst, calcifying odonto-
    genic
  giant cell — *see also* Neoplasm, uncertain behavior,
    by site
    bone D48.0
      malignant — *see* Neoplasm, bone, malignant
      chondromatous — *see* Neoplasm, bone, benign
    malignant — *see* Neoplasm, malignant, by site
    soft parts — *see* Neoplasm, connective tissue, un-
      certain behavior
      malignant — *see* Neoplasm, connective tissue,
        malignant
  glomus D18.00
    intra-abdominal D18.03
    intracranial D18.02
    jugulare D44.7
      malignant C75.5
    skin D18.01
    specified site NEC D18.09
  gonadal stromal — *see* Neoplasm, uncertain behavior,
    by site
  granular cell — *see also* Neoplasm, connective tissue,
    benign
    malignant — *see* Neoplasm, connective tissue, ma-
      lignant
  granulosa cell D39.1- ☑
    juvenile D39.1- ☑
    malignant C56- ☑
  granulosa cell-theca cell D39.1- ☑
    malignant C56- ☑
  Grawitz's C64- ☑
  hemorrhoidal — *see* Hemorrhoids
  hilar cell D27- ☑
  hilus cell D27- ☑
  Hurthle cell (benign) D34
    malignant C73
  hydatid — *see* Echinococcus
  hypernephroid — *see also* Neoplasm, uncertain behav-
    ior, by site
  interstitial cell — *see also* Neoplasm, uncertain behav-
    ior, by site
    benign — *see* Neoplasm, benign, by site
    malignant — *see* Neoplasm, malignant, by site
  intravascular bronchial alveolar D38.1
  islet cell — *see* Neoplasm, benign, by site
    malignant — *see* Neoplasm, malignant, by site
      pancreas C25.4
      specified site NEC — *see* Neoplasm, malignant,
        by site
      unspecified site C25.4
    pancreas D13.7
    specified site NEC — *see* Neoplasm, benign, by site
    unspecified site D13.7
  juxtaglomerular D41.0- ☑
  Klatskin's C22.1
  Krukenberg's C79.6- ☑
  Leydig cell — *see* Neoplasm, uncertain behavior, by
    site
    benign — *see* Neoplasm, benign, by site
      specified site — *see* Neoplasm, benign, by site
      unspecified site
        female D27.9
        male D29.20
    malignant — *see* Neoplasm, malignant, by site
      specified site — *see* Neoplasm, malignant, by
        site
      unspecified site
        female C56.9
        male C62.90
    specified site — *see* Neoplasm, uncertain behavior,
      by site
    unspecified site
      female D39.10
      male D40.10
  lipid cell, ovary D27- ☑
  lipoid cell, ovary D27- ☑
  malignant — *see also* Neoplasm, malignant, by site
    C80.1
    fusiform cell (type) C80.1
    giant cell (type) C80.1
    localized, plasma cell — *see* Plasmacytoma, solitary
    mixed NEC C80.1
    small cell (type) C80.1
    spindle cell (type) C80.1

Tumor — *continued*
  malignant — *see also* Neoplasm, malignant, by site —
    continued
    unclassified C80.1
  mast cell D47.09
  melanotic, neuroectodermal — *see* Neoplasm, benign,
    by site
  Merkel cell — *see* Carcinoma, Merkel cell
  mesenchymal
    malignant — *see* Neoplasm, connective tissue, ma-
      lignant
    mixed — *see* Neoplasm, connective tissue, uncertain
      behavior
  mesodermal, mixed — *see also* Neoplasm, malignant,
    by site
    liver C22.4
  mesonephric — *see also* Neoplasm, uncertain behavior,
    by site
    malignant — *see* Neoplasm, malignant, by site
  metastatic
    from specified site — *see* Neoplasm, malignant, by
      site
    of specified site — *see* Neoplasm, malignant, by site
    to specified site — *see* Neoplasm, secondary, by site
  mixed NEC — *see also* Neoplasm, benign, by site
    malignant — *see* Neoplasm, malignant, by site
  mucinous of low malignant potential
    specified site — *see* Neoplasm, malignant, by site
    unspecified site C56.9
  mucocarcinoid
    specified site — *see* Neoplasm, malignant, by site
    unspecified site C18.1
  mucoepidermoid — *see* Neoplasm, uncertain behavior,
    by site
  Müllerian, mixed
    specified site — *see* Neoplasm, malignant, by site
    unspecified site C54.9
  myoepithelial — *see* Neoplasm, benign, by site
  neuroectodermal (peripheral) — *see* Neoplasm, malig-
    nant, by site
    primitive
      specified site — *see* Neoplasm, malignant, by
        site
      unspecified site C71.9
  neuroendocrine D3A.8 (*following* D36)
    malignant poorly differentiated C7A.1 (*following*
      C75)
    secondary NEC C7B.8 (*following* C75)
    specified NEC C7A.8 (*following* C75)
  neurogenic olfactory C30.0
  nonencapsulated sclerosing C73
  odontogenic (adenomatoid) (benign) (calcifying epithe-
    lial) (keratocystic) (squamous) — *see* Cyst, calci-
    fying odontogenic
    malignant C41.1
      upper jaw (bone) C41.0
  ovarian stromal D39.1- ☑
  ovary, in pregnancy — *see* Pregnancy, complicated by
  pacinian — *see* Neoplasm, skin, benign
  Pancoast's — *see* Pancoast's syndrome
  papillary — *see also* Papilloma
    cystic D37.9
    mucinous of low malignant potential C56- ☑
      specified site — *see* Neoplasm, malignant, by
        site
      unspecified site C56.9
    serous of low malignant potential
      specified site — *see* Neoplasm, malignant, by
        site
      unspecified site C56.9
  pelvic, in pregnancy or childbirth — *see* Pregnancy,
    complicated by
  phantom F45.8
  phyllodes D48.6- ☑
    benign D24- ☑
    malignant — *see* Neoplasm, breast, malignant
  Pindborg — *see* Cyst, calcifying odontogenic
  placental site trophoblastic D39.2
  plasma cell (malignant) (localized) — *see* Plasmacy-
    toma, solitary
  polyvesicular vitelline
    specified site — *see* Neoplasm, malignant, by site
    unspecified site
      female C56.9
      male C62.90
  Pott's puffy — *see* Osteomyelitis, specified NEC
  Rathke's pouch D44.3
  retinal anlage — *see* Neoplasm, benign, by site

Tumor — *continued*
  salivary gland type, mixed — *see* Neoplasm, salivary
    gland, benign
    malignant — *see* Neoplasm, salivary gland, malig-
      nant
  Sampson's N80.1
  Schmincke's — *see* Neoplasm, nasopharynx, malignant
  sclerosing stromal D27- ☑
  sebaceous — *see* Cyst, sebaceous
  secondary — *see* Neoplasm, secondary, by site
    carcinoid C7B.00 (*following* C75)
      bone C7B.03 (*following* C75)
      distant lymph nodes C7B.01 (*following* C75)
      liver C7B.02 (*following* C75)
      peritoneum C7B.04 (*following* C75)
      specified NEC C7B.09 (*following* C75)
    neuroendocrine NEC C7B.8 (*following* C75)
  serous of low malignant potential
    specified site — *see* Neoplasm, malignant, by site
    unspecified site C56.9
  Sertoli cell — *see* Neoplasm, benign, by site
    with lipid storage
      specified site — *see* Neoplasm, benign, by site
      unspecified site
        female D27.9
        male D29.20
    specified site — *see* Neoplasm, benign, by site
    unspecified site
      female D27.9
      male D29.20
  Sertoli-Leydig cell — *see* Neoplasm, benign, by site
    specified site — *see* Neoplasm, benign, by site
    unspecified site
      female D27.9
      male D29.20
  sex cord (-stromal) — *see* Neoplasm, uncertain behav-
    ior, by site
    with annular tubules D39.1- ☑
  skin appendage — *see* Neoplasm, skin, benign
  smooth muscle — *see* Neoplasm, connective tissue,
    uncertain behavior
  soft tissue
    benign — *see* Neoplasm, connective tissue, benign
    malignant — *see* Neoplasm, connective tissue, ma-
      lignant
  sternomastoid (congenital) Q68.0
  stromal
    endometrial D39.0
    gastric D48.1
      benign D21.4
      malignant C16.9
      uncertain behavior D48.1
    gastrointestinal C49.A- ☑
      benign D21.4
      esophagus C49.A1
      malignant C49.A0
        colon C49.A4
        duodenum C49.A3
        esophagus C49.A1
        ileum C49.A3
        jejunum C49.A3
        large intestine C49.A4
        Meckel diverticulum C49.A3
        omentum C49.A9
        peritoneum C49.A9
        rectum C49.A5
        small intestine C49.A3
        specified site NEC C49.A9
        stomach C49.A2
      rectum C49.A5
      small intestine C49.A3
      specified site NEC C49.A9
      stomach C49.A2
      uncertain behavior D48.1
    intestine
      benign D21.4
      malignant
        large C49.A4
        small C49.A3
      uncertain behavior D48.1
    ovarian D39.1- ☑
    stomach C49.A2
      benign D21.4
      malignant C49.A2
      uncertain behavior D48.1
  sweat gland — *see also* Neoplasm, skin, uncertain be-
    havior
    benign — *see* Neoplasm, skin, benign

Tumor — *continued*
sweat gland — *see also* Neoplasm, skin, uncertain behavior — *continued*
    malignant — *see* Neoplasm, skin, malignant
syphilitic, brain A52.17
testicular D40.10
testicular stromal D40.1- ☑
theca cell D27.- ☑
theca cell-granulosa cell D39.1- ☑
Triton, malignant — *see* Neoplasm, nerve, malignant
trophoblastic, placental site D39.2
turban D23.4
uterus (body), in pregnancy or childbirth — *see* Pregnancy, complicated by, tumor, uterus
vagina, in pregnancy or childbirth — *see* Pregnancy, complicated by
varicose — *see* Varix
von Recklinghausen's — *see* Neurofibromatosis
vulva or perineum, in pregnancy or childbirth — *see* Pregnancy, complicated by
    causing obstructed labor O65.5
Warthin's — *see* Neoplasm, salivary gland, benign
Wilms' C64- ☑
yolk sac — *see* Neoplasm, malignant, by site
    specified site — *see* Neoplasm, malignant, by site
    unspecified site
      female C56.9
      male C62.90
Tumor lysis syndrome (following antineoplastic chemotherapy) (spontaneous) NEC E88.3
Tumorlet — *see* Neoplasm, uncertain behavior, by site
Tungiasis B88.1
Tunica vasculosa lentis Q12.2
Turban tumor D23.4
Türck's trachoma J37.0
Turner-Kieser syndrome Q87.2
Turner-like syndrome Q87.19
Turner's
hypoplasia (tooth) K00.4
syndrome Q96.9
    specified NEC Q96.8
tooth K00.4
Turner-Ullrich syndrome Q96.9
Tussis convulsiva — *see* Whooping cough
Twiddler's syndrome (due to)
automatic implantable defibrillator T82.198
cardiac pacemaker T82.198 ☑
Twilight state
epileptic F05
psychogenic F44.89
Twin (newborn) — *see also* Newborn, twin
conjoined Q89.4
pregnancy — *see* Pregnancy, twin
Twinning, teeth K00.2
Twist, twisted
bowel, colon or intestine K56.2
hair (congenital) Q84.1
mesentery K56.2
omentum K56.2
organ or site, congenital NEC — *see* Anomaly, by site
ovarian pedicle — *see* Torsion, ovary
Twitching R25.3
Tylosis (acquired) L84
buccalis K13.29
linguae K13.29
palmaris et plantaris (congenital) (inherited) Q82.8
    acquired L85.1
Tympanism R14.0
Tympanites (abdominal) (intestinal) R14.0
Tympanitis — *see* Myringitis
Tympanosclerosis H74.0 ☑
Tympanum — *see* condition
Tympany
abdomen R14.0
chest R09.89
Type A behavior pattern Z73.1
Typhlitis — *see* Appendicitis
Typhoenteritis — *see* Typhoid
Typhoid (abortive) (ambulant) (any site) (clinical) (fever) (hemorrhagic) (infection) (intermittent) (malignant) (rheumatic) (Widal negative) A01.00
with pneumonia A01.03
abdominal A01.09
arthritis A01.04
carrier (suspected) of Z22.0
cholecystitis (current) A01.09
endocarditis A01.02

Typhoid — *continued*
heart involvement A01.02
inoculation reaction — *see* Complications, vaccination
meningitis A01.01
mesenteric lymph nodes A01.09
myocarditis A01.02
osteomyelitis A01.05
perichondritis, larynx A01.09
pneumonia A01.03
specified NEC A01.09
spine A01.05
ulcer (perforating) A01.09
Typhomalaria (fever) — *see* Malaria
Typhomania A01.00
Typhoperitonitis A01.09
Typhus (fever) A75.9
abdominal, abdominalis — *see* Typhoid
African tick A77.1
amarillic A95.9
brain A75.9 *[G94]*
cerebral A75.9 *[G94]*
classical A75.0
due to Rickettsia
    prowazekii A75.0
      recrudescent A75.1
    tsutsugamushi A75.3
    typhi A75.2
endemic (flea-borne) A75.2
epidemic (louse-borne) A75.0
exanthematicus SAI A75.0
    brillii SAI A75.1
    mexicanus SAI A75.2
    typhus murinus A75.2
exanthematic NEC A75.0
flea-borne A75.2
India tick A77.1
Kenya (tick) A77.1
louse-borne A75.0
Mexican A75.2
mite-borne A75.3
murine A75.2
North Asian tick-borne A77.2
Orientia Tsutsugamushi (scrub typhus) A75.3
petechial A75.9
Queensland tick A77.3
rat A75.2
recrudescent A75.1
recurrens — *see* Fever, relapsing
Sao Paulo A77.0
scrub (China) (India) (Malaysia) (New Guinea) A75.3
shop (of Malaysia) A75.2
Siberian tick A77.2
tick-borne A77.9
tropical (mite-borne) A75.3
Tyrosinemia E70.21
newborn, transitory P74.5
Tyrosinosis E70.21
Tyrosinuria E70.29

U

Uhl's anomaly or disease Q24.8
Ulcer, ulcerated, ulcerating, ulceration, ulcerative
alveolar process M27.3
amebic (intestine) A06.1
    skin A06.7
anastomotic — *see* Ulcer, gastrojejunal
anorectal K62.6
antral — *see* Ulcer, stomach
anus (sphincter) (solitary) K62.6
aorta — *see* Aneurysm
aphthous (oral) (recurrent) K12.0
    genital organ(s)
      female N76.6
      male N50.89
artery I77.2
atrophic — *see* Ulcer, skin
    decubitus — *see* Ulcer, pressure, by site
back L98.429
    with
      bone involvement without evidence of necrosis L98.426
      bone necrosis L98.424
      exposed fat layer L98.422
      muscle involvement without evidence of necrosis L98.425
      muscle necrosis L98.423
      skin breakdown only L98.421

Ulcer, ulcerated, ulcerating, ulceration, ulcerative — *continued*
back — *continued*
    with — *continued*
      specified severity NEC L98.428
Barrett's (esophagus) K22.10
    with bleeding K22.11
bile duct (common) (hepatic) K83.8
bladder (solitary) (sphincter) NEC N32.89
    bilharzial B65.9 *[N33]*
    in schistosomiasis (bilharzial) B65.9 *[N33]*
    submucosal — *see* Cystitis, interstitial
    tuberculous A18.12
bleeding K27.4
bone — *see* Osteomyelitis, specified type NEC
bowel — *see* Ulcer, intestine
breast N61.1
bronchus J98.09
buccal (cavity) (traumatic) K12.1
Buruli A31.1
buttock L98.419
    with
      bone involvement without evidence of necrosis L98.416
      bone necrosis L98.414
      exposed fat layer L98.412
      muscle involvement without evidence of necrosis L98.415
      muscle necrosis L98.413
      skin breakdown only L98.411
      specified severity NEC L98.418
cancerous — *see* Neoplasm, malignant, by site
cardia K22.10
    with bleeding K22.11
cardioesophageal (peptic) K22.10
    with bleeding K22.11
cecum — *see* Ulcer, intestine
cervix (uteri) (decubitus) (trophic) N86
    with cervicitis N72
chancroidal A57
chiclero B55.1
chronic (cause unknown) — *see* Ulcer, skin
Cochin-China B55.1
colon — *see* Ulcer, intestine
conjunctiva H10.89
cornea H16.00- ☑
    with hypopyon H16.03- ☑
    central H16.01- ☑
    dendritic (herpes simplex) B00.52
    marginal H16.04- ☑
    Mooren's H16.05- ☑
    mycotic H16.06- ☑
    perforated H16.07- ☑
    ring H16.02- ☑
    tuberculous (phlyctenular) A18.52
corpus cavernosum (chronic) N48.5
crural — *see* Ulcer, lower limb
Curling's — *see* Ulcer, peptic, acute
Cushing's — *see* Ulcer, peptic, acute
cystic duct K82.8
cystitis (interstitial) — *see* Cystitis, interstitial
decubitus — *see* Ulcer, pressure, by site
dendritic, cornea (herpes simplex) B00.52
diabetes, diabetic — *see* Diabetes, ulcer
Dieulafoy's K25.0
due to
    infection NEC — *see* Ulcer, skin
    radiation NEC L59.8
    trophic disturbance (any region) — *see* Ulcer, skin
    X-ray L58.1
duodenum, duodenal (eroded) (peptic) K26.9
    with
      hemorrhage K26.4
        and perforation K26.6
      perforation K26.5
    acute K26.3
      with
        hemorrhage K26.0
          and perforation K26.2
        perforation K26.1
    chronic K26.7
      with
        hemorrhage K26.4
          and perforation K26.6
        perforation K26.5
dysenteric A09
elusive — *see* Cystitis, interstitial
endocarditis (acute) (chronic) (subacute) I28.8

☑ **Additional Character Required — Refer to the Tabular List for Character Selection**
▽ **Subterms under main terms may continue to next column or page**

Ulcer, ulcerated, ulcerating, ulceration, ulcerative
— continued
  epiglottis J38.7
  esophagus (peptic) K22.10
    with bleeding K22.11
    due to
      aspirin K22.10
        with bleeding K22.11
      gastrointestinal reflux disease (without bleeding)
        K21.00
        with bleeding K21.01
      ingestion of chemical or medicament K22.10
        with bleeding K22.11
    fungal K22.10
      with bleeding K22.11
    infective K22.10
      with bleeding K22.11
    varicose — see Varix, esophagus
  eyelid (region) H01.8
  fauces J39.2
  Fenwick (-Hunner) (solitary) — see Cystitis, interstitial
  fistulous — see Ulcer, skin
  foot (indolent) (trophic) — see Ulcer, lower limb
  frambesial, initial A66.0
  frenum (tongue) K14.0
  gallbladder or duct K82.8
  gangrenous — see Gangrene
  gastric — see Ulcer, stomach
  gastrocolic — see Ulcer, gastrojejunal
  gastroduodenal — see Ulcer, peptic
  gastroesophageal — see Ulcer, stomach
  gastrointestinal — see Ulcer, gastrojejunal
  gastrojejunal (peptic) K28.9
    with
      hemorrhage K28.4
        and perforation K28.6
      perforation K28.5
    acute K28.3
      with
        hemorrhage K28.0
          and perforation K28.2
        perforation K28.1
    chronic K28.7
      with
        hemorrhage K28.4
          and perforation K28.6
        perforation K28.5
  gastrojejunocolic — see Ulcer, gastrojejunal
  gingiva K06.8
  gingivitis K05.10
    nonplaque induced K05.11
    plaque induced K05.10
  glottis J38.7
  granuloma of pudenda A58
  gum K06.8
  gumma, due to yaws A66.4
  heel — see Ulcer, lower limb
  hemorrhoid — see also Hemorrhoids, by degree K64.8
  Hunner's — see Cystitis, interstitial
  hypopharynx J39.2
  hypopyon (chronic) (subacute) — see Ulcer, cornea,
    with hypopyon
  hypostaticum — see Ulcer, varicose
  ileum — see Ulcer, intestine
  intestine, intestinal K63.3
    with perforation K63.1
    amebic A06.1
    duodenal — see Ulcer, duodenum
    granulocytopenic (with hemorrhage) — see Neu-
      tropenia
    marginal — see Ulcer, gastrojejunal
    perforating K63.1
      newborn P78.0
    primary, small intestine K63.3
    rectum K62.6
    stercoraceous, stercoral K63.3
    tuberculous A18.32
    typhoid (fever) — see Typhoid
    varicose I86.8
  jejunum, jejunal — see Ulcer, gastrojejunal
  keratitis — see Ulcer, cornea
  knee — see Ulcer, lower limb
  labium (majus) (minus) N76.6
  laryngitis — see Laryngitis
  larynx (aphthous) (contact) J38.7
    diphtheritic A36.2
  leg — see Ulcer, lower limb
  lip K13.0

Ulcer, ulcerated, ulcerating, ulceration, ulcerative
— continued
  Lipschütz's N76.6
  lower limb (atrophic) (chronic) (neurogenic) (perforat-
    ing) (pyogenic) (trophic) (tropical) L97.909
    with
      bone involvement without evidence of necrosis
        L97.906
      bone necrosis L97.904
      exposed fat layer L97.902
      muscle involvement without evidence of necrosis
        L97.905
      muscle necrosis L97.903
      skin breakdown only L97.901
      specified severity NEC L97.908
    ankle L97.309
      with
        bone involvement without evidence of
          necrosis L97.306
        bone necrosis L97.304
        exposed fat layer L97.302
        muscle involvement without evidence of
          necrosis L97.305
        muscle necrosis L97.303
        skin breakdown only L97.301
        specified severity NEC L97.308
      left L97.329
        with
          bone involvement without evidence of
            necrosis L97.326
          bone necrosis L97.324
          exposed fat layer L97.322
          muscle involvement without evidence of
            necrosis L97.325
          muscle necrosis L97.323
          skin breakdown only L97.321
          specified severity NEC L97.328
      right L97.319
        with
          bone involvement without evidence of
            necrosis L97.316
          bone necrosis L97.314
          exposed fat layer L97.312
          muscle involvement without evidence of
            necrosis L97.315
          muscle necrosis L97.313
          skin breakdown only L97.311
          specified severity NEC L97.318
    calf L97.209
      with
        bone involvement without evidence of
          necrosis L97.206
        bone necrosis L97.204
        exposed fat layer L97.202
        muscle involvement without evidence of
          necrosis L97.205
        muscle necrosis L97.203
        skin breakdown only L97.201
        specified severity NEC L97.208
      left L97.229
        with
          bone involvement without evidence of
            necrosis L97.226
          bone necrosis L97.224
          exposed fat layer L97.222
          muscle involvement without evidence of
            necrosis L97.225
          muscle necrosis L97.223
          skin breakdown only L97.221
          specified severity NEC L97.228
      right L97.219
        with
          bone involvement without evidence of
            necrosis L97.216
          bone necrosis L97.214
          exposed fat layer L97.212
          muscle involvement without evidence of
            necrosis L97.215
          muscle necrosis L97.213
          skin breakdown only L97.211
          specified severity NEC L97.218
    decubitus — see Ulcer, pressure, by site
    foot specified NEC L97.509
      with
        bone involvement without evidence of
          necrosis L97.506
        bone necrosis L97.504
        exposed fat layer L97.502

Ulcer, ulcerated, ulcerating, ulceration, ulcerative
— continued
  lower limb — continued
    foot specified — continued
      with — continued
        muscle involvement without evidence of
          necrosis L97.505
        muscle necrosis L97.503
        skin breakdown only L97.501
        specified severity NEC L97.508
      left L97.529
        with
          bone involvement without evidence of
            necrosis L97.526
          bone necrosis L97.524
          exposed fat layer L97.522
          muscle involvement without evidence of
            necrosis L97.525
          muscle necrosis L97.523
          skin breakdown only L97.521
          specified severity NEC L97.528
      right L97.519
        with
          bone involvement without evidence of
            necrosis L97.516
          bone necrosis L97.514
          exposed fat layer L97.512
          muscle involvement without evidence of
            necrosis L97.515
          muscle necrosis L97.513
          skin breakdown only L97.511
          specified severity NEC L97.518
    heel L97.409
      with
        bone involvement without evidence of
          necrosis L97.406
        bone necrosis L97.404
        exposed fat layer L97.402
        muscle involvement without evidence of
          necrosis L97.405
        muscle necrosis L97.403
        skin breakdown only L97.401
        specified severity NEC L97.408
      left L97.429
        with
          bone involvement without evidence of
            necrosis L97.426
          bone necrosis L97.424
          exposed fat layer L97.422
          muscle involvement without evidence of
            necrosis L97.425
          muscle necrosis L97.423
          skin breakdown only L97.421
          specified severity NEC L97.428
      right L97.419
        with
          bone involvement without evidence of
            necrosis L97.416
          bone necrosis L97.414
          exposed fat layer L97.412
          muscle involvement without evidence of
            necrosis L97.415
          muscle necrosis L97.413
          skin breakdown only L97.411
          specified severity NEC L97.418
    left L97.929
      with
        bone involvement without evidence of
          necrosis L97.926
        bone necrosis L97.924
        exposed fat layer L97.922
        muscle involvement without evidence of
          necrosis L97.925
        muscle necrosis L97.923
        skin breakdown only L97.921
        specified severity NEC L97.928
    leprous A30.1
    lower leg NOS L97.909
      with
        bone involvement without evidence of
          necrosis L97.906
        bone necrosis L97.904
        exposed fat layer L97.902
        muscle involvement without evidence of
          necrosis L97.905
        muscle necrosis L97.903
        skin breakdown only L97.901
        specified severity NEC L97.908
    left L97.929

Ulcer, ulcerated, ulcerating, ulceration, ulcerative
— continued
  lower limb — continued
    lower leg — continued
      left — continued
        with
          bone involvement without evidence of necrosis L97.926
          bone necrosis L97.924
          exposed fat layer L97.922
          muscle involvement without evidence of necrosis L97.925
          muscle necrosis L97.923
          skin breakdown only L97.921
          specified severity NEC L97.928
       right L97.919
        with
          bone involvement without evidence of necrosis L97.916
          bone necrosis L97.914
          exposed fat layer L97.912
          muscle involvement without evidence of necrosis L97.915
          muscle necrosis L97.913
          skin breakdown only L97.911
          specified severity NEC L97.918
      specified site NEC L97.809
        with
          bone involvement without evidence of necrosis L97.806
          bone necrosis L97.804
          exposed fat layer L97.802
          muscle involvement without evidence of necrosis L97.805
          muscle necrosis L97.803
          skin breakdown only L97.801
          specified severity NEC L97.808
      left L97.829
        with
          bone involvement without evidence of necrosis L97.826
          bone necrosis L97.824
          exposed fat layer L97.822
          muscle involvement without evidence of necrosis L97.825
          muscle necrosis L97.823
          skin breakdown only L97.821
          specified severity NEC L97.828
      right L97.819
        with
          bone involvement without evidence of necrosis L97.816
          bone necrosis L97.814
          exposed fat layer L97.812
          muscle involvement without evidence of necrosis L97.815
          muscle necrosis L97.813
          skin breakdown only L97.811
          specified severity NEC L97.818
    midfoot L97.409
      with
        bone involvement without evidence of necrosis L97.406
        bone necrosis L97.404
        exposed fat layer L97.402
        muscle involvement without evidence of necrosis L97.405
        muscle necrosis L97.403
        skin breakdown only L97.401
        specified severity NEC L97.408
      left L97.429
        with
          bone involvement without evidence of necrosis L97.426
          bone necrosis L97.424
          exposed fat layer L97.422
          muscle involvement without evidence of necrosis L97.425
          muscle necrosis L97.423
          skin breakdown only L97.421
          specified severity NEC L97.428
      right L97.419
        with
          bone involvement without evidence of necrosis L97.416
          bone necrosis L97.414
          exposed fat layer L97.412
          muscle involvement without evidence of necrosis L97.415

Ulcer, ulcerated, ulcerating, ulceration, ulcerative
— continued
  lower limb — continued
    midfoot — continued
      right — continued
        with — continued
          muscle necrosis L97.413
          skin breakdown only L97.411
          specified severity NEC L97.418
    right L97.919
      with
        bone involvement without evidence of necrosis L97.916
        bone necrosis L97.914
        exposed fat layer L97.912
        muscle involvement without evidence of necrosis L97.915
        muscle necrosis L97.913
        skin breakdown only L97.911
        specified severity NEC L97.918
    syphilitic A52.19
    thigh L97.109
      with
        bone involvement without evidence of necrosis L97.106
        bone necrosis L97.104
        exposed fat layer L97.102
        muscle involvement without evidence of necrosis L97.105
        muscle necrosis L97.103
        skin breakdown only L97.101
        specified severity NEC L97.108
      left L97.129
        with
          bone involvement without evidence of necrosis L97.126
          bone necrosis L97.124
          exposed fat layer L97.122
          muscle involvement without evidence of necrosis L97.125
          muscle necrosis L97.123
          skin breakdown only L97.121
          specified severity NEC L97.128
      right L97.119
        with
          bone involvement without evidence of necrosis L97.116
          bone necrosis L97.114
          exposed fat layer L97.112
          muscle involvement without evidence of necrosis L97.115
          muscle necrosis L97.113
          skin breakdown only L97.111
          specified severity NEC L97.118
    toe L97.509
      with
        bone involvement without evidence of necrosis L97.506
        bone necrosis L97.504
        exposed fat layer L97.502
        muscle involvement without evidence of necrosis L97.505
        muscle necrosis L97.503
        skin breakdown only L97.501
        specified severity NEC L97.508
      left L97.529
        with
          bone involvement without evidence of necrosis L97.526
          bone necrosis L97.524
          exposed fat layer L97.522
          muscle involvement without evidence of necrosis L97.525
          muscle necrosis L97.523
          skin breakdown only L97.521
          specified severity NEC L97.528
      right L97.519
        with
          bone involvement without evidence of necrosis L97.516
          bone necrosis L97.514
          exposed fat layer L97.512
          muscle involvement without evidence of necrosis L97.515
          muscle necrosis L97.513
          skin breakdown only L97.511
          specified severity NEC L97.518
  varicose — see Varix, leg, with, ulcer
  luetic — see Ulcer, syphilitic

Ulcer, ulcerated, ulcerating, ulceration, ulcerative
— continued
  lung J98.4
    tuberculous — see Tuberculosis, pulmonary
  malignant — see Neoplasm, malignant, by site
  marginal NEC — see Ulcer, gastrojejunal
  meatus (urinarius) N34.2
  Meckel's diverticulum Q43.0
    malignant — see Table of Neoplasms, small intestine, malignant
  Meleney's (chronic undermining) — see Ulcer, skin
  Mooren's (cornea) — see Ulcer, cornea, Mooren's
  mycobacterial (skin) A31.1
  nasopharynx J39.2
  neck, uterus N86
  neurogenic NEC — see Ulcer, skin
  nose, nasal (passage) (infective) (septum) J34.0
    skin — see Ulcer, skin
    spirochetal A69.8
    varicose (bleeding) I86.8
  oral mucosa (traumatic) K12.1
  palate (soft) K12.1
  penis (chronic) N48.5
  peptic (site unspecified) K27.9
    with
      hemorrhage K27.4
        and perforation K27.6
      perforation K27.5
    acute K27.3
      with
        hemorrhage K27.0
          and perforation K27.2
        perforation K27.1
    chronic K27.7
      with
        hemorrhage K27.4
          and perforation K27.6
        perforation K27.5
    esophagus K22.10
      with bleeding K22.11
    newborn P78.82
  perforating K27.5
    skin — see Ulcer, skin
  peritonsillar J35.8
  phagedenic (tropical) — see Ulcer, skin
  pharynx J39.2
  phlebitis — see Phlebitis
  plaster — see Ulcer, pressure, by site
  popliteal space — see Ulcer, lower limb
  postpyloric — see Ulcer, duodenum
  prepuce N47.7
  prepyloric — see Ulcer, stomach
  pressure (pressure area) L89.9- ☑
    ankle L89.5- ☑
    back L89.1- ☑
    buttock L89.3- ☑
    coccyx L89.15- ☑
    contiguous site of back, buttock, hip L89.4- ☑
    elbow L89.0- ☑
    face L89.81- ☑
    head L89.81- ☑
    heel L89.6- ☑
    hip L89.2- ☑
    sacral region (tailbone) L89.15- ☑
    specified site NEC L89.89- ☑
    stage 1 (healing) (pre-ulcer skin changes limited to persistent focal edema)
      ankle L89.5- ☑
      back L89.1- ☑
      buttock L89.3- ☑
      coccyx L89.15- ☑
      contiguous site of back, buttock, hip L89.4- ☑
      elbow L89.0- ☑
      face L89.81- ☑
      head L89.81- ☑
      heel L89.6- ☑
      hip L89.2- ☑
      sacral region (tailbone) L89.15- ☑
      specified site NEC L89.89- ☑
    stage 2 (healing) (abrasion, blister, partial thickness skin loss involving epidermis and/or dermis)
      ankle L89.5- ☑
      back L89.1- ☑
      buttock L89.3- ☑
      coccyx L89.15- ☑
      contiguous site of back, buttock, hip L89.4- ☑
      elbow L89.0- ☑

Ulcer, ulcerated, ulcerating, ulceration, ulcerative
  — *continued*
  pressure — *continued*
    stage 2 — *continued*
      face L89.81- ☑
      head L89.81- ☑
      heel L89.6- ☑
      hip L89.2- ☑
      sacral region (tailbone) L89.15- ☑
      specified site NEC L89.89- ☑
    stage 3 (healing) (full thickness skin loss involving damage or necrosis of subcutaneous tissue)
      ankle L89.5- ☑
      back L89.1- ☑
      buttock L89.3- ☑
      coccyx L89.15- ☑
      contiguous site of back, buttock, hip L89.4- ☑
      elbow L89.0- ☑
      face L89.81- ☑
      head L89.81- ☑
      heel L89.6- ☑
      hip L89.2- ☑
      sacral region (tailbone) L89.15- ☑
      specified site NEC L89.89- ☑
    stage 4 (healing) (necrosis of soft tissues through to underlying muscle, tendon, or bone)
      ankle L89.5- ☑
      back L89.1- ☑
      buttock L89.3- ☑
      coccyx L89.15- ☑
      contiguous site of back, buttock, hip L89.4- ☑
      elbow L89.0- ☑
      face L89.81- ☑
      head L89.81- ☑
      heel L89.6- ☑
      hip L89.2- ☑
      sacral region (tailbone) L89.15- ☑
      specified site NEC L89.89- ☑
    unspecified stage
      ankle L89.5- ☑
      back L89.1- ☑
      buttock L89.3- ☑
      coccyx L89.15- ☑
      contiguous site of back, buttock, hip L89.4- ☑
      elbow L89.0- ☑
      face L89.81- ☑
      head L89.81- ☑
      heel L89.6- ☑
      hip L89.2- ☑
      sacral region (tailbone) L89.15- ☑
      specified site NEC L89.89- ☑
    unstageable
      ankle L89.5- ☑
      back L89.1- ☑
      buttock L89.3- ☑
      coccyx L89.15- ☑
      contiguous site of back, buttock, hip L89.4- ☑
      elbow L89.0- ☑
      face L89.81- ☑
      head L89.81- ☑
      heel L89.6- ☑
      hip L89.2- ☑
      sacral region (tailbone) L89.15- ☑
      specified site NEC L89.89- ☑
  primary of intestine K63.3
    with perforation K63.1
  prostate N41.9
  pyloric — *see* Ulcer, stomach
  rectosigmoid K63.3
    with perforation K63.1
  rectum (sphincter) (solitary) K62.6
    stercoraceous, stercoral K62.6
  retina — *see* Inflammation, chorioretinal
  rodent — *see also* Neoplasm, skin, malignant
  sclera — *see* Scleritis
  scrofulous (tuberculous) A18.2
  scrotum N50.89
    tuberculous A18.15
    varicose I86.1
  seminal vesicle N50.89
  sigmoid — *see* Ulcer, intestine
  skin (atrophic) (chronic) (neurogenic) (non-healing) (perforating) (pyogenic) (trophic) (tropical) L98.499
    with gangrene — *see* Gangrene
    amebic A06.7

Ulcer, ulcerated, ulcerating, ulceration, ulcerative
  — *continued*
  skin — *continued*
    back — *see* Ulcer, back
    buttock — *see* Ulcer, buttock
    decubitus — *see* Ulcer, pressure
    lower limb — *see* Ulcer, lower limb
    mycobacterial A31.1
    specified site NEC L98.499
      with
        bone involvement without evidence of necrosis L98.496
        bone necrosis L98.494
        exposed fat layer L98.492
        muscle involvement without evidence of necrosis L98.495
        muscle necrosis L98.493
        skin breakdown only L98.491
        specified severity NEC L98.498
    tuberculous (primary) A18.4
    varicose — *see* Ulcer, varicose
  sloughing — *see* Ulcer, skin
  solitary, anus or rectum (sphincter) K62.6
  sore throat J02.9
    streptococcal J02.0
  spermatic cord N50.89
  spine (tuberculous) A18.01
  stasis (venous) — *see* Varix, leg, with, ulcer
    without varicose veins I87.2
  stercoraceous, stercoral K63.3
    with perforation K63.1
    anus or rectum K62.6
  stoma, stomal — *see* Ulcer, gastrojejunal
  stomach (eroded) (peptic) (round) K25.9
    with
      hemorrhage K25.4
        and perforation K25.6
      perforation K25.5
    acute K25.3
      with
        hemorrhage K25.0
          and perforation K25.2
        perforation K25.1
    chronic K25.7
      with
        hemorrhage K25.4
          and perforation K25.6
        perforation K25.5
  stomal — *see* Ulcer, gastrojejunal
  stomatitis K12.1
  stress — *see* Ulcer, peptic
  strumous (tuberculous) A18.2
  submucosal, bladder — *see* Cystitis, interstitial
  syphilitic (any site) (early) (secondary) A51.39
    late A52.79
      perforating A52.79
        foot A52.11
  testis N50.89
  thigh — *see* Ulcer, lower limb
  throat J39.2
    diphtheritic A36.0
  toe — *see* Ulcer, lower limb
  tongue (traumatic) K14.0
  tonsil J35.8
    diphtheritic A36.0
  trachea J39.8
  trophic — *see* Ulcer, skin
  tropical — *see* Ulcer, skin
  tuberculous — *see* Tuberculosis, ulcer
  tunica vaginalis N50.89
  turbinate J34.89
  typhoid (perforating) — *see* Typhoid
  unspecified site — *see* Ulcer, skin
  urethra (meatus) — *see* Urethritis
  uterus N85.8
    cervix N86
      with cervicitis N72
    neck N86
      with cervicitis N72
  vagina N76.5
    in Behçet's disease M35.2 *[N77.0]*
    pessary N89.8
  valve, heart I33.0
  varicose (lower limb, any part) — *see also* Varix, leg, with, ulcer
    broad ligament I86.2
    esophagus — *see* Varix, esophagus

Ulcer, ulcerated, ulcerating, ulceration, ulcerative
  — *continued*
  varicose — *see also* Varix, leg, with, ulcer — *continued*
    inflamed or infected — *see* Varix, leg, with ulcer, with inflammation
    nasal septum I86.8
    perineum I86.3
    scrotum I86.1
    specified site NEC I86.8
    sublingual I86.0
    vulva I86.3
  vas deferens N50.89
  vulva (acute) (infectional) N76.6
    in (due to)
      Behçet's disease M35.2 *[N77.0]*
      herpesviral (herpes simplex) infection A60.04
      tuberculosis A18.18
  vulvobuccal, recurring N76.6
  X-ray L58.1
  yaws A66.4
Ulcerosa scarlatina A38.8
Ulcus — *see also* Ulcer
  cutis tuberculosum A18.4
  duodeni — *see* Ulcer, duodenum
  durum (syphilitic) A51.0
    extragenital A51.2
  gastrojejunale — *see* Ulcer, gastrojejunal
  hypostaticum — *see* Ulcer, varicose
  molle (cutis) (skin) A57
  serpens corneae — *see* Ulcer, cornea, central
  ventriculi — *see* Ulcer, stomach
Ulegyria Q04.8
Ulerythema
  ophryogenes, congenital Q84.2
  sycosiforme L73.8
Ullrich (-Bonnevie)(-Turner) **syndrome** — *see also* Turner's syndrome Q87.19
Ullrich-Feichtiger syndrome Q87.0
Ulnar — *see* condition
Ulorrhagia, ulorrhea K06.8
Umbilicus, umbilical — *see* condition
Unacceptable
  contours of tooth K08.54
  morphology of tooth K08.54
Unavailability (of)
  bed at medical facility Z75.1
  health service-related agencies Z75.4
  medical facilities (at) Z75.3
    due to
      investigation by social service agency Z75.2
      lack of services at home Z75.0
      remoteness from facility Z75.3
      waiting list Z75.1
    home Z75.0
    outpatient clinic Z75.3
  schooling Z55.1
  social service agencies Z75.4
Uncinaria americana infestation B76.1
Uncinariasis B76.9
Uncongenial work Z56.5
Unconscious (ness) — *see* Coma
Under observation — *see* Observation
Underachievement in school Z55.3
Underdevelopment — *see also* Undeveloped
  nose Q30.1
  sexual E30.0
Underdosing — *see also* Table of Drugs and Chemicals, categories T36-T50, with final character 6 Z91.14
  intentional NEC Z91.128
    due to financial hardship of patient Z91.120
  unintentional NEC Z91.138
    due to patient's age related debility Z91.130
Underfeeding, newborn P92.3
Underfill, endodontic M27.53
Underimmunization status Z28.3
Undernourishment — *see* Malnutrition
Undernutrition — *see* Malnutrition
Underweight R63.6
  for gestational age — *see* Light for dates
Underwood's disease P83.0
Undescended — *see also* Malposition, congenital
  cecum Q43.3
  colon Q43.3
  testicle — *see* Cryptorchid
Undeveloped, undevelopment — *see also* Hypoplasia
  brain (congenital) Q02
  cerebral (congenital) Q02

Undeveloped, undevelopment — *continued*
heart Q24.8
lung Q33.6
testis E29.1
uterus E30.0
Undiagnosed (disease) R69
Undulant fever — *see* Brucellosis
Unemployment, anxiety concerning Z56.0
threatened Z56.2
Unequal length (acquired) (limb) — *see also* Deformity,
limb, unequal length
leg — *see also* Deformity, limb, unequal length
congenital Q72.9- ☑
Unextracted dental root K08.3
Unguis incarnatus L60.0
Unhappiness R45.2
Unicornate uterus Q51.4
in pregnancy or childbirth O34.00
Unilateral — *see also* condition
development, breast N64.89
organ or site, congenital NEC — *see* Agenesis, by site
Unilocular heart Q20.8
Union, abnormal — *see also* Fusion
larynx and trachea Q34.8
Universal mesentery Q43.3
Unrepairable overhanging of dental restorative
materials K08.52
Unsatisfactory
restoration of tooth K08.50
specified NEC K08.59
sample of cytologic smear
anus R85.615
cervix R87.615
vagina R87.625
surroundings Z59.1
work Z56.5
Unsoundness of mind — *see* Psychosis
Unstable
back NEC — *see* Instability, joint, spine
hip (congenital) Q65.6
acquired — *see* Derangement, joint, specified type
NEC, hip
joint — *see* Instability, joint
secondary to removal of joint prosthesis M96.89
lie (mother) O32.0 ☑
lumbosacral joint (congenital) — *see* subcategory
M53.2
sacroiliac — *see* subcategory M53.2 ☑
spine NEC — *see* Instability, joint, spine
Unsteadiness on feet R26.81
Untruthfulness, child problem F91.8
Unverricht (-Lundborg) **disease or epilepsy** — *see*
Epilepsy, generalized, idiopathic
Unwanted pregnancy Z64.0
Upbringing, institutional Z62.22
away from parents NEC Z62.29
in care of non-parental family member Z62.21
in foster care Z62.21
in orphanage or group home Z62.22
in welfare custody Z62.21
Upper respiratory — *see* condition
Upset
gastric K30
gastrointestinal K30
psychogenic F45.8
intestinal (large) (small) K59.9
psychogenic F45.8
menstruation N93.9
mental F48.9
stomach K30
psychogenic F45.8
Urachus — *see also* condition
patent or persistent Q64.4
Urbach-Oppenheim disease (necrobiosis lipoidica dia-
beticorum) — *see* E08-E13 with .620
Urbach's lipoid proteinosis E78.89
Urbach-Wiethe disease E78.89
Urban yellow fever A95.1
Urea
blood, high — *see* Uremia
cycle metabolism disorder — *see* Disorder, urea cycle
metabolism
Uremia, uremic N19
with
ectopic or molar pregnancy O08.4
polyneuropathy N18.9 *[G63]*
chronic NOS — *see also* Disease, kidney, chronic N18.9

Uremia, uremic — *continued*
chronic — *see also* Disease, kidney, chronic — *contin-*
ued
due to hypertension — *see* Hypertensive, kidney
complicating
ectopic or molar pregnancy O08.4
congenital P96.0
extrarenal R39.2
following ectopic or molar pregnancy O08.4
newborn P96.0
prerenal R39.2
Ureter, ureteral — *see* condition
Ureteralgia N23
Ureterectasis — *see* Hydroureter
Ureteritis N28.89
cystica N28.86
due to calculus N20.1
with calculus, kidney N20.2
with hydronephrosis N13.2
gonococcal (acute) (chronic) A54.21
nonspecific N28.89
Ureterocele N28.89
congenital (orthotopic) Q62.31
ectopic Q62.32
Ureterolith, ureterolithiasis — *see* Calculus, ureter
Ureterostomy
attention to Z43.6
status Z93.6
Urethra, urethral — *see* condition
Urethralgia R39.89
Urethritis (anterior) (posterior) N34.2
calculous N21.1
candidal B37.41
chlamydial A56.01
diplococcal (gonococcal) A54.01
with abscess (accessory gland) (periurethral) A54.1
gonococcal A54.01
with abscess (accessory gland) (periurethral) A54.1
nongonococcal N34.1
Reiter's — *see* Reiter's disease
nonspecific N34.1
nonvenereal N34.1
postmenopausal N34.2
puerperal O86.22
Reiter's — *see* Reiter's disease
specified NEC N34.2
trichomonal or due to Trichomonas (vaginalis) A59.03
Urethrocele N81.0
with
cystocele — *see* Cystocele
prolapse of uterus — *see* Prolapse, uterus
Urethrolithiasis (with colic or infection) N21.1
Urethrorectal — *see* condition
Urethrorrhagia N36.8
Urethrorrhea R36.9
Urethrostomy
attention to Z43.6
status Z93.6
Urethrotrigonitis — *see* Trigonitis
Urethrovaginal — *see* condition
Urgency
fecal R15.2
hypertensive — *see* Hypertension
urinary R39.15
Urhidrosis, uridrosis L74.8
Uric acid in blood (increased) E79.0
Uricacidemia (asymptomatic) E79.0
Uricemia (asymptomatic) E79.0
Uricosuria R82.998
Urinary — *see* condition
Urination
frequent R35.0
painful R30.9
Urine
blood in — *see* Hematuria
discharge, excessive R35.8
enuresis, nonorganic origin F98.0
extravasation R39.0
frequency R35.0
incontinence R32
nonorganic origin F98.0
intermittent stream R39.198
pus in N39.0
retention or stasis R33.9
organic R33.8
drug-induced R33.0
psychogenic F45.8

Urine — *continued*
secretion
deficient R34
excessive R35.8
frequency R35.0
stream
intermittent R39.198
slowing R39.198
splitting R39.13
weak R39.12
Urinemia — *see* Uremia
Urinoma, urethra N36.8
Uroarthritis, infectious (Reiter's) — *see* Reiter's disease
Urodialysis R34
Urolithiasis — *see* Calculus, urinary
Uronephrosis — *see* Hydronephrosis
Uropathy N39.9
obstructive N13.9
specified NEC N13.8
reflux N13.9
specified NEC N13.8
vesicoureteral reflux-associated — *see* Reflux, vesicoureteral
Urosepsis — *code to* condition
Urticaria L50.9
with angioneurotic edema T78.3 ☑
hereditary D84.1
allergic L50.0
cholinergic L50.5
chronic L50.8
cold, familial L50.2
contact L50.6
dermatographic L50.3
due to
cold or heat L50.2
drugs L50.0
food L50.0
inhalants L50.0
plants L50.6
serum — *see also* Reaction, serum T80.69 ☑
factitial L50.3
familial cold M04.2
giant T78.3 ☑
hereditary D84.1
gigantea T78.3 ☑
idiopathic L50.1
larynx T78.3 ☑
hereditary D84.1
neonatorum P83.88
nonallergic L50.1
papulosa (Hebra) L28.2
pigmentosa D47.01
congenital Q82.2
of neonatal onset Q82.2
of newborn onset Q82.2
recurrent periodic L50.8
serum — *see also* Reaction, serum T80.69 ☑
solar L56.3
specified type NEC L50.8
thermal (cold) (heat) L50.2
vibratory L50.4
xanthelasmoidea — *see* Urticaria pigmentosa
Use (of)
alcohol Z72.89
with
intoxication F10.929
sleep disorder F10.982
withdrawal F10.939
with
perceptual disturbance F10.932
delirium F10.931
uncomplicated F10.930
harmful — *see* Abuse, alcohol
amphetamines — *see* Use, stimulant NEC
caffeine — *see* Use, stimulant NEC
cannabis F12.90
with
anxiety disorder F12.980
intoxication F12.929
with
delirium F12.921
perceptual disturbance F12.922
uncomplicated F12.920
other specified disorder F12.988
psychosis F12.959
delusions F12.950
hallucinations F12.951
unspecified disorder F12.99

Use — *continued*
  cannabis — *continued*
    with — *continued*
      withdrawal F12.93
  cocaine F14.90
    with
      anxiety disorder F14.980
      intoxication F14.929
        with
          delirium F14.921
          perceptual disturbance F14.922
        uncomplicated F14.920
      other specified disorder F14.988
      psychosis F14.959
        delusions F14.950
        hallucinations F14.951
      sexual dysfunction F14.981
      sleep disorder F14.982
      unspecified disorder F14.99
      withdrawal F14.93
    harmful — *see* Abuse, drug, cocaine
  drug(s) NEC F19.90
    with sleep disorder F19.982
    harmful — *see* Abuse, drug, by type
  hallucinogen NEC F16.90
    with
      anxiety disorder F16.980
      intoxication F16.929
        with
          delirium F16.921
        uncomplicated F16.920
      mood disorder F16.94
      other specified disorder F16.988
      perception disorder (flashbacks) F16.983
      psychosis F16.959
        delusions F16.950
        hallucinations F16.951
      unspecified disorder F16.99
    harmful — *see* Abuse, drug, hallucinogen NEC
  inhalants F18.90
    with
      anxiety disorder F18.980
      intoxication F18.929
        with delirium F18.921
        uncomplicated F18.920
      mood disorder F18.94
      other specified disorder F18.988
      persisting dementia F18.97
      psychosis F18.959
        delusions F18.950
        hallucinations F18.951
      unspecified disorder F18.99
    harmful — *see* Abuse, drug, inhalant
  methadone — *see* Use, opioid
  nonprescribed drugs F19.90
    harmful — *see* Abuse, non-psychoactive substance
  opioid F11.90
    with
      disorder F11.99
        mood F11.94
        sleep F11.982
        specified type NEC F11.988
      intoxication F11.929
        with
          delirium F11.921
          perceptual disturbance F11.922
        uncomplicated F11.920
      withdrawal F11.93
    harmful — *see* Abuse, drug, opioid
  patent medicines F19.90
    harmful — *see* Abuse, non-psychoactive substance
  psychoactive drug NEC F19.90
    with
      anxiety disorder F19.980
      intoxication F19.929
        with
          delirium F19.921
          perceptual disturbance F19.922
        uncomplicated F19.920
      mood disorder F19.94
      other specified disorder F19.988
      persisting
        amnestic disorder F19.96
        dementia F19.97
      psychosis F19.959
        delusions F19.950
        hallucinations F19.951
      sexual dysfunction F19.981

Use — *continued*
  psychoactive drug — *continued*
    with — *continued*
      sleep disorder F19.982
      unspecified disorder F19.99
      withdrawal F19.939
        with
          delirium F19.931
          perceptual disturbance F19.932
        uncomplicated F19.930
    harmful — *see* Abuse, drug NEC, psychoactive NEC
  sedative, hypnotic, or anxiolytic F13.90
    with
      anxiety disorder F13.980
      intoxication F13.929
        with
          delirium F13.921
        uncomplicated F13.920
      other specified disorder F13.988
      persisting
        amnestic disorder F13.96
        dementia F13.97
      psychosis F13.959
        delusions F13.950
        hallucinations F13.951
      sexual dysfunction F13.981
      sleep disorder F13.982
      unspecified disorder F13.99
    harmful — *see* Abuse, drug, sedative, hypnotic, or
        anxiolytic
  stimulant NEC F15.90
    with
      anxiety disorder F15.980
      intoxication F15.929
        with
          delirium F15.921
          perceptual disturbance F15.922
        uncomplicated F15.920
      mood disorder F15.94
      other specified disorder F15.988
      psychosis F15.959
        delusions F15.950
        hallucinations F15.951
      sexual dysfunction F15.981
      sleep disorder F15.982
      unspecified disorder F15.99
      withdrawal F15.93
    harmful — *see* Abuse, drug, stimulant NEC
  tobacco Z72.0
    with dependence — *see* Dependence, drug, nicotine
  volatile solvents — *see also* Use, inhalant F18.90
    harmful — *see* Abuse, drug, inhalant

Usher-Senear disease or syndrome L10.4
Uta B55.1
Uteromegaly N85.2
Uterovaginal — *see* condition
Uterovesical — *see* condition
Uveal — *see* condition
Uveitis (anterior) — *see also* Iridocyclitis
  acute — *see* Iridocyclitis, acute
  chronic — *see* Iridocyclitis, chronic
  due to toxoplasmosis (acquired) B58.09
    congenital P37.1
  granulomatous — *see* Iridocyclitis, chronic
  heterochromic — *see* Cyclitis, Fuchs' heterochromic
  lens-induced — *see* Iridocyclitis, lens-induced
  posterior — *see* Chorioretinitis
  sympathetic H44.13- ☑
  syphilitic (secondary) A51.43
    congenital (early) A50.01
    late A52.71
  tuberculous A18.54
Uveoencephalitis — *see* Inflammation, chorioretinal
Uveokeratitis — *see* Iridocyclitis
Uveoparotitis D86.89
Uvula — *see* condition
Uvulitis (acute) (catarrhal) (chronic) (membranous)
  (suppurative) (ulcerative) K12.2

V

Vaccination (prophylactic)
  complication or reaction — *see* Complications, vacci-
    nation
  delayed Z28.9
  encounter for Z23
  not done — *see* Immunization, not done, because of)
Vaccinia (generalized) (localized) T88.1 ☑

Vaccinia — *continued*
  congenital P35.8
  without vaccination B08.011
Vacuum, in sinus (accessory) (nasal) J34.89
Vagabond, vagabondage Z59.0
Vagabond's disease B85.1
Vagina, vaginal — *see* condition
Vaginalitis (tunica) (testis) N49.1
Vaginismus (reflex) N94.2
  functional F52.5
  nonorganic F52.5
  psychogenic F52.5
  secondary N94.2
Vaginitis (acute) (circumscribed) (diffuse) (emphysematous) (nonvenereal) (ulcerative) N76.0
  with ectopic or molar pregnancy O08.0
  amebic A06.82
  atrophic, postmenopausal N95.2
  bacterial N76.0
  blennorrhagic (gonococcal) A54.02
  candidal B37.3
  chlamydial A56.02
  chronic N76.1
  due to Trichomonas (vaginalis) A59.01
  following ectopic or molar pregnancy O08.0
  gonococcal A54.02
    with abscess (accessory gland) (periurethral) A54.1
  granuloma A58
  in (due to)
    candidiasis B37.3
    herpesviral (herpes simplex) infection A60.04
    pinworm infection B80 *[N77.1]*
  monilial B37.3
  mycotic (candidal) B37.3
  postmenopausal atrophic N95.2
  puerperal (postpartum) O86.13
  senile (atrophic) N95.2
  subacute or chronic N76.1
  syphilitic (early) A51.0
    late A52.76
  trichomonal A59.01
  tuberculous A18.18
Vaginosis — *see* Vaginitis
Vagotonia G52.2
Vagrancy Z59.0
VAIN — *see* Neoplasia, intraepithelial, vagina
Vallecula — *see* condition
Valley fever B38.0
Valsuani's disease — *see* Anemia, obstetric
Valve, valvular (formation) — *see also* condition
  cerebral ventricle (communicating) in situ Z98.2
  cervix, internal os Q51.828
  congenital NEC — *see* Atresia, by site
  ureter (pelvic junction) (vesical orifice) Q62.39
  urethra (congenital) (posterior) Q64.2
Valvulitis (chronic) — *see* Endocarditis
Valvulopathy — *see* Endocarditis
Van Bogaert's leukoencephalopathy (sclerosing)
  (subacute) A81.1
Van Bogaert-Scherer-Epstein disease or syndrome
  E75.5
Van Buchem's syndrome M85.2
Van Creveld-von Gierke disease E74.01
Van der Hoeve (-de Kleyn) **syndrome** Q78.0
Van der Woude's syndrome Q38.0
Van Neck's disease or osteochondrosis M91.0
Vanishing lung J44.9
Vapor asphyxia or suffocation T59.9 ☑
  specified agent — *see* Table of Drugs and Chemicals
Variance, lethal ball, prosthetic heart valve T82.09 ☑
Variants, thalassemic D56.8
Variations in hair color L67.1
Varicella B01.9
  with
    complications NEC B01.89
    encephalitis B01.11
    encephalomyelitis B01.11
    meningitis B01.0
    myelitis B01.12
    pneumonia B01.2
  congenital P35.8
Varices — *see* Varix
Varicocele (scrotum) (thrombosed) I86.1
  ovary I86.2
  perineum I86.3
  spermatic cord (ulcerated) I86.1
Varicose
  aneurysm (ruptured) I77.0

Subterms under main terms may continue to next column or page   ☑ Additional Character Required — Refer to the Tabular List for Character Selection   327

Use — Varicose

Varicose — *continued*
  dermatitis — *see* Varix, leg, with, inflammation
  eczema — *see* Varix, leg, with, inflammation
  phlebitis — *see* Varix, with, inflammation
  tumor — *see* Varix
  ulcer (lower limb, any part) — *see also* Varix, leg, with, ulcer
    anus — *see also* Hemorrhoids K64.8
    esophagus — *see* Varix, esophagus
    inflamed or infected — *see* Varix, leg, with ulcer, with inflammation
    nasal septum I86.8
    perineum I86.3
    scrotum I86.1
    specified site NEC I86.8
  vein — *see* Varix
  vessel — *see* Varix, leg
Varicosis, varicosities, varicosity — *see* Varix
Variola (major) (minor) B03
Varioloid B03
Varix (lower limb) I83.90
  with
    bleeding I83.899
    edema I83.899
    inflammation I83.10
      with ulcer (venous) I83.209
    pain I83.819
    rupture I83.899
    specified complication NEC I83.899
    stasis dermatitis I83.10
      with ulcer (venous) I83.209
    swelling I83.899
    ulcer I83.009
      with inflammation I83.209
  aneurysmal I77.0
  asymptomatic I83.9- ☑
  bladder I86.2
  broad ligament I86.2
  complicating
    childbirth (lower extremity) O87.4
      anus or rectum O87.2
      genital (vagina, vulva or perineum) O87.8
    pregnancy (lower extremity) O22.0- ☑
      anus or rectum O22.4- ☑
      genital (vagina, vulva or perineum) O22.1- ☑
    puerperium (lower extremity) O87.4
      anus or rectum O87.2
      genital (vagina, vulva, perineum) O87.8
  congenital (any site) Q27.8
  esophagus (idiopathic) (primary) (ulcerated) I85.00
    bleeding I85.01
    congenital Q27.8
    in (due to)
      alcoholic liver disease I85.10
        bleeding I85.11
      cirrhosis of liver I85.10
        bleeding I85.11
      portal hypertension I85.10
        bleeding I85.11
      schistosomiasis I85.10
        bleeding I85.11
      toxic liver disease I85.10
        bleeding I85.11
    secondary I85.10
      bleeding I85.11
  gastric I86.4
  inflamed or infected I83.10
    ulcerated I83.209
  labia (majora) I86.3
  leg (asymptomatic) I83.90
    with
      edema I83.899
      inflammation I83.10
        with ulcer — *see* Varix, leg, with, ulcer, with inflammation by site
      pain I83.819
      specified complication NEC I83.899
      swelling I83.899
      ulcer I83.009
        with inflammation I83.209
        ankle I83.003
          with inflammation I83.203
        calf I83.002
          with inflammation I83.202
        foot NEC I83.005
          with inflammation I83.205
        heel I83.004
          with inflammation I83.204

Varix — *continued*
  leg — *continued*
    with — *continued*
      ulcer — *continued*
        lower leg NEC I83.008
          with inflammation I83.208
        midfoot I83.004
          with inflammation I83.204
        thigh I83.001
          with inflammation I83.201
    bilateral (asymptomatic) I83.93
      with
        edema I83.893
        pain I83.813
        specified complication NEC I83.893
        swelling I83.893
        ulcer I83.0- ☑
          with inflammation I83.209
    left (asymptomatic) I83.92
      with
        edema I83.892
        inflammation I83.12
          with ulcer — *see* Varix, leg, with, ulcer, with inflammation by site
        pain I83.812
        specified complication NEC I83.892
        swelling I83.892
        ulcer I83.029
          with inflammation I83.229
          ankle I83.023
            with inflammation I83.223
          calf I83.022
            with inflammation I83.222
          foot NEC I83.025
            with inflammation I83.225
          heel I83.024
            with inflammation I83.224
          lower leg NEC I83.028
            with inflammation I83.228
          midfoot I83.024
            with inflammation I83.224
          thigh I83.021
            with inflammation I83.221
    right (asymptomatic) I83.91
      with
        edema I83.891
        inflammation I83.11
          with ulcer — *see* Varix, leg, with, ulcer, with inflammation by site
        pain I83.811
        specified complication NEC I83.891
        swelling I83.891
        ulcer I83.019
          with inflammation I83.219
          ankle I83.013
            with inflammation I83.213
          calf I83.012
            with inflammation I83.212
          foot NEC I83.015
            with inflammation I83.215
          heel I83.014
            with inflammation I83.214
          lower leg NEC I83.018
            with inflammation I83.218
          midfoot I83.014
            with inflammation I83.214
          thigh I83.011
            with inflammation I83.211
  nasal septum I86.8
  orbit I86.8
    congenital Q27.8
  ovary I86.2
  papillary I78.1
  pelvis I86.2
  perineum I86.3
  pharynx I86.8
  placenta O43.89- ☑
  renal papilla I86.8
  retina H35.09
  scrotum (ulcerated) I86.1
  sigmoid colon I86.8
  specified site NEC I86.8
  spinal (cord) (vessels) I86.8
  spleen, splenic (vein) (with phlebolith) I86.8
  stomach I86.4
  sublingual I86.0
  ulcerated I83.009
    inflamed or infected I83.209
  uterine ligament I86.2

Varix — *continued*
  vagina I86.8
  vocal cord I86.8
  vulva I86.3
Vas deferens — *see* condition
Vas deferentitis N49.1
Vasa previa O69.4 ☑
  hemorrhage from, affecting newborn P50.0
Vascular — *see also* condition
  loop on optic papilla Q14.2
  spasm I73.9
  spider I78.1
Vascularization, cornea — *see* Neovascularization, cornea
Vasculitis I77.6
  allergic D69.0
  cryoglobulinemic D89.1
  disseminated I77.6
  hypocomplementemic M31.8
  kidney I77.89
  livedoid L95.0
  nodular L95.8
  retina H35.06- ☑
  rheumatic — *see* Fever, rheumatic
  rheumatoid — *see* Rheumatoid, vasculitis
  skin (limited to) L95.9
    specified NEC L95.8
  systemic M31.8
Vasculopathy, necrotizing M31.9
  cardiac allograft T86.290
  specified NEC M31.8
Vasitis (nodosa) N49.1
  tuberculous A18.15
Vasodilation I73.9
Vasomotor — *see* condition
Vasoplasty, after previous sterilization Z31.0
  aftercare Z31.42
Vasospasm (vasoconstriction) I73.9
  cerebral (cerebrovascular) (artery) I67.848
    reversible I67.841
  coronary I20.1
  nerve
    arm — *see* Mononeuropathy, upper limb
    brachial plexus G54.0
    cervical plexus G54.2
    leg — *see* Mononeuropathy, lower limb
  peripheral NOS I73.9
  retina (artery) — *see* Occlusion, artery, retina
Vasospastic — *see* condition
Vasovagal attack (paroxysmal) R55
  psychogenic F45.8
VATER syndrome Q87.2
Vater's ampulla — *see* condition
Vegetation, vegetative
  adenoid (nasal fossa) J35.8
  endocarditis (acute) (any valve) (subacute) I33.0
  heart (mycotic) (valve) I33.0
Veil
  Jackson's Q43.3
Vein, venous — *see* condition
Veldt sore — *see* Ulcer, skin
Velpeau's hernia — *see* Hernia, femoral
Venereal
  bubo A55
  disease A64
  granuloma inguinale A58
  lymphogranuloma (Durand-Nicolas-Favre) A55
Venofibrosis I87.8
Venom, venomous — *see* Table of Drugs and Chemicals, by animal or substance, poisoning
Venous — *see* condition
Ventilator lung, newborn P27.8
Ventral — *see* condition
Ventricle, ventricular — *see also* condition
  escape I49.3
  inversion Q20.5
Ventriculitis (cerebral) — *see also* Encephalitis G04.90
Ventriculostomy status Z98.2
Vernet's syndrome G52.7
Verneuil's disease (syphilitic bursitis) A52.78
Verruca (due to HPV) (filiformis) (simplex) (viral) (vulgaris)☑ B07.9
  acuminata A63.0
  necrogenica (primary) (tuberculosa) A18.4
  plana B07.8
  plantaris B07.0
  seborrheica L82.1

☑ Additional Character Required — Refer to the Tabular List for Character Selection　　　☑ Subterms under main terms may continue to next column or page

Verruca — *continued*
  seborrheica — *continued*
    inflamed L82.0
    senile (seborrheic) L82.1
      inflamed L82.0
  tuberculosa (primary) A18.4
  venereal A63.0
Verrucosities — *see* Verruca
Verruga peruana, peruviana A44.1
Version
  cervix — *see* Malposition, uterus
  uterus (postinfectional) (postpartal, old) — *see* Malposition, uterus
Vertebra, vertebral — *see* condition
Vertical talus (congenital) Q66.80
  left foot Q66.82
  right foot Q66.81
Vertigo R42
  auditory — *see* Vertigo, aural
  aural H81.31- ☑
  benign paroxysmal (positional) H81.1- ☑
  central (origin) H81.4
  cerebral H81.4
  Dix and Hallpike (epidemic) — *see* Neuronitis, vestibular
  due to infrasound T75.23 ☑
  epidemic A88.1
    Dix and Hallpike — *see* Neuronitis, vestibular
    Pedersen's — *see* Neuronitis, vestibular
    vestibular neuronitis — *see* Neuronitis, vestibular
  hysterical F44.89
  infrasound T75.23 ☑
  labyrinthine — *see* subcategory H81.0 ☑
  laryngeal R05
  malignant positional H81.4
  Ménière's — *see* subcategory H81.0 ☑
  menopausal N95.1
  otogenic — *see* Vertigo, aural
  paroxysmal positional, benign — *see* Vertigo, benign paroxysmal
  Pedersen's (epidemic) — *see* Neuronitis, vestibular
  peripheral NEC H81.39- ☑
  positional
    benign paroxysmal — *see* Vertigo, benign paroxysmal
    malignant H81.4
Very-low-density-lipoprotein-type (VLDL) **hyperlipoproteinemia** E78.1
Vesania — *see* Psychosis
Vesical — *see* condition
Vesicle
  cutaneous R23.8
  seminal — *see* condition
  skin R23.8
Vesicocolic — *see* condition
Vesicoperineal — *see* condition
Vesicorectal — *see* condition
Vesicourethrorectal — *see* condition
Vesicovaginal — *see* condition
Vesicular — *see* condition
Vesiculitis (seminal) N49.0
  amebic A06.82
  gonorrheal (acute) (chronic) A54.23
  trichomonal A59.09
  tuberculous A18.15
Vestibulitis (ear) — *see also* subcategory H83.0 ☑
  nose (external) J34.89
  vulvar N94.810
Vestibulopathy , acute peripheral (recurrent) — *see* Neuronitis, vestibular
Vestige, vestigial — *see also* Persistence
  branchial Q18.0
  structures in vitreous Q14.0
Vibration
  adverse effects T75.20 ☑
    pneumatic hammer syndrome T75.21 ☑
    specified effect NEC T75.29 ☑
    vasospastic syndrome T75.22 ☑
    vertigo from infrasound T75.23 ☑
  exposure (occupational) Z57.7
  vertigo T75.23 ☑
Vibriosis A28.9
Victim (of)
  crime Z65.4
  disaster Z65.5
  terrorism Z65.4
  torture Z65.4

Victim — *continued*
  war Z65.5
Vidal's disease L28.0
Villaret's syndrome G52.7
Villous — *see* condition
VIN — *see* Neoplasia, intraepithelial, vulva
Vincent's infection (angina) (gingivitis) A69.1
  stomatitis NEC A69.1
Vinson-Plummer syndrome D50.1
Violence, physical R45.6
Viosterol deficiency — *see* Deficiency, calciferol
Vipoma — *see* Neoplasm, malignant, by site
Viremia B34.9
Virilism (adrenal) E25.9
  congenital E25.0
Virilization (female) (suprarenal) E25.9
  congenital E25.0
  isosexual E28.2
Virulent bubo A57
Virus, viral — *see also* condition
  as cause of disease classified elsewhere B97.89
    respiratory syncytial virus (RSV) — *see* Virus, infection, respiratory syncytial (RSV)
  cytomegalovirus B25.9
  human immunodeficiency (HIV) — *see* Human, immunodeficiency virus (HIV) disease
  infection — *see* Infection, virus
  respiratory syncytial (RSV)
    as cause of disease classified elsewhere B97.4
    bronchiolitis J21.0
    bronchitis J20.5
    bronchopneumonia J12.1
    otitis media H65.- ☑ *[B97.4]*
    pneumonia J12.1
    upper respiratory infection J06.9 *[B97.4]*
  specified NEC B34.8
  swine influenza (viruses that normally cause infections in pigs) — *see also* Influenza, due to, identified novel influenza A virus J09.X2
  West Nile (fever) A92.30
    with
      complications NEC A92.39
      cranial nerve disorders A92.32
      encephalitis A92.31
      encephalomyelitis A92.31
      neurologic manifestation NEC A92.32
      optic neuritis A92.32
      polyradiculitis A92.32
Viscera, visceral — *see* condition
Visceroptosis K63.4
Visible peristalsis R19.2
Vision, visual
  binocular, suppression H53.34
  blurred, blurring H53.8
    hysterical F44.6
  defect, defective NEC H54.7
  disorientation (syndrome) H53.8
  disturbance H53.9
    hysterical F44.6
  double H53.2
  examination Z01.00
    with abnormal findings Z01.01
    following failed vision screening Z01.020
      with abnormal findings Z01.021
  field, limitation (defect) — *see* Defect, visual field
  hallucinations R44.1
  halos H53.19
  loss — *see* Loss, vision
    sudden — *see* Disturbance, vision, subjective, loss, sudden
  low (both eyes) — *see* Low, vision
  perception, simultaneous without fusion H53.33
Vitality, lack or want of R53.83
  newborn P96.89
Vitamin deficiency — *see* Deficiency, vitamin
Vitelline duct, persistent Q43.0
Vitiligo L80
  eyelid H02.739
    left H02.736
      lower H02.735
      upper H02.734
    right H02.733
      lower H02.732
      upper H02.731
  pinta A67.2
  vulva N90.89
Vitreal corneal syndrome H59.01- ☑

Vitreoretinopathy, proliferative — *see also* Retinopathy, proliferative
  with retinal detachment — *see* Detachment, retina, traction
Vitreous — *see also* condition
  touch syndrome — *see* Complication, postprocedural, following cataract surgery
Vocal cord — *see* condition
Vogt-Koyanagi syndrome H20.82- ☑
Vogt's disease or syndrome G80.3
Vogt-Spielmeyer amaurotic idiocy or disease E75.4
Voice
  change R49.9
    specified NEC R49.8
  loss — *see* Aphonia
Volhynian fever A79.0
Volkmann's ischemic contracture or paralysis (complicating trauma) T79.6 ☑
Volvulus (bowel) (colon) (intestine) K56.2
  with perforation K56.2
  congenital Q43.8
  duodenum K31.5
  fallopian tube — *see* Torsion, fallopian tube
  oviduct — *see* Torsion, fallopian tube
  stomach (due to absence of gastrocolic ligament) K31.89
Vomiting R11.10
  with nausea R11.2
  asphyxia — *see* Foreign body, by site, causing asphyxia, gastric contents
  bilious (cause unknown) R11.14
    following gastro-intestinal surgery K91.0
    in newborn P92.01
  blood — *see* Hematemesis
  causing asphyxia, choking, or suffocation — *see* Foreign body, by site
  cyclical, in migraine G43.A0 (*following* G43.7)
    with refractory migraine G43.A1 (*following* G43.7)
    intractable G43.A1 (*following* G43.7)
    not intractable G43.A0 (*following* G43.7)
    psychogenic F50.89
    without refractory migraine G43.A0 (*following* G43.7)
  cyclical syndrome NOS (unrelated to migraine) R11.15
  fecal mater R11.13
  following gastrointestinal surgery K91.0
    psychogenic F50.89
  functional K31.89
  hysterical F50.89
  nervous F50.89
  neurotic F50.89
  newborn NEC P92.09
    bilious P92.01
  periodic R11.10
    psychogenic F50.89
  persistent R11.15
  projectile R11.12
  psychogenic F50.89
  uremic — *see* Uremia
  without nausea R11.11
Vomito negro — *see* Fever, yellow
Von Bezold's abscess — *see* Mastoiditis, acute
Von Economo-Cruchet disease A85.8
Von Eulenburg's disease G71.19
Von Gierke's disease E74.01
Von Hippel (-Lindau) **disease or syndrome** Q85.8
Von Jaksch's anemia or disease D64.89
Von Recklinghausen
  disease (neurofibromatosis) Q85.01
    bones E21.0
Von Schroetter's syndrome I82.890
Von Willebrand (-Jurgens)(-Minot) **disease or syndrome** D68.0
Von Zumbusch's disease L40.1
Voyeurism F65.3
Vrolik's disease Q78.0
Vulva — *see* condition
Vulvismus N94.2
Vulvitis (acute) (allergic) (atrophic) (hypertrophic) (intertriginous) (senile) N76.2
  with ectopic or molar pregnancy O08.0
  adhesive, congenital Q52.79
  blennorrhagic (gonococcal) A54.02
  candidal B37.3
  chlamydial A56.02
  due to Haemophilus ducreyi A57
  following ectopic or molar pregnancy O08.0
  gonococcal A54.02
    with abscess (accessory gland) (periurethral) A54.1

Vulvitis — *continued*
　herpesviral A60.04
　leukoplakic N90.4
　monilial B37.3
　puerperal (postpartum) O86.19
　subacute or chronic N76.3
　syphilitic (early) A51.0
　　late A52.76
　trichomonal A59.01
　tuberculous A18.18
Vulvodynia N94.819
　specified NEC N94.818
Vulvorectal — *see* condition
Vulvovaginitis (acute) — *see* Vaginitis

W

Waiting list, person on Z75.1
　for organ transplant Z76.82
　undergoing social agency investigation Z75.2
Waldenström
　hypergammaglobulinemia D89.0
　syndrome or macroglobulinemia C88.0
Waldenström-Kjellberg syndrome D50.1
Walking
　difficulty R26.2
　　psychogenic F44.4
　sleep F51.3
　　hysterical F44.89
Wall, abdominal — *see* condition
Wallenberg's disease or syndrome G46.3
Wallgren's disease I87.8
Wandering
　gallbladder, congenital Q44.1
　in diseases classified elsewhere Z91.83
　kidney, congenital Q63.8
　organ or site, congenital NEC — *see* Malposition, congenital, by site
　pacemaker (heart) I49.8
　spleen D73.89
War neurosis F48.8
Wart (due to HPV) (filiform) (infectious) (viral) B07.9
　anogenital region (venereal) A63.0
　common B07.8
　external genital organs (venereal) A63.0
　flat B07.8
　Hassal-Henle's (of cornea) H18.49
　Peruvian A44.1
　plantar B07.0
　prosector (tuberculous) A18.4
　seborrheic L82.1
　　inflamed L82.0
　senile (seborrheic) L82.1
　　inflamed L82.0
　tuberculous A18.4
　venereal A63.0
Warthin's tumor — *see* Neoplasm, salivary gland, benign
Wassilieff's disease A27.0
Wasting
　disease R64
　　due to malnutrition E41
　extreme (due to malnutrition) E41
　muscle NEC — *see* Atrophy, muscle
Water
　clefts (senile cataract) — *see* Cataract, senile, incipient
　deprivation of T73.1 ☑
　intoxication E87.79
　itch B76.9
　lack of T73.1 ☑
　loading E87.70
　on
　　brain — *see* Hydrocephalus
　　chest J94.8
　poisoning E87.79
Waterbrash R12
Waterhouse (-Friderichsen) **syndrome or disease** (meningococcal) A39.1
Water-losing nephritis N25.89
Watermelon stomach K31.819
　with hemorrhage K31.811
　without hemorrhage K31.819
Watsoniasis B66.8
Wax in ear — *see* Impaction, cerumen
Weak, weakening, weakness (generalized) R53.1
　arches (acquired) — *see also* Deformity, limb, flat foot
　bladder (sphincter) R32
　facial R29.810

Weak, weakening, weakness — *continued*
　facial — *continued*
　　following
　　　cerebrovascular disease I69.992
　　　　cerebral infarction I69.392
　　　　intracerebral hemorrhage I69.192
　　　　nontraumatic intracranial hemorrhage NEC I69.292
　　　　specified disease NEC I69.892
　　　　stroke I69.392
　　　　subarachnoid hemorrhage I69.092
　foot (double) — *see also* Weak, arches
　heart, cardiac — *see* Failure, heart
　mind F70
　muscle M62.81
　myocardium — *see* Failure, heart
　newborn P96.89
　pelvic fundus N81.89
　pubocervical tissue N81.82
　rectovaginal tissue N81.83
　senile R54
　urinary stream R39.12
　valvular — *see* Endocarditis
Wear, worn (with normal or routine use)
　articular bearing surface of internal joint prosthesis — *see* Complications, joint prosthesis, mechanical, wear of articular bearing surfaces, by site
　device, implant or graft — *see* Complications, by site, mechanical complication
　tooth, teeth (approximal) (hard tissues) (interproximal) (occlusal) K03.0
Weather, weathered
　effects of
　　cold T69.9 ☑
　　　specified effect NEC T69.8 ☑
　　hot — *see* Heat
　　skin L57.8
Weaver's syndrome Q87.3
Web, webbed (congenital)
　duodenal Q43.8
　esophagus Q39.4
　fingers Q70.1- ☑
　larynx (glottic) (subglottic) Q31.0
　neck (pterygium colli) Q18.3
　Paterson-Kelly D50.1
　popliteal syndrome Q87.89
　toes Q70.3- ☑
Weber-Christian disease M35.6
Weber-Cockayne syndrome (epidermolysis bullosa) Q81.8
Weber-Gubler syndrome G46.3
Weber-Leyden syndrome G46.3
Weber-Osler syndrome I78.0
Weber's paralysis or syndrome G46.3
Wedge-shaped or wedging vertebra — *see* Collapse, vertebra NEC
Wegener's granulomatosis or syndrome M31.30
　with
　　kidney involvement M31.31
　　lung involvement M31.30
　　　with kidney involvement M31.31
Wegner's disease A50.02
Weight
　1000-2499 grams at birth (low) — *see* Low, birthweight
　999 grams or less at birth (extremely low) — *see* Low, birthweight, extreme
　and length below 10th percentile for gestational age P05.1- ☑
　below but length above 10th percentile for gestational age P05.0- ☑
　gain (abnormal) (excessive) R63.5
　　in pregnancy — *see* Pregnancy, complicated by, excessive weight gain
　　low — *see* Pregnancy, complicated by, insufficient, weight gain
　loss (abnormal) (cause unknown) R63.4
Weightlessness (effect of) T75.82 ☑
Weil (l)-**Marchesani syndrome** Q87.19
Weil's disease A27.0
Weingarten's syndrome J82.89
Weir Mitchell's disease I73.81
Weiss-Baker syndrome G90.09
Wells' disease L98.3
Wen — *see* Cyst, sebaceous
Wenckebach's block or phenomenon I44.1
Werdnig-Hoffmann syndrome (muscular atrophy) G12.0

Werlhof's disease D69.3
Wermer's disease or syndrome E31.21
Werner-His disease A79.0
Werner's disease or syndrome E34.8
Wernicke-Korsakoff's syndrome or psychosis (alcoholic) F10.96
　with dependence F10.26
　drug-induced
　　due to drug abuse — *see* Abuse, drug, by type, with amnestic disorder
　　due to drug dependence — *see* Dependence, drug, by type, with amnestic disorder
　nonalcoholic F04
Wernicke-Posadas disease B38.9
Wernicke's
　developmental aphasia F80.2
　disease or syndrome E51.2
　encephalopathy E51.2
　polioencephalitis, superior E51.2
West African fever B50.8
Westphal-Strümpell syndrome E83.01
West's syndrome — *see* Epilepsy, spasms
Wet
　feet, tropical (maceration) (syndrome) — *see* Immersion, foot
　lung (syndrome), newborn P22.1
Wharton's duct — *see* condition
Wheal — *see* Urticaria
Wheezing R06.2
Whiplash injury S13.4 ☑
Whipple's disease — *see also* subcategory M14.8- K90.81
Whipworm (disease) (infection) (infestation) B79
Whistling face Q87.0
White — *see also* condition
　kidney, small N03.9
　leg, puerperal, postpartum, childbirth O87.1
　mouth B37.0
　patches of mouth K13.29
　spot lesions, teeth
　　chewing surface K02.51
　　pit and fissure surface K02.51
　　smooth surface K02.61
Whitehead L70.0
Whitlow — *see also* Cellulitis, digit
　with lymphangitis — *see* Lymphangitis, acute, digit
　herpesviral B00.89
Whitmore's disease or fever — *see* Melioidosis
Whooping cough A37.90
　with pneumonia A37.91
　　due to Bordetella
　　　bronchiseptica A37.81
　　　parapertussis A37.11
　　　pertussis A37.01
　　specified organism NEC A37.81
　due to
　　Bordetella
　　　bronchiseptica A37.80
　　　　with pneumonia A37.81
　　　parapertussis A37.10
　　　　with pneumonia A37.11
　　　pertussis A37.00
　　　　with pneumonia A37.01
　　specified NEC A37.80
　　　with pneumonia A37.81
Wichman's asthma J38.5
Wide cranial sutures, newborn P96.3
Widening aorta — *see* Ectasia, aorta
　with aneurysm — *see* Aneurysm, aorta
Wilkie's disease or syndrome K55.1
Wilkinson-Sneddon disease or syndrome L13.1
Willebrand (-Jürgens) **thrombopathy** D68.0
Williams syndrome Q93.82
Willige-Hunt disease or syndrome G23.1
Wilms' tumor C64- ☑
Wilson-Mikity syndrome P27.0
Wilson's
　disease or syndrome E83.01
　hepatolenticular degeneration E83.01
　lichen ruber L43.9
Window — *see also* Imperfect, closure
　aorticopulmonary Q21.4
Winter — *see* condition
Wiskott-Aldrich syndrome D82.0
Withdrawal state — *see also* Dependence, drug by type
　with withdrawal
　alcohol
　　with perceptual disturbances F10.232

☑ **Additional Character Required** — Refer to the Tabular List for Character Selection　　　　Subterms under main terms may continue to next column or page

Withdrawal state — *continued*
  alcohol — *continued*
    without perceptual disturbances F10.239
  caffeine F15.93
  cannabis F12.23
  newborn
    correct therapeutic substance properly administered P96.2
    infant of dependent mother P96.1
  therapeutic substance, neonatal P96.2
Witts' anemia D50.8
Witzelsucht F07.0
Woakes' ethmoiditis or syndrome J33.1
Wolff-Hirschorn syndrome Q93.3
Wolff-Parkinson-White syndrome I45.6
Wolhynian fever A79.0
Wolman's disease E75.5
Wood lung or pneumonitis J67.8
Woolly, wooly hair (congenital) (nevus) Q84.1
Woolsorter's disease A22.1
Word
  blindness (congenital) (developmental) F81.0
  deafness (congenital) (developmental) H93.25
Worm(s) (infection) (infestation) — *see also* Infestation, helminth
  guinea B72
  in intestine NEC B82.0
Worm-eaten soles A66.3
Worn out — *see* Exhaustion
  cardiac
    defibrillator (with synchronous cardiac pacemaker) Z45.02
    pacemaker
      battery Z45.010
      lead Z45.018
  device, implant or graft — *see* Complications, by site, mechanical
Worried well Z71.1
Worries R45.82
Wound check Z48.0- ☑
  due to injury — *code to* Injury, by site, using appropriate seventh character for subsequent encounter
Wound, open T14.8- ☑
  abdomen, abdominal
    wall S31.109 ☑
      with penetration into peritoneal cavity S31.609 ☑
      bite — *see* Bite, abdomen, wall
      epigastric region S31.102 ☑
        with penetration into peritoneal cavity S31.602 ☑
        bite — *see* Bite, abdomen, wall, epigastric region
        laceration — *see* Laceration, abdomen, wall, epigastric region
        puncture — *see* Puncture, abdomen, wall, epigastric region
      laceration — *see* Laceration, abdomen, wall
      left
        lower quadrant S31.104 ☑
          with penetration into peritoneal cavity S31.604 ☑
          bite — *see* Bite, abdomen, wall, left, lower quadrant
          laceration — *see* Laceration, abdomen, wall, left, lower quadrant
          puncture — *see* Puncture, abdomen, wall, left, lower quadrant
        upper quadrant S31.101 ☑
          with penetration into peritoneal cavity S31.601 ☑
          bite — *see* Bite, abdomen, wall, left, upper quadrant
          laceration — *see* Laceration, abdomen, wall, left, upper quadrant
          puncture — *see* Puncture, abdomen, wall, left, upper quadrant
      periumbilic region S31.105 ☑
        with penetration into peritoneal cavity S31.605 ☑
        bite — *see* Bite, abdomen, wall, periumbilic region
        laceration — *see* Laceration, abdomen, wall, periumbilic region
        puncture — *see* Puncture, abdomen, wall, periumbilic region

Wound, open — *continued*
  abdomen, abdominal — *continued*
    wall — *continued*
      right
        lower quadrant S31.103 ☑
          with penetration into peritoneal cavity S31.603 ☑
          bite — *see* Bite, abdomen, wall, right, lower quadrant
          laceration — *see* Laceration, abdomen, wall, right, lower quadrant
          puncture — *see* Puncture, abdomen, wall, right, lower quadrant
        upper quadrant S31.100 ☑
          with penetration into peritoneal cavity S31.600 ☑
          bite — *see* Bite, abdomen, wall, right, upper quadrant
          laceration — *see* Laceration, abdomen, wall, right, upper quadrant
          puncture — *see* Puncture, abdomen, wall, right, upper quadrant
  alveolar (process) — *see* Wound, open, oral cavity
  ankle S91.00- ☑
    bite — *see* Bite, ankle
    laceration — *see* Laceration, ankle
    puncture — *see* Puncture, ankle
  antecubital space — *see* Wound, open, elbow
  anterior chamber, eye — *see* Wound, open, ocular
  anus S31.839 ☑
    bite S31.835 ☑
    laceration — *see* Laceration, anus
    puncture — *see* Puncture, anus
  arm (upper) S41.10- ☑
    with amputation — *see* Amputation, traumatic, arm
    bite — *see* Bite, arm
    forearm — *see* Wound, open, forearm
    laceration — *see* Laceration, arm
    puncture — *see* Puncture, arm
  auditory canal (external) (meatus) — *see* Wound, open, ear
  auricle, ear — *see* Wound, open, ear
  axilla — *see* Wound, open, arm
  back — *see also* Wound, open, thorax, back
    lower S31.000 ☑
      with penetration into retroperitoneal space S31.001 ☑
      bite — *see* Bite, back, lower
      laceration — *see* Laceration, back, lower
      puncture — *see* Puncture, back, lower
  bite — *see* Bite
  blood vessel — *see* Injury, blood vessel
  breast S21.00- ☑
    with amputation — *see* Amputation, traumatic, breast
    bite — *see* Bite, breast
    laceration — *see* Laceration, breast
    puncture — *see* Puncture, breast
  buttock S31.809 ☑
    bite — *see* Bite, buttock
    laceration — *see* Laceration, buttock
    left S31.829 ☑
    puncture — *see* Puncture, buttock
    right S31.819 ☑
  calf — *see* Wound, open, leg
  canaliculus lacrimalis — *see* Wound, open, eyelid
  canthus, eye — *see* Wound, open, eyelid
  cervical esophagus S11.20 ☑
    bite S11.25 ☑
    laceration — *see* Laceration, esophagus, traumatic, cervical
    puncture — *see* Puncture, cervical esophagus
  cheek (external) S01.40- ☑
    bite — *see* Bite, cheek
    internal — *see* Wound, open, oral cavity
    laceration — *see* Laceration, cheek
    puncture — *see* Puncture, cheek
  chest wall — *see* Wound, open, thorax
  chin — *see* Wound, open, head, specified site NEC
  choroid — *see* Wound, open, ocular
  ciliary body (eye) — *see* Wound, open, ocular
  clitoris S31.40 ☑
    with amputation — *see* Amputation, traumatic, clitoris
    bite S31.45 ☑
    laceration — *see* Laceration, vulva

Wound, open — *continued*
  clitoris — *continued*
    puncture — *see* Puncture, vulva
  conjunctiva — *see* Wound, open, ocular
  cornea — *see* Wound, open, ocular
  costal region — *see* Wound, open, thorax
  Descemet's membrane — *see* Wound, open, ocular
  digit(s)
    foot — *see* Wound, open, toe
    hand — *see* Wound, open, finger
  ear (canal) (external) S01.30- ☑
    with amputation — *see* Amputation, traumatic, ear
    bite — *see* Bite, ear
    drum S09.2- ☑
    laceration — *see* Laceration, ear
    puncture — *see* Puncture, ear
  elbow S51.00- ☑
    bite — *see* Bite, elbow
    laceration — *see* Laceration, elbow
    puncture — *see* Puncture, elbow
  epididymis — *see* Wound, open, testis
  epigastric region S31.102 ☑
    with penetration into peritoneal cavity S31.602 ☑
    bite — *see* Bite, abdomen, wall, epigastric region
    laceration — *see* Laceration, abdomen, wall, epigastric region
    puncture — *see* Puncture, abdomen, wall, epigastric region
  epiglottis — *see* Wound, open, neck, specified site NEC
  esophagus (thoracic) S27.819 ☑
    cervical — *see* Wound, open, cervical esophagus
    laceration S27.813 ☑
    specified type NEC S27.818 ☑
  eye — *see* Wound, open, ocular
  eyeball — *see* Wound, open, ocular
  eyebrow — *see* Wound, open, eyelid
  eyelid S01.10- ☑
    bite — *see* Bite, eyelid
    laceration — *see* Laceration, eyelid
    puncture — *see* Puncture, eyelid
  face NEC — *see* Wound, open, head, specified site NEC
  finger(s) S61.209 ☑
    with
      amputation — *see* Amputation, traumatic, finger
      damage to nail S61.309 ☑
    bite — *see* Bite, finger
    index S61.208 ☑
      with
        damage to nail S61.308 ☑
      left S61.201 ☑
        with
          damage to nail S61.301 ☑
      right S61.200 ☑
        with
          damage to nail S61.300 ☑
    laceration — *see* Laceration, finger
    little S61.208 ☑
      with
        damage to nail S61.308 ☑
      left S61.207 ☑
        with damage to nail S61.307 ☑
      right S61.206 ☑
        with damage to nail S61.306 ☑
    middle S61.208 ☑
      with
        damage to nail S61.308 ☑
      left S61.203 ☑
        with damage to nail S61.303 ☑
      right S61.202 ☑
        with damage to nail S61.302 ☑
    puncture — *see* Puncture, finger
    ring S61.208 ☑
      with
        damage to nail S61.308 ☑
      left S61.205 ☑
        with damage to nail S61.305 ☑
      right S61.204 ☑
        with damage to nail S61.304 ☑
  flank — *see* Wound, open, abdomen, wall
  foot (except toe(s) alone) S91.30- ☑
    with amputation — *see* Amputation, traumatic, foot
    bite — *see* Bite, foot
    laceration — *see* Laceration, foot
    puncture — *see* Puncture, foot
    toe — *see* Wound, open, toe
  forearm S51.80- ☑

Wound, open — *continued*
  forearm — *continued*
    with
      amputation — *see* Amputation, traumatic, fore-
        arm
    bite — *see* Bite, forearm
    elbow only — *see* Wound, open, elbow
    laceration — *see* Laceration, forearm
    puncture — *see* Puncture, forearm
  forehead — *see* Wound, open, head, specified site NEC
  genital organs, external
    with amputation — *see* Amputation, traumatic,
      genital organs
    bite — *see* Bite, genital organ
    female S31.502 ☑
      vagina S31.40 ☑
      vulva S31.40 ☑
    laceration — *see* Laceration, genital organ
    male S31.501 ☑
      penis S31.20 ☑
      scrotum S31.30 ☑
      testes S31.30 ☑
    puncture — *see* Puncture, genital organ
  globe (eye) — *see* Wound, open, ocular
  groin — *see* Wound, open, abdomen, wall
  gum — *see* Wound, open, oral cavity
  hand S61.40- ☑
    with
      amputation — *see* Amputation, traumatic, hand
    bite — *see* Bite, hand
    finger(s) — *see* Wound, open, finger
    laceration — *see* Laceration, hand
    puncture — *see* Puncture, hand
    thumb — *see* Wound, open, thumb
  head S01.90 ☑
    bite — *see* Bite, head
    cheek — *see* Wound, open, cheek
    ear — *see* Wound, open, ear
    eyelid — *see* Wound, open, eyelid
    laceration — *see* Laceration, head
    lip — *see* Wound, open, lip
    nose S01.20 ☑
    oral cavity — *see* Wound, open, oral cavity
    puncture — *see* Puncture, head
    scalp — *see* Wound, open, scalp
    specified site NEC S01.80 ☑
    temporomandibular area — *see* Wound, open,
      cheek
  heel — *see* Wound, open, foot
  hip S71.00- ☑
    with amputation — *see* Amputation, traumatic, hip
    bite — *see* Bite, hip
    laceration — *see* Laceration, hip
    puncture — *see* Puncture, hip
  hymen S31.40 ☑
    bite — *see* Bite, vulva
    laceration — *see* Laceration, vagina
    puncture — *see* Puncture, vagina
  hypochondrium S31.109 ☑
    bite — *see* Bite, hypochondrium
    laceration — *see* Laceration, hypochondrium
    puncture — *see* Puncture, hypochondrium
  hypogastric region S31.109 ☑
    bite — *see* Bite, hypogastric region
    laceration — *see* Laceration, hypogastric region
    puncture — *see* Puncture, hypogastric region
  iliac (region) — *see* Wound, open, inguinal region
  inguinal region S31.109 ☑
    bite — *see* Bite, abdomen, wall, lower quadrant
    laceration — *see* Laceration, inguinal region
    puncture — *see* Puncture, inguinal region
  instep — *see* Wound, open, foot
  interscapular region — *see* Wound, open, thorax, back
  intraocular — *see* Wound, open, ocular
  iris — *see* Wound, open, ocular
  jaw — *see* Wound, open, head, specified site NEC
  knee S81.00- ☑
    bite — *see* Bite, knee
    laceration — *see* Laceration, knee
    puncture — *see* Puncture, knee
  labium (majus) (minus) — *see* Wound, open, vulva
  laceration — *see* Laceration, by site
  lacrimal duct — *see* Wound, open, eyelid
  larynx S11.019 ☑
    bite — *see* Bite, larynx
    laceration — *see* Laceration, larynx

Wound, open — *continued*
  larynx — *continued*
    puncture — *see* Puncture, larynx
  left
    lower quadrant S31.104 ☑
      with penetration into peritoneal cavity
        S31.604 ☑
      bite — *see* Bite, abdomen, wall, left, lower
        quadrant
      laceration — *see* Laceration, abdomen, wall, left,
        lower quadrant
      puncture — *see* Puncture, abdomen, wall, left,
        lower quadrant
    upper quadrant S31.101 ☑
      with penetration into peritoneal cavity
        S31.601 ☑
      bite — *see* Bite, abdomen, wall, left, upper
        quadrant
      laceration — *see* Laceration, abdomen, wall, left,
        upper quadrant
      puncture — *see* Puncture, abdomen, wall, left,
        upper quadrant
  leg (lower) S81.80- ☑
    with amputation — *see* Amputation, traumatic, leg
    ankle — *see* Wound, open, ankle
    bite — *see* Bite, leg
    foot — *see* Wound, open, foot
    knee — *see* Wound, open, knee
    laceration — *see* Laceration, leg
    puncture — *see* Puncture, leg
    toe — *see* Wound, open, toe
    upper — *see* Wound, open, thigh
  lip S01.501 ☑
    bite — *see* Bite, lip
    laceration — *see* Laceration, lip
    puncture — *see* Puncture, lip
  loin S31.109 ☑
    bite — *see* Bite, abdomen, wall
    laceration — *see* Laceration, loin
    puncture — *see* Puncture, loin
  lower back — *see* Wound, open, back, lower
  lumbar region — *see* Wound, open, back, lower
  malar region — *see* Wound, open, head, specified site
    NEC
  mammary — *see* Wound, open, breast
  mastoid region — *see* Wound, open, head, specified
    site NEC
  mouth — *see* Wound, open, oral cavity
  nail
    finger — *see* Wound, open, finger, with damage to
      nail
    toe — *see* Wound, open, toe, with damage to nail
  nape (neck) — *see* Wound, open, neck
  nasal (septum) (sinus) — *see* Wound, open, nose
  nasopharynx — *see* Wound, open, head, specified site
    NEC
  neck S11.90 ☑
    bite — *see* Bite, neck
    involving
      cervical esophagus S11.20 ☑
      larynx — *see* Wound, open, larynx
      pharynx S11.20 ☑
      thyroid S11.10 ☑
      trachea (cervical) S11.029 ☑
        bite — *see* Bite, trachea
        laceration S11.021 ☑
          with foreign body S11.022 ☑
        puncture S11.023 ☑
          with foreign body S11.024 ☑
    laceration — *see* Laceration, neck
    puncture — *see* Puncture, neck
    specified site NEC S11.80 ☑
      specified type NEC S11.89 ☑
  nose (septum) (sinus) S01.20 ☑
    with amputation — *see* Amputation, traumatic,
      nose
    bite — *see* Bite, nose
    laceration — *see* Laceration, nose
    puncture — *see* Puncture, nose
  ocular S05.90 ☑
    avulsion (traumatic enucleation) S05.7- ☑
    eyeball S05.6- ☑
      with foreign body S05.5- ☑
    eyelid — *see* Wound, open, eyelid
    laceration and rupture S05.3- ☑

Wound, open — *continued*
  ocular — *continued*
    laceration and rupture — *continued*
      with prolapse or loss of intraocular tissue
        S05.2- ☑
      orbit (penetrating) (with or without foreign body)
        S05.4- ☑
      periocular area — *see* Wound, open, eyelid
      specified NEC S05.8X- ☑
  oral cavity S01.502 ☑
    bite S01.552 ☑
    laceration — *see* Laceration, oral cavity
    puncture — *see* Puncture, oral cavity
  orbit — *see* Wound, open, ocular, orbit
  palate — *see* Wound, open, oral cavity
  palm — *see* Wound, open, hand
  pelvis, pelvic — *see also* Wound, open, back, lower
    girdle — *see* Wound, open, hip
  penetrating — *see* Puncture, by site
  penis S31.20 ☑
    with amputation — *see* Amputation, traumatic,
      penis
    bite S31.25 ☑
    laceration — *see* Laceration, penis
    puncture — *see* Puncture, penis
  perineum
    bite — *see* Bite, perineum
    female S31.502 ☑
    laceration — *see* Laceration, perineum
    male S31.501 ☑
    puncture — *see* Puncture, perineum
  periocular area (with or without lacrimal passages) —
    see Wound, open, eyelid
  periumbilic region S31.105 ☑
    with penetration into peritoneal cavity S31.605 ☑
    bite — *see* Bite, abdomen, wall, periumbilic region
    laceration — *see* Laceration, abdomen, wall, peri-
      umbilic region
    puncture — *see* Puncture, abdomen, wall, perium-
      bilic region
  phalanges
    finger — *see* Wound, open, finger
    toe — *see* Wound, open, toe
  pharynx S11.20 ☑
  pinna — *see* Wound, open, ear
  popliteal space — *see* Wound, open, knee
  prepuce — *see* Wound, open, penis
  pubic region — *see* Wound, open, back, lower
  pudendum — *see* Wound, open, genital organs, exter-
    nal
  puncture wound — *see* Puncture
  rectovaginal septum — *see* Wound, open, vagina
  right
    lower quadrant S31.103 ☑
      with penetration into peritoneal cavity
        S31.603 ☑
      bite — *see* Bite, abdomen, wall, right, lower
        quadrant
      laceration — *see* Laceration, abdomen, wall,
        right, lower quadrant
      puncture — *see* Puncture, abdomen, wall, right
        lower quadrant
    upper quadrant S31.100 ☑
      with penetration into peritoneal cavity
        S31.600 ☑
      bite — *see* Bite, abdomen, wall, right, upper
        quadrant
      laceration — *see* Laceration, abdomen, wall,
        right, upper quadrant
      puncture — *see* Puncture, abdomen, wall, right
        upper quadrant
  sacral region — *see* Wound, open, back, lower
  sacroiliac region — *see* Wound, open, back, lower
  salivary gland — *see* Wound, open, oral cavity
  scalp S01.00 ☑
    bite S01.05 ☑
    laceration — *see* Laceration, scalp
    puncture — *see* Puncture, scalp
  scalpel, newborn (birth injury) P15.8
  scapular region — *see* Wound, open, shoulder
  sclera — *see* Wound, open, ocular
  scrotum S31.30 ☑
    with amputation — *see* Amputation, traumatic,
      scrotum
    bite S31.35 ☑
    laceration — *see* Laceration, scrotum
    puncture — *see* Puncture, scrotum

☑ Additional Character Required — Refer to the Tabular List for Character Selection   ﹀ Subterms under main terms may continue to next column or page

Wound, open — *continued*
  shin — *see* Wound, open, leg
  shoulder S41.00- ☑
    with amputation — *see* Amputation, traumatic, arm
    bite — *see* Bite, shoulder
    laceration — *see* Laceration, shoulder
    puncture — *see* Puncture, shoulder
  skin NOS T14.8 ☑
  spermatic cord — *see* Wound, open, testis
  sternal region — *see* Wound, open, thorax, front wall
  submaxillary region — *see* Wound, open, head, specified site NEC
  submental region — *see* Wound, open, head, specified site NEC
  subungual
    finger(s) — *see* Wound, open, finger
    toe(s) — *see* Wound, open, toe
  supraclavicular region — *see* Wound, open, neck, specified site NEC
  temple, temporal region — *see* Wound, open, head, specified site NEC
  temporomandibular area — *see* Wound, open, cheek
  testis S31.30 ☑
    with amputation — *see* Amputation, traumatic, testes
    bite S31.35 ☑
    laceration — *see* Laceration, testis
    puncture — *see* Puncture, testis
  thigh S71.10- ☑
    with amputation — *see* Amputation, traumatic, hip
    bite — *see* Bite, thigh
    laceration — *see* Laceration, thigh
    puncture — *see* Puncture, thigh
  thorax, thoracic (wall) S21.90 ☑
    back S21.20- ☑
      with penetration S21.40 ☑
    bite — *see* Bite, thorax
    breast — *see* Wound, open, breast
    front S21.10- ☑
      with penetration S21.30 ☑
    laceration — *see* Laceration, thorax
    puncture — *see* Puncture, thorax
  throat — *see* Wound, open, neck
  thumb S61.009 ☑
    with
      amputation — *see* Amputation, traumatic, thumb
      damage to nail S61.109 ☑
    bite — *see* Bite, thumb
    laceration — *see* Laceration, thumb
    left S61.002 ☑
      with
        damage to nail S61.102 ☑
    puncture — *see* Puncture, thumb
    right S61.001 ☑
      with
        damage to nail S61.101 ☑
  thyroid (gland) — *see* Wound, open, neck, thyroid
  toe(s) S91.109 ☑
    with
      amputation — *see* Amputation, traumatic, toe
      damage to nail S91.209 ☑
    bite — *see* Bite, toe
    great S91.103 ☑
      with
        damage to nail S91.203 ☑
      left S91.102 ☑
        with
          damage to nail S91.202 ☑
      right S91.101 ☑
        with
          damage to nail S91.201 ☑
    laceration — *see* Laceration, toe
    lesser S91.106 ☑
      with
        damage to nail S91.206 ☑
      left S91.105 ☑
        with
          damage to nail S91.205 ☑
      right S91.104 ☑
        with
          damage to nail S91.204 ☑
    puncture — *see* Puncture, toe
  tongue — *see* Wound, open, oral cavity
  trachea (cervical region) — *see* Wound, open, neck, trachea

Wound, open — *continued*
  tunica vaginalis — *see* Wound, open, testis
  tympanum, tympanic membrane S09.2- ☑
    laceration — *see* Laceration, ear, drum
    puncture — *see* Puncture, tympanum
  umbilical region — *see* Wound, open, abdomen, wall, periumbilic region
  uvula — *see* Wound, open, oral cavity
  vagina S31.40 ☑
    bite S31.45 ☑
    laceration — *see* Laceration, vagina
    puncture — *see* Puncture, vagina
  vitreous (humor) — *see* Wound, open, ocular
  vocal cord S11.039 ☑
    bite — *see* Bite, vocal cord
    laceration S11.031 ☑
      with foreign body S11.032 ☑
    puncture S11.033 ☑
      with foreign body S11.034 ☑
  vulva S31.40 ☑
    with amputation — *see* Amputation, traumatic, vulva
    bite S31.45 ☑
    laceration — *see* Laceration, vulva
    puncture — *see* Puncture, vulva
  wrist S61.50- ☑
    bite — *see* Bite, wrist
    laceration — *see* Laceration, wrist
    puncture — *see* Puncture, wrist
Wound, superficial — *see* Injury — *see also* specified injury type
Wright's syndrome G54.0
Wrist — *see* condition
Wrong drug (by accident) (given in error) — *see* Table of Drugs and Chemicals, by drug, poisoning
Wry neck — *see* Torticollis
Wuchereria (bancrofti) **infestation** B74.0
Wuchereriasis B74.0
Wuchernde Struma Langhans C73

X

Xanthelasma (eyelid) (palpebrarum) H02.60
  left H02.66
    lower H02.65
    upper H02.64
  right H02.63
    lower H02.62
    upper H02.61
Xanthelasmatosis (essential) E78.2
Xanthinuria, hereditary E79.8
Xanthoastrocytoma
  specified site — *see* Neoplasm, malignant, by site
  unspecified site C71.9
Xanthofibroma — *see* Neoplasm, connective tissue, benign
Xanthogranuloma D76.3
Xanthoma(s), xanthomatosis (primary) (familial) (hereditary) E75.5
  with
    hyperlipoproteinemia
      Type I E78.3
      Type III E78.2
      Type IV E78.1
      Type V E78.3
  bone (generalisata) C96.5
  cerebrotendinous E75.5
  cutaneotendinous E75.5
  disseminatum (skin) E78.2
  eruptive E78.2
  hypercholesterinemic E78.00
  hypercholesterolemic E78.00
  hyperlipidemic E78.5
  joint E75.5
  multiple (skin) E78.2
  tendon (sheath) E75.5
  tuberosum E78.2
  tuberous E78.2
  tubo-eruptive E78.2
  verrucous, oral mucosa K13.4
Xanthosis R23.8
Xenophobia F40.10
Xeroderma — *see also* Ichthyosis
  acquired L85.0
    eyelid H01.149
      left H01.146
        lower H01.145

Xeroderma — *continued*
  acquired — *continued*
    eyelid — *continued*
      left — *continued*
        upper H01.144
      right H01.143
        lower H01.142
        upper H01.141
  pigmentosum Q82.1
  vitamin A deficiency E50.8
Xerophthalmia (vitamin A deficiency) E50.7
  unrelated to vitamin A deficiency — *see* Keratoconjunctivitis
Xerosis
  conjunctiva H11.14- ☑
    with Bitot's spots — *see also* Pigmentation, conjunctiva
      vitamin A deficiency E50.1
    vitamin A deficiency E50.0
  cornea H18.89- ☑
    with ulceration — *see* Ulcer, cornea
      vitamin A deficiency E50.3
    vitamin A deficiency E50.2
  cutis L85.3
  skin L85.3
Xerostomia K11.7
Xiphopagus Q89.4
XO syndrome Q96.9
X-ray (of)
  abnormal findings — *see* Abnormal, diagnostic imaging
  breast (mammogram) (routine) Z12.31
  chest
    routine (as part of a general medical examination) Z00.00
      with abnormal findings Z00.01
    routine (as part of a general medical examination) Z00.00
      with abnormal findings Z00.01
XXXXY syndrome Q98.1
XXY syndrome Q98.0

Y

Yaba pox (virus disease) B08.72
Yatapoxvirus B08.70
  specified NEC B08.79
Yawning R06.89
  psychogenic F45.8
Yaws A66.9
  bone lesions A66.6
  butter A66.1
  chancre A66.0
  cutaneous, less than five years after infection A66.2
  early (cutaneous) (macular) (maculopapular) (micropapular) (papular) A66.2
    frambeside A66.2
    skin lesions NEC A66.2
  eyelid A66.2
  ganglion A66.6
  gangosis, gangosa A66.5
  gumma, gummata A66.4
    bone A66.6
  gummatous
    frambeside A66.4
    osteitis A66.6
    periostitis A66.6
  hydrarthrosis — *see also* subcategory M14.8- A66.6
  hyperkeratosis (early) (late) A66.3
  initial lesions A66.0
  joint lesions — *see also* subcategory M14.8- A66.6
  juxta-articular nodules A66.7
  late nodular (ulcerated) A66.4
  latent (without clinical manifestations) (with positive serology) A66.8
  mother A66.0
  mucosal A66.7
  multiple papillomata A66.1
  nodular, late (ulcerated) A66.4
  osteitis A66.6
  papilloma, plantar or palmar A66.1
  periostitis (hypertrophic) A66.6
  specified NEC A66.7
  ulcers A66.4
  wet crab A66.1
Yeast infection — *see also* Candidiasis B37.9
Yellow
  atrophy (liver) — *see* Failure, hepatic
  fever — *see* Fever, yellow

Yellow — *continued*
  jack — *see* Fever, yellow
  jaundice — *see* Jaundice
  nail syndrome L60.5
Yersiniosis — *see also* Infection, Yersinia
  extraintestinal A28.2
  intestinal A04.6

Z

Zahorsky's syndrome (herpangina) B08.5
Zellweger's syndrome E71.510
Zenker's diverticulum (esophagus) K22.5
Ziehen-Oppenheim disease G24.1
Zieve's syndrome K70.0
Zika NOS A92.5
  congenital P35.4

Zinc
  deficiency, dietary E60
  metabolism disorder E83.2
Zollinger-Ellison syndrome E16.4
Zona — *see* Herpes, zoster
Zoophobia F40.218
Zoster (herpes) — *see* Herpes, zoster
Zygomycosis B46.9
  specified NEC B46.8
Zymotic — *see* condition

Yellow — Zymotic

334   ☑ **Additional Character Required** — Refer to the Tabular List for Character Selection   ▽ **Subterms under main terms may continue to next column or page**

Note: The list below gives the code number for neoplasms by anatomical site. For each site there are six possible code numbers according to whether the neoplasm in question is malignant, benign, in situ, of uncertain behavior, or of unspecified nature. The description of the neoplasm will often indicate which of the six columns is appropriate; e.g., malignant melanoma of skin, benign fibroadenoma of breast, carcinoma in situ of cervix uteri. Where such descriptors are not present, the remainder of the Index should be consulted where guidance is given to the appropriate column for each morphological (histological) variety listed; e.g., Mesonephroma – see Neoplasm, malignant; Embryoma — see also Neoplasm, uncertain behavior; Disease, Bowen's – see Neoplasm, skin, in situ. However, the guidance in the Index can be overridden if one of the descriptors mentioned above is present; e.g., malignant adenoma of colon is coded to C18.9 and not to D12.6 as the adjective "malignant" overrides the Index entry "Adenoma — see also Neoplasm, benign, by site." Codes listed with a dash -, following the code have a required additional character for laterality. The tabular list must be reviewed for the complete code.

	Malignant Primary	Malignant Secondary	Ca in situ	Benign	Uncertain Behavior	Unspecified Behavior
Neoplasm, neoplastic	C80.1	C79.9	D09.9	D36.9	D48.9	D49.9
abdomen, abdominal	C76.2	C79.8-☑	D09.8	D36.7	D48.7	D49.89
cavity	C76.2	C79.8-☑	D09.8	D36.7	D48.7	D49.89
organ	C76.2	C79.8-☑	D09.8	D36.7	D48.7	D49.89
viscera	C76.2	C79.8-☑	D09.8	D36.7	D48.7	D49.89
wall — see also Neoplasm, abdomen, wall, skin	C44.509	C79.2	D04.5	D23.5	D48.5	D49.2
connective tissue	C49.4	C79.8-☑	—	D21.4	D48.1	D49.2
skin	C44.509					
basal cell carcinoma	C44.519	—	—	—	—	—
specified type NEC	C44.599	—	—	—	—	—
squamous cell carcinoma	C44.529	—	—	—	—	—
abdominopelvic	C76.8	C79.8-☑		D36.7	D48.7	D49.89
accessory sinus — see Neoplasm, sinus						
acoustic nerve	C72.4-☑	C79.49	—	D33.3	D43.3	D49.7
adenoid (pharynx) (tissue)	C11.1	C79.89	D00.08	D10.6	D37.05	D49.0
adipose tissue — see also Neoplasm, connective tissue	C49.4	C79.89	—	D21.9	D48.1	D49.2
adnexa (uterine)	C57.4	C79.89	D07.39	D28.7	D39.8	D49.59
adrenal	C74.9-☑	C79.7-☑	D09.3	D35.0-☑	D44.1-☑	D49.7
capsule	C74.9-☑	C79.7-☑	D09.3	D35.0-☑	D44.1-☑	D49.7
cortex	C74.0-☑	C79.7-☑	D09.3	D35.0-☑	D44.1-☑	D49.7
gland	C74.9-☑	C79.7-☑	D09.3	D35.0-☑	D44.1-☑	D49.7
medulla	C74.1-☑	C79.7-☑	D09.3	D35.0-☑	D44.1-☑	D49.7
ala nasi (external) — see also Neoplasm, skin, nose	C44.301	C79.2	D04.39	D23.39	D48.5	D49.2
alimentary canal or tract NEC	C26.9	C78.80	D01.9	D13.9	D37.9	D49.0
alveolar	C03.9	C79.89	D00.03	D10.39	D37.09	D49.0
mucosa	C03.9	C79.89	D00.03	D10.39	D37.09	D49.0
lower	C03.1	C79.89	D00.03	D10.39	D37.09	D49.0
upper	C03.0	C79.89	D00.03	D10.39	D37.09	D49.0
ridge or process	C41.1	C79.51	—	D16.5	D48.0	D49.2
carcinoma	C03.9	C79.8-☑	—	—	—	—
lower	C03.1	C79.8-☑	—	—	—	—
upper	C03.0	C79.8-☑	—	—	—	—
lower	C41.1	C79.51	—	D16.5	D48.0	D49.2
mucosa	C03.9	C79.89	D00.03	D10.39	D37.09	D49.0
lower	C03.1	C79.89	D00.03	D10.39	D37.09	D49.0
upper	C03.0	C79.89	D00.03	D10.39	D37.09	D49.0
upper	C41.0	C79.51	—	D16.4	D48.0	D49.2
sulcus	C06.1	C79.89	D00.02	D10.39	D37.09	D49.0
alveolus	C03.9	C79.89	D00.03	D10.39	D37.09	D49.0
lower	C03.1	C79.89	D00.03	D10.39	D37.09	D49.0
upper	C03.0	C79.89	D00.03	D10.39	D37.09	D49.0
ampulla of Vater	C24.1	C78.89	D01.5	D13.5	D37.6	D49.0
ankle NEC	C76.5-☑	C79.89	D04.7-☑	D36.7	D48.7	D49.89
anorectum, anorectal (junction)	C21.8	C78.5	D01.3	D12.9	D37.8	D49.0
antecubital fossa or space	C76.4-☑	C79.89	D04.6-☑	D36.7	D48.7	D49.89

	Malignant Primary	Malignant Secondary	Ca in situ	Benign	Uncertain Behavior	Unspecified Behavior
Neoplasm, neoplastic — continued						
antrum (Highmore) (maxillary)	C31.0	C78.39	D02.3	D14.0	D38.5	D49.1
pyloric	C16.3	C78.89	D00.2	D13.1	D37.1	D49.0
tympanicum	C30.1	C78.39	D02.3	D14.0	D38.5	D49.1
anus, anal	C21.0	C78.5	D01.3	D12.9	D37.8	D49.0
canal	C21.1	C78.5	D01.3	D12.9	D37.8	D49.0
cloacogenic zone	C21.2	C78.5	D01.3	D12.9	D37.8	D49.0
margin — see also Neoplasm, anus, skin	C44.500	C79.2	D04.5	D23.5	D48.5	D49.2
overlapping lesion with rectosigmoid junction or rectum	C21.8	—	—	—	—	—
skin	C44.500	C79.2	D04.5	D23.5	D48.5	D49.2
basal cell carcinoma	C44.510	—	—	—	—	—
specified type NEC	C44.590	—	—	—	—	—
squamous cell carcinoma	C44.520	—	—	—	—	—
sphincter	C21.1	C78.5	D01.3	D12.9	D37.8	D49.0
aorta (thoracic)	C49.3	C79.89	—	D21.3	D48.1	D49.2
abdominal	C49.4	C79.89	—	D21.4	D48.1	D49.2
aortic body	C75.5	C79.89	—	D35.6	D44.7	D49.7
aponeurosis	C49.9	C79.89	—	D21.9	D48.1	D49.2
palmar	C49.1-☑	C79.89	—	D21.1-☑	D48.1	D49.2
plantar	C49.2-☑	C79.89	—	D21.2-☑	D48.1	D49.2
appendix	C18.1	C78.5	D01.0	D12.1	D37.3	D49.0
arachnoid	C70.9	C79.49	—	D32.9	D42.9	D49.7
cerebral	C70.0	C79.32	—	D32.0	D42.0	D49.7
spinal	C70.1	C79.49	—	D32.1	D42.1	D49.7
areola	C50.0-☑	C79.81	D05-☑	D24-☑	D48.6-☑	D49.3
arm NEC	C76.4-☑	C79.89	D04.6-☑	D36.7	D48.7	D49.89
artery — see Neoplasm, connective tissue						
aryepiglottic fold	C13.1	C79.89	D00.08	D10.7	D37.05	D49.0
hypopharyngeal aspect	C13.1	C79.89	D00.08	D10.7	D37.05	D49.0
laryngeal aspect	C32.1	C78.39	D02.0	D14.1	D38.0	D49.1
marginal zone	C13.1	C79.89	D00.08	D10.7	D37.05	D49.0
arytenoid (cartilage)	C32.3	C78.39	D02.0	D14.1	D38.0	D49.1
fold — see Neoplasm, aryepiglottic						
associated with transplanted organ	C80.2	—	—	—	—	—
atlas	C41.2	C79.51	—	D16.6	D48.0	D49.2
atrium, cardiac	C38.0	C79.89	—	D15.1	D48.7	D49.89
auditory						
canal (external) (skin)	C44.20-☑	C79.2	D04.2-☑	D23.2-☑	D48.5	D49.2
internal	C30.1	C78.39	D02.3	D14.0	D38.5	D49.1
nerve	C72.4-☑	C79.49	—	D33.3	D43.3	D49.7
tube	C30.1	C78.39	D02.3	D14.0	D38.5	D49.1
opening	C11.2	C79.89	D00.08	D10.6	D37.05	D49.0
auricle, ear — see also Neoplasm, skin, ear	C44.20-☑	C79.2	D04.2-☑	D23.2-☑	D48.5	D49.2
auricular canal (external) — see also Neoplasm, skin, ear	C44.20-☑	C79.2	D04.2-☑	D23.2-☑	D48.5	D49.2
internal	C30.1	C78.39	D02.3	D14.0	D38.5	D49.2
autonomic nerve or nervous system NEC (see Neoplasm, nerve, peripheral)						
axilla, axillary	C76.1	C79.89	D09.8	D36.7	D48.7	D49.89
fold — see also Neoplasm, skin, trunk	C44.509	C79.2	D04.5	D23.5	D48.5	D49.2
back NEC	C76.8	C79.89	D04.5	D36.7	D48.7	D49.89
Bartholin's gland	C51.0	C79.82	D07.1	D28.0	D39.8	D49.59
basal ganglia	C71.0	C79.31	—	D33.0	D43.0	D49.6
basis pedunculi	C71.7	C79.31	—	D33.1	D43.1	D49.6
bile or biliary (tract)	C24.9	C78.89	D01.5	D13.5	D37.6	D49.0

	Malignant Primary	Malignant Secondary	Ca in situ	Benign	Uncertain Behavior	Unspecified Behavior
Neoplasm, neoplastic — *continued*						
bile or biliary — *continued*						
canaliculi (biliferi) (intrahepatic)	C22.1	C78.7	D01.5	D13.4	D37.6	D49.0
canals, interlobular	C22.1	C78.89	D01.5	D13.4	D37.6	D49.0
duct or passage (common) (cystic) (extrahepatic)	C24.0	C78.89	D01.5	D13.5	D37.6	D49.0
interlobular	C22.1	C78.89	D01.5	D13.4	D37.6	D49.0
intrahepatic	C22.1	C78.7	D01.5	D13.4	D37.6	D49.0
and extrahepatic	C24.8	C78.89	D01.5	D13.5	D37.6	D49.0
bladder (urinary)	C67.9	C79.11	D09.0	D30.3	D41.4	D49.4
dome	C67.1	C79.11	D09.0	D30.3	D41.4	D49.4
neck	C67.5	C79.11	D09.0	D30.3	D41.4	D49.4
orifice	C67.9	C79.11	D09.0	D30.3	D41.4	D49.4
ureteric	C67.6	C79.11	D09.0	D30.3	D41.4	D49.4
urethral	C67.5	C79.11	D09.0	D30.3	D41.4	D49.4
overlapping lesion	C67.8	—	—	—	—	—
sphincter	C67.8	C79.11	D09.0	D30.3	D41.4	D49.4
trigone	C67.0	C79.11	D09.0	D30.3	D41.4	D49.4
urachus	C67.7	C79.11	D09.0	D30.3	D41.4	D49.4
wall	C67.9	C79.11	D09.0	D30.3	D41.4	D49.4
anterior	C67.3	C79.11	D09.0	D30.3	D41.4	D49.4
lateral	C67.2	C79.11	D09.0	D30.3	D41.4	D49.4
posterior	C67.4	C79.11	D09.0	D30.3	D41.4	D49.4
blood vessel — *see* Neoplasm, connective tissue						
bone (periosteum)	C41.9	C79.51	—	D16.9-	D48.0	D49.2
acetabulum						
ankle	C40.3-☑	C79.51	—	D16.3-☑	—	—
arm NEC	C40.0-☑	C79.51	—	D16.0-☑	—	—
astragalus	C40.3-☑	C79.51	—	D16.3-☑	—	—
atlas	C41.2	C79.51	—	D16.6	D48.0	D49.2
axis	C41.2	C79.51	—	D16.6	D48.0	D49.2
back NEC	C41.2	C79.51	—	D16.6	D48.0	D49.2
calcaneus	C40.3-☑	C79.51	—	D16.3-☑	—	—
calvarium	C41.0	C79.51	—	D16.4	D48.0	D49.2
carpus (any)	C40.1-☑	C79.51	—	D16.1-☑	—	—
cartilage NEC	C41.9	C79.51	—	D16.9	D48.0	D49.2
clavicle	C41.3	C79.51	—	D16.7	D48.0	D49.2
clivus	C41.0	C79.51	—	D16.4	D48.0	D49.2
coccygeal vertebra	C41.4	C79.51	—	D16.8	D48.0	D49.2
coccyx	C41.4	C79.51	—	D16.8	D48.0	D49.2
costal cartilage	C41.3	C79.51	—	D16.7	D48.0	D49.2
costovertebral joint	C41.3	C79.51	—	D16.7	D48.0	D49.2
cranial	C41.0	C79.51	—	D16.4	D48.0	D49.2
cuboid	C40.3-☑	C79.51	—	D16.3-☑	—	—
cuneiform	C41.9	C79.51	—	D16.9	D48.0	D49.2
elbow	C40.0-☑	C79.51	—	D16.0-☑	—	—
ethmoid (labyrinth)	C41.0	C79.51	—	D16.4	D48.0	D49.2
face	C41.0	C79.51	—	D16.4	D48.0	D49.2
femur (any part)	C40.2-☑	C79.51	—	D16.2-☑	—	—
fibula (any part)	C40.2-☑	C79.51	—	D16.2-☑	—	—
finger (any)	C40.1-☑	C79.51	—	D16.1-☑	—	—
foot	C40.3-☑	C79.51	—	D16.3-☑	—	—
forearm	C40.0-☑	C79.51	—	D16.0-☑	—	—
frontal	C41.0	C79.51	—	D16.4	D48.0	D49.2
hand	C40.1-☑	C79.51	—	D16.1-☑	—	—
heel	C40.3-☑	C79.51	—	D16.3-☑	—	—
hip	C41.4	C79.51	—	D16.8	D48.0	D49.2
humerus (any part)	C40.0-☑	C79.51	—	D16.0-☑	—	—
hyoid	C41.0	C79.51	—	D16.4	D48.0	D49.2
ilium	C41.4	C79.51	—	D16.8	D48.0	D49.2
innominate	C41.4	C79.51	—	D16.8	D48.0	D49.2
intervertebral cartilage or disc	C41.2	C79.51	—	D16.6	D48.0	D49.2
ischium	C41.4	C79.51	—	D16.8	D48.0	D49.2
jaw (lower)	C41.1	C79.51	—	D16.5	D48.0	D49.2
knee	C40.2-☑	C79.51	—	D16.2-☑	—	—
leg NEC	C40.2-☑	C79.51	—	D16.2-☑	—	—
limb NEC	C40.9-☑	C79.51	—	D16.9	—	—

	Malignant Primary	Malignant Secondary	Ca in situ	Benign	Uncertain Behavior	Unspecified Behavior
Neoplasm, neoplastic — *continued*						
bone — *continued*						
limb — *continued*						
lower (long bones)	C40.2-☑	C79.51	—	D16.2-☑	—	—
short bones	C40.3-☑	C79.51	—	D16.3-☑	—	—
upper (long bones)	C40.0-☑	C79.51	—	D16.0-☑	—	—
short bones	C40.1-☑	C79.51	—	D16.1-☑	—	—
malar	C41.0	C79.51	—	D16.4	D48.0	D49.2
mandible	C41.1	C79.51	—	D16.5	D48.0	D49.2
marrow NEC (any bone)	C96.9	C79.52	—	—	D47.9	D49.89
mastoid	C41.0	C79.51	—	D16.4	D48.0	D49.2
maxilla, maxillary (superior)	C41.0	C79.51	—	D16.4	D48.0	D49.2
inferior	C41.1	C79.51	—	D16.5	D48.0	D49.2
metacarpus (any)	C40.1-☑	C79.51	—	D16.1-☑	—	—
metatarsus (any)	C40.3-☑	C79.51	—	D16.3-☑	—	—
navicular						
ankle	C40.3-☑	C79.51	—	—	—	—
hand	C40.1-☑	C79.51	—	—	—	—
nose, nasal	C41.0	C79.51	—	D16.4	D48.0	D49.2
occipital	C41.0	C79.51	—	D16.4	D48.0	D49.2
orbit	C41.0	C79.51	—	D16.4	D48.0	D49.2
overlapping sites	C40.8-☑	—	—	—	—	—
parietal	C41.0	C79.51	—	D16.4	D48.0	D49.2
patella	C40.2-☑	C79.51	—	—	—	—
pelvic	C41.4	C79.51	—	D16.8	D48.0	D49.2
phalanges						
foot	C40.3-☑	C79.51	—	—	—	—
hand	C40.1-☑	C79.51	—	—	—	—
pubic	C41.4	C79.51	—	D16.8	D48.0	D49.2
radius (any part)	C40.0-☑	C79.51	—	D16.0-☑	—	—
rib	C41.3	C79.51	—	D16.7	D48.0	D49.2
sacral vertebra	C41.4	C79.51	—	D16.8	D48.0	D49.2
sacrum	C41.4	C79.51	—	D16.8	D48.0	D49.2
scaphoid						
of ankle	C40.3-☑	C79.51	—	—	—	—
of hand	C40.1-☑	C79.51	—	—	—	—
scapula (any part)	C40.0-☑	C79.51	—	D16.0-☑	—	—
sella turcica	C41.0	C79.51	—	D16.4	D48.0	D49.2
shoulder	C40.0-☑	C79.51	—	D16.0-☑	—	—
skull	C41.0	C79.51	—	D16.4	D48.0	D49.2
sphenoid	C41.0	C79.51	—	D16.4	D48.0	D49.2
spine, spinal (column)	C41.2	C79.51	—	D16.6	D48.0	D49.2
coccyx	C41.4	C79.51	—	D16.8	D48.0	D49.2
sacrum	C41.4	C79.51	—	D16.8	D48.0	D49.2
sternum	C41.3	C79.51	—	D16.7	D48.0	D49.2
tarsus (any)	C40.3-☑	C79.51	—	—	—	—
temporal	C41.0	C79.51	—	D16.4	D48.0	D49.2
thumb	C40.1-☑	C79.51	—	—	—	—
tibia (any part)	C40.2-☑	C79.51	—	—	—	—
toe (any)	C40.3-☑	C79.51	—	—	—	—
trapezium	C40.1-☑	C79.51	—	—	—	—
trapezoid	C40.1-☑	C79.51	—	—	—	—
turbinate	C41.0	C79.51	—	D16.4	D48.0	D49.2
ulna (any part)	C40.0-☑	C79.51	—	D16.0-☑	—	—
unciform	C40.1-☑	C79.51	—	—	—	—
vertebra (column)	C41.2	C79.51	—	D16.6	D48.0	D49.2
coccyx	C41.4	C79.51	—	D16.8	D48.0	D49.2
sacrum	C41.4	C79.51	—	D16.8	D48.0	D49.2
vomer	C41.0	C79.51	—	D16.4	D48.0	D49.2
wrist	C40.1-☑	C79.51	—	—	—	—
xiphoid process	C41.3	C79.51	—	D16.7	D48.0	D49.2
zygomatic	C41.0	C79.51	—	D16.4	D48.0	D49.2
book-leaf (mouth) — *ventral surface of tongue and floor of mouth*	C06.89	C79.89	D00.00	D10.39	D37.09	D49.0
bowel — *see* Neoplasm, intestine						
brachial plexus	C47.1-☑	C79.89	—	D36.12	D48.2	D49.2
brain NEC	C71.9	C79.31	—	D33.2	D43.2	D49.6

☑ Additional Character Required — Refer to the Tabular List for Character Selection

Subterms under main terms may continue to next column or page

Neoplasm, neoplastic — continued

brain — continued

	Malignant Primary	Malignant Secondary	Ca in situ	Benign	Uncertain Behavior	Unspecified Behavior
basal ganglia	C71.0	C79.31	—	D33.0	D43.0	D49.6
cerebellopontine angle	C71.6	C79.31	—	D33.1	D43.1	D49.6
cerebellum NOS	C71.6	C79.31	—	D33.1	D43.1	D49.6
cerebrum	C71.0	C79.31	—	D33.0	D43.0	D49.6
choroid plexus	C71.7	C79.31	—	D33.1	D43.1	D49.6
corpus callosum	C71.8	C79.31	—	D33.2	D43.2	D49.6
corpus striatum	C71.0	C79.31	—	D33.0	D43.0	D49.6
cortex (cerebral)	C71.0	C79.31	—	D33.0	D43.0	D49.6
frontal lobe	C71.1	C79.31	—	D33.0	D43.0	D49.6
globus pallidus	C71.0	C79.31	—	D33.0	D43.0	D49.6
hippocampus	C71.2	C79.31	—	D33.0	D43.0	D49.6
hypothalamus	C71.0	C79.31	—	D33.0	D43.0	D49.6
internal capsule	C71.0	C79.31	—	D33.0	D43.0	D49.6
medulla oblongata	C71.7	C79.31	—	D33.1	D43.1	D49.6
meninges	C70.0	C79.32	—	D32.0	D42.0	D49.7
midbrain	C71.7	C79.31	—	D33.1	D43.1	D49.6
occipital lobe	C71.4	C79.31	—	D33.0	D43.0	D49.6
overlapping lesion	C71.8	C79.31	—	—	—	—
parietal lobe	C71.3	C79.31	—	D33.0	D43.0	D49.6
peduncle	C71.7	C79.31	—	D33.1	D43.1	D49.6
pons	C71.7	C79.31	—	D33.1	D43.1	D49.6
stem	C71.7	C79.31	—	D33.1	D43.1	D49.6
tapetum	C71.8	C79.31	—	D33.2	D43.2	D49.6
temporal lobe	C71.2	C79.31	—	D33.0	D43.0	D49.6
thalamus	C71.0	C79.31	—	D33.0	D43.0	D49.6
uncus	C71.2	C79.31	—	D33.0	D43.0	D49.6
ventricle (floor)	C71.5	C79.31	—	D33.0	D43.0	D49.6
fourth	C71.7	C79.31	—	D33.1	D43.1	D49.6
branchial (cleft) (cyst) (vestiges)	C10.4	C79.89	D00.08	D10.5	D37.05	D49.0
breast (connective tissue) (glandular tissue) (soft parts)	C50.9-✓	C79.81	D05.-✓	D24.-✓	D48.6-✓	D49.3
areola	C50.0-✓	C79.81	D05.-✓	D24.-✓	D48.6-✓	D49.3
axillary tail	C50.6-✓	C79.81	D05.-✓	D24.-✓	D48.6-✓	D49.3
central portion	C50.1-✓	C79.81	D05.-✓	D24.-✓	D48.6-✓	D49.3
inner	C50.8-✓	C79.81	D05.-✓	D24.-✓	D48.6-✓	D49.3
lower	C50.8-✓	C79.81	D05.-✓	D24.-✓	D48.6-✓	D49.3
lower-inner quadrant	C50.3-✓	C79.81	D05.-✓	D24.-✓	D48.6-✓	D49.3
lower-outer quadrant	C50.5-✓	C79.81	D05.-✓	D24.-✓	D48.6-✓	D49.3
mastectomy site (skin) — see also Neoplasm, breast, skin	C44.501	C79.2	—	—	—	—
specified as breast tissue	C50.8-✓	C79.81	—	—	—	—
midline	C50.8-✓	C79.81	D05.-✓	D24.-✓	D48.6-✓	D49.3
nipple	C50.0-✓	C79.81	D05.-✓	D24.-✓	D48.6-✓	D49.3
outer	C50.8-✓	C79.81	D05.-✓	D24.-✓	D48.6-✓	D49.3
overlapping lesion	C50.8-✓	—	—	—	—	—
skin	C44.501	C79.2	D04.5	D23.5	D48.5	D49.2
basal cell carcinoma	C44.511	—	—	—	—	—
specified type NEC	C44.591	—	—	—	—	—
squamous cell carcinoma	C44.521	—	—	—	—	—
tail (axillary)	C50.6-✓	C79.81	D05.-✓	D24.-✓	D48.6-✓	D49.3
upper	C50.8-✓	C79.81	D05.-✓	D24.-✓	D48.6-✓	D49.3
upper-inner quadrant	C50.2-✓	C79.81	D05.-✓	D24.-✓	D48.6-✓	D49.3
upper-outer quadrant	C50.4-✓	C79.81	D05.-✓	D24.-✓	D48.6-✓	D49.3
broad ligament	C57.1-✓	C79.82	D07.39	D28.2	D39.8	D49.59
bronchiogenic, bronchogenic (lung)	C34.9-✓	C78.0-✓	D02.2-✓	D14.3-✓	D38.1	D49.1
bronchiole	C34.9-✓	C78.0-✓	D02.2-✓	D14.3-✓	D38.1	D49.1
bronchus	C34.9-✓	C78.0-✓	D02.2-✓	D14.3-✓	D38.1	D49.1
carina	C34.0-✓	C78.0-✓	D02.2-✓	D14.3-✓	D38.1	D49.1
lower lobe of lung	C34.3-✓	C78.0-✓	D02.2-✓	D14.3-✓	D38.1	D49.1

Neoplasm, neoplastic — continued

bronchus — continued

	Malignant Primary	Malignant Secondary	Ca in situ	Benign	Uncertain Behavior	Unspecified Behavior
main	C34.0-✓	C78.0-✓	D02.2-✓	D14.3-✓	D38.1	D49.1
middle lobe of lung	C34.2	C78.0-✓	D02.21	D14.31	D38.1	D49.1
overlapping lesion	C34.8-✓	—	—	—	—	—
upper lobe of lung	C34.1-✓	C78.0-✓	D02.2-✓	D14.3-✓	D38.1	D49.1
brow	C44.309	C79.2	D04.39	D23.39	D48.5	D49.2
basal cell carcinoma	C44.319	—	—	—	—	—
specified type NEC	C44.399	—	—	—	—	—
squamous cell carcinoma	C44.329	—	—	—	—	—
buccal (cavity)	C06.9	C79.89	D00.00	D10.39	D37.09	D49.0
commissure	C06.0	C79.89	D00.02	D10.39	D37.09	D49.0
groove (lower) (upper)	C06.1	C79.89	D00.02	D10.39	D37.09	D49.0
mucosa	C06.0	C79.89	D00.02	D10.39	D37.09	D49.0
sulcus (lower) (upper)	C06.1	C79.89	D00.02	D10.39	D37.09	D49.0
bulbourethral gland	C68.0	C79.19	D09.19	D30.4	D41.3	D49.59
bursa — see Neoplasm, connective tissue						
buttock NEC	C76.3	C79.89	D04.5	D36.7	D48.7	D49.89
calf	C76.5-✓	C79.89	D04.7-✓	D36.7	D48.7	D49.89
calvarium	C41.0	C79.51	—	D16.4	D48.0	D49.2
calyx, renal	C65.-✓	C79.0-✓	D09.19	D30.1-✓	D41.1-✓	D49.51-✓
canal anal	C21.1	C78.5	D01.3	D12.9	D37.8	D49.0
auditory (external) — see also Neoplasm, skin, ear	C44.20-✓	C79.2	D04.2-✓	D23.2-✓	D48.5	D49.2
auricular (external) — see also Neoplasm, skin, ear	C44.20-✓	C79.2	D04.2-✓	D23.2-✓	D48.5	D49.2
canaliculi, biliary (biliferi) (intrahepatic)	C22.1	C78.7	D01.5	D13.4	D37.6	D49.0
canthus (eye) (inner) (outer)	C44.10-✓	C79.2	D04.1-✓	D23.1-✓	D48.5	D49.2
basal cell carcinoma	C44.11-✓	—	—	—	—	—
sebaceous cell	C44.13-✓	—	—	—	—	—
specified type NEC	C44.19-✓	—	—	—	—	—
squamous cell carcinoma	C44.12-✓	—	—	—	—	—
capillary — see Neoplasm, connective tissue						
caput coli	C18.0	C78.5	D01.0	D12.0	D37.4	D49.0
carcinoid — see Tumor, carcinoid						
cardia (gastric)	C16.0	C78.89	D00.2	D13.1	D37.1	D49.0
cardiac orifice (stomach)	C16.0	C78.89	D00.2	D13.1	D37.1	D49.0
cardio-esophageal junction	C16.0	C78.89	D00.2	D13.1	D37.1	D49.0
cardio-esophagus	C16.0	C78.89	D00.2	D13.1	D37.1	D49.0
carina (bronchus)	C34.0-✓	C78.0-✓	D02.2-✓	D14.3-✓	D38.1	D49.1
carotid (artery)	C49.0	C79.89	—	D21.0	D48.1	D49.2
body	C75.4	C79.89	—	D35.5	D44.6	D49.7
carpus (any bone)	C40.1-✓	C79.51	—	D16.1-✓	—	—
cartilage (articular) (joint) NEC — see also Neoplasm, bone	C41.9	C79.51	—	D16.9	D48.0	D49.2
arytenoid	C32.3	C78.39	D02.0	D14.1	D38.0	D49.1
auricular	C49.0	C79.89	—	D21.0	D48.1	D49.2
bronchi	C34.0-✓	C78.39	—	D14.3-✓	D38.1	D49.1
costal	C41.3	C79.51	—	D16.7	D48.0	D49.2
cricoid	C32.3	C78.39	D02.0	D14.1	D38.0	D49.1
cuneiform	C32.3	C78.39	D02.0	D14.1	D38.0	D49.1
ear (external)	C49.0	C79.89	—	D21.0	D48.1	D49.2
ensiform	C41.3	C79.51	—	D16.7	D48.0	D49.2
epiglottis	C32.1	C78.39	D02.0	D14.1	D38.0	D49.1

Neoplasm, neoplastic

	Malignant Primary	Malignant Secondary	Ca in situ	Benign	Uncertain Behavior	Unspecified Behavior
Neoplasm, neoplastic						
— *continued*						
cartilage — *see also*						
Neoplasm, bone —						
continued						
epiglottis —						
continued						
anterior						
surface	C10.1	C79.89	D00.08	D10.5	D37.05	D49.0
eyelid	C49.0	C79.89	—	D21.0	D48.1	D49.2
intervertebral	C41.2	C79.51	—	D16.6	D48.0	D49.2
larynx, laryngeal	C32.3	C78.39	D02.0	D14.1	D38.0	D49.1
nose, nasal	C30.0	C78.39	D02.3	D14.0	D38.5	D49.1
pinna	C49.0	C79.89	—	D21.0	D48.1	D49.2
rib	C41.3	C79.51	—	D16.7	D48.0	D49.2
semilunar						
(knee)	C40.2-☑	C79.51	—	D16.2-☑	D48.0	D49.2
thyroid	C32.3	C78.39	D02.0	D14.1	D38.0	D49.1
trachea	C33	C78.39	D02.1	D14.2	D38.1	D49.1
cauda equina	C72.1	C79.49	—	D33.4	D43.4	D49.7
cavity						
buccal	C06.9	C79.89	D00.00	D10.30	D37.09	D49.0
nasal	C30.0	C78.39	D02.3	D14.0	D38.5	D49.1
oral	C06.9	C79.89	D00.00	D10.30	D37.09	D49.0
peritoneal	C48.2	C78.6	—	D20.1	D48.4	D49.0
tympanic	C30.1	C78.39	D02.3	D14.0	D38.5	D49.1
cecum	C18.0	C78.5	D01.0	D12.0	D37.4	D49.0
central nervous						
system	C72.9	C79.40	—	—	—	—
cerebellopontine						
(angle)	C71.6	C79.31	—	D33.1	D43.1	D49.6
cerebellum,						
cerebellar	C71.6	C79.31	—	D33.1	D43.1	D49.6
cerebrum, cerebra						
(cortex)						
(hemisphere)						
(white matter)	C71.0	C79.31	—	D33.0	D43.0	D49.6
meninges	C70.0	C79.32	—	D32.0	D42.0	D49.7
peduncle	C71.7	C79.31	—	D33.1	D43.1	D49.6
ventricle	C71.5	C79.31	—	D33.0	D43.0	D49.6
fourth	C71.7	C79.31	—	D33.1	D43.1	D49.6
cervical region	C76.0	C79.89	D09.8	D36.7	D48.7	D49.89
cervix (cervical) (uteri)						
(uterus)	C53.9	C79.82	D06.9	D26.0	D39.0	D49.59
canal	C53.0	C79.82	D06.0	D26.0	D39.0	D49.59
endocervix (canal)						
(gland)	C53.0	C79.82	D06.0	D26.0	D39.0	D49.59
exocervix	C53.1	C79.82	D06.1	D26.0	D39.0	D49.59
external os	C53.1	C79.82	D06.1	D26.0	D39.0	D49.59
internal os	C53.0	C79.82	D06.0	D26.0	D39.0	D49.59
nabothian gland	C53.0	C79.82	D06.0	D26.0	D39.0	D49.59
overlapping						
lesion	C53.8	—	—	—	—	—
squamocolumnar						
junction	C53.8	C79.82	D06.7	D26.0	D39.0	D49.59
stump	C53.8	C79.82	D06.7	D26.0	D39.0	D49.59
cheek	C76.0	C79.89	D09.8	D36.7	D48.7	D49.89
external	C44.309	C79.2	D04.39	D23.39	D48.5	D49.2
basal cell						
carcinoma	C44.319	—	—	—	—	—
specified type						
NEC	C44.399	—	—	—	—	—
squamous cell						
carcinoma	C44.329	—	—	—	—	—
inner aspect	C06.0	C79.89	D00.02	D10.39	D37.09	D49.0
internal	C06.0	C79.89	D00.02	D10.39	D37.09	D49.0
mucosa	C06.0	C79.89	D00.02	D10.39	D37.09	D49.0
chest (wall) NEC	C76.1	C79.89	D09.8	D36.7	D48.7	D49.89
chiasma opticum	C72.3-☑	C79.49	—	D33.3	D43.3	D49.7
chin	C44.309	C79.2	D04.39	D23.39	D48.5	D49.2
basal cell						
carcinoma	C44.319	—	—	—	—	—
specified type						
NEC	C44.399	—	—	—	—	—
squamous cell						
carcinoma	C44.329	—	—	—	—	—
choana	C11.3	C79.89	D00.08	D10.6	D37.05	D49.0
cholangiole	C22.1	C78.89	D01.5	D13.4	D37.6	D49.0
choledochal duct	C24.0	C78.89	D01.5	D13.5	D37.6	D49.0
choroid	C69.3-☑	C79.49	D09.2-☑	D31.3-☑	D48.7	D49.81
plexus	C71.5	C79.31	—	D33.0	D43.0	D49.6
ciliary body	C69.4-☑	C79.49	D09.2-☑	D31.4-☑	D48.7	D49.89
clavicle	C41.3	C79.51	—	D16.7	D48.0	D49.2

Neoplasm, neoplastic

	Malignant Primary	Malignant Secondary	Ca in situ	Benign	Uncertain Behavior	Unspecified Behavior
Neoplasm, neoplastic						
— *continued*						
clitoris	C51.2	C79.82	D07.1	D28.0	D39.8	D49.59
clivus	C41.0	C79.51	—	D16.4	D48.0	D49.2
cloacogenic zone	C21.2	C78.5	D01.3	D12.9	D37.8	D49.0
coccygeal						
body or glomus	C49.5	C79.89	—	D21.5	D48.1	D49.2
vertebra	C41.4	C79.51	—	D16.8	D48.0	D49.2
coccyx	C41.4	C79.51	—	D16.8	D48.0	D49.2
colon — *see also*						
Neoplasm,						
intestine,						
large	C18.9	C78.5	—	—	—	—
with rectum	C19	C78.5	D01.1	D12.7	D37.5	D49.0
columnella — *see also*						
Neoplasm, skin,						
face	C44.390	C79.2	D04.39	D23.39	D48.5	D49.2
column, spinal — *see*						
Neoplasm, spine						
commissure						
labial, lip	C00.6	C79.89	D00.01	D10.39	D37.01	D49.0
laryngeal	C32.0	C78.39	D02.0	D14.1	D38.0	D49.1
common (bile)						
duct	C24.0	C78.89	D01.5	D13.5	D37.6	D49.0
concha — *see also*						
Neoplasm, skin,						
ear	C44.20-☑	C79.2	D04.2-☑	D23.2-☑	D48.5	D49.2
nose	C30.0	C78.39	D02.3	D14.0	D38.5	D49.1
conjunctiva	C69.0-☑	C79.49	D09.2-☑	D31.0-☑	D48.7	D49.89
connective tissue						
NEC	C49.9	C79.89	—	D21.9	D48.1	D49.2

Note: For neoplasms of connective tissue (blood vessel, bursa, fascia, ligament, muscle, peripheral nerves, sympathetic and parasympathetic nerves and ganglia, synovia, tendon, etc.) or of morphological types that indicate connective tissue, code according to the list under "Neoplasm, connective tissue". For sites that do not appear in this list, code to neoplasm of that site; e.g., fibrosarcoma, pancreas (C25.9)

Note: Morphological types that indicate connective tissue appear in their proper place in the alphabetic index with the instruction "see Neoplasm, connective tissue ...."

	Malignant Primary	Malignant Secondary	Ca in situ	Benign	Uncertain Behavior	Unspecified Behavior
abdomen	C49.4	C79.89	—	D21.4	D48.1	D49.2
abdominal wall	C49.4	C79.89	—	D21.4	D48.1	D49.2
ankle	C49.2-☑	C79.89	—	D21.2-☑	D48.1	D49.2
antecubital fossa or						
space	C49.1-☑	C79.89	—	D21.1-☑	D48.1	D49.2
arm	C49.1-☑	C79.89	—	D21.1-☑	D48.1	D49.2
auricle (ear)	C49.0	C79.89	—	D21.0	D48.1	D49.2
axilla	C49.3	C79.89	—	D21.3	D48.1	D49.2
back	C49.6	C79.89	—	D21.6	D48.1	D49.2
breast — *see*						
Neoplasm,						
breast						
buttock	C49.5	C79.89	—	D21.5	D48.1	D49.2
calf	C49.2-☑	C79.89	—	D21.2-☑	D48.1	D49.2
cervical region	C49.0	C79.89	—	D21.0	D48.1	D49.2
cheek	C49.0	C79.89	—	D21.0	D48.1	D49.2
chest (wall)	C49.3	C79.89	—	D21.3	D48.1	D49.2
chin	C49.0	C79.89	—	D21.0	D48.1	D49.2
diaphragm	C49.3	C79.89	—	D21.3	D48.1	D49.2
ear (external)	C49.0	C79.89	—	D21.0	D48.1	D49.2
elbow	C49.1-☑	C79.89	—	D21.1-☑	D48.1	D49.2
extrarectal	C49.5	C79.89	—	D21.5	D48.1	D49.2
extremity	C49.9	C79.89	—	D21.9	D48.1	D49.2
lower	C49.2-☑	C79.89	—	D21.2-☑	D48.1	D49.2
upper	C49.1-☑	C79.89	—	D21.1-☑	D48.1	D49.2
eyelid	C49.0	C79.89	—	D21.0	D48.1	D49.2
face	C49.0	C79.89	—	D21.0	D48.1	D49.2
finger	C49.1-☑	C79.89	—	D21.1-☑	D48.1	D49.2
flank	C49.6	C79.89	—	D21.6	D48.1	D49.2
foot	C49.2-☑	C79.89	—	D21.2-☑	D48.1	D49.2
forearm	C49.1-☑	C79.89	—	D21.1-☑	D48.1	D49.2
forehead	C49.0	C79.89	—	D21.0	D48.1	D49.2
gastric	C49.4	C79.89	—	D21.4	D48.1	D49.2
gastrointestinal	C49.4	C79.89	—	D21.4	D48.1	D49.2
gluteal region	C49.5	C79.89	—	D21.5	D48.1	D49.2
great vessels						
NEC	C49.3	C79.89	—	D21.3	D48.1	D49.2
groin	C49.5	C79.89	—	D21.5	D48.1	D49.2
hand	C49.1-☑	C79.89	—	D21.1-☑	D48.1	D49.2
head	C49.0	C79.89	—	D21.0	D48.1	D49.2

338

☑ **Additional Character Required** — Refer to the Tabular List for Character Selection   ▽ **Subterms under main terms may continue to next column or page**

Neoplasm, neoplastic — continued	Malignant Primary	Malignant Secondary	Ca in situ	Benign	Uncertain Behavior	Unspecified Behavior
connective tissue — continued						
heel	C49.2-☑	C79.89	—	D21.2-☑	D48.1	D49.2
hip	C49.2-☑	C79.89	—	D21.2-☑	D48.1	D49.2
hypochondrium	C49.4	C79.89	—	D21.4	D48.1	D49.2
iliopsoas muscle	C49.5	C79.89	—	D21.5	D48.1	D49.2
infraclavicular region	C49.3	C79.89	—	D21.3	D48.1	D49.2
inguinal (canal) (region)	C49.5	C79.89	—	D21.5	D48.1	D49.2
intestinal	C49.4	C79.89	—	D21.4	D48.1	D49.2
intrathoracic	C49.3	C79.89	—	D21.3	D48.1	D49.2
ischiorectal fossa	C49.5	C79.89	—	D21.5	D48.1	D49.2
jaw	C03.9	C79.89	D00.03	D10.39	D48.1	D49.0
knee	C49.2-☑	C79.89	—	D21.2-☑	D48.1	D49.2
leg	C49.2-☑	C79.89	—	D21.2-☑	D48.1	D49.2
limb NEC	C49.9	C79.89	—	D21.9	D48.1	D49.2
lower	C49.2-☑	C79.89	—	D21.2-☑	D48.1	D49.2
upper	C49.1-☑	C79.89	—	D21.1-☑	D48.1	D49.2
nates	C49.5	C79.89	—	D21.5	D48.1	D49.2
neck	C49.0	C79.89	—	D21.0	D48.1	D49.2
orbit	C69.6-☑	C79.49	D09.2-☑	D31.6-☑	D48.1	D49.89
overlapping lesion	C49.8	—	—	—	—	—
pararectal	C49.5	C79.89	—	D21.5	D48.1	D49.2
para-urethral	C49.5	C79.89	—	D21.5	D48.1	D49.2
paravaginal	C49.5	C79.89	—	D21.5	D48.1	D49.2
pelvis (floor)	C49.5	C79.89	—	D21.5	D48.1	D49.2
pelvo-abdominal	C49.8	C79.89	—	D21.6	D48.1	D49.2
perineum	C49.5	C79.89	—	D21.5	D48.1	D49.2
perirectal (tissue)	C49.5	C79.89	—	D21.5	D48.1	D49.2
periurethral (tissue)	C49.5	C79.89	—	D21.5	D48.1	D49.2
popliteal fossa or space	C49.2-☑	C79.89	—	D21.2-☑	D48.1	D49.2
presacral	C49.5	C79.89	—	D21.5	D48.1	D49.2
psoas muscle	C49.4	C79.89	—	D21.4	D48.1	D49.2
pterygoid fossa	C49.0	C79.89	—	D21.0	D48.1	D49.2
rectovaginal septum or wall	C49.5	C79.89	—	D21.5	D48.1	D49.2
rectovesical	C49.5	C79.89	—	D21.5	D48.1	D49.2
retroperitoneum	C48.0	C78.6	—	D20.0	D48.3	D49.0
sacrococcygeal region	C49.5	C79.89	—	D21.5	D48.1	D49.2
scalp	C49.0	C79.89	—	D21.0	D48.1	D49.2
scapular region	C49.3	C79.89	—	D21.3	D48.1	D49.2
shoulder	C49.1-☑	C79.89	—	D21.1-☑	D48.1	D49.2
skin (dermis) NEC — see also Neoplasm, skin, by site	C44.90	C79.2	D04.9	D23.9	D48.5	D49.2
stomach	C49.4	C79.89	—	D21.4	D48.1	D49.2
submental	C49.0	C79.89	—	D21.0	D48.1	D49.2
supraclavicular region	C49.0	C79.89	—	D21.0	D48.1	D49.2
temple	C49.0	C79.89	—	D21.0	D48.1	D49.2
temporal region	C49.0	C79.89	—	D21.0	D48.1	D49.2
thigh	C49.2-☑	C79.89	—	D21.2-☑	D48.1	D49.2
thoracic (duct) (wall)	C49.3	C79.89	—	D21.3	D48.1	D49.2
thorax	C49.3	C79.89	—	D21.3	D48.1	D49.2
thumb	C49.1-☑	C79.89	—	D21.1-☑	D48.1	D49.2
toe	C49.2-☑	C79.89	—	D21.2-☑	D48.1	D49.2
trunk	C49.6	C79.89	—	D21.6	D48.1	D49.2
umbilicus	C49.4	C79.89	—	D21.4	D48.1	D49.2
vesicorectal	C49.5	C79.89	—	D21.5	D48.1	D49.2
wrist	C49.1-☑	C79.89	—	D21.1-☑	D48.1	D49.2
conus medullaris	C72.0	C79.49	—	D33.4	D43.4	D49.7
cord (true) (vocal)	C32.0	C78.39	D02.0	D14.1	D38.0	D49.1
false	C32.1	C78.39	D02.0	D14.1	D38.0	D49.1
spermatic	C63.1-☑	C79.82	D07.69	D29.8	D40.8	D49.59
spinal (cervical) (lumbar) (thoracic)	C72.0	C79.49	—	D33.4	D43.4	D49.7
cornea (limbus)	C69.1-☑	C79.49	D09.2-☑	D31.1-☑	D48.7	D49.89
corpus						
albicans	C56.-☑	C79.6-☑	D07.39	D27.-☑	D39.1-☑	D49.59
callosum, brain	C71.0	C79.31	—	D33.2	D43.2	D49.6

Neoplasm, neoplastic — continued	Malignant Primary	Malignant Secondary	Ca in situ	Benign	Uncertain Behavior	Unspecified Behavior
corpus — continued						
cavernosum	C60.2	C79.82	D07.4	D29.0	D40.8	D49.59
gastric	C16.2	C78.89	D00.2	D13.1	D37.1	D49.0
overlapping sites	C54.8	—	—	—	—	—
penis	C60.2	C79.82	D07.4	D29.0	D40.8	D49.59
striatum, cerebrum	C71.0	C79.31	—	D33.0	D43.0	D49.6
uteri	C54.9	C79.82	D07.0	D26.1	D39.0	D49.59
isthmus	C54.0	C79.82	D07.0	D26.1	D39.0	D49.59
cortex						
adrenal	C74.0-☑	C79.7-☑	D09.3	D35.0-☑	D44.1-☑	D49.7
cerebral	C71.0	C79.31	—	D33.0	D43.0	D49.6
costal cartilage	C41.3	C79.51	—	D16.7	D48.0	D49.2
costovertebral joint	C41.3	C79.51	—	D16.7	D48.0	D49.2
Cowper's gland	C68.0	C79.19	D09.19	D30.4	D41.3	D49.59
cranial (fossa, any)	C71.9	C79.31	—	D33.2	D43.2	D49.6
meninges	C70.0	C79.32	—	D32.0	D42.0	D49.7
nerve	C72.50	C79.49	—	D33.3	D43.3	D49.7
specified NEC	C72.59	C79.49	—	D33.3	D43.3	D49.7
craniobuccal pouch	C75.2	C79.89	D09.3	D35.2	D44.3	D49.7
craniopharyngeal (duct) (pouch)	C75.2	C79.89	D09.3	D35.3	D44.4	D49.7
cricoid	C13.0	C79.89	D00.08	D10.7	D37.05	D49.0
cartilage	C32.3	C78.39	D02.0	D14.1	D38.0	D49.1
cricopharynx	C13.0	C79.89	D00.08	D10.7	D37.05	D49.0
crypt of Morgagni	C21.8	C78.5	D01.3	D12.9	D37.8	D49.0
crystalline lens	C69.4-☑	C79.49	D09.2-☑	D31.4-☑	D48.7	D49.89
cul-de-sac (Douglas')	C48.1	C78.6	—	D20.1	D48.4	D49.0
cuneiform cartilage	C32.3	C78.39	D02.0	D14.1	D38.0	D49.1
cutaneous — see Neoplasm, skin						
cutis — see Neoplasm, skin						
cystic (bile) duct (common)	C24.0	C78.89	D01.5	D13.5	D37.6	D49.0
dermis — see Neoplasm, skin						
diaphragm	C49.3	C79.89	—	D21.3	D48.1	D49.2
digestive organs, system, tube, or tract NEC	C26.9	C78.89	D01.9	D13.9	D37.9	D49.0
disc, intervertebral	C41.2	C79.51	—	D16.6	D48.0	D49.2
disease, generalized	C80.0	—	—	—	—	—
disseminated	C80.0	—	—	—	—	—
Douglas' cul-de-sac or pouch	C48.1	C78.6	—	D20.1	D48.4	D49.0
duodenojejunal junction	C17.8	C78.4	D01.49	D13.39	D37.2	D49.0
duodenum	C17.0	C78.4	D01.49	D13.2	D37.2	D49.0
dura (cranial) (mater)	C70.9	C79.49	—	D32.9	D42.9	D49.7
cerebral	C70.0	C79.32	—	D32.0	D42.0	D49.7
spinal	C70.1	C79.49	—	D32.1	D42.1	D49.7
ear (external) — see also Neoplasm, skin, ear	C44.20-☑	C79.2	D04.2-☑	D23.2-☑	D48.5	D49.2
auricle or auris — see also Neoplasm, skin, ear	C44.20-☑	C79.2	D04.2-☑	D23.2-☑	D48.5	D49.2
canal, external — see also Neoplasm, skin, ear	C44.20-☑	C79.2	D04.2-☑	D23.2-☑	D48.5	D49.2
cartilage	C49.0	C79.89	—	D21.0	D48.1	D49.2
external meatus — see also Neoplasm, skin, ear	C44.20-☑	C79.2	D04.2-☑	D23.2-☑	D48.5	D49.2
inner	C30.1	C78.39	D02.3	D14.0	D38.5	D49.1
lobule — see also Neoplasm, skin, ear	C44.20-☑	C79.2	D04.2-☑	D23.2-☑	D48.5	D49.2
middle	C30.1	C78.39	D02.3	D14.0	D38.5	D49.1
overlapping lesion with accessory sinuses	C31.8	—	—	—	—	—

Neoplasm, ear — Neoplasm, frenulum

	Malignant Primary	Malignant Secondary	Ca in situ	Benign	Uncertain Behavior	Unspecified Behavior
Neoplasm, neoplastic						
— *continued*						
ear — *see also*						
Neoplasm, skin, ear						
— *continued*						
skin	C44.20-☑	C79.2	D04.2-☑	D23.2-☑	D48.5	D49.2
basal cell						
carcinoma	C44.21-☑	—	—	—	—	—
specified type						
NEC	C44.29-☑	—	—	—	—	—
squamous cell						
carcinoma	C44.22-☑	—	—	—	—	—
earlobe	C44.20-☑	C79.2	D04.2-☑	D23.2-☑	D48.5	D49.2
basal cell						
carcinoma	C44.21-☑	—	—	—	—	—
specified type						
NEC	C44.29-☑	—	—	—	—	—
squamous cell						
carcinoma	C44.22-☑	—	—	—	—	—
ejaculatory duct	C63.7	C79.82	D07.69	D29.8	D40.8	D49.59
elbow NEC	C76.4-☑	C79.89	D04.6-☑	D36.7	D48.7	D49.89
endocardium	C38.0	C79.89	—	D15.1	D48.7	D49.89
endocervix (canal)						
(gland)	C53.0	C79.82	D06.0	D26.0	D39.0	D49.59
endocrine gland						
NEC	C75.9	C79.89	D09.3	D35.9	D44.9	D49.7
pluriglandular	C75.8	C79.89	D09.3	D35.7	D44.9	D49.7
endometrium (gland)						
(stroma)	C54.1	C79.82	D07.0	D26.1	D39.0	D49.59
ensiform cartilage	C41.3	C79.51	—	D16.7	D48.0	D49.2
enteric — *see*						
Neoplasm,						
intestine						
ependyma (brain)	C71.5	C79.31	—	D33.0	D43.0	D49.6
fourth ventricle	C71.7	C79.31	—	D33.1	D43.1	D49.6
epicardium	C38.0	C79.89	—	D15.1	D48.7	D49.89
epididymis	C63.0-☑	C79.82	D07.69	D29.3-☑	D40.8	D49.59
epidural	C72.9	C79.49	—	D33.9	D43.9	D49.7
epiglottis	C32.1	C78.39	D02.0	D14.1	D38.0	D49.1
anterior aspect or						
surface	C10.1	C79.89	D00.08	D10.5	D37.05	D49.0
cartilage	C32.3	C78.39	D02.0	D14.1	D38.0	D49.1
free border						
(margin)	C10.1	C79.89	D00.08	D10.5	D37.05	D49.0
junctional						
region	C10.8	C79.89	D00.08	D10.5	D37.05	D49.0
posterior (laryngeal)						
surface	C32.1	C78.39	D02.0	D14.1	D38.0	D49.1
suprahyoid						
portion	C32.1	C78.39	D02.0	D14.1	D38.0	D49.1
esophagogastric						
junction	C16.0	C78.89	D00.2	D13.1	D37.1	D49.0
esophagus	C15.9	C78.89	D00.1	D13.0	D37.8	D49.0
abdominal	C15.5	C78.89	D00.1	D13.0	D37.8	D49.0
cervical	C15.3	C78.89	D00.1	D13.0	D37.8	D49.0
distal (third)	C15.5	C78.89	D00.1	D13.0	D37.8	D49.0
lower (third)	C15.5	C78.89	D00.1	D13.0	D37.8	D49.0
middle (third)	C15.4	C78.89	D00.1	D13.0	D37.8	D49.0
overlapping						
lesion	C15.8	—	—	—	—	—
proximal (third)	C15.3	C78.89	D00.1	D13.0	D37.8	D49.0
thoracic	C15.4	C78.89	D00.1	D13.0	D37.8	D49.0
upper (third)	C15.3	C78.89	D00.1	D13.0	D37.8	D49.0
ethmoid (sinus)	C31.1	C78.39	D02.3	D14.0	D38.5	D49.1
bone or						
labyrinth	C41.0	C79.51	—	D16.4	D48.0	D49.2
eustachian tube	C30.1	C78.39	D02.3	D14.0	D38.5	D49.1
exocervix	C53.1	C79.82	D06.1	D26.0	D39.0	D49.59
external						
meatus (ear) — *see also* Neoplasm,						
skin, ear	C44.20-☑	C79.2	D04.2-☑	D23.2-☑	D48.5	D49.2
os, cervix uteri	C53.1	C79.82	D06.1	D26.0	D39.0	D49.59
extradural	C72.9	C79.49	—	D33.9	D43.9	D49.7
extrahepatic (bile)						
duct	C24.0	C78.89	D01.5	D13.5	D37.6	D49.0
overlapping lesion						
with						
gallbladder	C24.8	—	—	—	—	—
extraocular						
muscle	C69.6-☑	C79.49	D09.2-☑	D31.6-☑	D48.7	D49.89
extrarectal	C76.3	C79.89	D09.8	D36.7	D48.7	D49.89
extremity	C76.8	C79.89	D04.8	D36.7	D48.7	D49.89

	Malignant Primary	Malignant Secondary	Ca in situ	Benign	Uncertain Behavior	Unspecified Behavior
Neoplasm, neoplastic						
— *continued*						
extremity — *continued*						
lower	C76.5-☑	C79.89	D04.7-☑	D36.7	D48.7	D49.89
upper	C76.4-☑	C79.89	D04.6-☑	D36.7	D48.7	D49.89
eyeball	C69.9-☑	C79.49	D09.2-☑	D31.9-☑	D48.7	D49.89
eyebrow	C44.309	C79.2	D04.39	D23.39	D48.5	D49.2
basal cell						
carcinoma	C44.319	—	—	—	—	—
specified type						
NEC	C44.399	—	—	—	—	—
squamous cell						
carcinoma	C44.329	—	—	—	—	—
eyelid (lower) (skin)						
(upper)	C44.10-☑					
basal cell						
carcinoma	C44.11-☑					
cartilage	C49.0	C79.89		D21.0	D48.1	D49.2
sebaceous cell	C44.13-☑					
specified type						
NEC	C44.19-☑					
squamous cell						
carcinoma	C44.12-☑					
eye NEC	C69.9-☑	C79.49	D09.2-☑	D31.9-☑	D48.7	D49.89
overlapping						
sites	C69.8-☑	—	—	—	—	—
face NEC	C76.0	C79.89	D04.39	D36.7	D48.7	D49.89
fallopian tube						
(accessory)	C57.0-☑	C79.82	D07.39	D28.2	D39.8	D49.59
falx (cerebella)						
(cerebri)	C70.0	C79.32	—	D32.0	D42.0	D49.7
fascia — *see also*						
Neoplasm,						
connective tissue						
palmar	C49.1-☑	C79.89	—	D21.1-☑	D48.1	D49.2
plantar	C49.2-☑	C79.89	—	D21.2-☑	D48.1	D49.2
fatty tissue — *see*						
Neoplasm,						
connective tissue						
fauces, faucial NEC	C10.9	C79.89	D00.08	D10.5	D37.05	D49.0
pillars	C09.1	C79.89	D00.08	D10.5	D37.05	D49.0
tonsil	C09.9	C79.89	D00.08	D10.4	D37.05	D49.0
femur (any part)	C40.2-☑	—	—	D16.2-☑	—	—
fetal membrane	C58	C79.82	D07.0	D26.7	D39.2	D49.59
fibrous tissue — *see*						
Neoplasm,						
connective tissue						
fibula (any part)	C40.2-☑	C79.51	—	D16.2-☑	—	—
filum terminale	C72.0	C79.49	—	D33.4	D43.4	D49.7
finger NEC	C76.4-☑	C79.89	D04.6-☑	D36.7	D48.7	D49.89
flank NEC	C76.8	C79.89	D04.5	D36.7	D48.7	D49.89
follicle, nabothian	C53.0	C79.82	D06.0	D26.0	D39.0	D49.59
foot NEC	C76.5-☑	C79.89	D04.7-☑	D36.7	D48.7	D49.89
forearm NEC	C76.4-☑	C79.89	D04.6-☑	D36.7	D48.7	D49.89
forehead (skin)	C44.309	C79.2	D04.39	D23.39	D48.5	D49.2
basal cell						
carcinoma	C44.319	—	—	—	—	—
specified type						
NEC	C44.399					
squamous cell						
carcinoma	C44.329	—	—	—	—	—
foreskin	C60.0	C79.82	D07.4	D29.0	D40.8	D49.59
fornix						
pharyngeal	C11.3	C79.89	D00.08	D10.6	D37.05	D49.0
vagina	C52	C79.82	D07.2	D28.1	D39.8	D49.59
fossa (of)						
anterior (cranial)	C71.9	C79.31	—	D33.2	D43.2	D49.6
cranial	C71.9	C79.31	—	D33.2	D43.2	D49.6
ischiorectal	C76.3	C79.89	D09.8	D36.7	D48.7	D49.89
middle (cranial)	C71.9	C79.31	—	D33.2	D43.2	D49.6
piriform	C12	C79.89	D00.08	D10.7	D37.05	D49.0
pituitary	C75.1	C79.89	D09.3	D35.2	D44.3	D49.7
posterior						
(cranial)	C71.9	C79.31	—	D33.2	D43.2	D49.6
pterygoid	C49.0	C79.89	—	D21.0	D48.1	D49.2
pyriform	C12	C79.89	D00.08	D10.7	D37.05	D49.0
Rosenmuller	C11.2	C79.89	D00.08	D10.6	D37.05	D49.0
tonsillar	C09.0	C79.89	D00.08	D10.5	D37.05	D49.0
fourchette	C51.9	C79.82	D07.1	D28.0	D39.8	D49.59
frenulum						
labii — *see*						
Neoplasm, lip,						
internal						

☑ **Additional Character Required — Refer to the Tabular List for Character Selection**   Subterms under main terms may continue to next column or page

Neoplasm, neoplastic — continued	Malignant Primary	Malignant Secondary	Ca in situ	Benign	Uncertain Behavior	Unspecified Behavior
frenulum — continued						
linguae	C02.2	C79.89	D00.07	D10.1	D37.02	D49.0
frontal						
bone	C41.0	C79.51	—	D16.4	D48.0	D49.2
lobe, brain	C71.1	C79.31	—	D33.0	D43.0	D49.6
pole	C71.1	C79.31	—	D33.0	D43.0	D49.6
sinus	C31.2	C78.39	D02.3	D14.0	D38.5	D49.1
fundus						
stomach	C16.1	C78.89	D00.2	D13.1	D37.1	D49.0
uterus	C54.3	C79.82	D07.0	D26.1	D39.0	D49.59
gallbladder	C23	C78.89	D01.5	D13.5	D37.6	D49.0
overlapping lesion with extrahepatic bile ducts	C24.8	—	—	—	—	—
gall duct						
(extrahepatic)	C24.0	C78.89	D01.5	D13.5	D37.6	D49.0
intrahepatic	C22.1	C78.7	D01.5	D13.4	D37.6	D49.0
ganglia — see also Neoplasm, nerve, peripheral	C47.9	C79.89	—	D36.10	D48.2	D49.2
basal	C71.0	C79.31	—	D33.0	D43.0	D49.6
cranial nerve	C72.50	C79.49	—	D33.3	D43.3	D49.7
Gartner's duct	C52	C79.82	D07.2	D28.1	D39.8	D49.59
gastric — see Neoplasm, stomach						
gastrocolic	C26.9	C78.89	D01.9	D13.9	D37.9	D49.0
gastroesophageal junction	C16.0	C78.89	D00.2	D13.1	D37.1	D49.0
gastrointestinal (tract) NEC	C26.9	C78.89	D01.9	D13.9	D37.9	D49.0
generalized	C80.0	—	—	—	—	—
genital organ or tract						
female NEC	C57.9	C79.82	D07.30	D28.9	D39.9	D49.59
overlapping lesion	C57.8	—	—	—	—	—
specified site NEC	C57.7	C79.82	D07.39	D28.7	D39.8	D49.59
male NEC	C63.9	C79.82	D07.60	D29.9	D40.9	D49.59
overlapping lesion	C63.8	—	—	—	—	—
specified site NEC	C63.7	C79.82	D07.69	D29.8	D40.8	D49.59
genitourinary tract						
female	C57.9	C79.82	D07.30	D28.9	D39.9	D49.59
male	C63.9	C79.82	D07.60	D29.9	D40.9	D49.59
gingiva (alveolar) (marginal)	C03.9	C79.89	D00.03	D10.39	D37.09	D49.0
lower	C03.1	C79.89	D00.03	D10.39	D37.09	D49.0
mandibular	C03.1	C79.89	D00.03	D10.39	D37.09	D49.0
maxillary	C03.0	C79.89	D00.03	D10.39	D37.09	D49.0
upper	C03.0	C79.89	D00.03	D10.39	D37.09	D49.0
gland, glandular (lymphatic) (system) — see also Neoplasm, lymph gland						
endocrine NEC	C75.9	C79.89	D09.3	D35.9	D44.9	D49.7
salivary — see Neoplasm, salivary gland						
glans penis	C60.1	C79.82	D07.4	D29.0	D40.8	D49.59
globus pallidus	C71.0	C79.31	—	D33.0	D43.0	D49.6
glomus						
coccygeal	C49.5	C79.89	—	D21.5	D48.1	D49.2
jugularis	C75.5	C79.89	—	D35.6	D44.7	D49.7
glosso-epiglottic fold(s)	C10.1	C79.89	D00.08	D10.5	D37.05	D49.0
glossopalatine fold	C09.1	C79.89	D00.08	D10.5	D37.05	D49.0
glossopharyngeal sulcus	C09.0	C79.89	D00.08	D10.5	D37.05	D49.0
glottis	C32.0	C78.39	D02.0	D14.1	D38.0	D49.1
gluteal region	C76.3	C79.89	D04.5	D36.7	D48.7	D49.89
great vessels NEC	C49.3	C79.89	—	D21.3	D48.1	D49.2
groin NEC	C76.3	C79.89	D04.5	D36.7	D48.7	D49.89
gum	C03.9	C79.89	D00.03	D10.39	D37.09	D49.0
lower	C03.1	C79.89	D00.03	D10.39	D37.09	D49.0
upper	C03.0	C79.89	D00.03	D10.39	D37.09	D49.0
hand NEC	C76.4-☑	C79.89	D04.6-☑	D36.7	D48.7	D49.89
head NEC	C76.0	C79.89	D04.4	D36.7	D48.7	D49.89
heart	C38.0	C79.89	—	D15.1	D48.7	D49.89

Neoplasm, neoplastic — continued	Malignant Primary	Malignant Secondary	Ca in situ	Benign	Uncertain Behavior	Unspecified Behavior
heel NEC	C76.5-☑	C79.89	D04.7-☑	D36.7	D48.7	D49.89
helix — see also Neoplasm, skin, ear	C44.20-☑	C79.2	D04.2-☑	D23.2-☑	D48.5	D49.2
hematopoietic, hemopoietic tissue NEC	C96.9	—	—	—	—	—
specified NEC	C96.Z	—	—	—	—	—
hemisphere, cerebral	C71.0	C79.31	—	D33.0	D43.0	D49.6
hemorrhoidal zone	C21.1	C78.5	D01.3	D12.9	D37.8	D49.0
hepatic — see also Index to disease, by histology	C22.9	C78.7	D01.5	D13.4	D37.6	D49.0
duct (bile)	C24.0	C78.89	D01.5	D13.5	D37.6	D49.0
flexure (colon)	C18.3	C78.5	D01.0	D12.3	D37.4	D49.0
primary	C22.8	C78.7	D01.5	D13.4	D37.6	D49.0
hepatobiliary	C24.9	C78.89	D01.5	D13.5	D37.6	D49.0
hepatoblastoma	C22.2	C78.7	D01.5	D13.4	D37.6	D49.0
hepatoma	C22.0	C78.7	D01.5	D13.4	D37.6	D49.0
hilus of lung	C34.0-☑	C78.0-☑	D02.2-☑	D14.3-☑	D38.1	D49.1
hippocampus, brain	C71.2	C79.31	—	D33.0	D43.0	D49.6
hip NEC	C76.5-☑	C79.89	D04.7-☑	D36.7	D48.7	D49.89
humerus (any part)	C40.0-☑	C79.51	—	D16.0-☑	—	—
hymen	C52	C79.82	D07.2	D28.1	D39.8	D49.59
hypopharynx, hypopharyngeal NEC	C13.9	C79.89	D00.08	D10.7	D37.05	D49.0
overlapping lesion	C13.8	—	—	—	—	—
postcricoid region	C13.0	C79.89	D00.08	D10.7	D37.05	D49.0
posterior wall	C13.2	C79.89	D00.08	D10.7	D37.05	D49.0
pyriform fossa (sinus)	C12	C79.89	D00.08	D10.7	D37.05	D49.0
hypophysis	C75.1	C79.89	D09.3	D35.2	D44.3	D49.7
hypothalamus	C71.0	C79.31	—	D33.0	D43.0	D49.6
ileocecum, ileocecal (coil) (junction) (valve)	C18.0	C78.5	D01.0	D12.0	D37.4	D49.0
ileum	C17.2	C78.4	D01.49	D13.39	D37.2	D49.0
ilium	C41.4	C79.51	—	D16.8	D48.0	D49.2
immunoproliferative NEC	C88.9	—	—	—	—	—
infraclavicular (region)	C76.1	C79.89	D04.5	D36.7	D48.7	D49.89
inguinal (region)	C76.3	C79.89	D04.5	D36.7	D48.7	D49.89
insula	C71.0	C79.31	—	D33.0	D43.0	D49.6
insular tissue (pancreas)	C25.4	C78.89	D01.7	D13.7	D37.8	D49.0
brain	C71.0	C79.31	—	D33.0	D43.0	D49.6
interarytenoid fold	C13.1	C78.39	D00.08	D10.7	D37.05	D49.0
hypopharyngeal aspect	C13.1	C79.89	D00.08	D10.7	D37.05	D49.0
laryngeal aspect	C32.1	C78.39	D02.0	D14.1	D38.0	D49.1
marginal zone	C13.1	C79.89	D00.08	D10.7	D37.05	D49.0
interdental papillae	C03.9	C79.89	D00.03	D10.39	D37.09	D49.0
lower	C03.1	C79.89	D00.03	D10.39	D37.09	D49.0
upper	C03.0	C79.89	D00.03	D10.39	D37.09	D49.0
internal						
capsule	C71.0	C79.31	—	D33.0	D43.0	D49.6
os (cervix)	C53.0	C79.82	D06.0	D26.0	D39.0	D49.59
intervertebral cartilage or disc	C41.2	C79.51	—	D16.6	D48.0	D49.2
intestine, intestinal	C26.0	C78.80	D01.40	D13.9	D37.9	D49.0
large	C18.9	C78.5	D01.0	D12.6	D37.4	D49.0
appendix	C18.1	C78.5	D01.0	D12.1	D37.3	D49.0
caput coli	C18.0	C78.5	D01.0	D12.0	D37.4	D49.0
cecum	C18.0	C78.5	D01.0	D12.0	D37.4	D49.0
colon	C18.9	C78.5	D01.0	D12.6	D37.4	D49.0
and rectum	C19	C78.5	D01.1	D12.7	D37.5	D49.0
ascending	C18.2	C78.5	D01.0	D12.2	D37.4	D49.0
caput	C18.0	C78.5	D01.0	D12.0	D37.4	D49.0
descending	C18.6	C78.5	D01.0	D12.4	D37.4	D49.0
distal	C18.6	C78.5	D01.0	D12.4	D37.4	D49.0

Neoplasm Table

Neoplasm, intestine, intestinal — Neoplasm, limbus of cornea

Neoplasm, neoplastic	Malignant Primary	Malignant Secondary	Ca in situ	Benign	Uncertain Behavior	Unspecified Behavior
— *continued*						
intestine, intestinal — *continued*						
large — *continued*						
colon — *continued*						
left	C18.6	C78.5	D01.0	D12.4	D37.4	D49.0
overlapping lesion	C18.8	—	—	—	—	—
pelvic	C18.7	C78.5	D01.0	D12.5	D37.4	D49.0
right	C18.2	C78.5	D01.0	D12.2	D37.4	D49.0
sigmoid (flexure)	C18.7	C78.5	D01.0	D12.5	D37.4	D49.0
transverse	C18.4	C78.5	D01.0	D12.3	D37.4	D49.0
hepatic flexure	C18.3	C78.5	D01.0	D12.3	D37.4	D49.0
ileocecum, ileocecal (coil) (valve)	C18.0	C78.5	D01.0	D12.0	D37.4	D49.0
overlapping lesion	C18.8	—	—	—	—	—
sigmoid flexure (lower) (upper)	C18.7	C78.5	D01.0	D12.5	D37.4	D49.0
splenic flexure	C18.5	C78.5	D01.0	D12.3	D37.4	D49.0
small	C17.9	C78.4	D01.40	D13.30	D37.2	D49.0
duodenum	C17.0	C78.4	D01.49	D13.2	D37.2	D49.0
ileum	C17.2	C78.4	D01.49	D13.39	D37.2	D49.0
jejunum	C17.1	C78.4	D01.49	D13.39	D37.2	D49.0
overlapping lesion	C17.8	—	—	—	—	—
tract NEC	C26.0	C78.89	D01.40	D13.9	D37.8	D49.0
intra-abdominal	C76.2	C79.89	D09.8	D36.7	D48.7	D49.89
intracranial NEC	C71.9	C79.31	—	D33.2	D43.2	D49.6
intrahepatic (bile) duct	C22.1	C78.7	D01.5	D13.4	D37.6	D49.0
intraocular	C69.9-☑	C79.49	D09.2-☑	D31.9-☑	D48.7	D49.89
intraorbital	C69.6-☑	C79.49	D09.2-☑	D31.6-☑	D48.7	D49.89
intrasellar	C75.1	C79.89	D09.3	D35.2	D44.3	D49.7
intrathoracic (cavity) (organs)	C76.1	C79.89	D09.8	D15.9	D48.7	D49.89
specified NEC	C76.1	C79.89	D09.8	D15.7	—	—
iris	C69.4-☑	C79.49	D09.2-☑	D31.4-☑	D48.7	D49.89
ischiorectal (fossa)	C76.3	C79.89	D09.8	D36.7	D48.7	D49.89
ischium	C41.4	C79.51	—	D16.8	D48.0	D49.2
island of Reil	C71.0	C79.31	—	D33.0	D43.0	D49.6
islands or islets of Langerhans	C25.4	C78.89	D01.7	D13.7	D37.8	D49.0
isthmus uteri	C54.0	C79.82	D07.0	D26.1	D39.0	D49.59
jaw	C76.0	C79.89	D09.8	D36.7	D48.7	D49.89
bone	C41.1	C79.51	—	D16.5	D48.0	D49.2
lower	C41.1	C79.51	—	D16.5	—	—
upper	C41.0	C79.51	—	D16.4	—	—
carcinoma (any type) (lower) (upper)	C76.0	C79.89	—	—	—	—
skin — *see also* Neoplasm, skin,						
face	C44.309	C79.2	D04.39	D23.39	D48.5	D49.2
soft tissues	C03.9	C79.89	D00.03	D10.39	D37.09	D49.0
lower	C03.1	C79.89	D00.03	D10.39	D37.09	D49.0
upper	C03.0	C79.89	D00.03	D10.39	D37.09	D49.0
jejunum	C17.1	C78.4	D01.49	D13.39	D37.2	D49.0
joint NEC — *see also* Neoplasm,						
bone	C41.9	C79.51	—	D16.9	D48.0	D49.2
acromioclavicular	C40.0-☑	C79.51	—	D16.0-☑	—	—
bursa or synovial membrane — *see* Neoplasm, connective tissue						
costovertebral	C41.3	C79.51	—	D16.7	D48.0	D49.2
sternocostal	C41.3	C79.51	—	D16.7	D48.0	D49.2
temporomandibular	C41.1	C79.51	—	D16.5	D48.0	D49.2
junction						
anorectal	C21.8	C78.5	D01.3	D12.9	D37.8	D49.0
cardioesophageal	C16.0	C78.89	D00.2	D13.1	D37.1	D49.0
esophagogastric	C16.0	C78.89	D00.2	D13.1	D37.1	D49.0
gastroesophageal	C16.0	C78.89	D00.2	D13.1	D37.1	D49.0
hard and soft palate	C05.9	C79.89	D00.00	D10.39	D37.09	D49.0
ileocecal	C18.0	C78.5	D01.0	D12.0	D37.4	D49.0

Neoplasm, neoplastic	Malignant Primary	Malignant Secondary	Ca in situ	Benign	Uncertain Behavior	Unspecified Behavior
— *continued*						
junction — *continued*						
pelvirectal	C19	C78.5	D01.1	D12.7	D37.5	D49.0
pelviureteric	C65.-☑	C79.0-☑	D09.19	D30.1-☑	D41.1-☑	D49.59
rectosigmoid	C19	C78.5	D01.1	D12.7	D37.5	D49.0
squamocolumnar, of cervix	C53.8	C79.82	D06.7	D26.0	D39.0	D49.59
Kaposi's sarcoma — *see* Kaposi's, sarcoma						
kidney (parenchymal)	C64.-☑	C79.0-☑	D09.19	D30.0-☑	D41.0-☑	D49.51-☑
calyx	C65.-☑	C79.0-☑	D09.19	D30.1-☑	D41.1-☑	D49.51-☑
hilus	C65.-☑	C79.0-☑	D09.19	D30.1-☑	D41.1-☑	D49.51-☑
pelvis	C65.-☑	C79.0-☑	D09.19	D30.1-☑	D41.1-☑	D49.51-☑
knee NEC	C76.5-☑	C79.89	D04.7-☑	D36.7	D48.7	D49.89
labia (skin)	C51.9	C79.82	D07.1	D28.0	D39.8	D49.59
majora	C51.0	C79.82	D07.1	D28.0	D39.8	D49.59
minora	C51.1	C79.82	D07.1	D28.0	D39.8	D49.59
labial — *see also* Neoplasm, lip	C00.9	C79.89	D00.01	D10.0	D37.01	D49.0
sulcus (lower) (upper)	C06.1	C79.89	D00.02	D10.39	D37.09	D49.0
labium (skin)	C51.9	C79.82	D07.1	D28.0	D39.8	D49.59
majus	C51.0	C79.82	D07.1	D28.0	D39.8	D49.59
minus	C51.1	C79.82	D07.1	D28.0	D39.8	D49.59
lacrimal						
canaliculi	C69.5-☑	C79.49	D09.2-☑	D31.5-☑	D48.7	D49.89
duct (nasal)	C69.5-☑	C79.49	D09.2-☑	D31.5-☑	D48.7	D49.89
gland	C69.5-☑	C79.49	D09.2-☑	D31.5-☑	D48.7	D49.89
punctum	C69.5-☑	C79.49	D09.2-☑	D31.5-☑	D48.7	D49.89
sac	C69.5-☑	C79.49	D09.2-☑	D31.5-☑	D48.7	D49.89
Langerhans, islands or islets	C25.4	C78.89	D01.7	D13.7	D37.8	D49.0
laryngopharynx	C13.9	C79.89	D00.08	D10.7	D37.05	D49.0
larynx, laryngeal NEC	C32.9	C78.39	D02.0	D14.1	D38.0	D49.1
aryepiglottic fold	C32.1	C78.39	D02.0	D14.1	D38.0	D49.1
cartilage (arytenoid) (cricoid) (cuneiform) (thyroid)	C32.3	C78.39	D02.0	D14.1	D38.0	D49.1
commissure (anterior) (posterior)	C32.0	C78.39	D02.0	D14.1	D38.0	D49.1
extrinsic NEC	C32.1	C78.39	D02.0	D14.1	D38.0	D49.1
meaning hypopharynx	C13.9	C79.89	D00.08	D10.7	D37.05	D49.0
interarytenoid fold	C32.1	C78.39	D02.0	D14.1	D38.0	D49.1
intrinsic	C32.0	C78.39	D02.0	D14.1	D38.0	D49.1
overlapping lesion	C32.8	—	—	—	—	—
ventricular band	C32.1	C78.39	D02.0	D14.1	D38.0	D49.1
leg NEC	C76.5-☑	C79.89	D04.7-☑	D36.7	D48.7	D49.89
lens, crystalline	C69.4-☑	C79.49	D09.2-☑	D31.4-☑	D48.7	D49.89
lid (lower) (upper)	C44.10-☑	C79.2	D04.1-☑	D23.1-☑	D48.5	D49.2
basal cell carcinoma	C44.11-☑	—	—	—	—	—
sebaceous cell	C44.13-☑	—	—	—	—	—
specified type NEC	C44.19-☑	—	—	—	—	—
squamous cell carcinoma	C44.12-☑	—	—	—	—	—
ligament — *see also* Neoplasm, connective tissue						
broad	C57.1-☑	C79.82	D07.39	D28.2	D39.8	D49.59
Mackenrodt's	C57.7	C79.82	D07.39	D28.7	D39.8	D49.59
non-uterine — *see* Neoplasm, connective tissue						
round	C57.2-☑	C79.82	—	D28.2	D39.8	D49.59
sacro-uterine	C57.3	C79.82	—	D28.2	D39.8	D49.59
uterine	C57.3	C79.82	—	D28.2	D39.8	D49.59
utero-ovarian	C57.7	C79.82	D07.39	D28.2	D39.8	D49.59
uterosacral	C57.3	C79.82	—	D28.2	D39.8	D49.59
limb	C76.8	C79.89	D04.8	D36.7	D48.7	D49.89
lower	C76.5-☑	C79.89	D04.7-☑	D36.7	D48.7	D49.89
upper	C76.4-☑	C79.89	D04.6-☑	D36.7	D48.7	D49.89
limbus of cornea	C69.1-☑	C79.49	D09.2-☑	D31.1-☑	D48.7	D49.89

	Malignant Primary	Malignant Secondary	Ca in situ	Benign	Uncertain Behavior	Unspecified Behavior
Neoplasm, neoplastic						
— *continued*						
lingual NEC — *see also*						
Neoplasm,						
tongue	C02.9	C79.89	D00.07	D10.1	D37.02	D49.0
lingula, lung	C34.1-☑	C78.0-☑	D02.2-☑	D14.3-☑	D38.1	D49.1
lip	C00.9	C79.89	D00.01	D10.0	D37.01	D49.0
buccal aspect — *see*						
Neoplasm, lip,						
internal						
commissure	C00.6	C79.89	D00.01	D10.0	D37.01	D49.0
external	C00.2	C79.89	D00.01	D10.0	D37.01	D49.0
lower	C00.1	C79.89	D00.01	D10.0	D37.01	D49.0
upper	C00.0	C79.89	D00.01	D10.0	D37.01	D49.0
frenulum — *see*						
Neoplasm, lip,						
internal						
inner aspect — *see*						
Neoplasm, lip,						
internal						
internal	C00.5	C79.89	D00.01	D10.0	D37.01	D49.0
lower	C00.4	C79.89	D00.01	D10.0	D37.01	D49.0
upper	C00.3	C79.89	D00.01	D10.0	D37.01	D49.0
lipstick area	C00.2	C79.89	D00.01	D10.0	D37.01	D49.0
lower	C00.1	C79.89	D00.01	D10.0	D37.01	D49.0
upper	C00.0	C79.89	D00.01	D10.0	D37.01	D49.0
lower	C00.1	C79.89	D00.01	D10.0	D37.01	D49.0
internal	C00.4	C79.89	D00.01	D10.0	D37.01	D49.0
mucosa — *see*						
Neoplasm, lip,						
internal						
oral aspect — *see*						
Neoplasm, lip,						
internal						
overlapping						
lesion	C00.8	—	—	—	—	—
with oral cavity or						
pharynx	C14.8	—	—	—	—	—
skin (commissure)						
(lower)						
(upper)	C44.00	C79.2	D04.0	D23.0	D48.5	D49.2
basal cell						
carcinoma	C44.01	—	—	—	—	—
specified type						
NEC	C44.09	—	—	—	—	—
squamous cell						
carcinoma	C44.02	—	—	—	—	—
upper	C00.0	C79.89	D00.01	D10.0	D37.01	D49.0
internal	C00.3	C79.89	D00.01	D10.0	D37.01	D49.0
vermilion						
border	C00.2	C79.89	D00.01	D10.0	D37.01	D49.0
lower	C00.1	C79.89	D00.01	D10.0	D37.01	D49.0
upper	C00.0	C79.89	D00.01	D10.0	D37.01	D49.0
lipomatous — *see*						
Lipoma, by site						
liver — *see also* Index						
to disease, by						
histology	C22.9	C78.7	D01.5	D13.4	D37.6	D49.0
primary	C22.8	C78.7	D01.5	D13.4	D37.6	D49.0
lumbosacral						
plexus	C47.5	C79.89	—	D36.16	D48.2	D49.2
lung	C34.9-☑	C78.0-☑	D02.2-☑	D14.3-☑	D38.1	D49.1
azygos lobe	C34.1-☑	C78.0-☑	D02.2-☑	D14.3-☑	D38.1	D49.1
carina	C34.0-☑	C78.0-☑	D02.2-☑	D14.3-☑	D38.1	D49.1
hilus	C34.0-☑	C78.0-☑	D02.2-☑	D14.3-☑	D38.1	D49.1
lingula	C34.1-☑	C78.0-☑	D02.2-☑	D14.3-☑	D38.1	D49.1
lobe NEC	C34.9-☑	C78.0-☑	D02.2-☑	D14.3-☑	D38.1	D49.1
lower lobe	C34.3-☑	C78.0-☑	D02.2-☑	D14.3-☑	D38.1	D49.1
main bronchus	C34.0-☑	C78.0-☑	D02.2-☑	D14.3-☑	D38.1	D49.1
mesothelioma — *see*						
Mesothelioma						
middle lobe	C34.2	C78.0-☑	D02.21	D14.31	D38.1	D49.1
overlapping						
lesion	C34.8-☑	—	—	—	—	—
upper lobe	C34.1-☑	C78.0-☑	D02.2-☑	D14.3-☑	D38.1	D49.1
lymph, lymphatic						
channel NEC	C49.9	C79.89	—	D21.9	D48.1	D49.2
gland						
(secondary)	—	C77.9	—	D36.0	D48.7	D49.89
abdominal	—	C77.2	—	D36.0	D48.7	D49.89
aortic	—	C77.2	—	D36.0	D48.7	D49.89
arm	—	C77.3	—	D36.0	D48.7	D49.89
Neoplasm, neoplastic						
— *continued*						
lymph, lymphatic						
channel —						
continued						
gland — *continued*						
auricular (anterior)						
(posterior)	—	C77.0	—	D36.0	D48.7	D49.89
axilla, axillary	—	C77.3	—	D36.0	D48.7	D49.89
brachial	—	C77.3	—	D36.0	D48.7	D49.89
bronchial	—	C77.1	—	D36.0	D48.7	D49.89
bronchopulmonary	—	C77.1	—	D36.0	D48.7	D49.89
celiac	—	C77.2	—	D36.0	D48.7	D49.89
cervical	—	C77.0	—	D36.0	D48.7	D49.89
cervicofacial	—	C77.0	—	D36.0	D48.7	D49.89
Cloquet	—	C77.4	—	D36.0	D48.7	D49.89
colic	—	C77.2	—	D36.0	D48.7	D49.89
common duct	—	C77.2	—	D36.0	D48.7	D49.89
cubital	—	C77.3	—	D36.0	D48.7	D49.89
diaphragmatic	—	C77.1	—	D36.0	D48.7	D49.89
epigastric,						
inferior	—	C77.1	—	D36.0	D48.7	D49.89
epitrochlear	—	C77.3	—	D36.0	D48.7	D49.89
esophageal	—	C77.1	—	D36.0	D48.7	D49.89
face	—	C77.0	—	D36.0	D48.7	D49.89
femoral	—	C77.4	—	D36.0	D48.7	D49.89
gastric	—	C77.2	—	D36.0	D48.7	D49.89
groin	—	C77.4	—	D36.0	D48.7	D49.89
head	—	C77.0	—	D36.0	D48.7	D49.89
hepatic	—	C77.2	—	D36.0	D48.7	D49.89
hilar						
(pulmonary)	—	C77.1	—	D36.0	D48.7	D49.89
splenic	—	C77.2	—	D36.0	D48.7	D49.89
hypogastric	—	C77.5	—	D36.0	D48.7	D49.89
ileocolic	—	C77.2	—	D36.0	D48.7	D49.89
iliac	—	C77.5	—	D36.0	D48.7	D49.89
infraclavicular	—	C77.3	—	D36.0	D48.7	D49.89
inguina,						
inguinal	—	C77.4	—	D36.0	D48.7	D49.89
innominate	—	C77.1	—	D36.0	D48.7	D49.89
intercostal	—	C77.1	—	D36.0	D48.7	D49.89
intestinal	—	C77.2	—	D36.0	D48.7	D49.89
intrabdominal	—	C77.2	—	D36.0	D48.7	D49.89
intrapelvic	—	C77.5	—	D36.0	D48.7	D49.89
intrathoracic	—	C77.1	—	D36.0	D48.7	D49.89
jugular	—	C77.0	—	D36.0	D48.7	D49.89
leg	—	C77.4	—	D36.0	D48.7	D49.89
limb						
lower	—	C77.4	—	D36.0	D48.7	D49.89
upper	—	C77.3	—	D36.0	D48.7	D49.89
lower limb	—	C77.4	—	D36.0	D48.7	D49.89
lumbar	—	C77.2	—	D36.0	D48.7	D49.89
mandibular	—	C77.0	—	D36.0	D48.7	D49.89
mediastinal	—	C77.1	—	D36.0	D48.7	D49.89
mesenteric						
(inferior)						
(superior)	—	C77.2	—	D36.0	D48.7	D49.89
midcolic	—	C77.2	—	D36.0	D48.7	D49.89
multiple sites in						
categories						
C77.0 -						
C77.5	—	C77.8	—	D36.0	D48.7	D49.89
neck	—	C77.0	—	D36.0	D48.7	D49.89
obturator	—	C77.5	—	D36.0	D48.7	D49.89
occipital	—	C77.0	—	D36.0	D48.7	D49.89
pancreatic	—	C77.2	—	D36.0	D48.7	D49.89
para-aortic	—	C77.2	—	D36.0	D48.7	D49.89
paracervical	—	C77.5	—	D36.0	D48.7	D49.89
parametrial	—	C77.5	—	D36.0	D48.7	D49.89
parasternal	—	C77.1	—	D36.0	D48.7	D49.89
parotid	—	C77.0	—	D36.0	D48.7	D49.89
pectoral	—	C77.3	—	D36.0	D48.7	D49.89
pelvic	—	C77.5	—	D36.0	D48.7	D49.89
peri-aortic	—	C77.2	—	D36.0	D48.7	D49.89
peripancreatic	—	C77.2	—	D36.0	D48.7	D49.89
popliteal	—	C77.4	—	D36.0	D48.7	D49.89
porta hepatis	—	C77.2	—	D36.0	D48.7	D49.89
portal	—	C77.2	—	D36.0	D48.7	D49.89
preauricular	—	C77.0	—	D36.0	D48.7	D49.89
prelaryngeal	—	C77.0	—	D36.0	D48.7	D49.89
presymphysial	—	C77.5	—	D36.0	D48.7	D49.89
pretracheal	—	C77.0	—	D36.0	D48.7	D49.89
primary (any site)						
NEC	C96.9	—	—	—	—	—

	Malignant Primary	Malignant Secondary	Ca in situ	Benign	Uncertain Behavior	Unspecified Behavior
Neoplasm, neoplastic — *continued*						
lymph, lymphatic channel — *continued*						
gland — *continued*						
pulmonary (hiler)	—	C77.1	—	D36.0	D48.7	D49.89
pyloric	—	C77.2	—	D36.0	D48.7	D49.89
retroperitoneal	—	C77.2	—	D36.0	D48.7	D49.89
retropharyngeal	—	C77.0	—	D36.0	D48.7	D49.89
Rosenmuller's	—	C77.4	—	D36.0	D48.7	D49.89
sacral	—	C77.5	—	D36.0	D48.7	D49.89
scalene	—	C77.0	—	D36.0	D48.7	D49.89
site NEC	—	C77.9	—	D36.0	D48.7	D49.89
splenic (hilar)	—	C77.2	—	D36.0	D48.7	D49.89
subclavicular	—	C77.3	—	D36.0	D48.7	D49.89
subinguinal	—	C77.4	—	D36.0	D48.7	D49.89
sublingual	—	C77.0	—	D36.0	D48.7	D49.89
submandibular	—	C77.0	—	D36.0	D48.7	D49.89
submaxillary	—	C77.0	—	D36.0	D48.7	D49.89
submental	—	C77.0	—	D36.0	D48.7	D49.89
subscapular	—	C77.3	—	D36.0	D48.7	D49.89
supraclavicular	—	C77.0	—	D36.0	D48.7	D49.89
thoracic	—	C77.1	—	D36.0	D48.7	D49.89
tibial	—	C77.4	—	D36.0	D48.7	D49.89
tracheal	—	C77.1	—	D36.0	D48.7	D49.89
tracheobronchial	—	C77.1	—	D36.0	D48.7	D49.89
upper limb	—	C77.3	—	D36.0	D48.7	D49.89
Virchow's	—	C77.0	—	D36.0	D48.7	D49.89
node — *see also* Neoplasm, lymph gland						
primary NEC	C96.9	—	—	—	—	—
vessel — *see also* Neoplasm, connective tissue	C49.9	C79.89	—	D21.9	D48.1	D49.2
Mackenrodt's ligament	C57.7	C79.82	D07.39	D28.7	D39.8	D49.59
malar	C41.0	C79.51	—	D16.4	D48.0	D49.2
region — *see* Neoplasm, cheek						
mammary gland — *see* Neoplasm, breast						
mandible	C41.1	C79.51	—	D16.5	D48.0	D49.2
alveolar						
mucosa (carcinoma)	C03.1	C79.89	D00.03	D10.39	D37.09	D49.0
ridge or process	C41.1	C79.51	—	D16.5	D48.0	D49.2
marrow (bone) NEC	C96.9	C79.52	—	—	D47.9	D49.89
mastectomy site (skin) — *see also* Neoplasm, breast, skin	C44.501	C79.2	—	—	—	—
specified as breast tissue	C50.8-☑	C79.81	—	—	—	—
mastoid (air cells) (antrum) (cavity)	C30.1	C78.39	D02.3	D14.0	D38.5	D49.1
bone or process	C41.0	C79.51	—	D16.4	D48.0	D49.2
maxilla, maxillary (superior)	C41.0	C79.51	—	D16.4	D48.0	D49.2
alveolar						
mucosa	C03.0	C79.89	D00.03	D10.39	D37.09	D49.0
ridge or process (carcinoma)	C41.0	C79.51	—	D16.4	D48.0	D49.2
antrum	C31.0	C78.39	D02.3	D14.0	D38.5	D49.1
carcinoma	C03.0	C79.51	—	—	—	—
inferior — *see* Neoplasm, mandible						
sinus	C31.0	C78.39	D02.3	D14.0	D38.5	D49.1
meatus external (ear) — *see also* Neoplasm, skin, ear	C44.20-☑	C79.2	D04.2-☑	D23.2-☑	D48.5	D49.2
Meckel diverticulum, malignant	C17.3	C78.4	D01.49	D13.39	D37.2	D49.0
mediastinum, mediastinal	C38.3	C78.1	—	D15.2	D38.3	D49.89
anterior	C38.1	C78.1	—	D15.2	D38.3	D49.89

	Malignant Primary	Malignant Secondary	Ca in situ	Benign	Uncertain Behavior	Unspecified Behavior
Neoplasm, neoplastic — *continued*						
mediastinum, mediastinal — *continued*						
posterior	C38.2	C78.1	—	D15.2	D38.3	D49.89
medulla						
adrenal	C74.1-☑	C79.7-☑	D09.3	D35.0-☑	D44.1-☑	D49.7
oblongata	C71.7	C79.31	—	D33.1	D43.1	D49.6
meibomian gland	C44.10-☑	C79.2	D04.1-☑	D23.1-☑	D48.5	D49.2
basal cell carcinoma	C44.11-☑	—	—	—	—	—
sebaceous cell	C44.13-☑	—	—	—	—	—
specified type NEC	C44.19-☑	—	—	—	—	—
squamous cell carcinoma	C44.12-☑	—	—	—	—	—
melanoma — *see* Melanoma						
meninges	C70.9	C79.49	—	D32.9	D42.9	D49.7
brain	C70.0	C79.32	—	D32.0	D42.0	D49.7
cerebral	C70.0	C79.32	—	D32.0	D42.0	D49.7
crainial	C70.0	C79.32	—	D32.0	D42.0	D49.7
intracranial	C70.0	C79.32	—	D32.0	D42.0	D49.7
spinal (cord)	C70.1	C79.49	—	D32.1	D42.1	D49.7
meniscus, knee joint (lateral) (medial)	C40.2-☑	C79.51	—	D16.2-☑	D48.0	D49.2
Merkel cell — *see* Carcinoma, Merkel cell						
mesentery, mesenteric	C48.1	C78.6	—	D20.1	D48.4	D49.0
mesoappendix	C48.1	C78.6	—	D20.1	D48.4	D49.0
mesocolon	C48.1	C78.6	—	D20.1	D48.4	D49.0
mesopharynx — *see* Neoplasm, oropharynx						
mesosalpinx	C57.1-☑	C79.82	D07.39	D28.2	D39.8	D49.59
mesothelial tissue — *see* Mesothelioma						
mesothelioma — *see* Mesothelioma						
mesovarium	C57.1-☑	C79.82	D07.39	D28.2	D39.8	D49.59
metacarpus (any bone)	C40.1-☑	C79.51	—	D16.1-☑	—	—
metastatic NEC — *see also* Neoplasm, by site, secondary	—	C79.9	—	—	—	—
metatarsus (any bone)	C40.3-☑	C79.51	—	D16.3-☑	—	—
midbrain	C71.7	C79.31	—	D33.1	D43.1	D49.6
milk duct — *see* Neoplasm, breast						
mons						
pubis	C51.9	C79.82	D07.1	D28.0	D39.8	D49.59
veneris	C51.9	C79.82	D07.1	D28.0	D39.8	D49.59
motor tract	C72.9	C79.49	—	D33.9	D43.9	D49.7
brain	C71.9	C79.31	—	D33.2	D43.2	D49.7
cauda equina	C72.1	C79.49	—	D33.4	D43.4	D49.7
spinal	C72.0	C79.49	—	D33.4	D43.4	D49.7
mouth	C06.9	C79.89	D00.00	D10.30	D37.09	D49.0
book-leaf	C06.89	C79.89	—	—	—	—
floor	C04.9	C79.89	D00.06	D10.2	D37.09	D49.0
anterior portion	C04.0	C79.89	D00.06	D10.2	D37.09	D49.0
lateral portion	C04.1	C79.89	D00.06	D10.2	D37.09	D49.0
overlapping lesion	C04.8	—	—	—	—	—
overlapping NEC	C06.80	—	—	—	—	—
roof	C05.9	C79.89	D00.00	D10.39	D37.09	D49.0
specified part NEC	C06.89	C79.89	D00.00	D10.39	D37.09	D49.0
vestibule	C06.1	C79.89	D00.00	D10.39	D37.09	D49.0
mucosa						
alveolar (ridge or process)	C03.9	C79.89	D00.03	D10.39	D37.09	D49.0
lower	C03.1	C79.89	D00.03	D10.39	D37.09	D49.0
upper	C03.0	C79.89	D00.03	D10.39	D37.09	D49.0
buccal	C06.0	C79.89	D00.02	D10.39	D37.09	D49.0
cheek	C06.0	C79.89	D00.02	D10.39	D37.09	D49.0

Neoplasm, neoplastic
— continued
mucosa — continued
lip — see Neoplasm, lip, internal

	Malignant Primary	Malignant Secondary	Ca in situ	Benign	Uncertain Behavior	Unspecified Behavior
nasal	C30.0	C78.39	D02.3	D14.0	D38.5	D49.1
oral	C06.0	C79.89	D00.02	D10.39	D37.09	D49.0
Mullerian duct						
female	C57.7	C79.82	D07.39	D28.7	D39.8	D49.59
male	C63.7	C79.82	D07.69	D29.8	D40.8	D49.59
muscle — see also Neoplasm, connective tissue						
extraocular	C69.6-✓	C79.49	D09.2-✓	D31.6-✓	D48.7	D49.89
myocardium	C38.0	C79.89	—	D15.1	D48.7	D49.89
myometrium	C54.2	C79.82	D07.0	D26.1	D39.0	D49.59
myopericardium	C38.0	C79.89	—	D15.1	D48.7	D49.89
nabothian gland (follicle)	C53.0	C79.82	D06.0	D26.0	D39.0	D49.59
nail — see also Neoplasm, skin, limb	C44.90	C79.2	D04.9	D23.9	D48.5	D49.2
finger — see also Neoplasm, skin, limb, upper	C44.60-✓	C79.2	D04.6-✓	D23.6-✓	D48.5	D49.2
toe — see also Neoplasm, skin, limb, lower	C44.70-✓	C79.2	D04.7-✓	D23.7-✓	D48.5	D49.2
nares, naris (anterior) (posterior)	C30.0	C78.39	D02.3	D14.0	D38.5	D49.1
nasal — see Neoplasm, nose						
nasolabial groove — see also Neoplasm, skin, face	C44.309	C79.2	D04.39	D23.39	D48.5	D49.2
nasolacrimal duct	C69.5-✓	C79.49	D09.2-✓	D31.5-✓	D48.7	D49.89
nasopharynx, nasopharyngeal	C11.9	C79.89	D00.08	D10.6	D37.05	D49.0
floor	C11.3	C79.89	D00.08	D10.6	D37.05	D49.0
overlapping lesion	C11.8	—	—	—	—	—
roof	C11.0	C79.89	D00.08	D10.6	D37.05	D49.0
wall	C11.9	C79.89	D00.08	D10.6	D37.05	D49.0
anterior	C11.3	C79.89	D00.08	D10.6	D37.05	D49.0
lateral	C11.2	C79.89	D00.08	D10.6	D37.05	D49.0
posterior	C11.1	C79.89	D00.08	D10.6	D37.05	D49.0
superior	C11.0	C79.89	D00.08	D10.6	D37.05	D49.0
nates — see also Neoplasm, skin, trunk	C44.509	C79.2	D04.5	D23.5	D48.5	D49.2
neck NEC	C76.0	C79.89	D09.8	D36.7	D48.7	D49.89
skin	C44.40	—	—	—	—	—
basal cell carcinoma	C44.41	—	—	—	—	—
specified type NEC	C44.49	—	—	—	—	—
squamous cell carcinoma	C44.42	—	—	—	—	—
nerve (ganglion)	C47.9	C79.89	—	D36.10	D48.2	D49.2
abducens	C72.59	C79.49	—	D33.3	D43.3	D49.7
accessory (spinal)	C72.59	C79.49	—	D33.3	D43.3	D49.7
acoustic	C72.4-✓	C79.49	—	D33.3	D43.3	D49.7
auditory	C72.4-✓	C79.49	—	D33.3	D43.3	D49.7
autonomic NEC — see also Neoplasm, nerve, peripheral	C47.9	C79.89	—	D36.10	D48.2	D49.2
brachial	C47.1-✓	C79.89	—	D36.12	D48.2	D49.2
cranial	C72.50	C79.49	—	D33.3	D43.3	D49.7
specified NEC	C72.59	C79.49	—	D33.3	D43.3	D49.7
facial	C72.59	C79.49	—	D33.3	D43.3	D49.7
femoral	C47.2-✓	C79.89	—	D36.13	D48.2	D49.2
ganglion NEC — see also Neoplasm, nerve, peripheral	C47.9	C79.89	—	D36.10	D48.2	D49.2
glossopharyngeal	C72.59	C79.49	—	D33.3	D43.3	D49.7
hypoglossal	C72.59	C79.49	—	D33.3	D43.3	D49.7
intercostal	C47.3	C79.89	—	D36.14	D48.2	D49.2
lumbar	C47.6	C79.89	—	D36.17	D48.2	D49.2
median	C47.1-✓	C79.89	—	D36.12	D48.2	D49.2
obturator	C47.2-✓	C79.89	—	D36.13	D48.2	D49.2

Neoplasm, neoplastic
— continued
nerve — continued

	Malignant Primary	Malignant Secondary	Ca in situ	Benign	Uncertain Behavior	Unspecified Behavior
oculomotor	C72.59	C79.49	—	D33.3	D43.3	D49.7
olfactory	C47.2-✓	C79.49	—	D33.3	D43.3	D49.7
optic	C72.3-✓	C79.49	—	D33.3	D43.3	D49.7
parasympathetic NEC	C47.9	C79.89	—	D36.10	D48.2	D49.2
peripheral NEC	C47.9	C79.89	—	D36.10	D48.2	D49.2
abdomen	C47.4	C79.89	—	D36.15	D48.2	D49.2
abdominal wall	C47.4	C79.89	—	D36.15	D48.2	D49.2
ankle	C47.2-✓	C79.89	—	D36.13	D48.2	D49.2
antecubital fossa or space	C47.1-✓	C79.89	—	D36.12	D48.2	D49.2
arm	C47.1-✓	C79.89	—	D36.12	D48.2	D49.2
auricle (ear)	C47.0	C79.89	—	D36.11	D48.2	D49.2
axilla	C47.3	C79.89	—	D36.12	D48.2	D49.2
back	C47.6	C79.89	—	D36.17	D48.2	D49.2
buttock	C47.5	C79.89	—	D36.16	D48.2	D49.2
calf	C47.2-✓	C79.89	—	D36.13	D48.2	D49.2
cervical region	C47.0	C79.89	—	D36.11	D48.2	D49.2
cheek	C47.0	C79.89	—	D36.11	D48.2	D49.2
chest (wall)	C47.3	C79.89	—	D36.14	D48.2	D49.2
chin	C47.0	C79.89	—	D36.11	D48.2	D49.2
ear (external)	C47.0	C79.89	—	D36.11	D48.2	D49.2
elbow	C47.1-✓	C79.89	—	D36.12	D48.2	D49.2
extrarectal	C47.5	C79.89	—	D36.16	D48.2	D49.2
extremity	C47.9	C79.89	—	D36.10	D48.2	D49.2
lower	C47.2-✓	C79.89	—	D36.13	D48.2	D49.2
upper	C47.1-✓	C79.89	—	D36.12	D48.2	D49.2
eyelid	C47.0	C79.89	—	D36.11	D48.2	D49.2
face	C47.0	C79.89	—	D36.11	D48.2	D49.2
finger	C47.1-✓	C79.89	—	D36.12	D48.2	D49.2
flank	C47.6	C79.89	—	D36.17	D48.2	D49.2
foot	C47.2-✓	C79.89	—	D36.13	D48.2	D49.2
forearm	C47.1-✓	C79.89	—	D36.12	D48.2	D49.2
forehead	C47.0	C79.89	—	D36.11	D48.2	D49.2
gluteal region	C47.5	C79.89	—	D36.16	D48.2	D49.2
groin	C47.5	C79.89	—	D36.16	D48.2	D49.2
hand	C47.1-✓	C79.89	—	D36.12	D48.2	D49.2
head	C47.0	C79.89	—	D36.11	D48.2	D49.2
heel	C47.2-✓	C79.89	—	D36.13	D48.2	D49.2
hip	C47.2-✓	C79.89	—	D36.13	D48.2	D49.2
infraclavicular region	C47.3	C79.89	—	D36.14	D48.2	D49.2
inguinal (canal) (region)	C47.5	C79.89	—	D36.16	D48.2	D49.2
intrathoracic	C47.3	C79.89	—	D36.14	D48.2	D49.2
ischiorectal fossa	C47.5	C79.89	—	D36.16	D48.2	D49.2
knee	C47.2-✓	C79.89	—	D36.13	D48.2	D49.2
leg	C47.2-✓	C79.89	—	D36.13	D48.2	D49.2
limb NEC	C47.9	C79.89	—	D36.10	D48.2	D49.2
lower	C47.2-✓	C79.89	—	D36.13	D48.2	D49.2
upper	C47.1-✓	C79.89	—	D36.12	D48.2	D49.2
nates	C47.5	C79.89	—	D36.16	D48.2	D49.2
neck	C47.0	C79.89	—	D36.11	D48.2	D49.2
orbit	C69.6-✓	C79.49	—	D31.6-✓	D48.7	D49.2
pararectal	C47.5	C79.89	—	D36.16	D48.2	D49.2
paraurethral	C47.5	C79.89	—	D36.16	D48.2	D49.2
paravaginal	C47.5	C79.89	—	D36.16	D48.2	D49.2
pelvis (floor)	C47.5	C79.89	—	D36.16	D48.2	D49.2
pelvoabdominal	C47.8	C79.89	—	D36.17	D48.2	D49.2
perineum	C47.5	C79.89	—	D36.16	D48.2	D49.2
perirectal (tissue)	C47.5	C79.89	—	D36.16	D48.2	D49.2
periurethral (tissue)	C47.5	C79.89	—	D36.16	D48.2	D49.2
popliteal fossa or space	C47.2-✓	C79.89	—	D36.13	D48.2	D49.2
presacral	C47.5	C79.89	—	D36.16	D48.2	D49.2
pterygoid fossa	C47.0	C79.89	—	D36.11	D48.2	D49.2
rectovaginal septum or wall	C47.5	C79.89	—	D36.16	D48.2	D49.2
rectovesical	C47.5	C79.89	—	D36.16	D48.2	D49.2
sacrococcygeal region	C47.5	C79.89	—	D36.16	D48.2	D49.2
scalp	C47.0	C79.89	—	D36.11	D48.2	D49.2

Neoplasm, neoplastic	Malignant Primary	Malignant Secondary	Ca in situ	Benign	Uncertain Behavior	Unspecified Behavior
— continued						
nerve — continued						
peripheral — continued						
scapular region	C47.3	C79.89	—	D36.14	D48.2	D49.2
shoulder	C47.1-☑	C79.89	—	D36.12	D48.2	D49.2
submental	C47.0	C79.89	—	D36.11	D48.2	D49.2
supraclavicular region	C47.0	C79.89	—	D36.11	D48.2	D49.2
temple	C47.0	C79.89	—	D36.11	D48.2	D49.2
temporal region	C47.0	C79.89	—	D36.11	D48.2	D49.2
thigh	C47.2-☑	C79.89	—	D36.13	D48.2	D49.2
thoracic (duct) (wall)	C47.3	C79.89	—	D36.14	D48.2	D49.2
thorax	C47.3	C79.89	—	D36.14	D48.2	D49.2
thumb	C47.1-☑	C79.89	—	D36.12	D48.2	D49.2
toe	C47.2-☑	C79.89	—	D36.13	D48.2	D49.2
trunk	C47.6	C79.89	—	D36.17	D48.2	D49.2
umbilicus	C47.4	C79.89	—	D36.15	D48.2	D49.2
vesicorectal	C47.5	C79.89	—	D36.16	D48.2	D49.2
wrist	C47.1-☑	C79.89	—	D36.12	D48.2	D49.2
radial	C47.1-☑	C79.89	—	D36.12	D48.2	D49.2
sacral	C47.5	C79.89	—	D36.16	D48.2	D49.2
sciatic	C47.2-☑	C79.89	—	D36.13	D48.2	D49.2
spinal NEC	C47.9	C79.89	—	D36.10	D48.2	D49.2
accessory	C72.59	C79.49		D33.3	D43.3	D49.7
sympathetic NEC — see also Neoplasm, nerve, peripheral	C47.9	C79.89	—	D36.10	D48.2	D49.2
trigeminal	C72.59	C79.49		D33.3	D43.3	D49.7
trochlear	C72.59	C79.49		D33.3	D43.3	D49.7
ulnar	C47.1-☑	C79.89	—	D36.12	D48.2	D49.2
vagus	C72.59	C79.49		D33.3	D43.3	D49.7
nervous system (central)	C72.9	C79.40		D33.9	D43.9	D49.7
autonomic — see Neoplasm, nerve, peripheral						
parasympathetic — see Neoplasm, nerve, peripheral						
specified site NEC	—	C79.49		D33.7	D43.8	—
sympathetic — see Neoplasm, nerve, peripheral						
nevus — see Nevus						
nipple	C50.0-☑	C79.81	D05.-☑	D24.-☑	—	—
nose, nasal	C76.0	C79.89	D09.8	D36.7	D48.7	D49.89
ala (external) (nasi) — see also Neoplasm, nose, skin	C44.301	C79.2	D04.39	D23.39	D48.5	D49.2
bone	C41.0	C79.51	—	D16.4	D48.0	D49.2
cartilage	C30.0	C78.39	D02.3	D14.0	D38.5	D49.1
cavity	C30.0	C78.39	D02.3	D14.0	D38.5	D49.1
choana	C11.3	C79.89	D00.08	D10.6	D37.05	D49.0
external (skin) — see also Neoplasm, nose, skin	C44.301	C79.2	D04.39	D23.39	D48.5	D49.2
fossa	C30.0	C78.39	D02.3	D14.0	D38.5	D49.1
internal	C30.0	C78.39	D02.3	D14.0	D38.5	D49.1
mucosa	C30.0	C78.39	D02.3	D14.0	D38.5	D49.1
septum	C30.0	C78.39	D02.3	D14.0	D38.5	D49.1
posterior margin	C11.3	C79.89	D00.08	D10.6	D37.05	D49.0
sinus — see Neoplasm, sinus						
skin	C44.301	C79.2	D04.39	D23.39	D48.5	D49.2
basal cell carcinoma	C44.311	—	—	—	—	—
specified type NEC	C44.391	—	—	—	—	—
squamous cell carcinoma	C44.321	—	—	—	—	—
turbinate (mucosa)	C30.0	C78.39	D02.3	D14.0	D38.5	D49.1
bone	C41.0	C79.51	—	D16.4	D48.0	D49.2
vestibule	C30.0	C78.39	D02.3	D14.0	D38.5	D49.1

Neoplasm, neoplastic	Malignant Primary	Malignant Secondary	Ca in situ	Benign	Uncertain Behavior	Unspecified Behavior
— continued						
nostril	C30.0	C78.39	D02.3	D14.0	D38.5	D49.1
nucleus pulposus	C41.2	C79.51	—	D16.6	D48.0	D49.2
occipital						
bone	C41.0	C79.51	—	D16.4	D48.0	D49.2
lobe or pole, brain	C71.4	C79.31		D33.0	D43.0	D49.6
odontogenic — see Neoplasm, jaw bone						
olfactory nerve or bulb	C72.2-☑	C79.49		D33.3	D43.3	D49.7
olive (brain)	C71.7	C79.31		D33.1	D43.1	D49.6
omentum	C48.1	C78.6		D20.1	D48.4	D49.0
operculum (brain)	C71.0	C79.31		D33.0	D43.0	D49.6
optic nerve, chiasm, or tract	C72.3-☑	C79.49	—	D33.3	D43.3	D49.7
oral (cavity)	C06.9	C79.89	D00.00	D10.30	D37.09	D49.0
ill-defined	C14.8	C79.89	D00.00	D10.30	D37.09	D49.0
mucosa	C06.0	C79.89	D00.02	D10.39	D37.09	D49.0
orbit	C69.6-☑	C79.49	D09.2-☑	D31.6-☑	D48.7	D49.89
autonomic nerve	C69.6-☑	C79.49		D31.6-☑	D48.7	D49.2
bone	C41.0	C79.51		D16.4	D48.0	D49.2
eye	C69.6-☑	C79.49	D09.2-☑	D31.6-☑	D48.7	D49.89
peripheral nerves	C69.6-☑	C79.49		D31.6-☑	D48.7	D49.2
soft parts	C69.6-☑	C79.49	D09.2-☑	D31.6-☑	D48.7	D49.89
organ of Zuckerkandl	C75.5	C79.89	—	D35.6	D44.7	D49.7
oropharynx	C10.9	C79.89	D00.08	D10.5	D37.05	D49.0
branchial cleft (vestige)	C10.4	C79.89	D00.08	D10.5	D37.05	D49.0
junctional region	C10.8	C79.89	D00.08	D10.5	D37.05	D49.0
lateral wall	C10.2	C79.89	D00.08	D10.5	D37.05	D49.0
overlapping lesion	C10.8	—	—	—	—	—
pillars or fauces	C09.1	C79.89	D00.08	D10.5	D37.05	D49.0
posterior wall	C10.3	C79.89	D00.08	D10.5	D37.05	D49.0
vallecula	C10.0	C79.89	D00.08	D10.5	D37.05	D49.0
os						
external	C53.1	C79.82	D06.1	D26.0	D39.0	D49.59
internal	C53.0	C79.82	D06.0	D26.0	D39.0	D49.59
ovary	C56.-☑	C79.6-☑	D07.39	D27.-☑	D39.1-☑	D49.59
oviduct	C57.0-☑	C79.82	D07.39	D28.2	D39.8	D49.59
palate	C05.9	C79.89	D00.00	D10.39	D37.09	D49.0
hard	C05.0	C79.89	D00.05	D10.39	D37.09	D49.0
junction of hard and soft palate	C05.9	C79.89	D00.00	D10.39	D37.09	D49.0
overlapping lesions	C05.8	—	—	—	—	—
soft	C05.1	C79.89	D00.04	D10.39	D37.09	D49.0
nasopharyngeal surface	C11.3	C79.89	D00.08	D10.6	D37.05	D49.0
posterior surface	C11.3	C79.89	D00.08	D10.6	D37.05	D49.0
superior surface	C11.3	C79.89	D00.08	D10.6	D37.05	D49.0
palatoglossal arch	C09.1	C79.89	D00.00	D10.5	D37.09	D49.0
palatopharyngeal arch	C09.1	C79.89	D00.00	D10.5	D37.09	D49.0
pallium	C71.0	C79.31		D33.0	D43.0	D49.6
palpebra	C44.10-☑	C79.2	D04.1-☑	D23.1-☑	D48.5	D49.2
basal cell carcinoma	C44.11-☑	—	—	—	—	—
sebaceous cell	C44.13-☑	—	—	—	—	—
specified type NEC	C44.19-☑	—	—	—	—	—
squamous cell carcinoma	C44.12-☑	—	—	—	—	—
pancreas	C25.9	C78.89	D01.7	D13.6	D37.8	D49.0
body	C25.1	C78.89	D01.7	D13.6	D37.8	D49.0
duct (of Santorini) (of Wirsung)	C25.3	C78.89	D01.7	D13.6	D37.8	D49.0
ectopic tissue	C25.7	C78.89	—	D13.6	D37.8	D49.0
head	C25.0	C78.89	D01.7	D13.6	D37.8	D49.0
islet cells	C25.4	C78.89	D01.7	D13.7	D37.8	D49.0
neck	C25.7	C78.89	D01.7	D13.6	D37.8	D49.0
overlapping lesion	C25.8	—	—	—	—	—
tail	C25.2	C78.89	D01.7	D13.6	D37.8	D49.0

Neoplasm, neoplastic — continued	Malignant Primary	Malignant Secondary	Ca in situ	Benign	Uncertain Behavior	Unspecified Behavior
para-aortic body	C75.5	C79.89	—	D35.6	D44.7	D49.7
paraganglion NEC	C75.5	C79.89	—	D35.6	D44.7	D49.7
parametrium	C57.3	C79.82	—	D28.2	D39.8	D49.59
paranephric	C48.0	C78.6	—	D20.0	D48.3	D49.0
pararectal	C76.3	C79.89	—	D36.7	D48.7	D49.89
parasagittal (region)	C76.0	C79.89	D09.8	D36.7	D48.7	D49.89
parasellar	C72.9	C79.49	—	D33.9	D43.8	D49.7
parathyroid (gland)	C75.0	C79.89	D09.3	D35.1	D44.2	D49.7
paraurethral	C76.3	C79.89	—	D36.7	D48.7	D49.89
gland	C68.1	C79.19	D09.19	D30.8	D41.8	D49.59
paravaginal	C76.3	C79.89	—	D36.7	D48.7	D49.89
parenchyma, kidney	C64.-✔	C79.0-✔	D09.19	D30.0-✔	D41.0-✔	D49.51-✔
parietal						
bone	C41.0	C79.51	—	D16.4	D48.0	D49.2
lobe, brain	C71.3	C79.31	—	D33.0	D43.0	D49.6
paroophoron	C57.1-✔	C79.82	D07.39	D28.2	D39.8	D49.59
parotid (duct) (gland)	C07	C79.89	D00.00	D11.0	D37.030	D49.0
parovarium	C57.1-✔	C79.82	D07.39	D28.2	D39.8	D49.59
patella	C40.20	C79.51	—	—	—	—
peduncle, cerebral	C71.7	C79.31	—	D33.1	D43.1	D49.6
pelvirectal junction	C19	C78.5	D01.1	D12.7	D37.5	D49.0
pelvis, pelvic	C76.3	C79.89	D09.8	D36.7	D48.7	D49.89
bone	C41.4	C79.51	—	D16.8	D48.0	D49.2
floor	C76.3	C79.89	D09.8	D36.7	D48.7	D49.89
renal	C65.-✔	C79.0-✔	D09.19	D30.1-✔	D41.1-✔	D49.51-✔
viscera	C76.3	C79.89	D09.8	D36.7	D48.7	D49.89
wall	C76.3	C79.89	D09.8	D36.7	D48.7	D49.89
pelvo-abdominal	C76.8	C79.89	D09.8	D36.7	D48.7	D49.89
penis	C60.9	C79.82	D07.4	D29.0	D40.8	D49.59
body	C60.2	C79.82	D07.4	D29.0	D40.8	D49.59
corpus (cavernosum)	C60.2	C79.82	D07.4	D29.0	D40.8	D49.59
glans	C60.1	C79.82	D07.4	D29.0	D40.8	D49.59
overlapping sites	C60.8	—	—	—	—	—
skin NEC	C60.9	C79.82	D07.4	D29.0	D40.8	D49.59
periadrenal (tissue)	C48.0	C78.6	—	D20.0	D48.3	D49.0
perianal (skin) — see also Neoplasm, anus, skin	C44.500	C79.2	D04.5	D23.5	D48.5	D49.2
pericardium	C38.0	C79.89	—	D15.1	D48.7	D49.89
perinephric	C48.0	C78.6	—	D20.0	D48.3	D49.0
perineum	C76.3	C79.89	D09.8	D36.7	D48.7	D49.89
periodontal tissue NEC	C03.9	C79.89	D00.03	D10.39	D37.09	D49.0
periosteum — see Neoplasm, bone						
peripancreatic	C48.0	C78.6	—	D20.0	D48.3	D49.0
peripheral nerve NEC	C47.9	C79.89	—	D36.10	D48.2	D49.2
perirectal (tissue)	C76.3	C79.89	—	D36.7	D48.7	D49.89
perirenal (tissue)	C48.0	C78.6	—	D20.0	D48.3	D49.0
peritoneum, peritoneal (cavity)	C48.2	C78.6	—	D20.1	D48.4	D49.0
benign mesothelial tissue — see Mesothelioma, benign						
overlapping lesion	C48.8	—	—	—	—	—
with digestive organs	C26.9	—	—	—	—	—
parietal	C48.1	C78.6	—	D20.1	D48.4	D49.0
pelvic	C48.1	C78.6	—	D20.1	D48.4	D49.0
specified part NEC	C48.1	C78.6	—	D20.1	D48.4	D49.0
peritonsillar (tissue)	C76.0	C79.89	D09.8	D36.7	D48.7	D49.89
periurethral tissue	C76.3	C79.89	—	D36.7	D48.7	D49.89
phalanges						
foot	C40.3-✔	C79.51	—	D16.3-✔	—	—
hand	C40.1-✔	C79.51	—	D16.1-✔	—	—
pharynx, pharyngeal	C14.0	C79.89	D00.08	D10.9	D37.05	D49.0
bursa	C11.1	C79.89	D00.08	D10.6	D37.05	D49.0

Neoplasm, neoplastic — continued	Malignant Primary	Malignant Secondary	Ca in situ	Benign	Uncertain Behavior	Unspecified Behavior
pharynx, pharyngeal — continued						
fornix	C11.3	C79.89	D00.08	D10.6	D37.05	D49.0
recess	C11.2	C79.89	D00.08	D10.6	D37.05	D49.0
region	C14.0	C79.89	D00.08	D10.9	D37.05	D49.0
tonsil	C11.1	C79.89	D00.08	D10.6	D37.05	D49.0
wall (lateral) (posterior)	C14.0	C79.89	D00.08	D10.9	D37.05	D49.0
pia mater	C70.9	C79.40	—	D32.9	D42.9	D49.7
cerebral	C70.0	C79.32	—	D32.0	D42.0	D49.7
cranial	C70.0	C79.32	—	D32.0	D42.0	D49.7
spinal	C70.1	C79.49	—	D32.1	D42.1	D49.7
pillars of fauces	C09.1	C79.89	D00.08	D10.5	D37.05	D49.0
pineal (body) (gland)	C75.3	C79.89	D09.3	D35.4	D44.5	D49.7
pinna (ear) NEC — see also Neoplasm, skin, ear	C44.20-✔	C79.2	D04.2-✔	D23.2-✔	D48.5	D49.2
piriform fossa or sinus	C12	C79.89	D00.08	D10.7	D37.05	D49.0
pituitary (body) (fossa) (gland) (lobe)	C75.1	C79.89	D09.3	D35.2	D44.3	D49.7
placenta	C58	C79.82	D07.0	D26.7	D39.2	D49.59
pleura, pleural (cavity)	C38.4	C78.2	—	D19.0	D38.2	D49.1
overlapping lesion with heart or mediastinum	C38.8	—	—	—	—	—
parietal	C38.4	C78.2	—	D19.0	D38.2	D49.1
visceral	C38.4	C78.2	—	D19.0	D38.2	D49.1
plexus						
brachial	C47.1-✔	C79.89	—	D36.12	D48.2	D49.2
cervical	C47.0	C79.89	—	D36.11	D48.2	D49.2
choroid	C71.5	C79.31	—	D33.0	D43.0	D49.6
lumbosacral	C47.5	C79.89	—	D36.16	D48.2	D49.2
sacral	C47.5	C79.89	—	D36.16	D48.2	D49.2
pluriendocrine	C75.8	C79.89	D09.3	D35.7	D44.9	D49.7
pole						
frontal	C71.1	C79.31	—	D33.0	D43.0	D49.6
occipital	C71.4	C79.31	—	D33.0	D43.0	D49.6
pons (varolii)	C71.7	C79.31	—	D33.1	D43.1	D49.6
popliteal fossa or space	C76.5-✔	C79.89	D04.7-✔	D36.7	D48.7	D49.89
postcricoid (region)	C13.0	C79.89	D00.08	D10.7	D37.05	D49.0
posterior fossa (cranial)	C71.9	C79.31	—	D33.2	D43.2	D49.6
postnasal space	C11.9	C79.89	D00.08	D10.6	D37.05	D49.0
prepuce	C60.0	C79.82	D07.4	D29.0	D40.8	D49.59
prepylorus	C16.4	C78.89	D00.2	D13.1	D37.1	D49.0
presacral (region)	C76.3	C79.89	—	D36.7	D48.7	D49.89
prostate (gland)	C61	C79.82	D07.5	D29.1	D40.0	D49.59
utricle	C68.0	C79.19	D09.19	D30.4	D41.3	D49.59
pterygoid fossa	C49.0	C79.89	—	D21.0	D48.1	D49.2
pubic bone	C41.4	C79.51	—	D16.8	D48.0	D49.2
pudenda, pudendum (female)	C51.9	C79.82	D07.1	D28.0	D39.8	D49.59
pulmonary — see also Neoplasm, lung	C34.9-✔	C78.0-✔	D02.2-✔	D14.3-✔	D38.1	D49.1
putamen	C71.0	C79.31	—	D33.0	D43.0	D49.6
pyloric						
antrum	C16.3	C78.89	D00.2	D13.1	D37.1	D49.0
canal	C16.4	C78.89	D00.2	D13.1	D37.1	D49.0
pylorus	C16.4	C78.89	D00.2	D13.1	D37.1	D49.0
pyramid (brain)	C71.7	C79.31	—	D33.1	D43.1	D49.6
pyriform fossa or sinus	C12	C79.89	D00.08	D10.7	D37.05	D49.0
radius (any part)	C40.0-✔	C79.51	—	D16.0-✔	—	—
Rathke's pouch	C75.1	C79.89	D09.3	D35.2	D44.3	D49.7
rectosigmoid (junction)	C19	C78.5	D01.1	D12.7	D37.5	D49.0
overlapping lesion with anus or rectum	C21.8	—	—	—	—	—
rectouterine pouch	C48.1	C78.6	—	D20.1	D48.4	D49.0
rectovaginal septum or wall	C76.3	C79.89	D09.8	D36.7	D48.7	D49.89
rectovesical septum	C76.3	C79.89	D09.8	D36.7	D48.7	D49.89
rectum (ampulla)	C20	C78.5	D01.2	D12.8	D37.5	D49.0

Neoplasm, neoplastic — continued	Malignant Primary	Malignant Secondary	Ca in situ	Benign	Uncertain Behavior	Unspecified Behavior
rectum — continued						
and colon	C19	C78.5	D01.1	D12.7	D37.5	D49.0
overlapping lesion with anus or rectosigmoid junction	C21.8	—	—	—	—	—
renal	C64.-☑	C79.0-☑	D09.19	D30.0-☑	D41.0-☑	D49.51-☑
calyx	C65.-☑	C79.0-☑	D09.19	D30.1-☑	D41.1-☑	D49.51-☑
hilus	C65.-☑	C79.0-☑	D09.19	D30.1-☑	D41.1-☑	D49.51-☑
parenchyma	C64.-☑	C79.0-☑	D09.19	D30.0-☑	D41.0-☑	D49.51-☑
pelvis	C65.-☑	C79.0-☑	D09.19	D30.1-☑	D41.1-☑	D49.51-☑
respiratory organs or system NEC	C39.9	C78.30	D02.4	D14.4	D38.6	D49.1
tract NEC	C39.9	C78.30	D02.4	D14.4	D38.5	D49.1
upper	C39.0	C78.30	D02.4	D14.4	D38.5	D49.1
retina	C69.2-☑	C79.49	D09.2-☑	D31.2-☑	D48.7	D49.81
retrobulbar	C69.6-☑	C79.49	—	D31.6-☑	D48.7	D49.89
retrocecal	C48.0	C78.6	—	D20.0	D48.3	D49.0
retromolar (area) (triangle) (trigone)	C06.2	C79.89	D00.00	D10.39	D37.09	D49.0
retro-orbital	C76.0	C79.89	D09.8	D36.7	D48.7	D49.89
retroperitoneal (space) (tissue)	C48.0	C78.6	—	D20.0	D48.3	D49.0
retroperitoneum	C48.0	C78.6	—	D20.0	D48.3	D49.0
retropharyngeal	C14.0	C79.89	D00.08	D10.9	D37.05	D49.0
retrovesical (septum)	C76.3	C79.89	D09.8	D36.7	D48.7	D49.89
rhinencephalon	C71.0	C79.31	—	D33.0	D43.0	D49.6
rib	C41.3	C79.51	—	D16.7	D48.0	D49.2
Rosenmuller's fossa	C11.2	C79.89	D00.08	D10.6	D37.05	D49.0
round ligament	C57.2-☑	C79.82	—	D28.2	D39.8	D49.59
sacrococcyx, sacrococcygeal	C41.4	C79.51	—	D16.8	D48.0	D49.2
region	C76.3	C79.89	D09.8	D36.7	D48.7	D49.89
sacrouterine ligament	C57.3	C79.82	—	D28.2	D39.8	D49.59
sacrum, sacral (vertebra)	C41.4	C79.51	—	D16.8	D48.0	D49.2
salivary gland or duct (major)	C08.9	C79.89	D00.00	D11.9	D37.039	D49.0
minor NEC	C06.9	C79.89	D00.00	D10.39	D37.04	D49.0
overlapping lesion	C08.9	—	—	—	—	—
parotid	C07	C79.89	D00.00	D11.0	D37.030	D49.0
pluriglandular	C08.9	C79.89	D00.00	D11.9	D37.039	D49.0
sublingual	C08.1	C79.89	D00.00	D11.7	D37.031	D49.0
submandibular	C08.0	C79.89	D00.00	D11.7	D37.032	D49.0
submaxillary	C08.0	C79.89	D00.00	D11.7	D37.032	D49.0
salpinx (uterine)	C57.0-☑	C79.82	D07.39	D28.2	D39.8	D49.59
Santorini's duct	C25.3	C78.89	D01.7	D13.6	D37.8	D49.0
scalp	C44.40	C79.2	D04.4	D23.4	D48.5	D49.2
basal cell carcinoma	C44.41	—	—	—	—	—
specified type NEC	C44.49	—	—	—	—	—
squamous cell carcinoma	C44.42	—	—	—	—	—
scapula (any part)	C40.0-☑	C79.51	—	D16.0-☑	D48.0	D49.2
scapular region	C76.1	C79.89	D09.8	D36.7	D48.7	D49.89
scar NEC — see also Neoplasm, skin, by site	C44.90	C79.2	D04.9	D23.9	D48.5	D49.2
sciatic nerve	C47.2-☑	C79.89	—	D36.13	D48.2	D49.2
sclera	C69.4-☑	C79.49	D09.2-☑	D31.4-☑	D48.7	D49.89
scrotum (skin)	C63.2	C79.82	D07.61	D29.4	D40.8	D49.59
sebaceous gland — see Neoplasm, skin						
sella turcica	C75.1	C79.89	D09.3	D35.2	D44.3	D49.7
bone	C41.0	C79.51	—	D16.4	D48.0	D49.2
semilunar cartilage (knee)	C40.2-☑	C79.51	—	D16.2-☑	D48.0	D49.2
seminal vesicle	C63.7	C79.82	D07.69	D29.8	D40.8	D49.59
septum						
nasal	C30.0	C78.39	D02.3	D14.0	D38.5	D49.1
posterior margin	C11.3	C79.89	D00.08	D10.6	D37.05	D49.0
rectovaginal	C76.3	C79.89	D09.8	D36.7	D48.7	D49.89
rectovesical	C76.3	C79.89	D09.8	D36.7	D48.7	D49.89

Neoplasm, neoplastic — continued	Malignant Primary	Malignant Secondary	Ca in situ	Benign	Uncertain Behavior	Unspecified Behavior
septum — continued						
urethrovaginal	C57.9	C79.82	D07.30	D28.9	D39.9	D49.59
vesicovaginal	C57.9	C79.82	D07.30	D28.9	D39.9	D49.59
shoulder NEC	C76.4-☑	C79.89	D04.6-☑	D36.7	D48.7	D49.89
sigmoid flexure (lower) (upper)	C18.7	C78.5	D01.0	D12.5	D37.4	D49.0
sinus (accessory)	C31.9	C78.39	D02.3	D14.0	D38.5	D49.1
bone (any)	C41.0	C79.51	—	D16.4	D48.0	D49.2
ethmoidal	C31.1	C78.39	D02.3	D14.0	D38.5	D49.1
frontal	C31.2	C78.39	D02.3	D14.0	D38.5	D49.1
maxillary	C31.0	C78.39	D02.3	D14.0	D38.5	D49.1
nasal, paranasal NEC	C31.9	C78.39	D02.3	D14.0	D38.5	D49.1
overlapping lesion	C31.8	—	—	—	—	—
pyriform	C12	C79.89	D00.08	D10.7	D37.05	D49.0
sphenoid	C31.3	C78.39	D02.3	D14.0	D38.5	D49.1
skeleton, skeletal NEC	C41.9	C79.51	—	D16.9	D48.0	D49.2
Skene's gland	C68.1	C79.19	D09.19	D30.8	D41.8	D49.59
skin NOS	C44.90	C79.2	D04.9	D23.9	D48.5	D49.2
abdominal wall	C44.509	C79.2	D04.5	D23.5	D48.5	D49.2
basal cell carcinoma	C44.519	—	—	—	—	—
specified type NEC	C44.599	—	—	—	—	—
squamous cell carcinoma	C44.529	—	—	—	—	—
ala nasi — see also Neoplasm, nose, skin	C44.301	C79.2	D04.39	D23.39	D48.5	D49.2
ankle — see also Neoplasm, skin, limb, lower	C44.70-☑	C79.2	D04.7-☑	D23.7-☑	D48.5	D49.2
antecubital space — see also Neoplasm, skin, limb, upper	C44.60-☑	C79.2	D04.6-☑	D23.6-☑	D48.5	D49.2
anus	C44.500	C79.2	D04.5	D23.5	D48.5	D49.2
basal cell carcinoma	C44.510	—	—	—	—	—
specified type NEC	C44.590	—	—	—	—	—
squamous cell carcinoma	C44.520	—	—	—	—	—
arm — see also Neoplasm, skin, limb, upper	C44.60-☑	C79.2	D04.6-☑	D23.6-☑	D48.5	D49.2
auditory canal (external) — see also Neoplasm, skin, ear	C44.20-☑	C79.2	D04.2-☑	D23.2-☑	D48.5	D49.2
auricle (ear) — see also Neoplasm, skin, ear	C44.20-☑	C79.2	D04.2-☑	D23.2-☑	D48.5	D49.2
auricular canal (external) — see also Neoplasm, skin, ear	C44.20-☑	C79.2	D04.2-☑	D23.2-☑	D48.5	D49.2
axilla, axillary fold — see also Neoplasm, skin, trunk	C44.509	C79.2	D04.5	D23.5	D48.5	D49.2
back — see also Neoplasm, skin, trunk	C44.509	C79.2	D04.5	D23.5	D48.5	D49.2
basal cell carcinoma	C44.91	—	—	—	—	—
breast	C44.501	C79.2	D04.5	D23.5	D48.5	D49.2
basal cell carcinoma	C44.511	—	—	—	—	—
specified type NEC	C44.591	—	—	—	—	—
squamous cell carcinoma	C44.521	—	—	—	—	—
brow — see also Neoplasm, skin, face	C44.309	C79.2	D04.39	D23.39	D48.5	D49.2
buttock — see also Neoplasm, skin, trunk	C44.509	C79.2	D04.5	D23.5	D48.5	D49.2

☑ Additional Character Required — Refer to the Tabular List for Character Selection   ▽ Subterms under main terms may continue to next column or page

Neoplasm, neoplastic — continued
skin — continued

	Malignant Primary	Malignant Secondary	Ca in situ	Benign	Uncertain Behavior	Unspecified Behavior
calf — see also Neoplasm, skin, limb, lower	C44.70-☑	C79.2	D04.7-☑	D23.7-☑	D48.5	D49.2
canthus (eye) (inner) (outer)	C44.10-☑	C79.2	D04.1-☑	D23.1-☑	D48.5	D49.2
basal cell carcinoma	C44.11-☑	—	—	—	—	—
sebaceous cell	C44.13-☑	—	—	—	—	—
specified type NEC	C44.19-☑	—	—	—	—	—
squamous cell carcinoma	C44.12-☑	—	—	—	—	—
cervical region — see also Neoplasm, skin, neck	C44.40	C79.2	D04.4	D23.4	D48.5	D49.2
cheek (external) — see also Neoplasm, skin, face	C44.309	C79.2	D04.39	D23.39	D48.5	D49.2
chest (wall) — see also Neoplasm, skin, trunk	C44.509	C79.2	D04.5	D23.5	D48.5	D49.2
chin — see also Neoplasm, skin, face	C44.309	C79.2	D04.39	D23.39	D48.5	D49.2
clavicular area — see also Neoplasm, skin, trunk	C44.509	C79.2	D04.5	D23.5	D48.5	D49.2
clitoris	C51.2	C79.82	D07.1	D28.0	D39.8	D49.59
columnella — see also Neoplasm, skin, face	C44.309	C79.2	D04.39	D23.39	D48.5	D49.2
concha — see also Neoplasm, skin, ear	C44.20-☑	C79.2	D04.2-☑	D23.2-☑	D48.5	D49.2
ear (external)	C44.20-☑	C79.2	D04.2-☑	D23.2-☑	D48.5	D49.2
basal cell carcinoma	C44.21-☑	—	—	—	—	—
specified type NEC	C44.29-☑	—	—	—	—	—
squamous cell carcinoma	C44.22-☑	—	—	—	—	—
elbow — see also Neoplasm, skin, limb, upper	C44.60-☑	C79.2	D04.6-☑	D23.6-☑	D48.5	D49.2
eyebrow — see also Neoplasm, skin, face	C44.309	C79.2	D04.39	D23.39	D48.5	D49.2
eyelid	C44.10-☑	C79.2	D04.1-☑	D23.1-☑	D48.5	D49.2
basal cell carcinoma	C44.11-☑	—	—	—	—	—
sebaceous cell	C44.13-☑	—	—	—	—	—
specified type NEC	C44.19-☑	—	—	—	—	—
squamous cell carcinoma	C44.12-☑	—	—	—	—	—
face NOS	C44.300	C79.2	D04.30	D23.30	D48.5	D49.2
basal cell carcinoma	C44.310	—	—	—	—	—
specified type NEC	C44.390	—	—	—	—	—
squamous cell carcinoma	C44.320	—	—	—	—	—
female genital organs (external)	C51.9	C79.82	D07.1	D28.0	D39.8	D49.59
clitoris	C51.2	C79.82	D07.1	D28.0	D39.8	D49.59
labium NEC	C51.9	C79.82	D07.1	D28.0	D39.8	D49.59
majus	C51.0	C79.82	D07.1	D28.0	D39.8	D49.59
minus	C51.1	C79.82	D07.1	D28.0	D39.8	D49.59
pudendum	C51.9	C79.82	D07.1	D28.0	D39.8	D49.59
vulva	C51.9	C79.82	D07.1	D28.0	D39.8	D49.59
finger — see also Neoplasm, skin, limb, upper	C44.60-☑	C79.2	D04.6-☑	D23.6-☑	D48.5	D49.2
flank — see also Neoplasm, skin, trunk	C44.509	C79.2	D04.5	D23.5	D48.5	D49.2
foot — see also Neoplasm, skin, limb, lower	C44.70-☑	C79.2	D04.7-☑	D23.7-☑	D48.5	D49.2

Neoplasm, neoplastic — continued
skin — continued

	Malignant Primary	Malignant Secondary	Ca in situ	Benign	Uncertain Behavior	Unspecified Behavior
forearm — see also Neoplasm, skin, limb, upper	C44.60-☑	C79.2	D04.6-☑	D23.6-☑	D48.5	D49.2
forehead — see also Neoplasm, skin, face	C44.309	C79.2	D04.39	D23.39	D48.5	D49.2
glabella — see also Neoplasm, skin, face	C44.309	C79.2	D04.39	D23.39	D48.5	D49.2
gluteal region — see also Neoplasm, skin, trunk	C44.509	C79.2	D04.5	D23.5	D48.5	D49.2
groin — see also Neoplasm, skin, trunk	C44.509	C79.2	D04.5	D23.5	D48.5	D49.2
hand — see also Neoplasm, skin, limb, upper	C44.60-☑	C79.2	D04.6-☑	D23.6-☑	D48.5	D49.2
head NEC — see also Neoplasm, skin, scalp	C44.40	C79.2	D04.4	D23.4	D48.5	D49.2
heel — see also Neoplasm, skin, limb, lower	C44.70-☑	C79.2	D04.7-☑	D23.7-☑	D48.5	D49.2
helix — see also Neoplasm, skin, ear	C44.20-☑	C79.2	D04.2-☑	D23.2-☑	D48.5	D49.2
hip — see also Neoplasm, skin, limb, lower	C44.70-☑	C79.2	D04.7-☑	D23.7-☑	D48.5	D49.2
infraclavicular region — see also Neoplasm, skin, trunk	C44.509	C79.2	D04.5	D23.5	D48.5	D49.2
inguinal region — see also Neoplasm, skin, trunk	C44.509	C79.2	D04.5	D23.5	D48.5	D49.2
jaw — see also Neoplasm, skin, face	C44.309	C79.2	D04.39	D23.39	D48.5	D49.2
Kaposi's sarcoma — see Kaposi's, sarcoma, skin						
knee — see also Neoplasm, skin, limb, lower	C44.70-☑	C79.2	D04.7-☑	D23.7-☑	D48.5	D49.2
labia						
majora	C51.0	C79.82	D07.1	D28.0	D39.8	D49.59
minora	C51.1	C79.82	D07.1	D28.0	D39.8	D49.59
leg — see also Neoplasm, skin, limb, lower	C44.70-☑	C79.2	D04.7-☑	D23.7-☑	D48.5	D49.2
lid (lower) (upper)	C44.10-☑	C79.2	D04.1-☑	D23.1-☑	D48.5	D49.2
basal cell carcinoma	C44.11-☑	—	—	—	—	—
sebaceous cell	C44.13-☑	—	—	—	—	—
specified type NEC	C44.19-☑	—	—	—	—	—
squamous cell carcinoma	C44.12-☑	—	—	—	—	—
limb NEC	C44.90	C79.2	D04.9	D23.9	D48.5	D49.2
basal cell carcinoma	C44.91	—	—	—	—	—
lower	C44.70-☑	C79.2	D04.7-☑	D23.7-☑	D48.5	D49.2
basal cell carcinoma	C44.71-☑	—	—	—	—	—
specified type NEC	C44.79-☑	—	—	—	—	—
squamous cell carcinoma	C44.72-☑	—	—	—	—	—
upper	C44.60-☑	C79.2	D04.6-☑	D23.6-☑	D48.5	D49.2
basal cell carcinoma	C44.61-☑	—	—	—	—	—
specified type NEC	C44.69-☑	—	—	—	—	—
squamous cell carcinoma	C44.62-☑	—	—	—	—	—
lip (lower) (upper)	C44.00	C79.2	D04.0	D23.0	D48.5	D49.2

	Malignant Primary	Malignant Secondary	Ca in situ	Benign	Uncertain Behavior	Unspecified Behavior
Neoplasm, neoplastic						
— *continued*						
skin — *continued*						
lip — *continued*						
basal cell carcinoma	C44.01	—	—	—	—	—
specified type NEC	C44.09	—	—	—	—	—
squamous cell carcinoma	C44.02	—	—	—	—	—
male genital organs	C63.9	C79.82	D07.60	D29.9	D40.8	D49.59
penis	C60.9	C79.82	D07.4	D29.0	D40.8	D49.59
prepuce	C60.0	C79.82	D07.4	D29.0	D40.8	D49.59
scrotum	C63.2	C79.82	D07.61	D29.4	D40.8	D49.59
mastectomy site (skin) — *see also* Neoplasm, skin, breast	C44.501	C79.2	—	—	—	—
specified as breast tissue	C50.8-✓	C79.81	—	—	—	—
meatus, acoustic (external) — *see also* Neoplasm, skin, ear	C44.20-✓	C79.2	D04.2-✓	D23.2-✓	D48.5	D49.2
melanotic — *see* Melanoma						
Merkel cell — *see* Carcinoma, Merkel cell						
nates — *see also* Neoplasm, skin, trunk	C44.509	C79.2	D04.5	D23.5	D48.5	D49.2
neck	C44.40	C79.2	D04.4	D23.4	D48.5	D49.2
basal cell carcinoma	C44.41	—	—	—	—	—
specified type NEC	C44.49	—	—	—	—	—
squamous cell carcinoma	C44.42	—	—	—	—	—
nevus — *see* Nevus, skin						
nose (external) — *see also* Neoplasm, nose, skin	C44.301	C79.2	D04.39	D23.39	D48.5	D49.2
overlapping lesion	C44.80	—	—	—	—	—
basal cell carcinoma	C44.81					
specified type NEC	C44.89					
squamous cell carcinoma	C44.82					
palm — *see also* Neoplasm, skin, limb, upper	C44.60-✓	C79.2	D04.6-✓	D23.6-✓	D48.5	D49.2
palpebra	C44.10-✓	C79.2	D04.1-✓	D23.1-✓	D48.5	D49.2
basal cell carcinoma	C44.11-✓	—	—	—	—	—
sebaceous cell	C44.13-✓	—	—	—	—	—
specified type NEC	C44.19-✓	—	—	—	—	—
squamous cell carcinoma	C44.12-✓	—	—	—	—	—
penis NEC	C60.9	C79.82	D07.4	D29.0	D40.8	D49.59
perianal — *see also* Neoplasm, skin, anus	C44.500	C79.2	D04.5	D23.5	D48.5	D49.2
perineum — *see also* Neoplasm, skin, anus	C44.500	C79.2	D04.5	D23.5	D48.5	D49.2
pinna — *see also* Neoplasm, skin, ear	C44.20-✓	C79.2	D04.2-✓	D23.2-✓	D48.5	D49.2
plantar — *see also* Neoplasm, skin, limb, lower	C44.70-✓	C79.2	D04.7-✓	D23.7-✓	D48.5	D49.2
popliteal fossa or space — *see also* Neoplasm, skin, limb, lower	C44.70-✓	C79.2	D04.7-✓	D23.7-✓	D48.5	D49.2
prepuce	C60.0	C79.82	D07.4	D29.0	D40.8	D49.59
Neoplasm, neoplastic						
— *continued*						
skin — *continued*						
pubes — *see also* Neoplasm, skin, trunk	C44.509	C79.2	D04.5	D23.5	D48.5	D49.2
sacrococcygeal region — *see also* Neoplasm, skin, trunk	C44.509	C79.2	D04.5	D23.5	D48.5	D49.2
scalp	C44.40	C79.2	D04.4	D23.4	D48.5	D49.2
basal cell carcinoma	C44.41	—	—	—	—	—
specified type NEC	C44.49	—	—	—	—	—
squamous cell carcinoma	C44.42	—	—	—	—	—
scapular region — *see also* Neoplasm, skin, trunk	C44.509	C79.2	D04.5	D23.5	D48.5	D49.2
scrotum	C63.2	C79.82	D07.61	D29.4	D40.8	D49.59
shoulder — *see also* Neoplasm, skin, limb, upper	C44.60-✓	C79.2	D04.6-✓	D23.6-✓	D48.5	D49.2
sole (foot) — *see also* Neoplasm, skin, limb, lower	C44.70-✓	C79.2	D04.7-✓	D23.7-✓	D48.5	D49.2
specified sites NEC	C44.80	C79.2	D04.8	D23.9	D48.5	D49.2
basal cell carcinoma	C44.81	—	—	—	—	—
specified type NEC	C44.89	—	—	—	—	—
squamous cell carcinoma	C44.82	—	—	—	—	—
specified type NEC	C44.99	—	—	—	—	—
squamous cell carcinoma	C44.92	—	—	—	—	—
submammary fold — *see also* Neoplasm, skin, trunk	C44.509	C79.2	D04.5	D23.5	D48.5	D49.2
supraclavicular region — *see also* Neoplasm, skin, neck	C44.40	C79.2	D04.4	D23.4	D48.5	D49.2
temple — *see also* Neoplasm, skin, face	C44.309	C79.2	D04.39	D23.39	D48.5	D49.2
thigh — *see also* Neoplasm, skin, limb, lower	C44.70-✓	C79.2	D04.7-✓	D23.7-✓	D48.5	D49.2
thoracic wall — *see also* Neoplasm, skin, trunk	C44.509	C79.2	D04.5	D23.5	D48.5	D49.2
thumb — *see also* Neoplasm, skin, limb, upper	C44.60-✓	C79.2	D04.6-✓	D23.6-✓	D48.5	D49.2
toe — *see also* Neoplasm, skin, limb, lower	C44.70-✓	C79.2	D04.7-✓	D23.7-✓	D48.5	D49.2
tragus — *see also* Neoplasm, skin, ear	C44.20-✓	C79.2	D04.2-✓	D23.2-✓	D48.5	D49.2
trunk	C44.509	C79.2	D04.5	D23.5	D48.5	D49.2
basal cell carcinoma	C44.519	—	—	—	—	—
specified type NEC	C44.599	—	—	—	—	—
squamous cell carcinoma	C44.529	—	—	—	—	—
umbilicus — *see also* Neoplasm, skin, trunk	C44.509	C79.2	D04.5	D23.5	D48.5	D49.2
vulva	C51.9	C79.82	D07.1	D28.0	D39.8	D49.59
overlapping lesion	C51.8					
wrist — *see also* Neoplasm, skin, limb, upper	C44.60-✓	C79.2	D04.6-✓	D23.6-✓	D48.5	D49.2
skull	C41.0	C79.51	—	D16.4	D48.0	D49.2

✓ Additional Character Required — Refer to the Tabular List for Character Selection ▽ Subterms under main terms may continue to next column or page

Neoplasm, neoplastic

	Malignant Primary	Malignant Secondary	Ca in situ	Benign	Uncertain Behavior	Unspecified Behavior
— *continued*						
soft parts or tissues — *see* Neoplasm, connective tissue						
specified site NEC	C76.8	C79.89	D09.8	D36.7	D48.7	D49.89
spermatic cord	C63.1-☑	C79.82	D07.69	D29.8	D40.8	D49.59
sphenoid	C31.3	C78.39	D02.3	D14.0	D38.5	D49.1
bone	C41.0	C79.51	—	D16.4	D48.0	D49.2
sinus	C31.3	C78.39	D02.3	D14.0	D38.5	D49.1
sphincter						
anal	C21.1	C78.5	D01.3	D12.9	D37.8	D49.0
of Oddi	C24.0	C78.89	D01.5	D13.5	D37.6	D49.0
spine, spinal						
(column)	C41.2	C79.51	—	D16.6	D48.0	D49.2
bulb	C71.7	C79.31	—	D33.1	D43.1	D49.6
coccyx	C41.4	C79.51	—	D16.8	D48.0	D49.2
cord (cervical) (lumbar) (sacral) (thoracic)	C72.0	C79.49		D33.4	D43.4	D49.7
dura mater	C70.1	C79.49	—	D32.1	D42.1	D49.7
lumbosacral	C41.2	C79.51	—	D16.6	D48.0	D49.2
marrow NEC	C96.9	C79.52	—	—		D49.89
membrane	C70.1	C79.49	—	D32.1	D42.1	D49.7
meninges	C70.1	C79.49	—	D32.1	D42.1	D49.7
nerve (root)	C47.9	C79.89	—	D36.10	D48.2	D49.2
pia mater	C70.1	C79.49	—	D32.1	D42.1	D49.7
root	C47.9	C79.89	—	D36.10	D48.2	D49.2
sacrum	C41.4	C79.51	—	D16.8	D48.0	D49.2
spleen, splenic NEC	C26.1	C78.89	D01.7	D13.9	D37.8	D49.0
flexure (colon)	C18.5	C78.5	D01.0	D12.3	D37.4	D49.0
stem, brain	C71.7	C79.31	—	D33.1	D43.1	D49.6
Stensen's duct	C07	C79.89	D00.00	D11.0	D37.030	D49.0
sternum	C41.3	C79.51	—	D16.7	D48.0	D49.2
stomach	C16.9	C78.89	D00.2	D13.1	D37.1	D49.0
antrum (pyloric)	C16.3	C78.89	D00.2	D13.1	D37.1	D49.0
body	C16.2	C78.89	D00.2	D13.1	D37.1	D49.0
cardia	C16.0	C78.89	D00.2	D13.1	D37.1	D49.0
cardiac orifice	C16.0	C78.89	D00.2	D13.1	D37.1	D49.0
corpus	C16.2	C78.89	D00.2	D13.1	D37.1	D49.0
fundus	C16.1	C78.89	D00.2	D13.1	D37.1	D49.0
greater curvature NEC	C16.6	C78.89	D00.2	D13.1	D37.1	D49.0
lesser curvature NEC	C16.5	C78.89	D00.2	D13.1	D37.1	D49.0
overlapping lesion	C16.8	—	—	—	—	—
prepylorus	C16.4	C78.89	D00.2	D13.1	D37.1	D49.0
pylorus	C16.4	C78.89	D00.2	D13.1	D37.1	D49.0
wall NEC	C16.9	C78.89	D00.2	D13.1	D37.1	D49.0
anterior NEC	C16.8	C78.89	D00.2	D13.1	D37.1	D49.0
posterior NEC	C16.8	C78.89	D00.2	D13.1	D37.1	D49.0
stroma, endometrial	C54.1	C79.82	D07.0	D26.1	D39.0	D49.59
stump, cervical	C53.8	C79.82	D06.7	D26.0	D39.0	D49.59
subcutaneous (nodule) (tissue) NEC — *see* Neoplasm, connective tissue						
subdural	C70.9	C79.32	—	D32.9	D42.9	D49.7
subglottis, subglottic	C32.2	C78.39	D02.0	D14.1	D38.0	D49.1
sublingual	C04.9	C79.89	D00.06	D10.2	D37.09	D49.0
gland or duct	C08.1	C79.89	D00.00	D11.7	D37.031	D49.0
submandibular gland	C08.0	C79.89	D00.00	D11.7	D37.032	D49.0
submaxillary gland or duct	C08.0	C79.89	D00.00	D11.7	D37.032	D49.0
submental	C76.0	C79.89	D09.8	D36.7	D48.7	D49.89
subpleural	C34.9-☑	C78.0-☑	D02.2-☑	D14.3-☑	D38.1	D49.1
substernal	C38.1	C78.1		D15.2	D38.3	D49.89
sudoriferous, sudoriparous gland, site unspecified	C44.90	C79.2	D04.9	D23.9	D48.5	D49.2
specified site — *see* Neoplasm, skin						
supraclavicular region	C76.0	C79.89	D09.8	D36.7	D48.7	D49.89
supraglottis	C32.1	C78.39	D02.0	D14.1	D38.0	D49.1
suprarenal	C74.9-☑	C79.7-☑	D09.3	D35.0-☑	D44.1-☑	D49.7
capsule	C74.9-☑	C79.7-☑	D09.3	D35.0-☑	D44.1-☑	D49.7

Neoplasm, neoplastic

	Malignant Primary	Malignant Secondary	Ca in situ	Benign	Uncertain Behavior	Unspecified Behavior
— *continued*						
suprarenal — *continued*						
cortex	C74.0-☑	C79.7-☑	D09.3	D35.0-☑	D44.1-☑	D49.7
gland	C74.9-☑	C79.7-☑	D09.3	D35.0-☑	D44.1-☑	D49.7
medulla	C74.1-☑	C79.7-☑	D09.3	D35.0-☑	D44.1-☑	D49.7
suprasellar (region)	C71.9	C79.31	—	D33.2	D43.2	D49.6
supratentorial (brain) NEC	C71.0	C79.31	—	D33.0	D43.0	D49.6
sweat gland (apocrine) (eccrine), site unspecified	C44.90	C79.2	D04.9	D23.9	D48.5	D49.2
specified site — *see* Neoplasm, skin						
sympathetic nerve or nervous system NEC	C47.9	C79.89	—	D36.10	D48.2	D49.2
symphysis pubis	C41.4	C79.51	—	D16.8	D48.0	D49.2
synovial membrane — *see* Neoplasm, connective tissue						
tapetum, brain	C71.8	C79.31	—	D33.2	D43.2	D49.6
tarsus (any bone)	C40.3-☑	C79.51		D16.3-☑	—	—
temple (skin) — *see also* Neoplasm, skin, face	C44.309	C79.2	D04.39	D23.39	D48.5	D49.2
temporal						
bone	C41.0	C79.51	—	D16.4	D48.0	D49.2
lobe or pole	C71.2	C79.31	—	D33.0	D43.0	D49.6
region	C76.0	C79.89	D09.8	D36.7	D48.7	D49.89
skin — *see also* Neoplasm, skin, face	C44.309	C79.2	D04.39	D23.39	D48.5	D49.2
tendon (sheath) — *see* Neoplasm, connective tissue						
tentorium (cerebelli)	C70.0	C79.32	—	D32.0	D42.0	D49.7
testis, testes	C62.9-☑	C79.82	D07.69	D29.2-☑	D40.1-☑	D49.59
descended	C62.1-☑	C79.82	D07.69	D29.2-☑	D40.1-☑	D49.59
ectopic	C62.0-☑	C79.82	D07.69	D29.2-☑	D40.1-☑	D49.59
retained	C62.0-☑	C79.82	D07.69	D29.2-☑	D40.1-☑	D49.59
scrotal	C62.1-☑	C79.82	D07.69	D29.2-☑	D40.1-☑	D49.59
undescended	C62.0-☑	C79.82	D07.69	D29.2-☑	D40.1-☑	D49.59
unspecified whether descended or undescended	C62.9-☑	C79.82	D07.69	D29.2-☑	D40.1-☑	D49.59
thalamus	C71.0	C79.31	—	D33.0	D43.0	D49.6
thigh NEC	C76.5-☑	C79.89	D04.7-☑	D36.7	D48.7	D49.89
thorax, thoracic (cavity) (organs NEC)	C76.1	C79.89	D09.8	D36.7	D48.7	D49.89
duct	C49.3	C79.89	—	D21.3	D48.1	D49.2
wall NEC	C76.1	C79.89	D09.8	D36.7	D48.7	D49.89
throat	C14.0	C79.89	D00.08	D10.9	D37.05	D49.0
thumb NEC	C76.4-☑	C79.89	D04.6-☑	D36.7	D48.7	D49.89
thymus (gland)	C37	C79.89	D09.3	D15.0	D38.4	D49.89
thyroglossal duct	C73	C79.89	D09.3	D34	D44.0	D49.7
thyroid (gland)	C73	C79.89	D09.3	D34	D44.0	D49.7
cartilage	C32.3	C78.39	D02.0	D14.1	D38.0	D49.1
tibia (any part)	C40.2-☑	C79.51	—	D16.2-☑	—	—
toe NEC	C76.5-☑	C79.89	D04.7-☑	D36.7	D48.7	D49.89
tongue	C02.9	C79.89	D00.07	D10.1	D37.02	D49.0
anterior (two-thirds) NEC	C02.3	C79.89	D00.07	D10.1	D37.02	D49.0
dorsal surface	C02.0	C79.89	D00.07	D10.1	D37.02	D49.0
ventral surface	C02.2	C79.89	D00.07	D10.1	D37.02	D49.0
base (dorsal surface)	C01	C79.89	D00.07	D10.1	D37.02	D49.0
border (lateral) dorsal surface NEC	C02.1	C79.89	D00.07	D10.1	D37.02	D49.0
	C02.0	C79.89	D00.07	D10.1	D37.02	D49.0
fixed part NEC	C01	C79.89	D00.07	D10.1	D37.02	D49.0
foreamen cecum	C02.0	C79.89	D00.07	D10.1	D37.02	D49.0
frenulum linguae	C02.2	C79.89	D00.07	D10.1	D37.02	D49.0
junctional zone	C02.8	C79.89	D00.07	D10.1	D37.02	D49.0
margin (lateral)	C02.1	C79.89	D00.07	D10.1	D37.02	D49.0
midline NEC	C02.0	C79.89	D00.07	D10.1	D37.02	D49.0
mobile part NEC	C02.3	C79.89	D00.07	D10.1	D37.02	D49.0

Neoplasm, neoplastic — continued

	Malignant Primary	Malignant Secondary	Ca in situ	Benign	Uncertain Behavior	Unspecified Behavior
tongue — *continued*						
overlapping lesion	C02.8	—	—	—	—	—
posterior (third)	C01	C79.89	D00.07	D10.1	D37.02	D49.0
root	C01	C79.89	D00.07	D10.1	D37.02	D49.0
surface (dorsal)	C02.0	C79.89	D00.07	D10.1	D37.02	D49.0
base	C01	C79.89	D00.07	D10.1	D37.02	D49.0
ventral	C02.2	C79.89	D00.07	D10.1	D37.02	D49.0
tip	C02.1	C79.89	D00.07	D10.1	D37.02	D49.0
tonsil	C02.4	C79.89	D00.07	D10.1	D37.02	D49.0
tonsil	C09.9	C79.89	D00.08	D10.4	D37.05	D49.0
fauces, faucial	C09.9	C79.89.	D00.08	D10.4	D37.05	D49.0
lingual	C02.4	C79.89	D00.07	D10.1	D37.02	D49.0
overlapping sites	C09.8	—	—	—	—	—
palatine	C09.9	C79.89	D00.08	D10.4	D37.05	D49.0
pharyngeal	C11.1	C79.89	D00.08	D10.6	D37.05	D49.0
pillar (anterior) (posterior)	C09.1	C79.89	D00.08	D10.5	D37.05	D49.0
tonsillar fossa	C09.0	C79.89	D00.08	D10.5	D37.05	D49.0
tooth socket NEC	C03.9	C79.89	D00.03	D10.39	D37.09	D49.0
trachea (cartilage) (mucosa)	C33	C78.39	D02.1	D14.2	D38.1	D49.1
overlapping lesion with bronchus or lung	C34.8-☑	—	—	—	—	—
tracheobronchial	C34.8-☑	C78.39	D02.1	D14.2	D38.1	D49.1
overlapping lesion with lung	C34.8-☑					
tragus — *see also* Neoplasm, skin, ear	C44.20-☑	C79.2	D04.2-☑	D23.2-☑	D48.5	D49.2
trunk NEC	C76.8	C79.89	D04.5	D36.7	D48.7	D49.89
tubo-ovarian	C57.8	C79.82	D07.39	D28.7	D39.8	D49.59
tunica vaginalis	C63.7	C79.82	D07.69	D29.8	D40.8	D49.59
turbinate (bone)	C41.0	C79.51		D16.4	D48.0	D49.2
nasal	C30.0	C78.39	D02.3	D14.0	D38.5	D49.1
tympanic cavity	C30.1	C78.39	D02.3	D14.0	D38.5	D49.1
ulna (any part)	C40.0-☑	C79.51		D16.0-☑	—	—
umbilicus, umbilical — *see also* Neoplasm, skin, trunk	C44.509	C79.2	D04.5	D23.5	D48.5	D49.2
uncus, brain	C71.2	C79.31	—	D33.0	D43.0	D49.6
unknown site or unspecified	C80.1	C79.9	D09.9	D36.9	D48.9	D49.9
urachus	C67.7	C79.11	D09.0	D30.3	D41.4	D49.4
ureter-bladder (junction)	C67.6	C79.11	D09.0	D30.3	D41.4	D49.4
ureter, ureteral	C66.-☑	C79.19	D09.19	D30.2-☑	D41.2-☑	D49.59
orifice (bladder)	C67.6	C79.11	D09.0	D30.3	D41.4	D49.4
urethra, urethral (gland)	C68.0	C79.19	D09.19	D30.4	D41.3	D49.59
orifice, internal	C67.5	C79.11	D09.0	D30.3	D41.4	D49.4
urethrovaginal (septum)	C57.9	C79.82	D07.30	D28.9	D39.8	D49.59
urinary organ or system	C68.9	C79.10	D09.10	D30.9	D41.9	D49.59
bladder — *see* Neoplasm, bladder						
overlapping lesion	C68.8	—	—	—	—	—
specified sites NEC	C68.8	C79.19	D09.19	D30.8	D41.8	D49.59
utero-ovarian	C57.8	C79.82	D07.39	D28.7	D39.8	D49.59
ligament	C57.1-☑	C79.82	D07.39	D28.2	D39.8	D49.59
uterosacral ligament	C57.3	C79.82		D28.2	D39.8	D49.59
uterus, uteri, uterine	C55	C79.82	D07.0	D26.9	D39.0	D49.59
adnexa NEC	C57.4	C79.82	D07.39	D28.7	D39.8	D49.59
body	C54.9	C79.82	D07.0	D26.1	D39.0	D49.59
cervix	C53.9	C79.82	D06.9	D26.0	D39.0	D49.59
cornu	C54.9	C79.82	D07.0	D26.1	D39.0	D49.59
corpus	C54.9	C79.82	D07.0	D26.1	D39.0	D49.59
endocervix (canal) (gland)	C53.0	C79.82	D06.0	D26.0	D39.0	D49.59
endometrium	C54.1	C79.82	D07.0	D26.1	D39.0	D49.59
exocervix	C53.1	C79.82	D06.1	D26.0	D39.0	D49.0
external os	C53.1	C79.82	D06.1	D26.0	D39.0	D49.0
fundus	C54.3	C79.82	D07.0	D26.1	D39.0	D49.59

Neoplasm, neoplastic — continued

	Malignant Primary	Malignant Secondary	Ca in situ	Benign	Uncertain Behavior	Unspecified Behavior
uterus, uteri, uterine — *continued*						
internal os	C53.0	C79.82	D06.0	D26.0	D39.0	D49.59
isthmus	C54.0	C79.82	D07.0	D26.1	D39.0	D49.59
ligament	C57.3	C79.82		D28.2	D39.8	D49.59
broad	C57.1-☑	C79.82	D07.39	D28.2	D39.8	D49.59
round	C57.2-☑	C79.82	—	D28.2	D39.8	D49.59
lower segment	C54.0	C79.82	D07.0	D26.1	D39.0	D49.59
myometrium	C54.2	C79.82	D07.0	D26.1	D39.0	D49.59
overlapping sites	C54.8	—	—	—	—	—
squamocolumnar junction	C53.8	C79.82	D06.7	D26.0	D39.0	D49.59
tube	C57.0-☑	C79.82	D07.39	D28.2	D39.8	D49.59
utricle, prostatic	C68.0	C79.19	D09.19	D30.4	D41.3	D49.59
uveal tract	C69.4-☑	C79.49	D09.2-☑	D31.4-☑	D48.7	D49.89
uvula	C05.2	C79.89	D00.04	D10.39	D37.09	D49.0
vagina, vaginal (fornix) (vault) (wall)	C52	C79.82	D07.2	D28.1	D39.8	D49.59
vaginovesical	C57.9	C79.82	D07.30	D28.9	D39.9	D49.59
septum	C57.9	C79.82	D07.30	D28.9	D39.9	D49.59
vallecula (epigiottis)	C10.0	C79.89	D00.08	D10.5	D37.05	D49.0
vascular — *see* Neoplasm, connective tissue						
vas deferens	C63.1-☑	C79.82	D07.69	D29.8	D40.8	D49.59
Vater's ampulla	C24.1	C78.89	D01.5	D13.5	D37.6	D49.0
vein, venous — *see* Neoplasm, connective tissue						
vena cava (abdominal) (inferior)	C49.4	C79.89	—	D21.4	D48.1	D49.2
superior	C49.3	C79.89	—	D21.3	D48.1	D49.2
ventricle (cerebral) (floor) (lateral) (third)	C71.5	C79.31	—	D33.0	D43.0	D49.6
cardiac (left) (right)	C38.0	C79.89	—	D15.1	D48.7	D49.89
fourth	C71.7	C79.31	—	D33.1	D43.1	D49.6
ventricular band of larynx	C32.1	C78.39	D02.0	D14.1	D38.0	D49.1
ventriculus — *see* Neoplasm, stomach						
vermillion border — *see* Neoplasm, lip						
vermis, cerebellum	C71.6	C79.31	—	D33.1	D43.1	D49.6
vertebra (column)	C41.2	C79.51	—	D16.6	D48.0	D49.2
coccyx	C41.4	C79.51	—	D16.8	D48.0	D49.2
marrow NEC	C96.9	C79.52	—	—	D47.9	D49.89
sacrum	C41.4	C79.51	—	D16.8	D48.0	D49.2
vesical — *see* Neoplasm, bladder						
vesicle, seminal	C63.7	C79.82	D07.69	D29.8	D40.8	D49.59
vesicocervical tissue	C57.9	C79.82	D07.30	D28.9	D39.9	D49.59
vesicorectal	C76.3	C79.82	D09.8	D36.7	D48.7	D49.89
vesicovaginal	C57.9	C79.82	D07.30	D28.9	D39.9	D49.59
septum	C57.9	C79.82	D07.30	D28.9	D39.8	D49.59
vessel (blood) — *see* Neoplasm, connective tissue						
vestibular gland, greater	C51.0	C79.82	D07.1	D28.0	D39.8	D49.59
vestibule						
mouth	C06.1	C79.89	D00.00	D10.39	D37.09	D49.0
nose	C30.0	C78.39	D02.3	D14.0	D38.5	D49.1
Virchow's gland	C77.0	C77.0	—	D36.0	D48.7	D49.89
viscera NEC	C76.8	C79.89	D09.8	D36.7	D48.7	D49.89
vocal cords (true)	C32.0	C78.39	D02.0	D14.1	D38.0	D49.1
false	C32.1	C78.39	D02.0	D14.1	D38.0	D49.1
vomer	C41.0	C79.51	—	D16.4	D48.0	D49.2
vulva	C51.9	C79.82	D07.1	D28.0	D39.8	D49.59
vulvovaginal gland	C51.0	C79.82	D07.1	D28.0	D39.8	D49.59
Waldeyer's ring	C14.2	C79.89	D00.08	D10.9	D37.05	D49.0
Wharton's duct	C08.0	C79.89	D00.00	D11.7	D37.032	D49.0
white matter (central) (cerebral)	C71.0	C79.31	—	D33.0	D43.0	D49.6

☑ **Additional Character Required — Refer to the Tabular List for Character Selection**   ▼ **Subterms under main terms may continue to next column or page**

	Malignant Primary	Malignant Secondary	Ca in situ	Benign	Uncertain Behavior	Unspecified Behavior
Neoplasm, neoplastic						
— *continued*						
windpipe	C33	C78.39	D02.1	D14.2	D38.1	D49.1
Wirsung's duct	C25.3	C78.89	D01.7	D13.6	D37.8	D49.0
wolffian (body) (duct)						
female	C57.7	C79.82	D07.39	D28.7	D39.8	D49.59
male	C63.7	C79.82	D07.69	D29.8	D40.8	D49.59
womb — *see*						
Neoplasm, uterus						
wrist NEC	C76.4-☑	C79.89	D04.6-☑	D36.7	D48.7	D49.89
xiphoid process	C41.3	C79.51	—	D16.7	D48.0	D49.2
Zuckerkandl						
organ	C75.5	C79.89	—	D35.6	D44.7	D49.7

Table of Drugs and Chemicals

14-hydroxydihydro-morphinone — Aerosporin

Substance	Poisoning, Accidental (unintentional)	Poisoning, Intentional Self-harm	Poisoning, Assault	Poisoning, Undetermined	Adverse Effect	Under-dosing
14-hydroxydihydro-morphinone	T40.2X1	T40.2X2	T40.2X3	T40.2X4	T40.2X5	T40.2X6
1-Propanol	T51.3X1	T51.3X2	T51.3X3	T51.3X4	—	—
2,3,7,8-Tetrachlorodibenzo-p-dioxin	T53.7X1	T53.7X2	T53.7X3	T53.7X4	—	—
2,4,5-T (trichloro-phenoxyacetic acid)	T60.1X1	T60.1X2	T60.1X3	T60.1X4	—	—
2,4,5-Trichlorophen-oxyacetic acid	T60.3X1	T60.3X2	T60.3X3	T60.3X4	—	—
2,4-D (dichlorophen-oxyacetic acid)	T60.3X1	T60.3X2	T60.3X3	T60.3X4	—	—
2,4-Toluene diisocyanate	T65.0X1	T65.0X2	T65.0X3	T65.0X4	—	—
2-Deoxy-5-fluorouridine	T45.1X1	T45.1X2	T45.1X3	T45.1X4	T45.1X5	T45.1X6
2-Ethoxyethanol	T52.3X1	T52.3X2	T52.3X3	T52.3X4	—	—
2-Methoxyethanol	T52.3X1	T52.3X2	T52.3X3	T52.3X4	—	—
2-Propanol	T51.2X1	T51.2X2	T51.2X3	T51.2X4	—	—
3,4-methylenedioxymeth-amphetamine	T43.641	T43.642	T43.643	T43.644	—	—
4-Aminobutyric acid	T43.8X1	T43.8X2	T43.8X3	T43.8X4	T43.8X5	T43.8X6
4-Aminophenol derivatives	T39.1X1	T39.1X2	T39.1X3	T39.1X4	T39.1X5	T39.1X6
5-Deoxy-5-fluorouridine	T45.1X1	T45.1X2	T45.1X3	T45.1X4	T45.1X5	T45.1X6
5-Methoxypsoralen (5-MOP)	T50.991	T50.992	T50.993	T50.994	T50.995	T50.996
8-Aminoquinoline drugs	T37.2X1	T37.2X2	T37.2X3	T37.2X4	T37.2X5	T37.2X6
8-Methoxypsoralen (8-MOP)	T50.991	T50.992	T50.993	T50.994	T50.995	T50.996
ABOB	T37.5X1	T37.5X2	T37.5X3	T37.5X4	T37.5X5	T37.5X6
Abrine	T62.2X1	T62.2X2	T62.2X3	T62.2X4	—	—
Abrus (seed)	T62.2X1	T62.2X2	T62.2X3	T62.2X4	—	—
Absinthe	T51.0X1	T51.0X2	T51.0X3	T51.0X4	—	—
beverage	T51.0X1	T51.0X2	T51.0X3	T51.0X4	—	—
Acaricide	T60.8X1	T60.8X2	T60.8X3	T60.8X4	—	—
Acebutolol	T44.7X1	T44.7X2	T44.7X3	T44.7X4	T44.7X5	T44.7X6
Acecarbromal	T42.6X1	T42.6X2	T42.6X3	T42.6X4	T42.6X5	T42.6X6
Aceclidine	T44.1X1	T44.1X2	T44.1X3	T44.1X4	T44.1X5	T44.1X6
Acedapsone	T37.0X1	T37.0X2	T37.0X3	T37.0X4	T37.0X5	T37.0X6
Acefylline piperazine	T48.6X1	T48.6X2	T48.6X3	T48.6X4	T48.6X5	T48.6X6
Acemorphan	T40.2X1	T40.2X2	T40.2X3	T40.2X4	T40.2X5	T40.2X6
Acenocoumarin	T45.511	T45.512	T45.513	T45.514	T45.515	T45.516
Acenocoumarol	T45.511	T45.512	T45.513	T45.514	T45.515	T45.516
Acepifylline	T48.6X1	T48.6X2	T48.6X3	T48.6X4	T48.6X5	T48.6X6
Acepromazine	T43.3X1	T43.3X2	T43.3X3	T43.3X4	T43.3X5	T43.3X6
Acesulfamethoxypyridazine	T37.0X1	T37.0X2	T37.0X3	T37.0X4	T37.0X5	T37.0X6
Acetal	T52.8X1	T52.8X2	T52.8X3	T52.8X4	—	—
Acetaldehyde (vapor)	T52.8X1	T52.8X2	T52.8X3	T52.8X4	—	—
liquid	T65.891	T65.892	T65.893	T65.894	—	—
Acetaminophen	T39.1X1	T39.1X2	T39.1X3	T39.1X4	T39.1X5	T39.1X6
Acetaminosalol	T39.1X1	T39.1X2	T39.1X3	T39.1X4	T39.1X5	T39.1X6
Acetanilide	T39.1X1	T39.1X2	T39.1X3	T39.1X4	T39.1X5	T39.1X6
Acetarsol	T37.3X1	T37.3X2	T37.3X3	T37.3X4	T37.3X5	T37.3X6
Acetazolamide	T50.2X1	T50.2X2	T50.2X3	T50.2X4	T50.2X5	T50.2X6
Acetiamine	T45.2X1	T45.2X2	T45.2X3	T45.2X4	T45.2X5	T45.2X6
Acetic						
acid	T54.2X1	T54.2X2	T54.2X3	T54.2X4	—	—
with sodium acetate (ointment)	T49.3X1	T49.3X2	T49.3X3	T49.3X4	T49.3X5	T49.3X6
ester (solvent)(vapor)	T52.8X1	T52.8X2	T52.8X3	T52.8X4	—	—
irrigating solution	T50.3X1	T50.3X2	T50.3X3	T50.3X4	T50.3X5	T50.3X6
medicinal (lotion)	T49.2X1	T49.2X2	T49.2X3	T49.2X4	T49.2X5	T49.2X6
anhydride	T65.891	T65.892	T65.893	T65.894	—	—
ether (vapor)	T52.8X1	T52.8X2	T52.8X3	T52.8X4	—	—
Acetohexamide	T38.3X1	T38.3X2	T38.3X3	T38.3X4	T38.3X5	T38.3X6
Acetohydroxamic acid	T50.991	T50.992	T50.993	T50.994	T50.995	T50.996
Acetomenaphthone	T45.7X1	T45.7X2	T45.7X3	T45.7X4	T45.7X5	T45.7X6
Acetomorphine	T40.1X1	T40.1X2	T40.1X3	T40.1X4	—	—
Acetone (oils)	T52.4X1	T52.4X2	T52.4X3	T52.4X4	—	—
chlorinated	T52.4X1	T52.4X2	T52.4X3	T52.4X4	—	—
vapor	T52.4X1	T52.4X2	T52.4X3	T52.4X4	—	—
Acetonitrile	T52.8X1	T52.8X2	T52.8X3	T52.8X4	—	—
Acetophenazine	T43.3X1	T43.3X2	T43.3X3	T43.3X4	T43.3X5	T43.3X6
Acetophenetedin	T39.1X1	T39.1X2	T39.1X3	T39.1X4	T39.1X5	T39.1X6
Acetophenone	T52.4X1	T52.4X2	T52.4X3	T52.4X4	—	—
Acetorphine	T40.2X1	T40.2X2	T40.2X3	T40.2X4	—	—
Acetosulfone (sodium)	T37.1X1	T37.1X2	T37.1X3	T37.1X4	T37.1X5	T37.1X6
Acetrizoate (sodium)	T50.8X1	T50.8X2	T50.8X3	T50.8X4	T50.8X5	T50.8X6
Acetrizoic acid	T50.8X1	T50.8X2	T50.8X3	T50.8X4	T50.8X5	T50.8X6
Acetyl						
bromide	T53.6X1	T53.6X2	T53.6X3	T53.6X4	—	—
chloride	T53.6X1	T53.6X2	T53.6X3	T53.6X4	—	—
Acetylcarbromal	T42.6X1	T42.6X2	T42.6X3	T42.6X4	T42.6X5	T42.6X6
Acetylcholine						
chloride	T44.1X1	T44.1X2	T44.1X3	T44.1X4	T44.1X5	T44.1X6
derivative	T44.1X1	T44.1X2	T44.1X3	T44.1X4	T44.1X5	T44.1X6

Substance	Poisoning, Accidental (unintentional)	Poisoning, Intentional Self-harm	Poisoning, Assault	Poisoning, Undetermined	Adverse Effect	Under-dosing
Acetylcysteine	T48.4X1	T48.4X2	T48.4X3	T48.4X4	T48.4X5	T48.4X6
Acetyldigitoxin	T46.0X1	T46.0X2	T46.0X3	T46.0X4	T46.0X5	T46.0X6
Acetyldigoxin	T46.0X1	T46.0X2	T46.0X3	T46.0X4	T46.0X5	T46.0X6
Acetyldihydrocodeine	T40.2X1	T40.2X2	T40.2X3	T40.2X4	—	—
Acetyldihydrocodeinone	T40.2X1	T40.2X2	T40.2X3	T40.2X4	—	—
Acetylene (gas)	T59.891	T59.892	T59.893	T59.894	—	—
dichloride	T53.6X1	T53.6X2	T53.6X3	T53.6X4	—	—
incomplete combustion of	T58.11	T58.12	T58.13	T58.14	—	—
industrial	T59.891	T59.892	T59.893	T59.894	—	—
tetrachloride	T53.6X1	T53.6X2	T53.6X3	T53.6X4	—	—
vapor	T53.6X1	T53.6X2	T53.6X3	T53.6X4	—	—
Acetylpheneturide	T42.6X1	T42.6X2	T42.6X3	T42.6X4	T42.6X5	T42.6X6
Acetylphenylhydrazine	T39.8X1	T39.8X2	T39.8X3	T39.8X4	T39.8X5	T39.8X6
Acetylsalicylic acid (salts)	T39.011	T39.012	T39.013	T39.014	T39.015	T39.016
enteric coated	T39.011	T39.012	T39.013	T39.014	T39.015	T39.016
Acetylsulfamethoxypyridazine	T37.0X1	T37.0X2	T37.0X3	T37.0X4	T37.0X5	T37.0X6
Achromycin	T36.4X1	T36.4X2	T36.4X3	T36.4X4	T36.4X5	T36.4X6
ophthalmic preparation	T49.5X1	T49.5X2	T49.5X3	T49.5X4	T49.5X5	T49.5X6
topical NEC	T49.0X1	T49.0X2	T49.0X3	T49.0X4	T49.0X5	T49.0X6
Aciclovir	T37.5X1	T37.5X2	T37.5X3	T37.5X4	T37.5X5	T37.5X6
Acidifying agent NEC	T50.901	T50.902	T50.903	T50.904	T50.905	T50.906
Acid (corrosive) NEC	T54.2X1	T54.2X2	T54.2X3	T54.2X4	—	—
Acipimox	T46.6X1	T46.6X2	T46.6X3	T46.6X4	T46.6X5	T46.6X6
Acitretin	T50.991	T50.992	T50.993	T50.994	T50.995	T50.996
Aclarubicin	T45.1X1	T45.1X2	T45.1X3	T45.1X4	T45.1X5	T45.1X6
Aclatonium napadisilate	T48.1X1	T48.1X2	T48.1X3	T48.1X4	T48.1X5	T48.1X6
Aconite (wild)	T46.991	T46.992	T46.993	T46.994	T46.995	T46.996
Aconitine	T46.991	T46.992	T46.993	T46.994	T46.995	T46.996
Aconitum ferox	T46.991	T46.992	T46.993	T46.994	T46.995	T46.996
Acridine	T65.6X1	T65.6X2	T65.6X3	T65.6X4	—	—
vapor	T59.891	T59.892	T59.893	T59.894	—	—
Acriflavine	T37.91	T37.92	T37.93	T37.94	T37.95	T37.96
Acriflavinium chloride	T49.0X1	T49.0X2	T49.0X3	T49.0X4	T49.0X5	T49.0X6
Acrinol	T49.0X1	T49.0X2	T49.0X3	T49.0X4	T49.0X5	T49.0X6
Acrisorcin	T49.0X1	T49.0X2	T49.0X3	T49.0X4	T49.0X5	T49.0X6
Acrivastine	T45.0X1	T45.0X2	T45.0X3	T45.0X4	T45.0X5	T45.0X6
Acrolein (gas)	T59.891	T59.892	T59.893	T59.894	—	—
liquid	T54.1X1	T54.1X2	T54.1X3	T54.1X4	—	—
Acrylamide	T65.891	T65.892	T65.893	T65.894	—	—
Acrylic resin	T49.3X1	T49.3X2	T49.3X3	T49.3X4	T49.3X5	T49.3X6
Acrylonitrile	T65.891	T65.892	T65.893	T65.894	—	—
Actaea spicata	T62.2X1	T62.2X2	T62.2X3	T62.2X4	—	—
berry	T62.1X1	T62.1X2	T62.1X3	T62.1X4	—	—
Acterol	T37.3X1	T37.3X2	T37.3X3	T37.3X4	T37.3X5	T37.3X6
ACTH	T38.811	T38.812	T38.813	T38.814	T38.815	T38.816
Actinomycin C	T45.1X1	T45.1X2	T45.1X3	T45.1X4	T45.1X5	T45.1X6
Actinomycin D	T45.1X1	T45.1X2	T45.1X3	T45.1X4	T45.1X5	T45.1X6
Activated charcoal — see also Charcoal, medicinal	T47.6X1	T47.6X2	T47.6X3	T47.6X4	T47.6X5	T47.6X6
Acyclovir	T37.5X1	T37.5X2	T37.5X3	T37.5X4	T37.5X5	T37.5X6
Adenine	T45.2X1	T45.2X2	T45.2X3	T45.2X4	T45.2X5	T45.2X6
arabinoside	T37.5X1	T37.5X2	T37.5X3	T37.5X4	T37.5X5	T37.5X6
Adenosine (phosphate)	T46.2X1	T46.2X2	T46.2X3	T46.2X4	T46.2X5	T46.2X6
ADH	T38.891	T38.892	T38.893	T38.894	T38.895	T38.896
Adhesive NEC	T65.891	T65.892	T65.893	T65.894	—	—
Adicillin	T36.0X1	T36.0X2	T36.0X3	T36.0X4	T36.0X5	T36.0X6
Adiphenine	T44.3X1	T44.3X2	T44.3X3	T44.3X4	T44.3X5	T44.3X6
Adipiodone	T50.8X1	T50.8X2	T50.8X3	T50.8X4	T50.8X5	T50.8X6
Adjunct, pharmaceutical	T50.901	T50.902	T50.903	T50.904	T50.905	T50.906
Adrenal (extract, cortex or medulla) (glucocorticoids) (hormones) (mineralocorticoids)	T38.0X1	T38.0X2	T38.0X3	T38.0X4	T38.0X5	T38.0X6
ENT agent	T49.6X1	T49.6X2	T49.6X3	T49.6X4	T49.6X5	T49.6X6
ophthalmic preparation	T49.5X1	T49.5X2	T49.5X3	T49.5X4	T49.5X5	T49.5X6
topical NEC	T49.0X1	T49.0X2	T49.0X3	T49.0X4	T49.0X5	T49.0X6
Adrenalin — see Adrenaline						
Adrenaline	T44.5X1	T44.5X2	T44.5X3	T44.5X4	T44.5X5	T44.5X6
Adrenergic NEC	T44.901	T44.902	T44.903	T44.904	T44.905	T44.906
blocking agent NEC	T44.8X1	T44.8X2	T44.8X3	T44.8X4	T44.8X5	T44.8X6
beta, heart	T44.7X1	T44.7X2	T44.7X3	T44.7X4	T44.7X5	T44.7X6
specified NEC	T44.991	T44.992	T44.993	T44.994	T44.995	T44.996
Adrenochrome						
derivative	T46.991	T46.992	T46.993	T46.994	T46.995	T46.996
(mono) semicarbazone	T46.991	T46.992	T46.993	T46.994	T46.995	T46.996
Adrenocorticotrophic hormone	T38.811	T38.812	T38.813	T38.814	T38.815	T38.816
Adrenocorticotrophin	T38.811	T38.812	T38.813	T38.814	T38.815	T38.816
Adriamycin	T45.1X1	T45.1X2	T45.1X3	T45.1X4	T45.1X5	T45.1X6
Aerosol spray NEC	T65.91	T65.92	T65.93	T65.94	—	—
Aerosporin	T36.8X1	T36.8X2	T36.8X3	T36.8X4	T36.8X5	T36.8X6
ENT agent	T49.6X1	T49.6X2	T49.6X3	T49.6X4	T49.6X5	T49.6X6
ophthalmic preparation	T49.5X1	T49.5X2	T49.5X3	T49.5X4	T49.5X5	T49.5X6

14-hydroxydihydro-morphinone — Aerosporin

Substance	Poisoning, Accidental (unintentional)	Poisoning, Intentional Self-harm	Poisoning, Assault	Poisoning, Undetermined	Adverse Effect	Under-dosing
Aerosporin — continued						
topical NEC	T49.0X1	T49.0X2	T49.0X3	T49.0X4	T49.0X5	T49.0X6
Aethusa cynapium	T62.2X1	T62.2X2	T62.2X3	T62.2X4	—	—
Afghanistan black	T40.7X1	T40.7X2	T40.7X3	T40.7X4	T40.7X5	T40.7X6
Aflatoxin	T64.01	T64.02	T64.03	T64.04	—	—
Afloqualone	T42.8X1	T42.8X2	T42.8X3	T42.8X4	T42.8X5	T42.8X6
African boxwood	T62.2X1	T62.2X2	T62.2X3	T62.2X4	—	—
Agar	T47.4X1	T47.4X2	T47.4X3	T47.4X4	T47.4X5	T47.4X6
Agonist						
predominantly						
alpha-adrenoreceptor	T44.4X1	T44.4X2	T44.4X3	T44.4X4	T44.4X5	T44.4X6
beta-adrenoreceptor	T44.5X1	T44.5X2	T44.5X3	T44.5X4	T44.5X5	T44.5X6
Agricultural agent NEC	T65.91	T65.92	T65.93	T65.94		
Agrypnal	T42.3X1	T42.3X2	T42.3X3	T42.3X4	T42.3X5	T42.3X6
AHLG	T50.Z11	T50.Z12	T50.Z13	T50.Z14	T50.Z15	T50.Z16
Air contaminant(s), source/type NOS	T65.91	T65.92	T65.93	T65.94		
Ajmaline	T46.2X1	T46.2X2	T46.2X3	T46.2X4	T46.2X5	T46.2X6
Akee	T62.1X1	T62.1X2	T62.1X3	T62.1X4		
Akrinol	T49.0X1	T49.0X2	T49.0X3	T49.0X4	T49.0X5	T49.0X6
Akritoin	T37.8X1	T37.8X2	T37.8X3	T37.8X4	T37.8X5	T37.8X6
Alacepril	T46.4X1	T46.4X2	T46.4X3	T46.4X4	T46.4X5	T46.4X6
Alantolactone	T37.4X1	T37.4X2	T37.4X3	T37.4X4	T37.4X5	T37.4X6
Albamycin	T36.8X1	T36.8X2	T36.8X3	T36.8X4	T36.8X5	T36.8X6
Albendazole	T37.4X1	T37.4X2	T37.4X3	T37.4X4	T37.4X5	T37.4X6
Albumin						
bovine	T45.8X1	T45.8X2	T45.8X3	T45.8X4	T45.8X5	T45.8X6
human serum	T45.8X1	T45.8X2	T45.8X3	T45.8X4	T45.8X5	T45.8X6
salt-poor	T45.8X1	T45.8X2	T45.8X3	T45.8X4	T45.8X5	T45.8X6
normal human serum	T45.8X1	T45.8X2	T45.8X3	T45.8X4	T45.8X5	T45.8X6
Albuterol	T48.6X1	T48.6X2	T48.6X3	T48.6X4	T48.6X5	T48.6X6
Albutoin	T42.0X1	T42.0X2	T42.0X3	T42.0X4	T42.0X5	T42.0X6
Alclometasone	T49.0X1	T49.0X2	T49.0X3	T49.0X4	T49.0X5	T49.0X6
Alcohol	T51.91	T51.92	T51.93	T51.94	—	—
absolute	T51.0X1	T51.0X2	T51.0X3	T51.0X4	—	—
beverage	T51.0X1	T51.0X2	T51.0X3	T51.0X4	—	—
allyl	T51.8X1	T51.8X2	T51.8X3	T51.8X4	—	—
amyl	T51.3X1	T51.3X2	T51.3X3	T51.3X4	—	—
antifreeze	T51.1X1	T51.1X2	T51.1X3	T51.1X4	—	—
beverage	T51.0X1	T51.0X2	T51.0X3	T51.0X4	—	—
butyl	T51.3X1	T51.3X2	T51.3X3	T51.3X4	—	—
dehydrated	T51.0X1	T51.0X2	T51.0X3	T51.0X4	—	—
beverage	T51.0X1	T51.0X2	T51.0X3	T51.0X4	—	—
denatured	T51.0X1	T51.0X2	T51.0X3	T51.0X4	—	—
deterrent NEC	T50.6X1	T50.6X2	T50.6X3	T50.6X4	T50.6X5	T50.6X6
diagnostic (gastric function)	T50.8X1	T50.8X2	T50.8X3	T50.8X4	T50.8X5	T50.8X6
ethyl	T51.0X1	T51.0X2	T51.0X3	T51.0X4	—	—
beverage	T51.0X1	T51.0X2	T51.0X3	T51.0X4	—	—
grain	T51.0X1	T51.0X2	T51.0X3	T51.0X4	—	—
beverage	T51.0X1	T51.0X2	T51.0X3	T51.0X4	—	—
industrial	T51.0X1	T51.0X2	T51.0X3	T51.0X4	—	—
isopropyl	T51.2X1	T51.2X2	T51.2X3	T51.2X4	—	—
methyl	T51.1X1	T51.1X2	T51.1X3	T51.1X4	—	—
preparation for consumption	T51.0X1	T51.0X2	T51.0X3	T51.0X4	—	—
propyl	T51.3X1	T51.3X2	T51.3X3	T51.3X4	—	—
secondary	T51.2X1	T51.2X2	T51.2X3	T51.2X4	—	—
radiator	T51.1X1	T51.1X2	T51.1X3	T51.1X4	—	—
rubbing	T51.2X1	T51.2X2	T51.2X3	T51.2X4	—	—
specified type NEC	T51.8X1	T51.8X2	T51.8X3	T51.8X4	—	—
surgical	T51.0X1	T51.0X2	T51.0X3	T51.0X4	—	—
vapor (from any type of Alcohol)	T59.891	T59.892	T59.893	T59.894	—	—
wood	T51.1X1	T51.1X2	T51.1X3	T51.1X4	—	—
Alcuronium (chloride)	T48.1X1	T48.1X2	T48.1X3	T48.1X4	T48.1X5	T48.1X6
Aldactone	T50.0X1	T50.0X2	T50.0X3	T50.0X4	T50.0X5	T50.0X6
Aldesulfone sodium	T37.1X1	T37.1X2	T37.1X3	T37.1X4	T37.1X5	T37.1X6
Aldicarb	T60.0X1	T60.0X2	T60.0X3	T60.0X4		
Aldomet	T46.5X1	T46.5X2	T46.5X3	T46.5X4	T46.5X5	T46.5X6
Aldosterone	T50.0X1	T50.0X2	T50.0X3	T50.0X4	T50.0X5	T50.0X6
Aldrin (dust)	T60.1X1	T60.1X2	T60.1X3	T60.1X4		
Aleve — see Naproxen						
Alexitol sodium	T47.1X1	T47.1X2	T47.1X3	T47.1X4	T47.1X5	T47.1X6
Alfacalcidol	T45.2X1	T45.2X2	T45.2X3	T45.2X4	T45.2X5	T45.2X6
Alfadolone	T41.1X1	T41.1X2	T41.1X3	T41.1X4	T41.1X5	T41.1X6
Alfaxalone	T41.1X1	T41.1X2	T41.1X3	T41.1X4	T41.1X5	T41.1X6
Alfentanil	T40.411	T40.412	T40.413	T40.414	T40.415	T40.416
Alfuzosin (hydrochloride)	T44.8X1	T44.8X2	T44.8X3	T44.8X4	T44.8X5	T44.8X6
Algae (harmful) (toxin)	T65.821	T65.822	T65.823	T65.824	—	—
Algeldrate	T47.1X1	T47.1X2	T47.1X3	T47.1X4	T47.1X5	T47.1X6
Algin	T47.8X1	T47.8X2	T47.8X3	T47.8X4	T47.8X5	T47.8X6
Alglucerase	T45.3X1	T45.3X2	T45.3X3	T45.3X4	T45.3X5	T45.3X6
Alidase	T45.3X1	T45.3X2	T45.3X3	T45.3X4	T45.3X5	T45.3X6
Alimemazine	T43.3X1	T43.3X2	T43.3X3	T43.3X4	T43.3X5	T43.3X6
Aliphatic thiocyanates	T65.0X1	T65.0X2	T65.0X3	T65.0X4	—	—
Alizapride	T45.0X1	T45.0X2	T45.0X3	T45.0X4	T45.0X5	T45.0X6
Alkali (caustic)	T54.3X1	T54.3X2	T54.3X3	T54.3X4		
Alkaline antiseptic solution (aromatic)	T49.6X1	T49.6X2	T49.6X3	T49.6X4	T49.6X5	T49.6X6
Alkalinizing agents (medicinal)	T50.901	T50.902	T50.903	T50.904	T50.905	T50.906
Alkalizing agent NEC	T50.901	T50.902	T50.903	T50.904	T50.905	T50.906
Alka-seltzer	T39.011	T39.012	T39.013	T39.014	T39.015	T39.016
Alkavervir	T46.5X1	T46.5X2	T46.5X3	T46.5X4	T46.5X5	T46.5X6
Alkonium (bromide)	T49.0X1	T49.0X2	T49.0X3	T49.0X4	T49.0X5	T49.0X6
Alkylating drug NEC	T45.1X1	T45.1X2	T45.1X3	T45.1X4	T45.1X5	T45.1X6
antimyeloproliferative	T45.1X1	T45.1X2	T45.1X3	T45.1X4	T45.1X5	T45.1X6
lymphatic	T45.1X1	T45.1X2	T45.1X3	T45.1X4	T45.1X5	T45.1X6
Alkylisocyanate	T65.0X1	T65.0X2	T65.0X3	T65.0X4	—	—
Allantoin	T49.4X1	T49.4X2	T49.4X3	T49.4X4	T49.4X5	T49.4X6
Allegron	T43.011	T43.012	T43.013	T43.014	T43.015	T43.016
Allethrin	T49.0X1	T49.0X2	T49.0X3	T49.0X4	T49.0X5	T49.0X6
Allobarbital	T42.3X1	T42.3X2	T42.3X3	T42.3X4	T42.3X5	T42.3X6
Allopurinol	T50.4X1	T50.4X2	T50.4X3	T50.4X4	T50.4X5	T50.4X6
Allyl						
alcohol	T51.8X1	T51.8X2	T51.8X3	T51.8X4	—	—
disulfide	T46.6X1	T46.6X2	T46.6X3	T46.6X4	T46.6X5	T46.6X6
Allylestrenol	T38.5X1	T38.5X2	T38.5X3	T38.5X4	T38.5X5	T38.5X6
Allylisopropylacetylurea	T42.6X1	T42.6X2	T42.6X3	T42.6X4	T42.6X5	T42.6X6
Allylisopropylmalonylurea	T42.3X1	T42.3X2	T42.3X3	T42.3X4	T42.3X5	T42.3X6
Allylthiourea	T49.3X1	T49.3X2	T49.3X3	T49.3X4	T49.3X5	T49.3X6
Allyltribromide	T42.6X1	T42.6X2	T42.6X3	T42.6X4	T42.6X5	T42.6X6
Allypropymal	T42.3X1	T42.3X2	T42.3X3	T42.3X4	T42.3X5	T42.3X6
Almagate	T47.1X1	T47.1X2	T47.1X3	T47.1X4	T47.1X5	T47.1X6
Almasilate	T47.1X1	T47.1X2	T47.1X3	T47.1X4	T47.1X5	T47.1X6
Almitrine	T50.7X1	T50.7X2	T50.7X3	T50.7X4	T50.7X5	T50.7X6
Aloes	T47.2X1	T47.2X2	T47.2X3	T47.2X4	T47.2X5	T47.2X6
Aloglutamol	T47.1X1	T47.1X2	T47.1X3	T47.1X4	T47.1X5	T47.1X6
Aloin	T47.2X1	T47.2X2	T47.2X3	T47.2X4	T47.2X5	T47.2X6
Aloxidone	T42.2X1	T42.2X2	T42.2X3	T42.2X4	T42.2X5	T42.2X6
Alpha						
acetyldigoxin	T46.0X1	T46.0X2	T46.0X3	T46.0X4	T46.0X5	T46.0X6
adrenergic blocking drug	T44.6X1	T44.6X2	T44.6X3	T44.6X4	T44.6X5	T44.6X6
amylase	T45.3X1	T45.3X2	T45.3X3	T45.3X4	T45.3X5	T45.3X6
tocoferol (acetate)	T45.2X1	T45.2X2	T45.2X3	T45.2X4	T45.2X5	T45.2X6
tocopherol	T45.2X1	T45.2X2	T45.2X3	T45.2X4	T45.2X5	T45.2X6
Alphadolone	T41.1X1	T41.1X2	T41.1X3	T41.1X4	T41.1X5	T41.1X6
Alphaprodine	T40.491	T40.492	T40.493	T40.494	T40.495	T40.496
Alphaxalone	T41.1X1	T41.1X2	T41.1X3	T41.1X4	T41.1X5	T41.1X6
Alprazolam	T42.4X1	T42.4X2	T42.4X3	T42.4X4	T42.4X5	T42.4X6
Alprenolol	T44.7X1	T44.7X2	T44.7X3	T44.7X4	T44.7X5	T44.7X6
Alprostadil	T46.7X1	T46.7X2	T46.7X3	T46.7X4	T46.7X5	T46.7X6
Alsactide	T38.811	T38.812	T38.813	T38.814	T38.815	T38.816
Alseroxylon	T46.5X1	T46.5X2	T46.5X3	T46.5X4	T46.5X5	T46.5X6
Alteplase	T45.611	T45.612	T45.613	T45.614	T45.615	T45.616
Altizide	T50.2X1	T50.2X2	T50.2X3	T50.2X4	T50.2X5	T50.2X6
Altretamine	T45.1X1	T45.1X2	T45.1X3	T45.1X4	T45.1X5	T45.1X6
Alum (medicinal)	T49.4X1	T49.4X2	T49.4X3	T49.4X4	T49.4X5	T49.4X6
nonmedicinal (ammonium) (potassium)	T56.891	T56.892	T56.893	T56.894		
Aluminium, aluminum						
acetate	T49.2X1	T49.2X2	T49.2X3	T49.2X4	T49.2X5	T49.2X6
solution	T49.0X1	T49.0X2	T49.0X3	T49.0X4	T49.0X5	T49.0X6
aspirin	T39.011	T39.012	T39.013	T39.014	T39.015	T39.016
bis (acetylsalicylate)	T39.011	T39.012	T39.013	T39.014	T39.015	T39.016
carbonate (gel, basic)	T47.1X1	T47.1X2	T47.1X3	T47.1X4	T47.1X5	T47.1X6
chlorhydroxide-complex	T47.1X1	T47.1X2	T47.1X3	T47.1X4	T47.1X5	T47.1X6
chloride	T49.2X1	T49.2X2	T49.2X3	T49.2X4	T49.2X5	T49.2X6
clofibrate	T46.6X1	T46.6X2	T46.6X3	T46.6X4	T46.6X5	T46.6X6
diacetate	T49.2X1	T49.2X2	T49.2X3	T49.2X4	T49.2X5	T49.2X6
glycinate	T47.1X1	T47.1X2	T47.1X3	T47.1X4	T47.1X5	T47.1X6
hydroxide (gel)	T47.1X1	T47.1X2	T47.1X3	T47.1X4	T47.1X5	T47.1X6
hydroxide-magnesium carb. gel	T47.1X1	T47.1X2	T47.1X3	T47.1X4	T47.1X5	T47.1X6
magnesium silicate	T47.1X1	T47.1X2	T47.1X3	T47.1X4	T47.1X5	T47.1X6
nicotinate	T46.7X1	T46.7X2	T46.7X3	T46.7X4	T46.7X5	T46.7X6
ointment (surgical) (topical)	T49.3X1	T49.3X2	T49.3X3	T49.3X4	T49.3X5	T49.3X6
phosphate	T47.1X1	T47.1X2	T47.1X3	T47.1X4	T47.1X5	T47.1X6
salicylate	T39.091	T39.092	T39.093	T39.094	T39.095	T39.096
silicate	T47.1X1	T47.1X2	T47.1X3	T47.1X4	T47.1X5	T47.1X6
sodium silicate	T47.1X1	T47.1X2	T47.1X3	T47.1X4	T47.1X5	T47.1X6
subacetate	T49.2X1	T49.2X2	T49.2X3	T49.2X4	T49.2X5	T49.2X6
sulfate	T49.0X1	T49.0X2	T49.0X3	T49.0X4	T49.0X5	T49.0X6
tannate	T47.6X1	T47.6X2	T47.6X3	T47.6X4	T47.6X5	T47.6X6

Substance	Poisoning, Accidental (unintentional)	Poisoning, Intentional Self-harm	Poisoning, Assault	Poisoning, Undetermined	Adverse Effect	Under-dosing
Aluminium, aluminum — *continued*						
topical NEC	T49.3X1	T49.3X2	T49.3X3	T49.3X4	T49.3X5	T49.3X6
Alurate	T42.3X1	T42.3X2	T42.3X3	T42.3X4	T42.3X5	T42.3X6
Alverine	T44.3X1	T44.3X2	T44.3X3	T44.3X4	T44.3X5	T44.3X6
Alvodine	T40.2X1	T40.2X2	T40.2X3	T40.2X4	T40.2X5	T40.2X6
Amanita phalloides	T62.0X1	T62.0X2	T62.0X3	T62.0X4	—	—
Amanitine	T62.0X1	T62.0X2	T62.0X3	T62.0X4	—	—
Amantadine	T42.8X1	T42.8X2	T42.8X3	T42.8X4	T42.8X5	T42.8X6
Ambazone	T49.6X1	T49.6X2	T49.6X3	T49.6X4	T49.6X5	T49.6X6
Ambenonium (chloride)	T44.0X1	T44.0X2	T44.0X3	T44.0X4	T44.0X5	T44.0X6
Ambroxol	T48.4X1	T48.4X2	T48.4X3	T48.4X4	T48.4X5	T48.4X6
Ambuphylline	T48.6X1	T48.6X2	T48.6X3	T48.6X4	T48.6X5	T48.6X6
Ambutonium bromide	T44.3X1	T44.3X2	T44.3X3	T44.3X4	T44.3X5	T44.3X6
Amcinonide	T49.0X1	T49.0X2	T49.0X3	T49.0X4	T49.0X5	T49.0X6
Amdinocilline	T36.0X1	T36.0X2	T36.0X3	T36.0X4	T36.0X5	T36.0X6
Ametazole	T50.8X1	T50.8X2	T50.8X3	T50.8X4	T50.8X5	T50.8X6
Amethocaine	T41.3X1	T41.3X2	T41.3X3	T41.3X4	T41.3X5	T41.3X6
regional	T41.3X1	T41.3X2	T41.3X3	T41.3X4	T41.3X5	T41.3X6
spinal	T41.3X1	T41.3X2	T41.3X3	T41.3X4	T41.3X5	T41.3X6
Amethopterin	T45.1X1	T45.1X2	T45.1X3	T45.1X4	T45.1X5	T45.1X6
Amezinium metilsulfate	T44.991	T44.992	T44.993	T44.994	T44.995	T44.996
Amfebutamone	T43.291	T43.292	T43.293	T43.294	T43.295	T43.296
Amfepramone	T50.5X1	T50.5X2	T50.5X3	T50.5X4	T50.5X5	T50.5X6
Amfetamine	T43.621	T43.622	T43.623	T43.624	T43.625	T43.626
Amfetaminil	T43.621	T43.622	T43.623	T43.624	T43.625	T43.626
Amfomycin	T36.8X1	T36.8X2	T36.8X3	T36.8X4	T36.8X5	T36.8X6
Amidefrine mesilate	T48.5X1	T48.5X2	T48.5X3	T48.5X4	T48.5X5	T48.5X6
Amidone	T40.3X1	T40.3X2	T40.3X3	T40.3X4	T40.3X5	T40.3X6
Amidopyrine	T39.2X1	T39.2X2	T39.2X3	T39.2X4	T39.2X5	T39.2X6
Amidotrizoate	T50.8X1	T50.8X2	T50.8X3	T50.8X4	T50.8X5	T50.8X6
Amiflamine	T43.1X1	T43.1X2	T43.1X3	T43.1X4	T43.1X5	T43.1X6
Amikacin	T36.5X1	T36.5X2	T36.5X3	T36.5X4	T36.5X5	T36.5X6
Amikhelline	T46.3X1	T46.3X2	T46.3X3	T46.3X4	T46.3X5	T46.3X6
Amiloride	T50.2X1	T50.2X2	T50.2X3	T50.2X4	T50.2X5	T50.2X6
Aminacrine	T49.0X1	T49.0X2	T49.0X3	T49.0X4	T49.0X5	T49.0X6
Amineptine	T43.011	T43.012	T43.013	T43.014	T43.015	T43.016
Aminitrozole	T37.3X1	T37.3X2	T37.3X3	T37.3X4	T37.3X5	T37.3X6
Aminoacetic acid (derivatives)	T50.3X1	T50.3X2	T50.3X3	T50.3X4	T50.3X5	T50.3X6
Amino acids	T50.3X1	T50.3X2	T50.3X3	T50.3X4	T50.3X5	T50.3X6
Aminoacridine	T49.0X1	T49.0X2	T49.0X3	T49.0X4	T49.0X5	T49.0X6
Aminobenzoic acid (-p)	T49.3X1	T49.3X2	T49.3X3	T49.3X4	T49.3X5	T49.3X6
Aminocaproic acid	T45.621	T45.622	T45.623	T45.624	T45.625	T45.626
Aminoethylisothiourium	T45.8X1	T45.8X2	T45.8X3	T45.8X4	T45.8X5	T45.8X6
Aminofenazone	T39.2X1	T39.2X2	T39.2X3	T39.2X4	T39.2X5	T39.2X6
Aminoglutethimide	T45.1X1	T45.1X2	T45.1X3	T45.1X4	T45.1X5	T45.1X6
Aminohippuric acid	T50.8X1	T50.8X2	T50.8X3	T50.8X4	T50.8X5	T50.8X6
Aminomethylbenzoic acid	T45.691	T45.692	T45.693	T45.694	T45.695	T45.696
Aminometradine	T50.2X1	T50.2X2	T50.2X3	T50.2X4	T50.2X5	T50.2X6
Aminopentamide	T44.3X1	T44.3X2	T44.3X3	T44.3X4	T44.3X5	T44.3X6
Aminophenazone	T39.2X1	T39.2X2	T39.2X3	T39.2X4	T39.2X5	T39.2X6
Aminophenol	T54.0X1	T54.0X2	T54.0X3	T54.0X4	—	—
Aminophenylpyridone	T43.591	T43.592	T43.593	T43.594	T43.595	T43.596
Aminophylline	T48.6X1	T48.6X2	T48.6X3	T48.6X4	T48.6X5	T48.6X6
Aminopterin sodium	T45.1X1	T45.1X2	T45.1X3	T45.1X4	T45.1X5	T45.1X6
Aminopyrine	T39.2X1	T39.2X2	T39.2X3	T39.2X4	T39.2X5	T39.2X6
Aminorex	T50.5X1	T50.5X2	T50.5X3	T50.5X4	T50.5X5	T50.5X6
Aminosalicylic acid	T37.1X1	T37.1X2	T37.1X3	T37.1X4	T37.1X5	T37.1X6
Aminosalylum	T37.1X1	T37.1X2	T37.1X3	T37.1X4	T37.1X5	T37.1X6
Amiodarone	T46.2X1	T46.2X2	T46.2X3	T46.2X4	T46.2X5	T46.2X6
Amiphenazole	T50.7X1	T50.7X2	T50.7X3	T50.7X4	T50.7X5	T50.7X6
Amiquinsin	T46.5X1	T46.5X2	T46.5X3	T46.5X4	T46.5X5	T46.5X6
Amisometradine	T50.2X1	T50.2X2	T50.2X3	T50.2X4	T50.2X5	T50.2X6
Amisulpride	T43.591	T43.592	T43.593	T43.594	T43.595	T43.596
Amitriptyline	T43.011	T43.012	T43.013	T43.014	T43.015	T43.016
Amitriptylinoxide	T43.011	T43.012	T43.013	T43.014	T43.015	T43.016
Amlexanox	T48.6X1	T48.6X2	T48.6X3	T48.6X4	T48.6X5	T48.6X6
Ammonia (fumes) (gas) (vapor)	T59.891	T59.892	T59.893	T59.894	—	—
aromatic spirit	T48.991	T48.992	T48.993	T48.994	T48.995	T48.996
liquid (household)	T54.3X1	T54.3X2	T54.3X3	T54.3X4	—	—
Ammoniated mercury	T49.0X1	T49.0X2	T49.0X3	T49.0X4	T49.0X5	T49.0X6
Ammonium						
acid tartrate	T49.5X1	T49.5X2	T49.5X3	T49.5X4	T49.5X5	T49.5X6
bromide	T42.6X1	T42.6X2	T42.6X3	T42.6X4	T42.6X5	T42.6X6
carbonate	T54.3X1	T54.3X2	T54.3X3	T54.3X4	—	—
chloride	T50.991	T50.992	T50.993	T50.994	T50.995	T50.996
expectorant	T48.4X1	T48.4X2	T48.4X3	T48.4X4	T48.4X5	T48.4X6
compounds (household)	T54.3X1	T54.3X2	T54.3X3	T54.3X4	—	—
NEC						
fumes (any usage)	T59.891	T59.892	T59.893	T59.894	—	—
industrial	T54.3X1	T54.3X2	T54.3X3	T54.3X4	—	—

Substance	Poisoning, Accidental (unintentional)	Poisoning, Intentional Self-harm	Poisoning, Assault	Poisoning, Undetermined	Adverse Effect	Under-dosing
Ammonium — *continued*						
ichthyosulronate	T49.4X1	T49.4X2	T49.4X3	T49.4X4	T49.4X5	T49.4X6
mandelate	T37.91	T37.92	T37.93	T37.94	T37.95	T37.96
sulfamate	T60.3X1	T60.3X2	T60.3X3	T60.3X4	—	—
sulfonate resin	T47.8X1	T47.8X2	T47.8X3	T47.8X4	T47.8X5	T47.8X6
Amobarbital (sodium)	T42.3X1	T42.3X2	T42.3X3	T42.3X4	T42.3X5	T42.3X6
Amodiaquine	T37.2X1	T37.2X2	T37.2X3	T37.2X4	T37.2X5	T37.2X6
Amopyroquin (e)	T37.2X1	T37.2X2	T37.2X3	T37.2X4	T37.2X5	T37.2X6
Amoxapine	T43.011	T43.012	T43.013	T43.014	T43.015	T43.016
Amoxicillin	T36.0X1	T36.0X2	T36.0X3	T36.0X4	T36.0X5	T36.0X6
Amperozide	T43.591	T43.592	T43.593	T43.594	T43.595	T43.596
Amphenidone	T43.591	T43.592	T43.593	T43.594	T43.595	T43.596
Amphetamine NEC	T43.621	T43.622	T43.623	T43.624	T43.625	T43.626
Amphomycin	T36.8X1	T36.8X2	T36.8X3	T36.8X4	T36.8X5	T36.8X6
Amphotalide	T37.4X1	T37.4X2	T37.4X3	T37.4X4	T37.4X5	T37.4X6
Amphotericin B	T36.7X1	T36.7X2	T36.7X3	T36.7X4	T36.7X5	T36.7X6
topical	T49.0X1	T49.0X2	T49.0X3	T49.0X4	T49.0X5	T49.0X6
Ampicillin	T36.0X1	T36.0X2	T36.0X3	T36.0X4	T36.0X5	T36.0X6
Amprotropine	T44.3X1	T44.3X2	T44.3X3	T44.3X4	T44.3X5	T44.3X6
Amsacrine	T45.1X1	T45.1X2	T45.1X3	T45.1X4	T45.1X5	T45.1X6
Amygdaline	T62.2X1	T62.2X2	T62.2X3	T62.2X4	—	—
Amyl						
acetate	T52.8X1	T52.8X2	T52.8X3	T52.8X4	—	—
vapor	T59.891	T59.892	T59.893	T59.894	—	—
alcohol	T51.3X1	T51.3X2	T51.3X3	T51.3X4	—	—
chloride	T53.6X1	T53.6X2	T53.6X3	T53.6X4	—	—
formate	T52.8X1	T52.8X2	T52.8X3	T52.8X4	—	—
nitrite	T46.3X1	T46.3X2	T46.3X3	T46.3X4	T46.3X5	T46.3X6
propionate	T65.891	T65.892	T65.893	T65.894	—	—
Amylase	T47.5X1	T47.5X2	T47.5X3	T47.5X4	T47.5X5	T47.5X6
Amyleine, regional	T41.3X1	T41.3X2	T41.3X3	T41.3X4	T41.3X5	T41.3X6
Amylene						
dichloride	T53.6X1	T53.6X2	T53.6X3	T53.6X4	—	—
hydrate	T51.3X1	T51.3X2	T51.3X3	T51.3X4	—	—
Amylmetacresol	T49.6X1	T49.6X2	T49.6X3	T49.6X4	T49.6X5	T49.6X6
Amylobarbitone	T42.3X1	T42.3X2	T42.3X3	T42.3X4	T42.3X5	T42.3X6
Amylocaine, regional	T41.3X1	T41.3X2	T41.3X3	T41.3X4	T41.3X5	T41.3X6
infiltration (subcutaneous)	T41.3X1	T41.3X2	T41.3X3	T41.3X4	T41.3X5	T41.3X6
nerve block (peripheral) (plexus)	T41.3X1	T41.3X2	T41.3X3	T41.3X4	T41.3X5	T41.3X6
spinal	T41.3X1	T41.3X2	T41.3X3	T41.3X4	T41.3X5	T41.3X6
topical (surface)	T41.3X1	T41.3X2	T41.3X3	T41.3X4	T41.3X5	T41.3X6
Amylopectin	T47.6X1	T47.6X2	T47.6X3	T47.6X4	T47.6X5	T47.6X6
Amytal (sodium)	T42.3X1	T42.3X2	T42.3X3	T42.3X4	T42.3X5	T42.3X6
Anabolic steroid	T38.7X1	T38.7X2	T38.7X3	T38.7X4	T38.7X5	T38.7X6
Analeptic NEC	T50.7X1	T50.7X2	T50.7X3	T50.7X4	T50.7X5	T50.7X6
Analgesic	T39.91	T39.92	T39.93	T39.94	T39.95	T39.96
anti-inflammatory NEC	T39.91	T39.92	T39.93	T39.94	T39.95	T39.96
propionic acid derivative	T39.311	T39.312	T39.313	T39.314	T39.315	T39.316
antirheumatic NEC	T39.4X1	T39.4X2	T39.4X3	T39.4X4	T39.4X5	T39.4X6
aromatic NEC	T39.1X1	T39.1X2	T39.1X3	T39.1X4	T39.1X5	T39.1X6
narcotic NEC	T40.601	T40.602	T40.603	T40.604	T40.605	T40.606
combination	T40.601	T40.602	T40.603	T40.604	T40.605	T40.606
obstetric	T40.601	T40.602	T40.603	T40.604	T40.605	T40.606
non-narcotic NEC	T39.91	T39.92	T39.93	T39.94	T39.95	T39.96
combination	T39.91	T39.92	T39.93	T39.94	T39.95	T39.96
pyrazole	T39.2X1	T39.2X2	T39.2X3	T39.2X4	T39.2X5	T39.2X6
specified NEC	T39.8X1	T39.8X2	T39.8X3	T39.8X4	T39.8X5	T39.8X6
Analgin	T39.2X1	T39.2X2	T39.2X3	T39.2X4	T39.2X5	T39.2X6
Anamirta cocculus	T62.1X1	T62.1X2	T62.1X3	T62.1X4	—	—
Ancillin	T36.0X1	T36.0X2	T36.0X3	T36.0X4	T36.0X5	T36.0X6
Ancrod	T45.691	T45.692	T45.693	T45.694	T45.695	T45.696
Androgen	T38.7X1	T38.7X2	T38.7X3	T38.7X4	T38.7X5	T38.7X6
Androgen-estrogen mixture	T38.7X1	T38.7X2	T38.7X3	T38.7X4	T38.7X5	T38.7X6
Androstalone	T38.7X1	T38.7X2	T38.7X3	T38.7X4	T38.7X5	T38.7X6
Androstanolone	T38.7X1	T38.7X2	T38.7X3	T38.7X4	T38.7X5	T38.7X6
Androsterone	T38.7X1	T38.7X2	T38.7X3	T38.7X4	T38.7X5	T38.7X6
Anemone pulsatilla	T62.2X1	T62.2X2	T62.2X3	T62.2X4	—	—
Anesthesia						
caudal	T41.3X1	T41.3X2	T41.3X3	T41.3X4	T41.3X5	T41.3X6
endotracheal	T41.0X1	T41.0X2	T41.0X3	T41.0X4	T41.0X5	T41.0X6
epidural	T41.3X1	T41.3X2	T41.3X3	T41.3X4	T41.3X5	T41.3X6
inhalation	T41.0X1	T41.0X2	T41.0X3	T41.0X4	T41.0X5	T41.0X6
local	T41.3X1	T41.3X2	T41.3X3	T41.3X4	T41.3X5	T41.3X6
mucosal	T41.3X1	T41.3X2	T41.3X3	T41.3X4	T41.3X5	T41.3X6
muscle relaxation	T48.1X1	T48.1X2	T48.1X3	T48.1X4	T48.1X5	T48.1X6
nerve blocking	T41.3X1	T41.3X2	T41.3X3	T41.3X4	T41.3X5	T41.3X6
plexus blocking	T41.3X1	T41.3X2	T41.3X3	T41.3X4	T41.3X5	T41.3X6
potentiated	T41.201	T41.202	T41.203	T41.204	T41.205	T41.206
rectal	T41.201	T41.202	T41.203	T41.204	T41.205	T41.206
general	T41.201	T41.202	T41.203	T41.204	T41.205	T41.206
local	T41.3X1	T41.3X2	T41.3X3	T41.3X4	T41.3X5	T41.3X6

Substance	Poisoning, Accidental (unintentional)	Poisoning, Intentional Self-harm	Poisoning, Assault	Poisoning, Undetermined	Adverse Effect	Under-dosing
Anesthesia — *continued*						
regional	T41.3X1	T41.3X2	T41.3X3	T41.3X4	T41.3X5	T41.3X6
surface	T41.3X1	T41.3X2	T41.3X3	T41.3X4	T41.3X5	T41.3X6
Anesthetic NEC — *see also* Anesthesia	T41.41	T41.42	T41.43	T41.44	T41.45	T41.46
with muscle relaxant	T41.201	T41.202	T41.203	T41.204	T41.205	T41.206
general	T41.201	T41.202	T41.203	T41.204	T41.205	T41.206
local	T41.3X1	T41.3X2	T41.3X3	T41.3X4	T41.3X5	T41.3X6
gaseous NEC	T41.0X1	T41.0X2	T41.0X3	T41.0X4	T41.0X5	T41.0X6
general NEC	T41.201	T41.202	T41.203	T41.204	T41.205	T41.206
halogenated hydrocarbon derivatives NEC	T41.0X1	T41.0X2	T41.0X3	T41.0X4	T41.0X5	T41.0X6
infiltration NEC	T41.3X1	T41.3X2	T41.3X3	T41.3X4	T41.3X5	T41.3X6
intravenous NEC	T41.1X1	T41.1X2	T41.1X3	T41.1X4	T41.1X5	T41.1X6
local NEC	T41.3X1	T41.3X2	T41.3X3	T41.3X4	T41.3X5	T41.3X6
rectal						
general	T41.201	T41.202	T41.203	T41.204	T41.205	T41.206
local	T41.3X1	T41.3X2	T41.3X3	T41.3X4	T41.3X5	T41.3X6
regional NEC	T41.3X1	T41.3X2	T41.3X3	T41.3X4	T41.3X5	T41.3X6
spinal NEC	T41.3X1	T41.3X2	T41.3X3	T41.3X4	T41.3X5	T41.3X6
thiobarbiturate	T41.1X1	T41.1X2	T41.1X3	T41.1X4	T41.1X5	T41.1X6
topical	T41.3X1	T41.3X2	T41.3X3	T41.3X4	T41.3X5	T41.3X6
Aneurine	T45.2X1	T45.2X2	T45.2X3	T45.2X4	T45.2X5	T45.2X6
Angio-Conray	T50.8X1	T50.8X2	T50.8X3	T50.8X4	T50.8X5	T50.8X6
Angiotensin	T44.5X1	T44.5X2	T44.5X3	T44.5X4	T44.5X5	T44.5X6
Angiotensinamide	T44.991	T44.992	T44.993	T44.994	T44.995	T44.996
Anhydrohydroxy-progesterone	T38.5X1	T38.5X2	T38.5X3	T38.5X4	T38.5X5	T38.5X6
Anhydron	T50.2X1	T50.2X2	T50.2X3	T50.2X4	T50.2X5	T50.2X6
Anileridine	T40.491	T40.492	T40.493	T40.494	T40.495	T40.496
Aniline (dye) (liquid)	T65.3X1	T65.3X2	T65.3X3	T65.3X4	—	—
analgesic	T39.1X1	T39.1X2	T39.1X3	T39.1X4	T39.1X5	T39.1X6
derivatives, therapeutic NEC	T39.1X1	T39.1X2	T39.1X3	T39.1X4	T39.1X5	T39.1X6
vapor	T65.3X1	T65.3X2	T65.3X3	T65.3X4	—	—
Aniscoropine	T44.3X1	T44.3X2	T44.3X3	T44.3X4	T44.3X5	T44.3X6
Anise oil	T47.5X1	T47.5X2	T47.5X3	T47.5X4	T47.5X5	T47.5X6
Anisidine	T65.3X1	T65.3X2	T65.3X3	T65.3X4	—	—
Anisindione	T45.511	T45.512	T45.513	T45.514	T45.515	T45.516
Anisotropine methyl-bromide	T44.3X1	T44.3X2	T44.3X3	T44.3X4	T44.3X5	T44.3X6
Anistreplase	T45.611	T45.612	T45.613	T45.614	T45.615	T45.616
Anorexiant (central)	T50.5X1	T50.5X2	T50.5X3	T50.5X4	T50.5X5	T50.5X6
Anorexic agents	T50.5X1	T50.5X2	T50.5X3	T50.5X4	T50.5X5	T50.5X6
Ansamycin	T36.6X1	T36.6X2	T36.6X3	T36.6X4	T36.6X5	T36.6X6
Ant (bite) (sting)	T63.421	T63.422	T63.423	T63.424	—	—
Antabuse	T50.6X1	T50.6X2	T50.6X3	T50.6X4	T50.6X5	T50.6X6
Antacid NEC	T47.1X1	T47.1X2	T47.1X3	T47.1X4	T47.1X5	T47.1X6
Antagonist						
Aldosterone	T50.0X1	T50.0X2	T50.0X3	T50.0X4	T50.0X5	T50.0X6
alpha-adrenoreceptor	T44.6X1	T44.6X2	T44.6X3	T44.6X4	T44.6X5	T44.6X6
anticoagulant	T45.7X1	T45.7X2	T45.7X3	T45.7X4	T45.7X5	T45.7X6
beta-adrenoreceptor	T44.7X1	T44.7X2	T44.7X3	T44.7X4	T44.7X5	T44.7X6
extrapyramidal NEC	T44.3X1	T44.3X2	T44.3X3	T44.3X4	T44.3X5	T44.3X6
folic acid	T45.1X1	T45.1X2	T45.1X3	T45.1X4	T45.1X5	T45.1X6
H2 receptor	T47.0X1	T47.0X2	T47.0X3	T47.0X4	T47.0X5	T47.0X6
heavy metal	T45.8X1	T45.8X2	T45.8X3	T45.8X4	T45.8X5	T45.8X6
narcotic analgesic	T50.7X1	T50.7X2	T50.7X3	T50.7X4	T50.7X5	T50.7X6
opiate	T50.7X1	T50.7X2	T50.7X3	T50.7X4	T50.7X5	T50.7X6
pyrimidine	T45.1X1	T45.1X2	T45.1X3	T45.1X4	T45.1X5	T45.1X6
serotonin	T46.5X1	T46.5X2	T46.5X3	T46.5X4	T46.5X5	T46.5X6
Antazoline	T45.0X1	T45.0X2	T45.0X3	T45.0X4	T45.0X5	T45.0X6
Anterior pituitary hormone NEC	T38.811	T38.812	T38.813	T38.814	T38.815	T38.816
Anthelmintic NEC	T37.4X1	T37.4X2	T37.4X3	T37.4X4	T37.4X5	T37.4X6
Anthiolimine	T37.4X1	T37.4X2	T37.4X3	T37.4X4	T37.4X5	T37.4X6
Anthralin	T49.4X1	T49.4X2	T49.4X3	T49.4X4	T49.4X5	T49.4X6
Anthramycin	T45.1X1	T45.1X2	T45.1X3	T45.1X4	T45.1X5	T45.1X6
Antiadrenergic NEC	T44.8X1	T44.8X2	T44.8X3	T44.8X4	T44.8X5	T44.8X6
Antiallergic NEC	T45.0X1	T45.0X2	T45.0X3	T45.0X4	T45.0X5	T45.0X6
Antiandrogen NEC	T38.6X1	T38.6X2	T38.6X3	T38.6X4	T38.6X5	T38.6X6
Anti-anemic (drug) (preparation)	T45.8X1	T45.8X2	T45.8X3	T45.8X4	T45.8X5	T45.8X6
Antianxiety drug NEC	T43.501	T43.502	T43.503	T43.504	T43.505	T43.506
Antiaris toxicaria	T65.891	T65.892	T65.893	T65.894	—	—
Antiarteriosclerotic drug	T46.6X1	T46.6X2	T46.6X3	T46.6X4	T46.6X5	T46.6X6
Antiasthmatic drug NEC	T48.6X1	T48.6X2	T48.6X3	T48.6X4	T48.6X5	T48.6X6
Antibiotic NEC	T36.91	T36.92	T36.93	T36.94	T36.95	T36.96
aminoglycoside	T36.5X1	T36.5X2	T36.5X3	T36.5X4	T36.5X5	T36.5X6
anticancer	T45.1X1	T45.1X2	T45.1X3	T45.1X4	T45.1X5	T45.1X6
antifungal	T36.7X1	T36.7X2	T36.7X3	T36.7X4	T36.7X5	T36.7X6
antimycobacterial	T36.5X1	T36.5X2	T36.5X3	T36.5X4	T36.5X5	T36.5X6
antineoplastic	T45.1X1	T45.1X2	T45.1X3	T45.1X4	T45.1X5	T45.1X6
b-lactam NEC	T36.1X1	T36.1X2	T36.1X3	T36.1X4	T36.1X5	T36.1X6

Substance	Poisoning, Accidental (unintentional)	Poisoning, Intentional Self-harm	Poisoning, Assault	Poisoning, Undetermined	Adverse Effect	Under-dosing
Antibiotic — *continued*						
cephalosporin (group)	T36.1X1	T36.1X2	T36.1X3	T36.1X4	T36.1X5	T36.1X6
chloramphenicol (group)	T36.2X1	T36.2X2	T36.2X3	T36.2X4	T36.2X5	T36.2X6
ENT	T49.6X1	T49.6X2	T49.6X3	T49.6X4	T49.6X5	T49.6X6
eye	T49.5X1	T49.5X2	T49.5X3	T49.5X4	T49.5X5	T49.5X6
fungicidal (local)	T49.0X1	T49.0X2	T49.0X3	T49.0X4	T49.0X5	T49.0X6
intestinal	T36.8X1	T36.8X2	T36.8X3	T36.8X4	T36.8X5	T36.8X6
local	T49.0X1	T49.0X2	T49.0X3	T49.0X4	T49.0X5	T49.0X6
macrolides	T36.3X1	T36.3X2	T36.3X3	T36.3X4	T36.3X5	T36.3X6
polypeptide	T36.8X1	T36.8X2	T36.8X3	T36.8X4	T36.8X5	T36.8X6
specified NEC	T36.8X1	T36.8X2	T36.8X3	T36.8X4	T36.8X5	T36.8X6
tetracycline (group)	T36.4X1	T36.4X2	T36.4X3	T36.4X4	T36.4X5	T36.4X6
throat	T49.6X1	T49.6X2	T49.6X3	T49.6X4	T49.6X5	T49.6X6
Anticancer agents NEC	T45.1X1	T45.1X2	T45.1X3	T45.1X4	T45.1X5	T45.1X6
Anticholesterolemic drug NEC	T46.6X1	T46.6X2	T46.6X3	T46.6X4	T46.6X5	T46.6X6
Anticholinergic NEC	T44.3X1	T44.3X2	T44.3X3	T44.3X4	T44.3X5	T44.3X6
Anticholinesterase	T44.0X1	T44.0X2	T44.0X3	T44.0X4	T44.0X5	T44.0X6
organophosphorus	T44.0X1	T44.0X2	T44.0X3	T44.0X4	T44.0X5	T44.0X6
insecticide	T60.0X1	T60.0X2	T60.0X3	T60.0X4		
nerve gas	T59.891	T59.892	T59.893	T59.894	—	—
reversible	T44.0X1	T44.0X2	T44.0X3	T44.0X4	T44.0X5	T44.0X6
ophthalmological	T49.5X1	T49.5X2	T49.5X3	T49.5X4	T49.5X5	T49.5X6
Anticoagulant NEC	T45.511	T45.512	T45.513	T45.514	T45.515	T45.516
Antagonist	T45.7X1	T45.7X2	T45.7X3	T45.7X4	T45.7X5	T45.7X6
Anti-common-cold drug NEC	T48.5X1	T48.5X2	T48.5X3	T48.5X4	T48.5X5	T48.5X6
Anticonvulsant	T42.71	T42.72	T42.73	T42.74	T42.75	T42.76
barbiturate	T42.3X1	T42.3X2	T42.3X3	T42.3X4	T42.3X5	T42.3X6
combination (with barbiturate)	T42.3X1	T42.3X2	T42.3X3	T42.3X4	T42.3X5	T42.3X6
hydantoin	T42.0X1	T42.0X2	T42.0X3	T42.0X4	T42.0X5	T42.0X6
hypnotic NEC	T42.6X1	T42.6X2	T42.6X3	T42.6X4	T42.6X5	T42.6X6
oxazolidinedione	T42.2X1	T42.2X2	T42.2X3	T42.2X4	T42.2X5	T42.2X6
pyrimidinedione	T42.6X1	T42.6X2	T42.6X3	T42.6X4	T42.6X5	T42.6X6
specified NEC	T42.6X1	T42.6X2	T42.6X3	T42.6X4	T42.6X5	T42.6X6
succinimide	T42.2X1	T42.2X2	T42.2X3	T42.2X4	T42.2X5	T42.2X6
Antidepressant	T43.201	T43.202	T43.203	T43.204	T43.205	T43.206
monoamine oxidase inhibitor	T43.1X1	T43.1X2	T43.1X3	T43.1X4	T43.1X5	T43.1X6
selective serotonin norepinephrine reuptake inhibitor	T43.211	T43.212	T43.213	T43.214	T43.215	T43.216
selective serotonin reuptake inhibitor	T43.221	T43.222	T43.223	T43.224	T43.225	T43.226
specified NEC	T43.291	T43.292	T43.293	T43.294	T43.295	T43.296
tetracyclic	T43.021	T43.022	T43.023	T43.024	T43.025	T43.026
triazolopyridine	T43.211	T43.212	T43.213	T43.214	T43.215	T43.216
tricyclic	T43.011	T43.012	T43.013	T43.014	T43.015	T43.016
Antidiabetic NEC	T38.3X1	T38.3X2	T38.3X3	T38.3X4	T38.3X5	T38.3X6
biguanide	T38.3X1	T38.3X2	T38.3X3	T38.3X4	T38.3X5	T38.3X6
and sulfonyl combined	T38.3X1	T38.3X2	T38.3X3	T38.3X4	T38.3X5	T38.3X6
combined	T38.3X1	T38.3X2	T38.3X3	T38.3X4	T38.3X5	T38.3X6
sulfonylurea	T38.3X1	T38.3X2	T38.3X3	T38.3X4	T38.3X5	T38.3X6
Antidiarrheal drug NEC	T47.6X1	T47.6X2	T47.6X3	T47.6X4	T47.6X5	T47.6X6
absorbent	T47.6X1	T47.6X2	T47.6X3	T47.6X4	T47.6X5	T47.6X6
Anti-D immunoglobulin (human)	T50.Z11	T50.Z12	T50.Z13	T50.Z14	T50.Z15	T50.Z16
Antidiphtheria serum	T50.Z11	T50.Z12	T50.Z13	T50.Z14	T50.Z15	T50.Z16
Antidiuretic hormone	T38.891	T38.892	T38.893	T38.894	T38.895	T38.896
Antidote NEC	T50.6X1	T50.6X2	T50.6X3	T50.6X4	T50.6X5	T50.6X6
heavy metal	T45.8X1	T45.8X2	T45.8X3	T45.8X4	T45.8X5	T45.8X6
Antidysrhythmic NEC	T46.2X1	T46.2X2	T46.2X3	T46.2X4	T46.2X5	T46.2X6
Antiemetic drug	T45.0X1	T45.0X2	T45.0X3	T45.0X4	T45.0X5	T45.0X6
Antiepilepsy agent	T42.71	T42.72	T42.73	T42.74	T42.75	T42.76
combination	T42.5X1	T42.5X2	T42.5X3	T42.5X4	T42.5X5	T42.5X6
mixed	T42.5X1	T42.5X2	T42.5X3	T42.5X4	T42.5X5	T42.5X6
specified, NEC	T42.6X1	T42.6X2	T42.6X3	T42.6X4	T42.6X5	T42.6X6
Antiestrogen NEC	T38.6X1	T38.6X2	T38.6X3	T38.6X4	T38.6X5	T38.6X6
Antifertility pill	T38.4X1	T38.4X2	T38.4X3	T38.4X4	T38.4X5	T38.4X6
Antifibrinolytic drug	T45.621	T45.622	T45.623	T45.624	T45.625	T45.626
Antifilarial drug	T37.4X1	T37.4X2	T37.4X3	T37.4X4	T37.4X5	T37.4X6
Antiflatulent	T47.5X1	T47.5X2	T47.5X3	T47.5X4	T47.5X5	T47.5X6
Antifreeze	T65.91	T65.92	T65.93	T65.94	—	—
alcohol	T51.1X1	T51.1X2	T51.1X3	T51.1X4	—	—
ethylene glycol	T51.8X1	T51.8X2	T51.8X3	T51.8X4	—	—
Antifungal						
antibiotic (systemic)	T36.7X1	T36.7X2	T36.7X3	T36.7X4	T36.7X5	T36.7X6
anti-infective NEC	T37.91	T37.92	T37.93	T37.94	T37.95	T37.96
disinfectant, local	T49.0X1	T49.0X2	T49.0X3	T49.0X4	T49.0X5	T49.0X6
nonmedicinal (spray)	T60.3X1	T60.3X2	T60.3X3	T60.3X4	—	—
topical	T49.0X1	T49.0X2	T49.0X3	T49.0X4	T49.0X5	T49.0X6

▽ Subterms under main terms may continue to next column or page — Additional Character May Be Required — Refer to the Tabular List for Character Selection — 357

Anesthesia — Antifungal

Table of Drugs and Chemicals

Anti-gastric-secretion drug NEC — Aristocort

Substance	Poisoning, Accidental (unintentional)	Poisoning, Intentional Self-harm	Poisoning, Assault	Poisoning, Undetermined	Adverse Effect	Under-dosing
Anti-gastric-secretion drug NEC	T47.1X1	T47.1X2	T47.1X3	T47.1X4	T47.1X5	T47.1X6
Antigonadotrophin NEC	T38.6X1	T38.6X2	T38.6X3	T38.6X4	T38.6X5	T38.6X6
Antihallucinogen	T43.501	T43.502	T43.503	T43.504	T43.505	T43.506
Antihelmintics	T37.4X1	T37.4X2	T37.4X3	T37.4X4	T37.4X5	T37.4X6
Antihemophilic						
factor	T45.8X1	T45.8X2	T45.8X3	T45.8X4	T45.8X5	T45.8X6
fraction	T45.8X1	T45.8X2	T45.8X3	T45.8X4	T45.8X5	T45.8X6
globulin concentrate	T45.7X1	T45.7X2	T45.7X3	T45.7X4	T45.7X5	T45.7X6
human plasma	T45.8X1	T45.8X2	T45.8X3	T45.8X4	T45.8X5	T45.8X6
plasma, dried	T45.7X1	T45.7X2	T45.7X3	T45.7X4	T45.7X5	T45.7X6
Antihemorrhoidal preparation	T49.2X1	T49.2X2	T49.2X3	T49.2X4	T49.2X5	T49.2X6
Antiheparin drug	T45.7X1	T45.7X2	T45.7X3	T45.7X4	T45.7X5	T45.7X6
Antihistamine	T45.0X1	T45.0X2	T45.0X3	T45.0X4	T45.0X5	T45.0X6
Antihookworm drug	T37.4X1	T37.4X2	T37.4X3	T37.4X4	T37.4X5	T37.4X6
Anti-human lymphocytic globulin	T50.Z11	T50.Z12	T50.Z13	T50.Z14	T50.Z15	T50.Z16
Antihyperlipidemic drug	T46.6X1	T46.6X2	T46.6X3	T46.6X4	T46.6X5	T46.6X6
Antihypertensive drug NEC	T46.5X1	T46.5X2	T46.5X3	T46.5X4	T46.5X5	T46.5X6
Anti-infective NEC	T37.91	T37.92	T37.93	T37.94	T37.95	T37.96
anthelmintic	T37.4X1	T37.4X2	T37.4X3	T37.4X4	T37.4X5	T37.4X6
antibiotics	T36.91	T36.92	T36.93	T36.94	T36.95	T36.96
specified NEC	T36.8X1	T36.8X2	T36.8X3	T36.8X4	T36.8X5	T36.8X6
antimalarial	T37.2X1	T37.2X2	T37.2X3	T37.2X4	T37.2X5	T37.2X6
antimycobacterial NEC	T37.1X1	T37.1X2	T37.1X3	T37.1X4	T37.1X5	T37.1X6
antibiotics	T36.5X1	T36.5X2	T36.5X3	T36.5X4	T36.5X5	T36.5X6
antiprotozoal NEC	T37.3X1	T37.3X2	T37.3X3	T37.3X4	T37.3X5	T37.3X6
blood	T37.2X1	T37.2X2	T37.2X3	T37.2X4	T37.2X5	T37.2X6
antiviral	T37.5X1	T37.5X2	T37.5X3	T37.5X4	T37.5X5	T37.5X6
arsenical	T37.8X1	T37.8X2	T37.8X3	T37.8X4	T37.8X5	T37.8X6
bismuth, local	T49.0X1	T49.0X2	T49.0X3	T49.0X4	T49.0X5	T49.0X6
ENT	T49.6X1	T49.6X2	T49.6X3	T49.6X4	T49.6X5	T49.6X6
eye NEC	T49.5X1	T49.5X2	T49.5X3	T49.5X4	T49.5X5	T49.5X6
heavy metals NEC	T37.8X1	T37.8X2	T37.8X3	T37.8X4	T37.8X5	T37.8X6
local NEC	T49.0X1	T49.0X2	T49.0X3	T49.0X4	T49.0X5	T49.0X6
specified NEC	T49.0X1	T49.0X2	T49.0X3	T49.0X4	T49.0X5	T49.0X6
mixed	T37.91	T37.92	T37.93	T37.94	T37.95	T37.96
ophthalmic preparation	T49.5X1	T49.5X2	T49.5X3	T49.5X4	T49.5X5	T49.5X6
topical NEC	T49.0X1	T49.0X2	T49.0X3	T49.0X4	T49.0X5	T49.0X6
Anti-inflammatory drug NEC	T39.391	T39.392	T39.393	T39.394	T39.395	T39.396
local	T49.0X1	T49.0X2	T49.0X3	T49.0X4	T49.0X5	T49.0X6
nonsteroidal NEC	T39.391	T39.392	T39.393	T39.394	T39.395	T39.396
propionic acid derivative	T39.311	T39.312	T39.313	T39.314	T39.315	T39.316
specified NEC	T39.391	T39.392	T39.393	T39.394	T39.395	T39.396
Antikaluretic	T50.3X1	T50.3X2	T50.3X3	T50.3X4	T50.3X5	T50.3X6
Antiknock (tetraethyl lead)	T56.0X1	T56.0X2	T56.0X3	T56.0X4	—	—
Antilipemic drug NEC	T46.6X1	T46.6X2	T46.6X3	T46.6X4	T46.6X5	T46.6X6
Antimalarial	T37.2X1	T37.2X2	T37.2X3	T37.2X4	T37.2X5	T37.2X6
prophylactic NEC	T37.2X1	T37.2X2	T37.2X3	T37.2X4	T37.2X5	T37.2X6
pyrimidine derivative	T37.2X1	T37.2X2	T37.2X3	T37.2X4	T37.2X5	T37.2X6
Antimetabolite	T45.1X1	T45.1X2	T45.1X3	T45.1X4	T45.1X5	T45.1X6
Antimitotic agent	T45.1X1	T45.1X2	T45.1X3	T45.1X4	T45.1X5	T45.1X6
Antimony (compounds) (vapor) NEC	T56.891	T56.892	T56.893	T56.894	—	—
anti-infectives	T37.8X1	T37.8X2	T37.8X3	T37.8X4	T37.8X5	T37.8X6
dimercaptosuccinate	T37.3X1	T37.3X2	T37.3X3	T37.3X4	T37.3X5	T37.3X6
hydride	T56.891	T56.892	T56.893	T56.894	—	—
pesticide (vapor)	T60.8X1	T60.8X2	T60.8X3	T60.8X4	—	—
potassium (sodium) tartrate	T37.8X1	T37.8X2	T37.8X3	T37.8X4	T37.8X5	T37.8X6
sodium	T37.3X1				T37.3X3	
dimercaptosuccinate						
tartrated	T37.8X1	T37.8X2	T37.8X3	T37.8X4	T37.8X5	T37.8X6
Antimuscarinic NEC	T44.3X1	T44.3X2	T44.3X3	T44.3X4	T44.3X5	T44.3X6
Antimycobacterial drug NEC	T37.1X1	T37.1X2	T37.1X3	T37.1X4	T37.1X5	T37.1X6
antibiotics	T36.5X1	T36.5X2	T36.5X3	T36.5X4	T36.5X5	T36.5X6
combination	T37.1X1	T37.1X2	T37.1X3	T37.1X4	T37.1X5	T37.1X6
Antinausea drug	T45.0X1	T45.0X2	T45.0X3	T45.0X4	T45.0X5	T45.0X6
Antinematode drug	T37.4X1	T37.4X2	T37.4X3	T37.4X4	T37.4X5	T37.4X6
Antineoplastic NEC	T45.1X1	T45.1X2	T45.1X3	T45.1X4	T45.1X5	T45.1X6
alkaloidal	T45.1X1	T45.1X2	T45.1X3	T45.1X4	T45.1X5	T45.1X6
antibiotics	T45.1X1	T45.1X2	T45.1X3	T45.1X4	T45.1X5	T45.1X6
combination	T45.1X1	T45.1X2	T45.1X3	T45.1X4	T45.1X5	T45.1X6
estrogen	T38.5X1	T38.5X2	T38.5X3	T38.5X4	T38.5X5	T38.5X6
steroid	T38.7X1	T38.7X2	T38.7X3	T38.7X4	T38.7X5	T38.7X6
Antiparasitic drug (systemic)	T37.91	T37.92	T37.93	T37.94	T37.95	T37.96
local	T49.0X1	T49.0X2	T49.0X3	T49.0X4	T49.0X5	T49.0X6
specified NEC	T37.8X1	T37.8X2	T37.8X3	T37.8X4	T37.8X5	T37.8X6
Antiparkinsonism drug NEC	T42.8X1	T42.8X2	T42.8X3	T42.8X4	T42.8X5	T42.8X6
Antiperspirant NEC	T49.2X1	T49.2X2	T49.2X3	T49.2X4	T49.2X5	T49.2X6
Antiphlogistic NEC	T39.4X1	T39.4X2	T39.4X3	T39.4X4	T39.4X5	T39.4X6
Antiplatyhelmintic drug	T37.4X1	T37.4X2	T37.4X3	T37.4X4	T37.4X5	T37.4X6
Antiprotozoal drug NEC	T37.3X1	T37.3X2	T37.3X3	T37.3X4	T37.3X5	T37.3X6
blood	T37.2X1	T37.2X2	T37.2X3	T37.2X4	T37.2X5	T37.2X6
local	T49.0X1	T49.0X2	T49.0X3	T49.0X4	T49.0X5	T49.0X6
Antipruritic drug NEC	T49.1X1	T49.1X2	T49.1X3	T49.1X4	T49.1X5	T49.1X6
Antipsychotic drug	T43.501	T43.502	T43.503	T43.504	T43.505	T43.506
specified NEC	T43.591	T43.592	T43.593	T43.594	T43.595	T43.596
Antipyretic	T39.91	T39.92	T39.93	T39.94	T39.95	T39.96
specified NEC	T39.8X1	T39.8X2	T39.8X3	T39.8X4	T39.8X5	T39.8X6
Antipyrine	T39.2X1	T39.2X2	T39.2X3	T39.2X4	T39.2X5	T39.2X6
Antirabies hyperimmune serum	T50.Z11	T50.Z12	T50.Z13	T50.Z14	T50.Z15	T50.Z16
Antirheumatic NEC	T39.4X1	T39.4X2	T39.4X3	T39.4X4	T39.4X5	T39.4X6
Antirigidity drug NEC	T42.8X1	T42.8X2	T42.8X3	T42.8X4	T42.8X5	T42.8X6
Antischistosomal drug	T37.4X1	T37.4X2	T37.4X3	T37.4X4	T37.4X5	T37.4X6
Antiscorpion sera	T50.Z11	T50.Z12	T50.Z13	T50.Z14	T50.Z15	T50.Z16
Antiseborrheics	T49.4X1	T49.4X2	T49.4X3	T49.4X4	T49.4X5	T49.4X6
Antiseptics (external) (medicinal)	T49.0X1	T49.0X2	T49.0X3	T49.0X4	T49.0X5	T49.0X6
Antistine	T45.0X1	T45.0X2	T45.0X3	T45.0X4	T45.0X5	T45.0X6
Antitapeworm drug	T37.4X1	T37.4X2	T37.4X3	T37.4X4	T37.4X5	T37.4X6
Antitetanus immunoglobulin	T50.Z11	T50.Z12	T50.Z13	T50.Z14	T50.Z15	T50.Z16
Antithrombotic	T45.521	T45.522	T45.523	T45.524	T45.525	T45.526
Antithyroid drug NEC	T38.2X1	T38.2X2	T38.2X3	T38.2X4	T38.2X5	T38.2X6
Antitoxin	T50.Z11	T50.Z12	T50.Z13	T50.Z14	T50.Z15	T50.Z16
diphtheria	T50.Z11	T50.Z12	T50.Z13	T50.Z14	T50.Z15	T50.Z16
gas gangrene	T50.Z11	T50.Z12	T50.Z13	T50.Z14	T50.Z15	T50.Z16
tetanus	T50.Z11	T50.Z12	T50.Z13	T50.Z14	T50.Z15	T50.Z16
Antitrichomonal drug	T37.3X1	T37.3X2	T37.3X3	T37.3X4	T37.3X5	T37.3X6
Antituberculars	T37.1X1	T37.1X2	T37.1X3	T37.1X4	T37.1X5	T37.1X6
antibiotics	T36.5X1	T36.5X2	T36.5X3	T36.5X4	T36.5X5	T36.5X6
Antitussive NEC	T48.3X1	T48.3X2	T48.3X3	T48.3X4	T48.3X5	T48.3X6
codeine mixture	T40.2X1	T40.2X2	T40.2X3	T40.2X4	T40.2X5	T40.2X6
opiate	T40.2X1	T40.2X2	T40.2X3	T40.2X4	T40.2X5	T40.2X6
Antivaricose drug	T46.8X1	T46.8X2	T46.8X3	T46.8X4	T46.8X5	T46.8X6
Antivenin, antivenom (sera)	T50.Z11	T50.Z12	T50.Z13	T50.Z14	T50.Z15	T50.Z16
crotaline	T50.Z11	T50.Z12	T50.Z13	T50.Z14	T50.Z15	T50.Z16
spider bite	T50.Z11	T50.Z12	T50.Z13	T50.Z14	T50.Z15	T50.Z16
Antivertigo drug	T45.0X1	T45.0X2	T45.0X3	T45.0X4	T45.0X5	T45.0X6
Antiviral drug NEC	T37.5X1	T37.5X2	T37.5X3	T37.5X4	T37.5X5	T37.5X6
eye	T49.5X1	T49.5X2	T49.5X3	T49.5X4	T49.5X5	T49.5X6
Antiwhipworm drug	T37.4X1	T37.4X2	T37.4X3	T37.4X4	T37.4X5	T37.4X6
Ant poison — see Insecticide						
Antrol — see also by specific chemical substance	T60.91	T60.92	T60.93	T60.94	—	—
fungicide	T60.91	T60.92	T60.93	T60.94	—	—
ANTU (alpha naphthylthiourea)	T60.4X1	T60.4X2	T60.4X3	T60.4X4	—	—
Apalcillin	T36.0X1	T36.0X2	T36.0X3	T36.0X4	T36.0X5	T36.0X6
APC	T48.5X1	T48.5X2	T48.5X3	T48.5X4	T48.5X5	T48.5X6
Aplonidine	T44.4X1	T44.4X2	T44.4X3	T44.4X4	T44.4X5	T44.4X6
Apomorphine	T47.7X1	T47.7X2	T47.7X3	T47.7X4	T47.7X5	T47.7X6
Appetite depressants, central	T50.5X1	T50.5X2	T50.5X3	T50.5X4	T50.5X5	T50.5X6
Apraclonidine (hydrochloride)	T44.4X1	T44.4X2	T44.4X3	T44.4X4	T44.4X5	T44.4X6
Apresoline	T46.5X1	T46.5X2	T46.5X3	T46.5X4	T46.5X5	T46.5X6
Aprindine	T46.2X1	T46.2X2	T46.2X3	T46.2X4	T46.2X5	T46.2X6
Aprobarbital	T42.3X1	T42.3X2	T42.3X3	T42.3X4	T42.3X5	T42.3X6
Apronalide	T42.6X1	T42.6X2	T42.6X3	T42.6X4	T42.6X5	T42.6X6
Aprotinin	T45.621	T45.622	T45.623	T45.624	T45.625	T45.626
Aptocaine	T41.3X1	T41.3X2	T41.3X3	T41.3X4	T41.3X5	T41.3X6
Aqua fortis	T54.2X1	T54.2X2	T54.2X3	T54.2X4	—	—
Ara-A	T37.5X1	T37.5X2	T37.5X3	T37.5X4	T37.5X5	T37.5X6
Ara-C	T45.1X1	T45.1X2	T45.1X3	T45.1X4	T45.1X5	T45.1X6
Arachis oil	T49.3X1	T49.3X2	T49.3X3	T49.3X4	T49.3X5	T49.3X6
cathartic	T47.4X1	T47.4X2	T47.4X3	T47.4X4	T47.4X5	T47.4X6
Aralen	T37.2X1	T37.2X2	T37.2X3	T37.2X4	T37.2X5	T37.2X6
Arecoline	T44.1X1	T44.1X2	T44.1X3	T44.1X4	T44.1X5	T44.1X6
Arginine	T50.991	T50.992	T50.993	T50.994	T50.995	T50.996
glutamate	T50.991	T50.992	T50.993	T50.994	T50.995	T50.996
Argyrol	T49.0X1	T49.0X2	T49.0X3	T49.0X4	T49.0X5	T49.0X6
ENT agent	T49.6X1	T49.6X2	T49.6X3	T49.6X4	T49.6X5	T49.6X6
ophthalmic preparation	T49.5X1	T49.5X2	T49.5X3	T49.5X4	T49.5X5	T49.5X6
Aristocort	T38.0X1	T38.0X2	T38.0X3	T38.0X4	T38.0X5	T38.0X6
ENT agent	T49.6X1	T49.6X2	T49.6X3	T49.6X4	T49.6X5	T49.6X6
ophthalmic preparation	T49.5X1	T49.5X2	T49.5X3	T49.5X4	T49.5X5	T49.5X6

Additional Character May Be Required — Refer to the Tabular List for Character Selection   ▽ Subterms under main terms may continue to next column or page

Substance	Poisoning, Accidental (unintentional)	Poisoning, Intentional Self-harm	Poisoning, Assault	Poisoning, Undetermined	Adverse Effect	Under-dosing
Aristocort — *continued*						
topical NEC	T49.0X1	T49.0X2	T49.0X3	T49.0X4	T49.0X5	T49.0X6
Aromatics, corrosive	T54.1X1	T54.1X2	T54.1X3	T54.1X4	—	—
disinfectants	T54.1X1	T54.1X2	T54.1X3	T54.1X4	—	—
Arsenate of lead	T57.0X1	T57.0X2	T57.0X3	T57.0X4	—	—
herbicide	T57.0X1	T57.0X2	T57.0X3	T57.0X4	—	—
Arsenic, arsenicals (compounds) (dust) (vapor) **NEC**	T57.0X1	T57.0X2	T57.0X3	T57.0X4	—	—
anti-infectives	T37.8X1	T37.8X2	T37.8X3	T37.8X4	T37.8X5	T37.8X6
pesticide (dust) (fumes)	T57.0X1	T57.0X2	T57.0X3	T57.0X4	—	—
Arsine (gas)	T57.0X1	T57.0X2	T57.0X3	T57.0X4	—	—
Arsphenamine (silver)	T37.8X1	T37.8X2	T37.8X3	T37.8X4	T37.8X5	T37.8X6
Arsthinol	T37.3X1	T37.3X2	T37.3X3	T37.3X4	T37.3X5	T37.3X6
Artane	T44.3X1	T44.3X2	T44.3X3	T44.3X4	T44.3X5	T44.3X6
Arthropod (venomous) **NEC**	T63.481	T63.482	T63.483	T63.484	—	—
Articaine	T41.3X1	T41.3X2	T41.3X3	T41.3X4	T41.3X5	T41.3X6
Asbestos	T57.8X1	T57.8X2	T57.8X3	T57.8X4	—	—
Ascaridole	T37.4X1	T37.4X2	T37.4X3	T37.4X4	T37.4X5	T37.4X6
Ascorbic acid	T45.2X1	T45.2X2	T45.2X3	T45.2X4	T45.2X5	T45.2X6
Asiaticoside	T49.0X1	T49.0X2	T49.0X3	T49.0X4	T49.0X5	T49.0X6
Asparaginase	T45.1X1	T45.1X2	T45.1X3	T45.1X4	T45.1X5	T45.1X6
Aspidium (oleoresin)	T37.4X1	T37.4X2	T37.4X3	T37.4X4	T37.4X5	T37.4X6
Aspirin (aluminum)	T39.011	T39.012	T39.013	T39.014	T39.015	T39.016
(soluble)						
Aspoxicillin	T36.0X1	T36.0X2	T36.0X3	T36.0X4	T36.0X5	T36.0X6
Astemizole	T45.0X1	T45.0X2	T45.0X3	T45.0X4	T45.0X5	T45.0X6
Astringent (local)	T49.2X1	T49.2X2	T49.2X3	T49.2X4	T49.2X5	T49.2X6
specified NEC	T49.2X1	T49.2X2	T49.2X3	T49.2X4	T49.2X5	T49.2X6
Astromicin	T36.5X1	T36.5X2	T36.5X3	T36.5X4	T36.5X5	T36.5X6
Ataractic drug NEC	T43.501	T43.502	T43.503	T43.504	T43.505	T43.506
Atenolol	T44.7X1	T44.7X2	T44.7X3	T44.7X4	T44.7X5	T44.7X6
Atonia drug, intestinal	T47.4X1	T47.4X2	T47.4X3	T47.4X4	T47.4X5	T47.4X6
Atophan	T50.4X1	T50.4X2	T50.4X3	T50.4X4	T50.4X5	T50.4X6
Atracurium besilate	T48.1X1	T48.1X2	T48.1X3	T48.1X4	T48.1X5	T48.1X6
Atropine	T44.3X1	T44.3X2	T44.3X3	T44.3X4	T44.3X5	T44.3X6
derivative	T44.3X1	T44.3X2	T44.3X3	T44.3X4	T44.3X5	T44.3X6
methonitrate	T44.3X1	T44.3X2	T44.3X3	T44.3X4	T44.3X5	T44.3X6
Attapulgite	T47.6X1	T47.6X2	T47.6X3	T47.6X4	T47.6X5	T47.6X6
Auramine	T65.891	T65.892	T65.893	T65.894	—	—
dye	T65.6X1	T65.6X2	T65.6X3	T65.6X4	—	—
fungicide	T60.3X1	T60.3X2	T60.3X3	T60.3X4	—	—
Auranofin	T39.4X1	T39.4X2	T39.4X3	T39.4X4	T39.4X5	T39.4X6
Aurantiin	T46.991	T46.992	T46.993	T46.994	T46.995	T46.996
Aureomycin	T36.4X1	T36.4X2	T36.4X3	T36.4X4	T36.4X5	T36.4X6
ophthalmic preparation	T49.5X1	T49.5X2	T49.5X3	T49.5X4	T49.5X5	T49.5X6
topical NEC	T49.0X1	T49.0X2	T49.0X3	T49.0X4	T49.0X5	T49.0X6
Aurothioglucose	T39.4X1	T39.4X2	T39.4X3	T39.4X4	T39.4X5	T39.4X6
Aurothioglycanide	T39.4X1	T39.4X2	T39.4X3	T39.4X4	T39.4X5	T39.4X6
Aurothiomalate sodium	T39.4X1	T39.4X2	T39.4X3	T39.4X4	T39.4X5	T39.4X6
Aurotioprol	T39.4X1	T39.4X2	T39.4X3	T39.4X4	T39.4X5	T39.4X6
Automobile fuel	T52.0X1	T52.0X2	T52.0X3	T52.0X4	—	—
Autonomic nervous system agent NEC	T44.901	T44.902	T44.903	T44.904	T44.905	T44.906
Avlosulfon	T37.1X1	T37.1X2	T37.1X3	T37.1X4	T37.1X5	T37.1X6
Avomine	T42.6X1	T42.6X2	T42.6X3	T42.6X4	T42.6X5	T42.6X6
Axerophthol	T45.2X1	T45.2X2	T45.2X3	T45.2X4	T45.2X5	T45.2X6
Azacitidine	T45.1X1	T45.1X2	T45.1X3	T45.1X4	T45.1X5	T45.1X6
Azacyclonol	T43.591	T43.592	T43.593	T43.594	T43.595	T43.596
Azadirachta	T60.2X1	T60.2X2	T60.2X3	T60.2X4	—	—
Azanidazole	T37.3X1	T37.3X2	T37.3X3	T37.3X4	T37.3X5	T37.3X6
Azapetine	T46.7X1	T46.7X2	T46.7X3	T46.7X4	T46.7X5	T46.7X6
Azapropazone	T39.2X1	T39.2X2	T39.2X3	T39.2X4	T39.2X5	T39.2X6
Azaribine	T45.1X1	T45.1X2	T45.1X3	T45.1X4	T45.1X5	T45.1X6
Azaserine	T45.1X1	T45.1X2	T45.1X3	T45.1X4	T45.1X5	T45.1X6
Azatadine	T45.0X1	T45.0X2	T45.0X3	T45.0X4	T45.0X5	T45.0X6
Azatepa	T45.1X1	T45.1X2	T45.1X3	T45.1X4	T45.1X5	T45.1X6
Azathioprine	T45.1X1	T45.1X2	T45.1X3	T45.1X4	T45.1X5	T45.1X6
Azelaic acid	T49.0X1	T49.0X2	T49.0X3	T49.0X4	T49.0X5	T49.0X6
Azelastine	T45.0X1	T45.0X2	T45.0X3	T45.0X4	T45.0X5	T45.0X6
Azidocillin	T36.0X1	T36.0X2	T36.0X3	T36.0X4	T36.0X5	T36.0X6
Azidothymidine	T37.5X1	T37.5X2	T37.5X3	T37.5X4	T37.5X5	T37.5X6
Azinphos (ethyl) (methyl)	T60.0X1	T60.0X2	T60.0X3	T60.0X4	—	—
Aziridine (chelating)	T54.1X1	T54.1X2	T54.1X3	T54.1X4	—	—
Azithromycin	T36.3X1	T36.3X2	T36.3X3	T36.3X4	T36.3X5	T36.3X6
Azlocillin	T36.0X1	T36.0X2	T36.0X3	T36.0X4	T36.0X5	T36.0X6
Azobenzene smoke	T65.3X1	T65.3X2	T65.3X3	T65.3X4	—	—
acaricide	T60.8X1	T60.8X2	T60.8X3	T60.8X4	—	—
Azosulfamide	T37.0X1	T37.0X2	T37.0X3	T37.0X4	T37.0X5	T37.0X6
AZT	T37.5X1	T37.5X2	T37.5X3	T37.5X4	T37.5X5	T37.5X6
Aztreonam	T36.1X1	T36.1X2	T36.1X3	T36.1X4	T36.1X5	T36.1X6
Azulfidine	T37.0X1	T37.0X2	T37.0X3	T37.0X4	T37.0X5	T37.0X6
Azuresin	T50.8X1	T50.8X2	T50.8X3	T50.8X4	T50.8X5	T50.8X6
b-acetyldigoxin	T46.0X1	T46.0X2	T46.0X3	T46.0X4	T46.0X5	T46.0X6
P-Acetamidophenol	T39.1X1	T39.1X2	T39.1X3	T39.1X4	T39.1X5	T39.1X6
Bacampicillin	T36.0X1	T36.0X2	T36.0X3	T36.0X4	T36.0X5	T36.0X6
Bacillus						
lactobacillus	T47.8X1	T47.8X2	T47.8X3	T47.8X4	T47.8X5	T47.8X6
subtilis	T47.6X1	T47.6X2	T47.6X3	T47.6X4	T47.6X5	T47.6X6
Bacimycin	T49.0X1	T49.0X2	T49.0X3	T49.0X4	T49.0X5	T49.0X6
ophthalmic preparation	T49.5X1	T49.5X2	T49.5X3	T49.5X4	T49.5X5	T49.5X6
Bacitracin zinc	T49.0X1	T49.0X2	T49.0X3	T49.0X4	T49.0X5	T49.0X6
with neomycin	T49.0X1	T49.0X2	T49.0X3	T49.0X4	T49.0X5	T49.0X6
ENT agent	T49.6X1	T49.6X2	T49.6X3	T49.6X4	T49.6X5	T49.6X6
ophthalmic preparation	T49.5X1	T49.5X2	T49.5X3	T49.5X4	T49.5X5	T49.5X6
topical NEC	T49.0X1	T49.0X2	T49.0X3	T49.0X4	T49.0X5	T49.0X6
Baclofen	T42.8X1	T42.8X2	T42.8X3	T42.8X4	T42.8X5	T42.8X6
Baking soda	T50.991	T50.992	T50.993	T50.994	T50.995	T50.996
BAL	T45.8X1	T45.8X2	T45.8X3	T45.8X4	T45.8X5	T45.8X6
Bambuterol	T48.6X1	T48.6X2	T48.6X3	T48.6X4	T48.6X5	T48.6X6
Bamethan (sulfate)	T46.7X1	T46.7X2	T46.7X3	T46.7X4	T46.7X5	T46.7X6
Bamifylline	T48.6X1	T48.6X2	T48.6X3	T48.6X4	T48.6X5	T48.6X6
Bamipine	T45.0X1	T45.0X2	T45.0X3	T45.0X4	T45.0X5	T45.0X6
Baneberry — *see Actaea spicata*						
Banewort — *see Belladonna*						
Barbenyl	T42.3X1	T42.3X2	T42.3X3	T42.3X4	T42.3X5	T42.3X6
Barbexaclone	T42.6X1	T42.6X2	T42.6X3	T42.6X4	T42.6X5	T42.6X6
Barbital	T42.3X1	T42.3X2	T42.3X3	T42.3X4	T42.3X5	T42.3X6
sodium	T42.3X1	T42.3X2	T42.3X3	T42.3X4	T42.3X5	T42.3X6
Barbitone	T42.3X1	T42.3X2	T42.3X3	T42.3X4	T42.3X5	T42.3X6
Barbiturate NEC	T42.3X1	T42.3X2	T42.3X3	T42.3X4	T42.3X5	T42.3X6
with tranquilizer	T42.3X1	T42.3X2	T42.3X3	T42.3X4	T42.3X5	T42.3X6
anesthetic (intravenous)	T41.1X1	T41.1X2	T41.1X3	T41.1X4	T41.1X5	T41.1X6
Barium (carbonate) (chloride) (sulfite)	T57.8X1	T57.8X2	T57.8X3	T57.8X4	—	—
diagnostic agent	T50.8X1	T50.8X2	T50.8X3	T50.8X4	T50.8X5	T50.8X6
pesticide	T60.4X1	T60.4X2	T60.4X3	T60.4X4	—	—
rodenticide	T60.4X1	T60.4X2	T60.4X3	T60.4X4	—	—
sulfate (medicinal)	T50.8X1	T50.8X2	T50.8X3	T50.8X4	T50.8X5	T50.8X6
Barrier cream	T49.3X1	T49.3X2	T49.3X3	T49.3X4	T49.3X5	T49.3X6
Basic fuchsin	T49.0X1	T49.0X2	T49.0X3	T49.0X4	T49.0X5	T49.0X6
Battery acid or fluid	T54.2X1	T54.2X2	T54.2X3	T54.2X4	—	—
Bay rum	T51.8X1	T51.8X2	T51.8X3	T51.8X4	—	—
b-benzalbutyramide	T46.6X1	T46.6X2	T46.6X3	T46.6X4	T46.6X5	T46.6X6
BCG (vaccine)	T50.A91	T50.A92	T50.A93	T50.A94	T50.A95	T50.A96
BCNU	T45.1X1	T45.1X2	T45.1X3	T45.1X4	T45.1X5	T45.1X6
Bearsfoot	T62.2X1	T62.2X2	T62.2X3	T62.2X4	—	—
Beclamide	T42.6X1	T42.6X2	T42.6X3	T42.6X4	T42.6X5	T42.6X6
Beclomethasone	T44.5X1	T44.5X2	T44.5X3	T44.5X4	T44.5X5	T44.5X6
Bee (sting) (venom)	T63.441	T63.442	T63.443	T63.444	—	—
Befunolol	T49.5X1	T49.5X2	T49.5X3	T49.5X4	T49.5X5	T49.5X6
Bekanamycin	T36.5X1	T36.5X2	T36.5X3	T36.5X4	T36.5X5	T36.5X6
Belladonna — *see also* Nightshade						
alkaloids	T44.3X1	T44.3X2	T44.3X3	T44.3X4	T44.3X5	T44.3X6
extract	T44.3X1	T44.3X2	T44.3X3	T44.3X4	T44.3X5	T44.3X6
herb	T44.3X1	T44.3X2	T44.3X3	T44.3X4	T44.3X5	T44.3X6
Bemegride	T50.7X1	T50.7X2	T50.7X3	T50.7X4	T50.7X5	T50.7X6
Benactyzine	T44.3X1	T44.3X2	T44.3X3	T44.3X4	T44.3X5	T44.3X6
Benadryl	T45.0X1	T45.0X2	T45.0X3	T45.0X4	T45.0X5	T45.0X6
Benaprizine	T44.3X1	T44.3X2	T44.3X3	T44.3X4	T44.3X5	T44.3X6
Benazepril	T46.4X1	T46.4X2	T46.4X3	T46.4X4	T46.4X5	T46.4X6
Bencyclane	T46.7X1	T46.7X2	T46.7X3	T46.7X4	T46.7X5	T46.7X6
Bendazol	T46.3X1	T46.3X2	T46.3X3	T46.3X4	T46.3X5	T46.3X6
Bendrofluazide	T50.2X1	T50.2X2	T50.2X3	T50.2X4	T50.2X5	T50.2X6
Bendroflumethiazide	T50.2X1	T50.2X2	T50.2X3	T50.2X4	T50.2X5	T50.2X6
Benemid	T50.4X1	T50.4X2	T50.4X3	T50.4X4	T50.4X5	T50.4X6
Benethamine penicillin	T36.0X1	T36.0X2	T36.0X3	T36.0X4	T36.0X5	T36.0X6
Benexate	T47.1X1	T47.1X2	T47.1X3	T47.1X4	T47.1X5	T47.1X6
Benfluorex	T46.6X1	T46.6X2	T46.6X3	T46.6X4	T46.6X5	T46.6X6
Benfotiamine	T45.2X1	T45.2X2	T45.2X3	T45.2X4	T45.2X5	T45.2X6
Benisone	T49.0X1	T49.0X2	T49.0X3	T49.0X4	T49.0X5	T49.0X6
Benomyl	T60.0X1	T60.0X2	T60.0X3	T60.0X4	—	—
Benoquin	T49.8X1	T49.8X2	T49.8X3	T49.8X4	T49.8X5	T49.8X6
Benoxinate	T41.3X1	T41.3X2	T41.3X3	T41.3X4	T41.3X5	T41.3X6
Benperidol	T43.4X1	T43.4X2	T43.4X3	T43.4X4	T43.4X5	T43.4X6
Benproperine	T48.3X1	T48.3X2	T48.3X3	T48.3X4	T48.3X5	T48.3X6
Benserazide	T42.8X1	T42.8X2	T42.8X3	T42.8X4	T42.8X5	T42.8X6
Bentazepam	T42.4X1	T42.4X2	T42.4X3	T42.4X4	T42.4X5	T42.4X6
Bentiromide	T50.8X1	T50.8X2	T50.8X3	T50.8X4	T50.8X5	T50.8X6
Bentonite	T49.3X1	T49.3X2	T49.3X3	T49.3X4	T49.3X5	T49.3X6
Benzalbutyramide	T46.6X1	T46.6X2	T46.6X3	T46.6X4	T46.6X5	T46.6X6
Benzalkonium (chloride)	T49.0X1	T49.0X2	T49.0X3	T49.0X4	T49.0X5	T49.0X6
ophthalmic preparation	T49.5X1	T49.5X2	T49.5X3	T49.5X4	T49.5X5	T49.5X6
Benzamidosalicylate (calcium)	T37.1X1	T37.1X2	T37.1X3	T37.1X4	T37.1X5	T37.1X6
Benzamine	T41.3X1	T41.3X2	T41.3X3	T41.3X4	T41.3X5	T41.3X6

Subterms under main terms may continue to next column or page   Additional Character May Be Required — Refer to the Tabular List for Character Selection

Substance	Poisoning, Accidental (unintentional)	Poisoning, Intentional Self-harm	Poisoning, Assault	Poisoning, Undetermined	Adverse Effect	Under-dosing
Benzamine — *continued*						
lactate	T49.1X1	T49.1X2	T49.1X3	T49.1X4	T49.1X5	T49.1X6
Benzamphetamine	T50.5X1	T50.5X2	T50.5X3	T50.5X4	T50.5X5	T50.5X6
Benzapril hydrochloride	T46.5X1	T46.5X2	T46.5X3	T46.5X4	T46.5X5	T46.5X6
Benzathine	T36.0X1	T36.0X2	T36.0X3	T36.0X4	T36.0X5	T36.0X6
benzylpenicillin						
Benzathine penicillin	T36.0X1	T36.0X2	T36.0X3	T36.0X4	T36.0X5	T36.0X6
Benzatropine	T42.8X1	T42.8X2	T42.8X3	T42.8X4	T42.8X5	T42.8X6
Benzbromarone	T50.4X1	T50.4X2	T50.4X3	T50.4X4	T50.4X5	T50.4X6
Benzcarbimine	T45.1X1	T45.1X2	T45.1X3	T45.1X4	T45.1X5	T45.1X6
Benzedrex	T44.991	T44.992	T44.993	T44.994	T44.995	T44.996
Benzedrine (amphetamine)	T43.621	T43.622	T43.623	T43.624	T43.625	T43.626
Benzenamine	T65.891	T65.892	T65.893	T65.894	—	—
Benzene	T52.1X1	T52.1X2	T52.1X3	T52.1X4	—	—
homologues (acetyl) (dimethyl) (methyl) (solvent)	T52.2X1	T52.2X2	T52.2X3	T52.2X4	—	—
Benzethonium (chloride)	T49.0X1	T49.0X2	T49.0X3	T49.0X4	T49.0X5	T49.0X6
Benzfetamine	T50.5X1	T50.5X2	T50.5X3	T50.5X4	T50.5X5	T50.5X6
Benzhexol	T44.3X1	T44.3X2	T44.3X3	T44.3X4	T44.3X5	T44.3X6
Benzhydramine (chloride)	T45.0X1	T45.0X2	T45.0X3	T45.0X4	T45.0X5	T45.0X6
Benzidine	T65.891	T65.892	T65.893	T65.894	—	—
Benzilonium bromide	T44.3X1	T44.3X2	T44.3X3	T44.3X4	T44.3X5	T44.3X6
Benzimidazole	T60.3X1	T60.3X2	T60.3X3	T60.3X4	—	—
Benzin (e) — *see* Ligroin						
Benziodarone	T46.3X1	T46.3X2	T46.3X3	T46.3X4	T46.3X5	T46.3X6
Benznidazole	T37.3X1	T37.3X2	T37.3X3	T37.3X4	T37.3X5	T37.3X6
Benzocaine	T41.3X1	T41.3X2	T41.3X3	T41.3X4	T41.3X5	T41.3X6
Benzodiapin	T42.4X1	T42.4X2	T42.4X3	T42.4X4	T42.4X5	T42.4X6
Benzodiazepine NEC	T42.4X1	T42.4X2	T42.4X3	T42.4X4	T42.4X5	T42.4X6
Benzoic acid	T49.0X1	T49.0X2	T49.0X3	T49.0X4	T49.0X5	T49.0X6
with salicylic acid	T49.0X1	T49.0X2	T49.0X3	T49.0X4	T49.0X5	T49.0X6
Benzoin (tincture)	T48.5X1	T48.5X2	T48.5X3	T48.5X4	T48.5X5	T48.5X6
Benzol (benzene)	T52.1X1	T52.1X2	T52.1X3	T52.1X4	—	—
vapor	T52.0X1	T52.0X2	T52.0X3	T52.0X4	—	—
Benzomorphan	T40.2X1	T40.2X2	T40.2X3	T40.2X4	T40.2X5	T40.2X6
Benzonatate	T48.3X1	T48.3X2	T48.3X3	T48.3X4	T48.3X5	T48.3X6
Benzophenones	T49.3X1	T49.3X2	T49.3X3	T49.3X4	T49.3X5	T49.3X6
Benzopyrone	T46.991	T46.992	T46.993	T46.994	T46.995	T46.996
Benzothiadiazides	T50.2X1	T50.2X2	T50.2X3	T50.2X4	T50.2X5	T50.2X6
Benzoxonium chloride	T49.0X1	T49.0X2	T49.0X3	T49.0X4	T49.0X5	T49.0X6
Benzoylpas calcium	T37.1X1	T37.1X2	T37.1X3	T37.1X4	T37.1X5	T37.1X6
Benzoyl peroxide	T49.0X1	T49.0X2	T49.0X3	T49.0X4	T49.0X5	T49.0X6
Benzperidin	T43.591	T43.592	T43.593	T43.594	T43.595	T43.596
Benzperidol	T43.591	T43.592	T43.593	T43.594	T43.595	T43.596
Benzphetamine	T50.5X1	T50.5X2	T50.5X3	T50.5X4	T50.5X5	T50.5X6
Benzpyrinium bromide	T44.1X1	T44.1X2	T44.1X3	T44.1X4	T44.1X5	T44.1X6
Benzquinamide	T45.0X1	T45.0X2	T45.0X3	T45.0X4	T45.0X5	T45.0X6
Benzthiazide	T50.2X1	T50.2X2	T50.2X3	T50.2X4	T50.2X5	T50.2X6
Benztropine						
anticholinergic	T44.3X1	T44.3X2	T44.3X3	T44.3X4	T44.3X5	T44.3X6
antiparkinson	T42.8X1	T42.8X2	T42.8X3	T42.8X4	T42.8X5	T42.8X6
Benzydamine	T49.0X1	T49.0X2	T49.0X3	T49.0X4	T49.0X5	T49.0X6
Benzyl						
acetate	T52.8X1	T52.8X2	T52.8X3	T52.8X4	—	—
alcohol	T49.0X1	T49.0X2	T49.0X3	T49.0X4	T49.0X5	T49.0X6
benzoate	T49.0X1	T49.0X2	T49.0X3	T49.0X4	T49.0X5	T49.0X6
Benzoic acid	T49.0X1	T49.0X2	T49.0X3	T49.0X4	T49.0X5	T49.0X6
morphine	T40.2X1	T40.2X2	T40.2X3	T40.2X4	—	—
nicotinate	T46.6X1	T46.6X2	T46.6X3	T46.6X4	T46.6X5	T46.6X6
penicillin	T36.0X1	T36.0X2	T36.0X3	T36.0X4	T36.0X5	T36.0X6
Benzylhydrochlorthiazide	T50.2X1	T50.2X2	T50.2X3	T50.2X4	T50.2X5	T50.2X6
Benzylpenicillin	T36.0X1	T36.0X2	T36.0X3	T36.0X4	T36.0X5	T36.0X6
Benzylthiouracil	T38.2X1	T38.2X2	T38.2X3	T38.2X4	T38.2X5	T38.2X6
Bephenium	T37.4X1	T37.4X2	T37.4X3	T37.4X4	T37.4X5	T37.4X6
hydroxynaphthoate						
Bepridil	T46.1X1	T46.1X2	T46.1X3	T46.1X4	T46.1X5	T46.1X6
Bergamot oil	T65.891	T65.892	T65.893	T65.894	—	—
Bergapten	T50.991	T50.992	T50.993	T50.994	T50.995	T50.996
Berries, poisonous	T62.1X1	T62.1X2	T62.1X3	T62.1X4	—	—
Beryllium (compounds)	T56.7X1	T56.7X2	T56.7X3	T56.7X4	—	—
beta adrenergic blocking agent, heart	T44.7X1	T44.7X2	T44.7X3	T44.7X4	T44.7X5	T44.7X6
Betacarotene	T45.2X1	T45.2X2	T45.2X3	T45.2X4	T45.2X5	T45.2X6
Beta-Chlor	T42.6X1	T42.6X2	T42.6X3	T42.6X4	T42.6X5	T42.6X6
Betahistine	T46.7X1	T46.7X2	T46.7X3	T46.7X4	T46.7X5	T46.7X6
Betaine	T47.5X1	T47.5X2	T47.5X3	T47.5X4	T47.5X5	T47.5X6
Betamethasone	T49.0X1	T49.0X2	T49.0X3	T49.0X4	T49.0X5	T49.0X6
topical	T49.0X1	T49.0X2	T49.0X3	T49.0X4	T49.0X5	T49.0X6
Betamicin	T36.8X1	T36.8X2	T36.8X3	T36.8X4	T36.8X5	T36.8X6
Betanidine	T46.5X1	T46.5X2	T46.5X3	T46.5X4	T46.5X5	T46.5X6
Betaxolol	T44.7X1	T44.7X2	T44.7X3	T44.7X4	T44.7X5	T44.7X6
Betazole	T50.8X1	T50.8X2	T50.8X3	T50.8X4	T50.8X5	T50.8X6
Bethanechol	T44.1X1	T44.1X2	T44.1X3	T44.1X4	T44.1X5	T44.1X6

Substance	Poisoning, Accidental (unintentional)	Poisoning, Intentional Self-harm	Poisoning, Assault	Poisoning, Undetermined	Adverse Effect	Under-dosing
Bethanechol — *continued*						
chloride	T44.1X1	T44.1X2	T44.1X3	T44.1X4	T44.1X5	T44.1X6
Bethanidine	T46.5X1	T46.5X2	T46.5X3	T46.5X4	T46.5X5	T46.5X6
Betoxycaine	T41.3X1	T41.3X2	T41.3X3	T41.3X4	T41.3X5	T41.3X6
Betula oil	T49.3X1	T49.3X2	T49.3X3	T49.3X4	T49.3X5	T49.3X6
Bevantolol	T44.7X1	T44.7X2	T44.7X3	T44.7X4	T44.7X5	T44.7X6
Bevonium metilsulfate	T44.3X1	T44.3X2	T44.3X3	T44.3X4	T44.3X5	T44.3X6
Bezafibrate	T46.6X1	T46.6X2	T46.6X3	T46.6X4	T46.6X5	T46.6X6
Bezitramide	T40.491	T40.492	T40.493	T40.494	T40.495	T40.496
BHA	T50.991	T50.992	T50.993	T50.994	T50.995	T50.996
Bhang	T40.7X1	T40.7X2	T40.7X3	T40.7X4	T40.7X5	T40.7X6
BHC (medicinal)	T49.0X1	T49.0X2	T49.0X3	T49.0X4	T49.0X5	T49.0X6
nonmedicinal (vapor)	T53.6X1	T53.6X2	T53.6X3	T53.6X4	—	—
Bialamicol	T37.3X1	T37.3X2	T37.3X3	T37.3X4	T37.3X5	T37.3X6
Bibenzonium bromide	T48.3X1	T48.3X2	T48.3X3	T48.3X4	T48.3X5	T48.3X6
Bibrocathol	T49.5X1	T49.5X2	T49.5X3	T49.5X4	T49.5X5	T49.5X6
Bichloride of mercury — *see* Mercury, chloride						
Bichromates (calcium) (potassium)(sodium) (crystals)	T57.8X1	T57.8X2	T57.8X3	T57.8X4	—	—
fumes	T56.2X1	T56.2X2	T56.2X3	T56.2X4	—	—
Biclotymol	T49.6X1	T49.6X2	T49.6X3	T49.6X4	T49.6X5	T49.6X6
Bicucculine	T50.7X1	T50.7X2	T50.7X3	T50.7X4	T50.7X5	T50.7X6
Bifemelane	T43.291	T43.292	T43.293	T43.294	T43.295	T43.296
Biguanide derivatives, oral	T38.3X1	T38.3X2	T38.3X3	T38.3X4	T38.3X5	T38.3X6
Bile salts	T47.5X1	T47.5X2	T47.5X3	T47.5X4	T47.5X5	T47.5X6
Biligrafin	T50.8X1	T50.8X2	T50.8X3	T50.8X4	T50.8X5	T50.8X6
Bilopaque	T50.8X1	T50.8X2	T50.8X3	T50.8X4	T50.8X5	T50.8X6
Binifibrate	T46.6X1	T46.6X2	T46.6X3	T46.6X4	T46.6X5	T46.6X6
Binitrobenzol	T65.3X1	T65.3X2	T65.3X3	T65.3X4	—	—
Bioflavonoid(s)	T46.991	T46.992	T46.993	T46.994	T46.995	T46.996
Biological substance NEC	T50.901	T50.902	T50.903	T50.904	T50.905	T50.906
Biotin	T45.2X1	T45.2X2	T45.2X3	T45.2X4	T45.2X5	T45.2X6
Biperiden	T44.3X1	T44.3X2	T44.3X3	T44.3X4	T44.3X5	T44.3X6
Bisacodyl	T47.2X1	T47.2X2	T47.2X3	T47.2X4	T47.2X5	T47.2X6
Bisbentiamine	T45.2X1	T45.2X2	T45.2X3	T45.2X4	T45.2X5	T45.2X6
Bisbutiamine	T45.2X1	T45.2X2	T45.2X3	T45.2X4	T45.2X5	T45.2X6
Bisdequalinium (salts) (diacetate)	T49.6X1	T49.6X2	T49.6X3	T49.6X4	T49.6X5	T49.6X6
Bishydroxycoumarin	T45.511	T45.512	T45.513	T45.514	T45.515	T45.516
Bismarsen	T37.8X1	T37.8X2	T37.8X3	T37.8X4	T37.8X5	T37.8X6
Bismuth salts	T47.6X1	T47.6X2	T47.6X3	T47.6X4	T47.6X5	T47.6X6
aluminate	T47.1X1	T47.1X2	T47.1X3	T47.1X4	T47.1X5	T47.1X6
anti-infectives	T37.8X1	T37.8X2	T37.8X3	T37.8X4	T37.8X5	T37.8X6
formic iodide	T49.0X1	T49.0X2	T49.0X3	T49.0X4	T49.0X5	T49.0X6
glycolylarsenate	T49.0X1	T49.0X2	T49.0X3	T49.0X4	T49.0X5	T49.0X6
nonmedicinal (compounds) NEC	T65.91	T65.92	T65.93	T65.94	—	—
subcarbonate	T47.6X1	T47.6X2	T47.6X3	T47.6X4	T47.6X5	T47.6X6
subsalicylate	T37.8X1	T37.8X2	T37.8X3	T37.8X4	T37.8X5	T37.8X6
sulfarsphenamine	T37.8X1	T37.8X2	T37.8X3	T37.8X4	T37.8X5	T37.8X6
Bisoprolol	T44.7X1	T44.7X2	T44.7X3	T44.7X4	T44.7X5	T44.7X6
Bisoxatin	T47.2X1	T47.2X2	T47.2X3	T47.2X4	T47.2X5	T47.2X6
Bisulepin (hydrochloride)	T45.0X1	T45.0X2	T45.0X3	T45.0X4	T45.0X5	T45.0X6
Bithionol	T37.8X1	T37.8X2	T37.8X3	T37.8X4	T37.8X5	T37.8X6
anthelminthic	T37.4X1	T37.4X2	T37.4X3	T37.4X4	T37.4X5	T37.4X6
Bitolterol	T48.6X1	T48.6X2	T48.6X3	T48.6X4	T48.6X5	T48.6X6
Bitoscanate	T37.4X1	T37.4X2	T37.4X3	T37.4X4	T37.4X5	T37.4X6
Bitter almond oil	T62.8X1	T62.8X2	T62.8X3	T62.8X4	—	—
Bittersweet	T62.2X1	T62.2X2	T62.2X3	T62.2X4	—	—
Black						
flag	T60.91	T60.92	T60.93	T60.94	—	—
henbane	T62.2X1	T62.2X2	T62.2X3	T62.2X4	—	—
leaf (40)	T60.91	T60.92	T60.93	T60.94	—	—
widow spider (bite)	T63.311	T63.312	T63.313	T63.314	—	—
Blast furnace gas (carbon monoxide from)	T58.8X1	T58.8X2	T58.8X3	T58.8X4	—	—
Bleach	T54.91	T54.92	T54.93	T54.94	—	—
Bleaching agent (medicinal)	T49.4X1	T49.4X2	T49.4X3	T49.4X4	T49.4X5	T49.4X6
Bleomycin	T45.1X1	T45.1X2	T45.1X3	T45.1X4	T45.1X5	T45.1X6
Blockain	T41.3X1	T41.3X2	T41.3X3	T41.3X4	T41.3X5	T41.3X6
infiltration (subcutaneous)	T41.3X1	T41.3X2	T41.3X3	T41.3X4	T41.3X5	T41.3X6
nerve block (peripheral) (plexus)	T41.3X1	T41.3X2	T41.3X3	T41.3X4	T41.3X5	T41.3X6
topical (surface)	T41.3X1	T41.3X2	T41.3X3	T41.3X4	T41.3X5	T41.3X6
Blockers, calcium channel	T46.1X1	T46.1X2	T46.1X3	T46.1X4	T46.1X5	T46.1X6
Blood (derivatives) (natural) (plasma) (whole)	T45.8X1	T45.8X2	T45.8X3	T45.8X4	T45.8X5	T45.8X6
dried	T45.8X1	T45.8X2	T45.8X3	T45.8X4	T45.8X5	T45.8X6

Note: Blocks continue — **Biotest**/**Bisulepin** entries also reference Z-codes:
| widow spider (bite) | T50.Z11 | T50.Z12 | T50.Z13 | T50.Z14 | T50.Z15 | T50.Z16 |

Substance	Poisoning, Accidental (unintentional)	Poisoning, Intentional Self-harm	Poisoning, Assault	Poisoning, Undetermined	Adverse Effect	Under-dosing
Blood — continued						
drug affecting NEC	T45.91	T45.92	T45.93	T45.94	T45.95	T45.96
expander NEC	T45.8X1	T45.8X2	T45.8X3	T45.8X4	T45.8X5	T45.8X6
fraction NEC	T45.8X1	T45.8X2	T45.8X3	T45.8X4	T45.8X5	T45.8X6
substitute (macromolecular)	T45.8X1	T45.8X2	T45.8X3	T45.8X4	T45.8X5	T45.8X6
Blue velvet	T40.2X1	T40.2X2	T40.2X3	T40.2X4	—	—
Bone meal	T62.8X1	T62.8X2	T62.8X3	T62.8X4	—	—
Bonine	T45.0X1	T45.0X2	T45.0X3	T45.0X4	T45.0X5	T45.0X6
Bopindolol	T44.7X1	T44.7X2	T44.7X3	T44.7X4	T44.7X5	T44.7X6
Boracic acid	T49.0X1	T49.0X2	T49.0X3	T49.0X4	T49.0X5	T49.0X6
ENT agent	T49.6X1	T49.6X2	T49.6X3	T49.6X4	T49.6X5	T49.6X6
ophthalmic preparation	T49.5X1	T49.5X2	T49.5X3	T49.5X4	T49.5X5	T49.5X6
Borane complex	T57.8X1	T57.8X2	T57.8X3	T57.8X4	—	—
Borate(s)	T57.8X1	T57.8X2	T57.8X3	T57.8X4	—	—
buffer	T50.991	T50.992	T50.993	T50.994	T50.995	T50.996
cleanser	T54.91	T54.92	T54.93	T54.94	—	—
sodium	T57.8X1	T57.8X2	T57.8X3	T57.8X4	—	—
Borax (cleanser)	T54.91	T54.92	T54.93	T54.94	—	—
Bordeaux mixture	T60.3X1	T60.3X2	T60.3X3	T60.3X4	—	—
Boric acid	T49.0X1	T49.0X2	T49.0X3	T49.0X4	T49.0X5	T49.0X6
ENT agent	T49.6X1	T49.6X2	T49.6X3	T49.6X4	T49.6X5	T49.6X6
ophthalmic preparation	T49.5X1	T49.5X2	T49.5X3	T49.5X4	T49.5X5	T49.5X6
Bornaprine	T44.3X1	T44.3X2	T44.3X3	T44.3X4	T44.3X5	T44.3X6
Boron	T57.8X1	T57.8X2	T57.8X3	T57.8X4	—	—
hydride NEC	T57.8X1	T57.8X2	T57.8X3	T57.8X4	—	—
fumes or gas	T57.8X1	T57.8X2	T57.8X3	T57.8X4	—	—
trifluoride	T59.891	T59.892	T59.893	T59.894	—	—
Botox	T48.291	T48.292	T48.293	T48.294	T48.295	T48.296
Botulinus anti-toxin (type A, B)	T50.Z11	T50.Z12	T50.Z13	T50.Z14	T50.Z15	T50.Z16
Brake fluid vapor	T59.891	T59.892	T59.893	T59.894	—	—
Brallobarbital	T42.3X1	T42.3X2	T42.3X3	T42.3X4	T42.3X5	T42.3X6
Bran (wheat)	T47.4X1	T47.4X2	T47.4X3	T47.4X4	T47.4X5	T47.4X6
Brass (fumes)	T56.891	T56.892	T56.893	T56.894	—	—
Brasso	T52.0X1	T52.0X2	T52.0X3	T52.0X4	—	—
Bretylium tosilate	T46.2X1	T46.2X2	T46.2X3	T46.2X4	T46.2X5	T46.2X6
Brevital (sodium)	T41.1X1	T41.1X2	T41.1X3	T41.1X4	T41.1X5	T41.1X6
Brinase	T45.3X1	T45.3X2	T45.3X3	T45.3X4	T45.3X5	T45.3X6
British antilewisite	T45.8X1	T45.8X2	T45.8X3	T45.8X4	T45.8X5	T45.8X6
Brodifacoum	T60.4X1	T60.4X2	T60.4X3	T60.4X4	—	—
Bromal (hydrate)	T42.6X1	T42.6X2	T42.6X3	T42.6X4	T42.6X5	T42.6X6
Bromazepam	T42.4X1	T42.4X2	T42.4X3	T42.4X4	T42.4X5	T42.4X6
Bromazine	T45.0X1	T45.0X2	T45.0X3	T45.0X4	T45.0X5	T45.0X6
Brombenzylcyanide	T59.3X1	T59.3X2	T59.3X3	T59.3X4	—	—
Bromelains	T45.3X1	T45.3X2	T45.3X3	T45.3X4	T45.3X5	T45.3X6
Bromethalin	T60.4X1	T60.4X2	T60.4X3	T60.4X4	—	—
Bromhexine	T48.4X1	T48.4X2	T48.4X3	T48.4X4	T48.4X5	T48.4X6
Bromide salts	T42.6X1	T42.6X2	T42.6X3	T42.6X4	T42.6X5	T42.6X6
Bromindione	T45.511	T45.512	T45.513	T45.514	T45.515	T45.516
Bromine						
compounds (medicinal)	T42.6X1	T42.6X2	T42.6X3	T42.6X4	T42.6X5	T42.6X6
sedative	T42.6X1	T42.6X2	T42.6X3	T42.6X4	T42.6X5	T42.6X6
vapor	T59.891	T59.892	T59.893	T59.894	—	—
Bromisoval	T42.6X1	T42.6X2	T42.6X3	T42.6X4	T42.6X5	T42.6X6
Bromisovalum	T42.6X1	T42.6X2	T42.6X3	T42.6X4	T42.6X5	T42.6X6
Bromobenzylcyanide	T59.3X1	T59.3X2	T59.3X3	T59.3X4	—	—
Bromochlorosalicylani-lide	T49.0X1	T49.0X2	T49.0X3	T49.0X4	T49.0X5	T49.0X6
Bromocriptine	T42.8X1	T42.8X2	T42.8X3	T42.8X4	T42.8X5	T42.8X6
Bromodiphenhydramine	T45.0X1	T45.0X2	T45.0X3	T45.0X4	T45.0X5	T45.0X6
Bromoform	T42.6X1	T42.6X2	T42.6X3	T42.6X4	T42.6X5	T42.6X6
Bromophenol blue reagent	T50.991	T50.992	T50.993	T50.994	T50.995	T50.996
Bromopride	T47.8X1	T47.8X2	T47.8X3	T47.8X4	T47.8X5	T47.8X6
Bromosalicylchloranitide	T49.0X1	T49.0X2	T49.0X3	T49.0X4	T49.0X5	T49.0X6
Bromosalicylhydroxamic acid	T37.1X1	T37.1X2	T37.1X3	T37.1X4	T37.1X5	T37.1X6
Bromo-seltzer	T39.1X1	T39.1X2	T39.1X3	T39.1X4	T39.1X5	T39.1X6
Bromoxynil	T60.3X1	T60.3X2	T60.3X3	T60.3X4	—	—
Bromperidol	T43.4X1	T43.4X2	T43.4X3	T43.4X4	T43.4X5	T43.4X6
Brompheniramine	T45.0X1	T45.0X2	T45.0X3	T45.0X4	T45.0X5	T45.0X6
Bromsulfophthalein	T50.8X1	T50.8X2	T50.8X3	T50.8X4	T50.8X5	T50.8X6
Bromural	T42.6X1	T42.6X2	T42.6X3	T42.6X4	T42.6X5	T42.6X6
Bromvaletone	T42.6X1	T42.6X2	T42.6X3	T42.6X4	T42.6X5	T42.6X6
Bronchodilator NEC	T48.6X1	T48.6X2	T48.6X3	T48.6X4	T48.6X5	T48.6X6
Brotizolam	T42.4X1	T42.4X2	T42.4X3	T42.4X4	T42.4X5	T42.4X6
Brovincamine	T46.7X1	T46.7X2	T46.7X3	T46.7X4	T46.7X5	T46.7X6
Brown recluse spider (bite) (venom)	T63.331	T63.332	T63.333	T63.334	—	—
Brown spider (bite) (venom)	T63.391	T63.392	T63.393	T63.394	—	—
Broxaterol	T48.6X1	T48.6X2	T48.6X3	T48.6X4	T48.6X5	T48.6X6
Broxuridine	T45.1X1	T45.1X2	T45.1X3	T45.1X4	T45.1X5	T45.1X6
Broxyquinoline	T37.8X1	T37.8X2	T37.8X3	T37.8X4	T37.8X5	T37.8X6
Bruceine	T48.291	T48.292	T48.293	T48.294	T48.295	T48.296
Brucia	T62.2X1	T62.2X2	T62.2X3	T62.2X4	—	—
Brucine	T65.1X1	T65.1X2	T65.1X3	T65.1X4	—	—
Brunswick green — see Copper						
Bruten — see Ibuprofen						
Bryonia	T47.2X1	T47.2X2	T47.2X3	T47.2X4	T47.2X5	T47.2X6
Buclizine	T45.0X1	T45.0X2	T45.0X3	T45.0X4	T45.0X5	T45.0X6
Buclosamide	T49.0X1	T49.0X2	T49.0X3	T49.0X4	T49.0X5	T49.0X6
Budesonide	T44.5X1	T44.5X2	T44.5X3	T44.5X4	T44.5X5	T44.5X6
Budralazine	T46.5X1	T46.5X2	T46.5X3	T46.5X4	T46.5X5	T46.5X6
Bufferin	T39.011	T39.012	T39.013	T39.014	T39.015	T39.016
Buflomedil	T46.7X1	T46.7X2	T46.7X3	T46.7X4	T46.7X5	T46.7X6
Buformin	T38.3X1	T38.3X2	T38.3X3	T38.3X4	T38.3X5	T38.3X6
Bufotenine	T40.991	T40.992	T40.993	T40.994	—	—
Bufrolin	T48.6X1	T48.6X2	T48.6X3	T48.6X4	T48.6X5	T48.6X6
Bufylline	T48.6X1	T48.6X2	T48.6X3	T48.6X4	T48.6X5	T48.6X6
Bulk filler	T50.5X1	T50.5X2	T50.5X3	T50.5X4	T50.5X5	T50.5X6
cathartic	T47.4X1	T47.4X2	T47.4X3	T47.4X4	T47.4X5	T47.4X6
Bumetanide	T50.1X1	T50.1X2	T50.1X3	T50.1X4	T50.1X5	T50.1X6
Bunaftine	T46.2X1	T46.2X2	T46.2X3	T46.2X4	T46.2X5	T46.2X6
Bunamiodyl	T50.8X1	T50.8X2	T50.8X3	T50.8X4	T50.8X5	T50.8X6
Bunazosin	T44.6X1	T44.6X2	T44.6X3	T44.6X4	T44.6X5	T44.6X6
Bunitrolol	T44.7X1	T44.7X2	T44.7X3	T44.7X4	T44.7X5	T44.7X6
Buphenine	T46.7X1	T46.7X2	T46.7X3	T46.7X4	T46.7X5	T46.7X6
Bupivacaine	T41.3X1	T41.3X2	T41.3X3	T41.3X4	T41.3X5	T41.3X6
infiltration (subcutaneous)	T41.3X1	T41.3X2	T41.3X3	T41.3X4	T41.3X5	T41.3X6
nerve block (peripheral) (plexus)	T41.3X1	T41.3X2	T41.3X3	T41.3X4	T41.3X5	T41.3X6
spinal	T41.3X1	T41.3X2	T41.3X3	T41.3X4	T41.3X5	T41.3X6
Bupranolol	T44.7X1	T44.7X2	T44.7X3	T44.7X4	T44.7X5	T44.7X6
Buprenorphine	T40.491	T40.492	T40.493	T40.494	T40.495	T40.496
Bupropion	T43.291	T43.292	T43.293	T43.294	T43.295	T43.296
Burimamide	T47.1X1	T47.1X2	T47.1X3	T47.1X4	T47.1X5	T47.1X6
Buserelin	T38.891	T38.892	T38.893	T38.894	T38.895	T38.896
Buspirone	T43.591	T43.592	T43.593	T43.594	T43.595	T43.596
Busulfan, busulphan	T45.1X1	T45.1X2	T45.1X3	T45.1X4	T45.1X5	T45.1X6
Butabarbital (sodium)	T42.3X1	T42.3X2	T42.3X3	T42.3X4	T42.3X5	T42.3X6
Butabarbitone	T42.3X1	T42.3X2	T42.3X3	T42.3X4	T42.3X5	T42.3X6
Butabarpal	T42.3X1	T42.3X2	T42.3X3	T42.3X4	T42.3X5	T42.3X6
Butacaine	T41.3X1	T41.3X2	T41.3X3	T41.3X4	T41.3X5	T41.3X6
Butalamine	T46.7X1	T46.7X2	T46.7X3	T46.7X4	T46.7X5	T46.7X6
Butalbital	T42.3X1	T42.3X2	T42.3X3	T42.3X4	T42.3X5	T42.3X6
Butallylonal	T42.3X1	T42.3X2	T42.3X3	T42.3X4	T42.3X5	T42.3X6
Butamben	T41.3X1	T41.3X2	T41.3X3	T41.3X4	T41.3X5	T41.3X6
Butamirate	T48.3X1	T48.3X2	T48.3X3	T48.3X4	T48.3X5	T48.3X6
Butane (distributed in mobile container)	T59.891	T59.892	T59.893	T59.894		
distributed through pipes	T59.891	T59.892	T59.893	T59.894	—	—
incomplete combustion	T58.11	T58.12	T58.13	T58.14	—	—
Butanilicaine	T41.3X1	T41.3X2	T41.3X3	T41.3X4	T41.3X5	T41.3X6
Butanol	T51.3X1	T51.3X2	T51.3X3	T51.3X4	—	—
Butanone, 2-butanone	T52.4X1	T52.4X2	T52.4X3	T52.4X4	—	—
Butantrone	T49.4X1	T49.4X2	T49.4X3	T49.4X4	T49.4X5	T49.4X6
Butaperazine	T43.3X1	T43.3X2	T43.3X3	T43.3X4	T43.3X5	T43.3X6
Butazolidin	T39.2X1	T39.2X2	T39.2X3	T39.2X4	T39.2X5	T39.2X6
Butetamate	T48.6X1	T48.6X2	T48.6X3	T48.6X4	T48.6X5	T48.6X6
Butethal	T42.3X1	T42.3X2	T42.3X3	T42.3X4	T42.3X5	T42.3X6
Butethamate	T44.3X1	T44.3X2	T44.3X3	T44.3X4	T44.3X5	T44.3X6
Buthalitone (sodium)	T41.1X1	T41.1X2	T41.1X3	T41.1X4	T41.1X5	T41.1X6
Butisol (sodium)	T42.3X1	T42.3X2	T42.3X3	T42.3X4	T42.3X5	T42.3X6
Butizide	T50.2X1	T50.2X2	T50.2X3	T50.2X4	T50.2X5	T50.2X6
Butobarbital	T42.3X1	T42.3X2	T42.3X3	T42.3X4	T42.3X5	T42.3X6
sodium	T42.3X1	T42.3X2	T42.3X3	T42.3X4	T42.3X5	T42.3X6
Butobarbitone	T42.3X1	T42.3X2	T42.3X3	T42.3X4	T42.3X5	T42.3X6
Butoconazole (nitrate)	T49.0X1	T49.0X2	T49.0X3	T49.0X4	T49.0X5	T49.0X6
Butorphanol	T40.491	T40.492	T40.493	T40.494	T40.495	T40.496
Butriptyline	T43.011	T43.012	T43.013	T43.014	T43.015	T43.016
Butropium bromide	T44.3X1	T44.3X2	T44.3X3	T44.3X4	T44.3X5	T44.3X6
Buttercups	T62.2X1	T62.2X2	T62.2X3	T62.2X4	—	—
Butter of antimony — see Antimony						
Butyl						
acetate (secondary)	T52.8X1	T52.8X2	T52.8X3	T52.8X4	—	—
alcohol	T51.3X1	T51.3X2	T51.3X3	T51.3X4	—	—
aminobenzoate	T41.3X1	T41.3X2	T41.3X3	T41.3X4	T41.3X5	T41.3X6
butyrate	T52.8X1	T52.8X2	T52.8X3	T52.8X4	—	—
carbinol	T51.3X1	T51.3X2	T51.3X3	T51.3X4	—	—
carbitol	T52.3X1	T52.3X2	T52.3X3	T52.3X4	—	—
cellosolve	T52.3X1	T52.3X2	T52.3X3	T52.3X4	—	—
chloral (hydrate)	T42.6X1	T42.6X2	T42.6X3	T42.6X4	T42.6X5	T42.6X6
formate	T52.8X1	T52.8X2	T52.8X3	T52.8X4	—	—
lactate	T52.8X1	T52.8X2	T52.8X3	T52.8X4	—	—

▽ Subterms under main terms may continue to next column or page   Additional Character May Be Required — Refer to the Tabular List for Character Selection   361

Blood — Butyl

Substance	Poisoning, Accidental (unintentional)	Poisoning, Intentional Self-harm	Poisoning, Assault	Poisoning, Undetermined	Adverse Effect	Under-dosing
Butyl — continued						
propionate	T52.8X1	T52.8X2	T52.8X3	T52.8X4	—	—
scopolamine bromide	T44.3X1	T44.3X2	T44.3X3	T44.3X4	T44.3X5	T44.3X6
thiobarbital sodium	T41.1X1	T41.1X2	T41.1X3	T41.1X4	T41.1X5	T41.1X6
Butylated hydroxyanisole	T50.992	T50.992	T50.993	T50.994	T50.995	T50.996
Butylchloral hydrate	T42.6X1	T42.6X2	T42.6X3	T42.6X4	T42.6X5	T42.6X6
Butyltoluene	T52.2X1	T52.2X2	T52.2X3	T52.2X4	—	—
Butyn	T41.3X1	T41.3X2	T41.3X3	T41.3X4	T41.3X5	T41.3X6
Butyrophenone (-based tranquilizers)	T43.4X1	T43.4X2	T43.4X3	T43.4X4	T43.4X5	T43.4X6
Cabergoline	T42.8X1	T42.8X2	T42.8X3	T42.8X4	T42.8X5	T42.8X6
Cacodyl, cacodylic acid	T57.0X1	T57.0X2	T57.0X3	T57.0X4	—	—
Cactinomycin	T45.1X1	T45.1X2	T45.1X3	T45.1X4	T45.1X5	T45.1X6
Cade oil	T49.4X1	T49.4X2	T49.4X3	T49.4X4	T49.4X5	T49.4X6
Cadexomer iodine	T49.0X1	T49.0X2	T49.0X3	T49.0X4	T49.0X5	T49.0X6
Cadmium (chloride) (fumes) (oxide)	T56.3X1	T56.3X2	T56.3X3	T56.3X4	—	—
sulfide (medicinal) NEC	T49.4X1	T49.4X2	T49.4X3	T49.4X4	T49.4X5	T49.4X6
Cadralazine	T46.5X1	T46.5X2	T46.5X3	T46.5X4	T46.5X5	T46.5X6
Caffeine	T43.611	T43.612	T43.613	T43.614	T43.615	T43.616
Calabar bean	T62.2X1	T62.2X2	T62.2X3	T62.2X4	—	—
Caladium seguinum	T62.2X1	T62.2X2	T62.2X3	T62.2X4	—	—
Calamine (lotion)	T49.3X1	T49.3X2	T49.3X3	T49.3X4	T49.3X5	T49.3X6
Calcifediol	T45.2X1	T45.2X2	T45.2X3	T45.2X4	T45.2X5	T45.2X6
Calciferol	T45.2X1	T45.2X2	T45.2X3	T45.2X4	T45.2X5	T45.2X6
Calcitonin	T50.991	T50.992	T50.993	T50.994	T50.995	T50.996
Calcitriol	T45.2X1	T45.2X2	T45.2X3	T45.2X4	T45.2X5	T45.2X6
Calcium	T50.3X1	T50.3X2	T50.3X3	T50.3X4	T50.3X5	T50.3X6
actylsalicylate	T39.011	T39.012	T39.013	T39.014	T39.015	T39.016
benzamidosalicylate	T37.1X1	T37.1X2	T37.1X3	T37.1X4	T37.1X5	T37.1X6
bromide	T42.6X1	T42.6X2	T42.6X3	T42.6X4	T42.6X5	T42.6X6
bromolactobionate	T42.6X1	T42.6X2	T42.6X3	T42.6X4	T42.6X5	T42.6X6
carbaspirin	T39.011	T39.012	T39.013	T39.014	T39.015	T39.016
carbimide	T50.6X1	T50.6X2	T50.6X3	T50.6X4	T50.6X5	T50.6X6
carbonate	T47.1X1	T47.1X2	T47.1X3	T47.1X4	T47.1X5	T47.1X6
chloride	T50.991	T50.992	T50.993	T50.994	T50.995	T50.996
anhydrous	T50.991	T50.992	T50.993	T50.994	T50.995	T50.996
cyanide	T57.8X1	T57.8X2	T57.8X3	T57.8X4	—	—
dioctyl sulfosuccinate	T47.4X1	T47.4X2	T47.4X3	T47.4X4	T47.4X5	T47.4X6
disodium edathamil	T45.8X1	T45.8X2	T45.8X3	T45.8X4	T45.8X5	T45.8X6
disodium edetate	T45.8X1	T45.8X2	T45.8X3	T45.8X4	T45.8X5	T45.8X6
dobesilate	T46.991	T46.992	T46.993	T46.994	T46.995	T46.996
EDTA	T45.8X1	T45.8X2	T45.8X3	T45.8X4	T45.8X5	T45.8X6
ferrous citrate	T45.4X1	T45.4X2	T45.4X3	T45.4X4	T45.4X5	T45.4X6
folinate	T45.8X1	T45.8X2	T45.8X3	T45.8X4	T45.8X5	T45.8X6
glubionate	T50.3X1	T50.3X2	T50.3X3	T50.3X4	T50.3X5	T50.3X6
gluconate	T50.3X1	T50.3X2	T50.3X3	T50.3X4	T50.3X5	T50.3X6
gluconogalactogluconate	T50.3X1	T50.3X2	T50.3X3	T50.3X4	T50.3X5	T50.3X6
hydrate, hydroxide	T54.3X1	T54.3X2	T54.3X3	T54.3X4	—	—
hypochlorite	T54.3X1	T54.3X2	T54.3X3	T54.3X4	—	—
iodide	T48.4X1	T48.4X2	T48.4X3	T48.4X4	T48.4X5	T48.4X6
ipodate	T50.8X1	T50.8X2	T50.8X3	T50.8X4	T50.8X5	T50.8X6
lactate	T50.3X1	T50.3X2	T50.3X3	T50.3X4	T50.3X5	T50.3X6
leucovorin	T45.8X1	T45.8X2	T45.8X3	T45.8X4	T45.8X5	T45.8X6
mandelate	T37.91	T37.92	T37.93	T37.94	T37.95	T37.96
oxide	T54.3X1	T54.3X2	T54.3X3	T54.3X4	—	—
pantothenate	T45.2X1	T45.2X2	T45.2X3	T45.2X4	T45.2X5	T45.2X6
phosphate	T50.3X1	T50.3X2	T50.3X3	T50.3X4	T50.3X5	T50.3X6
salicylate	T39.091	T39.092	T39.093	T39.094	T39.095	T39.096
salts	T50.3X1	T50.3X2	T50.3X3	T50.3X4	T50.3X5	T50.3X6
Calculus-dissolving drug	T50.991	T50.992	T50.993	T50.994	T50.995	T50.996
Calomel	T49.0X1	T49.0X2	T49.0X3	T49.0X4	T49.0X5	T49.0X6
Caloric agent	T50.3X1	T50.3X2	T50.3X3	T50.3X4	T50.3X5	T50.3X6
Calusterone	T38.7X1	T38.7X2	T38.7X3	T38.7X4	T38.7X5	T38.7X6
Camazepam	T42.4X1	T42.4X2	T42.4X3	T42.4X4	T42.4X5	T42.4X6
Camomile	T49.0X1	T49.0X2	T49.0X3	T49.0X4	T49.0X5	T49.0X6
Camoquin	T37.2X1	T37.2X2	T37.2X3	T37.2X4	T37.2X5	T37.2X6
Camphor						
insecticide	T60.2X1	T60.2X2	T60.2X3	T60.2X4	—	—
medicinal	T49.8X1	T49.8X2	T49.8X3	T49.8X4	T49.8X5	T49.8X6
Camylofin	T44.3X1	T44.3X2	T44.3X3	T44.3X4	T44.3X5	T44.3X6
Cancer chemotherapy drug regimen	T45.1X1	T45.1X2	T45.1X3	T45.1X4	T45.1X5	T45.1X6
Candeptin	T49.0X1	T49.0X2	T49.0X3	T49.0X4	T49.0X5	T49.0X6
Candicidin	T49.0X1	T49.0X2	T49.0X3	T49.0X4	T49.0X5	T49.0X6
Cannabinol	T40.7X1	T40.7X2	T40.7X3	T40.7X4	T40.7X5	T40.7X6
Cannabis (derivatives)	T40.7X1	T40.7X2	T40.7X3	T40.7X4	T40.7X5	T40.7X6
Canned heat	T51.1X1	T51.1X2	T51.1X3	T51.1X4	—	—
Canrenoic acid	T50.0X1	T50.0X2	T50.0X3	T50.0X4	T50.0X5	T50.0X6
Canrenone	T50.0X1	T50.0X2	T50.0X3	T50.0X4	T50.0X5	T50.0X6
Cantharides, cantharidin, cantharis	T49.8X1	T49.8X2	T49.8X3	T49.8X4	T49.8X5	T49.8X6
Canthaxanthin	T50.991	T50.992	T50.993	T50.994	T50.995	T50.996

Substance	Poisoning, Accidental (unintentional)	Poisoning, Intentional Self-harm	Poisoning, Assault	Poisoning, Undetermined	Adverse Effect	Under-dosing
Capillary-active drug NEC	T46.901	T46.902	T46.903	T46.904	T46.905	T46.906
Capreomycin	T36.8X1	T36.8X2	T36.8X3	T36.8X4	T36.8X5	T36.8X6
Capsicum	T49.4X1	T49.4X2	T49.4X3	T49.4X4	T49.4X5	T49.4X6
Captafol	T60.3X1	T60.3X2	T60.3X3	T60.3X4	—	—
Captan	T60.3X1	T60.3X2	T60.3X3	T60.3X4	—	—
Captodiame, captodiamine	T43.591	T43.592	T43.593	T43.594	T43.595	T43.596
Captopril	T46.4X1	T46.4X2	T46.4X3	T46.4X4	T46.4X5	T46.4X6
Caramiphen	T44.3X1	T44.3X2	T44.3X3	T44.3X4	T44.3X5	T44.3X6
Carazolol	T44.7X1	T44.7X2	T44.7X3	T44.7X4	T44.7X5	T44.7X6
Carbachol	T44.1X1	T44.1X2	T44.1X3	T44.1X4	T44.1X5	T44.1X6
Carbacrylamine (resin)	T50.3X1	T50.3X2	T50.3X3	T50.3X4	T50.3X5	T50.3X6
Carbamate (insecticide)	T60.0X1	T60.0X2	T60.0X3	T60.0X4	—	—
Carbamate (sedative)	T42.6X1	T42.6X2	T42.6X3	T42.6X4	T42.6X5	T42.6X6
herbicide	T60.0X1	T60.0X2	T60.0X3	T60.0X4	—	—
insecticide	T60.0X1	T60.0X2	T60.0X3	T60.0X4	—	—
Carbamazepine	T42.1X1	T42.1X2	T42.1X3	T42.1X4	T42.1X5	T42.1X6
Carbamide	T47.3X1	T47.3X2	T47.3X3	T47.3X4	T47.3X5	T47.3X6
peroxide	T49.0X1	T49.0X2	T49.0X3	T49.0X4	T49.0X5	T49.0X6
topical	T49.8X1	T49.8X2	T49.8X3	T49.8X4	T49.8X5	T49.8X6
Carbamylcholine chloride	T44.1X1	T44.1X2	T44.1X3	T44.1X4	T44.1X5	T44.1X6
Carbaril	T60.0X1	T60.0X2	T60.0X3	T60.0X4	—	—
Carbarsone	T37.3X1	T37.3X2	T37.3X3	T37.3X4	T37.3X5	T37.3X6
Carbaryl	T60.0X1	T60.0X2	T60.0X3	T60.0X4	—	—
Carbaspirin	T39.011	T39.012	T39.013	T39.014	T39.015	T39.016
Carbazochrome (salicylate) (sodium sulfonate)	T49.4X1	T49.4X2	T49.4X3	T49.4X4	T49.4X5	T49.4X6
Carbenicillin	T36.0X1	T36.0X2	T36.0X3	T36.0X4	T36.0X5	T36.0X6
Carbenoxolone	T47.1X1	T47.1X2	T47.1X3	T47.1X4	T47.1X5	T47.1X6
Carbetapentane	T48.3X1	T48.3X2	T48.3X3	T48.3X4	T48.3X5	T48.3X6
Carbethyl salicylate	T39.091	T39.092	T39.093	T39.094	T39.095	T39.096
Carbidopa (with levodopa)	T42.8X1	T42.8X2	T42.8X3	T42.8X4	T42.8X5	T42.8X6
Carbimazole	T38.2X1	T38.2X2	T38.2X3	T38.2X4	T38.2X5	T38.2X6
Carbinol	T51.1X1	T51.1X2	T51.1X3	T51.1X4	—	—
Carbinoxamine	T45.0X1	T45.0X2	T45.0X3	T45.0X4	T45.0X5	T45.0X6
Carbiphene	T39.8X1	T39.8X2	T39.8X3	T39.8X4	T39.8X5	T39.8X6
Carbitol	T52.3X1	T52.3X2	T52.3X3	T52.3X4	—	—
Carbocaine	T41.3X1	T41.3X2	T41.3X3	T41.3X4	T41.3X5	T41.3X6
infiltration (subcutaneous)	T41.3X1	T41.3X2	T41.3X3	T41.3X4	T41.3X5	T41.3X6
nerve block (peripheral) (plexus)	T41.3X1	T41.3X2	T41.3X3	T41.3X4	T41.3X5	T41.3X6
topical (surface)	T41.3X1	T41.3X2	T41.3X3	T41.3X4	T41.3X5	T41.3X6
Carbocisteine	T48.4X1	T48.4X2	T48.4X3	T48.4X4	T48.4X5	T48.4X6
Carbocromen	T46.3X1	T46.3X2	T46.3X3	T46.3X4	T46.3X5	T46.3X6
Carbol fuchsin	T49.0X1	T49.0X2	T49.0X3	T49.0X4	T49.0X5	T49.0X6
Carbolic acid — see also Phenol	T54.0X1	T54.0X2	T54.0X3	T54.0X4	—	—
Carbolonium (bromide)	T48.1X1	T48.1X2	T48.1X3	T48.1X4	T48.1X5	T48.1X6
Carbo medicinalis	T47.6X1	T47.6X2	T47.6X3	T47.6X4	T47.6X5	T47.6X6
Carbomycin	T36.8X1	T36.8X2	T36.8X3	T36.8X4	T36.8X5	T36.8X6
Carbon						
bisulfide (liquid)	T65.4X1	T65.4X2	T65.4X3	T65.4X4	—	—
vapor	T65.4X1	T65.4X2	T65.4X3	T65.4X4	—	—
dioxide (gas)	T59.7X1	T59.7X2	T59.7X3	T59.7X4	—	—
medicinal	T41.5X1	T41.5X2	T41.5X3	T41.5X4	T41.5X5	T41.5X6
nonmedicinal	T59.7X1	T59.7X2	T59.7X3	T59.7X4	—	—
snow	T49.4X1	T49.4X2	T49.4X3	T49.4X4	T49.4X5	T49.4X6
disulfide (liquid)	T65.4X1	T65.4X2	T65.4X3	T65.4X4	—	—
vapor	T65.4X1	T65.4X2	T65.4X3	T65.4X4	—	—
monoxide (from incomplete combustion)	T58.91	T58.92	T58.93	T58.94	—	—
blast furnace gas	T58.8X1	T58.8X2	T58.8X3	T58.8X4	—	—
butane (distributed in mobile container)	T58.11	T58.12	T58.13	T58.14	—	—
distributed through pipes	T58.11	T58.12	T58.13	T58.14	—	—
charcoal fumes	T58.2X1	T58.2X2	T58.2X3	T58.2X4	—	—
coal	T58.2X1	T58.2X2	T58.2X3	T58.2X4	—	—
coke (in domestic stoves, fireplaces)	T58.2X1	T58.2X2	T58.2X3	T58.2X4	—	—
exhaust gas (motor) not in transit	T58.01	T58.02	T58.03	T58.04	—	—
combustion engine, any not in watercraft	T58.01	T58.02	T58.03	T58.04	—	—
farm tractor, not in transit	T58.01	T58.02	T58.03	T58.04	—	—
gas engine	T58.01	T58.02	T58.03	T58.04	—	—
motor pump	T58.01	T58.02	T58.03	T58.04	—	—
motor vehicle, not in transit	T58.01	T58.02	T58.03	T58.04	—	—
fuel (in domestic use)	T58.2X1	T58.2X2	T58.2X3	T58.2X4	—	—
gas (piped)	T58.11	T58.12	T58.13	T58.14	—	—
in mobile container	T58.11	T58.12	T58.13	T58.14	—	—

Substance	Poisoning, Accidental (unintentional)	Poisoning, Intentional Self-harm	Poisoning, Assault	Poisoning, Undetermined	Adverse Effect	Under-dosing
Carbon — *continued*						
monoxide — *continued*						
fuel — *continued*						
piped (natural)	T58.11	T58.12	T58.13	T58.14	—	—
utility	T58.11	T58.12	T58.13	T58.14	—	—
in mobile container	T58.11	T58.12	T58.13	T58.14	—	—
gas (piped)	T58.11	T58.12	T58.13	T58.14	—	—
illuminating gas	T58.11	T58.12	T58.13	T58.14	—	—
industrial fuels or gases, any	T58.8X1	T58.8X2	T58.8X3	T58.8X4	—	—
kerosene (in domestic stoves, fireplaces)	T58.2X1	T58.2X2	T58.2X3	T58.2X4	—	—
kiln gas or vapor	T58.8X1	T58.8X2	T58.8X3	T58.8X4	—	—
motor exhaust gas, not in transit	T58.01	T58.02	T58.03	T58.04	—	—
piped gas (manufactured) (natural)	T58.11	T58.12	T58.13	T58.14	—	—
producer gas	T58.8X1	T58.8X2	T58.8X3	T58.8X4	—	—
propane (distributed in mobile container)	T58.11	T58.12	T58.13	T58.14	—	—
distributed through pipes	T58.11	T58.12	T58.13	T58.14	—	—
solid (in domestic stoves, fireplaces)	T58.2X1	T58.2X2	T58.2X3	T58.2X4	—	—
specified source NEC	T58.8X1	T58.8X2	T58.8X3	T58.8X4	—	—
stove gas	T58.11	T58.12	T58.13	T58.14	—	—
piped	T58.11	T58.12	T58.13	T58.14	—	—
utility gas	T58.11	T58.12	T58.13	T58.14	—	—
piped	T58.11	T58.12	T58.13	T58.14	—	—
water gas	T58.11	T58.12	T58.13	T58.14	—	—
wood (in domestic stoves, fireplaces)	T58.2X1	T58.2X2	T58.2X3	T58.2X4	—	—
tetrachloride (vapor) NEC	T53.0X1	T53.0X2	T53.0X3	T53.0X4	—	—
liquid (cleansing agent) NEC	T53.0X1	T53.0X2	T53.0X3	T53.0X4	—	—
solvent	T53.0X1	T53.0X2	T53.0X3	T53.0X4	—	—
Carbonic acid gas	T59.7X1	T59.7X2	T59.7X3	T59.7X4	—	—
anhydrase inhibitor NEC	T50.2X1	T50.2X2	T50.2X3	T50.2X4	T50.2X5	T50.2X6
Carbophenothion	T60.0X1	T60.0X2	T60.0X3	T60.0X4	—	—
Carboplatin	T45.1X1	T45.1X2	T45.1X3	T45.1X4	T45.1X5	T45.1X6
Carboprost	T48.0X1	T48.0X2	T48.0X3	T48.0X4	T48.0X5	T48.0X6
Carboquone	T45.1X1	T45.1X2	T45.1X3	T45.1X4	T45.1X5	T45.1X6
Carbowax	T49.3X1	T49.3X2	T49.3X3	T49.3X4	T49.3X5	T49.3X6
Carboxymethylcellulose	T47.4X1	T47.4X2	T47.4X3	T47.4X4	T47.4X5	T47.4X6
Carbrital	T42.3X1	T42.3X2	T42.3X3	T42.3X4	T42.3X5	T42.3X6
Carbromal	T42.6X1	T42.6X2	T42.6X3	T42.6X4	T42.6X5	T42.6X6
Carbutamide	T38.3X1	T38.3X2	T38.3X3	T38.3X4	T38.3X5	T38.3X6
Carbuterol	T48.6X1	T48.6X2	T48.6X3	T48.6X4	T48.6X5	T48.6X6
Cardiac						
depressants	T46.2X1	T46.2X2	T46.2X3	T46.2X4	T46.2X5	T46.2X6
rhythm regulator	T46.2X1	T46.2X2	T46.2X3	T46.2X4	T46.2X5	T46.2X6
specified NEC	T46.2X1	T46.2X2	T46.2X3	T46.2X4	T46.2X5	T46.2X6
Cardiografin	T50.8X1	T50.8X2	T50.8X3	T50.8X4	T50.8X5	T50.8X6
Cardiogreen	T50.8X1	T50.8X2	T50.8X3	T50.8X4	T50.8X5	T50.8X6
Cardiotonic (glycoside) **NEC**	T46.0X1	T46.0X2	T46.0X3	T46.0X4	T46.0X5	T46.0X6
Cardiovascular drug NEC	T46.901	T46.902	T46.903	T46.904	T46.905	T46.906
Cardrase	T50.2X1	T50.2X2	T50.2X3	T50.2X4	T50.2X5	T50.2X6
Carfecillin	T36.0X1	T36.0X2	T36.0X3	T36.0X4	T36.0X5	T36.0X6
Carfenazine	T43.3X1	T43.3X2	T43.3X3	T43.3X4	T43.3X5	T43.3X6
Carfusin	T49.0X1	T49.0X2	T49.0X3	T49.0X4	T49.0X5	T49.0X6
Carindacillin	T36.0X1	T36.0X2	T36.0X3	T36.0X4	T36.0X5	T36.0X6
Carisoprodol	T42.8X1	T42.8X2	T42.8X3	T42.8X4	T42.8X5	T42.8X6
Carmellose	T47.4X1	T47.4X2	T47.4X3	T47.4X4	T47.4X5	T47.4X6
Carminative	T47.5X1	T47.5X2	T47.5X3	T47.5X4	T47.5X5	T47.5X6
Carmofur	T45.1X1	T45.1X2	T45.1X3	T45.1X4	T45.1X5	T45.1X6
Carmustine	T45.1X1	T45.1X2	T45.1X3	T45.1X4	T45.1X5	T45.1X6
Carotene	T45.2X1	T45.2X2	T45.2X3	T45.2X4	T45.2X5	T45.2X6
Carphenazine	T43.3X1	T43.3X2	T43.3X3	T43.3X4	T43.3X5	T43.3X6
Carpipramine	T42.4X1	T42.4X2	T42.4X3	T42.4X4	T42.4X5	T42.4X6
Carprofen	T39.311	T39.312	T39.313	T39.314	T39.315	T39.316
Carpronium chloride	T44.3X1	T44.3X2	T44.3X3	T44.3X4	T44.3X5	T44.3X6
Carrageenan	T47.8X1	T47.8X2	T47.8X3	T47.8X4	T47.8X5	T47.8X6
Carteolol	T44.7X1	T44.7X2	T44.7X3	T44.7X4	T44.7X5	T44.7X6
Carter's Little Pills	T47.2X1	T47.2X2	T47.2X3	T47.2X4	T47.2X5	T47.2X6
Cascara (sagrada)	T47.2X1	T47.2X2	T47.2X3	T47.2X4	T47.2X5	T47.2X6
Cassava	T62.2X1	T62.2X2	T62.2X3	T62.2X4	—	—
Castellani's paint	T49.0X1	T49.0X2	T49.0X3	T49.0X4	T49.0X5	T49.0X6
Castor						
bean	T62.2X1	T62.2X2	T62.2X3	T62.2X4	—	—
oil	T47.2X1	T47.2X2	T47.2X3	T47.2X4	T47.2X5	T47.2X6
Catalase	T45.3X1	T45.3X2	T45.3X3	T45.3X4	T45.3X5	T45.3X6
Caterpillar (sting)	T63.431	T63.432	T63.433	T63.434		
Catha (edulis) (tea)	T43.691	T43.692	T43.693	T43.694	—	—

Substance	Poisoning, Accidental (unintentional)	Poisoning, Intentional Self-harm	Poisoning, Assault	Poisoning, Undetermined	Adverse Effect	Under-dosing
Cathartic NEC	T47.4X1	T47.4X2	T47.4X3	T47.4X4	T47.4X5	T47.4X6
anthacene derivative	T47.2X1	T47.2X2	T47.2X3	T47.2X4	T47.2X5	T47.2X6
bulk	T47.4X1	T47.4X2	T47.4X3	T47.4X4	T47.4X5	T47.4X6
contact	T47.2X1	T47.2X2	T47.2X3	T47.2X4	T47.2X5	T47.2X6
emollient NEC	T47.4X1	T47.4X2	T47.4X3	T47.4X4	T47.4X5	T47.4X6
irritant NEC	T47.2X1	T47.2X2	T47.2X3	T47.2X4	T47.2X5	T47.2X6
mucilage	T47.4X1	T47.4X2	T47.4X3	T47.4X4	T47.4X5	T47.4X6
saline	T47.3X1	T47.3X2	T47.3X3	T47.3X4	T47.3X5	T47.3X6
vegetable	T47.2X1	T47.2X2	T47.2X3	T47.2X4	T47.2X5	T47.2X6
Cathine	T50.5X1	T50.5X2	T50.5X3	T50.5X4	T50.5X5	T50.5X6
Cathomycin	T36.8X1	T36.8X2	T36.8X3	T36.8X4	T36.8X5	T36.8X6
Cation exchange resin	T50.3X1	T50.3X2	T50.3X3	T50.3X4	T50.3X5	T50.3X6
Caustic(s) NEC	T54.91	T54.92	T54.93	T54.94	—	—
alkali	T54.3X1	T54.3X2	T54.3X3	T54.3X4	—	—
hydroxide	T54.3X1	T54.3X2	T54.3X3	T54.3X4	—	—
potash	T54.3X1	T54.3X2	T54.3X3	T54.3X4	—	—
soda	T54.3X1	T54.3X2	T54.3X3	T54.3X4	—	—
specified NEC	T54.91	T54.92	T54.93	T54.94	—	—
Ceepryn	T49.0X1	T49.0X2	T49.0X3	T49.0X4	T49.0X5	T49.0X6
ENT agent	T49.6X1	T49.6X2	T49.6X3	T49.6X4	T49.6X5	T49.6X6
lozenges	T49.6X1	T49.6X2	T49.6X3	T49.6X4	T49.6X5	T49.6X6
Cefacetrile	T36.1X1	T36.1X2	T36.1X3	T36.1X4	T36.1X5	T36.1X6
Cefaclor	T36.1X1	T36.1X2	T36.1X3	T36.1X4	T36.1X5	T36.1X6
Cefadroxil	T36.1X1	T36.1X2	T36.1X3	T36.1X4	T36.1X5	T36.1X6
Cefalexin	T36.1X1	T36.1X2	T36.1X3	T36.1X4	T36.1X5	T36.1X6
Cefaloglycin	T36.1X1	T36.1X2	T36.1X3	T36.1X4	T36.1X5	T36.1X6
Cefaloridine	T36.1X1	T36.1X2	T36.1X3	T36.1X4	T36.1X5	T36.1X6
Cefalosporins	T36.1X1	T36.1X2	T36.1X3	T36.1X4	T36.1X5	T36.1X6
Cefalotin	T36.1X1	T36.1X2	T36.1X3	T36.1X4	T36.1X5	T36.1X6
Cefamandole	T36.1X1	T36.1X2	T36.1X3	T36.1X4	T36.1X5	T36.1X6
Cefamycin antibiotic	T36.1X1	T36.1X2	T36.1X3	T36.1X4	T36.1X5	T36.1X6
Cefapirin	T36.1X1	T36.1X2	T36.1X3	T36.1X4	T36.1X5	T36.1X6
Cefatrizine	T36.1X1	T36.1X2	T36.1X3	T36.1X4	T36.1X5	T36.1X6
Cefazedone	T36.1X1	T36.1X2	T36.1X3	T36.1X4	T36.1X5	T36.1X6
Cefazolin	T36.1X1	T36.1X2	T36.1X3	T36.1X4	T36.1X5	T36.1X6
Cefbuperazone	T36.1X1	T36.1X2	T36.1X3	T36.1X4	T36.1X5	T36.1X6
Cefetamet	T36.1X1	T36.1X2	T36.1X3	T36.1X4	T36.1X5	T36.1X6
Cefixime	T36.1X1	T36.1X2	T36.1X3	T36.1X4	T36.1X5	T36.1X6
Cefmenoxime	T36.1X1	T36.1X2	T36.1X3	T36.1X4	T36.1X5	T36.1X6
Cefmetazole	T36.1X1	T36.1X2	T36.1X3	T36.1X4	T36.1X5	T36.1X6
Cefminox	T36.1X1	T36.1X2	T36.1X3	T36.1X4	T36.1X5	T36.1X6
Cefonicid	T36.1X1	T36.1X2	T36.1X3	T36.1X4	T36.1X5	T36.1X6
Cefoperazone	T36.1X1	T36.1X2	T36.1X3	T36.1X4	T36.1X5	T36.1X6
Ceforanide	T36.1X1	T36.1X2	T36.1X3	T36.1X4	T36.1X5	T36.1X6
Cefotaxime	T36.1X1	T36.1X2	T36.1X3	T36.1X4	T36.1X5	T36.1X6
Cefotetan	T36.1X1	T36.1X2	T36.1X3	T36.1X4	T36.1X5	T36.1X6
Cefotiam	T36.1X1	T36.1X2	T36.1X3	T36.1X4	T36.1X5	T36.1X6
Cefoxitin	T36.1X1	T36.1X2	T36.1X3	T36.1X4	T36.1X5	T36.1X6
Cefpimizole	T36.1X1	T36.1X2	T36.1X3	T36.1X4	T36.1X5	T36.1X6
Cefpiramide	T36.1X1	T36.1X2	T36.1X3	T36.1X4	T36.1X5	T36.1X6
Cefradine	T36.1X1	T36.1X2	T36.1X3	T36.1X4	T36.1X5	T36.1X6
Cefroxadine	T36.1X1	T36.1X2	T36.1X3	T36.1X4	T36.1X5	T36.1X6
Cefsulodin	T36.1X1	T36.1X2	T36.1X3	T36.1X4	T36.1X5	T36.1X6
Ceftazidime	T36.1X1	T36.1X2	T36.1X3	T36.1X4	T36.1X5	T36.1X6
Cefteram	T36.1X1	T36.1X2	T36.1X3	T36.1X4	T36.1X5	T36.1X6
Ceftezole	T36.1X1	T36.1X2	T36.1X3	T36.1X4	T36.1X5	T36.1X6
Ceftizoxime	T36.1X1	T36.1X2	T36.1X3	T36.1X4	T36.1X5	T36.1X6
Ceftriaxone	T36.1X1	T36.1X2	T36.1X3	T36.1X4	T36.1X5	T36.1X6
Cefuroxime	T36.1X1	T36.1X2	T36.1X3	T36.1X4	T36.1X5	T36.1X6
Cefuzonam	T36.1X1	T36.1X2	T36.1X3	T36.1X4	T36.1X5	T36.1X6
Celestone	T38.0X1	T38.0X2	T38.0X3	T38.0X4	T38.0X5	T38.0X6
topical	T49.0X1	T49.0X2	T49.0X3	T49.0X4	T49.0X5	T49.0X6
Celiprolol	T44.7X1	T44.7X2	T44.7X3	T44.7X4	T44.7X5	T44.7X6
Cellosolve	T52.91	T52.92	T52.93	T52.94	—	—
Cell stimulants and proliferants	T49.8X1	T49.8X2	T49.8X3	T49.8X4	T49.8X5	T49.8X6
Cellulose						
cathartic	T47.4X1	T47.4X2	T47.4X3	T47.4X4	T47.4X5	T47.4X6
hydroxyethyl	T47.4X1	T47.4X2	T47.4X3	T47.4X4	T47.4X5	T47.4X6
nitrates (topical)	T49.3X1	T49.3X2	T49.3X3	T49.3X4	T49.3X5	T49.3X6
oxidized	T49.4X1	T49.4X2	T49.4X3	T49.4X4	T49.4X5	T49.4X6
Centipede (bite)	T63.411	T63.412	T63.413	T63.414	—	—
Central nervous system						
depressants	T42.71	T42.72	T42.73	T42.74	T42.75	T42.76
anesthetic (general) NEC	T41.201	T41.202	T41.203	T41.204	T41.205	T41.206
gases NEC	T41.0X1	T41.0X2	T41.0X3	T41.0X4	T41.0X5	T41.0X6
intravenous	T41.1X1	T41.1X2	T41.1X3	T41.1X4	T41.1X5	T41.1X6
barbiturates	T42.3X1	T42.3X2	T42.3X3	T42.3X4	T42.3X5	T42.3X6
benzodiazepines	T42.4X1	T42.4X2	T42.4X3	T42.4X4	T42.4X5	T42.4X6
bromides	T42.6X1	T42.6X2	T42.6X3	T42.6X4	T42.6X5	T42.6X6
cannabis sativa	T40.7X1	T40.7X2	T40.7X3	T40.7X4	T40.7X5	T40.7X6
chloral hydrate	T42.6X1	T42.6X2	T42.6X3	T42.6X4	T42.6X5	T42.6X6
ethanol	T51.0X1	T51.0X2	T51.0X3	T51.0X4	—	—

Substance	Poisoning, Accidental (unintentional)	Poisoning, Intentional Self-harm	Poisoning, Assault	Poisoning, Undetermined	Adverse Effect	Under-dosing
Central nervous system — continued						
depressants — continued						
hallucinogenics	T40.901	T40.902	T40.903	T40.904	T40.905	T40.906
hypnotics	T42.71	T42.72	T42.73	T42.74	T42.75	T42.76
specified NEC	T42.6X1	T42.6X2	T42.6X3	T42.6X4	T42.6X5	T42.6X6
muscle relaxants	T42.8X1	T42.8X2	T42.8X3	T42.8X4	T42.8X5	T42.8X6
paraldehyde	T42.6X1	T42.6X2	T42.6X3	T42.6X4	T42.6X5	T42.6X6
sedatives;	T42.71	T42.72	T42.73	T42.74	T42.75	T42.76
sedative-hypnotics						
mixed NEC	T42.6X1	T42.6X2	T42.6X3	T42.6X4	T42.6X5	T42.6X6
specified NEC	T42.6X1	T42.6X2	T42.6X3	T42.6X4	T42.6X5	T42.6X6
muscle-tone depressants	T42.8X1	T42.8X2	T42.8X3	T42.8X4	T42.8X5	T42.8X6
stimulants	T43.601	T43.602	T43.603	T43.604	T43.605	T43.606
amphetamines	T43.621	T43.622	T43.623	T43.624	T43.625	T43.626
analeptics	T50.7X1	T50.7X2	T50.7X3	T50.7X4	T50.7X5	T50.7X6
antidepressants	T43.201	T43.202	T43.203	T43.204	T43.205	T43.206
opiate antagonists	T50.7X1	T50.7X2	T50.7X3	T50.7X4	T50.7X5	T50.7X6
specified NEC	T43.691	T43.692	T43.693	T43.694	T43.695	T43.696
Cephalexin	T36.1X1	T36.1X2	T36.1X3	T36.1X4	T36.1X5	T36.1X6
Cephaloglycin	T36.1X1	T36.1X2	T36.1X3	T36.1X4	T36.1X5	T36.1X6
Cephaloridine	T36.1X1	T36.1X2	T36.1X3	T36.1X4	T36.1X5	T36.1X6
Cephalosporins	T36.1X1	T36.1X2	T36.1X3	T36.1X4	T36.1X5	T36.1X6
N (adicillin)	T36.0X1	T36.0X2	T36.0X3	T36.0X4	T36.0X5	T36.0X6
Cephalothin	T36.1X1	T36.1X2	T36.1X3	T36.1X4	T36.1X5	T36.1X6
Cephalotin	T36.1X1	T36.1X2	T36.1X3	T36.1X4	T36.1X5	T36.1X6
Cephradine	T36.1X1	T36.1X2	T36.1X3	T36.1X4	T36.1X5	T36.1X6
Cerbera (odallam)	T62.2X1	T62.2X2	T62.2X3	T62.2X4	—	—
Cerberin	T46.0X1	T46.0X2	T46.0X3	T46.0X4	T46.0X5	T46.0X6
Cerebral stimulants	T43.601	T43.602	T43.603	T43.604	T43.605	T43.606
psychotherapeutic	T43.601	T43.602	T43.603	T43.604	T43.605	T43.606
specified NEC	T43.691	T43.692	T43.693	T43.694	T43.695	T43.696
Cerium oxalate	T45.0X1	T45.0X2	T45.0X3	T45.0X4	T45.0X5	T45.0X6
Cerous oxalate	T45.0X1	T45.0X2	T45.0X3	T45.0X4	T45.0X5	T45.0X6
Ceruletide	T50.8X1	T50.8X2	T50.8X3	T50.8X4	T50.8X5	T50.8X6
Cetalkonium (chloride)	T49.0X1	T49.0X2	T49.0X3	T49.0X4	T49.0X5	T49.0X6
Cethexonium chloride	T49.0X1	T49.0X2	T49.0X3	T49.0X4	T49.0X5	T49.0X6
Cetiedil	T46.7X1	T46.7X2	T46.7X3	T46.7X4	T46.7X5	T46.7X6
Cetirizine	T45.0X1	T45.0X2	T45.0X3	T45.0X4	T45.0X5	T45.0X6
Cetomacrogol	T50.991	T50.992	T50.993	T50.994	T50.995	T50.996
Cetotiamine	T45.2X1	T45.2X2	T45.2X3	T45.2X4	T45.2X5	T45.2X6
Cetoxime	T45.0X1	T45.0X2	T45.0X3	T45.0X4	T45.0X5	T45.0X6
Cetraxate	T47.1X1	T47.1X2	T47.1X3	T47.1X4	T47.1X5	T47.1X6
Cetrimide	T49.0X1	T49.0X2	T49.0X3	T49.0X4	T49.0X5	T49.0X6
Cetrimonium (bromide)	T49.0X1	T49.0X2	T49.0X3	T49.0X4	T49.0X5	T49.0X6
Cetylpyridinium chloride	T49.0X1	T49.0X2	T49.0X3	T49.0X4	T49.0X5	T49.0X6
ENT agent	T49.6X1	T49.6X2	T49.6X3	T49.6X4	T49.6X5	T49.6X6
lozenges	T49.6X1	T49.6X2	T49.6X3	T49.6X4	T49.6X5	T49.6X6
Cevadilla — see Sabadilla						
Cevitamic acid	T45.2X1	T45.2X2	T45.2X3	T45.2X4	T45.2X5	T45.2X6
Chalk, precipitated	T47.1X1	T47.1X2	T47.1X3	T47.1X4	T47.1X5	T47.1X6
Chamomile	T49.0X1	T49.0X2	T49.0X3	T49.0X4	T49.0X5	T49.0X6
Ch'an su	T46.0X1	T46.0X2	T46.0X3	T46.0X4	T46.0X5	T46.0X6
Charcoal	T47.6X1	T47.6X2	T47.6X3	T47.6X4	T47.6X5	T47.6X6
activated — see also Charcoal, medicinal	T47.6X1	T47.6X2	T47.6X3	T47.6X4	T47.6X5	T47.6X6
fumes (Carbon monoxide)	T58.2X1	T58.2X2	T58.2X3	T58.2X4	—	—
industrial	T58.8X1	T58.8X2	T58.8X3	T58.8X4	—	—
medicinal (activated)	T47.6X1	T47.6X2	T47.6X3	T47.6X4	T47.6X5	T47.6X6
antidiarrheal	T47.6X1	T47.6X2	T47.6X3	T47.6X4	T47.6X5	T47.6X6
poison control	T47.8X1	T47.8X2	T47.8X3	T47.8X4	T47.8X5	T47.8X6
specified use other than for diarrhea	T47.8X1	T47.8X2	T47.8X3	T47.8X4	T47.8X5	T47.8X6
topical	T49.8X1	T49.8X2	T49.8X3	T49.8X4	T49.8X5	T49.8X6
Chaulmosulfone	T37.1X1	T37.1X2	T37.1X3	T37.1X4	T37.1X5	T37.1X6
Chelating agent NEC	T50.6X1	T50.6X2	T50.6X3	T50.6X4	T50.6X5	T50.6X6
Chelidonium majus	T62.2X1	T62.2X2	T62.2X3	T62.2X4	—	—
Chemical substance NEC	T65.91	T65.92	T65.93	T65.94	—	—
Chenodeoxycholic acid	T47.5X1	T47.5X2	T47.5X3	T47.5X4	T47.5X5	T47.5X6
Chenodiol	T47.5X1	T47.5X2	T47.5X3	T47.5X4	T47.5X5	T47.5X6
Chenopodium	T37.4X1	T37.4X2	T37.4X3	T37.4X4	T37.4X5	T37.4X6
Cherry laurel	T62.2X1	T62.2X2	T62.2X3	T62.2X4	—	—
Chinidin (e)	T46.2X1	T46.2X2	T46.2X3	T46.2X4	T46.2X5	T46.2X6
Chiniofon	T37.8X1	T37.8X2	T37.8X3	T37.8X4	T37.8X5	T37.8X6
Chlophedianol	T48.3X1	T48.3X2	T48.3X3	T48.3X4	T48.3X5	T48.3X6
Chloral	T42.6X1	T42.6X2	T42.6X3	T42.6X4	T42.6X5	T42.6X6
derivative	T42.6X1	T42.6X2	T42.6X3	T42.6X4	T42.6X5	T42.6X6
hydrate	T42.6X1	T42.6X2	T42.6X3	T42.6X4	T42.6X5	T42.6X6
Chloralamide	T42.6X1	T42.6X2	T42.6X3	T42.6X4	T42.6X5	T42.6X6
Chloralodol	T42.6X1	T42.6X2	T42.6X3	T42.6X4	T42.6X5	T42.6X6
Chloralose	T60.4X1	T60.4X2	T60.4X3	T60.4X4	—	—
Chlorambucil	T45.1X1	T45.1X2	T45.1X3	T45.1X4	T45.1X5	T45.1X6
Chloramine	T57.8X1	T57.8X2	T57.8X3	T57.8X4	—	—
Chloramine — continued						
T	T49.0X1	T49.0X2	T49.0X3	T49.0X4	T49.0X5	T49.0X6
topical	T49.0X1	T49.0X2	T49.0X3	T49.0X4	T49.0X5	T49.0X6
Chloramphenicol	T36.2X1	T36.2X2	T36.2X3	T36.2X4	T36.2X5	T36.2X6
ENT agent	T49.6X1	T49.6X2	T49.6X3	T49.6X4	T49.6X5	T49.6X6
ophthalmic preparation	T49.5X1	T49.5X2	T49.5X3	T49.5X4	T49.5X5	T49.5X6
topical NEC	T49.0X1	T49.0X2	T49.0X3	T49.0X4	T49.0X5	T49.0X6
Chlorate (potassium) (sodium) NEC	T60.3X1	T60.3X2	T60.3X3	T60.3X4	—	—
herbicide	T60.3X1	T60.3X2	T60.3X3	T60.3X4	—	—
Chlorazanil	T50.2X1	T50.2X2	T50.2X3	T50.2X4	T50.2X5	T50.2X6
Chlorbenzene, chlorbenzol	T53.7X1	T53.7X2	T53.7X3	T53.7X4	—	—
Chlorbenzoxamine	T44.3X1	T44.3X2	T44.3X3	T44.3X4	T44.3X5	T44.3X6
Chlorbutol	T42.6X1	T42.6X2	T42.6X3	T42.6X4	T42.6X5	T42.6X6
Chlorcyclizine	T45.0X1	T45.0X2	T45.0X3	T45.0X4	T45.0X5	T45.0X6
Chlordan (e) (dust)	T60.1X1	T60.1X2	T60.1X3	T60.1X4	—	—
Chlordantoin	T49.0X1	T49.0X2	T49.0X3	T49.0X4	T49.0X5	T49.0X6
Chlordiazepoxide	T42.4X1	T42.4X2	T42.4X3	T42.4X4	T42.4X5	T42.4X6
Chlordiethyl benzamide	T49.3X1	T49.3X2	T49.3X3	T49.3X4	T49.3X5	T49.3X6
Chloresium	T49.8X1	T49.8X2	T49.8X3	T49.8X4	T49.8X5	T49.8X6
Chlorethiazol	T42.6X1	T42.6X2	T42.6X3	T42.6X4	T42.6X5	T42.6X6
Chlorethyl — see Ethyl chloride						
Chloretone	T42.6X1	T42.6X2	T42.6X3	T42.6X4	T42.6X5	T42.6X6
Chlorex	T53.6X1	T53.6X2	T53.6X3	T53.6X4	—	—
insecticide	T60.1X1	T60.1X2	T60.1X3	T60.1X4	—	—
Chlorfenvinphos	T60.0X1	T60.0X2	T60.0X3	T60.0X4	—	—
Chlorhexadol	T42.6X1	T42.6X2	T42.6X3	T42.6X4	T42.6X5	T42.6X6
Chlorhexamide	T45.1X1	T45.1X2	T45.1X3	T45.1X4	T45.1X5	T45.1X6
Chlorhexidine	T49.0X1	T49.0X2	T49.0X3	T49.0X4	T49.0X5	T49.0X6
Chlorhydroxyquinolin	T49.0X1	T49.0X2	T49.0X3	T49.0X4	T49.0X5	T49.0X6
Chloride of lime (bleach)	T54.3X1	T54.3X2	T54.3X3	T54.3X4	—	—
Chlorimipramine	T43.011	T43.012	T43.013	T43.014	T43.015	T43.016
Chlorinated						
camphene	T53.6X1	T53.6X2	T53.6X3	T53.6X4	—	—
diphenyl	T53.7X1	T53.7X2	T53.7X3	T53.7X4	—	—
hydrocarbons NEC	T53.91	T53.92	T53.93	T53.94	—	—
solvents	T53.91	T53.92	T53.93	T53.94	—	—
lime (bleach)	T54.3X1	T54.3X2	T54.3X3	T54.3X4	—	—
and boric acid solution	T49.0X1	T49.0X2	T49.0X3	T49.0X4	T49.0X5	T49.0X6
naphthalene (insecticide)	T60.1X1	T60.1X2	T60.1X3	T60.1X4	—	—
industrial (non-pesticide)	T53.7X1	T53.7X2	T53.7X3	T53.7X4	—	—
pesticide NEC	T60.8X1	T60.8X2	T60.8X3	T60.8X4	—	—
soda — see also sodium hypochlorite						
solution	T49.0X1	T49.0X2	T49.0X3	T49.0X4	T49.0X5	T49.0X6
Chlorine (fumes) (gas)	T59.4X1	T59.4X2	T59.4X3	T59.4X4	—	—
bleach	T54.3X1	T54.3X2	T54.3X3	T54.3X4	—	—
compound gas NEC	T59.4X1	T59.4X2	T59.4X3	T59.4X4	—	—
disinfectant	T59.4X1	T59.4X2	T59.4X3	T59.4X4	—	—
releasing agents NEC	T59.4X1	T59.4X2	T59.4X3	T59.4X4	—	—
Chlorisondamine chloride	T46.991	T46.992	T46.993	T46.994	T46.995	T46.996
Chlormadinone	T38.5X1	T38.5X2	T38.5X3	T38.5X4	T38.5X5	T38.5X6
Chlormephos	T60.0X1	T60.0X2	T60.0X3	T60.0X4	—	—
Chlormerodrin	T50.2X1	T50.2X2	T50.2X3	T50.2X4	T50.2X5	T50.2X6
Chlormethiazole	T42.6X1	T42.6X2	T42.6X3	T42.6X4	T42.6X5	T42.6X6
Chlormethine	T45.1X1	T45.1X2	T45.1X3	T45.1X4	T45.1X5	T45.1X6
Chlormethylenecycline	T36.4X1	T36.4X2	T36.4X3	T36.4X4	T36.4X5	T36.4X6
Chlormezanone	T42.6X1	T42.6X2	T42.6X3	T42.6X4	T42.6X5	T42.6X6
Chloroacetic acid	T60.3X1	T60.3X2	T60.3X3	T60.3X4	—	—
Chloroacetone	T59.3X1	T59.3X2	T59.3X3	T59.3X4	—	—
Chloroacetophenone	T59.3X1	T59.3X2	T59.3X3	T59.3X4	—	—
Chloroaniline	T53.7X1	T53.7X2	T53.7X3	T53.7X4	—	—
Chlorobenzene, chlorobenzol	T53.7X1	T53.7X2	T53.7X3	T53.7X4	—	—
Chlorobromomethane (fire extinguisher)	T53.6X1	T53.6X2	T53.6X3	T53.6X4	—	—
Chlorobutanol	T49.0X1	T49.0X2	T49.0X3	T49.0X4	T49.0X5	T49.0X6
Chlorocresol	T49.0X1	T49.0X2	T49.0X3	T49.0X4	T49.0X5	T49.0X6
Chlorodehydromethyltestosterone	T38.7X1	T38.7X2	T38.7X3	T38.7X4	T38.7X5	T38.7X6
Chlorodinitrobenzene	T53.7X1	T53.7X2	T53.7X3	T53.7X4	—	—
dust or vapor	T53.7X1	T53.7X2	T53.7X3	T53.7X4	—	—
Chlorodiphenyl	T53.7X1	T53.7X2	T53.7X3	T53.7X4	—	—
Chloroethane — see Ethyl chloride						
Chloroethylene	T53.6X1	T53.6X2	T53.6X3	T53.6X4	—	—
Chlorofluorocarbons	T53.5X1	T53.5X2	T53.5X3	T53.5X4	—	—
Chloroform (fumes) (vapor)	T53.1X1	T53.1X2	T53.1X3	T53.1X4	—	—
anesthetic	T41.0X1	T41.0X2	T41.0X3	T41.0X4	T41.0X5	T41.0X6
solvent	T53.1X1	T53.1X2	T53.1X3	T53.1X4	—	—
water, concentrated	T41.0X1	T41.0X2	T41.0X3	T41.0X4	T41.0X5	T41.0X6
Chloroguanide	T37.2X1	T37.2X2	T37.2X3	T37.2X4	T37.2X5	T37.2X6

Substance	Poisoning, Accidental (unintentional)	Poisoning, Intentional Self-harm	Poisoning, Assault	Poisoning, Undetermined	Adverse Effect	Under-dosing
Chloromycetin	T36.2X1	T36.2X2	T36.2X3	T36.2X4	T36.2X5	T36.2X6
ENT agent	T49.6X1	T49.6X2	T49.6X3	T49.6X4	T49.6X5	T49.6X6
ophthalmic preparation	T49.5X1	T49.5X2	T49.5X3	T49.5X4	T49.5X5	T49.5X6
otic solution	T49.6X1	T49.6X2	T49.6X3	T49.6X4	T49.6X5	T49.6X6
topical NEC	T49.0X1	T49.0X2	T49.0X3	T49.0X4	T49.0X5	T49.0X6
Chloronitrobenzene	T53.7X1	T53.7X2	T53.7X3	T53.7X4	—	—
dust or vapor	T53.7X1	T53.7X2	T53.7X3	T53.7X4	—	—
Chlorophacinone	T60.4X1	T60.4X2	T60.4X3	T60.4X4	—	—
Chlorophenol	T53.7X1	T53.7X2	T53.7X3	T53.7X4	—	—
Chlorophenothane	T60.1X1	T60.1X2	T60.1X3	T60.1X4	—	—
Chlorophyll	T50.991	T50.992	T50.993	T50.994	T50.995	T50.996
Chloropicrin (fumes)	T53.6X1	T53.6X2	T53.6X3	T53.6X4	—	—
fumigant	T60.8X1	T60.8X2	T60.8X3	T60.8X4	—	—
fungicide	T60.3X1	T60.3X2	T60.3X3	T60.3X4	—	—
pesticide	T60.8X1	T60.8X2	T60.8X3	T60.8X4	—	—
Chloroprocaine	T41.3X1	T41.3X2	T41.3X3	T41.3X4	T41.3X5	T41.3X6
infiltration (subcutaneous)	T41.3X1	T41.3X2	T41.3X3	T41.3X4	T41.3X5	T41.3X6
nerve block (peripheral) (plexus)	T41.3X1	T41.3X2	T41.3X3	T41.3X4	T41.3X5	T41.3X6
spinal	T41.3X1	T41.3X2	T41.3X3	T41.3X4	T41.3X5	T41.3X6
Chloroptic	T49.5X1	T49.5X2	T49.5X3	T49.5X4	T49.5X5	T49.5X6
Chloropurine	T45.1X1	T45.1X2	T45.1X3	T45.1X4	T45.1X5	T45.1X6
Chloropyramine	T45.0X1	T45.0X2	T45.0X3	T45.0X4	T45.0X5	T45.0X6
Chloropyrifos	T60.0X1	T60.0X2	T60.0X3	T60.0X4	—	—
Chloropyrilene	T45.0X1	T45.0X2	T45.0X3	T45.0X4	T45.0X5	T45.0X6
Chloroquine	T37.2X1	T37.2X2	T37.2X3	T37.2X4	T37.2X5	T37.2X6
Chlorothalonil	T60.3X1	T60.3X2	T60.3X3	T60.3X4	—	—
Chlorothen	T45.0X1	T45.0X2	T45.0X3	T45.0X4	T45.0X5	T45.0X6
Chlorothiazide	T50.2X1	T50.2X2	T50.2X3	T50.2X4	T50.2X5	T50.2X6
Chlorothymol	T49.4X1	T49.4X2	T49.4X3	T49.4X4	T49.4X5	T49.4X6
Chlorotrianisene	T38.5X1	T38.5X2	T38.5X3	T38.5X4	T38.5X5	T38.5X6
Chlorovinyldichloroarsine, not in war	T57.0X1	T57.0X2	T57.0X3	T57.0X4	—	—
Chloroxine	T49.4X1	T49.4X2	T49.4X3	T49.4X4	T49.4X5	T49.4X6
Chloroxylenol	T49.0X1	T49.0X2	T49.0X3	T49.0X4	T49.0X5	T49.0X6
Chlorphenamine	T45.0X1	T45.0X2	T45.0X3	T45.0X4	T45.0X5	T45.0X6
Chlorphenesin	T42.8X1	T42.8X2	T42.8X3	T42.8X4	T42.8X5	T42.8X6
topical (antifungal)	T49.0X1	T49.0X2	T49.0X3	T49.0X4	T49.0X5	T49.0X6
Chlorpheniramine	T45.0X1	T45.0X2	T45.0X3	T45.0X4	T45.0X5	T45.0X6
Chlorphenoxamine	T45.0X1	T45.0X2	T45.0X3	T45.0X4	T45.0X5	T45.0X6
Chlorphentermine	T50.5X1	T50.5X2	T50.5X3	T50.5X4	T50.5X5	T50.5X6
Chlorprocaine — *see* Chloroprocaine						
Chlorproguanil	T37.2X1	T37.2X2	T37.2X3	T37.2X4	T37.2X5	T37.2X6
Chlorpromazine	T43.3X1	T43.3X2	T43.3X3	T43.3X4	T43.3X5	T43.3X6
Chlorpropamide	T38.3X1	T38.3X2	T38.3X3	T38.3X4	T38.3X5	T38.3X6
Chlorprothixene	T43.4X1	T43.4X2	T43.4X3	T43.4X4	T43.4X5	T43.4X6
Chlorquinaldol	T49.0X1	T49.0X2	T49.0X3	T49.0X4	T49.0X5	T49.0X6
Chlorquinol	T49.0X1	T49.0X2	T49.0X3	T49.0X4	T49.0X5	T49.0X6
Chlortalidone	T50.2X1	T50.2X2	T50.2X3	T50.2X4	T50.2X5	T50.2X6
Chlortetracycline	T36.4X1	T36.4X2	T36.4X3	T36.4X4	T36.4X5	T36.4X6
Chlorthalidone	T50.2X1	T50.2X2	T50.2X3	T50.2X4	T50.2X5	T50.2X6
Chlorthion	T60.0X1	T60.0X2	T60.0X3	T60.0X4	—	—
Chlorthiophos	T60.0X1	T60.0X2	T60.0X3	T60.0X4	—	—
Chlortrianisene	T38.5X1	T38.5X2	T38.5X3	T38.5X4	T38.5X5	T38.5X6
Chlor-Trimeton	T45.0X1	T45.0X2	T45.0X3	T45.0X4	T45.0X5	T45.0X6
Chlorzoxazone	T42.8X1	T42.8X2	T42.8X3	T42.8X4	T42.8X5	T42.8X6
Choke damp	T59.7X1	T59.7X2	T59.7X3	T59.7X4	—	—
Cholagogues	T47.5X1	T47.5X2	T47.5X3	T47.5X4	T47.5X5	T47.5X6
Cholebrine	T50.8X1	T50.8X2	T50.8X3	T50.8X4	T50.8X5	T50.8X6
Cholecalciferol	T45.2X1	T45.2X2	T45.2X3	T45.2X4	T45.2X5	T45.2X6
Cholecystokinin	T50.8X1	T50.8X2	T50.8X3	T50.8X4	T50.8X5	T50.8X6
Cholera vaccine	T50.A91	T50.A92	T50.A93	T50.A94	T50.A95	T50.A96
Choleretic	T47.5X1	T47.5X2	T47.5X3	T47.5X4	T47.5X5	T47.5X6
Cholesterol-lowering agents	T46.6X1	T46.6X2	T46.6X3	T46.6X4	T46.6X5	T46.6X6
Cholestyramine (resin)	T46.6X1	T46.6X2	T46.6X3	T46.6X4	T46.6X5	T46.6X6
Cholic acid	T47.5X1	T47.5X2	T47.5X3	T47.5X4	T47.5X5	T47.5X6
Choline	T48.6X1	T48.6X2	T48.6X3	T48.6X4	T48.6X5	T48.6X6
chloride	T50.991	T50.992	T50.993	T50.994	T50.995	T50.996
dihydrogen citrate	T50.991	T50.992	T50.993	T50.994	T50.995	T50.996
salicylate	T39.091	T39.092	T39.093	T39.094	T39.095	T39.096
theophyllinate	T48.6X1	T48.6X2	T48.6X3	T48.6X4	T48.6X5	T48.6X6
Cholinergic (drug) **NEC**	T44.1X1	T44.1X2	T44.1X3	T44.1X4	T44.1X5	T44.1X6
muscle tone enhancer	T44.1X1	T44.1X2	T44.1X3	T44.1X4	T44.1X5	T44.1X6
organophosphorus	T44.0X1	T44.0X2	T44.0X3	T44.0X4	T44.0X5	T44.0X6
insecticide	T60.0X1	T60.0X2	T60.0X3	T60.0X4	—	—
nerve gas	T59.891	T59.892	T59.893	T59.894	—	—
trimethyl ammonium propanediol	T44.1X1	T44.1X2	T44.1X3	T44.1X4	T44.1X5	T44.1X6
Cholinesterase reactivator	T50.6X1	T50.6X2	T50.6X3	T50.6X4	T50.6X5	T50.6X6
Cholografin	T50.8X1	T50.8X2	T50.8X3	T50.8X4	T50.8X5	T50.8X6
Chorionic gonadotropin	T38.891	T38.892	T38.893	T38.894	T38.895	T38.896
Chromate	T56.2X1	T56.2X2	T56.2X3	T56.2X4	—	—
dust or mist	T56.2X1	T56.2X2	T56.2X3	T56.2X4	—	—
lead — *see also* lead	T56.0X1	T56.0X2	T56.0X3	T56.0X4	—	—
paint	T56.0X1	T56.0X2	T56.0X3	T56.0X4	—	—
Chromic						
acid	T56.2X1	T56.2X2	T56.2X3	T56.2X4	—	—
dust or mist	T56.2X1	T56.2X2	T56.2X3	T56.2X4	—	—
phosphate 32P	T45.1X1	T45.1X2	T45.1X3	T45.1X4	T45.1X5	T45.1X6
Chromium	T56.2X1	T56.2X2	T56.2X3	T56.2X4	—	—
compounds — *see* Chromate						
sesquioxide	T50.8X1	T50.8X2	T50.8X3	T50.8X4	T50.8X5	T50.8X6
Chromomycin A3	T45.1X1	T45.1X2	T45.1X3	T45.1X4	T45.1X5	T45.1X6
Chromonar	T46.3X1	T46.3X2	T46.3X3	T46.3X4	T46.3X5	T46.3X6
Chromyl chloride	T56.2X1	T56.2X2	T56.2X3	T56.2X4	—	—
Chrysarobin	T49.4X1	T49.4X2	T49.4X3	T49.4X4	T49.4X5	T49.4X6
Chrysazin	T47.2X1	T47.2X2	T47.2X3	T47.2X4	T47.2X5	T47.2X6
Chymar	T45.3X1	T45.3X2	T45.3X3	T45.3X4	T45.3X5	T45.3X6
ophthalmic preparation	T49.5X1	T49.5X2	T49.5X3	T49.5X4	T49.5X5	T49.5X6
Chymopapain	T45.3X1	T45.3X2	T45.3X3	T45.3X4	T45.3X5	T45.3X6
Chymotrypsin	T45.3X1	T45.3X2	T45.3X3	T45.3X4	T45.3X5	T45.3X6
ophthalmic preparation	T49.5X1	T49.5X2	T49.5X3	T49.5X4	T49.5X5	T49.5X6
Cianidanol	T50.991	T50.992	T50.993	T50.994	T50.995	T50.996
Cianopramine	T43.011	T43.012	T43.013	T43.014	T43.015	T43.016
Cibenzoline	T46.2X1	T46.2X2	T46.2X3	T46.2X4	T46.2X5	T46.2X6
Ciclacillin	T36.0X1	T36.0X2	T36.0X3	T36.0X4	T36.0X5	T36.0X6
Ciclobarbital — *see* Hexobarbital						
Ciclonicate	T46.7X1	T46.7X2	T46.7X3	T46.7X4	T46.7X5	T46.7X6
Ciclopirox (olamine)	T49.0X1	T49.0X2	T49.0X3	T49.0X4	T49.0X5	T49.0X6
Ciclosporin	T45.1X1	T45.1X2	T45.1X3	T45.1X4	T45.1X5	T45.1X6
Cicuta maculata or virosa	T62.2X1	T62.2X2	T62.2X3	T62.2X4	—	—
Cicutoxin	T62.2X1	T62.2X2	T62.2X3	T62.2X4	—	—
Cigarette lighter fluid	T52.0X1	T52.0X2	T52.0X3	T52.0X4	—	—
Cigarettes (tobacco)	T65.221	T65.222	T65.223	T65.224	—	—
Ciguatoxin	T61.01	T61.02	T61.03	T61.04	—	—
Cilazapril	T46.4X1	T46.4X2	T46.4X3	T46.4X4	T46.4X5	T46.4X6
Cimetidine	T47.0X1	T47.0X2	T47.0X3	T47.0X4	T47.0X5	T47.0X6
Cimetropium bromide	T44.3X1	T44.3X2	T44.3X3	T44.3X4	T44.3X5	T44.3X6
Cinchocaine	T41.3X1	T41.3X2	T41.3X3	T41.3X4	T41.3X5	T41.3X6
topical (surface)	T41.3X1	T41.3X2	T41.3X3	T41.3X4	T41.3X5	T41.3X6
Cinchona	T37.2X1	T37.2X2	T37.2X3	T37.2X4	T37.2X5	T37.2X6
Cinchonine alkaloids	T37.2X1	T37.2X2	T37.2X3	T37.2X4	T37.2X5	T37.2X6
Cinchophen	T50.4X1	T50.4X2	T50.4X3	T50.4X4	T50.4X5	T50.4X6
Cinepazide	T46.7X1	T46.7X2	T46.7X3	T46.7X4	T46.7X5	T46.7X6
Cinnamedrine	T48.5X1	T48.5X2	T48.5X3	T48.5X4	T48.5X5	T48.5X6
Cinnarizine	T45.0X1	T45.0X2	T45.0X3	T45.0X4	T45.0X5	T45.0X6
Cinoxacin	T37.8X1	T37.8X2	T37.8X3	T37.8X4	T37.8X5	T37.8X6
Ciprofibrate	T46.6X1	T46.6X2	T46.6X3	T46.6X4	T46.6X5	T46.6X6
Ciprofloxacin	T36.8X1	T36.8X2	T36.8X3	T36.8X4	T36.8X5	T36.8X6
Cisapride	T47.8X1	T47.8X2	T47.8X3	T47.8X4	T47.8X5	T47.8X6
Cisplatin	T45.1X1	T45.1X2	T45.1X3	T45.1X4	T45.1X5	T45.1X6
Citalopram	T43.221	T43.222	T43.223	T43.224	T43.225	T43.226
Citanest	T41.3X1	T41.3X2	T41.3X3	T41.3X4	T41.3X5	T41.3X6
infiltration (subcutaneous)	T41.3X1	T41.3X2	T41.3X3	T41.3X4	T41.3X5	T41.3X6
nerve block (peripheral) (plexus)	T41.3X1	T41.3X2	T41.3X3	T41.3X4	T41.3X5	T41.3X6
Citric acid	T47.5X1	T47.5X2	T47.5X3	T47.5X4	T47.5X5	T47.5X6
Citrovorum (factor)	T45.8X1	T45.8X2	T45.8X3	T45.8X4	T45.8X5	T45.8X6
Claviceps purpurea	T62.2X1	T62.2X2	T62.2X3	T62.2X4	—	—
Clavulanic acid	T36.1X1	T36.1X2	T36.1X3	T36.1X4	T36.1X5	T36.1X6
Cleaner, cleansing agent, type not specified	T65.891	T65.892	T65.893	T65.894	—	—
of paint or varnish	T52.91	T52.92	T52.93	T52.94	—	—
specified type NEC	T65.891	T65.892	T65.893	T65.894	—	—
Clebopride	T47.8X1	T47.8X2	T47.8X3	T47.8X4	T47.8X5	T47.8X6
Clefamide	T37.3X1	T37.3X2	T37.3X3	T37.3X4	T37.3X5	T37.3X6
Clemastine	T45.0X1	T45.0X2	T45.0X3	T45.0X4	T45.0X5	T45.0X6
Clematis vitalba	T62.2X1	T62.2X2	T62.2X3	T62.2X4	—	—
Clemizole	T45.0X1	T45.0X2	T45.0X3	T45.0X4	T45.0X5	T45.0X6
penicillin	T36.0X1	T36.0X2	T36.0X3	T36.0X4	T36.0X5	T36.0X6
Clenbuterol	T48.6X1	T48.6X2	T48.6X3	T48.6X4	T48.6X5	T48.6X6
Clidinium bromide	T44.3X1	T44.3X2	T44.3X3	T44.3X4	T44.3X5	T44.3X6
Clindamycin	T36.8X1	T36.8X2	T36.8X3	T36.8X4	T36.8X5	T36.8X6
Clinofibrate	T46.6X1	T46.6X2	T46.6X3	T46.6X4	T46.6X5	T46.6X6
Clioquinol	T37.8X1	T37.8X2	T37.8X3	T37.8X4	T37.8X5	T37.8X6
Cliradon	T40.2X1	T40.2X2	T40.2X3	T40.2X4	—	—
Clobazam	T42.4X1	T42.4X2	T42.4X3	T42.4X4	T42.4X5	T42.4X6
Clobenzorex	T50.5X1	T50.5X2	T50.5X3	T50.5X4	T50.5X5	T50.5X6
Clobetasol	T49.0X1	T49.0X2	T49.0X3	T49.0X4	T49.0X5	T49.0X6
Clobetasone	T49.0X1	T49.0X2	T49.0X3	T49.0X4	T49.0X5	T49.0X6
Clobutinol	T48.3X1	T48.3X2	T48.3X3	T48.3X4	T48.3X5	T48.3X6
Clocortolone	T38.0X1	T38.0X2	T38.0X3	T38.0X4	T38.0X5	T38.0X6
Clodantoin	T49.0X1	T49.0X2	T49.0X3	T49.0X4	T49.0X5	T49.0X6

Chloromycetin — Clodantoin

Table of Drugs and Chemicals

Substance	Poisoning, Accidental (unintentional)	Poisoning, Intentional Self-harm	Poisoning, Assault	Poisoning, Undetermined	Adverse Effect	Under-dosing
Clodronic acid	T50.991	T50.992	T50.993	T50.994	T50.995	T50.996
Clofazimine	T37.1X1	T37.1X2	T37.1X3	T37.1X4	T37.1X5	T37.1X6
Clofedanol	T48.3X1	T48.3X2	T48.3X3	T48.3X4	T48.3X5	T48.3X6
Clofenamide	T50.2X1	T50.2X2	T50.2X3	T50.2X4	T50.2X5	T50.2X6
Clofenotane	T49.0X1	T49.0X2	T49.0X3	T49.0X4	T49.0X5	T49.0X6
Clofezone	T39.2X1	T39.2X2	T39.2X3	T39.2X4	T39.2X5	T39.2X6
Clofibrate	T46.6X1	T46.6X2	T46.6X3	T46.6X4	T46.6X5	T46.6X6
Clofibride	T46.6X1	T46.6X2	T46.6X3	T46.6X4	T46.6X5	T46.6X6
Cloforex	T50.5X1	T50.5X2	T50.5X3	T50.5X4	T50.5X5	T50.5X6
Clomethiazole	T42.6X1	T42.6X2	T42.6X3	T42.6X4	T42.6X5	T42.6X6
Clometocillin	T36.0X1	T36.0X2	T36.0X3	T36.0X4	T36.0X5	T36.0X6
Clomifene	T38.5X1	T38.5X2	T38.5X3	T38.5X4	T38.5X5	T38.5X6
Clomiphene	T38.5X1	T38.5X2	T38.5X3	T38.5X4	T38.5X5	T38.5X6
Clomipramine	T43.011	T43.012	T43.013	T43.014	T43.015	T43.016
Clomocycline	T36.4X1	T36.4X2	T36.4X3	T36.4X4	T36.4X5	T36.4X6
Clonazepam	T42.4X1	T42.4X2	T42.4X3	T42.4X4	T42.4X5	T42.4X6
Clonidine	T46.5X1	T46.5X2	T46.5X3	T46.5X4	T46.5X5	T46.5X6
Clonixin	T39.8X1	T39.8X2	T39.8X3	T39.8X4	T39.8X5	T39.8X6
Clopamide	T50.2X1	T50.2X2	T50.2X3	T50.2X4	T50.2X5	T50.2X6
Clopenthixol	T43.4X1	T43.4X2	T43.4X3	T43.4X4	T43.4X5	T43.4X6
Cloperastine	T48.3X1	T48.3X2	T48.3X3	T48.3X4	T48.3X5	T48.3X6
Clophedianol	T48.3X1	T48.3X2	T48.3X3	T48.3X4	T48.3X5	T48.3X6
Cloponone	T36.2X1	T36.2X2	T36.2X3	T36.2X4	T36.2X5	T36.2X6
Cloprednol	T38.0X1	T38.0X2	T38.0X3	T38.0X4	T38.0X5	T38.0X6
Cloral betaine	T42.6X1	T42.6X2	T42.6X3	T42.6X4	T42.6X5	T42.6X6
Cloramfenicol	T36.2X1	T36.2X2	T36.2X3	T36.2X4	T36.2X5	T36.2X6
Clorazepate (dipotassium)	T42.4X1	T42.4X2	T42.4X3	T42.4X4	T42.4X5	T42.4X6
Clorexolone	T50.2X1	T50.2X2	T50.2X3	T50.2X4	T50.2X5	T50.2X6
Clorfenamine	T45.0X1	T45.0X2	T45.0X3	T45.0X4	T45.0X5	T45.0X6
Clorgiline	T43.1X1	T43.1X2	T43.1X3	T43.1X4	T43.1X5	T43.1X6
Clorotepine	T44.3X1	T44.3X2	T44.3X3	T44.3X4	T44.3X5	T44.3X6
Clorox (bleach)	T54.91	T54.92	T54.93	T54.94	—	—
Clorprenaline	T48.6X1	T48.6X2	T48.6X3	T48.6X4	T48.6X5	T48.6X6
Clortermine	T50.5X1	T50.5X2	T50.5X3	T50.5X4	T50.5X5	T50.5X6
Clotiapine	T43.591	T43.592	T43.593	T43.594	T43.595	T43.596
Clotiazepam	T42.4X1	T42.4X2	T42.4X3	T42.4X4	T42.4X5	T42.4X6
Clotibric acid	T46.6X1	T46.6X2	T46.6X3	T46.6X4	T46.6X5	T46.6X6
Clotrimazole	T49.0X1	T49.0X2	T49.0X3	T49.0X4	T49.0X5	T49.0X6
Cloxacillin	T36.0X1	T36.0X2	T36.0X3	T36.0X4	T36.0X5	T36.0X6
Cloxazolam	T42.4X1	T42.4X2	T42.4X3	T42.4X4	T42.4X5	T42.4X6
Cloxiquine	T49.0X1	T49.0X2	T49.0X3	T49.0X4	T49.0X5	T49.0X6
Clozapine	T42.4X1	T42.4X2	T42.4X3	T42.4X4	T42.4X5	T42.4X6
Coagulant NEC	T45.7X1	T45.7X2	T45.7X3	T45.7X4	T45.7X5	T45.7X6
Coal (carbon monoxide from) —	T58.2X1	T58.2X2	T58.2X3	T58.2X4	—	—
see also Carbon, monoxide, coal						
oil — see Kerosene						
tar	T49.1X1	T49.1X2	T49.1X3	T49.1X4	T49.1X5	T49.1X6
fumes	T59.891	T59.892	T59.893	T59.894	—	—
medicinal (ointment)	T49.4X1	T49.4X2	T49.4X3	T49.4X4	T49.4X5	T49.4X6
analgesics NEC	T39.2X1	T39.2X2	T39.2X3	T39.2X4	T39.2X5	T39.2X6
naphtha (solvent)	T52.0X1	T52.0X2	T52.0X3	T52.0X4	—	—
Cobalamine	T45.2X1	T45.2X2	T45.2X3	T45.2X4	T45.2X5	T45.2X6
Cobalt (nonmedicinal) (fumes) (industrial)	T56.891	T56.892	T56.893	T56.894	—	—
medicinal (trace) (chloride)	T45.8X1	T45.8X2	T45.8X3	T45.8X4	T45.8X5	T45.8X6
Cobra (venom)	T63.041	T63.042	T63.043	T63.044	—	—
Coca (leaf)	T40.5X1	T40.5X2	T40.5X3	T40.5X4	T40.5X5	T40.5X6
Cocaine	T40.5X1	T40.5X2	T40.5X3	T40.5X4	T40.5X5	T40.5X6
topical anesthetic	T41.3X1	T41.3X2	T41.3X3	T41.3X4	T41.3X5	T41.3X6
Cocarboxylase	T45.3X1	T45.3X2	T45.3X3	T45.3X4	T45.3X5	T45.3X6
Coccidioidin	T50.8X1	T50.8X2	T50.8X3	T50.8X4	T50.8X5	T50.8X6
Cocculus indicus	T62.1X1	T62.1X2	T62.1X3	T62.1X4	—	—
Cochineal	T65.6X1	T65.6X2	T65.6X3	T65.6X4	—	—
medicinal products	T50.991	T50.992	T50.993	T50.994	T50.995	T50.996
Codeine	T40.2X1	T40.2X2	T40.2X3	T40.2X4	T40.2X5	T40.2X6
Cod-liver oil	T45.2X1	T45.2X2	T45.2X3	T45.2X4	T45.2X5	T45.2X6
Coenzyme A	T50.991	T50.992	T50.993	T50.994	T50.995	T50.996
Coffee	T62.8X1	T62.8X2	T62.8X3	T62.8X4	—	—
Cogalactoisomerase	T50.991	T50.992	T50.993	T50.994	T50.995	T50.996
Cogentin	T44.3X1	T44.3X2	T44.3X3	T44.3X4	T44.3X5	T44.3X6
Coke fumes or gas (carbon monoxide)	T58.2X1	T58.2X2	T58.2X3	T58.2X4	—	—
industrial use	T58.8X1	T58.8X2	T58.8X3	T58.8X4	—	—
Colace	T47.4X1	T47.4X2	T47.4X3	T47.4X4	T47.4X5	T47.4X6
Colaspase	T45.1X1	T45.1X2	T45.1X3	T45.1X4	T45.1X5	T45.1X6
Colchicine	T50.4X1	T50.4X2	T50.4X3	T50.4X4	T50.4X5	T50.4X6
Colchicum	T62.2X1	T62.2X2	T62.2X3	T62.2X4	—	—
Cold cream	T49.3X1	T49.3X2	T49.3X3	T49.3X4	T49.3X5	T49.3X6
Colecalciferol	T45.2X1	T45.2X2	T45.2X3	T45.2X4	T45.2X5	T45.2X6
Colestipol	T46.6X1	T46.6X2	T46.6X3	T46.6X4	T46.6X5	T46.6X6
Colestyramine	T46.6X1	T46.6X2	T46.6X3	T46.6X4	T46.6X5	T46.6X6
Colimycin	T36.8X1	T36.8X2	T36.8X3	T36.8X4	T36.8X5	T36.8X6
Colistimethate	T36.8X1	T36.8X2	T36.8X3	T36.8X4	T36.8X5	T36.8X6
Colistin	T36.8X1	T36.8X2	T36.8X3	T36.8X4	T36.8X5	T36.8X6
sulfate (eye preparation)	T49.5X1	T49.5X2	T49.5X3	T49.5X4	T49.5X5	T49.5X6
Collagen	T50.991	T50.992	T50.993	T50.994	T50.995	T50.996
Collagenase	T49.4X1	T49.4X2	T49.4X3	T49.4X4	T49.4X5	T49.4X6
Collodion	T49.3X1	T49.3X2	T49.3X3	T49.3X4	T49.3X5	T49.3X6
Colocynth	T47.2X1	T47.2X2	T47.2X3	T47.2X4	T47.2X5	T47.2X6
Colophony adhesive	T49.3X1	T49.3X2	T49.3X3	T49.3X4	T49.3X5	T49.3X6
Colorant — see also Dye						
Coloring matter — see Dye(s)						
Combustion gas (after combustion) — see Carbon, monoxide						
prior to combustion	T59.891	T59.892	T59.893	T59.894	—	—
Compazine	T43.3X1	T43.3X2	T43.3X3	T43.3X4	T43.3X5	T43.3X6
Compound						
1080 (sodium fluoroacetate)	T60.4X1	T60.4X2	T60.4X3	T60.4X4	—	—
269 (endrin)	T60.1X1	T60.1X2	T60.1X3	T60.1X4	—	—
3422 (parathion)	T60.0X1	T60.0X2	T60.0X3	T60.0X4	—	—
3911 (phorate)	T60.0X1	T60.0X2	T60.0X3	T60.0X4	—	—
3956 (toxaphene)	T60.1X1	T60.1X2	T60.1X3	T60.1X4	—	—
4049 (malathion)	T60.0X1	T60.0X2	T60.0X3	T60.0X4	—	—
4069 (malathion)	T60.0X1	T60.0X2	T60.0X3	T60.0X4	—	—
4124 (dicapthon)	T60.0X1	T60.0X2	T60.0X3	T60.0X4	—	—
42 (warfarin)	T60.4X1	T60.4X2	T60.4X3	T60.4X4	—	—
497 (dieldrin)	T60.1X1	T60.1X2	T60.1X3	T60.1X4	—	—
E (cortisone)	T38.0X1	T38.0X2	T38.0X3	T38.0X4	T38.0X5	T38.0X6
F (hydrocortisone)	T38.0X1	T38.0X2	T38.0X3	T38.0X4	T38.0X5	T38.0X6
Congener, anabolic	T38.7X1	T38.7X2	T38.7X3	T38.7X4	T38.7X5	T38.7X6
Congo red	T50.8X1	T50.8X2	T50.8X3	T50.8X4	T50.8X5	T50.8X6
Coniine, conine	T62.2X1	T62.2X2	T62.2X3	T62.2X4	—	—
Conium (maculatum)	T62.2X1	T62.2X2	T62.2X3	T62.2X4	—	—
Conjugated estrogenic substances	T38.5X1	T38.5X2	T38.5X3	T38.5X4	T38.5X5	T38.5X6
Contac	T48.5X1	T48.5X2	T48.5X3	T48.5X4	T48.5X5	T48.5X6
Contact lens solution	T49.5X1	T49.5X2	T49.5X3	T49.5X4	T49.5X5	T49.5X6
Contraceptive (oral)	T38.4X1	T38.4X2	T38.4X3	T38.4X4	T38.4X5	T38.4X6
vaginal	T49.8X1	T49.8X2	T49.8X3	T49.8X4	T49.8X5	T49.8X6
Contrast medium, radiography	T50.8X1	T50.8X2	T50.8X3	T50.8X4	T50.8X5	T50.8X6
Convallaria glycosides	T46.0X1	T46.0X2	T46.0X3	T46.0X4	T46.0X5	T46.0X6
Convallaria majalis	T62.2X1	T62.2X2	T62.2X3	T62.2X4	—	—
berry	T62.1X1	T62.1X2	T62.1X3	T62.1X4	—	—
Copperhead snake (bite) (venom)	T63.061	T63.062	T63.063	T63.064	—	—
Copper (dust) (fumes) (nonmedicinal) NEC	T56.4X1	T56.4X2	T56.4X3	T56.4X4	—	—
arsenate, arsenite	T57.0X1	T57.0X2	T57.0X3	T57.0X4	—	—
insecticide	T60.2X1	T60.2X2	T60.2X3	T60.2X4	—	—
emetic	T47.7X1	T47.7X2	T47.7X3	T47.7X4	T47.7X5	T47.7X6
fungicide	T60.3X1	T60.3X2	T60.3X3	T60.3X4	—	—
gluconate	T49.0X1	T49.0X2	T49.0X3	T49.0X4	T49.0X5	T49.0X6
insecticide	T60.2X1	T60.2X2	T60.2X3	T60.2X4	—	—
medicinal (trace)	T45.8X1	T45.8X2	T45.8X3	T45.8X4	T45.8X5	T45.8X6
oleate	T49.0X1	T49.0X2	T49.0X3	T49.0X4	T49.0X5	T49.0X6
sulfate	T56.4X1	T56.4X2	T56.4X3	T56.4X4	—	—
cupric	T56.4X1	T56.4X2	T56.4X3	T56.4X4	—	—
fungicide	T60.3X1	T60.3X2	T60.3X3	T60.3X4	—	—
medicinal						
ear	T49.6X1	T49.6X2	T49.6X3	T49.6X4	T49.6X5	T49.6X6
emetic	T47.7X1	T47.7X2	T47.7X3	T47.7X4	T47.7X5	T47.7X6
eye	T49.5X1	T49.5X2	T49.5X3	T49.5X4	T49.5X5	T49.5X6
cuprous	T56.4X1	T56.4X2	T56.4X3	T56.4X4	—	—
fungicide	T60.3X1	T60.3X2	T60.3X3	T60.3X4	—	—
medicinal						
ear	T49.6X1	T49.6X2	T49.6X3	T49.6X4	T49.6X5	T49.6X6
emetic	T47.7X1	T47.7X2	T47.7X3	T47.7X4	T47.7X5	T47.7X6
eye	T49.5X1	T49.5X2	T49.5X3	T49.5X4	T49.5X5	T49.5X6
Coral (sting)	T63.691	T63.692	T63.693	T63.694	—	—
snake (bite) (venom)	T63.021	T63.022	T63.023	T63.024	—	—
Corbadrine	T49.6X1	T49.6X2	T49.6X3	T49.6X4	T49.6X5	T49.6X6
Cordite	T65.891	T65.892	T65.893	T65.894	—	—
vapor	T59.891	T59.892	T59.893	T59.894	—	—
Cordran	T49.0X1	T49.0X2	T49.0X3	T49.0X4	T49.0X5	T49.0X6
Corn cures	T49.4X1	T49.4X2	T49.4X3	T49.4X4	T49.4X5	T49.4X6
Cornhusker's lotion	T49.3X1	T49.3X2	T49.3X3	T49.3X4	T49.3X5	T49.3X6
Corn starch	T49.3X1	T49.3X2	T49.3X3	T49.3X4	T49.3X5	T49.3X6
Coronary vasodilator NEC	T46.3X1	T46.3X2	T46.3X3	T46.3X4	T46.3X5	T46.3X6
Corrosive NEC	T54.91	T54.92	T54.93	T54.94	—	—
acid NEC	T54.2X1	T54.2X2	T54.2X3	T54.2X4	—	—
aromatics	T54.1X1	T54.1X2	T54.1X3	T54.1X4	—	—
disinfectant	T54.1X1	T54.1X2	T54.1X3	T54.1X4	—	—

Clodronic acid — Corrosive NEC

Substance	Poisoning, Accidental (unintentional)	Poisoning, Intentional Self-harm	Poisoning, Assault	Poisoning, Undetermined	Adverse Effect	Under-dosing
Corrosive — *continued*						
fumes NEC	T54.91	T54.92	T54.93	T54.94	—	—
specified NEC	T54.91	T54.92	T54.93	T54.94	—	—
sublimate	T56.1X1	T56.1X2	T56.1X3	T56.1X4	—	—
Cortate	T38.0X1	T38.0X2	T38.0X3	T38.0X4	T38.0X5	T38.0X6
Cort-Dome	T38.0X1	T38.0X2	T38.0X3	T38.0X4	T38.0X5	T38.0X6
ENT agent	T49.6X1	T49.6X2	T49.6X3	T49.6X4	T49.6X5	T49.6X6
ophthalmic preparation	T49.5X1	T49.5X2	T49.5X3	T49.5X4	T49.5X5	T49.5X6
topical NEC	T49.0X1	T49.0X2	T49.0X3	T49.0X4	T49.0X5	T49.0X6
Cortef	T38.0X1	T38.0X2	T38.0X3	T38.0X4	T38.0X5	T38.0X6
ENT agent	T49.6X1	T49.6X2	T49.6X3	T49.6X4	T49.6X5	T49.6X6
ophthalmic preparation	T49.5X1	T49.5X2	T49.5X3	T49.5X4	T49.5X5	T49.5X6
topical NEC	T49.0X1	T49.0X2	T49.0X3	T49.0X4	T49.0X5	T49.0X6
Corticosteroid	T38.0X1	T38.0X2	T38.0X3	T38.0X4	T38.0X5	T38.0X6
ENT agent	T49.6X1	T49.6X2	T49.6X3	T49.6X4	T49.6X5	T49.6X6
mineral	T50.0X1	T50.0X2	T50.0X3	T50.0X4	T50.0X5	T50.0X6
ophthalmic	T49.5X1	T49.5X2	T49.5X3	T49.5X4	T49.5X5	T49.5X6
topical NEC	T49.0X1	T49.0X2	T49.0X3	T49.0X4	T49.0X5	T49.0X6
Corticotropin	T38.811	T38.812	T38.813	T38.814	T38.815	T38.816
Cortisol	T49.0X1	T49.0X2	T49.0X3	T49.0X4	T49.0X5	T49.0X6
ENT agent	T49.6X1	T49.6X2	T49.6X3	T49.6X4	T49.6X5	T49.6X6
ophthalmic preparation	T49.5X1	T49.5X2	T49.5X3	T49.5X4	T49.5X5	T49.5X6
topical NEC	T49.0X1	T49.0X2	T49.0X3	T49.0X4	T49.0X5	T49.0X6
Cortisone (acetate)	T38.0X1	T38.0X2	T38.0X3	T38.0X4	T38.0X5	T38.0X6
ENT agent	T49.6X1	T49.6X2	T49.6X3	T49.6X4	T49.6X5	T49.6X6
ophthalmic preparation	T49.5X1	T49.5X2	T49.5X3	T49.5X4	T49.5X5	T49.5X6
topical NEC	T49.0X1	T49.0X2	T49.0X3	T49.0X4	T49.0X5	T49.0X6
Cortivazol	T38.0X1	T38.0X2	T38.0X3	T38.0X4	T38.0X5	T38.0X6
Cortogen	T38.0X1	T38.0X2	T38.0X3	T38.0X4	T38.0X5	T38.0X6
ENT agent	T49.6X1	T49.6X2	T49.6X3	T49.6X4	T49.6X5	T49.6X6
ophthalmic preparation	T49.5X1	T49.5X2	T49.5X3	T49.5X4	T49.5X5	T49.5X6
Cortone	T38.0X1	T38.0X2	T38.0X3	T38.0X4	T38.0X5	T38.0X6
ENT agent	T49.6X1	T49.6X2	T49.6X3	T49.6X4	T49.6X5	T49.6X6
ophthalmic preparation	T49.5X1	T49.5X2	T49.5X3	T49.5X4	T49.5X5	T49.5X6
Cortril	T38.0X1	T38.0X2	T38.0X3	T38.0X4	T38.0X5	T38.0X6
ENT agent	T49.6X1	T49.6X2	T49.6X3	T49.6X4	T49.6X5	T49.6X6
ophthalmic preparation	T49.5X1	T56.5X2	T49.5X3	T49.5X4	T49.5X5	T49.5X6
topical NEC	T49.0X1	T49.0X2	T49.0X3	T49.0X4	T49.0X5	T49.0X6
Corynebacterium parvum	T45.1X1	T45.1X2	T45.1X3	T45.1X4	T45.1X5	T45.1X6
Cosmetic preparation	T49.8X1	T49.8X2	T49.8X3	T49.8X4	T49.8X5	T49.8X6
Cosmetics	T49.8X1	T49.8X2	T49.8X3	T49.8X4	T49.8X5	T49.8X6
Cosyntropin	T38.811	T38.812	T38.813	T38.814	T38.815	T38.816
Cotarnine	T45.7X1	T45.7X2	T45.7X3	T45.7X4	T45.7X5	T45.7X6
Co-trimoxazole	T36.8X1	T36.8X2	T36.8X3	T36.8X4	T36.8X5	T36.8X6
Cottonseed oil	T49.3X1	T49.3X2	T49.3X3	T49.3X4	T49.3X5	T49.3X6
Cough mixture (syrup)	T48.4X1	T48.4X2	T48.4X3	T48.4X4	T48.4X5	T48.4X6
containing opiates	T40.2X1	T40.2X2	T40.2X3	T40.2X4	T40.2X5	T40.2X6
expectorants	T48.4X1	T48.4X2	T48.4X3	T48.4X4	T48.4X5	T48.4X6
Coumadin	T45.511	T45.512	T45.513	T45.514	T45.515	T45.516
rodenticide	T60.4X1	T60.4X2	T60.4X3	T60.4X4	—	—
Coumaphos	T60.0X1	T60.0X2	T60.0X3	T60.0X4	—	—
Coumarin	T45.511	T45.512	T45.513	T45.514	T45.515	T45.516
Coumetarol	T45.511	T45.512	T45.513	T45.514	T45.515	T45.516
Cowbane	T62.2X1	T62.2X2	T62.2X3	T62.2X4	—	—
Cozyme	T45.2X1	T45.2X2	T45.2X3	T45.2X4	T45.2X5	T45.2X6
Crack	T40.5X1	T40.5X2	T40.5X3	T40.5X4	—	—
Crataegus extract	T46.0X1	T46.0X2	T46.0X3	T46.0X4	T46.0X5	T46.0X6
Creolin	T54.1X1	T54.1X2	T54.1X3	T54.1X4	—	—
disinfectant	T54.1X1	T54.1X2	T54.1X3	T54.1X4	—	—
Creosol (compound)	T49.0X1	T49.0X2	T49.0X3	T49.0X4	T49.0X5	T49.0X6
Creosote (coal tar) (beechwood)	T49.0X1	T49.0X2	T49.0X3	T49.0X4	T49.0X5	T49.0X6
medicinal (expectorant)	T48.4X1	T48.4X2	T48.4X3	T48.4X4	T48.4X5	T48.4X6
syrup	T48.4X1	T48.4X2	T48.4X3	T48.4X4	T48.4X5	T48.4X6
Cresol(s)	T49.0X1	T49.0X2	T49.0X3	T49.0X4	T49.0X5	T49.0X6
and soap solution	T49.0X1	T49.0X2	T49.0X3	T49.0X4	T49.0X5	T49.0X6
Cresyl acetate	T49.0X1	T49.0X2	T49.0X3	T49.0X4	T49.0X5	T49.0X6
Cresylic acid	T49.0X1	T49.0X2	T49.0X3	T49.0X4	T49.0X5	T49.0X6
Crimidine	T60.4X1	T60.4X2	T60.4X3	T60.4X4	—	—
Croconazole	T37.8X1	T37.8X2	T37.8X3	T37.8X4	T37.8X5	T37.8X6
Cromoglicic acid	T48.6X1	T48.6X2	T48.6X3	T48.6X4	T48.6X5	T48.6X6
Cromolyn	T48.6X1	T48.6X2	T48.6X3	T48.6X4	T48.6X5	T48.6X6
Cromonar	T46.3X1	T46.3X2	T46.3X3	T46.3X4	T46.3X5	T46.3X6
Cropropamide	T39.8X1	T39.8X2	T39.8X3	T39.8X4	T39.8X5	T39.8X6
with crotethamide	T50.7X1	T50.7X2	T50.7X3	T50.7X4	T50.7X5	T50.7X6
Crotamiton	T49.0X1	T49.0X2	T49.0X3	T49.0X4	T49.0X5	T49.0X6
Crotethamide	T39.8X1	T39.8X2	T39.8X3	T39.8X4	T39.8X5	T39.8X6
with cropropamide	T50.7X1	T50.7X2	T50.7X3	T50.7X4	T50.7X5	T50.7X6
Croton (oil)	T47.2X1	T47.2X2	T47.2X3	T47.2X4	T47.2X5	T47.2X6
chloral	T42.6X1	T42.6X2	T42.6X3	T42.6X4	T42.6X5	T42.6X6
Crude oil	T52.0X1	T52.0X2	T52.0X3	T52.0X4	—	—
Cryogenine	T39.8X1	T39.8X2	T39.8X3	T39.8X4	T39.8X5	T39.8X6
Cryolite (vapor)	T60.1X1	T60.1X2	T60.1X3	T60.1X4	—	—

Substance	Poisoning, Accidental (unintentional)	Poisoning, Intentional Self-harm	Poisoning, Assault	Poisoning, Undetermined	Adverse Effect	Under-dosing
Cryolite — *continued*						
insecticide	T60.1X1	T60.1X2	T60.1X3	T60.1X4	—	—
Cryptenamine (tannates)	T46.5X1	T46.5X2	T46.5X3	T46.5X4	T46.5X5	T46.5X6
Crystal violet	T49.0X1	T49.0X2	T49.0X3	T49.0X4	T49.0X5	T49.0X6
Cuckoopint	T62.2X1	T62.2X2	T62.2X3	T62.2X4	—	—
Cumetharol	T45.511	T45.512	T45.513	T45.514	T45.515	T45.516
Cupric						
acetate	T60.3X1	T60.3X2	T60.3X3	T60.3X4	—	—
acetoarsenite	T57.0X1	T57.0X2	T57.0X3	T57.0X4	—	—
arsenate	T57.0X1	T57.0X2	T57.0X3	T57.0X4	—	—
gluconate	T49.0X1	T49.0X2	T49.0X3	T49.0X4	T49.0X5	T49.0X6
oleate	T49.0X1	T49.0X2	T49.0X3	T49.0X4	T49.0X5	T49.0X6
sulfate	T56.4X1	T56.4X2	T56.4X3	T56.4X4	—	—
Cuprous sulfate — *see also* Copper sulfate	T56.4X1	T56.4X2	T56.4X3	T56.4X4	—	—
Curare, curarine	T48.1X1	T48.1X2	T48.1X3	T48.1X4	T48.1X5	T48.1X6
Cyamemazine	T43.3X1	T43.3X2	T43.3X3	T43.3X4	T43.3X5	T43.3X6
Cyamopsis tetragonoloba	T46.6X1	T46.6X2	T46.6X3	T46.6X4	T46.6X5	T46.6X6
Cyanacetyl hydrazide	T37.1X1	T37.1X2	T37.1X3	T37.1X4	T37.1X5	T37.1X6
Cyanic acid (gas)	T59.891	T59.892	T59.893	T59.894	—	—
Cyanide(s) (compounds) (potassium) (sodium) NEC	T65.0X1	T65.0X2	T65.0X3	T65.0X4	—	—
dust or gas (inhalation) NEC	T57.3X1	T57.3X2	T57.3X3	T57.3X4	—	—
fumigant	T65.0X1	T65.0X2	T65.0X3	T65.0X4	—	—
hydrogen	T57.3X1	T57.3X2	T57.3X3	T57.3X4	—	—
mercuric — *see* Mercury						
pesticide (dust) (fumes)	T65.0X1	T65.0X2	T65.0X3	T65.0X4	—	—
Cyanoacrylate adhesive	T49.3X1	T49.3X2	T49.3X3	T49.3X4	T49.3X5	T49.3X6
Cyanocobalamin	T45.8X1	T45.8X2	T45.8X3	T45.8X4	T45.8X5	T45.8X6
Cyanogen (chloride) (gas) NEC	T59.891	T59.892	T59.893	T59.894	—	—
Cyclacillin	T36.0X1	T36.0X2	T36.0X3	T36.0X4	T36.0X5	T36.0X6
Cyclaine	T41.3X1	T41.3X2	T41.3X3	T41.3X4	T41.3X5	T41.3X6
Cyclamate	T50.991	T50.992	T50.993	T50.994	T50.995	T50.996
Cyclamen europaeum	T62.2X1	T62.2X2	T62.2X3	T62.2X4	—	—
Cyclandelate	T46.7X1	T46.7X2	T46.7X3	T46.7X4	T46.7X5	T46.7X6
Cyclazocine	T50.7X1	T50.7X2	T50.7X3	T50.7X4	T50.7X5	T50.7X6
Cyclizine	T45.0X1	T45.0X2	T45.0X3	T45.0X4	T45.0X5	T45.0X6
Cyclobarbital	T42.3X1	T42.3X2	T42.3X3	T42.3X4	T42.3X5	T42.3X6
Cyclobarbitone	T42.3X1	T42.3X2	T42.3X3	T42.3X4	T42.3X5	T42.3X6
Cyclobenzaprine	T48.1X1	T48.1X2	T48.1X3	T48.1X4	T48.1X5	T48.1X6
Cyclodrine	T44.3X1	T44.3X2	T44.3X3	T44.3X4	T44.3X5	T44.3X6
Cycloguanil embonate	T37.2X1	T37.2X2	T37.2X3	T37.2X4	T37.2X5	T37.2X6
Cyclohexane	T52.8X1	T52.8X2	T52.8X3	T52.8X4	—	—
Cyclohexanol	T51.8X1	T51.8X2	T51.8X3	T51.8X4	—	—
Cyclohexanone	T52.4X1	T52.4X2	T52.4X3	T52.4X4	—	—
Cycloheximide	T60.3X1	T60.3X2	T60.3X3	T60.3X4	—	—
Cyclohexyl acetate	T52.8X1	T52.8X2	T52.8X3	T52.8X4	—	—
Cycloleucin	T45.1X1	T45.1X2	T45.1X3	T45.1X4	T45.1X5	T45.1X6
Cyclomethycaine	T41.3X1	T41.3X2	T41.3X3	T41.3X4	T41.3X5	T41.3X6
Cyclopentamine	T44.4X1	T44.4X2	T44.4X3	T44.4X4	T44.4X5	T44.4X6
Cyclopenthiazide	T50.2X1	T50.2X2	T50.2X3	T50.2X4	T50.2X5	T50.2X6
Cyclopentolate	T44.3X1	T44.3X2	T44.3X3	T44.3X4	T44.3X5	T44.3X6
Cyclophosphamide	T45.1X1	T45.1X2	T45.1X3	T45.1X4	T45.1X5	T45.1X6
Cycloplegic drug	T49.5X1	T49.5X2	T49.5X3	T49.5X4	T49.5X5	T49.5X6
Cyclopropane	T41.291	T41.292	T41.293	T41.294	T41.295	T41.296
Cyclopyrabital	T39.8X1	T39.8X2	T39.8X3	T39.8X4	T39.8X5	T39.8X6
Cycloserine	T37.1X1	T37.1X2	T37.1X3	T37.1X4	T37.1X5	T37.1X6
Cyclosporin	T45.1X1	T45.1X2	T45.1X3	T45.1X4	T45.1X5	T45.1X6
Cyclothiazide	T50.2X1	T50.2X2	T50.2X3	T50.2X4	T50.2X5	T50.2X6
Cycrimine	T44.3X1	T44.3X2	T44.3X3	T44.3X4	T44.3X5	T44.3X6
Cyhalothrin	T60.1X1	T60.1X2	T60.1X3	T60.1X4	—	—
Cymarin	T46.0X1	T46.0X2	T46.0X3	T46.0X4	T46.0X5	T46.0X6
Cypermethrin	T60.1X1	T60.1X2	T60.1X3	T60.1X4	—	—
Cyphenothrin	T60.2X1	T60.2X2	T60.2X3	T60.2X4	—	—
Cyproheptadine	T45.0X1	T45.0X2	T45.0X3	T45.0X4	T45.0X5	T45.0X6
Cyproterone	T38.6X1	T38.6X2	T38.6X3	T38.6X4	T38.6X5	T38.6X6
Cysteamine	T50.6X1	T50.6X2	T50.6X3	T50.6X4	T50.6X5	T50.6X6
Cytarabine	T45.1X1	T45.1X2	T45.1X3	T45.1X4	T45.1X5	T45.1X6
Cytisus						
laburnum	T62.2X1	T62.2X2	T62.2X3	T62.2X4	—	—
scoparius	T62.2X1	T62.2X2	T62.2X3	T62.2X4	—	—
Cytochrome C	T47.5X1	T47.5X2	T47.5X3	T47.5X4	T47.5X5	T47.5X6
Cytomel	T38.1X1	T38.1X2	T38.1X3	T38.1X4	T38.1X5	T38.1X6
Cytosine arabinoside	T45.1X1	T45.1X2	T45.1X3	T45.1X4	T45.1X5	T45.1X6
Cytoxan	T45.1X1	T45.1X2	T45.1X3	T45.1X4	T45.1X5	T45.1X6
Cytozyme	T45.7X1	T45.7X2	T45.7X3	T45.7X4	T45.7X5	T45.7X6
S-Carboxymethylcysteine	T48.4X1	T48.4X2	T48.4X3	T48.4X4	T48.4X5	T48.4X6
Dacarbazine	T45.1X1	T45.1X2	T45.1X3	T45.1X4	T45.1X5	T45.1X6
Dactinomycin	T45.1X1	T45.1X2	T45.1X3	T45.1X4	T45.1X5	T45.1X6
DADPS	T37.1X1	T37.1X2	T37.1X3	T37.1X4	T37.1X5	T37.1X6

Substance	Poisoning, Accidental (unintentional)	Poisoning, Intentional Self-harm	Poisoning, Assault	Poisoning, Undetermined	Adverse Effect	Under-dosing
Dakin's solution	T49.0X1	T49.0X2	T49.0X3	T49.0X4	T49.0X5	T49.0X6
Dalapon (sodium)	T60.3X1	T60.3X2	T60.3X3	T60.3X4	—	—
Dalmane	T42.4X1	T42.4X2	T42.4X3	T42.4X4	T42.4X5	T42.4X6
Danazol	T38.6X1	T38.6X2	T38.6X3	T38.6X4	T38.6X5	T38.6X6
Danilone	T45.511	T45.512	T45.513	T45.514	T45.515	T45.516
Danthron	T47.2X1	T47.2X2	T47.2X3	T47.2X4	T47.2X5	T47.2X6
Dantrolene	T42.8X1	T42.8X2	T42.8X3	T42.8X4	T42.8X5	T42.8X6
Dantron	T47.2X1	T47.2X2	T47.2X3	T47.2X4	T47.2X5	T47.2X6
Daphne (gnidium) (mezereum)	T62.2X1	T62.2X2	T62.2X3	T62.2X4	—	—
berry	T62.1X1	T62.1X2	T62.1X3	T62.1X4	—	—
Dapsone	T37.1X1	T37.1X2	T37.1X3	T37.1X4	T37.1X5	T37.1X6
Daraprim	T37.2X1	T37.2X2	T37.2X3	T37.2X4	T37.2X5	T37.2X6
Darnel	T62.2X1	T62.2X2	T62.2X3	T62.2X4	—	—
Darvon	T39.8X1	T39.8X2	T39.8X3	T39.8X4	T39.8X5	T39.8X6
Daunomycin	T45.1X1	T45.1X2	T45.1X3	T45.1X4	T45.1X5	T45.1X6
Daunorubicin	T45.1X1	T45.1X2	T45.1X3	T45.1X4	T45.1X5	T45.1X6
DBI	T38.3X1	T38.3X2	T38.3X3	T38.3X4	T38.3X5	T38.3X6
D-Con	T60.91	T60.92	T60.93	T60.94	—	—
insecticide	T60.2X1	T60.2X2	T60.2X3	T60.2X4	—	—
rodenticide	T60.4X1	T60.4X2	T60.4X3	T60.4X4	—	—
DDAVP	T38.891	T38.892	T38.893	T38.894	T38.895	T38.896
DDE (bis(chlorophenyl)-dichloroethylene)	T60.2X1	T60.2X2	T60.2X3	T60.2X4	—	—
DDS	T37.1X1	T37.1X2	T37.1X3	T37.1X4	T37.1X5	T37.1X6
DDT (dust)	T60.1X1	T60.1X2	T60.1X3	T60.1X4	—	—
Deadly nightshade — see also Belladonna						
berry	T62.1X1	T62.1X2	T62.1X3	T62.1X4	—	—
Deamino-D-arginine vasopressin	T38.891	T38.892	T38.893	T38.894	T38.895	T38.896
Deanol (aceglumate)	T50.991	T50.992	T50.993	T50.994	T50.995	T50.996
Debrisoquine	T46.5X1	T46.5X2	T46.5X3	T46.5X4	T46.5X5	T46.5X6
Decaborane	T57.8X1	T57.8X2	T57.8X3	T57.8X4	—	—
fumes	T59.891	T59.892	T59.893	T59.894	—	—
Decadron	T38.0X1	T38.0X2	T38.0X3	T38.0X4	T38.0X5	T38.0X6
ENT agent	T49.6X1	T49.6X2	T49.6X3	T49.6X4	T49.6X5	T49.6X6
ophthalmic preparation	T49.5X1	T49.5X2	T49.5X3	T49.5X4	T49.5X5	T49.5X6
topical NEC	T49.0X1	T49.0X2	T49.0X3	T49.0X4	T49.0X5	T49.0X6
Decahydronaphthalene	T52.8X1	T52.8X2	T52.8X3	T52.8X4	—	—
Decalin	T52.8X1	T52.8X2	T52.8X3	T52.8X4	—	—
Decamethonium (bromide)	T48.1X1	T48.1X2	T48.1X3	T48.1X4	T48.1X5	T48.1X6
Decholin	T47.5X1	T47.5X2	T47.5X3	T47.5X4	T47.5X5	T47.5X6
Declomycin	T36.4X1	T36.4X2	T36.4X3	T36.4X4	T36.4X5	T36.4X6
Decongestant, nasal (mucosa)	T48.5X1	T48.5X2	T48.5X3	T48.5X4	T48.5X5	T48.5X6
combination	T48.5X1	T48.5X2	T48.5X3	T48.5X4	T48.5X5	T48.5X6
Deet	T60.8X1	T60.8X2	T60.8X3	T60.8X4	—	—
Deferoxamine	T45.8X1	T45.8X2	T45.8X3	T45.8X4	T45.8X5	T45.8X6
Deflazacort	T38.0X1	T38.0X2	T38.0X3	T38.0X4	T38.0X5	T38.0X6
Deglycyrrhizinized extract of licorice	T48.4X1	T48.4X2	T48.4X3	T48.4X4	T48.4X5	T48.4X6
Dehydrocholic acid	T47.5X1	T47.5X2	T47.5X3	T47.5X4	T47.5X5	T47.5X6
Dehydroemetine	T37.3X1	T37.3X2	T37.3X3	T37.3X4	T37.3X5	T37.3X6
Dekalin	T52.8X1	T52.8X2	T52.8X3	T52.8X4	—	—
Delalutin	T38.5X1	T38.5X2	T38.5X3	T38.5X4	T38.5X5	T38.5X6
Delorazepam	T42.4X1	T42.4X2	T42.4X3	T42.4X4	T42.4X5	T42.4X6
Delphinium	T62.2X1	T62.2X2	T62.2X3	T62.2X4	—	—
Deltamethrin	T60.1X1	T60.1X2	T60.1X3	T60.1X4	—	—
Deltasone	T38.0X1	T38.0X2	T38.0X3	T38.0X4	T38.0X5	T38.0X6
Deltra	T38.0X1	T38.0X2	T38.0X3	T38.0X4	T38.0X5	T38.0X6
Delvinal	T42.3X1	T42.3X2	T42.3X3	T42.3X4	T42.3X5	T42.3X6
Demecarium (bromide)	T49.5X1	T49.5X2	T49.5X3	T49.5X4	T49.5X5	T49.5X6
Demeclocycline	T36.4X1	T36.4X2	T36.4X3	T36.4X4	T36.4X5	T36.4X6
Demecolcine	T45.1X1	T45.1X2	T45.1X3	T45.1X4	T45.1X5	T45.1X6
Demegestone	T38.5X1	T38.5X2	T38.5X3	T38.5X4	T38.5X5	T38.5X6
Demelanizing agents	T49.8X1	T49.8X2	T49.8X3	T49.8X4	T49.8X5	T49.8X6
Demephion -O and -S	T60.0X1	T60.0X2	T60.0X3	T60.0X4	—	—
Demerol	T40.2X1	T40.2X2	T40.2X3	T40.2X4	T40.2X5	T40.2X6
Demethylchlortetracycline	T36.4X1	T36.4X2	T36.4X3	T36.4X4	T36.4X5	T36.4X6
Demethyltetracycline	T36.4X1	T36.4X2	T36.4X3	T36.4X4	T36.4X5	T36.4X6
Demeton -O and -S	T60.0X1	T60.0X2	T60.0X3	T60.0X4	—	—
Demulcent (external)	T49.3X1	T49.3X2	T49.3X3	T49.3X4	T49.3X5	T49.3X6
specified NEC	T49.3X1	T49.3X2	T49.3X3	T49.3X4	T49.3X5	T49.3X6
Demulen	T38.4X1	T38.4X2	T38.4X3	T38.4X4	T38.4X5	T38.4X6
Denatured alcohol	T51.0X1	T51.0X2	T51.0X3	T51.0X4	—	—
Dendrid	T49.5X1	T49.5X2	T49.5X3	T49.5X4	T49.5X5	T49.5X6
Dental drug, topical application NEC	T49.7X1	T49.7X2	T49.7X3	T49.7X4	T49.7X5	T49.7X6
Dentifrice	T49.7X1	T49.7X2	T49.7X3	T49.7X4	T49.7X5	T49.7X6
Deodorant spray (feminine hygiene)	T49.8X1	T49.8X2	T49.8X3	T49.8X4	T49.8X5	T49.8X6
Deoxycortone	T50.0X1	T50.0X2	T50.0X3	T50.0X4	T50.0X5	T50.0X6
Deoxyribonuclease (pancreatic)	T45.3X1	T45.3X2	T45.3X3	T45.3X4	T45.3X5	T45.3X6
Depilatory	T49.4X1	T49.4X2	T49.4X3	T49.4X4	T49.4X5	T49.4X6
Deprenalin	T42.8X1	T42.8X2	T42.8X3	T42.8X4	T42.8X5	T42.8X6
Deprenyl	T42.8X1	T42.8X2	T42.8X3	T42.8X4	T42.8X5	T42.8X6
Depressant						
appetite (central)	T50.5X1	T50.5X2	T50.5X3	T50.5X4	T50.5X5	T50.5X6
cardiac	T46.2X1	T46.2X2	T46.2X3	T46.2X4	T46.2X5	T46.2X6
central nervous system (anesthetic) — see also Central nervous system, depressants	T42.71	T42.72	T42.73	T42.74	T42.75	T42.76
general anesthetic	T41.201	T41.202	T41.203	T41.204	T41.205	T41.206
muscle tone	T42.8X1	T42.8X2	T42.8X3	T42.8X4	T42.8X5	T42.8X6
muscle tone, central	T42.8X1	T42.8X2	T42.8X3	T42.8X4	T42.8X5	T42.8X6
psychotherapeutic	T43.501	T43.502	T43.503	T43.504	T43.505	T43.506
Depressant, appetite	T50.5X1	T50.5X2	T50.5X3	T50.5X4	T50.5X5	T50.5X6
Deptropine	T45.0X1	T45.0X2	T45.0X3	T45.0X4	T45.0X5	T45.0X6
Dequalinium (chloride)	T49.0X1	T49.0X2	T49.0X3	T49.0X4	T49.0X5	T49.0X6
Derris root	T60.2X1	T60.2X2	T60.2X3	T60.2X4	—	—
Deserpidine	T46.5X1	T46.5X2	T46.5X3	T46.5X4	T46.5X5	T46.5X6
Desferrioxamine	T45.8X1	T45.8X2	T45.8X3	T45.8X4	T45.8X5	T45.8X6
Desipramine	T43.011	T43.012	T43.013	T43.014	T43.015	T43.016
Deslanoside	T46.0X1	T46.0X2	T46.0X3	T46.0X4	T46.0X5	T46.0X6
Desloughing agent	T49.4X1	T49.4X2	T49.4X3	T49.4X4	T49.4X5	T49.4X6
Desmethylimipramine	T43.011	T43.012	T43.013	T43.014	T43.015	T43.016
Desmopressin	T38.891	T38.892	T38.893	T38.894	T38.895	T38.896
Desocodeine	T40.2X1	T40.2X2	T40.2X3	T40.2X4	T40.2X5	T40.2X6
Desogestrel	T38.5X1	T38.5X2	T38.5X3	T38.5X4	T38.5X5	T38.5X6
Desomorphine	T40.2X1	T40.2X2	T40.2X3	T40.2X4	—	—
Desonide	T49.0X1	T49.0X2	T49.0X3	T49.0X4	T49.0X5	T49.0X6
Desoximetasone	T49.0X1	T49.0X2	T49.0X3	T49.0X4	T49.0X5	T49.0X6
Desoxycorticosteroid	T50.0X1	T50.0X2	T50.0X3	T50.0X4	T50.0X5	T50.0X6
Desoxycortone	T50.0X1	T50.0X2	T50.0X3	T50.0X4	T50.0X5	T50.0X6
Desoxyephedrine	T43.621	T43.622	T43.623	T43.624	T43.625	T43.626
Detaxtran	T46.6X1	T46.6X2	T46.6X3	T46.6X4	T46.6X5	T46.6X6
Detergent	T49.2X1	T49.2X2	T49.2X3	T49.2X4	T49.2X5	T49.2X6
external medication	T49.2X1	T49.2X2	T49.2X3	T49.2X4	T49.2X5	T49.2X6
local	T49.2X1	T49.2X2	T49.2X3	T49.2X4	T49.2X5	T49.2X6
medicinal	T49.2X1	T49.2X2	T49.2X3	T49.2X4	T49.2X5	T49.2X6
nonmedicinal	T55.1X1	T55.1X2	T55.1X3	T55.1X4	—	—
specified NEC	T55.1X1	T55.1X2	T55.1X3	T55.1X4	—	—
Deterrent, alcohol	T50.6X1	T50.6X2	T50.6X3	T50.6X4	T50.6X5	T50.6X6
Detoxifying agent	T50.6X1	T50.6X2	T50.6X3	T50.6X4	T50.6X5	T50.6X6
Detrothyronine	T38.1X1	T38.1X2	T38.1X3	T38.1X4	T38.1X5	T38.1X6
Dettol (external medication)	T49.0X1	T49.0X2	T49.0X3	T49.0X4	T49.0X5	T49.0X6
Dexamethasone	T38.0X1	T38.0X2	T38.0X3	T38.0X4	T38.0X5	T38.0X6
ENT agent	T49.6X1	T49.6X2	T49.6X3	T49.6X4	T49.6X5	T49.6X6
ophthalmic preparation	T49.5X1	T49.5X2	T49.5X3	T49.5X4	T49.5X5	T49.5X6
topical NEC	T49.0X1	T49.0X2	T49.0X3	T49.0X4	T49.0X5	T49.0X6
Dexamfetamine	T43.621	T43.622	T43.623	T43.624	T43.625	T43.626
Dexamphetamine	T43.621	T43.622	T43.623	T43.624	T43.625	T43.626
Dexbrompheniramine	T45.0X1	T45.0X2	T45.0X3	T45.0X4	T45.0X5	T45.0X6
Dexchlorpheniramine	T45.0X1	T45.0X2	T45.0X3	T45.0X4	T45.0X5	T45.0X6
Dexedrine	T43.621	T43.622	T43.623	T43.624	T43.625	T43.626
Dexetimide	T44.3X1	T44.3X2	T44.3X3	T44.3X4	T44.3X5	T44.3X6
Dexfenfluramine	T50.5X1	T50.5X2	T50.5X3	T50.5X4	T50.5X5	T50.5X6
Dexpanthenol	T45.2X1	T45.2X2	T45.2X3	T45.2X4	T45.2X5	T45.2X6
Dextran (40) (70) (150)	T45.8X1	T45.8X2	T45.8X3	T45.8X4	T45.8X5	T45.8X6
Dextriferron	T45.4X1	T45.4X2	T45.4X3	T45.4X4	T45.4X5	T45.4X6
Dextroamphetamine	T43.621	T43.622	T43.623	T43.624	T43.625	T43.626
Dextro calcium pantothenate	T45.2X1	T45.2X2	T45.2X3	T45.2X4	T45.2X5	T45.2X6
Dextromethorphan	T48.3X1	T48.3X2	T48.3X3	T48.3X4	T48.3X5	T48.3X6
Dextromoramide	T40.491	T40.492	T40.493	T40.494	—	—
topical	T49.8X1	T49.8X2	T49.8X3	T49.8X4	T49.8X5	T49.8X6
Dextro pantothenyl alcohol	T45.2X1	T45.2X2	T45.2X3	T45.2X4	T45.2X5	T45.2X6
Dextropropoxyphene	T40.491	T40.492	T40.493	T40.494	T40.495	T40.496
Dextrorphan	T40.2X1	T40.2X2	T40.2X3	T40.2X4	T40.2X5	T40.2X6
Dextrose	T50.3X1	T50.3X2	T50.3X3	T50.3X4	T50.3X5	T50.3X6
concentrated solution, intravenous	T46.8X1	T46.8X2	T46.8X3	T46.8X4	T46.8X5	T46.8X6
Dextrothyroxin	T38.1X1	T38.1X2	T38.1X3	T38.1X4	T38.1X5	T38.1X6
Dextrothyroxine sodium	T38.1X1	T38.1X2	T38.1X3	T38.1X4	T38.1X5	T38.1X6
DFP	T44.0X1	T44.0X2	T44.0X3	T44.0X4	T44.0X5	T44.0X6
DHE	T37.3X1	T37.3X2	T37.3X3	T37.3X4	T37.3X5	T37.3X6
45	T46.5X1	T46.5X2	T46.5X3	T46.5X4	T46.5X5	T46.5X6
Diabinese	T38.3X1	T38.3X2	T38.3X3	T38.3X4	T38.3X5	T38.3X6
Diacetone alcohol	T52.4X1	T52.4X2	T52.4X3	T52.4X4	—	—
Diacetyl monoxime	T50.991	T50.992	T50.993	T50.994	—	—
Diacetylmorphine	T40.1X1	T40.1X2	T40.1X3	T40.1X4	—	—
Diachylon plaster	T49.4X1	T49.4X2	T49.4X3	T49.4X4	T49.4X5	T49.4X6

Substance	Poisoning, Accidental (unintentional)	Poisoning, Intentional Self-harm	Poisoning, Assault	Poisoning, Undetermined	Adverse Effect	Under-dosing
Diaethylstilboestrolum	T38.5X1	T38.5X2	T38.5X3	T38.5X4	T38.5X5	T38.5X6
Diagnostic agent NEC	T50.8X1	T50.8X2	T50.8X3	T50.8X4	T50.8X5	T50.8X6
Dial (soap)	T49.2X1	T49.2X2	T49.2X3	T49.2X4	T49.2X5	T49.2X6
sedative	T42.3X1	T42.3X2	T42.3X3	T42.3X4	T42.3X5	T42.3X6
Dialkyl carbonate	T52.91	T52.92	T52.93	T52.94	—	—
Diallylbarbituric acid	T42.3X1	T42.3X2	T42.3X3	T42.3X4	T42.3X5	T42.3X6
Diallymal	T42.3X1	T42.3X2	T42.3X3	T42.3X4	T42.3X5	T42.3X6
Dialysis solution (intraperitoneal)	T50.3X1	T50.3X2	T50.3X3	T50.3X4	T50.3X5	T50.3X6
Diaminodiphenylsulfone	T37.1X1	T37.1X2	T37.1X3	T37.1X4	T37.1X5	T37.1X6
Diamorphine	T40.1X1	T40.1X2	T40.1X3	T40.1X4	—	—
Diamox	T50.2X1	T50.2X2	T50.2X3	T50.2X4	T50.2X5	T50.2X6
Diamthazole	T49.0X1	T49.0X2	T49.0X3	T49.0X4	T49.0X5	T49.0X6
Dianthone	T47.2X1	T47.2X2	T47.2X3	T47.2X4	T47.2X5	T47.2X6
Diaphenylsulfone	T37.0X1	T37.0X2	T37.0X3	T37.0X4	T37.0X5	T37.0X6
Diasone (sodium)	T37.1X1	T37.1X2	T37.1X3	T37.1X4	T37.1X5	T37.1X6
Diastase	T47.5X1	T47.5X2	T47.5X3	T47.5X4	T47.5X5	T47.5X6
Diatrizoate	T50.8X1	T50.8X2	T50.8X3	T50.8X4	T50.8X5	T50.8X6
Diazepam	T42.4X1	T42.4X2	T42.4X3	T42.4X4	T42.4X5	T42.4X6
Diazinon	T60.0X1	T60.0X2	T60.0X3	T60.0X4	—	—
Diazomethane (gas)	T59.891	T59.892	T59.893	T59.894	—	—
Diazoxide	T46.5X1	T46.5X2	T46.5X3	T46.5X4	T46.5X5	T46.5X6
Dibekacin	T36.5X1	T36.5X2	T36.5X3	T36.5X4	T36.5X5	T36.5X6
Dibenamine	T44.6X1	T44.6X2	T44.6X3	T44.6X4	T44.6X5	T44.6X6
Dibenzepin	T43.011	T43.012	T43.013	T43.014	T43.015	T43.016
Dibenzheptropine	T45.0X1	T45.0X2	T45.0X3	T45.0X4	T45.0X5	T45.0X6
Dibenzyline	T44.6X1	T44.6X2	T44.6X3	T44.6X4	T44.6X5	T44.6X6
Diborane (gas)	T59.891	T59.892	T59.893	T59.894	—	—
Dibromochloropropane	T60.8X1	T60.8X2	T60.8X3	T60.8X4	—	—
Dibromodulcitol	T45.1X1	T45.1X2	T45.1X3	T45.1X4	T45.1X5	T45.1X6
Dibromoethane	T53.6X1	T53.6X2	T53.6X3	T53.6X4	—	—
Dibromomannitol	T45.1X1	T45.1X2	T45.1X3	T45.1X4	T45.1X5	T45.1X6
Dibromopropamidine isethionate	T49.0X1	T49.0X2	T49.0X3	T49.0X4	T49.0X5	T49.0X6
Dibrompropamidine	T49.0X1	T49.0X2	T49.0X3	T49.0X4	T49.0X5	T49.0X6
Dibucaine	T41.3X1	T41.3X2	T41.3X3	T41.3X4	T41.3X5	T41.3X6
topical (surface)	T41.3X1	T41.3X2	T41.3X3	T41.3X4	T41.3X5	T41.3X6
Dibunate sodium	T48.3X1	T48.3X2	T48.3X3	T48.3X4	T48.3X5	T48.3X6
Dibutoline sulfate	T44.3X1	T44.3X2	T44.3X3	T44.3X4	T44.3X5	T44.3X6
Dicamba	T60.3X1	T60.3X2	T60.3X3	T60.3X4	—	—
Dicapthon	T60.0X1	T60.0X2	T60.0X3	T60.0X4	—	—
Dichlobenil	T60.3X1	T60.3X2	T60.3X3	T60.3X4	—	—
Dichlone	T60.3X1	T60.3X2	T60.3X3	T60.3X4	—	—
Dichloralphenozone	T42.6X1	T42.6X2	T42.6X3	T42.6X4	T42.6X5	T42.6X6
Dichlorbenzidine	T65.3X1	T65.3X2	T65.3X3	T65.3X4	—	—
Dichlorhydrin	T52.8X1	T52.8X2	T52.8X3	T52.8X4	—	—
Dichlorhydroxyquinoline	T37.8X1	T37.8X2	T37.8X3	T37.8X4	T37.8X5	T37.8X6
Dichlorobenzene	T53.7X1	T53.7X2	T53.7X3	T53.7X4	—	—
Dichlorobenzyl alcohol	T49.6X1	T49.6X2	T49.6X3	T49.6X4	T49.6X5	T49.6X6
Dichlorodifluoromethane	T53.5X1	T53.5X2	T53.5X3	T53.5X4	—	—
Dichloroethane	T52.8X1	T52.8X2	T52.8X3	T52.8X4	—	—
Dichloroethylene	T53.6X1	T53.6X2	T53.6X3	T53.6X4	—	—
Dichloroethyl sulfide, not in war	T59.891	T59.892	T59.893	T59.894	—	—
Dichloroformoxine, not in war	T59.891	T59.892	T59.893	T59.894	—	—
Dichlorohydrin, alpha-dichlorohydrin	T52.8X1	T52.8X2	T52.8X3	T52.8X4	—	—
Dichloromethane (solvent)	T53.4X1	T53.4X2	T53.4X3	T53.4X4	—	—
vapor	T53.4X1	T53.4X2	T53.4X3	T53.4X4	—	—
Dichloronaphthoquinone	T60.3X1	T60.3X2	T60.3X3	T60.3X4	—	—
Dichlorophen	T37.4X1	T37.4X2	T37.4X3	T37.4X4	T37.4X5	T37.4X6
Dichloropropene	T60.3X1	T60.3X2	T60.3X3	T60.3X4	—	—
Dichloropropionic acid	T60.3X1	T60.3X2	T60.3X3	T60.3X4	—	—
Dichlorphenamide	T50.2X1	T50.2X2	T50.2X3	T50.2X4	T50.2X5	T50.2X6
Dichlorvos	T60.0X1	T60.0X2	T60.0X3	T60.0X4	—	—
Diclofenac	T39.391	T39.392	T39.393	T39.394	T39.395	T39.396
Diclofenamide	T50.2X1	T50.2X2	T50.2X3	T50.2X4	T50.2X5	T50.2X6
Diclofensine	T43.291	T43.292	T43.293	T43.294	T43.295	T43.296
Diclonixine	T39.8X1	T39.8X2	T39.8X3	T39.8X4	T39.8X5	T39.8X6
Dicloxacillin	T36.0X1	T36.0X2	T36.0X3	T36.0X4	T36.0X5	T36.0X6
Dicophane	T49.0X1	T49.0X2	T49.0X3	T49.0X4	T49.0X5	T49.0X6
Dicoumarol, dicoumarin, dicumarol	T45.511	T45.512	T45.513	T45.514	T45.515	T45.516
Dicrotophos	T60.0X1	T60.0X2	T60.0X3	T60.0X4	—	—
Dicyanogen (gas)	T65.0X1	T65.0X2	T65.0X3	T65.0X4	—	—
Dicyclomine	T44.3X1	T44.3X2	T44.3X3	T44.3X4	T44.3X5	T44.3X6
Dicycloverine	T44.3X1	T44.3X2	T44.3X3	T44.3X4	T44.3X5	T44.3X6
Dideoxycytidine	T37.5X1	T37.5X2	T37.5X3	T37.5X4	T37.5X5	T37.5X6
Dideoxyinosine	T37.5X1	T37.5X2	T37.5X3	T37.5X4	T37.5X5	T37.5X6
Dieldrin (vapor)	T60.1X1	T60.1X2	T60.1X3	T60.1X4	—	—
Diemal	T42.3X1	T42.3X2	T42.3X3	T42.3X4	T42.3X5	T42.3X6
Dienestrol	T38.5X1	T38.5X2	T38.5X3	T38.5X4	T38.5X5	T38.5X6
Dienoestrol	T38.5X1	T38.5X2	T38.5X3	T38.5X4	T38.5X5	T38.5X6
Dietetic drug NEC	T50.901	T50.902	T50.903	T50.904	T50.905	T50.906
Diethazine	T42.8X1	T42.8X2	T42.8X3	T42.8X4	T42.8X5	T42.8X6
Diethyl						
barbituric acid	T42.3X1	T42.3X2	T42.3X3	T42.3X4	T42.3X5	T42.3X6
carbamazine	T37.4X1	T37.4X2	T37.4X3	T37.4X4	T37.4X5	T37.4X6
carbinol	T51.3X1	T51.3X2	T51.3X3	T51.3X4	—	—
carbonate	T52.8X1	T52.8X2	T52.8X3	T52.8X4	—	—
ether (vapor) — see also ether	T41.0X1	T41.0X2	T41.0X3	T41.0X4	T41.0X5	T41.0X6
oxide	T52.8X1	T52.8X2	T52.8X3	T52.8X4	—	—
propion	T50.5X1	T50.5X2	T50.5X3	T50.5X4	T50.5X5	T50.5X6
stilbestrol	T38.5X1	T38.5X2	T38.5X3	T38.5X4	T38.5X5	T38.5X6
toluamide (nonmedicinal)	T60.8X1	T60.8X2	T60.8X3	T60.8X4	—	—
medicinal	T49.3X1	T49.3X2	T49.3X3	T49.3X4	T49.3X5	T49.3X6
Diethylcarbamazine	T37.4X1	T37.4X2	T37.4X3	T37.4X4	T37.4X5	T37.4X6
Diethylene						
dioxide	T52.8X1	T52.8X2	T52.8X3	T52.8X4	—	—
glycol (monoacetate) (monobutyl ether) (monoethyl ether)	T52.3X1	T52.3X2	T52.3X3	T52.3X4	—	—
Diethylhexylphthalate	T65.891	T65.892	T65.893	T65.894	—	—
Diethylpropion	T50.5X1	T50.5X2	T50.5X3	T50.5X4	T50.5X5	T50.5X6
Diethylstilbestrol	T38.5X1	T38.5X2	T38.5X3	T38.5X4	T38.5X5	T38.5X6
Diethylstilboestrol	T38.5X1	T38.5X2	T38.5X3	T38.5X4	T38.5X5	T38.5X6
Diethylsulfone-diethylmethane	T42.6X1	T42.6X2	T42.6X3	T42.6X4	T42.6X5	T42.6X6
Diethyltoluamide	T49.0X1	T49.0X2	T49.0X3	T49.0X4	T49.0X5	T49.0X6
Diethyltryptamine (DET)	T40.991	T40.992	T40.993	T40.994	—	—
Difebarbamate	T42.3X1	T42.3X2	T42.3X3	T42.3X4	T42.3X5	T42.3X6
Difencloxazine	T40.2X1	T40.2X2	T40.2X3	T40.2X4	T40.2X5	T40.2X6
Difenidol	T45.0X1	T45.0X2	T45.0X3	T45.0X4	T45.0X5	T45.0X6
Difenoxin	T47.6X1	T47.6X2	T47.6X3	T47.6X4	T47.6X5	T47.6X6
Difetarsone	T37.3X1	T37.3X2	T37.3X3	T37.3X4	T37.3X5	T37.3X6
Diffusin	T45.3X1	T45.3X2	T45.3X3	T45.3X4	T45.3X5	T45.3X6
Diflorasone	T49.0X1	T49.0X2	T49.0X3	T49.0X4	T49.0X5	T49.0X6
Diflos	T44.0X1	T44.0X2	T44.0X3	T44.0X4	T44.0X5	T44.0X6
Diflubenzuron	T60.1X1	T60.1X2	T60.1X3	T60.1X4	—	—
Diflucortolone	T49.0X1	T49.0X2	T49.0X3	T49.0X4	T49.0X5	T49.0X6
Diflunisal	T39.091	T39.092	T39.093	T39.094	T39.095	T39.096
Difluoromethyldopa	T42.8X1	T42.8X2	T42.8X3	T42.8X4	T42.8X5	T42.8X6
Difluorophate	T44.0X1	T44.0X2	T44.0X3	T44.0X4	T44.0X5	T44.0X6
Digestant NEC	T47.5X1	T47.5X2	T47.5X3	T47.5X4	T47.5X5	T47.5X6
Digitalin (e)	T46.0X1	T46.0X2	T46.0X3	T46.0X4	T46.0X5	T46.0X6
Digitalis (leaf)(glycoside)	T46.0X1	T46.0X2	T46.0X3	T46.0X4	T46.0X5	T46.0X6
lanata	T46.0X1	T46.0X2	T46.0X3	T46.0X4	T46.0X5	T46.0X6
purpurea	T46.0X1	T46.0X2	T46.0X3	T46.0X4	T46.0X5	T46.0X6
Digitoxin	T46.0X1	T46.0X2	T46.0X3	T46.0X4	T46.0X5	T46.0X6
Digitoxose	T46.0X1	T46.0X2	T46.0X3	T46.0X4	T46.0X5	T46.0X6
Digoxin	T46.0X1	T46.0X2	T46.0X3	T46.0X4	T46.0X5	T46.0X6
Digoxine	T46.0X1	T46.0X2	T46.0X3	T46.0X4	T46.0X5	T46.0X6
Dihydralazine	T46.5X1	T46.5X2	T46.5X3	T46.5X4	T46.5X5	T46.5X6
Dihydrazine	T46.5X1	T46.5X2	T46.5X3	T46.5X4	T46.5X5	T46.5X6
Dihydrocodeine	T40.2X1	T40.2X2	T40.2X3	T40.2X4	T40.2X5	T40.2X6
Dihydrocodeinone	T40.2X1	T40.2X2	T40.2X3	T40.2X4	T40.2X5	T40.2X6
Dihydroergocornine	T46.7X1	T46.7X2	T46.7X3	T46.7X4	T46.7X5	T46.7X6
Dihydroergocristine (mesilate)	T46.7X1	T46.7X2	T46.7X3	T46.7X4	T46.7X5	T46.7X6
Dihydroergokryptine	T46.7X1	T46.7X2	T46.7X3	T46.7X4	T46.7X5	T46.7X6
Dihydroergotamine	T46.5X1	T46.5X2	T46.5X3	T46.5X4	T46.5X5	T46.5X6
Dihydroergotoxine mesilate	T46.7X1	T46.7X2	T46.7X3	T46.7X4	T46.7X5	T46.7X6
Dihydrohydroxycodeinone	T40.2X1	T40.2X2	T40.2X3	T40.2X4	T40.2X5	T40.2X6
Dihydrohydroxymorphinone	T40.2X1	T40.2X2	T40.2X3	T40.2X4	T40.2X5	T40.2X6
Dihydroisocodeine	T40.2X1	T40.2X2	T40.2X3	T40.2X4	T40.2X5	T40.2X6
Dihydromorphine	T40.2X1	T40.2X2	T40.2X3	T40.2X4	—	—
Dihydromorphinone	T40.2X1	T40.2X2	T40.2X3	T40.2X4	T40.2X5	T40.2X6
Dihydrostreptomycin	T36.5X1	T36.5X2	T36.5X3	T36.5X4	T36.5X5	T36.5X6
Dihydrotachysterol	T45.2X1	T45.2X2	T45.2X3	T45.2X4	T45.2X5	T45.2X6
Dihydroxyaluminum aminoacetate	T47.1X1	T47.1X2	T47.1X3	T47.1X4	T47.1X5	T47.1X6
Dihydroxyaluminum sodium carbonate	T47.1X1	T47.1X2	T47.1X3	T47.1X4	T47.1X5	T47.1X6
Dihydroxyanthraquinone	T47.2X1	T47.2X2	T47.2X3	T47.2X4	T47.2X5	T47.2X6
Dihydroxycodeinone	T40.2X1	T40.2X2	T40.2X3	T40.2X4	T40.2X5	T40.2X6
Dihydroxypropyl theophylline	T50.2X1	T50.2X2	T50.2X3	T50.2X4	T50.2X5	T50.2X6
Diiodohydroxyquin	T37.8X1	T37.8X2	T37.8X3	T37.8X4	T37.8X5	T37.8X6
topical	T49.0X1	T49.0X2	T49.0X3	T49.0X4	T49.0X5	T49.0X6
Diiodohydroxyquinoline	T37.8X1	T37.8X2	T37.8X3	T37.8X4	T37.8X5	T37.8X6
Diiodotyrosine	T38.2X1	T38.2X2	T38.2X3	T38.2X4	T38.2X5	T38.2X6
Diisopromine	T44.3X1	T44.3X2	T44.3X3	T44.3X4	T44.3X5	T44.3X6
Diisopropylamine	T46.3X1	T46.3X2	T46.3X3	T46.3X4	T46.3X5	T46.3X6
Diisopropylfluorophosphonate	T44.0X1	T44.0X2	T44.0X3	T44.0X4	T44.0X5	T44.0X6

▼ Subterms under main terms may continue to next column or page   Additional Character May Be Required — Refer to the Tabular List for Character Selection   369

Diaethylstilboestrolum — Diisopropylfluorophosphonate

Substance	Poisoning, Accidental (unintentional)	Poisoning, Intentional Self-harm	Poisoning, Assault	Poisoning, Undetermined	Adverse Effect	Under-dosing
Dilantin	T42.0X1	T42.0X2	T42.0X3	T42.0X4	T42.0X5	T42.0X6
Dilaudid	T40.2X1	T40.2X2	T40.2X3	T40.2X4	T40.2X5	T40.2X6
Dilazep	T46.3X1	T46.3X2	T46.3X3	T46.3X4	T46.3X5	T46.3X6
Dill	T47.5X1	T47.5X2	T47.5X3	T47.5X4	T47.5X5	T47.5X6
Diloxanide	T37.3X1	T37.3X2	T37.3X3	T37.3X4	T37.3X5	T37.3X6
Diltiazem	T46.1X1	T46.1X2	T46.1X3	T46.1X4	T46.1X5	T46.1X6
Dimazole	T49.0X1	T49.0X2	T49.0X3	T49.0X4	T49.0X5	T49.0X6
Dimefline	T50.7X1	T50.7X2	T50.7X3	T50.7X4	T50.7X5	T50.7X6
Dimefox	T60.0X1	T60.0X2	T60.0X3	T60.0X4	—	—
Dimemorfan	T48.3X1	T48.3X2	T48.3X3	T48.3X4	T48.3X5	T48.3X6
Dimenhydrinate	T45.0X1	T45.0X2	T45.0X3	T45.0X4	T45.0X5	T45.0X6
Dimercaprol (British anti-lewisite)	T45.8X1	T45.8X2	T45.8X3	T45.8X4	T45.8X5	T45.8X6
Dimercaptopropanol	T45.8X1	T45.8X2	T45.8X3	T45.8X4	T45.8X5	T45.8X6
Dimestrol	T38.5X1	T38.5X2	T38.5X3	T38.5X4	T38.5X5	T38.5X6
Dimetane	T45.0X1	T45.0X2	T45.0X3	T45.0X4	T45.0X5	T45.0X6
Dimethicone	T47.1X1	T47.1X2	T47.1X3	T47.1X4	T47.1X5	T47.1X6
Dimethindene	T45.0X1	T45.0X2	T45.0X3	T45.0X4	T45.0X5	T45.0X6
Dimethisoquin	T49.1X1	T49.1X2	T49.1X3	T49.1X4	T49.1X5	T49.1X6
Dimethisterone	T38.5X1	T38.5X2	T38.5X3	T38.5X4	T38.5X5	T38.5X6
Dimethoate	T60.0X1	T60.0X2	T60.0X3	T60.0X4	—	—
Dimethocaine	T41.3X1	T41.3X2	T41.3X3	T41.3X4	T41.3X5	T41.3X6
Dimethoxanate	T48.3X1	T48.3X2	T48.3X3	T48.3X4	T48.3X5	T48.3X6
Dimethyl						
arsine, arsinic acid	T57.0X1	T57.0X2	T57.0X3	T57.0X4	—	—
carbinol	T51.2X1	T51.2X2	T51.2X3	T51.2X4	—	—
carbonate	T52.8X1	T52.8X2	T52.8X3	T52.8X4	—	—
diguanide	T38.3X1	T38.3X2	T38.3X3	T38.3X4	T38.3X5	T38.3X6
ketone	T52.4X1	T52.4X2	T52.4X3	T52.4X4	—	—
vapor	T52.4X1	T52.4X2	T52.4X3	T52.4X4	—	—
meperidine	T40.2X1	T40.2X2	T40.2X3	T40.2X4	T40.2X5	T40.2X6
parathion	T60.0X1	T60.0X2	T60.0X3	T60.0X4	—	—
phthlate	T49.3X1	T49.3X2	T49.3X3	T49.3X4	T49.3X5	T49.3X6
polysiloxane	T47.8X1	T47.8X2	T47.8X3	T47.8X4	T47.8X5	T47.8X6
sulfate (fumes)	T59.891	T59.892	T59.893	T59.894	—	—
liquid	T65.891	T65.892	T65.893	T65.894	—	—
sulfoxide (nonmedicinal)	T52.8X1	T52.8X2	T52.8X3	T52.8X4	—	—
medicinal	T49.4X1	T49.4X2	T49.4X3	T49.4X4	T49.4X5	T49.4X6
tryptamine	T40.991	T40.992	T40.993	T40.994	—	—
tubocurarine	T48.1X1	T48.1X2	T48.1X3	T48.1X4	T48.1X5	T48.1X6
Dimethylamine sulfate	T49.4X1	T49.4X2	T49.4X3	T49.4X4	T49.4X5	T49.4X6
Dimethylformamide	T52.8X1	T52.8X2	T52.8X3	T52.8X4	—	—
Dimethyltubocurarinium chloride	T48.1X1	T48.1X2	T48.1X3	T48.1X4	T48.1X5	T48.1X6
Dimeticone	T47.1X1	T47.1X2	T47.1X3	T47.1X4	T47.1X5	T47.1X6
Dimetilan	T60.0X1	T60.0X2	T60.0X3	T60.0X4	—	—
Dimetindene	T45.0X1	T45.0X2	T45.0X3	T45.0X4	T45.0X5	T45.0X6
Dimetotiazine	T43.3X1	T43.3X2	T43.3X3	T43.3X4	T43.3X5	T43.3X6
Dimorpholamine	T50.7X1	T50.7X2	T50.7X3	T50.7X4	T50.7X5	T50.7X6
Dimoxyline	T46.3X1	T46.3X2	T46.3X3	T46.3X4	T46.3X5	T46.3X6
Dinitrobenzene	T65.3X1	T65.3X2	T65.3X3	T65.3X4	—	—
vapor	T59.891	T59.892	T59.893	T59.894	—	—
Dinitrobenzol	T65.3X1	T65.3X2	T65.3X3	T65.3X4	—	—
vapor	T59.891	T59.892	T59.893	T59.894	—	—
Dinitrobutylphenol	T65.3X1	T65.3X2	T65.3X3	T65.3X4	—	—
Dinitro (-ortho-)cresol (pesticide) (spray)	T65.3X1	T65.3X2	T65.3X3	T65.3X4	—	—
Dinitrocyclohexylphenol	T65.3X1	T65.3X2	T65.3X3	T65.3X4	—	—
Dinitrophenol	T65.3X1	T65.3X2	T65.3X3	T65.3X4	—	—
Dinoprost	T48.0X1	T48.0X2	T48.0X3	T48.0X4	T48.0X5	T48.0X6
Dinoprostone	T48.0X1	T48.0X2	T48.0X3	T48.0X4	T48.0X5	T48.0X6
Dinoseb	T60.3X1	T60.3X2	T60.3X3	T60.3X4	—	—
Dioctyl sulfosuccinate (calcium) (sodium)	T47.4X1	T47.4X2	T47.4X3	T47.4X4	T47.4X5	T47.4X6
Diodone	T50.8X1	T50.8X2	T50.8X3	T50.8X4	T50.8X5	T50.8X6
Diodoquin	T37.8X1	T37.8X2	T37.8X3	T37.8X4	T37.8X5	T37.8X6
Dionin	T40.2X1	T40.2X2	T40.2X3	T40.2X4	T40.2X5	T40.2X6
Diosmin	T46.991	T46.992	T46.993	T46.994	T46.995	T46.996
Dioxane	T52.8X1	T52.8X2	T52.8X3	T52.8X4	—	—
Dioxathion	T60.0X1	T60.0X2	T60.0X3	T60.0X4	—	—
Dioxin	T53.7X1	T53.7X2	T53.7X3	T53.7X4	—	—
Dioxopromethazine	T43.3X1	T43.3X2	T43.3X3	T43.3X4	T43.3X5	T43.3X6
Dioxyline	T46.3X1	T46.3X2	T46.3X3	T46.3X4	T46.3X5	T46.3X6
Dipentene	T52.8X1	T52.8X2	T52.8X3	T52.8X4	—	—
Diperodon	T41.3X1	T41.3X2	T41.3X3	T41.3X4	T41.3X5	T41.3X6
Diphacinone	T60.4X1	T60.4X2	T60.4X3	T60.4X4	—	—
Diphemanil	T44.3X1	T44.3X2	T44.3X3	T44.3X4	T44.3X5	T44.3X6
metilsulfate	T44.3X1	T44.3X2	T44.3X3	T44.3X4	T44.3X5	T44.3X6
Diphenadione	T45.511	T45.512	T45.513	T45.514	T45.515	T45.516
rodenticide	T60.4X1	T60.4X2	T60.4X3	T60.4X4	—	—
Diphenhydramine	T45.0X1	T45.0X2	T45.0X3	T45.0X4	T45.0X5	T45.0X6
Diphenidol	T45.0X1	T45.0X2	T45.0X3	T45.0X4	T45.0X5	T45.0X6
Diphenoxylate	T47.6X1	T47.6X2	T47.6X3	T47.6X4	T47.6X5	T47.6X6

Substance	Poisoning, Accidental (unintentional)	Poisoning, Intentional Self-harm	Poisoning, Assault	Poisoning, Undetermined	Adverse Effect	Under-dosing
Diphenylamine	T65.3X1	T65.3X2	T65.3X3	T65.3X4	—	—
Diphenylbutazone	T39.2X1	T39.2X2	T39.2X3	T39.2X4	T39.2X5	T39.2X6
Diphenylchloroarsine, not in war	T57.0X1	T57.0X2	T57.0X3	T57.0X4	—	—
Diphenylhydantoin	T42.0X1	T42.0X2	T42.0X3	T42.0X4	T42.0X5	T42.0X6
Diphenylmethane dye	T52.1X1	T52.1X2	T52.1X3	T52.1X4	—	—
Diphenylpyraline	T45.0X1	T45.0X2	T45.0X3	T45.0X4	T45.0X5	T45.0X6
Diphtheria						
antitoxin	T50.Z11	T50.Z12	T50.Z13	T50.Z14	T50.Z15	T50.Z16
toxoid	T50.A91	T50.A92	T50.A93	T50.A94	T50.A95	T50.A96
with tetanus toxoid	T50.A21	T50.A22	T50.A23	T50.A24	T50.A25	T50.A26
with pertussis component	T50.A11	T50.A12	T50.A13	T50.A14	T50.A15	T50.A16
vaccine	T50.A91	T50.A92	T50.A93	T50.A94	T50.A95	T50.A96
combination						
without pertussis	T50.A21	T50.A22	T50.A23	T50.A24	T50.A25	T50.A26
including pertussis	T50.A11	T50.A12	T50.A13	T50.A14	T50.A15	T50.A16
Diphylline	T50.2X1	T50.2X2	T50.2X3	T50.2X4	T50.2X5	T50.2X6
Dipipanone	T40.491	T40.492	T40.493	T40.494	—	—
Dipivefrine	T49.5X1	T49.5X2	T49.5X3	T49.5X4	T49.5X5	T49.5X6
Diplovax	T50.B91	T50.B92	T50.B93	T50.B94	T50.B95	T50.B96
Diprophylline	T50.2X1	T50.2X2	T50.2X3	T50.2X4	T50.2X5	T50.2X6
Dipropyline	T48.291	T48.292	T48.293	T48.294	T48.295	T48.296
Dipyridamole	T46.3X1	T46.3X2	T46.3X3	T46.3X4	T46.3X5	T46.3X6
Dipyrone	T39.2X1	T39.2X2	T39.2X3	T39.2X4	T39.2X5	T39.2X6
Diquat (dibromide)	T60.3X1	T60.3X2	T60.3X3	T60.3X4	—	—
Disinfectant	T65.891	T65.892	T65.893	T65.894	—	—
alkaline	T54.3X1	T54.3X2	T54.3X3	T54.3X4	—	—
aromatic	T54.1X1	T54.1X2	T54.1X3	T54.1X4	—	—
intestinal	T37.8X1	T37.8X2	T37.8X3	T37.8X4	T37.8X5	T37.8X6
Disipal	T42.8X1	T42.8X2	T42.8X3	T42.8X4	T42.8X5	T42.8X6
Disodium edetate	T50.6X1	T50.6X2	T50.6X3	T50.6X4	T50.6X5	T50.6X6
Disoprofol	T41.291	T41.292	T41.293	T41.294	T41.295	T41.296
Disopyramide	T46.2X1	T46.2X2	T46.2X3	T46.2X4	T46.2X5	T46.2X6
Distigmine (bromide)	T44.0X1	T44.0X2	T44.0X3	T44.0X4	T44.0X5	T44.0X6
Disulfamide	T50.2X1	T50.2X2	T50.2X3	T50.2X4	T50.2X5	T50.2X6
Disulfanilamide	T37.0X1	T37.0X2	T37.0X3	T37.0X4	T37.0X5	T37.0X6
Disulfiram	T50.6X1	T50.6X2	T50.6X3	T50.6X4	T50.6X5	T50.6X6
Disulfoton	T60.0X1	T60.0X2	T60.0X3	T60.0X4	—	—
Dithiazanine iodide	T37.4X1	T37.4X2	T37.4X3	T37.4X4	T37.4X5	T37.4X6
Dithiocarbamate	T60.0X1	T60.0X2	T60.0X3	T60.0X4	—	—
Dithranol	T49.4X1	T49.4X2	T49.4X3	T49.4X4	T49.4X5	T49.4X6
Diucardin	T50.2X1	T50.2X2	T50.2X3	T50.2X4	T50.2X5	T50.2X6
Diupres	T50.2X1	T50.2X2	T50.2X3	T50.2X4	T50.2X5	T50.2X6
Diuretic NEC	T50.2X1	T50.2X2	T50.2X3	T50.2X4	T50.2X5	T50.2X6
benzothiadiazine	T50.2X1	T50.2X2	T50.2X3	T50.2X4	T50.2X5	T50.2X6
carbonic acid anhydrase inhibitors	T50.2X1	T50.2X2	T50.2X3	T50.2X4	T50.2X5	T50.2X6
furfuryl NEC	T50.2X1	T50.2X2	T50.2X3	T50.2X4	T50.2X5	T50.2X6
loop (high-ceiling)	T50.1X1	T50.1X2	T50.1X3	T50.1X4	T50.1X5	T50.1X6
mercurial NEC	T50.2X1	T50.2X2	T50.2X3	T50.2X4	T50.2X5	T50.2X6
osmotic	T50.2X1	T50.2X2	T50.2X3	T50.2X4	T50.2X5	T50.2X6
purine NEC	T50.2X1	T50.2X2	T50.2X3	T50.2X4	T50.2X5	T50.2X6
saluretic NEC	T50.2X1	T50.2X2	T50.2X3	T50.2X4	T50.2X5	T50.2X6
sulfonamide	T50.2X1	T50.2X2	T50.2X3	T50.2X4	T50.2X5	T50.2X6
thiazide NEC	T50.2X1	T50.2X2	T50.2X3	T50.2X4	T50.2X5	T50.2X6
xanthine	T50.2X1	T50.2X2	T50.2X3	T50.2X4	T50.2X5	T50.2X6
Diurgin	T50.2X1	T50.2X2	T50.2X3	T50.2X4	T50.2X5	T50.2X6
Diuril	T50.2X1	T50.2X2	T50.2X3	T50.2X4	T50.2X5	T50.2X6
Diuron	T60.3X1	T60.3X2	T60.3X3	T60.3X4	—	—
Divalproex	T42.6X1	T42.6X2	T42.6X3	T42.6X4	T42.6X5	T42.6X6
Divinyl ether	T41.0X1	T41.0X2	T41.0X3	T41.0X4	T41.0X5	T41.0X6
Dixanthogen	T49.0X1	T49.0X2	T49.0X3	T49.0X4	T49.0X5	T49.0X6
Dixyrazine	T43.3X1	T43.3X2	T43.3X3	T43.3X4	T43.3X5	T43.3X6
D-lysergic acid diethylamide	T40.8X1	T40.8X2	T40.8X3	T40.8X4	—	—
DMCT	T36.4X1	T36.4X2	T36.4X3	T36.4X4	T36.4X5	T36.4X6
DMSO — see Dimethyl sulfoxide						
DNBP	T60.3X1	T60.3X2	T60.3X3	T60.3X4	—	—
DNOC	T65.3X1	T65.3X2	T65.3X3	T65.3X4	—	—
Dobutamine	T44.5X1	T44.5X2	T44.5X3	T44.5X4	T44.5X5	T44.5X6
DOCA	T38.0X1	T38.0X2	T38.0X3	T38.0X4	T38.0X5	T38.0X6
Docusate sodium	T47.4X1	T47.4X2	T47.4X3	T47.4X4	T47.4X5	T47.4X6
Dodicin	T49.0X1	T49.0X2	T49.0X3	T49.0X4	T49.0X5	T49.0X6
Dofamium chloride	T49.0X1	T49.0X2	T49.0X3	T49.0X4	T49.0X5	T49.0X6
Dolophine	T40.3X1	T40.3X2	T40.3X3	T40.3X4	T40.3X5	T40.3X6
Doloxene	T39.8X1	T39.8X2	T39.8X3	T39.8X4	T39.8X5	T39.8X6
Domestic gas (after combustion) — see Gas, utility						
prior to combustion	T59.891	T59.892	T59.893	T59.894	—	—
Domiodol	T48.4X1	T48.4X2	T48.4X3	T48.4X4	T48.4X5	T48.4X6
Domiphen (bromide)	T49.0X1	T49.0X2	T49.0X3	T49.0X4	T49.0X5	T49.0X6
Domperidone	T45.0X1	T45.0X2	T45.0X3	T45.0X4	T45.0X5	T45.0X6

370

Additional Character May Be Required — Refer to the Tabular List for Character Selection   Subterms under main terms may continue to next column or page

Substance	Poisoning, Accidental (unintentional)	Poisoning, Intentional Self-harm	Poisoning, Assault	Poisoning, Undetermined	Adverse Effect	Under-dosing
Dopa	T42.8X1	T42.8X2	T42.8X3	T42.8X4	T42.8X5	T42.8X6
Dopamine	T44.991	T44.992	T44.993	T44.994	T44.995	T44.996
Doriden	T42.6X1	T42.6X2	T42.6X3	T42.6X4	T42.6X5	T42.6X6
Dormiral	T42.3X1	T42.3X2	T42.3X3	T42.3X4	T42.3X5	T42.3X6
Dormison	T42.6X1	T42.6X2	T42.6X3	T42.6X4	T42.6X5	T42.6X6
Dornase	T48.4X1	T48.4X2	T48.4X3	T48.4X4	T48.4X5	T48.4X6
Dorsacaine	T41.3X1	T41.3X2	T41.3X3	T41.3X4	T41.3X5	T41.3X6
Dosulepin	T43.011	T43.012	T43.013	T43.014	T43.015	T43.016
Dothiepin	T43.011	T43.012	T43.013	T43.014	T43.015	T43.016
Doxantrazole	T48.6X1	T48.6X2	T48.6X3	T48.6X4	T48.6X5	T48.6X6
Doxapram	T50.7X1	T50.7X2	T50.7X3	T50.7X4	T50.7X5	T50.7X6
Doxazosin	T44.6X1	T44.6X2	T44.6X3	T44.6X4	T44.6X5	T44.6X6
Doxepin	T43.011	T43.012	T43.013	T43.014	T43.015	T43.016
Doxifluridine	T45.1X1	T45.1X2	T45.1X3	T45.1X4	T45.1X5	T45.1X6
Doxorubicin	T45.1X1	T45.1X2	T45.1X3	T45.1X4	T45.1X5	T45.1X6
Doxycycline	T36.4X1	T36.4X2	T36.4X3	T36.4X4	T36.4X5	T36.4X6
Doxylamine	T45.0X1	T45.0X2	T45.0X3	T45.0X4	T45.0X5	T45.0X6
Dramamine	T45.0X1	T45.0X2	T45.0X3	T45.0X4	T45.0X5	T45.0X6
Drano (drain cleaner)	T54.3X1	T54.3X2	T54.3X3	T54.3X4	—	—
Dressing, live pulp	T49.7X1	T49.7X2	T49.7X3	T49.7X4	T49.7X5	T49.7X6
Drocode	T40.2X1	T40.2X2	T40.2X3	T40.2X4	T40.2X5	T40.2X6
Dromoran	T40.2X1	T40.2X2	T40.2X3	T40.2X4	T40.2X5	T40.2X6
Dromostanolone	T38.7X1	T38.7X2	T38.7X3	T38.7X4	T38.7X5	T38.7X6
Dronabinol	T40.7X1	T40.7X2	T40.7X3	T40.7X4	T40.7X5	T40.7X6
Droperidol	T43.591	T43.592	T43.593	T43.594	T43.595	T43.596
Dropropizine	T48.3X1	T48.3X2	T48.3X3	T48.3X4	T48.3X5	T48.3X6
Drostanolone	T38.7X1	T38.7X2	T38.7X3	T38.7X4	T38.7X5	T38.7X6
Drotaverine	T44.3X1	T44.3X2	T44.3X3	T44.3X4	T44.3X5	T44.3X6
Drotrecogin alfa	T45.511	T45.512	T45.513	T45.514	T45.515	T45.516
Drug NEC	T50.901	T50.902	T50.903	T50.904	T50.905	T50.906
specified NEC	T50.991	T50.992	T50.993	T50.994	T50.995	T50.996
DTIC	T45.1X1	T45.1X2	T45.1X3	T45.1X4	T45.1X5	T45.1X6
Duboisine	T44.3X1	T44.3X2	T44.3X3	T44.3X4	T44.3X5	T44.3X6
Dulcolax	T47.2X1	T47.2X2	T47.2X3	T47.2X4	T47.2X5	T47.2X6
Duponol (C) (EP)	T49.2X1	T49.2X2	T49.2X3	T49.2X4	T49.2X5	T49.2X6
Durabolin	T38.7X1	T38.7X2	T38.7X3	T38.7X4	T38.7X5	T38.7X6
Dyclone	T41.3X1	T41.3X2	T41.3X3	T41.3X4	T41.3X5	T41.3X6
Dyclonine	T41.3X1	T41.3X2	T41.3X3	T41.3X4	T41.3X5	T41.3X6
Dydrogesterone	T38.5X1	T38.5X2	T38.5X3	T38.5X4	T38.5X5	T38.5X6
Dye NEC	T65.6X1	T65.6X2	T65.6X3	T65.6X4	—	—
antiseptic	T49.0X1	T49.0X2	T49.0X3	T49.0X4	T49.0X5	T49.0X6
diagnostic agents	T50.8X1	T50.8X2	T50.8X3	T50.8X4	T50.8X5	T50.8X6
pharmaceutical NEC	T50.901	T50.902	T50.903	T50.904	T50.905	T50.906
Dyflos	T44.0X1	T44.0X2	T44.0X3	T44.0X4	T44.0X5	T44.0X6
Dymelor	T38.3X1	T38.3X2	T38.3X3	T38.3X4	T38.3X5	T38.3X6
Dynamite	T65.3X1	T65.3X2	T65.3X3	T65.3X4	—	—
fumes	T59.891	T59.892	T59.893	T59.894	—	—
Dyphylline	T44.3X1	T44.3X2	T44.3X3	T44.3X4	T44.3X5	T44.3X6
b-eucaine	T49.1X1	T49.1X2	T49.1X3	T49.1X4	T49.1X5	T49.1X6
Ear drug NEC	T49.6X1	T49.6X2	T49.6X3	T49.6X4	T49.6X5	T49.6X6
Ear preparations	T49.6X1	T49.6X2	T49.6X3	T49.6X4	T49.6X5	T49.6X6
Echothiophate, echothiopate, ecothiopate	T49.5X1	T49.5X2	T49.5X3	T49.5X4	T49.5X5	T49.5X6
Econazole	T49.0X1	T49.0X2	T49.0X3	T49.0X4	T49.0X5	T49.0X6
Ecothiopate iodide	T49.5X1	T49.5X2	T49.5X3	T49.5X4	T49.5X5	T49.5X6
Ecstasy	T43.641	T43.642	T43.643	T43.644	—	—
Ectylurea	T42.6X1	T42.6X2	T42.6X3	T42.6X4	T42.6X5	T42.6X6
Edathamil disodium	T45.8X1	T45.8X2	T45.8X3	T45.8X4	T45.8X5	T45.8X6
Edecrin	T50.1X1	T50.1X2	T50.1X3	T50.1X4	T50.1X5	T50.1X6
Edetate, disodium (calcium)	T45.8X1	T45.8X2	T45.8X3	T45.8X4	T45.8X5	T45.8X6
Edoxudine	T49.5X1	T49.5X2	T49.5X3	T49.5X4	T49.5X5	T49.5X6
Edrophonium	T44.0X1	T44.0X2	T44.0X3	T44.0X4	T44.0X5	T44.0X6
chloride	T44.0X1	T44.0X2	T44.0X3	T44.0X4	T44.0X5	T44.0X6
EDTA	T50.6X1	T50.6X2	T50.6X3	T50.6X4	T50.6X5	T50.6X6
Eflornithine	T37.2X1	T37.2X2	T37.2X3	T37.2X4	T37.2X5	T37.2X6
Efloxate	T46.3X1	T46.3X2	T46.3X3	T46.3X4	T46.3X5	T46.3X6
Elase	T49.8X1	T49.8X2	T49.8X3	T49.8X4	T49.8X5	T49.8X6
Elastase	T47.5X1	T47.5X2	T47.5X3	T47.5X4	T47.5X5	T47.5X6
Elaterium	T47.2X1	T47.2X2	T47.2X3	T47.2X4	T47.2X5	T47.2X6
Elcatonin	T50.991	T50.992	T50.993	T50.994	T50.995	T50.996
Elder	T62.2X1	T62.2X2	T62.2X3	T62.2X4	—	—
berry, (unripe)	T62.1X1	T62.1X2	T62.1X3	T62.1X4	—	—
Electrolyte balance drug	T50.3X1	T50.3X2	T50.3X3	T50.3X4	T50.3X5	T50.3X6
Electrolytes NEC	T50.3X1	T50.3X2	T50.3X3	T50.3X4	T50.3X5	T50.3X6
Electrolytic agent NEC	T50.3X1	T50.3X2	T50.3X3	T50.3X4	T50.3X5	T50.3X6
Elemental diet	T50.901	T50.902	T50.903	T50.904	T50.905	T50.906
Elliptinium acetate	T45.1X1	T45.1X2	T45.1X3	T45.1X4	T45.1X5	T45.1X6
Embramine	T45.0X1	T45.0X2	T45.0X3	T45.0X4	T45.0X5	T45.0X6
Emepronium (salts)	T44.3X1	T44.3X2	T44.3X3	T44.3X4	T44.3X5	T44.3X6
bromide	T44.3X1	T44.3X2	T44.3X3	T44.3X4	T44.3X5	T44.3X6
Emetic NEC	T47.7X1	T47.7X2	T47.7X3	T47.7X4	T47.7X5	T47.7X6
Emetine	T37.3X1	T37.3X2	T37.3X3	T37.3X4	T37.3X5	T37.3X6

Substance	Poisoning, Accidental (unintentional)	Poisoning, Intentional Self-harm	Poisoning, Assault	Poisoning, Undetermined	Adverse Effect	Under-dosing
Emollient NEC	T49.3X1	T49.3X2	T49.3X3	T49.3X4	T49.3X5	T49.3X6
Emorfazone	T39.8X1	T39.8X2	T39.8X3	T39.8X4	T39.8X5	T39.8X6
Emylcamate	T43.591	T43.592	T43.593	T43.594	T43.595	T43.596
Enalapril	T46.4X1	T46.4X2	T46.4X3	T46.4X4	T46.4X5	T46.4X6
Enalaprilat	T46.4X1	T46.4X2	T46.4X3	T46.4X4	T46.4X5	T46.4X6
Encainide	T46.2X1	T46.2X2	T46.2X3	T46.2X4	T46.2X5	T46.2X6
Endocaine	T41.3X1	T41.3X2	T41.3X3	T41.3X4	T41.3X5	T41.3X6
Endosulfan	T60.2X1	T60.2X2	T60.2X3	T60.2X4	—	—
Endothall	T60.3X1	T60.3X2	T60.3X3	T60.3X4	—	—
Endralazine	T46.5X1	T46.5X2	T46.5X3	T46.5X4	T46.5X5	T46.5X6
Endrin	T60.1X1	T60.1X2	T60.1X3	T60.1X4	—	—
Enflurane	T41.0X1	T41.0X2	T41.0X3	T41.0X4	T41.0X5	T41.0X6
Enhexymal	T42.3X1	T42.3X2	T42.3X3	T42.3X4	T42.3X5	T42.3X6
Enocitabine	T45.1X1	T45.1X2	T45.1X3	T45.1X4	T45.1X5	T45.1X6
Enovid	T38.4X1	T38.4X2	T38.4X3	T38.4X4	T38.4X5	T38.4X6
Enoxacin	T36.8X1	T36.8X2	T36.8X3	T36.8X4	T36.8X5	T36.8X6
Enoxaparin (sodium)	T45.511	T45.512	T45.513	T45.514	T45.515	T45.516
Enpiprazole	T43.591	T43.592	T43.593	T43.594	T43.595	T43.596
Enprofylline	T48.6X1	T48.6X2	T48.6X3	T48.6X4	T48.6X5	T48.6X6
Enprostil	T47.1X1	T47.1X2	T47.1X3	T47.1X4	T47.1X5	T47.1X6
Enterogastrone	T38.891	T38.892	T38.893	T38.894	T38.895	T38.896
ENT preparations (anti-infectives)	T49.6X1	T49.6X2	T49.6X3	T49.6X4	T49.6X5	T49.6X6
Enviomycin	T36.8X1	T36.8X2	T36.8X3	T36.8X4	T36.8X5	T36.8X6
Enzodase	T45.3X1	T45.3X2	T45.3X3	T45.3X4	T45.3X5	T45.3X6
Enzyme NEC	T45.3X1	T45.3X2	T45.3X3	T45.3X4	T45.3X5	T45.3X6
depolymerizing	T49.8X1	T49.8X2	T49.8X3	T49.8X4	T49.8X5	T49.8X6
fibrolytic	T45.3X1	T45.3X2	T45.3X3	T45.3X4	T45.3X5	T45.3X6
gastric	T47.5X1	T47.5X2	T47.5X3	T47.5X4	T47.5X5	T47.5X6
intestinal	T47.5X1	T47.5X2	T47.5X3	T47.5X4	T47.5X5	T47.5X6
local action	T49.4X1	T49.4X2	T49.4X3	T49.4X4	T49.4X5	T49.4X6
proteolytic	T49.4X1	T49.4X2	T49.4X3	T49.4X4	T49.4X5	T49.4X6
thrombolytic	T45.3X1	T45.3X2	T45.3X3	T45.3X4	T45.3X5	T45.3X6
EPAB	T41.3X1	T41.3X2	T41.3X3	T41.3X4	T41.3X5	T41.3X6
Epanutin	T42.0X1	T42.0X2	T42.0X3	T42.0X4	T42.0X5	T42.0X6
Ephedra	T44.991	T44.992	T44.993	T44.994	T44.995	T44.996
Ephedrine	T44.991	T44.992	T44.993	T44.994	T44.995	T44.996
Epichlorhydrin, epichlorohydrin	T52.8X1	T52.8X2	T52.8X3	T52.8X4	—	—
Epicillin	T36.0X1	T36.0X2	T36.0X3	T36.0X4	T36.0X5	T36.0X6
Epiestriol	T38.5X1	T38.5X2	T38.5X3	T38.5X4	T38.5X5	T38.5X6
Epilim — *see* Sodium valproate						
Epimestrol	T38.5X1	T38.5X2	T38.5X3	T38.5X4	T38.5X5	T38.5X6
Epinephrine	T44.5X1	T44.5X2	T44.5X3	T44.5X4	T44.5X5	T44.5X6
Epirubicin	T45.1X1	T45.1X2	T45.1X3	T45.1X4	T45.1X5	T45.1X6
Epitiostanol	T38.7X1	T38.7X2	T38.7X3	T38.7X4	T38.7X5	T38.7X6
Epitizide	T50.2X1	T50.2X2	T50.2X3	T50.2X4	T50.2X5	T50.2X6
EPN	T60.0X1	T60.0X2	T60.0X3	T60.0X4	—	—
EPO	T45.8X1	T45.8X2	T45.8X3	T45.8X4	T45.8X5	T45.8X6
Epoetin alpha	T45.8X1	T45.8X2	T45.8X3	T45.8X4	T45.8X5	T45.8X6
Epomediol	T50.991	T50.992	T50.993	T50.994	T50.995	T50.996
Epoprostenol	T45.521	T45.522	T45.523	T45.524	T45.525	T45.526
Epoxy resin	T65.891	T65.892	T65.893	T65.894	—	—
Eprazinone	T48.4X1	T48.4X2	T48.4X3	T48.4X4	T48.4X5	T48.4X6
Epsilon aminocaproic acid	T45.621	T45.622	T45.623	T45.624	T45.625	T45.626
Epsom salt	T47.3X1	T47.3X2	T47.3X3	T47.3X4	T47.3X5	T47.3X6
Eptazocine	T40.491	T40.492	T40.493	T40.494	T40.495	T40.496
Equanil	T43.591	T43.592	T43.593	T43.594	T43.595	T43.596
Equisetum	T62.2X1	T62.2X2	T62.2X3	T62.2X4	—	—
diuretic	T50.2X1	T50.2X2	T50.2X3	T50.2X4	T50.2X5	T50.2X6
Ergobasine	T48.0X1	T48.0X2	T48.0X3	T48.0X4	T48.0X5	T48.0X6
Ergocalciferol	T45.2X1	T45.2X2	T45.2X3	T45.2X4	T45.2X5	T45.2X6
Ergoloid mesylates	T46.7X1	T46.7X2	T46.7X3	T46.7X4	T46.7X5	T46.7X6
Ergometrine	T48.0X1	T48.0X2	T48.0X3	T48.0X4	T48.0X5	T48.0X6
Ergonovine	T48.0X1	T48.0X2	T48.0X3	T48.0X4	T48.0X5	T48.0X6
Ergotamine	T46.5X1	T46.5X2	T46.5X3	T46.5X4	T46.5X5	T46.5X6
Ergotocine	T48.0X1	T48.0X2	T48.0X3	T48.0X4	T48.0X5	T48.0X6
Ergotrate	T48.0X1	T48.0X2	T48.0X3	T48.0X4	T48.0X5	T48.0X6
Ergot NEC	T64.81	T64.82	T64.83	T64.84	—	—
derivative	T48.0X1	T48.0X2	T48.0X3	T48.0X4	T48.0X5	T48.0X6
medicinal (alkaloids)	T48.0X1	T48.0X2	T48.0X3	T48.0X4	T48.0X5	T48.0X6
prepared	T48.0X1	T48.0X2	T48.0X3	T48.0X4	T48.0X5	T48.0X6
Eritrityl tetranitrate	T46.3X1	T46.3X2	T46.3X3	T46.3X4	T46.3X5	T46.3X6
Erythrityl tetranitrate	T46.3X1	T46.3X2	T46.3X3	T46.3X4	T46.3X5	T46.3X6
Erythrol tetranitrate	T46.3X1	T46.3X2	T46.3X3	T46.3X4	T46.3X5	T46.3X6
Erythromycin (salts)	T36.3X1	T36.3X2	T36.3X3	T36.3X4	T36.3X5	T36.3X6
ophthalmic preparation	T49.5X1	T49.5X2	T49.5X3	T49.5X4	T49.5X5	T49.5X6
topical NEC	T49.0X1	T49.0X2	T49.0X3	T49.0X4	T49.0X5	T49.0X6
Erythropoietin	T45.8X1	T45.8X2	T45.8X3	T45.8X4	T45.8X5	T45.8X6
human	T45.8X1	T45.8X2	T45.8X3	T45.8X4	T45.8X5	T45.8X6
Escin	T46.991	T46.992	T46.993	T46.994	T46.995	T46.996
Esculin	T45.2X1	T45.2X2	T45.2X3	T45.2X4	T45.2X5	T45.2X6
Esculoside	T45.2X1	T45.2X2	T45.2X3	T45.2X4	T45.2X5	T45.2X6

Table of Drugs and Chemicals

Substance	Poisoning, Accidental (unintentional)	Poisoning, Intentional Self-harm	Poisoning, Assault	Poisoning, Undetermined	Adverse Effect	Under-dosing
ESDT (ether-soluble tar distillate)	T49.1X1	T49.1X2	T49.1X3	T49.1X4	T49.1X5	T49.1X6
Eserine	T49.5X1	T49.5X2	T49.5X3	T49.5X4	T49.5X5	T49.5X6
Esflurbiprofen	T39.311	T39.312	T39.313	T39.314	T39.315	T39.316
Eskabarb	T42.3X1	T42.3X2	T42.3X3	T42.3X4	T42.3X5	T42.3X6
Eskalith	T43.8X1	T43.8X2	T43.8X3	T43.8X4	T43.8X5	T43.8X6
Esmolol	T44.7X1	T44.7X2	T44.7X3	T44.7X4	T44.7X5	T44.7X6
Estanozolol	T38.7X1	T38.7X2	T38.7X3	T38.7X4	T38.7X5	T38.7X6
Estazolam	T42.4X1	T42.4X2	T42.4X3	T42.4X4	T42.4X5	T42.4X6
Estradiol	T38.5X1	T38.5X2	T38.5X3	T38.5X4	T38.5X5	T38.5X6
with testosterone	T38.7X1	T38.7X2	T38.7X3	T38.7X4	T38.7X5	T38.7X6
benzoate	T38.5X1	T38.5X2	T38.5X3	T38.5X4	T38.5X5	T38.5X6
Estramustine	T45.1X1	T45.1X2	T45.1X3	T45.1X4	T45.1X5	T45.1X6
Estriol	T38.5X1	T38.5X2	T38.5X3	T38.5X4	T38.5X5	T38.5X6
Estrogen	T38.5X1	T38.5X2	T38.5X3	T38.5X4	T38.5X5	T38.5X6
with progesterone	T38.5X1	T38.5X2	T38.5X3	T38.5X4	T38.5X5	T38.5X6
conjugated	T38.5X1	T38.5X2	T38.5X3	T38.5X4	T38.5X5	T38.5X6
Estrone	T38.5X1	T38.5X2	T38.5X3	T38.5X4	T38.5X5	T38.5X6
Estropipate	T38.5X1	T38.5X2	T38.5X3	T38.5X4	T38.5X5	T38.5X6
Etacrynate sodium	T50.1X1	T50.1X2	T50.1X3	T50.1X4	T50.1X5	T50.1X6
Etacrynic acid	T50.1X1	T50.1X2	T50.1X3	T50.1X4	T50.1X5	T50.1X6
Etafedrine	T48.6X1	T48.6X2	T48.6X3	T48.6X4	T48.6X5	T48.6X6
Etafenone	T46.3X1	T46.3X2	T46.3X3	T46.3X4	T46.3X5	T46.3X6
Etambutol	T37.1X1	T37.1X2	T37.1X3	T37.1X4	T37.1X5	T37.1X6
Etamiphyllin	T48.6X1	T48.6X2	T48.6X3	T48.6X4	T48.6X5	T48.6X6
Etamivan	T50.7X1	T50.7X2	T50.7X3	T50.7X4	T50.7X5	T50.7X6
Etamsylate	T45.7X1	T45.7X2	T45.7X3	T45.7X4	T45.7X5	T45.7X6
Etebenecid	T50.4X1	T50.4X2	T50.4X3	T50.4X4	T50.4X5	T50.4X6
Ethacridine	T49.0X1	T49.0X2	T49.0X3	T49.0X4	T49.0X5	T49.0X6
Ethacrynic acid	T50.1X1	T50.1X2	T50.1X3	T50.1X4	T50.1X5	T50.1X6
Ethadione	T42.2X1	T42.2X2	T42.2X3	T42.2X4	T42.2X5	T42.2X6
Ethambutol	T37.1X1	T37.1X2	T37.1X3	T37.1X4	T37.1X5	T37.1X6
Ethamide	T50.2X1	T50.2X2	T50.2X3	T50.2X4	T50.2X5	T50.2X6
Ethamivan	T50.7X1	T50.7X2	T50.7X3	T50.7X4	T50.7X5	T50.7X6
Ethamsylate	T45.7X1	T45.7X2	T45.7X3	T45.7X4	T45.7X5	T45.7X6
Ethanol	T51.0X1	T51.0X2	T51.0X3	T51.0X4	—	—
beverage	T51.0X1	T51.0X2	T51.0X3	T51.0X4	—	—
Ethanolamine oleate	T46.8X1	T46.8X2	T46.8X3	T46.8X4	T46.8X5	T46.8X6
Ethaverine	T44.3X1	T44.3X2	T44.3X3	T44.3X4	T44.3X5	T44.3X6
Ethchlorvynol	T42.6X1	T42.6X2	T42.6X3	T42.6X4	T42.6X5	T42.6X6
Ethebenecid	T50.4X1	T50.4X2	T50.4X3	T50.4X4	T50.4X5	T50.4X6
Ether (vapor)	T41.0X1	T41.0X2	T41.0X3	T41.0X4	T41.0X5	T41.0X6
anesthetic	T41.0X1	T41.0X2	T41.0X3	T41.0X4	T41.0X5	T41.0X6
divinyl	T41.0X1	T41.0X2	T41.0X3	T41.0X4	T41.0X5	T41.0X6
ethyl (medicinal)	T41.0X1	T41.0X2	T41.0X3	T41.0X4	T41.0X5	T41.0X6
nonmedicinal	T52.8X1	T52.8X2	T52.8X3	T52.8X4	—	—
petroleum — see Ligroin						
solvent	T52.8X1	T52.8X2	T52.8X3	T52.8X4	—	—
Ethiazide	T50.2X1	T50.2X2	T50.2X3	T50.2X4	T50.2X5	T50.2X6
Ethidium chloride (vapor)	T59.891	T59.892	T59.893	T59.894	—	—
Ethinamate	T42.6X1	T42.6X2	T42.6X3	T42.6X4	T42.6X5	T42.6X6
Ethinylestradiol, ethinyloestradiol	T38.5X1	T38.5X2	T38.5X3	T38.5X4	T38.5X5	T38.5X6
with						
levonorgestrel	T38.4X1	T38.4X2	T38.4X3	T38.4X4	T38.4X5	T38.4X6
norethisterone	T38.4X1	T38.4X2	T38.4X3	T38.4X4	T38.4X5	T38.4X6
Ethiodized oil (131 I)	T50.8X1	T50.8X2	T50.8X3	T50.8X4	T50.8X5	T50.8X6
Ethion	T60.0X1	T60.0X2	T60.0X3	T60.0X4	—	—
Ethionamide	T37.1X1	T37.1X2	T37.1X3	T37.1X4	T37.1X5	T37.1X6
Ethioniamide	T37.1X1	T37.1X2	T37.1X3	T37.1X4	T37.1X5	T37.1X6
Ethisterone	T38.5X1	T38.5X2	T38.5X3	T38.5X4	T38.5X5	T38.5X6
Ethobral	T42.3X1	T42.3X2	T42.3X3	T42.3X4	T42.3X5	T42.3X6
Ethocaine (infiltration) (topical)	T41.3X1	T41.3X2	T41.3X3	T41.3X4	T41.3X5	T41.3X6
nerve block (peripheral) (plexus)	T41.3X1	T41.3X2	T41.3X3	T41.3X4	T41.3X5	T41.3X6
spinal	T41.3X1	T41.3X2	T41.3X3	T41.3X4	T41.3X5	T41.3X6
Ethoheptazine	T40.491	T40.492	T40.493	T40.494	T40.495	T40.496
Ethopropazine	T44.3X1	T44.3X2	T44.3X3	T44.3X4	T44.3X5	T44.3X6
Ethosuximide	T42.2X1	T42.2X2	T42.2X3	T42.2X4	T42.2X5	T42.2X6
Ethotoin	T42.0X1	T42.0X2	T42.0X3	T42.0X4	T42.0X5	T42.0X6
Ethoxazene	T37.91	T37.92	T37.93	T37.94	T37.95	T37.96
Ethoxazorutoside	T46.991	T46.992	T46.993	T46.994	T46.995	T46.996
Ethoxzolamide	T50.2X1	T50.2X2	T50.2X3	T50.2X4	T50.2X5	T50.2X6
Ethyl						
acetate	T52.8X1	T52.8X2	T52.8X3	T52.8X4	—	—
alcohol	T51.0X1	T51.0X2	T51.0X3	T51.0X4	—	—
beverage	T51.0X1	T51.0X2	T51.0X3	T51.0X4	—	—
aldehyde (vapor)	T59.891	T59.892	T59.893	T59.894	—	—
liquid	T52.8X1	T52.8X2	T52.8X3	T52.8X4	—	—
aminobenzoate	T41.3X1	T41.3X2	T41.3X3	T41.3X4	T41.3X5	T41.3X6
aminophenothiazine	T43.3X1	T43.3X2	T43.3X3	T43.3X4	T43.3X5	T43.3X6
benzoate	T52.8X1	T52.8X2	T52.8X3	T52.8X4	—	—

Substance	Poisoning, Accidental (unintentional)	Poisoning, Intentional Self-harm	Poisoning, Assault	Poisoning, Undetermined	Adverse Effect	Under-dosing
Ethyl — continued						
biscoumacetate	T45.511	T45.512	T45.513	T45.514	T45.515	T45.516
bromide (anesthetic)	T41.0X1	T41.0X2	T41.0X3	T41.0X4	T41.0X5	T41.0X6
carbamate	T45.1X1	T45.1X2	T45.1X3	T45.1X4	T45.1X5	T45.1X6
carbinol	T51.3X1	T51.3X2	T51.3X3	T51.3X4	—	—
carbonate	T52.8X1	T52.8X2	T52.8X3	T52.8X4	—	—
chaulmoograte	T37.1X1	T37.1X2	T37.1X3	T37.1X4	T37.1X5	T37.1X6
chloride (anesthetic)	T41.0X1	T41.0X2	T41.0X3	T41.0X4	T41.0X5	T41.0X6
anesthetic (local)	T41.3X1	T41.3X2	T41.3X3	T41.3X4	T41.3X5	T41.3X6
inhaled	T41.0X1	T41.0X2	T41.0X3	T41.0X4	T41.0X5	T41.0X6
local	T49.4X1	T49.4X2	T49.4X3	T49.4X4	T49.4X5	T49.4X6
solvent	T53.6X1	T53.6X2	T53.6X3	T53.6X4	—	—
dibunate	T48.3X1	T48.3X2	T48.3X3	T48.3X4	T48.3X5	T48.3X6
dichloroarsine (vapor)	T57.0X1	T57.0X2	T57.0X3	T57.0X4	—	—
estranol	T38.7X1	T38.7X2	T38.7X3	T38.7X4	T38.7X5	T38.7X6
ether — see also ether	T52.8X1	T52.8X2	T52.8X3	T52.8X4	—	—
formate NEC (solvent)	T52.0X1	T52.0X2	T52.0X3	T52.0X4	—	—
fumarate	T49.4X1	T49.4X2	T49.4X3	T49.4X4	T49.4X5	T49.4X6
hydroxyisobutyrate NEC (solvent)	T52.8X1	T52.8X2	T52.8X3	T52.8X4	—	—
iodoacetate	T59.3X1	T59.3X2	T59.3X3	T59.3X4	—	—
lactate NEC (solvent)	T52.8X1	T52.8X2	T52.8X3	T52.8X4	—	—
loflazepate	T42.4X1	T42.4X2	T42.4X3	T42.4X4	T42.4X5	T42.4X6
mercuric chloride	T56.1X1	T56.1X2	T56.1X3	T56.1X4	—	—
methylcarbinol	T51.8X1	T51.8X2	T51.8X3	T51.8X4	—	—
morphine	T40.2X1	T40.2X2	T40.2X3	T40.2X4	T40.2X5	T40.2X6
noradrenaline	T48.6X1	T48.6X2	T48.6X3	T48.6X4	T48.6X5	T48.6X6
oxybutyrate NEC (solvent)	T52.8X1	T52.8X2	T52.8X3	T52.8X4	—	—
Ethylene (gas)	T59.891	T59.892	T59.893	T59.894	—	—
anesthetic (general)	T41.0X1	T41.0X2	T41.0X3	T41.0X4	T41.0X5	T41.0X6
chlorohydrin	T52.8X1	T52.8X2	T52.8X3	T52.8X4	—	—
vapor	T53.6X1	T53.6X2	T53.6X3	T53.6X4	—	—
dichloride	T52.8X1	T52.8X2	T52.8X3	T52.8X4	—	—
vapor	T53.6X1	T53.6X2	T53.6X3	T53.6X4	—	—
dinitrate	T52.3X1	T52.3X2	T52.3X3	T52.3X4	—	—
glycol(s)	T52.8X1	T52.8X2	T52.8X3	T52.8X4	—	—
dinitrate	T52.3X1	T52.3X2	T52.3X3	T52.3X4	—	—
monobutyl ether	T52.3X1	T52.3X2	T52.3X3	T52.3X4	—	—
imine	T54.1X1	T54.1X2	T54.1X3	T54.1X4	—	—
oxide (fumigant) (nonmedicinal)	T59.891	T59.892	T59.893	T59.894	—	—
medicinal	T49.0X1	T49.0X2	T49.0X3	T49.0X4	T49.0X5	T49.0X6
Ethylenediaminetetra-acetic acid	T50.6X1	T50.6X2	T50.6X3	T50.6X4	T50.6X5	T50.6X6
Ethylenediamine theophylline	T48.6X1	T48.6X2	T48.6X3	T48.6X4	T48.6X5	T48.6X6
Ethylenedinitrilotetra-acetate	T50.6X1	T50.6X2	T50.6X3	T50.6X4	T50.6X5	T50.6X6
Ethylestrenol	T38.7X1	T38.7X2	T38.7X3	T38.7X4	T38.7X5	T38.7X6
Ethylhydroxycellulose	T47.4X1	T47.4X2	T47.4X3	T47.4X4	T47.4X5	T47.4X6
Ethylidene						
chloride NEC	T53.6X1	T53.6X2	T53.6X3	T53.6X4	—	—
diacetate	T60.3X1	T60.3X2	T60.3X3	T60.3X4	—	—
dicoumarin	T45.511	T45.512	T45.513	T45.514	T45.515	T45.516
dicoumarol	T45.511	T45.512	T45.513	T45.514	T45.515	T45.516
diethyl ether	T52.0X1	T52.0X2	T52.0X3	T52.0X4	—	—
Ethylmorphine	T40.2X1	T40.2X2	T40.2X3	T40.2X4	T40.2X5	T40.2X6
Ethylnorepinephrine	T48.6X1	T48.6X2	T48.6X3	T48.6X4	T48.6X5	T48.6X6
Ethylparachlorophen-oxyisobutyrate	T46.6X1	T46.6X2	T46.6X3	T46.6X4	T46.6X5	T46.6X6
Ethynodiol	T38.4X1	T38.4X2	T38.4X3	T38.4X4	T38.4X5	T38.4X6
with mestranol diacetate	T38.4X1	T38.4X2	T38.4X3	T38.4X4	T38.4X5	T38.4X6
Etidocaine	T41.3X1	T41.3X2	T41.3X3	T41.3X4	T41.3X5	T41.3X6
infiltration (subcutaneous)	T41.3X1	T41.3X2	T41.3X3	T41.3X4	T41.3X5	T41.3X6
nerve (peripheral) (plexus)	T41.3X1	T41.3X2	T41.3X3	T41.3X4	T41.3X5	T41.3X6
Etidronate	T50.991	T50.992	T50.993	T50.994	T50.995	T50.996
Etidronic acid (disodium salt)	T50.991	T50.992	T50.993	T50.994	T50.995	T50.996
Etifoxine	T42.6X1	T42.6X2	T42.6X3	T42.6X4	T42.6X5	T42.6X6
Etilefrine	T44.4X1	T44.4X2	T44.4X3	T44.4X4	T44.4X5	T44.4X6
Etilfen	T42.3X1	T42.3X2	T42.3X3	T42.3X4	T42.3X5	T42.3X6
Etinodiol	T38.4X1	T38.4X2	T38.4X3	T38.4X4	T38.4X5	T38.4X6
Etiroxate	T46.6X1	T46.6X2	T46.6X3	T46.6X4	T46.6X5	T46.6X6
Etizolam	T42.4X1	T42.4X2	T42.4X3	T42.4X4	T42.4X5	T42.4X6
Etodolac	T39.391	T39.392	T39.393	T39.394	T39.395	T39.396
Etofamide	T37.3X1	T37.3X2	T37.3X3	T37.3X4	T37.3X5	T37.3X6
Etofibrate	T46.6X1	T46.6X2	T46.6X3	T46.6X4	T46.6X5	T46.6X6
Etofylline	T46.7X1	T46.7X2	T46.7X3	T46.7X4	T46.7X5	T46.7X6
clofibrate	T46.6X1	T46.6X2	T46.6X3	T46.6X4	T46.6X5	T46.6X6
Etoglucid	T45.1X1	T45.1X2	T45.1X3	T45.1X4	T45.1X5	T45.1X6
Etomidate	T41.1X1	T41.1X2	T41.1X3	T41.1X4	T41.1X5	T41.1X6
Etomide	T39.8X1	T39.8X2	T39.8X3	T39.8X4	T39.8X5	T39.8X6
Etomidoline	T44.3X1	T44.3X2	T44.3X3	T44.3X4	T44.3X5	T44.3X6
Etoposide	T45.1X1	T45.1X2	T45.1X3	T45.1X4	T45.1X5	T45.1X6

Additional Character May Be Required — Refer to the Tabular List for Character Selection ▼ Subterms under main terms may continue to next column or page

Substance	Poisoning, Accidental (unintentional)	Poisoning, Intentional Self-harm	Poisoning, Assault	Poisoning, Undetermined	Adverse Effect	Under-dosing
Etorphine	T40.2X1	T40.2X2	T40.2X3	T40.2X4	T40.2X5	T40.2X6
Etoval	T42.3X1	T42.3X2	T42.3X3	T42.3X4	T42.3X5	T42.3X6
Etozolin	T50.1X1	T50.1X2	T50.1X3	T50.1X4	T50.1X5	T50.1X6
Etretinate	T50.991	T50.992	T50.993	T50.994	T50.995	T50.996
Etryptamine	T43.691	T43.692	T43.693	T43.694	T43.695	T43.696
Etybenzatropine	T44.3X1	T44.3X2	T44.3X3	T44.3X4	T44.3X5	T44.3X6
Etynodiol	T38.4X1	T38.4X2	T38.4X3	T38.4X4	T38.4X5	T38.4X6
Eucaine	T41.3X1	T41.3X2	T41.3X3	T41.3X4	T41.3X5	T41.3X6
Eucalyptus oil	T49.7X1	T49.7X2	T49.7X3	T49.7X4	T49.7X5	T49.7X6
Eucatropine	T49.5X1	T49.5X2	T49.5X3	T49.5X4	T49.5X5	T49.5X6
Eucodal	T40.2X1	T40.2X2	T40.2X3	T40.2X4	T40.2X5	T40.2X6
Euneryl	T42.3X1	T42.3X2	T42.3X3	T42.3X4	T42.3X5	T42.3X6
Euphthalmine	T44.3X1	T44.3X2	T44.3X3	T44.3X4	T44.3X5	T44.3X6
Eurax	T49.0X1	T49.0X2	T49.0X3	T49.0X4	T49.0X5	T49.0X6
Euresol	T49.4X1	T49.4X2	T49.4X3	T49.4X4	T49.4X5	T49.4X6
Euthroid	T38.1X1	T38.1X2	T38.1X3	T38.1X4	T38.1X5	T38.1X6
Evans blue	T50.8X1	T50.8X2	T50.8X3	T50.8X4	T50.8X5	T50.8X6
Evipal	T42.3X1	T42.3X2	T42.3X3	T42.3X4	T42.3X5	T42.3X6
sodium	T41.1X1	T41.1X2	T41.1X3	T41.1X4	T41.1X5	T41.1X6
Evipan	T42.3X1	T42.3X2	T42.3X3	T42.3X4	T42.3X5	T42.3X6
sodium	T41.1X1	T41.1X2	T41.1X3	T41.1X4	T41.1X5	T41.1X6
Exalamide	T49.0X1	T49.0X2	T49.0X3	T49.0X4	T49.0X5	T49.0X6
Exalgin	T39.1X1	T39.1X2	T39.1X3	T39.1X4	T39.1X5	T39.1X6
Excipients, pharmaceutical	T50.901	T50.902	T50.903	T50.904	T50.905	T50.906
Exhaust gas (engine) (motor vehicle)	T58.01	T58.02	T58.03	T58.04	—	—
Ex-Lax (phenolphthalein)	T47.2X1	T47.2X2	T47.2X3	T47.2X4	T47.2X5	T47.2X6
Expectorant NEC	T48.4X1	T48.4X2	T48.4X3	T48.4X4	T48.4X5	T48.4X6
Extended insulin zinc suspension	T38.3X1	T38.3X2	T38.3X3	T38.3X4	T38.3X5	T38.3X6
External medications (skin) (mucous membrane)	T49.91	T49.92	T49.93	T49.94	T49.95	T49.96
dental agent	T49.7X1	T49.7X2	T49.7X3	T49.7X4	T49.7X5	T49.7X6
ENT agent	T49.6X1	T49.6X2	T49.6X3	T49.6X4	T49.6X5	T49.6X6
ophthalmic preparation	T49.5X1	T49.5X2	T49.5X3	T49.5X4	T49.5X5	T49.5X6
specified NEC	T49.8X1	T49.8X2	T49.8X3	T49.8X4	T49.8X5	T49.8X6
Extrapyramidal antagonist NEC	T44.3X1	T44.3X2	T44.3X3	T44.3X4	T44.3X5	T44.3X6
Eye agents (anti-infective)	T49.5X1	T49.5X2	T49.5X3	T49.5X4	T49.5X5	T49.5X6
Eye drug NEC	T49.5X1	T49.5X2	T49.5X3	T49.5X4	T49.5X5	T49.5X6
FAC (fluorouracil + doxorubicin + cyclophosphamide)	T45.1X1	T45.1X2	T45.1X3	T45.1X4	T45.1X5	T45.1X6
Factor						
I (fibrinogen)	T45.8X1	T45.8X2	T45.8X3	T45.8X4	T45.8X5	T45.8X6
III (thromboplastin)	T45.8X1	T45.8X2	T45.8X3	T45.8X4	T45.8X5	T45.8X6
IX complex	T45.7X1	T45.7X2	T45.7X3	T45.7X4	T45.7X5	T45.7X6
human	T45.8X1	T45.8X2	T45.8X3	T45.8X4	T45.8X5	T45.8X6
VIII (antihemophilic Factor) (concentrate)	T45.8X1	T45.8X2	T45.8X3	T45.8X4	T45.8X5	T45.8X6
Famotidine	T47.0X1	T47.0X2	T47.0X3	T47.0X4	T47.0X5	T47.0X6
Fat suspension, intravenous	T50.991	T50.992	T50.993	T50.994	T50.995	T50.996
Fazadinium bromide	T48.1X1	T48.1X2	T48.1X3	T48.1X4	T48.1X5	T48.1X6
Febarbamate	T42.3X1	T42.3X2	T42.3X3	T42.3X4	T42.3X5	T42.3X6
Fecal softener	T47.4X1	T47.4X2	T47.4X3	T47.4X4	T47.4X5	T47.4X6
Fedrilate	T48.3X1	T48.3X2	T48.3X3	T48.3X4	T48.3X5	T48.3X6
Felodipine	T46.1X1	T46.1X2	T46.1X3	T46.1X4	T46.1X5	T46.1X6
Felypressin	T38.891	T38.892	T38.893	T38.894	T38.895	T38.896
Femoxetine	T43.221	T43.222	T43.223	T43.224	T43.225	T43.226
Fenalcomine	T46.3X1	T46.3X2	T46.3X3	T46.3X4	T46.3X5	T46.3X6
Fenamisal	T37.1X1	T37.1X2	T37.1X3	T37.1X4	T37.1X5	T37.1X6
Fenazone	T39.2X1	T39.2X2	T39.2X3	T39.2X4	T39.2X5	T39.2X6
Fenbendazole	T37.4X1	T37.4X2	T37.4X3	T37.4X4	T37.4X5	T37.4X6
Fenbutrazate	T50.5X1	T50.5X2	T50.5X3	T50.5X4	T50.5X5	T50.5X6
Fencamfamine	T43.691	T43.692	T43.693	T43.694	T43.695	T43.696
Fendiline	T46.1X1	T46.1X2	T46.1X3	T46.1X4	T46.1X5	T46.1X6
Fenetylline	T43.691	T43.692	T43.693	T43.694	T43.695	T43.696
Fenflumizole	T39.391	T39.392	T39.393	T39.394	T39.395	T39.396
Fenfluramine	T50.5X1	T50.5X2	T50.5X3	T50.5X4	T50.5X5	T50.5X6
Fenobarbital	T42.3X1	T42.3X2	T42.3X3	T42.3X4	T42.3X5	T42.3X6
Fenofibrate	T46.6X1	T46.6X2	T46.6X3	T46.6X4	T46.6X5	T46.6X6
Fenoprofen	T39.311	T39.312	T39.313	T39.314	T39.315	T39.316
Fenoterol	T48.6X1	T48.6X2	T48.6X3	T48.6X4	T48.6X5	T48.6X6
Fenoverine	T44.3X1	T44.3X2	T44.3X3	T44.3X4	T44.3X5	T44.3X6
Fenoxazoline	T48.5X1	T48.5X2	T48.5X3	T48.5X4	T48.5X5	T48.5X6
Fenproporex	T50.5X1	T50.5X2	T50.5X3	T50.5X4	T50.5X5	T50.5X6
Fenquizone	T50.2X1	T50.2X2	T50.2X3	T50.2X4	T50.2X5	T50.2X6
Fentanyl (analogs)	T40.411	T40.412	T40.413	T40.414	T40.415	T40.416
Fentazin	T43.3X1	T43.3X2	T43.3X3	T43.3X4	T43.3X5	T43.3X6
Fenthion	T60.0X1	T60.0X2	T60.0X3	T60.0X4	—	—
Fenticlor	T49.0X1	T49.0X2	T49.0X3	T49.0X4	T49.0X5	T49.0X6
Fenylbutazone	T39.2X1	T39.2X2	T39.2X3	T39.2X4	T39.2X5	T39.2X6

Substance	Poisoning, Accidental (unintentional)	Poisoning, Intentional Self-harm	Poisoning, Assault	Poisoning, Undetermined	Adverse Effect	Under-dosing
Feprazone	T39.2X1	T39.2X2	T39.2X3	T39.2X4	T39.2X5	T39.2X6
Fer de lance (bite) (venom)	T63.061	T63.062	T63.063	T63.064	—	—
Ferric — see also Iron						
chloride	T45.4X1	T45.4X2	T45.4X3	T45.4X4	T45.4X5	T45.4X6
citrate	T45.4X1	T45.4X2	T45.4X3	T45.4X4	T45.4X5	T45.4X6
hydroxide						
colloidal	T45.4X1	T45.4X2	T45.4X3	T45.4X4	T45.4X5	T45.4X6
polymaltose	T45.4X1	T45.4X2	T45.4X3	T45.4X4	T45.4X5	T45.4X6
pyrophosphate	T45.4X1	T45.4X2	T45.4X3	T45.4X4	T45.4X5	T45.4X6
Ferritin	T45.4X1	T45.4X2	T45.4X3	T45.4X4	T45.4X5	T45.4X6
Ferrocholinate	T45.4X1	T45.4X2	T45.4X3	T45.4X4	T45.4X5	T45.4X6
Ferrodextrane	T45.4X1	T45.4X2	T45.4X3	T45.4X4	T45.4X5	T45.4X6
Ferropolimaler	T45.4X1	T45.4X2	T45.4X3	T45.4X4	T45.4X5	T45.4X6
Ferrous — see also Iron						
phosphate	T45.4X1	T45.4X2	T45.4X3	T45.4X4	T45.4X5	T45.4X6
salt	T45.4X1	T45.4X2	T45.4X3	T45.4X4	T45.4X5	T45.4X6
with folic acid	T45.4X1	T45.4X2	T45.4X3	T45.4X4	T45.4X5	T45.4X6
Ferrous fumerate, gluconate, lactate, salt NEC, sulfate (medicinal)	T45.4X1	T45.4X2	T45.4X3	T45.4X4	T45.4X5	T45.4X6
Ferrovanadium (fumes)	T59.891	T59.892	T59.893	T59.894	—	—
Ferrum — see Iron						
Fertilizers NEC	T65.891	T65.892	T65.893	T65.894	—	—
with herbicide mixture	T60.3X1	T60.3X2	T60.3X3	T60.3X4	—	—
Fetoxilate	T47.6X1	T47.6X2	T47.6X3	T47.6X4	T47.6X5	T47.6X6
Fiber, dietary	T47.4X1	T47.4X2	T47.4X3	T47.4X4	T47.4X5	T47.4X6
Fiberglass	T65.831	T65.832	T65.833	T65.834	—	—
Fibrinogen (human)	T45.8X1	T45.8X2	T45.8X3	T45.8X4	T45.8X5	T45.8X6
Fibrinolysin (human)	T45.691	T45.692	T45.693	T45.694	T45.695	T45.696
Fibrinolysis						
affecting drug	T45.601	T45.602	T45.603	T45.604	T45.605	T45.606
inhibitor NEC	T45.621	T45.622	T45.623	T45.624	T45.625	T45.626
Fibrinolytic drug	T45.611	T45.612	T45.613	T45.614	T45.615	T45.616
Filix mas	T37.4X1	T37.4X2	T37.4X3	T37.4X4	T37.4X5	T37.4X6
Filtering cream	T49.3X1	T49.3X2	T49.3X3	T49.3X4	T49.3X5	T49.3X6
Fiorinal	T39.011	T39.012	T39.013	T39.014	T39.015	T39.016
Firedamp	T59.891	T59.892	T59.893	T59.894	—	—
Fish, noxious, nonbacterial	T61.91	T61.92	T61.93	T61.94	—	—
ciguatera	T61.01	T61.02	T61.03	T61.04	—	—
scombroid	T61.11	T61.12	T61.13	T61.14	—	—
shell	T61.781	T61.782	T61.783	T61.784	—	—
specified NEC	T61.771	T61.772	T61.773	T61.774	—	—
Flagyl	T37.3X1	T37.3X2	T37.3X3	T37.3X4	T37.3X5	T37.3X6
Flavine adenine dinucleotide	T45.2X1	T45.2X2	T45.2X3	T45.2X4	T45.2X5	T45.2X6
Flavodic acid	T46.991	T46.992	T46.993	T46.994	T46.995	T46.996
Flavoxate	T44.3X1	T44.3X2	T44.3X3	T44.3X4	T44.3X5	T44.3X6
Flaxedil	T48.1X1	T48.1X2	T48.1X3	T48.1X4	T48.1X5	T48.1X6
Flaxseed (medicinal)	T49.3X1	T49.3X2	T49.3X3	T49.3X4	T49.3X5	T49.3X6
Flecainide	T46.2X1	T46.2X2	T46.2X3	T46.2X4	T46.2X5	T46.2X6
Fleroxacin	T36.8X1	T36.8X2	T36.8X3	T36.8X4	T36.8X5	T36.8X6
Floctafenine	T39.8X1	T39.8X2	T39.8X3	T39.8X4	T39.8X5	T39.8X6
Flomax	T44.6X1	T44.6X2	T44.6X3	T44.6X4	T44.6X5	T44.6X6
Flomoxef	T36.1X1	T36.1X2	T36.1X3	T36.1X4	T36.1X5	T36.1X6
Flopropione	T44.3X1	T44.3X2	T44.3X3	T44.3X4	T44.3X5	T44.3X6
Florantyrone	T47.5X1	T47.5X2	T47.5X3	T47.5X4	T47.5X5	T47.5X6
Floraquin	T37.8X1	T37.8X2	T37.8X3	T37.8X4	T37.8X5	T37.8X6
Florinef	T38.0X1	T38.0X2	T38.0X3	T38.0X4	T38.0X5	T38.0X6
ENT agent	T49.6X1	T49.6X2	T49.6X3	T49.6X4	T49.6X5	T49.6X6
ophthalmic preparation	T49.5X1	T49.5X2	T49.5X3	T49.5X4	T49.5X5	T49.5X6
topical NEC	T49.0X1	T49.0X2	T49.0X3	T49.0X4	T49.0X5	T49.0X6
Flowers of sulfur	T49.4X1	T49.4X2	T49.4X3	T49.4X4	T49.4X5	T49.4X6
Floxuridine	T45.1X1	T45.1X2	T45.1X3	T45.1X4	T45.1X5	T45.1X6
Fluanisone	T43.4X1	T43.4X2	T43.4X3	T43.4X4	T43.4X5	T43.4X6
Flubendazole	T37.4X1	T37.4X2	T37.4X3	T37.4X4	T37.4X5	T37.4X6
Fluclorolone acetonide	T49.0X1	T49.0X2	T49.0X3	T49.0X4	T49.0X5	T49.0X6
Flucloxacillin	T36.0X1	T36.0X2	T36.0X3	T36.0X4	T36.0X5	T36.0X6
Fluconazole	T37.8X1	T37.8X2	T37.8X3	T37.8X4	T37.8X5	T37.8X6
Flucytosine	T37.8X1	T37.8X2	T37.8X3	T37.8X4	T37.8X5	T37.8X6
Fludeoxyglucose (18F)	T50.8X1	T50.8X2	T50.8X3	T50.8X4	T50.8X5	T50.8X6
Fludiazepam	T42.4X1	T42.4X2	T42.4X3	T42.4X4	T42.4X5	T42.4X6
Fludrocortisone	T50.0X1	T50.0X2	T50.0X3	T50.0X4	T50.0X5	T50.0X6
ENT agent	T49.6X1	T49.6X2	T49.6X3	T49.6X4	T49.6X5	T49.6X6
ophthalmic preparation	T49.5X1	T49.5X2	T49.5X3	T49.5X4	T49.5X5	T49.5X6
topical NEC	T49.0X1	T49.0X2	T49.0X3	T49.0X4	T49.0X5	T49.0X6
Fludroxycortide	T49.0X1	T49.0X2	T49.0X3	T49.0X4	T49.0X5	T49.0X6
Flufenamic acid	T39.391	T39.392	T39.393	T39.394	T39.395	T39.396
Fluindione	T45.511	T45.512	T45.513	T45.514	T45.515	T45.516
Flumequine	T37.8X1	T37.8X2	T37.8X3	T37.8X4	T37.8X5	T37.8X6
Flumethasone	T49.0X1	T49.0X2	T49.0X3	T49.0X4	T49.0X5	T49.0X6
Flumethiazide	T50.2X1	T50.2X2	T50.2X3	T50.2X4	T50.2X5	T50.2X6
Flumidin	T37.5X1	T37.5X2	T37.5X3	T37.5X4	T37.5X5	T37.5X6

▽ Subterms under main terms may continue to next column or page   Additional Character May Be Required — Refer to the Tabular List for Character Selection   373

Etorphine — Flumidin

Substance	Poisoning, Accidental (unintentional)	Poisoning, Intentional Self-harm	Poisoning, Assault	Poisoning, Undetermined	Adverse Effect	Under-dosing
Flunarizine	T46.7X1	T46.7X2	T46.7X3	T46.7X4	T46.7X5	T46.7X6
Flunidazole	T37.8X1	T37.8X2	T37.8X3	T37.8X4	T37.8X5	T37.8X6
Flunisolide	T48.6X1	T48.6X2	T48.6X3	T48.6X4	T48.6X5	T48.6X6
Flunitrazepam	T42.4X1	T42.4X2	T42.4X3	T42.4X4	T42.4X5	T42.4X6
Fluocinolone (acetonide)	T49.0X1	T49.0X2	T49.0X3	T49.0X4	T49.0X5	T49.0X6
Fluocinonide	T49.0X1	T49.0X2	T49.0X3	T49.0X4	T49.0X5	T49.0X6
Fluocortin (butyl)	T49.0X1	T49.0X2	T49.0X3	T49.0X4	T49.0X5	T49.0X6
Fluocortolone	T49.0X1	T49.0X2	T49.0X3	T49.0X4	T49.0X5	T49.0X6
Fluohydrocortisone	T38.0X1	T38.0X2	T38.0X3	T38.0X4	T38.0X5	T38.0X6
ENT agent	T49.6X1	T49.6X2	T49.6X3	T49.6X4	T49.6X5	T49.6X6
ophthalmic preparation	T49.5X1	T49.5X2	T49.5X3	T49.5X4	T49.5X5	T49.5X6
topical NEC	T49.0X1	T49.0X2	T49.0X3	T49.0X4	T49.0X5	T49.0X6
Fluonid	T49.0X1	T49.0X2	T49.0X3	T49.0X4	T49.0X5	T49.0X6
Fluopromazine	T43.3X1	T43.3X2	T43.3X3	T43.3X4	T43.3X5	T43.3X6
Fluoracetate	T60.8X1	T60.8X2	T60.8X3	T60.8X4	—	—
Fluorescein	T50.8X1	T50.8X2	T50.8X3	T50.8X4	T50.8X5	T50.8X6
Fluorhydrocortisone	T50.0X1	T50.0X2	T50.0X3	T50.0X4	T50.0X5	T50.0X6
Fluoride (nonmedicinal) (pesticide) (sodium) NEC	T60.8X1	T60.8X2	T60.8X3	T60.8X4	—	—
hydrogen — see Hydrofluoric acid						
medicinal NEC	T50.991	T50.992	T50.993	T50.994	T50.995	T50.996
dental use	T49.7X1	T49.7X2	T49.7X3	T49.7X4	T49.7X5	T49.7X6
not pesticide NEC	T54.91	T54.92	T54.93	T54.94	—	—
stannous	T49.7X1	T49.7X2	T49.7X3	T49.7X4	T49.7X5	T49.7X6
Fluorinated corticosteroids	T38.0X1	T38.0X2	T38.0X3	T38.0X4	T38.0X5	T38.0X6
Fluorine (gas)	T59.5X1	T59.5X2	T59.5X3	T59.5X4	—	—
salt — see Fluoride(s)						
Fluoristan	T49.7X1	T49.7X2	T49.7X3	T49.7X4	T49.7X5	T49.7X6
Fluormetholone	T49.0X1	T49.0X2	T49.0X3	T49.0X4	T49.0X5	T49.0X6
Fluoroacetate	T60.8X1	T60.8X2	T60.8X3	T60.8X4	—	—
Fluorocarbon monomer	T53.6X1	T53.6X2	T53.6X3	T53.6X4	—	—
Fluorocytosine	T37.8X1	T37.8X2	T37.8X3	T37.8X4	T37.8X5	T37.8X6
Fluorodeoxyuridine	T45.1X1	T45.1X2	T45.1X3	T45.1X4	T45.1X5	T45.1X6
Fluorometholone	T49.0X1	T49.0X2	T49.0X3	T49.0X4	T49.0X5	T49.0X6
ophthalmic preparation	T49.5X1	T49.5X2	T49.5X3	T49.5X4	T49.5X5	T49.5X6
Fluorophosphate insecticide	T60.0X1	T60.0X2	T60.0X3	T60.0X4	—	—
Fluorosol	T46.3X1	T46.3X2	T46.3X3	T46.3X4	T46.3X5	T46.3X6
Fluorouracil	T45.1X1	T45.1X2	T45.1X3	T45.1X4	T45.1X5	T45.1X6
Fluorphenylalanine	T49.5X1	T49.5X2	T49.5X3	T49.5X4	T49.5X5	T49.5X6
Fluothane	T41.0X1	T41.0X2	T41.0X3	T41.0X4	T41.0X5	T41.0X6
Fluoxetine	T43.221	T43.222	T43.223	T43.224	T43.225	T43.226
Fluoxymesterone	T38.7X1	T38.7X2	T38.7X3	T38.7X4	T38.7X5	T38.7X6
Flupenthixol	T43.4X1	T43.4X2	T43.4X3	T43.4X4	T43.4X5	T43.4X6
Flupentixol	T43.4X1	T43.4X2	T43.4X3	T43.4X4	T43.4X5	T43.4X6
Fluphenazine	T43.3X1	T43.3X2	T43.3X3	T43.3X4	T43.3X5	T43.3X6
Fluprednidene	T49.0X1	T49.0X2	T49.0X3	T49.0X4	T49.0X5	T49.0X6
Fluprednisolone	T38.0X1	T38.0X2	T38.0X3	T38.0X4	T38.0X5	T38.0X6
Fluradoline	T39.8X1	T39.8X2	T39.8X3	T39.8X4	T39.8X5	T39.8X6
Flurandrenolide	T49.0X1	T49.0X2	T49.0X3	T49.0X4	T49.0X5	T49.0X6
Flurandrenolone	T49.0X1	T49.0X2	T49.0X3	T49.0X4	T49.0X5	T49.0X6
Flurazepam	T42.4X1	T42.4X2	T42.4X3	T42.4X4	T42.4X5	T42.4X6
Flurbiprofen	T39.311	T39.312	T39.313	T39.314	T39.315	T39.316
Flurobate	T49.0X1	T49.0X2	T49.0X3	T49.0X4	T49.0X5	T49.0X6
Fluroxene	T41.0X1	T41.0X2	T41.0X3	T41.0X4	T41.0X5	T41.0X6
Fluspirilene	T43.591	T43.592	T43.593	T43.594	T43.595	T43.596
Flutamide	T38.6X1	T38.6X2	T38.6X3	T38.6X4	T38.6X5	T38.6X6
Flutazolam	T38.0X1	T38.0X2	T38.0X3	T38.0X4	T38.0X5	T38.0X6
Fluticasone propionate	T38.0X1	T38.0X2	T38.0X3	T38.0X4	T38.0X5	T38.0X6
Flutoprazepam	T42.4X1	T42.4X2	T42.4X3	T42.4X4	T42.4X5	T42.4X6
Flutropium bromide	T48.6X1	T48.6X2	T48.6X3	T48.6X4	T48.6X5	T48.6X6
Fluvoxamine	T43.221	T43.222	T43.223	T43.224	T43.225	T43.226
Folacin	T45.8X1	T45.8X2	T45.8X3	T45.8X4	T45.8X5	T45.8X6
Folic acid	T45.8X1	T45.8X2	T45.8X3	T45.8X4	T45.8X5	T45.8X6
with ferrous salt	T45.2X1	T45.2X2	T45.2X3	T45.2X4	T45.2X5	T45.2X6
antagonist	T45.1X1	T45.1X2	T45.1X3	T45.1X4	T45.1X5	T45.1X6
Folinic acid	T45.8X1	T45.8X2	T45.8X3	T45.8X4	T45.8X5	T45.8X6
Folium stramoniae	T48.6X1	T48.6X2	T48.6X3	T48.6X4	T48.6X5	T48.6X6
Follicle-stimulating hormone, human	T38.811	T38.812	T38.813	T38.814	T38.815	T38.816
Folpet	T60.3X1	T60.3X2	T60.3X3	T60.3X4	—	—
Fominoben	T48.3X1	T48.3X2	T48.3X3	T48.3X4	T48.3X5	T48.3X6
Food, foodstuffs, noxious, nonbacterial, NEC	T62.91	T62.92	T62.93	T62.94	—	—
berries	T62.1X1	T62.1X2	T62.1X3	T62.1X4	—	—
fish — see also Fish	T61.91	T61.92	T61.93	T61.94	—	—
mushrooms	T62.0X1	T62.0X2	T62.0X3	T62.0X4	—	—
plants	T62.2X1	T62.2X2	T62.2X3	T62.2X4	—	—
seafood	T61.91	T61.92	T61.93	T61.94	—	—
specified NEC	T61.8X1	T61.8X2	T61.8X3	T61.8X4	—	—
seeds	T62.2X1	T62.2X2	T62.2X3	T62.2X4	—	—
Food, foodstuffs, noxious, nonbacterial, — continued						
shellfish	T61.781	T61.782	T61.783	T61.784	—	—
specified NEC	T62.8X1	T62.8X2	T62.8X3	T62.8X4	—	—
Fool's parsley	T62.2X1	T62.2X2	T62.2X3	T62.2X4	—	—
Formaldehyde (solution), gas or vapor	T59.2X1	T59.2X2	T59.2X3	T59.2X4	—	—
fungicide	T60.3X1	T60.3X2	T60.3X3	T60.3X4	—	—
Formalin	T59.2X1	T59.2X2	T59.2X3	T59.2X4	—	—
fungicide	T60.3X1	T60.3X2	T60.3X3	T60.3X4	—	—
vapor	T59.2X1	T59.2X2	T59.2X3	T59.2X4	—	—
Formic acid	T54.2X1	T54.2X2	T54.2X3	T54.2X4	—	—
vapor	T59.891	T59.892	T59.893	T59.894	—	—
Foscarnet sodium	T37.5X1	T37.5X2	T37.5X3	T37.5X4	T37.5X5	T37.5X6
Fosfestrol	T38.5X1	T38.5X2	T38.5X3	T38.5X4	T38.5X5	T38.5X6
Fosfomycin	T36.8X1	T36.8X2	T36.8X3	T36.8X4	T36.8X5	T36.8X6
Fosfonet sodium	T37.5X1	T37.5X2	T37.5X3	T37.5X4	T37.5X5	T37.5X6
Fosinopril	T46.4X1	T46.4X2	T46.4X3	T46.4X4	T46.4X5	T46.4X6
sodium	T46.4X1	T46.4X2	T46.4X3	T46.4X4	T46.4X5	T46.4X6
Fowler's solution	T57.0X1	T57.0X2	T57.0X3	T57.0X4	—	—
Foxglove	T62.2X1	T62.2X2	T62.2X3	T62.2X4	—	—
Framycetin	T36.5X1	T36.5X2	T36.5X3	T36.5X4	T36.5X5	T36.5X6
Frangula	T47.2X1	T47.2X2	T47.2X3	T47.2X4	T47.2X5	T47.2X6
extract	T47.2X1	T47.2X2	T47.2X3	T47.2X4	T47.2X5	T47.2X6
Frei antigen	T50.8X1	T50.8X2	T50.8X3	T50.8X4	T50.8X5	T50.8X6
Freon	T53.5X1	T53.5X2	T53.5X3	T53.5X4	—	—
Fructose	T50.3X1	T50.3X2	T50.3X3	T50.3X4	T50.3X5	T50.3X6
Frusemide	T50.1X1	T50.1X2	T50.1X3	T50.1X4	T50.1X5	T50.1X6
FSH	T38.811	T38.812	T38.813	T38.814	T38.815	T38.816
Ftorafur	T45.1X1	T45.1X2	T45.1X3	T45.1X4	T45.1X5	T45.1X6
Fuel						
automobile	T52.0X1	T52.0X2	T52.0X3	T52.0X4	—	—
exhaust gas, not in transit	T58.01	T58.02	T58.03	T58.04	—	—
vapor NEC	T52.0X1	T52.0X2	T52.0X3	T52.0X4	—	—
gas (domestic use) — see also Carbon, monoxide, fuel, utility	T59.891	T59.892	T59.893	T59.894	—	—
utility	T59.891	T59.892	T59.893	T59.894	—	—
incomplete combustion of — see Carbon, monoxide, fuel, utility						
in mobile container	T59.891	T59.892	T59.893	T59.894	—	—
piped (natural)	T59.891	T59.892	T59.893	T59.894	—	—
industrial, incomplete combustion	T58.8X1	T58.8X2	T58.8X3	T58.8X4	—	—
Fugillin	T36.8X1	T36.8X2	T36.8X3	T36.8X4	T36.8X5	T36.8X6
Fulminate of mercury	T56.1X1	T56.1X2	T56.1X3	T56.1X4	—	—
Fulvicin	T36.7X1	T36.7X2	T36.7X3	T36.7X4	T36.7X5	T36.7X6
Fumadil	T36.8X1	T36.8X2	T36.8X3	T36.8X4	T36.8X5	T36.8X6
Fumagillin	T36.8X1	T36.8X2	T36.8X3	T36.8X4	T36.8X5	T36.8X6
Fumaric acid	T49.4X1	T49.4X2	T49.4X3	T49.4X4	T49.4X5	T49.4X6
Fumes (from)	T59.91	T59.92	T59.93	T59.94	—	—
carbon monoxide — see Carbon, monoxide						
charcoal (domestic use) — see Charcoal, fumes						
chloroform — see Chloroform						
coke (in domestic stoves, fireplaces) — see Coke fumes						
corrosive NEC	T54.91	T54.92	T54.93	T54.94	—	—
ether — see ether						
freons	T53.5X1	T53.5X2	T53.5X3	T53.5X4	—	—
hydrocarbons	T59.891	T59.892	T59.893	T59.894	—	—
petroleum (liquefied)	T59.891	T59.892	T59.893	T59.894	—	—
distributed through pipes (pure or mixed with air)	T59.891	T59.892	T59.893	T59.894	—	—
lead — see lead						
metal — see Metals, or the specified metal						
nitrogen dioxide	T59.0X1	T59.0X2	T59.0X3	T59.0X4	—	—
pesticides — see Pesticides						
petroleum (liquefied)	T59.891	T59.892	T59.893	T59.894	—	—
distributed through pipes (pure or mixed with air)	T59.891	T59.892	T59.893	T59.894	—	—
polyester	T59.891	T59.892	T59.893	T59.894	—	—
specified source NEC — see also substance specified	T59.891	T59.892	T59.893	T59.894	—	—
sulfur dioxide	T59.1X1	T59.1X2	T59.1X3	T59.1X4	—	—
Fumigant NEC	T60.91	T60.92	T60.93	T60.94	—	—

Additional Character May Be Required — Refer to the Tabular List for Character Selection ▽ Subterms under main terms may continue to next column or page

Substance	Poisoning, Accidental (unintentional)	Poisoning, Intentional Self-harm	Poisoning, Assault	Poisoning, Undetermined	Adverse Effect	Under-dosing
Fungicide NEC	T60.3X1	T60.3X2	T60.3X3	T60.3X4	—	—
(nonmedicinal)						
Fungi, noxious, used as food	T62.0X1	T62.0X2	T62.0X3	T62.0X4	—	—
Fungizone	T36.7X1	T36.7X2	T36.7X3	T36.7X4	T36.7X5	T36.7X6
topical	T49.0X1	T49.0X2	T49.0X3	T49.0X4	T49.0X5	T49.0X6
Furacin	T49.0X1	T49.0X2	T49.0X3	T49.0X4	T49.0X5	T49.0X6
Furadantin	T37.91	T37.92	T37.93	T37.94	T37.95	T37.96
Furazolidone	T37.8X1	T37.8X2	T37.8X3	T37.8X4	T37.8X5	T37.8X6
Furazolium chloride	T49.0X1	T49.0X2	T49.0X3	T49.0X4	T49.0X5	T49.0X6
Furfural	T52.8X1	T52.8X2	T52.8X3	T52.8X4	—	—
Furnace (coal burning) (domestic), gas from	T58.2X1	T58.2X2	T58.2X3	T58.2X4	—	—
industrial	T58.8X1	T58.8X2	T58.8X3	T58.8X4	—	—
Furniture polish	T65.891	T65.892	T65.893	T65.894	—	—
Furosemide	T50.1X1	T50.1X2	T50.1X3	T50.1X4	T50.1X5	T50.1X6
Furoxone	T37.91	T37.92	T37.93	T37.94	T37.95	T37.96
Fursultiamine	T45.2X1	T45.2X2	T45.2X3	T45.2X4	T45.2X5	T45.2X6
Fusafungine	T36.8X1	T36.8X2	T36.8X3	T36.8X4	T36.8X5	T36.8X6
Fusel oil (any) (amyl) (butyl) (propyl), vapor	T51.3X1	T51.3X2	T51.3X3	T51.3X4	—	—
Fusidate (ethanolamine) (sodium)	T36.8X1	T36.8X2	T36.8X3	T36.8X4	T36.8X5	T36.8X6
Fusidic acid	T36.8X1	T36.8X2	T36.8X3	T36.8X4	T36.8X5	T36.8X6
Fytic acid, nonasodium	T50.6X1	T50.6X2	T50.6X3	T50.6X4	T50.6X5	T50.6X6
b-Galactosidase	T47.5X1	T47.5X2	T47.5X3	T47.5X4	T47.5X5	T47.5X6
GABA	T43.8X1	T43.8X2	T43.8X3	T43.8X4	T43.8X5	T43.8X6
Gadopentetic acid	T50.8X1	T50.8X2	T50.8X3	T50.8X4	T50.8X5	T50.8X6
Galactose	T50.3X1	T50.3X2	T50.3X3	T50.3X4	T50.3X5	T50.3X6
Galantamine	T44.0X1	T44.0X2	T44.0X3	T44.0X4	T44.0X5	T44.0X6
Gallamine (triethiodide)	T48.1X1	T48.1X2	T48.1X3	T48.1X4	T48.1X5	T48.1X6
Gallium citrate	T50.991	T50.992	T50.993	T50.994	T50.995	T50.996
Gallopamil	T46.1X1	T46.1X2	T46.1X3	T46.1X4	T46.1X5	T46.1X6
Gamboge	T47.2X1	T47.2X2	T47.2X3	T47.2X4	T47.2X5	T47.2X6
Gamimune	T50.Z11	T50.Z12	T50.Z13	T50.Z14	T50.Z15	T50.Z16
Gamma-aminobutyric acid	T43.8X1	T43.8X2	T43.8X3	T43.8X4	T43.8X5	T43.8X6
Gamma-benzene hexachloride (medicinal)	T49.0X1	T49.0X2	T49.0X3	T49.0X4	T49.0X5	T49.0X6
nonmedicinal, vapor	T53.6X1	T53.6X2	T53.6X3	T53.6X4	—	—
Gamma-BHC (medicinal) — see also Gamma-benzene hexachloride	T49.0X1	T49.0X2	T49.0X3	T49.0X4	T49.0X5	T49.0X6
Gamma globulin	T50.Z11	T50.Z12	T50.Z13	T50.Z14	T50.Z15	T50.Z16
Gamulin	T50.Z11	T50.Z12	T50.Z13	T50.Z14	T50.Z15	T50.Z16
Ganciclovir (sodium)	T37.5X1	T37.5X2	T37.5X3	T37.5X4	T37.5X5	T37.5X6
Ganglionic blocking drug NEC	T44.2X1	T44.2X2	T44.2X3	T44.2X4	T44.2X5	T44.2X6
specified NEC	T44.2X1	T44.2X2	T44.2X3	T44.2X4	T44.2X5	T44.2X6
Ganja	T40.7X1	T40.7X2	T40.7X3	T40.7X4	T40.7X5	T40.7X6
Garamycin	T36.5X1	T36.5X2	T36.5X3	T36.5X4	T36.5X5	T36.5X6
ophthalmic preparation	T49.5X1	T49.5X2	T49.5X3	T49.5X4	T49.5X5	T49.5X6
topical NEC	T49.0X1	T49.0X2	T49.0X3	T49.0X4	T49.0X5	T49.0X6
Gardenal	T42.3X1	T42.3X2	T42.3X3	T42.3X4	T42.3X5	T42.3X6
Gardepanyl	T42.3X1	T42.3X2	T42.3X3	T42.3X4	T42.3X5	T42.3X6
Gaseous substance — see Gas						
Gasoline	T52.0X1	T52.0X2	T52.0X3	T52.0X4	—	—
vapor	T52.0X1	T52.0X2	T52.0X3	T52.0X4	—	—
Gastric enzymes	T47.5X1	T47.5X2	T47.5X3	T47.5X4	T47.5X5	T47.5X6
Gastrografin	T50.8X1	T50.8X2	T50.8X3	T50.8X4	T50.8X5	T50.8X6
Gastrointestinal drug	T47.91	T47.92	T47.93	T47.94	T47.95	T47.96
biological	T47.8X1	T47.8X2	T47.8X3	T47.8X4	T47.8X5	T47.8X6
specified NEC	T47.8X1	T47.8X2	T47.8X3	T47.8X4	T47.8X5	T47.8X6
Gas NEC	T59.91	T59.92	T59.93	T59.94		
acetylene	T59.891	T59.892	T59.893	T59.894	—	—
incomplete combustion of	T58.11	T58.12	T58.13	T58.14	—	—
air contaminants, source or type not specified	T59.91	T59.92	T59.93	T59.94	—	—
anesthetic	T41.0X1	T41.0X2	T41.0X3	T41.0X4	T41.0X5	T41.0X6
blast furnace	T58.8X1	T58.8X2	T58.8X3	T58.8X4	—	—
butane — see butane						
carbon monoxide — see Carbon, monoxide						
chlorine	T59.4X1	T59.4X2	T59.4X3	T59.4X4	—	—
coal	T58.2X1	T58.2X2	T58.2X3	T58.2X4	—	—
cyanide	T57.3X1	T57.3X2	T57.3X3	T57.3X4	—	—
dicyanogen	T65.0X1	T65.0X2	T65.0X3	T65.0X4	—	—
domestic — see Domestic gas						
exhaust	T58.01	T58.02	T58.03	T58.04		
from utility (for cooking, heating, or lighting) (after combustion) — see Carbon, monoxide, fuel, utility						

Substance	Poisoning, Accidental (unintentional)	Poisoning, Intentional Self-harm	Poisoning, Assault	Poisoning, Undetermined	Adverse Effect	Under-dosing
Gas — continued						
from utility — see Carbon, monoxide, fuel, utility — continued						
prior to combustion	T59.891	T59.892	T59.893	T59.894		
from wood- or coal-burning stove or fireplace	T58.2X1	T58.2X2	T58.2X3	T58.2X4		
fuel (domestic use) (after combustion) — see also Carbon, monoxide, fuel						
industrial use	T58.8X1	T58.8X2	T58.8X3	T58.8X4		
prior to combustion	T59.891	T59.892	T59.893	T59.894		
utility	T59.891	T59.892	T59.893	T59.894		
incomplete combustion of — see Carbon, monoxide, fuel, utility						
in mobile container	T59.891	T59.892	T59.893	T59.894		
piped (natural)	T59.891	T59.892	T59.893	T59.894		
garage	T58.01	T58.02	T58.03	T58.04		
hydrocarbon NEC	T59.891	T59.892	T59.893	T59.894		
incomplete combustion of — see Carbon, monoxide, fuel, utility						
liquefied — see butane						
piped	T59.891	T59.892	T59.893	T59.894		
hydrocyanic acid	T65.0X1	T65.0X2	T65.0X3	T65.0X4		
illuminating (after combustion)	T58.11	T58.12	T58.13	T58.14		
prior to combustion	T59.891	T59.892	T59.893	T59.894		
incomplete combustion, any — see Carbon, monoxide						
kiln	T58.8X1	T58.8X2	T58.8X3	T58.8X4		
lacrimogenic	T59.3X1	T59.3X2	T59.3X3	T59.3X4		
liquefied petroleum — see butane						
marsh	T59.891	T59.892	T59.893	T59.894		
motor exhaust, not in transit	T58.01	T58.02	T58.03	T58.04		
mustard, not in war	T59.891	T59.892	T59.893	T59.894		
natural	T59.891	T59.892	T59.893	T59.894		
nerve, not in war	T59.91	T59.92	T59.93	T59.94		
oil	T52.0X1	T52.0X2	T52.0X3	T52.0X4		
petroleum (liquefied) (distributed in mobile containers)	T59.891	T59.892	T59.893	T59.894		
piped (pure or mixed with air)	T59.891	T59.892	T59.893	T59.894		
piped (manufactured) (natural) NEC	T59.891	T59.892	T59.893	T59.894		
producer	T58.8X1	T58.8X2	T58.8X3	T58.8X4		
propane — see propane						
refrigerant (chlorofluoro-carbon)	T53.5X1	T53.5X2	T53.5X3	T53.5X4		
not chlorofluoro-carbon	T59.891	T59.892	T59.893	T59.894		
sewer	T59.91	T59.92	T59.93	T59.94		
specified source NEC	T59.91	T59.92	T59.93	T59.94		
stove (after combustion)	T58.11	T58.12	T58.13	T58.14		
prior to combustion	T59.891	T59.892	T59.893	T59.894		
tear	T59.3X1	T59.3X2	T59.3X3	T59.3X4		
therapeutic	T41.5X1	T41.5X2	T41.5X3	T41.5X4	T41.5X5	T41.5X6
utility (for cooking, heating, or lighting) (piped) NEC	T59.891	T59.892	T59.893	T59.894		
incomplete combustion of — see Carbon, monoxide, fuel, utility						
in mobile container	T59.891	T59.892	T59.893	T59.894		
piped (natural)	T59.891	T59.892	T59.893	T59.894		
water	T58.11	T58.12	T58.13	T58.14	—	—
incomplete combustion of — see Carbon, monoxide, fuel, utility						
Gaultheria procumbens	T62.2X1	T62.2X2	T62.2X3	T62.2X4	—	—
Gefarnate	T44.3X1	T44.3X2	T44.3X3	T44.3X4	T44.3X5	T44.3X6
Gelatin (intravenous)	T45.8X1	T45.8X2	T45.8X3	T45.8X4	T45.8X5	T45.8X6
absorbable (sponge)	T45.7X1	T45.7X2	T45.7X3	T45.7X4	T45.7X5	T45.7X6
Gelfilm	T49.8X1	T49.8X2	T49.8X3	T49.8X4	T49.8X5	T49.8X6
Gelfoam	T45.7X1	T45.7X2	T45.7X3	T45.7X4	T45.7X5	T45.7X6
Gelsemine	T50.991	T50.992	T50.993	T50.994	T50.995	T50.996
Gelsemium (sempervirens)	T62.2X1	T62.2X2	T62.2X3	T62.2X4	—	—
Gemeprost	T48.0X1	T48.0X2	T48.0X3	T48.0X4	T48.0X5	T48.0X6
Gemfibrozil	T46.6X1	T46.6X2	T46.6X3	T46.6X4	T46.6X5	T46.6X6
Gemonil	T42.3X1	T42.3X2	T42.3X3	T42.3X4	T42.3X5	T42.3X6
Gentamicin	T36.5X1	T36.5X2	T36.5X3	T36.5X4	T36.5X5	T36.5X6

Substance	Poisoning, Accidental (unintentional)	Poisoning, Intentional Self-harm	Poisoning, Assault	Poisoning, Undetermined	Adverse Effect	Under-dosing
Gentamicin — *continued*						
ophthalmic preparation	T49.5X1	T49.5X2	T49.5X3	T49.5X4	T49.5X5	T49.5X6
topical NEC	T49.0X1	T49.0X2	T49.0X3	T49.0X4	T49.0X5	T49.0X6
Gentian	T47.5X1	T47.5X2	T47.5X3	T47.5X4	T47.5X5	T47.5X6
violet	T49.0X1	T49.0X2	T49.0X3	T49.0X4	T49.0X5	T49.0X6
Gepefrine	T44.4X1	T44.4X2	T44.4X3	T44.4X4	T44.4X5	T44.4X6
Gestonorone caproate	T38.5X1	T38.5X2	T38.5X3	T38.5X4	T38.5X5	T38.5X6
Gexane	T49.0X1	T49.0X2	T49.0X3	T49.0X4	T49.0X5	T49.0X6
Gila monster (venom)	T63.111	T63.112	T63.113	T63.114	—	—
Ginger	T47.5X1	T47.5X2	T47.5X3	T47.5X4	T47.5X5	T47.5X6
Jamaica — *see* Jamaica, ginger						
Gitalin	T46.0X1	T46.0X2	T46.0X3	T46.0X4	T46.0X5	T46.0X6
amorphous	T46.0X1	T46.0X2	T46.0X3	T46.0X4	T46.0X5	T46.0X6
Gitaloxin	T46.0X1	T46.0X2	T46.0X3	T46.0X4	T46.0X5	T46.0X6
Gitoxin	T46.0X1	T46.0X2	T46.0X3	T46.0X4	T46.0X5	T46.0X6
Glafenine	T39.8X1	T39.8X2	T39.8X3	T39.8X4	T39.8X5	T39.8X6
Glandular extract (medicinal) NEC	T50.Z91	T50.Z92	T50.Z93	T50.Z94	T50.Z95	T50.Z96
Glaucarubin	T37.3X1	T37.3X2	T37.3X3	T37.3X4	T37.3X5	T37.3X6
Glibenclamide	T38.3X1	T38.3X2	T38.3X3	T38.3X4	T38.3X5	T38.3X6
Glibornuride	T38.3X1	T38.3X2	T38.3X3	T38.3X4	T38.3X5	T38.3X6
Gliclazide	T38.3X1	T38.3X2	T38.3X3	T38.3X4	T38.3X5	T38.3X6
Glimidine	T38.3X1	T38.3X2	T38.3X3	T38.3X4	T38.3X5	T38.3X6
Glipizide	T38.3X1	T38.3X2	T38.3X3	T38.3X4	T38.3X5	T38.3X6
Gliquidone	T38.3X1	T38.3X2	T38.3X3	T38.3X4	T38.3X5	T38.3X6
Glisolamide	T38.3X1	T38.3X2	T38.3X3	T38.3X4	T38.3X5	T38.3X6
Glisoxepide	T38.3X1	T38.3X2	T38.3X3	T38.3X4	T38.3X5	T38.3X6
Globin zinc insulin	T38.3X1	T38.3X2	T38.3X3	T38.3X4	T38.3X5	T38.3X6
Globulin						
antilymphocytic	T50.Z11	T50.Z12	T50.Z13	T50.Z14	T50.Z15	T50.Z16
antirhesus	T50.Z11	T50.Z12	T50.Z13	T50.Z14	T50.Z15	T50.Z16
antivenin	T50.Z11	T50.Z12	T50.Z13	T50.Z14	T50.Z15	T50.Z16
antiviral	T50.Z11	T50.Z12	T50.Z13	T50.Z14	T50.Z15	T50.Z16
Glucagon	T38.3X1	T38.3X2	T38.3X3	T38.3X4	T38.3X5	T38.3X6
Glucocorticoids	T38.0X1	T38.0X2	T38.0X3	T38.0X4	T38.0X5	T38.0X6
Glucocorticosteroid	T38.0X1	T38.0X2	T38.0X3	T38.0X4	T38.0X5	T38.0X6
Gluconic acid	T50.991	T50.992	T50.993	T50.994	T50.995	T50.996
Glucosamine sulfate	T39.4X1	T39.4X2	T39.4X3	T39.4X4	T39.4X5	T39.4X6
Glucose	T50.3X1	T50.3X2	T50.3X3	T50.3X4	T50.3X5	T50.3X6
with sodium chloride	T50.3X1	T50.3X2	T50.3X3	T50.3X4	T50.3X5	T50.3X6
Glucosulfone sodium	T37.1X1	T37.1X2	T37.1X3	T37.1X4	T37.1X5	T37.1X6
Glucurolactone	T47.8X1	T47.8X2	T47.8X3	T47.8X4	T47.8X5	T47.8X6
Glue NEC	T52.8X1	T52.8X2	T52.8X3	T52.8X4	—	—
Glutamic acid	T47.5X1	T47.5X2	T47.5X3	T47.5X4	T47.5X5	T47.5X6
Glutaral (medicinal)	T49.0X1	T49.0X2	T49.0X3	T49.0X4	T49.0X5	T49.0X6
nonmedicinal	T65.891	T65.892	T65.893	T65.894	—	—
Glutaraldehyde (nonmedicinal)	T65.891	T65.892	T65.893	T65.894	—	—
medicinal	T49.0X1	T49.0X2	T49.0X3	T49.0X4	T49.0X5	T49.0X6
Glutathione	T50.6X1	T50.6X2	T50.6X3	T50.6X4	T50.6X5	T50.6X6
Glutethimide	T42.6X1	T42.6X2	T42.6X3	T42.6X4	T42.6X5	T42.6X6
Glyburide	T38.3X1	T38.3X2	T38.3X3	T38.3X4	T38.3X5	T38.3X6
Glycerin	T47.4X1	T47.4X2	T47.4X3	T47.4X4	T47.4X5	T47.4X6
Glycerol	T47.4X1	T47.4X2	T47.4X3	T47.4X4	T47.4X5	T47.4X6
borax	T49.6X1	T49.6X2	T49.6X3	T49.6X4	T49.6X5	T49.6X6
intravenous	T50.3X1	T50.3X2	T50.3X3	T50.3X4	T50.3X5	T50.3X6
iodinated	T48.4X1	T48.4X2	T48.4X3	T48.4X4	T48.4X5	T48.4X6
Glycerophosphate	T50.991	T50.992	T50.993	T50.994	T50.995	T50.996
Glyceryl						
gualacolate	T48.4X1	T48.4X2	T48.4X3	T48.4X4	T48.4X5	T48.4X6
nitrate	T46.3X1	T46.3X2	T46.3X3	T46.3X4	T46.3X5	T46.3X6
triacetate (topical)	T49.0X1	T49.0X2	T49.0X3	T49.0X4	T49.0X5	T49.0X6
trinitrate	T46.3X1	T46.3X2	T46.3X3	T46.3X4	T46.3X5	T46.3X6
Glycine	T50.3X1	T50.3X2	T50.3X3	T50.3X4	T50.3X5	T50.3X6
Glyclopyramide	T38.3X1	T38.3X2	T38.3X3	T38.3X4	T38.3X5	T38.3X6
Glycobiarsol	T37.3X1	T37.3X2	T37.3X3	T37.3X4	T37.3X5	T37.3X6
Glycols (ether)	T52.3X1	T52.3X2	T52.3X3	T52.3X4	—	—
Glyconiazide	T37.1X1	T37.1X2	T37.1X3	T37.1X4	T37.1X5	T37.1X6
Glycopyrrolate	T44.3X1	T44.3X2	T44.3X3	T44.3X4	T44.3X5	T44.3X6
Glycopyrronium	T44.3X1	T44.3X2	T44.3X3	T44.3X4	T44.3X5	T44.3X6
bromide	T44.3X1	T44.3X2	T44.3X3	T44.3X4	T44.3X5	T44.3X6
Glycoside, cardiac (stimulant)	T46.0X1	T46.0X2	T46.0X3	T46.0X4	T46.0X5	T46.0X6
Glycyclamide	T38.3X1	T38.3X2	T38.3X3	T38.3X4	T38.3X5	T38.3X6
Glycyrrhiza extract	T48.4X1	T48.4X2	T48.4X3	T48.4X4	T48.4X5	T48.4X6
Glycyrrhizic acid	T48.4X1	T48.4X2	T48.4X3	T48.4X4	T48.4X5	T48.4X6
Glycyrrhizinate potassium	T48.4X1	T48.4X2	T48.4X3	T48.4X4	T48.4X5	T48.4X6
Glymidine sodium	T38.3X1	T38.3X2	T38.3X3	T38.3X4	T38.3X5	T38.3X6
Glyphosate	T60.3X1	T60.3X2	T60.3X3	T60.3X4	—	—
Glyphylline	T48.6X1	T48.6X2	T48.6X3	T48.6X4	T48.6X5	T48.6X6
Gold						
colloidal (l98Au)	T45.1X1	T45.1X2	T45.1X3	T45.1X4	T45.1X5	T45.1X6
salts	T39.4X1	T39.4X2	T39.4X3	T39.4X4	T39.4X5	T39.4X6

Substance	Poisoning, Accidental (unintentional)	Poisoning, Intentional Self-harm	Poisoning, Assault	Poisoning, Undetermined	Adverse Effect	Under-dosing
Golden sulfide of antimony	T56.891	T56.892	T56.893	T56.894	—	—
Goldylocks	T62.2X1	T62.2X2	T62.2X3	T62.2X4	—	—
Gonadal tissue extract	T38.901	T38.902	T38.903	T38.904	T38.905	T38.906
female	T38.5X1	T38.5X2	T38.5X3	T38.5X4	T38.5X5	T38.5X6
male	T38.7X1	T38.7X2	T38.7X3	T38.7X4	T38.7X5	T38.7X6
Gonadorelin	T38.891	T38.892	T38.893	T38.894	T38.895	T38.896
Gonadotropin	T38.891	T38.892	T38.893	T38.894	T38.895	T38.896
chorionic	T38.891	T38.892	T38.893	T38.894	T38.895	T38.896
pituitary	T38.811	T38.812	T38.813	T38.814	T38.815	T38.816
Goserelin	T45.1X1	T45.1X2	T45.1X3	T45.1X4	T45.1X5	T45.1X6
Grain alcohol	T51.0X1	T51.0X2	T51.0X3	T51.0X4	—	—
Gramicidin	T49.0X1	T49.0X2	T49.0X3	T49.0X4	T49.0X5	T49.0X6
Granisetron	T45.0X1	T45.0X2	T45.0X3	T45.0X4	T45.0X5	T45.0X6
Gratiola officinalis	T62.2X1	T62.2X2	T62.2X3	T62.2X4	—	—
Grease	T65.891	T65.892	T65.893	T65.894	—	—
Green hellebore	T62.2X1	T62.2X2	T62.2X3	T62.2X4	—	—
Green soap	T49.2X1	T49.2X2	T49.2X3	T49.2X4	T49.2X5	T49.2X6
Grifulvin	T36.7X1	T36.7X2	T36.7X3	T36.7X4	T36.7X5	T36.7X6
Griseofulvin	T36.7X1	T36.7X2	T36.7X3	T36.7X4	T36.7X5	T36.7X6
Growth hormone	T38.811	T38.812	T38.813	T38.814	T38.815	T38.816
Guaiacol derivatives	T48.4X1	T48.4X2	T48.4X3	T48.4X4	T48.4X5	T48.4X6
Guaiac reagent	T50.991	T50.992	T50.993	T50.994	T50.995	T50.996
Guaifenesin	T48.4X1	T48.4X2	T48.4X3	T48.4X4	T48.4X5	T48.4X6
Guaimesal	T48.4X1	T48.4X2	T48.4X3	T48.4X4	T48.4X5	T48.4X6
Guaiphenesin	T48.4X1	T48.4X2	T48.4X3	T48.4X4	T48.4X5	T48.4X6
Guamecycline	T36.4X1	T36.4X2	T36.4X3	T36.4X4	T36.4X5	T36.4X6
Guanabenz	T46.5X1	T46.5X2	T46.5X3	T46.5X4	T46.5X5	T46.5X6
Guanacline	T46.5X1	T46.5X2	T46.5X3	T46.5X4	T46.5X5	T46.5X6
Guanadrel	T46.5X1	T46.5X2	T46.5X3	T46.5X4	T46.5X5	T46.5X6
Guanatol	T37.2X1	T37.2X2	T37.2X3	T37.2X4	T37.2X5	T37.2X6
Guanethidine	T46.5X1	T46.5X2	T46.5X3	T46.5X4	T46.5X5	T46.5X6
Guanfacine	T46.5X1	T46.5X2	T46.5X3	T46.5X4	T46.5X5	T46.5X6
Guano	T65.891	T65.892	T65.893	T65.894	—	—
Guanochlor	T46.5X1	T46.5X2	T46.5X3	T46.5X4	T46.5X5	T46.5X6
Guanoclor	T46.5X1	T46.5X2	T46.5X3	T46.5X4	T46.5X5	T46.5X6
Guanoctine	T46.5X1	T46.5X2	T46.5X3	T46.5X4	T46.5X5	T46.5X6
Guanoxabenz	T46.5X1	T46.5X2	T46.5X3	T46.5X4	T46.5X5	T46.5X6
Guanoxan	T46.5X1	T46.5X2	T46.5X3	T46.5X4	T46.5X5	T46.5X6
Guar gum (medicinal)	T46.6X1	T46.6X2	T46.6X3	T46.6X4	T46.6X5	T46.6X6
Guaymycin	T36.7X1	T36.7X2	T36.7X3	T36.7X4	T36.7X5	T36.7X6
Hair						
dye	T49.4X1	T49.4X2	T49.4X3	T49.4X4	T49.4X5	T49.4X6
preparation NEC	T49.4X1	T49.4X2	T49.4X3	T49.4X4	T49.4X5	T49.4X6
Halazepam	T42.4X1	T42.4X2	T42.4X3	T42.4X4	T42.4X5	T42.4X6
Halcinolone	T49.0X1	T49.0X2	T49.0X3	T49.0X4	T49.0X5	T49.0X6
Halcinonide	T49.0X1	T49.0X2	T49.0X3	T49.0X4	T49.0X5	T49.0X6
Halethazole	T49.0X1	T49.0X2	T49.0X3	T49.0X4	T49.0X5	T49.0X6
Hallucinogen NOS	T40.901	T40.902	T40.903	T40.904	T40.905	T40.906
specified NEC	T40.991	T40.992	T40.993	T40.994	T40.995	T40.996
Halofantrine	T37.2X1	T37.2X2	T37.2X3	T37.2X4	T37.2X5	T37.2X6
Halofenate	T46.6X1	T46.6X2	T46.6X3	T46.6X4	T46.6X5	T46.6X6
Halometasone	T49.0X1	T49.0X2	T49.0X3	T49.0X4	T49.0X5	T49.0X6
Haloperidol	T43.4X1	T43.4X2	T43.4X3	T43.4X4	T43.4X5	T43.4X6
Haloprogin	T49.0X1	T49.0X2	T49.0X3	T49.0X4	T49.0X5	T49.0X6
Halotex	T49.0X1	T49.0X2	T49.0X3	T49.0X4	T49.0X5	T49.0X6
Halothane	T41.0X1	T41.0X2	T41.0X3	T41.0X4	T41.0X5	T41.0X6
Haloxazolam	T42.4X1	T42.4X2	T42.4X3	T42.4X4	T42.4X5	T42.4X6
Halquinols	T49.0X1	T49.0X2	T49.0X3	T49.0X4	T49.0X5	T49.0X6
Hamamelis	T49.2X1	T49.2X2	T49.2X3	T49.2X4	T49.2X5	T49.2X6
Haptendextran	T45.8X1	T45.8X2	T45.8X3	T45.8X4	T45.8X5	T45.8X6
Harmonyl	T46.5X1	T46.5X2	T46.5X3	T46.5X4	T46.5X5	T46.5X6
Hartmann's solution	T50.3X1	T50.3X2	T50.3X3	T50.3X4	T50.3X5	T50.3X6
Hashish	T40.7X1	T40.7X2	T40.7X3	T40.7X4	T40.7X5	T40.7X6
Hawaiian Woodrose seeds	T40.991	T40.992	T40.993	T40.994	—	—
HCB	T60.3X1	T60.3X2	T60.3X3	T60.3X4	—	—
HCH	T53.6X1	T53.6X2	T53.6X3	T53.6X4	—	—
medicinal	T49.0X1	T49.0X2	T49.0X3	T49.0X4	T49.0X5	T49.0X6
HCN	T57.3X1	T57.3X2	T57.3X3	T57.3X4	—	—
Headache cures, drugs, powders NEC	T50.901	T50.902	T50.903	T50.904	T50.905	T50.906
Heavenly Blue (morning glory)	T40.991	T40.992	T40.993	T40.994	—	—
Heavy metal antidote	T45.8X1	T45.8X2	T45.8X3	T45.8X4	T45.8X5	T45.8X6
Hedaquinium	T49.0X1	T49.0X2	T49.0X3	T49.0X4	T49.0X5	T49.0X6
Hedge hyssop	T62.2X1	T62.2X2	T62.2X3	T62.2X4	—	—
Heet	T49.8X1	T49.8X2	T49.8X3	T49.8X4	T49.8X5	T49.8X6
Helenin	T37.4X1	T37.4X2	T37.4X3	T37.4X4	T37.4X5	T37.4X6
Helium (nonmedicinal) NEC	T59.891	T59.892	T59.893	T59.894	—	—
medicinal	T48.991	T48.992	T48.993	T48.994	T48.995	T48.996
Hellebore (black) (green) (white)	T62.2X1	T62.2X2	T62.2X3	T62.2X4	—	—
Hematin	T45.8X1	T45.8X2	T45.8X3	T45.8X4	T45.8X5	T45.8X6

Additional Character May Be Required — Refer to the Tabular List for Character Selection   ▽ Subterms under main terms may continue to next column or page

Substance	Poisoning, Accidental (unintentional)	Poisoning, Intentional Self-harm	Poisoning, Assault	Poisoning, Undetermined	Adverse Effect	Under-dosing
Hematinic preparation	T45.8X1	T45.8X2	T45.8X3	T45.8X4	T45.8X5	T45.8X6
Hematological agent	T45.91	T45.92	T45.93	T45.94	T45.95	T45.96
specified NEC	T45.8X1	T45.8X2	T45.8X3	T45.8X4	T45.8X5	T45.8X6
Hemlock	T62.2X1	T62.2X2	T62.2X3	T62.2X4	—	—
Hemostatic	T45.621	T45.622	T45.623	T45.624	T45.625	T45.626
drug, systemic	T45.621	T45.622	T45.623	T45.624	T45.625	T45.626
Hemostyptic	T49.4X1	T49.4X2	T49.4X3	T49.4X4	T49.4X5	T49.4X6
Henbane	T62.2X1	T62.2X2	T62.2X3	T62.2X4	—	—
Heparin (sodium)	T45.511	T45.512	T45.513	T45.514	T45.515	T45.516
action reverser	T45.7X1	T45.7X2	T45.7X3	T45.7X4	T45.7X5	T45.7X6
Heparin-fraction	T45.511	T45.512	T45.513	T45.514	T45.515	T45.516
Heparinoid (systemic)	T45.511	T45.512	T45.513	T45.514	T45.515	T45.516
Hepatic secretion stimulant	T47.8X1	T47.8X2	T47.8X3	T47.8X4	T47.8X5	T47.8X6
Hepatitis B						
immune globulin	T50.Z11	T50.Z12	T50.Z13	T50.Z14	T50.Z15	T50.Z16
vaccine	T50.B91	T50.B92	T50.B93	T50.B94	T50.B95	T50.B96
Hepronicate	T46.7X1	T46.7X2	T46.7X3	T46.7X4	T46.7X5	T46.7X6
Heptabarb	T42.3X1	T42.3X2	T42.3X3	T42.3X4	T42.3X5	T42.3X6
Heptabarbital	T42.3X1	T42.3X2	T42.3X3	T42.3X4	T42.3X5	T42.3X6
Heptabarbitone	T42.3X1	T42.3X2	T42.3X3	T42.3X4	T42.3X5	T42.3X6
Heptachlor	T60.1X1	T60.1X2	T60.1X3	T60.1X4	—	—
Heptalgin	T40.2X1	T40.2X2	T40.2X3	T40.2X4	T40.2X5	T40.2X6
Heptaminol	T46.3X1	T46.3X2	T46.3X3	T46.3X4	T46.3X5	T46.3X6
Herbicide NEC	T60.3X1	T60.3X2	T60.3X3	T60.3X4	—	—
Heroin	T40.1X1	T40.1X2	T40.1X3	T40.1X4	—	—
Herplex	T49.5X1	T49.5X2	T49.5X3	T49.5X4	T49.5X5	T49.5X6
HES	T45.8X1	T45.8X2	T45.8X3	T45.8X4	T45.8X5	T45.8X6
Hesperidin	T46.991	T46.992	T46.993	T46.994	T46.995	T46.996
Hetacillin	T36.0X1	T36.0X2	T36.0X3	T36.0X4	T36.0X5	T36.0X6
Hetastarch	T45.8X1	T45.8X2	T45.8X3	T45.8X4	T45.8X5	T45.8X6
HETP	T60.0X1	T60.0X2	T60.0X3	T60.0X4	—	—
Hexachlorobenzene (vapor)	T60.3X1	T60.3X2	T60.3X3	T60.3X4	—	—
Hexachlorocyclohexane	T53.6X1	T53.6X2	T53.6X3	T53.6X4	—	—
Hexachlorophene	T49.0X1	T49.0X2	T49.0X3	T49.0X4	T49.0X5	T49.0X6
Hexadiline	T46.3X1	T46.3X2	T46.3X3	T46.3X4	T46.3X5	T46.3X6
Hexadimethrine (bromide)	T45.7X1	T45.7X2	T45.7X3	T45.7X4	T45.7X5	T45.7X6
Hexadylamine	T46.3X1	T46.3X2	T46.3X3	T46.3X4	T46.3X5	T46.3X6
Hexaethyl tetraphosphate	T60.0X1	T60.0X2	T60.0X3	T60.0X4	—	—
Hexafluorenium bromide	T48.1X1	T48.1X2	T48.1X3	T48.1X4	T48.1X5	T48.1X6
Hexafluronium (bromide)	T48.1X1	T48.1X2	T48.1X3	T48.1X4	T48.1X5	T48.1X6
Hexa-germ	T49.2X1	T49.2X2	T49.2X3	T49.2X4	T49.2X5	T49.2X6
Hexahydrobenzol	T52.8X1	T52.8X2	T52.8X3	T52.8X4	—	—
Hexahydrocresol(s)	T51.8X1	T51.8X2	T51.8X3	T51.8X4	—	—
arsenide	T57.0X1	T57.0X2	T57.0X3	T57.0X4	—	—
arseniurated	T57.0X1	T57.0X2	T57.0X3	T57.0X4	—	—
cyanide	T57.3X1	T57.3X2	T57.3X3	T57.3X4	—	—
gas	T59.891	T59.892	T59.893	T59.894	—	—
Fluoride (liquid)	T57.8X1	T57.8X2	T57.8X3	T57.8X4	—	—
vapor	T59.891	T59.892	T59.893	T59.894	—	—
phophorated	T60.0X1	T60.0X2	T60.0X3	T60.0X4	—	—
sulfate	T57.8X1	T57.8X2	T57.8X3	T57.8X4	—	—
sulfide (gas)	T59.6X1	T59.6X2	T59.6X3	T59.6X4	—	—
arseniurated	T57.0X1	T57.0X2	T57.0X3	T57.0X4	—	—
sulfurated	T57.8X1	T57.8X2	T57.8X3	T57.8X4	—	—
Hexahydrophenol	T51.8X1	T51.8X2	T51.8X3	T51.8X4	—	—
Hexalen	T51.8X1	T51.8X2	T51.8X3	T51.8X4	—	—
Hexamethonium bromide	T44.2X1	T44.2X2	T44.2X3	T44.2X4	T44.2X5	T44.2X6
Hexamethylene	T52.8X1	T52.8X2	T52.8X3	T52.8X4	—	—
Hexamethylmelamine	T45.1X1	T45.1X2	T45.1X3	T45.1X4	T45.1X5	T45.1X6
Hexamidine	T49.0X1	T49.0X2	T49.0X3	T49.0X4	T49.0X5	T49.0X6
Hexamine (mandelate)	T37.8X1	T37.8X2	T37.8X3	T37.8X4	T37.8X5	T37.8X6
Hexanone, 2-hexanone	T52.4X1	T52.4X2	T52.4X3	T52.4X4	—	—
Hexanuorenium	T48.1X1	T48.1X2	T48.1X3	T48.1X4	T48.1X5	T48.1X6
Hexapropymate	T42.6X1	T42.6X2	T42.6X3	T42.6X4	T42.6X5	T42.6X6
Hexasonium iodide	T44.3X1	T44.3X2	T44.3X3	T44.3X4	T44.3X5	T44.3X6
Hexcarbacholine bromide	T48.1X1	T48.1X2	T48.1X3	T48.1X4	T48.1X5	T48.1X6
Hexemal	T42.3X1	T42.3X2	T42.3X3	T42.3X4	T42.3X5	T42.3X6
Hexestrol	T38.5X1	T38.5X2	T38.5X3	T38.5X4	T38.5X5	T38.5X6
Hexethal (sodium)	T42.3X1	T42.3X2	T42.3X3	T42.3X4	T42.3X5	T42.3X6
Hexetidine	T37.8X1	T37.8X2	T37.8X3	T37.8X4	T37.8X5	T37.8X6
Hexobarbital	T42.3X1	T42.3X2	T42.3X3	T42.3X4	T42.3X5	T42.3X6
rectal	T41.291	T41.292	T41.293	T41.294	T41.295	T41.296
sodium	T41.1X1	T41.1X2	T41.1X3	T41.1X4	T41.1X5	T41.1X6
Hexobendine	T46.3X1	T46.3X2	T46.3X3	T46.3X4	T46.3X5	T46.3X6
Hexocyclium	T44.3X1	T44.3X2	T44.3X3	T44.3X4	T44.3X5	T44.3X6
metilsulfate	T44.3X1	T44.3X2	T44.3X3	T44.3X4	T44.3X5	T44.3X6
Hexoestrol	T38.5X1	T38.5X2	T38.5X3	T38.5X4	T38.5X5	T38.5X6
Hexone	T52.4X1	T52.4X2	T52.4X3	T52.4X4	—	—
Hexoprenaline	T48.6X1	T48.6X2	T48.6X3	T48.6X4	T48.6X5	T48.6X6
Hexylcaine	T41.3X1	T41.3X2	T41.3X3	T41.3X4	T41.3X5	T41.3X6
Hexylresorcinol	T52.2X1	T52.2X2	T52.2X3	T52.2X4	—	—
HGH (human growth hormone)	T38.811	T38.812	T38.813	T38.814	T38.815	T38.816
Hinkle's pills	T47.2X1	T47.2X2	T47.2X3	T47.2X4	T47.2X5	T47.2X6
Histalog	T50.8X1	T50.8X2	T50.8X3	T50.8X4	T50.8X5	T50.8X6
Histamine (phosphate)	T50.8X1	T50.8X2	T50.8X3	T50.8X4	T50.8X5	T50.8X6
Histoplasmin	T50.8X1	T50.8X2	T50.8X3	T50.8X4	T50.8X5	T50.8X6
Holly berries	T62.2X1	T62.2X2	T62.2X3	T62.2X4	—	—
Homatropine	T44.3X1	T44.3X2	T44.3X3	T44.3X4	T44.3X5	T44.3X6
methylbromide	T44.3X1	T44.3X2	T44.3X3	T44.3X4	T44.3X5	T44.3X6
Homochlorcyclizine	T45.0X1	T45.0X2	T45.0X3	T45.0X4	T45.0X5	T45.0X6
Homosalate	T49.3X1	T49.3X2	T49.3X3	T49.3X4	T49.3X5	T49.3X6
Homo-tet	T50.Z11	T50.Z12	T50.Z13	T50.Z14	T50.Z15	T50.Z16
Hormone	T38.801	T38.802	T38.803	T38.804	T38.805	T38.806
adrenal cortical steroids	T38.0X1	T38.0X2	T38.0X3	T38.0X4	T38.0X5	T38.0X6
androgenic	T38.7X1	T38.7X2	T38.7X3	T38.7X4	T38.7X5	T38.7X6
anterior pituitary NEC	T38.811	T38.812	T38.813	T38.814	T38.815	T38.816
antidiabetic agents	T38.3X1	T38.3X2	T38.3X3	T38.3X4	T38.3X5	T38.3X6
antidiuretic	T38.891	T38.892	T38.893	T38.894	T38.895	T38.896
cancer therapy	T45.1X1	T45.1X2	T45.1X3	T45.1X4	T45.1X5	T45.1X6
follicle stimulating	T38.811	T38.812	T38.813	T38.814	T38.815	T38.816
gonadotropic	T38.891	T38.892	T38.893	T38.894	T38.895	T38.896
pituitary	T38.811	T38.812	T38.813	T38.814	T38.815	T38.816
growth	T38.811	T38.812	T38.813	T38.814	T38.815	T38.816
luteinizing	T38.811	T38.812	T38.813	T38.814	T38.815	T38.816
ovarian	T38.5X1	T38.5X2	T38.5X3	T38.5X4	T38.5X5	T38.5X6
oxytocic	T48.0X1	T48.0X2	T48.0X3	T48.0X4	T48.0X5	T48.0X6
parathyroid (derivatives)	T50.991	T50.992	T50.993	T50.994	T50.995	T50.996
pituitary (posterior) NEC	T38.891	T38.892	T38.893	T38.894	T38.895	T38.896
anterior	T38.811	T38.812	T38.813	T38.814	T38.815	T38.816
specified, NEC	T38.891	T38.892	T38.893	T38.894	T38.895	T38.896
thyroid	T38.1X1	T38.1X2	T38.1X3	T38.1X4	T38.1X5	T38.1X6
Hornet (sting)	T63.451	T63.452	T63.453	T63.454	—	—
Horse anti-human lymphocytic serum	T50.Z11	T50.Z12	T50.Z13	T50.Z14	T50.Z15	T50.Z16
Horticulture agent NEC	T65.91	T65.92	T65.93	T65.94	—	—
with pesticide	T60.91	T60.92	T60.93	T60.94	—	—
Human						
albumin	T45.8X1	T45.8X2	T45.8X3	T45.8X4	T45.8X5	T45.8X6
growth hormone (HGH)	T38.811	T38.812	T38.813	T38.814	T38.815	T38.816
immune serum	T50.Z11	T50.Z12	T50.Z13	T50.Z14	T50.Z15	T50.Z16
Hyaluronidase	T45.3X1	T45.3X2	T45.3X3	T45.3X4	T45.3X5	T45.3X6
Hyazyme	T45.3X1	T45.3X2	T45.3X3	T45.3X4	T45.3X5	T45.3X6
Hycodan	T40.2X1	T40.2X2	T40.2X3	T40.2X4	T40.2X5	T40.2X6
Hydantoin derivative NEC	T42.0X1	T42.0X2	T42.0X3	T42.0X4	T42.0X5	T42.0X6
Hydeltra	T38.0X1	T38.0X2	T38.0X3	T38.0X4	T38.0X5	T38.0X6
Hydergine	T44.6X1	T44.6X2	T44.6X3	T44.6X4	T44.6X5	T44.6X6
Hydrabamine penicillin	T36.0X1	T36.0X2	T36.0X3	T36.0X4	T36.0X5	T36.0X6
Hydralazine	T46.5X1	T46.5X2	T46.5X3	T46.5X4	T46.5X5	T46.5X6
Hydrargaphen	T49.0X1	T49.0X2	T49.0X3	T49.0X4	T49.0X5	T49.0X6
Hydrargyri aminochloridum	T49.0X1	T49.0X2	T49.0X3	T49.0X4	T49.0X5	T49.0X6
Hydrastine	T48.291	T48.292	T48.293	T48.294	T48.295	T48.296
Hydrazine	T54.1X1	T54.1X2	T54.1X3	T54.1X4	—	—
monoamine oxidase inhibitors	T43.1X1	T43.1X2	T43.1X3	T43.1X4	T43.1X5	T43.1X6
Hydrazoic acid, azides	T54.2X1	T54.2X2	T54.2X3	T54.2X4	—	—
Hydriodic acid	T48.4X1	T48.4X2	T48.4X3	T48.4X4	T48.4X5	T48.4X6
Hydrocarbon gas	T59.891	T59.892	T59.893	T59.894	—	—
incomplete combustion of — see Carbon, monoxide, fuel, utility						
liquefied (mobile container)	T59.891	T59.892	T59.893	T59.894	—	—
piped (natural)	T59.891	T59.892	T59.893	T59.894	—	—
Hydrochloric acid (liquid)	T54.2X1	T54.2X2	T54.2X3	T54.2X4	—	—
medicinal (digestant)	T47.5X1	T47.5X2	T47.5X3	T47.5X4	T47.5X5	T47.5X6
vapor	T59.891	T59.892	T59.893	T59.894	—	—
Hydrochlorothiazide	T50.2X1	T50.2X2	T50.2X3	T50.2X4	T50.2X5	T50.2X6
Hydrocodone	T40.2X1	T40.2X2	T40.2X3	T40.2X4	T40.2X5	T40.2X6
Hydrocortisone (derivatives)	T38.0X1	T38.0X2	T38.0X3	T38.0X4	T38.0X5	T38.0X6
aceponate	T49.0X1	T49.0X2	T49.0X3	T49.0X4	T49.0X5	T49.0X6
ENT agent	T49.6X1	T49.6X2	T49.6X3	T49.6X4	T49.6X5	T49.6X6
ophthalmic preparation	T49.5X1	T49.5X2	T49.5X3	T49.5X4	T49.5X5	T49.5X6
topical NEC	T49.0X1	T49.0X2	T49.0X3	T49.0X4	T49.0X5	T49.0X6
Hydrocortone	T38.0X1	T38.0X2	T38.0X3	T38.0X4	T38.0X5	T38.0X6
ENT agent	T49.6X1	T49.6X2	T49.6X3	T49.6X4	T49.6X5	T49.6X6
ophthalmic preparation	T49.5X1	T49.5X2	T49.5X3	T49.5X4	T49.5X5	T49.5X6
topical NEC	T49.0X1	T49.0X2	T49.0X3	T49.0X4	T49.0X5	T49.0X6
Hydrocyanic acid (liquid)	T57.3X1	T57.3X2	T57.3X3	T57.3X4	—	—
gas	T65.0X1	T65.0X2	T65.0X3	T65.0X4	—	—
Hydroflumethiazide	T50.2X1	T50.2X2	T50.2X3	T50.2X4	T50.2X5	T50.2X6
Hydrofluoric acid (liquid)	T54.2X1	T54.2X2	T54.2X3	T54.2X4	—	—

⚕ Subterms under main terms may continue to next column or page   Additional Character May Be Required — Refer to the Tabular List for Character Selection   377

Hematinic preparation — Hydrofluoric acid

Table of Drugs and Chemicals

Hydrofluoric acid — Insulin

Substance	Poisoning, Accidental (unintentional)	Poisoning, Intentional Self-harm	Poisoning, Assault	Poisoning, Undetermined	Adverse Effect	Under-dosing
Hydrofluoric acid — *continued*						
vapor	T59.891	T59.892	T59.893	T59.894	—	—
Hydrogen	T59.891	T59.892	T59.893	T59.894	—	—
arsenide	T57.0X1	T57.0X2	T57.0X3	T57.0X4	—	—
arseniureted	T57.0X1	T57.0X2	T57.0X3	T57.0X4	—	—
chloride	T57.8X1	T57.8X2	T57.8X3	T57.8X4	—	—
cyanide (salts)	T57.3X1	T57.3X2	T57.3X3	T57.3X4	—	—
gas	T57.3X1	T57.3X2	T57.3X3	T57.3X4	—	—
Fluoride	T59.5X1	T59.5X2	T59.5X3	T59.5X4	—	—
vapor	T59.5X1	T59.5X2	T59.5X3	T59.5X4	—	—
peroxide	T49.0X1	T49.0X2	T49.0X3	T49.0X4	T49.0X5	T49.0X6
phosphureted	T57.1X1	T57.1X2	T57.1X3	T57.1X4	—	—
sulfide	T59.6X1	T59.6X2	T59.6X3	T59.6X4	—	—
arseniureted	T57.0X1	T57.0X2	T57.0X3	T57.0X4	—	—
sulfureted	T59.6X1	T59.6X2	T59.6X3	T59.6X4	—	—
Hydromethylpyridine	T46.7X1	T46.7X2	T46.7X3	T46.7X4	T46.7X5	T46.7X6
Hydromorphinol	T40.2X1	T40.2X2	T40.2X3	T40.2X4	—	—
Hydromorphinone	T40.2X1	T40.2X2	T40.2X3	T40.2X4	T40.2X5	T40.2X6
Hydromorphone	T40.2X1	T40.2X2	T40.2X3	T40.2X4	T40.2X5	T40.2X6
Hydromox	T50.2X1	T50.2X2	T50.2X3	T50.2X4	T50.2X5	T50.2X6
Hydrophilic lotion	T49.3X1	T49.3X2	T49.3X3	T49.3X4	T49.3X5	T49.3X6
Hydroquinidine	T46.2X1	T46.2X2	T46.2X3	T46.2X4	T46.2X5	T46.2X6
Hydroquinone	T52.2X1	T52.2X2	T52.2X3	T52.2X4	—	—
vapor	T59.891	T59.892	T59.893	T59.894	—	—
Hydrosulfuric acid (gas)	T59.6X1	T59.6X2	T59.6X3	T59.6X4	—	—
Hydrotalcite	T47.1X1	T47.1X2	T47.1X3	T47.1X4	T47.1X5	T47.1X6
Hydrous wool fat	T49.3X1	T49.3X2	T49.3X3	T49.3X4	T49.3X5	T49.3X6
Hydroxide, caustic	T54.3X1	T54.3X2	T54.3X3	T54.3X4	—	—
Hydroxocobalamin	T45.8X1	T45.8X2	T45.8X3	T45.8X4	T45.8X5	T45.8X6
Hydroxyamphetamine	T49.5X1	T49.5X2	T49.5X3	T49.5X4	T49.5X5	T49.5X6
Hydroxycarbamide	T45.1X1	T45.1X2	T45.1X3	T45.1X4	T45.1X5	T45.1X6
Hydroxychloroquine	T37.8X1	T37.8X2	T37.8X3	T37.8X4	T37.8X5	T37.8X6
Hydroxydihydrocodeinone	T40.2X1	T40.2X2	T40.2X3	T40.2X4	T40.2X5	T40.2X6
Hydroxyestrone	T38.5X1	T38.5X2	T38.5X3	T38.5X4	T38.5X5	T38.5X6
Hydroxyethyl starch	T45.8X1	T45.8X2	T45.8X3	T45.8X4	T45.8X5	T45.8X6
Hydroxymethylpentanone	T52.4X1	T52.4X2	T52.4X3	T52.4X4	—	—
Hydroxyphenamate	T43.591	T43.592	T43.593	T43.594	T43.595	T43.596
Hydroxyphenylbutazone	T39.2X1	T39.2X2	T39.2X3	T39.2X4	T39.2X5	T39.2X6
Hydroxyprogesterone	T38.5X1	T38.5X2	T38.5X3	T38.5X4	T38.5X5	T38.5X6
caproate	T38.5X1	T38.5X2	T38.5X3	T38.5X4	T38.5X5	T38.5X6
Hydroxyquinoline (derivatives) NEC	T37.8X1	T37.8X2	T37.8X3	T37.8X4	T37.8X5	T37.8X6
Hydroxystilbamidine	T37.3X1	T37.3X2	T37.3X3	T37.3X4	T37.3X5	T37.3X6
Hydroxytoluene (nonmedicinal)	T54.0X1	T54.0X2	T54.0X3	T54.0X4	—	—
medicinal	T49.0X1	T49.0X2	T49.0X3	T49.0X4	T49.0X5	T49.0X6
Hydroxyurea	T45.1X1	T45.1X2	T45.1X3	T45.1X4	T45.1X5	T45.1X6
Hydroxyzine	T43.591	T43.592	T43.593	T43.594	T43.595	T43.596
Hyoscine	T44.3X1	T44.3X2	T44.3X3	T44.3X4	T44.3X5	T44.3X6
Hyoscyamine	T44.3X1	T44.3X2	T44.3X3	T44.3X4	T44.3X5	T44.3X6
Hyoscyamus	T44.3X1	T44.3X2	T44.3X3	T44.3X4	T44.3X5	T44.3X6
dry extract	T44.3X1	T44.3X2	T44.3X3	T44.3X4	T44.3X5	T44.3X6
Hypaque	T50.8X1	T50.8X2	T50.8X3	T50.8X4	T50.8X5	T50.8X6
Hypertussis	T50.Z11	T50.Z12	T50.Z13	T50.Z14	T50.Z15	T50.Z16
Hypnotic	T42.71	T42.72	T42.73	T42.74	T42.75	T42.76
anticonvulsant	T42.71	T42.72	T42.73	T42.74	T42.75	T42.76
specified NEC	T42.6X1	T42.6X2	T42.6X3	T42.6X4	T42.6X5	T42.6X6
Hypochlorite	T49.0X1	T49.0X2	T49.0X3	T49.0X4	T49.0X5	T49.0X6
Hypophysis, posterior	T38.891	T38.892	T38.893	T38.894	T38.895	T38.896
Hypotensive NEC	T46.5X1	T46.5X2	T46.5X3	T46.5X4	T46.5X5	T46.5X6
Hypromellose	T49.5X1	T49.5X2	T49.5X3	T49.5X4	T49.5X5	T49.5X6
Ibacitabine	T37.5X1	T37.5X2	T37.5X3	T37.5X4	T37.5X5	T37.5X6
Ibopamine	T44.991	T44.992	T44.993	T44.994	T44.995	T44.996
Ibufenac	T39.311	T39.312	T39.313	T39.314	T39.315	T39.316
Ibuprofen	T39.311	T39.312	T39.313	T39.314	T39.315	T39.316
Ibuproxam	T39.311	T39.312	T39.313	T39.314	T39.315	T39.316
Ibuterol	T48.6X1	T48.6X2	T48.6X3	T48.6X4	T48.6X5	T48.6X6
Ichthammol	T49.0X1	T49.0X2	T49.0X3	T49.0X4	T49.0X5	T49.0X6
Ichthyol	T49.4X1	T49.4X2	T49.4X3	T49.4X4	T49.4X5	T49.4X6
Idarubicin	T45.1X1	T45.1X2	T45.1X3	T45.1X4	T45.1X5	T45.1X6
Idrocilamide	T42.8X1	T42.8X2	T42.8X3	T42.8X4	T42.8X5	T42.8X6
Ifenprodil	T46.7X1	T46.7X2	T46.7X3	T46.7X4	T46.7X5	T46.7X6
Ifosfamide	T45.1X1	T45.1X2	T45.1X3	T45.1X4	T45.1X5	T45.1X6
Iletin	T38.3X1	T38.3X2	T38.3X3	T38.3X4	T38.3X5	T38.3X6
Ilex	T62.2X1	T62.2X2	T62.2X3	T62.2X4	—	—
Illuminating gas (after combustion)	T58.11	T58.12	T58.13	T58.14	—	—
prior to combustion	T59.891	T59.892	T59.893	T59.894	—	—
Ilopan	T45.2X1	T45.2X2	T45.2X3	T45.2X4	T45.2X5	T45.2X6
Iloprost	T46.7X1	T46.7X2	T46.7X3	T46.7X4	T46.7X5	T46.7X6
Ilotycin	T36.3X1	T36.3X2	T36.3X3	T36.3X4	T36.3X5	T36.3X6
ophthalmic preparation	T49.5X1	T49.5X2	T49.5X3	T49.5X4	T49.5X5	T49.5X6
topical NEC	T49.0X1	T49.0X2	T49.0X3	T49.0X4	T49.0X5	T49.0X6

Substance	Poisoning, Accidental (unintentional)	Poisoning, Intentional Self-harm	Poisoning, Assault	Poisoning, Undetermined	Adverse Effect	Under-dosing
Imidazole-4-carboxamide	T45.1X1	T45.1X2	T45.1X3	T45.1X4	T45.1X5	T45.1X6
Iminostilbene	T42.1X1	T42.1X2	T42.1X3	T42.1X4	T42.1X5	T42.1X6
Imipenem	T36.0X1	T36.0X2	T36.0X3	T36.0X4	T36.0X5	T36.0X6
Imipramine	T43.011	T43.012	T43.013	T43.014	T43.015	T43.016
Immu-G	T50.Z11	T50.Z12	T50.Z13	T50.Z14	T50.Z15	T50.Z16
Immuglobin	T50.Z11	T50.Z12	T50.Z13	T50.Z14	T50.Z15	T50.Z16
Immune						
globulin	T50.Z11	T50.Z12	T50.Z13	T50.Z14	T50.Z15	T50.Z16
serum globulin	T50.Z11	T50.Z12	T50.Z13	T50.Z14	T50.Z15	T50.Z16
Immunoglobin human (intravenous) (normal)	T50.Z11	T50.Z12	T50.Z13	T50.Z14	T50.Z15	T50.Z16
unmodified	T50.Z11	T50.Z12	T50.Z13	T50.Z14	T50.Z15	T50.Z16
Immunosuppressive drug	T45.1X1	T45.1X2	T45.1X3	T45.1X4	T45.1X5	T45.1X6
Immu-tetanus	T50.Z11	T50.Z12	T50.Z13	T50.Z14	T50.Z15	T50.Z16
Indalpine	T43.221	T43.222	T43.223	T43.224	T43.225	T43.226
Indanazoline	T48.5X1	T48.5X2	T48.5X3	T48.5X4	T48.5X5	T48.5X6
Indandione (derivatives)	T45.511	T45.512	T45.513	T45.514	T45.515	T45.516
Indapamide	T46.5X1	T46.5X2	T46.5X3	T46.5X4	T46.5X5	T46.5X6
Indendione (derivatives)	T45.511	T45.512	T45.513	T45.514	T45.515	T45.516
Indenolol	T44.7X1	T44.7X2	T44.7X3	T44.7X4	T44.7X5	T44.7X6
Inderal	T44.7X1	T44.7X2	T44.7X3	T44.7X4	T44.7X5	T44.7X6
Indian						
hemp	T40.7X1	T40.7X2	T40.7X3	T40.7X4	T40.7X5	T40.7X6
tobacco	T62.2X1	T62.2X2	T62.2X3	T62.2X4	—	—
Indigo carmine	T50.8X1	T50.8X2	T50.8X3	T50.8X4	T50.8X5	T50.8X6
Indobufen	T45.521	T45.522	T45.523	T45.524	T45.525	T45.526
Indocin	T39.2X1	T39.2X2	T39.2X3	T39.2X4	T39.2X5	T39.2X6
Indocyanine green	T50.8X1	T50.8X2	T50.8X3	T50.8X4	T50.8X5	T50.8X6
Indometacin	T39.391	T39.392	T39.393	T39.394	T39.395	T39.396
Indomethacin	T39.391	T39.392	T39.393	T39.394	T39.395	T39.396
farnesil	T39.4X1	T39.4X2	T39.4X3	T39.4X4	T39.4X5	T39.4X6
Indoramin	T44.6X1	T44.6X2	T44.6X3	T44.6X4	T44.6X5	T44.6X6
Industrial						
alcohol	T51.0X1	T51.0X2	T51.0X3	T51.0X4	—	—
fumes	T59.891	T59.892	T59.893	T59.894	—	—
solvents (fumes) (vapors)	T52.91	T52.92	T52.93	T52.94	—	—
Influenza vaccine	T50.B91	T50.B92	T50.B93	T50.B94	T50.B95	T50.B96
Ingested substance NEC	T65.91	T65.92	T65.93	T65.94	—	—
INH	T37.1X1	T37.1X2	T37.1X3	T37.1X4	T37.1X5	T37.1X6
Inhalation, gas (noxious) — *see* Gas						
Inhibitor						
angiotensin-converting enzyme	T46.4X1	T46.4X2	T46.4X3	T46.4X4	T46.4X5	T46.4X6
carbonic anhydrase	T50.2X1	T50.2X2	T50.2X3	T50.2X4	T50.2X5	T50.2X6
fibrinolysis	T45.621	T45.622	T45.623	T45.624	T45.625	T45.626
monoamine oxidase NEC	T43.1X1	T43.1X2	T43.1X3	T43.1X4	T43.1X5	T43.1X6
hydrazine	T43.1X1	T43.1X2	T43.1X3	T43.1X4	T43.1X5	T43.1X6
postsynaptic	T43.8X1	T43.8X2	T43.8X3	T43.8X4	T43.8X5	T43.8X6
prothrombin synthesis	T45.511	T45.512	T45.513	T45.514	T45.515	T45.516
Ink	T65.891	T65.892	T65.893	T65.894	—	—
Inorganic substance NEC	T57.91	T57.92	T57.93	T57.94	—	—
Inosine pranobex	T37.5X1	T37.5X2	T37.5X3	T37.5X4	T37.5X5	T37.5X6
Inositol	T50.991	T50.992	T50.993	T50.994	T50.995	T50.996
nicotinate	T46.7X1	T46.7X2	T46.7X3	T46.7X4	T46.7X5	T46.7X6
Inproquone	T45.1X1	T45.1X2	T45.1X3	T45.1X4	T45.1X5	T45.1X6
Insecticide NEC	T60.91	T60.92	T60.93	T60.94	—	—
carbamate	T60.0X1	T60.0X2	T60.0X3	T60.0X4	—	—
chlorinated	T60.1X1	T60.1X2	T60.1X3	T60.1X4	—	—
mixed	T60.91	T60.92	T60.93	T60.94	—	—
organochlorine	T60.1X1	T60.1X2	T60.1X3	T60.1X4	—	—
organophosphorus	T60.0X1	T60.0X2	T60.0X3	T60.0X4	—	—
Insect (sting), venomous	T63.481	T63.482	T63.483	T63.484	—	—
ant	T63.421	T63.422	T63.423	T63.424	—	—
bee	T63.441	T63.442	T63.443	T63.444	—	—
caterpillar	T63.431	T63.432	T63.433	T63.434	—	—
hornet	T63.451	T63.452	T63.453	T63.454	—	—
wasp	T63.461	T63.462	T63.463	T63.464	—	—
Insular tissue extract	T38.3X1	T38.3X2	T38.3X3	T38.3X4	T38.3X5	T38.3X6
Insulin (amorphous) (globin) (isophane) (Lente) (NPH) (Semilente) (Ultralente)	T38.3X1	T38.3X2	T38.3X3	T38.3X4	T38.3X5	T38.3X6
defalan	T38.3X1	T38.3X2	T38.3X3	T38.3X4	T38.3X5	T38.3X6
human	T38.3X1	T38.3X2	T38.3X3	T38.3X4	T38.3X5	T38.3X6
injection, soluble	T38.3X1	T38.3X2	T38.3X3	T38.3X4	T38.3X5	T38.3X6
biphasic	T38.3X1	T38.3X2	T38.3X3	T38.3X4	T38.3X5	T38.3X6
intermediate acting	T38.3X1	T38.3X2	T38.3X3	T38.3X4	T38.3X5	T38.3X6
protamine zinc	T38.3X1	T38.3X2	T38.3X3	T38.3X4	T38.3X5	T38.3X6
slow acting	T38.3X1	T38.3X2	T38.3X3	T38.3X4	T38.3X5	T38.3X6
zinc						
protamine injection	T38.3X1	T38.3X2	T38.3X3	T38.3X4	T38.3X5	T38.3X6
suspension (amorphous) (crystalline)	T38.3X1	T38.3X2	T38.3X3	T38.3X4	T38.3X5	T38.3X6

Additional Character May Be Required — Refer to the Tabular List for Character Selection ▼ Subterms under main terms may continue to next column or page

Substance	Poisoning, Accidental (unintentional)	Poisoning, Intentional Self-harm	Poisoning, Assault	Poisoning, Undetermined	Adverse Effect	Under-dosing
Interferon (alpha) (beta) (gamma)	T37.5X1	T37.5X2	T37.5X3	T37.5X4	T37.5X5	T37.5X6
Intestinal motility control drug	T47.6X1	T47.6X2	T47.6X3	T47.6X4	T47.6X5	T47.6X6
biological	T47.8X1	T47.8X2	T47.8X3	T47.8X4	T47.8X5	T47.8X6
Intranarcon	T41.1X1	T41.1X2	T41.1X3	T41.1X4	T41.1X5	T41.1X6
Intravenous						
amino acids	T50.991	T50.992	T50.993	T50.994	T50.995	T50.996
fat suspension	T50.991	T50.992	T50.993	T50.994	T50.995	T50.996
Inulin	T50.8X1	T50.8X2	T50.8X3	T50.8X4	T50.8X5	T50.8X6
Invert sugar	T50.3X1	T50.3X2	T50.3X3	T50.3X4	T50.3X5	T50.3X6
Inza — see Naproxen						
Iobenzamic acid	T50.8X1	T50.8X2	T50.8X3	T50.8X4	T50.8X5	T50.8X6
Iocarmic acid	T50.8X1	T50.8X2	T50.8X3	T50.8X4	T50.8X5	T50.8X6
Iocetamic acid	T50.8X1	T50.8X2	T50.8X3	T50.8X4	T50.8X5	T50.8X6
Iodamide	T50.8X1	T50.8X2	T50.8X3	T50.8X4	T50.8X5	T50.8X6
Iodide NEC — see also	T49.0X1	T49.0X2	T49.0X3	T49.0X4	T49.0X5	T49.0X6
Iodine						
mercury (ointment)	T49.0X1	T49.0X2	T49.0X3	T49.0X4	T49.0X5	T49.0X6
methylate	T49.0X1	T49.0X2	T49.0X3	T49.0X4	T49.0X5	T49.0X6
potassium (expectorant) NEC	T48.4X1	T48.4X2	T48.4X3	T48.4X4	T48.4X5	T48.4X6
Iodinated						
contrast medium	T50.8X1	T50.8X2	T50.8X3	T50.8X4	T50.8X5	T50.8X6
glycerol	T48.4X1	T48.4X2	T48.4X3	T48.4X4	T48.4X5	T48.4X6
human serum albumin (131I)	T50.8X1	T50.8X2	T50.8X3	T50.8X4	T50.8X5	T50.8X6
Iodine (antiseptic, external) (tincture) NEC	T49.0X1	T49.0X2	T49.0X3	T49.0X4	T49.0X5	T49.0X6
125 — see also Radiation sickness, and Exposure to radioactive isotopes						
therapeutic	T50.991	T50.992	T50.993	T50.994	T50.995	T50.996
131 — see also Radiation sickness, and Exposure to radioactive isotopes	T50.8X1	T50.8X2	T50.8X3	T50.8X4	T50.8X5	T50.8X6
therapeutic	T38.2X1	T38.2X2	T38.2X3	T38.2X4	T38.2X5	T38.2X6
diagnostic	T50.8X1	T50.8X2	T50.8X3	T50.8X4	T50.8X5	T50.8X6
for thyroid conditions (antithyroid)	T38.2X1	T38.2X2	T38.2X3	T38.2X4	T38.2X5	T38.2X6
solution	T49.0X1	T49.0X2	T49.0X3	T49.0X4	T49.0X5	T49.0X6
vapor	T59.891	T59.892	T59.893	T59.894	—	—
Iodipamide	T50.8X1	T50.8X2	T50.8X3	T50.8X4	T50.8X5	T50.8X6
Iodized (poppy seed) oil	T50.8X1	T50.8X2	T50.8X3	T50.8X4	T50.8X5	T50.8X6
Iodobismitol	T37.8X1	T37.8X2	T37.8X3	T37.8X4	T37.8X5	T37.8X6
Iodochlorhydroxyquin	T37.8X1	T37.8X2	T37.8X3	T37.8X4	T37.8X5	T37.8X6
topical	T49.0X1	T49.0X2	T49.0X3	T49.0X4	T49.0X5	T49.0X6
Iodochlorhydroxyquinoline	T37.8X1	T37.8X2	T37.8X3	T37.8X4	T37.8X5	T37.8X6
Iodocholesterol (131I)	T50.8X1	T50.8X2	T50.8X3	T50.8X4	T50.8X5	T50.8X6
Iodoform	T49.0X1	T49.0X2	T49.0X3	T49.0X4	T49.0X5	T49.0X6
Iodohippuric acid	T50.8X1	T50.8X2	T50.8X3	T50.8X4	T50.8X5	T50.8X6
Iodopanoic acid	T50.8X1	T50.8X2	T50.8X3	T50.8X4	T50.8X5	T50.8X6
Iodophthalein (sodium)	T50.8X1	T50.8X2	T50.8X3	T50.8X4	T50.8X5	T50.8X6
Iodopyracet	T50.8X1	T50.8X2	T50.8X3	T50.8X4	T50.8X5	T50.8X6
Iodoquinol	T37.8X1	T37.8X2	T37.8X3	T37.8X4	T37.8X5	T37.8X6
Iodoxamic acid	T50.8X1	T50.8X2	T50.8X3	T50.8X4	T50.8X5	T50.8X6
Iofendylate	T50.8X1	T50.8X2	T50.8X3	T50.8X4	T50.8X5	T50.8X6
Ioglycamic acid	T50.8X1	T50.8X2	T50.8X3	T50.8X4	T50.8X5	T50.8X6
Iohexol	T50.8X1	T50.8X2	T50.8X3	T50.8X4	T50.8X5	T50.8X6
Ion exchange resin						
anion	T47.8X1	T47.8X2	T47.8X3	T47.8X4	T47.8X5	T47.8X6
cation	T50.3X1	T50.3X2	T50.3X3	T50.3X4	T50.3X5	T50.3X6
cholestyramine	T46.6X1	T46.6X2	T46.6X3	T46.6X4	T46.6X5	T46.6X6
intestinal	T47.8X1	T47.8X2	T47.8X3	T47.8X4	T47.8X5	T47.8X6
Iopamidol	T50.8X1	T50.8X2	T50.8X3	T50.8X4	T50.8X5	T50.8X6
Iopanoic acid	T50.8X1	T50.8X2	T50.8X3	T50.8X4	T50.8X5	T50.8X6
Iophenoic acid	T50.8X1	T50.8X2	T50.8X3	T50.8X4	T50.8X5	T50.8X6
Iopodate, sodium	T50.8X1	T50.8X2	T50.8X3	T50.8X4	T50.8X5	T50.8X6
Iopodic acid	T50.8X1	T50.8X2	T50.8X3	T50.8X4	T50.8X5	T50.8X6
Iopromide	T50.8X1	T50.8X2	T50.8X3	T50.8X4	T50.8X5	T50.8X6
Iopydol	T50.8X1	T50.8X2	T50.8X3	T50.8X4	T50.8X5	T50.8X6
Iotalamic acid	T50.8X1	T50.8X2	T50.8X3	T50.8X4	T50.8X5	T50.8X6
Iothalamate	T50.8X1	T50.8X2	T50.8X3	T50.8X4	T50.8X5	T50.8X6
Iothiouracil	T38.2X1	T38.2X2	T38.2X3	T38.2X4	T38.2X5	T38.2X6
Iotrol	T50.8X1	T50.8X2	T50.8X3	T50.8X4	T50.8X5	T50.8X6
Iotrolan	T50.8X1	T50.8X2	T50.8X3	T50.8X4	T50.8X5	T50.8X6
Iotroxate	T50.8X1	T50.8X2	T50.8X3	T50.8X4	T50.8X5	T50.8X6
Iotroxic acid	T50.8X1	T50.8X2	T50.8X3	T50.8X4	T50.8X5	T50.8X6
Ioversol	T50.8X1	T50.8X2	T50.8X3	T50.8X4	T50.8X5	T50.8X6
Ioxaglate	T50.8X1	T50.8X2	T50.8X3	T50.8X4	T50.8X5	T50.8X6
Ioxaglic acid	T50.8X1	T50.8X2	T50.8X3	T50.8X4	T50.8X5	T50.8X6
Ioxitalamic acid	T50.8X1	T50.8X2	T50.8X3	T50.8X4	T50.8X5	T50.8X6
Ipecac	T47.7X1	T47.7X2	T47.7X3	T47.7X4	T47.7X5	T47.7X6

Substance	Poisoning, Accidental (unintentional)	Poisoning, Intentional Self-harm	Poisoning, Assault	Poisoning, Undetermined	Adverse Effect	Under-dosing
Ipecacuanha	T48.4X1	T48.4X2	T48.4X3	T48.4X4	T48.4X5	T48.4X6
Ipodate, calcium	T50.8X1	T50.8X2	T50.8X3	T50.8X4	T50.8X5	T50.8X6
Ipral	T42.3X1	T42.3X2	T42.3X3	T42.3X4	T42.3X5	T42.3X6
Ipratropium (bromide)	T48.6X1	T48.6X2	T48.6X3	T48.6X4	T48.6X5	T48.6X6
Ipriflavone	T46.3X1	T46.3X2	T46.3X3	T46.3X4	T46.3X5	T46.3X6
Iprindole	T43.011	T43.012	T43.013	T43.014	T43.015	T43.016
Iproclozide	T43.1X1	T43.1X2	T43.1X3	T43.1X4	T43.1X5	T43.1X6
Iprofenin	T50.8X1	T50.8X2	T50.8X3	T50.8X4	T50.8X5	T50.8X6
Iproheptine	T49.2X1	T49.2X2	T49.2X3	T49.2X4	T49.2X5	T49.2X6
Iproniazid	T43.1X1	T43.1X2	T43.1X3	T43.1X4	T43.1X5	T43.1X6
Iproplatin	T45.1X1	T45.1X2	T45.1X3	T45.1X4	T45.1X5	T45.1X6
Iproveratril	T46.1X1	T46.1X2	T46.1X3	T46.1X4	T46.1X5	T46.1X6
Iron (compounds) (medicinal) NEC	T45.4X1	T45.4X2	T45.4X3	T45.4X4	T45.4X5	T45.4X6
ammonium	T45.4X1	T45.4X2	T45.4X3	T45.4X4	T45.4X5	T45.4X6
dextran injection	T45.4X1	T45.4X2	T45.4X3	T45.4X4	T45.4X5	T45.4X6
nonmedicinal	T56.891	T56.892	T56.893	T56.894	—	—
salts	T45.4X1	T45.4X2	T45.4X3	T45.4X4	T45.4X5	T45.4X6
sorbitex	T45.4X1	T45.4X2	T45.4X3	T45.4X4	T45.4X5	T45.4X6
sorbitol citric acid complex	T45.4X1	T45.4X2	T45.4X3	T45.4X4	T45.4X5	T45.4X6
Irrigating fluid (vaginal)	T49.8X1	T49.8X2	T49.8X3	T49.8X4	T49.8X5	T49.8X6
eye	T49.5X1	T49.5X2	T49.5X3	T49.5X4	T49.5X5	T49.5X6
Isepamicin	T36.5X1	T36.5X2	T36.5X3	T36.5X4	T36.5X5	T36.5X6
Isoaminile (citrate)	T48.3X1	T48.3X2	T48.3X3	T48.3X4	T48.3X5	T48.3X6
Isoamyl nitrite	T46.3X1	T46.3X2	T46.3X3	T46.3X4	T46.3X5	T46.3X6
Isobenzan	T60.1X1	T60.1X2	T60.1X3	T60.1X4	—	—
Isobutyl acetate	T52.8X1	T52.8X2	T52.8X3	T52.8X4	—	—
Isocarboxazid	T43.1X1	T43.1X2	T43.1X3	T43.1X4	T43.1X5	T43.1X6
Isoconazole	T49.0X1	T49.0X2	T49.0X3	T49.0X4	T49.0X5	T49.0X6
Isocyanate	T65.0X1	T65.0X2	T65.0X3	T65.0X4	—	—
Isoephedrine	T44.991	T44.992	T44.993	T44.994	T44.995	T44.996
Isoetarine	T48.6X1	T48.6X2	T48.6X3	T48.6X4	T48.6X5	T48.6X6
Isoethadione	T42.2X1	T42.2X2	T42.2X3	T42.2X4	T42.2X5	T42.2X6
Isoetharine	T44.5X1	T44.5X2	T44.5X3	T44.5X4	T44.5X5	T44.5X6
Isoflurane	T41.0X1	T41.0X2	T41.0X3	T41.0X4	T41.0X5	T41.0X6
Isoflurophate	T44.0X1	T44.0X2	T44.0X3	T44.0X4	T44.0X5	T44.0X6
Isomaltose, ferric complex	T45.4X1	T45.4X2	T45.4X3	T45.4X4	T45.4X5	T45.4X6
Isometheptene	T44.3X1	T44.3X2	T44.3X3	T44.3X4	T44.3X5	T44.3X6
Isoniazid	T37.1X1	T37.1X2	T37.1X3	T37.1X4	T37.1X5	T37.1X6
with						
rifampicin	T36.6X1	T36.6X2	T36.6X3	T36.6X4	T36.6X5	T36.6X6
thioacetazone	T37.1X1	T37.1X2	T37.1X3	T37.1X4	T37.1X5	T37.1X6
Isonicotinic acid hydrazide	T37.1X1	T37.1X2	T37.1X3	T37.1X4	T37.1X5	T37.1X6
Isonipecaine	T40.491	T40.492	T40.493	T40.494	T40.495	T40.496
Isopentaquine	T37.2X1	T37.2X2	T37.2X3	T37.2X4	T37.2X5	T37.2X6
Isophane insulin	T38.3X1	T38.3X2	T38.3X3	T38.3X4	T38.3X5	T38.3X6
Isophorone	T65.891	T65.892	T65.893	T65.894	—	—
Isophosphamide	T45.1X1	T45.1X2	T45.1X3	T45.1X4	T45.1X5	T45.1X6
Isopregnenone	T38.5X1	T38.5X2	T38.5X3	T38.5X4	T38.5X5	T38.5X6
Isoprenaline	T48.6X1	T48.6X2	T48.6X3	T48.6X4	T48.6X5	T48.6X6
Isopromethazine	T43.3X1	T43.3X2	T43.3X3	T43.3X4	T43.3X5	T43.3X6
Isopropamide	T44.3X1	T44.3X2	T44.3X3	T44.3X4	T44.3X5	T44.3X6
iodide	T44.3X1	T44.3X2	T44.3X3	T44.3X4	T44.3X5	T44.3X6
Isopropanol	T51.2X1	T51.2X2	T51.2X3	T51.2X4	—	—
Isopropyl						
acetate	T52.8X1	T52.8X2	T52.8X3	T52.8X4	—	—
alcohol	T51.2X1	T51.2X2	T51.2X3	T51.2X4	—	—
medicinal	T49.4X1	T49.4X2	T49.4X3	T49.4X4	T49.4X5	T49.4X6
ether	T52.8X1	T52.8X2	T52.8X3	T52.8X4	—	—
Isopropylaminophenazone	T39.2X1	T39.2X2	T39.2X3	T39.2X4	T39.2X5	T39.2X6
Isoproterenol	T48.6X1	T48.6X2	T48.6X3	T48.6X4	T48.6X5	T48.6X6
Isosorbide dinitrate	T46.3X1	T46.3X2	T46.3X3	T46.3X4	T46.3X5	T46.3X6
Isothipendyl	T45.0X1	T45.0X2	T45.0X3	T45.0X4	T45.0X5	T45.0X6
Isotretinoin	T50.991	T50.992	T50.993	T50.994	T50.995	T50.996
Isoxazolyl penicillin	T36.0X1	T36.0X2	T36.0X3	T36.0X4	T36.0X5	T36.0X6
Isoxicam	T39.391	T39.392	T39.393	T39.394	T39.395	T39.396
Isoxsuprine	T46.7X1	T46.7X2	T46.7X3	T46.7X4	T46.7X5	T46.7X6
Ispagula	T47.4X1	T47.4X2	T47.4X3	T47.4X4	T47.4X5	T47.4X6
husk	T47.4X1	T47.4X2	T47.4X3	T47.4X4	T47.4X5	T47.4X6
Isradipine	T46.1X1	T46.1X2	T46.1X3	T46.1X4	T46.1X5	T46.1X6
I-thyroxine sodium	T38.1X1	T38.1X2	T38.1X3	T38.1X4	T38.1X5	T38.1X6
Itraconazole	T37.8X1	T37.8X2	T37.8X3	T37.8X4	T37.8X5	T37.8X6
Itramin tosilate	T46.3X1	T46.3X2	T46.3X3	T46.3X4	T46.3X5	T46.3X6
Ivermectin	T37.4X1	T37.4X2	T37.4X3	T37.4X4	T37.4X5	T37.4X6
Izoniazid	T37.1X1	T37.1X2	T37.1X3	T37.1X4	T37.1X5	T37.1X6
with thioacetazone	T37.1X1	T37.1X2	T37.1X3	T37.1X4	T37.1X5	T37.1X6
Jalap	T47.2X1	T47.2X2	T47.2X3	T47.2X4	T47.2X5	T47.2X6
Jamaica						
dogwood (bark)	T39.8X1	T39.8X2	T39.8X3	T39.8X4	T39.8X5	T39.8X6
ginger	T65.891	T65.892	T65.893	T65.894	—	—
root	T62.2X1	T62.2X2	T62.2X3	T62.2X4	—	—
Jatropha	T62.2X1	T62.2X2	T62.2X3	T62.2X4	—	—
curcas	T62.2X1	T62.2X2	T62.2X3	T62.2X4	—	—

Substance	Poisoning, Accidental (unintentional)	Poisoning, Intentional Self-harm	Poisoning, Assault	Poisoning, Undetermined	Adverse Effect	Under-dosing
Jectofer	T45.4X1	T45.4X2	T45.4X3	T45.4X4	T45.4X5	T45.4X6
Jellyfish (sting)	T63.621	T63.622	T63.623	T63.624	—	—
Jequirity (bean)	T62.2X1	T62.2X2	T62.2X3	T62.2X4	—	—
Jimson weed (stramonium)	T62.2X1	T62.2X2	T62.2X3	T62.2X4	—	—
seeds	T62.2X1	T62.2X2	T62.2X3	T62.2X4	—	—
Josamycin	T36.3X1	T36.3X2	T36.3X3	T36.3X4	T36.3X5	T36.3X6
Juniper tar	T49.1X1	T49.1X2	T49.1X3	T49.1X4	T49.1X5	T49.1X6
Kallidinogenase	T46.7X1	T46.7X2	T46.7X3	T46.7X4	T46.7X5	T46.7X6
Kallikrein	T46.7X1	T46.7X2	T46.7X3	T46.7X4	T46.7X5	T46.7X6
Kanamycin	T36.5X1	T36.5X2	T36.5X3	T36.5X4	T36.5X5	T36.5X6
Kantrex	T36.5X1	T36.5X2	T36.5X3	T36.5X4	T36.5X5	T36.5X6
Kaolin	T47.6X1	T47.6X2	T47.6X3	T47.6X4	T47.6X5	T47.6X6
light	T47.6X1	T47.6X2	T47.6X3	T47.6X4	T47.6X5	T47.6X6
Karaya (gum)	T47.4X1	T47.4X2	T47.4X3	T47.4X4	T47.4X5	T47.4X6
Kebuzone	T39.2X1	T39.2X2	T39.2X3	T39.2X4	T39.2X5	T39.2X6
Kelevan	T60.1X1	T60.1X2	T60.1X3	T60.1X4	—	—
Kemithal	T41.1X1	T41.1X2	T41.1X3	T41.1X4	T41.1X5	T41.1X6
Kenacort	T38.0X1	T38.0X2	T38.0X3	T38.0X4	T38.0X5	T38.0X6
Keratolytic drug NEC	T49.4X1	T49.4X2	T49.4X3	T49.4X4	T49.4X5	T49.4X6
anthracene	T49.4X1	T49.4X2	T49.4X3	T49.4X4	T49.4X5	T49.4X6
Keratoplastic NEC	T49.4X1	T49.4X2	T49.4X3	T49.4X4	T49.4X5	T49.4X6
Kerosene, kerosine (fuel) (solvent) NEC	T52.0X1	T52.0X2	T52.0X3	T52.0X4	—	—
insecticide	T52.0X1	T52.0X2	T52.0X3	T52.0X4	—	—
vapor	T52.0X1	T52.0X2	T52.0X3	T52.0X4	—	—
Ketamine	T41.291	T41.292	T41.293	T41.294	T41.295	T41.296
Ketazolam	T42.4X1	T42.4X2	T42.4X3	T42.4X4	T42.4X5	T42.4X6
Ketazon	T39.2X1	T39.2X2	T39.2X3	T39.2X4	T39.2X5	T39.2X6
Ketobemidone	T40.491	T40.492	T40.493	T40.494	—	—
Ketoconazole	T49.0X1	T49.0X2	T49.0X3	T49.0X4	T49.0X5	T49.0X6
Ketols	T52.4X1	T52.4X2	T52.4X3	T52.4X4	—	—
Ketone oils	T52.4X1	T52.4X2	T52.4X3	T52.4X4	—	—
Ketoprofen	T39.311	T39.312	T39.313	T39.314	T39.315	T39.316
Ketorolac	T39.8X1	T39.8X2	T39.8X3	T39.8X4	T39.8X5	T39.8X6
Ketotifen	T45.0X1	T45.0X2	T45.0X3	T45.0X4	T45.0X5	T45.0X6
Khat	T43.691	T43.692	T43.693	T43.694	—	—
Khellin	T46.3X1	T46.3X2	T46.3X3	T46.3X4	T46.3X5	T46.3X6
Khelloside	T46.3X1	T46.3X2	T46.3X3	T46.3X4	T46.3X5	T46.3X6
Kiln gas or vapor (carbon monoxide)	T58.8X1	T58.8X2	T58.8X3	T58.8X4	—	—
Kitasamycin	T36.3X1	T36.3X2	T36.3X3	T36.3X4	T36.3X5	T36.3X6
Konsyl	T47.4X1	T47.4X2	T47.4X3	T47.4X4	T47.4X5	T47.4X6
Kosam seed	T62.2X1	T62.2X2	T62.2X3	T62.2X4	—	—
Krait (venom)	T63.091	T63.092	T63.093	T63.094	—	—
Kwell (insecticide)	T60.1X1	T60.1X2	T60.1X3	T60.1X4	—	—
anti-infective (topical)	T49.0X1	T49.0X2	T49.0X3	T49.0X4	T49.0X5	T49.0X6
Labetalol	T44.8X1	T44.8X2	T44.8X3	T44.8X4	T44.8X5	T44.8X6
Laburnum (seeds)	T62.2X1	T62.2X2	T62.2X3	T62.2X4	—	—
leaves	T62.2X1	T62.2X2	T62.2X3	T62.2X4	—	—
Lachesine	T49.5X1	T49.5X2	T49.5X3	T49.5X4	T49.5X5	T49.5X6
Lacidipine	T46.5X1	T46.5X2	T46.5X3	T46.5X4	T46.5X5	T46.5X6
Lacquer	T65.6X1	T65.6X2	T65.6X3	T65.6X4	—	—
Lacrimogenic gas	T59.3X1	T59.3X2	T59.3X3	T59.3X4	—	—
Lactated potassic saline	T50.3X1	T50.3X2	T50.3X3	T50.3X4	T50.3X5	T50.3X6
Lactic acid	T49.8X1	T49.8X2	T49.8X3	T49.8X4	T49.8X5	T49.8X6
Lactobacillus						
acidophilus	T47.6X1	T47.6X2	T47.6X3	T47.6X4	T47.6X5	T47.6X6
compound	T47.6X1	T47.6X2	T47.6X3	T47.6X4	T47.6X5	T47.6X6
bifidus, lyophilized	T47.6X1	T47.6X2	T47.6X3	T47.6X4	T47.6X5	T47.6X6
bulgaricus	T47.6X1	T47.6X2	T47.6X3	T47.6X4	T47.6X5	T47.6X6
sporogenes	T47.6X1	T47.6X2	T47.6X3	T47.6X4	T47.6X5	T47.6X6
Lactoflavin	T45.2X1	T45.2X2	T45.2X3	T45.2X4	T45.2X5	T45.2X6
Lactose (as excipient)	T50.901	T50.902	T50.903	T50.904	T50.905	T50.906
Lactuca (virosa) (extract)	T42.6X1	T42.6X2	T42.6X3	T42.6X4	T42.6X5	T42.6X6
Lactucarium	T42.6X1	T42.6X2	T42.6X3	T42.6X4	T42.6X5	T42.6X6
Lactulose	T47.3X1	T47.3X2	T47.3X3	T47.3X4	T47.3X5	T47.3X6
Laevo — see Levo-						
Lanatosides	T46.0X1	T46.0X2	T46.0X3	T46.0X4	T46.0X5	T46.0X6
Lanolin	T49.3X1	T49.3X2	T49.3X3	T49.3X4	T49.3X5	T49.3X6
Largactil	T43.3X1	T43.3X2	T43.3X3	T43.3X4	T43.3X5	T43.3X6
Larkspur	T62.2X1	T62.2X2	T62.2X3	T62.2X4	—	—
Laroxyl	T43.011	T43.012	T43.013	T43.014	T43.015	T43.016
Lasix	T50.1X1	T50.1X2	T50.1X3	T50.1X4	T50.1X5	T50.1X6
Lassar's paste	T49.4X1	T49.4X2	T49.4X3	T49.4X4	T49.4X5	T49.4X6
Latamoxef	T36.1X1	T36.1X2	T36.1X3	T36.1X4	T36.1X5	T36.1X6
Latex	T65.811	T65.812	T65.813	T65.814	—	—
Lathyrus (seed)	T62.2X1	T62.2X2	T62.2X3	T62.2X4	—	—
Laudanum	T40.0X1	T40.0X2	T40.0X3	T40.0X4	T40.0X5	T40.0X6
Laudexium	T48.1X1	T48.1X2	T48.1X3	T48.1X4	T48.1X5	T48.1X6
Laughing gas	T41.0X1	T41.0X2	T41.0X3	T41.0X4	T41.0X5	T41.0X6
Laurel, black or cherry	T62.2X1	T62.2X2	T62.2X3	T62.2X4	—	—
Laurolinium	T49.0X1	T49.0X2	T49.0X3	T49.0X4	T49.0X5	T49.0X6
Lauryl sulfoacetate	T49.2X1	T49.2X2	T49.2X3	T49.2X4	T49.2X5	T49.2X6

Substance	Poisoning, Accidental (unintentional)	Poisoning, Intentional Self-harm	Poisoning, Assault	Poisoning, Undetermined	Adverse Effect	Under-dosing
Laxative NEC	T47.4X1	T47.4X2	T47.4X3	T47.4X4	T47.4X5	T47.4X6
osmotic	T47.3X1	T47.3X2	T47.3X3	T47.3X4	T47.3X5	T47.3X6
saline	T47.3X1	T47.3X2	T47.3X3	T47.3X4	T47.3X5	T47.3X6
stimulant	T47.2X1	T47.2X2	T47.2X3	T47.2X4	T47.2X5	T47.2X6
L-dopa	T42.8X1	T42.8X2	T42.8X3	T42.8X4	T42.8X5	T42.8X6
Lead (dust) (fumes) (vapor)	T56.0X1	T56.0X2	T56.0X3	T56.0X4	—	—
NEC						
acetate	T49.2X1	T49.2X2	T49.2X3	T49.2X4	T49.2X5	T49.2X6
alkyl (fuel additive)	T56.0X1	T56.0X2	T56.0X3	T56.0X4	—	—
anti-infectives	T37.8X1	T37.8X2	T37.8X3	T37.8X4	T37.8X5	T37.8X6
antiknock compound (tetraethyl)	T56.0X1	T56.0X2	T56.0X3	T56.0X4	—	—
arsenate, arsenite (dust)(arsenic) (insecticide) (vapor)	T57.0X1	T57.0X2	T57.0X3	T57.0X4	—	—
carbonate	T56.0X1	T56.0X2	T56.0X3	T56.0X4	—	—
paint	T56.0X1	T56.0X2	T56.0X3	T56.0X4	—	—
chromate	T56.0X1	T56.0X2	T56.0X3	T56.0X4	—	—
paint	T56.0X1	T56.0X2	T56.0X3	T56.0X4	—	—
dioxide	T56.0X1	T56.0X2	T56.0X3	T56.0X4	—	—
inorganic	T56.0X1	T56.0X2	T56.0X3	T56.0X4	—	—
iodide	T56.0X1	T56.0X2	T56.0X3	T56.0X4	—	—
pigment (paint)	T56.0X1	T56.0X2	T56.0X3	T56.0X4	—	—
monoxide (dust)	T56.0X1	T56.0X2	T56.0X3	T56.0X4	—	—
paint	T56.0X1	T56.0X2	T56.0X3	T56.0X4	—	—
organic	T56.0X1	T56.0X2	T56.0X3	T56.0X4	—	—
oxide	T56.0X1	T56.0X2	T56.0X3	T56.0X4	—	—
paint	T56.0X1	T56.0X2	T56.0X3	T56.0X4	—	—
paint	T56.0X1	T56.0X2	T56.0X3	T56.0X4	—	—
salts	T56.0X1	T56.0X2	T56.0X3	T56.0X4	—	—
specified compound NEC	T56.0X1	T56.0X2	T56.0X3	T56.0X4	—	—
tetra-ethyl	T56.0X1	T56.0X2	T56.0X3	T56.0X4	—	—
Lebanese red	T40.7X1	T40.7X2	T40.7X3	T40.7X4	T40.7X5	T40.7X6
Lefetamine	T39.8X1	T39.8X2	T39.8X3	T39.8X4	T39.8X5	T39.8X6
Lenperone	T43.4X1	T43.4X2	T43.4X3	T43.4X4	T43.4X5	T43.4X6
Lente lietin (insulin)	T38.3X1	T38.3X2	T38.3X3	T38.3X4	T38.3X5	T38.3X6
Leptazol	T50.7X1	T50.7X2	T50.7X3	T50.7X4	T50.7X5	T50.7X6
Leptophos	T60.0X1	T60.0X2	T60.0X3	T60.0X4	—	—
Leritine	T40.2X1	T40.2X2	T40.2X3	T40.2X4	T40.2X5	T40.2X6
Letosteine	T48.4X1	T48.4X2	T48.4X3	T48.4X4	T48.4X5	T48.4X6
Letter	T38.1X1	T38.1X2	T38.1X3	T38.1X4	T38.1X5	T38.1X6
Lettuce opium	T42.6X1	T42.6X2	T42.6X3	T42.6X4	T42.6X5	T42.6X6
Leucinocaine	T41.3X1	T41.3X2	T41.3X3	T41.3X4	T41.3X5	T41.3X6
Leucocianidol	T46.991	T46.992	T46.993	T46.994	T46.995	T46.996
Leucovorin (factor)	T45.8X1	T45.8X2	T45.8X3	T45.8X4	T45.8X5	T45.8X6
Leukeran	T45.1X1	T45.1X2	T45.1X3	T45.1X4	T45.1X5	T45.1X6
Leuprolide	T38.891	T38.892	T38.893	T38.894	T38.895	T38.896
Levalbuterol	T48.6X1	T48.6X2	T48.6X3	T48.6X4	T48.6X5	T48.6X6
Levallorphan	T50.7X1	T50.7X2	T50.7X3	T50.7X4	T50.7X5	T50.7X6
Levamisole	T37.4X1	T37.4X2	T37.4X3	T37.4X4	T37.4X5	T37.4X6
Levanil	T42.6X1	T42.6X2	T42.6X3	T42.6X4	T42.6X5	T42.6X6
Levarterenol	T44.4X1	T44.4X2	T44.4X3	T44.4X4	T44.4X5	T44.4X6
Levdropropizine	T48.3X1	T48.3X2	T48.3X3	T48.3X4	T48.3X5	T48.3X6
Levobunolol	T49.5X1	T49.5X2	T49.5X3	T49.5X4	T49.5X5	T49.5X6
Levocabastine (hydrochloride)	T45.0X1	T45.0X2	T45.0X3	T45.0X4	T45.0X5	T45.0X6
Levocarnitine	T50.991	T50.992	T50.993	T50.994	T50.995	T50.996
Levodopa	T42.8X1	T42.8X2	T42.8X3	T42.8X4	T42.8X5	T42.8X6
with carbidopa	T42.8X1	T42.8X2	T42.8X3	T42.8X4	T42.8X5	T42.8X6
Levo-dromoran	T40.2X1	T40.2X2	T40.2X3	T40.2X4	T40.2X5	T40.2X6
Levoglutamide	T50.991	T50.992	T50.993	T50.994	T50.995	T50.996
Levoid	T38.1X1	T38.1X2	T38.1X3	T38.1X4	T38.1X5	T38.1X6
Levo-isomethadone	T40.3X1	T40.3X2	T40.3X3	T40.3X4	T40.3X5	T40.3X6
Levomepromazine	T43.3X1	T43.3X2	T43.3X3	T43.3X4	T43.3X5	T43.3X6
Levonordefrin	T49.6X1	T49.6X2	T49.6X3	T49.6X4	T49.6X5	T49.6X6
Levonorgestrel	T38.4X1	T38.4X2	T38.4X3	T38.4X4	T38.4X5	T38.4X6
with ethinylestradiol	T38.5X1	T38.5X2	T38.5X3	T38.5X4	T38.5X5	T38.5X6
Levopromazine	T43.3X1	T43.3X2	T43.3X3	T43.3X4	T43.3X5	T43.3X6
Levoprome	T42.6X1	T42.6X2	T42.6X3	T42.6X4	T42.6X5	T42.6X6
Levopropoxyphene	T40.491	T40.492	T40.493	T40.494	T40.495	T40.496
Levopropylhexedrine	T50.5X1	T50.5X2	T50.5X3	T50.5X4	T50.5X5	T50.5X6
Levoproxyphylline	T48.6X1	T48.6X2	T48.6X3	T48.6X4	T48.6X5	T48.6X6
Levorphanol	T40.491	T40.492	T40.493	T40.494	T40.495	T40.496
Levothyroxine	T38.1X1	T38.1X2	T38.1X3	T38.1X4	T38.1X5	T38.1X6
sodium	T38.1X1	T38.1X2	T38.1X3	T38.1X4	T38.1X5	T38.1X6
Levsin	T44.3X1	T44.3X2	T44.3X3	T44.3X4	T44.3X5	T44.3X6
Levulose	T50.3X1	T50.3X2	T50.3X3	T50.3X4	T50.3X5	T50.3X6
Lewisite (gas), not in war	T57.0X1	T57.0X2	T57.0X3	T57.0X4	—	—
Librium	T42.4X1	T42.4X2	T42.4X3	T42.4X4	T42.4X5	T42.4X6
Lidex	T49.0X1	T49.0X2	T49.0X3	T49.0X4	T49.0X5	T49.0X6
Lidocaine	T41.3X1	T41.3X2	T41.3X3	T41.3X4	T41.3X5	T41.3X6
regional	T41.3X1	T41.3X2	T41.3X3	T41.3X4	T41.3X5	T41.3X6
spinal	T41.3X1	T41.3X2	T41.3X3	T41.3X4	T41.3X5	T41.3X6

380

Additional Character May Be Required — Refer to the Tabular List for Character Selection ▼ Subterms under main terms may continue to next column or page

Substance	Poisoning, Accidental (unintentional)	Poisoning, Intentional Self-harm	Poisoning, Assault	Poisoning, Undetermined	Adverse Effect	Under-dosing
Lidofenin	T50.8X1	T50.8X2	T50.8X3	T50.8X4	T50.8X5	T50.8X6
Lidoflazine	T46.1X1	T46.1X2	T46.1X3	T46.1X4	T46.1X5	T46.1X6
Lighter fluid	T52.0X1	T52.0X2	T52.0X3	T52.0X4	—	—
Lignin hemicellulose	T47.6X1	T47.6X2	T47.6X3	T47.6X4	T47.6X5	T47.6X6
Lignocaine	T41.3X1	T41.3X2	T41.3X3	T41.3X4	T41.3X5	T41.3X6
regional	T41.3X1	T41.3X2	T41.3X3	T41.3X4	T41.3X5	T41.3X6
spinal	T41.3X1	T41.3X2	T41.3X3	T41.3X4	T41.3X5	T41.3X6
Ligroin (e) (solvent)	T52.0X1	T52.0X2	T52.0X3	T52.0X4	—	—
vapor	T59.891	T59.892	T59.893	T59.894	—	—
Ligustrum vulgare	T62.2X1	T62.2X2	T62.2X3	T62.2X4	—	—
Lily of the valley	T62.2X1	T62.2X2	T62.2X3	T62.2X4	—	—
Lime (chloride)	T54.3X1	T54.3X2	T54.3X3	T54.3X4	—	—
Limonene	T52.8X1	T52.8X2	T52.8X3	T52.8X4	—	—
Lincomycin	T36.8X1	T36.8X2	T36.8X3	T36.8X4	T36.8X5	T36.8X6
Lindane (insecticide) (nonmedicinal) (vapor)	T53.6X1	T53.6X2	T53.6X3	T53.6X4	—	—
medicinal	T49.0X1	T49.0X2	T49.0X3	T49.0X4	T49.0X5	T49.0X6
Liniments NEC	T49.91	T49.92	T49.93	T49.94	T49.95	T49.96
Linoleic acid	T46.6X1	T46.6X2	T46.6X3	T46.6X4	T46.6X5	T46.6X6
Linolenic acid	T46.6X1	T46.6X2	T46.6X3	T46.6X4	T46.6X5	T46.6X6
Linseed	T47.4X1	T47.4X2	T47.4X3	T47.4X4	T47.4X5	T47.4X6
Liothyronine	T38.1X1	T38.1X2	T38.1X3	T38.1X4	T38.1X5	T38.1X6
Liotrix	T38.1X1	T38.1X2	T38.1X3	T38.1X4	T38.1X5	T38.1X6
Lipancreatin	T47.5X1	T47.5X2	T47.5X3	T47.5X4	T47.5X5	T47.5X6
Lipo-alprostadil	T46.7X1	T46.7X2	T46.7X3	T46.7X4	T46.7X5	T46.7X6
Lipo-Lutin	T38.5X1	T38.5X2	T38.5X3	T38.5X4	T38.5X5	T38.5X6
Lipotropic drug NEC	T50.901	T50.902	T50.903	T50.904	T50.905	T50.906
Liquefied petroleum gases	T59.891	T59.892	T59.893	T59.894	—	—
piped (pure or mixed with air)	T59.891	T59.892	T59.893	T59.894	—	—
Liquid						
paraffin	T47.4X1	T47.4X2	T47.4X3	T47.4X4	T47.4X5	T47.4X6
petrolatum	T47.4X1	T47.4X2	T47.4X3	T47.4X4	T47.4X5	T47.4X6
topical	T49.3X1	T49.3X2	T49.3X3	T49.3X4	T49.3X5	T49.3X6
specified NEC	T65.891	T65.892	T65.893	T65.894	—	—
substance	T65.91	T65.92	T65.93	T65.94	—	—
Liquor creosolis compositus	T65.891	T65.892	T65.893	T65.894	—	—
Liquorice	T48.4X1	T48.4X2	T48.4X3	T48.4X4	T48.4X5	T48.4X6
extract	T47.8X1	T47.8X2	T47.8X3	T47.8X4	T47.8X5	T47.8X6
Lisinopril	T46.4X1	T46.4X2	T46.4X3	T46.4X4	T46.4X5	T46.4X6
Lisuride	T42.8X1	T42.8X2	T42.8X3	T42.8X4	T42.8X5	T42.8X6
Lithane	T43.8X1	T43.8X2	T43.8X3	T43.8X4	T43.8X5	T43.8X6
Lithium	T56.891	T56.892	T56.893	T56.894	—	—
gluconate	T43.591	T43.592	T43.593	T43.594	T43.595	T43.596
salts (carbonate)	T43.591	T43.592	T43.593	T43.594	T43.595	T43.596
Lithonate	T43.8X1	T43.8X2	T43.8X3	T43.8X4	T43.8X5	T43.8X6
Liver						
extract	T45.8X1	T45.8X2	T45.8X3	T45.8X4	T45.8X5	T45.8X6
for parenteral use	T45.8X1	T45.8X2	T45.8X3	T45.8X4	T45.8X5	T45.8X6
fraction 1	T45.8X1	T45.8X2	T45.8X3	T45.8X4	T45.8X5	T45.8X6
hydrolysate	T45.8X1	T45.8X2	T45.8X3	T45.8X4	T45.8X5	T45.8X6
Lizard (bite) (venom)	T63.121	T63.122	T63.123	T63.124	—	—
LMD	T45.8X1	T45.8X2	T45.8X3	T45.8X4	T45.8X5	T45.8X6
Lobelia	T62.2X1	T62.2X2	T62.2X3	T62.2X4	—	—
Lobeline	T50.7X1	T50.7X2	T50.7X3	T50.7X4	T50.7X5	T50.7X6
Local action drug NEC	T49.8X1	T49.8X2	T49.8X3	T49.8X4	T49.8X5	T49.8X6
Locorten	T49.0X1	T49.0X2	T49.0X3	T49.0X4	T49.0X5	T49.0X6
Lofepramine	T43.011	T43.012	T43.013	T43.014	T43.015	T43.016
Lolium temulentum	T62.2X1	T62.2X2	T62.2X3	T62.2X4	—	—
Lomotil	T47.6X1	T47.6X2	T47.6X3	T47.6X4	T47.6X5	T47.6X6
Lomustine	T45.1X1	T45.1X2	T45.1X3	T45.1X4	T45.1X5	T45.1X6
Lonidamine	T45.1X1	T45.1X2	T45.1X3	T45.1X4	T45.1X5	T45.1X6
Loperamide	T47.6X1	T47.6X2	T47.6X3	T47.6X4	T47.6X5	T47.6X6
Loprazolam	T42.4X1	T42.4X2	T42.4X3	T42.4X4	T42.4X5	T42.4X6
Lorajmine	T46.2X1	T46.2X2	T46.2X3	T46.2X4	T46.2X5	T46.2X6
Loratidine	T45.0X1	T45.0X2	T45.0X3	T45.0X4	T45.0X5	T45.0X6
Lorazepam	T42.4X1	T42.4X2	T42.4X3	T42.4X4	T42.4X5	T42.4X6
Lorcainide	T46.2X1	T46.2X2	T46.2X3	T46.2X4	T46.2X5	T46.2X6
Lormetazepam	T42.4X1	T42.4X2	T42.4X3	T42.4X4	T42.4X5	T42.4X6
Lotions NEC	T49.91	T49.92	T49.93	T49.94	T49.95	T49.96
Lotusate	T42.3X1	T42.3X2	T42.3X3	T42.3X4	T42.3X5	T42.3X6
Lovastatin	T46.6X1	T46.6X2	T46.6X3	T46.6X4	T46.6X5	T46.6X6
Lowila	T49.2X1	T49.2X2	T49.2X3	T49.2X4	T49.2X5	T49.2X6
Loxapine	T43.591	T43.592	T43.593	T43.594	T43.595	T43.596
Lozenges (throat)	T49.6X1	T49.6X2	T49.6X3	T49.6X4	T49.6X5	T49.6X6
LSD	T40.8X1	T40.8X2	T40.8X3	T40.8X4	—	—
L-Tryptophan — see amino acid						
Lubricant, eye	T49.5X1	T49.5X2	T49.5X3	T49.5X4	T49.5X5	T49.5X6
Lubricating oil NEC	T52.0X1	T52.0X2	T52.0X3	T52.0X4	—	—
Lucanthone	T37.4X1	T37.4X2	T37.4X3	T37.4X4	T37.4X5	T37.4X6
Luminal	T42.3X1	T42.3X2	T42.3X3	T42.3X4	T42.3X5	T42.3X6
Lung irritant (gas) NEC	T59.91	T59.92	T59.93	T59.94	—	—
Luteinizing hormone	T38.811	T38.812	T38.813	T38.814	T38.815	T38.816
Lutocylol	T38.5X1	T38.5X2	T38.5X3	T38.5X4	T38.5X5	T38.5X6
Lutromone	T38.5X1	T38.5X2	T38.5X3	T38.5X4	T38.5X5	T38.5X6
Lututrin	T48.291	T48.292	T48.293	T48.294	T48.295	T48.296
Lye (concentrated)	T54.3X1	T54.3X2	T54.3X3	T54.3X4	—	—
Lygranum (skin test)	T50.8X1	T50.8X2	T50.8X3	T50.8X4	T50.8X5	T50.8X6
Lymecycline	T36.4X1	T36.4X2	T36.4X3	T36.4X4	T36.4X5	T36.4X6
Lymphogranuloma venereum antigen	T50.8X1	T50.8X2	T50.8X3	T50.8X4	T50.8X5	T50.8X6
Lynestrenol	T38.4X1	T38.4X2	T38.4X3	T38.4X4	T38.4X5	T38.4X6
Lyovac Sodium Edecrin	T50.1X1	T50.1X2	T50.1X3	T50.1X4	T50.1X5	T50.1X6
Lypressin	T38.891	T38.892	T38.893	T38.894	T38.895	T38.896
Lysergic acid diethylamide	T40.8X1	T40.8X2	T40.8X3	T40.8X4	—	—
Lysergide	T40.8X1	T40.8X2	T40.8X3	T40.8X4	—	—
Lysine vasopressin	T38.891	T38.892	T38.893	T38.894	T38.895	T38.896
Lysol	T54.1X1	T54.1X2	T54.1X3	T54.1X4	—	—
Lysozyme	T49.0X1	T49.0X2	T49.0X3	T49.0X4	T49.0X5	T49.0X6
Lytta (vitatta)	T49.8X1	T49.8X2	T49.8X3	T49.8X4	T49.8X5	T49.8X6
Mace	T59.3X1	T59.3X2	T59.3X3	T59.3X4	—	—
Macrogol	T50.991	T50.992	T50.993	T50.994	T50.995	T50.996
Macrolide						
anabolic drug	T38.7X1	T38.7X2	T38.7X3	T38.7X4	T38.7X5	T38.7X6
antibiotic	T36.3X1	T36.3X2	T36.3X3	T36.3X4	T36.3X5	T36.3X6
Mafenide	T49.0X1	T49.0X2	T49.0X3	T49.0X4	T49.0X5	T49.0X6
Magaldrate	T47.1X1	T47.1X2	T47.1X3	T47.1X4	T47.1X5	T47.1X6
Magic mushroom	T40.991	T40.992	T40.993	T40.994	—	—
Magnamycin	T36.8X1	T36.8X2	T36.8X3	T36.8X4	T36.8X5	T36.8X6
Magnesia magma	T47.1X1	T47.1X2	T47.1X3	T47.1X4	T47.1X5	T47.1X6
Magnesium NEC	T56.891	T56.892	T56.893	T56.894	—	—
carbonate	T47.1X1	T47.1X2	T47.1X3	T47.1X4	T47.1X5	T47.1X6
citrate	T47.4X1	T47.4X2	T47.4X3	T47.4X4	T47.4X5	T47.4X6
hydroxide	T47.1X1	T47.1X2	T47.1X3	T47.1X4	T47.1X5	T47.1X6
oxide	T47.1X1	T47.1X2	T47.1X3	T47.1X4	T47.1X5	T47.1X6
peroxide	T49.0X1	T49.0X2	T49.0X3	T49.0X4	T49.0X5	T49.0X6
salicylate	T39.091	T39.092	T39.093	T39.094	T39.095	T39.096
silicofluoride	T50.3X1	T50.3X2	T50.3X3	T50.3X4	T50.3X5	T50.3X6
sulfate	T47.4X1	T47.4X2	T47.4X3	T47.4X4	T47.4X5	T47.4X6
thiosulfate	T45.0X1	T45.0X2	T45.0X3	T45.0X4	T45.0X5	T45.0X6
trisilicate	T47.1X1	T47.1X2	T47.1X3	T47.1X4	T47.1X5	T47.1X6
Malathion (medicinal)	T49.0X1	T49.0X2	T49.0X3	T49.0X4	T49.0X5	T49.0X6
insecticide	T60.0X1	T60.0X2	T60.0X3	T60.0X4	—	—
Male fern extract	T37.4X1	T37.4X2	T37.4X3	T37.4X4	T37.4X5	T37.4X6
M-AMSA	T45.1X1	T45.1X2	T45.1X3	T45.1X4	T45.1X5	T45.1X6
Mandelic acid	T37.8X1	T37.8X2	T37.8X3	T37.8X4	T37.8X5	T37.8X6
Manganese (dioxide) (salts)	T57.2X1	T57.2X2	T57.2X3	T57.2X4	—	—
medicinal	T50.991	T50.992	T50.993	T50.994	T50.995	T50.996
Mannitol	T47.3X1	T47.3X2	T47.3X3	T47.3X4	T47.3X5	T47.3X6
hexanitrate	T46.3X1	T46.3X2	T46.3X3	T46.3X4	T46.3X5	T46.3X6
Mannomustine	T45.1X1	T45.1X2	T45.1X3	T45.1X4	T45.1X5	T45.1X6
MAO inhibitors	T43.1X1	T43.1X2	T43.1X3	T43.1X4	T43.1X5	T43.1X6
Mapharsen	T37.8X1	T37.8X2	T37.8X3	T37.8X4	T37.8X5	T37.8X6
Maphenide	T49.0X1	T49.0X2	T49.0X3	T49.0X4	T49.0X5	T49.0X6
Maprotiline	T43.021	T43.022	T43.023	T43.024	T43.025	T43.026
Marcaine	T41.3X1	T41.3X2	T41.3X3	T41.3X4	T41.3X5	T41.3X6
infiltration (subcutaneous)	T41.3X1	T41.3X2	T41.3X3	T41.3X4	T41.3X5	T41.3X6
nerve block (peripheral) (plexus)	T41.3X1	T41.3X2	T41.3X3	T41.3X4	T41.3X5	T41.3X6
Marezine	T45.0X1	T45.0X2	T45.0X3	T45.0X4	T45.0X5	T45.0X6
Marihuana	T40.7X1	T40.7X2	T40.7X3	T40.7X4	T40.7X5	T40.7X6
Marijuana	T40.7X1	T40.7X2	T40.7X3	T40.7X4	T40.7X5	T40.7X6
Marine (sting)	T63.691	T63.692	T63.693	T63.694	—	—
animals (sting)	T63.691	T63.692	T63.693	T63.694	—	—
plants (sting)	T63.711	T63.712	T63.713	T63.714	—	—
Marplan	T43.1X1	T43.1X2	T43.1X3	T43.1X4	T43.1X5	T43.1X6
Marsh gas	T59.891	T59.892	T59.893	T59.894	—	—
Marsilid	T43.1X1	T43.1X2	T43.1X3	T43.1X4	T43.1X5	T43.1X6
Matulane	T45.1X1	T45.1X2	T45.1X3	T45.1X4	T45.1X5	T45.1X6
Mazindol	T50.5X1	T50.5X2	T50.5X3	T50.5X4	T50.5X5	T50.5X6
MCPA	T60.3X1	T60.3X2	T60.3X3	T60.3X4	—	—
MDMA	T43.641	T43.642	T43.643	T43.644	—	—
Meadow saffron	T62.2X1	T62.2X2	T62.2X3	T62.2X4	—	—
Measles virus vaccine (attenuated)	T50.B91	T50.B92	T50.B93	T50.B94	T50.B95	T50.B96
Meat, noxious	T62.8X1	T62.8X2	T62.8X3	T62.8X4	—	—
Meballymal	T42.3X1	T42.3X2	T42.3X3	T42.3X4	T42.3X5	T42.3X6
Mebanazine	T43.1X1	T43.1X2	T43.1X3	T43.1X4	T43.1X5	T43.1X6
Mebaral	T42.3X1	T42.3X2	T42.3X3	T42.3X4	T42.3X5	T42.3X6
Mebendazole	T37.4X1	T37.4X2	T37.4X3	T37.4X4	T37.4X5	T37.4X6
Mebeverine	T44.3X1	T44.3X2	T44.3X3	T44.3X4	T44.3X5	T44.3X6
Mebhydrolin	T45.0X1	T45.0X2	T45.0X3	T45.0X4	T45.0X5	T45.0X6
Mebumal	T42.3X1	T42.3X2	T42.3X3	T42.3X4	T42.3X5	T42.3X6
Mebutamate	T43.591	T43.592	T43.593	T43.594	T43.595	T43.596
Mecamylamine	T44.2X1	T44.2X2	T44.2X3	T44.2X4	T44.2X5	T44.2X6

Substance	Poisoning, Accidental (unintentional)	Poisoning, Intentional Self-harm	Poisoning, Assault	Poisoning, Undetermined	Adverse Effect	Under-dosing
Mechlorethamine	T45.1X1	T45.1X2	T45.1X3	T45.1X4	T45.1X5	T45.1X6
Mecillinam	T36.0X1	T36.0X2	T36.0X3	T36.0X4	T36.0X5	T36.0X6
Meclizine (hydrochloride)	T45.0X1	T45.0X2	T45.0X3	T45.0X4	T45.0X5	T45.0X6
Meclocycline	T36.4X1	T36.4X2	T36.4X3	T36.4X4	T36.4X5	T36.4X6
Meclofenamate	T39.391	T39.392	T39.393	T39.394	T39.395	T39.396
Meclofenamic acid	T39.391	T39.392	T39.393	T39.394	T39.395	T39.396
Meclofenoxate	T43.691	T43.692	T43.693	T43.694	T43.695	T43.696
Meclozine	T45.0X1	T45.0X2	T45.0X3	T45.0X4	T45.0X5	T45.0X6
Mecobalamin	T45.8X1	T45.8X2	T45.8X3	T45.8X4	T45.8X5	T45.8X6
Mecoprop	T60.3X1	T60.3X2	T60.3X3	T60.3X4	—	—
Mecrilate	T49.3X1	T49.3X2	T49.3X3	T49.3X4	T49.3X5	T49.3X6
Mecysteine	T48.4X1	T48.4X2	T48.4X3	T48.4X4	T48.4X5	T48.4X6
Medazepam	T42.4X1	T42.4X2	T42.4X3	T42.4X4	T42.4X5	T42.4X6
Medicament NEC	T50.901	T50.902	T50.903	T50.904	T50.905	T50.906
Medinal	T42.3X1	T42.3X2	T42.3X3	T42.3X4	T42.3X5	T42.3X6
Medomin	T42.3X1	T42.3X2	T42.3X3	T42.3X4	T42.3X5	T42.3X6
Medrogestone	T38.5X1	T38.5X2	T38.5X3	T38.5X4	T38.5X5	T38.5X6
Medroxalol	T44.8X1	T44.8X2	T44.8X3	T44.8X4	T44.8X5	T44.8X6
Medroxyprogesterone acetate (depot)	T38.5X1	T38.5X2	T38.5X3	T38.5X4	T38.5X5	T38.5X6
Medrysone	T49.0X1	T49.0X2	T49.0X3	T49.0X4	T49.0X5	T49.0X6
Mefenamic acid	T39.391	T39.392	T39.393	T39.394	T39.395	T39.396
Mefenorex	T50.5X1	T50.5X2	T50.5X3	T50.5X4	T50.5X5	T50.5X6
Mefloquine	T37.2X1	T37.2X2	T37.2X3	T37.2X4	T37.2X5	T37.2X6
Mefruside	T50.2X1	T50.2X2	T50.2X3	T50.2X4	T50.2X5	T50.2X6
Megahallucinogen	T40.901	T40.902	T40.903	T40.904	T40.905	T40.906
Megestrol	T38.5X1	T38.5X2	T38.5X3	T38.5X4	T38.5X5	T38.5X6
Meglumine						
antimoniate	T37.8X1	T37.8X2	T37.8X3	T37.8X4	T37.8X5	T37.8X6
diatrizoate	T50.8X1	T50.8X2	T50.8X3	T50.8X4	T50.8X5	T50.8X6
iodipamide	T50.8X1	T50.8X2	T50.8X3	T50.8X4	T50.8X5	T50.8X6
iotroxate	T50.8X1	T50.8X2	T50.8X3	T50.8X4	T50.8X5	T50.8X6
MEK (methyl ethyl ketone)	T52.4X1	T52.4X2	T52.4X3	T52.4X4	—	—
Meladinin	T49.3X1	T49.3X2	T49.3X3	T49.3X4	T49.3X5	T49.3X6
Meladrazine	T44.3X1	T44.3X2	T44.3X3	T44.3X4	T44.3X5	T44.3X6
Melaleuca alternifolia oil	T49.0X1	T49.0X2	T49.0X3	T49.0X4	T49.0X5	T49.0X6
Melanizing agents	T49.3X1	T49.3X2	T49.3X3	T49.3X4	T49.3X5	T49.3X6
Melanocyte-stimulating hormone	T38.891	T38.892	T38.893	T38.894	T38.895	T38.896
Melarsonyl potassium	T37.3X1	T37.3X2	T37.3X3	T37.3X4	T37.3X5	T37.3X6
Melarsoprol	T37.3X1	T37.3X2	T37.3X3	T37.3X4	T37.3X5	T37.3X6
Melia azedarach	T62.2X1	T62.2X2	T62.2X3	T62.2X4	—	—
Melitracen	T43.011	T43.012	T43.013	T43.014	T43.015	T43.016
Mellaril	T43.3X1	T43.3X2	T43.3X3	T43.3X4	T43.3X5	T43.3X6
Meloxine	T49.3X1	T49.3X2	T49.3X3	T49.3X4	T49.3X5	T49.3X6
Melperone	T43.4X1	T43.4X2	T43.4X3	T43.4X4	T43.4X5	T43.4X6
Melphalan	T45.1X1	T45.1X2	T45.1X3	T45.1X4	T45.1X5	T45.1X6
Memantine	T43.8X1	T43.8X2	T43.8X3	T43.8X4	T43.8X5	T43.8X6
Menadiol	T45.7X1	T45.7X2	T45.7X3	T45.7X4	T45.7X5	T45.7X6
sodium sulfate	T45.7X1	T45.7X2	T45.7X3	T45.7X4	T45.7X5	T45.7X6
Menadione	T45.7X1	T45.7X2	T45.7X3	T45.7X4	T45.7X5	T45.7X6
sodium bisulfite	T45.7X1	T45.7X2	T45.7X3	T45.7X4	T45.7X5	T45.7X6
Menaphthone	T45.7X1	T45.7X2	T45.7X3	T45.7X4	T45.7X5	T45.7X6
Menaquinone	T45.7X1	T45.7X2	T45.7X3	T45.7X4	T45.7X5	T45.7X6
Menatetrenone	T45.7X1	T45.7X2	T45.7X3	T45.7X4	T45.7X5	T45.7X6
Meningococcal vaccine	T50.A91	T50.A92	T50.A93	T50.A94	T50.A95	T50.A96
Menningovax (-AC) (-C)	T50.A91	T50.A92	T50.A93	T50.A94	T50.A95	T50.A96
Menotropins	T38.811	T38.812	T38.813	T38.814	T38.815	T38.816
Menthol	T48.5X1	T48.5X2	T48.5X3	T48.5X4	T48.5X5	T48.5X6
Mepacrine	T37.2X1	T37.2X2	T37.2X3	T37.2X4	T37.2X5	T37.2X6
Meparfynol	T42.6X1	T42.6X2	T42.6X3	T42.6X4	T42.6X5	T42.6X6
Mepartricin	T36.7X1	T36.7X2	T36.7X3	T36.7X4	T36.7X5	T36.7X6
Mepazine	T43.3X1	T43.3X2	T43.3X3	T43.3X4	T43.3X5	T43.3X6
Mepenzolate	T44.3X1	T44.3X2	T44.3X3	T44.3X4	T44.3X5	T44.3X6
bromide	T44.3X1	T44.3X2	T44.3X3	T44.3X4	T44.3X5	T44.3X6
Meperidine	T40.491	T40.492	T40.493	T40.494	T40.495	T40.496
Mephebarbital	T42.3X1	T42.3X2	T42.3X3	T42.3X4	T42.3X5	T42.3X6
Mephenamin (e)	T42.8X1	T42.8X2	T42.8X3	T42.8X4	T42.8X5	T42.8X6
Mephenesin	T42.8X1	T42.8X2	T42.8X3	T42.8X4	T42.8X5	T42.8X6
Mephenhydramine	T45.0X1	T45.0X2	T45.0X3	T45.0X4	T45.0X5	T45.0X6
Mephenoxalone	T42.8X1	T42.8X2	T42.8X3	T42.8X4	T42.8X5	T42.8X6
Mephentermine	T44.991	T44.992	T44.993	T44.994	T44.995	T44.996
Mephenytoin	T42.0X1	T42.0X2	T42.0X3	T42.0X4	T42.0X5	T42.0X6
with phenobarbital	T42.3X1	T42.3X2	T42.3X3	T42.3X4	T42.3X5	T42.3X6
Mephobarbital	T42.3X1	T42.3X2	T42.3X3	T42.3X4	T42.3X5	T42.3X6
Mephosfolan	T60.0X1	T60.0X2	T60.0X3	T60.0X4	—	—
Mepindolol	T44.7X1	T44.7X2	T44.7X3	T44.7X4	T44.7X5	T44.7X6
Mepiperphenidol	T44.3X1	T44.3X2	T44.3X3	T44.3X4	T44.3X5	T44.3X6
Mepitiostane	T38.7X1	T38.7X2	T38.7X3	T38.7X4	T38.7X5	T38.7X6
Mepivacaine	T41.3X1	T41.3X2	T41.3X3	T41.3X4	T41.3X5	T41.3X6
epidural	T41.3X1	T41.3X2	T41.3X3	T41.3X4	T41.3X5	T41.3X6
Meprednisone	T38.0X1	T38.0X2	T38.0X3	T38.0X4	T38.0X5	T38.0X6
Meprobam	T43.591	T43.592	T43.593	T43.594	T43.595	T43.596
Meprobamate	T43.591	T43.592	T43.593	T43.594	T43.595	T43.596
Meproscillarin	T46.0X1	T46.0X2	T46.0X3	T46.0X4	T46.0X5	T46.0X6
Meprylcaine	T41.3X1	T41.3X2	T41.3X3	T41.3X4	T41.3X5	T41.3X6
Meptazinol	T39.8X1	T39.8X2	T39.8X3	T39.8X4	T39.8X5	T39.8X6
Mepyramine	T45.0X1	T45.0X2	T45.0X3	T45.0X4	T45.0X5	T45.0X6
Mequitazine	T43.3X1	T43.3X2	T43.3X3	T43.3X4	T43.3X5	T43.3X6
Meralluride	T50.2X1	T50.2X2	T50.2X3	T50.2X4	T50.2X5	T50.2X6
Merbaphen	T50.2X1	T50.2X2	T50.2X3	T50.2X4	T50.2X5	T50.2X6
Merbromin	T49.0X1	T49.0X2	T49.0X3	T49.0X4	T49.0X5	T49.0X6
Mercaptobenzothiazole salts	T49.0X1	T49.0X2	T49.0X3	T49.0X4	T49.0X5	T49.0X6
Mercaptomerin	T50.2X1	T50.2X2	T50.2X3	T50.2X4	T50.2X5	T50.2X6
Mercaptopurine	T45.1X1	T45.1X2	T45.1X3	T45.1X4	T45.1X5	T45.1X6
Mercumatilin	T50.2X1	T50.2X2	T50.2X3	T50.2X4	T50.2X5	T50.2X6
Mercuramide	T50.2X1	T50.2X2	T50.2X3	T50.2X4	T50.2X5	T50.2X6
Mercurochrome	T49.0X1	T49.0X2	T49.0X3	T49.0X4	T49.0X5	T49.0X6
Mercurophylline	T50.2X1	T50.2X2	T50.2X3	T50.2X4	T50.2X5	T50.2X6
Mercury, mercurial, mercuric, mercurous (compounds) (cyanide) (fumes) (nonmedicinal) (vapor) NEC	T56.1X1	T56.1X2	T56.1X3	T56.1X4	—	—
ammoniated	T49.0X1	T49.0X2	T49.0X3	T49.0X4	T49.0X5	T49.0X6
anti-infective						
local	T49.0X1	T49.0X2	T49.0X3	T49.0X4	T49.0X5	T49.0X6
systemic	T37.8X1	T37.8X2	T37.8X3	T37.8X4	T37.8X5	T37.8X6
topical	T49.0X1	T49.0X2	T49.0X3	T49.0X4	T49.0X5	T49.0X6
chloride (ammoniated)	T49.0X1	T49.0X2	T49.0X3	T49.0X4	T49.0X5	T49.0X6
fungicide	T56.1X1	T56.1X2	T56.1X3	T56.1X4	—	—
diuretic NEC	T50.2X1	T50.2X2	T50.2X3	T50.2X4	T50.2X5	T50.2X6
fungicide	T56.1X1	T56.1X2	T56.1X3	T56.1X4	—	—
organic (fungicide)	T56.1X1	T56.1X2	T56.1X3	T56.1X4	—	—
oxide, yellow	T49.0X1	T49.0X2	T49.0X3	T49.0X4	T49.0X5	T49.0X6
Mersalyl	T50.2X1	T50.2X2	T50.2X3	T50.2X4	T50.2X5	T50.2X6
Merthiolate	T49.0X1	T49.0X2	T49.0X3	T49.0X4	T49.0X5	T49.0X6
ophthalmic preparation	T49.5X1	T49.5X2	T49.5X3	T49.5X4	T49.5X5	T49.5X6
Meruvax	T50.B91	T50.B92	T50.B93	T50.B94	T50.B95	T50.B96
Mesalazine	T47.8X1	T47.8X2	T47.8X3	T47.8X4	T47.8X5	T47.8X6
Mescal buttons	T40.991	T40.992	T40.993	T40.994	—	—
Mescaline	T40.991	T40.992	T40.993	T40.994	—	—
Mesna	T48.4X1	T48.4X2	T48.4X3	T48.4X4	T48.4X5	T48.4X6
Mesoglycan	T46.6X1	T46.6X2	T46.6X3	T46.6X4	T46.6X5	T46.6X6
Mesoridazine	T43.3X1	T43.3X2	T43.3X3	T43.3X4	T43.3X5	T43.3X6
Mestanolone	T38.7X1	T38.7X2	T38.7X3	T38.7X4	T38.7X5	T38.7X6
Mesterolone	T38.7X1	T38.7X2	T38.7X3	T38.7X4	T38.7X5	T38.7X6
Mestranol	T38.5X1	T38.5X2	T38.5X3	T38.5X4	T38.5X5	T38.5X6
Mesulergine	T42.8X1	T42.8X2	T42.8X3	T42.8X4	T42.8X5	T42.8X6
Mesulfen	T49.0X1	T49.0X2	T49.0X3	T49.0X4	T49.0X5	T49.0X6
Mesuximide	T42.2X1	T42.2X2	T42.2X3	T42.2X4	T42.2X5	T42.2X6
Metabutethamine	T41.3X1	T41.3X2	T41.3X3	T41.3X4	T41.3X5	T41.3X6
Metactesylacetate	T49.0X1	T49.0X2	T49.0X3	T49.0X4	T49.0X5	T49.0X6
Metacycline	T36.4X1	T36.4X2	T36.4X3	T36.4X4	T36.4X5	T36.4X6
Metaldehyde (snail killer) NEC	T60.8X1	T60.8X2	T60.8X3	T60.8X4	—	—
Metals (heavy) (nonmedicinal)	T56.91	T56.92	T56.93	T56.94	—	—
dust, fumes, or vapor NEC	T56.91	T56.92	T56.93	T56.94	—	—
light NEC	T56.91	T56.92	T56.93	T56.94	—	—
dust, fumes, or vapor NEC	T56.91	T56.92	T56.93	T56.94	—	—
specified NEC	T56.891	T56.892	T56.893	T56.894	—	—
thallium	T56.811	T56.812	T56.813	T56.814	—	—
Metamfetamine	T43.621	T43.622	T43.623	T43.624	T43.625	T43.626
Metamizole sodium	T39.2X1	T39.2X2	T39.2X3	T39.2X4	T39.2X5	T39.2X6
Metampicillin	T36.0X1	T36.0X2	T36.0X3	T36.0X4	T36.0X5	T36.0X6
Metamucil	T47.4X1	T47.4X2	T47.4X3	T47.4X4	T47.4X5	T47.4X6
Metandienone	T38.7X1	T38.7X2	T38.7X3	T38.7X4	T38.7X5	T38.7X6
Metandrostenolone	T38.7X1	T38.7X2	T38.7X3	T38.7X4	T38.7X5	T38.7X6
Metaphen	T49.0X1	T49.0X2	T49.0X3	T49.0X4	T49.0X5	T49.0X6
Metaphos	T60.0X1	T60.0X2	T60.0X3	T60.0X4	—	—
Metapramine	T43.011	T43.012	T43.013	T43.014	T43.015	T43.016
Metaproterenol	T48.291	T48.292	T48.293	T48.294	T48.295	T48.296
Metaraminol	T44.4X1	T44.4X2	T44.4X3	T44.4X4	T44.4X5	T44.4X6
Metaxalone	T42.8X1	T42.8X2	T42.8X3	T42.8X4	T42.8X5	T42.8X6
Metenolone	T38.7X1	T38.7X2	T38.7X3	T38.7X4	T38.7X5	T38.7X6
Metergoline	T42.8X1	T42.8X2	T42.8X3	T42.8X4	T42.8X5	T42.8X6
Metescufylline	T46.991	T46.992	T46.993	T46.994	T46.995	T46.996
Metetoin	T42.0X1	T42.0X2	T42.0X3	T42.0X4	T42.0X5	T42.0X6
Metformin	T38.3X1	T38.3X2	T38.3X3	T38.3X4	T38.3X5	T38.3X6
Methacholine	T44.1X1	T44.1X2	T44.1X3	T44.1X4	T44.1X5	T44.1X6
Methacycline	T36.4X1	T36.4X2	T36.4X3	T36.4X4	T36.4X5	T36.4X6
Methadone	T40.3X1	T40.3X2	T40.3X3	T40.3X4	T40.3X5	T40.3X6
Methallenestril	T38.5X1	T38.5X2	T38.5X3	T38.5X4	T38.5X5	T38.5X6

Additional Character May Be Required — Refer to the Tabular List for Character Selection ▼ Subterms under main terms may continue to next column or page

Substance	Poisoning, Accidental (unintentional)	Poisoning, Intentional Self-harm	Poisoning, Assault	Poisoning, Undetermined	Adverse Effect	Under-dosing
Methallenoestril	T38.5X1	T38.5X2	T38.5X3	T38.5X4	T38.5X5	T38.5X6
Methamphetamine	T43.621	T43.622	T43.623	T43.624	T43.625	T43.626
Methampyrone	T39.2X1	T39.2X2	T39.2X3	T39.2X4	T39.2X5	T39.2X6
Methandienone	T38.7X1	T38.7X2	T38.7X3	T38.7X4	T38.7X5	T38.7X6
Methandriol	T38.7X1	T38.7X2	T38.7X3	T38.7X4	T38.7X5	T38.7X6
Methandrostenolone	T38.7X1	T38.7X2	T38.7X3	T38.7X4	T38.7X5	T38.7X6
Methane	T59.891	T59.892	T59.893	T59.894	—	—
Methanethiol	T59.891	T59.892	T59.893	T59.894	—	—
Methaniazide	T37.1X1	T37.1X2	T37.1X3	T37.1X4	T37.1X5	T37.1X6
Methanol (vapor)	T51.1X1	T51.1X2	T51.1X3	T51.1X4	—	—
Methantheline	T44.3X1	T44.3X2	T44.3X3	T44.3X4	T44.3X5	T44.3X6
Methanthelinium bromide	T44.3X1	T44.3X2	T44.3X3	T44.3X4	T44.3X5	T44.3X6
Methaphenilene	T45.0X1	T45.0X2	T45.0X3	T45.0X4	T45.0X5	T45.0X6
Methapyrilene	T45.0X1	T45.0X2	T45.0X3	T45.0X4	T45.0X5	T45.0X6
Methaqualone (compound)	T42.6X1	T42.6X2	T42.6X3	T42.6X4	T42.6X5	T42.6X6
Metharbital	T42.3X1	T42.3X2	T42.3X3	T42.3X4	T42.3X5	T42.3X6
Methazolamide	T50.2X1	T50.2X2	T50.2X3	T50.2X4	T50.2X5	T50.2X6
Methdilazine	T43.3X1	T43.3X2	T43.3X3	T43.3X4	T43.3X5	T43.3X6
Methedrine	T43.621	T43.622	T43.623	T43.624	T43.625	T43.626
Methenamine (mandelate)	T37.8X1	T37.8X2	T37.8X3	T37.8X4	T37.8X5	T37.8X6
Methenolone	T38.7X1	T38.7X2	T38.7X3	T38.7X4	T38.7X5	T38.7X6
Methergine	T48.0X1	T48.0X2	T48.0X3	T48.0X4	T48.0X5	T48.0X6
Methetoin	T42.0X1	T42.0X2	T42.0X3	T42.0X4	T42.0X5	T42.0X6
Methiacil	T38.2X1	T38.2X2	T38.2X3	T38.2X4	T38.2X5	T38.2X6
Methicillin	T36.0X1	T36.0X2	T36.0X3	T36.0X4	T36.0X5	T36.0X6
Methimazole	T38.2X1	T38.2X2	T38.2X3	T38.2X4	T38.2X5	T38.2X6
Methiodal sodium	T50.8X1	T50.8X2	T50.8X3	T50.8X4	T50.8X5	T50.8X6
Methionine	T50.991	T50.992	T50.993	T50.994	T50.995	T50.996
Methisazone	T37.5X1	T37.5X2	T37.5X3	T37.5X4	T37.5X5	T37.5X6
Methisoprinol	T37.5X1	T37.5X2	T37.5X3	T37.5X4	T37.5X5	T37.5X6
Methitural	T42.3X1	T42.3X2	T42.3X3	T42.3X4	T42.3X5	T42.3X6
Methixene	T44.3X1	T44.3X2	T44.3X3	T44.3X4	T44.3X5	T44.3X6
Methobarbital, methobarbitone	T42.3X1	T42.3X2	T42.3X3	T42.3X4	T42.3X5	T42.3X6
Methocarbamol	T42.8X1	T42.8X2	T42.8X3	T42.8X4	T42.8X5	T42.8X6
skeletal muscle relaxant	T48.1X1	T48.1X2	T48.1X3	T48.1X4	T48.1X5	T48.1X6
Methohexital	T41.1X1	T41.1X2	T41.1X3	T41.1X4	T41.1X5	T41.1X6
Methohexitone	T41.1X1	T41.1X2	T41.1X3	T41.1X4	T41.1X5	T41.1X6
Methoin	T42.0X1	T42.0X2	T42.0X3	T42.0X4	T42.0X5	T42.0X6
Methopholine	T39.8X1	T39.8X2	T39.8X3	T39.8X4	T39.8X5	T39.8X6
Methopromazine	T43.3X1	T43.3X2	T43.3X3	T43.3X4	T43.3X5	T43.3X6
Methorate	T48.3X1	T48.3X2	T48.3X3	T48.3X4	T48.3X5	T48.3X6
Methoserpidine	T46.5X1	T46.5X2	T46.5X3	T46.5X4	T46.5X5	T46.5X6
Methotrexate	T45.1X1	T45.1X2	T45.1X3	T45.1X4	T45.1X5	T45.1X6
Methotrimeprazine	T43.3X1	T43.3X2	T43.3X3	T43.3X4	T43.3X5	T43.3X6
Methoxa-Dome	T49.3X1	T49.3X2	T49.3X3	T49.3X4	T49.3X5	T49.3X6
Methoxamine	T44.4X1	T44.4X2	T44.4X3	T44.4X4	T44.4X5	T44.4X6
Methoxsalen	T50.991	T50.992	T50.993	T50.994	T50.995	T50.996
Methoxyaniline	T65.3X1	T65.3X2	T65.3X3	T65.3X4	—	—
Methoxybenzyl penicillin	T36.0X1	T36.0X2	T36.0X3	T36.0X4	T36.0X5	T36.0X6
Methoxychlor	T53.7X1	T53.7X2	T53.7X3	T53.7X4	—	—
Methoxy-DDT	T53.7X1	T53.7X2	T53.7X3	T53.7X4	—	—
Methoxyflurane	T41.0X1	T41.0X2	T41.0X3	T41.0X4	T41.0X5	T41.0X6
Methoxyphenamine	T48.6X1	T48.6X2	T48.6X3	T48.6X4	T48.6X5	T48.6X6
Methoxypromazine	T43.3X1	T43.3X2	T43.3X3	T43.3X4	T43.3X5	T43.3X6
Methscopolamine bromide	T44.3X1	T44.3X2	T44.3X3	T44.3X4	T44.3X5	T44.3X6
Methsuximide	T42.2X1	T42.2X2	T42.2X3	T42.2X4	T42.2X5	T42.2X6
Methyclothiazide	T50.2X1	T50.2X2	T50.2X3	T50.2X4	T50.2X5	T50.2X6
Methyl						
acetate	T52.4X1	T52.4X2	T52.4X3	T52.4X4	—	—
acetone	T52.4X1	T52.4X2	T52.4X3	T52.4X4	—	—
acrylate	T65.891	T65.892	T65.893	T65.894	—	—
alcohol	T51.1X1	T51.1X2	T51.1X3	T51.1X4	—	—
aminophenol	T65.3X1	T65.3X2	T65.3X3	T65.3X4	—	—
amphetamine	T43.621	T43.622	T43.623	T43.624	T43.625	T43.626
androstanolone	T38.7X1	T38.7X2	T38.7X3	T38.7X4	T38.7X5	T38.7X6
atropine	T44.3X1	T44.3X2	T44.3X3	T44.3X4	T44.3X5	T44.3X6
benzene	T52.2X1	T52.2X2	T52.2X3	T52.2X4	—	—
benzoate	T52.8X1	T52.8X2	T52.8X3	T52.8X4	—	—
benzol	T52.2X1	T52.2X2	T52.2X3	T52.2X4	—	—
bromide (gas)	T59.891	T59.892	T59.893	T59.894	—	—
fumigant	T60.8X1	T60.8X2	T60.8X3	T60.8X4	—	—
butanol	T51.3X1	T51.3X2	T51.3X3	T51.3X4	—	—
carbinol	T51.1X1	T51.1X2	T51.1X3	T51.1X4	—	—
carbonate	T52.8X1	T52.8X2	T52.8X3	T52.8X4	—	—
CCNU	T45.1X1	T45.1X2	T45.1X3	T45.1X4	T45.1X5	T45.1X6
cellosolve	T52.91	T52.92	T52.93	T52.94	—	—
cellulose	T47.4X1	T47.4X2	T47.4X3	T47.4X4	T47.4X5	T47.4X6
chloride (gas)	T59.891	T59.892	T59.893	T59.894	—	—
chloroformate	T59.3X1	T59.3X2	T59.3X3	T59.3X4	—	—
cyclohexane	T52.8X1	T52.8X2	T52.8X3	T52.8X4	—	—
cyclohexanol	T51.8X1	T51.8X2	T51.8X3	T51.8X4	—	—

Substance	Poisoning, Accidental (unintentional)	Poisoning, Intentional Self-harm	Poisoning, Assault	Poisoning, Undetermined	Adverse Effect	Under-dosing
Methyl — *continued*						
cyclohexanone	T52.8X1	T52.8X2	T52.8X3	T52.8X4	—	—
cyclohexyl acetate	T52.8X1	T52.8X2	T52.8X3	T52.8X4	—	—
demeton	T60.0X1	T60.0X2	T60.0X3	T60.0X4	—	—
dihydromorphinone	T40.2X1	T40.2X2	T40.2X3	T40.2X4	T40.2X5	T40.2X6
ergometrine	T48.0X1	T48.0X2	T48.0X3	T48.0X4	T48.0X5	T48.0X6
ergonovine	T48.0X1	T48.0X2	T48.0X3	T48.0X4	T48.0X5	T48.0X6
ethyl ketone	T52.4X1	T52.4X2	T52.4X3	T52.4X4	—	—
glucamine antimonate	T37.8X1	T37.8X2	T37.8X3	T37.8X4	T37.8X5	T37.8X6
hydrazine	T65.891	T65.892	T65.893	T65.894	—	—
iodide	T65.891	T65.892	T65.893	T65.894	—	—
isobutyl ketone	T52.4X1	T52.4X2	T52.4X3	T52.4X4	—	—
isothiocyanate	T60.3X1	T60.3X2	T60.3X3	T60.3X4	—	—
mercaptan	T59.891	T59.892	T59.893	T59.894	—	—
morphine NEC	T40.2X1	T40.2X2	T40.2X3	T40.2X4	T40.2X5	T40.2X6
nicotinate	T49.4X1	T49.4X2	T49.4X3	T49.4X4	T49.4X5	T49.4X6
paraben	T49.0X1	T49.0X2	T49.0X3	T49.0X4	T49.0X5	T49.0X6
parafynol	T42.6X1	T42.6X2	T42.6X3	T42.6X4	T42.6X5	T42.6X6
parathion	T60.0X1	T60.0X2	T60.0X3	T60.0X4	—	—
peridol	T43.4X1	T43.4X2	T43.4X3	T43.4X4	T43.4X5	T43.4X6
phenidate	T43.631	T43.632	T43.633	T43.634	T43.635	T43.636
prednisolone	T38.0X1	T38.0X2	T38.0X3	T38.0X4	T38.0X5	T38.0X6
ENT agent	T49.6X1	T49.6X2	T49.6X3	T49.6X4	T49.6X5	T49.6X6
ophthalmic preparation	T49.5X1	T49.5X2	T49.5X3	T49.5X4	T49.5X5	T49.5X6
topical NEC	T49.0X1	T49.0X2	T49.0X3	T49.0X4	T49.0X5	T49.0X6
propylcarbinol	T51.3X1	T51.3X2	T51.3X3	T51.3X4	—	—
rosaniline NEC	T49.0X1	T49.0X2	T49.0X3	T49.0X4	T49.0X5	T49.0X6
salicylate	T49.2X1	T49.2X2	T49.2X3	T49.2X4	T49.2X5	T49.2X6
sulfate (fumes)	T59.891	T59.892	T59.893	T59.894	—	—
liquid	T52.8X1	T52.8X2	T52.8X3	T52.8X4	—	—
sulfonal	T42.6X1	T42.6X2	T42.6X3	T42.6X4	T42.6X5	T42.6X6
testosterone	T38.7X1	T38.7X2	T38.7X3	T38.7X4	T38.7X5	T38.7X6
thiouracil	T38.2X1	T38.2X2	T38.2X3	T38.2X4	T38.2X5	T38.2X6
Methylamphetamine	T43.621	T43.622	T43.623	T43.624	T43.625	T43.626
Methylated spirit	T51.1X1	T51.1X2	T51.1X3	T51.1X4	—	—
Methylatropine nitrate	T44.3X1	T44.3X2	T44.3X3	T44.3X4	T44.3X5	T44.3X6
Methylbenactyzium bromide	T44.3X1	T44.3X2	T44.3X3	T44.3X4	T44.3X5	T44.3X6
Methylbenzethonium chloride	T49.0X1	T49.0X2	T49.0X3	T49.0X4	T49.0X5	T49.0X6
Methylcellulose	T47.4X1	T47.4X2	T47.4X3	T47.4X4	T47.4X5	T47.4X6
laxative	T47.4X1	T47.4X2	T47.4X3	T47.4X4	T47.4X5	T47.4X6
Methylchlorophenoxyacetic acid	T60.3X1	T60.3X2	T60.3X3	T60.3X4	—	—
Methyldopa	T46.5X1	T46.5X2	T46.5X3	T46.5X4	T46.5X5	T46.5X6
Methyldopate	T46.5X1	T46.5X2	T46.5X3	T46.5X4	T46.5X5	T46.5X6
Methylene						
blue	T50.6X1	T50.6X2	T50.6X3	T50.6X4	T50.6X5	T50.6X6
chloride or dichloride (solvent) NEC	T53.4X1	T53.4X2	T53.4X3	T53.4X4	—	—
Methylenedioxyamphetamine	T43.621	T43.622	T43.623	T43.624	T43.625	T43.626
Methylenedioxymeth-amphetamine	T43.641	T43.642	T43.643	T43.644	—	—
Methylergometrine	T48.0X1	T48.0X2	T48.0X3	T48.0X4	T48.0X5	T48.0X6
Methylergonovine	T48.0X1	T48.0X2	T48.0X3	T48.0X4	T48.0X5	T48.0X6
Methylestrenolone	T38.5X1	T38.5X2	T38.5X3	T38.5X4	T38.5X5	T38.5X6
Methylethyl cellulose	T50.991	T50.992	T50.993	T50.994	T50.995	T50.996
Methylhexabital	T42.3X1	T42.3X2	T42.3X3	T42.3X4	T42.3X5	T42.3X6
Methylmorphine	T40.2X1	T40.2X2	T40.2X3	T40.2X4	T40.2X5	T40.2X6
Methylparaben (ophthalmic)	T49.5X1	T49.5X2	T49.5X3	T49.5X4	T49.5X5	T49.5X6
Methylparafynol	T42.6X1	T42.6X2	T42.6X3	T42.6X4	T42.6X5	T42.6X6
Methylpentynol, methylpenthynol	T42.6X1	T42.6X2	T42.6X3	T42.6X4	T42.6X5	T42.6X6
Methylphenidate	T43.631	T43.632	T43.633	T43.634	T43.635	T43.636
Methylphenobarbital	T42.3X1	T42.3X2	T42.3X3	T42.3X4	T42.3X5	T42.3X6
Methylpolysiloxane	T47.1X1	T47.1X2	T47.1X3	T47.1X4	T47.1X5	T47.1X6
Methylprednisolone — *see Methyl, prednisolone*						
Methylrosaniline	T49.0X1	T49.0X2	T49.0X3	T49.0X4	T49.0X5	T49.0X6
Methylrosanilinium chloride	T49.0X1	T49.0X2	T49.0X3	T49.0X4	T49.0X5	T49.0X6
Methyltestosterone	T38.7X1	T38.7X2	T38.7X3	T38.7X4	T38.7X5	T38.7X6
Methylthionine chloride	T50.6X1	T50.6X2	T50.6X3	T50.6X4	T50.6X5	T50.6X6
Methylthioninium chloride	T50.6X1	T50.6X2	T50.6X3	T50.6X4	T50.6X5	T50.6X6
Methylthiouracil	T38.2X1	T38.2X2	T38.2X3	T38.2X4	T38.2X5	T38.2X6
Methyprylon	T42.6X1	T42.6X2	T42.6X3	T42.6X4	T42.6X5	T42.6X6
Methysergide	T46.5X1	T46.5X2	T46.5X3	T46.5X4	T46.5X5	T46.5X6
Metiamide	T47.1X1	T47.1X2	T47.1X3	T47.1X4	T47.1X5	T47.1X6
Meticillin	T36.0X1	T36.0X2	T36.0X3	T36.0X4	T36.0X5	T36.0X6
Meticrane	T50.2X1	T50.2X2	T50.2X3	T50.2X4	T50.2X5	T50.2X6
Metildigoxin	T46.0X1	T46.0X2	T46.0X3	T46.0X4	T46.0X5	T46.0X6

Substance	Poisoning, Accidental (unintentional)	Poisoning, Intentional Self-harm	Poisoning, Assault	Poisoning, Undetermined	Adverse Effect	Under-dosing
Metipranolol	T49.5X1	T49.5X2	T49.5X3	T49.5X4	T49.5X5	T49.5X6
Metirosine	T46.5X1	T46.5X2	T46.5X3	T46.5X4	T46.5X5	T46.5X6
Metisazone	T37.5X1	T37.5X2	T37.5X3	T37.5X4	T37.5X5	T37.5X6
Metixene	T44.3X1	T44.3X2	T44.3X3	T44.3X4	T44.3X5	T44.3X6
Metizoline	T48.5X1	T48.5X2	T48.5X3	T48.5X4	T48.5X5	T48.5X6
Metoclopramide	T45.0X1	T45.0X2	T45.0X3	T45.0X4	T45.0X5	T45.0X6
Metofenazate	T43.3X1	T43.3X2	T43.3X3	T43.3X4	T43.3X5	T43.3X6
Metofoline	T39.8X1	T39.8X2	T39.8X3	T39.8X4	T39.8X5	T39.8X6
Metolazone	T50.2X1	T50.2X2	T50.2X3	T50.2X4	T50.2X5	T50.2X6
Metopon	T40.2X1	T40.2X2	T40.2X3	T40.2X4	T40.2X5	T40.2X6
Metoprine	T45.1X1	T45.1X2	T45.1X3	T45.1X4	T45.1X5	T45.1X6
Metoprolol	T44.7X1	T44.7X2	T44.7X3	T44.7X4	T44.7X5	T44.7X6
Metrifonate	T60.0X1	T60.0X2	T60.0X3	T60.0X4	—	—
Metrizamide	T50.8X1	T50.8X2	T50.8X3	T50.8X4	T50.8X5	T50.8X6
Metrizoic acid	T50.8X1	T50.8X2	T50.8X3	T50.8X4	T50.8X5	T50.8X6
Metronidazole	T37.8X1	T37.8X2	T37.8X3	T37.8X4	T37.8X5	T37.8X6
Metycaine	T41.3X1	T41.3X2	T41.3X3	T41.3X4	T41.3X5	T41.3X6
infiltration (subcutaneous)	T41.3X1	T41.3X2	T41.3X3	T41.3X4	T41.3X5	T41.3X6
nerve block (peripheral) (plexus)	T41.3X1	T41.3X2	T41.3X3	T41.3X4	T41.3X5	T41.3X6
topical (surface)	T41.3X1	T41.3X2	T41.3X3	T41.3X4	T41.3X5	T41.3X6
Metyrapone	T50.8X1	T50.8X2	T50.8X3	T50.8X4	T50.8X5	T50.8X6
Mevinphos	T60.0X1	T60.0X2	T60.0X3	T60.0X4	—	—
Mexazolam	T42.4X1	T42.4X2	T42.4X3	T42.4X4	T42.4X5	T42.4X6
Mexenone	T49.3X1	T49.3X2	T49.3X3	T49.3X4	T49.3X5	T49.3X6
Mexiletine	T46.2X1	T46.2X2	T46.2X3	T46.2X4	T46.2X5	T46.2X6
Mezereon	T62.2X1	T62.2X2	T62.2X3	T62.2X4	—	—
berries	T62.1X1	T62.1X2	T62.1X3	T62.1X4	—	—
Mezlocillin	T36.0X1	T36.0X2	T36.0X3	T36.0X4	T36.0X5	T36.0X6
Mianserin	T43.021	T43.022	T43.023	T43.024	T43.025	T43.026
Micatin	T49.0X1	T49.0X2	T49.0X3	T49.0X4	T49.0X5	T49.0X6
Miconazole	T49.0X1	T49.0X2	T49.0X3	T49.0X4	T49.0X5	T49.0X6
Micronomicin	T36.5X1	T36.5X2	T36.5X3	T36.5X4	T36.5X5	T36.5X6
Midazolam	T42.4X1	T42.4X2	T42.4X3	T42.4X4	T42.4X5	T42.4X6
Midecamycin	T36.3X1	T36.3X2	T36.3X3	T36.3X4	T36.3X5	T36.3X6
Mifepristone	T38.6X1	T38.6X2	T38.6X3	T38.6X4	T38.6X5	T38.6X6
Milk of magnesia	T47.1X1	T47.1X2	T47.1X3	T47.1X4	T47.1X5	T47.1X6
Millipede (tropical) (venomous)	T63.411	T63.412	T63.413	T63.414	—	—
Miltown	T43.591	T43.592	T43.593	T43.594	T43.595	T43.596
Milverine	T44.3X1	T44.3X2	T44.3X3	T44.3X4	T44.3X5	T44.3X6
Minaprine	T43.291	T43.292	T43.293	T43.294	T43.295	T43.296
Minaxolone	T41.291	T41.292	T41.293	T41.294	T41.295	T41.296
Mineral						
acids	T54.2X1	T54.2X2	T54.2X3	T54.2X4	—	—
oil (laxative)(medicinal)	T47.4X1	T47.4X2	T47.4X3	T47.4X4	T47.4X5	T47.4X6
emulsion	T47.2X1	T47.2X2	T47.2X3	T47.2X4	T47.2X5	T47.2X6
nonmedicinal	T52.0X1	T52.0X2	T52.0X3	T52.0X4	—	—
topical	T49.3X1	T49.3X2	T49.3X3	T49.3X4	T49.3X5	T49.3X6
salt NEC	T50.3X1	T50.3X2	T50.3X3	T50.3X4	T50.3X5	T50.3X6
spirits	T52.0X1	T52.0X2	T52.0X3	T52.0X4	—	—
Mineralocorticosteroid	T50.0X1	T50.0X2	T50.0X3	T50.0X4	T50.0X5	T50.0X6
Minocycline	T36.4X1	T36.4X2	T36.4X3	T36.4X4	T36.4X5	T36.4X6
Minoxidil	T46.7X1	T46.7X2	T46.7X3	T46.7X4	T46.7X5	T46.7X6
Miokamycin	T36.3X1	T36.3X2	T36.3X3	T36.3X4	T36.3X5	T36.3X6
Miotic drug	T49.5X1	T49.5X2	T49.5X3	T49.5X4	T49.5X5	T49.5X6
Mipafox	T60.0X1	T60.0X2	T60.0X3	T60.0X4	—	—
Mirex	T60.1X1	T60.1X2	T60.1X3	T60.1X4	—	—
Mirtazapine	T43.021	T43.022	T43.023	T43.024	T43.025	T43.026
Misonidazole	T37.3X1	T37.3X2	T37.3X3	T37.3X4	T37.3X5	T37.3X6
Misoprostol	T47.1X1	T47.1X2	T47.1X3	T47.1X4	T47.1X5	T47.1X6
Mithramycin	T45.1X1	T45.1X2	T45.1X3	T45.1X4	T45.1X5	T45.1X6
Mitobronitol	T45.1X1	T45.1X2	T45.1X3	T45.1X4	T45.1X5	T45.1X6
Mitoguazone	T45.1X1	T45.1X2	T45.1X3	T45.1X4	T45.1X5	T45.1X6
Mitolactol	T45.1X1	T45.1X2	T45.1X3	T45.1X4	T45.1X5	T45.1X6
Mitomycin	T45.1X1	T45.1X2	T45.1X3	T45.1X4	T45.1X5	T45.1X6
Mitopodozide	T45.1X1	T45.1X2	T45.1X3	T45.1X4	T45.1X5	T45.1X6
Mitotane	T45.1X1	T45.1X2	T45.1X3	T45.1X4	T45.1X5	T45.1X6
Mitoxantrone	T45.1X1	T45.1X2	T45.1X3	T45.1X4	T45.1X5	T45.1X6
Mivacurium chloride	T48.1X1	T48.1X2	T48.1X3	T48.1X4	T48.1X5	T48.1X6
Miyari bacteria	T47.6X1	T47.6X2	T47.6X3	T47.6X4	T47.6X5	T47.6X6
Moclobemide	T43.1X1	T43.1X2	T43.1X3	T43.1X4	T43.1X5	T43.1X6
Moderil	T46.5X1	T46.5X2	T46.5X3	T46.5X4	T46.5X5	T46.5X6
Mofebutazone	T39.2X1	T39.2X2	T39.2X3	T39.2X4	T39.2X5	T39.2X6
Mogadon — *see* Nitrazepam						
Molindone	T43.591	T43.592	T43.593	T43.594	T43.595	T43.596
Molsidomine	T46.3X1	T46.3X2	T46.3X3	T46.3X4	T46.3X5	T46.3X6
Mometasone	T49.0X1	T49.0X2	T49.0X3	T49.0X4	T49.0X5	T49.0X6
Monistat	T49.0X1	T49.0X2	T49.0X3	T49.0X4	T49.0X5	T49.0X6
Monkshood	T62.2X1	T62.2X2	T62.2X3	T62.2X4	—	—
Monoamine oxidase inhibitor NEC	T43.1X1	T43.1X2	T43.1X3	T43.1X4	T43.1X5	T43.1X6
hydrazine	T43.1X1	T43.1X2	T43.1X3	T43.1X4	T43.1X5	T43.1X6

Substance	Poisoning, Accidental (unintentional)	Poisoning, Intentional Self-harm	Poisoning, Assault	Poisoning, Undetermined	Adverse Effect	Under-dosing
Monobenzone	T49.4X1	T49.4X2	T49.4X3	T49.4X4	T49.4X5	T49.4X6
Monochloroacetic acid	T60.3X1	T60.3X2	T60.3X3	T60.3X4	—	—
Monochlorobenzene	T53.7X1	T53.7X2	T53.7X3	T53.7X4	—	—
Monoethanolamine	T46.8X1	T46.8X2	T46.8X3	T46.8X4	T46.8X5	T46.8X6
oleate	T46.8X1	T46.8X2	T46.8X3	T46.8X4	T46.8X5	T46.8X6
Monooctanoin	T50.991	T50.992	T50.993	T50.994	T50.995	T50.996
Monophenylbutazone	T39.2X1	T39.2X2	T39.2X3	T39.2X4	T39.2X5	T39.2X6
Monosodium glutamate	T65.891	T65.892	T65.893	T65.894	—	—
Monosulfiram	T49.0X1	T49.0X2	T49.0X3	T49.0X4	T49.0X5	T49.0X6
Monoxide, carbon — *see* Carbon, monoxide						
Monoxidine hydrochloride	T46.1X1	T46.1X2	T46.1X3	T46.1X4	T46.1X5	T46.1X6
Monuron	T60.3X1	T60.3X2	T60.3X3	T60.3X4	—	—
Moperone	T43.4X1	T43.4X2	T43.4X3	T43.4X4	T43.4X5	T43.4X6
Mopidamol	T45.1X1	T45.1X2	T45.1X3	T45.1X4	T45.1X5	T45.1X6
MOPP (mechloreth-amine + vincristine + prednisone + procarba-zine)	T45.1X1	T45.1X2	T45.1X3	T45.1X4	T45.1X5	T45.1X6
Morfin	T40.2X1	T40.2X2	T40.2X3	T40.2X4	T40.2X5	T40.2X6
Morinamide	T37.1X1	T37.1X2	T37.1X3	T37.1X4	T37.1X5	T37.1X6
Morning glory seeds	T40.991	T40.992	T40.993	T40.994	—	—
Moroxydine	T37.5X1	T37.5X2	T37.5X3	T37.5X4	T37.5X5	T37.5X6
Morphazinamide	T37.1X1	T37.1X2	T37.1X3	T37.1X4	T37.1X5	T37.1X6
Morphine	T40.2X1	T40.2X2	T40.2X3	T40.2X4	T40.2X5	T40.2X6
antagonist	T50.7X1	T50.7X2	T50.7X3	T50.7X4	T50.7X5	T50.7X6
Morpholinylethylmorphine	T40.2X1	T40.2X2	T40.2X3	T40.2X4		
Morsuximide	T42.2X1	T42.2X2	T42.2X3	T42.2X4	T42.2X5	T42.2X6
Mosapramine	T43.591	T43.592	T43.593	T43.594	T43.595	T43.596
Moth balls — *see also* Pesticides	T60.2X1	T60.2X2	T60.2X3	T60.2X4	—	—
naphthalene	T60.2X1	T60.2X2	T60.2X3	T60.2X4	—	—
paradichlorobenzene	T60.1X1	T60.1X2	T60.1X3	T60.1X4	—	—
Motor exhaust gas	T58.01	T58.02	T58.03	T58.04	—	—
Mouthwash (antiseptic) (zinc chloride)	T49.6X1	T49.6X2	T49.6X3	T49.6X4	T49.6X5	T49.6X6
Moxastine	T45.0X1	T45.0X2	T45.0X3	T45.0X4	T45.0X5	T45.0X6
Moxaverine	T44.3X1	T44.3X2	T44.3X3	T44.3X4	T44.3X5	T44.3X6
Moxisylyte	T46.7X1	T46.7X2	T46.7X3	T46.7X4	T46.7X5	T46.7X6
Mucilage, plant	T47.4X1	T47.4X2	T47.4X3	T47.4X4	T47.4X5	T47.4X6
Mucolytic drug	T48.4X1	T48.4X2	T48.4X3	T48.4X4	T48.4X5	T48.4X6
Mucomyst	T48.4X1	T48.4X2	T48.4X3	T48.4X4	T48.4X5	T48.4X6
Mucous membrane agents (external)	T49.91	T49.92	T49.93	T49.94	T49.95	T49.96
specified NEC	T49.8X1	T49.8X2	T49.8X3	T49.8X4	T49.8X5	T49.8X6
Multiple unspecified drugs, medicaments and biological substances	T50.911	T50.912	T50.913	T50.914	T50.915	T50.916
Mumps						
immune globulin (human)	T50.Z11	T50.Z12	T50.Z13	T50.Z14	T50.Z15	T50.Z16
skin test antigen	T50.8X1	T50.8X2	T50.8X3	T50.8X4	T50.8X5	T50.8X6
vaccine	T50.B91	T50.B92	T50.B93	T50.B94	T50.B95	T50.B96
Mumpsvax	T50.B91	T50.B92	T50.B93	T50.B94	T50.B95	T50.B96
Mupirocin	T49.0X1	T49.0X2	T49.0X3	T49.0X4	T49.0X5	T49.0X6
Muriatic acid — *see* Hydrochloric acid						
Muromonab-CD3	T45.1X1	T45.1X2	T45.1X3	T45.1X4	T45.1X5	T45.1X6
Muscle-action drug NEC	T48.201	T48.202	T48.203	T48.204	T48.205	T48.206
Muscle affecting agents NEC	T48.201	T48.202	T48.203	T48.204	T48.205	T48.206
oxytocic	T48.0X1	T48.0X2	T48.0X3	T48.0X4	T48.0X5	T48.0X6
relaxants	T48.201	T48.202	T48.203	T48.204	T48.205	T48.206
central nervous system	T42.8X1	T42.8X2	T42.8X3	T42.8X4	T42.8X5	T42.8X6
skeletal	T48.1X1	T48.1X2	T48.1X3	T48.1X4	T48.1X5	T48.1X6
smooth	T44.3X1	T44.3X2	T44.3X3	T44.3X4	T44.3X5	T44.3X6
Muscle relaxant — *see* Relaxant, muscle						
Muscle-tone depressant, central NEC	T42.8X1	T42.8X2	T42.8X3	T42.8X4	T42.8X5	T42.8X6
specified NEC	T42.8X1	T42.8X2	T42.8X3	T42.8X4	T42.8X5	T42.8X6
Mushroom, noxious	T62.0X1	T62.0X2	T62.0X3	T62.0X4	—	—
Mussel, noxious	T61.781	T61.782	T61.783	T61.784	—	—
Mustard (emetic)	T47.7X1	T47.7X2	T47.7X3	T47.7X4	T47.7X5	T47.7X6
black	T47.7X1	T47.7X2	T47.7X3	T47.7X4	T47.7X5	T47.7X6
gas, not in war	T59.91	T59.92	T59.93	T59.94	—	—
nitrogen	T45.1X1	T45.1X2	T45.1X3	T45.1X4	T45.1X5	T45.1X6
Mustine	T45.1X1	T45.1X2	T45.1X3	T45.1X4	T45.1X5	T45.1X6
M-vac	T45.1X1	T45.1X2	T45.1X3	T45.1X4	T45.1X5	T45.1X6
Mycifradin	T36.5X1	T36.5X2	T36.5X3	T36.5X4	T36.5X5	T36.5X6
topical	T49.0X1	T49.0X2	T49.0X3	T49.0X4	T49.0X5	T49.0X6
Mycitracin	T36.8X1	T36.8X2	T36.8X3	T36.8X4	T36.8X5	T36.8X6
ophthalmic preparation	T49.5X1	T49.5X2	T49.5X3	T49.5X4	T49.5X5	T49.5X6
Mycostatin	T36.7X1	T36.7X2	T36.7X3	T36.7X4	T36.7X5	T36.7X6
topical	T49.0X1	T49.0X2	T49.0X3	T49.0X4	T49.0X5	T49.0X6

Substance	Poisoning, Accidental (unintentional)	Poisoning, Intentional Self-harm	Poisoning, Assault	Poisoning, Undetermined	Adverse Effect	Under-dosing
Mycotoxins	T64.81	T64.82	T64.83	T64.84	—	—
aflatoxin	T64.01	T64.02	T64.03	T64.04	—	—
specified NEC	T64.81	T64.82	T64.83	T64.84	—	—
Mydriacyl	T44.3X1	T44.3X2	T44.3X3	T44.3X4	T44.3X5	T44.3X6
Mydriatic drug	T49.5X1	T49.5X2	T49.5X3	T49.5X4	T49.5X5	T49.5X6
Myelobromal	T45.1X1	T45.1X2	T45.1X3	T45.1X4	T45.1X5	T45.1X6
Myleran	T45.1X1	T45.1X2	T45.1X3	T45.1X4	T45.1X5	T45.1X6
Myochrysin (e)	T39.2X1	T39.2X2	T39.2X3	T39.2X4	T39.2X5	T39.2X6
Myoneural blocking agents	T48.1X1	T48.1X2	T48.1X3	T48.1X4	T48.1X5	T48.1X6
Myralact	T49.0X1	T49.0X2	T49.0X3	T49.0X4	T49.0X5	T49.0X6
Myristica fragrans	T62.2X1	T62.2X2	T62.2X3	T62.2X4	—	—
Myristicin	T65.891	T65.892	T65.893	T65.894	—	—
Mysoline	T42.3X1	T42.3X2	T42.3X3	T42.3X4	T42.3X5	T42.3X6
Nabilone	T40.7X1	T40.7X2	T40.7X3	T40.7X4	T40.7X5	T40.7X6
Nabumetone	T39.391	T39.392	T39.393	T39.394	T39.395	T39.396
Nadolol	T44.7X1	T44.7X2	T44.7X3	T44.7X4	T44.7X5	T44.7X6
Nafcillin	T36.0X1	T36.0X2	T36.0X3	T36.0X4	T36.0X5	T36.0X6
Nafoxidine	T38.6X1	T38.6X2	T38.6X3	T38.6X4	T38.6X5	T38.6X6
Naftazone	T46.991	T46.992	T46.993	T46.994	T46.995	T46.996
Naftidrofuryl (oxalate)	T46.7X1	T46.7X2	T46.7X3	T46.7X4	T46.7X5	T46.7X6
Naftifine	T49.0X1	T49.0X2	T49.0X3	T49.0X4	T49.0X5	T49.0X6
Nail polish remover	T52.91	T52.92	T52.93	T52.94	—	—
Nalbuphine	T40.491	T40.492	T40.493	T40.494	T40.495	T40.496
Naled	T60.0X1	T60.0X2	T60.0X3	T60.0X4	—	—
Nalidixic acid	T37.8X1	T37.8X2	T37.8X3	T37.8X4	T37.8X5	T37.8X6
Nalorphine	T50.7X1	T50.7X2	T50.7X3	T50.7X4	T50.7X5	T50.7X6
Naloxone	T50.7X1	T50.7X2	T50.7X3	T50.7X4	T50.7X5	T50.7X6
Naltrexone	T50.7X1	T50.7X2	T50.7X3	T50.7X4	T50.7X5	T50.7X6
Namenda	T43.8X1	T43.8X2	T43.8X3	T43.8X4	T43.8X5	T43.8X6
Nandrolone	T38.7X1	T38.7X2	T38.7X3	T38.7X4	T38.7X5	T38.7X6
Naphazoline	T48.5X1	T48.5X2	T48.5X3	T48.5X4	T48.5X5	T48.5X6
Naphtha (painters')	T52.0X1	T52.0X2	T52.0X3	T52.0X4	—	—
(petroleum)						
solvent	T52.0X1	T52.0X2	T52.0X3	T52.0X4	—	—
vapor	T52.0X1	T52.0X2	T52.0X3	T52.0X4	—	—
Naphthalene	T60.2X1	T60.2X2	T60.2X3	T60.2X4	—	—
(non-chlorinated)						
chlorinated	T60.1X1	T60.1X2	T60.1X3	T60.1X4	—	—
vapor	T60.1X1	T60.1X2	T60.1X3	T60.1X4	—	—
insecticide or moth repellent	T60.2X1	T60.2X2	T60.2X3	T60.2X4	—	—
chlorinated	T60.1X1	T60.1X2	T60.1X3	T60.1X4	—	—
vapor	T60.2X1	T60.2X2	T60.2X3	T60.2X4	—	—
chlorinated	T60.1X1	T60.1X2	T60.1X3	T60.1X4	—	—
Naphthol	T65.891	T65.892	T65.893	T65.894	—	—
Naphthylamine	T65.891	T65.892	T65.893	T65.894	—	—
Naphthylthiourea (ANTU)	T60.4X1	T60.4X2	T60.4X3	T60.4X4	—	—
Naprosyn — see Naproxen						
Naproxen	T39.311	T39.312	T39.313	T39.314	T39.315	T39.316
Narcotic (drug)	T40.601	T40.602	T40.603	T40.604	T40.605	T40.606
analgesic NEC	T40.601	T40.602	T40.603	T40.604	T40.605	T40.606
antagonist	T50.7X1	T50.7X2	T50.7X3	T50.7X4	T50.7X5	T50.7X6
specified NEC	T40.691	T40.692	T40.693	T40.694	T40.695	T40.696
synthetic	T40.491	T40.492	T40.493	T40.494	T40.495	T40.496
Narcotine	T48.3X1	T48.3X2	T48.3X3	T48.3X4	T48.3X5	T48.3X6
Nardil	T43.1X1	T43.1X2	T43.1X3	T43.1X4	T43.1X5	T43.1X6
Nasal drug NEC	T49.6X1	T49.6X2	T49.6X3	T49.6X4	T49.6X5	T49.6X6
Natamycin	T49.0X1	T49.0X2	T49.0X3	T49.0X4	T49.0X5	T49.0X6
Natrium cyanide — see Cyanide(s)						
Natural						
blood (product)	T45.8X1	T45.8X2	T45.8X3	T45.8X4	T45.8X5	T45.8X6
gas (piped)	T59.891	T59.892	T59.893	T59.894	—	—
incomplete combustion	T58.11	T58.12	T58.13	T58.14	—	—
Nealbarbital	T42.3X1	T42.3X2	T42.3X3	T42.3X4	T42.3X5	T42.3X6
Nectadon	T48.3X1	T48.3X2	T48.3X3	T48.3X4	T48.3X5	T48.3X6
Nedocromil	T48.6X1	T48.6X2	T48.6X3	T48.6X4	T48.6X5	T48.6X6
Nefopam	T39.8X1	T39.8X2	T39.8X3	T39.8X4	T39.8X5	T39.8X6
Nematocyst (sting)	T63.691	T63.692	T63.693	T63.694	—	—
Nembutal	T42.3X1	T42.3X2	T42.3X3	T42.3X4	T42.3X5	T42.3X6
Nemonapride	T43.591	T43.592	T43.593	T43.594	T43.595	T43.596
Neoarsphenamine	T37.8X1	T37.8X2	T37.8X3	T37.8X4	T37.8X5	T37.8X6
Neocinchophen	T50.4X1	T50.4X2	T50.4X3	T50.4X4	T50.4X5	T50.4X6
Neomycin (derivatives)	T36.5X1	T36.5X2	T36.5X3	T36.5X4	T36.5X5	T36.5X6
with						
bacitracin	T49.0X1	T49.0X2	T49.0X3	T49.0X4	T49.0X5	T49.0X6
neostigmine	T44.0X1	T44.0X2	T44.0X3	T44.0X4	T44.0X5	T44.0X6
ENT agent	T49.6X1	T49.6X2	T49.6X3	T49.6X4	T49.6X5	T49.6X6
ophthalmic preparation	T49.5X1	T49.5X2	T49.5X3	T49.5X4	T49.5X5	T49.5X6
topical NEC	T49.0X1	T49.0X2	T49.0X3	T49.0X4	T49.0X5	T49.0X6
Neonal	T42.3X1	T42.3X2	T42.3X3	T42.3X4	T42.3X5	T42.3X6
Neoprontosil	T37.0X1	T37.0X2	T37.0X3	T37.0X4	T37.0X5	T37.0X6

Substance	Poisoning, Accidental (unintentional)	Poisoning, Intentional Self-harm	Poisoning, Assault	Poisoning, Undetermined	Adverse Effect	Under-dosing
Neosalvarsan	T37.8X1	T37.8X2	T37.8X3	T37.8X4	T37.8X5	T37.8X6
Neosilversalvarsan	T37.8X1	T37.8X2	T37.8X3	T37.8X4	T37.8X5	T37.8X6
Neosporin	T36.8X1	T36.8X2	T36.8X3	T36.8X4	T36.8X5	T36.8X6
ENT agent	T49.6X1	T49.6X2	T49.6X3	T49.6X4	T49.6X5	T49.6X6
opthalmic preparation	T49.5X1	T49.5X2	T49.5X3	T49.5X4	T49.5X5	T49.5X6
topical NEC	T49.0X1	T49.0X2	T49.0X3	T49.0X4	T49.0X5	T49.0X6
Neostigmine bromide	T44.0X1	T44.0X2	T44.0X3	T44.0X4	T44.0X5	T44.0X6
Neraval	T42.3X1	T42.3X2	T42.3X3	T42.3X4	T42.3X5	T42.3X6
Neravan	T42.3X1	T42.3X2	T42.3X3	T42.3X4	T42.3X5	T42.3X6
Nerium oleander	T62.2X1	T62.2X2	T62.2X3	T62.2X4	—	—
Nerve gas, not in war	T59.91	T59.92	T59.93	T59.94	—	—
Nesacaine	T41.3X1	T41.3X2	T41.3X3	T41.3X4	T41.3X5	T41.3X6
infiltration (subcutaneous)	T41.3X1	T41.3X2	T41.3X3	T41.3X4	T41.3X5	T41.3X6
nerve block (peripheral) (plexus)	T41.3X1	T41.3X2	T41.3X3	T41.3X4	T41.3X5	T41.3X6
Netilmicin	T36.5X1	T36.5X2	T36.5X3	T36.5X4	T36.5X5	T36.5X6
Neurobarb	T42.3X1	T42.3X2	T42.3X3	T42.3X4	T42.3X5	T42.3X6
Neuroleptic drug NEC	T43.501	T43.502	T43.503	T43.504	T43.505	T43.506
Neuromuscular blocking drug	T48.1X1	T48.1X2	T48.1X3	T48.1X4	T48.1X5	T48.1X6
Neutral insulin injection	T38.3X1	T38.3X2	T38.3X3	T38.3X4	T38.3X5	T38.3X6
Neutral spirits	T51.0X1	T51.0X2	T51.0X3	T51.0X4	—	—
beverage	T51.0X1	T51.0X2	T51.0X3	T51.0X4	—	—
Niacin	T46.7X1	T46.7X2	T46.7X3	T46.7X4	T46.7X5	T46.7X6
Niacinamide	T45.2X1	T45.2X2	T45.2X3	T45.2X4	T45.2X5	T45.2X6
Nialamide	T43.1X1	T43.1X2	T43.1X3	T43.1X4	T43.1X5	T43.1X6
Niaprazine	T42.6X1	T42.6X2	T42.6X3	T42.6X4	T42.6X5	T42.6X6
Nicametate	T46.7X1	T46.7X2	T46.7X3	T46.7X4	T46.7X5	T46.7X6
Nicardipine	T46.1X1	T46.1X2	T46.1X3	T46.1X4	T46.1X5	T46.1X6
Nicergoline	T46.7X1	T46.7X2	T46.7X3	T46.7X4	T46.7X5	T46.7X6
Nickel (carbonyl) (tetra-carbonyl) (fumes) (vapor)	T56.891	T56.892	T56.893	T56.894	—	—
Nickelocene	T56.891	T56.892	T56.893	T56.894	—	—
Niclosamide	T37.4X1	T37.4X2	T37.4X3	T37.4X4	T37.4X5	T37.4X6
Nicofuranose	T46.7X1	T46.7X2	T46.7X3	T46.7X4	T46.7X5	T46.7X6
Nicomorphine	T40.2X1	T40.2X2	T40.2X3	T40.2X4	—	—
Nicorandil	T46.3X1	T46.3X2	T46.3X3	T46.3X4	T46.3X5	T46.3X6
Nicotiana (plant)	T62.2X1	T62.2X2	T62.2X3	T62.2X4	—	—
Nicotinamide	T45.2X1	T45.2X2	T45.2X3	T45.2X4	T45.2X5	T45.2X6
Nicotine (insecticide) (spray) (sulfate) **NEC**	T60.2X1	T60.2X2	T60.2X3	T60.2X4	—	—
from tobacco	T65.291	T65.292	T65.293	T65.294	—	—
cigarettes	T65.221	T65.222	T65.223	T65.224	—	—
not insecticide	T65.291	T65.292	T65.293	T65.294	—	—
Nicotinic acid	T46.7X1	T46.7X2	T46.7X3	T46.7X4	T46.7X5	T46.7X6
Nicotinyl alcohol	T46.7X1	T46.7X2	T46.7X3	T46.7X4	T46.7X5	T46.7X6
Nicoumalone	T45.511	T45.512	T45.513	T45.514	T45.515	T45.516
Nifedipine	T46.1X1	T46.1X2	T46.1X3	T46.1X4	T46.1X5	T46.1X6
Nifenazone	T39.2X1	T39.2X2	T39.2X3	T39.2X4	T39.2X5	T39.2X6
Nifuraldezone	T37.91	T37.92	T37.93	T37.94	T37.95	T37.96
Nifuratel	T37.8X1	T37.8X2	T37.8X3	T37.8X4	T37.8X5	T37.8X6
Nifurtimox	T37.3X1	T37.3X2	T37.3X3	T37.3X4	T37.3X5	T37.3X6
Nifurtoinol	T37.8X1	T37.8X2	T37.8X3	T37.8X4	T37.8X5	T37.8X6
Nightshade, deadly (solanum) — see also Belladonna	T62.2X1	T62.2X2	T62.2X3	T62.2X4	—	—
berry	T62.1X1	T62.1X2	T62.1X3	T62.1X4	—	—
Nikethamide	T50.7X1	T50.7X2	T50.7X3	T50.7X4	T50.7X5	T50.7X6
Nilstat	T36.7X1	T36.7X2	T36.7X3	T36.7X4	T36.7X5	T36.7X6
topical	T49.0X1	T49.0X2	T49.0X3	T49.0X4	T49.0X5	T49.0X6
Nilutamide	T38.6X1	T38.6X2	T38.6X3	T38.6X4	T38.6X5	T38.6X6
Nimesulide	T39.391	T39.392	T39.393	T39.394	T39.395	T39.396
Nimetazepam	T42.4X1	T42.4X2	T42.4X3	T42.4X4	T42.4X5	T42.4X6
Nimodipine	T46.1X1	T46.1X2	T46.1X3	T46.1X4	T46.1X5	T46.1X6
Nimorazole	T37.3X1	T37.3X2	T37.3X3	T37.3X4	T37.3X5	T37.3X6
Nimustine	T45.1X1	T45.1X2	T45.1X3	T45.1X4	T45.1X5	T45.1X6
Niridazole	T37.4X1	T37.4X2	T37.4X3	T37.4X4	T37.4X5	T37.4X6
Nisentil	T40.2X1	T40.2X2	T40.2X3	T40.2X4	T40.2X5	T40.2X6
Nisoldipine	T46.1X1	T46.1X2	T46.1X3	T46.1X4	T46.1X5	T46.1X6
Nitramine	T65.3X1	T65.3X2	T65.3X3	T65.3X4	—	—
Nitrate, organic	T46.3X1	T46.3X2	T46.3X3	T46.3X4	T46.3X5	T46.3X6
Nitrazepam	T42.4X1	T42.4X2	T42.4X3	T42.4X4	T42.4X5	T42.4X6
Nitrefazole	T50.6X1	T50.6X2	T50.6X3	T50.6X4	T50.6X5	T50.6X6
Nitrendipine	T46.1X1	T46.1X2	T46.1X3	T46.1X4	T46.1X5	T46.1X6
Nitric						
acid (liquid)	T54.2X1	T54.2X2	T54.2X3	T54.2X4	—	—
vapor	T59.891	T59.892	T59.893	T59.894	—	—
oxide (gas)	T59.0X1	T59.0X2	T59.0X3	T59.0X4	—	—
Nitrimidazine	T37.3X1	T37.3X2	T37.3X3	T37.3X4	T37.3X5	T37.3X6
Nitrite, amyl (medicinal) (vapor)	T46.3X1	T46.3X2	T46.3X3	T46.3X4	T46.3X5	T46.3X6
Nitroaniline	T65.3X1	T65.3X2	T65.3X3	T65.3X4	—	—
vapor	T59.891	T59.892	T59.893	T59.894	—	—
Nitrobenzene, nitrobenzol	T65.3X1	T65.3X2	T65.3X3	T65.3X4	—	—

Substance	Poisoning, Accidental (unintentional)	Poisoning, Intentional Self-harm	Poisoning, Assault	Poisoning, Undetermined	Adverse Effect	Under-dosing
Nitrobenzene, nitrobenzol — continued						
vapor	T65.3X1	T65.3X2	T65.3X3	T65.3X4	—	—
Nitrocellulose	T65.891	T65.892	T65.893	T65.894	—	—
lacquer	T65.891	T65.892	T65.893	T65.894	—	—
Nitrodiphenyl	T65.3X1	T65.3X2	T65.3X3	T65.3X4	—	—
Nitrofural	T49.0X1	T49.0X2	T49.0X3	T49.0X4	T49.0X5	T49.0X6
Nitrofurantoin	T37.8X1	T37.8X2	T37.8X3	T37.8X4	T37.8X5	T37.8X6
Nitrofurazone	T49.0X1	T49.0X2	T49.0X3	T49.0X4	T49.0X5	T49.0X6
Nitrogen	T59.0X1	T59.0X2	T59.0X3	T59.0X4	—	—
mustard	T45.1X1	T45.1X2	T45.1X3	T45.1X4	T45.1X5	T45.1X6
Nitroglycerin, nitroglycerol (medicinal)	T46.3X1	T46.3X2	T46.3X3	T46.3X4	T46.3X5	T46.3X6
nonmedicinal	T65.5X1	T65.5X2	T65.5X3	T65.5X4	—	—
fumes	T65.5X1	T65.5X2	T65.5X3	T65.5X4	—	—
Nitroglycol	T52.3X1	T52.3X2	T52.3X3	T52.3X4	—	—
Nitrohydrochloric acid	T54.2X1	T54.2X2	T54.2X3	T54.2X4	—	—
Nitromersol	T49.0X1	T49.0X2	T49.0X3	T49.0X4	T49.0X5	T49.0X6
Nitronaphthalene	T65.891	T65.892	T65.893	T65.894	—	—
Nitrophenol	T54.0X1	T54.0X2	T54.0X3	T54.0X4	—	—
Nitropropane	T52.8X1	T52.8X2	T52.8X3	T52.8X4	—	—
Nitroprusside	T46.5X1	T46.5X2	T46.5X3	T46.5X4	T46.5X5	T46.5X6
Nitrosodimethylamine	T65.3X1	T65.3X2	T65.3X3	T65.3X4	—	—
Nitrothiazol	T37.4X1	T37.4X2	T37.4X3	T37.4X4	T37.4X5	T37.4X6
Nitrotoluene, nitrotoluol	T65.3X1	T65.3X2	T65.3X3	T65.3X4	—	—
vapor	T65.3X1	T65.3X2	T65.3X3	T65.3X4	—	—
Nitrous						
acid (liquid)	T54.2X1	T54.2X2	T54.2X3	T54.2X4	—	—
fumes	T59.891	T59.892	T59.893	T59.894	—	—
ether spirit	T46.3X1	T46.3X2	T46.3X3	T46.3X4	T46.3X5	T46.3X6
oxide	T41.0X1	T41.0X2	T41.0X3	T41.0X4	T41.0X5	T41.0X6
Nitroxoline	T37.8X1	T37.8X2	T37.8X3	T37.8X4	T37.8X5	T37.8X6
Nitrozone	T49.0X1	T49.0X2	T49.0X3	T49.0X4	T49.0X5	T49.0X6
Nizatidine	T47.0X1	T47.0X2	T47.0X3	T47.0X4	T47.0X5	T47.0X6
Nizofenone	T43.8X1	T43.8X2	T43.8X3	T43.8X4	T43.8X5	T43.8X6
Noctec	T42.6X1	T42.6X2	T42.6X3	T42.6X4	T42.6X5	T42.6X6
Noludar	T42.6X1	T42.6X2	T42.6X3	T42.6X4	T42.6X5	T42.6X6
Nomegestrol	T38.5X1	T38.5X2	T38.5X3	T38.5X4	T38.5X5	T38.5X6
Nomifensine	T43.291	T43.292	T43.293	T43.294	T43.295	T43.296
Nonoxinol	T49.8X1	T49.8X2	T49.8X3	T49.8X4	T49.8X5	T49.8X6
Nonylphenoxy (polyethoxyethanol)	T49.8X1	T49.8X2	T49.8X3	T49.8X4	T49.8X5	T49.8X6
Noptil	T42.3X1	T42.3X2	T42.3X3	T42.3X4	T42.3X5	T42.3X6
Noradrenaline	T44.4X1	T44.4X2	T44.4X3	T44.4X4	T44.4X5	T44.4X6
Noramidopyrine	T39.2X1	T39.2X2	T39.2X3	T39.2X4	T39.2X5	T39.2X6
methanesulfonate sodium	T39.2X1	T39.2X2	T39.2X3	T39.2X4	T39.2X5	T39.2X6
Norbormide	T60.4X1	T60.4X2	T60.4X3	T60.4X4	—	—
Nordazepam	T42.4X1	T42.4X2	T42.4X3	T42.4X4	T42.4X5	T42.4X6
Norepinephrine	T44.4X1	T44.4X2	T44.4X3	T44.4X4	T44.4X5	T44.4X6
Norethandrolone	T38.7X1	T38.7X2	T38.7X3	T38.7X4	T38.7X5	T38.7X6
Norethindrone	T38.4X1	T38.4X2	T38.4X3	T38.4X4	T38.4X5	T38.4X6
Norethisterone (acetate)	T38.4X1	T38.4X2	T38.4X3	T38.4X4	T38.4X5	T38.4X6
(enantate)						
with ethinylestradiol	T38.5X1	T38.5X2	T38.5X3	T38.5X4	T38.5X5	T38.5X6
Noretynodrel	T38.5X1	T38.5X2	T38.5X3	T38.5X4	T38.5X5	T38.5X6
Norfenefrine	T44.4X1	T44.4X2	T44.4X3	T44.4X4	T44.4X5	T44.4X6
Norfloxacin	T36.8X1	T36.8X2	T36.8X3	T36.8X4	T36.8X5	T36.8X6
Norgestrel	T38.4X1	T38.4X2	T38.4X3	T38.4X4	T38.4X5	T38.4X6
Norgestrienone	T38.4X1	T38.4X2	T38.4X3	T38.4X4	T38.4X5	T38.4X6
Norlestrin	T38.4X1	T38.4X2	T38.4X3	T38.4X4	T38.4X5	T38.4X6
Norlutin	T38.4X1	T38.4X2	T38.4X3	T38.4X4	T38.4X5	T38.4X6
Normal serum albumin (human), salt-poor	T45.8X1	T45.8X2	T45.8X3	T45.8X4	T45.8X5	T45.8X6
Normethandrone	T38.5X1	T38.5X2	T38.5X3	T38.5X4	T38.5X5	T38.5X6
Normison — see Benzodiazepines						
Normorphine	T40.2X1	T40.2X2	T40.2X3	T40.2X4	—	—
Norpseudoephedrine	T50.5X1	T50.5X2	T50.5X3	T50.5X4	T50.5X5	T50.5X6
Nortestosterone (furanpropionate)	T38.7X1	T38.7X2	T38.7X3	T38.7X4	T38.7X5	T38.7X6
Nortriptyline	T43.011	T43.012	T43.013	T43.014	T43.015	T43.016
Noscapine	T48.3X1	T48.3X2	T48.3X3	T48.3X4	T48.3X5	T48.3X6
Nose preparations	T49.6X1	T49.6X2	T49.6X3	T49.6X4	T49.6X5	T49.6X6
Novobiocin	T36.5X1	T36.5X2	T36.5X3	T36.5X4	T36.5X5	T36.5X6
Novocain (infiltration)	T41.3X1	T41.3X2	T41.3X3	T41.3X4	T41.3X5	T41.3X6
(topical)						
nerve block (peripheral) (plexus)	T41.3X1	T41.3X2	T41.3X3	T41.3X4	T41.3X5	T41.3X6
spinal	T41.3X1	T41.3X2	T41.3X3	T41.3X4	T41.3X5	T41.3X6
Noxious foodstuff	T62.91	T62.92	T62.93	T62.94	—	—
specified NEC	T62.8X1	T62.8X2	T62.8X3	T62.8X4	—	—
Noxiptiline	T43.011	T43.012	T43.013	T43.014	T43.015	T43.016
Noxytiolin	T49.0X1	T49.0X2	T49.0X3	T49.0X4	T49.0X5	T49.0X6

Substance	Poisoning, Accidental (unintentional)	Poisoning, Intentional Self-harm	Poisoning, Assault	Poisoning, Undetermined	Adverse Effect	Under-dosing
NPH Iletin (insulin)	T38.3X1	T38.3X2	T38.3X3	T38.3X4	T38.3X5	T38.3X6
Numorphan	T40.2X1	T40.2X2	T40.2X3	T40.2X4	T40.2X5	T40.2X6
Nunol	T42.3X1	T42.3X2	T42.3X3	T42.3X4	T42.3X5	T42.3X6
Nupercaine (spinal anesthetic)	T41.3X1	T41.3X2	T41.3X3	T41.3X4	T41.3X5	T41.3X6
topical (surface)	T41.3X1	T41.3X2	T41.3X3	T41.3X4	T41.3X5	T41.3X6
Nutmeg oil (liniment)	T49.3X1	T49.3X2	T49.3X3	T49.3X4	T49.3X5	T49.3X6
Nutritional supplement	T50.901	T50.902	T50.903	T50.904	T50.905	T50.906
Nux vomica	T65.1X1	T65.1X2	T65.1X3	T65.1X4	—	—
Nydrazid	T37.1X1	T37.1X2	T37.1X3	T37.1X4	T37.1X5	T37.1X6
Nylidrin	T46.7X1	T46.7X2	T46.7X3	T46.7X4	T46.7X5	T46.7X6
Nystatin	T36.7X1	T36.7X2	T36.7X3	T36.7X4	T36.7X5	T36.7X6
topical	T49.0X1	T49.0X2	T49.0X3	T49.0X4	T49.0X5	T49.0X6
Nytol	T45.0X1	T45.0X2	T45.0X3	T45.0X4	T45.0X5	T45.0X6
Obidoxime chloride	T50.6X1	T50.6X2	T50.6X3	T50.6X4	T50.6X5	T50.6X6
Octafonium (chloride)	T49.3X1	T49.3X2	T49.3X3	T49.3X4	T49.3X5	T49.3X6
Octamethyl pyrophosphoramide	T60.0X1	T60.0X2	T60.0X3	T60.0X4	—	—
Octanoin	T50.991	T50.992	T50.993	T50.994	T50.995	T50.996
Octatropine methylbromide	T44.3X1	T44.3X2	T44.3X3	T44.3X4	T44.3X5	T44.3X6
Octotiamine	T45.2X1	T45.2X2	T45.2X3	T45.2X4	T45.2X5	T45.2X6
Octoxinol (9)	T49.8X1	T49.8X2	T49.8X3	T49.8X4	T49.8X5	T49.8X6
Octreotide	T38.991	T38.992	T38.993	T38.994	T38.995	T38.996
Octyl nitrite	T46.3X1	T46.3X2	T46.3X3	T46.3X4	T46.3X5	T46.3X6
Oestradiol	T38.5X1	T38.5X2	T38.5X3	T38.5X4	T38.5X5	T38.5X6
Oestriol	T38.5X1	T38.5X2	T38.5X3	T38.5X4	T38.5X5	T38.5X6
Oestrogen	T38.5X1	T38.5X2	T38.5X3	T38.5X4	T38.5X5	T38.5X6
Oestrone	T38.5X1	T38.5X2	T38.5X3	T38.5X4	T38.5X5	T38.5X6
Ofloxacin	T36.8X1	T36.8X2	T36.8X3	T36.8X4	T36.8X5	T36.8X6
Oil (of)	T65.891	T65.892	T65.893	T65.894	—	—
bitter almond	T62.8X1	T62.8X2	T62.8X3	T62.8X4	—	—
cloves	T49.7X1	T49.7X2	T49.7X3	T49.7X4	T49.7X5	T49.7X6
colors	T65.6X1	T65.6X2	T65.6X3	T65.6X4	—	—
fumes	T59.891	T59.892	T59.893	T59.894	—	—
lubricating	T52.0X1	T52.0X2	T52.0X3	T52.0X4	—	—
Niobe	T52.8X1	T52.8X2	T52.8X3	T52.8X4	—	—
vitriol (liquid)	T54.2X1	T54.2X2	T54.2X3	T54.2X4	—	—
fumes	T54.2X1	T54.2X2	T54.2X3	T54.2X4	—	—
wintergreen (bitter) NEC	T49.3X1	T49.3X2	T49.3X3	T49.3X4	T49.3X5	T49.3X6
Oily preparation (for skin)	T49.3X1	T49.3X2	T49.3X3	T49.3X4	T49.3X5	T49.3X6
Ointment NEC	T49.3X1	T49.3X2	T49.3X3	T49.3X4	T49.3X5	T49.3X6
Olanzapine	T43.591	T43.592	T43.593	T43.594	T43.595	T43.596
Oleander	T62.2X1	T62.2X2	T62.2X3	T62.2X4	—	—
Oleandomycin	T36.3X1	T36.3X2	T36.3X3	T36.3X4	T36.3X5	T36.3X6
Oleandrin	T46.0X1	T46.0X2	T46.0X3	T46.0X4	T46.0X5	T46.0X6
Oleic acid	T46.6X1	T46.6X2	T46.6X3	T46.6X4	T46.6X5	T46.6X6
Oleovitamin A	T45.2X1	T45.2X2	T45.2X3	T45.2X4	T45.2X5	T45.2X6
Oleum ricini	T47.2X1	T47.2X2	T47.2X3	T47.2X4	T47.2X5	T47.2X6
Olive oil (medicinal) NEC	T47.4X1	T47.4X2	T47.4X3	T47.4X4	T47.4X5	T47.4X6
Olivomycin	T45.1X1	T45.1X2	T45.1X3	T45.1X4	T45.1X5	T45.1X6
Olsalazine	T47.8X1	T47.8X2	T47.8X3	T47.8X4	T47.8X5	T47.8X6
Omeprazole	T47.1X1	T47.1X2	T47.1X3	T47.1X4	T47.1X5	T47.1X6
OMPA	T60.0X1	T60.0X2	T60.0X3	T60.0X4	—	—
Oncovin	T45.1X1	T45.1X2	T45.1X3	T45.1X4	T45.1X5	T45.1X6
Ondansetron	T45.0X1	T45.0X2	T45.0X3	T45.0X4	T45.0X5	T45.0X6
Ophthaine	T41.3X1	T41.3X2	T41.3X3	T41.3X4	T41.3X5	T41.3X6
Ophthetic	T41.3X1	T41.3X2	T41.3X3	T41.3X4	T41.3X5	T41.3X6
Opiate NEC	T40.601	T40.602	T40.603	T40.604	T40.605	T40.606
antagonists	T50.7X1	T50.7X2	T50.7X3	T50.7X4	T50.7X5	T50.7X6
Opioid NEC	T40.2X1	T40.2X2	T40.2X3	T40.2X4	T40.2X5	T40.2X6
Opipramol	T43.011	T43.012	T43.013	T43.014	T43.015	T43.016
Opium alkaloids (total)	T40.0X1	T40.0X2	T40.0X3	T40.0X4	T40.0X5	T40.0X6
standardized powdered	T40.0X1	T40.0X2	T40.0X3	T40.0X4	T40.0X5	T40.0X6
tincture (camphorated)	T40.0X1	T40.0X2	T40.0X3	T40.0X4	T40.0X5	T40.0X6
Oracon	T38.4X1	T38.4X2	T38.4X3	T38.4X4	T38.4X5	T38.4X6
Oragrafin	T50.8X1	T50.8X2	T50.8X3	T50.8X4	T50.8X5	T50.8X6
Oral contraceptives	T38.4X1	T38.4X2	T38.4X3	T38.4X4	T38.4X5	T38.4X6
Oral rehydration salts	T50.3X1	T50.3X2	T50.3X3	T50.3X4	T50.3X5	T50.3X6
Orazamide	T50.991	T50.992	T50.993	T50.994	T50.995	T50.996
Orciprenaline	T48.291	T48.292	T48.293	T48.294	T48.295	T48.296
Organidin	T48.4X1	T48.4X2	T48.4X3	T48.4X4	T48.4X5	T48.4X6
Organonitrate NEC	T46.3X1	T46.3X2	T46.3X3	T46.3X4	T46.3X5	T46.3X6
Organophosphates	T60.0X1	T60.0X2	T60.0X3	T60.0X4	—	—
Orimune	T50.B91	T50.B92	T50.B93	T50.B94	T50.B95	T50.B96
Orinase	T38.3X1	T38.3X2	T38.3X3	T38.3X4	T38.3X5	T38.3X6
Ormeloxifene	T38.6X1	T38.6X2	T38.6X3	T38.6X4	T38.6X5	T38.6X6
Ornidazole	T37.3X1	T37.3X2	T37.3X3	T37.3X4	T37.3X5	T37.3X6
Ornithine aspartate	T50.991	T50.992	T50.993	T50.994	T50.995	T50.996
Ornoprostil	T47.1X1	T47.1X2	T47.1X3	T47.1X4	T47.1X5	T47.1X6
Orphenadrine (hydrochloride)	T42.8X1	T42.8X2	T42.8X3	T42.8X4	T42.8X5	T42.8X6
Ortal (sodium)	T42.3X1	T42.3X2	T42.3X3	T42.3X4	T42.3X5	T42.3X6

Additional Character May Be Required — Refer to the Tabular List for Character Selection ▽ Subterms under main terms may continue to next column or page

Table of Drugs and Chemicals

Substance	Poisoning, Accidental (unintentional)	Poisoning, Intentional Self-harm	Poisoning, Assault	Poisoning, Undetermined	Adverse Effect	Under-dosing
Orthoboric acid	T49.0X1	T49.0X2	T49.0X3	T49.0X4	T49.0X5	T49.0X6
ENT agent	T49.6X1	T49.6X2	T49.6X3	T49.6X4	T49.6X5	T49.6X6
ophthalmic preparation	T49.5X1	T49.5X2	T49.5X3	T49.5X4	T49.5X5	T49.5X6
Orthocaine	T41.3X1	T41.3X2	T41.3X3	T41.3X4	T41.3X5	T41.3X6
Orthodichlorobenzene	T53.7X1	T53.7X2	T53.7X3	T53.7X4	—	—
Ortho-Novum	T38.4X1	T38.4X2	T38.4X3	T38.4X4	T38.4X5	T38.4X6
Orthotolidine (reagent)	T54.2X1	T54.2X2	T54.2X3	T54.2X4	—	—
Osmic acid (liquid)	T54.2X1	T54.2X2	T54.2X3	T54.2X4	—	—
fumes	T54.2X1	T54.2X2	T54.2X3	T54.2X4	—	—
Osmotic diuretics	T50.2X1	T50.2X2	T50.2X3	T50.2X4	T50.2X5	T50.2X6
Otilonium bromide	T44.3X1	T44.3X2	T44.3X3	T44.3X4	T44.3X5	T44.3X6
Otorhinolaryngological drug NEC	T49.6X1	T49.6X2	T49.6X3	T49.6X4	T49.6X5	T49.6X6
Ouabain (e)	T46.0X1	T46.0X2	T46.0X3	T46.0X4	T46.0X5	T46.0X6
Ovarian						
hormone	T38.5X1	T38.5X2	T38.5X3	T38.5X4	T38.5X5	T38.5X6
stimulant	T38.5X1	T38.5X2	T38.5X3	T38.5X4	T38.5X5	T38.5X6
Ovral	T38.4X1	T38.4X2	T38.4X3	T38.4X4	T38.4X5	T38.4X6
Ovulen	T38.4X1	T38.4X2	T38.4X3	T38.4X4	T38.4X5	T38.4X6
Oxacillin	T36.0X1	T36.0X2	T36.0X3	T36.0X4	T36.0X5	T36.0X6
Oxalic acid	T54.2X1	T54.2X2	T54.2X3	T54.2X4	—	—
ammonium salt	T50.991	T50.992	T50.993	T50.994	T50.995	T50.996
Oxamniquine	T37.4X1	T37.4X2	T37.4X3	T37.4X4	T37.4X5	T37.4X6
Oxanamide	T43.591	T43.592	T43.593	T43.594	T43.595	T43.596
Oxandrolone	T38.7X1	T38.7X2	T38.7X3	T38.7X4	T38.7X5	T38.7X6
Oxantel	T37.4X1	T37.4X2	T37.4X3	T37.4X4	T37.4X5	T37.4X6
Oxapium iodide	T44.3X1	T44.3X2	T44.3X3	T44.3X4	T44.3X5	T44.3X6
Oxaprotiline	T43.021	T43.022	T43.023	T43.024	T43.025	T43.026
Oxaprozin	T39.311	T39.312	T39.313	T39.314	T39.315	T39.316
Oxatomide	T45.0X1	T45.0X2	T45.0X3	T45.0X4	T45.0X5	T45.0X6
Oxazepam	T42.4X1	T42.4X2	T42.4X3	T42.4X4	T42.4X5	T42.4X6
Oxazimedrine	T50.5X1	T50.5X2	T50.5X3	T50.5X4	T50.5X5	T50.5X6
Oxazolam	T42.4X1	T42.4X2	T42.4X3	T42.4X4	T42.4X5	T42.4X6
Oxazolidine derivatives	T42.2X1	T42.2X2	T42.2X3	T42.2X4	T42.2X5	T42.2X6
Oxazolidinedione (derivative)	T42.2X1	T42.2X2	T42.2X3	T42.2X4	T42.2X5	T42.2X6
Ox bile extract	T47.5X1	T47.5X2	T47.5X3	T47.5X4	T47.5X5	T47.5X6
Oxcarbazepine	T42.1X1	T42.1X2	T42.1X3	T42.1X4	T42.1X5	T42.1X6
Oxedrine	T44.4X1	T44.4X2	T44.4X3	T44.4X4	T44.4X5	T44.4X6
Oxeladin (citrate)	T48.3X1	T48.3X2	T48.3X3	T48.3X4	T48.3X5	T48.3X6
Oxendolone	T38.5X1	T38.5X2	T38.5X3	T38.5X4	T38.5X5	T38.5X6
Oxetacaine	T41.3X1	T41.3X2	T41.3X3	T41.3X4	T41.3X5	T41.3X6
Oxethazine	T41.3X1	T41.3X2	T41.3X3	T41.3X4	T41.3X5	T41.3X6
Oxetorone	T39.8X1	T39.8X2	T39.8X3	T39.8X4	T39.8X5	T39.8X6
Oxiconazole	T49.0X1	T49.0X2	T49.0X3	T49.0X4	T49.0X5	T49.0X6
Oxidizing agent NEC	T54.91	T54.92	T54.93	T54.94	—	—
Oxipurinol	T50.4X1	T50.4X2	T50.4X3	T50.4X4	T50.4X5	T50.4X6
Oxitriptan	T43.291	T43.292	T43.293	T43.294	T43.295	T43.296
Oxitropium bromide	T48.6X1	T48.6X2	T48.6X3	T48.6X4	T48.6X5	T48.6X6
Oxodipine	T46.1X1	T46.1X2	T46.1X3	T46.1X4	T46.1X5	T46.1X6
Oxolamine	T48.3X1	T48.3X2	T48.3X3	T48.3X4	T48.3X5	T48.3X6
Oxolinic acid	T37.8X1	T37.8X2	T37.8X3	T37.8X4	T37.8X5	T37.8X6
Oxomemazine	T43.3X1	T43.3X2	T43.3X3	T43.3X4	T43.3X5	T43.3X6
Oxophenarsine	T37.3X1	T37.3X2	T37.3X3	T37.3X4	T37.3X5	T37.3X6
Oxprenolol	T44.7X1	T44.7X2	T44.7X3	T44.7X4	T44.7X5	T44.7X6
Oxsoralen	T49.3X1	T49.3X2	T49.3X3	T49.3X4	T49.3X5	T49.3X6
Oxtriphylline	T48.6X1	T48.6X2	T48.6X3	T48.6X4	T48.6X5	T48.6X6
Oxybate sodium	T41.291	T41.292	T41.293	T41.294	T41.295	T41.296
Oxybuprocaine	T41.3X1	T41.3X2	T41.3X3	T41.3X4	T41.3X5	T41.3X6
Oxybutynin	T44.3X1	T44.3X2	T44.3X3	T44.3X4	T44.3X5	T44.3X6
Oxychlorosene	T49.0X1	T49.0X2	T49.0X3	T49.0X4	T49.0X5	T49.0X6
Oxycodone	T40.2X1	T40.2X2	T40.2X3	T40.2X4	T40.2X5	T40.2X6
Oxyfedrine	T46.3X1	T46.3X2	T46.3X3	T46.3X4	T46.3X5	T46.3X6
Oxygen	T41.5X1	T41.5X2	T41.5X3	T41.5X4	T41.5X5	T41.5X6
Oxylone	T49.0X1	T49.0X2	T49.0X3	T49.0X4	T49.0X5	T49.0X6
ophthalmic preparation	T49.5X1	T49.5X2	T49.5X3	T49.5X4	T49.5X5	T49.5X6
Oxymesterone	T38.7X1	T38.7X2	T38.7X3	T38.7X4	T38.7X5	T38.7X6
Oxymetazoline	T48.5X1	T48.5X2	T48.5X3	T48.5X4	T48.5X5	T48.5X6
Oxymetholone	T38.7X1	T38.7X2	T38.7X3	T38.7X4	T38.7X5	T38.7X6
Oxymorphone	T40.2X1	T40.2X2	T40.2X3	T40.2X4	T40.2X5	T40.2X6
Oxypertine	T43.591	T43.592	T43.593	T43.594	T43.595	T43.596
Oxyphenbutazone	T39.2X1	T39.2X2	T39.2X3	T39.2X4	T39.2X5	T39.2X6
Oxyphencyclimine	T44.3X1	T44.3X2	T44.3X3	T44.3X4	T44.3X5	T44.3X6
Oxyphenisatine	T47.2X1	T47.2X2	T47.2X3	T47.2X4	T47.2X5	T47.2X6
Oxyphenonium bromide	T44.3X1	T44.3X2	T44.3X3	T44.3X4	T44.3X5	T44.3X6
Oxypolygelatin	T45.8X1	T45.8X2	T45.8X3	T45.8X4	T45.8X5	T45.8X6
Oxyquinoline (derivatives)	T37.8X1	T37.8X2	T37.8X3	T37.8X4	T37.8X5	T37.8X6
Oxytetracycline	T36.4X1	T36.4X2	T36.4X3	T36.4X4	T36.4X5	T36.4X6
Oxytocic drug NEC	T48.0X1	T48.0X2	T48.0X3	T48.0X4	T48.0X5	T48.0X6
Oxytocin (synthetic)	T48.0X1	T48.0X2	T48.0X3	T48.0X4	T48.0X5	T48.0X6
Ozone	T59.891	T59.892	T59.893	T59.894	—	—
PABA	T49.3X1	T49.3X2	T49.3X3	T49.3X4	T49.3X5	T49.3X6
Packed red cells	T45.8X1	T45.8X2	T45.8X3	T45.8X4	T45.8X5	T45.8X6
Padimate	T49.3X1	T49.3X2	T49.3X3	T49.3X4	T49.3X5	T49.3X6
Paint NEC	T65.6X1	T65.6X2	T65.6X3	T65.6X4	—	—
cleaner	T52.91	T52.92	T52.93	T52.94	—	—
fumes NEC	T59.891	T59.892	T59.893	T59.894	—	—
lead (fumes)	T56.0X1	T56.0X2	T56.0X3	T56.0X4	—	—
solvent NEC	T52.8X1	T52.8X2	T52.8X3	T52.8X4	—	—
stripper	T52.8X1	T52.8X2	T52.8X3	T52.8X4	—	—
Palfium	T40.2X1	T40.2X2	T40.2X3	T40.2X4	—	—
Palm kernel oil	T50.991	T50.992	T50.993	T50.994	T50.995	T50.996
Paludrine	T37.2X1	T37.2X2	T37.2X3	T37.2X4	T37.2X5	T37.2X6
PAM (pralidoxime)	T50.6X1	T50.6X2	T50.6X3	T50.6X4	T50.6X5	T50.6X6
Pamaquine (naphthoute)	T37.2X1	T37.2X2	T37.2X3	T37.2X4	T37.2X5	T37.2X6
Panadol	T39.1X1	T39.1X2	T39.1X3	T39.1X4	T39.1X5	T39.1X6
Pancreatic						
digestive secretion stimulant	T47.8X1	T47.8X2	T47.8X3	T47.8X4	T47.8X5	T47.8X6
dornase	T45.3X1	T45.3X2	T45.3X3	T45.3X4	T45.3X5	T45.3X6
Pancreatin	T47.5X1	T47.5X2	T47.5X3	T47.5X4	T47.5X5	T47.5X6
Pancrelipase	T47.5X1	T47.5X2	T47.5X3	T47.5X4	T47.5X5	T47.5X6
Pancuronium (bromide)	T48.1X1	T48.1X2	T48.1X3	T48.1X4	T48.1X5	T48.1X6
Pangamic acid	T45.2X1	T45.2X2	T45.2X3	T45.2X4	T45.2X5	T45.2X6
Panthenol	T45.2X1	T45.2X2	T45.2X3	T45.2X4	T45.2X5	T45.2X6
topical	T49.8X1	T49.8X2	T49.8X3	T49.8X4	T49.8X5	T49.8X6
Pantopon	T40.0X1	T40.0X2	T40.0X3	T40.0X4	T40.0X5	T40.0X6
Pantothenic acid	T45.2X1	T45.2X2	T45.2X3	T45.2X4	T45.2X5	T45.2X6
Panwarfin	T45.511	T45.512	T45.513	T45.514	T45.515	T45.516
Papain	T47.5X1	T47.5X2	T47.5X3	T47.5X4	T47.5X5	T47.5X6
digestant	T47.5X1	T47.5X2	T47.5X3	T47.5X4	T47.5X5	T47.5X6
Papaveretum	T40.0X1	T40.0X2	T40.0X3	T40.0X4	T40.0X5	T40.0X6
Papaverine	T44.3X1	T44.3X2	T44.3X3	T44.3X4	T44.3X5	T44.3X6
Para-acetamidophenol	T39.1X1	T39.1X2	T39.1X3	T39.1X4	T39.1X5	T39.1X6
Para-aminobenzoic acid	T49.3X1	T49.3X2	T49.3X3	T49.3X4	T49.3X5	T49.3X6
Para-aminophenol derivatives	T39.1X1	T39.1X2	T39.1X3	T39.1X4	T39.1X5	T39.1X6
Para-aminosalicylic acid	T37.1X1	T37.1X2	T37.1X3	T37.1X4	T37.1X5	T37.1X6
Paracetaldehyde	T42.6X1	T42.6X2	T42.6X3	T42.6X4	T42.6X5	T42.6X6
Paracetamol	T39.1X1	T39.1X2	T39.1X3	T39.1X4	T39.1X5	T39.1X6
Parachlorophenol (camphorated)	T49.0X1	T49.0X2	T49.0X3	T49.0X4	T49.0X5	T49.0X6
Paracodin	T40.2X1	T40.2X2	T40.2X3	T40.2X4	T40.2X5	T40.2X6
Paradione	T42.2X1	T42.2X2	T42.2X3	T42.2X4	T42.2X5	T42.2X6
Paraffin(s) (wax)	T52.0X1	T52.0X2	T52.0X3	T52.0X4	—	—
liquid (medicinal)	T47.4X1	T47.4X2	T47.4X3	T47.4X4	T47.4X5	T47.4X6
nonmedicinal	T52.0X1	T52.0X2	T52.0X3	T52.0X4	—	—
Paraformaldehyde	T60.3X1	T60.3X2	T60.3X3	T60.3X4	—	—
Paraldehyde	T42.6X1	T42.6X2	T42.6X3	T42.6X4	T42.6X5	T42.6X6
Paramethadione	T42.2X1	T42.2X2	T42.2X3	T42.2X4	T42.2X5	T42.2X6
Paramethasone	T38.0X1	T38.0X2	T38.0X3	T38.0X4	T38.0X5	T38.0X6
acetate	T49.0X1	T49.0X2	T49.0X3	T49.0X4	T49.0X5	T49.0X6
Paraoxon	T60.0X1	T60.0X2	T60.0X3	T60.0X4	—	—
Paraquat	T60.3X1	T60.3X2	T60.3X3	T60.3X4	—	—
Parasympatholytic NEC	T44.3X1	T44.3X2	T44.3X3	T44.3X4	T44.3X5	T44.3X6
Parasympathomimetic drug NEC	T44.1X1	T44.1X2	T44.1X3	T44.1X4	T44.1X5	T44.1X6
Parathion	T60.0X1	T60.0X2	T60.0X3	T60.0X4	—	—
Parathormone	T50.991	T50.992	T50.993	T50.994	T50.995	T50.996
Parathyroid extract	T50.991	T50.992	T50.993	T50.994	T50.995	T50.996
Paratyphoid vaccine	T50.A91	T50.A92	T50.A93	T50.A94	T50.A95	T50.A96
Paredrine	T44.4X1	T44.4X2	T44.4X3	T44.4X4	T44.4X5	T44.4X6
Paregoric	T40.0X1	T40.0X2	T40.0X3	T40.0X4	T40.0X5	T40.0X6
Pargyline	T46.5X1	T46.5X2	T46.5X3	T46.5X4	T46.5X5	T46.5X6
Paris green	T57.0X1	T57.0X2	T57.0X3	T57.0X4	—	—
insecticide	T57.0X1	T57.0X2	T57.0X3	T57.0X4	—	—
Parnate	T43.1X1	T43.1X2	T43.1X3	T43.1X4	T43.1X5	T43.1X6
Paromomycin	T36.5X1	T36.5X2	T36.5X3	T36.5X4	T36.5X5	T36.5X6
Paroxypropione	T45.1X1	T45.1X2	T45.1X3	T45.1X4	T45.1X5	T45.1X6
Parzone	T40.2X1	T40.2X2	T40.2X3	T40.2X4	T40.2X5	T40.2X6
PAS	T37.1X1	T37.1X2	T37.1X3	T37.1X4	T37.1X5	T37.1X6
Pasiniazid	T37.1X1	T37.1X2	T37.1X3	T37.1X4	T37.1X5	T37.1X6
PBB (polybrominated biphenyls)	T65.891	T65.892	T65.893	T65.894	—	—
PCB	T65.891	T65.892	T65.893	T65.894	—	—
PCP						
meaning pentachlorophenol	T60.1X1	T60.1X2	T60.1X3	T60.1X4	—	—
fungicide	T60.3X1	T60.3X2	T60.3X3	T60.3X4	—	—
herbicide	T60.3X1	T60.3X2	T60.3X3	T60.3X4	—	—
insecticide	T60.1X1	T60.1X2	T60.1X3	T60.1X4	—	—
meaning phencyclidine	T40.991	T40.992	T40.993	T40.994	—	—
Peach kernel oil (emulsion)	T47.4X1	T47.4X2	T47.4X3	T47.4X4	T47.4X5	T47.4X6
Peanut oil (emulsion) NEC	T47.4X1	T47.4X2	T47.4X3	T47.4X4	T47.4X5	T47.4X6
topical	T49.3X1	T49.3X2	T49.3X3	T49.3X4	T49.3X5	T49.3X6

Orthoboric acid — Peanut oil

Table of Drugs and Chemicals

Pearly Gates — Phenformin

Substance	Poisoning, Accidental (unintentional)	Poisoning, Intentional Self-harm	Poisoning, Assault	Poisoning, Undetermined	Adverse Effect	Under-dosing
Pearly Gates (morning glory seeds)	T40.991	T40.992	T40.993	T40.994	—	—
Pecazine	T43.3X1	T43.3X2	T43.3X3	T43.3X4	T43.3X5	T43.3X6
Pectin	T47.6X1	T47.6X2	T47.6X3	T47.6X4	T47.6X5	T47.6X6
Pefloxacin	T37.8X1	T37.8X2	T37.8X3	T37.8X4	T37.8X5	T37.8X6
Pegademase, bovine	T50.Z91	T50.Z92	T50.Z93	T50.Z94	T50.Z95	T50.Z96
Pelletierine tannate	T37.4X1	T37.4X2	T37.4X3	T37.4X4	T37.4X5	T37.4X6
Pemirolast (potassium)	T48.6X1	T48.6X2	T48.6X3	T48.6X4	T48.6X5	T48.6X6
Pemoline	T50.7X1	T50.7X2	T50.7X3	T50.7X4	T50.7X5	T50.7X6
Pempidine	T44.2X1	T44.2X2	T44.2X3	T44.2X4	T44.2X5	T44.2X6
Penamecillin	T36.0X1	T36.0X2	T36.0X3	T36.0X4	T36.0X5	T36.0X6
Penbutolol	T44.7X1	T44.7X2	T44.7X3	T44.7X4	T44.7X5	T44.7X6
Penethamate	T36.0X1	T36.0X2	T36.0X3	T36.0X4	T36.0X5	T36.0X6
Penfluridol	T43.591	T43.592	T43.593	T43.594	T43.595	T43.596
Penflutizide	T50.2X1	T50.2X2	T50.2X3	T50.2X4	T50.2X5	T50.2X6
Pengitoxin	T46.0X1	T46.0X2	T46.0X3	T46.0X4	T46.0X5	T46.0X6
Penicillamine	T50.6X1	T50.6X2	T50.6X3	T50.6X4	T50.6X5	T50.6X6
Penicillin (any)	T36.0X1	T36.0X2	T36.0X3	T36.0X4	T36.0X5	T36.0X6
Penicillinase	T45.3X1	T45.3X2	T45.3X3	T45.3X4	T45.3X5	T45.3X6
Penicilloyl polylysine	T50.8X1	T50.8X2	T50.8X3	T50.8X4	T50.8X5	T50.8X6
Penimepicycline	T36.4X1	T36.4X2	T36.4X3	T36.4X4	T36.4X5	T36.4X6
Pentachloroethane	T53.6X1	T53.6X2	T53.6X3	T53.6X4	—	—
Pentachloronaphthalene	T53.7X1	T53.7X2	T53.7X3	T53.7X4	—	—
Pentachlorophenol (pesticide)	T60.1X1	T60.1X2	T60.1X3	T60.1X4	—	—
fungicide	T60.3X1	T60.3X2	T60.3X3	T60.3X4	—	—
herbicide	T60.3X1	T60.3X2	T60.3X3	T60.3X4	—	—
insecticide	T60.1X1	T60.1X2	T60.1X3	T60.1X4	—	—
Pentaerythritol	T46.3X1	T46.3X2	T46.3X3	T46.3X4	T46.3X5	T46.3X6
chloral	T42.6X1	T42.6X2	T42.6X3	T42.6X4	T42.6X5	T42.6X6
tetranitrate NEC	T46.3X1	T46.3X2	T46.3X3	T46.3X4	T46.3X5	T46.3X6
Pentaerythrityl tetranitrate	T46.3X1	T46.3X2	T46.3X3	T46.3X4	T46.3X5	T46.3X6
Pentagastrin	T50.8X1	T50.8X2	T50.8X3	T50.8X4	T50.8X5	T50.8X6
Pentalin	T53.6X1	T53.6X2	T53.6X3	T53.6X4	—	—
Pentamethonium bromide	T44.2X1	T44.2X2	T44.2X3	T44.2X4	T44.2X5	T44.2X6
Pentamidine	T37.3X1	T37.3X2	T37.3X3	T37.3X4	T37.3X5	T37.3X6
Pentanol	T51.3X1	T51.3X2	T51.3X3	T51.3X4	—	—
Pentapyrrolinium (bitartrate)	T44.2X1	T44.2X2	T44.2X3	T44.2X4	T44.2X5	T44.2X6
Pentaquine	T37.2X1	T37.2X2	T37.2X3	T37.2X4	T37.2X5	T37.2X6
Pentazocine	T40.491	T40.492	T40.493	T40.494	T40.495	T40.496
Pentetrazole	T50.7X1	T50.7X2	T50.7X3	T50.7X4	T50.7X5	T50.7X6
Penthienate bromide	T44.3X1	T44.3X2	T44.3X3	T44.3X4	T44.3X5	T44.3X6
Pentifylline	T46.7X1	T46.7X2	T46.7X3	T46.7X4	T46.7X5	T46.7X6
Pentobarbital	T42.3X1	T42.3X2	T42.3X3	T42.3X4	T42.3X5	T42.3X6
sodium	T42.3X1	T42.3X2	T42.3X3	T42.3X4	T42.3X5	T42.3X6
Pentobarbitone	T42.3X1	T42.3X2	T42.3X3	T42.3X4	T42.3X5	T42.3X6
Pentolonium tartrate	T44.2X1	T44.2X2	T44.2X3	T44.2X4	T44.2X5	T44.2X6
Pentosan polysulfate (sodium)	T39.8X1	T39.8X2	T39.8X3	T39.8X4	T39.8X5	T39.8X6
Pentostatin	T45.1X1	T45.1X2	T45.1X3	T45.1X4	T45.1X5	T45.1X6
Pentothal	T41.1X1	T41.1X2	T41.1X3	T41.1X4	T41.1X5	T41.1X6
Pentoxifylline	T46.7X1	T46.7X2	T46.7X3	T46.7X4	T46.7X5	T46.7X6
Pentoxyverine	T48.3X1	T48.3X2	T48.3X3	T48.3X4	T48.3X5	T48.3X6
Pentrinat	T46.3X1	T46.3X2	T46.3X3	T46.3X4	T46.3X5	T46.3X6
Pentylenetetrazole	T50.7X1	T50.7X2	T50.7X3	T50.7X4	T50.7X5	T50.7X6
Pentylsalicylamide	T37.1X1	T37.1X2	T37.1X3	T37.1X4	T37.1X5	T37.1X6
Pentymal	T42.3X1	T42.3X2	T42.3X3	T42.3X4	T42.3X5	T42.3X6
Peplomycin	T45.1X1	T45.1X2	T45.1X3	T45.1X4	T45.1X5	T45.1X6
Peppermint (oil)	T47.5X1	T47.5X2	T47.5X3	T47.5X4	T47.5X5	T47.5X6
Pepsin	T47.5X1	T47.5X2	T47.5X3	T47.5X4	T47.5X5	T47.5X6
digestant	T47.5X1	T47.5X2	T47.5X3	T47.5X4	T47.5X5	T47.5X6
Pepstatin	T47.1X1	T47.1X2	T47.1X3	T47.1X4	T47.1X5	T47.1X6
Peptavlon	T50.8X1	T50.8X2	T50.8X3	T50.8X4	T50.8X5	T50.8X6
Perazine	T43.3X1	T43.3X2	T43.3X3	T43.3X4	T43.3X5	T43.3X6
Percaine (spinal)	T41.3X1	T41.3X2	T41.3X3	T41.3X4	T41.3X5	T41.3X6
topical (surface)	T41.3X1	T41.3X2	T41.3X3	T41.3X4	T41.3X5	T41.3X6
Perchloroethylene	T53.3X1	T53.3X2	T53.3X3	T53.3X4	—	—
medicinal	T37.4X1	T37.4X2	T37.4X3	T37.4X4	T37.4X5	T37.4X6
vapor	T53.3X1	T53.3X2	T53.3X3	T53.3X4	—	—
Percodan	T40.2X1	T40.2X2	T40.2X3	T40.2X4	T40.2X5	T40.2X6
Percogesic — *see also* acetaminophen	T45.0X1	T45.0X2	T45.0X3	T45.0X4	T45.0X5	T45.0X6
Percorten	T38.0X1	T38.0X2	T38.0X3	T38.0X4	T38.0X5	T38.0X6
Pergolide	T42.8X1	T42.8X2	T42.8X3	T42.8X4	T42.8X5	T42.8X6
Pergonal	T38.811	T38.812	T38.813	T38.814	T38.815	T38.816
Perhexilene	T46.3X1	T46.3X2	T46.3X3	T46.3X4	T46.3X5	T46.3X6
Perhexiline (maleate)	T46.3X1	T46.3X2	T46.3X3	T46.3X4	T46.3X5	T46.3X6
Periactin	T45.0X1	T45.0X2	T45.0X3	T45.0X4	T45.0X5	T45.0X6
Periciazine	T43.3X1	T43.3X2	T43.3X3	T43.3X4	T43.3X5	T43.3X6
Periclor	T42.6X1	T42.6X2	T42.6X3	T42.6X4	T42.6X5	T42.6X6
Perindopril	T46.4X1	T46.4X2	T46.4X3	T46.4X4	T46.4X5	T46.4X6
Perisoxal	T39.8X1	T39.8X2	T39.8X3	T39.8X4	T39.8X5	T39.8X6
Peritoneal dialysis solution	T50.3X1	T50.3X2	T50.3X3	T50.3X4	T50.3X5	T50.3X6
Peritrate	T46.3X1	T46.3X2	T46.3X3	T46.3X4	T46.3X5	T46.3X6
Perlapine	T42.4X1	T42.4X2	T42.4X3	T42.4X4	T42.4X5	T42.4X6
Permanganate	T65.891	T65.892	T65.893	T65.894	—	—
Permethrin	T60.1X1	T60.1X2	T60.1X3	T60.1X4	—	—
Pernocton	T42.3X1	T42.3X2	T42.3X3	T42.3X4	T42.3X5	T42.3X6
Pernoston	T42.3X1	T42.3X2	T42.3X3	T42.3X4	T42.3X5	T42.3X6
Peronine	T40.2X1	T40.2X2	T40.2X3	T40.2X4	—	—
Perphenazine	T43.3X1	T43.3X2	T43.3X3	T43.3X4	T43.3X5	T43.3X6
Pertofrane	T43.011	T43.012	T43.013	T43.014	T43.015	T43.016
Pertussis						
immune serum (human)	T50.Z11	T50.Z12	T50.Z13	T50.Z14	T50.Z15	T50.Z16
vaccine (with diphtheria toxoid) (with tetanus toxoid)	T50.A11	T50.A12	T50.A13	T50.A14	T50.A15	T50.A16
Peruvian balsam	T49.0X1	T49.0X2	T49.0X3	T49.0X4	T49.0X5	T49.0X6
Peruvoside	T46.0X1	T46.0X2	T46.0X3	T46.0X4	T46.0X5	T46.0X6
Pesticide (dust) (fumes) (vapor) NEC	T60.91	T60.92	T60.93	T60.94		
arsenic	T57.0X1	T57.0X2	T57.0X3	T57.0X4		
chlorinated	T60.1X1	T60.1X2	T60.1X3	T60.1X4		
cyanide	T65.0X1	T65.0X2	T65.0X3	T65.0X4		
kerosene	T52.0X1	T52.0X2	T52.0X3	T52.0X4		
mixture (of compounds)	T60.91	T60.92	T60.93	T60.94		
naphthalene	T60.2X1	T60.2X2	T60.2X3	T60.2X4		
organochlorine (compounds)	T60.1X1	T60.1X2	T60.1X3	T60.1X4		
petroleum (distillate) (products) NEC	T60.8X1	T60.8X2	T60.8X3	T60.8X4		
specified ingredient NEC	T60.8X1	T60.8X2	T60.8X3	T60.8X4		
strychnine	T65.1X1	T65.1X2	T65.1X3	T65.1X4		
thallium	T60.4X1	T60.4X2	T60.4X3	T60.4X4		
Pethidine	T40.491	T40.492	T40.493	T40.494	T40.495	T40.496
Petrichloral	T42.6X1	T42.6X2	T42.6X3	T42.6X4	T42.6X5	T42.6X6
Petrol	T52.0X1	T52.0X2	T52.0X3	T52.0X4		
vapor	T52.0X1	T52.0X2	T52.0X3	T52.0X4		
Petrolatum	T49.3X1	T49.3X2	T49.3X3	T49.3X4	T49.3X5	T49.3X6
hydrophilic	T49.3X1	T49.3X2	T49.3X3	T49.3X4	T49.3X5	T49.3X6
liquid	T47.4X1	T47.4X2	T47.4X3	T47.4X4	T47.4X5	T47.4X6
topical	T49.3X1	T49.3X2	T49.3X3	T49.3X4	T49.3X5	T49.3X6
nonmedicinal	T52.0X1	T52.0X2	T52.0X3	T52.0X4		
red veterinary	T49.3X1	T49.3X2	T49.3X3	T49.3X4	T49.3X5	T49.3X6
white	T49.3X1	T49.3X2	T49.3X3	T49.3X4	T49.3X5	T49.3X6
Petroleum (products) NEC	T52.0X1	T52.0X2	T52.0X3	T52.0X4		
benzine(s) — *see* Ligroin						
ether — *see* Ligroin						
jelly — *see* Petrolatum						
naphtha — *see* Ligroin						
pesticide	T60.8X1	T60.8X2	T60.8X3	T60.8X4		
solids	T52.0X1	T52.0X2	T52.0X3	T52.0X4		
solvents	T52.0X1	T52.0X2	T52.0X3	T52.0X4		
vapor	T52.0X1	T52.0X2	T52.0X3	T52.0X4		
Peyote	T40.991	T40.992	T40.993	T40.994		
Phanodorm, phanodorn	T42.3X1	T42.3X2	T42.3X3	T42.3X4	T42.3X5	T42.3X6
Phanquinone	T37.3X1	T37.3X2	T37.3X3	T37.3X4	T37.3X5	T37.3X6
Phanquone	T37.3X1	T37.3X2	T37.3X3	T37.3X4	T37.3X5	T37.3X6
Pharmaceutical						
adjunct NEC	T50.901	T50.902	T50.903	T50.904	T50.905	T50.906
excipient NEC	T50.901	T50.902	T50.903	T50.904	T50.905	T50.906
sweetener	T50.901	T50.902	T50.903	T50.904	T50.905	T50.906
viscous agent	T50.901	T50.902	T50.903	T50.904	T50.905	T50.906
Phemitone	T42.3X1	T42.3X2	T42.3X3	T42.3X4	T42.3X5	T42.3X6
Phenacaine	T41.3X1	T41.3X2	T41.3X3	T41.3X4	T41.3X5	T41.3X6
Phenacemide	T42.6X1	T42.6X2	T42.6X3	T42.6X4	T42.6X5	T42.6X6
Phenacetin	T39.1X1	T39.1X2	T39.1X3	T39.1X4	T39.1X5	T39.1X6
Phenadoxone	T40.2X1	T40.2X2	T40.2X3	T40.2X4	—	—
Phenaglycodol	T43.591	T43.592	T43.593	T43.594	T43.595	T43.596
Phenantoin	T42.0X1	T42.0X2	T42.0X3	T42.0X4	T42.0X5	T42.0X6
Phenaphthazine reagent	T50.991	T50.992	T50.993	T50.994	T50.995	T50.996
Phenazocine	T40.491	T40.492	T40.493	T40.494	T40.495	T40.496
Phenazone	T39.2X1	T39.2X2	T39.2X3	T39.2X4	T39.2X5	T39.2X6
Phenazopyridine	T39.8X1	T39.8X2	T39.8X3	T39.8X4	T39.8X5	T39.8X6
Phenbenicillin	T36.0X1	T36.0X2	T36.0X3	T36.0X4	T36.0X5	T36.0X6
Phenbutrazate	T50.5X1	T50.5X2	T50.5X3	T50.5X4	T50.5X5	T50.5X6
Phencyclidine	T40.991	T40.992	T40.993	T40.994	T40.995	T40.996
Phendimetrazine	T50.5X1	T50.5X2	T50.5X3	T50.5X4	T50.5X5	T50.5X6
Phenelzine	T43.1X1	T43.1X2	T43.1X3	T43.1X4	T43.1X5	T43.1X6
Phenemal	T42.3X1	T42.3X2	T42.3X3	T42.3X4	T42.3X5	T42.3X6
Phenergan	T42.6X1	T42.6X2	T42.6X3	T42.6X4	T42.6X5	T42.6X6
Pheneticillin	T36.0X1	T36.0X2	T36.0X3	T36.0X4	T36.0X5	T36.0X6
Pheneturide	T42.6X1	T42.6X2	T42.6X3	T42.6X4	T42.6X5	T42.6X6
Phenformin	T38.3X1	T38.3X2	T38.3X3	T38.3X4	T38.3X5	T38.3X6

Additional Character May Be Required — Refer to the Tabular List for Character Selection ▽ Subterms under main terms may continue to next column or page

Substance	Poisoning, Accidental (unintentional)	Poisoning, Intentional Self-harm	Poisoning, Assault	Poisoning, Undetermined	Adverse Effect	Under-dosing
Phenglutarimide	T44.3X1	T44.3X2	T44.3X3	T44.3X4	T44.3X5	T44.3X6
Phenicarbazide	T39.8X1	T39.8X2	T39.8X3	T39.8X4	T39.8X5	T39.8X6
Phenindamine	T45.0X1	T45.0X2	T45.0X3	T45.0X4	T45.0X5	T45.0X6
Phenindione	T45.511	T45.512	T45.513	T45.514	T45.515	T45.516
Pheniprazine	T43.1X1	T43.1X2	T43.1X3	T43.1X4	T43.1X5	T43.1X6
Pheniramine	T45.0X1	T45.0X2	T45.0X3	T45.0X4	T45.0X5	T45.0X6
Phenisatin	T47.2X1	T47.2X2	T47.2X3	T47.2X4	T47.2X5	T47.2X6
Phenmetrazine	T50.5X1	T50.5X2	T50.5X3	T50.5X4	T50.5X5	T50.5X6
Phenobal	T42.3X1	T42.3X2	T42.3X3	T42.3X4	T42.3X5	T42.3X6
Phenobarbital	T42.3X1	T42.3X2	T42.3X3	T42.3X4	T42.3X5	T42.3X6
with						
mephenytoin	T42.3X1	T42.3X2	T42.3X3	T42.3X4	T42.3X5	T42.3X6
phenytoin	T42.3X1	T42.3X2	T42.3X3	T42.3X4	T42.3X5	T42.3X6
sodium	T42.3X1	T42.3X2	T42.3X3	T42.3X4	T42.3X5	T42.3X6
Phenobarbitone	T42.3X1	T42.3X2	T42.3X3	T42.3X4	T42.3X5	T42.3X6
Phenobutiodil	T50.8X1	T50.8X2	T50.8X3	T50.8X4	T50.8X5	T50.8X6
Phenoctide	T49.0X1	T49.0X2	T49.0X3	T49.0X4	T49.0X5	T49.0X6
Phenol	T49.0X1	T49.0X2	T49.0X3	T49.0X4	T49.0X5	T49.0X6
disinfectant	T54.0X1	T54.0X2	T54.0X3	T54.0X4	—	—
in oil injection	T46.8X1	T46.8X2	T46.8X3	T46.8X4	T46.8X5	T46.8X6
medicinal	T49.1X1	T49.1X2	T49.1X3	T49.1X4	T49.1X5	T49.1X6
nonmedicinal NEC	T54.0X1	T54.0X2	T54.0X3	T54.0X4	—	—
pesticide	T60.8X1	T60.8X2	T60.8X3	T60.8X4	—	—
red	T50.8X1	T50.8X2	T50.8X3	T50.8X4	T50.8X5	T50.8X6
Phenolic preparation	T49.1X1	T49.1X2	T49.1X3	T49.1X4	T49.1X5	T49.1X6
Phenolphthalein	T47.2X1	T47.2X2	T47.2X3	T47.2X4	T47.2X5	T47.2X6
Phenolsulfonphthalein	T50.8X1	T50.8X2	T50.8X3	T50.8X4	T50.8X5	T50.8X6
Phenomorphan	T40.2X1	T40.2X2	T40.2X3	T40.2X4		
Phenonyl	T42.3X1	T42.3X2	T42.3X3	T42.3X4	T42.3X5	T42.3X6
Phenoperidine	T40.491	T40.492	T40.493	T40.494		
Phenopyrazone	T46.991	T46.992	T46.993	T46.994	T46.995	T46.996
Phenoquin	T50.4X1	T50.4X2	T50.4X3	T50.4X4	T50.4X5	T50.4X6
Phenothiazine (psychotropic) NEC	T43.3X1	T43.3X2	T43.3X3	T43.3X4	T43.3X5	T43.3X6
insecticide	T60.2X1	T60.2X2	T60.2X3	T60.2X4	—	—
Phenothrin	T49.0X1	T49.0X2	T49.0X3	T49.0X4	T49.0X5	T49.0X6
Phenoxybenzamine	T46.7X1	T46.7X2	T46.7X3	T46.7X4	T46.7X5	T46.7X6
Phenoxyethanol	T49.0X1	T49.0X2	T49.0X3	T49.0X4	T49.0X5	T49.0X6
Phenoxymethyl penicillin	T36.0X1	T36.0X2	T36.0X3	T36.0X4	T36.0X5	T36.0X6
Phenprobamate	T42.8X1	T42.8X2	T42.8X3	T42.8X4	T42.8X5	T42.8X6
Phenprocoumon	T45.511	T45.512	T45.513	T45.514	T45.515	T45.516
Phensuximide	T42.2X1	T42.2X2	T42.2X3	T42.2X4	T42.2X5	T42.2X6
Phentermine	T50.5X1	T50.5X2	T50.5X3	T50.5X4	T50.5X5	T50.5X6
Phenthicillin	T36.0X1	T36.0X2	T36.0X3	T36.0X4	T36.0X5	T36.0X6
Phentolamine	T46.7X1	T46.7X2	T46.7X3	T46.7X4	T46.7X5	T46.7X6
Phenyl						
butazone	T39.2X1	T39.2X2	T39.2X3	T39.2X4	T39.2X5	T39.2X6
enediamine	T65.3X1	T65.3X2	T65.3X3	T65.3X4	—	—
hydrazine	T65.3X1	T65.3X2	T65.3X3	T65.3X4	—	—
antineoplastic	T45.1X1	T45.1X2	T45.1X3	T45.1X4	T45.1X5	T45.1X6
mercuric compounds — see Mercury						
salicylate	T49.3X1	T49.3X2	T49.3X3	T49.3X4	T49.3X5	T49.3X6
Phenylalanine mustard	T45.1X1	T45.1X2	T45.1X3	T45.1X4	T45.1X5	T45.1X6
Phenylbutazone	T39.2X1	T39.2X2	T39.2X3	T39.2X4	T39.2X5	T39.2X6
Phenylenediamine	T65.3X1	T65.3X2	T65.3X3	T65.3X4	—	—
Phenylephrine	T44.4X1	T44.4X2	T44.4X3	T44.4X4	T44.4X5	T44.4X6
Phenylethylbiguanide	T38.3X1	T38.3X2	T38.3X3	T38.3X4	T38.3X5	T38.3X6
Phenylmercuric						
acetate	T49.0X1	T49.0X2	T49.0X3	T49.0X4	T49.0X5	T49.0X6
borate	T49.0X1	T49.0X2	T49.0X3	T49.0X4	T49.0X5	T49.0X6
nitrate	T49.0X1	T49.0X2	T49.0X3	T49.0X4	T49.0X5	T49.0X6
Phenylmethylbarbitone	T42.3X1	T42.3X2	T42.3X3	T42.3X4	T42.3X5	T42.3X6
Phenylpropanol	T47.5X1	T47.5X2	T47.5X3	T47.5X4	T47.5X5	T47.5X6
Phenylpropanolamine	T44.991	T44.992	T44.993	T44.994	T44.995	T44.996
Phenylsulfthion	T60.0X1	T60.0X2	T60.0X3	T60.0X4	—	—
Phenyltoloxamine	T45.0X1	T45.0X2	T45.0X3	T45.0X4	T45.0X5	T45.0X6
Phenyramidol, phenyramidon	T39.8X1	T39.8X2	T39.8X3	T39.8X4	T39.8X5	T39.8X6
Phenytoin	T42.0X1	T42.0X2	T42.0X3	T42.0X4	T42.0X5	T42.0X6
with Phenobarbital	T42.3X1	T42.3X2	T42.3X3	T42.3X4	T42.3X5	T42.3X6
pHisoHex	T49.2X1	T49.2X2	T49.2X3	T49.2X4	T49.2X5	T49.2X6
Pholcodine	T48.3X1	T48.3X2	T48.3X3	T48.3X4	T48.3X5	T48.3X6
Pholedrine	T46.991	T46.992	T46.993	T46.994	T46.995	T46.996
Phorate	T60.0X1	T60.0X2	T60.0X3	T60.0X4	—	—
Phosdrin	T60.0X1	T60.0X2	T60.0X3	T60.0X4	—	—
Phosfolan	T60.0X1	T60.0X2	T60.0X3	T60.0X4	—	—
Phosgene (gas)	T59.891	T59.892	T59.893	T59.894	—	—
Phosphamidon	T60.0X1	T60.0X2	T60.0X3	T60.0X4	—	—
Phosphate	T65.891	T65.892	T65.893	T65.894	—	—
laxative	T47.4X1	T47.4X2	T47.4X3	T47.4X4	T47.4X5	T47.4X6
organic	T60.0X1	T60.0X2	T60.0X3	T60.0X4	—	—
solvent	T52.91	T52.92	T52.93	T52.94	—	—

Substance	Poisoning, Accidental (unintentional)	Poisoning, Intentional Self-harm	Poisoning, Assault	Poisoning, Undetermined	Adverse Effect	Under-dosing
Phosphate — continued						
tricresyl	T65.891	T65.892	T65.893	T65.894	—	—
Phosphine	T57.1X1	T57.1X2	T57.1X3	T57.1X4	—	—
fumigant	T57.1X1	T57.1X2	T57.1X3	T57.1X4	—	—
Phospholine	T49.5X1	T49.5X2	T49.5X3	T49.5X4	T49.5X5	T49.5X6
Phosphoric acid	T54.2X1	T54.2X2	T54.2X3	T54.2X4	—	—
Phosphorus (compound) NEC	T57.1X1	T57.1X2	T57.1X3	T57.1X4	—	—
pesticide	T60.0X1	T60.0X2	T60.0X3	T60.0X4	—	—
Phthalates	T65.891	T65.892	T65.893	T65.894	—	—
Phthalic anhydride	T65.891	T65.892	T65.893	T65.894	—	—
Phthalimidoglutarimide	T42.6X1	T42.6X2	T42.6X3	T42.6X4	T42.6X5	T42.6X6
Phthalylsulfathiazole	T37.0X1	T37.0X2	T37.0X3	T37.0X4	T37.0X5	T37.0X6
Phylloquinone	T45.7X1	T45.7X2	T45.7X3	T45.7X4	T45.7X5	T45.7X6
Physeptone	T40.3X1	T40.3X2	T40.3X3	T40.3X4	T40.3X5	T40.3X6
Physostigma venenosum	T62.2X1	T62.2X2	T62.2X3	T62.2X4	—	—
Physostigmine	T49.5X1	T49.5X2	T49.5X3	T49.5X4	T49.5X5	T49.5X6
Phytolacca decandra	T62.2X1	T62.2X2	T62.2X3	T62.2X4	—	—
berries	T62.1X1	T62.1X2	T62.1X3	T62.1X4	—	—
Phytomenadione	T45.7X1	T45.7X2	T45.7X3	T45.7X4	T45.7X5	T45.7X6
Phytonadione	T45.7X1	T45.7X2	T45.7X3	T45.7X4	T45.7X5	T45.7X6
Picoperine	T48.3X1	T48.3X2	T48.3X3	T48.3X4	T48.3X5	T48.3X6
Picosulfate (sodium)	T47.2X1	T47.2X2	T47.2X3	T47.2X4	T47.2X5	T47.2X6
Picric (acid)	T54.2X1	T54.2X2	T54.2X3	T54.2X4	—	—
Picrotoxin	T50.7X1	T50.7X2	T50.7X3	T50.7X4	T50.7X5	T50.7X6
Piketoprofen	T49.0X1	T49.0X2	T49.0X3	T49.0X4	T49.0X5	T49.0X6
Pilocarpine	T44.1X1	T44.1X2	T44.1X3	T44.1X4	T44.1X5	T44.1X6
Pilocarpus (jaborandi) extract	T44.1X1	T44.1X2	T44.1X3	T44.1X4	T44.1X5	T44.1X6
Pilsicainide (hydrochloride)	T46.2X1	T46.2X2	T46.2X3	T46.2X4	T46.2X5	T46.2X6
Pimaricin	T36.7X1	T36.7X2	T36.7X3	T36.7X4	T36.7X5	T36.7X6
Pimeclone	T50.7X1	T50.7X2	T50.7X3	T50.7X4	T50.7X5	T50.7X6
Pimelic ketone	T52.8X1	T52.8X2	T52.8X3	T52.8X4	—	—
Pimethixene	T45.0X1	T45.0X2	T45.0X3	T45.0X4	T45.0X5	T45.0X6
Piminodine	T40.2X1	T40.2X2	T40.2X3	T40.2X4	T40.2X5	T40.2X6
Pimozide	T43.591	T43.592	T43.593	T43.594	T43.595	T43.596
Pinacidil	T46.5X1	T46.5X2	T46.5X3	T46.5X4	T46.5X5	T46.5X6
Pinaverium bromide	T44.3X1	T44.3X2	T44.3X3	T44.3X4	T44.3X5	T44.3X6
Pinazepam	T42.4X1	T42.4X2	T42.4X3	T42.4X4	T42.4X5	T42.4X6
Pindolol	T44.7X1	T44.7X2	T44.7X3	T44.7X4	T44.7X5	T44.7X6
Pindone	T60.4X1	T60.4X2	T60.4X3	T60.4X4	—	—
Pine oil (disinfectant)	T65.891	T65.892	T65.893	T65.894	—	—
Pinkroot	T37.4X1	T37.4X2	T37.4X3	T37.4X4	T37.4X5	T37.4X6
Pipadone	T40.2X1	T40.2X2	T40.2X3	T40.2X4		
Pipamazine	T45.0X1	T45.0X2	T45.0X3	T45.0X4	T45.0X5	T45.0X6
Pipamperone	T43.4X1	T43.4X2	T43.4X3	T43.4X4	T43.4X5	T43.4X6
Pipazetate	T48.3X1	T48.3X2	T48.3X3	T48.3X4	T48.3X5	T48.3X6
Pipemidic acid	T37.8X1	T37.8X2	T37.8X3	T37.8X4	T37.8X5	T37.8X6
Pipenzolate bromide	T44.3X1	T44.3X2	T44.3X3	T44.3X4	T44.3X5	T44.3X6
Piperacetazine	T43.3X1	T43.3X2	T43.3X3	T43.3X4	T43.3X5	T43.3X6
Piperacillin	T36.0X1	T36.0X2	T36.0X3	T36.0X4	T36.0X5	T36.0X6
Piperazine	T37.4X1	T37.4X2	T37.4X3	T37.4X4	T37.4X5	T37.4X6
estrone sulfate	T38.5X1	T38.5X2	T38.5X3	T38.5X4	T38.5X5	T38.5X6
Piper cubeba	T62.2X1	T62.2X2	T62.2X3	T62.2X4	—	—
Piperidine	T48.3X1	T48.3X2	T48.3X3	T48.3X4	T48.3X5	T48.3X6
Piperidolate	T44.3X1	T44.3X2	T44.3X3	T44.3X4	T44.3X5	T44.3X6
Piperocaine	T41.3X1	T41.3X2	T41.3X3	T41.3X4	T41.3X5	T41.3X6
infiltration (subcutaneous)	T41.3X1	T41.3X2	T41.3X3	T41.3X4	T41.3X5	T41.3X6
nerve block (peripheral) (plexus)	T41.3X1	T41.3X2	T41.3X3	T41.3X4	T41.3X5	T41.3X6
topical (surface)	T41.3X1	T41.3X2	T41.3X3	T41.3X4	T41.3X5	T41.3X6
Piperonyl butoxide	T60.8X1	T60.8X2	T60.8X3	T60.8X4		
Pipethanate	T44.3X1	T44.3X2	T44.3X3	T44.3X4	T44.3X5	T44.3X6
Pipobroman	T45.1X1	T45.1X2	T45.1X3	T45.1X4	T45.1X5	T45.1X6
Pipotiazine	T43.3X1	T43.3X2	T43.3X3	T43.3X4	T43.3X5	T43.3X6
Pipoxizine	T45.0X1	T45.0X2	T45.0X3	T45.0X4	T45.0X5	T45.0X6
Pipradrol	T43.691	T43.692	T43.693	T43.694	T43.695	T43.696
Piprinhydrinate	T45.0X1	T45.0X2	T45.0X3	T45.0X4	T45.0X5	T45.0X6
Pirarubicin	T45.1X1	T45.1X2	T45.1X3	T45.1X4	T45.1X5	T45.1X6
Pirazinamide	T37.1X1	T37.1X2	T37.1X3	T37.1X4	T37.1X5	T37.1X6
Pirbuterol	T48.6X1	T48.6X2	T48.6X3	T48.6X4	T48.6X5	T48.6X6
Pirenzepine	T47.1X1	T47.1X2	T47.1X3	T47.1X4	T47.1X5	T47.1X6
Piretanide	T50.1X1	T50.1X2	T50.1X3	T50.1X4	T50.1X5	T50.1X6
Piribedil	T42.8X1	T42.8X2	T42.8X3	T42.8X4	T42.8X5	T42.8X6
Piridoxilate	T46.3X1	T46.3X2	T46.3X3	T46.3X4	T46.3X5	T46.3X6
Piritramide	T40.491	T40.492	T40.493	T40.494		
Piromidic acid	T37.8X1	T37.8X2	T37.8X3	T37.8X4	T37.8X5	T37.8X6
Piroxicam	T39.391	T39.392	T39.393	T39.394	T39.395	T39.396
beta-cyclodextrin complex	T39.8X1	T39.8X2	T39.8X3	T39.8X4	T39.8X5	T39.8X6
Pirozadil	T46.6X1	T46.6X2	T46.6X3	T46.6X4	T46.6X5	T46.6X6
Piscidia (bark) (erythrina)	T39.8X1	T39.8X2	T39.8X3	T39.8X4	T39.8X5	T39.8X6
Pitch	T65.891	T65.892	T65.893	T65.894	—	—
Pitkin's solution	T41.3X1	T41.3X2	T41.3X3	T41.3X4	T41.3X5	T41.3X6

Substance	Poisoning, Accidental (unintentional)	Poisoning, Intentional Self-harm	Poisoning, Assault	Poisoning, Undetermined	Adverse Effect	Under-dosing
Pitocin	T48.0X1	T48.0X2	T48.0X3	T48.0X4	T48.0X5	T48.0X6
Pitressin (tannate)	T38.891	T38.892	T38.893	T38.894	T38.895	T38.896
Pituitary extracts	T38.891	T38.892	T38.893	T38.894	T38.895	T38.896
(posterior)						
anterior	T38.811	T38.812	T38.813	T38.814	T38.815	T38.816
Pituitrin	T38.891	T38.892	T38.893	T38.894	T38.895	T38.896
Pivampicillin	T36.0X1	T36.0X2	T36.0X3	T36.0X4	T36.0X5	T36.0X6
Pivmecillinam	T36.0X1	T36.0X2	T36.0X3	T36.0X4	T36.0X5	T36.0X6
Placental hormone	T38.891	T38.892	T38.893	T38.894	T38.895	T38.896
Placidyl	T42.6X1	T42.6X2	T42.6X3	T42.6X4	T42.6X5	T42.6X6
Plague vaccine	T50.A91	T50.A92	T50.A93	T50.A94	T50.A95	T50.A96
Plant						
food or fertilizer NEC	T65.891	T65.892	T65.893	T65.894	—	—
containing herbicide	T60.3X1	T60.3X2	T60.3X3	T60.3X4	—	—
noxious, used as food	T62.2X1	T62.2X2	T62.2X3	T62.2X4	—	—
berries	T62.1X1	T62.1X2	T62.1X3	T62.1X4	—	—
seeds	T62.2X1	T62.2X2	T62.2X3	T62.2X4	—	—
specified type NEC	T62.2X1	T62.2X2	T62.2X3	T62.2X4	—	—
Plasma	T45.8X1	T45.8X2	T45.8X3	T45.8X4	T45.8X5	T45.8X6
expander NEC	T45.8X1	T45.8X2	T45.8X3	T45.8X4	T45.8X5	T45.8X6
protein fraction (human)	T45.8X1	T45.8X2	T45.8X3	T45.8X4	T45.8X5	T45.8X6
Plasmanate	T45.8X1	T45.8X2	T45.8X3	T45.8X4	T45.8X5	T45.8X6
Plasminogen (tissue)	T45.611	T45.612	T45.613	T45.614	T45.615	T45.616
activator						
Plaster dressing	T49.3X1	T49.3X2	T49.3X3	T49.3X4	T49.3X5	T49.3X6
Plastic dressing	T49.3X1	T49.3X2	T49.3X3	T49.3X4	T49.3X5	T49.3X6
Plegicil	T43.3X1	T43.3X2	T43.3X3	T43.3X4	T43.3X5	T43.3X6
Plicamycin	T45.1X1	T45.1X2	T45.1X3	T45.1X4	T45.1X5	T45.1X6
Podophyllotoxin	T49.8X1	T49.8X2	T49.8X3	T49.8X4	T49.8X5	T49.8X6
Podophyllum (resin)	T49.4X1	T49.4X2	T49.4X3	T49.4X4	T49.4X5	T49.4X6
Poisonous berries	T62.1X1	T62.1X2	T62.1X3	T62.1X4	—	—
Poison NEC	T65.91	T65.92	T65.93	T65.94	—	—
Pokeweed (any part)	T62.2X1	T62.2X2	T62.2X3	T62.2X4	—	—
Poldine metilsulfate	T44.3X1	T44.3X2	T44.3X3	T44.3X4	T44.3X5	T44.3X6
Polidexide (sulfate)	T46.6X1	T46.6X2	T46.6X3	T46.6X4	T46.6X5	T46.6X6
Polidocanol	T46.8X1	T46.8X2	T46.8X3	T46.8X4	T46.8X5	T46.8X6
Poliomyelitis vaccine	T50.B91	T50.B92	T50.B93	T50.B94	T50.B95	T50.B96
Polish (car) (floor) (furniture)	T65.891	T65.892	T65.893	T65.894	—	—
(metal) (porcelain)						
(silver)						
abrasive	T65.891	T65.892	T65.893	T65.894	—	—
porcelain	T65.891	T65.892	T65.893	T65.894	—	—
Poloxalkol	T47.4X1	T47.4X2	T47.4X3	T47.4X4	T47.4X5	T47.4X6
Poloxamer	T47.4X1	T47.4X2	T47.4X3	T47.4X4	T47.4X5	T47.4X6
Polyaminostyrene resins	T50.3X1	T50.3X2	T50.3X3	T50.3X4	T50.3X5	T50.3X6
Polycarbophil	T47.4X1	T47.4X2	T47.4X3	T47.4X4	T47.4X5	T47.4X6
Polychlorinated biphenyl	T65.891	T65.892	T65.893	T65.894	—	—
Polycycline	T36.4X1	T36.4X2	T36.4X3	T36.4X4	T36.4X5	T36.4X6
Polyester fumes	T59.891	T59.892	T59.893	T59.894	—	—
Polyester resin hardener	T52.91	T52.92	T52.93	T52.94	—	—
fumes	T59.891	T59.892	T59.893	T59.894	—	—
Polyestradiol phosphate	T38.5X1	T38.5X2	T38.5X3	T38.5X4	T38.5X5	T38.5X6
Polyethanolamine alkyl	T49.2X1	T49.2X2	T49.2X3	T49.2X4	T49.2X5	T49.2X6
sulfate						
Polyethylene adhesive	T49.3X1	T49.3X2	T49.3X3	T49.3X4	T49.3X5	T49.3X6
Polyferose	T45.4X1	T45.4X2	T45.4X3	T45.4X4	T45.4X5	T45.4X6
Polygeline	T45.8X1	T45.8X2	T45.8X3	T45.8X4	T45.8X5	T45.8X6
Polymyxin	T36.8X1	T36.8X2	T36.8X3	T36.8X4	T36.8X5	T36.8X6
B	T36.8X1	T36.8X2	T36.8X3	T36.8X4	T36.8X5	T36.8X6
ENT agent	T49.6X1	T49.6X2	T49.6X3	T49.6X4	T49.6X5	T49.6X6
ophthalmic preparation	T49.5X1	T49.5X2	T49.5X3	T49.5X4	T49.5X5	T49.5X6
topical NEC	T49.0X1	T49.0X2	T49.0X3	T49.0X4	T49.0X5	T49.0X6
E sulfate (eye preparation)	T49.5X1	T49.5X2	T49.5X3	T49.5X4	T49.5X5	T49.5X6
Polynoxylin	T49.0X1	T49.0X2	T49.0X3	T49.0X4	T49.0X5	T49.0X6
Polyoestradiol phosphate	T38.5X1	T38.5X2	T38.5X3	T38.5X4	T38.5X5	T38.5X6
Polyoxymethyleneurea	T49.0X1	T49.0X2	T49.0X3	T49.0X4	T49.0X5	T49.0X6
Polysilane	T47.8X1	T47.8X2	T47.8X3	T47.8X4	T47.8X5	T47.8X6
Polytetrafluoroethylene	T59.891	T59.892	T59.893	T59.894	—	—
(inhaled)						
Polythiazide	T50.2X1	T50.2X2	T50.2X3	T50.2X4	T50.2X5	T50.2X6
Polyvidone	T45.8X1	T45.8X2	T45.8X3	T45.8X4	T45.8X5	T45.8X6
Polyvinylpyrrolidone	T45.8X1	T45.8X2	T45.8X3	T45.8X4	T45.8X5	T45.8X6
Pontocaine (hydrochloride)	T41.3X1	T41.3X2	T41.3X3	T41.3X4	T41.3X5	T41.3X6
(infiltration) (topical)						
nerve block (peripheral)	T41.3X1	T41.3X2	T41.3X3	T41.3X4	T41.3X5	T41.3X6
(plexus)						
spinal	T41.3X1	T41.3X2	T41.3X3	T41.3X4	T41.3X5	T41.3X6
Porfiromycin	T45.1X1	T45.1X2	T45.1X3	T45.1X4	T45.1X5	T45.1X6
Posterior pituitary hormone NEC	T38.891	T38.892	T38.893	T38.894	T38.895	T38.896
Pot	T40.7X1	T40.7X2	T40.7X3	T40.7X4	T40.7X5	T40.7X6
Potash (caustic)	T54.3X1	T54.3X2	T54.3X3	T54.3X4	—	—

Substance	Poisoning, Accidental (unintentional)	Poisoning, Intentional Self-harm	Poisoning, Assault	Poisoning, Undetermined	Adverse Effect	Under-dosing
Potassic saline injection	T50.3X1	T50.3X2	T50.3X3	T50.3X4	T50.3X5	T50.3X6
(lactated)						
Potassium (salts) **NEC**	T50.3X1	T50.3X2	T50.3X3	T50.3X4	T50.3X5	T50.3X6
aminobenzoate	T45.8X1	T45.8X2	T45.8X3	T45.8X4	T45.8X5	T45.8X6
aminosalicylate	T37.1X1	T37.1X2	T37.1X3	T37.1X4	T37.1X5	T37.1X6
antimony ' tartrate'	T37.8X1	T37.8X2	T37.8X3	T37.8X4	T37.8X5	T37.8X6
arsenite (solution)	T57.0X1	T57.0X2	T57.0X3	T57.0X4	—	—
bichromate	T56.2X1	T56.2X2	T56.2X3	T56.2X4	—	—
bisulfate	T47.3X1	T47.3X2	T47.3X3	T47.3X4	T47.3X5	T47.3X6
bromide	T42.6X1	T42.6X2	T42.6X3	T42.6X4	T42.6X5	T42.6X6
canrenoate	T50.0X1	T50.0X2	T50.0X3	T50.0X4	T50.0X5	T50.0X6
carbonate	T54.3X1	T54.3X2	T54.3X3	T54.3X4	—	—
chlorate NEC	T65.891	T65.892	T65.893	T65.894	—	—
chloride	T50.3X1	T50.3X2	T50.3X3	T50.3X4	T50.3X5	T50.3X6
citrate	T50.991	T50.992	T50.993	T50.994	T50.995	T50.996
cyanide	T65.0X1	T65.0X2	T65.0X3	T65.0X4	—	—
ferric hexacyanoferrate	T50.6X1	T50.6X2	T50.6X3	T50.6X4	T50.6X5	T50.6X6
(medicinal)						
nonmedicinal	T65.891	T65.892	T65.893	T65.894	—	—
Fluoride	T57.8X1	T57.8X2	T57.8X3	T57.8X4	—	—
glucaldrate	T47.1X1	T47.1X2	T47.1X3	T47.1X4	T47.1X5	T47.1X6
hydroxide	T54.3X1	T54.3X2	T54.3X3	T54.3X4	—	—
iodate	T49.0X1	T49.0X2	T49.0X3	T49.0X4	T49.0X5	T49.0X6
iodide	T48.4X1	T48.4X2	T48.4X3	T48.4X4	T48.4X5	T48.4X6
nitrate	T57.8X1	T57.8X2	T57.8X3	T57.8X4	—	—
oxalate	T65.891	T65.892	T65.893	T65.894	—	—
perchlorate (nonmedicinal)	T65.891	T65.892	T65.893	T65.894	—	—
NEC						
antithyroid	T38.2X1	T38.2X2	T38.2X3	T38.2X4	T38.2X5	T38.2X6
medicinal	T38.2X1	T38.2X2	T38.2X3	T38.2X4	T38.2X5	T38.2X6
Permanganate	T65.891	T65.892	T65.893	T65.894	—	—
(nonmedicinal)						
medicinal	T49.0X1	T49.0X2	T49.0X3	T49.0X4	T49.0X5	T49.0X6
sulfate	T47.2X1	T47.2X2	T47.2X3	T47.2X4	T47.2X5	T47.2X6
Potassium-removing resin	T50.3X1	T50.3X2	T50.3X3	T50.3X4	T50.3X5	T50.3X6
Potassium-retaining drug	T50.3X1	T50.3X2	T50.3X3	T50.3X4	T50.3X5	T50.3X6
Povidone	T45.8X1	T45.8X2	T45.8X3	T45.8X4	T45.8X5	T45.8X6
iodine	T49.0X1	T49.0X2	T49.0X3	T49.0X4	T49.0X5	T49.0X6
Practolol	T44.7X1	T44.7X2	T44.7X3	T44.7X4	T44.7X5	T44.7X6
Prajmalium bitartrate	T46.2X1	T46.2X2	T46.2X3	T46.2X4	T46.2X5	T46.2X6
Pralidoxime (iodide)	T50.6X1	T50.6X2	T50.6X3	T50.6X4	T50.6X5	T50.6X6
chloride	T50.6X1	T50.6X2	T50.6X3	T50.6X4	T50.6X5	T50.6X6
Pramiverine	T44.3X1	T44.3X2	T44.3X3	T44.3X4	T44.3X5	T44.3X6
Pramocaine	T49.1X1	T49.1X2	T49.1X3	T49.1X4	T49.1X5	T49.1X6
Pramoxine	T49.1X1	T49.1X2	T49.1X3	T49.1X4	T49.1X5	T49.1X6
Prasterone	T38.7X1	T38.7X2	T38.7X3	T38.7X4	T38.7X5	T38.7X6
Pravastatin	T46.6X1	T46.6X2	T46.6X3	T46.6X4	T46.6X5	T46.6X6
Prazepam	T42.4X1	T42.4X2	T42.4X3	T42.4X4	T42.4X5	T42.4X6
Praziquantel	T37.4X1	T37.4X2	T37.4X3	T37.4X4	T37.4X5	T37.4X6
Prazitone	T43.291	T43.292	T43.293	T43.294	T43.295	T43.296
Prazosin	T44.6X1	T44.6X2	T44.6X3	T44.6X4	T44.6X5	T44.6X6
Prednicarbate	T49.0X1	T49.0X2	T49.0X3	T49.0X4	T49.0X5	T49.0X6
Prednimustine	T45.1X1	T45.1X2	T45.1X3	T45.1X4	T45.1X5	T45.1X6
Prednisolone	T38.0X1	T38.0X2	T38.0X3	T38.0X4	T38.0X5	T38.0X6
ENT agent	T49.6X1	T49.6X2	T49.6X3	T49.6X4	T49.6X5	T49.6X6
ophthalmic preparation	T49.5X1	T49.5X2	T49.5X3	T49.5X4	T49.5X5	T49.5X6
steaglate	T49.0X1	T49.0X2	T49.0X3	T49.0X4	T49.0X5	T49.0X6
topical NEC	T49.0X1	T49.0X2	T49.0X3	T49.0X4	T49.0X5	T49.0X6
Prednisone	T38.0X1	T38.0X2	T38.0X3	T38.0X4	T38.0X5	T38.0X6
Prednylidene	T38.0X1	T38.0X2	T38.0X3	T38.0X4	T38.0X5	T38.0X6
Pregnandiol	T38.5X1	T38.5X2	T38.5X3	T38.5X4	T38.5X5	T38.5X6
Pregneninolone	T38.5X1	T38.5X2	T38.5X3	T38.5X4	T38.5X5	T38.5X6
Preludin	T43.691	T43.692	T43.693	T43.694	T43.695	T43.696
Premarin	T38.5X1	T38.5X2	T38.5X3	T38.5X4	T38.5X5	T38.5X6
Premedication anesthetic	T41.201	T41.202	T41.203	T41.204	T41.205	T41.206
Prenalterol	T44.5X1	T44.5X2	T44.5X3	T44.5X4	T44.5X5	T44.5X6
Prenoxdiazine	T48.3X1	T48.3X2	T48.3X3	T48.3X4	T48.3X5	T48.3X6
Prenylamine	T46.3X1	T46.3X2	T46.3X3	T46.3X4	T46.3X5	T46.3X6
Preparation H	T49.8X1	T49.8X2	T49.8X3	T49.8X4	T49.8X5	T49.8X6
Preparation, local	T49.4X1	T49.4X2	T49.4X3	T49.4X4	T49.4X5	T49.4X6
Preservative	T65.891	T65.892	T65.893	T65.894	—	—
(nonmedicinal)						
medicinal	T50.901	T50.902	T50.903	T50.904	T50.905	T50.906
wood	T60.91	T60.92	T60.93	T60.94	—	—
Prethcamide	T50.7X1	T50.7X2	T50.7X3	T50.7X4	T50.7X5	T50.7X6
Pride of China	T62.2X1	T62.2X2	T62.2X3	T62.2X4	—	—
Pridinol	T44.3X1	T44.3X2	T44.3X3	T44.3X4	T44.3X5	T44.3X6
Prifinium bromide	T44.3X1	T44.3X2	T44.3X3	T44.3X4	T44.3X5	T44.3X6
Prilocaine	T41.3X1	T41.3X2	T41.3X3	T41.3X4	T41.3X5	T41.3X6
infiltration (subcutaneous)	T41.3X1	T41.3X2	T41.3X3	T41.3X4	T41.3X5	T41.3X6
nerve block (peripheral)	T41.3X1	T41.3X2	T41.3X3	T41.3X4	T41.3X5	T41.3X6
(plexus)						
regional	T41.3X1	T41.3X2	T41.3X3	T41.3X4	T41.3X5	T41.3X6

Substance	Poisoning, Accidental (unintentional)	Poisoning, Intentional Self-harm	Poisoning, Assault	Poisoning, Undetermined	Adverse Effect	Under-dosing
Primaquine	T37.2X1	T37.2X2	T37.2X3	T37.2X4	T37.2X5	T37.2X6
Primidone	T42.6X1	T42.6X2	T42.6X3	T42.6X4	T42.6X5	T42.6X6
Primula (veris)	T62.2X1	T62.2X2	T62.2X3	T62.2X4	—	—
Prinadol	T40.2X1	T40.2X2	T40.2X3	T40.2X4	T40.2X5	T40.2X6
Priscol, Priscoline	T44.6X1	T44.6X2	T44.6X3	T44.6X4	T44.6X5	T44.6X6
Pristinamycin	T36.3X1	T36.3X2	T36.3X3	T36.3X4	T36.3X5	T36.3X6
Privet	T62.2X1	T62.2X2	T62.2X3	T62.2X4	—	—
berries	T62.1X1	T62.1X2	T62.1X3	T62.1X4	—	—
Privine	T44.4X1	T44.4X2	T44.4X3	T44.4X4	T44.4X5	T44.4X6
Pro-Banthine	T44.3X1	T44.3X2	T44.3X3	T44.3X4	T44.3X5	T44.3X6
Probarbital	T42.3X1	T42.3X2	T42.3X3	T42.3X4	T42.3X5	T42.3X6
Probenecid	T50.4X1	T50.4X2	T50.4X3	T50.4X4	T50.4X5	T50.4X6
Probucol	T46.6X1	T46.6X2	T46.6X3	T46.6X4	T46.6X5	T46.6X6
Procainamide	T46.2X1	T46.2X2	T46.2X3	T46.2X4	T46.2X5	T46.2X6
Procaine	T41.3X1	T41.3X2	T41.3X3	T41.3X4	T41.3X5	T41.3X6
benzylpenicillin	T36.0X1	T36.0X2	T36.0X3	T36.0X4	T36.0X5	T36.0X6
nerve block (periphreal) (plexus)	T41.3X1	T41.3X2	T41.3X3	T41.3X4	T41.3X5	T41.3X6
penicillin G	T36.0X1	T36.0X2	T36.0X3	T36.0X4	T36.0X5	T36.0X6
regional	T41.3X1	T41.3X2	T41.3X3	T41.3X4	T41.3X5	T41.3X6
spinal	T41.3X1	T41.3X2	T41.3X3	T41.3X4	T41.3X5	T41.3X6
Procalmidol	T43.591	T43.592	T43.593	T43.594	T43.595	T43.596
Procarbazine	T45.1X1	T45.1X2	T45.1X3	T45.1X4	T45.1X5	T45.1X6
Procaterol	T44.5X1	T44.5X2	T44.5X3	T44.5X4	T44.5X5	T44.5X6
Prochlorperazine	T43.3X1	T43.3X2	T43.3X3	T43.3X4	T43.3X5	T43.3X6
Procyclidine	T44.3X1	T44.3X2	T44.3X3	T44.3X4	T44.3X5	T44.3X6
Producer gas	T58.8X1	T58.8X2	T58.8X3	T58.8X4	—	—
Profadol	T40.491	T40.492	T40.493	T40.494	T40.495	T40.496
Profenamine	T44.3X1	T44.3X2	T44.3X3	T44.3X4	T44.3X5	T44.3X6
Profenil	T44.3X1	T44.3X2	T44.3X3	T44.3X4	T44.3X5	T44.3X6
Proflavine	T49.0X1	T49.0X2	T49.0X3	T49.0X4	T49.0X5	T49.0X6
Progabide	T42.6X1	T42.6X2	T42.6X3	T42.6X4	T42.6X5	T42.6X6
Progesterone	T38.5X1	T38.5X2	T38.5X3	T38.5X4	T38.5X5	T38.5X6
Progestin	T38.5X1	T38.5X2	T38.5X3	T38.5X4	T38.5X5	T38.5X6
oral contraceptive	T38.4X1	T38.4X2	T38.4X3	T38.4X4	T38.4X5	T38.4X6
Progestogen NEC	T38.5X1	T38.5X2	T38.5X3	T38.5X4	T38.5X5	T38.5X6
Progestone	T38.5X1	T38.5X2	T38.5X3	T38.5X4	T38.5X5	T38.5X6
Proglumide	T47.1X1	T47.1X2	T47.1X3	T47.1X4	T47.1X5	T47.1X6
Proguanil	T37.2X1	T37.2X2	T37.2X3	T37.2X4	T37.2X5	T37.2X6
Prolactin	T38.811	T38.812	T38.813	T38.814	T38.815	T38.816
Prolintane	T43.691	T43.692	T43.693	T43.694	T43.695	T43.696
Proloid	T38.1X1	T38.1X2	T38.1X3	T38.1X4	T38.1X5	T38.1X6
Proluton	T38.5X1	T38.5X2	T38.5X3	T38.5X4	T38.5X5	T38.5X6
Promacetin	T37.1X1	T37.1X2	T37.1X3	T37.1X4	T37.1X5	T37.1X6
Promazine	T43.3X1	T43.3X2	T43.3X3	T43.3X4	T43.3X5	T43.3X6
Promedol	T40.2X1	T40.2X2	T40.2X3	T40.2X4	—	—
Promegestone	T38.5X1	T38.5X2	T38.5X3	T38.5X4	T38.5X5	T38.5X6
Promethazine (teoclate)	T43.3X1	T43.3X2	T43.3X3	T43.3X4	T43.3X5	T43.3X6
Promin	T37.1X1	T37.1X2	T37.1X3	T37.1X4	T37.1X5	T37.1X6
Pronase	T45.3X1	T45.3X2	T45.3X3	T45.3X4	T45.3X5	T45.3X6
Pronestyl (hydrochloride)	T46.2X1	T46.2X2	T46.2X3	T46.2X4	T46.2X5	T46.2X6
Pronetalol	T44.7X1	T44.7X2	T44.7X3	T44.7X4	T44.7X5	T44.7X6
Prontosil	T37.0X1	T37.0X2	T37.0X3	T37.0X4	T37.0X5	T37.0X6
Propachlor	T60.3X1	T60.3X2	T60.3X3	T60.3X4	—	—
Propafenone	T46.2X1	T46.2X2	T46.2X3	T46.2X4	T46.2X5	T46.2X6
Propallylonal	T42.3X1	T42.3X2	T42.3X3	T42.3X4	T42.3X5	T42.3X6
Propamidine	T49.0X1	T49.0X2	T49.0X3	T49.0X4	T49.0X5	T49.0X6
Propane (distributed in mobile container)	T59.891	T59.892	T59.893	T59.894	—	—
distributed through pipes	T59.891	T59.892	T59.893	T59.894	—	—
incomplete combustion	T58.11	T58.12	T58.13	T58.14	—	—
Propanidid	T41.291	T41.292	T41.293	T41.294	T41.295	T41.296
Propanil	T60.3X1	T60.3X2	T60.3X3	T60.3X4	—	—
Propantheline	T44.3X1	T44.3X2	T44.3X3	T44.3X4	T44.3X5	T44.3X6
bromide	T44.3X1	T44.3X2	T44.3X3	T44.3X4	T44.3X5	T44.3X6
Proparacaine	T41.3X1	T41.3X2	T41.3X3	T41.3X4	T41.3X5	T41.3X6
Propatylnitrate	T46.3X1	T46.3X2	T46.3X3	T46.3X4	T46.3X5	T46.3X6
Propicillin	T36.0X1	T36.0X2	T36.0X3	T36.0X4	T36.0X5	T36.0X6
Propiolactone	T49.0X1	T49.0X2	T49.0X3	T49.0X4	T49.0X5	T49.0X6
Propiomazine	T45.0X1	T45.0X2	T45.0X3	T45.0X4	T45.0X5	T45.0X6
Propionaldehyde (medicinal)	T42.6X1	T42.6X2	T42.6X3	T42.6X4	T42.6X5	T42.6X6
Propionate (calcium) (sodium)	T49.0X1	T49.0X2	T49.0X3	T49.0X4	T49.0X5	T49.0X6
Propion gel	T49.0X1	T49.0X2	T49.0X3	T49.0X4	T49.0X5	T49.0X6
Propitocaine	T41.3X1	T41.3X2	T41.3X3	T41.3X4	T41.3X5	T41.3X6
infiltration (subcutaneous)	T41.3X1	T41.3X2	T41.3X3	T41.3X4	T41.3X5	T41.3X6
nerve block (peripheral) (plexus)	T41.3X1	T41.3X2	T41.3X3	T41.3X4	T41.3X5	T41.3X6
Propofol	T41.291	T41.292	T41.293	T41.294	T41.295	T41.296
Propoxur	T60.0X1	T60.0X2	T60.0X3	T60.0X4	—	—
Propoxycaine	T41.3X1	T41.3X2	T41.3X3	T41.3X4	T41.3X5	T41.3X6
infiltration (subcutaneous)	T41.3X1	T41.3X2	T41.3X3	T41.3X4	T41.3X5	T41.3X6

Substance	Poisoning, Accidental (unintentional)	Poisoning, Intentional Self-harm	Poisoning, Assault	Poisoning, Undetermined	Adverse Effect	Under-dosing
Propoxycaine — *continued*						
nerve block (peripheral) (plexus)	T41.3X1	T41.3X2	T41.3X3	T41.3X4	T41.3X5	T41.3X6
topical (surface)	T41.3X1	T41.3X2	T41.3X3	T41.3X4	T41.3X5	T41.3X6
Propoxyphene	T40.491	T40.492	T40.493	T40.494	T40.495	T40.496
Propranolol	T44.7X1	T44.7X2	T44.7X3	T44.7X4	T44.7X5	T44.7X6
Propyl						
alcohol	T51.3X1	T51.3X2	T51.3X3	T51.3X4	—	—
carbinol	T51.3X1	T51.3X2	T51.3X3	T51.3X4	—	—
hexadrine	T44.4X1	T44.4X2	T44.4X3	T44.4X4	T44.4X5	T44.4X6
iodone	T50.8X1	T50.8X2	T50.8X3	T50.8X4	T50.8X5	T50.8X6
thiouracil	T38.2X1	T38.2X2	T38.2X3	T38.2X4	T38.2X5	T38.2X6
Propylaminophenothiazine	T43.3X1	T43.3X2	T43.3X3	T43.3X4	T43.3X5	T43.3X6
Propylene	T59.891	T59.892	T59.893	T59.894	—	—
Propylhexedrine	T48.5X1	T48.5X2	T48.5X3	T48.5X4	T48.5X5	T48.5X6
Propyliodone	T50.8X1	T50.8X2	T50.8X3	T50.8X4	T50.8X5	T50.8X6
Propylparaben (ophthalmic)	T49.5X1	T49.5X2	T49.5X3	T49.5X4	T49.5X5	T49.5X6
Propylthiouracil	T38.2X1	T38.2X2	T38.2X3	T38.2X4	T38.2X5	T38.2X6
Propyphenazone	T39.2X1	T39.2X2	T39.2X3	T39.2X4	T39.2X5	T39.2X6
Proquazone	T39.391	T39.392	T39.393	T39.394	T39.395	T39.396
Proscillaridin	T46.0X1	T46.0X2	T46.0X3	T46.0X4	T46.0X5	T46.0X6
Prostacyclin	T45.521	T45.522	T45.523	T45.524	T45.525	T45.526
Prostaglandin (I2)	T45.521	T45.522	T45.523	T45.524	T45.525	T45.526
E1	T46.7X1	T46.7X2	T46.7X3	T46.7X4	T46.7X5	T46.7X6
E2	T48.0X1	T48.0X2	T48.0X3	T48.0X4	T48.0X5	T48.0X6
F2 alpha	T48.0X1	T48.0X2	T48.0X3	T48.0X4	T48.0X5	T48.0X6
Prostigmin	T44.0X1	T44.0X2	T44.0X3	T44.0X4	T44.0X5	T44.0X6
Prosultiamine	T45.2X1	T45.2X2	T45.2X3	T45.2X4	T45.2X5	T45.2X6
Protamine sulfate	T45.7X1	T45.7X2	T45.7X3	T45.7X4	T45.7X5	T45.7X6
zinc insulin	T38.3X1	T38.3X2	T38.3X3	T38.3X4	T38.3X5	T38.3X6
Protease	T47.5X1	T47.5X2	T47.5X3	T47.5X4	T47.5X5	T47.5X6
Protectant, skin NEC	T49.3X1	T49.3X2	T49.3X3	T49.3X4	T49.3X5	T49.3X6
Protein hydrolysate	T50.991	T50.992	T50.993	T50.994	T50.995	T50.996
Prothiaden — *see* Dothiepin hydrochloride						
Prothionamide	T37.1X1	T37.1X2	T37.1X3	T37.1X4	T37.1X5	T37.1X6
Prothipendyl	T43.591	T43.592	T43.593	T43.594	T43.595	T43.596
Prothoate	T60.0X1	T60.0X2	T60.0X3	T60.0X4	—	—
Prothrombin						
activator	T45.7X1	T45.7X2	T45.7X3	T45.7X4	T45.7X5	T45.7X6
synthesis inhibitor	T45.511	T45.512	T45.513	T45.514	T45.515	T45.516
Protionamide	T37.1X1	T37.1X2	T37.1X3	T37.1X4	T37.1X5	T37.1X6
Protirelin	T38.891	T38.892	T38.893	T38.894	T38.895	T38.896
Protokylol	T48.6X1	T48.6X2	T48.6X3	T48.6X4	T48.6X5	T48.6X6
Protopam	T50.6X1	T50.6X2	T50.6X3	T50.6X4	T50.6X5	T50.6X6
Protoveratrine(s) (A) (B)	T46.5X1	T46.5X2	T46.5X3	T46.5X4	T46.5X5	T46.5X6
Protriptyline	T43.011	T43.012	T43.013	T43.014	T43.015	T43.016
Provera	T38.5X1	T38.5X2	T38.5X3	T38.5X4	T38.5X5	T38.5X6
Provitamin A	T45.2X1	T45.2X2	T45.2X3	T45.2X4	T45.2X5	T45.2X6
Proxibarbal	T42.3X1	T42.3X2	T42.3X3	T42.3X4	T42.3X5	T42.3X6
Proxymetacaine	T41.3X1	T41.3X2	T41.3X3	T41.3X4	T41.3X5	T41.3X6
Proxyphylline	T48.6X1	T48.6X2	T48.6X3	T48.6X4	T48.6X5	T48.6X6
Prozac — *see* Fluoxetine hydrochloride						
Prunus						
laurocerasus	T62.2X1	T62.2X2	T62.2X3	T62.2X4	—	—
virginiana	T62.2X1	T62.2X2	T62.2X3	T62.2X4	—	—
Prussian blue						
commercial	T65.891	T65.892	T65.893	T65.894	—	—
therapeutic	T50.6X1	T50.6X2	T50.6X3	T50.6X4	T50.6X5	T50.6X6
Prussic acid	T65.0X1	T65.0X2	T65.0X3	T65.0X4	—	—
vapor	T57.3X1	T57.3X2	T57.3X3	T57.3X4	—	—
Pseudoephedrine	T44.991	T44.992	T44.993	T44.994	T44.995	T44.996
Psilocin	T40.991	T40.992	T40.993	T40.994	—	—
Psilocybin	T40.991	T40.992	T40.993	T40.994	—	—
Psilocybine	T40.991	T40.992	T40.993	T40.994	—	—
Psoralene (nonmedicinal)	T65.891	T65.892	T65.893	T65.894		
Psoralens (medicinal)	T50.991	T50.992	T50.993	T50.994	T50.995	T50.996
PSP (phenolsulfonphthalein)	T50.8X1	T50.8X2	T50.8X3	T50.8X4	T50.8X5	T50.8X6
Psychodysleptic drug NOS	T40.901	T40.902	T40.903	T40.904	T40.905	T40.906
specified NEC	T40.991	T40.992	T40.993	T40.994	T40.995	T40.996
Psychostimulant	T43.601	T43.602	T43.603	T43.604	T43.605	T43.606
amphetamine	T43.621	T43.622	T43.623	T43.624	T43.625	T43.626
caffeine	T43.611	T43.612	T43.613	T43.614	T43.615	T43.616
methylphenidate	T43.631	T43.632	T43.633	T43.634	T43.635	T43.636
specified NEC	T43.691	T43.692	T43.693	T43.694	T43.695	T43.696
Psychotherapeutic drug NEC	T43.91	T43.92	T43.93	T43.94	T43.95	T43.96
antidepressants — *see also* Antidepressant	T43.201	T43.202	T43.203	T43.204	T43.205	T43.206
specified NEC	T43.8X1	T43.8X2	T43.8X3	T43.8X4	T43.8X5	T43.8X6

Table of Drugs and Chemicals

Psychotherapeutic drug NEC — Rifampin

Substance	Poisoning, Accidental (unintentional)	Poisoning, Intentional Self-harm	Poisoning, Assault	Poisoning, Undetermined	Adverse Effect	Under-dosing
Psychotherapeutic drug — continued						
tranquilizers NEC	T43.501	T43.502	T43.503	T43.504	T43.505	T43.506
Psychotomimetic agents	T40.901	T40.902	T40.903	T40.904	T40.905	T40.906
Psychotropic drug NEC	T43.91	T43.92	T43.93	T43.94	T43.95	T43.96
specified NEC	T43.8X1	T43.8X2	T43.8X3	T43.8X4	T43.8X5	T43.8X6
Psyllium hydrophilic mucilloid	T47.4X1	T47.4X2	T47.4X3	T47.4X4	T47.4X5	T47.4X6
Pteroylglutamic acid	T45.8X1	T45.8X2	T45.8X3	T45.8X4	T45.8X5	T45.8X6
Pteroyltriglutamate	T45.1X1	T45.1X2	T45.1X3	T45.1X4	T45.1X5	T45.1X6
PTFE — see Polytetrafluoroethylene						
Pulp						
devitalizing paste	T49.7X1	T49.7X2	T49.7X3	T49.7X4	T49.7X5	T49.7X6
dressing	T49.7X1	T49.7X2	T49.7X3	T49.7X4	T49.7X5	T49.7X6
Pulsatilla	T62.2X1	T62.2X2	T62.2X3	T62.2X4	—	—
Pumpkin seed extract	T37.4X1	T37.4X2	T37.4X3	T37.4X4	T37.4X5	T37.4X6
Purex (bleach)	T54.91	T54.92	T54.93	T54.94	—	—
Purgative NEC — see also Cathartic	T47.4X1	T47.4X2	T47.4X3	T47.4X4	T47.4X5	T47.4X6
Purine analogue (antineoplastic)	T45.1X1	T45.1X2	T45.1X3	T45.1X4	T45.1X5	T45.1X6
Purine diuretics	T50.2X1	T50.2X2	T50.2X3	T50.2X4	T50.2X5	T50.2X6
Purinethol	T45.1X1	T45.1X2	T45.1X3	T45.1X4	T45.1X5	T45.1X6
PVP	T45.8X1	T45.8X2	T45.8X3	T45.8X4	T45.8X5	T45.8X6
Pyrabital	T39.8X1	T39.8X2	T39.8X3	T39.8X4	T39.8X5	T39.8X6
Pyramidon	T39.2X1	T39.2X2	T39.2X3	T39.2X4	T39.2X5	T39.2X6
Pyrantel	T37.4X1	T37.4X2	T37.4X3	T37.4X4	T37.4X5	T37.4X6
Pyrathiazine	T45.0X1	T45.0X2	T45.0X3	T45.0X4	T45.0X5	T45.0X6
Pyrazinamide	T37.1X1	T37.1X2	T37.1X3	T37.1X4	T37.1X5	T37.1X6
Pyrazinoic acid (amide)	T37.1X1	T37.1X2	T37.1X3	T37.1X4	T37.1X5	T37.1X6
Pyrazole (derivatives)	T39.2X1	T39.2X2	T39.2X3	T39.2X4	T39.2X5	T39.2X6
Pyrazolone analgesic NEC	T39.2X1	T39.2X2	T39.2X3	T39.2X4	T39.2X5	T39.2X6
Pyrethrin, pyrethrum (nonmedicinal)	T60.2X1	T60.2X2	T60.2X3	T60.2X4	—	—
Pyrethrum extract	T49.0X1	T49.0X2	T49.0X3	T49.0X4	T49.0X5	T49.0X6
Pyribenzamine	T45.0X1	T45.0X2	T45.0X3	T45.0X4	T45.0X5	T45.0X6
Pyridine	T52.8X1	T52.8X2	T52.8X3	T52.8X4	—	—
aldoxime methiodide	T50.6X1	T50.6X2	T50.6X3	T50.6X4	T50.6X5	T50.6X6
aldoxime methyl chloride	T50.6X1	T50.6X2	T50.6X3	T50.6X4	T50.6X5	T50.6X6
vapor	T59.891	T59.892	T59.893	T59.894	—	—
Pyridium	T39.8X1	T39.8X2	T39.8X3	T39.8X4	T39.8X5	T39.8X6
Pyridostigmine bromide	T44.0X1	T44.0X2	T44.0X3	T44.0X4	T44.0X5	T44.0X6
Pyridoxal phosphate	T45.2X1	T45.2X2	T45.2X3	T45.2X4	T45.2X5	T45.2X6
Pyridoxine	T45.2X1	T45.2X2	T45.2X3	T45.2X4	T45.2X5	T45.2X6
Pyrilamine	T45.0X1	T45.0X2	T45.0X3	T45.0X4	T45.0X5	T45.0X6
Pyrimethamine	T37.2X1	T37.2X2	T37.2X3	T37.2X4	T37.2X5	T37.2X6
with sulfadoxine	T37.2X1	T37.2X2	T37.2X3	T37.2X4	T37.2X5	T37.2X6
Pyrimidine antagonist	T45.1X1	T45.1X2	T45.1X3	T45.1X4	T45.1X5	T45.1X6
Pyriminil	T60.4X1	T60.4X2	T60.4X3	T60.4X4	—	—
Pyrithione zinc	T49.4X1	T49.4X2	T49.4X3	T49.4X4	T49.4X5	T49.4X6
Pyrithyldione	T42.6X1	T42.6X2	T42.6X3	T42.6X4	T42.6X5	T42.6X6
Pyrogallic acid	T49.0X1	T49.0X2	T49.0X3	T49.0X4	T49.0X5	T49.0X6
Pyrogallol	T49.0X1	T49.0X2	T49.0X3	T49.0X4	T49.0X5	T49.0X6
Pyroxylin	T49.3X1	T49.3X2	T49.3X3	T49.3X4	T49.3X5	T49.3X6
Pyrrobutamine	T45.0X1	T45.0X2	T45.0X3	T45.0X4	T45.0X5	T45.0X6
Pyrrolizidine alkaloids	T62.8X1	T62.8X2	T62.8X3	T62.8X4	—	—
Pyrvinium chloride	T37.4X1	T37.4X2	T37.4X3	T37.4X4	T37.4X5	T37.4X6
PZI	T38.3X1	T38.3X2	T38.3X3	T38.3X4	T38.3X5	T38.3X6
Quaalude	T42.6X1	T42.6X2	T42.6X3	T42.6X4	T42.6X5	T42.6X6
Quarternary ammonium						
anti-infective	T49.0X1	T49.0X2	T49.0X3	T49.0X4	T49.0X5	T49.0X6
ganglion blocking	T44.2X1	T44.2X2	T44.2X3	T44.2X4	T44.2X5	T44.2X6
parasympatholytic	T44.3X1	T44.3X2	T44.3X3	T44.3X4	T44.3X5	T44.3X6
Quazepam	T42.4X1	T42.4X2	T42.4X3	T42.4X4	T42.4X5	T42.4X6
Quicklime	T54.3X1	T54.3X2	T54.3X3	T54.3X4	—	—
Quillaja extract	T48.4X1	T48.4X2	T48.4X3	T48.4X4	T48.4X5	T48.4X6
Quinacrine	T37.2X1	T37.2X2	T37.2X3	T37.2X4	T37.2X5	T37.2X6
Quinaglute	T46.2X1	T46.2X2	T46.2X3	T46.2X4	T46.2X5	T46.2X6
Quinalbarbital	T42.3X1	T42.3X2	T42.3X3	T42.3X4	T42.3X5	T42.3X6
Quinalbarbitone sodium	T42.3X1	T42.3X2	T42.3X3	T42.3X4	T42.3X5	T42.3X6
Quinalphos	T60.0X1	T60.0X2	T60.0X3	T60.0X4	—	—
Quinapril	T46.4X1	T46.4X2	T46.4X3	T46.4X4	T46.4X5	T46.4X6
Quinestradiol	T38.5X1	T38.5X2	T38.5X3	T38.5X4	T38.5X5	T38.5X6
Quinestradol	T38.5X1	T38.5X2	T38.5X3	T38.5X4	T38.5X5	T38.5X6
Quinestrol	T38.5X1	T38.5X2	T38.5X3	T38.5X4	T38.5X5	T38.5X6
Quinethazone	T50.2X1	T50.2X2	T50.2X3	T50.2X4	T50.2X5	T50.2X6
Quingestanol	T38.4X1	T38.4X2	T38.4X3	T38.4X4	T38.4X5	T38.4X6
Quinidine	T46.2X1	T46.2X2	T46.2X3	T46.2X4	T46.2X5	T46.2X6
Quinine	T37.2X1	T37.2X2	T37.2X3	T37.2X4	T37.2X5	T37.2X6
Quiniobine	T37.8X1	T37.8X2	T37.8X3	T37.8X4	T37.8X5	T37.8X6
Quinisocaine	T49.1X1	T49.1X2	T49.1X3	T49.1X4	T49.1X5	T49.1X6
Quinocide	T37.2X1	T37.2X2	T37.2X3	T37.2X4	T37.2X5	T37.2X6
Quinoline (derivatives) NEC	T37.8X1	T37.8X2	T37.8X3	T37.8X4	T37.8X5	T37.8X6
Quinupramine	T43.011	T43.012	T43.013	T43.014	T43.015	T43.016
Quotane	T41.3X1	T41.3X2	T41.3X3	T41.3X4	T41.3X5	T41.3X6
Rabies						
immune globulin (human)	T50.Z11	T50.Z12	T50.Z13	T50.Z14	T50.Z15	T50.Z16
vaccine	T50.B91	T50.B92	T50.B93	T50.B94	T50.B95	T50.B96
Racemoramide	T40.2X1	T40.2X2	T40.2X3	T40.2X4	—	—
Racemorphan	T40.2X1	T40.2X2	T40.2X3	T40.2X4	T40.2X5	T40.2X6
Racepinefrin	T44.5X1	T44.5X2	T44.5X3	T44.5X4	T44.5X5	T44.5X6
Raclopride	T43.591	T43.592	T43.593	T43.594	T43.595	T43.596
Radiator alcohol	T51.1X1	T51.1X2	T51.1X3	T51.1X4	—	—
Radioactive drug NEC	T50.8X1	T50.8X2	T50.8X3	T50.8X4	T50.8X5	T50.8X6
Radio-opaque (drugs) (materials)	T50.8X1	T50.8X2	T50.8X3	T50.8X4	T50.8X5	T50.8X6
Ramifenazone	T39.2X1	T39.2X2	T39.2X3	T39.2X4	T39.2X5	T39.2X6
Ramipril	T46.4X1	T46.4X2	T46.4X3	T46.4X4	T46.4X5	T46.4X6
Ranitidine	T47.0X1	T47.0X2	T47.0X3	T47.0X4	T47.0X5	T47.0X6
Ranunculus	T62.2X1	T62.2X2	T62.2X3	T62.2X4	—	—
Rat poison NEC	T60.4X1	T60.4X2	T60.4X3	T60.4X4	—	—
Rattlesnake (venom)	T63.011	T63.012	T63.013	T63.014	—	—
Raubasine	T46.7X1	T46.7X2	T46.7X3	T46.7X4	T46.7X5	T46.7X6
Raudixin	T46.5X1	T46.5X2	T46.5X3	T46.5X4	T46.5X5	T46.5X6
Rautensin	T46.5X1	T46.5X2	T46.5X3	T46.5X4	T46.5X5	T46.5X6
Rautina	T46.5X1	T46.5X2	T46.5X3	T46.5X4	T46.5X5	T46.5X6
Rautotal	T46.5X1	T46.5X2	T46.5X3	T46.5X4	T46.5X5	T46.5X6
Rauwiloid	T46.5X1	T46.5X2	T46.5X3	T46.5X4	T46.5X5	T46.5X6
Rauwoldin	T46.5X1	T46.5X2	T46.5X3	T46.5X4	T46.5X5	T46.5X6
Rauwolfia (alkaloids)	T46.5X1	T46.5X2	T46.5X3	T46.5X4	T46.5X5	T46.5X6
Razoxane	T45.1X1	T45.1X2	T45.1X3	T45.1X4	T45.1X5	T45.1X6
Realgar	T57.0X1	T57.0X2	T57.0X3	T57.0X4	—	—
Recombinant (R) — see specific protein						
Red blood cells, packed	T45.8X1	T45.8X2	T45.8X3	T45.8X4	T45.8X5	T45.8X6
Red squill (scilliroside)	T60.4X1	T60.4X2	T60.4X3	T60.4X4	—	—
Reducing agent, industrial NEC	T65.891	T65.892	T65.893	T65.894	—	—
Refrigerant gas (chlorofluorocarbon)	T53.5X1	T53.5X2	T53.5X3	T53.5X4	—	—
not chlorofluorocarbon	T59.891	T59.892	T59.893	T59.894	—	—
Regroton	T50.2X1	T50.2X2	T50.2X3	T50.2X4	T50.2X5	T50.2X6
Rehydration salts (oral)	T50.3X1	T50.3X2	T50.3X3	T50.3X4	T50.3X5	T50.3X6
Rela	T42.8X1	T42.8X2	T42.8X3	T42.8X4	T42.8X5	T42.8X6
Relaxant, muscle						
anesthetic	T48.1X1	T48.1X2	T48.1X3	T48.1X4	T48.1X5	T48.1X6
central nervous system	T42.8X1	T42.8X2	T42.8X3	T42.8X4	T42.8X5	T42.8X6
skeletal NEC	T48.1X1	T48.1X2	T48.1X3	T48.1X4	T48.1X5	T48.1X6
smooth NEC	T44.3X1	T44.3X2	T44.3X3	T44.3X4	T44.3X5	T44.3X6
Remoxipride	T43.591	T43.592	T43.593	T43.594	T43.595	T43.596
Renese	T50.2X1	T50.2X2	T50.2X3	T50.2X4	T50.2X5	T50.2X6
Renografin	T50.8X1	T50.8X2	T50.8X3	T50.8X4	T50.8X5	T50.8X6
Replacement solution	T50.3X1	T50.3X2	T50.3X3	T50.3X4	T50.3X5	T50.3X6
Reproterol	T48.6X1	T48.6X2	T48.6X3	T48.6X4	T48.6X5	T48.6X6
Rescinnamine	T46.5X1	T46.5X2	T46.5X3	T46.5X4	T46.5X5	T46.5X6
Reserpin (e)	T46.5X1	T46.5X2	T46.5X3	T46.5X4	T46.5X5	T46.5X6
Resorcin, resorcinol (nonmedicinal)	T65.891	T65.892	T65.893	T65.894	—	—
medicinal	T49.4X1	T49.4X2	T49.4X3	T49.4X4	T49.4X5	T49.4X6
Respaire	T48.4X1	T48.4X2	T48.4X3	T48.4X4	T48.4X5	T48.4X6
Respiratory drug NEC	T48.901	T48.902	T48.903	T48.904	T48.905	T48.906
antiasthmatic NEC	T48.6X1	T48.6X2	T48.6X3	T48.6X4	T48.6X5	T48.6X6
anti-common-cold NEC	T48.5X1	T48.5X2	T48.5X3	T48.5X4	T48.5X5	T48.5X6
expectorant NEC	T48.4X1	T48.4X2	T48.4X3	T48.4X4	T48.4X5	T48.4X6
stimulant	T48.901	T48.902	T48.903	T48.904	T48.905	T48.906
Retinoic acid	T49.0X1	T49.0X2	T49.0X3	T49.0X4	T49.0X5	T49.0X6
Retinol	T45.2X1	T45.2X2	T45.2X3	T45.2X4	T45.2X5	T45.2X6
Rh (D) immune globulin (human)	T50.Z11	T50.Z12	T50.Z13	T50.Z14	T50.Z15	T50.Z16
Rhodine	T39.011	T39.012	T39.013	T39.014	T39.015	T39.016
RhoGAM	T50.Z11	T50.Z12	T50.Z13	T50.Z14	T50.Z15	T50.Z16
Rhubarb						
dry extract	T47.2X1	T47.2X2	T47.2X3	T47.2X4	T47.2X5	T47.2X6
tincture, compound	T47.2X1	T47.2X2	T47.2X3	T47.2X4	T47.2X5	T47.2X6
Ribavirin	T37.5X1	T37.5X2	T37.5X3	T37.5X4	T37.5X5	T37.5X6
Riboflavin	T45.2X1	T45.2X2	T45.2X3	T45.2X4	T45.2X5	T45.2X6
Ribostamycin	T36.5X1	T36.5X2	T36.5X3	T36.5X4	T36.5X5	T36.5X6
Ricin	T62.2X1	T62.2X2	T62.2X3	T62.2X4	—	—
Ricinus communis	T62.2X1	T62.2X2	T62.2X3	T62.2X4	—	—
Rickettsial vaccine NEC	T50.A91	T50.A92	T50.A93	T50.A94	T50.A95	T50.A96
Rifabutin	T36.6X1	T36.6X2	T36.6X3	T36.6X4	T36.6X5	T36.6X6
Rifamide	T36.6X1	T36.6X2	T36.6X3	T36.6X4	T36.6X5	T36.6X6
Rifampicin	T36.6X1	T36.6X2	T36.6X3	T36.6X4	T36.6X5	T36.6X6
with isoniazid	T37.1X1	T37.1X2	T37.1X3	T37.1X4	T37.1X5	T37.1X6
Rifampin	T36.6X1	T36.6X2	T36.6X3	T36.6X4	T36.6X5	T36.6X6

Substance	Poisoning, Accidental (unintentional)	Poisoning, Intentional Self-harm	Poisoning, Assault	Poisoning, Undetermined	Adverse Effect	Under-dosing
Rifamycin	T36.6X1	T36.6X2	T36.6X3	T36.6X4	T36.6X5	T36.6X6
Rifaximin	T36.6X1	T36.6X2	T36.6X3	T36.6X4	T36.6X5	T36.6X6
Rimantadine	T37.5X1	T37.5X2	T37.5X3	T37.5X4	T37.5X5	T37.5X6
Rimazolium metilsulfate	T39.8X1	T39.8X2	T39.8X3	T39.8X4	T39.8X5	T39.8X6
Rimifon	T37.1X1	T37.1X2	T37.1X3	T37.1X4	T37.1X5	T37.1X6
Rimiterol	T48.6X1	T48.6X2	T48.6X3	T48.6X4	T48.6X5	T48.6X6
Ringer (lactate) **solution**	T50.3X1	T50.3X2	T50.3X3	T50.3X4	T50.3X5	T50.3X6
Ristocetin	T36.8X1	T36.8X2	T36.8X3	T36.8X4	T36.8X5	T36.8X6
Ritalin	T43.631	T43.632	T43.633	T43.634	T43.635	T43.636
Ritodrine	T44.5X1	T44.5X2	T44.5X3	T44.5X4	T44.5X5	T44.5X6
Roach killer — *see* Insecticide						
Rociverine	T44.3X1	T44.3X2	T44.3X3	T44.3X4	T44.3X5	T44.3X6
Rocky Mountain spotted fever vaccine	T50.A91	T50.A92	T50.A93	T50.A94	T50.A95	T50.A96
Rodenticide NEC	T60.4X1	T60.4X2	T60.4X3	T60.4X4	—	—
Rohypnol	T42.4X1	T42.4X2	T42.4X3	T42.4X4	T42.4X5	T42.4X6
Rokitamycin	T36.3X1	T36.3X2	T36.3X3	T36.3X4	T36.3X5	T36.3X6
Rolaids	T47.1X1	T47.1X2	T47.1X3	T47.1X4	T47.1X5	T47.1X6
Rolitetracycline	T36.4X1	T36.4X2	T36.4X3	T36.4X4	T36.4X5	T36.4X6
Romilar	T48.3X1	T48.3X2	T48.3X3	T48.3X4	T48.3X5	T48.3X6
Ronifibrate	T46.6X1	T46.6X2	T46.6X3	T46.6X4	T46.6X5	T46.6X6
Rosaprostol	T47.1X1	T47.1X2	T47.1X3	T47.1X4	T47.1X5	T47.1X6
Rose bengal sodium (131I)	T50.8X1	T50.8X2	T50.8X3	T50.8X4	T50.8X5	T50.8X6
Rose water ointment	T49.3X1	T49.3X2	T49.3X3	T49.3X4	T49.3X5	T49.3X6
Rosoxacin	T37.8X1	T37.8X2	T37.8X3	T37.8X4	T37.8X5	T37.8X6
Rotenone	T60.2X1	T60.2X2	T60.2X3	T60.2X4	—	—
Rotoxamine	T45.0X1	T45.0X2	T45.0X3	T45.0X4	T45.0X5	T45.0X6
Rough-on-rats	T60.4X1	T60.4X2	T60.4X3	T60.4X4	—	—
Roxatidine	T47.0X1	T47.0X2	T47.0X3	T47.0X4	T47.0X5	T47.0X6
Roxithromycin	T36.3X1	T36.3X2	T36.3X3	T36.3X4	T36.3X5	T36.3X6
Rt-PA	T45.611	T45.612	T45.613	T45.614	T45.615	T45.616
Rubbing alcohol	T51.2X1	T51.2X2	T51.2X3	T51.2X4	—	—
Rubefacient	T49.4X1	T49.4X2	T49.4X3	T49.4X4	T49.4X5	T49.4X6
Rubella vaccine	T50.B91	T50.B92	T50.B93	T50.B94	T50.B95	T50.B96
Rubeola vaccine	T50.B91	T50.B92	T50.B93	T50.B94	T50.B95	T50.B96
Rubidium chloride Rb82	T50.8X1	T50.8X2	T50.8X3	T50.8X4	T50.8X5	T50.8X6
Rubidomycin	T45.1X1	T45.1X2	T45.1X3	T45.1X4	T45.1X5	T45.1X6
Rue	T62.2X1	T62.2X2	T62.2X3	T62.2X4	—	—
Rufocromomycin	T45.1X1	T45.1X2	T45.1X3	T45.1X4	T45.1X5	T45.1X6
Russel's viper venin	T45.7X1	T45.7X2	T45.7X3	T45.7X4	T45.7X5	T45.7X6
Ruta (graveolens)	T62.2X1	T62.2X2	T62.2X3	T62.2X4	—	—
Rutinum	T46.991	T46.992	T46.993	T46.994	T46.995	T46.996
Rutoside	T46.991	T46.992	T46.993	T46.994	T46.995	T46.996
b-sitosterol(s)	T46.6X1	T46.6X2	T46.6X3	T46.6X4	T46.6X5	T46.6X6
Sabadilla (plant)	T62.2X1	T62.2X2	T62.2X3	T62.2X4	—	—
pesticide	T60.2X1	T60.2X2	T60.2X3	T60.2X4	—	—
Saccharated iron oxide	T45.8X1	T45.8X2	T45.8X3	T45.8X4	T45.8X5	T45.8X6
Saccharin	T50.901	T50.902	T50.903	T50.904	T50.905	T50.906
Saccharomyces boulardii	T47.6X1	T47.6X2	T47.6X3	T47.6X4	T47.6X5	T47.6X6
Safflower oil	T46.6X1	T46.6X2	T46.6X3	T46.6X4	T46.6X5	T46.6X6
Safrazine	T43.1X1	T43.1X2	T43.1X3	T43.1X4	T43.1X5	T43.1X6
Salazosulfapyridine	T37.0X1	T37.0X2	T37.0X3	T37.0X4	T37.0X5	T37.0X6
Salbutamol	T48.6X1	T48.6X2	T48.6X3	T48.6X4	T48.6X5	T48.6X6
Salicylamide	T39.091	T39.092	T39.093	T39.094	T39.095	T39.096
Salicylate NEC	T39.091	T39.092	T39.093	T39.094	T39.095	T39.096
methyl	T49.3X1	T49.3X2	T49.3X3	T49.3X4	T49.3X5	T49.3X6
theobromine calcium	T50.2X1	T50.2X2	T50.2X3	T50.2X4	T50.2X5	T50.2X6
Salicylazosulfapyridine	T37.0X1	T37.0X2	T37.0X3	T37.0X4	T37.0X5	T37.0X6
Salicylhydroxamic acid	T49.0X1	T49.0X2	T49.0X3	T49.0X4	T49.0X5	T49.0X6
Salicylic acid	T49.4X1	T49.4X2	T49.4X3	T49.4X4	T49.4X5	T49.4X6
with benzoic acid	T49.4X1	T49.4X2	T49.4X3	T49.4X4	T49.4X5	T49.4X6
congeners	T39.091	T39.092	T39.093	T39.094	T39.095	T39.096
derivative	T39.091	T39.092	T39.093	T39.094	T39.095	T39.096
salts	T39.091	T39.092	T39.093	T39.094	T39.095	T39.096
Salinazid	T37.1X1	T37.1X2	T37.1X3	T37.1X4	T37.1X5	T37.1X6
Salmeterol	T48.6X1	T48.6X2	T48.6X3	T48.6X4	T48.6X5	T48.6X6
Salol	T49.3X1	T49.3X2	T49.3X3	T49.3X4	T49.3X5	T49.3X6
Salsalate	T39.091	T39.092	T39.093	T39.094	T39.095	T39.096
Salt-replacing drug	T50.901	T50.902	T50.903	T50.904	T50.905	T50.906
Salt-retaining mineralocorticoid	T50.0X1	T50.0X2	T50.0X3	T50.0X4	T50.0X5	T50.0X6
Salt substitute	T50.901	T50.902	T50.903	T50.904	T50.905	T50.906
Saluretic NEC	T50.2X1	T50.2X2	T50.2X3	T50.2X4	T50.2X5	T50.2X6
Saluron	T50.2X1	T50.2X2	T50.2X3	T50.2X4	T50.2X5	T50.2X6
Salvarsan 606 (neosilver) (silver)	T37.8X1	T37.8X2	T37.8X3	T37.8X4	T37.8X5	T37.8X6
Sambucus canadensis	T62.2X1	T62.2X2	T62.2X3	T62.2X4	—	—
berry	T62.1X1	T62.1X2	T62.1X3	T62.1X4	—	—
Sandril	T46.5X1	T46.5X2	T46.5X3	T46.5X4	T46.5X5	T46.5X6
Sanguinaria canadensis	T62.2X1	T62.2X2	T62.2X3	T62.2X4	—	—
Saniflush (cleaner)	T54.2X1	T54.2X2	T54.2X3	T54.2X4	—	—
Santonin	T37.4X1	T37.4X2	T37.4X3	T37.4X4	T37.4X5	T37.4X6
Santyl	T49.8X1	T49.8X2	T49.8X3	T49.8X4	T49.8X5	T49.8X6

Substance	Poisoning, Accidental (unintentional)	Poisoning, Intentional Self-harm	Poisoning, Assault	Poisoning, Undetermined	Adverse Effect	Under-dosing
Saralasin	T46.5X1	T46.5X2	T46.5X3	T46.5X4	T46.5X5	T46.5X6
Sarcolysin	T45.1X1	T45.1X2	T45.1X3	T45.1X4	T45.1X5	T45.1X6
Sarkomycin	T45.1X1	T45.1X2	T45.1X3	T45.1X4	T45.1X5	T45.1X6
Saroten	T43.011	T43.012	T43.013	T43.014	T43.015	T43.016
Saturnine — *see* Lead						
Savin (oil)	T49.4X1	T49.4X2	T49.4X3	T49.4X4	T49.4X5	T49.4X6
Scammony	T47.2X1	T47.2X2	T47.2X3	T47.2X4	T47.2X5	T47.2X6
Scarlet red	T49.8X1	T49.8X2	T49.8X3	T49.8X4	T49.8X5	T49.8X6
Scheele's green	T57.0X1	T57.0X2		T57.0X4		
insecticide	T57.0X1	T57.0X2	T57.0X3	T57.0X4		
Schizontozide (blood)	T37.2X1	T37.2X2	T37.2X3	T37.2X4	T37.2X5	T37.2X6
(tissue)						
Schradan	T60.0X1	T60.0X2	T60.0X3	T60.0X4		
Schweinfurth green	T57.0X1	T57.0X2	T57.0X3	T57.0X4		
insecticide	T57.0X1	T57.0X2	T57.0X3	T57.0X4		
Scilla, rat poison	T60.4X1	T60.4X2	T60.4X3	T60.4X4		
Scillaren	T60.4X1	T60.4X2	T60.4X3	T60.4X4		
Sclerosing agent	T46.8X1	T46.8X2	T46.8X3	T46.8X4	T46.8X5	T46.8X6
Scombrotoxin	T61.11	T61.12	T61.13	T61.14		
Scopolamine	T44.3X1	T44.3X2	T44.3X3	T44.3X4	T44.3X5	T44.3X6
Scopolia extract	T44.3X1	T44.3X2	T44.3X3	T44.3X4	T44.3X5	T44.3X6
Scouring powder	T65.891	T65.892	T65.893	T65.894		
Sea						
anemone (sting)	T63.631	T63.632	T63.633	T63.634		
cucumber (sting)	T63.691	T63.692	T63.693	T63.694		
snake (bite) (venom)	T63.091	T63.092	T63.093	T63.094		
urchin spine (puncture)	T63.691	T63.692	T63.693	T63.694		
Seafood	T61.91	T61.92	T61.93	T61.94		
specified NEC	T61.8X1	T61.8X2	T61.8X3	T61.8X4		
Secbutabarbital	T42.3X1	T42.3X2	T42.3X3	T42.3X4	T42.3X5	T42.3X6
Secbutabarbitone	T42.3X1	T42.3X2	T42.3X3	T42.3X4	T42.3X5	T42.3X6
Secnidazole	T37.3X1	T37.3X2	T37.3X3	T37.3X4	T37.3X5	T37.3X6
Secobarbital	T42.3X1	T42.3X2	T42.3X3	T42.3X4	T42.3X5	T42.3X6
Seconal	T42.3X1	T42.3X2	T42.3X3	T42.3X4	T42.3X5	T42.3X6
Secretin	T50.8X1	T50.8X2	T50.8X3	T50.8X4	T50.8X5	T50.8X6
Sedative NEC	T42.71	T42.72	T42.73	T42.74	T42.75	T42.76
mixed NEC	T42.6X1	T42.6X2	T42.6X3	T42.6X4	T42.6X5	T42.6X6
Sedormid	T42.6X1	T42.6X2	T42.6X3	T42.6X4	T42.6X5	T42.6X6
Seed disinfectant or dressing	T60.8X1	T60.8X2	T60.8X3	T60.8X4		
Seeds (poisonous)	T62.2X1	T62.2X2	T62.2X3	T62.2X4		
Selegiline	T42.8X1	T42.8X2	T42.8X3	T42.8X4	T42.8X5	T42.8X6
Selenium NEC	T56.891	T56.892	T56.893	T56.894		
disulfide or sulfide	T49.4X1	T49.4X2	T49.4X3	T49.4X4	T49.4X5	T49.4X6
fumes	T59.891	T59.892	T59.893	T59.894		
sulfide	T49.4X1	T49.4X2	T49.4X3	T49.4X4	T49.4X5	T49.4X6
Selenomethionine (75Se)	T50.8X1	T50.8X2	T50.8X3	T50.8X4	T50.8X5	T50.8X6
Selsun	T49.4X1	T49.4X2	T49.4X3	T49.4X4	T49.4X5	T49.4X6
Semustine	T45.1X1	T45.1X2	T45.1X3	T45.1X4	T45.1X5	T45.1X6
Senega syrup	T48.4X1	T48.4X2	T48.4X3	T48.4X4	T48.4X5	T48.4X6
Senna	T47.2X1	T47.2X2	T47.2X3	T47.2X4	T47.2X5	T47.2X6
Sennoside A+B	T47.2X1	T47.2X2	T47.2X3	T47.2X4	T47.2X5	T47.2X6
Septisol	T49.2X1	T49.2X2	T49.2X3	T49.2X4	T49.2X5	T49.2X6
Seractide	T38.811	T38.812	T38.813	T38.814	T38.815	T38.816
Serax	T42.4X1	T42.4X2	T42.4X3	T42.4X4	T42.4X5	T42.4X6
Serenesil	T42.6X1	T42.6X2	T42.6X3	T42.6X4	T42.6X5	T42.6X6
Serenium (hydrochloride)	T37.91	T37.92	T37.93	T37.94	T37.95	T37.96
Serepax — *see* Oxazepam						
Sermorelin	T38.891	T38.892	T38.893	T38.894	T38.895	T38.896
Sernyl	T41.1X1	T41.1X2	T41.1X3	T41.1X4	T41.1X5	T41.1X6
Serotonin	T50.991	T50.992	T50.993	T50.994	T50.995	T50.996
Serpasil	T46.5X1	T46.5X2	T46.5X3	T46.5X4	T46.5X5	T46.5X6
Serrapeptase	T45.3X1	T45.3X2	T45.3X3	T45.3X4	T45.3X5	T45.3X6
Serum						
antibotulinus	T50.Z11	T50.Z12	T50.Z13	T50.Z14	T50.Z15	T50.Z16
anticytotoxic	T50.Z11	T50.Z12	T50.Z13	T50.Z14	T50.Z15	T50.Z16
antidiphtheria	T50.Z11	T50.Z12	T50.Z13	T50.Z14	T50.Z15	T50.Z16
antimeningococcus	T50.Z11	T50.Z12	T50.Z13	T50.Z14	T50.Z15	T50.Z16
anti-Rh	T50.Z11	T50.Z12	T50.Z13	T50.Z14	T50.Z15	T50.Z16
anti-snake-bite	T50.Z11	T50.Z12	T50.Z13	T50.Z14	T50.Z15	T50.Z16
antitetanic	T50.Z11	T50.Z12	T50.Z13	T50.Z14	T50.Z15	T50.Z16
antitoxic	T50.Z11	T50.Z12	T50.Z13	T50.Z14	T50.Z15	T50.Z16
complement (inhibitor)	T45.8X1	T45.8X2	T45.8X3	T45.8X4	T45.8X5	T45.8X6
convalescent	T50.Z11	T50.Z12	T50.Z13	T50.Z14	T50.Z15	T50.Z16
hemolytic complement	T45.8X1	T45.8X2	T45.8X3	T45.8X4	T45.8X5	T45.8X6
immune (human)	T50.Z11	T50.Z12	T50.Z13	T50.Z14	T50.Z15	T50.Z16
protective NEC	T50.Z11	T50.Z12	T50.Z13	T50.Z14	T50.Z15	T50.Z16
Setastine	T45.0X1	T45.0X2	T45.0X3	T45.0X4	T45.0X5	T45.0X6
Setoperone	T43.591	T43.592	T43.593	T43.594	T43.595	T43.596
Sewer gas	T59.91	T59.92	T59.93	T59.94		
Shampoo	T55.0X1	T55.0X2	T55.0X3	T55.0X4		
Shellfish, noxious, nonbacterial	T61.781	T61.782	T61.783	T61.784		

▽ Subterms under main terms may continue to next column or page   **Additional Character May Be Required** — Refer to the Tabular List for Character Selection

Table of Drugs and Chemicals

Substance	Poisoning, Accidental (unintentional)	Poisoning, Intentional Self-harm	Poisoning, Assault	Poisoning, Undetermined	Adverse Effect	Under-dosing
Sildenafil	T46.7X1	T46.7X2	T46.7X3	T46.7X4	T46.7X5	T46.7X6
Silibinin	T50.991	T50.992	T50.993	T50.994	T50.995	T50.996
Silicone NEC	T65.891	T65.892	T65.893	T65.894	—	—
medicinal	T49.3X1	T49.3X2	T49.3X3	T49.3X4	T49.3X5	T49.3X6
Silvadene	T49.0X1	T49.0X2	T49.0X3	T49.0X4	T49.0X5	T49.0X6
Silver	T49.0X1	T49.0X2	T49.0X3	T49.0X4	T49.0X5	T49.0X6
anti-infectives	T49.0X1	T49.0X2	T49.0X3	T49.0X4	T49.0X5	T49.0X6
arsphenamine	T37.8X1	T37.8X2	T37.8X3	T37.8X4	T37.8X5	T37.8X6
colloidal	T49.0X1	T49.0X2	T49.0X3	T49.0X4	T49.0X5	T49.0X6
nitrate	T49.0X1	T49.0X2	T49.0X3	T49.0X4	T49.0X5	T49.0X6
ophthalmic preparation	T49.5X1	T49.5X2	T49.5X3	T49.5X4	T49.5X5	T49.5X6
toughened (keratolytic)	T49.4X1	T49.4X2	T49.4X3	T49.4X4	T49.4X5	T49.4X6
nonmedicinal (dust)	T56.891	T56.892	T56.893	T56.894	—	—
protein	T49.5X1	T49.5X2	T49.5X3	T49.5X4	T49.5X5	T49.5X6
salvarsan	T37.8X1	T37.8X2	T37.8X3	T37.8X4	T37.8X5	T37.8X6
sulfadiazine	T49.4X1	T49.4X2	T49.4X3	T49.4X4	T49.4X5	T49.4X6
Silymarin	T50.991	T50.992	T50.993	T50.994	T50.995	T50.996
Simaldrate	T47.1X1	T47.1X2	T47.1X3	T47.1X4	T47.1X5	T47.1X6
Simazine	T60.3X1	T60.3X2	T60.3X3	T60.3X4	—	—
Simethicone	T47.1X1	T47.1X2	T47.1X3	T47.1X4	T47.1X5	T47.1X6
Simfibrate	T46.6X1	T46.6X2	T46.6X3	T46.6X4	T46.6X5	T46.6X6
Simvastatin	T46.6X1	T46.6X2	T46.6X3	T46.6X4	T46.6X5	T46.6X6
Sincalide	T50.8X1	T50.8X2	T50.8X3	T50.8X4	T50.8X5	T50.8X6
Sinequan	T43.011	T43.012	T43.013	T43.014	T43.015	T43.016
Singoserp	T46.5X1	T46.5X2	T46.5X3	T46.5X4	T46.5X5	T46.5X6
Sintrom	T45.511	T45.512	T45.513	T45.514	T45.515	T45.516
Sisomicin	T36.5X1	T36.5X2	T36.5X3	T36.5X4	T36.5X5	T36.5X6
Sitosterols	T46.6X1	T46.6X2	T46.6X3	T46.6X4	T46.6X5	T46.6X6
Skeletal muscle relaxants	T48.1X1	T48.1X2	T48.1X3	T48.1X4	T48.1X5	T48.1X6
Skin						
agents (external)	T49.91	T49.92	T49.93	T49.94	T49.95	T49.96
specified NEC	T49.8X1	T49.8X2	T49.8X3	T49.8X4	T49.8X5	T49.8X6
test antigen	T50.8X1	T50.8X2	T50.8X3	T50.8X4	T50.8X5	T50.8X6
Sleep-eze	T45.0X1	T45.0X2	T45.0X3	T45.0X4	T45.0X5	T45.0X6
Sleeping draught, pill	T42.71	T42.72	T42.73	T42.74	T42.75	T42.76
Smallpox vaccine	T50.B11	T50.B12	T50.B13	T50.B14	T50.B15	T50.B16
Smelter fumes NEC	T56.91	T56.92	T56.93	T56.94	—	—
Smog	T59.1X1	T59.1X2	T59.1X3	T59.1X4	—	—
Smoke NEC	T59.811	T59.812	T59.813	T59.814	—	—
Smooth muscle relaxant	T44.3X1	T44.3X2	T44.3X3	T44.3X4	T44.3X5	T44.3X6
Snail killer NEC	T60.8X1	T60.8X2	T60.8X3	T60.8X4	—	—
Snake venom or bite	T63.001	T63.002	T63.003	T63.004	—	—
hemocoagulase	T45.7X1	T45.7X2	T45.7X3	T45.7X4	T45.7X5	T45.7X6
Snuff	T65.211	T65.212	T65.213	T65.214	—	—
Soap (powder) (product)	T55.0X1	T55.0X2	T55.0X3	T55.0X4	—	—
enema	T47.4X1	T47.4X2	T47.4X3	T47.4X4	T47.4X5	T47.4X6
medicinal, soft	T49.2X1	T49.2X2	T49.2X3	T49.2X4	T49.2X5	T49.2X6
superfatted	T49.2X1	T49.2X2	T49.2X3	T49.2X4	T49.2X5	T49.2X6
Sobrerol	T48.4X1	T48.4X2	T48.4X3	T48.4X4	T48.4X5	T48.4X6
Soda (caustic)	T54.3X1	T54.3X2	T54.3X3	T54.3X4	—	—
bicarb	T47.1X1	T47.1X2	T47.1X3	T47.1X4	T47.1X5	T47.1X6
chlorinated — *see* Sodium, hypochlorite						
Sodium						
acetosulfone	T37.1X1	T37.1X2	T37.1X3	T37.1X4	T37.1X5	T37.1X6
acetrizoate	T50.8X1	T50.8X2	T50.8X3	T50.8X4	T50.8X5	T50.8X6
acid phosphate	T50.3X1	T50.3X2	T50.3X3	T50.3X4	T50.3X5	T50.3X6
alginate	T47.8X1	T47.8X2	T47.8X3	T47.8X4	T47.8X5	T47.8X6
amidotrizoate	T50.8X1	T50.8X2	T50.8X3	T50.8X4	T50.8X5	T50.8X6
aminopterin	T45.1X1	T45.1X2	T45.1X3	T45.1X4	T45.1X5	T45.1X6
amylosulfate	T47.8X1	T47.8X2	T47.8X3	T47.8X4	T47.8X5	T47.8X6
amytal	T42.3X1	T42.3X2	T42.3X3	T42.3X4	T42.3X5	T42.3X6
antimony gluconate	T37.3X1	T37.3X2	T37.3X3	T37.3X4	T37.3X5	T37.3X6
arsenate	T57.0X1	T57.0X2	T57.0X3	T57.0X4	—	—
aurothiomalate	T39.4X1	T39.4X2	T39.4X3	T39.4X4	T39.4X5	T39.4X6
aurothiosulfate	T39.4X1	T39.4X2	T39.4X3	T39.4X4	T39.4X5	T39.4X6
barbiturate	T42.3X1	T42.3X2	T42.3X3	T42.3X4	T42.3X5	T42.3X6
basic phosphate	T47.4X1	T47.4X2	T47.4X3	T47.4X4	T47.4X5	T47.4X6
bicarbonate	T47.1X1	T47.1X2	T47.1X3	T47.1X4	T47.1X5	T47.1X6
bichromate	T57.8X1	T57.8X2	T57.8X3	T57.8X4	—	—
biphosphate	T50.3X1	T50.3X2	T50.3X3	T50.3X4	T50.3X5	T50.3X6
bisulfate	T65.891	T65.892	T65.893	T65.894	—	—
borate						
cleanser	T57.8X1	T57.8X2	T57.8X3	T57.8X4	—	—
eye	T49.5X1	T49.5X2	T49.5X3	T49.5X4	T49.5X5	T49.5X6
therapeutic	T49.8X1	T49.8X2	T49.8X3	T49.8X4	T49.8X5	T49.8X6
bromide	T42.6X1	T42.6X2	T42.6X3	T42.6X4	T42.6X5	T42.6X6
cacodylate (nonmedicinal) NEC	T50.8X1	T50.8X2	T50.8X3	T50.8X4	T50.8X5	T50.8X6
anti-infective	T37.8X1	T37.8X2	T37.8X3	T37.8X4	T37.8X5	T37.8X6
herbicide	T60.3X1	T60.3X2	T60.3X3	T60.3X4	—	—
calcium edetate	T45.8X1	T45.8X2	T45.8X3	T45.8X4	T45.8X5	T45.8X6
carbonate NEC	T54.3X1	T54.3X2	T54.3X3	T54.3X4	—	—

Substance	Poisoning, Accidental (unintentional)	Poisoning, Intentional Self-harm	Poisoning, Assault	Poisoning, Undetermined	Adverse Effect	Under-dosing
Sodium — *continued*						
chlorate NEC	T65.891	T65.892	T65.893	T65.894	—	—
herbicide	T54.91	T54.92	T54.93	T54.94	—	—
chloride	T50.3X1	T50.3X2	T50.3X3	T50.3X4	T50.3X5	T50.3X6
with glucose	T50.3X1	T50.3X2	T50.3X3	T50.3X4	T50.3X5	T50.3X6
chromate	T65.891	T65.892	T65.893	T65.894	—	—
citrate	T50.991	T50.992	T50.993	T50.994	T50.995	T50.996
cromoglicate	T48.6X1	T48.6X2	T48.6X3	T48.6X4	T48.6X5	T48.6X6
cyanide	T65.0X1	T65.0X2	T65.0X3	T65.0X4	—	—
cyclamate	T50.3X1	T50.3X2	T50.3X3	T50.3X4	T50.3X5	T50.3X6
dehydrocholate	T45.8X1	T45.8X2	T45.8X3	T45.8X4	T45.8X5	T45.8X6
diatrizoate	T50.8X1	T50.8X2	T50.8X3	T50.8X4	T50.8X5	T50.8X6
dibunate	T48.4X1	T48.4X2	T48.4X3	T48.4X4	T48.4X5	T48.4X6
dioctyl sulfosuccinate	T47.4X1	T47.4X2	T47.4X3	T47.4X4	T47.4X5	T47.4X6
dipantoyl ferrate	T45.8X1	T45.8X2	T45.8X3	T45.8X4	T45.8X5	T45.8X6
edetate	T45.8X1	T45.8X2	T45.8X3	T45.8X4	T45.8X5	T45.8X6
ethacrynate	T50.1X1	T50.1X2	T50.1X3	T50.1X4	T50.1X5	T50.1X6
feredetate	T45.8X1	T45.8X2	T45.8X3	T45.8X4	T45.8X5	T45.8X6
Fluoride — *see* Fluoride						
fluoroacetate (dust) (pesticide)	T60.4X1	T60.4X2	T60.4X3	T60.4X4	—	—
free salt	T50.3X1	T50.3X2	T50.3X3	T50.3X4	T50.3X5	T50.3X6
fusidate	T36.8X1	T36.8X2	T36.8X3	T36.8X4	T36.8X5	T36.8X6
glucaldrate	T47.1X1	T47.1X2	T47.1X3	T47.1X4	T47.1X5	T47.1X6
glucosulfone	T37.1X1	T37.1X2	T37.1X3	T37.1X4	T37.1X5	T37.1X6
glutamate	T45.8X1	T45.8X2	T45.8X3	T45.8X4	T45.8X5	T45.8X6
hydrogen carbonate	T50.3X1	T50.3X2	T50.3X3	T50.3X4	T50.3X5	T50.3X6
hydroxide	T54.3X1	T54.3X2	T54.3X3	T54.3X4	—	—
hypochlorite (bleach) NEC	T54.3X1	T54.3X2	T54.3X3	T54.3X4	—	—
disinfectant	T54.3X1	T54.3X2	T54.3X3	T54.3X4	—	—
medicinal (anti-infective) (external)	T49.0X1	T49.0X2	T49.0X3	T49.0X4	T49.0X5	T49.0X6
vapor	T54.3X1	T54.3X2	T54.3X3	T54.3X4	—	—
hyposulfite	T49.0X1	T49.0X2	T49.0X3	T49.0X4	T49.0X5	T49.0X6
indigotin disulfonate	T50.8X1	T50.8X2	T50.8X3	T50.8X4	T50.8X5	T50.8X6
iodide	T50.991	T50.992	T50.993	T50.994	T50.995	T50.996
I-131	T50.8X1	T50.8X2	T50.8X3	T50.8X4	T50.8X5	T50.8X6
therapeutic	T38.2X1	T38.2X2	T38.2X3	T38.2X4	T38.2X5	T38.2X6
iodohippurate (131I)	T50.8X1	T50.8X2	T50.8X3	T50.8X4	T50.8X5	T50.8X6
iopodate	T50.8X1	T50.8X2	T50.8X3	T50.8X4	T50.8X5	T50.8X6
iothalamate	T50.8X1	T50.8X2	T50.8X3	T50.8X4	T50.8X5	T50.8X6
iron edetate	T45.4X1	T45.4X2	T45.4X3	T45.4X4	T45.4X5	T45.4X6
lactate (compound solution)	T45.8X1	T45.8X2	T45.8X3	T45.8X4	T45.8X5	T45.8X6
lauryl (sulfate)	T49.2X1	T49.2X2	T49.2X3	T49.2X4	T49.2X5	T49.2X6
L-triiodothyronine	T38.1X1	T38.1X2	T38.1X3	T38.1X4	T38.1X5	T38.1X6
magnesium citrate	T50.991	T50.992	T50.993	T50.994	T50.995	T50.996
mersalate	T50.2X1	T50.2X2	T50.2X3	T50.2X4	T50.2X5	T50.2X6
metasilicate	T65.891	T65.892	T65.893	T65.894	—	—
metrizoate	T50.8X1	T50.8X2	T50.8X3	T50.8X4	T50.8X5	T50.8X6
monofluoroacetate (pesticide)	T60.1X1	T60.1X2	T60.1X3	T60.1X4	—	—
morrhuate	T46.8X1	T46.8X2	T46.8X3	T46.8X4	T46.8X5	T46.8X6
nafcillin	T36.0X1	T36.0X2	T36.0X3	T36.0X4	T36.0X5	T36.0X6
nitrate (oxidizing agent)	T65.891	T65.892	T65.893	T65.894	—	—
nitrite	T50.6X1	T50.6X2	T50.6X3	T50.6X4	T50.6X5	T50.6X6
nitroferricyanide	T46.5X1	T46.5X2	T46.5X3	T46.5X4	T46.5X5	T46.5X6
nitroprusside	T46.5X1	T46.5X2	T46.5X3	T46.5X4	T46.5X5	T46.5X6
oxalate	T65.891	T65.892	T65.893	T65.894	—	—
oxide/peroxide	T65.891	T65.892	T65.893	T65.894	—	—
oxybate	T41.291	T41.292	T41.293	T41.294	T41.295	T41.296
para-aminohippurate	T50.8X1	T50.8X2	T50.8X3	T50.8X4	T50.8X5	T50.8X6
perborate (nonmedicinal) NEC	T65.891	T65.892	T65.893	T65.894	—	—
medicinal	T49.0X1	T49.0X2	T49.0X3	T49.0X4	T49.0X5	T49.0X6
soap	T55.0X1	T55.0X2	T55.0X3	T55.0X4	—	—
percarbonate — *see* Sodium, perborate						
pertechnetate Tc99m	T50.8X1	T50.8X2	T50.8X3	T50.8X4	T50.8X5	T50.8X6
phosphate						
cellulose	T45.8X1	T45.8X2	T45.8X3	T45.8X4	T45.8X5	T45.8X6
dibasic	T47.2X1	T47.2X2	T47.2X3	T47.2X4	T47.2X5	T47.2X6
monobasic	T47.2X1	T47.2X2	T47.2X3	T47.2X4	T47.2X5	T47.2X6
phytate	T50.6X1	T50.6X2	T50.6X3	T50.6X4	T50.6X5	T50.6X6
picosulfate	T47.2X1	T47.2X2	T47.2X3	T47.2X4	T47.2X5	T47.2X6
polyhydroxyaluminium monocarbonate	T47.1X1	T47.1X2	T47.1X3	T47.1X4	T47.1X5	T47.1X6
polystyrene sulfonate	T50.3X1	T50.3X2	T50.3X3	T50.3X4	T50.3X5	T50.3X6
propionate	T49.0X1	T49.0X2	T49.0X3	T49.0X4	T49.0X5	T49.0X6
propyl hydroxybenzoate	T50.991	T50.992	T50.993	T50.994	T50.995	T50.996
psylliate	T46.8X1	T46.8X2	T46.8X3	T46.8X4	T46.8X5	T46.8X6
removing resins	T50.3X1	T50.3X2	T50.3X3	T50.3X4	T50.3X5	T50.3X6
salicylate	T39.091	T39.092	T39.093	T39.094	T39.095	T39.096

Sildenafil — Sodium

Substance	Poisoning, Accidental (unintentional)	Poisoning, Intentional Self-harm	Poisoning, Assault	Poisoning, Undetermined	Adverse Effect	Under-dosing
Sodium — continued						
salt NEC	T50.3X1	T50.3X2	T50.3X3	T50.3X4	T50.3X5	T50.3X6
selenate	T60.2X1	T60.2X2	T60.2X3	T60.2X4	—	—
stibogluconate	T37.3X1	T37.3X2	T37.3X3	T37.3X4	T37.3X5	T37.3X6
sulfate	T47.4X1	T47.4X2	T47.4X3	T47.4X4	T47.4X5	T47.4X6
sulfoxone	T37.1X1	T37.1X2	T37.1X3	T37.1X4	T37.1X5	T37.1X6
tetradecyl sulfate	T46.8X1	T46.8X2	T46.8X3	T46.8X4	T46.8X5	T46.8X6
thiopental	T41.1X1	T41.1X2	T41.1X3	T41.1X4	T41.1X5	T41.1X6
thiosalicylate	T39.091	T39.092	T39.093	T39.094	T39.095	T39.096
thiosulfate	T50.6X1	T50.6X2	T50.6X3	T50.6X4	T50.6X5	T50.6X6
tolbutamide	T38.3X1	T38.3X2	T38.3X3	T38.3X4	T38.3X5	T38.3X6
(L)-triiodothyronine	T38.1X1	T38.1X2	T38.1X3	T38.1X4	T38.1X5	T38.1X6
tyropanoate	T50.8X1	T50.8X2	T50.8X3	T50.8X4	T50.8X5	T50.8X6
valproate	T42.6X1	T42.6X2	T42.6X3	T42.6X4	T42.6X5	T42.6X6
versenate	T50.6X1	T50.6X2	T50.6X3	T50.6X4	T50.6X5	T50.6X6
Sodium-free salt	T50.901	T50.902	T50.903	T50.904	T50.905	T50.906
Sodium-removing resin	T50.3X1	T50.3X2	T50.3X3	T50.3X4	T50.3X5	T50.3X6
Soft soap	T55.0X1	T55.0X2	T55.0X3	T55.0X4	—	—
Solanine	T62.2X1	T62.2X2	T62.2X3	T62.2X4	—	—
berries	T62.1X1	T62.1X2	T62.1X3	T62.1X4	—	—
Solanum dulcamara	T62.2X1	T62.2X2	T62.2X3	T62.2X4	—	—
berries	T62.1X1	T62.1X2	T62.1X3	T62.1X4	—	—
Solapsone	T37.1X1	T37.1X2	T37.1X3	T37.1X4	T37.1X5	T37.1X6
Solar lotion	T49.3X1	T49.3X2	T49.3X3	T49.3X4	T49.3X5	T49.3X6
Solasulfone	T37.1X1	T37.1X2	T37.1X3	T37.1X4	T37.1X5	T37.1X6
Soldering fluid	T65.891	T65.892	T65.893	T65.894	—	—
Solid substance	T65.91	T65.92	T65.93	T65.94	—	—
specified NEC	T65.891	T65.892	T65.893	T65.894	—	—
Solvent, industrial NEC	T52.91	T52.92	T52.93	T52.94	—	—
naphtha	T52.0X1	T52.0X2	T52.0X3	T52.0X4	—	—
petroleum	T52.0X1	T52.0X2	T52.0X3	T52.0X4	—	—
specified NEC	T52.8X1	T52.8X2	T52.8X3	T52.8X4	—	—
Soma	T42.8X1	T42.8X2	T42.8X3	T42.8X4	T42.8X5	T42.8X6
Somatorelin	T38.891	T38.892	T38.893	T38.894	T38.895	T38.896
Somatostatin	T38.991	T38.992	T38.993	T38.994	T38.995	T38.996
Somatotropin	T38.811	T38.812	T38.813	T38.814	T38.815	T38.816
Somatrem	T38.811	T38.812	T38.813	T38.814	T38.815	T38.816
Somatropin	T38.811	T38.812	T38.813	T38.814	T38.815	T38.816
Sominex	T45.0X1	T45.0X2	T45.0X3	T45.0X4	T45.0X5	T45.0X6
Somnos	T42.6X1	T42.6X2	T42.6X3	T42.6X4	T42.6X5	T42.6X6
Somonal	T42.3X1	T42.3X2	T42.3X3	T42.3X4	T42.3X5	T42.3X6
Soneryl	T42.3X1	T42.3X2	T42.3X3	T42.3X4	T42.3X5	T42.3X6
Soothing syrup	T50.901	T50.902	T50.903	T50.904	T50.905	T50.906
Sopor	T42.6X1	T42.6X2	T42.6X3	T42.6X4	T42.6X5	T42.6X6
Soporific	T42.71	T42.72	T42.73	T42.74	T42.75	T42.76
Soporific drug	T42.71	T42.72	T42.73	T42.74	T42.75	T42.76
specified type NEC	T42.6X1	T42.6X2	T42.6X3	T42.6X4	T42.6X5	T42.6X6
Sorbide nitrate	T46.3X1	T46.3X2	T46.3X3	T46.3X4	T46.3X5	T46.3X6
Sorbitol	T47.4X1	T47.4X2	T47.4X3	T47.4X4	T47.4X5	T47.4X6
Sotalol	T44.7X1	T44.7X2	T44.7X3	T44.7X4	T44.7X5	T44.7X6
Sotradecol	T46.8X1	T46.8X2	T46.8X3	T46.8X4	T46.8X5	T46.8X6
Soysterol	T46.6X1	T46.6X2	T46.6X3	T46.6X4	T46.6X5	T46.6X6
Spacoline	T44.3X1	T44.3X2	T44.3X3	T44.3X4	T44.3X5	T44.3X6
Spanish fly	T49.8X1	T49.8X2	T49.8X3	T49.8X4	T49.8X5	T49.8X6
Sparine	T43.3X1	T43.3X2	T43.3X3	T43.3X4	T43.3X5	T43.3X6
Sparteine	T48.0X1	T48.0X2	T48.0X3	T48.0X4	T48.0X5	T48.0X6
Spasmolytic						
anticholinergics	T44.3X1	T44.3X2	T44.3X3	T44.3X4	T44.3X5	T44.3X6
autonomic	T44.3X1	T44.3X2	T44.3X3	T44.3X4	T44.3X5	T44.3X6
bronchial NEC	T48.6X1	T48.6X2	T48.6X3	T48.6X4	T48.6X5	T48.6X6
quaternary ammonium	T44.3X1	T44.3X2	T44.3X3	T44.3X4	T44.3X5	T44.3X6
skeletal muscle NEC	T48.1X1	T48.1X2	T48.1X3	T48.1X4	T48.1X5	T48.1X6
Spectinomycin	T36.5X1	T36.5X2	T36.5X3	T36.5X4	T36.5X5	T36.5X6
Speed	T43.621	T43.622	T43.623	T43.624	T43.625	T43.626
Spermicide	T49.8X1	T49.8X2	T49.8X3	T49.8X4	T49.8X5	T49.8X6
Spider (bite) (venom)	T63.391	T63.392	T63.393	T63.394	—	—
antivenin	T50.Z11	T50.Z12	T50.Z13	T50.Z14	T50.Z15	T50.Z16
Spigelia (root)	T37.4X1	T37.4X2	T37.4X3	T37.4X4	T37.4X5	T37.4X6
Spindle inactivator	T50.4X1	T50.4X2	T50.4X3	T50.4X4	T50.4X5	T50.4X6
Spiperone	T43.4X1	T43.4X2	T43.4X3	T43.4X4	T43.4X5	T43.4X6
Spiramycin	T36.3X1	T36.3X2	T36.3X3	T36.3X4	T36.3X5	T36.3X6
Spirapril	T46.4X1	T46.4X2	T46.4X3	T46.4X4	T46.4X5	T46.4X6
Spirilene	T43.591	T43.592	T43.593	T43.594	T43.595	T43.596
Spirit(s) (neutral) NEC	T51.0X1	T51.0X2	T51.0X3	T51.0X4	—	—
beverage	T51.0X1	T51.0X2	T51.0X3	T51.0X4	—	—
industrial	T51.0X1	T51.0X2	T51.0X3	T51.0X4	—	—
mineral	T52.0X1	T52.0X2	T52.0X3	T52.0X4	—	—
of salt — see Hydrochloric acid						
surgical	T51.0X1	T51.0X2	T51.0X3	T51.0X4	—	—
Spironolactone	T50.0X1	T50.0X2	T50.0X3	T50.0X4	T50.0X5	T50.0X6
Spiroperidol	T43.4X1	T43.4X2	T43.4X3	T43.4X4	T43.4X5	T43.4X6
Sponge, absorbable (gelatin)	T45.7X1	T45.7X2	T45.7X3	T45.7X4	T45.7X5	T45.7X6

Substance	Poisoning, Accidental (unintentional)	Poisoning, Intentional Self-harm	Poisoning, Assault	Poisoning, Undetermined	Adverse Effect	Under-dosing
Sporostacin	T49.0X1	T49.0X2	T49.0X3	T49.0X4	T49.0X5	T49.0X6
Spray (aerosol)	T65.91	T65.92	T65.93	T65.94	—	—
cosmetic	T65.891	T65.892	T65.893	T65.894	—	—
medicinal NEC	T50.901	T50.902	T50.903	T50.904	T50.905	T50.906
pesticides — see Pesticides						
specified content — see specific substance						
Spurge flax	T62.2X1	T62.2X2	T62.2X3	T62.2X4	—	—
Spurges	T62.2X1	T62.2X2	T62.2X3	T62.2X4	—	—
Sputum viscosity-lowering drug	T48.4X1	T48.4X2	T48.4X3	T48.4X4	T48.4X5	T48.4X6
Squill	T46.0X1	T46.0X2	T46.0X3	T46.0X4	T46.0X5	T46.0X6
rat poison	T60.4X1	T60.4X2	T60.4X3	T60.4X4	—	—
Squirting cucumber (cathartic)	T47.2X1	T47.2X2	T47.2X3	T47.2X4	T47.2X5	T47.2X6
Stains	T65.6X1	T65.6X2	T65.6X3	T65.6X4	—	—
Stannous fluoride	T49.7X1	T49.7X2	T49.7X3	T49.7X4	T49.7X5	T49.7X6
Stanolone	T38.7X1	T38.7X2	T38.7X3	T38.7X4	T38.7X5	T38.7X6
Stanozolol	T38.7X1	T38.7X2	T38.7X3	T38.7X4	T38.7X5	T38.7X6
Staphisagria or stavesacre (pediculicide)	T49.0X1	T49.0X2	T49.0X3	T49.0X4	T49.0X5	T49.0X6
Starch	T50.901	T50.902	T50.903	T50.904	T50.905	T50.906
Stelazine	T43.3X1	T43.3X2	T43.3X3	T43.3X4	T43.3X5	T43.3X6
Stemetil	T43.3X1	T43.3X2	T43.3X3	T43.3X4	T43.3X5	T43.3X6
Stepronin	T48.4X1	T48.4X2	T48.4X3	T48.4X4	T48.4X5	T48.4X6
Sterculia	T47.4X1	T47.4X2	T47.4X3	T47.4X4	T47.4X5	T47.4X6
Sternutator gas	T59.891	T59.892	T59.893	T59.894	—	—
Steroid	T38.0X1	T38.0X2	T38.0X3	T38.0X4	T38.0X5	T38.0X6
anabolic	T38.7X1	T38.7X2	T38.7X3	T38.7X4	T38.7X5	T38.7X6
androgenic	T38.7X1	T38.7X2	T38.7X3	T38.7X4	T38.7X5	T38.7X6
antineoplastic, hormone	T38.7X1	T38.7X2	T38.7X3	T38.7X4	T38.7X5	T38.7X6
estrogen	T38.5X1	T38.5X2	T38.5X3	T38.5X4	T38.5X5	T38.5X6
ENT agent	T49.6X1	T49.6X2	T49.6X3	T49.6X4	T49.6X5	T49.6X6
ophthalmic preparation	T49.5X1	T49.5X2	T49.5X3	T49.5X4	T49.5X5	T49.5X6
topical NEC	T49.0X1	T49.0X2	T49.0X3	T49.0X4	T49.0X5	T49.0X6
Stibine	T56.891	T56.892	T56.893	T56.894	—	—
Stibogluconate	T37.3X1	T37.3X2	T37.3X3	T37.3X4	T37.3X5	T37.3X6
Stibophen	T37.4X1	T37.4X2	T37.4X3	T37.4X4	T37.4X5	T37.4X6
Stilbamidine (isetionate)	T37.3X1	T37.3X2	T37.3X3	T37.3X4	T37.3X5	T37.3X6
Stilbestrol	T38.5X1	T38.5X2	T38.5X3	T38.5X4	T38.5X5	T38.5X6
Stilboestrol	T38.5X1	T38.5X2	T38.5X3	T38.5X4	T38.5X5	T38.5X6
Stimulant						
central nervous system — see also Psychostimulant	T43.601	T43.602	T43.603	T43.604	T43.605	T43.606
analeptics	T50.7X1	T50.7X2	T50.7X3	T50.7X4	T50.7X5	T50.7X6
opiate antagonist	T50.7X1	T50.7X2	T50.7X3	T50.7X4	T50.7X5	T50.7X6
psychotherapeutic NEC — see also Psychotherapeutic drug	T43.601	T43.602	T43.603	T43.604	T43.605	T43.606
specified NEC	T43.691	T43.692	T43.693	T43.694	T43.695	T43.696
respiratory	T48.901	T48.902	T48.903	T48.904	T48.905	T48.906
Stone-dissolving drug	T50.901	T50.902	T50.903	T50.904	T50.905	T50.906
Storage battery (cells) (acid)	T54.2X1	T54.2X2	T54.2X3	T54.2X4	—	—
Stovaine	T41.3X1	T41.3X2	T41.3X3	T41.3X4	T41.3X5	T41.3X6
infiltration (subcutaneous)	T41.3X1	T41.3X2	T41.3X3	T41.3X4	T41.3X5	T41.3X6
nerve block (peripheral) (plexus)	T41.3X1	T41.3X2	T41.3X3	T41.3X4	T41.3X5	T41.3X6
spinal	T41.3X1	T41.3X2	T41.3X3	T41.3X4	T41.3X5	T41.3X6
topical (surface)	T41.3X1	T41.3X2	T41.3X3	T41.3X4	T41.3X5	T41.3X6
Stovarsal	T37.8X1	T37.8X2	T37.8X3	T37.8X4	T37.8X5	T37.8X6
Stove gas — see Gas, stove						
Stoxil	T49.5X1	T49.5X2	T49.5X3	T49.5X4	T49.5X5	T49.5X6
Stramonium	T48.6X1	T48.6X2	T48.6X3	T48.6X4	T48.6X5	T48.6X6
natural state	T62.2X1	T62.2X2	T62.2X3	T62.2X4	—	—
Streptodornase	T45.3X1	T45.3X2	T45.3X3	T45.3X4	T45.3X5	T45.3X6
Streptoduocin	T36.5X1	T36.5X2	T36.5X3	T36.5X4	T36.5X5	T36.5X6
Streptokinase	T45.611	T45.612	T45.613	T45.614	T45.615	T45.616
Streptomycin (derivative)	T36.5X1	T36.5X2	T36.5X3	T36.5X4	T36.5X5	T36.5X6
Streptonivicin	T36.5X1	T36.5X2	T36.5X3	T36.5X4	T36.5X5	T36.5X6
Streptovarycin	T36.5X1	T36.5X2	T36.5X3	T36.5X4	T36.5X5	T36.5X6
Streptozocin	T45.1X1	T45.1X2	T45.1X3	T45.1X4	T45.1X5	T45.1X6
Streptozotocin	T45.1X1	T45.1X2	T45.1X3	T45.1X4	T45.1X5	T45.1X6
Stripper (paint) (solvent)	T52.8X1	T52.8X2	T52.8X3	T52.8X4	—	—
Strobane	T60.1X1	T60.1X2	T60.1X3	T60.1X4	—	—
Strofantina	T46.0X1	T46.0X2	T46.0X3	T46.0X4	T46.0X5	T46.0X6
Strophanthin (g) (k)	T46.0X1	T46.0X2	T46.0X3	T46.0X4	T46.0X5	T46.0X6
Strophanthus	T46.0X1	T46.0X2	T46.0X3	T46.0X4	T46.0X5	T46.0X6
Strophantin	T46.0X1	T46.0X2	T46.0X3	T46.0X4	T46.0X5	T46.0X6
Strophantin-g	T46.0X1	T46.0X2	T46.0X3	T46.0X4	T46.0X5	T46.0X6
Strychnine (nonmedicinal) (pesticide) (salts)	T65.1X1	T65.1X2	T65.1X3	T65.1X4	—	—
medicinal	T48.291	T48.292	T48.293	T48.294	T48.295	T48.296

Table of Drugs and Chemicals

Substance	Poisoning, Accidental (unintentional)	Poisoning, Intentional Self-harm	Poisoning, Assault	Poisoning, Undetermined	Adverse Effect	Under-dosing
Strychnos (ignatii) — see Strychnine						
Styramate	T42.8X1	T42.8X2	T42.8X3	T42.8X4	T42.8X5	T42.8X6
Styrene	T65.891	T65.892	T65.893	T65.894	—	—
Succinimide, antiepileptic or anticonvulsant	T42.2X1	T42.2X2	T42.2X3	T42.2X4	T42.2X5	T42.2X6
mercuric — see Mercury						
Succinylcholine	T48.1X1	T48.1X2	T48.1X3	T48.1X4	T48.1X5	T48.1X6
Succinylsulfathiazole	T37.0X1	T37.0X2	T37.0X3	T37.0X4	T37.0X5	T37.0X6
Sucralfate	T47.1X1	T47.1X2	T47.1X3	T47.1X4	T47.1X5	T47.1X6
Sucrose	T50.3X1	T50.3X2	T50.3X3	T50.3X4	T50.3X5	T50.3X6
Sufentanil	T40.411	T40.412	T40.413	T40.414	T40.415	T40.416
Sulbactam	T36.0X1	T36.0X2	T36.0X3	T36.0X4	T36.0X5	T36.0X6
Sulbenicillin	T36.0X1	T36.0X2	T36.0X3	T36.0X4	T36.0X5	T36.0X6
Sulbentine	T49.0X1	T49.0X2	T49.0X3	T49.0X4	T49.0X5	T49.0X6
Sulfacetamide	T49.0X1	T49.0X2	T49.0X3	T49.0X4	T49.0X5	T49.0X6
ophthalmic preparation	T49.5X1	T49.5X2	T49.5X3	T49.5X4	T49.5X5	T49.5X6
Sulfachlorpyridazine	T37.0X1	T37.0X2	T37.0X3	T37.0X4	T37.0X5	T37.0X6
Sulfacitine	T37.0X1	T37.0X2	T37.0X3	T37.0X4	T37.0X5	T37.0X6
Sulfadiasulfone sodium	T37.0X1	T37.0X2	T37.0X3	T37.0X4	T37.0X5	T37.0X6
Sulfadiazine	T37.0X1	T37.0X2	T37.0X3	T37.0X4	T37.0X5	T37.0X6
silver (topical)	T49.0X1	T49.0X2	T49.0X3	T49.0X4	T49.0X5	T49.0X6
Sulfadimethoxine	T37.0X1	T37.0X2	T37.0X3	T37.0X4	T37.0X5	T37.0X6
Sulfadimidine	T37.0X1	T37.0X2	T37.0X3	T37.0X4	T37.0X5	T37.0X6
Sulfadoxine	T37.0X1	T37.0X2	T37.0X3	T37.0X4	T37.0X5	T37.0X6
with pyrimethamine	T37.2X1	T37.2X2	T37.2X3	T37.2X4	T37.2X5	T37.2X6
Sulfaethidole	T37.0X1	T37.0X2	T37.0X3	T37.0X4	T37.0X5	T37.0X6
Sulfafurazole	T37.0X1	T37.0X2	T37.0X3	T37.0X4	T37.0X5	T37.0X6
Sulfaguanidine	T37.0X1	T37.0X2	T37.0X3	T37.0X4	T37.0X5	T37.0X6
Sulfalene	T37.0X1	T37.0X2	T37.0X3	T37.0X4	T37.0X5	T37.0X6
Sulfaloxate	T37.0X1	T37.0X2	T37.0X3	T37.0X4	T37.0X5	T37.0X6
Sulfaloxic acid	T37.0X1	T37.0X2	T37.0X3	T37.0X4	T37.0X5	T37.0X6
Sulfamazone	T39.2X1	T39.2X2	T39.2X3	T39.2X4	T39.2X5	T39.2X6
Sulfamerazine	T37.0X1	T37.0X2	T37.0X3	T37.0X4	T37.0X5	T37.0X6
Sulfameter	T37.0X1	T37.0X2	T37.0X3	T37.0X4	T37.0X5	T37.0X6
Sulfamethazine	T37.0X1	T37.0X2	T37.0X3	T37.0X4	T37.0X5	T37.0X6
Sulfamethizole	T37.0X1	T37.0X2	T37.0X3	T37.0X4	T37.0X5	T37.0X6
Sulfamethoxazole	T37.0X1	T37.0X2	T37.0X3	T37.0X4	T37.0X5	T37.0X6
with trimethoprim	T36.8X1	T36.8X2	T36.8X3	T36.8X4	T36.8X5	T36.8X6
Sulfamethoxydiazine	T37.0X1	T37.0X2	T37.0X3	T37.0X4	T37.0X5	T37.0X6
Sulfamethoxypyridazine	T37.0X1	T37.0X2	T37.0X3	T37.0X4	T37.0X5	T37.0X6
Sulfamethylthiazole	T37.0X1	T37.0X2	T37.0X3	T37.0X4	T37.0X5	T37.0X6
Sulfametoxydiazine	T37.0X1	T37.0X2	T37.0X3	T37.0X4	T37.0X5	T37.0X6
Sulfamidopyrine	T39.2X1	T39.2X2	T39.2X3	T39.2X4	T39.2X5	T39.2X6
Sulfamonomethoxine	T37.0X1	T37.0X2	T37.0X3	T37.0X4	T37.0X5	T37.0X6
Sulfamoxole	T37.0X1	T37.0X2	T37.0X3	T37.0X4	T37.0X5	T37.0X6
Sulfamylon	T49.0X1	T49.0X2	T49.0X3	T49.0X4	T49.0X5	T49.0X6
Sulfan blue (diagnostic dye)	T50.8X1	T50.8X2	T50.8X3	T50.8X4	T50.8X5	T50.8X6
Sulfanilamide	T37.0X1	T37.0X2	T37.0X3	T37.0X4	T37.0X5	T37.0X6
Sulfanilylguanidine	T37.0X1	T37.0X2	T37.0X3	T37.0X4	T37.0X5	T37.0X6
Sulfaperin	T37.0X1	T37.0X2	T37.0X3	T37.0X4	T37.0X5	T37.0X6
Sulfaphenazole	T37.0X1	T37.0X2	T37.0X3	T37.0X4	T37.0X5	T37.0X6
Sulfaphenylthiazole	T37.0X1	T37.0X2	T37.0X3	T37.0X4	T37.0X5	T37.0X6
Sulfaproxyline	T37.0X1	T37.0X2	T37.0X3	T37.0X4	T37.0X5	T37.0X6
Sulfapyridine	T37.0X1	T37.0X2	T37.0X3	T37.0X4	T37.0X5	T37.0X6
Sulfapyrimidine	T37.0X1	T37.0X2	T37.0X3	T37.0X4	T37.0X5	T37.0X6
Sulfarsphenamine	T37.8X1	T37.8X2	T37.8X3	T37.8X4	T37.8X5	T37.8X6
Sulfasalazine	T37.0X1	T37.0X2	T37.0X3	T37.0X4	T37.0X5	T37.0X6
Sulfasuxidine	T37.0X1	T37.0X2	T37.0X3	T37.0X4	T37.0X5	T37.0X6
Sulfasymazine	T37.0X1	T37.0X2	T37.0X3	T37.0X4	T37.0X5	T37.0X6
Sulfated amylopectin	T47.8X1	T47.8X2	T47.8X3	T47.8X4	T47.8X5	T47.8X6
Sulfathiazole	T37.0X1	T37.0X2	T37.0X3	T37.0X4	T37.0X5	T37.0X6
Sulfatostearate	T49.2X1	T49.2X2	T49.2X3	T49.2X4	T49.2X5	T49.2X6
Sulfinpyrazone	T50.4X1	T50.4X2	T50.4X3	T50.4X4	T50.4X5	T50.4X6
Sulfiram	T49.0X1	T49.0X2	T49.0X3	T49.0X4	T49.0X5	T49.0X6
Sulfisomidine	T37.0X1	T37.0X2	T37.0X3	T37.0X4	T37.0X5	T37.0X6
Sulfisoxazole	T37.0X1	T37.0X2	T37.0X3	T37.0X4	T37.0X5	T37.0X6
ophthalmic preparation	T49.5X1	T49.5X2	T49.5X3	T49.5X4	T49.5X5	T49.5X6
Sulfobromophthalein (sodium)	T50.8X1	T50.8X2	T50.8X3	T50.8X4	T50.8X5	T50.8X6
Sulfobromphthalein	T50.8X1	T50.8X2	T50.8X3	T50.8X4	T50.8X5	T50.8X6
Sulfogaiacol	T48.4X1	T48.4X2	T48.4X3	T48.4X4	T48.4X5	T48.4X6
Sulfomyxin	T36.8X1	T36.8X2	T36.8X3	T36.8X4	T36.8X5	T36.8X6
Sulfonal	T42.6X1	T42.6X2	T42.6X3	T42.6X4	T42.6X5	T42.6X6
Sulfonamide NEC	T37.0X1	T37.0X2	T37.0X3	T37.0X4	T37.0X5	T37.0X6
eye	T49.5X1	T49.5X2	T49.5X3	T49.5X4	T49.5X5	T49.5X6
Sulfonazide	T37.1X1	T37.1X2	T37.1X3	T37.1X4	T37.1X5	T37.1X6
Sulfones	T37.1X1	T37.1X2	T37.1X3	T37.1X4	T37.1X5	T37.1X6
Sulfonethylmethane	T42.6X1	T42.6X2	T42.6X3	T42.6X4	T42.6X5	T42.6X6
Sulfonmethane	T42.6X1	T42.6X2	T42.6X3	T42.6X4	T42.6X5	T42.6X6
Sulfonphthal, sulfonphthol	T50.8X1	T50.8X2	T50.8X3	T50.8X4	T50.8X5	T50.8X6

Substance	Poisoning, Accidental (unintentional)	Poisoning, Intentional Self-harm	Poisoning, Assault	Poisoning, Undetermined	Adverse Effect	Under-dosing
Sulfonylurea derivatives, oral	T38.3X1	T38.3X2	T38.3X3	T38.3X4	T38.3X5	T38.3X6
Sulforidazine	T43.3X1	T43.3X2	T43.3X3	T43.3X4	T43.3X5	T43.3X6
Sulfoxone	T37.1X1	T37.1X2	T37.1X3	T37.1X4	T37.1X5	T37.1X6
Sulfuric acid	T54.2X1	T54.2X2	T54.2X3	T54.2X4	—	—
Sulfur, sulfurated, sulfuric, sulfurous, sulfuryl (compounds NEC) (medicinal)	T49.4X1	T49.4X2	T49.4X3	T49.4X4	T49.4X5	T49.4X6
acid	T54.2X1	T54.2X2	T54.2X3	T54.2X4	—	—
dioxide (gas)	T59.1X1	T59.1X2	T59.1X3	T59.1X4		
ether — see Ether(s)						
hydrogen	T59.6X1	T59.6X2	T59.6X3	T59.6X4	—	—
medicinal (keratolytic) (ointment) NEC	T49.4X1	T49.4X2	T49.4X3	T49.4X4	T49.4X5	T49.4X6
ointment	T49.0X1	T49.0X2	T49.0X3	T49.0X4	T49.0X5	T49.0X6
pesticide (vapor)	T60.91	T60.92	T60.93	T60.94	—	—
vapor NEC	T59.891	T59.892	T59.893	T59.894		
Sulglicotide	T47.1X1	T47.1X2	T47.1X3	T47.1X4	T47.1X5	T47.1X6
Sulindac	T39.391	T39.392	T39.393	T39.394	T39.395	T39.396
Sulisatin	T47.2X1	T47.2X2	T47.2X3	T47.2X4	T47.2X5	T47.2X6
Sulisobenzone	T49.3X1	T49.3X2	T49.3X3	T49.3X4	T49.3X5	T49.3X6
Sulkowitch's reagent	T50.8X1	T50.8X2	T50.8X3	T50.8X4	T50.8X5	T50.8X6
Sulmetozine	T44.3X1	T44.3X2	T44.3X3	T44.3X4	T44.3X5	T44.3X6
Suloctidil	T46.7X1	T46.7X2	T46.7X3	T46.7X4	T46.7X5	T46.7X6
Sulph- — see also Sulf-						
Sulphadiazine	T37.0X1	T37.0X2	T37.0X3	T37.0X4	T37.0X5	T37.0X6
Sulphadimethoxine	T37.0X1	T37.0X2	T37.0X3	T37.0X4	T37.0X5	T37.0X6
Sulphadimidine	T37.0X1	T37.0X2	T37.0X3	T37.0X4	T37.0X5	T37.0X6
Sulphadione	T37.1X1	T37.1X2	T37.1X3	T37.1X4	T37.1X5	T37.1X6
Sulphafurazole	T37.0X1	T37.0X2	T37.0X3	T37.0X4	T37.0X5	T37.0X6
Sulphamethizole	T37.0X1	T37.0X2	T37.0X3	T37.0X4	T37.0X5	T37.0X6
Sulphamethoxazole	T37.0X1	T37.0X2	T37.0X3	T37.0X4	T37.0X5	T37.0X6
Sulphan blue	T50.8X1	T50.8X2	T50.8X3	T50.8X4	T50.8X5	T50.8X6
Sulphaphenazole	T37.0X1	T37.0X2	T37.0X3	T37.0X4	T37.0X5	T37.0X6
Sulphapyridine	T37.0X1	T37.0X2	T37.0X3	T37.0X4	T37.0X5	T37.0X6
Sulphasalazine	T37.0X1	T37.0X2	T37.0X3	T37.0X4	T37.0X5	T37.0X6
Sulphinpyrazone	T50.4X1	T50.4X2	T50.4X3	T50.4X4	T50.4X5	T50.4X6
Sulpiride	T43.591	T43.592	T43.593	T43.594	T43.595	T43.596
Sulprostone	T48.0X1	T48.0X2	T48.0X3	T48.0X4	T48.0X5	T48.0X6
Sulpyrine	T39.2X1	T39.2X2	T39.2X3	T39.2X4	T39.2X5	T39.2X6
Sultamicillin	T36.0X1	T36.0X2	T36.0X3	T36.0X4	T36.0X5	T36.0X6
Sulthiame	T42.6X1	T42.6X2	T42.6X3	T42.6X4	T42.6X5	T42.6X6
Sultiame	T42.6X1	T42.6X2	T42.6X3	T42.6X4	T42.6X5	T42.6X6
Sultopride	T43.591	T43.592	T43.593	T43.594	T43.595	T43.596
Sumatriptan	T39.8X1	T39.8X2	T39.8X3	T39.8X4	T39.8X5	T39.8X6
Sunflower seed oil	T46.6X1	T46.6X2	T46.6X3	T46.6X4	T46.6X5	T46.6X6
Superinone	T48.4X1	T48.4X2	T48.4X3	T48.4X4	T48.4X5	T48.4X6
Suprofen	T39.311	T39.312	T39.313	T39.314	T39.315	T39.316
Suramin (sodium)	T37.4X1	T37.4X2	T37.4X3	T37.4X4	T37.4X5	T37.4X6
Surfacaine	T41.3X1	T41.3X2	T41.3X3	T41.3X4	T41.3X5	T41.3X6
Surital	T41.1X1	T41.1X2	T41.1X3	T41.1X4	T41.1X5	T41.1X6
Sutilains	T45.3X1	T45.3X2	T45.3X3	T45.3X4	T45.3X5	T45.3X6
Suxamethonium (chloride)	T48.1X1	T48.1X2	T48.1X3	T48.1X4	T48.1X5	T48.1X6
Suxethonium (chloride)	T48.1X1	T48.1X2	T48.1X3	T48.1X4	T48.1X5	T48.1X6
Suxibuzone	T39.2X1	T39.2X2	T39.2X3	T39.2X4	T39.2X5	T39.2X6
Sweetener	T50.901	T50.902	T50.903	T50.904	T50.905	T50.906
Sweet niter spirit	T46.3X1	T46.3X2	T46.3X3	T46.3X4	T46.3X5	T46.3X6
Sweet oil (birch)	T49.3X1	T49.3X2	T49.3X3	T49.3X4	T49.3X5	T49.3X6
Sym-dichloroethyl ether	T53.6X1	T53.6X2	T53.6X3	T53.6X4	—	—
Sympatholytic NEC	T44.8X1	T44.8X2	T44.8X3	T44.8X4	T44.8X5	T44.8X6
haloalkylamine	T44.8X1	T44.8X2	T44.8X3	T44.8X4	T44.8X5	T44.8X6
Sympathomimetic NEC	T44.901	T44.902	T44.903	T44.904	T44.905	T44.906
anti-common-cold	T48.5X1	T48.5X2	T48.5X3	T48.5X4	T48.5X5	T48.5X6
bronchodilator	T48.6X1	T48.6X2	T48.6X3	T48.6X4	T48.6X5	T48.6X6
specified NEC	T44.991	T44.992	T44.993	T44.994	T44.995	T44.996
Synagis	T50.B91	T50.B92	T50.B93	T50.B94	T50.B95	T50.B96
Synalar	T49.0X1	T49.0X2	T49.0X3	T49.0X4	T49.0X5	T49.0X6
Synthroid	T38.1X1	T38.1X2	T38.1X3	T38.1X4	T38.1X5	T38.1X6
Syntocinon	T48.0X1	T48.0X2	T48.0X3	T48.0X4	T48.0X5	T48.0X6
Syrosingopine	T46.5X1	T46.5X2	T46.5X3	T46.5X4	T46.5X5	T46.5X6
Systemic drug	T45.91	T45.92	T45.93	T45.94	T45.95	T45.96
specified NEC	T45.8X1	T45.8X2	T45.8X3	T45.8X4	T45.8X5	T45.8X6
Tablets — see also specified substance	T50.901	T50.902	T50.903	T50.904	T50.905	T50.906
Tace	T38.5X1	T38.5X2	T38.5X3	T38.5X4	T38.5X5	T38.5X6
Tacrine	T44.0X1	T44.0X2	T44.0X3	T44.0X4	T44.0X5	T44.0X6
Tadalafil	T46.7X1	T46.7X2	T46.7X3	T46.7X4	T46.7X5	T46.7X6
Talampicillin	T36.0X1	T36.0X2	T36.0X3	T36.0X4	T36.0X5	T36.0X6
Talbutal	T42.3X1	T42.3X2	T42.3X3	T42.3X4	T42.3X5	T42.3X6
Talc powder	T49.3X1	T49.3X2	T49.3X3	T49.3X4	T49.3X5	T49.3X6
Talcum	T49.3X1	T49.3X2	T49.3X3	T49.3X4	T49.3X5	T49.3X6
Taleranol	T38.6X1	T38.6X2	T38.6X3	T38.6X4	T38.6X5	T38.6X6

Strychnos — Taleranol

Substance	Poisoning, Accidental (unintentional)	Poisoning, Intentional Self-harm	Poisoning, Assault	Poisoning, Undetermined	Adverse Effect	Under-dosing
Tamoxifen	T38.6X1	T38.6X2	T38.6X3	T38.6X4	T38.6X5	T38.6X6
Tamsulosin	T44.6X1	T44.6X2	T44.6X3	T44.6X4	T44.6X5	T44.6X6
Tandearil, tanderil	T39.2X1	T39.2X2	T39.2X3	T39.2X4	T39.2X5	T39.2X6
Tannic acid	T49.2X1	T49.2X2	T49.2X3	T49.2X4	T49.2X5	T49.2X6
medicinal (astringent)	T49.2X1	T49.2X2	T49.2X3	T49.2X4	T49.2X5	T49.2X6
Tannin — see Tannic acid						
Tansy	T62.2X1	T62.2X2	T62.2X3	T62.2X4	—	—
TAO	T36.3X1	T36.3X2	T36.3X3	T36.3X4	T36.3X5	T36.3X6
Tapazole	T38.2X1	T38.2X2	T38.2X3	T38.2X4	T38.2X5	T38.2X6
Taractan	T43.591	T43.592	T43.593	T43.594	T43.595	T43.596
Tarantula (venomous)	T63.321	T63.322	T63.323	T63.324	—	—
Tartar emetic	T37.8X1	T37.8X2	T37.8X3	T37.8X4	T37.8X5	T37.8X6
Tartaric acid	T65.891	T65.892	T65.893	T65.894	—	—
Tartrated antimony (anti-infective)	T37.8X1	T37.8X2	T37.8X3	T37.8X4	T37.8X5	T37.8X6
Tartrate, laxative	T47.4X1	T47.4X2	T47.4X3	T47.4X4	T47.4X5	T47.4X6
Tar NEC	T52.0X1	T52.0X2	T52.0X3	T52.0X4	—	—
camphor	T60.1X1	T60.1X2	T60.1X3	T60.1X4	—	—
distillate	T49.1X1	T49.1X2	T49.1X3	T49.1X4	T49.1X5	T49.1X6
fumes	T59.891	T59.892	T59.893	T59.894	—	—
medicinal	T49.1X1	T49.1X2	T49.1X3	T49.1X4	T49.1X5	T49.1X6
ointment	T49.1X1	T49.1X2	T49.1X3	T49.1X4	T49.1X5	T49.1X6
Tauromustine	T45.1X1	T45.1X2	T45.1X3	T45.1X4	T45.1X5	T45.1X6
TCA — see Trichloroacetic acid						
TCDD	T53.7X1	T53.7X2	T53.7X3	T53.7X4	—	—
TDI (vapor)	T65.0X1	T65.0X2	T65.0X3	T65.0X4	—	—
Tear						
gas	T59.3X1	T59.3X2	T59.3X3	T59.3X4	—	—
solution	T49.5X1	T49.5X2	T49.5X3	T49.5X4	T49.5X5	T49.5X6
Teclothiazide	T50.2X1	T50.2X2	T50.2X3	T50.2X4	T50.2X5	T50.2X6
Teclozan	T37.3X1	T37.3X2	T37.3X3	T37.3X4	T37.3X5	T37.3X6
Tegafur	T45.1X1	T45.1X2	T45.1X3	T45.1X4	T45.1X5	T45.1X6
Tegretol	T42.1X1	T42.1X2	T42.1X3	T42.1X4	T42.1X5	T42.1X6
Teicoplanin	T36.8X1	T36.8X2	T36.8X3	T36.8X4	T36.8X5	T36.8X6
Telepaque	T50.8X1	T50.8X2	T50.8X3	T50.8X4	T50.8X5	T50.8X6
Tellurium	T56.891	T56.892	T56.893	T56.894	—	—
fumes	T56.891	T56.892	T56.893	T56.894	—	—
TEM	T45.1X1	T45.1X2	T45.1X3	T45.1X4	T45.1X5	T45.1X6
Temazepam	T42.4X1	T42.4X2	T42.4X3	T42.4X4	T42.4X5	T42.4X6
Temocillin	T36.0X1	T36.0X2	T36.0X3	T36.0X4	T36.0X5	T36.0X6
Tenamfetamine	T43.621	T43.622	T43.623	T43.624	T43.625	T43.626
Teniposide	T45.1X1	T45.1X2	T45.1X3	T45.1X4	T45.1X5	T45.1X6
Tenitramine	T46.3X1	T46.3X2	T46.3X3	T46.3X4	T46.3X5	T46.3X6
Tenoglicin	T48.4X1	T48.4X2	T48.4X3	T48.4X4	T48.4X5	T48.4X6
Tenonitrozole	T37.3X1	T37.3X2	T37.3X3	T37.3X4	T37.3X5	T37.3X6
Tenoxicam	T39.391	T39.392	T39.393	T39.394	T39.395	T39.396
TEPA	T45.1X1	T45.1X2	T45.1X3	T45.1X4	T45.1X5	T45.1X6
TEPP	T60.0X1	T60.0X2	T60.0X3	T60.0X4	—	—
Teprotide	T46.5X1	T46.5X2	T46.5X3	T46.5X4	T46.5X5	T46.5X6
Terazosin	T44.6X1	T44.6X2	T44.6X3	T44.6X4	T44.6X5	T44.6X6
Terbufos	T60.0X1	T60.0X2	T60.0X3	T60.0X4	—	—
Terbutaline	T48.6X1	T48.6X2	T48.6X3	T48.6X4	T48.6X5	T48.6X6
Terconazole	T49.0X1	T49.0X2	T49.0X3	T49.0X4	T49.0X5	T49.0X6
Terfenadine	T45.0X1	T45.0X2	T45.0X3	T45.0X4	T45.0X5	T45.0X6
Teriparatide (acetate)	T50.991	T50.992	T50.993	T50.994	T50.995	T50.996
Terizidone	T37.1X1	T37.1X2	T37.1X3	T37.1X4	T37.1X5	T37.1X6
Terlipressin	T38.891	T38.892	T38.893	T38.894	T38.895	T38.896
Terodiline	T46.3X1	T46.3X2	T46.3X3	T46.3X4	T46.3X5	T46.3X6
Teroxalene	T37.4X1	T37.4X2	T37.4X3	T37.4X4	T37.4X5	T37.4X6
Terpin (cis) hydrate	T48.4X1	T48.4X2	T48.4X3	T48.4X4	T48.4X5	T48.4X6
Terramycin	T36.4X1	T36.4X2	T36.4X3	T36.4X4	T36.4X5	T36.4X6
Tertatolol	T44.7X1	T44.7X2	T44.7X3	T44.7X4	T44.7X5	T44.7X6
Tessalon	T48.3X1	T48.3X2	T48.3X3	T48.3X4	T48.3X5	T48.3X6
Testolactone	T38.7X1	T38.7X2	T38.7X3	T38.7X4	T38.7X5	T38.7X6
Testosterone	T38.7X1	T38.7X2	T38.7X3	T38.7X4	T38.7X5	T38.7X6
Tetanus toxoid or vaccine	T50.A91	T50.A92	T50.A93	T50.A94	T50.A95	T50.A96
antitoxin	T50.Z11	T50.Z12	T50.Z13	T50.Z14	T50.Z15	T50.Z16
immune globulin (human)	T50.Z11	T50.Z12	T50.Z13	T50.Z14	T50.Z15	T50.Z16
toxoid	T50.A91	T50.A92	T50.A93	T50.A94	T50.A95	T50.A96
with diphtheria toxoid	T50.A21	T50.A22	T50.A23	T50.A24	T50.A25	T50.A26
with pertussis	T50.A11	T50.A12	T50.A13	T50.A14	T50.A15	T50.A16
Tetrabenazine	T43.591	T43.592	T43.593	T43.594	T43.595	T43.596
Tetracaine	T41.3X1	T41.3X2	T41.3X3	T41.3X4	T41.3X5	T41.3X6
nerve block (peripheral) (plexus)	T41.3X1	T41.3X2	T41.3X3	T41.3X4	T41.3X5	T41.3X6
regional	T41.3X1	T41.3X2	T41.3X3	T41.3X4	T41.3X5	T41.3X6
spinal	T41.3X1	T41.3X2	T41.3X3	T41.3X4	T41.3X5	T41.3X6
Tetrachlorethylene — see Tetrachloroethylene						
Tetrachlormethiazide	T50.2X1	T50.2X2	T50.2X3	T50.2X4	T50.2X5	T50.2X6
Tetrachloroethane	T53.6X1	T53.6X2	T53.6X3	T53.6X4	—	—
vapor	T53.6X1	T53.6X2	T53.6X3	T53.6X4	—	—
paint or varnish	T53.6X1	T53.6X2	T53.6X3	T53.6X4	—	—
Tetrachloroethylene (liquid)	T53.3X1	T53.3X2	T53.3X3	T53.3X4	—	—
medicinal	T37.4X1	T37.4X2	T37.4X3	T37.4X4	T37.4X5	T37.4X6
vapor	T53.3X1	T53.3X2	T53.3X3	T53.3X4	—	—
Tetrachloromethane — see Carbon tetrachloride						
Tetracosactide	T38.811	T38.812	T38.813	T38.814	T38.815	T38.816
Tetracosactrin	T38.811	T38.812	T38.813	T38.814	T38.815	T38.816
Tetracycline	T36.4X1	T36.4X2	T36.4X3	T36.4X4	T36.4X5	T36.4X6
ophthalmic preparation	T49.5X1	T49.5X2	T49.5X3	T49.5X4	T49.5X5	T49.5X6
topical NEC	T49.0X1	T49.0X2	T49.0X3	T49.0X4	T49.0X5	T49.0X6
Tetradifon	T60.8X1	T60.8X2	T60.8X3	T60.8X4	—	—
Tetradotoxin	T61.771	T61.772	T61.773	T61.774	—	—
Tetraethyl						
lead	T56.0X1	T56.0X2	T56.0X3	T56.0X4	—	—
pyrophosphate	T60.0X1	T60.0X2	T60.0X3	T60.0X4	—	—
Tetraethylammonium chloride	T44.2X1	T44.2X2	T44.2X3	T44.2X4	T44.2X5	T44.2X6
Tetraethylthiuram disulfide	T50.6X1	T50.6X2	T50.6X3	T50.6X4	T50.6X5	T50.6X6
Tetrahydroaminoacridine	T44.0X1	T44.0X2	T44.0X3	T44.0X4	T44.0X5	T44.0X6
Tetrahydrocannabinol	T40.7X1	T40.7X2	T40.7X3	T40.7X4	T40.7X5	T40.7X6
Tetrahydrofuran	T52.8X1	T52.8X2	T52.8X3	T52.8X4	—	—
Tetrahydronaphthalene	T52.8X1	T52.8X2	T52.8X3	T52.8X4	—	—
Tetrahydrozoline	T49.5X1	T49.5X2	T49.5X3	T49.5X4	T49.5X5	T49.5X6
Tetralin	T52.8X1	T52.8X2	T52.8X3	T52.8X4	—	—
Tetramethrin	T60.2X1	T60.2X2	T60.2X3	T60.2X4	—	—
Tetramethylthiuram (disulfide) NEC	T60.3X1	T60.3X2	T60.3X3	T60.3X4	—	—
medicinal	T49.0X1	T49.0X2	T49.0X3	T49.0X4	T49.0X5	T49.0X6
Tetramisole	T37.4X1	T37.4X2	T37.4X3	T37.4X4	T37.4X5	T37.4X6
Tetranicotinoyl fructose	T46.7X1	T46.7X2	T46.7X3	T46.7X4	T46.7X5	T46.7X6
Tetrazepam	T42.4X1	T42.4X2	T42.4X3	T42.4X4	T42.4X5	T42.4X6
Tetronal	T42.6X1	T42.6X2	T42.6X3	T42.6X4	T42.6X5	T42.6X6
Tetryl	T65.3X1	T65.3X2	T65.3X3	T65.3X4	—	—
Tetrylammonium chloride	T44.2X1	T44.2X2	T44.2X3	T44.2X4	T44.2X5	T44.2X6
Tetryzoline	T49.5X1	T49.5X2	T49.5X3	T49.5X4	T49.5X5	T49.5X6
Thalidomide	T45.1X1	T45.1X2	T45.1X3	T45.1X4	T45.1X5	T45.1X6
Thallium (compounds) (dust) NEC	T56.811	T56.812	T56.813	T56.814	—	—
pesticide	T60.4X1	T60.4X2	T60.4X3	T60.4X4	—	—
THC	T40.7X1	T40.7X2	T40.7X3	T40.7X4	T40.7X5	T40.7X6
Thebacon	T48.3X1	T48.3X2	T48.3X3	T48.3X4	T48.3X5	T48.3X6
Thebaine	T40.2X1	T40.2X2	T40.2X3	T40.2X4	T40.2X5	T40.2X6
Thenoic acid	T49.6X1	T49.6X2	T49.6X3	T49.6X4	T49.6X5	T49.6X6
Thenyldiamine	T45.0X1	T45.0X2	T45.0X3	T45.0X4	T45.0X5	T45.0X6
Theobromine (calcium salicylate)	T48.6X1	T48.6X2	T48.6X3	T48.6X4	T48.6X5	T48.6X6
sodium salicylate	T48.6X1	T48.6X2	T48.6X3	T48.6X4	T48.6X5	T48.6X6
Theophyllamine	T48.6X1	T48.6X2	T48.6X3	T48.6X4	T48.6X5	T48.6X6
Theophylline	T48.6X1	T48.6X2	T48.6X3	T48.6X4	T48.6X5	T48.6X6
aminobenzoic acid	T48.6X1	T48.6X2	T48.6X3	T48.6X4	T48.6X5	T48.6X6
ethylenediamine	T48.6X1	T48.6X2	T48.6X3	T48.6X4	T48.6X5	T48.6X6
piperazine p-amino-benzoate	T48.6X1	T48.6X2	T48.6X3	T48.6X4	T48.6X5	T48.6X6
Thiabendazole	T37.4X1	T37.4X2	T37.4X3	T37.4X4	T37.4X5	T37.4X6
Thialbarbital	T41.1X1	T41.1X2	T41.1X3	T41.1X4	T41.1X5	T41.1X6
Thiamazole	T38.2X1	T38.2X2	T38.2X3	T38.2X4	T38.2X5	T38.2X6
Thiambutosine	T37.1X1	T37.1X2	T37.1X3	T37.1X4	T37.1X5	T37.1X6
Thiamine	T45.2X1	T45.2X2	T45.2X3	T45.2X4	T45.2X5	T45.2X6
Thiamphenicol	T36.2X1	T36.2X2	T36.2X3	T36.2X4	T36.2X5	T36.2X6
Thiamylal	T41.1X1	T41.1X2	T41.1X3	T41.1X4	T41.1X5	T41.1X6
sodium	T41.1X1	T41.1X2	T41.1X3	T41.1X4	T41.1X5	T41.1X6
Thiazesim	T43.291	T43.292	T43.293	T43.294	T43.295	T43.296
Thiazides (diuretics)	T50.2X1	T50.2X2	T50.2X3	T50.2X4	T50.2X5	T50.2X6
Thiazinamium metilsulfate	T43.3X1	T43.3X2	T43.3X3	T43.3X4	T43.3X5	T43.3X6
Thiethylperazine	T43.3X1	T43.3X2	T43.3X3	T43.3X4	T43.3X5	T43.3X6
Thimerosal	T49.0X1	T49.0X2	T49.0X3	T49.0X4	T49.0X5	T49.0X6
ophthalmic preparation	T49.5X1	T49.5X2	T49.5X3	T49.5X4	T49.5X5	T49.5X6
Thioacetazone	T37.1X1	T37.1X2	T37.1X3	T37.1X4	T37.1X5	T37.1X6
with isoniazid	T37.1X1	T37.1X2	T37.1X3	T37.1X4	T37.1X5	T37.1X6
Thiobarbital sodium	T41.1X1	T41.1X2	T41.1X3	T41.1X4	T41.1X5	T41.1X6
Thiobarbiturate anesthetic	T41.1X1	T41.1X2	T41.1X3	T41.1X4	T41.1X5	T41.1X6
Thiobismol	T37.8X1	T37.8X2	T37.8X3	T37.8X4	T37.8X5	T37.8X6
Thiobutabarbital sodium	T41.1X1	T41.1X2	T41.1X3	T41.1X4	T41.1X5	T41.1X6
Thiocarbamate (insecticide)	T60.0X1	T60.0X2	T60.0X3	T60.0X4	—	—
Thiocarbamide	T38.2X1	T38.2X2	T38.2X3	T38.2X4	T38.2X5	T38.2X6
Thiocarbarsone	T37.8X1	T37.8X2	T37.8X3	T37.8X4	T37.8X5	T37.8X6
Thiocarlide	T37.1X1	T37.1X2	T37.1X3	T37.1X4	T37.1X5	T37.1X6
Thioctamide	T50.991	T50.992	T50.993	T50.994	T50.995	T50.996

Substance	Poisoning, Accidental (unintentional)	Poisoning, Intentional Self-harm	Poisoning, Assault	Poisoning, Undetermined	Adverse Effect	Under-dosing
Thioctic acid	T50.991	T50.992	T50.993	T50.994	T50.995	T50.996
Thiofos	T60.0X1	T60.0X2	T60.0X3	T60.0X4	—	—
Thioglycolate	T49.4X1	T49.4X2	T49.4X3	T49.4X4	T49.4X5	T49.4X6
Thioglycolic acid	T65.891	T65.892	T65.893	T65.894	—	—
Thioguanine	T45.1X1	T45.1X2	T45.1X3	T45.1X4	T45.1X5	T45.1X6
Thiomercaptomerin	T50.2X1	T50.2X2	T50.2X3	T50.2X4	T50.2X5	T50.2X6
Thiomerin	T50.2X1	T50.2X2	T50.2X3	T50.2X4	T50.2X5	T50.2X6
Thiomersal	T49.0X1	T49.0X2	T49.0X3	T49.0X4	T49.0X5	T49.0X6
Thionazin	T60.0X1	T60.0X2	T60.0X3	T60.0X4	—	—
Thiopental (sodium)	T41.1X1	T41.1X2	T41.1X3	T41.1X4	T41.1X5	T41.1X6
Thiopentone (sodium)	T41.1X1	T41.1X2	T41.1X3	T41.1X4	T41.1X5	T41.1X6
Thiopropazate	T43.3X1	T43.3X2	T43.3X3	T43.3X4	T43.3X5	T43.3X6
Thioproperazine	T43.3X1	T43.3X2	T43.3X3	T43.3X4	T43.3X5	T43.3X6
Thioridazine	T43.3X1	T43.3X2	T43.3X3	T43.3X4	T43.3X5	T43.3X6
Thiosinamine	T49.3X1	T49.3X2	T49.3X3	T49.3X4	T49.3X5	T49.3X6
Thiotepa	T45.1X1	T45.1X2	T45.1X3	T45.1X4	T45.1X5	T45.1X6
Thiothixene	T43.4X1	T43.4X2	T43.4X3	T43.4X4	T43.4X5	T43.4X6
Thiouracil (benzyl) (methyl)	T38.2X1	T38.2X2	T38.2X3	T38.2X4	T38.2X5	T38.2X6
(propyl)						
Thiourea	T38.2X1	T38.2X2	T38.2X3	T38.2X4	T38.2X5	T38.2X6
Thiphenamil	T44.3X1	T44.3X2	T44.3X3	T44.3X4	T44.3X5	T44.3X6
Thiram	T60.3X1	T60.3X2	T60.3X3	T60.3X4	—	—
medicinal	T49.2X1	T49.2X2	T49.2X3	T49.2X4	T49.2X5	T49.2X6
Thonzylamine (systemic)	T45.0X1	T45.0X2	T45.0X3	T45.0X4	T45.0X5	T45.0X6
mucosal decongestant	T48.5X1	T48.5X2	T48.5X3	T48.5X4	T48.5X5	T48.5X6
Thorazine	T43.3X1	T43.3X2	T43.3X3	T43.3X4	T43.3X5	T43.3X6
Thorium dioxide	T50.8X1	T50.8X2	T50.8X3	T50.8X4	T50.8X5	T50.8X6
suspension						
Thornapple	T62.2X1	T62.2X2	T62.2X3	T62.2X4	—	—
Throat drug NEC	T49.6X1	T49.6X2	T49.6X3	T49.6X4	T49.6X5	T49.6X6
Thrombin	T45.7X1	T45.7X2	T45.7X3	T45.7X4	T45.7X5	T45.7X6
Thrombolysin	T45.611	T45.612	T45.613	T45.614	T45.615	T45.616
Thromboplastin	T45.7X1	T45.7X2	T45.7X3	T45.7X4	T45.7X5	T45.7X6
Thurfyl nicotinate	T46.7X1	T46.7X2	T46.7X3	T46.7X4	T46.7X5	T46.7X6
Thymol	T49.0X1	T49.0X2	T49.0X3	T49.0X4	T49.0X5	T49.0X6
Thymopentin	T37.5X1	T37.5X2	T37.5X3	T37.5X4	T37.5X5	T37.5X6
Thymoxamine	T46.7X1	T46.7X2	T46.7X3	T46.7X4	T46.7X5	T46.7X6
Thymus extract	T38.891	T38.892	T38.893	T38.894	T38.895	T38.896
Thyreotrophic hormone	T38.811	T38.812	T38.813	T38.814	T38.815	T38.816
Thyroglobulin	T38.1X1	T38.1X2	T38.1X3	T38.1X4	T38.1X5	T38.1X6
Thyroid (hormone)	T38.1X1	T38.1X2	T38.1X3	T38.1X4	T38.1X5	T38.1X6
Thyrolar	T38.1X1	T38.1X2	T38.1X3	T38.1X4	T38.1X5	T38.1X6
Thyrotrophin	T38.811	T38.812	T38.813	T38.814	T38.815	T38.816
Thyrotropic hormone	T38.811	T38.812	T38.813	T38.814	T38.815	T38.816
Thyroxine	T38.1X1	T38.1X2	T38.1X3	T38.1X4	T38.1X5	T38.1X6
Tiabendazole	T37.4X1	T37.4X2	T37.4X3	T37.4X4	T37.4X5	T37.4X6
Tiamizide	T50.2X1	T50.2X2	T50.2X3	T50.2X4	T50.2X5	T50.2X6
Tianeptine	T43.291	T43.292	T43.293	T43.294	T43.295	T43.296
Tiapamil	T46.1X1	T46.1X2	T46.1X3	T46.1X4	T46.1X5	T46.1X6
Tiapride	T43.591	T43.592	T43.593	T43.594	T43.595	T43.596
Tiaprofenic acid	T39.311	T39.312	T39.313	T39.314	T39.315	T39.316
Tiaramide	T39.8X1	T39.8X2	T39.8X3	T39.8X4	T39.8X5	T39.8X6
Ticarcillin	T36.0X1	T36.0X2	T36.0X3	T36.0X4	T36.0X5	T36.0X6
Ticlatone	T49.0X1	T49.0X2	T49.0X3	T49.0X4	T49.0X5	T49.0X6
Ticlopidine	T45.521	T45.522	T45.523	T45.524	T45.525	T45.526
Ticrynafen	T50.1X1	T50.1X2	T50.1X3	T50.1X4	T50.1X5	T50.1X6
Tidiacic	T50.991	T50.992	T50.993	T50.994	T50.995	T50.996
Tiemonium	T44.3X1	T44.3X2	T44.3X3	T44.3X4	T44.3X5	T44.3X6
iodide	T44.3X1	T44.3X2	T44.3X3	T44.3X4	T44.3X5	T44.3X6
Tienilic acid	T50.1X1	T50.1X2	T50.1X3	T50.1X4	T50.1X5	T50.1X6
Tifenamil	T44.3X1	T44.3X2	T44.3X3	T44.3X4	T44.3X5	T44.3X6
Tigan	T45.0X1	T45.0X2	T45.0X3	T45.0X4	T45.0X5	T45.0X6
Tigloidine	T44.3X1	T44.3X2	T44.3X3	T44.3X4	T44.3X5	T44.3X6
Tilactase	T47.5X1	T47.5X2	T47.5X3	T47.5X4	T47.5X5	T47.5X6
Tiletamine	T41.291	T41.292	T41.293	T41.294	T41.295	T41.296
Tilidine	T40.491	T40.492	T40.493	T40.494	—	—
Timepidium bromide	T44.3X1	T44.3X2	T44.3X3	T44.3X4	T44.3X5	T44.3X6
Timiperone	T43.4X1	T43.4X2	T43.4X3	T43.4X4	T43.4X5	T43.4X6
Timolol	T44.7X1	T44.7X2	T44.7X3	T44.7X4	T44.7X5	T44.7X6
Tincture, iodine — see Iodine						
Tindal	T43.3X1	T43.3X2	T43.3X3	T43.3X4	T43.3X5	T43.3X6
Tinidazole	T37.3X1	T37.3X2	T37.3X3	T37.3X4	T37.3X5	T37.3X6
Tin (chloride) (dust) (oxide)	T56.6X1	T56.6X2	T56.6X3	T56.6X4	—	—
NEC						
anti-infectives	T37.8X1	T37.8X2	T37.8X3	T37.8X4	T37.8X5	T37.8X6
Tinoridine	T39.8X1	T39.8X2	T39.8X3	T39.8X4	T39.8X5	T39.8X6
Tiocarlide	T37.1X1	T37.1X2	T37.1X3	T37.1X4	T37.1X5	T37.1X6
Tioclomarol	T45.511	T45.512	T45.513	T45.514	T45.515	T45.516
Tioconazole	T49.0X1	T49.0X2	T49.0X3	T49.0X4	T49.0X5	T49.0X6
Tioguanine	T45.1X1	T45.1X2	T45.1X3	T45.1X4	T45.1X5	T45.1X6
Tiopronin	T50.991	T50.992	T50.993	T50.994	T50.995	T50.996
Tiotixene	T43.4X1	T43.4X2	T43.4X3	T43.4X4	T43.4X5	T43.4X6
Tioxolone	T49.4X1	T49.4X2	T49.4X3	T49.4X4	T49.4X5	T49.4X6

Substance	Poisoning, Accidental (unintentional)	Poisoning, Intentional Self-harm	Poisoning, Assault	Poisoning, Undetermined	Adverse Effect	Under-dosing
Tipepidine	T48.3X1	T48.3X2	T48.3X3	T48.3X4	T48.3X5	T48.3X6
Tiquizium bromide	T44.3X1	T44.3X2	T44.3X3	T44.3X4	T44.3X5	T44.3X6
Tiratricol	T38.1X1	T38.1X2	T38.1X3	T38.1X4	T38.1X5	T38.1X6
Tisopurine	T50.4X1	T50.4X2	T50.4X3	T50.4X4	T50.4X5	T50.4X6
Titanium (compounds)	T56.891	T56.892	T56.893	T56.894	—	—
(vapor)						
dioxide	T49.3X1	T49.3X2	T49.3X3	T49.3X4	T49.3X5	T49.3X6
ointment	T49.3X1	T49.3X2	T49.3X3	T49.3X4	T49.3X5	T49.3X6
oxide	T49.3X1	T49.3X2	T49.3X3	T49.3X4	T49.3X5	T49.3X6
tetrachloride	T56.891	T56.892	T56.893	T56.894	—	—
Titanocene	T56.891	T56.892	T56.893	T56.894	—	—
Titroid	T38.1X1	T38.1X2	T38.1X3	T38.1X4	T38.1X5	T38.1X6
Tizanidine	T42.8X1	T42.8X2	T42.8X3	T42.8X4	T42.8X5	T42.8X6
TMTD	T60.3X1	T60.3X2	T60.3X3	T60.3X4	—	—
TNT (fumes)	T65.3X1	T65.3X2	T65.3X3	T65.3X4	—	—
Toadstool	T62.0X1	T62.0X2	T62.0X3	T62.0X4	—	—
Tobacco NEC	T65.291	T65.292	T65.293	T65.294	—	—
cigarettes	T65.221	T65.222	T65.223	T65.224	—	—
Indian	T62.2X1	T62.2X2	T62.2X3	T62.2X4	—	—
smoke, second-hand	T65.221	T65.222	T65.223	T65.224	—	—
Tobramycin	T36.5X1	T36.5X2	T36.5X3	T36.5X4	T36.5X5	T36.5X6
Tocainide	T46.2X1	T46.2X2	T46.2X3	T46.2X4	T46.2X5	T46.2X6
Tocoferol	T45.2X1	T45.2X2	T45.2X3	T45.2X4	T45.2X5	T45.2X6
Tocopherol	T45.2X1	T45.2X2	T45.2X3	T45.2X4	T45.2X5	T45.2X6
acetate	T45.2X1	T45.2X2	T45.2X3	T45.2X4	T45.2X5	T45.2X6
Tocosamine	T48.0X1	T48.0X2	T48.0X3	T48.0X4	T48.0X5	T48.0X6
Todralazine	T46.5X1	T46.5X2	T46.5X3	T46.5X4	T46.5X5	T46.5X6
Tofisopam	T42.4X1	T42.4X2	T42.4X3	T42.4X4	T42.4X5	T42.4X6
Tofranil	T43.011	T43.012	T43.013	T43.014	T43.015	T43.016
Toilet deodorizer	T65.891	T65.892	T65.893	T65.894	—	—
Tolamolol	T44.7X1	T44.7X2	T44.7X3	T44.7X4	T44.7X5	T44.7X6
Tolazamide	T38.3X1	T38.3X2	T38.3X3	T38.3X4	T38.3X5	T38.3X6
Tolazoline	T46.7X1	T46.7X2	T46.7X3	T46.7X4	T46.7X5	T46.7X6
Tolbutamide (sodium)	T38.3X1	T38.3X2	T38.3X3	T38.3X4	T38.3X5	T38.3X6
Tolciclate	T49.0X1	T49.0X2	T49.0X3	T49.0X4	T49.0X5	T49.0X6
Tolmetin	T39.391	T39.392	T39.393	T39.394	T39.395	T39.396
Tolnaftate	T49.0X1	T49.0X2	T49.0X3	T49.0X4	T49.0X5	T49.0X6
Tolonidine	T46.5X1	T46.5X2	T46.5X3	T46.5X4	T46.5X5	T46.5X6
Toloxatone	T42.6X1	T42.6X2	T42.6X3	T42.6X4	T42.6X5	T42.6X6
Tolperisone	T44.3X1	T44.3X2	T44.3X3	T44.3X4	T44.3X5	T44.3X6
Tolserol	T42.8X1	T42.8X2	T42.8X3	T42.8X4	T42.8X5	T42.8X6
Toluene (liquid)	T52.2X1	T52.2X2	T52.2X3	T52.2X4	—	—
diisocyanate	T65.0X1	T65.0X2	T65.0X3	T65.0X4	—	—
Toluidine	T65.891	T65.892	T65.893	T65.894	—	—
vapor	T59.891	T59.892	T59.893	T59.894	—	—
Toluol (liquid)	T52.2X1	T52.2X2	T52.2X3	T52.2X4	—	—
vapor	T52.2X1	T52.2X2	T52.2X3	T52.2X4	—	—
Toluylenediamine	T65.3X1	T65.3X2	T65.3X3	T65.3X4	—	—
Tolylene-2,4-diisocyanate	T65.0X1	T65.0X2	T65.0X3	T65.0X4	—	—
Tonic NEC	T50.901	T50.902	T50.903	T50.904	T50.905	T50.906
Topical action drug NEC	T49.91	T49.92	T49.93	T49.94	T49.95	T49.96
ear, nose or throat	T49.6X1	T49.6X2	T49.6X3	T49.6X4	T49.6X5	T49.6X6
eye	T49.5X1	T49.5X2	T49.5X3	T49.5X4	T49.5X5	T49.5X6
skin	T49.91	T49.92	T49.93	T49.94	T49.95	T49.96
specified NEC	T49.8X1	T49.8X2	T49.8X3	T49.8X4	T49.8X5	T49.8X6
Toquizine	T44.3X1	T44.3X2	T44.3X3	T44.3X4	T44.3X5	T44.3X6
Toremifene	T38.6X1	T38.6X2	T38.6X3	T38.6X4	T38.6X5	T38.6X6
Tosylchloramide sodium	T49.8X1	T49.8X2	T49.8X3	T49.8X4	T49.8X5	T49.8X6
Toxaphene (dust) (spray)	T60.1X1	T60.1X2	T60.1X3	T60.1X4	—	—
Toxin, diphtheria (Schick	T50.8X1	T50.8X2	T50.8X3	T50.8X4	T50.8X5	T50.8X6
Test)						
Toxoid						
combined	T50.A21	T50.A22	T50.A23	T50.A24	T50.A25	T50.A26
diphtheria	T50.A91	T50.A92	T50.A93	T50.A94	T50.A95	T50.A96
tetanus	T50.A91	T50.A92	T50.A93	T50.A94	T50.A95	T50.A96
Trace element NEC	T45.8X1	T45.8X2	T45.8X3	T45.8X4	T45.8X5	T45.8X6
Tractor fuel NEC	T52.0X1	T52.0X2	T52.0X3	T52.0X4	—	—
Tragacanth	T50.991	T50.992	T50.993	T50.994	T50.995	T50.996
Tramadol	T40.421	T40.422	T40.423	T40.424	T40.425	T40.426
Tramazoline	T48.5X1	T48.5X2	T48.5X3	T48.5X4	T48.5X5	T48.5X6
Tranexamic acid	T45.621	T45.622	T45.623	T45.624	T45.625	T45.626
Tranilast	T45.0X1	T45.0X2	T45.0X3	T45.0X4	T45.0X5	T45.0X6
Tranquilizer NEC	T43.501	T43.502	T43.503	T43.504	T43.505	T43.506
with hypnotic or sedative	T42.6X1	T42.6X2	T42.6X3	T42.6X4	T42.6X5	T42.6X6
benzodiazepine NEC	T42.4X1	T42.4X2	T42.4X3	T42.4X4	T42.4X5	T42.4X6
butyrophenone NEC	T43.4X1	T43.4X2	T43.4X3	T43.4X4	T43.4X5	T43.4X6
carbamate	T43.591	T43.592	T43.593	T43.594	T43.595	T43.596
dimethylamine	T43.3X1	T43.3X2	T43.3X3	T43.3X4	T43.3X5	T43.3X6
ethylamine	T43.3X1	T43.3X2	T43.3X3	T43.3X4	T43.3X5	T43.3X6
hydroxyzine	T43.591	T43.592	T43.593	T43.594	T43.595	T43.596
major NEC	T43.501	T43.502	T43.503	T43.504	T43.505	T43.506
penothiazine NEC	T43.3X1	T43.3X2	T43.3X3	T43.3X4	T43.3X5	T43.3X6
phenothiazine-based	T43.3X1	T43.3X2	T43.3X3	T43.3X4	T43.3X5	T43.3X6

Substance	Poisoning, Accidental (unintentional)	Poisoning, Intentional Self-harm	Poisoning, Assault	Poisoning, Undetermined	Adverse Effect	Under-dosing
Tranquilizer — *continued*						
piperazine NEC	T43.3X1	T43.3X2	T43.3X3	T43.3X4	T43.3X5	T43.3X6
piperidine	T43.3X1	T43.3X2	T43.3X3	T43.3X4	T43.3X5	T43.3X6
propylamine	T43.3X1	T43.3X2	T43.3X3	T43.3X4	T43.3X5	T43.3X6
specified NEC	T43.591	T43.592	T43.593	T43.594	T43.595	T43.596
thioxanthene NEC	T43.591	T43.592	T43.593	T43.594	T43.595	T43.596
Tranxene	T42.4X1	T42.4X2	T42.4X3	T42.4X4	T42.4X5	T42.4X6
Tranylcypromine	T43.1X1	T43.1X2	T43.1X3	T43.1X4	T43.1X5	T43.1X6
Trapidil	T46.3X1	T46.3X2	T46.3X3	T46.3X4	T46.3X5	T46.3X6
Trasentine	T44.3X1	T44.3X2	T44.3X3	T44.3X4	T44.3X5	T44.3X6
Travert	T50.3X1	T50.3X2	T50.3X3	T50.3X4	T50.3X5	T50.3X6
Trazodone	T43.211	T43.212	T43.213	T43.214	T43.215	T43.216
Trecator	T37.1X1	T37.1X2	T37.1X3	T37.1X4	T37.1X5	T37.1X6
Treosulfan	T45.1X1	T45.1X2	T45.1X3	T45.1X4	T45.1X5	T45.1X6
Tretamine	T45.1X1	T45.1X2	T45.1X3	T45.1X4	T45.1X5	T45.1X6
Tretinoin	T49.0X1	T49.0X2	T49.0X3	T49.0X4	T49.0X5	T49.0X6
Tretoquinol	T48.6X1	T48.6X2	T48.6X3	T48.6X4	T48.6X5	T48.6X6
Triacetin	T49.0X1	T49.0X2	T49.0X3	T49.0X4	T49.0X5	T49.0X6
Triacetoxyanthracene	T49.4X1	T49.4X2	T49.4X3	T49.4X4	T49.4X5	T49.4X6
Triacetyloleandomycin	T36.3X1	T36.3X2	T36.3X3	T36.3X4	T36.3X5	T36.3X6
Triamcinolone	T38.0X1	T38.0X2	T38.0X3	T38.0X4	T38.0X5	T38.0X6
ENT agent	T49.6X1	T49.6X2	T49.6X3	T49.6X4	T49.6X5	T49.6X6
hexacetonide	T49.0X1	T49.0X2	T49.0X3	T49.0X4	T49.0X5	T49.0X6
ophthalmic preparation	T49.5X1	T49.5X2	T49.5X3	T49.5X4	T49.5X5	T49.5X6
topical NEC	T49.0X1	T49.0X2	T49.0X3	T49.0X4	T49.0X5	T49.0X6
Triampyzine	T44.3X1	T44.3X2	T44.3X3	T44.3X4	T44.3X5	T44.3X6
Triamterene	T50.2X1	T50.2X2	T50.2X3	T50.2X4	T50.2X5	T50.2X6
Triazine (herbicide)	T60.3X1	T60.3X2	T60.3X3	T60.3X4	—	—
Triaziquone	T45.1X1	T45.1X2	T45.1X3	T45.1X4	T45.1X5	T45.1X6
Triazolam	T42.4X1	T42.4X2	T42.4X3	T42.4X4	T42.4X5	T42.4X6
Triazole (herbicide)	T60.3X1	T60.3X2	T60.3X3	T60.3X4	—	—
Tribenoside	T46.991	T46.992	T46.993	T46.994	T46.995	T46.996
Tribromacetaldehyde	T42.6X1	T42.6X2	T42.6X3	T42.6X4	T42.6X5	T42.6X6
Tribromoethanol, rectal	T41.291	T41.292	T41.293	T41.294	T41.295	T41.296
Tribromomethane	T42.6X1	T42.6X2	T42.6X3	T42.6X4	T42.6X5	T42.6X6
Trichlorethane	T53.2X1	T53.2X2	T53.2X3	T53.2X4	—	—
Trichlorethylene	T53.2X1	T53.2X2	T53.2X3	T53.2X4	—	—
Trichlorfon	T60.0X1	T60.0X2	T60.0X3	T60.0X4	—	—
Trichlormethiazide	T50.2X1	T50.2X2	T50.2X3	T50.2X4	T50.2X5	T50.2X6
Trichlormethine	T45.1X1	T45.1X2	T45.1X3	T45.1X4	T45.1X5	T45.1X6
Trichloroacetic acid, Trichloracetic acid	T54.2X1	T54.2X2	T54.2X3	T54.2X4	—	—
medicinal	T49.4X1	T49.4X2	T49.4X3	T49.4X4	T49.4X5	T49.4X6
Trichloroethane	T53.2X1	T53.2X2	T53.2X3	T53.2X4	—	—
Trichloroethanol	T42.6X1	T42.6X2	T42.6X3	T42.6X4	T42.6X5	T42.6X6
Trichloroethylene (liquid) (vapor)	T53.2X1	T53.2X2	T53.2X3	T53.2X4	—	—
anesthetic (gas)	T41.0X1	T41.0X2	T41.0X3	T41.0X4	T41.0X5	T41.0X6
vapor NEC	T53.2X1	T53.2X2	T53.2X3	T53.2X4	—	—
Trichloroethyl phosphate	T42.6X1	T42.6X2	T42.6X3	T42.6X4	T42.6X5	T42.6X6
Trichlorofluoromethane NEC	T53.5X1	T53.5X2	T53.5X3	T53.5X4	—	—
Trichloronate	T60.0X1	T60.0X2	T60.0X3	T60.0X4	—	—
Trichloropropane	T53.6X1	T53.6X2	T53.6X3	T53.6X4	—	—
Trichlorotriethylamine	T45.1X1	T45.1X2	T45.1X3	T45.1X4	T45.1X5	T45.1X6
Trichomonacides NEC	T37.3X1	T37.3X2	T37.3X3	T37.3X4	T37.3X5	T37.3X6
Trichomycin	T36.7X1	T36.7X2	T36.7X3	T36.7X4	T36.7X5	T36.7X6
Triclobisonium chloride	T49.0X1	T49.0X2	T49.0X3	T49.0X4	T49.0X5	T49.0X6
Triclocarban	T49.0X1	T49.0X2	T49.0X3	T49.0X4	T49.0X5	T49.0X6
Triclofos	T42.6X1	T42.6X2	T42.6X3	T42.6X4	T42.6X5	T42.6X6
Triclosan	T49.0X1	T49.0X2	T49.0X3	T49.0X4	T49.0X5	T49.0X6
Tricresyl phosphate	T65.891	T65.892	T65.893	T65.894	—	—
solvent	T52.91	T52.92	T52.93	T52.94	—	—
Tricyclamol chloride	T44.3X1	T44.3X2	T44.3X3	T44.3X4	T44.3X5	T44.3X6
Tridesilon	T49.0X1	T49.0X2	T49.0X3	T49.0X4	T49.0X5	T49.0X6
Tridihexethyl iodide	T44.3X1	T44.3X2	T44.3X3	T44.3X4	T44.3X5	T44.3X6
Tridione	T42.2X1	T42.2X2	T42.2X3	T42.2X4	T42.2X5	T42.2X6
Trientine	T45.8X1	T45.8X2	T45.8X3	T45.8X4	T45.8X5	T45.8X6
Triethanolamine NEC	T54.3X1	T54.3X2	T54.3X3	T54.3X4	—	—
detergent	T54.3X1	T54.3X2	T54.3X3	T54.3X4	—	—
trinitrate (biphosphate)	T46.3X1	T46.3X2	T46.3X3	T46.3X4	T46.3X5	T46.3X6
Triethanomelamine	T45.1X1	T45.1X2	T45.1X3	T45.1X4	T45.1X5	T45.1X6
Triethylenemelamine	T45.1X1	T45.1X2	T45.1X3	T45.1X4	T45.1X5	T45.1X6
Triethylenephosphoramide	T45.1X1	T45.1X2	T45.1X3	T45.1X4	T45.1X5	T45.1X6
Triethylenethiophosphoramide	T45.1X1	T45.1X2	T45.1X3	T45.1X4	T45.1X5	T45.1X6
Trifluoperazine	T43.3X1	T43.3X2	T43.3X3	T43.3X4	T43.3X5	T43.3X6
Trifluoroethyl vinyl ether	T41.0X1	T41.0X2	T41.0X3	T41.0X4	T41.0X5	T41.0X6
Trifluperidol	T43.4X1	T43.4X2	T43.4X3	T43.4X4	T43.4X5	T43.4X6
Triflupromazine	T43.3X1	T43.3X2	T43.3X3	T43.3X4	T43.3X5	T43.3X6
Trifluridine	T37.5X1	T37.5X2	T37.5X3	T37.5X4	T37.5X5	T37.5X6
Triflusal	T45.521	T45.522	T45.523	T45.524	T45.525	T45.526
Trihexyphenidyl	T44.3X1	T44.3X2	T44.3X3	T44.3X4	T44.3X5	T44.3X6
Triiodothyronine	T38.1X1	T38.1X2	T38.1X3	T38.1X4	T38.1X5	T38.1X6
Trilene	T41.0X1	T41.0X2	T41.0X3	T41.0X4	T41.0X5	T41.0X6
Trilostane	T38.991	T38.992	T38.993	T38.994	T38.995	T38.996
Trimebutine	T44.3X1	T44.3X2	T44.3X3	T44.3X4	T44.3X5	T44.3X6
Trimecaine	T41.3X1	T41.3X2	T41.3X3	T41.3X4	T41.3X5	T41.3X6
Trimeprazine (tartrate)	T44.3X1	T44.3X2	T44.3X3	T44.3X4	T44.3X5	T44.3X6
Trimetaphan camsilate	T44.2X1	T44.2X2	T44.2X3	T44.2X4	T44.2X5	T44.2X6
Trimetazidine	T46.7X1	T46.7X2	T46.7X3	T46.7X4	T46.7X5	T46.7X6
Trimethadione	T42.2X1	T42.2X2	T42.2X3	T42.2X4	T42.2X5	T42.2X6
Trimethaphan	T44.2X1	T44.2X2	T44.2X3	T44.2X4	T44.2X5	T44.2X6
Trimethidinium	T44.2X1	T44.2X2	T44.2X3	T44.2X4	T44.2X5	T44.2X6
Trimethobenzamide	T45.0X1	T45.0X2	T45.0X3	T45.0X4	T45.0X5	T45.0X6
Trimethoprim	T37.8X1	T37.8X2	T37.8X3	T37.8X4	T37.8X5	T37.8X6
with sulfamethoxazole	T36.8X1	T36.8X2	T36.8X3	T36.8X4	T36.8X5	T36.8X6
Trimethylcarbinol	T51.3X1	T51.3X2	T51.3X3	T51.3X4	—	—
Trimethylpsoralen	T49.3X1	T49.3X2	T49.3X3	T49.3X4	T49.3X5	T49.3X6
Trimeton	T45.0X1	T45.0X2	T45.0X3	T45.0X4	T45.0X5	T45.0X6
Trimetrexate	T45.1X1	T45.1X2	T45.1X3	T45.1X4	T45.1X5	T45.1X6
Trimipramine	T43.011	T43.012	T43.013	T43.014	T43.015	T43.016
Trimustine	T45.1X1	T45.1X2	T45.1X3	T45.1X4	T45.1X5	T45.1X6
Trinitrine	T46.3X1	T46.3X2	T46.3X3	T46.3X4	T46.3X5	T46.3X6
Trinitrobenzol	T65.3X1	T65.3X2	T65.3X3	T65.3X4	—	—
Trinitrophenol	T65.3X1	T65.3X2	T65.3X3	T65.3X4	—	—
Trinitrotoluene (fumes)	T65.3X1	T65.3X2	T65.3X3	T65.3X4	—	—
Trional	T42.6X1	T42.6X2	T42.6X3	T42.6X4	T42.6X5	T42.6X6
Triorthocresyl phosphate	T65.891	T65.892	T65.893	T65.894	—	—
Trioxide of arsenic	T57.0X1	T57.0X2	T57.0X3	T57.0X4	—	—
Trioxysalen	T49.4X1	T49.4X2	T49.4X3	T49.4X4	T49.4X5	T49.4X6
Tripamide	T50.2X1	T50.2X2	T50.2X3	T50.2X4	T50.2X5	T50.2X6
Triparanol	T46.6X1	T46.6X2	T46.6X3	T46.6X4	T46.6X5	T46.6X6
Tripelennamine	T45.0X1	T45.0X2	T45.0X3	T45.0X4	T45.0X5	T45.0X6
Triperiden	T44.3X1	T44.3X2	T44.3X3	T44.3X4	T44.3X5	T44.3X6
Triperidol	T43.4X1	T43.4X2	T43.4X3	T43.4X4	T43.4X5	T43.4X6
Triphenylphosphate	T65.891	T65.892	T65.893	T65.894	—	—
Triple						
bromides	T42.6X1	T42.6X2	T42.6X3	T42.6X4	T42.6X5	T42.6X6
carbonate	T47.1X1	T47.1X2	T47.1X3	T47.1X4	T47.1X5	T47.1X6
vaccine						
DPT	T50.A11	T50.A12	T50.A13	T50.A14	T50.A15	T50.A16
including pertussis	T50.A11	T50.A12	T50.A13	T50.A14	T50.A15	T50.A16
MMR	T50.B91	T50.B92	T50.B93	T50.B94	T50.B95	T50.B96
Triprolidine	T45.0X1	T45.0X2	T45.0X3	T45.0X4	T45.0X5	T45.0X6
Trisodium hydrogen edetate	T50.6X1	T50.6X2	T50.6X3	T50.6X4	T50.6X5	T50.6X6
Trisoralen	T49.3X1	T49.3X2	T49.3X3	T49.3X4	T49.3X5	T49.3X6
Trisulfapyrimidines	T37.0X1	T37.0X2	T37.0X3	T37.0X4	T37.0X5	T37.0X6
Trithiozine	T44.3X1	T44.3X2	T44.3X3	T44.3X4	T44.3X5	T44.3X6
Tritiozine	T44.3X1	T44.3X2	T44.3X3	T44.3X4	T44.3X5	T44.3X6
Tritoqualine	T45.0X1	T45.0X2	T45.0X3	T45.0X4	T45.0X5	T45.0X6
Trofosfamide	T45.1X1	T45.1X2	T45.1X3	T45.1X4	T45.1X5	T45.1X6
Troleandomycin	T36.3X1	T36.3X2	T36.3X3	T36.3X4	T36.3X5	T36.3X6
Trolnitrate (phosphate)	T46.3X1	T46.3X2	T46.3X3	T46.3X4	T46.3X5	T46.3X6
Tromantadine	T37.5X1	T37.5X2	T37.5X3	T37.5X4	T37.5X5	T37.5X6
Trometamol	T50.2X1	T50.2X2	T50.2X3	T50.2X4	T50.2X5	T50.2X6
Tromethamine	T50.2X1	T50.2X2	T50.2X3	T50.2X4	T50.2X5	T50.2X6
Tronothane	T41.3X1	T41.3X2	T41.3X3	T41.3X4	T41.3X5	T41.3X6
Tropacine	T44.3X1	T44.3X2	T44.3X3	T44.3X4	T44.3X5	T44.3X6
Tropatepine	T44.3X1	T44.3X2	T44.3X3	T44.3X4	T44.3X5	T44.3X6
Tropicamide	T44.3X1	T44.3X2	T44.3X3	T44.3X4	T44.3X5	T44.3X6
Trospium chloride	T44.3X1	T44.3X2	T44.3X3	T44.3X4	T44.3X5	T44.3X6
Troxerutin	T46.991	T46.992	T46.993	T46.994	T46.995	T46.996
Troxidone	T42.2X1	T42.2X2	T42.2X3	T42.2X4	T42.2X5	T42.2X6
Tryparsamide	T37.3X1	T37.3X2	T37.3X3	T37.3X4	T37.3X5	T37.3X6
Trypsin	T45.3X1	T45.3X2	T45.3X3	T45.3X4	T45.3X5	T45.3X6
Tryptizol	T43.011	T43.012	T43.013	T43.014	T43.015	T43.016
TSH	T38.811	T38.812	T38.813	T38.814	T38.815	T38.816
Tuaminoheptane	T48.5X1	T48.5X2	T48.5X3	T48.5X4	T48.5X5	T48.5X6
Tuberculin, purified protein derivative (PPD)	T50.8X1	T50.8X2	T50.8X3	T50.8X4	T50.8X5	T50.8X6
Tubocurare	T48.1X1	T48.1X2	T48.1X3	T48.1X4	T48.1X5	T48.1X6
Tubocurarine (chloride)	T48.1X1	T48.1X2	T48.1X3	T48.1X4	T48.1X5	T48.1X6
Tulobuterol	T48.6X1	T48.6X2	T48.6X3	T48.6X4	T48.6X5	T48.6X6
Turpentine (spirits of)	T52.8X1	T52.8X2	T52.8X3	T52.8X4	—	—
vapor	T52.8X1	T52.8X2	T52.8X3	T52.8X4	—	—
Tybamate	T43.591	T43.592	T43.593	T43.594	T43.595	T43.596
Tyloxapol	T48.4X1	T48.4X2	T48.4X3	T48.4X4	T48.4X5	T48.4X6
Tymazoline	T48.5X1	T48.5X2	T48.5X3	T48.5X4	T48.5X5	T48.5X6
Typhoid-paratyphoid vaccine	T50.A91	T50.A92	T50.A93	T50.A94	T50.A95	T50.A96
Typhus vaccine	T50.A91	T50.A92	T50.A93	T50.A94	T50.A95	T50.A96
Tyropanoate	T50.8X1	T50.8X2	T50.8X3	T50.8X4	T50.8X5	T50.8X6
Tyrothricin	T49.6X1	T49.6X2	T49.6X3	T49.6X4	T49.6X5	T49.6X6
ENT agent	T49.6X1	T49.6X2	T49.6X3	T49.6X4	T49.6X5	T49.6X6
ophthalmic preparation	T49.5X1	T49.5X2	T49.5X3	T49.5X4	T49.5X5	T49.5X6

▽ **Subterms under main terms may continue to next column or page**   **Additional Character May Be Required — Refer to the Tabular List for Character Selection**

Table of Drugs and Chemicals

Substance	Poisoning, Accidental (unintentional)	Poisoning, Intentional Self-harm	Poisoning, Assault	Poisoning, Undetermined	Adverse Effect	Under-dosing
Ufenamate	T39.391	T39.392	T39.393	T39.394	T39.395	T39.396
Ultraviolet light	T49.3X1	T49.3X2	T49.3X3	T49.3X4	T49.3X5	T49.3X6
protectant						
Undecenoic acid	T49.0X1	T49.0X2	T49.0X3	T49.0X4	T49.0X5	T49.0X6
Undecoylium	T49.0X1	T49.0X2	T49.0X3	T49.0X4	T49.0X5	T49.0X6
Undecylenic acid	T49.0X1	T49.0X2	T49.0X3	T49.0X4	T49.0X5	T49.0X6
(derivatives)						
Unna's boot	T49.3X1	T49.3X2	T49.3X3	T49.3X4	T49.3X5	T49.3X6
Unsaturated fatty acid	T46.6X1	T46.6X2	T46.6X3	T46.6X4	T46.6X5	T46.6X6
Uracil mustard	T45.1X1	T45.1X2	T45.1X3	T45.1X4	T45.1X5	T45.1X6
Uramustine	T45.1X1	T45.1X2	T45.1X3	T45.1X4	T45.1X5	T45.1X6
Urapidil	T46.5X1	T46.5X2	T46.5X3	T46.5X4	T46.5X5	T46.5X6
Urari	T48.1X1	T48.1X2	T48.1X3	T48.1X4	T48.1X5	T48.1X6
Urate oxidase	T50.4X1	T50.4X2	T50.4X3	T50.4X4	T50.4X5	T50.4X6
Urea	T47.3X1	T47.3X2	T47.3X3	T47.3X4	T47.3X5	T47.3X6
peroxide	T49.0X1	T49.0X2	T49.0X3	T49.0X4	T49.0X5	T49.0X6
stibamine	T37.4X1	T37.4X2	T37.4X3	T37.4X4	T37.4X5	T37.4X6
topical	T49.8X1	T49.8X2	T49.8X3	T49.8X4	T49.8X5	T49.8X6
Urethane	T45.1X1	T45.1X2	T45.1X3	T45.1X4	T45.1X5	T45.1X6
Urginea (maritima) (scilla) — see Squill						
Uric acid metabolism drug NEC	T50.4X1	T50.4X2	T50.4X3	T50.4X4	T50.4X5	T50.4X6
Uricosuric agent	T50.4X1	T50.4X2	T50.4X3	T50.4X4	T50.4X5	T50.4X6
Urinary anti-infective	T37.8X1	T37.8X2	T37.8X3	T37.8X4	T37.8X5	T37.8X6
Urofollitropin	T38.812	T38.813	T38.813	T38.814	T38.815	T38.816
Urokinase	T45.611	T45.612	T45.613	T45.614	T45.615	T45.616
Urokon	T50.8X1	T50.8X2	T50.8X3	T50.8X4	T50.8X5	T50.8X6
Ursodeoxycholic acid	T50.991	T50.992	T50.993	T50.994	T50.995	T50.996
Ursodiol	T50.991	T50.992	T50.993	T50.994	T50.995	T50.996
Urtica	T62.2X1	T62.2X2	T62.2X3	T62.2X4	—	—
Utility gas — see Gas, utility						
Vaccine NEC	T50.Z91	T50.Z92	T50.Z93	T50.Z94	T50.Z95	T50.Z96
antineoplastic	T50.Z91	T50.Z92	T50.Z93	T50.Z94	T50.Z95	T50.Z96
bacterial NEC	T50.A91	T50.A92	T50.A93	T50.A94	T50.A95	T50.A96
with						
other bacterial component	T50.A21	T50.A22	T50.A23	T50.A24	T50.A25	T50.A26
pertussis component	T50.A11	T50.A12	T50.A13	T50.A14	T50.A15	T50.A16
viral-rickettsial component	T50.A21	T50.A22	T50.A23	T50.A24	T50.A25	T50.A26
mixed NEC	T50.A21	T50.A22	T50.A23	T50.A24	T50.A25	T50.A26
BCG	T50.A91	T50.A92	T50.A93	T50.A94	T50.A95	T50.A96
cholera	T50.A91	T50.A92	T50.A93	T50.A94	T50.A95	T50.A96
diphtheria	T50.A91	T50.A92	T50.A93	T50.A94	T50.A95	T50.A96
with tetanus	T50.A21	T50.A22	T50.A23	T50.A24	T50.A25	T50.A26
and pertussis	T50.A11	T50.A12	T50.A13	T50.A14	T50.A15	T50.A16
influenza	T50.B91	T50.B92	T50.B93	T50.B94	T50.B95	T50.B96
measles	T50.B91	T50.B92	T50.B93	T50.B94	T50.B95	T50.B96
with mumps and rubella	T50.B91	T50.B92	T50.B93	T50.B94	T50.B95	T50.B96
meningococcal	T50.A91	T50.A92	T50.A93	T50.A94	T50.A95	T50.A96
mumps	T50.B91	T50.B92	T50.B93	T50.B94	T50.B95	T50.B96
paratyphoid	T50.A91	T50.A92	T50.A93	T50.A94	T50.A95	T50.A96
pertussis	T50.A11	T50.A12	T50.A13	T50.A14	T50.A15	T50.A16
with diphtheria	T50.A11	T50.A12	T50.A13	T50.A14	T50.A15	T50.A16
and tetanus	T50.A11	T50.A12	T50.A13	T50.A14	T50.A15	T50.A16
with other component	T50.A11	T50.A12	T50.A13	T50.A14	T50.A15	T50.A16
plague	T50.A91	T50.A92	T50.A93	T50.A94	T50.A95	T50.A96
poliomyelitis	T50.B91	T50.B92	T50.B93	T50.B94	T50.B95	T50.B96
poliovirus	T50.B91	T50.B92	T50.B93	T50.B94	T50.B95	T50.B96
rabies	T50.B91	T50.B92	T50.B93	T50.B94	T50.B95	T50.B96
respiratory syncytial virus	T50.B91	T50.B92	T50.B93	T50.B94	T50.B95	T50.B96
rickettsial NEC	T50.A91	T50.A92	T50.A93	T50.A94	T50.A95	T50.A96
with						
bacterial component	T50.A21	T50.A22	T50.A23	T50.A24	T50.A25	T50.A26
Rocky Mountain spotted fever	T50.A91	T50.A92	T50.A93	T50.A94	T50.A95	T50.A96
rubella	T50.B91	T50.B92	T50.B93	T50.B94	T50.B95	T50.B96
sabin oral	T50.B91	T50.B92	T50.B93	T50.B94	T50.B95	T50.B96
smallpox	T50.B11	T50.B12	T50.B13	T50.B14	T50.B15	T50.B16
TAB	T50.A91	T50.A92	T50.A93	T50.A94	T50.A95	T50.A96
tetanus	T50.A91	T50.A92	T50.A93	T50.A94	T50.A95	T50.A96
typhoid	T50.A91	T50.A92	T50.A93	T50.A94	T50.A95	T50.A96
typhus	T50.A91	T50.A92	T50.A93	T50.A94	T50.A95	T50.A96
viral NEC	T50.B91	T50.B92	T50.B93	T50.B94	T50.B95	T50.B96
yellow fever	T50.B91	T50.B92	T50.B93	T50.B94	T50.B95	T50.B96
Vaccinia immune globulin	T50.Z11	T50.Z12	T50.Z13	T50.Z14	T50.Z15	T50.Z16
Vaginal contraceptives	T49.8X1	T49.8X2	T49.8X3	T49.8X4	T49.8X5	T49.8X6
Valerian						
root	T42.6X1	T42.6X2	T42.6X3	T42.6X4	T42.6X5	T42.6X6
tincture	T42.6X1	T42.6X2	T42.6X3	T42.6X4	T42.6X5	T42.6X6
Valethamate bromide	T44.3X1	T44.3X2	T44.3X3	T44.3X4	T44.3X5	T44.3X6
Valisone	T49.0X1	T49.0X2	T49.0X3	T49.0X4	T49.0X5	T49.0X6

Substance	Poisoning, Accidental (unintentional)	Poisoning, Intentional Self-harm	Poisoning, Assault	Poisoning, Undetermined	Adverse Effect	Under-dosing
Valium	T42.4X1	T42.4X2	T42.4X3	T42.4X4	T42.4X5	T42.4X6
Valmid	T42.6X1	T42.6X2	T42.6X3	T42.6X4	T42.6X5	T42.6X6
Valnoctamide	T42.6X1	T42.6X2	T42.6X3	T42.6X4	T42.6X5	T42.6X6
Valproate (sodium)	T42.6X1	T42.6X2	T42.6X3	T42.6X4	T42.6X5	T42.6X6
Valproic acid	T42.6X1	T42.6X2	T42.6X3	T42.6X4	T42.6X5	T42.6X6
Valpromide	T42.6X1	T42.6X2	T42.6X3	T42.6X4	T42.6X5	T42.6X6
Vanadium	T56.891	T56.892	T56.893	T56.894	—	—
Vancomycin	T36.8X1	T36.8X2	T36.8X3	T36.8X4	T36.8X5	T36.8X6
Vapor — see also Gas	T59.91	T59.92	T59.93	T59.94	—	—
kiln (carbon monoxide)	T58.8X1	T58.8X2	T58.8X3	T58.8X4		
lead — see lead						
specified source NEC	T59.891	T59.892	T59.893	T59.894		
Vardenafil	T46.7X1	T46.7X2	T46.7X3	T46.7X4	T46.7X5	T46.7X6
Varicose reduction drug	T46.8X1	T46.8X2	T46.8X3	T46.8X4	T46.8X5	T46.8X6
Varnish	T65.4X1	T65.4X2	T65.4X3	T65.4X4	—	—
cleaner	T52.91	T52.92	T52.93	T52.94	—	—
Vaseline	T49.3X1	T49.3X2	T49.3X3	T49.3X4	T49.3X5	T49.3X6
Vasodilan	T46.7X1	T46.7X2	T46.7X3	T46.7X4	T46.7X5	T46.7X6
Vasodilator						
coronary NEC	T46.3X1	T46.3X2	T46.3X3	T46.3X4	T46.3X5	T46.3X6
peripheral NEC	T46.7X1	T46.7X2	T46.7X3	T46.7X4	T46.7X5	T46.7X6
Vasopressin	T38.891	T38.892	T38.893	T38.894	T38.895	T38.896
Vasopressor drugs	T38.891	T38.892	T38.893	T38.894	T38.895	T38.896
Vecuronium bromide	T48.1X1	T48.1X2	T48.1X3	T48.1X4	T48.1X5	T48.1X6
Vegetable extract, astringent	T49.2X1	T49.2X2	T49.2X3	T49.2X4	T49.2X5	T49.2X6
Venlafaxine	T43.211	T43.212	T43.213	T43.214	T43.215	T43.216
Venom, venomous (bite) (sting)	T63.91	T63.92	T63.93	T63.94	—	—
amphibian NEC	T63.831	T63.832	T63.833	T63.834	—	—
animal NEC	T63.891	T63.892	T63.893	T63.894	—	—
ant	T63.421	T63.422	T63.423	T63.424	—	—
arthropod NEC	T63.481	T63.482	T63.483	T63.484	—	—
bee	T63.441	T63.442	T63.443	T63.444	—	—
centipede	T63.411	T63.412	T63.413	T63.414	—	—
fish	T63.591	T63.592	T63.593	T63.594	—	—
frog	T63.811	T63.812	T63.813	T63.814	—	—
hornet	T63.451	T63.452	T63.453	T63.454	—	—
insect NEC	T63.481	T63.482	T63.483	T63.484	—	—
lizard	T63.121	T63.122	T63.123	T63.124	—	—
marine						
animals	T63.691	T63.692	T63.693	T63.694	—	—
bluebottle	T63.611	T63.612	T63.613	T63.614	—	—
jellyfish NEC	T63.621	T63.622	T63.623	T63.624	—	—
Portugese Man-o-war	T63.611	T63.612	T63.613	T63.614	—	—
sea anemone	T63.631	T63.632	T63.633	T63.634	—	—
specified NEC	T63.691	T63.692	T63.693	T63.694	—	—
fish	T63.591	T63.592	T63.593	T63.594	—	—
plants	T63.711	T63.712	T63.713	T63.714	—	—
sting ray	T63.511	T63.512	T63.513	T63.514	—	—
millipede (tropical)	T63.411	T63.412	T63.413	T63.414	—	—
plant NEC	T63.791	T63.792	T63.793	T63.794	—	—
marine	T63.711	T63.712	T63.713	T63.714	—	—
reptile	T63.191	T63.192	T63.193	T63.194	—	—
gila monster	T63.111	T63.112	T63.113	T63.114	—	—
lizard NEC	T63.121	T63.122	T63.123	T63.124	—	—
scorpion	T63.2X1	T63.2X2	T63.2X3	T63.2X4	—	—
snake	T63.001	T63.002	T63.003	T63.004	—	—
African NEC	T63.081	T63.082	T63.083	T63.084	—	—
American (North) (South) NEC	T63.061	T63.062	T63.063	T63.064	—	—
Asian	T63.081	T63.082	T63.083	T63.084	—	—
Australian	T63.071	T63.072	T63.073	T63.074	—	—
cobra	T63.041	T63.042	T63.043	T63.044	—	—
coral snake	T63.021	T63.022	T63.023	T63.024	—	—
rattlesnake	T63.011	T63.012	T63.013	T63.014	—	—
specified NEC	T63.091	T63.092	T63.093	T63.094	—	—
taipan	T63.031	T63.032	T63.033	T63.034	—	—
specified NEC	T63.891	T63.892	T63.893	T63.894	—	—
spider	T63.301	T63.302	T63.303	T63.304	—	—
black widow	T63.311	T63.312	T63.313	T63.314	—	—
brown recluse	T63.331	T63.332	T63.333	T63.334	—	—
specified NEC	T63.391	T63.392	T63.393	T63.394	—	—
tarantula	T63.321	T63.322	T63.323	T63.324	—	—
sting ray	T63.511	T63.512	T63.513	T63.514	—	—
toad	T63.821	T63.822	T63.823	T63.824	—	—
wasp	T63.461	T63.462	T63.463	T63.464	—	—
Venous sclerosing drug NEC	T46.8X1	T46.8X2	T46.8X3	T46.8X4	T46.8X5	T46.8X6
Ventolin — see Albuterol						
Veramon	T42.3X1	T42.3X2	T42.3X3	T42.3X4	T42.3X5	T42.3X6
Verapamil	T46.1X1	T46.1X2	T46.1X3	T46.1X4	T46.1X5	T46.1X6
Veratrine	T46.5X1	T46.5X2	T46.5X3	T46.5X4	T46.5X5	T46.5X6

Substance	Poisoning, Accidental (unintentional)	Poisoning, Intentional Self-harm	Poisoning, Assault	Poisoning, Undetermined	Adverse Effect	Under-dosing
Veratrum						
album	T62.2X1	T62.2X2	T62.2X3	T62.2X4	—	—
alkaloids	T46.5X1	T46.5X2	T46.5X3	T46.5X4	T46.5X5	T46.5X6
viride	T62.2X1	T62.2X2	T62.2X3	T62.2X4	—	—
Verdigris	T60.3X1	T60.3X2	T60.3X3	T60.3X4		
Veronal	T42.3X1	T42.3X2	T42.3X3	T42.3X4	T42.3X5	T42.3X6
Veroxil	T37.4X1	T37.4X2	T37.4X3	T37.4X4	T37.4X5	T37.4X6
Versenate	T50.6X1	T50.6X2	T50.6X3	T50.6X4	T50.6X5	T50.6X6
Versidyne	T39.8X1	T39.8X2	T39.8X3	T39.8X4	T39.8X5	T39.8X6
Vetrabutine	T48.0X1	T48.0X2	T48.0X3	T48.0X4	T48.0X5	T48.0X6
Vidarabine	T37.5X1	T37.5X2	T37.5X3	T37.5X4	T37.5X5	T37.5X6
Vienna						
green	T57.0X1	T57.0X2	T57.0X3	T57.0X4	—	—
insecticide	T60.2X1	T60.2X2	T60.2X3	T60.2X4	—	—
red	T57.0X1	T57.0X2	T57.0X3	T57.0X4	—	—
pharmaceutical dye	T50.991	T50.992	T50.993	T50.994	T50.995	T50.996
Vigabatrin	T42.6X1	T42.6X2	T42.6X3	T42.6X4	T42.6X5	T42.6X6
Viloxazine	T43.291	T43.292	T43.293	T43.294	T43.295	T43.296
Viminol	T39.8X1	T39.8X2	T39.8X3	T39.8X4	T39.8X5	T39.8X6
Vinbarbital, vinbarbitone	T42.3X1	T42.3X2	T42.3X3	T42.3X4	T42.3X5	T42.3X6
Vinblastine	T45.1X1	T45.1X2	T45.1X3	T45.1X4	T45.1X5	T45.1X6
Vinburnine	T46.7X1	T46.7X2	T46.7X3	T46.7X4	T46.7X5	T46.7X6
Vincamine	T45.1X1	T45.1X2	T45.1X3	T45.1X4	T45.1X5	T45.1X6
Vincristine	T45.1X1	T45.1X2	T45.1X3	T45.1X4	T45.1X5	T45.1X6
Vindesine	T45.1X1	T45.1X2	T45.1X3	T45.1X4	T45.1X5	T45.1X6
Vinesthene, vinethene	T41.0X1	T41.0X2	T41.0X3	T41.0X4	T41.0X5	T41.0X6
Vinorelbine tartrate	T45.1X1	T45.1X2	T45.1X3	T45.1X4	T45.1X5	T45.1X6
Vinpocetine	T46.7X1	T46.7X2	T46.7X3	T46.7X4	T46.7X5	T46.7X6
Vinyl						
acetate	T65.891	T65.892	T65.893	T65.894	—	—
bital	T42.3X1	T42.3X2	T42.3X3	T42.3X4	T42.3X5	T42.3X6
bromide	T65.891	T65.892	T65.893	T65.894	—	—
chloride	T59.891	T59.892	T59.893	T59.894	—	—
ether	T41.0X1	T41.0X2	T41.0X3	T41.0X4	T41.0X5	T41.0X6
Vinylbital	T42.3X1	T42.3X2	T42.3X3	T42.3X4	T42.3X5	T42.3X6
Vinylidene chloride	T65.891	T65.892	T65.893	T65.894	—	—
Vioform	T37.8X1	T37.8X2	T37.8X3	T37.8X4	T37.8X5	T37.8X6
topical	T49.0X1	T49.0X2	T49.0X3	T49.0X4	T49.0X5	T49.0X6
Viomycin	T36.8X1	T36.8X2	T36.8X3	T36.8X4	T36.8X5	T36.8X6
Viosterol	T45.2X1	T45.2X2	T45.2X3	T45.2X4	T45.2X5	T45.2X6
Viper (venom)	T63.091	T63.092	T63.093	T63.094	—	—
Viprynium	T37.4X1	T37.4X2	T37.4X3	T37.4X4	T37.4X5	T37.4X6
Viquidil	T46.7X1	T46.7X2	T46.7X3	T46.7X4	T46.7X5	T46.7X6
Viral vaccine NEC	T50.B91	T50.B92	T50.B93	T50.B94	T50.B95	T50.B96
Virginiamycin	T36.8X1	T36.8X2	T36.8X3	T36.8X4	T36.8X5	T36.8X6
Virugon	T37.5X1	T37.5X2	T37.5X3	T37.5X4	T37.5X5	T37.5X6
Viscous agent	T50.901	T50.902	T50.903	T50.904	T50.905	T50.906
Visine	T49.5X1	T49.5X2	T49.5X3	T49.5X4	T49.5X5	T49.5X6
Visnadine	T46.3X1	T46.3X2	T46.3X3	T46.3X4	T46.3X5	T46.3X6
Vitamin NEC	T45.2X1	T45.2X2	T45.2X3	T45.2X4	T45.2X5	T45.2X6
A	T45.2X1	T45.2X2	T45.2X3	T45.2X4	T45.2X5	T45.2X6
B1	T45.2X1	T45.2X2	T45.2X3	T45.2X4	T45.2X5	T45.2X6
B2	T45.2X1	T45.2X2	T45.2X3	T45.2X4	T45.2X5	T45.2X6
B6	T45.2X1	T45.2X2	T45.2X3	T45.2X4	T45.2X5	T45.2X6
B12	T45.2X1	T45.2X2	T45.2X3	T45.2X4	T45.2X5	T45.2X6
B15	T45.2X1	T45.2X2	T45.2X3	T45.2X4	T45.2X5	T45.2X6
B NEC	T45.2X1	T45.2X2	T45.2X3	T45.2X4	T45.2X5	T45.2X6
nicotinic acid	T46.7X1	T46.7X2	T46.7X3	T46.7X4	T46.7X5	T46.7X6
C	T45.2X1	T45.2X2	T45.2X3	T45.2X4	T45.2X5	T45.2X6
D	T45.2X1	T45.2X2	T45.2X3	T45.2X4	T45.2X5	T45.2X6
D2	T45.2X1	T45.2X2	T45.2X3	T45.2X4	T45.2X5	T45.2X6
D3	T45.2X1	T45.2X2	T45.2X3	T45.2X4	T45.2X5	T45.2X6
E	T45.2X1	T45.2X2	T45.2X3	T45.2X4	T45.2X5	T45.2X6
E acetate	T45.2X1	T45.2X2	T45.2X3	T45.2X4	T45.2X5	T45.2X6
hematopoietic	T45.8X1	T45.8X2	T45.8X3	T45.8X4	T45.8X5	T45.8X6
K1	T45.7X1	T45.7X2	T45.7X3	T45.7X4	T45.7X5	T45.7X6
K2	T45.7X1	T45.7X2	T45.7X3	T45.7X4	T45.7X5	T45.7X6
K NEC	T45.7X1	T45.7X2	T45.7X3	T45.7X4	T45.7X5	T45.7X6
PP	T45.2X1	T45.2X2	T45.2X3	T45.2X4	T45.2X5	T45.2X6
ulceroprotectant	T47.1X1	T47.1X2	T47.1X3	T47.1X4	T47.1X5	T47.1X6
Vleminckx's solution	T49.4X1	T49.4X2	T49.4X3	T49.4X4	T49.4X5	T49.4X6
Voltaren — see Diclofenac						
Warfarin	T45.511	T45.512	T45.513	T45.514	T45.515	T45.516
rodenticide	T60.4X1-	T60.4X2-	T60.4X3-	T60.4X4-	—	—
sodium	T45.511	T45.512	T45.513	T45.514	T45.515	T45.516
Wasp (sting)	T63.461	T63.462	T63.463	T63.464	—	—
Water						
balance drug	T50.3X1	T50.3X2	T50.3X3	T50.3X4	T50.3X5	T50.3X6
distilled	T50.3X1	T50.3X2	T50.3X3	T50.3X4	T50.3X5	T50.3X6
gas — see Gas, water						

Substance	Poisoning, Accidental (unintentional)	Poisoning, Intentional Self-harm	Poisoning, Assault	Poisoning, Undetermined	Adverse Effect	Under-dosing
Water — continued						
gas — see Gas, water — continued						
incomplete combustion of — see Carbon, monoxide, fuel, utility						
hemlock	T62.2X1	T62.2X2	T62.2X3	T62.2X4	—	—
moccasin (venom)	T63.061	T63.062	T63.063	T63.064	—	—
purified	T50.3X1	T50.3X2	T50.3X3	T50.3X4	T50.3X5	T50.3X6
Wax (paraffin) (petroleum)	T52.0X1	T52.0X2	T52.0X3	T52.0X4	—	—
automobile	T65.891	T65.892	T65.893	T65.894	—	—
floor	T52.0X1	T52.0X2	T52.0X3	T52.0X4	—	—
Weed killers NEC	T60.3X1	T60.3X2	T60.3X3	T60.3X4	—	—
Welldorm	T42.6X1	T42.6X2	T42.6X3	T42.6X4	T42.6X5	T42.6X6
White						
arsenic	T57.0X1	T57.0X2	T57.0X3	T57.0X4	—	—
hellebore	T62.2X1	T62.2X2	T62.2X3	T62.2X4	—	—
lotion (keratolytic)	T49.4X1	T49.4X2	T49.4X3	T49.4X4	T49.4X5	T49.4X6
spirit	T52.0X1	T52.0X2	T52.0X3	T52.0X4	—	—
Whitewash	T65.891	T65.892	T65.893	T65.894	—	—
Whole blood (human)	T45.8X1	T45.8X2	T45.8X3	T45.8X4	T45.8X5	T45.8X6
Wild						
black cherry	T62.2X1	T62.2X2	T62.2X3	T62.2X4	—	—
poisonous plants NEC	T62.2X1	T62.2X2	T62.2X3	T62.2X4	—	—
Window cleaning fluid	T65.891	T65.892	T65.893	T65.894	—	—
Wintergreen (oil)	T49.3X1	T49.3X2	T49.3X3	T49.3X4	T49.3X5	T49.3X6
Wisterine	T62.2X1	T62.2X2	T62.2X3	T62.2X4	—	—
Witch hazel	T49.2X1	T49.2X2	T49.2X3	T49.2X4	T49.2X5	T49.2X6
Wood alcohol or spirit	T51.1X1	T51.1X2	T51.1X3	T51.1X4	—	—
Wool fat (hydrous)	T49.3X1	T49.3X2	T49.3X3	T49.3X4	T49.3X5	T49.3X6
Woorali	T48.1X1	T48.1X2	T48.1X3	T48.1X4	T48.1X5	T48.1X6
Wormseed, American	T37.4X1	T37.4X2	T37.4X3	T37.4X4	T37.4X5	T37.4X6
Xamoterol	T44.5X1	T44.5X2	T44.5X3	T44.5X4	T44.5X5	T44.5X6
Xanthine diuretics	T50.2X1	T50.2X2	T50.2X3	T50.2X4	T50.2X5	T50.2X6
Xanthinol nicotinate	T46.7X1	T46.7X2	T46.7X3	T46.7X4	T46.7X5	T46.7X6
Xanthotoxin	T49.3X1	T49.3X2	T49.3X3	T49.3X4	T49.3X5	T49.3X6
Xantinol nicotinate	T46.7X1	T46.7X2	T46.7X3	T46.7X4	T46.7X5	T46.7X6
Xantocillin	T36.0X1	T36.0X2	T36.0X3	T36.0X4	T36.0X5	T36.0X6
Xenon (127Xe) (133Xe)	T50.8X1	T50.8X2	T50.8X3	T50.8X4	T50.8X5	T50.8X6
Xenysalate	T49.4X1	T49.4X2	T49.4X3	T49.4X4	T49.4X5	T49.4X6
Xibornol	T37.8X1	T37.8X2	T37.8X3	T37.8X4	T37.8X5	T37.8X6
Xigris	T45.511	T45.512	T45.513	T45.514	T45.515	T45.516
Xipamide	T50.2X1	T50.2X2	T50.2X3	T50.2X4	T50.2X5	T50.2X6
Xylene (vapor)	T52.2X1	T52.2X2	T52.2X3	T52.2X4	—	—
Xylocaine (infiltration) (topical)	T41.3X1	T41.3X2	T41.3X3	T41.3X4	T41.3X5	T41.3X6
nerve block (peripheral) (plexus)	T41.3X1	T41.3X2	T41.3X3	T41.3X4	T41.3X5	T41.3X6
spinal	T41.3X1	T41.3X2	T41.3X3	T41.3X4	T41.3X5	T41.3X6
Xylol (vapor)	T52.2X1	T52.2X2	T52.2X3	T52.2X4	—	—
Xylometazoline	T48.5X1	T48.5X2	T48.5X3	T48.5X4	T48.5X5	T48.5X6
Yeast	T45.2X1	T45.2X2	T45.2X3	T45.2X4	T45.2X5	T45.2X6
dried	T45.2X1	T45.2X2	T45.2X3	T45.2X4	T45.2X5	T45.2X6
Yellow						
fever vaccine	T50.B91	T50.B92	T50.B93	T50.B94	T50.B95	T50.B96
jasmine	T62.2X1	T62.2X2	T62.2X3	T62.2X4	—	—
phenolphthalein	T47.2X1	T47.2X2	T47.2X3	T47.2X4	T47.2X5	T47.2X6
Yew	T62.2X1	T62.2X2	T62.2X3	T62.2X4	—	—
Yohimbic acid	T40.991	T40.992	T40.993	T40.994	T40.995	T40.996
Zactane	T39.8X1	T39.8X2	T39.8X3	T39.8X4	T39.8X5	T39.8X6
Zalcitabine	T37.5X1	T37.5X2	T37.5X3	T37.5X4	T37.5X5	T37.5X6
Zaroxolyn	T50.2X1	T50.2X2	T50.2X3	T50.2X4	T50.2X5	T50.2X6
Zephiran (topical)	T49.0X1	T49.0X2	T49.0X3	T49.0X4	T49.0X5	T49.0X6
ophthalmic preparation	T49.5X1	T49.5X2	T49.5X3	T49.5X4	T49.5X5	T49.5X6
Zeranol	T38.7X1	T38.7X2	T38.7X3	T38.7X4	T38.7X5	T38.7X6
Zerone	T51.1X1	T51.1X2	T51.1X3	T51.1X4	—	—
Zidovudine	T37.5X1	T37.5X2	T37.5X3	T37.5X4	T37.5X5	T37.5X6
Zimeldine	T43.221	T43.222	T43.223	T43.224	T43.225	T43.226
Zinc (compounds) (fumes) (vapor)	T56.5X1	T56.5X2	T56.5X3	T56.5X4	—	—
NEC						
anti-infectives	T49.0X1	T49.0X2	T49.0X3	T49.0X4	T49.0X5	T49.0X6
antivaricose	T46.8X1	T46.8X2	T46.8X3	T46.8X4	T46.8X5	T46.8X6
bacitracin	T49.0X1	T49.0X2	T49.0X3	T49.0X4	T49.0X5	T49.0X6
chloride (mouthwash)	T49.6X1	T49.6X2	T49.6X3	T49.6X4	T49.6X5	T49.6X6
chromate	T56.5X1	T56.5X2	T56.5X3	T56.5X4	—	—
gelatin	T49.3X1	T49.3X2	T49.3X3	T49.3X4	T49.3X5	T49.3X6
oxide	T49.3X1	T49.3X2	T49.3X3	T49.3X4	T49.3X5	T49.3X6
plaster	T49.3X1	T49.3X2	T49.3X3	T49.3X4	T49.3X5	T49.3X6
peroxide	T49.0X1	T49.0X2	T49.0X3	T49.0X4	T49.0X5	T49.0X6
pesticides	T56.5X1	T56.5X2	T56.5X3	T56.5X4	—	—
phosphide	T60.4X1	T60.4X2	T60.4X3	T60.4X4	—	—
pyrithionate	T49.4X1	T49.4X2	T49.4X3	T49.4X4	T49.4X5	T49.4X6
stearate	T49.3X1	T49.3X2	T49.3X3	T49.3X4	T49.3X5	T49.3X6

▽ Subterms under main terms may continue to next column or page   Additional Character May Be Required — Refer to the Tabular List for Character Selection   401

Veratrum — Zinc

Substance	Poisoning, Accidental (unintentional)	Poisoning, Intentional Self-harm	Poisoning, Assault	Poisoning, Undetermined	Adverse Effect	Under-dosing
Zinc (compounds) (fumes) (vapor) **NEC** — *continued*						
sulfate	T49.5X1	T49.5X2	T49.5X3	T49.5X4	T49.5X5	T49.5X6
ENT agent	T49.6X1	T49.6X2	T49.6X3	T49.6X4	T49.6X5	T49.6X6
ophthalmic solution	T49.5X1	T49.5X2	T49.5X3	T49.5X4	T49.5X5	T49.5X6
topical NEC	T49.0X1	T49.0X2	T49.0X3	T49.0X4	T49.0X5	T49.0X6
undecylenate	T49.0X1	T49.0X2	T49.0X3	T49.0X4	T49.0X5	T49.0X6
Zineb	T60.0X1	T60.0X2	T60.0X3	T60.0X4	—	—
Zinostatin	T45.1X1	T45.1X2	T45.1X3	T45.1X4	T45.1X5	T45.1X6
Zipeprol	T48.3X1	T48.3X2	T48.3X3	T48.3X4	T48.3X5	T48.3X6
Zofenopril	T46.4X1	T46.4X2	T46.4X3	T46.4X4	T46.4X5	T46.4X6
Zolpidem	T42.6X1	T42.6X2	T42.6X3	T42.6X4	T42.6X5	T42.6X6
Zomepirac	T39.391	T39.392	T39.393	T39.394	T39.395	T39.396
Zopiclone	T42.6X1	T42.6X2	T42.6X3	T42.6X4	T42.6X5	T42.6X6
Zorubicin	T45.1X1	T45.1X2	T45.1X3	T45.1X4	T45.1X5	T45.1X6
Zotepine	T43.591	T43.592	T43.593	T43.594	T43.595	T43.596
Zovant	T45.511	T45.512	T45.513	T45.514	T45.515	T45.516
Zoxazolamine	T42.8X1	T42.8X2	T42.8X3	T42.8X4	T42.8X5	T42.8X6
Zuclopenthixol	T43.4X1	T43.4X2	T43.4X3	T43.4X4	T43.4X5	T43.4X6
Zygadenus (venenosus)	T62.2X1	T62.2X2	T62.2X3	T62.2X4	—	—
Zyprexa	T43.591	T43.592	T43.593	T43.594	T43.595	T43.596

A

Abandonment (causing exposure to weather conditions) (with intent to injure or kill) NEC X58 ☑

Abuse (adult) (child) (mental) (physical) (sexual) X58 ☑

Accident (to) X58 ☑
  aircraft (in transit) (powered) — *see also* Accident, transport, aircraft
    due to, caused by cataclysm — *see* Forces of nature, by type
  animal-drawn vehicle — *see* Accident, transport, animal-drawn vehicle occupant
  animal-rider — *see* Accident, transport, animal-rider
  automobile — *see* Accident, transport, car occupant
  bare foot water skier V94.4 ☑
  boat, boating — *see also* Accident, watercraft
    striking swimmer
      powered V94.11 ☑
      unpowered V94.12 ☑
  bus — *see* Accident, transport, bus occupant
  cable car, not on rails V98.0 ☑
    on rails — *see* Accident, transport, streetcar occupant
  car — *see* Accident, transport, car occupant
  caused by, due to
    animal NEC W64 ☑
    chain hoist W24.0 ☑
    cold (excessive) — *see* Exposure, cold
    corrosive liquid, substance — *see* Table of Drugs and Chemicals
    cutting or piercing instrument — *see* Contact, with, by type of instrument
    drive belt W24.0 ☑
    electric
      current — *see* Exposure, electric current
      motor — *see also* Contact, with, by type of machine W31.3 ☑
      current (of) W86.8 ☑
    environmental factor NEC X58 ☑
    explosive material — *see* Explosion
    fire, flames — *see* Exposure, fire
    firearm missile — *see* Discharge, firearm by type
    heat (excessive) — *see* Heat
    hot — *see* Contact, with, hot
    ignition — *see* Ignition
    lifting device W24.0 ☑
    lightning — *see* subcategory T75.0 ☑
      causing fire — *see* Exposure, fire
    machine, machinery — *see* Contact, with, by type of machine
    natural factor NEC X58 ☑
    pulley (block) W24.0 ☑
    radiation — *see* Radiation
    steam X13.1 ☑
      inhalation X13.0 ☑
      pipe X16 ☑
    thunderbolt — *see* subcategory T75.0 ☑
      causing fire — *see* Exposure, fire
    transmission device W24.1 ☑
  coach — *see* Accident, transport, bus occupant
  coal car — *see* Accident, transport, industrial vehicle occupant
  diving — *see also* Fall, into, water
    with
      drowning or submersion — *see* Drowning
  forklift — *see* Accident, transport, industrial vehicle occupant
  heavy transport vehicle NOS — *see* Accident, transport, truck occupant
  ice yacht V98.2 ☑
  in
    medical, surgical procedure
      as, or due to misadventure — *see* Misadventure
      causing an abnormal reaction or later complication without mention of misadventure — *see also* Complication of or following, by type of procedure Y84.9
  land yacht V98.1 ☑
  late effect of — *see* W00-X58 with 7th character S
  logging car — *see* Accident, transport, industrial vehicle occupant
  machine, machinery — *see also* Contact, with, by type of machine
    on board watercraft V93.69 ☑
      explosion — *see* Explosion, in, watercraft

Accident — *continued*
  machine, machinery — *see also* Contact, with, by type of machine — *continued*
    on board watercraft — *continued*
      fire — *see* Burn, on board watercraft
      powered craft V93.63 ☑
        ferry boat V93.61 ☑
        fishing boat V93.62 ☑
        jetskis V93.63 ☑
        liner V93.61 ☑
        merchant ship V93.60 ☑
        passenger ship V93.61 ☑
        sailboat V93.64 ☑
  mine tram — *see* Accident, transport, industrial vehicle occupant
  mobility scooter (motorized) — *see* Accident, transport, pedestrian, conveyance, specified type NEC
  motor scooter — *see* Accident, transport, motorcyclist
  motor vehicle NOS (traffic) — *see also* Accident, transport V89.2 ☑
    nontraffic V89.0 ☑
    three-wheeled NOS — *see* Accident, transport, three-wheeled motor vehicle occupant
  motorcycle NOS — *see* Accident, transport, motorcyclist
  nonmotor vehicle NOS (nontraffic) — *see also* Accident, transport V89.1 ☑
    traffic NOS V89.3 ☑
  nontraffic (victim's mode of transport NOS) V88.9 ☑
    collision (between) V88.7 ☑
      bus and truck V88.5 ☑
      car and:
        bus V88.3 ☑
        pickup V88.2 ☑
        three-wheeled motor vehicle V88.0 ☑
        train V88.6 ☑
        truck V88.4 ☑
        two-wheeled motor vehicle V88.0 ☑
        van V88.2 ☑
      specified vehicle NEC and:
        three-wheeled motor vehicle V88.1 ☑
        two-wheeled motor vehicle V88.1 ☑
    known mode of transport — *see* Accident, transport, by type of vehicle
    noncollision V88.8 ☑
  on board watercraft V93.89 ☑
    powered craft V93.83 ☑
      ferry boat V93.81 ☑
      fishing boat V93.82 ☑
      jetskis V93.83 ☑
      liner V93.81 ☑
      merchant ship V93.80 ☑
      passenger ship V93.81 ☑
    unpowered craft V93.88 ☑
      canoe V93.85 ☑
      inflatable V93.86 ☑
      in tow
        recreational V94.31 ☑
        specified NEC V94.32 ☑
      kayak V93.85 ☑
      sailboat V93.84 ☑
      surf-board V93.88 ☑
      water skis V93.87 ☑
      windsurfer V93.88 ☑
  parachutist V97.29 ☑
    entangled in object V97.21 ☑
    injured on landing V97.22 ☑
  pedal cycle — *see* Accident, transport, pedal cyclist
  pedestrian (on foot)
    with
      another pedestrian W51 ☑
        on pedestrian conveyance NEC V00.09 ☑
      with fall W03 ☑
        due to ice or snow W00.0 ☑
      rider of
        hoverboard V00.038 ☑
        Segway V00.038 ☑
        standing
          electric scooter V00.031 ☑
          micro-mobility pedestrian conveyance NEC V00.038 ☑
      roller skater (in-line) V00.01 ☑
      skate boarder V00.02 ☑
      transport vehicle — *see* Accident, transport
    on pedestrian conveyance — *see* Accident, transport, pedestrian, conveyance

Accident — *continued*
  pick-up truck or van — *see* Accident, transport, pickup truck occupant
  quarry truck — *see* Accident, transport, industrial vehicle occupant
  railway vehicle (any) (in motion) — *see* Accident, transport, railway vehicle occupant
    due to cataclysm — *see* Forces of nature, by type
  scooter (non-motorized) — *see* Accident, transport, pedestrian, conveyance, scooter
  sequelae of — *see* categories W00-X58 with 7th character S
  skateboard — *see* Accident, transport, pedestrian, conveyance, skateboard
  ski(ing) — *see* Accident, transport, pedestrian, conveyance
    lift V98.3 ☑
  specified cause NEC X58 ☑
  streetcar — *see* Accident, transport, streetcar occupant
  traffic (victim's mode of transport NOS) V87.9 ☑
    collision (between) V87.7 ☑
      bus and truck V87.5 ☑
      car and:
        bus V87.3 ☑
        pickup V87.2 ☑
        three-wheeled motor vehicle V87.0 ☑
        train V87.6 ☑
        truck V87.4 ☑
        two-wheeled motor vehicle V87.0 ☑
        van V87.2 ☑
      specified vehicle NEC V86.39 ☑
      and
        three-wheeled motor vehicle V87.1 ☑
        two-wheeled motor vehicle V87.1 ☑
      driver V86.09 ☑
      passenger V86.19 ☑
      person on outside V86.29 ☑
      while boarding or alighting V86.49 ☑
    known mode of transport — *see* Accident, transport, by type of vehicle
    noncollision V87.8 ☑
  transport (involving injury to) V99
    18 wheeler — *see* Accident, transport, truck occupant
    agricultural vehicle occupant (nontraffic) V84.9 ☑
      driver V84.5 ☑
      hanger-on V84.7 ☑
      passenger V84.6 ☑
      traffic V84.3 ☑
        driver V84.0 ☑
        hanger-on V84.2 ☑
        passenger V84.1 ☑
      while boarding or alighting V84.4 ☑
    aircraft NEC V97.89 ☑
      military NEC V97.818 ☑
        civilian injured by V97.811 ☑
        with civilian aircraft V97.810 ☑
      occupant injured (in)
        nonpowered craft accident V96.9 ☑
          balloon V96.00 ☑
            collision V96.03 ☑
            crash V96.01 ☑
            explosion V96.05 ☑
            fire V96.04 ☑
            forced landing V96.02 ☑
            specified type NEC V96.09 ☑
          glider V96.20 ☑
            collision V96.23 ☑
            crash V96.21 ☑
            explosion V96.25 ☑
            fire V96.24 ☑
            forced landing V96.22 ☑
            specified type NEC V96.29 ☑
          hang glider V96.10 ☑
            collision V96.13 ☑
            crash V96.11 ☑
            explosion V96.15 ☑
            fire V96.14 ☑
            forced landing V96.12 ☑
            specified type NEC V96.19 ☑
          specified craft NEC V96.8 ☑
        powered craft accident V95.9 ☑
          fixed wing NEC
            commercial V95.30 ☑
              collision V95.33 ☑
              crash V95.31 ☑

Accident — *continued*
  transport — *continued*
    aircraft — *continued*
      occupant injured — *continued*
        powered craft accident — *continued*
          fixed wing — *continued*
            commercial — *continued*
              explosion V95.35 ☑
              fire V95.34 ☑
              forced landing V95.32 ☑
              specified type NEC V95.39 ☑
            private V95.20 ☑
              collision V95.23 ☑
              crash V95.21 ☑
              explosion V95.25 ☑
              fire V95.24 ☑
              forced landing V95.22 ☑
              specified type NEC V95.29 ☑
          glider V95.10 ☑
            collision V95.13 ☑
            crash V95.11 ☑
            explosion V95.15 ☑
            fire V95.14 ☑
            forced landing V95.12 ☑
            specified type NEC V95.19 ☑
          helicopter V95.00 ☑
            collision V95.03 ☑
            crash V95.01 ☑
            explosion V95.05 ☑
            fire V95.04 ☑
            forced landing V95.02 ☑
            specified type NEC V95.09 ☑
          spacecraft V95.40 ☑
            collision V95.43 ☑
            crash V95.41 ☑
            explosion V95.45 ☑
            fire V95.44 ☑
            forced landing V95.42 ☑
            specified type NEC V95.49 ☑
          specified craft NEC V95.8 ☑
         ultralight V95.10 ☑
            collision V95.13 ☑
            crash V95.11 ☑
            explosion V95.15 ☑
            fire V95.14 ☑
            forced landing V95.12 ☑
            specified type NEC V95.19 ☑
      specified accident NEC V97.0 ☑
      while boarding or alighting V97.1 ☑
    person (injured by)
      falling from, in or on aircraft V97.0 ☑
      machinery on aircraft V97.89 ☑
      on ground with aircraft involvement
        V97.39 ☑
      rotating propeller V97.32 ☑
      struck by object falling from aircraft V97.31 ☑
      sucked into aircraft jet V97.33 ☑
      while boarding or alighting aircraft V97.1 ☑
    airport (battery-powered) passenger vehicle — *see*
      Accident, transport, industrial vehicle occu-
      pant
    all-terrain vehicle occupant (nontraffic) V86.95 ☑
      driver V86.55 ☑
      dune buggy — *see* Accident, transport, dune
        buggy occupant
      hanger-on V86.75 ☑
      passenger V86.65 ☑
      snowmobile — *see* Accident, transport, snowmo-
        bile occupant
      specified type NEC V86.99 ☑
        driver V86.59 ☑
        passenger V86.69 ☑
        person on outside V86.79 ☑
      traffic V86.35 ☑
        driver V86.05 ☑
        hanger-on V86.25 ☑
        passenger V86.15 ☑
      while boarding or alighting V86.45 ☑
    ambulance occupant (traffic) V86.31 ☑
      driver V86.01 ☑
      hanger-on V86.21 ☑
      nontraffic V86.91 ☑
        driver V86.51 ☑
        hanger-on V86.71 ☑
        passenger V86.61 ☑
      passenger V86.11 ☑

Accident — *continued*
  transport — *continued*
    ambulance occupant — *continued*
      while boarding or alighting V86.41 ☑
    animal-drawn vehicle occupant (in) V80.929 ☑
      collision (with)
        animal V80.12 ☑
          being ridden V80.711 ☑
        animal-drawn vehicle V80.721 ☑
        bus V80.42 ☑
        car V80.42 ☑
        fixed or stationary object V80.82 ☑
        military vehicle V80.920 ☑
        nonmotor vehicle V80.791 ☑
        pedal cycle V80.22 ☑
        pedestrian V80.12 ☑
        pickup V80.42 ☑
        railway train or vehicle V80.62 ☑
        specified motor vehicle NEC V80.52 ☑
        streetcar V80.731 ☑
        truck V80.42 ☑
        two- or three-wheeled motor vehicle
          V80.32 ☑
        van V80.42 ☑
      noncollision V80.02 ☑
      specified circumstance NEC V80.928 ☑
    animal-rider V80.919 ☑
      collision (with)
        animal V80.11 ☑
          being ridden V80.710 ☑
        animal-drawn vehicle V80.720 ☑
        bus V80.41 ☑
        car V80.41 ☑
        fixed or stationary object V80.81 ☑
        military vehicle V80.910 ☑
        nonmotor vehicle V80.790 ☑
        pedal cycle V80.21 ☑
        pedestrian V80.11 ☑
        pickup V80.41 ☑
        railway train or vehicle V80.61 ☑
        specified motor vehicle NEC V80.51 ☑
        streetcar V80.730 ☑
        truck V80.41 ☑
        two- or three-wheeled motor vehicle
          V80.31 ☑
        van V80.41 ☑
      noncollision V80.018 ☑
        specified as horse rider V80.010 ☑
      specified circumstance NEC V80.918 ☑
    armored car — *see* Accident, transport, truck occu-
      pant
    battery-powered truck (baggage) (mail) — *see* Ac-
      cident, transport, industrial vehicle occupant
    bus occupant V79.9 ☑
      collision (with)
        animal (traffic) V70.9 ☑
          being ridden (traffic) V76.9 ☑
            nontraffic V76.3 ☑
            while boarding or alighting V76.4 ☑
          nontraffic V70.3 ☑
            while boarding or alighting V70.4 ☑
        animal-drawn vehicle (traffic) V76.9 ☑
          nontraffic V76.3 ☑
          while boarding or alighting V76.4 ☑
        bus (traffic) V74.9 ☑
          nontraffic V74.3 ☑
          while boarding or alighting V74.4 ☑
        car (traffic) V73.9 ☑
          nontraffic V73.3 ☑
          while boarding or alighting V73.4 ☑
        motor vehicle NOS (traffic) V79.60 ☑
          nontraffic V79.20 ☑
          specified type NEC (traffic) V79.69 ☑
            nontraffic V79.29 ☑
        pedal cycle (traffic) V71.9 ☑
          nontraffic V71.3 ☑
          while boarding or alighting V71.4 ☑
        pickup truck (traffic) V73.9 ☑
          nontraffic V73.3 ☑
          while boarding or alighting V73.4 ☑
        railway vehicle (traffic) V75.9 ☑
          nontraffic V75.3 ☑
          while boarding or alighting V75.4 ☑
        specified vehicle NEC (traffic) V76.9 ☑
          nontraffic V76.3 ☑
          while boarding or alighting V76.4 ☑

Accident — *continued*
  transport — *continued*
    bus occupant — *continued*
      collision — *continued*
        stationary object (traffic) V77.9 ☑
          nontraffic V77.3 ☑
          while boarding or alighting V77.4 ☑
        streetcar (traffic) V76.9 ☑
          nontraffic V76.3 ☑
          while boarding or alighting V76.4 ☑
        three wheeled motor vehicle (traffic) V72.9 ☑
          nontraffic V72.3 ☑
          while boarding or alighting V72.4 ☑
        truck (traffic) V74.9 ☑
          nontraffic V74.3 ☑
          while boarding or alighting V74.4 ☑
        two wheeled motor vehicle (traffic) V72.9 ☑
          nontraffic V72.3 ☑
          while boarding or alighting V72.4 ☑
        van (traffic) V73.9 ☑
          nontraffic V73.3 ☑
          while boarding or alighting V73.4 ☑
      driver
        collision (with)
          animal (traffic) V70.5 ☑
            being ridden (traffic) V76.5 ☑
              nontraffic V76.0 ☑
            nontraffic V70.0 ☑
          animal-drawn vehicle (traffic) V76.5 ☑
            nontraffic V76.0 ☑
          bus (traffic) V74.5 ☑
            nontraffic V74.0 ☑
          car (traffic) V73.5 ☑
            nontraffic V73.0 ☑
          motor vehicle NOS (traffic) V79.40 ☑
            nontraffic V79.00 ☑
            specified type NEC (traffic) V79.49 ☑
              nontraffic V79.09 ☑
          pedal cycle (traffic) V71.5 ☑
            nontraffic V71.0 ☑
          pickup truck (traffic) V73.5 ☑
            nontraffic V73.0 ☑
          railway vehicle (traffic) V75.5 ☑
            nontraffic V75.0 ☑
          specified vehicle NEC (traffic) V76.5 ☑
            nontraffic V76.0 ☑
          stationary object (traffic) V77.5 ☑
            nontraffic V77.0 ☑
          streetcar (traffic) V76.5 ☑
            nontraffic V76.0 ☑
          three wheeled motor vehicle (traffic)
            V72.5 ☑
            nontraffic V72.0 ☑
          truck (traffic) V74.5 ☑
            nontraffic V74.0 ☑
          two wheeled motor vehicle (traffic)
            V72.5 ☑
            nontraffic V72.0 ☑
          van (traffic) V73.5 ☑
            nontraffic V73.0 ☑
        noncollision accident (traffic) V78.5 ☑
          nontraffic V78.0 ☑
      hanger-on
        collision (with)
          animal (traffic) V70.7 ☑
            being ridden (traffic) V76.7 ☑
              nontraffic V76.2 ☑
            nontraffic V70.2 ☑
          animal-drawn vehicle (traffic) V76.7 ☑
            nontraffic V76.2 ☑
          bus (traffic) V74.7 ☑
            nontraffic V74.2 ☑
          car (traffic) V73.7 ☑
            nontraffic V73.2 ☑
          pedal cycle (traffic) V71.7 ☑
            nontraffic V71.2 ☑
          pickup truck (traffic) V73.7 ☑
            nontraffic V73.2 ☑
          railway vehicle (traffic) V75.7 ☑
            nontraffic V75.2 ☑
          specified vehicle NEC (traffic) V76.7 ☑
            nontraffic V76.2 ☑
          stationary object (traffic) V77.7 ☑
            nontraffic V77.2 ☑
          streetcar (traffic) V76.7 ☑
            nontraffic V76.2 ☑

☑ **Additional Character Required** — Refer to the Tabular List for Character Selection   ▽ Subterms under main terms may continue to next column or page

Accident — *continued*
  transport — *continued*
    bus occupant — *continued*
      hanger-on — *continued*
        collision — *continued*
          three wheeled motor vehicle (traffic)
            V72.7 ☑
            nontraffic V72.2 ☑
          truck (traffic) V74.7 ☑
            nontraffic V74.2 ☑
          two wheeled motor vehicle (traffic)
            V72.7 ☑
            nontraffic V72.2 ☑
          van (traffic) V73.7 ☑
            nontraffic V73.2 ☑
        noncollision accident (traffic) V78.7 ☑
          nontraffic V78.2 ☑
      noncollision accident (traffic) V78.9 ☑
        nontraffic V78.3 ☑
        while boarding or alighting V78.4 ☑
      nontraffic V79.3 ☑
      passenger
        collision (with)
          animal (traffic) V70.6 ☑
            being ridden (traffic) V76.6 ☑
              nontraffic V76.1 ☑
            nontraffic V70.1 ☑
          animal-drawn vehicle (traffic) V76.6 ☑
            nontraffic V76.1 ☑
          bus (traffic) V74.6 ☑
            nontraffic V74.1 ☑
          car (traffic) V73.6 ☑
            nontraffic V73.1 ☑
          motor vehicle NOS (traffic) V79.50 ☑
            nontraffic V79.10 ☑
              specified type NEC (traffic) V79.59 ☑
                nontraffic V79.19 ☑
          pedal cycle (traffic) V71.6 ☑
            nontraffic V71.1 ☑
          pickup truck (traffic) V73.6 ☑
            nontraffic V73.1 ☑
          railway vehicle (traffic) V75.6 ☑
            nontraffic V75.1 ☑
          specified vehicle NEC (traffic) V76.6 ☑
            nontraffic V76.1 ☑
          stationary object (traffic) V77.6 ☑
            nontraffic V77.1 ☑
          streetcar (traffic) V76.6 ☑
            nontraffic V76.1 ☑
          three wheeled motor vehicle (traffic)
            V72.6 ☑
            nontraffic V72.1 ☑
          truck (traffic) V74.6 ☑
            nontraffic V74.1 ☑
          two wheeled motor vehicle (traffic)
            V72.6 ☑
            nontraffic V72.1 ☑
          van (traffic) V73.6 ☑
            nontraffic V73.1 ☑
        noncollision accident (traffic) V78.6 ☑
          nontraffic V78.1 ☑
    specified type NEC V79.88 ☑
      military vehicle V79.81 ☑
    cable car, not on rails V98.0 ☑
      on rails — *see* Accident, transport, streetcar oc-
        cupant
    car occupant V49.9 ☑
      ambulance occupant — *see* Accident, transport,
        ambulance occupant
      collision (with)
        animal (traffic) V40.9 ☑
          being ridden (traffic) V46.9 ☑
            nontraffic V46.3 ☑
              while boarding or alighting V46.4 ☑
          nontraffic V40.3 ☑
          while boarding or alighting V40.4 ☑
        animal-drawn vehicle (traffic) V46.9 ☑
          nontraffic V46.3 ☑
          while boarding or alighting V46.4 ☑
        bus (traffic) V44.9 ☑
          nontraffic V44.3 ☑
          while boarding or alighting V44.4 ☑
        car (traffic) V43.92 ☑
          nontraffic V43.32 ☑
          while boarding or alighting V43.42 ☑
        motor vehicle NOS (traffic) V49.60 ☑

Accident — *continued*
  transport — *continued*
    car occupant — *continued*
      collision — *continued*
        motor vehicle — *continued*
          nontraffic V49.20 ☑
            specified type NEC (traffic) V49.69 ☑
              nontraffic V49.29 ☑
        pedal cycle (traffic) V41.9 ☑
          nontraffic V41.3 ☑
          while boarding or alighting V41.4 ☑
        pickup truck (traffic) V43.93 ☑
          nontraffic V43.33 ☑
          while boarding or alighting V43.43 ☑
        railway vehicle (traffic) V45.9 ☑
          nontraffic V45.3 ☑
          while boarding or alighting V45.4 ☑
        specified vehicle NEC (traffic) V46.9 ☑
          nontraffic V46.3 ☑
          while boarding or alighting V46.4 ☑
        sport utility vehicle (traffic) V43.91 ☑
          nontraffic V43.31 ☑
          while boarding or alighting V43.41 ☑
        stationary object (traffic) V47.9 ☑
          nontraffic V47.3 ☑
          while boarding or alighting V47.4 ☑
        streetcar (traffic) V46.9 ☑
          nontraffic V46.3 ☑
          while boarding or alighting V46.4 ☑
        three wheeled motor vehicle (traffic) V42.9 ☑
          nontraffic V42.3 ☑
          while boarding or alighting V42.4 ☑
        truck (traffic) V44.9 ☑
          nontraffic V44.3 ☑
          while boarding or alighting V44.4 ☑
        two wheeled motor vehicle (traffic) V42.9 ☑
          nontraffic V42.3 ☑
          while boarding or alighting V42.4 ☑
        van (traffic) V43.94 ☑
          nontraffic V43.34 ☑
          while boarding or alighting V43.44 ☑
      driver
        collision (with)
          animal (traffic) V40.5 ☑
            being ridden (traffic) V46.5 ☑
              nontraffic V46.0 ☑
            nontraffic V40.0 ☑
          animal-drawn vehicle (traffic) V46.5 ☑
            nontraffic V46.0 ☑
          bus (traffic) V44.5 ☑
            nontraffic V44.0 ☑
          car (traffic) V43.52 ☑
            nontraffic V43.02 ☑
          motor vehicle NOS (traffic) V49.40 ☑
            nontraffic V49.00 ☑
              specified type NEC (traffic) V49.49 ☑
                nontraffic V49.09 ☑
          pedal cycle (traffic) V41.5 ☑
            nontraffic V41.0 ☑
          pickup truck (traffic) V43.53 ☑
            nontraffic V43.03 ☑
          railway vehicle (traffic) V45.5 ☑
            nontraffic V45.0 ☑
          specified vehicle NEC (traffic) V46.5 ☑
            nontraffic V46.0 ☑
          sport utility vehicle (traffic) V43.51 ☑
            nontraffic V43.01 ☑
          stationary object (traffic) V47.5 ☑
            nontraffic V47.0 ☑
          streetcar (traffic) V46.5 ☑
            nontraffic V46.0 ☑
          three wheeled motor vehicle (traffic)
            V42.5 ☑
            nontraffic V42.0 ☑
          truck (traffic) V44.5 ☑
            nontraffic V44.0 ☑
          two wheeled motor vehicle (traffic)
            V42.5 ☑
            nontraffic V42.0 ☑
          van (traffic) V43.54 ☑
            nontraffic V43.04 ☑
        noncollision accident (traffic) V48.5 ☑
          nontraffic V48.0 ☑
      hanger-on
        collision (with)
          animal (traffic) V40.7 ☑

Accident — *continued*
  transport — *continued*
    car occupant — *continued*
      hanger-on — *continued*
        collision — *continued*
          animal — *continued*
            being ridden (traffic) V46.7 ☑
              nontraffic V46.2 ☑
            nontraffic V40.2 ☑
          animal-drawn vehicle (traffic) V46.7 ☑
            nontraffic V46.2 ☑
          bus (traffic) V44.7 ☑
            nontraffic V44.2 ☑
          car (traffic) V43.72 ☑
            nontraffic V43.22 ☑
          pedal cycle (traffic) V41.7 ☑
            nontraffic V41.2 ☑
          pickup truck (traffic) V43.73 ☑
            nontraffic V43.23 ☑
          railway vehicle (traffic) V45.7 ☑
            nontraffic V45.2 ☑
          specified vehicle NEC (traffic) V46.7 ☑
            nontraffic V46.2 ☑
          sport utility vehicle (traffic) V43.71 ☑
            nontraffic V43.21 ☑
          stationary object (traffic) V47.7 ☑
            nontraffic V47.2 ☑
          streetcar (traffic) V46.7 ☑
            nontraffic V46.2 ☑
          three wheeled motor vehicle (traffic)
            V42.7 ☑
            nontraffic V42.2 ☑
          truck (traffic) V44.7 ☑
            nontraffic V44.2 ☑
          two wheeled motor vehicle (traffic)
            V42.7 ☑
            nontraffic V42.2 ☑
          van (traffic) V43.74 ☑
            nontraffic V43.24 ☑
        noncollision accident (traffic) V48.7 ☑
          nontraffic V48.2 ☑
      noncollision accident (traffic) V48.9 ☑
        nontraffic V48.3 ☑
        while boarding or alighting V48.4 ☑
      nontraffic V49.3 ☑
      passenger
        collision (with)
          animal (traffic) V40.6 ☑
            being ridden (traffic) V46.6 ☑
              nontraffic V46.1 ☑
            nontraffic V40.1 ☑
          animal-drawn vehicle (traffic) V46.6 ☑
            nontraffic V46.1 ☑
          bus (traffic) V44.6 ☑
            nontraffic V44.1 ☑
          car (traffic) V43.62 ☑
            nontraffic V43.12 ☑
          motor vehicle NOS (traffic) V49.50 ☑
            nontraffic V49.10 ☑
              specified type NEC (traffic) V49.59 ☑
                nontraffic V49.19 ☑
          pedal cycle (traffic) V41.6 ☑
            nontraffic V41.1 ☑
          pickup truck (traffic) V43.63 ☑
            nontraffic V43.13 ☑
          railway vehicle (traffic) V45.6 ☑
            nontraffic V45.1 ☑
          specified vehicle NEC (traffic) V46.6 ☑
            nontraffic V46.1 ☑
          sport utility vehicle (traffic) V43.61 ☑
            nontraffic V43.11 ☑
          stationary object (traffic) V47.6 ☑
            nontraffic V47.1 ☑
          streetcar (traffic) V46.6 ☑
            nontraffic V46.1 ☑
          three wheeled motor vehicle (traffic)
            V42.6 ☑
            nontraffic V42.1 ☑
          truck (traffic) V44.6 ☑
            nontraffic V44.1 ☑
          two wheeled motor vehicle (traffic)
            V42.6 ☑
            nontraffic V42.1 ☑
          van (traffic) V43.64 ☑
            nontraffic V43.14 ☑
        noncollision accident (traffic) V48.6 ☑

Accident — *continued*
  transport — *continued*
    car occupant — *continued*
      passenger — *continued*
        noncollision accident — *continued*
          nontraffic V48.1 ☑
        specified type NEC V49.88 ☑
        military vehicle V49.81 ☑
    coal car — *see* Accident, transport, industrial vehicle occupant
    construction vehicle occupant (nontraffic) V85.9 ☑
      driver V85.5 ☑
      hanger-on V85.7 ☑
      passenger V85.6 ☑
      traffic V85.3 ☑
        driver V85.0 ☑
        hanger-on V85.2 ☑
        passenger V85.1 ☑
      while boarding or alighting V85.4 ☑
    dirt bike rider (nontraffic) V86.96 ☑
      driver V86.56 ☑
      hanger-on V86.76 ☑
      passenger V86.66 ☑
      traffic V86.36 ☑
        driver V86.06 ☑
        hanger-on V86.26 ☑
        passenger V86.16 ☑
      while boarding or alighting V86.46 ☑
    due to cataclysm — *see* Forces of nature, by type
    dune buggy occupant (nontraffic) V86.93 ☑
      driver V86.53 ☑
      hanger-on V86.73 ☑
      passenger V86.63 ☑
      traffic V86.33 ☑
        driver V86.03 ☑
        hanger-on V86.23 ☑
        passenger V86.13 ☑
      while boarding or alighting V86.43 ☑
    forklift — *see* Accident, transport, industrial vehicle occupant
    go cart — *see* Accident, transport, all-terrain vehicle occupant
    golf cart — *see* Accident, transport, all-terrain vehicle occupant
    heavy transport vehicle occupant — *see* Accident, transport, truck occupant
    hoverboard V00.848 ☑
    ice yacht V98.2 ☑
    industrial vehicle occupant (nontraffic) V83.9 ☑
      driver V83.5 ☑
      hanger-on V83.7 ☑
      passenger V83.6 ☑
      traffic V83.3 ☑
        driver V83.0 ☑
        hanger-on V83.2 ☑
        passenger V83.1 ☑
      while boarding or alighting V83.4 ☑
    interurban electric car — *see* Accident, transport, streetcar
    land yacht V98.1 ☑
    logging car — *see* Accident, transport, industrial vehicle occupant
    military vehicle occupant (traffic) V86.34 ☑
      driver V86.04 ☑
      hanger-on V86.24 ☑
      nontraffic V86.94 ☑
        driver V86.54 ☑
        hanger-on V86.74 ☑
        passenger V86.64 ☑
      passenger V86.14 ☑
      while boarding or alighting V86.44 ☑
    mine tram — *see* Accident, transport, industrial vehicle occupant
    motor vehicle NEC occupant (traffic) V89.2 ☑
    motorcoach — *see* Accident, transport, bus occupant
    motor/cross bike rider — *see also* Accident, transport, dirt bike rider V86.96 ☑
    motorcyclist V29.9 ☑
      collision (with)
        animal (traffic) V20.9 ☑
          being ridden (traffic) V26.9 ☑
            nontraffic V26.2 ☑
            while boarding or alighting V26.3 ☑
          nontraffic V20.2 ☑
          while boarding or alighting V20.3 ☑

Accident — *continued*
  transport — *continued*
    motorcyclist — *continued*
      collision — *continued*
        animal-drawn vehicle (traffic) V26.9 ☑
          nontraffic V26.2 ☑
          while boarding or alighting V26.3 ☑
        bus (traffic) V24.9 ☑
          nontraffic V24.2 ☑
          while boarding or alighting V24.3 ☑
        car (traffic) V23.9 ☑
          nontraffic V23.2 ☑
          while boarding or alighting V23.3 ☑
        motor vehicle NOS (traffic) V29.60 ☑
          nontraffic V29.20 ☑
          specified type NEC (traffic) V29.69 ☑
            nontraffic V29.29 ☑
        pedal cycle (traffic) V21.9 ☑
          nontraffic V21.2 ☑
          while boarding or alighting V21.3 ☑
        pickup truck (traffic) V23.9 ☑
          nontraffic V23.2 ☑
          while boarding or alighting V23.3 ☑
        railway vehicle (traffic) V25.9 ☑
          nontraffic V25.2 ☑
          while boarding or alighting V25.3 ☑
        specified vehicle NEC (traffic) V26.9 ☑
          nontraffic V26.2 ☑
          while boarding or alighting V26.3 ☑
        stationary object (traffic) V27.9 ☑
          nontraffic V27.2 ☑
          while boarding or alighting V27.3 ☑
        streetcar (traffic) V26.9 ☑
          nontraffic V26.2 ☑
          while boarding or alighting V26.3 ☑
        three wheeled motor vehicle (traffic) V22.9 ☑
          nontraffic V22.2 ☑
          while boarding or alighting V22.3 ☑
        truck (traffic) V24.9 ☑
          nontraffic V24.2 ☑
          while boarding or alighting V24.3 ☑
        two wheeled motor vehicle (traffic) V22.9 ☑
          nontraffic V22.2 ☑
          while boarding or alighting V22.3 ☑
        van (traffic) V23.9 ☑
          nontraffic V23.2 ☑
          while boarding or alighting V23.3 ☑
      driver
        collision (with)
          animal (traffic) V20.4 ☑
            being ridden (traffic) V26.4 ☑
              nontraffic V26.0 ☑
            nontraffic V20.0 ☑
          animal-drawn vehicle (traffic) V26.4 ☑
            nontraffic V26.0 ☑
          bus (traffic) V24.4 ☑
            nontraffic V24.0 ☑
          car (traffic) V23.4 ☑
            nontraffic V23.0 ☑
          motor vehicle NOS (traffic) V29.40 ☑
            nontraffic V29.00 ☑
            specified type NEC (traffic) V29.49 ☑
              nontraffic V29.09 ☑
          pedal cycle (traffic) V21.4 ☑
            nontraffic V21.0 ☑
          pickup truck (traffic) V23.4 ☑
            nontraffic V23.0 ☑
          railway vehicle (traffic) V25.4 ☑
            nontraffic V25.0 ☑
          specified vehicle NEC (traffic) V26.4 ☑
            nontraffic V26.0 ☑
          stationary object (traffic) V27.4 ☑
            nontraffic V27.0 ☑
          streetcar (traffic) V26.4 ☑
            nontraffic V26.0 ☑
          three wheeled motor vehicle (traffic) V22.4 ☑
            nontraffic V22.0 ☑
          truck (traffic) V24.4 ☑
            nontraffic V24.0 ☑
          two wheeled motor vehicle (traffic) V22.4 ☑
            nontraffic V22.0 ☑
          van (traffic) V23.4 ☑
            nontraffic V23.0 ☑
        noncollision accident (traffic) V28.4 ☑

Accident — *continued*
  transport — *continued*
    motorcyclist — *continued*
      driver — *continued*
        noncollision accident — *continued*
          nontraffic V28.0 ☑
        noncollision accident (traffic) V28.9 ☑
          nontraffic V28.2 ☑
          while boarding or alighting V28.3 ☑
      nontraffic V29.3 ☑
      passenger
        collision (with)
          animal (traffic) V20.5 ☑
            being ridden (traffic) V26.5 ☑
              nontraffic V26.1 ☑
            nontraffic V20.1 ☑
          animal-drawn vehicle (traffic) V26.5 ☑
            nontraffic V26.1 ☑
          bus (traffic) V24.5 ☑
            nontraffic V24.1 ☑
          car (traffic) V23.5 ☑
            nontraffic V23.1 ☑
          motor vehicle NOS (traffic) V29.50 ☑
            nontraffic V29.10 ☑
            specified type NEC (traffic) V29.59 ☑
              nontraffic V29.19 ☑
          pedal cycle (traffic) V21.5 ☑
            nontraffic V21.1 ☑
          pickup truck (traffic) V23.5 ☑
            nontraffic V23.1 ☑
          railway vehicle (traffic) V25.5 ☑
            nontraffic V25.1 ☑
          specified vehicle NEC (traffic) V26.5 ☑
            nontraffic V26.1 ☑
          stationary object (traffic) V27.5 ☑
            nontraffic V27.1 ☑
          streetcar (traffic) V26.5 ☑
            nontraffic V26.1 ☑
          three wheeled motor vehicle (traffic) V22.5 ☑
            nontraffic V22.1 ☑
          truck (traffic) V24.5 ☑
            nontraffic V24.1 ☑
          two wheeled motor vehicle (traffic) V22.5 ☑
            nontraffic V22.1 ☑
          van (traffic) V23.5 ☑
            nontraffic V23.1 ☑
        noncollision accident (traffic) V28.5 ☑
          nontraffic V28.1 ☑
      specified type NEC V29.88 ☑
      military vehicle V29.81 ☑
    occupant (of)
      aircraft (powered) V95.9 ☑
        fixed wing
          commercial — *see* Accident, transport, aircraft, occupant, powered, fixed wing, commercial
          private — *see* Accident, transport, aircraft, occupant, powered, fixed wing, private
        nonpowered V96.9 ☑
        specified NEC V95.8 ☑
      airport battery-powered vehicle — *see* Accident, transport, industrial vehicle occupant
      all-terrain vehicle (ATV) — *see* Accident, transport, all-terrain vehicle occupant
      animal-drawn vehicle — *see* Accident, transport, animal-drawn vehicle occupant
      automobile — *see* Accident, transport, car occupant
      balloon V96.00 ☑
      battery-powered vehicle — *see* Accident, transport, industrial vehicle occupant
      bicycle — *see* Accident, transport, pedal cyclist
        motorized — *see* Accident, transport, motorcycle rider
      boat NEC — *see* Accident, watercraft
      bulldozer — *see* Accident, transport, construction vehicle occupant
      bus — *see* Accident, transport, bus occupant
      cable car (on rails) — *see also* Accident, transport, streetcar occupant
        not on rails V98.0 ☑
      car — *see also* Accident, transport, car occupant

Accident — *continued*
  transport — *continued*
    occupant — *continued*
      car — *see also* Accident, transport, car occupant
          — *continued*
        cable (on rails) — *see also* Accident, transport,
            streetcar occupant
          not on rails V98.0 ☑
        coach — *see* Accident, transport, bus occupant
        coal-car — *see* Accident, transport, industrial
            vehicle occupant
        digger — *see* Accident, transport, construction
            vehicle occupant
        dump truck — *see* Accident, transport, construc-
            tion vehicle occupant
        earth-leveler — *see* Accident, transport, construc-
            tion vehicle occupant
        farm machinery (self-propelled) — *see* Accident,
            transport, agricultural vehicle occupant
        forklift — *see* Accident, transport, industrial ve-
            hicle occupant
        glider (unpowered) V96.20 ☑
          hang V96.10 ☑
          powered (microlight) (ultralight) — *see* Acci-
              dent, transport, aircraft, occupant,
              powered, glider
        glider (unpowered) NEC V96.20 ☑
        hang-glider V96.10 ☑
        harvester — *see* Accident, transport, agricultural
            vehicle occupant
        heavy (transport) vehicle — *see* Accident, trans-
            port, truck occupant
        helicopter — *see* Accident, transport, aircraft,
            occupant, helicopter
        ice-yacht V98.2 ☑
        kite (carrying person) V96.8 ☑
        land-yacht V98.1 ☑
        logging car — *see* Accident, transport, industrial
            vehicle occupant
        mechanical shovel — *see* Accident, transport,
            construction vehicle occupant
        microlight — *see* Accident, transport, aircraft,
            occupant, powered, glider
        minibus — *see* Accident, transport, pickup truck
            occupant
        minivan — *see* Accident, transport, pickup truck
            occupant
        moped — *see* Accident, transport, motorcycle
        motor scooter — *see* Accident, transport, motor-
            cycle
        motorcycle (with sidecar) — *see* Accident,
            transport, motorcycle
        off-road motor-vehicle — *see also* Accident,
            transport, all-terrain vehicle occupant
            V86.99 ☑
        pedal cycle — *see also* Accident, transport, pedal
            cyclist
        pick-up (truck) — *see* Accident, transport, pickup
            truck occupant
        railway (train) (vehicle) (subterranean) (elevated)
            — *see* Accident, transport, railway vehicle
            occupant
        rickshaw — *see* Accident, transport, pedal cycle
          motorized — *see* Accident, transport, three-
              wheeled motor vehicle
          pedal driven — *see* Accident, transport, pedal
              cyclist
        road-roller — *see* Accident, transport, construc-
            tion vehicle occupant
        ship NOS V94.9 ☑
        ski-lift (chair) (gondola) V98.3 ☑
        snowmobile — *see* Accident, transport, snowmo-
            bile occupant
        spacecraft, spaceship — *see* Accident, transport,
            aircraft, occupant, spacecraft
        sport utility vehicle — *see* Accident, transport,
            pickup truck occupant
        streetcar (interurban) (operating on public street
            or highway) — *see* Accident, transport,
            streetcar occupant
        SUV — *see* Accident, transport, pickup truck oc-
            cupant
        téléférique V98.0 ☑
        three-wheeled vehicle (motorized) — *see also*
            Accident, transport, three-wheeled motor
            vehicle occupant

Accident — *continued*
  transport — *continued*
    occupant — *continued*
      three-wheeled vehicle — *see also* Accident,
          transport, three-wheeled motor vehicle
          occupant — *continued*
        nonmotorized — *see* Accident, transport,
            pedal cycle
      tractor (farm) (and trailer) — *see* Accident,
          transport, agricultural vehicle occupant
      train — *see* Accident, transport, railway vehicle
          occupant
      tram — *see* Accident, transport, streetcar occu-
          pant
        in mine or quarry — *see* Accident, transport,
            industrial vehicle occupant
      tricycle — *see* Accident, transport, pedal cycle
        motorized — *see* Accident, transport, three-
            wheeled motor vehicle
      trolley — *see* Accident, transport, streetcar occu-
          pant
        in mine or quarry — *see* Accident, transport,
            industrial vehicle occupant
      tub, in mine or quarry — *see* Accident, transport,
          industrial vehicle occupant
      ultralight — *see* Accident, transport, aircraft, oc-
          cupant, powered, glider
      van — *see* Accident, transport, van occupant
      vehicle NEC V89.9 ☑
        heavy transport — *see* Accident, transport,
            truck occupant
        motor (traffic) NEC V89.2 ☑
          nontraffic NEC V89.0 ☑
      watercraft NOS V94.9 ☑
        causing drowning — *see* Drowning, resulting
            from accident to boat
    off-road motor-vehicle — *see also* Accident, trans-
        port, all-terrain vehicle occupant V86.99 ☑
    parachutist V97.29 ☑
      after accident to aircraft — *see* Accident, trans-
          port, aircraft
      entangled in object V97.21 ☑
      injured on landing V97.22 ☑
    pedal cyclist V19.9 ☑
      collision (with)
        animal (traffic) V10.9 ☑
          being ridden (traffic) V16.9 ☑
            nontraffic V16.2 ☑
            while boarding or alighting V16.3 ☑
          nontraffic V10.2 ☑
          while boarding or alighting V10.3 ☑
        animal-drawn vehicle (traffic) V16.9 ☑
          nontraffic V16.2 ☑
          while boarding or alighting V16.3 ☑
        bus (traffic) V14.9 ☑
          nontraffic V14.2 ☑
          while boarding or alighting V14.3 ☑
        car (traffic) V13.9 ☑
          nontraffic V13.2 ☑
          while boarding or alighting V13.3 ☑
        motor vehicle NOS (traffic) V19.60 ☑
          nontraffic V19.20 ☑
          specified type NEC (traffic) V19.69 ☑
            nontraffic V19.29 ☑
        pedal cycle (traffic) V11.9 ☑
          nontraffic V11.2 ☑
          while boarding or alighting V11.3 ☑
        pickup truck (traffic) V13.9 ☑
          nontraffic V13.2 ☑
          while boarding or alighting V13.3 ☑
        railway vehicle (traffic) V15.9 ☑
          nontraffic V15.2 ☑
          while boarding or alighting V15.3 ☑
        specified vehicle NEC (traffic) V16.9 ☑
          nontraffic V16.2 ☑
          while boarding or alighting V16.3 ☑
        stationary object (traffic) V17.9 ☑
          nontraffic V17.2 ☑
          while boarding or alighting V17.3 ☑
        streetcar (traffic) V16.9 ☑
          nontraffic V16.2 ☑
          while boarding or alighting V16.3 ☑
        three wheeled motor vehicle (traffic) V12.9 ☑
          nontraffic V12.2 ☑
          while boarding or alighting V12.3 ☑
        truck (traffic) V14.9 ☑

Accident — *continued*
  transport — *continued*
    pedal cyclist — *continued*
      collision — *continued*
        truck — *continued*
          nontraffic V14.2 ☑
          while boarding or alighting V14.3 ☑
        two wheeled motor vehicle (traffic) V12.9 ☑
          nontraffic V12.2 ☑
          while boarding or alighting V12.3 ☑
        van (traffic) V13.9 ☑
          nontraffic V13.2 ☑
          while boarding or alighting V13.3 ☑
      driver
        collision (with)
          animal (traffic) V10.4 ☑
            being ridden (traffic) V16.4 ☑
              nontraffic V16.0 ☑
            nontraffic V10.0 ☑
          animal-drawn vehicle (traffic) V16.4 ☑
            nontraffic V16.0 ☑
          bus (traffic) V14.4 ☑
            nontraffic V14.0 ☑
          car (traffic) V13.4 ☑
            nontraffic V13.0 ☑
          motor vehicle NOS (traffic) V19.40 ☑
            nontraffic V19.00 ☑
            specified type NEC (traffic) V19.49 ☑
              nontraffic V19.09 ☑
          pedal cycle (traffic) V11.4 ☑
            nontraffic V11.0 ☑
          pickup truck (traffic) V13.4 ☑
            nontraffic V13.0 ☑
          railway vehicle (traffic) V15.4 ☑
            nontraffic V15.0 ☑
          specified vehicle NEC (traffic) V16.4 ☑
            nontraffic V16.0 ☑
          stationary object (traffic) V17.4 ☑
            nontraffic V17.0 ☑
          streetcar (traffic) V16.4 ☑
            nontraffic V16.0 ☑
          three wheeled motor vehicle (traffic)
              V12.4 ☑
            nontraffic V12.0 ☑
          truck (traffic) V14.4 ☑
            nontraffic V14.0 ☑
          two wheeled motor vehicle (traffic)
              V12.4 ☑
            nontraffic V12.0 ☑
          van (traffic) V13.4 ☑
            nontraffic V13.0 ☑
        noncollision accident (traffic) V18.4 ☑
          nontraffic V18.0 ☑
      noncollision accident (traffic) V18.9 ☑
        nontraffic V18.2 ☑
        while boarding or alighting V18.3 ☑
      nontraffic V19.3 ☑
      passenger
        collision (with)
          animal (traffic) V10.5 ☑
            being ridden (traffic) V16.5 ☑
              nontraffic V16.1 ☑
            nontraffic V10.1 ☑
          animal-drawn vehicle (traffic) V16.5 ☑
            nontraffic V16.1 ☑
          bus (traffic) V14.5 ☑
            nontraffic V14.1 ☑
          car (traffic) V13.5 ☑
            nontraffic V13.1 ☑
          motor vehicle NOS (traffic) V19.50 ☑
            nontraffic V19.10 ☑
            specified type NEC (traffic) V19.59 ☑
              nontraffic V19.19 ☑
          pedal cycle (traffic) V11.5 ☑
            nontraffic V11.1 ☑
          pickup truck (traffic) V13.5 ☑
            nontraffic V13.1 ☑
          railway vehicle (traffic) V15.5 ☑
            nontraffic V15.1 ☑
          specified vehicle NEC (traffic) V16.5 ☑
            nontraffic V16.1 ☑
          stationary object (traffic) V17.5 ☑
            nontraffic V17.1 ☑
          streetcar (traffic) V16.5 ☑
            nontraffic V16.1 ☑

Accident — *continued*
  transport — *continued*
    pedal cyclist — *continued*
      passenger — *continued*
        collision — *continued*
          three wheeled motor vehicle (traffic)
            V12.5 ☑
            nontraffic V12.1 ☑
          truck (traffic) V14.5 ☑
            nontraffic V14.1 ☑
          two wheeled motor vehicle (traffic)
            V12.5 ☑
            nontraffic V12.1 ☑
          van (traffic) V13.5 ☑
            nontraffic V13.1 ☑
          noncollision accident (traffic) V18.5 ☑
            nontraffic V18.1 ☑
        specified type NEC V19.88 ☑
        military vehicle V19.81 ☑
    pedestrian
      conveyance (occupant) V09.9 ☑
        baby stroller V00.828 ☑
          collision (with) V09.9 ☑
            animal being ridden or animal drawn
              vehicle V06.99 ☑
              nontraffic V06.09 ☑
              traffic V06.19 ☑
            bus or heavy transport V04.99 ☑
              nontraffic V04.09 ☑
              traffic V04.19 ☑
            car V03.99 ☑
              nontraffic V03.09 ☑
              traffic V03.19 ☑
            pedal cycle V01.99 ☑
              nontraffic V01.09 ☑
              traffic V01.19 ☑
            pick-up truck or van V03.99 ☑
              nontraffic V03.09 ☑
              traffic V03.19 ☑
            railway (train) (vehicle) V05.99 ☑
              nontraffic V05.09 ☑
              traffic V05.19 ☑
            stationary object V00.822 ☑
            streetcar V06.99 ☑
              nontraffic V06.09 ☑
              traffic V06.19 ☑
            two- or three-wheeled motor vehicle
              V02.99 ☑
              nontraffic V02.09 ☑
              traffic V02.19 ☑
            vehicle V09.9 ☑
              animal-drawn V06.99 ☑
                nontraffic V06.09 ☑
                traffic V06.19 ☑
              motor
                nontraffic V09.00 ☑
                traffic V09.20 ☑
           fall V00.821 ☑
          nontraffic V09.1 ☑
            involving motor vehicle NEC V09.00 ☑
          traffic V09.3 ☑
            involving motor vehicle NEC V09.20 ☑
        flat-bottomed NEC V00.388 ☑
          collision (with) V09.9 ☑
            animal being ridden or animal drawn
              vehicle V06.99 ☑
              nontraffic V06.09 ☑
              traffic V06.19 ☑
            bus or heavy transport V04.99 ☑
              nontraffic V04.09 ☑
              traffic V04.19 ☑
            car V03.99 ☑
              nontraffic V03.09 ☑
              traffic V03.19 ☑
            pedal cycle V01.99 ☑
              nontraffic V01.09 ☑
              traffic V01.19 ☑
            pick-up truck or van V03.99 ☑
              nontraffic V03.09 ☑
              traffic V03.19 ☑
            railway (train) (vehicle) V05.99 ☑
              nontraffic V05.09 ☑
              traffic V05.19 ☑
            stationary object V00.382 ☑
            streetcar V06.99 ☑
              nontraffic V06.09 ☑

Accident — *continued*
  transport — *continued*
    pedestrian — *continued*
      conveyance — *continued*
        flat-bottomed — *continued*
          collision — *continued*
           streetcar — *continued*
           two- or three-wheeled motor vehicle
            V02.99 ☑
            nontraffic V02.09 ☑
            traffic V02.19 ☑
           vehicle V09.9 ☑
            animal-drawn V06.99 ☑
              nontraffic V06.09 ☑
              traffic V06.19 ☑
            motor
              nontraffic V09.00 ☑
              traffic V09.20 ☑
         fall V00.381 ☑
        nontraffic V09.1 ☑
          involving motor vehicle NEC V09.00 ☑
        snow
          board — *see* Accident, transport,
            pedestrian, conveyance, snow
            board
          ski — *see* Accident, transport, pedes-
            trian, conveyance, skis (snow)
        traffic V09.3 ☑
          involving motor vehicle NEC V09.20 ☑
        gliding type NEC V00.288 ☑
          collision (with) V09.9 ☑
            animal being ridden or animal drawn
              vehicle V06.99 ☑
              nontraffic V06.09 ☑
              traffic V06.19 ☑
            bus or heavy transport V04.99 ☑
              nontraffic V04.09 ☑
              traffic V04.19 ☑
            car V03.99 ☑
              nontraffic V03.09 ☑
              traffic V03.19 ☑
            pedal cycle V01.99 ☑
              nontraffic V01.09 ☑
              traffic V01.19 ☑
            pick-up truck or van V03.99 ☑
              nontraffic V03.09 ☑
              traffic V03.19 ☑
            railway (train) (vehicle) V05.99 ☑
              nontraffic V05.09 ☑
              traffic V05.19 ☑
            stationary object V00.282 ☑
            streetcar V06.99 ☑
              nontraffic V06.09 ☑
              traffic V02.19 ☑
            two- or three-wheeled motor vehicle
            V02.99 ☑
            nontraffic V02.09 ☑
            traffic V02.19 ☑
           vehicle V09.9 ☑
            animal-drawn V06.99 ☑
              nontraffic V06.09 ☑
              traffic V06.19 ☑
            motor
              nontraffic V09.00 ☑
              traffic V09.20 ☑
        fall V00.281 ☑
        heelies — *see* Accident, transport,
          pedestrian, conveyance, heelies
        ice skate — *see* Accident, transport,
          pedestrian, conveyance, ice skate
        nontraffic V09.1 ☑
          involving motor vehicle NEC V09.00 ☑
        sled — *see* Accident, transport, pedestri-
          an, conveyance, sled
        traffic V09.3 ☑
          involving motor vehicle NEC V09.20 ☑
        wheelies — *see* Accident, transport,
          pedestrian, conveyance, heelies
        heelies V00.158 ☑
          colliding with stationary object
            V00.152 ☑
          fall V00.151 ☑

Accident — *continued*
  transport — *continued*
    pedestrian — *continued*
      conveyance — *continued*
        hoverboard
          collision with
           animal being ridden or animal drawn
             vehicle V06.938 ☑
             nontraffic V06.038 ☑
             traffic V06.138 ☑
           bus or heavy transport V04.938 ☑
            nontraffic V04.038 ☑
            traffic V04.138 ☑
           car V03.938 ☑
            nontraffic V03.038 ☑
            traffic V03.138 ☑
           pedal cycle V01.938 ☑
            nontraffic V01.038 ☑
            traffic V01.138 ☑
           pick-up or van V03.938 ☑
            nontraffic V03.038 ☑
            traffic V03.138 ☑
           railway (train) (vehicle) V05.938 ☑
            nontraffic V05.038 ☑
            traffic V05.138 ☑
           streetcar V06.938 ☑
            nontraffic V06.038 ☑
            traffic V06.138 ☑
           three-wheeled motor vehicle
            V02.938 ☑
            nontraffic V02.038 ☑
            traffic V02.138 ☑
           two-wheeled motor vehicle
            V02.938 ☑
            nontraffic V02.038 ☑
            traffic V02.138 ☑
           vehicle, nonmotor, specified NEC
            V06.938 ☑
            nontraffic V06.038 ☑
            traffic V06.138 ☑
          fall V00.848 ☑
        ice skates V00.218 ☑
          collision (with) V09.9 ☑
           animal being ridden or animal drawn
            vehicle V06.99 ☑
            nontraffic V06.09 ☑
            traffic V06.19 ☑
           bus or heavy transport V04.99 ☑
            nontraffic V04.09 ☑
            traffic V04.19 ☑
           car V03.99 ☑
            nontraffic V03.09 ☑
            traffic V03.19 ☑
           pedal cycle V01.99 ☑
            nontraffic V01.09 ☑
            traffic V01.19 ☑
           pick-up truck or van V03.99 ☑
            nontraffic V03.09 ☑
            traffic V03.19 ☑
           railway (train) (vehicle) V05.99 ☑
            nontraffic V05.09 ☑
            traffic V05.19 ☑
           stationary object V00.212 ☑
           streetcar V06.99 ☑
            nontraffic V06.09 ☑
            traffic V06.19 ☑
           two- or three-wheeled motor vehicle
            V02.99 ☑
            nontraffic V02.09 ☑
            traffic V02.19 ☑
           vehicle V09.9 ☑
            animal-drawn V06.99 ☑
             nontraffic V06.09 ☑
             traffic V06.19 ☑
            motor
             nontraffic V09.00 ☑
             traffic V09.20 ☑
        fall V00.211 ☑
        nontraffic V09.1 ☑
          involving motor vehicle NEC V09.00 ☑
        traffic V09.3 ☑
          involving motor vehicle NEC V09.20 ☑
        motorized mobility scooter V00.838 ☑
          collision with stationary object
           V00.832 ☑
          fall from V00.831 ☑

Accident — *continued*
  transport — *continued*
    pedestrian — *continued*
      conveyance — *continued*
        nontraffic V09.1 ☑
          involving motor vehicle V09.00 ☑
            military V09.01 ☑
            specified type NEC V09.09 ☑
        roller skates (non in-line) V00.128 ☑
          collision (with) V09.9 ☑
            animal being ridden or animal drawn
              vehicle V06.91 ☑
              nontraffic V06.01 ☑
              traffic V06.11 ☑
            bus or heavy transport V04.91 ☑
              nontraffic V04.01 ☑
              traffic V04.11 ☑
            car V03.91 ☑
              nontraffic V03.01 ☑
              traffic V03.11 ☑
            pedal cycle V01.91 ☑
              nontraffic V01.01 ☑
              traffic V01.11 ☑
            pick-up truck or van V03.91 ☑
              nontraffic V03.01 ☑
              traffic V03.11 ☑
            railway (train) (vehicle) V05.91 ☑
              nontraffic V05.01 ☑
              traffic V05.11 ☑
            stationary object V00.122 ☑
            streetcar V06.91 ☑
              nontraffic V06.01 ☑
              traffic V06.11 ☑
            two- or three-wheeled motor vehicle
              V02.91 ☑
              nontraffic V02.01 ☑
              traffic V02.11 ☑
            vehicle V09.9 ☑
              animal-drawn V06.91 ☑
                nontraffic V06.01 ☑
                traffic V06.11 ☑
              motor
                nontraffic V09.00 ☑
                traffic V09.20 ☑
         fall V00.121 ☑
        in-line V00.118 ☑
          collision — *see also* Accident, trans-
            port, pedestrian, conveyance
            occupant, roller skates, collision
            with stationary object V00.112 ☑
          fall V00.111 ☑
          nontraffic V09.1 ☑
            involving motor vehicle NEC V09.00 ☑
          traffic V09.3 ☑
            involving motor vehicle NEC V09.20 ☑
        rolling shoes V00.158 ☑
          colliding with stationary object
            V00.152 ☑
          fall V00.151 ☑
        rolling type NEC V00.188 ☑
          collision (with) V09.9 ☑
            animal being ridden or animal drawn
              vehicle V06.99 ☑
              nontraffic V06.09 ☑
              traffic V06.19 ☑
            bus or heavy transport V04.99 ☑
              nontraffic V04.09 ☑
              traffic V04.19 ☑
            car V03.99 ☑
              nontraffic V03.09 ☑
              traffic V03.19 ☑
            pedal cycle V01.99 ☑
              nontraffic V01.09 ☑
              traffic V01.19 ☑
            pick-up truck or van V03.99 ☑
              nontraffic V03.09 ☑
              traffic V03.19 ☑
            railway (train) (vehicle) V05.99 ☑
              nontraffic V05.09 ☑
              traffic V05.19 ☑
            stationary object V00.182 ☑
            streetcar V06.99 ☑
              nontraffic V06.09 ☑
              traffic V06.19 ☑
            two- or three-wheeled motor vehicle
              V02.99 ☑

Accident — *continued*
  transport — *continued*
    pedestrian — *continued*
      conveyance — *continued*
        rolling type — *continued*
          collision — *continued*
            two- or three-wheeled motor vehicle
              — *continued*
              nontraffic V02.09 ☑
              traffic V02.19 ☑
            vehicle V09.9 ☑
              animal-drawn V06.99 ☑
                nontraffic V06.09 ☑
                traffic V06.19 ☑
              motor
                nontraffic V09.00 ☑
                traffic V09.20 ☑
          fall V00.181 ☑
          in-line roller skate — *see* Accident,
            transport, pedestrian, conveyance,
            roller skate, in-line
          nontraffic V09.1 ☑
            involving motor vehicle NEC V09.00 ☑
          roller skate — *see* Accident, transport,
            pedestrian, conveyance, roller
            skate
          scooter (non-motorized) — *see* Accident,
            transport, pedestrian, conveyance,
            scooter
          skateboard — *see* Accident, transport,
            pedestrian, conveyance, skate-
            board
          traffic V09.3 ☑
            involving motor vehicle NEC V09.20 ☑
        scooter (non-motorized) V00.148 ☑
          collision (with) V09.9 ☑
            animal being ridden or animal drawn
              vehicle V06.99 ☑
              nontraffic V06.09 ☑
              traffic V06.19 ☑
            bus or heavy transport V04.99 ☑
              nontraffic V04.09 ☑
              traffic V04.19 ☑
            car V03.99 ☑
              nontraffic V03.09 ☑
              traffic V03.19 ☑
            pedal cycle V01.99 ☑
              nontraffic V01.09 ☑
              traffic V01.19 ☑
            pick-up truck or van V03.99 ☑
              nontraffic V03.09 ☑
              traffic V03.19 ☑
            railway (train) (vehicle) V05.99 ☑
              nontraffic V05.09 ☑
              traffic V05.19 ☑
            stationary object V00.142 ☑
            streetcar V06.99 ☑
              nontraffic V06.09 ☑
              traffic V06.19 ☑
            two- or three-wheeled motor vehicle
              V02.99 ☑
              nontraffic V02.09 ☑
              traffic V02.19 ☑
            vehicle V09.9 ☑
              animal-drawn V06.99 ☑
                nontraffic V06.09 ☑
                traffic V06.19 ☑
              motor
                nontraffic V09.00 ☑
                traffic V09.20 ☑
          fall V00.141 ☑
          nontraffic V09.1 ☑
            involving motor vehicle NEC V09.00 ☑
          traffic V09.3 ☑
            involving motor vehicle NEC V09.20 ☑
        Segway
          collision with
            animal being ridden or animal drawn
              vehicle V06.938 ☑
              nontraffic V06.038 ☑
              traffic V06.138 ☑
            bus or heavy transport V04.938 ☑
              nontraffic V04.038 ☑
              traffic V04.138 ☑
            car V03.938 ☑
              nontraffic V03.038 ☑

Accident — *continued*
  transport — *continued*
    pedestrian — *continued*
      conveyance — *continued*
        Segway — *continued*
          collision with — *continued*
            car — *continued*
              traffic V03.138 ☑
            pedal cycle V01.938 ☑
              nontraffic V01.038 ☑
              traffic V01.138 ☑
            pick-up or van V03.938 ☑
              nontraffic V03.038 ☑
              traffic V03.138 ☑
            railway (train) (vehicle) V05.938 ☑
              nontraffic V05.038 ☑
              traffic V05.138 ☑
            streetcar V06.938 ☑
              nontraffic V06.038 ☑
              traffic V06.138 ☑
            three-wheeled vehicle V02.938 ☑
              nontraffic V02.038 ☑
              traffic V02.138 ☑
            two-wheeled vehicle V02.938 ☑
              nontraffic V02.038 ☑
              traffic V02.138 ☑
            vehicle, nonmotor, specified NEC
              V06.938 ☑
              nontraffic V06.038 ☑
              traffic V06.138 ☑
          fall V00.848 ☑
        skate board V00.138 ☑
          collision (with) V09.9 ☑
            animal being ridden or animal drawn
              vehicle V06.92 ☑
              nontraffic V06.02 ☑
              traffic V06.12 ☑
            bus or heavy transport V04.92 ☑
              nontraffic V04.02 ☑
              traffic V04.12 ☑
            car V03.92 ☑
              nontraffic V03.02 ☑
              traffic V03.12 ☑
            pedal cycle V01.92 ☑
              nontraffic V01.02 ☑
              traffic V01.12 ☑
            pick-up truck or van V03.92 ☑
              nontraffic V03.02 ☑
              traffic V03.12 ☑
            railway (train) (vehicle) V05.92 ☑
              nontraffic V05.02 ☑
              traffic V05.12 ☑
            stationary object V00.132 ☑
            streetcar V06.92 ☑
              nontraffic V06.02 ☑
              traffic V06.12 ☑
            two- or three-wheeled motor vehicle
              V02.92 ☑
              nontraffic V02.02 ☑
              traffic V02.12 ☑
            vehicle V09.9 ☑
              animal-drawn V06.92 ☑
                nontraffic V06.02 ☑
                traffic V06.12 ☑
              motor
                nontraffic V09.00 ☑
                traffic V09.20 ☑
         fall V00.131 ☑
          nontraffic V09.1 ☑
            involving motor vehicle NEC V09.00 ☑
          traffic V09.3 ☑
            involving motor vehicle NEC V09.20 ☑
        skis (snow) V00.328 ☑
          collision (with) V09.9 ☑
            animal being ridden or animal drawn
              vehicle V06.99 ☑
              nontraffic V06.09 ☑
              traffic V06.19 ☑
            bus or heavy transport V04.99 ☑
              nontraffic V04.09 ☑
              traffic V04.19 ☑
            car V03.99 ☑
              nontraffic V03.09 ☑
              traffic V03.19 ☑
            pedal cycle V01.99 ☑
              nontraffic V01.09 ☑

Accident — *continued*
  transport — *continued*
    pedestrian — *continued*
      conveyance — *continued*
        skis — *continued*
          collision — *continued*
            pedal cycle — *continued*
              traffic V01.19 ☑
            pick-up truck or van V03.99 ☑
              nontraffic V03.09 ☑
              traffic V03.19 ☑
            railway (train) (vehicle) V05.99 ☑
              nontraffic V05.09 ☑
              traffic V05.19 ☑
            stationary object V00.322 ☑
            streetcar V06.99 ☑
              nontraffic V06.09 ☑
              traffic V06.19 ☑
            two- or three-wheeled motor vehicle V02.99 ☑
              nontraffic V02.09 ☑
              traffic V02.19 ☑
            vehicle V09.9 ☑
              animal-drawn V06.99 ☑
                nontraffic V06.09 ☑
                traffic V06.19 ☑
              motor•
                nontraffic V09.00 ☑
                traffic V09.20 ☑
           fall V00.321 ☑
          nontraffic V09.1 ☑
            involving motor vehicle NEC V09.00 ☑
          traffic V09.3 ☑
            involving motor vehicle NEC V09.20 ☑
         sled V00.228 ☑
          collision (with) V09.9 ☑
            animal being ridden or animal drawn vehicle V06.99 ☑
              nontraffic V06.09 ☑
              traffic V06.19 ☑
            bus or heavy transport V04.99 ☑
              nontraffic V04.09 ☑
              traffic V04.19 ☑
            car V03.99 ☑
              nontraffic V03.09 ☑
              traffic V03.19 ☑
            pedal cycle V01.99 ☑
              nontraffic V01.09 ☑
              traffic V01.19 ☑
            pick-up truck or van V03.99 ☑
              nontraffic V03.09 ☑
              traffic V03.19 ☑
            railway (train) (vehicle) V05.99 ☑
              nontraffic V05.09 ☑
              traffic V05.19 ☑
            stationary object V00.222 ☑
            streetcar V06.99 ☑
              nontraffic V06.09 ☑
              traffic V06.19 ☑
            two- or three-wheeled motor vehicle V02.99 ☑
              nontraffic V02.09 ☑
              traffic V02.19 ☑
            vehicle V09.9 ☑
              animal-drawn V06.99 ☑
                nontraffic V06.09 ☑
                traffic V06.19 ☑
              motor
                nontraffic V09.00 ☑
                traffic V09.20 ☑
           fall V00.221 ☑
          nontraffic V09.1 ☑
            involving motor vehicle NEC V09.00 ☑
          traffic V09.3 ☑
            involving motor vehicle NEC V09.20 ☑
         snow board V00.318 ☑
          collision (with) V09.9 ☑
            animal being ridden or animal drawn vehicle V06.99 ☑
              nontraffic V06.09 ☑
              traffic V06.19 ☑
            bus or heavy transport V04.99 ☑
              nontraffic V04.09 ☑
              traffic V04.19 ☑
            car V03.99 ☑
              nontraffic V03.09 ☑

Accident — *continued*
  transport — *continued*
    pedestrian — *continued*
      conveyance — *continued*
        snow board — *continued*
          collision — *continued*
            car — *continued*
              traffic V03.19 ☑
            pedal cycle V01.99 ☑
              nontraffic V01.09 ☑
              traffic V01.19 ☑
            pick-up truck or van V03.99 ☑
              nontraffic V03.09 ☑
              traffic V03.19 ☑
            railway (train) (vehicle) V05.99 ☑
              nontraffic V05.09 ☑
              traffic V05.19 ☑
            stationary object V00.312 ☑
            streetcar V06.99 ☑
              nontraffic V06.09 ☑
              traffic V06.19 ☑
            two- or three-wheeled motor vehicle V02.99 ☑
              nontraffic V02.09 ☑
              traffic V02.19 ☑
            vehicle V09.9 ☑
              animal-drawn V06.99 ☑
                nontraffic V06.09 ☑
                traffic V06.19 ☑
              motor
                nontraffic V09.00 ☑
                traffic V09.20 ☑
           fall V00.311 ☑
          nontraffic V09.1 ☑
            involving motor vehicle NEC V09.00 ☑
          traffic V09.3 ☑
            involving motor vehicle NEC V09.20 ☑
         specified type NEC V00.898 ☑
          collision (with) V09.9 ☑
            animal being ridden or animal drawn vehicle V06.99 ☑
              nontraffic V06.09 ☑
              traffic V06.19 ☑
            bus or heavy transport V04.99 ☑
              nontraffic V04.09 ☑
              traffic V04.19 ☑
            car V03.99 ☑
              nontraffic V03.09 ☑
              traffic V03.19 ☑
            pedal cycle V01.99 ☑
              nontraffic V01.09 ☑
              traffic V01.19 ☑
            pick-up truck or van V03.99 ☑
              nontraffic V03.09 ☑
              traffic V03.19 ☑
            railway (train) (vehicle) V05.99 ☑
              nontraffic V05.09 ☑
              traffic V05.19 ☑
            stationary object V00.892 ☑
            streetcar V06.99 ☑
              nontraffic V06.09 ☑
              traffic V06.19 ☑
            two- or three-wheeled motor vehicle V02.99 ☑
              nontraffic V02.09 ☑
              traffic V02.19 ☑
            vehicle V09.9 ☑
              animal-drawn V06.99 ☑
                nontraffic V06.09 ☑
                traffic V06.19 ☑
              motor
                nontraffic V09.00 ☑
                traffic V09.20 ☑
           fall V00.891 ☑
          nontraffic V09.1 ☑
            involving motor vehicle NEC V09.00 ☑
          traffic V09.3 ☑
            involving motor vehicle NEC V09.20 ☑
        standing
          electric scooter
            collsion with
              animal being ridden or animal drawn vehicle V06.931 ☑
                nontraffic V06.031 ☑
                traffic V06.131 ☑
              bus or heavy transport V04.931 ☑

Accident — *continued*
  transport — *continued*
    pedestrian — *continued*
      conveyance — *continued*
        standing — *continued*
          electric scooter — *continued*
            collsion with — *continued*
              bus or heavy transport — *continued*
                nontraffic V04.031 ☑
                traffic V04.131 ☑
              car V03.931 ☑
                nontraffic V04.031 ☑
                traffic V04.131 ☑
              pedal cycle V01.931 ☑
                nontraffic V01.031 ☑
                traffic V01.131 ☑
              pick-up or van V03.931 ☑
                nontraffic V03.031 ☑
                traffic V03.131 ☑
              railway (train) (vehicle) V05.931 ☑
                nontraffic V05.031 ☑
                traffic V05.131 ☑
              streetcar V06.931 ☑
                nontraffic V06.031 ☑
                traffic V06.131 ☑
              three-wheeled motor vehicle V02.931 ☑
                nontraffic V02.031 ☑
                traffic V02.131 ☑
              two-wheeled motor vehicle V02.931 ☑
                nontraffic V02.031 ☑
                traffic V02.131 ☑
              vehicle, nonmotor, specified NEC V06.931 ☑
                nontraffic V06.031 ☑
                traffic V06.131 ☑
           fall V00.841 ☑
          micro-mobility pedestrian conveyance
            collision with
              animal being ridden or animal drawn vehicle V06.938 ☑
                nontraffic V06.038 ☑
                traffic V06.138 ☑
              bus or heavy transport V04.938 ☑
                nontraffic V04.038 ☑
                traffic V04.138 ☑
              car V03.938 ☑
                nontraffic V03.038 ☑
                traffic V03.138 ☑
              pedal cycle V01.938 ☑
                nontraffic V01.038 ☑
                traffic V01.138 ☑
              pick-up or van V03.938 ☑
                nontraffic V03.038 ☑
                traffic V03.138 ☑
              railway (train) (vehicle) V05.938 ☑
                nontraffic V05.038 ☑
                traffic V05.138 ☑
              stationary object V00.842 ☑
              streetcar V06.938 ☑
                nontraffic V06.038 ☑
                traffic V06.138 ☑
              three-wheeled motor vehicle V02.938 ☑
                nontraffic V02.038 ☑
                traffic V02.138 ☑
              two-wheeled motor vehicle V02.938 ☑
                nontraffic V02.038 ☑
                traffic V02.138 ☑
              vehicle, nonmotor, specified NEC V06.938 ☑
                nontraffic V06.038 ☑
                traffic V06.138 ☑
           fall V00.848 ☑
        traffic V09.3 ☑
          involving motor vehicle V09.20 ☑
           military V09.21 ☑
           specified type NEC V09.29 ☑
        wheelchair (powered) V00.818 ☑
          collision (with) V09.9 ☑
            animal being ridden or animal drawn vehicle V06.99 ☑
              nontraffic V06.09 ☑

☑ **Additional Character Required — Refer to the Tabular List for Character Selection**   🔽 Subterms under main terms may continue to next column or page

Accident — *continued*
  transport — *continued*
    pedestrian — *continued*
      conveyance — *continued*
        wheelchair — *continued*
          collision — *continued*
            animal being ridden or animal drawn
              vehicle — *continued*
              traffic V06.19 ☑
            bus or heavy transport V04.99 ☑
              nontraffic V04.09 ☑
              traffic V04.19 ☑
            car V03.99 ☑
              nontraffic V03.09 ☑
              traffic V03.19 ☑
            pedal cycle V01.99 ☑
              nontraffic V01.09 ☑
              traffic V01.19 ☑
            pick-up truck or van V03.99 ☑
              nontraffic V03.09 ☑
              traffic V03.19 ☑
            railway (train) (vehicle) V05.99 ☑
              nontraffic V05.09 ☑
              traffic V05.19 ☑
            stationary object V00.812 ☑
            streetcar V06.99 ☑
              nontraffic V06.09 ☑
              traffic V06.19 ☑
            two- or three-wheeled motor vehicle
              V02.99 ☑
              nontraffic V02.09 ☑
              traffic V02.19 ☑
            vehicle V09.9 ☑
              animal-drawn V06.99 ☑
                nontraffic V06.09 ☑
                traffic V06.19 ☑
              motor
                nontraffic V09.00 ☑
                traffic V09.20 ☑
           fall V00.811 ☑
          nontraffic V09.1 ☑
            involving motor vehicle NEC V09.00 ☑
          traffic V09.3 ☑
            involving motor vehicle NEC V09.20 ☑
        wheeled shoe V00.158 ☑
          colliding with stationary object
            V00.152 ☑
          fall V00.151 ☑
    on foot — *see also* Accident, pedestrian
      collision (with)
        animal being ridden or animal drawn ve-
          hicle V06.90 ☑
          nontraffic V06.00 ☑
          traffic V06.10 ☑
        bus or heavy transport V04.90 ☑
          nontraffic V04.00 ☑
          traffic V04.10 ☑
        car V03.90 ☑
          nontraffic V03.00 ☑
          traffic V03.10 ☑
        pedal cycle V01.90 ☑
          nontraffic V01.00 ☑
          traffic V01.10 ☑
        pick-up truck or van V03.90 ☑
          nontraffic V03.00 ☑
          traffic V03.10 ☑
        railway (train) (vehicle) V05.90 ☑
          nontraffic V05.00 ☑
          traffic V05.10 ☑
        streetcar V06.90 ☑
          nontraffic V06.00 ☑
          traffic V06.10 ☑
        two- or three-wheeled motor vehicle
          V02.90 ☑
          nontraffic V02.00 ☑
          traffic V02.10 ☑
        vehicle V09.9 ☑
          animal-drawn V06.90 ☑
            nontraffic V06.00 ☑
            traffic V06.10 ☑
          motor
            nontraffic V09.1 ☑
            involving motor vehicle V09.00 ☑
              military V09.01 ☑
              specified type NEC V09.09 ☑
          traffic V09.3 ☑

Accident — *continued*
  transport — *continued*
    pedestrian — *continued*
      on foot — *see also* Accident, pedestrian — con-
        tinued
        traffic — *continued*
          involving motor vehicle V09.20 ☑
            military V09.21 ☑
            specified type NEC V09.29 ☑
      person NEC (unknown way or transportation) V99 ☑
        collision (between)
          bus (with)
            heavy transport vehicle (traffic) V87.5 ☑
              nontraffic V88.5 ☑
          car (with)
            bus (traffic) V87.3 ☑
              nontraffic V88.3 ☑
            heavy transport vehicle (traffic) V87.4 ☑
              nontraffic V88.4 ☑
            nontraffic V88.5 ☑
            pick-up truck or van (traffic) V87.2 ☑
              nontraffic V88.2 ☑
            train or railway vehicle (traffic) V87.6 ☑
              nontraffic V88.6 ☑
            two-or three-wheeled motor vehicle
              (traffic) V87.0 ☑
              nontraffic V88.0 ☑
          motor vehicle (traffic) NEC V87.7 ☑
            nontraffic V88.7 ☑
          two-or three-wheeled vehicle (with) (traffic)
            motor vehicle NEC V87.1 ☑
            nontraffic V88.1 ☑
          nonmotor vehicle (collision) (noncollision) (traf-
            fic) V87.9 ☑
            nontraffic V88.9 ☑
    pickup truck occupant V59.9 ☑
      collision (with)
        animal (traffic) V50.9 ☑
          being ridden (traffic) V56.9 ☑
            nontraffic V56.3 ☑
            while boarding or alighting V56.4 ☑
          nontraffic V50.3 ☑
          while boarding or alighting V50.4 ☑
        animal-drawn vehicle (traffic) V56.9 ☑
          nontraffic V56.3 ☑
          while boarding or alighting V56.4 ☑
        bus (traffic) V54.9 ☑
          nontraffic V54.3 ☑
          while boarding or alighting V54.4 ☑
        car (traffic) V53.9 ☑
          nontraffic V53.3 ☑
          while boarding or alighting V53.4 ☑
        motor vehicle NOS (traffic) V59.60 ☑
          nontraffic V59.20 ☑
          specified type NEC (traffic) V59.69 ☑
            nontraffic V59.29 ☑
        pedal cycle (traffic) V51.9 ☑
          nontraffic V51.3 ☑
          while boarding or alighting V51.4 ☑
        pickup truck (traffic) V53.9 ☑
          nontraffic V53.3 ☑
          while boarding or alighting V53.4 ☑
        railway vehicle (traffic) V55.9 ☑
          nontraffic V55.3 ☑
          while boarding or alighting V55.4 ☑
        specified vehicle NEC (traffic) V56.9 ☑
          nontraffic V56.3 ☑
          while boarding or alighting V56.4 ☑
        stationary object (traffic) V57.9 ☑
          nontraffic V57.3 ☑
          while boarding or alighting V57.4 ☑
        streetcar (traffic) V56.9 ☑
          nontraffic V56.3 ☑
          while boarding or alighting V56.4 ☑
        three wheeled motor vehicle (traffic) V52.9 ☑
          nontraffic V52.3 ☑
          while boarding or alighting V52.4 ☑
        truck (traffic) V54.9 ☑
          nontraffic V54.3 ☑
          while boarding or alighting V54.4 ☑
        two wheeled motor vehicle (traffic) V52.9 ☑
          nontraffic V52.3 ☑
          while boarding or alighting V52.4 ☑
        van (traffic) V53.9 ☑
          nontraffic V53.3 ☑
          while boarding or alighting V53.4 ☑

Accident — *continued*
  transport — *continued*
    pickup truck occupant — *continued*
      driver
        collision (with)
          animal (traffic) V50.5 ☑
            being ridden (traffic) V56.5 ☑
              nontraffic V56.0 ☑
            nontraffic V50.0 ☑
          animal-drawn vehicle (traffic) V56.5 ☑
            nontraffic V56.0 ☑
          bus (traffic) V54.5 ☑
            nontraffic V54.0 ☑
          car (traffic) V53.5 ☑
            nontraffic V53.0 ☑
          motor vehicle NOS (traffic) V59.40 ☑
            nontraffic V59.00 ☑
            specified type NEC (traffic) V59.49 ☑
              nontraffic V59.09 ☑
          pedal cycle (traffic) V51.5 ☑
            nontraffic V51.0 ☑
          pickup truck (traffic) V53.5 ☑
            nontraffic V53.0 ☑
          railway vehicle (traffic) V55.5 ☑
            nontraffic V55.0 ☑
          specified vehicle NEC (traffic) V56.5 ☑
            nontraffic V56.0 ☑
          stationary object (traffic) V57.5 ☑
            nontraffic V57.0 ☑
          streetcar (traffic) V56.5 ☑
            nontraffic V56.0 ☑
          three wheeled motor vehicle (traffic)
            V52.5 ☑
            nontraffic V52.0 ☑
          truck (traffic) V54.5 ☑
            nontraffic V54.0 ☑
          two wheeled motor vehicle (traffic)
            V52.5 ☑
            nontraffic V52.0 ☑
          van (traffic) V53.5 ☑
            nontraffic V53.0 ☑
        noncollision accident (traffic) V58.5 ☑
          nontraffic V58.0 ☑
      hanger-on
        collision (with)
          animal (traffic) V50.7 ☑
            being ridden (traffic) V56.7 ☑
              nontraffic V56.2 ☑
            nontraffic V50.2 ☑
          animal-drawn vehicle (traffic) V56.7 ☑
            nontraffic V56.2 ☑
          bus (traffic) V54.7 ☑
            nontraffic V54.2 ☑
          car (traffic) V53.7 ☑
            nontraffic V53.2 ☑
          pedal cycle (traffic) V51.7 ☑
            nontraffic V51.2 ☑
          pickup truck (traffic) V53.7 ☑
            nontraffic V53.2 ☑
          railway vehicle (traffic) V55.7 ☑
            nontraffic V55.2 ☑
          specified vehicle NEC (traffic) V56.7 ☑
            nontraffic V56.2 ☑
          stationary object (traffic) V57.7 ☑
            nontraffic V57.2 ☑
          streetcar (traffic) V56.7 ☑
            nontraffic V56.2 ☑
          three wheeled motor vehicle (traffic)
            V52.7 ☑
            nontraffic V52.2 ☑
          truck (traffic) V54.7 ☑
            nontraffic V54.2 ☑
          two wheeled motor vehicle (traffic)
            V52.7 ☑
            nontraffic V52.2 ☑
          van (traffic) V53.7 ☑
            nontraffic V53.2 ☑
        noncollision accident (traffic) V58.7 ☑
          nontraffic V58.2 ☑
      noncollision accident (traffic) V58.9 ☑
        nontraffic V58.3 ☑
        while boarding or alighting V58.4 ☑
      nontraffic V59.3 ☑
      passenger
        collision (with)
          animal (traffic) V50.6 ☑

Accident — *continued*
  transport — *continued*
    pickup truck occupant — *continued*
      passenger — *continued*
        collision — *continued*
          animal — *continued*
            being ridden (traffic) V56.6 ☑
              nontraffic V56.1 ☑
              nontraffic V50.1 ☑
            animal-drawn vehicle (traffic) V56.6 ☑
              nontraffic V56.1 ☑
            bus (traffic) V54.6 ☑
              nontraffic V54.1 ☑
            car (traffic) V53.6 ☑
              nontraffic V53.1 ☑
            motor vehicle NOS (traffic) V59.50 ☑
              nontraffic V59.10 ☑
              specified type NEC (traffic) V59.59 ☑
                nontraffic V59.19 ☑
            pedal cycle (traffic) V51.6 ☑
              nontraffic V51.1 ☑
            pickup truck (traffic) V53.6 ☑
              nontraffic V53.1 ☑
            railway vehicle (traffic) V55.6 ☑
              nontraffic V55.1 ☑
            specified vehicle NEC (traffic) V56.6 ☑
              nontraffic V56.1 ☑
            stationary object (traffic) V57.6 ☑
              nontraffic V57.1 ☑
            streetcar (traffic) V56.6 ☑
              nontraffic V56.1 ☑
            three wheeled motor vehicle (traffic) V52.6 ☑
              nontraffic V52.1 ☑
            truck (traffic) V54.6 ☑
              nontraffic V54.1 ☑
            two wheeled motor vehicle (traffic) V52.6 ☑
              nontraffic V52.1 ☑
            van (traffic) V53.6 ☑
              nontraffic V53.1 ☑
        noncollision accident (traffic) V58.6 ☑
          nontraffic V58.1 ☑
      specified type NEC V59.88 ☑
      military vehicle V59.81 ☑
    quarry truck — *see* Accident, transport, industrial vehicle occupant
    race car — *see* Accident, transport, motor vehicle NEC occupant
    railway vehicle occupant V81.9 ☑
      collision (with) V81.3 ☑
        motor vehicle (non-military) (traffic) V81.1 ☑
          military V81.83 ☑
          nontraffic V81.0 ☑
        rolling stock V81.2 ☑
        specified object NEC V81.3 ☑
      during derailment V81.7 ☑
        with antecedent collision — *see* Accident, transport, railway vehicle occupant, collision
      explosion V81.81 ☑
      fall (in railway vehicle) V81.5 ☑
        during derailment V81.7 ☑
          with antecedent collision — *see* Accident, transport, railway vehicle occupant, collision
        from railway vehicle V81.6 ☑
          during derailment V81.7 ☑
            with antecedent collision — *see* Accident, transport, railway vehicle occupant, collision
        while boarding or alighting V81.4 ☑
      fire V81.81 ☑
      object falling onto train V81.82 ☑
      specified type NEC V81.89 ☑
      while boarding or alighting V81.4 ☑
    Segway V00.848 ☑
    ski lift V98.3 ☑
    snowmobile occupant (nontraffic) V86.92 ☑
      driver V86.52 ☑
      hanger-on V86.72 ☑
      passenger V86.62 ☑
      traffic V86.32 ☑
        driver V86.02 ☑
        hanger-on V86.22 ☑
        passenger V86.12 ☑

Accident — *continued*
  transport — *continued*
    snowmobile occupant — *continued*
      while boarding or alighting V86.42 ☑
    specified NEC V98.8 ☑
    sport utility vehicle occupant — *see also* Accident, transport, pickup truck occupant
    streetcar occupant V82.9 ☑
      collision (with) V82.3 ☑
        motor vehicle (traffic) V82.1 ☑
          nontraffic V82.0 ☑
        rolling stock V82.2 ☑
      during derailment V82.7 ☑
        with antecedent collision — *see* Accident, transport, streetcar occupant, collision
      fall (in streetcar) V82.5 ☑
        during derailment V82.7 ☑
          with antecedent collision — *see* Accident, transport, streetcar occupant, collision
      from streetcar V82.6 ☑
        during derailment V82.7 ☑
          with antecedent collision — *see* Accident, transport, streetcar occupant, collision
        while boarding or alighting V82.4 ☑
      while boarding or alighting V82.4 ☑
      specified type NEC V82.8 ☑
      while boarding or alighting V82.4 ☑
    three-wheeled motor vehicle occupant V39.9 ☑
      collision (with)
        animal (traffic) V30.9 ☑
          being ridden (traffic) V36.9 ☑
            nontraffic V36.3 ☑
            while boarding or alighting V36.4 ☑
          nontraffic V30.3 ☑
          while boarding or alighting V30.4 ☑
        animal-drawn vehicle (traffic) V36.9 ☑
          nontraffic V36.3 ☑
          while boarding or alighting V36.4 ☑
        bus (traffic) V34.9 ☑
          nontraffic V34.3 ☑
          while boarding or alighting V34.4 ☑
        car (traffic) V33.9 ☑
          nontraffic V33.3 ☑
          while boarding or alighting V33.4 ☑
        motor vehicle NOS (traffic) V39.60 ☑
          nontraffic V39.20 ☑
          specified type NEC (traffic) V39.69 ☑
            nontraffic V39.29 ☑
        pedal cycle (traffic) V31.9 ☑
          nontraffic V31.3 ☑
          while boarding or alighting V31.4 ☑
        pickup truck (traffic) V33.9 ☑
          nontraffic V33.3 ☑
          while boarding or alighting V33.4 ☑
        railway vehicle (traffic) V35.9 ☑
          nontraffic V35.3 ☑
          while boarding or alighting V35.4 ☑
        specified vehicle NEC (traffic) V36.9 ☑
          nontraffic V36.3 ☑
          while boarding or alighting V36.4 ☑
        stationary object (traffic) V37.9 ☑
          nontraffic V37.3 ☑
          while boarding or alighting V37.4 ☑
        streetcar (traffic) V36.9 ☑
          nontraffic V36.3 ☑
          while boarding or alighting V36.4 ☑
        three wheeled motor vehicle (traffic) V32.9 ☑
          nontraffic V32.3 ☑
          while boarding or alighting V32.4 ☑
        truck (traffic) V34.9 ☑
          nontraffic V34.3 ☑
          while boarding or alighting V34.4 ☑
        two wheeled motor vehicle (traffic) V32.9 ☑
          nontraffic V32.3 ☑
          while boarding or alighting V32.4 ☑
        van (traffic) V33.9 ☑
          nontraffic V33.3 ☑
          while boarding or alighting V33.4 ☑
      driver
        collision (with)
          animal (traffic) V30.5 ☑
            being ridden (traffic) V36.5 ☑
              nontraffic V36.0 ☑
            nontraffic V30.0 ☑

Accident — *continued*
  transport — *continued*
    three-wheeled motor vehicle occupant — *continued*
      driver — *continued*
        collision — *continued*
          animal-drawn vehicle (traffic) V36.5 ☑
            nontraffic V36.0 ☑
          bus (traffic) V34.5 ☑
            nontraffic V34.0 ☑
          car (traffic) V33.5 ☑
            nontraffic V33.0 ☑
          motor vehicle NOS (traffic) V39.40 ☑
            nontraffic V39.00 ☑
            specified type NEC (traffic) V39.49 ☑
              nontraffic V39.09 ☑
          pedal cycle (traffic) V31.5 ☑
            nontraffic V31.0 ☑
          pickup truck (traffic) V33.5 ☑
            nontraffic V33.0 ☑
          railway vehicle (traffic) V35.5 ☑
            nontraffic V35.0 ☑
          specified vehicle NEC (traffic) V36.5 ☑
            nontraffic V36.0 ☑
          stationary object (traffic) V37.5 ☑
            nontraffic V37.0 ☑
          streetcar (traffic) V36.5 ☑
            nontraffic V36.0 ☑
          three wheeled motor vehicle (traffic) V32.5 ☑
            nontraffic V32.0 ☑
          truck (traffic) V34.5 ☑
            nontraffic V34.0 ☑
          two wheeled motor vehicle (traffic) V32.5 ☑
            nontraffic V32.0 ☑
          van (traffic) V33.5 ☑
            nontraffic V33.0 ☑
        noncollision accident (traffic) V38.5 ☑
          nontraffic V38.0 ☑
      hanger-on
        collision (with)
          animal (traffic) V30.7 ☑
            being ridden (traffic) V36.7 ☑
              nontraffic V36.2 ☑
            nontraffic V30.2 ☑
          animal-drawn vehicle (traffic) V36.7 ☑
            nontraffic V36.2 ☑
          bus (traffic) V34.7 ☑
            nontraffic V34.2 ☑
          car (traffic) V33.7 ☑
            nontraffic V33.2 ☑
          pedal cycle (traffic) V31.7 ☑
            nontraffic V31.2 ☑
          pickup truck (traffic) V33.7 ☑
            nontraffic V33.2 ☑
          railway vehicle (traffic) V35.7 ☑
            nontraffic V35.2 ☑
          specified vehicle NEC (traffic) V36.7 ☑
            nontraffic V36.2 ☑
          stationary object (traffic) V37.7 ☑
            nontraffic V37.2 ☑
          streetcar (traffic) V36.7 ☑
            nontraffic V36.2 ☑
          three wheeled motor vehicle (traffic) V32.7 ☑
            nontraffic V32.2 ☑
          truck (traffic) V34.7 ☑
            nontraffic V34.2 ☑
          two wheeled motor vehicle (traffic) V32.7 ☑
            nontraffic V32.2 ☑
          van (traffic) V33.7 ☑
            nontraffic V33.2 ☑
        noncollision accident (traffic) V38.7 ☑
          nontraffic V38.2 ☑
      noncollision accident (traffic) V38.9 ☑
        nontraffic V38.3 ☑
        while boarding or alighting V38.4 ☑
      nontraffic V39.3 ☑
      passenger
        collision (with)
          animal (traffic) V30.6 ☑
            being ridden (traffic) V36.6 ☑
              nontraffic V36.1 ☑
            nontraffic V30.1 ☑

Accident — *continued*
  transport — *continued*
    three-wheeled motor vehicle occupant — *continued*
      passenger — *continued*
        collision — *continued*
          animal-drawn vehicle (traffic) V36.6 ☑
            nontraffic V36.1 ☑
          bus (traffic) V34.6 ☑
            nontraffic V34.1 ☑
          car (traffic) V33.6 ☑
            nontraffic V33.1 ☑
          motor vehicle NOS (traffic) V39.50 ☑
            nontraffic V39.10 ☑
            specified type NEC (traffic) V39.59 ☑
              nontraffic V39.19 ☑
          pedal cycle (traffic) V31.6 ☑
            nontraffic V31.1 ☑
          pickup truck (traffic) V33.6 ☑
            nontraffic V33.1 ☑
          railway vehicle (traffic) V35.6 ☑
            nontraffic V35.1 ☑
          specified vehicle NEC (traffic) V36.6 ☑
            nontraffic V36.1 ☑
          stationary object (traffic) V37.6 ☑
            nontraffic V37.1 ☑
          streetcar (traffic) V36.6 ☑
            nontraffic V36.1 ☑
          three wheeled motor vehicle (traffic) V32.6 ☑
            nontraffic V32.1 ☑
          truck (traffic) V34.6 ☑
            nontraffic V34.1 ☑
          two wheeled motor vehicle (traffic) V32.6 ☑
            nontraffic V32.1 ☑
          van (traffic) V33.6 ☑
            nontraffic V33.1 ☑
        noncollision accident (traffic) V38.6 ☑
          nontraffic V38.1 ☑
        specified type NEC V39.89 ☑
        military vehicle V39.81 ☑
    tractor (farm) (and trailer) — *see* Accident, transport, agricultural vehicle occupant
    tram — *see* Accident, transport, streetcar
      in mine or quarry — *see* Accident, transport, industrial vehicle occupant
    trolley — *see* Accident, transport, streetcar
      in mine or quarry — *see* Accident, transport, industrial vehicle occupant
    truck (heavy) occupant V69.9 ☑
      collision (with)
        animal (traffic) V60.9 ☑
          being ridden (traffic) V66.9 ☑
            nontraffic V66.3 ☑
            while boarding or alighting V66.4 ☑
          nontraffic V60.3 ☑
          while boarding or alighting V60.4 ☑
        animal-drawn vehicle (traffic) V66.9 ☑
          nontraffic V66.3 ☑
          while boarding or alighting V66.4 ☑
        bus (traffic) V64.9 ☑
          nontraffic V64.3 ☑
          while boarding or alighting V64.4 ☑
        car (traffic) V63.9 ☑
          nontraffic V63.3 ☑
          while boarding or alighting V63.4 ☑
        motor vehicle NOS (traffic) V69.60 ☑
          nontraffic V69.20 ☑
          specified type NEC (traffic) V69.69 ☑
            nontraffic V69.29 ☑
        pedal cycle (traffic) V61.9 ☑
          nontraffic V61.3 ☑
          while boarding or alighting V61.4 ☑
        pickup truck (traffic) V63.9 ☑
          nontraffic V63.3 ☑
          while boarding or alighting V63.4 ☑
        railway vehicle (traffic) V65.9 ☑
          nontraffic V65.3 ☑
          while boarding or alighting V65.4 ☑
        specified vehicle NEC (traffic) V66.9 ☑
          nontraffic V66.3 ☑
          while boarding or alighting V66.4 ☑
        stationary object (traffic) V67.9 ☑
          nontraffic V67.3 ☑
          while boarding or alighting V67.4 ☑

Accident — *continued*
  transport — *continued*
    truck occupant — *continued*
      collision — *continued*
        streetcar (traffic) V66.9 ☑
          nontraffic V66.3 ☑
          while boarding or alighting V66.4 ☑
        three wheeled motor vehicle (traffic) V62.9 ☑
          nontraffic V62.3 ☑
          while boarding or alighting V62.4 ☑
        truck (traffic) V64.9 ☑
          nontraffic V64.3 ☑
          while boarding or alighting V64.4 ☑
        two wheeled motor vehicle (traffic) V62.9 ☑
          nontraffic V62.3 ☑
          while boarding or alighting V62.4 ☑
        van (traffic) V63.9 ☑
          nontraffic V63.3 ☑
          while boarding or alighting V63.4 ☑
      driver
        collision (with)
          animal (traffic) V60.5 ☑
            being ridden (traffic) V66.5 ☑
              nontraffic V66.0 ☑
            nontraffic V60.0 ☑
          animal-drawn vehicle (traffic) V66.5 ☑
            nontraffic V66.0 ☑
          bus (traffic) V64.5 ☑
            nontraffic V64.0 ☑
          car (traffic) V63.5 ☑
            nontraffic V63.0 ☑
          motor vehicle NOS (traffic) V69.40 ☑
            nontraffic V69.00 ☑
            specified type NEC (traffic) V69.49 ☑
              nontraffic V69.09 ☑
          pedal cycle (traffic) V61.5 ☑
            nontraffic V61.0 ☑
          pickup truck (traffic) V63.5 ☑
            nontraffic V63.0 ☑
          railway vehicle (traffic) V65.5 ☑
          specified vehicle NEC (traffic) V66.5 ☑
            nontraffic V66.0 ☑
          stationary object (traffic) V67.5 ☑
            nontraffic V67.0 ☑
          streetcar (traffic) V66.5 ☑
            nontraffic V66.0 ☑
          three wheeled motor vehicle (traffic) V62.5 ☑
            nontraffic V62.0 ☑
          truck (traffic) V64.5 ☑
            nontraffic V64.0 ☑
          two wheeled motor vehicle (traffic) V62.5 ☑
            nontraffic V62.0 ☑
          van (traffic) V63.5 ☑
            nontraffic V63.0 ☑
        noncollision accident (traffic) V68.5 ☑
          nontraffic V68.0 ☑
      dump — *see* Accident, transport, construction vehicle occupant
      hanger-on
        collision (with)
          animal (traffic) V60.7 ☑
            being ridden (traffic) V66.7 ☑
              nontraffic V66.2 ☑
            nontraffic V60.2 ☑
          animal-drawn vehicle (traffic) V66.7 ☑
            nontraffic V66.2 ☑
          bus (traffic) V64.7 ☑
            nontraffic V64.2 ☑
          car (traffic) V63.7 ☑
            nontraffic V63.2 ☑
          pedal cycle (traffic) V61.7 ☑
            nontraffic V61.2 ☑
          pickup truck (traffic) V63.7 ☑
            nontraffic V63.2 ☑
          railway vehicle (traffic) V65.7 ☑
            nontraffic V65.2 ☑
          specified vehicle NEC (traffic) V66.7 ☑
            nontraffic V66.2 ☑
          stationary object (traffic) V67.7 ☑
            nontraffic V67.2 ☑
          streetcar (traffic) V66.7 ☑
            nontraffic V66.2 ☑

Accident — *continued*
  transport — *continued*
    truck occupant — *continued*
      hanger-on — *continued*
        collision — *continued*
          three wheeled motor vehicle (traffic) V62.7 ☑
            nontraffic V62.2 ☑
          truck (traffic) V64.7 ☑
            nontraffic V64.2 ☑
          two wheeled motor vehicle (traffic) V62.7 ☑
            nontraffic V62.2 ☑
          van (traffic) V63.7 ☑
            nontraffic V63.2 ☑
        noncollision accident (traffic) V68.7 ☑
          nontraffic V68.2 ☑
      noncollision accident (traffic) V68.9 ☑
        nontraffic V68.3 ☑
        while boarding or alighting V68.4 ☑
      nontraffic V69.3 ☑
      passenger
        collision (with)
          animal (traffic) V60.6 ☑
            being ridden (traffic) V66.6 ☑
              nontraffic V66.1-
            nontraffic V60.1 ☑
          animal-drawn vehicle (traffic) V66.6 ☑
            nontraffic V66.1 ☑
          bus (traffic) V64.6 ☑
            nontraffic V64.1 ☑
          car (traffic) V63.6 ☑
            nontraffic V63.1 ☑
          motor vehicle NOS (traffic) V69.50 ☑
            nontraffic V69.10 ☑
            specified type NEC (traffic) V69.59 ☑
              nontraffic V69.19 ☑
          pedal cycle (traffic) V61.6 ☑
            nontraffic V61.1 ☑
          pickup truck (traffic) V63.6 ☑
            nontraffic V63.1 ☑
          railway vehicle (traffic) V65.6 ☑
            nontraffic V65.1 ☑
          specified vehicle NEC (traffic) V66.6 ☑
            nontraffic V66.1 ☑
          stationary object (traffic) V67.6 ☑
            nontraffic V67.1 ☑
          streetcar (traffic) V66.6 ☑
            nontraffic V66.1 ☑
          three wheeled motor vehicle (traffic) V62.6 ☑
            nontraffic V62.1 ☑
          truck (traffic) V64.6 ☑
            nontraffic V64.1 ☑
          two wheeled motor vehicle (traffic) V62.6 ☑
            nontraffic V62.1 ☑
          van (traffic) V63.6 ☑
            nontraffic V63.1 ☑
        noncollision accident (traffic) V68.6 ☑
          nontraffic V68.1 ☑
      pickup — *see* Accident, transport, pickup truck occupant
      specified type NEC V69.88 ☑
      military vehicle V69.81 ☑
    van occupant V59.9 ☑
      collision (with)
        animal (traffic) V50.9 ☑
          being ridden (traffic) V56.9 ☑
            nontraffic V56.3 ☑
            while boarding or alighting V56.4 ☑
          nontraffic V50.3 ☑
          while boarding or alighting V50.4 ☑
        animal-drawn vehicle (traffic) V56.9 ☑
          nontraffic V56.3 ☑
          while boarding or alighting V56.4 ☑
        bus (traffic) V54.9 ☑
          nontraffic V54.3 ☑
          while boarding or alighting V54.4 ☑
        car (traffic) V53.9 ☑
          nontraffic V53.3 ☑
          while boarding or alighting V53.4 ☑
        motor vehicle NOS (traffic) V59.60 ☑
          nontraffic V59.20 ☑
          specified type NEC (traffic) V59.69 ☑
            nontraffic V59.29 ☑

Accident — *continued*
  transport — *continued*
    van occupant — *continued*
      collision — *continued*
        pedal cycle (traffic) V51.9 ☑
          nontraffic V51.3 ☑
          while boarding or alighting V51.4 ☑
        pickup truck (traffic) V53.9 ☑
          nontraffic V53.3 ☑
          while boarding or alighting V53.4 ☑
        railway vehicle (traffic) V55.9 ☑
          nontraffic V55.3 ☑
          while boarding or alighting V55.4 ☑
        specified vehicle NEC (traffic) V56.9 ☑
          nontraffic V56.3 ☑
          while boarding or alighting V56.4 ☑
        stationary object (traffic) V57.9 ☑
          nontraffic V57.3 ☑
          while boarding or alighting V57.4 ☑
        streetcar (traffic) V56.9 ☑
          nontraffic V56.3 ☑
          while boarding or alighting V56.4 ☑
        three wheeled motor vehicle (traffic) V52.9 ☑
          nontraffic V52.3 ☑
          while boarding or alighting V52.4 ☑
        truck (traffic) V54.9 ☑
          nontraffic V54.3 ☑
          while boarding or alighting V54.4 ☑
        two wheeled motor vehicle (traffic) V52.9 ☑
          nontraffic V52.3 ☑
          while boarding or alighting V52.4 ☑
        van (traffic) V53.9 ☑
          nontraffic V53.3 ☑
          while boarding or alighting V53.4 ☑
    driver
      collision (with)
        animal (traffic) V50.5 ☑
          being ridden (traffic) V56.5 ☑
            nontraffic V56.0 ☑
          nontraffic V50.0 ☑
        animal-drawn vehicle (traffic) V56.5 ☑
          nontraffic V56.0 ☑
        bus (traffic) V54.5 ☑
          nontraffic V54.0 ☑
        car (traffic) V53.5 ☑
          nontraffic V53.0 ☑
        motor vehicle NOS (traffic) V59.40 ☑
          nontraffic V59.00 ☑
          specified type NEC (traffic) V59.49 ☑
            nontraffic V59.09 ☑
        pedal cycle (traffic) V51.5 ☑
          nontraffic V51.0 ☑
        pickup truck (traffic) V53.5 ☑
          nontraffic V53.0 ☑
        railway vehicle (traffic) V55.5 ☑
          nontraffic V55.0 ☑
        specified vehicle NEC (traffic) V56.5 ☑
          nontraffic V56.0 ☑
        stationary object (traffic) V57.5 ☑
          nontraffic V57.0 ☑
        streetcar (traffic) V56.5 ☑
          nontraffic V56.0 ☑
        three wheeled motor vehicle (traffic) V52.5 ☑
          nontraffic V52.0 ☑
        truck (traffic) V54.5 ☑
          nontraffic V54.0 ☑
        two wheeled motor vehicle (traffic) V52.5 ☑
          nontraffic V52.0 ☑
        van (traffic) V53.5 ☑
          nontraffic V53.0 ☑
      noncollision accident (traffic) V58.5 ☑
        nontraffic V58.0 ☑
    hanger-on
      collision (with)
        animal (traffic) V50.7 ☑
          being ridden (traffic) V56.7 ☑
            nontraffic V56.2 ☑
          nontraffic V50.2 ☑
        animal-drawn vehicle (traffic) V56.7 ☑
          nontraffic V56.2 ☑
        bus (traffic) V54.7 ☑
          nontraffic V54.2 ☑
        car (traffic) V53.7 ☑
          nontraffic V53.2 ☑

Accident — *continued*
  transport — *continued*
    van occupant — *continued*
      hanger-on — *continued*
        collision — *continued*
          pedal cycle (traffic) V51.7 ☑
            nontraffic V51.2 ☑
          pickup truck (traffic) V53.7 ☑
            nontraffic V53.2 ☑
          railway vehicle (traffic) V55.7 ☑
            nontraffic V55.2 ☑
          specified vehicle NEC (traffic) V56.7 ☑
            nontraffic V56.2 ☑
          stationary object (traffic) V57.7 ☑
            nontraffic V57.2 ☑
          streetcar (traffic) V56.7 ☑
            nontraffic V56.2 ☑
          three wheeled motor vehicle (traffic) V52.7 ☑
            nontraffic V52.2 ☑
          truck (traffic) V54.7 ☑
            nontraffic V54.2 ☑
          two wheeled motor vehicle (traffic) V52.7 ☑
            nontraffic V52.2 ☑
          van (traffic) V53.7 ☑
            nontraffic V53.2 ☑
        noncollision accident (traffic) V58.7 ☑
          nontraffic V58.2 ☑
      noncollision accident (traffic) V58.9 ☑
        nontraffic V58.3 ☑
        while boarding or alighting V58.4 ☑
      nontraffic V59.3 ☑
      passenger
        collision (with)
          animal (traffic) V50.6 ☑
            being ridden (traffic) V56.6 ☑
              nontraffic V56.1 ☑
            nontraffic V50.1 ☑
          animal-drawn vehicle (traffic) V56.6 ☑
            nontraffic V56.1 ☑
          bus (traffic) V54.6 ☑
            nontraffic V54.1 ☑
          car (traffic) V53.6 ☑
            nontraffic V53.1 ☑
          motor vehicle NOS (traffic) V59.50 ☑
            nontraffic V59.10 ☑
            specified type NEC (traffic) V59.59 ☑
              nontraffic V59.19 ☑
          pedal cycle (traffic) V51.6 ☑
            nontraffic V51.1 ☑
          pickup truck (traffic) V53.6 ☑
            nontraffic V53.1 ☑
          railway vehicle (traffic) V55.6 ☑
            nontraffic V55.1 ☑
          specified vehicle NEC (traffic) V56.6 ☑
            nontraffic V56.1 ☑
          stationary object (traffic) V57.6 ☑
            nontraffic V57.1 ☑
          streetcar (traffic) V56.6 ☑
            nontraffic V56.1 ☑
          three wheeled motor vehicle (traffic) V52.6 ☑
            nontraffic V52.1 ☑
          truck (traffic) V54.6 ☑
            nontraffic V54.1 ☑
          two wheeled motor vehicle (traffic) V52.6 ☑
            nontraffic V52.1 ☑
          van (traffic) V53.6 ☑
            nontraffic V53.1 ☑
        noncollision accident (traffic) V58.6 ☑
          nontraffic V58.1 ☑
      specified type NEC V59.88 ☑
      military vehicle V59.81 ☑
    watercraft occupant — *see* Accident, watercraft
  vehicle NEC V89.9 ☑
    animal-drawn NEC — *see* Accident, transport, animal-drawn vehicle occupant
    special
      agricultural — *see* Accident, transport, agricultural vehicle occupant
      construction — *see* Accident, transport, construction vehicle occupant
      industrial — *see* Accident, transport, industrial vehicle occupant

Accident — *continued*
  vehicle — *continued*
    three-wheeled NEC (motorized) — *see* Accident, transport, three-wheeled motor vehicle occupant
  watercraft V94.9 ☑
    causing
      drowning — *see* Drowning, due to, accident to, watercraft
      injury NEC V91.89 ☑
        crushed between craft and object V91.19 ☑
          powered craft V91.13 ☑
            ferry boat V91.11 ☑
            fishing boat V91.12 ☑
            jetskis V91.13 ☑
            liner V91.11 ☑
            merchant ship V91.10 ☑
            passenger ship V91.11 ☑
          unpowered craft V91.18 ☑
            canoe V91.15 ☑
            inflatable V91.16 ☑
            kayak V91.15 ☑
            sailboat V91.14 ☑
            surf-board V91.18 ☑
            windsurfer V91.18 ☑
        fall on board V91.29 ☑
          powered craft V91.23 ☑
            ferry boat V91.21 ☑
            fishing boat V91.22 ☑
            jetskis V91.23 ☑
            liner V91.21 ☑
            merchant ship V91.20 ☑
            passenger ship V91.21 ☑
          unpowered craft
            canoe V91.25 ☑
            inflatable V91.26 ☑
            kayak V91.25 ☑
            sailboat V91.24 ☑
        fire on board causing burn V91.09 ☑
          powered craft V91.03 ☑
            ferry boat V91.01 ☑
            fishing boat V91.02 ☑
            jetskis V91.03 ☑
            liner V91.01 ☑
            merchant ship V91.00 ☑
            passenger ship V91.01 ☑
          unpowered craft V91.08 ☑
            canoe V91.05 ☑
            inflatable V91.06 ☑
            kayak V91.05 ☑
            sailboat V91.04 ☑
            surf-board V91.08 ☑
            water skis V91.07 ☑
            windsurfer V91.08 ☑
        hit by falling object V91.39 ☑
          powered craft V91.33 ☑
            ferry boat V91.31 ☑
            fishing boat V91.32 ☑
            jetskis V91.33 ☑
            liner V91.31 ☑
            merchant ship V91.30 ☑
            passenger ship V91.31 ☑
          unpowered craft V91.38 ☑
            canoe V91.35 ☑
            inflatable V91.36 ☑
            kayak V91.35 ☑
            sailboat V91.34 ☑
            surf-board V91.38 ☑
            water skis V91.37 ☑
            windsurfer V91.38 ☑
        specified type NEC V91.89 ☑
          powered craft V91.83 ☑
            ferry boat V91.81 ☑
            fishing boat V91.82 ☑
            jetskis V91.83 ☑
            liner V91.81 ☑
            merchant ship V91.80 ☑
            passenger ship V91.81 ☑
          unpowered craft V91.88 ☑
            canoe V91.85 ☑
            inflatable V91.86 ☑
            kayak V91.85 ☑
            sailboat V91.84 ☑
            surf-board V91.88 ☑
            water skis V91.87 ☑
            windsurfer V91.88 ☑

Accident — *continued*
  watercraft — *continued*
    due to, caused by cataclysm — *see* Forces of nature, by type
    military NEC V94.818 ☑
      civilian in water injured by V94.811 ☑
      with civilian watercraft V94.810 ☑
    nonpowered, struck by
      nonpowered vessel V94.22 ☑
      powered vessel V94.21 ☑
    specified type NEC V94.89 ☑
    striking swimmer
      powered V94.11 ☑
      unpowered V94.12 ☑
Acid throwing (assault) Y08.89 ☑
Activity (involving) (of victim at time of event) Y93.9
  aerobic and step exercise (class) Y93.A3 (*following* Y93.7)
  alpine skiing Y93.23
  animal care NEC Y93.K9 (*following* Y93.7)
  arts and handcrafts NEC Y93.D9 (*following* Y93.7)
  athletics played as a team or group NEC Y93.69
  athletics played individually NEC Y93.59
  athletics NEC Y93.79
  baking Y93.G3 (*following* Y93.7)
  ballet Y93.41
  barbells Y93.B3 (*following* Y93.7)
  BASE (Building, Antenna, Span, Earth) jumping Y93.33
  baseball Y93.64
  basketball Y93.67
  bathing (personal) Y93.E1 (*following* Y93.7)
  beach volleyball Y93.68
  bike riding Y93.55
  blackout game Y93.85
  boogie boarding Y93.18
  bowling Y93.54
  boxing Y93.71
  brass instrument playing Y93.J4 (*following* Y93.7)
  building construction Y93.H3 (*following* Y93.7)
  bungee jumping Y93.34
  calisthenics Y93.A2 (*following* Y93.7)
  canoeing (in calm and turbulent water) Y93.16
  capture the flag Y93.6A
  cardiorespiratory exercise NEC Y93.A9 (*following* Y93.7)
  caregiving (providing) NEC Y93.F9 (*following* Y93.7)
    bathing Y93.F1 (*following* Y93.7)
    lifting Y93.F2 (*following* Y93.7)
  cellular
    communication device Y93.C2 (*following* Y93.7)
    telephone Y93.C2 (*following* Y93.7)
  challenge course Y93.A5 (*following* Y93.7)
  cheerleading Y93.45
  choking game Y93.85
  circuit training Y93.A4 (*following* Y93.7)
  cleaning
    floor Y93.E5 (*following* Y93.7)
  climbing NEC Y93.39
    mountain Y93.31
    rock Y93.31
    wall Y93.31
  clothing care and maintenance NEC Y93.E9 (*following* Y93.7)
  combatives Y93.75
  computer
    keyboarding Y93.C1 (*following* Y93.7)
    technology NEC Y93.C9 (*following* Y93.7)
  confidence course Y93.A5 (*following* Y93.7)
  construction (building) Y93.H3 (*following* Y93.7)
  cooking and baking Y93.G3 (*following* Y93.7)
  cool down exercises Y93.A2 (*following* Y93.7)
  cricket Y93.69
  crocheting Y93.D1 (*following* Y93.7)
  cross country skiing Y93.24
  dancing (all types) Y93.41
  digging
    dirt Y93.H1 (*following* Y93.7)
  dirt digging Y93.H1 (*following* Y93.7)
  dishwashing Y93.G1 (*following* Y93.7)
  diving (platform) (springboard) Y93.12
    underwater Y93.15
  dodge ball Y93.6A
  downhill skiing Y93.23
  drum playing Y93.J2 (*following* Y93.7)
  dumbbells Y93.B3 (*following* Y93.7)
  electronic
    devices NEC Y93.C9 (*following* Y93.7)
      hand held interactive Y93.C2 (*following* Y93.7)

Activity — *continued*
  electronic — *continued*
    game playing (using) (with)
      interactive device Y93.C2 (*following* Y93.7)
      keyboard or other stationary device Y93.C1 (*following* Y93.7)
  elliptical machine Y93.A1 (*following* Y93.7)
  exercise(s)
    machines ((primarily) for)
      cardiorespiratory conditioning Y93.A1 (*following* Y93.7)
      muscle strengthening Y93.B1 (*following* Y93.7)
    muscle strengthening (non-machine) NEC Y93.B9 (*following* Y93.7)
  external motion NEC Y93.I9 (*following* Y93.7)
    rollercoaster Y93.I1 (*following* Y93.7)
  fainting game Y93.85
  field hockey Y93.65
  figure skating (pairs) (singles) Y93.21
  flag football Y93.62
  floor mopping and cleaning Y93.E5 (*following* Y93.7)
  food preparation and clean up Y93.G1 (*following* Y93.7)
  football (American) NOS Y93.61
    flag Y93.62
    tackle Y93.61
    touch Y93.62
  four square Y93.6A
  free weights Y93.B3 (*following* Y93.7)
  frisbee (ultimate) Y93.74
  furniture
    building Y93.D3 (*following* Y93.7)
    finishing Y93.D3 (*following* Y93.7)
    repair Y93.D3 (*following* Y93.7)
  game playing (electronic)
    using interactive device Y93.C2 (*following* Y93.7)
    using keyboard or other stationary device Y93.C1 (*following* Y93.7)
  gardening Y93.H2 (*following* Y93.7)
  golf Y93.53
  grass drills Y93.A6 (*following* Y93.7)
  grilling and smoking food Y93.G2 (*following* Y93.7)
  grooming and shearing an animal Y93.K3 (*following* Y93.7)
  guerilla drills Y93.A6 (*following* Y93.7)
  gymnastics (rhythmic) Y93.43
  hand held interactive electronic device Y93.C2 (*following* Y93.7)
  handball Y93.73
  handcrafts NEC Y93.D9 (*following* Y93.7)
  hang gliding Y93.35
  hiking (on level or elevated terrain) Y93.Ø1
  hockey (ice) Y93.22
    field Y93.65
  horseback riding Y93.52
  household (interior) maintenance NEC Y93.E9 (*following* Y93.7)
  ice NEC Y93.29
    dancing Y93.21
    hockey Y93.22
    skating Y93.21
  inline roller skating Y93.51
  ironing Y93.E4 (*following* Y93.7)
  judo Y93.75
  jumping jacks Y93.A2 (*following* Y93.7)
  jumping rope Y93.56
  jumping (off) NEC Y93.39
    BASE (Building, Antenna, Span, Earth) Y93.33
    bungee Y93.34
    jacks Y93.A2 (*following* Y93.7)
    rope Y93.56
  karate Y93.75
  kayaking (in calm and turbulent water) Y93.16
  keyboarding (computer) Y93.C1 (*following* Y93.7)
  kickball Y93.6A
  knitting Y93.D1 (*following* Y93.7)
  lacrosse Y93.65
  land maintenance NEC Y93.H9 (*following* Y93.7)
  landscaping Y93.H2 (*following* Y93.7)
  laundry Y93.E2 (*following* Y93.7)
  machines (exercise)
    primarily for cardiorespiratory conditioning Y93.A1 (*following* Y93.7)
    primarily for muscle strengthening Y93.B1 (*following* Y93.7)
  maintenance
    exterior building NEC Y93.H9 (*following* Y93.7)
    household (interior) NEC Y93.E9 (*following* Y93.7)
    land Y93.H9 (*following* Y93.7)
    property Y93.H9 (*following* Y93.7)

Activity — *continued*
  marching (on level or elevated terrain) Y93.Ø1
  martial arts Y93.75
  microwave oven Y93.G3 (*following* Y93.7)
  milking an animal Y93.K2 (*following* Y93.7)
  mopping (floor) Y93.E5 (*following* Y93.7)
  mountain climbing Y93.31
  muscle strengthening
    exercises (non-machine) NEC Y93.B9 (*following* Y93.7)
    machines Y93.B1 (*following* Y93.7)
  musical keyboard (electronic) playing Y93.J1 (*following* Y93.7)
  nordic skiing Y93.24
  obstacle course Y93.A5 (*following* Y93.7)
  oven (microwave) Y93.G3 (*following* Y93.7)
  packing up and unpacking in moving to a new residence Y93.E6 (*following* Y93.7)
  parasailing Y93.19
  pass out game Y93.85
  percussion instrument playing NEC Y93.J2 (*following* Y93.7)
  personal
    bathing and showering Y93.E1 (*following* Y93.7)
    hygiene NEC Y93.E8 (*following* Y93.7)
    showering Y93.E1 (*following* Y93.7)
  physical games generally associated with school recess, summer camp and children Y93.6A
  physical training NEC Y93.A9 (*following* Y93.7)
  piano playing Y93.J1 (*following* Y93.7)
  pilates Y93.B4 (*following* Y93.7)
  platform diving Y93.12
  playing musical instrument
    brass instrument Y93.J4 (*following* Y93.7)
    drum Y93.J2 (*following* Y93.7)
    musical keyboard (electronic) Y93.J1 (*following* Y93.7)
    percussion instrument NEC Y93.J2 (*following* Y93.7)
    piano Y93.J1 (*following* Y93.7)
    string instrument Y93.J3 (*following* Y93.7)
    winds instrument Y93.J4 (*following* Y93.7)
  property maintenance
    exterior NEC Y93.H9 (*following* Y93.7)
    interior NEC Y93.E9 (*following* Y93.7)
  pruning (garden and lawn) Y93.H2 (*following* Y93.7)
  pull-ups Y93.B2 (*following* Y93.7)
  push-ups Y93.B2 (*following* Y93.7)
  racquetball Y93.73
  rafting (in calm and turbulent water) Y93.16
  raking (leaves) Y93.H1 (*following* Y93.7)
  rappelling Y93.32
  refereeing a sports activity Y93.81
  residential relocation Y93.E6 (*following* Y93.7)
  rhythmic gymnastics Y93.43
  rhythmic movement NEC Y93.49
  riding
    horseback Y93.52
    rollercoaster Y93.I1 (*following* Y93.7)
  rock climbing Y93.31
  roller skating (inline) Y93.51
  rollercoaster riding Y93.I1 (*following* Y93.7)
  rough housing and horseplay Y93.83
  rowing (in calm and turbulent water) Y93.16
  rugby Y93.63
  running Y93.Ø2
  SCUBA diving Y93.15
  sewing Y93.D2 (*following* Y93.7)
  shoveling Y93.H1 (*following* Y93.7)
    dirt Y93.H1 (*following* Y93.7)
    snow Y93.H1 (*following* Y93.7)
  showering (personal) Y93.E1 (*following* Y93.7)
  sit-ups Y93.B2 (*following* Y93.7)
  skateboarding Y93.51
  skating (ice) Y93.21
    roller Y93.51
  skiing (alpine) (downhill) Y93.23
    cross country Y93.24
    nordic Y93.24
    water Y93.17
  sledding (snow) Y93.23
  sleeping (sleep) Y93.84
  smoking and grilling food Y93.G2 (*following* Y93.7)
  snorkeling Y93.15
  snow NEC Y93.29
    boarding Y93.23
    shoveling Y93.H1 (*following* Y93.7)
    sledding Y93.23
    tubing Y93.23
  soccer Y93.66

▼ Subterms under main terms may continue to next column or page   ☑ **Additional Character Required** — Refer to the Tabular List for Character Selection

Activity — continued
  softball Y93.64
  specified NEC Y93.89
  spectator at an event Y93.82
  sports NEC Y93.79
    sports played as a team or group NEC Y93.69
    sports played individually NEC Y93.59
  springboard diving Y93.12
  squash Y93.73
  stationary bike Y93.A1 (following Y93.7)
  step (stepping) exercise (class) Y93.A3 (following Y93.7)
  stepper machine Y93.A1 (following Y93.7)
  stove Y93.G3 (following Y93.7)
  string instrument playing Y93.J3 (following Y93.7)
  surfing Y93.18
    wind Y93.18
  swimming Y93.11
  tackle football Y93.61
  tap dancing Y93.41
  tennis Y93.73
  tobogganing Y93.23
  touch football Y93.62
  track and field events (non-running) Y93.57
    running Y93.02
  trampoline Y93.44
  treadmill Y93.A1 (following Y93.7)
  trimming shrubs Y93.H2 (following Y93.7)
  tubing (in calm and turbulent water) Y93.16
    snow Y93.23
  ultimate frisbee Y93.74
  underwater diving Y93.15
  unpacking in moving to a new residence Y93.E6 (following Y93.7)
  use of stove, oven and microwave oven Y93.G3 (following Y93.7)
  vacuuming Y93.E3 (following Y93.7)
  volleyball (beach) (court) Y93.68
  wake boarding Y93.17
  walking (on level or elevated terrain) Y93.01
    an animal Y93.K1 (following Y93.7)
  walking an animal Y93.K1 (following Y93.7)
  wall climbing Y93.31
  warm up and cool down exercises Y93.A2 (following Y93.7)
  water NEC Y93.19
    aerobics Y93.14
    craft NEC Y93.19
    exercise Y93.14
    polo Y93.13
    skiing Y93.17
    sliding Y93.18
    survival training and testing Y93.19
  weeding (garden and lawn) Y93.H2 (following Y93.7)
  wind instrument playing Y93.J4 (following Y93.7)
  windsurfing Y93.18
  wrestling Y93.72
  yoga Y93.42
Adverse effect of drugs — see Table of Drugs and Chemicals
Aerosinusitis — see Air, pressure
After-effect, late — see Sequelae
Air
  blast in war operations — see War operations, air blast
  pressure
    change, rapid
      during
        ascent W94.29 ☑
          while (in) (surfacing from)
            aircraft W94.23 ☑
            deep water diving W94.21 ☑
            underground W94.22 ☑
        descent W94.39 ☑
          in
            aircraft W94.31 ☑
            water W94.32 ☑
      high, prolonged W94.0 ☑
      low, prolonged W94.12 ☑
        due to residence or long visit at high altitude W94.11 ☑
Alpine sickness W94.11 ☑
Altitude sickness W94.11 ☑
Anaphylactic shock, anaphylaxis — see Table of Drugs and Chemicals
Andes disease W94.11 ☑
Arachnidism, arachnoidism X58 ☑
Arson (with intent to injure or kill) X97 ☑

Asphyxia, asphyxiation
  by
    food (bone) (seed) — see categories T17 and T18 ☑
    gas — see also Table of Drugs and Chemicals
      legal
        execution — see Legal, intervention, gas
        intervention — see Legal, intervention, gas
  from
    fire — see also Exposure, fire
      in war operations — see War operations, fire
    ignition — see Ignition
    vomitus T17.81 ☑
  in war operations — see War operations, restriction of airway
Aspiration
  food (any type) (into respiratory tract) (with asphyxia, obstruction respiratory tract, suffocation) — see categories T17 and T18 ☑
  foreign body — see Foreign body, aspiration
  vomitus (with asphyxia, obstruction respiratory tract, suffocation) T17.81 ☑
Assassination (attempt) — see Assault
Assault (homicidal) (by) (in) Y09
  arson X97 ☑
  bite (of human being) Y04.1 ☑
  bodily force Y04.8 ☑
    bite Y04.1 ☑
    bumping into Y04.2 ☑
    sexual — see subcategories T74.0, T76.0 ☑
    unarmed fight Y04.0 ☑
  bomb X96.9 ☑
    antipersonnel X96.0 ☑
    fertilizer X96.3 ☑
    gasoline X96.1 ☑
    letter X96.2 ☑
    petrol X96.1 ☑
    pipe X96.3 ☑
    specified NEC X96.8 ☑
  brawl (hand) (fists) (foot) (unarmed) Y04.0 ☑
  burning, burns (by fire) NEC X97 ☑
    acid Y08.89 ☑
    caustic, corrosive substance Y08.89 ☑
    chemical from swallowing caustic, corrosive substance — see Table of Drugs and Chemicals
    cigarette(s) X97 ☑
    hot object X98.9 ☑
      fluid NEC X98.2 ☑
      household appliance X98.3 ☑
      specified NEC X98.8 ☑
      steam X98.0 ☑
      tap water X98.1 ☑
      vapors X98.0 ☑
    scalding — see Assault, burning
    steam X98.0 ☑
    vitriol Y08.89 ☑
  caustic, corrosive substance (gas) Y08.89 ☑
  crashing of
    aircraft Y08.81 ☑
    motor vehicle Y03.8 ☑
      pushed in front of Y02.0 ☑
      run over Y03.0 ☑
      specified NEC Y03.8 ☑
  cutting or piercing instrument X99.9 ☑
    dagger X99.2 ☑
    glass X99.0 ☑
    knife X99.1 ☑
    specified NEC X99.8 ☑
    sword X99.2 ☑
  dagger X99.2 ☑
  drowning (in) X92.9 ☑
    bathtub X92.0 ☑
    natural water X92.3 ☑
    specified NEC X92.8 ☑
    swimming pool X92.1 ☑
      following fall X92.2 ☑
  dynamite X96.8 ☑
  explosive(s) (material) X96.9 ☑
  fight (hand) (fists) (foot) (unarmed) Y04.0 ☑
    with weapon — see Assault, by type of weapon
  fire X97 ☑
  firearm X95.9 ☑
    airgun X95.01 ☑
    handgun X93 ☑
    hunting rifle X94.1 ☑
    larger X94.9 ☑
      specified NEC X94.8 ☑

Assault — continued
  firearm — continued
    machine gun X94.2 ☑
    shotgun X94.0 ☑
    specified NEC X95.8 ☑
  from high place Y01 ☑
  gunshot (wound) NEC — see Assault, firearm, by type
  incendiary device X97 ☑
  injury Y09
    to child due to criminal abortion attempt NEC Y08.89 ☑
  knife X99.1 ☑
  late effect of — see categories X92-Y08 with 7th character S
  placing before moving object NEC Y02.8 ☑
    motor vehicle Y02.0 ☑
  poisoning — see categories T36-T65 with 7th character S
  puncture, any part of body — see Assault, cutting or piercing instrument
  pushing
    before moving object NEC Y02.8 ☑
      motor vehicle Y02.0 ☑
      subway train Y02.1 ☑
      train Y02.1 ☑
    from high place Y01 ☑
  rape T74.2- ☑
  scalding — see Assault, burning
  sequelae of — see categories X92-Y08 with 7th character S
  sexual (by bodily force) T74.2- ☑
  shooting — see Assault, firearm
  specified means NEC Y08.89 ☑
  stab, any part of body — see Assault, cutting or piercing instrument
  steam X98.0 ☑
  striking against
    other person Y04.2 ☑
    sports equipment Y08.09 ☑
      baseball bat Y08.02 ☑
      hockey stick Y08.01 ☑
  struck by
    sports equipment Y08.09 ☑
      baseball bat Y08.02 ☑
      hockey stick Y08.01 ☑
  submersion — see Assault, drowning
  violence Y09
  weapon Y09
    blunt Y00 ☑
    cutting or piercing — see Assault, cutting or piercing instrument
    firearm — see Assault, firearm
  wound Y09
    cutting — see Assault, cutting or piercing instrument
    gunshot — see Assault, firearm
    knife X99.1 ☑
    piercing — see Assault, cutting or piercing instrument
    puncture — see Assault, cutting or piercing instrument
    stab — see Assault, cutting or piercing instrument
Attack by mammals NEC W55.89 ☑
Avalanche — see Landslide
Aviator's disease — see Air, pressure

B

Barotitis, barodontalgia, barosinusitis, barotrauma (otitic) (sinus) — see Air, pressure
Battered (baby) (child) (person) (syndrome) X58 ☑
Bayonet wound W26.1 ☑
  in
    legal intervention — see Legal, intervention, sharp object, bayonet
    war operations — see War operations, combat
  stated as undetermined whether accidental or intentional Y28.8 ☑
  suicide (attempt) X78.2 ☑
Bean in nose — see categories T17 and T18 ☑
Bed set on fire NEC — see Exposure, fire, uncontrolled, building, bed
Beheading (by guillotine)
  homicide X99.9 ☑
  legal execution — see Legal, intervention
Bending, injury in (prolonged) (static) X50.1 ☑

Bends — see Air, pressure, change
Bite, bitten by
  alligator W58.01 ☑
  arthropod (nonvenomous) NEC W57 ☑
  bull W55.21 ☑
  cat W55.01 ☑
  cow W55.21 ☑
  crocodile W58.11 ☑
  dog W54.0 ☑
  goat W55.31 ☑
  hoof stock NEC W55.31 ☑
  horse W55.11 ☑
  human being (accidentally) W50.3 ☑
    with intent to injure or kill Y04.1 ☑
    as, or caused by, a crowd or human stampede (with
        fall) W52 ☑
    assault Y04.1 ☑
    homicide (attempt) Y04.1 ☑
    in
        fight Y04.1 ☑
  insect (nonvenomous) W57 ☑
  lizard (nonvenomous) W59.01 ☑
  mammal NEC W55.81 ☑
    marine W56.31 ☑
  marine animal (nonvenomous) W56.81 ☑
  millipede W57 ☑
  moray eel W56.51 ☑
  mouse W53.01 ☑
  person(s) (accidentally) W50.3 ☑
    with intent to injure or kill Y04.1 ☑
    as, or caused by, a crowd or human stampede (with
        fall) W52 ☑
    assault Y04.1 ☑
    homicide (attempt) Y04.1 ☑
    in
        fight Y04.1 ☑
  pig W55.41 ☑
  raccoon W55.51 ☑
  rat W53.11 ☑
  reptile W59.81 ☑
    lizard W59.01 ☑
    snake W59.11 ☑
    turtle W59.21 ☑
        terrestrial W59.81 ☑
  rodent W53.81 ☑
    mouse W53.01 ☑
    rat W53.11 ☑
    specified NEC W53.81 ☑
    squirrel W53.21 ☑
  shark W56.41 ☑
  sheep W55.31 ☑
  snake (nonvenomous) W59.11 ☑
  spider (nonvenomous) W57 ☑
  squirrel W53.21 ☑
Blast (air) in war operations — see War operations, blast
Blizzard X37.2 ☑
Blood alcohol level Y90.9
  less than 20mg/100ml Y90.0
  presence in blood, level not specified Y90.9
  20-39mg/100ml Y90.1
  40-59mg/100ml Y90.2
  60-79mg/100ml Y90.3
  80-99mg/100ml Y90.4
  100-119mg/100ml Y90.5
  120-199mg/100ml Y90.6
  200-239mg/100ml Y90.7
Blow X58 ☑
  by law-enforcing agent, police (on duty) — see Legal,
      intervention, manhandling
    blunt object — see Legal, intervention, blunt object
Blowing up — see Explosion
Brawl (hand) (fists) (foot) Y04.0 ☑
Breakage (accidental) (part of)
  ladder (causing fall) W11 ☑
  scaffolding (causing fall) W12 ☑
Broken
  glass, contact with — see Contact, with, glass
  power line (causing electric shock) W85 ☑
Bumping against, into (accidentally)
  object NEC W22.8 ☑
    caused by crowd or human stampede (with fall)
        W52 ☑
    sports equipment W21.9 ☑
    with fall — see Fall, due to, bumping against, object
  person(s) W51 ☑
    with fall W03 ☑

Bumping against, into — continued
  person(s) — continued
    with fall — continued
        due to ice or snow W00.0 ☑
    assault Y04.2 ☑
    caused by, a crowd or human stampede (with fall)
        W52 ☑
    homicide (attempt) Y04.2 ☑
  sports equipment W21.9 ☑
Burn, burned, burning (accidental) (by) (from) (on)
  acid NEC — see Table of Drugs and Chemicals
  bed linen — see Exposure, fire, uncontrolled, in build-
      ing, bed
  blowtorch X08.8 ☑
    with ignition of clothing NEC X06.2 ☑
        nightwear X05 ☑
  bonfire, campfire (controlled) — see also Exposure,
      fire, controlled, not in building)
    uncontrolled — see Exposure, fire, uncontrolled,
        not in building
  candle X08.8 ☑
    with ignition of clothing NEC X06.2 ☑
        nightwear X05 ☑
  caustic liquid, substance (external) (internal) NEC —
      see Table of Drugs and Chemicals
  chemical (external) (internal) — see also Table of Drugs
      and Chemicals
    in war operations — see War operations. fire
  cigar(s) or cigarette(s) X08.8 ☑
    with ignition of clothing NEC X06.2 ☑
        nightwear X05 ☑
  clothes, clothing NEC (from controlled fire) X06.2 ☑
    with conflagration — see Exposure, fire, uncon-
        trolled, building
        not in building or structure — see Exposure, fire,
            uncontrolled, not in building
  cooker (hot) X15.8 ☑
    stated as undetermined whether accidental or inten-
        tional Y27.3 ☑
    suicide (attempt) X77.3 ☑
  electric blanket X16 ☑
  engine (hot) X17 ☑
  fire, flames — see Exposure, fire
  flare, Very pistol — see Discharge, firearm NEC
  heat
    from appliance (electrical) (household) X15.8 ☑
        cooker X15.8 ☑
        hotplate X15.2 ☑
        kettle X15.8 ☑
        light bulb X15.8 ☑
        saucepan X15.3 ☑
        skillet X15.3 ☑
        stated as undetermined whether accidental or
            intentional Y27.3 ☑
        stove X15.0 ☑
        suicide (attempt) X77.3 ☑
        toaster X15.1 ☑
    in local application or packing during medical or
        surgical procedure Y63.5
  heating
    appliance, radiator or pipe X16 ☑
  homicide (attempt) — see Assault, burning
  hot
    air X14.1 ☑
    cooker X15.8 ☑
    drink X10.0 ☑
    engine X17 ☑
    fat X10.2 ☑
    fluid NEC X12 ☑
    food X10.1 ☑
    gases X14.1 ☑
    heating appliance X16 ☑
    household appliance NEC X15.8 ☑
    kettle X15.8 ☑
    liquid NEC X12 ☑
    machinery X17 ☑
    metal (molten) (liquid) NEC X18 ☑
    object (not producing fire or flames) NEC X19 ☑
    oil (cooking) X10.2 ☑
    pipe(s) X16 ☑
    radiator X16 ☑
    saucepan (glass) (metal) X15.3 ☑
    stove (kitchen) X15.0 ☑
    substance NEC X19 ☑
        caustic or corrosive NEC — see Table of Drugs
            and Chemicals

Burn, burned, burning — continued
  hot — continued
    toaster X15.1 ☑
    tool X17 ☑
    vapor X13.1 ☑
    water (tap) — see Contact, with, hot, tap water
  hotplate X15.2 ☑
    suicide (attempt) X77.3 ☑
  ignition — see Ignition
  in war operations — see War operations, fire
  inflicted by other person X97 ☑
    by hot objects, hot vapor, and steam — see Assault,
        burning, hot object
  internal, from swallowed caustic, corrosive liquid, sub-
      stance — see Table of Drugs and Chemicals
  iron (hot) X15.8 ☑
    stated as undetermined whether accidental or inten-
        tional Y27.3 ☑
    suicide (attempt) X77.3 ☑
  kettle (hot) X15.8 ☑
    stated as undetermined whether accidental or inten-
        tional Y27.3 ☑
    suicide (attempt) X77.3 ☑
  lamp (flame) X08.8 ☑
    with ignition of clothing NEC X06.2 ☑
        nightwear X05 ☑
  lighter (cigar) (cigarette) X08.8 ☑
    with ignition of clothing NEC X06.2 ☑
        nightwear X05 ☑
  lightning — see subcategory T75.0 ☑
    causing fire — see Exposure, fire
  liquid (boiling) (hot) NEC X12 ☑
    stated as undetermined whether accidental or inten-
        tional Y27.2 ☑
    suicide (attempt) X77.2 ☑
  local application of externally applied substance in
      medical or surgical care Y63.5
  machinery (hot) X17 ☑
  matches X08.8 ☑
    with ignition of clothing NEC X06.2 ☑
        nightwear X05 ☑
  mattress — see Exposure, fire, uncontrolled, building,
      bed
  medicament, externally applied Y63.5
  metal (hot) (liquid) (molten) NEC X18 ☑
  nightwear (nightclothes, nightdress, gown, pajamas,
      robe) X05 ☑
  object (hot) NEC X19 ☑
  on board watercraft
    due to
        accident to watercraft V91.09 ☑
            powered craft V91.03 ☑
                ferry boat V91.01 ☑
                fishing boat V91.02 ☑
                jetskis V91.03 ☑
                liner V91.01 ☑
                merchant ship V91.00 ☑
                passenger ship V91.01 ☑
            unpowered craft V91.08 ☑
                canoe V91.05 ☑
                inflatable V91.06 ☑
                kayak V91.05 ☑
                sailboat V91.04 ☑
                surf-board V91.08 ☑
                water skis V91.07 ☑
                windsurfer V91.08 ☑
        fire on board V93.09 ☑
            ferry boat V93.01 ☑
            fishing boat V93.02 ☑
            jetskis V93.03 ☑
            liner V93.01 ☑
            merchant ship V93.00 ☑
            passenger ship V93.01 ☑
            powered craft NEC V93.03 ☑
            sailboat V93.04 ☑
        specified heat source NEC on board V93.19 ☑
            ferry boat V93.11 ☑
            fishing boat V93.12 ☑
            jetskis V93.13 ☑
            liner V93.11 ☑
            merchant ship V93.10 ☑
            passenger ship V93.11 ☑
            powered craft NEC V93.13 ☑
            sailboat V93.14 ☑
    pipe (hot) X16 ☑
        smoking X08.8 ☑

Burn, burned, burning — *continued*
- pipe — *continued*
  - smoking — *continued*
    - with ignition of clothing NEC X06.2 ☑
      - nightwear X05 ☑
- powder — *see* Powder burn
- radiator (hot) X16 ☑
- saucepan (hot) (glass) (metal) X15.3 ☑
  - stated as undetermined whether accidental or intentional Y27.3 ☑
  - suicide (attempt) X77.3 ☑
- self-inflicted X76 ☑
  - stated as undetermined whether accidental or intentional Y26 ☑
- stated as undetermined whether accidental or intentional Y27.0 ☑
- steam X13.1 ☑
  - pipe X16 ☑
    - stated as undetermined whether accidental or intentional Y27.8 ☑
- stated as undetermined whether accidental or intentional Y27.0 ☑
- suicide (attempt) X77.0 ☑
- stove (hot) (kitchen) X15.0 ☑
  - stated as undetermined whether accidental or intentional Y27.3 ☑
  - suicide (attempt) X77.3 ☑
- substance (hot) NEC X19 ☑
  - boiling X12 ☑
    - stated as undetermined whether accidental or intentional Y27.2 ☑
    - suicide (attempt) X77.2 ☑
  - molten (metal) X18 ☑
- suicide (attempt) NEC X76 ☑
  - hot
    - household appliance X77.3 ☑
    - object X77.9 ☑
- therapeutic misadventure
  - heat in local application or packing during medical or surgical procedure Y63.5
  - overdose of radiation Y63.2
- toaster (hot) X15.1 ☑
  - stated as undetermined whether accidental or intentional Y27.3 ☑
  - suicide (attempt) X77.3 ☑
- tool (hot) X17 ☑
- torch, welding X08.8 ☑
  - with ignition of clothing NEC X06.2 ☑
    - nightwear X05 ☑
- trash fire (controlled) — *see* Exposure, fire, controlled, not in building
  - uncontrolled — *see* Exposure, fire, uncontrolled, not in building
- vapor (hot) X13.1 ☑
  - stated as undetermined whether accidental or intentional Y27.0 ☑
  - suicide (attempt) X77.0 ☑
- Very pistol — *see* Discharge, firearm NEC

Butted by animal W55.82 ☑
- bull W55.22 ☑
- cow W55.22 ☑
- goat W55.32 ☑
- horse W55.12 ☑
- pig W55.42 ☑
- sheep W55.32 ☑

C

Caisson disease — *see* Air, pressure, change
Campfire (exposure to) (controlled) — *see also* Exposure, fire, controlled, not in building
- uncontrolled — *see* Exposure, fire, uncontrolled, not in building
Capital punishment (any means) — *see* Legal, intervention
Car sickness T75.3 ☑
Casualty (not due to war) NEC X58 ☑
- war — *see* War operations
Cat
- bite W55.01 ☑
- scratch W55.03 ☑
Cataclysm, cataclysmic (any injury) NEC — *see* Forces of nature
Catching fire — *see* Exposure, fire

Caught
- between
  - folding object W23.0 ☑
  - objects (moving) (stationary and moving) W23.0 ☑
    - and machinery — *see* Contact, with, by type of machine
    - stationary W23.1 ☑
  - sliding door and door frame W23.0 ☑
- by, in
  - machinery (moving parts of) — *see* Contact, with, by type of machine
  - washing-machine wringer W23.0 ☑
  - under packing crate (due to losing grip) W23.1 ☑
Cave-in caused by cataclysmic earth surface movement or eruption — *see* Landslide
Change(s) in air pressure — *see* Air, pressure, change
Choked, choking (on) (any object except food or vomitus)
- food (bone) (seed) — *see* categories T17 and T18 ☑
- vomitus T17.81- ☑
Civil insurrection — *see* War operations
Cloudburst (any injury) X37.8 ☑
Cold, exposure to (accidental) (excessive) (extreme) (natural) (place) NEC — *see* Exposure, cold
Collapse
- building W20.1 ☑
  - burning (uncontrolled fire) X00.2 ☑
- dam or man-made structure (causing earth movement) X36.0 ☑
- machinery — *see* Contact, with, by type of machine
- structure W20.1 ☑
  - burning (uncontrolled fire) X00.2 ☑
Collision (accidental) NEC — *see also* Accident, transport V89.9 ☑
- pedestrian W51 ☑
  - with fall W03 ☑
    - due to ice or snow W00.0 ☑
    - involving pedestrian conveyance — *see* Accident, transport, pedestrian, conveyance
  - and
    - crowd or human stampede (with fall) W52 ☑
    - object W22.8 ☑
      - with fall — *see* Fall, due to, bumping against, object
- person(s) — *see* Collision, pedestrian
- transport vehicle NEC V89.9 ☑
  - and
    - avalanche, fallen or not moving — *see* Accident, transport
      - falling or moving — *see* Landslide
    - landslide, fallen or not moving — *see* Accident, transport
      - falling or moving — *see* Landslide
  - due to cataclysm — *see* Forces of nature, by type
  - intentional, purposeful suicide (attempt) — *see* Suicide, collision
Combustion, spontaneous — *see* Ignition
Complication (delayed) **of or following** (medical or surgical procedure) Y84.9
- with misadventure — *see* Misadventure
- amputation of limb(s) Y83.5
- anastomosis (arteriovenous) (blood vessel) (gastrojejunal) (tendon) (natural or artificial material) Y83.2
- aspiration (of fluid) Y84.4
  - tissue Y84.8
- biopsy Y84.8
- blood
  - sampling Y84.7
  - transfusion
    - procedure Y84.8
- bypass Y83.2
- catheterization (urinary) Y84.6
  - cardiac Y84.0
- colostomy Y83.3
- cystostomy Y83.3
- dialysis (kidney) Y84.1
- drug — *see* Table of Drugs and Chemicals
- due to misadventure — *see* Misadventure
- duodenostomy Y83.3
- electroshock therapy Y84.3
- external stoma, creation of Y83.3
- formation of external stoma Y83.3
- gastrostomy Y83.3
- graft Y83.2
- hypothermia (medically-induced) Y84.8

Complication (delayed) **of or following** — *continued*
- implant, implantation (of)
  - artificial
    - internal device (cardiac pacemaker) (electrodes in brain) (heart valve prosthesis) (orthopedic) Y83.1
    - material or tissue (for anastomosis or bypass) Y83.2
      - with creation of external stoma Y83.3
  - natural tissues (for anastomosis or bypass) Y83.2
    - with creation of external stoma Y83.3
- infusion
  - procedure Y84.8
- injection — *see* Table of Drugs and Chemicals
  - procedure Y84.8
- insertion of gastric or duodenal sound Y84.5
- insulin-shock therapy Y84.3
- paracentesis (abdominal) (thoracic) (aspirative) Y84.4
- procedures other than surgical operation — *see* Complication of or following, by type of procedure
- radiological procedure or therapy Y84.2
- removal of organ (partial) (total) NEC Y83.6
- sampling
  - blood Y84.7
  - fluid NEC Y84.4
  - tissue Y84.8
- shock therapy Y84.3
- surgical operation NEC — *see also* Complication of or following, by type of operation Y83.9
  - reconstructive NEC Y83.4
    - with
      - anastomosis, bypass or graft Y83.2
      - formation of external stoma Y83.3
  - specified NEC Y83.8
- transfusion — *see also* Table of Drugs and Chemicals
  - procedure Y84.8
- transplant, transplantation (heart) (kidney) (liver) (whole organ, any) Y83.0
  - partial organ Y83.4
- ureterostomy Y83.3
- vaccination — *see also* Table of Drugs and Chemicals
  - procedure Y84.8
Compression
- divers' squeeze — *see* Air, pressure, change
- trachea by
  - food (lodged in esophagus) — *see* categories T17 and T18 ☑
  - vomitus (lodged in esophagus) T17.81- ☑
Conflagration — *see* Exposure, fire, uncontrolled
Constriction (external)
- hair W49.01 ☑
- jewelry W49.04 ☑
- ring W49.04 ☑
- rubber band W49.03 ☑
- specified item NEC W49.09 ☑
- string W49.02 ☑
- thread W49.02 ☑
Contact (accidental)
- with
  - abrasive wheel (metalworking) W31.1 ☑
  - alligator W58.09 ☑
    - bite W58.01 ☑
    - crushing W58.03 ☑
    - strike W58.02 ☑
  - amphibian W62.9 ☑
    - frog W62.0 ☑
    - toad W62.1 ☑
  - animal (nonvenomous) NEC W64 ☑
    - marine W56.89 ☑
      - bite W56.81 ☑
      - dolphin — *see* Contact, with, dolphin
      - fish NEC — *see* Contact, with, fish
      - mammal — *see* Contact, with, mammal, marine
      - orca — *see* Contact, with, orca
      - sea lion — *see* Contact, with, sea lion
      - shark — *see* Contact, with, shark
      - strike W56.82 ☑
  - animate mechanical force NEC W64 ☑
  - arrow W21.89 ☑
    - not thrown, projected or falling W45.8 ☑
  - arthropods (nonvenomous) W57 ☑
  - axe W27.0 ☑
  - band-saw (industrial) W31.2 ☑
  - bayonet — *see* Bayonet wound
  - bee(s) X58 ☑

☑ **Additional Character Required** — Refer to the Tabular List for Character Selection ▽ **Subterms under main terms may continue to next column or page**

Contact — *continued*
  with — *continued*
    bench-saw (industrial) W31.2 ☑
    bird W61.99 ☑
      bite W61.91 ☑
      chicken — *see* Contact, with, chicken
      duck — *see* Contact, with, duck
      goose — *see* Contact, with, goose
      macaw — *see* Contact, with, macaw
      parrot — *see* Contact, with, parrot
      psittacine — *see* Contact, with, psittacine
      strike W61.92 ☑
      turkey — *see* Contact, with, turkey
    blender W29.0 ☑
    boiling water X12 ☑
      stated as undetermined whether accidental or
        intentional Y27.2 ☑
      suicide (attempt) X77.2 ☑
    bore, earth-drilling or mining (land) (seabed)
      W31.0 ☑
    buffalo — *see* Contact, with, hoof stock NEC
    bull W55.29 ☑
      bite W55.21 ☑
      gored W55.22 ☑
      strike W55.22 ☑
    bumper cars W31.81 ☑
    camel — *see* Contact, with, hoof stock NEC
    can
      lid W26.8 ☑
      opener W27.4 ☑
        powered W29.0 ☑
    cat W55.09 ☑
      bite W55.01 ☑
      scratch W55.03 ☑
    caterpillar (venomous) X58 ☑
    centipede (venomous) X58 ☑
    chain
      hoist W24.0 ☑
        agricultural operations W30.89 ☑
      saw W29.3 ☑
    chicken W61.39 ☑
      peck W61.33 ☑
      strike W61.32 ☑
    chisel W27.0 ☑
    circular saw W31.2 ☑
    cobra X58 ☑
    combine (harvester) W30.0 ☑
    conveyer belt W24.1 ☑
    cooker (hot) X15.8 ☑
      stated as undetermined whether accidental or
        intentional Y27.3 ☑
      suicide (attempt) X77.3 ☑
    coral X58 ☑
    cotton gin W31.82 ☑
    cow W55.29 ☑
      bite W55.21 ☑
      strike W55.22 ☑
    crane W24.0 ☑
      agricultural operations W30.89 ☑
    crocodile W58.19 ☑
      bite W58.11 ☑
      crushing W58.13 ☑
      strike W58.12 ☑
    dagger W26.1 ☑
      stated as undetermined whether accidental or
        intentional Y28.2 ☑
      suicide (attempt) X78.2 ☑
    dairy equipment W31.82 ☑
    dart W21.89 ☑
      not thrown, projected or falling W45.8 ☑
    deer — *see* Contact, with, hoof stock NEC
    derrick W24.0 ☑
      agricultural operations W30.89 ☑
        hay W30.2 ☑
    dog W54.8 ☑
      bite W54.0 ☑
      strike W54.1 ☑
    dolphin W56.09 ☑
      bite W56.01 ☑
      strike W56.02 ☑
    donkey — *see* Contact, with, hoof stock NEC
    drill (powered) W29.8 ☑
      earth (land) (seabed) W31.0 ☑
      nonpowered W27.8 ☑
    drive belt W24.0 ☑
      agricultural operations W30.89 ☑

Contact — *continued*
  with — *continued*
    dry ice — *see* Exposure, cold, man-made
    dryer (clothes) (powered) (spin) W29.2 ☑
    duck W61.69 ☑
      bite W61.61 ☑
      strike W61.62 ☑
    earth (-)
      drilling machine (industrial) W31.0 ☑
      scraping machine in stationary use W31.83 ☑
    edge of stiff paper W26.2 ☑
    electric
      beater W29.0 ☑
      blanket X16 ☑
      fan W29.2 ☑
        commercial W31.82 ☑
      knife W29.1 ☑
      mixer W29.0 ☑
    elevator (building) W24.0 ☑
      agricultural operations W30.89 ☑
        grain W30.3 ☑
    engine(s), hot NEC X17 ☑
    excavating machine W31.0 ☑
    farm machine W30.9 ☑
    feces — *see* Contact, with, by type of animal
    fer de lance X58 ☑
    fish W56.59 ☑
      bite W56.51 ☑
      shark — *see* Contact, with, shark
      strike W56.52 ☑
    flying horses W31.81 ☑
    forging (metalworking) machine W31.1 ☑
    fork W27.4 ☑
    forklift (truck) W24.0 ☑
      agricultural operations W30.89 ☑
    frog W62.0 ☑
    garden
      cultivator (powered) W29.3 ☑
        riding W30.89 ☑
      fork W27.1 ☑
    gas turbine W31.3 ☑
    Gila monster X58 ☑
    giraffe — *see* Contact, with, hoof stock NEC
    glass (sharp) (broken) W25 ☑
      assault X99.0 ☑
      due to fall — *see* Fall, by type
      stated as undetermined whether accidental or
        intentional Y28.0 ☑
      suicide (attempt) X78.0 ☑
      with subsequent fall W18.02 ☑
    goat W55.39 ☑
      bite W55.31 ☑
      strike W55.32 ☑
    goose W61.59 ☑
      bite W61.51 ☑
      strike W61.52 ☑
    hand
      saw W27.0 ☑
      tool (not powered) NEC W27.8 ☑
        powered W29.8 ☑
    harvester W30.0 ☑
    hay-derrick W30.2 ☑
    heating
      appliance (hot) X16 ☑
      pad (electric) X16 ☑
    heat NEC X19 ☑
      from appliance (electrical) (household) — *see*
        Contact, with, hot, household appliance
      heating appliance X16 ☑
    hedge-trimmer (powered) W29.3 ☑
    hoe W27.1 ☑
    hoist (chain) (shaft) NEC W24.0 ☑
      agricultural W30.89 ☑
    hoof stock NEC W55.39 ☑
      bite W55.31 ☑
      strike W55.32 ☑
    hornet(s) X58 ☑
    horse W55.19 ☑
      bite W55.11 ☑
      strike W55.12 ☑
    hot
      air X14.1 ☑
        inhalation X14.0 ☑
      cooker X15.8 ☑
      drinks X10.0 ☑
      engine X17 ☑

Contact — *continued*
  with — *continued*
    hot — *continued*
      fats X10.2 ☑
      fluids NEC X12 ☑
        assault X98.2 ☑
        suicide (attempt) X77.2 ☑
        undetermined whether accidental or inten-
          tional Y27.2 ☑
      food X10.1 ☑
      gases X14.1 ☑
        inhalation X14.0 ☑
      heating appliance X16 ☑
      household appliance X15.8 ☑
        assault X98.3 ☑
        cooker X15.8 ☑
        hotplate X15.2 ☑
        kettle X15.8 ☑
        light bulb X15.8 ☑
        object NEC X19 ☑
          assault X98.8 ☑
          stated as undetermined whether acciden-
            tal or intentional Y27.9 ☑
          suicide (attempt) X77.8 ☑
        saucepan X15.3 ☑
        skillet X15.3 ☑
        stated as undetermined whether accidental
          or intentional Y27.3 ☑
        stove X15.0 ☑
        suicide (attempt) X77.3 ☑
        toaster X15.1 ☑
      kettle X15.8 ☑
      light bulb X15.8 ☑
      liquid NEC — *see also* Burn X12 ☑
        drinks X10.0 ☑
        stated as undetermined whether accidental
          or intentional Y27.2 ☑
        suicide (attempt) X77.2 ☑
        tap water X11.8 ☑
          stated as undetermined whether acciden-
            tal or intentional Y27.1 ☑
          suicide (attempt) X77.1 ☑
      machinery X17 ☑
      metal (molten) (liquid) NEC X18 ☑
      object (not producing fire or flames) NEC X19 ☑
      oil (cooking) X10.2 ☑
      pipe X16 ☑
      plate X15.2 ☑
      radiator X16 ☑
      saucepan (glass) (metal) X15.3 ☑
      skillet X15.3 ☑
      stove (kitchen) X15.0 ☑
      substance NEC X19 ☑
      tap-water X11.8 ☑
        assault X98.1 ☑
        heated on stove X12 ☑
          stated as undetermined whether acciden-
            tal or intentional Y27.2 ☑
          suicide (attempt) X77.2 ☑
        in bathtub X11.0 ☑
        running X11.1 ☑
        stated as undetermined whether accidental
          or intentional Y27.1 ☑
        suicide (attempt) X77.1 ☑
      toaster X15.1 ☑
      tool X17 ☑
      vapors X13.1 ☑
        inhalation X13.0 ☑
      water (tap) X11.8 ☑
        boiling X12 ☑
          stated as undetermined whether acciden-
            tal or intentional Y27.2 ☑
          suicide (attempt) X77.2 ☑
        heated on stove X12 ☑
          stated as undetermined whether acciden-
            tal or intentional Y27.2 ☑
          suicide (attempt) X77.2 ☑
        in bathtub X11.0 ☑
        running X11.1 ☑
        stated as undetermined whether accidental
          or intentional Y27.1 ☑
        suicide (attempt) X77.1 ☑
    hotplate X15.2 ☑
    ice-pick W27.4 ☑
    insect (nonvenomous) NEC W57 ☑
    kettle (hot) X15.8 ☑

Contact — *continued*
with — *continued*
  knife W26.0 ☑
    assault X99.1 ☑
    electric W29.1 ☑
    stated as undetermined whether accidental or
      intentional Y28.1 ☑
    suicide (attempt) X78.1 ☑
  lathe (metalworking) W31.1 ☑
    turnings W45.8 ☑
    woodworking W31.2 ☑
  lawnmower (powered) (ridden) W28 ☑
    causing electrocution W86.8 ☑
      suicide (attempt) X83.1 ☑
    unpowered W27.1 ☑
  lift, lifting (devices) W24.0 ☑
    agricultural operations W30.89 ☑
    shaft W24.0 ☑
  liquefied gas — *see* Exposure, cold, man-made
  liquid air, hydrogen, nitrogen — *see* Exposure, cold, man-made
  lizard (nonvenomous) W59.09 ☑
    bite W59.01 ☑
    strike W59.02 ☑
  llama — *see* Contact, with, hoof stock NEC
  macaw W61.19 ☑
    bite W61.11 ☑
    strike W61.12 ☑
  machine, machinery W31.9 ☑
    abrasive wheel W31.1 ☑
    agricultural including animal-powered W30.9 ☑
      combine harvester W30.0 ☑
      grain storage elevator W30.3 ☑
      hay derrick W30.2 ☑
      power take-off device W30.1 ☑
      reaper W30.0 ☑
      specified NEC W30.89 ☑
      thresher W30.0 ☑
      transport vehicle, stationary W30.81 ☑
    band saw W31.2 ☑
    bench saw W31.2 ☑
    circular saw W31.2 ☑
    commercial NEC W31.82 ☑
    drilling, metal (industrial) W31.1 ☑
    earth-drilling W31.0 ☑
    earthmoving or scraping W31.89 ☑
    excavating W31.89 ☑
    forging machine W31.1 ☑
    gas turbine W31.3 ☑
    hot X17 ☑
    internal combustion engine W31.3 ☑
    land drill W31.0 ☑
    lathe W31.1 ☑
    lifting (devices) W24.0 ☑
    metal drill W31.1 ☑
    metalworking (industrial) W31.1 ☑
    milling, metal W31.1 ☑
    mining W31.0 ☑
    molding W31.2 ☑
    overhead plane W31.2 ☑
    power press, metal W31.1 ☑
    prime mover W31.3 ☑
    printing W31.89 ☑
    radial saw W31.2 ☑
    recreational W31.81 ☑
    roller-coaster W31.81 ☑
    rolling mill, metal W31.1 ☑
    sander W31.2 ☑
    seabed drill W31.0 ☑
    shaft
      hoist W31.0 ☑
      lift W31.0 ☑
    specified NEC W31.89 ☑
    spinning W31.89 ☑
    steam engine W31.3 ☑
    transmission W24.1 ☑
    undercutter W31.0 ☑
    water driven turbine W31.3 ☑
    weaving W31.89 ☑
    woodworking or forming (industrial) W31.2 ☑
  mammal (feces) (urine) W55.89 ☑
    bull — *see* Contact, with, bull
    cat — *see* Contact, with, cat
    cow — *see* Contact, with, cow
    goat — *see* Contact, with, goat
    hoof stock — *see* Contact, with, hoof stock

Contact — *continued*
with — *continued*
  mammal — *continued*
    horse — *see* Contact, with, horse
    marine W56.39 ☑
      dolphin — *see* Contact, with, dolphin
      orca — *see* Contact, with, orca
      sea lion — *see* Contact, with, sea lion
      specified NEC W56.39 ☑
        bite W56.31 ☑
        strike W56.32 ☑
    pig — *see* Contact, with, pig
    raccoon — *see* Contact, with, raccoon
    rodent — *see* Contact, with, rodent
    sheep — *see* Contact, with, sheep
    specified NEC W55.89 ☑
      bite W55.81 ☑
      strike W55.82 ☑
  marine
    animal W56.89 ☑
      bite W56.81 ☑
      dolphin — *see* Contact, with, dolphin
      fish NEC — *see* Contact, with, fish
      mammal — *see* Contact, with, mammal, marine
      orca — *see* Contact, with, orca
      sea lion — *see* Contact, with, sea lion
      shark — *see* Contact, with, shark
      strike W56.82 ☑
  meat
    grinder (domestic) W29.0 ☑
      industrial W31.82 ☑
      nonpowered W27.4 ☑
    slicer (domestic) W29.0 ☑
      industrial W31.82 ☑
  merry go round W31.81 ☑
  metal, hot (liquid) (molten) NEC X18 ☑
  millipede W57 ☑
  nail W45.0 ☑
    gun W29.4 ☑
  needle (sewing) W27.3 ☑
    hypodermic W46.0 ☑
      contaminated W46.1 ☑
  object (blunt) NEC
    hot NEC X19 ☑
    legal intervention — *see* Legal, intervention, blunt object
    sharp NEC W45.8 ☑
      inflicted by other person NEC W45.8 ☑
        stated as
          intentional homicide (attempt) — *see* Assault, cutting or piercing instrument
      legal intervention — *see* Legal, intervention, sharp object
      self-inflicted X78.9 ☑
  orca W56.29 ☑
    bite W56.21 ☑
    strike W56.22 ☑
  overhead plane W31.2 ☑
  paper (as sharp object) W26.2 ☑
  paper-cutter W27.5 ☑
  parrot W61.09 ☑
    bite W61.01 ☑
    strike W61.02 ☑
  pig W55.49 ☑
    bite W55.41 ☑
    strike W55.42 ☑
  pipe, hot X16 ☑
  pitchfork W27.1 ☑
  plane (metal) (wood) W27.0 ☑
    overhead W31.2 ☑
  plant thorns, spines, sharp leaves or other mechanisms W60 ☑
  powered
    garden cultivator W29.3 ☑
    household appliance, implement, or machine W29.8 ☑
    saw (industrial) W31.2 ☑
      hand W29.8 ☑
  printing machine W31.89 ☑
  psittacine bird W61.29 ☑
    bite W61.21 ☑
    macaw — *see* Contact, with, macaw
    parrot — *see* Contact, with, parrot
    strike W61.22 ☑

Contact — *continued*
with — *continued*
  pulley (block) (transmission) W24.0 ☑
    agricultural operations W30.89 ☑
  raccoon W55.59 ☑
    bite W55.51 ☑
    strike W55.52 ☑
  radial-saw (industrial) W31.2 ☑
  radiator (hot) X16 ☑
  rake W27.1 ☑
  rattlesnake X58 ☑
  reaper W30.0 ☑
  reptile W59.89 ☑
    lizard — *see* Contact, with, lizard
    snake — *see* Contact, with, snake
    specified NEC W59.89 ☑
      bite W59.81 ☑
      crushing W59.83 ☑
      strike W59.82 ☑
    turtle — *see* Contact, with, turtle
  rivet gun (powered) W29.4 ☑
  road scraper — *see* Accident, transport, construction vehicle
  rodent (feces) (urine) W53.89 ☑
    bite W53.81 ☑
    mouse W53.09 ☑
      bite W53.01 ☑
    rat W53.19 ☑
      bite W53.11 ☑
    specified NEC W53.89 ☑
      bite W53.81 ☑
    squirrel W53.29 ☑
      bite W53.21 ☑
  roller coaster W31.81 ☑
  rope NEC W24.0 ☑
    agricultural operations W30.89 ☑
  saliva — *see* Contact, with, by type of animal
  sander W29.8 ☑
    industrial W31.2 ☑
  saucepan (hot) (glass) (metal) X15.3 ☑
  saw W27.0 ☑
    band (industrial) W31.2 ☑
    bench (industrial) W31.2 ☑
    chain W29.3 ☑
    hand W27.0 ☑
  sawing machine, metal W31.1 ☑
  scissors W27.2 ☑
  scorpion X58 ☑
  screwdriver W27.0 ☑
    powered W29.8 ☑
  sea
    anemone, cucumber or urchin (spine) X58 ☑
    lion W56.19 ☑
      bite W56.11 ☑
      strike W56.12 ☑
  serpent — *see* Contact, with, snake, by type
  sewing-machine (electric) (powered) W29.2 ☑
    not powered W27.8 ☑
  shaft (hoist) (lift) (transmission) NEC W24.0 ☑
    agricultural W30.89 ☑
  shark W56.49 ☑
    bite W56.41 ☑
    strike W56.42 ☑
  sharp object(s) W26.9 ☑
    specified NEC W26.8 ☑
  shears (hand) W27.2 ☑
    powered (industrial) W31.1 ☑
      domestic W29.2 ☑
  sheep W55.39 ☑
    bite W55.31 ☑
    strike W55.32 ☑
  shovel W27.8 ☑
    steam — *see* Accident, transport, construction vehicle
  snake (nonvenomous) W59.19 ☑
    bite W59.11 ☑
    crushing W59.13 ☑
    strike W59.12 ☑
  spade W27.1 ☑
  spider (venomous) X58 ☑
  spin-drier W29.2 ☑
  spinning machine W31.89 ☑
  splinter W45.8 ☑
  sports equipment W21.9 ☑
  staple gun (powered) W29.8 ☑
  steam X13.1 ☑

☑ **Additional Character Required** — Refer to the Tabular List for Character Selection
☑ Subterms under main terms may continue to next column or page

Contact — *continued*
  with — *continued*
    steam — *continued*
      engine W31.3 ☑
      inhalation X13.0 ☑
      pipe X16 ☑
      shovel W31.89 ☑
    stove (hot) (kitchen) X15.0 ☑
    substance, hot NEC X19 ☑
      molten (metal) X18 ☑
    sword W26.1 ☑
      assault X99.2 ☑
      stated as undetermined whether accidental or
        intentional Y28.2 ☑
      suicide (attempt) X78.2 ☑
    tarantula X58 ☑
    thresher W30.0 ☑
    tin can lid W26.8 ☑
    toad W62.1 ☑
    toaster (hot) X15.1 ☑
    tool W27.8 ☑
      hand (not powered) W27.8 ☑
        auger W27.0 ☑
        axe W27.0 ☑
        can opener W27.4 ☑
        chisel W27.0 ☑
        fork W27.4 ☑
        garden W27.1 ☑
        handsaw W27.0 ☑
        hoe W27.1 ☑
        ice-pick W27.4 ☑
        kitchen utensil W27.4 ☑
        manual
          lawn mower W27.1 ☑
          sewing machine W27.8 ☑
        meat grinder W27.4 ☑
        needle (sewing) W27.3 ☑
          hypodermic W46.0 ☑
            contaminated W46.1 ☑
        paper cutter W27.5 ☑
        pitchfork W27.1 ☑
        rake W27.1 ☑
        scissors W27.2 ☑
        screwdriver W27.0 ☑
        specified NEC W27.8 ☑
        workbench W27.0 ☑
      hot X17 ☑
      powered W29.8 ☑
        blender W29.0 ☑
          commercial W31.82 ☑
        can opener W29.0 ☑
          commercial W31.82 ☑
        chainsaw W29.3 ☑
        clothes dryer W29.2 ☑
          commercial W31.82 ☑
        dishwasher W29.2 ☑
          commercial W31.82 ☑
        edger W29.3 ☑
        electric fan W29.2 ☑
          commercial W31.82 ☑
        electric knife W29.1 ☑
        food processor W29.0 ☑
          commercial W31.82 ☑
        garbage disposal W29.0 ☑
          commercial W31.82 ☑
        garden tool W29.3 ☑
        hedge trimmer W29.3 ☑
        ice maker W29.0 ☑
          commercial W31.82 ☑
        kitchen appliance W29.0 ☑
          commercial W31.82 ☑
        lawn mower W28 ☑
        meat grinder W29.0 ☑
          commercial W31.82 ☑
        mixer W29.0 ☑
          commercial W31.82 ☑
        rototiller W29.3 ☑
        sewing machine W29.2 ☑
          commercial W31.82 ☑
        washing machine W29.2 ☑
          commercial W31.82 ☑
    transmission device (belt, cable, chain, gear, pinion,
      shaft) W24.1 ☑
        agricultural operations W30.89 ☑
    turbine (gas) (water-driven) W31.3 ☑
    turkey W61.49 ☑

Contact — *continued*
  with — *continued*
    turkey — *continued*
      peck W61.43 ☑
      strike W61.42 ☑
    turtle (nonvenomous) W59.29 ☑
      bite W59.21 ☑
      strike W59.22 ☑
      terrestrial W59.89 ☑
        bite W59.81 ☑
        crushing W59.83 ☑
        strike W59.82 ☑
      under-cutter W31.0 ☑
    urine — *see* Contact, with, by type of animal
    vehicle
      agricultural use (transport) — *see* Accident,
        transport, agricultural vehicle
        not on public highway W30.81 ☑
      industrial use (transport) — *see* Accident, trans-
        port, industrial vehicle
        not on public highway W31.83 ☑
      off-road use (transport) — *see* Accident, trans-
        port, all-terrain or off-road vehicle
        not on public highway W31.83 ☑
      special construction use (transport) — *see* Acci-
        dent, transport, construction vehicle
        not on public highway W31.83 ☑
    venomous
      animal X58 ☑
      arthropods X58 ☑
      lizard X58 ☑
      marine animal NEC X58 ☑
      marine plant NEC X58 ☑
      millipedes (tropical) X58 ☑
      plant(s) X58 ☑
      snake X58 ☑
      spider X58 ☑
      viper X58 ☑
    washing-machine (powered) W29.2 ☑
    wasp X58 ☑
    weaving-machine W31.89 ☑
    winch W24.0 ☑
      agricultural operations W30.89 ☑
    wire NEC W24.0 ☑
      agricultural operations W30.89 ☑
    wood slivers W45.8 ☑
    yellow jacket X58 ☑
    zebra — *see* Contact, with, hoof stock NEC
  pressure X50.9 ☑
  stress X50.9 ☑
Coup de soleil X32 ☑
Crash
  aircraft (in transit) (powered) V95.9 ☑
    balloon V96.01 ☑
    fixed wing NEC (private) V95.21 ☑
      commercial V95.31 ☑
    glider V96.21 ☑
      hang V96.11 ☑
      powered V95.11 ☑
    helicopter V95.01 ☑
    in war operations — *see* War operations, destruction
      of aircraft
    microlight V95.11 ☑
    nonpowered V96.9 ☑
      specified NEC V96.8 ☑
    powered NEC V95.8 ☑
    stated as
      homicide (attempt) Y08.81 ☑
      suicide (attempt) X83.0 ☑
    ultralight V95.11 ☑
  spacecraft V95.41 ☑
  transport vehicle NEC — *see also* Accident, transport
    V89.9 ☑
    homicide (attempt) Y03.8 ☑
    motor NEC (traffic) V89.2 ☑
      homicide (attempt) Y03.8 ☑
      suicide (attempt) — *see* Suicide, collision
Cruelty (mental) (physical) (sexual) X58 ☑
Crushed (accidentally) X58 ☑
  between objects (moving) (stationary and moving)
    W23.0 ☑
    stationary W23.1 ☑
  by
    alligator W58.03 ☑
    avalanche NEC — *see* Landslide
    cave-in W20.0 ☑

Crushed — *continued*
  by — *continued*
    cave-in — *continued*
      caused by cataclysmic earth surface movement
        — *see* Landslide
    crocodile W58.13 ☑
    crowd or human stampede W52 ☑
    falling
      aircraft V97.39 ☑
        in war operations — *see* War operations, de-
          struction of aircraft
      earth, material W20.0 ☑
        caused by cataclysmic earth surface move-
          ment — *see* Landslide
      object NEC W20.8 ☑
    landslide NEC — *see* Landslide
    lizard (nonvenomous) W59.09 ☑
    machinery — *see* Contact, with, by type of machine
    reptile NEC W59.89 ☑
    snake (nonvenomous) W59.13 ☑
  in
    machinery — *see* Contact, with, by type of machine
Cut, cutting (any part of body) (accidental) — *see also*
  Contact, with, by object or machine
  during medical or surgical treatment as misadventure
    — *see* Index to Diseases and Injuries, Complica-
    tions
  homicide (attempt) — *see* Assault, cutting or piercing
    instrument
  inflicted by other person — *see* Assault, cutting or
    piercing instrument
  legal
    execution — *see* Legal, intervention
    intervention — *see* Legal, intervention, sharp object
  machine NEC — *see also* Contact, with, by type of ma-
    chine W31.9 ☑
  self-inflicted — *see* Suicide, cutting or piercing instru-
    ment
  suicide (attempt) — *see* Suicide, cutting or piercing
    instrument
Cyclone (any injury) X37.1 ☑

D

Decapitation (accidental circumstances) NEC X58 ☑
  homicide X99.9 ☑
  legal execution — *see* Legal, intervention
Dehydration from lack of water X58 ☑
Deprivation X58 ☑
Derailment (accidental)
  railway (rolling stock) (train) (vehicle) (without an-
    tecedent collision) V81.7 ☑
    with antecedent collision — *see* Accident, transport,
      railway vehicle occupant
  streetcar (without antecedent collision) V82.7 ☑
    with antecedent collision — *see* Accident, transport,
      streetcar occupant
Descent
  parachute (voluntary) (without accident to aircraft)
    V97.29 ☑
    due to accident to aircraft — *see* Accident, transport,
      aircraft
Desertion X58 ☑
Destitution X58 ☑
Disability, late effect or sequela of injury — *see* Se-
  quelae
Discharge (accidental)
  airgun W34.010 ☑
    assault X95.01 ☑
    homicide (attempt) X95.01 ☑
    stated as undetermined whether accidental or inten-
      tional Y24.0 ☑
    suicide (attempt) X74.01 ☑
  BB gun — *see* Discharge, airgun
  firearm (accidental) W34.00 ☑
    assault X95.9 ☑
    handgun (pistol) (revolver) W32.0 ☑
      assault X93 ☑
      homicide (attempt) X93 ☑
      legal intervention — *see* Legal, intervention,
        firearm, handgun
      stated as undetermined whether accidental or
        intentional Y22 ☑
      suicide (attempt) X72 ☑
    homicide (attempt) X95.9 ☑
    hunting rifle W33.02 ☑

Discharge — continued
- firearm — continued
  - hunting rifle — continued
    - assault X94.1 ☑
    - homicide (attempt) X94.1 ☑
    - legal intervention
      - injuring
        - bystander Y35.032 ☑
        - law enforcement personnel Y35.031 ☑
        - suspect Y35.033 ☑
        - unspecified person Y35.039 ☑
    - stated as undetermined whether accidental or intentional Y23.1 ☑
    - suicide (attempt) X73.1 ☑
  - larger W33.00 ☑
    - assault X94.9 ☑
    - homicide (attempt) X94.9 ☑
    - hunting rifle — see Discharge, firearm, hunting rifle
    - legal intervention — see Legal, intervention, firearm by type of firearm
    - machine gun — see Discharge, firearm, machine gun
    - shotgun — see Discharge, firearm, shotgun
    - specified NEC W33.09 ☑
      - assault X94.8 ☑
      - homicide (attempt) X94.8 ☑
      - legal intervention
        - injuring
          - bystander Y35.092 ☑
          - law enforcement personnel Y35.091 ☑
          - suspect Y35.093 ☑
          - unspecified person Y35.099 ☑
      - stated as undetermined whether accidental or intentional Y23.8 ☑
      - suicide (attempt) X73.8 ☑
    - stated as undetermined whether accidental or intentional Y23.9 ☑
    - suicide (attempt) X73.9 ☑
  - legal intervention
    - injuring
      - bystander Y35.002 ☑
      - law enforcement personnel Y35.001 ☑
      - suspect Y35.03 ☑
      - unspecified person Y35.009 ☑
    - using rubber bullet
      - injuring
        - bystander Y35.042 ☑
        - law enforcement personnel Y35.041 ☑
        - suspect Y35.043 ☑
        - unspecified person Y35.049 ☑
  - machine gun W33.03 ☑
    - assault X94.2 ☑
    - homicide (attempt) X94.2 ☑
    - legal intervention — see Legal, intervention, firearm, machine gun
    - stated as undetermined whether accidental or intentional Y23.3 ☑
    - suicide (attempt) X73.2 ☑
  - pellet gun — see Discharge, airgun
  - shotgun W33.01 ☑
    - assault X94.0 ☑
    - homicide (attempt) X94.0 ☑
    - legal intervention — see Legal, intervention, firearm, specified NEC
    - stated as undetermined whether accidental or intentional Y23.0 ☑
    - suicide (attempt) X73.0 ☑
  - specified NEC W34.09 ☑
    - assault X95.8 ☑
    - homicide (attempt) X95.8 ☑
    - legal intervention — see Legal, intervention, firearm, specified NEC
    - stated as undetermined whether accidental or intentional Y24.8 ☑
    - suicide (attempt) X74.8 ☑
  - stated as undetermined whether accidental or intentional Y24.9 ☑
  - suicide (attempt) X74.9 ☑
  - Very pistol W34.09 ☑
    - assault X95.8 ☑
    - homicide (attempt) X95.8 ☑
    - stated as undetermined whether accidental or intentional Y24.8 ☑
    - suicide (attempt) X74.8 ☑

Discharge — continued
- firework(s) W39 ☑
  - stated as undetermined whether accidental or intentional Y25 ☑
- gas-operated gun NEC W34.018 ☑
  - airgun — see Discharge, airgun
  - assault X95.09 ☑
  - homicide (attempt) X95.09 ☑
  - paintball gun — see Discharge, paintball gun
  - stated as undetermined whether accidental or intentional Y24.8 ☑
  - suicide (attempt) X74.09 ☑
- gun NEC — see also Discharge, firearm NEC
  - air — see Discharge, airgun
  - BB — see Discharge, airgun
  - for single hand use — see Discharge, firearm, handgun
  - hand — see Discharge, firearm, handgun
  - machine — see Discharge, firearm, machine gun
  - other specified — see Discharge, firearm NEC
  - paintball — see Discharge, paintball gun
  - pellet — see Discharge, airgun
- handgun — see Discharge, firearm, handgun
- machine gun — see Discharge, firearm, machine gun
- paintball gun W34.011 ☑
  - assault X95.02 ☑
  - homicide (attempt) X95.02 ☑
  - stated as undetermined whether accidental or intentional Y24.8 ☑
  - suicide (attempt) X74.02 ☑
- pistol — see Discharge, firearm, handgun
  - flare — see Discharge, firearm, Very pistol
  - pellet — see Discharge, airgun
  - Very — see Discharge, firearm, Very pistol
- revolver — see Discharge, firearm, handgun
- rifle (hunting) — see Discharge, firearm, hunting rifle
- shotgun — see Discharge, firearm, shotgun
- spring-operated gun NEC W34.018 ☑
  - assault X95.09 ☑
  - homicide (attempt) X95.09 ☑
  - stated as undetermined whether accidental or intentional Y24.8 ☑
  - suicide (attempt) X74.09 ☑

Disease
- Andes W94.11 ☑
- aviator's — see Air, pressure
- range W94.11 ☑

Diver's disease, palsy, paralysis, squeeze — see Air, pressure

Diving (into water) — see Accident, diving

Dog bite W54.0 ☑

Dragged by transport vehicle NEC — see also Accident, transport V09.9 ☑

Drinking poison (accidental) — see Table of Drugs and Chemicals

Dropped (accidentally) **while being carried or supported by other person** W04 ☑

Drowning (accidental) W74 ☑
- assault X92.9 ☑
- due to
  - accident (to)
    - machinery — see Contact, with, by type of machine
    - watercraft V90.89 ☑
      - burning V90.29 ☑
        - powered V90.23 ☑
          - fishing boat V90.22 ☑
          - jetskis V90.23 ☑
          - merchant ship V90.20 ☑
          - passenger ship V90.21 ☑
        - unpowered V90.28 ☑
          - canoe V90.25 ☑
          - inflatable V90.26 ☑
          - kayak V90.25 ☑
          - sailboat V90.24 ☑
          - water skis V90.27 ☑
      - crushed V90.39 ☑
        - powered V90.33 ☑
          - fishing boat V90.32 ☑
          - jetskis V90.33 ☑
          - merchant ship V90.30 ☑
          - passenger ship V90.31 ☑
        - unpowered V90.38 ☑
          - canoe V90.35 ☑
          - inflatable V90.36 ☑
          - kayak V90.35 ☑

Drowning — continued
- due to — continued
  - accident — continued
    - watercraft — continued
      - crushed — continued
        - unpowered — continued
          - sailboat V90.34 ☑
          - water skis V90.37 ☑
      - overturning V90.09 ☑
        - powered V90.03 ☑
          - fishing boat V90.02 ☑
          - jetskis V90.03 ☑
          - merchant ship V90.00 ☑
          - passenger ship V90.01 ☑
        - unpowered V90.08 ☑
          - canoe V90.05 ☑
          - inflatable V90.06 ☑
          - kayak V90.05 ☑
          - sailboat V90.04 ☑
      - sinking V90.19 ☑
        - powered V90.13 ☑
          - fishing boat V90.12 ☑
          - jetskis V90.13 ☑
          - merchant ship V90.10 ☑
          - passenger ship V90.11 ☑
        - unpowered V90.18 ☑
          - canoe V90.15 ☑
          - inflatable V90.16 ☑
          - kayak V90.15 ☑
          - sailboat V90.14 ☑
      - specified type NEC V90.89 ☑
        - powered V90.83 ☑
          - fishing boat V90.82 ☑
          - jetskis V90.83 ☑
          - merchant ship V90.80 ☑
          - passenger ship V90.81 ☑
        - unpowered V90.88 ☑
          - canoe V90.85 ☑
          - inflatable V90.86 ☑
          - kayak V90.85 ☑
          - sailboat V90.84 ☑
          - water skis V90.87 ☑
  - avalanche — see Landslide
  - cataclysmic
    - earth surface movement NEC — see Forces of nature, earth movement
    - storm — see Forces of nature, cataclysmic storm
  - cloudburst X37.8 ☑
  - cyclone X37.1 ☑
  - fall overboard (from) V92.09 ☑
    - powered craft V92.03 ☑
      - ferry boat V92.01 ☑
      - fishing boat V92.02 ☑
      - jetskis V92.03 ☑
      - liner V92.01 ☑
      - merchant ship V92.00 ☑
      - passenger ship V92.01 ☑
  - resulting from
    - accident to watercraft — see Drowning, due to, accident to, watercraft
    - being washed overboard (from) V92.29 ☑
      - powered craft V92.23 ☑
        - ferry boat V92.21 ☑
        - fishing boat V92.22 ☑
        - jetskis V92.23 ☑
        - liner V92.21 ☑
        - merchant ship V92.20 ☑
        - passenger ship V92.21 ☑
      - unpowered craft V92.28 ☑
        - canoe V92.25 ☑
        - inflatable V92.26 ☑
        - kayak V92.25 ☑
        - sailboat V92.24 ☑
        - surf-board V92.28 ☑
        - water skis V92.27 ☑
        - windsurfer V92.28 ☑
    - motion of watercraft V92.19 ☑
      - powered craft V92.13 ☑
        - ferry boat V92.11 ☑
        - fishing boat V92.12 ☑
        - jetskis V92.13 ☑
        - liner V92.11 ☑
        - merchant ship V92.10 ☑
        - passenger ship V92.11 ☑
      - unpowered craft
        - canoe V92.15 ☑

Drowning — continued
  due to — continued
    fall overboard — continued
      resulting from — continued
        motion of watercraft — continued
          unpowered craft — continued
            inflatable V92.16 ☑
            kayak V92.15 ☑
            sailboat V92.14 ☑
        unpowered craft V92.08 ☑
          canoe V92.05 ☑
          inflatable V92.06 ☑
          kayak V92.05 ☑
          sailboat V92.04 ☑
          surf-board V92.08 ☑
          water skis V92.07 ☑
          windsurfer V92.08 ☑
    hurricane X37.0 ☑
    jumping into water from watercraft (involved in
      accident) — see also Drowning, due to, acci-
      dent to, watercraft
      without accident to or on watercraft W16.711 ☑
    tidal wave NEC — see Forces of nature, tidal wave
    torrential rain X37.8 ☑
  following
    fall
      into
        bathtub W16.211 ☑
        bucket W16.221 ☑
        fountain — see Drowning, following, fall, into,
          water, specified NEC
        quarry — see Drowning, following, fall, into,
          water, specified NEC
        reservoir — see Drowning, following, fall, into,
          water, specified NEC
        swimming-pool W16.011 ☑
          stated as undetermined whether acciden-
            tal or intentional Y21.3 ☑
          striking
            bottom W16.021 ☑
            wall W16.031 ☑
          suicide (attempt) X71.2 ☑
        water NOS W16.41 ☑
          natural (lake) (open sea) (river) (stream)
            (pond) W16.111 ☑
            striking
              bottom W16.121 ☑
              side W16.131 ☑
          specified NEC W16.311 ☑
            striking
              bottom W16.321 ☑
              wall W16.331 ☑
    overboard NEC — see Drowning, due to, fall
      overboard
    jump or dive
      from boat W16.711 ☑
        striking bottom W16.721 ☑
      into
        fountain — see Drowning, following, jump
          or dive, into, water, specified NEC
        quarry — see Drowning, following, jump or
          dive, into, water, specified NEC
        reservoir — see Drowning, following, jump
          or dive, into, water, specified NEC
        swimming-pool W16.511 ☑
          striking
            bottom W16.521 ☑
            wall W16.531 ☑
          suicide (attempt) X71.2 ☑
        water NOS W16.91 ☑
          natural (lake) (open sea) (river) (stream)
            (pond) W16.611 ☑
          specified NEC W16.811 ☑
            bottom W16.821 ☑
            striking
              bottom W16.821 ☑
              wall W16.831 ☑
          striking
            bottom W16.821 ☑
            wall W16.831 ☑
          striking bottom W16.621 ☑
  homicide (attempt) X92.9 ☑
  in
    bathtub (accidental) W65 ☑
      assault X92.0 ☑
      following fall W16.211 ☑

Drowning — continued
  in — continued
    bathtub — continued
      following fall — continued
        stated as undetermined whether accidental
          or intentional Y21.1 ☑
      stated as undetermined whether accidental or
        intentional Y21.0 ☑
      suicide (attempt) X71.0 ☑
    lake — see Drowning, in, natural water
    natural water (lake) (open sea) (river) (stream)
      (pond) W69 ☑
      assault X92.3 ☑
      following
        dive or jump W16.611 ☑
          striking bottom W16.621 ☑
        fall W16.111 ☑
          striking
            bottom W16.121 ☑
            side W16.131 ☑
      stated as undetermined whether accidental or
        intentional Y21.4 ☑
      suicide (attempt) X71.3 ☑
    quarry — see Drowning, in, specified place NEC
    quenching tank — see Drowning, in, specified place
      NEC
    reservoir — see Drowning, in, specified place NEC
    river — see Drowning, in, natural water
    sea — see Drowning, in, natural water
    specified place NEC W73 ☑
      assault X92.8 ☑
      following
        dive or jump W16.811 ☑
          striking
            bottom W16.821 ☑
            wall W16.831 ☑
        fall W16.311 ☑
          striking
            bottom W16.321 ☑
            wall W16.331 ☑
      stated as undetermined whether accidental or
        intentional Y21.8 ☑
      suicide (attempt) X71.8 ☑
    stream — see Drowning, in, natural water
    swimming-pool W67 ☑
      assault X92.1 ☑
        following fall X92.2 ☑
      following
        dive or jump W16.511 ☑
          striking
            bottom W16.521 ☑
            wall W16.531 ☑
        fall W16.011 ☑
          striking
            bottom W16.021 ☑
            wall W16.031 ☑
      stated as undetermined whether accidental or
        intentional Y21.2 ☑
        following fall Y21.3 ☑
      suicide (attempt) X71.1 ☑
        following fall X71.2 ☑
    war operations — see War operations, restriction
      of airway
  resulting from accident to watercraft — see Drowning,
    due to, accident, watercraft
  self-inflicted X71.9 ☑
  stated as undetermined whether accidental or inten-
    tional Y21.9 ☑
  suicide (attempt) X71.9 ☑

E

Earth falling (on) W20.0 ☑
  caused by cataclysmic earth surface movement or
    eruption — see Landslide
Earth (surface) **movement NEC** — see Forces of nature,
  earth movement
Earthquake (any injury) X34 ☑
Effect(s) (adverse) **of**
  air pressure (any) — see Air, pressure
  cold, excessive (exposure to) — see Exposure, cold
  heat (excessive) — see Heat
  hot place (weather) — see Heat
  insolation X30 ☑
  late — see Sequelae
  motion — see Motion

Effect(s) (adverse) **of** — continued
  nuclear explosion or weapon in war operations — see
    War operations, nuclear weapon
  radiation — see Radiation
  travel — see Travel
Electric shock (accidental) (by) (in) — see Exposure,
  electric current
Electrocution (accidental) — see Exposure, electric current
Endotracheal tube wrongly placed during anesthetic
  procedure
Entanglement
  in
    bed linen, causing suffocation T71 ☑
    wheel of pedal cycle V19.88 ☑
Entry of foreign body or material — see Foreign body
Environmental pollution related condition — see
  category Z57
Execution, legal (any method) — see Legal, intervention
Exhaustion
  cold — see Exposure, cold
  due to excessive exertion — see also Overexertion
    X50.9 ☑
  heat — see Heat
Explosion (accidental) (of) (with secondary fire) W40.9 ☑
  acetylene W40.1 ☑
  aerosol can W36.1 ☑
  air tank (compressed) (in machinery) W36.2 ☑
  aircraft (in transit) (powered) NEC V95.9 ☑
    balloon V96.05 ☑
    fixed wing NEC (private) V95.25 ☑
      commercial V95.35 ☑
    glider V96.25 ☑
      hang V96.15 ☑
      powered V95.15 ☑
    helicopter V95.05 ☑
    in war operations — see War operations, destruction
      of aircraft
    microlight V95.15 ☑
    nonpowered V96.9 ☑
      specified NEC V96.8 ☑
    powered NEC V95.8 ☑
    stated as
      homicide (attempt) Y03.8 ☑
      suicide (attempt) X83.0 ☑
    ultralight V95.15 ☑
  anesthetic gas in operating room W40.1 ☑
  antipersonnel bomb W40.8 ☑
    assault X96.0 ☑
    homicide (attempt) X96.0 ☑
    suicide (attempt) X75 ☑
  assault X96.9 ☑
  bicycle tire W37.0 ☑
  blasting (cap) (materials) W40.0 ☑
  boiler (machinery), not on transport vehicle W35 ☑
    on watercraft — see Explosion, in, watercraft
  butane W40.1 ☑
  caused by other person X96.9 ☑
  coal gas W40.1 ☑
  detonator W40.0 ☑
  dump (munitions) W40.8 ☑
  dynamite W40.0 ☑
    in
      assault X96.8 ☑
      homicide (attempt) X96.8 ☑
      legal intervention
        injuring
          bystander Y35.112 ☑
          law enforcement personnel Y35.111 ☑
          suspect Y35.113 ☑
          unspecified person Y35.119 ☑
      suicide (attempt) X75 ☑
  explosive (material) W40.9 ☑
    gas W40.1 ☑
    in blasting operation W40.0 ☑
    specified NEC W40.8 ☑
      in
        assault X96.8 ☑
        homicide (attempt) X96.8 ☑
        legal intervention
          injuring
            bystander Y35.192 ☑
            law enforcement personnel
              Y35.191 ☑
            suspect Y35.193 ☑
            unspecified person Y35.199 ☑

Explosion — *continued*
  explosive — *continued*
    specified — *continued*
      in — *continued*
        suicide (attempt) X75 ☑
  factory (munitions) W40.8 ☑
  fertilizer bomb W40.8 ☑
    assault X96.3 ☑
    homicide (attempt) X96.3 ☑
    suicide (attempt) X75 ☑
  firearm (parts) NEC W34.19 ☑
    airgun W34.110 ☑
    BB gun W34.110 ☑
    gas, air or spring-operated gun NEC W34.118 ☑
    hangun W32.1 ☑
    hunting rifle W33.12 ☑
    larger firearm W33.10 ☑
      specified NEC W33.19 ☑
    machine gun W33.13 ☑
    paintball gun W34.111 ☑
    pellet gun W34.110 ☑
    shotgun W33.11 ☑
    Very pistol [flare] W34.19 ☑
  fire-damp W40.1 ☑
  fireworks W39 ☑
  gas (coal) (explosive) W40.1 ☑
    cylinder W36.9 ☑
      aerosol can W36.1 ☑
      air tank W36.2 ☑
      pressurized W36.3 ☑
      specified NEC W36.8 ☑
  gasoline (fumes) (tank) not in moving motor vehicle W40.1 ☑
    bomb W40.8 ☑
      assault X96.1 ☑
      homicide (attempt) X96.1 ☑
      suicide (attempt) X75 ☑
    in motor vehicle — *see* Accident, transport, by type of vehicle
  grain store W40.8 ☑
  grenade W40.8 ☑
    in
      assault X96.8 ☑
      homicide (attempt) X96.8 ☑
      legal intervention
        injuring
          bystander Y35.192 ☑
          law enforcement personnel Y35.191 ☑
          suspect Y35.193 ☑
          unspecified person Y35.199 ☑
      suicide (attempt) X75 ☑
  handgun (parts) — *see* Explosion, firearm, hangun (parts)
  homicide (attempt) X96.9 ☑
    antipersonnel bomb — *see* Explosion, antipersonnel bomb
    fertilizer bomb — *see* Explosion, fertilizer bomb
    gasoline bomb — *see* Explosion, gasoline bomb
    letter bomb — *see* Explosion, letter bomb
    pipe bomb — *see* Explosion, pipe bomb
    specified NEC X96.8 ☑
  hose, pressurized W37.8 ☑
  hot water heater, tank (in machinery) W35 ☑
    on watercraft — *see* Explosion, in, watercraft
  in, on
    dump W40.8 ☑
    factory W40.8 ☑
    mine (of explosive gases) NEC W40.1 ☑
    watercraft V93.59 ☑
      powered craft V93.53 ☑
        ferry boat V93.51 ☑
        fishing boat V93.52 ☑
        jetskis V93.53 ☑
        liner V93.51 ☑
        merchant ship V93.50 ☑
        passenger ship V93.51 ☑
        sailboat V93.54 ☑
  letter bomb W40.8 ☑
    assault X96.2 ☑
    homicide (attempt) X96.2 ☑
    suicide (attempt) X75 ☑
  machinery — *see also* Contact, with, by type of machine
    on board watercraft — *see* Explosion, in, watercraft
    pressure vessel — *see* Explosion, by type of vessel
  methane W40.1 ☑

Explosion — *continued*
  mine W40.1 ☑
  missile NEC W40.8 ☑
  mortar bomb W40.8 ☑
    in
      assault X96.8 ☑
      homicide (attempt) X96.8 ☑
      legal intervention
        injuring
          bystander Y35.192 ☑
          law enforcement personnel Y35.191 ☑
          suspect Y35.193 ☑
          unspecified person Y35.199 ☑
      suicide (attempt) X75 ☑
  munitions (dump) (factory) W40.8 ☑
  pipe, pressurized W37.8 ☑
    bomb W40.8 ☑
      assault X96.4 ☑
      homicide (attempt) X96.4 ☑
      suicide (attempt) X75 ☑
  pressure, pressurized
    cooker W38 ☑
    gas tank (in machinery) W36.3 ☑
    hose W37.8 ☑
    pipe W37.8 ☑
    specified device NEC W38 ☑
    tire W37.8 ☑
      bicycle W37.0 ☑
    vessel (in machinery) W38 ☑
  propane W40.1 ☑
  self-inflicted X75 ☑
  shell (artillery) NEC W40.8 ☑
    during war operations — *see* War operations, explosion
    in
      legal intervention
        injuring
          bystander Y35.122 ☑
          law enforcement personnel Y35.121 ☑
          suspect Y35.123 ☑
          unspecified person Y35.129 ☑
    war — *see* War operations, explosion
  spacecraft V95.45 ☑
  stated as undetermined whether accidental or intentional Y25 ☑
  steam or water lines (in machinery) W37.8 ☑
  stove W40.9 ☑
  suicide (attempt) X75 ☑
  tire, pressurized W37.8 ☑
    bicycle W37.0 ☑
  undetermined whether accidental or intentional Y25 ☑
  vehicle tire NEC W37.8 ☑
    bicycle W37.0 ☑
  war operations — *see* War operations, explosion

Exposure (to) X58 ☑
  air pressure change — *see* Air, pressure
  cold (accidental) (excessive) (extreme) (natural) (place) X31 ☑
    assault Y08.89 ☑
    due to
      man-made conditions W93.8 ☑
        dry ice (contact) W93.01 ☑
          inhalation W93.02 ☑
        liquid air (contact) (hydrogen) (nitrogen) W93.11 ☑
          inhalation W93.12 ☑
        refrigeration unit (deep freeze) W93.2 ☑
        suicide (attempt) X83.2 ☑
      weather (conditions) X31 ☑
    homicide (attempt) Y08.89 ☑
    self-inflicted X83.2 ☑
  due to abandonment or neglect X58 ☑
  electric current W86.8 ☑
    appliance (faulty) W86.8 ☑
      domestic W86.0 ☑
    caused by other person Y08.89 ☑
    conductor (faulty) W86.1 ☑
    control apparatus (faulty) W86.1 ☑
    electric power generating plant, distribution station W86.1 ☑
    electroshock gun — *see* Exposure, electric current, taser
    high-voltage cable W85 ☑
    homicide (attempt) Y08.89 ☑
    legal execution — *see* Legal, intervention, specified means NEC

Exposure — *continued*
  electric current — *continued*
    lightning — *see* subcategory T75.0 ☑
    live rail W86.8 ☑
    misadventure in medical or surgical procedure in electroshock therapy Y63.4
    motor (electric) (faulty) W86.8 ☑
      domestic W86.0 ☑
    self-inflicted X83.1 ☑
    specified NEC W86.8 ☑
      domestic W86.0 ☑
    stun gun — *see* Exposure, electric current, taser
    suicide (attempt) X83.1 ☑
    taser W86.8 ☑
      assault Y08.89 ☑
      legal intervention — *see* category Y35
      self-harm (intentional) X83.8 ☑
      undetermined intent Y33 ☑
    third rail W86.8 ☑
    transformer (faulty) W86.1 ☑
    transmission lines W85 ☑
  environmental tobacco smoke X58 ☑
  excessive
    cold — *see* Exposure, cold
    heat (natural) NEC X30 ☑
      man-made W92 ☑
  factor(s) NOS X58 ☑
    environmental NEC X58 ☑
    man-made NEC W99 ☑
    natural NEC — *see* Forces of nature
    specified NEC X58 ☑
  fire, flames (accidental) X08.8 ☑
    assault X97 ☑
    campfire — *see* Exposure, fire, controlled, not in building
    controlled (in)
      with ignition (of) clothing — *see also* Ignition, clothes X06.2 ☑
      nightwear X05 ☑
    bonfire — *see* Exposure, fire, controlled, not in building
    brazier (in building or structure) — *see also* Exposure, fire, controlled, building
      not in building or structure — *see* Exposure, fire, controlled, not in building
    building or structure X02.0 ☑
      with
        fall from building X02.3 ☑
        from building X02.5 ☑
        injury due to building collapse X02.2 ☑
        smoke inhalation X02.1 ☑
        hit by object from building X02.4 ☑
        specified mode of injury NEC X02.8 ☑
    fireplace, furnace or stove — *see* Exposure, fire, controlled, building
    not in building or structure X03.0 ☑
      with
        fall X03.3 ☑
        smoke inhalation X03.1 ☑
        hit by object X03.4 ☑
        specified mode of injury NEC X03.8 ☑
    trash — *see* Exposure, fire, controlled, not in building
    fireplace — *see* Exposure, fire, controlled, building
    fittings or furniture (in building or structure) (uncontrolled) — *see* Exposure, fire, uncontrolled, building
    forest (uncontrolled) — *see* Exposure, fire, uncontrolled, not in building
    grass (uncontrolled) — *see* Exposure, fire, uncontrolled, not in building
    hay (uncontrolled) — *see* Exposure, fire, uncontrolled, not in building
    homicide (attempt) X97 ☑
    ignition of highly flammable material X04 ☑
    in, of, on, starting in
      machinery — *see* Contact, with, by type of machine
      motor vehicle (in motion) — *see also* Accident, transport, occupant by type of vehicle V87.8 ☑
        with collision — *see* Collision
      railway rolling stock, train, vehicle V81.81 ☑
        with collision — *see* Accident, transport, railway vehicle occupant
      street car (in motion) V82.8 ☑

☑ **Additional Character Required** — Refer to the Tabular List for Character Selection
◬ **Subterms under main terms may continue to next column or page**

Exposure — *continued*
  fire, flames — *continued*
    in, of, on, starting in — *continued*
      street car — *continued*
        with collision — *see* Accident, transport,
          streetcar occupant
        transport vehicle NEC — *see also* Accident,
          transport
          with collision — *see* Collision
      war operations — *see also* War operations, fire
        from nuclear explosion — *see* War operations,
          nuclear weapons
      watercraft (in transit) (not in transit) V91.09 ☑
        localized — *see* Burn, on board watercraft,
          due to, fire on board
        powered craft V91.03 ☑
          ferry boat V91.01 ☑
          fishing boat V91.02 ☑
          jet skis V91.03 ☑
          liner V91.01 ☑
          merchant ship V91.00 ☑
          passenger ship V91.01 ☑
        unpowered craft V91.08 ☑
          canoe V91.05 ☑
          inflatable V91.06 ☑
          kayak V91.05 ☑
          sailboat V91.04 ☑
          surf-board V91.08 ☑
          waterskis V91.07 ☑
          windsurfer V91.08 ☑
    lumber (uncontrolled) — *see* Exposure, fire, uncon-
      trolled, not in building
    mine (uncontrolled) — *see* Exposure, fire, uncon-
      trolled, not in building
    prairie (uncontrolled) — *see* Exposure, fire, uncon-
      trolled, not in building
    resulting from
      explosion — *see* Explosion
      lightning X08.8 ☑
    self-inflicted X76 ☑
    specified NEC X08.8 ☑
    started by other person X97 ☑
    stated as undetermined whether accidental or inten-
      tional Y26 ☑
    stove — *see* Exposure, fire, controlled, building
    suicide (attempt) X76 ☑
    tunnel (uncontrolled) — *see* Exposure, fire, uncon-
      trolled, not in building
    uncontrolled
      in building or structure X00.0 ☑
        with
          fall from building X00.3 ☑
          injury due to building collapse X00.2 ☑
          jump from building X00.5 ☑
          smoke inhalation X00.1 ☑
        bed X08.00 ☑
          due to
            cigarette X08.01 ☑
            specified material NEC X08.09 ☑
          furniture NEC X08.20 ☑
            due to
              cigarette X08.21 ☑
              specified material NEC X08.29 ☑
          hit by object from building X00.4 ☑
          sofa X08.10 ☑
            due to
              cigarette X08.11 ☑
              specified material NEC X08.19 ☑
          specified mode of injury NEC X00.8 ☑
      not in building or structure (any) X01.0 ☑
        with
          fall X01.3 ☑
          smoke inhalation X01.1 ☑
          hit by object X01.4 ☑
          specified mode of injury NEC X01.8 ☑
        undetermined whether accidental or intentional
          Y26 ☑
  forces of nature NEC — *see* Forces of nature
  G-forces (abnormal) W49.9 ☑
  gravitational forces (abnormal) W49.9 ☑
  heat (natural) NEC — *see* Heat
  high-pressure jet (hydraulic) (pneumatic) W49.9 ☑
  hydraulic jet W49.9 ☑
  inanimate mechanical force W49.9 ☑
  jet, high-pressure (hydraulic) (pneumatic) W49.9 ☑
  lightning — *see* subcategory T75.0 ☑

Exposure — *continued*
  lightning — *see* subcategory — *continued*
    causing fire — *see* Exposure, fire
  mechanical forces NEC W49.9 ☑
    animate NEC W64 ☑
    inanimate NEC W49.9 ☑
  noise W42.9 ☑
    supersonic W42.0 ☑
  noxious substance — *see* Table of Drugs and Chemicals
  pneumatic jet W49.9 ☑
  prolonged in deep-freeze unit or refrigerator W93.2 ☑
  radiation — *see* Radiation
  smoke — *see also* Exposure, fire
    tobacco, second hand Z77.22
  specified factors NEC X58 ☑
  sunlight X32 ☑
    man-made (sun lamp) W89.8 ☑
      tanning bed W89.1 ☑
  supersonic waves W42.0 ☑
  transmission line(s), electric W85 ☑
  vibration W49.9 ☑
  waves
    infrasound W49.9 ☑
    sound W42.9 ☑
    supersonic W42.0 ☑
  weather NEC — *see* Forces of nature
External cause status Y99.9
  child assisting in compensated work for family Y99.8
  civilian activity done for financial or other compensa-
    tion Y99.0
  civilian activity done for income or pay Y99.0
  family member assisting in compensated work for
    other family member Y99.8
  hobby not done for income Y99.8
  leisure activity Y99.8
  military activity Y99.1
  off-duty activity of military personnel Y99.8
  recreation or sport not for income or while a student
    Y99.8
  specified NEC Y99.8
  student activity Y99.8
  volunteer activity Y99.2

F

Factors, supplemental
  alcohol
    blood level
      less than 20mg/100ml Y90.0
      presence in blood, level not specified Y90.9
      20-39mg/100ml Y90.1
      40-59mg/100ml Y90.2
      60-79mg/100ml Y90.3
      80-99mg/100ml Y90.4
      100-119mg/100ml Y90.5
      120-199mg/100ml Y90.6
      200-239mg/100ml Y90.7
      240mg/100ml or more Y90.8
    presence in blood, but level not specified Y90.9
  environmental-pollution-related condition- *see* Z57
  nosocomial condition Y95
  work-related condition Y99.0
Failure
  in suture or ligature during surgical procedure Y65.2
  mechanical, of instrument or apparatus (any) (during
    any medical or surgical procedure) Y65.8
  sterile precautions (during medical and surgical care)
    — *see* Misadventure, failure, sterile precautions,
    by type of procedure
  to
    introduce tube or instrument Y65.4
      endotracheal tube during anesthesia Y65.3
    make curve (transport vehicle) NEC — *see* Accident,
      transport
    remove tube or instrument Y65.4
Fall, falling (accidental) W19 ☑
  building W20.1 ☑
    burning (uncontrolled fire) X00.3 ☑
  down
    embankment W17.81 ☑
    escalator W10.0 ☑
    hill W17.81 ☑
    ladder W11 ☑
    ramp W10.2 ☑
    stairs, steps W10.9 ☑

Fall, falling — *continued*
  due to
    bumping against
      object W18.00 ☑
        sharp glass W18.02 ☑
        specified NEC W18.09 ☑
        sports equipment W18.01 ☑
      person W03 ☑
        due to ice or snow W00.0 ☑
        on pedestrian conveyance — *see* Accident,
          transport, pedestrian, conveyance
    collision with another person W03 ☑
      due to ice or snow W00.0 ☑
      involving pedestrian conveyance — *see* Acci-
        dent, transport, pedestrian, conveyance
    grocery cart tipping over W17.82 ☑
    ice or snow W00.9 ☑
      from one level to another W00.2 ☑
        on stairs or steps W00.1 ☑
      involving pedestrian conveyance — *see* Acci-
        dent, transport, pedestrian, conveyance
      on same level W00.0 ☑
    slipping (on moving sidewalk) W01.0 ☑
      with subsequent striking against object
        W01.10 ☑
        furniture W01.190 ☑
        sharp object W01.119 ☑
          glass W01.110 ☑
          power tool or machine W01.111 ☑
          specified NEC W01.118 ☑
        specified NEC W01.198 ☑
    striking against
      object W18.00 ☑
        sharp glass W18.02 ☑
        specified NEC W18.09 ☑
        sports equipment W18.01 ☑
      person W03 ☑
        due to ice or snow W00.0 ☑
        on pedestrian conveyance — *see* Accident,
          transport, pedestrian, conveyance
  earth (with asphyxia or suffocation (by pressure)) —
    see Earth, falling
  from, off, out of
    aircraft NEC (with accident to aircraft NEC) V97.0 ☑
      while boarding or alighting V97.1 ☑
    balcony W13.0 ☑
    bed W06 ☑
    boat, ship, watercraft NEC (with drowning or sub-
      mersion) — *see* Drowning, due to, fall over-
      board
      with hitting bottom or object V94.0 ☑
    bridge W13.1 ☑
    building W13.9 ☑
      burning (uncontrolled fire) X00.3 ☑
    cavity W17.2 ☑
    chair W07 ☑
    cherry picker W17.89 ☑
    cliff W15 ☑
    dock W17.4 ☑
    embankment W17.81 ☑
    escalator W10.0 ☑
    flagpole W13.8 ☑
    furniture NEC W08 ☑
    grocery cart W17.82 ☑
    haystack W17.89 ☑
    high place NEC W17.89 ☑
      stated as undetermined whether accidental or
        intentional Y30 ☑
    hole W17.2 ☑
    incline W10.2 ☑
    ladder W11 ☑
    lifting device W17.89 ☑
    machine, machinery — *see also* Contact, with, by
      type of machine
      not in operation W17.89 ☑
    manhole W17.1 ☑
    mobile elevated work platform [MEWP] W17.89 ☑
    motorized mobility scooter W05.2 ☑
    one level to another NEC W17.89 ☑
      intentional, purposeful, suicide (attempt) X80 ☑
      stated as undetermined whether accidental or
        intentional Y30 ☑
    pit W17.2 ☑
    playground equipment W09.8 ☑
      jungle gym W09.2 ☑
      slide W09.0 ☑

Fall, falling — *continued*
from, off, out of — *continued*
  playground equipment — *continued*
    swing W09.1 ☑
  quarry W17.89 ☑
  railing W13.9 ☑
  ramp W10.2 ☑
  roof W13.2 ☑
  scaffolding W12 ☑
  scooter (nonmotorized) W05.1 ☑
    motorized mobility W05.2 ☑
  sky lift W17.89 ☑
  stairs, steps W10.9 ☑
    curb W10.1 ☑
    due to ice or snow W00.1 ☑
    escalator W10.0 ☑
    incline W10.2 ☑
    ramp W10.2 ☑
    sidewalk curb W10.1 ☑
    specified NEC W10.8 ☑
    standing
      electric scooter V00.841 ☑
      micro-mobility pedestrian conveyance V00.848 ☑
  stepladder W11 ☑
  storm drain W17.1 ☑
  streetcar NEC W82.6 ☑
    while boarding or alighting V82.4 ☑
    with antecedent collision — *see* Accident, transport, streetcar occupant
  structure NEC W13.8 ☑
    burning (uncontrolled fire) X00.3 ☑
  table W08 ☑
  toilet W18.11 ☑
    with subsequent striking against object W18.12 ☑
  train NEC V81.6 ☑
    during derailment (without antecedent collision) V81.7 ☑
    with antecedent collision — *see* Accident, transport, railway vehicle occupant
    while boarding or alighting V81.4 ☑
  transport vehicle after collision — *see* Accident, transport, by type of vehicle, collision
  tree W14 ☑
  vehicle (in motion) NEC — *see also* Accident, transport V89.9 ☑
    motor NEC — *see also* Accident, transport, occupant, by type of vehicle V87.8 ☑
    stationary W17.89 ☑
      while boarding or alighting — *see* Accident, transport, by type of vehicle, while boarding or alighting
  viaduct W13.8 ☑
  wall W13.8 ☑
  watercraft — *see also* Drowning, due to, fall overboard
    with hitting bottom or object V94.0 ☑
  well W17.0 ☑
  wheelchair, non-moving W05.0 ☑
    powered — *see* Accident, transport, pedestrian, conveyance occupant, specified type NEC
  window W13.4 ☑
in, on
  aircraft NEC V97.0 ☑
    while boarding or alighting V97.1 ☑
    with accident to aircraft V97.0 ☑
  bathtub (empty) W18.2 ☑
    filled W16.212 ☑
      causing drowning W16.211 ☑
  escalator W10.0 ☑
  incline W10.2 ☑
  ladder W11 ☑
  machine, machinery — *see* Contact, with, by type of machine
  object, edged, pointed or sharp (with cut) — *see* Fall, by type
  playground equipment W09.8 ☑
    jungle gym W09.2 ☑
    slide W09.0 ☑
    swing W09.1 ☑
  ramp W10.2 ☑
  scaffolding W12 ☑
  shower W18.2 ☑
    causing drowning W16.211 ☑
  staircase, stairs, steps W10.9 ☑

Fall, falling — *continued*
in, on — *continued*
  staircase, stairs, steps — *continued*
    curb W10.1 ☑
    due to ice or snow W00.1 ☑
    escalator W10.0 ☑
    incline W10.2 ☑
    specified NEC W10.8 ☑
  streetcar (without antecedent collision) V82.5 ☑
    with antecedent collision — *see* Accident, transport, streetcar occupant
    while boarding or alighting V82.4 ☑
  train (without antecedent collision) V81.5 ☑
    with antecedent collision — *see* Accident, transport, railway vehicle occupant
    during derailment (without antecedent collision) V81.7 ☑
    with antecedent collision — *see* Accident, transport, railway vehicle occupant
    while boarding or alighting V81.4 ☑
  transport vehicle after collision — *see* Accident, transport, by type of vehicle, collision
  watercraft W93.39 ☑
    due to
      accident to craft V91.29 ☑
        powered craft V91.23 ☑
          ferry boat V91.21 ☑
          fishing boat V91.22 ☑
          jetskis V91.23 ☑
          liner V91.21 ☑
          merchant ship V91.20 ☑
          passenger ship V91.21 ☑
        unpowered craft
          canoe V91.25 ☑
          inflatable V91.26 ☑
          kayak V91.25 ☑
          sailboat V91.24 ☑
      powered craft V93.33 ☑
        ferry boat V93.31 ☑
        fishing boat V93.32 ☑
        jetskis V93.33 ☑
        liner V93.31 ☑
        merchant ship V93.30 ☑
        passenger ship V93.31 ☑
      unpowered craft V93.38 ☑
        canoe V93.35 ☑
        inflatable V93.36 ☑
        kayak V93.35 ☑
        sailboat V93.34 ☑
        surf-board V93.38 ☑
        windsurfer V93.38 ☑
into
  cavity W17.2 ☑
  dock W17.4 ☑
  fire — *see* Exposure, fire, by type
  haystack W17.89 ☑
  hole W17.2 ☑
  lake — *see* Fall, into, water
  manhole W17.1 ☑
  moving part of machinery — *see* Contact, with, by type of machine
  ocean — *see* Fall, into, water
  opening in surface NEC W17.89 ☑
  pit W17.2 ☑
  pond — *see* Fall, into, water
  quarry W17.89 ☑
  river — *see* Fall, into, water
  shaft W17.89 ☑
  storm drain W17.1 ☑
  stream — *see* Fall, into, water
  swimming pool — *see also* Fall, into, water, in, swimming pool
    empty W17.3 ☑
  tank W17.89 ☑
  water W16.42 ☑
    causing drowning W16.41 ☑
    from watercraft — *see* Drowning, due to, fall overboard
    hitting diving board W21.4 ☑
    in
      bathtub W16.212 ☑
        causing drowning W16.211 ☑
      bucket W16.222 ☑
        causing drowning W16.221 ☑
      natural body of water W16.112 ☑
        causing drowning W16.111 ☑

Fall, falling — *continued*
into — *continued*
  water — *continued*
    in — *continued*
      natural body of water — *continued*
        striking
          bottom W16.122 ☑
            causing drowning W16.121 ☑
          side W16.132 ☑
            causing drowning W16.131 ☑
      specified water NEC W16.312 ☑
        causing drowning W16.311 ☑
        striking
          bottom W16.322 ☑
            causing drowning W16.321 ☑
          wall W16.332 ☑
            causing drowning W16.331 ☑
      swimming pool W16.012 ☑
        causing drowning W16.011 ☑
        striking
          bottom W16.022 ☑
            causing drowning W16.031 ☑
          wall W16.032 ☑
            causing drowning W16.021 ☑
      utility bucket W16.222 ☑
        causing drowning W16.221 ☑
    well W17.0 ☑
involving
  bed W06 ☑
  chair W07 ☑
  furniture NEC W08 ☑
  glass — *see* Fall, by type
  playground equipment W09.8 ☑
    jungle gym W09.2 ☑
    slide W09.0 ☑
    swing W09.1 ☑
  roller blades — *see* Accident, transport, pedestrian, conveyance
  skateboard(s) — *see* Accident, transport, pedestrian, conveyance
  skates (ice) (in line) (roller) — *see* Accident, transport, pedestrian, conveyance
  skis — *see* Accident, transport, pedestrian, conveyance
  table W08 ☑
  wheelchair, non-moving W05.0 ☑
    powered — *see* Accident, transport, pedestrian, conveyance, specified type NEC
object — *see* Struck by, object, falling
off
  toilet W18.11 ☑
    with subsequent striking against object W18.12 ☑
on same level W18.30 ☑
  due to
    specified NEC W18.39 ☑
    stepping on an object W18.31 ☑
out of
  bed W06 ☑
  building NEC W13.8 ☑
  chair W07 ☑
  furniture NEC W08 ☑
  wheelchair, non-moving W05.0 ☑
    powered — *see* Accident, transport, pedestrian, conveyance, specified type NEC
  window W13.4 ☑
over
  animal W01.0 ☑
  cliff W15 ☑
  embankment W17.81 ☑
  small object W01.0 ☑
rock W20.8 ☑
same level W18.30 ☑
  from
    being crushed, pushed, or stepped on by a crowd or human stampede W52 ☑
    collision, pushing, shoving, by or with other person W03 ☑
    slipping, stumbling, tripping W01.0 ☑
  involving ice or snow W00.0 ☑
    involving skates (ice) (roller), skateboard, skis — *see* Accident, transport, pedestrian, conveyance
snowslide (avalanche) — *see* Landslide
stone W20.8 ☑
structure W20.1 ☑

☑ **Additional Character Required** — Refer to the Tabular List for Character Selection   🖝 **Subterms under main terms may continue to next column or page**

Fall, falling — *continued*
  structure — *continued*
    burning (uncontrolled fire) X00.3 ☑
  through
    bridge W13.1 ☑
    floor W13.3 ☑
    roof W13.2 ☑
    wall W13.8 ☑
    window W13.4 ☑
  timber W20.8 ☑
  tree (caused by lightning) W20.8 ☑
  while being carried or supported by other person(s) W04 ☑
Fallen on by
  animal (not being ridden) NEC W55.89 ☑
Felo-de-se — *see* Suicide
Fight (hand) (fists) (foot) — *see* Assault, fight
Fire (accidental) — *see* Exposure, fire
Firearm discharge — *see* Discharge, firearm
Fireball effects from nuclear explosion in war operations — *see* War operations, nuclear weapons
Fireworks (explosion) W39 ☑
Flash burns from explosion — *see* Explosion
Flood (any injury) (caused by) X38 ☑
  collapse of man-made structure causing earth movement X36.0 ☑
  tidal wave — *see* Forces of nature, tidal wave
Food (any type) **in**
  air passages (with asphyxia, obstruction, or suffocation) — *see* categories T17 and T18 ☑
  alimentary tract causing asphyxia (due to compression of trachea) — *see* categories T17 and T18 ☑
Forces of nature X39.8 ☑
  avalanche X36.1 ☑
    causing transport accident — *see* Accident, transport, by type of vehicle
  blizzard X37.2 ☑
  cataclysmic storm X37.9 ☑
    with flood X38 ☑
    blizzard X37.2 ☑
    cloudburst X37.8 ☑
    cyclone X37.1 ☑
    dust storm X37.3 ☑
    hurricane X37.0 ☑
    specified storm NEC X37.8 ☑
    storm surge X37.0 ☑
    tornado X37.1 ☑
    twister X37.1 ☑
    typhoon X37.0 ☑
  cloudburst X37.8 ☑
  cold (natural) X31 ☑
  cyclone X37.1 ☑
  dam collapse causing earth movement X36.0 ☑
  dust storm X37.3 ☑
  earth movement X36.1 ☑
    caused by dam or structure collapse X36.0 ☑
    earthquake X34 ☑
  earthquake X34 ☑
  flood (caused by) X38 ☑
    dam collapse X36.0 ☑
    tidal wave — *see* Forces of nature, tidal wave
  heat (natural) X30 ☑
  hurricane X37.0 ☑
  landslide X36.1 ☑
    causing transport accident — *see* Accident, transport, by type of vehicle
  lightning — *see* subcategory T75.0 ☑
    causing fire — *see* Exposure, fire
  mudslide X36.1 ☑
    causing transport accident — *see* Accident, transport, by type of vehicle
  radiation (natural) X39.08 ☑
    radon X39.01 ☑
  radon X39.01 ☑
  specified force NEC X39.8 ☑
  storm surge X37.0 ☑
  structure collapse causing earth movement X36.0 ☑
  sunlight X32 ☑
  tidal wave X37.41 ☑
    due to
      earthquake X37.41 ☑
      landslide X37.43 ☑
      storm X37.42 ☑
      volcanic eruption X37.41 ☑
  tornado X37.1 ☑
  tsunami X37.41 ☑

Forces of nature — *continued*
  twister X37.1 ☑
  typhoon X37.0 ☑
  volcanic eruption X35 ☑
Foreign body
  aspiration — *see* Index to Diseases and Injuries, Foreign body, respiratory tract
  embedded in skin W45 ☑
  entering through skin W45.8 ☑
    can lid W26.8 ☑
    nail W45.0 ☑
    paper W26.2 ☑
    specified NEC W45.8 ☑
    splinter W45.8 ☑
Forest fire (exposure to) — *see* Exposure, fire, uncontrolled, not in building
Found injured X58 ☑
  from exposure (to) — *see* Exposure
  on
    highway, road(way), street V89.9 ☑
    railway right of way V81.9 ☑
Fracture (circumstances unknown or unspecified) X58 ☑
  due to specified cause NEC X58 ☑
Freezing — *see* Exposure, cold
Frostbite X31 ☑
  due to man-made conditions — *see* Exposure, cold, man-made
Frozen — *see* Exposure, cold

G

Gored by bull W55.22 ☑
Gunshot wound W34.00 ☑

H

Hailstones, injured by X39.8 ☑
Hanged herself or himself — *see* Hanging, self-inflicted
Hanging (accidental) — *see also* category T71 ☑
  legal execution — *see* Legal, intervention, specified means NEC
Heat (effects of) (excessive) X30 ☑
  due to
    man-made conditions W92 ☑
      on board watercraft V93.29 ☑
        fishing boat V93.22 ☑
        merchant ship V93.20 ☑
        passenger ship V93.21 ☑
        sailboat V93.24 ☑
        specified powered craft NEC V93.23 ☑
    weather (conditions) X30 ☑
  from
    electric heating apparatus causing burning X16 ☑
    nuclear explosion in war operations — *see* War operations, nuclear weapons
  inappropriate in local application or packing in medical or surgical procedure Y63.5
Hemorrhage
  delayed following medical or surgical treatment without mention of misadventure — *see* Index to Diseases and Injuries, Complication(s)
  during medical or surgical treatment as misadventure — *see* Index to Diseases and Injuries, Complication(s)
High
  altitude (effects) — *see* Air, pressure, low
  level of radioactivity, effects — *see* Radiation
  pressure (effects) — *see* Air, pressure, high
  temperature, effects — *see* Heat
Hit, hitting (accidental) by — *see* Struck by
Hitting against — *see* Striking against
Homicide (attempt) (justifiable) — *see* Assault
Hot
  place, effects — *see also* Heat
  weather, effects X30 ☑
House fire (uncontrolled) — *see* Exposure, fire, uncontrolled, building
Humidity, causing problem X39.8 ☑
Hunger X58 ☑
Hurricane (any injury) X37.0 ☑
Hypobarism, hypobaropathy — *see* Air, pressure, low

I

Ictus
  caloris — *see also* Heat

Ictus — *continued*
  solaris X30 ☑
Ignition (accidental) — *see also* Exposure, fire X08.8 ☑
  anesthetic gas in operating room W40.1 ☑
  apparel X06.2 ☑
    from highly flammable material X04 ☑
    nightwear X05 ☑
  bed linen (sheets) (spreads) (pillows) (mattress) — *see* Exposure, fire, uncontrolled, building, bed
  benzine X04 ☑
  clothes, clothing NEC (from controlled fire) X06.2 ☑
    from
      highly flammable material X04 ☑
  ether X04 ☑
    in operating room W40.1 ☑
  explosive material — *see* Explosion
  gasoline X04 ☑
  jewelry (plastic) (any) X06.0 ☑
  kerosene X04 ☑
  material
    explosive — *see* Explosion
    highly flammable with secondary explosion X04 ☑
  nightwear X05 ☑
  paraffin X04 ☑
  petrol X04 ☑
Immersion (accidental) — *see also* Drowning
  hand or foot due to cold (excessive) X31 ☑
Implantation of quills of porcupine W55.89 ☑
Inanition (from) (hunger) X58 ☑
  thirst X58 ☑
Inappropriate operation performed
  correct operation on wrong side or body part (wrong side) (wrong site) Y65.53
  operation intended for another patient done on wrong patient Y65.52
  wrong operation performed on correct patient Y65.51
Inattention after, at birth (homicidal intent) (infanticidal intent) X58 ☑
Incident, adverse
  device
    anesthesiology Y70.8
      accessory Y70.2
      diagnostic Y70.0
      miscellaneous Y70.8
      monitoring Y70.0
      prosthetic Y70.2
      rehabilitative Y70.1
      surgical Y70.3
      therapeutic Y70.1
    cardiovascular Y71.8
      accessory Y71.2
      diagnostic Y71.0
      miscellaneous Y71.8
      monitoring Y71.0
      prosthetic Y71.2
      rehabilitative Y71.1
      surgical Y71.3
      therapeutic Y71.1
    gastroenterology Y73.8
      accessory Y73.2
      diagnostic Y73.0
      miscellaneous Y73.8
      monitoring Y73.0
      prosthetic Y73.2
      rehabilitative Y73.1
      surgical Y73.3
      therapeutic Y73.1
    general
      hospital Y74.8
        accessory Y74.2
        diagnostic Y74.0
        miscellaneous Y74.8
        monitoring Y74.0
        prosthetic Y74.2
        rehabilitative Y74.1
        surgical Y74.3
        therapeutic Y74.1
      surgical Y81.8
        accessory Y81.2
        diagnostic Y81.0
        miscellaneous Y81.8
        monitoring Y81.0
        prosthetic Y81.2
        rehabilitative Y81.1
        surgical Y81.3
        therapeutic Y81.1
    gynecological Y76.8
      accessory Y76.2

Incident, adverse — *continued*
  device — *continued*
    gynecological — *continued*
      diagnostic Y76.0
      miscellaneous Y76.8
      monitoring Y76.0
      prosthetic Y76.2
      rehabilitative Y76.1
      surgical Y76.3
      therapeutic Y76.1
    medical Y82.9
      specified type NEC Y82.8
    neurological Y75.8
      accessory Y75.2
      diagnostic Y75.0
      miscellaneous Y75.8
      monitoring Y75.0
      prosthetic Y75.2
      rehabilitative Y75.1
      surgical Y75.3
      therapeutic Y75.1
    obstetrical Y76.8
      accessory Y76.2
      diagnostic Y76.0
      miscellaneous Y76.8
      monitoring Y76.0
      prosthetic Y76.2
      rehabilitative Y76.1
      surgical Y76.3
      therapeutic Y76.1
    ophthalmic Y77.8
      accessory Y77.2
      contact lens (rigid gas permeable) (soft (hydrophilic)) Y77.11
      diagnostic Y77.0
      miscellaneous Y77.8
      monitoring Y77.0
      prosthetic Y77.2
      rehabilitative Y77.19
      surgical Y77.3
      therapeutic Y77.19
    orthopedic Y79.8
      accessory Y79.2
      diagnostic Y79.0
      miscellaneous Y79.8
      monitoring Y79.0
      prosthetic Y79.2
      rehabilitative Y79.1
      surgical Y79.3
      therapeutic Y79.1
    otorhinolaryngological Y72.8
      accessory Y72.2
      diagnostic Y72.0
      miscellaneous Y72.8
      monitoring Y72.0
      prosthetic Y72.2
      rehabilitative Y72.1
      surgical Y72.3
      therapeutic Y72.1
    personal use Y74.8
      accessory Y74.2
      diagnostic Y74.0
      miscellaneous Y74.8
      monitoring Y74.0
      prosthetic Y74.2
      rehabilitative Y74.1
      surgical Y74.3
      therapeutic Y74.1
    physical medicine Y80.8
      accessory Y80.2
      diagnostic Y80.0
      miscellaneous Y80.8
      monitoring Y80.0
      prosthetic Y80.2
      rehabilitative Y80.1
      surgical Y80.3
      therapeutic Y80.1
    plastic surgical Y81.8
      accessory Y81.2
      diagnostic Y81.0
      miscellaneous Y81.8
      monitoring Y81.0
      prosthetic Y81.2
      rehabilitative Y81.1
      surgical Y81.3
      therapeutic Y81.1
    radiological Y78.8
      accessory Y78.2
      diagnostic Y78.0

Incident, adverse — *continued*
  device — *continued*
    radiological — *continued*
      miscellaneous Y78.8
      monitoring Y78.0
      prosthetic Y78.2
      rehabilitative Y78.1
      surgical Y78.3
      therapeutic Y78.1
    urology Y73.8
      accessory Y73.2
      diagnostic Y73.0
      miscellaneous Y73.8
      monitoring Y73.0
      prosthetic Y73.2
      rehabilitative Y73.1
      surgical Y73.3
      therapeutic Y73.1
Incineration (accidental) — *see* Exposure, fire
Infanticide — *see* Assault
Infrasound waves (causing injury) W49.9 ☑
Ingestion
  foreign body (causing injury) (with obstruction) — *see* Foreign body, alimentary canal
  poisonous
    plant(s) X58 ☑
    substance NEC — *see* Table of Drugs and Chemicals
Inhalation
  excessively cold substance, man-made — *see* Exposure, cold, man-made
  food (any type) (into respiratory tract) (with asphyxia, obstruction respiratory tract, suffocation) — *see* categories T17 and T18 ☑
  foreign body — *see* Foreign body, aspiration
  gastric contents (with asphyxia, obstruction respiratory passage, suffocation) T17.81- ☑
  hot air or gases X14.0 ☑
  liquid air, hydrogen, nitrogen W93.12 ☑
    suicide (attempt) X83.2 ☑
  steam X13.0 ☑
    assault X98.0 ☑
    stated as undetermined whether accidental or intentional Y27.0 ☑
  suicide (attempt) X77.0 ☑
  toxic gas — *see* Table of Drugs and Chemicals
  vomitus (with asphyxia, obstruction respiratory passage, suffocation) T17.81- ☑
Injury, injured (accidental(ly)) NOS X58 ☑
  by, caused by, from
    assault — *see* Assault
    law-enforcing agent, police, in course of legal intervention — *see* Legal intervention
    suicide (attempt) X83.8 ☑
  due to, in
    civil insurrection — *see* War operations
    fight — *see also* Assault, fight Y04.0 ☑
    war operations — *see* War operations
  homicide — *see also* Assault Y09
  inflicted (by)
    in course of arrest (attempted), suppression of disturbance, maintenance of order, by law-enforcing agents — *see* Legal intervention
    other person
      stated as
        accidental X58 ☑
        intentional, homicide (attempt) — *see* Assault
        undetermined whether accidental or intentional Y33 ☑
    purposely (inflicted) by other person(s) — *see* Assault
    self-inflicted X83.8 ☑
      stated as accidental X58 ☑
    specified cause NEC X58 ☑
    undetermined whether accidental or intentional Y33 ☑
Insolation, effects X30 ☑
Insufficient nourishment X58 ☑
Interruption of respiration (by)
  food (lodged in esophagus) — *see* categories T17 and T18 ☑
  vomitus (lodged in esophagus) T17.81- ☑
Intervention, legal — *see* Legal intervention
Intoxication
  drug — *see* Table of Drugs and Chemicals
  poison — *see* Table of Drugs and Chemicals

J

Jammed (accidentally)
  between objects (moving) (stationary and moving) W23.0 ☑
    stationary W23.1 ☑
Jumped, jumping
  before moving object NEC X81.8 ☑
    motor vehicle X81.0 ☑
    subway train X81.1 ☑
    train X81.1 ☑
    undetermined whether accidental or intentional Y31 ☑
  from
    boat (into water) voluntarily, without accident (to or on boat) W16.712 ☑
      striking bottom W16.722 ☑
        causing drowning W16.721 ☑
      with
        accident to or on boat — *see* Accident, watercraft
        drowning or submersion W16.711 ☑
          suicide (attempt) X71.3 ☑
    building — *see also* Jumped, from, high place W13.9 ☑
      burning (uncontrolled fire) X00.5 ☑
    high place NEC W17.89 ☑
      suicide (attempt) X80 ☑
      undetermined whether accidental or intentional Y30 ☑
    structure — *see also* Jumped, from, high place W13.9 ☑
      burning (uncontrolled fire) X00.5 ☑
  into water W16.92 ☑
    causing drowning W16.91 ☑
    from, off watercraft — *see* Jumped, from, boat
    in
      natural body W16.612 ☑
        causing drowning W16.611 ☑
        striking bottom W16.622 ☑
          causing drowning W16.621 ☑
      specified place NEC W16.812 ☑
        causing drowning W16.811 ☑
        striking
          bottom W16.822 ☑
            causing drowning W16.821 ☑
          wall W16.832 ☑
            causing drowning W16.831 ☑
      swimming pool W16.512 ☑
        causing drowning W16.511 ☑
        striking
          bottom W16.522 ☑
            causing drowning W16.521 ☑
          wall W16.532 ☑
            causing drowning W16.531 ☑
    suicide (attempt) X71.3 ☑

K

Kicked by
  animal NEC W55.82 ☑
  person(s) (accidentally) W50.1 ☑
    with intent to injure or kill Y04.0 ☑
    as, or caused by, a crowd or human stampede (with fall) W52 ☑
    assault Y04.0 ☑
    homicide (attempt) Y04.0 ☑
    in
      fight Y04.0 ☑
      legal intervention
        injuring
          bystander Y35.812 ☑
          law enforcement personnel Y35.811 ☑
          suspect Y35.813 ☑
          unspecified person Y35.819 ☑
Kicking
  against
    object W22.8 ☑
      sports equipment W21.9 ☑
      stationary W22.09 ☑
        sports equipment W21.89 ☑
    person — *see* Striking against, person
    sports equipment W21.9 ☑
  carpet stretcher with knee X50.3 ☑
Killed, killing (accidentally) NOS — *see also* Injury X58 ☑

Killed, killing — *continued*

  in

    action — *see* War operations

    brawl, fight (hand) (fists) (foot) Y04.0 ☑

      by weapon — *see also* Assault

        cutting, piercing — *see* Assault, cutting or piercing instrument

        firearm — *see* Discharge, firearm, by type, homicide

  self

    stated as

      accident NOS X58 ☑

      suicide — *see* Suicide

      undetermined whether accidental or intentional Y33 ☑

Kneeling (prolonged (static)) X50.1 ☑

Knocked down (accidentally) (by) NOS X58 ☑

  animal (not being ridden) NEC — *see also* Struck by, by type of animal

  crowd or human stampede W52 ☑

  person W51 ☑

    in brawl, fight Y04.0 ☑

  transport vehicle NEC — *see also* Accident, transport V09.9 ☑

L

Laceration NEC — *see* Injury

Lack of

  care (helpless person) (infant) (newborn) X58 ☑

  food except as result of abandonment or neglect X58 ☑

    due to abandonment or neglect X58 ☑

  water except as result of transport accident X58 ☑

    due to transport accident — *see* Accident, transport, by type

  helpless person, infant, newborn X58 ☑

Landslide (falling on transport vehicle) X36.1 ☑

  caused by collapse of man-made structure X36.0 ☑

Late effect — *see* Sequelae

Legal

  execution (any method) — *see* Legal, intervention

  intervention (by)

    baton — *see* Legal, intervention, blunt object, baton

    bayonet — *see* Legal, intervention, sharp object, bayonet

    blow — *see* Legal, intervention, manhandling

    blunt object

      baton

        injuring

          bystander Y35.312 ☑

          law enforcement personnel Y35.311 ☑

          suspect Y35.313 ☑

          unspecified person Y35.319 ☑

      injuring

        bystander Y35.302 ☑

        law enforcement personnel Y35.301 ☑

        suspect Y35.303 ☑

        unspecified person Y35.309 ☑

      specified NEC

        injuring

          bystander Y35.392 ☑

          law enforcement personnel Y35.391 ☑

          suspect Y35.393 ☑

          unspecified person Y35.399 ☑

      stave

        injuring

          bystander Y35.392 ☑

          law enforcement personnel Y35.391 ☑

          suspect Y35.393 ☑

          unspecified person Y35.399 ☑

    bomb — *see* Legal, intervention, explosive

    conducted energy device

      injuring

        bystander Y35.832 ☑

        law enforcement personnel Y35.831 ☑

        suspect Y35.833 ☑

        unspecified person Y35.839 ☑

    cutting or piercing instrument — *see* Legal, intervention, sharp object

    dynamite — *see* Legal, intervention, explosive, dynamite

    electroshock device (taser)

      injuring

        bystander Y35.832 ☑

        law enforcement personnel Y35.831 ☑

Legal — *continued*

  intervention — *continued*

    electroshock device — *continued*

      injuring — *continued*

        suspect Y35.833 ☑

        unspecified person Y35.839 ☑

    explosive(s)

      dynamite

        injuring

          bystander Y35.112 ☑

          law enforcement personnel Y35.111 ☑

          suspect Y35.113 ☑

          unspecified person Y35.119 ☑

      grenade

        injuring

          bystander Y35.192 ☑

          law enforcement personnel Y35.191 ☑

          suspect Y35.193 ☑

          unspecified person Y35.199 ☑

      injuring

        bystander Y35.102 ☑

        law enforcement personnel Y35.101 ☑

        suspect Y35.103 ☑

        unspecified person Y35.109 ☑

      mortar bomb

        injuring

          bystander Y35.192 ☑

          law enforcement personnel Y35.191 ☑

          suspect Y35.193 ☑

          unspecified person Y35.199 ☑

      shell

        injuring

          bystander Y35.122 ☑

          law enforcement personnel Y35.121 ☑

          suspect Y35.123 ☑

          unspecified person Y35.129 ☑

      specified NEC

        injuring

          bystander Y35.192 ☑

          law enforcement personnel Y35.191 ☑

          suspect Y35.193 ☑

          unspecified person Y35.199 ☑

    firearm(s) (discharge)

      handgun

        injuring

          bystander Y35.022 ☑

          law enforcement personnel Y35.021 ☑

          suspect Y35.023 ☑

          unspecified person Y35.029 ☑

      injuring

        bystander Y35.002 ☑

        law enforcement personnel Y35.001 ☑

        suspect Y35.003 ☑

        unspecified person Y35.009 ☑

      machine gun

        injuring

          bystander Y35.012 ☑

          law enforcement personnel Y35.011 ☑

          suspect Y35.013 ☑

          unspecified person Y35.019 ☑

      rifle pellet

        injuring

          bystander Y35.032 ☑

          law enforcement personnel Y35.031 ☑

          suspect Y35.033 ☑

          unspecified person Y35.039 ☑

      rubber bullet

        injuring

          bystander Y35.042 ☑

          law enforcement personnel Y35.041 ☑

          suspect Y35.043 ☑

          unspecified person Y35.049 ☑

      shotgun — *see* Legal, intervention, firearm, specified NEC

      specified NEC

        injuring

          bystander Y35.092 ☑

          law enforcement personnel Y35.091 ☑

          suspect Y35.093 ☑

          unspecified person Y35.099 ☑

    gas (asphyxiation) (poisoning)

      injuring

        bystander Y35.202 ☑

        law enforcement personnel Y35.201 ☑

        suspect Y35.203 ☑

        unspecified person Y35.209 ☑

Legal — *continued*

  intervention — *continued*

    gas — *continued*

      specified NEC

        injuring

          bystander Y35.292 ☑

          law enforcement personnel Y35.291 ☑

          suspect Y35.293 ☑

          unspecified person Y35.299 ☑

      tear gas

        injuring

          bystander Y35.212 ☑

          law enforcement personnel Y35.211 ☑

          suspect Y35.213 ☑

          unspecified person Y35.219 ☑

    grenade — *see* Legal, intervention, explosive, grenade

    injuring

      bystander Y35.92 ☑

      law enforcement personnel Y35.91 ☑

      suspect Y35.93 ☑

      unspecified person Y35.99 ☑

    late effect (of) — *see* with 7th character S Y35 ☑

    manhandling

      injuring

        bystander Y35.812 ☑

        law enforcement personnel Y35.811 ☑

        suspect Y35.813 ☑

        unspecified person Y35.819 ☑

    sequelae (of) — *see* with 7th character S Y35 ☑

    sharp objects

      bayonet

        injuring

          bystander Y35.412 ☑

          law enforcement personnel Y35.411 ☑

          suspect Y35.413 ☑

          unspecified person Y35.419 ☑

      injuring

        bystander Y35.402 ☑

        law enforcement personnel Y35.401 ☑

        suspect Y35.403 ☑

        unspecified person Y35.409 ☑

      specified NEC

        injuring

          bystander Y35.492 ☑

          law enforcement personnel Y35.491 ☑

          suspect Y35.493 ☑

          unspecified person Y35.499 ☑

    specified means NEC

      injuring

        bystander Y35.892 ☑

        law enforcement personnel Y35.891 ☑

        suspect Y35.893 ☑

    stabbing — *see* Legal, intervention, sharp object

    stave — *see* Legal, intervention, blunt object, stave

    stun gun

      injuring

        bystander Y35.832 ☑

        law enforcement personnel Y35.831 ☑

        suspect Y35.833 ☑

        unspecified person Y35.839 ☑

    taser

      injuring

        bystander Y35.832 ☑

        law enforcement personnel Y35.831 ☑

        suspect Y35.833 ☑

        unspecified person Y35.839 ☑

    tear gas — *see* Legal, intervention, gas, tear gas

    truncheon — *see* Legal, intervention, blunt object, stave

Lifting — *see also* Overexertion

  heavy objects X50.0 ☑

  weights X50.0 ☑

Lightning (shock) (stroke) (struck by) — *see* subcategory T75.0 ☑

  causing fire — *see* Exposure, fire

Loss of control (transport vehicle) NEC — *see* Accident, transport

Lost at sea NOS — *see* Drowning, due to, fall overboard

Low

  pressure (effects) — *see* Air, pressure, low

  temperature (effects) — *see* Exposure, cold

Lying before train, vehicle or other moving object X81.8 ☑

  subway train X81.1 ☑

  train X81.1 ☑

Lying before train, vehicle or other moving object
Lying before train, vehicle or other moving object
— *continued*
undetermined whether accidental or intentional Y31 ☑
Lynching — *see* Assault

M

Malfunction (mechanism or component) (of)
firearm W34.1Ø ☑
airgun W34.11Ø ☑
BB gun W34.11Ø ☑
gas, air or spring-operated gun NEC W34.118 ☑
handgun W32.1 ☑
hunting rifle W33.12 ☑
larger firearm W33.1Ø ☑
specified NEC W33.19 ☑
machine gun W33.13 ☑
paintball gun W34.111 ☑
pellet gun W34.11Ø ☑
shotgun W33.11 ☑
specified NEC W34.19 ☑
Very pistol [flare] W34.19 ☑
handgun — *see* Malfunction, firearm, handgun
Maltreatment — *see* Perpetrator
Mangled (accidentally) NOS X58 ☑
Manhandling (in brawl, fight) YØ4.Ø ☑
legal intervention — *see* Legal, intervention, manhandling
Manslaughter (nonaccidental) — *see* Assault
Mauled by animal NEC W55.89 ☑
Medical procedure, complication of (delayed or as an abnormal reaction without mention of misadventure) — *see* Complication of or following, by specified type of procedure
due to or as a result of misadventure — *see* Misadventure
Melting (due to fire) — *see also* Exposure, fire
apparel NEC XØ6.3 ☑
clothes, clothing NEC XØ6.3 ☑
nightwear XØ5 ☑
fittings or furniture (burning building) (uncontrolled fire) XØØ.8 ☑
nightwear XØ5 ☑
plastic jewelry XØ6.1 ☑
Mental cruelty X58 ☑
Military operations (injuries to military and civilians occuring during peacetime on military property and during routine military exercises and operations) (by) (from) (involving) Y37.9Ø- ☑
air blast Y37.2Ø- ☑
aircraft
destruction — *see* Military operations, destruction of aircraft
airway restriction — *see* Military operations, restriction of airways
asphyxiation — *see* Military operations, restriction of airways
biological weapons Y37.6X- ☑
blast Y37.2Ø- ☑
blast fragments Y37.2Ø- ☑
blast wave Y37.2Ø- ☑
blast wind Y37.2Ø- ☑
bomb Y37.2Ø- ☑
dirty Y37.5Ø- ☑
gasoline Y37.31- ☑
incendiary Y37.31- ☑
petrol Y37.31- ☑
bullet Y37.43- ☑
incendiary Y37.32- ☑
rubber Y37.41- ☑
chemical weapons Y37.7X- ☑
combat
hand to hand (unarmed) combat Y37.44- ☑
using blunt or piercing object Y37.45- ☑
conflagration — *see* Military operations, fire
conventional warfare NEC Y37.49- ☑
depth-charge Y37.Ø1- ☑
destruction of aircraft Y37.1Ø- ☑
due to
air to air missile Y37.11- ☑
collision with other aircraft Y37.12- ☑
detonation (accidental) of onboard munitions and explosives Y37.14- ☑
enemy fire or explosives Y37.11- ☑
explosive placed on aircraft Y37.11- ☑
onboard fire Y37.13- ☑

Military operations — *continued*
destruction of aircraft — *continued*
due to — *continued*
rocket propelled grenade [RPG] Y37.11- ☑
small arms fire Y37.11- ☑
surface to air missile Y37.11- ☑
specified NEC Y37.19- ☑
detonation (accidental) of
onboard marine weapons Y37.Ø5- ☑
own munitions or munitions launch device Y37.24- ☑
dirty bomb Y37.5Ø- ☑
explosion (of) Y37.2Ø- ☑
aerial bomb Y37.21- ☑
bomb NOS — *see also* Military operations, bomb(s) Y37.2Ø- ☑
fragments Y37.2Ø- ☑
grenade Y37.29- ☑
guided missile Y37.22- ☑
improvised explosive device [IED] (person-borne) (roadside) (vehicle-borne) Y37.23- ☑
land mine Y37.29- ☑
marine mine (at sea) (in harbor) Y37.Ø2- ☑
marine weapon Y37.ØØ- ☑
specified NEC Y37.Ø9- ☑
own munitions or munitions launch device (accidental) Y37.24- ☑
sea-based artillery shell Y37.Ø3- ☑
specified NEC Y37.29- ☑
torpedo Y37.Ø4- ☑
fire Y37.3Ø- ☑
specified NEC Y37.39- ☑
firearms
discharge Y37.43- ☑
pellets Y37.42- ☑
flamethrower Y37.33- ☑
fragments (from) (of)
improvised explosive device [IED] (person-borne) (roadside) (vehicle-borne) Y37.26- ☑
munitions Y37.25- ☑
specified NEC Y37.29- ☑
weapons Y37.27- ☑
friendly fire Y37.92- ☑
hand to hand (unarmed) combat Y37.44- ☑
hot substances — *see* Military operations, fire
incendiary bullet Y37.32- ☑
nuclear weapon (effects of) Y37.5Ø- ☑
acute radiation exposure Y37.54- ☑
blast pressure Y37.51- ☑
direct blast Y37.51- ☑
direct heat Y37.53- ☑
fallout exposure Y37.54- ☑
fireball Y37.53- ☑
indirect blast (struck or crushed by blast debris) (being thrown by blast) Y37.52- ☑
ionizing radiation (immediate exposure) Y37.54- ☑
nuclear radiation Y37.54- ☑
radiation
ionizing (immediate exposure) Y37.54- ☑
nuclear Y37.54- ☑
thermal Y37.53- ☑
secondary effects Y37.54- ☑
specified NEC Y37.59- ☑
thermal radiation Y37.53- ☑
restriction of air (airway)
intentional Y37.46- ☑
unintentional Y37.47- ☑
rubber bullets Y37.41- ☑
shrapnel NOS Y37.29- ☑
suffocation — *see* Military operations, restriction of airways
unconventional warfare NEC Y37.7X- ☑
underwater blast NOS Y37.ØØ- ☑
warfare
conventional NEC Y37.49- ☑
unconventional NEC Y37.7X- ☑
weapon of mass destruction [WMD] Y37.91- ☑
weapons
biological weapons Y37.6X- ☑
chemical Y37.7X- ☑
nuclear (effects of) Y37.5Ø- ☑
acute radiation exposure Y37.54- ☑
blast pressure Y37.51- ☑
direct blast Y37.51- ☑
direct heat Y37.53- ☑
fallout exposure Y37.54- ☑

Military operations — *continued*
weapons — *continued*
nuclear — *continued*
fireball Y37.53- ☑
radiation
ionizing (immediate exposure) Y37.54- ☑
nuclear Y37.54- ☑
thermal Y37.53- ☑
secondary effects Y37.54- ☑
specified NEC Y37.59- ☑
of mass destruction [WMD] Y37.91- ☑
Misadventure(s) **to patient**(s) **during surgical or medical care** Y69
contaminated medical or biological substance (blood, drug, fluid) Y64.9
administered (by) NEC Y64.9
immunization Y64.1
infusion Y64.Ø
injection Y64.1
specified means NEC Y64.8
transfusion Y64.Ø
vaccination Y64.1
excessive amount of blood or other fluid during transfusion or infusion Y63.Ø
failure
in dosage Y63.9
electroshock therapy Y63.4
inappropriate temperature (too hot or too cold) in local application and packing Y63.5
infusion
excessive amount of fluid Y63.Ø
incorrect dilution of fluid Y63.1
insulin-shock therapy Y63.4
nonadministration of necessary drug or biological substance Y63.6
overdose — *see* Table of Drugs and Chemicals
radiation, in therapy Y63.2
radiation
overdose Y63.2
specified procedure NEC Y63.8
transfusion
excessive amount of blood Y63.Ø
mechanical, of instrument or apparatus (any) (during any procedure) Y65.8
sterile precautions (during procedure) Y62.9
aspiration of fluid or tissue (by puncture or catheterization, except heart) Y62.6
biopsy (except needle aspiration) Y62.8
needle (aspirating) Y62.6
blood sampling Y62.6
catheterization Y62.6
heart Y62.5
dialysis (kidney) Y62.2
endoscopic examination Y62.4
enema Y62.8
immunization Y62.3
infusion Y62.1
injection Y62.3
needle biopsy Y62.6
paracentesis (abdominal) (thoracic) Y62.6
perfusion Y62.2
puncture (lumbar) Y62.6
removal of catheter or packing Y62.8
specified procedure NEC Y62.8
surgical operation Y62.Ø
transfusion Y62.1
vaccination Y62.3
suture or ligature during surgical procedure Y65.2
to introduce or to remove tube or instrument — *see* Failure, to
hemorrhage — *see* Index to Diseases and Injuries, Complication(s)
inadvertent exposure of patient to radiation Y63.3
inappropriate
operation performed — *see* Inappropriate operation performed
temperature (too hot or too cold) in local application or packing Y63.5
infusion — *see also* Misadventure, by type, infusion Y69
excessive amount of fluid Y63.Ø
incorrect dilution of fluid Y63.1
wrong fluid Y65.1
mismatched blood in transfusion Y65.Ø
nonadministration of necessary drug or biological substance Y63.6
overdose — *see* Table of Drugs and Chemicals
radiation (in therapy) Y63.2

☑ Additional Character Required — Refer to the Tabular List for Character Selection ⬇ Subterms under main terms may continue to next column or page

Misadventure(s) **to patient**(s) **during surgical or medical care** — *continued*
  perforation — *see* Index to Diseases and Injuries, Complication(s)
  performance of inappropriate operation — *see* Inappropriate operation performed
  puncture — *see* Index to Diseases and Injuries, Complication(s)
  specified type NEC Y65.8
    failure
      suture or ligature during surgical operation Y65.2
      to introduce or to remove tube or instrument — *see* Failure, to
    infusion of wrong fluid Y65.1
    performance of inappropriate operation — *see* Inappropriate operation performed
    transfusion of mismatched blood Y65.0
    wrong
      fluid in infusion Y65.1
      placement of endotracheal tube during anesthetic procedure Y65.3
  transfusion — *see* Misadventure, by type, transfusion
    excessive amount of blood Y63.0
    mismatched blood Y65.0
  wrong
    drug given in error — *see* Table of Drugs and Chemicals
    fluid in infusion Y65.1
    placement of endotracheal tube during anesthetic procedure Y65.3
Mismatched blood in transfusion Y65.0
Motion sickness T75.3 ☑
Mountain sickness W94.11 ☑
Mudslide (of cataclysmic nature) — *see* Landslide
Murder (attempt) — *see* Assault

N

Nail
  contact with W45.0 ☑
    gun W29.4 ☑
  embedded in skin W45.0 ☑
Neglect (criminal) (homicidal intent) X58 ☑
Noise (causing injury) (pollution) W42.9 ☑
  supersonic W42.0 ☑
Nonadministration (of)
  drug or biological substance (necessary) Y63.6
  surgical and medical care Y66
Nosocomial condition Y95

O

Object
  falling
    from, in, on, hitting
      machinery — *see* Contact, with, by type of machine
    set in motion by
      accidental explosion or rupture of pressure vessel W38 ☑
      firearm — *see* Discharge, firearm, by type
      machine(ry) — *see* Contact, with, by type of machine
Overdose (drug) — *see* Table of Drugs and Chemicals
  radiation Y63.2
Overexertion X50.9 ☑
  from
    prolonged static or awkward postures X50.1 ☑
    repetitive movements X50.3 ☑
    specified strenuous movements or postures NEC X50.9 ☑
    strenuous movement or load X50.0 ☑
Overexposure (accidental) (to)
  cold — *see also* Exposure, cold X31 ☑
    due to man-made conditions — *see* Exposure, cold, man-made
  heat — *see also* Heat X30 ☑
  radiation — *see* Radiation
  radioactivity W88.0 ☑
  sun (sunburn) X32 ☑
  weather NEC — *see* Forces of nature
  wind NEC — *see* Forces of nature
Overheated — *see* Heat
Overturning (accidental)
  machinery — *see* Contact, with, by type of machine
  transport vehicle NEC — *see also* Accident, transport V89.9 ☑

Overturning — *continued*
  watercraft (causing drowning, submersion) — *see also* Drowning, due to, accident to, watercraft, overturning
    causing injury except drowning or submersion — *see* Accident, watercraft, causing, injury NEC

P

Parachute descent (voluntary) (without accident to aircraft) V97.29 ☑
  due to accident to aircraft — *see* Accident, transport, aircraft
Pecked by bird W61.99 ☑
Perforation during medical or surgical treatment as misadventure — *see* Index to Diseases and Injuries, Complication(s)
Perpetrator, perpetration, of assault, maltreatment and neglect (by) Y07.9
  boyfriend Y07.03
  brother Y07.410
    stepbrother Y07.435
  coach Y07.53
  cousin
    female Y07.491
    male Y07.490
  daycare provider Y07.519
    at-home
      adult care Y07.512
      childcare Y07.510
    care center
      adult care Y07.513
      childcare Y07.511
  family member NEC Y07.499
  father Y07.11
    adoptive Y07.13
    foster Y07.420
    stepfather Y07.430
  foster father Y07.420
  foster mother Y07.421
  girl friend Y07.04
  healthcare provider Y07.529
    mental health Y07.521
    specified NEC Y07.528
  husband Y07.01
  instructor Y07.53
  mother Y07.12
    adoptive Y07.14
    foster Y07.421
    stepmother Y07.433
  multiple perpetrators Y07.6
  nonfamily member Y07.50
    specified NEC Y07.59
  nurse Y07.528
  occupational therapist Y07.528
  partner of parent
    female Y07.434
    male Y07.432
  physical therapist Y07.528
  sister Y07.411
  speech therapist Y07.528
  stepbrother Y07.435
  stepfather Y07.430
  stepmother Y07.433
  stepsister Y07.436
  teacher Y07.53
  wife Y07.02
Piercing — *see* Contact, with, by type of object or machine
Pinched
  between objects (moving) (stationary and moving) W23.0 ☑
    stationary W23.1 ☑
Pinned under machine(ry) — *see* Contact, with, by type of machine
Place of occurrence Y92.9
  abandoned house Y92.89
  airplane Y92.813
  airport Y92.520
  ambulatory health services establishment NEC Y92.538
  ambulatory surgery center Y92.530
  amusement park Y92.831
  apartment (co-op) — *see* Place of occurrence, residence, apartment
  assembly hall Y92.29
  bank Y92.510
  barn Y92.71
  baseball field Y92.320

Place of occurrence — *continued*
  basketball court Y92.310
  beach Y92.832
  boarding house — *see* Place of occurrence, residence, boarding house
  boat Y92.814
  bowling alley Y92.39
  bridge Y92.89
  building under construction Y92.61
  bus Y92.811
    station Y92.521
  cafe Y92.511
  campsite Y92.833
  campus — *see* Place of occurrence, school
  canal Y92.89
  car Y92.810
  casino Y92.59
  children's home — *see* Place of occurrence, residence, institutional, orphanage
  church Y92.22
  cinema Y92.26
  clubhouse Y92.29
  coal pit Y92.64
  college (community) Y92.214
  condominium — *see* Place of occurrence, residence, apartment
  construction area — *see* Place of occurrence, industrial and construction area
  convalescent home — *see* Place of occurrence, residence, institutional, nursing home
  court-house Y92.240
  cricket ground Y92.328
  cultural building Y92.258
    art gallery Y92.250
    museum Y92.251
    music hall Y92.252
    opera house Y92.253
    specified NEC Y92.258
    theater Y92.254
  dancehall Y92.252
  day nursery Y92.210
  dentist office Y92.531
  derelict house Y92.89
  desert Y92.820
  dockyard Y92.62
  dock NOS Y92.89
  doctor's office Y92.531
  dormitory — *see* Place of occurrence, residence, institutional, school dormitory
  dry dock Y92.62
  factory (building) (premises) Y92.63
  farm (land under cultivation) (outbuildings) Y92.79
    barn Y92.71
    chicken coop Y92.72
    field Y92.73
    hen house Y92.72
    house — *see* Place of occurrence, residence, house
    orchard Y92.74
    specified NEC Y92.79
  football field Y92.321
  forest Y92.821
  freeway Y92.411
  gallery Y92.250
  garage (commercial) Y92.59
    boarding house Y92.044
    military base Y92.135
    mobile home Y92.025
    nursing home Y92.124
    orphanage Y92.114
    private house Y92.015
    reform school Y92.155
  gas station Y92.524
  gasworks Y92.69
  golf course Y92.39
  gravel pit Y92.64
  grocery Y92.512
  gymnasium Y92.39
  handball court Y92.318
  harbor Y92.89
  harness racing course Y92.39
  healthcare provider office Y92.531
  highway (interstate) Y92.411
  hill Y92.828
  hockey rink Y92.330
  home — *see* Place of occurrence, residence
  hospice — *see* Place of occurrence, residence, institutional, nursing home
  hospital Y92.239

▽ Subterms under main terms may continue to next column or page   ☑ Additional Character Required — Refer to the Tabular List for Character Selection   431

Misadventure — Place of occurrence

Place of occurrence — *continued*
  hospital — *continued*
    cafeteria Y92.233
    corridor Y92.232
    operating room Y92.234
    patient
      bathroom Y92.231
      room Y92.230
    specified NEC Y92.238
  hotel Y92.59
  house — *see also* Place of occurrence, residence
    abandoned Y92.89
    under construction Y92.61
  industrial and construction area (yard) Y92.69
    building under construction Y92.61
    dock Y92.62
    dry dock Y92.62
    factory Y92.63
    gasworks Y92.69
    mine Y92.64
    oil rig Y92.65
    pit Y92.64
    power station Y92.69
    shipyard Y92.62
    specified NEC Y92.69
    tunnel under construction Y92.69
    workshop Y92.69
  kindergarten Y92.211
  lacrosse field Y92.328
  lake Y92.828
  library Y92.241
  mall Y92.59
  market Y92.512
  marsh Y92.828
  military
    base — *see* Place of occurrence, residence, institutional, military base
    training ground Y92.84
  mine Y92.64
  mosque Y92.22
  motel Y92.59
  motorway (interstate) Y92.411
  mountain Y92.828
  movie-house Y92.26
  museum Y92.251
  music-hall Y92.252
  not applicable Y92.9
  nuclear power station Y92.69
  nursing home — *see* Place of occurrence, residence, institutional, nursing home
  office building Y92.59
  offshore installation Y92.65
  oil rig Y92.65
  old people's home — *see* Place of occurrence, residence, institutional, specified NEC
  opera-house Y92.253
  orphanage — *see* Place of occurrence, residence, institutional, orphanage
  outpatient surgery center Y92.530
  park (public) Y92.830
    amusement Y92.831
  parking garage Y92.89
    lot Y92.481
  pavement Y92.480
  physician office Y92.531
  polo field Y92.328
  pond Y92.828
  post office Y92.242
  power station Y92.69
  prairie Y92.828
  prison — *see* Place of occurrence, residence, institutional, prison
  public
    administration building Y92.248
      city hall Y92.243
      courthouse Y92.240
      library Y92.241
      post office Y92.242
      specified NEC Y92.248
    building NEC Y92.29
    hall Y92.29
    place NOS Y92.89
  race course Y92.39
  radio station Y92.59
  railway line (bridge) Y92.85
  ranch (outbuildings) — *see* Place of occurrence, farm
  recreation area Y92.838
    amusement park Y92.831

Place of occurrence — *continued*
  recreation area — *continued*
    beach Y92.832
    campsite Y92.833
    park (public) Y92.830
    seashore Y92.832
    specified NEC Y92.838
  reform school - — *see* Place of occurrence, residence, institutional, reform school
  religious institution Y92.22
  residence (non-institutional) (private) Y92.009
    apartment Y92.039
      bathroom Y92.031
      bedroom Y92.032
      kitchen Y92.030
      specified NEC Y92.038
    bathroom Y92.002
    bedroom Y92.003
    boarding house Y92.049
      bathroom Y92.041
      bedroom Y92.042
      driveway Y92.043
      garage Y92.044
      garden Y92.046
      kitchen Y92.040
      specified NEC Y92.048
      swimming pool Y92.045
      yard Y92.046
    dining room Y92.001
    garden Y92.007
    home Y92.009
    house, single family Y92.019
      bathroom Y92.012
      bedroom Y92.013
      dining room Y92.011
      driveway Y92.014
      garage Y92.015
      garden Y92.017
      kitchen Y92.010
      specified NEC Y92.018
      swimming pool Y92.016
      yard Y92.017
    institutional Y92.10
      children's home — *see* Place of occurrence, residence, institutional, orphanage
      hospice — *see* Place of occurrence, residence, institutional, nursing home
      military base Y92.139
        barracks Y92.133
        garage Y92.135
        garden Y92.137
        kitchen Y92.130
        mess hall Y92.131
        specified NEC Y92.138
        swimming pool Y92.136
        yard Y92.137
      nursing home Y92.129
        bathroom Y92.121
        bedroom Y92.122
        driveway Y92.123
        garage Y92.124
        garden Y92.126
        kitchen Y92.120
        specified NEC Y92.128
        swimming pool Y92.125
        yard Y92.126
      orphanage Y92.119
        bathroom Y92.111
        bedroom Y92.112
        driveway Y92.113
        garage Y92.114
        garden Y92.116
        kitchen Y92.110
        specified NEC Y92.118
        swimming pool Y92.115
        yard Y92.116
      prison Y92.149
        bathroom Y92.142
        cell Y92.143
        courtyard Y92.147
        dining room Y92.141
        kitchen Y92.140
        specified NEC Y92.148
        swimming pool Y92.146
      reform school Y92.159
        bathroom Y92.152
        bedroom Y92.153
        dining room Y92.151
        driveway Y92.154

Place of occurrence — *continued*
  residence — *continued*
    institutional — *continued*
      reform school — *continued*
        garage Y92.155
        garden Y92.157
        kitchen Y92.150
        specified NEC Y92.158
        swimming pool Y92.156
        yard Y92.157
      school dormitory Y92.169
        bathroom Y92.162
        bedroom Y92.163
        dining room Y92.161
        kitchen Y92.160
        specified NEC Y92.168
      specified NEC Y92.199
        bathroom Y92.192
        bedroom Y92.193
        dining room Y92.191
        driveway Y92.194
        garage Y92.195
        garden Y92.197
        kitchen Y92.190
        specified NEC Y92.198
        swimming pool Y92.196
        yard Y92.197
    kitchen Y92.000
    mobile home Y92.029
      bathroom Y92.022
      bedroom Y92.023
      dining room Y92.021
      driveway Y92.024
      garage Y92.025
      garden Y92.027
      kitchen Y92.020
      specified NEC Y92.028
      swimming pool Y92.026
      yard Y92.027
    specified place in residence NEC Y92.008
    specified residence type NEC Y92.099
      bathroom Y92.091
      bedroom Y92.092
      driveway Y92.093
      garage Y92.094
      garden Y92.096
      kitchen Y92.090
      specified NEC Y92.098
      swimming pool Y92.095
      yard Y92.096
  restaurant Y92.511
  riding school Y92.39
  river Y92.828
  road Y92.410
  rodeo ring Y92.39
  rugby field Y92.328
  same day surgery center Y92.530
  sand pit Y92.64
  school (private) (public) (state) Y92.219
    college Y92.214
    daycare center Y92.210
    elementary school Y92.211
    high school Y92.213
    kindergarten Y92.211
    middle school Y92.212
    specified NEC Y92.218
    trace school Y92.215
    university Y92.214
    vocational school Y92.215
  sea (shore) Y92.832
  senior citizen center Y92.29
  service area
    airport Y92.520
    bus station Y92.521
    gas station Y92.524
    highway rest stop Y92.523
    railway station Y92.522
  shipyard Y92.62
  shop (commercial) Y92.513
  sidewalk Y92.480
  silo Y92.79
  skating rink (roller) Y92.331
    ice Y92.330
  slaughter house Y92.86
  soccer field Y92.322
  specified place NEC Y92.89
  sports area Y92.39
    athletic
      court Y92.318

Place of occurrence — *continued*
  sports area — *continued*
    athletic — *continued*
      court — *continued*
        basketball Y92.310
        specified NEC Y92.318
        squash Y92.311
        tennis Y92.312
      field Y92.328
        baseball Y92.320
        cricket ground Y92.328
        football Y92.321
        hockey Y92.328
        soccer Y92.322
        specified NEC Y92.328
    golf course Y92.39
    gymnasium Y92.39
    riding school Y92.39
    skating rink (roller) Y92.331
      ice Y92.330
    stadium Y92.39
    swimming pool Y92.34
  squash court Y92.311
  stadium Y92.39
  steeplechasing course Y92.39
  store Y92.512
  stream Y92.828
  street and highway Y92.410
    bike path Y92.482
    freeway Y92.411
    highway ramp Y92.415
    interstate highway Y92.411
    local residential or business street Y92.414
    motorway Y92.411
    parking lot Y92.481
    parkway Y92.412
    sidewalk Y92.480
    specified NEC Y92.488
    state road Y92.413
  subway car Y92.816
  supermarket Y92.512
  swamp Y92.828
  swimming pool (public) Y92.34
    private (at) Y92.095
      boarding house Y92.045
      military base Y92.136
      mobile home Y92.026
      nursing home Y92.125
      orphanage Y92.115
      prison Y92.146
      reform school Y92.156
      single family residence Y92.016
  synagogue Y92.22
  television station Y92.59
  tennis court Y92.312
  theater Y92.254
  trade area Y92.59
    bank Y92.510
    cafe Y92.511
    casino Y92.59
    garage Y92.59
    hotel Y92.59
    market Y92.512
    office building Y92.59
    radio station Y92.59
    restaurant Y92.511
    shop Y92.513
    shopping mall Y92.59
    store Y92.512
    supermarket Y92.512
    television station Y92.59
    warehouse Y92.59
  trailer park, residential — *see* Place of occurrence, residence, mobile home
  trailer site NOS Y92.89
  train Y92.815
    station Y92.522
  truck Y92.812
  tunnel under construction Y92.69
  university Y92.214
  urgent (health) care center Y92.532
  vehicle (transport) Y92.818
    airplane Y92.813
    boat Y92.814
    bus Y92.811
    car Y92.810
    specified NEC Y92.818
    subway car Y92.816
    train Y92.815

Place of occurrence — *continued*
  vehicle — *continued*
    truck Y92.812
  warehouse Y92.59
  water reservoir Y92.89
  wilderness area Y92.828
    desert Y92.820
    forest Y92.821
    marsh Y92.828
    mountain Y92.828
    prairie Y92.828
    specified NEC Y92.828
    swamp Y92.828
  workshop Y92.69
  yard, private Y92.096
    boarding house Y92.046
    mobile home Y92.027
    single family house Y92.017
  youth center Y92.29
  zoo (zoological garden) Y92.834
Plumbism — *see* Table of Drugs and Chemicals, lead
Poisoning (accidental) (by) — *see also* Table of Drugs and Chemicals
  by plant, thorns, spines, sharp leaves or other mechanisms NEC X58 ☑
  carbon monoxide
    generated by
      motor vehicle — *see* Accident, transport
      watercraft (in transit) (not in transit) V93.89 ☑
        ferry boat V93.81 ☑
        fishing boat V93.82 ☑
        jet skis V93.83 ☑
        liner V93.81 ☑
        merchant ship V93.80 ☑
        passenger ship V93.81 ☑
        powered craft NEC V93.83 ☑
  caused by injection of poisons into skin by plant thorns, spines, sharp leaves X58 ☑
  marine or sea plants (venomous) X58 ☑
  execution — *see* Legal, intervention, gas
    intervention
      by gas — *see* Legal, intervention, gas
      other specified means — *see* Legal, intervention, specified means NEC
  exhaust gas
    generated by
      motor vehicle — *see* Accident, transport
      watercraft (in transit) (not in transit) V93.89 ☑
        ferry boat V93.81 ☑
        fishing boat V93.82 ☑
        jet skis V93.83 ☑
        liner V93.81 ☑
        merchant ship V93.80 ☑
        passenger ship V93.81 ☑
        powered craft NEC V93.83 ☑
  fumes or smoke due to
    explosion — *see also* Explosion W40.9 ☑
    fire — *see* Exposure, fire
    ignition — *see* Ignition
  gas
    in legal intervention — *see* Legal, intervention, gas
    legal execution — *see* Legal, intervention, gas
  in war operations — *see* War operations
  legal
Powder burn (by) (from)
  airgun W34.110 ☑
  BB gun W34.110 ☑
  firearm NEC W34.19 ☑
  gas, air or spring-operated gun NEC W34.118 ☑
  handgun W32.1 ☑
  hunting rifle W33.12 ☑
  larger firearm W33.10 ☑
    specified NEC W33.19 ☑
  machine gun W33.13 ☑
  paintball gun W34.111 ☑
  pellet gun W34.110 ☑
  shotgun W33.11 ☑
  Very pistol [flare] W34.19 ☑
Premature cessation (of) **surgical and medical care** Y66
Privation (food) (water) X58 ☑
Procedure (operation)
  correct, on wrong side or body part (wrong side) (wrong site) Y65.53
  intended for another patient done on wrong patient Y65.52
  performed on patient not scheduled for surgery Y65.52

Procedure — *continued*
  performed on wrong patient Y65.52
  wrong, performed on correct patient Y65.51
Prolonged
  sitting in transport vehicle — *see* Travel, by type of vehicle
  stay in
    high altitude as cause of anoxia, barodontalgia, barotitis or hypoxia W94.11 ☑
    weightless environment X52 ☑
Pulling, excessive — *see also* Overexertion X50.9- ☑
Puncture, puncturing — *see also* Contact, with, by type of object or machine
  by
    plant thorns, spines, sharp leaves or other mechanisms NEC W60 ☑
  during medical or surgical treatment as misadventure — *see* Index to Diseases and Injuries, Complication(s)
Pushed, pushing (accidental) (injury in)
  by other person(s) (accidental) W51 ☑
    as, or caused by, a crowd or human stampede (with fall) W52 ☑
    before moving object NEC Y02.8 ☑
      motor vehicle Y02.0 ☑
      subway train Y02.1 ☑
      train Y02.1 ☑
    from
      high place NEC
        in accidental circumstances W17.89 ☑
        stated as
          intentional, homicide (attempt) Y01 ☑
          undetermined whether accidental or intentional Y30 ☑
      transport vehicle NEC — *see also* Accident, transport V89.9 ☑
        stated as
          intentional, homicide (attempt) Y08.89 ☑
    with fall W03 ☑
      due to ice or snow W00.0 ☑
  overexertion X50.9 ☑

R

Radiation (exposure to)
  arc lamps W89.0 ☑
  atomic power plant (malfunction) NEC W88.1 ☑
  complication of or abnormal reaction to medical radiotherapy Y84.2
  electromagnetic, ionizing W88.0 ☑
  gamma rays W88.1 ☑
  in
    war operations (from or following nuclear explosion) — *see* War operations
  inadvertent exposure of patient (receiving test or therapy) Y63.3
  infrared (heaters and lamps) W90.1 ☑
    excessive heat from W92 ☑
  ionized, ionizing (particles, artificially accelerated)
    radioisotopes W88.1 ☑
    specified NEC W88.8 ☑
    x-rays W88.0 ☑
  isotopes, radioactive — *see* Radiation, radioactive isotopes
  laser(s) W90.2 ☑
    in war operations — *see* War operations
    misadventure in medical care Y63.2
  light sources (man-made visible and ultraviolet) W89.9 ☑
    natural X32 ☑
    specified NEC W89.8 ☑
    tanning bed W89.1 ☑
    welding light W89.0 ☑
  man-made visible light W89.9 ☑
    specified NEC W89.8 ☑
    tanning bed W89.1 ☑
    welding light W89.0 ☑
  microwave W90.8 ☑
  misadventure in medical or surgical procedure Y63.2
  natural NEC X39.08 ☑
    radon X39.01 ☑
  overdose (in medical or surgical procedure) Y63.2
  radar W90.0 ☑
  radioactive isotopes (any) W88.1 ☑
    atomic power plant malfunction W88.1 ☑
    misadventure in medical or surgical treatment Y63.2

Radiation — *continued*
  radiofrequency W90.0 ☑
  radium NEC W88.1 ☑
  sun X32 ☑
  ultraviolet (light) (man-made) W89.9 ☑
    natural X32 ☑
    specified NEC W89.8 ☑
    tanning bed W89.1 ☑
    welding light W89.0 ☑
  welding arc, torch, or light W89.0 ☑
    excessive heat from W92 ☑
  x-rays (hard) (soft) W88.0 ☑
Range disease W94.11 ☑
Rape (attempted) T74.2- ☑
Rat bite W53.11 ☑
Reaching (prolonged) (static) X50.1 ☑
Reaction, abnormal to medical procedure — *see also*
  Complication of or following, by type of procedure
  Y84.9
  biologicals — *see* Table of Drugs and Chemicals
  drugs — *see* Table of Drugs and Chemicals
  vaccine — *see* Table of Drugs and Chemicals
  with misadventure — *see* Misadventure
Recoil
  airgun W34.110 ☑
  BB gun W34.110 ☑
  firearm NEC W34.19 ☑
  gas, air or spring-operated gun NEC W34.118 ☑
  handgun W32.1 ☑
  hunting rifle W33.12 ☑
  larger firearm W33.10 ☑
    specified NEC W33.19 ☑
  machine gun W33.13 ☑
  paintball gun W34.111 ☑
  pellet W34.110 ☑
  shotgun W33.11 ☑
  Very pistol [flare] W34.19 ☑
Reduction in
  atmospheric pressure — *see* Air, pressure, change
Rock falling on or hitting (accidentally) (person)
  W20.8 ☑
  in cave-in W20.0 ☑
Run over (accidentally) (by)
  animal (not being ridden) NEC W55.89 ☑
  machinery — *see* Contact, with, by specified type of
  machine
  transport vehicle NEC — *see also* Accident, transport
  V09.9 ☑
    intentional homicide (attempt) Y03.0 ☑
    motor NEC V09.20 ☑
      intentional homicide (attempt) Y03.0 ☑
Running
  before moving object X81.8 ☑
  motor vehicle X81.0 ☑
Running off, away
  animal (being ridden) — *see also* Accident, transport
  V80.918 ☑
  not being ridden W55.89 ☑
  animal-drawn vehicle NEC — *see also* Accident, transport V80.928 ☑
  highway, road(way), street
    transport vehicle NEC — *see also* Accident, transport
    V89.9 ☑
Rupture pressurized devices — *see* Explosion, by type
  of device

S

Saturnism — *see* Table of Drugs and Chemicals, lead
Scald, scalding (accidental) (by) (from) (in) X19 ☑
  air (hot) X14.1 ☑
  gases (hot) X14.1 ☑
  homicide (attempt) — *see* Assault, burning, hot object
  inflicted by other person
    stated as intentional, homicide (attempt) — *see*
      Assault, burning, hot object
  liquid (boiling) (hot) NEC X12 ☑
    stated as undetermined whether accidental or inten-
      tional Y27.2 ☑
    suicide (attempt) X77.2 ☑
  local application of externally applied substance in
    medical or surgical care Y63.5
  metal (molten) (liquid) (hot) NEC X18 ☑
  self-inflicted X77.9 ☑
  stated as undetermined whether accidental or inten-
    tional Y27.8 ☑

Scald, scalding — *continued*
  steam X13.1 ☑
    assault X98.0 ☑
    stated as undetermined whether accidental or inten-
      tional Y27.0 ☑
    suicide (attempt) X77.0 ☑
  suicide (attempt) X77.9 ☑
  vapor (hot) X13.1 ☑
    assault X98.0 ☑
    stated as undetermined whether accidental or inten-
      tional Y27.0 ☑
    suicide (attempt) X77.0 ☑
Scratched by
  cat W55.03 ☑
  person(s) (accidentally) W50.4 ☑
    with intent to injure or kill Y04.0 ☑
    as, or caused by, a crowd or human stampede (with
      fall) W52 ☑
    assault Y04.0 ☑
    homicide (attempt) Y04.0 ☑
    in
      fight Y04.0 ☑
      legal intervention
        injuring
          bystander Y35.892 ☑
          law enforcement personnel Y35.891 ☑
          suspect Y35.893 ☑
Seasickness T75.3 ☑
Self-harm NEC — *see also* External cause by type, undetermined whether accidental or intentional
  intentional — *see* Suicide
  poisoning NEC — *see* Table of Drugs and Chemicals,
    poisoning, accidental
Self-inflicted (injury) **NEC** — *see also* External cause by
  type, undetermined whether accidental or intentional
  intentional — *see* Suicide
  poisoning NEC — *see* Table of Drugs and Chemicals,
    poisoning, accidental
Sequelae (of)
  accident NEC — *see* W00-X58 with 7th character S
  assault (homicidal) (any means) — *see* X92-Y08 with
    7th character S
  homicide, attempt (any means) — *see* X92-Y08 with
    7th character S
  injury undetermined whether accidentally or purposely
    inflicted — *see* Y21-Y33 with 7th character S
  intentional self-harm (classifiable to X71-X83) — *see*
    X71-X83 with 7th character S
  legal intervention — *see* with 7th character S Y35 ☑
  motor vehicle accident — *see* V00-V99 with 7th char-
    acter S
  suicide, attempt (any means) — *see* X71-X83 with 7th
    character S
  transport accident — *see* V00-V99 with 7th character
    S
  war operations — *see* War operations
Shock
  electric — *see* Exposure, electric current
  from electric appliance (any) (faulty) W86.8 ☑
    domestic W86.0 ☑
    suicide (attempt) X83.1 ☑
Shooting, shot (accidental(ly)) — *see also* Discharge,
  firearm, by type
  herself or himself — *see* Discharge, firearm by type,
    self-inflicted
  homicide (attempt) — *see* Discharge, firearm by type,
    homicide
  in war operations — *see* War operations
  inflicted by other person — *see* Discharge, firearm by
    type, homicide
    accidental — *see* Discharge, firearm, by type of
      firearm
  legal
    execution — *see* Legal, intervention, firearm
    intervention — *see* Legal, intervention, firearm
  self-inflicted — *see* Discharge, firearm by type, suicide
    accidental — *see* Discharge, firearm, by type of
      firearm
  suicide (attempt) — *see* Discharge, firearm by type,
    suicide
Shoving (accidentally) **by other person** — *see* Pushed,
  by other person
Sickness
  alpine W94.11 ☑
  motion — *see* Motion
  mountain W94.11 ☑

Sinking (accidental)
  watercraft (causing drowning, submersion) — *see also*
    Drowning, due to, accident to, watercraft, sinking
    causing injury except drowning or submersion —
      see Accident, watercraft, causing, injury NEC
Siriasis X32 ☑
Sitting (prolonged) (static) X50.1 ☑
Slashed wrists — *see* Cut, self-inflicted
Slipping (accidental) (on same level) (with fall) W01.0 ☑
  on
    ice W00.0 ☑
      with skates — *see* Accident, transport, pedestri-
        an, conveyance
    mud W01.0 ☑
    oil W01.0 ☑
    snow W00.0 ☑
      with skis — *see* Accident, transport, pedestrian,
        conveyance
    surface (slippery) (wet) NEC W01.0 ☑
  without fall W18.40 ☑
    due to
      specified NEC W18.49 ☑
      stepping from one level to another W18.43 ☑
      stepping into hole or opening W18.42 ☑
      stepping on object W18.41 ☑
Sliver, wood, contact with W45.8 ☑
Smoldering (due to fire) — *see* Exposure, fire
Sodomy (attempted) **by force** T74.2 ☑
Sound waves (causing injury) W42.9 ☑
  supersonic W42.0 ☑
Splinter, contact with W45.8 ☑
Stab, stabbing — *see* Cut
Standing (prolonged) (static) X50.1 ☑
Starvation X58 ☑
Status of external cause Y99.9
  child assisting in compensated work for family Y99.8
  civilian activity done for financial or other compensa-
    tion Y99.0
  civilian activity done for income or pay Y99.0
  family member assisting in compensated work for
    other family member Y99.8
  hobby not done for income Y99.8
  leisure activity Y99.8
  military activity Y99.1
  off-duty activity of military personnel Y99.8
  recreation or sport not for income or while a student
    Y99.8
  specified NEC Y99.8
  student activity Y99.8
  volunteer activity Y99.2
Stepped on
  by
    animal (not being ridden) NEC W55.89 ☑
    crowd or human stampede W52 ☑
    person W50.0 ☑
Stepping on
  object W22.8 ☑
    sports equipment W21.9 ☑
    stationary W22.09 ☑
      sports equipment W21.89 ☑
    with fall W18.31 ☑
  person W51 ☑
    by crowd or human stampede W52 ☑
  sports equipment W21.9 ☑
Sting
  arthropod, nonvenomous W57 ☑
  insect, nonvenomous W57 ☑
Storm (cataclysmic) — *see* Forces of nature, cataclysmic
  storm
Straining, excessive — *see also* Overexertion X50.9 ☑
Strangling — *see* Strangulation
Strangulation (accidental) T71 ☑
Strenuous movements — *see also* Overexertion
  X50.9 ☑
Striking against
  airbag (automobile) W22.10 ☑
    driver side W22.11 ☑
    front passenger side W22.12 ☑
    specified NEC W22.19 ☑
  bottom when
    diving or jumping into water (in) W16.822 ☑
      causing drowning W16.821 ☑
      from boat W16.722 ☑
        causing drowning W16.721 ☑
      natural body W16.622 ☑
        causing drowning W16.821 ☑

Striking against — *continued*
  bottom when — *continued*
    diving or jumping into water — *continued*
      swimming pool W16.522 ☑
        causing drowning W16.521 ☑
    falling into water (in) W16.322 ☑
      causing drowning W16.321 ☑
      fountain — *see* Striking against, bottom when, falling into water, specified NEC
      natural body W16.122 ☑
        causing drowning W16.121 ☑
      reservoir — *see* Striking against, bottom when, falling into water, specified NEC
      specified NEC W16.322 ☑
        causing drowning W16.321 ☑
      swimming pool W16.022 ☑
        causing drowning W16.021 ☑
  diving board (swimming-pool) W21.4 ☑
  object W22.8 ☑
    caused by crowd or human stampede (with fall) W52 ☑
    furniture W22.03 ☑
    lamppost W22.02 ☑
    sports equipment W21.9 ☑
    stationary W22.09 ☑
      sports equipment W21.89 ☑
    wall W22.01 ☑
    with
      drowning or submersion — *see* Drowning
      fall — *see* Fall, due to, bumping against, object
  person(s) W51 ☑
    as, or caused by, a crowd or human stampede (with fall) W52 ☑
    assault Y04.2 ☑
    homicide (attempt) Y04.2 ☑
    with fall W03 ☑
      due to ice or snow W00.0 ☑
  sports equipment W21.9 ☑
  wall (when) W22.01 ☑
    diving or jumping into water (in) W16.832 ☑
      causing drowning W16.831 ☑
      swimming pool W16.532 ☑
        causing drowning W16.531 ☑
    falling into water (in) W16.332 ☑
      causing drowning W16.331 ☑
      fountain — *see* Striking against, wall when, falling into water, specified NEC
      natural body W16.132 ☑
        causing drowning W16.131 ☑
      reservoir — *see* Striking against, wall when, falling into water, specified NEC
      specified NEC W16.332 ☑
        causing drowning W16.331 ☑
      swimming pool W16.032 ☑
        causing drowning W16.031 ☑
    swimming pool (when) W22.042 ☑
      causing drowning W22.041 ☑
      diving or jumping into water W16.532 ☑
        causing drowning W16.531 ☑
      falling into water W16.032 ☑
        causing drowning W16.031 ☑

Struck (accidentally) **by**
  airbag (automobile) W22.10 ☑
    driver side W22.11 ☑
    front passenger side W22.12 ☑
    specified NEC W22.19 ☑
  alligator W58.02 ☑
  animal (not being ridden) NEC W55.89 ☑
  avalanche — *see* Landslide
  ball (hit) (thrown) W21.00 ☑
    assault Y08.09 ☑
    baseball W21.03 ☑
    basketball W21.05 ☑
    football W21.01 ☑
    golf ball W21.04 ☑
    soccer W21.02 ☑
    softball W21.07 ☑
    specified NEC W21.09 ☑
    volleyball W21.06 ☑
  bat or racquet
    baseball bat W21.11 ☑
      assault Y08.02 ☑
    golf club W21.13 ☑
      assault Y08.09 ☑
    specified NEC W21.19 ☑
      assault Y08.09 ☑

Struck (accidentally) **by** — *continued*
  bat or racquet — *continued*
    tennis racquet W21.12 ☑
      assault Y08.09 ☑
  bullet — *see also* Discharge, firearm by type
    in war operations — *see* War operations
  crocodile W58.12 ☑
  dog W54.1 ☑
  flare, Very pistol — *see* Discharge, firearm NEC
  hailstones X39.8 ☑
  hockey (ice)
    field
      puck W21.221 ☑
      stick W21.211 ☑
    puck W21.220 ☑
    stick W21.210 ☑
      assault Y08.01 ☑
  landslide — *see* Landslide
  law-enforcement agent (on duty) — *see* Legal, intervention, manhandling
    with blunt object — *see* Legal, intervention, blunt object
  lightning T75.0 ☑
    causing fire — *see* Exposure, fire
  machine — *see* Contact, with, by type of machine
  mammal NEC W55.89 ☑
    marine W56.32 ☑
  marine animal W56.82 ☑
  missile
    firearm — *see* Discharge, firearm by type
    in war operations — *see* War operations, missile
  object W22.8 ☑
    blunt W22.8 ☑
      assault Y00 ☑
      suicide (attempt) X79 ☑
      undetermined whether accidental or intentional Y29 ☑
    falling W20.8 ☑
      from, in, on
        building W20.1 ☑
          burning (uncontrolled fire) X00.4 ☑
        cataclysmic
          earth surface movement NEC — *see* Landslide
          storm — *see* Forces of nature, cataclysmic storm
        cave-in W20.0 ☑
        earthquake X34 ☑
        machine (in operation) — *see* Contact, with, by type of machine
        structure W20.1 ☑
          burning X00.4 ☑
        transport vehicle (in motion) — *see* Accident, transport, by type of vehicle
        watercraft V93.49 ☑
          due to
            accident to craft V91.39 ☑
              powered craft V91.33 ☑
                ferry boat V91.31 ☑
                fishing boat V91.32 ☑
                jetskis V91.33 ☑
                liner V91.31 ☑
                merchant ship V91.30 ☑
                passenger ship V91.31 ☑
              unpowered craft V91.38 ☑
                canoe V91.35 ☑
                inflatable V91.36 ☑
                kayak V91.35 ☑
                sailboat V91.34 ☑
                surf-board V91.38 ☑
                windsurfer V91.38 ☑
            powered craft V93.43 ☑
              ferry boat V93.41 ☑
              fishing boat V93.42 ☑
              jetskis V93.43 ☑
              liner V93.41 ☑
              merchant ship V93.40 ☑
              passenger ship V93.41 ☑
            unpowered craft V93.48 ☑
              sailboat V93.44 ☑
              surf-board V93.48 ☑
              windsurfer V93.48 ☑
      moving NEC W20.8 ☑
    projected W20.8 ☑
      assault Y00 ☑
      in sports W21.9 ☑

Struck (accidentally) **by** — *continued*
  object — *continued*
    projected — *continued*
      in sports — *continued*
        assault Y08.09 ☑
        ball W21.00 ☑
          baseball W21.03 ☑
          basketball W21.05 ☑
          football W21.01 ☑
          golf ball W21.04 ☑
          soccer W21.02 ☑
          softball W21.07 ☑
          specified NEC W21.09 ☑
          volleyball W21.06 ☑
        bat or racquet
          baseball bat W21.11 ☑
            assault Y08.02 ☑
          golf club W21.13 ☑
            assault Y08.09 ☑
          specified NEC W21.19 ☑
            assault Y08.09 ☑
          tennis racquet W21.12 ☑
            assault Y08.09 ☑
        hockey (ice)
          field
            puck W21.221 ☑
            stick W21.211 ☑
          puck W21.220 ☑
          stick W21.210 ☑
            assault Y08.01 ☑
          specified NEC W21.89 ☑
      set in motion by explosion — *see* Explosion
    thrown W20.8 ☑
      assault Y00 ☑
      in sports W21.9 ☑
        assault Y08.09 ☑
        ball W21.00 ☑
          baseball W21.03 ☑
          basketball W21.05 ☑
          football W21.01 ☑
          golf ball W21.04 ☑
          soccer W21.02 ☑
          soft ball W21.07 ☑
          specified NEC W21.09 ☑
          volleyball W21.06 ☑
        bat or racquet
          baseball bat W21.11 ☑
            assault Y08.02 ☑
          golf club W21.13 ☑
            assault Y08.09 ☑
          specified NEC W21.19 ☑
            assault Y08.09 ☑
          tennis racquet W21.12 ☑
            assault Y08.09 ☑
        hockey (ice)
          field
            puck W21.221 ☑
            stick W21.211 ☑
          puck W21.220 ☑
          stick W21.210 ☑
            assault Y08.01 ☑
          specified NEC W21.89 ☑
  other person(s) W50.0 ☑
    with
      blunt object W22.8 ☑
        intentional, homicide (attempt) Y00 ☑
        sports equipment W21.9 ☑
        undetermined whether accidental or intentional Y29 ☑
      fall W03 ☑
        due to ice or snow W00.0 ☑
    as, or caused by, a crowd or human stampede (with fall) W52 ☑
    assault Y04.2 ☑
    homicide (attempt) Y04.2 ☑
    in legal intervention
      injuring
        bystander Y35.812 ☑
        law enforcement personnel Y35.811 ☑
        suspect Y35.813 ☑
        unspecified person Y35.819 ☑
    sports equipment W21.9 ☑
  police (on duty) — *see* Legal, intervention, manhandling
    with blunt object — *see* Legal, intervention, blunt object

☑ Subterms under main terms may continue to next column or page   ☑ Additional Character Required — Refer to the Tabular List for Character Selection

435

Striking against — Struck

Struck (accidentally) **by** — *continued*
  sports equipment W21.9 ☑
    assault Y08.09 ☑
    ball W21.00 ☑
      baseball W21.03 ☑
      basketball W21.05 ☑
      football W21.01 ☑
      golf ball W21.04 ☑
      soccer W21.02 ☑
      soft ball W21.07 ☑
      specified NEC W21.09 ☑
      volleyball W21.06 ☑
    bat or racquet
      baseball bat W21.11 ☑
        assault Y08.02 ☑
      golf club W21.13 ☑
        assault Y08.09 ☑
      specified NEC W21.19 ☑
      tennis racquet W21.12 ☑
        assault Y08.09 ☑
    cleats (shoe) W21.31 ☑
    foot wear NEC W21.39 ☑
    football helmet W21.81 ☑
    hockey (ice)
      field
        puck W21.221 ☑
        stick W21.211 ☑
      puck W21.220 ☑
      stick W21.210 ☑
        assault Y08.01 ☑
    skate blades W21.32 ☑
    specified NEC W21.89 ☑
      assault Y08.09 ☑
  thunderbolt — *see* subcategory T75.0 ☑
    causing fire — *see* Exposure, fire
  transport vehicle NEC — *see also* Accident, transport
      V09.9 ☑
    intentional, homicide (attempt) Y03.0 ☑
    motor NEC — *see also* Accident, transport V09.20 ☑
      homicide Y03.0 ☑
  vehicle (transport) NEC — *see* Accident, transport, by
      type of vehicle
    stationary (falling from jack, hydraulic lift, ramp)
      W20.8 ☑
Stumbling
  over
    animal NEC W01.0 ☑
      with fall W18.09 ☑
    carpet, rug or (small) object W22.8 ☑
      with fall W18.09 ☑
    person W51 ☑
      with fall W03 ☑
        due to ice or snow W00.0 ☑
  without fall W18.40 ☑
    due to
      specified NEC W18.49 ☑
      stepping from one level to another W18.43 ☑
      stepping into hole or opening W18.42 ☑
      stepping on object W18.41 ☑
Submersion (accidental) — *see* Drowning
Suffocation (accidental) (by external means) (by pressure)
    (mechanical) — *see also* category T71 ☑
  due to, by
    avalanche — *see* Landslide
    explosion — *see* Explosion
    fire — *see* Exposure, fire
    food, any type (aspiration) (ingestion) (inhalation)
        — *see* categories T17 and T18 ☑
    ignition — *see* Ignition
    landslide — *see* Landslide
    machine(ry) — *see* Contact, with, by type of machine
    vomitus (aspiration) (inhalation) T17.81- ☑
  in
    burning building X00.8 ☑
Suicide, suicidal (attempted) (by) X83.8 ☑
  blunt object X79 ☑
  burning, burns X76 ☑
    hot object X77.9 ☑
      fluid NEC X77.2 ☑
      household appliance X77.3 ☑
      specified NEC X77.8 ☑
      steam X77.0 ☑
      tap water X77.1 ☑
      vapors X77.0 ☑
    caustic substance — *see* Table of Drugs and Chemicals

Suicide, suicidal — *continued*
  cold, extreme X83.2 ☑
  collision of motor vehicle with
    motor vehicle X82.0 ☑
    specified NEC X82.8 ☑
    train X82.1 ☑
    tree X82.2 ☑
  crashing of aircraft X83.0 ☑
  cut (any part of body) X78.9 ☑
  cutting or piercing instrument X78.9 ☑
    dagger X78.2 ☑
    glass X78.0 ☑
    knife X78.1 ☑
    specified NEC X78.8 ☑
    sword X78.2 ☑
  drowning (in) X71.9 ☑
    bathtub X71.0 ☑
    natural water X71.3 ☑
    specified NEC X71.8 ☑
    swimming pool X71.1 ☑
      following fall X71.2 ☑
  electrocution X83.1 ☑
  explosive(s) (material) X75 ☑
  fire, flames X76 ☑
  firearm X74.9 ☑
    airgun X74.01 ☑
    handgun X72 ☑
    hunting rifle X73.1 ☑
    larger X73.9 ☑
      specified NEC X73.8 ☑
    machine gun X73.2 ☑
    shotgun X73.0 ☑
    specified NEC X74.8 ☑
  hanging X83.8 ☑
  hot object — *see* Suicide, burning, hot object
  jumping
    before moving object X81.8 ☑
      motor vehicle X81.0 ☑
      subway train X81.1 ☑
      train X81.1 ☑
    from high place X80 ☑
  late effect of attempt — *see* X71-X83 with 7th character
      S
  lying before moving object, train, vehicle X81.8 ☑
  poisoning — *see* Table of Drugs and Chemicals
  puncture (any part of body) — *see* Suicide, cutting or
      piercing instrument
  scald — *see* Suicide, burning, hot object
  sequelae of attempt — *see* X71-X83 with 7th character
      S
  sharp object (any) — *see* Suicide, cutting or piercing
      instrument
  shooting — *see* Suicide, firearm
  specified means NEC X83.8 ☑
  stab (any part of body) — *see* Suicide, cutting or
      piercing instrument
  steam, hot vapors X77.0 ☑
  strangulation X83.8 ☑
  submersion — *see* Suicide, drowning
  suffocation X83.8 ☑
  wound NEC X83.8 ☑
Sunstroke X32 ☑
Supersonic waves (causing injury) W42.0 ☑
Surgical procedure, complication of (delayed or as an
    abnormal reaction without mention of misadven-
    ture) — *see also* Complication of or following, by
    type of procedure
  due to or as a result of misadventure — *see* Misadven-
      ture
Swallowed, swallowing
  foreign body — *see* Foreign body, alimentary canal
  poison — *see* Table of Drugs and Chemicals
  substance
    caustic or corrosive — *see* Table of Drugs and
        Chemicals
    poisonous — *see* Table of Drugs and Chemicals

T

Tackle in sport W03 ☑
Terrorism (involving) Y38.80 ☑
  biological weapons Y38.6X- ☑
  chemical weapons Y38.7X- ☑
  conflagration Y38.3X- ☑
  drowning and submersion Y38.89- ☑
  explosion Y38.2X- ☑

Terrorism — *continued*
  explosion — *continued*
    destruction of aircraft Y38.1X- ☑
    marine weapons Y38.0X- ☑
  fire Y38.3X- ☑
  firearms Y38.4X- ☑
  hot substances Y38.3X- ☑
  lasers Y38.89- ☑
  nuclear weapons Y38.5X- ☑
  piercing or stabbing instruments Y38.89- ☑
  secondary effects Y38.9X- ☑
  specified method NEC Y38.89- ☑
  suicide bomber Y38.81- ☑
Thirst X58 ☑
Threat to breathing
  aspiration — *see* Aspiration
  due to cave-in, falling earth or substance NEC T71 ☑
Thrown (accidentally)
  against part (any) of or object in transport vehicle (in
      motion) NEC — *see also* Accident, transport
  from
    high place, homicide (attempt) Y01 ☑
    machinery — *see* Contact, with, by type of machine
    transport vehicle NEC — *see also* Accident, transport
        V89.9 ☑
  off — *see* Thrown, from
Thunderbolt — *see* subcategory T75.0 ☑
  causing fire — *see* Exposure, fire
Tidal wave (any injury) **NEC** — *see* Forces of nature, tidal
    wave
Took
  overdose (drug) — *see* Table of Drugs and Chemicals
  poison — *see* Table of Drugs and Chemicals
Tornado (any injury) X37.1 ☑
Torrential rain (any injury) X37.8 ☑
Torture X58 ☑
Trampled by animal NEC W55.89 ☑
Trapped (accidentally)
  between objects (moving) (stationary and moving) —
      see Caught
  by part (any) of
    motorcycle V29.88 ☑
    pedal cycle V19.88 ☑
    transport vehicle NEC — *see also* Accident, transport
        V89.9 ☑
Travel (effects) (sickness) T75.3 ☑
Tree falling on or hitting (accidentally) (person)
    W20.8 ☑
Tripping
  over
    animal W01.0 ☑
      with fall W01.0 ☑
    carpet, rug or (small) object W22.8 ☑
      with fall W18.09 ☑
    person W51 ☑
      with fall W03 ☑
        due to ice or snow W00.0 ☑
  without fall W18.40 ☑
    due to
      specified NEC W18.49 ☑
      stepping from one level to another W18.43 ☑
      stepping into hole or opening W18.42 ☑
      stepping on object W18.41 ☑
Twisted by person(s) (accidentally) W50.2 ☑
  with intent to injure or kill Y04.0 ☑
  as, or caused by, a crowd or human stampede (with
      fall) W52 ☑
  assault Y04.0 ☑
  homicide (attempt) Y04.0 ☑
  in
    fight Y04.0 ☑
    legal intervention — *see* Legal, intervention, man-
        handling
Twisting (prolonged) (static) X50.1- ☑

U

**Underdosing of necessary drugs, medicaments or
    biological substances** Y63.6
Undetermined intent (contact) (exposure)
  automobile collision Y32 ☑
  blunt object Y29 ☑
  drowning (submersion) (in) Y21.9 ☑
    bathtub Y21.0 ☑
      after fall Y21.1 ☑

Undetermined intent — *continued*
  drowning — *continued*
    natural water (lake) (ocean) (pond) (river) (stream) Y21.4 ☑
    specified place NEC Y21.8 ☑
    swimming pool Y21.2 ☑
      after fall Y21.3 ☑
  explosive material Y25 ☑
  fall, jump or push from high place Y30 ☑
  falling, lying or running before moving object Y31 ☑
  fire Y26 ☑
  firearm discharge Y24.9 ☑
    airgun (BB) (pellet) Y24.0 ☑
    handgun (pistol) (revolver) Y22 ☑
    hunting rifle Y23.1 ☑
    larger Y23.9 ☑
      hunting rifle Y23.1 ☑
      machine gun Y23.3 ☑
      military Y23.2 ☑
      shotgun Y23.0 ☑
      specified type NEC Y23.8 ☑
    machine gun Y23.3 ☑
    military Y23.2 ☑
    shotgun Y23.0 ☑
    specified type NEC Y24.8 ☑
    Very pistol Y24.8 ☑
  hot object Y27.9 ☑
    fluid NEC Y27.2 ☑
    household appliance Y27.3 ☑
    specified object NEC Y27.8 ☑
    steam Y27.0 ☑
    tap water Y27.1 ☑
    vapor Y27.0 ☑
  jump, fall or push from high place Y30 ☑
  lying, falling or running before moving object Y31 ☑
  motor vehicle crash Y32 ☑
  push, fall or jump from high place Y30 ☑
  running, falling or lying before moving object Y31 ☑
  sharp object Y28.9 ☑
    dagger Y28.2 ☑
    glass Y28.0 ☑
    knife Y28.1 ☑
    specified object NEC Y28.8 ☑
    sword Y28.2 ☑
  smoke Y26 ☑
  specified event NEC Y33 ☑
Use of hand as hammer X50.3 ☑

V

Vibration (causing injury) W49.9 ☑
Victim (of)
  avalanche — *see* Landslide
  earth movements NEC — *see* Forces of nature, earth movement
  earthquake X34 ☑
  flood — *see* Flood
  landslide — *see* Landslide
  lightning — *see* subcategory T75.0 ☑
    causing fire — *see* Exposure, fire
  storm (cataclysmic) NEC — *see* Forces of nature, cataclysmic storm
  volcanic eruption X35 ☑
Volcanic eruption (any injury) X35 ☑
Vomitus, gastric contents in air passages (with asphyxia, obstruction or suffocation) T17.81- ☑

W

Walked into stationary object (any) W22.09 ☑
  furniture W22.03 ☑
  lamppost W22.02 ☑
  wall W22.01 ☑
War operations (injuries to military personnel and civilians during war, civil insurrection and peacekeeping missions) (by) (from) (involving) Y36.90 ☑
  after cessation of hostilities Y36.89- ☑

War operations — *continued*
  after cessation of hostilities — *continued*
    explosion (of)
      bomb placed during war operations Y36.82- ☑
      mine placed during war operations Y36.81- ☑
      specified NEC Y36.88- ☑
  air blast Y36.20- ☑
  aircraft
    destruction — *see* War operations, destruction of aircraft
  airway restriction — *see* War operations, restriction of airways
  asphyxiation — *see* War operations, restriction of airways
  biological weapons Y36.6X- ☑
  blast Y36.20- ☑
  blast fragments Y36.20- ☑
  blast wave Y36.20- ☑
  blast wind Y36.20- ☑
  bomb Y36.20- ☑
    dirty Y36.50- ☑
    gasoline Y36.31- ☑
    incendiary Y36.31- ☑
    petrol Y36.31- ☑
  bullet Y36.43- ☑
    incendiary Y36.32- ☑
    rubber Y36.41- ☑
  chemical weapons Y36.7X- ☑
  combat
    hand to hand (unarmed) combat Y36.44- ☑
    using blunt or piercing object Y36.45- ☑
  conflagration — *see* War operations, fire
  conventional warfare NEC Y36.49- ☑
  depth-charge Y36.01- ☑
  destruction of aircraft Y36.10- ☑
    due to
      air to air missile Y36.11- ☑
      collision with other aircraft Y36.12- ☑
      detonation (accidental) of onboard munitions and explosives Y36.14- ☑
      enemy fire or explosives Y36.11- ☑
      explosive placed on aircraft Y36.11- ☑
      onboard fire Y36.13- ☑
      rocket propelled grenade [RPG] Y36.11- ☑
      small arms fire Y36.11- ☑
      surface to air missile Y36.11- ☑
    specified NEC Y36.19- ☑
  detonation (accidental) of
    onboard marine weapons Y36.05- ☑
    own munitions or munitions launch device Y36.24- ☑
  dirty bomb Y36.50- ☑
  explosion (of) Y36.20- ☑
    aerial bomb Y36.21- ☑
    after cessation of hostilities
      bomb placed during war operations Y36.82- ☑
      mine placed during war operations Y36.81- ☑
    bomb NOS — *see also* War operations, bomb(s) Y36.20- ☑
    fragments Y36.20- ☑
    grenade Y36.29- ☑
    guided missile Y36.22- ☑
    improvised explosive device [IED] (person-borne) (roadside) (vehicle-borne) Y36.23- ☑
    land mine Y36.29- ☑
    marine mine (at sea) (in harbor) Y36.02- ☑
    marine weapon Y36.00- ☑
      specified NEC Y36.09- ☑
    own munitions or munitions launch device (accidental) Y36.24- ☑
    sea-based artillery shell Y36.03- ☑
    specified NEC Y36.29- ☑
    torpedo Y36.04- ☑
  fire Y36.30- ☑
    specified NEC Y36.39- ☑
  firearms
    discharge Y36.43- ☑
    pellets Y36.42- ☑

War operations — *continued*
  flamethrower Y36.33- ☑
  fragments (from) (of)
    improvised explosive device [IED] (person-borne) (roadside) (vehicle-borne) Y36.26- ☑
    munitions Y36.25- ☑
    specified NEC Y36.29- ☑
    weapons Y36.27- ☑
  friendly fire Y36.92 ☑
  hand to hand (unarmed) combat Y36.44- ☑
  hot substances — *see* War operations, fire
  incendiary bullet Y36.32- ☑
  nuclear weapon (effects of) Y36.50- ☑
    acute radiation exposure Y36.54- ☑
    blast pressure Y36.51- ☑
    direct blast Y36.51- ☑
    direct heat Y36.53- ☑
    fallout exposure Y36.54- ☑
    fireball Y36.53- ☑
    indirect blast (struck or crushed by blast debris) (being thrown by blast) Y36.52- ☑
    ionizing radiation (immediate exposure) Y36.54- ☑
    nuclear radiation Y36.54- ☑
    radiation
      ionizing (immediate exposure) Y36.54- ☑
      nuclear Y36.54- ☑
      thermal Y36.53- ☑
    secondary effects Y36.54- ☑
    specified NEC Y36.59- ☑
    thermal radiation Y36.53- ☑
  restriction of air (airway)
    intentional Y36.46- ☑
    unintentional Y36.47- ☑
  rubber bullets Y36.41- ☑
  shrapnel NOS Y36.29- ☑
  suffocation — *see* War operations, restriction of airways
  unconventional warfare NEC Y36.7X- ☑
  underwater blast NOS Y36.00- ☑
  warfare
    conventional NEC Y36.49- ☑
    unconventional NEC Y36.7X- ☑
  weapon of mass destruction [WMD] Y36.91 ☑
  weapons
    biological weapons Y36.6X- ☑
    chemical Y36.7X- ☑
    nuclear (effects of) Y36.50- ☑
      acute radiation exposure Y36.54- ☑
      blast pressure Y36.51- ☑
      direct blast Y36.51- ☑
      direct heat Y36.53- ☑
      fallout exposure Y36.54- ☑
      fireball Y36.53- ☑
      radiation
        ionizing (immediate exposure) Y36.54- ☑
        nuclear Y36.54- ☑
        thermal Y36.53- ☑
      secondary effects Y36.54- ☑
      specified NEC Y36.59- ☑
    of mass destruction [WMD] Y36.91 ☑
Washed
  away by flood — *see* Flood
  off road by storm (transport vehicle) — *see* Forces of nature, cataclysmic storm
Weather exposure NEC — *see* Forces of nature
Weightlessness (causing injury) (effects of) (in spacecraft, real or simulated) X52 ☑
Work related condition Y99.0
Wound (accidental) NEC — *see also* Injury X58 ☑
  battle — *see also* War operations Y36.90 ☑
  gunshot — *see* Discharge, firearm by type
Wreck transport vehicle NEC — *see also* Accident, transport V89.9 ☑
Wrong
  device implanted into correct surgical site Y65.51
  fluid in infusion Y65.1
  patient, procedure performed on Y65.52
  procedure (operation) on correct patient Y65.51

Chapter 1. Certain Infectious and Parasitic Diseases (A00–B99), U07.1

Chapter-specific Guidelines with Coding Examples

The chapter-specific guidelines from the ICD-10-CM Official Guidelines for Coding and Reporting have been provided below. Along with these guidelines are coding examples, contained in the shaded boxes, that have been developed to help illustrate the coding and/or sequencing guidance found in these guidelines.

a. Human immunodeficiency virus (HIV) infections

1) Code only confirmed cases

Code only confirmed cases of HIV infection/illness. This is an exception to the hospital inpatient guideline Section II, H.

In this context, "confirmation" does not require documentation of positive serology or culture for HIV; the provider's diagnostic statement that the patient is HIV positive, or has an HIV-related illness is sufficient.

> Patient admitted with anemia with possible HIV infection
>
> **D64.9   Anemia, unspecified**
>
> *Explanation:* Only the anemia is coded in this scenario because it has not been confirmed that an HIV infection is present. This is an exception to the guideline Section II, H for hospital inpatient coding.

2) Selection and sequencing of HIV codes

(a) Patient admitted for HIV-related condition

If a patient is admitted for an HIV-related condition, the principal diagnosis should be B20, Human immunodeficiency virus [HIV] disease followed by additional diagnosis codes for all reported HIV-related conditions.

(b) Patient with HIV disease admitted for unrelated condition

If a patient with HIV disease is admitted for an unrelated condition (such as a traumatic injury), the code for the unrelated condition (e.g., the nature of injury code) should be the principal diagnosis. Other diagnoses would be B20 followed by additional diagnosis codes for all reported HIV-related conditions.

> Unstable angina, native coronary artery atherosclerosis, HIV
>
> **I25.110   Atherosclerotic heart disease of native coronary artery with unstable angina pectoris**
>
> **B20   Human immunodeficiency virus [HIV] disease**
>
> *Explanation:* The arteriosclerotic coronary artery disease and the unstable angina are not related to HIV, so those conditions are reported first using a combination code, and HIV is reported secondarily.

(c) Whether the patient is newly diagnosed

Whether the patient is newly diagnosed or has had previous admissions/encounters for HIV conditions is irrelevant to the sequencing decision.

(d) Asymptomatic human immunodeficiency virus

Z21, Asymptomatic human immunodeficiency virus [HIV] infection status, is to be applied when the patient without any documentation of symptoms is listed as being "HIV positive," "known HIV," "HIV test positive," or similar terminology. Do not use this code if the term "AIDS" is used or if the patient is treated for any HIV-related illness or is described as having any condition(s) resulting from his/her HIV positive status; use B20 in these cases.

> Patient admitted with acute appendicitis. Status positive HIV test on Atripla, with no prior symptoms
>
> **K35.80   Unspecified acute appendicitis**
>
> **Z21   Asymptomatic human immunodeficiency virus [HIV] infection status**
>
> *Explanation:* Code Z21 is sequenced second since documentation indicates that the patient has had a positive HIV test but has been asymptomatic. Being on medication for HIV is not an indication that code B20 is used instead of Z21. Unless there has been documentation that the patient has had current or prior symptoms or HIV-related complications, code B20 is not used. The appendicitis is not an AIDS-related complication and is sequenced first.

(e) Patients with inconclusive HIV serology

Patients with inconclusive HIV serology, but no definitive diagnosis or manifestations of the illness, may be assigned code R75, Inconclusive laboratory evidence of human immunodeficiency virus [HIV].

(f) Previously diagnosed HIV-related illness

Patients with any known prior diagnosis of an HIV-related illness should be coded to B20. Once a patient has developed an HIV-related illness, the patient should always be assigned code B20 on every subsequent admission/encounter. Patients previously diagnosed with any HIV illness (B20) should never be assigned to R75 or Z21, Asymptomatic human immunodeficiency virus [HIV] infection status.

(g) HIV infection in pregnancy, childbirth and the puerperium

During pregnancy, childbirth or the puerperium, a patient admitted (or presenting for a health care encounter) because of an HIV-related illness should receive a principal diagnosis code of O98.7-, Human immunodeficiency [HIV] disease complicating pregnancy, childbirth and the puerperium, followed by B20 and the code(s) for the HIV-related illness(es). Codes from Chapter 15 always take sequencing priority.

Patients with asymptomatic HIV infection status admitted (or presenting for a health care encounter) during pregnancy, childbirth, or the puerperium should receive codes of O98.7- and Z21.

(h) Encounters for testing for HIV

If a patient is being seen to determine his/her HIV status, use code Z11.4, Encounter for screening for human immunodeficiency virus [HIV]. Use additional codes for any associated high-risk behavior.

If a patient with signs or symptoms is being seen for HIV testing, code the signs and symptoms. An additional counseling code Z71.7, Human immunodeficiency virus [HIV] counseling, may be used if counseling is provided during the encounter for the test.

When a patient returns to be informed of his/her HIV test results and the test result is negative, use code Z71.7, Human immunodeficiency virus [HIV] counseling.

If the results are positive, see previous guidelines and assign codes as appropriate.

b. Infectious agents as the cause of diseases classified to other chapters

Certain infections are classified in chapters other than Chapter 1 and no organism is identified as part of the infection code. In these instances, it is necessary to use an additional code from Chapter 1 to identify the organism. A code from category B95, Streptococcus, Staphylococcus, and Enterococcus as the cause of diseases classified to other chapters, B96, Other bacterial agents as the cause of diseases classified to other chapters, or B97, Viral agents as the cause of diseases classified to other chapters, is to be used as an additional code to identify the organism. An instructional note will be found at the infection code advising that an additional organism code is required.

> E. coli UTI
>
> **N39.0   Urinary tract infection, site not specified**
>
> **B96.20   Unspecified Escherichia coli [E.coli] as the cause of diseases classified elsewhere**
>
> *Explanation:* An instructional note under the code for the urinary tract infection indicates to code also the specific organism.

c. Infections resistant to antibiotics

Many bacterial infections are resistant to current antibiotics. It is necessary to identify all infections documented as antibiotic resistant. Assign a code from category Z16, Resistance to antimicrobial drugs, following the infection code only if the infection code does not identify drug resistance.

d. Sepsis, severe sepsis, and septic shock

1) Coding of sepsis and severe sepsis

(a) Sepsis

For a diagnosis of sepsis, assign the appropriate code for the underlying systemic infection. If the type of infection or causal organism is not further specified, assign code A41.9, Sepsis, unspecified organism.

A code from subcategory R65.2, Severe sepsis, should not be assigned unless severe sepsis or an associated acute organ dysfunction is documented.

(i) Negative or inconclusive blood cultures and sepsis

Negative or inconclusive blood cultures do not preclude a diagnosis of sepsis in patients with clinical evidence of the condition; however, the provider should be queried.

(ii) Urosepsis

The term urosepsis is a nonspecific term. It is not to be considered synonymous with sepsis. It has no default code in the Alphabetic Index. Should a provider use this term, he/she must be queried for clarification.

(iii) Sepsis with organ dysfunction

If a patient has sepsis and associated acute organ dysfunction or multiple organ dysfunction (MOD), follow the instructions for coding severe sepsis.

(iv) Acute organ dysfunction that is not clearly associated with the sepsis

If a patient has sepsis and an acute organ dysfunction, but the medical record documentation indicates that the acute organ dysfunction is related to a medical condition other than the sepsis, do not assign a code from subcategory R65.2, Severe sepsis. An acute organ dysfunction must be associated with the sepsis in order to assign the severe sepsis code. If the documentation is not clear as to whether an acute organ dysfunction is related to the sepsis or another medical condition, query the provider.

Sepsis and acute respiratory failure due to COPD exacerbation	
A41.9	Sepsis, unspecified organism
J44.1	Chronic obstructive pulmonary disease with (acute) exacerbation
J96.00	Acute respiratory failure, unspecified whether with hypoxia or hypercapnia

Explanation: Although acute organ dysfunction is present in the form of acute respiratory failure, severe sepsis (R65.2) is not coded in this example, as the acute respiratory failure is attributed to the COPD exacerbation rather than the sepsis. Sequencing of these codes would be determined by the circumstances of the admission.

(b) Severe sepsis

The coding of severe sepsis requires a minimum of 2 codes: first a code for the underlying systemic infection, followed by a code from subcategory R65.2, Severe sepsis. If the causal organism is not documented, assign code A41.9, Sepsis, unspecified organism, for the infection. Additional code(s) for the associated acute organ dysfunction are also required.

Due to the complex nature of severe sepsis, some cases may require querying the provider prior to assignment of the codes.

2) Septic shock

(a) Septic shock generally refers to circulatory failure associated with severe sepsis, and therefore, it represents a type of acute organ dysfunction.

For cases of septic shock, the code for the systemic infection should be sequenced first, followed by code R65.21, Severe sepsis with septic shock or code T81.12, Postprocedural septic shock. Any additional codes for the other acute organ dysfunctions should also be assigned. As noted in the sequencing instructions in the Tabular List, the code for septic shock cannot be assigned as a principal diagnosis.

Sepsis with septic shock	
A41.9	Sepsis, unspecified organism
R65.21	Severe sepsis with septic shock

Explanation: Documentation of septic shock automatically implies severe sepsis as it is a form of acute organ dysfunction. Septic shock is not coded as the principal diagnosis; it is always preceded by the code for the systemic infection.

3) Sequencing of severe sepsis

If severe sepsis is present on admission, and meets the definition of principal diagnosis, the underlying systemic infection should be assigned as principal diagnosis followed by the appropriate code from subcategory R65.2 as required by the sequencing rules in the Tabular List. A code from subcategory R65.2 can never be assigned as a principal diagnosis.

When severe sepsis develops during an encounter (it was not present on admission), the underlying systemic infection and the appropriate code from subcategory R65.2 should be assigned as secondary diagnoses.

Severe sepsis may be present on admission, but the diagnosis may not be confirmed until sometime after admission. If the documentation is not clear whether severe sepsis was present on admission, the provider should be queried.

4) Sepsis or severe sepsis with a localized infection

If the reason for admission is sepsis or severe sepsis and a localized infection, such as pneumonia or cellulitis, a code(s) for the underlying systemic infection should be assigned first and the code for the localized infection should be assigned as a secondary diagnosis. If the patient has severe sepsis, a code from subcategory R65.2 should also be assigned as a secondary diagnosis. If the patient is admitted with a localized infection, such as pneumonia, and sepsis/severe sepsis doesn't develop until after admission, the localized infection should be assigned first, followed by the appropriate sepsis/severe sepsis codes.

Patient presents with acute renal failure due to severe sepsis from *Pseudomonas* pneumonia	
A41.52	Sepsis due to Pseudomonas
J15.1	Pneumonia due to Pseudomonas
R65.20	Severe sepsis without septic shock
N17.9	Acute kidney failure, unspecified

Explanation: If all conditions are present on admission, the systemic infection (sepsis) is sequenced first followed by the codes for the localized infection (pneumonia), severe sepsis and any organ dysfunction. If only the pneumonia was present on admission with the sepsis and resulting renal failure developing later in the admission, then the pneumonia would be sequenced first.

5) Sepsis due to a postprocedural infection
(a) Documentation of causal relationship

As with all postprocedural complications, code assignment is based on the provider's documentation of the relationship between the infection and the procedure.

(b) Sepsis due to a postprocedural infection

For infections following a procedure, a code from T81.40, to T81.43 Infection following a procedure, or a code from O86.00 to O86.03, Infection of obstetric surgical wound, that identifies the site of the infection should be coded first, if known. Assign an additional code for sepsis following a procedure (T81.44) or sepsis following an obstetrical procedure (O86.04). Use an additional code to identify the infectious agent. If the patient has severe sepsis, the appropriate code from subcategory R65.2 should also be assigned with the additional code(s) for any acute organ dysfunction.

For infections following infusion, transfusion, therapeutic injection, or immunization, a code from subcategory T80.2, Infections following infusion, transfusion, and therapeutic injection, or code T88.0-, Infection following immunization, should be coded first, followed by the code for the specific infection. If the patient has severe sepsis, the appropriate code from subcategory R65.2 should also be assigned, with the additional codes(s) for any acute organ dysfunction.

(c) Postprocedural infection and postprocedural septic shock

If a postprocedural infection has resulted in postprocedural septic shock, assign the codes indicated above for sepsis due to a postprocedural infection, followed by code T81.12-, Postprocedural septic shock. Do not assign code R65.21, Severe sepsis with septic shock. Additional code(s) should be assigned for any acute organ dysfunction.

Septic shock following abdominal procedure with intramuscular abscess	
T81.42XA	Infection following a procedure, deep incisional surgical site, initial encounter
T81.44XA	Sepsis following a procedure, initial encounter
A41.9	Sepsis, unspecified organism
T81.12XA	Postprocedural septic shock, initial encounter

Explanation: The first code reported identifies the site of the postprocedural infection with intramuscular abscess coded to "deep incisional surgical site." If sepsis occurred as a result of the postprocedural infection, code T81.44- should be coded as a secondary diagnosis, followed by a code for the specific type of sepsis. Postprocedural septic shock is captured by code T81.12- and not with code R65.21. If any other acute organ dysfunction was documented as associated with the postprocedural sepsis, additional codes could be assigned to represent those conditions.

6) Sepsis and severe sepsis associated with a noninfectious process (condition)

In some cases, a noninfectious process (condition) such as trauma, may lead to an infection which can result in sepsis or severe sepsis. If sepsis or severe sepsis is documented as associated with a noninfectious condition, such as a burn or serious injury, and this condition meets the definition for principal diagnosis, the code for the noninfectious condition should be sequenced first, followed by the code for the resulting infection. If severe sepsis is present, a code from subcategory R65.2 should also be assigned with any associated organ dysfunction(s) codes. It is not necessary to assign a code from subcategory R65.1, Systemic inflammatory response syndrome (SIRS) of non-infectious origin, for these cases.

If the infection meets the definition of principal diagnosis, it should be sequenced before the non-infectious condition. When both the associated non-infectious condition and the infection meet the definition of principal diagnosis, either may be assigned as principal diagnosis.

Only one code from category R65, Symptoms and signs specifically associated with systemic inflammation and infection, should be assigned. Therefore, when a non-infectious condition leads to an infection resulting in severe sepsis, assign the appropriate code from subcategory R65.2, Severe sepsis. Do not additionally assign a code from subcategory R65.1, Systemic inflammatory response syndrome (SIRS) of non-infectious origin.

See Section I.C.18. SIRS due to non-infectious process

> Patient admitted with multiple third-degree burns of right upper arm develops severe MSSA sepsis with septic shock, three days into admission
>
> **T22.391A**   **Burn of third degree of multiple sites of right shoulder and upper arm limb, except wrist and hand, initial encounter**
>
> **A41.01**   **Sepsis due to Methicillin susceptible Staphylococcus aureus**
>
> **R65.21**   **Severe sepsis with septic shock**
>
> *Explanation:* Severe sepsis is coded rather than SIRS from R65 because it is documented as a severe systemic infectious response with septic shock to a noninfectious condition. The code for the systemic infection is not used as the principal diagnosis because it was not present on admission. The patient was admitted for the burn injury.

7) Sepsis and septic shock complicating abortion, pregnancy, childbirth, and the puerperium

See Section I.C.15. Sepsis and septic shock complicating abortion, pregnancy, childbirth and the puerperium

8) Newborn sepsis

See Section I.C.16. f. Bacterial sepsis of Newborn

e. Methicillin resistant Staphylococcus aureus (MRSA) conditions

1) Selection and sequencing of MRSA codes

(a) Combination codes for MRSA infection

When a patient is diagnosed with an infection that is due to methicillin resistant *Staphylococcus aureus* (MRSA), and that infection has a combination code that includes the causal organism (e.g., sepsis, pneumonia) assign the appropriate combination code for the condition (e.g., code A41.02, Sepsis due to Methicillin resistant Staphylococcus aureus or code J15.212, Pneumonia due to Methicillin resistant Staphylococcus aureus). Do not assign code B95.62, Methicillin resistant Staphylococcus aureus infection as the cause of diseases classified elsewhere, as an additional code, because the combination code includes the type of infection and the MRSA organism. Do not assign a code from subcategory Z16.11, Resistance to penicillins, as an additional diagnosis.

See Section C.1. for instructions on coding and sequencing of sepsis and severe sepsis.

(b) Other codes for MRSA infection

When there is documentation of a current infection (e.g., wound infection, stitch abscess, urinary tract infection) due to MRSA, and that infection does not have a combination code that includes the causal organism, assign the appropriate code to identify the condition along with code B95.62, Methicillin resistant Staphylococcus aureus infection as the cause of diseases classified elsewhere for the MRSA infection. Do not assign a code from subcategory Z16.11, Resistance to penicillins.

(c) Methicillin susceptible Staphylococcus aureus (MSSA) and MRSA colonization

The condition or state of being colonized or carrying MSSA or MRSA is called colonization or carriage, while an individual person is described as being colonized or being a carrier. Colonization means that MSSA or MSRA is present on or in the body without necessarily causing illness. A positive MRSA colonization test might be documented by the provider as "MRSA screen positive" or "MRSA nasal swab positive".

Assign code Z22.322, Carrier or suspected carrier of Methicillin resistant Staphylococcus aureus, for patients documented as having MRSA colonization. Assign code Z22.321, Carrier or suspected carrier of Methicillin susceptible Staphylococcus aureus, for patient**s** documented as having MSSA colonization. Colonization is not necessarily indicative of a disease process or as the cause of a specific condition the patient may have unless documented as such by the provider.

(d) MRSA colonization and infection

If a patient is documented as having both MRSA colonization and infection during a hospital admission, code Z22.322, Carrier or suspected carrier of Methicillin resistant Staphylococcus aureus, and a code for the MRSA infection may both be assigned.

f. Zika virus infections

1) Code only confirmed cases

Code only a confirmed diagnosis of Zika virus (A92.5, Zika virus disease) as documented by the provider. This is an exception to the hospital inpatient guideline Section II, H. In this context, "confirmation" does not require documentation of the type of test performed; the provider's diagnostic statement that the condition is confirmed is sufficient. This code should be assigned regardless of the stated mode of transmission.

If the provider documents "suspected", "possible" or "probable" Zika, do not assign code A92.5. Assign a code(s) explaining the reason for encounter (such as fever, rash, or joint pain) or Z20.821, Contact with and (suspected) exposure to Zika virus.

> A 45-year-old female recently returned from a Caribbean vacation complaining of fever, headache, joint and muscle aches and is admitted for suspected influenza. Infectious Disease consult diagnoses Zika virus. Patient discharged with Zika virus disease and instructions for hydration, rest, acetaminophen, and follow-up with Infectious Disease.
>
> **A92.5**   **Zika virus disease**
>
> *Explanation:* Although only a confirmed diagnosis should be coded, when a provider documents a diagnosis of Zika virus, code A92.5 Zika virus disease, is reported whether or not there is any indication of the type of tests performed. If the patient is pregnant, code first a code from category O98.5- Other viral diseases complicating pregnancy, childbirth and the puerperium, followed by code (A92.5) for the confirmed Zika virus. See also guideline 1.C.15.a.1.

g. Coronavirus infections

1) COVID-19 infection (infection due to SARS-CoV-2)

(a) Code only confirmed cases

Code only a confirmed diagnosis of the 2019 novel coronavirus disease (COVID-19) as documented by the provider or documentation of a positive COVID-19 test result. For a confirmed diagnosis, assign code U07.1, COVID-19. This is an exception to the hospital inpatient guideline Section II, H. In this context, "confirmation" does not require documentation of a positive test result for COVID-19; the provider's documentation that the individual has COVID-19 is sufficient.

If the provider documents "suspected," "possible," "probable," or "inconclusive" COVID-19, do not assign code U07.1. Instead, code the signs and symptoms reported. See guideline I.C.1.g.1.g.

> An elderly patient who is a former smoker is admitted with a productive cough, fatigue, and chest discomfort. CXR and PFTs indicate acute bronchitis. Treatment includes cough suppressants and anti-inflammatory medication, along with isolation precautions. The provider documents acute bronchitis likely due to COVID-19. Laboratory tests were inconclusive.
>
> **J20.9**   **Acute bronchitis, unspecified**
>
> **Z87.891**   **History of tobacco dependence**
>
> *Explanation:* Because the COVID-19 diagnosis was documented as likely by the provider, code U07.1 cannot be assigned. Instead a code explaining the reason for the encounter is used, in this case the acute bronchitis. Code J20.9 Acute bronchitis, unspecified, is used because the causative organism, specifically that which causes COVID-19, is not confirmed. Without further documentation of COVID-19 or another causative organism being present, code J20.8 Acute bronchitis due to other specified organisms, does not apply.

A 75-year-old male from a nursing home presents with shortness of breath and fever of 102.7. Patient was diagnosed with pneumonia, confirmed on CXR. Laboratory tests come back positive for COVID-19.

U07.1   **COVID-19**

J12.89   **Other viral pneumonia**

Explanation: The provider does not need to explicitly link the test result to the respiratory condition, nor does the provider need to explicitly document a diagnosis of COVID-19; the positive test result alone can be used to assign code U07.1. This advice is limited to laboratory tests for COVID-19 only. The significance of all other laboratory test results must be documented by the provider. According to guideline I.C.1.b, code U07.1 should be sequenced before the pneumonia code (J12.89).

(b) Sequencing of codes

When COVID-19 meets the definition of principal diagnosis, code U07.1, COVID-19, should be sequenced first, followed by the appropriate codes for associated manifestations, except when another guideline requires that certain codes be sequenced first, such as obstetrics, sepsis, or transplant complications.

The patient presents with acute hypoxic respiratory failure due to sepsis from COVID-19 related pneumonia.

A41.89   **Other specified sepsis**

U07.1   **COVID-19**

J12.89   **Other viral pneumonia**

J96.01   **Acute respiratory failure with hypoxia**

R65.20   **Severe sepsis without septic shock**

Explanation: If all conditions are present on admission, the systemic infection (sepsis) is sequenced first, followed by the code(s) for the localized infection (COVID-19 and pneumonia). The acute respiratory failure (acute organ dysfunction) is clearly documented as being associated with the sepsis, and therefore a severe sepsis code from subcategory R65.2- can also be assigned. If the sepsis had developed later in the admission, with or without any associated respiratory failure, the COVID-19 code would be sequenced first.

For a COVID-19 infection that progresses to sepsis, see Section I.C.1.d. Sepsis, Severe Sepsis, and Septic Shock

See Section I.C.15.s. for COVID-19 infection in pregnancy, childbirth, and the puerperium

See Section I.C.16.h. for COVID-19 infection in newborn

For a COVID-19 infection in a lung transplant patient, see Section I.C.19.g.3.a. Transplant complications other than kidney.

(c) Acute respiratory manifestations of COVID-19

When the reason for the encounter/admission is a respiratory manifestation of COVID-19, assign code U07.1, COVID-19, as the principal/first-listed diagnosis and assign code(s) for the respiratory manifestation(s) as additional diagnoses.

The following conditions are examples of common respiratory manifestations of COVID-19.

(i) Pneumonia

For a patient with pneumonia confirmed as due to COVID-19, assign codes U07.1, COVID-19, and J12.89, Other viral pneumonia.

(ii) Acute bronchitis

For a patient with acute bronchitis confirmed as due to COVID-19, assign codes U07.1, and J20.8, Acute bronchitis due to other specified organisms.

Bronchitis not otherwise specified (NOS) due to COVID-19 should be coded using code U07.1 and J40, Bronchitis, not specified as acute or chronic.

(iii) Lower respiratory infection

If the COVID-19 is documented as being associated with a lower respiratory infection, not otherwise specified (NOS), or an acute respiratory infection, NOS, codes U07.1 and J22, Unspecified acute lower respiratory infection, should be assigned.

If the COVID-19 is documented as being associated with a respiratory infection, NOS, codes U07.1 and J98.8, Other specified respiratory disorders, should be assigned.

(iv) Acute respiratory distress syndrome

For acute respiratory distress syndrome (ARDS) due to COVID-19, assign codes U07.1, and J80, Acute respiratory distress syndrome.

(v) Acute respiratory failure

For acute respiratory failure due to COVID-19, assign code U07.1, and code J96.0-, Acute respiratory failure.

(d) Non-respiratory manifestations of COVID-19

When the reason for the encounter/admission is a non-respiratory manifestation (e.g., viral enteritis) of COVID-19, assign code U07.1, COVID-19, as the principal/first-listed diagnosis and assign code(s) for the manifestation(s) as additional diagnoses.

(e) Exposure to COVID-19

For asymptomatic individuals with actual or suspected exposure to COVID-19, assign code Z20.828, Contact with and (suspected) exposure to other viral communicable diseases.

For symptomatic individuals with actual or suspected exposure to COVID-19 and the infection has been ruled out, or test results are inconclusive or unknown, assign code Z20.828, Contact with and (suspected) exposure to other viral communicable diseases. See guideline I.C.21.c.1, Contact/Exposure, for additional guidance regarding the use of category Z20 codes.

If COVID-19 is confirmed, see guideline I.C.1.g.1.a.

(f) Screening for COVID-19

During the COVID-19 pandemic, a screening code is generally not appropriate. For encounters for COVID-19 testing, including preoperative testing, code as exposure to COVID-19 (guideline I.C.1.g.1.e).

Coding guidance will be updated as new information concerning any changes in the pandemic status becomes available.

(g) Signs and symptoms without definitive diagnosis of COVID-19

For patients presenting with any signs/symptoms associated with COVID-19 (such as fever, etc.) but a definitive diagnosis has not been established, assign the appropriate code(s) for each of the presenting signs and symptoms such as:

- **R05 Cough**
- **R06.02 Shortness of breath**
- **R50.9 Fever, unspecified**

If a patient with signs/symptoms associated with COVID-19 also has an actual or suspected contact with or exposure to COVID-19, assign Z20.828, Contact with and (suspected) exposure to other viral communicable diseases, as an additional code.

(h) Asymptomatic individuals who test positive for COVID-19

For asymptomatic individuals who test positive for COVID-19, see guideline I.C.1.g.1.a. Although the individual is asymptomatic, the individual has tested positive and is considered to have the COVID-19 infection.

(i) Personal history of COVID-19

For patients with a history of COVID-19, assign code Z86.19, Personal history of other infectious and parasitic diseases.

(j) Follow-up visits after COVID-19 infection has resolved

For individuals who previously had COVID-19 and are being seen for follow-up evaluation, and COVID-19 test results are negative, assign codes Z09, Encounter for follow-up examination after completed treatment for conditions other than malignant neoplasm, and Z86.19, Personal history of other infectious and parasitic diseases.

(k) Encounter for antibody testing

For an encounter for antibody testing that is not being performed to confirm a current COVID-19 infection, nor is a follow-up test after resolution of COVID-19, assign Z01.84, Encounter for antibody response examination.

Follow the applicable guidelines above if the individual is being tested to confirm a current COVID-19 infection.

For follow-up testing after a COVID-19 infection, see guideline I.C.1.g.1.j.

Chapter 1. Certain Infectious and Parasitic Diseases (A00-B99)

INCLUDES   diseases generally recognized as communicable or transmissible

Use additional code to identify resistance to antimicrobial drugs (Z16.-)

EXCLUDES 1   certain localized infections — see body system-related chapters

EXCLUDES 2   carrier or suspected carrier of infectious disease (Z22.-)
infectious and parasitic diseases complicating pregnancy, childbirth and the puerperium (O98.-)
infectious and parasitic diseases specific to the perinatal period (P35-P39)
influenza and other acute respiratory infections (J00-J22)

This chapter contains the following blocks:

A00-A09   Intestinal infectious diseases
A15-A19   Tuberculosis
A20-A28   Certain zoonotic bacterial diseases
A30-A49   Other bacterial diseases
A50-A64   Infections with a predominantly sexual mode of transmission
A65-A69   Other spirochetal diseases
A70-A74   Other diseases caused by chlamydiae
A75-A79   Rickettsioses
A80-A89   Viral and prion infections of the central nervous system
A90-A99   Arthropod-borne viral fevers and viral hemorrhagic fevers
B00-B09   Viral infections characterized by skin and mucous membrane lesions
B10   Other human herpesviruses
B15-B19   Viral hepatitis
B20   Human immunodeficiency virus [HIV] disease
B25-B34   Other viral diseases
B35-B49   Mycoses
B50-B64   Protozoal diseases
B65-B83   Helminthiases
B85-B89   Pediculosis, acariasis and other infestations
B90-B94   Sequelae of infectious and parasitic diseases
B95-B97   Bacterial and viral infectious agents
B99   Other infectious diseases

Intestinal infectious diseases (A00-A09)

✓4ᵗʰ A00   Cholera

DEF: Acute infection of the bowel due to vibrio cholerae that presents with profuse diarrhea, cramps, and vomiting, resulting in severe dehydration, electrolyte imbalance, and death. It is spread through ingestion of food or water contaminated with feces of infected persons.

A00.0   **Cholera due to Vibrio cholerae 01, biovar cholerae**   `CC`
Classical cholera

A00.1   **Cholera due to Vibrio cholerae 01, biovar eltor**   `CC`
Cholera eltor

A00.9   **Cholera, unspecified**   `CC`

✓4ᵗʰ A01   Typhoid and paratyphoid fevers

DEF: Typhoid fever: Acute generalized illness caused by *Salmonella typhi*. Clinical features include fever, headache, abdominal pain, cough, toxemia, leukopenia, abnormal pulse, rose spots on the skin, bacteremia, hyperplasia of intestinal lymph nodes, mesenteric lymphadenopathy, and Peyer's patches in the intestines.
DEF: Paratyphoid fever: Prolonged febrile illness, caused by *Salmonella* serotypes other than *S. typhi*, especially *S. enterica* serotypes paratyphi A, B, and C.

✓5ᵗʰ A01.0   **Typhoid fever**
Infection due to Salmonella typhi

    A01.00   **Typhoid fever, unspecified**   `CC`
    A01.01   **Typhoid meningitis**   `CC`
    A01.02   **Typhoid fever with heart involvement**   `CC`
      Typhoid endocarditis
      Typhoid myocarditis
    A01.03   **Typhoid pneumonia**   `CC` `HCC`
    A01.04   **Typhoid arthritis**   `CC` `HCC`
    A01.05   **Typhoid osteomyelitis**   `CC` `HCC`
    A01.09   **Typhoid fever with other complications**   `CC`

A01.1   **Paratyphoid fever A**   `CC`
A01.2   **Paratyphoid fever B**   `CC`
A01.3   **Paratyphoid fever C**   `CC`
A01.4   **Paratyphoid fever, unspecified**   `CC`
Infection due to Salmonella paratyphi NOS

✓4ᵗʰ A02   Other salmonella infections

INCLUDES   infection or foodborne intoxication due to any Salmonella species other than S. typhi and S. paratyphi

A02.0   **Salmonella enteritis**   `CC`
Salmonellosis
TIP: Dehydration (E86.0) is a complication of salmonella enteritis and may be reported separately.

A02.1   **Salmonella sepsis**   `HIV` `MCC` `HCC`

✓5ᵗʰ A02.2   **Localized salmonella infections**

    A02.20   **Localized salmonella infection, unspecified**   `HIV`
    A02.21   **Salmonella meningitis**   `HIV` `MCC`
    A02.22   **Salmonella pneumonia**   `HIV` `MCC` `HCC`
    A02.23   **Salmonella arthritis**   `HIV` `CC` `HCC`
    A02.24   **Salmonella osteomyelitis**   `HIV` `CC` `HCC`
    A02.25   **Salmonella pyelonephritis**   `HIV` `CC`
      Salmonella tubulo-interstitial nephropathy
    A02.29   **Salmonella with other localized infection**   `HIV` `CC`

A02.8   **Other specified salmonella infections**   `HIV` `CC`
A02.9   **Salmonella infection, unspecified**   `HIV` `CC`

✓4ᵗʰ A03   Shigellosis

DEF: Infection caused by the genus *Shigella*, of the family *Enterobacteriaceae* that is known to cause an acute dysenteric infection of the bowel with fever, drowsiness, anorexia, nausea, vomiting, bloody diarrhea, abdominal cramps, and distention.

A03.0   **Shigellosis due to Shigella dysenteriae**   `CC`
Group A shigellosis [Shiga-Kruse dysentery]

A03.1   **Shigellosis due to Shigella flexneri**
Group B shigellosis

A03.2   **Shigellosis due to Shigella boydii**
Group C shigellosis

A03.3   **Shigellosis due to Shigella sonnei**
Group D shigellosis

A03.8   **Other shigellosis**
A03.9   **Shigellosis, unspecified**
Bacillary dysentery NOS

✓4ᵗʰ A04   Other bacterial intestinal infections

EXCLUDES 1   bacterial foodborne intoxications, NEC (A05.-)
tuberculous enteritis (A18.32)

DEF: Escherichia coli: Gram negative, anaerobic of the family *Enterobacteriaceae* found in the large intestine of warm-blooded animals, generally as a nonpathologic entity aiding in digestion. They become pathogenic when an opportunity to grow somewhere outside this relationship presents itself, such as ingestion of fecal contaminated food or water.

A04.0   **Enteropathogenic Escherichia coli infection**   `CC`
A04.1   **Enterotoxigenic Escherichia coli infection**   `CC`
A04.2   **Enteroinvasive Escherichia coli infection**   `CC`
A04.3   **Enterohemorrhagic Escherichia coli infection**   `CC`
DEF: *E. coli* infection penetrating the intestinal mucosa, producing microscopic ulceration and bleeding.

A04.4   **Other intestinal Escherichia coli infections**   `CC`
Escherichia coli enteritis NOS

A04.5   **Campylobacter enteritis**   `CC`
TIP: For Guillain-Barre syndrome occurring as a sequela of *Campylobacter enteritis*, assign code G61.0 as the first-listed diagnosis followed by B94.8 for the sequelae.

A04.6   **Enteritis due to Yersinia enterocolitica**   `CC`
EXCLUDES 1   extraintestinal yersiniosis (A28.2)

✓5ᵗʰ A04.7   **Enterocolitis due to Clostridium difficile**
Foodborne intoxication by Clostridium difficile
Pseudomembraneous colitis
AHA: 2017,4Q,4

    A04.71   **Enterocolitis due to Clostridium difficile, recurrent**
      AHA: 2020,1Q,18
    A04.72   **Enterocolitis due to Clostridium difficile, not specified as recurrent**   `CC`

A04.8   **Other specified bacterial intestinal infections**   `CC`
A04.9   **Bacterial intestinal infection, unspecified**   `CC`
Bacterial enteritis NOS

✔ Additional Character Required   ✓x7ᵗʰ Placeholder   Unacceptable PDx   Questionable PDx   Manifestation   Unspecified Dx   `M1`-`H14` HAC   `HCC` CMS-HCC Dx   `HIV` HIV Dx

✓4th A05 Other bacterial foodborne intoxications, not elsewhere classified

EXCLUDES 1   Clostridium difficile foodborne intoxication and infection (A04.7-)
    Escherichia coli infection (A04.0-A04.4)
    listeriosis (A32.-)
    salmonella foodborne intoxication and infection (A02.-)
    toxic effect of noxious foodstuffs (T61-T62)

A05.0 Foodborne staphylococcal intoxication   CC
TIP: Assign code A04.8 to report a staphylococcal infection when it is caused by the ingestion of contaminated food but not caused by *S. aureus* toxins.

A05.1 Botulism food poisoning   CC
Botulism NOS
Classical foodborne intoxication due to Clostridium botulinum
EXCLUDES 1   infant botulism (A48.51)
    wound botulism (A48.52)
DEF: Muscle-paralyzing neurotoxic disease caused by ingesting pre-formed toxin from the bacterium *Clostridium botulinum*. It causes vomiting and diarrhea, vision problems, slurred speech, difficulty swallowing, paralysis, and death.

A05.2 Foodborne Clostridium perfringens [Clostridium welchii] intoxication   CC
Enteritis necroticans
Pig-bel

A05.3 Foodborne Vibrio parahaemolyticus intoxication   CC
A05.4 Foodborne Bacillus cereus intoxication   CC
A05.5 Foodborne Vibrio vulnificus intoxication   CC
A05.8 Other specified bacterial foodborne intoxications   CC
A05.9 Bacterial foodborne intoxication, unspecified

✓4th A06 Amebiasis

INCLUDES   infection due to Entamoeba histolytica
EXCLUDES 1   other protozoal intestinal diseases (A07.-)
EXCLUDES 2   acanthamebiasis (B60.1-)
    Naegleriasis (B60.2)
DEF: Infection with a single cell protozoan known as the amoeba. Transmission occurs through ingestion of feces, contaminated food or water, use of human feces as fertilizer, or person-to-person contact.

A06.0 Acute amebic dysentery   CC
Acute amebiasis
Intestinal amebiasis NOS

A06.1 Chronic intestinal amebiasis   CC
A06.2 Amebic nondysenteric colitis   CC
A06.3 Ameboma of intestine   CC
Ameboma NOS
A06.4 Amebic liver abscess   MCC
Hepatic amebiasis
A06.5 Amebic lung abscess   MCC HCC
Amebic abscess of lung (and liver)
A06.6 Amebic brain abscess   MCC
Amebic abscess of brain (and liver) (and lung)
A06.7 Cutaneous amebiasis
✓5th A06.8 Amebic infection of other sites
A06.81 Amebic cystitis   CC
A06.82 Other amebic genitourinary infections   CC
Amebic balanitis
Amebic vesiculitis
Amebic vulvovaginitis
A06.89 Other amebic infections   CC
Amebic appendicitis
Amebic splenic abscess
A06.9 Amebiasis, unspecified

✓4th A07 Other protozoal intestinal diseases
DEF: Protozoa: Group comprised of the simplest, single celled organisms, ranging in size from micro to macroscopic. They can live alone or in colonies, and do not show any differentiation in tissues. Most are motile and can live free in nature, but some are parasitic, causing disease in the variety of hosts they inhabit.

A07.0 Balantidiasis
Balantidial dysentery
A07.1 Giardiasis [lambliasis]   CC
DEF: Infection caused by the flagellate protozoan *Giardia lamblia* causing gastrointestinal problems such as vomiting, chronic diarrhea, and weight loss. The most common parasite in the US, this is usually transmitted by ingesting contaminated water while in the cyst state and latches onto the wall of the small intestine.

A07.2 Cryptosporidiosis   CC HCC
DEF: Microscopic parasite found in water and one of the most common causes of waterborne gastrointestinal infectious disease in the United States. It is usually transmitted by ingesting contaminated drinking water or recreational water and causes profuse watery diarrhea, flatulence, abdominal pain, and cramping.

A07.3 Isosporiasis   HIV CC
Infection due to Isospora belli and Isospora hominis
Intestinal coccidiosis
Isosporosis

A07.4 Cyclosporiasis   CC
A07.8 Other specified protozoal intestinal diseases   CC
Intestinal microsporidiosis
Intestinal trichomoniasis
Sarcocystosis
Sarcosporidiosis

A07.9 Protozoal intestinal disease, unspecified   CC
Flagellate diarrhea
Protozoal colitis
Protozoal diarrhea
Protozoal dysentery

✓4th A08 Viral and other specified intestinal infections
EXCLUDES 1   influenza with involvement of gastrointestinal tract (J09.X3, J10.2, J11.2)

A08.0 Rotaviral enteritis   CC
✓5th A08.1 Acute gastroenteropathy due to Norwalk agent and other small round viruses
A08.11 Acute gastroenteropathy due to Norwalk agent
Acute gastroenteropathy due to Norovirus
Acute gastroenteropathy due to Norwalk-like agent
A08.19 Acute gastroenteropathy due to other small round viruses   CC
Acute gastroenteropathy due to small round virus [SRV] NOS

A08.2 Adenoviral enteritis   CC
✓5th A08.3 Other viral enteritis
A08.31 Calicivirus enteritis   CC
A08.32 Astrovirus enteritis   CC
A08.39 Other viral enteritis   CC
Coxsackie virus enteritis
Echovirus enteritis
Enterovirus enteritis NEC
Torovirus enteritis

A08.4 Viral intestinal infection, unspecified
Viral enteritis NOS
Viral gastroenteritis NOS
Viral gastroenteropathy NOS
AHA: 2016,3Q,12

A08.8 Other specified intestinal infections

A09 Infectious gastroenteritis and colitis, unspecified   CC
Infectious colitis NOS
Infectious enteritis NOS
Infectious gastroenteritis NOS
EXCLUDES 1   colitis NOS (K52.9)
    diarrhea NOS (R19.7)
    enteritis NOS (K52.9)
    gastroenteritis NOS (K52.9)
    noninfective gastroenteritis and colitis, unspecified (K52.9)
DEF: Colitis: Inflammation of mucous membranes of the colon.
DEF: Enteritis: Inflammation of mucous membranes of the small intestine.
DEF: Gastroenteritis: Inflammation of mucous membranes of the stomach and intestines.

N Newborn: 0   P Pediatric: 0-17   M Maternity: 9-64   A Adult: 15-124   MCC Major Complication/Comorbidity   CC Complication/Comorbidity   SW Severe Wound Dx

444   ICD-10-CM 2021

Tuberculosis (A15-A19)

INCLUDES	infections due to Mycobacterium tuberculosis and Mycobacterium bovis
EXCLUDES 1	congenital tuberculosis (P37.0)
	nonspecific reaction to test for tuberculosis without active tuberculosis (R76.1-)
	pneumoconiosis associated with tuberculosis, any type in A15 (J65)
	positive PPD (R76.11)
	positive tuberculin skin test without active tuberculosis (R76.11)
	sequelae of tuberculosis (B90.-)
	silicotuberculosis (J65)

DEF: Bacterial infection that typically spreads by inhalation of an airborne agent that usually attacks the lungs, but may also affect other organs.

✓4th **A15 Respiratory tuberculosis**

A15.0 Tuberculosis of lung `HIV` `CC`
  Tuberculous bronchiectasis
  Tuberculous fibrosis of lung
  Tuberculous pneumonia
  Tuberculous pneumothorax

Tuberculosis of Lung

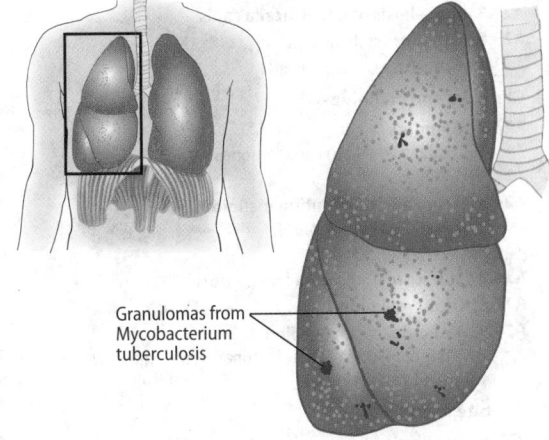

Granulomas from
Mycobacterium
tuberculosis

A15.4 Tuberculosis of intrathoracic lymph nodes `HIV` `CC`
  Tuberculosis of hilar lymph nodes
  Tuberculosis of mediastinal lymph nodes
  Tuberculosis of tracheobronchial lymph nodes
  EXCLUDES 1 *tuberculosis specified as primary (A15.7)*

A15.5 Tuberculosis of larynx, trachea and bronchus `HIV` `CC`
  Tuberculosis of bronchus
  Tuberculosis of glottis
  Tuberculosis of larynx
  Tuberculosis of trachea

A15.6 Tuberculous pleurisy `HIV` `CC`
  Tuberculosis of pleura Tuberculous empyema
  EXCLUDES 1 *primary respiratory tuberculosis (A15.7)*

A15.7 Primary respiratory tuberculosis `HIV` `CC`

A15.8 Other respiratory tuberculosis `HIV` `CC`
  Mediastinal tuberculosis
  Nasopharyngeal tuberculosis
  Tuberculosis of nose
  Tuberculosis of sinus [any nasal]

A15.9 Respiratory tuberculosis unspecified `HIV` `CC`

✓4th **A17 Tuberculosis of nervous system**

A17.0 Tuberculous meningitis `HIV` `MCC`
  Tuberculosis of meninges (cerebral)(spinal)
  Tuberculous leptomeningitis
  EXCLUDES 1 *tuberculous meningoencephalitis (A17.82)*

A17.1 Meningeal tuberculoma `HIV` `MCC`
  Tuberculoma of meninges (cerebral) (spinal)
  EXCLUDES 2 *tuberculoma of brain and spinal cord (A17.81)*

✓5th **A17.8 Other tuberculosis of nervous system**

  A17.81 Tuberculoma of brain and spinal cord `HIV` `MCC`
    Tuberculous abscess of brain and spinal cord

  A17.82 Tuberculous meningoencephalitis `HIV` `MCC`
    Tuberculous myelitis

  A17.83 Tuberculous neuritis `HIV` `MCC`
    Tuberculous mononeuropathy

  A17.89 Other tuberculosis of nervous system `HIV` `MCC`
    Tuberculous polyneuropathy

A17.9 Tuberculosis of nervous system, unspecified `HIV` `CC`

✓4th **A18 Tuberculosis of other organs**

✓5th **A18.0 Tuberculosis of bones and joints**

  A18.01 Tuberculosis of spine `HIV` `CC`
    Pott's disease or curvature of spine
    Tuberculous arthritis
    Tuberculous osteomyelitis of spine
    Tuberculous spondylitis

  A18.02 Tuberculous arthritis of other joints `HIV` `CC`
    Tuberculosis of hip (joint)
    Tuberculosis of knee (joint)

  A18.03 Tuberculosis of other bones `HIV` `CC`
    Tuberculous mastoiditis
    Tuberculous osteomyelitis

  A18.09 Other musculoskeletal tuberculosis `HIV` `CC`
    Tuberculous myositis
    Tuberculous synovitis
    Tuberculous tenosynovitis

✓5th **A18.1 Tuberculosis of genitourinary system**

  A18.10 Tuberculosis of genitourinary system, unspecified `HIV` `CC`

  A18.11 Tuberculosis of kidney and ureter `HIV` `CC`

  A18.12 Tuberculosis of bladder `HIV` `CC`

  A18.13 Tuberculosis of other urinary organs `HIV` `CC`
    Tuberculous urethritis

  A18.14 Tuberculosis of prostate `HIV` `CC` `A` ♂

  A18.15 Tuberculosis of other male genital organs `HIV` `CC` ♂

  A18.16 Tuberculosis of cervix `HIV` `CC` ♀

  A18.17 Tuberculous female pelvic inflammatory disease `HIV` `CC` ♀
    Tuberculous endometritis
    Tuberculous oophoritis and salpingitis

  A18.18 Tuberculosis of other female genital organs `HIV` `CC` ♀
    Tuberculous ulceration of vulva

A18.2 Tuberculous peripheral lymphadenopathy `HIV` `CC`
  Tuberculous adenitis
  EXCLUDES 2 *tuberculosis of bronchial and mediastinal lymph nodes (A15.4)*
    tuberculosis of mesenteric and retroperitoneal lymph nodes (A18.39)
    tuberculous tracheobronchial adenopathy (A15.4)

✓5th **A18.3 Tuberculosis of intestines, peritoneum and mesenteric glands**

  A18.31 Tuberculous peritonitis `HIV` `MCC`
    Tuberculous ascites
    DEF: Tuberculous inflammation of the membrane lining the abdomen.

  A18.32 Tuberculous enteritis `HIV` `CC`
    Tuberculosis of anus and rectum
    Tuberculosis of intestine (large) (small)

  A18.39 Retroperitoneal tuberculosis `HIV` `CC`
    Tuberculosis of mesenteric glands
    Tuberculosis of retroperitoneal (lymph glands)

A18.4 Tuberculosis of skin and subcutaneous tissue `HIV` `CC`
  Erythema induratum, tuberculous
  Lupus excedens
  Lupus vulgaris NOS
  Lupus vulgaris of eyelid
  Scrofuloderma
  Tuberculosis of external ear
  EXCLUDES 2 *lupus erythematosus (L93.-)*
    systemic lupus erythematosus (M32.-)

✓5th **A18.5 Tuberculosis of eye**
  EXCLUDES 2 *lupus vulgaris of eyelid (A18.4)*

  A18.50 Tuberculosis of eye, unspecified `HIV` `CC`

  A18.51 Tuberculous episcleritis `HIV` `CC`

A18.52 Tuberculous keratitis `HIV` `CC`
Tuberculous interstitial keratitis
Tuberculous keratoconjunctivitis (interstitial) (phlyctenular)

A18.53 Tuberculous chorioretinitis `HIV` `CC`

A18.54 Tuberculous iridocyclitis `HIV` `CC`

A18.59 Other tuberculosis of eye `HIV` `CC`
Tuberculous conjunctivitis

A18.6 Tuberculosis of (inner) (middle) ear `HIV` `CC`
Tuberculous otitis media
> `EXCLUDES 2`   tuberculosis of external ear (A18.4)
> tuberculous mastoiditis (A18.03)

A18.7 Tuberculosis of adrenal glands `HIV` `CC`
Tuberculous Addison's disease

`√5th` **A18.8 Tuberculosis of other specified organs**

A18.81 Tuberculosis of thyroid gland `HIV` `CC`

A18.82 Tuberculosis of other endocrine glands `HIV` `CC`
Tuberculosis of pituitary gland
Tuberculosis of thymus gland

A18.83 Tuberculosis of digestive tract organs, not elsewhere classified `HIV` `CC`
> `EXCLUDES 1`   tuberculosis of intestine (A18.32)

A18.84 Tuberculosis of heart `HIV` `CC`
Tuberculous cardiomyopathy
Tuberculous endocarditis
Tuberculous myocarditis
Tuberculous pericarditis

A18.85 Tuberculosis of spleen `HIV` `CC`

A18.89 Tuberculosis of other sites `HIV` `CC`
Tuberculosis of muscle
Tuberculous cerebral arteritis

`√4th` **A19 Miliary tuberculosis**
> `INCLUDES`   disseminated tuberculosis
> generalized tuberculosis
> tuberculous polyserositis

A19.0 Acute miliary tuberculosis of a single specified site `HIV` `MCC`

A19.1 Acute miliary tuberculosis of multiple sites `HIV` `MCC`

A19.2 Acute miliary tuberculosis, unspecified `HIV` `MCC`

A19.8 Other miliary tuberculosis `HIV` `MCC`

A19.9 Miliary tuberculosis, unspecified `HIV` `MCC`

Certain zoonotic bacterial diseases (A20-A28)

`√4th` **A20 Plague**
> `INCLUDES`   infection due to Yersinia pestis

A20.0 Bubonic plague `MCC`

A20.1 Cellulocutaneous plague `MCC`

A20.2 Pneumonic plague `MCC` `HCC`

A20.3 Plague meningitis `MCC`

A20.7 Septicemic plague `MCC` `HCC`

A20.8 Other forms of plague `MCC`
Abortive plague
Asymptomatic plague
Pestis minor

A20.9 Plague, unspecified `MCC`

`√4th` **A21 Tularemia**
> `INCLUDES`   deer-fly fever
> infection due to Francisella tularensis
> rabbit fever

DEF: Febrile disease transmitted to humans by the bites of deer flies, fleas, and ticks, by inhaling aerosolized *F. tularensis*, or by ingesting contaminated food or water. Patients quickly develop fever, chills, weakness, headache, backache, and malaise.

A21.0 Ulceroglandular tularemia `CC`

A21.1 Oculoglandular tularemia `CC`
Ophthalmic tularemia

A21.2 Pulmonary tularemia `CC` `HCC`

A21.3 Gastrointestinal tularemia `CC`
Abdominal tularemia

A21.7 Generalized tularemia `CC`

A21.8 Other forms of tularemia `CC`

A21.9 Tularemia, unspecified `CC`

`√4th` **A22 Anthrax**
> `INCLUDES`   infection due to Bacillus anthracis

A22.0 Cutaneous anthrax `CC`
Malignant carbuncle
Malignant pustule

A22.1 Pulmonary anthrax `MCC` `HCC`
Inhalation anthrax
Ragpicker's disease
Woolsorter's disease

A22.2 Gastrointestinal anthrax `CC`

A22.7 Anthrax sepsis `MCC` `HCC`

A22.8 Other forms of anthrax `CC`
Anthrax meningitis

A22.9 Anthrax, unspecified `CC`

`√4th` **A23 Brucellosis**
> `INCLUDES`   Malta fever
> Mediterranean fever
> undulant fever

A23.0 Brucellosis due to Brucella melitensis

A23.1 Brucellosis due to Brucella abortus

A23.2 Brucellosis due to Brucella suis

A23.3 Brucellosis due to Brucella canis

A23.8 Other brucellosis `CC`

A23.9 Brucellosis, unspecified `CC`

`√4th` **A24 Glanders and melioidosis**

A24.0 Glanders `CC`
Infection due to Pseudomonas mallei
Malleus

A24.1 Acute and fulminating melioidosis `CC`
Melioidosis pneumonia
Melioidosis sepsis

A24.2 Subacute and chronic melioidosis `CC`

A24.3 Other melioidosis `CC`

A24.9 Melioidosis, unspecified `CC`
Infection due to Pseudomonas pseudomallei NOS
Whitmore's disease

`√4th` **A25 Rat-bite fevers**

A25.0 Spirillosis `CC`
Sodoku

A25.1 Streptobacillosis `CC`
Epidemic arthritic erythema
Haverhill fever
Streptobacillary rat-bite fever

A25.9 Rat-bite fever, unspecified `CC`

`√4th` **A26 Erysipeloid**
DEF: Acute cutaneous infection typically caused by trauma to the skin. Presenting as cellulitis, it may become systemic affecting other organs. It is gram positive bacillus and mainly acquired by those who routinely handle meat.

A26.0 Cutaneous erysipeloid
Erythema migrans

A26.7 Erysipelothrix sepsis `MCC` `HCC`

A26.8 Other forms of erysipeloid

A26.9 Erysipeloid, unspecified

`√4th` **A27 Leptospirosis**

A27.0 Leptospirosis icterohemorrhagica `CC`
Leptospiral or spirochetal jaundice (hemorrhagic)
Weil's disease

`√5th` **A27.8 Other forms of leptospirosis**

A27.81 Aseptic meningitis in leptospirosis `MCC`

A27.89 Other forms of leptospirosis `CC`

A27.9 Leptospirosis, unspecified `CC`

`√4th` **A28 Other zoonotic bacterial diseases, not elsewhere classified**

A28.0 Pasteurellosis `CC`

A28.1 Cat-scratch disease `CC`
Cat-scratch fever

A28.2 Extraintestinal yersiniosis `CC`
> `EXCLUDES 1`   enteritis due to Yersinia enterocolitica (A04.6)
> plague (A20.-)

A28.8 Other specified zoonotic bacterial diseases, not elsewhere classified `CC`

A28.9 Zoonotic bacterial disease, unspecified `CC`

`N` Newborn: 0   `P` Pediatric: 0-17   `M` Maternity: 9-64   `A` Adult: 15-124   `MCC` Major Complication/Comorbidity   `CC` Complication/Comorbidity   `SW` Severe Wound Dx

446   ICD-10-CM 2021

Other bacterial diseases (A30-A49)

AHA: 2016,3Q,8-14

√4ᵗʰ **A30 Leprosy [Hansen's disease]**
- **INCLUDES**   infection due to Mycobacterium leprae
- **EXCLUDES 1**   sequelae of leprosy (B92)

    A30.0 Indeterminate leprosy   CC
       I leprosy

    A30.1 Tuberculoid leprosy   CC
       TT leprosy

    A30.2 Borderline tuberculoid leprosy   CC
       BT leprosy

    A30.3 Borderline leprosy   CC
       BB leprosy

    A30.4 Borderline lepromatous leprosy   CC
       BL leprosy

    A30.5 Lepromatous leprosy   CC
       LL leprosy

    A30.8 Other forms of leprosy   CC
    A30.9 Leprosy, unspecified   CC

√4ᵗʰ **A31 Infection due to other mycobacteria**
- **EXCLUDES 2**   leprosy (A30.-)
-            tuberculosis (A15-A19)

    A31.0 Pulmonary mycobacterial infection   CC HCC
       Infection due to Mycobacterium avium
       Infection due to Mycobacterium intracellulare [Battey bacillus]
       Infection due to Mycobacterium kansasii

    A31.1 Cutaneous mycobacterial infection   CC
       Buruli ulcer
       Infection due to Mycobacterium marinum
       Infection due to Mycobacterium ulcerans

    A31.2 Disseminated mycobacterium avium-intracellulare complex (DMAC)   HIV CC HCC
       MAC sepsis

    A31.8 Other mycobacterial infections   HIV CC
    A31.9 Mycobacterial infection, unspecified   HIV CC
       Atypical mycobacterial infection NOS
       Mycobacteriosis NOS

√4ᵗʰ **A32 Listeriosis**
- **INCLUDES**   listerial foodborne infection
- **EXCLUDES 1**   neonatal (disseminated) listeriosis (P37.2)

    A32.0 Cutaneous listeriosis   CC
√5ᵗʰ   **A32.1 Listerial meningitis and meningoencephalitis**
       A32.11 Listerial meningitis   CC
       A32.12 Listerial meningoencephalitis   CC
    A32.7 Listerial sepsis   MCC HCC
√5ᵗʰ   **A32.8 Other forms of listeriosis**
       A32.81 Oculoglandular listeriosis   CC
       A32.82 Listerial endocarditis   CC
       A32.89 Other forms of listeriosis   CC
           Listerial cerebral arteritis
    A32.9 Listeriosis, unspecified   CC

A33 Tetanus neonatorum   MCC N

A34 Obstetrical tetanus   CC M ♀

A35 Other tetanus   MCC
    Tetanus NOS
- **EXCLUDES 1**   obstetrical tetanus (A34)
-            tetanus neonatorum (A33)

DEF: Tetanus: Acute, often fatal, infectious disease caused by the anaerobic, spore-forming bacillus *Clostridium tetani*. The bacillus enters the body through a contaminated wound, burns, surgical wounds, or cutaneous ulcers. Symptoms include lockjaw, spasms, seizures, and paralysis.

√4ᵗʰ **A36 Diphtheria**

    A36.0 Pharyngeal diphtheria   CC
       Diphtheritic membranous angina
       Tonsillar diphtheria

    A36.1 Nasopharyngeal diphtheria   CC
    A36.2 Laryngeal diphtheria   CC
       Diphtheritic laryngotracheitis

    A36.3 Cutaneous diphtheria
- **EXCLUDES 2**   erythrasma (L08.1)

√5ᵗʰ   **A36.8 Other diphtheria**
       A36.81 Diphtheritic cardiomyopathy   CC HCC
           Diphtheritic myocarditis
       A36.82 Diphtheritic radiculomyelitis   CC
       A36.83 Diphtheritic polyneuritis   CC
       A36.84 Diphtheritic tubulo-interstitial nephropathy   CC
       A36.85 Diphtheritic cystitis   CC
       A36.86 Diphtheritic conjunctivitis   CC
       A36.89 Other diphtheritic complications   CC
           Diphtheritic peritonitis
    A36.9 Diphtheria, unspecified   CC

√4ᵗʰ **A37 Whooping cough**
   DEF: Acute, highly contagious respiratory tract infection caused by *Bordetella pertussis* and *B. bronchiseptica*. Whooping cough is known by its characteristic paroxysmal cough.

√5ᵗʰ   **A37.0 Whooping cough due to Bordetella pertussis**
       A37.00 Whooping cough due to Bordetella pertussis without pneumonia   CC
       A37.01 Whooping cough due to Bordetella pertussis with pneumonia   MCC
√5ᵗʰ   **A37.1 Whooping cough due to Bordetella parapertussis**
       A37.10 Whooping cough due to Bordetella parapertussis without pneumonia   CC
       A37.11 Whooping cough due to Bordetella parapertussis with pneumonia   MCC
√5ᵗʰ   **A37.8 Whooping cough due to other Bordetella species**
       A37.80 Whooping cough due to other Bordetella species without pneumonia   CC
       A37.81 Whooping cough due to other Bordetella species with pneumonia   MCC
√5ᵗʰ   **A37.9 Whooping cough, unspecified species**
       A37.90 Whooping cough, unspecified species without pneumonia   CC
       A37.91 Whooping cough, unspecified species with pneumonia   MCC

√4ᵗʰ **A38 Scarlet fever**
- **INCLUDES**   scarlatina
- **EXCLUDES 2**   streptococcal sore throat (J02.0)

DEF: Acute contagious disease caused by Group A bacteria, the same bacterium that causes strep throat. Individuals with strep throat can develop scarlet fever particularly if the infection is not treated with antibiotics. It is characterized by a red blush to the skin of the chest and abdomen and swelling of the nose, throat, and mouth.

    A38.0 Scarlet fever with otitis media   CC
    A38.1 Scarlet fever with myocarditis   CC
    A38.8 Scarlet fever with other complications   CC
    A38.9 Scarlet fever, uncomplicated   CC
       Scarlet fever, NOS

√4ᵗʰ **A39 Meningococcal infection**
   DEF: Condition caused by *Neisseria meningitidis*, a bacteria that may invade the spinal cord, brain, heart, joints, optic nerve, or bloodstream.

    A39.0 Meningococcal meningitis   MCC
    A39.1 Waterhouse-Friderichsen syndrome   MCC HCC
       Meningococcal hemorrhagic adrenalitis
       Meningococcic adrenal syndrome
    A39.2 Acute meningococcemia   MCC HCC
    A39.3 Chronic meningococcemia   MCC HCC
    A39.4 Meningococcemia, unspecified   MCC HCC
√5ᵗʰ   **A39.5 Meningococcal heart disease**
       A39.50 Meningococcal carditis, unspecified   MCC
       A39.51 Meningococcal endocarditis   MCC
       A39.52 Meningococcal myocarditis   MCC
       A39.53 Meningococcal pericarditis   MCC
√5ᵗʰ   **A39.8 Other meningococcal infections**
       A39.81 Meningococcal encephalitis   MCC
       A39.82 Meningococcal retrobulbar neuritis   CC
       A39.83 Meningococcal arthritis   CC HCC
       A39.84 Postmeningococcal arthritis   CC HCC
       A39.89 Other meningococcal infections   CC
           Meningococcal conjunctivitis

✔ Additional Character Required   √x7ᵗʰ Placeholder   Unacceptable PDx   Questionable PDx   Manifestation   Unspecified Dx   H1-H14 HAC   HCC CMS-HCC Dx   HIV HIV Dx

ICD-10-CM 2021   447

A39.9   **Meningococcal infection, unspecified**   `CC`
    Meningococcal disease NOS

√4ᵗʰ **A40**   **Streptococcal sepsis**
    Code first:
     postprocedural streptococcal sepsis (T81.4-)
     streptococcal sepsis during labor (O75.3)
     streptococcal sepsis following abortion or ectopic or molar pregnancy
     (O03-O07, O08.0)
     streptococcal sepsis following immunization (T88.0)
     streptococcal sepsis following infusion, transfusion or therapeutic
     injection (T80.2-)
    EXCLUDES 1   neonatal (P36.0-P36.1)
          puerperal sepsis (O85)
          sepsis due to Streptococcus, group D (A41.81)
    AHA: 2020,2Q,8,28; 2019,4Q,65; 2018,4Q,89; 2018,1Q,16; 2016,1Q,32

   A40.0   **Sepsis due to streptococcus, group A**   `MCC` `HCC`
   A40.1   **Sepsis due to streptococcus, group B**   `MCC` `HCC`
       AHA: 2019,1Q,14
   A40.3   **Sepsis due to Streptococcus pneumoniae**   `MCC` `HCC`
       Pneumococcal sepsis
   A40.8   **Other streptococcal sepsis**   `MCC` `HCC`
   A40.9   **Streptococcal sepsis, unspecified**   `HIV` `MCC` `HCC`

√4ᵗʰ **A41**   **Other sepsis**
    Code first:
     postprocedural sepsis (T81.4-)
     sepsis during labor (O75.3)
     sepsis following abortion, ectopic or molar pregnancy (O03-O07,
     O08.0)
     sepsis following immunization (T88.0)
     sepsis following infusion, transfusion or therapeutic injection (T80.2-)
    EXCLUDES 1   bacteremia NOS (R78.81)
          neonatal (P36.-)
          puerperal sepsis (O85)
          streptococcal sepsis (A40.-)
    EXCLUDES 2   sepsis (due to) (in) actinomycotic (A42.7)
          sepsis (due to) (in) anthrax (A22.7)
          sepsis (due to) (in) candidal (B37.7)
          sepsis (due to) (in) Erysipelothrix (A26.7)
          sepsis (due to) (in) extraintestinal yersiniosis (A28.2)
          sepsis (due to) (in) gonococcal (A54.86)
          sepsis (due to) (in) herpesviral (B00.7)
          sepsis (due to) (in) listerial (A32.7)
          sepsis (due to) (in) melioidosis (A24.1)
          sepsis (due to) (in) meningococcal (A39.2-A39.4)
          sepsis (due to) (in) plague (A20.7)
          sepsis (due to) (in) tularemia (A21.7)
          toxic shock syndrome (A48.3)
    AHA: 2020,2Q,8,28; 2019,4Q,65; 2019,3Q,17; 2018,4Q,18; 2018,1Q,16;
    2016,1Q,32; 2014,2Q,13

√5ᵗʰ   **A41.0**   **Sepsis due to Staphylococcus aureus**
     A41.01   **Sepsis due to Methicillin susceptible Staphylococcus
           aureus**   `HIV` `MCC` `HCC`
           MSSA sepsis
           Staphylococcus aureus sepsis NOS
           AHA: 2020,2Q,17
     A41.02   **Sepsis due to Methicillin resistant Staphylococcus
           aureus**   `HIV` `MCC` `HCC`
   A41.1   **Sepsis due to other specified staphylococcus**   `HIV` `MCC` `HCC`
       Coagulase negative staphylococcus sepsis
   A41.2   **Sepsis due to unspecified staphylococcus**   `HIV` `MCC` `HCC`
   A41.3   **Sepsis due to Hemophilus influenzae**   `HIV` `MCC` `HCC`
   A41.4   **Sepsis due to anaerobes**   `HIV` `MCC` `HCC`
       EXCLUDES 1   gas gangrene (A48.0)
√5ᵗʰ   **A41.5**   **Sepsis due to other Gram-negative organisms**
     A41.50   **Gram-negative sepsis, unspecified**   `HIV` `MCC` `HCC`
           Gram-negative sepsis NOS
           AHA: 2020,2Q,28
     A41.51   **Sepsis due to Escherichia coli [E. coli]**   `HIV` `MCC` `HCC`
           AHA: 2020,2Q,17
     A41.52   **Sepsis due to Pseudomonas**   `HIV` `MCC` `HCC`
           Pseudomonas aeroginosa
     A41.53   **Sepsis due to Serratia**   `HIV` `MCC` `HCC`
     A41.59   **Other Gram-negative sepsis**   `HIV` `MCC` `HCC`

√5ᵗʰ **A41.8**   **Other specified sepsis**
   A41.81   **Sepsis due to Enterococcus**   `HIV` `MCC` `HCC`
       TIP: *E. faecium,* is a species of *Enterococcus* that is
       highly resistant to multiple antibiotics. Assign a code
       from category Z16 when resistance to antimicrobial
       drugs is documented.
   A41.89   **Other specified sepsis**   `HIV` `MCC` `HCC`
       AHA: 2020,2Q,8; 2017,1Q,51; 2016,3Q,8-14
       TIP: Viral sepsis is coded here; assign an additional code
       to identify the specific viral agent or illness.
   A41.9   **Sepsis, unspecified organism**   `HIV` `MCC` `HCC`
       Septicemia NOS
       AHA: 2020,2Q,28

√4ᵗʰ **A42**   **Actinomycosis**
    EXCLUDES 1   actinomycetoma (B47.1)
   A42.0   **Pulmonary actinomycosis**   `HIV` `CC` `HCC`
   A42.1   **Abdominal actinomycosis**   `HIV` `CC`
   A42.2   **Cervicofacial actinomycosis**   `HIV` `CC`
   A42.7   **Actinomycotic sepsis**   `HIV` `MCC` `HCC`
√5ᵗʰ   **A42.8**   **Other forms of actinomycosis**
     A42.81   **Actinomycotic meningitis**   `HIV` `CC`
     A42.82   **Actinomycotic encephalitis**   `HIV` `CC`
     A42.89   **Other forms of actinomycosis**   `HIV` `CC`
   A42.9   **Actinomycosis, unspecified**   `HIV` `CC`

√4ᵗʰ **A43**   **Nocardiosis**
    DEF: Rare bacterial infection occurring most often in those with weakened
    immune systems. Can be acquired in soil, decaying plants, or standing
    water. It typically begins in the lungs and has a tendency to spread to
    other body systems.
   A43.0   **Pulmonary nocardiosis**   `HIV` `CC` `HCC`
   A43.1   **Cutaneous nocardiosis**   `HIV` `CC`
   A43.8   **Other forms of nocardiosis**   `HIV` `CC`
   A43.9   **Nocardiosis, unspecified**   `HIV` `CC`

√4ᵗʰ **A44**   **Bartonellosis**
   A44.0   **Systemic bartonellosis**   `CC`
       Oroya fever
   A44.1   **Cutaneous and mucocutaneous bartonellosis**   `CC`
       Verruga peruana
   A44.8   **Other forms of bartonellosis**   `CC`
   A44.9   **Bartonellosis, unspecified**   `CC`

A46   **Erysipelas**
    EXCLUDES 1   postpartum or puerperal erysipelas (O86.89)
    DEF: Skin infection affecting the upper dermis and superficial dermal
    lymphatics. Lesion edges are well-demarcated with distinct raised borders.
    It is often caused by group A *Streptococci.*

√4ᵗʰ **A48**   **Other bacterial diseases, not elsewhere classified**
    EXCLUDES 1   actinomycetoma (B47.1)
   A48.0   **Gas gangrene**   `MCC` `HCC`
       Clostridial cellulitis
       Clostridial myonecrosis
       AHA: 2017,4Q,102
   A48.1   **Legionnaires' disease**   `HIV` `MCC` `HCC`
       DEF: Severe and often fatal infection by *Legionella pneumophila.*
       Symptoms include high fever, gastrointestinal pain, headache,
       myalgia, dry cough, and pneumonia and it is usually transmitted
       through airborne water droplets via air conditioning systems or
       hot tubs.
   A48.2   **Nonpneumonic Legionnaires' disease [Pontiac fever]**
   A48.3   **Toxic shock syndrome**   `MCC` `HCC`
       Use additional code to identify the organism (B95, B96)
       EXCLUDES 1   endotoxic shock NOS (R57.8)
              sepsis NOS (A41.9)
       DEF: Bacteria producing an endotoxin, such as *Staphylococci,*
       flood the body with the toxins producing a high fever, vomiting
       and diarrhea, decreasing blood pressure, a skin rash, and shock.
       Synonym(s): TSS.
   A48.4   **Brazilian purpuric fever**
       Systemic Hemophilus aegyptius infection
√5ᵗʰ   **A48.5**   **Other specified botulism**
       Non-foodborne intoxication due to toxins of Clostridium
       botulinum [C. botulinum]
       EXCLUDES 1   food poisoning due to toxins of Clostridium
              botulinum (A05.1)
     A48.51   **Infant botulism**   `CC` `P`

N Newborn: 0   P Pediatric: 0-17   M Maternity: 9-64   A Adult: 15-124   `MCC` Major Complication/Comorbidity   `CC` Complication/Comorbidity   `SW` Severe Wound Dx

448   ICD-10-CM 2021

A48.52 **Wound botulism**   `CC`
     Non-foodborne botulism NOS
     Use additional code for associated wound

A48.8 **Other specified bacterial diseases**

✓4ᵗʰ A49 **Bacterial infection of unspecified site**
     EXCLUDES 1   *bacterial agents as the cause of diseases classified elsewhere (B95-B96)*
         chlamydial infection NOS (A74.9)
         meningococcal infection NOS (A39.9)
         rickettsial infection NOS (A79.9)
         spirochetal infection NOS (A69.9)

✓5ᵗʰ A49.0 **Staphylococcal infection, unspecified site**

     A49.01 **Methicillin susceptible Staphylococcus aureus infection, unspecified site**
         Methicillin susceptible Staphylococcus aureus (MSSA) infection
         Staphylococcus aureus infection NOS

     A49.02 **Methicillin resistant Staphylococcus aureus infection, unspecified site**
         Methicillin resistant Staphylococcus aureus (MRSA) infection

A49.1 **Streptococcal infection, unspecified site**

A49.2 **Hemophilus influenzae infection, unspecified site**

A49.3 **Mycoplasma infection, unspecified site**

A49.8 **Other bacterial infections of unspecified site**

A49.9 **Bacterial infection, unspecified**
     EXCLUDES 1   *bacteremia NOS (R78.81)*

Infections with a predominantly sexual mode of transmission (A50-A64)

EXCLUDES 1   *human immunodeficiency virus [HIV] disease (B20)*
         nonspecific and nongonococcal urethritis (N34.1)
         Reiter's disease (M02.3-)

✓4ᵗʰ A50 **Congenital syphilis**

✓5ᵗʰ A50.0 **Early congenital syphilis, symptomatic**
     Any congenital syphilitic condition specified as early or manifest less than two years after birth.

     A50.01 **Early congenital syphilitic oculopathy**   `CC`

     A50.02 **Early congenital syphilitic osteochondropathy**   `CC`

     A50.03 **Early congenital syphilitic pharyngitis**   `CC`
         Early congenital syphilitic laryngitis

     A50.04 **Early congenital syphilitic pneumonia**   `CC`

     A50.05 **Early congenital syphilitic rhinitis**   `CC`

     A50.06 **Early cutaneous congenital syphilis**   `CC`

     A50.07 **Early mucocutaneous congenital syphilis**   `CC`

     A50.08 **Early visceral congenital syphilis**   `CC`

     A50.09 **Other early congenital syphilis, symptomatic**   `CC`

A50.1 **Early congenital syphilis, latent**
     Congenital syphilis without clinical manifestations, with positive serological reaction and negative spinal fluid test, less than two years after birth.

A50.2 **Early congenital syphilis, unspecified**   `CC`
     Congenital syphilis NOS less than two years after birth.

✓5ᵗʰ A50.3 **Late congenital syphilitic oculopathy**
     EXCLUDES 1   *Hutchinson's triad (A50.53)*

     A50.30 **Late congenital syphilitic oculopathy, unspecified**   `CC`

     A50.31 **Late congenital syphilitic interstitial keratitis**   `CC`

     A50.32 **Late congenital syphilitic chorioretinitis**   `CC`

     A50.39 **Other late congenital syphilitic oculopathy**   `CC`

✓5ᵗʰ A50.4 **Late congenital neurosyphilis [juvenile neurosyphilis]**
     Use additional code to identify any associated mental disorder
     EXCLUDES 1   *Hutchinson's triad (A50.53)*

     A50.40 **Late congenital neurosyphilis, unspecified**   `CC`
         Juvenile neurosyphilis NOS

     A50.41 **Late congenital syphilitic meningitis**   `MCC`

     A50.42 **Late congenital syphilitic encephalitis**   `MCC`

     A50.43 **Late congenital syphilitic polyneuropathy**   `CC`

     A50.44 **Late congenital syphilitic optic nerve atrophy**   `CC`

     A50.45 **Juvenile general paresis**   `CC`
         Dementia paralytica juvenilis
         Juvenile tabetoparetic neurosyphilis

     A50.49 **Other late congenital neurosyphilis**   `CC`
         Juvenile tabes dorsalis

✓5ᵗʰ A50.5 **Other late congenital syphilis, symptomatic**
     Any congenital syphilitic condition specified as late or manifest two years or more after birth.

     A50.51 **Clutton's joints**   `CC`

     A50.52 **Hutchinson's teeth**   `CC`

     A50.53 **Hutchinson's triad**   `CC`

     A50.54 **Late congenital cardiovascular syphilis**   `CC`

     A50.55 **Late congenital syphilitic arthropathy**   `CC` `HCC`

     A50.56 **Late congenital syphilitic osteochondropathy**   `CC`

     A50.57 **Syphilitic saddle nose**   `CC`

     A50.59 **Other late congenital syphilis, symptomatic**   `CC`

A50.6 **Late congenital syphilis, latent**
     Congenital syphilis without clinical manifestations, with positive serological reaction and negative spinal fluid test, two years or more after birth.

A50.7 **Late congenital syphilis, unspecified**
     Congenital syphilis NOS two years or more after birth.

A50.9 **Congenital syphilis, unspecified**

✓4ᵗʰ A51 **Early syphilis**
     DEF: Syphilis: Sexually transmitted disease caused by the treponema pallidum spirochete. Syphilis usually exhibits cutaneous manifestations and may exist for years without symptoms.

A51.0 **Primary genital syphilis**
     Syphilitic chancre NOS

A51.1 **Primary anal syphilis**

A51.2 **Primary syphilis of other sites**

✓5ᵗʰ A51.3 **Secondary syphilis of skin and mucous membranes**
     DEF: Transitory or chronic cutaneous eruptions that present within two to 10 weeks following an initial syphilis infection that may include nontender lymphadenopathy along with alopecia and condylomata lata.

     A51.31 **Condyloma latum**   `CC`

     A51.32 **Syphilitic alopecia**   `CC`

     A51.39 **Other secondary syphilis of skin**   `CC`
         Syphilitic leukoderma
         Syphilitic mucous patch
         EXCLUDES 1   *late syphilitic leukoderma (A52.79)*

✓5ᵗʰ A51.4 **Other secondary syphilis**

     A51.41 **Secondary syphilitic meningitis**   `MCC`

     A51.42 **Secondary syphilitic female pelvic disease**   `CC` ♀

     A51.43 **Secondary syphilitic oculopathy**   `CC`
         Secondary syphilitic chorioretinitis
         Secondary syphilitic iridocyclitis, iritis
         Secondary syphilitic uveitis

     A51.44 **Secondary syphilitic nephritis**   `CC`

     A51.45 **Secondary syphilitic hepatitis**   `CC`

     A51.46 **Secondary syphilitic osteopathy**   `CC`

     A51.49 **Other secondary syphilitic conditions**   `CC`
         Secondary syphilitic lymphadenopathy
         Secondary syphilitic myositis

A51.5 **Early syphilis, latent**
     Syphilis (acquired) without clinical manifestations, with positive serological reaction and negative spinal fluid test, less than two years after infection.

A51.9 **Early syphilis, unspecified**

✓4ᵗʰ A52 **Late syphilis**

✓5ᵗʰ A52.0 **Cardiovascular and cerebrovascular syphilis**

     A52.00 **Cardiovascular syphilis, unspecified**   `CC`

     A52.01 **Syphilitic aneurysm of aorta**   `CC`

     A52.02 **Syphilitic aortitis**   `CC`

     A52.03 **Syphilitic endocarditis**   `CC`
         Syphilitic aortic valve incompetence or stenosis
         Syphilitic mitral valve stenosis
         Syphilitic pulmonary valve regurgitation

     A52.04 **Syphilitic cerebral arteritis**   `CC`

     A52.05 **Other cerebrovascular syphilis**   `CC`
         Syphilitic cerebral aneurysm (ruptured) (non-ruptured)
         Syphilitic cerebral thrombosis

A52.06 Other syphilitic heart involvement `CC`
Syphilitic coronary artery disease
Syphilitic myocarditis
Syphilitic pericarditis

A52.09 Other cardiovascular syphilis `CC`

✓5ᵗʰ **A52.1 Symptomatic neurosyphilis**

A52.10 Symptomatic neurosyphilis, unspecified `CC`

A52.11 Tabes dorsalis `CC`
Locomotor ataxia (progressive)
Tabetic neurosyphilis

A52.12 Other cerebrospinal syphilis `CC`

A52.13 Late syphilitic meningitis `MCC`

A52.14 Late syphilitic encephalitis `MCC`

A52.15 Late syphilitic neuropathy `CC`
Late syphilitic acoustic neuritis
Late syphilitic optic (nerve) atrophy
Late syphilitic polyneuropathy
Late syphilitic retrobulbar neuritis

A52.16 Charcôt's arthropathy (tabetic) `CC`
DEF: Progressive neurologic arthropathy in which chronic degeneration of joints in the weight-bearing areas with peripheral hypertrophy occurs as a complication of a neuropathy disorder. Supporting structures relax from a loss of sensation resulting in chronic joint instability.

A52.17 General paresis `CC`
Dementia paralytica

A52.19 Other symptomatic neurosyphilis `CC`
Syphilitic parkinsonism

A52.2 Asymptomatic neurosyphilis `CC`

A52.3 Neurosyphilis, unspecified `CC`
Gumma (syphilitic)
Syphilis (late)
Syphiloma

✓5ᵗʰ **A52.7 Other symptomatic late syphilis**

A52.71 Late syphilitic oculopathy `CC`
Late syphilitic chorioretinitis
Late syphilitic episcleritis

A52.72 Syphilis of lung and bronchus `CC`

A52.73 Symptomatic late syphilis of other respiratory organs `CC`

A52.74 Syphilis of liver and other viscera `CC`
Late syphilitic peritonitis

A52.75 Syphilis of kidney and ureter `CC`
Syphilitic glomerular disease

A52.76 Other genitourinary symptomatic late syphilis `CC`
Late syphilitic female pelvic inflammatory disease

A52.77 Syphilis of bone and joint `CC`

A52.78 Syphilis of other musculoskeletal tissue `CC`
Late syphilitic bursitis
Syphilis [stage unspecified] of bursa
Syphilis [stage unspecified] of muscle
Syphilis [stage unspecified] of synovium
Syphilis [stage unspecified] of tendon

A52.79 Other symptomatic late syphilis `CC`
Late syphilitic leukoderma
Syphilis of adrenal gland
Syphilis of pituitary gland
Syphilis of thyroid gland
Syphilitic splenomegaly
EXCLUDES 1 syphilitic leukoderma (secondary) (A51.39)

A52.8 Late syphilis, latent
Syphilis (acquired) without clinical manifestations, with positive serological reaction and negative spinal fluid test, two years or more after infection

A52.9 Late syphilis, unspecified

✓4ᵗʰ **A53 Other and unspecified syphilis**

A53.0 Latent syphilis, unspecified as early or late
Latent syphilis NOS
Positive serological reaction for syphilis

A53.9 Syphilis, unspecified
Infection due to Treponema pallidum NOS
Syphilis (acquired) NOS
EXCLUDES 1 syphilis NOS under two years of age (A50.2)

✓4ᵗʰ **A54 Gonococcal infection**
DEF: Sexually transmitted bacterial infection caused by *Neisseria gonorrhoeae*. Women are often asymptomatic, while men tend to develop urinary symptoms quickly.

✓5ᵗʰ **A54.0 Gonococcal infection of lower genitourinary tract without periurethral or accessory gland abscess**
EXCLUDES 1 gonococcal infection with genitourinary gland abscess (A54.1)
gonococcal infection with periurethral abscess (A54.1)

A54.00 Gonococcal infection of lower genitourinary tract, unspecified `CC`

A54.01 Gonococcal cystitis and urethritis, unspecified `CC`

A54.02 Gonococcal vulvovaginitis, unspecified `CC` ♀

A54.03 Gonococcal cervicitis, unspecified `CC` ♀

A54.09 Other gonococcal infection of lower genitourinary tract `CC`

A54.1 Gonococcal infection of lower genitourinary tract with periurethral and accessory gland abscess `CC`
Gonococcal Bartholin's gland abscess

✓5ᵗʰ **A54.2 Gonococcal pelviperitonitis and other gonococcal genitourinary infection**

A54.21 Gonococcal infection of kidney and ureter `CC`

A54.22 Gonococcal prostatitis `CC` ♂

A54.23 Gonococcal infection of other male genital organs `CC` ♂
Gonococcal epididymitis
Gonococcal orchitis

A54.24 Gonococcal female pelvic inflammatory disease `CC` ♀
Gonococcal pelviperitonitis
EXCLUDES 1 gonococcal peritonitis (A54.85)

A54.29 Other gonococcal genitourinary infections `CC`

✓5ᵗʰ **A54.3 Gonococcal infection of eye**

A54.30 Gonococcal infection of eye, unspecified `CC`

A54.31 Gonococcal conjunctivitis `CC`
Ophthalmia neonatorum due to gonococcus

A54.32 Gonococcal iridocyclitis `CC`

A54.33 Gonococcal keratitis `CC`

A54.39 Other gonococcal eye infection `CC`
Gonococcal endophthalmia

✓5ᵗʰ **A54.4 Gonococcal infection of musculoskeletal system**

A54.40 Gonococcal infection of musculoskeletal system, unspecified `CC` `HCC`

A54.41 Gonococcal spondylopathy `CC` `HCC`

A54.42 Gonococcal arthritis `CC` `HCC`
EXCLUDES 2 gonococcal infection of spine (A54.41)

A54.43 Gonococcal osteomyelitis `CC` `HCC`
EXCLUDES 2 gonococcal infection of spine (A54.41)

A54.49 Gonococcal infection of other musculoskeletal tissue `CC` `HCC`
Gonococcal bursitis
Gonococcal myositis
Gonococcal synovitis
Gonococcal tenosynovitis

A54.5 Gonococcal pharyngitis

A54.6 Gonococcal infection of anus and rectum

✓5ᵗʰ **A54.8 Other gonococcal infections**

A54.81 Gonococcal meningitis `MCC`

A54.82 Gonococcal brain abscess `CC`

A54.83 Gonococcal heart infection `CC`
Gonococcal endocarditis
Gonococcal myocarditis
Gonococcal pericarditis

A54.84 Gonococcal pneumonia `CC` `HCC`

A54.85 Gonococcal peritonitis `CC` `HCC`
EXCLUDES 1 gonococcal pelviperitonitis (A54.24)

A54.86 Gonococcal sepsis `MCC` `HCC`

A54.89 Other gonococcal infections `CC`
Gonococcal keratoderma
Gonococcal lymphadenitis

A54.9 Gonococcal infection, unspecified `CC`

A55   Chlamydial lymphogranuloma (venereum)
     Climatic or tropical bubo
     Durand-Nicolas-Favre disease
     Esthiomene
     Lymphogranuloma inguinale

✓4ᵗʰ **A56   Other sexually transmitted chlamydial diseases**
     INCLUDES   sexually transmitted diseases due to Chlamydia trachomatis
     EXCLUDES 1   neonatal chlamydial conjunctivitis (P39.1)
         neonatal chlamydial pneumonia (P23.1)
     EXCLUDES 2   chlamydial lymphogranuloma (A55)
         conditions classified to A74.-
     DEF: Chlamydia trachomatis: Bacterium that causes a common venereal disease. Symptoms of chlamydia are usually mild or absent, however, serious complications may cause irreversible damage, including cystitis, pelvic inflammatory disease, and infertility in women and discharge from the penis, prostatitis, and infertility in men. Genital chlamydial infection can cause arthritis, skin lesions, and inflammation of the eye and urethra.
     Synonym(s): Reiter's syndrome.

   ✓5ᵗʰ **A56.0   Chlamydial infection of lower genitourinary tract**
       A56.00   Chlamydial infection of lower genitourinary tract, unspecified
       A56.01   Chlamydial cystitis and urethritis
       A56.02   Chlamydial vulvovaginitis   ♀
       A56.09   Other chlamydial infection of lower genitourinary tract
           Chlamydial cervicitis

   ✓5ᵗʰ **A56.1   Chlamydial infection of pelviperitoneum and other genitourinary organs**
       A56.11   Chlamydial female pelvic inflammatory disease   ♀
       A56.19   Other chlamydial genitourinary infection
           Chlamydial epididymitis
           Chlamydial orchitis

   A56.2   Chlamydial infection of genitourinary tract, unspecified
   A56.3   Chlamydial infection of anus and rectum
   A56.4   Chlamydial infection of pharynx
   A56.8   Sexually transmitted chlamydial infection of other sites

A57   Chancroid
     Ulcus molle
     DEF: Localized infection by *Haemophilus ducreyi,* causing genital ulcers and infecting the inguinal lymph nodes.

A58   Granuloma inguinale
     Donovanosis

✓4ᵗʰ **A59   Trichomoniasis**
     EXCLUDES 2   intestinal trichomoniasis (A07.8)
     DEF: Infection with the parasitic, flagellated protozoa of the genus *Trichomonas.* This protozoon is found in the intestinal and genitourinary tracts of humans and in the mouth around tartar, cavities, and areas of periodontal disease.

   ✓5ᵗʰ **A59.0   Urogenital trichomoniasis**
       A59.00   Urogenital trichomoniasis, unspecified
           Fluor (vaginalis) due to Trichomonas
           Leukorrhea (vaginalis) due to Trichomonas
       A59.01   Trichomonal vulvovaginitis   ♀
       A59.02   Trichomonal prostatitis   ♂
       A59.03   Trichomonal cystitis and urethritis
       A59.09   Other urogenital trichomoniasis
           Trichomonas cervicitis
   A59.8   Trichomoniasis of other sites
   A59.9   Trichomoniasis, unspecified

✓4ᵗʰ **A60   Anogenital herpesviral [herpes simplex] infections**
   ✓5ᵗʰ **A60.0   Herpesviral infection of genitalia and urogenital tract**
       A60.00   Herpesviral infection of urogenital system, unspecified   HIV
       A60.01   Herpesviral infection of penis   HIV ♂
       A60.02   Herpesviral infection of other male genital organs   ♂
       A60.03   Herpesviral cervicitis   ♀
       A60.04   Herpesviral vulvovaginitis   HIV ♀
           Herpesviral [herpes simplex] ulceration
           Herpesviral [herpes simplex] vaginitis
           Herpesviral [herpes simplex] vulvitis

       A60.09   Herpesviral infection of other urogenital tract   HIV
           AHA: 2020,1Q,20
   A60.1   Herpesviral infection of perianal skin and rectum   HIV
   A60.9   Anogenital herpesviral infection, unspecified   HIV

✓4ᵗʰ **A63   Other predominantly sexually transmitted diseases, not elsewhere classified**
     EXCLUDES 2   molluscum contagiosum (B08.1)
         papilloma of cervix (D26.0)
   A63.0   Anogenital (venereal) warts
       Anogenital warts due to (human) papillomavirus [HPV]
       Condyloma acuminatum
   A63.8   Other specified predominantly sexually transmitted diseases

A64   Unspecified sexually transmitted disease

Other spirochetal diseases (A65-A69)

     EXCLUDES 2   leptospirosis (A27.-)
         syphilis (A50-A53)

A65   Nonvenereal syphilis
     Bejel
     Endemic syphilis
     Njovera

✓4ᵗʰ **A66   Yaws**
     INCLUDES   bouba
         frambesia (tropica)
         pian
   A66.0   Initial lesions of yaws
       Chancre of yaws
       Frambesia, initial or primary
       Initial frambesial ulcer
       Mother yaw
   A66.1   Multiple papillomata and wet crab yaws
       Frambesioma
       Pianoma
       Plantar or palmar papilloma of yaws
   A66.2   Other early skin lesions of yaws
       Cutaneous yaws, less than five years after infection
       Early yaws (cutaneous) (macular) (maculopapular) (micropapular) (papular)
       Frambeside of early yaws
   A66.3   Hyperkeratosis of yaws
       Ghoul hand
       Hyperkeratosis, palmar or plantar (early) (late) due to yaws
       Worm-eaten soles
   A66.4   Gummata and ulcers of yaws
       Gummatous frambeside
       Nodular late yaws (ulcerated)
   A66.5   Gangosa
       Rhinopharyngitis mutilans
   A66.6   Bone and joint lesions of yaws   HCC
       Yaws ganglion
       Yaws goundou
       Yaws gumma, bone
       Yaws gummatous osteitis or periostitis
       Yaws hydrarthrosis
       Yaws osteitis
       Yaws periostitis (hypertrophic)
   A66.7   Other manifestations of yaws
       Juxta-articular nodules of yaws
       Mucosal yaws
   A66.8   Latent yaws
       Yaws without clinical manifestations, with positive serology
   A66.9   Yaws, unspecified

✓4ᵗʰ **A67   Pinta [carate]**
   A67.0   Primary lesions of pinta
       Chancre (primary) of pinta
       Papule (primary) of pinta
   A67.1   Intermediate lesions of pinta
       Erythematous plaques of pinta
       Hyperchromic lesions of pinta
       Hyperkeratosis of pinta
       Pintids

✓ Additional Character Required   ✓x7ᵗʰ Placeholder   Unacceptable PDx   Questionable PDx   Manifestation   Unspecified Dx   H1-H14 HAC   HCC CMS-HCC Dx   HIV HIV Dx

ICD-10-CM 2021   451

Chapter 1. Certain Infectious and Parasitic Diseases

A67.2   **Late lesions of pinta**
Achromic skin lesions of pinta
Cicatricial skin lesions of pinta
Dyschromic skin lesions of pinta

A67.3   **Mixed lesions of pinta**
Achromic with hyperchromic skin lesions of pinta [carate]

A67.9   **Pinta, unspecified**

✓4ᵗʰ **A68 Relapsing fevers**

INCLUDES   recurrent fever
EXCLUDES 2   Lyme disease (A69.2-)

A68.0   **Louse-borne relapsing fever**   CC
Relapsing fever due to Borrelia recurrentis

A68.1   **Tick-borne relapsing fever**   CC
Relapsing fever due to any Borrelia species other than Borrelia recurrentis

A68.9   **Relapsing fever, unspecified**   CC

✓4ᵗʰ **A69 Other spirochetal infections**

A69.0   **Necrotizing ulcerative stomatitis**
Cancrum oris
Fusospirochetal gangrene
Noma
Stomatitis gangrenosa

A69.1   **Other Vincent's infections**   CC
Fusospirochetal pharyngitis
Necrotizing ulcerative (acute) gingivitis
Necrotizing ulcerative (acute) gingivostomatitis
Spirochetal stomatitis
Trench mouth
Vincent's angina
Vincent's gingivitis

✓5ᵗʰ **A69.2**   **Lyme disease**
Erythema chronicum migrans due to Borrelia burgdorferi
DEF: Recurrent multisystem disorder through tick bites that begins with lesions of erythema chronicum migrans and is followed by arthritis of the large joints, myalgia, malaise, and neurological and cardiac manifestations.

    A69.20   **Lyme disease, unspecified**   CC
    A69.21   **Meningitis due to Lyme disease**   CC
    A69.22   **Other neurologic disorders in Lyme disease**   CC
      Cranial neuritis
      Meningoencephalitis
      Polyneuropathy
    A69.23   **Arthritis due to Lyme disease**   CC HCC
    A69.29   **Other conditions associated with Lyme disease**   CC
      Myopericarditis due to Lyme disease
      AHA: 2016,3Q,12

A69.8   **Other specified spirochetal infections**
A69.9   **Spirochetal infection, unspecified**

Other diseases caused by chlamydiae (A70-A74)

EXCLUDES 1   sexually transmitted chlamydial diseases (A55-A56)

A70 Chlamydia psittaci infections   CC
Ornithosis
Parrot fever
Psittacosis

✓4ᵗʰ **A71 Trachoma**

EXCLUDES 1   sequelae of trachoma (B94.0)

A71.0   **Initial stage of trachoma**
Trachoma dubium

A71.1   **Active stage of trachoma**
Granular conjunctivitis (trachomatous)
Trachomatous follicular conjunctivitis
Trachomatous pannus

A71.9   **Trachoma, unspecified**

✓4ᵗʰ **A74 Other diseases caused by chlamydiae**

EXCLUDES 1   neonatal chlamydial conjunctivitis (P39.1)
          neonatal chlamydial pneumonia (P23.1)
          Reiter's disease (M02.3-)
          sexually transmitted chlamydial diseases (A55-A56)
EXCLUDES 2   chlamydial pneumonia (J16.0)

A74.0   **Chlamydial conjunctivitis**
Paratrachoma

✓5ᵗʰ **A74.8**   **Other chlamydial diseases**
    A74.81   **Chlamydial peritonitis**
    A74.89   **Other chlamydial diseases**

A74.9   **Chlamydial infection, unspecified**
Chlamydiosis NOS

Rickettsioses (A75-A79)

DEF: Rickettsia: Condition caused by bacteria that live in lice/ticks transmitted to humans through bites.

✓4ᵗʰ **A75 Typhus fever**

EXCLUDES 1   rickettsiosis due to Ehrlichia sennetsu (A79.81)

A75.0   **Epidemic louse-borne typhus fever due to Rickettsia prowazekii**   CC
Classical typhus (fever)
Epidemic (louse-borne) typhus

A75.1   **Recrudescent typhus [Brill's disease]**   CC
Brill-Zinsser disease

A75.2   **Typhus fever due to Rickettsia typhi**   CC
Murine (flea-borne) typhus

A75.3   **Typhus fever due to Rickettsia tsutsugamushi**   CC
Scrub (mite-borne) typhus
Tsutsugamushi fever
▶Typhus fever due to Orientia Tsutsugamushi (scrub typhus)◀

A75.9   **Typhus fever, unspecified**   CC
Typhus (fever) NOS

✓4ᵗʰ **A77 Spotted fever [tick-borne rickettsioses]**

A77.0   **Spotted fever due to Rickettsia rickettsii**   CC
Rocky Mountain spotted fever
Sao Paulo fever

A77.1   **Spotted fever due to Rickettsia conorii**   CC
African tick typhus
Boutonneuse fever
India tick typhus
Kenya tick typhus
Marseilles fever
Mediterranean tick fever

A77.2   **Spotted fever due to Rickettsia siberica**   CC
North Asian tick fever
Siberian tick typhus

A77.3   **Spotted fever due to Rickettsia australis**   CC
Queensland tick typhus

✓5ᵗʰ **A77.4**   **Ehrlichiosis**

EXCLUDES 1   Rickettsiosis due to Ehrlichia sennetsu (A79.81)

    A77.40   **Ehrlichiosis, unspecified**   CC
    A77.41   **Ehrlichiosis chafeensis [E. chafeensis]**   CC
    A77.49   **Other ehrlichiosis**   CC
      ▶Ehrlichiosis due to E. ewingii◀
      ▶Ehrlichiosis due to E. muris euclairensis◀

A77.8   **Other spotted fevers**   CC
▶Rickettsia 364D/R. philipii (Pacific Coast tick fever)◀
▶Spotted fever due to Rickettsia africae (African tick bite fever)◀
▶Spotted fever due to Rickettsia parkeri◀

A77.9   **Spotted fever, unspecified**   CC
Tick-borne typhus NOS

A78 Q fever   CC
Infection due to Coxiella burnetii
Nine Mile fever
Quadrilateral fever

✓4ᵗʰ **A79 Other rickettsioses**

A79.0   **Trench fever**   CC
Quintan fever
Wolhynian fever

A79.1   **Rickettsialpox due to Rickettsia akari**   CC
Kew Garden fever
Vesicular rickettsiosis

✓5ᵗʰ **A79.8**   **Other specified rickettsioses**
    A79.81   **Rickettsiosis due to Ehrlichia sennetsu**   CC
      ▶Rickettsiosis due to Neorickettsia sennetsu◀
    A79.89   **Other specified rickettsioses**   CC

A79.9   **Rickettsiosis, unspecified**   CC
Rickettsial infection NOS

Viral and prion infections of the central nervous system (A80-A89)

EXCLUDES 1   postpolio syndrome (G14)
       sequelae of poliomyelitis (B91)
       sequelae of viral encephalitis (B94.1)

✓4ᵗʰ **A80**   **Acute poliomyelitis**

   A80.0   Acute paralytic poliomyelitis, vaccine-associated   `MCC`

   A80.1   Acute paralytic poliomyelitis, wild virus, imported   `MCC`

   A80.2   Acute paralytic poliomyelitis, wild virus, indigenous   `MCC`

   ✓5ᵗʰ **A80.3**   Acute paralytic poliomyelitis, other and unspecified

      A80.30   Acute paralytic poliomyelitis, unspecified   `MCC`

      A80.39   Other acute paralytic poliomyelitis   `MCC`

   A80.4   Acute nonparalytic poliomyelitis

   A80.9   Acute poliomyelitis, unspecified

✓4ᵗʰ **A81**   **Atypical virus infections of central nervous system**

   INCLUDES   diseases of the central nervous system caused by prions

   Use additional code to identify:
   dementia with behavioral disturbance (F02.81)
   dementia without behavioral disturbance (F02.80)

   ✓5ᵗʰ **A81.0**   Creutzfeldt-Jakob disease

      DEF: Communicable, rare spongiform encephalopathy occurring later in life with progressive destruction of the pyramidal and extrapyramidal systems eventually leading to death. Progressive dementia, wasting of muscles, tremor, and other symptoms are present.

      A81.00   Creutzfeldt-Jakob disease, unspecified   `CC` `HCC`
        Jakob-Creutzfeldt disease, unspecified

      A81.01   Variant Creutzfeldt-Jakob disease   `CC` `HCC`
        vCJD

      A81.09   Other Creutzfeldt-Jakob disease   `CC` `HCC`
        CJD
        Familial Creutzfeldt-Jakob disease
        Iatrogenic Creutzfeldt-Jakob disease
        Sporadic Creutzfeldt-Jakob disease
        Subacute spongiform encephalopathy (with dementia)

   A81.1   Subacute sclerosing panencephalitis   `CC` `HCC`
      Dawson's inclusion body encephalitis
      Van Bogaert's sclerosing leukoencephalopathy

   A81.2   Progressive multifocal leukoencephalopathy   `HIV` `CC` `HCC`
      Multifocal leukoencephalopathy NOS

   ✓5ᵗʰ **A81.8**   Other atypical virus infections of central nervous system

      A81.81   Kuru   `CC` `HCC`

      A81.82   Gerstmann-Sträussler-Scheinker syndrome   `HIV` `CC` `HCC`
        GSS syndrome

      A81.83   Fatal familial insomnia   `HIV` `CC` `HCC`
        FFI

      A81.89   Other atypical virus infections of central nervous system   `HIV` `CC` `HCC`

   A81.9   Atypical virus infection of central nervous system, unspecified   `HIV` `CC` `HCC`
      Prion diseases of the central nervous system NOS

✓4ᵗʰ **A82**   **Rabies**

   A82.0   Sylvatic rabies   `CC`

   A82.1   Urban rabies   `CC`

   A82.9   Rabies, unspecified   `CC`

✓4ᵗʰ **A83**   **Mosquito-borne viral encephalitis**

   INCLUDES   mosquito-borne viral meningoencephalitis
   EXCLUDES 2   Venezuelan equine encephalitis (A92.2)
       West Nile fever (A92.3-)
       West Nile virus (A92.3-)

   A83.0   Japanese encephalitis   `MCC`

   A83.1   Western equine encephalitis   `MCC`

   A83.2   Eastern equine encephalitis   `MCC`

   A83.3   St Louis encephalitis   `MCC`

   A83.4   Australian encephalitis   `MCC`
      Kunjin virus disease

   A83.5   California encephalitis   `MCC`
      California meningoencephalitis
      La Crosse encephalitis

   A83.6   Rocio virus disease   `MCC`

   A83.8   Other mosquito-borne viral encephalitis   `MCC`

   A83.9   Mosquito-borne viral encephalitis, unspecified   `MCC`

✓4ᵗʰ **A84**   **Tick-borne viral encephalitis**

   INCLUDES   tick-borne viral meningoencephalitis

   A84.0   Far Eastern tick-borne encephalitis [Russian spring-summer encephalitis]   `MCC`

   A84.1   Central European tick-borne encephalitis   `MCC`

▲   ✓5ᵗʰ **A84.8**   Other tick-borne viral encephalitis
      ~~Louping ill~~
      ~~Powassan virus disease~~

●   **A84.81**   Powassan virus disease   `MCC`

●   **A84.89**   Other tick-borne viral encephalitis   `MCC`
        Louping ill
        Code first, if applicable, transfusion related infection (T80.22-)

   A84.9   Tick-borne viral encephalitis, unspecified   `MCC`

✓4ᵗʰ **A85**   **Other viral encephalitis, not elsewhere classified**

   INCLUDES   specified viral encephalomyelitis NEC
       specified viral meningoencephalitis NEC
   EXCLUDES 1   benign myalgic encephalomyelitis (G93.3)
       encephalitis due to cytomegalovirus (B25.8)
       encephalitis due to herpesvirus NEC (B10.0-)
       encephalitis due to herpesvirus [herpes simplex] (B00.4)
       encephalitis due to measles virus (B05.0)
       encephalitis due to mumps virus (B26.2)
       encephalitis due to poliomyelitis virus (A80.-)
       encephalitis due to zoster (B02.0)
       lymphocytic choriomeningitis (A87.2)

   A85.0   Enteroviral encephalitis   `HIV` `CC`
      Enteroviral encephalomyelitis

   A85.1   Adenoviral encephalitis   `HIV` `CC`
      Adenoviral meningoencephalitis

   A85.2   Arthropod-borne viral encephalitis, unspecified   `MCC`
      EXCLUDES 1   West nile virus with encephalitis (A92.31)

   A85.8   Other specified viral encephalitis   `HIV` `CC`
      Encephalitis lethargica
      Von Economo-Cruchet disease

A86   **Unspecified viral encephalitis**   `HIV` `CC`
   Viral encephalomyelitis NOS
   Viral meningoencephalitis NOS

✓4ᵗʰ **A87**   **Viral meningitis**

   EXCLUDES 1   meningitis due to herpesvirus [herpes simplex] (B00.3)
       meningitis due to measles virus (B05.1)
       meningitis due to mumps virus (B26.1)
       meningitis due to poliomyelitis virus (A80.-)
       meningitis due to zoster (B02.1)

   DEF: Meningitis: Inflammation of the meningeal layers of the brain and spine.

   A87.0   Enteroviral meningitis   `CC`
      Coxsackievirus meningitis
      Echovirus meningitis

   A87.1   Adenoviral meningitis   `CC`

   A87.2   Lymphocytic choriomeningitis   `CC`
      Lymphocytic meningoencephalitis

   A87.8   Other viral meningitis   `CC`

   A87.9   Viral meningitis, unspecified   `CC`

✓4ᵗʰ **A88**   **Other viral infections of central nervous system, not elsewhere classified**

   EXCLUDES 1   viral encephalitis NOS (A86)
       viral meningitis NOS (A87.9)

   A88.0   Enteroviral exanthematous fever [Boston exanthem]   `CC`

   A88.1   Epidemic vertigo

   A88.8   Other specified viral infections of central nervous system   `HIV` `CC`

A89   **Unspecified viral infection of central nervous system**   `HIV` `CC`

Arthropod-borne viral fevers and viral hemorrhagic fevers (A90-A99)

A90   **Dengue fever [classical dengue]**   `CC`
   EXCLUDES 1   dengue hemorrhagic fever (A91)
   AHA: 2016,3Q,13

A91   **Dengue hemorrhagic fever**   `CC`

✓ Additional Character Required   ✓x7ᵗʰ Placeholder   Unacceptable PDx   Questionable PDx   Manifestation   Unspecified Dx   `H1`-`H4` HAC   `HCC` CMS-HCC Dx   `HIV` HIV Dx

ICD-10-CM 2021   453

✓4ᵗʰ A92 Other mosquito-borne viral fevers

> EXCLUDES 1   Ross River disease (B33.1)

A92.0 Chikungunya virus disease   CC
Chikungunya (hemorrhagic) fever

A92.1 O'nyong-nyong fever   CC

A92.2 Venezuelan equine fever   CC
Venezuelan equine encephalitis
Venezuelan equine encephalomyelitis virus disease

✓5ᵗʰ A92.3 West Nile virus infection
West Nile fever
AHA: 2016,3Q,12

A92.30 West Nile virus infection, unspecified   MCC
West Nile fever NOS
West Nile fever without complications
West Nile virus NOS

A92.31 West Nile virus infection with encephalitis   MCC
West Nile encephalitis
West Nile encephalomyelitis

A92.32 West Nile virus infection with other neurologic manifestation   MCC
Use additional code to specify the neurologic manifestation

A92.39 West Nile virus infection with other complications   MCC
Use additional code to specify the other conditions

A92.4 Rift Valley fever   CC

A92.5 Zika virus disease   CC
Zika virus fever
Zika virus infection
Zika NOS

> EXCLUDES 1   congenital Zika virus disease (P35.4)

AHA: 2016,4Q,4-7
DEF: Virus transmitted via a bite from an infected Aedes species mosquito. Common symptoms of the virus include fever, rash, joint pain, and conjunctivitis; they are usually mild in nature and may last from several days to a week. Most people who have the Zika virus do not require medical attention; however, in pregnant women, the Zika virus can cause a serious birth defect called microcephaly, as well as other severe fetal brain defects.
TIP: Code only confirmed diagnoses of Zika virus; documentation by the physician that the disease is confirmed is sufficient.

A92.8 Other specified mosquito-borne viral fevers   CC

A92.9 Mosquito-borne viral fever, unspecified   CC

✓4ᵗʰ A93 Other arthropod-borne viral fevers, not elsewhere classified

A93.0 Oropouche virus disease   CC
Oropouche fever

A93.1 Sandfly fever   CC
Pappataci fever
Phlebotomus fever

A93.2 Colorado tick fever   CC

A93.8 Other specified arthropod-borne viral fevers   CC
Piry virus disease
Vesicular stomatitis virus disease [Indiana fever]

A94 Unspecified arthropod-borne viral fever   CC
Arboviral fever NOS
Arbovirus infection NOS

✓4ᵗʰ A95 Yellow fever

A95.0 Sylvatic yellow fever   CC
Jungle yellow fever

A95.1 Urban yellow fever   CC

A95.9 Yellow fever, unspecified   CC

✓4ᵗʰ A96 Arenaviral hemorrhagic fever

A96.0 Junin hemorrhagic fever   CC
Argentinian hemorrhagic fever

A96.1 Machupo hemorrhagic fever   CC
Bolivian hemorrhagic fever

A96.2 Lassa fever

A96.8 Other arenaviral hemorrhagic fevers   CC

A96.9 Arenaviral hemorrhagic fever, unspecified   CC

✓4ᵗʰ A98 Other viral hemorrhagic fevers, not elsewhere classified

> EXCLUDES 1   chikungunya hemorrhagic fever (A92.0)
> dengue hemorrhagic fever (A91)

A98.0 Crimean-Congo hemorrhagic fever   CC
Central Asian hemorrhagic fever

A98.1 Omsk hemorrhagic fever   CC

A98.2 Kyasanur Forest disease

A98.3 Marburg virus disease

A98.4 Ebola virus disease

A98.5 Hemorrhagic fever with renal syndrome   CC
Epidemic hemorrhagic fever
Korean hemorrhagic fever
Russian hemorrhagic fever
Hantaan virus disease
Hantavirus disease with renal manifestations
Nephropathia epidemica
Songo fever

> EXCLUDES 1   hantavirus (cardio)-pulmonary syndrome (B33.4)

A98.8 Other specified viral hemorrhagic fevers   CC

A99 Unspecified viral hemorrhagic fever   CC

Viral infections characterized by skin and mucous membrane lesions (B00-B09)

✓4ᵗʰ B00 Herpesviral [herpes simplex] infections

> EXCLUDES 1   congenital herpesviral infections (P35.2)
> EXCLUDES 2   anogenital herpesviral infection (A60.-)
> gammaherpesviral mononucleosis (B27.0-)
> herpangina (B08.5)

B00.0 Eczema herpeticum   HIV
Kaposi's varicelliform eruption

B00.1 Herpesviral vesicular dermatitis   HIV
Herpes simplex facialis
Herpes simplex labialis
Herpes simplex otitis externa
Vesicular dermatitis of ear
Vesicular dermatitis of lip

B00.2 Herpesviral gingivostomatitis and pharyngotonsillitis   HIV CC
Herpesviral pharyngitis

B00.3 Herpesviral meningitis   HIV MCC

B00.4 Herpesviral encephalitis   HIV MCC
Herpesviral meningoencephalitis
Simian B disease

> EXCLUDES 1   herpesviral encephalitis due to herpesvirus 6 and 7 (B10.01, B10.09)
> non-simplex herpesviral encephalitis (B10.0-)

✓5ᵗʰ B00.5 Herpesviral ocular disease

B00.50 Herpesviral ocular disease, unspecified   HIV CC

B00.51 Herpesviral iridocyclitis   HIV CC
Herpesviral iritis
Herpesviral uveitis, anterior

B00.52 Herpesviral keratitis   HIV CC
Herpesviral keratoconjunctivitis

B00.53 Herpesviral conjunctivitis   HIV CC

B00.59 Other herpesviral disease of eye   HIV CC
Herpesviral dermatitis of eyelid

B00.7 Disseminated herpesviral disease   HIV MCC HCC
Herpesviral sepsis

✓5ᵗʰ B00.8 Other forms of herpesviral infections

B00.81 Herpesviral hepatitis   HIV CC

B00.82 Herpes simplex myelitis   MCC HCC

B00.89 Other herpesviral infection   HIV CC
Herpesviral whitlow

B00.9 Herpesviral infection, unspecified   HIV
Herpes simplex infection NOS

✓4ᵗʰ B01 Varicella [chickenpox]

B01.0 Varicella meningitis   CC

✓5ᵗʰ B01.1 Varicella encephalitis, myelitis and encephalomyelitis
Postchickenpox encephalitis, myelitis and encephalomyelitis

B01.11 Varicella encephalitis and encephalomyelitis   MCC
Postchickenpox encephalitis and encephalomyelitis

N Newborn: 0   P Pediatric: 0-17   M Maternity: 9-64   A Adult: 15-124   MCC Major Complication/Comorbidity   CC Complication/Comorbidity   SW Severe Wound Dx

454   ICD-10-CM 2021

      B01.12   **Varicella** myelitis   `MCC` `HCC`
                Postchickenpox myelitis
    B01.2   **Varicella** pneumonia   `MCC`
 ✓5ᵗʰ **B01.8**   **Varicella with other complications**
      B01.81   **Varicella** keratitis   `CC`
      B01.89   **Other varicella complications**   `CC`
    B01.9   **Varicella without complication**   `CC`
           Varicella NOS

✓4ᵗʰ **B02** **Zoster [herpes zoster]**
      `INCLUDES`   shingles
               zona
    B02.0   **Zoster** encephalitis   `HIV` `CC`
           Zoster meningoencephalitis
    B02.1   **Zoster** meningitis   `HIV` `MCC`
           AHA: 2019,1Q,18
 ✓5ᵗʰ **B02.2**   **Zoster with other nervous system involvement**
      B02.21   **Postherpetic** geniculate ganglionitis   `HIV` `CC`
      B02.22   **Postherpetic** trigeminal neuralgia   `HIV` `CC`
      B02.23   **Postherpetic** polyneuropathy   `HIV` `CC`
      B02.24   **Postherpetic** myelitis   `MCC` `HCC`
                Herpes zoster myelitis
      B02.29   **Other postherpetic nervous system involvement**   `HIV` `CC`
                Postherpetic radiculopathy
 ✓5ᵗʰ **B02.3**   **Zoster** ocular disease
      B02.30   **Zoster ocular disease, unspecified**   `HIV` `CC`
      B02.31   **Zoster** conjunctivitis   `HIV` `CC`
      B02.32   **Zoster** iridocyclitis   `HIV` `CC`
      B02.33   **Zoster** keratitis   `HIV` `CC`
                Herpes zoster keratoconjunctivitis
      B02.34   **Zoster** scleritis   `HIV` `CC`
      B02.39   **Other herpes zoster eye disease**   `HIV` `CC`
                Zoster blepharitis
    B02.7   **Disseminated** zoster   `HIV` `CC`
    B02.8   **Zoster with other complications**   `HIV` `CC`
           Herpes zoster otitis externa
    B02.9   **Zoster without complications**   `HIV`
           Zoster NOS

   B03 **Smallpox**   `CC`
      `NOTE`   In 1980 the 33rd World Health Assembly declared that smallpox had been eradicated.
            The classification is maintained for surveillance purposes.

   B04 **Monkeypox**   `CC`

✓4ᵗʰ **B05** **Measles**
      `INCLUDES`   morbilli
      `EXCLUDES 1`   *subacute sclerosing panencephalitis (A81.1)*
    B05.0   **Measles complicated by** encephalitis   `MCC`
           Postmeasles encephalitis
    B05.1   **Measles complicated by** meningitis   `CC`
           Postmeasles meningitis
    B05.2   **Measles complicated by** pneumonia   `MCC`
           Postmeasles pneumonia
    B05.3   **Measles complicated by** otitis media
           Postmeasles otitis media
    B05.4   **Measles with intestinal complications**   `CC`
 ✓5ᵗʰ **B05.8**   **Measles with other complications**
      B05.81   **Measles** keratitis and keratoconjunctivitis   `CC`
      B05.89   **Other measles complications**   `CC`
    B05.9   **Measles without complication**
           Measles NOS

✓4ᵗʰ **B06** **Rubella [German measles]**
      `EXCLUDES 1`   *congenital rubella (P35.0)*
      DEF: Highly contagious virus in which the symptoms are mild and short-lived in most people. Rubella during pregnancy, however, can result in abortion, stillbirth, or congenital defects.
 ✓5ᵗʰ **B06.0**   **Rubella with** neurological complications
      B06.00   **Rubella with neurological complication, unspecified**   `CC`
      B06.01   **Rubella** encephalitis   `MCC`
                Rubella meningoencephalitis
      B06.02   **Rubella** meningitis   `CC`
      B06.09   **Other neurological complications of rubella**   `CC`

 ✓5ᵗʰ **B06.8**   **Rubella with other complications**
      B06.81   **Rubella** pneumonia   `CC`
      B06.82   **Rubella** arthritis   `CC` `HCC`
      B06.89   **Other rubella complications**   `CC`
    B06.9   **Rubella without complication**
           Rubella NOS

✓4ᵗʰ **B07** **Viral warts**
      `INCLUDES`   verruca simplex
                verruca vulgaris
                viral warts due to human papillomavirus
      `EXCLUDES 2`   *anogenital (venereal) warts (A63.0)*
                papilloma of bladder (D41.4)
                papilloma of cervix (D26.0)
                papilloma larynx (D14.1)
    B07.0   **Plantar wart**
           Verruca plantaris
    B07.8   **Other viral warts**
           Common wart
           Flat wart
           Verruca plana
    B07.9   **Viral wart, unspecified**

✓4ᵗʰ **B08** **Other viral infections characterized by skin and mucous membrane lesions, not elsewhere classified**
      `EXCLUDES 1`   *vesicular stomatitis virus disease (A93.8)*
 ✓5ᵗʰ **B08.0**   **Other orthopoxvirus infections**
        `EXCLUDES 2`   *monkeypox (B04)*
  ✓6ᵗʰ **B08.01**   **Cowpox and vaccinia not from vaccine**
         B08.010   **Cowpox**
                DEF: Disease contracted by milking infected cows. The vesicles usually appear on the fingers, hands, and adjacent areas and usually disappear without scarring. Other symptoms include local edema, lymphangitis, and regional lymphadenitis with or without fever.
         B08.011   **Vaccinia not from vaccine**
                `EXCLUDES 1`   *vaccinia (from vaccination) (generalized) (T88.1)*
      B08.02   **Orf virus disease**
                Contagious pustular dermatitis
                Ecthyma contagiosum
      B08.03   **Pseudocowpox [milker's node]**
      B08.04   **Paravaccinia, unspecified**
      B08.09   **Other orthopoxvirus infections**
                Orthopoxvirus infection NOS
    B08.1   **Molluscum contagiosum**
           DEF: Benign poxvirus infection causing small bumps on the skin or conjunctiva and is transmitted by close contact.
 ✓5ᵗʰ **B08.2**   **Exanthema subitum [sixth disease]**
           Roseola infantum
      B08.20   **Exanthema subitum [sixth disease], unspecified**   `P`
                Roseola infantum, unspecified
      B08.21   **Exanthema subitum [sixth disease] due to** human herpesvirus 6   `P`
                Roseola infantum due to human herpesvirus 6
      B08.22   **Exanthema subitum [sixth disease] due to** human herpesvirus 7   `P`
                Roseola infantum due to human herpesvirus 7
    B08.3   **Erythema infectiosum [fifth disease]**   `CC`
           DEF: Infection with human parvovirus B19, mainly occurring in children. Symptoms include a low-grade fever, malaise, or a "cold" a few days before the appearance of a mild rash illness that presents as a "slapped-cheek" rash on the face and a lacy red rash on the trunk and limbs.
    B08.4   **Enteroviral vesicular stomatitis with exanthem**
           Hand, foot and mouth disease
    B08.5   **Enteroviral vesicular pharyngitis**
           Herpangina
           DEF: Acute infectious Coxsackie virus infection causing throat lesions, fever, and vomiting that generally affects children in the summer.
 ✓5ᵗʰ **B08.6**   **Parapoxvirus infections**
      B08.60   **Parapoxvirus infection, unspecified**
      B08.61   **Bovine stomatitis**
      B08.62   **Sealpox**
      B08.69   **Other parapoxvirus infections**

☑ Additional Character Required   ✓x7ᵗʰ Placeholder   Unacceptable PDx   Questionable PDx   Manifestation   Unspecified Dx   `H1`-`H14` HAC   `HCC` CMS-HCC Dx   `HIV` HIV Dx

ICD-10-CM 2021   455

✓5ᵗʰ B08.7 Yatapoxvirus infections

    B08.70 Yatapoxvirus infection, unspecified

    B08.71 Tanapox virus disease `CC`

    B08.72 Yaba pox virus disease
       Yaba monkey tumor disease

    B08.79 Other yatapoxvirus infections

B08.8 Other specified viral infections characterized by skin and mucous membrane lesions
    Enteroviral lymphonodular pharyngitis
    Foot-and-mouth disease
    Poxvirus NEC

B09 Unspecified viral infection characterized by skin and mucous membrane lesions
    Viral enanthema NOS
    Viral exanthema NOS

Other human herpesviruses (B10)

✓4ᵗʰ B10 Other human herpesviruses

    EXCLUDES 2   cytomegalovirus (B25.9)
       Epstein-Barr virus (B27.0-)
       herpes NOS (B00.9)
       herpes simplex (B00.-)
       herpes zoster (B02.-)
       human herpesvirus NOS (B00.-)
       human herpesvirus 1 and 2 (B00.-)
       human herpesvirus 3 (B01.-, B02.-)
       human herpesvirus 4 (B27.0-)
       human herpesvirus 5 (B25.-)
       varicella (B01.-)
       zoster (B02.-)

    ✓5ᵗʰ B10.0 Other human herpesvirus encephalitis

       EXCLUDES 2   herpes encephalitis NOS (B00.4)
          herpes simplex encephalitis (B00.4)
          human herpesvirus encephalitis (B00.4)
          simian B herpes virus encephalitis (B00.4)

       B10.01 Human herpesvirus 6 encephalitis `HIV` `MCC`

       B10.09 Other human herpesvirus encephalitis `HIV` `MCC`
          Human herpesvirus 7 encephalitis

    ✓5ᵗʰ B10.8 Other human herpesvirus infection

       B10.81 Human herpesvirus 6 infection

       B10.82 Human herpesvirus 7 infection

       B10.89 Other human herpesvirus infection
          Human herpesvirus 8 infection
          Kaposi's sarcoma-associated herpesvirus infection

Viral hepatitis (B15-B19)

    EXCLUDES 1   sequelae of viral hepatitis (B94.2)
    EXCLUDES 2   cytomegaloviral hepatitis (B25.1)
       herpesviral [herpes simplex] hepatitis (B00.81)

DEF: Hepatitis A: HAV infection that is self-limiting with flulike symptoms. Transmission is fecal-oral.
DEF: Hepatitis B: HBV infection that can be chronic and systemic. Transmission is bodily fluids.
DEF: Hepatitis C: HCV infection that can be chronic and systemic. Transmission is blood transfusion and unidentified agents.
DEF: Hepatitis D (delta): HDV that occurs only in the presence of hepatitis B virus. Transmission is contaminated blood in contact with mucous membranes.
DEF: Hepatitis E: HEV is an epidemic form. Transmission is fecal-oral, most often from contaminated water.

✓4ᵗʰ B15 Acute hepatitis A

    B15.0 Hepatitis A with hepatic coma `MCC`

    B15.9 Hepatitis A without hepatic coma `CC`
       Hepatitis A (acute)(viral) NOS

✓4ᵗʰ B16 Acute hepatitis B

    AHA: 2016,3Q,13

    B16.0 Acute hepatitis B with delta-agent with hepatic coma `MCC`

    B16.1 Acute hepatitis B with delta-agent without hepatic coma `CC`

    B16.2 Acute hepatitis B without delta-agent with hepatic coma `MCC`

    B16.9 Acute hepatitis B without delta-agent and without hepatic coma `CC`
       Hepatitis B (acute) (viral) NOS

✓4ᵗʰ B17 Other acute viral hepatitis

    B17.0 Acute delta-(super) infection of hepatitis B carrier `CC`

✓5ᵗʰ B17.1 Acute hepatitis C

    B17.10 Acute hepatitis C without hepatic coma `CC`
       Acute hepatitis C NOS

    B17.11 Acute hepatitis C with hepatic coma `MCC`

B17.2 Acute hepatitis E `CC`

B17.8 Other specified acute viral hepatitis `CC`
    Hepatitis non-A non-B (acute) (viral) NEC

B17.9 Acute viral hepatitis, unspecified `CC`
    Acute hepatitis NOS
    Acute infectious hepatitis NOS

✓4ᵗʰ B18 Chronic viral hepatitis

    INCLUDES   carrier of viral hepatitis

    AHA: 2017,1Q,41

    B18.0 Chronic viral hepatitis B with delta-agent `CC` `HCC`

    B18.1 Chronic viral hepatitis B without delta-agent `CC` `HCC`
       Carrier of viral hepatitis B
       Chronic (viral) hepatitis B

    B18.2 Chronic viral hepatitis C `HCC`
       Carrier of viral hepatitis C
       AHA: 2018,1Q,4

    B18.8 Other chronic viral hepatitis `CC` `HCC`
       Carrier of other viral hepatitis

    B18.9 Chronic viral hepatitis, unspecified `CC` `HCC`
       Carrier of unspecified viral hepatitis

✓4ᵗʰ B19 Unspecified viral hepatitis

    B19.0 Unspecified viral hepatitis with hepatic coma `MCC`

    ✓5ᵗʰ B19.1 Unspecified viral hepatitis B

       B19.10 Unspecified viral hepatitis B without hepatic coma `CC`
          Unspecified viral hepatitis B NOS

       B19.11 Unspecified viral hepatitis B with hepatic coma `MCC`

    ✓5ᵗʰ B19.2 Unspecified viral hepatitis C

       B19.20 Unspecified viral hepatitis C without hepatic coma
          Viral hepatitis C NOS

       B19.21 Unspecified viral hepatitis C with hepatic coma `MCC`

    B19.9 Unspecified viral hepatitis without hepatic coma `CC`
       Viral hepatitis NOS

Human immunodeficiency virus [HIV] disease (B20)

B20 Human immunodeficiency virus [HIV] disease `CC` `HCC`

    INCLUDES   acquired immune deficiency syndrome [AIDS]
          AIDS-related complex [ARC]
          HIV infection, symptomatic

    Code first Human immunodeficiency virus [HIV] disease complicating pregnancy, childbirth and the puerperium, if applicable (O98.7-)
    Use additional code(s) to identify all manifestations of HIV infection

    EXCLUDES 1   asymptomatic human immunodeficiency virus [HIV] infection status (Z21)
       exposure to HIV virus (Z20.6)
       inconclusive serologic evidence of HIV (R75)

    AHA: 2020,2Q,12; 2019,1Q,8-11

Other viral diseases (B25-B34)

✓4ᵗʰ B25 Cytomegaloviral disease

    EXCLUDES 1   congenital cytomegalovirus infection (P35.1)
       cytomegaloviral mononucleosis (B27.1-)

    B25.0 Cytomegaloviral pneumonitis `MCC` `HCC`

    B25.1 Cytomegaloviral hepatitis `CC` `HCC`

    B25.2 Cytomegaloviral pancreatitis `MCC` `HCC`

    B25.8 Other cytomegaloviral diseases `HIV` `CC` `HCC`
       Cytomegaloviral encephalitis

    B25.9 Cytomegaloviral disease, unspecified `HIV` `CC` `HCC`

✓4ᵗʰ B26 Mumps

    INCLUDES   epidemic parotitis
       infectious parotitis

    B26.0 Mumps orchitis `CC` ♂

    B26.1 Mumps meningitis `MCC`

    B26.2 Mumps encephalitis `MCC`

    B26.3 Mumps pancreatitis `CC`

N Newborn: 0   P Pediatric: 0-17   M Maternity: 9-64   A Adult: 15-124   MCC Major Complication/Comorbidity   CC Complication/Comorbidity   SW Severe Wound Dx

456   ICD-10-CM 2021

✓5ᵗʰ **B26.8** **Mumps with other complications**

    B26.81 **Mumps** hepatitis `CC`

    B26.82 **Mumps** myocarditis `CC`

    B26.83 **Mumps** nephritis `CC`

    B26.84 **Mumps** polyneuropathy `CC`

    B26.85 **Mumps** arthritis `CC` `HCC`

    B26.89 **Other mumps complications** `CC`

B26.9 **Mumps without complication**
    Mumps NOS
    Mumps parotitis NOS

✓4ᵗʰ **B27** **Infectious mononucleosis**

  INCLUDES glandular fever
        monocytic angina
        Pfeiffer's disease

✓5ᵗʰ **B27.0** **Gammaherpesviral mononucleosis**
    Mononucleosis due to Epstein-Barr virus

    B27.00 **Gammaherpesviral mononucleosis** without complication

    B27.01 **Gammaherpesviral mononucleosis** with polyneuropathy

    B27.02 **Gammaherpesviral mononucleosis** with meningitis

    B27.09 **Gammaherpesviral mononucleosis** with other complications
        Hepatomegaly in gammaherpesviral mononucleosis

✓5ᵗʰ **B27.1** **Cytomegaloviral mononucleosis**

    B27.10 **Cytomegaloviral mononucleosis** without complications

    B27.11 **Cytomegaloviral mononucleosis** with polyneuropathy

    B27.12 **Cytomegaloviral mononucleosis** with meningitis

    B27.19 **Cytomegaloviral mononucleosis** with other complication
        Hepatomegaly in cytomegaloviral mononucleosis

✓5ᵗʰ **B27.8** **Other infectious mononucleosis**

    B27.80 **Other infectious mononucleosis** without complication

    B27.81 **Other infectious mononucleosis** with polyneuropathy

    B27.82 **Other infectious mononucleosis** with meningitis

    B27.89 **Other infectious mononucleosis** with other complication
        Hepatomegaly in other infectious mononucleosis

✓5ᵗʰ **B27.9** **Infectious mononucleosis, unspecified**

    B27.90 **Infectious mononucleosis, unspecified** without complication

    B27.91 **Infectious mononucleosis, unspecified** with polyneuropathy

    B27.92 **Infectious mononucleosis, unspecified** with meningitis

    B27.99 **Infectious mononucleosis, unspecified** with other complication
        Hepatomegaly in unspecified infectious mononucleosis

✓4ᵗʰ **B30** **Viral conjunctivitis**

  EXCLUDES 1 herpesviral [herpes simplex] ocular disease (B00.5)
        ocular zoster (B02.3)

Viral Conjunctivitis

Normal conjunctiva

Inflamed conjunctiva

B30.0 **Keratoconjunctivitis due to adenovirus**
    Epidemic keratoconjunctivitis
    Shipyard eye

B30.1 **Conjunctivitis due to adenovirus**
    Acute adenoviral follicular conjunctivitis
    Swimming-pool conjunctivitis

B30.2 **Viral pharyngoconjunctivitis**

B30.3 **Acute epidemic hemorrhagic conjunctivitis (enteroviral)**
    Conjunctivitis due to coxsackievirus 24
    Conjunctivitis due to enterovirus 70
    Hemorrhagic conjunctivitis (acute)(epidemic)

B30.8 **Other viral conjunctivitis**
    Newcastle conjunctivitis

B30.9 **Viral conjunctivitis, unspecified**

✓4ᵗʰ **B33** **Other viral diseases, not elsewhere classified**

B33.0 **Epidemic myalgia**
    Bornholm disease

B33.1 **Ross River disease** `CC`
    Epidemic polyarthritis and exanthema
    Ross River fever

✓5ᵗʰ **B33.2** **Viral carditis**
    Coxsackie (virus) carditis

    B33.20 **Viral carditis, unspecified** `CC`

    B33.21 **Viral endocarditis** `CC`

    B33.22 **Viral myocarditis** `CC`

    B33.23 **Viral pericarditis** `CC`

    B33.24 **Viral cardiomyopathy** `HCC`

B33.3 **Retrovirus infections, not elsewhere classified**
    Retrovirus infection NOS

B33.4 **Hantavirus (cardio)-pulmonary syndrome [HPS] [HCPS]** `CC`
    Hantavirus disease with pulmonary manifestations
    Sin nombre virus disease
    Use additional code to identify any associated acute kidney failure (N17.9)
    EXCLUDES 1 hantavirus disease with renal manifestations (A98.5)
        hemorrhagic fever with renal manifestations (A98.5)

B33.8 **Other specified viral diseases**
    EXCLUDES 1 anogenital human papillomavirus infection (A63.0)
        viral warts due to human papillomavirus infection (B07)

✓4ᵗʰ **B34** **Viral infection of unspecified site**

  EXCLUDES 1 anogenital human papillomavirus infection (A63.0)
        cytomegaloviral disease NOS (B25.9)
        herpesvirus [herpes simplex] infection NOS (B00.9)
        retrovirus infection NOS (B33.3)
        viral agents as the cause of diseases classified elsewhere (B97.-)
        viral warts due to human papillomavirus infection (B07)

B34.0 **Adenovirus infection, unspecified**

✓ Additional Character Required ✓x7ᵗʰ Placeholder Unacceptable PDx Questionable PDx Manifestation Unspecified Dx H1-H14 HAC HCC CMS-HCC Dx HIV HIV Dx

ICD-10-CM 2021   **457**

B34.1 Enterovirus infection, unspecified
Coxsackievirus infection NOS
Echovirus infection NOS

B34.2 Coronavirus infection, unspecified
EXCLUDES 1 ▶COVID-19 (U07.1)◀
pneumonia due to SARS-associated coronavirus (J12.81)
AHA: 2020,1Q,34-36
TIP: Do not report this code for COVID-19; refer to U07.1.

B34.3 Parvovirus infection, unspecified   CC

B34.4 Papovavirus infection, unspecified

B34.8 Other viral infections of unspecified site

B34.9 Viral infection, unspecified
Viremia NOS
AHA: 2016,3Q,10

Mycoses (B35-B49)

EXCLUDES 2   hypersensitivity pneumonitis due to organic dust (J67.-)
mycosis fungoides (C84.0-)

✓4ᵗʰ **B35 Dermatophytosis**
INCLUDES   favus
infections due to species of Epidermophyton, Micro-sporum and Trichophyton
tinea, any type except those in B36.-
DEF: Contagious superficial fungal infection of the skin that invades and grows in dead keratin.

B35.0 Tinea barbae and tinea capitis
Beard ringworm
Kerion
Scalp ringworm
Sycosis, mycotic

B35.1 Tinea unguium
Dermatophytic onychia
Dermatophytosis of nail
Onychomycosis
Ringworm of nails

B35.2 Tinea manuum
Dermatophytosis of hand
Hand ringworm

B35.3 Tinea pedis
Athlete's foot
Dermatophytosis of foot
Foot ringworm

B35.4 Tinea corporis
Ringworm of the body

B35.5 Tinea imbricata
Tokelau

B35.6 Tinea cruris
Dhobi itch
Groin ringworm
Jock itch

B35.8 Other dermatophytoses
Disseminated dermatophytosis
Granulomatous dermatophytosis

B35.9 Dermatophytosis, unspecified
Ringworm NOS

✓4ᵗʰ **B36 Other superficial mycoses**

B36.0 Pityriasis versicolor
Tinea flava
Tinea versicolor

B36.1 Tinea nigra
Keratomycosis nigricans palmaris
Microsporosis nigra
Pityriasis nigra

B36.2 White piedra
Tinea blanca

B36.3 Black piedra

B36.8 Other specified superficial mycoses

B36.9 Superficial mycosis, unspecified

✓4ᵗʰ **B37 Candidiasis**
INCLUDES   candidosis
moniliasis
EXCLUDES 1   neonatal candidiasis (P37.5)
DEF: Candida: Genus of yeast-like fungi that are commonly found in the mouth, skin, intestinal tract, and vagina. It may cause a white, cheesy discharge.

B37.0 Candidal stomatitis   HIV   CC
Oral thrush

B37.1 Pulmonary candidiasis   HIV   MCC   HCC
Candidal bronchitis
Candidal pneumonia

B37.2 Candidiasis of skin and nail   HIV
Candidal onychia
Candidal paronychia
EXCLUDES 2   diaper dermatitis (L22)

B37.3 Candidiasis of vulva and vagina   ♀
Candidal vulvovaginitis
Monilial vulvovaginitis
Vaginal thrush

✓5ᵗʰ **B37.4 Candidiasis of other urogenital sites**

B37.41 Candidal cystitis and urethritis   CC   H6

B37.42 Candidal balanitis   ♂

B37.49 Other urogenital candidiasis   CC   H6
Candidal pyelonephritis

B37.5 Candidal meningitis   HIV   MCC

B37.6 Candidal endocarditis   HIV   MCC

B37.7 Candidal sepsis   MCC   HCC
Disseminated candidiasis
Systemic candidiasis
AHA: 2014,4Q,46
TIP: This code is assigned when sepsis is documented as due to any Candida type. If non-Candida albicans is documented, code B48.8 Other specified mycoses, is assigned.

✓5ᵗʰ **B37.8 Candidiasis of other sites**

B37.81 Candidal esophagitis   HIV   CC   HCC

B37.82 Candidal enteritis   HIV   CC
Candidal proctitis

B37.83 Candidal cheilitis   HIV   CC

B37.84 Candidal otitis externa   HIV   CC

B37.89 Other sites of candidiasis   HIV   CC
Candidal osteomyelitis

B37.9 Candidiasis, unspecified   HIV
Thrush NOS

✓4ᵗʰ **B38 Coccidioidomycosis**

B38.0 Acute pulmonary coccidioidomycosis   HIV   CC   HCC

B38.1 Chronic pulmonary coccidioidomycosis   HIV   CC   HCC

B38.2 Pulmonary coccidioidomycosis, unspecified   HIV   CC   HCC

B38.3 Cutaneous coccidioidomycosis   HIV   CC

B38.4 Coccidioidomycosis meningitis   HIV   MCC
DEF: Coccidioides immitis infection of the lining of the brain and/or spinal cord.

B38.7 Disseminated coccidioidomycosis   HIV   CC
Generalized coccidioidomycosis

✓5ᵗʰ **B38.8 Other forms of coccidioidomycosis**

B38.81 Prostatic coccidioidomycosis   HIV   CC   ♂

B38.89 Other forms of coccidioidomycosis   HIV   CC

B38.9 Coccidioidomycosis, unspecified   HIV   CC

N Newborn: 0   P Pediatric: 0-17   M Maternity: 9-64   A Adult: 15-124   MCC Major Complication/Comorbidity   CC Complication/Comorbidity   SW Severe Wound Dx

458   ICD-10-CM 2021

B34.1–B38.9

✓4ᵗʰ **B39 Histoplasmosis**

Code first associated AIDS (B20)

Use additional code for any associated manifestations, such as:

endocarditis (I39)
meningitis (G02)
pericarditis (I32)
retinitis (H32)

DEF: Type of lung infection caused by breathing in fungal spores often found in the droppings of bats and birds or soil contaminated by their droppings.

Histoplasmosis

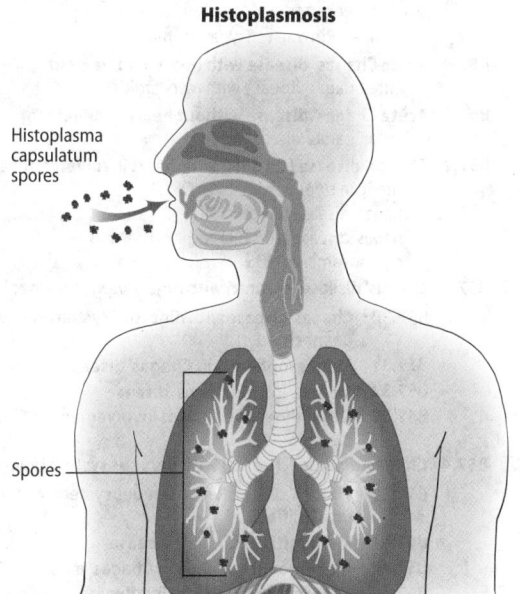

Histoplasma capsulatum spores

Spores

B39.0 Acute pulmonary histoplasmosis capsulati   `HIV` `MCC` `HCC`
B39.1 Chronic pulmonary histoplasmosis capsulati   `HIV` `MCC` `HCC`
B39.2 Pulmonary histoplasmosis capsulati, unspecified   `HIV` `MCC` `HCC`
B39.3 Disseminated histoplasmosis capsulati   `HIV` `CC`
     Generalized histoplasmosis capsulati
B39.4 Histoplasmosis capsulati, unspecified   `HIV`
     American histoplasmosis
B39.5 Histoplasmosis duboisii   `HIV`
     African histoplasmosis
B39.9 Histoplasmosis, unspecified   `HIV`

✓4ᵗʰ **B40 Blastomycosis**

     EXCLUDES 1   *Brazilian blastomycosis (B41.-)*
               keloidal blastomycosis (B48.0)

B40.0 Acute pulmonary blastomycosis   `CC` `HCC`
B40.1 Chronic pulmonary blastomycosis   `CC` `HCC`
B40.2 Pulmonary blastomycosis, unspecified   `CC` `HCC`
B40.3 Cutaneous blastomycosis   `CC`
B40.7 Disseminated blastomycosis   `CC`
     Generalized blastomycosis
✓5ᵗʰ **B40.8 Other forms of blastomycosis**

     B40.81 Blastomycotic meningoencephalitis   `CC`
           Meningomyelitis due to blastomycosis
     B40.89 Other forms of blastomycosis   `CC`
B40.9 Blastomycosis, unspecified   `CC`

✓4ᵗʰ **B41 Paracoccidioidomycosis**

     INCLUDES   Brazilian blastomycosis
            Lutz' disease

B41.0 Pulmonary paracoccidioidomycosis   `CC` `HCC`
B41.7 Disseminated paracoccidioidomycosis   `CC`
     Generalized paracoccidioidomycosis
B41.8 Other forms of paracoccidioidomycosis   `CC`
B41.9 Paracoccidioidomycosis, unspecified   `CC`

✓4ᵗʰ **B42 Sporotrichosis**

B42.0 Pulmonary sporotrichosis
B42.1 Lymphocutaneous sporotrichosis

B42.7 Disseminated sporotrichosis
     Generalized sporotrichosis
✓5ᵗʰ **B42.8 Other forms of sporotrichosis**

     B42.81 Cerebral sporotrichosis
           Meningitis due to sporotrichosis
     B42.82 Sporotrichosis arthritis   `HCC`
     B42.89 Other forms of sporotrichosis
B42.9 Sporotrichosis, unspecified

✓4ᵗʰ **B43 Chromomycosis and pheomycotic abscess**

B43.0 Cutaneous chromomycosis
     Dermatitis verrucosa
B43.1 Pheomycotic brain abscess
     Cerebral chromomycosis
B43.2 Subcutaneous pheomycotic abscess and cyst
B43.8 Other forms of chromomycosis
B43.9 Chromomycosis, unspecified

✓4ᵗʰ **B44 Aspergillosis**

     INCLUDES   aspergilloma

B44.0 Invasive pulmonary aspergillosis   `MCC` `HCC`
B44.1 Other pulmonary aspergillosis   `CC` `HCC`
B44.2 Tonsillar aspergillosis   `CC` `HCC`
B44.7 Disseminated aspergillosis   `CC` `HCC`
     Generalized aspergillosis
✓5ᵗʰ **B44.8 Other forms of aspergillosis**

     B44.81 Allergic bronchopulmonary aspergillosis   `CC` `HCC`
     B44.89 Other forms of aspergillosis   `CC` `HCC`
B44.9 Aspergillosis, unspecified   `CC` `HCC`

✓4ᵗʰ **B45 Cryptococcosis**

B45.0 Pulmonary cryptococcosis   `HIV` `CC` `HCC`
B45.1 Cerebral cryptococcosis   `MCC` `HCC`
     Cryptococcal meningitis
     Cryptococcosis meningocerebralis
B45.2 Cutaneous cryptococcosis   `HIV` `CC` `HCC`
B45.3 Osseous cryptococcosis   `HIV` `CC` `HCC`
B45.7 Disseminated cryptococcosis   `HIV` `CC` `HCC`
     Generalized cryptococcosis
B45.8 Other forms of cryptococcosis   `HIV` `CC` `HCC`
B45.9 Cryptococcosis, unspecified   `HIV` `CC` `HCC`

✓4ᵗʰ **B46 Zygomycosis**

B46.0 Pulmonary mucormycosis   `MCC` `HCC`
B46.1 Rhinocerebral mucormycosis   `MCC` `HCC`
B46.2 Gastrointestinal mucormycosis   `MCC` `HCC`
B46.3 Cutaneous mucormycosis   `MCC` `HCC`
     Subcutaneous mucormycosis
B46.4 Disseminated mucormycosis   `MCC` `HCC`
     Generalized mucormycosis
B46.5 Mucormycosis, unspecified   `MCC` `HCC`
B46.8 Other zygomycoses   `MCC` `HCC`
     Entomophthoromycosis
B46.9 Zygomycosis, unspecified   `MCC` `HCC`
     Phycomycosis NOS

✓4ᵗʰ **B47 Mycetoma**

B47.0 Eumycetoma   `CC`
     Madura foot, mycotic
     Maduromycosis
B47.1 Actinomycetoma   `HIV` `CC`
B47.9 Mycetoma, unspecified   `HIV` `CC`
     Madura foot NOS

✓4ᵗʰ **B48 Other mycoses, not elsewhere classified**

B48.0 Lobomycosis
     Keloidal blastomycosis
     Lobo's disease
B48.1 Rhinosporidiosis
B48.2 Allescheriasis   `CC`
     Infection due to Pseudallescheria boydii
     EXCLUDES 1   *eumycetoma (B47.0)*
B48.3 Geotrichosis   `CC`
     Geotrichum stomatitis
B48.4 Penicillosis   `CC` `HCC`
     ▶Talaromycosis◀

☑ Additional Character Required   ✓x7ᵗʰ Placeholder   Unacceptable PDx   Questionable PDx   Manifestation   Unspecified Dx   `H1`-`H4` HAC   `HCC` CMS-HCC Dx   `HIV` HIV Dx

ICD-10-CM 2021   **459**

B48.8 Other specified mycoses `HIV` `CC` `HCC`
Adiaspiromycosis
Infection of tissue and organs by Alternaria
Infection of tissue and organs by Drechslera
Infection of tissue and organs by Fusarium
Infection of tissue and organs by saprophytic fungi NEC
AHA: 2014,4Q,46; 2014,2Q,13
TIP: This code is assigned when sepsis is documented as due to non-*Candida albicans*. If sepsis is due to any *Candida* type, code B37.7 Candidal sepsis, is assigned.

B49 Unspecified mycosis `CC`
Fungemia NOS

Protozoal diseases (B50-B64)

`EXCLUDES 1`   *amebiasis (A06.-)*
other protozoal intestinal diseases (A07.-)

✓4ᵗʰ **B50 Plasmodium falciparum malaria**
`INCLUDES`   mixed infections of Plasmodium falciparum with any other Plasmodium species

B50.0 Plasmodium falciparum malaria with cerebral complications `CC`
Cerebral malaria NOS

B50.8 Other severe and complicated Plasmodium falciparum malaria `CC`
Severe or complicated Plasmodium falciparum malaria NOS

B50.9 Plasmodium falciparum malaria, unspecified `MCC`

✓4ᵗʰ **B51 Plasmodium vivax malaria**
`INCLUDES`   mixed infections of Plasmodium vivax with other Plasmodium species, except Plasmodium falciparum
`EXCLUDES 1`   *Plasmodium vivax with Plasmodium falciparum (B50.-)*

B51.0 Plasmodium vivax malaria with rupture of spleen `CC`
B51.8 Plasmodium vivax malaria with other complications `CC`
B51.9 Plasmodium vivax malaria without complication `CC`
Plasmodium vivax malaria NOS

✓4ᵗʰ **B52 Plasmodium malariae malaria**
`INCLUDES`   mixed infections of Plasmodium malariae with other Plasmodium species, except Plasmodium falciparum and Plasmodium vivax
`EXCLUDES 1`   *Plasmodium falciparum (B50.-)*
Plasmodium vivax (B51.-)

B52.0 Plasmodium malariae malaria with nephropathy `CC`
B52.8 Plasmodium malariae malaria with other complications `CC`
B52.9 Plasmodium malariae malaria without complication `CC`
Plasmodium malariae malaria NOS

✓4ᵗʰ **B53 Other specified malaria**

B53.0 Plasmodium ovale malaria `CC`
`EXCLUDES 1`   *Plasmodium ovale with Plasmodium falciparum (B50.-)*
Plasmodium ovale with Plasmodium malariae (B52.-)
Plasmodium ovale with Plasmodium vivax (B51.-)

B53.1 Malaria due to simian plasmodia `CC`
`EXCLUDES 1`   *malaria due to simian plasmodia with Plasmodium falciparum (B50.-)*
malaria due to simian plasmodia with Plasmodium malariae (B52.-)
malaria due to simian plasmodia with Plasmodium ovale (B53.0)
malaria due to simian plasmodia with Plasmodium vivax (B51.-)

B53.8 Other malaria, not elsewhere classified `CC`

B54 Unspecified malaria `CC`

✓4ᵗʰ **B55 Leishmaniasis**

B55.0 Visceral leishmaniasis `CC`
Kala-azar
Post-kala-azar dermal leishmaniasis

B55.1 Cutaneous leishmaniasis `CC`
B55.2 Mucocutaneous leishmaniasis `CC`
B55.9 Leishmaniasis, unspecified `CC`

✓4ᵗʰ **B56 African trypanosomiasis**

B56.0 Gambiense trypanosomiasis `CC`
Infection due to Trypanosoma brucei gambiense
West African sleeping sickness

B56.1 Rhodesiense trypanosomiasis `CC`
East African sleeping sickness
Infection due to Trypanosoma brucei rhodesiense

B56.9 African trypanosomiasis, unspecified `CC`
Sleeping sickness NOS

✓4ᵗʰ **B57 Chagas' disease**
`INCLUDES`   American trypanosomiasis
infection due to Trypanosoma cruzi

B57.0 Acute Chagas' disease with heart involvement `CC`
Acute Chagas' disease with myocarditis

B57.1 Acute Chagas' disease without heart involvement `CC`
Acute Chagas' disease NOS

B57.2 Chagas' disease (chronic) with heart involvement `CC`
American trypanosomiasis NOS
Chagas' disease (chronic) NOS
Chagas' disease (chronic) with myocarditis
Trypanosomiasis NOS

✓5ᵗʰ **B57.3 Chagas' disease (chronic) with digestive system involvement**

B57.30 Chagas' disease with digestive system involvement, unspecified `CC`
B57.31 Megaesophagus in Chagas' disease `CC`
B57.32 Megacolon in Chagas' disease `CC`
B57.39 Other digestive system involvement in Chagas' disease `CC`

✓5ᵗʰ **B57.4 Chagas' disease (chronic) with nervous system involvement**

B57.40 Chagas' disease with nervous system involvement, unspecified `CC`
B57.41 Meningitis in Chagas' disease `CC`
B57.42 Meningoencephalitis in Chagas' disease `CC`
B57.49 Other nervous system involvement in Chagas' disease `CC`

B57.5 Chagas' disease (chronic) with other organ involvement `CC`

✓4ᵗʰ **B58 Toxoplasmosis**
`INCLUDES`   infection due to Toxoplasma gondii
`EXCLUDES 1`   *congenital toxoplasmosis (P37.1)*

✓5ᵗʰ **B58.0 Toxoplasma oculopathy**

B58.00 Toxoplasma oculopathy, unspecified `HIV` `CC`
B58.01 Toxoplasma chorioretinitis `HIV` `CC`
B58.09 Other toxoplasma oculopathy `HIV` `CC`
Toxoplasma uveitis

B58.1 Toxoplasma hepatitis `HIV` `CC`
B58.2 Toxoplasma meningoencephalitis `HIV` `MCC` `HCC`
B58.3 Pulmonary toxoplasmosis `HIV` `MCC` `HCC`

✓5ᵗʰ **B58.8 Toxoplasmosis with other organ involvement**

B58.81 Toxoplasma myocarditis `HIV` `MCC`
B58.82 Toxoplasma myositis `HIV` `CC`
B58.83 Toxoplasma tubulo-interstitial nephropathy `HIV` `CC`
Toxoplasma pyelonephritis
B58.89 Toxoplasmosis with other organ involvement `HIV` `CC`

B58.9 Toxoplasmosis, unspecified `HIV` `CC`

B59 Pneumocystosis `HIV` `MCC` `HCC`
Pneumonia due to Pneumocystis carinii
Pneumonia due to Pneumocystis jiroveci

✓4ᵗʰ **B60 Other protozoal diseases, not elsewhere classified**
`EXCLUDES 1`   *cryptosporidiosis (A07.2)*
intestinal microsporidiosis (A07.8)
isosporiasis (A07.3)

▲ ✓5ᵗʰ **B60.0 Babesiosis**
Piroplasmosis

● **B60.00 Babesiosis, unspecified** `CC`
Babesiosis due to unspecified Babesia species
Piroplasmosis, unspecified

● **B60.01 Babesiosis due to Babesia microti** `CC`
Infection due to B. microti

●   **B60.02**   **Babesiosis due to** Babesia duncani   `CC`
Infection due to B. duncani and B. duncani-type species

●   **B60.03**   **Babesiosis due to** Babesia divergens   `CC`
Babesiosis due to Babesia MO-1
Infection due to B. divergens and B. divergens-like strains

●   **B60.09**   **Other babesiosis**   `CC`
Babesiosis due to Babesia KO-1
Babesiosis due to Babesia venatorum
Infection due to other Babesia species
Infection due to other protozoa of the order Piroplasmida
Other piroplasmosis

√5ᵗʰ **B60.1**   **Acanthamebiasis**

     B60.10   **Acanthamebiasis, unspecified**   `CC`

     B60.11   **Meningoencephalitis due to Acanthamoeba (culbertsoni)**

     B60.12   **Conjunctivitis due to Acanthamoeba**

     B60.13   **Keratoconjunctivitis due to Acanthamoeba**

     B60.19   **Other acanthamebic disease**   `CC`

B60.2   **Naegleriasis**
Primary amebic meningoencephalitis

B60.8   **Other specified protozoal diseases**   `HIV`
Microsporidiosis

B64   **Unspecified protozoal disease**

Helminthiases (B65-B83)

√4ᵗʰ **B65**   **Schistosomiasis [bilharziasis]**

   `INCLUDES`   snail fever

B65.0   **Schistosomiasis due to** Schistosoma haematobium **[urinary schistosomiasis]**   `CC`

B65.1   **Schistosomiasis due to** Schistosoma mansoni **[intestinal schistosomiasis]**   `CC`

B65.2   **Schistosomiasis due to** Schistosoma japonicum   `CC`
Asiatic schistosomiasis

B65.3   **Cercarial dermatitis**   `CC`
Swimmer's itch

B65.8   **Other schistosomiasis**   `CC`
Infection due to Schistosoma intercalatum
Infection due to Schistosoma mattheei
Infection due to Schistosoma mekongi

B65.9   **Schistosomiasis, unspecified**   `CC`

√4ᵗʰ **B66**   **Other fluke infections**

B66.0   **Opisthorchiasis**   `CC`
Infection due to cat liver fluke
Infection due to Opisthorchis (felineus)(viverrini)

B66.1   **Clonorchiasis**   `CC`
Chinese liver fluke disease
Infection due to Clonorchis sinensis
Oriental liver fluke disease

B66.2   **Dicroceliasis**   `CC`
Infection due to Dicrocoelium dendriticum
Lancet fluke infection

B66.3   **Fascioliasis**   `CC`
Infection due to Fasciola gigantica
Infection due to Fasciola hepatica
Infection due to Fasciola indica
Sheep liver fluke disease

B66.4   **Paragonimiasis**   `CC` `HCC`
Infection due to Paragonimus species
Lung fluke disease
Pulmonary distomiasis

B66.5   **Fasciolopsiasis**   `CC`
Infection due to Fasciolopsis buski
Intestinal distomiasis

B66.8   **Other specified fluke infections**   `CC`
Echinostomiasis
Heterophyiasis
Metagonimiasis
Nanophyetiasis
Watsoniasis

B66.9   **Fluke infection, unspecified**

√4ᵗʰ **B67**   **Echinococcosis**

   `INCLUDES`   hydatidosis

B67.0   **Echinococcus granulosus infection of liver**   `CC`

B67.1   **Echinococcus granulosus infection of lung**   `CC` `HCC`

B67.2   **Echinococcus granulosus infection of bone**   `CC`

√5ᵗʰ **B67.3**   **Echinococcus granulosus infection, other and multiple sites**

     B67.31   **Echinococcus granulosus infection, thyroid gland**   `CC`

     B67.32   **Echinococcus granulosus infection, multiple sites**   `CC`

     B67.39   **Echinococcus granulosus infection, other sites**   `CC`

B67.4   **Echinococcus granulosus infection, unspecified**   `CC`
Dog tapeworm (infection)

B67.5   **Echinococcus multilocularis infection of liver**   `CC`

√5ᵗʰ **B67.6**   **Echinococcus multilocularis infection, other and multiple sites**

     B67.61   **Echinococcus multilocularis infection, multiple sites**   `CC`

     B67.69   **Echinococcus multilocularis infection, other sites**   `CC`

B67.7   **Echinococcus multilocularis infection, unspecified**   `CC`

B67.8   **Echinococcosis, unspecified, of liver**   `CC`

√5ᵗʰ **B67.9**   **Echinococcosis, other and unspecified**

     B67.90   **Echinococcosis, unspecified**   `CC`
Echinococcosis NOS

     B67.99   **Other echinococcosis**   `CC`

√4ᵗʰ **B68**   **Taeniasis**

   `EXCLUDES 1`   cysticercosis (B69.-)

B68.0   **Taenia solium taeniasis**   `CC`
Pork tapeworm (infection)

B68.1   **Taenia saginata taeniasis**   `CC`
Beef tapeworm (infection)
Infection due to adult tapeworm Taenia saginata

B68.9   **Taeniasis, unspecified**   `CC`

√4ᵗʰ **B69**   **Cysticercosis**

   `INCLUDES`   cysticerciasis infection due to larval form of Taenia solium
DEF: Condition that is developed when larvae or eggs of the tapeworm *Taenia solium* are ingested, most commonly in fecally contaminated water or undercooked pork.

B69.0   **Cysticercosis of central nervous system**   `CC`

B69.1   **Cysticercosis of eye**   `CC`

√5ᵗʰ **B69.8**   **Cysticercosis of other sites**

     B69.81   **Myositis in cysticercosis**   `CC`

     B69.89   **Cysticercosis of other sites**   `CC`

B69.9   **Cysticercosis, unspecified**   `CC`

√4ᵗʰ **B70**   **Diphyllobothriasis and sparganosis**

B70.0   **Diphyllobothriasis**   `CC`
Diphyllobothrium (adult) (latum) (pacificum) infection
Fish tapeworm (infection)
   `EXCLUDES 2`   larval diphyllobothriasis (B70.1)

B70.1   **Sparganosis**   `CC`
Infection due to Sparganum (mansoni) (proliferum)
Infection due to Spirometra larva
Larval diphyllobothriasis
Spirometrosis

√4ᵗʰ **B71**   **Other cestode infections**

B71.0   **Hymenolepiasis**   `CC`
Dwarf tapeworm infection
Rat tapeworm (infection)

B71.1   **Dipylidiasis**   `CC`

B71.8   **Other specified cestode infections**   `CC`
Coenurosis

B71.9   **Cestode infection, unspecified**
Tapeworm (infection) NOS

B72   **Dracunculiasis**   `CC`
   `INCLUDES`   guinea worm infection
infection due to Dracunculus medinensis

☑ Additional Character Required   √x7ᵗʰ Placeholder   Unacceptable PDx   Questionable PDx   Manifestation   Unspecified Dx   H1-H14 HAC   HCC CMS-HCC Dx   HIV HIV Dx

ICD-10-CM 2021   **461**

Chapter 1. Certain Infectious and Parasitic Diseases

B60.02–B72

Chapter 1. Certain Infectious and Parasitic Diseases

✓4ᵗʰ B73 Onchocerciasis
    INCLUDES   onchocerca volvulus infection
      onchocercosis
      river blindness
   ✓5ᵗʰ B73.0 Onchocerciasis with eye disease
    B73.00 Onchocerciasis with eye involvement, unspecified CC
    B73.01 Onchocerciasis with endophthalmitis CC
    B73.02 Onchocerciasis with glaucoma CC
    B73.09 Onchocerciasis with other eye involvement CC
      Infestation of eyelid due to onchocerciasis
   B73.1 Onchocerciasis without eye disease CC

✓4ᵗʰ B74 Filariasis
    EXCLUDES 2   onchocerciasis (B73)
      tropical (pulmonary) eosinophilia NOS (J82)
   B74.0 Filariasis due to Wuchereria bancrofti CC
      Bancroftian elephantiasis
      Bancroftian filariasis
   B74.1 Filariasis due to Brugia malayi CC
   B74.2 Filariasis due to Brugia timori CC
   B74.3 Loiasis CC
      Calabar swelling
      Eyeworm disease of Africa
      Loa loa infection
   B74.4 Mansonelliasis CC
      Infection due to Mansonella ozzardi
      Infection due to Mansonella perstans
      Infection due to Mansonella streptocerca
   B74.8 Other filariases CC
      Dirofilariasis
   B74.9 Filariasis, unspecified CC

B75 Trichinellosis CC
    INCLUDES   infection due to Trichinella species
      trichiniasis
    DEF: Infection by *Trichinella spiralis,* the smallest of the parasitic nematodes, that is transmitted by eating undercooked pork or bear meat. **Synonym(s):** *Trichinosis.*

✓4ᵗʰ B76 Hookworm diseases
    INCLUDES   uncinariasis
   B76.0 Ancylostomiasis CC
      Infection due to Ancylostoma species
   B76.1 Necatoriasis CC
      Infection due to Necator americanus
   B76.8 Other hookworm diseases CC
   B76.9 Hookworm disease, unspecified CC
      Cutaneous larva migrans NOS

✓4ᵗʰ B77 Ascariasis
    INCLUDES   ascaridiasis
      roundworm infection
   B77.0 Ascariasis with intestinal complications CC
   ✓5ᵗʰ B77.8 Ascariasis with other complications
    B77.81 Ascariasis pneumonia MCC
    B77.89 Ascariasis with other complications CC
   B77.9 Ascariasis, unspecified CC

✓4ᵗʰ B78 Strongyloidiasis
    EXCLUDES 1   trichostrongyliasis (B81.2)
   B78.0 Intestinal strongyloidiasis HIV CC
   B78.1 Cutaneous strongyloidiasis
   B78.7 Disseminated strongyloidiasis HIV CC
   B78.9 Strongyloidiasis, unspecified HIV CC

B79 Trichuriasis CC
    INCLUDES   trichocephaliasis
      whipworm (disease)(infection)

B80 Enterobiasis CC
    INCLUDES   oxyuriasis
      pinworm infection
      threadworm infection

✓4ᵗʰ B81 Other intestinal helminthiases, not elsewhere classified
    EXCLUDES 1   angiostrongyliasis due to:
      angiostrongylus cantonensis (B83.2)
      parastrongylus cantonensis (B83.2)
   B81.0 Anisakiasis CC
      Infection due to Anisakis larva
   B81.1 Intestinal capillariasis CC
      Capillariasis NOS
      Infection due to Capillaria philippinensis
    EXCLUDES 2   hepatic capillariasis (B83.8)
   B81.2 Trichostrongyliasis CC
   B81.3 Intestinal angiostrongyliasis
      Angiostrongyliasis due to:
      angiostrongylus costaricensis
      parastrongylus costaricensis
   B81.4 Mixed intestinal helminthiases CC
      Infection due to intestinal helminths classified to more than one of the categories B65.0-B81.3 and B81.8
      Mixed helminthiasis NOS
   B81.8 Other specified intestinal helminthiases CC
      Infection due to Oesophagostomum species [esophagostomiasis]
      Infection due to Ternidens diminutus [ternidensiasis]

✓4ᵗʰ B82 Unspecified intestinal parasitism
   B82.0 Intestinal helminthiasis, unspecified CC
   B82.9 Intestinal parasitism, unspecified

✓4ᵗʰ B83 Other helminthiases
    EXCLUDES 1   capillariasis NOS (B81.1)
    EXCLUDES 2   intestinal capillariasis (B81.1)
   B83.0 Visceral larva migrans
      Toxocariasis
   B83.1 Gnathostomiasis
      Wandering swelling
   B83.2 Angiostrongyliasis due to Parastrongylus cantonensis
      Eosinophilic meningoencephalitis due to Parastrongylus cantonensis
    EXCLUDES 2   intestinal angiostrongyliasis (B81.3)
   B83.3 Syngamiasis
      Syngamosis
   B83.4 Internal hirudiniasis
    EXCLUDES 2   external hirudiniasis (B88.3)
   B83.8 Other specified helminthiases
      Acanthocephaliasis
      Gongylonemiasis
      Hepatic capillariasis
      Metastrongyliasis
      Thelaziasis
   B83.9 Helminthiasis, unspecified
      Worms NOS
    EXCLUDES 1   intestinal helminthiasis NOS (B82.0)

Pediculosis, acariasis and other infestations (B85-B89)

✓4ᵗʰ B85 Pediculosis and phthiriasis
   B85.0 Pediculosis due to Pediculus humanus capitis
      Head-louse infestation
   B85.1 Pediculosis due to Pediculus humanus corporis
      Body-louse infestation
   B85.2 Pediculosis, unspecified
   B85.3 Phthiriasis
      Infestation by crab-louse
      Infestation by Phthirus pubis
   B85.4 Mixed pediculosis and phthiriasis
      Infestation classifiable to more than one of the categories B85.0-B85.3

B86 Scabies
      Sarcoptic itch
    DEF: Mite infestation that is caused by *Sarcoptes scabiei.* Scabies causes intense itching and sometimes secondary infection.

✓4ᵗʰ B87 Myiasis
    INCLUDES   infestation by larva of flies
   B87.0 Cutaneous myiasis
      Creeping myiasis

B87.1   **Wound myiasis**
Traumatic myiasis

B87.2   **Ocular myiasis**

B87.3   **Nasopharyngeal myiasis**
Laryngeal myiasis

B87.4   **Aural myiasis**

☑5ᵗʰ **B87.8**   **Myiasis of other sites**

    B87.81   **Genitourinary myiasis**

    B87.82   **Intestinal myiasis**

    B87.89   **Myiasis of other sites**

B87.9   **Myiasis, unspecified**

☑4ᵗʰ **B88**   **Other infestations**

B88.0   **Other acariasis**
Acarine dermatitis
Dermatitis due to Demodex species
Dermatitis due to Dermanyssus gallinae
Dermatitis due to Liponyssoides sanguineus
Trombiculosis
EXCLUDES 2   scabies (B86)

B88.1   **Tungiasis [sandflea infestation]**

B88.2   **Other arthropod infestations**
Scarabiasis

B88.3   **External hirudiniasis**
Leech infestation NOS
EXCLUDES 2   internal hirudiniasis (B83.4)

B88.8   **Other specified infestations**
Ichthyoparasitism due to Vandellia cirrhosa
Linguatulosis
Porocephaliasis

B88.9   **Infestation, unspecified**
Infestation (skin) NOS
Infestation by mites NOS
Skin parasites NOS

B89   **Unspecified parasitic disease**

Sequelae of infectious and parasitic diseases (B90-B94)

NOTE   Categories B90-B94 are to be used to indicate conditions in categories A00-B89 as the cause of sequelae, which are themselves classified elsewhere. The "sequelae" include conditions specified as such; they also include residuals of diseases classifiable to the above categories if there is evidence that the disease itself is no longer present. Codes from these categories are not to be used for chronic infections. Code chronic current infections to active infectious disease as appropriate.

Code first condition resulting from (sequela) the infectious or parasitic disease

☑4ᵗʰ **B90**   **Sequelae of tuberculosis**

B90.0   **Sequelae of central nervous system tuberculosis**

B90.1   **Sequelae of genitourinary tuberculosis**

B90.2   **Sequelae of tuberculosis of bones and joints**

B90.8   **Sequelae of tuberculosis of other organs**
EXCLUDES 2   sequelae of respiratory tuberculosis (B90.9)

B90.9   **Sequelae of respiratory and unspecified tuberculosis**
Sequelae of tuberculosis NOS

B91   **Sequelae of poliomyelitis**
EXCLUDES 1   postpolio syndrome (G14)

B92   **Sequelae of leprosy**

☑4ᵗʰ **B94**   **Sequelae of other and unspecified infectious and parasitic diseases**

B94.0   **Sequelae of trachoma**

B94.1   **Sequelae of viral encephalitis**

B94.2   **Sequelae of viral hepatitis**

B94.8   **Sequelae of other specified infectious and parasitic diseases**
AHA: 2017,4Q,109

B94.9   **Sequelae of unspecified infectious and parasitic disease**

Bacterial and viral infectious agents (B95-B97)

NOTE   These categories are provided for use as supplementary or additional codes to identify the infectious agent(s) in diseases classified elsewhere.

AHA: 2020,2Q,18; 2018,4Q,34; 2018,1Q,16

☑4ᵗʰ **B95**   **Streptococcus, Staphylococcus, and Enterococcus as the cause of diseases classified elsewhere**

B95.0   **Streptococcus, group A, as the cause of diseases classified elsewhere**

B95.1   **Streptococcus, group B, as the cause of diseases classified elsewhere**
AHA: 2020,1Q,10; 2019,2Q,8-10

B95.2   **Enterococcus as the cause of diseases classified elsewhere**

B95.3   **Streptococcus pneumoniae as the cause of diseases classified elsewhere**

B95.4   **Other streptococcus as the cause of diseases classified elsewhere**

B95.5   **Unspecified streptococcus as the cause of diseases classified elsewhere**

☑5ᵗʰ **B95.6**   **Staphylococcus aureus as the cause of diseases classified elsewhere**

    B95.61   **Methicillin susceptible Staphylococcus aureus infection as the cause of diseases classified elsewhere**
Methicillin susceptible Staphylococcus aureus (MSSA) infection as the cause of diseases classified elsewhere
Staphylococcus aureus infection NOS as the cause of diseases classified elsewhere

    B95.62   **Methicillin resistant Staphylococcus aureus infection as the cause of diseases classified elsewhere**
Methicillin resistant staphylococcus aureus (MRSA) infection as the cause of diseases classified elsewhere
AHA: 2016,1Q,12

B95.7   **Other staphylococcus as the cause of diseases classified elsewhere**

B95.8   **Unspecified staphylococcus as the cause of diseases classified elsewhere**

☑4ᵗʰ **B96**   **Other bacterial agents as the cause of diseases classified elsewhere**

B96.0   **Mycoplasma pneumoniae [M. pneumoniae] as the cause of diseases classified elsewhere**
Pleuro-pneumonia-like-organism [PPLO]

B96.1   **Klebsiella pneumoniae [K. pneumoniae] as the cause of diseases classified elsewhere**

☑5ᵗʰ **B96.2**   **Escherichia coli [E. coli] as the cause of diseases classified elsewhere**

    B96.20   **Unspecified Escherichia coli [E. coli] as the cause of diseases classified elsewhere**
Escherichia coli [E. coli] NOS

    B96.21   **Shiga toxin-producing Escherichia coli [E. coli] [STEC] O157 as the cause of diseases classified elsewhere**
E. coli O157:H- (nonmotile) with confirmation of Shiga toxin
E. coli O157 with confirmation of Shiga toxin when H antigen is unknown, or is not H7
O157:H7 Escherichia coli [E.coli] with or without confirmation of Shiga toxin-production
Shiga toxin-producing Escherichia coli [E.coli] O157:H7 with or without confirmation of Shiga toxin-production
STEC O157:H7 with or without confirmation of Shiga toxin-production

    B96.22   **Other specified Shiga toxin-producing Escherichia coli [E. coli] [STEC] as the cause of diseases classified elsewhere**
Non-O157 Shiga toxin-producing Escherichia coli [E.coli]
Non-O157 Shiga toxin-producing Escherichia coli [E.coli] with known O group

    B96.23   **Unspecified Shiga toxin-producing Escherichia coli [E. coli] [STEC] as the cause of diseases classified elsewhere**
Shiga toxin-producing Escherichia coli [E. coli] with unspecified O group
STEC NOS

    B96.29   **Other Escherichia coli [E. coli] as the cause of diseases classified elsewhere**
Non-Shiga toxin-producing E. coli

B96.3   **Hemophilus influenzae [H. influenzae] as the cause of diseases classified elsewhere**

B96.4   **Proteus (mirabilis) (morganii) as the cause of diseases classified elsewhere**

B96.5   **Pseudomonas (aeruginosa) (mallei) (pseudomallei) as the cause of diseases classified elsewhere**
AHA: 2015,1Q,18

Chapter 1. Certain Infectious and Parasitic Diseases

B96.6   Bacteroides fragilis [B. fragilis] as the cause of diseases classified elsewhere

B96.7   Clostridium perfringens [C. perfringens] as the cause of diseases classified elsewhere

√5ᵗʰ **B96.8**   Other specified bacterial agents as the cause of diseases classified elsewhere

     B96.81   Helicobacter pylori [H. pylori] as the cause of diseases classified elsewhere

     B96.82   Vibrio vulnificus as the cause of diseases classified elsewhere

     B96.89   Other specified bacterial agents as the cause of diseases classified elsewhere

√4ᵗʰ **B97**   **Viral agents as the cause of diseases classified elsewhere**

     AHA: 2016,3Q,8-10,14

B97.0   Adenovirus as the cause of diseases classified elsewhere

√5ᵗʰ **B97.1**   Enterovirus as the cause of diseases classified elsewhere

     B97.10   Unspecified enterovirus as the cause of diseases classified elsewhere

     B97.11   Coxsackievirus as the cause of diseases classified elsewhere

     B97.12   Echovirus as the cause of diseases classified elsewhere

     B97.19   Other enterovirus as the cause of diseases classified elsewhere

√5ᵗʰ **B97.2**   Coronavirus as the cause of diseases classified elsewhere

     TIP: Do not report a code from this subcategory for COVID-19; refer to U07.1.

     B97.21   SARS-associated coronavirus as the cause of diseases classified elsewhere   CC

         EXCLUDES 1   *pneumonia due to SARS-associated coronavirus (J12.81)*

     B97.29   Other coronavirus as the cause of diseases classified elsewhere

         AHA: 2020,2Q,5; 2020,1Q,34-36

√5ᵗʰ **B97.3**   Retrovirus as the cause of diseases classified elsewhere

     EXCLUDES 1   *human immunodeficiency virus [HIV] disease (B20)*

     B97.30   Unspecified retrovirus as the cause of diseases classified elsewhere

     B97.31   Lentivirus as the cause of diseases classified elsewhere

     B97.32   Oncovirus as the cause of diseases classified elsewhere

     B97.33   Human T-cell lymphotrophic virus, type I [HTLV-I] as the cause of diseases classified elsewhere   CC

     B97.34   Human T-cell lymphotrophic virus, type II [HTLV-II] as the cause of diseases classified elsewhere   CC

     B97.35   Human immunodeficiency virus, type 2 [HIV 2] as the cause of diseases classified elsewhere   CC   HCC

     B97.39   Other retrovirus as the cause of diseases classified elsewhere

B97.4   Respiratory syncytial virus as the cause of diseases classified elsewhere

     RSV as the cause of diseases classified elsewhere

     Code first related disorders, such as:

       otitis media (H65.-)

       upper respiratory infection (J06.9)

     EXCLUDES 2   *acute bronchiolitis due to respiratory syncytial virus (RSV) (J21.0)*

         acute bronchitis due to respiratory syncytial virus (RSV) (J20.5)

         respiratory syncytial virus (RSV) pneumonia (J12.1)

B97.5   Reovirus as the cause of diseases classified elsewhere

B97.6   Parvovirus as the cause of diseases classified elsewhere

B97.7   Papillomavirus as the cause of diseases classified elsewhere

√5ᵗʰ **B97.8**   Other viral agents as the cause of diseases classified elsewhere

     B97.81   Human metapneumovirus as the cause of diseases classified elsewhere

     B97.89   Other viral agents as the cause of diseases classified elsewhere

Other infectious diseases (B99)

√4ᵗʰ **B99**   **Other and unspecified infectious diseases**

B99.8   Other infectious disease   HIV

B99.9   Unspecified infectious disease

N Newborn: 0   P Pediatric: 0-17   M Maternity: 9-64   A Adult: 15-124   MCC Major Complication/Comorbidity   CC Complication/Comorbidity   SW Severe Wound Dx

464   ICD-10-CM 2021

Chapter 2. Neoplasms (C00–D49)

Chapter-specific Guidelines with Coding Examples

The chapter-specific guidelines from the ICD-10-CM Official Guidelines for Coding and Reporting have been provided below. Along with these guidelines are coding examples, contained in the shaded boxes, that have been developed to help illustrate the coding and/or sequencing guidance found in these guidelines.

General guidelines

Chapter 2 of the ICD-10-CM contains the codes for most benign and all malignant neoplasms. Certain benign neoplasms, such as prostatic adenomas, may be found in the specific body system chapters. To properly code a neoplasm, it is necessary to determine from the record if the neoplasm is benign, in-situ, malignant, or of uncertain histologic behavior. If malignant, any secondary (metastatic) sites should also be determined.

Primary malignant neoplasms overlapping site boundaries

A primary malignant neoplasm that overlaps two or more contiguous (next to each other) sites should be classified to the subcategory/code .8 ('overlapping lesion'), unless the combination is specifically indexed elsewhere. For multiple neoplasms of the same site that are not contiguous such as tumors in different quadrants of the same breast, codes for each site should be assigned.

> A 73-year-old white female with a large rapidly growing malignant tumor in the left breast extending from the upper outer quadrant into the axillary tail
>
> **C50.812   Malignant neoplasm of overlapping sites of left female breast**
>
> *Explanation*: Because this is a single large tumor that overlaps two contiguous sites, a single code for overlapping sites is assigned.

> A 52-year old white female with two distinct lesions of the right breast, one (0.5 cm) in the upper outer quadrant and a second (1.5 cm) in the lower outer quadrant; path report indicates both lesions are malignant
>
> **C50.411   Malignant neoplasm of upper-outer quadrant of right female breast**
>
> **C50.511   Malignant neoplasm of lower-outer quadrant of right female breast**
>
> *Explanation*: This patient has two distinct malignant lesions of right breast in adjacent quadrants. Because the lesions are not contiguous, two codes are reported.

Malignant neoplasm of ectopic tissue

Malignant neoplasms of ectopic tissue are to be coded to the site of origin mentioned, e.g., ectopic pancreatic malignant neoplasms involving the stomach are coded to malignant neoplasm of pancreas, unspecified (C25.9).

The neoplasm table in the Alphabetic Index should be referenced first. However, if the histological term is documented, that term should be referenced first, rather than going immediately to the Neoplasm Table, in order to determine which column in the Neoplasm Table is appropriate. For example, if the documentation indicates "adenoma," refer to the term in the Alphabetic Index to review the entries under this term and the instructional note to "see also neoplasm, by site, benign." The table provides the proper code based on the type of neoplasm and the site. It is important to select the proper column in the table that corresponds to the type of neoplasm. The Tabular List should then be referenced to verify that the correct code has been selected from the table and that a more specific site code does not exist.

See Section I.C.21. Factors influencing health status and contact with health services, Status, for information regarding Z15.0, codes for genetic susceptibility to cancer.

a. Treatment directed at the malignancy

If the treatment is directed at the malignancy, designate the malignancy as the principal diagnosis.

The only exception to this guideline is if a patient admission/encounter is solely for the administration of chemotherapy, immunotherapy or external beam radiation therapy, assign the appropriate Z51.-- code as the first-listed or principal diagnosis, and the diagnosis or problem for which the service is being performed as a secondary diagnosis.

b. Treatment of secondary site

When a patient is admitted because of a primary neoplasm with metastasis and treatment is directed toward the secondary site only, the secondary neoplasm is designated as the principal diagnosis even though the primary malignancy is still present.

> Patient with primary prostate cancer with metastasis to lungs admitted for wedge resection of mass in right lung
>
> **C78.01   Secondary malignant neoplasm of right lung**
>
> **C61   Malignant neoplasm of prostate**
>
> *Explanation*: Since the admission is for treatment of the lung metastasis, the secondary lung metastasis is sequenced before the primary prostate cancer.

c. Coding and sequencing of complications

Coding and sequencing of complications associated with the malignancies or with the therapy thereof are subject to the following guidelines:

1) Anemia associated with malignancy

When admission/encounter is for management of an anemia associated with the malignancy, and the treatment is only for anemia, the appropriate code for the malignancy is sequenced as the principal or first-listed diagnosis followed by the appropriate code for the anemia (such as code D63.0, Anemia in neoplastic disease).

> Patient is admitted for treatment of anemia in advanced colon cancer
>
> **C18.9   Malignant neoplasm of colon, unspecified**
>
> **D63.0   Anemia in neoplastic disease**
>
> *Explanation*: Even though the admission was solely to treat the anemia, this guideline indicates that the code for the malignancy is sequenced first.

2) Anemia associated with chemotherapy, immunotherapy and radiation therapy

When the admission/encounter is for management of an anemia associated with an adverse effect of the administration of chemotherapy or immunotherapy and the only treatment is for the anemia, the anemia code is sequenced first followed by the appropriate codes for the neoplasm and the adverse effect (T45.1X5, Adverse effect of antineoplastic and immunosuppressive drugs).

> A 56-year-old Hispanic male with grade II follicular lymphoma involving multiple lymph node sites referred for blood transfusion to treat anemia due to chemotherapy
>
> **D64.81   Anemia due to antineoplastic chemotherapy**
>
> **C82.18   Follicular lymphoma grade II, lymph nodes of multiple sites**
>
> **T45.1X5A   Adverse effect of antineoplastic and immunosuppressive drugs, initial encounter**
>
> *Explanation*: The code for the anemia is sequenced first followed by the code for the malignant neoplasm and lastly the code for the adverse effect.

When the admission/encounter is for management of an anemia associated with an adverse effect of radiotherapy, the anemia code should be sequenced first, followed by the appropriate neoplasm code and code Y84.2, Radiological procedure and radiotherapy as the cause of abnormal reaction of the patient, or of later complication, without mention of misadventure at the time of the procedure.

A 55-year-old male with a large malignant rectal tumor has been receiving external radiation therapy to shrink the tumor prior to planned surgery. He is admitted today for a blood transfusion to treat anemia related to radiation therapy.

D64.89	**Other specified anemias**
C20	**Malignant neoplasm of rectum**
Y84.2	**Radiological procedure and radiotherapy as the cause of abnormal reaction of the patient, or of later complication, without mention of misadventure at the time of the procedure**

Explanation: The code for the anemia is sequenced first, followed by the code for the malignancy, and lastly the code for the abnormal reaction due to radiotherapy.

3) Management of dehydration due to the malignancy

When the admission/encounter is for management of dehydration due to the malignancy and only the dehydration is being treated (intravenous rehydration), the dehydration is sequenced first, followed by the code(s) for the malignancy.

4) Treatment of a complication resulting from a surgical procedure

When the admission/encounter is for treatment of a complication resulting from a surgical procedure, designate the complication as the principal or first-listed diagnosis if treatment is directed at resolving the complication.

d. Primary malignancy previously excised

When a primary malignancy has been previously excised or eradicated from its site and there is no further treatment directed to that site and there is no evidence of any existing primary malignancy at that site, a code from category Z85, Personal history of malignant neoplasm, should be used to indicate the former site of the malignancy. Any mention of extension, invasion, or metastasis to another site is coded as a secondary malignant neoplasm to that site. The secondary site may be the principal or first-listed diagnosis with the Z85 code used as a secondary code.

History of breast cancer, left radical mastectomy 18 months ago with no current treatment; bronchoscopy with lung biopsy shows metastatic disease in the right lung

C78.01	**Secondary malignant neoplasm of right lung**
Z85.3	**Personal history of malignant neoplasm of breast**

Explanation: The patient has undergone a diagnostic procedure that revealed metastatic breast cancer in the right lung. The code for the secondary (metastatic) site is sequenced first followed by a personal history code to identify the former site of the primary malignancy.

e. Admissions/encounters involving chemotherapy, immunotherapy and radiation therapy

1) Episode of care involves surgical removal of neoplasm

When an episode of care involves the surgical removal of a neoplasm, primary or secondary site, followed by adjunct chemotherapy or radiation treatment during the same episode of care, the code for the neoplasm should be assigned as principal or first-listed diagnosis.

2) Patient admission/encounter solely for administration of chemotherapy, immunotherapy and radiation therapy

If a patient admission/encounter is solely for the administration of chemotherapy, immunotherapy or external beam radiation therapy assign code Z51.0, Encounter for antineoplastic radiation therapy, or Z51.11, Encounter for antineoplastic chemotherapy, or Z51.12, Encounter for antineoplastic immunotherapy as the first-listed or principal diagnosis. If a patient receives more than one of these therapies during the same admission more than one of these codes may be assigned, in any sequence.

The malignancy for which the therapy is being administered should be assigned as a secondary diagnosis.

If a patient admission/encounter is for the insertion or implantation of radioactive elements (e.g., brachytherapy) the appropriate code for the malignancy is sequenced as the principal or first-listed diagnosis. Code Z51.0 should not be assigned.

3) Patient admitted for radiation therapy, chemotherapy or immunotherapy and develops complications

When a patient is admitted for the purpose of external beam radiotherapy, immunotherapy or chemotherapy and develops complications such as uncontrolled nausea and vomiting or dehydration, the principal or first-listed diagnosis is Z51.0, Encounter for antineoplastic radiation therapy, or Z51.11, Encounter for antineoplastic chemotherapy, or Z51.12, Encounter for antineoplastic immunotherapy followed by any codes for the complications.

When a patient is admitted for the purpose of insertion or implantation of radioactive elements (e.g., brachytherapy) and develops complications such as uncontrolled nausea and vomiting or dehydration, the principal or first-listed diagnosis is the appropriate code for the malignancy followed by any codes for the complications.

A patient with prostate cancer was admitted for brachytherapy seed implantation and consequently developed urinary retention.

C61	**Malignant neoplasm of prostate**
R33.9	**Retention of urine, unspecified**

Explanation: A code for the malignancy should be listed as the principal diagnosis when insertion of a radioactive element is the reason for admission, even when a complication related to that radioactive element occurs. Codes describing the complications should be listed as secondary codes.

f. Admission/encounter to determine extent of malignancy

When the reason for admission/encounter is to determine the extent of the malignancy, or for a procedure such as paracentesis or thoracentesis, the primary malignancy or appropriate metastatic site is designated as the principal or first-listed diagnosis, even though chemotherapy or radiotherapy is administered.

Patient with left lung cancer with malignant pleural effusion admitted for paracentesis and initiation/administration of chemotherapy

C34.92	**Malignant neoplasm of unspecified part of left bronchus or lung**
J91.0	**Malignant pleural effusion**
Z51.11	**Encounter for antineoplastic chemotherapy**

Explanation: The lung cancer is sequenced before the chemotherapy in this instance because the paracentesis for the malignant effusion is also being performed. An instructional note under the malignant effusion instructs that the lung cancer be sequenced first.

g. Symptoms, signs, and abnormal findings listed in Chapter 18 associated with neoplasms

Symptoms, signs, and ill-defined conditions listed in Chapter 18 characteristic of, or associated with, an existing primary or secondary site malignancy cannot be used to replace the malignancy as principal or first-listed diagnosis, regardless of the number of admissions or encounters for treatment and care of the neoplasm.

See Section I.C.21. Factors influencing health status and contact with health services, Encounter for prophylactic organ removal.

h. Admission/encounter for pain control/management

See Section I.C.6. for information on coding admission/encounter for pain control/management.

i. Malignancy in two or more noncontiguous sites

A patient may have more than one malignant tumor in the same organ. These tumors may represent different primaries or metastatic disease, depending on the site. Should the documentation be unclear, the provider should be queried as to the status of each tumor so that the correct codes can be assigned.

j. Disseminated malignant neoplasm, unspecified

Code C80.0, Disseminated malignant neoplasm, unspecified, is for use only in those cases where the patient has advanced metastatic disease and no known primary or secondary sites are specified. It should not be used in place of assigning codes for the primary site and all known secondary sites.

Patient who has had no medical care for many years is seen today and diagnosed with carcinomatosis

C80.0	**Disseminated malignant neoplasm, unspecified**

Explanation: Carcinomatosis NOS is an "includes" note under this code. Should seldom be used but is available for use in cases such as this.

k. Malignant neoplasm without specification of site

Code C80.1, Malignant (primary) neoplasm, unspecified, equates to Cancer, unspecified. This code should only be used when no determination can be made as to the primary site of a malignancy. This code should rarely be used in the inpatient setting.

l. Sequencing of neoplasm codes

1) Encounter for treatment of primary malignancy

If the reason for the encounter is for treatment of a primary malignancy, assign the malignancy as the principal/first-listed diagnosis. The primary site is to be sequenced first, followed by any metastatic sites.

2) Encounter for treatment of secondary malignancy

When an encounter is for a primary malignancy with metastasis and treatment is directed toward the metastatic (secondary) site(s) only, the metastatic site(s) is designated as the principal/first-listed diagnosis. The primary malignancy is coded as an additional code.

> Patient has primary colon cancer with metastasis to rib and is evaluated for possible excision of portion of rib bone
>
> **C79.51**   **Secondary malignant neoplasm of bone**
>
> **C18.9**   **Malignant neoplasm of colon, unspecified**
>
> *Explanation*: The treatment for this encounter is focused on the metastasis to the rib bone rather than the primary colon cancer, thus indicating that the bone metastasis is sequenced as the first-listed code.

3) Malignant neoplasm in a pregnant patient

When a pregnant woman has a malignant neoplasm, a code from subcategory O9A.1-, Malignant neoplasm complicating pregnancy, childbirth, and the puerperium, should be sequenced first, followed by the appropriate code from Chapter 2 to indicate the type of neoplasm.

> A 30-year-old pregnant female in second trimester evaluated for thyroid malignancy
>
> **O9A.112**   **Malignant neoplasm complicating pregnancy, second trimester**
>
> **C73**   **Malignant neoplasm of thyroid gland**
>
> *Explanation*: Codes from chapter 15 describing complications of pregnancy are sequenced as first-listed codes, further specified by codes from other chapters such as neoplastic, unless the pregnancy is documented as incidental to the condition. See also guideline 1.C.15.a.1.

4) Encounter for complication associated with a neoplasm

When an encounter is for management of a complication associated with a neoplasm, such as dehydration, and the treatment is only for the complication, the complication is coded first, followed by the appropriate code(s) for the neoplasm.

The exception to this guideline is anemia. When the admission/encounter is for management of an anemia associated with the malignancy, and the treatment is only for anemia, the appropriate code for the malignancy is sequenced as the principal or first-listed diagnosis followed by code D63.0, Anemia in neoplastic disease.

> Patient with pancreatic cancer is seen for initiation of TPN for cancer-related moderate protein-calorie malnutrition
>
> **E44.0**   **Moderate protein-calorie malnutrition**
>
> **C25.9**   **Malignant neoplasm of pancreas, unspecified**
>
> *Explanation*: The encounter is to initiate treatment for malnutrition, a common complication of many types of neoplasms, and is sequenced first.

5) Complication from surgical procedure for treatment of a neoplasm

When an encounter is for treatment of a complication resulting from a surgical procedure performed for the treatment of the neoplasm, designate the complication as the principal/first-listed diagnosis. See the guideline regarding the coding of a current malignancy versus personal history to determine if the code for the neoplasm should also be assigned.

6) Pathologic fracture due to a neoplasm

When an encounter is for a pathological fracture due to a neoplasm, and the focus of treatment is the fracture, a code from subcategory M84.5, Pathological fracture in neoplastic disease, should be sequenced first, followed by the code for the neoplasm.

If the focus of treatment is the neoplasm with an associated pathological fracture, the neoplasm code should be sequenced first, followed by a code from M84.5 for the pathological fracture.

m. Current malignancy versus personal history of malignancy

When a primary malignancy has been excised but further treatment, such as an additional surgery for the malignancy, radiation therapy or chemotherapy is directed to that site, the primary malignancy code should be used until treatment is completed.

> Female patient with ongoing chemotherapy after right mastectomy for breast cancer
>
> **C50.911**   **Malignant neoplasm of unspecified site of right female breast**
>
> **Z90.11**   **Acquired absence of right breast and nipple**
>
> *Explanation*: Even though the breast has been removed, the breast cancer is still being treated with chemotherapy and therefore is still coded as a current condition rather than personal history.

When a primary malignancy has been previously excised or eradicated from its site, there is no further treatment (of the malignancy) directed to that site, and there is no evidence of any existing primary malignancy at that site, a code from category Z85, Personal history of malignant neoplasm, should be used to indicate the former site of the malignancy.

Codes from subcategories Z85.0–Z85.85 should only be assigned for the former site of a primary malignancy, not the site of a secondary malignancy. **Code Z85.89** may be assigned for the former site(s) of either a primary or secondary malignancy.

See Section I.C.21. Factors influencing health status and contact with health services, History (of)

n. Leukemia, multiple myeloma, and malignant plasma cell neoplasms in remission versus personal history

The categories for leukemia, and category C90, Multiple myeloma and malignant plasma cell neoplasms, have codes indicating whether or not the leukemia has achieved remission. There are also codes Z85.6, Personal history of leukemia, and Z85.79, Personal history of other malignant neoplasms of lymphoid, hematopoietic and related tissues. If the documentation is unclear as to whether the leukemia has achieved remission, the provider should be queried.

See Section I.C.21. Factors influencing health status and contact with health services, History (of)

o. Aftercare following surgery for neoplasm

See Section I.C.21. Factors influencing health status and contact with health services, Aftercare

p. Follow-up care for completed treatment of a malignancy

See Section I.C.21. Factors influencing health status and contact with health services, Follow-up

q. Prophylactic organ removal for prevention of malignancy

See Section I.C. 21, Factors influencing health status and contact with health services, Prophylactic organ removal

r. Malignant neoplasm associated with transplanted organ

A malignant neoplasm of a transplanted organ should be coded as a transplant complication. Assign first the appropriate code from category T86.-, Complications of transplanted organs and tissue, followed by code C80.2, Malignant neoplasm associated with transplanted organ. Use an additional code for the specific malignancy.

Chapter 2. Neoplasms (C00-D49)

NOTE

Functional activity

All neoplasms are classified in this chapter, whether they are functionally active or not. An additional code from Chapter 4 may be used, to identify functional activity associated with any neoplasm.

Morphology [Histology]

Chapter 2 classifies neoplasms primarily by site (topography), with broad groupings for behavior, malignant, in situ, benign, etc. The Table of Neoplasms should be used to identify the correct topography code. In a few cases, such as for malignant melanoma and certain neuroendocrine tumors, the morphology (histologic type) is included in the category and codes.

Primary malignant neoplasms overlapping site boundaries

A primary malignant neoplasm that overlaps two or more contiguous (next to each other) sites should be classified to the subcategory/code .8 ("overlapping lesion"), unless the combination is specifically indexed elsewhere. For multiple neoplasms of the same site that are not contiguous, such as tumors in different quadrants of the same breast, codes for each site should be assigned.

Malignant neoplasm of ectopic tissue

Malignant neoplasms of ectopic tissue are to be coded to the site mentioned, e.g., ectopic pancreatic malignant neoplasms are coded to pancreas, unspecified (C25.9).

AHA: 2017,4Q,103; 2017,1Q,4,5-6,8

This chapter contains the following blocks:

C00-C14   Malignant neoplasms of lip, oral cavity and pharynx
C15-C26   Malignant neoplasms of digestive organs
C30-C39   Malignant neoplasms of respiratory and intrathoracic organs
C40-C41   Malignant neoplasms of bone and articular cartilage
C43-C44   Melanoma and other malignant neoplasms of skin
C45-C49   Malignant neoplasms of mesothelial and soft tissue
C50   Malignant neoplasms of breast
C51-C58   Malignant neoplasms of female genital organs
C60-C63   Malignant neoplasms of male genital organs
C64-C68   Malignant neoplasms of urinary tract
C69-C72   Malignant neoplasms of eye, brain and other parts of central nervous system
C73-C75   Malignant neoplasms of thyroid and other endocrine glands
C7A   Malignant neuroendocrine tumors
C7B   Secondary neuroendocrine tumors
C76-C80   Malignant neoplasms of ill-defined, other secondary and unspecified sites
C81-C96   Malignant neoplasms of lymphoid, hematopoietic and related tissue
D00-D09   In situ neoplasms
D10-D36   Benign neoplasms, except benign neuroendocrine tumors
D3A   Benign neuroendocrine tumors
D37-D48   Neoplasms of uncertain behavior, polycythemia vera and myelodysplastic syndromes
D49   Neoplasms of unspecified behavior

MALIGNANT NEOPLASMS(C00-C96)

Malignant neoplasms, stated or presumed to be primary (of specified sites), and certain specified histologies, except neuroendocrine, and of lymphoid, hematopoietic and related tissue (C00-C75)

Malignant neoplasms of lip, oral cavity and pharynx (C00-C14)

☑4ᵗʰ C00 Malignant neoplasm of lip

Use additional code to identify:
    alcohol abuse and dependence (F10.-)
    history of tobacco dependence (Z87.891)
    tobacco dependence (F17.-)
    tobacco use (Z72.0)
      EXCLUDES 1   *malignant melanoma of lip (C43.0)*
                Merkel cell carcinoma of lip (C4A.0)
                other and unspecified malignant neoplasm of skin of lip (C44.0-)

C00.0   Malignant neoplasm of external upper lip
    Malignant neoplasm of lipstick area of upper lip
    Malignant neoplasm of upper lip NOS
    Malignant neoplasm of vermilion border of upper lip

C00.1   Malignant neoplasm of external lower lip
    Malignant neoplasm of lower lip NOS
    Malignant neoplasm of lipstick area of lower lip
    Malignant neoplasm of vermilion border of lower lip

C00.2   Malignant neoplasm of external lip, unspecified
    Malignant neoplasm of vermilion border of lip NOS

C00.3   Malignant neoplasm of upper lip, inner aspect
    Malignant neoplasm of buccal aspect of upper lip
    Malignant neoplasm of frenulum of upper lip
    Malignant neoplasm of mucosa of upper lip
    Malignant neoplasm of oral aspect of upper lip

C00.4   Malignant neoplasm of lower lip, inner aspect
    Malignant neoplasm of buccal aspect of lower lip
    Malignant neoplasm of frenulum of lower lip
    Malignant neoplasm of mucosa of lower lip
    Malignant neoplasm of oral aspect of lower lip

C00.5   Malignant neoplasm of lip, unspecified, inner aspect
    Malignant neoplasm of buccal aspect of lip, unspecified
    Malignant neoplasm of frenulum of lip, unspecified
    Malignant neoplasm of mucosa of lip, unspecified
    Malignant neoplasm of oral aspect of lip, unspecified

C00.6   Malignant neoplasm of commissure of lip, unspecified

C00.8   Malignant neoplasm of overlapping sites of lip

C00.9   Malignant neoplasm of lip, unspecified

C01   Malignant neoplasm of base of tongue   `HCC`
    Malignant neoplasm of dorsal surface of base of tongue
    Malignant neoplasm of fixed part of tongue NOS
    Malignant neoplasm of posterior third of tongue
    Use additional code to identify:
       alcohol abuse and dependence (F10.-)
       history of tobacco dependence (Z87.891)
       tobacco dependence (F17.-)
       tobacco use (Z72.0)

Malignant Neoplasm of Tongue

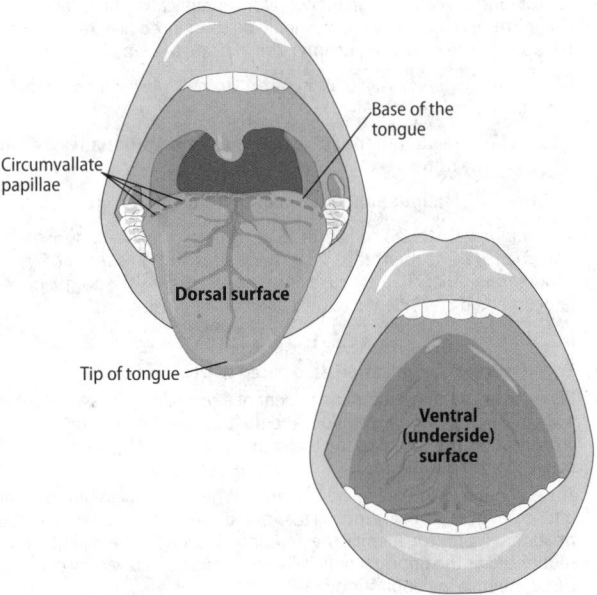

Circumvallate papillae

Base of the tongue

Dorsal surface

Tip of tongue

Ventral (underside) surface

☑4ᵗʰ C02 Malignant neoplasm of other and unspecified parts of tongue

Use additional code to identify:
    alcohol abuse and dependence (F10.-)
    history of tobacco dependence (Z87.891)
    tobacco dependence (F17.-)
    tobacco use (Z72.0)

C02.0   Malignant neoplasm of dorsal surface of tongue   `HCC`
    Malignant neoplasm of anterior two-thirds of tongue, dorsal surface
      EXCLUDES 2   *malignant neoplasm of dorsal surface of base of tongue (C01)*

C02.1   Malignant neoplasm of border of tongue   `HCC`
    Malignant neoplasm of tip of tongue

C02.2   Malignant neoplasm of ventral surface of tongue   `HCC`
    Malignant neoplasm of anterior two-thirds of tongue, ventral surface
    Malignant neoplasm of frenulum linguae

C02.3   Malignant neoplasm of anterior two-thirds of tongue, part unspecified   `HCC`
    Malignant neoplasm of middle third of tongue NOS
    Malignant neoplasm of mobile part of tongue NOS

N Newborn: 0   **P** Pediatric: 0-17   **M** Maternity: 9-64   **A** Adult: 15-124   **MCC** Major Complication/Comorbidity   **CC** Complication/Comorbidity   **SW** Severe Wound Dx

468   ICD-10-CM 2021

C02.4 Malignant neoplasm of lingual tonsil HCC
  EXCLUDES 2 *malignant neoplasm of tonsil NOS (C09.9)*

C02.8 Malignant neoplasm of overlapping sites of tongue HCC
  Malignant neoplasm of two or more contiguous sites of tongue

C02.9 Malignant neoplasm of tongue, unspecified HCC

✓4ᵗʰ **C03 Malignant neoplasm of gum**
  INCLUDES malignant neoplasm of alveolar (ridge) mucosa
    malignant neoplasm of gingiva
  Use additional code to identify:
    alcohol abuse and dependence (F10.-)
    history of tobacco dependence (Z87.891)
    tobacco dependence (F17.-)
    tobacco use (Z72.0)
  EXCLUDES 2 *malignant odontogenic neoplasms (C41.0-C41.1)*

  C03.0 Malignant neoplasm of upper gum HCC
  C03.1 Malignant neoplasm of lower gum HCC
  C03.9 Malignant neoplasm of gum, unspecified HCC

✓4ᵗʰ **C04 Malignant neoplasm of floor of mouth**
  Use additional code to identify:
    alcohol abuse and dependence (F10.-)
    history of tobacco dependence (Z87.891)
    tobacco dependence (F17.-)
    tobacco use (Z72.0)

  C04.0 Malignant neoplasm of anterior floor of mouth HCC
    Malignant neoplasm of anterior to the premolar-canine junction
  C04.1 Malignant neoplasm of lateral floor of mouth HCC
  C04.8 Malignant neoplasm of overlapping sites of floor of mouth HCC
  C04.9 Malignant neoplasm of floor of mouth, unspecified HCC

✓4ᵗʰ **C05 Malignant neoplasm of palate**
  Use additional code to identify:
    alcohol abuse and dependence (F10.-)
    history of tobacco dependence (Z87.891)
    tobacco dependence (F17.-)
    tobacco use (Z72.0)
  EXCLUDES 1 *Kaposi's sarcoma of palate (C46.2)*

  C05.0 Malignant neoplasm of hard palate HCC
  C05.1 Malignant neoplasm of soft palate HCC
    EXCLUDES 2 *malignant neoplasm of nasopharyngeal surface of soft palate (C11.3)*
  C05.2 Malignant neoplasm of uvula HCC
  C05.8 Malignant neoplasm of overlapping sites of palate HCC
  C05.9 Malignant neoplasm of palate, unspecified HCC
    Malignant neoplasm of roof of mouth

✓4ᵗʰ **C06 Malignant neoplasm of other and unspecified parts of mouth**
  Use additional code to identify:
    alcohol abuse and dependence (F10.-)
    history of tobacco dependence (Z87.891)
    tobacco dependence (F17.-)
    tobacco use (Z72.0)

  C06.0 Malignant neoplasm of cheek mucosa HCC
    Malignant neoplasm of buccal mucosa NOS
    Malignant neoplasm of internal cheek
  C06.1 Malignant neoplasm of vestibule of mouth HCC
    Malignant neoplasm of buccal sulcus (upper) (lower)
    Malignant neoplasm of labial sulcus (upper) (lower)
  C06.2 Malignant neoplasm of retromolar area HCC
  ✓5ᵗʰ **C06.8 Malignant neoplasm of overlapping sites of other and unspecified parts of mouth**
    C06.80 Malignant neoplasm of overlapping sites of unspecified parts of mouth HCC
    C06.89 Malignant neoplasm of overlapping sites of other parts of mouth HCC
      "book leaf" neoplasm [ventral surface of tongue and floor of mouth]
  C06.9 Malignant neoplasm of mouth, unspecified HCC
    Malignant neoplasm of minor salivary gland, unspecified site
    Malignant neoplasm of oral cavity NOS

C07 Malignant neoplasm of parotid gland HCC
  Use additional code to identify:
    alcohol abuse and dependence (F10.-)
    exposure to environmental tobacco smoke (Z77.22)
    exposure to tobacco smoke in the perinatal period (P96.81)
    history of tobacco dependence (Z87.891)
    occupational exposure to environmental tobacco smoke (Z57.31)
    tobacco dependence (F17.-)
    tobacco use (Z72.0)

✓4ᵗʰ **C08 Malignant neoplasm of other and unspecified major salivary glands**
  INCLUDES malignant neoplasm of salivary ducts
  Use additional code to identify:
    alcohol abuse and dependence (F10.-)
    exposure to environmental tobacco smoke (Z77.22)
    exposure to tobacco smoke in the perinatal period (P96.81)
    history of tobacco dependence (Z87.891)
    occupational exposure to environmental tobacco smoke (Z57.31)
    tobacco dependence (F17.-)
    tobacco use (Z72.0)
  EXCLUDES 1 *malignant neoplasms of specified minor salivary glands which are classified according to their anatomical location*
  EXCLUDES 2 *malignant neoplasms of minor salivary glands NOS (C06.9)*
    malignant neoplasm of parotid gland (C07)

  C08.0 Malignant neoplasm of submandibular gland HCC
    Malignant neoplasm of submaxillary gland
  C08.1 Malignant neoplasm of sublingual gland HCC
  C08.9 Malignant neoplasm of major salivary gland, unspecified HCC
    Malignant neoplasm of salivary gland (major) NOS

✓4ᵗʰ **C09 Malignant neoplasm of tonsil**
  Use additional code to identify:
    alcohol abuse and dependence (F10.-)
    exposure to environmental tobacco smoke (Z77.22)
    exposure to tobacco smoke in the perinatal period (P96.81)
    history of tobacco dependence (Z87.891)
    occupational exposure to environmental tobacco smoke (Z57.31)
    tobacco dependence (F17.-)
    tobacco use (Z72.0)
  EXCLUDES 2 *malignant neoplasm of lingual tonsil (C02.4)*
    malignant neoplasm of pharyngeal tonsil (C11.1)

  C09.0 Malignant neoplasm of tonsillar fossa HCC
  C09.1 Malignant neoplasm of tonsillar pillar (anterior) (posterior) HCC
  C09.8 Malignant neoplasm of overlapping sites of tonsil HCC
  C09.9 Malignant neoplasm of tonsil, unspecified HCC
    Malignant neoplasm of tonsil NOS
    Malignant neoplasm of faucial tonsils
    Malignant neoplasm of palatine tonsils

✓4ᵗʰ **C10 Malignant neoplasm of oropharynx**
  Use additional code to identify:
    alcohol abuse and dependence (F10.-)
    exposure to environmental tobacco smoke (Z77.22)
    exposure to tobacco smoke in the perinatal period (P96.81)
    history of tobacco dependence (Z87.891)
    occupational exposure to environmental tobacco smoke (Z57.31)
    tobacco dependence (F17.-)
    tobacco use (Z72.0)
  EXCLUDES 2 *malignant neoplasm of tonsil (C09.-)*
  DEF: Oropharynx: Middle portion of pharynx (throat); communicates with the oral cavity, nasopharynx and laryngopharynx.

  C10.0 Malignant neoplasm of vallecula HCC
  C10.1 Malignant neoplasm of anterior surface of epiglottis HCC
    Malignant neoplasm of epiglottis, free border [margin]
    Malignant neoplasm of glossoepiglottic fold(s)
    EXCLUDES 2 *malignant neoplasm of epiglottis (suprahyoid portion) NOS (C32.1)*
  C10.2 Malignant neoplasm of lateral wall of oropharynx HCC
  C10.3 Malignant neoplasm of posterior wall of oropharynx HCC
  C10.4 Malignant neoplasm of branchial cleft HCC
    Malignant neoplasm of branchial cyst [site of neoplasm]
  C10.8 Malignant neoplasm of overlapping sites of oropharynx HCC
    Malignant neoplasm of junctional region of oropharynx
  C10.9 Malignant neoplasm of oropharynx, unspecified HCC

Chapter 2. Neoplasms

C02.4–C10.9

✓ Additional Character Required ✓x7ᵗʰ Placeholder Unacceptable PDx Questionable PDx Manifestation Unspecified Dx H1-H14 HAC HCC CMS-HCC Dx HIV HIV Dx

✓4ᵗʰ **C11 Malignant neoplasm of nasopharynx**

Use additional code to identify:
exposure to environmental tobacco smoke (Z77.22)
exposure to tobacco smoke in the perinatal period (P96.81)
history of tobacco dependence (Z87.891)
occupational exposure to environmental tobacco smoke (Z57.31)
tobacco dependence (F17.-)
tobacco use (Z72.0)
DEF: Nasopharynx: Upper portion of pharynx (throat); communicates with the nasal cavities, oropharynx and tympanic cavities.

C11.0 Malignant neoplasm of superior wall of nasopharynx HCC
Malignant neoplasm of roof of nasopharynx

C11.1 Malignant neoplasm of posterior wall of nasopharynx HCC
Malignant neoplasm of adenoid
Malignant neoplasm of pharyngeal tonsil

C11.2 Malignant neoplasm of lateral wall of nasopharynx HCC
Malignant neoplasm of fossa of Rosenmüller
Malignant neoplasm of opening of auditory tube
Malignant neoplasm of pharyngeal recess

C11.3 Malignant neoplasm of anterior wall of nasopharynx HCC
Malignant neoplasm of floor of nasopharynx
Malignant neoplasm of nasopharyngeal (anterior) (posterior) surface of soft palate
Malignant neoplasm of posterior margin of nasal choana
Malignant neoplasm of posterior margin of nasal septum

C11.8 Malignant neoplasm of overlapping sites of nasopharynx HCC

C11.9 Malignant neoplasm of nasopharynx, unspecified HCC
Malignant neoplasm of nasopharyngeal wall NOS

C12 Malignant neoplasm of pyriform sinus HCC
Malignant neoplasm of pyriform fossa
Use additional code to identify:
exposure to environmental tobacco smoke (Z77.22)
exposure to tobacco smoke in the perinatal period (P96.81)
history of tobacco dependence (Z87.891)
occupational exposure to environmental tobacco smoke (Z57.31)
tobacco dependence (F17.-)
tobacco use (Z72.0)

✓4ᵗʰ **C13 Malignant neoplasm of hypopharynx**

Use additional code to identify:
exposure to environmental tobacco smoke (Z77.22)
exposure to tobacco smoke in the perinatal period (P96.81)
history of tobacco dependence (Z87.891)
occupational exposure to environmental tobacco smoke (Z57.31)
tobacco dependence (F17.-)
tobacco use (Z72.0)
EXCLUDES 2   *malignant neoplasm of pyriform sinus (C12)*
DEF: Hypopharynx: Lower portion of pharynx (throat); communicates with the oropharynx and the esophagus. *Synonyms: laryngopharynx.*

C13.0 Malignant neoplasm of postcricoid region HCC

C13.1 Malignant neoplasm of aryepiglottic fold, hypopharyngeal aspect HCC
Malignant neoplasm of aryepiglottic fold, marginal zone
Malignant neoplasm of aryepiglottic fold NOS
Malignant neoplasm of interarytenoid fold, marginal zone
Malignant neoplasm of interarytenoid fold NOS
EXCLUDES 2   *malignant neoplasm of aryepiglottic fold or interarytenoid fold, laryngeal aspect (C32.1)*

C13.2 Malignant neoplasm of posterior wall of hypopharynx HCC

C13.8 Malignant neoplasm of overlapping sites of hypopharynx HCC

C13.9 Malignant neoplasm of hypopharynx, unspecified HCC
Malignant neoplasm of hypopharyngeal wall NOS

✓4ᵗʰ **C14 Malignant neoplasm of other and ill-defined sites in the lip, oral cavity and pharynx**

Use additional code to identify:
alcohol abuse and dependence (F10.-)
exposure to environmental tobacco smoke (Z77.22)
exposure to tobacco smoke in the perinatal period (P96.81)
history of tobacco dependence (Z87.891)
occupational exposure to environmental tobacco smoke (Z57.31)
tobacco dependence (F17.-)
tobacco use (Z72.0)
EXCLUDES 1   *malignant neoplasm of oral cavity NOS (C06.9)*

C14.0 Malignant neoplasm of pharynx, unspecified HCC

C14.2 Malignant neoplasm of Waldeyer's ring HCC
DEF: Waldeyer's ring: Ring of lymphoid tissue that is made up of the two palatine tonsils, the pharyngeal tonsil (adenoid), and the lingual tonsil. It functions as the defense against infection and assists with the development of the immune system.

C14.8 Malignant neoplasm of overlapping sites of lip, oral cavity and pharynx HCC
Primary malignant neoplasm of two or more contiguous sites of lip, oral cavity and pharynx
EXCLUDES 1   *"book leaf" neoplasm [ventral surface of tongue and floor of mouth] (C06.89)*

Malignant neoplasms of digestive organs (C15-C26)

EXCLUDES 1   *Kaposi's sarcoma of gastrointestinal sites (C46.4)*
EXCLUDES 2   *gastrointestinal stromal tumors (C49.A-)*

✓4ᵗʰ **C15 Malignant neoplasm of esophagus**

Use additional code to identify:
alcohol abuse and dependence (F10.-)

C15.3 Malignant neoplasm of upper third of esophagus CC HCC
C15.4 Malignant neoplasm of middle third of esophagus CC HCC
C15.5 Malignant neoplasm of lower third of esophagus CC HCC
EXCLUDES 1   *malignant neoplasm of cardio-esophageal junction (C16.0)*

C15.8 Malignant neoplasm of overlapping sites of esophagus CC HCC
C15.9 Malignant neoplasm of esophagus, unspecified CC HCC

✓4ᵗʰ **C16 Malignant neoplasm of stomach**

Use additional code to identify:
alcohol abuse and dependence (F10.-)
EXCLUDES 2   *malignant carcinoid tumor of the stomach (C7A.092)*

C16.0 Malignant neoplasm of cardia CC HCC
Malignant neoplasm of cardiac orifice
Malignant neoplasm of cardio-esophageal junction
Malignant neoplasm of esophagus and stomach
Malignant neoplasm of gastro-esophageal junction

C16.1 Malignant neoplasm of fundus of stomach CC HCC
C16.2 Malignant neoplasm of body of stomach CC HCC
C16.3 Malignant neoplasm of pyloric antrum CC HCC
Malignant neoplasm of gastric antrum

C16.4 Malignant neoplasm of pylorus CC HCC
Malignant neoplasm of prepylorus
Malignant neoplasm of pyloric canal

C16.5 Malignant neoplasm of lesser curvature of stomach, unspecified CC HCC
Malignant neoplasm of lesser curvature of stomach, not classifiable to C16.1-C16.4

C16.6 Malignant neoplasm of greater curvature of stomach, unspecified CC HCC
Malignant neoplasm of greater curvature of stomach, not classifiable to C16.0-C16.4

C16.8 Malignant neoplasm of overlapping sites of stomach CC HCC
C16.9 Malignant neoplasm of stomach, unspecified CC HCC
Gastric cancer NOS

✓4ᵗʰ **C17 Malignant neoplasm of small intestine**
EXCLUDES 1   *malignant carcinoid tumors of the small intestine (C7A.01)*
AHA: 2016,1Q,19

C17.0 Malignant neoplasm of duodenum CC HCC
C17.1 Malignant neoplasm of jejunum CC HCC
C17.2 Malignant neoplasm of ileum CC HCC
EXCLUDES 1   *malignant neoplasm of ileocecal valve (C18.0)*

C17.3 Meckel's diverticulum, malignant CC HCC
EXCLUDES 1   *Meckel's diverticulum, congenital (Q43.0)*
DEF: Congenital, abnormal remnant of embryonic digestive system development that leaves a sacculation or outpouching from the wall of the small intestine near the terminal part of the ileum made of acid-secreting tissue as in the stomach.

C17.8 Malignant neoplasm of overlapping sites of small intestine CC HCC
C17.9 Malignant neoplasm of small intestine, unspecified CC HCC

✓4ᵗʰ **C18 Malignant neoplasm of colon**
> **EXCLUDES 1** *malignant carcinoid tumors of the colon (C7A.02-)*

Colon

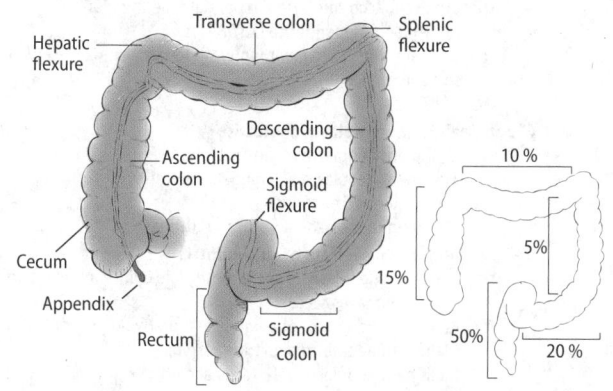

Anatomical distribution
of large bowel cancers

C18.0 Malignant neoplasm of cecum   CC HCC
Malignant neoplasm of ileocecal valve

C18.1 Malignant neoplasm of appendix   CC HCC

C18.2 Malignant neoplasm of ascending colon   CC HCC

C18.3 Malignant neoplasm of hepatic flexure   CC HCC

C18.4 Malignant neoplasm of transverse colon   CC HCC

C18.5 Malignant neoplasm of splenic flexure   CC HCC

C18.6 Malignant neoplasm of descending colon   CC HCC

C18.7 Malignant neoplasm of sigmoid colon   CC HCC
Malignant neoplasm of sigmoid (flexure)
> **EXCLUDES 1** *malignant neoplasm of rectosigmoid junction (C19)*

C18.8 Malignant neoplasm of overlapping sites of colon   CC HCC

C18.9 Malignant neoplasm of colon, unspecified   CC HCC
Malignant neoplasm of large intestine NOS

C19 Malignant neoplasm of rectosigmoid junction   CC HCC
Malignant neoplasm of colon with rectum
Malignant neoplasm of rectosigmoid (colon)
> **EXCLUDES 1** *malignant carcinoid tumors of the colon (C7A.02-)*

C20 Malignant neoplasm of rectum   CC HCC
Malignant neoplasm of rectal ampulla
> **EXCLUDES 1** *malignant carcinoid tumor of the rectum (C7A.026)*

✓4ᵗʰ **C21 Malignant neoplasm of anus and anal canal**
> **EXCLUDES 2** *malignant carcinoid tumors of the colon (C7A.02-)*
> *malignant melanoma of anal margin (C43.51)*
> *malignant melanoma of anal skin (C43.51)*
> *malignant melanoma of perianal skin (C43.51)*
> *other and unspecified malignant neoplasm of anal margin*
> *(C44.500, C44.510, C44.520, C44.590)*
> *other and unspecified malignant neoplasm of anal skin*
> *(C44.500, C44.510, C44.520, C44.590)*
> *other and unspecified malignant neoplasm of perianal skin*
> *(C44.500, C44.510, C44.520, C44.590)*

C21.0 Malignant neoplasm of anus, unspecified   CC HCC

C21.1 Malignant neoplasm of anal canal   CC HCC
Malignant neoplasm of anal sphincter

C21.2 Malignant neoplasm of cloacogenic zone   CC HCC

C21.8 Malignant neoplasm of overlapping sites of rectum, anus and anal canal   CC HCC
Malignant neoplasm of anorectal junction
Malignant neoplasm of anorectum
Primary malignant neoplasm of two or more contiguous sites
of rectum, anus and anal canal

✓4ᵗʰ **C22 Malignant neoplasm of liver and intrahepatic bile ducts**
> **EXCLUDES 1** *malignant neoplasm of biliary tract NOS (C24.9)*
> *secondary malignant neoplasm of liver and intrahepatic bile*
> *duct (C78.7)*

Use additional code to identify:
alcohol abuse and dependence (F10.-)
hepatitis B (B16.-, B18.0-B18.1)
hepatitis C (B17.1-, B18.2)

C22.0 Liver cell carcinoma   CC HCC
Hepatocellular carcinoma
Hepatoma
AHA: 2016,1Q,18

C22.1 Intrahepatic bile duct carcinoma   CC HCC
Cholangiocarcinoma
> **EXCLUDES 1** *malignant neoplasm of hepatic duct (C24.0)*

C22.2 Hepatoblastoma   CC HCC

C22.3 Angiosarcoma of liver   CC HCC
Kupffer cell sarcoma

C22.4 Other sarcomas of liver   CC HCC

C22.7 Other specified carcinomas of liver   CC HCC

C22.8 Malignant neoplasm of liver, primary, unspecified as to type   CC HCC

C22.9 Malignant neoplasm of liver, not specified as primary or secondary   CC HCC

C23 Malignant neoplasm of gallbladder   CC HCC

✓4ᵗʰ **C24 Malignant neoplasm of other and unspecified parts of biliary tract**
> **EXCLUDES 1** *malignant neoplasm of intrahepatic bile duct (C22.1)*

C24.0 Malignant neoplasm of extrahepatic bile duct   CC HCC
Malignant neoplasm of biliary duct or passage NOS
Malignant neoplasm of common bile duct
Malignant neoplasm of cystic duct
Malignant neoplasm of hepatic duct

C24.1 Malignant neoplasm of ampulla of Vater   CC HCC
DEF: Malignant neoplasm in the area of dilation at the juncture
of the common bile and pancreatic ducts near the opening into
the lumen of the duodenum.

C24.8 Malignant neoplasm of overlapping sites of biliary tract   CC HCC
Malignant neoplasm involving both intrahepatic and
extrahepatic bile ducts
Primary malignant neoplasm of two or more contiguous sites
of biliary tract

C24.9 Malignant neoplasm of biliary tract, unspecified   CC HCC

✓4ᵗʰ **C25 Malignant neoplasm of pancreas**
Code also exocrine pancreatic insufficiency (K86.81)
Use additional code to identify:
alcohol abuse and dependence (F10.-)

Pancreas

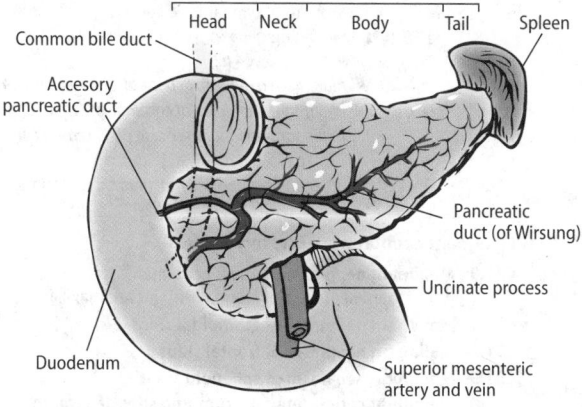

C25.0 Malignant neoplasm of head of pancreas   CC HCC
C25.1 Malignant neoplasm of body of pancreas   CC HCC
C25.2 Malignant neoplasm of tail of pancreas   CC HCC
C25.3 Malignant neoplasm of pancreatic duct   CC HCC

C25.4 Malignant neoplasm of endocrine pancreas `CC` `HCC`
Malignant neoplasm of islets of Langerhans
Use additional code to identify any functional activity

C25.7 Malignant neoplasm of other parts of pancreas `CC` `HCC`
Malignant neoplasm of neck of pancreas

C25.8 Malignant neoplasm of overlapping sites of pancreas `CC` `HCC`

C25.9 Malignant neoplasm of pancreas, unspecified `CC` `HCC`

✓4ᵗʰ **C26 Malignant neoplasm of other and ill-defined digestive organs**
> *EXCLUDES 1*   malignant neoplasm of peritoneum and retroperitoneum (C48.-)

C26.0 Malignant neoplasm of intestinal tract, part unspecified `HCC`
Malignant neoplasm of intestine NOS

C26.1 Malignant neoplasm of spleen `HCC`
> *EXCLUDES 1*   Hodgkin lymphoma (C81.-)
> non-Hodgkin lymphoma (C82-C85)

C26.9 Malignant neoplasm of ill-defined sites within the digestive system `HCC`
Malignant neoplasm of alimentary canal or tract NOS
Malignant neoplasm of gastrointestinal tract NOS
> *EXCLUDES 1*   malignant neoplasm of abdominal NOS (C76.2)
> malignant neoplasm of intra-abdominal NOS (C76.2)

Malignant neoplasms of respiratory and intrathoracic organs (C30-C39)

`INCLUDES`   malignant neoplasm of middle ear
`EXCLUDES 1`   mesothelioma (C45.-)

✓4ᵗʰ **C30 Malignant neoplasm of nasal cavity and middle ear**

C30.0 Malignant neoplasm of nasal cavity `HCC`
Malignant neoplasm of cartilage of nose
Malignant neoplasm of nasal concha
Malignant neoplasm of internal nose
Malignant neoplasm of septum of nose
Malignant neoplasm of vestibule of nose
> *EXCLUDES 1*   malignant neoplasm of nasal bone (C41.0)
> malignant neoplasm of nose NOS (C76.0)
> malignant neoplasm of olfactory bulb (C72.2-)
> malignant neoplasm of posterior margin of nasal septum and choana (C11.3)
> malignant melanoma of skin of nose (C43.31)
> malignant neoplasm of turbinates (C41.0)
> other and unspecified malignant neoplasm of skin of nose (C44.301, C44.311, C44.321, C44.391)

C30.1 Malignant neoplasm of middle ear `HCC`
Malignant neoplasm of antrum tympanicum
Malignant neoplasm of auditory tube
Malignant neoplasm of eustachian tube
Malignant neoplasm of inner ear
Malignant neoplasm of mastoid air cells
Malignant neoplasm of tympanic cavity
> *EXCLUDES 1*   malignant neoplasm of auricular canal (external) (C43.2-,C44.2-)
> malignant neoplasm of bone of ear (meatus) (C41.0)
> malignant neoplasm of cartilage of ear (C49.0)
> malignant melanoma of skin of (external) ear (C43.2-)
> other and unspecified malignant neoplasm of skin of (external) ear (C44.2-)

✓4ᵗʰ **C31 Malignant neoplasm of accessory sinuses**

C31.0 Malignant neoplasm of maxillary sinus `HCC`
Malignant neoplasm of antrum (Highmore) (maxillary)

C31.1 Malignant neoplasm of ethmoidal sinus `HCC`

C31.2 Malignant neoplasm of frontal sinus `HCC`

C31.3 Malignant neoplasm of sphenoid sinus `HCC`

C31.8 Malignant neoplasm of overlapping sites of accessory sinuses `HCC`

C31.9 Malignant neoplasm of accessory sinus, unspecified `HCC`

✓4ᵗʰ **C32 Malignant neoplasm of larynx**
Use additional code to identify:
alcohol abuse and dependence (F10.-)
exposure to environmental tobacco smoke (Z77.22)
exposure to tobacco smoke in the perinatal period (P96.81)
history of tobacco dependence (Z87.891)
occupational exposure to environmental tobacco smoke (Z57.31)
tobacco dependence (F17.-)
tobacco use (Z72.0)

C32.0 Malignant neoplasm of glottis `HCC`
Malignant neoplasm of intrinsic larynx
Malignant neoplasm of laryngeal commissure (anterior)(posterior)
Malignant neoplasm of vocal cord (true) NOS

C32.1 Malignant neoplasm of supraglottis `HCC`
Malignant neoplasm of aryepiglottic fold or interarytenoid fold, laryngeal aspect
Malignant neoplasm of epiglottis (suprahyoid portion) NOS
Malignant neoplasm of extrinsic larynx
Malignant neoplasm of false vocal cord
Malignant neoplasm of posterior (laryngeal) surface of epiglottis
Malignant neoplasm of ventricular bands
> *EXCLUDES 2*   malignant neoplasm of anterior surface of epiglottis (C10.1)
> malignant neoplasm of aryepiglottic fold or interarytenoid fold, hypopharyngeal aspect (C13.1)
> malignant neoplasm of aryepiglottic fold or interarytenoid fold, marginal zone (C13.1)
> malignant neoplasm of aryepiglottic fold or interarytenoid fold NOS (C13.1)

C32.2 Malignant neoplasm of subglottis `HCC`

C32.3 Malignant neoplasm of laryngeal cartilage `HCC`

C32.8 Malignant neoplasm of overlapping sites of larynx `HCC`

C32.9 Malignant neoplasm of larynx, unspecified `HCC`

C33 Malignant neoplasm of trachea `CC` `HCC`
Use additional code to identify:
exposure to environmental tobacco smoke (Z77.22)
exposure to tobacco smoke in the perinatal period (P96.81)
history of tobacco dependence (Z87.891)
occupational exposure to environmental tobacco smoke (Z57.31)
tobacco dependence (F17.-)
tobacco use (Z72.0)

✓4ᵗʰ **C34 Malignant neoplasm of bronchus and lung**
Use additional code to identify:
exposure to environmental tobacco smoke (Z77.22)
exposure to tobacco smoke in the perinatal period (P96.81)
history of tobacco dependence (Z87.891)
occupational exposure to environmental tobacco smoke (Z57.31)
tobacco dependence (F17.-)
tobacco use (Z72.0)
> *EXCLUDES 1*   Kaposi's sarcoma of lung (C46.5-)
> malignant carcinoid tumor of the bronchus and lung (C7A.090)

AHA: 2019,1Q,16
TIP: When documented, assign code I31.3 for associated malignant pericardial effusion. If the sole reason for admission is to treat the effusion with no treatment of the lung malignancy rendered, code I31.3 may be sequenced first.

✓5ᵗʰ **C34.0 Malignant neoplasm of main bronchus**
Malignant neoplasm of carina
Malignant neoplasm of hilus (of lung)

C34.00 Malignant neoplasm of unspecified main bronchus `CC` `HCC`

C34.01 Malignant neoplasm of right main bronchus `CC` `HCC`

C34.02 Malignant neoplasm of left main bronchus `CC` `HCC`

✓5ᵗʰ **C34.1 Malignant neoplasm of upper lobe, bronchus or lung**

C34.10 Malignant neoplasm of upper lobe, unspecified bronchus or lung `CC` `HCC`

C34.11 Malignant neoplasm of upper lobe, right bronchus or lung `CC` `HCC`

C34.12 Malignant neoplasm of upper lobe, left bronchus or lung `CC` `HCC`

C34.2 Malignant neoplasm of middle lobe, bronchus or lung `CC` `HCC`

√5ᵗʰ **C34.3 Malignant neoplasm of lower lobe, bronchus or lung**

C34.30 Malignant neoplasm of lower lobe, unspecified bronchus or lung `CC` `HCC`

C34.31 Malignant neoplasm of lower lobe, right bronchus or lung `CC` `HCC`

C34.32 Malignant neoplasm of lower lobe, left bronchus or lung `CC` `HCC`

√5ᵗʰ **C34.8 Malignant neoplasm of overlapping sites of bronchus and lung**

C34.80 Malignant neoplasm of overlapping sites of unspecified bronchus and lung `CC` `HCC`

C34.81 Malignant neoplasm of overlapping sites of right bronchus and lung `CC` `HCC`

C34.82 Malignant neoplasm of overlapping sites of left bronchus and lung `CC` `HCC`

√5ᵗʰ **C34.9 Malignant neoplasm of unspecified part of bronchus or lung**

C34.90 Malignant neoplasm of unspecified part of unspecified bronchus or lung `CC` `HCC`
Lung cancer NOS

C34.91 Malignant neoplasm of unspecified part of right bronchus or lung `CC` `HCC`

C34.92 Malignant neoplasm of unspecified part of left bronchus or lung `CC` `HCC`

C37 Malignant neoplasm of thymus `CC` `HCC`
EXCLUDES 1   *malignant carcinoid tumor of the thymus (C7A.091)*

√4ᵗʰ **C38 Malignant neoplasm of heart, mediastinum and pleura**
EXCLUDES 1   *mesothelioma (C45.-)*

C38.0 Malignant neoplasm of heart `CC` `HCC`
Malignant neoplasm of pericardium
EXCLUDES 1   *malignant neoplasm of great vessels (C49.3)*

C38.1 Malignant neoplasm of anterior mediastinum `CC` `HCC`

C38.2 Malignant neoplasm of posterior mediastinum `CC` `HCC`

C38.3 Malignant neoplasm of mediastinum, part unspecified `CC` `HCC`

C38.4 Malignant neoplasm of pleura `CC` `HCC`

C38.8 Malignant neoplasm of overlapping sites of heart, mediastinum and pleura `CC` `HCC`

√4ᵗʰ **C39 Malignant neoplasm of other and ill-defined sites in the respiratory system and intrathoracic organs**
Use additional code to identify:
exposure to environmental tobacco smoke (Z77.22)
exposure to tobacco smoke in the perinatal period (P96.81)
history of tobacco dependence (Z87.891)
occupational exposure to environmental tobacco smoke (Z57.31)
tobacco dependence (F17.-)
tobacco use (Z72.0)
EXCLUDES 1   *intrathoracic malignant neoplasm NOS (C76.1)*
thoracic malignant neoplasm NOS (C76.1)

C39.0 Malignant neoplasm of upper respiratory tract, part unspecified `HCC`

C39.9 Malignant neoplasm of lower respiratory tract, part unspecified `HCC`
Malignant neoplasm of respiratory tract NOS

Malignant neoplasms of bone and articular cartilage (C40-C41)

INCLUDES   malignant neoplasm of cartilage (articular) (joint)
malignant neoplasm of periosteum
EXCLUDES 1   *malignant neoplasm of bone marrow NOS (C96.9)*
malignant neoplasm of synovia (C49.-)

√4ᵗʰ **C40 Malignant neoplasm of bone and articular cartilage of limbs**
Use additional code to identify major osseous defect, if applicable (M89.7-)

√5ᵗʰ **C40.0 Malignant neoplasm of scapula and long bones of upper limb**

C40.00 Malignant neoplasm of scapula and long bones of unspecified upper limb `CC` `HCC`

C40.01 Malignant neoplasm of scapula and long bones of right upper limb `CC` `HCC`

C40.02 Malignant neoplasm of scapula and long bones of left upper limb `CC` `HCC`

√5ᵗʰ **C40.1 Malignant neoplasm of short bones of upper limb**

C40.10 Malignant neoplasm of short bones of unspecified upper limb `CC` `HCC`

C40.11 Malignant neoplasm of short bones of right upper limb `CC` `HCC`

C40.12 Malignant neoplasm of short bones of left upper limb `CC` `HCC`

√5ᵗʰ **C40.2 Malignant neoplasm of long bones of lower limb**

C40.20 Malignant neoplasm of long bones of unspecified lower limb `CC` `HCC`

C40.21 Malignant neoplasm of long bones of right lower limb `CC` `HCC`

C40.22 Malignant neoplasm of long bones of left lower limb `CC` `HCC`

√5ᵗʰ **C40.3 Malignant neoplasm of short bones of lower limb**

C40.30 Malignant neoplasm of short bones of unspecified lower limb `CC` `HCC`

C40.31 Malignant neoplasm of short bones of right lower limb `CC` `HCC`

C40.32 Malignant neoplasm of short bones of left lower limb `CC` `HCC`

√5ᵗʰ **C40.8 Malignant neoplasm of overlapping sites of bone and articular cartilage of limb**

C40.80 Malignant neoplasm of overlapping sites of bone and articular cartilage of unspecified limb `CC` `HCC`

C40.81 Malignant neoplasm of overlapping sites of bone and articular cartilage of right limb `CC` `HCC`

C40.82 Malignant neoplasm of overlapping sites of bone and articular cartilage of left limb `CC` `HCC`

√5ᵗʰ **C40.9 Malignant neoplasm of unspecified bones and articular cartilage of limb**

C40.90 Malignant neoplasm of unspecified bones and articular cartilage of unspecified limb `CC` `HCC`

C40.91 Malignant neoplasm of unspecified bones and articular cartilage of right limb `CC` `HCC`

C40.92 Malignant neoplasm of unspecified bones and articular cartilage of left limb `CC` `HCC`

√4ᵗʰ **C41 Malignant neoplasm of bone and articular cartilage of other and unspecified sites**
EXCLUDES 1   *malignant neoplasm of bones of limbs (C40.-)*
malignant neoplasm of cartilage of ear (C49.0)
malignant neoplasm of cartilage of eyelid (C49.0)
malignant neoplasm of cartilage of larynx (C32.3)
malignant neoplasm of cartilage of limbs (C40.-)
malignant neoplasm of cartilage of nose (C30.0)

C41.0 Malignant neoplasm of bones of skull and face `CC` `HCC`
Malignant neoplasm of maxilla (superior)
Malignant neoplasm of orbital bone
EXCLUDES 2   *carcinoma, any type except intraosseous or odontogenic of:*
maxillary sinus (C31.0)
upper jaw (C03.0)
malignant neoplasm of jaw bone (lower) (C41.1)

C41.1 Malignant neoplasm of mandible `CC` `HCC`
Malignant neoplasm of inferior maxilla
Malignant neoplasm of lower jaw bone
EXCLUDES 2   *carcinoma, any type except intraosseous or odontogenic of:*
jaw NOS (C03.9)
lower (C03.1)
malignant neoplasm of upper jaw bone (C41.0)

C41.2 Malignant neoplasm of vertebral column `CC` `HCC`
EXCLUDES 1   *malignant neoplasm of sacrum and coccyx (C41.4)*

C41.3 Malignant neoplasm of ribs, sternum and clavicle `CC` `HCC`

C41.4 Malignant neoplasm of pelvic bones, sacrum and coccyx `CC` `HCC`

C41.9 Malignant neoplasm of bone and articular cartilage, unspecified `CC` `HCC`

Melanoma and other malignant neoplasms of skin (C43-C44)

√4ᵗʰ **C43 Malignant melanoma of skin**
EXCLUDES 1   *melanoma in situ (D03.-)*
EXCLUDES 2   *malignant melanoma of skin of genital organs (C51-C52, C60.-, C63.-)*
Merkel cell carcinoma (C4A.-)
sites other than skin - code to malignant neoplasm of the site

C43.0 Malignant melanoma of lip `HCC`
EXCLUDES 1   *malignant neoplasm of vermilion border of lip (C00.0-C00.2)*

√5ᵗʰ **C43.1** **Malignant melanoma of** eyelid, including canthus

AHA: 2018,4Q,4

    C43.10 **Malignant melanoma of unspecified eyelid, including canthus**   HCC

√6ᵗʰ **C43.11** **Malignant melanoma of** right **eyelid, including canthus**

      C43.111 **Malignant melanoma of right** upper **eyelid, including canthus**

      C43.112 **Malignant melanoma of right** lower **eyelid, including canthus**   HCC

√6ᵗʰ **C43.12** **Malignant melanoma of** left **eyelid, including canthus**

      C43.121 **Malignant melanoma of left** upper **eyelid, including canthus**   HCC

      C43.122 **Malignant melanoma of left** lower **eyelid, including canthus**   HCC

√5ᵗʰ **C43.2** **Malignant melanoma of** ear and external auricular canal

    C43.20 **Malignant melanoma of unspecified ear and external auricular canal**   HCC

    C43.21 **Malignant melanoma of** right **ear and external auricular canal**

    C43.22 **Malignant melanoma of** left **ear and external auricular canal**   HCC

√5ᵗʰ **C43.3** **Malignant melanoma of** other and unspecified parts of face

    C43.30 **Malignant melanoma of unspecified part of face**   HCC

    C43.31 **Malignant melanoma of** nose   HCC

    C43.39 **Malignant melanoma of other parts of face**   HCC

C43.4 **Malignant melanoma of** scalp and neck

√5ᵗʰ **C43.5** **Malignant melanoma of** trunk

    EXCLUDES 2   *malignant neoplasm of anus NOS (C21.0)*

                  malignant neoplasm of scrotum (C63.2)

    C43.51 **Malignant melanoma of** anal skin   HCC

       Malignant melanoma of anal margin

       Malignant melanoma of perianal skin

    C43.52 **Malignant melanoma of** skin of breast   HCC

    C43.59 **Malignant melanoma of other part of trunk**   HCC

√5ᵗʰ **C43.6** **Malignant melanoma of** upper limb, including shoulder

    C43.60 **Malignant melanoma of unspecified upper limb, including shoulder**   HCC

    C43.61 **Malignant melanoma of** right **upper limb, including shoulder**   HCC

    C43.62 **Malignant melanoma of** left **upper limb, including shoulder**   HCC

√5ᵗʰ **C43.7** **Malignant melanoma of** lower limb, including hip

    C43.70 **Malignant melanoma of unspecified lower limb, including hip**   HCC

    C43.71 **Malignant melanoma of** right **lower limb, including hip**   HCC

    C43.72 **Malignant melanoma of** left **lower limb, including hip**   HCC

C43.8 **Malignant melanoma of** overlapping sites **of skin**   HCC

C43.9 **Malignant melanoma of skin, unspecified**   HCC

    Malignant melanoma of unspecified site of skin

    Melanoma (malignant) NOS

√4ᵗʰ **C4A** **Merkel cell carcinoma**

    DEF: Malignant cutaneous cancer predominantly found in elderly patients with sun exposure that usually presents as a flesh-colored or bluish-red lump typically seen on the neck, head, and face.

C4A.0 **Merkel cell carcinoma of** lip   HCC

    EXCLUDES 1   *malignant neoplasm of vermilion border of lip (C00.0–C00.2)*

√5ᵗʰ **C4A.1** **Merkel cell carcinoma of** eyelid, including canthus

AHA: 2018,4Q,4

    C4A.10 **Merkel cell carcinoma of unspecified eyelid, including canthus**   HCC

√6ᵗʰ **C4A.11** **Merkel cell carcinoma of** right **eyelid, including canthus**

      C4A.111 **Merkel cell carcinoma of right** upper **eyelid, including canthus**   HCC

      C4A.112 **Merkel cell carcinoma of right** lower **eyelid, including canthus**   HCC

√6ᵗʰ **C4A.12** **Merkel cell carcinoma of** left **eyelid, including canthus**

      C4A.121 **Merkel cell carcinoma of left** upper **eyelid, including canthus**   HCC

      C4A.122 **Merkel cell carcinoma of left** lower **eyelid, including canthus**   HCC

√5ᵗʰ **C4A.2** **Merkel cell carcinoma of** ear and external auricular canal

    C4A.20 **Merkel cell carcinoma of unspecified ear and external auricular canal**   HCC

    C4A.21 **Merkel cell carcinoma of** right **ear and external auricular canal**

    C4A.22 **Merkel cell carcinoma of** left **ear and external auricular canal**   HCC

√5ᵗʰ **C4A.3** **Merkel cell carcinoma of other and unspecified** parts of face

    C4A.30 **Merkel cell carcinoma of unspecified part of face**   HCC

    C4A.31 **Merkel cell carcinoma of** nose   HCC

    C4A.39 **Merkel cell carcinoma of other parts of face**   HCC

C4A.4 **Merkel cell carcinoma of** scalp and neck   HCC

√5ᵗʰ **C4A.5** **Merkel cell carcinoma of** trunk

    EXCLUDES 2   *malignant neoplasm of anus NOS (C21.0)*

                  malignant neoplasm of scrotum (C63.2)

    C4A.51 **Merkel cell carcinoma of** anal skin   HCC

       Merkel cell carcinoma of anal margin

       Merkel cell carcinoma of perianal skin

    C4A.52 **Merkel cell carcinoma of** skin of breast   HCC

    C4A.59 **Merkel cell carcinoma of other part of trunk**   HCC

√5ᵗʰ **C4A.6** **Merkel cell carcinoma of** upper limb, including shoulder

    C4A.60 **Merkel cell carcinoma of unspecified upper limb, including shoulder**   HCC

    C4A.61 **Merkel cell carcinoma of** right **upper limb, including shoulder**   HCC

    C4A.62 **Merkel cell carcinoma of** left **upper limb, including shoulder**   HCC

√5ᵗʰ **C4A.7** **Merkel cell carcinoma of** lower limb, including hip

    C4A.70 **Merkel cell carcinoma of unspecified lower limb, including hip**   HCC

    C4A.71 **Merkel cell carcinoma of** right **lower limb, including hip**   HCC

    C4A.72 **Merkel cell carcinoma of** left **lower limb, including hip**   HCC

C4A.8 **Merkel cell carcinoma of** overlapping sites   HCC

C4A.9 **Merkel cell carcinoma, unspecified**   HCC

    Merkel cell carcinoma of unspecified site

    Merkel cell carcinoma NOS

√4ᵗʰ **C44** **Other and unspecified malignant neoplasm** of skin

    INCLUDES   malignant neoplasm of sebaceous glands

               malignant neoplasm of sweat glands

    EXCLUDES 1   *Kaposi's sarcoma of skin (C46.0)*

              malignant melanoma of skin (C43.-)

              malignant neoplasm of skin of genital organs (C51-C52, C60.-, C63.2)

              Merkel cell carcinoma (C4A.-)

    DEF: Basal cell carcinoma: Abnormal growth of skin cells that arises from the deepest layer of the epidermis and may present as an open sore, red patches, pink growth, or scar. Typically caused by sun exposure, it is one of the most common forms of skin cancer.

    DEF: Squamous cell carcinoma: Uncontrolled growth of abnormal skin cells that arises from the outer layers of the skin (epidermis) and may present as an open sore. It is characterized by a firm, red nodule, elevated growth with a central depression, or a flat sore with a scaly crust.

√5ᵗʰ **C44.0** **Other and unspecified malignant neoplasm of skin of** lip

    EXCLUDES 1   *malignant neoplasm of lip (C00.-)*

    C44.00 **Unspecified malignant neoplasm of skin of lip**

    C44.01 **Basal cell carcinoma of skin of lip**

    C44.02 **Squamous cell carcinoma of skin of lip**

    C44.09 **Other specified malignant neoplasm of skin of lip**

√5ᵗʰ **C44.1** **Other and unspecified malignant neoplasm of skin of** eyelid, including canthus

    EXCLUDES 1   *connective tissue of eyelid (C49.0)*

    AHA: 2018,4Q,4

√6ᵗʰ **C44.10** **Unspecified malignant neoplasm of skin of eyelid, including canthus**

      C44.101 **Unspecified malignant neoplasm of skin of unspecified eyelid, including canthus**

√7ᵗʰ   **C44.102** **Unspecified malignant neoplasm of skin of right eyelid, including canthus**

        C44.1021 **Unspecified malignant neoplasm of skin of right** upper **eyelid, including canthus**

N Newborn: 0   P Pediatric: 0-17   M Maternity: 9-64   A Adult: 15-124   MCC Major Complication/Comorbidity   CC Complication/Comorbidity   SW Severe Wound Dx

474   ICD-10-CM 2021

        C44.1022 Unspecified malignant neoplasm of skin of right lower eyelid, including canthus

    √7ʰ **C44.109** Unspecified malignant neoplasm of skin of left eyelid, including canthus

        C44.1091 Unspecified malignant neoplasm of skin of left upper eyelid, including canthus

        C44.1092 Unspecified malignant neoplasm of skin of left lower eyelid, including canthus

√6ʰ **C44.11** Basal cell carcinoma of skin of eyelid, including canthus

    C44.111 Basal cell carcinoma of skin of unspecified eyelid, including canthus

    √7ʰ **C44.112** Basal cell carcinoma of skin of right eyelid, including canthus

        C44.1121 Basal cell carcinoma of skin of right upper eyelid, including canthus

        C44.1122 Basal cell carcinoma of skin of right lower eyelid, including canthus

    √7ʰ **C44.119** Basal cell carcinoma of skin of left eyelid, including canthus

        C44.1191 Basal cell carcinoma of skin of left upper eyelid, including canthus

        C44.1192 Basal cell carcinoma of skin of left lower eyelid, including canthus

√6ʰ **C44.12** Squamous cell carcinoma of skin of eyelid, including canthus

    C44.121 Squamous cell carcinoma of skin of unspecified eyelid, including canthus

    √7ʰ **C44.122** Squamous cell carcinoma of skin of right eyelid, including canthus

        C44.1221 Squamous cell carcinoma of skin of right upper eyelid, including canthus

        C44.1222 Squamous cell carcinoma of skin of right lower eyelid, including canthus

    √7ʰ **C44.129** Squamous cell carcinoma of skin of left eyelid, including canthus

        C44.1291 Squamous cell carcinoma of skin of left upper eyelid, including canthus

        C44.1292 Squamous cell carcinoma of skin of left lower eyelid, including canthus

√6ʰ **C44.13** Sebaceous cell carcinoma of skin of eyelid, including canthus

    C44.131 Sebaceous cell carcinoma of skin of unspecified eyelid, including canthus

    √7ʰ **C44.132** Sebaceous cell carcinoma of skin of right eyelid, including canthus

        C44.1321 Sebaceous cell carcinoma of skin of right upper eyelid, including canthus

        C44.1322 Sebaceous cell carcinoma of skin of right lower eyelid, including canthus

    √7ʰ **C44.139** Sebaceous cell carcinoma of skin of left eyelid, including canthus

        C44.1391 Sebaceous cell carcinoma of skin of left upper eyelid, including canthus

        C44.1392 Sebaceous cell carcinoma of skin of left lower eyelid, including canthus

√6ʰ **C44.19** Other specified malignant neoplasm of skin of eyelid, including canthus

    C44.191 Other specified malignant neoplasm of skin of unspecified eyelid, including canthus

    √7ʰ **C44.192** Other specified malignant neoplasm of skin of right eyelid, including canthus

        C44.1921 Other specified malignant neoplasm of skin of right upper eyelid, including canthus

        C44.1922 Other specified malignant neoplasm of skin of right lower eyelid, including canthus

    √7ʰ **C44.199** Other specified malignant neoplasm of skin of left eyelid, including canthus

        C44.1991 Other specified malignant neoplasm of skin of left upper eyelid, including canthus

        C44.1992 Other specified malignant neoplasm of skin of left lower eyelid, including canthus

√5ʰ **C44.2** Other and unspecified malignant neoplasm of skin of ear and external auricular canal

    EXCLUDES 1 *connective tissue of ear (C49.0)*

    √6ʰ **C44.20** Unspecified malignant neoplasm of skin of ear and external auricular canal

        C44.201 Unspecified malignant neoplasm of skin of unspecified ear and external auricular canal

        C44.202 Unspecified malignant neoplasm of skin of right ear and external auricular canal

        C44.209 Unspecified malignant neoplasm of skin of left ear and external auricular canal

    √6ʰ **C44.21** Basal cell carcinoma of skin of ear and external auricular canal

        C44.211 Basal cell carcinoma of skin of unspecified ear and external auricular canal

        C44.212 Basal cell carcinoma of skin of right ear and external auricular canal

        C44.219 Basal cell carcinoma of skin of left ear and external auricular canal

    √6ʰ **C44.22** Squamous cell carcinoma of skin of ear and external auricular canal

        C44.221 Squamous cell carcinoma of skin of unspecified ear and external auricular canal

        C44.222 Squamous cell carcinoma of skin of right ear and external auricular canal

        C44.229 Squamous cell carcinoma of skin of left ear and external auricular canal

    √6ʰ **C44.29** Other specified malignant neoplasm of skin of ear and external auricular canal

        C44.291 Other specified malignant neoplasm of skin of unspecified ear and external auricular canal

        C44.292 Other specified malignant neoplasm of skin of right ear and external auricular canal

        C44.299 Other specified malignant neoplasm of skin of left ear and external auricular canal

√5ʰ **C44.3** Other and unspecified malignant neoplasm of skin of other and unspecified parts of face

    √6ʰ **C44.30** Unspecified malignant neoplasm of skin of other and unspecified parts of face

        C44.300 Unspecified malignant neoplasm of skin of unspecified part of face

        C44.301 Unspecified malignant neoplasm of skin of nose

        C44.309 Unspecified malignant neoplasm of skin of other parts of face

    √6ʰ **C44.31** Basal cell carcinoma of skin of other and unspecified parts of face

        C44.310 Basal cell carcinoma of skin of unspecified parts of face

        C44.311 Basal cell carcinoma of skin of nose

        C44.319 Basal cell carcinoma of skin of other parts of face

    √6ʰ **C44.32** Squamous cell carcinoma of skin of other and unspecified parts of face

        C44.320 Squamous cell carcinoma of skin of unspecified parts of face

        C44.321 Squamous cell carcinoma of skin of nose

        C44.329 Squamous cell carcinoma of skin of other parts of face

    √6ʰ **C44.39** Other specified malignant neoplasm of skin of other and unspecified parts of face

        C44.390 Other specified malignant neoplasm of skin of unspecified parts of face

        C44.391 Other specified malignant neoplasm of skin of nose

        C44.399 Other specified malignant neoplasm of skin of other parts of face

☑ Additional Character Required   √x7ʰ Placeholder   Unacceptable PDx   Questionable PDx   Manifestation   Unspecified Dx   **H1**-**H14** HAC   **HCC** CMS-HCC Dx   **HIV** HIV Dx

ICD-10-CM 2021   475

✓5ᵗʰ **C44.4 Other and unspecified malignant neoplasm of skin of scalp and neck**
    C44.40 Unspecified malignant neoplasm of skin of scalp and neck
    C44.41 Basal cell carcinoma **of skin of scalp and neck**
    C44.42 Squamous cell carcinoma **of skin of scalp and neck**
    C44.49 Other specified malignant neoplasm of skin of scalp and neck

✓5ᵗʰ **C44.5 Other and unspecified malignant neoplasm of skin of trunk**
    EXCLUDES 1   *anus NOS (C21.0)*
                scrotum (C63.2)
  ✓6ᵗʰ **C44.50 Unspecified malignant neoplasm of skin of trunk**
    C44.500 Unspecified malignant neoplasm of anal skin
         Unspecified malignant neoplasm of anal margin
         Unspecified malignant neoplasm of perianal skin
    C44.501 Unspecified malignant neoplasm of skin of breast
    C44.509 Unspecified malignant neoplasm of skin of other part of trunk
  ✓6ᵗʰ **C44.51** Basal cell carcinoma **of skin of trunk**
    C44.510 Basal cell carcinoma of anal skin
         Basal cell carcinoma of anal margin
         Basal cell carcinoma of perianal skin
    C44.511 Basal cell carcinoma of skin of breast
    C44.519 Basal cell carcinoma of skin of other part of trunk
  ✓6ᵗʰ **C44.52** Squamous cell carcinoma **of skin of trunk**
    C44.520 Squamous cell carcinoma of anal skin
         Squamous cell carcinoma of anal margin
         Squamous cell carcinoma of perianal skin
    C44.521 Squamous cell carcinoma of skin of breast
    C44.529 Squamous cell carcinoma of skin of other part of trunk
  ✓6ᵗʰ **C44.59 Other specified malignant neoplasm of skin of trunk**
    C44.590 Other specified malignant neoplasm of anal skin
         Other specified malignant neoplasm of anal margin
         Other specified malignant neoplasm of perianal skin
    C44.591 Other specified malignant neoplasm of skin of breast
    C44.599 Other specified malignant neoplasm of skin of other part of trunk

✓5ᵗʰ **C44.6 Other and unspecified malignant neoplasm of skin of upper limb, including shoulder**
  ✓6ᵗʰ **C44.60 Unspecified malignant neoplasm of skin of upper limb, including shoulder**
    C44.601 Unspecified malignant neoplasm of skin of unspecified upper limb, including shoulder
    C44.602 Unspecified malignant neoplasm of skin of right upper limb, including shoulder
    C44.609 Unspecified malignant neoplasm of skin of left upper limb, including shoulder
  ✓6ᵗʰ **C44.61** Basal cell carcinoma **of skin of upper limb, including shoulder**
    C44.611 Basal cell carcinoma of skin of unspecified upper limb, including shoulder
    C44.612 Basal cell carcinoma of skin of right upper limb, including shoulder
    C44.619 Basal cell carcinoma of skin of left upper limb, including shoulder
  ✓6ᵗʰ **C44.62** Squamous cell carcinoma **of skin of upper limb, including shoulder**
    C44.621 Squamous cell carcinoma of skin of unspecified upper limb, including shoulder
    C44.622 Squamous cell carcinoma of skin of right upper limb, including shoulder
    C44.629 Squamous cell carcinoma of skin of left upper limb, including shoulder
  ✓6ᵗʰ **C44.69 Other specified malignant neoplasm of skin of upper limb, including shoulder**
    C44.691 Other specified malignant neoplasm of skin of unspecified upper limb, including shoulder

    C44.692 Other specified malignant neoplasm of skin of right upper limb, including shoulder
    C44.699 Other specified malignant neoplasm of skin of left upper limb, including shoulder

✓5ᵗʰ **C44.7 Other and unspecified malignant neoplasm of skin of lower limb, including hip**
  ✓6ᵗʰ **C44.70 Unspecified malignant neoplasm of skin of lower limb, including hip**
    C44.701 Unspecified malignant neoplasm of skin of unspecified lower limb, including hip
    C44.702 Unspecified malignant neoplasm of skin of right lower limb, including hip
    C44.709 Unspecified malignant neoplasm of skin of left lower limb, including hip
  ✓6ᵗʰ **C44.71** Basal cell carcinoma **of skin of lower limb, including hip**
    C44.711 Basal cell carcinoma of skin of unspecified lower limb, including hip
    C44.712 Basal cell carcinoma of skin of right lower limb, including hip
    C44.719 Basal cell carcinoma of skin of left lower limb, including hip
  ✓6ᵗʰ **C44.72** Squamous cell carcinoma **of skin of lower limb, including hip**
    C44.721 Squamous cell carcinoma of skin of unspecified lower limb, including hip
    C44.722 Squamous cell carcinoma of skin of right lower limb, including hip
    C44.729 Squamous cell carcinoma of skin of left lower limb, including hip
  ✓6ᵗʰ **C44.79 Other specified malignant neoplasm of skin of lower limb, including hip**
    C44.791 Other specified malignant neoplasm of skin of unspecified lower limb, including hip
    C44.792 Other specified malignant neoplasm of skin of right lower limb, including hip
    C44.799 Other specified malignant neoplasm of skin of left lower limb, including hip

✓5ᵗʰ **C44.8 Other and unspecified malignant neoplasm of overlapping sites of skin**
    C44.80 Unspecified malignant neoplasm of overlapping sites of skin
    C44.81 Basal cell carcinoma **of overlapping sites of skin**
    C44.82 Squamous cell carcinoma **of overlapping sites of skin**
    C44.89 Other specified malignant neoplasm of overlapping sites of skin

✓5ᵗʰ **C44.9 Other and unspecified malignant neoplasm of skin, unspecified**
    C44.90 Unspecified malignant neoplasm of skin, unspecified
         Malignant neoplasm of unspecified site of skin
    C44.91 Basal cell carcinoma **of skin, unspecified**
    C44.92 Squamous cell carcinoma **of skin, unspecified**
    C44.99 Other specified malignant neoplasm of skin, unspecified

Malignant neoplasms of mesothelial and soft tissue (C45-C49)

✓4ᵗʰ **C45 Mesothelioma**
    DEF: Rare type of cancer that forms in the thin layer of protective tissue that covers the majority of internal organs (mesothelium).

    C45.0 Mesothelioma of pleura   CC HCC
         EXCLUDES 1   *other malignant neoplasm of pleura (C38.4)*
         AHA: 2017,2Q,11
         TIP: For pleural mesothelioma that has metastasized to the chest wall, assign this code for the primary site along with C79.89 for metastatic cancer in the chest wall.

    C45.1 Mesothelioma of peritoneum   CC HCC
         Mesothelioma of cul-de-sac
         Mesothelioma of mesentery
         Mesothelioma of mesocolon
         Mesothelioma of omentum
         Mesothelioma of peritoneum (parietal) (pelvic)
         EXCLUDES 1   *other malignant neoplasm of soft tissue of peritoneum (C48.-)*

    C45.2 Mesothelioma of pericardium   CC HCC
         EXCLUDES 1   *other malignant neoplasm of pericardium (C38.0)*

    C45.7 Mesothelioma of other sites   HCC

C45.9   **Mesothelioma, unspecified**   `HCC`

✓4ᵗʰ **C46** **Kaposi's sarcoma**

Code first any human immunodeficiency virus [HIV] disease (B2Ø)

DEF: Malignant neoplasm that causes patches of abnormal tissue to grow under the skin, in the lining of the mouth, nose, and throat, in lymph nodes, or in other visceral organs. Kaposi's sarcoma is caused by human herpesvirus8 (HHV8).

C46.Ø   **Kaposi's sarcoma of skin**   `HIV` `CC` `HCC`

C46.1   **Kaposi's sarcoma of soft tissue**   `HIV` `CC` `HCC`
     Kaposi's sarcoma of blood vessel
     Kaposi's sarcoma of connective tissue
     Kaposi's sarcoma of fascia
     Kaposi's sarcoma of ligament
     Kaposi's sarcoma of lymphatic(s) NEC
     Kaposi's sarcoma of muscle
     EXCLUDES 2   *Kaposi's sarcoma of lymph glands and nodes (C46.3)*

C46.2   **Kaposi's sarcoma of palate**   `HIV` `CC` `HCC`

C46.3   **Kaposi's sarcoma of lymph nodes**   `HIV` `CC` `HCC`

C46.4   **Kaposi's sarcoma of gastrointestinal sites**   `HIV` `CC` `HCC`

✓5ᵗʰ **C46.5**   **Kaposi's sarcoma of lung**
     AHA: 2019,1Q,16
     TIP: When associated malignant pericardial effusion is documented, assign code I31.3. If the sole reason for admission is to treat the effusion with no treatment of the lung malignancy rendered, code I31.3 may be sequenced first.

     C46.5Ø   **Kaposi's sarcoma of unspecified lung**   `HIV` `CC` `HCC`
     C46.51   **Kaposi's sarcoma of right lung**   `HIV` `CC` `HCC`
     C46.52   **Kaposi's sarcoma of left lung**   `HIV` `CC` `HCC`

C46.7   **Kaposi's sarcoma of other sites**   `HIV` `CC` `HCC`

C46.9   **Kaposi's sarcoma, unspecified**   `HIV` `CC` `HCC`
     Kaposi's sarcoma of unspecified site

✓4ᵗʰ **C47** **Malignant neoplasm of peripheral nerves and autonomic nervous system**

     INCLUDES   malignant neoplasm of sympathetic and parasympathetic nerves and ganglia

     EXCLUDES 1   *Kaposi's sarcoma of soft tissue (C46.1)*

C47.Ø   **Malignant neoplasm of peripheral nerves of head, face and neck**   `CC` `HCC`
     EXCLUDES 1   *malignant neoplasm of peripheral nerves of orbit (C69.6-)*

✓5ᵗʰ **C47.1**   **Malignant neoplasm of peripheral nerves of upper limb, including shoulder**

     C47.1Ø   **Malignant neoplasm of peripheral nerves of unspecified upper limb, including shoulder**   `CC` `HCC`
     C47.11   **Malignant neoplasm of peripheral nerves of right upper limb, including shoulder**   `CC` `HCC`
     C47.12   **Malignant neoplasm of peripheral nerves of left upper limb, including shoulder**   `CC` `HCC`

✓5ᵗʰ **C47.2**   **Malignant neoplasm of peripheral nerves of lower limb, including hip**

     C47.2Ø   **Malignant neoplasm of peripheral nerves of unspecified lower limb, including hip**   `CC` `HCC`
     C47.21   **Malignant neoplasm of peripheral nerves of right lower limb, including hip**   `CC` `HCC`
     C47.22   **Malignant neoplasm of peripheral nerves of left lower limb, including hip**   `CC` `HCC`

C47.3   **Malignant neoplasm of peripheral nerves of thorax**   `CC` `HCC`

C47.4   **Malignant neoplasm of peripheral nerves of abdomen**   `CC` `HCC`

C47.5   **Malignant neoplasm of peripheral nerves of pelvis**   `CC` `HCC`

C47.6   **Malignant neoplasm of peripheral nerves of trunk, unspecified**   `CC` `HCC`
     Malignant neoplasm of peripheral nerves of unspecified part of trunk

C47.8   **Malignant neoplasm of overlapping sites of peripheral nerves and autonomic nervous system**   `CC` `HCC`

C47.9   **Malignant neoplasm of peripheral nerves and autonomic nervous system, unspecified**   `CC` `HCC`
     Malignant neoplasm of unspecified site of peripheral nerves and autonomic nervous system

✓4ᵗʰ **C48** **Malignant neoplasm of retroperitoneum and peritoneum**

     EXCLUDES 1   *Kaposi's sarcoma of connective tissue (C46.1)*
     mesothelioma (C45.-)

C48.Ø   **Malignant neoplasm of retroperitoneum**   `CC` `HCC`

C48.1   **Malignant neoplasm of specified parts of peritoneum**   `CC` `HCC`
     Malignant neoplasm of cul-de-sac
     Malignant neoplasm of mesentery
     Malignant neoplasm of mesocolon
     Malignant neoplasm of omentum
     Malignant neoplasm of parietal peritoneum
     Malignant neoplasm of pelvic peritoneum

C48.2   **Malignant neoplasm of peritoneum, unspecified**   `CC` `HCC`

C48.8   **Malignant neoplasm of overlapping sites of retroperitoneum and peritoneum**   `CC` `HCC`

✓4ᵗʰ **C49** **Malignant neoplasm of other connective and soft tissue**

     INCLUDES   malignant neoplasm of blood vessel
     malignant neoplasm of bursa
     malignant neoplasm of cartilage
     malignant neoplasm of fascia
     malignant neoplasm of fat
     malignant neoplasm of ligament, except uterine
     malignant neoplasm of lymphatic vessel
     malignant neoplasm of muscle
     malignant neoplasm of synovia
     malignant neoplasm of tendon (sheath)

     EXCLUDES 1   *malignant neoplasm of cartilage (of):*
         articular (C4Ø-C41)
         larynx (C32.3)
         nose (C3Ø.Ø)
     malignant neoplasm of connective tissue of breast (C5Ø.-)

     EXCLUDES 2   *Kaposi's sarcoma of soft tissue (C46.1)*
     malignant neoplasm of heart (C38.Ø)
     malignant neoplasm of peripheral nerves and autonomic nervous system (C47.-)
     malignant neoplasm of peritoneum (C48.2)
     malignant neoplasm of retroperitoneum (C48.Ø)
     malignant neoplasm of uterine ligament (C57.3)
     mesothelioma (C45.-)

C49.Ø   **Malignant neoplasm of connective and soft tissue of head, face and neck**   `CC` `HCC`
     Malignant neoplasm of connective tissue of ear
     Malignant neoplasm of connective tissue of eyelid
     EXCLUDES 1   *connective tissue of orbit (C69.6-)*

✓5ᵗʰ **C49.1**   **Malignant neoplasm of connective and soft tissue of upper limb, including shoulder**

     C49.1Ø   **Malignant neoplasm of connective and soft tissue of unspecified upper limb, including shoulder**   `CC` `HCC`
     C49.11   **Malignant neoplasm of connective and soft tissue of right upper limb, including shoulder**   `CC` `HCC`
     C49.12   **Malignant neoplasm of connective and soft tissue of left upper limb, including shoulder**   `CC` `HCC`

✓5ᵗʰ **C49.2**   **Malignant neoplasm of connective and soft tissue of lower limb, including hip**

     C49.2Ø   **Malignant neoplasm of connective and soft tissue of unspecified lower limb, including hip**   `CC` `HCC`
     C49.21   **Malignant neoplasm of connective and soft tissue of right lower limb, including hip**   `CC` `HCC`
     C49.22   **Malignant neoplasm of connective and soft tissue of left lower limb, including hip**   `CC` `HCC`

C49.3   **Malignant neoplasm of connective and soft tissue of thorax**   `CC` `HCC`
     Malignant neoplasm of axilla
     Malignant neoplasm of diaphragm
     Malignant neoplasm of great vessels
     EXCLUDES 1   *malignant neoplasm of breast (C5Ø.-)*
         malignant neoplasm of heart (C38.Ø)
         malignant neoplasm of mediastinum (C38.1-C38.3)
         malignant neoplasm of thymus (C37)

     AHA: 2015,3Q,19

C49.4   **Malignant neoplasm of connective and soft tissue of abdomen**   `CC` `HCC`
     Malignant neoplasm of abdominal wall
     Malignant neoplasm of hypochondrium

C49.5   **Malignant neoplasm of connective and soft tissue of pelvis**   `CC` `HCC`
     Malignant neoplasm of buttock
     Malignant neoplasm of groin
     Malignant neoplasm of perineum

☑ Additional Character Required   ✓x7ᵗʰ Placeholder   Unacceptable PDx   Questionable PDx   Manifestation   Unspecified Dx   H1-H14 HAC   HCC CMS-HCC Dx   HIV HIV Dx

ICD-10-CM 2021   477

C49.6   **Malignant neoplasm of connective and soft tissue of trunk, unspecified** `CC` `HCC`

Malignant neoplasm of back NOS

C49.8   **Malignant neoplasm of overlapping sites of connective and soft tissue** `CC` `HCC`

Primary malignant neoplasm of two or more contiguous sites of connective and soft tissue

C49.9   **Malignant neoplasm of connective and soft tissue, unspecified** `CC` `HCC`

√5ᵗʰ **C49.A**   **Gastrointestinal stromal tumor**

AHA: 2016,4Q,8
DEF: Uncommon malignant tumor found in the GI tract that originates from interstitial cells of the autonomic nervous system. Most occur in the stomach or small intestine but can originate anywhere in the GI tract.

C49.A0   **Gastrointestinal stromal tumor, unspecified site** `CC` `HCC`

C49.A1   **Gastrointestinal stromal tumor of esophagus** `CC` `HCC`

C49.A2   **Gastrointestinal stromal tumor of stomach** `CC` `HCC`

C49.A3   **Gastrointestinal stromal tumor of small intestine** `CC` `HCC`

C49.A4   **Gastrointestinal stromal tumor of large intestine** `CC` `HCC`

C49.A5   **Gastrointestinal stromal tumor of rectum** `CC` `HCC`

C49.A9   **Gastrointestinal stromal tumor of other sites** `CC` `HCC`

Malignant neoplasms of breast (C50)

√4ᵗʰ **C50**   **Malignant neoplasm of breast**

INCLUDES   connective tissue of breast
Paget's disease of breast
Paget's disease of nipple

Use additional code to identify estrogen receptor status (Z17.0, Z17.1)

EXCLUDES 1   skin of breast (C44.501, C44.511, C44.521, C44.591)

AHA: 2017,4Q,19

Female Breast

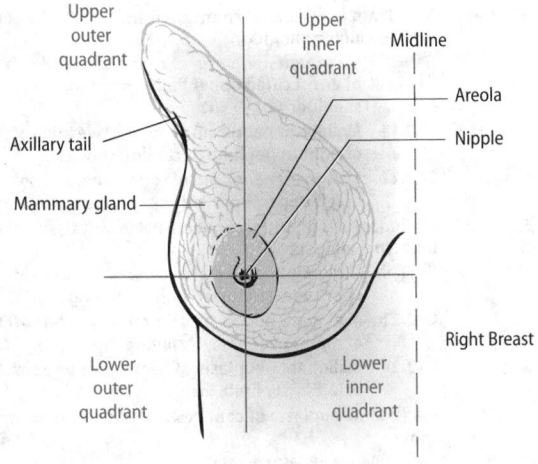

Upper outer quadrant — Upper inner quadrant — Midline — Areola — Nipple — Axillary tail — Mammary gland — Lower outer quadrant — Lower inner quadrant — Right Breast

√5ᵗʰ **C50.0**   **Malignant neoplasm of nipple and areola**

√6ᵗʰ **C50.01**   **Malignant neoplasm of nipple and areola, female**

C50.011   Malignant neoplasm of nipple and areola, right female breast `HCC` ♀

C50.012   Malignant neoplasm of nipple and areola, left female breast `HCC` ♀

C50.019   Malignant neoplasm of nipple and areola, unspecified female breast `HCC` ♀

√6ᵗʰ **C50.02**   **Malignant neoplasm of nipple and areola, male**

C50.021   Malignant neoplasm of nipple and areola, right male breast `HCC` ♂

C50.022   Malignant neoplasm of nipple and areola, left male breast `HCC` ♂

C50.029   Malignant neoplasm of nipple and areola, unspecified male breast `HCC` ♂

√5ᵗʰ **C50.1**   **Malignant neoplasm of central portion of breast**

√6ᵗʰ **C50.11**   **Malignant neoplasm of central portion of breast, female**

C50.111   Malignant neoplasm of central portion of right female breast `HCC` ♀

C50.112   Malignant neoplasm of central portion of left female breast `HCC` ♀

C50.119   Malignant neoplasm of central portion of unspecified female breast `HCC` ♀

√6ᵗʰ **C50.12**   **Malignant neoplasm of central portion of breast, male**

C50.121   Malignant neoplasm of central portion of right male breast `HCC` ♂

C50.122   Malignant neoplasm of central portion of left male breast `HCC` ♂

C50.129   Malignant neoplasm of central portion of unspecified male breast `HCC` ♂

√5ᵗʰ **C50.2**   **Malignant neoplasm of upper-inner quadrant of breast**

√6ᵗʰ **C50.21**   **Malignant neoplasm of upper-inner quadrant of breast, female**

C50.211   Malignant neoplasm of upper-inner quadrant of right female breast `HCC` ♀

C50.212   Malignant neoplasm of upper-inner quadrant of left female breast `HCC` ♀

C50.219   Malignant neoplasm of upper-inner quadrant of unspecified female breast `HCC` ♀

√6ᵗʰ **C50.22**   **Malignant neoplasm of upper-inner quadrant of breast, male**

C50.221   Malignant neoplasm of upper-inner quadrant of right male breast `HCC` ♂

C50.222   Malignant neoplasm of upper-inner quadrant of left male breast `HCC` ♂

C50.229   Malignant neoplasm of upper-inner quadrant of unspecified male breast `HCC` ♂

√5ᵗʰ **C50.3**   **Malignant neoplasm of lower-inner quadrant of breast**

√6ᵗʰ **C50.31**   **Malignant neoplasm of lower-inner quadrant of breast, female**

C50.311   Malignant neoplasm of lower-inner quadrant of right female breast `HCC` ♀

C50.312   Malignant neoplasm of lower-inner quadrant of left female breast `HCC` ♀

C50.319   Malignant neoplasm of lower-inner quadrant of unspecified female breast `HCC` ♀

√6ᵗʰ **C50.32**   **Malignant neoplasm of lower-inner quadrant of breast, male**

C50.321   Malignant neoplasm of lower-inner quadrant of right male breast `HCC` ♂

C50.322   Malignant neoplasm of lower-inner quadrant of left male breast `HCC` ♂

C50.329   Malignant neoplasm of lower-inner quadrant of unspecified male breast `HCC` ♂

√5ᵗʰ **C50.4**   **Malignant neoplasm of upper-outer quadrant of breast**

√6ᵗʰ **C50.41**   **Malignant neoplasm of upper-outer quadrant of breast, female**

C50.411   Malignant neoplasm of upper-outer quadrant of right female breast `HCC` ♀

C50.412   Malignant neoplasm of upper-outer quadrant of left female breast `HCC` ♀

C50.419   Malignant neoplasm of upper-outer quadrant of unspecified female breast `HCC` ♀

√6ᵗʰ **C50.42**   **Malignant neoplasm of upper-outer quadrant of breast, male**

C50.421   Malignant neoplasm of upper-outer quadrant of right male breast `HCC` ♂

C50.422   Malignant neoplasm of upper-outer quadrant of left male breast `HCC` ♂

C50.429   Malignant neoplasm of upper-outer quadrant of unspecified male breast `HCC` ♂

√5ᵗʰ **C50.5**   **Malignant neoplasm of lower-outer quadrant of breast**

√6ᵗʰ **C50.51**   **Malignant neoplasm of lower-outer quadrant of breast, female**

C50.511   Malignant neoplasm of lower-outer quadrant of right female breast `HCC` ♀

C50.512   Malignant neoplasm of lower-outer quadrant of left female breast `HCC` ♀

C50.519   Malignant neoplasm of lower-outer quadrant of unspecified female breast   HCC ♀

√6ᵗʰ   **C50.52**   Malignant neoplasm of lower-outer quadrant of breast, male

C50.521   Malignant neoplasm of lower-outer quadrant of right male breast   HCC ♂

C50.522   Malignant neoplasm of lower-outer quadrant of left male breast   HCC ♂

C50.529   Malignant neoplasm of lower-outer quadrant of unspecified male breast   HCC ♂

√5ᵗʰ   **C50.6**   Malignant neoplasm of axillary tail of breast

√6ᵗʰ   **C50.61**   Malignant neoplasm of axillary tail of breast, female

C50.611   Malignant neoplasm of axillary tail of right female breast   HCC ♀

C50.612   Malignant neoplasm of axillary tail of left female breast   HCC ♀

C50.619   Malignant neoplasm of axillary tail of unspecified female breast   HCC ♀

√6ᵗʰ   **C50.62**   Malignant neoplasm of axillary tail of breast, male

C50.621   Malignant neoplasm of axillary tail of right male breast   HCC ♂

C50.622   Malignant neoplasm of axillary tail of left male breast   HCC ♂

C50.629   Malignant neoplasm of axillary tail of unspecified male breast   HCC ♂

√5ᵗʰ   **C50.8**   Malignant neoplasm of overlapping sites of breast

√6ᵗʰ   **C50.81**   Malignant neoplasm of overlapping sites of breast, female

C50.811   Malignant neoplasm of overlapping sites of right female breast   HCC ♀

C50.812   Malignant neoplasm of overlapping sites of left female breast   HCC ♀

C50.819   Malignant neoplasm of overlapping sites of unspecified female breast   HCC ♀

√6ᵗʰ   **C50.82**   Malignant neoplasm of overlapping sites of breast, male

C50.821   Malignant neoplasm of overlapping sites of right male breast   HCC ♂

C50.822   Malignant neoplasm of overlapping sites of left male breast   HCC ♂

C50.829   Malignant neoplasm of overlapping sites of unspecified male breast   HCC ♂

√5ᵗʰ   **C50.9**   Malignant neoplasm of breast of unspecified site

√6ᵗʰ   **C50.91**   Malignant neoplasm of breast of unspecified site, female

C50.911   Malignant neoplasm of unspecified site of right female breast   HCC ♀

C50.912   Malignant neoplasm of unspecified site of left female breast   HCC ♀

C50.919   Malignant neoplasm of unspecified site of unspecified female breast   HCC ♀

√6ᵗʰ   **C50.92**   Malignant neoplasm of breast of unspecified site, male

C50.921   Malignant neoplasm of unspecified site of right male breast   HCC ♂

C50.922   Malignant neoplasm of unspecified site of left male breast   HCC ♂

C50.929   Malignant neoplasm of unspecified site of unspecified male breast   HCC ♂

Malignant neoplasms of female genital organs (C51-C58)

INCLUDES   malignant neoplasm of skin of female genital organs

√4ᵗʰ   **C51**   **Malignant neoplasm of vulva**

EXCLUDES 1   carcinoma in situ of vulva (D07.1)

C51.0   Malignant neoplasm of labium majus   HCC ♀
Malignant neoplasm of Bartholin's [greater vestibular] gland

C51.1   Malignant neoplasm of labium minus   HCC ♀

C51.2   Malignant neoplasm of clitoris   HCC ♀

C51.8   Malignant neoplasm of overlapping sites of vulva   HCC ♀

C51.9   Malignant neoplasm of vulva, unspecified   HCC ♀
Malignant neoplasm of external female genitalia NOS
Malignant neoplasm of pudendum

C52   **Malignant neoplasm of vagina**   HCC ♀
EXCLUDES 1   carcinoma in situ of vagina (D07.2)

√4ᵗʰ   **C53**   **Malignant neoplasm of cervix uteri**

EXCLUDES 1   carcinoma in situ of cervix uteri (D06.-)

AHA: 2017,4Q,103

C53.0   Malignant neoplasm of endocervix   HCC ♀

C53.1   Malignant neoplasm of exocervix   HCC ♀

C53.8   Malignant neoplasm of overlapping sites of cervix uteri   HCC ♀

C53.9   Malignant neoplasm of cervix uteri, unspecified   HCC ♀

√4ᵗʰ   **C54**   **Malignant neoplasm of corpus uteri**

C54.0   Malignant neoplasm of isthmus uteri   HCC ♀
Malignant neoplasm of lower uterine segment

C54.1   Malignant neoplasm of endometrium   HCC ♀

C54.2   Malignant neoplasm of myometrium   HCC ♀

C54.3   Malignant neoplasm of fundus uteri   HCC ♀

C54.8   Malignant neoplasm of overlapping sites of corpus uteri   HCC ♀

C54.9   Malignant neoplasm of corpus uteri, unspecified   HCC ♀

C55   **Malignant neoplasm of uterus, part unspecified**   HCC ♀

√4ᵗʰ   **C56**   **Malignant neoplasm of ovary**

Use additional code to identify any functional activity

C56.1   Malignant neoplasm of right ovary   CC HCC ♀

C56.2   Malignant neoplasm of left ovary   CC HCC ♀

C56.9   Malignant neoplasm of unspecified ovary   CC HCC ♀

√4ᵗʰ   **C57**   **Malignant neoplasm of other and unspecified female genital organs**

√5ᵗʰ   **C57.0**   Malignant neoplasm of fallopian tube
Malignant neoplasm of oviduct
Malignant neoplasm of uterine tube

C57.00   Malignant neoplasm of unspecified fallopian tube   HCC ♀

C57.01   Malignant neoplasm of right fallopian tube   HCC ♀

C57.02   Malignant neoplasm of left fallopian tube   HCC ♀

√5ᵗʰ   **C57.1**   Malignant neoplasm of broad ligament

C57.10   Malignant neoplasm of unspecified broad ligament   HCC ♀

C57.11   Malignant neoplasm of right broad ligament   HCC ♀

C57.12   Malignant neoplasm of left broad ligament   HCC ♀

√5ᵗʰ   **C57.2**   Malignant neoplasm of round ligament

C57.20   Malignant neoplasm of unspecified round ligament   HCC ♀

C57.21   Malignant neoplasm of right round ligament   HCC ♀

C57.22   Malignant neoplasm of left round ligament   HCC ♀

C57.3   Malignant neoplasm of parametrium   HCC ♀
Malignant neoplasm of uterine ligament NOS

C57.4   Malignant neoplasm of uterine adnexa, unspecified   HCC ♀

C57.7   Malignant neoplasm of other specified female genital organs   HCC ♀
Malignant neoplasm of wolffian body or duct

C57.8   Malignant neoplasm of overlapping sites of female genital organs   HCC ♀
Primary malignant neoplasm of two or more contiguous sites of the female genital organs whose point of origin cannot be determined
Primary tubo-ovarian malignant neoplasm whose point of origin cannot be determined
Primary utero-ovarian malignant neoplasm whose point of origin cannot be determined

C57.9   Malignant neoplasm of female genital organ, unspecified   HCC ♀
Malignant neoplasm of female genitourinary tract NOS

C58   **Malignant neoplasm of placenta**   HCC M ♀
INCLUDES   choriocarcinoma NOS
chorionepithelioma NOS
EXCLUDES 1   chorioadenoma (destruens) (D39.2)
hydatidiform mole NOS (O01.9)
invasive hydatidiform mole (D39.2)
male choriocarcinoma NOS (C62.9-)
malignant hydatidiform mole (D39.2)

✔ Additional Character Required   √x7ᵗʰ Placeholder   Unacceptable PDx   Questionable PDx   Manifestation   Unspecified Dx   H1-H14 HAC   HCC CMS-HCC Dx   HIV HIV Dx
ICD-10-CM 2021   479
C50.519-C58

Chapter 2. Neoplasms

C60–C69.12

Malignant neoplasms of male genital organs (C60-C63)

INCLUDES   malignant neoplasm of skin of male genital organs

✓4ᵗʰ **C60 Malignant neoplasm of penis**

   C60.0 Malignant neoplasm of prepuce   HCC ♂
     Malignant neoplasm of foreskin

   C60.1 Malignant neoplasm of glans penis   HCC ♂

   C60.2 Malignant neoplasm of body of penis   HCC ♂
     Malignant neoplasm of corpus cavernosum

   C60.8 Malignant neoplasm of overlapping sites of penis   HCC ♂

   C60.9 Malignant neoplasm of penis, unspecified   HCC ♂
     Malignant neoplasm of skin of penis NOS

C61 Malignant neoplasm of prostate   HCC ♂
   Use additional code to identify:
   hormone sensitivity status (Z19.1-Z19.2)
   rising PSA following treatment for malignant neoplasm of prostate (R97.21)
     EXCLUDES 1   malignant neoplasm of seminal vesicle (C63.7)
   AHA: 2017,1Q,17

✓4ᵗʰ **C62 Malignant neoplasm of testis**
   Use additional code to identify any functional activity

   ✓5ᵗʰ **C62.0 Malignant neoplasm of undescended testis**
     Malignant neoplasm of ectopic testis
     Malignant neoplasm of retained testis

     C62.00 Malignant neoplasm of unspecified undescended testis   HCC ♂

     C62.01 Malignant neoplasm of undescended right testis   HCC ♂

     C62.02 Malignant neoplasm of undescended left testis   HCC ♂

   ✓5ᵗʰ **C62.1 Malignant neoplasm of descended testis**
     Malignant neoplasm of scrotal testis

     C62.10 Malignant neoplasm of unspecified descended testis   HCC ♂

     C62.11 Malignant neoplasm of descended right testis   HCC ♂

     C62.12 Malignant neoplasm of descended left testis   HCC ♂

   ✓5ᵗʰ **C62.9 Malignant neoplasm of testis, unspecified whether descended or undescended**

     C62.90 Malignant neoplasm of unspecified testis, unspecified whether descended or undescended   HCC ♂
      Malignant neoplasm of testis NOS

     C62.91 Malignant neoplasm of right testis, unspecified whether descended or undescended   HCC ♂

     C62.92 Malignant neoplasm of left testis, unspecified whether descended or undescended   HCC ♂

✓4ᵗʰ **C63 Malignant neoplasm of other and unspecified male genital organs**

   ✓5ᵗʰ **C63.0 Malignant neoplasm of epididymis**

     C63.00 Malignant neoplasm of unspecified epididymis   HCC ♂

     C63.01 Malignant neoplasm of right epididymis   HCC ♂

     C63.02 Malignant neoplasm of left epididymis   HCC ♂

   ✓5ᵗʰ **C63.1 Malignant neoplasm of spermatic cord**

     C63.10 Malignant neoplasm of unspecified spermatic cord   HCC ♂

     C63.11 Malignant neoplasm of right spermatic cord   HCC ♂

     C63.12 Malignant neoplasm of left spermatic cord   HCC ♂

   C63.2 Malignant neoplasm of scrotum   HCC ♂
     Malignant neoplasm of skin of scrotum

   C63.7 Malignant neoplasm of other specified male genital organs   HCC ♂
     Malignant neoplasm of seminal vesicle
     Malignant neoplasm of tunica vaginalis

   C63.8 Malignant neoplasm of overlapping sites of male genital organs   HCC ♂
     Primary malignant neoplasm of two or more contiguous sites of male genital organs whose point of origin cannot be determined

C63.9 Malignant neoplasm of male genital organ, unspecified   HCC ♂
   Malignant neoplasm of male genitourinary tract NOS

Malignant neoplasms of urinary tract (C64-C68)

✓4ᵗʰ **C64 Malignant neoplasm of kidney, except renal pelvis**
   EXCLUDES 1   malignant carcinoid tumor of the kidney (C7A.093)
     malignant neoplasm of renal calyces (C65.-)
     malignant neoplasm of renal pelvis (C65.-)

   C64.1 Malignant neoplasm of right kidney, except renal pelvis   CC HCC

   C64.2 Malignant neoplasm of left kidney, except renal pelvis   CC HCC

   C64.9 Malignant neoplasm of unspecified kidney, except renal pelvis   CC HCC

✓4ᵗʰ **C65 Malignant neoplasm of renal pelvis**
   INCLUDES   malignant neoplasm of pelviureteric junction
     malignant neoplasm of renal calyces

   C65.1 Malignant neoplasm of right renal pelvis   CC HCC

   C65.2 Malignant neoplasm of left renal pelvis   CC HCC

   C65.9 Malignant neoplasm of unspecified renal pelvis   CC HCC

✓4ᵗʰ **C66 Malignant neoplasm of ureter**
   EXCLUDES 1   malignant neoplasm of ureteric orifice of bladder (C67.6)

   C66.1 Malignant neoplasm of right ureter   CC HCC

   C66.2 Malignant neoplasm of left ureter   CC HCC

   C66.9 Malignant neoplasm of unspecified ureter   CC HCC

✓4ᵗʰ **C67 Malignant neoplasm of bladder**

   C67.0 Malignant neoplasm of trigone of bladder   HCC

   C67.1 Malignant neoplasm of dome of bladder   HCC

   C67.2 Malignant neoplasm of lateral wall of bladder   HCC

   C67.3 Malignant neoplasm of anterior wall of bladder   HCC

   C67.4 Malignant neoplasm of posterior wall of bladder   HCC

   C67.5 Malignant neoplasm of bladder neck   HCC
     Malignant neoplasm of internal urethral orifice

   C67.6 Malignant neoplasm of ureteric orifice   HCC

   C67.7 Malignant neoplasm of urachus   HCC

   C67.8 Malignant neoplasm of overlapping sites of bladder   HCC

   C67.9 Malignant neoplasm of bladder, unspecified   HCC
     AHA: 2016,1Q,19

✓4ᵗʰ **C68 Malignant neoplasm of other and unspecified urinary organs**
   EXCLUDES 1   malignant neoplasm of female genitourinary tract NOS (C57.9)
     malignant neoplasm of male genitourinary tract NOS (C63.9)

   C68.0 Malignant neoplasm of urethra   CC HCC
     EXCLUDES 1   malignant neoplasm of urethral orifice of bladder (C67.5)

   C68.1 Malignant neoplasm of paraurethral glands   CC HCC

   C68.8 Malignant neoplasm of overlapping sites of urinary organs   CC HCC
     Primary malignant neoplasm of two or more contiguous sites of urinary organs whose point of origin cannot be determined

   C68.9 Malignant neoplasm of urinary organ, unspecified   CC HCC
     Malignant neoplasm of urinary system NOS

Malignant neoplasms of eye, brain and other parts of central nervous system (C69-C72)

✓4ᵗʰ **C69 Malignant neoplasm of eye and adnexa**
   EXCLUDES 1   malignant neoplasm of connective tissue of eyelid (C49.0)
     malignant neoplasm of eyelid (skin) (C43.1-, C44.1-)
     malignant neoplasm of optic nerve (C72.3-)

   ✓5ᵗʰ **C69.0 Malignant neoplasm of conjunctiva**

     C69.00 Malignant neoplasm of unspecified conjunctiva   HCC

     C69.01 Malignant neoplasm of right conjunctiva   HCC

     C69.02 Malignant neoplasm of left conjunctiva   HCC

   ✓5ᵗʰ **C69.1 Malignant neoplasm of cornea**

     C69.10 Malignant neoplasm of unspecified cornea   HCC

     C69.11 Malignant neoplasm of right cornea   HCC

     C69.12 Malignant neoplasm of left cornea   HCC

N Newborn: 0   P Pediatric: 0-17   M Maternity: 9-64   A Adult: 15-124   MCC Major Complication/Comorbidity   CC Complication/Comorbidity   SW Severe Wound Dx

480   ICD-10-CM 2021

√5ᵗʰ **C69.2 Malignant neoplasm of retina**

> EXCLUDES 1   *dark area on retina (D49.81)*
> *neoplasm of unspecified behavior of retina and choroid (D49.81)*
> *retinal freckle (D49.81)*

C69.20 Malignant neoplasm of unspecified retina `HCC`
C69.21 Malignant neoplasm of right retina `HCC`
C69.22 Malignant neoplasm of left retina `HCC`

√5ᵗʰ **C69.3 Malignant neoplasm of choroid**

C69.30 Malignant neoplasm of unspecified choroid `HCC`
C69.31 Malignant neoplasm of right choroid `HCC`
C69.32 Malignant neoplasm of left choroid `HCC`

√5ᵗʰ **C69.4 Malignant neoplasm of ciliary body**

C69.40 Malignant neoplasm of unspecified ciliary body `HCC`
C69.41 Malignant neoplasm of right ciliary body `HCC`
C69.42 Malignant neoplasm of left ciliary body `HCC`

√5ᵗʰ **C69.5 Malignant neoplasm of lacrimal gland and duct**

Malignant neoplasm of lacrimal sac
Malignant neoplasm of nasolacrimal duct

C69.50 Malignant neoplasm of unspecified lacrimal gland and duct `HCC`
C69.51 Malignant neoplasm of right lacrimal gland and duct `HCC`
C69.52 Malignant neoplasm of left lacrimal gland and duct `HCC`

√5ᵗʰ **C69.6 Malignant neoplasm of orbit**

Malignant neoplasm of connective tissue of orbit
Malignant neoplasm of extraocular muscle
Malignant neoplasm of peripheral nerves of orbit
Malignant neoplasm of retrobulbar tissue
Malignant neoplasm of retro-ocular tissue

> EXCLUDES 1   *malignant neoplasm of orbital bone (C41.0)*

C69.60 Malignant neoplasm of unspecified orbit `HCC`
C69.61 Malignant neoplasm of right orbit `HCC`
C69.62 Malignant neoplasm of left orbit `HCC`

√5ᵗʰ **C69.8 Malignant neoplasm of overlapping sites of eye and adnexa**

C69.80 Malignant neoplasm of overlapping sites of unspecified eye and adnexa `HCC`
C69.81 Malignant neoplasm of overlapping sites of right eye and adnexa `HCC`
C69.82 Malignant neoplasm of overlapping sites of left eye and adnexa `HCC`

√5ᵗʰ **C69.9 Malignant neoplasm of unspecified site of eye**

Malignant neoplasm of eyeball

C69.90 Malignant neoplasm of unspecified site of unspecified eye `HCC`
C69.91 Malignant neoplasm of unspecified site of right eye `HCC`
C69.92 Malignant neoplasm of unspecified site of left eye `HCC`

√4ᵗʰ **C70 Malignant neoplasm of meninges**

C70.0 Malignant neoplasm of cerebral meninges `CC` `HCC`
C70.1 Malignant neoplasm of spinal meninges `CC` `HCC`
C70.9 Malignant neoplasm of meninges, unspecified `CC` `HCC`

√4ᵗʰ **C71 Malignant neoplasm of brain**

> EXCLUDES 1   *malignant neoplasm of cranial nerves (C72.2-C72.5)*
> *retrobulbar malignant neoplasm (C69.6-)*

Lobes of the Brain

C71.0 Malignant neoplasm of cerebrum, except lobes and ventricles `CC` `HCC`
     Malignant neoplasm of supratentorial NOS
C71.1 Malignant neoplasm of frontal lobe `CC` `HCC`
C71.2 Malignant neoplasm of temporal lobe `CC` `HCC`
C71.3 Malignant neoplasm of parietal lobe `CC` `HCC`
C71.4 Malignant neoplasm of occipital lobe `CC` `HCC`
C71.5 Malignant neoplasm of cerebral ventricle `CC` `HCC`
> EXCLUDES 1   *malignant neoplasm of fourth cerebral ventricle (C71.7)*
C71.6 Malignant neoplasm of cerebellum `CC` `HCC`
C71.7 Malignant neoplasm of brain stem `CC` `HCC`
     Malignant neoplasm of fourth cerebral ventricle
     Infratentorial malignant neoplasm NOS
C71.8 Malignant neoplasm of overlapping sites of brain `CC` `HCC`
C71.9 Malignant neoplasm of brain, unspecified `CC` `HCC`
     AHA: 2014,3Q,3

√4ᵗʰ **C72 Malignant neoplasm of spinal cord, cranial nerves and other parts of central nervous system**

> EXCLUDES 1   *malignant neoplasm of meninges (C70.-)*
> *malignant neoplasm of peripheral nerves and autonomic nervous system (C47.-)*

C72.0 Malignant neoplasm of spinal cord `CC` `HCC`
C72.1 Malignant neoplasm of cauda equina `CC` `HCC`

√5ᵗʰ **C72.2 Malignant neoplasm of olfactory nerve**

Malignant neoplasm of olfactory bulb

C72.20 Malignant neoplasm of unspecified olfactory nerve `CC` `HCC`
C72.21 Malignant neoplasm of right olfactory nerve `CC` `HCC`
C72.22 Malignant neoplasm of left olfactory nerve `CC` `HCC`

√5ᵗʰ **C72.3 Malignant neoplasm of optic nerve**

C72.30 Malignant neoplasm of unspecified optic nerve `CC` `HCC`
C72.31 Malignant neoplasm of right optic nerve `CC` `HCC`
C72.32 Malignant neoplasm of left optic nerve `CC` `HCC`

√5ᵗʰ **C72.4 Malignant neoplasm of acoustic nerve**

C72.40 Malignant neoplasm of unspecified acoustic nerve `CC` `HCC`
C72.41 Malignant neoplasm of right acoustic nerve `CC` `HCC`
C72.42 Malignant neoplasm of left acoustic nerve `CC` `HCC`

√5ᵗʰ **C72.5 Malignant neoplasm of other and unspecified cranial nerves**

C72.50 Malignant neoplasm of unspecified cranial nerve `CC` `HCC`
     Malignant neoplasm of cranial nerve NOS
C72.59 Malignant neoplasm of other cranial nerves `CC` `HCC`

C72.9   **Malignant neoplasm of central nervous system, unspecified**   CC HCC

> Malignant neoplasm of unspecified site of central nervous system
>
> Malignant neoplasm of nervous system NOS

Malignant neoplasms of thyroid and other endocrine glands (C73-C75)

C73   **Malignant neoplasm of thyroid gland**   HCC

> Use additional code to identify any functional activity

✓4ᵗʰ **C74**   **Malignant neoplasm of adrenal gland**

> **TIP:** If an adrenal gland tumor is described as functioning (producing too much of a hormone), additional codes should be assigned to report the functional activity.

✓5ᵗʰ **C74.0**   **Malignant neoplasm of cortex of adrenal gland**

     C74.00   **Malignant neoplasm of cortex of unspecified adrenal gland**   CC HCC

     C74.01   **Malignant neoplasm of cortex of right adrenal gland**   CC HCC

     C74.02   **Malignant neoplasm of cortex of left adrenal gland**   CC HCC

✓5ᵗʰ **C74.1**   **Malignant neoplasm of medulla of adrenal gland**

     C74.10   **Malignant neoplasm of medulla of unspecified adrenal gland**   CC HCC

     C74.11   **Malignant neoplasm of medulla of right adrenal gland**   CC HCC

     C74.12   **Malignant neoplasm of medulla of left adrenal gland**   CC HCC

✓5ᵗʰ **C74.9**   **Malignant neoplasm of unspecified part of adrenal gland**

     C74.90   **Malignant neoplasm of unspecified part of unspecified adrenal gland**   CC HCC

     C74.91   **Malignant neoplasm of unspecified part of right adrenal gland**   CC HCC

     C74.92   **Malignant neoplasm of unspecified part of left adrenal gland**   CC HCC

✓4ᵗʰ **C75**   **Malignant neoplasm of other endocrine glands and related structures**

     EXCLUDES 1   malignant carcinoid tumors (C7A.0-)

               malignant neoplasm of adrenal gland (C74.-)

               malignant neoplasm of endocrine pancreas (C25.4)

               malignant neoplasm of islets of Langerhans (C25.4)

               malignant neoplasm of ovary (C56.-)

               malignant neoplasm of testis (C62.-)

               malignant neoplasm of thymus (C37)

               malignant neoplasm of thyroid gland (C73)

               malignant neuroendocrine tumors (C7A.-)

     C75.0   **Malignant neoplasm of parathyroid gland**   CC HCC

     C75.1   **Malignant neoplasm of pituitary gland**   CC HCC

     C75.2   **Malignant neoplasm of craniopharyngeal duct**   CC HCC

     C75.3   **Malignant neoplasm of pineal gland**   CC HCC

     C75.4   **Malignant neoplasm of carotid body**   CC HCC

     C75.5   **Malignant neoplasm of aortic body and other paraganglia**   CC HCC

     C75.8   **Malignant neoplasm with pluriglandular involvement, unspecified**   CC HCC

     C75.9   **Malignant neoplasm of endocrine gland, unspecified**   CC HCC

Malignant neuroendocrine tumors (C7A)

✓4ᵗʰ **C7A**   **Malignant neuroendocrine tumors**

> Code also any associated multiple endocrine neoplasia [MEN] syndromes (E31.2-)
>
> Use additional code to identify any associated endocrine syndrome, such as:
>
> carcinoid syndrome (E34.0)
>
> EXCLUDES 2   malignant pancreatic islet cell tumors (C25.4)
>
>   Merkel cell carcinoma (C4A.-)
>
> **AHA:** 2019,3Q,7
>
> **DEF:** Tumors comprised of cells that are capable of producing hormonal syndromes in which the normal hormonal balance required to support body system functions is adversely affected.

✓5ᵗʰ **C7A.0**   **Malignant carcinoid tumors**

> **AHA:** 2019,3Q,7
>
> **DEF:** Specific type of slow-growing benign or malignant neuroendocrine tumors. Carcinoid tumors occur most commonly in the hormone producing cells of the gastrointestinal tracts and can also occur in the pancreas, testes, ovaries, or lungs.

     C7A.00   **Malignant carcinoid tumor of unspecified site**   CC HCC

✓6ᵗʰ   **C7A.01**   **Malignant carcinoid tumors of the small intestine**

         C7A.010   **Malignant carcinoid tumor of the duodenum**   CC HCC

         C7A.011   **Malignant carcinoid tumor of the jejunum**   CC HCC

         C7A.012   **Malignant carcinoid tumor of the ileum**   CC HCC

         C7A.019   **Malignant carcinoid tumor of the small intestine, unspecified portion**   CC HCC

✓6ᵗʰ   **C7A.02**   **Malignant carcinoid tumors of the appendix, large intestine, and rectum**

         C7A.020   **Malignant carcinoid tumor of the appendix**   CC HCC

         C7A.021   **Malignant carcinoid tumor of the cecum**   CC HCC

         C7A.022   **Malignant carcinoid tumor of the ascending colon**   CC HCC

         C7A.023   **Malignant carcinoid tumor of the transverse colon**   CC HCC

         C7A.024   **Malignant carcinoid tumor of the descending colon**   CC HCC

         C7A.025   **Malignant carcinoid tumor of the sigmoid colon**   CC HCC

         C7A.026   **Malignant carcinoid tumor of the rectum**   CC HCC

         C7A.029   **Malignant carcinoid tumor of the large intestine, unspecified portion**   CC HCC

                Malignant carcinoid tumor of the colon NOS

✓6ᵗʰ   **C7A.09**   **Malignant carcinoid tumors of other sites**

         C7A.090   **Malignant carcinoid tumor of the bronchus and lung**   CC HCC

                AHA: 2019,1Q,16

                TIP: When associated malignant pericardial effusion is documented, assign code I31.3. If the sole reason for admission is to treat the effusion with no treatment of the lung malignancy rendered, code I31.3 may be sequenced first.

         C7A.091   **Malignant carcinoid tumor of the thymus**   CC HCC

         C7A.092   **Malignant carcinoid tumor of the stomach**   CC HCC

         C7A.093   **Malignant carcinoid tumor of the kidney**   CC HCC

         C7A.094   **Malignant carcinoid tumor of the foregut, unspecified**   CC HCC

         C7A.095   **Malignant carcinoid tumor of the midgut, unspecified**   CC HCC

         C7A.096   **Malignant carcinoid tumor of the hindgut, unspecified**   CC HCC

         C7A.098   **Malignant carcinoid tumors of other sites**   CC HCC

N Newborn: 0   P Pediatric: 0-17   M Maternity: 9-64   A Adult: 15-124   MCC Major Complication/Comorbidity   CC Complication/Comorbidity   SW Severe Wound Dx

482   ICD-10-CM 2021

C7A.1 Malignant poorly differentiated neuroendocrine tumors `CC` `HCC`
Malignant poorly differentiated neuroendocrine tumor NOS
Malignant poorly differentiated neuroendocrine carcinoma, any site
High grade neuroendocrine carcinoma, any site

C7A.8 Other malignant neuroendocrine tumors `CC` `HCC`
AHA: 2019,3Q,7

Secondary neuroendocrine tumors (C7B)

✓4ᵗʰ **C7B** Secondary neuroendocrine tumors
Use additional code to identify any functional activity

✓5ᵗʰ **C7B.0** Secondary carcinoid tumors
AHA: 2019,3Q,7

C7B.00 Secondary carcinoid tumors, unspecified site `HCC`

C7B.01 Secondary carcinoid tumors of distant lymph nodes `CC` `HCC`

C7B.02 Secondary carcinoid tumors of liver `CC` `HCC`

C7B.03 Secondary carcinoid tumors of bone `CC` `HCC`

C7B.04 Secondary carcinoid tumors of peritoneum `CC` `HCC`
Mesentary metastasis of carcinoid tumor

C7B.09 Secondary carcinoid tumors of other sites `CC` `HCC`

C7B.1 Secondary Merkel cell carcinoma `HCC`
Merkel cell carcinoma nodal presentation
Merkel cell carcinoma visceral metastatic presentation

C7B.8 Other secondary neuroendocrine tumors `CC` `HCC`
AHA: 2019,3Q,7

Malignant neoplasms of ill-defined, other secondary and unspecified sites (C76-C80)

✓4ᵗʰ **C76** Malignant neoplasm of other and ill-defined sites
EXCLUDES 1 malignant neoplasm of female genitourinary tract NOS (C57.9)
malignant neoplasm of male genitourinary tract NOS (C63.9)
malignant neoplasm of lymphoid, hematopoietic and related tissue (C81-C96)
malignant neoplasm of skin (C44.-)
malignant neoplasm of unspecified site NOS (C80.1)

C76.0 Malignant neoplasm of head, face and neck `HCC`
Malignant neoplasm of cheek NOS
Malignant neoplasm of nose NOS

C76.1 Malignant neoplasm of thorax `HCC`
Intrathoracic malignant neoplasm NOS
Malignant neoplasm of axilla NOS
Thoracic malignant neoplasm NOS

C76.2 Malignant neoplasm of abdomen `HCC`

C76.3 Malignant neoplasm of pelvis `HCC`
Malignant neoplasm of groin NOS
Malignant neoplasm of sites overlapping systems within the pelvis
Rectovaginal (septum) malignant neoplasm
Rectovesical (septum) malignant neoplasm

✓5ᵗʰ **C76.4** Malignant neoplasm of upper limb

C76.40 Malignant neoplasm of unspecified upper limb `HCC`

C76.41 Malignant neoplasm of right upper limb `HCC`

C76.42 Malignant neoplasm of left upper limb `HCC`

✓5ᵗʰ **C76.5** Malignant neoplasm of lower limb

C76.50 Malignant neoplasm of unspecified lower limb `HCC`

C76.51 Malignant neoplasm of right lower limb `HCC`

C76.52 Malignant neoplasm of left lower limb `HCC`

C76.8 Malignant neoplasm of other specified ill-defined sites `HCC`
Malignant neoplasm of overlapping ill-defined sites

✓4ᵗʰ **C77** Secondary and unspecified malignant neoplasm of lymph nodes
EXCLUDES 1 malignant neoplasm of lymph nodes, specified as primary (C81-C86, C88, C96.-)
mesentary metastasis of carcinoid tumor (C7B.04)
secondary carcinoid tumors of distant lymph nodes (C7B.01)

C77.0 Secondary and unspecified malignant neoplasm of lymph nodes of head, face and neck `CC` `HCC`
Secondary and unspecified malignant neoplasm of supraclavicular lymph nodes

C77.1 Secondary and unspecified malignant neoplasm of intrathoracic lymph nodes `CC` `HCC`

C77.2 Secondary and unspecified malignant neoplasm of intra-abdominal lymph nodes `CC` `HCC`

C77.3 Secondary and unspecified malignant neoplasm of axilla and upper limb lymph nodes `CC` `HCC`
Secondary and unspecified malignant neoplasm of pectoral lymph nodes

C77.4 Secondary and unspecified malignant neoplasm of inguinal and lower limb lymph nodes `CC` `HCC`

C77.5 Secondary and unspecified malignant neoplasm of intrapelvic lymph nodes `CC` `HCC`

C77.8 Secondary and unspecified malignant neoplasm of lymph nodes of multiple regions `CC` `HCC`

C77.9 Secondary and unspecified malignant neoplasm of lymph node, unspecified `CC` `HCC`

✓4ᵗʰ **C78** Secondary malignant neoplasm of respiratory and digestive organs
EXCLUDES 1 secondary carcinoid tumors of liver (C7B.02)
secondary carcinoid tumors of peritoneum (C7B.04)
EXCLUDES 2 lymph node metastases (C77.0)

✓5ᵗʰ **C78.0** Secondary malignant neoplasm of lung
AHA: 2019,1Q,16

C78.00 Secondary malignant neoplasm of unspecified lung `CC` `HCC`

C78.01 Secondary malignant neoplasm of right lung `CC` `HCC`

C78.02 Secondary malignant neoplasm of left lung `CC` `HCC`

C78.1 Secondary malignant neoplasm of mediastinum `CC` `HCC`

C78.2 Secondary malignant neoplasm of pleura `CC` `HCC`

✓5ᵗʰ **C78.3** Secondary malignant neoplasm of other and unspecified respiratory organs

C78.30 Secondary malignant neoplasm of unspecified respiratory organ `CC` `HCC`

C78.39 Secondary malignant neoplasm of other respiratory organs `CC` `HCC`

C78.4 Secondary malignant neoplasm of small intestine `CC` `HCC`

C78.5 Secondary malignant neoplasm of large intestine and rectum `CC` `HCC`

C78.6 Secondary malignant neoplasm of retroperitoneum and peritoneum `CC` `HCC`
AHA: 2017,2Q,12

C78.7 Secondary malignant neoplasm of liver and intrahepatic bile duct `CC` `HCC`

✓5ᵗʰ **C78.8** Secondary malignant neoplasm of other and unspecified digestive organs

C78.80 Secondary malignant neoplasm of unspecified digestive organ `CC` `HCC`

C78.89 Secondary malignant neoplasm of other digestive organs `CC` `HCC`
Code also exocrine pancreatic insufficiency (K86.81)

✓4ᵗʰ **C79** Secondary malignant neoplasm of other and unspecified sites
EXCLUDES 1 secondary carcinoid tumors (C7B.-)
secondary neuroendocrine tumors (C7B.-)

✓5ᵗʰ **C79.0** Secondary malignant neoplasm of kidney and renal pelvis

C79.00 Secondary malignant neoplasm of unspecified kidney and renal pelvis `CC` `HCC`

C79.01 Secondary malignant neoplasm of right kidney and renal pelvis `CC` `HCC`

C79.02 Secondary malignant neoplasm of left kidney and renal pelvis `CC` `HCC`

✓5ᵗʰ **C79.1** Secondary malignant neoplasm of bladder and other and unspecified urinary organs

C79.10 Secondary malignant neoplasm of unspecified urinary organs `CC` `HCC`

C79.11 **Secondary malignant neoplasm of bladder** cc hcc

EXCLUDES 2 lymph node metastases (C77.0)

C79.19 **Secondary malignant neoplasm of other urinary organs** cc hcc

C79.2 **Secondary malignant neoplasm of skin** cc hcc

EXCLUDES 1 secondary Merkel cell carcinoma (C7B.1)

✓5ᵗʰ **C79.3** **Secondary malignant neoplasm of brain and cerebral meninges**

C79.31 **Secondary malignant neoplasm of brain** cc hcc

C79.32 **Secondary malignant neoplasm of cerebral meninges** cc hcc

AHA: 2020,1Q,13

✓5ᵗʰ **C79.4** **Secondary malignant neoplasm of other and unspecified parts of nervous system**

C79.40 **Secondary malignant neoplasm of unspecified part of nervous system** cc hcc

C79.49 **Secondary malignant neoplasm of other parts of nervous system** cc hcc

✓5ᵗʰ **C79.5** **Secondary malignant neoplasm of bone and bone marrow**

EXCLUDES 1 secondary carcinoid tumors of bone (C7B.03)

C79.51 **Secondary malignant neoplasm of bone** cc hcc

TIP: Do not assign in addition to a code from subcategory C90.0 when multiple myeloma is described as metastatic to the bone; bone involvement is integral to multiple myeloma.

C79.52 **Secondary malignant neoplasm of bone marrow** cc hcc

✓5ᵗʰ **C79.6** **Secondary malignant neoplasm of ovary**

C79.60 **Secondary malignant neoplasm of unspecified ovary** cc hcc ♀

C79.61 **Secondary malignant neoplasm of right ovary** cc hcc ♀

C79.62 **Secondary malignant neoplasm of left ovary** cc hcc ♀

✓5ᵗʰ **C79.7** **Secondary malignant neoplasm of adrenal gland**

C79.70 **Secondary malignant neoplasm of unspecified adrenal gland** cc hcc

C79.71 **Secondary malignant neoplasm of right adrenal gland** cc hcc

C79.72 **Secondary malignant neoplasm of left adrenal gland** cc hcc

✓5ᵗʰ **C79.8** **Secondary malignant neoplasm of other specified sites**

C79.81 **Secondary malignant neoplasm of breast** cc hcc

C79.82 **Secondary malignant neoplasm of genital organs** cc hcc

C79.89 **Secondary malignant neoplasm of other specified sites** cc hcc

AHA: 2017,2Q,11

C79.9 **Secondary malignant neoplasm of unspecified site** cc hcc

Metastatic cancer NOS
Metastatic disease NOS

EXCLUDES 1 carcinomatosis NOS (C80.0)

generalized cancer NOS (C80.0)

malignant (primary) neoplasm of unspecified site (C80.1)

✓4ᵗʰ **C80** **Malignant neoplasm without specification of site**

EXCLUDES 1 malignant carcinoid tumor of unspecified site (C7A.00)

malignant neoplasm of specified multiple sites — code to each site

C80.0 **Disseminated malignant neoplasm, unspecified** cc hcc

Carcinomatosis NOS
Generalized cancer, unspecified site (primary) (secondary)
Generalized malignancy, unspecified site (primary) (secondary)

C80.1 **Malignant (primary) neoplasm, unspecified** hcc

Cancer NOS
Cancer unspecified site (primary)
Carcinoma unspecified site (primary)
Malignancy unspecified site (primary)

EXCLUDES 1 secondary malignant neoplasm of unspecified site (C79.9)

C80.2 **Malignant neoplasm associated with transplanted organ** cc hcc

Code first complication of transplanted organ (T86.-)
Use additional code to identify the specific malignancy

Malignant neoplasms of lymphoid, hematopoietic and related tissue (C81-C96)

EXCLUDES 2 Kaposi's sarcoma of lymph nodes (C46.3)

secondary and unspecified neoplasm of lymph nodes (C77.-)

secondary neoplasm of bone marrow (C79.52)

secondary neoplasm of spleen (C78.89)

✓4ᵗʰ **C81** **Hodgkin lymphoma**

EXCLUDES 1 personal history of Hodgkin lymphoma (Z85.71)

DEF: Malignant disorder of lymphoid cells characterized by the presence of progressively swollen lymph nodes and spleen that may also involve the liver. A diagnosis of Hodgkin's lymphoma can be confirmed by the presence of Reed-Sternberg cells. Synonym(s): Hodgkin disease.

✓5ᵗʰ **C81.0** **Nodular lymphocyte predominant Hodgkin lymphoma**

C81.00 **Nodular lymphocyte predominant Hodgkin lymphoma, unspecified site** cc hcc

C81.01 **Nodular lymphocyte predominant Hodgkin lymphoma, lymph nodes of head, face, and neck** cc hcc

C81.02 **Nodular lymphocyte predominant Hodgkin lymphoma, intrathoracic lymph nodes** cc hcc

C81.03 **Nodular lymphocyte predominant Hodgkin lymphoma, intra-abdominal lymph nodes** cc hcc

C81.04 **Nodular lymphocyte predominant Hodgkin lymphoma, lymph nodes of axilla and upper limb** cc hcc

C81.05 **Nodular lymphocyte predominant Hodgkin lymphoma, lymph nodes of inguinal region and lower limb** cc hcc

C81.06 **Nodular lymphocyte predominant Hodgkin lymphoma, intrapelvic lymph nodes** cc hcc

C81.07 **Nodular lymphocyte predominant Hodgkin lymphoma, spleen** cc hcc

C81.08 **Nodular lymphocyte predominant Hodgkin lymphoma, lymph nodes of multiple sites** cc hcc

C81.09 **Nodular lymphocyte predominant Hodgkin lymphoma, extranodal and solid organ sites** cc hcc

✓5ᵗʰ **C81.1** **Nodular sclerosis Hodgkin lymphoma**

Nodular sclerosis classical Hodgkin lymphoma

C81.10 **Nodular sclerosis Hodgkin lymphoma, unspecified site** cc hcc

C81.11 **Nodular sclerosis Hodgkin lymphoma, lymph nodes of head, face, and neck** cc hcc

C81.12 **Nodular sclerosis Hodgkin lymphoma, intrathoracic lymph nodes** cc hcc

C81.13 **Nodular sclerosis Hodgkin lymphoma, intra-abdominal lymph nodes** cc hcc

C81.14 **Nodular sclerosis Hodgkin lymphoma, lymph nodes of axilla and upper limb** cc hcc

C81.15 **Nodular sclerosis Hodgkin lymphoma, lymph nodes of inguinal region and lower limb** cc hcc

C81.16 **Nodular sclerosis Hodgkin lymphoma, intrapelvic lymph nodes** cc hcc

C81.17 **Nodular sclerosis Hodgkin lymphoma, spleen** cc hcc

C81.18 **Nodular sclerosis Hodgkin lymphoma, lymph nodes of multiple sites** cc hcc

C81.19 **Nodular sclerosis Hodgkin lymphoma, extranodal and solid organ sites** cc hcc

✓5ᵗʰ **C81.2** **Mixed cellularity Hodgkin lymphoma**

Mixed cellularity classical Hodgkin lymphoma

C81.20 **Mixed cellularity Hodgkin lymphoma, unspecified site** cc hcc

C81.21 **Mixed cellularity Hodgkin lymphoma, lymph nodes of head, face, and neck** cc hcc

C81.22 **Mixed cellularity Hodgkin lymphoma, intrathoracic lymph nodes** cc hcc

C81.23 **Mixed cellularity Hodgkin lymphoma, intra-abdominal lymph nodes** cc hcc

C81.24 **Mixed cellularity Hodgkin lymphoma, lymph nodes of axilla and upper limb** cc hcc

C81.25 **Mixed cellularity Hodgkin lymphoma, lymph nodes of inguinal region and lower limb** cc hcc

C81.26 **Mixed cellularity Hodgkin lymphoma, intrapelvic lymph nodes** cc hcc

C81.27 **Mixed cellularity Hodgkin lymphoma, spleen** cc hcc

N Newborn: 0   P Pediatric: 0-17   M Maternity: 9-64   A Adult: 15-124   MCC Major Complication/Comorbidity   CC Complication/Comorbidity   SW Severe Wound Dx

484   ICD-10-CM 2021

C81.28   **Mixed cellularity Hodgkin lymphoma, lymph nodes of multiple sites** `CC` `HCC`

C81.29   **Mixed cellularity Hodgkin lymphoma, extranodal and solid organ sites** `CC` `HCC`

√5ᵗʰ **C81.3 Lymphocyte depleted Hodgkin lymphoma**

Lymphocyte depleted classical Hodgkin lymphoma

C81.30   **Lymphocyte depleted Hodgkin lymphoma, unspecified site** `CC` `HCC`

C81.31   **Lymphocyte depleted Hodgkin lymphoma, lymph nodes of head, face, and neck** `CC` `HCC`

C81.32   **Lymphocyte depleted Hodgkin lymphoma, intrathoracic lymph nodes** `CC` `HCC`

C81.33   **Lymphocyte depleted Hodgkin lymphoma, intra-abdominal lymph nodes** `CC` `HCC`

C81.34   **Lymphocyte depleted Hodgkin lymphoma, lymph nodes of axilla and upper limb** `CC` `HCC`

C81.35   **Lymphocyte depleted Hodgkin lymphoma, lymph nodes of inguinal region and lower limb** `CC` `HCC`

C81.36   **Lymphocyte depleted Hodgkin lymphoma, intrapelvic lymph nodes** `CC` `HCC`

C81.37   **Lymphocyte depleted Hodgkin lymphoma, spleen** `CC` `HCC`

C81.38   **Lymphocyte depleted Hodgkin lymphoma, lymph nodes of multiple sites** `CC` `HCC`

C81.39   **Lymphocyte depleted Hodgkin lymphoma, extranodal and solid organ sites** `CC` `HCC`

√5ᵗʰ **C81.4 Lymphocyte-rich Hodgkin lymphoma**

Lymphocyte-rich classical Hodgkin lymphoma

EXCLUDES 1   *nodular lymphocyte predominant Hodgkin lymphoma (C81.0-)*

C81.40   **Lymphocyte-rich Hodgkin lymphoma, unspecified site** `CC` `HCC`

C81.41   **Lymphocyte-rich Hodgkin lymphoma, lymph nodes of head, face, and neck** `CC` `HCC`

C81.42   **Lymphocyte-rich Hodgkin lymphoma, intrathoracic lymph nodes** `CC` `HCC`

C81.43   **Lymphocyte-rich Hodgkin lymphoma, intra-abdominal lymph nodes** `CC` `HCC`

C81.44   **Lymphocyte-rich Hodgkin lymphoma, lymph nodes of axilla and upper limb** `CC` `HCC`

C81.45   **Lymphocyte-rich Hodgkin lymphoma, lymph nodes of inguinal region and lower limb** `CC` `HCC`

C81.46   **Lymphocyte-rich Hodgkin lymphoma, intrapelvic lymph nodes** `CC` `HCC`

C81.47   **Lymphocyte-rich Hodgkin lymphoma, spleen** `CC` `HCC`

C81.48   **Lymphocyte-rich Hodgkin lymphoma, lymph nodes of multiple sites** `CC` `HCC`

C81.49   **Lymphocyte-rich Hodgkin lymphoma, extranodal and solid organ sites** `CC` `HCC`

√5ᵗʰ **C81.7 Other Hodgkin lymphoma**

Classical Hodgkin lymphoma NOS
Other classical Hodgkin lymphoma

C81.70   **Other Hodgkin lymphoma, unspecified site** `CC` `HCC`

C81.71   **Other Hodgkin lymphoma, lymph nodes of head, face, and neck** `CC` `HCC`

C81.72   **Other Hodgkin lymphoma, intrathoracic lymph nodes** `CC` `HCC`

C81.73   **Other Hodgkin lymphoma, intra-abdominal lymph nodes** `CC` `HCC`

C81.74   **Other Hodgkin lymphoma, lymph nodes of axilla and upper limb** `CC` `HCC`

C81.75   **Other Hodgkin lymphoma, lymph nodes of inguinal region and lower limb** `CC` `HCC`

C81.76   **Other Hodgkin lymphoma, intrapelvic lymph nodes** `CC` `HCC`

C81.77   **Other Hodgkin lymphoma, spleen** `CC` `HCC`

C81.78   **Other Hodgkin lymphoma, lymph nodes of multiple sites** `CC` `HCC`

C81.79   **Other Hodgkin lymphoma, extranodal and solid organ sites** `CC` `HCC`

√5ᵗʰ **C81.9 Hodgkin lymphoma, unspecified**

C81.90   **Hodgkin lymphoma, unspecified, unspecified site** `CC` `HCC`

C81.91   **Hodgkin lymphoma, unspecified, lymph nodes of head, face, and neck** `CC` `HCC`

C81.92   **Hodgkin lymphoma, unspecified, intrathoracic lymph nodes** `CC` `HCC`

C81.93   **Hodgkin lymphoma, unspecified, intra-abdominal lymph nodes** `CC` `HCC`

C81.94   **Hodgkin lymphoma, unspecified, lymph nodes of axilla and upper limb** `CC` `HCC`

C81.95   **Hodgkin lymphoma, unspecified, lymph nodes of inguinal region and lower limb** `CC` `HCC`

C81.96   **Hodgkin lymphoma, unspecified, intrapelvic lymph nodes** `CC` `HCC`

C81.97   **Hodgkin lymphoma, unspecified, spleen** `CC` `HCC`

C81.98   **Hodgkin lymphoma, unspecified, lymph nodes of multiple sites** `CC` `HCC`

C81.99   **Hodgkin lymphoma, unspecified, extranodal and solid organ sites** `CC` `HCC`

√4ᵗʰ **C82 Follicular lymphoma**

INCLUDES   follicular lymphoma with or without diffuse areas

EXCLUDES 1   *mature T/NK-cell lymphomas (C84.-)*
personal history of non-Hodgkin lymphoma (Z85.72)

DEF: Most common subgroup of non-Hodgkin lymphomas (NHL), accounting for 20 to 30 percent of all NHLs. NHL is a B-cell lymphoma that is slow growing and characterized by the circular pattern of malignant cell growth with the cells clustered into identifiable nodules or follicles.

√5ᵗʰ **C82.0 Follicular lymphoma grade I**

C82.00   **Follicular lymphoma grade I, unspecified site** `CC` `HCC`

C82.01   **Follicular lymphoma grade I, lymph nodes of head, face, and neck** `CC` `HCC`

C82.02   **Follicular lymphoma grade I, intrathoracic lymph nodes** `CC` `HCC`

C82.03   **Follicular lymphoma grade I, intra-abdominal lymph nodes** `CC` `HCC`

C82.04   **Follicular lymphoma grade I, lymph nodes of axilla and upper limb** `CC` `HCC`

C82.05   **Follicular lymphoma grade I, lymph nodes of inguinal region and lower limb** `CC` `HCC`

C82.06   **Follicular lymphoma grade I, intrapelvic lymph nodes** `CC` `HCC`

C82.07   **Follicular lymphoma grade I, spleen** `CC` `HCC`

C82.08   **Follicular lymphoma grade I, lymph nodes of multiple sites** `CC` `HCC`

C82.09   **Follicular lymphoma grade I, extranodal and solid organ sites** `CC` `HCC`

√5ᵗʰ **C82.1 Follicular lymphoma grade II**

C82.10   **Follicular lymphoma grade II, unspecified site** `CC` `HCC`

C82.11   **Follicular lymphoma grade II, lymph nodes of head, face, and neck** `CC` `HCC`

C82.12   **Follicular lymphoma grade II, intrathoracic lymph nodes** `CC` `HCC`

C82.13   **Follicular lymphoma grade II, intra-abdominal lymph nodes** `CC` `HCC`

C82.14   **Follicular lymphoma grade II, lymph nodes of axilla and upper limb** `CC` `HCC`

C82.15   **Follicular lymphoma grade II, lymph nodes of inguinal region and lower limb** `CC` `HCC`

C82.16   **Follicular lymphoma grade II, intrapelvic lymph nodes** `CC` `HCC`

C82.17   **Follicular lymphoma grade II, spleen** `CC` `HCC`

C82.18   **Follicular lymphoma grade II, lymph nodes of multiple sites** `CC` `HCC`

C82.19   **Follicular lymphoma grade II, extranodal and solid organ sites** `CC` `HCC`

√5ᵗʰ **C82.2 Follicular lymphoma grade III, unspecified**

C82.20   **Follicular lymphoma grade III, unspecified, unspecified site** `CC` `HCC`

C82.21   **Follicular lymphoma grade III, unspecified, lymph nodes of head, face, and neck** `CC` `HCC`

C82.22   **Follicular lymphoma grade III, unspecified, intrathoracic lymph nodes** `CC` `HCC`

C82.23   **Follicular lymphoma grade III, unspecified, intra-abdominal lymph nodes** `CC` `HCC`

C82.24   **Follicular lymphoma grade III, unspecified, lymph nodes of axilla and upper limb** `CC` `HCC`

C82.25   **Follicular lymphoma grade III, unspecified, lymph nodes of inguinal region and lower limb** `CC` `HCC`

C82.26   **Follicular lymphoma grade III, unspecified, intrapelvic lymph nodes** `CC` `HCC`

C82.27   **Follicular lymphoma grade III, unspecified, spleen** `CC` `HCC`

✓ Additional Character Required   √x7ᵗʰ Placeholder   Unacceptable PDx   Questionable PDx   Manifestation   Unspecified Dx   H1-H14 HAC   HCC CMS-HCC Dx   HIV HIV Dx

ICD-10-CM 2021   485

C81.28–C82.27

C82.28 Follicular lymphoma grade III, unspecified, lymph nodes of multiple sites `CC` `HCC`

C82.29 Follicular lymphoma grade III, unspecified, extranodal and solid organ sites `CC` `HCC`

√5ᵗʰ **C82.3** Follicular lymphoma grade IIIa

C82.30 Follicular lymphoma grade IIIa, unspecified site `CC` `HCC`

C82.31 Follicular lymphoma grade IIIa, lymph nodes of head, face, and neck `CC` `HCC`

C82.32 Follicular lymphoma grade IIIa, intrathoracic lymph nodes `CC` `HCC`

C82.33 Follicular lymphoma grade IIIa, intra-abdominal lymph nodes `CC` `HCC`

C82.34 Follicular lymphoma grade IIIa, lymph nodes of axilla and upper limb `CC` `HCC`

C82.35 Follicular lymphoma grade IIIa, lymph nodes of inguinal region and lower limb `CC` `HCC`

C82.36 Follicular lymphoma grade IIIa, intrapelvic lymph nodes `CC` `HCC`

C82.37 Follicular lymphoma grade IIIa, spleen `CC` `HCC`

C82.38 Follicular lymphoma grade IIIa, lymph nodes of multiple sites `CC` `HCC`

C82.39 Follicular lymphoma grade IIIa, extranodal and solid organ sites `CC` `HCC`

√5ᵗʰ **C82.4** Follicular lymphoma grade IIIb

C82.40 Follicular lymphoma grade IIIb, unspecified site `CC` `HCC`

C82.41 Follicular lymphoma grade IIIb, lymph nodes of head, face, and neck `CC` `HCC`

C82.42 Follicular lymphoma grade IIIb, intrathoracic lymph nodes `CC` `HCC`

C82.43 Follicular lymphoma grade IIIb, intra-abdominal lymph nodes `CC` `HCC`

C82.44 Follicular lymphoma grade IIIb, lymph nodes of axilla and upper limb `CC` `HCC`

C82.45 Follicular lymphoma grade IIIb, lymph nodes of inguinal region and lower limb `CC` `HCC`

C82.46 Follicular lymphoma grade IIIb, intrapelvic lymph nodes `CC` `HCC`

C82.47 Follicular lymphoma grade IIIb, spleen `CC` `HCC`

C82.48 Follicular lymphoma grade IIIb, lymph nodes of multiple sites `CC` `HCC`

C82.49 Follicular lymphoma grade IIIb, extranodal and solid organ sites `CC` `HCC`

√5ᵗʰ **C82.5** Diffuse follicle center lymphoma

C82.50 Diffuse follicle center lymphoma, unspecified site `HIV` `CC` `HCC`

C82.51 Diffuse follicle center lymphoma, lymph nodes of head, face, and neck `HIV` `CC` `HCC`

C82.52 Diffuse follicle center lymphoma, intrathoracic lymph nodes `HIV` `CC` `HCC`

C82.53 Diffuse follicle center lymphoma, intra-abdominal lymph nodes `HIV` `CC` `HCC`

C82.54 Diffuse follicle center lymphoma, lymph nodes of axilla and upper limb `HIV` `CC` `HCC`

C82.55 Diffuse follicle center lymphoma, lymph nodes of inguinal region and lower limb `HIV` `CC` `HCC`

C82.56 Diffuse follicle center lymphoma, intrapelvic lymph nodes `HIV` `CC` `HCC`

C82.57 Diffuse follicle center lymphoma, spleen `HIV` `CC` `HCC`

C82.58 Diffuse follicle center lymphoma, lymph nodes of multiple sites `HIV` `CC` `HCC`

C82.59 Diffuse follicle center lymphoma, extranodal and solid organ sites `HIV` `CC` `HCC`

√5ᵗʰ **C82.6** Cutaneous follicle center lymphoma

C82.60 Cutaneous follicle center lymphoma, unspecified site `CC` `HCC`

C82.61 Cutaneous follicle center lymphoma, lymph nodes of head, face, and neck `CC` `HCC`

C82.62 Cutaneous follicle center lymphoma, intrathoracic lymph nodes `CC` `HCC`

C82.63 Cutaneous follicle center lymphoma, intra-abdominal lymph nodes `CC` `HCC`

C82.64 Cutaneous follicle center lymphoma, lymph nodes of axilla and upper limb `CC` `HCC`

C82.65 Cutaneous follicle center lymphoma, lymph nodes of inguinal region and lower limb `CC` `HCC`

C82.66 Cutaneous follicle center lymphoma, intrapelvic lymph nodes `CC` `HCC`

C82.67 Cutaneous follicle center lymphoma, spleen `CC` `HCC`

C82.68 Cutaneous follicle center lymphoma, lymph nodes of multiple sites `CC` `HCC`

C82.69 Cutaneous follicle center lymphoma, extranodal and solid organ sites `CC` `HCC`

√5ᵗʰ **C82.8** Other types of follicular lymphoma

C82.80 Other types of follicular lymphoma, unspecified site `CC` `HCC`

C82.81 Other types of follicular lymphoma, lymph nodes of head, face, and neck `CC` `HCC`

C82.82 Other types of follicular lymphoma, intrathoracic lymph nodes `CC` `HCC`

C82.83 Other types of follicular lymphoma, intra-abdominal lymph nodes `CC` `HCC`

C82.84 Other types of follicular lymphoma, lymph nodes of axilla and upper limb `CC` `HCC`

C82.85 Other types of follicular lymphoma, lymph nodes of inguinal region and lower limb `CC` `HCC`

C82.86 Other types of follicular lymphoma, intrapelvic lymph nodes `CC` `HCC`

C82.87 Other types of follicular lymphoma, spleen `CC` `HCC`

C82.88 Other types of follicular lymphoma, lymph nodes of multiple sites `CC` `HCC`

C82.89 Other types of follicular lymphoma, extranodal and solid organ sites `CC` `HCC`

√5ᵗʰ **C82.9** Follicular lymphoma, unspecified

C82.90 Follicular lymphoma, unspecified, unspecified site `CC` `HCC`

C82.91 Follicular lymphoma, unspecified, lymph nodes of head, face, and neck `CC` `HCC`

C82.92 Follicular lymphoma, unspecified, intrathoracic lymph nodes `CC` `HCC`

C82.93 Follicular lymphoma, unspecified, intra-abdominal lymph nodes `CC` `HCC`

C82.94 Follicular lymphoma, unspecified, lymph nodes of axilla and upper limb `CC` `HCC`

C82.95 Follicular lymphoma, unspecified, lymph nodes of inguinal region and lower limb `CC` `HCC`

C82.96 Follicular lymphoma, unspecified, intrapelvic lymph nodes `CC` `HCC`

C82.97 Follicular lymphoma, unspecified, spleen `CC` `HCC`

C82.98 Follicular lymphoma, unspecified, lymph nodes of multiple sites `CC` `HCC`

C82.99 Follicular lymphoma, unspecified, extranodal and solid organ sites `CC` `HCC`

√4ᵗʰ **C83** Non-follicular lymphoma

EXCLUDES 1 personal history of non-Hodgkin lymphoma (Z85.72)

√5ᵗʰ **C83.0** Small cell B-cell lymphoma

Lymphoplasmacytic lymphoma
Nodal marginal zone lymphoma
Non-leukemic variant of B-CLL
Splenic marginal zone lymphoma

EXCLUDES 1 chronic lymphocytic leukemia (C91.1)
mature T/NK-cell lymphomas (C84.-)
Waldenström macroglobulinemia (C88.0)

DEF: Nonfollicular lymphoma that is rare, slow growing, and usually found in the older population.

C83.00 Small cell B-cell lymphoma, unspecified site `HIV` `CC` `HCC`

C83.01 Small cell B-cell lymphoma, lymph nodes of head, face, and neck `HIV` `CC` `HCC`

C83.02 Small cell B-cell lymphoma, intrathoracic lymph nodes `HIV` `CC` `HCC`

C83.03 Small cell B-cell lymphoma, intra-abdominal lymph nodes `HIV` `CC` `HCC`

C83.04 Small cell B-cell lymphoma, lymph nodes of axilla and upper limb `HIV` `CC` `HCC`

C83.05 Small cell B-cell lymphoma, lymph nodes of inguinal region and lower limb `HIV` `CC` `HCC`

C83.06 Small cell B-cell lymphoma, intrapelvic lymph nodes `HIV` `CC` `HCC`

C83.07 Small cell B-cell lymphoma, spleen `HIV` `CC` `HCC`

C83.08 Small cell B-cell lymphoma, lymph nodes of multiple sites `HIV` `CC` `HCC`

N Newborn: 0 | P Pediatric: 0-17 | M Maternity: 9-64 | A Adult: 15-124 | MCC Major Complication/Comorbidity | CC Complication/Comorbidity | SW Severe Wound Dx

486 | ICD-10-CM 2021

C83.09   Small cell B-cell lymphoma, extranodal and solid organ sites `HIV` `CC` `HCC`

√5ᵗʰ **C83.1**   Mantle cell lymphoma

Centrocytic lymphoma
Malignant lymphomatous polyposis
DEF: Rare form of B-cell non-Hodgkin lymphoma named for the location of the tumor cell production, the mantle zone of the lymph nodes.

C83.10   Mantle cell lymphoma, unspecified site `HIV` `CC` `HCC`

C83.11   Mantle cell lymphoma, lymph nodes of head, face, and neck `HIV` `CC` `HCC`

C83.12   Mantle cell lymphoma, intrathoracic lymph nodes `HIV` `CC` `HCC`

C83.13   Mantle cell lymphoma, intra-abdominal lymph nodes `HIV` `CC` `HCC`

C83.14   Mantle cell lymphoma, lymph nodes of axilla and upper limb `HIV` `CC` `HCC`

C83.15   Mantle cell lymphoma, lymph nodes of inguinal region and lower limb `HIV` `CC` `HCC`

C83.16   Mantle cell lymphoma, intrapelvic lymph nodes `HIV` `CC` `HCC`

C83.17   Mantle cell lymphoma, spleen `HIV` `CC` `HCC`

C83.18   Mantle cell lymphoma, lymph nodes of multiple sites `HIV` `CC` `HCC`

C83.19   Mantle cell lymphoma, extranodal and solid organ sites `HIV` `CC` `HCC`

√5ᵗʰ **C83.3**   Diffuse large B-cell lymphoma

Anaplastic diffuse large B-cell lymphoma
CD30-positive diffuse large B-cell lymphoma
Centroblastic diffuse large B-cell lymphoma
Diffuse large B-cell lymphoma, subtype not specified
Immunoblastic diffuse large B-cell lymphoma
Plasmablastic diffuse large B-cell lymphoma
T-cell rich diffuse large B-cell lymphoma
EXCLUDES 1   mediastinal (thymic) large B-cell lymphoma (C85.2-)
    mature T/NK-cell lymphomas (C84.-)
DEF: Nonfollicular lymphoma that is one of the more common types of lymphoma. This cancer is fast growing and affects any age but is found mostly in the older population.

C83.30   Diffuse large B-cell lymphoma, unspecified site `HIV` `CC` `HCC`

C83.31   Diffuse large B-cell lymphoma, lymph nodes of head, face, and neck `HIV` `CC` `HCC`

C83.32   Diffuse large B-cell lymphoma, intrathoracic lymph nodes `HIV` `CC` `HCC`

C83.33   Diffuse large B-cell lymphoma, intra-abdominal lymph nodes `HIV` `CC` `HCC`

C83.34   Diffuse large B-cell lymphoma, lymph nodes of axilla and upper limb `HIV` `CC` `HCC`

C83.35   Diffuse large B-cell lymphoma, lymph nodes of inguinal region and lower limb `HIV` `CC` `HCC`

C83.36   Diffuse large B-cell lymphoma, intrapelvic lymph nodes `HIV` `CC` `HCC`

C83.37   Diffuse large B-cell lymphoma, spleen `HIV` `CC` `HCC`

C83.38   Diffuse large B-cell lymphoma, lymph nodes of multiple sites `HIV` `CC` `HCC`

C83.39   Diffuse large B-cell lymphoma, extranodal and solid organ sites `HIV` `CC` `HCC`

√5ᵗʰ **C83.5**   Lymphoblastic (diffuse) lymphoma

B-precursor lymphoma
Lymphoblastic B-cell lymphoma
Lymphoblastic lymphoma NOS
Lymphoblastic T-cell lymphoma
T-precursor lymphoma
DEF: Type of non-Hodgkin lymphoma considered lymphoma or leukemia—the determination is made based on the amount of bone marrow involvement. The cells are small to medium immature T-cells that often originate in the thymus where many of the T-cells are made.

C83.50   Lymphoblastic (diffuse) lymphoma, unspecified site `CC` `HCC`

C83.51   Lymphoblastic (diffuse) lymphoma, lymph nodes of head, face, and neck `CC` `HCC`

C83.52   Lymphoblastic (diffuse) lymphoma, intrathoracic lymph nodes `CC` `HCC`

C83.53   Lymphoblastic (diffuse) lymphoma, intra-abdominal lymph nodes `CC` `HCC`

C83.54   Lymphoblastic (diffuse) lymphoma, lymph nodes of axilla and upper limb `CC` `HCC`

C83.55   Lymphoblastic (diffuse) lymphoma, lymph nodes of inguinal region and lower limb `CC` `HCC`

C83.56   Lymphoblastic (diffuse) lymphoma, intrapelvic lymph nodes `CC` `HCC`

C83.57   Lymphoblastic (diffuse) lymphoma, spleen `CC` `HCC`

C83.58   Lymphoblastic (diffuse) lymphoma, lymph nodes of multiple sites `CC` `HCC`

C83.59   Lymphoblastic (diffuse) lymphoma, extranodal and solid organ sites `CC` `HCC`

√5ᵗʰ **C83.7**   Burkitt lymphoma

Atypical Burkitt lymphoma
Burkitt-like lymphoma
EXCLUDES 1   mature B-cell leukemia Burkitt type (C91.A-)
DEF: Malignancy of the lymphatic system, most often seen as a large bone-deteriorating lesion within the jaw or as an abdominal mass. It is a form of non-Hodgkin's lymphoma and is recognized as the fastest growing human tumor.

C83.70   Burkitt lymphoma, unspecified site `HIV` `CC` `HCC`

C83.71   Burkitt lymphoma, lymph nodes of head, face, and neck `HIV` `CC` `HCC`

C83.72   Burkitt lymphoma, intrathoracic lymph nodes `HIV` `CC` `HCC`

C83.73   Burkitt lymphoma, intra-abdominal lymph nodes `HIV` `CC` `HCC`

C83.74   Burkitt lymphoma, lymph nodes of axilla and upper limb `HIV` `CC` `HCC`

C83.75   Burkitt lymphoma, lymph nodes of inguinal region and lower limb `HIV` `CC` `HCC`

C83.76   Burkitt lymphoma, intrapelvic lymph nodes `HIV` `CC` `HCC`

C83.77   Burkitt lymphoma, spleen `HIV` `CC` `HCC`

C83.78   Burkitt lymphoma, lymph nodes of multiple sites `HIV` `CC` `HCC`

C83.79   Burkitt lymphoma, extranodal and solid organ sites `HIV` `CC` `HCC`

√5ᵗʰ **C83.8**   Other non-follicular lymphoma

Intravascular large B-cell lymphoma
Lymphoid granulomatosis
Primary effusion B-cell lymphoma
EXCLUDES 1   mediastinal (thymic) large B-cell lymphoma (C85.2-)
    T-cell rich B-cell lymphoma (C83.3-)

C83.80   Other non-follicular lymphoma, unspecified site `HIV` `CC` `HCC`

C83.81   Other non-follicular lymphoma, lymph nodes of head, face, and neck `HIV` `CC` `HCC`

C83.82   Other non-follicular lymphoma, intrathoracic lymph nodes `HIV` `CC` `HCC`

C83.83   Other non-follicular lymphoma, intra-abdominal lymph nodes `HIV` `CC` `HCC`

C83.84   Other non-follicular lymphoma, lymph nodes of axilla and upper limb `HIV` `CC` `HCC`

C83.85   Other non-follicular lymphoma, lymph nodes of inguinal region and lower limb `HIV` `CC` `HCC`

C83.86   Other non-follicular lymphoma, intrapelvic lymph nodes `HIV` `CC` `HCC`

C83.87   Other non-follicular lymphoma, spleen `HIV` `CC` `HCC`

C83.88   Other non-follicular lymphoma, lymph nodes of multiple sites `HIV` `CC` `HCC`

C83.89   Other non-follicular lymphoma, extranodal and solid organ sites `HIV` `CC` `HCC`

√5ᵗʰ **C83.9**   Non-follicular (diffuse) lymphoma, unspecified

C83.90   Non-follicular (diffuse) lymphoma, unspecified, unspecified site `HIV` `CC` `HCC`

C83.91   Non-follicular (diffuse) lymphoma, unspecified, lymph nodes of head, face, and neck `HIV` `CC` `HCC`

C83.92   Non-follicular (diffuse) lymphoma, unspecified, intrathoracic lymph nodes `HIV` `CC` `HCC`

C83.93   Non-follicular (diffuse) lymphoma, unspecified, intra-abdominal lymph nodes `HIV` `CC` `HCC`

C83.94   Non-follicular (diffuse) lymphoma, unspecified, lymph nodes of axilla and upper limb `HIV` `CC` `HCC`

C83.95   Non-follicular (diffuse) lymphoma, unspecified, lymph nodes of inguinal region and lower limb `HIV` `CC` `HCC`

Chapter 2. Neoplasms

C83.96 Non-follicular (diffuse) lymphoma, unspecified, **intrapelvic** lymph nodes `HIV` `CC` `HCC`

C83.97 Non-follicular (diffuse) lymphoma, unspecified, **spleen** `HIV` `CC` `HCC`

C83.98 Non-follicular (diffuse) lymphoma, unspecified, lymph nodes of **multiple sites** `HIV` `CC` `HCC`

C83.99 Non-follicular (diffuse) lymphoma, unspecified, **extranodal and solid organ sites** `HIV` `CC` `HCC`

√4th **C84** **Mature T/NK-cell lymphomas**

    `EXCLUDES 1`   personal history of non-Hodgkin lymphoma (Z85.72)

√5th **C84.0** **Mycosis fungoides**

    `EXCLUDES 1`   peripheral T-cell lymphoma, not classified (C84.4-)

    DEF: Most common form of cutaneous T-cell lymphoma. A type of non-Hodgkin lymphoma in which white blood cells become cancerous and affect the skin and sometimes internal organs.

    Synonym(s): *Alibert-Bazin syndrome.*

C84.00 **Mycosis fungoides, unspecified site** `CC` `HCC`

C84.01 Mycosis fungoides, lymph nodes of **head, face, and neck** `CC` `HCC`

C84.02 Mycosis fungoides, **intrathoracic** lymph nodes `CC` `HCC`

C84.03 Mycosis fungoides, **intra-abdominal** lymph nodes `CC` `HCC`

C84.04 Mycosis fungoides, lymph nodes of **axilla and upper limb** `CC` `HCC`

C84.05 Mycosis fungoides, lymph nodes of **inguinal region and lower limb** `CC` `HCC`

C84.06 Mycosis fungoides, **intrapelvic** lymph nodes `CC` `HCC`

C84.07 Mycosis fungoides, **spleen** `CC` `HCC`

C84.08 Mycosis fungoides, lymph nodes of **multiple sites** `CC` `HCC`

C84.09 Mycosis fungoides, **extranodal and solid organ sites** `CC` `HCC`

√5th **C84.1** **Sézary disease**

    DEF: Extension of mycosis fungoides that affects the blood and all of the skin, appearing as sunburn, rather than patches. It spreads to the lymph nodes and is often linked to a weakened immune system.

C84.10 **Sézary disease, unspecified site** `CC` `HCC`

C84.11 Sézary disease, lymph nodes of **head, face, and neck** `CC` `HCC`

C84.12 Sézary disease, **intrathoracic** lymph nodes `CC` `HCC`

C84.13 Sézary disease, **intra-abdominal** lymph nodes `CC` `HCC`

C84.14 Sézary disease, lymph nodes of **axilla and upper limb** `CC` `HCC`

C84.15 Sézary disease, lymph nodes of **inguinal region and lower limb** `CC` `HCC`

C84.16 Sézary disease, **intrapelvic** lymph nodes `CC` `HCC`

C84.17 Sézary disease, **spleen** `CC` `HCC`

C84.18 Sézary disease, lymph nodes of **multiple sites** `CC` `HCC`

C84.19 Sézary disease, **extranodal and solid organ sites** `CC` `HCC`

√5th **C84.4** **Peripheral T-cell lymphoma, not classified**

    Lennert's lymphoma

    Lymphoepithelioid lymphoma

    Mature T-cell lymphoma, not elsewhere classified

C84.40 **Peripheral T-cell lymphoma, not classified, unspecified site** `HIV` `CC` `HCC`

C84.41 Peripheral T-cell lymphoma, not classified, lymph nodes of **head, face, and neck** `HIV` `CC` `HCC`

C84.42 Peripheral T-cell lymphoma, not classified, **intrathoracic** lymph nodes `HIV` `CC` `HCC`

C84.43 Peripheral T-cell lymphoma, not classified, **intra-abdominal** lymph nodes `HIV` `CC` `HCC`

C84.44 Peripheral T-cell lymphoma, not classified, lymph nodes of **axilla and upper limb** `HIV` `CC` `HCC`

C84.45 Peripheral T-cell lymphoma, not classified, lymph nodes of **inguinal region and lower limb** `HIV` `CC` `HCC`

C84.46 Peripheral T-cell lymphoma, not classified, **intrapelvic** lymph nodes `HIV` `CC` `HCC`

C84.47 Peripheral T-cell lymphoma, not classified, **spleen** `HIV` `CC` `HCC`

C84.48 Peripheral T-cell lymphoma, not classified, lymph nodes of **multiple sites** `HIV` `CC` `HCC`

C84.49 Peripheral T-cell lymphoma, not classified, **extranodal and solid organ sites** `HIV` `CC` `HCC`

√5th **C84.6** **Anaplastic large cell lymphoma, ALK-positive**

    Anaplastic large cell lymphoma, CD30-positive

C84.60 **Anaplastic large cell lymphoma, ALK-positive, unspecified site** `HIV` `CC` `HCC`

C84.61 Anaplastic large cell lymphoma, ALK-positive, lymph nodes of **head, face, and neck** `HIV` `CC` `HCC`

C84.62 Anaplastic large cell lymphoma, ALK-positive, **intrathoracic** lymph nodes `HIV` `CC` `HCC`

C84.63 Anaplastic large cell lymphoma, ALK-positive, **intra-abdominal** lymph nodes `HIV` `CC` `HCC`

C84.64 Anaplastic large cell lymphoma, ALK-positive, lymph nodes of **axilla and upper limb** `HIV` `CC` `HCC`

C84.65 Anaplastic large cell lymphoma, ALK-positive, lymph nodes of **inguinal region and lower limb** `HIV` `CC` `HCC`

C84.66 Anaplastic large cell lymphoma, ALK-positive, **intrapelvic** lymph nodes `HIV` `CC` `HCC`

C84.67 Anaplastic large cell lymphoma, ALK-positive, **spleen** `HIV` `CC` `HCC`

C84.68 Anaplastic large cell lymphoma, ALK-positive, lymph nodes of **multiple sites** `HIV` `CC` `HCC`

C84.69 Anaplastic large cell lymphoma, ALK-positive, **extranodal and solid organ sites** `HIV` `CC` `HCC`

√5th **C84.7** **Anaplastic large cell lymphoma, ALK-negative**

    `EXCLUDES 1`   primary cutaneous CD30-positive T-cell proliferations (C86.6-)

C84.70 **Anaplastic large cell lymphoma, ALK-negative, unspecified site** `HIV` `CC` `HCC`

C84.71 Anaplastic large cell lymphoma, ALK-negative, lymph nodes of **head, face, and neck** `HIV` `CC` `HCC`

C84.72 Anaplastic large cell lymphoma, ALK-negative, **intrathoracic** lymph nodes `HIV` `CC` `HCC`

C84.73 Anaplastic large cell lymphoma, ALK-negative, **intra-abdominal** lymph nodes `HIV` `CC` `HCC`

C84.74 Anaplastic large cell lymphoma, ALK-negative, lymph nodes of **axilla and upper limb** `HIV` `CC` `HCC`

C84.75 Anaplastic large cell lymphoma, ALK-negative, lymph nodes of **inguinal region and lower limb** `HIV` `CC` `HCC`

C84.76 Anaplastic large cell lymphoma, ALK-negative, **intrapelvic** lymph nodes `HIV` `CC` `HCC`

C84.77 Anaplastic large cell lymphoma, ALK-negative, **spleen** `HIV` `CC` `HCC`

C84.78 Anaplastic large cell lymphoma, ALK-negative, lymph nodes of **multiple sites** `HIV` `CC` `HCC`

C84.79 Anaplastic large cell lymphoma, ALK-negative, **extranodal and solid organ sites** `HIV` `CC` `HCC`

√5th **C84.A** **Cutaneous T-cell lymphoma, unspecified**

C84.A0 **Cutaneous T-cell lymphoma, unspecified, unspecified site** `HIV` `CC` `HCC`

C84.A1 Cutaneous T-cell lymphoma, unspecified lymph nodes of **head, face, and neck** `HIV` `CC` `HCC`

C84.A2 Cutaneous T-cell lymphoma, unspecified, **intrathoracic** lymph nodes `HIV` `CC` `HCC`

C84.A3 Cutaneous T-cell lymphoma, unspecified, **intra-abdominal** lymph nodes `HIV` `CC` `HCC`

C84.A4 Cutaneous T-cell lymphoma, unspecified, lymph nodes of **axilla and upper limb** `HIV` `CC` `HCC`

C84.A5 Cutaneous T-cell lymphoma, unspecified, lymph nodes of **inguinal region and lower limb** `HIV` `CC` `HCC`

C84.A6 Cutaneous T-cell lymphoma, unspecified, **intrapelvic** lymph nodes `HIV` `CC` `HCC`

C84.A7 Cutaneous T-cell lymphoma, unspecified, **spleen** `HIV` `CC` `HCC`

C84.A8 Cutaneous T-cell lymphoma, unspecified, lymph nodes of **multiple sites** `HIV` `CC` `HCC`

C84.A9 Cutaneous T-cell lymphoma, unspecified, **extranodal and solid organ sites** `HIV` `CC` `HCC`

`N` Newborn: 0   `P` Pediatric: 0-17   `M` Maternity: 9-64   `A` Adult: 15-124   `MCC` Major Complication/Comorbidity   `CC` Complication/Comorbidity   `SW` Severe Wound Dx

488   ICD-10-CM 2021

√5ᵗʰ **C84.Z** **Other mature T/NK-cell lymphomas**

> NOTE   If T-cell lineage or involvement is mentioned in conjunction with a specific lymphoma, code to the more specific description.
>
> EXCLUDES 1   *angioimmunoblastic T-cell lymphoma (C86.5)*
> *blastic NK-cell lymphoma (C86.4)*
> *enteropathy-type T-cell lymphoma (C86.2)*
> *extranodal NK-cell lymphoma, nasal type (C86.0)*
> *hepatosplenic T-cell lymphoma (C86.1)*
> *primary cutaneous CD30-positive T-cell proliferations (C86.6)*
> *subcutaneous panniculitis-like T-cell lymphoma (C86.3)*
> *T-cell leukemia (C91.1-)*

C84.Z0 **Other mature T/NK-cell lymphomas, unspecified site**   HIV CC HCC

C84.Z1 **Other mature T/NK-cell lymphomas, lymph nodes of** head, face, and neck   HIV CC HCC

C84.Z2 **Other mature T/NK-cell lymphomas, intrathoracic lymph nodes**   HIV CC HCC

C84.Z3 **Other mature T/NK-cell lymphomas, intra-abdominal lymph nodes**   HIV CC HCC

C84.Z4 **Other mature T/NK-cell lymphomas, lymph nodes of** axilla and upper limb   HIV CC HCC

C84.Z5 **Other mature T/NK-cell lymphomas, lymph nodes of** inguinal region and lower limb   HIV CC HCC

C84.Z6 **Other mature T/NK-cell lymphomas, intrapelvic lymph nodes**   HIV CC HCC

C84.Z7 **Other mature T/NK-cell lymphomas, spleen**   HIV CC HCC

C84.Z8 **Other mature T/NK-cell lymphomas, lymph nodes of** multiple sites   HIV CC HCC

C84.Z9 **Other mature T/NK-cell lymphomas, extranodal and solid organ sites**   HIV CC HCC

√5ᵗʰ **C84.9** **Mature T/NK-cell lymphomas, unspecified**

NK/T cell lymphoma NOS

> EXCLUDES 1   *mature T-cell lymphoma, not elsewhere classified (C84.4-)*

C84.90 **Mature T/NK-cell lymphomas, unspecified, unspecified site**   HIV CC HCC

C84.91 **Mature T/NK-cell lymphomas, unspecified, lymph nodes of** head, face, and neck   HIV CC HCC

C84.92 **Mature T/NK-cell lymphomas, unspecified, intrathoracic lymph nodes**   HIV CC HCC

C84.93 **Mature T/NK-cell lymphomas, unspecified, intra-abdominal lymph nodes**   HIV CC HCC

C84.94 **Mature T/NK-cell lymphomas, unspecified, lymph nodes of** axilla and upper limb   HIV CC HCC

C84.95 **Mature T/NK-cell lymphomas, unspecified, lymph nodes of** inguinal region and lower limb   HIV CC HCC

C84.96 **Mature T/NK-cell lymphomas, unspecified, intrapelvic lymph nodes**   HIV CC HCC

C84.97 **Mature T/NK-cell lymphomas, unspecified, spleen**   HIV CC HCC

C84.98 **Mature T/NK-cell lymphomas, unspecified, lymph nodes of** multiple sites   HIV CC HCC

C84.99 **Mature T/NK-cell lymphomas, unspecified, extranodal and solid organ sites**   HIV CC HCC

√4ᵗʰ **C85** **Other specified and unspecified types of** non-Hodgkin lymphoma

> EXCLUDES 1   *other specified types of T/NK-cell lymphoma (C86.-)*
> *personal history of non-Hodgkin lymphoma (Z85.72)*

√5ᵗʰ **C85.1** **Unspecified B-cell lymphoma**

> NOTE   If B-cell lineage or involvement is mentioned in conjunction with a specific lymphoma, code to the more specific description.

C85.10 **Unspecified B-cell lymphoma, unspecified site**

C85.11 **Unspecified B-cell lymphoma, lymph nodes of** head, face, and neck   HIV CC HCC

C85.12 **Unspecified B-cell lymphoma, intrathoracic lymph nodes**   HIV CC HCC

C85.13 **Unspecified B-cell lymphoma, intra-abdominal lymph nodes**   HIV CC HCC

C85.14 **Unspecified B-cell lymphoma, lymph nodes of** axilla and upper limb   HIV CC HCC

C85.15 **Unspecified B-cell lymphoma, lymph nodes of** inguinal region and lower limb   HIV CC HCC

C85.16 **Unspecified B-cell lymphoma, intrapelvic lymph nodes**   HIV CC HCC

C85.17 **Unspecified B-cell lymphoma,** spleen   HIV CC HCC

C85.18 **Unspecified B-cell lymphoma, lymph nodes of** multiple sites   HIV CC HCC

C85.19 **Unspecified B-cell lymphoma, extranodal and solid organ sites**   HIV CC HCC

√5ᵗʰ **C85.2** **Mediastinal (thymic) large B-cell lymphoma**

C85.20 **Mediastinal (thymic) large B-cell lymphoma, unspecified site**   HIV CC HCC

C85.21 **Mediastinal (thymic) large B-cell lymphoma, lymph nodes of** head, face, and neck   HIV CC HCC

C85.22 **Mediastinal (thymic) large B-cell lymphoma, intrathoracic lymph nodes**   HIV CC HCC

C85.23 **Mediastinal (thymic) large B-cell lymphoma, intra-abdominal lymph nodes**   HIV CC HCC

C85.24 **Mediastinal (thymic) large B-cell lymphoma, lymph nodes of** axilla and upper limb   HIV CC HCC

C85.25 **Mediastinal (thymic) large B-cell lymphoma, lymph nodes of** inguinal region and lower limb   HIV CC HCC

C85.26 **Mediastinal (thymic) large B-cell lymphoma, intrapelvic lymph nodes**   HIV CC HCC

C85.27 **Mediastinal (thymic) large B-cell lymphoma, spleen**   HIV CC HCC

C85.28 **Mediastinal (thymic) large B-cell lymphoma, lymph nodes of** multiple sites   HIV CC HCC

C85.29 **Mediastinal (thymic) large B-cell lymphoma, extranodal and solid organ sites**   HIV CC HCC

√5ᵗʰ **C85.8** **Other specified types of non-Hodgkin lymphoma**

C85.80 **Other specified types of non-Hodgkin lymphoma, unspecified site**   HIV CC HCC

C85.81 **Other specified types of non-Hodgkin lymphoma, lymph nodes of** head, face, and neck   HIV CC HCC

C85.82 **Other specified types of non-Hodgkin lymphoma, intrathoracic lymph nodes**   HIV CC HCC

C85.83 **Other specified types of non-Hodgkin lymphoma, intra-abdominal lymph nodes**   HIV CC HCC

C85.84 **Other specified types of non-Hodgkin lymphoma, lymph nodes of** axilla and upper limb   HIV CC HCC

C85.85 **Other specified types of non-Hodgkin lymphoma, lymph nodes of** inguinal region and lower limb   HIV CC HCC

C85.86 **Other specified types of non-Hodgkin lymphoma, intrapelvic lymph nodes**   HIV CC HCC

C85.87 **Other specified types of non-Hodgkin lymphoma, spleen**   HIV CC HCC

C85.88 **Other specified types of non-Hodgkin lymphoma, lymph nodes of** multiple sites   HIV CC HCC

C85.89 **Other specified types of non-Hodgkin lymphoma, extranodal and solid organ sites**   HIV CC HCC

√5ᵗʰ **C85.9** **Non-Hodgkin lymphoma, unspecified**

Lymphoma NOS
Malignant lymphoma NOS
Non-Hodgkin lymphoma NOS

C85.90 **Non-Hodgkin lymphoma, unspecified, unspecified site**   HIV CC HCC

C85.91 **Non-Hodgkin lymphoma, unspecified, lymph nodes of** head, face, and neck   HIV CC HCC

C85.92 **Non-Hodgkin lymphoma, unspecified, intrathoracic lymph nodes**   HIV CC HCC

C85.93 **Non-Hodgkin lymphoma, unspecified, intra-abdominal lymph nodes**   HIV CC HCC

C85.94 **Non-Hodgkin lymphoma, unspecified, lymph nodes of** axilla and upper limb   HIV CC HCC

C85.95 **Non-Hodgkin lymphoma, unspecified, lymph nodes of** inguinal region and lower limb   HIV CC HCC

C85.96 **Non-Hodgkin lymphoma, unspecified, intrapelvic lymph nodes**   HIV CC HCC

C85.97 **Non-Hodgkin lymphoma, unspecified, spleen**   HIV CC HCC

C85.98 **Non-Hodgkin lymphoma, unspecified, lymph nodes of** multiple sites   HIV CC HCC

C85.99 **Non-Hodgkin lymphoma, unspecified, extranodal and solid organ sites**   HIV CC HCC

Chapter 2. Neoplasms

√4ᵗʰ **C86 Other specified types of T/NK-cell lymphoma**

EXCLUDES 1   anaplastic large cell lymphoma, ALK negative (C84.7-)
anaplastic large cell lymphoma, ALK positive (C84.6-)
mature T/NK-cell lymphomas (C84.-)
other specified types of non-Hodgkin lymphoma (C85.8-)

C86.0 Extranodal NK/T-cell lymphoma, nasal type   HIV CC HCC

C86.1 Hepatosplenic T-cell lymphoma   HIV CC HCC
Alpha-beta and gamma delta types

C86.2 Enteropathy-type (intestinal) T-cell lymphoma   HIV CC HCC
Enteropathy associated T-cell lymphoma

C86.3 Subcutaneous panniculitis-like T-cell lymphoma   HIV CC HCC

C86.4 Blastic NK-cell lymphoma   HIV CC HCC
Blastic plasmacytoid dendritic cell neoplasm (BPDCN)

C86.5 Angioimmunoblastic T-cell lymphoma   HIV CC HCC
Angioimmunoblastic lymphadenopathy with dysproteinemia (AILD)

C86.6 Primary cutaneous CD30-positive T-cell proliferations   HIV CC HCC
Lymphomatoid papulosis
Primary cutaneous anaplastic large cell lymphoma
Primary cutaneous CD30-positive large cell lymphoma

√4ᵗʰ **C88 Malignant immunoproliferative diseases and certain other B-cell lymphomas**

EXCLUDES 1   B-cell lymphoma, unspecified (C85.1-)
personal history of other malignant neoplasms of lymphoid, hematopoietic and related tissues (Z85.79)

C88.0 Waldenström macroglobulinemia   HCC
Lymphoplasmacytic lymphoma with IgM-production
Macroglobulinemia (idiopathic) (primary)
EXCLUDES 1   small cell B-cell lymphoma (C83.0)

C88.2 Heavy chain disease   CC HCC
Franklin disease
Gamma heavy chain disease
Mu heavy chain disease

C88.3 Immunoproliferative small intestinal disease   CC HCC
Alpha heavy chain disease
Mediterranean lymphoma

C88.4 Extranodal marginal zone B-cell lymphoma of mucosa-associated lymphoid tissue [MALT-lymphoma]   HIV CC HCC
Lymphoma of skin-associated lymphoid tissue [SALT-lymphoma]
Lymphoma of bronchial-associated lymphoid tissue [BALT-lymphoma]
EXCLUDES 1   high malignant (diffuse large B-cell) lymphoma (C83.3-)

C88.8 Other malignant immunoproliferative diseases   CC HCC

C88.9 Malignant immunoproliferative disease, unspecified   CC HCC
Immunoproliferative disease NOS

√4ᵗʰ **C90 Multiple myeloma and malignant plasma cell neoplasms**

EXCLUDES 1   personal history of other malignant neoplasms of lymphoid, hematopoietic and related tissues (Z85.79)

AHA: 2019,2Q,30

√5ᵗʰ **C90.0 Multiple myeloma**
Kahler's disease
Medullary plasmacytoma
Myelomatosis
Plasma cell myeloma
EXCLUDES 1   solitary myeloma (C90.3-)
solitary plasmacytoma (C90.3-)
TIP: Do not assign an additional code for bone metastasis (C79.51) when multiple myeloma is described as metastatic to the bone; bone involvement is integral to this disease process.

C90.00 Multiple myeloma not having achieved remission   CC HCC
Multiple myeloma with failed remission
Multiple myeloma NOS

C90.01 Multiple myeloma in remission   CC HCC

C90.02 Multiple myeloma in relapse   CC HCC

√5ᵗʰ **C90.1 Plasma cell leukemia**
Plasmacytic leukemia
AHA: 2019,2Q,30

C90.10 Plasma cell leukemia not having achieved remission   CC HCC
Plasma cell leukemia with failed remission
Plasma cell leukemia NOS

C90.11 Plasma cell leukemia in remission   CC HCC

C90.12 Plasma cell leukemia in relapse   CC HCC

√5ᵗʰ **C90.2 Extramedullary plasmacytoma**

C90.20 Extramedullary plasmacytoma not having achieved remission   CC HCC
Extramedullary plasmacytoma with failed remission
Extramedullary plasmacytoma NOS

C90.21 Extramedullary plasmacytoma in remission   CC HCC

C90.22 Extramedullary plasmacytoma in relapse   CC HCC

√5ᵗʰ **C90.3 Solitary plasmacytoma**
Localized malignant plasma cell tumor NOS
Plasmacytoma NOS
Solitary myeloma

C90.30 Solitary plasmacytoma not having achieved remission   CC HCC
Solitary plasmacytoma with failed remission
Solitary plasmacytoma NOS

C90.31 Solitary plasmacytoma in remission   CC HCC

C90.32 Solitary plasmacytoma in relapse   CC HCC

√4ᵗʰ **C91 Lymphoid leukemia**

EXCLUDES 1   personal history of leukemia (Z85.6)

AHA: 2020,1Q,13
DEF: Malignant proliferation of immature lymphocytes (white blood cells that make up lymphoid tissue), called lymphoblasts, that originate in the bone marrow. Can be acute (ALL) or chronic (CLL).

√5ᵗʰ **C91.0 Acute lymphoblastic leukemia [ALL]**

NOTE   Codes in subcategory C91.0- should only be used for T-cell and B-cell precursor leukemia

C91.00 Acute lymphoblastic leukemia not having achieved remission   CC HCC
Acute lymphoblastic leukemia with failed remission
Acute lymphoblastic leukemia NOS

C91.01 Acute lymphoblastic leukemia, in remission   CC HCC

C91.02 Acute lymphoblastic leukemia, in relapse   CC HCC

√5ᵗʰ **C91.1 Chronic lymphocytic leukemia of B-cell type**
Lymphoplasmacytic leukemia
Richter syndrome
EXCLUDES 1   lymphoplasmacytic lymphoma (C83.0-)

C91.10 Chronic lymphocytic leukemia of B-cell type not having achieved remission   CC HCC
Chronic lymphocytic leukemia of B-cell type with failed remission
Chronic lymphocytic leukemia of B-cell type NOS

C91.11 Chronic lymphocytic leukemia of B-cell type in remission   CC HCC

C91.12 Chronic lymphocytic leukemia of B-cell type in relapse   CC HCC

√5ᵗʰ **C91.3 Prolymphocytic leukemia of B-cell type**

C91.30 Prolymphocytic leukemia of B-cell type not having achieved remission   CC HCC
Prolymphocytic leukemia of B-cell type with failed remission
Prolymphocytic leukemia of B-cell type NOS

C91.31 Prolymphocytic leukemia of B-cell type, in remission   CC HCC

C91.32 Prolymphocytic leukemia of B-cell type, in relapse   CC HCC

✓5ᵗʰ **C91.4** Hairy cell leukemia

Leukemic reticuloendotheliosis

DEF: Rare type of leukemia that is slow growing and often also considered a type of lymphoma. The small B-cell lymphocytes appear with "hairy" projections under a microscope and are found mostly in the bone marrow, spleen, and blood.

    C91.40 Hairy cell leukemia not having achieved remission   CC HCC

        Hairy cell leukemia with failed remission

        Hairy cell leukemia NOS

    C91.41 Hairy cell leukemia, in remission   CC HCC

    C91.42 Hairy cell leukemia, in relapse   CC HCC

✓5ᵗʰ **C91.5** Adult T-cell lymphoma/leukemia (HTLV-1-associated)

Acute variant of adult T-cell lymphoma/leukemia (HTLV-1-associated)

Chronic variant of adult T-cell lymphoma/leukemia (HTLV-1-associated)

Lymphomatoid variant of adult T-cell lymphoma/leukemia (HTLV-1-associated)

Smouldering variant of adult T-cell lymphoma/leukemia (HTLV-1-associated)

    C91.50 Adult T-cell lymphoma/leukemia (HTLV-1-associated) not having achieved remission   CC HCC A

        Adult T-cell lymphoma/leukemia (HTLV-1-associated) with failed remission

        Adult T-cell lymphoma/leukemia (HTLV-1-associated) NOS

    C91.51 Adult T-cell lymphoma/leukemia (HTLV-1-associated), in remission   CC HCC A

    C91.52 Adult T-cell lymphoma/leukemia (HTLV-1-associated), in relapse   CC HCC A

✓5ᵗʰ **C91.6** Prolymphocytic leukemia of T-cell type

    C91.60 Prolymphocytic leukemia of T-cell type not having achieved remission   CC HCC

        Prolymphocytic leukemia of T-cell type with failed remission

        Prolymphocytic leukemia of T-cell type NOS

    C91.61 Prolymphocytic leukemia of T-cell type, in remission   CC HCC

    C91.62 Prolymphocytic leukemia of T-cell type, in relapse   CC HCC

✓5ᵗʰ **C91.A** Mature B-cell leukemia Burkitt-type

    EXCLUDES 1   Burkitt lymphoma (C83.7-)

    C91.A0 Mature B-cell leukemia Burkitt-type not having achieved remission   CC HCC

        Mature B-cell leukemia Burkitt-type with failed remission

        Mature B-cell leukemia Burkitt-type NOS

    C91.A1 Mature B-cell leukemia Burkitt-type, in remission   CC HCC

    C91.A2 Mature B-cell leukemia Burkitt-type, in relapse   CC HCC

✓5ᵗʰ **C91.Z** Other lymphoid leukemia

T-cell large granular lymphocytic leukemia (associated with rheumatoid arthritis)

    C91.Z0 Other lymphoid leukemia not having achieved remission   CC HCC

        Other lymphoid leukemia with failed remission

        Other lymphoid leukemia NOS

    C91.Z1 Other lymphoid leukemia, in remission   CC HCC

    C91.Z2 Other lymphoid leukemia, in relapse   CC HCC

✓5ᵗʰ **C91.9** Lymphoid leukemia, unspecified

    C91.90 Lymphoid leukemia, unspecified not having achieved remission   CC HCC

        Lymphoid leukemia with failed remission

        Lymphoid leukemia NOS

    C91.91 Lymphoid leukemia, unspecified, in remission   CC HCC

    C91.92 Lymphoid leukemia, unspecified, in relapse   CC HCC

✓4ᵗʰ **C92** Myeloid leukemia

INCLUDES   granulocytic leukemia

        myelogenous leukemia

EXCLUDES 1   personal history of leukemia (Z85.6)

AHA: 2020,1Q,13; 2019,1Q,16

DEF: Cancer that develops in immature myelocytes called myeloblasts. These are the cells that become white blood cells (except lymphocytes), red blood cells, or platelet making cells. Can be acute (AML) or chronic (CML).

TIP: Pancytopenia, although common in some types of myeloid leukemias, is not always inherent. When it is documented, code D61.818 can be assigned in addition to a code from this category.

✓5ᵗʰ **C92.0** Acute myeloblastic leukemia

Acute myeloblastic leukemia, minimal differentiation

Acute myeloblastic leukemia (with maturation)

Acute myeloblastic leukemia 1/ETO

Acute myeloblastic leukemia M0

Acute myeloblastic leukemia M1

Acute myeloblastic leukemia M2

Acute myeloblastic leukemia with t(8;21)

Acute myeloblastic leukemia (without a FAB classification) NOS

Refractory anemia with excess blasts in transformation [RAEBT]

    EXCLUDES 1   acute exacerbation of chronic myeloid leukemia (C92.10)

        refractory anemia with excess of blasts not in transformation (D46.2-)

    AHA: 2018,4Q,87

    C92.00 Acute myeloblastic leukemia, not having achieved remission   CC HCC

        Acute myeloblastic leukemia with failed remission

        Acute myeloblastic leukemia NOS

    C92.01 Acute myeloblastic leukemia, in remission   CC HCC

    C92.02 Acute myeloblastic leukemia, in relapse   CC HCC

✓5ᵗʰ **C92.1** Chronic myeloid leukemia, BCR/ABL-positive

Chronic myelogenous leukemia, Philadelphia chromosome (Ph1) positive

Chronic myelogenous leukemia, t(9;22) (q34;q11)

Chronic myelogenous leukemia with crisis of blast cells

    EXCLUDES 1   atypical chronic myeloid leukemia BCR/ABL-negative (C92.2-)

        chronic myelomonocytic leukemia (C93.1-)

        chronic myeloproliferative disease (D47.1)

    C92.10 Chronic myeloid leukemia, BCR/ABL-positive, not having achieved remission   CC HCC

        Chronic myeloid leukemia, BCR/ABL-positive with failed remission

        Chronic myeloid leukemia, BCR/ABL-positive NOS

    C92.11 Chronic myeloid leukemia, BCR/ABL-positive, in remission   CC HCC

    C92.12 Chronic myeloid leukemia, BCR/ABL-positive, in relapse   CC HCC

✓5ᵗʰ **C92.2** Atypical chronic myeloid leukemia, BCR/ABL-negative

    C92.20 Atypical chronic myeloid leukemia, BCR/ABL-negative, not having achieved remission   CC HCC

        Atypical chronic myeloid leukemia, BCR/ABL-negative with failed remission

        Atypical chronic myeloid leukemia, BCR/ABL-negative NOS

    C92.21 Atypical chronic myeloid leukemia, BCR/ABL-negative, in remission   CC HCC

    C92.22 Atypical chronic myeloid leukemia, BCR/ABL-negative, in relapse   CC HCC

✓5ᵗʰ **C92.3** Myeloid sarcoma

A malignant tumor of immature myeloid cells

Chloroma

Granulocytic sarcoma

    C92.30 Myeloid sarcoma, not having achieved remission   CC HCC

        Myeloid sarcoma with failed remission

        Myeloid sarcoma NOS

    C92.31 Myeloid sarcoma, in remission   CC HCC

    C92.32 Myeloid sarcoma, in relapse   CC HCC

✅ Additional Character Required   ✓x7ᵗʰ Placeholder   Unacceptable PDx   Questionable PDx   Manifestation   Unspecified Dx   H1-H14 HAC   HCC CMS-HCC Dx   HIV HIV Dx

ICD-10-CM 2021   491

√5th **C92.4** **Acute promyelocytic** leukemia

AML M3

AML Me with t(15;17) and variants

C92.40 **Acute promyelocytic leukemia,** not having achieved remission CC HCC

Acute promyelocytic leukemia with failed remission

Acute promyelocytic leukemia NOS

C92.41 **Acute promyelocytic leukemia,** in remission CC HCC

C92.42 **Acute promyelocytic leukemia,** in relapse CC HCC

√5th **C92.5** **Acute myelomonocytic** leukemia

AML M4

AML M4 Eo with inv(16) or t(16;16)

C92.50 **Acute myelomonocytic leukemia,** not having achieved remission CC HCC

Acute myelomonocytic leukemia with failed remission

Acute myelomonocytic leukemia NOS

C92.51 **Acute myelomonocytic leukemia,** in remission CC HCC

C92.52 **Acute myelomonocytic leukemia,** in relapse CC HCC

√5th **C92.6** **Acute myeloid** leukemia with **11q23-abnormality**

Acute myeloid leukemia with variation of MLL-gene

C92.60 **Acute myeloid leukemia with 11q23-abnormality** not having achieved remission CC HCC

Acute myeloid leukemia with 11q23-abnormality with failed remission

Acute myeloid leukemia with 11q23-abnormality NOS

C92.61 **Acute myeloid leukemia with 11q23-abnormality** in remission CC HCC

C92.62 **Acute myeloid leukemia with 11q23-abnormality** in relapse CC HCC

√5th **C92.A** **Acute myeloid** leukemia with **multilineage dysplasia**

Acute myeloid leukemia with dysplasia of remaining hematopoesis and/or myelodysplastic disease in its history

C92.A0 **Acute myeloid leukemia with multilineage dysplasia,** not having achieved remission CC HCC

Acute myeloid leukemia with multilineage dysplasia with failed remission

Acute myeloid leukemia with multilineage dysplasia NOS

C92.A1 **Acute myeloid leukemia with multilineage dysplasia,** in remission CC HCC

C92.A2 **Acute myeloid leukemia with multilineage dysplasia,** in relapse CC HCC

√5th **C92.Z** **Other myeloid leukemia**

C92.Z0 **Other myeloid leukemia** not having achieved remission CC HCC

Myeloid leukemia NEC with failed remission

Myeloid leukemia NEC

C92.Z1 **Other myeloid leukemia,** in remission CC HCC

C92.Z2 **Other myeloid leukemia,** in relapse CC HCC

√5th **C92.9** **Myeloid leukemia, unspecified**

C92.90 **Myeloid leukemia, unspecified,** not having achieved remission CC HCC

Myeloid leukemia, unspecified with failed remission

Myeloid leukemia, unspecified NOS

C92.91 **Myeloid leukemia, unspecified** in remission CC HCC

C92.92 **Myeloid leukemia, unspecified** in relapse CC HCC

√4th **C93** **Monocytic leukemia**

INCLUDES monocytoid leukemia

EXCLUDES 1 personal history of leukemia (Z85.6)

AHA: 2020,1Q,13

√5th **C93.0** **Acute monoblastic/monocytic leukemia**

AML M5

AML M5a

AML M5b

C93.00 **Acute monoblastic/monocytic leukemia,** not having achieved remission CC HCC

Acute monoblastic/monocytic leukemia with failed remission

Acute monoblastic/monocytic leukemia NOS

C93.01 **Acute monoblastic/monocytic leukemia,** in remission CC HCC

C93.02 **Acute monoblastic/monocytic leukemia,** in relapse CC HCC

√5th **C93.1** **Chronic myelomonocytic** leukemia

Chronic monocytic leukemia

CMML-1

CMML-2

CMML with eosinophilia

►Code also, if applicable, eosinophilia (D72.18)◄

C93.10 **Chronic myelomonocytic leukemia** not having achieved remission CC HCC

Chronic myelomonocytic leukemia with failed remission

Chronic myelomonocytic leukemia NOS

C93.11 **Chronic myelomonocytic leukemia,** in remission CC HCC

C93.12 **Chronic myelomonocytic leukemia,** in relapse CC HCC

√5th **C93.3** **Juvenile myelomonocytic leukemia**

C93.30 **Juvenile myelomonocytic leukemia,** not having achieved remission CC HCC P

Juvenile myelomonocytic leukemia with failed remission

Juvenile myelomonocytic leukemia NOS

C93.31 **Juvenile myelomonocytic leukemia,** in remission CC HCC P

C93.32 **Juvenile myelomonocytic leukemia,** in relapse CC HCC P

√5th **C93.Z** **Other monocytic leukemia**

C93.Z0 **Other monocytic leukemia,** not having achieved remission CC HCC

Other monocytic leukemia NOS

C93.Z1 **Other monocytic leukemia,** in remission CC HCC

C93.Z2 **Other monocytic leukemia,** in relapse CC HCC

√5th **C93.9** **Monocytic leukemia, unspecified**

C93.90 **Monocytic leukemia, unspecified,** not having achieved remission CC HCC

Monocytic leukemia, unspecified with failed remission

Monocytic leukemia, unspecified NOS

C93.91 **Monocytic leukemia, unspecified** in remission CC HCC

C93.92 **Monocytic leukemia, unspecified** in relapse CC HCC

√4th **C94** **Other leukemias of** specified cell type

EXCLUDES 1 leukemic reticuloendotheliosis (C91.4-)

myelodysplastic syndromes (D46.-)

personal history of leukemia (Z85.6)

plasma cell leukemia (C90.1-)

AHA: 2020,1Q,13

√5th **C94.0** **Acute erythroid leukemia**

Acute myeloid leukemia M6(a)(b)

Erythroleukemia

DEF: Erythroleukemia: Malignant blood dyscrasia (a myeloproliferative disorder).

C94.00 **Acute erythroid leukemia,** not having achieved remission CC HCC

Acute erythroid leukemia with failed remission

Acute erythroid leukemia NOS

C94.01 **Acute erythroid leukemia,** in remission CC HCC

C94.02 **Acute erythroid leukemia,** in relapse CC HCC

√5th **C94.2** **Acute megakaryoblastic leukemia**

Acute myeloid leukemia M7

Acute megakaryocytic leukemia

C94.20 **Acute megakaryoblastic leukemia** not having achieved remission CC HCC

Acute megakaryoblastic leukemia with failed remission

Acute megakaryoblastic leukemia NOS

C94.21 **Acute megakaryoblastic leukemia,** in remission CC HCC

C94.22 **Acute megakaryoblastic leukemia,** in relapse CC HCC

N Newborn: 0 | P Pediatric: 0-17 | M Maternity: 9-64 | A Adult: 15-124 | MCC Major Complication/Comorbidity | CC Complication/Comorbidity | SW Severe Wound Dx

492 | ICD-10-CM 2021

√5ᵗʰ **C94.3** **Mast cell leukemia**

     AHA: 2017,4Q,5

     C94.30 **Mast cell leukemia** not having achieved
             remission   `CC` `HCC`
           Mast cell leukemia with failed remission
           Mast cell leukemia NOS

     C94.31 **Mast cell leukemia,** in remission   `CC` `HCC`
     C94.32 **Mast cell leukemia,** in relapse   `CC` `HCC`

√5ᵗʰ **C94.4** **Acute panmyelosis with myelofibrosis**

     Acute myelofibrosis

     EXCLUDES 1   myelofibrosis NOS (D75.81)
                  secondary myelofibrosis NOS (D75.81)

     C94.40 **Acute panmyelosis with myelofibrosis** not having
             achieved remission   `CC` `HCC`
           Acute myelofibrosis NOS
           Acute panmyelosis with myelofibrosis with failed
              remission
           Acute panmyelosis NOS

     C94.41 **Acute panmyelosis with myelofibrosis,** in
             remission   `CC` `HCC`

     C94.42 **Acute panmyelosis with myelofibrosis,** in
             relapse   `CC` `HCC`

C94.6 **Myelodysplastic disease, not classified**   `CC` `HCC`

     Myeloproliferative disease, not classified

√5ᵗʰ **C94.8** **Other specified leukemias**

     Aggressive NK-cell leukemia
     Acute basophilic leukemia

     C94.80 **Other specified leukemias** not having achieved
             remission   `CC` `HCC`
           Other specified leukemia with failed remission
           Other specified leukemias NOS

     C94.81 **Other specified leukemias,** in remission   `CC` `HCC`
     C94.82 **Other specified leukemias,** in relapse   `CC` `HCC`

√4ᵗʰ **C95** **Leukemia of unspecified cell type**

     EXCLUDES 1   personal history of leukemia (Z85.6)

     AHA: 2020,1Q,13

√5ᵗʰ **C95.0** **Acute leukemia of unspecified cell type**

     Acute bilineal leukemia
     Acute mixed lineage leukemia
     Biphenotypic acute leukemia
     Stem cell leukemia of unclear lineage

     EXCLUDES 1   acute exacerbation of unspecified chronic leukemia
                  (C95.10)

     C95.00 **Acute leukemia of unspecified cell type** not having
             achieved remission   `CC` `HCC`
           Acute leukemia of unspecified cell type with failed
              remission
           Acute leukemia NOS

     C95.01 **Acute leukemia of unspecified cell type,** in
             remission   `CC` `HCC`

     C95.02 **Acute leukemia of unspecified cell type,** in
             relapse   `CC` `HCC`

√5ᵗʰ **C95.1** **Chronic leukemia of unspecified cell type**

     C95.10 **Chronic leukemia of unspecified cell type** not
             having achieved remission   `CC` `HCC`
           Chronic leukemia of unspecified cell type with failed
              remission
           Chronic leukemia NOS

     C95.11 **Chronic leukemia of unspecified cell type,** in
             remission   `CC` `HCC`

     C95.12 **Chronic leukemia of unspecified cell type,** in
             relapse   `CC` `HCC`

√5ᵗʰ **C95.9** **Leukemia, unspecified**

     C95.90 **Leukemia, unspecified** not having achieved
             remission   `CC` `HCC`
           Leukemia, unspecified with failed remission
           Leukemia NOS

     C95.91 **Leukemia, unspecified,** in remission   `CC` `HCC`
     C95.92 **Leukemia, unspecified,** in relapse   `CC` `HCC`

√4ᵗʰ **C96** **Other and unspecified malignant neoplasms of lymphoid,
hematopoietic and related tissue**

     EXCLUDES 1   personal history of other malignant neoplasms of lymphoid,
                  hematopoietic and related tissues (Z85.79)

     C96.0 **Multifocal and multisystemic (disseminated) Langerhans-cell
histiocytosis**   `CC` `HCC`
           Histiocytosis X, multisystemic
           Letterer-Siwe disease

           EXCLUDES 1   adult pulmonary Langerhans cell histiocytosis
                       (J84.82)
                      multifocal and unisysemic Langerhans-cell
                         histiocytosis (C96.5)
                      unifocal Langerhans-cell histiocytosis (C96.6)

     √5ᵗʰ **C96.2** **Malignant mast cell neoplasm**

           EXCLUDES 1   indolent mastocytosis (D47.02)
                      mast cell leukemia (C94.30)
                      mastocytosis (congenital) (cutaneous) (Q82.2)

           AHA: 2017,4Q,5
           DEF: Mast cell: Type of white blood cell found in the loose
           connective tissue of blood vessels and bronchioles responsible
           for acute hypersensitivity reactions, including anaphylactic shock.
           The IgE receptors on these cells bind with allergens causing cell
           degranulation and diffuse, widespread histamine release that
           results in airway constriction and vasodilation with decreased
           systemic blood pressure.

           C96.20 **Malignant mast cell neoplasm,**
                 unspecified   `CC` `HCC`

           C96.21 **Aggressive systemic mastocytosis**   `CC` `HCC`
           C96.22 **Mast cell sarcoma**   `CC` `HCC`
           C96.29 **Other malignant mast cell neoplasm**   `CC` `HCC`

     C96.4 **Sarcoma of dendritic cells (accessory cells)**   `CC` `HCC`
           Follicular dendritic cell sarcoma
           Interdigitating dendritic cell sarcoma
           Langerhans cell sarcoma

     C96.5 **Multifocal and unisystemic Langerhans-cell
histiocytosis**   `CC` `HCC`
           Hand-Schüller-Christian disease
           Histiocytosis X, multifocal

           EXCLUDES 1   multifocal and multisystemic (disseminated)
                         Langerhans-cell histiocytosis (C96.0)
                      unifocal Langerhans-cell histiocytosis (C96.6)

     C96.6 **Unifocal Langerhans-cell histiocytosis**   `CC` `HCC`
           Eosinophilic granuloma
           Histiocytosis X, unifocal
           Histiocytosis X NOS
           Langerhans-cell histiocytosis NOS

           EXCLUDES 1   multifocal and multisysemic (disseminated)
                         Langerhans-cell histiocytosis (C96.0)
                      multifocal and unisystemic Langerhans-cell
                         histiocytosis (C96.5)

     C96.A **Histiocytic sarcoma**   `CC` `HCC`
           Malignant histiocytosis

     C96.Z **Other specified malignant neoplasms of lymphoid,
hematopoietic and related tissue**   `CC` `HCC`

     C96.9 **Malignant neoplasm of lymphoid, hematopoietic and related
tissue, unspecified**   `CC` `HCC`

✔ Additional Character Required   √x7ᵗʰ Placeholder   Unacceptable PDx   Questionable PDx   Manifestation   Unspecified Dx   `H1`-`H14` HAC   `HCC` CMS-HCC Dx   `HIV` HIV Dx

In situ neoplasms (D00-D09)

INCLUDES	Bowen's disease
	erythroplasia
	grade III intraepithelial neoplasia
	Queyrat's erythroplasia

✓4ᵗʰ **D00** **Carcinoma in situ of oral cavity, esophagus and stomach**

    EXCLUDES 1   melanoma in situ (D03.-)

✓5ᵗʰ **D00.0** **Carcinoma in situ of lip, oral cavity and pharynx**

       Use additional code to identify:

       exposure to environmental tobacco smoke (Z77.22)

       exposure to tobacco smoke in the perinatal period (P96.81)

       history of tobacco dependence (Z87.891)

       occupational exposure to environmental tobacco smoke (Z57.31)

       tobacco dependence (F17.-)

       tobacco use (Z72.0)

      EXCLUDES 1   carcinoma in situ of aryepiglottic fold or interarytenoid fold, laryngeal aspect (D02.0)

          carcinoma in situ of epiglottis NOS (D02.0)

          carcinoma in situ of epiglottis suprahyoid portion (D02.0)

          carcinoma in situ of skin of lip (D03.0, D04.0)

       D00.00 **Carcinoma in situ of oral cavity, unspecified site**

       D00.01 **Carcinoma in situ of labial mucosa and vermilion border**

       D00.02 **Carcinoma in situ of buccal mucosa**

       D00.03 **Carcinoma in situ of gingiva and edentulous alveolar ridge**

       D00.04 **Carcinoma in situ of soft palate**

       D00.05 **Carcinoma in situ of hard palate**

       D00.06 **Carcinoma in situ of floor of mouth**

       D00.07 **Carcinoma in situ of tongue**

       D00.08 **Carcinoma in situ of pharynx**

          Carcinoma in situ of aryepiglottic fold NOS

          Carcinoma in situ of hypopharyngeal aspect of aryepiglottic fold

          Carcinoma in situ of marginal zone of aryepiglottic fold

     D00.1 **Carcinoma in situ of esophagus**

     D00.2 **Carcinoma in situ of stomach**

✓4ᵗʰ **D01** **Carcinoma in situ of other and unspecified digestive organs**

    EXCLUDES 1   melanoma in situ (D03.-)

     D01.0 **Carcinoma in situ of colon**

      EXCLUDES 1   carcinoma in situ of rectosigmoid junction (D01.1)

     D01.1 **Carcinoma in situ of rectosigmoid junction**

     D01.2 **Carcinoma in situ of rectum**

     D01.3 **Carcinoma in situ of anus and anal canal**

       Anal intraepithelial neoplasia III [AIN III]

       Severe dysplasia of anus

      EXCLUDES 1   anal intraepithelial neoplasia I and II [AIN I and AIN II] (K62.82)

          carcinoma in situ of anal margin (D04.5)

          carcinoma in situ of anal skin (D04.5)

          carcinoma in situ of perianal skin (D04.5)

✓5ᵗʰ **D01.4** **Carcinoma in situ of other and unspecified parts of intestine**

      EXCLUDES 1   carcinoma in situ of ampulla of Vater (D01.5)

       D01.40 **Carcinoma in situ of unspecified part of intestine**

       D01.49 **Carcinoma in situ of other parts of intestine**

     D01.5 **Carcinoma in situ of liver, gallbladder and bile ducts**

       Carcinoma in situ of ampulla of Vater

     D01.7 **Carcinoma in situ of other specified digestive organs**

       Carcinoma in situ of pancreas

     D01.9 **Carcinoma in situ of digestive organ, unspecified**

✓4ᵗʰ **D02** **Carcinoma in situ of middle ear and respiratory system**

       Use additional code to identify:

       exposure to environmental tobacco smoke (Z77.22)

       exposure to tobacco smoke in the perinatal period (P96.81)

       history of tobacco dependence (Z87.891)

       occupational exposure to environmental tobacco smoke (Z57.31)

       tobacco dependence (F17.-)

       tobacco use (Z72.0)

      EXCLUDES 1   melanoma in situ (D03.-)

     D02.0 **Carcinoma in situ of larynx**

       Carcinoma in situ of aryepiglottic fold or interarytenoid fold, laryngeal aspect

       Carcinoma in situ of epiglottis (suprahyoid portion)

      EXCLUDES 1   carcinoma in situ of aryepiglottic fold or interarytenoid fold NOS (D00.08)

          carcinoma in situ of hypopharyngeal aspect (D00.08)

          carcinoma in situ of marginal zone (D00.08)

     D02.1 **Carcinoma in situ of trachea**

✓5ᵗʰ **D02.2** **Carcinoma in situ of bronchus and lung**

       D02.20 **Carcinoma in situ of unspecified bronchus and lung**

       D02.21 **Carcinoma in situ of right bronchus and lung**

       D02.22 **Carcinoma in situ of left bronchus and lung**

     D02.3 **Carcinoma in situ of other parts of respiratory system**

       Carcinoma in situ of accessory sinuses

       Carcinoma in situ of middle ear

       Carcinoma in situ of nasal cavities

      EXCLUDES 1   carcinoma in situ of ear (external) (skin) (D04.2-)

          carcinoma in situ of nose NOS (D09.8)

          carcinoma in situ of skin of nose (D04.3)

     D02.4 **Carcinoma in situ of respiratory system, unspecified**

✓4ᵗʰ **D03** **Melanoma in situ**

     D03.0 **Melanoma in situ of lip**   HCC

✓5ᵗʰ **D03.1** **Melanoma in situ of eyelid, including canthus**

       AHA: 2018,4Q,4

       D03.10 **Melanoma in situ of unspecified eyelid, including canthus**   HCC

✓6ᵗʰ   **D03.11** **Melanoma in situ of right eyelid, including canthus**

          D03.111 **Melanoma in situ of right upper eyelid, including canthus**   HCC

          D03.112 **Melanoma in situ of right lower eyelid, including canthus**   HCC

✓6ᵗʰ   **D03.12** **Melanoma in situ of left eyelid, including canthus**

          D03.121 **Melanoma in situ of left upper eyelid, including canthus**   HCC

          D03.122 **Melanoma in situ of left lower eyelid, including canthus**   HCC

✓5ᵗʰ **D03.2** **Melanoma in situ of ear and external auricular canal**

       D03.20 **Melanoma in situ of unspecified ear and external auricular canal**   HCC

       D03.21 **Melanoma in situ of right ear and external auricular canal**   HCC

       D03.22 **Melanoma in situ of left ear and external auricular canal**   HCC

✓5ᵗʰ **D03.3** **Melanoma in situ of other and unspecified parts of face**

       D03.30 **Melanoma in situ of unspecified part of face**   HCC

       D03.39 **Melanoma in situ of other parts of face**   HCC

     D03.4 **Melanoma in situ of scalp and neck**   HCC

✓5ᵗʰ **D03.5** **Melanoma in situ of trunk**

       D03.51 **Melanoma in situ of anal skin**   HCC

          Melanoma in situ of anal margin

          Melanoma in situ of perianal skin

       D03.52 **Melanoma in situ of breast (skin) (soft tissue)**   HCC

       D03.59 **Melanoma in situ of other part of trunk**   HCC

✓5ᵗʰ **D03.6** **Melanoma in situ of upper limb, including shoulder**

       D03.60 **Melanoma in situ of unspecified upper limb, including shoulder**   HCC

       D03.61 **Melanoma in situ of right upper limb, including shoulder**   HCC

       D03.62 **Melanoma in situ of left upper limb, including shoulder**   HCC

✓5ᵗʰ **D03.7** **Melanoma in situ of lower limb, including hip**

       D03.70 **Melanoma in situ of unspecified lower limb, including hip**   HCC

N Newborn: 0   P Pediatric: 0-17   M Maternity: 9-64   A Adult: 15-124   MCC Major Complication/Comorbidity   CC Complication/Comorbidity   SW Severe Wound Dx

494   ICD-10-CM 2021

D03.71 Melanoma in situ of right lower limb, including hip `HCC`

D03.72 Melanoma in situ of left lower limb, including hip `HCC`

D03.8 Melanoma in situ of other sites `HCC`
Melanoma in situ of scrotum
EXCLUDES 1 *carcinoma in situ of scrotum (D07.61)*

D03.9 Melanoma in situ, unspecified `HCC`

√4ᵗʰ **D04** Carcinoma in situ of skin
EXCLUDES 1 *erythroplasia of Queyrat (penis) NOS (D07.4)*
melanoma in situ (D03.-)

D04.0 Carcinoma in situ of skin of lip
EXCLUDES 2 *carcinoma in situ of vermilion border of lip (D00.01)*

√5ᵗʰ **D04.1** Carcinoma in situ of skin of eyelid, including canthus
AHA: 2018,4Q,4

D04.10 Carcinoma in situ of skin of unspecified eyelid, including canthus

√6ᵗʰ **D04.11** Carcinoma in situ of skin of right eyelid, including canthus
D04.111 Carcinoma in situ of skin of right upper eyelid, including canthus
D04.112 Carcinoma in situ of skin of right lower eyelid, including canthus

√6ᵗʰ **D04.12** Carcinoma in situ of skin of left eyelid, including canthus
D04.121 Carcinoma in situ of skin of left upper eyelid, including canthus
D04.122 Carcinoma in situ of skin of left lower eyelid, including canthus

√5ᵗʰ **D04.2** Carcinoma in situ of skin of ear and external auricular canal
D04.20 Carcinoma in situ of skin of unspecified ear and external auricular canal
D04.21 Carcinoma in situ of skin of right ear and external auricular canal
D04.22 Carcinoma in situ of skin of left ear and external auricular canal

√5ᵗʰ **D04.3** Carcinoma in situ of skin of other and unspecified parts of face
D04.30 Carcinoma in situ of skin of unspecified part of face
D04.39 Carcinoma in situ of skin of other parts of face

D04.4 Carcinoma in situ of skin of scalp and neck

D04.5 Carcinoma in situ of skin of trunk
Carcinoma in situ of anal margin
Carcinoma in situ of anal skin
Carcinoma in situ of perianal skin
Carcinoma in situ of skin of breast
EXCLUDES 1 *carcinoma in situ of anus NOS (D01.3)*
carcinoma in situ of scrotum (D07.61)
carcinoma in situ of skin of genital organs (D07.-)

√5ᵗʰ **D04.6** Carcinoma in situ of skin of upper limb, including shoulder
D04.60 Carcinoma in situ of skin of unspecified upper limb, including shoulder
D04.61 Carcinoma in situ of skin of right upper limb, including shoulder
D04.62 Carcinoma in situ of skin of left upper limb, including shoulder

√5ᵗʰ **D04.7** Carcinoma in situ of skin of lower limb, including hip
D04.70 Carcinoma in situ of skin of unspecified lower limb, including hip
D04.71 Carcinoma in situ of skin of right lower limb, including hip
D04.72 Carcinoma in situ of skin of left lower limb, including hip

D04.8 Carcinoma in situ of skin of other sites
D04.9 Carcinoma in situ of skin, unspecified

√4ᵗʰ **D05** Carcinoma in situ of breast
EXCLUDES 1 *carcinoma in situ of skin of breast (D04.5)*
melanoma in situ of breast (skin) (D03.5)
Paget's disease of breast or nipple (C50.-)

√5ᵗʰ **D05.0** Lobular carcinoma in situ of breast
D05.00 Lobular carcinoma in situ of unspecified breast
D05.01 Lobular carcinoma in situ of right breast
D05.02 Lobular carcinoma in situ of left breast

√5ᵗʰ **D05.1** Intraductal carcinoma in situ of breast
D05.10 Intraductal carcinoma in situ of unspecified breast
D05.11 Intraductal carcinoma in situ of right breast

D05.12 Intraductal carcinoma in situ of left breast

√5ᵗʰ **D05.8** Other specified type of carcinoma in situ of breast
D05.80 Other specified type of carcinoma in situ of unspecified breast
D05.81 Other specified type of carcinoma in situ of right breast
D05.82 Other specified type of carcinoma in situ of left breast

√5ᵗʰ **D05.9** Unspecified type of carcinoma in situ of breast
D05.90 Unspecified type of carcinoma in situ of unspecified breast
D05.91 Unspecified type of carcinoma in situ of right breast
D05.92 Unspecified type of carcinoma in situ of left breast

√4ᵗʰ **D06** Carcinoma in situ of cervix uteri
INCLUDES cervical adenocarcinoma in situ
cervical intraepithelial glandular neoplasia
cervical intraepithelial neoplasia III [CIN III]
severe dysplasia of cervix uteri
EXCLUDES 1 *cervical intraepithelial neoplasia II [CIN II] (N87.1)*
cytologic evidence of malignancy of cervix without histologic confirmation (R87.614)
high grade squamous intraepithelial lesion (HGSIL) of cervix (R87.613)
melanoma in situ of cervix (D03.5)
moderate cervical dysplasia (N87.1)

D06.0 Carcinoma in situ of endocervix ♀
D06.1 Carcinoma in situ of exocervix ♀
D06.7 Carcinoma in situ of other parts of cervix ♀
D06.9 Carcinoma in situ of cervix, unspecified ♀

√4ᵗʰ **D07** Carcinoma in situ of other and unspecified genital organs
EXCLUDES 1 *melanoma in situ of trunk (D03.5)*

D07.0 Carcinoma in situ of endometrium ♀
D07.1 Carcinoma in situ of vulva ♀
Severe dysplasia of vulva
Vulvar intraepithelial neoplasia III [VIN III]
EXCLUDES 1 *moderate dysplasia of vulva (N90.1)*
vulvar intraepithelial neoplasia II [VIN II] (N90.1)

D07.2 Carcinoma in situ of vagina ♀
Severe dysplasia of vagina
Vaginal intraepithelial neoplasia III [VAIN III]
EXCLUDES 1 *moderate dysplasia of vagina (N89.1)*
vaginal intraepithelial neoplasia II [VIN II] (N89.1)

√5ᵗʰ **D07.3** Carcinoma in situ of other and unspecified female genital organs
D07.30 Carcinoma in situ of unspecified female genital organs ♀
D07.39 Carcinoma in situ of other female genital organs ♀

D07.4 Carcinoma in situ of penis ♂
Erythroplasia of Queyrat NOS

D07.5 Carcinoma in situ of prostate ♂
Prostatic intraepithelial neoplasia III (PIN III)
Severe dysplasia of prostate
EXCLUDES 1 *dysplasia (mild) (moderate) of prostate (N42.3-)*
prostatic intraepithelial neoplasia II [PIN II] (N42.3-)

√5ᵗʰ **D07.6** Carcinoma in situ of other and unspecified male genital organs
D07.60 Carcinoma in situ of unspecified male genital organs ♂
D07.61 Carcinoma in situ of scrotum ♂
D07.69 Carcinoma in situ of other male genital organs ♂

√4ᵗʰ **D09** Carcinoma in situ of other and unspecified sites
EXCLUDES 1 *melanoma in situ (D03.-)*

D09.0 Carcinoma in situ of bladder

√5ᵗʰ **D09.1** Carcinoma in situ of other and unspecified urinary organs
D09.10 Carcinoma in situ of unspecified urinary organ
D09.19 Carcinoma in situ of other urinary organs

√5ᵗʰ **D09.2** Carcinoma in situ of eye
EXCLUDES 1 *carcinoma in situ of skin of eyelid (D04.1-)*
D09.20 Carcinoma in situ of unspecified eye
D09.21 Carcinoma in situ of right eye
D09.22 Carcinoma in situ of left eye

✓ Additional Character Required   √x7ᵗʰ Placeholder   Unacceptable PDx   Questionable PDx   Manifestation   Unspecified Dx   H1-H14 HAC   HCC CMS-HCC Dx   HIV HIV Dx
ICD-10-CM 2021
495

Chapter 2. Neoplasms

D03.71–D09.22

Chapter 2. Neoplasms

D09.3 Carcinoma in situ of thyroid and other endocrine glands
> EXCLUDES 1   *carcinoma in situ of endocrine pancreas (D01.7)*
> *carcinoma in situ of ovary (D07.39)*
> *carcinoma in situ of testis (D07.69)*

D09.8 Carcinoma in situ of other specified sites

D09.9 Carcinoma in situ, unspecified

Benign neoplasms, except benign neuroendocrine tumors (D10-D36)

✓4ᵗʰ **D10 Benign neoplasm of mouth and pharynx**

D10.0 Benign neoplasm of lip
> Benign neoplasm of lip (frenulum) (inner aspect) (mucosa) (vermilion border)
> EXCLUDES 1   *benign neoplasm of skin of lip (D22.0, D23.0)*

D10.1 Benign neoplasm of tongue
> Benign neoplasm of lingual tonsil

D10.2 Benign neoplasm of floor of mouth

✓5ᵗʰ **D10.3 Benign neoplasm of other and unspecified parts of mouth**

> **D10.30 Benign neoplasm of unspecified part of mouth**
> **D10.39 Benign neoplasm of other parts of mouth**
>> Benign neoplasm of minor salivary gland NOS
>> EXCLUDES 1   *benign odontogenic neoplasms (D16.4-D16.5)*
>> *benign neoplasm of mucosa of lip (D10.0)*
>> *benign neoplasm of nasopharyngeal surface of soft palate (D10.6)*

D10.4 Benign neoplasm of tonsil
> Benign neoplasm of tonsil (faucial) (palatine)
> EXCLUDES 1   *benign neoplasm of lingual tonsil (D10.1)*
> *benign neoplasm of pharyngeal tonsil (D10.6)*
> *benign neoplasm of tonsillar fossa (D10.5)*
> *benign neoplasm of tonsillar pillars (D10.5)*

D10.5 Benign neoplasm of other parts of oropharynx
> Benign neoplasm of epiglottis, anterior aspect
> Benign neoplasm of tonsillar fossa
> Benign neoplasm of tonsillar pillars
> Benign neoplasm of vallecula
> EXCLUDES 1   *benign neoplasm of epiglottis NOS (D14.1)*
> *benign neoplasm of epiglottis, suprahyoid portion (D14.1)*
> **DEF:** Oropharynx: Middle portion of pharynx (throat); communicates with the oral cavity, nasopharynx and laryngopharynx.

D10.6 Benign neoplasm of nasopharynx
> Benign neoplasm of pharyngeal tonsil
> Benign neoplasm of posterior margin of septum and choanae
> **DEF:** Nasopharynx: Upper portion of pharynx (throat); communicates with the nasal cavities, oropharynx and tympanic cavities.

D10.7 Benign neoplasm of hypopharynx
> **DEF:** Hypopharynx: Lower portion of pharynx (throat); communicates with the oropharynx and the esophagus.
> *Synonyms: laryngopharynx.*

D10.9 Benign neoplasm of pharynx, unspecified

✓4ᵗʰ **D11 Benign neoplasm of major salivary glands**
> EXCLUDES 1   *benign neoplasms of specified minor salivary glands which are classified according to their anatomical location*
> *benign neoplasms of minor salivary glands NOS (D10.39)*

D11.0 Benign neoplasm of parotid gland

D11.7 Benign neoplasm of other major salivary glands
> Benign neoplasm of sublingual salivary gland
> Benign neoplasm of submandibular salivary gland

D11.9 Benign neoplasm of major salivary gland, unspecified

✓4ᵗʰ **D12 Benign neoplasm of colon, rectum, anus and anal canal**
> EXCLUDES 1   *benign carcinoid tumors of the large intestine, and rectum (D3A.02-)*
> *polyp of colon NOS (K63.5)*
> **AHA:** 2018,2Q,14; 2017,1Q,15; 2015,2Q,14
> **TIP:** Code K63.5 Polyp of colon, is assigned when documentation states hyperplastic colon polyps, regardless of the site in the colon. Slow-growing, hyperplastic polyps are not precancerous and are classified differently from benign or adenomatous polyps.

D12.0 Benign neoplasm of cecum
> Benign neoplasm of ileocecal valve

D12.1 Benign neoplasm of appendix
> EXCLUDES 1   *benign carcinoid tumor of the appendix (D3A.020)*

D12.2 Benign neoplasm of ascending colon

D12.3 Benign neoplasm of transverse colon
> Benign neoplasm of hepatic flexure
> Benign neoplasm of splenic flexure
> **AHA:** 2017,1Q,16

D12.4 Benign neoplasm of descending colon

D12.5 Benign neoplasm of sigmoid colon

D12.6 Benign neoplasm of colon, unspecified
> Adenomatosis of colon
> Benign neoplasm of large intestine NOS
> Polyposis (hereditary) of colon
> EXCLUDES 1   *inflammatory polyp of colon (K51.4-)*

D12.7 Benign neoplasm of rectosigmoid junction

D12.8 Benign neoplasm of rectum
> EXCLUDES 1   *benign carcinoid tumor of the rectum (D3A.026)*
> **AHA:** 2018,1Q,6

D12.9 Benign neoplasm of anus and anal canal
> Benign neoplasm of anus NOS
> EXCLUDES 1   *benign neoplasm of anal margin (D22.5, D23.5)*
> *benign neoplasm of anal skin (D22.5, D23.5)*
> *benign neoplasm of perianal skin (D22.5, D23.5)*

✓4ᵗʰ **D13 Benign neoplasm of other and ill-defined parts of digestive system**
> EXCLUDES 1   *benign stromal tumors of digestive system (D21.4)*

D13.0 Benign neoplasm of esophagus

D13.1 Benign neoplasm of stomach
> EXCLUDES 1   *benign carcinoid tumor of the stomach (D3A.092)*

D13.2 Benign neoplasm of duodenum
> EXCLUDES 1   *benign carcinoid tumor of the duodenum (D3A.010)*

✓5ᵗʰ **D13.3 Benign neoplasm of other and unspecified parts of small intestine**
> EXCLUDES 1   *benign carcinoid tumors of the small intestine (D3A.01-)*
> *benign neoplasm of ileocecal valve (D12.0)*

> **D13.30 Benign neoplasm of unspecified part of small intestine**
> **D13.39 Benign neoplasm of other parts of small intestine**

D13.4 Benign neoplasm of liver
> Benign neoplasm of intrahepatic bile ducts

D13.5 Benign neoplasm of extrahepatic bile ducts

D13.6 Benign neoplasm of pancreas
> EXCLUDES 1   *benign neoplasm of endocrine pancreas (D13.7)*

D13.7 Benign neoplasm of endocrine pancreas
> Benign neoplasm of islets of Langerhans
> Islet cell tumor
> Use additional code to identify any functional activity

D13.9 Benign neoplasm of ill-defined sites within the digestive system
> Benign neoplasm of digestive system NOS
> Benign neoplasm of intestine NOS
> Benign neoplasm of spleen

✓4ᵗʰ **D14 Benign neoplasm of middle ear and respiratory system**

D14.0 Benign neoplasm of middle ear, nasal cavity and accessory sinuses
> Benign neoplasm of cartilage of nose
> EXCLUDES 1   *benign neoplasm of auricular canal (external) (D22.2-, D23.2-)*
> *benign neoplasm of bone of ear (D16.4)*
> *benign neoplasm of bone of nose (D16.4)*
> *benign neoplasm of cartilage of ear (D21.0)*
> *benign neoplasm of ear (external)(skin) (D22.2-, D23.2-)*
> *benign neoplasm of nose NOS (D36.7)*
> *benign neoplasm of skin of nose (D22.39, D23.39)*
> *benign neoplasm of olfactory bulb (D33.3)*
> *benign neoplasm of posterior margin of septum and choanae (D10.6)*
> *polyp of accessory sinus (J33.8)*
> *polyp of ear (middle) (H74.4)*
> *polyp of nasal (cavity) (J33.-)*

Ⓝ Newborn: 0   Ⓟ Pediatric: 0-17   Ⓜ Maternity: 9-64   Ⓐ Adult: 15-124   **MCC** Major Complication/Comorbidity   **CC** Complication/Comorbidity   **SW** Severe Wound Dx

496   ICD-10-CM 2021

D14.1 **Benign neoplasm of** larynx
Adenomatous polyp of larynx
Benign neoplasm of epiglottis (suprahyoid portion)
　EXCLUDES 1　*benign neoplasm of epiglottis, anterior aspect (D10.5)*
　　　　　　polyp (nonadenomatous) of vocal cord or larynx
　　　　　　(J38.1)

D14.2 **Benign neoplasm of** trachea

✓5ᵗʰ **D14.3** **Benign neoplasm of** bronchus and lung
　EXCLUDES 1　*benign carcinoid tumor of the bronchus and lung*
　　　　　　(D3A.090)
　　　D14.30 **Benign neoplasm of unspecified bronchus and lung**
　　　D14.31 **Benign neoplasm of** right **bronchus and lung**
　　　D14.32 **Benign neoplasm of** left **bronchus and lung**

D14.4 **Benign neoplasm of respiratory system, unspecified**

✓4ᵗʰ **D15** **Benign neoplasm of other and unspecified** intrathoracic organs
　EXCLUDES 1　*benign neoplasm of mesothelial tissue (D19.-)*

D15.0 **Benign neoplasm of** thymus
　EXCLUDES 1　*benign carcinoid tumor of the thymus (D3A.091)*

D15.1 **Benign neoplasm of** heart
　EXCLUDES 1　*benign neoplasm of great vessels (D21.3)*

D15.2 **Benign neoplasm of** mediastinum
D15.7 **Benign neoplasm of other specified intrathoracic organs**
D15.9 **Benign neoplasm of intrathoracic organ, unspecified**

✓4ᵗʰ **D16** **Benign neoplasm of** bone and articular cartilage
　EXCLUDES 1　*benign neoplasm of connective tissue of ear (D21.0)*
　　　　　　benign neoplasm of connective tissue of eyelid (D21.0)
　　　　　　benign neoplasm of connective tissue of larynx (D14.1)
　　　　　　benign neoplasm of connective tissue of nose (D14.0)
　　　　　　benign neoplasm of synovia (D21.-)

✓5ᵗʰ **D16.0** **Benign neoplasm of** scapula and long bones of upper limb
　　　D16.00 **Benign neoplasm of scapula and long bones of unspecified upper limb**
　　　D16.01 **Benign neoplasm of scapula and long bones of** right **upper limb**
　　　D16.02 **Benign neoplasm of scapula and long bones of** left **upper limb**

✓5ᵗʰ **D16.1** **Benign neoplasm of** short bones of upper limb
　　　D16.10 **Benign neoplasm of short bones of unspecified upper limb**
　　　D16.11 **Benign neoplasm of short bones of** right **upper limb**
　　　D16.12 **Benign neoplasm of short bones of** left **upper limb**

✓5ᵗʰ **D16.2** **Benign neoplasm of** long bones of lower limb
　　　D16.20 **Benign neoplasm of long bones of unspecified lower limb**
　　　D16.21 **Benign neoplasm of long bones of** right **lower limb**
　　　D16.22 **Benign neoplasm of long bones of** left **lower limb**

✓5ᵗʰ **D16.3** **Benign neoplasm of** short bones of lower limb
　　　D16.30 **Benign neoplasm of short bones of unspecified lower limb**
　　　D16.31 **Benign neoplasm of short bones of** right **lower limb**
　　　D16.32 **Benign neoplasm of short bones of** left **lower limb**

D16.4 **Benign neoplasm of bones of** skull and face
Benign neoplasm of maxilla (superior)
Benign neoplasm of orbital bone
Keratocyst of maxilla
Keratocystic odontogenic tumor of maxilla
　EXCLUDES 2　*benign neoplasm of lower jaw bone (D16.5)*

D16.5 **Benign neoplasm of** lower jaw bone
Keratocyst of mandible
Keratocystic odontogenic tumor of mandible

D16.6 **Benign neoplasm of** vertebral column
　EXCLUDES 1　*benign neoplasm of sacrum and coccyx (D16.8)*

D16.7 **Benign neoplasm of** ribs, sternum and clavicle
D16.8 **Benign neoplasm of** pelvic bones, sacrum and coccyx
D16.9 **Benign neoplasm of bone and articular cartilage, unspecified**

✓4ᵗʰ **D17** **Benign** lipomatous **neoplasm**

D17.0 **Benign lipomatous neoplasm of** skin and subcutaneous tissue of head, face and neck
D17.1 **Benign lipomatous neoplasm of** skin and subcutaneous tissue of trunk

✓5ᵗʰ **D17.2** **Benign lipomatous neoplasm of** skin and subcutaneous tissue of limb
　　　D17.20 **Benign lipomatous neoplasm of skin and subcutaneous tissue of unspecified limb**

　　　D17.21 **Benign lipomatous neoplasm of skin and subcutaneous tissue of** right arm
　　　D17.22 **Benign lipomatous neoplasm of skin and subcutaneous tissue of** left arm
　　　D17.23 **Benign lipomatous neoplasm of skin and subcutaneous tissue of** right leg
　　　D17.24 **Benign lipomatous neoplasm of skin and subcutaneous tissue of** left leg

✓5ᵗʰ **D17.3** **Benign lipomatous neoplasm of** skin and subcutaneous tissue of other and unspecified sites
　　　D17.30 **Benign lipomatous neoplasm of skin and subcutaneous tissue of unspecified sites**
　　　D17.39 **Benign lipomatous neoplasm of skin and subcutaneous tissue of other sites**

D17.4 **Benign lipomatous neoplasm of** intrathoracic organs
D17.5 **Benign lipomatous neoplasm of** intra-abdominal organs
　EXCLUDES 1　*benign lipomatous neoplasm of peritoneum and retroperitoneum (D17.79)*

D17.6 **Benign lipomatous neoplasm of** spermatic cord　　　♂

✓5ᵗʰ **D17.7** **Benign lipomatous neoplasm of other sites**
　　　D17.71 **Benign lipomatous neoplasm of** kidney
　　　D17.72 **Benign lipomatous neoplasm of other** genitourinary organ
　　　D17.79 **Benign lipomatous neoplasm of other sites**
　　　　Benign lipomatous neoplasm of peritoneum
　　　　Benign lipomatous neoplasm of retroperitoneum

D17.9 **Benign lipomatous neoplasm, unspecified**
Lipoma NOS

✓4ᵗʰ **D18** **Hemangioma and lymphangioma, any site**
　EXCLUDES 1　*benign neoplasm of glomus jugulare (D35.6)*
　　　　　　blue or pigmented nevus (D22.-)
　　　　　　nevus NOS (D22.-)
　　　　　　vascular nevus (Q82.5)

✓5ᵗʰ **D18.0** **Hemangioma**
Angioma NOS
Cavernous nevus
DEF: Common benign tumor usually occurring in infancy that is composed of newly formed blood vessels due to malformation of the angioblastic tissue.
　　　D18.00 **Hemangioma unspecified site**
　　　D18.01 **Hemangioma of** skin and subcutaneous tissue
　　　D18.02 **Hemangioma of** intracranial structures　　HCC
　　　D18.03 **Hemangioma of** intra-abdominal structures
　　　D18.09 **Hemangioma of other sites**

D18.1 **Lymphangioma, any site**
AHA: 2018,3Q,31; 2018,2Q,13

✓4ᵗʰ **D19** **Benign neoplasm of** mesothelial tissue

D19.0 **Benign neoplasm of mesothelial tissue of** pleura
D19.1 **Benign neoplasm of mesothelial tissue of** peritoneum
D19.7 **Benign neoplasm of mesothelial tissue of other sites**
D19.9 **Benign neoplasm of mesothelial tissue, unspecified**
Benign mesothelioma NOS

✓4ᵗʰ **D20** **Benign neoplasm of soft tissue of** retroperitoneum and peritoneum
　EXCLUDES 1　*benign lipomatous neoplasm of peritoneum and retroperitoneum (D17.79)*
　　　　　　benign neoplasm of mesothelial tissue (D19.-)

D20.0 **Benign neoplasm of soft tissue of** retroperitoneum
D20.1 **Benign neoplasm of soft tissue of** peritoneum

✓ Additional Character Required　✓x7ᵗʰ Placeholder　Unacceptable PDx　Questionable PDx　Manifestation　Unspecified Dx　H1-H14 HAC　HCC CMS-HCC Dx　HIV HIV Dx
ICD-10-CM 2021　　　　　　　　　　　　　　　　　　　　　　　497

D14.1–D20.1

✓4ᵗʰ **D21 Other benign neoplasms of connective and other soft tissue**

INCLUDES benign neoplasm of blood vessel
benign neoplasm of bursa
benign neoplasm of cartilage
benign neoplasm of fascia
benign neoplasm of fat
benign neoplasm of ligament, except uterine
benign neoplasm of lymphatic channel
benign neoplasm of muscle
benign neoplasm of synovia
benign neoplasm of tendon (sheath)
benign stromal tumors

EXCLUDES 1 *benign neoplasm of articular cartilage (D16.-)*
benign neoplasm of cartilage of larynx (D14.1)
benign neoplasm of cartilage of nose (D14.0)
benign neoplasm of connective tissue of breast (D24.-)
benign neoplasm of peripheral nerves and autonomic nervous system (D36.1-)
benign neoplasm of peritoneum (D20.1)
benign neoplasm of retroperitoneum (D20.0)
benign neoplasm of uterine ligament, any (D28.2)
benign neoplasm of vascular tissue (D18.-)
hemangioma (D18.0-)
lipomatous neoplasm (D17.-)
lymphangioma (D18.1)
uterine leiomyoma (D25.-)

D21.0 Benign neoplasm of connective and other soft tissue of head, face and neck
Benign neoplasm of connective tissue of ear
Benign neoplasm of connective tissue of eyelid
EXCLUDES 1 *benign neoplasm of connective tissue of orbit (D31.6-)*

✓5ᵗʰ **D21.1 Benign neoplasm of connective and other soft tissue of upper limb, including shoulder**
D21.10 Benign neoplasm of connective and other soft tissue of unspecified upper limb, including shoulder
D21.11 Benign neoplasm of connective and other soft tissue of right upper limb, including shoulder
D21.12 Benign neoplasm of connective and other soft tissue of left upper limb, including shoulder

✓5ᵗʰ **D21.2 Benign neoplasm of connective and other soft tissue of lower limb, including hip**
D21.20 Benign neoplasm of connective and other soft tissue of unspecified lower limb, including hip
D21.21 Benign neoplasm of connective and other soft tissue of right lower limb, including hip
D21.22 Benign neoplasm of connective and other soft tissue of left lower limb, including hip

D21.3 Benign neoplasm of connective and other soft tissue of thorax
Benign neoplasm of axilla
Benign neoplasm of diaphragm
Benign neoplasm of great vessels
EXCLUDES 1 *benign neoplasm of heart (D15.1)*
benign neoplasm of mediastinum (D15.2)
benign neoplasm of thymus (D15.0)

D21.4 Benign neoplasm of connective and other soft tissue of abdomen
Benign stromal tumors of abdomen

D21.5 Benign neoplasm of connective and other soft tissue of pelvis
EXCLUDES 1 *benign neoplasm of any uterine ligament (D28.2)*
uterine leiomyoma (D25.-)

D21.6 Benign neoplasm of connective and other soft tissue of trunk, unspecified
▶Benign neoplasm of connective and other soft tissue of back NOS◀

D21.9 Benign neoplasm of connective and other soft tissue, unspecified

✓4ᵗʰ **D22 Melanocytic nevi**
INCLUDES atypical nevus
blue hairy pigmented nevus
nevus NOS

D22.0 Melanocytic nevi of lip

✓5ᵗʰ **D22.1 Melanocytic nevi of eyelid, including canthus**
AHA: 2018,4Q,4
D22.10 Melanocytic nevi of unspecified eyelid, including canthus

✓6ᵗʰ **D22.11 Melanocytic nevi of right eyelid, including canthus**
D22.111 Melanocytic nevi of right upper eyelid, including canthus
D22.112 Melanocytic nevi of right lower eyelid, including canthus

✓6ᵗʰ **D22.12 Melanocytic nevi of left eyelid, including canthus**
D22.121 Melanocytic nevi of left upper eyelid, including canthus
D22.122 Melanocytic nevi of left lower eyelid, including canthus

✓5ᵗʰ **D22.2 Melanocytic nevi of ear and external auricular canal**
D22.20 Melanocytic nevi of unspecified ear and external auricular canal
D22.21 Melanocytic nevi of right ear and external auricular canal
D22.22 Melanocytic nevi of left ear and external auricular canal

✓5ᵗʰ **D22.3 Melanocytic nevi of other and unspecified parts of face**
D22.30 Melanocytic nevi of unspecified part of face
D22.39 Melanocytic nevi of other parts of face

D22.4 Melanocytic nevi of scalp and neck

D22.5 Melanocytic nevi of trunk
Melanocytic nevi of anal margin
Melanocytic nevi of anal skin
Melanocytic nevi of perianal skin
Melanocytic nevi of skin of breast

✓5ᵗʰ **D22.6 Melanocytic nevi of upper limb, including shoulder**
D22.60 Melanocytic nevi of unspecified upper limb, including shoulder
D22.61 Melanocytic nevi of right upper limb, including shoulder
D22.62 Melanocytic nevi of left upper limb, including shoulder

✓5ᵗʰ **D22.7 Melanocytic nevi of lower limb, including hip**
D22.70 Melanocytic nevi of unspecified lower limb, including hip
D22.71 Melanocytic nevi of right lower limb, including hip
D22.72 Melanocytic nevi of left lower limb, including hip

D22.9 Melanocytic nevi, unspecified

✓4ᵗʰ **D23 Other benign neoplasms of skin**
INCLUDES benign neoplasm of hair follicles
benign neoplasm of sebaceous glands
benign neoplasm of sweat glands
EXCLUDES 1 *benign lipomatous neoplasms of skin (D17.0-D17.3)*
EXCLUDES 2 *melanocytic nevi (D22.-)*

D23.0 Other benign neoplasm of skin of lip
EXCLUDES 1 *benign neoplasm of vermilion border of lip (D10.0)*

✓5ᵗʰ **D23.1 Other benign neoplasm of skin of eyelid, including canthus**
AHA: 2018,4Q,4
D23.10 Other benign neoplasm of skin of unspecified eyelid, including canthus
✓6ᵗʰ **D23.11 Other benign neoplasm of skin of right eyelid, including canthus**
D23.111 Other benign neoplasm of skin of right upper eyelid, including canthus
D23.112 Other benign neoplasm of skin of right lower eyelid, including canthus
✓6ᵗʰ **D23.12 Other benign neoplasm of skin of left eyelid, including canthus**
D23.121 Other benign neoplasm of skin of left upper eyelid, including canthus
D23.122 Other benign neoplasm of skin of left lower eyelid, including canthus

✓5ᵗʰ **D23.2 Other benign neoplasm of skin of ear and external auricular canal**
D23.20 Other benign neoplasm of skin of unspecified ear and external auricular canal
D23.21 Other benign neoplasm of skin of right ear and external auricular canal
D23.22 Other benign neoplasm of skin of left ear and external auricular canal

✓5ᵗʰ **D23.3 Other benign neoplasm of skin of other and unspecified parts of face**
D23.30 Other benign neoplasm of skin of unspecified part of face
D23.39 Other benign neoplasm of skin of other parts of face

D23.4 Other benign neoplasm of skin of scalp and neck

D23.5 Other benign neoplasm of skin of trunk
    Other benign neoplasm of anal margin
    Other benign neoplasm of anal skin
    Other benign neoplasm of perianal skin
    Other benign neoplasm of skin of breast
    EXCLUDES 1   *benign neoplasm of anus NOS (D12.9)*

✓5th **D23.6** Other benign neoplasm of skin of upper limb, including shoulder
    D23.60 Other benign neoplasm of skin of unspecified upper limb, including shoulder
    D23.61 Other benign neoplasm of skin of right upper limb, including shoulder
    D23.62 Other benign neoplasm of skin of left upper limb, including shoulder

✓5th **D23.7** Other benign neoplasm of skin of lower limb, including hip
    D23.70 Other benign neoplasm of skin of unspecified lower limb, including hip
    D23.71 Other benign neoplasm of skin of right lower limb, including hip
    D23.72 Other benign neoplasm of skin of left lower limb, including hip

D23.9 Other benign neoplasm of skin, unspecified

✓4th **D24** Benign neoplasm of breast
    INCLUDES   benign neoplasm of connective tissue of breast
         benign neoplasm of soft parts of breast
         fibroadenoma of breast
    EXCLUDES 2   *adenofibrosis of breast (N60.2)*
         benign cyst of breast (N60.-)
         benign mammary dysplasia (N60.-)
         benign neoplasm of skin of breast (D22.5, D23.5)
         fibrocystic disease of breast (N60.-)

    D24.1 Benign neoplasm of right breast
    D24.2 Benign neoplasm of left breast
    D24.9 Benign neoplasm of unspecified breast

✓4th **D25** Leiomyoma of uterus
    INCLUDES   uterine fibroid
         uterine fibromyoma
         uterine myoma

Uterine Leiomyomas (Fibroids)

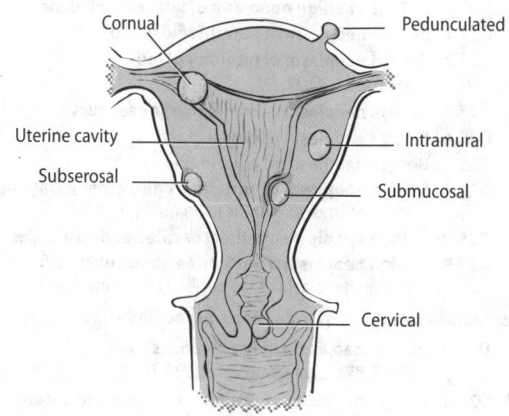

Cornual   Pedunculated
Uterine cavity   Intramural
Subserosal   Submucosal
Cervical

    D25.0 Submucous leiomyoma of uterus ♀
    D25.1 Intramural leiomyoma of uterus ♀
         Interstitial leiomyoma of uterus
    D25.2 Subserosal leiomyoma of uterus ♀
         Subperitoneal leiomyoma of uterus
    D25.9 Leiomyoma of uterus, unspecified ♀

✓4th **D26** Other benign neoplasms of uterus
    D26.0 Other benign neoplasm of cervix uteri ♀
    D26.1 Other benign neoplasm of corpus uteri ♀
    D26.7 Other benign neoplasm of other parts of uterus ♀
    D26.9 Other benign neoplasm of uterus, unspecified ♀

✓4th **D27** Benign neoplasm of ovary
    Use additional code to identify any functional activity
    EXCLUDES 2   *corpus albicans cyst (N83.2-)*
         corpus luteum cyst (N83.1-)
         endometrial cyst (N80.1)
         follicular (atretic) cyst (N83.0-)
         graafian follicle cyst (N83.0-)
         ovarian cyst NEC (N83.2-)
         ovarian retention cyst (N83.2-)

    D27.0 Benign neoplasm of right ovary ♀
    D27.1 Benign neoplasm of left ovary ♀
    D27.9 Benign neoplasm of unspecified ovary ♀

✓4th **D28** Benign neoplasm of other and unspecified female genital organs
    INCLUDES   adenomatous polyp
         benign neoplasm of skin of female genital organs
         benign teratoma
    EXCLUDES 1   *epoophoron cyst (Q50.5)*
         fimbrial cyst (Q50.4)
         Gartner's duct cyst (Q52.4)
         parovarian cyst (Q50.5)

    D28.0 Benign neoplasm of vulva ♀
    D28.1 Benign neoplasm of vagina ♀
    D28.2 Benign neoplasm of uterine tubes and ligaments ♀
         Benign neoplasm of fallopian tube
         Benign neoplasm of uterine ligament (broad) (round)
    D28.7 Benign neoplasm of other specified female genital organs ♀
    D28.9 Benign neoplasm of female genital organ, unspecified ♀

✓4th **D29** Benign neoplasm of male genital organs
    INCLUDES   benign neoplasm of skin of male genital organs
    D29.0 Benign neoplasm of penis ♂
    D29.1 Benign neoplasm of prostate ♂
         EXCLUDES 1   *enlarged prostate (N40.-)*
    ✓5th **D29.2** Benign neoplasm of testis
         Use additional code to identify any functional activity
         D29.20 Benign neoplasm of unspecified testis ♂
         D29.21 Benign neoplasm of right testis ♂
         D29.22 Benign neoplasm of left testis ♂
    ✓5th **D29.3** Benign neoplasm of epididymis
         D29.30 Benign neoplasm of unspecified epididymis ♂
         D29.31 Benign neoplasm of right epididymis ♂
         D29.32 Benign neoplasm of left epididymis ♂
    D29.4 Benign neoplasm of scrotum ♂
         Benign neoplasm of skin of scrotum
    D29.8 Benign neoplasm of other specified male genital organs ♂
         Benign neoplasm of seminal vesicle
         Benign neoplasm of spermatic cord
         Benign neoplasm of tunica vaginalis
    D29.9 Benign neoplasm of male genital organ, unspecified ♂

✓4th **D30** Benign neoplasm of urinary organs
    ✓5th **D30.0** Benign neoplasm of kidney
         EXCLUDES 1   *benign carcinoid tumor of the kidney (D3A.093)*
         benign neoplasm of renal calyces (D30.1-)
         benign neoplasm of renal pelvis (D30.1-)
         D30.00 Benign neoplasm of unspecified kidney
         D30.01 Benign neoplasm of right kidney
         D30.02 Benign neoplasm of left kidney
    ✓5th **D30.1** Benign neoplasm of renal pelvis
         D30.10 Benign neoplasm of unspecified renal pelvis
         D30.11 Benign neoplasm of right renal pelvis
         D30.12 Benign neoplasm of left renal pelvis
    ✓5th **D30.2** Benign neoplasm of ureter
         EXCLUDES 1   *benign neoplasm of ureteric orifice of bladder (D30.3)*
         D30.20 Benign neoplasm of unspecified ureter
         D30.21 Benign neoplasm of right ureter
         D30.22 Benign neoplasm of left ureter
    D30.3 Benign neoplasm of bladder
         Benign neoplasm of ureteric orifice of bladder
         Benign neoplasm of urethral orifice of bladder

✓ Additional Character Required   ✓x7th Placeholder   Unacceptable PDx   Questionable PDx   Manifestation   Unspecified Dx   H1-H14 HAC   HCC CMS-HCC Dx   HIV HIV Dx

Chapter 2. Neoplasms

D30.4 Benign neoplasm of urethra
> **EXCLUDES 1**   *benign neoplasm of urethral orifice of bladder (D30.3)*

D30.8 Benign neoplasm of other specified urinary organs
Benign neoplasm of paraurethral glands

D30.9 Benign neoplasm of urinary organ, unspecified
Benign neoplasm of urinary system NOS

✓4ᵗʰ **D31 Benign neoplasm of eye and adnexa**
> **EXCLUDES 1**   *benign neoplasm of connective tissue of eyelid (D21.0)*
> *benign neoplasm of optic nerve (D33.3)*
> *benign neoplasm of skin of eyelid (D22.1-, D23.1-)*

✓5ᵗʰ **D31.0 Benign neoplasm of conjunctiva**
> **D31.00 Benign neoplasm of unspecified conjunctiva**
> **D31.01 Benign neoplasm of right conjunctiva**
> **D31.02 Benign neoplasm of left conjunctiva**

✓5ᵗʰ **D31.1 Benign neoplasm of cornea**
> **D31.10 Benign neoplasm of unspecified cornea**
> **D31.11 Benign neoplasm of right cornea**
> **D31.12 Benign neoplasm of left cornea**

✓5ᵗʰ **D31.2 Benign neoplasm of retina**
> **EXCLUDES 1**   *dark area on retina (D49.81)*
> *hemangioma of retina (D49.81)*
> *neoplasm of unspecified behavior of retina and choroid (D49.81)*
> *retinal freckle (D49.81)*

> **D31.20 Benign neoplasm of unspecified retina**
> **D31.21 Benign neoplasm of right retina**
> **D31.22 Benign neoplasm of left retina**

✓5ᵗʰ **D31.3 Benign neoplasm of choroid**
> **D31.30 Benign neoplasm of unspecified choroid**
> **D31.31 Benign neoplasm of right choroid**
> **D31.32 Benign neoplasm of left choroid**

✓5ᵗʰ **D31.4 Benign neoplasm of ciliary body**
> **D31.40 Benign neoplasm of unspecified ciliary body**
> **D31.41 Benign neoplasm of right ciliary body**
> **D31.42 Benign neoplasm of left ciliary body**

✓5ᵗʰ **D31.5 Benign neoplasm of lacrimal gland and duct**
Benign neoplasm of lacrimal sac
Benign neoplasm of nasolacrimal duct
> **D31.50 Benign neoplasm of unspecified lacrimal gland and duct**
> **D31.51 Benign neoplasm of right lacrimal gland and duct**
> **D31.52 Benign neoplasm of left lacrimal gland and duct**

✓5ᵗʰ **D31.6 Benign neoplasm of unspecified site of orbit**
Benign neoplasm of connective tissue of orbit
Benign neoplasm of extraocular muscle
Benign neoplasm of peripheral nerves of orbit
Benign neoplasm of retrobulbar tissue
Benign neoplasm of retro-ocular tissue
> **EXCLUDES 1**   *benign neoplasm of orbital bone (D16.4)*

> **D31.60 Benign neoplasm of unspecified site of unspecified orbit**
> **D31.61 Benign neoplasm of unspecified site of right orbit**
> **D31.62 Benign neoplasm of unspecified site of left orbit**

✓5ᵗʰ **D31.9 Benign neoplasm of unspecified part of eye**
Benign neoplasm of eyeball
> **D31.90 Benign neoplasm of unspecified part of unspecified eye**
> **D31.91 Benign neoplasm of unspecified part of right eye**
> **D31.92 Benign neoplasm of unspecified part of left eye**

✓4ᵗʰ **D32 Benign neoplasm of meninges**
D32.0 Benign neoplasm of cerebral meninges   HCC
D32.1 Benign neoplasm of spinal meninges   HCC
D32.9 Benign neoplasm of meninges, unspecified   HCC
Meningioma NOS

✓4ᵗʰ **D33 Benign neoplasm of brain and other parts of central nervous system**
> **EXCLUDES 1**   *angioma (D18.0-)*
> *benign neoplasm of meninges (D32.-)*
> *benign neoplasm of peripheral nerves and autonomic nervous system (D36.1-)*
> *hemangioma (D18.0-)*
> *neurofibromatosis (Q85.0-)*
> *retro-ocular benign neoplasm (D31.6-)*

D33.0 Benign neoplasm of brain, supratentorial   HCC
Benign neoplasm of cerebral ventricle
Benign neoplasm of cerebrum
Benign neoplasm of frontal lobe
Benign neoplasm of occipital lobe
Benign neoplasm of parietal lobe
Benign neoplasm of temporal lobe
> **EXCLUDES 1**   *benign neoplasm of fourth ventricle (D33.1)*

D33.1 Benign neoplasm of brain, infratentorial   HCC
Benign neoplasm of brain stem
Benign neoplasm of cerebellum
Benign neoplasm of fourth ventricle

D33.2 Benign neoplasm of brain, unspecified   HCC
D33.3 Benign neoplasm of cranial nerves   HCC
Benign neoplasm of olfactory bulb
D33.4 Benign neoplasm of spinal cord   HCC
D33.7 Benign neoplasm of other specified parts of central nervous system   HCC
D33.9 Benign neoplasm of central nervous system, unspecified   HCC
Benign neoplasm of nervous system (central) NOS

D34 Benign neoplasm of thyroid gland
Use additional code to identify any functional activity

✓4ᵗʰ **D35 Benign neoplasm of other and unspecified endocrine glands**
Use additional code to identify any functional activity
> **EXCLUDES 1**   *benign neoplasm of endocrine pancreas (D13.7)*
> *benign neoplasm of ovary (D27.-)*
> *benign neoplasm of testis (D29.2.-)*
> *benign neoplasm of thymus (D15.0)*

✓5ᵗʰ **D35.0 Benign neoplasm of adrenal gland**
> **D35.00 Benign neoplasm of unspecified adrenal gland**
> **D35.01 Benign neoplasm of right adrenal gland**
> **D35.02 Benign neoplasm of left adrenal gland**

D35.1 Benign neoplasm of parathyroid gland
D35.2 Benign neoplasm of pituitary gland   HCC
   AHA: 2014,3Q,22
D35.3 Benign neoplasm of craniopharyngeal duct   HCC
D35.4 Benign neoplasm of pineal gland   HCC
D35.5 Benign neoplasm of carotid body
D35.6 Benign neoplasm of aortic body and other paraganglia
Benign tumor of glomus jugulare
D35.7 Benign neoplasm of other specified endocrine glands
D35.9 Benign neoplasm of endocrine gland, unspecified
Benign neoplasm of unspecified endocrine gland

✓4ᵗʰ **D36 Benign neoplasm of other and unspecified sites**
D36.0 Benign neoplasm of lymph nodes
> **EXCLUDES 1**   *lymphangioma (D18.1)*

✓5ᵗʰ **D36.1 Benign neoplasm of peripheral nerves and autonomic nervous system**
> **EXCLUDES 1**   *benign neoplasm of peripheral nerves of orbit (D31.6-)*
> *neurofibromatosis (Q85.0-)*

> **D36.10 Benign neoplasm of peripheral nerves and autonomic nervous system, unspecified**
> **D36.11 Benign neoplasm of peripheral nerves and autonomic nervous system of face, head, and neck**
> **D36.12 Benign neoplasm of peripheral nerves and autonomic nervous system, upper limb, including shoulder**
> **D36.13 Benign neoplasm of peripheral nerves and autonomic nervous system of lower limb, including hip**
> **D36.14 Benign neoplasm of peripheral nerves and autonomic nervous system of thorax**
> **D36.15 Benign neoplasm of peripheral nerves and autonomic nervous system of abdomen**

N Newborn: 0   P Pediatric: 0-17   M Maternity: 9-64   A Adult: 15-124   MCC Major Complication/Comorbidity   CC Complication/Comorbidity   SW Severe Wound Dx

500   ICD-10-CM 2021

    D36.16   **Benign neoplasm of peripheral nerves and autonomic nervous system of** pelvis

    D36.17   **Benign neoplasm of peripheral nerves and autonomic nervous system of** trunk, **unspecified**

D36.7   **Benign neoplasm of other specified sites**
    Benign neoplasm of back NOS
    Benign neoplasm of nose NOS

D36.9   **Benign neoplasm, unspecified site**

Benign neuroendocrine tumors (D3A)

√4ᵗʰ **D3A**   **Benign neuroendocrine tumors**
    Code also any associated multiple endocrine neoplasia [MEN] syndromes (E31.2-)
    Use additional code to identify any associated endocrine syndrome, such as:
    carcinoid syndrome (E34.0)
    EXCLUDES 2   *benign pancreatic islet cell tumors (D13.7)*

√5ᵗʰ **D3A.0**   **Benign** carcinoid tumors

    D3A.00   **Benign carcinoid tumor of unspecified site**
        Carcinoid tumor NOS

  √6ᵗʰ   **D3A.01**   **Benign carcinoid tumors of the** small intestine

    D3A.010   **Benign carcinoid tumor of the** duodenum
    D3A.011   **Benign carcinoid tumor of the** jejunum
    D3A.012   **Benign carcinoid tumor of the** ileum
    D3A.019   **Benign carcinoid tumor of the small intestine, unspecified portion**

  √6ᵗʰ   **D3A.02**   **Benign carcinoid tumors of the** appendix, large intestine, and rectum

    D3A.020   **Benign carcinoid tumor of the** appendix
    D3A.021   **Benign carcinoid tumor of the** cecum
    D3A.022   **Benign carcinoid tumor of the** ascending colon
    D3A.023   **Benign carcinoid tumor of the** transverse colon
    D3A.024   **Benign carcinoid tumor of the** descending colon
    D3A.025   **Benign carcinoid tumor of the** sigmoid colon
    D3A.026   **Benign carcinoid tumor of the** rectum
    D3A.029   **Benign carcinoid tumor of the large intestine, unspecified portion**
        Benign carcinoid tumor of the colon NOS

  √6ᵗʰ   **D3A.09**   **Benign carcinoid tumors of other sites**

    D3A.090   **Benign carcinoid tumor of the** bronchus and lung
    D3A.091   **Benign carcinoid tumor of the** thymus
    D3A.092   **Benign carcinoid tumor of the** stomach
    D3A.093   **Benign carcinoid tumor of the** kidney
    D3A.094   **Benign carcinoid tumor of the** foregut, **unspecified**
    D3A.095   **Benign carcinoid tumor of the** midgut, **unspecified**
    D3A.096   **Benign carcinoid tumor of the** hindgut, **unspecified**
    D3A.098   **Benign carcinoid tumors of other sites**

D3A.8   **Other benign neuroendocrine tumors**
    Neuroendocrine tumor NOS

Neoplasms of uncertain behavior, polycythemia vera and myelodysplastic syndromes (D37-D48)

NOTE   Categories D37-D44, and D48 classify by site neoplasms of uncertain behavior, i.e., histologic confirmation whether the neoplasm is malignant or benign cannot be made.

EXCLUDES 1   *neoplasms of unspecified behavior (D49.-)*

√4ᵗʰ **D37**   **Neoplasm of uncertain behavior of** oral cavity and digestive organs

    EXCLUDES 1   *stromal tumors of uncertain behavior of digestive system (D48.1)*

√5ᵗʰ **D37.0**   **Neoplasm of uncertain behavior of** lip, oral cavity and pharynx

    EXCLUDES 1   *neoplasm of uncertain behavior of aryepiglottic fold or interarytenoid fold, laryngeal aspect (D38.0)*
        neoplasm of uncertain behavior of epiglottis NOS (D38.0)
        neoplasm of uncertain behavior of skin of lip (D48.5)
        neoplasm of uncertain behavior of suprahyoid portion of epiglottis (D38.0)

    D37.01   **Neoplasm of uncertain behavior of** lip
        Neoplasm of uncertain behavior of vermilion border of lip

    D37.02   **Neoplasm of uncertain behavior of** tongue

  √6ᵗʰ   **D37.03**   **Neoplasm of uncertain behavior of the** major salivary glands

    D37.030   **Neoplasm of uncertain behavior of the** parotid **salivary glands**
    D37.031   **Neoplasm of uncertain behavior of the** sublingual **salivary glands**
    D37.032   **Neoplasm of uncertain behavior of the** submandibular **salivary glands**
    D37.039   **Neoplasm of uncertain behavior of the** major salivary glands, unspecified

    D37.04   **Neoplasm of uncertain behavior of the** minor salivary glands
        Neoplasm of uncertain behavior of submucosal salivary glands of lip
        Neoplasm of uncertain behavior of submucosal salivary glands of cheek
        Neoplasm of uncertain behavior of submucosal salivary glands of hard palate
        Neoplasm of uncertain behavior of submucosal salivary glands of soft palate

    D37.05   **Neoplasm of uncertain behavior of** pharynx
        Neoplasm of uncertain behavior of aryepiglottic fold of pharynx NOS
        Neoplasm of uncertain behavior of hypopharyngeal aspect of aryepiglottic fold of pharynx
        Neoplasm of uncertain behavior of marginal zone of aryepiglottic fold of pharynx

    D37.09   **Neoplasm of uncertain behavior of other specified sites of the oral cavity**

D37.1   **Neoplasm of uncertain behavior of** stomach

D37.2   **Neoplasm of uncertain behavior of** small intestine

D37.3   **Neoplasm of uncertain behavior of** appendix

D37.4   **Neoplasm of uncertain behavior of** colon

D37.5   **Neoplasm of uncertain behavior of** rectum
    Neoplasm of uncertain behavior of rectosigmoid junction

D37.6   **Neoplasm of uncertain behavior of** liver, gallbladder and bile ducts
    Neoplasm of uncertain behavior of ampulla of Vater

D37.8   **Neoplasm of uncertain behavior of other specified digestive organs**
    Neoplasm of uncertain behavior of anal canal
    Neoplasm of uncertain behavior of anal sphincter
    Neoplasm of uncertain behavior of anus NOS
    Neoplasm of uncertain behavior of esophagus
    Neoplasm of uncertain behavior of intestine NOS
    Neoplasm of uncertain behavior of pancreas
    EXCLUDES 1   *neoplasm of uncertain behavior of anal margin (D48.5)*
        neoplasm of uncertain behavior of anal skin (D48.5)
        neoplasm of uncertain behavior of perianal skin (D48.5)

D37.9   **Neoplasm of uncertain behavior of digestive organ, unspecified**

☑ Additional Character Required   √x7ᵗʰ Placeholder   Unacceptable PDx   Questionable PDx   Manifestation   Unspecified Dx   H1-H14 HAC   HCC CMS-HCC Dx   HIV HIV Dx

ICD-10-CM 2021   501

Chapter 2. Neoplasms

D38–D44.9

✓4ᵗʰ **D38 Neoplasm of uncertain behavior of middle ear and respiratory and intrathoracic organs**
     EXCLUDES 1   *neoplasm of uncertain behavior of heart (D48.7)*

   D38.0 Neoplasm of uncertain behavior of larynx
     Neoplasm of uncertain behavior of aryepiglottic fold or interarytenoid fold, laryngeal aspect
     Neoplasm of uncertain behavior of epiglottis (suprahyoid portion)
     EXCLUDES 1   *neoplasm of uncertain behavior of aryepiglottic fold or interarytenoid fold NOS (D37.05)*
         neoplasm of uncertain behavior of hypopharyngeal aspect of aryepiglottic fold (D37.05)
         neoplasm of uncertain behavior of marginal zone of aryepiglottic fold (D37.05)

   D38.1 Neoplasm of uncertain behavior of trachea, bronchus and lung

   D38.2 Neoplasm of uncertain behavior of pleura

   D38.3 Neoplasm of uncertain behavior of mediastinum

   D38.4 Neoplasm of uncertain behavior of thymus

   D38.5 Neoplasm of uncertain behavior of other respiratory organs
     Neoplasm of uncertain behavior of accessory sinuses
     Neoplasm of uncertain behavior of cartilage of nose
     Neoplasm of uncertain behavior of middle ear
     Neoplasm of uncertain behavior of nasal cavities
     EXCLUDES 1   *neoplasm of uncertain behavior of ear (external) (skin) (D48.5)*
         neoplasm of uncertain behavior of nose NOS (D48.7)
         neoplasm of uncertain behavior of skin of nose (D48.5)

   D38.6 Neoplasm of uncertain behavior of respiratory organ, unspecified

✓4ᵗʰ **D39 Neoplasm of uncertain behavior of female genital organs**

   D39.0 Neoplasm of uncertain behavior of uterus ♀

✓5ᵗʰ   **D39.1 Neoplasm of uncertain behavior of ovary**
     Use additional code to identify any functional activity

     D39.10 Neoplasm of uncertain behavior of unspecified ovary ♀

     D39.11 Neoplasm of uncertain behavior of right ovary ♀

     D39.12 Neoplasm of uncertain behavior of left ovary ♀

   D39.2 Neoplasm of uncertain behavior of placenta Ⓜ ♀
     Chorioadenoma destruens
     Invasive hydatidiform mole
     Malignant hydatidiform mole
     EXCLUDES 1   *hydatidiform mole NOS (O01.9)*

   D39.8 Neoplasm of uncertain behavior of other specified female genital organs ♀
     Neoplasm of uncertain behavior of skin of female genital organs

   D39.9 Neoplasm of uncertain behavior of female genital organ, unspecified ♀

✓4ᵗʰ **D40 Neoplasm of uncertain behavior of male genital organs**

   D40.0 Neoplasm of uncertain behavior of prostate ♂

✓5ᵗʰ   **D40.1 Neoplasm of uncertain behavior of testis**

     D40.10 Neoplasm of uncertain behavior of unspecified testis ♂

     D40.11 Neoplasm of uncertain behavior of right testis ♂

     D40.12 Neoplasm of uncertain behavior of left testis ♂

   D40.8 Neoplasm of uncertain behavior of other specified male genital organs ♂
     Neoplasm of uncertain behavior of skin of male genital organs

   D40.9 Neoplasm of uncertain behavior of male genital organ, unspecified ♂

✓4ᵗʰ **D41 Neoplasm of uncertain behavior of urinary organs**

✓5ᵗʰ   **D41.0 Neoplasm of uncertain behavior of kidney**
     EXCLUDES 1   *neoplasm of uncertain behavior of renal pelvis (D41.1-)*

     D41.00 Neoplasm of uncertain behavior of unspecified kidney

     D41.01 Neoplasm of uncertain behavior of right kidney

     D41.02 Neoplasm of uncertain behavior of left kidney

✓5ᵗʰ   **D41.1 Neoplasm of uncertain behavior of renal pelvis**

     D41.10 Neoplasm of uncertain behavior of unspecified renal pelvis

     D41.11 Neoplasm of uncertain behavior of right renal pelvis

     D41.12 Neoplasm of uncertain behavior of left renal pelvis

✓5ᵗʰ   **D41.2 Neoplasm of uncertain behavior of ureter**

     D41.20 Neoplasm of uncertain behavior of unspecified ureter

     D41.21 Neoplasm of uncertain behavior of right ureter

     D41.22 Neoplasm of uncertain behavior of left ureter

   D41.3 Neoplasm of uncertain behavior of urethra

   D41.4 Neoplasm of uncertain behavior of bladder

   D41.8 Neoplasm of uncertain behavior of other specified urinary organs

   D41.9 Neoplasm of uncertain behavior of unspecified urinary organ

✓4ᵗʰ **D42 Neoplasm of uncertain behavior of meninges**

   D42.0 Neoplasm of uncertain behavior of cerebral meninges ᴴᶜᶜ

   D42.1 Neoplasm of uncertain behavior of spinal meninges ᴴᶜᶜ

   D42.9 Neoplasm of uncertain behavior of meninges, unspecified ᴴᶜᶜ

✓4ᵗʰ **D43 Neoplasm of uncertain behavior of brain and central nervous system**
     EXCLUDES 1   *neoplasm of uncertain behavior of peripheral nerves and autonomic nervous system (D48.2)*

   D43.0 Neoplasm of uncertain behavior of brain, supratentorial ᴴᶜᶜ
     Neoplasm of uncertain behavior of cerebral ventricle
     Neoplasm of uncertain behavior of cerebrum
     Neoplasm of uncertain behavior of frontal lobe
     Neoplasm of uncertain behavior of occipital lobe
     Neoplasm of uncertain behavior of parietal lobe
     Neoplasm of uncertain behavior of temporal lobe
     EXCLUDES 1   *neoplasm of uncertain behavior of fourth ventricle (D43.1)*

   D43.1 Neoplasm of uncertain behavior of brain, infratentorial ᴴᶜᶜ
     Neoplasm of uncertain behavior of brain stem
     Neoplasm of uncertain behavior of cerebellum
     Neoplasm of uncertain behavior of fourth ventricle

   D43.2 Neoplasm of uncertain behavior of brain, unspecified ᴴᶜᶜ

   D43.3 Neoplasm of uncertain behavior of cranial nerves ᴴᶜᶜ

   D43.4 Neoplasm of uncertain behavior of spinal cord ᴴᶜᶜ

   D43.8 Neoplasm of uncertain behavior of other specified parts of central nervous system ᴴᶜᶜ

   D43.9 Neoplasm of uncertain behavior of central nervous system, unspecified ᴴᶜᶜ
     Neoplasm of uncertain behavior of nervous system (central) NOS

✓4ᵗʰ **D44 Neoplasm of uncertain behavior of endocrine glands**
     EXCLUDES 1   *multiple endocrine adenomatosis (E31.2-)*
         multiple endocrine neoplasia (E31.2-)
         neoplasm of uncertain behavior of endocrine pancreas (D37.8)
         neoplasm of uncertain behavior of ovary (D39.1-)
         neoplasm of uncertain behavior of testis (D40.1-)
         neoplasm of uncertain behavior of thymus (D38.4)

   D44.0 Neoplasm of uncertain behavior of thyroid gland

✓5ᵗʰ   **D44.1 Neoplasm of uncertain behavior of adrenal gland**
     Use additional code to identify any functional activity

     D44.10 Neoplasm of uncertain behavior of unspecified adrenal gland

     D44.11 Neoplasm of uncertain behavior of right adrenal gland

     D44.12 Neoplasm of uncertain behavior of left adrenal gland

   D44.2 Neoplasm of uncertain behavior of parathyroid gland

   D44.3 Neoplasm of uncertain behavior of pituitary gland ᴴᶜᶜ
     Use additional code to identify any functional activity

   D44.4 Neoplasm of uncertain behavior of craniopharyngeal duct ᴴᶜᶜ

   D44.5 Neoplasm of uncertain behavior of pineal gland ᴴᶜᶜ

   D44.6 Neoplasm of uncertain behavior of carotid body ᴴᶜᶜ

   D44.7 Neoplasm of uncertain behavior of aortic body and other paraganglia ᴴᶜᶜ
     AHA: 2016,4Q,26

   D44.9 Neoplasm of uncertain behavior of unspecified endocrine gland

Ⓝ Newborn: 0   Ⓟ Pediatric: 0-17   Ⓜ Maternity: 9-64   Ⓐ Adult: 15-124   **ᴹᶜᶜ** Major Complication/Comorbidity   **ᶜᶜ** Complication/Comorbidity   **ˢᵂ** Severe Wound Dx

502   ICD-10-CM 2021

D45 Polycythemia vera   HCC
> EXCLUDES 1   familial polycythemia (D75.0)
>   secondary polycythemia (D75.1)

DEF: Abnormal proliferation of all bone marrow elements, increased red cell mass, and total blood volume. The etiology is unknown, but it is frequently associated with splenomegaly, leukocytosis, and thrombocythemia.

✓4ᵗʰ D46 Myelodysplastic syndromes

Use additional code for adverse effect, if applicable, to identify drug (T36-T50 with fifth or sixth character 5)
> EXCLUDES 2   drug-induced aplastic anemia (D61.1)

D46.0 Refractory anemia without ring sideroblasts, so stated   HCC
Refractory anemia without sideroblasts, without excess of blasts

D46.1 Refractory anemia with ring sideroblasts   HCC
RARS

✓5ᵗʰ D46.2 Refractory anemia with excess of blasts [RAEB]

D46.20 Refractory anemia with excess of blasts, unspecified   HCC
RAEB NOS

D46.21 Refractory anemia with excess of blasts 1   HCC
RAEB 1

D46.22 Refractory anemia with excess of blasts 2   CC HCC
RAEB 2

D46.A Refractory cytopenia with multilineage dysplasia   HCC

D46.B Refractory cytopenia with multilineage dysplasia and ring sideroblasts   HCC
RCMD RS

D46.C Myelodysplastic syndrome with isolated del(5q) chromosomal abnormality   CC HCC
Myelodysplastic syndrome with 5q deletion
5q minus syndrome NOS

D46.4 Refractory anemia, unspecified   HCC

D46.Z Other myelodysplastic syndromes   HCC
> EXCLUDES 1   chronic myelomonocytic leukemia (C93.1-)

D46.9 Myelodysplastic syndrome, unspecified   HCC
Myelodysplasia NOS

✓4ᵗʰ D47 Other neoplasms of uncertain behavior of lymphoid, hematopoietic and related tissue

✓5ᵗʰ D47.0 Mast cell neoplasms of uncertain behavior
> EXCLUDES 1   congenital cutaneous mastocytosis (Q82.2)
>   histiocytic neoplasms of uncertain behavior (D47.Z9)
>   malignant mast cell neoplasm (C96.2-)

AHA: 2017,4Q,5

D47.01 Cutaneous mastocytosis   CC
Diffuse cutaneous mastocytosis
Maculopapular cutaneous mastocytosis
Solitary mastocytoma
Telangiectasia macularis eruptiva perstans
Urticaria pigmentosa
> EXCLUDES 1   congenital (diffuse) (maculopapular) cutaneous mastocytosis (Q82.2)
>   congenital urticaria pigmentosa (Q82.2)
>   extracutaneous mastocytoma (D47.09)

D47.02 Systemic mastocytosis   CC
Indolent systemic mastocytosis
Isolated bone marrow mastocytosis
Smoldering systemic mastocytosis
Systemic mastocytosis, with an associated hematological non-mast cell lineage disease (SM-AHNMD)
Code also, if applicable, any associated hematological non-mast cell lineage disease, such as:
    acute myeloid leukemia (C92.6-, C92.A-)
    chronic myelomonocytic leukemia (C93.1-)
    essential thrombocytosis (D47.3)
    hypereosinophilic syndrome (D72.1)
    myelodysplastic syndrome (D46.9)
    myeloproliferative syndrome (D47.1)
    non-Hodgkin lymphoma (C82-C85)
    plasma cell myeloma (C90.0-)
    polycythemia vera (D45)
> EXCLUDES 1   aggressive systemic mastocytosis (C96.21)
>   mast cell leukemia (C94.3-)

D47.09 Other mast cell neoplasms of uncertain behavior   CC
Extracutaneous mastocytoma
Mast cell tumor NOS
Mastocytoma NOS
Mastocytosis NOS

D47.1 Chronic myeloproliferative disease   CC HCC
Chronic neutrophilic leukemia
Myeloproliferative disease, unspecified
> EXCLUDES 1   atypical chronic myeloid leukemia BCR/ABL-negative (C92.2-)
>   chronic myeloid leukemia BCR/ABL-positive (C92.1-)
>   myelofibrosis NOS (D75.81)
>   myelophthisic anemia (D61.82)
>   myelophthisis (D61.82)
>   secondary myelofibrosis NOS (D75.81)

D47.2 Monoclonal gammopathy
Monoclonal gammopathy of undetermined significance [MGUS]

D47.3 Essential (hemorrhagic) thrombocythemia   HCC
Essential thrombocytosis
Idiopathic hemorrhagic thrombocythemia
DEF: Chronic myeloproliferative neoplasm involving production of excess blood platelets that may result in abnormal clotting or hemorrhaging.

D47.4 Osteomyelofibrosis   HCC
Chronic idiopathic myelofibrosis
Myelofibrosis (idiopathic) (with myeloid metaplasia)
Myelosclerosis (megakaryocytic) with myeloid metaplasia
Secondary myelofibrosis in myeloproliferative disease
> EXCLUDES 1   acute myelofibrosis (C94.4-)

✓5ᵗʰ D47.Z Other specified neoplasms of uncertain behavior of lymphoid, hematopoietic and related tissue
AHA: 2016,4Q,8

D47.Z1 Post-transplant lymphoproliferative disorder (PTLD)   CC HCC
Code first complications of transplanted organs and tissue (T86.-)
DEF: Excessive proliferation of B-cell lymphocytes following Epstein-Barr virus infection in organ transplant patients. It may progress to non-Hodgkin lymphoma.

D47.Z2 Castleman disease   CC HCC
Code also if applicable human herpesvirus 8 infection (B10.89)
> EXCLUDES 2   Kaposi's sarcoma ▶(C46.-)◄
DEF: Rare disease of the lymph nodes and lymphoid tissues that closely mimics lymphoma.

D47.Z9 Other specified neoplasms of uncertain behavior of lymphoid, hematopoietic and related tissue   CC HCC
Histiocytic tumors of uncertain behavior

D47.9 Neoplasm of uncertain behavior of lymphoid, hematopoietic and related tissue, unspecified   CC HCC
Lymphoproliferative disease NOS

✓4ᵗʰ D48 Neoplasm of uncertain behavior of other and unspecified sites
> EXCLUDES 1   neurofibromatosis (nonmalignant) (Q85.0-)

D48.0 Neoplasm of uncertain behavior of bone and articular cartilage
> EXCLUDES 1   neoplasm of uncertain behavior of cartilage of ear (D48.1)
>   neoplasm of uncertain behavior of cartilage of larynx (D38.0)
>   neoplasm of uncertain behavior of cartilage of nose (D38.5)
>   neoplasm of uncertain behavior of connective tissue of eyelid (D48.1)
>   neoplasm of uncertain behavior of synovia (D48.1)

✔ Additional Character Required   ✓x7ᵗʰ Placeholder   Unacceptable PDx   Questionable PDx   Manifestation   Unspecified Dx   H1-H14 HAC   HCC CMS-HCC Dx   HIV HIV Dx

ICD-10-CM 2021   503

D45–D48.0

D48.1 Neoplasm of uncertain behavior of connective and other soft tissue

Neoplasm of uncertain behavior of connective tissue of ear

Neoplasm of uncertain behavior of connective tissue of eyelid

Stromal tumors of uncertain behavior of digestive system

> **EXCLUDES 1** *neoplasm of uncertain behavior of articular cartilage (D48.0)*
>
> *neoplasm of uncertain behavior of cartilage of larynx (D38.0)*
>
> *neoplasm of uncertain behavior of cartilage of nose (D38.5)*
>
> *neoplasm of uncertain behavior of connective tissue of breast (D48.6-)*

D48.2 Neoplasm of uncertain behavior of peripheral nerves and autonomic nervous system

> **EXCLUDES 1** *neoplasm of uncertain behavior of peripheral nerves of orbit (D48.7)*

D48.3 Neoplasm of uncertain behavior of retroperitoneum

D48.4 Neoplasm of uncertain behavior of peritoneum

D48.5 Neoplasm of uncertain behavior of skin

Neoplasm of uncertain behavior of anal margin

Neoplasm of uncertain behavior of anal skin

Neoplasm of uncertain behavior of perianal skin

Neoplasm of uncertain behavior of skin of breast

> **EXCLUDES 1** *neoplasm of uncertain behavior of anus NOS (D37.8)*
>
> *neoplasm of uncertain behavior of skin of genital organs (D39.8, D40.8)*
>
> *neoplasm of uncertain behavior of vermilion border of lip (D37.0)*

✓5ᵗʰ D48.6 Neoplasm of uncertain behavior of breast

Neoplasm of uncertain behavior of connective tissue of breast

Cystosarcoma phyllodes

> **EXCLUDES 1** *neoplasm of uncertain behavior of skin of breast (D48.5)*

D48.60 Neoplasm of uncertain behavior of unspecified breast

D48.61 Neoplasm of uncertain behavior of right **breast**

D48.62 Neoplasm of uncertain behavior of left **breast**

D48.7 Neoplasm of uncertain behavior of other specified sites

Neoplasm of uncertain behavior of eye

Neoplasm of uncertain behavior of heart

Neoplasm of uncertain behavior of peripheral nerves of orbit

> **EXCLUDES 1** *neoplasm of uncertain behavior of connective tissue (D48.1)*
>
> *neoplasm of uncertain behavior of skin of eyelid (D48.5)*

D48.9 Neoplasm of uncertain behavior, unspecified

Neoplasms of unspecified behavior (D49)

✓4ᵗʰ D49 Neoplasms of unspecified behavior

> **NOTE** Category D49 classifies by site neoplasms of unspecified morphology and behavior. The term "mass", unless otherwise stated, is not to be regarded as a neoplastic growth.
>
> **INCLUDES** "growth" NOS
> neoplasm NOS
> new growth NOS
> tumor NOS
>
> **EXCLUDES 1** *neoplasms of uncertain behavior (D37-D44, D48)*

D49.0 Neoplasm of unspecified behavior of digestive system

> **EXCLUDES 1** *neoplasm of unspecified behavior of margin of anus (D49.2)*
>
> *neoplasm of unspecified behavior of perianal skin (D49.2)*
>
> *neoplasm of unspecified behavior of skin of anus (D49.2)*

D49.1 Neoplasm of unspecified behavior of respiratory system

D49.2 Neoplasm of unspecified behavior of bone, soft tissue, and skin

> **EXCLUDES 1** *neoplasm of unspecified behavior of anal canal (D49.0)*
>
> *neoplasm of unspecified behavior of anus NOS (D49.0)*
>
> *neoplasm of unspecified behavior of bone marrow (D49.89)*
>
> *neoplasm of unspecified behavior of cartilage of larynx (D49.1)*
>
> *neoplasm of unspecified behavior of cartilage of nose (D49.1)*
>
> *neoplasm of unspecified behavior of connective tissue of breast (D49.3)*
>
> *neoplasm of unspecified behavior of skin of genital organs (D49.59)*
>
> *neoplasm of unspecified behavior of vermilion border of lip (D49.0)*

D49.3 Neoplasm of unspecified behavior of breast

> **EXCLUDES 1** *neoplasm of unspecified behavior of skin of breast (D49.2)*

D49.4 Neoplasm of unspecified behavior of bladder

✓5ᵗʰ D49.5 Neoplasm of unspecified behavior of other genitourinary organs

AHA: 2016,4Q,9

✓6ᵗʰ D49.51 Neoplasm of unspecified behavior of kidney

D49.511 Neoplasm of unspecified behavior of right **kidney**

D49.512 Neoplasm of unspecified behavior of left **kidney**

D49.519 Neoplasm of unspecified behavior of unspecified kidney

D49.59 Neoplasm of unspecified behavior of other genitourinary organ

D49.6 Neoplasm of unspecified behavior of brain **HCC**

> **EXCLUDES 1** *neoplasm of unspecified behavior of cerebral meninges (D49.7)*
>
> *neoplasm of unspecified behavior of cranial nerves (D49.7)*

D49.7 Neoplasm of unspecified behavior of endocrine glands and other parts of nervous system

> **EXCLUDES 1** *neoplasm of unspecified behavior of peripheral, sympathetic, and parasympathetic nerves and ganglia (D49.2)*

✓5ᵗʰ D49.8 Neoplasm of unspecified behavior of other specified sites

> **EXCLUDES 1** *neoplasm of unspecified behavior of eyelid (skin) (D49.2)*
>
> *neoplasm of unspecified behavior of eyelid cartilage (D49.2)*
>
> *neoplasm of unspecified behavior of great vessels (D49.2)*
>
> *neoplasm of unspecified behavior of optic nerve (D49.7)*

D49.81 Neoplasm of unspecified behavior of retina and choroid

Dark area on retina

Retinal freckle

D49.89 Neoplasm of unspecified behavior of other specified sites

D49.9 Neoplasm of unspecified behavior of unspecified site

Ⓝ Newborn: 0 **Ⓟ** Pediatric: 0-17 **Ⓜ** Maternity: 9-64 **Ⓐ** Adult: 15-124 **MCC** Major Complication/Comorbidity **CC** Complication/Comorbidity **SW** Severe Wound Dx

504 ICD-10-CM 2021

Chapter 3. Diseases of the Blood and Blood-forming Organs and Certain Disorders Involving the Immune Mechanism (D5Ø–D89)

Chapter-specific Guidelines with Coding Examples
Reserved for future guideline expansion

Chapter 3. Diseases of the Blood and Blood-forming Organs and Certain Disorders Involving the Immune Mechanism (D50-D89)

EXCLUDES 2   autoimmune disease (systemic) NOS (M35.9)
certain conditions originating in the perinatal period (P00-P96)
complications of pregnancy, childbirth and the puerperium (O00-O9A)
congenital malformations, deformations and chromosomal abnormalities (Q00-Q99)
endocrine, nutritional and metabolic diseases (E00-E88)
human immunodeficiency virus [HIV] disease (B20)
injury, poisoning and certain other consequences of external causes (S00-T88)
neoplasms (C00-D49)
symptoms, signs and abnormal clinical and laboratory findings, not elsewhere classified (R00-R94)

This chapter contains the following blocks:

D50-D53   Nutritional anemias
D55-D59   Hemolytic anemias
D60-D64   Aplastic and other anemias and other bone marrow failure syndromes
D65-D69   Coagulation defects, purpura and other hemorrhagic conditions
D70-D77   Other disorders of blood and blood-forming organs
D78   Intraoperative and postprocedural complications of the spleen
D80-D89   Certain disorders involving the immune mechanism

Nutritional anemias (D50-D53)

DEF: Nutritional anemia: The result of inadequate intake or absorption of a vitamin or mineral that impacts the production of red blood cells or causes them to develop abnormally affecting the size and shape.
TIP: Documentation must identify a link between anemia and the nutritional deficiency; low levels of a particular nutrient may occur concurrently with anemia but not cause the anemia.

✓4th **D50**   **Iron deficiency anemia**

    INCLUDES   asiderotic anemia
               hypochromic anemia

    D50.0   **Iron deficiency anemia secondary to blood loss (chronic)**
       Posthemorrhagic anemia (chronic)
       EXCLUDES 1   acute posthemorrhagic anemia (D62)
                  congenital anemia from fetal blood loss (P61.3)
       AHA: 2019,3Q,17

    D50.1   **Sideropenic dysphagia**
       Kelly-Paterson syndrome
       Plummer-Vinson syndrome

    D50.8   **Other iron deficiency anemias**
       Iron deficiency anemia due to inadequate dietary iron intake

    D50.9   **Iron deficiency anemia, unspecified**

✓4th **D51**   **Vitamin B12 deficiency anemia**

    EXCLUDES 1   vitamin B12 deficiency (E53.8)

    D51.0   **Vitamin B12 deficiency anemia due to intrinsic factor deficiency**
       Addison anemia
       Biermer anemia
       Pernicious (congenital) anemia
       Congenital intrinsic factor deficiency
       DEF: Chronic progressive anemia due to vitamin B12 malabsorption, caused by lack of secretion of intrinsic factor, which is produced by the gastric mucosa of the stomach.

    D51.1   **Vitamin B12 deficiency anemia due to selective vitamin B12 malabsorption with proteinuria**
       Imerslund (Gräsbeck) syndrome
       Megaloblastic hereditary anemia

    D51.2   **Transcobalamin II deficiency**

    D51.3   **Other dietary vitamin B12 deficiency anemia**
       Vegan anemia

    D51.8   **Other vitamin B12 deficiency anemias**

    D51.9   **Vitamin B12 deficiency anemia, unspecified**

✓4th **D52**   **Folate deficiency anemia**

    EXCLUDES 1   folate deficiency without anemia (E53.8)
    DEF: Deficiency in a B complex vitamin needed for the production of healthy red blood cells. Lack of folate, or folic acid, and other absorption conditions can cause anemia resulting in large, misshapen red blood cells called megaloblasts.

    D52.0   **Dietary folate deficiency anemia**
       Nutritional megaloblastic anemia
       DEF: Result of a poor diet with inadequate intake of folate, which is needed to produce healthy red blood cells.

    D52.1   **Drug-induced folate deficiency anemia**
       Use additional code for adverse effect, if applicable, to identify drug (T36-T50 with fifth or sixth character 5)

    D52.8   **Other folate deficiency anemias**

    D52.9   **Folate deficiency anemia, unspecified**
       Folic acid deficiency anemia NOS

✓4th **D53**   **Other nutritional anemias**

    INCLUDES   megaloblastic anemia unresponsive to vitamin B12 or folate therapy

    D53.0   **Protein deficiency anemia**
       Amino-acid deficiency anemia
       Orotaciduric anemia
       EXCLUDES 1   Lesch-Nyhan syndrome (E79.1)

    D53.1   **Other megaloblastic anemias, not elsewhere classified**
       Megaloblastic anemia NOS
       EXCLUDES 1   Di Guglielmo's disease (C94.0)

    D53.2   **Scorbutic anemia**
       EXCLUDES 1   scurvy (E54)

    D53.8   **Other specified nutritional anemias**
       Anemia associated with deficiency of copper
       Anemia associated with deficiency of molybdenum
       Anemia associated with deficiency of zinc
       EXCLUDES 1   nutritional deficiencies without anemia, such as:
                 copper deficiency NOS (E61.0)
                 molybdenum deficiency NOS (E61.5)
                 zinc deficiency NOS (E60)

    D53.9   **Nutritional anemia, unspecified**
       Simple chronic anemia
       EXCLUDES 1   anemia NOS (D64.9)
       AHA: 2018,4Q,88

Hemolytic anemias (D55-D59)

✓4th **D55**   **Anemia due to enzyme disorders**

    EXCLUDES 1   drug-induced enzyme deficiency anemia (D59.2)

    D55.0   **Anemia due to glucose-6-phosphate dehydrogenase [G6PD] deficiency**   HCC
       Favism
       G6PD deficiency anemia
       EXCLUDES 1   glucose-6-phosphate dehydrogenase (G6PD) deficiency without anemia (D75.A)

    D55.1   **Anemia due to other disorders of glutathione metabolism**   HCC
       Anemia (due to) enzyme deficiencies, except G6PD, related to the hexose monophosphate [HMP] shunt pathway
       Anemia (due to) hemolytic nonspherocytic (hereditary), type I

    D55.2   **Anemia due to disorders of glycolytic enzymes**   HCC
       Hemolytic nonspherocytic (hereditary) anemia, type II
       Hexokinase deficiency anemia
       Pyruvate kinase [PK] deficiency anemia
       Triose-phosphate isomerase deficiency anemia
       EXCLUDES 1   disorders of glycolysis not associated with anemia ▶(E74.81-)◄

    D55.3   **Anemia due to disorders of nucleotide metabolism**   HCC

    D55.8   **Other anemias due to enzyme disorders**   HCC

    D55.9   **Anemia due to enzyme disorder, unspecified**   HCC

N Newborn: 0   P Pediatric: 0-17   M Maternity: 9-64   A Adult: 15-124   MCC Major Complication/Comorbidity   CC Complication/Comorbidity   SW Severe Wound Dx

506   ICD-10-CM 2021

✔4ᵗʰ **D56 Thalassemia**

EXCLUDES 1   sickle-cell thalassemia (D57.4-)

DEF: Group of inherited disorders of hemoglobin metabolism causing mild to severe anemia. It is usually found in people of Mediterranean, African, Chinese, or Asian descent.

Thalassemia

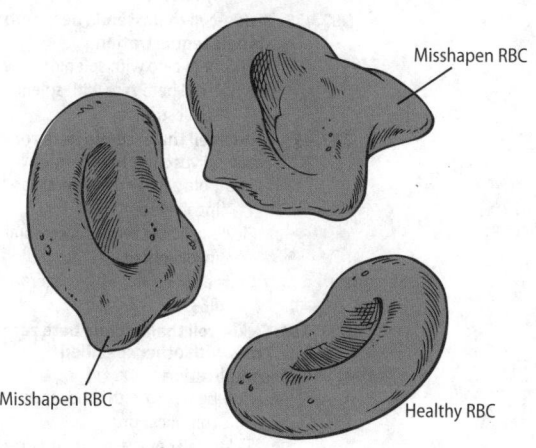

Misshapen RBC

Misshapen RBC

Healthy RBC

D56.0 Alpha thalassemia   HCC
Alpha thalassemia major
Hemoglobin H Constant Spring
Hemoglobin H disease
Hydrops fetalis due to alpha thalassemia
Severe alpha thalassemia
Triple gene defect alpha thalassemia
Use additional code, if applicable, for hydrops fetalis due to alpha thalassemia (P56.99)

EXCLUDES 1   alpha thalassemia trait or minor (D56.3)
asymptomatic alpha thalassemia (D56.3)
hydrops fetalis due to isoimmunization (P56.0)
hydrops fetalis not due to immune hemolysis (P83.2)

DEF: HBA1 and HBA2 genetic variant of chromosome 16 prevalent among those of African and Southeast Asian descent. Alpha thalassemia is associated with a wide spectrum of anemic presentation and includes hemoglobin H disease subtypes.

D56.1 Beta thalassemia   HCC
Beta thalassemia major
Cooley's anemia
Homozygous beta thalassemia
Severe beta thalassemia
Thalassemia intermedia
Thalassemia major

EXCLUDES 1   beta thalassemia minor (D56.3)
beta thalassemia trait (D56.3)
delta-beta thalassemia (D56.2)
hemoglobin E-beta thalassemia (D56.5)
sickle-cell beta thalassemia (D57.4-)

D56.2 Delta-beta thalassemia   HCC
Homozygous delta-beta thalassemia

EXCLUDES 1   delta-beta thalassemia minor (D56.3)
delta-beta thalassemia trait (D56.3)

D56.3 Thalassemia minor
Alpha thalassemia minor
Alpha thalassemia silent carrier
Alpha thalassemia trait
Beta thalassemia minor
Beta thalassemia trait
Delta-beta thalassemia minor
Delta-beta thalassemia trait
Thalassemia trait NOS

EXCLUDES 1   alpha thalassemia (D56.0)
beta thalassemia (D56.1)
delta-beta thalassemia (D56.2)
hemoglobin E-beta thalassemia (D56.5)
sickle-cell trait (D57.3)

DEF: Solitary abnormal gene that identifies a carrier of the disease, yet with an absence of symptoms or a clinically mild anemic presentation.

D56.4 Hereditary persistence of fetal hemoglobin [HPFH]   HCC

D56.5 Hemoglobin E-beta thalassemia   HCC

EXCLUDES 1   beta thalassemia (D56.1)
beta thalassemia minor (D56.3)
beta thalassemia trait (D56.3)
delta-beta thalassemia (D56.2)
delta-beta thalassemia trait (D56.3)
hemoglobin E disease (D58.2)
other hemoglobinopathies (D58.2)
sickle-cell beta thalassemia (D57.4-)

D56.8 Other thalassemias   HCC
Dominant thalassemia
Hemoglobin C thalassemia
Mixed thalassemia
Thalassemia with other hemoglobinopathy

EXCLUDES 1   hemoglobin C disease (D58.2)
hemoglobin E disease (D58.2)
other hemoglobinopathies (D58.2)
sickle-cell anemia (D57.-)
sickle-cell thalassemia (D57.4)

D56.9 Thalassemia, unspecified
Mediterranean anemia (with other hemoglobinopathy)

✔4ᵗʰ **D57 Sickle-cell disorders**
Use additional code for any associated fever (R50.81)

EXCLUDES 1   other hemoglobinopathies (D58.-)

DEF: Severe, chronic inherited diseases caused by a genetic variation in hemoglobin protein of the red blood cell. The gene mutation causes the red blood cell to become hard, sticky, and crescent or sickle shaped making it harder for red blood cells to travel through the bloodstream disrupting blood flow and decreasing oxygen transport to tissues.

Sickle cell

Sickle cells

Normal RBCs

✔5ᵗʰ **D57.0 Hb-SS disease with crisis**
▶Sickle-cell disease with crisis◀
Hb-SS disease with vasoocclusive pain

D57.00 Hb-SS disease with crisis, unspecified   MCC HCC
▶Hb-SS disease with (painful) crisis NOS◀
▶Hb-SS disease with vasoocclusive pain NOS◀

D57.01 Hb-SS disease with acute chest syndrome   MCC HCC

D57.02 Hb-SS disease with splenic sequestration   MCC HCC

✔ Additional Character Required   ✔x7ᵗʰ Placeholder   Unacceptable PDx   Questionable PDx   Manifestation   Unspecified Dx   H1 - H14 HAC   HCC CMS-HCC Dx   HIV HIV Dx

ICD-10-CM 2021   507

Chapter 3. Diseases of the Blood and Blood-forming Organs

D57.03 Hb-SS disease with cerebral vascular involvement `MCC`
Code also, if applicable, cerebral infarction (I63.-)

D57.09 Hb-SS disease with crisis with other specified complication `MCC`
Use additional code to identify complications, such as:
cholelithiasis (K80.-)
priapism (N48.32)

D57.1 Sickle-cell disease without crisis `HCC`
Hb-SS disease without crisis
Sickle-cell anemia NOS
Sickle-cell disease NOS
Sickle-cell disorder NOS

√5ᵗʰ **D57.2** Sickle-cell/Hb-C disease
Hb-SC disease
Hb-S/Hb-C disease

D57.20 Sickle-cell/Hb-C disease without crisis `HCC`

√6ᵗʰ **D57.21** Sickle-cell/Hb-C disease with crisis

D57.211 Sickle-cell/Hb-C disease with acute chest syndrome `MCC` `HCC`

D57.212 Sickle-cell/Hb-C disease with splenic sequestration `MCC` `HCC`

D57.213 Sickle-cell/Hb-C disease with cerebral vascular involvement `MCC`
Code also, if applicable, cerebral infarction (I63.-)

D57.218 Sickle-cell/Hb-C disease with crisis with other specified complication `MCC`
Use additional code to identify complications, such as:
cholelithiasis (K80.-)
priapism (N48.32)

D57.219 Sickle-cell/Hb-C disease with crisis, unspecified `MCC` `HCC`
Sickle-cell/Hb-C disease with crisis NOS
►Sickle-cell/Hb-C disease with vasoocclusive pain NOS◄

D57.3 Sickle-cell trait `HCC`
Hb-S trait
Heterozygous hemoglobin S
DEF: Heterozygous genetic makeup characterized by one gene for normal hemoglobin and one for sickle-cell hemoglobin. The clinical disease is rarely present.

√5ᵗʰ **D57.4** Sickle-cell thalassemia
Sickle-cell beta thalassemia
Thalassemia Hb-S disease

D57.40 Sickle-cell thalassemia without crisis `HCC`
Microdrepanocytosis
Sickle-cell thalassemia NOS

▲ √6ᵗʰ **D57.41** Sickle-cell thalassemia, unspecified, with crisis
►Sickle-cell thalassemia with (painful) crisis NOS◄
►Sickle-cell thalassemia with vasoocclusive pain NOS◄

▲ **D57.411** Sickle-cell thalassemia, unspecified, with acute chest syndrome `MCC` `HCC`

▲ **D57.412** Sickle-cell thalassemia, unspecified, with splenic sequestration `MCC` `HCC`

● **D57.413** Sickle-cell thalassemia, unspecified, with cerebral vascular involvement `MCC`
Code also, if applicable cerebral infarction (I63.-)

● **D57.418** Sickle-cell thalassemia, unspecified, with crisis with other specified complication `MCC`
Use additional code to identify complications, such as:
cholelithiasis (K80.-)
priapism (N48.32)

▲ **D57.419** Sickle-cell thalassemia, unspecified, with crisis `MCC` `HCC`
►Sickle-cell thalassemia with (painful) crisis NOS◄
►Sickle-cell thalassemia with vasoocclusive pain◄

● **D57.42** Sickle-cell thalassemia beta zero without crisis
HbS-beta zero without crisis
Sickle-cell beta zero without crisis

√6ᵗʰ **D57.43** Sickle-cell thalassemia beta zero with crisis
HbS-beta zero with crisis
Sickle-cell beta zero with crisis

D57.431 Sickle-cell thalassemia beta zero with acute chest syndrome `MCC`
HbS-beta zero with acute chest syndrome
Sickle-cell beta zero with acute chest syndrome

D57.432 Sickle-cell thalassemia beta zero with splenic sequestration `MCC`
HbS-beta zero with splenic sequestration
Sickle-cell beta zero with splenic sequestration

D57.433 Sickle-cell thalassemia beta zero with cerebral vascular involvement `MCC`
HbS-beta zero with cerebral vascular involvement
Sickle-cell beta zero with cerebral vascular involvement
Code also, if applicable cerebral infarction (I63.-)

D57.438 Sickle-cell thalassemia beta zero with crisis with other specified complication `MCC`
HbS-beta zero with other specified complication
Sickle-cell beta zero with other specified complication
Use additional code to identify complications, such as:
cholelithiasis (K80.-)
priapism (N48.32)

D57.439 Sickle-cell thalassemia beta zero with crisis, unspecified `MCC`
HbS-beta zero with other specified complication
Sickle-cell beta zero with crisis unspecified
Sickle-cell thalassemia beta zero with (painful) crisis NOS
Sickle-cell thalassemia beta zero with vasoocclusive pain

● **D57.44** Sickle-cell thalassemia beta plus without crisis
HbS-beta plus without crisis
Sickle-cell beta plus without crisis

√6ᵗʰ **D57.45** Sickle-cell thalassemia beta plus with crisis
HbS-beta plus with crisis
Sickle-cell beta plus with crisis

D57.451 Sickle-cell thalassemia beta plus with acute chest syndrome `MCC`
HbS-beta plus with acute chest syndrome
Sickle-cell beta plus with acute chest syndrome

D57.452 Sickle-cell thalassemia beta plus with splenic sequestration `MCC`
HbS-beta plus with splenic sequestration
Sickle-cell beta plus with splenic sequestration

D57.453 Sickle-cell thalassemia beta plus with cerebral vascular involvement `MCC`
HbS-beta plus with cerebral vascular involvement
Sickle-cell beta plus with cerebral vascular involvement
Code also, if applicable cerebral infarction (I63.-)

D57.458 Sickle-cell thalassemia beta plus with crisis with other specified complication `MCC`
HbS-beta plus with crisis with other specified complication
Sickle-cell beta plus with crisis with other specified complication
Use additional code to identify complications, such as:
cholelithiasis (K80.-)
priapism (N48.32)

N Newborn: 0   P Pediatric: 0-17   M Maternity: 9-64   A Adult: 15-124   `MCC` Major Complication/Comorbidity   `CC` Complication/Comorbidity   `SW` Severe Wound Dx

508   ICD-10-CM 2021

●   **D57.459**   **Sickle-cell thalassemia beta plus with crisis, unspecified**   `MCC`
       HbS-beta plus with crisis with unspecified complication
       Sickle-cell beta plus with crisis with unspecified complication
       Sickle-cell thalassemia beta plus with (painful) crisis NOS
       Sickle-cell thalassemia beta plus with vasoocclusive pain

√5ᵗʰ   **D57.8**   **Other sickle-cell disorders**
     Hb-SD disease
     Hb-SE disease

     D57.80   **Other sickle-cell disorders** without crisis   `HCC`

√6ᵗʰ   **D57.81**   **Other sickle-cell disorders** with crisis

       D57.811   **Other sickle-cell disorders** with acute chest syndrome   `MCC` `HCC`

       D57.812   **Other sickle-cell disorders** with splenic sequestration   `MCC` `HCC`

●   **D57.813**   **Other sickle-cell disorders** with cerebral vascular involvement   `MCC`
         Code also, if applicable: cerebral infarction (I63.-)

●   **D57.818**   **Other sickle-cell disorders with crisis with other specified complication**   `MCC`
         Use additional code to identify complications, such as:
           cholelithiasis (K80.-)
           priapism (N48.32)

       D57.819   **Other sickle-cell disorders with crisis, unspecified**   `MCC` `HCC`
         Other sickle-cell disorders with crisis NOS
         ▶Other sickle-cell disorders with vasooclusive pain NOS◀

√4ᵗʰ   **D58**   **Other** hereditary **hemolytic anemias**
     `EXCLUDES 1`   hemolytic anemia of the newborn (P55.-)

     D58.0   **Hereditary** spherocytosis   `HCC`
       Acholuric (familial) jaundice
       Congenital (spherocytic) hemolytic icterus
       Minkowski-Chauffard syndrome
       DEF: Inherited condition caused by mutations to genes responsible for the production of proteins that form the membranes of red blood cells. The shape and flexibility of the red blood cell membrane is altered diminishing the cells ability to traverse the spleen, therefore becoming trapped and destroyed before the red blood cell has reached maturity.

     D58.1   **Hereditary** elliptocytosis   `HCC`
       Elliptocytosis (congenital)
       Ovalocytosis (congenital) (hereditary)

     D58.2   **Other** hemoglobinopathies   `HCC`
       Abnormal hemoglobin NOS
       Congenital Heinz body anemia
       Hb-C disease
       Hb-D disease
       Hb-E disease
       Hemoglobinopathy NOS
       Unstable hemoglobin hemolytic disease
       `EXCLUDES 1`   familial polycythemia (D75.0)
           Hb-M disease (D74.0)
           hemoglobin E-beta thalassemia (D56.5)
           hereditary persistence of fetal hemoglobin [HPFH] (D56.4)
           high-altitude polycythemia (D75.1)
           methemoglobinemia (D74.-)
           other hemoglobinopathies with thalassemia (D56.8)

     D58.8   **Other specified hereditary hemolytic anemias**   `CC` `HCC`
       Stomatocytosis

     D58.9   **Hereditary hemolytic anemia, unspecified**   `CC` `HCC`

√4ᵗʰ   **D59**   **Acquired** hemolytic anemia
     DEF: Non-hereditary anemia characterized by premature destruction of red blood cells caused by infectious organisms, poisons, and physical agents.

     D59.0   **Drug-induced autoimmune** hemolytic anemia   `CC` `HCC`
       Use additional code for adverse effect, if applicable, to identify drug (T36-T50 with fifth or sixth character 5)

▲   √5ᵗʰ   **D59.1**   **Other** autoimmune **hemolytic anemias**
     ~~Autoimmune hemolytic disease (cold type) (warm type)~~
     ~~Chronic cold hemagglutinin disease~~
     ~~Cold agglutinin disease~~
     ~~Cold agglutinin hemoglobinuria~~
     ~~Cold type (secondary) (symptomatic) hemolytic anemia~~
     ~~Warm type (secondary) (symptomatic) hemolytic anemia~~
     `EXCLUDES 1`   *Evans syndrome (D69.41)*
         hemolytic disease of newborn (P55.-)
         paroxysmal cold hemoglobinuria (D59.6)
     `EXCLUDES 2`   ▶*Evans syndrome (D69.41)*◀
         ▶*hemolytic disease of newborn (P55.-)*◀
         ▶*paroxysmal cold hemoglobinuria (D59.6)*◀

●   **D59.10**   **Autoimmune hemolytic anemia, unspecified**   `CC`

●   **D59.11**   **Warm autoimmune hemolytic anemia**   `CC`
       Warm type (primary) (secondary) (symptomatic) autoimmune hemolytic anemia
       Warm type autoimmune hemolytic disease

●   **D59.12**   **Cold autoimmune hemolytic anemia**   `CC`
       Chronic cold hemagglutinin disease
       Cold agglutinin disease
       Cold agglutinin hemoglobinuria
       Cold type (primary) (secondary) (symptomatic) autoimmune hemolytic anemia
       Cold type autoimmune hemolytic disease

●   **D59.13**   **Mixed type autoimmune hemolytic anemia**   `CC`
       Mixed type autoimmune hemolytic disease
       Mixed type, cold and warm, (primary) (secondary) (symptomatic) autoimmune hemolytic anemia

●   **D59.19**   **Other autoimmune hemolytic anemia**   `CC`

     D59.2   **Drug-induced nonautoimmune** hemolytic anemia   `CC` `HCC`
       Drug-induced enzyme deficiency anemia
       Use additional code for adverse effect, if applicable, to identify drug (T36-T50 with fifth or sixth character 5)

     D59.3   **Hemolytic-uremic syndrome**   `MCC` `HCC`
       Use additional code to identify associated:
         E. coli infection (B96.2-)
         Pneumococcal pneumonia (J13)
         Shigella dysenteriae (A03.9)
       DEF: Condition typically precipitated by infection causing low platelets and destruction of red blood cells resulting in hemolytic anemia. This cell damage and blockage of renal capillaries lead to kidney failure. Mainly affects children.

     D59.4   **Other** nonautoimmune **hemolytic anemias**   `CC` `HCC`
       Mechanical hemolytic anemia
       Microangiopathic hemolytic anemia
       Toxic hemolytic anemia

     D59.5   **Paroxysmal nocturnal hemoglobinuria [Marchiafava-Micheli]**   `HCC`
       `EXCLUDES 1`   hemoglobinuria NOS (R82.3)

     D59.6   **Hemoglobinuria** due to hemolysis from other external causes   `HCC`
       Hemoglobinuria from exertion
       March hemoglobinuria
       Paroxysmal cold hemoglobinuria
       Use additional code (Chapter 20) to identify external cause
       `EXCLUDES 1`   hemoglobinuria NOS (R82.3)

     D59.8   **Other acquired hemolytic anemias**   `HCC`

     D59.9   **Acquired hemolytic anemia, unspecified**   `CC` `HCC`
       Idiopathic hemolytic anemia, chronic

Aplastic and other anemias and other bone marrow failure syndromes (D60-D64)

√4ᵗʰ   **D60**   **Acquired pure red cell aplasia [erythroblastopenia]**
     `INCLUDES`   red cell aplasia (acquired) (adult) (with thymoma)
     `EXCLUDES 1`   congenital red cell aplasia (D61.01)
     DEF: Bone marrow failure characterized by underproduction of red blood cells while white blood cell and platelet production remains normal.

     D60.0   **Chronic acquired pure red cell aplasia**   `MCC` `HCC`
     D60.1   **Transient acquired pure red cell aplasia**   `MCC` `HCC`
     D60.8   **Other acquired pure red cell aplasias**   `MCC` `HCC`
     D60.9   **Acquired pure red cell aplasia, unspecified**   `MCC` `HCC`

Chapter 3. Diseases of the Blood and Blood-forming Organs

D61–D64.4

✓4ᵗʰ **D61 Other aplastic anemias and other bone marrow failure syndromes**

     EXCLUDES 1   *neutropenia (D70.-)*

     EXCLUDES 2   ▶*neutropenia (D70.-)*◀

     AHA: 2014,4Q,22

     DEF: Aplastic anemia: Bone marrow failure characterized by underproduction of red bloods cells, white blood cells and platelets.

✓5ᵗʰ **D61.0 Constitutional** aplastic anemia

     D61.01 Constitutional (pure) red blood cell aplasia   CC HCC

        Blackfan-Diamond syndrome
        Congenital (pure) red cell aplasia
        Familial hypoplastic anemia
        Primary (pure) red cell aplasia
        Red cell (pure) aplasia of infants
        EXCLUDES 1   *acquired red cell aplasia (D60.9)*

     D61.09 Other constitutional aplastic anemia   CC HCC
        Fanconi's anemia
        Pancytopenia with malformations

D61.1 Drug-induced aplastic anemia   MCC HCC
     Use additional code for adverse effect, if applicable, to identify drug (T36-T50 with fifth or sixth character 5)

D61.2 Aplastic anemia due to other external agents   MCC HCC
     Code first, if applicable, toxic effects of substances chiefly nonmedicinal as to source (T51-T65)

D61.3 Idiopathic aplastic anemia   MCC HCC

✓5ᵗʰ **D61.8 Other specified aplastic anemias and other bone marrow failure syndromes**

     ✓6ᵗʰ **D61.81 Pancytopenia**

        EXCLUDES 1   *pancytopenia (due to) (with) aplastic anemia (D61.9)*
        pancytopenia (due to) (with) bone marrow infiltration (D61.82)
        pancytopenia (due to) (with) congenital (pure) red cell aplasia (D61.01)
        pancytopenia (due to) (with) hairy cell leukemia (C91.4-)
        pancytopenia (due to) (with) human immunodeficiency virus disease (B20)
        pancytopenia (due to) (with) leukoerythroblastic anemia (D61.82)
        pancytopenia (due to) (with) myeloproliferative disease (D47.1)
        EXCLUDES 2   *pancytopenia (due to) (with) myelodysplastic syndromes (D46.-)*

        DEF: Shortage of all three blood cells: white, red, and platelets.

        D61.810 Antineoplastic chemotherapy induced pancytopenia   MCC HCC
           EXCLUDES 2   *aplastic anemia due to antineoplastic chemotherapy (D61.1)*

        D61.811 Other drug-induced pancytopenia   MCC HCC
           EXCLUDES 2   *aplastic anemia due to drugs (D61.1)*

        D61.818 Other pancytopenia   CC HCC
           AHA: 2019,1Q,16
           TIP: Assign this code in addition to myeloid leukemia codes (C92.-) when pancytopenia is documented. Although common in some types of myeloid leukemia, pancytopenia is not always inherent.

     D61.82 Myelophthisis   CC HCC
        Leukoerythroblastic anemia
        Myelophthisic anemia
        Panmyelophthisis
        Code also the underlying disorder, such as:
           malignant neoplasm of breast (C50.-)
           tuberculosis (A15.-)
        EXCLUDES 1   *idiopathic myelofibrosis (D47.1)*
           myelofibrosis NOS (D75.81)
           myelofibrosis with myeloid metaplasia (D47.4)
           primary myelofibrosis (D47.1)
           secondary myelofibrosis (D75.81)

        DEF: Condition that occurs when normal hematopoietic tissue in the bone marrow is replaced with abnormal tissue, such as fibrous tissue or tumors. Most commonly seen during the advanced stages of cancer.

     D61.89 Other specified aplastic anemias and other bone marrow failure syndromes   MCC HCC

D61.9 Aplastic anemia, unspecified   CC HCC
     Hypoplastic anemia NOS
     Medullary hypoplasia

D62 Acute posthemorrhagic anemia   CC
     EXCLUDES 1   *anemia due to chronic blood loss (D50.0)*
        blood loss anemia NOS (D50.0)
        congenital anemia from fetal blood loss (P61.3)
     AHA: 2019,3Q,11,17

✓4ᵗʰ **D63 Anemia in chronic diseases classified elsewhere**

     D63.0 Anemia in neoplastic disease
        Code first neoplasm (C00-D49)
        EXCLUDES 1   *aplastic anemia due to antineoplastic chemotherapy (D61.1)*
        EXCLUDES 2   *anemia due to antineoplastic chemotherapy (D64.81)*

     D63.1 Anemia in chronic kidney disease
        Erythropoietin resistant anemia (EPO resistant anemia)
        Code first underlying chronic kidney disease (CKD) (N18.-)

     D63.8 Anemia in other chronic diseases classified elsewhere
        Code first underlying disease, such as:
           diphyllobothriasis (B70.0)
           hookworm disease (B76.0-B76.9)
           hypothyroidism (E00.0-E03.9)
           malaria (B50.0-B54)
           symptomatic late syphilis (A52.79)
           tuberculosis (A18.89)

✓4ᵗʰ **D64 Other anemias**
     EXCLUDES 1   *refractory anemia (D46.-)*
        refractory anemia with excess blasts in transformation [RAEB T] (C92.0-)

     DEF: Sideroblastic anemia: Hereditary or secondary disorder in which the red blood cells cannot effectively use iron, a nutrient needed to make hemoglobin. Although the iron can enter the red blood cell it is not assimilated into the hemoglobin molecule and builds up ringed sideroblasts around the cell nucleus.

     D64.0 Hereditary sideroblastic anemia   HCC
        Sex-linked hypochromic sideroblastic anemia

     D64.1 Secondary sideroblastic anemia due to disease   HCC
        Code first underlying disease

     D64.2 Secondary sideroblastic anemia due to drugs and toxins   HCC
        Code first poisoning due to drug or toxin, if applicable (T36-T65 with fifth or sixth character 1-4 or 6)
        Use additional code for adverse effect, if applicable, to identify drug (T36-T50 with fifth or sixth character 5)

     D64.3 Other sideroblastic anemias   HCC
        Sideroblastic anemia NOS
        Pyridoxine-responsive sideroblastic anemia NEC

     D64.4 Congenital dyserythropoietic anemia
        Dyshematopoietic anemia (congenital)
        EXCLUDES 1   *Blackfan-Diamond syndrome (D61.01)*
           Di Guglielmo's disease (C94.0)

N Newborn: 0   P Pediatric: 0-17   M Maternity: 9-64   A Adult: 15-124   MCC Major Complication/Comorbidity   CC Complication/Comorbidity   SW Severe Wound Dx

510   ICD-10-CM 2021

✓5ᵗʰ D64.8 Other specified anemias

   D64.81 Anemia due to antineoplastic chemotherapy
      Antineoplastic chemotherapy induced anemia
      EXCLUDES 1   *aplastic anemia due to antineoplastic chemotherapy (D61.1)*
      EXCLUDES 2   *anemia in neoplastic disease (D63.0)*
      AHA: 2014,4Q,22
      DEF: Reversible adverse effect of chemotherapy, causing inhibition of bone marrow production. A decrease in red blood cell production prevents adequate oxygenation of the tissues and organs causing fatigue, shortness of breath (SOB), and exacerbation of other medical conditions.

   D64.89 Other specified anemias
      Infantile pseudoleukemia

D64.9 Anemia, unspecified
      AHA: 2018,4Q,88; 2017,1Q,7

Coagulation defects, purpura and other hemorrhagic conditions (D65-D69)

D65 Disseminated intravascular coagulation [defibrination syndrome]   MCC HCC
   Afibrinogenemia, acquired
   Consumption coagulopathy
   Diffuse or disseminated intravascular coagulation [DIC]
   Fibrinolytic hemorrhage, acquired
   Fibrinolytic purpura
   Purpura fulminans
   EXCLUDES 1   *disseminated intravascular coagulation (complicating):*
      abortion or ectopic or molar pregnancy (O00-O07, O08.1)
      in newborn (P60)
      pregnancy, childbirth and the puerperium (O45.0, O46.0, O67.0, O72.3)

Coagulation

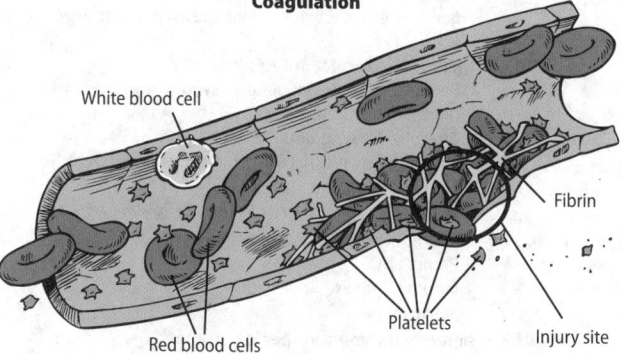

White blood cell
Fibrin
Red blood cells
Platelets
Injury site

D66 Hereditary factor VIII deficiency   MCC HCC
   Classical hemophilia
   Deficiency factor VIII (with functional defect)
   Hemophilia A
   Hemophilia NOS
   EXCLUDES 1   *factor VIII deficiency with vascular defect (D68.0)*
   DEF: Hereditary, sex-linked lack of antihemophilic globulin (AHG) (factor VIII) that causes abnormal coagulation characterized by increased bleeding; large bruises of skin; bleeding in the mouth, nose, and gastrointestinal tract; and hemorrhages into joints, resulting in swelling and impaired function.

D67 Hereditary factor IX deficiency   MCC HCC
   Christmas disease
   Factor IX deficiency (with functional defect)
   Hemophilia B
   Plasma thromboplastin component [PTC] deficiency

✓4ᵗʰ D68 Other coagulation defects

   EXCLUDES 1   *abnormal coagulation profile (R79.1)*
      coagulation defects complicating abortion or ectopic or molar pregnancy (O00-O07, O08.1)
      coagulation defects complicating pregnancy, childbirth and the puerperium (O45.0, O46.0, O67.0, O72.3)
   AHA: 2016,1Q,14

D68.0 Von Willebrand's disease   CC HCC
   Angiohemophilia
   Factor VIII deficiency with vascular defect
   Vascular hemophilia
   EXCLUDES 1   *capillary fragility (hereditary) (D69.8)*
      factor VIII deficiency NOS (D66)
      factor VIII deficiency with functional defect (D66)
   DEF: Congenital, abnormal blood coagulation caused by deficient blood factor VII. Symptoms include excess or prolonged bleeding.

D68.1 Hereditary factor XI deficiency   CC HCC
   Hemophilia C
   Plasma thromboplastin antecedent [PTA] deficiency
   Rosenthal's disease

D68.2 Hereditary deficiency of other clotting factors   CC HCC
   AC globulin deficiency
   Congenital afibrinogenemia
   Deficiency of factor I [fibrinogen]
   Deficiency of factor II [prothrombin]
   Deficiency of factor V [labile]
   Deficiency of factor VII [stable]
   Deficiency of factor X [Stuart-Prower]
   Deficiency of factor XII [Hageman]
   Deficiency of factor XIII [fibrin stabilizing]
   Dysfibrinogenemia (congenital)
   Hypoproconvertinemia
   Owren's disease
   Proaccelerin deficiency

✓5ᵗʰ D68.3 Hemorrhagic disorder due to circulating anticoagulants

  ✓6ᵗʰ D68.31 Hemorrhagic disorder due to intrinsic circulating anticoagulants, antibodies, or inhibitors

     D68.311 Acquired hemophilia   CC HCC
        Autoimmune hemophilia
        Autoimmune inhibitors to clotting factors
        Secondary hemophilia

     D68.312 Antiphospholipid antibody with hemorrhagic disorder   CC HCC
        Lupus anticoagulant (LAC) with hemorrhagic disorder
        Systemic lupus erythematosus [SLE] inhibitor with hemorrhagic disorder
        EXCLUDES 1   *antiphospholipid antibody, finding without diagnosis (R76.0)*
          antiphospholipid antibody syndrome (D68.61)
          antiphospholipid antibody with hypercoagulable state (D68.61)
          lupus anticoagulant (LAC) finding without diagnosis (R76.0)
          lupus anticoagulant (LAC) with hypercoagulable state (D68.62)
          systemic lupus erythematosus [SLE] inhibitor finding without diagnosis (R76.0)
          systemic lupus erythematosus [SLE] inhibitor with hypercoagulable state (D68.62)

Chapter 3. Diseases of the Blood and Blood-forming Organs

D68.318   **Other hemorrhagic disorder due to intrinsic circulating anticoagulants, antibodies, or inhibitors** `CC` `HCC`
Antithromboplastinemia
Antithromboplastinogenemia
Hemorrhagic disorder due to intrinsic increase in antithrombin
Hemorrhagic disorder due to intrinsic increase in anti-VIIIa
Hemorrhagic disorder due to intrinsic increase in anti-IXa
Hemorrhagic disorder due to intrinsic increase in anti-XIa

D68.32   **Hemorrhagic disorder due to extrinsic circulating anticoagulants** `CC` `HCC`
Drug-induced hemorrhagic disorder
Hemorrhagic disorder due to increase in anti-IIa
Hemorrhagic disorder due to increase in anti-Xa
Hyperheparinemia
Use additional code for adverse effect, if applicable, to identify drug (T45.515, T45.525)
AHA: 2016,1Q,14-15
TIP: Do not assign to identify routine therapeutic anticoagulation effects; assign only for documented adverse effects.

D68.4   **Acquired coagulation factor deficiency** `CC` `HCC`
Deficiency of coagulation factor due to liver disease
Deficiency of coagulation factor due to vitamin K deficiency
   EXCLUDES 1   *vitamin K deficiency of newborn (P53)*

✓5ᵗʰ **D68.5**   **Primary thrombophilia**
Primary hypercoagulable states
   EXCLUDES 1   *antiphospholipid syndrome (D68.61)*
     lupus anticoagulant (D68.62)
     secondary activated protein C resistance (D68.69)
     secondary antiphospholipid antibody syndrome (D68.69)
     secondary lupus anticoagulant with hypercoagulable state (D68.69)
     secondary systemic lupus erythematosus [SLE] inhibitor with hypercoagulable state (D68.69)
     systemic lupus erythematosus [SLE] inhibitor finding without diagnosis (R76.0)
     systemic lupus erythematosus [SLE] inhibitor with hemorrhagic disorder (D68.312)
     thrombotic thrombocytopenic purpura (M31.1)
DEF: Thrombophilia: Increased tendency of the blood to clot, which can lead to thrombus or embolus formation.

D68.51   **Activated protein C resistance** `CC` `HCC`
Factor V Leiden mutation

D68.52   **Prothrombin gene mutation** `CC` `HCC`

D68.59   **Other primary thrombophilia** `CC` `HCC`
Antithrombin III deficiency
Hypercoagulable state NOS
Primary hypercoagulable state NEC
Primary thrombophilia NEC
Protein C deficiency
Protein S deficiency
Thrombophilia NOS

✓5ᵗʰ **D68.6**   **Other thrombophilia**
Other hypercoagulable states
   EXCLUDES 1   *diffuse or disseminated intravascular coagulation [DIC] (D65)*
     heparin induced thrombocytopenia (HIT) (D75.82)
     hyperhomocysteinemia (E72.11)

D68.61   **Antiphospholipid syndrome** `CC` `HCC`
Anticardiolipin syndrome
Antiphospholipid antibody syndrome
   EXCLUDES 1   *anti-phospholipid antibody, finding without diagnosis (R76.0)*
     anti-phospholipid antibody with hemorrhagic disorder (D68.312)
     lupus anticoagulant syndrome (D68.62)

D68.62   **Lupus anticoagulant syndrome** `CC` `HCC`
Lupus anticoagulant
Presence of systemic lupus erythematosus [SLE] inhibitor
   EXCLUDES 1   *anticardiolipin syndrome (D68.61)*
     antiphospholipid syndrome (D68.61)
     lupus anticoagulant (LAC) finding without diagnosis (R76.0)
     lupus anticoagulant (LAC) with hemorrhagic disorder (D68.312)

D68.69   **Other thrombophilia** `CC` `HCC`
Hypercoagulable states NEC
Secondary hypercoagulable state NOS

D68.8   **Other specified coagulation defects** `CC` `HCC`
   EXCLUDES 1   *hemorrhagic disease of newborn (P53)*

D68.9   **Coagulation defect, unspecified** `CC` `HCC`

✓4ᵗʰ **D69**   **Purpura and other hemorrhagic conditions**
   EXCLUDES 1   *benign hypergammaglobulinemic purpura (D89.0)*
     cryoglobulinemic purpura (D89.1)
     essential (hemorrhagic) thrombocythemia (D47.3)
     hemorrhagic thrombocythemia (D47.3)
     purpura fulminans (D65)
     thrombotic thrombocytopenic purpura (M31.1)
     Waldenström hypergammaglobulinemic purpura (D89.0)

D69.0   **Allergic purpura** `CC` `HCC`
Allergic vasculitis
Nonthrombocytopenic hemorrhagic purpura
Nonthrombocytopenic idiopathic purpura
Purpura anaphylactoid
Purpura Henoch(-Schönlein)
Purpura rheumatica
Vascular purpura
   EXCLUDES 1   *thrombocytopenic hemorrhagic purpura (D69.3)*
DEF: Any hemorrhagic condition, thrombocytic or nonthrombocytopenic in origin, caused by a presumed allergic reaction.

D69.1   **Qualitative platelet defects** `HCC`
Bernard-Soulier [giant platelet] syndrome
Glanzmann's disease
Grey platelet syndrome
Thromboasthenia (hemorrhagic) (hereditary)
Thrombocytopathy
   EXCLUDES 1   *von Willebrand's disease (D68.0)*

D69.2   **Other nonthrombocytopenic purpura** `HCC`
Purpura NOS
Purpura simplex
Senile purpura

D69.3   **Immune thrombocytopenic purpura** `CC` `HCC`
Hemorrhagic (thrombocytopenic) purpura
Idiopathic thrombocytopenic purpura
Tidal platelet dysgenesis
DEF: Tidal platelet dysgenesis: Fluctuation of platelet counts from normal to very low within periods of 20 to 40 days and may involve autoimmune platelet destruction.

✓5ᵗʰ **D69.4**   **Other primary thrombocytopenia**
   EXCLUDES 1   *transient neonatal thrombocytopenia (P61.0)*
     Wiskott-Aldrich syndrome (D82.0)

D69.41   **Evans syndrome** `CC` `HCC`

D69.42   **Congenital and hereditary thrombocytopenia purpura** `CC` `HCC`
Congenital thrombocytopenia
Hereditary thrombocytopenia
Code first congenital or hereditary disorder, such as:
   thrombocytopenia with absent radius (TAR syndrome) (Q87.2)

D69.49   **Other primary thrombocytopenia** `HCC`
Megakaryocytic hypoplasia
Primary thrombocytopenia NOS

✓5ᵗʰ **D69.5**   **Secondary thrombocytopenia**
   EXCLUDES 1   *heparin induced thrombocytopenia (HIT) (D75.82)*
     transient thrombocytopenia of newborn (P61.0)

D69.51   **Posttransfusion purpura**
Posttransfusion purpura from whole blood (fresh) or blood products
PTP

N Newborn: 0   P Pediatric: 0-17   M Maternity: 9-64   A Adult: 15-124   MCC Major Complication/Comorbidity   CC Complication/Comorbidity   SW Severe Wound Dx

512   ICD-10-CM 2021

D69.59 Other secondary thrombocytopenia
AHA: 2014,4Q,22

D69.6 Thrombocytopenia, unspecified   HCC

D69.8 Other specified hemorrhagic conditions   HCC
Capillary fragility (hereditary)
Vascular pseudohemophilia

D69.9 Hemorrhagic condition, unspecified   HCC

Other disorders of blood and blood-forming organs (D70-D77)

✓4ᵗʰ D70 Neutropenia

INCLUDES   agranulocytosis
decreased absolute neurophile count (ANC)
Use additional code for any associated:
fever (R50.81)
mucositis (J34.81, K12.3-, K92.81, N76.81)
EXCLUDES 1   neutropenic splenomegaly (D73.81)
transient neonatal neutropenia (P61.5)
DEF: Abnormally low number of neutrophils. Neutrophils are phagocytic, meaning they surround and consume harmful pathogens, primarily bacteria. When neutrophil counts decrease the risk of infection increases.

D70.0 Congenital agranulocytosis   HCC
Congenital neutropenia
Infantile genetic agranulocytosis
Kostmann's disease

D70.1 Agranulocytosis secondary to cancer chemotherapy   HCC
Code also underlying neoplasm
Use additional code for adverse effect, if applicable, to identify drug (T45.1X5)
AHA: 2014,4Q,22

D70.2 Other drug-induced agranulocytosis   HCC
Use additional code for adverse effect, if applicable, to identify drug (T36-T50 with fifth or sixth character 5)

D70.3 Neutropenia due to infection   HCC

D70.4 Cyclic neutropenia   HCC
Cyclic hematopoiesis
Periodic neutropenia

D70.8 Other neutropenia   HCC

D70.9 Neutropenia, unspecified   HCC

D71 Functional disorders of polymorphonuclear neutrophils   HCC
Cell membrane receptor complex [CR3] defect
Chronic (childhood) granulomatous disease
Congenital dysphagocytosis
Progressive septic granulomatosis

✓4ᵗʰ D72 Other disorders of white blood cells
EXCLUDES 1   basophilia (D72.824)
immunity disorders (D80-D89)
neutropenia (D70)
preleukemia (syndrome) (D46.9)

D72.0 Genetic anomalies of leukocytes   HCC
Alder (granulation) (granulocyte) anomaly
Alder syndrome
Hereditary leukocytic hypersegmentation
Hereditary leukocytic hyposegmentation
Hereditary leukomelanopathy
May-Hegglin (granulation) (granulocyte) anomaly
May-Hegglin syndrome
Pelger-Huët (granulation) (granulocyte) anomaly
Pelger-Huët syndrome
EXCLUDES 1   Chédiak (-Steinbrinck)-Higashi syndrome (E70.330)

▲ ✓5ᵗʰ **D72.1** Eosinophilia
~~Allergic eosinophilia~~
~~Hereditary eosinophilia~~
EXCLUDES 1   ~~Löffler's syndrome (J82)~~
~~pulmonary eosinophilia (J82)~~
EXCLUDES 2   ▶Löffler's syndrome (J82)◀
▶pulmonary eosinophilia (J82)◀

● **D72.10** Eosinophilia, unspecified

● ✓6ᵗʰ **D72.11** Hypereosinophilic syndrome [HES]

● **D72.110** Idiopathic hypereosinophilic syndrome [IHES]

D72.111 Lymphocytic Variant Hypereosinophilic Syndrome [LHES]
Lymphocyte variant hypereosinophilia
Code also, if applicable, any associated lymphocytic neoplastic disorder

D72.118 Other hypereosinophilic syndrome
Episodic angioedema with eosinophilia
Gleich's syndrome

D72.119 Hypereosinophilic syndrome [HES], unspecified

D72.12 Drug rash with eosinophilia and systemic symptoms syndrome
DRESS syndrome
Use additional code for adverse effect, if applicable, to identify drug (T36-T50 with fifth or sixth character 5)

D72.18 *Eosinophilia in diseases classified elsewhere*
Code first underlying disease, such as:
chronic myelomonocytic leukemia (C93.1-)

D72.19 Other eosinophilia
Familial eosinophilia
Hereditary eosinophilia

✓5ᵗʰ D72.8 Other specified disorders of white blood cells
EXCLUDES 1   leukemia (C91-C95)

✓6ᵗʰ **D72.81** Decreased white blood cell count
EXCLUDES 1   neutropenia (D70.-)

D72.810 Lymphocytopenia
Decreased lymphocytes

D72.818 Other decreased white blood cell count
Basophilic leukopenia
Eosinophilic leukopenia
Monocytopenia
Other decreased leukocytes
Plasmacytopenia

D72.819 Decreased white blood cell count, unspecified
Decreased leukocytes, unspecified
Leukocytopenia, unspecified
Leukopenia
EXCLUDES 1   malignant leukopenia (D70.9)

✓6ᵗʰ **D72.82** Elevated white blood cell count
EXCLUDES 1   eosinophilia (D72.1)

D72.820 Lymphocytosis (symptomatic)
Elevated lymphocytes

D72.821 Monocytosis (symptomatic)
EXCLUDES 1   infectious mononucleosis (B27.-)

D72.822 Plasmacytosis

D72.823 Leukemoid reaction
Basophilic leukemoid reaction
Leukemoid reaction NOS
Lymphocytic leukemoid reaction
Monocytic leukemoid reaction
Myelocytic leukemoid reaction
Neutrophilic leukemoid reaction

D72.824 Basophilia
DEF: Increase in the basophils of the blood, a type of white blood cell, often seen in conjunction with neoplastic disorders.

D72.825 Bandemia
Bandemia without diagnosis of specific infection
EXCLUDES 1   confirmed infection — code to infection
leukemia (C91.-, C92.-, C93.-, C94.-, C95.-)
DEF: Increase in early neutrophil cells, called band cells that may indicate infection.

D72.828 Other elevated white blood cell count

D72.829 Elevated white blood cell count, unspecified
Elevated leukocytes, unspecified
Leukocytosis, unspecified

D72.89 Other specified disorders of white blood cells
Abnormality of white blood cells NEC

D72.9 Disorder of white blood cells, unspecified
Abnormal leukocyte differential NOS

☑ Additional Character Required   ✓x7ᵗʰ Placeholder   Unacceptable PDx   Questionable PDx   Manifestation   Unspecified Dx   H1 - H14 HAC   HCC CMS-HCC Dx   HIV HIV Dx

✓4ᵗʰ D73 Diseases of spleen

D73.0 Hyposplenism
Atrophy of spleen
> **EXCLUDES 1**   asplenia (congenital) (Q89.01)
> postsurgical absence of spleen (Z90.81)

D73.1 Hypersplenism
> **EXCLUDES 1**   neutropenic splenomegaly (D73.81)
> primary splenic neutropenia (D73.81)
> splenitis, splenomegaly in late syphilis (A52.79)
> splenitis, splenomegaly in tuberculosis (A18.85)
> splenomegaly NOS (R16.1)
> splenomegaly congenital (Q89.0)

D73.2 Chronic congestive splenomegaly

D73.3 Abscess of spleen

D73.4 Cyst of spleen

D73.5 Infarction of spleen
Splenic rupture, nontraumatic
Torsion of spleen
> **EXCLUDES 1**   rupture of spleen due to Plasmodium vivax malaria (B51.0)
> traumatic rupture of spleen (S36.03-)

✓5ᵗʰ D73.8 Other diseases of spleen

D73.81 Neutropenic splenomegaly
Werner-Schultz disease

D73.89 Other diseases of spleen
Fibrosis of spleen NOS
Perisplenitis
Splenitis NOS

D73.9 Disease of spleen, unspecified

✓4ᵗʰ D74 Methemoglobinemia

D74.0 Congenital methemoglobinemia   `CC`
Congenital NADH-methemoglobin reductase deficiency
Hemoglobin-M [Hb-M] disease
Methemoglobinemia, hereditary

D74.8 Other methemoglobinemias   `CC`
Acquired methemoglobinemia (with sulfhemoglobinemia)
Toxic methemoglobinemia

D74.9 Methemoglobinemia, unspecified   `CC`

✓4ᵗʰ D75 Other and unspecified diseases of blood and blood-forming organs
> **EXCLUDES 2**   acute lymphadenitis (L04.-)
> chronic lymphadenitis (I88.1)
> enlarged lymph nodes (R59.-)
> hypergammaglobulinemia NOS (D89.2)
> lymphadenitis NOS (I88.9)
> mesenteric lymphadenitis (acute) (chronic) (I88.0)

D75.0 Familial erythrocytosis
Benign polycythemia
Familial polycythemia
> **EXCLUDES 1**   hereditary ovalocytosis (D58.1)

D75.1 Secondary polycythemia
Acquired polycythemia
Emotional polycythemia
Erythrocytosis NOS
Hypoxemic polycythemia
Nephrogenous polycythemia
Polycythemia due to erythropoietin
Polycythemia due to fall in plasma volume
Polycythemia due to high altitude
Polycythemia due to stress
Polycythemia NOS
Relative polycythemia
> **EXCLUDES 1**   polycythemia neonatorum (P61.1)
> polycythemia vera (D45)

DEF: Elevated number of red blood cells in circulating blood as a result of reduced oxygen supply to the tissues.

✓5ᵗʰ D75.8 Other specified diseases of blood and blood-forming organs

D75.81 Myelofibrosis   `CC` `HCC`
Myelofibrosis NOS
Secondary myelofibrosis NOS
Code first the underlying disorder, such as:
    malignant neoplasm of breast (C50.-)
Use additional code, if applicable, for associated therapy-related myelodysplastic syndrome (D46.-)
Use additional code for adverse effect, if applicable, to identify drug (T45.1X5)
> **EXCLUDES 1**   acute myelofibrosis (C94.4-)
> idiopathic myelofibrosis (D47.1)
> leukoerythroblastic anemia (D61.82)
> myelofibrosis with myeloid metaplasia (D47.4) •
> myelophthisic anemia (D61.82)
> myelophthisis (D61.82)
> primary myelofibrosis (D47.1)

D75.82 Heparin induced thrombocytopenia (HIT)   `HCC`
DEF: Immune-mediated reaction to heparin therapy causing an abrupt fall in platelet count and serious complications such as pulmonary embolism, stroke, AMI, or DVT.

D75.89 Other specified diseases of blood and blood-forming organs

D75.9 Disease of blood and blood-forming organs, unspecified

D75.A Glucose-6-phosphate dehydrogenase (G6PD) deficiency without anemia
> **EXCLUDES 1**   glucose-6-phosphate dehydrogenase (G6PD) deficiency with anemia (D55.0)

AHA: 2019,4Q,4-5

✓4ᵗʰ D76 Other specified diseases with participation of lymphoreticular and reticulohistiocytic tissue
> **EXCLUDES 1**   (Abt-) Letterer-Siwe disease (C96.0)
> eosinophilic granuloma (C96.6)
> Hand-Schüller-Christian disease (C96.5)
> histiocytic medullary reticulosis (C96.9)
> histiocytic sarcoma (C96.A)
> histiocytosis X, multifocal (C96.5)
> histiocytosis X, unifocal (C96.6)
> Langerhans-cell histiocytosis, multifocal (C96.5)
> Langerhans-cell histiocytosis NOS (C96.6)
> Langerhans-cell histiocytosis, unifocal (C96.6)
> leukemic reticuloendotheliosis (C91.4-)
> lipomelanotic reticulosis (I89.8)
> malignant histiocytosis (C96.A)
> malignant reticulosis (C86.0)
> nonlipid reticuloendotheliosis (C96.0)

D76.1 Hemophagocytic lymphohistiocytosis   `CC` `HCC`
Familial hemophagocytic reticulosis
Histiocytoses of mononuclear phagocytes

D76.2 Hemophagocytic syndrome, infection-associated   `CC` `HCC`
Use additional code to identify infectious agent or disease

D76.3 Other histiocytosis syndromes   `CC` `HCC`
Reticulohistiocytoma (giant-cell)
Sinus histiocytosis with massive lymphadenopathy
Xanthogranuloma

D77 Other disorders of blood and blood-forming organs in diseases classified elsewhere
Code first underlying disease, such as:
    amyloidosis (E85.-)
    congenital early syphilis (A50.0)
    echinococcosis (B67.0-B67.9)
    malaria (B50.0-B54)
    schistosomiasis [bilharziasis] (B65.0-B65.9)
    vitamin C deficiency (E54)
> **EXCLUDES 1**   rupture of spleen due to Plasmodium vivax malaria (B51.0)
> splenitis, splenomegaly in late syphilis (A52.79)
> splenitis, splenomegaly in tuberculosis (A18.85)

N Newborn: 0   P Pediatric: 0-17   M Maternity: 9-64   A Adult: 15-124   MCC Major Complication/Comorbidity   CC Complication/Comorbidity   SW Severe Wound Dx

514   ICD-10-CM 2021

Intraoperative and postprocedural complications of the spleen (D78)

√4ᵗʰ **D78 Intraoperative and postprocedural complications of the spleen**

AHA: 2016,4Q,9-10

√5ᵗʰ **D78.0 Intraoperative hemorrhage and hematoma of the spleen complicating a procedure**

EXCLUDES 1   *intraoperative hemorrhage and hematoma of the spleen due to accidental puncture or laceration during a procedure (D78.1-)*

D78.01 Intraoperative hemorrhage and hematoma of the spleen complicating a procedure on the spleen CC

D78.02 Intraoperative hemorrhage and hematoma of the spleen complicating other procedure CC

√5ᵗʰ **D78.1 Accidental puncture and laceration of the spleen during a procedure**

D78.11 Accidental puncture and laceration of the spleen during a procedure on the spleen CC

D78.12 Accidental puncture and laceration of the spleen during other procedure CC

√5ᵗʰ **D78.2 Postprocedural hemorrhage of the spleen following a procedure**

D78.21 Postprocedural hemorrhage of the spleen following a procedure on the spleen CC

D78.22 Postprocedural hemorrhage of the spleen following other procedure CC

√5ᵗʰ **D78.3 Postprocedural hematoma and seroma of the spleen following a procedure**

D78.31 Postprocedural hematoma of the spleen following a procedure on the spleen CC

D78.32 Postprocedural hematoma of the spleen following other procedure CC

D78.33 Postprocedural seroma of the spleen following a procedure on the spleen CC

D78.34 Postprocedural seroma of the spleen following other procedure CC

√5ᵗʰ **D78.8 Other intraoperative and postprocedural complications of the spleen**

Use additional code, if applicable, to further specify disorder

D78.81 Other intraoperative complications of the spleen CC

D78.89 Other postprocedural complications of the spleen CC

Certain disorders involving the immune mechanism (D80-D89)

INCLUDES   defects in the complement system
immunodeficiency disorders, except human immunodeficiency virus [HIV] disease
sarcoidosis

EXCLUDES 1   *autoimmune disease (systemic) NOS (M35.9)*
functional disorders of polymorphonuclear neutrophils (D71)
human immunodeficiency virus [HIV] disease (B20)

√4ᵗʰ **D80 Immunodeficiency with predominantly antibody defects**

D80.0 Hereditary hypogammaglobulinemia CC HCC
Autosomal recessive agammaglobulinemia (Swiss type)
X-linked agammaglobulinemia [Bruton] (with growth hormone deficiency)

D80.1 Nonfamilial hypogammaglobulinemia CC HCC
Agammaglobulinemia with immunoglobulin-bearing B-lymphocytes
Common variable agammaglobulinemia [CVAgamma]
Hypogammaglobulinemia NOS

D80.2 Selective deficiency of immunoglobulin A [IgA] CC HCC

D80.3 Selective deficiency of immunoglobulin G [IgG] subclasses CC HCC

D80.4 Selective deficiency of immunoglobulin M [IgM] CC HCC

D80.5 Immunodeficiency with increased immunoglobulin M [IgM] CC HCC

D80.6 Antibody deficiency with near-normal immunoglobulins or with hyperimmunoglobulinemia CC HCC

D80.7 Transient hypogammaglobulinemia of infancy CC HCC

D80.8 Other immunodeficiencies with predominantly antibody defects CC HCC
Kappa light chain deficiency

D80.9 Immunodeficiency with predominantly antibody defects, unspecified CC HCC

√4ᵗʰ **D81 Combined immunodeficiencies**

EXCLUDES 1   *autosomal recessive agammaglobulinemia (Swiss type) (D80.0)*

D81.0 Severe combined immunodeficiency [SCID] with reticular dysgenesis CC HCC

D81.1 Severe combined immunodeficiency [SCID] with low T- and B-cell numbers CC HCC

D81.2 Severe combined immunodeficiency [SCID] with low or normal B-cell numbers CC HCC

√5ᵗʰ **D81.3 Adenosine deaminase [ADA] deficiency**

AHA: 2019,4Q,5-6

D81.30 Adenosine deaminase deficiency, unspecified CC HCC
ADA deficiency NOS

D81.31 Severe combined immunodeficiency due to adenosine deaminase deficiency CC HCC
ADA deficiency with SCID
Adenosine deaminase [ADA] deficiency with severe combined immunodeficiency

D81.32 Adenosine deaminase 2 deficiency CC HCC
ADA2 deficiency
Adenosine deaminase deficiency type 2
Code also, if applicable, any associated manifestations, such as:
polyarteritis nodosa (M30.0)
stroke (I63.-)

D81.39 Other adenosine deaminase deficiency CC HCC
Adenosine deaminase [ADA] deficiency type 1, NOS
Adenosine deaminase [ADA] deficiency type 1, without SCID
Adenosine deaminase [ADA] deficiency type 1, without severe combined immunodeficiency
Partial ADA deficiency (type 1)
Partial adenosine deaminase deficiency (type 1)

D81.4 Nezelof's syndrome CC HCC

D81.5 Purine nucleoside phosphorylase [PNP] deficiency CC HCC

D81.6 Major histocompatibility complex class I deficiency CC HCC
Bare lymphocyte syndrome

D81.7 Major histocompatibility complex class II deficiency CC HCC

√5ᵗʰ **D81.8 Other combined immunodeficiencies**

√6ᵗʰ **D81.81 Biotin-dependent carboxylase deficiency**
Multiple carboxylase deficiency

EXCLUDES 1   *biotin-dependent carboxylase deficiency due to dietary deficiency of biotin (E53.8)*

D81.810 Biotinidase deficiency

D81.818 Other biotin-dependent carboxylase deficiency
Holocarboxylase synthetase deficiency
Other multiple carboxylase deficiency

D81.819 Biotin-dependent carboxylase deficiency, unspecified
Multiple carboxylase deficiency, unspecified

D81.89 Other combined immunodeficiencies CC HCC

D81.9 Combined immunodeficiency, unspecified CC HCC
Severe combined immunodeficiency disorder [SCID] NOS

√4ᵗʰ **D82 Immunodeficiency associated with other major defects**

EXCLUDES 1   *ataxia telangiectasia [Louis-Bar] (G11.3)*

D82.0 Wiskott-Aldrich syndrome CC HCC
Immunodeficiency with thrombocytopenia and eczema

D82.1 Di George's syndrome CC HCC
Pharyngeal pouch syndrome
Thymic alymphoplasia
Thymic aplasia or hypoplasia with immunodeficiency
AHA: 2019,3Q,14

D82.2 Immunodeficiency with short-limbed stature HCC

D82.3 Immunodeficiency following hereditary defective response to Epstein-Barr virus HCC
X-linked lymphoproliferative disease

D82.4 Hyperimmunoglobulin E [IgE] syndrome HCC

D82.8 Immunodeficiency associated with other specified major defects HCC

D82.9 Immunodeficiency associated with major defect, unspecified HCC

✔ Additional Character Required   √x7ᵗʰ Placeholder   Unacceptable PDx   Questionable PDx   Manifestation   Unspecified Dx   H1-H14 HAC   HCC CMS-HCC Dx   HIV HIV Dx

ICD-10-CM 2021   515

√4th **D83 Common variable immunodeficiency**

D83.0 Common variable immunodeficiency with predominant abnormalities of B-cell numbers and function `CC` `HCC`

D83.1 Common variable immunodeficiency with predominant immunoregulatory T-cell disorders `CC` `HCC`

D83.2 Common variable immunodeficiency with autoantibodies to B- or T-cells `CC` `HCC`

D83.8 Other common variable immunodeficiencies `CC` `HCC`

D83.9 Common variable immunodeficiency, unspecified `CC` `HCC`

√4th **D84 Other immunodeficiencies**

D84.0 Lymphocyte function antigen-1 [LFA-1] defect `HCC`

D84.1 Defects in the complement system `HCC`
　　C1 esterase inhibitor [C1-INH] deficiency

▲　√5th **D84.8 Other specified immunodeficiencies**

●　　**D84.81 Immunodeficiency due to conditions classified elsewhere** `CC`
　　　　Code first underlying condition, such as:
　　　　　chromosomal abnormalities (Q90-Q99)
　　　　　diabetes mellitus (E08-E13)
　　　　　malignant neoplasms (C00-C96)
　　　　　EXCLUDES 1　certain disorders involving the immune mechanism (D80-D83, D84.0, D84.1, D84.9)
　　　　　　　human immunodeficiency virus [HIV] disease (B20)

●　　√6th **D84.82 Immunodeficiency due to drugs and external causes**

●　　　**D84.821 Immunodeficiency due to** drugs `CC`
　　　　　Immunodeficiency due to (current or past) medication
　　　　　Use additional code for adverse effect if applicable, to identify adverse effect of drug (T36-T50 with fifth or six character 5)
　　　　　Use additional code, if applicable, for associated long term (current) drug therapy drug or medication such as:
　　　　　long term (current) drug therapy systemic steroids (Z79.52)
　　　　　　other long term (current) drug therapy (Z79.899)

●　　　**D84.822 Immunodeficiency due to external causes** `CC`
　　　　　Code also, if applicable, radiological procedure and radiotherapy (Y84.2)
　　　　　Use additional code for external cause such as:
　　　　　exposure to ionizing radiation (W88)

●　　**D84.89 Other immunodeficiencies** `CC`

D84.9 Immunodeficiency, unspecified `CC` `HCC`
　　▶Immunocompromised NOS◀
　　▶Immunodeficient NOS◀
　　▶Immunosuppressed NOS◀

√4th **D86 Sarcoidosis**
　　DEF: Clustering of immune cells resulting in granuloma formation. Often affects the lungs and lymphatic system but can occur in other body sites.

D86.0 Sarcoidosis of lung `HCC`

D86.1 Sarcoidosis of lymph nodes

D86.2 Sarcoidosis of lung with sarcoidosis of lymph nodes `HCC`

D86.3 Sarcoidosis of skin

√5th **D86.8 Sarcoidosis of other sites**

D86.81 Sarcoid meningitis

D86.82 Multiple cranial nerve palsies in sarcoidosis `HCC`

D86.83 Sarcoid iridocyclitis

D86.84 Sarcoid pyelonephritis
　　Tubulo-interstitial nephropathy in sarcoidosis

D86.85 Sarcoid myocarditis

D86.86 Sarcoid arthropathy
　　Polyarthritis in sarcoidosis

D86.87 Sarcoid myositis

D86.89 Sarcoidosis of other sites
　　Hepatic granuloma
　　Uveoparotid fever [Heerfordt]

D86.9 Sarcoidosis, unspecified

√4th **D89 Other disorders involving the immune mechanism, not elsewhere classified**
　　EXCLUDES 1　hyperglobulinemia NOS (R77.1)
　　　　monoclonal gammopathy (of undetermined significance) (D47.2)
　　EXCLUDES 2　transplant failure and rejection (T86.-)

D89.0 Polyclonal hypergammaglobulinemia
　　Benign hypergammaglobulinemic purpura
　　Polyclonal gammopathy NOS

D89.1 Cryoglobulinemia `HCC`
　　Cryoglobulinemic purpura
　　Cryoglobulinemic vasculitis
　　Essential cryoglobulinemia
　　Idiopathic cryoglobulinemia
　　Mixed cryoglobulinemia
　　Primary cryoglobulinemia
　　Secondary cryoglobulinemia

D89.2 Hypergammaglobulinemia, unspecified

D89.3 Immune reconstitution syndrome `HCC`
　　Immune reconstitution inflammatory syndrome [IRIS]
　　Use additional code for adverse effect, if applicable, to identify drug (T36-T50 with fifth or sixth character 5)

√5th **D89.4 Mast cell activation syndrome and related disorders**
　　EXCLUDES 1　aggressive systemic mastocytosis (C96.21)
　　　　congenital cutaneous mastocytosis (Q82.2)
　　　　(non-congenital) cutaneous mastocytosis (D47.01)
　　　　(indolent) systemic mastocytosis (D47.02)
　　　　malignant mast cell neoplasm (C96.2-)
　　　　malignant mastocytoma (C96.29)
　　　　mast cell leukemia (C94.3-)
　　　　mast cell sarcoma (C96.22)
　　　　mastocytoma NOS (D47.09)
　　　　other mast cell neoplasms of uncertain behavior (D47.09)
　　　　systemic mastocytosis associated with a clonal hematologic non-mast cell lineage disease (SM-AHNMD) (D47.02)

AHA: 2016,4Q,11

D89.40 Mast cell activation, unspecified `HCC`
　　Mast cell activation disorder, unspecified
　　Mast cell activation syndrome, NOS

D89.41 Monoclonal mast cell activation syndrome `HCC`

D89.42 Idiopathic mast cell activation syndrome `HCC`

D89.43 Secondary mast cell activation `HCC`
　　Secondary mast cell activation syndrome
　　Code also underlying etiology, if known

D89.49 Other mast cell activation disorder `HCC`
　　Other mast cell activation syndrome

√5th **D89.8 Other specified disorders involving the immune mechanism, not elsewhere classified**

√6th **D89.81 Graft-versus-host disease**
　　Code first underlying cause, such as:
　　　complications of transplanted organs and tissue (T86.-)
　　　complications of blood transfusion (T80.89)
　　Use additional code to identify associated manifestations, such as:
　　　desquamative dermatitis (L30.8)
　　　diarrhea (R19.7)
　　　elevated bilirubin (R17)
　　　hair loss (L65.9)

D89.810 Acute graft-versus-host disease `CC` `HCC`

D89.811 Chronic graft-versus-host disease `CC` `HCC`

D89.812 Acute on chronic graft-versus-host disease `CC` `HCC`

D89.813 Graft-versus-host disease, unspecified `CC` `HCC`

D89.82 Autoimmune lymphoproliferative syndrome [ALPS] `HCC`
　　DEF: Rare genetic alteration of the Fas protein that impairs normal cellular apoptosis (normal cell death), causing abnormal accumulation of lymphocytes in the lymph glands, liver, and spleen. Symptoms include neutropenia, anemia, and thrombocytopenia.

N Newborn: 0　**P** Pediatric: 0-17　**M** Maternity: 9-64　**A** Adult: 15-124　**MCC** Major Complication/Comorbidity　**CC** Complication/Comorbidity　**SW** Severe Wound Dx

516　　ICD-10-CM 2021

●   ✓6ᵗʰ   **D89.83**   **Cytokine release syndrome**

Code first underlying cause, such as:
 complications following infusion, transfusion and therapeutic injection (T80.89-)
 complications of transplanted organs and tissue (T86.-)
Use additional code to identify associated manifestations

●   **D89.831**   **Cytokine release syndrome, grade 1**

●   **D89.832**   **Cytokine release syndrome, grade 2**

●   **D89.833**   **Cytokine release syndrome, grade 3**

●   **D89.834**   **Cytokine release syndrome, grade 4**

●   **D89.835**   **Cytokine release syndrome, grade 5**

●   **D89.839**   **Cytokine release syndrome, grade unspecified**

      D89.89   **Other specified disorders involving the immune mechanism, not elsewhere classified**   HCC

           EXCLUDES 1   *human immunodeficiency virus disease (B20)*

           AHA: 2017,4Q,109

   D89.9   **Disorder involving the immune mechanism, unspecified**   HCC

Immune disease NOS

AHA: 2015,3Q,22

☑ Additional Character Required   ✓x7ᵗʰ Placeholder   Unacceptable PDx   Questionable PDx   Manifestation   Unspecified Dx   H1-H14 HAC   HCC CMS-HCC Dx   HIV HIV Dx

ICD-10-CM 2021   **517**

Chapter 4. Endocrine, Nutritional and Metabolic Diseases (E00–E89)

Chapter-specific Guidelines with Coding Examples

The chapter-specific guidelines from the ICD-10-CM Official Guidelines for Coding and Reporting have been provided below. Along with these guidelines are coding examples, contained in the shaded boxes, that have been developed to help illustrate the coding and/or sequencing guidance found in these guidelines.

a. Diabetes mellitus

The diabetes mellitus codes are combination codes that include the type of diabetes mellitus, the body system affected, and the complications affecting that body system. As many codes within a particular category as are necessary to describe all of the complications of the disease may be used. They should be sequenced based on the reason for a particular encounter. Assign as many codes from categories E08–E13 as needed to identify all of the associated conditions that the patient has.

> Patient is seen for poorly controlled diabetes, type 2, with diabetic polyneuropathy and diabetic retinopathy with macular edema
>
> **E11.65**   **Type 2 diabetes mellitus with hyperglycemia**
>
> **E11.311**   **Type 2 diabetes mellitus with unspecified diabetic retinopathy with macular edema**
>
> **E11.42**   **Type 2 diabetes mellitus with diabetic polyneuropathy**
>
> *Explanation*: Use as many codes to describe the diabetic complications as needed. Many are combination codes that describe more than one condition. Code first the reason for the encounter. "Poorly controlled" is described as "with hyperglycemia." Diabetes documented as "uncontrolled" is not assumed to be hyperglycemic but can be classified to either hyperglycemia or hypoglycemia. If documentation is not clear, the provider must be queried so that the appropriate code can be reported.

1) Type of diabetes

The age of a patient is not the sole determining factor, though most type 1 diabetics develop the condition before reaching puberty. For this reason type 1 diabetes mellitus is also referred to as juvenile diabetes.

> A 45-year-old patient is diagnosed with type 1 diabetes
>
> **E10.9**   **Type 1 diabetes mellitus without complications**
>
> *Explanation*: Although most type 1 diabetics are diagnosed in childhood or adolescence, it can also begin in adults.

2) Type of diabetes mellitus not documented

If the type of diabetes mellitus is not documented in the medical record the default is E11.-, Type 2 diabetes mellitus.

> H & P lists diabetes and hypertension on patient problem list
>
> **E11.9**   **Type 2 diabetes mellitus without complications**
>
> **I10**   **Essential (primary) hypertension**
>
> *Explanation*: Since the type of diabetes was not documented and no complications were noted, the default code is E11.9.

3) Diabetes mellitus and the use of insulin, oral hypoglycemics, and injectable non-insulin drugs

If the documentation in a medical record does not indicate the type of diabetes but does indicate that the patient uses insulin, code E11.-, Type 2 diabetes mellitus, should be assigned. An additional code should be assigned from category Z79 to identify the long-term (current) use of insulin or oral hypoglycemic drugs. If the patient is treated with both oral medications and insulin, only the code for long-term (current) use of insulin should be assigned. **If the patient is treated with both insulin and an injectable non-insulin antidiabetic drug, assign codes Z79.4, Long-term (current) use of insulin, and Z79.899, Other long term (current) drug therapy. If the patient is treated with both oral hypoglycemic drugs and an injectable non-insulin antidiabetic drug, assign codes Z79.84, Long-term (current) use of oral hypoglycemic drugs, and Z79.899, Other long-term (current) drug therapy.** Code Z79.4 should not be assigned if insulin is given temporarily to bring a type 2 patient's blood sugar under control during an encounter.

> Type 2 diabetic patient on daily metformin and Victoza is admitted in ketoacidosis, insulin given to stabilize blood sugars and discontinued at discharge
>
> **E11.10**   **Type 2 diabetes mellitus with ketoacidosis without coma**
>
> **Z79.84**   **Long term (current) use of oral hypoglycemic drugs**
>
> **Z79.899**   **Other long term (current) drug therapy**
>
> *Explanation*: Documentation indicates the patient is on an oral antidiabetic medication (metformin) and an injectable noninsulin antidiabetic medication (Victoza). Although insulin was given to the patient during the encounter, it was discontinued at discharge, indicating that the patient does not regularly use insulin. A Z code representing long-term use of the oral drug and long-term use of the injectable medication can be applied. Applying code Z79.4 to represent long-term use of insulin would be inappropriate.

4) Diabetes mellitus in pregnancy and gestational diabetes

See Section I.C.15. Diabetes mellitus in pregnancy.

See Section I.C.15. Gestational (pregnancy induced) diabetes

5) Complications due to insulin pump malfunction

(a) Underdose of insulin due to insulin pump failure

An underdose of insulin due to an insulin pump failure should be assigned to a code from subcategory T85.6, Mechanical complication of other specified internal and external prosthetic devices, implants and grafts, that specifies the type of pump malfunction, as the principal or first-listed code, followed by code T38.3X6-, Underdosing of insulin and oral hypoglycemic [antidiabetic] drugs. Additional codes for the type of diabetes mellitus and any associated complications due to the underdosing should also be assigned.

> A 24-year-old type 1 diabetic male treated in ED for hyperglycemia; insulin pump found to be malfunctioning and underdosing
>
> **T85.614A**   **Breakdown (mechanical) of insulin pump, initial encounter**
>
> **T38.3X6A**   **Underdosing of insulin and oral hypoglycemic [antidiabetic] drugs, initial encounter**
>
> **E10.65**   **Type 1 diabetes mellitus with hyperglycemia**
>
> *Explanation*: The complication code for the mechanical breakdown of the pump is sequenced first, followed by the underdosing code and type of diabetes with complication. Code all other diabetic complication codes necessary to describe the patient's condition.

(b) Overdose of insulin due to insulin pump failure

The principal or first-listed code for an encounter due to an insulin pump malfunction resulting in an overdose of insulin, should also be T85.6-, Mechanical complication of other specified internal and external prosthetic devices, implants and grafts, followed by code T38.3X1-, Poisoning by insulin and oral hypoglycemic [antidiabetic] drugs, accidental (unintentional).

> A 24-year-old type 1 diabetic male found down with diabetic coma, brought into ED and treated for hypoglycemia; insulin pump found to be malfunctioning and overdosing
>
> **T85.614A**   **Breakdown (mechanical) of insulin pump, initial encounter**
>
> **T38.3X1A**   **Poisoning by insulin and oral hypoglycemic [antidiabetic] drugs, accidental (unintentional), initial encounter**
>
> **E10.641**   **Type 1 diabetes mellitus with hypoglycemia with coma**
>
> *Explanation*: The complication code for the mechanical breakdown of the pump is sequenced first, followed by the poisoning code and type of diabetes with complication. All the characters in the combination code must be used to form a valid code and to fully describe the type of diabetes, the hypoglycemia, and the coma.

Chapter 4. Endocrine, Nutritional and Metabolic Diseases

6) **Secondary diabetes mellitus**

Codes under categories E08, Diabetes mellitus due to underlying condition, E09, Drug or chemical induced diabetes mellitus, and E13, Other specified diabetes mellitus, identify complications/manifestations associated with secondary diabetes mellitus. Secondary diabetes is always caused by another condition or event (e.g., cystic fibrosis, malignant neoplasm of pancreas, pancreatectomy, adverse effect of drug, or poisoning).

(a) **Secondary diabetes mellitus and the use of insulin or oral hypoglycemic drugs**

For patients with secondary diabetes mellitus who routinely use insulin or oral hypoglycemic drugs, an additional code from category Z79 should be assigned to identify the long-term (current) use of insulin or oral hypoglycemic drugs. If the patient is treated with both oral medications and insulin, only the code for long-term (current) use of insulin should be assigned. **If the patient is treated with both insulin and an injectable non-insulin antidiabetic drug, assign codes Z79.4, Long-term (current) use of insulin, and Z79.899, Other long term (current) drug therapy. If the patient is treated with both oral hypoglycemic drugs and an injectable non-insulin antidiabetic drug, assign codes Z79.84, Long-term (current) use of oral hypoglycemic drugs, and Z79.899, Other long-term (current) drug therapy.** Code Z79.4 should not be assigned if insulin is given temporarily to bring a secondary diabetic patient's blood sugar under control during an encounter.

> The patient, maintained on metformin and insulin, was admitted for treatment of diabetic gangrene. The patient developed diabetes secondary to Nelson's syndrome.
>
> **E24.1**   **Nelson's syndrome**
>
> **E08.52**   **Diabetes mellitus due to underlying condition with diabetic peripheral angiopathy with gangrene**
>
> **Z79.4**   **Long term (current) use of insulin**
>
> *Explanation*: When diabetes is caused by an underlying condition, the underlying condition should always be sequenced before any codes representing the diabetes. Patients with secondary diabetes may be maintained on both insulin and an oral hypoglycemic. Report only the code for the long-term use of insulin when both oral hypoglycemic and insulin are prescribed.

(b) **Assigning and sequencing secondary diabetes codes and its causes**

The sequencing of the secondary diabetes codes in relationship to codes for the cause of the diabetes is based on the Tabular List instructions for categories E08, E09 and E13.

(i) **Secondary diabetes mellitus due to pancreatectomy**

For postpancreatectomy diabetes mellitus (lack of insulin due to the surgical removal of all or part of the pancreas), assign code E89.1, Postprocedural hypoinsulinemia. Assign a code from category E13 and a code from subcategory Z90.41, Acquired absence of pancreas, as additional codes.

> Patient with newly diagnosed diabetes after surgical removal of part of pancreas is discharged with referral for consult to initiate insulin.
>
> **E89.1**   **Postprocedural hypoinsulinemia**
>
> **E13.9**   **Other specified diabetes mellitus without complications**
>
> **Z90.411**   **Acquired partial absence of pancreas**
>
> *Explanation*: Sequence the postprocedural complication of the hypoinsulinemia due to the partial removal of the pancreas as the first-listed code, followed by the other specified diabetes (NEC) with or without complications and the partial or total acquired absence of the pancreas. Code Z79.4 Long term (current) use of insulin, is not added because the insulin has not yet been started.

(ii) **Secondary diabetes due to drugs**

Secondary diabetes may be caused by an adverse effect of correctly administered medications, poisoning or sequela of poisoning.

See section I.C.19.e for coding of adverse effects and poisoning, and section I.C.20 for external cause code reporting.

> Initial encounter for corticosteroid-induced diabetes mellitus
>
> **E09.9**   **Drug or chemical induced diabetes mellitus without complications**
>
> **T38.0X5A**   **Adverse effect of glucocorticoids and synthetic analogues, initial encounter**
>
> *Explanation*: If the diabetes is caused by an adverse effect of a drug, the diabetic condition is coded first. If it occurs from a poisoning or overdose, the poisoning code causing the diabetes is sequenced first.

Chapter 4. Endocrine, Nutritional and Metabolic Diseases (E00-E89)

> **NOTE** All neoplasms, whether functionally active or not, are classified in Chapter 2. Appropriate codes in this chapter (i.e. E05.8, E07.0, E16-E31, E34.-) may be used as additional codes to indicate either functional activity by neoplasms and ectopic endocrine tissue or hyperfunction and hypofunction of endocrine glands associated with neoplasms and other conditions classified elsewhere.

> **EXCLUDES 1** *transitory endocrine and metabolic disorders specific to newborn (P70-P74)*

AHA: 2018,2Q,6

This chapter contains the following blocks:

E00-E07   Disorders of thyroid gland
E08-E13   Diabetes mellitus
E15-E16   Other disorders of glucose regulation and pancreatic internal secretion
E20-E35   Disorders of other endocrine glands
E36   Intraoperative complications of endocrine system
E40-E46   Malnutrition
E50-E64   Other nutritional deficiencies
E65-E68   Overweight, obesity and other hyperalimentation
E70-E88   Metabolic disorders
E89   Postprocedural endocrine and metabolic complications and disorders, not elsewhere classified

Disorders of thyroid gland (E00-E07)

✓4ᵗʰ E00 Congenital iodine-deficiency syndrome

Use additional code (F70-F79) to identify associated intellectual disabilities

> **EXCLUDES 1** *subclinical iodine-deficiency hypothyroidism (E02)*

E00.0 Congenital iodine-deficiency syndrome, neurological type
Endemic cretinism, neurological type

E00.1 Congenital iodine-deficiency syndrome, myxedematous type
Endemic hypothyroid cretinism
Endemic cretinism, myxedematous type

E00.2 Congenital iodine-deficiency syndrome, mixed type
Endemic cretinism, mixed type

E00.9 Congenital iodine-deficiency syndrome, unspecified
Congenital iodine-deficiency hypothyroidism NOS
Endemic cretinism NOS

✓4ᵗʰ E01 Iodine-deficiency related thyroid disorders and allied conditions

> **EXCLUDES 1** *congenital iodine-deficiency syndrome (E00.-)*
> *subclinical iodine-deficiency hypothyroidism (E02)*

E01.0 Iodine-deficiency related diffuse (endemic) goiter

E01.1 Iodine-deficiency related multinodular (endemic) goiter
Iodine-deficiency related nodular goiter

E01.2 Iodine-deficiency related (endemic) goiter, unspecified
Endemic goiter NOS

E01.8 Other iodine-deficiency related thyroid disorders and allied conditions
Acquired iodine-deficiency hypothyroidism NOS

E02 Subclinical iodine-deficiency hypothyroidism

✓4ᵗʰ E03 Other hypothyroidism

> **EXCLUDES 1** *iodine-deficiency related hypothyroidism (E00-E02)*
> *postprocedural hypothyroidism (E89.0)*

DEF: Hypothyroidism: Underproduction of thyroid hormone.

E03.0 Congenital hypothyroidism with diffuse goiter
Congenital parenchymatous goiter (nontoxic)
Congenital goiter (nontoxic) NOS

> **EXCLUDES 1** *transitory congenital goiter with normal function (P72.0)*

E03.1 Congenital hypothyroidism without goiter
Aplasia of thyroid (with myxedema)
Congenital atrophy of thyroid
Congenital hypothyroidism NOS

E03.2 Hypothyroidism due to medicaments and other exogenous substances
Code first poisoning due to drug or toxin, if applicable (T36-T65 with fifth or sixth character 1-4 or 6)
Use additional code for adverse effect, if applicable, to identify drug (T36-T50 with fifth or sixth character 5)

E03.3 Postinfectious hypothyroidism

E03.4 Atrophy of thyroid (acquired)

> **EXCLUDES 1** *congenital atrophy of thyroid (E03.1)*

E03.5 Myxedema coma   `MCC` `HCC`

E03.8 Other specified hypothyroidism

E03.9 Hypothyroidism, unspecified
Myxedema NOS

✓4ᵗʰ E04 Other nontoxic goiter

> **EXCLUDES 1** *congenital goiter (NOS) (diffuse) (parenchymatous) (E03.0)*
> *iodine-deficiency related goiter (E00-E02)*

E04.0 Nontoxic diffuse goiter
Diffuse (colloid) nontoxic goiter
Simple nontoxic goiter

E04.1 Nontoxic single thyroid nodule
Colloid nodule (cystic) (thyroid)
Nontoxic uninodular goiter
Thyroid (cystic) nodule NOS
DEF: Enlarged thyroid, commonly due to decreased thyroid production, with a single nodule. No clinical hypothyroidism.

E04.2 Nontoxic multinodular goiter
Cystic goiter NOS
Multinodular (cystic) goiter NOS
DEF: Enlarged thyroid, commonly due to decreased thyroid production with multiple nodules. No clinical hypothyroidism.

E04.8 Other specified nontoxic goiter

E04.9 Nontoxic goiter, unspecified
Goiter NOS
Nodular goiter (nontoxic) NOS

✓4ᵗʰ E05 Thyrotoxicosis [hyperthyroidism]

> **EXCLUDES 1** *chronic thyroiditis with transient thyrotoxicosis (E06.2)*
> *neonatal thyrotoxicosis (P72.1)*

DEF: Excessive quantities of hormones from the thyroid gland caused by overproduction or loss of storage ability.

✓5ᵗʰ E05.0 Thyrotoxicosis with diffuse goiter
Exophthalmic or toxic goiter NOS
Graves' disease
Toxic diffuse goiter
DEF: Diffuse thyroid enlargement accompanied by hyperthyroidism, bulging eyes, and dermopathy.

E05.00 Thyrotoxicosis with diffuse goiter without thyrotoxic crisis or storm

E05.01 Thyrotoxicosis with diffuse goiter with thyrotoxic crisis or storm   `MCC`

Goiter

Pyramidal lobe
Thyroid cartilage
Healthy thyroid
Goiter (hyperfunctioning thyroid)

✓5ᵗʰ E05.1 Thyrotoxicosis with toxic single thyroid nodule
Thyrotoxicosis with toxic uninodular goiter
DEF: Symptomatic hyperthyroidism with a single nodule on the enlarged thyroid gland. Onset of symptoms can be abrupt and include extreme nervousness, insomnia, weight loss, tremors, and psychosis or coma.

E05.10 Thyrotoxicosis with toxic single thyroid nodule without thyrotoxic crisis or storm

E05.11 Thyrotoxicosis with toxic single thyroid nodule with thyrotoxic crisis or storm   `MCC`

✓5ᵗʰ E05.2 Thyrotoxicosis with toxic multinodular goiter
Toxic nodular goiter NOS

E05.20 Thyrotoxicosis with toxic multinodular goiter without thyrotoxic crisis or storm

E05.21 Thyrotoxicosis with toxic multinodular goiter with thyrotoxic crisis or storm   `MCC`

✓5ᵗʰ E05.3 Thyrotoxicosis from ectopic thyroid tissue

E05.30 Thyrotoxicosis from ectopic thyroid tissue without thyrotoxic crisis or storm

E05.31 Thyrotoxicosis from ectopic thyroid tissue with thyrotoxic crisis or storm   `MCC`

✓ Additional Character Required   ✓x7ᵗʰ Placeholder   Unacceptable PDx   Questionable PDx   Manifestation   Unspecified Dx   H1-H14 HAC   HCC CMS-HCC Dx   HIV HIV Dx

ICD-10-CM 2021   521

√5ᵗʰ **E05.4** Thyrotoxicosis factitia

E05.40 **Thyrotoxicosis factitia** without thyrotoxic crisis or storm

E05.41 **Thyrotoxicosis factitia** with thyrotoxic crisis or storm   MCC

√5ᵗʰ **E05.8** **Other thyrotoxicosis**
Overproduction of thyroid-stimulating hormone

E05.80 **Other thyrotoxicosis** without thyrotoxic crisis or storm

E05.81 **Other thyrotoxicosis** with thyrotoxic crisis or storm   MCC

√5ᵗʰ **E05.9** **Thyrotoxicosis, unspecified**
Hyperthyroidism NOS

E05.90 **Thyrotoxicosis, unspecified** without thyrotoxic crisis or storm

E05.91 **Thyrotoxicosis, unspecified** with thyrotoxic crisis or storm   MCC

√4ᵗʰ **E06** **Thyroiditis**
EXCLUDES 1   postpartum thyroiditis (O90.5)
DEF: Inflammation of the thyroid gland.

E06.0 **Acute thyroiditis**   CC
Abscess of thyroid
Pyogenic thyroiditis
Suppurative thyroiditis
Use additional code (B95-B97) to identify infectious agent

E06.1 **Subacute thyroiditis**
de Quervain thyroiditis
Giant-cell thyroiditis
Granulomatous thyroiditis
Nonsuppurative thyroiditis
Viral thyroiditis
EXCLUDES 1   autoimmune thyroiditis (E06.3)

E06.2 **Chronic thyroiditis with transient thyrotoxicosis**
EXCLUDES 1   autoimmune thyroiditis (E06.3)

E06.3 **Autoimmune thyroiditis**
Hashimoto's thyroiditis
Hashitoxicosis (transient)
Lymphadenoid goiter
Lymphocytic thyroiditis
Struma lymphomatosa

E06.4 **Drug-induced thyroiditis**
Use additional code for adverse effect, if applicable, to identify drug (T36-T50 with fifth or sixth character 5)

E06.5 **Other chronic thyroiditis**
Chronic fibrous thyroiditis
Chronic thyroiditis NOS
Ligneous thyroiditis
Riedel thyroiditis

E06.9 **Thyroiditis, unspecified**

√4ᵗʰ **E07** **Other disorders of thyroid**

E07.0 **Hypersecretion of calcitonin**
C-cell hyperplasia of thyroid
Hypersecretion of thyrocalcitonin

E07.1 **Dyshormogenetic goiter**
Familial dyshormogenetic goiter
Pendred's syndrome
EXCLUDES 1   transitory congenital goiter with normal function (P72.0)

√5ᵗʰ **E07.8** **Other specified disorders of thyroid**

E07.81 **Sick-euthyroid syndrome**
Euthyroid sick-syndrome
DEF: Thyroid dysfunction caused by abnormal levels of thyroid hormones T3 and/or T4. This syndrome is often associated with starvation or critical illness.

E07.89 **Other specified disorders of thyroid**
Abnormality of thyroid-binding globulin
Hemorrhage of thyroid
Infarction of thyroid

E07.9 **Disorder of thyroid, unspecified**

Diabetes mellitus (E08-E13)

AHA: 2020,1Q,12; 2018,2Q,6; 2017,4Q,100-101; 2016,2Q,36; 2016,1Q,11-13; 2013,4Q,114; 2013,3Q,20

√4ᵗʰ **E08** **Diabetes mellitus** due to underlying condition
Code first the underlying condition, such as:
    congenital rubella (P35.0)
    Cushing's syndrome (E24.-)
    cystic fibrosis (E84.-)
    malignant neoplasm (C00-C96)
    malnutrition (E40-E46)
    pancreatitis and other diseases of the pancreas (K85-K86.-)
Use additional code to identify control using:
    insulin (Z79.4)
    oral antidiabetic drugs (Z79.84)
    oral hypoglycemic drugs (Z79.84)
EXCLUDES 1   drug or chemical induced diabetes mellitus (E09.-)
    gestational diabetes (O24.4-)
    neonatal diabetes mellitus (P70.2)
    postpancreatectomy diabetes mellitus (E13.-)
    postprocedural diabetes mellitus (E13.-)
    secondary diabetes mellitus NEC (E13.-)
    type 1 diabetes mellitus (E10.-)
    type 2 diabetes mellitus (E11.-)

√5ᵗʰ **E08.0** **Diabetes mellitus due to underlying condition with hyperosmolarity**
DEF: Diabetic hyperosmolarity: Extremely high levels of glucose in the blood without ketones.

E08.00 **Diabetes mellitus due to underlying condition with hyperosmolarity** without nonketotic hyperglycemic-hyperosmolar coma (NKHHC)   MCC H9 HCC

E08.01 **Diabetes mellitus due to underlying condition with hyperosmolarity** with coma   MCC H9 HCC

√5ᵗʰ **E08.1** **Diabetes mellitus due to underlying condition with ketoacidosis**
DEF: Diabetic ketoacidosis: Potentially life-threatening complication due to a shortage of insulin in which the body switches to burning fatty acids and producing acidic ketone bodies.

E08.10 **Diabetes mellitus due to underlying condition with ketoacidosis** without coma   MCC H9 HCC

E08.11 **Diabetes mellitus due to underlying condition with ketoacidosis** with coma   MCC HCC

√5ᵗʰ **E08.2** **Diabetes mellitus due to underlying condition with kidney complications**
AHA: 2019,3Q,3; 2018,4Q,88

E08.21 **Diabetes mellitus due to underlying condition with diabetic nephropathy**   HCC
Diabetes mellitus due to underlying condition with intercapillary glomerulosclerosis
Diabetes mellitus due to underlying condition with intracapillary glomerulonephrosis
Diabetes mellitus due to underlying condition with Kimmelstiel-Wilson disease

E08.22 **Diabetes mellitus due to underlying condition with diabetic chronic kidney disease**   HCC
Use additional code to identify stage of chronic kidney disease (N18.1-N18.6)

E08.29 **Diabetes mellitus due to underlying condition with other diabetic kidney complication**   HCC
Renal tubular degeneration in diabetes mellitus due to underlying condition

N Newborn: 0   P Pediatric: 0-17   M Maternity: 9-64   A Adult: 15-124   MCC Major Complication/Comorbidity   CC Complication/Comorbidity   SW Severe Wound Dx

522   ICD-10-CM 2021

√5ᵗʰ **E08.3** **Diabetes mellitus due to underlying condition with ophthalmic complications**
AHA: 2016,4Q,11-13

One of the following 7th characters is to be assigned to codes in subcategories E08.32, E08.33, E08.34, E08.35, and E08.37 to designate laterality of the disease:
1 right eye
2 left eye
3 bilateral
9 unspecified eye

√6ᵗʰ **E08.31** **Diabetes mellitus due to underlying condition with unspecified diabetic retinopathy**
DEF: Diabetic retinopathy: Diabetic complication from damage to the retinal vessels resulting in vision problems that can progress to blindness.

E08.311 *Diabetes mellitus due to underlying condition with unspecified diabetic retinopathy with macular edema* HCC

E08.319 *Diabetes mellitus due to underlying condition with unspecified diabetic retinopathy without macular edema* HCC

√6ᵗʰ **E08.32** **Diabetes mellitus due to underlying condition with mild nonproliferative diabetic retinopathy**
Diabetes mellitus due to underlying condition with nonproliferative diabetic retinopathy NOS

√7ᵗʰ *E08.321* *Diabetes mellitus due to underlying condition with mild nonproliferative diabetic retinopathy with macular edema* HCC

√7ᵗʰ *E08.329* *Diabetes mellitus due to underlying condition with mild nonproliferative diabetic retinopathy without macular edema* HCC

√6ᵗʰ **E08.33** **Diabetes mellitus due to underlying condition with moderate nonproliferative diabetic retinopathy**

√7ᵗʰ *E08.331* *Diabetes mellitus due to underlying condition with moderate nonproliferative diabetic retinopathy with macular edema* HCC

√7ᵗʰ *E08.339* *Diabetes mellitus due to underlying condition with moderate nonproliferative diabetic retinopathy without macular edema* HCC

√6ᵗʰ **E08.34** **Diabetes mellitus due to underlying condition with severe nonproliferative diabetic retinopathy**

√7ᵗʰ *E08.341* *Diabetes mellitus due to underlying condition with severe nonproliferative diabetic retinopathy with macular edema* HCC

√7ᵗʰ *E08.349* *Diabetes mellitus due to underlying condition with severe nonproliferative diabetic retinopathy without macular edema* HCC

√6ᵗʰ **E08.35** **Diabetes mellitus due to underlying condition with proliferative diabetic retinopathy**

√7ᵗʰ *E08.351* *Diabetes mellitus due to underlying condition with proliferative diabetic retinopathy with macular edema* HCC

√7ᵗʰ *E08.352* *Diabetes mellitus due to underlying condition with proliferative diabetic retinopathy with traction retinal detachment involving the macula* HCC

√7ᵗʰ *E08.353* *Diabetes mellitus due to underlying condition with proliferative diabetic retinopathy with traction retinal detachment not involving the macula* HCC

√7ᵗʰ *E08.354* *Diabetes mellitus due to underlying condition with proliferative diabetic retinopathy with combined traction retinal detachment and rhegmatogenous retinal detachment* HCC

√7ᵗʰ *E08.355* *Diabetes mellitus due to underlying condition with stable proliferative diabetic retinopathy* HCC

√7ᵗʰ *E08.359* *Diabetes mellitus due to underlying condition with proliferative diabetic retinopathy without macular edema* HCC

E08.36 *Diabetes mellitus due to underlying condition with diabetic cataract* HCC
AHA: 2019,2Q,30-31; 2016,4Q,142

√x7ᵗʰ **E08.37** *Diabetes mellitus due to underlying condition with diabetic macular edema, resolved following treatment* HCC

E08.39 *Diabetes mellitus due to underlying condition with other diabetic ophthalmic complication* HCC
Use additional code to identify manifestation, such as:
diabetic glaucoma (H40-H42)

√5ᵗʰ **E08.4** **Diabetes mellitus due to underlying condition with neurological complications**

E08.40 *Diabetes mellitus due to underlying condition with diabetic neuropathy, unspecified* HCC

E08.41 *Diabetes mellitus due to underlying condition with diabetic mononeuropathy* HCC

E08.42 *Diabetes mellitus due to underlying condition with diabetic polyneuropathy*
Diabetes mellitus due to underlying condition with diabetic neuralgia

E08.43 *Diabetes mellitus due to underlying condition with diabetic autonomic (poly)neuropathy* HCC
Diabetes mellitus due to underlying condition with diabetic gastroparesis
AHA: 2013,4Q,114

E08.44 *Diabetes mellitus due to underlying condition with diabetic amyotrophy* HCC

E08.49 *Diabetes mellitus due to underlying condition with other diabetic neurological complication* HCC

√5ᵗʰ **E08.5** **Diabetes mellitus due to underlying condition with circulatory complications**

E08.51 *Diabetes mellitus due to underlying condition with diabetic peripheral angiopathy without gangrene* HCC
AHA: 2018,3Q,3-4; 2018,2Q,7

E08.52 *Diabetes mellitus due to underlying condition with diabetic peripheral angiopathy with gangrene* CC HCC
Diabetes mellitus due to underlying condition with diabetic gangrene
AHA: 2020,2Q,18; 2018,3Q,3; 2018,2Q,7; 2017,4Q,102

E08.59 *Diabetes mellitus due to underlying condition with other circulatory complications* HCC

√5ᵗʰ **E08.6** **Diabetes mellitus due to underlying condition with other specified complications**

√6ᵗʰ **E08.61** **Diabetes mellitus due to underlying condition with diabetic arthropathy**

E08.610 *Diabetes mellitus due to underlying condition with diabetic neuropathic arthropathy* HCC
Diabetes mellitus due to underlying condition with Charcôt's joints
DEF: Charcot's joint: Progressive neurologic arthropathy in which chronic degeneration of joints in the weight-bearing areas with peripheral hypertrophy occurs as a complication of a neuropathy disorder. Supporting structures relax from a loss of sensation resulting in chronic joint instability.

E08.618 *Diabetes mellitus due to underlying condition with other diabetic arthropathy* HCC
AHA: 2018,2Q,6

√6ᵗʰ **E08.62** **Diabetes mellitus due to underlying condition with skin complications**

E08.620 *Diabetes mellitus due to underlying condition with diabetic dermatitis* HCC
Diabetes mellitus due to underlying condition with diabetic necrobiosis lipoidica

E08.621 *Diabetes mellitus due to underlying condition with foot ulcer* HCC
Use additional code to identify site of ulcer (L97.4-, L97.5-)
AHA: 2020,2Q,19

Chapter 4. Endocrine, Nutritional and Metabolic Diseases

E08.622   **Diabetes mellitus due to underlying condition with other skin ulcer**   HCC
Use additional code to identify site of ulcer (L97.1-L97.9, L98.41-L98.49)
AHA: 2017,4Q,17

E08.628   **Diabetes mellitus due to underlying condition with other skin complications**   HCC

√6ᵗʰ **E08.63**   **Diabetes mellitus due to underlying condition with oral complications**

E08.630   **Diabetes mellitus due to underlying condition with periodontal disease**

E08.638   **Diabetes mellitus due to underlying condition with other oral complications**   HCC

√6ᵗʰ **E08.64**   **Diabetes mellitus due to underlying condition with hypoglycemia**
AHA: 2017,1Q,42

E08.641   **Diabetes mellitus due to underlying condition with hypoglycemia with coma**   MCC HCC

E08.649   **Diabetes mellitus due to underlying condition with hypoglycemia without coma**   HCC
AHA: 2016,3Q,42; 2015,3Q,21

E08.65   **Diabetes mellitus due to underlying condition with hyperglycemia**   HCC
AHA: 2017,1Q,42; 2013,3Q,20

E08.69   **Diabetes mellitus due to underlying condition with other specified complication**   HCC
Use additional code to identify complication
AHA: 2016,4Q,141; 2016,1Q,13

E08.8   **Diabetes mellitus due to underlying condition with unspecified complications**   HCC

E08.9   **Diabetes mellitus due to underlying condition without complications**   HCC
AHA: 2020,2Q,18

√4ᵗʰ **E09**   **Drug or chemical induced diabetes mellitus**
Code first poisoning due to drug or toxin, if applicable (T36-T65 with fifth or sixth character 1-4 or 6)
Use additional code for adverse effect, if applicable, to identify drug (T36-T50 with fifth or sixth character 5)
Use additional code to identify control using:
    insulin (Z79.4)
    oral antidiabetic drugs (Z79.84)
    oral hypoglycemic drugs (Z79.84)
EXCLUDES 1   diabetes mellitus due to underlying condition (E08.-)
    gestational diabetes (O24.4-)
    neonatal diabetes mellitus (P70.2)
    postpancreatectomy diabetes mellitus (E13.-)
    postprocedural diabetes mellitus (E13.-)
    secondary diabetes mellitus NEC (E13.-)
    type 1 diabetes mellitus (E10.-)
    type 2 diabetes mellitus (E11.-)

√5ᵗʰ **E09.0**   **Drug or chemical induced diabetes mellitus with hyperosmolarity**
DEF: Diabetic hyperosmolarity: Extremely high levels of glucose in the blood without ketones.

E09.00   **Drug or chemical induced diabetes mellitus with hyperosmolarity without nonketotic hyperglycemic-hyperosmolar coma (NKHHC)**   MCC H9 HCC

E09.01   **Drug or chemical induced diabetes mellitus with hyperosmolarity with coma**   MCC H9 HCC

√5ᵗʰ **E09.1**   **Drug or chemical induced diabetes mellitus with ketoacidosis**
DEF: Diabetic ketoacidosis: Potentially life-threatening complication due to a shortage of insulin in which the body switches to burning fatty acids and producing acidic ketone bodies.

E09.10   **Drug or chemical induced diabetes mellitus with ketoacidosis without coma**   MCC H9 HCC

E09.11   **Drug or chemical induced diabetes mellitus with ketoacidosis with coma**   MCC HCC

√5ᵗʰ **E09.2**   **Drug or chemical induced diabetes mellitus with kidney complications**
AHA: 2019,3Q,3; 2018,4Q,88

E09.21   **Drug or chemical induced diabetes mellitus with diabetic nephropathy**   HCC
Drug or chemical induced diabetes mellitus with intercapillary glomerulosclerosis
Drug or chemical induced diabetes mellitus with intracapillary glomerulonephrosis
Drug or chemical induced diabetes mellitus with Kimmelstiel-Wilson disease

E09.22   **Drug or chemical induced diabetes mellitus with diabetic chronic kidney disease**   HCC
Use additional code to identify stage of chronic kidney disease (N18.1-N18.6)

E09.29   **Drug or chemical induced diabetes mellitus with other diabetic kidney complication**   HCC
Drug or chemical induced diabetes mellitus with renal tubular degeneration

√5ᵗʰ **E09.3**   **Drug or chemical induced diabetes mellitus with ophthalmic complications**
AHA: 2016,4Q,11-13

> One of the following 7th characters is to be assigned to codes in subcategories E09.32, E09.33, E09.34, E09.35, and E09.37 to designate laterality of the disease:
> 1   right eye
> 2   left eye
> 3   bilateral
> 9   unspecified eye

√6ᵗʰ **E09.31**   **Drug or chemical induced diabetes mellitus with unspecified diabetic retinopathy**
DEF: Diabetic retinopathy: Diabetic complication from damage to the retinal vessels resulting in vision problems that can progress to blindness.

E09.311   **Drug or chemical induced diabetes mellitus with unspecified diabetic retinopathy with macular edema**   HCC

E09.319   **Drug or chemical induced diabetes mellitus with unspecified diabetic retinopathy without macular edema**   HCC

√6ᵗʰ **E09.32**   **Drug or chemical induced diabetes mellitus with mild nonproliferative diabetic retinopathy**
Drug or chemical induced diabetes mellitus with nonproliferative diabetic retinopathy NOS

√7ᵗʰ **E09.321**   **Drug or chemical induced diabetes mellitus with mild nonproliferative diabetic retinopathy with macular edema**   HCC

√7ᵗʰ **E09.329**   **Drug or chemical induced diabetes mellitus with mild nonproliferative diabetic retinopathy without macular edema**   HCC

√6ᵗʰ **E09.33**   **Drug or chemical induced diabetes mellitus with moderate nonproliferative diabetic retinopathy**

√7ᵗʰ **E09.331**   **Drug or chemical induced diabetes mellitus with moderate nonproliferative diabetic retinopathy with macular edema**   HCC

√7ᵗʰ **E09.339**   **Drug or chemical induced diabetes mellitus with moderate nonproliferative diabetic retinopathy without macular edema**   HCC

√6ᵗʰ **E09.34**   **Drug or chemical induced diabetes mellitus with severe nonproliferative diabetic retinopathy**

√7ᵗʰ **E09.341**   **Drug or chemical induced diabetes mellitus with severe nonproliferative diabetic retinopathy with macular edema**   HCC

√7ᵗʰ **E09.349**   **Drug or chemical induced diabetes mellitus with severe nonproliferative diabetic retinopathy without macular edema**   HCC

√6ᵗʰ **E09.35**   **Drug or chemical induced diabetes mellitus with proliferative diabetic retinopathy**

√7ᵗʰ **E09.351**   **Drug or chemical induced diabetes mellitus with proliferative diabetic retinopathy with macular edema**   HCC

√7ᵗʰ **E09.352**   **Drug or chemical induced diabetes mellitus with proliferative diabetic retinopathy with traction retinal detachment involving the macula**   HCC

√7ᵗʰ **E09.353** **Drug or chemical induced diabetes mellitus with proliferative diabetic retinopathy** with traction retinal detachment not involving the macula   HCC

√7ᵗʰ **E09.354** **Drug or chemical induced diabetes mellitus with proliferative diabetic retinopathy** with combined traction retinal detachment and rhegmatogenous retinal detachment   HCC

√7ᵗʰ **E09.355** **Drug or chemical induced diabetes mellitus** with stable **proliferative diabetic retinopathy**   HCC

√7ᵗʰ **E09.359** **Drug or chemical induced diabetes mellitus with proliferative diabetic retinopathy** without macular edema   HCC

E09.36 **Drug or chemical induced diabetes mellitus with diabetic** cataract   HCC
> **AHA:** 2019,2Q,30-31; 2016,4Q,142

√x7ᵗʰ **E09.37** **Drug or chemical induced diabetes mellitus with diabetic** macular edema, resolved following treatment   HCC

E09.39 **Drug or chemical induced diabetes mellitus with other diabetic ophthalmic complication**   HCC
> Use additional code to identify manifestation, such as:
> diabetic glaucoma (H40-H42)

√5ᵗʰ **E09.4** **Drug or chemical induced diabetes mellitus with** neurological complications

E09.40 **Drug or chemical induced diabetes mellitus with neurological complications with diabetic neuropathy, unspecified**   HCC

E09.41 **Drug or chemical induced diabetes mellitus with neurological complications with diabetic mononeuropathy**   HCC

E09.42 **Drug or chemical induced diabetes mellitus with neurological complications with diabetic polyneuropathy**   HCC
> Drug or chemical induced diabetes mellitus with diabetic neuralgia

E09.43 **Drug or chemical induced diabetes mellitus with neurological complications with diabetic** autonomic (poly)neuropathy   HCC
> Drug or chemical induced diabetes mellitus with diabetic gastroparesis
> **AHA:** 2013,4Q,114

E09.44 **Drug or chemical induced diabetes mellitus with neurological complications with diabetic amyotrophy**   HCC

E09.49 **Drug or chemical induced diabetes mellitus with neurological complications with other diabetic neurological complication**   HCC

√5ᵗʰ **E09.5** **Drug or chemical induced diabetes mellitus with** circulatory complications

E09.51 **Drug or chemical induced diabetes mellitus with diabetic** peripheral angiopathy without gangrene   HCC
> **AHA:** 2018,3Q,3-4; 2018,2Q,7

E09.52 **Drug or chemical induced diabetes mellitus with diabetic** peripheral angiopathy with gangrene   CC HCC
> Drug or chemical induced diabetes mellitus with diabetic gangrene
> **AHA:** 2020,2Q,18; 2018,3Q,3; 2018,2Q,7; 2017,4Q,102

E09.59 **Drug or chemical induced diabetes mellitus with other circulatory complications**   HCC

√5ᵗʰ **E09.6** **Drug or chemical induced diabetes mellitus with other specified complications**

√6ᵗʰ **E09.61** **Drug or chemical induced diabetes mellitus with diabetic** arthropathy

E09.610 **Drug or chemical induced diabetes mellitus with diabetic** neuropathic arthropathy   HCC
> Drug or chemical induced diabetes mellitus with Charcôt's joints
> **DEF:** Charcot's joint: Progressive neurologic arthropathy in which chronic degeneration of joints in the weight-bearing areas with peripheral hypertrophy occurs as a complication of a neuropathy disorder. Supporting structures relax from a loss of sensation resulting in chronic joint instability.

E09.618 **Drug or chemical induced diabetes mellitus with other diabetic arthropathy**   HCC
> **AHA:** 2018,2Q,6

√6ᵗʰ **E09.62** **Drug or chemical induced diabetes mellitus with** skin complications

E09.620 **Drug or chemical induced diabetes mellitus with** diabetic dermatitis   HCC
> Drug or chemical induced diabetes mellitus with diabetic necrobiosis lipoidica

E09.621 **Drug or chemical induced diabetes mellitus with** foot ulcer   HCC
> Use additional code to identify site of ulcer (L97.4-, L97.5-)
> **AHA:** 2020,2Q,19

E09.622 **Drug or chemical induced diabetes mellitus with other skin ulcer**   HCC
> Use additional code to identify site of ulcer (L97.1-L97.9, L98.41-L98.49)
> **AHA:** 2017,4Q,17

E09.628 **Drug or chemical induced diabetes mellitus with other skin complications**   HCC

√6ᵗʰ **E09.63** **Drug or chemical induced diabetes mellitus with** oral complications

E09.630 **Drug or chemical induced diabetes mellitus with** periodontal disease   HCC

E09.638 **Drug or chemical induced diabetes mellitus with other oral complications**   HCC

√6ᵗʰ **E09.64** **Drug or chemical induced diabetes mellitus with** hypoglycemia
> **AHA:** 2017,1Q,42

E09.641 **Drug or chemical induced diabetes mellitus with hypoglycemia** with coma   MCC HCC

E09.649 **Drug or chemical induced diabetes mellitus with hypoglycemia** without coma   HCC
> **AHA:** 2016,3Q,42; 2015,3Q,21

E09.65 **Drug or chemical induced diabetes mellitus with** hyperglycemia   HCC
> **AHA:** 2017,1Q,42; 2013,3Q,20

E09.69 **Drug or chemical induced diabetes mellitus with other specified complication**   HCC
> Use additional code to identify complication
> **AHA:** 2016,4Q,141; 2016,1Q,13

E09.8 **Drug or chemical induced diabetes mellitus with unspecified complications**   HCC

E09.9 **Drug or chemical induced diabetes mellitus** without complications   HCC
> **AHA:** 2020,2Q,18

☑ Additional Character Required   √x7ᵗʰ Placeholder   Unacceptable PDx   Questionable PDx   Manifestation   Unspecified Dx   H1 - H14 HAC   HCC CMS-HCC Dx   HIV HIV Dx

ICD-10-CM 2021   525

√4ᵗʰ **E10** **Type 1 diabetes mellitus**

> INCLUDES brittle diabetes (mellitus)
> diabetes (mellitus) due to autoimmune process
> diabetes (mellitus) due to immune mediated pancreatic
> islet beta-cell destruction
> idiopathic diabetes (mellitus)
> juvenile onset diabetes (mellitus)
> ketosis-prone diabetes (mellitus)
>
> EXCLUDES 1 *diabetes mellitus due to underlying condition (E08.-)*
> *drug or chemical induced diabetes mellitus (E09.-)*
> *gestational diabetes (O24.4-)*
> *hyperglycemia NOS (R73.9)*
> *neonatal diabetes mellitus (P70.2)*
> *postpancreatectomy diabetes mellitus (E13.-)*
> *postprocedural diabetes mellitus (E13.-)*
> *secondary diabetes mellitus NEC (E13.-)*
> *type 2 diabetes mellitus (E11.-)*

√5ᵗʰ **E10.1** **Type 1 diabetes mellitus with ketoacidosis**

> **AHA:** 2013,3Q,20
> **DEF:** Diabetic ketoacidosis: Potentially life-threatening complication due to a shortage of insulin in which the body switches to burning fatty acids and producing acidic ketone bodies.

    E10.10 **Type 1 diabetes mellitus with ketoacidosis without coma** MCC H9 HCC

    E10.11 **Type 1 diabetes mellitus with ketoacidosis with coma** MCC HCC

√5ᵗʰ **E10.2** **Type 1 diabetes mellitus with kidney complications**

> **AHA:** 2019,3Q,3; 2018,4Q,88

    E10.21 **Type 1 diabetes mellitus with diabetic nephropathy** HCC

> Type 1 diabetes mellitus with intercapillary glomerulosclerosis
> Type 1 diabetes mellitus with intracapillary glomerulonephrosis
> Type 1 diabetes mellitus with Kimmelstiel-Wilson disease

    E10.22 **Type 1 diabetes mellitus with diabetic chronic kidney disease** HCC

> Use additional code to identify stage of chronic kidney disease (N18.1-N18.6)

    E10.29 **Type 1 diabetes mellitus with other diabetic kidney complication** HCC

> Type 1 diabetes mellitus with renal tubular degeneration
> **AHA:** 2016,1Q,13

√5ᵗʰ **E10.3** **Type 1 diabetes mellitus with ophthalmic complications**

> **AHA:** 2016,4Q,11-13
>
> One of the following 7th characters is to be assigned to codes in subcategories E10.32, E10.33, E10.34, E10.35, and E10.37 to designate laterality of the disease:
> 1   right eye
> 2   left eye
> 3   bilateral
> 9   unspecified eye

√6ᵗʰ **E10.31** **Type 1 diabetes mellitus with unspecified diabetic retinopathy**

> **DEF:** Diabetic retinopathy: Diabetic complication from damage to the retinal vessels resulting in vision problems that can progress to blindness.

    E10.311 **Type 1 diabetes mellitus with unspecified diabetic retinopathy with macular edema** HCC

    E10.319 **Type 1 diabetes mellitus with unspecified diabetic retinopathy without macular edema** HCC

√6ᵗʰ **E10.32** **Type 1 diabetes mellitus with mild nonproliferative diabetic retinopathy**

> Type 1 diabetes mellitus with nonproliferative diabetic retinopathy NOS

    √7ᵗʰ **E10.321** **Type 1 diabetes mellitus with mild nonproliferative diabetic retinopathy with macular edema** HCC

    √7ᵗʰ **E10.329** **Type 1 diabetes mellitus with mild nonproliferative diabetic retinopathy without macular edema** HCC

√6ᵗʰ **E10.33** **Type 1 diabetes mellitus with moderate nonproliferative diabetic retinopathy**

    √7ᵗʰ **E10.331** **Type 1 diabetes mellitus with moderate nonproliferative diabetic retinopathy with macular edema** HCC

    √7ᵗʰ **E10.339** **Type 1 diabetes mellitus with moderate nonproliferative diabetic retinopathy without macular edema** HCC

√6ᵗʰ **E10.34** **Type 1 diabetes mellitus with severe nonproliferative diabetic retinopathy**

    √7ᵗʰ **E10.341** **Type 1 diabetes mellitus with severe nonproliferative diabetic retinopathy with macular edema** HCC

    √7ᵗʰ **E10.349** **Type 1 diabetes mellitus with severe nonproliferative diabetic retinopathy without macular edema** HCC

√6ᵗʰ **E10.35** **Type 1 diabetes mellitus with proliferative diabetic retinopathy**

    √7ᵗʰ **E10.351** **Type 1 diabetes mellitus with proliferative diabetic retinopathy with macular edema** HCC

    √7ᵗʰ **E10.352** **Type 1 diabetes mellitus with proliferative diabetic retinopathy with traction retinal detachment involving the macula** HCC

    √7ᵗʰ **E10.353** **Type 1 diabetes mellitus with proliferative diabetic retinopathy with traction retinal detachment not involving the macula** HCC

    √7ᵗʰ **E10.354** **Type 1 diabetes mellitus with proliferative diabetic retinopathy with combined traction retinal detachment and rhegmatogenous retinal detachment** HCC

    √7ᵗʰ **E10.355** **Type 1 diabetes mellitus with stable proliferative diabetic retinopathy** HCC

    √7ᵗʰ **E10.359** **Type 1 diabetes mellitus with proliferative diabetic retinopathy without macular edema** HCC

    E10.36 **Type 1 diabetes mellitus with diabetic cataract** HCC

> **AHA:** 2019,2Q,30-31; 2016,4Q,142

√x7ᵗʰ **E10.37** **Type 1 diabetes mellitus with diabetic macular edema, resolved following treatment** HCC

    E10.39 **Type 1 diabetes mellitus with other diabetic ophthalmic complication** HCC

> Use additional code to identify manifestation, such as:
> diabetic glaucoma (H40-H42)

√5ᵗʰ **E10.4** **Type 1 diabetes mellitus with neurological complications**

    E10.40 **Type 1 diabetes mellitus with diabetic neuropathy, unspecified** HCC

    E10.41 **Type 1 diabetes mellitus with diabetic mononeuropathy** HCC

    E10.42 **Type 1 diabetes mellitus with diabetic polyneuropathy** HCC

> Type 1 diabetes mellitus with diabetic neuralgia

    E10.43 **Type 1 diabetes mellitus with diabetic autonomic (poly)neuropathy** HCC

> Type 1 diabetes mellitus with diabetic gastroparesis
> **AHA:** 2013,4Q,114

    E10.44 **Type 1 diabetes mellitus with diabetic amyotrophy** HCC

    E10.49 **Type 1 diabetes mellitus with other diabetic neurological complication** HCC

√5ᵗʰ **E10.5** **Type 1 diabetes mellitus with circulatory complications**

    E10.51 **Type 1 diabetes mellitus with diabetic peripheral angiopathy without gangrene** HCC

> **AHA:** 2018,3Q,3-4; 2018,2Q,7

    E10.52 **Type 1 diabetes mellitus with diabetic peripheral angiopathy with gangrene** CC HCC

> Type 1 diabetes mellitus with diabetic gangrene
> **AHA:** 2020,2Q,18; 2018,3Q,3; 2018,2Q,7; 2017,4Q,102

    E10.59 **Type 1 diabetes mellitus with other circulatory complications** HCC

N Newborn: 0   P Pediatric: 0-17   M Maternity: 9-64   A Adult: 15-124   MCC Major Complication/Comorbidity   CC Complication/Comorbidity   SW Severe Wound Dx

526   ICD-10-CM 2021

✓5ᵗʰ **E10.6 Type 1 diabetes mellitus with other specified complications**

✓6ᵗʰ   **E10.61 Type 1 diabetes mellitus with diabetic arthropathy**

       E10.610 Type 1 diabetes mellitus with diabetic neuropathic arthropathy `HCC`

         Type 1 diabetes mellitus with Charcôt's joints

         DEF: Charcot's joint: Progressive neurologic arthropathy in which chronic degeneration of joints in the weight-bearing areas with peripheral hypertrophy occurs as a complication of a neuropathy disorder. Supporting structures relax from a loss of sensation resulting in chronic joint instability.

       E10.618 Type 1 diabetes mellitus with other diabetic arthropathy `HCC`

         AHA: 2018,2Q,6

✓6ᵗʰ   **E10.62 Type 1 diabetes mellitus with skin complications**

       E10.620 Type 1 diabetes mellitus with diabetic dermatitis `HCC`

         Type 1 diabetes mellitus with diabetic necrobiosis lipoidica

       E10.621 Type 1 diabetes mellitus with foot ulcer `HCC`

         Use additional code to identify site of ulcer (L97.4-, L97.5-)

         AHA: 2020,2Q,19

       E10.622 Type 1 diabetes mellitus with other skin ulcer `HCC`

         Use additional code to identify site of ulcer (L97.1-L97.9, L98.41-L98.49)

         AHA: 2017,4Q,17

       E10.628 Type 1 diabetes mellitus with other skin complications `HCC`

✓6ᵗʰ   **E10.63 Type 1 diabetes mellitus with oral complications**

       E10.630 Type 1 diabetes mellitus with periodontal disease `HCC`

       E10.638 Type 1 diabetes mellitus with other oral complications `HCC`

✓6ᵗʰ   **E10.64 Type 1 diabetes mellitus with hypoglycemia**

     AHA: 2017,1Q,42

       E10.641 Type 1 diabetes mellitus with hypoglycemia with coma `MCC` `HCC`

       E10.649 Type 1 diabetes mellitus with hypoglycemia without coma `HCC`

         AHA: 2016,3Q,42; 2016,1Q,13; 2015,3Q,21

       E10.65 Type 1 diabetes mellitus with hyperglycemia `HCC`

         AHA: 2017,1Q,42; 2013,3Q,20

       E10.69 Type 1 diabetes mellitus with other specified complication `HCC`

         Use additional code to identify complication

         AHA: 2016,4Q,141; 2016,1Q,13

E10.8 Type 1 diabetes mellitus with unspecified complications `HCC`

E10.9 Type 1 diabetes mellitus without complications `HCC`

   AHA: 2020,2Q,18

✓4ᵗʰ **E11 Type 2 diabetes mellitus**

   `INCLUDES`   diabetes (mellitus) due to insulin secretory defect

          diabetes NOS

          insulin resistant diabetes (mellitus)

   Use additional code to identify control using:

     insulin (Z79.4)

     oral antidiabetic drugs (Z79.84)

     oral hypoglycemic drugs (Z79.84)

   `EXCLUDES 1`   *diabetes mellitus due to underlying condition (E08.-)*

          drug or chemical induced diabetes mellitus (E09.-)

          gestational diabetes (O24.4-)

          neonatal diabetes mellitus (P70.2)

          postpancreatectomy diabetes mellitus (E13.-)

          postprocedural diabetes mellitus (E13.-)

          secondary diabetes mellitus NEC (E13.-)

          type 1 diabetes mellitus (E10.-)

   AHA: 2020,1Q,12; 2016,2Q,10; 2013,1Q,26

✓5ᵗʰ **E11.0 Type 2 diabetes mellitus with hyperosmolarity**

   DEF: Diabetic hyperosmolarity: Extremely high levels of glucose in the blood without ketones.

     E11.00 Type 2 diabetes mellitus with hyperosmolarity without nonketotic hyperglycemic-hyperosmolar coma (NKHHC) `MCC` `H9` `HCC`

     E11.01 Type 2 diabetes mellitus with hyperosmolarity with coma `MCC` `H9` `HCC`

✓5ᵗʰ **E11.1 Type 2 diabetes mellitus with ketoacidosis**

   AHA: 2017,4Q,6

   DEF: Diabetic ketoacidosis: Potentially life-threatening complication due to a shortage of insulin in which the body switches to burning fatty acids and producing acidic ketone bodies.

     E11.10 Type 2 diabetes mellitus with ketoacidosis without coma `MCC` `HCC`

     E11.11 Type 2 diabetes mellitus with ketoacidosis with coma `MCC` `HCC`

✓5ᵗʰ **E11.2 Type 2 diabetes mellitus with kidney complications**

   AHA: 2019,3Q,3; 2018,4Q,88

     E11.21 Type 2 diabetes mellitus with diabetic nephropathy `HCC`

         Type 2 diabetes mellitus with intercapillary glomerulosclerosis

         Type 2 diabetes mellitus with intracapillary glomerulonephrosis

         Type 2 diabetes mellitus with Kimmelstiel-Wilson disease

     E11.22 Type 2 diabetes mellitus with diabetic chronic kidney disease `HCC`

         Use additional code to identify stage of chronic kidney disease (N18.1-N18.6)

     E11.29 Type 2 diabetes mellitus with other diabetic kidney complication `HCC`

         Type 2 diabetes mellitus with renal tubular degeneration

✓5ᵗʰ **E11.3 Type 2 diabetes mellitus with ophthalmic complications**

   AHA: 2016,4Q,11-13

> One of the following 7th characters is to be assigned to codes in subcategories E11.32, E11.33, E11.34, E11.35, and E11.37 to designate laterality of the disease:
>
> 1   right eye
> 2   left eye
> 3   bilateral
> 9   unspecified eye

✓6ᵗʰ **E11.31 Type 2 diabetes mellitus with unspecified diabetic retinopathy**

     DEF: Diabetic retinopathy: Diabetic complication from damage to the retinal vessels resulting in vision problems that can progress to blindness.

     E11.311 Type 2 diabetes mellitus with unspecified diabetic retinopathy with macular edema `HCC`

     E11.319 Type 2 diabetes mellitus with unspecified diabetic retinopathy without macular edema `HCC`

Chapter 4. Endocrine, Nutritional and Metabolic Diseases

√6ᵗʰ **E11.32** **Type 2 diabetes mellitus with** mild nonproliferative diabetic retinopathy
Type 2 diabetes mellitus with nonproliferative diabetic retinopathy NOS

   √7ᵗʰ **E11.321** **Type 2 diabetes mellitus with mild nonproliferative diabetic retinopathy with macular edema** HCC

   √7ᵗʰ **E11.329** **Type 2 diabetes mellitus with mild nonproliferative diabetic retinopathy without macular edema** HCC

√6ᵗʰ **E11.33** **Type 2 diabetes mellitus with** moderate nonproliferative diabetic retinopathy

   √7ᵗʰ **E11.331** **Type 2 diabetes mellitus with moderate nonproliferative diabetic retinopathy with macular edema** HCC

   √7ᵗʰ **E11.339** **Type 2 diabetes mellitus with moderate nonproliferative diabetic retinopathy without macular edema** HCC

√6ᵗʰ **E11.34** **Type 2 diabetes mellitus with** severe nonproliferative diabetic retinopathy

   √7ᵗʰ **E11.341** **Type 2 diabetes mellitus with severe nonproliferative diabetic retinopathy with macular edema** HCC

   √7ᵗʰ **E11.349** **Type 2 diabetes mellitus with severe nonproliferative diabetic retinopathy without macular edema** HCC

√6ᵗʰ **E11.35** **Type 2 diabetes mellitus with** proliferative **diabetic retinopathy**

   √7ᵗʰ **E11.351** **Type 2 diabetes mellitus with proliferative diabetic retinopathy with macular edema** HCC

   √7ᵗʰ **E11.352** **Type 2 diabetes mellitus with proliferative diabetic retinopathy with traction retinal detachment involving the macula** HCC

   √7ᵗʰ **E11.353** **Type 2 diabetes mellitus with proliferative diabetic retinopathy with traction retinal detachment not involving the macula** HCC

   √7ᵗʰ **E11.354** **Type 2 diabetes mellitus with proliferative diabetic retinopathy with combined traction retinal detachment and rhegmatogenous retinal detachment** HCC

   √7ᵗʰ **E11.355** **Type 2 diabetes mellitus with** stable **proliferative diabetic retinopathy** HCC

   √7ᵗʰ **E11.359** **Type 2 diabetes mellitus with proliferative diabetic retinopathy without macular edema** HCC

E11.36 **Type 2 diabetes mellitus with diabetic cataract** HCC
   AHA: 2019,2Q,30-31; 2016,4Q,142

√x7ᵗʰ **E11.37** **Type 2 diabetes mellitus with diabetic** macular **edema, resolved following treatment** HCC

E11.39 **Type 2 diabetes mellitus with other diabetic ophthalmic complication** HCC
   Use additional code to identify manifestation, such as:
     diabetic glaucoma (H40-H42)

√5ᵗʰ **E11.4** **Type 2 diabetes mellitus with** neurological complications

   E11.40 **Type 2 diabetes mellitus with diabetic** neuropathy, **unspecified** HCC
   AHA: 2013,4Q,129

   E11.41 **Type 2 diabetes mellitus with diabetic mononeuropathy** HCC

   E11.42 **Type 2 diabetes mellitus with diabetic polyneuropathy** HCC
   Type 2 diabetes mellitus with diabetic neuralgia
   AHA: 2020,1Q,12

   E11.43 **Type 2 diabetes mellitus with diabetic** autonomic **(poly)neuropathy** HCC
   Type 2 diabetes mellitus with diabetic gastroparesis
   AHA: 2013,4Q,114

   E11.44 **Type 2 diabetes mellitus with diabetic amyotrophy** HCC

   E11.49 **Type 2 diabetes mellitus with other diabetic neurological complication** HCC

√5ᵗʰ **E11.5** **Type 2 diabetes mellitus with** circulatory complications

   E11.51 **Type 2 diabetes mellitus with diabetic** peripheral **angiopathy without gangrene** HCC
   AHA: 2018,3Q,3-4; 2018,2Q,7

   E11.52 **Type 2 diabetes mellitus with diabetic** peripheral **angiopathy with gangrene** CC HCC
   Type 2 diabetes mellitus with diabetic gangrene
   AHA: 2020,2Q,18; 2018,3Q,3; 2018,2Q,7; 2017,4Q,102

   E11.59 **Type 2 diabetes mellitus with other circulatory complications** HCC

√5ᵗʰ **E11.6** **Type 2 diabetes mellitus with other specified complications**

  √6ᵗʰ **E11.61** **Type 2 diabetes mellitus with diabetic** arthropathy

    E11.610 **Type 2 diabetes mellitus with diabetic** neuropathic **arthropathy** HCC
    Type 2 diabetes mellitus with Charcôt's joints
    DEF: Charcot's joint: Progressive neurologic arthropathy in which chronic degeneration of joints in the weight-bearing areas with peripheral hypertrophy occurs as a complication of a neuropathy disorder. Supporting structures relax from a loss of sensation resulting in chronic joint instability.

    E11.618 **Type 2 diabetes mellitus with other diabetic arthropathy** HCC
    AHA: 2018,2Q,6

  √6ᵗʰ **E11.62** **Type 2 diabetes mellitus with** skin complications

    E11.620 **Type 2 diabetes mellitus with** diabetic **dermatitis** HCC
    Type 2 diabetes mellitus with diabetic necrobiosis lipoidica

    E11.621 **Type 2 diabetes mellitus with** foot **ulcer** HCC
    Use additional code to identify site of ulcer (L97.4-, L97.5-)
    AHA: 2020,2Q,19; 2020,1Q,12

    E11.622 **Type 2 diabetes mellitus with other skin ulcer** HCC
    Use additional code to identify site of ulcer (L97.1-L97.9, L98.41-L98.49)
    AHA: 2017,4Q,17

    E11.628 **Type 2 diabetes mellitus with other skin complications** HCC

  √6ᵗʰ **E11.63** **Type 2 diabetes mellitus with** oral complications

    E11.630 **Type 2 diabetes mellitus with** periodontal **disease** HCC

    E11.638 **Type 2 diabetes mellitus with other oral complications** HCC

  √6ᵗʰ **E11.64** **Type 2 diabetes mellitus with** hypoglycemia
    AHA: 2017,1Q,42

    E11.641 **Type 2 diabetes mellitus with hypoglycemia** with coma MCC HCC

    E11.649 **Type 2 diabetes mellitus with hypoglycemia** without coma HCC
    AHA: 2016,3Q,42; 2015,3Q,21

   E11.65 **Type 2 diabetes mellitus with hyperglycemia** HCC
   AHA: 2017,1Q,42; 2013,3Q,20

   E11.69 **Type 2 diabetes mellitus with other specified complication** HCC
   Use additional code to identify complication
   AHA: 2020,1Q,12; 2016,4Q,141; 2016,1Q,13

E11.8 **Type 2 diabetes mellitus with unspecified complications** HCC

E11.9 **Type 2 diabetes mellitus** without complications HCC
   AHA: 2020,2Q,18

☑4ᵗʰ **E13　Other specified diabetes mellitus**

INCLUDES　　diabetes mellitus due to genetic defects of beta-cell function
　　　　　　　diabetes mellitus due to genetic defects in insulin action
　　　　　　　postpancreatectomy diabetes mellitus
　　　　　　　postprocedural diabetes mellitus
　　　　　　　secondary diabetes mellitus NEC

Use additional code to identify control using:
insulin (Z79.4)
oral antidiabetic drugs (Z79.84)
oral hypoglycemic drugs (Z79.84)

EXCLUDES 1　diabetes (mellitus) due to autoimmune process (E10.-)
　　　　　　　diabetes (mellitus) due to immune mediated pancreatic islet beta-cell destruction (E10.-)
　　　　　　　diabetes mellitus due to underlying condition (E08.-)
　　　　　　　drug or chemical induced diabetes mellitus (E09.-)
　　　　　　　gestational diabetes (O24.4-)
　　　　　　　neonatal diabetes mellitus (P70.2)
　　　　　　　type 1 diabetes mellitus (E10.-)

AHA: 2018,3Q,4; 2016,1Q,11-13
TIP: Use this category when the diabetes is documented as diabetes type 1.5. Synonymous terms used in the documentation may also include combined diabetes type 1 and type 2, latent autoimmune diabetes of adults (LADA), slow-progressing type 1 diabetes, or double diabetes.
TIP: When postprocedural or postpancreatectomy hypoinsulinemia (E89.1) is documented with postprocedural or postpancreatectomy diabetes mellitus (E13.-), code E89.1 should be sequenced first.

☑5ᵗʰ **E13.0　Other specified diabetes mellitus with hyperosmolarity**
DEF: Diabetic hyperosmolarity: Extremely high levels of glucose in the blood without ketones.

E13.00　Other specified diabetes mellitus with hyperosmolarity without nonketotic hyperglycemic-hyperosmolar coma (NKHHC)　MCC H9 HCC
EXCLUDES 2　type 2 diabetes mellitus (E11.-)

E13.01　Other specified diabetes mellitus with hyperosmolarity with coma　MCC H9 HCC

☑5ᵗʰ **E13.1　Other specified diabetes mellitus with ketoacidosis**
AHA: 2016,2Q,10; 2013,1Q,26
DEF: Diabetic ketoacidosis: Potentially life-threatening complication due to a shortage of insulin in which the body switches to burning fatty acids and producing acidic ketone bodies.

E13.10　Other specified diabetes mellitus with ketoacidosis without coma　MCC H9 HCC

E13.11　Other specified diabetes mellitus with ketoacidosis with coma　MCC HCC

☑5ᵗʰ **E13.2　Other specified diabetes mellitus with kidney complications**
AHA: 2019,3Q,3; 2018,4Q,88

E13.21　Other specified diabetes mellitus with diabetic nephropathy　HCC
Other specified diabetes mellitus with intercapillary glomerulosclerosis
Other specified diabetes mellitus with intracapillary glomerulonephrosis
Other specified diabetes mellitus with Kimmelstiel-Wilson disease

E13.22　Other specified diabetes mellitus with diabetic chronic kidney disease　HCC
Use additional code to identify stage of chronic kidney disease (N18.1-N18.6)

E13.29　Other specified diabetes mellitus with other diabetic kidney complication　HCC
Other specified diabetes mellitus with renal tubular degeneration

☑5ᵗʰ **E13.3　Other specified diabetes mellitus with ophthalmic complications**
AHA: 2016,4Q,11-13

One of the following 7th characters is to be assigned to codes in subcategories E13.32, E13.33, E13.34, E13.35, and E13.37 to designate laterality of the disease:
1　right eye
2　left eye
3　bilateral
9　unspecified eye

☑6ᵗʰ **E13.31　Other specified diabetes mellitus with unspecified diabetic retinopathy**
DEF: Diabetic retinopathy: Diabetic complication from damage to the retinal vessels resulting in vision problems that can progress to blindness.

E13.311　Other specified diabetes mellitus with unspecified diabetic retinopathy with macular edema　HCC

E13.319　Other specified diabetes mellitus with unspecified diabetic retinopathy without macular edema　HCC

☑6ᵗʰ **E13.32　Other specified diabetes mellitus with mild nonproliferative diabetic retinopathy**
Other specified diabetes mellitus with nonproliferative diabetic retinopathy NOS

☑7ᵗʰ **E13.321　Other specified diabetes mellitus with mild nonproliferative diabetic retinopathy with macular edema**　HCC

☑7ᵗʰ **E13.329　Other specified diabetes mellitus with mild nonproliferative diabetic retinopathy without macular edema**　HCC

☑6ᵗʰ **E13.33　Other specified diabetes mellitus with moderate nonproliferative diabetic retinopathy**

☑7ᵗʰ **E13.331　Other specified diabetes mellitus with moderate nonproliferative diabetic retinopathy with macular edema**　HCC

☑7ᵗʰ **E13.339　Other specified diabetes mellitus with moderate nonproliferative diabetic retinopathy without macular edema**　HCC

☑6ᵗʰ **E13.34　Other specified diabetes mellitus with severe nonproliferative diabetic retinopathy**

☑7ᵗʰ **E13.341　Other specified diabetes mellitus with severe nonproliferative diabetic retinopathy with macular edema**　HCC

☑7ᵗʰ **E13.349　Other specified diabetes mellitus with severe nonproliferative diabetic retinopathy without macular edema**　HCC

☑6ᵗʰ **E13.35　Other specified diabetes mellitus with proliferative diabetic retinopathy**

☑7ᵗʰ **E13.351　Other specified diabetes mellitus with proliferative diabetic retinopathy with macular edema**　HCC

☑7ᵗʰ **E13.352　Other specified diabetes mellitus with proliferative diabetic retinopathy with traction retinal detachment involving the macula**　HCC

☑7ᵗʰ **E13.353　Other specified diabetes mellitus with proliferative diabetic retinopathy with traction retinal detachment not involving the macula**　HCC

☑7ᵗʰ **E13.354　Other specified diabetes mellitus with proliferative diabetic retinopathy with combined traction retinal detachment and rhegmatogenous retinal detachment**　HCC

☑7ᵗʰ **E13.355　Other specified diabetes mellitus with stable proliferative diabetic retinopathy**　HCC

☑7ᵗʰ **E13.359　Other specified diabetes mellitus with proliferative diabetic retinopathy without macular edema**　HCC

E13.36　Other specified diabetes mellitus with diabetic cataract　HCC
AHA: 2019,2Q,30-31; 2016,4Q,142

☑x7ᵗʰ **E13.37　Other specified diabetes mellitus with diabetic macular edema, resolved following treatment**　HCC

E13.39 **Other specified diabetes mellitus with other diabetic ophthalmic complication** `HCC`
Use additional code to identify manifestation, such as:
diabetic glaucoma (H40-H42)

√5th E13.4 **Other specified diabetes mellitus with neurological complications**

E13.40 **Other specified diabetes mellitus with diabetic neuropathy, unspecified** `HCC`

E13.41 **Other specified diabetes mellitus with diabetic mononeuropathy** `HCC`

E13.42 **Other specified diabetes mellitus with diabetic polyneuropathy** `HCC`
Other specified diabetes mellitus with diabetic neuralgia

E13.43 **Other specified diabetes mellitus with diabetic autonomic (poly)neuropathy** `HCC`
Other specified diabetes mellitus with diabetic gastroparesis
AHA: 2013,4Q,114

E13.44 **Other specified diabetes mellitus with diabetic amyotrophy** `HCC`

E13.49 **Other specified diabetes mellitus with other diabetic neurological complication** `HCC`

√5th E13.5 **Other specified diabetes mellitus with circulatory complications**

E13.51 **Other specified diabetes mellitus with diabetic peripheral angiopathy without gangrene** `HCC`
AHA: 2018,3Q,3-4; 2018,2Q,7

E13.52 **Other specified diabetes mellitus with diabetic peripheral angiopathy with gangrene** `CC` `HCC`
Other specified diabetes mellitus with diabetic gangrene
AHA: 2020,2Q,18; 2018,3Q,3; 2018,2Q,7; 2017,4Q,102

E13.59 **Other specified diabetes mellitus with other circulatory complications** `HCC`

√5th E13.6 **Other specified diabetes mellitus with other specified complications**

√6th E13.61 **Other specified diabetes mellitus with diabetic arthropathy**

E13.610 **Other specified diabetes mellitus with diabetic neuropathic arthropathy** `HCC`
Other specified diabetes mellitus with Charcôt's joints
DEF: Charcôt's joint: Progressive neurologic arthropathy in which chronic degeneration of joints in the weight-bearing areas with peripheral hypertrophy occurs as a complication of a neuropathy disorder. Supporting structures relax from a loss of sensation resulting in chronic joint instability.

E13.618 **Other specified diabetes mellitus with other diabetic arthropathy** `HCC`
AHA: 2018,2Q,6

√6th E13.62 **Other specified diabetes mellitus with skin complications**

E13.620 **Other specified diabetes mellitus with diabetic dermatitis** `HCC`
Other specified diabetes mellitus with diabetic necrobiosis lipoidica

E13.621 **Other specified diabetes mellitus with foot ulcer** `HCC`
Use additional code to identify site of ulcer (L97.4-, L97.5-)
AHA: 2020,2Q,19

E13.622 **Other specified diabetes mellitus with other skin ulcer** `HCC`
Use additional code to identify site of ulcer (L97.1-L97.9, L98.41-L98.49)
AHA: 2017,4Q,17

E13.628 **Other specified diabetes mellitus with other skin complications** `HCC`

√6th E13.63 **Other specified diabetes mellitus with oral complications**

E13.630 **Other specified diabetes mellitus with periodontal disease** `HCC`

E13.638 **Other specified diabetes mellitus with other oral complications** `HCC`

√6th E13.64 **Other specified diabetes mellitus with hypoglycemia**
AHA: 2017,1Q,42

E13.641 **Other specified diabetes mellitus with hypoglycemia with coma** `MCC` `HCC`

E13.649 **Other specified diabetes mellitus with hypoglycemia without coma** `HCC`
AHA: 2016,3Q,42; 2015,3Q,21

E13.65 **Other specified diabetes mellitus with hyperglycemia** `HCC`
AHA: 2017,1Q,42; 2013,3Q,20

E13.69 **Other specified diabetes mellitus with other specified complication** `HCC`
Use additional code to identify complication
AHA: 2016,4Q,141; 2016,1Q,13

E13.8 **Other specified diabetes mellitus with unspecified complications** `HCC`

E13.9 **Other specified diabetes mellitus without complications** `HCC`
AHA: 2020,2Q,18

Other disorders of glucose regulation and pancreatic internal secretion (E15-E16)

E15 **Nondiabetic hypoglycemic coma** `CC` `H9` `HCC`
`INCLUDES` drug-induced insulin coma in nondiabetic hyperinsulinism with hypoglycemic coma
hypoglycemic coma NOS

√4th E16 **Other disorders of pancreatic internal secretion**

E16.0 **Drug-induced hypoglycemia without coma**
`EXCLUDES 1` diabetes with hypoglycemia without coma (E09.649)
Use additional code for adverse effect, if applicable, to identify drug (T36-T50 with fifth or sixth character 5)

E16.1 **Other hypoglycemia**
Functional hyperinsulinism
Functional nonhyperinsulinemic hypoglycemia
Hyperinsulinism NOS
Hyperplasia of pancreatic islet beta cells NOS
`EXCLUDES 1` diabetes with hypoglycemia (E08.649, E10.649, E11.649, E13.649)
hypoglycemia in infant of diabetic mother (P70.1)
neonatal hypoglycemia (P70.4)

E16.2 **Hypoglycemia, unspecified**
`EXCLUDES 1` diabetes with hypoglycemia (E08.649, E10.649, E11.649, E13.649)
AHA: 2016,3Q,42
TIP: Assign for nondiabetic hypoglycemic encephalopathy not further clarified in the documentation.

E16.3 **Increased secretion of glucagon**
Hyperplasia of pancreatic endocrine cells with glucagon excess

E16.4 **Increased secretion of gastrin**
Hypergastrinemia
Hyperplasia of pancreatic endocrine cells with gastrin excess
Zollinger-Ellison syndrome

E16.8 **Other specified disorders of pancreatic internal secretion**
Increased secretion from endocrine pancreas of growth hormone-releasing hormone
Increased secretion from endocrine pancreas of pancreatic polypeptide
Increased secretion from endocrine pancreas of somatostatin
Increased secretion from endocrine pancreas of vasoactive-intestinal polypeptide

E16.9 **Disorder of pancreatic internal secretion, unspecified**
Islet-cell hyperplasia NOS
Pancreatic endocrine cell hyperplasia NOS

Disorders of other endocrine glands (E20-E35)

> **EXCLUDES 1**　galactorrhea (N64.3)
> gynecomastia (N62)

✓4ᵗʰ E20　Hypoparathyroidism

> **EXCLUDES 1**　Di George's syndrome (D82.1)
> postprocedural hypoparathyroidism (E89.2)
> tetany NOS (R29.0)
> transitory neonatal hypoparathyroidism (P71.4)

E20.0　Idiopathic hypoparathyroidism　　　HCC
> **DEF:** Abnormally low secretion of parathyroid hormones, with unknown cause, which causes decreased calcium and increased phosphorus in the blood, resulting in muscle cramps, tetany, tingling, or burning in the lips, fingers, and toes, and cataracts.

E20.1　Pseudohypoparathyroidism

E20.8　Other hypoparathyroidism　　　HCC

E20.9　Hypoparathyroidism, unspecified　　　HCC
> Parathyroid tetany

✓4ᵗʰ E21　Hyperparathyroidism and other disorders of parathyroid gland

> **EXCLUDES 1**　adult osteomalacia (M83.-)
> ectopic hyperparathyroidism (E34.2)
> familial hypocalciuric hypercalcemia (E83.52)
> hungry bone syndrome (E83.81)
> infantile and juvenile osteomalacia (E55.0)

E21.0　Primary hyperparathyroidism　　　HCC
> Hyperplasia of parathyroid
> Osteitis fibrosa cystica generalisata [von Recklinghausen's disease of bone]
> **DEF:** Parathyroid dysfunction commonly caused by hyperplasia of two or more glands. Symptoms include hypercalcemia and increased parathyroid hormone levels.

E21.1　Secondary hyperparathyroidism, not elsewhere classified　　　HCC
> **EXCLUDES 1**　secondary hyperparathyroidism of renal origin (N25.81)

E21.2　Other hyperparathyroidism　　　HCC
> Tertiary hyperparathyroidism
> **EXCLUDES 1**　familial hypocalciuric hypercalcemia (E83.52)

E21.3　Hyperparathyroidism, unspecified　　　HCC

E21.4　Other specified disorders of parathyroid gland　　　HCC

E21.5　Disorder of parathyroid gland, unspecified　　　HCC

✓4ᵗʰ E22　Hyperfunction of pituitary gland

> **EXCLUDES 1**　Cushing's syndrome (E24.-)
> Nelson's syndrome (E24.1)
> overproduction of ACTH not associated with Cushing's disease (E27.0)
> overproduction of pituitary ACTH (E24.0)
> overproduction of thyroid-stimulating hormone (E05.8-)

E22.0　Acromegaly and pituitary gigantism　　　HCC
> Overproduction of growth hormone
> **EXCLUDES 1**　constitutional gigantism (E34.4)
> constitutional tall stature (E34.4)
> increased secretion from endocrine pancreas of growth hormone-releasing hormone (E16.8)
> **DEF:** Acromegaly: Chronic condition caused by overproduction of the pituitary growth hormone resulting in enlarged skeletal parts and facial features.

E22.1　Hyperprolactinemia　　　CC HCC
> Use additional code for adverse effect, if applicable, to identify drug (T36-T50 with fifth or sixth character 5)

E22.2　Syndrome of inappropriate secretion of antidiuretic hormone　　　CC HCC

E22.8　Other hyperfunction of pituitary gland　　　CC HCC
> Central precocious puberty

E22.9　Hyperfunction of pituitary gland, unspecified　　　CC HCC

✓4ᵗʰ E23　Hypofunction and other disorders of the pituitary gland

> **INCLUDES**　the listed conditions whether the disorder is in the pituitary or the hypothalamus
> **EXCLUDES 1**　postprocedural hypopituitarism (E89.3)

E23.0　Hypopituitarism　　　CC HCC
> Fertile eunuch syndrome
> Hypogonadotropic hypogonadism
> Idiopathic growth hormone deficiency
> Isolated deficiency of gonadotropin
> Isolated deficiency of growth hormone
> Isolated deficiency of pituitary hormone
> Kallmann's syndrome
> Lorain-Levi short stature
> Necrosis of pituitary gland (postpartum)
> Panhypopituitarism
> Pituitary cachexia
> Pituitary insufficiency NOS
> Pituitary short stature
> Sheehan's syndrome
> Simmonds' disease

E23.1　Drug-induced hypopituitarism　　　HCC
> Use additional code for adverse effect, if applicable, to identify drug (T36-T50 with fifth or sixth character 5)

E23.2　Diabetes insipidus　　　CC HCC
> **EXCLUDES 1**　nephrogenic diabetes insipidus (N25.1)

E23.3　Hypothalamic dysfunction, not elsewhere classified　　　HCC
> **EXCLUDES 1**　Prader-Willi syndrome (Q87.11)
> Russell-Silver syndrome (Q87.19)

E23.6　Other disorders of pituitary gland　　　HCC
> Abscess of pituitary
> Adiposogenital dystrophy

E23.7　Disorder of pituitary gland, unspecified　　　HCC

✓4ᵗʰ E24　Cushing's syndrome

> **EXCLUDES 1**　congenital adrenal hyperplasia (E25.0)
> **DEF:** Abdominal striae, acne, hypertension, decreased carbohydrate tolerance, moon face, obesity, protein catabolism, and psychiatric disturbances resulting from increased adrenocortical secretion of cortisol caused by ACTH-dependent adrenocortical hyperplasia or tumor, or by steroid effects.

E24.0　Pituitary-dependent Cushing's disease　　　CC HCC
> Overproduction of pituitary ACTH
> Pituitary-dependent hypercorticalism

E24.1　Nelson's syndrome　　　HCC

E24.2　Drug-induced Cushing's syndrome　　　CC HCC
> Use additional code for adverse effect, if applicable, to identify drug (T36-T50 with fifth or sixth character 5)

E24.3　Ectopic ACTH syndrome　　　CC HCC

E24.4　Alcohol-induced pseudo-Cushing's syndrome　　　CC HCC

E24.8　Other Cushing's syndrome　　　CC HCC

E24.9　Cushing's syndrome, unspecified　　　CC HCC

✓4ᵗʰ E25　Adrenogenital disorders

> **INCLUDES**　adrenogenital syndromes, virilizing or feminizing, whether acquired or due to adrenal hyperplasia
> consequent on inborn enzyme defects in hormone synthesis
> female adrenal pseudohermaphroditism
> female heterosexual precocious pseudopuberty
> male isosexual precocious pseudopuberty
> male macrogenitosomia praecox
> male sexual precocity with adrenal hyperplasia
> male virilization (female)
> **EXCLUDES 1**　indeterminate sex and pseudohermaphroditism (Q56)
> chromosomal abnormalities (Q90-Q99)

E25.0　Congenital adrenogenital disorders associated with enzyme deficiency　　　HCC
> Congenital adrenal hyperplasia
> 21-Hydroxylase deficiency
> Salt-losing congenital adrenal hyperplasia

E25.8　Other adrenogenital disorders　　　HCC
> Idiopathic adrenogenital disorder
> Use additional code for adverse effect, if applicable, to identify drug (T36-T50 with fifth or sixth character 5)

E25.9　Adrenogenital disorder, unspecified　　　HCC
> Adrenogenital syndrome NOS

☑ Additional Character Required　✓x7ᵗʰ Placeholder　Unacceptable PDx　Questionable PDx　Manifestation　Unspecified Dx　H1-H14 HAC　HCC CMS-HCC Dx　HIV HIV Dx

ICD-10-CM 2021　　　　　　　　　　　　　　　　　　　　　　　　531

Chapter 4. Endocrine, Nutritional and Metabolic Diseases

√4ᵗʰ **E26 Hyperaldosteronism**

  √5ᵗʰ **E26.0 Primary hyperaldosteronism**

    E26.01 Conn's syndrome   HCC
      Code also adrenal adenoma (D35.0-)

    E26.02 Glucocorticoid-remediable aldosteronism   HCC
      Familial aldosteronism type I
      DEF: Rare autosomal dominant familial form of primary aldosteronism in which the secretion of aldosterone is under the influence of adrenocorticotrophic hormone (ACTH) rather than the renin-angiotensin mechanism. Moderate hypersecretion of aldosterone and suppressed plasma renin activity that are rapidly reversed by administration of glucosteroids. Symptoms include hypertension and mild hypokalemia.

    E26.09 Other primary hyperaldosteronism   HCC
      Primary aldosteronism due to adrenal hyperplasia (bilateral)

  E26.1 Secondary hyperaldosteronism   HCC

  √5ᵗʰ **E26.8 Other hyperaldosteronism**

    E26.81 Bartter's syndrome   HCC
    E26.89 Other hyperaldosteronism   HCC

  E26.9 Hyperaldosteronism, unspecified   HCC
    Aldosteronism NOS
    Hyperaldosteronism NOS

√4ᵗʰ **E27 Other disorders of adrenal gland**

  E27.0 Other adrenocortical overactivity   CC HCC
    Overproduction of ACTH, not associated with Cushing's disease
    Premature adrenarche
    EXCLUDES 1   *Cushing's syndrome (E24.-)*

  E27.1 Primary adrenocortical insufficiency   CC HCC
    Addison's disease
    Autoimmune adrenalitis
    EXCLUDES 1   *Addison only phenotype adrenoleukodystrophy (E71.528)*
      amyloidosis (E85.-)
      tuberculous Addison's disease (A18.7)
      Waterhouse-Friderichsen syndrome (A39.1)

  E27.2 Addisonian crisis   CC HCC
    Adrenal crisis
    Adrenocortical crisis
    DEF: Life-threatening condition that occurs when there is not enough cortisol excreted from the adrenal glands. This condition may be due to injury to the adrenal glands or to the pituitary gland, which controls adrenal hormone secretion, or when a patient stops hydrocortisone treatment too quickly or too early.

  E27.3 Drug-induced adrenocortical insufficiency   CC HCC
    Use additional code for adverse effect, if applicable, to identify drug (T36-T50 with fifth or sixth character 5)

  √5ᵗʰ **E27.4 Other and unspecified adrenocortical insufficiency**
    EXCLUDES 1   *adrenoleukodystrophy [Addison-Schilder] (E71.528)*
      Waterhouse-Friderichsen syndrome (A39.1)

    E27.40 Unspecified adrenocortical insufficiency   CC HCC
      Adrenocortical insufficiency NOS
      Hypoaldosteronism

    E27.49 Other adrenocortical insufficiency   CC HCC
      Adrenal hemorrhage
      Adrenal infarction

  E27.5 Adrenomedullary hyperfunction   CC HCC
    Adrenomedullary hyperplasia
    Catecholamine hypersecretion

  E27.8 Other specified disorders of adrenal gland   HCC
    Abnormality of cortisol-binding globulin

  E27.9 Disorder of adrenal gland, unspecified   HCC

√4ᵗʰ **E28 Ovarian dysfunction**
    EXCLUDES 1   *isolated gonadotropin deficiency (E23.0)*
      postprocedural ovarian failure (E89.4-)

  E28.0 Estrogen excess   ♀
    Use additional code for adverse effect, if applicable, to identify drug (T36-T50 with fifth or sixth character 5)

  E28.1 Androgen excess   ♀
    Hypersecretion of ovarian androgens
    Use additional code for adverse effect, if applicable, to identify drug (T36-T50 with fifth or sixth character 5)

  E28.2 Polycystic ovarian syndrome   ♀
    Sclerocystic ovary syndrome
    Stein-Leventhal syndrome
    DEF: Common hormonal disorder among women of reproductive age that involves enlarged ovaries with numerous small cysts located along the outer ovarian edge.

  √5ᵗʰ **E28.3 Primary ovarian failure**
    EXCLUDES 1   *pure gonadal dysgenesis (Q99.1)*
      Turner's syndrome (Q96.-)

    √6ᵗʰ **E28.31 Premature menopause**

      E28.310 Symptomatic premature menopause   A ♀
        Symptoms such as flushing, sleeplessness, headache, lack of concentration, associated with premature menopause

      E28.319 Asymptomatic premature menopause   A ♀
        Premature menopause NOS

    E28.39 Other primary ovarian failure   ♀
      Decreased estrogen
      Resistant ovary syndrome

  E28.8 Other ovarian dysfunction   ♀
    Ovarian hyperfunction NOS
    EXCLUDES 1   *postprocedural ovarian failure (E89.4-)*

  E28.9 Ovarian dysfunction, unspecified   ♀

√4ᵗʰ **E29 Testicular dysfunction**
    EXCLUDES 1   *androgen insensitivity syndrome (E34.5-)*
      azoospermia or oligospermia NOS (N46.0-N46.1)
      isolated gonadotropin deficiency (E23.0)
      Klinefelter's syndrome (Q98.0-Q98.1, Q98.4)

  E29.0 Testicular hyperfunction   ♂
    Hypersecretion of testicular hormones

  E29.1 Testicular hypofunction   ♂
    Defective biosynthesis of testicular androgen NOS
    5-delta-Reductase deficiency (with male pseudohermaphroditism)
    Testicular hypogonadism NOS
    Use additional code for adverse effect, if applicable, to identify drug (T36-T50 with fifth or sixth character 5)
    EXCLUDES 1   *postprocedural testicular hypofunction (E89.5)*

  E29.8 Other testicular dysfunction   ♂
  E29.9 Testicular dysfunction, unspecified   ♂

√4ᵗʰ **E30 Disorders of puberty, not elsewhere classified**

  E30.0 Delayed puberty
    Constitutional delay of puberty
    Delayed sexual development

  E30.1 Precocious puberty   P
    Precocious menstruation
    EXCLUDES 1   *Albright (-McCune) (-Sternberg) syndrome (Q78.1)*
      central precocious puberty (E22.8)
      congenital adrenal hyperplasia (E25.0)
      female heterosexual precocious pseudopuberty (E25.-)
      male isosexual precocious pseudopuberty (E25.-)

  E30.8 Other disorders of puberty   P
    Premature thelarche

  E30.9 Disorder of puberty, unspecified

√4ᵗʰ **E31 Polyglandular dysfunction**
    EXCLUDES 1   *ataxia telangiectasia [Louis-Bar] (G11.3)*
      dystrophia myotonica [Steinert] (G71.11)
      pseudohypoparathyroidism (E20.1)

  E31.0 Autoimmune polyglandular failure   HCC
    Schmidt's syndrome

  E31.1 Polyglandular hyperfunction   HCC
    EXCLUDES 1   *multiple endocrine adenomatosis (E31.2-)*
      multiple endocrine neoplasia (E31.2-)

N Newborn: 0   P Pediatric: 0-17   M Maternity: 9-64   A Adult: 15-124   MCC Major Complication/Comorbidity   CC Complication/Comorbidity   SW Severe Wound Dx

532   ICD-10-CM 2021

√5ᵗʰ **E31.2 Multiple endocrine neoplasia [MEN] syndromes**

Multiple endocrine adenomatosis

Code also any associated malignancies and other conditions associated with the syndromes

DEF: Group of conditions in which several endocrine glands grow excessively (such as in adenomatous hyperplasia) and/or develop benign or malignant tumors. Tumors and hyperplasia associated with MEN often produce excess hormones, which impede normal physiology. There is no comprehensive cure known for MEN syndrome. Treatment is directed at the hyperplasia or tumors in each individual gland. Tumors are usually surgically removed and oral medications or hormonal injections are used to correct hormone imbalances.

E31.20 Multiple endocrine neoplasia [MEN] syndrome, unspecified HCC

Multiple endocrine adenomatosis NOS

Multiple endocrine neoplasia [MEN] syndrome NOS

E31.21 Multiple endocrine neoplasia [MEN] type I HCC

Wermer's syndrome

E31.22 Multiple endocrine neoplasia [MEN] type IIA HCC

Sipple's syndrome

E31.23 Multiple endocrine neoplasia [MEN] type IIB HCC

E31.8 Other polyglandular dysfunction HCC

E31.9 Polyglandular dysfunction, unspecified HCC

√4ᵗʰ **E32 Diseases of thymus**

EXCLUDES 1   *aplasia or hypoplasia of thymus with immunodeficiency (D82.1)*

myasthenia gravis (G70.0)

E32.0 Persistent hyperplasia of thymus HCC

Hypertrophy of thymus

E32.1 Abscess of thymus CC HCC

E32.8 Other diseases of thymus HCC

EXCLUDES 1   *aplasia or hypoplasia with immunodeficiency (D82.1)*

thymoma (D15.0)

E32.9 Disease of thymus, unspecified HCC

√4ᵗʰ **E34 Other endocrine disorders**

EXCLUDES 1   *pseudohypoparathyroidism (E20.1)*

E34.0 Carcinoid syndrome CC HCC

NOTE   May be used as an additional code to identify functional activity associated with a carcinoid tumor.

E34.1 Other hypersecretion of intestinal hormones

E34.2 Ectopic hormone secretion, not elsewhere classified

EXCLUDES 1   *ectopic ACTH syndrome (E24.3)*

E34.3 Short stature due to endocrine disorder

Constitutional short stature

Laron-type short stature

EXCLUDES 1   *achondroplastic short stature (Q77.4)*

hypochondroplastic short stature (Q77.4)

nutritional short stature (E45)

pituitary short stature (E23.0)

progeria (E34.8)

renal short stature (N25.0)

Russell-Silver syndrome (Q87.19)

short-limbed stature with immunodeficiency (D82.2)

short stature in specific dysmorphic syndromes — code to syndrome — see Alphabetical Index

short stature NOS (R62.52)

E34.4 Constitutional tall stature HCC

Constitutional gigantism

√5ᵗʰ **E34.5 Androgen insensitivity syndrome**

DEF: X-linked recessive condition in which individuals that are chromosomally male fail to develop normal male external genitalia due to an abnormality on the X chromosome that prohibits the body, completely or in part, from recognizing the androgens produced. *Synonym(s): AIS*

E34.50 Androgen insensitivity syndrome, unspecified

Androgen insensitivity NOS

E34.51 Complete androgen insensitivity syndrome

Complete androgen insensitivity

de Quervain syndrome

Goldberg-Maxwell syndrome

E34.52 Partial androgen insensitivity syndrome

Partial androgen insensitivity

Reifenstein syndrome

E34.8 Other specified endocrine disorders

Pineal gland dysfunction

Progeria

EXCLUDES 2   *pseudohypoparathyroidism (E20.1)*

E34.9 Endocrine disorder, unspecified

Endocrine disturbance NOS

Hormone disturbance NOS

E35 *Disorders of endocrine glands in diseases classified elsewhere*

Code first underlying disease, such as:

late congenital syphilis of thymus gland [Dubois disease] (A50.5)

Use additional code, if applicable, to identify:

sequelae of tuberculosis of other organs (B90.8)

EXCLUDES 1   *Echinococcus granulosus infection of thyroid gland (B67.3)*

meningococcal hemorrhagic adrenalitis (A39.1)

syphilis of endocrine gland (A52.79)

tuberculosis of adrenal gland, except calcification (A18.7)

tuberculosis of endocrine gland NEC (A18.82)

tuberculosis of thyroid gland (A18.81)

Waterhouse-Friderichsen syndrome (A39.1)

Intraoperative complications of endocrine system (E36)

√4ᵗʰ **E36 Intraoperative complications of endocrine system**

EXCLUDES 2   *postprocedural endocrine and metabolic complications and disorders, not elsewhere classified (E89.-)*

√5ᵗʰ **E36.0 Intraoperative hemorrhage and hematoma of an endocrine system organ or structure complicating a procedure**

EXCLUDES 1   *intraoperative hemorrhage and hematoma of an endocrine system organ or structure due to accidental puncture or laceration during a procedure (E36.1-)*

E36.01 Intraoperative hemorrhage and hematoma of an endocrine system organ or structure complicating an endocrine system procedure CC

AHA: 2020,1Q,19

E36.02 Intraoperative hemorrhage and hematoma of an endocrine system organ or structure complicating other procedure CC

√5ᵗʰ **E36.1 Accidental puncture and laceration of an endocrine system organ or structure during a procedure**

E36.11 Accidental puncture and laceration of an endocrine system organ or structure during an endocrine system procedure CC

E36.12 Accidental puncture and laceration of an endocrine system organ or structure during other procedure CC

E36.8 Other intraoperative complications of endocrine system

Use additional code, if applicable, to further specify disorder

Malnutrition (E40-E46)

EXCLUDES 1   *intestinal malabsorption (K90.-)*

sequelae of protein-calorie malnutrition (E64.0)

EXCLUDES 2   *nutritional anemias (D50-D53)*

starvation (T73.0)

AHA: 2020,1Q,4-7; 2017,4Q,108; 2017,3Q,25

TIP: Assign additional code for BMI from category Z68, when documented. BMI can be based on documentation from clinicians who are not the patient's provider.

TIP: Malnutrition is not considered integral to cancer; assign the appropriate code in addition to the code for the specific type of cancer.

E40 Kwashiorkor MCC HCC

Severe malnutrition with nutritional edema with dyspigmentation of skin and hair

EXCLUDES 1   *marasmic kwashiorkor (E42)*

E41 Nutritional marasmus MCC HCC

Severe malnutrition with marasmus

EXCLUDES 1   *marasmic kwashiorkor (E42)*

AHA: 2017,3Q,24

DEF: Protein-calorie malabsorption or malnutrition in children characterized by tissue wasting, dehydration, and subcutaneous fat depletion. It may occur with infectious disease.

E42 Marasmic kwashiorkor MCC HCC

Intermediate form severe protein-calorie malnutrition

Severe protein-calorie malnutrition with signs of both kwashiorkor and marasmus

E43 Unspecified severe protein-calorie malnutrition MCC HCC

Starvation edema

AHA: 2020,1Q,5,6; 2017,4Q,108

Chapter 4. Endocrine, Nutritional and Metabolic Diseases

E44–E61.9

✓4ᵗʰ **E44** **Protein-calorie malnutrition of moderate and mild degree**
> **AHA:** 2020,1Q,5

E44.0 Moderate protein-calorie malnutrition   CC HCC

E44.1 Mild protein-calorie malnutrition   CC HCC

E45 **Retarded development following protein-calorie malnutrition**   CC HCC
> Nutritional short stature
> Nutritional stunting
> Physical retardation due to malnutrition

E46 **Unspecified protein-calorie malnutrition**   CC HCC
> Malnutrition NOS
> Protein-calorie imbalance NOS
> **EXCLUDES 1**   nutritional deficiency NOS (E63.9)
> **AHA:** 2018,4Q,82

Other nutritional deficiencies (E50-E64)

> **EXCLUDES 2**   nutritional anemias (D50-D53)

✓4ᵗʰ **E50** **Vitamin A deficiency**
> **EXCLUDES 1**   sequelae of vitamin A deficiency (E64.1)

E50.0 Vitamin A deficiency with conjunctival xerosis

E50.1 Vitamin A deficiency with Bitot's spot and conjunctival xerosis
> Bitot's spot in the young child
> **DEF:** Vitamin A deficiency with conjunctival dryness and superficial spots of keratinized epithelium.

E50.2 Vitamin A deficiency with corneal xerosis

E50.3 Vitamin A deficiency with corneal ulceration and xerosis

E50.4 Vitamin A deficiency with keratomalacia
> **DEF:** Vitamin A deficiency creating corneal dryness that progresses to corneal insensitivity, softness, and necrosis. It is usually bilateral.

E50.5 Vitamin A deficiency with night blindness

E50.6 Vitamin A deficiency with xerophthalmic scars of cornea

E50.7 Other ocular manifestations of vitamin A deficiency
> Xerophthalmia NOS

E50.8 Other manifestations of vitamin A deficiency
> Follicular keratosis
> Xeroderma

E50.9 Vitamin A deficiency, unspecified
> Hypovitaminosis A NOS

✓4ᵗʰ **E51** **Thiamine deficiency**
> **EXCLUDES 1**   sequelae of thiamine deficiency (E64.8)

✓5ᵗʰ **E51.1** Beriberi

E51.11 Dry beriberi   CC
> Beriberi NOS
> Beriberi with polyneuropathy

E51.12 Wet beriberi   CC
> Beriberi with cardiovascular manifestations
> Cardiovascular beriberi
> Shoshin disease

E51.2 Wernicke's encephalopathy   CC
> **DEF:** Deficiency of vitamin B1 resulting in a triad of acute mental confusion, ataxia, and ophthalmoplegia. The vast majority of affected patients are alcoholics.

E51.8 Other manifestations of thiamine deficiency   CC

E51.9 Thiamine deficiency, unspecified   CC

E52 **Niacin deficiency [pellagra]**
> Niacin (-tryptophan) deficiency
> Nicotinamide deficiency
> Pellagra (alcoholic)
> **EXCLUDES 1**   sequelae of niacin deficiency (E64.8)

✓4ᵗʰ **E53** **Deficiency of other B group vitamins**
> **EXCLUDES 1**   sequelae of vitamin B deficiency (E64.8)

E53.0 Riboflavin deficiency   CC
> Ariboflavinosis
> Vitamin B2 deficiency

E53.1 Pyridoxine deficiency
> Vitamin B6 deficiency
> **EXCLUDES 1**   pyridoxine-responsive sideroblastic anemia (D64.3)

E53.8 **Deficiency of other specified B group vitamins**
> Biotin deficiency
> Cyanocobalamin deficiency
> Folate deficiency
> Folic acid deficiency
> Pantothenic acid deficiency
> Vitamin B12 deficiency
> **EXCLUDES 1**   folate deficiency anemia (D52.-)
>   vitamin B12 deficiency anemia (D51.-)

E53.9 Vitamin B deficiency, unspecified

E54 **Ascorbic acid deficiency**
> Deficiency of vitamin C
> Scurvy
> **EXCLUDES 1**   scorbutic anemia (D53.2)
>   sequelae of vitamin C deficiency (E64.2)
> **DEF:** Vitamin C deficiency causing swollen gums, myalgia, weight loss, and weakness.

✓4ᵗʰ **E55** **Vitamin D deficiency**
> **EXCLUDES 1**   adult osteomalacia (M83.-)
>   osteoporosis (M80.-)
>   sequelae of rickets (E64.3)

E55.0 Rickets, active   CC
> Infantile osteomalacia
> Juvenile osteomalacia
> **EXCLUDES 1**   celiac rickets (K90.0)
>   Crohn's rickets (K50.-)
>   hereditary vitamin D-dependent rickets (E83.32)
>   inactive rickets (E64.3)
>   renal rickets (N25.0)
>   sequelae of rickets (E64.3)
>   vitamin D-resistant rickets (E83.31)
> **DEF:** Rickets: Softening or weakening of the bones due to a lack of vitamin D, calcium, and phosphate.

E55.9 Vitamin D deficiency, unspecified
> Avitaminosis D

✓4ᵗʰ **E56** **Other vitamin deficiencies**
> **EXCLUDES 1**   sequelae of other vitamin deficiencies (E64.8)

E56.0 Deficiency of vitamin E

E56.1 Deficiency of vitamin K
> **EXCLUDES 1**   deficiency of coagulation factor due to vitamin K deficiency (D68.4)
>   vitamin K deficiency of newborn (P53)

E56.8 Deficiency of other vitamins

E56.9 Vitamin deficiency, unspecified

E58 **Dietary calcium deficiency**
> **EXCLUDES 1**   disorders of calcium metabolism (E83.5-)
>   sequelae of calcium deficiency (E64.8)

E59 **Dietary selenium deficiency**
> Keshan disease
> **EXCLUDES 1**   sequelae of selenium deficiency (E64.8)

E60 **Dietary zinc deficiency**

✓4ᵗʰ **E61** **Deficiency of other nutrient elements**
> Use additional code for adverse effect, if applicable, to identify drug (T36-T50 with fifth or sixth character 5)
> **EXCLUDES 1**   disorders of mineral metabolism (E83.-)
>   iodine deficiency related thyroid disorders (E00-E02)
>   sequelae of malnutrition and other nutritional deficiencies (E64.-)

E61.0 Copper deficiency

E61.1 Iron deficiency
> **EXCLUDES 1**   iron deficiency anemia (D50.-)

E61.2 Magnesium deficiency

E61.3 Manganese deficiency

E61.4 Chromium deficiency

E61.5 Molybdenum deficiency

E61.6 Vanadium deficiency

E61.7 Deficiency of multiple nutrient elements

E61.8 Deficiency of other specified nutrient elements

E61.9 Deficiency of nutrient element, unspecified

N Newborn: 0   P Pediatric: 0-17   M Maternity: 9-64   A Adult: 15-124   MCC Major Complication/Comorbidity   CC Complication/Comorbidity   SW Severe Wound Dx

534   ICD-10-CM 2021

✓4ᵗʰ **E63 Other nutritional deficiencies**

     EXCLUDES 1   *dehydration (E86.0)*
                  failure to thrive, adult (R62.7)
                  failure to thrive, child (R62.51)
                  feeding problems in newborn (P92.-)
                  sequelae of malnutrition and other nutritional deficiencies
                  (E64.-)

     E63.0 Essential fatty acid [EFA] deficiency
     E63.1 Imbalance of constituents of food intake
     E63.8 Other specified nutritional deficiencies
     E63.9 Nutritional deficiency, unspecified

✓4ᵗʰ **E64 Sequelae of malnutrition and other nutritional deficiencies**

     NOTE   This category is to be used to indicate conditions in categories E43, E44, E46, E50-E63 as the cause of sequelae, which are themselves classified elsewhere. The 'sequelae' include conditions specified as such; they also include the late effects of diseases classifiable to the above categories if the disease itself is no longer present

     Code first condition resulting from (sequela) of malnutrition and other nutritional deficiencies

     E64.0 Sequelae of protein-calorie malnutrition CC HCC
         EXCLUDES 2   *retarded development following protein-calorie malnutrition (E45)*
     E64.1 Sequelae of vitamin A deficiency
     E64.2 Sequelae of vitamin C deficiency
     E64.3 Sequelae of rickets
     E64.8 Sequelae of other nutritional deficiencies
     E64.9 Sequelae of unspecified nutritional deficiency

Overweight, obesity and other hyperalimentation (E65-E68)

E65 Localized adiposity
     Fat pad

✓4ᵗʰ **E66 Overweight and obesity**

     Code first obesity complicating pregnancy, childbirth and the puerperium, if applicable (O99.21-)
     Use additional code to identify body mass index (BMI), if known (Z68.-)
     EXCLUDES 1   *adiposogenital dystrophy (E23.6)*
                  lipomatosis NOS (E88.2)
                  lipomatosis dolorosa [Dercum] (E88.2)
                  Prader-Willi syndrome (Q87.11)
     AHA: 2018,4Q,77,79-80
     TIP: Do not assign a BMI code (Z68.-) when a pregnant patient is documented as being overweight or obese. Only a code from subcategory O99.21- and a code from this category should be assigned.

     ✓5ᵗʰ **E66.0 Obesity due to excess calories**

         E66.01 Morbid (severe) obesity due to excess calories H11 HCC
             EXCLUDES 1   *morbid (severe) obesity with alveolar hypoventilation (E66.2)*

         E66.09 Other obesity due to excess calories
     E66.1 Drug-induced obesity
         Use additional code for adverse effect, if applicable, to identify drug (T36-T50 with fifth or sixth character 5)
     E66.2 Morbid (severe) obesity with alveolar hypoventilation CC HCC
         Obesity hypoventilation syndrome (OHS)
         Pickwickian syndrome
     E66.3 Overweight
         AHA: 2018,4Q,78
     E66.8 Other obesity
     E66.9 Obesity, unspecified
         Obesity NOS

✓4ᵗʰ **E67 Other hyperalimentation**

     EXCLUDES 1   *hyperalimentation NOS (R63.2)*
                  sequelae of hyperalimentation (E68)
     E67.0 Hypervitaminosis A
     E67.1 Hypercarotenemia
         DEF: Elevated blood carotene level as a result of excessive carotenoid ingestion or an inability to convert carotenoids to vitamin A. Characteristics often include yellow discoloration of the skin, which may follow overeating of carotenoid-rich foods such as carrots, sweet potatoes, or squash.
     E67.2 Megavitamin-B6 syndrome
     E67.3 Hypervitaminosis D
     E67.8 Other specified hyperalimentation

E68 Sequelae of hyperalimentation
     Code first condition resulting from (sequela) of hyperalimentation

Metabolic disorders (E70-E88)

     EXCLUDES 1   *androgen insensitivity syndrome (E34.5-)*
                  congenital adrenal hyperplasia (E25.0)
                  ▶*Ehlers-Danlos syndromes◀ (Q79.6-)*
                  hemolytic anemias attributable to enzyme disorders (D55.-)
                  Marfan's syndrome (Q87.4)
                  5-alpha-reductase deficiency (E29.1)
     AHA: 2018,2Q,6

✓4ᵗʰ **E70 Disorders of aromatic amino-acid metabolism**

     E70.0 Classical phenylketonuria CC HCC
     E70.1 Other hyperphenylalaninemias CC HCC
     ✓5ᵗʰ **E70.2 Disorders of tyrosine metabolism**

         EXCLUDES 1   *transitory tyrosinemia of newborn (P74.5)*
         E70.20 Disorder of tyrosine metabolism, unspecified CC HCC
         E70.21 Tyrosinemia CC HCC
             Hypertyrosinemia
         E70.29 Other disorders of tyrosine metabolism CC HCC
             Alkaptonuria
             Ochronosis

     ✓5ᵗʰ **E70.3 Albinism**
         DEF: Absence of pigment in skin, hair, and eyes. This genetic condition is often accompanied by astigmatism, photophobia, and nystagmus.
         E70.30 Albinism, unspecified CC HCC
     ✓6ᵗʰ **E70.31 Ocular albinism**

         E70.310 X-linked ocular albinism CC HCC
         E70.311 Autosomal recessive ocular albinism CC HCC
         E70.318 Other ocular albinism CC HCC
         E70.319 Ocular albinism, unspecified CC HCC
     ✓6ᵗʰ **E70.32 Oculocutaneous albinism**

         EXCLUDES 1   *Chediak-Higashi syndrome (E70.330)*
                  Hermansky-Pudlak syndrome (E70.331)
         E70.320 Tyrosinase negative oculocutaneous albinism CC HCC
             Albinism I
             Oculocutaneous albinism ty-neg
         E70.321 Tyrosinase positive oculocutaneous albinism CC HCC
             Albinism II
             Oculocutaneous albinism ty-pos
         E70.328 Other oculocutaneous albinism CC HCC
             Cross syndrome
         E70.329 Oculocutaneous albinism, unspecified CC HCC
     ✓6ᵗʰ **E70.33 Albinism with hematologic abnormality**

         E70.330 Chediak-Higashi syndrome CC HCC
         E70.331 Hermansky-Pudlak syndrome CC HCC
         E70.338 Other albinism with hematologic abnormality CC HCC
         E70.339 Albinism with hematologic abnormality, unspecified CC HCC
         E70.39 Other specified albinism CC HCC
             Piebaldism

     ✓5ᵗʰ **E70.4 Disorders of histidine metabolism**

         E70.40 Disorders of histidine metabolism, unspecified CC HCC
         E70.41 Histidinemia CC HCC
         E70.49 Other disorders of histidine metabolism CC HCC
     E70.5 Disorders of tryptophan metabolism CC HCC
▲ ✓5ᵗʰ **E70.8 Other disorders of aromatic amino-acid metabolism**
●   **E70.81 Aromatic L-amino acid decarboxylase deficiency** CC
             AADC deficiency
●   **E70.89 Other disorders of aromatic amino-acid metabolism** CC
     E70.9 Disorder of aromatic amino-acid metabolism, unspecified CC HCC

✓4ᵗʰ **E71 Disorders of branched-chain amino-acid metabolism and fatty-acid metabolism**

     E71.0 Maple-syrup-urine disease CC HCC

✓5ᵗʰ **E71.1 Other disorders of branched-chain amino-acid metabolism**

     ✓6ᵗʰ **E71.11 Branched-chain organic acidurias**

         E71.110 Isovaleric acidemia CC HCC

         E71.111 3-methylglutaconic aciduria CC HCC

         E71.118 Other branched-chain organic acidurias CC HCC

     ✓6ᵗʰ **E71.12 Disorders of propionate metabolism**

         E71.120 Methylmalonic acidemia CC HCC

         E71.121 Propionic acidemia CC HCC

         E71.128 Other disorders of propionate metabolism CC HCC

     E71.19 Other disorders of branched-chain amino-acid metabolism CC HCC

         Hyperleucine-isoleucinemia

         Hypervalinemia

E71.2 Disorder of branched-chain amino-acid metabolism, unspecified CC HCC

✓5ᵗʰ **E71.3 Disorders of fatty-acid metabolism**

     EXCLUDES 1   *peroxisomal disorders (E71.5)*

         Refsum's disease (G60.1)

         Schilder's disease (G37.0)

     EXCLUDES 2   *carnitine deficiency due to inborn error of metabolism (E71.42)*

     E71.30 Disorder of fatty-acid metabolism, unspecified

     ✓6ᵗʰ **E71.31 Disorders of fatty-acid oxidation**

         E71.310 Long chain/very long chain acyl CoA dehydrogenase deficiency CC HCC

            LCAD

            VLCAD

         E71.311 Medium chain acyl CoA dehydrogenase deficiency CC HCC

            MCAD

         E71.312 Short chain acyl CoA dehydrogenase deficiency CC HCC

            SCAD

         E71.313 Glutaric aciduria type II CC HCC

            Glutaric aciduria type II A

            Glutaric aciduria type II B

            Glutaric aciduria type II C

            EXCLUDES 1   *glutaric aciduria (type 1) NOS (E72.3)*

         E71.314 Muscle carnitine palmitoyltransferase deficiency CC HCC

         E71.318 Other disorders of fatty-acid oxidation CC HCC

     E71.32 Disorders of ketone metabolism CC HCC

     E71.39 Other disorders of fatty-acid metabolism CC HCC

✓5ᵗʰ **E71.4 Disorders of carnitine metabolism**

     EXCLUDES 1   *muscle carnitine palmitoyltransferase deficiency (E71.314)*

     E71.40 Disorder of carnitine metabolism, unspecified HCC

     E71.41 Primary carnitine deficiency HCC

     E71.42 Carnitine deficiency due to inborn errors of metabolism HCC

         Code also associated inborn error or metabolism

     E71.43 Iatrogenic carnitine deficiency HCC

         Carnitine deficiency due to hemodialysis

         Carnitine deficiency due to Valproic acid therapy

     ✓6ᵗʰ **E71.44 Other secondary carnitine deficiency**

         E71.440 Ruvalcaba-Myhre-Smith syndrome HCC

         E71.448 Other secondary carnitine deficiency HCC

✓5ᵗʰ **E71.5 Peroxisomal disorders**

     EXCLUDES 1   *Schilder's disease (G37.0)*

     E71.50 Peroxisomal disorder, unspecified CC HCC

     ✓6ᵗʰ **E71.51 Disorders of peroxisome biogenesis**

         Group 1 peroxisomal disorders

         EXCLUDES 1   *Refsum's disease (G60.1)*

         E71.510 Zellweger syndrome CC HCC

         E71.511 Neonatal adrenoleukodystrophy CC HCC

            EXCLUDES 1   *X-linked adrenoleukodystrophy (E71.42-)*

         E71.518 Other disorders of peroxisome biogenesis CC HCC

     ✓6ᵗʰ **E71.52 X-linked adrenoleukodystrophy**

         E71.520 Childhood cerebral X-linked adrenoleukodystrophy CC HCC

         E71.521 Adolescent X-linked adrenoleukodystrophy CC HCC

         E71.522 Adrenomyeloneuropathy CC HCC

         E71.528 Other X-linked adrenoleukodystrophy CC HCC

            Addison only phenotype adrenoleukodystrophy

            Addison-Schilder adrenoleukodystrophy

         E71.529 X-linked adrenoleukodystrophy, unspecified type CC HCC

     E71.53 Other group 2 peroxisomal disorders CC HCC

     ✓6ᵗʰ **E71.54 Other peroxisomal disorders**

         E71.540 Rhizomelic chondrodysplasia punctata CC HCC

            EXCLUDES 1   *chondrodysplasia punctata NOS (Q77.3)*

         E71.541 Zellweger-like syndrome CC HCC

         E71.542 Other group 3 peroxisomal disorders CC HCC

         E71.548 Other peroxisomal disorders CC HCC

✓4ᵗʰ **E72 Other disorders of amino-acid metabolism**

     EXCLUDES 1   *disorders of:*

         aromatic amino-acid metabolism (E70.-)

         branched-chain amino-acid metabolism (E71.0-E71.2)

         fatty-acid metabolism (E71.3)

         purine and pyrimidine metabolism (E79.-)

         gout (M1A.-, M10.-)

✓5ᵗʰ **E72.0 Disorders of amino-acid transport**

     EXCLUDES 1   *disorders of tryptophan metabolism (E70.5)*

     E72.00 Disorders of amino-acid transport, unspecified CC HCC

     E72.01 Cystinuria CC HCC

     E72.02 Hartnup's disease CC HCC

     E72.03 Lowe's syndrome CC HCC

         Use additional code for associated glaucoma (H42)

     E72.04 Cystinosis CC HCC

         Fanconi (-de Toni) (-Debré) syndrome with cystinosis

         EXCLUDES 1   *Fanconi (-de Toni) (-Debré) syndrome without cystinosis (E72.09)*

     E72.09 Other disorders of amino-acid transport CC HCC

         Fanconi (-de Toni) (-Debré) syndrome, unspecified

✓5ᵗʰ **E72.1 Disorders of sulfur-bearing amino-acid metabolism**

     EXCLUDES 1   *cystinosis (E72.04)*

         cystinuria (E72.01)

         transcobalamin II deficiency (D51.2)

     E72.10 Disorders of sulfur-bearing amino-acid metabolism, unspecified CC HCC

     E72.11 Homocystinuria CC HCC

         Cystathionine synthase deficiency

     E72.12 Methylenetetrahydrofolate reductase deficiency CC HCC

     E72.19 Other disorders of sulfur-bearing amino-acid metabolism CC HCC

         Cystathioninuria

         Methioninemia

         Sulfite oxidase deficiency

✓6ᵗʰ **E72.2 Disorders of urea cycle metabolism**

     EXCLUDES 1   *disorders of ornithine metabolism (E72.4)*

     E72.20 Disorder of urea cycle metabolism, unspecified CC HCC

         Hyperammonemia

         EXCLUDES 1   *hyperammonemia- hyperornithinemia-homocitrullinemia syndrome E72.4*

            transient hyperammonemia of newborn (P74.6)

     E72.21 Argininemia CC HCC

     E72.22 Arginosuccinic aciduria CC HCC

     E72.23 Citrullinemia CC HCC

     E72.29 Other disorders of urea cycle metabolism CC HCC

N Newborn: 0   P Pediatric: 0-17   M Maternity: 9-64   A Adult: 15-124   MCC Major Complication/Comorbidity   CC Complication/Comorbidity   SW Severe Wound Dx

536   ICD-10-CM 2021

E72.3 **Disorders of lysine and hydroxylysine metabolism** `CC` `HCC`
Glutaric aciduria NOS
Glutaric aciduria (type I)
Hydroxylysinemia
Hyperlysinemia
> **EXCLUDES 1**   glutaric aciduria type II (E71.313)
> Refsum's disease (G60.1)
> Zellweger syndrome (E71.510)

E72.4 **Disorders of ornithine metabolism** `CC` `HCC`
Hyperammonemia-Hyperornithinemia-Homocitrullinemia syndrome
Ornithinemia (types I, II)
Ornithine transcarbamylase deficiency
> **EXCLUDES 1**   hereditary choroidal dystrophy (H31.2-)

√5ᵗʰ **E72.5** **Disorders of glycine metabolism**

     E72.50 **Disorder of glycine metabolism, unspecified** `CC` `HCC`

     E72.51 **Non-ketotic hyperglycinemia** `CC` `HCC`

     E72.52 **Trimethylaminuria** `CC` `HCC`

     E72.53 **Primary hyperoxaluria** `CC` `HCC`
         Oxalosis
         Oxaluria
         AHA: 2018,4Q,29

     E72.59 **Other disorders of glycine metabolism** `CC` `HCC`
         D-glycericacidemia
         Hyperhydroxyprolinemia
         Hyperprolinemia (types I, II)
         Sarcosinemia

√5ᵗʰ **E72.8** **Other specified disorders of amino-acid metabolism**
AHA: 2018,4Q,5

     E72.81 **Disorders of gamma aminobutyric acid metabolism** `CC` `HCC`
         4-hydroxybutyric aciduria
         Disorders of GABA metabolism
         GABA metabolic defect
         GABA transaminase deficiency
         GABA-T deficiency
         Gamma-hydroxybutyric aciduria
         SSADHD
         Succinic semialdehyde dehydrogenase deficiency

     E72.89 **Other specified disorders of amino-acid metabolism** `CC` `HCC`
         Disorders of beta-amino-acid metabolism
         Disorders of gamma-glutamyl cycle

     E72.9 **Disorder of amino-acid metabolism, unspecified** `CC` `HCC`

√4ᵗʰ **E73** **Lactose intolerance**
DEF: Inability to break down sugar in dairy products due to a deficiency in the enzyme lactase.

     E73.0 **Congenital lactase deficiency**

     E73.1 **Secondary lactase deficiency**

     E73.8 **Other lactose intolerance**

     E73.9 **Lactose intolerance, unspecified**

√4ᵗʰ **E74** **Other disorders of carbohydrate metabolism**
> **EXCLUDES 1**   diabetes mellitus (E08-E13)
> hypoglycemia NOS (E16.2)
> increased secretion of glucagon (E16.3)
> mucopolysaccharidosis (E76.0-E76.3)

√5ᵗʰ **E74.0** **Glycogen storage disease**

     E74.00 **Glycogen storage disease, unspecified** `CC` `HCC`

     E74.01 **von Gierke disease** `CC` `HCC`
         Type I glycogen storage disease

     E74.02 **Pompe disease** `CC` `HCC`
         Cardiac glycogenosis
         Type II glycogen storage disease

     E74.03 **Cori disease** `CC` `HCC`
         Forbes disease
         Type III glycogen storage disease

     E74.04 **McArdle disease** `CC` `HCC`
         Type V glycogen storage disease

     E74.09 **Other glycogen storage disease** `CC` `HCC`
         Andersen disease
         Hers disease
         Tauri disease
         Glycogen storage disease, types 0, IV, VI-XI
         Liver phosphorylase deficiency
         Muscle phosphofructokinase deficiency

√5ᵗʰ **E74.1** **Disorders of fructose metabolism**
> **EXCLUDES 1**   muscle phosphofructokinase deficiency (E74.09)

     E74.10 **Disorder of fructose metabolism, unspecified**

     E74.11 **Essential fructosuria**
         Fructokinase deficiency

     E74.12 **Hereditary fructose intolerance**
         Fructosemia

     E74.19 **Other disorders of fructose metabolism**
         Fructose-1, 6-diphosphatase deficiency

√5ᵗʰ **E74.2** **Disorders of galactose metabolism**

     E74.20 **Disorders of galactose metabolism, unspecified** `CC` `HCC`

     E74.21 **Galactosemia** `CC` `HCC`
         DEF: Any of three genetic disorders caused by a defective galactose metabolism. Symptoms include failure to thrive in infancy, jaundice, liver and spleen damage, cataracts, and mental retardation.

     E74.29 **Other disorders of galactose metabolism** `CC` `HCC`
         Galactokinase deficiency

√5ᵗʰ **E74.3** **Other disorders of intestinal carbohydrate absorption**
> **EXCLUDES 2**   lactose intolerance (E73.-)

     E74.31 **Sucrase-isomaltase deficiency**

     E74.39 **Other disorders of intestinal carbohydrate absorption**
         Disorder of intestinal carbohydrate absorption NOS
         Glucose-galactose malabsorption
         Sucrase deficiency

E74.4 **Disorders of pyruvate metabolism and gluconeogenesis** `CC` `HCC`
Deficiency of phosphoenolpyruvate carboxykinase
Deficiency of pyruvate carboxylase
Deficiency of pyruvate dehydrogenase
> **EXCLUDES 1**   disorders of pyruvate metabolism and gluconeogenesis with anemia (D55.-)
> Leigh's syndrome (G31.82)

▲ √5ᵗʰ **E74.8** **Other specified disorders of carbohydrate metabolism**
~~Essential pentosuria~~
~~Renal glycosuria~~

●   √6ᵗʰ **E74.81** **Disorders of glucose transport, not elsewhere classified**

●   **E74.810** **Glucose transporter protein type 1 deficiency** `CC`
           De Vivo syndrome
           Glucose transport defect, blood-brain barrier
           Glut1 deficiency
           GLUT1 deficiency syndrome 1, infantile onset
           GLUT1 deficiency syndrome 2, childhood onset

●   **E74.818** **Other disorders of glucose transport** `CC`
           (Familial) renal glycosuria

●   **E74.819** **Disorders of glucose transport, unspecified** `CC`

●   **E74.89** **Other specified disorders of carbohydrate metabolism** `CC`
         Essential pentosuria

     E74.9 **Disorder of carbohydrate metabolism, unspecified** `HCC`

√4ᵗʰ **E75** **Disorders of sphingolipid metabolism and other lipid storage disorders**
> **EXCLUDES 1**   mucolipidosis, types I-III (E77.0-E77.1)
> Refsum's disease (G60.1)

√5ᵗʰ **E75.0** **GM2 gangliosidosis**

     E75.00 **GM2 gangliosidosis, unspecified** `CC` `HCC`

     E75.01 **Sandhoff disease** `CC` `HCC`

E75.02 Tay-Sachs disease `CC` `HCC`
DEF: Genetic mutation of the HEXA gene that inhibits the breakdown of a toxic substance called ganglioside. The accumulation of ganglioside results in destruction of the neurons in the brain and spinal cord.

Tay-Sachs Disease

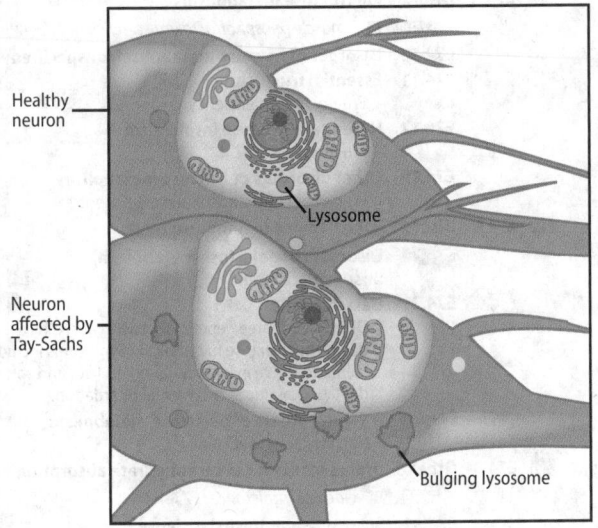

Healthy neuron
Lysosome
Neuron affected by Tay-Sachs
Bulging lysosome

E75.09 Other GM2 gangliosidosis `CC` `HCC`
Adult GM2 gangliosidosis
Juvenile GM2 gangliosidosis

✓5ᵗʰ **E75.1 Other and unspecified gangliosidosis**

E75.10 Unspecified gangliosidosis `CC` `HCC`
Gangliosidosis NOS

E75.11 Mucolipidosis IV `CC` `HCC`

E75.19 Other gangliosidosis `CC` `HCC`
GM1 gangliosidosis
GM3 gangliosidosis

✓5ᵗʰ **E75.2 Other sphingolipidosis**
EXCLUDES 1 adrenoleukodystrophy [Addison-Schilder] (E71.528)

E75.21 Fabry (-Anderson) disease `HCC`

E75.22 Gaucher disease `HCC`

E75.23 Krabbe disease `CC` `HCC`

✓6ᵗʰ **E75.24 Niemann-Pick disease**

E75.240 Niemann-Pick disease type A `HCC`
E75.241 Niemann-Pick disease type B `HCC`
E75.242 Niemann-Pick disease type C `HCC`
E75.243 Niemann-Pick disease type D `HCC`
E75.248 Other Niemann-Pick disease `HCC`
E75.249 Niemann-Pick disease, unspecified `HCC`

E75.25 Metachromatic leukodystrophy `CC` `HCC`

E75.26 Sulfatase deficiency `CC` `HCC`
Multiple sulfatase deficiency (MSD)
AHA: 2018,4Q,5-6

E75.29 Other sphingolipidosis `CC` `HCC`
Farber's syndrome
Sulfatide lipidosis

E75.3 Sphingolipidosis, unspecified `HCC`

E75.4 Neuronal ceroid lipofuscinosis `CC` `HCC`
Batten disease
Bielschowsky-Jansky disease
Kufs disease
Spielmeyer-Vogt disease

E75.5 Other lipid storage disorders
Cerebrotendinous cholesterosis [van Bogaert-Scherer-Epstein]
Wolman's disease

E75.6 Lipid storage disorder, unspecified

✓4ᵗʰ **E76 Disorders of glycosaminoglycan metabolism**

✓5ᵗʰ **E76.0 Mucopolysaccharidosis, type I**

E76.01 Hurler's syndrome `CC` `HCC`
E76.02 Hurler-Scheie syndrome `CC` `HCC`
E76.03 Scheie's syndrome `CC` `HCC`

E76.1 Mucopolysaccharidosis, type II `CC` `HCC`
Hunter's syndrome

✓5ᵗʰ **E76.2 Other mucopolysaccharidoses**

✓6ᵗʰ **E76.21 Morquio mucopolysaccharidoses**

E76.210 Morquio A mucopolysaccharidoses `CC` `HCC`
Classic Morquio syndrome
Morquio syndrome A
Mucopolysaccharidosis, type IVA

E76.211 Morquio B mucopolysaccharidoses `CC` `HCC`
Morquio-like mucopolysaccharidoses
Morquio-like syndrome
Morquio syndrome B
Mucopolysaccharidosis, type IVB

E76.219 Morquio mucopolysaccharidoses, unspecified `CC` `HCC`
Morquio syndrome
Mucopolysaccharidosis, type IV

E76.22 Sanfilippo mucopolysaccharidoses `CC` `HCC`
Mucopolysaccharidosis, type III (A) (B) (C) (D)
Sanfilippo A syndrome
Sanfilippo B syndrome
Sanfilippo C syndrome
Sanfilippo D syndrome

E76.29 Other mucopolysaccharidoses `CC` `HCC`
beta-Glucuronidase deficiency
Maroteaux-Lamy (mild) (severe) syndrome
Mucopolysaccharidosis, types VI, VII

E76.3 Mucopolysaccharidosis, unspecified `CC` `HCC`

E76.8 Other disorders of glucosaminoglycan metabolism `CC` `HCC`

E76.9 Glucosaminoglycan metabolism disorder, unspecified `CC` `HCC`

✓4ᵗʰ **E77 Disorders of glycoprotein metabolism**

E77.0 Defects in post-translational modification of lysosomal enzymes `HCC`
Mucolipidosis II [I-cell disease]
Mucolipidosis III [pseudo-Hurler polydystrophy]

E77.1 Defects in glycoprotein degradation `HCC`
Aspartylglucosaminuria
Fucosidosis
Mannosidosis
Sialidosis [mucolipidosis I]

E77.8 Other disorders of glycoprotein metabolism `HCC`

E77.9 Disorder of glycoprotein metabolism, unspecified `HCC`

✓4ᵗʰ **E78 Disorders of lipoprotein metabolism and other lipidemias**
EXCLUDES 1 sphingolipidosis (E75.0-E75.3)

✓5ᵗʰ **E78.0 Pure hypercholesterolemia**
AHA: 2016,4Q,13-14

E78.00 Pure hypercholesterolemia, unspecified
Fredrickson's hyperlipoproteinemia, type IIa
Hyperbetalipoproteinemia
Low-density-lipoprotein-type [LDL] hyperlipoproteinemia
(Pure) hypercholesterolemia NOS

E78.01 Familial hypercholesterolemia

E78.1 Pure hyperglyceridemia
Elevated fasting triglycerides
Endogenous hyperglyceridemia
Fredrickson's hyperlipoproteinemia, type IV
Hyperlipidemia, group B
Hyperprebetalipoproteinemia
Very-low-density-lipoprotein-type [VLDL] hyperlipoproteinemia

E78.2   **Mixed hyperlipidemia**
Broad- or floating-betalipoproteinemia
Combined hyperlipidemia NOS
Elevated cholesterol with elevated triglycerides NEC
Fredrickson's hyperlipoproteinemia, type IIb or III
Hyperbetalipoproteinemia with prebetalipoproteinemia
Hypercholesteremia with endogenous hyperglyceridemia
Hyperlipidemia, group C
Tubo-eruptive xanthoma
Xanthoma tuberosum
> EXCLUDES 1   cerebrotendinous cholesterosis [van Bogaert-Scherer-Epstein] (E75.5)
> familial combined hyperlipidemia (E78.49)

E78.3   **Hyperchylomicronemia**
Chylomicron retention disease
Fredrickson's hyperlipoproteinemia, type I or V
Hyperlipidemia, group D
Mixed hyperglyceridemia

√5ᵗʰ E78.4   **Other hyperlipidemia**
AHA: 2018,4Q,6
    E78.41   **Elevated Lipoprotein(a)**
       Elevated Lp(a)
    E78.49   **Other hyperlipidemia**
       Familial combined hyperlipidemia

E78.5   **Hyperlipidemia, unspecified**

E78.6   **Lipoprotein deficiency**
Abetalipoproteinemia
Depressed HDL cholesterol
High-density lipoprotein deficiency
Hypoalphalipoproteinemia
Hypobetalipoproteinemia (familial)
Lecithin cholesterol acyltransferase deficiency
Tangier disease

√5ᵗʰ E78.7   **Disorders of bile acid and cholesterol metabolism**
> EXCLUDES 1   Niemann-Pick disease type C (E75.242)

    E78.70   **Disorder of bile acid and cholesterol metabolism, unspecified**
    E78.71   **Barth syndrome**   CC
    E78.72   **Smith-Lemli-Opitz syndrome**   CC
    E78.79   **Other disorders of bile acid and cholesterol metabolism**

√5ᵗʰ E78.8   **Other disorders of lipoprotein metabolism**
    E78.81   **Lipoid dermatoarthritis**
    E78.89   **Other lipoprotein metabolism disorders**

E78.9   **Disorder of lipoprotein metabolism, unspecified**

√4ᵗʰ E79   **Disorders of purine and pyrimidine metabolism**
> EXCLUDES 1   Ataxia-telangiectasia (Q87.19)
> Bloom's syndrome (Q82.8)
> Cockayne's syndrome (Q87.19)
> calculus of kidney (N20.0)
> combined immunodeficiency disorders (D81.-)
> Fanconi's anemia (D61.09)
> gout (M1A.-, M10.-)
> orotaciduric anemia (D53.0)
> progeria (E34.8)
> Werner's syndrome (E34.8)
> xeroderma pigmentosum (Q82.1)

E79.0   **Hyperuricemia without signs of inflammatory arthritis and tophaceous disease**
Asymptomatic hyperuricemia

E79.1   **Lesch-Nyhan syndrome**   CC HCC
HGPRT deficiency

E79.2   **Myoadenylate deaminase deficiency**   CC HCC

E79.8   **Other disorders of purine and pyrimidine metabolism**   CC HCC
Hereditary xanthinuria

E79.9   **Disorder of purine and pyrimidine metabolism, unspecified**   CC HCC

√4ᵗʰ E80   **Disorders of porphyrin and bilirubin metabolism**
> INCLUDES   defects of catalase and peroxidase

E80.0   **Hereditary erythropoietic porphyria**   CC HCC
Congenital erythropoietic porphyria
Erythropoietic protoporphyria

E80.1   **Porphyria cutanea tarda**   CC HCC

√5ᵗʰ E80.2   **Other and unspecified porphyria**
    E80.20   **Unspecified porphyria**   CC HCC
       Porphyria NOS
    E80.21   **Acute intermittent (hepatic) porphyria**   CC HCC
    E80.29   **Other porphyria**   CC HCC
       Hereditary coproporphyria

E80.3   **Defects of catalase and peroxidase**   CC HCC
Acatalasia [Takahara]

E80.4   **Gilbert syndrome**

E80.5   **Crigler-Najjar syndrome**

E80.6   **Other disorders of bilirubin metabolism**
Dubin-Johnson syndrome
Rotor's syndrome

E80.7   **Disorder of bilirubin metabolism, unspecified**

√4ᵗʰ E83   **Disorders of mineral metabolism**
> EXCLUDES 1   dietary mineral deficiency (E58-E61)
> parathyroid disorders (E20-E21)
> vitamin D deficiency (E55.-)

√5ᵗʰ E83.0   **Disorders of copper metabolism**
    E83.00   **Disorder of copper metabolism, unspecified**
    E83.01   **Wilson's disease**
       Code also associated Kayser Fleischer ring (H18.04-)
    E83.09   **Other disorders of copper metabolism**
       Menkes' (kinky hair) (steely hair) disease

√5ᵗʰ E83.1   **Disorders of iron metabolism**
> EXCLUDES 1   iron deficiency anemia (D50.-)
> sideroblastic anemia (D64.0-D64.3)

    E83.10   **Disorder of iron metabolism, unspecified**
    √6ᵗʰ E83.11   **Hemochromatosis**
> EXCLUDES 1   GALD (P78.84)
> gestational alloimmune liver disease (P78.84)
> neonatal hemochromatosis (P78.84)

       E83.110   **Hereditary hemochromatosis**   HCC
          Bronzed diabetes
          Pigmentary cirrhosis (of liver)
          Primary (hereditary) hemochromatosis
       E83.111   **Hemochromatosis due to repeated red blood cell transfusions**
          Iron overload due to repeated red blood cell transfusions
          Transfusion (red blood cell) associated hemochromatosis
       E83.118   **Other hemochromatosis**
       E83.119   **Hemochromatosis, unspecified**
    E83.19   **Other disorders of iron metabolism**
       Use additional code, if applicable, for idiopathic pulmonary hemosiderosis (J84.03)

E83.2   **Disorders of zinc metabolism**
Acrodermatitis enteropathica

√5ᵗʰ E83.3   **Disorders of phosphorus metabolism and phosphatases**
> EXCLUDES 1   adult osteomalacia (M83.-)
> osteoporosis (M80.-)

    E83.30   **Disorder of phosphorus metabolism, unspecified**
    E83.31   **Familial hypophosphatemia**
       Vitamin D-resistant osteomalacia
       Vitamin D-resistant rickets
> EXCLUDES 1   vitamin D-deficiency rickets (E55.0)

    E83.32   **Hereditary vitamin D-dependent rickets (type 1) (type 2)**
       25-hydroxyvitamin D 1-alpha-hydroxylase deficiency
       Pseudovitamin D deficiency
       Vitamin D receptor defect
    E83.39   **Other disorders of phosphorus metabolism**
       Acid phosphatase deficiency
       Hypophosphatasia

√5ᵗʰ E83.4   **Disorders of magnesium metabolism**
    E83.40   **Disorders of magnesium metabolism, unspecified**
    E83.41   **Hypermagnesemia**
       AHA: 2016,4Q,54
    E83.42   **Hypomagnesemia**
    E83.49   **Other disorders of magnesium metabolism**

√ Additional Character Required   √x7ᵗʰ Placeholder   Unacceptable PDx   Questionable PDx   Manifestation   Unspecified Dx   H1-H14 HAC   HCC CMS-HCC Dx   HIV HIV Dx

ICD-10-CM 2021   539

Chapter 4. Endocrine, Nutritional and Metabolic Diseases

E83.5–E87.8

√5ᵗʰ **E83.5** **Disorders of calcium metabolism**

> EXCLUDES 1   chondrocalcinosis (M11.1-M11.2)
> hungry bone syndrome (E83.81)
> hyperparathyroidism (E21.0-E21.3)

    E83.50 **Unspecified disorder of calcium metabolism**
    E83.51 **Hypocalcemia**
    E83.52 **Hypercalcemia**
       Familial hypocalciuric hypercalcemia
    E83.59 **Other disorders of calcium metabolism**

√5ᵗʰ **E83.8** **Other disorders of mineral metabolism**

    E83.81 **Hungry bone syndrome**
    E83.89 **Other disorders of mineral metabolism**

E83.9 **Disorder of mineral metabolism, unspecified**

√4ᵗʰ **E84** **Cystic fibrosis**

> INCLUDES   mucoviscidosis

Code also exocrine pancreatic insufficiency (K86.81)
DEF: Genetic disorder affecting the respiratory, digestive, and reproductive systems in infants to young adults by disturbing exocrine gland function and causing chronic pulmonary disease with excess mucus production and pancreatic deficiency.

E84.0 **Cystic fibrosis with pulmonary manifestations**   MCC HCC
      Use additional code to identify any infectious organism present, such as:
      Pseudomonas (B96.5)

√5ᵗʰ **E84.1** **Cystic fibrosis with intestinal manifestations**

    E84.11 **Meconium ileus in cystic fibrosis**   MCC HCC N
>   EXCLUDES 1   meconium ileus not due to cystic fibrosis (P76.0)

    E84.19 **Cystic fibrosis with other intestinal manifestations**   CC HCC
       Distal intestinal obstruction syndrome

E84.8 **Cystic fibrosis with other manifestations**   CC HCC

E84.9 **Cystic fibrosis, unspecified**   CC HCC

√4ᵗʰ **E85** **Amyloidosis**

> EXCLUDES 2   Alzheimer's disease (G30.0-)

DEF: Conditions of diverse etiologies characterized by the accumulation of insoluble fibrillar proteins (amyloid) in various organs and tissues of the body, compromising vital functions.

E85.0 **Non-neuropathic heredofamilial amyloidosis**   CC HCC
      Hereditary amyloid nephropathy
      Code also associated disorders, such as:
        autoinflammatory syndromes (M04.-)
>   EXCLUDES 2   transthyretin-related (ATTR) familial amyloid cardiomyopathy (E85.4)

E85.1 **Neuropathic heredofamilial amyloidosis**   CC HCC
      Amyloid polyneuropathy (Portuguese)
      Transthyretin-related (ATTR) familial amyloid polyneuropathy
      AHA: 2012,4Q,99

E85.2 **Heredofamilial amyloidosis, unspecified**   CC HCC

E85.3 **Secondary systemic amyloidosis**   CC HCC
      Hemodialysis-associated amyloidosis

E85.4 **Organ-limited amyloidosis**   CC HCC
      Localized amyloidosis
      Transthyretin-related (ATTR) familial amyloid cardiomyopathy

√5ᵗʰ **E85.8** **Other amyloidosis**
      AHA: 2017,4Q,7

    E85.81 **Light chain (AL) amyloidosis**   CC HCC
    E85.82 **Wild-type transthyretin-related (ATTR) amyloidosis**   CC HCC
       Senile systemic amyloidosis (SSA)
    E85.89 **Other amyloidosis**   CC HCC

E85.9 **Amyloidosis, unspecified**   CC HCC

√4ᵗʰ **E86** **Volume depletion**

Use additional code(s) for any associated disorders of electrolyte and acid-base balance (E87.-)

> EXCLUDES 1   dehydration of newborn (P74.1)
> hypovolemic shock NOS (R57.1)
> postprocedural hypovolemic shock (T81.19)
> traumatic hypovolemic shock (T79.4)
> EXCLUDES 2   ▶hypovolemic shock NOS (R57.1)◀

AHA: 2019,2Q,7; 2018,2Q,6

E86.0 **Dehydration**
      AHA: 2019,2Q,7; 2019,1Q,12; 2014,1Q,7
      TIP: Can be assigned in addition to hypernatremia (E87.0) or hyponatremia (E87.1), when documented.

E86.1 **Hypovolemia**
      Depletion of volume of plasma

E86.9 **Volume depletion, unspecified**
      DEF: Depletion of total body water (dehydration) and/or contraction of total intravascular plasma (hypovolemia).

√4ᵗʰ **E87** **Other disorders of fluid, electrolyte and acid-base balance**

> EXCLUDES 1   diabetes insipidus (E23.2)
> electrolyte imbalance associated with hyperemesis gravidarum (O21.1)
> electrolyte imbalance following ectopic or molar pregnancy (O08.5)
> familial periodic paralysis (G72.3)

AHA: 2018,2Q,6

E87.0 **Hyperosmolality and hypernatremia**   CC
      Sodium [Na] excess
      Sodium [Na] overload
      AHA: 2014,1Q,7
      TIP: Assign an additional code for dehydration (E86.0), when documented.

E87.1 **Hypo-osmolality and hyponatremia**   CC
      Sodium [Na] deficiency
>   EXCLUDES 1   syndrome of inappropriate secretion of antidiuretic hormone (E22.2)

      AHA: 2014,1Q,7
      TIP: Assign an additional code for dehydration (E86.0), when documented.

E87.2 **Acidosis**   CC
      Acidosis NOS
      Lactic acidosis
      Metabolic acidosis
      Respiratory acidosis
>   EXCLUDES 1   diabetic acidosis — see categories E08-E10, E13 with ketoacidosis

      DEF: Reduction of alkaline in the blood and tissues caused by an increase in acid and decrease in bicarbonate.

E87.3 **Alkalosis**   CC
      Alkalosis NOS
      Metabolic alkalosis
      Respiratory alkalosis

E87.4 **Mixed disorder of acid-base balance**   CC

E87.5 **Hyperkalemia**
      Potassium [K] excess
      Potassium [K] overload

E87.6 **Hypokalemia**
      Potassium [K] deficiency

√5ᵗʰ **E87.7** **Fluid overload**

>   EXCLUDES 1   edema NOS (R60.9)
> fluid retention (R60.9)

    E87.70 **Fluid overload, unspecified**
    E87.71 **Transfusion associated circulatory overload**
       Fluid overload due to transfusion (blood) (blood components)
       TACO
    E87.79 **Other fluid overload**

E87.8 **Other disorders of electrolyte and fluid balance, not elsewhere classified**
      Electrolyte imbalance NOS
      Hyperchloremia
      Hypochloremia

N Newborn: 0   P Pediatric: 0-17   M Maternity: 9-64   A Adult: 15-124   MCC Major Complication/Comorbidity   CC Complication/Comorbidity   SW Severe Wound Dx

540   ICD-10-CM 2021

☑4ᵗʰ **E88 Other and unspecified metabolic disorders**

     Use additional codes for associated conditions

     EXCLUDES 1   *histiocytosis X (chronic) (C96.6)*

☑5ᵗʰ   **E88.0 Disorders of plasma-protein metabolism, not elsewhere classified**

     EXCLUDES 1   *disorder of lipoprotein metabolism (E78.-)*

         monoclonal gammopathy (of undetermined significance) (D47.2)

         polyclonal hypergammaglobulinemia (D89.0)

         Waldenström macroglobulinemia (C88.0)

     EXCLUDES 2   ▶*disorder of lipoprotein metabolism (E78.-)*◀

     E88.01 Alpha-1-antitrypsin deficiency   `HCC`

         AAT deficiency

     E88.02 Plasminogen deficiency   `CC`

         Dysplasminogenemia

         Hypoplasminogenemia

         Type 1 plasminogen deficiency

         Type 2 plasminogen deficiency

         Code also, if applicable, ligneous conjunctivitis (H10.51)

         Use additional code for associated findings, such as:

         hydrocephalus (G91.4)

         otitis media (H67.-)

         respiratory disorder related to plasminogen deficiency (J99)

         AHA: 2018,4Q,6-7

     E88.09 Other disorders of plasma-protein metabolism, not elsewhere classified

         Bisalbuminemia

   E88.1 Lipodystrophy, not elsewhere classified

     Lipodystrophy NOS

     EXCLUDES 1   *Whipple's disease (K90.81)*

   E88.2 Lipomatosis, not elsewhere classified

     Lipomatosis NOS

     Lipomatosis (Check) dolorosa [Dercum]

   E88.3 Tumor lysis syndrome   `MCC`

     Tumor lysis syndrome (spontaneous)

     Tumor lysis syndrome following antineoplastic drug chemotherapy

     Use additional code for adverse effect, if applicable, to identify drug (T45.1X5)

     AHA: 2020,1Q,37; 2019,2Q,24

     DEF: Potentially fatal metabolic complication of tumor necrosis caused by spontaneous or treatment-related accumulation of byproducts from dying cancer cells. Symptoms include hyperkalemia, hyperphosphatemia, hypocalcemia, hyperuricemia, and hyperuricosuria.

☑5ᵗʰ   **E88.4 Mitochondrial metabolism disorders**

     EXCLUDES 1   *disorders of pyruvate metabolism (E74.4)*

         Kearns-Sayre syndrome (H49.81)

         Leber's disease (H47.22)

         Leigh's encephalopathy (G31.82)

         mitochondrial myopathy, NEC (G71.3)

         Reye's syndrome (G93.7)

     E88.40 Mitochondrial metabolism disorder, unspecified   `CC` `HCC`

     E88.41 MELAS syndrome   `CC` `HCC`

         Mitochondrial myopathy, encephalopathy, lactic acidosis and stroke-like episodes

     E88.42 MERRF syndrome   `CC` `HCC`

         Myoclonic epilepsy associated with ragged-red fibers

         Code also progressive myoclonic epilepsy (G40.3-)

     E88.49 Other mitochondrial metabolism disorders   `CC` `HCC`

☑5ᵗʰ   **E88.8 Other specified metabolic disorders**

     E88.81 Metabolic syndrome

         Dysmetabolic syndrome X

         Use additional codes for associated manifestations, such as:

         obesity (E66.-)

         DEF: Group of health risks that increase the likelihood of developing heart disease, stroke, and diabetes. These risks include certain parameters for blood pressure, cholesterol, and glucose levels.

     E88.89 Other specified metabolic disorders   `HCC`

         Launois-Bensaude adenolipomatosis

         EXCLUDES 1   *adult pulmonary Langerhans cell histiocytosis (J84.82)*

   E88.9 Metabolic disorder, unspecified

Postprocedural endocrine and metabolic complications and disorders, not elsewhere classified (E89)

☑4ᵗʰ **E89 Postprocedural endocrine and metabolic complications and disorders, not elsewhere classified**

     EXCLUDES 2   *intraoperative complications of endocrine system organ or structure (E36.0-, E36.1-, E36.8)*

   E89.0 Postprocedural hypothyroidism

     Postirradiation hypothyroidism

     Postsurgical hypothyroidism

   E89.1 Postprocedural hypoinsulinemia   `CC`

     Postpancreatectomy hyperglycemia

     Postsurgical hypoinsulinemia

     Use additional code, if applicable, to identify:

     acquired absence of pancreas (Z90.41-)

     diabetes mellitus (postpancreatectomy) (postprocedural) (E13.-)

     insulin use (Z79.4)

     EXCLUDES 1   *transient postprocedural hyperglycemia (R73.9)*

         transient postprocedural hypoglycemia (E16.2)

   E89.2 Postprocedural hypoparathyroidism   `HCC`

     Parathyroprival tetany

   E89.3 Postprocedural hypopituitarism   `HCC`

     Postirradiation hypopituitarism

☑5ᵗʰ   **E89.4 Postprocedural ovarian failure**

     E89.40 Asymptomatic postprocedural ovarian failure   ♀

         Postprocedural ovarian failure NOS

     E89.41 Symptomatic postprocedural ovarian failure   ♀

         Symptoms such as flushing, sleeplessness, headache, lack of concentration, associated with postprocedural menopause

   E89.5 Postprocedural testicular hypofunction   ♂

   E89.6 Postprocedural adrenocortical (-medullary) hypofunction   `CC` `HCC`

☑5ᵗʰ   **E89.8 Other postprocedural endocrine and metabolic complications and disorders**

     AHA: 2016,4Q,9-10

☑6ᵗʰ   **E89.81 Postprocedural hemorrhage of an endocrine system organ or structure following a procedure**

     E89.810 Postprocedural hemorrhage of an endocrine system organ or structure following an endocrine system procedure   `CC`

     E89.811 Postprocedural hemorrhage of an endocrine system organ or structure following other procedure   `CC`

☑6ᵗʰ   **E89.82 Postprocedural hematoma and seroma of an endocrine system organ or structure**

     E89.820 Postprocedural hematoma of an endocrine system organ or structure following an endocrine system procedure   `CC`

     E89.821 Postprocedural hematoma of an endocrine system organ or structure following other procedure   `CC`

     E89.822 Postprocedural seroma of an endocrine system organ or structure following an endocrine system procedure   `CC`

     E89.823 Postprocedural seroma of an endocrine system organ or structure following other procedure   `CC`

     E89.89 Other postprocedural endocrine and metabolic complications and disorders   `CC`

         Use additional code, if applicable, to further specify disorder

☑ Additional Character Required   ✓x7ᵗʰ Placeholder   Unacceptable PDx   Questionable PDx   Manifestation   Unspecified Dx   H1-H14 HAC   HCC CMS-HCC Dx   HIV HIV Dx

ICD-10-CM 2021   541

Chapter 5. Mental, Behavioral and Neurodevelopmental Disorders (F01–F99)

Chapter-specific Guidelines with Coding Examples

The chapter-specific guidelines from the ICD-10-CM Official Guidelines for Coding and Reporting have been provided below. Along with these guidelines are coding examples, contained in the shaded boxes, that have been developed to help illustrate the coding and/or sequencing guidance found in these guidelines.

a. Pain disorders related to psychological factors

Assign code F45.41, for pain that is exclusively related to psychological disorders. As indicated by the Excludes 1 note under category G89, a code from category G89 should not be assigned with code F45.41.

> Perceived abdominal pain determined to be persistent somatoform pain disorder
>
> **F45.41   Pain disorder exclusively related to psychological factors**
>
> *Explanation*: This pain was diagnosed as being exclusively psychological; therefore, no code from category G89 is added.

Code F45.42, Pain disorders with related psychological factors, should be used with a code from category G89, Pain, not elsewhere classified, if there is documentation of a psychological component for a patient with acute or chronic pain.

See Section I.C.6. Pain

b. Mental and behavioral disorders due to psychoactive substance use

1) In remission

Selection of codes for "in remission" for categories F10-F19, Mental and behavioral disorders due to psychoactive substance use (categories F10-F19 with -11, -.21) requires the provider's clinical judgment. The appropriate codes for "in remission" are assigned only on the basis of provider documentation (as defined in the Official Guidelines for Coding and Reporting), unless otherwise instructed by the classification.

Mild substance use disorders in early or sustained remission are classified to the appropriate codes for substance abuse in remission, and moderate or severe substance use disorders in early or sustained remission are classified to the appropriate codes for substance dependence in remission.

> Insomnia in patient with history of methamphetamine abuse; lab results indicate no current drug use
>
> **G47.00   Insomnia, unspecified**
>
> **F15.10   Other stimulant abuse, uncomplicated**
>
> *Explanation*: Insomnia is a common side-effect of stimulant use, such as methamphetamines. Although lab tests do not indicate that the patient is currently using methamphetamines, there is no specific documentation stating that the stimulant abuse is in remission. "History of" abuse does not equate to "in remission" in this instance.

2) Psychoactive substance use, abuse and dependence

When the provider documentation refers to use, abuse and dependence of the same substance (e.g. alcohol, opioid, cannabis, etc.), only one code should be assigned to identify the pattern of use based on the following hierarchy:

- If both use and abuse are documented, assign only the code for abuse
- If both abuse and dependence are documented, assign only the code for dependence
- If use, abuse and dependence are all documented, assign only the code for dependence
- If both use and dependence are documented, assign only the code for dependence.

> History and physical notes cannabis dependence; progress note says cannabis abuse
>
> **F12.20   Cannabis dependence, uncomplicated**
>
> *Explanation*: In the hierarchy, the dependence code is used if both abuse and dependence are documented.

> Discharge summary says cocaine abuse; progress notes list cocaine use
>
> **F14.10   Cocaine abuse, uncomplicated**
>
> *Explanation*: In the hierarchy, the abuse code is used if both abuse and use are documented.

3) Psychoactive substance use, unspecified

As with all other unspecified diagnoses, the codes for unspecified psychoactive substance use disorders (F10.9-, F11.9-, F12.9-, F13.9-, F14.9-, F15.9-, F16.9-, F18.9-, F19.9-) should only be assigned based on provider documentation and when they meet the definition of a reportable diagnosis (see Section III, Reporting Additional Diagnoses). These codes are to be used only when the psychoactive substance use is associated with a physical **disorder included in chapter 5 (such as sexual dysfunction and sleep disorder), or a** mental or behavioral disorder, and such a relationship is documented by the provider.

c. Factitious disorder

Factitious disorder imposed on self or Munchausen's syndrome is a disorder in which a person falsely reports or causes his or her own physical or psychological signs or symptoms. For patients with documented factitious disorder on self or Munchausen's syndrome, assign the appropriate code from subcategory F68.1-, Factitious disorder imposed on self.

Munchausen's syndrome by proxy (MSBP) is a disorder in which a caregiver (perpetrator) falsely reports or causes an illness or injury in another person (victim) under his or her care, such as a child, an elderly adult, or a person who has a disability. The condition is also referred to as "factitious disorder imposed on another" or "factitious disorder by proxy." The perpetrator, not the victim, receives this diagnosis. Assign code F68.A, Factitious disorder imposed on another, to the perpetrator's record. For the victim of a patient suffering from MSBP, assign the appropriate code from categories T74, Adult and child abuse, neglect and other maltreatment, confirmed, or T76, Adult and child abuse, neglect and other maltreatment, suspected.

See Section I.C.19.f. Adult and child abuse, neglect and other maltreatment

Chapter 5. Mental, Behavioral and Neurodevelopmental Disorders

Chapter 5. Mental, Behavioral and Neurodevelopmental Disorders (F01-F99)

INCLUDES   disorders of psychological development

EXCLUDES 2   *symptoms, signs and abnormal clinical laboratory findings, not elsewhere classified (R00-R99)*

This chapter contains the following blocks:

F01-F09	Mental disorders due to known physiological conditions
F10-F19	Mental and behavioral disorders due to psychoactive substance use
F20-F29	Schizophrenia, schizotypal, delusional, and other non-mood psychotic disorders
F30-F39	Mood [affective] disorders
F40-F48	Anxiety, dissociative, stress-related, somatoform and other nonpsychotic mental disorders
F50-F59	Behavioral syndromes associated with physiological disturbances and physical factors
F60-F69	Disorders of adult personality and behavior
F70-F79	Intellectual disabilities
F80-F89	Pervasive and specific developmental disorders
F90-F98	Behavioral and emotional disorders with onset usually occurring in childhood and adolescence
F99	Unspecified mental disorder

Mental disorders due to known physiological conditions (F01-F09)

NOTE   This block comprises a range of mental disorders grouped together on the basis of their having in common a demonstrable etiology in cerebral disease, brain injury, or other insult leading to cerebral dysfunction. The dysfunction may be primary, as in diseases, injuries, and insults that affect the brain directly and selectively; or secondary, as in systemic diseases and disorders that attack the brain only as one of the multiple organs or systems of the body that are involved.

✓4ᵗʰ F01   Vascular dementia

Vascular dementia as a result of infarction of the brain due to vascular disease, including hypertensive cerebrovascular disease.

INCLUDES   arteriosclerotic dementia

Code first the underlying physiological condition or sequelae of cerebrovascular disease.

✓5ᵗʰ F01.5   Vascular dementia

F01.50   **Vascular dementia** without behavioral disturbance   **HCC** **A**

Major neurocognitive disorder without behavioral disturbance

F01.51   **Vascular dementia** with behavioral disturbance   **CC** **HCC** **A**

Major neurocognitive disorder due to vascular disease, with behavioral disturbance

Major neurocognitive disorder with aggressive behavior

Major neurocognitive disorder with combative behavior

Major neurocognitive disorder with violent behavior

Vascular dementia with aggressive behavior

Vascular dementia with combative behavior

Vascular dementia with violent behavior

Use additional code, if applicable, to identify wandering in vascular dementia (Z91.83)

✓4ᵗʰ F02   Dementia in other diseases classified elsewhere

INCLUDES   major neurocognitive disorder in other diseases classified elsewhere

Code first the underlying physiological condition, such as:

Alzheimer's (G30.-)
cerebral lipidosis (E75.4)
Creutzfeldt-Jakob disease (A81.0-)
dementia with Lewy bodies (G31.83)
dementia with Parkinsonism (G31.83)
epilepsy and recurrent seizures (G40.-)
frontotemporal dementia (G31.09)
hepatolenticular degeneration (E83.0)
human immunodeficiency virus [HIV] disease (B20)
Huntington's disease (G10)
hypercalcemia (E83.52)
hypothyroidism, acquired (E00-E03.-)
intoxications (T36-T65)
Jakob-Creutzfeldt disease (A81.0-)
multiple sclerosis (G35)
neurosyphilis (A52.17)
niacin deficiency [pellagra] (E52)
Parkinson's disease (G20)
Pick's disease (G31.01)
polyarteritis nodosa (M30.0)
prion disease (A81.9)
systemic lupus erythematosus (M32.-)
traumatic brain injury (S06.-)
trypanosomiasis (B56.-, B57.-)
vitamin B deficiency (E53.8)

EXCLUDES 2   *dementia in alcohol and psychoactive substance disorders (F10-F19, with .17, .27, .97)*

vascular dementia (F01.5-)

✓5ᵗʰ F02.8   Dementia in other diseases classified elsewhere

AHA: 2017,2Q,7; 2016,4Q,141; 2016,2Q,6

TIP: A code from this subcategory should always be assigned with a code from category G30 when Alzheimer's disease is documented, even in the absence of documented dementia.

F02.80   *Dementia in other diseases classified elsewhere without behavioral disturbance*   **HCC**

Dementia in other diseases classified elsewhere NOS

Major neurocognitive disorder in other diseases classified elsewhere

F02.81   *Dementia in other diseases classified elsewhere with behavioral disturbance*   **CC** **HCC**

Dementia in other diseases classified elsewhere with aggressive behavior

Dementia in other diseases classified elsewhere with combative behavior

Dementia in other diseases classified elsewhere with violent behavior

Major neurocognitive disorder in other diseases classified elsewhere with aggressive behavior

Major neurocognitive disorder in other diseases classified elsewhere with combative behavior

Major neurocognitive disorder in other diseases classified elsewhere with violent behavior

Use additional code, if applicable, to identify wandering in dementia in conditions classified elsewhere (Z91.83)

✓4ᵗʰ F03   Unspecified dementia

Presenile dementia NOS
Presenile psychosis NOS
Primary degenerative dementia NOS
Senile dementia NOS
Senile dementia depressed or paranoid type
Senile psychosis NOS

EXCLUDES 1   *senility NOS (R41.81)*

EXCLUDES 2   *mild memory disturbance due to known physiological condition (F06.8)*

senile dementia with delirium or acute confusional state (F05)

✓5ᵗʰ F03.9   Unspecified dementia

F03.90   **Unspecified dementia** without behavioral disturbance   **HIV** **HCC** **A**

Dementia NOS

AHA: 2012,4Q,92

N Newborn: 0   **P** Pediatric: 0-17   **M** Maternity: 9-64   **A** Adult: 15-124   **MCC** Major Complication/Comorbidity   **CC** Complication/Comorbidity   **SW** Severe Wound Dx

544   ICD-10-CM 2021

F03.91   **Unspecified dementia** with behavioral disturbance   `CC` `HCC` `A`

Unspecified dementia with aggressive behavior
Unspecified dementia with combative behavior
Unspecified dementia with violent behavior
Use additional code, if applicable, to identify wandering in unspecified dementia (Z91.83)

F04   **Amnestic disorder due to known physiological condition**   `HCC`

Korsakov's psychosis or syndrome, nonalcoholic
Code first the underlying physiological condition

EXCLUDES 1   amnesia NOS (R41.3)
anterograde amnesia (R41.1)
dissociative amnesia (F44.0)
retrograde amnesia (R41.2)

EXCLUDES 2   alcohol-induced or unspecified Korsakov's syndrome (F10.26, F10.96)
Korsakov's syndrome induced by other psychoactive substances (F13.26, F13.96, F19.16, F19.26, F19.96)

F05   **Delirium due to known physiological condition**   `CC`

Acute or subacute brain syndrome
Acute or subacute confusional state (nonalcoholic)
Acute or subacute infective psychosis
Acute or subacute organic reaction
Acute or subacute psycho-organic syndrome
Delirium of mixed etiology
Delirium superimposed on dementia
Sundowning
Code first the underlying physiological condition

EXCLUDES 1   delirium NOS (R41.0)

EXCLUDES 2   delirium tremens alcohol-induced or unspecified (F10.231, F10.921)

AHA: 2019,2Q,34

`√4ᵗʰ` **F06**   **Other mental disorders due to known physiological condition**

INCLUDES   mental disorders due to endocrine disorder
mental disorders due to exogenous hormone
mental disorders due to exogenous toxic substance
mental disorders due to primary cerebral disease
mental disorders due to somatic illness
mental disorders due to systemic disease affecting the brain

Code first the underlying physiological condition

EXCLUDES 1   unspecified dementia (F03)

EXCLUDES 2   delirium due to known physiological condition (F05)
dementia as classified in F01-F02
other mental disorders associated with alcohol and other psychoactive substances (F10-F19)

F06.0   **Psychotic disorder** with hallucinations **due to known physiological condition**   `CC`

Organic hallucinatory state (nonalcoholic)

EXCLUDES 2   hallucinations and perceptual disturbance induced by alcohol and other psychoactive substances (F10-F19 with .151, .251, .951)
schizophrenia (F20.-)

F06.1   **Catatonic disorder due to known physiological condition**

Catatonia associated with another mental disorder
Catatonia NOS

EXCLUDES 1   catatonic stupor (R40.1)
stupor NOS (R40.1)

EXCLUDES 2   catatonic schizophrenia (F20.2)
dissociative stupor (F44.2)

DEF: Catatonic: Abnormal neuropsychiatric state characterized by stupor, immobility or purposeless movements, or unresponsiveness in a person who otherwise appears awake.

F06.2   **Psychotic disorder** with delusions **due to known physiological condition**   `CC`

Paranoid and paranoid-hallucinatory organic states
Schizophrenia-like psychosis in epilepsy

EXCLUDES 2   alcohol and drug-induced psychotic disorder (F10-F19 with .150, .250, .950)
brief psychotic disorder (F23)
delusional disorder (F22)
schizophrenia (F20.-)

`√5ᵗʰ` **F06.3**   **Mood disorder due to known physiological condition**

EXCLUDES 2   mood disorders due to alcohol and other psychoactive substances (F10-F19 with .14, .24, .94)
mood disorders, not due to known physiological condition or unspecified (F30-F39)

F06.30   **Mood disorder due to known physiological condition, unspecified**

F06.31   **Mood disorder due to known physiological condition with** depressive features

Depressive disorder due to known physiological condition, with depressive features

F06.32   **Mood disorder due to known physiological condition with** major depressive-like episode

Depressive disorder due to known physiological condition, with major depressive-like episode

F06.33   **Mood disorder due to known physiological condition with** manic features

Bipolar and related disorder due to a known physiological condition, with manic features
Bipolar and related disorder due to known physiological condition, with manic- or hypomanic-like episodes

F06.34   **Mood disorder due to known physiological condition with** mixed features

Bipolar and related disorder due to known physiological condition, with mixed features
Depressive disorder due to known physiological condition, with mixed features

F06.4   **Anxiety disorder due to known physiological condition**

EXCLUDES 2   anxiety disorders due to alcohol and other psychoactive substances (F10-F19 with .180, .280, .980)
anxiety disorders, not due to known physiological condition or unspecified (F40.-, F41.-)

F06.8   **Other specified mental disorders due to known physiological condition**   `HIV`

Epileptic psychosis NOS
Obsessive-compulsive and related disorder due to a known physiological condition
Organic dissociative disorder
Organic emotionally labile [asthenic] disorder

`√4ᵗʰ` **F07**   **Personality and behavioral disorders due to known physiological condition**

Code first the underlying physiological condition

F07.0   **Personality** change **due to known physiological condition**

Frontal lobe syndrome
Limbic epilepsy personality syndrome
Lobotomy syndrome
Organic personality disorder
Organic pseudopsychopathic personality
Organic pseudoretarded personality
Postleucotomy syndrome
Code first underlying physiological condition

EXCLUDES 1   mild cognitive impairment (G31.84)
postconcussional syndrome (F07.81)
postencephalitic syndrome (F07.89)
signs and symptoms involving emotional state (R45.-)

EXCLUDES 2   specific personality disorder (F60.-)

`√5ᵗʰ` **F07.8**   **Other personality and behavioral disorders due to known physiological condition**

F07.81   **Postconcussional syndrome**

Postcontusional syndrome (encephalopathy)
Post-traumatic brain syndrome, nonpsychotic
Use additional code to identify associated post-traumatic headache, if applicable (G44.3-)

EXCLUDES 1   current concussion (brain) (S06.0-)
postencephalitic syndrome (F07.89)

DEF: Concussion symptoms that persist for weeks or months after a head injury. These symptoms may include headache, giddiness, fatigue, insomnia, mood fluctuation, and a subjective feeling of impaired intellectual function with extreme reaction to normal stressors.

F07.89   **Other personality and behavioral disorders due to known physiological condition**

Postencephalitic syndrome
Right hemispheric organic affective disorder

☑ Additional Character Required   `√x7ᵗʰ` Placeholder   Unacceptable PDx   Questionable PDx   Manifestation   Unspecified Dx   `H1`-`H14` HAC   `HCC` CMS-HCC Dx   `HIV` HIV Dx

ICD-10-CM 2021   545

Chapter 5. Mental, Behavioral and Neurodevelopmental Disorders

F07.9   **Unspecified personality and behavioral disorder due to known physiological condition**   HIV
· Organic psychosyndrome

F09   **Unspecified mental disorder due to known physiological condition**   HIV
Mental disorder NOS due to known physiological condition
Organic brain syndrome NOS
Organic mental disorder NOS
Organic psychosis NOS
Symptomatic psychosis NOS
Code first the underlying physiological condition
EXCLUDES 1   psychosis NOS (F29)

Mental and behavioral disorders due to psychoactive substance use (F10-F19)

AHA: 2020,1Q,9; 2018,4Q,69-70; 2017,4Q,8; 2017,2Q,27

✓4ᵗʰ **F10**   **Alcohol related disorders**
Use additional code for blood alcohol level, if applicable (Y90.-)
AHA: 2019,3Q,8

✓5ᵗʰ **F10.1**   **Alcohol abuse**
EXCLUDES 1   alcohol dependence (F10.2-)
alcohol use, unspecified (F10.9-)
AHA: 2018,1Q,16; 2015,2Q,15
TIP: Alcohol withdrawal is classified to dependence only (F10.23-); there is no combination code for alcohol abuse with withdrawal. When alcohol abuse and alcohol withdrawal are documented for the same encounter, query the provider for clarification.
TIP: Assign when documentation indicates alcohol withdrawal without dependence; do not assign an additional code for withdrawal.

F10.10   **Alcohol abuse, uncomplicated**
Alcohol use disorder, mild

F10.11   **Alcohol abuse, in remission**
Alcohol use disorder, mild, in early remission
Alcohol use disorder, mild, in sustained remission

✓6ᵗʰ **F10.12**   **Alcohol abuse with intoxication**

     F10.120   **Alcohol abuse with intoxication, uncomplicated**   HCC

     F10.121   **Alcohol abuse with intoxication delirium**   CC HCC

     F10.129   **Alcohol abuse with intoxication, unspecified**   HCC

· ✓6ᵗʰ **F10.13**   **Alcohol abuse, with withdrawal**

·   **F10.130**   **Alcohol abuse with withdrawal, uncomplicated**   CC

·   **F10.131**   **Alcohol abuse with withdrawal delirium**   CC

·   **F10.132**   **Alcohol abuse with withdrawal with perceptual disturbance**   CC

·   **F10.139**   **Alcohol abuse with withdrawal, unspecified**   CC

F10.14   **Alcohol abuse with alcohol-induced mood disorder**   CC HCC
Alcohol use disorder, mild, with alcohol-induced bipolar or related disorder
Alcohol use disorder, mild, with alcohol-induced depressive disorder

✓6ᵗʰ **F10.15**   **Alcohol abuse with alcohol-induced psychotic disorder**

     F10.150   **Alcohol abuse with alcohol-induced psychotic disorder with delusions**   HCC

     F10.151   **Alcohol abuse with alcohol-induced psychotic disorder with hallucinations**   CC HCC
       DEF: Psychosis lasting less than six months with slight or no clouding of consciousness in which auditory hallucinations predominate.

     F10.159   **Alcohol abuse with alcohol-induced psychotic disorder, unspecified**   CC HCC

✓6ᵗʰ **F10.18**   **Alcohol abuse with other alcohol-induced disorders**

     F10.180   **Alcohol abuse with alcohol-induced anxiety disorder**   CC HCC

     F10.181   **Alcohol abuse with alcohol-induced sexual dysfunction**   CC HCC

     F10.182   **Alcohol abuse with alcohol-induced sleep disorder**   HCC

     F10.188   **Alcohol abuse with other alcohol-induced disorder**   CC HCC

F10.19   **Alcohol abuse with unspecified alcohol-induced disorder**   CC HCC

✓5ᵗʰ **F10.2**   **Alcohol dependence**
EXCLUDES 1   alcohol abuse (F10.1-)
alcohol use, unspecified (F10.9-)
EXCLUDES 2   toxic effect of alcohol (T51.0-)

F10.20   **Alcohol dependence, uncomplicated**   HCC
Alcohol use disorder, moderate
Alcohol use disorder, severe
AHA: 2020,1Q,9

F10.21   **Alcohol dependence, in remission**   HCC
Alcohol use disorder, moderate, in early remission
Alcohol use disorder, moderate, in sustained remission
Alcohol use disorder, severe, in early remission
Alcohol use disorder, severe, in sustained remission

✓6ᵗʰ **F10.22**   **Alcohol dependence with intoxication**
Acute drunkenness (in alcoholism)
EXCLUDES 2   alcohol dependence with withdrawal (F10.23-)

     F10.220   **Alcohol dependence with intoxication, uncomplicated**   HCC

     F10.221   **Alcohol dependence with intoxication delirium**   CC HCC

     F10.229   **Alcohol dependence with intoxication, unspecified**   HCC

✓6ᵗʰ **F10.23**   **Alcohol dependence with withdrawal**
EXCLUDES 2   alcohol dependence with intoxication (F10.22-)
AHA: 2018,1Q,16; 2015,2Q,15
TIP: Do not assign a code from this subcategory when documentation indicates alcohol withdrawal without dependence.

     F10.230   **Alcohol dependence with withdrawal, uncomplicated**   CC HCC

     F10.231   **Alcohol dependence with withdrawal delirium**   CC HCC

     F10.232   **Alcohol dependence with withdrawal with perceptual disturbance**   CC HCC

     F10.239   **Alcohol dependence with withdrawal, unspecified**   CC HCC

F10.24   **Alcohol dependence with alcohol-induced mood disorder**   CC HCC
Alcohol use disorder, moderate, with alcohol-induced bipolar or related disorder
Alcohol use disorder, moderate, with alcohol-induced depressive disorder
Alcohol use disorder, severe, with alcohol-induced bipolar or related disorder
Alcohol use disorder, severe, with alcohol-induced depressive disorder

✓6ᵗʰ **F10.25**   **Alcohol dependence with alcohol-induced psychotic disorder**

     F10.250   **Alcohol dependence with alcohol-induced psychotic disorder with delusions**   HCC

     F10.251   **Alcohol dependence with alcohol-induced psychotic disorder with hallucinations**   CC HCC

     F10.259   **Alcohol dependence with alcohol-induced psychotic disorder, unspecified**   CC HCC

F10.26   **Alcohol dependence with alcohol-induced persisting amnestic disorder**   HCC
Alcohol use disorder, moderate, with alcohol-induced major neurocognitive disorder, amnestic-confabulatory type
Alcohol use disorder, severe, with alcohol-induced major neurocognitive disorder, amnestic-confabulatory type
DEF: Prominent and lasting reduced memory span and disordered time appreciation and confabulation that occurs in alcoholics as sequel to acute alcoholic psychosis.

F10.27   **Alcohol dependence with alcohol-induced persisting dementia**   `CC` `HCC`
> Alcohol use disorder, moderate, with alcohol-induced major neurocognitive disorder, nonamnestic-confabulatory type
> Alcohol use disorder, severe, with alcohol-induced major neurocognitive disorder, nonamnestic-confabulatory type

√6ᵗʰ **F10.28**   **Alcohol dependence with other alcohol-induced disorders**

> **F10.280**   **Alcohol dependence with alcohol-induced anxiety disorder**   `CC` `HCC`

> **F10.281**   **Alcohol dependence with alcohol-induced sexual dysfunction**   `CC` `HCC`

> **F10.282**   **Alcohol dependence with alcohol-induced sleep disorder**   `HCC`

> **F10.288**   **Alcohol dependence with other alcohol-induced disorder**   `CC` `HCC`
> > Alcohol use disorder, moderate, with alcohol-induced mild neurocognitive disorder
> > Alcohol use disorder, severe, with alcohol-induced mild neurocognitive disorder
> > **AHA:** 2020,1Q,9

F10.29   **Alcohol dependence with unspecified alcohol-induced disorder**   `CC` `HCC`

√5ᵗʰ **F10.9**   **Alcohol use, unspecified**
> `EXCLUDES 1`   alcohol abuse (F10.1-)
> > alcohol dependence (F10.2-)
> **AHA:** 2018,2Q,10-11
> **TIP:** Assign a substance use code only when the provider documents a relationship between the use and an associated physical, mental, or behavioral disorder. As with all diagnoses, substance use codes must meet the definition of a reportable diagnosis.

√6ᵗʰ **F10.92**   **Alcohol use, unspecified with intoxication**

> **F10.920**   **Alcohol use, unspecified with intoxication, uncomplicated**   `HCC`
> > **AHA:** 2018,2Q,10-11

> **F10.921**   **Alcohol use, unspecified with intoxication delirium**   `CC` `HCC`

> **F10.929**   **Alcohol use, unspecified with intoxication, unspecified**   `HCC`

● √6ᵗʰ **F10.93**   **Alcohol use, unspecified with withdrawal**

● > **F10.930**   **Alcohol use, unspecified with withdrawal, uncomplicated**   `CC`

● > **F10.931**   **Alcohol use, unspecified with withdrawal delirium**   `CC`

● > **F10.932**   **Alcohol use, unspecified with withdrawal with perceptual disturbance**   `CC`

● > **F10.939**   **Alcohol use, unspecified with withdrawal, unspecified**   `CC`

F10.94   **Alcohol use, unspecified with alcohol-induced mood disorder**   `CC` `HCC`
> Alcohol induced bipolar or related disorder, without use disorder
> Alcohol induced depressive disorder, without use disorder

√6ᵗʰ **F10.95**   **Alcohol use, unspecified with alcohol-induced psychotic disorder**

> **F10.950**   **Alcohol use, unspecified with alcohol-induced psychotic disorder with delusions**   `HCC`

> **F10.951**   **Alcohol use, unspecified with alcohol-induced psychotic disorder with hallucinations**   `CC` `HCC`

> **F10.959**   **Alcohol use, unspecified with alcohol-induced psychotic disorder, unspecified**   `CC` `HCC`
> > Alcohol-induced psychotic disorder without use disorder

F10.96   **Alcohol use, unspecified with alcohol-induced persisting amnestic disorder**   `HCC`
> Alcohol-induced major neurocognitive disorder, amnestic-confabulatory type, without use disorder

F10.97   **Alcohol use, unspecified with alcohol-induced persisting dementia**   `HCC`
> Alcohol-induced major neurocognitive disorder, nonamnestic-confabulatory type, without use disorder

√6ᵗʰ **F10.98**   **Alcohol use, unspecified with other alcohol-induced disorders**

> **F10.980**   **Alcohol use, unspecified with alcohol-induced anxiety disorder**   `CC` `HCC`
> > Alcohol induced anxiety disorder, without use disorder

> **F10.981**   **Alcohol use, unspecified with alcohol-induced sexual dysfunction**   `CC` `HCC`
> > Alcohol induced sexual dysfunction, without use disorder

> **F10.982**   **Alcohol use, unspecified with alcohol-induced sleep disorder**   `HCC`
> > Alcohol induced sleep disorder, without use disorder

> **F10.988**   **Alcohol use, unspecified with other alcohol-induced disorder**   `CC` `HCC`
> > Alcohol induced mild neurocognitive disorder, without use disorder

F10.99   **Alcohol use, unspecified with unspecified alcohol-induced disorder**   `CC` `HCC`

√4ᵗʰ **F11**   **Opioid related disorders**

√5ᵗʰ **F11.1**   **Opioid abuse**
> `EXCLUDES 1`   opioid dependence (F11.2-)
> > opioid use, unspecified (F11.9-)

> **F11.10**   **Opioid abuse, uncomplicated**   `HCC`
> > Opioid use disorder, mild

> **F11.11**   **Opioid abuse, in remission**   `HCC`
> > Opioid use disorder, mild, in early remission
> > Opioid use disorder, mild, in sustained remission

√6ᵗʰ **F11.12**   **Opioid abuse with intoxication**

> **F11.120**   **Opioid abuse with intoxication, uncomplicated**   `HCC`

> **F11.121**   **Opioid abuse with intoxication delirium**   `CC` `HCC`

> **F11.122**   **Opioid abuse with intoxication with perceptual disturbance**   `HCC`

> **F11.129**   **Opioid abuse with intoxication, unspecified**   `HCC`

● > **F11.13**   **Opioid abuse with withdrawal**   `CC`

> **F11.14**   **Opioid abuse with opioid-induced mood disorder**   `HCC`
> > Opioid use disorder, mild, with opioid-induced depressive disorder

√6ᵗʰ **F11.15**   **Opioid abuse with opioid-induced psychotic disorder**

> **F11.150**   **Opioid abuse with opioid-induced psychotic disorder with delusions**   `CC` `HCC`

> **F11.151**   **Opioid abuse with opioid-induced psychotic disorder with hallucinations**   `CC` `HCC`

> **F11.159**   **Opioid abuse with opioid-induced psychotic disorder, unspecified**   `HCC`

√6ᵗʰ **F11.18**   **Opioid abuse with other opioid-induced disorder**

> **F11.181**   **Opioid abuse with opioid-induced sexual dysfunction**   `HCC`

> **F11.182**   **Opioid abuse with opioid-induced sleep disorder**   `HCC`

> **F11.188**   **Opioid abuse with other opioid-induced disorder**   `HCC`

F11.19   **Opioid abuse with unspecified opioid-induced disorder**   `HCC`

√5ᵗʰ **F11.2**   **Opioid dependence**
> `EXCLUDES 1`   opioid abuse (F11.1-)
> > opioid use, unspecified (F11.9-)
> `EXCLUDES 2`   opioid poisoning (T40.0-T40.2-)

> **F11.20**   **Opioid dependence, uncomplicated**   `CC` `HCC`
> > Opioid use disorder, moderate
> > Opioid use disorder, severe

☑ Additional Character Required   √x7ᵗʰ Placeholder   Unacceptable PDx   Questionable PDx   Manifestation   Unspecified Dx   `H1`-`H14` HAC   `HCC` CMS-HCC Dx   `HIV` HIV Dx

ICD-10-CM 2021

547

Chapter 5. Mental, Behavioral and Neurodevelopmental Disorders

F11.21   **Opioid dependence, in remission**   HCC
- Opioid use disorder, moderate, in early remission
- Opioid use disorder, moderate, in sustained remission
- Opioid use disorder, severe, in early remission
- Opioid use disorder, severe, in sustained remission

√6ᵗʰ **F11.22**   **Opioid dependence with intoxication**

> EXCLUDES 1   opioid dependence with withdrawal (F11.23)

F11.220   **Opioid dependence with intoxication, uncomplicated**   HCC

F11.221   **Opioid dependence with intoxication delirium**   CC HCC

F11.222   **Opioid dependence with intoxication with perceptual disturbance**   CC HCC

F11.229   **Opioid dependence with intoxication, unspecified**   HCC

F11.23   **Opioid dependence with withdrawal**   CC HCC

> EXCLUDES 1   opioid dependence with intoxication (F11.22-)

F11.24   **Opioid dependence with opioid-induced mood disorder**   HCC
- Opioid use disorder, moderate, with opioid induced depressive disorder

√6ᵗʰ **F11.25**   **Opioid dependence with opioid-induced psychotic disorder**

F11.250   **Opioid dependence with opioid-induced psychotic disorder with delusions**   CC HCC

F11.251   **Opioid dependence with opioid-induced psychotic disorder with hallucinations**   CC HCC

F11.259   **Opioid dependence with opioid-induced psychotic disorder, unspecified**   CC HCC

√6ᵗʰ **F11.28**   **Opioid dependence with other opioid-induced disorder**

F11.281   **Opioid dependence with opioid-induced sexual dysfunction**   CC HCC

F11.282   **Opioid dependence with opioid-induced sleep disorder**   CC HCC

F11.288   **Opioid dependence with other opioid-induced disorder**   CC HCC

F11.29   **Opioid dependence with unspecified opioid-induced disorder**   HCC

√5ᵗʰ **F11.9**   **Opioid use, unspecified**

> EXCLUDES 1   opioid abuse (F11.1-)
> opioid dependence (F11.2-)

> **TIP:** Assign a substance use code only when the provider documents a relationship between the use and an associated physical, mental, or behavioral disorder. As with all diagnoses, substance use codes must meet the definition of a reportable diagnosis.

F11.90   **Opioid use, unspecified, uncomplicated**
> AHA: 2018,2Q,10-11

√6ᵗʰ **F11.92**   **Opioid use, unspecified with intoxication**

> EXCLUDES 1   opioid use, unspecified with withdrawal (F11.93)

F11.920   **Opioid use, unspecified with intoxication, uncomplicated**   HCC

F11.921   **Opioid use, unspecified with intoxication delirium**   CC HCC
- Opioid-induced delirium

F11.922   **Opioid use, unspecified with intoxication with perceptual disturbance**   HCC

F11.929   **Opioid use, unspecified with intoxication, unspecified**   HCC

F11.93   **Opioid use, unspecified with withdrawal**   CC HCC

> EXCLUDES 1   opioid use, unspecified with intoxication (F11.92-)

F11.94   **Opioid use, unspecified with opioid-induced mood disorder**   HCC
- Opioid induced depressive disorder, without use disorder

√6ᵗʰ **F11.95**   **Opioid use, unspecified with opioid-induced psychotic disorder**

F11.950   **Opioid use, unspecified with opioid-induced psychotic disorder with delusions**   CC HCC

F11.951   **Opioid use, unspecified with opioid-induced psychotic disorder with hallucinations**   CC HCC

F11.959   **Opioid use, unspecified with opioid-induced psychotic disorder, unspecified**   HCC

√6ᵗʰ **F11.98**   **Opioid use, unspecified with other specified opioid-induced disorder**

F11.981   **Opioid use, unspecified with opioid-induced sexual dysfunction**   HCC
- Opioid induced sexual dysfunction, without use disorder

F11.982   **Opioid use, unspecified with opioid-induced sleep disorder**   HCC
- Opioid induced sleep disorder, without use disorder

F11.988   **Opioid use, unspecified with other opioid-induced disorder**   HCC
- Opioid induced anxiety disorder, without use disorder

F11.99   **Opioid use, unspecified with unspecified opioid-induced disorder**   HCC

√4ᵗʰ **F12**   **Cannabis related disorders**

> INCLUDES   marijuana
> AHA: 2020,1Q,8

√5ᵗʰ **F12.1**   **Cannabis abuse**

> EXCLUDES 1   cannabis dependence (F12.2-)
> cannabis use, unspecified (F12.9-)

F12.10   **Cannabis abuse, uncomplicated**
- Cannabis use disorder, mild

F12.11   **Cannabis abuse, in remission**
- Cannabis use disorder, mild, in early remission
- Cannabis use disorder, mild, in sustained remission

√6ᵗʰ **F12.12**   **Cannabis abuse with intoxication**

F12.120   **Cannabis abuse with intoxication, uncomplicated**   HCC

F12.121   **Cannabis abuse with intoxication delirium**   CC HCC

F12.122   **Cannabis abuse with intoxication with perceptual disturbance**   HCC

F12.129   **Cannabis abuse with intoxication, unspecified**   HCC

F12.13   **Cannabis abuse with withdrawal**

√6ᵗʰ **F12.15**   **Cannabis abuse with psychotic disorder**

F12.150   **Cannabis abuse with psychotic disorder with delusions**   CC HCC

F12.151   **Cannabis abuse with psychotic disorder with hallucinations**   CC HCC

F12.159   **Cannabis abuse with psychotic disorder, unspecified**   HCC

√6ᵗʰ **F12.18**   **Cannabis abuse with other cannabis-induced disorder**

F12.180   **Cannabis abuse with cannabis-induced anxiety disorder**   HCC

F12.188   **Cannabis abuse with other cannabis-induced disorder**   HCC
- Cannabis use disorder, mild, with cannabis-induced sleep disorder

F12.19   **Cannabis abuse with unspecified cannabis-induced disorder**   HCC

√5ᵗʰ **F12.2**   **Cannabis dependence**

> EXCLUDES 1   cannabis abuse (F12.1-)
> cannabis use, unspecified (F12.9-)
> EXCLUDES 2   cannabis poisoning (T40.7-)

F12.20   **Cannabis dependence, uncomplicated**   HCC
- Cannabis use disorder, moderate
- Cannabis use disorder, severe

F12.21   **Cannabis dependence, in remission**   HCC
- Cannabis use disorder, moderate, in early remission
- Cannabis use disorder, moderate, in sustained remission
- Cannabis use disorder, severe, in early remission
- Cannabis use disorder, severe, in sustained remission

√6ᵗʰ **F12.22**   **Cannabis dependence with intoxication**

F12.220   **Cannabis dependence with intoxication, uncomplicated**   HCC

F12.221   **Cannabis dependence with intoxication delirium**   CC HCC

F12.222   **Cannabis dependence with intoxication with perceptual disturbance**   HCC

F12.229 **Cannabis dependence with intoxication, unspecified** `HCC`

F12.23 **Cannabis dependence with** withdrawal `HCC`
     AHA: 2018,4Q,7

√6ᵗʰ F12.25 **Cannabis dependence with** psychotic disorder
     F12.250 **Cannabis dependence with psychotic disorder with** delusions `CC` `HCC`
     F12.251 **Cannabis dependence with psychotic disorder with** hallucinations `CC` `HCC`
     F12.259 **Cannabis dependence with psychotic disorder, unspecified** `HCC`

√6ᵗʰ F12.28 **Cannabis dependence with other cannabis-induced disorder**
     F12.280 **Cannabis dependence with cannabis-induced** anxiety disorder `HCC`
     F12.288 **Cannabis dependence with other cannabis-induced disorder** `HCC`
         Cannabis use disorder, moderate, with cannabis-induced sleep disorder
         Cannabis use disorder, severe, with cannabis-induced sleep disorder

F12.29 **Cannabis dependence with unspecified cannabis-induced disorder** `HCC`

√5ᵗʰ F12.9 **Cannabis use, unspecified**
     EXCLUDES 1   cannabis abuse (F12.1-)
              cannabis dependence (F12.2-)
     TIP: Assign a substance use code only when the provider documents a relationship between the use and an associated physical, mental, or behavioral disorder. As with all diagnoses, substance use codes must meet the definition of a reportable diagnosis.
     F12.90 **Cannabis use, unspecified,** uncomplicated
         AHA: 2018,2Q,10-11

√6ᵗʰ F12.92 **Cannabis use, unspecified with** intoxication
     F12.920 **Cannabis use, unspecified with intoxication,** uncomplicated `HCC`
     F12.921 **Cannabis use, unspecified with intoxication** delirium `CC` `HCC`
     F12.922 **Cannabis use, unspecified with intoxication with** perceptual disturbance `HCC`
     F12.929 **Cannabis use, unspecified with intoxication, unspecified** `HCC`

F12.93 **Cannabis use, unspecified with** withdrawal `HCC`
     AHA: 2018,4Q,7

√6ᵗʰ F12.95 **Cannabis use, unspecified with** psychotic disorder
     F12.950 **Cannabis use, unspecified with psychotic disorder with** delusions `CC` `HCC`
     F12.951 **Cannabis use, unspecified with psychotic disorder with** hallucinations `CC` `HCC`
     F12.959 **Cannabis use, unspecified with psychotic disorder, unspecified** `HCC`
         Cannabis induced psychotic disorder, without use disorder

√6ᵗʰ F12.98 **Cannabis use, unspecified with other cannabis-induced disorder**
     F12.980 **Cannabis use, unspecified with** anxiety disorder `HCC`
         Cannabis induced anxiety disorder, without use disorder
     F12.988 **Cannabis use, unspecified with other cannabis-induced disorder** `HCC`
         Cannabis induced sleep disorder, without use disorder

F12.99 **Cannabis use, unspecified with unspecified cannabis-induced disorder** `HCC`

√4ᵗʰ **F13 Sedative, hypnotic, or anxiolytic related disorders**

√5ᵗʰ F13.1 **Sedative, hypnotic or anxiolytic-related** abuse
     EXCLUDES 1   sedative, hypnotic or anxiolytic-related dependence (F13.2-)
              sedative, hypnotic, or anxiolytic use, unspecified (F13.9-)
     F13.10 **Sedative, hypnotic or anxiolytic abuse,** uncomplicated `HCC`
         Sedative, hypnotic, or anxiolytic use disorder, mild

F13.11 **Sedative, hypnotic or anxiolytic abuse,** in remission `HCC`
     Sedative, hypnotic or anxiolytic use disorder, mild, in early remission
     Sedative, hypnotic or anxiolytic use disorder, mild, in sustained remission

√6ᵗʰ F13.12 **Sedative, hypnotic or anxiolytic abuse with** intoxication
     F13.120 **Sedative, hypnotic or anxiolytic abuse with intoxication,** uncomplicated `HCC`
     F13.121 **Sedative, hypnotic or anxiolytic abuse with intoxication** delirium `CC` `HCC`
     F13.129 **Sedative, hypnotic or anxiolytic abuse with intoxication, unspecified** `HCC`

√6ᵗʰ F13.13 **Sedative, hypnotic or anxiolytic abuse with** withdrawal
     F13.130 **Sedative, hypnotic or anxiolytic abuse with withdrawal,** uncomplicated `CC`
     F13.131 **Sedative, hypnotic or anxiolytic abuse with withdrawal** delirium `CC`
     F13.132 **Sedative, hypnotic or anxiolytic abuse with withdrawal with** perceptual disturbance `CC`
     F13.139 **Sedative, hypnotic or anxiolytic abuse with withdrawal, unspecified** `CC`

F13.14 **Sedative, hypnotic or anxiolytic abuse with sedative, hypnotic or anxiolytic-induced** mood disorder `HCC`
     Sedative, hypnotic, or anxiolytic use disorder, mild, with sedative, hypnotic, or anxiolytic-induced bipolar or related disorder
     Sedative, hypnotic, or anxiolytic use disorder, mild, with sedative, hypnotic, or anxiolytic-induced depressive disorder

√6ᵗʰ F13.15 **Sedative, hypnotic or anxiolytic abuse with sedative, hypnotic or anxiolytic-induced** psychotic disorder
     F13.150 **Sedative, hypnotic or anxiolytic abuse with sedative, hypnotic or anxiolytic-induced psychotic disorder with** delusions `CC` `HCC`
     F13.151 **Sedative, hypnotic or anxiolytic abuse with sedative, hypnotic or anxiolytic-induced psychotic disorder with** hallucinations `CC` `HCC`
     F13.159 **Sedative, hypnotic or anxiolytic abuse with sedative, hypnotic or anxiolytic-induced psychotic disorder, unspecified** `HCC`

√6ᵗʰ F13.18 **Sedative, hypnotic or anxiolytic abuse with other sedative, hypnotic or anxiolytic-induced disorders**
     F13.180 **Sedative, hypnotic or anxiolytic abuse with sedative, hypnotic or anxiolytic-induced** anxiety disorder `HCC`
     F13.181 **Sedative, hypnotic or anxiolytic abuse with sedative, hypnotic or anxiolytic-induced** sexual dysfunction `HCC`
     F13.182 **Sedative, hypnotic or anxiolytic abuse with sedative, hypnotic or anxiolytic-induced** sleep disorder `HCC`
     F13.188 **Sedative, hypnotic or anxiolytic abuse with other sedative, hypnotic or anxiolytic-induced disorder** `HCC`

F13.19 **Sedative, hypnotic or anxiolytic abuse with unspecified sedative, hypnotic or anxiolytic-induced disorder** `HCC`

√5ᵗʰ F13.2 **Sedative, hypnotic or anxiolytic-related** dependence
     EXCLUDES 1   sedative, hypnotic or anxiolytic-related abuse (F13.1-)
              sedative, hypnotic, or anxiolytic use, unspecified (F13.9-)
     EXCLUDES 2   sedative, hypnotic, or anxiolytic poisoning (T42.-)
     F13.20 **Sedative, hypnotic or anxiolytic dependence,** uncomplicated `CC` `HCC`

✓ Additional Character Required   √x7ᵗʰ Placeholder   Unacceptable PDx   Questionable PDx   Manifestation   Unspecified Dx   **H1**-**H4** HAC   `HCC` CMS-HCC Dx   **HIV** HIV Dx

ICD-10-CM 2021   **549**

Chapter 5. Mental, Behavioral and Neurodevelopmental Disorders

F13.21–F13.931

F13.21 **Sedative, hypnotic or anxiolytic dependence, in remission** `HCC`

Sedative, hypnotic or anxiolytic use disorder, moderate, in early remission

Sedative, hypnotic or anxiolytic use disorder, moderate, in sustained remission

Sedative, hypnotic or anxiolytic use disorder, severe, in early remission

Sedative, hypnotic or anxiolytic use disorder, severe, in sustained remission

√6ᵗʰ F13.22 **Sedative, hypnotic or anxiolytic dependence with intoxication**

     `EXCLUDES 1` *sedative, hypnotic or anxiolytic dependence with withdrawal (F13.23-)*

F13.220 **Sedative, hypnotic or anxiolytic dependence with intoxication, uncomplicated** `HCC`

F13.221 **Sedative, hypnotic or anxiolytic dependence with intoxication delirium** `CC` `HCC`

F13.229 **Sedative, hypnotic or anxiolytic dependence with intoxication, unspecified** `HCC`

√6ᵗʰ F13.23 **Sedative, hypnotic or anxiolytic dependence with withdrawal**

Sedative, hypnotic, or anxiolytic use disorder, moderate

Sedative, hypnotic, or anxiolytic use disorder, severe

     `EXCLUDES 1` *sedative, hypnotic or anxiolytic dependence with intoxication (F13.22-)*

F13.230 **Sedative, hypnotic or anxiolytic dependence with withdrawal, uncomplicated** `CC` `HCC`

F13.231 **Sedative, hypnotic or anxiolytic dependence with withdrawal delirium** `CC` `HCC`

F13.232 **Sedative, hypnotic or anxiolytic dependence with withdrawal with perceptual disturbance** `CC` `HCC`

Sedative, hypnotic, or anxiolytic withdrawal with perceptual disturbances

F13.239 **Sedative, hypnotic or anxiolytic dependence with withdrawal, unspecified** `CC` `HCC`

Sedative, hypnotic, or anxiolytic withdrawal without perceptual disturbances

F13.24 **Sedative, hypnotic or anxiolytic dependence with sedative, hypnotic or anxiolytic-induced mood disorder** `HCC`

Sedative, hypnotic, or anxiolytic use disorder, moderate, with sedative, hypnotic, or anxiolytic-induced bipolar or related disorder

Sedative, hypnotic, or anxiolytic use disorder, moderate, with sedative, hypnotic, or anxiolytic-induced depressive disorder

Sedative, hypnotic, or anxiolytic use disorder, severe, with sedative, hypnotic, or anxiolytic-induced bipolar or related disorder

Sedative, hypnotic, or anxiolytic use disorder, severe, with sedative, hypnotic, or anxiolytic-induced depressive disorder

√6ᵗʰ F13.25 **Sedative, hypnotic or anxiolytic dependence with sedative, hypnotic or anxiolytic-induced psychotic disorder**

F13.250 **Sedative, hypnotic or anxiolytic dependence with sedative, hypnotic or anxiolytic-induced psychotic disorder with delusions** `CC` `HCC`

F13.251 **Sedative, hypnotic or anxiolytic dependence with sedative, hypnotic or anxiolytic-induced psychotic disorder with hallucinations** `CC` `HCC`

F13.259 **Sedative, hypnotic or anxiolytic dependence with sedative, hypnotic or anxiolytic-induced psychotic disorder, unspecified** `CC` `HCC`

F13.26 **Sedative, hypnotic or anxiolytic dependence with sedative, hypnotic or anxiolytic-induced persisting amnestic disorder** `CC` `HCC`

F13.27 **Sedative, hypnotic or anxiolytic dependence with sedative, hypnotic or anxiolytic-induced persisting dementia** `CC` `HCC`

Sedative, hypnotic, or anxiolytic use disorder, moderate, with sedative, hypnotic, or anxiolytic induced major neurocognitive disorder

Sedative, hypnotic, or anxiolytic use disorder, severe, with sedative, hypnotic, or anxiolytic-induced major neurocognitive disorder

√6ᵗʰ F13.28 **Sedative, hypnotic or anxiolytic dependence with other sedative, hypnotic or anxiolytic-induced disorders**

F13.280 **Sedative, hypnotic or anxiolytic dependence with sedative, hypnotic or anxiolytic-induced anxiety disorder** `CC` `HCC`

F13.281 **Sedative, hypnotic or anxiolytic dependence with sedative, hypnotic or anxiolytic-induced sexual dysfunction** `CC` `HCC`

F13.282 **Sedative, hypnotic or anxiolytic dependence with sedative, hypnotic or anxiolytic-induced sleep disorder** `CC` `HCC`

F13.288 **Sedative, hypnotic or anxiolytic dependence with other sedative, hypnotic or anxiolytic-induced disorder** `CC` `HCC`

Sedative, hypnotic, or anxiolytic use disorder, moderate, with sedative, hypnotic, or anxiolytic-induced mild neurocognitive disorder

Sedative, hypnotic, or anxiolytic use disorder, severe, with sedative, hypnotic, or anxiolytic-induced mild neurocognitive disorder

F13.29 **Sedative, hypnotic or anxiolytic dependence with unspecified sedative, hypnotic or anxiolytic-induced disorder** `HCC`

√5ᵗʰ F13.9 **Sedative, hypnotic or anxiolytic-related use, unspecified**

     `EXCLUDES 1` *sedative, hypnotic or anxiolytic-related abuse (F13.1-)*
sedative, hypnotic or anxiolytic-related dependence (F13.2-)

TIP: Assign a substance use code only when the provider documents a relationship between the use and an associated physical, mental, or behavioral disorder. As with all diagnoses, substance use codes must meet the definition of a reportable diagnosis.

F13.90 **Sedative, hypnotic, or anxiolytic use, unspecified, uncomplicated**

     AHA: 2018,2Q,10-11

√6ᵗʰ F13.92 **Sedative, hypnotic or anxiolytic use, unspecified with intoxication**

     `EXCLUDES 1` *sedative, hypnotic or anxiolytic use, unspecified with withdrawal (F13.93-)*

F13.920 **Sedative, hypnotic or anxiolytic use, unspecified with intoxication, uncomplicated** `HCC`

F13.921 **Sedative, hypnotic or anxiolytic use, unspecified with intoxication delirium** `CC` `HCC`

Sedative, hypnotic, or anxiolytic-induced delirium

F13.929 **Sedative, hypnotic or anxiolytic use, unspecified with intoxication, unspecified** `HCC`

√6ᵗʰ F13.93 **Sedative, hypnotic or anxiolytic use, unspecified with withdrawal**

     `EXCLUDES 1` *sedative, hypnotic or anxiolytic use, unspecified with intoxication (F13.92-)*

F13.930 **Sedative, hypnotic or anxiolytic use, unspecified with withdrawal, uncomplicated** `CC` `HCC`

F13.931 **Sedative, hypnotic or anxiolytic use, unspecified with withdrawal delirium** `CC` `HCC`

N Newborn: 0   P Pediatric: 0-17   M Maternity: 9-64   A Adult: 15-124   `MCC` Major Complication/Comorbidity   `CC` Complication/Comorbidity   `SW` Severe Wound Dx

550   ICD-10-CM 2021

F13.932 **Sedative, hypnotic or anxiolytic use, unspecified with withdrawal with perceptual disturbances** `CC` `HCC`

F13.939 **Sedative, hypnotic or anxiolytic use, unspecified with withdrawal, unspecified** `CC` `HCC`

F13.94 **Sedative, hypnotic or anxiolytic use, unspecified with sedative, hypnotic or anxiolytic-induced** mood disorder `HCC`

    Sedative, hypnotic, or anxiolytic-induced bipolar or related disorder, without use disorder

    Sedative, hypnotic, or anxiolytic-induced depressive disorder, without use disorder

√6th F13.95 **Sedative, hypnotic or anxiolytic use, unspecified with sedative, hypnotic or anxiolytic-induced** psychotic disorder

F13.950 **Sedative, hypnotic or anxiolytic use, unspecified with sedative, hypnotic or anxiolytic-induced psychotic disorder with** delusions `CC` `HCC`

F13.951 **Sedative, hypnotic or anxiolytic use, unspecified with sedative, hypnotic or anxiolytic-induced psychotic disorder with** hallucinations `CC` `HCC`

F13.959 **Sedative, hypnotic or anxiolytic use, unspecified with sedative, hypnotic or anxiolytic-induced psychotic disorder, unspecified** `HCC`

    Sedative, hypnotic, or anxiolytic-induced psychotic disorder, without use disorder

F13.96 **Sedative, hypnotic or anxiolytic use, unspecified with sedative, hypnotic or anxiolytic-induced** persisting amnestic disorder `HCC`

F13.97 **Sedative, hypnotic or anxiolytic use, unspecified with sedative, hypnotic or anxiolytic-induced** persisting dementia `CC` `HCC`

    Sedative, hypnotic, or anxiolytic-induced major neurocognitive disorder, without use disorder

√6th F13.98 **Sedative, hypnotic or anxiolytic use, unspecified with other sedative, hypnotic or anxiolytic-induced disorders**

F13.980 **Sedative, hypnotic or anxiolytic use, unspecified with sedative, hypnotic or anxiolytic-induced** anxiety disorder `HCC`

    Sedative, hypnotic, or anxiolytic-induced anxiety disorder, without use disorder

F13.981 **Sedative, hypnotic or anxiolytic use, unspecified with sedative, hypnotic or anxiolytic-induced** sexual dysfunction `HCC`

    Sedative, hypnotic, or anxiolytic-induced sexual dysfunction disorder, without use disorder

F13.982 **Sedative, hypnotic or anxiolytic use, unspecified with sedative, hypnotic or anxiolytic-induced** sleep disorder `HCC`

    Sedative, hypnotic, or anxiolytic-induced sleep disorder, without use disorder

F13.988 **Sedative, hypnotic or anxiolytic use, unspecified with other sedative, hypnotic or anxiolytic-induced disorder** `HCC`

    Sedative, hypnotic, or anxiolytic-induced mild neurocognitive disorder

F13.99 **Sedative, hypnotic or anxiolytic use, unspecified with unspecified sedative, hypnotic or anxiolytic-induced disorder** `HCC`

√4th **F14 Cocaine related disorders**

    EXCLUDES 2   *other stimulant-related disorders (F15.-)*

√5th **F14.1 Cocaine** abuse

    EXCLUDES 1   *cocaine dependence (F14.2-)*

             cocaine use, unspecified (F14.9-)

F14.10 **Cocaine abuse, uncomplicated** `HCC`

    Cocaine use disorder, mild

F14.11 **Cocaine abuse, in remission** `HCC`

    Cocaine use disorder, mild, in early remission

    Cocaine use disorder, mild, in sustained remission

√6th F14.12 **Cocaine abuse with** intoxication

F14.120 **Cocaine abuse with intoxication, uncomplicated** `HCC`

F14.121 **Cocaine abuse with intoxication with** delirium `CC` `HCC`

F14.122 **Cocaine abuse with intoxication with** perceptual disturbance `HCC`

F14.129 **Cocaine abuse with intoxication, unspecified** `HCC`

● F14.13 **Cocaine abuse, unspecified with** withdrawal `CC`

F14.14 **Cocaine abuse with cocaine-induced** mood disorder `HCC`

    Cocaine use disorder, mild, with cocaine-induced bipolar or related disorder

    Cocaine use disorder, mild, with cocaine-induced depressive disorder

√6th F14.15 **Cocaine abuse with cocaine-induced** psychotic disorder

F14.150 **Cocaine abuse with cocaine-induced psychotic disorder with** delusions `CC` `HCC`

F14.151 **Cocaine abuse with cocaine-induced psychotic disorder with** hallucinations `CC` `HCC`

F14.159 **Cocaine abuse with cocaine-induced psychotic disorder, unspecified** `HCC`

√6th F14.18 **Cocaine abuse with other cocaine-induced disorder**

F14.180 **Cocaine abuse with cocaine-induced** anxiety disorder `HCC`

F14.181 **Cocaine abuse with cocaine-induced** sexual dysfunction `HCC`

F14.182 **Cocaine abuse with cocaine-induced** sleep disorder `HCC`

F14.188 **Cocaine abuse with other cocaine-induced disorder** `HCC`

    Cocaine use disorder, mild, with cocaine-induced obsessive compulsive or related disorder

F14.19 **Cocaine abuse with unspecified cocaine-induced disorder** `HCC`

√5th **F14.2 Cocaine** dependence

    EXCLUDES 1   *cocaine abuse (F14.1-)*

             cocaine use, unspecified (F14.9-)

    EXCLUDES 2   *cocaine poisoning (T40.5-)*

F14.20 **Cocaine dependence, uncomplicated** `CC` `HCC`

    Cocaine use disorder, moderate

    Cocaine use disorder, severe

F14.21 **Cocaine dependence, in remission** `HCC`

    Cocaine use disorder, moderate, in early remission

    Cocaine use disorder, moderate, in sustained remission

    Cocaine use disorder, severe, in early remission

    Cocaine use disorder, severe, in sustained remission

√6th F14.22 **Cocaine dependence with** intoxication

    EXCLUDES 1   *cocaine dependence with withdrawal (F14.23)*

F14.220 **Cocaine dependence with intoxication, uncomplicated** `HCC`

F14.221 **Cocaine dependence with intoxication delirium** `CC` `HCC`

F14.222 **Cocaine dependence with intoxication with** perceptual disturbance `CC` `HCC`

F14.229 **Cocaine dependence with intoxication, unspecified** `CC` `HCC`

F14.23 **Cocaine dependence with** withdrawal `CC` `HCC`

    EXCLUDES 1   *cocaine dependence with intoxication (F14.22-)*

F14.24 **Cocaine dependence with cocaine-induced** mood disorder `HCC`

    Cocaine use disorder, moderate, with cocaine-induced bipolar or related disorder

    Cocaine use disorder, moderate, with cocaine-induced depressive disorder

    Cocaine use disorder, severe, with cocaine-induced bipolar or related disorder

    Cocaine use disorder, severe, with cocaine-induced depressive disorder

√6th F14.25 **Cocaine dependence with cocaine-induced** psychotic disorder

F14.250 **Cocaine dependence with cocaine-induced psychotic disorder with** delusions `CC` `HCC`

☑ Additional Character Required   √x7th Placeholder   Unacceptable PDx   Questionable PDx   Manifestation   Unspecified Dx   H1 - H14 HAC   HCC CMS-HCC Dx   HIV HIV Dx

ICD-10-CM 2021   551

F14.251 Cocaine dependence with cocaine-induced psychotic disorder with hallucinations `CC` `HCC`

F14.259 Cocaine dependence with cocaine-induced psychotic disorder, unspecified `CC` `HCC`

√6ᵗʰ **F14.28 Cocaine dependence with other cocaine-induced disorder**

F14.280 Cocaine dependence with cocaine-induced anxiety disorder `CC` `HCC`

F14.281 Cocaine dependence with cocaine-induced sexual dysfunction `CC` `HCC`

F14.282 Cocaine dependence with cocaine-induced sleep disorder `CC` `HCC`

F14.288 Cocaine dependence with other cocaine-induced disorder `CC` `HCC`

Cocaine use disorder, moderate, with cocaine-induced obsessive compulsive or related disorder

Cocaine use disorder, severe, with cocaine-induced obsessive compulsive or related disorder

F14.29 Cocaine dependence with unspecified cocaine-induced disorder `HCC`

√5ᵗʰ **F14.9 Cocaine use, unspecified**

EXCLUDES 1 cocaine abuse (F14.1-)
cocaine dependence (F14.2-)

TIP: Assign a substance use code only when the provider documents a relationship between the use and an associated physical, mental, or behavioral disorder. As with all diagnoses, substance use codes must meet the definition of a reportable diagnosis.

F14.90 Cocaine use, unspecified, uncomplicated
AHA: 2018,2Q,10-11

√6ᵗʰ **F14.92 Cocaine use, unspecified with intoxication**

F14.920 Cocaine use, unspecified with intoxication, uncomplicated `HCC`

F14.921 Cocaine use, unspecified with intoxication delirium `CC` `HCC`

F14.922 Cocaine use, unspecified with intoxication with perceptual disturbance `HCC`

F14.929 Cocaine use, unspecified with intoxication, unspecified `HCC`

F14.93 Cocaine use, unspecified with withdrawal `CC`

F14.94 Cocaine use, unspecified with cocaine-induced mood disorder `HCC`

Cocaine induced bipolar or related disorder, without use disorder

Cocaine induced depressive disorder, without use disorder

√6ᵗʰ **F14.95 Cocaine use, unspecified with cocaine-induced psychotic disorder**

F14.950 Cocaine use, unspecified with cocaine-induced psychotic disorder with delusions `CC` `HCC`

F14.951 Cocaine use, unspecified with cocaine-induced psychotic disorder with hallucinations `CC` `HCC`

F14.959 Cocaine use, unspecified with cocaine-induced psychotic disorder, unspecified `HCC`

Cocaine induced psychotic disorder, without use disorder

√6ᵗʰ **F14.98 Cocaine use, unspecified with other specified cocaine-induced disorder**

F14.980 Cocaine use, unspecified with cocaine-induced anxiety disorder `HCC`

Cocaine induced anxiety disorder, without use disorder

F14.981 Cocaine use, unspecified with cocaine-induced sexual dysfunction `HCC`

Cocaine induced sexual dysfunction, without use disorder

F14.982 Cocaine use, unspecified with cocaine-induced sleep disorder `HCC`

Cocaine induced sleep disorder, without use disorder

F14.988 Cocaine use, unspecified with other cocaine-induced disorder `HCC`

Cocaine induced obsessive compulsive or related disorder

F14.99 Cocaine use, unspecified with unspecified cocaine-induced disorder `HCC`

√4ᵗʰ **F15 Other stimulant related disorders**

INCLUDES amphetamine-related disorders
caffeine

EXCLUDES 2 cocaine-related disorders (F14.-)

√5ᵗʰ **F15.1 Other stimulant abuse**

EXCLUDES 1 other stimulant dependence (F15.2-)
other stimulant use, unspecified (F15.9-)

F15.10 Other stimulant abuse, uncomplicated `HCC`

Amphetamine type substance use disorder, mild
Other or unspecified stimulant use disorder, mild

F15.11 Other stimulant abuse, in remission `HCC`

Amphetamine type substance use disorder, mild, in early remission

Amphetamine type substance use disorder, mild, in sustained remission

Other or unspecified stimulant use disorder, mild, in early remission

Other or unspecified stimulant use disorder, mild, in sustained remission

√6ᵗʰ **F15.12 Other stimulant abuse with intoxication**

F15.120 Other stimulant abuse with intoxication, uncomplicated `HCC`

F15.121 Other stimulant abuse with intoxication delirium `CC` `HCC`

F15.122 Other stimulant abuse with intoxication with perceptual disturbance `HCC`

Amphetamine or other stimulant use disorder, mild, with amphetamine or other stimulant intoxication, with perceptual disturbances

F15.129 Other stimulant abuse with intoxication, unspecified `HCC`

Amphetamine or other stimulant use disorder, mild, with amphetamine or other stimulant intoxication, without perceptual disturbances

F15.13 Other stimulant abuse with withdrawal `CC`

F15.14 Other stimulant abuse with stimulant-induced mood disorder `HCC`

Amphetamine or other stimulant use disorder, mild, with amphetamine or other stimulant induced bipolar or related disorder

Amphetamine or other stimulant use disorder, mild, with amphetamine or other stimulant induced depressive disorder

√6ᵗʰ **F15.15 Other stimulant abuse with stimulant-induced psychotic disorder**

F15.150 Other stimulant abuse with stimulant-induced psychotic disorder with delusions `CC` `HCC`

F15.151 Other stimulant abuse with stimulant-induced psychotic disorder with hallucinations `CC` `HCC`

F15.159 Other stimulant abuse with stimulant-induced psychotic disorder, unspecified `HCC`

√6ᵗʰ **F15.18 Other stimulant abuse with other stimulant-induced disorder**

F15.180 Other stimulant abuse with stimulant-induced anxiety disorder `HCC`

F15.181 Other stimulant abuse with stimulant-induced sexual dysfunction `HCC`

F15.182 Other stimulant abuse with stimulant-induced sleep disorder `HCC`

F15.188 Other stimulant abuse with other stimulant-induced disorder `HCC`
Amphetamine or other stimulant use disorder, mild, with amphetamine or other stimulant induced obsessive-compulsive or related disorder

F15.19 Other stimulant abuse with unspecified stimulant-induced disorder `HCC`

√5ᵗʰ **F15.2 Other stimulant dependence**

     EXCLUDES 1   other stimulant abuse (F15.1-)
                  other stimulant use, unspecified (F15.9-)

F15.20 Other stimulant dependence, uncomplicated `CC` `HCC`
Amphetamine type substance use disorder, moderate
Amphetamine type substance use disorder, severe
Other or unspecified stimulant use disorder, moderate
Other or unspecified stimulant use disorder, severe

F15.21 Other stimulant dependence, in remission `HCC`
Amphetamine type substance use disorder, moderate, in early remission
Amphetamine type substance use disorder, moderate, in sustained remission
Amphetamine type substance use disorder, severe, in early remission
Amphetamine type substance use disorder, severe, in sustained remission
Other or unspecified stimulant use disorder, moderate, in early remission
Other or unspecified stimulant use disorder, moderate, in sustained remission
Other or unspecified stimulant use disorder, severe, in early remission
Other or unspecified stimulant use disorder, severe, in sustained remission

√6ᵗʰ **F15.22 Other stimulant dependence with intoxication**

     EXCLUDES 1   other stimulant dependence with withdrawal (F15.23)

F15.220 Other stimulant dependence with intoxication, uncomplicated `HCC`

F15.221 Other stimulant dependence with intoxication delirium `CC` `HCC`

F15.222 Other stimulant dependence with intoxication with perceptual disturbance `CC` `HCC`
Amphetamine or other stimulant use disorder, moderate, with amphetamine or other stimulant intoxication, with perceptual disturbances
Amphetamine or other stimulant use disorder, severe, with amphetamine or other stimulant intoxication, with perceptual disturbances

F15.229 Other stimulant dependence with intoxication, unspecified `HCC`
Amphetamine or other stimulant use disorder, moderate, with amphetamine or other stimulant intoxication, without perceptual disturbances
Amphetamine or other stimulant use disorder, severe, with amphetamine or other stimulant intoxication, without perceptual disturbances

F15.23 Other stimulant dependence with withdrawal `CC` `HCC`
Amphetamine or other stimulant withdrawal
     EXCLUDES 1   other stimulant dependence with intoxication (F15.22-)

F15.24 Other stimulant dependence with stimulant-induced mood disorder `HCC`
Amphetamine or other stimulant use disorder, moderate, with amphetamine or other stimulant-induced bipolar or related disorder
Amphetamine or other stimulant use disorder, moderate, with amphetamine or other stimulant induced depressive disorder
Amphetamine or other stimulant use disorder, severe, with amphetamine or other stimulant-induced bipolar or related disorder
Amphetamine or other stimulant use disorder, severe, with amphetamine or other stimulant-induced depressive disorder

√6ᵗʰ **F15.25 Other stimulant dependence with stimulant-induced psychotic disorder**

F15.250 Other stimulant dependence with stimulant-induced psychotic disorder with delusions `CC` `HCC`

F15.251 Other stimulant dependence with stimulant-induced psychotic disorder with hallucinations `CC` `HCC`

F15.259 Other stimulant dependence with stimulant-induced psychotic disorder, unspecified `CC` `HCC`

√6ᵗʰ **F15.28 Other stimulant dependence with other stimulant-induced disorder**

F15.280 Other stimulant dependence with stimulant-induced anxiety disorder `CC` `HCC`

F15.281 Other stimulant dependence with stimulant-induced sexual dysfunction `CC` `HCC`

F15.282 Other stimulant dependence with stimulant-induced sleep disorder `CC` `HCC`

F15.288 Other stimulant dependence with other stimulant-induced disorder `CC` `HCC`
Amphetamine or other stimulant use disorder, moderate, with amphetamine orother stimulant induced obsessive compulsive or related disorder
Amphetamine or other stimulant use disorder, severe, with amphetamine or otherstimulant induced obsessive compulsive or related disorder

F15.29 Other stimulant dependence with unspecified stimulant-induced disorder `HCC`

√5ᵗʰ **F15.9 Other stimulant use, unspecified**

     EXCLUDES 1   other stimulant abuse (F15.1-)
                  other stimulant dependence (F15.2-)

TIP: Assign a substance use code only when the provider documents a relationship between the use and an associated physical, mental, or behavioral disorder. As with all diagnoses, substance use codes must meet the definition of a reportable diagnosis.

F15.90 Other stimulant use, unspecified, uncomplicated
AHA: 2018,2Q,10-11

√6ᵗʰ **F15.92 Other stimulant use, unspecified with intoxication**

     EXCLUDES 1   other stimulant use, unspecified with withdrawal (F15.93)

F15.920 Other stimulant use, unspecified with intoxication, uncomplicated `HCC`

F15.921 Other stimulant use, unspecified with intoxication delirium `CC` `HCC`
Amphetamine or other stimulant-induced delirium

F15.922 Other stimulant use, unspecified with intoxication with perceptual disturbance `HCC`

F15.929 Other stimulant use, unspecified with intoxication, unspecified `HCC`
Caffeine intoxication

F15.93 Other stimulant use, unspecified with withdrawal `CC` `HCC`
Caffeine withdrawal
     EXCLUDES 1   other stimulant use, unspecified with intoxication (F15.92-)

F15.94 Other stimulant use, unspecified with stimulant-induced mood disorder HCC
Amphetamine or other stimulant-induced bipolar or related disorder, without use disorder
Amphetamine or other stimulant-induced depressive disorder, without use disorder

✓6ᵗʰ **F15.95 Other stimulant use, unspecified with stimulant-induced psychotic disorder**
F15.950 Other stimulant use, unspecified with stimulant-induced psychotic disorder with delusions CC HCC
F15.951 Other stimulant use, unspecified with stimulant-induced psychotic disorder with hallucinations CC HCC
F15.959 Other stimulant use, unspecified with stimulant-induced psychotic disorder, unspecified HCC
Amphetamine or other stimulant-induced psychotic disorder, without use disorder

✓6ᵗʰ **F15.98 Other stimulant use, unspecified with other stimulant-induced disorder**
F15.980 Other stimulant use, unspecified with stimulant-induced anxiety disorder HCC
Amphetamine or other stimulant-induced anxiety disorder, without use disorder
Caffeine induced anxiety disorder, without use disorder
F15.981 Other stimulant use, unspecified with stimulant-induced sexual dysfunction HCC
Amphetamine or other stimulant-induced sexual dysfunction, without use disorder
F15.982 Other stimulant use, unspecified with stimulant-induced sleep disorder HCC
Amphetamine or other stimulant-induced sleep disorder, without use disorder
Caffeine induced sleep disorder, without use disorder
F15.988 Other stimulant use, unspecified with other stimulant-induced disorder HCC
Amphetamine or other stimulant-induced obsessive compulsive or related disorder, without use disorder

F15.99 Other stimulant use, unspecified with unspecified stimulant-induced disorder HCC

✓4ᵗʰ **F16 Hallucinogen related disorders**
INCLUDES   ecstasy
PCP
phencyclidine
AHA: 2018,4Q,31

✓5ᵗʰ **F16.1 Hallucinogen abuse**
EXCLUDES 1   *hallucinogen dependence (F16.2-)*
hallucinogen use, unspecified (F16.9-)

F16.10 Hallucinogen abuse, uncomplicated HCC
Other hallucinogen use disorder, mild
Phencyclidine use disorder, mild
F16.11 Hallucinogen abuse, in remission HCC
Other hallucinogen use disorder, mild, in early remission
Other hallucinogen use disorder, mild, in sustained remission
Phencyclidine use disorder, mild, in early remission
Phencyclidine use disorder, mild, in sustained remission

✓6ᵗʰ **F16.12 Hallucinogen abuse with intoxication**
F16.120 Hallucinogen abuse with intoxication, uncomplicated HCC
F16.121 Hallucinogen abuse with intoxication with delirium CC HCC
F16.122 Hallucinogen abuse with intoxication with perceptual disturbance HCC
F16.129 Hallucinogen abuse with intoxication, unspecified HCC

F16.14 Hallucinogen abuse with hallucinogen-induced mood disorder HCC
Other hallucinogen use disorder, mild, with other hallucinogen induced bipolar or related disorder
Other hallucinogen use disorder, mild, with other hallucinogen induced depressive disorder
Phencyclidine use disorder, mild, with phencyclidine induced bipolar or related disorder
Phencyclidine use disorder, mild, with phencyclidine induced depressive disorder

✓6ᵗʰ **F16.15 Hallucinogen abuse with hallucinogen-induced psychotic disorder**
F16.150 Hallucinogen abuse with hallucinogen-induced psychotic disorder with delusions CC HCC
F16.151 Hallucinogen abuse with hallucinogen-induced psychotic disorder with hallucinations CC HCC
F16.159 Hallucinogen abuse with hallucinogen-induced psychotic disorder, unspecified HCC

✓6ᵗʰ **F16.18 Hallucinogen abuse with other hallucinogen-induced disorder**
F16.180 Hallucinogen abuse with hallucinogen-induced anxiety disorder HCC
F16.183 Hallucinogen abuse with hallucinogen persisting perception disorder (flashbacks) HCC
F16.188 Hallucinogen abuse with other hallucinogen-induced disorder HCC

F16.19 Hallucinogen abuse with unspecified hallucinogen-induced disorder HCC

✓5ᵗʰ **F16.2 Hallucinogen dependence**
EXCLUDES 1   *hallucinogen abuse (F16.1-)*
hallucinogen use, unspecified (F16.9-)

F16.20 Hallucinogen dependence, uncomplicated CC HCC
Other hallucinogen use disorder, moderate
Other hallucinogen use disorder, severe
Phencyclidine use disorder, moderate
Phencyclidine use disorder, severe
F16.21 Hallucinogen dependence, in remission HCC
Other hallucinogen use disorder, moderate, in early remission
Other hallucinogen use disorder, moderate, in sustained remission
Other hallucinogen use disorder, severe, in early remission
Other hallucinogen use disorder, severe, in sustained remission
Phencyclidine use disorder, moderate, in early remission
Phencyclidine use disorder, moderate, in sustained remission
Phencyclidine use disorder, severe, in early remission
Phencyclidine use disorder, severe, in sustained remission

✓6ᵗʰ **F16.22 Hallucinogen dependence with intoxication**
F16.220 Hallucinogen dependence with intoxication, uncomplicated HCC
F16.221 Hallucinogen dependence with intoxication with delirium CC HCC
F16.229 Hallucinogen dependence with intoxication, unspecified HCC

N Newborn: 0   P Pediatric: 0-17   M Maternity: 9-64   A Adult: 15-124   MCC Major Complication/Comorbidity   CC Complication/Comorbidity   SW Severe Wound Dx

554   ICD-10-CM 2021

F16.24 **Hallucinogen dependence with hallucinogen-induced** mood disorder   HCC

    Other hallucinogen use disorder, moderate, with other hallucinogen induced bipolar or related disorder

    Other hallucinogen use disorder, moderate, with other hallucinogen induced depressive disorder

    Other hallucinogen use disorder, severe, with other hallucinogen-induced bipolar or related disorder

    Other hallucinogen use disorder, severe, with other hallucinogen-induced depressive disorder

    Phencyclidine use disorder, moderate, with phencyclidine induced bipolar or related disorder

    Phencyclidine use disorder, moderate, with phencyclidine induced depressive disorder

    Phencyclidine use disorder, severe, with phencyclidine induced bipolar or related disorder

    Phencyclidine use disorder, severe, with phencyclidine-induced depressive disorder

✓6ᵗʰ **F16.25** **Hallucinogen dependence with hallucinogen-induced** psychotic disorder

    F16.250 **Hallucinogen dependence with hallucinogen-induced psychotic disorder with** delusions   CC HCC

    F16.251 **Hallucinogen dependence with hallucinogen-induced psychotic disorder with** hallucinations   CC HCC

    F16.259 **Hallucinogen dependence with hallucinogen-induced psychotic disorder, unspecified**   CC HCC

✓6ᵗʰ **F16.28** **Hallucinogen dependence with** other **hallucinogen-induced disorder**

    F16.280 **Hallucinogen dependence with hallucinogen-induced** anxiety disorder   CC HCC

    F16.283 **Hallucinogen dependence with hallucinogen** persisting perception disorder (flashbacks)   CC HCC

    F16.288 **Hallucinogen dependence with other hallucinogen-induced disorder**   CC HCC

    F16.29 **Hallucinogen dependence with unspecified hallucinogen-induced disorder**   HCC

✓5ᵗʰ **F16.9** **Hallucinogen** use, unspecified

    EXCLUDES 1   *hallucinogen abuse (F16.1-)*

        hallucinogen dependence (F16.2-)

    TIP: Assign a substance use code only when the provider documents a relationship between the use and an associated physical, mental, or behavioral disorder. As with all diagnoses, substance use codes must meet the definition of a reportable diagnosis.

    F16.90 **Hallucinogen use, unspecified, uncomplicated**

        AHA: 2018,2Q,10-11

✓6ᵗʰ **F16.92** **Hallucinogen use, unspecified with** intoxication

    F16.920 **Hallucinogen use, unspecified with intoxication,** uncomplicated   HCC

    F16.921 **Hallucinogen use, unspecified with intoxication with** delirium   CC HCC

        Other hallucinogen intoxication delirium

    F16.929 **Hallucinogen use, unspecified with intoxication, unspecified**   HCC

    F16.94 **Hallucinogen use, unspecified with hallucinogen-induced** mood disorder   HCC

        Other hallucinogen induced bipolar or related disorder, without use disorder

        Other hallucinogen induced depressive disorder, without use disorder

        Phencyclidine induced bipolar or related disorder, without use disorder

        Phencyclidine induced depressive disorder, without use disorder

✓6ᵗʰ **F16.95** **Hallucinogen use, unspecified with hallucinogen-induced** psychotic disorder

    F16.950 **Hallucinogen use, unspecified with hallucinogen-induced psychotic disorder with** delusions   CC HCC

    F16.951 **Hallucinogen use, unspecified with hallucinogen-induced psychotic disorder with** hallucinations   CC HCC

    F16.959 **Hallucinogen use, unspecified with hallucinogen-induced psychotic disorder, unspecified**   HCC

        Other hallucinogen induced psychotic disorder, without use disorder

        Phencyclidine induced psychotic disorder, without use disorder

✓6ᵗʰ **F16.98** **Hallucinogen use, unspecified with other specified hallucinogen-induced disorder**

    F16.980 **Hallucinogen use, unspecified with hallucinogen-induced** anxiety disorder   HCC

        Other hallucinogen-induced anxiety disorder, without use disorder

        Phencyclidine induced anxiety disorder, without use disorder

    F16.983 **Hallucinogen use, unspecified with hallucinogen** persisting perception disorder (flashbacks)   HCC

    F16.988 **Hallucinogen use, unspecified with other hallucinogen-induced disorder**   HCC

    F16.99 **Hallucinogen use, unspecified with unspecified hallucinogen-induced disorder**   HCC

✓4ᵗʰ **F17** **Nicotine** dependence

    EXCLUDES 1   *history of tobacco dependence (Z87.891)*

        tobacco use NOS (Z72.0)

    EXCLUDES 2   *tobacco use (smoking) during pregnancy, childbirth and the puerperium (O99.33-)*

        toxic effect of nicotine (T65.2-)

    AHA: 2013,4Q,108-109

✓5ᵗʰ **F17.2** **Nicotine** dependence

    ✓6ᵗʰ **F17.20** **Nicotine dependence, unspecified**

        F17.200 **Nicotine dependence, unspecified, uncomplicated**

            Tobacco use disorder, mild

            Tobacco use disorder, moderate

            Tobacco use disorder, severe

            AHA: 2016,1Q,36

            TIP: Assign when provider documentation indicates "smoker" without further specification.

        F17.201 **Nicotine dependence, unspecified, in remission**

            Tobacco use disorder, mild, in early remission

            Tobacco use disorder, mild, in sustained remission

            Tobacco use disorder, moderate, in early remission

            Tobacco use disorder, moderate, in sustained remission

            Tobacco use disorder, severe, in early remission

            Tobacco use disorder, severe, in sustained remission

        F17.203 **Nicotine dependence unspecified, with** withdrawal   CC

            Tobacco withdrawal

        F17.208 **Nicotine dependence, unspecified, with other nicotine-induced disorders**

        F17.209 **Nicotine dependence, unspecified, with unspecified nicotine-induced disorders**

    ✓6ᵗʰ **F17.21** **Nicotine dependence,** cigarettes

        F17.210 **Nicotine dependence, cigarettes, uncomplicated**

            AHA: 2017,2Q,28-29

F17.211 Nicotine dependence, cigarettes, in remission
Tobacco use disorder, cigarettes, mild, in early remission
Tobacco use disorder, cigarettes, mild, in sustained remission
Tobacco use disorder, cigarettes, moderate, in early remission
Tobacco use disorder, cigarettes, moderate, in sustained remission
Tobacco use disorder, cigarettes, severe, in early remission
Tobacco use disorder, cigarettes, severe, in sustained remission

F17.213 Nicotine dependence, cigarettes, with withdrawal CC

F17.218 Nicotine dependence, cigarettes, with other nicotine-induced disorders

F17.219 Nicotine dependence, cigarettes, with unspecified nicotine-induced disorders

√6ᵗʰ **F17.22 Nicotine dependence, chewing tobacco**

F17.220 Nicotine dependence, chewing tobacco, uncomplicated

F17.221 Nicotine dependence, chewing tobacco, in remission
Tobacco use disorder, chewing tobacco, mild, in early remission
Tobacco use disorder, chewing tobacco, mild, in sustained remission
Tobacco use disorder, chewing tobacco, moderate, in early remission
Tobacco use disorder, chewing tobacco, moderate, in sustained remission
Tobacco use disorder, chewing tobacco, severe, in early remission
Tobacco use disorder, chewing tobacco, severe, in sustained remission

F17.223 Nicotine dependence, chewing tobacco, with withdrawal CC

F17.228 Nicotine dependence, chewing tobacco, with other nicotine-induced disorders

F17.229 Nicotine dependence, chewing tobacco, with unspecified nicotine-induced disorders

√6ᵗʰ **F17.29 Nicotine dependence, other tobacco product**

F17.290 Nicotine dependence, other tobacco product, uncomplicated
AHA: 2017,2Q,28-29

F17.291 Nicotine dependence, other tobacco product, in remission
Tobacco use disorder, other tobacco product, mild, in early remission
Tobacco use disorder, other tobacco product, mild, in sustained remission
Tobacco use disorder, other tobacco product, moderate, in early remission
Tobacco use disorder, other tobacco product, moderate, in sustained remission
Tobacco use disorder, other tobacco product, severe, in early remission
Tobacco use disorder, other tobacco product, severe, in sustained remission

F17.293 Nicotine dependence, other tobacco product, with withdrawal CC

F17.298 Nicotine dependence, other tobacco product, with other nicotine-induced disorders

F17.299 Nicotine dependence, other tobacco product, with unspecified nicotine-induced disorders

√4ᵗʰ **F18 Inhalant related disorders**
INCLUDES   volatile solvents

√5ᵗʰ **F18.1 Inhalant abuse**
EXCLUDES 1   *inhalant dependence (F18.2-)*
inhalant use, unspecified (F18.9-)

F18.10 Inhalant abuse, uncomplicated HCC
Inhalant use disorder, mild

F18.11 Inhalant abuse, in remission HCC
Inhalant use disorder, mild, in early remission
Inhalant use disorder, mild, in sustained remission

√6ᵗʰ **F18.12 Inhalant abuse with intoxication**

F18.120 Inhalant abuse with intoxication, uncomplicated HCC

F18.121 Inhalant abuse with intoxication delirium CC HCC

F18.129 Inhalant abuse with intoxication, unspecified HCC

F18.14 Inhalant abuse with inhalant-induced mood disorder HCC
Inhalant use disorder, mild, with inhalant induced depressive disorder

√6ᵗʰ **F18.15 Inhalant abuse with inhalant-induced psychotic disorder**

F18.150 Inhalant abuse with inhalant-induced psychotic disorder with delusions CC HCC

F18.151 Inhalant abuse with inhalant-induced psychotic disorder with hallucinations CC HCC

F18.159 Inhalant abuse with inhalant-induced psychotic disorder, unspecified HCC

F18.17 Inhalant abuse with inhalant-induced dementia CC HCC
Inhalant use disorder, mild, with inhalant induced major neurocognitive disorder

√6ᵗʰ **F18.18 Inhalant abuse with other inhalant-induced disorders**

F18.180 Inhalant abuse with inhalant-induced anxiety disorder HCC

F18.188 Inhalant abuse with other inhalant-induced disorder HCC
Inhalant use disorder, mild, with inhalant induced mild neurocognitive disorder

F18.19 Inhalant abuse with unspecified inhalant-induced disorder HCC

√5ᵗʰ **F18.2 Inhalant dependence**
EXCLUDES 1   *inhalant abuse (F18.1-)*
inhalant use, unspecified (F18.9-)

F18.20 Inhalant dependence, uncomplicated CC HCC
Inhalant use disorder, moderate
Inhalant use disorder, severe

F18.21 Inhalant dependence, in remission HCC
Inhalant use disorder, moderate, in early remission
Inhalant use disorder, moderate, in sustained remission
Inhalant use disorder, severe, in early remission
Inhalant use disorder, severe, in sustained remission

√6ᵗʰ **F18.22 Inhalant dependence with intoxication**

F18.220 Inhalant dependence with intoxication, uncomplicated HCC

F18.221 Inhalant dependence with intoxication delirium CC HCC

F18.229 Inhalant dependence with intoxication, unspecified HCC

F18.24 Inhalant dependence with inhalant-induced mood disorder HCC
Inhalant use disorder, moderate, with inhalant induced depressive disorder
Inhalant use disorder, severe, with inhalant induced depressive disorder

√6ᵗʰ **F18.25 Inhalant dependence with inhalant-induced psychotic disorder**

F18.250 Inhalant dependence with inhalant-induced psychotic disorder with delusions CC HCC

F18.251 Inhalant dependence with inhalant-induced psychotic disorder with hallucinations CC HCC

F18.259 Inhalant dependence with inhalant-induced psychotic disorder, unspecified `CC` `HCC`

F18.27 Inhalant dependence with inhalant-induced dementia `CC` `HCC`
Inhalant use disorder, moderate, with inhalant induced major neurocognitive disorder
Inhalant use disorder, severe, with inhalant induced major neurocognitive disorder

✓6ᵗʰ **F18.28** Inhalant dependence with other inhalant-induced disorders

F18.280 Inhalant dependence with inhalant-induced anxiety disorder `CC` `HCC`

F18.288 Inhalant dependence with other inhalant-induced disorder `CC` `HCC`
Inhalant use disorder, moderate, with inhalant-induced mild neurocognitive disorder
Inhalant use disorder, severe, with inhalant-induced mild neurocognitive disorder

F18.29 Inhalant dependence with unspecified inhalant-induced disorder `HCC`

✓5ᵗʰ **F18.9** Inhalant use, unspecified
EXCLUDES 1 inhalant abuse (F18.1-)
           inhalant dependence (F18.2-)
TIP: Assign a substance use code only when the provider documents a relationship between the use and an associated physical, mental, or behavioral disorder. As with all diagnoses, substance use codes must meet the definition of a reportable diagnosis.

F18.90 Inhalant use, unspecified, uncomplicated
AHA: 2018,2Q,10-11

✓6ᵗʰ **F18.92** Inhalant use, unspecified with intoxication

F18.920 Inhalant use, unspecified with intoxication, uncomplicated `HCC`

F18.921 Inhalant use, unspecified with intoxication with delirium `CC` `HCC`

F18.929 Inhalant use, unspecified with intoxication, unspecified `HCC`

F18.94 Inhalant use, unspecified with inhalant-induced mood disorder `HCC`
Inhalant induced depressive disorder

✓6ᵗʰ **F18.95** Inhalant use, unspecified with inhalant-induced psychotic disorder

F18.950 Inhalant use, unspecified with inhalant-induced psychotic disorder with delusions `CC` `HCC`

F18.951 Inhalant use, unspecified with inhalant-induced psychotic disorder with hallucinations `CC` `HCC`

F18.959 Inhalant use, unspecified with inhalant-induced psychotic disorder, unspecified `HCC`

F18.97 Inhalant use, unspecified with inhalant-induced persisting dementia `CC` `HCC`
Inhalant-induced major neurocognitive disorder

✓6ᵗʰ **F18.98** Inhalant use, unspecified with other inhalant-induced disorders

F18.980 Inhalant use, unspecified with inhalant-induced anxiety disorder `HCC`

F18.988 Inhalant use, unspecified with other inhalant-induced disorder `HCC`
Inhalant-induced mild neurocognitive disorder

F18.99 Inhalant use, unspecified with unspecified inhalant-induced disorder `HCC`

✓4ᵗʰ **F19** Other psychoactive substance related disorders
INCLUDES polysubstance drug use (indiscriminate drug use)

✓5ᵗʰ **F19.1** Other psychoactive substance abuse
EXCLUDES 1 other psychoactive substance dependence (F19.2-)
           other psychoactive substance use, unspecified (F19.9-)

F19.10 Other psychoactive substance abuse, uncomplicated `HCC`
Other (or unknown) substance use disorder, mild

F19.11 Other psychoactive substance abuse, in remission `HCC`
Other (or unknown) substance use disorder, mild, in early remission
Other (or unknown) substance use disorder, mild, in sustained remission

✓6ᵗʰ **F19.12** Other psychoactive substance abuse with intoxication

F19.120 Other psychoactive substance abuse with intoxication, uncomplicated `HCC`

F19.121 Other psychoactive substance abuse with intoxication delirium `CC` `HCC`

F19.122 Other psychoactive substance abuse with intoxication with perceptual disturbances `HCC`

F19.129 Other psychoactive substance abuse with intoxication, unspecified `HCC`

✓6ᵗʰ **F19.13** Other psychoactive substance abuse with withdrawal

● **F19.130** Other psychoactive substance abuse with withdrawal, uncomplicated `CC`

● **F19.131** Other psychoactive substance abuse with withdrawal delirium `CC`

● **F19.132** Other psychoactive substance abuse with withdrawal with perceptual disturbance `CC`

● **F19.139** Other psychoactive substance abuse with withdrawal, unspecified `CC`

F19.14 Other psychoactive substance abuse with psychoactive substance-induced mood disorder `HCC`
Other (or unknown) substance use disorder, mild, with other (or unknown) substance-induced bipolar or related disorder
Other (or unknown) substance use disorder, mild, with other (or unknown) substance-induced depressive disorder

✓6ᵗʰ **F19.15** Other psychoactive substance abuse with psychoactive substance-induced psychotic disorder

F19.150 Other psychoactive substance abuse with psychoactive substance-induced psychotic disorder with delusions `CC` `HCC`

F19.151 Other psychoactive substance abuse with psychoactive substance-induced psychotic disorder with hallucinations `CC` `HCC`

F19.159 Other psychoactive substance abuse with psychoactive substance-induced psychotic disorder, unspecified `HCC`

F19.16 Other psychoactive substance abuse with psychoactive substance-induced persisting amnestic disorder `HCC`

F19.17 Other psychoactive substance abuse with psychoactive substance-induced persisting dementia `CC` `HCC`
Other (or unknown) substance use disorder, mild, with other (or unknown) substance-induced major neurocognitive disorder

✓6ᵗʰ **F19.18** Other psychoactive substance abuse with other psychoactive substance-induced disorders

F19.180 Other psychoactive substance abuse with psychoactive substance-induced anxiety disorder `HCC`

F19.181 Other psychoactive substance abuse with psychoactive substance-induced sexual dysfunction `HCC`

F19.182 Other psychoactive substance abuse with psychoactive substance-induced sleep disorder `HCC`

☑ Additional Character Required   ✓x7ᵗʰ Placeholder   Unacceptable PDx   Questionable PDx   Manifestation   Unspecified Dx   `H1`-`H14` HAC   `HCC` CMS-HCC Dx   `HIV` HIV Dx

Chapter 5. Mental, Behavioral and Neurodevelopmental Disorders

F19.188   **Other psychoactive substance abuse with other psychoactive substance-induced disorder** HCC
- Other (or unknown) substance use disorder, mild, with other (or unknown) substance induced mild neurocognitive disorder
- Other (or unknown) substance use disorder, mild, with other (or unknown) substance induced obsessive-compulsive or related disorder

F19.19   **Other psychoactive substance abuse with unspecified psychoactive substance-induced disorder** HCC

√5ᵗʰ **F19.2**   **Other psychoactive substance dependence**
> EXCLUDES 1   *other psychoactive substance abuse (F19.1-)*
> *other psychoactive substance use, unspecified (F19.9-)*

F19.20   **Other psychoactive substance dependence, uncomplicated** CC HCC
- Other (or unknown) substance use disorder, moderate
- Other (or unknown) substance use disorder, severe

F19.21   **Other psychoactive substance dependence, in remission** HCC
- Other (or unknown) substance use disorder, moderate, in early remission
- Other (or unknown) substance use disorder, moderate, in sustained remission
- Other (or unknown) substance use disorder, severe, in early remission
- Other (or unknown) substance use disorder, severe, in sustained remission

√6ᵗʰ **F19.22**   **Other psychoactive substance dependence with intoxication**
> EXCLUDES 1   *other psychoactive substance dependence with withdrawal (F19.23-)*

F19.220   **Other psychoactive substance dependence with intoxication, uncomplicated** HCC

F19.221   **Other psychoactive substance dependence with intoxication delirium** CC HCC

F19.222   **Other psychoactive substance dependence with intoxication with perceptual disturbance** CC HCC

F19.229   **Other psychoactive substance dependence with intoxication, unspecified** HCC

√6ᵗʰ **F19.23**   **Other psychoactive substance dependence with withdrawal**
> EXCLUDES 1   *other psychoactive substance dependence with intoxication (F19.22-)*

F19.230   **Other psychoactive substance dependence with withdrawal, uncomplicated** CC HCC

F19.231   **Other psychoactive substance dependence with withdrawal delirium** CC HCC

F19.232   **Other psychoactive substance dependence with withdrawal with perceptual disturbance** CC HCC

F19.239   **Other psychoactive substance dependence with withdrawal, unspecified** CC HCC

F19.24   **Other psychoactive substance dependence with psychoactive substance-induced mood disorder** HCC
- Other (or unknown) substance use disorder, moderate, with other (or unknown) substance induced bipolar or related disorder
- Other (or unknown) substance use disorder, moderate, with other (or unknown) substance induced depressive disorder
- Other (or unknown) substance use disorder, severe, with other (or unknown) substance induced bipolar or related disorder
- Other (or unknown) substance use disorder, severe, with other (or unknown) substance induced depressive disorder

√6ᵗʰ **F19.25**   **Other psychoactive substance dependence with psychoactive substance-induced psychotic disorder**

F19.250   **Other psychoactive substance dependence with psychoactive substance-induced psychotic disorder with delusions** CC HCC

F19.251   **Other psychoactive substance dependence with psychoactive substance-induced psychotic disorder with hallucinations** CC HCC

F19.259   **Other psychoactive substance dependence with psychoactive substance-induced psychotic disorder, unspecified** CC HCC

F19.26   **Other psychoactive substance dependence with psychoactive substance-induced persisting amnestic disorder** CC HCC

F19.27   **Other psychoactive substance dependence with psychoactive substance-induced persisting dementia** CC HCC
- Other (or unknown) substance use disorder, moderate, with other (or unknown) substance induced major neurocognitive disorder
- Other (or unknown) substance use disorder, severe, with other (or unknown) substance induced major neurocognitive disorder

√6ᵗʰ **F19.28**   **Other psychoactive substance dependence with other psychoactive substance-induced disorders**

F19.280   **Other psychoactive substance dependence with psychoactive substance-induced anxiety disorder** CC HCC

F19.281   **Other psychoactive substance dependence with psychoactive substance-induced sexual dysfunction** CC HCC

F19.282   **Other psychoactive substance dependence with psychoactive substance-induced sleep disorder** CC HCC

F19.288   **Other psychoactive substance dependence with other psychoactive substance-induced disorder** CC HCC
- Other (or unknown) substance use disorder, moderate, with other (or unknown) substance induced mild neurocognitive disorder
- Other (or unknown) substance use disorder, severe, with other (or unknown) substance induced mild neurocognitive disorder
- Other (or unknown) substance use disorder, moderate, with other (or unknown) substance induced obsessive compulsive or related disorder
- Other (or unknown) substance use disorder, severe, with other (or unknown) substance induced obsessive-compulsive or related disorder

F19.29   **Other psychoactive substance dependence with unspecified psychoactive substance-induced disorder** HCC

N Newborn: 0   P Pediatric: 0-17   M Maternity: 9-64   A Adult: 15-124   MCC Major Complication/Comorbidity   CC Complication/Comorbidity   SW Severe Wound Dx

558   ICD-10-CM 2021

✓5ᵗʰ **F19.9**   **Other psychoactive substance use, unspecified**

> **EXCLUDES 1**   *other psychoactive substance abuse (F19.1-)*
>
> *other psychoactive substance dependence (F19.2-)*

TIP: Assign a substance use code only when the provider documents a relationship between the use and an associated physical, mental, or behavioral disorder. As with all diagnoses, substance use codes must meet the definition of a reportable diagnosis.

  F19.90   **Other psychoactive substance use, unspecified, uncomplicated**
> AHA: 2018,2Q,10-11

✓6ᵗʰ **F19.92**   **Other psychoactive substance use, unspecified with intoxication**

> **EXCLUDES 1**   *other psychoactive substance use, unspecified with withdrawal (F19.93)*

  F19.920   **Other psychoactive substance use, unspecified with intoxication, uncomplicated**   HCC

  F19.921   **Other psychoactive substance use, unspecified with intoxication with delirium**   CC HCC
> Other (or unknown) substance-induced delirium

  F19.922   **Other psychoactive substance use, unspecified with intoxication with perceptual disturbance**   HCC

  F19.929   **Other psychoactive substance use, unspecified with intoxication, unspecified**   HCC

✓6ᵗʰ **F19.93**   **Other psychoactive substance use, unspecified with withdrawal**

> **EXCLUDES 1**   *other psychoactive substance use, unspecified with intoxication (F19.92-)*

  F19.930   **Other psychoactive substance use, unspecified with withdrawal, uncomplicated**   CC HCC

  F19.931   **Other psychoactive substance use, unspecified with withdrawal delirium**   CC HCC

  F19.932   **Other psychoactive substance use, unspecified with withdrawal with perceptual disturbance**   CC HCC

  F19.939   **Other psychoactive substance use, unspecified with withdrawal, unspecified**   CC HCC

  F19.94   **Other psychoactive substance use, unspecified with psychoactive substance-induced mood disorder**   HCC
> Other (or unknown) substance-induced bipolar or related disorder, without use disorder
>
> Other (or unknown) substance-induced depressive disorder, without use disorder

✓6ᵗʰ **F19.95**   **Other psychoactive substance use, unspecified with psychoactive substance-induced psychotic disorder**

  F19.950   **Other psychoactive substance use, unspecified with psychoactive substance-induced psychotic disorder with delusions**   CC HCC

  F19.951   **Other psychoactive substance use, unspecified with psychoactive substance-induced psychotic disorder with hallucinations**   CC HCC

  F19.959   **Other psychoactive substance use, unspecified with psychoactive substance-induced psychotic disorder, unspecified**   HCC
> Other or unknown substance-induced psychotic disorder, without use disorder

  F19.96   **Other psychoactive substance use, unspecified with psychoactive substance-induced persisting amnestic disorder**   HCC

  F19.97   **Other psychoactive substance use, unspecified with psychoactive substance-induced persisting dementia**   CC HCC
> Other (or unknown) substance-induced major neurocognitive disorder, without use disorder

✓6ᵗʰ **F19.98**   **Other psychoactive substance use, unspecified with other psychoactive substance-induced disorders**

  F19.980   **Other psychoactive substance use, unspecified with psychoactive substance-induced anxiety disorder**   HCC
> Other (or unknown) substance-induced anxiety disorder, without use disorder

  F19.981   **Other psychoactive substance use, unspecified with psychoactive substance-induced sexual dysfunction**   HCC
> Other (or unknown) substance-induced sexual dysfunction, without use disorder

  F19.982   **Other psychoactive substance use, unspecified with psychoactive substance-induced sleep disorder**   HCC
> Other (or unknown) substance-induced sleep disorder, without use disorder

  F19.988   **Other psychoactive substance use, unspecified with other psychoactive substance-induced disorder**   HCC
> Other (or unknown) substance-induced mild neurocognitive disorder, without use disorder
>
> Other (or unknown) substance-induced obsessive-compulsive or related disorder, without use disorder

  F19.99   **Other psychoactive substance use, unspecified with unspecified psychoactive substance-induced disorder**   HCC

Schizophrenia, schizotypal, delusional, and other non-mood psychotic disorders (F20-F29)

✓4ᵗʰ **F20**   **Schizophrenia**

> **EXCLUDES 1**   *brief psychotic disorder (F23)*
>
> *cyclic schizophrenia (F25.0)*
>
> *mood [affective] disorders with psychotic symptoms (F30.2, F31.2, F31.5, F31.64, F32.3, F33.3)*
>
> *schizoaffective disorder (F25.-)*
>
> *schizophrenic reaction NOS (F23)*

> **EXCLUDES 2**   *schizophrenic reaction in:*
>
> *alcoholism (F10.15-, F10.25-, F10.95-)*
>
> *brain disease (F06.2)*
>
> *epilepsy (F06.2)*
>
> *psychoactive drug use (F11-F19 with .15, .25, .95)*
>
> *schizotypal disorder (F21)*

DEF: Group of disorders with disturbances in thought (delusions, hallucinations), mood (blunted, flattened, inappropriate affect), and sense of self. Schizophrenia also includes bizarre, purposeless behavior, repetitive activity, or inactivity.

  F20.0   **Paranoid schizophrenia**   CC HCC
> Paraphrenic schizophrenia

> **EXCLUDES 1**   *involutional paranoid state (F22)*
>
> *paranoia (F22)*

DEF: Preoccupied with delusional suspicions and auditory hallucinations related to a single theme. This type of schizophrenia is usually hostile, grandiose, threatening, persecutory, and occasionally hypochondriacal.

  F20.1   **Disorganized schizophrenia**   CC HCC
> Hebephrenic schizophrenia
>
> Hebephrenia

  F20.2   **Catatonic schizophrenia**   CC HCC
> Schizophrenic catalepsy
>
> Schizophrenic catatonia
>
> Schizophrenic flexibilitas cerea

> **EXCLUDES 1**   *catatonic stupor (R40.1)*

DEF: Extreme changes in motor activity. One extreme is a decreased response or reaction to the environment and the other is spontaneous activity.

  F20.3   **Undifferentiated schizophrenia**   HCC
> Atypical schizophrenia

> **EXCLUDES 1**   *acute schizophrenia-like psychotic disorder (F23)*

> **EXCLUDES 2**   *post-schizophrenic depression (F32.89)*

✔ Additional Character Required   ✗7ᵗʰ Placeholder   Unacceptable PDx   Questionable PDx   Manifestation   Unspecified Dx   H1-H14 HAC   HCC CMS-HCC Dx   HIV HIV Dx

ICD-10-CM 2021   **559**

F20.5   **Residual** schizophrenia   `CC` `HCC`
    Restzustand (schizophrenic)
    Schizophrenic residual state

√5ᵗʰ **F20.8**   **Other schizophrenia**

    F20.81   **Schizophreniform disorder**   `CC` `HCC`
        Schizophreniform psychosis NOS

    F20.89   **Other schizophrenia**   `CC` `HCC`
        Cenesthopathic schizophrenia
        Simple schizophrenia

F20.9   **Schizophrenia, unspecified**   `HCC`
    AHA: 2019,2Q,32

F21   **Schizotypal disorder**   `HCC`
    Borderline schizophrenia
    Latent schizophrenia
    Latent schizophrenic reaction
    Prepsychotic schizophrenia
    Prodromal schizophrenia
    Pseudoneurotic schizophrenia
    Pseudopsychopathic schizophrenia
    Schizotypal personality disorder
    EXCLUDES 2   *Asperger's syndrome (F84.5)*
               schizoid personality disorder (F60.1)
    DEF: Disorder characterized by various oddities of thinking, perception, communication, and behavior that may be manifested as magical thinking, ideas of reference, paranoid ideation, recurrent illusions and derealization (depersonalization), or social isolation.

F22   **Delusional disorders**   `HCC`
    Delusional dysmorphophobia
    Involutional paranoid state
    Paranoia
    Paranoia querulans
    Paranoid psychosis
    Paranoid state
    Paraphrenia (late)
    Sensitiver Beziehungswahn
    EXCLUDES 1   *mood [affective] disorders with psychotic symptoms (F30.2,*
               F31.2, F31.5, F31.64, F32.3, F33.3)
               paranoid schizophrenia (F20.0)
    EXCLUDES 2   *paranoid personality disorder (F60.0)*
               paranoid psychosis, psychogenic (F23)
               paranoid reaction (F23)

F23   **Brief psychotic disorder**   `CC` `HCC`
    Paranoid reaction
    Psychogenic paranoid psychosis
    EXCLUDES 2   *mood [affective] disorders with psychotic symptoms (F30.2,*
               F31.2, F31.5, F31.64, F32.3, F33.3)
    AHA: 2019,2Q,32

F24   **Shared psychotic disorder**   `HCC`
    Folie à deux
    Induced paranoid disorder
    Induced psychotic disorder

√4ᵗʰ **F25**   **Schizoaffective disorders**
    EXCLUDES 1   *mood [affective] disorders with psychotic symptoms (F30.2,*
               F31.2, F31.5, F31.64, F32.3, F33.3)
               schizophrenia (F20.-)

    F25.0   **Schizoaffective disorder, bipolar type**   `HCC`
        Cyclic schizophrenia
        Schizoaffective disorder, manic type
        Schizoaffective disorder, mixed type
        Schizoaffective psychosis, bipolar type

    F25.1   **Schizoaffective disorder, depressive type**   `HCC`
        Schizoaffective psychosis, depressive type

    F25.8   **Other schizoaffective disorders**   `HCC`

    F25.9   **Schizoaffective disorder, unspecified**   `HCC`
        Schizoaffective psychosis NOS

F28   **Other psychotic disorder not due to a substance or known physiological condition**   `HIV` `HCC`
    Chronic hallucinatory psychosis
    Other specified schizophrenia spectrum and other psychotic disorder

F29   **Unspecified psychosis not due to a substance or known physiological condition**   `HIV` `HCC`
    Psychosis NOS
    Unspecified schizophrenia spectrum and other psychotic disorder
    EXCLUDES 1   *mental disorder NOS (F99)*
               unspecified mental disorder due to known physiological
               condition (F09)

Mood [affective] disorders (F30-F39)

√4ᵗʰ **F30**   **Manic episode**
    INCLUDES   bipolar disorder, single manic episode
             mixed affective episode
    EXCLUDES 1   *bipolar disorder (F31.-)*
               major depressive disorder, recurrent (F33.-)
               major depressive disorder, single episode (F32.-)
    DEF: Mania: Characterized by abnormal states of elation or excitement out of keeping with the individual's circumstances and varying from enhanced liveliness (hypomania) to violent, almost uncontrollable, excitement. Aggression and anger, flight of ideas, distractibility, impaired judgment, and grandiose ideas are common.

  √5ᵗʰ **F30.1**   **Manic episode without psychotic symptoms**

    F30.10   **Manic episode without psychotic symptoms, unspecified**   `CC` `HCC`

    F30.11   **Manic episode without psychotic symptoms, mild**   `CC` `HCC`

    F30.12   **Manic episode without psychotic symptoms, moderate**   `CC` `HCC`

    F30.13   **Manic episode, severe, without psychotic symptoms**   `CC` `HCC`

  F30.2   **Manic episode, severe with psychotic symptoms**   `CC` `HCC`
    Manic stupor
    Mania with mood-congruent psychotic symptoms
    Mania with mood-incongruent psychotic symptoms

  F30.3   **Manic episode in partial remission**   `HCC`

  F30.4   **Manic episode in full remission**   `HCC`

  F30.8   **Other manic episodes**   `HCC`
    Hypomania

  F30.9   **Manic episode, unspecified**   `CC` `HCC`
    Mania NOS

√4ᵗʰ **F31**   **Bipolar disorder**
    INCLUDES   bipolar I disorder
             bipolar type I disorder
             manic-depressive illness
             manic-depressive psychosis
             manic-depressive reaction
    EXCLUDES 1   *bipolar disorder, single manic episode (F30.-)*
               major depressive disorder, recurrent (F33.-)
               major depressive disorder, single episode (F32.-)
    EXCLUDES 2   *cyclothymia (F34.0)*
    AHA: 2020,1Q,23

  F31.0   **Bipolar disorder, current episode hypomanic**   `CC` `HCC`

  √5ᵗʰ **F31.1**   **Bipolar disorder, current episode manic without psychotic features**

    F31.10   **Bipolar disorder, current episode manic without psychotic features, unspecified**   `CC` `HCC`

    F31.11   **Bipolar disorder, current episode manic without psychotic features, mild**   `CC` `HCC`

    F31.12   **Bipolar disorder, current episode manic without psychotic features, moderate**   `CC` `HCC`

    F31.13   **Bipolar disorder, current episode manic without psychotic features, severe**   `CC` `HCC`

  F31.2   **Bipolar disorder, current episode manic severe with psychotic features**   `CC` `HCC`
    Bipolar disorder, current episode manic with mood-congruent psychotic symptoms
    Bipolar disorder, current episode manic with mood-incongruent psychotic symptoms
    Bipolar I disorder, current or most recent episode manic with psychotic features

  √5ᵗʰ **F31.3**   **Bipolar disorder, current episode depressed, mild or moderate severity**

    F31.30   **Bipolar disorder, current episode depressed, mild or moderate severity, unspecified**   `CC` `HCC`

    F31.31   **Bipolar disorder, current episode depressed, mild**   `CC` `HCC`

    F31.32   **Bipolar disorder, current episode depressed, moderate**   `CC` `HCC`

F31.4 **Bipolar disorder, current episode** depressed, severe, without psychotic features   CC HCC

F31.5 **Bipolar disorder, current episode** depressed, severe, with psychotic features   CC HCC
Bipolar disorder, current episode depressed with mood-congruent psychotic symptoms
Bipolar disorder, current episode depressed with mood-incongruent psychotic symptoms
Bipolar I disorder, current or most recent episode depressed, with psychotic features

√5ᵗʰ **F31.6** **Bipolar disorder, current episode** mixed

    F31.60 **Bipolar disorder, current episode mixed, unspecified**   CC HCC

    F31.61 **Bipolar disorder, current episode mixed,** mild   CC HCC

    F31.62 **Bipolar disorder, current episode mixed,** moderate   CC HCC

    F31.63 **Bipolar disorder, current episode mixed,** severe, without psychotic features   CC HCC

    F31.64 **Bipolar disorder, current episode mixed,** severe, with psychotic features   CC HCC
Bipolar disorder, current episode mixed with mood-congruent psychotic symptoms
Bipolar disorder, current episode mixed with mood-incongruent psychotic symptoms

√5ᵗʰ **F31.7** **Bipolar disorder, currently** in remission

    F31.70 **Bipolar disorder, currently in remission, most recent episode unspecified**   HCC

    F31.71 **Bipolar disorder, in partial remission, most recent episode** hypomanic   HCC

    F31.72 **Bipolar disorder, in full remission, most recent episode** hypomanic   HCC

    F31.73 **Bipolar disorder, in partial remission, most recent episode** manic   HCC

    F31.74 **Bipolar disorder, in full remission, most recent episode** manic   HCC

    F31.75 **Bipolar disorder, in partial remission, most recent episode** depressed   HCC

    F31.76 **Bipolar disorder, in full remission, most recent episode** depressed   HCC

    F31.77 **Bipolar disorder, in partial remission, most recent episode** mixed   HCC

    F31.78 **Bipolar disorder, in full remission, most recent episode** mixed   HCC

√5ᵗʰ **F31.8** **Other bipolar disorders**

    F31.81 **Bipolar II disorder**   CC HCC
Bipolar disorder, type 2

    F31.89 **Other bipolar disorder**   CC HCC
Recurrent manic episodes NOS

F31.9 **Bipolar disorder, unspecified**   HCC
Manic depression
AHA: 2020,1Q,23

√4ᵗʰ **F32** **Major depressive disorder,** single episode

    INCLUDES single episode of agitated depression
single episode of depressive reaction
single episode of major depression
single episode of psychogenic depression
single episode of reactive depression
single episode of vital depression

    EXCLUDES 1 *bipolar disorder (F31.-)*
manic episode (F30.-)
recurrent depressive disorder (F33.-)

    EXCLUDES 2 *adjustment disorder (F43.2)*

AHA: 2020,1Q,23
DEF: Mood disorder that produces depression that may exhibit as sadness, low self-esteem, or guilt feelings. Other manifestations may be withdrawal from friends and family and interrupted sleep.

F32.0 **Major depressive disorder, single episode,** mild   CC HCC

F32.1 **Major depressive disorder, single episode,** moderate   CC HCC

F32.2 **Major depressive disorder, single episode,** severe without psychotic features   CC HCC

F32.3 **Major depressive disorder, single episode,** severe with psychotic features   CC HCC
Single episode of major depression with mood-congruent psychotic symptoms
Single episode of major depression with mood-incongruent psychotic symptoms
Single episode of major depression with psychotic symptoms
Single episode of psychogenic depressive psychosis
Single episode of psychotic depression
Single episode of reactive depressive psychosis

F32.4 **Major depressive disorder, single episode,** in partial remission   HCC

F32.5 **Major depressive disorder, single episode,** in full remission   HCC

√5ᵗʰ **F32.8** **Other depressive episodes**
AHA: 2016,4Q,14

    F32.81 **Premenstrual dysphoric disorder**   ♀
        EXCLUDES 1 *premenstrual tension syndrome (N94.3)*
        DEF: Severe manifestation of premenstrual syndrome (PMS) that can be disabling and destructive to day-to-day activities. It can exacerbate pre-existing emotional disorders, like depression and anxiety, and cause feelings of loss of control, fatigue, and irritability.

    F32.89 **Other specified depressive episodes**
Atypical depression
Post-schizophrenic depression
Single episode of 'masked' depression NOS

F32.9 **Major depressive disorder, single episode, unspecified**
Depression NOS
Depressive disorder NOS
Major depression NOS
AHA: 2013,4Q,107

√4ᵗʰ **F33** **Major depressive disorder,** recurrent

    INCLUDES recurrent episodes of depressive reaction
recurrent episodes of endogenous depression
recurrent episodes of major depression
recurrent episodes of psychogenic depression
recurrent episodes of reactive depression
recurrent episodes of seasonal depressive disorder
recurrent episodes of vital depression

    EXCLUDES 1 *bipolar disorder (F31.-)*
manic episode (F30.-)

AHA: 2020,1Q,23
DEF: Mood disorder that produces depression that may exhibit as sadness, low self-esteem, or guilt feelings. Other manifestations may be withdrawal from friends and family and interrupted sleep.

F33.0 **Major depressive disorder, recurrent,** mild   CC HCC

F33.1 **Major depressive disorder, recurrent,** moderate   CC HCC

F33.2 **Major depressive disorder, recurrent,** severe without psychotic features   CC HCC

F33.3 **Major depressive disorder, recurrent,** severe with psychotic symptoms   CC HCC
Endogenous depression with psychotic symptoms
Major depressive disorder, recurrent, with psychotic features
Recurrent severe episodes of major depression with mood-congruent psychotic symptoms
Recurrent severe episodes of major depression with mood-incongruent psychotic symptoms
Recurrent severe episodes of major depression with psychotic symptoms
Recurrent severe episodes of psychogenic depressive psychosis
Recurrent severe episodes of psychotic depression
Recurrent severe episodes of reactive depressive psychosis

√5ᵗʰ **F33.4** **Major depressive disorder, recurrent,** in remission

    F33.40 **Major depressive disorder, recurrent, in remission, unspecified**   CC HCC

    F33.41 **Major depressive disorder, recurrent, in** partial remission   HCC

    F33.42 **Major depressive disorder, recurrent, in** full remission   HCC

F33.8 **Other recurrent depressive disorders**   CC HCC
Recurrent brief depressive episodes

F33.9 **Major depressive disorder, recurrent, unspecified**   CC HCC
Monopolar depression NOS

✓4ᵗʰ **F34 Persistent mood [affective] disorders**

F34.0 Cyclothymic disorder
Affective personality disorder
Cycloid personality
Cyclothymia
Cyclothymic personality
DEF: Mood disorder characterized by fast and repeated alterations between hypomanic and depressed moods.

F34.1 Dysthymic disorder
Depressive neurosis
Depressive personality disorder
Dysthymia
Neurotic depression
Persistent anxiety depression
Persistent depressive disorder
EXCLUDES 2 anxiety depression (mild or not persistent) (F41.8)
DEF: Depression without psychosis. It is a less severe but persistent depression and is considered a mild to moderate chronic form of depression.

✓5ᵗʰ **F34.8 Other persistent mood [affective] disorders**
AHA: 2016,4Q,14
F34.81 Disruptive mood dysregulation disorder CC HCC
F34.89 Other specified persistent mood disorders CC HCC

F34.9 Persistent mood [affective] disorder, unspecified CC HCC

F39 Unspecified mood [affective] disorder HCC
Affective psychosis NOS

Anxiety, dissociative, stress-related, somatoform and other nonpsychotic mental disorders (F40-F48)

✓4ᵗʰ **F40 Phobic anxiety disorders**
DEF: Phobia: Broad-range anxiety with abnormally intense dread of certain objects or specific situations that would not normally have that effect.

✓5ᵗʰ **F40.0 Agoraphobia**
DEF: Profound anxiety or fear of leaving familiar settings like home, or being in unfamiliar locations or with strangers or crowds. Agoraphobia may or may not be preceded by recurrent panic attacks.
F40.00 Agoraphobia, unspecified
F40.01 Agoraphobia with panic disorder
Panic disorder with agoraphobia
EXCLUDES 1 panic disorder without agoraphobia (F41.0)
F40.02 Agoraphobia without panic disorder

✓5ᵗʰ **F40.1 Social phobias**
Anthropophobia
Social anxiety disorder
Social anxiety disorder of childhood
Social neurosis
F40.10 Social phobia, unspecified
F40.11 Social phobia, generalized

✓5ᵗʰ **F40.2 Specific (isolated) phobias**
EXCLUDES 2 dysmorphophobia (nondelusional) (F45.22)
nosophobia (F45.22)

✓6ᵗʰ **F40.21 Animal type phobia**
F40.210 Arachnophobia
Fear of spiders
F40.218 Other animal type phobia
✓6ᵗʰ **F40.22 Natural environment type phobia**
F40.220 Fear of thunderstorms
F40.228 Other natural environment type phobia
✓6ᵗʰ **F40.23 Blood, injection, injury type phobia**
F40.230 Fear of blood
F40.231 Fear of injections and transfusions
F40.232 Fear of other medical care
F40.233 Fear of injury
✓6ᵗʰ **F40.24 Situational type phobia**
F40.240 Claustrophobia
F40.241 Acrophobia
F40.242 Fear of bridges
F40.243 Fear of flying
F40.248 Other situational type phobia

✓6ᵗʰ **F40.29 Other specified phobia**
F40.290 Androphobia
Fear of men
F40.291 Gynephobia
Fear of women
F40.298 Other specified phobia
F40.8 Other phobic anxiety disorders
Phobic anxiety disorder of childhood
F40.9 Phobic anxiety disorder, unspecified
Phobia NOS
Phobic state NOS

✓4ᵗʰ **F41 Other anxiety disorders**
EXCLUDES 2 anxiety in:
acute stress reaction (F43.0)
neurasthenia (F48.8)
psychophysiologic disorders (F45.-)
transient adjustment reaction (F43.2)
separation anxiety (F93.0)

F41.0 Panic disorder [episodic paroxysmal anxiety]
Panic attack
Panic state
EXCLUDES 1 panic disorder with agoraphobia (F40.01)
DEF: Neurotic disorder characterized by recurrent panic or anxiety, apprehension, fear, or terror. Symptoms include shortness of breath, palpitations, dizziness, and shakiness; fear of dying may persist.

F41.1 Generalized anxiety disorder
Anxiety neurosis
Anxiety reaction
Anxiety state
Overanxious disorder
EXCLUDES 2 neurasthenia (F48.8)

F41.3 Other mixed anxiety disorders
F41.8 Other specified anxiety disorders
Anxiety depression (mild or not persistent)
Anxiety hysteria
Mixed anxiety and depressive disorder
F41.9 Anxiety disorder, unspecified
Anxiety NOS

✓4ᵗʰ **F42 Obsessive-compulsive disorder**
EXCLUDES 2 obsessive-compulsive personality (disorder) (F60.5)
obsessive-compulsive symptoms occurring in depression (F32-F33)
obsessive-compulsive symptoms occurring in schizophrenia (F20.-)
AHA: 2016,4Q,14-15
F42.2 Mixed obsessional thoughts and acts
F42.3 Hoarding disorder
F42.4 Excoriation (skin-picking) disorder
EXCLUDES 1 factitial dermatitis (L98.1)
other specified behavioral and emotional disorders with onset usually occurring in early childhood and adolescence (F98.8)
F42.8 Other obsessive-compulsive disorder
Anancastic neurosis
Obsessive-compulsive neurosis
F42.9 Obsessive-compulsive disorder, unspecified

✓4ᵗʰ **F43 Reaction to severe stress, and adjustment disorders**
F43.0 Acute stress reaction
Acute crisis reaction
Acute reaction to stress
Combat and operational stress reaction
Combat fatigue
Crisis state
Psychic shock
✓5ᵗʰ **F43.1 Post-traumatic stress disorder (PTSD)**
Traumatic neurosis
DEF: Preoccupation with traumatic events beyond normal experience (i.e., rape, personal assault, etc.) that may also include recurring flashbacks of the trauma. Symptoms include difficulty remembering, sleeping, or concentrating, and guilt feelings for surviving.
F43.10 Post-traumatic stress disorder, unspecified
F43.11 Post-traumatic stress disorder, acute
F43.12 Post-traumatic stress disorder, chronic

✓5ᵗʰ **F43.2 Adjustment disorders**
     Culture shock
     Grief reaction
     Hospitalism in children
     EXCLUDES 2   *separation anxiety disorder of childhood (F93.0)*

     F43.20 Adjustment disorder, unspecified
     F43.21 Adjustment disorder with depressed mood
         AHA: 2014,1Q,25
     F43.22 Adjustment disorder with anxiety
     F43.23 Adjustment disorder with mixed anxiety and depressed mood
     F43.24 Adjustment disorder with disturbance of conduct
     F43.25 Adjustment disorder with mixed disturbance of emotions and conduct
     F43.29 Adjustment disorder with other symptoms

F43.8 Other reactions to severe stress
     Other specified trauma and stressor-related disorder

F43.9 Reaction to severe stress, unspecified
     Trauma and stressor-related disorder, NOS

✓4ᵗʰ **F44 Dissociative and conversion disorders**
     INCLUDES   conversion hysteria
               conversion reaction
               hysteria
               hysterical psychosis
     EXCLUDES 2   *malingering [conscious simulation] (Z76.5)*

F44.0 Dissociative amnesia   HCC
     EXCLUDES 1   *amnesia NOS (R41.3)*
            anterograde amnesia (R41.1)
            dissociative amnesia with dissociative fugue (F44.1)
            retrograde amnesia (R41.2)
     EXCLUDES 2   *alcohol-or other psychoactive substance-induced amnestic disorder (F10, F13, F19 with .26, .96)*
            amnestic disorder due to known physiological condition (F04)
            postictal amnesia in epilepsy (G40.-)

F44.1 Dissociative fugue   HCC
     Dissociative amnesia with dissociative fugue
     EXCLUDES 2   *postictal fugue in epilepsy (G40.-)*
     DEF: Dissociative hysteria identified by memory loss and flight from familiar surroundings to a completely separate environment. Episodes may last hours or days. Conscious activity is not associated with perception of surroundings and there is no later memory of the episode.

F44.2 Dissociative stupor
     EXCLUDES 1   *catatonic stupor (R40.1)*
            stupor NOS (R40.1)
     EXCLUDES 2   *catatonic disorder due to known physiological condition (F06.1)*
            depressive stupor (F32, F33)
            manic stupor (F30, F31)

F44.4 Conversion disorder with motor symptom or deficit
     Conversion disorder with abnormal movement
     Conversion disorder with speech symptoms
     Conversion disorder with swallowing symptoms
     Conversion disorder with weakness/paralysis
     Dissociative motor disorders
     Psychogenic aphonia
     Psychogenic dysphonia

F44.5 Conversion disorder with seizures or convulsions
     Conversion disorder with attacks or seizures
     Dissociative convulsions
     AHA: 2019,1Q,19

F44.6 Conversion disorder with sensory symptom or deficit
     Conversion disorder with anesthesia or sensory loss
     Conversion disorder with special sensory symptoms
     Dissociative anesthesia and sensory loss
     Psychogenic deafness

F44.7 Conversion disorder with mixed symptom presentation

✓5ᵗʰ **F44.8 Other dissociative and conversion disorders**
     F44.81 Dissociative identity disorder   HCC
         Multiple personality disorder

     F44.89 Other dissociative and conversion disorders
         Ganser's syndrome
         Psychogenic confusion
         Psychogenic twilight state
         Trance and possession disorders

F44.9 Dissociative and conversion disorder, unspecified
     Dissociative disorder NOS

✓4ᵗʰ **F45 Somatoform disorders**
     EXCLUDES 2   *dissociative and conversion disorders (F44.-)*
            factitious disorders (F68.1-, F68.A)
            hair-plucking (F63.3)
            lalling (F80.0)
            lisping (F80.0)
            malingering [conscious simulation] (Z76.5)
            nail-biting (F98.8)
            psychological or behavioral factors associated with disorders or diseases classified elsewhere (F54)
            sexual dysfunction, not due to a substance or known physiological condition (F52.-)
            thumb-sucking (F98.8)
            tic disorders (in childhood and adolescence) (F95.-)
            Tourette's syndrome (F95.2)
            trichotillomania (F63.3)
     DEF: Types of disorders causing inconsistent physical symptoms that cannot be explained.

F45.0 Somatization disorder
     Briquet's disorder
     Multiple psychosomatic disorder

F45.1 Undifferentiated somatoform disorder
     Somatic symptom disorder
     Undifferentiated psychosomatic disorder

✓5ᵗʰ **F45.2 Hypochondriacal disorders**
     EXCLUDES 2   *delusional dysmorphophobia (F22)*
            fixed delusions about bodily functions or shape (F22)

     F45.20 Hypochondriacal disorder, unspecified
     F45.21 Hypochondriasis
         Hypochondriacal neurosis
         Illness anxiety disorder
     F45.22 Body dysmorphic disorder
         Dysmorphophobia (nondelusional)
         Nosophobia
     F45.29 Other hypochondriacal disorders

✓5ᵗʰ **F45.4 Pain disorders related to psychological factors**
     EXCLUDES 1   *pain NOS (R52)*

     F45.41 Pain disorder exclusively related to psychological factors
         Somatoform pain disorder (persistent)
     F45.42 Pain disorder with related psychological factors
         Code also associated acute or chronic pain (G89.-)

F45.8 Other somatoform disorders
     Psychogenic dysmenorrhea
     Psychogenic dysphagia, including 'globus hystericus'
     Psychogenic pruritus
     Psychogenic torticollis
     Somatoform autonomic dysfunction
     Teeth grinding
     EXCLUDES 1   *sleep related teeth grinding (G47.63)*

F45.9 Somatoform disorder, unspecified
     Psychosomatic disorder NOS

✓4ᵗʰ **F48 Other nonpsychotic mental disorders**
     F48.1 Depersonalization-derealization syndrome   HCC
     F48.2 Pseudobulbar affect
         Involuntary emotional expression disorder
         Code first underlying cause, if known, such as:
            amyotrophic lateral sclerosis (G12.21)
            multiple sclerosis (G35)
            sequelae of cerebrovascular disease (I69.-)
            sequelae of traumatic intracranial injury (S06.-)

     F48.8 Other specified nonpsychotic mental disorders
         Dhat syndrome
         Neurasthenia
         Occupational neurosis, including writer's cramp
         Psychasthenia
         Psychasthenic neurosis
         Psychogenic syncope

Chapter 5. Mental, Behavioral and Neurodevelopmental Disorders

F48.9   Nonpsychotic mental disorder, unspecified
Neurosis NOS

Behavioral syndromes associated with physiological disturbances and physical factors (F50-F59)

✓4ᵗʰ **F50   Eating disorders**
EXCLUDES 1   anorexia NOS (R63.0)
feeding difficulties (R63.3)
feeding problems of newborn (P92.-)
polyphagia (R63.2)
EXCLUDES 2   feeding disorder in infancy or childhood (F98.2-)
AHA: 2018,4Q,82
TIP: Assign additional code for BMI from category Z68, when documented. BMI can be based on documentation from clinicians who are not the patient's provider.

✓5ᵗʰ **F50.0   Anorexia nervosa**
EXCLUDES 1   loss of appetite (R63.0)
psychogenic loss of appetite (F50.89)
DEF: Psychological eating disorder characterized by an intense fear of gaining weight and an unrealistic perception of body image that perpetuates the feeling of being fat or having too much fat. Avoidance of food and restrictive or unhealthy eating are common.

     F50.00   Anorexia nervosa, unspecified   CC
     F50.01   Anorexia nervosa, restricting type   CC
     F50.02   Anorexia nervosa, binge eating/purging type   CC
       EXCLUDES 1   bulimia nervosa (F50.2)

F50.2   Bulimia nervosa   CC
Bulimia NOS
Hyperorexia nervosa
EXCLUDES 1   anorexia nervosa, binge eating/purging type (F50.02)
DEF: Episodic pattern of overeating (binge eating) followed by purging or extreme exercise accompanied by an awareness of the abnormal eating pattern with a fear of not being able to stop eating.

✓5ᵗʰ **F50.8   Other eating disorders**
EXCLUDES 2   pica of infancy and childhood (F98.3)
AHA: 2017,4Q,9; 2016,4Q,15-16
     F50.81   Binge eating disorder
     F50.82   Avoidant/restrictive food intake disorder
     F50.89   Other specified eating disorder
       Pica in adults
       Psychogenic loss of appetite

     F50.9   Eating disorder, unspecified
Atypical anorexia nervosa
Atypical bulimia nervosa
Feeding or eating disorder, unspecified
Other specified feeding disorder

✓4ᵗʰ **F51   Sleep disorders not due to a substance or known physiological condition**
EXCLUDES 2   organic sleep disorders (G47.-)

✓5ᵗʰ **F51.0   Insomnia not due to a substance or known physiological condition**
EXCLUDES 2   alcohol related insomnia (F10.182, F10.282, F10.982)
drug-related insomnia (F11.182, F11.282, F11.982, F13.182, F13.282, F13.982, F14.182, F14.282, F14.982, F15.182, F15.282, F15.982, F19.182, F19.282, F19.982)
insomnia NOS (G47.0-)
insomnia due to known physiological condition (G47.0-)
organic insomnia (G47.0-)
sleep deprivation (Z72.820)
     F51.01   Primary insomnia
       Idiopathic insomnia
     F51.02   Adjustment insomnia
     F51.03   Paradoxical insomnia
     F51.04   Psychophysiologic insomnia
     F51.05   Insomnia due to other mental disorder
       Code also associated mental disorder
     F51.09   Other insomnia not due to a substance or known physiological condition

✓5ᵗʰ **F51.1   Hypersomnia not due to a substance or known physiological condition**
EXCLUDES 2   alcohol related hypersomnia (F10.182, F10.282, F10.982)
drug-related hypersomnia (F11.182, F11.282, F11.982, F13.182, F13.282, F13.982, F14.182, F14.282, F14.982, F15.182, F15.282, F15.982, F19.182, F19.282, F19.982)
hypersomnia NOS (G47.10)
hypersomnia due to known physiological condition (G47.10)
idiopathic hypersomnia (G47.11, G47.12)
narcolepsy (G47.4-)
     F51.11   Primary hypersomnia
     F51.12   Insufficient sleep syndrome
       EXCLUDES 1   sleep deprivation (Z72.820)
     F51.13   Hypersomnia due to other mental disorder
       Code also associated mental disorder
     F51.19   Other hypersomnia not due to a substance or known physiological condition

F51.3   Sleepwalking [somnambulism]
Non-rapid eye movement sleep arousal disorders, sleepwalking type

F51.4   Sleep terrors [night terrors]
Non-rapid eye movement sleep arousal disorders, sleep terror type

F51.5   Nightmare disorder
Dream anxiety disorder

F51.8   Other sleep disorders not due to a substance or known physiological condition

F51.9   Sleep disorder not due to a substance or known physiological condition, unspecified
Emotional sleep disorder NOS

✓4ᵗʰ **F52   Sexual dysfunction not due to a substance or known physiological condition**
EXCLUDES 2   Dhat syndrome (F48.8)

F52.0   Hypoactive sexual desire disorder
Lack or loss of sexual desire
Male hypoactive sexual desire disorder
Sexual anhedonia
EXCLUDES 1   decreased libido (R68.82)

F52.1   Sexual aversion disorder
Sexual aversion and lack of sexual enjoyment

✓5ᵗʰ **F52.2   Sexual arousal disorders**
Failure of genital response
     F52.21   Male erectile disorder   ♂
       Erectile disorder
       Psychogenic impotence
       EXCLUDES 1   impotence of organic origin (N52.-)
         impotence NOS (N52.-)
     F52.22   Female sexual arousal disorder   ♀
       Female sexual interest/arousal disorder

✓5ᵗʰ **F52.3   Orgasmic disorder**
Inhibited orgasm
Psychogenic anorgasmy
     F52.31   Female orgasmic disorder   ♀
     F52.32   Male orgasmic disorder   ♂
       Delayed ejaculation

F52.4   Premature ejaculation   ♂

F52.5   Vaginismus not due to a substance or known physiological condition   ♀
Psychogenic vaginismus
EXCLUDES 2   vaginismus (due to a known physiological condition) (N94.2)
DEF: Psychogenic response resulting in painful contractions of the vaginal canal muscles. This condition can be severe enough to prevent sexual intercourse.

F52.6   Dyspareunia not due to a substance or known physiological condition
Genito-pelvic pain penetration disorder
Psychogenic dyspareunia
EXCLUDES 2   dyspareunia (due to a known physiological condition) (N94.1-)

F52.8 Other sexual dysfunction not due to a substance or known physiological condition
Excessive sexual drive
Nymphomania
Satyriasis

F52.9 Unspecified sexual dysfunction not due to a substance or known physiological condition
Sexual dysfunction NOS

✓4ᵗʰ **F53 Mental and behavioral disorders associated with the puerperium, not elsewhere classified**
EXCLUDES 1   *mood disorders with psychotic features (F30.2, F31.2, F31.5, F31.64, F32.3, F33.3)*
postpartum dysphoria (O90.6)
psychosis in schizophrenia, schizotypal, delusional, and other psychotic disorders (F20-F29)

AHA: 2018,4Q,8

F53.0 Postpartum depression   M ♀
Postnatal depression, NOS
Postpartum depression, NOS

F53.1 Puerperal psychosis   HCC M ♀
Postpartum psychosis
Puerperal psychosis, NOS

F54 Psychological and behavioral factors associated with disorders or diseases classified elsewhere
Psychological factors affecting physical conditions
Code first the associated physical disorder, such as:
asthma (J45.-)
dermatitis (L23-L25)
gastric ulcer (K25.-)
mucous colitis (K58.-)
ulcerative colitis (K51.-)
urticaria (L50.-)
EXCLUDES 2   *tension-type headache (G44.2)*

✓4ᵗʰ **F55 Abuse of non-psychoactive substances**
EXCLUDES 2   *abuse of psychoactive substances (F10-F19)*

F55.0 Abuse of antacids
F55.1 Abuse of herbal or folk remedies
F55.2 Abuse of laxatives
F55.3 Abuse of steroids or hormones
F55.4 Abuse of vitamins
F55.8 Abuse of other non-psychoactive substances

F59 Unspecified behavioral syndromes associated with physiological disturbances and physical factors
Psychogenic physiological dysfunction NOS

Disorders of adult personality and behavior (F60-F69)

✓4ᵗʰ **F60 Specific personality disorders**

F60.0 Paranoid personality disorder   HCC
Expansive paranoid personality (disorder)
Fanatic personality (disorder)
Paranoid personality (disorder)
Querulant personality (disorder)
Sensitive paranoid personality (disorder)
EXCLUDES 2   *paranoia (F22)*
paranoia querulans (F22)
paranoid psychosis (F22)
paranoid schizophrenia (F20.0)
paranoid state (F22)

F60.1 Schizoid personality disorder   HCC
EXCLUDES 2   *Asperger's syndrome (F84.5)*
delusional disorder (F22)
schizoid disorder of childhood (F84.5)
schizophrenia (F20.-)
schizotypal disorder (F21)

F60.2 Antisocial personality disorder   HCC
Amoral personality (disorder)
Asocial personality (disorder)
Dissocial personality disorder
Psychopathic personality (disorder)
Sociopathic personality (disorder)
EXCLUDES 1   *conduct disorders (F91.-)*
EXCLUDES 2   *borderline personality disorder (F60.3)*

F60.3 Borderline personality disorder   HCC
Aggressive personality (disorder)
Emotionally unstable personality disorder
Explosive personality (disorder)
EXCLUDES 2   *antisocial personality disorder (F60.2)*

F60.4 Histrionic personality disorder   HCC
Hysterical personality (disorder)
Psychoinfantile personality (disorder)

F60.5 Obsessive-compulsive personality disorder   HCC
Anankastic personality (disorder)
Compulsive personality (disorder)
Obsessional personality (disorder)
EXCLUDES 2   *obsessive-compulsive disorder ▶(F42.-)◀*

F60.6 Avoidant personality disorder   HCC
Anxious personality disorder

F60.7 Dependent personality disorder   HCC
Asthenic personality (disorder)
Inadequate personality (disorder)
Passive personality (disorder)
DEF: Lack of self-confidence, fear of abandonment, and an obsessive need to be taken care of.

✓5ᵗʰ **F60.8 Other specific personality disorders**

F60.81 Narcissistic personality disorder   HCC
F60.89 Other specific personality disorders   HCC
Eccentric personality disorder
"Haltlose" type personality disorder
Immature personality disorder
Passive-aggressive personality disorder
Psychoneurotic personality disorder
Self-defeating personality disorder

F60.9 Personality disorder, unspecified   HCC
Character disorder NOS
Character neurosis NOS
Pathological personality NOS

✓4ᵗʰ **F63 Impulse disorders**
EXCLUDES 2   *habitual excessive use of alcohol or psychoactive substances (F10-F19)*
impulse disorders involving sexual behavior (F65.-)

F63.0 Pathological gambling
Compulsive gambling
Gambling disorder
EXCLUDES 1   *gambling and betting NOS (Z72.6)*
EXCLUDES 2   *excessive gambling by manic patients (F30, F31)*
gambling in antisocial personality disorder (F60.2)

F63.1 Pyromania
Pathological fire-setting
EXCLUDES 2   *fire-setting (by) (in):*
adult with antisocial personality disorder (F60.2)
alcohol or psychoactive substance intoxication (F10-F19)
conduct disorders (F91.-)
mental disorders due to known physiological condition (F01-F09)
schizophrenia (F20.-)

F63.2 Kleptomania
Pathological stealing
EXCLUDES 1   *shoplifting as the reason for observation for suspected mental disorder (Z03.8)*
EXCLUDES 2   *depressive disorder with stealing (F31-F33)*
stealing due to underlying mental condition - code to mental condition
stealing in mental disorders due to known physiological condition (F01-F09)

F63.3 Trichotillomania
Hair plucking
EXCLUDES 2   *other stereotyped movement disorder (F98.4)*

✓5ᵗʰ **F63.8 Other impulse disorders**

F63.81 Intermittent explosive disorder
F63.89 Other impulse disorders
F63.9 Impulse disorder, unspecified
Impulse control disorder NOS

Chapter 5. Mental, Behavioral and Neurodevelopmental Disorders

F64–F80.4

✓4ᵗʰ **F64 Gender identity disorders**
    AHA: 2016,4Q,16

F64.0 Transsexualism
    Gender identity disorder in adolescence and adulthood
    Gender dysphoria in adolescents and adults

F64.1 Dual role transvestism
    Use additional code to identify sex reassignment status
    (Z87.890)
    EXCLUDES 1   *gender identity disorder in childhood (F64.2)*
    EXCLUDES 2   *fetishistic transvestism (F65.1)*

F64.2 Gender identity disorder of childhood   P
    Gender dysphoria in children
    EXCLUDES 1   *gender identity disorder in adolescence and*
             adulthood (F64.0)
    EXCLUDES 2   *sexual maturation disorder (F66)*

F64.8 Other gender identity disorders
    Other specified gender dysphoria

F64.9 Gender identity disorder, unspecified
    Gender dysphoria, unspecified
    Gender-role disorder NOS

✓4ᵗʰ **F65 Paraphilias**

F65.0 Fetishism
    Fetishistic disorder

F65.1 Transvestic fetishism
    Fetishistic transvestism
    Transvestic disorder

F65.2 Exhibitionism
    Exhibitionistic disorder

F65.3 Voyeurism
    Voyeuristic disorder

F65.4 Pedophilia
    Pedophilic disorder

✓5ᵗʰ **F65.5 Sadomasochism**

    F65.50 Sadomasochism, unspecified
    F65.51 Sexual masochism
        Sexual masochism disorder
    F65.52 Sexual sadism
        Sexual sadism disorder

✓5ᵗʰ **F65.8 Other paraphilias**

    F65.81 Frotteurism
        Frotteuristic disorder
    F65.89 Other paraphilias
        Necrophilia
        Other specified paraphilic disorder

F65.9 Paraphilia, unspecified
    Paraphilic disorder, unspecified
    Sexual deviation NOS

F66 Other sexual disorders
    Sexual maturation disorder
    Sexual relationship disorder

✓4ᵗʰ **F68 Other disorders of adult personality and behavior**
    AHA: 2018,4Q,9,65

✓5ᵗʰ **F68.1 Factitious disorder imposed on self**
    Compensation neurosis
    Elaboration of physical symptoms for psychological reasons
    Hospital hopper syndrome
    Münchausen's syndrome
    Peregrinating patient
    EXCLUDES 2   *factitial dermatitis (L98.1)*
               person feigning illness (with obvious motivation)
               (Z76.5)

    F68.10 Factitious disorder imposed on self, unspecified   CC
    F68.11 Factitious disorder imposed on self, with predominantly psychological signs and symptoms
    F68.12 Factitious disorder imposed on self, with predominantly physical signs and symptoms   CC
    F68.13 Factitious disorder imposed on self, with combined psychological and physical signs and symptoms

F68.A Factitious disorder imposed on another   CC
    Factitious disorder by proxy
    Münchausen's by proxy

F68.8 Other specified disorders of adult personality and behavior

F69 Unspecified disorder of adult personality and behavior   A

Intellectual disabilities (F70-F79)

Code first any associated physical or developmental disorders
EXCLUDES 1   *borderline intellectual functioning, IQ above 70 to 84 (R41.83)*

F70 Mild intellectual disabilities
    IQ level 50-55 to approximately 70
    Mild mental subnormality

F71 Moderate intellectual disabilities
    IQ level 35-40 to 50-55
    Moderate mental subnormality

F72 Severe intellectual disabilities   CC
    IQ 20-25 to 35-40
    Severe mental subnormality

F73 Profound intellectual disabilities   CC
    IQ level below 20-25
    Profound mental subnormality

F78 Other intellectual disabilities

F79 Unspecified intellectual disabilities
    Mental deficiency NOS
    Mental subnormality NOS

Pervasive and specific developmental disorders (F80-F89)

✓4ᵗʰ **F80 Specific developmental disorders of speech and language**

F80.0 Phonological disorder
    Dyslalia
    Functional speech articulation disorder
    Lalling
    Lisping
    Phonological developmental disorder
    Speech articulation developmental disorder
    Speech-sound disorder
    EXCLUDES 1   *speech articulation impairment due to aphasia NOS*
               (R47.01)
               speech articulation impairment due to apraxia
               (R48.2)
    EXCLUDES 2   *speech articulation impairment due to hearing loss*
               (F80.4)
               speech articulation impairment due to intellectual
               disabilities (F70-F79)
               speech articulation impairment with expressive
               language developmental disorder (F80.1)
               speech articulation impairment with mixed receptive
               expressive language developmental disorder
               (F80.2)

F80.1 Expressive language disorder
    Developmental dysphasia or aphasia, expressive type
    EXCLUDES 1   *mixed receptive-expressive language disorder (F80.2)*
               dysphasia and aphasia NOS (R47.-)
    EXCLUDES 2   *acquired aphasia with epilepsy [Landau-Kleffner]*
               (G40.80-)
               selective mutism (F94.0)
               intellectual disabilities (F70-F79)
               pervasive developmental disorders (F84.-)

F80.2 Mixed receptive-expressive language disorder
    Developmental dysphasia or aphasia, receptive type
    Developmental Wernicke's aphasia
    EXCLUDES 1   *central auditory processing disorder (H93.25)*
               dysphasia or aphasia NOS (R47.-)
               expressive language disorder (F80.1)
               expressive type dysphasia or aphasia (F80.1)
               word deafness (H93.25)
    EXCLUDES 2   *acquired aphasia with epilepsy [Landau-Kleffner]*
               (G40.80-)
               pervasive developmental disorders (F84.-)
               selective mutism (F94.0)
               intellectual disabilities (F70-F79)

F80.4 Speech and language development delay due to hearing loss
    Code also type of hearing loss (H90.-, H91.-)

N Newborn: 0   P Pediatric: 0-17   M Maternity: 9-64   A Adult: 15-124   MCC Major Complication/Comorbidity   CC Complication/Comorbidity   SW Severe Wound Dx

566   ICD-10-CM 2021

√5ᵗʰ **F80.8 Other developmental disorders of speech and language**
     AHA: 2017,1Q,27

F80.81 Childhood onset fluency disorder
     Cluttering NOS
     Stuttering NOS
     EXCLUDES 1   *adult onset fluency disorder (F98.5)*
         fluency disorder in conditions classified elsewhere (R47.82)
         fluency disorder (stuttering) following cerebrovascular disease (I69. with final characters -23)

F80.82 Social pragmatic communication disorder
     EXCLUDES 1   *Asperger's syndrome (F84.5)*
         autistic disorder (F84.0)
     AHA: 2016,4Q,16

F80.89 Other developmental disorders of speech and language

F80.9 Developmental disorder of speech and language, unspecified
     Communication disorder NOS
     Language disorder NOS

√4ᵗʰ **F81 Specific developmental disorders of scholastic skills**

F81.0 Specific reading disorder
     "Backward reading"
     Developmental dyslexia
     Specific learning disorder, with impairment in reading
     Specific reading retardation
     EXCLUDES 1   *alexia NOS (R48.0)*
         dyslexia NOS (R48.0)
     DEF: Serious impairment of reading skills unexplained in relation to general intelligence and teaching processes.

F81.2 Mathematics disorder
     Developmental acalculia
     Developmental arithmetical disorder
     Developmental Gerstmann's syndrome
     Specific learning disorder, with impairment in mathematics
     EXCLUDES 1   *acalculia NOS (R48.8)*
     EXCLUDES 2   *arithmetical difficulties associated with a reading disorder (F81.0)*
         arithmetical difficulties associated with a spelling disorder (F81.81)
         arithmetical difficulties due to inadequate teaching (Z55.8)

√5ᵗʰ **F81.8 Other developmental disorders of scholastic skills**

F81.81 Disorder of written expression
     Specific learning disorder, with impairment in written expression
     Specific spelling disorder

F81.89 Other developmental disorders of scholastic skills

F81.9 Developmental disorder of scholastic skills, unspecified
     Knowledge acquisition disability NOS
     Learning disability NOS
     Learning disorder NOS

F82 Specific developmental disorder of motor function
     Clumsy child syndrome
     Developmental coordination disorder
     Developmental dyspraxia
     EXCLUDES 1   *abnormalities of gait and mobility (R26.-)*
         lack of coordination (R27.-)
     EXCLUDES 2   *lack of coordination secondary to intellectual disabilities (F70-F79)*

√4ᵗʰ **F84 Pervasive developmental disorders**
     Use additional code to identify any associated medical condition and intellectual disabilities.

F84.0 Autistic disorder   CC
     Autism spectrum disorder
     Infantile autism
     Infantile psychosis
     Kanner's syndrome
     EXCLUDES 1   *Asperger's syndrome (F84.5)*
     AHA: 2017,1Q,27

F84.2 Rett's syndrome   CC
     EXCLUDES 1   *Asperger's syndrome (F84.5)*
         autistic disorder (F84.0)
         other childhood disintegrative disorder (F84.3)

F84.3 Other childhood disintegrative disorder   CC P
     Dementia infantilis
     Disintegrative psychosis
     Heller's syndrome
     Symbiotic psychosis
     Use additional code to identify any associated neurological condition
     EXCLUDES 1   *Asperger's syndrome (F84.5)*
         autistic disorder (F84.0)
         Rett's syndrome (F84.2)

F84.5 Asperger's syndrome   CC
     Asperger's disorder
     Autistic psychopathy
     Schizoid disorder of childhood
     DEF: High-functioning form of autism. Children with this syndrome usually develop speech on schedule, are generally very intelligent, and communicate well, but have considerable social shortcomings. *Synonym(s): AS.*

F84.8 Other pervasive developmental disorders   CC
     Overactive disorder associated with intellectual disabilities and stereotyped movements

F84.9 Pervasive developmental disorder, unspecified   CC
     Atypical autism

F88 Other disorders of psychological development
     Developmental agnosia
     Global developmental delay
     Other specified neurodevelopmental disorder

F89 Unspecified disorder of psychological development
     Developmental disorder NOS
     Neurodevelopmental disorder NOS

Behavioral and emotional disorders with onset usually occurring in childhood and adolescence (F90-F98)

NOTE   Codes within categories F90-F98 may be used regardless of the age of a patient. These disorders generally have onset within the childhood or adolescent years, but may continue throughout life or not be diagnosed until adulthood

√4ᵗʰ **F90 Attention-deficit hyperactivity disorders**
     INCLUDES   attention deficit disorder with hyperactivity
         attention deficit syndrome with hyperactivity
     EXCLUDES 2   *anxiety disorders (F40.-, F41.-)*
         mood [affective] disorders (F30-F39)
         pervasive developmental disorders (F84.-)
         schizophrenia (F20.-)

F90.0 Attention-deficit hyperactivity disorder, predominantly inattentive type
     Attention-deficit/hyperactivity disorder, predominantly inattentive presentation

F90.1 Attention-deficit hyperactivity disorder, predominantly hyperactive type
     Attention-deficit/hyperactivity disorder, predominantly hyperactive impulsive presentation

F90.2 Attention-deficit hyperactivity disorder, combined type
     Attention-deficit/hyperactivity disorder, combined presentation

F90.8 Attention-deficit hyperactivity disorder, other type

F90.9 Attention-deficit hyperactivity disorder, unspecified type
     Attention-deficit hyperactivity disorder of childhood or adolescence NOS
     Attention-deficit hyperactivity disorder NOS

√4ᵗʰ **F91 Conduct disorders**
     EXCLUDES 1   *antisocial behavior (Z72.81-)*
         antisocial personality disorder (F60.2)
     EXCLUDES 2   *conduct problems associated with attention-deficit hyperactivity disorder (F90.-)*
         mood [affective] disorders (F30-F39)
         pervasive developmental disorders (F84.-)
         schizophrenia (F20.-)

F91.0 Conduct disorder confined to family context

F91.1 Conduct disorder, childhood-onset type
     Unsocialized conduct disorder
     Conduct disorder, solitary aggressive type
     Unsocialized aggressive disorder

F91.2 Conduct disorder, adolescent-onset type
     Socialized conduct disorder
     Conduct disorder, group type

F91.3 Oppositional defiant disorder

F91.8   **Other conduct disorders**
Other specified conduct disorder
Other specified disruptive disorder

✓**F91.9**   **Conduct disorder, unspecified**
Behavioral disorder NOS
Conduct disorder NOS
Disruptive behavior disorder NOS
Disruptive disorder NOS

✓4ᵗʰ **F93**   **Emotional disorders with onset specific to childhood**

F93.0   **Separation anxiety disorder of childhood**
    EXCLUDES 2   *mood [affective] disorders (F30-F39)*
               nonpsychotic mental disorders (F40-F48)
               phobic anxiety disorder of childhood (F40.8)
               social phobia (F40.1)

F93.8   **Other childhood emotional disorders**
Identity disorder
    EXCLUDES 2   *gender identity disorder of childhood (F64.2)*

✓**F93.9**   **Childhood emotional disorder, unspecified**

✓4ᵗʰ **F94**   **Disorders of social functioning with onset specific to childhood and adolescence**

F94.0   **Selective mutism**
Elective mutism
    EXCLUDES 2   *pervasive developmental disorders (F84.-)*
               schizophrenia (F20.-)
               specific developmental disorders of speech and language (F80.-)
               transient mutism as part of separation anxiety in young children (F93.0)

F94.1   **Reactive attachment disorder of childhood**
Use additional code to identify any associated failure to thrive or growth retardation
    EXCLUDES 1   *disinhibited attachment disorder of childhood (F94.2)*
               normal variation in pattern of selective attachment
    EXCLUDES 2   *Asperger's syndrome (F84.5)*
               maltreatment syndromes (T74.-)
               sexual or physical abuse in childhood, resulting in psychosocial problems (Z62.81-)

F94.2   **Disinhibited attachment disorder of childhood**
Affectionless psychopathy
Institutional syndrome
    EXCLUDES 1   *reactive attachment disorder of childhood (F94.1)*
    EXCLUDES 2   *Asperger's syndrome (F84.5)*
               attention-deficit hyperactivity disorders (F90.-)
               hospitalism in children (F43.2-)

F94.8   **Other childhood disorders of social functioning**

✓**F94.9**   **Childhood disorder of social functioning, unspecified**

✓4ᵗʰ **F95**   **Tic disorder**

F95.0   **Transient tic disorder**
Provisional tic disorder

F95.1   **Chronic motor or vocal tic disorder**

F95.2   **Tourette's disorder**
Combined vocal and multiple motor tic disorder [de la Tourette]
Tourette's syndrome

F95.8   **Other tic disorders**

✓**F95.9**   **Tic disorder, unspecified**
Tic NOS

✓4ᵗʰ **F98**   **Other behavioral and emotional disorders with onset usually occurring in childhood and adolescence**
    EXCLUDES 2   *breath-holding spells (R06.89)*
               gender identity disorder of childhood (F64.2)
               Kleine-Levin syndrome (G47.13)
               obsessive-compulsive disorder ▶*(F42.-)*◀
               sleep disorders not due to a substance or known physiological condition (F51.-)

F98.0   **Enuresis not due to a substance or known physiological condition**
Enuresis (primary) (secondary) of nonorganic origin
Functional enuresis
Psychogenic enuresis
Urinary incontinence of nonorganic origin
    EXCLUDES 1   *enuresis NOS (R32)*

F98.1   **Encopresis not due to a substance or known physiological condition**
Functional encopresis
Incontinence of feces of nonorganic origin
Psychogenic encopresis
Use additional code to identify the cause of any coexisting constipation
    EXCLUDES 1   *encopresis NOS (R15.-)*

✓5ᵗʰ **F98.2**   **Other feeding disorders of infancy and childhood**
    EXCLUDES 1   *feeding difficulties (R63.3)*
    EXCLUDES 2   *anorexia nervosa and other eating disorders (F50.-)*
               feeding problems of newborn (P92.-)
               pica of infancy or childhood (F98.3)

   F98.21   **Rumination disorder of infancy**
   F98.29   **Other feeding disorders of infancy and early childhood**

F98.3   **Pica of infancy and childhood**

F98.4   **Stereotyped movement disorders**
Stereotype/habit disorder
    EXCLUDES 1   *abnormal involuntary movements (R25.-)*
    EXCLUDES 2   *compulsions in obsessive-compulsive disorder* ▶*(F42.-)*◀
               hair plucking (F63.3)
               movement disorders of organic origin (G20-G25)
               nail-biting (F98.8)
               nose-picking (F98.8)
               stereotypies that are part of a broader psychiatric condition (F01-F95)
               thumb-sucking (F98.8)
               tic disorders (F95.-)
               trichotillomania (F63.3)

F98.5   **Adult onset fluency disorder**
    EXCLUDES 1   *childhood onset fluency disorder (F80.81)*
               dysphasia (R47.02)
               fluency disorder in conditions classified elsewhere (R47.82)
               fluency disorder (stuttering) following cerebrovascular disease (I69. with final characters -23)
               tic disorders (F95.-)

F98.8   **Other specified behavioral and emotional disorders with onset usually occurring in childhood and adolescence**
Excessive masturbation
Nail-biting
Nose-picking
Thumb-sucking

✓**F98.9**   **Unspecified behavioral and emotional disorders with onset usually occurring in childhood and adolescence**

Unspecified mental disorder (F99)

F99   **Mental disorder, not otherwise specified**
Mental illness NOS
    EXCLUDES 1   *unspecified mental disorder due to known physiological condition (F09)*

Chapter 6. Diseases of the Nervous System (GØØ-G99)

Chapter-specific Guidelines with Coding Examples

The chapter-specific guidelines from the ICD-10-CM Official Guidelines for Coding and Reporting have been provided below. Along with these guidelines are coding examples, contained in the shaded boxes, that have been developed to help illustrate the coding and/or sequencing guidance found in these guidelines.

a. Dominant/nondominant side

Codes from category G81, Hemiplegia and hemiparesis, and subcategories G83.1, Monoplegia of lower limb, G83.2, Monoplegia of upper limb, and G83.3, Monoplegia, unspecified, identify whether the dominant or nondominant side is affected. Should the affected side be documented, but not specified as dominant or nondominant, and the classification system does not indicate a default, code selection is as follows:

- For ambidextrous patients, the default should be dominant.
- If the left side is affected, the default is non-dominant.
- If the right side is affected, the default is dominant.

> Hemiplegia affecting left side of ambidextrous patient
>
> **G81.92   Hemiplegia, unspecified affecting left dominant side**
>
> *Explanation*: Documentation states that the left side is affected and dominant is used for ambidextrous persons.

> Right spastic hemiplegia, unknown whether patient is right- or left-handed
>
> **G81.11   Spastic hemiplegia affecting right dominant side**
>
> *Explanation*: Since it is unknown whether the patient is right- or left-handed, if the right side is affected, the default is dominant.

b. Pain—category G89

1) General coding information

Codes in category G89, Pain, not elsewhere classified, may be used in conjunction with codes from other categories and chapters to provide more detail about acute or chronic pain and neoplasm-related pain, unless otherwise indicated below.

If the pain is not specified as acute or chronic, post-thoracotomy, postprocedural, or neoplasm-related, do not assign codes from category G89.

A code from category G89 should not be assigned if the underlying (definitive) diagnosis is known, unless the reason for the encounter is pain control/ management and not management of the underlying condition.

When an admission or encounter is for a procedure aimed at treating the underlying condition (e.g., spinal fusion, kyphoplasty), a code for the underlying condition (e.g., vertebral fracture, spinal stenosis) should be assigned as the principal diagnosis. No code from category G89 should be assigned.

> Elderly patient with back pain is admitted for kyphoplasty for age-related osteopathic compression fracture at vertebra T3
>
> **M8Ø.Ø8XA   Age-related osteoporosis with current pathological fracture, vertebra(e), initial encounter for fracture**
>
> *Explanation*: No code is assigned for the pain as it is inherent in the underlying condition being treated.

(a) Category G89 codes as principal or first-listed diagnosis

Category G89 codes are acceptable as principal diagnosis or the first-listed code:

- When pain control or pain management is the reason for the admission/encounter (e.g., a patient with displaced intervertebral disc, nerve impingement and severe back pain presents for injection of steroid into the spinal canal). The underlying cause of the pain should be reported as an additional diagnosis, if known.

- When a patient is admitted for the insertion of a neurostimulator for pain control, assign the appropriate pain code as the principal or first-listed diagnosis. When an admission or encounter is for a procedure aimed at treating the underlying condition and a neurostimulator is inserted for pain control during the same admission/encounter, a code for the underlying condition should be assigned as the principal diagnosis and the appropriate pain code should be assigned as a secondary diagnosis.

> Patient with chronic pain from lumbar spondylosis with radiculopathy not relieved by surgery is admitted for insertion of neurostimulator.
>
> **G89.29   Other chronic pain**
>
> **M47.26   Other spondylosis with radiculopathy, lumbar region**
>
> *Explanation*: Since the patient is admitted specifically for a neurostimulator implantation for pain management and not to treat the underlying spondylosis, the chronic pain code is sequenced first, followed by the underlying condition. Neither code M54.16 nor M54.5 is necessary because M47.26 describes the radiculopathy and the site.

(b) Use of category G89 codes in conjunction with site specific pain codes

(i) Assigning category G89 and site-specific pain codes

Codes from category G89 may be used in conjunction with codes that identify the site of pain (including codes from chapter 18) if the category G89 code provides additional information. For example, if the code describes the site of the pain, but does not fully describe whether the pain is acute or chronic, then both codes should be assigned.

> During hospital stay, patient is seen by orthopaedics to evaluate chronic left shoulder pain.
>
> **M25.512   Pain in left shoulder**
>
> **G89.29   Other chronic pain**
>
> *Explanation*: No underlying condition has been determined yet so the pain would be the reason for the visit. The M25 code in this instance does not fully describe the condition as it does not represent that the pain is chronic. The G89 chronic pain code is assigned to provide specificity.

(ii) Sequencing of category G89 codes with site-specific pain codes

The sequencing of category G89 codes with site-specific pain codes (including chapter 18 codes), is dependent on the circumstances of the encounter/admission as follows:

- If the encounter is for pain control or pain management, assign the code from category G89 followed by the code identifying the specific site of pain (e.g., encounter for pain management for acute neck pain from trauma is assigned code G89.11, Acute pain due to trauma, followed by code M54.2, Cervicalgia, to identify the site of pain).

> Management of acute, traumatic right knee pain
>
> **G89.11   Acute pain due to trauma**
>
> **M25.561   Pain in right knee**
>
> *Explanation*: The reason for the encounter is to manage or control the pain, not to treat or evaluate an underlying condition. The G89 pain code is assigned as the principal diagnosis but in this instance does not fully describe the condition as it does not include the site and laterality. The M25 pain code is added to provide this information.

- If the encounter is for any other reason except pain control or pain management, and a related definitive diagnosis has not been established (confirmed) by the provider, assign the code for the specific site of pain first, followed by the appropriate code from category G89.

> Tests are performed to investigate the source of the patient's chronic epigastric abdominal pain
>
> **R1Ø.13   Epigastric pain**
>
> **G89.29   Other chronic pain**
>
> *Explanation*: In this instance the patient's epigastric pain is not being treated; rather the source of the pain is being investigated. A code from chapter 18 for epigastric pain is sequenced before the additional specificity of the G89 code for the chronic pain.

2) Pain due to devices, implants and grafts
See Section I.C.19. Pain due to medical devices

3) Postoperative pain
The provider's documentation should be used to guide the coding of postoperative pain, as well as *Section III. Reporting Additional Diagnoses* and *Section IV. Diagnostic Coding and Reporting in the Outpatient Setting*.

The default for post-thoracotomy and other postoperative pain not specified as acute or chronic is the code for the acute form.

Routine or expected postoperative pain immediately after surgery should not be coded.

> Pain pump dose is increased for the patient's unexpected, extreme pain post-thoracotomy
>
> **G89.12   Acute post-thoracotomy pain**
>
> *Explanation*: When acute or chronic is not documented, default to acute. The use of "unexpected, extreme" and the increase of medication dosage indicate that the pain was more than routine or expected.

(a) Postoperative pain not associated with specific postoperative complication

Postoperative pain not associated with a specific postoperative complication is assigned to the appropriate postoperative pain code in category G89.

(b) Postoperative pain associated with specific postoperative complication

Postoperative pain associated with a specific postoperative complication (such as painful wire sutures) is assigned to the appropriate code(s) found in Chapter 19, Injury, poisoning, and certain other consequences of external causes. If appropriate, use additional code(s) from category G89 to identify acute or chronic pain (G89.18 or G89.28).

4) Chronic pain
Chronic pain is classified to subcategory G89.2. There is no time frame defining when pain becomes chronic pain. The provider's documentation should be used to guide use of these codes.

5) Neoplasm related pain
Code G89.3 is assigned to pain documented as being related, associated or due to cancer, primary or secondary malignancy, or tumor. This code is assigned regardless of whether the pain is acute or chronic.

This code may be assigned as the principal or first-listed code when the stated reason for the admission/encounter is documented as pain control/pain management. The underlying neoplasm should be reported as an additional diagnosis.

> Pain medication adjustment for chronic pain from bone metastasis
>
> **G89.3   Neoplasm related pain (acute)(chronic)**
>
> **C79.51   Secondary malignant neoplasm of bone**
>
> *Explanation*: Since the encounter was for pain medication management, the pain, rather than the neoplasm, was the reason for the encounter and is sequenced first. This "neoplasm-related pain" code includes both acute and chronic pain.

When the reason for the admission/encounter is management of the neoplasm and the pain associated with the neoplasm is also documented, code G89.3 may be assigned as an additional diagnosis. It is not necessary to assign an additional code for the site of the pain.

See Section I.C.2 for instructions on the sequencing of neoplasms for all other stated reasons for the admission/encounter (except for pain control/pain management).

> Patient with lung cancer presents with acute hip pain and is evaluated and found to have iliac bone metastasis
>
> **C79.51   Secondary malignant neoplasm of bone**
>
> **C34.9Ø   Malignant neoplasm of unspecified part of unspecified bronchus or lung**
>
> **G89.3   Neoplasm related pain (acute)(chronic)**
>
> *Explanation*: The reason for the encounter was the evaluation and diagnosis of the bone metastasis, whose code would be assigned as first-listed, followed by codes for the primary neoplasm and the pain due to the iliac bone metastasis.

6) Chronic pain syndrome
Central pain syndrome (G89.Ø) and chronic pain syndrome (G89.4) are different than the term "chronic pain," and therefore codes should only be used when the provider has specifically documented this condition.
See Section I.C.5. Pain disorders related to psychological factors

Chapter 6. Diseases of the Nervous System (G00–G99)

EXCLUDES 2   certain conditions originating in the perinatal period (P04-P96)
certain infectious and parasitic diseases (A00-B99)
complications of pregnancy, childbirth and the puerperium (O00-O9A)
congenital malformations, deformations, and chromosomal abnormalities (Q00-Q99)
endocrine, nutritional and metabolic diseases (E00-E88)
injury, poisoning and certain other consequences of external causes (S00-T88)
neoplasms (C00-D49)
symptoms, signs and abnormal clinical and laboratory findings, not elsewhere classified (R00-R94)

This chapter contains the following blocks:

G00-G09   Inflammatory diseases of the central nervous system
G10-G14   Systemic atrophies primarily affecting the central nervous system
G20-G26   Extrapyramidal and movement disorders
G30-G32   Other degenerative diseases of the nervous system
G35-G37   Demyelinating diseases of the central nervous system
G40-G47   Episodic and paroxysmal disorders
G50-G59   Nerve, nerve root and plexus disorders
G60-G65   Polyneuropathies and other disorders of the peripheral nervous system
G70-G73   Diseases of myoneural junction and muscle
G80-G83   Cerebral palsy and other paralytic syndromes
G89-G99   Other disorders of the nervous system

Inflammatory diseases of the central nervous system (G00–G09)

✓4ᵗʰ G00   Bacterial meningitis, not elsewhere classified

INCLUDES   bacterial arachnoiditis
bacterial leptomeningitis
bacterial meningitis
bacterial pachymeningitis

EXCLUDES 1   bacterial meningoencephalitis (G04.2)
bacterial meningomyelitis (G04.2)

DEF: Inflammation of meningeal layers of the brain and spinal cord due to a bacterial infection.

G00.0   Hemophilus meningitis   MCC
Meningitis due to Hemophilus influenzae

G00.1   Pneumococcal meningitis   MCC
Meningtitis due to Streptococcal pneumoniae

G00.2   Streptococcal meningitis   MCC
Use additional code to further identify organism (B95.0-B95.5)

G00.3   Staphylococcal meningitis   MCC
Use additional code to further identify organism (B95.61-B95.8)

G00.8   Other bacterial meningitis   MCC
Meningitis due to Escherichia coli
Meningitis due to Friedländer's bacillus
Meningitis due to Klebsiella
Use additional code to further identify organism (B96.-)

G00.9   Bacterial meningitis, unspecified   MCC
Meningitis due to gram-negative bacteria, unspecified
Purulent meningitis NOS
Pyogenic meningitis NOS
Suppurative meningitis NOS

G01   Meningitis in bacterial diseases classified elsewhere   MCC
Code first underlying disease

EXCLUDES 1   meningitis (in):
gonococcal (A54.81)
leptospirosis (A27.81)
listeriosis (A32.11)
Lyme disease (A69.21)
meningococcal (A39.0)
neurosyphilis (A52.13)
tuberculosis (A17.0)
meningoencephalitis and meningomyelitis in bacterial diseases classified elsewhere (G05)

G02   Meningitis in other infectious and parasitic diseases classified elsewhere   MCC
Code first underlying disease, such as:
African trypanosomiasis (B56.-)
poliovirus infection (A80.-)

EXCLUDES 1   candidal meningitis (B37.5)
coccidioidomycosis meningitis (B38.4)
cryptococcal meningitis (B45.1)
herpesviral [herpes simplex] meningitis (B00.3)
infectious mononucleosis complicated by meningitis (B27.- with fourth character 2)
measles complicated by meningitis (B05.1)
meningoencephalitis and meningomyelitis in other infectious and parasitic diseases classified elsewhere (G05)
mumps meningitis (B26.1)
rubella meningitis (B06.02)
varicella [chickenpox] meningitis (B01.0)
zoster meningitis (B02.1)

✓4ᵗʰ G03   Meningitis due to other and unspecified causes

INCLUDES   arachnoiditis NOS
leptomeningitis NOS
meningitis NOS
pachymeningitis NOS

EXCLUDES 1   meningoencephalitis (G04.-)
meningomyelitis (G04.-)

G03.0   Nonpyogenic meningitis   MCC
Aseptic meningitis
Nonbacterial meningitis
DEF: Type of meningitis where no bacterial, viral, or other infectious source exists that explains the meningitis symptomology.

G03.1   Chronic meningitis   CC

G03.2   Benign recurrent meningitis [Mollaret]   CC
DEF: Aseptic or noninfectious inflammation of the meninges with the presence of Mollaret cells in the spinal fluid. The patient experiences recurrent bouts of inflammation, lasting anywhere from two to five days.

G03.8   Meningitis due to other specified causes   MCC

G03.9   Meningitis, unspecified   MCC
Arachnoiditis (spinal) NOS

✓4ᵗʰ G04   Encephalitis, myelitis and encephalomyelitis

INCLUDES   acute ascending myelitis
meningoencephalitis
meningomyelitis

EXCLUDES 1   encephalopathy NOS (G93.40)

EXCLUDES 2   acute transverse myelitis (G37.3-)
alcoholic encephalopathy (G31.2)
benign myalgic encephalomyelitis (G93.3)
multiple sclerosis (G35)
subacute necrotizing myelitis (G37.4)
toxic encephalitis (G92)
toxic encephalopathy (G92)

DEF: Encephalitis: Inflammation of the brain, often caused by viral or bacterial infection.
DEF: Encephalomyelitis: Inflammatory disease, often viral in nature, that affects the brain and spinal cord.
DEF: Myelitis: Inflammation of the spinal cord.

✓5ᵗʰ G04.0   Acute disseminated encephalitis and encephalomyelitis (ADEM)

EXCLUDES 1   acute necrotizing hemorrhagic encephalopathy (G04.3-)
other noninfectious acute disseminated encephalomyelitis (noninfectious ADEM) (G04.81)

G04.00   Acute disseminated encephalitis and encephalomyelitis, unspecified   MCC

G04.01   Postinfectious acute disseminated encephalitis and encephalomyelitis (postinfectious ADEM)   MCC

EXCLUDES 1   post chickenpox encephalitis (B01.1)
post measles encephalitis (B05.0)
post measles myelitis (B05.1)

✔ Additional Character Required   ✓x7ᵗʰ Placeholder   Unacceptable PDx   Questionable PDx   Manifestation   Unspecified Dx   H1-H14 HAC   HCC CMS-HCC Dx   HIV HIV Dx

ICD-10-CM 2021   571

Chapter 6. Diseases of the Nervous System

G04.02   **Postimmunization acute disseminated encephalitis, myelitis and encephalomyelitis**   `MCC`
Encephalitis, post immunization
Encephalomyelitis, post immunization
Use additional code to identify the vaccine (T50.A-, T50.B-, T50.Z-)

G04.1   **Tropical spastic paraplegia**   `CC` `HCC`

G04.2   **Bacterial meningoencephalitis and meningomyelitis, not elsewhere classified**   `MCC`

✓5ᵗʰ **G04.3**   **Acute necrotizing hemorrhagic encephalopathy**
> **EXCLUDES 1**   *acute disseminated encephalitis and encephalomyelitis (G04.0-)*

   G04.30   **Acute necrotizing hemorrhagic encephalopathy, unspecified**   `MCC`

   G04.31   **Postinfectious acute necrotizing hemorrhagic encephalopathy**   `MCC`

   G04.32   **Postimmunization acute necrotizing hemorrhagic encephalopathy**   `MCC`
Use additional code to identify the vaccine (T50.A-, T50.B-, T50.Z-)

   G04.39   **Other acute necrotizing hemorrhagic encephalopathy**   `MCC`
Code also underlying etiology, if applicable

✓5ᵗʰ **G04.8**   **Other encephalitis, myelitis and encephalomyelitis**
Code also any associated seizure (G40.-, R56.9)

   G04.81   **Other encephalitis and encephalomyelitis**   `HIV` `MCC`
Noninfectious acute disseminated encephalomyelitis (noninfectious ADEM)

   G04.89   **Other myelitis**   `HIV` `MCC` `HCC`
AHA: 2020,1Q,14
TIP: Report for acute flaccid myelitis.

✓5ᵗʰ **G04.9**   **Encephalitis, myelitis and encephalomyelitis, unspecified**

   G04.90   **Encephalitis and encephalomyelitis, unspecified**   `HIV` `MCC`
Ventriculitis (cerebral) NOS

   G04.91   **Myelitis, unspecified**   `HIV` `MCC` `HCC`

✓4ᵗʰ **G05**   **Encephalitis, myelitis and encephalomyelitis in diseases classified elsewhere**
Code first underlying disease, such as:
human immunodeficiency virus [HIV] disease (B20)
poliovirus (A80.-)
suppurative otitis media (H66.01-H66.4)
trichinellosis (B75)
> **EXCLUDES 1**   *adenoviral encephalitis, myelitis and encephalomyelitis (A85.1)*
> *congenital toxoplasmosis encephalitis, myelitis and encephalomyelitis (P37.1)*
> *cytomegaloviral encephalitis, myelitis and encephalomyelitis (B25.8)*
> *encephalitis, myelitis and encephalomyelitis (in) measles (B05.0)*
> *encephalitis, myelitis and encephalomyelitis (in) systemic lupus erythematosus (M32.19)*
> *enteroviral encephalitis, myelitis and encephalomyelitis (A85.0)*
> *eosinophilic meningoencephalitis (B83.2)*
> *herpesviral [herpes simplex] encephalitis, myelitis and encephalomyelitis (B00.4)*
> *listerial encephalitis, myelitis and encephalomyelitis (A32.12)*
> *meningococcal encephalitis, myelitis and encephalomyelitis (A39.81)*
> *mumps encephalitis, myelitis and encephalomyelitis (B26.2)*
> *postchickenpox encephalitis, myelitis and encephalomyelitis (B01.1-)*
> *rubella encephalitis, myelitis and encephalomyelitis (B06.01)*
> *toxoplasmosis encephalitis, myelitis and encephalomyelitis (B58.2)*
> *zoster encephalitis, myelitis and encephalomyelitis (B02.0)*

   G05.3   *Encephalitis and encephalomyelitis in diseases classified elsewhere*   `MCC`
Meningoencephalitis in diseases classified elsewhere

   G05.4   *Myelitis in diseases classified elsewhere*   `MCC` `HCC`
Meningomyelitis in diseases classified elsewhere

✓4ᵗʰ **G06**   **Intracranial and intraspinal abscess and granuloma**
Use additional code (B95-B97) to identify infectious agent
DEF: Abscess: Circumscribed collection of pus resulting from bacteria, frequently associated with swelling and other signs of inflammation.
DEF: Granuloma: Abnormal, dense collections or cells forming a mass or nodule of chronically inflamed tissue with granulations that is usually associated with an infective process.

   G06.0   **Intracranial abscess and granuloma**   `MCC`
Brain [any part] abscess (embolic)
Cerebellar abscess (embolic)
Cerebral abscess (embolic)
Intracranial epidural abscess or granuloma
Intracranial extradural abscess or granuloma
Intracranial subdural abscess or granuloma
Otogenic abscess (embolic)
> **EXCLUDES 1**   *tuberculous intracranial abscess and granuloma (A17.81)*

   G06.1   **Intraspinal abscess and granuloma**   `MCC`
Abscess (embolic) of spinal cord [any part]
Intraspinal epidural abscess or granuloma
Intraspinal extradural abscess or granuloma
Intraspinal subdural abscess or granuloma
> **EXCLUDES 1**   *tuberculous intraspinal abscess and granuloma (A17.81)*

   G06.2   **Extradural and subdural abscess, unspecified**   `MCC`

G07   *Intracranial and intraspinal abscess and granuloma in diseases classified elsewhere*   `MCC`
Code first underlying disease, such as:
schistosomiasis granuloma of brain (B65.-)
> **EXCLUDES 1**   *abscess of brain:*
>   *amebic (A06.6)*
>   *chromomycotic (B43.1)*
>   *gonococcal (A54.82)*
>   *tuberculous (A17.81)*
>   *tuberculoma of meninges (A17.1)*

G08   **Intracranial and intraspinal phlebitis and thrombophlebitis**   `MCC`
Septic embolism of intracranial or intraspinal venous sinuses and veins
Septic endophlebitis of intracranial or intraspinal venous sinuses and veins
Septic phlebitis of intracranial or intraspinal venous sinuses and veins
Septic thrombophlebitis of intracranial or intraspinal venous sinuses and veins
Septic thrombosis of intracranial or intraspinal venous sinuses and veins
> **EXCLUDES 1**   *intracranial phlebitis and thrombophlebitis complicating:*
> *abortion, ectopic or molar pregnancy (O00-O07, O08.7)*
> *pregnancy, childbirth and the puerperium (O22.5, O87.3)*
> *nonpyogenic intracranial phlebitis and thrombophlebitis (I67.6)*
> **EXCLUDES 2**   *intracranial phlebitis and thrombophlebitis complicating*
> *nonpyogenic intraspinal phlebitis and thrombophlebitis (G95.1)*

DEF: Inflammation and formation of a blood clot in a vein within the brain or spine, or their linings.

G09   **Sequelae of inflammatory diseases of central nervous system**
   `NOTE`   Category G09 is to be used to indicate conditions whose primary classification is to G00-G08 as the cause of sequelae, themselves classifiable elsewhere. The "sequelae" include conditions specified as residuals.
Code first condition resulting from (sequela) of inflammatory diseases of central nervous system

Systemic atrophies primarily affecting the central nervous system (G10-G14)

G10   **Huntington's disease**   `CC` `HCC`
Huntington's chorea
Huntington's dementia
Code also dementia in other diseases classified elsewhere without behavioral disturbance (F02.80)
DEF: Genetic disease caused by degeneration of nerve cells in the brain, characterized by chronic progressive mental deterioration. Dementia and death occur within 15 to 20 years of onset.

N Newborn: 0   P Pediatric: 0-17   M Maternity: 9-64   A Adult: 15-124   `MCC` Major Complication/Comorbidity   `CC` Complication/Comorbidity   `SW` Severe Wound Dx

572   ICD-10-CM 2021

G11 Hereditary ataxia

EXCLUDES 2   cerebral palsy (G80.-)
hereditary and idiopathic neuropathy (G60.-)
metabolic disorders (E70-E88)

DEF: Ataxia: Defect in muscular control or coordination due to a central nervous system disorder, particularly when voluntary muscular movements are attempted.

G11.0 Congenital nonprogressive ataxia   CC HCC

G11.1 Early-onset cerebellar ataxia   ✓5ᵗʰ

~~Early-onset cerebellar ataxia with essential tremor~~
~~Early-onset cerebellar ataxia with myoclonus [Hunt's ataxia]~~
~~Early-onset cerebellar ataxia with retained tendon reflexes~~
~~Friedreich's ataxia (autosomal recessive)~~
~~X-linked recessive spinocerebellar ataxia~~

G11.10 Early-onset cerebellar ataxia, unspecified   CC

G11.11 Friedreich ataxia   CC
Autosomal recessive Friedreich ataxia
Friedreich ataxia with retained reflexes

G11.19 Other early-onset cerebellar ataxia   CC
Early-onset cerebellar ataxia with essential tremor
Early-onset cerebellar ataxia with myoclonus [Hunt's ataxia]
Early-onset cerebellar ataxia with retained tendon reflexes
X-linked recessive spinocerebellar ataxia

G11.2 Late-onset cerebellar ataxia   CC HCC A

G11.3 Cerebellar ataxia with defective DNA repair   CC HCC
Ataxia telangiectasia [Louis-Bar]
EXCLUDES 2   Cockayne's syndrome (Q87.19)
other disorders of purine and pyrimidine metabolism (E79.-)
xeroderma pigmentosum (Q82.1)

G11.4 Hereditary spastic paraplegia   CC HCC

G11.8 Other hereditary ataxias   CC HCC

G11.9 Hereditary ataxia, unspecified   CC HCC
Hereditary cerebellar ataxia NOS
Hereditary cerebellar degeneration
Hereditary cerebellar disease
Hereditary cerebellar syndrome

G12 Spinal muscular atrophy and related syndromes   ✓4ᵗʰ

G12.0 Infantile spinal muscular atrophy, type I [Werdnig-Hoffman]   CC HCC

G12.1 Other inherited spinal muscular atrophy   CC HCC
Adult form spinal muscular atrophy
Childhood form, type II spinal muscular atrophy
Distal spinal muscular atrophy
Juvenile form, type III spinal muscular atrophy [Kugelberg-Welander]
Progressive bulbar palsy of childhood [Fazio-Londe]
Scapuloperoneal form spinal muscular atrophy

G12.2 Motor neuron disease   ✓5ᵗʰ
AHA: 2017,4Q,9-10

G12.20 Motor neuron disease, unspecified   CC HCC
G12.21 Amyotrophic lateral sclerosis   CC HCC A
G12.22 Progressive bulbar palsy   CC HCC
G12.23 Primary lateral sclerosis   CC HCC
G12.24 Familial motor neuron disease   CC HCC
G12.25 Progressive spinal muscle atrophy   CC HCC
G12.29 Other motor neuron disease   CC HCC

G12.8 Other spinal muscular atrophies and related syndromes   CC HCC

G12.9 Spinal muscular atrophy, unspecified   CC HCC

G13 Systemic atrophies primarily affecting central nervous system in diseases classified elsewhere   ✓4ᵗʰ

G13.0 Paraneoplastic neuromyopathy and neuropathy   HCC
Carcinomatous neuromyopathy
Sensorial paraneoplastic neuropathy [Denny Brown]
Code first underlying neoplasm (C00-D49)

G13.1 Other systemic atrophy primarily affecting central nervous system in neoplastic disease   HCC
Paraneoplastic limbic encephalopathy
Code first underlying neoplasm (C00-D49)

G13.2 Systemic atrophy primarily affecting the central nervous system in myxedema   HCC
Code first underlying disease, such as:
hypothyroidism (E03.-)
myxedematous congenital iodine deficiency (E00.1)

G13.8 Systemic atrophy primarily affecting central nervous system in other diseases classified elsewhere   HCC
Code first underlying disease

G14 Postpolio syndrome

INCLUDES   postpolio myelitic syndrome
EXCLUDES 1   sequelae of poliomyelitis (B91)

Extrapyramidal and movement disorders (G20-G26)

G20 Parkinson's disease   HCC
Hemiparkinsonism
Idiopathic Parkinsonism or Parkinson's disease
Paralysis agitans
Parkinsonism or Parkinson's disease NOS
Primary Parkinsonism or Parkinson's disease
▶Use additional code to identify:◀
▶dementia with behavioral disturbance (F02.81)◀
▶dementia without behavioral disturbance (F02.80)◀
EXCLUDES 1   dementia with Parkinsonism (G31.83)
AHA: 2017,2Q,7; 2016,2Q,6
TIP: Repeated falls (R29.6) are not integral to Parkinson's disease and can be separately coded.

G21 Secondary parkinsonism   ✓4ᵗʰ

EXCLUDES 1   dementia with Parkinsonism (G31.83)
Huntington's disease (G10)
Shy-Drager syndrome (G90.3)
syphilitic Parkinsonism (A52.19)

G21.0 Malignant neuroleptic syndrome   MCC
Use additional code for adverse effect, if applicable, to identify drug (T43.3X5, T43.4X5, T43.505, T43.595)
EXCLUDES 1   neuroleptic induced parkinsonism (G21.11)

G21.1 Other drug-induced secondary parkinsonism   ✓5ᵗʰ

G21.11 Neuroleptic induced parkinsonism   CC HCC
Use additional code for adverse effect, if applicable, to identify drug (T43.3X5, T43.4X5, T43.505, T43.595)
EXCLUDES 1   malignant neuroleptic syndrome (G21.0)

G21.19 Other drug induced secondary parkinsonism   CC HCC
Other medication-induced parkinsonism
Use additional code for adverse effect, if applicable, to identify drug (T36-T50 with fifth or sixth character 5)

G21.2 Secondary parkinsonism due to other external agents   CC HCC
Code first (T51-T65) to identify external agent

G21.3 Postencephalitic parkinsonism   CC HCC

G21.4 Vascular parkinsonism   HCC

G21.8 Other secondary parkinsonism   CC HCC

G21.9 Secondary parkinsonism, unspecified   CC HCC

G23 Other degenerative diseases of basal ganglia   ✓4ᵗʰ

EXCLUDES 2   multi-system degeneration of the autonomic nervous system (G90.3)

G23.0 Hallervorden-Spatz disease   CC HCC
Pigmentary pallidal degeneration

G23.1 Progressive supranuclear ophthalmoplegia [Steele-Richardson-Olszewski]   CC HCC
Progressive supranuclear palsy

G23.2 Striatonigral degeneration   CC HCC

G23.8 Other specified degenerative diseases of basal ganglia   CC HCC
Calcification of basal ganglia

G23.9 Degenerative disease of basal ganglia, unspecified   CC HCC

✔ Additional Character Required   ✓x7ᵗʰ Placeholder   Unacceptable PDx   Questionable PDx   Manifestation   Unspecified Dx   H1-H14 HAC   HCC CMS-HCC Dx   HIV HIV Dx

✓4ᵗʰ **G24 Dystonia**

INCLUDES dyskinesia

EXCLUDES 2 athetoid cerebral palsy (G80.3)

DEF: Disorder of abnormal muscle tone, excessive or inadequate. Involuntary movements and prolonged muscle contractions result in tremors, abnormalities in posture, and twisting body motions that affect an isolated area or the whole body.

✓5ᵗʰ **G24.0 Drug induced dystonia**

Use additional code for adverse effect, if applicable, to identify drug (T36-T50 with fifth or sixth character 5)

G24.01 Drug induced subacute dyskinesia
Drug induced blepharospasm
Drug induced orofacial dyskinesia
Neuroleptic induced tardive dyskinesia
Tardive dyskinesia

G24.02 Drug induced acute dystonia CC
Acute dystonic reaction to drugs
Neuroleptic induced acute dystonia

G24.09 Other drug induced dystonia CC

G24.1 Genetic torsion dystonia
Dystonia deformans progressiva
Dystonia musculorum deformans
Familial torsion dystonia
Idiopathic familial dystonia
Idiopathic (torsion) dystonia NOS
(Schwalbe-) Ziehen-Oppenheim disease

G24.2 Idiopathic nonfamilial dystonia CC

G24.3 Spasmodic torticollis

EXCLUDES 1 congenital torticollis (Q68.0)
hysterical torticollis (F44.4)
ocular torticollis (R29.891)
psychogenic torticollis (F45.8)
torticollis NOS (M43.6)
traumatic recurrent torticollis (S13.4)

DEF: Twisted, unnatural position of the neck due to contracted cervical muscles that pull the head to one side or cause involuntary shaking of the head.

G24.4 Idiopathic orofacial dystonia
Orofacial dyskinesia

EXCLUDES 1 drug induced orofacial dyskinesia (G24.01)

G24.5 Blepharospasm

EXCLUDES 1 drug induced blepharospasm (G24.01)

DEF: Involuntary contraction of the orbicularis oculi muscle, resulting in the eyelids being completely closed.

G24.8 Other dystonia CC
Acquired torsion dystonia NOS

G24.9 Dystonia, unspecified
Dyskinesia NOS

✓4ᵗʰ **G25 Other extrapyramidal and movement disorders**

EXCLUDES 2 sleep related movement disorders (G47.6-)

G25.0 Essential tremor
Familial tremor

EXCLUDES 1 tremor NOS (R25.1)

G25.1 Drug-induced tremor
Use additional code for adverse effect, if applicable, to identify drug (T36-T50 with fifth or sixth character 5)

G25.2 Other specified forms of tremor
Intention tremor

G25.3 Myoclonus
Drug-induced myoclonus
Palatal myoclonus
Use additional code for adverse effect, if applicable, to identify drug (T36-T50 with fifth or sixth character 5)

EXCLUDES 1 facial myokymia (G51.4)
myoclonic epilepsy (G40.-)

DEF: Spasmodic, brief, involuntary muscle contractions that can be due to an undetermined etiology, drug-induced, or caused by a disease process.

G25.4 Drug-induced chorea
Use additional code for adverse effect, if applicable, to identify drug (T36-T50 with fifth or sixth character 5)

G25.5 Other chorea
Chorea NOS

EXCLUDES 1 chorea NOS with heart involvement (I02.0)
Huntington's chorea (G10)
rheumatic chorea (I02.-)
Sydenham's chorea (I02.-)

✓5ᵗʰ **G25.6 Drug induced tics and other tics of organic origin**

G25.61 Drug induced tics
Use additional code for adverse effect, if applicable, to identify drug (T36-T50 with fifth or sixth character 5)

G25.69 Other tics of organic origin

EXCLUDES 1 habit spasm (F95.9)
tic NOS (F95.9)
Tourette's syndrome (F95.2)

✓5ᵗʰ **G25.7 Other and unspecified drug induced movement disorders**
Use additional code for adverse effect, if applicable, to identify drug (T36-T50 with fifth or sixth character 5)

G25.70 Drug induced movement disorder, unspecified

G25.71 Drug induced akathisia
Drug induced acathisia
Neuroleptic induced acute akathisia
Tardive akathisia

G25.79 Other drug induced movement disorders

✓5ᵗʰ **G25.8 Other specified extrapyramidal and movement disorders**

G25.81 Restless legs syndrome

DEF: Neurological disorder of unknown etiology creating an irresistible urge to move the legs, which may temporarily relieve the symptoms. This syndrome is accompanied by motor restlessness and sensations of pain, burning, prickling, or tingling.

G25.82 Stiff-man syndrome CC

G25.83 Benign shuddering attacks

G25.89 Other specified extrapyramidal and movement disorders

G25.9 Extrapyramidal and movement disorder, unspecified CC

G26 Extrapyramidal and movement disorders in diseases classified elsewhere
Code first underlying disease

Other degenerative diseases of the nervous system (G30-G32)

✓4ᵗʰ **G30 Alzheimer's disease**

INCLUDES Alzheimer's dementia senile and presenile forms

Use additional code to identify:
delirium, if applicable (F05)
dementia with behavioral disturbance (F02.81)
dementia without behavioral disturbance (F02.80)

EXCLUDES 1 senile degeneration of brain NEC (G31.1)
senile dementia NOS (F03)
senility NOS (R41.81)

AHA: 2017,1Q,43

TIP: A code from subcategory F02.8 should always be assigned with a code from this category, even in the absence of documented dementia.

TIP: Functional quadriplegia (R53.2) is not integral to Alzheimer's disease and can be coded in addition to codes from category G30.

G30.0 Alzheimer's disease with early onset HCC

G30.1 Alzheimer's disease with late onset HCC A

G30.8 Other Alzheimer's disease HCC

G30.9 Alzheimer's disease, unspecified HCC

AHA: 2016,2Q,6; 2012,4Q,95

☑️4ᵗʰ **G31 Other degenerative diseases of nervous system, not elsewhere classified**

For codes G31.0–G31.83, G31.85–G31.9, use additional code to identify:
dementia with behavioral disturbance (F02.81)
dementia without behavioral disturbance (F02.80)

EXCLUDES 2   *Reye's syndrome (G93.7)*

☑️5ᵗʰ **G31.0 Frontotemporal dementia**

G31.01 Pick's disease   HCC

Primary progressive aphasia
Progressive isolated aphasia
DEF: Progressive frontotemporal dementia with asymmetrical atrophy of the frontal and temporal regions of the cerebral cortex and abnormal rounded brain cells called Pick cells with the presence of abnormal staining of protein (called tau). Symptoms include prominent apathy, behavioral changes such as disinhibition and restlessness, echolalia, impairment of language, memory, and intellect, increased carelessness, poor personal hygiene, and decreased attention span.

G31.09 Other frontotemporal dementia   HCC

Frontal dementia

G31.1 Senile degeneration of brain, not elsewhere classified   HCC

EXCLUDES 1   *Alzheimer's disease (G30.-)*
senility NOS (R41.81)

G31.2 Degeneration of nervous system due to alcohol   HCC

Alcoholic cerebellar ataxia
Alcoholic cerebellar degeneration
Alcoholic cerebral degeneration
Alcoholic encephalopathy
Dysfunction of the autonomic nervous system due to alcohol
Code also associated alcoholism (F10.-)

☑️5ᵗʰ **G31.8 Other specified degenerative diseases of nervous system**

G31.81 Alpers disease   CC HCC

Grey-matter degeneration

G31.82 Leigh's disease   CC HCC

Subacute necrotizing encephalopathy

G31.83 Dementia with Lewy bodies   HCC

Dementia with Parkinsonism
Lewy body dementia
Lewy body disease
AHA: 2017,2Q,7; 2016,4Q,141
DEF: Cerebral dementia with neurophysiologic changes, increased hippocampal volume, hypoperfusion in the occipital lobes, beta amyloid deposits with neurofibrillary tangles, and atrophy of the cortex and brainstem. Hallmark neuropsychological characteristics include fluctuating cognition with pronounced variation in attention and alertness, recurrent hallucinations, and Parkinsonism.

G31.84 Mild cognitive impairment, so stated

Mild neurocognitive disorder

EXCLUDES 1   *age related cognitive decline (R41.81)*
altered mental status (R41.82)
cerebral degeneration (G31.9)
change in mental status (R41.82)
cognitive deficits following (sequelae of) cerebral hemorrhage or infarction (I69.01-, I69.11-, I69.21-, I69.31-, I69.81-, I69.91-)
cognitive impairment due to intracranial or head injury (S06.-)
dementia (F01.-, F02.-, F03)
mild memory disturbance (F06.8)
neurologic neglect syndrome (R41.4)
personality change, nonpsychotic (F68.8)

G31.85 Corticobasal degeneration   HCC

G31.89 Other specified degenerative diseases of nervous system   HCC

G31.9 Degenerative disease of nervous system, unspecified   HCC

☑️4ᵗʰ **G32 Other degenerative disorders of nervous system in diseases classified elsewhere**

G32.0 **Subacute combined degeneration of spinal cord in diseases classified elsewhere**   CC HCC

Dana-Putnam syndrome
Sclerosis of spinal cord (combined) (dorsolateral) (posterolateral)
Code first underlying disease, such as:
anemia (D51.9)
dietary (D51.3)
pernicious (D51.0)
vitamin B12 deficiency (E53.8)

EXCLUDES 1   *syphilitic combined degeneration of spinal cord (A52.11)*

☑️5ᵗʰ **G32.8 Other specified degenerative disorders of nervous system in diseases classified elsewhere**

Code first underlying disease, such as:
amyloidosis cerebral degeneration (E85.-)
cerebral degeneration (due to) hypothyroidism (E00.0-E03.9)
cerebral degeneration (due to) neoplasm (C00-D49)
cerebral degeneration (due to) vitamin B deficiency, except thiamine (E52-E53.-)

EXCLUDES 1   *superior hemorrhagic polioencephalitis [Wernicke's encephalopathy] (E51.2)*

G32.81 **Cerebellar ataxia in diseases classified elsewhere**   CC HCC

Code first underlying disease, such as:
celiac disease (with gluten ataxia) (K90.0)
cerebellar ataxia (in) neoplastic disease (paraneoplastic cerebellar degeneration) (C00-D49)
non-celiac gluten ataxia (M35.9)

EXCLUDES 1   *systemic atrophy primarily affecting the central nervous system in alcoholic cerebellar ataxia (G31.2)*
systemic atrophy primarily affecting the central nervous system in myxedema (G13.2)

G32.89 **Other specified degenerative disorders of nervous system in diseases classified elsewhere**

Degenerative encephalopathy in diseases classified elsewhere

Demyelinating diseases of the central nervous system (G35-G37)

G35 Multiple sclerosis   HCC

Disseminated multiple sclerosis
Generalized multiple sclerosis
Multiple sclerosis NOS
Multiple sclerosis of brain stem
Multiple sclerosis of cord

☑️4ᵗʰ **G36 Other acute disseminated demyelination**

EXCLUDES 1   *postinfectious encephalitis and encephalomyelitis NOS (G04.01)*

DEF: Demyelination: Abnormal loss of myelin, the protective white matter that insulates nerve endings and facilitates neuroreception and neurotransmission. When this substance is damaged, the nerve is short-circuited, resulting in impaired or loss of function.

G36.0 Neuromyelitis optica [Devic]   CC HCC

Demyelination in optic neuritis

EXCLUDES 1   *optic neuritis NOS (H46)*

G36.1 Acute and subacute hemorrhagic leukoencephalitis [Hurst]   CC HCC

G36.8 Other specified acute disseminated demyelination   CC HCC

G36.9 Acute disseminated demyelination, unspecified   HIV CC HCC

☑️4ᵗʰ **G37 Other demyelinating diseases of central nervous system**

G37.0 Diffuse sclerosis of central nervous system   CC HCC

Periaxial encephalitis
Schilder's disease

EXCLUDES 1   *X linked adrenoleukodystrophy (E71.52-)*

G37.1 Central demyelination of corpus callosum   CC HCC

G37.2 Central pontine myelinolysis   CC HCC

☑️ Additional Character Required   ✓ₓ7ᵗʰ Placeholder   Unacceptable PDx   Questionable PDx   Manifestation   Unspecified Dx   H1 - H14 HAC   HCC CMS-HCC Dx   HIV HIV Dx

ICD-10-CM 2021   **575**

G37.3 **Acute transverse myelitis in demyelinating disease of central nervous system**   CC HCC
    Acute transverse myelitis NOS
    Acute transverse myelopathy
    EXCLUDES 1 *multiple sclerosis (G35)*
        neuromyelitis optica [Devic] (G36.0)

G37.4 **Subacute necrotizing myelitis of central nervous system**   HIV MCC HCC

G37.5 **Concentric sclerosis [Balo] of central nervous system**   CC HCC

G37.8 **Other specified demyelinating diseases of central nervous system**   CC HCC

G37.9 **Demyelinating disease of central nervous system, unspecified**   HIV CC HCC

Episodic and paroxysmal disorders (G40-G47)

✓4th **G40 Epilepsy and recurrent seizures**

    NOTE The following terms are to be considered equivalent to intractable: pharmacoresistant (pharmacologically resistant), treatment resistant, refractory (medically) and poorly controlled

    EXCLUDES 1 *conversion disorder with seizures (F44.5)*
        convulsions NOS (R56.9)
        post traumatic seizures (R56.1)
        seizure (convulsive) NOS (R56.9)
        seizure of newborn (P90)
    EXCLUDES 2 *hippocampal sclerosis (G93.81)*
        mesial temporal sclerosis (G93.81)
        temporal sclerosis (G93.81)
        Todd's paralysis (G83.84)

✓5th **G40.0 Localization-related (focal) (partial) idiopathic epilepsy and epileptic syndromes with seizures of localized onset**
    Benign childhood epilepsy with centrotemporal EEG spikes
    Childhood epilepsy with occipital EEG paroxysms
    EXCLUDES 1 *adult onset localization-related epilepsy (G40.1-, G40.2-)*

    ✓6th **G40.00 Localization-related (focal) (partial) idiopathic epilepsy and epileptic syndromes with seizures of localized onset, not intractable**
        Localization-related (focal) (partial) idiopathic epilepsy and epileptic syndromes with seizures of localized onset without intractability

        G40.001 Localization-related (focal) (partial) idiopathic epilepsy and epileptic syndromes with seizures of localized onset, not intractable, with status epilepticus   CC HCC

        G40.009 Localization-related (focal) (partial) idiopathic epilepsy and epileptic syndromes with seizures of localized onset, not intractable, without status epilepticus   CC HCC
          Localization-related (focal) (partial) idiopathic epilepsy and epileptic syndromes with seizures of localized onset NOS

    ✓6th **G40.01 Localization-related (focal) (partial) idiopathic epilepsy and epileptic syndromes with seizures of localized onset, intractable**
        G40.011 Localization-related (focal) (partial) idiopathic epilepsy and epileptic syndromes with seizures of localized onset, intractable, with status epilepticus   CC HCC

        G40.019 Localization-related (focal) (partial) idiopathic epilepsy and epileptic syndromes with seizures of localized onset, intractable, without status epilepticus   CC HCC

✓5th **G40.1 Localization-related (focal) (partial) symptomatic epilepsy and epileptic syndromes with simple partial seizures**
    Attacks without alteration of consciousness
    Epilepsia partialis continua [Kozhevnikof]
    Simple partial seizures developing into secondarily generalized seizures

    ✓6th **G40.10 Localization-related (focal) (partial) symptomatic epilepsy and epileptic syndromes with simple partial seizures, not intractable**
        Localization-related (focal) (partial) symptomatic epilepsy and epileptic syndromes with simple partial seizures without intractability

        G40.101 Localization-related (focal) (partial) symptomatic epilepsy and epileptic syndromes with simple partial seizures, not intractable, with status epilepticus   CC HCC

        G40.109 Localization-related (focal) (partial) symptomatic epilepsy and epileptic syndromes with simple partial seizures, not intractable, without status epilepticus   CC HCC
          Localization-related (focal) (partial) symptomatic epilepsy and epileptic syndromes with simple partial seizures NOS

    ✓6th **G40.11 Localization-related (focal) (partial) symptomatic epilepsy and epileptic syndromes with simple partial seizures, intractable**
        G40.111 Localization-related (focal) (partial) symptomatic epilepsy and epileptic syndromes with simple partial seizures, intractable, with status epilepticus   CC HCC

        G40.119 Localization-related (focal) (partial) symptomatic epilepsy and epileptic syndromes with simple partial seizures, intractable, without status epilepticus   CC HCC

✓5th **G40.2 Localization-related (focal) (partial) symptomatic epilepsy and epileptic syndromes with complex partial seizures**
    Attacks with alteration of consciousness, often with automatisms
    Complex partial seizures developing into secondarily generalized seizures

    ✓6th **G40.20 Localization-related (focal) (partial) symptomatic epilepsy and epileptic syndromes with complex partial seizures, not intractable**
        Localization-related (focal) (partial) symptomatic epilepsy and epileptic syndromes with complex partial seizures without intractability

        G40.201 Localization-related (focal) (partial) symptomatic epilepsy and epileptic syndromes with complex partial seizures, not intractable, with status epilepticus   CC HCC

        G40.209 Localization-related (focal) (partial) symptomatic epilepsy and epileptic syndromes with complex partial seizures, not intractable, without status epilepticus   CC HCC
          Localization-related (focal) (partial) symptomatic epilepsy and epileptic syndromes with complex partial seizures NOS

    ✓6th **G40.21 Localization-related (focal) (partial) symptomatic epilepsy and epileptic syndromes with complex partial seizures, intractable**
        G40.211 Localization-related (focal) (partial) symptomatic epilepsy and epileptic syndromes with complex partial seizures, intractable, with status epilepticus   CC HCC

        G40.219 Localization-related (focal) (partial) symptomatic epilepsy and epileptic syndromes with complex partial seizures, intractable, without status epilepticus   CC HCC

✓5ᵗʰ **G40.3** Generalized idiopathic epilepsy and epileptic syndromes
Code also MERRF syndrome, if applicable (E88.42)

✓6ᵗʰ **G40.30** Generalized idiopathic epilepsy and epileptic syndromes, not intractable
Generalized idiopathic epilepsy and epileptic syndromes without intractability

G40.301 Generalized idiopathic epilepsy and epileptic syndromes, not intractable, with status epilepticus `MCC` `HCC`

G40.309 Generalized idiopathic epilepsy and epileptic syndromes, not intractable, without status epilepticus `HCC`
Generalized idiopathic epilepsy and epileptic syndromes NOS

✓6ᵗʰ **G40.31** Generalized idiopathic epilepsy and epileptic syndromes, intractable

G40.311 Generalized idiopathic epilepsy and epileptic syndromes, intractable, with status epilepticus `MCC` `HCC`

G40.319 Generalized idiopathic epilepsy and epileptic syndromes, intractable, without status epilepticus `MCC` `HCC`

✓5ᵗʰ **G40.A** Absence epileptic syndrome
Childhood absence epilepsy [pyknolepsy]
Juvenile absence epilepsy
Absence epileptic syndrome, NOS

✓6ᵗʰ **G40.A0** Absence epileptic syndrome, not intractable

G40.A01 Absence epileptic syndrome, not intractable, with status epilepticus `HCC`

G40.A09 Absence epileptic syndrome, not intractable, without status epilepticus `HCC`

✓6ᵗʰ **G40.A1** Absence epileptic syndrome, intractable

G40.A11 Absence epileptic syndrome, intractable, with status epilepticus `CC` `HCC`

G40.A19 Absence epileptic syndrome, intractable, without status epilepticus `CC` `HCC`

✓5ᵗʰ **G40.B** Juvenile myoclonic epilepsy [impulsive petit mal]

✓6ᵗʰ **G40.B0** Juvenile myoclonic epilepsy, not intractable

G40.B01 Juvenile myoclonic epilepsy, not intractable, with status epilepticus `CC` `HCC`

G40.B09 Juvenile myoclonic epilepsy, not intractable, without status epilepticus `CC` `HCC`

✓6ᵗʰ **G40.B1** Juvenile myoclonic epilepsy, intractable

G40.B11 Juvenile myoclonic epilepsy, intractable, with status epilepticus `CC` `HCC`

G40.B19 Juvenile myoclonic epilepsy, intractable, without status epilepticus `CC` `HCC`

✓5ᵗʰ **G40.4** Other generalized epilepsy and epileptic syndromes
Epilepsy with grand mal seizures on awakening
Epilepsy with myoclonic absences
Epilepsy with myoclonic-astatic seizures
Grand mal seizure NOS
Nonspecific atonic epileptic seizures
Nonspecific clonic epileptic seizures
Nonspecific myoclonic epileptic seizures
Nonspecific tonic epileptic seizures
Nonspecific tonic-clonic epileptic seizures
Symptomatic early myoclonic encephalopathy

✓6ᵗʰ **G40.40** Other generalized epilepsy and epileptic syndromes, not intractable
Other generalized epilepsy and epileptic syndromes without intractability
Other generalized epilepsy and epileptic syndromes NOS

G40.401 Other generalized epilepsy and epileptic syndromes, not intractable, with status epilepticus `HCC`

G40.409 Other generalized epilepsy and epileptic syndromes, not intractable, without status epilepticus `HCC`

✓6ᵗʰ **G40.41** Other generalized epilepsy and epileptic syndromes, intractable

G40.411 Other generalized epilepsy and epileptic syndromes, intractable, with status epilepticus `CC` `HCC`

G40.419 Other generalized epilepsy and epileptic syndromes, intractable, without status epilepticus `CC` `HCC`

● **G40.42** Cyclin-Dependent Kinase-Like 5 Deficiency Disorder
CDKL5
Use additional code, if known, to identify associated manifestations, such as:
cortical blindness (H47.61-)
global development delay (F88)

✓5ᵗʰ **G40.5** Epileptic seizures related to external causes
Epileptic seizures related to alcohol
Epileptic seizures related to drugs
Epileptic seizures related to hormonal changes
Epileptic seizures related to sleep deprivation
Epileptic seizures related to stress
Code also, if applicable, associated epilepsy and recurrent seizures (G40.-)
Use additional code for adverse effect, if applicable, to identify drug (T36-T50 with fifth or sixth character 5)

✓6ᵗʰ **G40.50** Epileptic seizures related to external causes, not intractable

G40.501 Epileptic seizures related to external causes, not intractable, with status epilepticus `CC` `HCC`

G40.509 Epileptic seizures related to external causes, not intractable, without status epilepticus `CC` `HCC`
Epileptic seizures related to external causes, NOS

✓5ᵗʰ **G40.8** Other epilepsy and recurrent seizures
Epilepsies and epileptic syndromes undetermined as to whether they are focal or generalized
Landau-Kleffner syndrome

✓6ᵗʰ **G40.80** Other epilepsy

G40.801 Other epilepsy, not intractable, with status epilepticus `CC` `HCC`
Other epilepsy without intractability with status epilepticus

G40.802 Other epilepsy, not intractable, without status epilepticus `CC` `HCC`
Other epilepsy NOS
Other epilepsy without intractability without status epilepticus

G40.803 Other epilepsy, intractable, with status epilepticus `CC` `HCC`

G40.804 Other epilepsy, intractable, without status epilepticus `CC` `HCC`

✓6ᵗʰ **G40.81** Lennox-Gastaut syndrome
DEF: Severe form of epilepsy with usual onset in early childhood. Seizures are frequent and difficult to treat, causing falls and intellectual impairment.

G40.811 Lennox-Gastaut syndrome, not intractable, with status epilepticus `CC` `HCC`

G40.812 Lennox-Gastaut syndrome, not intractable, without status epilepticus `CC` `HCC`

G40.813 Lennox-Gastaut syndrome, intractable, with status epilepticus `CC` `HCC`

G40.814 Lennox-Gastaut syndrome, intractable, without status epilepticus `CC` `HCC`

✓6ᵗʰ **G40.82** Epileptic spasms
Infantile spasms
Salaam attacks
West's syndrome

G40.821 Epileptic spasms, not intractable, with status epilepticus `CC` `HCC`

G40.822 Epileptic spasms, not intractable, without status epilepticus `CC` `HCC`

G40.823 Epileptic spasms, intractable, with status epilepticus `CC` `HCC`

G40.824 Epileptic spasms, intractable, without status epilepticus `CC` `HCC`

● ✓6ᵗʰ **G40.83** Dravet syndrome
Polymorphic epilepsy in infancy (PMEI)
Severe myoclonic epilepsy in infancy (SMEI)

● **G40.833** Dravet syndrome, intractable, with status epilepticus `CC`

G40.834 **Dravet syndrome,** intractable, without status epilepticus   `CC`
     Dravet syndrome NOS

G40.89 **Other seizures**   `CC` `HCC`
     EXCLUDES 1   post traumatic seizures (R56.1)
           recurrent seizures NOS (G40.909)
           seizure NOS (R56.9)

√5ᵗʰ **G40.9** **Epilepsy, unspecified**
     AHA: 2019, 1Q, 19

     √6ᵗʰ **G40.90** **Epilepsy, unspecified,** not intractable
         Epilepsy, unspecified, without intractability
         G40.901 **Epilepsy, unspecified, not intractable, with status epilepticus**   `HCC`
         G40.909 **Epilepsy, unspecified, not intractable, without status epilepticus**   `HCC`
            Epilepsy NOS
            Epileptic convulsions NOS
            Epileptic fits NOS
            Epileptic seizures NOS
            Recurrent seizures NOS
            Seizure disorder NOS

     √6ᵗʰ **G40.91** **Epilepsy, unspecified,** intractable
         Intractable seizure disorder NOS
         G40.911 **Epilepsy, unspecified, intractable, with status epilepticus**   `CC` `HCC`
         G40.919 **Epilepsy, unspecified, intractable, without status epilepticus**   `CC` `HCC`

√4ᵗʰ **G43** **Migraine**

     NOTE   The following terms are to be considered equivalent to intractable: pharmacoresistant (pharmacologically resistant), treatment resistant, refractory (medically) and poorly controlled

     Use additional code for adverse effect, if applicable, to identify drug (T36-T50 with fifth or sixth character 5)
     EXCLUDES 1   headache NOS ▶(R51.9)◀
           lower half migraine (G44.00)
     EXCLUDES 2   headache syndromes (G44.-)
     DEF: Headaches that occur periodically on one or both sides of the head that may be associated with nausea and vomiting, sensitivity to light and sound, dizziness, distorted vision, and cognitive disturbances.

√5ᵗʰ **G43.0** **Migraine** without aura
     Common migraine
     EXCLUDES 1   chronic migraine without aura (G43.7-)

     √6ᵗʰ **G43.00** **Migraine without aura,** not intractable
         Migraine without aura without mention of refractory migraine
         G43.001 **Migraine without aura, not intractable, with status migrainosus**
         G43.009 **Migraine without aura, not intractable, without status migrainosus**
            Migraine without aura NOS

     √6ᵗʰ **G43.01** **Migraine without aura,** intractable
         Migraine without aura with refractory migraine
         G43.011 **Migraine without aura, intractable, with status migrainosus**
         G43.019 **Migraine without aura, intractable, without status migrainosus**

√5ᵗʰ **G43.1** **Migraine** with aura
     Basilar migraine
     Classical migraine
     Migraine equivalents
     Migraine preceded or accompanied by transient focal neurological phenomena
     Migraine triggered seizures
     Migraine with acute-onset aura
     Migraine with aura without headache (migraine equivalents)
     Migraine with prolonged aura
     Migraine with typical aura
     Retinal migraine
     Code also any associated seizure (G40.-, R56.9)
     EXCLUDES 1   persistent migraine aura (G43.5-, G43.6-)

     √6ᵗʰ **G43.10** **Migraine with aura,** not intractable
         Migraine with aura without mention of refractory migraine
         G43.101 **Migraine with aura, not intractable, with status migrainosus**

G43.109 **Migraine with aura, not intractable, without status migrainosus**
     Migraine with aura NOS

     √6ᵗʰ **G43.11** **Migraine with aura,** intractable
         Migraine with aura with refractory migraine
         G43.111 **Migraine with aura, intractable, with status migrainosus**
         G43.119 **Migraine with aura, intractable, without status migrainosus**

√5ᵗʰ **G43.4** **Hemiplegic migraine**
     Familial migraine
     Sporadic migraine

     √6ᵗʰ **G43.40** **Hemiplegic migraine,** not intractable
         Hemiplegic migraine without refractory migraine
         G43.401 **Hemiplegic migraine, not intractable, with status migrainosus**
         G43.409 **Hemiplegic migraine, not intractable, without status migrainosus**
            Hemiplegic migraine NOS

     √6ᵗʰ **G43.41** **Hemiplegic migraine,** intractable
         Hemiplegic migraine with refractory migraine
         G43.411 **Hemiplegic migraine, intractable, with status migrainosus**
         G43.419 **Hemiplegic migraine, intractable, without status migrainosus**

√5ᵗʰ **G43.5** **Persistent** migraine aura without cerebral infarction

     √6ᵗʰ **G43.50** **Persistent migraine aura without cerebral infarction,** not intractable
         Persistent migraine aura without cerebral infarction, without refractory migraine
         G43.501 **Persistent migraine aura without cerebral infarction, not intractable, with status migrainosus**
         G43.509 **Persistent migraine aura without cerebral infarction, not intractable, without status migrainosus**
            Persistent migraine aura NOS

     √6ᵗʰ **G43.51** **Persistent migraine aura without cerebral infarction,** intractable
         Persistent migraine aura without cerebral infarction, with refractory migraine
         G43.511 **Persistent migraine aura without cerebral infarction, intractable, with status migrainosus**
         G43.519 **Persistent migraine aura without cerebral infarction, intractable, without status migrainosus**

√5ᵗʰ **G43.6** **Persistent** migraine aura with cerebral infarction
     Code also the type of cerebral infarction (I63.-)

     √6ᵗʰ **G43.60** **Persistent migraine aura with cerebral infarction,** not intractable
         Persistent migraine aura with cerebral infarction, without refractory migraine
         G43.601 **Persistent migraine aura with cerebral infarction, not intractable, with status migrainosus**   `CC`
         G43.609 **Persistent migraine aura with cerebral infarction, not intractable, without status migrainosus**   `CC`

     √6ᵗʰ **G43.61** **Persistent migraine aura with cerebral infarction,** intractable
         Persistent migraine aura with cerebral infarction, with refractory migraine
         G43.611 **Persistent migraine aura with cerebral infarction, intractable, with status migrainosus**   `CC`
         G43.619 **Persistent migraine aura with cerebral infarction, intractable, without status migrainosus**   `CC`

√5ᵗʰ **G43.7** **Chronic** migraine without aura
     Transformed migraine
     EXCLUDES 1   migraine without aura (G43.0-)

     √6ᵗʰ **G43.70** **Chronic migraine without aura,** not intractable
         Chronic migraine without aura, without refractory migraine
         G43.701 **Chronic migraine without aura, not intractable, with status migrainosus**

N Newborn: 0   P Pediatric: 0-17   M Maternity: 9-64   A Adult: 15-124   `MCC` Major Complication/Comorbidity   `CC` Complication/Comorbidity   `SW` Severe Wound Dx

578   ICD-10-CM 2021

G43.709 **Chronic migraine without aura, not intractable,** without status migrainosus
Chronic migraine without aura NOS

✓6ᵗʰ G43.71 **Chronic migraine without aura, intractable**
Chronic migraine without aura, with refractory migraine

G43.711 **Chronic migraine without aura, intractable, with status migrainosus**

G43.719 **Chronic migraine without aura, intractable, without status migrainosus**

✓5ᵗʰ G43.A **Cyclical vomiting**

EXCLUDES 1   *cyclical vomiting syndrome unrelated to migraine (R11.15)*

AHA: 2019,4Q,15

G43.A0 **Cyclical vomiting, in migraine, not intractable**
Cyclical vomiting, without refractory migraine

G43.A1 **Cyclical vomiting, in migraine, intractable**
Cyclical vomiting, with refractory migraine

✓5ᵗʰ G43.B **Ophthalmoplegic migraine**

G43.B0 **Ophthalmoplegic migraine, not intractable**
Ophthalmoplegic migraine, without refractory migraine

G43.B1 **Ophthalmoplegic migraine, intractable**
Ophthalmoplegic migraine, with refractory migraine

✓5ᵗʰ G43.C **Periodic headache syndromes in child or adult**

G43.C0 **Periodic headache syndromes in child or adult, not intractable**
Periodic headache syndromes in child or adult, without refractory migraine

G43.C1 **Periodic headache syndromes in child or adult, intractable**
Periodic headache syndromes in child or adult, with refractory migraine

✓5ᵗʰ G43.D **Abdominal migraine**

G43.D0 **Abdominal migraine, not intractable**
Abdominal migraine, without refractory migraine

G43.D1 **Abdominal migraine, intractable**
Abdominal migraine, with refractory migraine

✓5ᵗʰ G43.8 **Other migraine**

✓6ᵗʰ G43.80 **Other migraine, not intractable**
Other migraine, without refractory migraine

G43.801 **Other migraine, not intractable, with status migrainosus**

G43.809 **Other migraine, not intractable, without status migrainosus**

✓6ᵗʰ G43.81 **Other migraine, intractable**
Other migraine, with refractory migraine

G43.811 **Other migraine, intractable, with status migrainosus**

G43.819 **Other migraine, intractable, without status migrainosus**

✓6ᵗʰ G43.82 **Menstrual migraine, not intractable**
Menstrual headache, not intractable
Menstrual migraine, without refractory migraine
Menstrually related migraine, not intractable
Pre-menstrual headache, not intractable
Pre-menstrual migraine, not intractable
Pure menstrual migraine, not intractable
Code also associated premenstrual tension syndrome (N94.3)

G43.821 **Menstrual migraine, not intractable, with status migrainosus** ♀

G43.829 **Menstrual migraine, not intractable, without status migrainosus** ♀
Menstrual migraine NOS

✓6ᵗʰ G43.83 **Menstrual migraine, intractable**
Menstrual headache, intractable
Menstrual migraine, with refractory migraine
Menstrually related migraine, intractable
Pre-menstrual headache, intractable
Pre-menstrual migraine, intractable
Pure menstrual migraine, intractable
Code also associated premenstrual tension syndrome (N94.3)

G43.831 **Menstrual migraine, intractable, with status migrainosus** ♀

G43.839 **Menstrual migraine, intractable, without status migrainosus** ♀

✓5ᵗʰ G43.9 **Migraine, unspecified**

✓6ᵗʰ G43.90 **Migraine, unspecified, not intractable**
Migraine, unspecified, without refractory migraine

G43.901 **Migraine, unspecified, not intractable, with status migrainosus**
Status migrainosus NOS

G43.909 **Migraine, unspecified, not intractable, without status migrainosus**
Migraine NOS

✓6ᵗʰ G43.91 **Migraine, unspecified, intractable**
Migraine, unspecified, with refractory migraine

G43.911 **Migraine, unspecified, intractable, with status migrainosus**

G43.919 **Migraine, unspecified, intractable, without status migrainosus**

✓4ᵗʰ **G44 Other headache syndromes**

EXCLUDES 1   *headache NOS ▶(R51.9)◀*
EXCLUDES 2   *atypical facial pain (G50.1)*
headache due to lumbar puncture (G97.1)
migraines (G43.-)
trigeminal neuralgia (G50.0)

✓5ᵗʰ **G44.0 Cluster headaches and other trigeminal autonomic cephalgias (TAC)**
DEF: Cluster headache: Characteristic grouping or clustering of headaches that can last for a number of weeks or months and then completely disappear for months or years. They are typically not associated with gastrointestinal upset or light sensitivity as experienced in migraines.

✓6ᵗʰ G44.00 **Cluster headache syndrome, unspecified**
Ciliary neuralgia
Cluster headache NOS
Histamine cephalgia
Lower half migraine
Migrainous neuralgia

G44.001 **Cluster headache syndrome, unspecified, intractable**

G44.009 **Cluster headache syndrome, unspecified, not intractable**
Cluster headache syndrome NOS

✓6ᵗʰ G44.01 **Episodic cluster headache**

G44.011 **Episodic cluster headache, intractable**

G44.019 **Episodic cluster headache, not intractable**
Episodic cluster headache NOS

✓6ᵗʰ G44.02 **Chronic cluster headache**

G44.021 **Chronic cluster headache, intractable**

G44.029 **Chronic cluster headache, not intractable**
Chronic cluster headache NOS

✓6ᵗʰ G44.03 **Episodic paroxysmal hemicrania**
Paroxysmal hemicrania NOS

G44.031 **Episodic paroxysmal hemicrania, intractable**

G44.039 **Episodic paroxysmal hemicrania, not intractable**
Episodic paroxysmal hemicrania NOS

✓6ᵗʰ G44.04 **Chronic paroxysmal hemicrania**

G44.041 **Chronic paroxysmal hemicrania, intractable**

G44.049 **Chronic paroxysmal hemicrania, not intractable**
Chronic paroxysmal hemicrania NOS

✓6ᵗʰ G44.05 **Short lasting unilateral neuralgiform headache with conjunctival injection and tearing (SUNCT)**

G44.051 **Short lasting unilateral neuralgiform headache with conjunctival injection and tearing (SUNCT), intractable**

G44.059 **Short lasting unilateral neuralgiform headache with conjunctival injection and tearing (SUNCT), not intractable**
Short lasting unilateral neuralgiform headache with conjunctival injection and tearing (SUNCT) NOS

✓6ᵗʰ G44.09 **Other trigeminal autonomic cephalgias (TAC)**

G44.091 **Other trigeminal autonomic cephalgias (TAC), intractable**

G44.099 **Other trigeminal autonomic cephalgias (TAC), not intractable**

✔ Additional Character Required   ✓x7ᵗʰ Placeholder   Unacceptable PDx   Questionable PDx   Manifestation   Unspecified Dx   H1 -H14 HAC   HCC CMS-HCC Dx   HIV HIV Dx

ICD-10-CM 2021   579

Chapter 6. Diseases of the Nervous System

G44.1 **Vascular** headache, not elsewhere classified

EXCLUDES 2   *cluster headache (G44.0)*
complicated headache syndromes (G44.5-)
drug-induced headache (G44.4-)
migraine (G43.-)
other specified headache syndromes (G44.8-)
post-traumatic headache (G44.3-)
tension-type headache (G44.2-)

✓5th **G44.2** **Tension-type** headache

✓6th   **G44.20** **Tension-type** headache, unspecified

G44.201 Tension-type headache, unspecified, intractable

G44.209 Tension-type headache, unspecified, not intractable
Tension headache NOS

✓6th   **G44.21** **Episodic** tension-type headache

G44.211 Episodic tension-type headache, intractable

G44.219 Episodic tension-type headache, not intractable
Episodic tension-type headache NOS

✓6th   **G44.22** **Chronic** tension-type headache

G44.221 Chronic tension-type headache, intractable

G44.229 Chronic tension-type headache, not intractable
Chronic tension-type headache NOS

✓5th **G44.3** **Post-traumatic** headache

✓6th   **G44.30** **Post-traumatic** headache, unspecified

G44.301 Post-traumatic headache, unspecified, intractable

G44.309 Post-traumatic headache, unspecified, not intractable
Post-traumatic headache NOS

✓6th   **G44.31** **Acute** post-traumatic headache

G44.311 Acute post-traumatic headache, intractable

G44.319 Acute post-traumatic headache, not intractable
Acute post-traumatic headache NOS

✓6th   **G44.32** **Chronic** post-traumatic headache

G44.321 Chronic post-traumatic headache, intractable

G44.329 Chronic post-traumatic headache, not intractable
Chronic post-traumatic headache NOS

✓5th **G44.4** **Drug-induced** headache, not elsewhere classified
Medication overuse headache
Use additional code for adverse effect, if applicable, to identify drug (T36-T50 with fifth or sixth character 5)

G44.40 **Drug-induced** headache, not elsewhere classified, not intractable

G44.41 **Drug-induced** headache, not elsewhere classified, intractable

✓5th **G44.5** **Complicated** headache syndromes

G44.51 **Hemicrania** continua
DEF: Persistent primary headache of unknown causation occurring on one side of the face and head. May last for more than three months, with daily and continuous pain of moderate intensity with severe exacerbations.

G44.52 **New daily persistent** headache (NDPH)

G44.53 **Primary thunderclap** headache

G44.59 **Other complicated** headache syndrome

✓5th **G44.8** **Other specified** headache syndromes

EXCLUDES 2   ▶*headache with orthostatic or positional component, not elsewhere classifed (R51.0)*◄

G44.81 **Hypnic** headache

G44.82 **Headache associated with** sexual activity
Orgasmic headache
Preorgasmic headache

G44.83 **Primary cough** headache

G44.84 **Primary exertional** headache

G44.85 **Primary stabbing** headache

G44.89 **Other** headache syndrome

✓4th **G45** **Transient cerebral ischemic attacks and related syndromes**

EXCLUDES 1   *neonatal cerebral ischemia (P91.0)*
transient retinal artery occlusion (H34.0-)

AHA: 2018,2Q,9
DEF: Transient cerebral ischemic attack: Intermittent or brief cerebral dysfunction from lack of oxygenation with no persistent neurological deficits associated with occlusive vascular disease. TIA may denote an impending cerebrovascular accident.

G45.0 **Vertebro-basilar** artery syndrome   CC

G45.1 **Carotid** artery syndrome (hemispheric)   CC

G45.2 **Multiple and bilateral** precerebral artery syndromes   CC

G45.3 **Amaurosis** fugax   CC

G45.4 **Transient global** amnesia

EXCLUDES 1   *amnesia NOS (R41.3)*

G45.8 **Other transient** cerebral ischemic attacks and related syndromes   CC

G45.9 **Transient** cerebral ischemic attack, unspecified   CC
Spasm of cerebral artery
TIA
Transient cerebral ischemia NOS

✓4th **G46** **Vascular syndromes of brain in cerebrovascular diseases**
Code first underlying cerebrovascular disease (I60-I69)

G46.0 **Middle cerebral** artery syndrome   CC

G46.1 **Anterior cerebral** artery syndrome   CC

G46.2 **Posterior cerebral** artery syndrome   CC

G46.3 **Brain stem stroke** syndrome
Benedikt syndrome
Claude syndrome
Foville syndrome
Millard-Gubler syndrome
Wallenberg syndrome
Weber syndrome

G46.4 **Cerebellar stroke** syndrome

G46.5 **Pure motor lacunar** syndrome

G46.6 **Pure sensory lacunar** syndrome

G46.7 **Other lacunar** syndromes

G46.8 **Other vascular** syndromes of brain in cerebrovascular diseases

✓4th **G47** **Sleep disorders**

EXCLUDES 2   *nightmares (F51.5)*
nonorganic sleep disorders (F51.-)
sleep terrors (F51.4)
sleepwalking (F51.3)

✓5th **G47.0** **Insomnia**

EXCLUDES 2   *alcohol related insomnia (F10.182, F10.282, F10.982)*
drug-related insomnia (F11.182, F11.282, F11.982, F13.182, F13.282, F13.982, F14.182, F14.282, F14.982, F15.182, F15.282, F15.982, F19.182, F19.282, F19.982)
idiopathic insomnia (F51.01)
insomnia due to a mental disorder (F51.05)
insomnia not due to a substance or known physiological condition (F51.0-)
nonorganic insomnia (F51.0-)
primary insomnia (F51.01)
sleep apnea (G47.3-)

G47.00 **Insomnia, unspecified**
Insomnia NOS

G47.01 **Insomnia due to medical condition**
Code also associated medical condition

G47.09 **Other insomnia**

N Newborn: 0   P Pediatric: 0-17   M Maternity: 9-64   A Adult: 15-124   MCC Major Complication/Comorbidity   CC Complication/Comorbidity   SW Severe Wound Dx

580   ICD-10-CM 2021

√5ᵗʰ **G47.1 Hypersomnia**

     EXCLUDES 2   alcohol-related hypersomnia (F10.182, F10.282, F10.982)

           drug-related hypersomnia (F11.182, F11.282, F11.982, F13.182, F13.282, F13.982, F14.182, F14.282, F14.982, F15.182, F15.282, F15.982, F19.182, F19.282, F19.982)

           hypersomnia due to a mental disorder (F51.13)

           hypersomnia not due to a substance or known physiological condition (F51.1-)

           primary hypersomnia (F51.11)

           sleep apnea (G47.3-)

     G47.10 Hypersomnia, unspecified
         Hypersomnia NOS

     G47.11 Idiopathic hypersomnia with long sleep time
         Idiopathic hypersomnia NOS

     G47.12 Idiopathic hypersomnia without long sleep time

     G47.13 Recurrent hypersomnia
         Kleine-Levin syndrome
         Menstrual related hypersomnia

     G47.14 Hypersomnia due to medical condition
         Code also associated medical condition

     G47.19 Other hypersomnia

√5ᵗʰ **G47.2 Circadian rhythm sleep disorders**

     Disorders of the sleep wake schedule
     Inversion of nyctohemeral rhythm
     Inversion of sleep rhythm
     DEF: Circadian rhythm: Daily cycle (24-hour period) of physical, mental and behavioral changes. It is largely influenced by environmental ques, such as changes in light or temperature.
     Synonyms: sleep/wake cycle.

     G47.20 Circadian rhythm sleep disorder, unspecified type
         Sleep wake schedule disorder NOS

     G47.21 Circadian rhythm sleep disorder, delayed sleep phase type
         Delayed sleep phase syndrome

     G47.22 Circadian rhythm sleep disorder, advanced sleep phase type

     G47.23 Circadian rhythm sleep disorder, irregular sleep wake type
         Irregular sleep-wake pattern

     G47.24 Circadian rhythm sleep disorder, free running type
         Circadian rhythm sleep disorder, non-24-hour sleep-wake type

     G47.25 Circadian rhythm sleep disorder, jet lag type

     G47.26 Circadian rhythm sleep disorder, shift work type

     G47.27 Circadian rhythm sleep disorder in conditions classified elsewhere
         Code first underlying condition

     G47.29 Other circadian rhythm sleep disorder

√5ᵗʰ **G47.3 Sleep apnea**

     Code also any associated underlying condition

     EXCLUDES 1   apnea NOS (R06.81)
           Cheyne-Stokes breathing (R06.3)
           pickwickian syndrome (E66.2)
           sleep apnea of newborn (P28.3)

     G47.30 Sleep apnea, unspecified
         Sleep apnea NOS

     G47.31 Primary central sleep apnea
         Idiopathic central sleep apnea

     G47.32 High altitude periodic breathing

     G47.33 Obstructive sleep apnea (adult) (pediatric)
         Obstructive sleep apnea hypopnea
         EXCLUDES 1   obstructive sleep apnea of newborn (P28.3)

     G47.34 Idiopathic sleep related nonobstructive alveolar hypoventilation
         Sleep related hypoxia

     G47.35 Congenital central alveolar hypoventilation syndrome

     G47.36 Sleep related hypoventilation in conditions classified elsewhere
         Sleep related hypoxemia in conditions classified elsewhere
         Code first underlying condition

     G47.37 Central sleep apnea in conditions classified elsewhere
         Code first underlying condition

     G47.39 Other sleep apnea

√5ᵗʰ **G47.4 Narcolepsy and cataplexy**

     √6ᵗʰ **G47.41 Narcolepsy**

         G47.411 Narcolepsy with cataplexy

         G47.419 Narcolepsy without cataplexy
            Narcolepsy NOS

     √6ᵗʰ **G47.42 Narcolepsy in conditions classified elsewhere**
         Code first underlying condition

         G47.421 Narcolepsy in conditions classified elsewhere with cataplexy

         G47.429 Narcolepsy in conditions classified elsewhere without cataplexy

√5ᵗʰ **G47.5 Parasomnia**

     EXCLUDES 1   alcohol induced parasomnia (F10.182, F10.282, F10.982)

           drug induced parasomnia (F11.182, F11.282, F11.982, F13.182, F13.282, F13.982, F14.182, F14.282, F14.982, F15.182, F15.282, F15.982, F19.182, F19.282, F19.982)

           parasomnia not due to a substance or known physiological condition (F51.8)

     G47.50 Parasomnia, unspecified
         Parasomnia NOS

     G47.51 Confusional arousals

     G47.52 REM sleep behavior disorder

     G47.53 Recurrent isolated sleep paralysis

     G47.54 Parasomnia in conditions classified elsewhere
         Code first underlying condition

     G47.59 Other parasomnia

√5ᵗʰ **G47.6 Sleep related movement disorders**

     EXCLUDES 2   restless legs syndrome (G25.81)

     G47.61 Periodic limb movement disorder

     G47.62 Sleep related leg cramps

     G47.63 Sleep related bruxism
         EXCLUDES 1   psychogenic bruxism (F45.8)

     G47.69 Other sleep related movement disorders

G47.8 Other sleep disorders
     Other specified sleep-wake disorder

G47.9 Sleep disorder, unspecified
     Sleep disorder NOS
     Unspecified sleep-wake disorder

☑ Additional Character Required   √x7ᵗʰ Placeholder   Unacceptable PDx   Questionable PDx   Manifestation   Unspecified Dx   H1-H4 HAC   HCC CMS-HCC Dx   HIV HIV Dx

ICD-10-CM 2021   581

Nerve, nerve root and plexus disorders (G50-G59)

> EXCLUDES 1   current traumatic nerve, nerve root and plexus disorders — see Injury, nerve by body region
> neuralgia NOS (M79.2)
> neuritis NOS (M79.2)
> peripheral neuritis in pregnancy (O26.82-)
> radiculitis NOS (M54.1-)

✓4ᵗʰ G50   Disorders of trigeminal nerve

> INCLUDES   disorders of 5th cranial nerve

Trigeminal and Facial Nerve Branches

Supratrochlear nerve
Supraorbital nerve
V2 branch
Infraorbital nerve
V1 branch
Trigeminal nerve (CN V) branches in infratemporal fossa
V3 branch
Mental nerve
Mental foramen

G50.0   Trigeminal neuralgia
Syndrome of paroxysmal facial pain
Tic douloureux

G50.1   Atypical facial pain

G50.8   Other disorders of trigeminal nerve

G50.9   Disorder of trigeminal nerve, unspecified

✓4ᵗʰ G51   Facial nerve disorders

> INCLUDES   disorders of 7th cranial nerve

G51.0   Bell's palsy
Facial palsy

G51.1   Geniculate ganglionitis
> EXCLUDES 1   postherpetic geniculate ganglionitis (B02.21)

G51.2   Melkersson's syndrome
Melkersson-Rosenthal syndrome

✓5ᵗʰ G51.3   Clonic hemifacial spasm
AHA: 2018,4Q,10
G51.31   Clonic hemifacial spasm, right
G51.32   Clonic hemifacial spasm, left
G51.33   Clonic hemifacial spasm, bilateral
G51.39   Clonic hemifacial spasm, unspecified

G51.4   Facial myokymia

G51.8   Other disorders of facial nerve

G51.9   Disorder of facial nerve, unspecified

✓4ᵗʰ G52   Disorders of other cranial nerves

> EXCLUDES 2   disorders of acoustic [8th] nerve (H93.3)
> disorders of optic [2nd] nerve (H46, H47.0)
> paralytic strabismus due to nerve palsy (H49.0-H49.2)

G52.0   Disorders of olfactory nerve
Disorders of 1st cranial nerve

G52.1   Disorders of glossopharyngeal nerve
Disorder of 9th cranial nerve
Glossopharyngeal neuralgia

G52.2   Disorders of vagus nerve
Disorders of pneumogastric [10th] nerve

G52.3   Disorders of hypoglossal nerve
Disorders of 12th cranial nerve

G52.7   Disorders of multiple cranial nerves
Polyneuritis cranialis

G52.8   Disorders of other specified cranial nerves

G52.9   Cranial nerve disorder, unspecified

G53   Cranial nerve disorders in diseases classified elsewhere

Code first underlying disease, such as:
neoplasm (C00-D49)

> EXCLUDES 1   multiple cranial nerve palsy in sarcoidosis (D86.82)
> multiple cranial nerve palsy in syphilis (A52.15)
> postherpetic geniculate ganglionitis (B02.21)
> postherpetic trigeminal neuralgia (B02.22)

✓4ᵗʰ G54   Nerve root and plexus disorders

> EXCLUDES 1   current traumatic nerve root and plexus disorders — see nerve injury by body region
> intervertebral disc disorders (M50-M51)
> neuralgia or neuritis NOS (M79.2)
> neuritis or radiculitis brachial NOS (M54.13)
> neuritis or radiculitis lumbar NOS (M54.16)
> neuritis or radiculitis lumbosacral NOS (M54.17)
> neuritis or radiculitis thoracic NOS (M54.14)
> radiculitis NOS (M54.10)
> radiculopathy NOS (M54.10)
> spondylosis (M47.-)

G54.0   Brachial plexus disorders
Thoracic outlet syndrome
DEF: Acquired disorder affecting the spinal nerves that send signals to the shoulder, arm, and hand, causing corresponding motor and sensory dysfunction. This disorder is characterized by regional paresthesia, pain, muscle weakness, and in severe cases paralysis.

G54.1   Lumbosacral plexus disorders

G54.2   Cervical root disorders, not elsewhere classified

G54.3   Thoracic root disorders, not elsewhere classified

G54.4   Lumbosacral root disorders, not elsewhere classified

G54.5   Neuralgic amyotrophy
Parsonage-Aldren-Turner syndrome
Shoulder-girdle neuritis
> EXCLUDES 1   neuralgic amyotrophy in diabetes mellitus (E08-E13 with .44)

G54.6   Phantom limb syndrome with pain   HCC

G54.7   Phantom limb syndrome without pain   HCC
Phantom limb syndrome NOS

G54.8   Other nerve root and plexus disorders

G54.9   Nerve root and plexus disorder, unspecified

G55   Nerve root and plexus compressions in diseases classified elsewhere

Code first underlying disease, such as:
neoplasm (C00-D49)

> EXCLUDES 1   nerve root compression (due to) (in) ankylosing spondylitis (M45.-)
> nerve root compression (due to) (in) dorsopathies (M53.-, M54.-)
> nerve root compression (due to) (in) intervertebral disc disorders (M50.1.-, M51.1.-)
> nerve root compression (due to) (in) spondylopathies (M46.-, M48.-)
> nerve root compression (due to) (in) spondylosis (M47.0-M47.2-)

✓4ᵗʰ G56   Mononeuropathies of upper limb

> **EXCLUDES 1**   current traumatic nerve disorder — see nerve injury by body region
>
> **AHA:** 2016,4Q,17-18

Nerves of Upper Limb

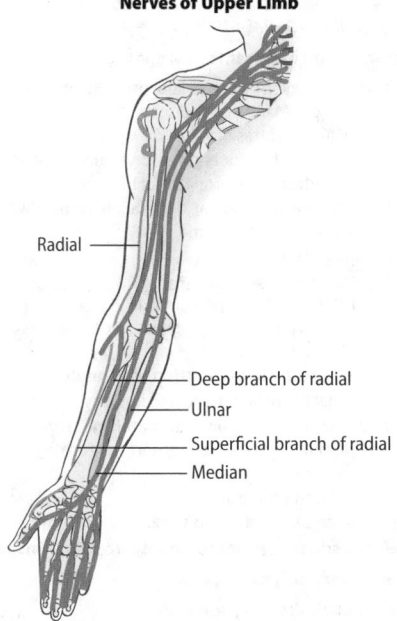

- Radial
- Deep branch of radial
- Ulnar
- Superficial branch of radial
- Median

✓5ᵗʰ G56.Ø   Carpal tunnel syndrome

DEF: Swelling and inflammation in the tendons or bursa surrounding the median nerve caused by repetitive activity. The resulting compression on the nerve causes pain, numbness, and tingling especially to the palm, index, middle finger, and thumb.

- **G56.ØØ**   Carpal tunnel syndrome, unspecified upper limb
- **G56.Ø1**   Carpal tunnel syndrome, right upper limb
- **G56.Ø2**   Carpal tunnel syndrome, left upper limb
- **G56.Ø3**   Carpal tunnel syndrome, bilateral upper limbs

✓5ᵗʰ G56.1   Other lesions of median nerve

- **G56.1Ø**   Other lesions of median nerve, unspecified upper limb
- **G56.11**   Other lesions of median nerve, right upper limb
- **G56.12**   Other lesions of median nerve, left upper limb
- **G56.13**   Other lesions of median nerve, bilateral upper limbs

✓5ᵗʰ G56.2   Lesion of ulnar nerve

Tardy ulnar nerve palsy

- **G56.2Ø**   Lesion of ulnar nerve, unspecified upper limb
- **G56.21**   Lesion of ulnar nerve, right upper limb
- **G56.22**   Lesion of ulnar nerve, left upper limb
- **G56.23**   Lesion of ulnar nerve, bilateral upper limbs

✓5ᵗʰ G56.3   Lesion of radial nerve

- **G56.3Ø**   Lesion of radial nerve, unspecified upper limb
- **G56.31**   Lesion of radial nerve, right upper limb
- **G56.32**   Lesion of radial nerve, left upper limb
- **G56.33**   Lesion of radial nerve, bilateral upper limbs

✓5ᵗʰ G56.4   Causalgia of upper limb

Complex regional pain syndrome II of upper limb

> **EXCLUDES 1**   complex regional pain syndrome I of lower limb (G9Ø.52-)
> complex regional pain syndrome I of upper limb (G9Ø.51-)
> complex regional pain syndrome II of lower limb (G57.7-)
> reflex sympathetic dystrophy of lower limb (G9Ø.52-)
> reflex sympathetic dystrophy of upper limb (G9Ø.51-)

- **G56.4Ø**   Causalgia of unspecified upper limb
- **G56.41**   Causalgia of right upper limb
- **G56.42**   Causalgia of left upper limb
- **G56.43**   Causalgia of bilateral upper limbs

✓5ᵗʰ G56.8   Other specified mononeuropathies of upper limb

Interdigital neuroma of upper limb

- **G56.8Ø**   Other specified mononeuropathies of unspecified upper limb

- **G56.81**   Other specified mononeuropathies of right upper limb
- **G56.82**   Other specified mononeuropathies of left upper limb
- **G56.83**   Other specified mononeuropathies of bilateral upper limbs

✓5ᵗʰ G56.9   Unspecified mononeuropathy of upper limb

- **G56.9Ø**   Unspecified mononeuropathy of unspecified upper limb
- **G56.91**   Unspecified mononeuropathy of right upper limb
- **G56.92**   Unspecified mononeuropathy of left upper limb
- **G56.93**   Unspecified mononeuropathy of bilateral upper limbs

✓4ᵗʰ G57   Mononeuropathies of lower limb

> **EXCLUDES 1**   current traumatic nerve disorder — see nerve injury by body region
>
> **AHA:** 2016,4Q,17-18

Nerves of Lower Limb

- Obturator nerve
- Sciatic nerve
- Femoral nerve
- Saphenous nerve
- Common fibular (peroneal) nerve
- Deep fibular (peroneal) nerve
- Tibial nerve
- Superficial fibular (peroneal) nerve

✓5ᵗʰ G57.Ø   Lesion of sciatic nerve

> **EXCLUDES 1**   sciatica NOS (M54.3-)
> **EXCLUDES 2**   sciatica attributed to intervertebral disc disorder (M51.1.-)

- **G57.ØØ**   Lesion of sciatic nerve, unspecified lower limb
- **G57.Ø1**   Lesion of sciatic nerve, right lower limb
- **G57.Ø2**   Lesion of sciatic nerve, left lower limb
- **G57.Ø3**   Lesion of sciatic nerve, bilateral lower limbs

✓5ᵗʰ G57.1   Meralgia paresthetica

Lateral cutaneous nerve of thigh syndrome

- **G57.1Ø**   Meralgia paresthetica, unspecified lower limb
- **G57.11**   Meralgia paresthetica, right lower limb
- **G57.12**   Meralgia paresthetica, left lower limb
- **G57.13**   Meralgia paresthetica, bilateral lower limbs

✓5ᵗʰ G57.2   Lesion of femoral nerve

- **G57.2Ø**   Lesion of femoral nerve, unspecified lower limb
- **G57.21**   Lesion of femoral nerve, right lower limb
- **G57.22**   Lesion of femoral nerve, left lower limb
- **G57.23**   Lesion of femoral nerve, bilateral lower limbs

✓5ᵗʰ G57.3   Lesion of lateral popliteal nerve

Peroneal nerve palsy

- **G57.3Ø**   Lesion of lateral popliteal nerve, unspecified lower limb
- **G57.31**   Lesion of lateral popliteal nerve, right lower limb
- **G57.32**   Lesion of lateral popliteal nerve, left lower limb
- **G57.33**   Lesion of lateral popliteal nerve, bilateral lower limbs

Chapter 6. Diseases of the Nervous System

✓5ᵗʰ **G57.4** **Lesion of** medial popliteal nerve
    G57.40 **Lesion of medial popliteal nerve, unspecified lower limb**
    G57.41 **Lesion of medial popliteal nerve,** right **lower limb**
    G57.42 **Lesion of medial popliteal nerve,** left **lower limb**
    G57.43 **Lesion of medial popliteal nerve,** bilateral **lower limbs**

✓5ᵗʰ **G57.5** **Tarsal tunnel syndrome**
    G57.50 **Tarsal tunnel syndrome, unspecified lower limb**
    G57.51 **Tarsal tunnel syndrome,** right **lower limb**
    G57.52 **Tarsal tunnel syndrome,** left **lower limb**
    G57.53 **Tarsal tunnel syndrome,** bilateral **lower limbs**

✓5ᵗʰ **G57.6** **Lesion of** plantar nerve
    Morton's metatarsalgia
    G57.60 **Lesion of plantar nerve, unspecified lower limb**
    G57.61 **Lesion of plantar nerve,** right **lower limb**
    G57.62 **Lesion of plantar nerve,** left **lower limb**
    G57.63 **Lesion of plantar nerve,** bilateral **lower limbs**

✓5ᵗʰ **G57.7** **Causalgia** of lower limb
    Complex regional pain syndrome II of lower limb
    EXCLUDES 1   *complex regional pain syndrome I of lower limb (G90.52-)*
        complex regional pain syndrome I of upper limb (G90.51-)
        complex regional pain syndrome II of upper limb (G56.4-)
        reflex sympathetic dystrophy of lower limb (G90.52-)
        reflex sympathetic dystrophy of upper limb (G90.51-)
    G57.70 **Causalgia of unspecified lower limb**
    G57.71 **Causalgia of** right **lower limb**
    G57.72 **Causalgia of** left **lower limb**
    G57.73 **Causalgia of** bilateral **lower limbs**

✓5ᵗʰ **G57.8** **Other specified mononeuropathies of lower limb**
    Interdigital neuroma of lower limb
    G57.80 **Other specified mononeuropathies of unspecified lower limb**
    G57.81 **Other specified mononeuropathies of** right **lower limb**
    G57.82 **Other specified mononeuropathies of** left **lower limb**
    G57.83 **Other specified mononeuropathies of** bilateral **lower limbs**

✓5ᵗʰ **G57.9** **Unspecified mononeuropathy of lower limb**
    G57.90 **Unspecified mononeuropathy of unspecified lower limb**
    G57.91 **Unspecified mononeuropathy of** right **lower limb**
    G57.92 **Unspecified mononeuropathy of** left **lower limb**
    G57.93 **Unspecified mononeuropathy of** bilateral **lower limbs**

✓4ᵗʰ **G58** **Other mononeuropathies**
    G58.0 **Intercostal neuropathy**
    G58.7 **Mononeuritis multiplex**
    G58.8 **Other specified mononeuropathies**
    G58.9 **Mononeuropathy, unspecified**

G59 ***Mononeuropathy in diseases classified elsewhere***
    Code first underlying disease
    EXCLUDES 1   *diabetic mononeuropathy (E08-E13 with .41)*
        syphilitic nerve paralysis (A52.19)
        syphilitic neuritis (A52.15)
        tuberculous mononeuropathy (A17.83)

Polyneuropathies and other disorders of the peripheral nervous system (G60-G65)

    EXCLUDES 1   *neuralgia NOS (M79.2)*
        neuritis NOS (M79.2)
        peripheral neuritis in pregnancy (O26.82-)
        radiculitis NOS (M54.10)

✓4ᵗʰ **G60** **Hereditary and idiopathic** neuropathy
    G60.0 **Hereditary** motor and sensory **neuropathy**
        Charcôt-Marie-Tooth disease
        Déjérine-Sottas disease
        Hereditary motor and sensory neuropathy, types I-IV
        Hypertrophic neuropathy of infancy
        Peroneal muscular atrophy (axonal type) (hypertrophic type)
        Roussy-Levy syndrome
    G60.1 **Refsum's disease**   `CC`
        Infantile Refsum disease
        DEF: Genetic disorder of the lipid metabolism characterized by retinitis pigmentosa, degenerative nerve disease, ataxia, and dry, rough, scaly skin.
    G60.2 **Neuropathy in association with hereditary ataxia**
    G60.3 **Idiopathic** progressive **neuropathy**
    G60.8 **Other hereditary and idiopathic neuropathies**
        Dominantly inherited sensory neuropathy
        Morvan's disease
        Nelaton's syndrome
        Recessively inherited sensory neuropathy
    G60.9 **Hereditary and idiopathic neuropathy, unspecified**

✓4ᵗʰ **G61** **Inflammatory** polyneuropathy
    G61.0 **Guillain-Barre syndrome**   `CC` `HCC`
        Acute (post-)infective polyneuritis
        Miller Fisher syndrome
        AHA: 2014,2Q,4
        DEF: Autoimmune disorder due to an immune response to foreign antigens with paraplegia of limbs, flaccid paralysis, ophthalmoplegia, ataxia, and areflexia. In most cases, this disorder is triggered by a mild viral infection, surgery, or following an immunization.
        TIP: Guillain-Barre syndrome can occur as a sequela of *Campylobacter enteritis*. Assign code B94.8 for the sequelae as an additional diagnosis.
    G61.1 **Serum neuropathy**   `HCC`
        Use additional code for adverse effect, if applicable, to identify serum (T50.-)
    ✓5ᵗʰ **G61.8** **Other inflammatory polyneuropathies**
        G61.81 **Chronic inflammatory demyelinating polyneuritis**   `CC` `HCC`
        G61.82 **Multifocal motor neuropathy**   `HCC`
           MMN
           AHA: 2016,4Q,18
        G61.89 **Other inflammatory polyneuropathies**   `HCC`
    G61.9 **Inflammatory polyneuropathy, unspecified**   `HCC`

✓4ᵗʰ **G62** **Other and unspecified polyneuropathies**
    G62.0 **Drug-induced** polyneuropathy   `HCC`
        Use additional code for adverse effect, if applicable, to identify drug (T36-T50 with fifth or sixth character 5)
    G62.1 **Alcoholic** polyneuropathy   `HCC`
        AHA: 2019,3Q,8
    G62.2 **Polyneuropathy due to other toxic agents**   `HCC`
        Code first (T51-T65) to identify toxic agent
    ✓5ᵗʰ **G62.8** **Other specified polyneuropathies**
        G62.81 **Critical illness polyneuropathy**   `CC` `HCC`
           Acute motor neuropathy
        G62.82 **Radiation-induced polyneuropathy**   `HCC`
           Use additional external cause code (W88-W90, X39.0-) to identify cause
        G62.89 **Other specified polyneuropathies**
           AHA: 2016,2Q,11
    G62.9 **Polyneuropathy, unspecified**
        Neuropathy NOS

G63 **Polyneuropathy in diseases classified elsewhere**   HCC

Code first underlying disease, such as:
- amyloidosis (E85.-)
- endocrine disease, except diabetes (E00-E07, E15-E16, E20-E34)
- metabolic diseases (E70-E88)
- neoplasm (C00-D49)
- nutritional deficiency (E40-E64)

   EXCLUDES 1   polyneuropathy (in):
- diabetes mellitus (E08-E13 with .42)
- diphtheria (A36.83)
- infectious mononucleosis (B27.0-B27.9 with 1)
- Lyme disease (A69.22)
- mumps (B26.84)
- postherpetic (B02.23)
- rheumatoid arthritis (M05.5-)
- scleroderma (M34.83)
- systemic lupus erythematosus (M32.19)

     AHA: 2012,4Q,99

G64 **Other disorders of peripheral nervous system**

Disorder of peripheral nervous system NOS

☑4ᵗʰ **G65** **Sequelae of inflammatory and toxic polyneuropathies**

Code first condition resulting from (sequela) of inflammatory and toxic polyneuropathies

  G65.0 **Sequelae of Guillain-Barré syndrome**   HCC

  G65.1 **Sequelae of other inflammatory polyneuropathy**   HCC

  G65.2 **Sequelae of toxic polyneuropathy**   HCC

Diseases of myoneural junction and muscle (G70-G73)

☑4ᵗʰ **G70** **Myasthenia gravis and other myoneural disorders**

   EXCLUDES 1   botulism (A05.1, A48.51-A48.52)
             transient neonatal myasthenia gravis (P94.0)

☑5ᵗʰ **G70.0** **Myasthenia gravis**

     DEF: Autoimmune neuromuscular disorder caused by antibodies to the acetylcholine receptors at the neuromuscular junction, interfering with proper binding of the neurotransmitter from the neuron to the target muscle, causing muscle weakness, fatigue, and exhaustion, without pain or atrophy.

    G70.00 **Myasthenia gravis without (acute) exacerbation**   HCC

         Myasthenia gravis NOS

    G70.01 **Myasthenia gravis with (acute) exacerbation**   MCC HCC

         Myasthenia gravis in crisis

  G70.1 **Toxic myoneural disorders**   HCC

     Code first (T51-T65) to identify toxic agent

  G70.2 **Congenital and developmental myasthenia**   HCC

☑5ᵗʰ **G70.8** **Other specified myoneural disorders**

    G70.80 **Lambert-Eaton syndrome, unspecified**   CC HCC

         Lambert-Eaton syndrome NOS

    G70.81 *Lambert-Eaton syndrome in disease classified elsewhere*   CC HCC

         Code first underlying disease

         EXCLUDES 1   Lambert-Eaton syndrome in neoplastic disease (G73.1)

    G70.89 **Other specified myoneural disorders**   HCC

  G70.9 **Myoneural disorder, unspecified**   HCC

☑4ᵗʰ **G71** **Primary disorders of muscles**

   EXCLUDES 2   arthrogryposis multiplex congenita (Q74.3)
             metabolic disorders (E70-E88)
             myositis (M60.-)

☑5ᵗʰ **G71.0** **Muscular dystrophy**

     AHA: 2018,4Q,11-12

    G71.00 **Muscular dystrophy, unspecified**   HCC

    G71.01 **Duchenne or Becker muscular dystrophy**   HCC

         Autosomal recessive, childhood type, muscular dystrophy resembling Duchenne or Becker muscular dystrophy

         Benign [Becker] muscular dystrophy

         Severe [Duchenne] muscular dystrophy

    G71.02 **Facioscapulohumeral muscular dystrophy**   HCC

         Scapulohumeral muscular dystrophy

    G71.09 **Other specified muscular dystrophies**   HCC

         Benign scapuloperoneal muscular dystrophy with early contractures [Emery-Dreifuss]

         Congenital muscular dystrophy NOS

         Congenital muscular dystrophy with specific morphological abnormalities of the muscle fiber

         Distal muscular dystrophy

         Limb-girdle muscular dystrophy

         Ocular muscular dystrophy

         Oculopharyngeal muscular dystrophy

         Scapuloperoneal muscular dystrophy

☑5ᵗʰ **G71.1** **Myotonic disorders**

    G71.11 **Myotonic muscular dystrophy**   HCC

         Dystrophia myotonica [Steinert]

         Myotonia atrophica

         Myotonic dystrophy

         Proximal myotonic myopathy (PROMM)

         Steinert disease

    G71.12 **Myotonia congenita**

         Acetazolamide responsive myotonia congenita

         Dominant myotonia congenita [Thomsen disease]

         Myotonia levior

         Recessive myotonia congenita [Becker disease]

    G71.13 **Myotonic chondrodystrophy**

         Chondrodystrophic myotonia

         Congenital myotonic chondrodystrophy

         Schwartz-Jampel disease

    G71.14 **Drug induced myotonia**

         Use additional code for adverse effect, if applicable, to identify drug (T36-T50 with fifth or sixth character 5)

    G71.19 **Other specified myotonic disorders**

         Myotonia fluctuans

         Myotonia permanens

         Neuromyotonia [Isaacs]

         Paramyotonia congenita (of von Eulenburg)

         Pseudomyotonia

         Symptomatic myotonia

▲ ☑5ᵗʰ **G71.2** **Congenital myopathies**

     ~~Central core disease~~

     ~~Fiber-type disproportion~~

     ~~Minicore disease~~

     ~~Multicore disease~~

     ~~Myotubular (centronuclear) myopathy~~

     ~~Nemaline myopathy~~

     EXCLUDES 1   ~~arthrogryposis multiplex congenita (Q74.3)~~

     EXCLUDES 2   ►arthrogryposis multiplex congenita (Q74.3)◄

 ●   **G71.20** **Congenital myopathy, unspecifed**   CC

 ●   **G71.21** **Nemaline myopathy**   CC

 ● ☑6ᵗʰ **G71.22** **Centronuclear myopathy**

 ●   **G71.220** **X-linked myotubular myopathy**   CC

             Myotubular (centronuclear) myopathy

        G71.228 **Other centronuclear myopathy**   CC

             Autosomal centronuclear myopathy

             Autosomal dominant centronuclear myopathy

             Autosomal recessive centronuclear myopathy

             Centronuclear myopathy, NOS

 ●   **G71.29** **Other congenital myopathy**   CC

         Central core disease

         Minicore disease

         Multicore disease

         Multiminicore disease

  G71.3 **Mitochondrial myopathy, not elsewhere classified**

     EXCLUDES 1   Kearns-Sayre syndrome (H49.81)
             Leber's disease (H47.21)
             Leigh's encephalopathy (G31.82)
             mitochondrial metabolism disorders (E88.4.-)
             Reye's syndrome (G93.7)

  G71.8 **Other primary disorders of muscles**

  G71.9 **Primary disorder of muscle, unspecified**

     Hereditary myopathy NOS

☑ Additional Character Required   ☑x7ᵗʰ Placeholder   Unacceptable PDx   Questionable PDx   Manifestation   Unspecified Dx   H1-H14 HAC   HCC CMS-HCC Dx   HIV HIV Dx

Chapter 6. Diseases of the Nervous System

G72–G82.52

✓4ᵗʰ **G72 Other and unspecified myopathies**

> EXCLUDES 1   arthrogryposis multiplex congenita (Q74.3)
> dermatopolymyositis (M33.-)
> ischemic infarction of muscle (M62.2-)
> myositis (M60.-)
> polymyositis (M33.2.-)

G72.0 Drug-induced myopathy   CC
> Use additional code for adverse effect, if applicable, to identify drug (T36-T50 with fifth or sixth character 5)

G72.1 Alcoholic myopathy   CC
> Use additional code to identify alcoholism (F10.-)

G72.2 Myopathy due to other toxic agents   CC
> Code first (T51-T65) to identify toxic agent

G72.3 Periodic paralysis
> Familial periodic paralysis
> Hyperkalemic periodic paralysis (familial)
> Hypokalemic periodic paralysis (familial)
> Myotonic periodic paralysis (familial)
> Normokalemic paralysis (familial)
> Potassium sensitive periodic paralysis
>> EXCLUDES 1   paramyotonia congenita (of von Eulenburg) (G71.19)

✓5ᵗʰ **G72.4 Inflammatory and immune myopathies, not elsewhere classified**

G72.41 Inclusion body myositis [IBM]

G72.49 Other inflammatory and immune myopathies, not elsewhere classified
> Inflammatory myopathy NOS

✓5ᵗʰ **G72.8 Other specified myopathies**

G72.81 Critical illness myopathy   CC
> Acute necrotizing myopathy
> Acute quadriplegic myopathy
> Intensive care (ICU) myopathy
> Myopathy of critical illness

G72.89 Other specified myopathies

G72.9 Myopathy, unspecified

✓4ᵗʰ **G73 Disorders of myoneural junction and muscle in diseases classified elsewhere**

G73.1 Lambert-Eaton syndrome in neoplastic disease   CC HCC
> Code first underlying neoplasm (C00-D49)
>> EXCLUDES 1   Lambert-Eaton syndrome not associated with neoplasm (G70.80-G70.81)

G73.3 Myasthenic syndromes in other diseases classified elsewhere   CC HCC
> Code first underlying disease, such as:
> neoplasm (C00-D49)
> thyrotoxicosis (E05.-)

G73.7 Myopathy in diseases classified elsewhere
> Code first underlying disease, such as:
> hyperparathyroidism (E21.0, E21.3)
> hypoparathyroidism (E20.-)
> glycogen storage disease (E74.0)
> lipid storage disorders (E75.-)
>> EXCLUDES 1   myopathy in:
>> rheumatoid arthritis (M05.32)
>> sarcoidosis (D86.87)
>> scleroderma (M34.82)
>> sicca syndrome [Sjögren] (M35.03)
>> systemic lupus erythematosus (M32.19)

Cerebral palsy and other paralytic syndromes (G80-G83)

✓4ᵗʰ **G80 Cerebral palsy**
> EXCLUDES 1   hereditary spastic paraplegia (G11.4)

G80.0 Spastic quadriplegic cerebral palsy   MCC HCC
> Congenital spastic paralysis (cerebral)

G80.1 Spastic diplegic cerebral palsy   CC HCC
> Spastic cerebral palsy NOS

G80.2 Spastic hemiplegic cerebral palsy   CC HCC

G80.3 Athetoid cerebral palsy   CC HCC
> Double athetosis (syndrome)
> Dyskinetic cerebral palsy
> Dystonic cerebral palsy
> Vogt disease

G80.4 Ataxic cerebral palsy   HCC

G80.8 Other cerebral palsy   HCC
> Mixed cerebral palsy syndromes

G80.9 Cerebral palsy, unspecified   HCC
> Cerebral palsy NOS

✓4ᵗʰ **G81 Hemiplegia and hemiparesis**

> NOTE   This category is to be used only when hemiplegia (complete)(incomplete) is reported without further specification, or is stated to be old or longstanding but of unspecified cause. The category is also for use in multiple coding to identify these types of hemiplegia resulting from any cause.

> EXCLUDES 1   congenital cerebral palsy (G80.-)
> hemiplegia and hemiparesis due to sequela of cerebrovascular disease (I69.05-, I69.15-, I69.25-, I69.35-, I69.85-, I69.95-)

AHA: 2015,1Q,25

TIP: If the documentation specifies the affected side but not whether it is the dominant or nondominant side, the default is as follows: for ambidextrous patients, the default is dominant; when the left side is affected, the default is nondominant; and when the right side is affected, the default is dominant.

✓5ᵗʰ **G81.0 Flaccid hemiplegia**

G81.00 Flaccid hemiplegia affecting unspecified side   CC HCC

G81.01 Flaccid hemiplegia affecting right dominant side   CC HCC

G81.02 Flaccid hemiplegia affecting left dominant side   CC HCC

G81.03 Flaccid hemiplegia affecting right nondominant side   CC HCC

G81.04 Flaccid hemiplegia affecting left nondominant side   CC HCC

✓5ᵗʰ **G81.1 Spastic hemiplegia**

G81.10 Spastic hemiplegia affecting unspecified side   CC HCC

G81.11 Spastic hemiplegia affecting right dominant side   CC HCC

G81.12 Spastic hemiplegia affecting left dominant side   CC HCC

G81.13 Spastic hemiplegia affecting right nondominant side   CC HCC

G81.14 Spastic hemiplegia affecting left nondominant side   CC HCC

✓5ᵗʰ **G81.9 Hemiplegia, unspecified**
> **AHA:** 2014,1Q,23

G81.90 Hemiplegia, unspecified affecting unspecified side   CC HCC

G81.91 Hemiplegia, unspecified affecting right dominant side   CC HCC

G81.92 Hemiplegia, unspecified affecting left dominant side   CC HCC

G81.93 Hemiplegia, unspecified affecting right nondominant side   CC HCC

G81.94 Hemiplegia, unspecified affecting left nondominant side   CC HCC

✓4ᵗʰ **G82 Paraplegia (paraparesis) and quadriplegia (quadriparesis)**

> NOTE   This category is to be used only when the listed conditions are reported without further specification, or are stated to be old or longstanding but of unspecified cause. The category is also for use in multiple coding to identify these conditions resulting from any cause

> EXCLUDES 1   congenital cerebral palsy (G80.-)
> functional quadriplegia (R53.2)
> hysterical paralysis (F44.4)

✓5ᵗʰ **G82.2 Paraplegia**
> Paralysis of both lower limbs NOS
> Paraparesis (lower) NOS
> Paraplegia (lower) NOS
> **AHA:** 2017,3Q,3

G82.20 Paraplegia, unspecified   CC HCC

G82.21 Paraplegia, complete   CC HCC

G82.22 Paraplegia, incomplete   CC HCC

✓5ᵗʰ **G82.5 Quadriplegia**

G82.50 Quadriplegia, unspecified   MCC HCC

G82.51 Quadriplegia, C1-C4 complete   MCC HCC

G82.52 Quadriplegia, C1-C4 incomplete   MCC HCC

N Newborn: 0   P Pediatric: 0-17   M Maternity: 9-64   A Adult: 15-124   MCC Major Complication/Comorbidity   CC Complication/Comorbidity   SW Severe Wound Dx

586

ICD-10-CM 2021

G82.53   **Quadriplegia, C5-C7 complete**   MCC HCC

G82.54   **Quadriplegia, C5-C7 incomplete**   MCC HCC

√4ᵗʰ **G83 Other paralytic syndromes**

> **NOTE**   This category is to be used only when the listed conditions are reported without further specification, or are stated to be old or longstanding but of unspecified cause. The category is also for use in multiple coding to identify these conditions resulting from any cause.

> **INCLUDES**   paralysis (complete) (incomplete), except as in G80-G82

G83.0 Diplegia of upper limbs   CC HCC
> Diplegia (upper)
> Paralysis of both upper limbs

√5ᵗʰ **G83.1 Monoplegia of lower limb**
> Paralysis of lower limb
> **EXCLUDES 1**   monoplegia of lower limbs due to sequela of cerebrovascular disease (I69.04-, I69.14-, I69.24-, I69.34-, I69.84-, I69.94-)

> **TIP:** If the documentation specifies the affected side but not whether it is the dominant or nondominant side, the default is as follows: for ambidextrous patients, the default is dominant; when the left side is affected, the default is nondominant; and when the right side is affected, the default is dominant.

> **G83.10 Monoplegia of lower limb affecting unspecified side**   HCC

> **G83.11 Monoplegia of lower limb affecting right dominant side**   HCC

> **G83.12 Monoplegia of lower limb affecting left dominant side**   HCC

> **G83.13 Monoplegia of lower limb affecting right nondominant side**   HCC

> **G83.14 Monoplegia of lower limb affecting left nondominant side**   HCC

√5ᵗʰ **G83.2 Monoplegia of upper limb**
> Paralysis of upper limb
> **EXCLUDES 1**   monoplegia of upper limbs due to sequela of cerebrovascular disease (I69.03-, I69.13-, I69.23-, I69.33-, I69.83-, I69.93-)

> **TIP:** If the documentation specifies the affected side but not whether it is the dominant or nondominant side, the default is as follows: for ambidextrous patients, the default is dominant; when the left side is affected, the default is nondominant; and when the right side is affected, the default is dominant.

> **G83.20 Monoplegia of upper limb affecting unspecified side**   HCC

> **G83.21 Monoplegia of upper limb affecting right dominant side**   HCC

> **G83.22 Monoplegia of upper limb affecting left dominant side**   HCC

> **G83.23 Monoplegia of upper limb affecting right nondominant side**   HCC

> **G83.24 Monoplegia of upper limb affecting left nondominant side**   HCC

√5ᵗʰ **G83.3 Monoplegia, unspecified**

> **TIP:** If the documentation specifies the affected side but not whether it is the dominant or nondominant side, the default is as follows: for ambidextrous patients, the default is dominant; when the left side is affected, the default is nondominant; and when the right side is affected, the default is dominant.

> **G83.30 Monoplegia, unspecified affecting unspecified side**   HCC

> **G83.31 Monoplegia, unspecified affecting right dominant side**   HCC

> **G83.32 Monoplegia, unspecified affecting left dominant side**   HCC

> **G83.33 Monoplegia, unspecified affecting right nondominant side**   HCC

> **G83.34 Monoplegia, unspecified affecting left nondominant side**   HCC

G83.4 Cauda equina syndrome   CC HCC
> Neurogenic bladder due to cauda equina syndrome
> **EXCLUDES 1**   cord bladder NOS (G95.89)
>   neurogenic bladder NOS (N31.9)

> **DEF:** Compression of the spinal nerve roots presenting with pain and tingling radiating down the buttocks, back of the thigh and calf, and into the foot in a sciatic manner with aching in the bladder, perineum, and sacrum. Loss of bowel and bladder control may also occur.

G83.5 Locked-in state   MCC HCC

√5ᵗʰ **G83.8 Other specified paralytic syndromes**
> **EXCLUDES 1**   paralytic syndromes due to current spinal cord injury — code to spinal cord injury (S14, S24, S34)

> **G83.81 Brown-Séquard syndrome**   HCC

> **G83.82 Anterior cord syndrome**   HCC

> **G83.83 Posterior cord syndrome**   HCC

> **G83.84 Todd's paralysis (postepileptic)**   HCC

> **G83.89 Other specified paralytic syndromes**   HCC

G83.9 Paralytic syndrome, unspecified   HCC

Other disorders of the nervous system (G89-G99)

√4ᵗʰ **G89 Pain, not elsewhere classified**
> Code also related psychological factors associated with pain (F45.42)
> **EXCLUDES 1**   generalized pain NOS (R52)
>   pain disorders exclusively related to psychological factors (F45.41)
>   pain NOS (R52)
> **EXCLUDES 2**   atypical face pain (G50.1)
>   headache syndromes (G44.-)
>   localized pain, unspecified type — code to pain by site, such as:
>   abdomen pain (R10.-)
>   back pain (M54.9)
>   breast pain (N64.4)
>   chest pain (R07.1-R07.9)
>   ear pain (H92.0-)
>   eye pain (H57.1)
>   headache ▶(R51.9)◀
>   joint pain (M25.5-)
>   limb pain (M79.6-)
>   lumbar region pain (M54.5)
>   painful urination (R30.9)
>   pelvic and perineal pain (R10.2)
>   renal colic (N23)
>   shoulder pain (M25.51-)
>   spine pain (M54.-)
>   throat pain (R07.0)
>   tongue pain (K14.6)
>   tooth pain (K08.8)
>   migraines (G43.-)
>   myalgia (M79.1-)
>   pain from prosthetic devices, implants, and grafts (T82.84, T83.84, T84.84, T85.84-)
>   phantom limb syndrome with pain (G54.6)
>   vulvar vestibulitis (N94.810)
>   vulvodynia (N94.81-)

G89.0 Central pain syndrome
> Déjérine-Roussy syndrome
> Myelopathic pain syndrome
> Thalamic pain syndrome (hyperesthetic)

√5ᵗʰ **G89.1 Acute pain, not elsewhere classified**

> **G89.11 Acute pain due to trauma**

> **G89.12 Acute post-thoracotomy pain**
> > Post-thoracotomy pain NOS

> **G89.18 Other acute postprocedural pain**
> > Postoperative pain NOS
> > Postprocedural pain NOS

√5ᵗʰ **G89.2 Chronic pain, not elsewhere classified**
> **EXCLUDES 1**   causalgia, lower limb (G57.7-)
>   causalgia, upper limb (G56.4-)
>   central pain syndrome (G89.0)
>   chronic pain syndrome (G89.4)
>   complex regional pain syndrome II, lower limb (G57.7-)
>   complex regional pain syndrome II, upper limb (G56.4-)
>   neoplasm related chronic pain (G89.3)
>   reflex sympathetic dystrophy (G90.5-)

> **G89.21 Chronic pain due to trauma**

> **G89.22 Chronic post-thoracotomy pain**

> **G89.28 Other chronic postprocedural pain**
> > Other chronic postoperative pain

> **G89.29 Other chronic pain**

☑ Additional Character Required   √x7ᵗʰ Placeholder   Unacceptable PDx   Questionable PDx   Manifestation   Unspecified Dx   H1-H14 HAC   HCC CMS-HCC Dx   HIV HIV Dx

ICD-10-CM 2021   587

Chapter 6. Diseases of the Nervous System

G89.3 Neoplasm related pain (acute) (chronic)
Cancer associated pain
Pain due to malignancy (primary) (secondary)
Tumor associated pain

G89.4 Chronic pain syndrome
Chronic pain associated with significant psychosocial dysfunction

✓4ᵗʰ G90 Disorders of autonomic nervous system
EXCLUDES 1   *dysfunction of the autonomic nervous system due to alcohol (G31.2)*

✓5ᵗʰ G90.0 Idiopathic peripheral autonomic neuropathy

     G90.01 Carotid sinus syncope
        Carotid sinus syndrome
        DEF: Vagal activation caused by pressure on the carotid sinus baroreceptors. Sympathetic nerve impulses may cause sinus arrest or AV block.

     G90.09 Other idiopathic peripheral autonomic neuropathy
        Idiopathic peripheral autonomic neuropathy NOS

G90.1 Familial dysautonomia [Riley-Day]   `HCC`

G90.2 Horner's syndrome
Bernard(-Horner) syndrome
Cervical sympathetic dystrophy or paralysis

G90.3 Multi-system degeneration of the autonomic nervous system   `CC` `HCC`
Neurogenic orthostatic hypotension [Shy-Drager]
    EXCLUDES 1   *orthostatic hypotension NOS (I95.1)*

G90.4 Autonomic dysreflexia
Use additional code to identify the cause, such as:
    fecal impaction (K56.41)
    pressure ulcer (pressure area) (L89.-)
    urinary tract infection (N39.0)

✓5ᵗʰ G90.5 Complex regional pain syndrome I (CRPS I)
Reflex sympathetic dystrophy
    EXCLUDES 1   *causalgia of lower limb (G57.7-)*
             causalgia of upper limb (G56.4-)
             complex regional pain syndrome II of lower limb (G57.7-)
             complex regional pain syndrome II of upper limb (G56.4-)

     G90.50 Complex regional pain syndrome I, unspecified   `CC`

     ✓6ᵗʰ G90.51 Complex regional pain syndrome I of upper limb

        G90.511 Complex regional pain syndrome I of right upper limb   `CC`

        G90.512 Complex regional pain syndrome I of left upper limb   `CC`

        G90.513 Complex regional pain syndrome I of upper limb, bilateral   `CC`

        G90.519 Complex regional pain syndrome I of unspecified upper limb   `CC`

     ✓6ᵗʰ G90.52 Complex regional pain syndrome I of lower limb

        G90.521 Complex regional pain syndrome I of right lower limb   `CC`

        G90.522 Complex regional pain syndrome I of left lower limb   `CC`

        G90.523 Complex regional pain syndrome I of lower limb, bilateral   `CC`

        G90.529 Complex regional pain syndrome I of unspecified lower limb   `CC`

     G90.59 Complex regional pain syndrome I of other specified site   `CC`

G90.8 Other disorders of autonomic nervous system

G90.9 Disorder of the autonomic nervous system, unspecified

✓4ᵗʰ G91 Hydrocephalus
INCLUDES   acquired hydrocephalus
EXCLUDES 1   *Arnold-Chiari syndrome with hydrocephalus (Q07.-)*
            congenital hydrocephalus (Q03.-)
            spina bifida with hydrocephalus (Q05.-)
DEF: Abnormal buildup of cerebrospinal fluid in the brain causing dilation of the ventricles.

Hydrocephalus (Acquired)

Normal ventricles   Hydrocephalic ventricles

G91.0 Communicating hydrocephalus   `CC` `HCC`
Secondary normal pressure hydrocephalus

G91.1 Obstructive hydrocephalus   `CC` `HCC`
DEF: Obstruction of the cerebrospinal fluid passage from the brain into the spinal canal characterized by headaches, drowsiness, poor coordination, urinary incontinence, nausea, vomiting, and papilledema.

G91.2 (Idiopathic) normal pressure hydrocephalus   `CC` `HCC`
Normal pressure hydrocephalus NOS

G91.3 Post-traumatic hydrocephalus, unspecified   `CC` `HCC`

G91.4 *Hydrocephalus in diseases classified elsewhere*   `HCC`
Code first underlying condition, such as:
    congenital syphilis (A50.4-)
    neoplasm (C00-D49)
    plasminogen deficiency (E88.02)
    EXCLUDES 1   *hydrocephalus due to congenital toxoplasmosis (P37.1)*
    AHA: 2014,3Q,3

G91.8 Other hydrocephalus   `CC` `HCC`

G91.9 Hydrocephalus, unspecified   `CC` `HCC`

G92 Toxic encephalopathy   `MCC`
Toxic encephalitis
Toxic metabolic encephalopathy
▶Code first, if applicable, drug induced (T36-T50) or use (T51-T65) to identify toxic agent◀
~~Code first (T51-T65) to identify toxic agent~~
AHA: 2017,1Q,39-40
DEF: Brain tissue degeneration due to a toxic substance.

✓4ᵗʰ G93 Other disorders of brain

G93.0 Cerebral cysts
Arachnoid cyst
Porencephalic cyst, acquired
    EXCLUDES 1   *acquired periventricular cysts of newborn (P91.1)*
            congenital cerebral cysts (Q04.6)

G93.1 Anoxic brain damage, not elsewhere classified   `CC` `HCC`
    EXCLUDES 1   *cerebral anoxia due to anesthesia during labor and delivery (O74.3)*
            cerebral anoxia due to anesthesia during the puerperium (O89.2)
            neonatal anoxia (P84)
DEF: Brain injury not resulting from birth trauma that is due to lack of oxygen. Brain cells, when deprived of oxygen; begin to expire after 4 minutes.

N Newborn: 0   P Pediatric: 0-17   M Maternity: 9-64   A Adult: 15-124   MCC Major Complication/Comorbidity   CC Complication/Comorbidity   SW Severe Wound Dx

588   ICD-10-CM 2021

G93.2 Benign intracranial hypertension
▶Pseudotumor◀
EXCLUDES 1   *hypertensive encephalopathy (I67.4)*
▶*obstructive hydrocephalus (G91.1)*◀

G93.3 Postviral fatigue syndrome
Benign myalgic encephalomyelitis
EXCLUDES 1   *chronic fatigue syndrome NOS (R53.82)*

√5ᵗʰ G93.4 Other and unspecified encephalopathy
EXCLUDES 1   *alcoholic encephalopathy (G31.2)*
encephalopathy in diseases classified elsewhere (G94)
hypertensive encephalopathy (I67.4)
toxic (metabolic) encephalopathy (G92)
EXCLUDES 2 ▶*toxic (metabolic) encephalopathy (G92)*◀

G93.40 Encephalopathy, unspecified   `HIV` `CC`
AHA: 2017,2Q,8

G93.41 Metabolic encephalopathy   `HIV` `MCC`
Septic encephalopathy
AHA: 2017,2Q,8; 2016,3Q,42; 2015,3Q,21
TIP: Assign separately when documented with diabetic hypoglycemia (E08.649, E09.649, E10.649, E11.649, E13.649).

G93.49 Other encephalopathy   `HIV` `CC`
Encephalopathy NEC
AHA: 2018,4Q,16; 2018,2Q,22,24; 2017,2Q,9

G93.5 Compression of brain   `MCC` `HCC`
Arnold-Chiari type 1 compression of brain
Compression of brain (stem)
Herniation of brain (stem)
EXCLUDES 1   *diffuse traumatic compression of brain (S06.2-)*
focal traumatic compression of brain (S06.3-)
AHA: 2020,2Q,31

G93.6 Cerebral edema   `MCC` `HCC`
EXCLUDES 1   *cerebral edema due to birth injury (P11.0)*
traumatic cerebral edema (S06.1-)

G93.7 Reye's syndrome   `MCC` `HCC` `P`
Code first poisoning due to salicylates, if applicable (T39.0-, with sixth character 1-4)
Use additional code for adverse effect due to salicylates, if applicable (T39.0-, with sixth character 5)
DEF: Rare childhood illness often developed after a viral upper respiratory infection. Symptoms include vomiting, elevated serum transaminase, brain swelling, disturbances of consciousness, seizures, and changes in liver and other viscera and it can be fatal.

√5ᵗʰ G93.8 Other specified disorders of brain

G93.81 Temporal sclerosis
Hippocampal sclerosis
Mesial temporal sclerosis

G93.82 Brain death   `MCC`

G93.89 Other specified disorders of brain
Postradiation encephalopathy
AHA: 2020,2Q,24; 2019,3Q,8

G93.9 Disorder of brain, unspecified   `HIV`

G94 Other disorders of brain in diseases classified elsewhere
Code first underlying disease
EXCLUDES 1   *encephalopathy in congenital syphilis (A50.49)*
encephalopathy in influenza (J09.X9, J10.81, J11.81)
encephalopathy in syphilis (A52.19)
hydrocephalus in diseases classified elsewhere (G91.4)
AHA: 2018,2Q,22; 2017,2Q,8-9

√4ᵗʰ G95 Other and unspecified diseases of spinal cord
EXCLUDES 2   *myelitis (G04.-)*

G95.0 Syringomyelia and syringobulbia   `CC` `HCC`

√5ᵗʰ G95.1 Vascular myelopathies
EXCLUDES 2   *intraspinal phlebitis and thrombophlebitis, except non-pyogenic (G08)*

G95.11 Acute infarction of spinal cord (embolic) (nonembolic)   `MCC` `HCC`
Anoxia of spinal cord
Arterial thrombosis of spinal cord

G95.19 Other vascular myelopathies   `MCC` `HCC`
Edema of spinal cord
Hematomyelia
Nonpyogenic intraspinal phlebitis and thrombophlebitis
Subacute necrotic myelopathy

√5ᵗʰ G95.2 Other and unspecified cord compression

G95.20 Unspecified cord compression   `HIV` `CC` `HCC`

G95.29 Other cord compression   `HIV` `CC` `HCC`

√5ᵗʰ G95.8 Other specified diseases of spinal cord
EXCLUDES 1   *neurogenic bladder NOS (N31.9)*
neurogenic bladder due to cauda equina syndrome (G83.4)
neuromuscular dysfunction of bladder without spinal cord lesion (N31.-)

G95.81 Conus medullaris syndrome   `CC` `HCC`

G95.89 Other specified diseases of spinal cord   `CC` `HCC`
Cord bladder NOS
Drug-induced myelopathy
Radiation-induced myelopathy
EXCLUDES 1   *myelopathy NOS (G95.9)*

G95.9 Disease of spinal cord, unspecified   `HIV` `CC` `HCC`
Myelopathy NOS

√4ᵗʰ G96 Other disorders of central nervous system
▶Code also if applicable:◀
▶intracranial hypotension (G96.81-)◀

▲ **√5ᵗʰ G96.0 Cerebrospinal fluid leak**
▶Code also if applicable:◀
▶intracranial hypotension (G96.81-)◀
EXCLUDES 1   *cerebrospinal fluid leak from spinal puncture (G97.0)*
AHA: 2018,2Q,13
DEF: Cerebrospinal fluid discharging from the nose or the ear caused by a fracture of the frontal bone with tearing of dura mater and arachnoid. It is characterized by watery drainage usually from only one side of the nose or one ear, headache, vision changes, and hearing loss.

G96.00 Cerebrospinal fluid leak, unspecified   `CC`
Code also if applicable:
head injury (S00.- to S09.-)

G96.01 Cranial cerebrospinal fluid leak, spontaneous   `CC`
Otorrhea due to spontaneous cerebrospinal fluid CSF leak
Rhinorrhea due to spontaneous cerebrospinal fluid CSF leak
Spontaneous cerebrospinal fluid leak from skull base

G96.02 Spinal cerebrospinal fluid leak, spontaneous   `CC`
Spontaneous cerebrospinal fluid leak from spine

G96.08 Other cranial cerebrospinal fluid leak   `CC`
Postoperative cranial cerebrospinal fluid leak
Traumatic cranial cerebrospinal fluid leak
Code also if applicable:
head injury (S00.- to S09.-)

G96.09 Other spinal cerebrospinal fluid leak   `CC`
Other spinal CSF leak
Postoperative spinal cerebrospinal fluid leak
Traumatic spinal cerebrospinal fluid leak
Code also if applicable:
head injury (S00.- to S09.-)

√5ᵗʰ G96.1 Disorders of meninges, not elsewhere classified

G96.11 Dural tear   `CC`
▶Code also intracranial hypotension, if applicable (G96.81-)◀
EXCLUDES 1   *accidental puncture or laceration of dura during a procedure (G97.41)*
AHA: 2014,4Q,24

G96.12 Meningeal adhesions (cerebral) (spinal)

▲ **√6ᵗʰ G96.19 Other disorders of meninges, not elsewhere classified**

G96.191 Perineural cyst
Cervical nerve root cyst
Lumbar nerve root cyst
Sacral nerve root cyst
Tarlov cyst
Thoracic nerve root cyst

☑ Additional Character Required   √x7ᵗʰ Placeholder   Unacceptable PDx   Questionable PDx   Manifestation   Unspecified Dx   H1-H14 HAC   HCC CMS-HCC Dx   HIV HIV Dx

ICD-10-CM 2021   589

- **G96.198** **Other disorders of meninges, not elsewhere classified**

▲ ✓5ᵗʰ **G96.8** **Other specified disorders of central nervous system**

- ✓6ᵗʰ **G96.81** Intracranial hypotension

  Code also any associated diagnoses, such as:
  brachial amyotrophy (G54.5)
  cerebrospinal fluid leak from spine (G96.02)
  cranial nerve disorders in diseases classified elsewhere (G53)
  nerve root and compressions in diseases classified elsewhere (G55)
  nonpyogenic thrombosis of intracranial venous system (I67.6)
  nontraumatic intracerebral hemorrhage (I61.-)
  nontraumatic subdural hemorrhage (I62.0-)
  other and unspecified cord compression (G95.2-)
  other secondary parkinsonism (G21.8)
  reversible cerebrovascular vasoconstriction syndrome (I67.841)
  spinal cord herniation (G95.89)
  stroke (I63.-)
  syringomyelia (G95.0)

- **G96.810** Intracranial hypotension, unspecified
- **G96.811** Intracranial hypotension, spontaneous
- **G96.819** Other intracranial hypotension

  G96.89 Other specified disorders of central nervous system

  G96.9 Disorder of central nervous system, unspecified `HIV`

✓4ᵗʰ **G97** **Intraoperative and postprocedural complications and disorders of nervous system, not elsewhere classified**

  `EXCLUDES 2` intraoperative and postprocedural cerebrovascular infarction (I97.81-, I97.82-)

  AHA: 2016,4Q,9-10

  G97.0 **Cerebrospinal fluid leak from spinal puncture** `CC`
  ▶Code also any associated diagnoses or complications, such as:◀
  ▶intracranial hypotension following a procedure (G97.83-G97.84)◀

Spinal Puncture

- Spinal cord
- Epidural space
- Subarachnoid space
- Vertebra
- Spinal needle

Lumbar area

  G97.1 **Other reaction to spinal and lumbar puncture**
  Headache due to lumbar puncture
  ▶Other reaction to spinal dural puncture◀
  ▶Code also, if applicable, any associated headache with orthostatic component (R51.0)◀

  G97.2 **Intracranial hypotension following ventricular shunting** `CC`
  ▶Code also any associated diagnoses or complications◀

✓5ᵗʰ **G97.3** **Intraoperative hemorrhage and hematoma of a nervous system organ or structure complicating a procedure**
  `EXCLUDES 1` intraoperative hemorrhage and hematoma of a nervous system organ or structure due to accidental puncture and laceration during a procedure (G97.4-)

  G97.31 **Intraoperative hemorrhage and hematoma of a nervous system organ or structure complicating a nervous system procedure** `CC`

  G97.32 **Intraoperative hemorrhage and hematoma of a nervous system organ or structure complicating other procedure** `CC`

✓5ᵗʰ **G97.4** **Accidental puncture and laceration of a nervous system organ or structure during a procedure**

  G97.41 **Accidental puncture or laceration of dura during a procedure** `CC`
  Incidental (inadvertent) durotomy
  ▶Code also any associated diagnoses or complications◀
  AHA: 2014,4Q,24

  G97.48 **Accidental puncture and laceration of other nervous system organ or structure during a nervous system procedure** `CC`

  G97.49 **Accidental puncture and laceration of other nervous system organ or structure during other procedure** `CC`

✓5ᵗʰ **G97.5** **Postprocedural hemorrhage of a nervous system organ or structure following a procedure**

  G97.51 **Postprocedural hemorrhage of a nervous system organ or structure following a nervous system procedure** `CC`

  G97.52 **Postprocedural hemorrhage of a nervous system organ or structure following other procedure** `CC`

✓5ᵗʰ **G97.6** **Postprocedural hematoma and seroma of a nervous system organ or structure following a procedure**

  G97.61 **Postprocedural hematoma of a nervous system organ or structure following a nervous system procedure** `CC`

  G97.62 **Postprocedural hematoma of a nervous system organ or structure following other procedure** `CC`

  G97.63 **Postprocedural seroma of a nervous system organ or structure following a nervous system procedure** `CC`

  G97.64 **Postprocedural seroma of a nervous system organ or structure following other procedure** `CC`

✓5ᵗʰ **G97.8** **Other intraoperative and postprocedural complications and disorders of nervous system**
  Use additional code to further specify disorder

  G97.81 **Other intraoperative complications of nervous system** `CC`

  G97.82 **Other postprocedural complications and disorders of nervous system** `CC`

- **G97.83** **Intracranial hypotension following lumbar cerebrospinal fluid shunting** `CC`
  Code also any associated diagnoses or complications

- **G97.84** **Intracranial hypotension following other procedure** `CC`
  Code also, if applicable:
  accidental puncture or laceration of dura during a procedure (G97.41)
  cerebrospinal fluid leak from spinal puncture (G97.0)

✓4ᵗʰ **G98** **Other disorders of nervous system not elsewhere classified**
  `INCLUDES` nervous system disorder NOS

  G98.0 **Neurogenic arthritis, not elsewhere classified**
  Nonsyphilitic neurogenic arthropathy NEC
  Nonsyphilitic neurogenic spondylopathy NEC
  `EXCLUDES 1` spondylopathy (in):
  syringomyelia and syringobulbia (G95.0)
  tabes dorsalis (A52.11)

  G98.8 **Other disorders of nervous system** `HIV`
  Nervous system disorder NOS

✓4ᵗʰ **G99** **Other disorders of nervous system in diseases classified elsewhere**

  G99.0 *Autonomic neuropathy in diseases classified elsewhere* `CC`
  Code first underlying disease, such as:
  amyloidosis (E85.-)
  gout (M1A.-, M10.-)
  hyperthyroidism (E05.-)
  `EXCLUDES 1` diabetic autonomic neuropathy (E08-E13 with .43)

`N` Newborn: 0 `P` Pediatric: 0-17 `M` Maternity: 9-64 `A` Adult: 15-124 `MCC` Major Complication/Comorbidity `CC` Complication/Comorbidity `SW` Severe Wound Dx

590   ICD-10-CM 2021

G99.2 **Myelopathy in diseases classified elsewhere**   `CC` `HCC`
Code first underlying disease, such as:
neoplasm (C00-D49)
EXCLUDES 1   myelopathy in:
intervertebral disease (M50.0-, M51.0-)
spondylosis (M47.0-, M47.1-)
AHA: 2018,3Q,18-19
TIP: Use this code in addition to a spondylolisthesis code (M43.1-)
or a spinal stenosis code (M48.0-) when either of these disorders
is documented as the cause of the myelopathy.

G99.8 **Other specified disorders of nervous system in diseases classified elsewhere**
Code first underlying disorder, such as:
amyloidosis (E85.-)
avitaminosis (E56.9)
EXCLUDES 1   nervous system involvement in:
cysticercosis (B69.0)
rubella (B06.0-)
syphilis (A52.1-)

G99.2 **Myelopathy in diseases classified elsewhere**   `CC` `HCC`

Chapter 7. Diseases of the Eye and Adnexa (H00–H59)

Chapter-specific Guidelines with Coding Examples

The chapter-specific guidelines from the ICD-10-CM Official Guidelines for Coding and Reporting have been provided below. Along with these guidelines are coding examples, contained in the shaded boxes, that have been developed to help illustrate the coding and/or sequencing guidance found in these guidelines.

a. Glaucoma

1) Assigning glaucoma codes

Assign as many codes from category H40, Glaucoma, as needed to identify the type of glaucoma, the affected eye, and the glaucoma stage.

2) Bilateral glaucoma with same type and stage

When a patient has bilateral glaucoma and both eyes are documented as being the same type and stage, and there is a code for bilateral glaucoma, report only the code for the type of glaucoma, bilateral, with the seventh character for the stage.

> Bilateral severe stage pigmentary glaucoma
>
> **H40.1333   Pigmentary glaucoma, bilateral, severe stage**
>
> *Explanation*: In this scenario, the patient has the same type and stage of glaucoma in both eyes. As this type of glaucoma has a code for bilateral, assign only the code for the bilateral glaucoma with the seventh character for the stage.

When a patient has bilateral glaucoma and both eyes are documented as being the same type and stage, and the classification does not provide a code for bilateral glaucoma (i.e. subcategories H40.10 and H40.20) report only one code for the type of glaucoma with the appropriate seventh character for the stage.

> Bilateral open-angle glaucoma; not specified as to type and stage indeterminate in both eyes
>
> **H40.10X4   Unspecified open-angle glaucoma, indeterminate stage**
>
> *Explanation*: In this scenario, the patient has glaucoma of the same type and stage of both eyes, but there is no code specifically for bilateral glaucoma. Only one code is assigned with the appropriate seventh character for the stage.

3) Bilateral glaucoma stage with different types or stages

When a patient has bilateral glaucoma and each eye is documented as having a different type or stage, and the classification distinguishes laterality, assign the appropriate code for each eye rather than the code for bilateral glaucoma.

When a patient has bilateral glaucoma and each eye is documented as having a different type, and the classification does not distinguish laterality (i.e. subcategories H40.10 and H40.20), assign one code for each type of glaucoma with the appropriate seventh character for the stage.

> Documentation relates mild, unspecified primary angle-closure glaucoma of the left eye with mild unspecified open-angle glaucoma of the right eye
>
> **H40.20X1   Unspecified primary angle-closure glaucoma, mild stage**
>
> **H40.10X1   Unspecified open-angle glaucoma, mild stage**
>
> *Explanation*: In this scenario the patient has a different type of glaucoma in each eye and the classification does not distinguish laterality. A code for each type of glaucoma is assigned, each with the appropriate seventh character for the stage.

When a patient has bilateral glaucoma and each eye is documented as having the same type, but different stage, and the classification does not distinguish laterality (i.e. subcategories H40.10 and H40.20), assign a code for the type of glaucoma for each eye with the seventh character for the specific glaucoma stage documented for each eye.

> Bilateral open-angle glaucoma, not specified as to type; the right eye is documented to be in mild stage and the left eye as being in moderate stage
>
> **H40.10X1   Unspecified open-angle glaucoma, mild stage**
>
> **H40.10X2   Unspecified open-angle glaucoma, moderate stage**
>
> *Explanation*: In this scenario the patient has the same type of glaucoma in each eye but each eye is at a different stage, and the classification does not distinguish laterality at this subcategory level. Two codes are assigned; both codes represent the same type of glaucoma but each has a different seventh character identifying the appropriate stage for each eye.

4) Patient admitted with glaucoma and stage evolves during the admission

If a patient is admitted with glaucoma and the stage progresses during the admission, assign the code for highest stage documented.

> Patient admitted with mild low-tension glaucoma of the right eye, which progresses to moderate stage during the patient's stay
>
> **H40.1212   Low-tension glaucoma, right eye, moderate stage**
>
> *Explanation*: When the glaucoma stage progresses during an admission, assign only the code for the highest stage documented.

5) Indeterminate stage glaucoma

Assignment of the seventh character "4" for "indeterminate stage" should be based on the clinical documentation. The seventh character "4" is used for glaucomas whose stage cannot be clinically determined. This seventh character should not be confused with the seventh character "0", unspecified, which should be assigned when there is no documentation regarding the stage of the glaucoma.

b. Blindness

If "blindness" or "low vision" of both eyes is documented but the visual impairment category is not documented, assign code H54.3, Unqualified visual loss, both eyes. If "blindness" or "low vision" in one eye is documented but the visual impairment category is not documented, assign a code from H54.6-, Unqualified visual loss, one eye. If "blindness" or "visual loss" is documented without any information about whether one or both eyes are affected, assign code H54.7, Unspecified visual loss.

> Blindness in 89-year-old male
>
> **H54.7   Unspecified visual loss**
>
> *Explanation*: Blindness is stated, but there is no mention of whether one or both eyes are affected or the severity of this visual impairment.

Chapter 7. Diseases of the Eye and Adnexa (H00-H59)

NOTE Use an external cause code following the code for the eye condition, if applicable, to identify the cause of the eye condition

EXCLUDES 2 certain conditions originating in the perinatal period (P04-P96)
certain infectious and parasitic diseases (A00-B99)
complications of pregnancy, childbirth and the puerperium (O00-O9A)
congenital malformations, deformations, and chromosomal abnormalities (Q00-Q99)
diabetes mellitus related eye conditions (E09.3-, E10.3-, E11.3-, E13.3-)
endocrine, nutritional and metabolic diseases (E00-E88)
injury (trauma) of eye and orbit (S05.-)
injury, poisoning and certain other consequences of external causes (S00-T88)
neoplasms (C00-D49)
symptoms, signs and abnormal clinical and laboratory findings, not elsewhere classified (R00-R94)
syphilis related eye disorders (A50.01, A50.3-, A51.43, A52.71)

This chapter contains the following blocks:

H00-H05 Disorders of eyelid, lacrimal system and orbit
H10-H11 Disorders of conjunctiva
H15-H22 Disorders of sclera, cornea, iris and ciliary body
H25-H28 Disorders of lens
H30-H36 Disorders of choroid and retina
H40-H42 Glaucoma
H43-H44 Disorders of vitreous body and globe
H46-H47 Disorders of optic nerve and visual pathways
H49-H52 Disorders of ocular muscles, binocular movement, accommodation and refraction
H53-H54 Visual disturbances and blindness
H55-H57 Other disorders of eye and adnexa
H59 Intraoperative and postprocedural complications and disorders of eye and adnexa, not elsewhere classified

Disorders of eyelid, lacrimal system and orbit (H00-H05)

EXCLUDES 2 open wound of eyelid (S01.1-)
superficial injury of eyelid (S00.1-, S00.2-)

✓4ᵗʰ H00 Hordeolum and chalazion

✓5ᵗʰ H00.0 Hordeolum (externum) (internum) of eyelid

DEF: Acute localized infection of the gland of Zeis (external hordeolum) or Molt or of the meibomian glands (internal hordeolum) of the orbit.

✓6ᵗʰ H00.01 Hordeolum externum

Hordeolum NOS
Stye

H00.011 Hordeolum externum right upper eyelid
H00.012 Hordeolum externum right lower eyelid
H00.013 Hordeolum externum right eye, unspecified eyelid
H00.014 Hordeolum externum left upper eyelid
H00.015 Hordeolum externum left lower eyelid
H00.016 Hordeolum externum left eye, unspecified eyelid
H00.019 Hordeolum externum unspecified eye, unspecified eyelid

✓6ᵗʰ H00.02 Hordeolum internum

Infection of meibomian gland

H00.021 Hordeolum internum right upper eyelid
H00.022 Hordeolum internum right lower eyelid
H00.023 Hordeolum internum right eye, unspecified eyelid
H00.024 Hordeolum internum left upper eyelid
H00.025 Hordeolum internum left lower eyelid
H00.026 Hordeolum internum left eye, unspecified eyelid
H00.029 Hordeolum internum unspecified eye, unspecified eyelid

✓6ᵗʰ H00.03 Abscess of eyelid

Furuncle of eyelid

H00.031 Abscess of right upper eyelid
H00.032 Abscess of right lower eyelid
H00.033 Abscess of eyelid right eye, unspecified eyelid
H00.034 Abscess of left upper eyelid
H00.035 Abscess of left lower eyelid
H00.036 Abscess of eyelid left eye, unspecified eyelid
H00.039 Abscess of eyelid unspecified eye, unspecified eyelid

✓5ᵗʰ H00.1 Chalazion

Meibomian (gland) cyst

EXCLUDES 2 infected meibomian gland (H00.02-)

DEF: Noninfectious, obstructive mass in the oil gland of the eyelid that results in a small chronic lump or inflammation.

H00.11 Chalazion right upper eyelid
H00.12 Chalazion right lower eyelid
H00.13 Chalazion right eye, unspecified eyelid
H00.14 Chalazion left upper eyelid
H00.15 Chalazion left lower eyelid
H00.16 Chalazion left eye, unspecified eyelid
H00.19 Chalazion unspecified eye, unspecified eyelid

✓4ᵗʰ H01 Other inflammation of eyelid

✓5ᵗʰ H01.0 Blepharitis

EXCLUDES 1 blepharoconjunctivitis (H10.5-)

✓6ᵗʰ H01.00 Unspecified blepharitis

AHA: 2018,4Q,13

H01.001 Unspecified blepharitis right upper eyelid
H01.002 Unspecified blepharitis right lower eyelid
H01.003 Unspecified blepharitis right eye, unspecified eyelid
H01.004 Unspecified blepharitis left upper eyelid
H01.005 Unspecified blepharitis left lower eyelid
H01.006 Unspecified blepharitis left eye, unspecified eyelid
H01.009 Unspecified blepharitis unspecified eye, unspecified eyelid
H01.00A Unspecified blepharitis right eye, upper and lower eyelids
H01.00B Unspecified blepharitis left eye, upper and lower eyelids

✓6ᵗʰ H01.01 Ulcerative blepharitis

AHA: 2018,4Q,13

H01.011 Ulcerative blepharitis right upper eyelid
H01.012 Ulcerative blepharitis right lower eyelid
H01.013 Ulcerative blepharitis right eye, unspecified eyelid
H01.014 Ulcerative blepharitis left upper eyelid
H01.015 Ulcerative blepharitis left lower eyelid
H01.016 Ulcerative blepharitis left eye, unspecified eyelid
H01.019 Ulcerative blepharitis unspecified eye, unspecified eyelid
H01.01A Ulcerative blepharitis right eye, upper and lower eyelids
H01.01B Ulcerative blepharitis left eye, upper and lower eyelids

✓6ᵗʰ H01.02 Squamous blepharitis

AHA: 2018,4Q,13

H01.021 Squamous blepharitis right upper eyelid
H01.022 Squamous blepharitis right lower eyelid
H01.023 Squamous blepharitis right eye, unspecified eyelid
H01.024 Squamous blepharitis left upper eyelid
H01.025 Squamous blepharitis left lower eyelid
H01.026 Squamous blepharitis left eye, unspecified eyelid
H01.029 Squamous blepharitis unspecified eye, unspecified eyelid
H01.02A Squamous blepharitis right eye, upper and lower eyelids
H01.02B Squamous blepharitis left eye, upper and lower eyelids

✓5ᵗʰ H01.1 Noninfectious dermatoses of eyelid

✓6ᵗʰ H01.11 Allergic dermatitis of eyelid

Contact dermatitis of eyelid

H01.111 Allergic dermatitis of right upper eyelid
H01.112 Allergic dermatitis of right lower eyelid
H01.113 Allergic dermatitis of right eye, unspecified eyelid
H01.114 Allergic dermatitis of left upper eyelid
H01.115 Allergic dermatitis of left lower eyelid
H01.116 Allergic dermatitis of left eye, unspecified eyelid
H01.119 Allergic dermatitis of unspecified eye, unspecified eyelid

✓6ᵗʰ **H01.12 Discoid lupus erythematosus of eyelid**
     H01.121 Discoid lupus erythematosus of right upper eyelid
     H01.122 Discoid lupus erythematosus of right lower eyelid
     H01.123 Discoid lupus erythematosus of right eye, unspecified eyelid
     H01.124 Discoid lupus erythematosus of left upper eyelid
     H01.125 Discoid lupus erythematosus of left lower eyelid
     H01.126 Discoid lupus erythematosus of left eye, unspecified eyelid
     H01.129 Discoid lupus erythematosus of unspecified eye, unspecified eyelid

✓6ᵗʰ **H01.13 Eczematous dermatitis of eyelid**
     H01.131 Eczematous dermatitis of right upper eyelid
     H01.132 Eczematous dermatitis of right lower eyelid
     H01.133 Eczematous dermatitis of right eye, unspecified eyelid
     H01.134 Eczematous dermatitis of left upper eyelid
     H01.135 Eczematous dermatitis of left lower eyelid
     H01.136 Eczematous dermatitis of left eye, unspecified eyelid
     H01.139 Eczematous dermatitis of unspecified eye, unspecified eyelid

✓6ᵗʰ **H01.14 Xeroderma of eyelid**
     H01.141 Xeroderma of right upper eyelid
     H01.142 Xeroderma of right lower eyelid
     H01.143 Xeroderma of right eye, unspecified eyelid
     H01.144 Xeroderma of left upper eyelid
     H01.145 Xeroderma of left lower eyelid
     H01.146 Xeroderma of left eye, unspecified eyelid
     H01.149 Xeroderma of unspecified eye, unspecified eyelid

H01.8 Other specified inflammations of eyelid

H01.9 Unspecified inflammation of eyelid
     Inflammation of eyelid NOS

✓4ᵗʰ **H02 Other disorders of eyelid**
     EXCLUDES 1   congenital malformations of eyelid (Q10.0-Q10.3)

Entropion and Ectropion

Normal eyelid   Entropion   Ectropion

✓5ᵗʰ **H02.0 Entropion and trichiasis of eyelid**
     DEF: Entropion: Inversion of the eyelid, turning the edge in toward the eyeball and causing irritation from contact of the lashes with the surface of the eye.
     DEF: Trichiasis: Condition wherein the eyelid is in a normal position but lashes are ingrown or misdirected in their growth so that they irritate the tissues of the eye.

✓6ᵗʰ **H02.00 Unspecified entropion of eyelid**
     H02.001 Unspecified entropion of right upper eyelid
     H02.002 Unspecified entropion of right lower eyelid
     H02.003 Unspecified entropion of right eye, unspecified eyelid
     H02.004 Unspecified entropion of left upper eyelid
     H02.005 Unspecified entropion of left lower eyelid
     H02.006 Unspecified entropion of left eye, unspecified eyelid

     H02.009 Unspecified entropion of unspecified eye, unspecified eyelid

✓6ᵗʰ **H02.01 Cicatricial entropion of eyelid**
     H02.011 Cicatricial entropion of right upper eyelid
     H02.012 Cicatricial entropion of right lower eyelid
     H02.013 Cicatricial entropion of right eye, unspecified eyelid
     H02.014 Cicatricial entropion of left upper eyelid
     H02.015 Cicatricial entropion of left lower eyelid
     H02.016 Cicatricial entropion of left eye, unspecified eyelid
     H02.019 Cicatricial entropion of unspecified eye, unspecified eyelid

✓6ᵗʰ **H02.02 Mechanical entropion of eyelid**
     H02.021 Mechanical entropion of right upper eyelid
     H02.022 Mechanical entropion of right lower eyelid
     H02.023 Mechanical entropion of right eye, unspecified eyelid
     H02.024 Mechanical entropion of left upper eyelid
     H02.025 Mechanical entropion of left lower eyelid
     H02.026 Mechanical entropion of left eye, unspecified eyelid
     H02.029 Mechanical entropion of unspecified eye, unspecified eyelid

✓6ᵗʰ **H02.03 Senile entropion of eyelid**
     H02.031 Senile entropion of right upper eyelid   Ⓐ
     H02.032 Senile entropion of right lower eyelid   Ⓐ
     H02.033 Senile entropion of right eye, unspecified eyelid   Ⓐ
     H02.034 Senile entropion of left upper eyelid   Ⓐ
     H02.035 Senile entropion of left lower eyelid   Ⓐ
     H02.036 Senile entropion of left eye, unspecified eyelid
     H02.039 Senile entropion of unspecified eye, unspecified eyelid   Ⓐ

✓6ᵗʰ **H02.04 Spastic entropion of eyelid**
     H02.041 Spastic entropion of right upper eyelid
     H02.042 Spastic entropion of right lower eyelid
     H02.043 Spastic entropion of right eye, unspecified eyelid
     H02.044 Spastic entropion of left upper eyelid
     H02.045 Spastic entropion of left lower eyelid
     H02.046 Spastic entropion of left eye, unspecified eyelid
     H02.049 Spastic entropion of unspecified eye, unspecified eyelid

✓6ᵗʰ **H02.05 Trichiasis without entropion**
     H02.051 Trichiasis without entropion right upper eyelid
     H02.052 Trichiasis without entropion right lower eyelid
     H02.053 Trichiasis without entropion right eye, unspecified eyelid
     H02.054 Trichiasis without entropion left upper eyelid
     H02.055 Trichiasis without entropion left lower eyelid
     H02.056 Trichiasis without entropion left eye, unspecified eyelid
     H02.059 Trichiasis without entropion unspecified eye, unspecified eyelid

✓5ᵗʰ **H02.1 Ectropion of eyelid**
     DEF: Drooping of the lower eyelid away from the eye or outward turning or eversion of the edge of the eyelid, exposing the palpebral conjunctiva and causing irritation.

✓6ᵗʰ **H02.10 Unspecified ectropion of eyelid**
     H02.101 Unspecified ectropion of right upper eyelid
     H02.102 Unspecified ectropion of right lower eyelid
     H02.103 Unspecified ectropion of right eye, unspecified eyelid
     H02.104 Unspecified ectropion of left upper eyelid
     H02.105 Unspecified ectropion of left lower eyelid

Chapter 7. Diseases of the Eye and Adnexa

H02.106–H02.36

H02.106   Unspecified ectropion of left eye, unspecified eyelid

H02.109   Unspecified ectropion of unspecified eye, unspecified eyelid

✓6ᵗʰ **H02.11**   Cicatricial ectropion of eyelid

H02.111   Cicatricial ectropion of right upper eyelid

H02.112   Cicatricial ectropion of right lower eyelid

H02.113   Cicatricial ectropion of right eye, unspecified eyelid

H02.114   Cicatricial ectropion of left upper eyelid

H02.115   Cicatricial ectropion of left lower eyelid

H02.116   Cicatricial ectropion of left eye, unspecified eyelid

H02.119   Cicatricial ectropion of unspecified eye, unspecified eyelid

✓6ᵗʰ **H02.12**   Mechanical ectropion of eyelid

H02.121   Mechanical ectropion of right upper eyelid

H02.122   Mechanical ectropion of right lower eyelid

H02.123   Mechanical ectropion of right eye, unspecified eyelid

H02.124   Mechanical ectropion of left upper eyelid

H02.125   Mechanical ectropion of left lower eyelid

H02.126   Mechanical ectropion of left eye, unspecified eyelid

H02.129   Mechanical ectropion of unspecified eye, unspecified eyelid

✓6ᵗʰ **H02.13**   Senile ectropion of eyelid

H02.131   Senile ectropion of right upper eyelid   A

H02.132   Senile ectropion of right lower eyelid   A

H02.133   Senile ectropion of right eye, unspecified eyelid   A

H02.134   Senile ectropion of left upper eyelid   A

H02.135   Senile ectropion of left lower eyelid   A

H02.136   Senile ectropion of left eye, unspecified eyelid   A

H02.139   Senile ectropion of unspecified eye, unspecified eyelid   A

✓6ᵗʰ **H02.14**   Spastic ectropion of eyelid

H02.141   Spastic ectropion of right upper eyelid

H02.142   Spastic ectropion of right lower eyelid

H02.143   Spastic ectropion of right eye, unspecified eyelid

H02.144   Spastic ectropion of left upper eyelid

H02.145   Spastic ectropion of left lower eyelid

H02.146   Spastic ectropion of left eye, unspecified eyelid

H02.149   Spastic ectropion of unspecified eye, unspecified eyelid

✓6ᵗʰ **H02.15**   Paralytic ectropion of eyelid

AHA: 2018,4Q,13

H02.151   Paralytic ectropion of right upper eyelid

H02.152   Paralytic ectropion of right lower eyelid

H02.153   Paralytic ectropion of right eye, unspecified eyelid

H02.154   Paralytic ectropion of left upper eyelid

H02.155   Paralytic ectropion of left lower eyelid

H02.156   Paralytic ectropion of left eye, unspecified eyelid

H02.159   Paralytic ectropion of unspecified eye, unspecified eyelid

✓5ᵗʰ **H02.2**   Lagophthalmos

AHA: 2018,4Q,14

DEF: Condition of the eye that prevents it from closing completely.

✓6ᵗʰ **H02.20**   Unspecified lagophthalmos

H02.201   Unspecified lagophthalmos right upper eyelid

H02.202   Unspecified lagophthalmos right lower eyelid

H02.203   Unspecified lagophthalmos right eye, unspecified eyelid

H02.204   Unspecified lagophthalmos left upper eyelid

H02.205   Unspecified lagophthalmos left lower eyelid

H02.206   Unspecified lagophthalmos left eye, unspecified eyelid

H02.209   Unspecified lagophthalmos unspecified eye, unspecified eyelid

H02.20A   Unspecified lagophthalmos right eye, upper and lower eyelids

H02.20B   Unspecified lagophthalmos left eye, upper and lower eyelids

H02.20C   Unspecified lagophthalmos, bilateral, upper and lower eyelids

✓6ᵗʰ **H02.21**   Cicatricial lagophthalmos

H02.211   Cicatricial lagophthalmos right upper eyelid

H02.212   Cicatricial lagophthalmos right lower eyelid

H02.213   Cicatricial lagophthalmos right eye, unspecified eyelid

H02.214   Cicatricial lagophthalmos left upper eyelid

H02.215   Cicatricial lagophthalmos left lower eyelid

H02.216   Cicatricial lagophthalmos left eye, unspecified eyelid

H02.219   Cicatricial lagophthalmos unspecified eye, unspecified eyelid

H02.21A   Cicatricial lagophthalmos right eye, upper and lower eyelids

H02.21B   Cicatricial lagophthalmos left eye, upper and lower eyelids

H02.21C   Cicatricial lagophthalmos, bilateral, upper and lower eyelids

✓6ᵗʰ **H02.22**   Mechanical lagophthalmos

H02.221   Mechanical lagophthalmos right upper eyelid

H02.222   Mechanical lagophthalmos right lower eyelid

H02.223   Mechanical lagophthalmos right eye, unspecified eyelid

H02.224   Mechanical lagophthalmos left upper eyelid

H02.225   Mechanical lagophthalmos left lower eyelid

H02.226   Mechanical lagophthalmos left eye, unspecified eyelid

H02.229   Mechanical lagophthalmos unspecified eye, unspecified eyelid

H02.22A   Mechanical lagophthalmos right eye, upper and lower eyelids

H02.22B   Mechanical lagophthalmos left eye, upper and lower eyelids

H02.22C   Mechanical lagophthalmos, bilateral, upper and lower eyelids

✓6ᵗʰ **H02.23**   Paralytic lagophthalmos

H02.231   Paralytic lagophthalmos right upper eyelid

H02.232   Paralytic lagophthalmos right lower eyelid

H02.233   Paralytic lagophthalmos right eye, unspecified eyelid

H02.234   Paralytic lagophthalmos left upper eyelid

H02.235   Paralytic lagophthalmos left lower eyelid

H02.236   Paralytic lagophthalmos left eye, unspecified eyelid

H02.239   Paralytic lagophthalmos unspecified eye, unspecified eyelid

H02.23A   Paralytic lagophthalmos right eye, upper and lower eyelids

H02.23B   Paralytic lagophthalmos left eye, upper and lower eyelids

H02.23C   Paralytic lagophthalmos, bilateral, upper and lower eyelids

✓5ᵗʰ **H02.3**   Blepharochalasis

Pseudoptosis

DEF: Loss of elasticity and relaxation of skin of the eyelid, thickened or indurated skin on the eyelid associated with recurrent episodes of edema, and intracellular atrophy.

H02.30   Blepharochalasis unspecified eye, unspecified eyelid

H02.31   Blepharochalasis right upper eyelid

H02.32   Blepharochalasis right lower eyelid

H02.33   Blepharochalasis right eye, unspecified eyelid

H02.34   Blepharochalasis left upper eyelid

H02.35   Blepharochalasis left lower eyelid

H02.36   Blepharochalasis left eye, unspecified eyelid

N Newborn: 0   P Pediatric: 0-17   M Maternity: 9-64   A Adult: 15-124   MCC Major Complication/Comorbidity   CC Complication/Comorbidity   SW Severe Wound Dx

596   ICD-10-CM 2021

✓5ᵗʰ **H02.4 Ptosis of eyelid**

  ✓6ᵗʰ **H02.40 Unspecified ptosis of eyelid**

    H02.401 Unspecified ptosis of right eyelid
    H02.402 Unspecified ptosis of left eyelid
    H02.403 Unspecified ptosis of bilateral eyelids
    H02.409 Unspecified ptosis of unspecified eyelid

  ✓6ᵗʰ **H02.41 Mechanical ptosis of eyelid**

    H02.411 Mechanical ptosis of right eyelid
    H02.412 Mechanical ptosis of left eyelid
    H02.413 Mechanical ptosis of bilateral eyelids
    H02.419 Mechanical ptosis of unspecified eyelid

  ✓6ᵗʰ **H02.42 Myogenic ptosis of eyelid**

    H02.421 Myogenic ptosis of right eyelid
    H02.422 Myogenic ptosis of left eyelid
    H02.423 Myogenic ptosis of bilateral eyelids
    H02.429 Myogenic ptosis of unspecified eyelid

  ✓6ᵗʰ **H02.43 Paralytic ptosis of eyelid**

    Neurogenic ptosis of eyelid
    H02.431 Paralytic ptosis of right eyelid
    H02.432 Paralytic ptosis of left eyelid
    H02.433 Paralytic ptosis of bilateral eyelids
    H02.439 Paralytic ptosis unspecified eyelid

✓5ᵗʰ **H02.5 Other disorders affecting eyelid function**

    EXCLUDES 2   blepharospasm (G24.5)
          organic tic (G25.69)
          psychogenic tic (F95.-)

  ✓6ᵗʰ **H02.51 Abnormal innervation syndrome**

    H02.511 Abnormal innervation syndrome right upper eyelid
    H02.512 Abnormal innervation syndrome right lower eyelid
    H02.513 Abnormal innervation syndrome right eye, unspecified eyelid
    H02.514 Abnormal innervation syndrome left upper eyelid
    H02.515 Abnormal innervation syndrome left lower eyelid
    H02.516 Abnormal innervation syndrome left eye, unspecified eyelid
    H02.519 Abnormal innervation syndrome unspecified eye, unspecified eyelid

  ✓6ᵗʰ **H02.52 Blepharophimosis**

    Ankyloblepharon
    H02.521 Blepharophimosis right upper eyelid
    H02.522 Blepharophimosis right lower eyelid
    H02.523 Blepharophimosis right eye, unspecified eyelid
    H02.524 Blepharophimosis left upper eyelid
    H02.525 Blepharophimosis left lower eyelid
    H02.526 Blepharophimosis left eye, unspecified eyelid
    H02.529 Blepharophimosis unspecified eye, unspecified lid

  ✓6ᵗʰ **H02.53 Eyelid retraction**

    Eyelid lag
    H02.531 Eyelid retraction right upper eyelid
    H02.532 Eyelid retraction right lower eyelid
    H02.533 Eyelid retraction right eye, unspecified eyelid
    H02.534 Eyelid retraction left upper eyelid
    H02.535 Eyelid retraction left lower eyelid
    H02.536 Eyelid retraction left eye, unspecified eyelid
    H02.539 Eyelid retraction unspecified eye, unspecified lid

  H02.59 Other disorders affecting eyelid function

    Deficient blink reflex
    Sensory disorders

✓5ᵗʰ **H02.6 Xanthelasma of eyelid**

    DEF: Condition in which there are small yellow tumors that occur on the eyelid, usually appearing near the nose.

    H02.60 Xanthelasma of unspecified eye, unspecified eyelid
    H02.61 Xanthelasma of right upper eyelid
    H02.62 Xanthelasma of right lower eyelid
    H02.63 Xanthelasma of right eye, unspecified eyelid
    H02.64 Xanthelasma of left upper eyelid
    H02.65 Xanthelasma of left lower eyelid
    H02.66 Xanthelasma of left eye, unspecified eyelid

✓5ᵗʰ **H02.7 Other and unspecified degenerative disorders of eyelid and periocular area**

    H02.70 Unspecified degenerative disorders of eyelid and periocular area

  ✓6ᵗʰ **H02.71 Chloasma of eyelid and periocular area**

    Dyspigmentation of eyelid
    Hyperpigmentation of eyelid
    H02.711 Chloasma of right upper eyelid and periocular area
    H02.712 Chloasma of right lower eyelid and periocular area
    H02.713 Chloasma of right eye, unspecified eyelid and periocular area
    H02.714 Chloasma of left upper eyelid and periocular area
    H02.715 Chloasma of left lower eyelid and periocular area
    H02.716 Chloasma of left eye, unspecified eyelid and periocular area
    H02.719 Chloasma of unspecified eye, unspecified eyelid and periocular area

  ✓6ᵗʰ **H02.72 Madarosis of eyelid and periocular area**

    Hypotrichosis of eyelid
    H02.721 Madarosis of right upper eyelid and periocular area
    H02.722 Madarosis of right lower eyelid and periocular area
    H02.723 Madarosis of right eye, unspecified eyelid and periocular area
    H02.724 Madarosis of left upper eyelid and periocular area
    H02.725 Madarosis of left lower eyelid and periocular area
    H02.726 Madarosis of left eye, unspecified eyelid and periocular area
    H02.729 Madarosis of unspecified eye, unspecified eyelid and periocular area

  ✓6ᵗʰ **H02.73 Vitiligo of eyelid and periocular area**

    Hypopigmentation of eyelid
    H02.731 Vitiligo of right upper eyelid and periocular area
    H02.732 Vitiligo of right lower eyelid and periocular area
    H02.733 Vitiligo of right eye, unspecified eyelid and periocular area
    H02.734 Vitiligo of left upper eyelid and periocular area
    H02.735 Vitiligo of left lower eyelid and periocular area
    H02.736 Vitiligo of left eye, unspecified eyelid and periocular area
    H02.739 Vitiligo of unspecified eye, unspecified eyelid and periocular area

    H02.79 Other degenerative disorders of eyelid and periocular area

✓5ᵗʰ **H02.8 Other specified disorders of eyelid**

  ✓6ᵗʰ **H02.81 Retained foreign body in eyelid**

    Use additional code to identify the type of retained foreign body (Z18.-)
    EXCLUDES 1   laceration of eyelid with foreign body (S01.12-)
          retained intraocular foreign body (H44.6-, H44.7-)
          superficial foreign body of eyelid and periocular area (S00.25-)
    H02.811 Retained foreign body in right upper eyelid
    H02.812 Retained foreign body in right lower eyelid
    H02.813 Retained foreign body in right eye, unspecified eyelid
    H02.814 Retained foreign body in left upper eyelid
    H02.815 Retained foreign body in left lower eyelid
    H02.816 Retained foreign body in left eye, unspecified eyelid
    H02.819 Retained foreign body in unspecified eye, unspecified eyelid

  ✓6ᵗʰ **H02.82 Cysts of eyelid**

    Sebaceous cyst of eyelid
    H02.821 Cysts of right upper eyelid
    H02.822 Cysts of right lower eyelid

☑ Additional Character Required   ✓x7ᵗʰ Placeholder   Unacceptable PDx   Questionable PDx   Manifestation   Unspecified Dx   H1-H14 HAC   HCC CMS-HCC Dx   HIV HIV Dx

ICD-10-CM 2021   597

Chapter 7. Diseases of the Eye and Adnexa

H02.823–H04.151

H02.823   Cysts of right eye, unspecified eyelid
H02.824   Cysts of left upper eyelid
H02.825   Cysts of left lower eyelid
H02.826   Cysts of left eye, unspecified eyelid
H02.829   Cysts of unspecified eye, unspecified eyelid

✓6th H02.83   **Dermatochalasis of eyelid**

DEF: Acquired form of connective tissue disorder associated with decreased elastic tissue and abnormal elastin formation, resulting in loss of elasticity of the skin of the eyelid. It is generally associated with aging.

H02.831   Dermatochalasis of right upper eyelid
H02.832   Dermatochalasis of right lower eyelid
H02.833   Dermatochalasis of right eye, unspecified eyelid
H02.834   Dermatochalasis of left upper eyelid
H02.835   Dermatochalasis of left lower eyelid
H02.836   Dermatochalasis of left eye, unspecified eyelid
H02.839   Dermatochalasis of unspecified eye, unspecified eyelid

✓6th H02.84   **Edema of eyelid**

Hyperemia of eyelid

H02.841   Edema of right upper eyelid
H02.842   Edema of right lower eyelid
H02.843   Edema of right eye, unspecified eyelid
H02.844   Edema of left upper eyelid
H02.845   Edema of left lower eyelid
H02.846   Edema of left eye, unspecified eyelid
H02.849   Edema of unspecified eye, unspecified eyelid

✓6th H02.85   **Elephantiasis of eyelid**

H02.851   Elephantiasis of right upper eyelid
H02.852   Elephantiasis of right lower eyelid
H02.853   Elephantiasis of right eye, unspecified eyelid
H02.854   Elephantiasis of left upper eyelid
H02.855   Elephantiasis of left lower eyelid
H02.856   Elephantiasis of left eye, unspecified eyelid
H02.859   Elephantiasis of unspecified eye, unspecified eyelid

✓6th H02.86   **Hypertrichosis of eyelid**

H02.861   Hypertrichosis of right upper eyelid
H02.862   Hypertrichosis of right lower eyelid
H02.863   Hypertrichosis of right eye, unspecified eyelid
H02.864   Hypertrichosis of left upper eyelid
H02.865   Hypertrichosis of left lower eyelid
H02.866   Hypertrichosis of left eye, unspecified eyelid
H02.869   Hypertrichosis of unspecified eye, unspecified eyelid

✓6th H02.87   **Vascular anomalies of eyelid**

H02.871   Vascular anomalies of right upper eyelid
H02.872   Vascular anomalies of right lower eyelid
H02.873   Vascular anomalies of right eye, unspecified eyelid
H02.874   Vascular anomalies of left upper eyelid
H02.875   Vascular anomalies of left lower eyelid
H02.876   Vascular anomalies of left eye, unspecified eyelid
H02.879   Vascular anomalies of unspecified eye, unspecified eyelid

✓6th H02.88   **Meibomian gland dysfunction of eyelid**

AHA: 2018,4Q,14-15

H02.881   Meibomian gland dysfunction right upper eyelid
H02.882   Meibomian gland dysfunction right lower eyelid
H02.883   Meibomian gland dysfunction of right eye, unspecified eyelid
H02.884   Meibomian gland dysfunction left upper eyelid
H02.885   Meibomian gland dysfunction left lower eyelid
H02.886   Meibomian gland dysfunction of left eye, unspecified eyelid
H02.889   Meibomian gland dysfunction of unspecified eye, unspecified eyelid

H02.88A   Meibomian gland dysfunction right eye, upper and lower eyelids
H02.88B   Meibomian gland dysfunction left eye, upper and lower eyelids

H02.89   **Other specified disorders of eyelid**

Hemorrhage of eyelid

H02.9   **Unspecified disorder of eyelid**

Disorder of eyelid NOS

✓4th **H04**   **Disorders of lacrimal system**

EXCLUDES 1   congenital malformations of lacrimal system (Q10.4-Q10.6)

✓5th **H04.0**   **Dacryoadenitis**

DEF: Inflammation of the lacrimal gland.

✓6th H04.00   **Unspecified dacryoadenitis**

H04.001   Unspecified dacryoadenitis, right lacrimal gland
H04.002   Unspecified dacryoadenitis, left lacrimal gland
H04.003   Unspecified dacryoadenitis, bilateral lacrimal glands
H04.009   Unspecified dacryoadenitis, unspecified lacrimal gland

✓6th H04.01   **Acute dacryoadenitis**

H04.011   Acute dacryoadenitis, right lacrimal gland
H04.012   Acute dacryoadenitis, left lacrimal gland
H04.013   Acute dacryoadenitis, bilateral lacrimal glands
H04.019   Acute dacryoadenitis, unspecified lacrimal gland

✓6th H04.02   **Chronic dacryoadenitis**

H04.021   Chronic dacryoadenitis, right lacrimal gland
H04.022   Chronic dacryoadenitis, left lacrimal gland
H04.023   Chronic dacryoadenitis, bilateral lacrimal gland
H04.029   Chronic dacryoadenitis, unspecified lacrimal gland

✓6th H04.03   **Chronic enlargement of lacrimal gland**

H04.031   Chronic enlargement of right lacrimal gland
H04.032   Chronic enlargement of left lacrimal gland
H04.033   Chronic enlargement of bilateral lacrimal glands
H04.039   Chronic enlargement of unspecified lacrimal gland

✓5th **H04.1**   **Other disorders of lacrimal gland**

✓6th H04.11   **Dacryops**

H04.111   Dacryops of right lacrimal gland
H04.112   Dacryops of left lacrimal gland
H04.113   Dacryops of bilateral lacrimal glands
H04.119   Dacryops of unspecified lacrimal gland

✓6th H04.12   **Dry eye syndrome**

Tear film insufficiency, NOS

H04.121   Dry eye syndrome of right lacrimal gland
H04.122   Dry eye syndrome of left lacrimal gland
H04.123   Dry eye syndrome of bilateral lacrimal glands
H04.129   Dry eye syndrome of unspecified lacrimal gland

✓6th H04.13   **Lacrimal cyst**

Lacrimal cystic degeneration

H04.131   Lacrimal cyst, right lacrimal gland
H04.132   Lacrimal cyst, left lacrimal gland
H04.133   Lacrimal cyst, bilateral lacrimal glands
H04.139   Lacrimal cyst, unspecified lacrimal gland

✓6th H04.14   **Primary lacrimal gland atrophy**

H04.141   Primary lacrimal gland atrophy, right lacrimal gland
H04.142   Primary lacrimal gland atrophy, left lacrimal gland
H04.143   Primary lacrimal gland atrophy, bilateral lacrimal glands
H04.149   Primary lacrimal gland atrophy, unspecified lacrimal gland

✓6th H04.15   **Secondary lacrimal gland atrophy**

H04.151   Secondary lacrimal gland atrophy, right lacrimal gland

N Newborn: 0   P Pediatric: 0-17   M Maternity: 9-64   A Adult: 15-124   MCC Major Complication/Comorbidity   CC Complication/Comorbidity   SW Severe Wound Dx

598   ICD-10-CM 2021

H04.152 **Secondary lacrimal gland atrophy, left lacrimal gland**

H04.153 **Secondary lacrimal gland atrophy, bilateral lacrimal glands**

H04.159 **Secondary lacrimal gland atrophy, unspecified lacrimal gland**

✓6ᵗʰ H04.16 **Lacrimal gland dislocation**

H04.161 **Lacrimal gland dislocation, right lacrimal gland**

H04.162 **Lacrimal gland dislocation, left lacrimal gland**

H04.163 **Lacrimal gland dislocation, bilateral lacrimal glands**

H04.169 **Lacrimal gland dislocation, unspecified lacrimal gland**

H04.19 **Other specified disorders of lacrimal gland**

✓5ᵗʰ H04.2 **Epiphora**

DEF: Excessive tearing or overflow of tears down the cheeks often due to a stricture in the lacrimal passages but can be caused by other conditions.

✓6ᵗʰ H04.20 **Unspecified epiphora**

H04.201 **Unspecified epiphora, right side**

H04.202 **Unspecified epiphora, left side**

H04.203 **Unspecified epiphora, bilateral**

H04.209 **Unspecified epiphora, unspecified side**

✓6ᵗʰ H04.21 **Epiphora due to excess lacrimation**

H04.211 **Epiphora due to excess lacrimation, right lacrimal gland**

H04.212 **Epiphora due to excess lacrimation, left lacrimal gland**

H04.213 **Epiphora due to excess lacrimation, bilateral lacrimal glands**

H04.219 **Epiphora due to excess lacrimation, unspecified lacrimal gland**

✓6ᵗʰ H04.22 **Epiphora due to insufficient drainage**

H04.221 **Epiphora due to insufficient drainage, right side**

H04.222 **Epiphora due to insufficient drainage, left side**

H04.223 **Epiphora due to insufficient drainage, bilateral**

H04.229 **Epiphora due to insufficient drainage, unspecified side**

✓5ᵗʰ H04.3 **Acute and unspecified inflammation of lacrimal passages**

EXCLUDES 1 neonatal dacryocystitis (P39.1)

✓6ᵗʰ H04.30 **Unspecified dacryocystitis**

H04.301 **Unspecified dacryocystitis of right lacrimal passage**

H04.302 **Unspecified dacryocystitis of left lacrimal passage**

H04.303 **Unspecified dacryocystitis of bilateral lacrimal passages**

H04.309 **Unspecified dacryocystitis of unspecified lacrimal passage**

✓6ᵗʰ H04.31 **Phlegmonous dacryocystitis**

H04.311 **Phlegmonous dacryocystitis of right lacrimal passage**

H04.312 **Phlegmonous dacryocystitis of left lacrimal passage**

H04.313 **Phlegmonous dacryocystitis of bilateral lacrimal passages**

H04.319 **Phlegmonous dacryocystitis of unspecified lacrimal passage**

✓6ᵗʰ H04.32 **Acute dacryocystitis**

Acute dacryopericystitis

H04.321 **Acute dacryocystitis of right lacrimal passage**

H04.322 **Acute dacryocystitis of left lacrimal passage**

H04.323 **Acute dacryocystitis of bilateral lacrimal passages**

H04.329 **Acute dacryocystitis of unspecified lacrimal passage**

✓6ᵗʰ H04.33 **Acute lacrimal canaliculitis**

H04.331 **Acute lacrimal canaliculitis of right lacrimal passage**

H04.332 **Acute lacrimal canaliculitis of left lacrimal passage**

H04.333 **Acute lacrimal canaliculitis of bilateral lacrimal passages**

H04.339 **Acute lacrimal canaliculitis of unspecified lacrimal passage**

✓5ᵗʰ H04.4 **Chronic inflammation of lacrimal passages**

✓6ᵗʰ H04.41 **Chronic dacryocystitis**

H04.411 **Chronic dacryocystitis of right lacrimal passage**

H04.412 **Chronic dacryocystitis of left lacrimal passage**

H04.413 **Chronic dacryocystitis of bilateral lacrimal passages**

H04.419 **Chronic dacryocystitis of unspecified lacrimal passage**

✓6ᵗʰ H04.42 **Chronic lacrimal canaliculitis**

H04.421 **Chronic lacrimal canaliculitis of right lacrimal passage**

H04.422 **Chronic lacrimal canaliculitis of left lacrimal passage**

H04.423 **Chronic lacrimal canaliculitis of bilateral lacrimal passages**

H04.429 **Chronic lacrimal canaliculitis of unspecified lacrimal passage**

✓6ᵗʰ H04.43 **Chronic lacrimal mucocele**

H04.431 **Chronic lacrimal mucocele of right lacrimal passage**

H04.432 **Chronic lacrimal mucocele of left lacrimal passage**

H04.433 **Chronic lacrimal mucocele of bilateral lacrimal passages**

H04.439 **Chronic lacrimal mucocele of unspecified lacrimal passage**

✓5ᵗʰ H04.5 **Stenosis and insufficiency of lacrimal passages**

✓6ᵗʰ H04.51 **Dacryolith**

H04.511 **Dacryolith of right lacrimal passage**

H04.512 **Dacryolith of left lacrimal passage**

H04.513 **Dacryolith of bilateral lacrimal passages**

H04.519 **Dacryolith of unspecified lacrimal passage**

✓6ᵗʰ H04.52 **Eversion of lacrimal punctum**

H04.521 **Eversion of right lacrimal punctum**

H04.522 **Eversion of left lacrimal punctum**

H04.523 **Eversion of bilateral lacrimal punctum**

H04.529 **Eversion of unspecified lacrimal punctum**

✓6ᵗʰ H04.53 **Neonatal obstruction of nasolacrimal duct**

EXCLUDES 1 congenital stenosis and stricture of lacrimal duct (Q10.5)

H04.531 **Neonatal obstruction of right nasolacrimal duct** Ⓝ

H04.532 **Neonatal obstruction of left nasolacrimal duct** Ⓝ

H04.533 **Neonatal obstruction of bilateral nasolacrimal duct** Ⓝ

H04.539 **Neonatal obstruction of unspecified nasolacrimal duct** Ⓝ

✓6ᵗʰ H04.54 **Stenosis of lacrimal canaliculi**

H04.541 **Stenosis of right lacrimal canaliculi**

H04.542 **Stenosis of left lacrimal canaliculi**

H04.543 **Stenosis of bilateral lacrimal canaliculi**

H04.549 **Stenosis of unspecified lacrimal canaliculi**

✓6ᵗʰ H04.55 **Acquired stenosis of nasolacrimal duct**

H04.551 **Acquired stenosis of right nasolacrimal duct**

H04.552 **Acquired stenosis of left nasolacrimal duct**

H04.553 **Acquired stenosis of bilateral nasolacrimal duct**

H04.559 **Acquired stenosis of unspecified nasolacrimal duct**

✓6ᵗʰ H04.56 **Stenosis of lacrimal punctum**

H04.561 **Stenosis of right lacrimal punctum**

H04.562 **Stenosis of left lacrimal punctum**

H04.563 **Stenosis of bilateral lacrimal punctum**

H04.569 **Stenosis of unspecified lacrimal punctum**

✓6ᵗʰ H04.57 **Stenosis of lacrimal sac**

H04.571 **Stenosis of right lacrimal sac**

H04.572 **Stenosis of left lacrimal sac**

H04.573 **Stenosis of bilateral lacrimal sac**

H04.579 **Stenosis of unspecified lacrimal sac**

☑ Additional Character Required ✓ˣ⁷ᵗʰ Placeholder Unacceptable PDx Questionable PDx Manifestation Unspecified Dx ⌗1-⌗6 HAC ⌗⌗ᴄ CMS-HCC Dx ⌗ⁱᵛ HIV Dx

ICD-10-CM 2021 599

✓5ᵗʰ **H04.6　Other changes of lacrimal passages**

　✓6ᵗʰ **H04.61　Lacrimal fistula**

　　　H04.611　Lacrimal fistula right lacrimal passage　　**SW**

　　　H04.612　Lacrimal fistula left lacrimal passage　　**SW**

　　　H04.613　Lacrimal fistula bilateral lacrimal passages　　**SW**

　　　H04.619　Lacrimal fistula unspecified lacrimal passage　　**SW**

　　H04.69　Other changes of lacrimal passages

✓5ᵗʰ **H04.8　Other disorders of lacrimal system**

　✓6ᵗʰ **H04.81　Granuloma of lacrimal passages**

　　　H04.811　Granuloma of right lacrimal passage

　　　H04.812　Granuloma of left lacrimal passage

　　　H04.813　Granuloma of bilateral lacrimal passages

　　　H04.819　Granuloma of unspecified lacrimal passage

　　H04.89　Other disorders of lacrimal system

　H04.9　Disorder of lacrimal system, unspecified

✓4ᵗʰ **H05　Disorders of orbit**

　EXCLUDES 1　congenital malformation of orbit (Q10.7)

　✓5ᵗʰ **H05.0　Acute inflammation of orbit**

　　H05.00　Unspecified acute inflammation of orbit

　　✓6ᵗʰ **H05.01　Cellulitis of orbit**

　　　　Abscess of orbit

　　　　H05.011　Cellulitis of right orbit　　**CC**

　　　　H05.012　Cellulitis of left orbit　　**CC**

　　　　H05.013　Cellulitis of bilateral orbits　　**CC**

　　　　H05.019　Cellulitis of unspecified orbit　　**CC**

　　✓6ᵗʰ **H05.02　Osteomyelitis of orbit**

　　　　H05.021　Osteomyelitis of right orbit　　**CC**

　　　　H05.022　Osteomyelitis of left orbit　　**CC**

　　　　H05.023　Osteomyelitis of bilateral orbits　　**CC**

　　　　H05.029　Osteomyelitis of unspecified orbit　　**CC**

　　✓6ᵗʰ **H05.03　Periostitis of orbit**

　　　　H05.031　Periostitis of right orbit　　**CC**

　　　　H05.032　Periostitis of left orbit　　**CC**

　　　　H05.033　Periostitis of bilateral orbits　　**CC**

　　　　H05.039　Periostitis of unspecified orbit　　**CC**

　　✓6ᵗʰ **H05.04　Tenonitis of orbit**

　　　　H05.041　Tenonitis of right orbit

　　　　H05.042　Tenonitis of left orbit

　　　　H05.043　Tenonitis of bilateral orbits

　　　　H05.049　Tenonitis of unspecified orbit

　✓5ᵗʰ **H05.1　Chronic inflammatory disorders of orbit**

　　H05.10　Unspecified chronic inflammatory disorders of orbit

　　✓6ᵗʰ **H05.11　Granuloma of orbit**

　　　　Pseudotumor (inflammatory) of orbit

　　　　H05.111　Granuloma of right orbit

　　　　H05.112　Granuloma of left orbit

　　　　H05.113　Granuloma of bilateral orbits

　　　　H05.119　Granuloma of unspecified orbit

　　✓6ᵗʰ **H05.12　Orbital myositis**

　　　　H05.121　Orbital myositis, right orbit

　　　　H05.122　Orbital myositis, left orbit

　　　　H05.123　Orbital myositis, bilateral

　　　　H05.129　Orbital myositis, unspecified orbit

　✓5ᵗʰ **H05.2　Exophthalmic conditions**

　　H05.20　Unspecified exophthalmos

　　✓6ᵗʰ **H05.21　Displacement (lateral) of globe**

　　　　H05.211　Displacement (lateral) of globe, right eye

　　　　H05.212　Displacement (lateral) of globe, left eye

　　　　H05.213　Displacement (lateral) of globe, bilateral

　　　　H05.219　Displacement (lateral) of globe, unspecified eye

　　✓6ᵗʰ **H05.22　Edema of orbit**

　　　　Orbital congestion

　　　　H05.221　Edema of right orbit

　　　　H05.222　Edema of left orbit

　　　　H05.223　Edema of bilateral orbit

　　　　H05.229　Edema of unspecified orbit

　　✓6ᵗʰ **H05.23　Hemorrhage of orbit**

　　　　H05.231　Hemorrhage of right orbit

　　　　H05.232　Hemorrhage of left orbit

　　　　H05.233　Hemorrhage of bilateral orbit

　　　　H05.239　Hemorrhage of unspecified orbit

　　✓6ᵗʰ **H05.24　Constant exophthalmos**

　　　　H05.241　Constant exophthalmos, right eye

　　　　H05.242　Constant exophthalmos, left eye

　　　　H05.243　Constant exophthalmos, bilateral

　　　　H05.249　Constant exophthalmos, unspecified eye

　　✓6ᵗʰ **H05.25　Intermittent exophthalmos**

　　　　H05.251　Intermittent exophthalmos, right eye

　　　　H05.252　Intermittent exophthalmos, left eye

　　　　H05.253　Intermittent exophthalmos, bilateral

　　　　H05.259　Intermittent exophthalmos, unspecified eye

　　✓6ᵗʰ **H05.26　Pulsating exophthalmos**

　　　　H05.261　Pulsating exophthalmos, right eye

　　　　H05.262　Pulsating exophthalmos, left eye

　　　　H05.263　Pulsating exophthalmos, bilateral

　　　　H05.269　Pulsating exophthalmos, unspecified eye

　✓5ᵗʰ **H05.3　Deformity of orbit**

　　EXCLUDES 1　congenital deformity of orbit (Q10.7)

　　　　　　　hypertelorism (Q75.2)

　　H05.30　Unspecified deformity of orbit

　　✓6ᵗʰ **H05.31　Atrophy of orbit**

　　　　H05.311　Atrophy of right orbit

　　　　H05.312　Atrophy of left orbit

　　　　H05.313　Atrophy of bilateral orbit

　　　　H05.319　Atrophy of unspecified orbit

　　✓6ᵗʰ **H05.32　Deformity of orbit due to bone disease**

　　　　Code also associated bone disease

　　　　H05.321　Deformity of right orbit due to bone disease

　　　　H05.322　Deformity of left orbit due to bone disease

　　　　H05.323　Deformity of bilateral orbits due to bone disease

　　　　H05.329　Deformity of unspecified orbit due to bone disease

　　✓6ᵗʰ **H05.33　Deformity of orbit due to trauma or surgery**

　　　　H05.331　Deformity of right orbit due to trauma or surgery

　　　　H05.332　Deformity of left orbit due to trauma or surgery

　　　　H05.333　Deformity of bilateral orbits due to trauma or surgery

　　　　H05.339　Deformity of unspecified orbit due to trauma or surgery

　　✓6ᵗʰ **H05.34　Enlargement of orbit**

　　　　H05.341　Enlargement of right orbit

　　　　H05.342　Enlargement of left orbit

　　　　H05.343　Enlargement of bilateral orbits

　　　　H05.349　Enlargement of unspecified orbit

　　✓6ᵗʰ **H05.35　Exostosis of orbit**

　　　　H05.351　Exostosis of right orbit

　　　　H05.352　Exostosis of left orbit

　　　　H05.353　Exostosis of bilateral orbits

　　　　H05.359　Exostosis of unspecified orbit

　✓5ᵗʰ **H05.4　Enophthalmos**

　　✓6ᵗʰ **H05.40　Unspecified enophthalmos**

　　　　H05.401　Unspecified enophthalmos, right eye

　　　　H05.402　Unspecified enophthalmos, left eye

　　　　H05.403　Unspecified enophthalmos, bilateral

　　　　H05.409　Unspecified enophthalmos, unspecified eye

　　✓6ᵗʰ **H05.41　Enophthalmos due to atrophy of orbital tissue**

　　　　H05.411　Enophthalmos due to atrophy of orbital tissue, right eye

　　　　H05.412　Enophthalmos due to atrophy of orbital tissue, left eye

　　　　H05.413　Enophthalmos due to atrophy of orbital tissue, bilateral

　　　　H05.419　Enophthalmos due to atrophy of orbital tissue, unspecified eye

　　✓6ᵗʰ **H05.42　Enophthalmos due to trauma or surgery**

　　　　H05.421　Enophthalmos due to trauma or surgery, right eye

　　　　H05.422　Enophthalmos due to trauma or surgery, left eye

N Newborn: 0　　**P** Pediatric: 0-17　　**M** Maternity: 9-64　　**A** Adult: 15-124　　**MCC** Major Complication/Comorbidity　　**CC** Complication/Comorbidity　　**SW** Severe Wound Dx

ICD-10-CM 2021

H05.423 Enophthalmos due to trauma or surgery, bilateral

H05.429 Enophthalmos due to trauma or surgery, unspecified eye

✓5ᵗʰ **H05.5 Retained (old) foreign body following penetrating wound of orbit**

Retrobulbar foreign body

Use additional code to identify the type of retained foreign body (Z18.-)

EXCLUDES 1 current penetrating wound of orbit (S05.4-)

EXCLUDES 2 retained foreign body of eyelid (H02.81-)

retained intraocular foreign body (H44.6-, H44.7-)

H05.50 Retained (old) foreign body following penetrating wound of unspecified orbit

H05.51 Retained (old) foreign body following penetrating wound of right orbit

H05.52 Retained (old) foreign body following penetrating wound of left orbit

H05.53 Retained (old) foreign body following penetrating wound of bilateral orbits

✓5ᵗʰ **H05.8 Other disorders of orbit**

✓6ᵗʰ **H05.81 Cyst of orbit**

Encephalocele of orbit

H05.811 Cyst of right orbit

H05.812 Cyst of left orbit

H05.813 Cyst of bilateral orbits

H05.819 Cyst of unspecified orbit

✓6ᵗʰ **H05.82 Myopathy of extraocular muscles**

H05.821 Myopathy of extraocular muscles, right orbit

H05.822 Myopathy of extraocular muscles, left orbit

H05.823 Myopathy of extraocular muscles, bilateral

H05.829 Myopathy of extraocular muscles, unspecified orbit

H05.89 Other disorders of orbit

H05.9 Unspecified disorder of orbit

Disorders of conjunctiva (H10-H11)

✓4ᵗʰ **H10 Conjunctivitis**

EXCLUDES 1 keratoconjunctivitis (H16.2-)

✓5ᵗʰ **H10.0 Mucopurulent conjunctivitis**

✓6ᵗʰ **H10.01 Acute follicular conjunctivitis**

H10.011 Acute follicular conjunctivitis, right eye

H10.012 Acute follicular conjunctivitis, left eye

H10.013 Acute follicular conjunctivitis, bilateral

H10.019 Acute follicular conjunctivitis, unspecified eye

✓6ᵗʰ **H10.02 Other mucopurulent conjunctivitis**

H10.021 Other mucopurulent conjunctivitis, right eye

H10.022 Other mucopurulent conjunctivitis, left eye

H10.023 Other mucopurulent conjunctivitis, bilateral

H10.029 Other mucopurulent conjunctivitis, unspecified eye

✓5ᵗʰ **H10.1 Acute atopic conjunctivitis**

Acute papillary conjunctivitis

H10.10 Acute atopic conjunctivitis, unspecified eye

H10.11 Acute atopic conjunctivitis, right eye

H10.12 Acute atopic conjunctivitis, left eye

H10.13 Acute atopic conjunctivitis, bilateral

✓5ᵗʰ **H10.2 Other acute conjunctivitis**

✓6ᵗʰ **H10.21 Acute toxic conjunctivitis**

Acute chemical conjunctivitis

Code first (T51-T65) to identify chemical and intent

EXCLUDES 1 burn and corrosion of eye and adnexa (T26.-)

H10.211 Acute toxic conjunctivitis, right eye

H10.212 Acute toxic conjunctivitis, left eye

H10.213 Acute toxic conjunctivitis, bilateral

H10.219 Acute toxic conjunctivitis, unspecified eye

✓6ᵗʰ **H10.22 Pseudomembranous conjunctivitis**

H10.221 Pseudomembranous conjunctivitis, right eye

H10.222 Pseudomembranous conjunctivitis, left eye

H10.223 Pseudomembranous conjunctivitis, bilateral

H10.229 Pseudomembranous conjunctivitis, unspecified eye

✓6ᵗʰ **H10.23 Serous conjunctivitis, except viral**

EXCLUDES 1 viral conjunctivitis (B30.-)

H10.231 Serous conjunctivitis, except viral, right eye

H10.232 Serous conjunctivitis, except viral, left eye

H10.233 Serous conjunctivitis, except viral, bilateral

H10.239 Serous conjunctivitis, except viral, unspecified eye

✓5ᵗʰ **H10.3 Unspecified acute conjunctivitis**

EXCLUDES 1 ophthalmia neonatorum NOS (P39.1)

H10.30 Unspecified acute conjunctivitis, unspecified eye

H10.31 Unspecified acute conjunctivitis, right eye

H10.32 Unspecified acute conjunctivitis, left eye

H10.33 Unspecified acute conjunctivitis, bilateral

✓5ᵗʰ **H10.4 Chronic conjunctivitis**

✓6ᵗʰ **H10.40 Unspecified chronic conjunctivitis**

H10.401 Unspecified chronic conjunctivitis, right eye

H10.402 Unspecified chronic conjunctivitis, left eye

H10.403 Unspecified chronic conjunctivitis, bilateral

H10.409 Unspecified chronic conjunctivitis, unspecified eye

✓6ᵗʰ **H10.41 Chronic giant papillary conjunctivitis**

H10.411 Chronic giant papillary conjunctivitis, right eye

H10.412 Chronic giant papillary conjunctivitis, left eye

H10.413 Chronic giant papillary conjunctivitis, bilateral

H10.419 Chronic giant papillary conjunctivitis, unspecified eye

✓6ᵗʰ **H10.42 Simple chronic conjunctivitis**

H10.421 Simple chronic conjunctivitis, right eye

H10.422 Simple chronic conjunctivitis, left eye

H10.423 Simple chronic conjunctivitis, bilateral

H10.429 Simple chronic conjunctivitis, unspecified eye

✓6ᵗʰ **H10.43 Chronic follicular conjunctivitis**

H10.431 Chronic follicular conjunctivitis, right eye

H10.432 Chronic follicular conjunctivitis, left eye

H10.433 Chronic follicular conjunctivitis, bilateral

H10.439 Chronic follicular conjunctivitis, unspecified eye

✓6ᵗʰ **H10.44 Vernal conjunctivitis**

EXCLUDES 1 vernal keratoconjunctivitis with limbar and corneal involvement (H16.26-)

H10.45 Other chronic allergic conjunctivitis

✓5ᵗʰ **H10.5 Blepharoconjunctivitis**

✓6ᵗʰ **H10.50 Unspecified blepharoconjunctivitis**

H10.501 Unspecified blepharoconjunctivitis, right eye

H10.502 Unspecified blepharoconjunctivitis, left eye

H10.503 Unspecified blepharoconjunctivitis, bilateral

H10.509 Unspecified blepharoconjunctivitis, unspecified eye

✓6ᵗʰ **H10.51 Ligneous conjunctivitis**

Code also underlying condition if known, such as: plasminogen deficiency (E88.02)

H10.511 Ligneous conjunctivitis, right eye

H10.512 Ligneous conjunctivitis, left eye

H10.513 Ligneous conjunctivitis, bilateral

H10.519 Ligneous conjunctivitis, unspecified eye

☑ Additional Character Required   ✓x 7ᵗʰ Placeholder   Unacceptable PDx   Questionable PDx   Manifestation   Unspecified Dx   H1-H14 HAC   HCC CMS-HCC Dx   HIV HIV Dx

ICD-10-CM 2021   601

✓6th **H10.52** Angular **blepharoconjunctivitis**
 H10.521 Angular blepharoconjunctivitis, right eye
 H10.522 Angular blepharoconjunctivitis, left eye
 H10.523 Angular blepharoconjunctivitis, bilateral
 H10.529 Angular blepharoconjunctivitis, unspecified eye

✓6th **H10.53** Contact **blepharoconjunctivitis**
 H10.531 Contact blepharoconjunctivitis, right eye
 H10.532 Contact blepharoconjunctivitis, left eye
 H10.533 Contact blepharoconjunctivitis, bilateral
 H10.539 Contact blepharoconjunctivitis, unspecified eye

✓5th **H10.8** **Other conjunctivitis**
 ✓6th **H10.81** **Pingueculitis**
  EXCLUDES 1 *pinguecula (H11.15-)*
  H10.811 Pingueculitis, right eye
  H10.812 Pingueculitis, left eye
  H10.813 Pingueculitis, bilateral
  H10.819 Pingueculitis, unspecified eye
 ✓6th **H10.82** Rosacea **conjunctivitis**
  Code first underlying rosacea dermatitis (L71.-)
  AHA: 2018,4Q,15
  H10.821 Rosacea conjunctivitis, right eye
  H10.822 Rosacea conjunctivitis, left eye
  H10.823 Rosacea conjunctivitis, bilateral
  H10.829 Rosacea conjunctivitis, unspecified eye
 H10.89 **Other conjunctivitis**

H10.9 **Unspecified conjunctivitis**

✓4th **H11** **Other disorders of conjunctiva**
 EXCLUDES 1 *keratoconjunctivitis (H16.2-)*

✓5th **H11.0** **Pterygium of eye**
 EXCLUDES 1 *pseudopterygium (H11.81-)*
 DEF: Benign, wedge-shaped, conjunctival thickening that advances from the inner corner of the eye toward the cornea.

Pterygium

Pterygium

✓6th **H11.00** **Unspecified pterygium of eye**
 H11.001 Unspecified pterygium of right eye
 H11.002 Unspecified pterygium of left eye
 H11.003 Unspecified pterygium of eye, bilateral
 H11.009 Unspecified pterygium of unspecified eye

✓6th **H11.01** Amyloid **pterygium**
 H11.011 Amyloid pterygium of right eye
 H11.012 Amyloid pterygium of left eye
 H11.013 Amyloid pterygium of eye, bilateral
 H11.019 Amyloid pterygium of unspecified eye

✓6th **H11.02** Central **pterygium of eye**
 H11.021 Central pterygium of right eye
 H11.022 Central pterygium of left eye
 H11.023 Central pterygium of eye, bilateral
 H11.029 Central pterygium of unspecified eye

✓6th **H11.03** Double **pterygium of eye**
 H11.031 Double pterygium of right eye
 H11.032 Double pterygium of left eye
 H11.033 Double pterygium of eye, bilateral
 H11.039 Double pterygium of unspecified eye

✓6th **H11.04** Peripheral **pterygium of eye, stationary**
 H11.041 Peripheral pterygium, stationary, right eye
 H11.042 Peripheral pterygium, stationary, left eye
 H11.043 Peripheral pterygium, stationary, bilateral
 H11.049 Peripheral pterygium, stationary, unspecified eye

✓6th **H11.05** Peripheral **pterygium of eye, progressive**
 H11.051 Peripheral pterygium, progressive, right eye
 H11.052 Peripheral pterygium, progressive, left eye
 H11.053 Peripheral pterygium, progressive, bilateral
 H11.059 Peripheral pterygium, progressive, unspecified eye

✓6th **H11.06** Recurrent **pterygium of eye**
 H11.061 Recurrent pterygium of right eye
 H11.062 Recurrent pterygium of left eye
 H11.063 Recurrent pterygium of eye, bilateral
 H11.069 Recurrent pterygium of unspecified eye

✓5th **H11.1** **Conjunctival degenerations and deposits**
 EXCLUDES 2 *pseudopterygium (H11.81)*
 H11.10 **Unspecified conjunctival degenerations**
 ✓6th **H11.11** Conjunctival **deposits**
  H11.111 Conjunctival deposits, right eye
  H11.112 Conjunctival deposits, left eye
  H11.113 Conjunctival deposits, bilateral
  H11.119 Conjunctival deposits, unspecified eye
 ✓6th **H11.12** Conjunctival **concretions**
  H11.121 Conjunctival concretions, right eye
  H11.122 Conjunctival concretions, left eye
  H11.123 Conjunctival concretions, bilateral
  H11.129 Conjunctival concretions, unspecified eye
 ✓6th **H11.13** Conjunctival **pigmentations**
  Conjunctival argyrosis [argyria]
  H11.131 Conjunctival pigmentations, right eye
  H11.132 Conjunctival pigmentations, left eye
  H11.133 Conjunctival pigmentations, bilateral
  H11.139 Conjunctival pigmentations, unspecified eye
 ✓6th **H11.14** **Conjunctival xerosis, unspecified**
  EXCLUDES 1 *xerosis of conjunctiva due to vitamin A deficiency (E50.0, E50.1)*
  DEF: Abnormal dryness of the conjunctiva due to lack of insufficient tears or conjunctival secretions.
  H11.141 Conjunctival xerosis, unspecified, right eye
  H11.142 Conjunctival xerosis, unspecified, left eye
  H11.143 Conjunctival xerosis, unspecified, bilateral
  H11.149 Conjunctival xerosis, unspecified, unspecified eye

N Newborn: 0 P Pediatric: 0-17 M Maternity: 9-64 A Adult: 15-124 MCC Major Complication/Comorbidity CC Complication/Comorbidity SW Severe Wound Dx

602 ICD-10-CM 2021

☑6ᵗʰ **H11.15 Pinguecula**

> **EXCLUDES 1**   *pingueculitis (H10.81-)*
>
> **DEF:** Proliferation on the conjunctiva near the sclerocorneal junction, usually of the side of the nose and usually in older patients.

Pinguecula

Pinguecula

H11.151 Pinguecula, **right** eye
H11.152 Pinguecula, **left** eye
H11.153 Pinguecula, **bilateral**
H11.159 Pinguecula, **unspecified** eye

☑5ᵗʰ **H11.2 Conjunctival scars**

   ☑6ᵗʰ **H11.21 Conjunctival adhesions and strands (localized)**

      H11.211 **Conjunctival adhesions and strands (localized), right** eye
      H11.212 **Conjunctival adhesions and strands (localized), left** eye
      H11.213 **Conjunctival adhesions and strands (localized), bilateral**
      H11.219 **Conjunctival adhesions and strands (localized), unspecified** eye

   ☑6ᵗʰ **H11.22 Conjunctival granuloma**

      H11.221 **Conjunctival granuloma, right** eye
      H11.222 **Conjunctival granuloma, left** eye
      H11.223 **Conjunctival granuloma, bilateral**
      H11.229 **Conjunctival granuloma, unspecified**

   ☑6ᵗʰ **H11.23 Symblepharon**

      H11.231 **Symblepharon, right** eye
      H11.232 **Symblepharon, left** eye
      H11.233 **Symblepharon, bilateral**
      H11.239 **Symblepharon, unspecified** eye

   ☑6ᵗʰ **H11.24 Scarring of conjunctiva**

      H11.241 **Scarring of conjunctiva, right** eye
      H11.242 **Scarring of conjunctiva, left** eye
      H11.243 **Scarring of conjunctiva, bilateral**
      H11.249 **Scarring of conjunctiva, unspecified** eye

☑5ᵗʰ **H11.3 Conjunctival hemorrhage**

   Subconjunctival hemorrhage

   H11.30 **Conjunctival hemorrhage, unspecified** eye
   H11.31 **Conjunctival hemorrhage, right** eye
   H11.32 **Conjunctival hemorrhage, left** eye
   H11.33 **Conjunctival hemorrhage, bilateral**

☑5ᵗʰ **H11.4 Other conjunctival vascular disorders and cysts**

   ☑6ᵗʰ **H11.41 Vascular abnormalities of conjunctiva**

      Conjunctival aneurysm

      H11.411 **Vascular abnormalities of conjunctiva, right eye**
      H11.412 **Vascular abnormalities of conjunctiva, left eye**
      H11.413 **Vascular abnormalities of conjunctiva, bilateral**
      H11.419 **Vascular abnormalities of conjunctiva, unspecified eye**

   ☑6ᵗʰ **H11.42 Conjunctival edema**

      H11.421 **Conjunctival edema, right** eye
      H11.422 **Conjunctival edema, left** eye
      H11.423 **Conjunctival edema, bilateral**
      H11.429 **Conjunctival edema, unspecified** eye

   ☑6ᵗʰ **H11.43 Conjunctival hyperemia**

      H11.431 **Conjunctival hyperemia, right** eye
      H11.432 **Conjunctival hyperemia, left eye**
      H11.433 **Conjunctival hyperemia, bilateral**
      H11.439 **Conjunctival hyperemia, unspecified eye**

   ☑6ᵗʰ **H11.44 Conjunctival cysts**

      H11.441 **Conjunctival cysts, right** eye
      H11.442 **Conjunctival cysts, left** eye
      H11.443 **Conjunctival cysts, bilateral**
      H11.449 **Conjunctival cysts, unspecified eye**

☑5ᵗʰ **H11.8 Other specified disorders of conjunctiva**

   ☑6ᵗʰ **H11.81 Pseudopterygium of conjunctiva**

      H11.811 **Pseudopterygium of conjunctiva, right eye**
      H11.812 **Pseudopterygium of conjunctiva, left eye**
      H11.813 **Pseudopterygium of conjunctiva, bilateral**
      H11.819 **Pseudopterygium of conjunctiva, unspecified eye**

   ☑6ᵗʰ **H11.82 Conjunctivochalasis**

      H11.821 **Conjunctivochalasis, right** eye
      H11.822 **Conjunctivochalasis, left** eye
      H11.823 **Conjunctivochalasis, bilateral**
      H11.829 **Conjunctivochalasis, unspecified eye**

   H11.89 **Other specified disorders of conjunctiva**

H11.9 Unspecified disorder of conjunctiva

Disorders of sclera, cornea, iris and ciliary body (H15-H22)

☑4ᵗʰ **H15 Disorders of sclera**

   ☑5ᵗʰ **H15.0 Scleritis**

     ☑6ᵗʰ **H15.00 Unspecified scleritis**

        H15.001 **Unspecified scleritis, right eye**
        H15.002 **Unspecified scleritis, left eye**
        H15.003 **Unspecified scleritis, bilateral**
        H15.009 **Unspecified scleritis, unspecified eye**

     ☑6ᵗʰ **H15.01 Anterior scleritis**

        H15.011 **Anterior scleritis, right** eye
        H15.012 **Anterior scleritis, left** eye
        H15.013 **Anterior scleritis, bilateral**
        H15.019 **Anterior scleritis, unspecified eye**

     ☑6ᵗʰ **H15.02 Brawny scleritis**

        H15.021 **Brawny scleritis, right** eye
        H15.022 **Brawny scleritis, left** eye
        H15.023 **Brawny scleritis, bilateral**
        H15.029 **Brawny scleritis, unspecified eye**

     ☑6ᵗʰ **H15.03 Posterior scleritis**

        Sclerotenonitis

        H15.031 **Posterior scleritis, right** eye
        H15.032 **Posterior scleritis, left** eye
        H15.033 **Posterior scleritis, bilateral**
        H15.039 **Posterior scleritis, unspecified eye**

     ☑6ᵗʰ **H15.04 Scleritis with corneal involvement**

        H15.041 **Scleritis with corneal involvement, right eye**
        H15.042 **Scleritis with corneal involvement, left eye**
        H15.043 **Scleritis with corneal involvement, bilateral**
        H15.049 **Scleritis with corneal involvement, unspecified eye**

     ☑6ᵗʰ **H15.05 Scleromalacia perforans**

        H15.051 **Scleromalacia perforans, right** eye
        H15.052 **Scleromalacia perforans, left** eye
        H15.053 **Scleromalacia perforans, bilateral**
        H15.059 **Scleromalacia perforans, unspecified eye**

     ☑6ᵗʰ **H15.09 Other scleritis**

        Scleral abscess

        H15.091 **Other scleritis, right** eye
        H15.092 **Other scleritis, left** eye
        H15.093 **Other scleritis, bilateral**
        H15.099 **Other scleritis, unspecified eye**

   ☑5ᵗʰ **H15.1 Episcleritis**

     ☑6ᵗʰ **H15.10 Unspecified episcleritis**

        H15.101 **Unspecified episcleritis, right eye**
        H15.102 **Unspecified episcleritis, left eye**
        H15.103 **Unspecified episcleritis, bilateral**
        H15.109 **Unspecified episcleritis, unspecified eye**

☑ Additional Character Required   ✓ₓ7ᵗʰ Placeholder   Unacceptable PDx   Questionable PDx   Manifestation   Unspecified Dx   H1-H14 HAC   HCC CMS-HCC Dx   HIV HIV Dx

ICD-10-CM 2021   **603**

✓6ᵗʰ **H15.11** Episcleritis periodica fugax

    H15.111 Episcleritis periodica fugax, right eye
    H15.112 Episcleritis periodica fugax, left eye
    H15.113 Episcleritis periodica fugax, bilateral
    H15.119 Episcleritis periodica fugax, unspecified eye

✓6ᵗʰ **H15.12** Nodular episcleritis

    H15.121 Nodular episcleritis, right eye
    H15.122 Nodular episcleritis, left eye
    H15.123 Nodular episcleritis, bilateral
    H15.129 Nodular episcleritis, unspecified eye

✓5ᵗʰ **H15.8** Other disorders of sclera

    EXCLUDES 2   blue sclera (Q13.5)
                  degenerative myopia (H44.2-)

  ✓6ᵗʰ **H15.81** Equatorial staphyloma

    H15.811 Equatorial staphyloma, right eye
    H15.812 Equatorial staphyloma, left eye
    H15.813 Equatorial staphyloma, bilateral
    H15.819 Equatorial staphyloma, unspecified eye

  ✓6ᵗʰ **H15.82** Localized anterior staphyloma

    H15.821 Localized anterior staphyloma, right eye
    H15.822 Localized anterior staphyloma, left eye
    H15.823 Localized anterior staphyloma, bilateral
    H15.829 Localized anterior staphyloma, unspecified eye

  ✓6ᵗʰ **H15.83** Staphyloma posticum

    H15.831 Staphyloma posticum, right eye
    H15.832 Staphyloma posticum, left eye
    H15.833 Staphyloma posticum, bilateral
    H15.839 Staphyloma posticum, unspecified eye

  ✓6ᵗʰ **H15.84** Scleral ectasia

    H15.841 Scleral ectasia, right eye
    H15.842 Scleral ectasia, left eye
    H15.843 Scleral ectasia, bilateral
    H15.849 Scleral ectasia, unspecified eye

  ✓6ᵗʰ **H15.85** Ring staphyloma

    H15.851 Ring staphyloma, right eye
    H15.852 Ring staphyloma, left eye
    H15.853 Ring staphyloma, bilateral
    H15.859 Ring staphyloma, unspecified eye

  H15.89 Other disorders of sclera

H15.9 Unspecified disorder of sclera

✓4ᵗʰ **H16** Keratitis

  DEF: Condition in which the cornea becomes inflamed and irritated.

✓5ᵗʰ **H16.0** Corneal ulcer

  ✓6ᵗʰ **H16.00** Unspecified corneal ulcer

    H16.001 Unspecified corneal ulcer, right eye
    H16.002 Unspecified corneal ulcer, left eye
    H16.003 Unspecified corneal ulcer, bilateral
    H16.009 Unspecified corneal ulcer, unspecified eye

  ✓6ᵗʰ **H16.01** Central corneal ulcer

    H16.011 Central corneal ulcer, right eye
    H16.012 Central corneal ulcer, left eye
    H16.013 Central corneal ulcer, bilateral
    H16.019 Central corneal ulcer, unspecified eye

  ✓6ᵗʰ **H16.02** Ring corneal ulcer

    H16.021 Ring corneal ulcer, right eye
    H16.022 Ring corneal ulcer, left eye
    H16.023 Ring corneal ulcer, bilateral
    H16.029 Ring corneal ulcer, unspecified eye

  ✓6ᵗʰ **H16.03** Corneal ulcer with hypopyon

    H16.031 Corneal ulcer with hypopyon, right eye
    H16.032 Corneal ulcer with hypopyon, left eye
    H16.033 Corneal ulcer with hypopyon, bilateral
    H16.039 Corneal ulcer with hypopyon, unspecified eye

  ✓6ᵗʰ **H16.04** Marginal corneal ulcer

    H16.041 Marginal corneal ulcer, right eye
    H16.042 Marginal corneal ulcer, left eye
    H16.043 Marginal corneal ulcer, bilateral
    H16.049 Marginal corneal ulcer, unspecified eye

  ✓6ᵗʰ **H16.05** Mooren's corneal ulcer

    H16.051 Mooren's corneal ulcer, right eye
    H16.052 Mooren's corneal ulcer, left eye

    H16.053 Mooren's corneal ulcer, bilateral
    H16.059 Mooren's corneal ulcer, unspecified eye

  ✓6ᵗʰ **H16.06** Mycotic corneal ulcer

    H16.061 Mycotic corneal ulcer, right eye
    H16.062 Mycotic corneal ulcer, left eye
    H16.063 Mycotic corneal ulcer, bilateral
    H16.069 Mycotic corneal ulcer, unspecified eye

  ✓6ᵗʰ **H16.07** Perforated corneal ulcer

    H16.071 Perforated corneal ulcer, right eye
    H16.072 Perforated corneal ulcer, left eye
    H16.073 Perforated corneal ulcer, bilateral
    H16.079 Perforated corneal ulcer, unspecified eye

✓5ᵗʰ **H16.1** Other and unspecified superficial keratitis without conjunctivitis

  ✓6ᵗʰ **H16.10** Unspecified superficial keratitis

    H16.101 Unspecified superficial keratitis, right eye
    H16.102 Unspecified superficial keratitis, left eye
    H16.103 Unspecified superficial keratitis, bilateral
    H16.109 Unspecified superficial keratitis, unspecified eye

  ✓6ᵗʰ **H16.11** Macular keratitis

    Areolar keratitis
    Nummular keratitis
    Stellate keratitis
    Striate keratitis
    H16.111 Macular keratitis, right eye
    H16.112 Macular keratitis, left eye
    H16.113 Macular keratitis, bilateral
    H16.119 Macular keratitis, unspecified eye

  ✓6ᵗʰ **H16.12** Filamentary keratitis

    H16.121 Filamentary keratitis, right eye
    H16.122 Filamentary keratitis, left eye
    H16.123 Filamentary keratitis, bilateral
    H16.129 Filamentary keratitis, unspecified eye

  ✓6ᵗʰ **H16.13** Photokeratitis

    Snow blindness
    Welders keratitis
    H16.131 Photokeratitis, right eye
    H16.132 Photokeratitis, left eye
    H16.133 Photokeratitis, bilateral
    H16.139 Photokeratitis, unspecified eye

  ✓6ᵗʰ **H16.14** Punctate keratitis

    H16.141 Punctate keratitis, right eye
    H16.142 Punctate keratitis, left eye
    H16.143 Punctate keratitis, bilateral
    H16.149 Punctate keratitis, unspecified eye

✓5ᵗʰ **H16.2** Keratoconjunctivitis

  ✓6ᵗʰ **H16.20** Unspecified keratoconjunctivitis

    Superficial keratitis with conjunctivitis NOS
    H16.201 Unspecified keratoconjunctivitis, right eye
    H16.202 Unspecified keratoconjunctivitis, left eye
    H16.203 Unspecified keratoconjunctivitis, bilateral
    H16.209 Unspecified keratoconjunctivitis, unspecified eye

  ✓6ᵗʰ **H16.21** Exposure keratoconjunctivitis

    H16.211 Exposure keratoconjunctivitis, right eye
    H16.212 Exposure keratoconjunctivitis, left eye
    H16.213 Exposure keratoconjunctivitis, bilateral
    H16.219 Exposure keratoconjunctivitis, unspecified eye

  ✓6ᵗʰ **H16.22** Keratoconjunctivitis sicca, not specified as Sjögren's

    EXCLUDES 1   Sjögren's syndrome (M35.01)

    H16.221 Keratoconjunctivitis sicca, not specified as Sjögren's, right eye
    H16.222 Keratoconjunctivitis sicca, not specified as Sjögren's, left eye
    H16.223 Keratoconjunctivitis sicca, not specified as Sjögren's, bilateral
    H16.229 Keratoconjunctivitis sicca, not specified as Sjögren's, unspecified eye

  ✓6ᵗʰ **H16.23** Neurotrophic keratoconjunctivitis

    H16.231 Neurotrophic keratoconjunctivitis, right eye
    H16.232 Neurotrophic keratoconjunctivitis, left eye

N Newborn: 0   **P** Pediatric: 0-17   **M** Maternity: 9-64   **A** Adult: 15-124   **MCC** Major Complication/Comorbidity   **CC** Complication/Comorbidity   **SW** Severe Wound Dx

604   ICD-10-CM 2021

           H16.233   Neurotrophic keratoconjunctivitis, bilateral

           H16.239   Neurotrophic keratoconjunctivitis, unspecified eye

☑6th   H16.24   Ophthalmia nodosa

           H16.241   Ophthalmia nodosa, right eye

           H16.242   Ophthalmia nodosa, left eye

           H16.243   Ophthalmia nodosa, bilateral

           H16.249   Ophthalmia nodosa, unspecified eye

☑6th   H16.25   Phlyctenular keratoconjunctivitis

           H16.251   Phlyctenular keratoconjunctivitis, right eye

           H16.252   Phlyctenular keratoconjunctivitis, left eye

           H16.253   Phlyctenular keratoconjunctivitis, bilateral

           H16.259   Phlyctenular keratoconjunctivitis, unspecified eye

☑6th   H16.26   Vernal keratoconjunctivitis, with limbar and corneal involvement

              EXCLUDES 1   *vernal conjunctivitis without limbar and corneal involvement (H10.44)*

           H16.261   Vernal keratoconjunctivitis, with limbar and corneal involvement, right eye

           H16.262   Vernal keratoconjunctivitis, with limbar and corneal involvement, left eye

           H16.263   Vernal keratoconjunctivitis, with limbar and corneal involvement, bilateral

           H16.269   Vernal keratoconjunctivitis, with limbar and corneal involvement, unspecified eye

☑6th   H16.29   Other keratoconjunctivitis

           H16.291   Other keratoconjunctivitis, right eye

           H16.292   Other keratoconjunctivitis, left eye

           H16.293   Other keratoconjunctivitis, bilateral

           H16.299   Other keratoconjunctivitis, unspecified eye

☑5th   H16.3   Interstitial and deep keratitis

☑6th   H16.30   Unspecified interstitial keratitis

           H16.301   Unspecified interstitial keratitis, right eye

           H16.302   Unspecified interstitial keratitis, left eye

           H16.303   Unspecified interstitial keratitis, bilateral

           H16.309   Unspecified interstitial keratitis, unspecified eye

☑6th   H16.31   Corneal abscess

           H16.311   Corneal abscess, right eye

           H16.312   Corneal abscess, left eye

           H16.313   Corneal abscess, bilateral

           H16.319   Corneal abscess, unspecified eye

☑6th   H16.32   Diffuse interstitial keratitis

             Cogan's syndrome

           H16.321   Diffuse interstitial keratitis, right eye

           H16.322   Diffuse interstitial keratitis, left eye

           H16.323   Diffuse interstitial keratitis, bilateral

           H16.329   Diffuse interstitial keratitis, unspecified eye

☑6th   H16.33   Sclerosing keratitis

           H16.331   Sclerosing keratitis, right eye

           H16.332   Sclerosing keratitis, left eye

           H16.333   Sclerosing keratitis, bilateral

           H16.339   Sclerosing keratitis, unspecified eye

☑6th   H16.39   Other interstitial and deep keratitis

           H16.391   Other interstitial and deep keratitis, right eye

           H16.392   Other interstitial and deep keratitis, left eye

           H16.393   Other interstitial and deep keratitis, bilateral

           H16.399   Other interstitial and deep keratitis, unspecified eye

☑5th   H16.4   Corneal neovascularization

☑6th   H16.40   Unspecified corneal neovascularization

           H16.401   Unspecified corneal neovascularization, right eye

           H16.402   Unspecified corneal neovascularization, left eye

           H16.403   Unspecified corneal neovascularization, bilateral

           H16.409   Unspecified corneal neovascularization, unspecified eye

☑6th   H16.41   Ghost vessels (corneal)

           H16.411   Ghost vessels (corneal), right eye

           H16.412   Ghost vessels (corneal), left eye

           H16.413   Ghost vessels (corneal), bilateral

           H16.419   Ghost vessels (corneal), unspecified eye

☑6th   H16.42   Pannus (corneal)

           H16.421   Pannus (corneal), right eye

           H16.422   Pannus (corneal), left eye

           H16.423   Pannus (corneal), bilateral

           H16.429   Pannus (corneal), unspecified eye

☑6th   H16.43   Localized vascularization of cornea

           H16.431   Localized vascularization of cornea, right eye

           H16.432   Localized vascularization of cornea, left eye

           H16.433   Localized vascularization of cornea, bilateral

           H16.439   Localized vascularization of cornea, unspecified eye

☑6th   H16.44   Deep vascularization of cornea

           H16.441   Deep vascularization of cornea, right eye

           H16.442   Deep vascularization of cornea, left eye

           H16.443   Deep vascularization of cornea, bilateral

           H16.449   Deep vascularization of cornea, unspecified eye

      H16.8   Other keratitis

      H16.9   Unspecified keratitis

☑4th   H17   Corneal scars and opacities

☑5th   H17.0   Adherent leukoma

        H17.00   Adherent leukoma, unspecified eye

        H17.01   Adherent leukoma, right eye

        H17.02   Adherent leukoma, left eye

        H17.03   Adherent leukoma, bilateral

☑5th   H17.1   Central corneal opacity

        H17.10   Central corneal opacity, unspecified eye

        H17.11   Central corneal opacity, right eye

        H17.12   Central corneal opacity, left eye

        H17.13   Central corneal opacity, bilateral

☑5th   H17.8   Other corneal scars and opacities

☑6th   H17.81   Minor opacity of cornea

             Corneal nebula

           H17.811   Minor opacity of cornea, right eye

           H17.812   Minor opacity of cornea, left eye

           H17.813   Minor opacity of cornea, bilateral

           H17.819   Minor opacity of cornea, unspecified eye

☑6th   H17.82   Peripheral opacity of cornea

           H17.821   Peripheral opacity of cornea, right eye

           H17.822   Peripheral opacity of cornea, left eye

           H17.823   Peripheral opacity of cornea, bilateral

           H17.829   Peripheral opacity of cornea, unspecified eye

        H17.89   Other corneal scars and opacities

      H17.9   Unspecified corneal scar and opacity

☑4th   H18   Other disorders of cornea

☑5th   H18.0   Corneal pigmentations and deposits

☑6th   H18.00   Unspecified corneal deposit

           H18.001   Unspecified corneal deposit, right eye

           H18.002   Unspecified corneal deposit, left eye

           H18.003   Unspecified corneal deposit, bilateral

           H18.009   Unspecified corneal deposit, unspecified eye

☑6th   H18.01   Anterior corneal pigmentations

             Staehli's line

           H18.011   Anterior corneal pigmentations, right eye

           H18.012   Anterior corneal pigmentations, left eye

           H18.013   Anterior corneal pigmentations, bilateral

           H18.019   Anterior corneal pigmentations, unspecified eye

☑6th   H18.02   Argentous corneal deposits

           H18.021   Argentous corneal deposits, right eye

           H18.022   Argentous corneal deposits, left eye

           H18.023   Argentous corneal deposits, bilateral

           H18.029   Argentous corneal deposits, unspecified eye

Chapter 7. Diseases of the Eye and Adnexa

H18.03–H18.529

√6ᵗʰ **H18.03 Corneal deposits in metabolic disorders**

Code also associated metabolic disorder

H18.031 **Corneal deposits in metabolic disorders, right eye**

H18.032 **Corneal deposits in metabolic disorders, left eye**

H18.033 **Corneal deposits in metabolic disorders, bilateral**

H18.039 **Corneal deposits in metabolic disorders, unspecified eye**

√6ᵗʰ **H18.04 Kayser-Fleischer ring**

Code also associated Wilson's disease (E83.01)

H18.041 **Kayser-Fleischer ring, right eye**

H18.042 **Kayser-Fleischer ring, left eye**

H18.043 **Kayser-Fleischer ring, bilateral**

H18.049 **Kayser-Fleischer ring, unspecified eye**

√6ᵗʰ **H18.05 Posterior corneal pigmentations**

Krukenberg's spindle

H18.051 **Posterior corneal pigmentations, right eye**

H18.052 **Posterior corneal pigmentations, left eye**

H18.053 **Posterior corneal pigmentations, bilateral**

H18.059 **Posterior corneal pigmentations, unspecified eye**

√6ᵗʰ **H18.06 Stromal corneal pigmentations**

Hematocornea

H18.061 **Stromal corneal pigmentations, right eye**

H18.062 **Stromal corneal pigmentations, left eye**

H18.063 **Stromal corneal pigmentations, bilateral**

H18.069 **Stromal corneal pigmentations, unspecified eye**

√5ᵗʰ **H18.1 Bullous keratopathy**

DEF: Corneal swelling due to a damaged corneal endothelium. Bullous keratopathy is characterized by recurring, rupturing epithelial blisters causing glaucoma, iridocyclitis, and Fuchs dystrophy.

H18.10 **Bullous keratopathy, unspecified eye**

H18.11 **Bullous keratopathy, right eye**

H18.12 **Bullous keratopathy, left eye**

H18.13 **Bullous keratopathy, bilateral**

√5ᵗʰ **H18.2 Other and unspecified corneal edema**

H18.20 **Unspecified corneal edema**

√6ᵗʰ **H18.21 Corneal edema secondary to contact lens**

EXCLUDES 2   *other corneal disorders due to contact lens (H18.82-)*

H18.211 **Corneal edema secondary to contact lens, right eye**

H18.212 **Corneal edema secondary to contact lens, left eye**

H18.213 **Corneal edema secondary to contact lens, bilateral**

H18.219 **Corneal edema secondary to contact lens, unspecified eye**

√6ᵗʰ **H18.22 Idiopathic corneal edema**

H18.221 **Idiopathic corneal edema, right eye**

H18.222 **Idiopathic corneal edema, left eye**

H18.223 **Idiopathic corneal edema, bilateral**

H18.229 **Idiopathic corneal edema, unspecified eye**

√6ᵗʰ **H18.23 Secondary corneal edema**

H18.231 **Secondary corneal edema, right eye**

H18.232 **Secondary corneal edema, left eye**

H18.233 **Secondary corneal edema, bilateral**

H18.239 **Secondary corneal edema, unspecified eye**

√5ᵗʰ **H18.3 Changes of corneal membranes**

H18.30 **Unspecified corneal membrane change**

√6ᵗʰ **H18.31 Folds and rupture in Bowman's membrane**

H18.311 **Folds and rupture in Bowman's membrane, right eye**

H18.312 **Folds and rupture in Bowman's membrane, left eye**

H18.313 **Folds and rupture in Bowman's membrane, bilateral**

H18.319 **Folds and rupture in Bowman's membrane, unspecified eye**

√6ᵗʰ **H18.32 Folds in Descemet's membrane**

H18.321 **Folds in Descemet's membrane, right eye**

H18.322 **Folds in Descemet's membrane, left eye**

H18.323 **Folds in Descemet's membrane, bilateral**

H18.329 **Folds in Descemet's membrane, unspecified eye**

√6ᵗʰ **H18.33 Rupture in Descemet's membrane**

H18.331 **Rupture in Descemet's membrane, right eye**

H18.332 **Rupture in Descemet's membrane, left eye**

H18.333 **Rupture in Descemet's membrane, bilateral**

H18.339 **Rupture in Descemet's membrane, unspecified eye**

√5ᵗʰ **H18.4 Corneal degeneration**

EXCLUDES 1   *Mooren's ulcer (H16.0-)*

recurrent erosion of cornea (H18.83-)

H18.40 **Unspecified corneal degeneration**

√6ᵗʰ **H18.41 Arcus senilis**

Senile corneal changes

H18.411 **Arcus senilis, right eye**

H18.412 **Arcus senilis, left eye**

H18.413 **Arcus senilis, bilateral**

H18.419 **Arcus senilis, unspecified eye**

√6ᵗʰ **H18.42 Band keratopathy**

H18.421 **Band keratopathy, right eye**

H18.422 **Band keratopathy, left eye**

H18.423 **Band keratopathy, bilateral**

H18.429 **Band keratopathy, unspecified eye**

H18.43 **Other calcerous corneal degeneration**

√6ᵗʰ **H18.44 Keratomalacia**

EXCLUDES 1   *keratomalacia due to vitamin A deficiency (E50.4)*

H18.441 **Keratomalacia, right eye**

H18.442 **Keratomalacia, left eye**

H18.443 **Keratomalacia, bilateral**

H18.449 **Keratomalacia, unspecified eye**

√6ᵗʰ **H18.45 Nodular corneal degeneration**

H18.451 **Nodular corneal degeneration, right eye**

H18.452 **Nodular corneal degeneration, left eye**

H18.453 **Nodular corneal degeneration, bilateral**

H18.459 **Nodular corneal degeneration, unspecified eye**

√6ᵗʰ **H18.46 Peripheral corneal degeneration**

H18.461 **Peripheral corneal degeneration, right eye**

H18.462 **Peripheral corneal degeneration, left eye**

H18.463 **Peripheral corneal degeneration, bilateral**

H18.469 **Peripheral corneal degeneration, unspecified eye**

H18.49 **Other corneal degeneration**

√5ᵗʰ **H18.5 Hereditary corneal dystrophies**

▲ √6ᵗʰ **H18.50 Unspecified hereditary corneal dystrophies**

● H18.501 **Unspecified hereditary corneal dystrophies, right eye**

● H18.502 **Unspecified hereditary corneal dystrophies, left eye**

● H18.503 **Unspecified hereditary corneal dystrophies, bilateral**

● H18.509 **Unspecified hereditary corneal dystrophies, unspecified eye**

▲ √6ᵗʰ **H18.51 Endothelial corneal dystrophy**

Fuchs' dystrophy

H18.511 **Endothelial corneal dystrophy, right eye**

H18.512 **Endothelial corneal dystrophy, left eye**

H18.513 **Endothelial corneal dystrophy, bilateral**

H18.519 **Endothelial corneal dystrophy, unspecified eye**

▲ √6ᵗʰ **H18.52 Epithelial (juvenile) corneal dystrophy**

● H18.521 **Epithelial (juvenile) corneal dystrophy, right eye**

● H18.522 **Epithelial (juvenile) corneal dystrophy, left eye**

● H18.523 **Epithelial (juvenile) corneal dystrophy, bilateral**

● H18.529 **Epithelial (juvenile) corneal dystrophy, unspecified eye**

N Newborn: 0   P Pediatric: 0-17   M Maternity: 9-64   A Adult: 15-124   MCC Major Complication/Comorbidity   CC Complication/Comorbidity   SW Severe Wound Dx

606   ICD-10-CM 2021

▲   ✓6ᵗʰ **H18.53** Granular corneal dystrophy
●   **H18.531** Granular corneal dystrophy, right eye
●   **H18.532** Granular corneal dystrophy, left eye
●   **H18.533** Granular corneal dystrophy, bilateral
●   **H18.539** Granular corneal dystrophy, unspecified eye

▲   ✓6ᵗʰ **H18.54** Lattice corneal dystrophy
●   **H18.541** Lattice corneal dystrophy, right eye
●   **H18.542** Lattice corneal dystrophy, left eye
●   **H18.543** Lattice corneal dystrophy, bilateral
●   **H18.549** Lattice corneal dystrophy, unspecified eye

▲   ✓6ᵗʰ **H18.55** Macular corneal dystrophy
●   **H18.551** Macular corneal dystrophy, right eye
●   **H18.552** Macular corneal dystrophy, left eye
●   **H18.553** Macular corneal dystrophy, bilateral
●   **H18.559** Macular corneal dystrophy, unspecified eye

▲   ✓6ᵗʰ **H18.59** Other hereditary corneal dystrophies
●   **H18.591** Other hereditary corneal dystrophies, right eye
●   **H18.592** Other hereditary corneal dystrophies, left eye
●   **H18.593** Other hereditary corneal dystrophies, bilateral
●   **H18.599** Other hereditary corneal dystrophies, unspecified eye

✓5ᵗʰ **H18.6 Keratoconus**

✓6ᵗʰ **H18.60** Keratoconus, unspecified
     H18.601 Keratoconus, unspecified, right eye
     H18.602 Keratoconus, unspecified, left eye
     H18.603 Keratoconus, unspecified, bilateral
     H18.609 Keratoconus, unspecified, unspecified eye

✓6ᵗʰ **H18.61** Keratoconus, stable
     H18.611 Keratoconus, stable, right eye
     H18.612 Keratoconus, stable, left eye
     H18.613 Keratoconus, stable, bilateral
     H18.619 Keratoconus, stable, unspecified eye

✓6ᵗʰ **H18.62** Keratoconus, unstable
     Acute hydrops
     H18.621 Keratoconus, unstable, right eye
     H18.622 Keratoconus, unstable, left eye
     H18.623 Keratoconus, unstable, bilateral
     H18.629 Keratoconus, unstable, unspecified eye

✓5ᵗʰ **H18.7 Other and unspecified corneal deformities**
     EXCLUDES 1   congenital malformations of cornea (Q13.3-Q13.4)
     H18.70 Unspecified corneal deformity

✓6ᵗʰ **H18.71** Corneal ectasia
     H18.711 Corneal ectasia, right eye
     H18.712 Corneal ectasia, left eye
     H18.713 Corneal ectasia, bilateral
     H18.719 Corneal ectasia, unspecified eye

✓6ᵗʰ **H18.72** Corneal staphyloma
     H18.721 Corneal staphyloma, right eye
     H18.722 Corneal staphyloma, left eye
     H18.723 Corneal staphyloma, bilateral
     H18.729 Corneal staphyloma, unspecified eye

✓6ᵗʰ **H18.73** Descemetocele
     H18.731 Descemetocele, right eye
     H18.732 Descemetocele, left eye
     H18.733 Descemetocele, bilateral
     H18.739 Descemetocele, unspecified eye

✓6ᵗʰ **H18.79** Other corneal deformities
     H18.791 Other corneal deformities, right eye
     H18.792 Other corneal deformities, left eye
     H18.793 Other corneal deformities, bilateral
     H18.799 Other corneal deformities, unspecified eye

✓5ᵗʰ **H18.8 Other specified disorders of cornea**

✓6ᵗʰ **H18.81** Anesthesia and hypoesthesia of cornea
     H18.811 Anesthesia and hypoesthesia of cornea, right eye
     H18.812 Anesthesia and hypoesthesia of cornea, left eye

     H18.813 Anesthesia and hypoesthesia of cornea, bilateral
     H18.819 Anesthesia and hypoesthesia of cornea, unspecified eye

✓6ᵗʰ **H18.82** Corneal disorder due to contact lens
     EXCLUDES 2   corneal edema due to contact lens (H18.21-)
     H18.821 Corneal disorder due to contact lens, right eye
     H18.822 Corneal disorder due to contact lens, left eye
     H18.823 Corneal disorder due to contact lens, bilateral
     H18.829 Corneal disorder due to contact lens, unspecified eye

✓6ᵗʰ **H18.83** Recurrent erosion of cornea
     H18.831 Recurrent erosion of cornea, right eye
     H18.832 Recurrent erosion of cornea, left eye
     H18.833 Recurrent erosion of cornea, bilateral
     H18.839 Recurrent erosion of cornea, unspecified eye

✓6ᵗʰ **H18.89** Other specified disorders of cornea
     H18.891 Other specified disorders of cornea, right eye
     H18.892 Other specified disorders of cornea, left eye
     H18.893 Other specified disorders of cornea, bilateral
     H18.899 Other specified disorders of cornea, unspecified eye

H18.9 Unspecified disorder of cornea

✓4ᵗʰ **H20 Iridocyclitis**

✓5ᵗʰ **H20.0 Acute and subacute iridocyclitis**
     Acute anterior uveitis
     Acute cyclitis
     Acute iritis
     Subacute anterior uveitis
     Subacute cyclitis
     Subacute iritis
     EXCLUDES 1   iridocyclitis, iritis, uveitis (due to) (in) diabetes mellitus (E08-E13 with .39)
         iridocyclitis, iritis, uveitis (due to) (in) diphtheria (A36.89)
         iridocyclitis, iritis, uveitis (due to) (in) gonococcal (A54.32)
         iridocyclitis, iritis, uveitis (due to) (in) herpes (simplex) (B00.51)
         iridocyclitis, iritis, uveitis (due to) (in) herpes zoster (B02.32)
         iridocyclitis, iritis, uveitis (due to) (in) late congenital syphilis (A50.39)
         iridocyclitis, iritis, uveitis (due to) (in) late syphilis (A52.71)
         iridocyclitis, iritis, uveitis (due to) (in) sarcoidosis (D86.83)
         iridocyclitis, iritis, uveitis (due to) (in) syphilis (A51.43)
         iridocyclitis, iritis, uveitis (due to) (in) toxoplasmosis (B58.09)
         iridocyclitis, iritis, uveitis (due to) (in) tuberculosis (A18.54)

     H20.00 Unspecified acute and subacute iridocyclitis   CC

✓6ᵗʰ **H20.01** Primary iridocyclitis
     H20.011 Primary iridocyclitis, right eye   CC
     H20.012 Primary iridocyclitis, left eye   CC
     H20.013 Primary iridocyclitis, bilateral   CC
     H20.019 Primary iridocyclitis, unspecified eye   CC

✓6ᵗʰ **H20.02** Recurrent acute iridocyclitis
     H20.021 Recurrent acute iridocyclitis, right eye   CC
     H20.022 Recurrent acute iridocyclitis, left eye   CC
     H20.023 Recurrent acute iridocyclitis, bilateral   CC
     H20.029 Recurrent acute iridocyclitis, unspecified eye   CC

Chapter 7. Diseases of the Eye and Adnexa *(side margin)*

  ✓6ᵗ **H20.03** Secondary infectious iridocyclitis

    H20.031 Secondary infectious iridocyclitis, right eye   CC

    H20.032 Secondary infectious iridocyclitis, left eye   CC

    H20.033 Secondary infectious iridocyclitis, bilateral   CC

    H20.039 Secondary infectious iridocyclitis, unspecified eye   CC

  ✓6ᵗ **H20.04** Secondary noninfectious iridocyclitis

    H20.041 Secondary noninfectious iridocyclitis, right eye

    H20.042 Secondary noninfectious iridocyclitis, left eye

    H20.043 Secondary noninfectious iridocyclitis, bilateral

    H20.049 Secondary noninfectious iridocyclitis, unspecified eye

  ✓6ᵗ **H20.05** Hypopyon

    H20.051 Hypopyon, right eye

    H20.052 Hypopyon, left eye

    H20.053 Hypopyon, bilateral

    H20.059 Hypopyon, unspecified eye

✓5ᵗ **H20.1** Chronic iridocyclitis

    Use additional code for any associated cataract (H26.21-)

    EXCLUDES 2   posterior cyclitis (H30.2-)

    H20.10 Chronic iridocyclitis, unspecified eye

    H20.11 Chronic iridocyclitis, right eye

    H20.12 Chronic iridocyclitis, left eye

    H20.13 Chronic iridocyclitis, bilateral

✓5ᵗ **H20.2** Lens-induced iridocyclitis

    H20.20 Lens-induced iridocyclitis, unspecified eye

    H20.21 Lens-induced iridocyclitis, right eye

    H20.22 Lens-induced iridocyclitis, left eye

    H20.23 Lens-induced iridocyclitis, bilateral

✓5ᵗ **H20.8** Other iridocyclitis

    EXCLUDES 2   glaucomatocyclitis crises (H40.4-)

              posterior cyclitis (H30.2-)

              sympathetic uveitis (H44.13-)

  ✓6ᵗ **H20.81** Fuchs' heterochromic cyclitis

    H20.811 Fuchs' heterochromic cyclitis, right eye

    H20.812 Fuchs' heterochromic cyclitis, left eye

    H20.813 Fuchs' heterochromic cyclitis, bilateral

    H20.819 Fuchs' heterochromic cyclitis, unspecified eye

  ✓6ᵗ **H20.82** Vogt-Koyanagi syndrome

    H20.821 Vogt-Koyanagi syndrome, right eye

    H20.822 Vogt-Koyanagi syndrome, left eye

    H20.823 Vogt-Koyanagi syndrome, bilateral

    H20.829 Vogt-Koyanagi syndrome, unspecified eye

H20.9 Unspecified iridocyclitis   CC

    Uveitis NOS

✓4ᵗ **H21** Other disorders of iris and ciliary body

    EXCLUDES 2   sympathetic uveitis (H44.1-)

✓5ᵗ **H21.0** Hyphema

    EXCLUDES 1   traumatic hyphema (S05.1-)

Hyphema

    — Iris
    — Cornea
    — Hyphema

    H21.00 Hyphema, unspecified eye

    H21.01 Hyphema, right eye

    H21.02 Hyphema, left eye

    H21.03 Hyphema, bilateral

✓5ᵗ **H21.1** Other vascular disorders of iris and ciliary body

    Neovascularization of iris or ciliary body

    Rubeosis iridis

    Rubeosis of iris

  ✓6ᵗ **H21.1X** Other vascular disorders of iris and ciliary body

    H21.1X1 Other vascular disorders of iris and ciliary body, right eye

    H21.1X2 Other vascular disorders of iris and ciliary body, left eye

    H21.1X3 Other vascular disorders of iris and ciliary body, bilateral

    H21.1X9 Other vascular disorders of iris and ciliary body, unspecified eye

✓5ᵗ **H21.2** Degeneration of iris and ciliary body

  ✓6ᵗ **H21.21** Degeneration of chamber angle

    H21.211 Degeneration of chamber angle, right eye

    H21.212 Degeneration of chamber angle, left eye

    H21.213 Degeneration of chamber angle, bilateral

    H21.219 Degeneration of chamber angle, unspecified eye

  ✓6ᵗ **H21.22** Degeneration of ciliary body

    H21.221 Degeneration of ciliary body, right eye

    H21.222 Degeneration of ciliary body, left eye

    H21.223 Degeneration of ciliary body, bilateral

    H21.229 Degeneration of ciliary body, unspecified eye

  ✓6ᵗ **H21.23** Degeneration of iris (pigmentary)

    Translucency of iris

    H21.231 Degeneration of iris (pigmentary), right eye

    H21.232 Degeneration of iris (pigmentary), left eye

    H21.233 Degeneration of iris (pigmentary), bilateral

    H21.239 Degeneration of iris (pigmentary), unspecified eye

  ✓6ᵗ **H21.24** Degeneration of pupillary margin

    H21.241 Degeneration of pupillary margin, right eye

    H21.242 Degeneration of pupillary margin, left eye

    H21.243 Degeneration of pupillary margin, bilateral

    H21.249 Degeneration of pupillary margin, unspecified eye

  ✓6ᵗ **H21.25** Iridoschisis

    H21.251 Iridoschisis, right eye

    H21.252 Iridoschisis, left eye

    H21.253 Iridoschisis, bilateral

    H21.259 Iridoschisis, unspecified eye

  ✓6ᵗ **H21.26** Iris atrophy (essential) (progressive)

    H21.261 Iris atrophy (essential) (progressive), right eye

    H21.262 Iris atrophy (essential) (progressive), left eye

    H21.263 Iris atrophy (essential) (progressive), bilateral

    H21.269 Iris atrophy (essential) (progressive), unspecified eye

  ✓6ᵗ **H21.27** Miotic pupillary cyst

    H21.271 Miotic pupillary cyst, right eye

    H21.272 Miotic pupillary cyst, left eye

    H21.273 Miotic pupillary cyst, bilateral

    H21.279 Miotic pupillary cyst, unspecified eye

    H21.29 Other iris atrophy

✓5ᵗ **H21.3** Cyst of iris, ciliary body and anterior chamber

    EXCLUDES 2   miotic pupillary cyst (H21.27-)

  ✓6ᵗ **H21.30** Idiopathic cysts of iris, ciliary body or anterior chamber

    Cyst of iris, ciliary body or anterior chamber NOS

    H21.301 Idiopathic cysts of iris, ciliary body or anterior chamber, right eye

    H21.302 Idiopathic cysts of iris, ciliary body or anterior chamber, left eye

    H21.303 Idiopathic cysts of iris, ciliary body or anterior chamber, bilateral

N Newborn: 0   P Pediatric: 0-17   M Maternity: 9-64   A Adult: 15-124   MCC Major Complication/Comorbidity   CC Complication/Comorbidity   SW Severe Wound Dx

608   ICD-10-CM 2021

H21.309 Idiopathic cysts of iris, ciliary body or anterior chamber, unspecified eye

✓6ᵗʰ **H21.31** Exudative cysts of iris or anterior chamber

H21.311 Exudative cysts of iris or anterior chamber, right eye

H21.312 Exudative cysts of iris or anterior chamber, left eye

H21.313 Exudative cysts of iris or anterior chamber, bilateral

H21.319 Exudative cysts of iris or anterior chamber, unspecified eye

✓6ᵗʰ **H21.32** Implantation cysts of iris, ciliary body or anterior chamber

H21.321 Implantation cysts of iris, ciliary body or anterior chamber, right eye

H21.322 Implantation cysts of iris, ciliary body or anterior chamber, left eye

H21.323 Implantation cysts of iris, ciliary body or anterior chamber, bilateral

H21.329 Implantation cysts of iris, ciliary body or anterior chamber, unspecified eye

✓6ᵗʰ **H21.33** Parasitic cyst of iris, ciliary body or anterior chamber

H21.331 Parasitic cyst of iris, ciliary body or anterior chamber, right eye `CC`

H21.332 Parasitic cyst of iris, ciliary body or anterior chamber, left eye `CC`

H21.333 Parasitic cyst of iris, ciliary body or anterior chamber, bilateral `CC`

H21.339 Parasitic cyst of iris, ciliary body or anterior chamber, unspecified eye `CC`

✓6ᵗʰ **H21.34** Primary cyst of pars plana

H21.341 Primary cyst of pars plana, right eye

H21.342 Primary cyst of pars plana, left eye

H21.343 Primary cyst of pars plana, bilateral

H21.349 Primary cyst of pars plana, unspecified eye

✓6ᵗʰ **H21.35** Exudative cyst of pars plana

DEF: Protein, fatty-filled bullous elevation of the nonpigmented outermost ciliary epithelium of pars plana, due to fluid leak from blood vessels.

H21.351 Exudative cyst of pars plana, right eye

H21.352 Exudative cyst of pars plana, left eye

H21.353 Exudative cyst of pars plana, bilateral

H21.359 Exudative cyst of pars plana, unspecified eye

✓5ᵗʰ **H21.4** Pupillary membranes

Iris bombé
Pupillary occlusion
Pupillary seclusion
EXCLUDES 1   congenital pupillary membranes (Q13.8)

H21.40 Pupillary membranes, unspecified eye

H21.41 Pupillary membranes, right eye

H21.42 Pupillary membranes, left eye

H21.43 Pupillary membranes, bilateral

✓5ᵗʰ **H21.5** Other and unspecified adhesions and disruptions of iris and ciliary body

EXCLUDES 1   corectopia (Q13.2)

✓6ᵗʰ **H21.50** Unspecified adhesions of iris

Synechia (iris) NOS

H21.501 Unspecified adhesions of iris, right eye

H21.502 Unspecified adhesions of iris, left eye

H21.503 Unspecified adhesions of iris, bilateral

H21.509 Unspecified adhesions of iris and ciliary body, unspecified eye

✓6ᵗʰ **H21.51** Anterior synechiae (iris)

H21.511 Anterior synechiae (iris), right eye

H21.512 Anterior synechiae (iris), left eye

H21.513 Anterior synechiae (iris), bilateral

H21.519 Anterior synechiae (iris), unspecified eye

✓6ᵗʰ **H21.52** Goniosynechiae

H21.521 Goniosynechiae, right eye

H21.522 Goniosynechiae, left eye

H21.523 Goniosynechiae, bilateral

H21.529 Goniosynechiae, unspecified eye

✓6ᵗʰ **H21.53** Iridodialysis

H21.531 Iridodialysis, right eye

H21.532 Iridodialysis, left eye

H21.533 Iridodialysis, bilateral

H21.539 Iridodialysis, unspecified eye

✓6ᵗʰ **H21.54** Posterior synechiae (iris)

H21.541 Posterior synechiae (iris), right eye

H21.542 Posterior synechiae (iris), left eye

H21.543 Posterior synechiae (iris), bilateral

H21.549 Posterior synechiae (iris), unspecified eye

✓6ᵗʰ **H21.55** Recession of chamber angle

H21.551 Recession of chamber angle, right eye

H21.552 Recession of chamber angle, left eye

H21.553 Recession of chamber angle, bilateral

H21.559 Recession of chamber angle, unspecified eye

✓6ᵗʰ **H21.56** Pupillary abnormalities

Deformed pupil
Ectopic pupil
Rupture of sphincter, pupil
EXCLUDES 1   congenital deformity of pupil (Q13.2-)

H21.561 Pupillary abnormality, right eye

H21.562 Pupillary abnormality, left eye

H21.563 Pupillary abnormality, bilateral

H21.569 Pupillary abnormality, unspecified eye

✓5ᵗʰ **H21.8** Other specified disorders of iris and ciliary body

H21.81 Floppy iris syndrome

Intraoperative floppy iris syndrome (IFIS)
Use additional code for adverse effect, if applicable, to identify drug (T36-T50 with fifth or sixth character 5)

H21.82 Plateau iris syndrome (post-iridectomy) (postprocedural)

H21.89 Other specified disorders of iris and ciliary body

H21.9 Unspecified disorder of iris and ciliary body

H22 *Disorders of iris and ciliary body in diseases classified elsewhere*

Code first underlying disease, such as:
gout (M1A.-, M10.-)
leprosy (A30.-)
parasitic disease (B89)

Disorders of lens (H25-H28)

✓4ᵗʰ **H25** **Age-related cataract**

Senile cataract
EXCLUDES 2   capsular glaucoma with pseudoexfoliation of lens (H40.1-)

Cataracts

Normal lens — Iris, Cornea, Pupil, Lens, Vitreous, Retina

Lens affected by cataracts — Clouded lens

✓5ᵗʰ **H25.0** Age-related incipient cataract

✓6ᵗʰ **H25.01** Cortical age-related cataract

H25.011 Cortical age-related cataract, right eye `A`

H25.012 Cortical age-related cataract, left eye `A`

H25.013 Cortical age-related cataract, bilateral `A`

H25.019 Cortical age-related cataract, unspecified eye `A`

✓6ᵗʰ **H25.03** Anterior subcapsular polar age-related cataract

H25.031 Anterior subcapsular polar age-related cataract, right eye `A`

☑ Additional Character Required   ✓x7ᵗʰ Placeholder   Unacceptable PDx   Questionable PDx   Manifestation   Unspecified Dx   H1-H14 HAC   HCC CMS-HCC Dx   HIV HIV Dx

ICD-10-CM 2021   609

H25.032   Anterior subcapsular polar age-related cataract, **left eye**   A

H25.033   Anterior subcapsular polar age-related cataract, **bilateral**   A

H25.039   Anterior subcapsular polar age-related cataract, **unspecified eye**   A

√6ᵗʰ **H25.04**   Posterior subcapsular polar **age-related cataract**

H25.041   Posterior subcapsular polar age-related cataract, **right eye**   A

H25.042   Posterior subcapsular polar age-related cataract, **left eye**   A

H25.043   Posterior subcapsular polar age-related cataract, **bilateral**   A

H25.049   Posterior subcapsular polar age-related cataract, **unspecified eye**   A

√6ᵗʰ **H25.09**   **Other age-related incipient cataract**

Coronary age-related cataract
Punctate age-related cataract
Water clefts

H25.091   Other age-related incipient cataract, **right eye**   A

H25.092   Other age-related incipient cataract, **left eye**   A

H25.093   Other age-related incipient cataract, **bilateral**   A

H25.099   Other age-related incipient cataract, **unspecified eye**   A

√5ᵗʰ **H25.1**   **Age-related nuclear cataract**

Cataracta brunescens
Nuclear sclerosis cataract
AHA: 2019,2Q,31; 2016,1Q,32

H25.10   **Age-related nuclear cataract, unspecified eye**   A

H25.11   **Age-related nuclear cataract, right eye**   A

H25.12   **Age-related nuclear cataract, left eye**   A

H25.13   **Age-related nuclear cataract, bilateral**   A

√5ᵗʰ **H25.2**   **Age-related cataract, morgagnian type**

Age-related hypermature cataract

H25.20   **Age-related cataract, morgagnian type, unspecified eye**   A

H25.21   **Age-related cataract, morgagnian type, right eye**   A

H25.22   **Age-related cataract, morgagnian type, left eye**   A

H25.23   **Age-related cataract, morgagnian type, bilateral**   A

√5ᵗʰ **H25.8**   **Other age-related cataract**

√6ᵗʰ **H25.81**   Combined forms of **age-related cataract**

AHA: 2019,2Q,30

H25.811   Combined forms of age-related cataract, **right eye**   A

H25.812   Combined forms of age-related cataract, **left eye**   A

H25.813   Combined forms of age-related cataract, **bilateral**   A

H25.819   Combined forms of age-related cataract, **unspecified eye**   A

H25.89   **Other age-related cataract**   A

H25.9   **Unspecified age-related cataract**   A

√4ᵗʰ **H26**   **Other cataract**

EXCLUDES 1   congenital cataract (Q12.0)

√5ᵗʰ **H26.0**   Infantile and juvenile **cataract**

√6ᵗʰ **H26.00**   **Unspecified infantile and juvenile cataract**

H26.001   Unspecified infantile and juvenile cataract, **right eye**   P

H26.002   Unspecified infantile and juvenile cataract, **left eye**   P

H26.003   Unspecified infantile and juvenile cataract, **bilateral**   P

H26.009   Unspecified infantile and juvenile cataract, **unspecified eye**   P

√6ᵗʰ **H26.01**   Infantile and juvenile **cortical, lamellar, or zonular cataract**

H26.011   Infantile and juvenile cortical, lamellar, or zonular cataract, **right eye**   P

H26.012   Infantile and juvenile cortical, lamellar, or zonular cataract, **left eye**   P

H26.013   Infantile and juvenile cortical, lamellar, or zonular cataract, **bilateral**   P

H26.019   Infantile and juvenile cortical, lamellar, or zonular cataract, **unspecified eye**   P

√6ᵗʰ **H26.03**   Infantile and juvenile **nuclear cataract**

H26.031   Infantile and juvenile nuclear cataract, **right eye**   P

H26.032   Infantile and juvenile nuclear cataract, **left eye**   P

H26.033   Infantile and juvenile nuclear cataract, **bilateral**   P

H26.039   Infantile and juvenile nuclear cataract, **unspecified eye**   P

√6ᵗʰ **H26.04**   Anterior subcapsular polar **infantile and juvenile cataract**

H26.041   Anterior subcapsular polar infantile and juvenile cataract, **right eye**   P

H26.042   Anterior subcapsular polar infantile and juvenile cataract, **left eye**   P

H26.043   Anterior subcapsular polar infantile and juvenile cataract, **bilateral**   P

H26.049   Anterior subcapsular polar infantile and juvenile cataract, **unspecified eye**   P

√6ᵗʰ **H26.05**   Posterior subcapsular polar **infantile and juvenile cataract**

H26.051   Posterior subcapsular polar infantile and juvenile cataract, **right eye**   P

H26.052   Posterior subcapsular polar infantile and juvenile cataract, **left eye**   P

H26.053   Posterior subcapsular polar infantile and juvenile cataract, **bilateral**   P

H26.059   Posterior subcapsular polar infantile and juvenile cataract, **unspecified eye**   P

√6ᵗʰ **H26.06**   **Combined forms of infantile and juvenile cataract**

H26.061   Combined forms of infantile and juvenile cataract, **right eye**   P

H26.062   Combined forms of infantile and juvenile cataract, **left eye**   P

H26.063   Combined forms of infantile and juvenile cataract, **bilateral**   P

H26.069   Combined forms of infantile and juvenile cataract, **unspecified eye**   P

H26.09   **Other infantile and juvenile cataract**   P

√5ᵗʰ **H26.1**   **Traumatic cataract**

Use additional code (Chapter 20) to identify external cause

√6ᵗʰ **H26.10**   **Unspecified traumatic cataract**

H26.101   Unspecified traumatic cataract, **right eye**

H26.102   Unspecified traumatic cataract, **left eye**

H26.103   Unspecified traumatic cataract, **bilateral**

H26.109   Unspecified traumatic cataract, **unspecified eye**

√6ᵗʰ **H26.11**   **Localized traumatic opacities**

H26.111   Localized traumatic opacities, **right eye**

H26.112   Localized traumatic opacities, **left eye**

H26.113   Localized traumatic opacities, **bilateral**

H26.119   Localized traumatic opacities, **unspecified eye**

√6ᵗʰ **H26.12**   **Partially resolved traumatic cataract**

H26.121   Partially resolved traumatic cataract, **right eye**

H26.122   Partially resolved traumatic cataract, **left eye**

H26.123   Partially resolved traumatic cataract, **bilateral**

H26.129   Partially resolved traumatic cataract, **unspecified eye**

√6ᵗʰ **H26.13**   **Total traumatic cataract**

H26.131   Total traumatic cataract, **right eye**

H26.132   Total traumatic cataract, **left eye**

H26.133   Total traumatic cataract, **bilateral**

H26.139   Total traumatic cataract, **unspecified eye**

√5ᵗʰ **H26.2**   **Complicated cataract**

H26.20   **Unspecified complicated cataract**

Cataracta complicata NOS

√6ᵗʰ **H26.21**   **Cataract with neovascularization**

Code also associated condition, such as:
chronic iridocyclitis (H20.1-)

H26.211   Cataract with neovascularization, **right eye**

N Newborn: 0   P Pediatric: 0-17   M Maternity: 9-64   A Adult: 15-124   MCC Major Complication/Comorbidity   CC Complication/Comorbidity   SW Severe Wound Dx

610

ICD-10-CM 2021

H26.212 Cataract with neovascularization, **left eye**

H26.213 Cataract with neovascularization, **bilateral**

H26.219 Cataract with neovascularization, **unspecified eye**

√6ᵗʰ **H26.22** Cataract secondary to ocular disorders (degenerative) (inflammatory)
  Code also associated ocular disorder

H26.221 Cataract secondary to ocular disorders (degenerative) (inflammatory), **right eye**

H26.222 Cataract secondary to ocular disorders (degenerative) (inflammatory), **left eye**

H26.223 Cataract secondary to ocular disorders (degenerative) (inflammatory), **bilateral**

H26.229 Cataract secondary to ocular disorders (degenerative) (inflammatory), **unspecified eye**

√6ᵗʰ **H26.23** Glaucomatous flecks (subcapsular)
  Code first underlying glaucoma (H40-H42)

H26.231 Glaucomatous flecks (subcapsular), **right eye**

H26.232 Glaucomatous flecks (subcapsular), **left eye**

H26.233 Glaucomatous flecks (subcapsular), **bilateral**

H26.239 Glaucomatous flecks (subcapsular), **unspecified eye**

√5ᵗʰ **H26.3** Drug-induced **cataract**
  Toxic cataract
  Use additional code for adverse effect, if applicable, to identify drug (T36-T50 with fifth or sixth character 5)

H26.30 Drug-induced cataract, **unspecified eye**

H26.31 Drug-induced cataract, **right eye**

H26.32 Drug-induced cataract, **left eye**

H26.33 Drug-induced cataract, **bilateral**

√5ᵗʰ **H26.4** Secondary cataract

H26.40 Unspecified secondary cataract

√6ᵗʰ **H26.41** Soemmering's ring

H26.411 Soemmering's ring, **right eye**

H26.412 Soemmering's ring, **left eye**

H26.413 Soemmering's ring, **bilateral**

H26.419 Soemmering's ring, **unspecified eye**

√6ᵗʰ **H26.49** Other secondary cataract
  AHA: 2018,2Q,14

H26.491 Other secondary cataract, **right eye**

H26.492 Other secondary cataract, **left eye**

H26.493 Other secondary cataract, **bilateral**

H26.499 Other secondary cataract, **unspecified eye**

H26.8 Other specified cataract

H26.9 Unspecified cataract

√4ᵗʰ **H27** Other disorders of lens

EXCLUDES 1 *congenital lens malformations (Q12.-)*
  mechanical complications of intraocular lens implant (T85.2)
  pseudophakia (Z96.1)

√5ᵗʰ **H27.0** Aphakia
  Acquired absence of lens
  Acquired aphakia
  Aphakia due to trauma
  EXCLUDES 1 *cataract extraction status (Z98.4-)*
    congenital absence of lens (Q12.3)
    congenital aphakia (Q12.3)

H27.00 Aphakia, **unspecified eye**

H27.01 Aphakia, **right eye**

H27.02 Aphakia, **left eye**

H27.03 Aphakia, **bilateral**

√5ᵗʰ **H27.1** Dislocation of lens

H27.10 Unspecified dislocation of lens

√6ᵗʰ **H27.11** Subluxation of lens

H27.111 Subluxation of lens, **right eye**

H27.112 Subluxation of lens, **left eye**

H27.113 Subluxation of lens, **bilateral**

H27.119 Subluxation of lens, **unspecified eye**

√6ᵗʰ **H27.12** Anterior dislocation of lens

H27.121 Anterior dislocation of lens, **right eye**

H27.122 Anterior dislocation of lens, **left eye**

H27.123 Anterior dislocation of lens, **bilateral**

H27.129 Anterior dislocation of lens, **unspecified eye**

√6ᵗʰ **H27.13** Posterior dislocation of lens

H27.131 Posterior dislocation of lens, **right eye**

H27.132 Posterior dislocation of lens, **left eye**

H27.133 Posterior dislocation of lens, **bilateral**

H27.139 Posterior dislocation of lens, **unspecified eye**

H27.8 Other specified disorders of lens

H27.9 Unspecified disorder of lens

H28 *Cataract in diseases classified elsewhere*
  Code first underlying disease, such as:
    hypoparathyroidism (E20.-)
    myotonia (G71.1-)
    myxedema (E03.-)
    protein-calorie malnutrition (E40-E46)
  EXCLUDES 1 *cataract in diabetes mellitus (E08.36, E09.36, E10.36, E11.36, E13.36)*

Disorders of choroid and retina (H30-H36)

√4ᵗʰ **H30** Chorioretinal inflammation

√5ᵗʰ **H30.0** Focal **chorioretinal inflammation**
  Focal chorioretinitis
  Focal choroiditis
  Focal retinitis
  Focal retinochoroiditis

√6ᵗʰ **H30.00** Unspecified focal chorioretinal inflammation
  Focal chorioretinitis NOS
  Focal choroiditis NOS
  Focal retinitis NOS
  Focal retinochoroiditis NOS

H30.001 Unspecified focal chorioretinal inflammation, **right eye**

H30.002 Unspecified focal chorioretinal inflammation, **left eye**

H30.003 Unspecified focal chorioretinal inflammation, **bilateral**

H30.009 Unspecified focal chorioretinal inflammation, **unspecified eye**

√6ᵗʰ **H30.01** Focal chorioretinal inflammation, **juxtapapillary**

H30.011 Focal chorioretinal inflammation, **juxtapapillary, right eye**

H30.012 Focal chorioretinal inflammation, **juxtapapillary, left eye**

H30.013 Focal chorioretinal inflammation, **juxtapapillary, bilateral**

H30.019 Focal chorioretinal inflammation, **juxtapapillary, unspecified eye**

√6ᵗʰ **H30.02** Focal chorioretinal inflammation of **posterior pole**

H30.021 Focal chorioretinal inflammation of posterior pole, **right eye**

H30.022 Focal chorioretinal inflammation of posterior pole, **left eye**

H30.023 Focal chorioretinal inflammation of posterior pole, **bilateral**

H30.029 Focal chorioretinal inflammation of posterior pole, **unspecified eye**

√6ᵗʰ **H30.03** Focal chorioretinal inflammation, **peripheral**

H30.031 Focal chorioretinal inflammation, **peripheral, right eye**

H30.032 Focal chorioretinal inflammation, **peripheral, left eye**

H30.033 Focal chorioretinal inflammation, **peripheral, bilateral**

H30.039 Focal chorioretinal inflammation, **peripheral, unspecified eye**

√6ᵗʰ **H30.04** Focal chorioretinal inflammation, **macular or paramacular**

H30.041 Focal chorioretinal inflammation, **macular or paramacular, right eye**

H30.042 Focal chorioretinal inflammation, **macular or paramacular, left eye**

H30.043 Focal chorioretinal inflammation, **macular or paramacular, bilateral**

H30.049 Focal chorioretinal inflammation, **macular or paramacular, unspecified eye**

✔ Additional Character Required   √x7ᵗʰ Placeholder   Unacceptable PDx   Questionable PDx   Manifestation   Unspecified Dx   H1-H14 HAC   HCC CMS-HCC Dx   HIV HIV Dx

ICD-10-CM 2021   **611**

✓5ᵗʰ **H30.1** Disseminated **chorioretinal inflammation**

Disseminated chorioretinitis
Disseminated choroiditis
Disseminated retinitis
Disseminated retinochoroiditis

EXCLUDES 2   *exudative retinopathy (H35.02-)*

✓6ᵗʰ **H30.10 Unspecified disseminated chorioretinal inflammation**

Disseminated chorioretinitis NOS
Disseminated choroiditis NOS
Disseminated retinitis NOS
Disseminated retinochoroiditis NOS

H30.101 Unspecified disseminated chorioretinal inflammation, **right** eye   `CC`

H30.102 Unspecified disseminated chorioretinal inflammation, **left** eye   `CC`

H30.103 Unspecified disseminated chorioretinal inflammation, **bilateral**   `CC`

H30.109 Unspecified disseminated chorioretinal inflammation, unspecified eye   `CC`

✓6ᵗʰ **H30.11** Disseminated chorioretinal inflammation of posterior pole

H30.111 Disseminated chorioretinal inflammation of posterior pole, **right** eye   `CC`

H30.112 Disseminated chorioretinal inflammation of posterior pole, **left** eye   `CC`

H30.113 Disseminated chorioretinal inflammation of posterior pole, **bilateral**   `CC`

H30.119 Disseminated chorioretinal inflammation of posterior pole, unspecified eye   `CC`

✓6ᵗʰ **H30.12** Disseminated chorioretinal inflammation, peripheral

H30.121 Disseminated chorioretinal inflammation, peripheral **right** eye   `CC`

H30.122 Disseminated chorioretinal inflammation, peripheral, **left** eye   `CC`

H30.123 Disseminated chorioretinal inflammation, peripheral, **bilateral**   `CC`

H30.129 Disseminated chorioretinal inflammation, peripheral, unspecified eye   `CC`

✓6ᵗʰ **H30.13** Disseminated chorioretinal inflammation, generalized

H30.131 Disseminated chorioretinal inflammation, generalized, **right** eye   `CC`

H30.132 Disseminated chorioretinal inflammation, generalized, **left** eye   `CC`

H30.133 Disseminated chorioretinal inflammation, generalized, **bilateral**   `CC`

H30.139 Disseminated chorioretinal inflammation, generalized, unspecified eye   `CC`

✓6ᵗʰ **H30.14** Acute posterior multifocal placoid pigment epitheliopathy

H30.141 Acute posterior multifocal placoid pigment epitheliopathy, **right** eye   `CC`

H30.142 Acute posterior multifocal placoid pigment epitheliopathy, **left** eye   `CC`

H30.143 Acute posterior multifocal placoid pigment epitheliopathy, **bilateral**   `CC`

H30.149 Acute posterior multifocal placoid pigment epitheliopathy, unspecified eye   `CC`

✓5ᵗʰ **H30.2** Posterior cyclitis

Pars planitis

H30.20 Posterior cyclitis, unspecified eye

H30.21 Posterior cyclitis, **right** eye

H30.22 Posterior cyclitis, **left** eye

H30.23 Posterior cyclitis, **bilateral**

✓5ᵗʰ **H30.8** Other chorioretinal inflammations

✓6ᵗʰ **H30.81** Harada's disease

H30.811 Harada's disease, **right** eye

H30.812 Harada's disease, **left** eye

H30.813 Harada's disease, **bilateral**

H30.819 Harada's disease, unspecified eye

✓6ᵗʰ **H30.89** Other chorioretinal inflammations

H30.891 Other chorioretinal inflammations, **right** eye   `CC`

H30.892 Other chorioretinal inflammations, **left** eye   `CC`

H30.893 Other chorioretinal inflammations, **bilateral**   `CC`

H30.899 Other chorioretinal inflammations, unspecified eye   `CC`

✓5ᵗʰ **H30.9** Unspecified chorioretinal inflammation

Chorioretinitis NOS
Choroiditis NOS
Neuroretinitis NOS
Retinitis NOS
Retinochoroiditis NOS

H30.90 Unspecified chorioretinal inflammation, unspecified eye   `CC`

H30.91 Unspecified chorioretinal inflammation, **right** eye   `CC`

H30.92 Unspecified chorioretinal inflammation, **left** eye   `CC`

H30.93 Unspecified chorioretinal inflammation, **bilateral**   `CC`

✓4ᵗʰ **H31 Other disorders of choroid**

✓5ᵗʰ **H31.0** Chorioretinal scars

EXCLUDES 2   *postsurgical chorioretinal scars (H59.81-)*

✓6ᵗʰ **H31.00** Unspecified chorioretinal scars

H31.001 Unspecified chorioretinal scars, **right** eye

H31.002 Unspecified chorioretinal scars, **left** eye

H31.003 Unspecified chorioretinal scars, **bilateral**

H31.009 Unspecified chorioretinal scars, unspecified eye

✓6ᵗʰ **H31.01** Macula scars of posterior pole (postinflammatory) (post-traumatic)

EXCLUDES 1   *postprocedural chorioretinal scar (H59.81-)*

H31.011 Macula scars of posterior pole (postinflammatory) (post-traumatic), **right** eye

H31.012 Macula scars of posterior pole (postinflammatory) (post-traumatic), **left** eye

H31.013 Macula scars of posterior pole (postinflammatory) (post-traumatic), **bilateral**

H31.019 Macula scars of posterior pole (postinflammatory) (post-traumatic), unspecified eye

✓6ᵗʰ **H31.02** Solar retinopathy

H31.021 Solar retinopathy, **right** eye

H31.022 Solar retinopathy, **left** eye

H31.023 Solar retinopathy, **bilateral**

H31.029 Solar retinopathy, unspecified eye

✓6ᵗʰ **H31.09** Other chorioretinal scars

H31.091 Other chorioretinal scars, **right** eye

H31.092 Other chorioretinal scars, **left** eye

H31.093 Other chorioretinal scars, **bilateral**

H31.099 Other chorioretinal scars, unspecified eye

✓5ᵗʰ **H31.1** Choroidal degeneration

EXCLUDES 2   *angioid streaks of macula (H35.33)*

✓6ᵗʰ **H31.10** Unspecified choroidal degeneration

Choroidal sclerosis NOS

H31.101 Choroidal degeneration, unspecified, **right** eye

H31.102 Choroidal degeneration, unspecified, **left** eye

H31.103 Choroidal degeneration, unspecified, **bilateral**

H31.109 Choroidal degeneration, unspecified, unspecified eye

✓6ᵗʰ **H31.11** Age-related choroidal atrophy

H31.111 Age-related choroidal atrophy, **right** eye   `A`

H31.112 Age-related choroidal atrophy, **left** eye   `A`

H31.113 Age-related choroidal atrophy, **bilateral**   `A`

H31.119 Age-related choroidal atrophy, unspecified eye   `A`

✓6ᵗʰ **H31.12** Diffuse secondary atrophy of choroid

H31.121 Diffuse secondary atrophy of choroid, **right** eye

| N Newborn: 0 | P Pediatric: 0-17 | M Maternity: 9-64 | A Adult: 15-124 | MCC Major Complication/Comorbidity | CC Complication/Comorbidity | SW Severe Wound Dx |

612

ICD-10-CM 2021

H31.122 Diffuse secondary atrophy of choroid, left eye

H31.123 Diffuse secondary atrophy of choroid, bilateral

H31.129 Diffuse secondary atrophy of choroid, unspecified eye

√5ᵗʰ **H31.2 Hereditary choroidal dystrophy**

EXCLUDES 2   *hyperornithinemia (E72.4)*

ornithinemia (E72.4)

H31.20 Hereditary choroidal dystrophy, unspecified

H31.21 Choroideremia

H31.22 Choroidal dystrophy (central areolar) (generalized) (peripapillary)

H31.23 Gyrate atrophy, choroid

H31.29 Other hereditary choroidal dystrophy

√5ᵗʰ **H31.3 Choroidal hemorrhage and rupture**

√6ᵗʰ **H31.30 Unspecified choroidal hemorrhage**

H31.301 Unspecified choroidal hemorrhage, right eye

H31.302 Unspecified choroidal hemorrhage, left eye

H31.303 Unspecified choroidal hemorrhage, bilateral

H31.309 Unspecified choroidal hemorrhage, unspecified eye

√6ᵗʰ **H31.31 Expulsive choroidal hemorrhage**

H31.311 Expulsive choroidal hemorrhage, right eye

H31.312 Expulsive choroidal hemorrhage, left eye

H31.313 Expulsive choroidal hemorrhage, bilateral

H31.319 Expulsive choroidal hemorrhage, unspecified eye

√6ᵗʰ **H31.32 Choroidal rupture**

H31.321 Choroidal rupture, right eye   CC

H31.322 Choroidal rupture, left eye   CC

H31.323 Choroidal rupture, bilateral   CC

H31.329 Choroidal rupture, unspecified eye   CC

√5ᵗʰ **H31.4 Choroidal detachment**

√6ᵗʰ **H31.40 Unspecified choroidal detachment**

H31.401 Unspecified choroidal detachment, right eye   CC

H31.402 Unspecified choroidal detachment, left eye   CC

H31.403 Unspecified choroidal detachment, bilateral   CC

H31.409 Unspecified choroidal detachment, unspecified eye   CC

√6ᵗʰ **H31.41 Hemorrhagic choroidal detachment**

H31.411 Hemorrhagic choroidal detachment, right eye   CC

H31.412 Hemorrhagic choroidal detachment, left eye   CC

H31.413 Hemorrhagic choroidal detachment, bilateral   CC

H31.419 Hemorrhagic choroidal detachment, unspecified eye   CC

√6ᵗʰ **H31.42 Serous choroidal detachment**

H31.421 Serous choroidal detachment, right eye   CC

H31.422 Serous choroidal detachment, left eye   CC

H31.423 Serous choroidal detachment, bilateral   CC

H31.429 Serous choroidal detachment, unspecified eye   CC

H31.8 Other specified disorders of choroid

H31.9 Unspecified disorder of choroid

H32 Chorioretinal disorders in diseases classified elsewhere

Code first underlying disease, such as:

congenital toxoplasmosis (P37.1)

histoplasmosis (B39.-)

leprosy (A30.-)

EXCLUDES 1   *chorioretinitis (in):*

toxoplasmosis (acquired) (B58.01)

tuberculosis (A18.53)

√4ᵗʰ **H33 Retinal detachments and breaks**

EXCLUDES 1   *detachment of retinal pigment epithelium (H35.72-, H35.73-)*

Retinal Detachment

Lens, Vitreous, Choroid, Area of detachment, Iris, Retina, Cornea, Sclera

√5ᵗʰ **H33.0 Retinal detachment with retinal break**

Rhegmatogenous retinal detachment

EXCLUDES 1   *serous retinal detachment (without retinal break) (H33.2-)*

√6ᵗʰ **H33.00 Unspecified retinal detachment with retinal break**

H33.001 Unspecified retinal detachment with retinal break, right eye

H33.002 Unspecified retinal detachment with retinal break, left eye

H33.003 Unspecified retinal detachment with retinal break, bilateral

H33.009 Unspecified retinal detachment with retinal break, unspecified eye

√6ᵗʰ **H33.01 Retinal detachment with single break**

H33.011 Retinal detachment with single break, right eye

H33.012 Retinal detachment with single break, left eye

H33.013 Retinal detachment with single break, bilateral

H33.019 Retinal detachment with single break, unspecified eye

√6ᵗʰ **H33.02 Retinal detachment with multiple breaks**

H33.021 Retinal detachment with multiple breaks, right eye

H33.022 Retinal detachment with multiple breaks, left eye

H33.023 Retinal detachment with multiple breaks, bilateral

H33.029 Retinal detachment with multiple breaks, unspecified eye

√6ᵗʰ **H33.03 Retinal detachment with giant retinal tear**

H33.031 Retinal detachment with giant retinal tear, right eye

H33.032 Retinal detachment with giant retinal tear, left eye

H33.033 Retinal detachment with giant retinal tear, bilateral

H33.039 Retinal detachment with giant retinal tear, unspecified eye

√6ᵗʰ **H33.04 Retinal detachment with retinal dialysis**

H33.041 Retinal detachment with retinal dialysis, right eye

H33.042 Retinal detachment with retinal dialysis, left eye

H33.043 Retinal detachment with retinal dialysis, bilateral

H33.049 Retinal detachment with retinal dialysis, unspecified eye

√6ᵗʰ **H33.05 Total retinal detachment**

H33.051 Total retinal detachment, right eye

H33.052 Total retinal detachment, left eye

H33.053 Total retinal detachment, bilateral

H33.059 Total retinal detachment, unspecified eye

☑ Additional Character Required   √x7ᵗʰ Placeholder   Unacceptable PDx   Questionable PDx   Manifestation   Unspecified Dx   H1-H14 HAC   HCC CMS-HCC Dx   HIV HIV Dx

ICD-10-CM 2021   613

Chapter 7. Diseases of the Eye and Adnexa

H33.1–H34.832

√5ᵗʰ **H33.1 Retinoschisis and retinal cysts**

  EXCLUDES 1   *congenital retinoschisis (Q14.1)*
         microcystoid degeneration of retina (H35.42-)

√6ᵗʰ **H33.10 Unspecified retinoschisis**

  H33.101 Unspecified retinoschisis, right eye
  H33.102 Unspecified retinoschisis, left eye
  H33.103 Unspecified retinoschisis, bilateral
  H33.109 Unspecified retinoschisis, unspecified eye

√6ᵗʰ **H33.11 Cyst of ora serrata**

  H33.111 Cyst of ora serrata, right eye
  H33.112 Cyst of ora serrata, left eye
  H33.113 Cyst of ora serrata, bilateral
  H33.119 Cyst of ora serrata, unspecified eye

√6ᵗʰ **H33.12 Parasitic cyst of retina**

  H33.121 Parasitic cyst of retina, right eye CC
  H33.122 Parasitic cyst of retina, left eye CC
  H33.123 Parasitic cyst of retina, bilateral CC
  H33.129 Parasitic cyst of retina, unspecified eye CC

√6ᵗʰ **H33.19 Other retinoschisis and retinal cysts**

  Pseudocyst of retina
  H33.191 Other retinoschisis and retinal cysts, right eye
  H33.192 Other retinoschisis and retinal cysts, left eye
  H33.193 Other retinoschisis and retinal cysts, bilateral
  H33.199 Other retinoschisis and retinal cysts, unspecified eye

√5ᵗʰ **H33.2 Serous retinal detachment**

  Retinal detachment NOS
  Retinal detachment without retinal break
  EXCLUDES 1   *central serous chorioretinopathy (H35.71-)*

  H33.20 Serous retinal detachment, unspecified eye CC
  H33.21 Serous retinal detachment, right eye CC
  H33.22 Serous retinal detachment, left eye CC
  H33.23 Serous retinal detachment, bilateral CC

√5ᵗʰ **H33.3 Retinal breaks without detachment**

  EXCLUDES 1   *chorioretinal scars after surgery for detachment (H59.81-)*
         peripheral retinal degeneration without break (H35.4-)

√6ᵗʰ **H33.30 Unspecified retinal break**

  H33.301 Unspecified retinal break, right eye
  H33.302 Unspecified retinal break, left eye
  H33.303 Unspecified retinal break, bilateral
  H33.309 Unspecified retinal break, unspecified eye

√6ᵗʰ **H33.31 Horseshoe tear of retina without detachment**

  Operculum of retina without detachment
  H33.311 Horseshoe tear of retina without detachment, right eye
  H33.312 Horseshoe tear of retina without detachment, left eye
  H33.313 Horseshoe tear of retina without detachment, bilateral
  H33.319 Horseshoe tear of retina without detachment, unspecified eye

√6ᵗʰ **H33.32 Round hole of retina without detachment**

  H33.321 Round hole, right eye
  H33.322 Round hole, left eye
  H33.323 Round hole, bilateral
  H33.329 Round hole, unspecified eye

√6ᵗʰ **H33.33 Multiple defects of retina without detachment**

  H33.331 Multiple defects of retina without detachment, right eye
  H33.332 Multiple defects of retina without detachment, left eye
  H33.333 Multiple defects of retina without detachment, bilateral
  H33.339 Multiple defects of retina without detachment, unspecified eye

√5ᵗʰ **H33.4 Traction detachment of retina**

  Proliferative vitreo-retinopathy with retinal detachment
  H33.40 Traction detachment of retina, unspecified eye CC
  H33.41 Traction detachment of retina, right eye CC

  H33.42 Traction detachment of retina, left eye CC
  H33.43 Traction detachment of retina, bilateral CC

H33.8 Other retinal detachments CC

√4ᵗʰ **H34 Retinal vascular occlusions**

  EXCLUDES 1   *amaurosis fugax (G45.3)*

√5ᵗʰ **H34.0 Transient retinal artery occlusion**

  H34.00 Transient retinal artery occlusion, unspecified eye CC
  H34.01 Transient retinal artery occlusion, right eye CC
  H34.02 Transient retinal artery occlusion, left eye CC
  H34.03 Transient retinal artery occlusion, bilateral CC

√5ᵗʰ **H34.1 Central retinal artery occlusion**

  H34.10 Central retinal artery occlusion, unspecified eye CC
  H34.11 Central retinal artery occlusion, right eye CC
  H34.12 Central retinal artery occlusion, left eye CC
  H34.13 Central retinal artery occlusion, bilateral CC

√5ᵗʰ **H34.2 Other retinal artery occlusions**

√6ᵗʰ **H34.21 Partial retinal artery occlusion**

  Hollenhorst's plaque
  Retinal microembolism
  H34.211 Partial retinal artery occlusion, right eye CC
  H34.212 Partial retinal artery occlusion, left eye CC
  H34.213 Partial retinal artery occlusion, bilateral CC
  H34.219 Partial retinal artery occlusion, unspecified eye CC

√6ᵗʰ **H34.23 Retinal artery branch occlusion**

  H34.231 Retinal artery branch occlusion, right eye CC
  H34.232 Retinal artery branch occlusion, left eye CC
  H34.233 Retinal artery branch occlusion, bilateral CC
  H34.239 Retinal artery branch occlusion, unspecified eye CC

√5ᵗʰ **H34.8 Other retinal vascular occlusions**

  AHA: 2016,4Q,19

√6ᵗʰ **H34.81 Central retinal vein occlusion**

> One of the following 7th characters is to be assigned to codes in subcategory H34.81 to designate the severity of the occlusion:
> 0   with macular edema
> 1   with retinal neovascularization
> 2   stable
>   old central retinal vein occlusion

  √7ᵗʰ **H34.811 Central retinal vein occlusion, right eye** CC
  √7ᵗʰ **H34.812 Central retinal vein occlusion, left eye** CC
  √7ᵗʰ **H34.813 Central retinal vein occlusion, bilateral** CC
  √7ᵗʰ **H34.819 Central retinal vein occlusion, unspecified eye** CC

√6ᵗʰ **H34.82 Venous engorgement**

  Incipient retinal vein occlusion
  Partial retinal vein occlusion
  H34.821 Venous engorgement, right eye
  H34.822 Venous engorgement, left eye
  H34.823 Venous engorgement, bilateral
  H34.829 Venous engorgement, unspecified eye

√6ᵗʰ **H34.83 Tributary (branch) retinal vein occlusion**

> One of the following 7th characters is to be assigned to codes in subcategory H34.83 to designate the severity of the occlusion:
> 0   with macular edema
> 1   with retinal neovascularization
> 2   stable
>   old tributary (branch) retinal vein occlusion

  √7ᵗʰ **H34.831 Tributary (branch) retinal vein occlusion, right eye**
  √7ᵗʰ **H34.832 Tributary (branch) retinal vein occlusion, left eye**

       ✓7ᵗʰ **H34.833** **Tributary (branch) retinal vein occlusion, bilateral**

       ✓7ᵗʰ **H34.839** **Tributary (branch) retinal vein occlusion, unspecified eye**

     H34.9 **Unspecified retinal vascular occlusion**   CC

✓4ᵗʰ **H35** **Other retinal disorders**

    EXCLUDES 2   *diabetic retinal disorders (E08.311-E08.359, E09.311-E09.359, E10.311-E10.359, E11.311-E11.359, E13.311-E13.359)*

✓5ᵗʰ **H35.0** **Background retinopathy and retinal vascular changes**

    Code also any associated hypertension (I10.-)

    H35.00 **Unspecified background retinopathy**

   ✓6ᵗʰ **H35.01** **Changes in retinal vascular appearance**

     Retinal vascular sheathing

     H35.011 **Changes in retinal vascular appearance, right eye**

     H35.012 **Changes in retinal vascular appearance, left eye**

     H35.013 **Changes in retinal vascular appearance, bilateral**

     H35.019 **Changes in retinal vascular appearance, unspecified eye**

   ✓6ᵗʰ **H35.02** **Exudative retinopathy**

     Coats retinopathy

     H35.021 **Exudative retinopathy, right eye**

     H35.022 **Exudative retinopathy, left eye**

     H35.023 **Exudative retinopathy, bilateral**

     H35.029 **Exudative retinopathy, unspecified eye**

   ✓6ᵗʰ **H35.03** **Hypertensive retinopathy**

     H35.031 **Hypertensive retinopathy, right eye**

     H35.032 **Hypertensive retinopathy, left eye**

     H35.033 **Hypertensive retinopathy, bilateral**

     H35.039 **Hypertensive retinopathy, unspecified eye**

   ✓6ᵗʰ **H35.04** **Retinal micro-aneurysms, unspecified**

     H35.041 **Retinal micro-aneurysms, unspecified, right eye**

     H35.042 **Retinal micro-aneurysms, unspecified, left eye**

     H35.043 **Retinal micro-aneurysms, unspecified, bilateral**

     H35.049 **Retinal micro-aneurysms, unspecified, unspecified eye**

   ✓6ᵗʰ **H35.05** **Retinal neovascularization, unspecified**

     H35.051 **Retinal neovascularization, unspecified, right eye**

     H35.052 **Retinal neovascularization, unspecified, left eye**

     H35.053 **Retinal neovascularization, unspecified, bilateral**

     H35.059 **Retinal neovascularization, unspecified, unspecified eye**

   ✓6ᵗʰ **H35.06** **Retinal vasculitis**

     Eales disease

     Retinal perivasculitis

     DEF: Sight-threatening intraocular inflammation of the retinal blood vessels that causes minimal, partial, or even complete blindness.

     H35.061 **Retinal vasculitis, right eye**

     H35.062 **Retinal vasculitis, left eye**

     H35.063 **Retinal vasculitis, bilateral**

     H35.069 **Retinal vasculitis, unspecified eye**

   ✓6ᵗʰ **H35.07** **Retinal telangiectasis**

     H35.071 **Retinal telangiectasis, right eye**

     H35.072 **Retinal telangiectasis, left eye**

     H35.073 **Retinal telangiectasis, bilateral**

     H35.079 **Retinal telangiectasis, unspecified eye**

    H35.09 **Other intraretinal microvascular abnormalities**

     Retinal varices

✓5ᵗʰ **H35.1** **Retinopathy of prematurity**

   ✓6ᵗʰ **H35.10** **Retinopathy of prematurity, unspecified**

     Retinopathy of prematurity NOS

     H35.101 **Retinopathy of prematurity, unspecified, right eye**

     H35.102 **Retinopathy of prematurity, unspecified, left eye**

     H35.103 **Retinopathy of prematurity, unspecified, bilateral**

     H35.109 **Retinopathy of prematurity, unspecified, unspecified eye**

   ✓6ᵗʰ **H35.11** **Retinopathy of prematurity, stage 0**

     H35.111 **Retinopathy of prematurity, stage 0, right eye**

     H35.112 **Retinopathy of prematurity, stage 0, left eye**

     H35.113 **Retinopathy of prematurity, stage 0, bilateral**

     H35.119 **Retinopathy of prematurity, stage 0, unspecified eye**

   ✓6ᵗʰ **H35.12** **Retinopathy of prematurity, stage 1**

     H35.121 **Retinopathy of prematurity, stage 1, right eye**

     H35.122 **Retinopathy of prematurity, stage 1, left eye**

     H35.123 **Retinopathy of prematurity, stage 1, bilateral**

     H35.129 **Retinopathy of prematurity, stage 1, unspecified eye**

   ✓6ᵗʰ **H35.13** **Retinopathy of prematurity, stage 2**

     H35.131 **Retinopathy of prematurity, stage 2, right eye**

     H35.132 **Retinopathy of prematurity, stage 2, left eye**

     H35.133 **Retinopathy of prematurity, stage 2, bilateral**

     H35.139 **Retinopathy of prematurity, stage 2, unspecified eye**

   ✓6ᵗʰ **H35.14** **Retinopathy of prematurity, stage 3**

     H35.141 **Retinopathy of prematurity, stage 3, right eye**

     H35.142 **Retinopathy of prematurity, stage 3, left eye**

     H35.143 **Retinopathy of prematurity, stage 3, bilateral**

     H35.149 **Retinopathy of prematurity, stage 3, unspecified eye**

   ✓6ᵗʰ **H35.15** **Retinopathy of prematurity, stage 4**

     H35.151 **Retinopathy of prematurity, stage 4, right eye**

     H35.152 **Retinopathy of prematurity, stage 4, left eye**

     H35.153 **Retinopathy of prematurity, stage 4, bilateral**

     H35.159 **Retinopathy of prematurity, stage 4, unspecified eye**

   ✓6ᵗʰ **H35.16** **Retinopathy of prematurity, stage 5**

     H35.161 **Retinopathy of prematurity, stage 5, right eye**

     H35.162 **Retinopathy of prematurity, stage 5, left eye**

     H35.163 **Retinopathy of prematurity, stage 5, bilateral**

     H35.169 **Retinopathy of prematurity, stage 5, unspecified eye**

   ✓6ᵗʰ **H35.17** **Retrolental fibroplasia**

     H35.171 **Retrolental fibroplasia, right eye**

     H35.172 **Retrolental fibroplasia, left eye**

     H35.173 **Retrolental fibroplasia, bilateral**

     H35.179 **Retrolental fibroplasia, unspecified eye**

✓5ᵗʰ **H35.2** **Other non-diabetic proliferative retinopathy**

    Proliferative vitreo-retinopathy

    EXCLUDES 1   *proliferative vitreo-retinopathy with retinal detachment (H33.4-)*

    H35.20 **Other non-diabetic proliferative retinopathy, unspecified eye**

    H35.21 **Other non-diabetic proliferative retinopathy, right eye**

    H35.22 **Other non-diabetic proliferative retinopathy, left eye**

    H35.23 **Other non-diabetic proliferative retinopathy, bilateral**

✓5ᵗʰ **H35.3** **Degeneration of macula and posterior pole**

    H35.30 **Unspecified macular degeneration**   A

     Age-related macular degeneration

✓ Additional Character Required   ✓x7ᵗʰ Placeholder   Unacceptable PDx   Questionable PDx   Manifestation   Unspecified Dx   H1 - H14 HAC   HCC CMS-HCC Dx   HIV HIV Dx

ICD-10-CM 2021   615

Chapter 7. Diseases of the Eye and Adnexa

H35.31–H35.51

✓6ᵗʰ **H35.31** **Nonexudative age-related macular degeneration**

Atrophic age-related macular degeneration
Dry age-related macular degeneration
AHA: 2016,4Q,20-21

One of the following 7th characters is to be assigned to each code in subcategory H35.31 to designate the stage of the disease:
Ø   stage unspecified
1   early dry stage
2   intermediate dry stage
3   advanced atrophic without subfoveal involvement
     advanced dry stage
4   advanced atrophic with subfoveal involvement

✓7ᵗʰ **H35.311** **Nonexudative age-related macular degeneration, right eye**   A

✓7ᵗʰ **H35.312** **Nonexudative age-related macular degeneration, left eye**   A

✓7ᵗʰ **H35.313** **Nonexudative age-related macular degeneration, bilateral**   A

✓7ᵗʰ **H35.319** **Nonexudative age-related macular degeneration, unspecified eye**   A

✓6ᵗʰ **H35.32** **Exudative age-related macular degeneration**

Wet age-related macular degeneration
AHA: 2016,4Q,20-21

One of the following 7th characters is to be assigned to each code in subcategory H35.32 to designate the stage of the disease:
Ø   stage unspecified
1   with active choroidal neovascularization
2   with inactive choroidal neovascularization
     with involuted or regressed neovascularization
3   with inactive scar

✓7ᵗʰ **H35.321** **Exudative age-related macular degeneration, right eye**   HCC A

✓7ᵗʰ **H35.322** **Exudative age-related macular degeneration, left eye**   HCC A

✓7ᵗʰ **H35.323** **Exudative age-related macular degeneration, bilateral**   HCC A

✓7ᵗʰ **H35.329** **Exudative age-related macular degeneration, unspecified eye**   HCC A

H35.33 **Angioid streaks of macula**
DEF: Degeneration of the choroid; characterized by broad, irregular, dark brown streaks radiating from optic disc; occurs with pseudoxanthoma elasticum or Paget's disease.

✓6ᵗʰ **H35.34** **Macular cyst, hole, or pseudohole**

H35.341 **Macular cyst, hole, or pseudohole, right eye**

H35.342 **Macular cyst, hole, or pseudohole, left eye**

H35.343 **Macular cyst, hole, or pseudohole, bilateral**

H35.349 **Macular cyst, hole, or pseudohole, unspecified eye**

✓6ᵗʰ **H35.35** **Cystoid macular degeneration**

EXCLUDES 1   *cystoid macular edema following cataract surgery (H59.Ø3-)*

H35.351 **Cystoid macular degeneration, right eye**

H35.352 **Cystoid macular degeneration, left eye**

H35.353 **Cystoid macular degeneration, bilateral**

H35.359 **Cystoid macular degeneration, unspecified eye**

✓6ᵗʰ **H35.36** **Drusen (degenerative) of macula**

AHA: 2017,1Q,51; 2016,4Q,21

H35.361 **Drusen (degenerative) of macula, right eye**

H35.362 **Drusen (degenerative) of macula, left eye**

H35.363 **Drusen (degenerative) of macula, bilateral**

H35.369 **Drusen (degenerative) of macula, unspecified eye**

✓6ᵗʰ **H35.37** **Puckering of macula**

H35.371 **Puckering of macula, right eye**

H35.372 **Puckering of macula, left eye**

H35.373 **Puckering of macula, bilateral**

H35.379 **Puckering of macula, unspecified eye**

✓6ᵗʰ **H35.38** **Toxic maculopathy**

Code first poisoning due to drug or toxin, if applicable (T36-T65 with fifth or sixth character 1-4 or 6)
Use additional code for adverse effect, if applicable, to identify drug (T36-T5Ø with fifth or sixth character 5)

H35.381 **Toxic maculopathy, right eye**

H35.382 **Toxic maculopathy, left eye**

H35.383 **Toxic maculopathy, bilateral**

H35.389 **Toxic maculopathy, unspecified eye**

✓6ᵗʰ **H35.4** **Peripheral retinal degeneration**

EXCLUDES 1   *hereditary retinal degeneration (dystrophy) (H35.5-)*
peripheral retinal degeneration with retinal break (H33.3-)

H35.40 **Unspecified peripheral retinal degeneration**

✓6ᵗʰ **H35.41** **Lattice degeneration of retina**

Palisade degeneration of retina
DEF: Degeneration of the retina, often bilateral, that is usually benign. It is characterized by lines intersecting at irregular intervals in the peripheral retina. Retinal thinning and retinal holes may occur.

H35.411 **Lattice degeneration of retina, right eye**

H35.412 **Lattice degeneration of retina, left eye**

H35.413 **Lattice degeneration of retina, bilateral**

H35.419 **Lattice degeneration of retina, unspecified eye**

✓6ᵗʰ **H35.42** **Microcystoid degeneration of retina**

H35.421 **Microcystoid degeneration of retina, right eye**

H35.422 **Microcystoid degeneration of retina, left eye**

H35.423 **Microcystoid degeneration of retina, bilateral**

H35.429 **Microcystoid degeneration of retina, unspecified eye**

✓6ᵗʰ **H35.43** **Paving stone degeneration of retina**

H35.431 **Paving stone degeneration of retina, right eye**

H35.432 **Paving stone degeneration of retina, left eye**

H35.433 **Paving stone degeneration of retina, bilateral**

H35.439 **Paving stone degeneration of retina, unspecified eye**

✓6ᵗʰ **H35.44** **Age-related reticular degeneration of retina**

H35.441 **Age-related reticular degeneration of retina, right eye**   A

H35.442 **Age-related reticular degeneration of retina, left eye**   A

H35.443 **Age-related reticular degeneration of retina, bilateral**   A

H35.449 **Age-related reticular degeneration of retina, unspecified eye**   A

✓6ᵗʰ **H35.45** **Secondary pigmentary degeneration**

H35.451 **Secondary pigmentary degeneration, right eye**

H35.452 **Secondary pigmentary degeneration, left eye**

H35.453 **Secondary pigmentary degeneration, bilateral**

H35.459 **Secondary pigmentary degeneration, unspecified eye**

✓6ᵗʰ **H35.46** **Secondary vitreoretinal degeneration**

H35.461 **Secondary vitreoretinal degeneration, right eye**

H35.462 **Secondary vitreoretinal degeneration, left eye**

H35.463 **Secondary vitreoretinal degeneration, bilateral**

H35.469 **Secondary vitreoretinal degeneration, unspecified eye**

✓5ᵗʰ **H35.5** **Hereditary retinal dystrophy**

EXCLUDES 1   *dystrophies primarily involving Bruch's membrane (H31.1-)*

H35.50 **Unspecified hereditary retinal dystrophy**

H35.51 **Vitreoretinal dystrophy**

N Newborn: 0   P Pediatric: 0-17   M Maternity: 9-64   A Adult: 15-124   MCC Major Complication/Comorbidity   CC Complication/Comorbidity   SW Severe Wound Dx

616   ICD-10-CM 2021

H35.52 **Pigmentary retinal dystrophy**
　　　　Albipunctate retinal dystrophy
　　　　Retinitis pigmentosa
　　　　Tapetoretinal dystrophy

H35.53 **Other dystrophies primarily involving the sensory retina**
　　　　Stargardt's disease

H35.54 **Dystrophies primarily involving the retinal pigment epithelium**
　　　　Vitelliform retinal dystrophy

✓5ᵗʰ **H35.6 Retinal hemorrhage**

　　H35.60 Retinal hemorrhage, unspecified eye
　　H35.61 **Retinal hemorrhage, right eye**
　　H35.62 **Retinal hemorrhage, left eye**
　　H35.63 **Retinal hemorrhage, bilateral**

✓5ᵗʰ **H35.7 Separation of retinal layers**
　　EXCLUDES 1　retinal detachment (serous) (H33.2-)
　　　　　　　　rhegmatogenous retinal detachment (H33.0-)

　　H35.70 Unspecified separation of retinal layers　CC
✓6ᵗʰ **H35.71 Central serous chorioretinopathy**

　　　H35.711 **Central serous chorioretinopathy, right eye**
　　　H35.712 **Central serous chorioretinopathy, left eye**
　　　H35.713 **Central serous chorioretinopathy, bilateral**
　　　H35.719 Central serous chorioretinopathy, unspecified eye

✓6ᵗʰ **H35.72 Serous detachment of retinal pigment epithelium**

　　　H35.721 **Serous detachment of retinal pigment epithelium, right eye**　CC
　　　H35.722 **Serous detachment of retinal pigment epithelium, left eye**　CC
　　　H35.723 **Serous detachment of retinal pigment epithelium, bilateral**　CC
　　　H35.729 Serous detachment of retinal pigment epithelium, unspecified eye　CC

✓6ᵗʰ **H35.73 Hemorrhagic detachment of retinal pigment epithelium**

　　　H35.731 **Hemorrhagic detachment of retinal pigment epithelium, right eye**　CC
　　　H35.732 **Hemorrhagic detachment of retinal pigment epithelium, left eye**　CC
　　　H35.733 **Hemorrhagic detachment of retinal pigment epithelium, bilateral**　CC
　　　H35.739 Hemorrhagic detachment of retinal pigment epithelium, unspecified eye　CC

✓5ᵗʰ **H35.8 Other specified retinal disorders**
　　EXCLUDES 2　retinal hemorrhage (H35.6-)

　　H35.81 **Retinal edema**
　　　　Retinal cotton wool spots
　　H35.82 **Retinal ischemia**　CC
　　H35.89 **Other specified retinal disorders**

H35.9 Unspecified retinal disorder

H36 *Retinal disorders in diseases classified elsewhere*
　　Code first underlying disease, such as:
　　　lipid storage disorders (E75.-)
　　　sickle-cell disorders (D57.-)
　　EXCLUDES 1　arteriosclerotic retinopathy (H35.0-)
　　　　　　　　diabetic retinopathy (E08.3-, E09.3-, E10.3-, E11.3-, E13.3-)

Glaucoma (H40–H42)

✓4ᵗʰ **H40 Glaucoma**
　　EXCLUDES 1　absolute glaucoma (H44.51-)
　　　　　　　　congenital glaucoma (Q15.0)
　　　　　　　　traumatic glaucoma due to birth injury (P15.3)

Open Angle/Angle Closure Glaucoma

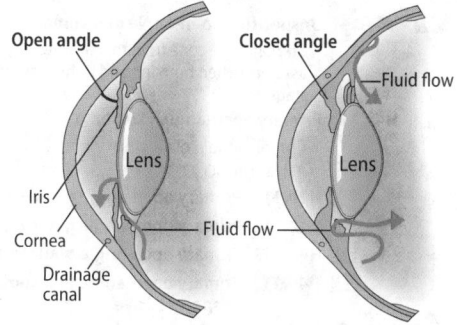

✓5ᵗʰ **H40.0 Glaucoma suspect**
　　✓6ᵗʰ **H40.00 Preglaucoma, unspecified**

　　　　H40.001 Preglaucoma, unspecified, right eye
　　　　H40.002 Preglaucoma, unspecified, left eye
　　　　H40.003 Preglaucoma, unspecified, bilateral
　　　　H40.009 Preglaucoma, unspecified, unspecified eye

　　✓6ᵗʰ **H40.01 Open angle with borderline findings, low risk**
　　　　Open angle, low risk
　　　　H40.011 **Open angle with borderline findings, low risk, right eye**
　　　　H40.012 **Open angle with borderline findings, low risk, left eye**
　　　　H40.013 **Open angle with borderline findings, low risk, bilateral**
　　　　H40.019 Open angle with borderline findings, low risk, unspecified eye

　　✓6ᵗʰ **H40.02 Open angle with borderline findings, high risk**
　　　　Open angle, high risk
　　　　H40.021 **Open angle with borderline findings, high risk, right eye**
　　　　H40.022 **Open angle with borderline findings, high risk, left eye**
　　　　H40.023 **Open angle with borderline findings, high risk, bilateral**
　　　　H40.029 Open angle with borderline findings, high risk, unspecified eye

　　✓6ᵗʰ **H40.03 Anatomical narrow angle**
　　　　Primary angle closure suspect
　　　　H40.031 **Anatomical narrow angle, right eye**
　　　　H40.032 **Anatomical narrow angle, left eye**
　　　　H40.033 **Anatomical narrow angle, bilateral**
　　　　H40.039 Anatomical narrow angle, unspecified eye

　　✓6ᵗʰ **H40.04 Steroid responder**
　　　　H40.041 **Steroid responder, right eye**
　　　　H40.042 **Steroid responder, left eye**
　　　　H40.043 **Steroid responder, bilateral**
　　　　H40.049 Steroid responder, unspecified eye

　　✓6ᵗʰ **H40.05 Ocular hypertension**
　　　　H40.051 **Ocular hypertension, right eye**
　　　　H40.052 **Ocular hypertension, left eye**
　　　　H40.053 **Ocular hypertension, bilateral**
　　　　H40.059 Ocular hypertension, unspecified eye

　　✓6ᵗʰ **H40.06 Primary angle closure without glaucoma damage**
　　　　H40.061 **Primary angle closure without glaucoma damage, right eye**
　　　　H40.062 **Primary angle closure without glaucoma damage, left eye**
　　　　H40.063 **Primary angle closure without glaucoma damage, bilateral**
　　　　H40.069 Primary angle closure without glaucoma damage, unspecified eye

Chapter 7. Diseases of the Eye and Adnexa

H40.1–H40.53

√5ᵗʰ **H40.1   Open-angle glaucoma**

> One of the following 7th characters is to be assigned to each code in subcategories H40.10, H40.11, H40.12, H40.13, and H40.14 to designate the stage of glaucoma.
> 0   stage unspecified
> 1   mild stage
> 2   moderate stage
> 3   severe stage
> 4   indeterminate stage

√x7ᵗʰ   **H40.10   Unspecified open-angle glaucoma**

> **TIP:** Only one code from this subcategory should be assigned when both left and right eyes are the same stage.

√6ᵗʰ   **H40.11   Primary open-angle glaucoma**

> Chronic simple glaucoma
> **AHA:** 2016,4Q,22

√7ᵗʰ   **H40.111   Primary open-angle glaucoma, right eye**

√7ᵗʰ   **H40.112   Primary open-angle glaucoma, left eye**

√7ᵗʰ   **H40.113   Primary open-angle glaucoma, bilateral**

√7ᵗʰ   **H40.119   Primary open-angle glaucoma, unspecified eye**

√6ᵗʰ   **H40.12   Low-tension glaucoma**

√7ᵗʰ   **H40.121   Low-tension glaucoma, right eye**

√7ᵗʰ   **H40.122   Low-tension glaucoma, left eye**

√7ᵗʰ   **H40.123   Low-tension glaucoma, bilateral**

√7ᵗʰ   **H40.129   Low-tension glaucoma, unspecified eye**

√6ᵗʰ   **H40.13   Pigmentary glaucoma**

√7ᵗʰ   **H40.131   Pigmentary glaucoma, right eye**

√7ᵗʰ   **H40.132   Pigmentary glaucoma, left eye**

√7ᵗʰ   **H40.133   Pigmentary glaucoma, bilateral**

√7ᵗʰ   **H40.139   Pigmentary glaucoma, unspecified eye**

√6ᵗʰ   **H40.14   Capsular glaucoma with pseudoexfoliation of lens**

√7ᵗʰ   **H40.141   Capsular glaucoma with pseudoexfoliation of lens, right eye**

√7ᵗʰ   **H40.142   Capsular glaucoma with pseudoexfoliation of lens, left eye**

√7ᵗʰ   **H40.143   Capsular glaucoma with pseudoexfoliation of lens, bilateral**

√7ᵗʰ   **H40.149   Capsular glaucoma with pseudoexfoliation of lens, unspecified eye**

√6ᵗʰ   **H40.15   Residual stage of open-angle glaucoma**

H40.151   Residual stage of open-angle glaucoma, right eye

H40.152   Residual stage of open-angle glaucoma, left eye

H40.153   Residual stage of open-angle glaucoma, bilateral

H40.159   Residual stage of open-angle glaucoma, unspecified eye

√5ᵗʰ **H40.2   Primary angle-closure glaucoma**

> **EXCLUDES 1**   aqueous misdirection (H40.83-)
> malignant glaucoma (H40.83-)

> One of the following 7th characters is to be assigned to code H40.20 and H40.22- to designate the stage of glaucoma.
> 0   stage unspecified
> 1   mild stage
> 2   moderate stage
> 3   severe stage
> 4   indeterminate stage

√x7ᵗʰ   **H40.20   Unspecified primary angle-closure glaucoma**

> **TIP:** Only one code from this subcategory should be assigned when both left and right eyes are the same stage.

√6ᵗʰ   **H40.21   Acute angle-closure glaucoma**

> Acute angle-closure glaucoma attack
> Acute angle-closure glaucoma crisis

H40.211   Acute angle-closure glaucoma, right eye   CC

H40.212   Acute angle-closure glaucoma, left eye   CC

H40.213   Acute angle-closure glaucoma, bilateral

H40.219   Acute angle-closure glaucoma, unspecified eye   CC

√6ᵗʰ   **H40.22   Chronic angle-closure glaucoma**

> Chronic primary angle closure glaucoma

√7ᵗʰ   **H40.221   Chronic angle-closure glaucoma, right eye**

√7ᵗʰ   **H40.222   Chronic angle-closure glaucoma, left eye**

√7ᵗʰ   **H40.223   Chronic angle-closure glaucoma, bilateral**

√7ᵗʰ   **H40.229   Chronic angle-closure glaucoma, unspecified eye**

√6ᵗʰ   **H40.23   Intermittent angle-closure glaucoma**

H40.231   Intermittent angle-closure glaucoma, right eye

H40.232   Intermittent angle-closure glaucoma, left eye

H40.233   Intermittent angle-closure glaucoma, bilateral

H40.239   Intermittent angle-closure glaucoma, unspecified eye

√6ᵗʰ   **H40.24   Residual stage of angle-closure glaucoma**

H40.241   Residual stage of angle-closure glaucoma, right eye

H40.242   Residual stage of angle-closure glaucoma, left eye

H40.243   Residual stage of angle-closure glaucoma, bilateral

H40.249   Residual stage of angle-closure glaucoma, unspecified eye

√5ᵗʰ **H40.3   Glaucoma secondary to eye trauma**

> Code also underlying condition

> One of the following 7th characters is to be assigned to each code in subcategory H40.3- to designate the stage of glaucoma.
> 0   stage unspecified
> 1   mild stage
> 2   moderate stage
> 3   severe stage
> 4   indeterminate stage

√x7ᵗʰ   **H40.30   Glaucoma secondary to eye trauma, unspecified eye**

√x7ᵗʰ   **H40.31   Glaucoma secondary to eye trauma, right eye**

√x7ᵗʰ   **H40.32   Glaucoma secondary to eye trauma, left eye**

√x7ᵗʰ   **H40.33   Glaucoma secondary to eye trauma, bilateral**

√5ᵗʰ **H40.4   Glaucoma secondary to eye inflammation**

> Code also underlying condition

> One of the following 7th characters is to be assigned to each code in subcategory H40.4- to designate the stage of glaucoma.
> 0   stage unspecified
> 1   mild stage
> 2   moderate stage
> 3   severe stage
> 4   indeterminate stage

√x7ᵗʰ   **H40.40   Glaucoma secondary to eye inflammation, unspecified eye**

√x7ᵗʰ   **H40.41   Glaucoma secondary to eye inflammation, right eye**

√x7ᵗʰ   **H40.42   Glaucoma secondary to eye inflammation, left eye**

√x7ᵗʰ   **H40.43   Glaucoma secondary to eye inflammation, bilateral**

√5ᵗʰ **H40.5   Glaucoma secondary to other eye disorders**

> Code also underlying eye disorder

> One of the following 7th characters is to be assigned to each code in subcategory H40.5- to designate the stage of glaucoma.
> 0   stage unspecified
> 1   mild stage
> 2   moderate stage
> 3   severe stage
> 4   indeterminate stage

√x7ᵗʰ   **H40.50   Glaucoma secondary to other eye disorders, unspecified eye**

√x7ᵗʰ   **H40.51   Glaucoma secondary to other eye disorders, right eye**

√x7ᵗʰ   **H40.52   Glaucoma secondary to other eye disorders, left eye**

√x7ᵗʰ   **H40.53   Glaucoma secondary to other eye disorders, bilateral**

N Newborn: 0   P Pediatric: 0-17   M Maternity: 9-64   A Adult: 15-124   MCC Major Complication/Comorbidity   CC Complication/Comorbidity   SW Severe Wound Dx

618   ICD-10-CM 2021

√5ᵗʰ **H40.6 Glaucoma** secondary to drugs

Use additional code for adverse effect, if applicable, to identify drug (T36-T50 with fifth or sixth character 5)

One of the following 7th characters is to be assigned to each code in subcategory H40.6- to designate the stage of glaucoma
- Ø stage unspecified
- 1 mild stage
- 2 moderate stage
- 3 severe stage
- 4 indeterminate stage

√x7ᵗʰ **H40.60 Glaucoma secondary to drugs, unspecified eye**

√x7ᵗʰ **H40.61 Glaucoma secondary to drugs, right eye**

√x7ᵗʰ **H40.62 Glaucoma secondary to drugs, left eye**

√x7ᵗʰ **H40.63 Glaucoma secondary to drugs, bilateral**

√5ᵗʰ **H40.8 Other glaucoma**

√6ᵗʰ **H40.81 Glaucoma with** increased episcleral venous pressure

    H40.811 Glaucoma with increased episcleral venous pressure, right eye

    H40.812 Glaucoma with increased episcleral venous pressure, left eye

    H40.813 Glaucoma with increased episcleral venous pressure, bilateral

    H40.819 Glaucoma with increased episcleral venous pressure, unspecified eye

√6ᵗʰ **H40.82 Hypersecretion glaucoma**

    H40.821 Hypersecretion glaucoma, right eye

    H40.822 Hypersecretion glaucoma, left eye

    H40.823 Hypersecretion glaucoma, bilateral

    H40.829 Hypersecretion glaucoma, unspecified eye

√6ᵗʰ **H40.83 Aqueous misdirection**

Malignant glaucoma

    H40.831 Aqueous misdirection, right eye

    H40.832 Aqueous misdirection, left eye

    H40.833 Aqueous misdirection, bilateral

    H40.839 Aqueous misdirection, unspecified eye

    H40.89 Other specified glaucoma

H40.9 Unspecified glaucoma

H42 *Glaucoma in diseases classified elsewhere*

Code first underlying condition, such as:
amyloidosis (E85.-)
aniridia (Q13.1)
glaucoma (in) diabetes mellitus (E08.39, E09.39, E10.39, E11.39, E13.39)
Lowe's syndrome (E72.03)
Reiger's anomaly (Q13.81)
specified metabolic disorder (E70-E88)

EXCLUDES 1   *glaucoma (in) onchocerciasis (B73.02)*
        glaucoma (in) syphilis (A52.71)
        glaucoma (in) tuberculous (A18.59)

Disorders of vitreous body and globe (H43-H44)

√4ᵗʰ **H43 Disorders of vitreous body**

√5ᵗʰ **H43.0 Vitreous prolapse**

EXCLUDES 1   *traumatic vitreous prolapse (S05.2-)*
        vitreous syndrome following cataract surgery (H59.0-)

    H43.00 Vitreous prolapse, unspecified eye

    H43.01 Vitreous prolapse, right eye

    H43.02 Vitreous prolapse, left eye

    H43.03 Vitreous prolapse, bilateral

√5ᵗʰ **H43.1 Vitreous hemorrhage**

    H43.10 Vitreous hemorrhage, unspecified eye   HCC

    H43.11 Vitreous hemorrhage, right eye   HCC

    H43.12 Vitreous hemorrhage, left eye   HCC

    H43.13 Vitreous hemorrhage, bilateral   HCC

√5ᵗʰ **H43.2 Crystalline deposits in vitreous body**

    H43.20 Crystalline deposits in vitreous body, unspecified eye

    H43.21 Crystalline deposits in vitreous body, right eye

    H43.22 Crystalline deposits in vitreous body, left eye

    H43.23 Crystalline deposits in vitreous body, bilateral

√5ᵗʰ **H43.3 Other vitreous opacities**

√6ᵗʰ **H43.31 Vitreous membranes and strands**

    H43.311 Vitreous membranes and strands, right eye

    H43.312 Vitreous membranes and strands, left eye

    H43.313 Vitreous membranes and strands, bilateral

    H43.319 Vitreous membranes and strands, unspecified eye

√6ᵗʰ **H43.39 Other vitreous opacities**

Vitreous floaters

    H43.391 Other vitreous opacities, right eye

    H43.392 Other vitreous opacities, left eye

    H43.393 Other vitreous opacities, bilateral

    H43.399 Other vitreous opacities, unspecified eye

√5ᵗʰ **H43.8 Other disorders of vitreous body**

EXCLUDES 1   *proliferative vitreo-retinopathy with retinal detachment (H33.4-)*

EXCLUDES 2   *vitreous abscess (H44.02-)*

√6ᵗʰ **H43.81 Vitreous degeneration**

Vitreous detachment

    H43.811 Vitreous degeneration, right eye

    H43.812 Vitreous degeneration, left eye

    H43.813 Vitreous degeneration, bilateral

    H43.819 Vitreous degeneration, unspecified eye

√6ᵗʰ **H43.82 Vitreomacular adhesion**

Vitreomacular traction

    H43.821 Vitreomacular adhesion, right eye   A

    H43.822 Vitreomacular adhesion, left eye   A

    H43.823 Vitreomacular adhesion, bilateral   A

    H43.829 Vitreomacular adhesion, unspecified eye   A

    H43.89 Other disorders of vitreous body

H43.9 Unspecified disorder of vitreous body

√4ᵗʰ **H44 Disorders of globe**

INCLUDES   disorders affecting multiple structures of eye

√5ᵗʰ **H44.0 Purulent endophthalmitis**

Use additional code to identify organism

EXCLUDES 1   *bleb associated endophthalmitis (H59.4-)*

√6ᵗʰ **H44.00 Unspecified purulent endophthalmitis**

    H44.001 Unspecified purulent endophthalmitis, right eye   CC

    H44.002 Unspecified purulent endophthalmitis, left eye   CC

    H44.003 Unspecified purulent endophthalmitis, bilateral   CC

    H44.009 Unspecified purulent endophthalmitis, unspecified eye   CC

√6ᵗʰ **H44.01 Panophthalmitis (acute)**

    H44.011 Panophthalmitis (acute), right eye   CC

    H44.012 Panophthalmitis (acute), left eye   CC

    H44.013 Panophthalmitis (acute), bilateral   CC

    H44.019 Panophthalmitis (acute), unspecified eye   CC

√6ᵗʰ **H44.02 Vitreous abscess (chronic)**

    H44.021 Vitreous abscess (chronic), right eye   CC

    H44.022 Vitreous abscess (chronic), left eye   CC

    H44.023 Vitreous abscess (chronic), bilateral   CC

    H44.029 Vitreous abscess (chronic), unspecified eye   CC

√5ᵗʰ **H44.1 Other endophthalmitis**

EXCLUDES 1   *bleb associated endophthalmitis (H59.4-)*

EXCLUDES 2   *ophthalmia nodosa (H16.2-)*

√6ᵗʰ **H44.11 Panuveitis**

DEF: Inflammation of all layers of the uvea of the eye, including the choroid, iris, and ciliary body. It also typically involves the lens, retina, optic nerve, and vitreous and causes reduced vision or blindness.

    H44.111 Panuveitis, right eye   CC

    H44.112 Panuveitis, left eye   CC

    H44.113 Panuveitis, bilateral   CC

    H44.119 Panuveitis, unspecified eye   CC

☑ Additional Character Required   √x7ᵗʰ Placeholder   Unacceptable PDx   Questionable PDx   Manifestation   Unspecified Dx   H1-H14 HAC   HCC CMS-HCC Dx   HIV HIV Dx

ICD-10-CM 2021   619

Chapter 7. Diseases of the Eye and Adnexa

H44.12–H44.539

✓6th **H44.12** Parasitic endophthalmitis, unspecified
- **H44.121** Parasitic endophthalmitis, unspecified, right eye `CC`
- **H44.122** Parasitic endophthalmitis, unspecified, left eye `CC`
- **H44.123** Parasitic endophthalmitis, unspecified, bilateral `CC`
- **H44.129** Parasitic endophthalmitis, unspecified, unspecified eye `CC`

✓6th **H44.13** Sympathetic uveitis
- **H44.131** Sympathetic uveitis, right eye `CC`
- **H44.132** Sympathetic uveitis, left eye `CC`
- **H44.133** Sympathetic uveitis, bilateral `CC`
- **H44.139** Sympathetic uveitis, unspecified eye `CC`

H44.19 Other endophthalmitis `CC`

✓5th **H44.2** Degenerative myopia
Malignant myopia
AHA: 2017,4Q,10-11
- **H44.20** Degenerative myopia, unspecified eye
- **H44.21** Degenerative myopia, right eye
- **H44.22** Degenerative myopia, left eye
- **H44.23** Degenerative myopia, bilateral

✓6th **H44.2A** Degenerative myopia with choroidal neovascularization
Use additional code for any associated choroid disorders (H31.-)
- **H44.2A1** Degenerative myopia with choroidal neovascularization, right eye
- **H44.2A2** Degenerative myopia with choroidal neovascularization, left eye
- **H44.2A3** Degenerative myopia with choroidal neovascularization, bilateral eye
- **H44.2A9** Degenerative myopia with choroidal neovascularization, unspecified eye

✓6th **H44.2B** Degenerative myopia with macular hole
- **H44.2B1** Degenerative myopia with macular hole, right eye
- **H44.2B2** Degenerative myopia with macular hole, left eye
- **H44.2B3** Degenerative myopia with macular hole, bilateral eye
- **H44.2B9** Degenerative myopia with macular hole, unspecified eye

✓6th **H44.2C** Degenerative myopia with retinal detachment
Use additional code to identify the retinal detachment (H33.-)
- **H44.2C1** Degenerative myopia with retinal detachment, right eye
- **H44.2C2** Degenerative myopia with retinal detachment, left eye
- **H44.2C3** Degenerative myopia with retinal detachment, bilateral eye
- **H44.2C9** Degenerative myopia with retinal detachment, unspecified eye

✓6th **H44.2D** Degenerative myopia with foveoschisis
- **H44.2D1** Degenerative myopia with foveoschisis, right eye
- **H44.2D2** Degenerative myopia with foveoschisis, left eye
- **H44.2D3** Degenerative myopia with foveoschisis, bilateral eye
- **H44.2D9** Degenerative myopia with foveoschisis, unspecified eye

✓6th **H44.2E** Degenerative myopia with other maculopathy
- **H44.2E1** Degenerative myopia with other maculopathy, right eye
- **H44.2E2** Degenerative myopia with other maculopathy, left eye
- **H44.2E3** Degenerative myopia with other maculopathy, bilateral eye
- **H44.2E9** Degenerative myopia with other maculopathy, unspecified eye

✓5th **H44.3** Other and unspecified degenerative disorders of globe
- **H44.30** Unspecified degenerative disorder of globe

✓6th **H44.31** Chalcosis
- **H44.311** Chalcosis, right eye
- **H44.312** Chalcosis, left eye
- **H44.313** Chalcosis, bilateral
- **H44.319** Chalcosis, unspecified eye

✓6th **H44.32** Siderosis of eye
DEF: Iron pigment deposits within tissue of the eyeball caused by high iron content of the blood. Symptoms include cataracts, rust-colored anterior subcapsular deposits, iris heterochromia, pupillary mydriasis, and depressed electroretinogram amplitudes.
- **H44.321** Siderosis of eye, right eye
- **H44.322** Siderosis of eye, left eye
- **H44.323** Siderosis of eye, bilateral
- **H44.329** Siderosis of eye, unspecified eye

✓6th **H44.39** Other degenerative disorders of globe
- **H44.391** Other degenerative disorders of globe, right eye
- **H44.392** Other degenerative disorders of globe, left eye
- **H44.393** Other degenerative disorders of globe, bilateral
- **H44.399** Other degenerative disorders of globe, unspecified eye

✓5th **H44.4** Hypotony of eye
- **H44.40** Unspecified hypotony of eye

✓6th **H44.41** Flat anterior chamber hypotony of eye
- **H44.411** Flat anterior chamber hypotony of right eye
- **H44.412** Flat anterior chamber hypotony of left eye
- **H44.413** Flat anterior chamber hypotony of eye, bilateral
- **H44.419** Flat anterior chamber hypotony of unspecified eye

✓6th **H44.42** Hypotony of eye due to ocular fistula
- **H44.421** Hypotony of right eye due to ocular fistula
- **H44.422** Hypotony of left eye due to ocular fistula
- **H44.423** Hypotony of eye due to ocular fistula, bilateral
- **H44.429** Hypotony of unspecified eye due to ocular fistula

✓6th **H44.43** Hypotony of eye due to other ocular disorders
- **H44.431** Hypotony of eye due to other ocular disorders, right eye
- **H44.432** Hypotony of eye due to other ocular disorders, left eye
- **H44.433** Hypotony of eye due to other ocular disorders, bilateral
- **H44.439** Hypotony of eye due to other ocular disorders, unspecified eye

✓6th **H44.44** Primary hypotony of eye
- **H44.441** Primary hypotony of right eye
- **H44.442** Primary hypotony of left eye
- **H44.443** Primary hypotony of eye, bilateral
- **H44.449** Primary hypotony of unspecified eye

✓5th **H44.5** Degenerated conditions of globe
- **H44.50** Unspecified degenerated conditions of globe

✓6th **H44.51** Absolute glaucoma
- **H44.511** Absolute glaucoma, right eye
- **H44.512** Absolute glaucoma, left eye
- **H44.513** Absolute glaucoma, bilateral
- **H44.519** Absolute glaucoma, unspecified eye

✓6th **H44.52** Atrophy of globe
Phthisis bulbi
- **H44.521** Atrophy of globe, right eye
- **H44.522** Atrophy of globe, left eye
- **H44.523** Atrophy of globe, bilateral
- **H44.529** Atrophy of globe, unspecified eye

✓6th **H44.53** Leucocoria
- **H44.531** Leucocoria, right eye
- **H44.532** Leucocoria, left eye
- **H44.533** Leucocoria, bilateral
- **H44.539** Leucocoria, unspecified eye

✓5ᵗʰ **H44.6** **Retained (old) intraocular foreign body, magnetic**

Use additional code to identify magnetic foreign body (Z18.11)

EXCLUDES 1 current intraocular foreign body (S05.-)

EXCLUDES 2 retained foreign body in eyelid (H02.81-)

retained (old) foreign body following penetrating wound of orbit (H05.5-)

retained (old) intraocular foreign body, nonmagnetic (H44.7-)

✓6ᵗʰ **H44.60** **Unspecified retained (old) intraocular foreign body, magnetic**

H44.601 Unspecified retained (old) intraocular foreign body, magnetic, right eye

H44.602 Unspecified retained (old) intraocular foreign body, magnetic, left eye

H44.603 Unspecified retained (old) intraocular foreign body, magnetic, bilateral

H44.609 Unspecified retained (old) intraocular foreign body, magnetic, unspecified eye

✓6ᵗʰ **H44.61** **Retained (old) magnetic foreign body in anterior chamber**

H44.611 Retained (old) magnetic foreign body in anterior chamber, right eye

H44.612 Retained (old) magnetic foreign body in anterior chamber, left eye

H44.613 Retained (old) magnetic foreign body in anterior chamber, bilateral

H44.619 Retained (old) magnetic foreign body in anterior chamber, unspecified eye

✓6ᵗʰ **H44.62** **Retained (old) magnetic foreign body in iris or ciliary body**

H44.621 Retained (old) magnetic foreign body in iris or ciliary body, right eye

H44.622 Retained (old) magnetic foreign body in iris or ciliary body, left eye

H44.623 Retained (old) magnetic foreign body in iris or ciliary body, bilateral

H44.629 Retained (old) magnetic foreign body in iris or ciliary body, unspecified eye

✓6ᵗʰ **H44.63** **Retained (old) magnetic foreign body in lens**

H44.631 Retained (old) magnetic foreign body in lens, right eye

H44.632 Retained (old) magnetic foreign body in lens, left eye

H44.633 Retained (old) magnetic foreign body in lens, bilateral

H44.639 Retained (old) magnetic foreign body in lens, unspecified eye

✓6ᵗʰ **H44.64** **Retained (old) magnetic foreign body in posterior wall of globe**

H44.641 Retained (old) magnetic foreign body in posterior wall of globe, right eye

H44.642 Retained (old) magnetic foreign body in posterior wall of globe, left eye

H44.643 Retained (old) magnetic foreign body in posterior wall of globe, bilateral

H44.649 Retained (old) magnetic foreign body in posterior wall of globe, unspecified eye

✓6ᵗʰ **H44.65** **Retained (old) magnetic foreign body in vitreous body**

H44.651 Retained (old) magnetic foreign body in vitreous body, right eye

H44.652 Retained (old) magnetic foreign body in vitreous body, left eye

H44.653 Retained (old) magnetic foreign body in vitreous body, bilateral

H44.659 Retained (old) magnetic foreign body in vitreous body, unspecified eye

✓6ᵗʰ **H44.69** **Retained (old) intraocular foreign body, magnetic, in other or multiple sites**

H44.691 Retained (old) intraocular foreign body, magnetic, in other or multiple sites, right eye

H44.692 Retained (old) intraocular foreign body, magnetic, in other or multiple sites, left eye

H44.693 Retained (old) intraocular foreign body, magnetic, in other or multiple sites, bilateral

H44.699 Retained (old) intraocular foreign body, magnetic, in other or multiple sites, unspecified eye

✓5ᵗʰ **H44.7** **Retained (old) intraocular foreign body, nonmagnetic**

Use additional code to identify nonmagnetic foreign body (Z18.01-Z18.10, Z18.12, Z18.2-Z18.9)

EXCLUDES 1 current intraocular foreign body (S05.-)

EXCLUDES 2 retained foreign body in eyelid (H02.81-)

retained (old) foreign body following penetrating wound of orbit (H05.5-)

retained (old) intraocular foreign body, magnetic (H44.6-)

✓6ᵗʰ **H44.70** **Unspecified retained (old) intraocular foreign body, nonmagnetic**

H44.701 Unspecified retained (old) intraocular foreign body, nonmagnetic, right eye

H44.702 Unspecified retained (old) intraocular foreign body, nonmagnetic, left eye

H44.703 Unspecified retained (old) intraocular foreign body, nonmagnetic, bilateral

H44.709 Unspecified retained (old) intraocular foreign body, nonmagnetic, unspecified eye

Retained (old) intraocular foreign body NOS

✓6ᵗʰ **H44.71** **Retained (nonmagnetic) (old) foreign body in anterior chamber**

H44.711 Retained (nonmagnetic) (old) foreign body in anterior chamber, right eye

H44.712 Retained (nonmagnetic) (old) foreign body in anterior chamber, left eye

H44.713 Retained (nonmagnetic) (old) foreign body in anterior chamber, bilateral

H44.719 Retained (nonmagnetic) (old) foreign body in anterior chamber, unspecified eye

✓6ᵗʰ **H44.72** **Retained (nonmagnetic) (old) foreign body in iris or ciliary body**

H44.721 Retained (nonmagnetic) (old) foreign body in iris or ciliary body, right eye

H44.722 Retained (nonmagnetic) (old) foreign body in iris or ciliary body, left eye

H44.723 Retained (nonmagnetic) (old) foreign body in iris or ciliary body, bilateral

H44.729 Retained (nonmagnetic) (old) foreign body in iris or ciliary body, unspecified eye

✓6ᵗʰ **H44.73** **Retained (nonmagnetic) (old) foreign body in lens**

H44.731 Retained (nonmagnetic) (old) foreign body in lens, right eye

H44.732 Retained (nonmagnetic) (old) foreign body in lens, left eye

H44.733 Retained (nonmagnetic) (old) foreign body in lens, bilateral

H44.739 Retained (nonmagnetic) (old) foreign body in lens, unspecified eye

✓6ᵗʰ **H44.74** **Retained (nonmagnetic) (old) foreign body in posterior wall of globe**

H44.741 Retained (nonmagnetic) (old) foreign body in posterior wall of globe, right eye

H44.742 Retained (nonmagnetic) (old) foreign body in posterior wall of globe, left eye

H44.743 Retained (nonmagnetic) (old) foreign body in posterior wall of globe, bilateral

H44.749 Retained (nonmagnetic) (old) foreign body in posterior wall of globe, unspecified eye

✓6ᵗʰ **H44.75** **Retained (nonmagnetic) (old) foreign body in vitreous body**

H44.751 Retained (nonmagnetic) (old) foreign body in vitreous body, right eye

H44.752 Retained (nonmagnetic) (old) foreign body in vitreous body, left eye

H44.753 Retained (nonmagnetic) (old) foreign body in vitreous body, bilateral

H44.759 Retained (nonmagnetic) (old) foreign body in vitreous body, unspecified eye

✓6ᵗʰ **H44.79** **Retained (old) intraocular foreign body, nonmagnetic, in other or multiple sites**

H44.791 Retained (old) intraocular foreign body, nonmagnetic, in other or multiple sites, right eye

H44.792 Retained (old) intraocular foreign body, nonmagnetic, in other or multiple sites, left eye

---

☑ Additional Character Required   ✓x7ᵗʰ Placeholder   Unacceptable PDx   Questionable PDx   Manifestation   Unspecified Dx   H1 - H14 HAC   HCC CMS-HCC Dx   HIV HIV Dx

        H44.793   **Retained (old) intraocular foreign body, nonmagnetic, in other or multiple sites, bilateral**

        H44.799   **Retained (old) intraocular foreign body, nonmagnetic, in other or multiple sites, unspecified eye**

√5ᵗʰ **H44.8**   **Other disorders of globe**

  √6ᵗʰ **H44.81**   **Hemophthalmos**

     DEF: Pool of blood within the eyeball, not from a current injury.

     H44.811   **Hemophthalmos, right eye**

     H44.812   **Hemophthalmos, left eye**

     H44.813   **Hemophthalmos, bilateral**

     H44.819   **Hemophthalmos, unspecified eye**

  √6ᵗʰ **H44.82**   **Luxation of globe**

     H44.821   **Luxation of globe, right eye**

     H44.822   **Luxation of globe, left eye**

     H44.823   **Luxation of globe, bilateral**

     H44.829   **Luxation of globe, unspecified eye**

    H44.89   **Other disorders of globe**

  H44.9   **Unspecified disorder of globe**

Disorders of optic nerve and visual pathways (H46-H47)

√4ᵗʰ **H46**   **Optic neuritis**

    EXCLUDES 2   *ischemic optic neuropathy (H47.01-)*
                neuromyelitis optica [Devic] (G36.0)

 √5ᵗʰ **H46.0**   **Optic papillitis**

    H46.00   **Optic papillitis, unspecified eye**   CC

    H46.01   **Optic papillitis, right eye**   CC

    H46.02   **Optic papillitis, left eye**   CC

    H46.03   **Optic papillitis, bilateral**   CC

 √5ᵗʰ **H46.1**   **Retrobulbar neuritis**

    Retrobulbar neuritis NOS

    EXCLUDES 1   *syphilitic retrobulbar neuritis (A52.15)*

    H46.10   **Retrobulbar neuritis, unspecified eye**   CC

    H46.11   **Retrobulbar neuritis, right eye**   CC

    H46.12   **Retrobulbar neuritis, left eye**   CC

    H46.13   **Retrobulbar neuritis, bilateral**   CC

  H46.2   **Nutritional optic neuropathy**

  H46.3   **Toxic optic neuropathy**

    Code first (T51-T65) to identify cause

  H46.8   **Other optic neuritis**   CC

  H46.9   **Unspecified optic neuritis**   CC

√4ᵗʰ **H47**   **Other disorders of optic [2nd] nerve and visual pathways**

 √5ᵗʰ **H47.0**   **Disorders of optic nerve, not elsewhere classified**

  √6ᵗʰ **H47.01**   **Ischemic optic neuropathy**

     H47.011   **Ischemic optic neuropathy, right eye**

     H47.012   **Ischemic optic neuropathy, left eye**

     H47.013   **Ischemic optic neuropathy, bilateral**

     H47.019   **Ischemic optic neuropathy, unspecified eye**

  √6ᵗʰ **H47.02**   **Hemorrhage in optic nerve sheath**

     H47.021   **Hemorrhage in optic nerve sheath, right eye**

     H47.022   **Hemorrhage in optic nerve sheath, left eye**

     H47.023   **Hemorrhage in optic nerve sheath, bilateral**

     H47.029   **Hemorrhage in optic nerve sheath, unspecified eye**

  √6ᵗʰ **H47.03**   **Optic nerve hypoplasia**

     H47.031   **Optic nerve hypoplasia, right eye**

     H47.032   **Optic nerve hypoplasia, left eye**

     H47.033   **Optic nerve hypoplasia, bilateral**

     H47.039   **Optic nerve hypoplasia, unspecified eye**

  √6ᵗʰ **H47.09**   **Other disorders of optic nerve, not elsewhere classified**

    Compression of optic nerve

     H47.091   **Other disorders of optic nerve, not elsewhere classified, right eye**

     H47.092   **Other disorders of optic nerve, not elsewhere classified, left eye**

     H47.093   **Other disorders of optic nerve, not elsewhere classified, bilateral**

     H47.099   **Other disorders of optic nerve, not elsewhere classified, unspecified eye**

 √5ᵗʰ **H47.1**   **Papilledema**

    DEF: Swelling of the optic papilla, the raised area connected to the optic disk made up of nerves that enter the eyeball. It may be caused by increased intracranial pressure, decreased ocular pressure, or a retinal disorder.

    H47.10   **Unspecified papilledema**   CC

    H47.11   **Papilledema associated with increased intracranial pressure**   CC

    H47.12   **Papilledema associated with decreased ocular pressure**

    H47.13   **Papilledema associated with retinal disorder**

  √6ᵗʰ **H47.14**   **Foster-Kennedy syndrome**

     H47.141   **Foster-Kennedy syndrome, right eye**

     H47.142   **Foster-Kennedy syndrome, left eye**

     H47.143   **Foster-Kennedy syndrome, bilateral**

     H47.149   **Foster-Kennedy syndrome, unspecified eye**

 √5ᵗʰ **H47.2**   **Optic atrophy**

    H47.20   **Unspecified optic atrophy**

  √6ᵗʰ **H47.21**   **Primary optic atrophy**

     H47.211   **Primary optic atrophy, right eye**

     H47.212   **Primary optic atrophy, left eye**

     H47.213   **Primary optic atrophy, bilateral**

     H47.219   **Primary optic atrophy, unspecified eye**

    H47.22   **Hereditary optic atrophy**

    Leber's optic atrophy

  √6ᵗʰ **H47.23**   **Glaucomatous optic atrophy**

     H47.231   **Glaucomatous optic atrophy, right eye**

     H47.232   **Glaucomatous optic atrophy, left eye**

     H47.233   **Glaucomatous optic atrophy, bilateral**

     H47.239   **Glaucomatous optic atrophy, unspecified eye**

  √6ᵗʰ **H47.29**   **Other optic atrophy**

    Temporal pallor of optic disc

     H47.291   **Other optic atrophy, right eye**

     H47.292   **Other optic atrophy, left eye**

     H47.293   **Other optic atrophy, bilateral**

     H47.299   **Other optic atrophy, unspecified eye**

 √5ᵗʰ **H47.3**   **Other disorders of optic disc**

  √6ᵗʰ **H47.31**   **Coloboma of optic disc**

     H47.311   **Coloboma of optic disc, right eye**

     H47.312   **Coloboma of optic disc, left eye**

     H47.313   **Coloboma of optic disc, bilateral**

     H47.319   **Coloboma of optic disc, unspecified eye**

  √6ᵗʰ **H47.32**   **Drusen of optic disc**

     H47.321   **Drusen of optic disc, right eye**

     H47.322   **Drusen of optic disc, left eye**

     H47.323   **Drusen of optic disc, bilateral**

     H47.329   **Drusen of optic disc, unspecified eye**

  √6ᵗʰ **H47.33**   **Pseudopapilledema of optic disc**

     H47.331   **Pseudopapilledema of optic disc, right eye**

     H47.332   **Pseudopapilledema of optic disc, left eye**

     H47.333   **Pseudopapilledema of optic disc, bilateral**

     H47.339   **Pseudopapilledema of optic disc, unspecified eye**

  √6ᵗʰ **H47.39**   **Other disorders of optic disc**

     H47.391   **Other disorders of optic disc, right eye**

     H47.392   **Other disorders of optic disc, left eye**

     H47.393   **Other disorders of optic disc, bilateral**

     H47.399   **Other disorders of optic disc, unspecified eye**

 √5ᵗʰ **H47.4**   **Disorders of optic chiasm**

    Code also underlying condition

    H47.41   **Disorders of optic chiasm in (due to) inflammatory disorders**   CC

    H47.42   **Disorders of optic chiasm in (due to) neoplasm**   CC

    H47.43   **Disorders of optic chiasm in (due to) vascular disorders**   CC

    H47.49   **Disorders of optic chiasm in (due to) other disorders**   CC

N Newborn: 0   P Pediatric: 0-17   M Maternity: 9-64   A Adult: 15-124   MCC Major Complication/Comorbidity   CC Complication/Comorbidity   SW Severe Wound Dx

622   ICD-10-CM 2021

✓5ᵗʰ **H47.5 Disorders of other visual pathways**

Disorders of optic tracts, geniculate nuclei and optic radiations
Code also underlying condition

✓6ᵗʰ **H47.51 Disorders of visual pathways in (due to) inflammatory disorders**

H47.511 Disorders of visual pathways in (due to) inflammatory disorders, **right** side   cc

H47.512 Disorders of visual pathways in (due to) inflammatory disorders, **left** side   cc

H47.519 Disorders of visual pathways in (due to) inflammatory disorders, unspecified side   cc

✓6ᵗʰ **H47.52 Disorders of visual pathways in (due to) neoplasm**

H47.521 Disorders of visual pathways in (due to) neoplasm, **right** side   cc

H47.522 Disorders of visual pathways in (due to) neoplasm, **left** side   cc

H47.529 Disorders of visual pathways in (due to) neoplasm, unspecified side   cc

✓6ᵗʰ **H47.53 Disorders of visual pathways in (due to) vascular disorders**

H47.531 Disorders of visual pathways in (due to) vascular disorders, **right** side   cc

H47.532 Disorders of visual pathways in (due to) vascular disorders, **left** side   cc

H47.539 Disorders of visual pathways in (due to) vascular disorders, unspecified side   cc

✓5ᵗʰ **H47.6 Disorders of visual cortex**

Code also underlying condition

EXCLUDES 1   injury to visual cortex S04.04-

✓6ᵗʰ **H47.61 Cortical blindness**

H47.611 Cortical blindness, **right** side of brain

H47.612 Cortical blindness, **left** side of brain

H47.619 Cortical blindness, unspecified side of brain

✓6ᵗʰ **H47.62 Disorders of visual cortex in (due to) inflammatory disorders**

H47.621 Disorders of visual cortex in (due to) inflammatory disorders, **right** side of brain   cc

H47.622 Disorders of visual cortex in (due to) inflammatory disorders, **left** side of brain   cc

H47.629 Disorders of visual cortex in (due to) inflammatory disorders, unspecified side of brain   cc

✓6ᵗʰ **H47.63 Disorders of visual cortex in (due to) neoplasm**

H47.631 Disorders of visual cortex in (due to) neoplasm, **right** side of brain   cc

H47.632 Disorders of visual cortex in (due to) neoplasm, **left** side of brain   cc

H47.639 Disorders of visual cortex in (due to) neoplasm, unspecified side of brain   cc

✓6ᵗʰ **H47.64 Disorders of visual cortex in (due to) vascular disorders**

H47.641 Disorders of visual cortex in (due to) vascular disorders, **right** side of brain   cc

H47.642 Disorders of visual cortex in (due to) vascular disorders, **left** side of brain   cc

H47.649 Disorders of visual cortex in (due to) vascular disorders, unspecified side of brain   cc

H47.9 Unspecified disorder of visual pathways

Disorders of ocular muscles, binocular movement, accommodation and refraction (H49-H52)

EXCLUDES 2   nystagmus and other irregular eye movements (H55)

✓4ᵗʰ **H49 Paralytic strabismus**

EXCLUDES 2   internal ophthalmoplegia (H52.51-)
internuclear ophthalmoplegia (H51.2-)
progressive supranuclear ophthalmoplegia (G23.1)

DEF: Strabismus: Misalignment of the eyes with the inability to move and focus in the same direction due to conditions affecting the muscles controlling them.

✓5ᵗʰ **H49.0 Third [oculomotor] nerve palsy**

H49.00 Third [oculomotor] nerve palsy, unspecified eye

H49.01 Third [oculomotor] nerve palsy, **right** eye

H49.02 Third [oculomotor] nerve palsy, **left** eye

H49.03 Third [oculomotor] nerve palsy, **bilateral**

✓5ᵗʰ **H49.1 Fourth [trochlear] nerve palsy**

H49.10 Fourth [trochlear] nerve palsy, unspecified eye

H49.11 Fourth [trochlear] nerve palsy, **right** eye

H49.12 Fourth [trochlear] nerve palsy, **left** eye

H49.13 Fourth [trochlear] nerve palsy, **bilateral**

✓5ᵗʰ **H49.2 Sixth [abducent] nerve palsy**

H49.20 Sixth [abducent] nerve palsy, unspecified eye

H49.21 Sixth [abducent] nerve palsy, **right** eye

H49.22 Sixth [abducent] nerve palsy, **left** eye

H49.23 Sixth [abducent] nerve palsy, **bilateral**

✓5ᵗʰ **H49.3 Total (external) ophthalmoplegia**

H49.30 Total (external) ophthalmoplegia, unspecified eye

H49.31 Total (external) ophthalmoplegia, **right** eye

H49.32 Total (external) ophthalmoplegia, **left** eye

H49.33 Total (external) ophthalmoplegia, **bilateral**

✓5ᵗʰ **H49.4 Progressive external ophthalmoplegia**

EXCLUDES 1   Kearns-Sayre syndrome (H49.81-)

H49.40 Progressive external ophthalmoplegia, unspecified eye

H49.41 Progressive external ophthalmoplegia, **right** eye

H49.42 Progressive external ophthalmoplegia, **left** eye

H49.43 Progressive external ophthalmoplegia, **bilateral**

✓5ᵗʰ **H49.8 Other paralytic strabismus**

✓6ᵗʰ **H49.81 Kearns-Sayre syndrome**

Progressive external ophthalmoplegia with pigmentary retinopathy
Use additional code for other manifestation, such as: heart block (I45.9)

H49.811 Kearns-Sayre syndrome, **right** eye   cc   HCC

H49.812 Kearns-Sayre syndrome, **left** eye   cc   HCC

H49.813 Kearns-Sayre syndrome, **bilateral**   cc   HCC

H49.819 Kearns-Sayre syndrome, unspecified eye   cc   HCC

✓6ᵗʰ **H49.88 Other paralytic strabismus**

External ophthalmoplegia NOS

H49.881 Other paralytic strabismus, **right** eye

H49.882 Other paralytic strabismus, **left** eye

H49.883 Other paralytic strabismus, **bilateral**

H49.889 Other paralytic strabismus, unspecified eye

H49.9 Unspecified paralytic strabismus

✓4ᵗʰ **H50 Other strabismus**

DEF: Strabismus: Misalignment of the eyes with the inability to move and focus in the same direction due to conditions affecting the muscles controlling them.

✓5ᵗʰ **H50.0 Esotropia**

Convergent concomitant strabismus

EXCLUDES 1   intermittent esotropia (H50.31-, H50.32)

H50.00 Unspecified esotropia

✓6ᵗʰ **H50.01 Monocular esotropia**

H50.011 Monocular esotropia, **right** eye

H50.012 Monocular esotropia, **left** eye

✓6ᵗʰ **H50.02 Monocular esotropia with A pattern**

H50.021 Monocular esotropia with A pattern, **right** eye

✓ Additional Character Required   ✓x7ᵗʰ Placeholder   Unacceptable PDx   Questionable PDx   Manifestation   Unspecified Dx   H1-H14 HAC   HCC CMS-HCC Dx   HIV HIV Dx

H50.022 Monocular esotropia with A pattern, left eye

✓6ᵗʰ **H50.03** Monocular esotropia with V pattern

H50.031 Monocular esotropia with V pattern, right eye

H50.032 Monocular esotropia with V pattern, left eye

✓6ᵗʰ **H50.04** Monocular esotropia with other noncomitancies

H50.041 Monocular esotropia with other noncomitancies, right eye

H50.042 Monocular esotropia with other noncomitancies, left eye

H50.05 Alternating esotropia

H50.06 Alternating esotropia with A pattern

H50.07 Alternating esotropia with V pattern

H50.08 Alternating esotropia with other noncomitancies

Eye Muscle Diseases

R.   L.
Monocular (one eye only) esotropia (inward)

Monocular exotropia (outward)

Monocular hypertropia (upward)

✓5ᵗʰ **H50.1** Exotropia

Divergent concomitant strabismus

EXCLUDES 1 *intermittent exotropia (H50.33-, H50.34)*

H50.10 Unspecified exotropia

✓6ᵗʰ **H50.11** Monocular exotropia

H50.111 Monocular exotropia, right eye

H50.112 Monocular exotropia, left eye

✓6ᵗʰ **H50.12** Monocular exotropia with A pattern

H50.121 Monocular exotropia with A pattern, right eye

H50.122 Monocular exotropia with A pattern, left eye

✓6ᵗʰ **H50.13** Monocular exotropia with V pattern

H50.131 Monocular exotropia with V pattern, right eye

H50.132 Monocular exotropia with V pattern, left eye

✓6ᵗʰ **H50.14** Monocular exotropia with other noncomitancies

H50.141 Monocular exotropia with other noncomitancies, right eye

H50.142 Monocular exotropia with other noncomitancies, left eye

H50.15 Alternating exotropia

H50.16 Alternating exotropia with A pattern

H50.17 Alternating exotropia with V pattern

H50.18 Alternating exotropia with other noncomitancies

✓5ᵗʰ **H50.2** Vertical strabismus

Hypertropia

H50.21 Vertical strabismus, right eye

H50.22 Vertical strabismus, left eye

✓5ᵗʰ **H50.3** Intermittent heterotropia

H50.30 Unspecified intermittent heterotropia

✓6ᵗʰ **H50.31** Intermittent monocular esotropia

H50.311 Intermittent monocular esotropia, right eye

H50.312 Intermittent monocular esotropia, left eye

H50.32 Intermittent alternating esotropia

✓6ᵗʰ **H50.33** Intermittent monocular exotropia

H50.331 Intermittent monocular exotropia, right eye

H50.332 Intermittent monocular exotropia, left eye

H50.34 Intermittent alternating exotropia

✓5ᵗʰ **H50.4** Other and unspecified heterotropia

H50.40 Unspecified heterotropia

✓6ᵗʰ **H50.41** Cyclotropia

H50.411 Cyclotropia, right eye

H50.412 Cyclotropia, left eye

H50.42 Monofixation syndrome

H50.43 Accommodative component in esotropia

✓5ᵗʰ **H50.5** Heterophoria

H50.50 Unspecified heterophoria

H50.51 Esophoria

H50.52 Exophoria

H50.53 Vertical heterophoria

H50.54 Cyclophoria

H50.55 Alternating heterophoria

✓5ᵗʰ **H50.6** Mechanical strabismus

H50.60 Mechanical strabismus, unspecified

✓6ᵗʰ **H50.61** Brown's sheath syndrome

H50.611 Brown's sheath syndrome, right eye

H50.612 Brown's sheath syndrome, left eye

H50.69 Other mechanical strabismus

Strabismus due to adhesions

Traumatic limitation of duction of eye muscle

✓5ᵗʰ **H50.8** Other specified strabismus

✓6ᵗʰ **H50.81** Duane's syndrome

H50.811 Duane's syndrome, right eye

H50.812 Duane's syndrome, left eye

H50.89 Other specified strabismus

H50.9 Unspecified strabismus

✓4ᵗʰ **H51** Other disorders of binocular movement

H51.0 Palsy (spasm) of conjugate gaze

✓5ᵗʰ **H51.1** Convergence insufficiency and excess

H51.11 Convergence insufficiency

H51.12 Convergence excess

✓5ᵗʰ **H51.2** Internuclear ophthalmoplegia

H51.20 Internuclear ophthalmoplegia, unspecified eye

H51.21 Internuclear ophthalmoplegia, right eye

H51.22 Internuclear ophthalmoplegia, left eye

H51.23 Internuclear ophthalmoplegia, bilateral

H51.8 Other specified disorders of binocular movement

H51.9 Unspecified disorder of binocular movement

✓4ᵗʰ **H52** Disorders of refraction and accommodation

✓5ᵗʰ **H52.0** Hypermetropia

H52.00 Hypermetropia, unspecified eye

H52.01 Hypermetropia, right eye

H52.02 Hypermetropia, left eye

H52.03 Hypermetropia, bilateral

✓5ᵗʰ **H52.1** Myopia

EXCLUDES 1 *degenerative myopia (H44.2-)*

H52.10 Myopia, unspecified eye

H52.11 Myopia, right eye

H52.12 Myopia, left eye

H52.13 Myopia, bilateral

✓5ᵗʰ **H52.2** Astigmatism

✓6ᵗʰ **H52.20** Unspecified astigmatism

H52.201 Unspecified astigmatism, right eye

H52.202 Unspecified astigmatism, left eye

H52.203 Unspecified astigmatism, bilateral

H52.209 Unspecified astigmatism, unspecified eye

✓6ᵗʰ **H52.21** Irregular astigmatism

H52.211 Irregular astigmatism, right eye

H52.212 Irregular astigmatism, left eye

H52.213 Irregular astigmatism, bilateral

H52.219 Irregular astigmatism, unspecified eye

N Newborn: 0   P Pediatric: 0-17   M Maternity: 9-64   A Adult: 15-124   **MCC** Major Complication/Comorbidity   **CC** Complication/Comorbidity   **SW** Severe Wound Dx

624   ICD-10-CM 2021

✓6ᵗʰ **H52.22** Regular **astigmatism**

    H52.221 Regular astigmatism, **right eye**
    H52.222 Regular astigmatism, **left eye**
    H52.223 Regular astigmatism, **bilateral**
    H52.229 Regular astigmatism, **unspecified eye**

✓5ᵗʰ **H52.3** Anisometropia and aniseikonia

    H52.31 Anisometropia
    H52.32 Aniseikonia

H52.4 Presbyopia

✓5ᵗʰ **H52.5** Disorders of accommodation

✓6ᵗʰ **H52.51** Internal **ophthalmoplegia (complete) (total)**

    H52.511 Internal ophthalmoplegia (complete) (total), **right eye**
    H52.512 Internal ophthalmoplegia (complete) (total), **left eye**
    H52.513 Internal ophthalmoplegia (complete) (total), **bilateral**
    H52.519 Internal ophthalmoplegia (complete) (total), **unspecified eye**

✓6ᵗʰ **H52.52** Paresis **of accommodation**

    H52.521 Paresis of accommodation, **right eye**
    H52.522 Paresis of accommodation, **left eye**
    H52.523 Paresis of accommodation, **bilateral**
    H52.529 Paresis of accommodation, **unspecified eye**

✓6ᵗʰ **H52.53** Spasm **of accommodation**

    H52.531 Spasm of accommodation, **right eye**
    H52.532 Spasm of accommodation, **left eye**
    H52.533 Spasm of accommodation, **bilateral**
    H52.539 Spasm of accommodation, **unspecified eye**

H52.6 Other disorders of refraction

H52.7 Unspecified disorder of refraction

Visual disturbances and blindness (H53-H54)

✓4ᵗʰ **H53** Visual disturbances

✓5ᵗʰ **H53.0** Amblyopia ex anopsia

    EXCLUDES 1   *amblyopia due to vitamin A deficiency (E50.5)*

✓6ᵗʰ **H53.00** Unspecified **amblyopia**

    H53.001 Unspecified amblyopia, **right eye**
    H53.002 Unspecified amblyopia, **left eye**
    H53.003 Unspecified amblyopia, **bilateral**
    H53.009 Unspecified amblyopia, **unspecified eye**

✓6ᵗʰ **H53.01** Deprivation **amblyopia**

    H53.011 Deprivation amblyopia, **right eye**
    H53.012 Deprivation amblyopia, **left eye**
    H53.013 Deprivation amblyopia, **bilateral**
    H53.019 Deprivation amblyopia, **unspecified eye**

✓6ᵗʰ **H53.02** Refractive **amblyopia**

    H53.021 Refractive amblyopia, **right eye**
    H53.022 Refractive amblyopia, **left eye**
    H53.023 Refractive amblyopia, **bilateral**
    H53.029 Refractive amblyopia, **unspecified eye**

✓6ᵗʰ **H53.03** Strabismic **amblyopia**

    EXCLUDES 1   *strabismus (H50.-)*

    H53.031 Strabismic amblyopia, **right eye**
    H53.032 Strabismic amblyopia, **left eye**
    H53.033 Strabismic amblyopia, **bilateral**
    H53.039 Strabismic amblyopia, **unspecified eye**

✓6ᵗʰ **H53.04** Amblyopia **suspect**

    AHA: 2016,4Q,22-23

    H53.041 Amblyopia suspect, **right eye**
    H53.042 Amblyopia suspect, **left eye**
    H53.043 Amblyopia suspect, **bilateral**
    H53.049 Amblyopia suspect, **unspecified eye**

✓5ᵗʰ **H53.1** Subjective visual disturbances

    EXCLUDES 1   *subjective visual disturbances due to vitamin A deficiency (E50.5)*
    visual hallucinations (R44.1)

    H53.10 Unspecified subjective visual disturbances
    H53.11 Day blindness
        Hemeralopia

✓6ᵗʰ **H53.12** Transient **visual loss**

    Scintillating scotoma
    EXCLUDES 1   *amaurosis fugax (G45.3-)*
        transient retinal artery occlusion (H34.0-)

    H53.121 Transient visual loss, **right eye** cc
    H53.122 Transient visual loss, **left eye** cc
    H53.123 Transient visual loss, **bilateral** cc
    H53.129 Transient visual loss, **unspecified eye** cc

✓6ᵗʰ **H53.13** Sudden **visual loss**

    H53.131 Sudden visual loss, **right eye** cc
    H53.132 Sudden visual loss, **left eye** cc
    H53.133 Sudden visual loss, **bilateral** cc
    H53.139 Sudden visual loss, **unspecified eye** cc

✓6ᵗʰ **H53.14** Visual **discomfort**

    Asthenopia
    Photophobia

    H53.141 Visual discomfort, **right eye**
    H53.142 Visual discomfort, **left eye**
    H53.143 Visual discomfort, **bilateral**
    H53.149 Visual discomfort, **unspecified**

    H53.15 Visual distortions **of shape and size**
        Metamorphopsia
    H53.16 Psychophysical **visual disturbances**
    H53.19 Other subjective visual disturbances
        Visual halos

H53.2 Diplopia

    Double vision

✓5ᵗʰ **H53.3** Other and unspecified disorders of binocular vision

    H53.30 Unspecified disorder of binocular vision
    H53.31 Abnormal retinal correspondence
    H53.32 Fusion with defective stereopsis
    H53.33 Simultaneous visual perception without fusion
    H53.34 Suppression of binocular vision

✓5ᵗʰ **H53.4** Visual field defects

    H53.40 Unspecified visual field defects

✓6ᵗʰ **H53.41** Scotoma involving **central area**

    Central scotoma

    H53.411 Scotoma involving central area, **right eye**
    H53.412 Scotoma involving central area, **left eye**
    H53.413 Scotoma involving central area, **bilateral**
    H53.419 Scotoma involving central area, **unspecified eye**

✓6ᵗʰ **H53.42** Scotoma of **blind spot area**

    Enlarged blind spot

    H53.421 Scotoma of blind spot area, **right eye**
    H53.422 Scotoma of blind spot area, **left eye**
    H53.423 Scotoma of blind spot area, **bilateral**
    H53.429 Scotoma of blind spot area, **unspecified eye**

✓6ᵗʰ **H53.43** Sector or arcuate **defects**

    Arcuate scotoma
    Bjerrum scotoma

    H53.431 Sector or arcuate defects, **right eye**
    H53.432 Sector or arcuate defects, **left eye**
    H53.433 Sector or arcuate defects, **bilateral**
    H53.439 Sector or arcuate defects, **unspecified eye**

✓6ᵗʰ **H53.45** Other localized visual field defect

    Peripheral visual field defect
    Ring scotoma NOS
    Scotoma NOS

    H53.451 Other localized visual field defect, **right eye**
    H53.452 Other localized visual field defect, **left eye**
    H53.453 Other localized visual field defect, **bilateral**
    H53.459 Other localized visual field defect, **unspecified eye**

✓6ᵗʰ **H53.46** Homonymous **bilateral field defects**

    Homonymous hemianopia
    Homonymous hemianopsia
    Quadrant anopia
    Quadrant anopsia

    H53.461 Homonymous bilateral field defects, **right side**

H53.462 **Homonymous bilateral field defects, left** side

H53.469 **Homonymous bilateral field defects, unspecified side**
Homonymous bilateral field defects NOS

H53.47 **Heteronymous bilateral field defects**
Heteronymous hemianop(s)ia

✓6ᵗʰ H53.48 **Generalized contraction of visual field**

H53.481 **Generalized contraction of visual field, right eye**

H53.482 **Generalized contraction of visual field, left eye**

H53.483 **Generalized contraction of visual field, bilateral**

H53.489 **Generalized contraction of visual field, unspecified eye**

✓5ᵗʰ H53.5 **Color vision deficiencies**
Color blindness
EXCLUDES 2 *day blindness (H53.11)*

H53.50 **Unspecified color vision deficiencies**
Color blindness NOS

H53.51 **Achromatopsia**
DEF: Nonprogressive genetic visual disorder characterized by complete color blindness, decreased vision, and light sensitivity.

H53.52 **Acquired color vision deficiency**

H53.53 **Deuteranomaly**
Deuteranopia
DEF: Male-only genetic disorder causing difficulty in distinguishing green and red; no shortened spectrum.

H53.54 **Protanomaly**
Protanopia

H53.55 **Tritanomaly**
Tritanopia

H53.59 **Other color vision deficiencies**

✓5ᵗʰ H53.6 **Night blindness**
EXCLUDES 1 *night blindness due to vitamin A deficiency (E50.5)*

H53.60 **Unspecified night blindness**
H53.61 **Abnormal dark adaptation curve**
H53.62 **Acquired night blindness**
H53.63 **Congenital night blindness**
H53.69 **Other night blindness**

✓5ᵗʰ H53.7 **Vision sensitivity deficiencies**
H53.71 **Glare sensitivity**
H53.72 **Impaired contrast sensitivity**

H53.8 **Other visual disturbances**
H53.9 **Unspecified visual disturbance**

✓4ᵗʰ H54 **Blindness and low vision**

NOTE For definition of visual impairment categories see table below

Code first any associated underlying cause of the blindness
EXCLUDES 1 *amaurosis fugax (G45.3)*
AHA: 2017,4Q,11-12

✓5ᵗʰ H54.0 **Blindness, both eyes**
Visual impairment categories 3, 4, 5 in both eyes.

✓6ᵗʰ H54.0X **Blindness, both eyes, different category levels**

✓7ᵗʰ H54.0X3 **Blindness right eye, category 3**

H54.0X33 **Blindness right eye category 3, blindness left eye category 3**

H54.0X34 **Blindness right eye category 3, blindness left eye category 4**

H54.0X35 **Blindness right eye category 3, blindness left eye category 5**

✓7ᵗʰ H54.0X4 **Blindness right eye, category 4**

H54.0X43 **Blindness right eye category 4, blindness left eye category 3**

H54.0X44 **Blindness right eye category 4, blindness left eye category 4**

H54.0X45 **Blindness right eye category 4, blindness left eye category 5**

✓7ᵗʰ H54.0X5 **Blindness right eye, category 5**

H54.0X53 **Blindness right eye category 5, blindness left eye category 3**

H54.0X54 **Blindness right eye category 5, blindness left eye category 4**

H54.0X55 **Blindness right eye category 5, blindness left eye category 5**

✓5ᵗʰ H54.1 **Blindness, one eye, low vision other eye**
Visual impairment categories 3, 4, 5 in one eye, with categories 1 or 2 in the other eye.

H54.10 **Blindness, one eye, low vision other eye, unspecified eyes**

✓6ᵗʰ H54.11 **Blindness, right eye, low vision left eye**

✓7ᵗʰ H54.113 **Blindness right eye category 3, low vision left eye**

H54.1131 **Blindness right eye category 3, low vision left eye category 1**

H54.1132 **Blindness right eye category 3, low vision left eye category 2**

✓7ᵗʰ H54.114 **Blindness right eye category 4, low vision left eye**

H54.1141 **Blindness right eye category 4, low vision left eye category 1**

H54.1142 **Blindness right eye category 4, low vision left eye category 2**

✓7ᵗʰ H54.115 **Blindness right eye category 5, low vision left eye**

H54.1151 **Blindness right eye category 5, low vision left eye category 1**

H54.1152 **Blindness right eye category 5, low vision left eye category 2**

✓6ᵗʰ H54.12 **Blindness, left eye, low vision right eye**

✓7ᵗʰ H54.121 **Low vision right eye category 1, blindness left eye**

H54.1213 **Low vision right eye category 1, blindness left eye category 3**

H54.1214 **Low vision right eye category 1, blindness left eye category 4**

H54.1215 **Low vision right eye category 1, blindness left eye category 5**

✓7ᵗʰ H54.122 **Low vision right eye category 2, blindness left eye**

H54.1223 **Low vision right eye category 2, blindness left eye category 3**

H54.1224 **Low vision right eye category 2, blindness left eye category 4**

H54.1225 **Low vision right eye category 2, blindness left eye category 5**

✓5ᵗʰ H54.2 **Low vision, both eyes**
Visual impairment categories 1 or 2 in both eyes.

✓6ᵗʰ H54.2X **Low vision, both eyes, different category levels**

✓7ᵗʰ H54.2X1 **Low vision, right eye, category 1**

H54.2X11 **Low vision right eye category 1, low vision left eye category 1**

H54.2X12 **Low vision right eye category 1, low vision left eye category 2**

✓7ᵗʰ H54.2X2 **Low vision right eye, category 2**

H54.2X21 **Low vision right eye category 2, low vision left eye category 1**

H54.2X22 **Low vision right eye category 2, low vision left eye category 2**

H54.3 **Unqualified visual loss, both eyes**
Visual impairment category 9 in both eyes.
TIP: Assign only when both eyes are documented as affected by blindness or low vision but the visual impairment category is not documented.

✓5ᵗʰ H54.4 **Blindness, one eye**
Visual impairment categories 3, 4, 5 in one eye [normal vision in other eye]

H54.40 **Blindness, one eye, unspecified eye**

✓6ᵗʰ H54.41 **Blindness, right eye, normal vision left eye**

✓7ᵗʰ H54.413 **Blindness, right eye, category 3**

H54.413A **Blindness right eye category 3, normal vision left eye**

✓7ᵗʰ H54.414 **Blindness, right eye, category 4**

H54.414A **Blindness right eye category 4, normal vision left eye**

  ☑7ᵗʰ **H54.415** **Blindness, right eye, category 5**

        H54.415A **Blindness right eye category 5, normal vision left eye**

 ☑6ᵗʰ **H54.42** Blindness, left eye, normal vision right eye

    ☑7ᵗʰ **H54.42A** **Blindness, left eye, category 3-5**

        H54.42A3 **Blindness left eye category 3, normal vision right eye**

        H54.42A4 **Blindness left eye category 4, normal vision right eye**

        H54.42A5 **Blindness left eye category 5, normal vision right eye**

☑5ᵗʰ **H54.5** **Low vision, one eye**

   Visual impairment categories 1 or 2 in one eye [normal vision in other eye].

   H54.50 **Low vision, one eye, unspecified eye**

 ☑6ᵗʰ **H54.51** Low vision, right eye, normal vision left eye

    ☑7ᵗʰ **H54.511** **Low vision, right eye, category 1-2**

        H54.511A **Low vision right eye category 1, normal vision left eye**

        H54.512A **Low vision right eye category 2, normal vision left eye**

  ☑7ᵗʰ **H54.52** Low vision, left eye, normal vision right eye

    ☑7ᵗʰ **H54.52A** **Low vision, left eye, category 1-2**

        H54.52A1 **Low vision left eye category 1, normal vision right eye**

        H54.52A2 **Low vision left eye category 2, normal vision right eye**

☑5ᵗʰ **H54.6** Unqualified visual loss, one eye

   Visual impairment category 9 in one eye [normal vision in other eye].

   TIP: Assign a code from this category only when one eye is documented as affected by blindness or low vision but the visual impairment category is not documented.

   H54.60 **Unqualified visual loss, one eye, unspecified**

   H54.61 **Unqualified visual loss, right eye, normal vision left eye**

   H54.62 **Unqualified visual loss, left eye, normal vision right eye**

H54.7 **Unspecified visual loss**

   Visual impairment category 9 NOS

   TIP: Assign only when documentation specifies blindness, visual loss, or low vision but not whether one or both eyes are affected or the visual impairment category.

 H54.8 Legal blindness, **as defined in USA**

   Blindness NOS according to USA definition

   EXCLUDES 1 *legal blindness with specification of impairment level (H54.0-H54.7)*

   NOTE The table below gives a classification of severity of visual impairment recommended by a WHO Study Group on the Prevention of Blindness, Geneva, 6-10 November 1972.

   The term "low vision" in category H54 comprises categories 1 and 2 of the table, the term "blindness" categories 3, 4 and 5, and the term "unqualified visual loss" category 9.

   If the extent of the visual field is taken into account, patients with a field no greater than 10 but greater than 5 around central fixation should be placed in category 3 and patients with a field no greater than 5 around central fixation should be placed in category 4, even if the central acuity is not impaired.

Category of visual impairment	Visual acuity with best possible correction	
	Maximum less than:	**Minimum equal to or better than:**
1	6/18 3/10 (0.3) 20/70	6/60 1/10 (0.1) 20/200
2	6/60 1/10 (0.1) 20/200	3/60 1/20 (0.05) 20/400
3	3/60 1/200 (0.05) 20/400	1/60 (finger counting at one meter) 1/50 (0.02) 5/300 (20/1200)
4	1/60 (finger counting at one meter) 1/50 (0.02) 5/300	Light perception
5	No light perception	
9	Undetermined or unspecified	

Other disorders of eye and adnexa (H55-H57)

☑4ᵗʰ **H55** **Nystagmus and other irregular eye movements**

 ☑5ᵗʰ **H55.0** **Nystagmus**

   DEF: Rapid, rhythmic, involuntary movements of the eyeball in vertical, horizontal, rotational, or mixed directions.

   H55.00 **Unspecified nystagmus**

   H55.01 Congenital **nystagmus**

   H55.02 Latent **nystagmus**

   H55.03 Visual deprivation **nystagmus**

   H55.04 Dissociated **nystagmus**

   H55.09 **Other forms of nystagmus**

 ☑5ᵗʰ **H55.8** **Other irregular eye movements**

▲   **H55.81** Deficient saccadic **eye movements**

●   **H55.82** Deficient smooth pursuit **eye movements**

   H55.89 **Other irregular eye movements**

☑4ᵗʰ **H57** **Other disorders of eye and adnexa**

 ☑5ᵗʰ **H57.0** **Anomalies of pupillary function**

   H57.00 **Unspecified anomaly of pupillary function**

   H57.01 **Argyll Robertson pupil, atypical**

     EXCLUDES 1 *syphilitic Argyll Robertson pupil (A52.19)*

   H57.02 **Anisocoria**

   H57.03 **Miosis**

   H57.04 **Mydriasis**

  ☑6ᵗʰ **H57.05** **Tonic pupil**

     H57.051 **Tonic pupil, right eye**

     H57.052 **Tonic pupil, left eye**

     H57.053 **Tonic pupil, bilateral**

     H57.059 **Tonic pupil, unspecified eye**

   H57.09 **Other anomalies of pupillary function**

 ☑5ᵗʰ **H57.1** **Ocular pain**

   H57.10 **Ocular pain, unspecified eye**

☑ Additional Character Required   ☑x7ᵗʰ Placeholder   Unacceptable PDx   Questionable PDx   Manifestation   Unspecified Dx   H1-H14 HAC   HCC CMS-HCC Dx   HIV HIV Dx

ICD-10-CM 2021   **627**

H57.11　　**Ocular pain, right** eye
H57.12　　**Ocular pain, left** eye
H57.13　　**Ocular pain, bilateral**
✓5ᵗʰ **H57.8** **Other specified disorders of eye and adnexa**
　　　AHA: 2018,4Q,15-16
　✓6ᵗʰ **H57.81** **Brow ptosis**
　　　H57.811　**Brow ptosis, right**
　　　H57.812　**Brow ptosis, left**
　　　H57.813　**Brow ptosis, bilateral**
　　　H57.819　**Brow ptosis, unspecified**
　　H57.89　**Other specified disorders of eye and adnexa**
✓ **H57.9** **Unspecified disorder of eye and adnexa**

Intraoperative and postprocedural complications and disorders of eye and adnexa, not elsewhere classified (H59)

✓4ᵗʰ **H59** **Intraoperative and postprocedural complications and disorders of eye and adnexa, not elsewhere classified**
　　　EXCLUDES 1　mechanical complication of intraocular lens (T85.2)
　　　　　　mechanical complication of other ocular prosthetic devices, implants and grafts (T85.3)
　　　　　　pseudophakia (Z96.1)
　　　　　　secondary cataracts (H26.4-)
　✓5ᵗʰ **H59.0** **Disorders of the eye** following cataract surgery
　　✓6ᵗʰ **H59.01** **Keratopathy (bullous aphakic) following cataract surgery**
　　　　Vitreal corneal syndrome
　　　　Vitreous (touch) syndrome
　　　　H59.011　**Keratopathy (bullous aphakic) following cataract surgery, right eye**　cc
　　　　H59.012　**Keratopathy (bullous aphakic) following cataract surgery, left eye**　cc
　　　　H59.013　**Keratopathy (bullous aphakic) following cataract surgery, bilateral**　cc
　　　　H59.019　**Keratopathy (bullous aphakic) following cataract surgery, unspecified eye**　cc
　　✓6ᵗʰ **H59.02** **Cataract (lens) fragments in eye following cataract surgery**
　　　　H59.021　**Cataract (lens) fragments in eye following cataract surgery, right eye**
　　　　H59.022　**Cataract (lens) fragments in eye following cataract surgery, left eye**
　　　　H59.023　**Cataract (lens) fragments in eye following cataract surgery, bilateral**
　　　　H59.029　**Cataract (lens) fragments in eye following cataract surgery, unspecified eye**
　　✓6ᵗʰ **H59.03** **Cystoid macular edema** following cataract surgery
　　　　H59.031　**Cystoid macular edema following cataract surgery, right eye**　cc
　　　　H59.032　**Cystoid macular edema following cataract surgery, left eye**　cc
　　　　H59.033　**Cystoid macular edema following cataract surgery, bilateral**　cc
　　　　H59.039　**Cystoid macular edema following cataract surgery, unspecified eye**　cc
　　✓6ᵗʰ **H59.09** **Other disorders of the eye following cataract surgery**
　　　　H59.091　**Other disorders of the right eye following cataract surgery**　cc
　　　　H59.092　**Other disorders of the left eye following cataract surgery**　cc
　　　　H59.093　**Other disorders of the eye following cataract surgery, bilateral**　cc
　　　　H59.099　**Other disorders of unspecified eye following cataract surgery**　cc
　✓5ᵗʰ **H59.1** **Intraoperative hemorrhage and hematoma** of eye and adnexa complicating a procedure
　　　EXCLUDES 1　intraoperative hemorrhage and hematoma of eye and adnexa due to accidental puncture or laceration during a procedure (H59.2-)
　　✓6ᵗʰ **H59.11** **Intraoperative hemorrhage and hematoma of eye and adnexa complicating an** ophthalmic procedure
　　　　H59.111　**Intraoperative hemorrhage and hematoma of right eye and adnexa complicating an ophthalmic procedure**　cc
　　　　H59.112　**Intraoperative hemorrhage and hematoma of left eye and adnexa complicating an ophthalmic procedure**　cc

H59.113　**Intraoperative hemorrhage and hematoma of eye and adnexa complicating an ophthalmic procedure, bilateral**　cc
H59.119　**Intraoperative hemorrhage and hematoma of unspecified eye and adnexa complicating an ophthalmic procedure**　cc
　✓6ᵗʰ **H59.12** **Intraoperative hemorrhage and hematoma of eye and adnexa complicating** other procedure
　　　H59.121　**Intraoperative hemorrhage and hematoma of right eye and adnexa complicating other procedure**　cc
　　　H59.122　**Intraoperative hemorrhage and hematoma of left eye and adnexa complicating other procedure**　cc
　　　H59.123　**Intraoperative hemorrhage and hematoma of eye and adnexa complicating other procedure, bilateral**　cc
　　　H59.129　**Intraoperative hemorrhage and hematoma of unspecified eye and adnexa complicating other procedure**　cc
✓5ᵗʰ **H59.2** **Accidental puncture and laceration** of eye and adnexa during a procedure
　✓6ᵗʰ **H59.21** **Accidental puncture and laceration of eye and adnexa during an** ophthalmic procedure
　　　H59.211　**Accidental puncture and laceration of right eye and adnexa during an ophthalmic procedure**　cc
　　　H59.212　**Accidental puncture and laceration of left eye and adnexa during an ophthalmic procedure**　cc
　　　H59.213　**Accidental puncture and laceration of eye and adnexa during an ophthalmic procedure, bilateral**　cc
　　　H59.219　**Accidental puncture and laceration of unspecified eye and adnexa during an ophthalmic procedure**　cc
　✓6ᵗʰ **H59.22** **Accidental puncture and laceration of eye and adnexa during** other procedure
　　　H59.221　**Accidental puncture and laceration of right eye and adnexa during other procedure**　cc
　　　H59.222　**Accidental puncture and laceration of left eye and adnexa during other procedure**　cc
　　　H59.223　**Accidental puncture and laceration of eye and adnexa during other procedure, bilateral**　cc
　　　H59.229　**Accidental puncture and laceration of unspecified eye and adnexa during other procedure**　cc
✓5ᵗʰ **H59.3** **Postprocedural hemorrhage, hematoma, and seroma** of eye and adnexa following a procedure
　　AHA: 2016,4Q,9-10
　✓6ᵗʰ **H59.31** **Postprocedural** hemorrhage **of eye and adnexa following an** ophthalmic procedure
　　　H59.311　**Postprocedural hemorrhage of right eye and adnexa following an ophthalmic procedure**　cc
　　　H59.312　**Postprocedural hemorrhage of left eye and adnexa following an ophthalmic procedure**　cc
　　　H59.313　**Postprocedural hemorrhage of eye and adnexa following an ophthalmic procedure, bilateral**　cc
　　　H59.319　**Postprocedural hemorrhage of unspecified eye and adnexa following an ophthalmic procedure**　cc
　✓6ᵗʰ **H59.32** **Postprocedural** hemorrhage **of eye and adnexa following** other procedure
　　　H59.321　**Postprocedural hemorrhage of right eye and adnexa following other procedure**　cc
　　　H59.322　**Postprocedural hemorrhage of left eye and adnexa following other procedure**　cc
　　　H59.323　**Postprocedural hemorrhage of eye and adnexa following other procedure, bilateral**　cc

        H59.329 Postprocedural hemorrhage of unspecified eye and adnexa following other procedure   `cc`

✓6ᵗʰ **H59.33** Postprocedural hematoma of eye and adnexa following an ophthalmic procedure

        H59.331 Postprocedural hematoma of right eye and adnexa following an ophthalmic procedure   `cc`

        H59.332 Postprocedural hematoma of left eye and adnexa following an ophthalmic procedure   `cc`

        H59.333 Postprocedural hematoma of eye and adnexa following an ophthalmic procedure, bilateral   `cc`

        H59.339 Postprocedural hematoma of unspecified eye and adnexa following an ophthalmic procedure   `cc`

✓6ᵗʰ **H59.34** Postprocedural hematoma of eye and adnexa following other procedure

        H59.341 Postprocedural hematoma of right eye and adnexa following other procedure   `cc`

        H59.342 Postprocedural hematoma of left eye and adnexa following other procedure   `cc`

        H59.343 Postprocedural hematoma of eye and adnexa following other procedure, bilateral   `cc`

        H59.349 Postprocedural hematoma of unspecified eye and adnexa following other procedure   `cc`

✓6ᵗʰ **H59.35** Postprocedural seroma of eye and adnexa following an ophthalmic procedure

        H59.351 Postprocedural seroma of right eye and adnexa following an ophthalmic procedure   `cc`

        H59.352 Postprocedural seroma of left eye and adnexa following an ophthalmic procedure   `cc`

        H59.353 Postprocedural seroma of eye and adnexa following an ophthalmic procedure, bilateral   `cc`

        H59.359 Postprocedural seroma of unspecified eye and adnexa following an ophthalmic procedure   `cc`

✓6ᵗʰ **H59.36** Postprocedural seroma of eye and adnexa following other procedure

        H59.361 Postprocedural seroma of right eye and adnexa following other procedure   `cc`

        H59.362 Postprocedural seroma of left eye and adnexa following other procedure   `cc`

        H59.363 Postprocedural seroma of eye and adnexa following other procedure, bilateral   `cc`

        H59.369 Postprocedural seroma of unspecified eye and adnexa following other procedure   `cc`

✓5ᵗʰ **H59.4** Inflammation (infection) of postprocedural bleb

    Postprocedural blebitis

    EXCLUDES 1   filtering (vitreous) bleb after glaucoma surgery status (Z98.83)

    H59.40 Inflammation (infection) of postprocedural bleb, unspecified

    H59.41 Inflammation (infection) of postprocedural bleb, stage 1

    H59.42 Inflammation (infection) of postprocedural bleb, stage 2

    H59.43 Inflammation (infection) of postprocedural bleb, stage 3

        Bleb endophthalmitis

✓5ᵗʰ **H59.8** Other intraoperative and postprocedural complications and disorders of eye and adnexa, not elsewhere classified

✓6ᵗʰ **H59.81** Chorioretinal scars after surgery for detachment

    H59.811 Chorioretinal scars after surgery for detachment, right eye   `cc`

    H59.812 Chorioretinal scars after surgery for detachment, left eye   `cc`

    H59.813 Chorioretinal scars after surgery for detachment, bilateral   `cc`

    H59.819 Chorioretinal scars after surgery for detachment, unspecified eye   `cc`

    H59.88 Other intraoperative complications of eye and adnexa, not elsewhere classified   `cc`

    H59.89 Other postprocedural complications and disorders of eye and adnexa, not elsewhere classified   `cc`

☑ Additional Character Required   ✓x7ᵗʰ Placeholder   Unacceptable PDx   Questionable PDx   Manifestation   Unspecified Dx   H1 -H14 HAC   HCC CMS-HCC Dx   HIV HIV Dx

Chapter 8. Diseases of the Ear and Mastoid Process (H60–H95)

Chapter-specific Guidelines with Coding Examples
Reserved for future guideline expansion.

Chapter 8. Diseases of the Ear and Mastoid Process (H60-H95)

NOTE Use an external cause code following the code for the ear condition, if applicable, to identify the cause of the ear condition

EXCLUDES 2
certain conditions originating in the perinatal period (P04-P96)
certain infectious and parasitic diseases (A00-B99)
complications of pregnancy, childbirth and the puerperium (O00-O9A)
congenital malformations, deformations and chromosomal abnormalities (Q00-Q99)
endocrine, nutritional and metabolic diseases (E00-E88)
injury, poisoning and certain other consequences of external causes (S00-T88)
neoplasms (C00-D49)
symptoms, signs and abnormal clinical and laboratory findings, not elsewhere classified (R00-R94)

This chapter contains the following blocks:
H60-H62   Diseases of external ear
H65-H75   Diseases of middle ear and mastoid
H80-H83   Diseases of inner ear
H90-H94   Other disorders of ear
H95   Intraoperative and postprocedural complications and disorders of ear and mastoid process, not elsewhere classified

Diseases of external ear (H60-H62)

H60 Otitis externa

TIP: When the specific infectious agent is identified, a code from Chapter 1 is assigned instead of a code from this category.

H60.0 Abscess of external ear

Boil of external ear
Carbuncle of auricle or external auditory canal
Furuncle of external ear

H60.00   Abscess of external ear, unspecified ear
H60.01   Abscess of right external ear
H60.02   Abscess of left external ear
H60.03   Abscess of external ear, bilateral

H60.1 Cellulitis of external ear

Cellulitis of auricle
Cellulitis of external auditory canal

H60.10   Cellulitis of external ear, unspecified ear
H60.11   Cellulitis of right external ear
H60.12   Cellulitis of left external ear
H60.13   Cellulitis of external ear, bilateral

H60.2 Malignant otitis externa

H60.20   Malignant otitis externa, unspecified ear   **CC**
H60.21   Malignant otitis externa, right ear   **CC**
H60.22   Malignant otitis externa, left ear   **CC**
H60.23   Malignant otitis externa, bilateral   **CC**

H60.3 Other infective otitis externa

H60.31   Diffuse otitis externa

    H60.311   Diffuse otitis externa, right ear
    H60.312   Diffuse otitis externa, left ear
    H60.313   Diffuse otitis externa, bilateral
    H60.319   Diffuse otitis externa, unspecified ear

H60.32   Hemorrhagic otitis externa

    H60.321   Hemorrhagic otitis externa, right ear
    H60.322   Hemorrhagic otitis externa, left ear
    H60.323   Hemorrhagic otitis externa, bilateral
    H60.329   Hemorrhagic otitis externa, unspecified ear

H60.33   Swimmer's ear

    DEF: Commonly occurs when water gets trapped in the ear after swimming.
    H60.331   Swimmer's ear, right ear
    H60.332   Swimmer's ear, left ear
    H60.333   Swimmer's ear, bilateral
    H60.339   Swimmer's ear, unspecified ear

H60.39   Other infective otitis externa

    H60.391   Other infective otitis externa, right ear
    H60.392   Other infective otitis externa, left ear
    H60.393   Other infective otitis externa, bilateral
    H60.399   Other infective otitis externa, unspecified ear

H60.4 Cholesteatoma of external ear

Keratosis obturans of external ear (canal)

EXCLUDES 2
cholesteatoma of middle ear (H71.-)
recurrent cholesteatoma of postmastoidectomy cavity (H95.0-)

DEF: Cholesteatoma: Noncancerous cyst-like mass of cell debris, including cholesterol and epithelial cells resulting from trauma, repeated or improperly healed infections, and congenital enclosure of epidermal cells.

H60.40   Cholesteatoma of external ear, unspecified ear
H60.41   Cholesteatoma of right external ear
H60.42   Cholesteatoma of left external ear
H60.43   Cholesteatoma of external ear, bilateral

H60.5 Acute noninfective otitis externa

H60.50   Unspecified acute noninfective otitis externa

    Acute otitis externa NOS
    H60.501   Unspecified acute noninfective otitis externa, right ear
    H60.502   Unspecified acute noninfective otitis externa, left ear
    H60.503   Unspecified acute noninfective otitis externa, bilateral
    H60.509   Unspecified acute noninfective otitis externa, unspecified ear

H60.51   Acute actinic otitis externa

    H60.511   Acute actinic otitis externa, right ear
    H60.512   Acute actinic otitis externa, left ear
    H60.513   Acute actinic otitis externa, bilateral
    H60.519   Acute actinic otitis externa, unspecified ear

H60.52   Acute chemical otitis externa

    H60.521   Acute chemical otitis externa, right ear
    H60.522   Acute chemical otitis externa, left ear
    H60.523   Acute chemical otitis externa, bilateral
    H60.529   Acute chemical otitis externa, unspecified ear

H60.53   Acute contact otitis externa

    H60.531   Acute contact otitis externa, right ear
    H60.532   Acute contact otitis externa, left ear
    H60.533   Acute contact otitis externa, bilateral
    H60.539   Acute contact otitis externa, unspecified ear

H60.54   Acute eczematoid otitis externa

    H60.541   Acute eczematoid otitis externa, right ear
    H60.542   Acute eczematoid otitis externa, left ear
    H60.543   Acute eczematoid otitis externa, bilateral
    H60.549   Acute eczematoid otitis externa, unspecified ear

H60.55   Acute reactive otitis externa

    H60.551   Acute reactive otitis externa, right ear
    H60.552   Acute reactive otitis externa, left ear
    H60.553   Acute reactive otitis externa, bilateral
    H60.559   Acute reactive otitis externa, unspecified ear

H60.59   Other noninfective acute otitis externa

    H60.591   Other noninfective acute otitis externa, right ear
    H60.592   Other noninfective acute otitis externa, left ear
    H60.593   Other noninfective acute otitis externa, bilateral
    H60.599   Other noninfective acute otitis externa, unspecified ear

H60.6 Unspecified chronic otitis externa

H60.60   Unspecified chronic otitis externa, unspecified ear
H60.61   Unspecified chronic otitis externa, right ear
H60.62   Unspecified chronic otitis externa, left ear
H60.63   Unspecified chronic otitis externa, bilateral

H60.8 Other otitis externa

H60.8X   Other otitis externa

    H60.8X1   Other otitis externa, right ear
    H60.8X2   Other otitis externa, left ear
    H60.8X3   Other otitis externa, bilateral
    H60.8X9   Other otitis externa, unspecified ear

H60.9 Unspecified otitis externa

H60.90   Unspecified otitis externa, unspecified ear
H60.91   Unspecified otitis externa, right ear

N Newborn: 0   **P** Pediatric: 0-17   **M** Maternity: 9-64   **A** Adult: 15-124   **MCC** Major Complication/Comorbidity   **CC** Complication/Comorbidity   **SW** Severe Wound Dx

632   ICD-10-CM 2021

H60.92   Unspecified otitis externa, **left** ear

H60.93   Unspecified otitis externa, **bilateral**

✓4ᵗʰ **H61**   **Other disorders of external ear**

     ✓5ᵗʰ **H61.0**   **Chondritis and perichondritis of external ear**

         Chondrodermatitis nodularis chronica helicis

         Perichondritis of auricle

         Perichondritis of pinna

         ✓6ᵗʰ **H61.00**   **Unspecified perichondritis of external ear**

             H61.001   **Unspecified perichondritis of right external ear**

             H61.002   **Unspecified perichondritis of left external ear**

             H61.003   **Unspecified perichondritis of external ear, bilateral**

             H61.009   **Unspecified perichondritis of external ear, unspecified ear**

         ✓6ᵗʰ **H61.01**   **Acute perichondritis of external ear**

             H61.011   **Acute perichondritis of right external ear**

             H61.012   **Acute perichondritis of left external ear**

             H61.013   **Acute perichondritis of external ear, bilateral**

             H61.019   **Acute perichondritis of external ear, unspecified ear**

         ✓6ᵗʰ **H61.02**   **Chronic perichondritis of external ear**

             H61.021   **Chronic perichondritis of right external ear**

             H61.022   **Chronic perichondritis of left external ear**

             H61.023   **Chronic perichondritis of external ear, bilateral**

             H61.029   **Chronic perichondritis of external ear, unspecified ear**

         ✓6ᵗʰ **H61.03**   **Chondritis of external ear**

             Chondritis of auricle

             Chondritis of pinna

             AHA: 2015,1Q,18

             DEF: Infection that has progressed into the cartilage and presents as indurated and edematous skin over the pinna. Vascular compromise occurs with tissue necrosis and deformity.

             H61.031   **Chondritis of right external ear**

             H61.032   **Chondritis of left external ear**

             H61.033   **Chondritis of external ear, bilateral**

             H61.039   **Chondritis of external ear, unspecified ear**

     ✓5ᵗʰ **H61.1**   **Noninfective disorders of pinna**

         EXCLUDES 2   cauliflower ear (M95.1-)

                       gouty tophi of ear (M1A.-)

         ✓6ᵗʰ **H61.10**   **Unspecified noninfective disorders of pinna**

             Disorder of pinna NOS

             H61.101   **Unspecified noninfective disorders of pinna, right ear**

             H61.102   **Unspecified noninfective disorders of pinna, left ear**

             H61.103   **Unspecified noninfective disorders of pinna, bilateral**

             H61.109   **Unspecified noninfective disorders of pinna, unspecified ear**

         ✓6ᵗʰ **H61.11**   **Acquired deformity of pinna**

             Acquired deformity of auricle

             EXCLUDES 2   cauliflower ear (M95.1-)

             H61.111   **Acquired deformity of pinna, right ear**

             H61.112   **Acquired deformity of pinna, left ear**

             H61.113   **Acquired deformity of pinna, bilateral**

             H61.119   **Acquired deformity of pinna, unspecified ear**

         ✓6ᵗʰ **H61.12**   **Hematoma of pinna**

             Hematoma of auricle

             H61.121   **Hematoma of pinna, right ear**

             H61.122   **Hematoma of pinna, left ear**

             H61.123   **Hematoma of pinna, bilateral**

             H61.129   **Hematoma of pinna, unspecified ear**

         ✓6ᵗʰ **H61.19**   **Other noninfective disorders of pinna**

             H61.191   **Noninfective disorders of pinna, right ear**

             H61.192   **Noninfective disorders of pinna, left ear**

             H61.193   **Noninfective disorders of pinna, bilateral**

             H61.199   **Noninfective disorders of pinna, unspecified ear**

     ✓5ᵗʰ **H61.2**   **Impacted cerumen**

         Wax in ear

         H61.20   **Impacted cerumen, unspecified ear**

         H61.21   **Impacted cerumen, right ear**

         H61.22   **Impacted cerumen, left ear**

         H61.23   **Impacted cerumen, bilateral**

     ✓5ᵗʰ **H61.3**   **Acquired stenosis of external ear canal**

         Collapse of external ear canal

         EXCLUDES 1   postprocedural stenosis of external ear canal (H95.81-)

         ✓6ᵗʰ **H61.30**   **Acquired stenosis of external ear canal, unspecified**

             H61.301   **Acquired stenosis of right external ear canal, unspecified**

             H61.302   **Acquired stenosis of left external ear canal, unspecified**

             H61.303   **Acquired stenosis of external ear canal, unspecified, bilateral**

             H61.309   **Acquired stenosis of external ear canal, unspecified, unspecified ear**

         ✓6ᵗʰ **H61.31**   **Acquired stenosis of external ear canal secondary to trauma**

             H61.311   **Acquired stenosis of right external ear canal secondary to trauma**

             H61.312   **Acquired stenosis of left external ear canal secondary to trauma**

             H61.313   **Acquired stenosis of external ear canal secondary to trauma, bilateral**

             H61.319   **Acquired stenosis of external ear canal secondary to trauma, unspecified ear**

         ✓6ᵗʰ **H61.32**   **Acquired stenosis of external ear canal secondary to inflammation and infection**

             DEF: Narrowing of the external ear canal due to chronic inflammation or infection.

             H61.321   **Acquired stenosis of right external ear canal secondary to inflammation and infection**

             H61.322   **Acquired stenosis of left external ear canal secondary to inflammation and infection**

             H61.323   **Acquired stenosis of external ear canal secondary to inflammation and infection, bilateral**

             H61.329   **Acquired stenosis of external ear canal secondary to inflammation and infection, unspecified ear**

         ✓6ᵗʰ **H61.39**   **Other acquired stenosis of external ear canal**

             H61.391   **Other acquired stenosis of right external ear canal**

             H61.392   **Other acquired stenosis of left external ear canal**

             H61.393   **Other acquired stenosis of external ear canal, bilateral**

             H61.399   **Other acquired stenosis of external ear canal, unspecified ear**

     ✓5ᵗʰ **H61.8**   **Other specified disorders of external ear**

         ✓6ᵗʰ **H61.81**   **Exostosis of external canal**

             H61.811   **Exostosis of right external canal**

             H61.812   **Exostosis of left external canal**

             H61.813   **Exostosis of external canal, bilateral**

             H61.819   **Exostosis of external canal, unspecified ear**

         ✓6ᵗʰ **H61.89**   **Other specified disorders of external ear**

             H61.891   **Other specified disorders of right external ear**

             H61.892   **Other specified disorders of left external ear**

             H61.893   **Other specified disorders of external ear, bilateral**

             H61.899   **Other specified disorders of external ear, unspecified ear**

     ✓5ᵗʰ **H61.9**   **Disorder of external ear, unspecified**

         H61.90   **Disorder of external ear, unspecified, unspecified ear**

         H61.91   **Disorder of right external ear, unspecified**

         H61.92   **Disorder of left external ear, unspecified**

         H61.93   **Disorder of external ear, unspecified, bilateral**

✓ Additional Character Required   ✓x7ᵗʰ Placeholder   Unacceptable PDx   Questionable PDx   Manifestation   Unspecified Dx   H1-H14 HAC   HCC CMS-HCC Dx   HIV HIV Dx

✓4ᵗʰ H62   Disorders of external ear in diseases classified elsewhere

  ✓5ᵗʰ H62.4   Otitis externa in other diseases classified elsewhere

Code first underlying disease, such as:
erysipelas (A46)
impetigo (L01.0)

    EXCLUDES 1   *otitis externa (in):*
candidiasis (B37.84)
herpes viral [herpes simplex] (B00.1)
herpes zoster (B02.8)

  H62.40   *Otitis externa in other diseases classified elsewhere, unspecified ear*

  H62.41   *Otitis externa in other diseases classified elsewhere, right ear*

  H62.42   *Otitis externa in other diseases classified elsewhere, left ear*

  H62.43   *Otitis externa in other diseases classified elsewhere, bilateral*

  ✓5ᵗʰ H62.8   Other disorders of external ear in diseases classified elsewhere

Code first underlying disease, such as:
gout (M1A.-, M10.-)

  ✓6ᵗʰ H62.8X   Other disorders of external ear in diseases classified elsewhere

  H62.8X1   *Other disorders of right external ear in diseases classified elsewhere*

  H62.8X2   *Other disorders of left external ear in diseases classified elsewhere*

  H62.8X3   *Other disorders of external ear in diseases classified elsewhere, bilateral*

  H62.8X9   *Other disorders of external ear in diseases classified elsewhere, unspecified ear*

Diseases of middle ear and mastoid (H65-H75)

✓4ᵗʰ H65   Nonsuppurative otitis media

  INCLUDES   nonsuppurative otitis media with myringitis

Use additional code for any associated perforated tympanic membrane (H72.-)

Use additional code, if applicable, to identify:
exposure to environmental tobacco smoke (Z77.22)
exposure to tobacco smoke in the perinatal period (P96.81)
history of tobacco dependence (Z87.891)
infectious agent (B95-B97)
occupational exposure to environmental tobacco smoke (Z57.31)
tobacco dependence (F17.-)
tobacco use (Z72.0)

  ✓5ᵗʰ H65.0   Acute serous otitis media

Acute and subacute secretory otitis

  H65.00   Acute serous otitis media, unspecified ear

  H65.01   Acute serous otitis media, right ear

  H65.02   Acute serous otitis media, left ear

  H65.03   Acute serous otitis media, bilateral

  H65.04   Acute serous otitis media, recurrent, right ear

  H65.05   Acute serous otitis media, recurrent, left ear

  H65.06   Acute serous otitis media, recurrent, bilateral

  H65.07   Acute serous otitis media, recurrent, unspecified ear

  ✓5ᵗʰ H65.1   Other acute nonsuppurative otitis media

  EXCLUDES 1   *otitic barotrauma (T70.0)*
otitis media (acute) NOS (H66.9)

  ✓6ᵗʰ H65.11   Acute and subacute allergic otitis media (mucoid) (sanguinous) (serous)

  H65.111   Acute and subacute allergic otitis media (mucoid) (sanguinous) (serous), right ear

  H65.112   Acute and subacute allergic otitis media (mucoid) (sanguinous) (serous), left ear

  H65.113   Acute and subacute allergic otitis media (mucoid) (sanguinous) (serous), bilateral

  H65.114   Acute and subacute allergic otitis media (mucoid) (sanguinous) (serous), recurrent, right ear

  H65.115   Acute and subacute allergic otitis media (mucoid) (sanguinous) (serous), recurrent, left ear

  H65.116   Acute and subacute allergic otitis media (mucoid) (sanguinous) (serous), recurrent, bilateral

  H65.117   Acute and subacute allergic otitis media (mucoid) (sanguinous) (serous), recurrent, unspecified ear

  H65.119   Acute and subacute allergic otitis media (mucoid) (sanguinous) (serous), unspecified ear

  ✓6ᵗʰ H65.19   Other acute nonsuppurative otitis media

Acute and subacute mucoid otitis media
Acute and subacute nonsuppurative otitis media NOS
Acute and subacute sanguinous otitis media
Acute and subacute seromucinous otitis media

  H65.191   Other acute nonsuppurative otitis media, right ear

  H65.192   Other acute nonsuppurative otitis media, left ear

  H65.193   Other acute nonsuppurative otitis media, bilateral

  H65.194   Other acute nonsuppurative otitis media, recurrent, right ear

  H65.195   Other acute nonsuppurative otitis media, recurrent, left ear

  H65.196   Other acute nonsuppurative otitis media, recurrent, bilateral

  H65.197   Other acute nonsuppurative otitis media recurrent, unspecified ear

  H65.199   Other acute nonsuppurative otitis media, unspecified ear

  ✓5ᵗʰ H65.2   Chronic serous otitis media

Chronic tubotympanal catarrh

  H65.20   Chronic serous otitis media, unspecified ear

  H65.21   Chronic serous otitis media, right ear

  H65.22   Chronic serous otitis media, left ear

  H65.23   Chronic serous otitis media, bilateral

  ✓5ᵗʰ H65.3   Chronic mucoid otitis media

Chronic mucinous otitis media
Chronic secretory otitis media
Chronic transudative otitis media
Glue ear

  EXCLUDES 1   *adhesive middle ear disease (H74.1)*

  H65.30   Chronic mucoid otitis media, unspecified ear

  H65.31   Chronic mucoid otitis media, right ear

  H65.32   Chronic mucoid otitis media, left ear .

  H65.33   Chronic mucoid otitis media, bilateral

  ✓5ᵗʰ H65.4   Other chronic nonsuppurative otitis media

  ✓6ᵗʰ H65.41   Chronic allergic otitis media

  H65.411   Chronic allergic otitis media, right ear

  H65.412   Chronic allergic otitis media, left ear

  H65.413   Chronic allergic otitis media, bilateral

  H65.419   Chronic allergic otitis media, unspecified ear

  ✓6ᵗʰ H65.49   Other chronic nonsuppurative otitis media

Chronic exudative otitis media
Chronic nonsuppurative otitis media NOS
Chronic otitis media with effusion (nonpurulent)
Chronic seromucinous otitis media

  H65.491   Other chronic nonsuppurative otitis media, right ear

  H65.492   Other chronic nonsuppurative otitis media, left ear

  H65.493   Other chronic nonsuppurative otitis media, bilateral

  H65.499   Other chronic nonsuppurative otitis media, unspecified ear

  ✓5ᵗʰ H65.9   Unspecified nonsuppurative otitis media

Allergic otitis media NOS
Catarrhal otitis media NOS
Exudative otitis media NOS
Mucoid otitis media NOS
Otitis media with effusion (nonpurulent) NOS
Secretory otitis media NOS
Seromucinous otitis media NOS
Serous otitis media NOS
Transudative otitis media NOS

  H65.90   Unspecified nonsuppurative otitis media, unspecified ear

  H65.91   Unspecified nonsuppurative otitis media, right ear

  H65.92   Unspecified nonsuppurative otitis media, left ear

  H65.93   Unspecified nonsuppurative otitis media, bilateral

N Newborn: 0   **P** Pediatric: 0-17   **M** Maternity: 9-64   **A** Adult: 15-124   **MCC** Major Complication/Comorbidity   **CC** Complication/Comorbidity   **SW** Severe Wound Dx

634   ICD-10-CM 2021

☑4ᵗʰ **H66 Suppurative and unspecified otitis media**

     INCLUDES   suppurative and unspecified otitis media with myringitis

     Use additional code to identify:

       exposure to environmental tobacco smoke (Z77.22)

       exposure to tobacco smoke in the perinatal period (P96.81)

       history of tobacco dependence (Z87.891)

       occupational exposure to environmental tobacco smoke (Z57.31)

       tobacco dependence (F17.-)

       tobacco use (Z72.0)

     AHA: 2016,1Q,34

☑5ᵗʰ **H66.0**   **Acute suppurative otitis media**

     ☑6ᵗʰ **H66.00**   **Acute suppurative otitis media** without spontaneous rupture of ear drum

       H66.001   **Acute suppurative otitis media without spontaneous rupture of ear drum, right ear**

       H66.002   **Acute suppurative otitis media without spontaneous rupture of ear drum, left ear**

       H66.003   **Acute suppurative otitis media without spontaneous rupture of ear drum, bilateral**

       H66.004   **Acute suppurative otitis media without spontaneous rupture of ear drum, recurrent, right ear**

       H66.005   **Acute suppurative otitis media without spontaneous rupture of ear drum, recurrent, left ear**

       H66.006   **Acute suppurative otitis media without spontaneous rupture of ear drum, recurrent, bilateral**

       H66.007   **Acute suppurative otitis media without spontaneous rupture of ear drum, recurrent, unspecified ear**

       H66.009   **Acute suppurative otitis media without spontaneous rupture of ear drum, unspecified ear**

     ☑6ᵗʰ **H66.01**   **Acute suppurative otitis media** with spontaneous rupture of ear drum

       DEF: Sudden, severe inflammation of the middle ear, causing pressure that perforates the ear drum tissue.

       H66.011   **Acute suppurative otitis media with spontaneous rupture of ear drum, right ear**

       H66.012   **Acute suppurative otitis media with spontaneous rupture of ear drum, left ear**

       H66.013   **Acute suppurative otitis media with spontaneous rupture of ear drum, bilateral**

       H66.014   **Acute suppurative otitis media with spontaneous rupture of ear drum, recurrent, right ear**

       H66.015   **Acute suppurative otitis media with spontaneous rupture of ear drum, recurrent, left ear**

       H66.016   **Acute suppurative otitis media with spontaneous rupture of ear drum, recurrent, bilateral**

       H66.017   **Acute suppurative otitis media with spontaneous rupture of ear drum, recurrent, unspecified ear**

       H66.019   **Acute suppurative otitis media with spontaneous rupture of ear drum, unspecified ear**

☑5ᵗʰ **H66.1**   **Chronic tubotympanic suppurative otitis media**

     Benign chronic suppurative otitis media

     Chronic tubotympanic disease

     Use additional code for any associated perforated tympanic membrane (H72.-)

     H66.10   **Chronic tubotympanic suppurative otitis media, unspecified**

     H66.11   **Chronic tubotympanic suppurative otitis media, right ear**

     H66.12   **Chronic tubotympanic suppurative otitis media, left ear**

     H66.13   **Chronic tubotympanic suppurative otitis media, bilateral**

☑5ᵗʰ **H66.2**   **Chronic atticoantral suppurative otitis media**

     Chronic atticoantral disease

     Use additional code for any associated perforated tympanic membrane (H72.-)

     H66.20   **Chronic atticoantral suppurative otitis media, unspecified ear**

     H66.21   **Chronic atticoantral suppurative otitis media, right ear**

     H66.22   **Chronic atticoantral suppurative otitis media, left ear**

     H66.23   **Chronic atticoantral suppurative otitis media, bilateral**

☑5ᵗʰ **H66.3**   **Other chronic suppurative otitis media**

     Chronic suppurative otitis media NOS

     Use additional code for any associated perforated tympanic membrane (H72.-)

     EXCLUDES 1   tuberculous otitis media (A18.6)

     ☑6ᵗʰ **H66.3X**   **Other chronic suppurative otitis media**

       H66.3X1   **Other chronic suppurative otitis media, right ear**

       H66.3X2   **Other chronic suppurative otitis media, left ear**

       H66.3X3   **Other chronic suppurative otitis media, bilateral**

       H66.3X9   **Other chronic suppurative otitis media, unspecified ear**

☑5ᵗʰ **H66.4**   **Suppurative otitis media, unspecified**

     Purulent otitis media NOS

     Use additional code for any associated perforated tympanic membrane (H72.-)

     H66.40   **Suppurative otitis media, unspecified, unspecified ear**

     H66.41   **Suppurative otitis media, unspecified, right ear**

     H66.42   **Suppurative otitis media, unspecified, left ear**

     H66.43   **Suppurative otitis media, unspecified, bilateral**

☑5ᵗʰ **H66.9**   **Otitis media, unspecified**

     Otitis media NOS

     Acute otitis media NOS

     Chronic otitis media NOS

     Use additional code for any associated perforated tympanic membrane (H72.-)

     H66.90   **Otitis media, unspecified, unspecified ear**

     H66.91   **Otitis media, unspecified, right ear**

     H66.92   **Otitis media, unspecified, left ear**

     H66.93   **Otitis media, unspecified, bilateral**

☑4ᵗʰ **H67 Otitis media in diseases classified elsewhere**

     Code first underlying disease, such as:

       plasminogen deficiency (E88.02)

       viral disease NEC (B00-B34)

     Use additional code for any associated perforated tympanic membrane (H72.-)

     EXCLUDES 1   otitis media in:

       influenza (J09.X9, J10.83, J11.83)

       measles (B05.3)

       scarlet fever (A38.0)

       tuberculosis (A18.6)

     H67.1   *Otitis media in diseases classified elsewhere, right ear*

     H67.2   *Otitis media in diseases classified elsewhere, left ear*

     H67.3   *Otitis media in diseases classified elsewhere, bilateral*

     H67.9   *Otitis media in diseases classified elsewhere, unspecified ear*

☑4ᵗʰ **H68 Eustachian salpingitis and obstruction**

     DEF: Eustachian tube: Internal channel between the tympanic cavity and the nasopharynx that equalizes internal pressure to the outside pressure and drains mucous production from the middle ear.

     ☑5ᵗʰ **H68.0**   **Eustachian salpingitis**

       ☑6ᵗʰ **H68.00**   **Unspecified Eustachian salpingitis**

         H68.001   **Unspecified Eustachian salpingitis, right ear**

         H68.002   **Unspecified Eustachian salpingitis, left ear**

         H68.003   **Unspecified Eustachian salpingitis, bilateral**

         H68.009   **Unspecified Eustachian salpingitis, unspecified ear**

       ☑6ᵗʰ **H68.01**   **Acute Eustachian salpingitis**

         H68.011   **Acute Eustachian salpingitis, right ear**

         H68.012   **Acute Eustachian salpingitis, left ear**

         H68.013   **Acute Eustachian salpingitis, bilateral**

         H68.019   **Acute Eustachian salpingitis, unspecified ear**

       ☑6ᵗʰ **H68.02**   **Chronic Eustachian salpingitis**

         H68.021   **Chronic Eustachian salpingitis, right ear**

         H68.022   **Chronic Eustachian salpingitis, left ear**

☑ Additional Character Required   ✓x7ᵗʰ Placeholder   Unacceptable PDx   Questionable PDx   Manifestation   Unspecified Dx   H1-H14 HAC   HCC CMS-HCC Dx   HIV HIV Dx

ICD-10-CM 2021   **635**

Chapter 8. Diseases of the Ear and Mastoid Process

H68.023–H70.93

        H68.023 Chronic Eustachian salpingitis, **bilateral**
        H68.029 Chronic Eustachian salpingitis, **unspecified ear**

✓5ᵗʰ **H68.1** **Obstruction** of Eustachian tube
    Stenosis of Eustachian tube
    Stricture of Eustachian tube

  ✓6ᵗʰ **H68.10** **Unspecified obstruction of Eustachian tube**
      H68.101 **Unspecified obstruction of Eustachian tube, right ear**
      H68.102 **Unspecified obstruction of Eustachian tube, left ear**
      H68.103 **Unspecified obstruction of Eustachian tube, bilateral**
      H68.109 **Unspecified obstruction of Eustachian tube, unspecified ear**

  ✓6ᵗʰ **H68.11** **Osseous** obstruction of Eustachian tube
      H68.111 **Osseous obstruction of Eustachian tube, right ear**
      H68.112 **Osseous obstruction of Eustachian tube, left ear**
      H68.113 **Osseous obstruction of Eustachian tube, bilateral**
      H68.119 **Osseous obstruction of Eustachian tube, unspecified ear**

  ✓6ᵗʰ **H68.12** **Intrinsic cartilagenous** obstruction of Eustachian tube
      H68.121 **Intrinsic cartilagenous obstruction of Eustachian tube, right ear**
      H68.122 **Intrinsic cartilagenous obstruction of Eustachian tube, left ear**
      H68.123 **Intrinsic cartilagenous obstruction of Eustachian tube, bilateral**
      H68.129 **Intrinsic cartilagenous obstruction of Eustachian tube, unspecified ear**

  ✓6ᵗʰ **H68.13** **Extrinsic cartilagenous** obstruction of Eustachian tube
    Compression of Eustachian tube
      H68.131 **Extrinsic cartilagenous obstruction of Eustachian tube, right ear**
      H68.132 **Extrinsic cartilagenous obstruction of Eustachian tube, left ear**
      H68.133 **Extrinsic cartilagenous obstruction of Eustachian tube, bilateral**
      H68.139 **Extrinsic cartilagenous obstruction of Eustachian tube, unspecified ear**

✓4ᵗʰ **H69** **Other and unspecified disorders of Eustachian tube**
    DEF: Eustachian tube: Internal channel between the tympanic cavity and the nasopharynx that equalizes internal pressure to the outside pressure and drains mucous production from the middle ear.

  ✓5ᵗʰ **H69.0** **Patulous** Eustachian tube
      H69.00 **Patulous Eustachian tube, unspecified ear**
      H69.01 **Patulous Eustachian tube, right ear**
      H69.02 **Patulous Eustachian tube, left ear**
      H69.03 **Patulous Eustachian tube, bilateral**

  ✓5ᵗʰ **H69.8** **Other specified disorders of Eustachian tube**
      H69.80 **Other specified disorders of Eustachian tube, unspecified ear**
      H69.81 **Other specified disorders of Eustachian tube, right ear**
      H69.82 **Other specified disorders of Eustachian tube, left ear**
      H69.83 **Other specified disorders of Eustachian tube, bilateral**

  ✓5ᵗʰ **H69.9** **Unspecified Eustachian tube disorder**
      H69.90 **Unspecified Eustachian tube disorder, unspecified ear**
      H69.91 **Unspecified Eustachian tube disorder, right ear**
      H69.92 **Unspecified Eustachian tube disorder, left ear**
      H69.93 **Unspecified Eustachian tube disorder, bilateral**

✓4ᵗʰ **H70** **Mastoiditis and related conditions**

  ✓5ᵗʰ **H70.0** **Acute** mastoiditis
    Abscess of mastoid
    Empyema of mastoid

    ✓6ᵗʰ **H70.00** **Acute mastoiditis** without complications
      H70.001 **Acute mastoiditis without complications, right ear** CC
      H70.002 **Acute mastoiditis without complications, left ear** CC

      H70.003 **Acute mastoiditis without complications, bilateral** CC
      H70.009 **Acute mastoiditis without complications, unspecified ear** CC

    ✓6ᵗʰ **H70.01** **Subperiosteal abscess** of mastoid
      H70.011 **Subperiosteal abscess of mastoid, right ear**
      H70.012 **Subperiosteal abscess of mastoid, left ear** CC
      H70.013 **Subperiosteal abscess of mastoid, bilateral**
      H70.019 **Subperiosteal abscess of mastoid, unspecified ear** CC

    ✓6ᵗʰ **H70.09** **Acute mastoiditis with other complications**
      H70.091 **Acute mastoiditis with other complications, right ear** CC
      H70.092 **Acute mastoiditis with other complications, left ear** CC
      H70.093 **Acute mastoiditis with other complications, bilateral** CC
      H70.099 **Acute mastoiditis with other complications, unspecified ear** CC

  ✓5ᵗʰ **H70.1** **Chronic mastoiditis**
    Caries of mastoid
    Fistula of mastoid
    EXCLUDES 1 *tuberculous mastoiditis (A18.03)*
      H70.10 **Chronic mastoiditis, unspecified ear**
      H70.11 **Chronic mastoiditis, right ear**
      H70.12 **Chronic mastoiditis, left ear**
      H70.13 **Chronic mastoiditis, bilateral**

  ✓5ᵗʰ **H70.2** **Petrositis**
    Inflammation of petrous bone

    ✓6ᵗʰ **H70.20** **Unspecified petrositis**
      H70.201 **Unspecified petrositis, right ear**
      H70.202 **Unspecified petrositis, left ear**
      H70.203 **Unspecified petrositis, bilateral**
      H70.209 **Unspecified petrositis, unspecified ear**

    ✓6ᵗʰ **H70.21** **Acute petrositis**
    DEF: Sudden, severe inflammation of the petrous temporal bone behind the ear, associated with a middle ear infection.
      H70.211 **Acute petrositis, right ear**
      H70.212 **Acute petrositis, left ear**
      H70.213 **Acute petrositis, bilateral**
      H70.219 **Acute petrositis, unspecified ear**

    ✓6ᵗʰ **H70.22** **Chronic petrositis**
      H70.221 **Chronic petrositis, right ear**
      H70.222 **Chronic petrositis, left ear**
      H70.223 **Chronic petrositis, bilateral**
      H70.229 **Chronic petrositis, unspecified ear**

  ✓5ᵗʰ **H70.8** **Other mastoiditis and related conditions**
    EXCLUDES 1 *preauricular sinus and cyst (Q18.1)*
        sinus, fistula, and cyst of branchial cleft (Q18.0)

    ✓6ᵗʰ **H70.81** **Postauricular fistula**
      H70.811 **Postauricular fistula, right ear** SW
      H70.812 **Postauricular fistula, left ear** SW
      H70.813 **Postauricular fistula, bilateral** SW
      H70.819 **Postauricular fistula, unspecified ear** SW

    ✓6ᵗʰ **H70.89** **Other mastoiditis and related conditions**
      H70.891 **Other mastoiditis and related conditions, right ear**
      H70.892 **Other mastoiditis and related conditions, left ear**
      H70.893 **Other mastoiditis and related conditions, bilateral**
      H70.899 **Other mastoiditis and related conditions, unspecified ear**

  ✓5ᵗʰ **H70.9** **Unspecified mastoiditis**
      H70.90 **Unspecified mastoiditis, unspecified ear**
      H70.91 **Unspecified mastoiditis, right ear**
      H70.92 **Unspecified mastoiditis, left ear**
      H70.93 **Unspecified mastoiditis, bilateral**

N Newborn: 0   P Pediatric: 0-17   M Maternity: 9-64   A Adult: 15-124   MCC Major Complication/Comorbidity   CC Complication/Comorbidity   SW Severe Wound Dx

636   ICD-10-CM 2021

☑️4ᵗʰ **H71 Cholesteatoma of middle ear**

> **EXCLUDES 2**   cholesteatoma of external ear (H60.4-)
> recurrent cholesteatoma of postmastoidectomy cavity
> (H95.0-)
>
> **DEF:** Cholesteatoma: Noncancerous cyst-like mass of cell debris, including cholesterol and epithelial cells resulting from trauma, repeated or improperly healed infections, and congenital enclosure of epidermal cells.

Cholesteatoma of Middle Ear

Middle ear chamber

Ear drum

Cholesteatoma sac

☑️5ᵗʰ **H71.0 Cholesteatoma of attic**

    H71.00 Cholesteatoma of attic, unspecified ear
    H71.01 Cholesteatoma of attic, right ear
    H71.02 Cholesteatoma of attic, left ear
    H71.03 Cholesteatoma of attic, bilateral

☑️5ᵗʰ **H71.1 Cholesteatoma of tympanum**

    H71.10 Cholesteatoma of tympanum, unspecified ear
    H71.11 Cholesteatoma of tympanum, right ear
    H71.12 Cholesteatoma of tympanum, left ear
    H71.13 Cholesteatoma of tympanum, bilateral

☑️5ᵗʰ **H71.2 Cholesteatoma of mastoid**

    H71.20 Cholesteatoma of mastoid, unspecified ear
    H71.21 Cholesteatoma of mastoid, right ear
    H71.22 Cholesteatoma of mastoid, left ear
    H71.23 Cholesteatoma of mastoid, bilateral

☑️5ᵗʰ **H71.3 Diffuse cholesteatosis**

    H71.30 Diffuse cholesteatosis, unspecified ear
    H71.31 Diffuse cholesteatosis, right ear
    H71.32 Diffuse cholesteatosis, left ear
    H71.33 Diffuse cholesteatosis, bilateral

☑️5ᵗʰ **H71.9 Unspecified cholesteatoma**

    H71.90 Unspecified cholesteatoma, unspecified ear
    H71.91 Unspecified cholesteatoma, right ear
    H71.92 Unspecified cholesteatoma, left ear
    H71.93 Unspecified cholesteatoma, bilateral

☑️4ᵗʰ **H72 Perforation of tympanic membrane**

> **INCLUDES**   persistent post-traumatic perforation of ear drum
> postinflammatory perforation of ear drum
>
> Code first any associated otitis media (H65.-, H66.1-, H66.2-, H66.3-, H66.4-, H66.9-, H67.-)
>
> **EXCLUDES 1**   acute suppurative otitis media with rupture of the tympanic membrane (H66.01-)
> traumatic rupture of ear drum (S09.2-)

☑️5ᵗʰ **H72.0 Central perforation of tympanic membrane**

    H72.00 Central perforation of tympanic membrane, unspecified ear
    H72.01 Central perforation of tympanic membrane, right ear
    H72.02 Central perforation of tympanic membrane, left ear
    H72.03 Central perforation of tympanic membrane, bilateral

☑️5ᵗʰ **H72.1 Attic perforation of tympanic membrane**

    Perforation of pars flaccida
    H72.10 Attic perforation of tympanic membrane, unspecified ear
    H72.11 Attic perforation of tympanic membrane, right ear
    H72.12 Attic perforation of tympanic membrane, left ear

    H72.13 Attic perforation of tympanic membrane, bilateral

☑️5ᵗʰ **H72.2 Other marginal perforations of tympanic membrane**

   ☑️6ᵗʰ **H72.2X** Other marginal perforations of tympanic membrane

     H72.2X1 Other marginal perforations of tympanic membrane, right ear
     H72.2X2 Other marginal perforations of tympanic membrane, left ear
     H72.2X3 Other marginal perforations of tympanic membrane, bilateral
     H72.2X9 Other marginal perforations of tympanic membrane, unspecified ear

☑️5ᵗʰ **H72.8 Other perforations of tympanic membrane**

   ☑️6ᵗʰ **H72.81** Multiple perforations of tympanic membrane

     H72.811 Multiple perforations of tympanic membrane, right ear
     H72.812 Multiple perforations of tympanic membrane, left ear
     H72.813 Multiple perforations of tympanic membrane, bilateral
     H72.819 Multiple perforations of tympanic membrane, unspecified ear

   ☑️6ᵗʰ **H72.82** Total perforations of tympanic membrane

     H72.821 Total perforations of tympanic membrane, right ear
     H72.822 Total perforations of tympanic membrane, left ear
     H72.823 Total perforations of tympanic membrane, bilateral
     H72.829 Total perforations of tympanic membrane, unspecified ear

☑️5ᵗʰ **H72.9 Unspecified perforation of tympanic membrane**

    H72.90 Unspecified perforation of tympanic membrane, unspecified ear
    H72.91 Unspecified perforation of tympanic membrane, right ear
    H72.92 Unspecified perforation of tympanic membrane, left ear
    H72.93 Unspecified perforation of tympanic membrane, bilateral

☑️4ᵗʰ **H73 Other disorders of tympanic membrane**

☑️5ᵗʰ **H73.0 Acute myringitis**

> **EXCLUDES 1**   acute myringitis with otitis media (H65, H66)

   ☑️6ᵗʰ **H73.00** Unspecified acute myringitis

     Acute tympanitis NOS
     H73.001 Acute myringitis, right ear
     H73.002 Acute myringitis, left ear
     H73.003 Acute myringitis, bilateral
     H73.009 Acute myringitis, unspecified ear

   ☑️6ᵗʰ **H73.01** Bullous myringitis

     DEF: Bacterial or viral otitis media that is characterized by the appearance of serous or hemorrhagic blebs on the ear drum and sudden onset of severe pain in ear.
     H73.011 Bullous myringitis, right ear
     H73.012 Bullous myringitis, left ear
     H73.013 Bullous myringitis, bilateral
     H73.019 Bullous myringitis, unspecified ear

   ☑️6ᵗʰ **H73.09** Other acute myringitis

     H73.091 Other acute myringitis, right ear
     H73.092 Other acute myringitis, left ear
     H73.093 Other acute myringitis, bilateral
     H73.099 Other acute myringitis, unspecified ear

☑️5ᵗʰ **H73.1 Chronic myringitis**

    Chronic tympanitis

> **EXCLUDES 1**   chronic myringitis with otitis media (H65, H66)

    H73.10 Chronic myringitis, unspecified ear
    H73.11 Chronic myringitis, right ear
    H73.12 Chronic myringitis, left ear
    H73.13 Chronic myringitis, bilateral

☑️5ᵗʰ **H73.2 Unspecified myringitis**

    H73.20 Unspecified myringitis, unspecified ear
    H73.21 Unspecified myringitis, right ear
    H73.22 Unspecified myringitis, left ear
    H73.23 Unspecified myringitis, bilateral

☑️5ᵗʰ **H73.8 Other specified disorders of tympanic membrane**

   ☑️6ᵗʰ **H73.81** Atrophic flaccid tympanic membrane

     H73.811 Atrophic flaccid tympanic membrane, right ear

☑️ Additional Character Required   ☑️x7ᵗʰ Placeholder   Unacceptable PDx   Questionable PDx   Manifestation   Unspecified Dx   H1–H14 HAC   HCC CMS-HCC Dx   HIV HIV Dx

ICD-10-CM 2021   **637**

H73.812 Atrophic flaccid tympanic membrane, left ear

H73.813 Atrophic flaccid tympanic membrane, bilateral

H73.819 Atrophic flaccid tympanic membrane, unspecified ear

✓6ᵗʰ **H73.82** Atrophic nonflaccid tympanic membrane

H73.821 Atrophic nonflaccid tympanic membrane, right ear

H73.822 Atrophic nonflaccid tympanic membrane, left ear

H73.823 Atrophic nonflaccid tympanic membrane, bilateral

H73.829 Atrophic nonflaccid tympanic membrane, unspecified ear

✓6ᵗʰ **H73.89** Other specified disorders of tympanic membrane

H73.891 Other specified disorders of tympanic membrane, right ear

H73.892 Other specified disorders of tympanic membrane, left ear

H73.893 Other specified disorders of tympanic membrane, bilateral

H73.899 Other specified disorders of tympanic membrane, unspecified ear

✓5ᵗʰ **H73.9** Unspecified disorder of tympanic membrane

H73.90 Unspecified disorder of tympanic membrane, unspecified ear

H73.91 Unspecified disorder of tympanic membrane, right ear

H73.92 Unspecified disorder of tympanic membrane, left ear

H73.93 Unspecified disorder of tympanic membrane, bilateral

✓4ᵗʰ **H74** Other disorders of middle ear mastoid

EXCLUDES 2   mastoiditis (H70.-)

✓5ᵗʰ **H74.0** Tympanosclerosis

DEF: Calcification of tissue in the ear drum, middle ear bones, and middle ear canal.

H74.01 Tympanosclerosis, right ear

H74.02 Tympanosclerosis, left ear

H74.03 Tympanosclerosis, bilateral

H74.09 Tympanosclerosis, unspecified ear

✓5ᵗʰ **H74.1** Adhesive middle ear disease

Adhesive otitis

EXCLUDES 1   glue ear (H65.3-)

H74.11 Adhesive right middle ear disease

H74.12 Adhesive left middle ear disease

H74.13 Adhesive middle ear disease, bilateral

H74.19 Adhesive middle ear disease, unspecified ear

✓5ᵗʰ **H74.2** Discontinuity and dislocation of ear ossicles

H74.20 Discontinuity and dislocation of ear ossicles, unspecified ear

H74.21 Discontinuity and dislocation of right ear ossicles

H74.22 Discontinuity and dislocation of left ear ossicles

H74.23 Discontinuity and dislocation of ear ossicles, bilateral

✓5ᵗʰ **H74.3** Other acquired abnormalities of ear ossicles

✓6ᵗʰ **H74.31** Ankylosis of ear ossicles

H74.311 Ankylosis of ear ossicles, right ear

H74.312 Ankylosis of ear ossicles, left ear

H74.313 Ankylosis of ear ossicles, bilateral

H74.319 Ankylosis of ear ossicles, unspecified ear

✓6ᵗʰ **H74.32** Partial loss of ear ossicles

H74.321 Partial loss of ear ossicles, right ear

H74.322 Partial loss of ear ossicles, left ear

H74.323 Partial loss of ear ossicles, bilateral

H74.329 Partial loss of ear ossicles, unspecified ear

✓6ᵗʰ **H74.39** Other acquired abnormalities of ear ossicles

H74.391 Other acquired abnormalities of right ear ossicles

H74.392 Other acquired abnormalities of left ear ossicles

H74.393 Other acquired abnormalities of ear ossicles, bilateral

H74.399 Other acquired abnormalities of ear ossicles, unspecified ear

✓5ᵗʰ **H74.4** Polyp of middle ear

H74.40 Polyp of middle ear, unspecified ear

H74.41 Polyp of right middle ear

H74.42 Polyp of left middle ear

H74.43 Polyp of middle ear, bilateral

✓5ᵗʰ **H74.8** Other specified disorders of middle ear and mastoid

✓6ᵗʰ **H74.8X** Other specified disorders of middle ear and mastoid

H74.8X1 Other specified disorders of right middle ear and mastoid

H74.8X2 Other specified disorders of left middle ear and mastoid

H74.8X3 Other specified disorders of middle ear and mastoid, bilateral

H74.8X9 Other specified disorders of middle ear and mastoid, unspecified ear

✓5ᵗʰ **H74.9** Unspecified disorder of middle ear and mastoid

H74.90 Unspecified disorder of middle ear and mastoid, unspecified ear

H74.91 Unspecified disorder of right middle ear and mastoid

H74.92 Unspecified disorder of left middle ear and mastoid

H74.93 Unspecified disorder of middle ear and mastoid, bilateral

✓4ᵗʰ **H75** Other disorders of middle ear and mastoid in diseases classified elsewhere

Code first underlying disease

✓5ᵗʰ **H75.0** Mastoiditis in infectious and parasitic diseases classified elsewhere

EXCLUDES 1   mastoiditis (in):
syphilis (A52.77)
tuberculosis (A18.03)

H75.00 *Mastoiditis in infectious and parasitic diseases classified elsewhere, unspecified ear*

H75.01 *Mastoiditis in infectious and parasitic diseases classified elsewhere, right ear*

H75.02 *Mastoiditis in infectious and parasitic diseases classified elsewhere, left ear*

H75.03 *Mastoiditis in infectious and parasitic diseases classified elsewhere, bilateral*

✓5ᵗʰ **H75.8** Other specified disorders of middle ear and mastoid in diseases classified elsewhere

H75.80 *Other specified disorders of middle ear and mastoid in diseases classified elsewhere, unspecified ear*

H75.81 *Other specified disorders of right middle ear and mastoid in diseases classified elsewhere*

H75.82 *Other specified disorders of left middle ear and mastoid in diseases classified elsewhere*

H75.83 *Other specified disorders of middle ear and mastoid in diseases classified elsewhere, bilateral*

Diseases of inner ear (H80-H83)

✓4ᵗʰ **H80** Otosclerosis

INCLUDES   otospongiosis

✓5ᵗʰ **H80.0** Otosclerosis involving oval window, nonobliterative

H80.00 Otosclerosis involving oval window, nonobliterative, unspecified ear

H80.01 Otosclerosis involving oval window, nonobliterative, right ear

H80.02 Otosclerosis involving oval window, nonobliterative, left ear

H80.03 Otosclerosis involving oval window, nonobliterative, bilateral

✓5ᵗʰ **H80.1** Otosclerosis involving oval window, obliterative

H80.10 Otosclerosis involving oval window, obliterative, unspecified ear

H80.11 Otosclerosis involving oval window, obliterative, right ear

H80.12 Otosclerosis involving oval window, obliterative, left ear

H80.13 Otosclerosis involving oval window, obliterative, bilateral

✓5ᵗʰ **H80.2** Cochlear otosclerosis

Otosclerosis involving otic capsule
Otosclerosis involving round window

H80.20 Cochlear otosclerosis, unspecified ear

H80.21 Cochlear otosclerosis, right ear

H80.22 Cochlear otosclerosis, left ear

H80.23 Cochlear otosclerosis, bilateral

N Newborn: 0   P Pediatric: 0-17   M Maternity: 9-64   A Adult: 15-124   MCC Major Complication/Comorbidity   CC Complication/Comorbidity   SW Severe Wound Dx

638   ICD-10-CM 2021

✓5ᵗʰ **H80.8 Other otosclerosis**

     H80.80 Other otosclerosis, unspecified ear
     H80.81 Other otosclerosis, right ear
     H80.82 Other otosclerosis, left ear
     H80.83 Other otosclerosis, bilateral

✓5ᵗʰ **H80.9 Unspecified otosclerosis**

     H80.90 Unspecified otosclerosis, unspecified ear
     H80.91 Unspecified otosclerosis, right ear
     H80.92 Unspecified otosclerosis, left ear
     H80.93 Unspecified otosclerosis, bilateral

✓4ᵗʰ **H81 Disorders of vestibular function**

     EXCLUDES 1   epidemic vertigo (A88.1)
                 vertigo NOS (R42)

✓5ᵗʰ **H81.0 Ménière's disease**

     Labyrinthine hydrops
     Ménière's syndrome or vertigo
     DEF: Distended membranous labyrinth of the middle ear from fluctuating pressure of fluid (hydrops) that causes vertigo, tinnitus, pressure, and hearing loss that may last on and off for several hours. Episodes may occur in clusters or may subside for weeks, months, or even years.

     H81.01 Ménière's disease, right ear
     H81.02 Ménière's disease, left ear
     H81.03 Ménière's disease, bilateral
     H81.09 Ménière's disease, unspecified ear

✓5ᵗʰ **H81.1 Benign paroxysmal vertigo**

     H81.10 Benign paroxysmal vertigo, unspecified ear
     H81.11 Benign paroxysmal vertigo, right ear
     H81.12 Benign paroxysmal vertigo, left ear
     H81.13 Benign paroxysmal vertigo, bilateral

✓5ᵗʰ **H81.2 Vestibular neuronitis**

     DEF: Transient benign vertigo caused by inflammation of the vestibular nerve. It is characterized by response to caloric stimulation on one side and nystagmus with rhythmic movement of the eyes. Normal auditory function is present.

     H81.20 Vestibular neuronitis, unspecified ear
     H81.21 Vestibular neuronitis, right ear
     H81.22 Vestibular neuronitis, left ear
     H81.23 Vestibular neuronitis, bilateral

✓5ᵗʰ **H81.3 Other peripheral vertigo**

     ✓6ᵗʰ **H81.31 Aural vertigo**

         H81.311 Aural vertigo, right ear
         H81.312 Aural vertigo, left ear
         H81.313 Aural vertigo, bilateral
         H81.319 Aural vertigo, unspecified ear

     ✓6ᵗʰ **H81.39 Other peripheral vertigo**

         Lermoyez' syndrome
         Otogenic vertigo
         Peripheral vertigo NOS
         H81.391 Other peripheral vertigo, right ear
         H81.392 Other peripheral vertigo, left ear
         H81.393 Other peripheral vertigo, bilateral
         H81.399 Other peripheral vertigo, unspecified ear

H81.4 Vertigo of central origin

     Central positional nystagmus
     H81.41 Vertigo of central origin, right ear
     H81.42 Vertigo of central origin, left ear
     H81.43 Vertigo of central origin, bilateral
     H81.49 Vertigo of central origin, unspecified ear

✓5ᵗʰ **H81.8 Other disorders of vestibular function**

     ✓6ᵗʰ **H81.8X Other disorders of vestibular function**

         H81.8X1 Other disorders of vestibular function, right ear
         H81.8X2 Other disorders of vestibular function, left ear
         H81.8X3 Other disorders of vestibular function, bilateral
         H81.8X9 Other disorders of vestibular function, unspecified ear

✓5ᵗʰ **H81.9 Unspecified disorder of vestibular function**

     Vertiginous syndrome NOS
     H81.90 Unspecified disorder of vestibular function, unspecified ear
     H81.91 Unspecified disorder of vestibular function, right ear
     H81.92 Unspecified disorder of vestibular function, left ear

     H81.93 Unspecified disorder of vestibular function, bilateral

✓4ᵗʰ **H82 Vertiginous syndromes in diseases classified elsewhere**

     Code first underlying disease
     EXCLUDES 1   epidemic vertigo (A88.1)

     H82.1 Vertiginous syndromes in diseases classified elsewhere, right ear
     H82.2 Vertiginous syndromes in diseases classified elsewhere, left ear
     H82.3 Vertiginous syndromes in diseases classified elsewhere, bilateral
     H82.9 Vertiginous syndromes in diseases classified elsewhere, unspecified ear

✓4ᵗʰ **H83 Other diseases of inner ear**

     ✓5ᵗʰ **H83.0 Labyrinthitis**

         DEF: Inflammation of the inner ear, or labyrinth, characterized by pus, vertigo, dizziness, nausea, and hearing loss.
         H83.01 Labyrinthitis, right ear
         H83.02 Labyrinthitis, left ear
         H83.03 Labyrinthitis, bilateral
         H83.09 Labyrinthitis, unspecified ear

     ✓5ᵗʰ **H83.1 Labyrinthine fistula**

         H83.11 Labyrinthine fistula, right ear
         H83.12 Labyrinthine fistula, left ear   SW
         H83.13 Labyrinthine fistula, bilateral   SW
         H83.19 Labyrinthine fistula, unspecified ear   SW

     ✓5ᵗʰ **H83.2 Labyrinthine dysfunction**

         Labyrinthine hypersensitivity
         Labyrinthine hypofunction
         Labyrinthine loss of function
         DEF: Decreased function of the labyrinth sensors.

         ✓6ᵗʰ **H83.2X Labyrinthine dysfunction**

             H83.2X1 Labyrinthine dysfunction, right ear
             H83.2X2 Labyrinthine dysfunction, left ear
             H83.2X3 Labyrinthine dysfunction, bilateral
             H83.2X9 Labyrinthine dysfunction, unspecified ear

     ✓5ᵗʰ **H83.3 Noise effects on inner ear**

         Acoustic trauma of inner ear
         Noise-induced hearing loss of inner ear

         ✓6ᵗʰ **H83.3X Noise effects on inner ear**

             H83.3X1 Noise effects on right inner ear
             H83.3X2 Noise effects on left inner ear
             H83.3X3 Noise effects on inner ear, bilateral
             H83.3X9 Noise effects on inner ear, unspecified ear

     ✓5ᵗʰ **H83.8 Other specified diseases of inner ear**

         ✓6ᵗʰ **H83.8X Other specified diseases of inner ear**

             H83.8X1 Other specified diseases of right inner ear
             H83.8X2 Other specified diseases of left inner ear
             H83.8X3 Other specified diseases of inner ear, bilateral
             H83.8X9 Other specified diseases of inner ear, unspecified ear

     ✓5ᵗʰ **H83.9 Unspecified disease of inner ear**

         H83.90 Unspecified disease of inner ear, unspecified ear
         H83.91 Unspecified disease of right inner ear
         H83.92 Unspecified disease of left inner ear
         H83.93 Unspecified disease of inner ear, bilateral

Other disorders of ear (H90-H94)

✓4ᵗʰ **H90 Conductive and sensorineural hearing loss**

     EXCLUDES 1   *deaf nonspeaking NEC (H91.3)*
                  deafness NOS (H91.9-)
                  hearing loss NOS (H91.9-)
                  noise-induced hearing loss (H83.3-)
                  ototoxic hearing loss (H91.0-)
                  sudden (idiopathic) hearing loss (H91.2-)

     AHA: 2015,2Q,7
     DEF: Conductive hearing loss: Hearing Loss due to the inability of sound waves to move from the outer (external ear) to the inner ear.
     DEF: Sensorineural hearing loss: Hearing loss that occurs from damage to the hair cells of the inner ear or problems with the nerve pathways from the inner ear to the brain.

     H90.0 Conductive hearing loss, bilateral

✓ Additional Character Required   ✓x7ᵗʰ Placeholder   Unacceptable PDx   Questionable PDx   Manifestation   Unspecified Dx   H1-H14 HAC   HCC CMS-HCC Dx   HIV HIV Dx

ICD-10-CM 2021   639

✓5ᵗʰ **H90.1** Conductive hearing loss, unilateral with unrestricted hearing on the contralateral side
 H90.11 Conductive hearing loss, unilateral, right ear, with unrestricted hearing on the contralateral side
 H90.12 Conductive hearing loss, unilateral, left ear, with unrestricted hearing on the contralateral side

H90.2 Conductive hearing loss, unspecified
 Conductive deafness NOS

H90.3 Sensorineural hearing loss, bilateral

✓5ᵗʰ **H90.4** Sensorineural hearing loss, unilateral with unrestricted hearing on the contralateral side
 H90.41 Sensorineural hearing loss, unilateral, right ear, with unrestricted hearing on the contralateral side
 H90.42 Sensorineural hearing loss, unilateral, left ear, with unrestricted hearing on the contralateral side

H90.5 Unspecified sensorineural hearing loss
 Central hearing loss NOS
 Congenital deafness NOS
 Neural hearing loss NOS
 Perceptive hearing loss NOS
 Sensorineural deafness NOS
 Sensory hearing loss NOS
 EXCLUDES 1 *abnormal auditory perception (H93.2-)*
    psychogenic deafness (F44.6)

H90.6 Mixed conductive and sensorineural hearing loss, bilateral
 AHA: 2015,2Q,7

✓5ᵗʰ **H90.7** Mixed conductive and sensorineural hearing loss, unilateral with unrestricted hearing on the contralateral side
 H90.71 Mixed conductive and sensorineural hearing loss, unilateral, right ear, with unrestricted hearing on the contralateral side
 H90.72 Mixed conductive and sensorineural hearing loss, unilateral, left ear, with unrestricted hearing on the contralateral side

H90.8 Mixed conductive and sensorineural hearing loss, unspecified

✓5ᵗʰ **H90.A** Conductive and sensorineural hearing loss with restricted hearing on the contralateral side
 AHA: 2016,4Q,23-25
 ✓6ᵗʰ **H90.A1** Conductive hearing loss, unilateral, with restricted hearing on the contralateral side
  H90.A11 Conductive hearing loss, unilateral, right ear with restricted hearing on the contralateral side
  H90.A12 Conductive hearing loss, unilateral, left ear with restricted hearing on the contralateral side
 ✓6ᵗʰ **H90.A2** Sensorineural hearing loss, unilateral, with restricted hearing on the contralateral side
  H90.A21 Sensorineural hearing loss, unilateral, right ear, with restricted hearing on the contralateral side
  H90.A22 Sensorineural hearing loss, unilateral, left ear, with restricted hearing on the contralateral side
 ✓6ᵗʰ **H90.A3** Mixed conductive and sensorineural hearing loss, unilateral with restricted hearing on the contralateral side
  H90.A31 Mixed conductive and sensorineural hearing loss, unilateral, right ear with restricted hearing on the contralateral side
  H90.A32 Mixed conductive and sensorineural hearing, unilateral, left ear with restricted hearing on the contralateral side

✓4ᵗʰ **H91** Other and unspecified hearing loss
 EXCLUDES 1 *abnormal auditory perception (H93.2-)*
    hearing loss as classified in H90.-
    impacted cerumen (H61.2-)
    noise-induced hearing loss (H83.3-)
    psychogenic deafness (F44.6)
    transient ischemic deafness (H93.01-)

✓5ᵗʰ **H91.0** Ototoxic hearing loss
 Code first poisoning due to drug or toxin, if applicable (T36-T65 with fifth or sixth character 1-4 or 6)
 Use additional code for adverse effect, if applicable, to identify drug (T36-T50 with fifth or sixth character 5)
 H91.01 Ototoxic hearing loss, right ear
 H91.02 Ototoxic hearing loss, left ear
 H91.03 Ototoxic hearing loss, bilateral
 H91.09 Ototoxic hearing loss, unspecified ear

✓5ᵗʰ **H91.1** Presbycusis
 Presbyacusia
 H91.10 Presbycusis, unspecified ear
 H91.11 Presbycusis, right ear
 H91.12 Presbycusis, left ear
 H91.13 Presbycusis, bilateral

✓5ᵗʰ **H91.2** Sudden idiopathic hearing loss
 Sudden hearing loss NOS
 H91.20 Sudden idiopathic hearing loss, unspecified ear
 H91.21 Sudden idiopathic hearing loss, right ear
 H91.22 Sudden idiopathic hearing loss, left ear
 H91.23 Sudden idiopathic hearing loss, bilateral

H91.3 Deaf nonspeaking, not elsewhere classified

✓5ᵗʰ **H91.8** Other specified hearing loss
 ✓6ᵗʰ **H91.8X** Other specified hearing loss
  H91.8X1 Other specified hearing loss, right ear
  H91.8X2 Other specified hearing loss, left ear
  H91.8X3 Other specified hearing loss, bilateral
  H91.8X9 Other specified hearing loss, unspecified ear

✓5ᵗʰ **H91.9** Unspecified hearing loss
 Deafness NOS
 High frequency deafness
 Low frequency deafness
 H91.90 Unspecified hearing loss, unspecified ear
 H91.91 Unspecified hearing loss, right ear
 H91.92 Unspecified hearing loss, left ear
 H91.93 Unspecified hearing loss, bilateral

✓4ᵗʰ **H92** Otalgia and effusion of ear

✓5ᵗʰ **H92.0** Otalgia
 H92.01 Otalgia, right ear
 H92.02 Otalgia, left ear
 H92.03 Otalgia, bilateral
 H92.09 Otalgia, unspecified ear

✓5ᵗʰ **H92.1** Otorrhea
 EXCLUDES 1 *leakage of cerebrospinal fluid through ear (G96.0)*
 H92.10 Otorrhea, unspecified ear
 H92.11 Otorrhea, right ear
 H92.12 Otorrhea, left ear
 H92.13 Otorrhea, bilateral

✓5ᵗʰ **H92.2** Otorrhagia
 EXCLUDES 1 *traumatic otorrhagia — code to injury*
 H92.20 Otorrhagia, unspecified ear
 H92.21 Otorrhagia, right ear
 H92.22 Otorrhagia, left ear
 H92.23 Otorrhagia, bilateral

✓4ᵗʰ **H93** Other disorders of ear, not elsewhere classified

✓5ᵗʰ **H93.0** Degenerative and vascular disorders of ear
 EXCLUDES 1 *presbycusis (H91.1)*
 ✓6ᵗʰ **H93.01** Transient ischemic deafness
  H93.011 Transient ischemic deafness, right ear
  H93.012 Transient ischemic deafness, left ear
  H93.013 Transient ischemic deafness, bilateral
  H93.019 Transient ischemic deafness, unspecified ear
 ✓6ᵗʰ **H93.09** Unspecified degenerative and vascular disorders of ear
  H93.091 Unspecified degenerative and vascular disorders of right ear
  H93.092 Unspecified degenerative and vascular disorders of left ear
  H93.093 Unspecified degenerative and vascular disorders of ear, bilateral
  H93.099 Unspecified degenerative and vascular disorders of unspecified ear

✓5ᵗʰ **H93.1** Tinnitus
 H93.11 Tinnitus, right ear
 H93.12 Tinnitus, left ear
 H93.13 Tinnitus, bilateral
 H93.19 Tinnitus, unspecified ear

✓5ᵗʰ **H93.A** Pulsatile tinnitus
 AHA: 2016,4Q,25-26
 H93.A1 Pulsatile tinnitus, right ear
 H93.A2 Pulsatile tinnitus, left ear
 H93.A3 Pulsatile tinnitus, bilateral

H93.A9   **Pulsatile tinnitus, unspecified ear**

√5ᵗʰ **H93.2**   **Other abnormal auditory perceptions**
    EXCLUDES 2   *auditory hallucinations (R44.0)*

   √6ᵗʰ **H93.21**   **Auditory recruitment**
      H93.211   **Auditory recruitment, right ear**
      H93.212   **Auditory recruitment, left ear**
      H93.213   **Auditory recruitment, bilateral**
      H93.219   **Auditory recruitment, unspecified ear**

   √6ᵗʰ **H93.22**   **Diplacusis**
      H93.221   **Diplacusis, right ear**
      H93.222   **Diplacusis, left ear**
      H93.223   **Diplacusis, bilateral**
      H93.229   **Diplacusis, unspecified ear**

   √6ᵗʰ **H93.23**   **Hyperacusis**
      DEF: Exceptionally acute sense of hearing caused by such conditions as Bell's palsy. This term may also refer to painful sensitivity to sounds.
      H93.231   **Hyperacusis, right ear**
      H93.232   **Hyperacusis, left ear**
      H93.233   **Hyperacusis, bilateral**
      H93.239   **Hyperacusis, unspecified ear**

   √6ᵗʰ **H93.24**   **Temporary auditory threshold shift**
      H93.241   **Temporary auditory threshold shift, right ear**
      H93.242   **Temporary auditory threshold shift, left ear**
      H93.243   **Temporary auditory threshold shift, bilateral**
      H93.249   **Temporary auditory threshold shift, unspecified ear**

   H93.25   **Central auditory processing disorder**
      Congenital auditory imperception
      Word deafness
      EXCLUDES 1   *mixed receptive-expressive language disorder (F80.2)*

   √6ᵗʰ **H93.29**   **Other abnormal auditory perceptions**
      H93.291   **Other abnormal auditory perceptions, right ear**
      H93.292   **Other abnormal auditory perceptions, left ear**
      H93.293   **Other abnormal auditory perceptions, bilateral**
      H93.299   **Other abnormal auditory perceptions, unspecified ear**

√5ᵗʰ **H93.3**   **Disorders of acoustic nerve**
    Disorder of 8th cranial nerve
    EXCLUDES 1   *acoustic neuroma (D33.3)*
               syphilitic acoustic neuritis (A52.15)

   √6ᵗʰ **H93.3X**   **Disorders of acoustic nerve**
      H93.3X1   **Disorders of right acoustic nerve**
      H93.3X2   **Disorders of left acoustic nerve**
      H93.3X3   **Disorders of bilateral acoustic nerves**
      H93.3X9   **Disorders of unspecified acoustic nerve**

√5ᵗʰ **H93.8**   **Other specified disorders of ear**

   √6ᵗʰ **H93.8X**   **Other specified disorders of ear**
      H93.8X1   **Other specified disorders of right ear**
      H93.8X2   **Other specified disorders of left ear**
      H93.8X3   **Other specified disorders of ear, bilateral**
      H93.8X9   **Other specified disorders of ear, unspecified ear**

√5ᵗʰ **H93.9**   **Unspecified disorder of ear**
      H93.90   **Unspecified disorder of ear, unspecified ear**
      H93.91   **Unspecified disorder of right ear**
      H93.92   **Unspecified disorder of left ear**
      H93.93   **Unspecified disorder of ear, bilateral**

√4ᵗʰ **H94**   **Other disorders of ear in diseases classified elsewhere**

   √5ᵗʰ **H94.0**   **Acoustic neuritis in infectious and parasitic diseases classified elsewhere**
      Code first underlying disease, such as:
      parasitic disease (B65-B89)
      EXCLUDES 1   *acoustic neuritis (in):*
               herpes zoster (B02.29)
               syphilis (A52.15)

      H94.00   *Acoustic neuritis in infectious and parasitic diseases classified elsewhere, unspecified ear*
      H94.01   *Acoustic neuritis in infectious and parasitic diseases classified elsewhere, right ear*

      H94.02   *Acoustic neuritis in infectious and parasitic diseases classified elsewhere, left ear*
      H94.03   *Acoustic neuritis in infectious and parasitic diseases classified elsewhere, bilateral*

   √5ᵗʰ **H94.8**   **Other specified disorders of ear in diseases classified elsewhere**
      Code first underlying disease, such as:
      congenital syphilis (A50.0)
      EXCLUDES 1   *aural myiasis (B87.4)*
               syphilitic labyrinthitis (A52.79)

      H94.80   *Other specified disorders of ear in diseases classified elsewhere, unspecified ear*
      H94.81   *Other specified disorders of right ear in diseases classified elsewhere*
      H94.82   *Other specified disorders of left ear in diseases classified elsewhere*
      H94.83   *Other specified disorders of ear in diseases classified elsewhere, bilateral*

Intraoperative and postprocedural complications and disorders of ear and mastoid process, not elsewhere classified (H95)

√4ᵗʰ **H95**   **Intraoperative and postprocedural complications and disorders of ear and mastoid process, not elsewhere classified**
    AHA: 2016,4Q,9-10

   √5ᵗʰ **H95.0**   **Recurrent cholesteatoma of postmastoidectomy cavity**
      H95.00   **Recurrent cholesteatoma of postmastoidectomy cavity, unspecified ear**
      H95.01   **Recurrent cholesteatoma of postmastoidectomy cavity, right ear**
      H95.02   **Recurrent cholesteatoma of postmastoidectomy cavity, left ear**
      H95.03   **Recurrent cholesteatoma of postmastoidectomy cavity, bilateral ears**

   √5ᵗʰ **H95.1**   **Other disorders of ear and mastoid process following mastoidectomy**

    √6ᵗʰ **H95.11**   **Chronic inflammation of postmastoidectomy cavity**
      H95.111   **Chronic inflammation of postmastoidectomy cavity, right ear**
      H95.112   **Chronic inflammation of postmastoidectomy cavity, left ear**
      H95.113   **Chronic inflammation of postmastoidectomy cavity, bilateral ears**
      H95.119   **Chronic inflammation of postmastoidectomy cavity, unspecified ear**

    √6ᵗʰ **H95.12**   **Granulation of postmastoidectomy cavity**
      H95.121   **Granulation of postmastoidectomy cavity, right ear**
      H95.122   **Granulation of postmastoidectomy cavity, left ear**
      H95.123   **Granulation of postmastoidectomy cavity, bilateral ears**
      H95.129   **Granulation of postmastoidectomy cavity, unspecified ear**

    √6ᵗʰ **H95.13**   **Mucosal cyst of postmastoidectomy cavity**
      H95.131   **Mucosal cyst of postmastoidectomy cavity, right ear**
      H95.132   **Mucosal cyst of postmastoidectomy cavity, left ear**
      H95.133   **Mucosal cyst of postmastoidectomy cavity, bilateral ears**
      H95.139   **Mucosal cyst of postmastoidectomy cavity, unspecified ear**

    √6ᵗʰ **H95.19**   **Other disorders following mastoidectomy**
      H95.191   **Other disorders following mastoidectomy, right ear**
      H95.192   **Other disorders following mastoidectomy, left ear**
      H95.193   **Other disorders following mastoidectomy, bilateral ears**
      H95.199   **Other disorders following mastoidectomy, unspecified ear**

Chapter 8. Diseases of the Ear and Mastoid Process

√5ᵗʰ **H95.2 Intraoperative hemorrhage and hematoma of ear and mastoid process complicating a procedure**

     EXCLUDES 1   *intraoperative hemorrhage and hematoma of ear and mastoid process due to accidental puncture or laceration during a procedure (H95.3-)*

     H95.21 Intraoperative hemorrhage and hematoma of ear and mastoid process complicating a procedure on the ear and mastoid process   CC

     H95.22 Intraoperative hemorrhage and hematoma of ear and mastoid process complicating other procedure   CC

√5ᵗʰ **H95.3 Accidental puncture and laceration of ear and mastoid process during a procedure**

     H95.31 Accidental puncture and laceration of the ear and mastoid process during a procedure on the ear and mastoid process   CC

     H95.32 Accidental puncture and laceration of the ear and mastoid process during other procedure   CC

√5ᵗʰ **H95.4 Postprocedural hemorrhage of ear and mastoid process following a procedure**

     H95.41 Postprocedural hemorrhage of ear and mastoid process following a procedure on the ear and mastoid process   CC

     H95.42 Postprocedural hemorrhage of ear and mastoid process following other procedure   CC

√5ᵗʰ **H95.5 Postprocedural hematoma and seroma of ear and mastoid process following a procedure**

     H95.51 Postprocedural hematoma of ear and mastoid process following a procedure on the ear and mastoid process   CC

     H95.52 Postprocedural hematoma of ear and mastoid process following other procedure   CC

     H95.53 Postprocedural seroma of ear and mastoid process following a procedure on the ear and mastoid process   CC

     H95.54 Postprocedural seroma of ear and mastoid process following other procedure   CC

√5ᵗʰ **H95.8 Other intraoperative and postprocedural complications and disorders of the ear and mastoid process, not elsewhere classified**

     EXCLUDES 2   *postprocedural complications and disorders following mastoidectomy (H95.Ø-, H95.1-)*

  √6ᵗʰ **H95.81** Postprocedural stenosis of external ear canal

       H95.811 Postprocedural stenosis of right external ear canal   CC

       H95.812 Postprocedural stenosis of left external ear canal   CC

       H95.813 Postprocedural stenosis of external ear canal, bilateral   CC

       H95.819 Postprocedural stenosis of unspecified external ear canal   CC

     H95.88 Other intraoperative complications and disorders of the ear and mastoid process, not elsewhere classified   CC

       Use additional code, if applicable, to further specify disorder

     H95.89 Other postprocedural complications and disorders of the ear and mastoid process, not elsewhere classified   CC

       Use additional code, if applicable, to further specify disorder

N Newborn: 0   P Pediatric: 0-17   M Maternity: 9-64   A Adult: 15-124   MCC Major Complication/Comorbidity   CC Complication/Comorbidity   SW Severe Wound Dx

642   ICD-10-CM 2021

Chapter 9. Diseases of the Circulatory System (IØØ–I99)

Chapter-specific Guidelines with Coding Examples

The chapter-specific guidelines from the ICD-10-CM Official Guidelines for Coding and Reporting have been provided below. Along with these guidelines are coding examples, contained in the shaded boxes, that have been developed to help illustrate the coding and/or sequencing guidance found in these guidelines.

a. Hypertension

The classification presumes a causal relationship between hypertension and heart involvement and between hypertension and kidney involvement, as the two conditions are linked by the term "with" in the Alphabetic Index. These conditions should be coded as related even in the absence of provider documentation explicitly linking them, unless the documentation clearly states the conditions are unrelated.

For hypertension and conditions not specifically linked by relational terms such as "with," "associated with" or "due to" in the classification, provider documentation must link the conditions in order to code them as related.

1) Hypertension with heart disease

Hypertension with heart conditions classified to I5Ø.- or I51.4-I51.7, I51.89, I51.9, are assigned to a code from category I11, Hypertensive heart disease. Use additional code(s) from category I5Ø, Heart failure, to identify the type(s) of heart failure in those patients with heart failure.

The same heart conditions (I5Ø.-, I51.4-I51.7, I51.89, I51.9) with hypertension are coded separately if the provider has documented they are unrelated to the hypertension. Sequence according to the circumstances of the admission/encounter.

> Patient is admitted in left heart failure. Patient also has a history of hypertension managed by medication.
>
> **I11.Ø**   **Hypertensive heart disease with heart failure**
>
> **I5Ø.1**   **Left ventricular failure, unspecified**
>
> *Explanation*: Without a diagnostic statement to the contrary, hypertension and heart failure have an assumed causal relationship, and a combination code should be used. An additional code to identify the type of heart failure (I5Ø.-) should also be provided.

2) Hypertensive chronic kidney disease

Assign codes from category I12, Hypertensive chronic kidney disease, when both hypertension and a condition classifiable to category N18, Chronic kidney disease (CKD), are present. CKD should not be coded as hypertensive if the provider indicates the CKD is not related to the hypertension.

The appropriate code from category N18 should be used as a secondary code with a code from category I12 to identify the stage of chronic kidney disease.

See Section I.C.14. Chronic kidney disease.

If a patient has hypertensive chronic kidney disease and acute renal failure, **the acute renal failure should also be coded. Sequence according to the circumstances of the admission/encounter.**

> Patient is admitted with stage IV chronic kidney disease (CKD) due to polycystic kidney disease. Patient also is on lisinopril for hypertension.
>
> **N18.4**   **Chronic kidney disease, stage 4 (severe)**
>
> **Q61.3**   **Polycystic kidney, unspecified**
>
> **I1Ø**   **Essential (primary) hypertension**
>
> *Explanation*: A combination code describing a relationship between hypertension and CKD is not used because the physician documentation identifies the polycystic kidney disease as the cause for the CKD.

3) Hypertensive heart and chronic kidney disease

Assign codes from combination category I13, Hypertensive heart and chronic kidney disease, when there is hypertension with both heart and kidney involvement. If heart failure is present, assign an additional code from category I5Ø to identify the type of heart failure.

The appropriate code from category N18, Chronic kidney disease, should be used as a secondary code with a code from category I13 to identify the stage of chronic kidney disease.

See Section I.C.14. Chronic kidney disease.

The codes in category I13, Hypertensive heart and chronic kidney disease, are combination codes that include hypertension, heart disease and chronic kidney disease. The Includes note at I13 specifies that the conditions included at I11 and I12 are included together in I13. If a patient

has hypertension, heart disease and chronic kidney disease, then a code from I13 should be used, not individual codes for hypertension, heart disease and chronic kidney disease, or codes from I11 or I12.

For patients with both acute renal failure and chronic kidney disease, **the acute renal failure should also be coded. Sequence according to the circumstances of the admission/encounter.**

> Patient admitted with acute tubular necrosis, history of hypertensive heart and kidney disease with congestive heart failure and stage 3a chronic kidney disease
>
> **N17.Ø**   **Acute kidney failure with tubular necrosis**
>
> **I13.Ø**   **Hypertensive heart and chronic kidney disease with heart failure and stage 1 through stage 4 chronic kidney disease, or unspecified chronic kidney disease**
>
> **I5Ø.9**   **Heart failure, unspecified**
>
> **N18.31**   **Chronic kidney disease, stage 3a**
>
> *Explanation*: It is appropriate to report an acute kidney failure code and a chronic kidney failure code when both conditions are treated during an encounter. In this instance, the acute renal failure was the focus of treatment and therefore sequenced as principal diagnosis. Combination codes in category I13 are used to report conditions classifiable to *both* categories I11 and I12. Do not report conditions classifiable to I11 and I12 separately. Use additional codes to report the type of heart failure and stage of CKD.

4) Hypertensive cerebrovascular disease

For hypertensive cerebrovascular disease, first assign the appropriate code from categories I6Ø-I69, followed by the appropriate hypertension code.

> Rupture of cerebral aneurysm caused by malignant hypertension
>
> **I6Ø.7**   **Nontraumatic subarachnoid hemorrhage from unspecified intracranial artery**
>
> **I1Ø**   **Essential (primary) hypertension**
>
> *Explanation*: Hypertensive cerebrovascular disease requires two codes: the appropriate I6Ø–I69 code followed by the appropriate hypertension code.

5) Hypertensive retinopathy

Subcategory H35.Ø, Background retinopathy and retinal vascular changes, should be used with a code from category I1Ø – I15, Hypertensive disease to include the systemic hypertension. The sequencing is based on the reason for the encounter.

6) Hypertension, secondary

Secondary hypertension is due to an underlying condition. Two codes are required: one to identify the underlying etiology and one from category I15 to identify the hypertension. Sequencing of codes is determined by the reason for admission/encounter.

> Renovascular hypertension due to renal artery atherosclerosis
>
> **I15.Ø**   **Renovascular hypertension**
>
> **I7Ø.1**   **Atherosclerosis of renal artery**
>
> *Explanation*: Secondary hypertension requires two codes: a code to identify the etiology and the appropriate I15 code.

7) Hypertension, transient

Assign code RØ3.Ø, Elevated blood pressure reading without diagnosis of hypertension, unless patient has an established diagnosis of hypertension. Assign code O13.-, Gestational [pregnancy-induced] hypertension without significant proteinuria, or O14.-, Pre-eclampsia, for transient hypertension of pregnancy.

8) Hypertension, controlled

This diagnostic statement usually refers to an existing state of hypertension under control by therapy. Assign the appropriate code from categories I1Ø-I15, Hypertensive diseases.

9) Hypertension, uncontrolled

Uncontrolled hypertension may refer to untreated hypertension or hypertension not responding to current therapeutic regimen. In either case, assign the appropriate code from categories I1Ø-I15, Hypertensive diseases.

10) Hypertensive crisis

Assign a code from category I16, Hypertensive crisis, for documented hypertensive urgency, hypertensive emergency or unspecified hypertensive crisis. Code also any identified hypertensive disease (I10-I15). The sequencing is based on the reason for the encounter.

11) Pulmonary hypertension

Pulmonary hypertension is classified to category I27, Other pulmonary heart diseases. For secondary pulmonary hypertension (I27.1, I27.2-), code also any associated conditions or adverse effects of drugs or toxins. The sequencing is based on the reason for the encounter, except for adverse effects of drugs (See Section I.C.19.e.).

b. Atherosclerotic coronary artery disease and angina

ICD-10-CM has combination codes for atherosclerotic heart disease with angina pectoris. The subcategories for these codes are I25.11, Atherosclerotic heart disease of native coronary artery with angina pectoris and I25.7, Atherosclerosis of coronary artery bypass graft(s) and coronary artery of transplanted heart with angina pectoris.

When using one of these combination codes it is not necessary to use an additional code for angina pectoris. A causal relationship can be assumed in a patient with both atherosclerosis and angina pectoris, unless the documentation indicates the angina is due to something other than the atherosclerosis.

If a patient with coronary artery disease is admitted due to an acute myocardial infarction (AMI), the AMI should be sequenced before the coronary artery disease.

See Section I.C.9. Acute myocardial infarction (AMI)

c. Intraoperative and postprocedural cerebrovascular accident

Medical record documentation should clearly specify the cause- and- effect relationship between the medical intervention and the cerebrovascular accident in order to assign a code for intraoperative or postprocedural cerebrovascular accident.

Proper code assignment depends on whether it was an infarction or hemorrhage and whether it occurred intraoperatively or postoperatively. If it was a cerebral hemorrhage, code assignment depends on the type of procedure performed.

Embolic cerebral infarction of the right middle cerebral artery that occurred during hip replacement surgery. The surgeon documented as due to the surgery.

I97.811	**Intraoperative cerebrovascular infarction during other surgery**
I63.411	**Cerebral infarction due to embolism of right middle cerebral artery**

Explanation: Code assignment for intraoperative or postprocedural cerebrovascular accident is based on the provider's documentation of a cause-and-effect relationship between the condition and the procedure. Proper code assignment also depends on whether the cerebrovascular accident was an infarction or hemorrhage, occurred intraoperatively or postoperatively, and the type of procedure performed.

---

d. Sequelae of cerebrovascular disease

1) Category I69, Sequelae of cerebrovascular disease

Category I69 is used to indicate conditions classifiable to categories I60-I67 as the causes of sequela (neurologic deficits), themselves classified elsewhere. These "late effects" include neurologic deficits that persist after initial onset of conditions classifiable to categories I60-I67. The neurologic deficits caused by cerebrovascular disease may be present from the onset or may arise at any time after the onset of the condition classifiable to categories I60-I67.

Codes from category I69, Sequelae of cerebrovascular disease, that specify hemiplegia, hemiparesis and monoplegia identify whether the dominant or nondominant side is affected. Should the affected side be documented, but not specified as dominant or nondominant, and the classification system does not indicate a default, code selection is as follows:

- For ambidextrous patients, the default should be dominant.
- If the left side is affected, the default is non-dominant.
- If the right side is affected, the default is dominant.

2) Codes from category I69 with codes from I60–I67

Codes from category I69 may be assigned on a health care record with codes from I60-I67, if the patient has a current cerebrovascular disease and deficits from an old cerebrovascular disease.

3) Codes from category I69 and personal history of transient ischemic attack (TIA) and cerebral infarction (Z86.73)

Codes from category I69 should not be assigned if the patient does not have neurologic deficits.

See Section I.C.21. 4. History (of) for use of personal history codes

e. Acute myocardial infarction (AMI)

1) Type 1 ST elevation myocardial infarction (STEMI) and non ST elevation myocardial infarction (NSTEMI)

The ICD-10-CM codes for type 1 acute myocardial infarction (AMI) identify the site, such as anterolateral wall or true posterior wall. Subcategories I21.0-I21.2 and code I21.3 are used for type 1 ST elevation myocardial infarction (STEMI). Code I21.4, Non-ST elevation (NSTEMI) myocardial infarction, is used for type 1 non-ST elevation myocardial infarction (NSTEMI) and nontransmural MIs.

If a type 1 NSTEMI evolves to STEMI, assign the STEMI code. If a type 1 STEMI converts to NSTEMI due to thrombolytic therapy, it is still coded as STEMI.

For encounters occurring while the myocardial infarction is equal to, or less than, four weeks old, including transfers to another acute setting or a postacute setting, and the myocardial infarction meets the definition for "other diagnoses" (see Section III, Reporting Additional Diagnoses), codes from category I21 may continue to be reported. For encounters after the 4 week time frame and the patient is still receiving care related to the myocardial infarction, the appropriate aftercare code should be assigned, rather than a code from category I21. For old or healed myocardial infarctions not requiring further care, code I25.2, Old myocardial infarction, may be assigned.

2) Acute myocardial infarction, unspecified

Code I21.9, Acute myocardial infarction, unspecified, is the default for unspecified acute myocardial infarction or unspecified type. If only type 1 STEMI or transmural MI without the site is documented, assign code I21.3, ST elevation (STEMI) myocardial infarction of unspecified site.

3) AMI documented as nontransmural or subendocardial but site provided

If an AMI is documented as nontransmural or subendocardial, but the site is provided, it is still coded as a subendocardial AMI.

See Section I.C.21.3 for information on coding status post administration of tPA in a different facility within the last 24 hours.

4) Subsequent acute myocardial infarction

A code from category I22, Subsequent ST elevation (STEMI) and non-ST elevation (NSTEMI) myocardial infarction, is to be used when a patient who has suffered a type 1 or unspecified AMI has a new AMI within the 4 week time frame of the initial AMI. A code from category I22 must be used in conjunction with a code from category I21. The sequencing of the I22 and I21 codes depends on the circumstances of the encounter.

Do not assign code I22 for subsequent myocardial infarctions other than type 1 or unspecified. For subsequent type 2 AMI assign only code I21.A1. For subsequent type 4 or type 5 AMI, assign only code I21.A9.

If a subsequent myocardial infarction of one type occurs within 4 weeks of a myocardial infarction of a different type, assign the appropriate codes from category I21 to identify each type. Do not assign a code from I22. Codes from category I22 should only be assigned if both the initial and subsequent myocardial infarctions are type 1 or unspecified.

5) Other types of myocardial infarction

The ICD-10-CM provides codes for different types of myocardial infarction. Type 1 myocardial infarctions are assigned to codes I21.0-I21.4.

Type 2 myocardial infarction (myocardial infarction due to demand ischemia or secondary to ischemic imbalance) is assigned to code I21.A1, Myocardial infarction type 2 with the underlying cause coded first. Do not assign code I24.8, Other forms of acute ischemic heart disease, for the demand ischemia. If a type 2 AMI is described as NSTEMI or STEMI, only assign code I21.A1. Codes I21.01-I21.4 should only be assigned for type 1 AMIs.

Acute myocardial infarctions type 3, 4a, 4b, 4c and 5 are assigned to code I21.A9, Other myocardial infarction type.

The "Code also" and "Code first" notes should be followed related to complications, and for coding of postprocedural myocardial infarctions during or following cardiac surgery.

Myocardial infarction involving the left circumflex artery occurring during PTCA with stent insertion to treat coronary artery disease

I25.10	**Atherosclerotic heart disease of native coronary artery without angina pectoris**
I97.790	**Other intraoperative cardiac functional disturbances during cardiac surgery**
I21.A9	**Other myocardial infarction type**

Explanation: A myocardial infarction occurring during a revascularization procedure is not considered a type 1 myocardial infarction (MI) and should not be coded to a type 1 MI code (I21.0-, I21.1-, I21.2-, I21.3) even when the specific site of the MI is documented. According to the code first instruction at I21.A9, the complication code (I97.790) should be sequenced before code I21.A9.

Chapter 9. Diseases of the Circulatory System (I00-I99)

EXCLUDES 2   *certain conditions originating in the perinatal period (P04-P96)*
certain infectious and parasitic diseases (A00-B99)
complications of pregnancy, childbirth and the puerperium (O00-O9A)
congenital malformations, deformations, and chromosomal abnormalities (Q00-Q99)
endocrine, nutritional and metabolic diseases (E00-E88)
injury, poisoning and certain other consequences of external causes (S00-T88)
neoplasms (C00-D49)
symptoms, signs and abnormal clinical and laboratory findings, not elsewhere classified (R00-R94)
systemic connective tissue disorders (M30-M36)
transient cerebral ischemic attacks and related syndromes (G45.-)

This chapter contains the following blocks:

I00-I02	Acute rheumatic fever
I05-I09	Chronic rheumatic heart diseases
I10-I16	Hypertensive diseases
I20-I25	Ischemic heart diseases
I26-I28	Pulmonary heart disease and diseases of pulmonary circulation
I30-I52	Other forms of heart disease
I60-I69	Cerebrovascular diseases
I70-I79	Diseases of arteries, arterioles and capillaries
I80-I89	Diseases of veins, lymphatic vessels and lymph nodes, not elsewhere classified
I95-I99	Other and unspecified disorders of the circulatory system

Acute rheumatic fever (I00-I02)

DEF: Inflammatory disease that can follow a throat infection by group A streptococci. Complications can involve the joints (arthritis), subcutaneous tissue (nodules), skin (erythema marginatum), heart (carditis), or brain (chorea).

I00   **Rheumatic fever without heart involvement**
    INCLUDES   arthritis, rheumatic, acute or subacute
    EXCLUDES 1   *rheumatic fever with heart involvement (I01.0-I01.9)*

✓4ᵗʰ I01   **Rheumatic fever with heart involvement**
    EXCLUDES 1   *chronic diseases of rheumatic origin (I05-I09) unless rheumatic fever is also present or there is evidence of reactivation or activity of the rheumatic process*

    I01.0   **Acute rheumatic pericarditis**   `CC`
       Any condition in I00 with pericarditis
       Rheumatic pericarditis (acute)
       EXCLUDES 1   *acute pericarditis not specified as rheumatic (I30.-)*

    I01.1   **Acute rheumatic endocarditis**   `CC`
       Any condition in I00 with endocarditis or valvulitis
       Acute rheumatic valvulitis

    I01.2   **Acute rheumatic myocarditis**   `CC`
       Any condition in I00 with myocarditis

    I01.8   **Other acute rheumatic heart disease**   `CC`
       Any condition in I00 with other or multiple types of heart involvement
       Acute rheumatic pancarditis

    I01.9   **Acute rheumatic heart disease, unspecified**   `CC`
       Any condition in I00 with unspecified type of heart involvement
       Rheumatic carditis, acute
       Rheumatic heart disease, active or acute

✓4ᵗʰ I02   **Rheumatic chorea**
    INCLUDES   Sydenham's chorea
    EXCLUDES 1   *chorea NOS (G25.5)*
              Huntington's chorea (G10)

    I02.0   **Rheumatic chorea with heart involvement**   `CC`
       Chorea NOS with heart involvement
       Rheumatic chorea with heart involvement of any type classifiable under I01.-

    I02.9   **Rheumatic chorea without heart involvement**   `CC`
       Rheumatic chorea NOS

Chronic rheumatic heart diseases (I05-I09)

✓4ᵗʰ I05   **Rheumatic mitral valve diseases**
    INCLUDES   conditions classifiable to both I05.0 and I05.2-I05.9, whether specified as rheumatic or not
    EXCLUDES 1   *mitral valve disease specified as nonrheumatic (I34.-)*
              mitral valve disease with aortic and/or tricuspid valve involvement (I08.-)

    I05.0   **Rheumatic mitral stenosis**
       Mitral (valve) obstruction (rheumatic)
       DEF: Narrowing of the mitral valve between the left atrium and left ventricle due to rheumatic fever. Symptoms include shortness of breath during or after exercise, fatigue, palpitations, chest discomfort, and swelling of feet or legs.

    I05.1   **Rheumatic mitral insufficiency**
       Rheumatic mitral incompetence
       Rheumatic mitral regurgitation
       EXCLUDES 1   *mitral insufficiency not specified as rheumatic (I34.0)*

    I05.2   **Rheumatic mitral stenosis with insufficiency**
       Rheumatic mitral stenosis with incompetence or regurgitation

    I05.8   **Other rheumatic mitral valve diseases**
       Rheumatic mitral (valve) failure

    I05.9   **Rheumatic mitral valve disease, unspecified**
       Rheumatic mitral (valve) disorder (chronic) NOS

✓4ᵗʰ I06   **Rheumatic aortic valve diseases**
    EXCLUDES 1   *aortic valve disease not specified as rheumatic (I35.-)*
              aortic valve disease with mitral and/or tricuspid valve involvement (I08.-)

    I06.0   **Rheumatic aortic stenosis**
       Rheumatic aortic (valve) obstruction

    I06.1   **Rheumatic aortic insufficiency**
       Rheumatic aortic incompetence
       Rheumatic aortic regurgitation

    I06.2   **Rheumatic aortic stenosis with insufficiency**
       Rheumatic aortic stenosis with incompetence or regurgitation

    I06.8   **Other rheumatic aortic valve diseases**

    I06.9   **Rheumatic aortic valve disease, unspecified**
       Rheumatic aortic (valve) disease NOS

✓4ᵗʰ I07   **Rheumatic tricuspid valve diseases**
    INCLUDES   rheumatic tricuspid valve diseases specified as rheumatic or unspecified
    EXCLUDES 1   *tricuspid valve disease specified as nonrheumatic (I36.-)*
              tricuspid valve disease with aortic and/or mitral valve involvement (I08.-)

    I07.0   **Rheumatic tricuspid stenosis**
       Tricuspid (valve) stenosis (rheumatic)

    I07.1   **Rheumatic tricuspid insufficiency**
       Tricuspid (valve) insufficiency (rheumatic)

    I07.2   **Rheumatic tricuspid stenosis and insufficiency**

    I07.8   **Other rheumatic tricuspid valve diseases**

    I07.9   **Rheumatic tricuspid valve disease, unspecified**
       Rheumatic tricuspid valve disorder NOS

✓4ᵗʰ I08   **Multiple valve diseases**
    INCLUDES   multiple valve diseases specified as rheumatic or unspecified
    EXCLUDES 1   *endocarditis, valve unspecified (I38)*
              multiple valve disease specified a nonrheumatic (I34.-, I35.-, I36.-, I37.-, I38.-, Q22.-, Q23.-, Q24.8-)
              rheumatic valve disease NOS (I09.1)

    I08.0   **Rheumatic disorders of both mitral and aortic valves**
       Involvement of both mitral and aortic valves specified as rheumatic or unspecified
       AHA: 2019,2Q,5

    I08.1   **Rheumatic disorders of both mitral and tricuspid valves**

    I08.2   **Rheumatic disorders of both aortic and tricuspid valves**

    I08.3   **Combined rheumatic disorders of mitral, aortic and tricuspid valves**

    I08.8   **Other rheumatic multiple valve diseases**

    I08.9   **Rheumatic multiple valve disease, unspecified**

✓4ᵗʰ I09   **Other rheumatic heart diseases**

    I09.0   **Rheumatic myocarditis**   `CC`
       EXCLUDES 1   *myocarditis not specified as rheumatic (I51.4)*

☑ Additional Character Required   ✓x7ᵗʰ Placeholder   Unacceptable PDx   Questionable PDx   Manifestation   Unspecified Dx   `H1`-`H14` HAC   `HCC` CMS-HCC Dx   `HIV` HIV Dx

ICD-10-CM 2021   645

I09.1 **Rheumatic diseases of endocardium, valve unspecified**
Rheumatic endocarditis (chronic)
Rheumatic valvulitis (chronic)
EXCLUDES 1   *endocarditis, valve unspecified (I38)*

I09.2 **Chronic rheumatic pericarditis**   CC
Adherent pericardium, rheumatic
Chronic rheumatic mediastinopericarditis
Chronic rheumatic myopericarditis
EXCLUDES 1   *chronic pericarditis not specified as rheumatic (I31.-)*

√5ᵗʰ **I09.8** **Other specified rheumatic heart diseases**

     I09.81 **Rheumatic heart failure**   CC HCC
       Use additional code to identify type of heart failure (I50.-)
       DEF: Decreased cardiac output, edema, and hypertension due to rheumatic heart disease.

     I09.89 **Other specified rheumatic heart diseases**
       Rheumatic disease of pulmonary valve

I09.9 **Rheumatic heart disease, unspecified**
Rheumatic carditis
EXCLUDES 1   *rheumatoid carditis (M05.31)*

Hypertensive diseases (I10-I16)

Use additional code to identify:
exposure to environmental tobacco smoke (Z77.22)
history of tobacco dependence (Z87.891)
occupational exposure to environmental tobacco smoke (Z57.31)
tobacco dependence (F17.-)
tobacco use (Z72.0)
EXCLUDES 1   *neonatal hypertension (P29.2)*
         primary pulmonary hypertension (I27.0)
EXCLUDES 2   *hypertensive disease complicating pregnancy, childbirth and the puerperium (O10-O11, O13-O16)*

I10 **Essential (primary) hypertension**
   INCLUDES   high blood pressure
       hypertension (arterial) (benign) (essential) (malignant) (primary) (systemic)
   EXCLUDES 1   *hypertensive disease complicating pregnancy, childbirth and the puerperium (O10-O11, O13-O16)*
   EXCLUDES 2   *essential (primary) hypertension involving vessels of brain (I60-I69)*
         essential (primary) hypertension involving vessels of eye (H35.0-)
   AHA: 2020,1Q,12; 2018,2Q,9; 2016,4Q,27

√4ᵗʰ **I11** **Hypertensive heart disease**
   INCLUDES   ►any condition in I50.- or I51.4-I51.7, I51.89, I51.9 due to hypertension◄
   AHA: 2018,2Q,9
   TIP: Do not assign a code from this category when provider documentation indicates the heart disease is attributable to another cause.

     I11.0 **Hypertensive heart disease with heart failure**   HCC
       Hypertensive heart failure
       Use additional code to identify type of heart failure (I50.-)
       AHA: 2017,1Q,47

     I11.9 **Hypertensive heart disease without heart failure**
       Hypertensive heart disease NOS

√4ᵗʰ **I12** **Hypertensive chronic kidney disease**
   INCLUDES   any condition in N18 and N26 — due to hypertension
       arteriosclerosis of kidney
       arteriosclerotic nephritis (chronic) (interstitial)
       hypertensive nephropathy
       nephrosclerosis
   EXCLUDES 1   *hypertension due to kidney disease (I15.0, I15.1)*
         renovascular hypertension (I15.0)
         secondary hypertension (I15.-)
   EXCLUDES 2   *acute kidney failure (N17.-)*
   AHA: 2019,3Q,3; 2018,4Q,88; 2016,3Q,22
   TIP: Do not assign a code from this category when provider documentation indicates the chronic kidney disease (CKD) is attributable to another cause.

     I12.0 **Hypertensive chronic kidney disease with stage 5 chronic kidney disease or end stage renal disease**   CC HCC
       Use additional code to identify the stage of chronic kidney disease (N18.5, N18.6)

     I12.9 **Hypertensive chronic kidney disease with stage 1 through stage 4 chronic kidney disease, or unspecified chronic kidney disease**
       Hypertensive chronic kidney disease NOS
       Hypertensive renal disease NOS
       Use additional code to identify the stage of chronic kidney disease (N18.1-N18.4, N18.9)

√4ᵗʰ **I13** **Hypertensive heart and chronic kidney disease**
   INCLUDES   any condition in I11.- with any condition in I12.-
       cardiorenal disease
       cardiovascular renal disease
   TIP: Do not assign a code from this category when provider documentation indicates the heart and/or chronic kidney disease is attributable to another cause.

     I13.0 **Hypertensive heart and chronic kidney disease with heart failure and stage 1 through stage 4 chronic kidney disease, or unspecified chronic kidney disease**   CC HCC
       Use additional code to identify type of heart failure (I50.-)
       Use additional code to identify stage of chronic kidney disease (N18.1-N18.4, N18.9)

√5ᵗʰ   **I13.1** **Hypertensive heart and chronic kidney disease without heart failure**

       I13.10 **Hypertensive heart and chronic kidney disease without heart failure, with stage 1 through stage 4 chronic kidney disease, or unspecified chronic kidney disease**
         Hypertensive heart disease and hypertensive chronic kidney disease NOS
         Use additional code to identify the stage of chronic kidney disease (N18.1-N18.4, N18.9)

       I13.11 **Hypertensive heart and chronic kidney disease without heart failure, with stage 5 chronic kidney disease, or end stage renal disease**   CC HCC
         Use additional code to identify the stage of chronic kidney disease (N18.5, N18.6)

     I13.2 **Hypertensive heart and chronic kidney disease with heart failure and with stage 5 chronic kidney disease, or end stage renal disease**   CC HCC
       Use additional code to identify type of heart failure (I50.-)
       Use additional code to identify the stage of chronic kidney disease (N18.5, N18.6)

√4ᵗʰ **I15** **Secondary hypertension**
   Code also underlying condition
   EXCLUDES 1   *postprocedural hypertension (I97.3)*
   EXCLUDES 2   *secondary hypertension involving vessels of brain (I60-I69)*
         secondary hypertension involving vessels of eye (H35.0-)

     I15.0 **Renovascular hypertension**
     I15.1 **Hypertension secondary to other renal disorders**
       AHA: 2016,3Q,22
     I15.2 **Hypertension secondary to endocrine disorders**
     I15.8 **Other secondary hypertension**
     I15.9 **Secondary hypertension, unspecified**

√4ᵗʰ **I16** **Hypertensive crisis**
   Code also any identified hypertensive disease (I10-I15)
   AHA: 2016,4Q,26-28
     I16.0 **Hypertensive urgency**
     I16.1 **Hypertensive emergency**   CC
     I16.9 **Hypertensive crisis, unspecified**   CC

Ischemic heart diseases (I20-I25)

Use additional code to identify presence of hypertension (I10-I16)

✓4ᵗʰ I20 Angina pectoris

Use additional code to identify:
exposure to environmental tobacco smoke (Z77.22)
history of tobacco dependence (Z87.891)
occupational exposure to environmental tobacco smoke (Z57.31)
tobacco dependence (F17.-)
tobacco use (Z72.0)

EXCLUDES 1 angina pectoris with atherosclerotic heart disease of native coronary arteries (I25.1-)
atherosclerosis of coronary artery bypass graft(s) and coronary artery of transplanted heart with angina pectoris (I25.7-)
postinfarction angina (I23.7)

DEF: Chest pain due to reduced blood flow resulting in a lack of oxygen to the heart muscles.

I20.0 Unstable angina CC HCC
Accelerated angina
Crescendo angina
De novo effort angina
Intermediate coronary syndrome
Preinfarction syndrome
Worsening effort angina
DEF: Condition representing an intermediate stage between angina of effort and acute myocardial infarction.

I20.1 Angina pectoris with documented spasm CC HCC
Angiospastic angina
Prinzmetal angina
Spasm-induced angina
Variant angina

I20.8 Other forms of angina pectoris HCC
Angina equivalent
Angina of effort
Coronary slow flow syndrome
Stable angina
Stenocardia
Use additional code(s) for symptoms associated with angina equivalent

I20.9 Angina pectoris, unspecified HCC
Angina NOS
Anginal syndrome
Cardiac angina
Ischemic chest pain

✓4ᵗʰ I21 Acute myocardial infarction

INCLUDES cardiac infarction
coronary (artery) embolism
coronary (artery) occlusion
coronary (artery) rupture
coronary (artery) thrombosis
infarction of heart, myocardium, or ventricle
myocardial infarction specified as acute or with a stated duration of 4 weeks (28 days) or less from onset

Use additional code, if applicable, to identify:
exposure to environmental tobacco smoke (Z77.22)
history of tobacco dependence (Z87.891)
occupational exposure to environmental tobacco smoke (Z57.31)
status post administration of tPA (rtPA) in a different facility within the last 24 hours prior to admission to current facility (Z92.82)
tobacco dependence (F17.-)
tobacco use (Z72.0)

EXCLUDES 2 old myocardial infarction (I25.2)
postmyocardial infarction syndrome (I24.1)
subsequent type 1 myocardial infarction (I22.-)

AHA: 2019,2Q,5; 2018,4Q,68; 2018,3Q,5; 2017,4Q,12-14; 2017,1Q,44-45; 2016,4Q,140; 2015,2Q,16; 2013,1Q,25; 2012,4Q,96,102-103

TIP: When chronic total occlusion and myocardial infarction are documented as being in different vessels, assign code I25.82 Chronic total occlusion of coronary artery, in addition to the myocardial infarction code.

✓5ᵗʰ I21.0 ST elevation (STEMI) myocardial infarction of anterior wall

Type 1 ST elevation myocardial infarction of anterior wall
DEF: ST elevation myocardial infarction: Complete obstruction of one or more coronary arteries causing decreased blood flow (ischemia) and necrosis of myocardial muscle cells.

I21.01 ST elevation (STEMI) myocardial infarction involving left main coronary artery MCC HCC

I21.02 ST elevation (STEMI) myocardial infarction involving left anterior descending coronary artery MCC HCC
ST elevation (STEMI) myocardial infarction involving diagonal coronary artery
AHA: 2013,1Q,25

I21.09 ST elevation (STEMI) myocardial infarction involving other coronary artery of anterior wall MCC HCC
Acute transmural myocardial infarction of anterior wall
Anteroapical transmural (Q wave) infarction (acute)
Anterolateral transmural (Q wave) infarction (acute)
Anteroseptal transmural (Q wave) infarction (acute)
Transmural (Q wave) infarction (acute) (of) anterior (wall) NOS
AHA: 2012,4Q,102-103

✓5ᵗʰ I21.1 ST elevation (STEMI) myocardial infarction of inferior wall

Type 1 ST elevation myocardial infarction of inferior wall
DEF: ST elevation myocardial infarction: Complete obstruction of one or more coronary arteries causing decreased blood flow (ischemia) and necrosis of myocardial muscle cells.

I21.11 ST elevation (STEMI) myocardial infarction involving right coronary artery MCC HCC
Inferoposterior transmural (Q wave) infarction (acute)

I21.19 ST elevation (STEMI) myocardial infarction involving other coronary artery of inferior wall MCC HCC
Acute transmural myocardial infarction of inferior wall
Inferolateral transmural (Q wave) infarction (acute)
Transmural (Q wave) infarction (acute) (of) diaphragmatic wall
Transmural (Q wave) infarction (acute) (of) inferior (wall) NOS
EXCLUDES 2 ST elevation (STEMI) myocardial infarction involving left circumflex coronary artery (I21.21)
AHA: 2012,4Q,96

✓5ᵗʰ I21.2 ST elevation (STEMI) myocardial infarction of other sites

Type 1 ST elevation myocardial infarction of other sites
DEF: ST elevation myocardial infarction: Complete obstruction of one or more coronary arteries causing decreased blood flow (ischemia) and necrosis of myocardial muscle cells.

I21.21 ST elevation (STEMI) myocardial infarction involving left circumflex coronary artery MCC HCC
ST elevation (STEMI) myocardial infarction involving oblique marginal coronary artery

I21.29 ST elevation (STEMI) myocardial infarction involving other sites MCC HCC
Acute transmural myocardial infarction of other sites
Apical-lateral transmural (Q wave) infarction (acute)
Basal-lateral transmural (Q wave) infarction (acute)
High lateral transmural (Q wave) infarction (acute)
Lateral (wall) NOS transmural (Q wave) infarction (acute)
Posterior (true) transmural (Q wave) infarction (acute)
Posterobasal transmural (Q wave) infarction (acute)
Posterolateral transmural (Q wave) infarction (acute)
Posteroseptal transmural (Q wave) infarction (acute)
Septal transmural (Q wave) infarction (acute) NOS

I21.3 ST elevation (STEMI) myocardial infarction of unspecified site MCC HCC

Acute transmural myocardial infarction of unspecified site
Transmural (Q wave) myocardial infarction NOS
Type 1 ST elevation myocardial infarction of unspecified site
DEF: ST elevation myocardial infarction: Complete obstruction of one or more coronary arteries causing decreased blood flow (ischemia) and necrosis of myocardial muscle cells.

I21.4 Non-ST elevation (NSTEMI) myocardial infarction MCC HCC

Acute subendocardial myocardial infarction
Non-Q wave myocardial infarction NOS
Nontransmural myocardial infarction NOS
Type 1 non-ST elevation myocardial infarction
AHA: 2019,2Q,33; 2017,1Q,44-45
DEF: Partial obstruction of one or more coronary arteries that causes decreased blood flow (ischemia) and may cause partial thickness necrosis of myocardial muscle cells.

I21.9   **Acute myocardial infarction, unspecified**   `MCC` `HCC`
     Myocardial infarction (acute) NOS

✓5ᵗʰ **I21.A**   **Other type of myocardial infarction**
     AHA: 2019,2Q,5

     I21.A1   **Myocardial infarction type 2**   `MCC` `HCC`
         Myocardial infarction due to demand ischemia
         Myocardial infarction secondary to ischemic
             imbalance
         Code first the underlying cause, such as:
             anemia (D50.0-D64.9)
             chronic obstructive pulmonary disease (J44.-)
             paroxysmal tachycardia (I47.0-I47.9)
             shock (R57.0-R57.9)
         AHA: 2019,4Q,53; 2017,4Q,13-14
         DEF: Often referred to as due to demand ischemia,
         myocardial infarction (MI) type 2 refers to an MI due to
         ischemia and necrosis resulting from an oxygen
         imbalance to the heart. This mismatch between oxygen
         decreased supply and increased demand is caused by
         conditions other than coronary artery disease such as
         vasospasm, embolism, anemia, hypertension,
         hypotension, or arrhythmias.

     I21.A9   **Other myocardial infarction type**   `MCC` `HCC`
         Myocardial infarction associated with
             revascularization procedure
         Myocardial infarction type 3
         Myocardial infarction type 4a
         Myocardial infarction type 4b
         Myocardial infarction type 4c
         Myocardial infarction type 5
         Code first, if applicable, postprocedural myocardial
             infarction following cardiac surgery (I97.190), or
             postprocedural myocardial infarction during
             cardiac surgery (I97.790)
         Code also complication, if known and applicable, such
             as:
             (acute) stent occlusion (T82.897-)
             (acute) stent stenosis (T82.855-)
             (acute) stent thrombosis (T82.867-)
             cardiac arrest due to underlying cardiac condition
                (I46.2)
             complication of percutaneous coronary intervention
                (PCI) (I97.89)
             occlusion of coronary artery bypass graft (T82.218-)
         AHA: 2019,2Q,33

✓4ᵗʰ **I22**   **Subsequent ST elevation (STEMI) and non-ST elevation (NSTEMI) myocardial infarction**
     `INCLUDES`   acute myocardial infarction occurring within four weeks
             (28 days) of a previous acute myocardial infarction,
             regardless of site
             cardiac infarction
             coronary (artery) embolism
             coronary (artery) occlusion
             coronary (artery) rupture
             coronary (artery) thrombosis
             infarction of heart, myocardium, or ventricle
             recurrent myocardial infarction
             reinfarction of myocardium
             rupture of heart, myocardium, or ventricle
             subsequent type 1 myocardial infarction
     Use additional code, if applicable, to identify:
         exposure to environmental tobacco smoke (Z77.22)
         history of tobacco dependence (Z87.891)
         occupational exposure to environmental tobacco smoke (Z57.31)
         status post administration of tPA (rtPA) in a different facility within
             the last 24 hours prior to admission to current facility (Z92.82)
         tobacco dependence (F17.-)
         tobacco use (Z72.0)
     `EXCLUDES 1`   subsequent myocardial infarction, type 2 (I21.A1)
             subsequent myocardial infarction of other type (type 3) (type
                4) (type 5) (I21.A9)
     AHA: 2018,4Q,68; 2018,3Q,5; 2017,4Q,12-13; 2017,2Q,11; 2013,1Q,25;
     2012,4Q,97,102-103
     DEF: Non-ST elevation myocardial infarction: Partial obstruction of one
     or more coronary arteries that causes decreased blood flow (ischemia)
     and may cause partial thickness necrosis of myocardial muscle cells.
     DEF: ST elevation myocardial infarction: Complete obstruction of one or
     more coronary arteries causing decreased blood flow (ischemia) and
     necrosis of myocardial muscle cells.
     TIP: When chronic total occlusion and myocardial infarction are
     documented as being in different vessels, assign code I25.82 Chronic total
     occlusion of coronary artery, in addition to the myocardial infarction code.

I22.0   **Subsequent ST elevation (STEMI) myocardial infarction of**
        anterior wall   `MCC` `HCC`
         Subsequent acute transmural myocardial infarction of anterior
             wall
         Subsequent transmural (Q wave) infarction (acute)(of) anterior
             (wall) NOS
         Subsequent anteroapical transmural (Q wave) infarction (acute)
         Subsequent anterolateral transmural (Q wave) infarction (acute)
         Subsequent anteroseptal transmural (Q wave) infarction (acute)

I22.1   **Subsequent ST elevation (STEMI) myocardial infarction of**
        inferior wall   `MCC` `HCC`
         Subsequent acute transmural myocardial infarction of inferior
             wall
         Subsequent transmural (Q wave) infarction (acute)(of)
             diaphragmatic wall
         Subsequent transmural (Q wave) infarction (acute)(of) inferior
             (wall) NOS
         Subsequent inferolateral transmural (Q wave) infarction (acute)
         Subsequent inferoposterior transmural (Q wave) infarction
             (acute)
         AHA: 2012,4Q,102

I22.2   **Subsequent non-ST elevation (NSTEMI) myocardial**
        infarction   `MCC` `HCC`
         Subsequent acute subendocardial myocardial infarction
         Subsequent non-Q wave myocardial infarction NOS
         Subsequent nontransmural myocardial infarction NOS

N Newborn: 0   P Pediatric: 0-17   M Maternity: 9-64   A Adult: 15-124   `MCC` Major Complication/Comorbidity   `CC` Complication/Comorbidity   `SW` Severe Wound Dx

648   ICD-10-CM 2021

I22.8 **Subsequent ST elevation (STEMI) myocardial infarction of other sites** `MCC` `HCC`

Subsequent acute transmural myocardial infarction of other sites

Subsequent apical-lateral transmural (Q wave) myocardial infarction (acute)

Subsequent basal-lateral transmural (Q wave) myocardial infarction (acute)

Subsequent high lateral transmural (Q wave) myocardial infarction (acute)

Subsequent transmural (Q wave) myocardial infarction (acute)(of) lateral (wall) NOS

Subsequent posterior (true) transmural (Q wave) myocardial infarction (acute)

Subsequent posterobasal transmural (Q wave) myocardial infarction (acute)

Subsequent posterolateral transmural (Q wave) myocardial infarction (acute)

Subsequent posteroseptal transmural (Q wave) myocardial infarction (acute)

Subsequent septal NOS transmural (Q wave) myocardial infarction (acute)

I22.9 **Subsequent ST elevation (STEMI) myocardial infarction of unspecified site** `MCC` `HCC`

Subsequent acute myocardial infarction of unspecified site

Subsequent myocardial infarction (acute) NOS

☑4ᵗʰ **I23** **Certain current complications following ST elevation (STEMI) and non-ST elevation (NSTEMI) myocardial infarction (within the 28 day period)**

AHA: 2017,2Q,11

DEF: ST elevation myocardial infarction: Complete obstruction of one or more coronary arteries causing decreased blood flow (ischemia) and necrosis of myocardial muscle cells.

DEF: Non-ST elevation myocardial infarction: Partial obstruction of one or more coronary arteries that causes decreased blood flow (ischemia) and may cause partial thickness necrosis of myocardial muscle cells.

I23.0 **Hemopericardium as current complication following acute myocardial infarction** `CC` `HCC` `A`

EXCLUDES 1   *hemopericardium not specified as current complication following acute myocardial infarction (I31.2)*

I23.1 **Atrial septal defect as current complication following acute myocardial infarction** `CC` `HCC` `A`

EXCLUDES 1   *acquired atrial septal defect not specified as current complication following acute myocardial infarction (I51.0)*

I23.2 **Ventricular septal defect as current complication following acute myocardial infarction** `CC` `HCC` `A`

EXCLUDES 1   *acquired ventricular septal defect not specified as current complication following acute myocardial infarction (I51.0)*

I23.3 **Rupture of cardiac wall without hemopericardium as current complication following acute myocardial infarction** `CC` `HCC` `A`

I23.4 **Rupture of chordae tendineae as current complication following acute myocardial infarction** `MCC` `HCC`

EXCLUDES 1   *rupture of chordae tendineae not specified as current complication following acute myocardial infarction (I51.1)*

I23.5 **Rupture of papillary muscle as current complication following acute myocardial infarction** `MCC` `HCC`

EXCLUDES 1   *rupture of papillary muscle not specified as current complication following acute myocardial infarction (I51.2)*

I23.6 **Thrombosis of atrium, auricular appendage, and ventricle as current complications following acute myocardial infarction** `CC` `HCC` `A`

EXCLUDES 1   *thrombosis of atrium, auricular appendage, and ventricle not specified as current complication following acute myocardial infarction (I51.3)*

I23.7 **Postinfarction angina** `CC` `HCC` `A`

AHA: 2015,2Q,16

TIP: When postinfarction angina occurs with atherosclerotic coronary artery disease, code both I23.7 and I25.118 for atherosclerotic disease with other forms of angina pectoris.

I23.8 **Other current complications following acute myocardial infarction** `CC` `HCC` `A`

☑4ᵗʰ **I24** **Other acute ischemic heart diseases**

EXCLUDES 1   *angina pectoris (I20.-)*

           transient myocardial ischemia in newborn (P29.4)

I24.0 **Acute coronary thrombosis not resulting in myocardial infarction** `CC` `HCC`

Acute coronary (artery) (vein) embolism not resulting in myocardial infarction

Acute coronary (artery) (vein) occlusion not resulting in myocardial infarction

Acute coronary (artery) (vein) thromboembolism not resulting in myocardial infarction

EXCLUDES 1   *atherosclerotic heart disease (I25.1-)*

AHA: 2013,1Q,24

I24.1 **Dressler's syndrome** `CC` `HCC`

Postmyocardial infarction syndrome

EXCLUDES 1   *postinfarction angina (I23.7)*

DEF: Fever, leukocytosis, chest pain, evidence of pericarditis, pleurisy, and pneumonia occurring days or weeks after a myocardial infarction.

I24.8 **Other forms of acute ischemic heart disease** `CC` `HCC`

EXCLUDES 1   *myocardial infarction due to demand ischemia (I21.A1)*

AHA: 2019,4Q,53; 2017,4Q,13

I24.9 **Acute ischemic heart disease, unspecified** `CC` `HCC`

EXCLUDES 1   *ischemic heart disease (chronic) NOS (I25.9)*

☑4ᵗʰ **I25** **Chronic ischemic heart disease**

Use additional code to identify:

chronic total occlusion of coronary artery (I25.82)

exposure to environmental tobacco smoke (Z77.22)

history of tobacco dependence (Z87.891)

occupational exposure to environmental tobacco smoke (Z57.31)

tobacco dependence (F17.-)

tobacco use (Z72.0)

☑5ᵗʰ **I25.1** **Atherosclerotic heart disease of native coronary artery**

Atherosclerotic cardiovascular disease

Coronary (artery) atheroma

Coronary (artery) atherosclerosis

Coronary (artery) disease

Coronary (artery) sclerosis

Use additional code, if applicable, to identify:

coronary atherosclerosis due to calcified coronary lesion (I25.84)

coronary atherosclerosis due to lipid rich plaque (I25.83)

EXCLUDES 2   *atheroembolism (I75.-)*

           atherosclerosis of coronary artery bypass graft(s) and transplanted heart (I25.7-)

Atheromas

Atheromas (fatty tissue and/or plaque)   Lumen

I25.10 **Atherosclerotic heart disease of native coronary artery without angina pectoris** `A`

Atherosclerotic heart disease NOS

AHA: 2015,2Q,16; 2012,4Q,92

☑6ᵗʰ **I25.11** **Atherosclerotic heart disease of native coronary artery with angina pectoris**

I25.110 **Atherosclerotic heart disease of native coronary artery with unstable angina pectoris** `CC` `HCC` `A`

EXCLUDES 1   *unstable angina without atherosclerotic heart disease (I20.0)*

☑ Additional Character Required   ☑x7ᵗʰ Placeholder   Unacceptable PDx   Questionable PDx   Manifestation   Unspecified Dx   `H1`-`H14` HAC   `HCC` CMS-HCC Dx   `HIV` HIV Dx

ICD-10-CM 2021   649

I25.111   Atherosclerotic heart disease of native coronary artery with angina pectoris with documented spasm   HCC A

     EXCLUDES 1   angina pectoris with documented spasm without atherosclerotic heart disease (I20.1)

I25.118   Atherosclerotic heart disease of native coronary artery with other forms of angina pectoris   HCC A

     EXCLUDES 1   other forms of angina pectoris without atherosclerotic heart disease (I20.8)

     AHA: 2015,2Q,16

     TIP: When postinfarction angina occurs with atherosclerotic coronary artery disease, code both I23.7 and I25.118 for atherosclerotic disease with other forms of angina pectoris.

I25.119   Atherosclerotic heart disease of native coronary artery with unspecified angina pectoris   HCC A

     Atherosclerotic heart disease with angina NOS

     Atherosclerotic heart disease with ischemic chest pain

     EXCLUDES 1   unspecified angina pectoris without atherosclerotic heart disease (I20.9)

I25.2   **Old myocardial infarction**

   Healed myocardial infarction

   Past myocardial infarction diagnosed by ECG or other investigation, but currently presenting no symptoms

I25.3   **Aneurysm of heart**   CC

   Mural aneurysm

   Ventricular aneurysm

✓5ᵗʰ **I25.4**   **Coronary artery aneurysm and dissection**

   I25.41   **Coronary artery aneurysm**

     Coronary arteriovenous fistula, acquired

     EXCLUDES 1   congenital coronary (artery) aneurysm (Q24.5)

   I25.42   **Coronary artery dissection**   MCC

     DEF: Tear in the intimal arterial wall of a coronary artery resulting in the sudden intrusion of blood within the layers of the wall.

I25.5   **Ischemic cardiomyopathy**

     EXCLUDES 2   coronary atherosclerosis (I25.1-, I25.7-)

I25.6   **Silent myocardial ischemia**

✓5ᵗʰ **I25.7**   **Atherosclerosis of coronary artery bypass graft(s) and coronary artery of transplanted heart with angina pectoris**

   Use additional code, if applicable, to identify:

     coronary atherosclerosis due to calcified coronary lesion (I25.84)

     coronary atherosclerosis due to lipid rich plaque (I25.83)

     EXCLUDES 1   atherosclerosis of bypass graft(s) of transplanted heart without angina pectoris (I25.812)

         atherosclerosis of coronary artery bypass graft(s) without angina pectoris (I25.810)

         atherosclerosis of native coronary artery of transplanted heart without angina pectoris (I25.811)

✓6ᵗʰ **I25.70**   **Atherosclerosis of coronary artery bypass graft(s), unspecified, with angina pectoris**

   I25.700   **Atherosclerosis of coronary artery bypass graft(s), unspecified, with unstable angina pectoris**   CC HCC A

     EXCLUDES 1   unstable angina pectoris without atherosclerosis of coronary artery bypass graft (I20.0)

   I25.701   **Atherosclerosis of coronary artery bypass graft(s), unspecified, with angina pectoris with documented spasm**   HCC A

     EXCLUDES 1   angina pectoris with documented spasm without atherosclerosis of coronary artery bypass graft (I20.1)

I25.708   **Atherosclerosis of coronary artery bypass graft(s), unspecified, with other forms of angina pectoris**   HCC A

     EXCLUDES 1   other forms of angina pectoris without atherosclerosis of coronary artery bypass graft (I20.8)

I25.709   **Atherosclerosis of coronary artery bypass graft(s), unspecified, with unspecified angina pectoris**   HCC A

     EXCLUDES 1   unspecified angina pectoris without atherosclerosis of coronary artery bypass graft (I20.9)

✓6ᵗʰ **I25.71**   **Atherosclerosis of autologous vein coronary artery bypass graft(s) with angina pectoris**

   I25.710   **Atherosclerosis of autologous vein coronary artery bypass graft(s) with unstable angina pectoris**   CC HCC A

     EXCLUDES 1   unstable angina without atherosclerosis of autologous vein coronary artery bypass graft(s) (I20.0)

     EXCLUDES 2   embolism or thrombus of coronary artery bypass graft(s) (T82.8-)

   I25.711   **Atherosclerosis of autologous vein coronary artery bypass graft(s) with angina pectoris with documented spasm**   CC HCC A

     EXCLUDES 1   angina pectoris with documented spasm without atherosclerosis of autologous vein coronary artery bypass graft(s) (I20.1)

   I25.718   **Atherosclerosis of autologous vein coronary artery bypass graft(s) with other forms of angina pectoris**   CC HCC A

     EXCLUDES 1   other forms of angina pectoris without atherosclerosis of autologous vein coronary artery bypass graft(s) (I20.8)

   I25.719   **Atherosclerosis of autologous vein coronary artery bypass graft(s) with unspecified angina pectoris**   CC HCC A

     EXCLUDES 1   unspecified angina pectoris without atherosclerosis of autologous vein coronary artery bypass graft(s) (I20.9)

✓6ᵗʰ **I25.72**   **Atherosclerosis of autologous artery coronary artery bypass graft(s) with angina pectoris**

   Atherosclerosis of internal mammary artery graft with angina pectoris

   I25.720   **Atherosclerosis of autologous artery coronary artery bypass graft(s) with unstable angina pectoris**   CC HCC A

     EXCLUDES 1   unstable angina without atherosclerosis of autologous artery coronary artery bypass graft(s) (I20.0)

   I25.721   **Atherosclerosis of autologous artery coronary artery bypass graft(s) with angina pectoris with documented spasm**   CC HCC A

     EXCLUDES 1   angina pectoris with documented spasm without atherosclerosis of autologous artery coronary artery bypass graft(s) (I20.1)

N Newborn: 0   P Pediatric: 0-17   M Maternity: 9-64   A Adult: 15-124   MCC Major Complication/Comorbidity   CC Complication/Comorbidity   SW Severe Wound Dx

650   ICD-10-CM 2021

I25.728 Atherosclerosis of autologous artery coronary artery bypass graft(s) with other forms of angina pectoris `CC` `HCC` `A`
> **EXCLUDES 1**   *other forms of angina pectoris without atherosclerosis of autologous artery coronary artery bypass graft(s) (I20.8)*

I25.729 Atherosclerosis of autologous artery coronary artery bypass graft(s) with unspecified angina pectoris `CC` `HCC` `A`
> **EXCLUDES 1**   *unspecified angina pectoris without atherosclerosis of autologous artery coronary artery bypass graft(s) (I20.9)*

√6ᵗʰ **I25.73** Atherosclerosis of nonautologous biological coronary artery bypass graft(s) with angina pectoris

I25.730 Atherosclerosis of nonautologous biological coronary artery bypass graft(s) with unstable angina pectoris `CC` `HCC` `A`
> **EXCLUDES 1**   *unstable angina without atherosclerosis of nonautologous biological coronary artery bypass graft(s) (I20.0)*

I25.731 Atherosclerosis of nonautologous biological coronary artery bypass graft(s) with angina pectoris with documented spasm `CC` `HCC` `A`
> **EXCLUDES 1**   *angina pectoris with documented spasm without atherosclerosis of nonautologous biological coronary artery bypass graft(s) (I20.1)*

I25.738 Atherosclerosis of nonautologous biological coronary artery bypass graft(s) with other forms of angina pectoris `CC` `HCC` `A`
> **EXCLUDES 1**   *other forms of angina pectoris without atherosclerosis of nonautologous biological coronary artery bypass graft(s) (I20.8)*

I25.739 Atherosclerosis of nonautologous biological coronary artery bypass graft(s) with unspecified angina pectoris `CC` `HCC` `A`
> **EXCLUDES 1**   *unspecified angina pectoris without atherosclerosis of nonautologous biological coronary artery bypass graft(s) (I20.9)*

√6ᵗʰ **I25.75** Atherosclerosis of native coronary artery of transplanted heart with angina pectoris
> **EXCLUDES 1**   *atherosclerosis of native coronary artery of transplanted heart without angina pectoris (I25.811)*

I25.750 Atherosclerosis of native coronary artery of transplanted heart with unstable angina `CC` `HCC`

I25.751 Atherosclerosis of native coronary artery of transplanted heart with angina pectoris with documented spasm `CC` `HCC`

I25.758 Atherosclerosis of native coronary artery of transplanted heart with other forms of angina pectoris `CC` `HCC`

I25.759 Atherosclerosis of native coronary artery of transplanted heart with unspecified angina pectoris `CC` `HCC`

√6ᵗʰ **I25.76** Atherosclerosis of bypass graft of coronary artery of transplanted heart with angina pectoris
> **EXCLUDES 1**   *atherosclerosis of bypass graft of coronary artery of transplanted heart without angina pectoris (I25.812)*

I25.760 Atherosclerosis of bypass graft of coronary artery of transplanted heart with unstable angina `CC` `HCC` `A`

I25.761 Atherosclerosis of bypass graft of coronary artery of transplanted heart with angina pectoris with documented spasm `CC` `HCC` `A`

I25.768 Atherosclerosis of bypass graft of coronary artery of transplanted heart with other forms of angina pectoris `CC` `HCC` `A`

I25.769 Atherosclerosis of bypass graft of coronary artery of transplanted heart with unspecified angina pectoris `CC` `HCC` `A`

√6ᵗʰ **I25.79** Atherosclerosis of other coronary artery bypass graft(s) with angina pectoris

I25.790 Atherosclerosis of other coronary artery bypass graft(s) with unstable angina pectoris `CC` `HCC` `A`
> **EXCLUDES 1**   *unstable angina without atherosclerosis of other coronary artery bypass graft(s) (I20.0)*

I25.791 Atherosclerosis of other coronary artery bypass graft(s) with angina pectoris with documented spasm `CC` `HCC` `A`
> **EXCLUDES 1**   *angina pectoris with documented spasm without atherosclerosis of other coronary artery bypass graft(s) (I20.1)*

I25.798 Atherosclerosis of other coronary artery bypass graft(s) with other forms of angina pectoris `CC` `HCC` `A`
> **EXCLUDES 1**   *other forms of angina pectoris without atherosclerosis of other coronary artery bypass graft(s) (I20.8)*

I25.799 Atherosclerosis of other coronary artery bypass graft(s) with unspecified angina pectoris `CC` `HCC` `A`
> **EXCLUDES 1**   *unspecified angina pectoris without atherosclerosis of other coronary artery bypass graft(s) (I20.9)*

√5ᵗʰ **I25.8** Other forms of chronic ischemic heart disease

√6ᵗʰ **I25.81** Atherosclerosis of other coronary vessels without angina pectoris
> Use additional code, if applicable, to identify:
> coronary atherosclerosis due to calcified coronary lesion (I25.84)
> coronary atherosclerosis due to lipid rich plaque (I25.83)
> **EXCLUDES 2**   *atherosclerotic heart disease of native coronary artery without angina pectoris (I25.10)*

I25.810 Atherosclerosis of coronary artery bypass graft(s) without angina pectoris `CC` `A`
> Atherosclerosis of coronary artery bypass graft NOS
> **EXCLUDES 1**   *atherosclerosis of coronary bypass graft(s) with angina pectoris (I25.70-I25.73-, I25.79-)*

I25.811 Atherosclerosis of native coronary artery of transplanted heart without angina pectoris `CC`
> Atherosclerosis of native coronary artery of transplanted heart NOS
> **EXCLUDES 1**   *atherosclerosis of native coronary artery of transplanted heart with angina pectoris (I25.75-)*

I25.812 Atherosclerosis of bypass graft of coronary artery of transplanted heart without angina pectoris `CC` `A`
> Atherosclerosis of bypass graft of transplanted heart NOS
> **EXCLUDES 1**   *atherosclerosis of bypass graft of transplanted heart with angina pectoris (I25.76)*

☑ Additional Character Required   √x7ᵗʰ Placeholder   Unacceptable PDx   Questionable PDx   Manifestation   Unspecified Dx   `H1`-`H14` HAC   `HCC` CMS-HCC Dx   `HIV` HIV Dx

ICD-10-CM 2021   651

I25.82   **Chronic total occlusion of coronary artery**
Complete occlusion of coronary artery
Total occlusion of coronary artery
Code first coronary atherosclerosis (I25.1-, I25.7-, I25.81-)

> **EXCLUDES 1**   *acute coronary occlusion with myocardial infarction (I21.0-I21.9, I22.-)*
> *acute coronary occlusion without myocardial infarction (I24.0)*

AHA: 2018,3Q,5
DEF: Complete blockage of the coronary artery due to plaque accumulation over an extended period of time, resulting in substantial reduction of blood flow. Symptoms include angina or chest pain.
TIP: Report this code in addition to a code from category I21 or I22 when the chronic total occlusion and the myocardial infarction are documented as being in different vessels.

I25.83   **Coronary atherosclerosis due to lipid rich plaque**   `A`
Code first coronary atherosclerosis (I25.1-, I25.7-, I25.81-)

I25.84   **Coronary atherosclerosis due to calcified coronary lesion**
Coronary atherosclerosis due to severely calcified coronary lesion
Code first coronary atherosclerosis (I25.1-, I25.7-, I25.81-)

I25.89   **Other forms of chronic ischemic heart disease**

I25.9   **Chronic ischemic heart disease, unspecified**
Ischemic heart disease (chronic) NOS

Pulmonary heart disease and diseases of pulmonary circulation (I26-I28)

✓4ᵗʰ I26 Pulmonary embolism

> **INCLUDES**   pulmonary (acute)(artery)(vein) infarction
> pulmonary (acute) (artery)(vein) thromboembolism
> pulmonary (acute)(artery)(vein) thrombosis
> **EXCLUDES 2**   *chronic pulmonary embolism (I27.82)*
> *personal history of pulmonary embolism (Z86.711)*
> *pulmonary embolism complicating abortion, ectopic or molar pregnancy (O00-O07, O08.2)*
> *pulmonary embolism complicating pregnancy, childbirth and the puerperium (O88.-)*
> *pulmonary embolism due to trauma (T79.0, T79.1)*
> *pulmonary embolism due to complications of surgical and medical care (T80.0, T81.7-, T82.8-)*
> *septic (non-pulmonary) arterial embolism (I76)*

✓5ᵗʰ I26.0   **Pulmonary embolism with acute cor pulmonale**
DEF: Cor pulmonale: Heart-lung disease appearing in identifiable forms as chronic or acute. The chronic form of this heart-lung disease is marked by dilation, hypertrophy and failure of the right ventricle due to a disease that has affected the function of the lungs, excluding congenital or left heart diseases and is also called chronic cardiopulmonary disease. The acute form is an overload of the right ventricle from a rapid onset of pulmonary hypertension, usually arising from a pulmonary embolism.

I26.01   **Septic pulmonary embolism with acute cor pulmonale**   `MCC` `HCC`
Code first underlying infection

I26.02   **Saddle embolus of pulmonary artery with acute cor pulmonale**   `MCC` `H10` `HCC`

I26.09   **Other pulmonary embolism with acute cor pulmonale**   `MCC` `H10` `HCC`
Acute cor pulmonale NOS
AHA: 2014,4Q,21

✓5ᵗʰ I26.9   **Pulmonary embolism without acute cor pulmonale**

I26.90   **Septic pulmonary embolism without acute cor pulmonale**   `MCC` `HCC`
Code first underlying infection

I26.92   **Saddle embolus of pulmonary artery without acute cor pulmonale**   `MCC` `H10` `HCC`

I26.93   **Single subsegmental pulmonary embolism without acute cor pulmonale**   `MCC` `H10` `HCC`
Subsegmental pulmonary embolism NOS
AHA: 2019,4Q,6-7

I26.94   **Multiple subsegmental pulmonary emboli without acute cor pulmonale**   `MCC` `H10` `HCC`
AHA: 2019,4Q,6-7

I26.99   **Other pulmonary embolism without acute cor pulmonale**   `MCC` `H10` `HCC`
Acute pulmonary embolism NOS
Pulmonary embolism NOS
AHA: 2019,2Q,22

✓4ᵗʰ I27 Other pulmonary heart diseases

I27.0   **Primary pulmonary hypertension**   `CC` `HCC`
Heritable pulmonary arterial hypertension
Idiopathic pulmonary arterial hypertension
Primary group 1 pulmonary hypertension
Primary pulmonary arterial hypertension

> **EXCLUDES 1**   *persistent pulmonary hypertension of newborn (P29.30)*
> *pulmonary hypertension NOS (I27.20)*
> *secondary pulmonary arterial hypertension (I27.21)*
> *secondary pulmonary hypertension (I27.29)*

DEF: Condition that occurs when pressure within the pulmonary artery is elevated and vascular resistance is observed in the lungs.

I27.1   **Kyphoscoliotic heart disease**   `CC` `HCC`

✓5ᵗʰ I27.2   **Other secondary pulmonary hypertension**
Code also associated underlying condition

> **EXCLUDES 1**   *Eisenmenger's syndrome (I27.83)*

AHA: 2017,4Q,14-15; 2014,4Q,21
DEF: Condition that occurs when pressure within the pulmonary artery is elevated and vascular resistance is observed in the lungs.

I27.20   **Pulmonary hypertension, unspecified**   `HCC`
Pulmonary hypertension NOS

I27.21   **Secondary pulmonary arterial hypertension**   `HCC`
(Associated) (drug-induced) (toxin-induced) pulmonary arterial hypertension NOS
(Associated) (drug-induced) (toxin-induced) (secondary) group 1 pulmonary hypertension
Code also associated conditions if applicable, or adverse effects of drugs or toxins, such as:
adverse effect of appetite depressants (T50.5X5)
congenital heart disease (Q20-Q28)
human immunodeficiency virus [HIV] disease (B20)
polymyositis (M33.2-)
portal hypertension (K76.6)
rheumatoid arthritis (M05.-)
schistosomiasis (B65.-)
Sjögren syndrome (M35.0-)
systemic sclerosis (M34.-)

I27.22   **Pulmonary hypertension due to left heart disease**   `HCC`
Group 2 pulmonary hypertension
Code also associated left heart disease, if known, such as:
multiple valve disease (I08.-)
rheumatic aortic valve diseases (I06.-)
rheumatic mitral valve diseases (I05.-)

I27.23   **Pulmonary hypertension due to lung diseases and hypoxia**   `HCC`
Group 3 pulmonary hypertension
Code also associated lung disease, if known, such as:
bronchiectasis (J47.-)
cystic fibrosis with pulmonary manifestations (E84.0)
interstitial lung disease (J84.-)
pleural effusion (J90)
sleep apnea (G47.3-)

I27.24   **Chronic thromboembolic pulmonary hypertension**   `HCC`
Group 4 pulmonary hypertension
Code also associated pulmonary embolism, if applicable (I26.-, I27.82)

N Newborn: 0   **P** Pediatric: 0-17   **M** Maternity: 9-64   **A** Adult: 15-124   **MCC** Major Complication/Comorbidity   **CC** Complication/Comorbidity   **SW** Severe Wound Dx

652   ICD-10-CM 2021

I27.29 Other secondary pulmonary hypertension `HCC`
Group 5 pulmonary hypertension
Pulmonary hypertension with unclear multifactorial
mechanisms
Pulmonary hypertension due to hematologic
disorders
Pulmonary hypertension due to metabolic disorders
Pulmonary hypertension due to other systemic
disorders
Code also other associated disorders, if known, such
as:
  chronic myeloid leukemia ▶(C92.10-C92.22)◀
  essential thrombocythemia (D47.3)
  Gaucher disease (E75.22)
  hypertensive chronic kidney disease with end stage
    renal disease (I12.0, I13.11, I13.2)
  hyperthyroidism (E05.-)
  hypothyroidism (E00-E03)
  polycythemia vera (D45)
  sarcoidosis (D86.-)
AHA: 2016,2Q,8

✓5ᵗʰ I27.8 Other specified pulmonary heart diseases

I27.81 Cor pulmonale (chronic) `HCC`
Cor pulmonale NOS
EXCLUDES 1   *acute cor pulmonale (I26.0-)*
AHA: 2014,4Q,21
DEF: Heart-lung disease appearing in identifiable forms
as chronic or acute. The chronic form of this heart-lung
disease is marked by dilation, hypertrophy and failure
of the right ventricle due to a disease that has affected
the function of the lungs, excluding congenital or left
heart diseases and is also called chronic
cardiopulmonary disease. The acute form is an overload
of the right ventricle from a rapid onset of pulmonary
hypertension, usually arising from a pulmonary
embolism.

I27.82 Chronic pulmonary embolism `CC` `HCC`
Use additional code, if applicable, for associated
long-term (current) use of anticoagulants
(Z79.01)
EXCLUDES 1   *personal history of pulmonary embolism
(Z86.711)*
DEF: Long-standing condition commonly associated
with pulmonary hypertension in which small blood
clots travel to the lungs repeatedly over many weeks,
months, or years, requiring continuation of established
anticoagulant or thrombolytic therapy.

I27.83 Eisenmenger's syndrome `HCC`
Eisenmenger's complex
(Irreversible) Eisenmenger's disease
Pulmonary hypertension with right to left shunt
related to congenital heart disease
Code also underlying heart defect, if known, such as:
  atrial septal defect (Q21.1)
  Eisenmenger's defect (Q21.8)
  patent ductus arteriosus (Q25.0)
  ventricular septal defect (Q21.0)
DEF: Pulmonary hypertension with congenital
communication between two circulations resulting in
a right to left shunt. This causes reduced oxygen
saturation in the arterial blood, leading to cyanosis and
organ damage. Once it develops, this life-threating
condition is irreversible.

I27.89 Other specified pulmonary heart diseases `HCC`

I27.9 Pulmonary heart disease, unspecified `HCC`
Chronic cardiopulmonary disease

✓4ᵗʰ I28 Other diseases of pulmonary vessels

I28.0 Arteriovenous fistula of pulmonary vessels `CC` `HCC`
EXCLUDES 1   *congenital arteriovenous fistula (Q25.72)*

I28.1 Aneurysm of pulmonary artery `CC` `HCC`
EXCLUDES 1   *congenital aneurysm (Q25.79)*
           congenital arteriovenous aneurysm (Q25.72)

I28.8 Other diseases of pulmonary vessels `HCC`
Pulmonary arteritis
Pulmonary endarteritis
Rupture of pulmonary vessels
Stenosis of pulmonary vessels
Stricture of pulmonary vessels

I28.9 Disease of pulmonary vessels, unspecified `HCC`

Other forms of heart disease (I30-I52)

✓4ᵗʰ I30 Acute pericarditis
INCLUDES   acute mediastinopericarditis
    acute myopericarditis
    acute pericardial effusion
    acute pleuropericarditis
    acute pneumopericarditis
EXCLUDES 1   *Dressler's syndrome (I24.1)*
    rheumatic pericarditis (acute) (I01.0)
    viral pericarditis due to Coxsakie virus (B33.23)
DEF: Pericarditis: Inflammation affecting the pericardium, the fibroserous
membrane that surrounds the heart.

I30.0 Acute nonspecific idiopathic pericarditis `CC`

I30.1 Infective pericarditis `CC`
Pneumococcal pericarditis
Pneumopyopericardium
Purulent pericarditis
Pyopericarditis
Pyopericardium
Pyopneumopericardium
Staphylococcal pericarditis
Streptococcal pericarditis
Suppurative pericarditis
Viral pericarditis
Use additional code (B95-B97) to identify infectious agent

I30.8 Other forms of acute pericarditis `CC`

I30.9 Acute pericarditis, unspecified `CC`

✓4ᵗʰ I31 Other diseases of pericardium
EXCLUDES 1   *diseases of pericardium specified as rheumatic (I09.2)*
    postcardiotomy syndrome (I97.0)
    traumatic injury to pericardium (S26.-)

I31.0 Chronic adhesive pericarditis `CC`
Accretio cordis
Adherent pericardium
Adhesive mediastinopericarditis

I31.1 Chronic constrictive pericarditis `CC`
Concretio cordis
Pericardial calcification

I31.2 Hemopericardium, not elsewhere classified `CC`
EXCLUDES 1   *hemopericardium as current complication following
acute myocardial infarction (I23.0)*
DEF: Presence of blood in the pericardial sac (pericardium). It can
lead to potentially fatal cardiac tamponade if enough blood enters
the pericardial cavity.

I31.3 Pericardial effusion (noninflammatory) `CC`
Chylopericardium
EXCLUDES 1   *acute pericardial effusion (I30.9)*
AHA: 2019,1Q,16
TIP: Assign this code for documented malignant pericardial
effusion. If the sole reason for admission is to treat the effusion
with no treatment rendered for the associated malignancy, this
code may be sequenced first.

I31.4   **Cardiac tamponade**   `CC`
Code first underlying cause
DEF: Life-threatening condition in which fluid or blood accumulates in the space between the muscle of the heart (myocardium) and the outer sac that covers the heart (pericardium), resulting in compression of the heart.

Cardiac Tamponade

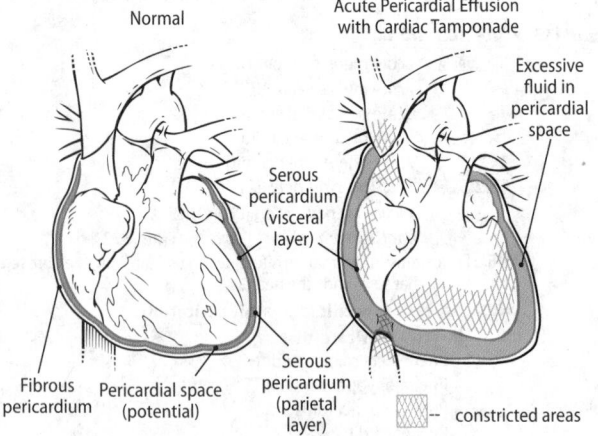

Normal   Acute Pericardial Effusion with Cardiac Tamponade

Excessive fluid in pericardial space

Serous pericardium (visceral layer)

Fibrous pericardium   Pericardial space (potential)

Serous pericardium (parietal layer)

-- constricted areas

I31.8   **Other specified diseases of pericardium**   `CC`
Epicardial plaques
Focal pericardial adhesions

I31.9   **Disease of pericardium, unspecified**   `CC`
Pericarditis (chronic) NOS

I32   *Pericarditis in diseases classified elsewhere*   `CC`
Code first underlying disease
EXCLUDES 1   *pericarditis (in):*
     coxsackie (virus) (B33.23)
     gonococcal (A54.83)
     meningococcal (A39.53)
     rheumatoid (arthritis) (M05.31)
     syphilitic (A52.06)
     systemic lupus erythematosus (M32.12)
     tuberculosis (A18.84)
DEF: Pericarditis: Inflammation affecting the pericardium, the fibroserous membrane that surrounds the heart.

✓4th **I33**   **Acute and subacute endocarditis**
EXCLUDES 1   *acute rheumatic endocarditis (I01.1)*
          endocarditis NOS (I38)
DEF: Endocarditis: Inflammatory disease of the interior lining of the heart chamber and heart valves.

I33.0   **Acute and subacute infective endocarditis**   `HIV` `MCC`
Bacterial endocarditis (acute) (subacute)
Infective endocarditis (acute) (subacute) NOS
Endocarditis lenta (acute) (subacute)
Malignant endocarditis (acute) (subacute)
Purulent endocarditis (acute) (subacute)
Septic endocarditis (acute) (subacute)
Ulcerative endocarditis (acute) (subacute)
Vegetative endocarditis (acute) (subacute)
Use additional code (B95-B97) to identify infectious agent

I33.9   **Acute and subacute endocarditis, unspecified**   `HIV` `MCC`
Acute endocarditis NOS
Acute myoendocarditis NOS
Acute periendocarditis NOS
Subacute endocarditis NOS
Subacute myoendocarditis NOS
Subacute periendocarditis NOS

✓4th **I34**   **Nonrheumatic mitral valve disorders**
EXCLUDES 1   *mitral valve disease (I05.9)*
     mitral valve failure (I05.8)
     mitral valve stenosis (I05.0)
     mitral valve disorder of unspecified cause with diseases of aortic and/or tricuspid valve(s) (I08.-)
     mitral valve disorder of unspecified cause with mitral stenosis or obstruction (I05.0)
     mitral valve disorder specified as congenital (Q23.2, Q23.9)
     mitral valve disorder specified as rheumatic (I05.-)

I34.0   **Nonrheumatic mitral (valve) insufficiency**
Nonrheumatic mitral (valve) incompetence NOS
Nonrheumatic mitral (valve) regurgitation NOS

I34.1   **Nonrheumatic mitral (valve) prolapse**
Floppy nonrheumatic mitral valve syndrome
EXCLUDES 1   *Marfan's syndrome (Q87.4-)*

I34.2   **Nonrheumatic mitral (valve) stenosis**

I34.8   **Other nonrheumatic mitral valve disorders**

I34.9   **Nonrheumatic mitral valve disorder, unspecified**

✓4th **I35**   **Nonrheumatic aortic valve disorders**
EXCLUDES 1   *aortic valve disorder of unspecified cause but with diseases of mitral and/or tricuspid valve(s) (I08.-)*
     aortic valve disorder specified as congenital (Q23.0, Q23.1)
     aortic valve disorder specified as rheumatic (I06.-)
     hypertrophic subaortic stenosis (I42.1)

I35.0   **Nonrheumatic aortic (valve) stenosis**

I35.1   **Nonrheumatic aortic (valve) insufficiency**
Nonrheumatic aortic (valve) incompetence NOS
Nonrheumatic aortic (valve) regurgitation NOS

I35.2   **Nonrheumatic aortic (valve) stenosis with insufficiency**

I35.8   **Other nonrheumatic aortic valve disorders**

I35.9   **Nonrheumatic aortic valve disorder, unspecified**

✓4th **I36**   **Nonrheumatic tricuspid valve disorders**
EXCLUDES 1   *tricuspid valve disorders of unspecified cause (I07.-)*
     tricuspid valve disorders specified as congenital (Q22.4, Q22.8, Q22.9)
     tricuspid valve disorders specified as rheumatic (I07.-)
     tricuspid valve disorders with aortic and/or mitral valve involvement (I08.-)

I36.0   **Nonrheumatic tricuspid (valve) stenosis**

I36.1   **Nonrheumatic tricuspid (valve) insufficiency**
Nonrheumatic tricuspid (valve) incompetence
Nonrheumatic tricuspid (valve) regurgitation

I36.2   **Nonrheumatic tricuspid (valve) stenosis with insufficiency**

I36.8   **Other nonrheumatic tricuspid valve disorders**

I36.9   **Nonrheumatic tricuspid valve disorder, unspecified**

✓4th **I37**   **Nonrheumatic pulmonary valve disorders**
EXCLUDES 1   *pulmonary valve disorder specified as congenital (Q22.1, Q22.2, Q22.3)*
     pulmonary valve disorder specified as rheumatic (I09.89)

I37.0   **Nonrheumatic pulmonary valve stenosis**

I37.1   **Nonrheumatic pulmonary valve insufficiency**
Nonrheumatic pulmonary valve incompetence
Nonrheumatic pulmonary valve regurgitation

I37.2   **Nonrheumatic pulmonary valve stenosis with insufficiency**

I37.8   **Other nonrheumatic pulmonary valve disorders**

I37.9   **Nonrheumatic pulmonary valve disorder, unspecified**

I38   **Endocarditis, valve unspecified**   `CC`
INCLUDES   endocarditis (chronic) NOS
     valvular incompetence NOS
     valvular insufficiency NOS
     valvular regurgitation NOS
     valvular stenosis NOS
     valvulitis (chronic) NOS
EXCLUDES 1   *congenital insufficiency of cardiac valve NOS (Q24.8)*
     congenital stenosis of cardiac valve NOS (Q24.8)
     endocardial fibroelastosis (I42.4)
     endocarditis specified as rheumatic (I09.1)
DEF: Endocarditis: Inflammatory disease of the interior lining of the heart chamber and heart valves.

I39   ***Endocarditis and heart valve disorders in diseases classified elsewhere***   `CC`

Code first underlying disease, such as:
Q fever (A78)

   `EXCLUDES 1`   *endocardial involvement in:*
       candidiasis (B37.6)
       gonococcal infection (A54.83)
       Libman-Sacks disease (M32.11)
       listerosis (A32.82)
       meningococcal infection (A39.51)
       rheumatoid arthritis (MØ5.31)
       syphilis (A52.Ø3)
       tuberculosis (A18.84)
       typhoid fever (AØ1.Ø2)

DEF: Endocarditis: Inflammatory disease of the interior lining of the heart chamber and heart valves.

`✓4ᵗʰ` **I4Ø**   **Acute myocarditis**

   `INCLUDES`   subacute myocarditis
   `EXCLUDES 1`   *acute rheumatic myocarditis (IØ1.2)*

DEF: Myocarditis: Inflammation of the middle layer of the heart, which is composed of muscle tissue.

I4Ø.Ø   **Infective myocarditis**   `HIV` `MCC`
     Septic myocarditis
     Use additional code (B95-B97) to identify infectious agent

I4Ø.1   **Isolated myocarditis**   `HIV` `MCC`
     Fiedler's myocarditis
     Giant cell myocarditis
     Idiopathic myocarditis

I4Ø.8   **Other acute myocarditis**   `HIV` `MCC`

I4Ø.9   **Acute myocarditis, unspecified**   `HIV` `MCC`

I41   ***Myocarditis in diseases classified elsewhere***   `MCC`

Code first underlying disease, such as:
typhus (A75.Ø-A75.9)

   `EXCLUDES 1`   *myocarditis (in):*
       Chagas' disease (chronic) (B57.2)
       acute (B57.Ø)
       coxsackie (virus) infection (B33.22)
       diphtheritic (A36.81)
       gonococcal (A54.83)
       influenzal (JØ9.X9, J1Ø.82, J11.82)
       meningococcal (A39.52)
       mumps (B26.82)
       rheumatoid arthritis (MØ5.31)
       sarcoid (D86.85)
       syphilis (A52.Ø6)
       toxoplasmosis (B58.81)
       tuberculous (A18.84)

DEF: Myocarditis: Inflammation of the middle layer of the heart, which is composed of muscle tissue.

`✓4ᵗʰ` **I42**   **Cardiomyopathy**

   `INCLUDES`   myocardiopathy

Code first pre-existing cardiomyopathy complicating pregnancy and puerperium (O99.4)

   `EXCLUDES 2`   *ischemic cardiomyopathy (I25.5)*
       peripartum cardiomyopathy (O9Ø.3)
       ventricular hypertrophy (I51.7)

I42.Ø   **Dilated cardiomyopathy**   `CC` `HCC`
     Congestive cardiomyopathy

I42.1   **Obstructive hypertrophic cardiomyopathy**   `CC` `HCC`
     Hypertrophic subaortic stenosis (idiopathic)
     DEF: Cardiomyopathy marked by left ventricle hypertrophy and an enlarged septum that result in obstructed blood flow, arrhythmias, mitral regurgitation, and sudden cardiac death.
     TIP: When this condition is described as inherited, assign code Q24.8.

I42.2   **Other hypertrophic cardiomyopathy**   `CC` `HCC`
     Nonobstructive hypertrophic cardiomyopathy

I42.3   **Endomyocardial (eosinophilic) disease**   `CC` `HCC`
     Endomyocardial (tropical) fibrosis
     Löffler's endocarditis

I42.4   **Endocardial fibroelastosis**   `CC` `HCC`
     Congenital cardiomyopathy
     Elastomyofibrosis

I42.5   **Other restrictive cardiomyopathy**   `CC` `HCC`
     Constrictive cardiomyopathy NOS

I42.6   **Alcoholic cardiomyopathy**   `CC` `HCC`
     Code also presence of alcoholism (F1Ø.-)

I42.7   **Cardiomyopathy due to drug and external agent**   `CC` `HCC`
     Code first poisoning due to drug or toxin, if applicable (T36-T65 with fifth or sixth character 1-4 or 6)
     Use additional code for adverse effect, if applicable, to identify drug (T36-T5Ø with fifth or sixth character 5)

I42.8   **Other cardiomyopathies**   `CC` `HCC`

I42.9   **Cardiomyopathy, unspecified**   `CC` `HCC`
     Cardiomyopathy (primary) (secondary) NOS

I43   ***Cardiomyopathy in diseases classified elsewhere***   `CC` `HCC`

Code first underlying disease, such as:
amyloidosis (E85.-)
glycogen storage disease (E74.Ø)
gout (M1Ø.Ø-)
thyrotoxicosis (EØ5.Ø-EØ5.9-)

   `EXCLUDES 1`   *cardiomyopathy (in):*
       coxsackie (virus) (B33.24)
       diphtheria (A36.81)
       sarcoidosis (D86.85)
       tuberculosis (A18.84)

`✓4ᵗʰ` **I44**   **Atrioventricular and left bundle-branch block**

I44.Ø   **Atrioventricular block, first degree**

I44.1   **Atrioventricular block, second degree**
     Atrioventricular block, type I and II
     Möbitz block, type I and II
     Second degree block, type I and II
     Wenckebach's block

I44.2   **Atrioventricular block, complete**   `CC` `HCC`
     Complete heart block NOS
     Third degree block
     AHA: 2019,2Q,4

`✓5ᵗʰ` **I44.3**   **Other and unspecified atrioventricular block**
     Atrioventricular block NOS

     I44.3Ø   **Unspecified atrioventricular block**
     I44.39   **Other atrioventricular block**

I44.4   **Left anterior fascicular block**

I44.5   **Left posterior fascicular block**

`✓5ᵗʰ` **I44.6**   **Other and unspecified fascicular block**

     I44.6Ø   **Unspecified fascicular block**
         Left bundle-branch hemiblock NOS

     I44.69   **Other fascicular block**

I44.7   **Left bundle-branch block, unspecified**

Conduction Disorders

`✓4ᵗʰ` **I45**   **Other conduction disorders**

I45.Ø   **Right fascicular block**

☑ Additional Character Required   `✓x7ᵗʰ` Placeholder   Unacceptable PDx   Questionable PDx   Manifestation   Unspecified Dx   `H1`-`H14` HAC   `HCC` CMS-HCC Dx   `HIV` HIV Dx

ICD-10-CM 2021   **655**

Chapter 9. Diseases of the Circulatory System

I45.1–I49.9

✓6th **I45.1** **Other and unspecified right bundle-branch block**

     I45.10 **Unspecified right bundle-branch block**
         Right bundle-branch block NOS

     I45.19 **Other right bundle-branch block**

I45.2 **Bifascicular block** `CC`

I45.3 **Trifascicular block** `CC`

I45.4 **Nonspecific intraventricular block**
     Bundle-branch block NOS

I45.5 **Other specified heart block**
     Sinoatrial block
     Sinoauricular block
     `EXCLUDES 1` *heart block NOS (I45.9)*

I45.6 **Pre-excitation syndrome**
     Accelerated atrioventricular conduction
     Accessory atrioventricular conduction
     Anomalous atrioventricular excitation
     Lown-Ganong-Levine syndrome
     Pre-excitation atrioventricular conduction
     Wolff-Parkinson-White syndrome

✓5th **I45.8** **Other specified conduction disorders**

     I45.81 **Long QT syndrome**
         DEF: Condition characterized by recurrent syncope, malignant arrhythmias, and sudden death. This syndrome has a characteristic prolonged Q-T interval on an electrocardiogram.

     I45.89 **Other specified conduction disorders** `CC`
         Atrioventricular [AV] dissociation
         Interference dissociation
         Isorhythmic dissociation
         Nonparoxysmal AV nodal tachycardia
         AHA: 2013,2Q,31

I45.9 **Conduction disorder, unspecified**
     Heart block NOS
     Stokes-Adams syndrome

✓4th **I46** **Cardiac arrest**
     `EXCLUDES 1` *cardiogenic shock (R57.0)*
     `EXCLUDES 2` ▶*cardiogenic shock (R57.0)*◀
     AHA: 2019,2Q,4-5

I46.2 **Cardiac arrest due to underlying cardiac condition** `MCC` `HCC`
     Code first underlying cardiac condition

I46.8 **Cardiac arrest due to other underlying condition** `MCC` `HCC`
     Code first underlying condition

I46.9 **Cardiac arrest, cause unspecified** `MCC` `HCC`

✓4th **I47** **Paroxysmal tachycardia**
     Code first tachycardia complicating:
         abortion or ectopic or molar pregnancy (O00-O07, O08.8)
         obstetric surgery and procedures (O75.4)
     `EXCLUDES 1` *tachycardia NOS (R00.0)*
         sinoauricular tachycardia NOS (R00.0)
         sinus [sinusal] tachycardia NOS (R00.0)

I47.0 **Re-entry ventricular arrhythmia** `CC` `HCC`

I47.1 **Supraventricular tachycardia** `CC` `HCC`
     Atrial (paroxysmal) tachycardia
     Atrioventricular [AV] (paroxysmal) tachycardia
     Atrioventricular re-entrant (nodal) tachycardia [AVNRT] [AVRT]
     Junctional (paroxysmal) tachycardia
     Nodal (paroxysmal) tachycardia

I47.2 **Ventricular tachycardia** `CC` `HCC`
     AHA: 2013,3Q,23

I47.9 **Paroxysmal tachycardia, unspecified** `HCC`
     Bouveret (-Hoffman) syndrome

✓4th **I48** **Atrial fibrillation and flutter**

I48.0 **Paroxysmal atrial fibrillation** `HCC`
     AHA: 2018,3Q,6

✓5th **I48.1** **Persistent atrial fibrillation**
     `EXCLUDES 1` *permanent atrial fibrillation (I48.21)*
     AHA: 2019,4Q,7; 2019,2Q,3; 2018,3Q,6

     I48.11 **Longstanding persistent atrial fibrillation** `CC` `HCC`

     I48.19 **Other persistent atrial fibrillation** `CC` `HCC`
         Chronic persistent atrial fibrillation
         Persistent atrial fibrillation, NOS
         AHA: 2019,4Q,7

✓5th **I48.2** **Chronic atrial fibrillation**
     AHA: 2019,4Q,7; 2019,2Q,3; 2018,3Q,6

     I48.20 **Chronic atrial fibrillation, unspecified** `CC` `HCC`
         `EXCLUDES 1` *chronic persistent atrial fibrillation (I48.19)*

     I48.21 **Permanent atrial fibrillation** `CC` `HCC`

I48.3 **Typical atrial flutter** `CC` `HCC`
     Type I atrial flutter

I48.4 **Atypical atrial flutter** `CC` `HCC`
     Type II atrial flutter

✓5th **I48.9** **Unspecified atrial fibrillation and atrial flutter**

     I48.91 **Unspecified atrial fibrillation** `HCC`

     I48.92 **Unspecified atrial flutter** `CC` `HCC`

✓4th **I49** **Other cardiac arrhythmias**
     Code first cardiac arrhythmia complicating:
         abortion or ectopic or molar pregnancy (O00-O07, O08.8)
         obstetric surgery and procedures (O75.4)
     `EXCLUDES 1` *neonatal dysrhythmia (P29.1-)*
         sinoatrial bradycardia (R00.1)
         sinus bradycardia (R00.1)
         vagal bradycardia (R00.1)
     `EXCLUDES 2` *bradycardia NOS (R00.1)*

✓5th **I49.0** **Ventricular fibrillation and flutter**

     I49.01 **Ventricular fibrillation** `MCC` `HCC`

     I49.02 **Ventricular flutter** `MCC` `HCC`

I49.1 **Atrial premature depolarization**
     Atrial premature beats

I49.2 **Junctional premature depolarization** `CC` `HCC`

I49.3 **Ventricular premature depolarization**
     AHA: 2020,2Q,23

✓5th **I49.4** **Other and unspecified premature depolarization**

     I49.40 **Unspecified premature depolarization**
         Premature beats NOS

     I49.49 **Other premature depolarization**
         Ectopic beats
         Extrasystoles
         Extrasystolic arrhythmias
         Premature contractions

I49.5 **Sick sinus syndrome** `HCC`
     Tachycardia-bradycardia syndrome
     AHA: 2019,1Q,33
     TIP: The presence of a pacemaker controls but does not cure sick sinus syndrome and therefore is considered a reportable chronic condition. When a pacemaker is evaluated by a provider, this code and code Z95.0 Presence of cardiac pacemaker, should be reported, even in the absence of any notable changes or management.

I49.8 **Other specified cardiac arrhythmias**
     Brugada syndrome
     Coronary sinus rhythm disorder
     Ectopic rhythm disorder
     Nodal rhythm disorder

I49.9 **Cardiac arrhythmia, unspecified**
     Arrhythmia (cardiac) NOS

`N` Newborn: 0   `P` Pediatric: 0-17   `M` Maternity: 9-64   `A` Adult: 15-124   `MCC` Major Complication/Comorbidity   `CC` Complication/Comorbidity   `SW` Severe Wound Dx

656   ICD-10-CM 2021

✓4ᵗʰ **I50 Heart failure**

Code first:

heart failure complicating abortion or ectopic or molar pregnancy (O00–O07, O08.8)

heart failure due to hypertension (I11.0)

heart failure due to hypertension with chronic kidney disease (I13.-)

heart failure following surgery (I97.13-)

obstetric surgery and procedures (O75.4)

rheumatic heart failure (I09.81)

EXCLUDES 1 *neonatal cardiac failure (P29.0)*

EXCLUDES 2 *cardiac arrest (I46.-)*

AHA: 2018,4Q,67; 2018,2Q,9; 2017,1Q,47; 2014,1Q,25; 2013,2Q,33

I50.1 Left ventricular failure, unspecified   CC HCC

Cardiac asthma

Edema of lung with heart disease NOS

Edema of lung with heart failure

Left heart failure

Pulmonary edema with heart disease NOS

Pulmonary edema with heart failure

EXCLUDES 1 *edema of lung without heart disease or heart failure (J81.-)*

pulmonary edema without heart disease or failure (J81.-)

✓5ᵗʰ **I50.2 Systolic (congestive) heart failure**

Heart failure with reduced ejection fraction [HFrEF]

Systolic left ventricular heart failure

Code also end stage heart failure, if applicable (I50.84)

EXCLUDES 1 *combined systolic (congestive) and diastolic (congestive) heart failure (I50.4-)*

AHA: 2017,1Q,46; 2016,1Q,10

I50.20 Unspecified systolic (congestive) heart failure   CC HCC

I50.21 Acute systolic (congestive) heart failure   MCC HCC

I50.22 Chronic systolic (congestive) heart failure   CC HCC

I50.23 Acute on chronic systolic (congestive) heart failure   MCC HCC

✓5ᵗʰ **I50.3 Diastolic (congestive) heart failure**

Diastolic left ventricular heart failure

Heart failure with normal ejection fraction

Heart failure with preserved ejection fraction [HFpEF]

Code also end stage heart failure, if applicable (I50.84)

EXCLUDES 1 *combined systolic (congestive) and diastolic (congestive) heart failure (I50.4-)*

AHA: 2017,1Q,46; 2016,1Q,10

I50.30 Unspecified diastolic (congestive) heart failure   CC HCC

I50.31 Acute diastolic (congestive) heart failure   MCC HCC

I50.32 Chronic diastolic (congestive) heart failure   CC HCC

I50.33 Acute on chronic diastolic (congestive) heart failure   MCC HCC

✓5ᵗʰ **I50.4 Combined systolic (congestive) and diastolic (congestive) heart failure**

Combined systolic and diastolic left ventricular heart failure

Heart failure with reduced ejection fraction and diastolic dysfunction

Code also end stage heart failure, if applicable (I50.84)

AHA: 2017,1Q,46; 2016,1Q,10

I50.40 Unspecified combined systolic (congestive) and diastolic (congestive) heart failure   CC HCC

I50.41 Acute combined systolic (congestive) and diastolic (congestive) heart failure   MCC HCC

I50.42 Chronic combined systolic (congestive) and diastolic (congestive) heart failure   CC HCC

I50.43 Acute on chronic combined systolic (congestive) and diastolic (congestive) heart failure   MCC HCC

✓5ᵗʰ **I50.8 Other heart failure**

AHA: 2017,4Q,15-16

✓6ᵗʰ **I50.81 Right heart failure**

Right ventricular failure

I50.810 Right heart failure, unspecified   HCC

Right heart failure without mention of left heart failure

Right ventricular failure NOS

I50.811 Acute right heart failure   HCC

Acute isolated right heart failure

Acute (isolated) right ventricular failure

I50.812 Chronic right heart failure   HCC

Chronic isolated right heart failure

Chronic (isolated) right ventricular failure

I50.813 Acute on chronic right heart failure   HCC

Acute on chronic isolated right heart failure

Acute on chronic (isolated) right ventricular failure

Acute decompensation of chronic (isolated) right ventricular failure

Acute exacerbation of chronic (isolated) right ventricular failure

I50.814 Right heart failure due to left heart failure   HCC

Right ventricular failure secondary to left ventricular failure

Code also the type of left ventricular failure, if known (I50.2-I50.43)

EXCLUDES 1 *right heart failure with but not due to left heart failure (I50.82)*

I50.82 Biventricular heart failure   HCC

Code also the type of left ventricular failure as systolic, diastolic, or combined, if known (I50.2-I50.43)

I50.83 High output heart failure

DEF: Occurs when the high demand for blood exceeds the capacity of a normally functioning heart to meet the demand.

I50.84 End stage heart failure   HCC

Stage D heart failure

Code also the type of heart failure as systolic, diastolic, or combined, if known (I50.2-I50.43)

I50.89 Other heart failure   HCC

I50.9 Heart failure, unspecified   HCC

Cardiac, heart or myocardial failure NOS

Congestive heart disease

Congestive heart failure NOS

EXCLUDES 2 *fluid overload unrelated to congestive heart failure (E87.70)*

AHA: 2017,4Q,15-16; 2017,1Q,45-46; 2014,4Q,21; 2012,4Q,92

✓4ᵗʰ **I51 Complications and ill-defined descriptions of heart disease**

EXCLUDES 1 *any condition in I51.4-I51.9 due to hypertension (I11.-)*

any condition in I51.4-I51.9 due to hypertension and chronic kidney disease (I13.-)

heart disease specified as rheumatic (I00-I09)

I51.0 Cardiac septal defect, acquired   CC A

Acquired septal atrial defect (old)

Acquired septal auricular defect (old)

Acquired septal ventricular defect (old)

EXCLUDES 1 *cardiac septal defect as current complication following acute myocardial infarction (I23.1, I23.2)*

DEF: Abnormal communication between opposite heart chambers due to a defect of the septum. It is not present at birth.

I51.1 Rupture of chordae tendineae, not elsewhere classified   MCC HCC

EXCLUDES 1 *rupture of chordae tendineae as current complication following acute myocardial infarction (I23.4)*

I51.2 Rupture of papillary muscle, not elsewhere classified   MCC HCC

EXCLUDES 1 *rupture of papillary muscle as current complication following acute myocardial infarction (I23.5)*

I51.3 Intracardiac thrombosis, not elsewhere classified

Apical thrombosis (old)

Atrial thrombosis (old)

Auricular thrombosis (old)

Mural thrombosis (old)

Ventricular thrombosis (old)

EXCLUDES 1 *intracardiac thrombosis as current complication following acute myocardial infarction (I23.6)*

AHA: 2013,1Q,24

✓ Additional Character Required   ✓x7ᵗʰ Placeholder   Unacceptable PDx   Questionable PDx   Manifestation   Unspecified Dx   H1-H14 HAC   HCC CMS-HCC Dx   HIV HIV Dx

Chapter 9. Diseases of the Circulatory System

I51.4 Myocarditis, unspecified `HCC`
Chronic (interstitial) myocarditis
Myocardial fibrosis
Myocarditis NOS
> `EXCLUDES 1` *acute or subacute myocarditis (I40.-)*
AHA: 2018,4Q,67; 2018,2Q,9

I51.5 Myocardial degeneration `HCC`
Fatty degeneration of heart or myocardium
Myocardial disease
Senile degeneration of heart or myocardium
AHA: 2018,4Q,67; 2018,2Q,9

I51.7 Cardiomegaly
Cardiac dilatation
Cardiac hypertrophy
Ventricular dilatation
AHA: 2018,4Q,67; 2018,2Q,9

✓5ᵗʰ **I51.8 Other ill-defined heart diseases**
AHA: 2018,2Q,9

I51.81 Takotsubo syndrome `CC`
Reversible left ventricular dysfunction following sudden emotional stress
Stress induced cardiomyopathy
Takotsubo cardiomyopathy
Transient left ventricular apical ballooning syndrome
DEF: Complex of symptoms mimicking myocardial infarct in absence of heart disease, with the majority of cases occurring in postmenopausal women. Heart muscles are temporarily weakened, and a sudden, massive surge of adrenalin stuns the heart, greatly reducing the ability to pump blood.

I51.89 Other ill-defined heart diseases
Carditis (acute)(chronic)
Pancarditis (acute)(chronic)
AHA: 2019,2Q,5; 2018,4Q,67

I51.9 Heart disease, unspecified
AHA: 2018,4Q,67; 2018,2Q,9

I52 Other heart disorders in diseases classified elsewhere
Code first underlying disease, such as:
congenital syphilis (A50.5)
mucopolysaccharidosis (E76.3)
schistosomiasis (B65.0-B65.9)
> `EXCLUDES 1` *heart disease (in):*
> *gonococcal infection (A54.83)*
> *meningococcal infection (A39.50)*
> *rheumatoid arthritis (M05.31)*
> *syphilis (A52.06)*

Cerebrovascular diseases (I60-I69)

Use additional code to identify presence of:
alcohol abuse and dependence (F10.-)
exposure to environmental tobacco smoke (Z77.22)
history of tobacco dependence (Z87.891)
hypertension (I10-I16)
occupational exposure to environmental tobacco smoke (Z57.31)
tobacco dependence (F17.-)
tobacco use (Z72.0)
> `EXCLUDES 1` *traumatic intracranial hemorrhage (S06.-)*
AHA: 2014,3Q,5; 2012,4Q,91-92

✓4ᵗʰ **I60 Nontraumatic subarachnoid hemorrhage**
> `EXCLUDES 1` *syphilitic ruptured cerebral aneurysm (A52.05)*
> `EXCLUDES 2` *sequelae of subarachnoid hemorrhage (I69.0-)*

✓5ᵗʰ **I60.0 Nontraumatic subarachnoid hemorrhage from carotid siphon and bifurcation**

I60.00 Nontraumatic subarachnoid hemorrhage from unspecified carotid siphon and bifurcation `MCC` `HCC`

I60.01 Nontraumatic subarachnoid hemorrhage from right carotid siphon and bifurcation `MCC` `HCC`

I60.02 Nontraumatic subarachnoid hemorrhage from left carotid siphon and bifurcation `MCC` `HCC`

✓5ᵗʰ **I60.1 Nontraumatic subarachnoid hemorrhage from middle cerebral artery**

I60.10 Nontraumatic subarachnoid hemorrhage from unspecified middle cerebral artery `MCC` `HCC`

I60.11 Nontraumatic subarachnoid hemorrhage from right middle cerebral artery `MCC` `HCC`

I60.12 Nontraumatic subarachnoid hemorrhage from left middle cerebral artery `MCC` `HCC`

I60.2 Nontraumatic subarachnoid hemorrhage from anterior communicating artery `MCC` `HCC`

✓5ᵗʰ **I60.3 Nontraumatic subarachnoid hemorrhage from posterior communicating artery**

I60.30 Nontraumatic subarachnoid hemorrhage from unspecified posterior communicating artery `MCC` `HCC`

I60.31 Nontraumatic subarachnoid hemorrhage from right posterior communicating artery `MCC` `HCC`

I60.32 Nontraumatic subarachnoid hemorrhage from left posterior communicating artery `MCC` `HCC`

I60.4 Nontraumatic subarachnoid hemorrhage from basilar artery `MCC` `HCC`

✓5ᵗʰ **I60.5 Nontraumatic subarachnoid hemorrhage from vertebral artery**

I60.50 Nontraumatic subarachnoid hemorrhage from unspecified vertebral artery `MCC` `HCC`

I60.51 Nontraumatic subarachnoid hemorrhage from right vertebral artery `MCC` `HCC`

I60.52 Nontraumatic subarachnoid hemorrhage from left vertebral artery `MCC` `HCC`

I60.6 Nontraumatic subarachnoid hemorrhage from other intracranial arteries `MCC` `HCC`

I60.7 Nontraumatic subarachnoid hemorrhage from unspecified intracranial artery `MCC` `HCC`
Ruptured (congenital) berry aneurysm
Ruptured (congenital) cerebral aneurysm
Subarachnoid hemorrhage (nontraumatic) from cerebral artery NOS
Subarachnoid hemorrhage (nontraumatic) from communicating artery NOS
> `EXCLUDES 1` *berry aneurysm, nonruptured (I67.1)*

I60.8 Other nontraumatic subarachnoid hemorrhage `MCC` `HCC`
Meningeal hemorrhage
Rupture of cerebral arteriovenous malformation

I60.9 Nontraumatic subarachnoid hemorrhage, unspecified `MCC` `HCC`

✓4ᵗʰ **I61 Nontraumatic intracerebral hemorrhage**
> `EXCLUDES 2` *sequelae of intracerebral hemorrhage (I69.1-)*
AHA: 2017,2Q,9-10

I61.0 Nontraumatic intracerebral hemorrhage in hemisphere, subcortical `MCC` `HCC`
Deep intracerebral hemorrhage (nontraumatic)
AHA: 2016,4Q,27

I61.1 Nontraumatic intracerebral hemorrhage in hemisphere, cortical `MCC` `HCC`
Cerebral lobe hemorrhage (nontraumatic)
Superficial intracerebral hemorrhage (nontraumatic)

I61.2 Nontraumatic intracerebral hemorrhage in hemisphere, unspecified `MCC` `HCC`

I61.3 Nontraumatic intracerebral hemorrhage in brain stem `MCC` `HCC`

I61.4 Nontraumatic intracerebral hemorrhage in cerebellum `MCC` `HCC`

I61.5 Nontraumatic intracerebral hemorrhage, intraventricular `MCC` `HCC`

I61.6 Nontraumatic intracerebral hemorrhage, multiple localized `MCC` `HCC`

I61.8 Other nontraumatic intracerebral hemorrhage `MCC` `HCC`

I61.9 Nontraumatic intracerebral hemorrhage, unspecified `MCC` `HCC`

✓4ᵗʰ **I62 Other and unspecified nontraumatic intracranial hemorrhage**
> `EXCLUDES 2` *sequelae of intracranial hemorrhage (I69.2)*

✓5ᵗʰ **I62.0 Nontraumatic subdural hemorrhage**

I62.00 Nontraumatic subdural hemorrhage, unspecified `MCC` `HCC`

I62.01 Nontraumatic acute subdural hemorrhage `MCC` `HCC`

I62.02 Nontraumatic subacute subdural hemorrhage `MCC` `HCC`

I62.03 Nontraumatic chronic subdural hemorrhage `MCC` `HCC`

I62.1 Nontraumatic extradural hemorrhage `MCC` `HCC`
Nontraumatic epidural hemorrhage

I62.9 Nontraumatic intracranial hemorrhage, unspecified `CC` `HCC`

`N` Newborn: 0   `P` Pediatric: 0-17   `M` Maternity: 9-64   `A` Adult: 15-124   `MCC` Major Complication/Comorbidity   `CC` Complication/Comorbidity   `SW` Severe Wound Dx

658   ICD-10-CM 2021

√4ᵗʰ I63 Cerebral infarction

    INCLUDES   occlusion and stenosis of cerebral and precerebral arteries, resulting in cerebral infarction

    Use additional code, if applicable, to identify status post administration of tPA (rtPA) in a different facility within the last 24 hours prior to admission to current facility (Z92.82)

    Use additional code, if known, to indicate National Institutes of Health Stroke Scale (NIHSS) score (R29.7-)

    EXCLUDES 1   ▶neonatal cerebral infarction (P91.82-)◀

    EXCLUDES 2   sequelae of cerebral infarction (I69.3-)

    AHA: 2017,2Q,9-10; 2016,4Q,28,61-62; 2014,1Q,23

    TIP: Weakness on one side of the body documented as secondary to stroke is synonymous with hemiparesis/hemiplegia (G81.-). Weakness of one limb documented as secondary to stroke is synonymous with monoplegia (G83.1-, G83.2-, G83.3-).

  √5ᵗʰ I63.0 Cerebral infarction due to thrombosis of precerebral arteries

    I63.00 Cerebral infarction due to thrombosis of unspecified precerebral artery   MCC HCC

    √6ᵗʰ I63.01 Cerebral infarction due to thrombosis of vertebral artery

        I63.011 Cerebral infarction due to thrombosis of right vertebral artery   MCC HCC

        I63.012 Cerebral infarction due to thrombosis of left vertebral artery   MCC HCC

        I63.013 Cerebral infarction due to thrombosis of bilateral vertebral arteries   MCC HCC

        I63.019 Cerebral infarction due to thrombosis of unspecified vertebral artery   MCC HCC

    I63.02 Cerebral infarction due to thrombosis of basilar artery   MCC HCC

    √6ᵗʰ I63.03 Cerebral infarction due to thrombosis of carotid artery

        I63.031 Cerebral infarction due to thrombosis of right carotid artery   MCC HCC

        I63.032 Cerebral infarction due to thrombosis of left carotid artery   MCC HCC

        I63.033 Cerebral infarction due to thrombosis of bilateral carotid arteries   MCC HCC

        I63.039 Cerebral infarction due to thrombosis of unspecified carotid artery   MCC HCC

    I63.09 Cerebral infarction due to thrombosis of other precerebral artery   MCC HCC

  √5ᵗʰ I63.1 Cerebral infarction due to embolism of precerebral arteries

    I63.10 Cerebral infarction due to embolism of unspecified precerebral artery   MCC HCC

    √6ᵗʰ I63.11 Cerebral infarction due to embolism of vertebral artery

        I63.111 Cerebral infarction due to embolism of right vertebral artery   MCC HCC

        I63.112 Cerebral infarction due to embolism of left vertebral artery   MCC HCC

        I63.113 Cerebral infarction due to embolism of bilateral vertebral arteries   MCC HCC

        I63.119 Cerebral infarction due to embolism of unspecified vertebral artery   MCC HCC

    I63.12 Cerebral infarction due to embolism of basilar artery   MCC HCC

    √6ᵗʰ I63.13 Cerebral infarction due to embolism of carotid artery

        I63.131 Cerebral infarction due to embolism of right carotid artery   MCC HCC

        I63.132 Cerebral infarction due to embolism of left carotid artery   MCC HCC

        I63.133 Cerebral infarction due to embolism of bilateral carotid arteries   MCC HCC

        I63.139 Cerebral infarction due to embolism of unspecified carotid artery   MCC HCC

    I63.19 Cerebral infarction due to embolism of other precerebral artery   MCC HCC

  √5ᵗʰ I63.2 Cerebral infarction due to unspecified occlusion or stenosis of precerebral arteries

    I63.20 Cerebral infarction due to unspecified occlusion or stenosis of unspecified precerebral arteries   MCC HCC

    √6ᵗʰ I63.21 Cerebral infarction due to unspecified occlusion or stenosis of vertebral arteries

        I63.211 Cerebral infarction due to unspecified occlusion or stenosis of right vertebral artery   MCC HCC

        I63.212 Cerebral infarction due to unspecified occlusion or stenosis of left vertebral artery   MCC HCC

        I63.213 Cerebral infarction due to unspecified occlusion or stenosis of bilateral vertebral arteries   MCC HCC

        I63.219 Cerebral infarction due to unspecified occlusion or stenosis of unspecified vertebral artery   MCC HCC

    I63.22 Cerebral infarction due to unspecified occlusion or stenosis of basilar artery   MCC HCC

    √6ᵗʰ I63.23 Cerebral infarction due to unspecified occlusion or stenosis of carotid arteries

        I63.231 Cerebral infarction due to unspecified occlusion or stenosis of right carotid arteries   MCC HCC

        I63.232 Cerebral infarction due to unspecified occlusion or stenosis of left carotid arteries   MCC HCC

        I63.233 Cerebral infarction due to unspecified occlusion or stenosis of bilateral carotid arteries   MCC HCC

        I63.239 Cerebral infarction due to unspecified occlusion or stenosis of unspecified carotid artery   MCC HCC

    I63.29 Cerebral infarction due to unspecified occlusion or stenosis of other precerebral arteries   MCC HCC

  √5ᵗʰ I63.3 Cerebral infarction due to thrombosis of cerebral arteries

    I63.30 Cerebral infarction due to thrombosis of unspecified cerebral artery   MCC HCC

    √6ᵗʰ I63.31 Cerebral infarction due to thrombosis of middle cerebral artery

        I63.311 Cerebral infarction due to thrombosis of right middle cerebral artery   MCC HCC

        I63.312 Cerebral infarction due to thrombosis of left middle cerebral artery   MCC HCC

        I63.313 Cerebral infarction due to thrombosis of bilateral middle cerebral arteries   MCC HCC

        I63.319 Cerebral infarction due to thrombosis of unspecified middle cerebral artery   MCC HCC

    √6ᵗʰ I63.32 Cerebral infarction due to thrombosis of anterior cerebral artery

        I63.321 Cerebral infarction due to thrombosis of right anterior cerebral artery   MCC HCC

        I63.322 Cerebral infarction due to thrombosis of left anterior cerebral artery   MCC HCC

        I63.323 Cerebral infarction due to thrombosis of bilateral anterior cerebral arteries   MCC HCC

        I63.329 Cerebral infarction due to thrombosis of unspecified anterior cerebral artery   MCC HCC

    √6ᵗʰ I63.33 Cerebral infarction due to thrombosis of posterior cerebral artery

        I63.331 Cerebral infarction due to thrombosis of right posterior cerebral artery   MCC HCC

        I63.332 Cerebral infarction due to thrombosis of left posterior cerebral artery   MCC HCC

        I63.333 Cerebral infarction due to thrombosis of bilateral posterior cerebral arteries   MCC HCC

        I63.339 Cerebral infarction due to thrombosis of unspecified posterior cerebral artery   MCC HCC

    √6ᵗʰ I63.34 Cerebral infarction due to thrombosis of cerebellar artery

        I63.341 Cerebral infarction due to thrombosis of right cerebellar artery   MCC HCC

        I63.342 Cerebral infarction due to thrombosis of left cerebellar artery   MCC HCC

        I63.343 Cerebral infarction due to thrombosis of bilateral cerebellar arteries   MCC HCC

        I63.349 Cerebral infarction due to thrombosis of unspecified cerebellar artery   MCC HCC

    I63.39 Cerebral infarction due to thrombosis of other cerebral artery   MCC HCC

  √5ᵗʰ I63.4 Cerebral infarction due to embolism of cerebral arteries

    I63.40 Cerebral infarction due to embolism of unspecified cerebral artery   MCC HCC

☑ Additional Character Required   √x7ᵗʰ Placeholder   Unacceptable PDx   Questionable PDx   Manifestation   Unspecified Dx   **H1**-**H14** HAC   **HCC** CMS-HCC Dx   **HIV** HIV Dx

ICD-10-CM 2021   659

Chapter 9. Diseases of the Circulatory System

✓6ᵗʰ **I63.41**   **Cerebral infarction due to embolism of middle cerebral artery**

     I63.411   **Cerebral infarction due to embolism of right middle cerebral artery** `MCC` `HCC`

     I63.412   **Cerebral infarction due to embolism of left middle cerebral artery** `MCC` `HCC`

     I63.413   **Cerebral infarction due to embolism of bilateral middle cerebral arteries** `MCC` `HCC`

     I63.419   **Cerebral infarction due to embolism of unspecified middle cerebral artery** `MCC` `HCC`

✓6ᵗʰ **I63.42**   **Cerebral infarction due to embolism of anterior cerebral artery**

     I63.421   **Cerebral infarction due to embolism of right anterior cerebral artery** `MCC` `HCC`

     I63.422   **Cerebral infarction due to embolism of left anterior cerebral artery** `MCC` `HCC`

     I63.423   **Cerebral infarction due to embolism of bilateral anterior cerebral arteries** `MCC` `HCC`

     I63.429   **Cerebral infarction due to embolism of unspecified anterior cerebral artery** `MCC` `HCC`

✓6ᵗʰ **I63.43**   **Cerebral infarction due to embolism of posterior cerebral artery**

     I63.431   **Cerebral infarction due to embolism of right posterior cerebral artery** `MCC` `HCC`

     I63.432   **Cerebral infarction due to embolism of left posterior cerebral artery** `MCC` `HCC`

     I63.433   **Cerebral infarction due to embolism of bilateral posterior cerebral arteries** `MCC` `HCC`

     I63.439   **Cerebral infarction due to embolism of unspecified posterior cerebral artery** `MCC` `HCC`

✓6ᵗʰ **I63.44**   **Cerebral infarction due to embolism of cerebellar artery**

     I63.441   **Cerebral infarction due to embolism of right cerebellar artery** `MCC` `HCC`

     I63.442   **Cerebral infarction due to embolism of left cerebellar artery** `MCC` `HCC`

     I63.443   **Cerebral infarction due to embolism of bilateral cerebellar arteries** `MCC` `HCC`

     I63.449   **Cerebral infarction due to embolism of unspecified cerebellar artery** `MCC` `HCC`

     I63.49   **Cerebral infarction due to embolism of other cerebral artery** `MCC` `HCC`

✓5ᵗʰ **I63.5**   **Cerebral infarction due to unspecified occlusion or stenosis of cerebral arteries**

     I63.50   **Cerebral infarction due to unspecified occlusion or stenosis of unspecified cerebral artery** `MCC` `HCC`

✓6ᵗʰ **I63.51**   **Cerebral infarction due to unspecified occlusion or stenosis of middle cerebral artery**

     I63.511   **Cerebral infarction due to unspecified occlusion or stenosis of right middle cerebral artery** `MCC` `HCC`

     I63.512   **Cerebral infarction due to unspecified occlusion or stenosis of left middle cerebral artery** `MCC` `HCC`

     I63.513   **Cerebral infarction due to unspecified occlusion or stenosis of bilateral middle cerebral arteries** `MCC` `HCC`

     I63.519   **Cerebral infarction due to unspecified occlusion or stenosis of unspecified middle cerebral artery** `MCC` `HCC`

✓6ᵗʰ **I63.52**   **Cerebral infarction due to unspecified occlusion or stenosis of anterior cerebral artery**

     I63.521   **Cerebral infarction due to unspecified occlusion or stenosis of right anterior cerebral artery** `MCC` `HCC`

     I63.522   **Cerebral infarction due to unspecified occlusion or stenosis of left anterior cerebral artery** `MCC` `HCC`

     I63.523   **Cerebral infarction due to unspecified occlusion or stenosis of bilateral anterior cerebral arteries** `MCC` `HCC`

     I63.529   **Cerebral infarction due to unspecified occlusion or stenosis of unspecified anterior cerebral artery** `MCC` `HCC`

✓6ᵗʰ **I63.53**   **Cerebral infarction due to unspecified occlusion or stenosis of posterior cerebral artery**

     I63.531   **Cerebral infarction due to unspecified occlusion or stenosis of right posterior cerebral artery** `MCC` `HCC`

     I63.532   **Cerebral infarction due to unspecified occlusion or stenosis of left posterior cerebral artery** `MCC` `HCC`

     I63.533   **Cerebral infarction due to unspecified occlusion or stenosis of bilateral posterior cerebral arteries** `MCC` `HCC`

     I63.539   **Cerebral infarction due to unspecified occlusion or stenosis of unspecified posterior cerebral artery** `MCC` `HCC`

✓6ᵗʰ **I63.54**   **Cerebral infarction due to unspecified occlusion or stenosis of cerebellar artery**

     I63.541   **Cerebral infarction due to unspecified occlusion or stenosis of right cerebellar artery** `MCC` `HCC`

     I63.542   **Cerebral infarction due to unspecified occlusion or stenosis of left cerebellar artery** `MCC` `HCC`

     I63.543   **Cerebral infarction due to unspecified occlusion or stenosis of bilateral cerebellar arteries** `MCC` `HCC`

     I63.549   **Cerebral infarction due to unspecified occlusion or stenosis of unspecified cerebellar artery** `MCC` `HCC`

     I63.59   **Cerebral infarction due to unspecified occlusion or stenosis of other cerebral artery** `MCC` `HCC`

I63.6   **Cerebral infarction due to cerebral venous thrombosis, nonpyogenic** `MCC` `HCC`

✓5ᵗʰ **I63.8**   **Other cerebral infarction**

     AHA: 2018,4Q,16

     I63.81   **Other cerebral infarction due to occlusion or stenosis of small artery** `MCC` `HCC`
           Lacunar infarction

     I63.89   **Other cerebral infarction** `MCC` `HCC`

I63.9   **Cerebral infarction, unspecified** `MCC` `HCC`
     Stroke NOS
     `EXCLUDES 2`   *transient cerebral ischemic attacks and related syndromes (G45.-)*
     AHA: 2020,2Q,29; 2015,1Q,25
     TIP: When provider documentation does not identify the location of an infarction, imaging reports can be used to pinpoint the location and lead to a more specific infarction code.

✓4ᵗʰ **I65**   **Occlusion and stenosis of precerebral arteries, not resulting in cerebral infarction**

     `INCLUDES`   embolism of precerebral artery
           narrowing of precerebral artery
           obstruction (complete) (partial) of precerebral artery
           thrombosis of precerebral artery
     `EXCLUDES 1`   *insufficiency, NOS, of precerebral artery (G45.-)*
           insufficiency of precerebral arteries causing cerebral infarction (I63.0-I63.2)
     AHA: 2018,2Q,9

✓5ᵗʰ **I65.0**   **Occlusion and stenosis of vertebral artery**

     I65.01   **Occlusion and stenosis of right vertebral artery**
     I65.02   **Occlusion and stenosis of left vertebral artery**
     I65.03   **Occlusion and stenosis of bilateral vertebral arteries**
     I65.09   **Occlusion and stenosis of unspecified vertebral artery**

I65.1   **Occlusion and stenosis of basilar artery**

✓5ᵗʰ **I65.2**   **Occlusion and stenosis of carotid artery**

     I65.21   **Occlusion and stenosis of right carotid artery**
     I65.22   **Occlusion and stenosis of left carotid artery**
     I65.23   **Occlusion and stenosis of bilateral carotid arteries**
     I65.29   **Occlusion and stenosis of unspecified carotid artery**

I65.8   **Occlusion and stenosis of other precerebral arteries**

I65.9   **Occlusion and stenosis of unspecified precerebral artery**
     Occlusion and stenosis of precerebral artery NOS

N Newborn: 0   P Pediatric: 0-17   M Maternity: 9-64   A Adult: 15-124   `MCC` Major Complication/Comorbidity   `CC` Complication/Comorbidity   `SW` Severe Wound Dx

660   ICD-10-CM 2021

☑4ᵗʰ **I66 Occlusion and stenosis of cerebral arteries, not resulting in cerebral infarction**

  INCLUDES   embolism of cerebral artery

              narrowing of cerebral artery

              obstruction (complete) (partial) of cerebral artery

              thrombosis of cerebral artery

  EXCLUDES 1   *occlusion and stenosis of cerebral artery causing cerebral infarction (I63.3-I63.5)*

  ☑5ᵗʰ **I66.0 Occlusion and stenosis of middle cerebral artery**

      I66.01 Occlusion and stenosis of right middle cerebral artery

      I66.02 Occlusion and stenosis of left middle cerebral artery

      I66.03 Occlusion and stenosis of bilateral middle cerebral arteries

      I66.09 Occlusion and stenosis of unspecified middle cerebral artery

  ☑5ᵗʰ **I66.1 Occlusion and stenosis of anterior cerebral artery**

      I66.11 Occlusion and stenosis of right anterior cerebral artery

      I66.12 Occlusion and stenosis of left anterior cerebral artery

      I66.13 Occlusion and stenosis of bilateral anterior cerebral arteries

      I66.19 Occlusion and stenosis of unspecified anterior cerebral artery

  ☑5ᵗʰ **I66.2 Occlusion and stenosis of posterior cerebral artery**

      I66.21 Occlusion and stenosis of right posterior cerebral artery

      I66.22 Occlusion and stenosis of left posterior cerebral artery

      I66.23 Occlusion and stenosis of bilateral posterior cerebral arteries

      I66.29 Occlusion and stenosis of unspecified posterior cerebral artery

  I66.3 Occlusion and stenosis of cerebellar arteries

  I66.8 Occlusion and stenosis of other cerebral arteries

    Occlusion and stenosis of perforating arteries

  I66.9 Occlusion and stenosis of unspecified cerebral artery

☑4ᵗʰ **I67 Other cerebrovascular diseases**

  EXCLUDES 2   *sequelae of the listed conditions (I69.8)*

  I67.0 Dissection of cerebral arteries, nonruptured   MCC HCC

    EXCLUDES 1   *ruptured cerebral arteries (I60.7)*

I67.1 Cerebral aneurysm, nonruptured

  Cerebral aneurysm NOS

  Cerebral arteriovenous fistula, acquired

  Internal carotid artery aneurysm, intracranial portion

  Internal carotid artery aneurysm, NOS

  EXCLUDES 1   *congenital cerebral aneurysm, nonruptured (Q28.-)*

                       ruptured cerebral aneurysm (I60.7)

Berry Aneurysm

Common sites of berry aneurysms in the circle of Willis arteries

I67.2 Cerebral atherosclerosis   A

  Atheroma of cerebral and precerebral arteries

I67.3 Progressive vascular leukoencephalopathy   HIV CC HCC

  Binswanger's disease

I67.4 Hypertensive encephalopathy   CC

  EXCLUDES 2   *insufficiency, NOS, of precerebral arteries (G45.2)*

I67.5 Moyamoya disease   CC

  DEF: Cerebrovascular ischemia. Vessels occlude and rupture, causing tiny hemorrhages at the base of brain. It affects predominantly Japanese people.

I67.6 Nonpyogenic thrombosis of intracranial venous system   CC

  Nonpyogenic thrombosis of cerebral vein

  Nonpyogenic thrombosis of intracranial venous sinus

  EXCLUDES 1   *nonpyogenic thrombosis of intracranial venous system causing infarction (I63.6)*

I67.7 Cerebral arteritis, not elsewhere classified   CC

  Granulomatous angiitis of the nervous system

  EXCLUDES 1   *allergic granulomatous angiitis (M30.1)*

☑5ᵗʰ **I67.8 Other specified cerebrovascular diseases**

  I67.81 Acute cerebrovascular insufficiency   CC

    Acute cerebrovascular insufficiency unspecified as to location or reversibility

  I67.82 Cerebral ischemia   CC

    Chronic cerebral ischemia

  I67.83 Posterior reversible encephalopathy syndrome   HIV MCC

    PRES

  ☑6ᵗʰ **I67.84 Cerebral vasospasm and vasoconstriction**

    I67.841 Reversible cerebrovascular vasoconstriction syndrome   CC

      Call-Fleming syndrome

      Code first underlying condition, if applicable, such as eclampsia (O15.00-O15.9)

    I67.848 Other cerebrovascular vasospasm and vasoconstriction   CC

☑ Additional Character Required   ☑x7ᵗʰ Placeholder   Unacceptable PDx   Questionable PDx   Manifestation   Unspecified Dx   H1-H4ᵗʰ HAC   HCC CMS-HCC Dx   HIV HIV Dx

ICD-10-CM 2021   661

√6ᵗʰ **I67.85 Hereditary cerebrovascular diseases**

AHA: 2018,4Q,17

I67.850 Cerebral autosomal dominant arteriopathy with subcortical infarcts and leukoencephalopathy CC

CADASIL

Code also any associated diagnoses, such as:

epilepsy (G40.-)

stroke (I63.-)

vascular dementia (F01.-)

I67.858 Other hereditary cerebrovascular disease CC

I67.89 Other cerebrovascular disease CC

I67.9 Cerebrovascular disease, unspecified

√4ᵗʰ **I68 Cerebrovascular disorders in diseases classified elsewhere**

I68.0 Cerebral amyloid angiopathy

Code first underlying amyloidosis (E85.-)

I68.2 Cerebral arteritis in other diseases classified elsewhere CC

Code first underlying disease

EXCLUDES 1 cerebral arteritis (in):

listerosis (A32.89)

syphilis (A52.04)

systemic lupus erythematosus (M32.19)

tuberculosis (A18.89)

I68.8 Other cerebrovascular disorders in diseases classified elsewhere

Code first underlying disease

EXCLUDES 1 syphilitic cerebral aneurysm (A52.05)

√4ᵗʰ **I69 Sequelae of cerebrovascular disease**

NOTE Category I69 is to be used to indicate conditions in I60-I67 as the cause of sequelae. The "sequelae" include conditions specified as such or as residuals which may occur at any time after the onset of the causal condition

EXCLUDES 1 personal history of cerebral infarction without residual deficit (Z86.73)

personal history of prolonged reversible ischemic neurologic deficit (PRIND) (Z86.73)

personal history of reversible ischemic neurologcial deficit (RIND) (Z86.73)

sequelae of traumatic intracranial injury (S06.-)

AHA: 2020,2Q,29; 2017,1Q,47; 2016,4Q,28; 2015,1Q,25; 2012,4Q,106

TIP: Weakness on one side of the body (unilateral weakness) documented as secondary to old cerebrovascular disease is synonymous with hemiparesis/hemiplegia. Weakness of one limb documented as secondary to old cerebrovascular disease is synonymous with monoplegia.

TIP: For codes describing hemiplegia, hemiparesis, and monoplegia; if the documentation identifies the affected side but not whether it is the dominant or nondominant side, the default is as follows: for ambidextrous patients, the default is dominant; when the left side is affected, the default is nondominant; and when the right side is affected, the default is dominant.

√5ᵗʰ **I69.0 Sequelae of nontraumatic subarachnoid hemorrhage**

I69.00 Unspecified sequelae of nontraumatic subarachnoid hemorrhage

√6ᵗʰ **I69.01 Cognitive deficits following nontraumatic subarachnoid hemorrhage**

I69.010 Attention and concentration deficit following nontraumatic subarachnoid hemorrhage

I69.011 Memory deficit following nontraumatic subarachnoid hemorrhage

I69.012 Visuospatial deficit and spatial neglect following nontraumatic subarachnoid hemorrhage

I69.013 Psychomotor deficit following nontraumatic subarachnoid hemorrhage

I69.014 Frontal lobe and executive function deficit following nontraumatic subarachnoid hemorrhage

I69.015 Cognitive social or emotional deficit following nontraumatic subarachnoid hemorrhage

I69.018 Other symptoms and signs involving cognitive functions following nontraumatic subarachnoid hemorrhage

I69.019 Unspecified symptoms and signs involving cognitive functions following nontraumatic subarachnoid hemorrhage

√6ᵗʰ **I69.02 Speech and language deficits following nontraumatic subarachnoid hemorrhage**

I69.020 Aphasia following nontraumatic subarachnoid hemorrhage

I69.021 Dysphasia following nontraumatic subarachnoid hemorrhage

I69.022 Dysarthria following nontraumatic subarachnoid hemorrhage

I69.023 Fluency disorder following nontraumatic subarachnoid hemorrhage

Stuttering following nontraumatic subarachnoid hemorrhage

I69.028 Other speech and language deficits following nontraumatic subarachnoid hemorrhage

√6ᵗʰ **I69.03 Monoplegia of upper limb following nontraumatic subarachnoid hemorrhage**

AHA: 2017,1Q,47

I69.031 Monoplegia of upper limb following nontraumatic subarachnoid hemorrhage affecting right dominant side HCC

I69.032 Monoplegia of upper limb following nontraumatic subarachnoid hemorrhage affecting left dominant side HCC

I69.033 Monoplegia of upper limb following nontraumatic subarachnoid hemorrhage affecting right non-dominant side HCC

I69.034 Monoplegia of upper limb following nontraumatic subarachnoid hemorrhage affecting left non-dominant side HCC

I69.039 Monoplegia of upper limb following nontraumatic subarachnoid hemorrhage affecting unspecified side HCC

√6ᵗʰ **I69.04 Monoplegia of lower limb following nontraumatic subarachnoid hemorrhage**

AHA: 2017,1Q,47

I69.041 Monoplegia of lower limb following nontraumatic subarachnoid hemorrhage affecting right dominant side HCC

I69.042 Monoplegia of lower limb following nontraumatic subarachnoid hemorrhage affecting left dominant side HCC

I69.043 Monoplegia of lower limb following nontraumatic subarachnoid hemorrhage affecting right non-dominant side HCC

I69.044 Monoplegia of lower limb following nontraumatic subarachnoid hemorrhage affecting left non-dominant side HCC

I69.049 Monoplegia of lower limb following nontraumatic subarachnoid hemorrhage affecting unspecified side HCC

√6ᵗʰ **I69.05 Hemiplegia and hemiparesis following nontraumatic subarachnoid hemorrhage**

AHA: 2015,1Q,25

I69.051 Hemiplegia and hemiparesis following nontraumatic subarachnoid hemorrhage affecting right dominant side CC HCC

I69.052 Hemiplegia and hemiparesis following nontraumatic subarachnoid hemorrhage affecting left dominant side CC HCC

I69.053 Hemiplegia and hemiparesis following nontraumatic subarachnoid hemorrhage affecting right non-dominant side CC HCC

I69.054 Hemiplegia and hemiparesis following nontraumatic subarachnoid hemorrhage affecting left non-dominant side CC HCC

I69.059 Hemiplegia and hemiparesis following nontraumatic subarachnoid hemorrhage affecting unspecified side CC HCC

N Newborn: 0 P Pediatric: 0-17 M Maternity: 9-64 A Adult: 15-124 MCC Major Complication/Comorbidity CC Complication/Comorbidity SW Severe Wound Dx

662

ICD-10-CM 2021

√6ᵗʰ **I69.06 Other paralytic syndrome following nontraumatic subarachnoid hemorrhage**
Use additional code to identify type of paralytic syndrome, such as:
locked-in state (G83.5)
quadriplegia (G82.5-)
EXCLUDES 1   *hemiplegia/hemiparesis following nontraumatic subarachnoid hemorrhage (I69.05-)*
monoplegia of lower limb following nontraumatic subarachnoid hemorrhage (I69.04-)
monoplegia of upper limb following nontraumatic subarachnoid hemorrhage (I69.03-)

     I69.061 Other paralytic syndrome following nontraumatic subarachnoid hemorrhage affecting right dominant side HCC

     I69.062 Other paralytic syndrome following nontraumatic subarachnoid hemorrhage affecting left dominant side HCC

     I69.063 Other paralytic syndrome following nontraumatic subarachnoid hemorrhage affecting right non-dominant side HCC

     I69.064 Other paralytic syndrome following nontraumatic subarachnoid hemorrhage affecting left non-dominant side HCC

     I69.065 Other paralytic syndrome following nontraumatic subarachnoid hemorrhage, bilateral HCC

     I69.069 Other paralytic syndrome following nontraumatic subarachnoid hemorrhage affecting unspecified side HCC

√6ᵗʰ **I69.09 Other sequelae of nontraumatic subarachnoid hemorrhage**

     I69.090 Apraxia following nontraumatic subarachnoid hemorrhage

     I69.091 Dysphagia following nontraumatic subarachnoid hemorrhage
Use additional code to identify the type of dysphagia, if known (R13.1-)

     I69.092 Facial weakness following nontraumatic subarachnoid hemorrhage
Facial droop following nontraumatic subarachnoid hemorrhage

     I69.093 Ataxia following nontraumatic subarachnoid hemorrhage

     I69.098 Other sequelae following nontraumatic subarachnoid hemorrhage
Alterations of sensation following nontraumatic subarachnoid hemorrhage
Disturbance of vision following nontraumatic subarachnoid hemorrhage
Use additional code to identify the sequelae

√5ᵗʰ **I69.1 Sequelae of nontraumatic intracerebral hemorrhage**

     I69.10 Unspecified sequelae of nontraumatic intracerebral hemorrhage

√6ᵗʰ **I69.11 Cognitive deficits following nontraumatic intracerebral hemorrhage**

     I69.110 Attention and concentration deficit following nontraumatic intracerebral hemorrhage

     I69.111 Memory deficit following nontraumatic intracerebral hemorrhage

     I69.112 Visuospatial deficit and spatial neglect following nontraumatic intracerebral hemorrhage

     I69.113 Psychomotor deficit following nontraumatic intracerebral hemorrhage

     I69.114 Frontal lobe and executive function deficit following nontraumatic intracerebral hemorrhage

     I69.115 Cognitive social or emotional deficit following nontraumatic intracerebral hemorrhage

     I69.118 Other symptoms and signs involving cognitive functions following nontraumatic intracerebral hemorrhage

     I69.119 Unspecified symptoms and signs involving cognitive functions following nontraumatic intracerebral hemorrhage

√6ᵗʰ **I69.12 Speech and language deficits following nontraumatic intracerebral hemorrhage**

     I69.120 Aphasia following nontraumatic intracerebral hemorrhage

     I69.121 Dysphasia following nontraumatic intracerebral hemorrhage

     I69.122 Dysarthria following nontraumatic intracerebral hemorrhage

     I69.123 Fluency disorder following nontraumatic intracerebral hemorrhage
Stuttering following nontraumatic intracerebral hemorrhage

     I69.128 Other speech and language deficits following nontraumatic intracerebral hemorrhage

√6ᵗʰ **I69.13 Monoplegia of upper limb following nontraumatic intracerebral hemorrhage**
AHA: 2017,1Q,47

     I69.131 Monoplegia of upper limb following nontraumatic intracerebral hemorrhage affecting right dominant side HCC

     I69.132 Monoplegia of upper limb following nontraumatic intracerebral hemorrhage affecting left dominant side HCC

     I69.133 Monoplegia of upper limb following nontraumatic intracerebral hemorrhage affecting right non-dominant side HCC

     I69.134 Monoplegia of upper limb following nontraumatic intracerebral hemorrhage affecting left non-dominant side HCC

     I69.139 Monoplegia of upper limb following nontraumatic intracerebral hemorrhage affecting unspecified side HCC

√6ᵗʰ **I69.14 Monoplegia of lower limb following nontraumatic intracerebral hemorrhage**
AHA: 2017,1Q,47

     I69.141 Monoplegia of lower limb following nontraumatic intracerebral hemorrhage affecting right dominant side HCC

     I69.142 Monoplegia of lower limb following nontraumatic intracerebral hemorrhage affecting left dominant side HCC

     I69.143 Monoplegia of lower limb following nontraumatic intracerebral hemorrhage affecting right non-dominant side HCC

     I69.144 Monoplegia of lower limb following nontraumatic intracerebral hemorrhage affecting left non-dominant side HCC

     I69.149 Monoplegia of lower limb following nontraumatic intracerebral hemorrhage affecting unspecified side HCC

√6ᵗʰ **I69.15 Hemiplegia and hemiparesis following nontraumatic intracerebral hemorrhage**
AHA: 2015,1Q,25

     I69.151 Hemiplegia and hemiparesis following nontraumatic intracerebral hemorrhage affecting right dominant side CC HCC

     I69.152 Hemiplegia and hemiparesis following nontraumatic intracerebral hemorrhage affecting left dominant side CC HCC

     I69.153 Hemiplegia and hemiparesis following nontraumatic intracerebral hemorrhage affecting right non-dominant side CC HCC

     I69.154 Hemiplegia and hemiparesis following nontraumatic intracerebral hemorrhage affecting left non-dominant side CC HCC

     I69.159 Hemiplegia and hemiparesis following nontraumatic intracerebral hemorrhage affecting unspecified side CC HCC

√6ᵗʰ **I69.16** **Other paralytic syndrome following nontraumatic intracerebral hemorrhage**
Use additional code to identify type of paralytic syndrome, such as:
locked-in state (G83.5)
quadriplegia (G82.5-)
> EXCLUDES 1 *hemiplegia/hemiparesis following nontraumatic intracerebral hemorrhage (I69.15-)*
> *monoplegia of lower limb following nontraumatic intracerebral hemorrhage (I69.14-)*
> *monoplegia of upper limb following nontraumatic intracerebral hemorrhage (I69.13-)*

I69.161 **Other paralytic syndrome following nontraumatic intracerebral hemorrhage affecting right dominant side** HCC

I69.162 **Other paralytic syndrome following nontraumatic intracerebral hemorrhage affecting left dominant side** HCC

I69.163 **Other paralytic syndrome following nontraumatic intracerebral hemorrhage affecting right non-dominant side** HCC

I69.164 **Other paralytic syndrome following nontraumatic intracerebral hemorrhage affecting left non-dominant side** HCC

I69.165 **Other paralytic syndrome following nontraumatic intracerebral hemorrhage, bilateral** HCC

I69.169 **Other paralytic syndrome following nontraumatic intracerebral hemorrhage affecting unspecified side** HCC

√6ᵗʰ **I69.19** **Other sequelae of nontraumatic intracerebral hemorrhage**

I69.190 **Apraxia following nontraumatic intracerebral hemorrhage**

I69.191 **Dysphagia following nontraumatic intracerebral hemorrhage**
Use additional code to identify the type of dysphagia, if known (R13.1-)

I69.192 **Facial weakness following nontraumatic intracerebral hemorrhage**
Facial droop following nontraumatic intracerebral hemorrhage

I69.193 **Ataxia following nontraumatic intracerebral hemorrhage**

I69.198 **Other sequelae of nontraumatic intracerebral hemorrhage**
Alteration of sensations following nontraumatic intracerebral hemorrhage
Disturbance of vision following nontraumatic intracerebral hemorrhage
Use additional code to identify the sequelae

√5ᵗʰ **I69.2** **Sequelae of other nontraumatic intracranial hemorrhage**

I69.20 **Unspecified sequelae of other nontraumatic intracranial hemorrhage**

√6ᵗʰ **I69.21** **Cognitive deficits following other nontraumatic intracranial hemorrhage**

I69.210 **Attention and concentration deficit following other nontraumatic intracranial hemorrhage**

I69.211 **Memory deficit following other nontraumatic intracranial hemorrhage**

I69.212 **Visuospatial deficit and spatial neglect following other nontraumatic intracranial hemorrhage**

I69.213 **Psychomotor deficit following other nontraumatic intracranial hemorrhage**

I69.214 **Frontal lobe and executive function deficit following other nontraumatic intracranial hemorrhage**

I69.215 **Cognitive social or emotional deficit following other nontraumatic intracranial hemorrhage**

I69.218 **Other symptoms and signs involving cognitive functions following other nontraumatic intracranial hemorrhage**

I69.219 **Unspecified symptoms and signs involving cognitive functions following other nontraumatic intracranial hemorrhage**

√6ᵗʰ **I69.22** **Speech and language deficits following other nontraumatic intracranial hemorrhage**

I69.220 **Aphasia following other nontraumatic intracranial hemorrhage**

I69.221 **Dysphasia following other nontraumatic intracranial hemorrhage**

I69.222 **Dysarthria following other nontraumatic intracranial hemorrhage**

I69.223 **Fluency disorder following other nontraumatic intracranial hemorrhage**
Stuttering following other nontraumatic intracranial hemorrhage

I69.228 **Other speech and language deficits following other nontraumatic intracranial hemorrhage**

√6ᵗʰ **I69.23** **Monoplegia of upper limb following other nontraumatic intracranial hemorrhage**
AHA: 2017,1Q,47

I69.231 **Monoplegia of upper limb following other nontraumatic intracranial hemorrhage affecting right dominant side** HCC

I69.232 **Monoplegia of upper limb following other nontraumatic intracranial hemorrhage affecting left dominant side** HCC

I69.233 **Monoplegia of upper limb following other nontraumatic intracranial hemorrhage affecting right non-dominant side** HCC

I69.234 **Monoplegia of upper limb following other nontraumatic intracranial hemorrhage affecting left non-dominant side** HCC

I69.239 **Monoplegia of upper limb following other nontraumatic intracranial hemorrhage affecting unspecified side** HCC

√6ᵗʰ **I69.24** **Monoplegia of lower limb following other nontraumatic intracranial hemorrhage**
AHA: 2017,1Q,47

I69.241 **Monoplegia of lower limb following other nontraumatic intracranial hemorrhage affecting right dominant side** HCC

I69.242 **Monoplegia of lower limb following other nontraumatic intracranial hemorrhage affecting left dominant side** HCC

I69.243 **Monoplegia of lower limb following other nontraumatic intracranial hemorrhage affecting right non-dominant side** HCC

I69.244 **Monoplegia of lower limb following other nontraumatic intracranial hemorrhage affecting left non-dominant side** HCC

I69.249 **Monoplegia of lower limb following other nontraumatic intracranial hemorrhage affecting unspecified side** HCC

√6ᵗʰ **I69.25** **Hemiplegia and hemiparesis following other nontraumatic intracranial hemorrhage**
AHA: 2015,1Q,25

I69.251 **Hemiplegia and hemiparesis following other nontraumatic intracranial hemorrhage affecting right dominant side** CC HCC

I69.252 **Hemiplegia and hemiparesis following other nontraumatic intracranial hemorrhage affecting left dominant side** CC HCC

I69.253 **Hemiplegia and hemiparesis following other nontraumatic intracranial hemorrhage affecting right non-dominant side** CC HCC

I69.254 **Hemiplegia and hemiparesis following other nontraumatic intracranial hemorrhage affecting left non-dominant side** CC HCC

I69.259 **Hemiplegia and hemiparesis following other nontraumatic intracranial hemorrhage affecting unspecified side** CC HCC

√6ᵗʰ **I69.26** **Other paralytic syndrome following other nontraumatic intracranial hemorrhage**

Use additional code to identify type of paralytic syndrome, such as:

locked-in state (G83.5)

quadriplegia (G82.5-)

EXCLUDES 1 *hemiplegia/hemiparesis following other nontraumatic intracranial hemorrhage (I69.25-)*

monoplegia of lower limb following other nontraumatic intracranial hemorrhage (I69.24-)

monoplegia of upper limb following other nontraumatic intracranial hemorrhage (I69.23-)

I69.261 **Other paralytic syndrome following other nontraumatic intracranial hemorrhage affecting right dominant side** HCC

I69.262 **Other paralytic syndrome following other nontraumatic intracranial hemorrhage affecting left dominant side** HCC

I69.263 **Other paralytic syndrome following other nontraumatic intracranial hemorrhage affecting right non-dominant side** HCC

I69.264 **Other paralytic syndrome following other nontraumatic intracranial hemorrhage affecting left non-dominant side** HCC

I69.265 **Other paralytic syndrome following other nontraumatic intracranial hemorrhage, bilateral** HCC

I69.269 **Other paralytic syndrome following other nontraumatic intracranial hemorrhage affecting unspecified side** HCC

√6ᵗʰ **I69.29** **Other sequelae of other nontraumatic intracranial hemorrhage**

I69.290 **Apraxia following other nontraumatic intracranial hemorrhage**

I69.291 **Dysphagia following other nontraumatic intracranial hemorrhage**

Use additional code to identify the type of dysphagia, if known (R13.1-)

I69.292 **Facial weakness following other nontraumatic intracranial hemorrhage**

Facial droop following other nontraumatic intracranial hemorrhage

I69.293 **Ataxia following other nontraumatic intracranial hemorrhage**

I69.298 **Other sequelae of other nontraumatic intracranial hemorrhage**

Alteration of sensation following other nontraumatic intracranial hemorrhage

Disturbance of vision following other nontraumatic intracranial hemorrhage

Use additional code to identify the sequelae

√5ᵗʰ **I69.3** **Sequelae of cerebral infarction**

Sequelae of stroke NOS

AHA: 2013,4Q,127-128; 2012,4Q,92,94

I69.30 **Unspecified sequelae of cerebral infarction**

√6ᵗʰ **I69.31** **Cognitive deficits following cerebral infarction**

I69.310 **Attention and concentration deficit following cerebral infarction**

I69.311 **Memory deficit following cerebral infarction**

I69.312 **Visuospatial deficit and spatial neglect following cerebral infarction**

I69.313 **Psychomotor deficit following cerebral infarction**

I69.314 **Frontal lobe and executive function deficit following cerebral infarction**

I69.315 **Cognitive social or emotional deficit following cerebral infarction**

I69.318 **Other symptoms and signs involving cognitive functions following cerebral infarction**

I69.319 **Unspecified symptoms and signs involving cognitive functions following cerebral infarction**

√6ᵗʰ **I69.32** **Speech and language deficits following cerebral infarction**

I69.320 **Aphasia following cerebral infarction**

I69.321 **Dysphasia following cerebral infarction**

AHA: 2012,4Q,91

I69.322 **Dysarthria following cerebral infarction**

EXCLUDES 2 *transient ischemic attack (TIA) (G45.9)*

I69.323 **Fluency disorder following cerebral infarction**

Stuttering following cerebral infarction

I69.328 **Other speech and language deficits following cerebral infarction**

√6ᵗʰ **I69.33** **Monoplegia of upper limb following cerebral infarction**

AHA: 2017,1Q,47

I69.331 **Monoplegia of upper limb following cerebral infarction affecting right dominant side** HCC

I69.332 **Monoplegia of upper limb following cerebral infarction affecting left dominant side** HCC

I69.333 **Monoplegia of upper limb following cerebral infarction affecting right non-dominant side** HCC

I69.334 **Monoplegia of upper limb following cerebral infarction affecting left non-dominant side** HCC

I69.339 **Monoplegia of upper limb following cerebral infarction affecting unspecified side** HCC

√6ᵗʰ **I69.34** **Monoplegia of lower limb following cerebral infarction**

AHA: 2017,1Q,47

I69.341 **Monoplegia of lower limb following cerebral infarction affecting right dominant side** HCC

I69.342 **Monoplegia of lower limb following cerebral infarction affecting left dominant side** HCC

I69.343 **Monoplegia of lower limb following cerebral infarction affecting right non-dominant side** HCC

I69.344 **Monoplegia of lower limb following cerebral infarction affecting left non-dominant side** HCC

I69.349 **Monoplegia of lower limb following cerebral infarction affecting unspecified side** HCC

√6ᵗʰ **I69.35** **Hemiplegia and hemiparesis following cerebral infarction**

AHA: 2015,1Q,25

I69.351 **Hemiplegia and hemiparesis following cerebral infarction affecting right dominant side** CC HCC

EXCLUDES 2 *transient ischemic attack (TIA) (G45.9)*

I69.352 **Hemiplegia and hemiparesis following cerebral infarction affecting left dominant side** CC HCC

I69.353 **Hemiplegia and hemiparesis following cerebral infarction affecting right non-dominant side** CC HCC

I69.354 **Hemiplegia and hemiparesis following cerebral infarction affecting left non-dominant side** CC HCC

AHA: 2012,4Q,91

I69.359 **Hemiplegia and hemiparesis following cerebral infarction affecting unspecified side** CC HCC

☑ Additional Character Required   √x7ᵗʰ Placeholder   Unacceptable PDx   Questionable PDx   Manifestation   Unspecified Dx   H1-H14 HAC   HCC CMS-HCC Dx   HIV HIV Dx

ICD-10-CM 2021   **665**

Chapter 9. Diseases of the Circulatory System

I69.36–I69.863

✓6ᵗʰ **I69.36 Other paralytic syndrome following cerebral infarction**

Use additional code to identify type of paralytic syndrome, such as:
locked-in state (G83.5)
quadriplegia (G82.5-)

EXCLUDES 1   *hemiplegia/hemiparesis following cerebral infarction (I69.35-)*
monoplegia of lower limb following cerebral infarction (I69.34-)
monoplegia of upper limb following cerebral infarction (I69.33-)

I69.361 **Other paralytic syndrome following cerebral infarction affecting** right **dominant side**   HCC

I69.362 **Other paralytic syndrome following cerebral infarction affecting** left **dominant side**   HCC

I69.363 **Other paralytic syndrome following cerebral infarction affecting** right **non-dominant side**   HCC

I69.364 **Other paralytic syndrome following cerebral infarction affecting** left **non-dominant side**   HCC

I69.365 **Other paralytic syndrome following cerebral infarction, bilateral**   HCC

I69.369 **Other paralytic syndrome following cerebral infarction affecting unspecified side**   HCC

✓6ᵗʰ **I69.39 Other sequelae of cerebral infarction**

I69.390 **Apraxia following cerebral infarction**

I69.391 **Dysphagia following cerebral infarction**

Use additional code to identify the type of dysphagia, if known (R13.1-)

I69.392 **Facial weakness following cerebral infarction**

Facial droop following cerebral infarction

I69.393 **Ataxia following cerebral infarction**

I69.398 **Other sequelae of cerebral infarction**

Alteration of sensation following cerebral infarction
Disturbance of vision following cerebral infarction
Use additional code to identify the sequelae
AHA: 2020,2Q,29

✓5ᵗʰ **I69.8 Sequelae of other cerebrovascular diseases**

EXCLUDES 1   *sequelae of traumatic intracranial injury (S06.-)*

I69.80 **Unspecified sequelae of other cerebrovascular disease**

✓6ᵗʰ **I69.81 Cognitive deficits following other cerebrovascular disease**

I69.810 **Attention and concentration deficit following other cerebrovascular disease**

I69.811 **Memory deficit following other cerebrovascular disease**

I69.812 **Visuospatial deficit and spatial neglect following other cerebrovascular disease**

I69.813 **Psychomotor deficit following other cerebrovascular disease**

I69.814 **Frontal lobe and executive function deficit following other cerebrovascular disease**

I69.815 **Cognitive social or emotional deficit following other cerebrovascular disease**

I69.818 **Other symptoms and signs involving cognitive functions following other cerebrovascular disease**

I69.819 **Unspecified symptoms and signs involving cognitive functions following other cerebrovascular disease**

✓6ᵗʰ **I69.82 Speech and language deficits following other cerebrovascular disease**

I69.820 **Aphasia following other cerebrovascular disease**

I69.821 **Dysphasia following other cerebrovascular disease**

I69.822 **Dysarthria following other cerebrovascular disease**

I69.823 **Fluency disorder following other cerebrovascular disease**

Stuttering following other cerebrovascular disease

I69.828 **Other speech and language deficits following other cerebrovascular disease**

AHA: 2019,3Q,8

✓6ᵗʰ **I69.83 Monoplegia of upper limb following other cerebrovascular disease**

AHA: 2017,1Q,47

I69.831 **Monoplegia of upper limb following other cerebrovascular disease affecting** right **dominant side**   HCC

I69.832 **Monoplegia of upper limb following other cerebrovascular disease affecting** left **dominant side**   HCC

I69.833 **Monoplegia of upper limb following other cerebrovascular disease affecting** right **non-dominant side**   HCC

I69.834 **Monoplegia of upper limb following other cerebrovascular disease affecting** left **non-dominant side**   HCC

I69.839 **Monoplegia of upper limb following other cerebrovascular disease affecting unspecified side**   HCC

✓6ᵗʰ **I69.84 Monoplegia of lower limb following other cerebrovascular disease**

AHA: 2017,1Q,47

I69.841 **Monoplegia of lower limb following other cerebrovascular disease affecting** right **dominant side**   HCC

I69.842 **Monoplegia of lower limb following other cerebrovascular disease affecting** left **dominant side**   HCC

I69.843 **Monoplegia of lower limb following other cerebrovascular disease affecting** right **non-dominant side**   HCC

I69.844 **Monoplegia of lower limb following other cerebrovascular disease affecting** left **non-dominant side**   HCC

I69.849 **Monoplegia of lower limb following other cerebrovascular disease affecting unspecified side**   HCC

✓6ᵗʰ **I69.85 Hemiplegia and hemiparesis following other cerebrovascular disease**

AHA: 2015,1Q,25

I69.851 **Hemiplegia and hemiparesis following other cerebrovascular disease affecting** right **dominant side**   CC HCC

I69.852 **Hemiplegia and hemiparesis following other cerebrovascular disease affecting** left **dominant side**   CC HCC

I69.853 **Hemiplegia and hemiparesis following other cerebrovascular disease affecting** right **non-dominant side**   CC HCC

I69.854 **Hemiplegia and hemiparesis following other cerebrovascular disease affecting** left **non-dominant side**   CC HCC

I69.859 **Hemiplegia and hemiparesis following other cerebrovascular disease affecting unspecified side**   CC HCC

✓6ᵗʰ **I69.86 Other paralytic syndrome following other cerebrovascular disease**

Use additional code to identify type of paralytic syndrome, such as:
locked-in state (G83.5)
quadriplegia (G82.5-)

EXCLUDES 1   *hemiplegia/hemiparesis following other cerebrovascular disease (I69.85-)*
monoplegia of lower limb following other cerebrovascular disease (I69.84-)
monoplegia of upper limb following other cerebrovascular disease (I69.83-)

I69.861 **Other paralytic syndrome following other cerebrovascular disease affecting** right **dominant side**   HCC

I69.862 **Other paralytic syndrome following other cerebrovascular disease affecting** left **dominant side**   HCC

I69.863 **Other paralytic syndrome following other cerebrovascular disease affecting** right **non-dominant side**   HCC

N Newborn: 0   P Pediatric: 0-17   M Maternity: 9-64   A Adult: 15-124   MCC Major Complication/Comorbidity   CC Complication/Comorbidity   SW Severe Wound Dx

666   ICD-10-CM 2021

I69.864 Other paralytic syndrome following other cerebrovascular disease affecting left non-dominant side   HCC

I69.865 Other paralytic syndrome following other cerebrovascular disease, bilateral   HCC

I69.869 Other paralytic syndrome following other cerebrovascular disease affecting unspecified side   HCC

√6ᵗʰ **I69.89** Other sequelae of other cerebrovascular disease

I69.890 Apraxia following other cerebrovascular disease

I69.891 Dysphagia following other cerebrovascular disease

Use additional code to identify the type of dysphagia, if known (R13.1-)

I69.892 Facial weakness following other cerebrovascular disease

Facial droop following other cerebrovascular disease

I69.893 Ataxia following other cerebrovascular disease

I69.898 Other sequelae of other cerebrovascular disease

Alteration of sensation following other cerebrovascular disease

Disturbance of vision following other cerebrovascular disease

Use additional code to identify the sequelae

√5ᵗʰ **I69.9** Sequelae of unspecified cerebrovascular diseases

EXCLUDES 1   sequelae of stroke (I69.3)

sequelae of traumatic intracranial injury (S06.-)

I69.90 Unspecified sequelae of unspecified cerebrovascular disease

√6ᵗʰ **I69.91** Cognitive deficits following unspecified cerebrovascular disease

I69.910 Attention and concentration deficit following unspecified cerebrovascular disease

I69.911 Memory deficit following unspecified cerebrovascular disease

I69.912 Visuospatial deficit and spatial neglect following unspecified cerebrovascular disease

I69.913 Psychomotor deficit following unspecified cerebrovascular disease

I69.914 Frontal lobe and executive function deficit following unspecified cerebrovascular disease

I69.915 Cognitive social or emotional deficit following unspecified cerebrovascular disease

I69.918 Other symptoms and signs involving cognitive functions following unspecified cerebrovascular disease

I69.919 Unspecified symptoms and signs involving cognitive functions following unspecified cerebrovascular disease

√6ᵗʰ **I69.92** Speech and language deficits following unspecified cerebrovascular disease

I69.920 Aphasia following unspecified cerebrovascular disease

I69.921 Dysphasia following unspecified cerebrovascular disease

I69.922 Dysarthria following unspecified cerebrovascular disease

I69.923 Fluency disorder following unspecified cerebrovascular disease

Stuttering following unspecified cerebrovascular disease

I69.928 Other speech and language deficits following unspecified cerebrovascular disease

√6ᵗʰ **I69.93** Monoplegia of upper limb following unspecified cerebrovascular disease

AHA: 2017,1Q,47

I69.931 Monoplegia of upper limb following unspecified cerebrovascular disease affecting right dominant side   HCC

I69.932 Monoplegia of upper limb following unspecified cerebrovascular disease affecting left dominant side   HCC

I69.933 Monoplegia of upper limb following unspecified cerebrovascular disease affecting right non-dominant side   HCC

I69.934 Monoplegia of upper limb following unspecified cerebrovascular disease affecting left non-dominant side   HCC

I69.939 Monoplegia of upper limb following unspecified cerebrovascular disease affecting unspecified side   HCC

√6ᵗʰ **I69.94** Monoplegia of lower limb following unspecified cerebrovascular disease

AHA: 2017,1Q,47

I69.941 Monoplegia of lower limb following unspecified cerebrovascular disease affecting right dominant side   HCC

I69.942 Monoplegia of lower limb following unspecified cerebrovascular disease affecting left dominant side   HCC

I69.943 Monoplegia of lower limb following unspecified cerebrovascular disease affecting right non-dominant side   HCC

I69.944 Monoplegia of lower limb following unspecified cerebrovascular disease affecting left non-dominant side   HCC

I69.949 Monoplegia of lower limb following unspecified cerebrovascular disease affecting unspecified side   HCC

√6ᵗʰ **I69.95** Hemiplegia and hemiparesis following unspecified cerebrovascular disease

AHA: 2015,1Q,25

I69.951 Hemiplegia and hemiparesis following unspecified cerebrovascular disease affecting right dominant side   CC   HCC

I69.952 Hemiplegia and hemiparesis following unspecified cerebrovascular disease affecting left dominant side   CC   HCC

I69.953 Hemiplegia and hemiparesis following unspecified cerebrovascular disease affecting right non-dominant side   CC   HCC

I69.954 Hemiplegia and hemiparesis following unspecified cerebrovascular disease affecting left non-dominant side   CC   HCC

I69.959 Hemiplegia and hemiparesis following unspecified cerebrovascular disease affecting unspecified side   CC   HCC

√6ᵗʰ **I69.96** Other paralytic syndrome following unspecified cerebrovascular disease

Use additional code to identify type of paralytic syndrome, such as:

locked-in state (G83.5)

quadriplegia (G82.5-)

EXCLUDES 1   hemiplegia/hemiparesis following unspecified cerebrovascular disease (I69.95-)

monoplegia of lower limb following unspecified cerebrovascular disease (I69.94-)

monoplegia of upper limb following unspecified cerebrovascular disease (I69.93-)

I69.961 Other paralytic syndrome following unspecified cerebrovascular disease affecting right dominant side   HCC

I69.962 Other paralytic syndrome following unspecified cerebrovascular disease affecting left dominant side   HCC

I69.963 Other paralytic syndrome following unspecified cerebrovascular disease affecting right non-dominant side   HCC

I69.964 Other paralytic syndrome following unspecified cerebrovascular disease affecting left non-dominant side   HCC

I69.965 Other paralytic syndrome following unspecified cerebrovascular disease, bilateral   HCC

I69.969 Other paralytic syndrome following unspecified cerebrovascular disease affecting unspecified side   HCC

✔ Additional Character Required   √x7ᵗʰ Placeholder   Unacceptable PDx   Questionable PDx   Manifestation   Unspecified Dx   H1 - H14 HAC   HCC CMS-HCC Dx   HIV HIV Dx

Chapter 9. Diseases of the Circulatory System

I69.99–I70.239

✓6ᵗʰ **I69.99 Other sequelae of unspecified cerebrovascular disease**

I69.990 Apraxia following unspecified cerebrovascular disease

I69.991 Dysphagia following unspecified cerebrovascular disease
Use additional code to identify the type of dysphagia, if known (R13.1-)

I69.992 Facial weakness following unspecified cerebrovascular disease
Facial droop following unspecified cerebrovascular disease

I69.993 Ataxia following unspecified cerebrovascular disease

I69.998 Other sequelae following unspecified cerebrovascular disease
Alteration in sensation following unspecified cerebrovascular disease
Disturbance of vision following unspecified cerebrovascular disease
Use additional code to identify the sequelae

Diseases of arteries, arterioles and capillaries (I70-I79)

✓4ᵗʰ **I70 Atherosclerosis**

INCLUDES   arterial degeneration
arteriolosclerosis
arteriosclerosis
arteriosclerotic vascular disease
arteriovascular degeneration
atheroma
endarteritis deformans or obliterans
senile arteritis
senile endarteritis
vascular degeneration

Use additional code to identify:
exposure to environmental tobacco smoke (Z77.22)
history of tobacco dependence (Z87.891)
occupational exposure to environmental tobacco smoke (Z57.31)
tobacco dependence (F17.-)
tobacco use (Z72.0)

EXCLUDES 2   *arteriosclerotic cardiovascular disease (I25.1-)*
arteriosclerotic heart disease (I25.1-)
atheroembolism (I75.-)
cerebral atherosclerosis (I67.2)
coronary atherosclerosis (I25.1-)
mesenteric atherosclerosis (K55.1)
precerebral atherosclerosis (I67.2)
primary pulmonary atherosclerosis (I27.0)

I70.0 Atherosclerosis of aorta   HCC A

I70.1 Atherosclerosis of renal artery   HCC A
Goldblatt's kidney
EXCLUDES 2   *atherosclerosis of renal arterioles (I12.-)*

✓5ᵗʰ **I70.2 Atherosclerosis of native arteries of the extremities**
Mönckeberg's (medial) sclerosis
Use additional code, if applicable, to identify chronic total occlusion of artery of extremity (I70.92)
EXCLUDES 2   *atherosclerosis of bypass graft of extremities (I70.30-I70.79)*
AHA: 2018,3Q,4; 2018,2Q,7

✓6ᵗʰ **I70.20 Unspecified atherosclerosis of native arteries of extremities**

I70.201 Unspecified atherosclerosis of native arteries of extremities, right leg   HCC A

I70.202 Unspecified atherosclerosis of native arteries of extremities, left leg   HCC A

I70.203 Unspecified atherosclerosis of native arteries of extremities, bilateral legs   HCC A

I70.208 Unspecified atherosclerosis of native arteries of extremities, other extremity   HCC A

I70.209 Unspecified atherosclerosis of native arteries of extremities, unspecified extremity   HCC A

✓6ᵗʰ **I70.21 Atherosclerosis of native arteries of extremities with intermittent claudication**

I70.211 Atherosclerosis of native arteries of extremities with intermittent claudication, right leg   HCC A

I70.212 Atherosclerosis of native arteries of extremities with intermittent claudication, left leg   HCC A

I70.213 Atherosclerosis of native arteries of extremities with intermittent claudication, bilateral legs   HCC A

I70.218 Atherosclerosis of native arteries of extremities with intermittent claudication, other extremity   HCC A

I70.219 Atherosclerosis of native arteries of extremities with intermittent claudication, unspecified extremity   HCC A

✓6ᵗʰ **I70.22 Atherosclerosis of native arteries of extremities with rest pain**
INCLUDES   any condition classifiable to I70.21-
▶chronic limb-threatening ischemia NOS of native arteries of extremities◀
▶chronic limb-threatening ischemia of native arteries of extremities with rest pain◀
▶critical limb ischemia NOS of native arteries of extremities◀
▶critical limb ischemia of native arteries of extremities with rest pain◀

I70.221 Atherosclerosis of native arteries of extremities with rest pain, right leg   HCC A

I70.222 Atherosclerosis of native arteries of extremities with rest pain, left leg   HCC A

I70.223 Atherosclerosis of native arteries of extremities with rest pain, bilateral legs   HCC A

I70.228 Atherosclerosis of native arteries of extremities with rest pain, other extremity   HCC A

I70.229 Atherosclerosis of native arteries of extremities with rest pain, unspecified extremity   HCC A

✓6ᵗʰ **I70.23 Atherosclerosis of native arteries of right leg with ulceration**
INCLUDES   any condition classifiable to I70.211 and I70.221
▶chronic limb-threatening ischemia of native arteries of right leg with ulceration◀
▶critical limb ischemia of native arteries of right leg with ulceration◀
Use additional code to identify severity of ulcer (L97.-)

I70.231 Atherosclerosis of native arteries of right leg with ulceration of thigh   HCC A

I70.232 Atherosclerosis of native arteries of right leg with ulceration of calf   HCC A

I70.233 Atherosclerosis of native arteries of right leg with ulceration of ankle   HCC A

I70.234 Atherosclerosis of native arteries of right leg with ulceration of heel and midfoot   HCC A
Atherosclerosis of native arteries of right leg with ulceration of plantar surface of midfoot

I70.235 Atherosclerosis of native arteries of right leg with ulceration of other part of foot   HCC A
Atherosclerosis of native arteries of right leg extremities with ulceration of toe

I70.238 Atherosclerosis of native arteries of right leg with ulceration of other part of lower leg   HCC A

I70.239 Atherosclerosis of native arteries of right leg with ulceration of unspecified site   HCC A

N Newborn: 0   P Pediatric: 0-17   M Maternity: 9-64   A Adult: 15-124   MCC Major Complication/Comorbidity   CC Complication/Comorbidity   SW Severe Wound Dx

668   ICD-10-CM 2021

✓6ᵗʰ **I70.24** **Atherosclerosis of native arteries of left leg with ulceration**

> INCLUDES   any condition classifiable to I70.212 and I70.222
>> ▶chronic limb-threatening ischemia of native arteries of left leg with ulceration◀
>> ▶critical limb ischemia of native arteries of left leg with ulceration◀
> Use additional code to identify severity of ulcer (L97.-)

     I70.241 **Atherosclerosis of native arteries of left leg with ulceration of thigh** HCC A

     I70.242 **Atherosclerosis of native arteries of left leg with ulceration of calf** HCC A

     I70.243 **Atherosclerosis of native arteries of left leg with ulceration of ankle** HCC A

     I70.244 **Atherosclerosis of native arteries of left leg with ulceration of heel and midfoot** HCC A
           Atherosclerosis of native arteries of left leg with ulceration of plantar surface of midfoot

     I70.245 **Atherosclerosis of native arteries of left leg with ulceration of other part of foot** HCC A
           Atherosclerosis of native arteries of left leg extremities with ulceration of toe

     I70.248 **Atherosclerosis of native arteries of left leg with ulceration of other part of lower leg** HCC A

     I70.249 **Atherosclerosis of native arteries of left leg with ulceration of unspecified site** HCC A

I70.25 **Atherosclerosis of native arteries of other extremities with ulceration** HCC A

> INCLUDES   any condition classifiable to I70.218 and I70.228
> Use additional code to identify the severity of the ulcer (L98.49-)

✓6ᵗʰ **I70.26** **Atherosclerosis of native arteries of extremities with gangrene**

> INCLUDES   any condition classifiable to I70.21-, I70.22-, I70.23-, I70.24-, and I70.25-
>> ▶chronic limb-threatening ischemia of native arteries of extremities with gangrene◀
>> ▶critical limb ischemia of native arteries of extremities with gangrene◀
> Use additional code to identify the severity of any ulcer (L97.-, L98.49-), if applicable

     I70.261 **Atherosclerosis of native arteries of extremities with gangrene, right leg** CC HCC A

     I70.262 **Atherosclerosis of native arteries of extremities with gangrene, left leg** CC HCC A

     I70.263 **Atherosclerosis of native arteries of extremities with gangrene, bilateral legs** CC HCC A

     I70.268 **Atherosclerosis of native arteries of extremities with gangrene, other extremity** CC HCC A

     I70.269 **Atherosclerosis of native arteries of extremities with gangrene, unspecified extremity** CC HCC A

✓6ᵗʰ **I70.29** **Other atherosclerosis of native arteries of extremities**

     I70.291 **Other atherosclerosis of native arteries of extremities, right leg** HCC A

     I70.292 **Other atherosclerosis of native arteries of extremities, left leg** HCC A

     I70.293 **Other atherosclerosis of native arteries of extremities, bilateral legs** HCC A

     I70.298 **Other atherosclerosis of native arteries of extremities, other extremity** HCC A

     I70.299 **Other atherosclerosis of native arteries of extremities, unspecified extremity** HCC A

✓5ᵗʰ **I70.3** **Atherosclerosis of unspecified type of bypass graft(s) of the extremities**

> Use additional code, if applicable, to identify chronic total occlusion of artery of extremity (I70.92)
> EXCLUDES 1   embolism or thrombus of bypass graft(s) of extremities (T82.8-)

✓6ᵗʰ **I70.30** **Unspecified atherosclerosis of unspecified type of bypass graft(s) of the extremities**

     I70.301 **Unspecified atherosclerosis of unspecified type of bypass graft(s) of the extremities, right leg** HCC A

     I70.302 **Unspecified atherosclerosis of unspecified type of bypass graft(s) of the extremities, left leg** HCC A

     I70.303 **Unspecified atherosclerosis of unspecified type of bypass graft(s) of the extremities, bilateral legs** HCC A

     I70.308 **Unspecified atherosclerosis of unspecified type of bypass graft(s) of the extremities, other extremity** HCC A

     I70.309 **Unspecified atherosclerosis of unspecified type of bypass graft(s) of the extremities, unspecified extremity** HCC A

✓6ᵗʰ **I70.31** **Atherosclerosis of unspecified type of bypass graft(s) of the extremities with intermittent claudication**

     I70.311 **Atherosclerosis of unspecified type of bypass graft(s) of the extremities with intermittent claudication, right leg** HCC A

     I70.312 **Atherosclerosis of unspecified type of bypass graft(s) of the extremities with intermittent claudication, left leg** HCC A

     I70.313 **Atherosclerosis of unspecified type of bypass graft(s) of the extremities with intermittent claudication, bilateral legs** HCC A

     I70.318 **Atherosclerosis of unspecified type of bypass graft(s) of the extremities with intermittent claudication, other extremity** HCC A

     I70.319 **Atherosclerosis of unspecified type of bypass graft(s) of the extremities with intermittent claudication, unspecified extremity** HCC A

✓6ᵗʰ **I70.32** **Atherosclerosis of unspecified type of bypass graft(s) of the extremities with rest pain**

> INCLUDES   any condition classifiable to I70.31-
>> ▶chronic limb-threatening ischemia NOS of unspecified type of bypass graft(s) of the extremities◀
>> ▶chronic limb-threatening ischemia of unspecified type of bypass graft(s) of the extremities with rest pain, right leg◀
>> ▶critical limb ischemia NOS of unspecified type of bypass graft(s) of the extremities◀
>> ▶critical limb ischemia of unspecified type of bypass graft(s) of the extremities with rest pain◀

     I70.321 **Atherosclerosis of unspecified type of bypass graft(s) of the extremities with rest pain, right leg** HCC A

     I70.322 **Atherosclerosis of unspecified type of bypass graft(s) of the extremities with rest pain, left leg** HCC A

     I70.323 **Atherosclerosis of unspecified type of bypass graft(s) of the extremities with rest pain, bilateral legs** HCC A

     I70.328 **Atherosclerosis of unspecified type of bypass graft(s) of the extremities with rest pain, other extremity** HCC A

     I70.329 **Atherosclerosis of unspecified type of bypass graft(s) of the extremities with rest pain, unspecified extremity** HCC A

Chapter 9. Diseases of the Circulatory System

✓6ᵗʰ **I70.33** **Atherosclerosis of unspecified type of bypass graft(s) of the right leg with ulceration**
INCLUDES any condition classifiable to I70.311 and I70.321
▶chronic limb-threatening ischemia of unspecified type of bypass graft(s) of the right leg with ulceration◀
▶critical limb ischemia of unspecified type of bypass graft(s) of the right leg with ulceration◀
Use additional code to identify severity of ulcer (L97.-)

I70.331 Atherosclerosis of unspecified type of bypass graft(s) of the right leg with ulceration of thigh CC HCC A

I70.332 Atherosclerosis of unspecified type of bypass graft(s) of the right leg with ulceration of calf CC HCC A

I70.333 Atherosclerosis of unspecified type of bypass graft(s) of the right leg with ulceration of ankle CC HCC A

I70.334 Atherosclerosis of unspecified type of bypass graft(s) of the right leg with ulceration of heel and midfoot CC HCC A
Atherosclerosis of unspecified type of bypass graft(s) of right leg with ulceration of plantar surface of midfoot

I70.335 Atherosclerosis of unspecified type of bypass graft(s) of the right leg with ulceration of other part of foot HCC A
Atherosclerosis of unspecified type of bypass graft(s) of the right leg with ulceration of toe

I70.338 Atherosclerosis of unspecified type of bypass graft(s) of the right leg with ulceration of other part of lower leg CC HCC A

I70.339 Atherosclerosis of unspecified type of bypass graft(s) of the right leg with ulceration of unspecified site CC HCC A

✓6ᵗʰ **I70.34** **Atherosclerosis of unspecified type of bypass graft(s) of the left leg with ulceration**
INCLUDES any condition classifiable to I70.312 and I70.322
▶chronic limb-threatening ischemia of unspecified type of bypass graft(s) of the left leg with ulceration◀
▶critical limb ischemia of unspecified type of bypass graft(s) of the left leg with ulceration◀
Use additional code to identify severity of ulcer (L97.-)

I70.341 Atherosclerosis of unspecified type of bypass graft(s) of the left leg with ulceration of thigh CC HCC A

I70.342 Atherosclerosis of unspecified type of bypass graft(s) of the left leg with ulceration of calf CC HCC A

I70.343 Atherosclerosis of unspecified type of bypass graft(s) of the left leg with ulceration of ankle CC HCC A

I70.344 Atherosclerosis of unspecified type of bypass graft(s) of the left leg with ulceration of heel and midfoot CC HCC A
Atherosclerosis of unspecified type of bypass graft(s) of left leg with ulceration of plantar surface of midfoot

I70.345 Atherosclerosis of unspecified type of bypass graft(s) of the left leg with ulceration of other part of foot HCC A
Atherosclerosis of unspecified type of bypass graft(s) of the left leg with ulceration of toe

I70.348 Atherosclerosis of unspecified type of bypass graft(s) of the left leg with ulceration of other part of lower leg CC HCC A

I70.349 Atherosclerosis of unspecified type of bypass graft(s) of the left leg with ulceration of unspecified site CC HCC A

I70.35 **Atherosclerosis of unspecified type of bypass graft(s) of other extremity with ulceration** HCC A
INCLUDES any condition classifiable to I70.318 and I70.328
Use additional code to identify severity of ulcer (L98.49-)

✓6ᵗʰ **I70.36** **Atherosclerosis of unspecified type of bypass graft(s) of the extremities with gangrene**
INCLUDES any condition classifiable to I70.31-, I70.32-, I70.33-, I70.34-, I70.35
▶chronic limb-threatening ischemia of unspecified type of bypass graft(s) of the extremities with gangrene◀
▶critical limb ischemia of unspecified type of bypass graft(s) of the extremities with gangrene◀
Use additional code to identify the severity of any ulcer (L97.-, L98.49-), if applicable

I70.361 Atherosclerosis of unspecified type of bypass graft(s) of the extremities with gangrene, right leg CC HCC A

I70.362 Atherosclerosis of unspecified type of bypass graft(s) of the extremities with gangrene, left leg CC HCC A

I70.363 Atherosclerosis of unspecified type of bypass graft(s) of the extremities with gangrene, bilateral legs CC HCC A

I70.368 Atherosclerosis of unspecified type of bypass graft(s) of the extremities with gangrene, other extremity CC HCC A

I70.369 Atherosclerosis of unspecified type of bypass graft(s) of the extremities with gangrene, unspecified extremity CC HCC A

✓6ᵗʰ **I70.39** **Other atherosclerosis of unspecified type of bypass graft(s) of the extremities**

I70.391 Other atherosclerosis of unspecified type of bypass graft(s) of the extremities, right leg HCC A

I70.392 Other atherosclerosis of unspecified type of bypass graft(s) of the extremities, left leg HCC A

I70.393 Other atherosclerosis of unspecified type of bypass graft(s) of the extremities, bilateral legs HCC A

I70.398 Other atherosclerosis of unspecified type of bypass graft(s) of the extremities, other extremity HCC A

I70.399 Other atherosclerosis of unspecified type of bypass graft(s) of the extremities, unspecified extremity HCC A

✓5ᵗʰ **I70.4** **Atherosclerosis of autologous vein bypass graft(s) of the extremities**
Use additional code, if applicable, to identify chronic total occlusion of artery of extremity (I70.92)

✓6ᵗʰ **I70.40** **Unspecified atherosclerosis of autologous vein bypass graft(s) of the extremities**

I70.401 Unspecified atherosclerosis of autologous vein bypass graft(s) of the extremities, right leg HCC A

I70.402 Unspecified atherosclerosis of autologous vein bypass graft(s) of the extremities, left leg HCC A

I70.403 Unspecified atherosclerosis of autologous vein bypass graft(s) of the extremities, bilateral legs HCC A

I70.408 Unspecified atherosclerosis of autologous vein bypass graft(s) of the extremities, other extremity HCC A

I70.409 Unspecified atherosclerosis of autologous vein bypass graft(s) of the extremities, unspecified extremity HCC A

✓6ᵗʰ **I70.41** **Atherosclerosis of autologous vein bypass graft(s) of the extremities with intermittent claudication**

I70.411 Atherosclerosis of autologous vein bypass graft(s) of the extremities with intermittent claudication, right leg HCC A

I70.412 Atherosclerosis of autologous vein bypass graft(s) of the extremities with intermittent claudication, left leg `HCC` `A`

I70.413 Atherosclerosis of autologous vein bypass graft(s) of the extremities with intermittent claudication, bilateral legs `HCC` `A`

I70.418 Atherosclerosis of autologous vein bypass graft(s) of the extremities with intermittent claudication, other extremity `HCC` `A`

I70.419 Atherosclerosis of autologous vein bypass graft(s) of the extremities with intermittent claudication, unspecified extremity `HCC` `A`

√6ᵗʰ **I70.42 Atherosclerosis of autologous vein bypass graft(s) of the extremities with rest pain**
> `INCLUDES` any condition classifiable to I70.41-
> ▸chronic limb-threatening ischemia NOS of autologous vein bypass graft(s) of the extremities◂
> ▸chronic limb-threatening ischemia of autologous vein bypass graft(s) of the extremities with rest pain◂
> ▸critical limb ischemia NOS of autologous vein bypass graft(s) of the extremities◂
> ▸critical limb ischemia of autologous vein bypass graft(s) of the extremities with rest pain◂

I70.421 Atherosclerosis of autologous vein bypass graft(s) of the extremities with rest pain, right leg `HCC` `A`

I70.422 Atherosclerosis of autologous vein bypass graft(s) of the extremities with rest pain, left leg `HCC` `A`

I70.423 Atherosclerosis of autologous vein bypass graft(s) of the extremities with rest pain, bilateral legs `HCC` `A`

I70.428 Atherosclerosis of autologous vein bypass graft(s) of the extremities with rest pain, other extremity `HCC` `A`

I70.429 Atherosclerosis of autologous vein bypass graft(s) of the extremities with rest pain, unspecified extremity `HCC` `A`

√6ᵗʰ **I70.43 Atherosclerosis of autologous vein bypass graft(s) of the right leg with ulceration**
> `INCLUDES` any condition classifiable to I70.411 and I70.421
> ▸chronic limb-threatening ischemia of autologous vein bypass graft(s) of the right leg with ulceration◂
> ▸critical limb ischemia of autologous vein bypass graft(s) of the right leg with ulceration◂

Use additional code to identify severity of ulcer (L97.-)

I70.431 Atherosclerosis of autologous vein bypass graft(s) of the right leg with ulceration of thigh `CC` `HCC` `A`

I70.432 Atherosclerosis of autologous vein bypass graft(s) of the right leg with ulceration of calf `CC` `HCC` `A`

I70.433 Atherosclerosis of autologous vein bypass graft(s) of the right leg with ulceration of ankle `CC` `HCC` `A`

I70.434 Atherosclerosis of autologous vein bypass graft(s) of the right leg with ulceration of heel and midfoot `CC` `HCC` `A`
> Atherosclerosis of autologous vein bypass graft(s) of right leg with ulceration of plantar surface of midfoot

I70.435 Atherosclerosis of autologous vein bypass graft(s) of the right leg with ulceration of other part of foot `HCC` `A`
> Atherosclerosis of autologous vein bypass graft(s) of right leg with ulceration of toe

I70.438 Atherosclerosis of autologous vein bypass graft(s) of the right leg with ulceration of other part of lower leg `CC` `HCC` `A`

I70.439 Atherosclerosis of autologous vein bypass graft(s) of the right leg with ulceration of unspecified site `CC` `HCC` `A`

√6ᵗʰ **I70.44 Atherosclerosis of autologous vein bypass graft(s) of the left leg with ulceration**
> `INCLUDES` any condition classifiable to I70.412 and I70.422
> ▸chronic limb-threatening ischemia of autologous vein bypass graft(s) of the left leg with ulceration◂
> ▸critical limb ischemia of autologous vein bypass graft(s) of the left leg with ulceration◂

Use additional code to identify severity of ulcer (L97.-)

I70.441 Atherosclerosis of autologous vein bypass graft(s) of the left leg with ulceration of thigh `CC` `HCC` `A`

I70.442 Atherosclerosis of autologous vein bypass graft(s) of the left leg with ulceration of calf `CC` `HCC` `A`

I70.443 Atherosclerosis of autologous vein bypass graft(s) of the left leg with ulceration of ankle `CC` `HCC` `A`

I70.444 Atherosclerosis of autologous vein bypass graft(s) of the left leg with ulceration of heel and midfoot `CC` `HCC` `A`
> Atherosclerosis of autologous vein bypass graft(s) of left leg with ulceration of plantar surface of midfoot

I70.445 Atherosclerosis of autologous vein bypass graft(s) of the left leg with ulceration of other part of foot `HCC` `A`
> Atherosclerosis of autologous vein bypass graft(s) of left leg with ulceration of toe

I70.448 Atherosclerosis of autologous vein bypass graft(s) of the left leg with ulceration of other part of lower leg `CC` `HCC` `A`

I70.449 Atherosclerosis of autologous vein bypass graft(s) of the left leg with ulceration of unspecified site `CC` `HCC` `A`

I70.45 Atherosclerosis of autologous vein bypass graft(s) of other extremity with ulceration `HCC` `A`
> `INCLUDES` any condition classifiable to I70.418, I70.428, and I70.438

Use additional code to identify severity of ulcer (L98.49)

√6ᵗʰ **I70.46 Atherosclerosis of autologous vein bypass graft(s) of the extremities with gangrene**
> `INCLUDES` any condition classifiable to I70.41-, I70.42-, and I70.43-, I70.44-, I70.45
> ▸chronic limb-threatening ischemia of autologous vein bypass graft(s) of the extremities with gangrene◂
> ▸critical limb ischemia of autologous vein bypass graft(s) of the extremities with gangrene◂

Use additional code to identify the severity of any ulcer (L97.-, L98.49-), if applicable

I70.461 Atherosclerosis of autologous vein bypass graft(s) of the extremities with gangrene, right leg `CC` `HCC` `A`

I70.462 Atherosclerosis of autologous vein bypass graft(s) of the extremities with gangrene, left leg `CC` `HCC` `A`

I70.463 Atherosclerosis of autologous vein bypass graft(s) of the extremities with gangrene, bilateral legs `CC` `HCC` `A`

I70.468 Atherosclerosis of autologous vein bypass graft(s) of the extremities with gangrene, other extremity `CC` `HCC` `A`

I70.469 Atherosclerosis of autologous vein bypass graft(s) of the extremities with gangrene, unspecified extremity `CC` `HCC` `A`

√6ᵗʰ **I70.49 Other atherosclerosis of autologous vein bypass graft(s) of the extremities**

I70.491 Other atherosclerosis of autologous vein bypass graft(s) of the extremities, right leg `HCC` `A`

I70.492 Other atherosclerosis of autologous vein bypass graft(s) of the extremities, left leg `HCC` `A`

I70.493   **Other atherosclerosis of autologous vein bypass graft(s) of the extremities, bilateral legs**   HCC A

I70.498   **Other atherosclerosis of autologous vein bypass graft(s) of the extremities, other extremity**   HCC A

I70.499   **Other atherosclerosis of autologous vein bypass graft(s) of the extremities, unspecified extremity**   HCC A

✓5th **I70.5**   **Atherosclerosis of nonautologous biological bypass graft(s) of the extremities**

Use additional code, if applicable, to identify chronic total occlusion of artery of extremity (I70.92)

✓6th **I70.50**   **Unspecified atherosclerosis of nonautologous biological bypass graft(s) of the extremities**

I70.501   **Unspecified atherosclerosis of nonautologous biological bypass graft(s) of the extremities, right leg**   HCC A

I70.502   **Unspecified atherosclerosis of nonautologous biological bypass graft(s) of the extremities, left leg**   HCC A

I70.503   **Unspecified atherosclerosis of nonautologous biological bypass graft(s) of the extremities, bilateral legs**   HCC A

I70.508   **Unspecified atherosclerosis of nonautologous biological bypass graft(s) of the extremities, other extremity**   HCC A

I70.509   **Unspecified atherosclerosis of nonautologous biological bypass graft(s) of the extremities, unspecified extremity**   HCC A

✓6th **I70.51**   **Atherosclerosis of nonautologous biological bypass graft(s) of the extremities intermittent claudication**

I70.511   **Atherosclerosis of nonautologous biological bypass graft(s) of the extremities with intermittent claudication, right leg**   HCC A

I70.512   **Atherosclerosis of nonautologous biological bypass graft(s) of the extremities with intermittent claudication, left leg**   HCC A

I70.513   **Atherosclerosis of nonautologous biological bypass graft(s) of the extremities with intermittent claudication, bilateral legs**   HCC A

I70.518   **Atherosclerosis of nonautologous biological bypass graft(s) of the extremities with intermittent claudication, other extremity**   HCC A

I70.519   **Atherosclerosis of nonautologous biological bypass graft(s) of the extremities with intermittent claudication, unspecified extremity**   HCC A

✓6th **I70.52**   **Atherosclerosis of nonautologous biological bypass graft(s) of the extremities with rest pain**

INCLUDES   any condition classifiable to I70.51-

▶chronic limb-threatening ischemia NOS of nonautologous biological bypass graft(s) of the extremities◀

▶chronic limb-threatening ischemia of nonautologous biological bypass graft(s) of the extremities with rest pain◀

▶critical limb ischemia NOS of nonautologous biological bypass graft(s) of the extremities◀

▶critical limb ischemia of nonautologous biological bypass graft(s) of the extremities with rest pain◀

I70.521   **Atherosclerosis of nonautologous biological bypass graft(s) of the extremities with rest pain, right leg**   HCC A

I70.522   **Atherosclerosis of nonautologous biological bypass graft(s) of the extremities with rest pain, left leg**   HCC A

I70.523   **Atherosclerosis of nonautologous biological bypass graft(s) of the extremities with rest pain, bilateral legs**   HCC A

I70.528   **Atherosclerosis of nonautologous biological bypass graft(s) of the extremities with rest pain, other extremity**   HCC A

I70.529   **Atherosclerosis of nonautologous biological bypass graft(s) of the extremities with rest pain, unspecified extremity**   HCC A

✓6th **I70.53**   **Atherosclerosis of nonautologous biological bypass graft(s) of the right leg with ulceration**

INCLUDES   any condition classifiable to I70.511 and I70.521

▶chronic limb-threatening ischemia of nonautologous biological bypass graft(s) of the right leg with ulceration◀

▶critical limb ischemia of nonautologous biological bypass graft(s) of the right leg with ulceration◀

Use additional code to identify severity of ulcer (L97.-)

I70.531   **Atherosclerosis of nonautologous biological bypass graft(s) of the right leg with ulceration of thigh**   CC HCC A

I70.532   **Atherosclerosis of nonautologous biological bypass graft(s) of the right leg with ulceration of calf**   CC HCC A

I70.533   **Atherosclerosis of nonautologous biological bypass graft(s) of the right leg with ulceration of ankle**   CC HCC A

I70.534   **Atherosclerosis of nonautologous biological bypass graft(s) of the right leg with ulceration of heel and midfoot**   CC HCC A

Atherosclerosis of nonautologous biological bypass graft(s) of right leg with ulceration of plantar surface of midfoot

I70.535   **Atherosclerosis of nonautologous biological bypass graft(s) of the right leg with ulceration of other part of foot**   HCC A

Atherosclerosis of nonautologous biological bypass graft(s) of the right leg with ulceration of toe

I70.538   **Atherosclerosis of nonautologous biological bypass graft(s) of the right leg with ulceration of other part of lower leg**   CC HCC A

I70.539   **Atherosclerosis of nonautologous biological bypass graft(s) of the right leg with ulceration of unspecified site**   CC HCC A

✓6th **I70.54**   **Atherosclerosis of nonautologous biological bypass graft(s) of the left leg with ulceration**

INCLUDES   any condition classifiable to I70.512 and I70.522

▶chronic limb-threatening ischemia of nonautologous biological bypass graft(s) of the left leg with ulceration◀

▶critical limb ischemia of nonautologous biological bypass graft(s) of the left leg with ulceration◀

Use additional code to identify severity of ulcer (L97.-)

I70.541   **Atherosclerosis of nonautologous biological bypass graft(s) of the left leg with ulceration of thigh**   CC HCC A

I70.542   **Atherosclerosis of nonautologous biological bypass graft(s) of the left leg with ulceration of calf**   CC HCC A

I70.543   **Atherosclerosis of nonautologous biological bypass graft(s) of the left leg with ulceration of ankle**   CC HCC A

I70.544   **Atherosclerosis of nonautologous biological bypass graft(s) of the left leg with ulceration of heel and midfoot**   CC HCC A

Atherosclerosis of nonautologous biological bypass graft(s) of left leg with ulceration of plantar surface of midfoot

N Newborn: 0   P Pediatric: 0-17   M Maternity: 9-64   A Adult: 15-124   MCC Major Complication/Comorbidity   CC Complication/Comorbidity   SW Severe Wound Dx

672   ICD-10-CM 2021

I70.545 Atherosclerosis of nonautologous biological bypass graft(s) of the left leg with ulceration of other part of foot `HCC` `A`

Atherosclerosis of nonautologous biological bypass graft(s) of the left leg with ulceration of toe

I70.548 Atherosclerosis of nonautologous biological bypass graft(s) of the left leg with ulceration of other part of lower leg `CC` `HCC` `A`

I70.549 Atherosclerosis of nonautologous biological bypass graft(s) of the left leg with ulceration of unspecified site `CC` `HCC` `A`

I70.55 Atherosclerosis of nonautologous biological bypass graft(s) of other extremity with ulceration `HCC` `A`

INCLUDES any condition classifiable to I70.518, I70.528, and I70.538

Use additional code to identify severity of ulcer (L98.49)

√6ᵗʰ **I70.56** Atherosclerosis of nonautologous biological bypass graft(s) of the extremities with gangrene

INCLUDES any condition classifiable to I70.51-, I70.52-, and I70.53-, I70.54-, I70.55
▶chronic limb-threatening ischemia of nonautologous biological bypass graft(s) of the extremities with gangrene◀
▶critical limb ischemia of nonautologous biological bypass graft(s) of the extremities with gangrene◀

Use additional code to identify the severity of any ulcer (L97.-, L98.49-), if applicable

I70.561 Atherosclerosis of nonautologous biological bypass graft(s) of the extremities with gangrene, right leg `CC` `HCC` `A`

I70.562 Atherosclerosis of nonautologous biological bypass graft(s) of the extremities with gangrene, left leg `CC` `HCC` `A`

I70.563 Atherosclerosis of nonautologous biological bypass graft(s) of the extremities with gangrene, bilateral legs `CC` `HCC` `A`

I70.568 Atherosclerosis of nonautologous biological bypass graft(s) of the extremities with gangrene, other extremity `CC` `HCC` `A`

I70.569 Atherosclerosis of nonautologous biological bypass graft(s) of the extremities with gangrene, unspecified extremity `CC` `HCC` `A`

√6ᵗʰ **I70.59** Other atherosclerosis of nonautologous biological bypass graft(s) of the extremities

I70.591 Other atherosclerosis of nonautologous biological bypass graft(s) of the extremities, right leg `HCC` `A`

I70.592 Other atherosclerosis of nonautologous biological bypass graft(s) of the extremities, left leg `HCC` `A`

I70.593 Other atherosclerosis of nonautologous biological bypass graft(s) of the extremities, bilateral legs `HCC` `A`

I70.598 Other atherosclerosis of nonautologous biological bypass graft(s) of the extremities, other extremity `HCC` `A`

I70.599 Other atherosclerosis of nonautologous biological bypass graft(s) of the extremities, unspecified extremity `HCC` `A`

√5ᵗʰ **I70.6** Atherosclerosis of nonbiological bypass graft(s) of the extremities

Use additional code, if applicable, to identify chronic total occlusion of artery of extremity (I70.92)

√6ᵗʰ **I70.60** Unspecified atherosclerosis of nonbiological bypass graft(s) of the extremities

I70.601 Unspecified atherosclerosis of nonbiological bypass graft(s) of the extremities, right leg `HCC` `A`

I70.602 Unspecified atherosclerosis of nonbiological bypass graft(s) of the extremities, left leg `HCC` `A`

I70.603 Unspecified atherosclerosis of nonbiological bypass graft(s) of the extremities, bilateral legs `HCC` `A`

I70.608 Unspecified atherosclerosis of nonbiological bypass graft(s) of the extremities, other extremity `HCC` `A`

I70.609 Unspecified atherosclerosis of nonbiological bypass graft(s) of the extremities, unspecified extremity `HCC` `A`

√6ᵗʰ **I70.61** Atherosclerosis of nonbiological bypass graft(s) of the extremities with intermittent claudication

I70.611 Atherosclerosis of nonbiological bypass graft(s) of the extremities with intermittent claudication, right leg `HCC` `A`

I70.612 Atherosclerosis of nonbiological bypass graft(s) of the extremities with intermittent claudication, left leg `HCC` `A`

I70.613 Atherosclerosis of nonbiological bypass graft(s) of the extremities with intermittent claudication, bilateral legs `HCC` `A`

I70.618 Atherosclerosis of nonbiological bypass graft(s) of the extremities with intermittent claudication, other extremity `HCC` `A`

I70.619 Atherosclerosis of nonbiological bypass graft(s) of the extremities with intermittent claudication, unspecified extremity `HCC` `A`

√6ᵗʰ **I70.62** Atherosclerosis of nonbiological bypass graft(s) of the extremities with rest pain

INCLUDES any condition classifiable to I70.61-
▶chronic limb-threatening ischemia NOS of nonbiological bypass graft(s) of the extremities◀
▶chronic limb-threatening ischemia of nonbiological bypass graft(s) of the extremities with rest pain◀
▶critical limb ischemia NOS of nonbiological bypass graft(s) of the extremities◀
▶critical limb ischemia of nonbiological bypass graft(s) of the extremities with rest pain◀

I70.621 Atherosclerosis of nonbiological bypass graft(s) of the extremities with rest pain, right leg `HCC` `A`

I70.622 Atherosclerosis of nonbiological bypass graft(s) of the extremities with rest pain, left leg `HCC` `A`

I70.623 Atherosclerosis of nonbiological bypass graft(s) of the extremities with rest pain, bilateral legs `HCC` `A`

I70.628 Atherosclerosis of nonbiological bypass graft(s) of the extremities with rest pain, other extremity `HCC` `A`

I70.629 Atherosclerosis of nonbiological bypass graft(s) of the extremities with rest pain, unspecified extremity `HCC` `A`

√6ᵗʰ **I70.63** Atherosclerosis of nonbiological bypass graft(s) of the right leg with ulceration

INCLUDES any condition classifiable to I70.611 and I70.621
▶chronic limb-threatening ischemia of nonbiological bypass graft(s) of the right leg with ulceration◀
▶critical limb ischemia of nonbiological bypass graft(s) of the right leg with ulceration◀

Use additional code to identify severity of ulcer (L97.-)

I70.631 Atherosclerosis of nonbiological bypass graft(s) of the right leg with ulceration of thigh `CC` `HCC` `A`

I70.632 Atherosclerosis of nonbiological bypass graft(s) of the right leg with ulceration of calf `CC` `HCC` `A`

☑ Additional Character Required   √x7ᵗʰ Placeholder   Unacceptable PDx   Questionable PDx   Manifestation   Unspecified Dx   H1-H4 HAC   HCC CMS-HCC Dx   HIV HIV Dx

ICD-10-CM 2021   673

I70.633 **Atherosclerosis of nonbiological bypass graft(s) of the right leg with ulceration of ankle** `CC` `HCC` `A`

I70.634 **Atherosclerosis of nonbiological bypass graft(s) of the right leg with ulceration of heel and midfoot** `CC` `HCC` `A`

Atherosclerosis of nonbiological bypass graft(s) of right leg with ulceration of plantar surface of midfoot

I70.635 **Atherosclerosis of nonbiological bypass graft(s) of the right leg with ulceration of other part of foot** `HCC` `A`

Atherosclerosis of nonbiological bypass graft(s) of the right leg with ulceration of toe

I70.638 **Atherosclerosis of nonbiological bypass graft(s) of the right leg with ulceration of other part of lower leg** `CC` `HCC` `A`

I70.639 **Atherosclerosis of nonbiological bypass graft(s) of the right leg with ulceration of unspecified site** `CC` `HCC` `A`

✓6th I70.64 **Atherosclerosis of nonbiological bypass graft(s) of the left leg with ulceration**

INCLUDES any condition classifiable to I70.612 and I70.622

▶chronic limb-threatening ischemia of nonbiological bypass graft(s) of the left leg with ulceration◀

▶critical limb ischemia of nonbiological bypass graft(s) of the left leg with ulceration◀

Use additional code to identify severity of ulcer (L97.-)

I70.641 **Atherosclerosis of nonbiological bypass graft(s) of the left leg with ulceration of thigh** `CC` `HCC` `A`

I70.642 **Atherosclerosis of nonbiological bypass graft(s) of the left leg with ulceration of calf** `CC` `HCC` `A`

I70.643 **Atherosclerosis of nonbiological bypass graft(s) of the left leg with ulceration of ankle** `CC` `HCC` `A`

I70.644 **Atherosclerosis of nonbiological bypass graft(s) of the left leg with ulceration of heel and midfoot** `CC` `HCC` `A`

Atherosclerosis of nonbiological bypass graft(s) of left leg with ulceration of plantar surface of midfoot

I70.645 **Atherosclerosis of nonbiological bypass graft(s) of the left leg with ulceration of other part of foot** `HCC` `A`

Atherosclerosis of nonbiological bypass graft(s) of the left leg with ulceration of toe

I70.648 **Atherosclerosis of nonbiological bypass graft(s) of the left leg with ulceration of other part of lower leg** `CC` `HCC` `A`

I70.649 **Atherosclerosis of nonbiological bypass graft(s) of the left leg with ulceration of unspecified site** `CC` `HCC` `A`

I70.65 **Atherosclerosis of nonbiological bypass graft(s) of other extremity with ulceration** `HCC` `A`

INCLUDES any condition classifiable to I70.618 and I70.628

Use additional code to identify severity of ulcer (L98.49)

✓6th I70.66 **Atherosclerosis of nonbiological bypass graft(s) of the extremities with gangrene**

INCLUDES any condition classifiable to I70.61-, I70.62-, I70.63-, I70.64-, I70.65

▶chronic limb-threatening ischemia of nonbiological bypass graft(s) of the extremities with gangrene◀

▶critical limb ischemia of nonbiological bypass graft(s) of the extremities with gangrene◀

Use additional code to identify the severity of any ulcer (L97.-, L98.49-), if applicable

I70.661 **Atherosclerosis of nonbiological bypass graft(s) of the extremities with gangrene, right leg** `CC` `HCC` `A`

I70.662 **Atherosclerosis of nonbiological bypass graft(s) of the extremities with gangrene, left leg** `CC` `HCC` `A`

I70.663 **Atherosclerosis of nonbiological bypass graft(s) of the extremities with gangrene, bilateral legs** `CC` `HCC` `A`

I70.668 **Atherosclerosis of nonbiological bypass graft(s) of the extremities with gangrene, other extremity** `CC` `HCC` `A`

I70.669 **Atherosclerosis of nonbiological bypass graft(s) of the extremities with gangrene, unspecified extremity** `CC` `HCC` `A`

✓6th I70.69 **Other atherosclerosis of nonbiological bypass graft(s) of the extremities**

I70.691 **Other atherosclerosis of nonbiological bypass graft(s) of the extremities, right leg** `HCC` `A`

I70.692 **Other atherosclerosis of nonbiological bypass graft(s) of the extremities, left leg** `HCC` `A`

I70.693 **Other atherosclerosis of nonbiological bypass graft(s) of the extremities, bilateral legs** `HCC` `A`

I70.698 **Other atherosclerosis of nonbiological bypass graft(s) of the extremities, other extremity** `HCC` `A`

I70.699 **Other atherosclerosis of nonbiological bypass graft(s) of the extremities, unspecified extremity** `HCC` `A`

✓5th I70.7 **Atherosclerosis of other type of bypass graft(s) of the extremities**

Use additional code, if applicable, to identify chronic total occlusion of artery of extremity (I70.92)

✓6th I70.70 **Unspecified atherosclerosis of other type of bypass graft(s) of the extremities**

I70.701 **Unspecified atherosclerosis of other type of bypass graft(s) of the extremities, right leg** `HCC` `A`

I70.702 **Unspecified atherosclerosis of other type of bypass graft(s) of the extremities, left leg** `HCC` `A`

I70.703 **Unspecified atherosclerosis of other type of bypass graft(s) of the extremities, bilateral legs** `HCC` `A`

I70.708 **Unspecified atherosclerosis of other type of bypass graft(s) of the extremities, other extremity** `HCC` `A`

I70.709 **Unspecified atherosclerosis of other type of bypass graft(s) of the extremities, unspecified extremity** `HCC` `A`

✓6th I70.71 **Atherosclerosis of other type of bypass graft(s) of the extremities with intermittent claudication**

I70.711 **Atherosclerosis of other type of bypass graft(s) of the extremities with intermittent claudication, right leg** `HCC` `A`

I70.712 **Atherosclerosis of other type of bypass graft(s) of the extremities with intermittent claudication, left leg** `HCC` `A`

I70.713 **Atherosclerosis of other type of bypass graft(s) of the extremities with intermittent claudication, bilateral legs** `HCC` `A`

I70.718 **Atherosclerosis of other type of bypass graft(s) of the extremities with intermittent claudication, other extremity** `HCC` `A`

I70.719 **Atherosclerosis of other type of bypass graft(s) of the extremities with intermittent claudication, unspecified extremity** `HCC` `A`

N Newborn: 0   P Pediatric: 0-17   M Maternity: 9-64   A Adult: 15-124   MCC Major Complication/Comorbidity   CC Complication/Comorbidity   SW Severe Wound Dx

674   ICD-10-CM 2021

✓6ᵗʰ **I70.72 Atherosclerosis of other type of bypass graft(s) of the extremities with rest pain**

    INCLUDES any condition classifiable to I70.71-

      ▶chronic limb-threatening ischemia NOS of other type of bypass graft(s) of the extremities◀

      ▶chronic limb-threatening ischemia of other type of bypass graft(s) of the extremities with rest pain◀

      ▶critical limb ischemia NOS of other type of bypass graft(s) of the extremities◀

      ▶critical limb ischemia of other type of bypass graft(s) of the extremities with rest pain◀

  I70.721 Atherosclerosis of other type of bypass graft(s) of the extremities with rest pain, right leg HCC A

  I70.722 Atherosclerosis of other type of bypass graft(s) of the extremities with rest pain, left leg HCC A

  I70.723 Atherosclerosis of other type of bypass graft(s) of the extremities with rest pain, bilateral legs HCC A

  I70.728 Atherosclerosis of other type of bypass graft(s) of the extremities with rest pain, other extremity HCC A

  I70.729 Atherosclerosis of other type of bypass graft(s) of the extremities with rest pain, unspecified extremity HCC A

✓6ᵗʰ **I70.73 Atherosclerosis of other type of bypass graft(s) of the right leg with ulceration**

    INCLUDES any condition classifiable to I70.711 and I70.721

      ▶chronic limb-threatening ischemia of other type of bypass graft(s) of the right leg with ulceration◀

      ▶critical limb ischemia of other type of bypass graft(s) of the right leg with ulceration◀

  Use additional code to identify severity of ulcer (L97.-)

  I70.731 Atherosclerosis of other type of bypass graft(s) of the right leg with ulceration of thigh CC HCC A

  I70.732 Atherosclerosis of other type of bypass graft(s) of the right leg with ulceration of calf CC HCC A

  I70.733 Atherosclerosis of other type of bypass graft(s) of the right leg with ulceration of ankle CC HCC A

  I70.734 Atherosclerosis of other type of bypass graft(s) of the right leg with ulceration of heel and midfoot CC HCC A

    Atherosclerosis of other type of bypass graft(s) of right leg with ulceration of plantar surface of midfoot

  I70.735 Atherosclerosis of other type of bypass graft(s) of the right leg with ulceration of other part of foot HCC A

    Atherosclerosis of other type of bypass graft(s) of right leg with ulceration of toe

  I70.738 Atherosclerosis of other type of bypass graft(s) of the right leg with ulceration of other part of lower leg CC HCC A

  I70.739 Atherosclerosis of other type of bypass graft(s) of the right leg with ulceration of unspecified site CC HCC A

✓6ᵗʰ **I70.74 Atherosclerosis of other type of bypass graft(s) of the left leg with ulceration**

    INCLUDES any condition classifiable to I70.712 and I70.722

      ▶chronic limb-threatening ischemia of other type of bypass graft(s) of the left leg with ulceration◀

      ▶critical limb ischemia of other type of bypass graft(s) of the left leg with ulceration◀

  Use additional code to identify severity of ulcer (L97.-)

  I70.741 Atherosclerosis of other type of bypass graft(s) of the left leg with ulceration of thigh CC HCC A

  I70.742 Atherosclerosis of other type of bypass graft(s) of the left leg with ulceration of calf CC HCC A

  I70.743 Atherosclerosis of other type of bypass graft(s) of the left leg with ulceration of ankle CC HCC A

  I70.744 Atherosclerosis of other type of bypass graft(s) of the left leg with ulceration of heel and midfoot CC HCC A

    Atherosclerosis of other type of bypass graft(s) of left leg with ulceration of plantar surface of midfoot

  I70.745 Atherosclerosis of other type of bypass graft(s) of the left leg with ulceration of other part of foot HCC A

    Atherosclerosis of other type of bypass graft(s) of left leg with ulceration of toe

  I70.748 Atherosclerosis of other type of bypass graft(s) of the left leg with ulceration of other part of lower leg CC HCC A

  I70.749 Atherosclerosis of other type of bypass graft(s) of the left leg with ulceration of unspecified site CC HCC A

I70.75 Atherosclerosis of other type of bypass graft(s) of other extremity with ulceration HCC A

    INCLUDES any condition classifiable to I70.718 and I70.728

  Use additional code to identify severity of ulcer (L98.49)

✓6ᵗʰ **I70.76 Atherosclerosis of other type of bypass graft(s) of the extremities with gangrene**

    INCLUDES any condition classifiable to I70.71-, I70.72-, I70.73-, I70.74-, I70.75

      ▶chronic limb-threatening ischemia of other type of bypass graft(s) of the extremities with gangrene◀

      ▶critical limb ischemia of other type of bypass graft(s) of the extremities with gangrene◀

  Use additional code to identify the severity of any ulcer (L97.-, L98.49-), if applicable

  I70.761 Atherosclerosis of other type of bypass graft(s) of the extremities with gangrene, right leg CC HCC A

  I70.762 Atherosclerosis of other type of bypass graft(s) of the extremities with gangrene, left leg CC HCC A

  I70.763 Atherosclerosis of other type of bypass graft(s) of the extremities with gangrene, bilateral legs CC HCC A

  I70.768 Atherosclerosis of other type of bypass graft(s) of the extremities with gangrene, other extremity CC HCC A

  I70.769 Atherosclerosis of other type of bypass graft(s) of the extremities with gangrene, unspecified extremity CC HCC A

✓6ᵗʰ **I70.79 Other atherosclerosis of other type of bypass graft(s) of the extremities**

  I70.791 Other atherosclerosis of other type of bypass graft(s) of the extremities, right leg HCC A

  I70.792 Other atherosclerosis of other type of bypass graft(s) of the extremities, left leg HCC A

  I70.793 Other atherosclerosis of other type of bypass graft(s) of the extremities, bilateral legs HCC A

  I70.798 Other atherosclerosis of other type of bypass graft(s) of the extremities, other extremity HCC A

  I70.799 Other atherosclerosis of other type of bypass graft(s) of the extremities, unspecified extremity HCC A

I70.8 Atherosclerosis of other arteries A

  TIP: Arteriosclerosis of the iliac arteries is coded here.

✓5ᵗʰ **I70.9 Other and unspecified atherosclerosis**

  I70.90 Unspecified atherosclerosis A

  I70.91 Generalized atherosclerosis A

✓ Additional Character Required   ✓x7ᵗʰ Placeholder   Unacceptable PDx   Questionable PDx   Manifestation   Unspecified Dx   H1-H14 HAC   HCC CMS-HCC Dx   HIV HIV Dx

ICD-10-CM 2021   675

Chapter 9. Diseases of the Circulatory System

I70.92   **Chronic total occlusion** of artery of the extremities   `CC` `HCC` `A`
Complete occlusion of artery of the extremities
Total occlusion of artery of the extremities
Code first atherosclerosis of arteries of the extremities (I70.2-, I70.3-, I70.4-, I70.5-, I70.6-, I70.7-)

✓4ᵗʰ **I71**   **Aortic aneurysm and dissection**
   `EXCLUDES 1`   *aortic ectasia (I77.81-)*
           syphilitic aortic aneurysm (A52.01)
           traumatic aortic aneurysm (S25.09, S35.09)

✓5ᵗʰ **I71.0**   **Dissection of aorta**
   I71.00   **Dissection of unspecified site of aorta**   `MCC` `HCC`
   I71.01   **Dissection of thoracic aorta**   `MCC` `HCC`
   I71.02   **Dissection of abdominal aorta**   `MCC` `HCC`
   I71.03   **Dissection of thoracoabdominal aorta**   `MCC` `HCC`

I71.1   **Thoracic aortic aneurysm, ruptured**   `MCC` `HCC`
I71.2   **Thoracic aortic aneurysm, without rupture**   `HCC`
I71.3   **Abdominal aortic aneurysm, ruptured**   `MCC` `HCC`
I71.4   **Abdominal aortic aneurysm, without rupture**   `HCC`
I71.5   **Thoracoabdominal aortic aneurysm, ruptured**   `MCC` `HCC`
I71.6   **Thoracoabdominal aortic aneurysm, without rupture**   `HCC`
I71.8   **Aortic aneurysm of unspecified site, ruptured**   `MCC` `HCC`
   Rupture of aorta NOS
I71.9   **Aortic aneurysm of unspecified site, without rupture**   `HCC`
   Aneurysm of aorta
   Dilatation of aorta
   Hyaline necrosis of aorta

✓4ᵗʰ **I72**   **Other aneurysm**
   `INCLUDES`   aneurysm (cirsoid) (false) (ruptured)
   `EXCLUDES 2`   *acquired aneurysm (I77.0)*
           aneurysm (of) aorta (I71.-)
           aneurysm (of) arteriovenous NOS (Q27.3-)
           carotid artery dissection (I77.71)
           cerebral (nonruptured) aneurysm (I67.1)
           coronary aneurysm (I25.4)
           coronary artery dissection (I25.42)
           dissection of artery NEC (I77.79)
           dissection of precerebral artery, congenital (nonruptured) (Q28.1)
           heart aneurysm (I25.3)
           iliac artery dissection (I77.72)
           precerebral artery, congenital (nonruptured) (Q28.1)
           pulmonary artery aneurysm (I28.1)
           renal artery dissection (I77.73)
           retinal aneurysm (H35.0)
           ruptured cerebral aneurysm (I60.7)
           varicose aneurysm (I77.0)
           vertebral artery dissection (I77.74)
   AHA: 2016,4Q,28-29

I72.0   **Aneurysm of carotid artery**   `HCC`
   Aneurysm of common carotid artery
   Aneurysm of external carotid artery
   Aneurysm of internal carotid artery, extracranial portion
   `EXCLUDES 1`   *aneurysm of internal carotid artery, intracranial portion (I67.1)*
           aneurysm of internal carotid artery NOS (I67.1)

I72.1   **Aneurysm of artery of upper extremity**   `HCC`
I72.2   **Aneurysm of renal artery**   `HCC`
I72.3   **Aneurysm of iliac artery**   `HCC`
I72.4   **Aneurysm of artery of lower extremity**   `HCC`
   AHA: 2019,2Q,21
I72.5   **Aneurysm of other precerebral arteries**   `HCC`
   Aneurysm of basilar artery (trunk)
   `EXCLUDES 2`   *aneurysm of carotid artery (I72.0)*
           aneurysm of vertebral artery (I72.6)
           dissection of carotid artery (I77.71)
           dissection of other precerebral arteries (I77.75)
           dissection of vertebral artery (I77.74)
I72.6   **Aneurysm of vertebral artery**   `HCC`
   `EXCLUDES 2`   *dissection of vertebral artery (I77.74)*
I72.8   **Aneurysm of other specified arteries**   `HCC`

I72.9   **Aneurysm of unspecified site**   `HCC`

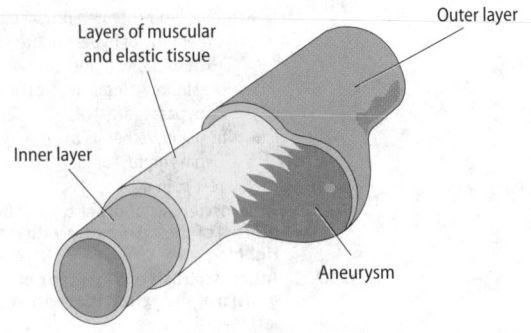

Aneurysm

Layers of muscular and elastic tissue

Outer layer

Inner layer

Aneurysm

✓4ᵗʰ **I73**   **Other peripheral vascular diseases**
   `EXCLUDES 2`   *chilblains (T69.1)*
           frostbite (T33-T34)
           immersion hand or foot (T69.0-)
           spasm of cerebral artery (G45.9)
   AHA: 2018,4Q,87

✓5ᵗʰ **I73.0**   **Raynaud's syndrome**
   Raynaud's disease
   Raynaud's phenomenon (secondary)
   DEF: Constriction of the arteries of the digits caused by cold or by nerve or arterial damage and can be prompted by stress or emotion. Blood cannot reach the skin and soft tissues and the skin turns white with blue mottling.
   I73.00   **Raynaud's syndrome without gangrene**
   I73.01   **Raynaud's syndrome with gangrene**   `CC` `HCC`

I73.1   **Thromboangiitis obliterans [Buerger's disease]**   `HCC`
   DEF: Inflammatory disease of the extremity blood vessels, mainly the lower blood vessels. This disease is associated with heavy tobacco use. The arteries are more affected than veins. It occurs primarily in young men and leads to tissue ischemia and gangrene.

✓5ᵗʰ **I73.8**   **Other specified peripheral vascular diseases**
   `EXCLUDES 1`   *diabetic (peripheral) angiopathy (E08-E13 with .51-.52)*
   I73.81   **Erythromelalgia**   `HCC`
   I73.89   **Other specified peripheral vascular diseases**   `HCC`
     Acrocyanosis
     Erythrocyanosis
     Simple acroparesthesia [Schultze's type]
     Vasomotor acroparesthesia [Nothnagel's type]

I73.9   **Peripheral vascular disease, unspecified**   `HCC`
   Intermittent claudication
   Peripheral angiopathy NOS
   Spasm of artery
   `EXCLUDES 1`   *atherosclerosis of the extremities (I70.2-I70.7-)*
   AHA: 2018,2Q,7

Chapter 9. Diseases of the Circulatory System

I74–I77.819

✓4ᵗʰ **I74** **Arterial embolism and thrombosis**

    INCLUDES   embolic infarction

               embolic occlusion

               thrombotic infarction

               thrombotic occlusion

    Code first:

        embolism and thrombosis complicating abortion or ectopic or molar pregnancy (O00-O07, O08.2)

        embolism and thrombosis complicating pregnancy, childbirth and the puerperium (O88.-)

    EXCLUDES 2   atheroembolism (I75.-)

               basilar embolism and thrombosis (I63.0-I63.2, I65.1)

               carotid embolism and thrombosis (I63.0-I63.2, I65.2)

               cerebral embolism and thrombosis (I63.3-I63.5, I66.-)

               coronary embolism and thrombosis (I21-I25)

               mesenteric embolism and thrombosis (K55.0-)

               ophthalmic embolism and thrombosis (H34.-)

               precerebral embolism and thrombosis NOS (I63.0-I63.2, I65.9)

               pulmonary embolism and thrombosis (I26.-)

               renal embolism and thrombosis (N28.0)

               retinal embolism and thrombosis (H34.-)

               septic embolism and thrombosis (I76)

               vertebral embolism and thrombosis (I63.0-I63.2, I65.0)

    ✓5ᵗʰ **I74.0** **Embolism and thrombosis of abdominal aorta**

        I74.01   **Saddle embolus of abdominal aorta**   `MCC` `HCC`

        I74.09   **Other arterial embolism and thrombosis of abdominal aorta**   `CC` `HCC`

            Aortic bifurcation syndrome

            Aortoiliac obstruction

            Leriche's syndrome

    ✓5ᵗʰ **I74.1** **Embolism and thrombosis of other and unspecified parts of aorta**

        I74.10   **Embolism and thrombosis of unspecified parts of aorta**   `CC` `HCC`

        I74.11   **Embolism and thrombosis of thoracic aorta**   `CC` `HCC`

        I74.19   **Embolism and thrombosis of other parts of aorta**   `CC` `HCC`

    I74.2 **Embolism and thrombosis of arteries of the upper extremities**   `CC` `HCC`

    I74.3 **Embolism and thrombosis of arteries of the lower extremities**   `CC` `HCC`

    I74.4 **Embolism and thrombosis of arteries of extremities, unspecified**   `CC` `HCC`

        Peripheral arterial embolism NOS

    I74.5 **Embolism and thrombosis of iliac artery**   `CC` `HCC`

    I74.8 **Embolism and thrombosis of other arteries**   `CC` `HCC`

    I74.9 **Embolism and thrombosis of unspecified artery**   `CC` `HCC`

✓4ᵗʰ **I75** **Atheroembolism**

    INCLUDES   atherothrombotic microembolism

               cholesterol embolism

    ✓5ᵗʰ **I75.0** **Atheroembolism of extremities**

        ✓6ᵗʰ **I75.01** **Atheroembolism of upper extremity**

            I75.011   **Atheroembolism of right upper extremity**   `CC` `HCC`

            I75.012   **Atheroembolism of left upper extremity**   `CC` `HCC`

            I75.013   **Atheroembolism of bilateral upper extremities**   `CC` `HCC`

            I75.019   **Atheroembolism of unspecified upper extremity**   `CC` `HCC`

        ✓6ᵗʰ **I75.02** **Atheroembolism of lower extremity**

            I75.021   **Atheroembolism of right lower extremity**   `CC` `HCC`

            I75.022   **Atheroembolism of left lower extremity**   `CC` `HCC`

            I75.023   **Atheroembolism of bilateral lower extremities**   `CC` `HCC`

            I75.029   **Atheroembolism of unspecified lower extremity**   `CC` `HCC`

    ✓5ᵗʰ **I75.8** **Atheroembolism of other sites**

        I75.81   **Atheroembolism of kidney**   `CC` `HCC`

            Use additional code for any associated acute kidney failure and chronic kidney disease (N17.-, N18.-)

        I75.89   **Atheroembolism of other site**   `CC` `HCC`

I76 **Septic arterial embolism**   `CC` `HCC`

    Code first underlying infection, such as:

        infective endocarditis (I33.0)

        lung abscess (J85.-)

    Use additional code to identify the site of the embolism (I74.-)

    EXCLUDES 2   septic pulmonary embolism (I26.01, I26.90)

✓4ᵗʰ **I77** **Other disorders of arteries and arterioles**

    EXCLUDES 2   collagen (vascular) diseases (M30-M36)

               hypersensitivity angiitis (M31.0)

               pulmonary artery (I28.-)

    I77.0 **Arteriovenous fistula, acquired**   `HCC`

        Aneurysmal varix

        Arteriovenous aneurysm, acquired

        EXCLUDES 1   arteriovenous aneurysm NOS (Q27.3-)

               presence of arteriovenous shunt (fistula) for dialysis (Z99.2)

               traumatic — see injury of blood vessel by body region

        EXCLUDES 2   cerebral (I67.1)

               coronary (I25.4)

        DEF: Communication between an artery and vein caused by trauma or invasive procedures.

    I77.1 **Stricture of artery**   `HCC`

        Narrowing of artery

    I77.2 **Rupture of artery**   `CC` `HCC`

        Erosion of artery

        Fistula of artery

        Ulcer of artery

        EXCLUDES 1   traumatic rupture of artery — see injury of blood vessel by body region

    I77.3 **Arterial fibromuscular dysplasia**   `HCC`

        Fibromuscular hyperplasia (of) carotid artery

        Fibromuscular hyperplasia (of) renal artery

    I77.4 **Celiac artery compression syndrome**   `CC` `HCC`

    I77.5 **Necrosis of artery**   `CC` `HCC`

    I77.6 **Arteritis, unspecified**   `HCC`

        Aortitis NOS

        Endarteritis NOS

        EXCLUDES 1   arteritis or endarteritis:

               aortic arch (M31.4)

               cerebral NEC (I67.7)

               coronary (I25.89)

               deformans (I70.-)

               giant cell (M31.5, M31.6)

               obliterans (I70.-)

               senile (I70.-)

    ✓5ᵗʰ **I77.7** **Other arterial dissection**

        EXCLUDES 2   dissection of aorta (I71.0-)

               dissection of coronary artery (I25.42)

        AHA: 2016,4Q,28-29

        I77.70   **Dissection of unspecified artery**   `MCC` `HCC`

        I77.71   **Dissection of carotid artery**   `MCC` `HCC`

        I77.72   **Dissection of iliac artery**   `MCC` `HCC`

        I77.73   **Dissection of renal artery**   `MCC` `HCC`

        I77.74   **Dissection of vertebral artery**   `MCC` `HCC`

            EXCLUDES 2   aneurysm of vertebral artery (I72.6)

        I77.75   **Dissection of other precerebral arteries**   `MCC` `HCC`

            Dissection of basilar artery (trunk)

            EXCLUDES 2   aneurysm of carotid artery (I72.0)

                  aneurysm of other precerebral arteries (I72.5)

                  aneurysm of vertebral artery (I72.6)

                  dissection of carotid artery (I77.71)

                  dissection of vertebral artery (I77.74)

        I77.76   **Dissection of artery of upper extremity**   `MCC` `HCC`

        I77.77   **Dissection of artery of lower extremity**   `MCC` `HCC`

        I77.79   **Dissection of other specified artery**   `MCC` `HCC`

    ✓5ᵗʰ **I77.8** **Other specified disorders of arteries and arterioles**

        ✓6ᵗʰ **I77.81** **Aortic ectasia**

            Ectasis aorta

            EXCLUDES 1   aortic aneurysm and dissection (I71.0-)

            I77.810   **Thoracic aortic ectasia**   `HCC`

            I77.811   **Abdominal aortic ectasia**   `HCC`

            I77.812   **Thoracoabdominal aortic ectasia**   `HCC`

            I77.819   **Aortic ectasia, unspecified site**   `HCC`

✓ Additional Character Required   ✓x7ᵗʰ Placeholder   Unacceptable PDx   Questionable PDx   Manifestation   Unspecified Dx   `H1`-`H14` HAC   `HCC` CMS-HCC Dx   `HIV` HIV Dx

ICD-10-CM 2021   **677**

I77.89   **Other specified disorders of arteries and arterioles** `HCC`

I77.9   **Disorder of arteries and arterioles, unspecified** `HCC`
AHA: 2018,2Q,7

✓4th **I78**   **Diseases of capillaries**

I78.0   **Hereditary hemorrhagic telangiectasia** `HCC`
Rendu-Osler-Weber disease

I78.1   **Nevus, non-neoplastic**
Araneus nevus
Senile nevus
Spider nevus
Stellar nevus
EXCLUDES 1   nevus NOS (D22.-)
    vascular NOS (Q82.5)
EXCLUDES 2   blue nevus (D22.-)
    flammeus nevus (Q82.5)
    hairy nevus (D22.-)
    melanocytic nevus (D22.-)
    pigmented nevus (D22.-)
    portwine nevus (Q82.5)
    sanguineous nevus (Q82.5)
    strawberry nevus (Q82.5)
    verrucous nevus (Q82.5)
AHA: 2019,1Q,21

I78.8   **Other diseases of capillaries**

I78.9   **Disease of capillaries, unspecified**

✓4th **I79**   **Disorders of arteries, arterioles and capillaries in diseases classified elsewhere**

I79.0   *Aneurysm of aorta in diseases classified elsewhere* `HCC`
Code first underlying disease
EXCLUDES 1   syphilitic aneurysm (A52.01)

I79.1   *Aortitis in diseases classified elsewhere* `HCC`
Code first underlying disease
EXCLUDES 1   syphilitic aortitis (A52.02)

I79.8   *Other disorders of arteries, arterioles and capillaries in diseases classified elsewhere* `HCC`
Code first underlying disease, such as:
amyloidosis (E85.-)
EXCLUDES 1   diabetic (peripheral) angiopathy (E08-E13 with .51-.52)
    syphilitic endarteritis (A52.09)
    tuberculous endarteritis (A18.89)

Diseases of veins, lymphatic vessels and lymph nodes, not elsewhere classified (I80-I89)

✓4th **I80**   **Phlebitis and thrombophlebitis**
INCLUDES   endophlebitis
    inflammation, vein
    periphlebitis
    suppurative phlebitis
Code first:
phlebitis and thrombophlebitis complicating abortion, ectopic or molar pregnancy (O00-O07, O08.7)
phlebitis and thrombophlebitis complicating pregnancy, childbirth and the puerperium (O22.-, O87.)
EXCLUDES 1   venous embolism and thrombosis of lower extremities (I82.4-, I82.5-, I82.81-)

✓5th **I80.0**   **Phlebitis and thrombophlebitis of superficial vessels of lower extremities**
Phlebitis and thrombophlebitis of femoropopliteal vein

I80.00   **Phlebitis and thrombophlebitis of superficial vessels of unspecified lower extremity**

I80.01   **Phlebitis and thrombophlebitis of superficial vessels of right lower extremity**

I80.02   **Phlebitis and thrombophlebitis of superficial vessels of left lower extremity**

I80.03   **Phlebitis and thrombophlebitis of superficial vessels of lower extremities, bilateral**

✓5th **I80.1**   **Phlebitis and thrombophlebitis of femoral vein**
Phlebitis and thrombophlebitis of common femoral vein
Phlebitis and thrombophlebitis of deep femoral vein

I80.10   **Phlebitis and thrombophlebitis of unspecified femoral vein** `CC` `HCC`

I80.11   **Phlebitis and thrombophlebitis of right femoral vein** `CC` `HCC`

I80.12   **Phlebitis and thrombophlebitis of left femoral vein** `CC` `HCC`

I80.13   **Phlebitis and thrombophlebitis of femoral vein, bilateral** `CC` `HCC`

✓5th **I80.2**   **Phlebitis and thrombophlebitis of other and unspecified deep vessels of lower extremities**

✓6th **I80.20**   **Phlebitis and thrombophlebitis of unspecified deep vessels of lower extremities**

I80.201   **Phlebitis and thrombophlebitis of unspecified deep vessels of right lower extremity** `CC` `HCC`

I80.202   **Phlebitis and thrombophlebitis of unspecified deep vessels of left lower extremity** `CC` `HCC`

I80.203   **Phlebitis and thrombophlebitis of unspecified deep vessels of lower extremities, bilateral** `CC` `HCC`

I80.209   **Phlebitis and thrombophlebitis of unspecified deep vessels of unspecified lower extremity** `CC` `HCC`

✓6th **I80.21**   **Phlebitis and thrombophlebitis of iliac vein**
Phlebitis and thrombophlebitis of common iliac vein
Phlebitis and thrombophlebitis of external iliac vein
Phlebitis and thrombophlebitis of internal iliac vein

I80.211   **Phlebitis and thrombophlebitis of right iliac vein** `CC` `HCC`

I80.212   **Phlebitis and thrombophlebitis of left iliac vein** `CC` `HCC`

I80.213   **Phlebitis and thrombophlebitis of iliac vein, bilateral** `CC` `HCC`

I80.219   **Phlebitis and thrombophlebitis of unspecified iliac vein** `CC` `HCC`

✓6th **I80.22**   **Phlebitis and thrombophlebitis of popliteal vein**

I80.221   **Phlebitis and thrombophlebitis of right popliteal vein** `CC` `HCC`

I80.222   **Phlebitis and thrombophlebitis of left popliteal vein** `CC` `HCC`

I80.223   **Phlebitis and thrombophlebitis of popliteal vein, bilateral** `CC` `HCC`

I80.229   **Phlebitis and thrombophlebitis of unspecified popliteal vein** `CC` `HCC`

✓6th **I80.23**   **Phlebitis and thrombophlebitis of tibial vein**
Phlebitis and thrombophlebitis of anterior tibial vein
Phlebitis and thrombophlebitis of posterior tibial vein

I80.231   **Phlebitis and thrombophlebitis of right tibial vein** `CC` `HCC`

I80.232   **Phlebitis and thrombophlebitis of left tibial vein** `CC` `HCC`

I80.233   **Phlebitis and thrombophlebitis of tibial vein, bilateral** `CC` `HCC`

I80.239   **Phlebitis and thrombophlebitis of unspecified tibial vein** `CC` `HCC`

✓6th **I80.24**   **Phlebitis and thrombophlebitis of peroneal vein**
AHA: 2019,4Q,8

I80.241   **Phlebitis and thrombophlebitis of right peroneal vein** `CC` `HCC`

I80.242   **Phlebitis and thrombophlebitis of left peroneal vein** `CC` `HCC`

I80.243   **Phlebitis and thrombophlebitis of peroneal vein, bilateral** `CC` `HCC`

I80.249   **Phlebitis and thrombophlebitis of unspecified peroneal vein** `CC` `HCC`

✓6th **I80.25**   **Phlebitis and thrombophlebitis of calf muscular vein**
Phlebitis and thrombophlebitis of calf muscular vein, NOS
Phlebitis and thrombophlebitis of gastrocnemial vein
Phlebitis and thrombophlebitis of soleal vein
AHA: 2019,4Q,8

I80.251   **Phlebitis and thrombophlebitis of right calf muscular vein** `HCC`

I80.252   **Phlebitis and thrombophlebitis of left calf muscular vein** `HCC`

I80.253   **Phlebitis and thrombophlebitis of calf muscular vein, bilateral** `HCC`

I80.259   **Phlebitis and thrombophlebitis of unspecified calf muscular vein** `HCC`

✓6ᵗʰ   **I80.29**   **Phlebitis and thrombophlebitis of other deep vessels of lower extremities**

    I80.291   **Phlebitis and thrombophlebitis of other deep vessels of right lower extremity**   CC   HCC

    I80.292   **Phlebitis and thrombophlebitis of other deep vessels of left lower extremity**   CC   HCC

    I80.293   **Phlebitis and thrombophlebitis of other deep vessels of lower extremity, bilateral**   CC   HCC

    I80.299   **Phlebitis and thrombophlebitis of other deep vessels of unspecified lower extremity**   CC   HCC

I80.3   **Phlebitis and thrombophlebitis of lower extremities, unspecified**

I80.8   **Phlebitis and thrombophlebitis of other sites**

I80.9   **Phlebitis and thrombophlebitis of unspecified site**

I81   **Portal vein thrombosis**   MCC

    Portal (vein) obstruction

    EXCLUDES 2   *hepatic vein thrombosis (I82.0)*

             phlebitis of portal vein (K75.1)

    AHA: 2019,4Q,68

✓4ᵗʰ   **I82**   **Other venous embolism and thrombosis**

    Code first venous embolism and thrombosis complicating:

      abortion, ectopic or molar pregnancy (O00-O07, O08.7)

      pregnancy, childbirth and the puerperium (O22.-, O87.-)

    EXCLUDES 2   *venous embolism and thrombosis (of):*

           cerebral (I63.6, I67.6)

           coronary (I21-I25)

           intracranial and intraspinal, septic or NOS (G08)

           intracranial, nonpyogenic (I67.6)

           intraspinal, nonpyogenic (G95.1)

           mesenteric (K55.0-)

           portal (I81)

           pulmonary (I26.-)

I82.0   **Budd-Chiari syndrome**   MCC   HCC

    Hepatic vein thrombosis

    DEF: Thrombosis or other obstruction of the hepatic veins. Symptoms include an enlarged liver, extensive collateral vessels, intractable ascites, and severe portal hypertension.

I82.1   **Thrombophlebitis migrans**   CC

✓5ᵗʰ   **I82.2**   **Embolism and thrombosis of vena cava and other thoracic veins**

   ✓6ᵗʰ   **I82.21**   **Embolism and thrombosis of superior vena cava**

      I82.210   **Acute embolism and thrombosis of superior vena cava**   CC   HCC

        Embolism and thrombosis of superior vena cava NOS

      I82.211   **Chronic embolism and thrombosis of superior vena cava**   CC   HCC

   ✓6ᵗʰ   **I82.22**   **Embolism and thrombosis of inferior vena cava**

      I82.220   **Acute embolism and thrombosis of inferior vena cava**   MCC   HCC

        Embolism and thrombosis of inferior vena cava NOS

      I82.221   **Chronic embolism and thrombosis of inferior vena cava**   MCC   HCC

   ✓6ᵗʰ   **I82.29**   **Embolism and thrombosis of other thoracic veins**

      Embolism and thrombosis of brachiocephalic (innominate) vein

      I82.290   **Acute embolism and thrombosis of other thoracic veins**   CC   HCC

      I82.291   **Chronic embolism and thrombosis of other thoracic veins**   CC   HCC

I82.3   **Embolism and thrombosis of renal vein**   CC   HCC

✓5ᵗʰ   **I82.4**   **Acute embolism and thrombosis of deep veins of lower extremity**

   ✓6ᵗʰ   **I82.40**   **Acute embolism and thrombosis of unspecified deep veins of lower extremity**

     Deep vein thrombosis NOS

     DVT NOS

     EXCLUDES 1   *acute embolism and thrombosis of unspecified deep veins of distal lower extremity (I82.4Z-)*

              acute embolism and thrombosis of unspecified deep veins of proximal lower extremity (I82.4Y-)

     I82.401   **Acute embolism and thrombosis of unspecified deep veins of right lower extremity**   CC   H10   HCC

     I82.402   **Acute embolism and thrombosis of unspecified deep veins of left lower extremity**   CC   H10   HCC

     I82.403   **Acute embolism and thrombosis of unspecified deep veins of lower extremity, bilateral**   CC   H10   HCC

     I82.409   **Acute embolism and thrombosis of unspecified deep veins of unspecified lower extremity**   CC   H10   HCC

   ✓6ᵗʰ   **I82.41**   **Acute embolism and thrombosis of femoral vein**

     Acute embolism and thrombosis of common femoral vein

     Acute embolism and thrombosis of deep femoral vein

     I82.411   **Acute embolism and thrombosis of right femoral vein**   CC   H10   HCC

     I82.412   **Acute embolism and thrombosis of left femoral vein**   CC   H10   HCC

     I82.413   **Acute embolism and thrombosis of femoral vein, bilateral**   CC   H10   HCC

     I82.419   **Acute embolism and thrombosis of unspecified femoral vein**   CC   H10   HCC

   ✓6ᵗʰ   **I82.42**   **Acute embolism and thrombosis of iliac vein**

     Acute embolism and thrombosis of common iliac vein

     Acute embolism and thrombosis of external iliac vein

     Acute embolism and thrombosis of internal iliac vein

     I82.421   **Acute embolism and thrombosis of right iliac vein**   CC   H10   HCC

     I82.422   **Acute embolism and thrombosis of left iliac vein**   CC   H10   HCC

     I82.423   **Acute embolism and thrombosis of iliac vein, bilateral**   CC   H10   HCC

     I82.429   **Acute embolism and thrombosis of unspecified iliac vein**   CC   H10   HCC

   ✓6ᵗʰ   **I82.43**   **Acute embolism and thrombosis of popliteal vein**

     I82.431   **Acute embolism and thrombosis of right popliteal vein**   CC   H10   HCC

     I82.432   **Acute embolism and thrombosis of left popliteal vein**   CC   H10   HCC

     I82.433   **Acute embolism and thrombosis of popliteal vein, bilateral**   CC   H10   HCC

     I82.439   **Acute embolism and thrombosis of unspecified popliteal vein**   CC   H10   HCC

   ✓6ᵗʰ   **I82.44**   **Acute embolism and thrombosis of tibial vein**

     Acute embolism and thrombosis of anterior tibial vein

     Acute embolism and thrombosis of posterior tibial vein

     I82.441   **Acute embolism and thrombosis of right tibial vein**   CC   H10   HCC

     I82.442   **Acute embolism and thrombosis of left tibial vein**   CC   H10   HCC

     I82.443   **Acute embolism and thrombosis of tibial vein, bilateral**   CC   H10   HCC

     I82.449   **Acute embolism and thrombosis of unspecified tibial vein**   CC   H10   HCC

   ✓6ᵗʰ   **I82.45**   **Acute embolism and thrombosis of peroneal vein**

     AHA: 2019,4Q,8-10

     I82.451   **Acute embolism and thrombosis of right peroneal vein**   CC   H10   HCC

     I82.452   **Acute embolism and thrombosis of left peroneal vein**   CC   H10   HCC

     I82.453   **Acute embolism and thrombosis of peroneal vein, bilateral**   CC   H10   HCC

     I82.459   **Acute embolism and thrombosis of unspecified peroneal vein**   CC   H10   HCC

☑ Additional Character Required   ✓x7ᵗʰ Placeholder   Unacceptable PDx   Questionable PDx   Manifestation   Unspecified Dx   H1 - H14 HAC   HCC CMS-HCC Dx   HIV HIV Dx

ICD-10-CM 2021   **679**

√6ᵗʰ **I82.46** **Acute embolism and thrombosis of calf muscular vein**

Acute embolism and thrombosis of calf muscular vein, NOS

Acute embolism and thrombosis of gastrocnemial vein

Acute embolism and thrombosis of soleal vein

AHA: 2019,4Q,8-10

I82.461 **Acute embolism and thrombosis of right calf muscular vein** `HCC`

I82.462 **Acute embolism and thrombosis of left calf muscular vein** `HCC`

I82.463 **Acute embolism and thrombosis of calf muscular vein, bilateral** `HCC`

I82.469 **Acute embolism and thrombosis of unspecified calf muscular vein** `HCC`

√6ᵗʰ **I82.49** **Acute embolism and thrombosis of other specified deep vein of lower extremity**

I82.491 **Acute embolism and thrombosis of other specified deep vein of right lower extremity** `CC` `H10` `HCC`

I82.492 **Acute embolism and thrombosis of other specified deep vein of left lower extremity** `CC` `H10` `HCC`

I82.493 **Acute embolism and thrombosis of other specified deep vein of lower extremity, bilateral** `CC` `H10` `HCC`

I82.499 **Acute embolism and thrombosis of other specified deep vein of unspecified lower extremity** `CC` `H10` `HCC`

√6ᵗʰ **I82.4Y** **Acute embolism and thrombosis of unspecified deep veins of proximal lower extremity**

Acute embolism and thrombosis of deep vein of thigh NOS

Acute embolism and thrombosis of deep vein of upper leg NOS

I82.4Y1 **Acute embolism and thrombosis of unspecified deep veins of right proximal lower extremity** `CC` `H10` `HCC`

I82.4Y2 **Acute embolism and thrombosis of unspecified deep veins of left proximal lower extremity** `CC` `H10` `HCC`

I82.4Y3 **Acute embolism and thrombosis of unspecified deep veins of proximal lower extremity, bilateral** `CC` `H10` `HCC`

I82.4Y9 **Acute embolism and thrombosis of unspecified deep veins of unspecified proximal lower extremity** `CC` `H10` `HCC`

√6ᵗʰ **I82.4Z** **Acute embolism and thrombosis of unspecified deep veins of distal lower extremity**

Acute embolism and thrombosis of deep vein of calf NOS

Acute embolism and thrombosis of deep vein of lower leg NOS

I82.4Z1 **Acute embolism and thrombosis of unspecified deep veins of right distal lower extremity** `CC` `H10` `HCC`

I82.4Z2 **Acute embolism and thrombosis of unspecified deep veins of left distal lower extremity** `CC` `H10` `HCC`

I82.4Z3 **Acute embolism and thrombosis of unspecified deep veins of distal lower extremity, bilateral** `CC` `H10` `HCC`

I82.4Z9 **Acute embolism and thrombosis of unspecified deep veins of unspecified distal lower extremity** `CC` `H10` `HCC`

√5ᵗʰ **I82.5** **Chronic embolism and thrombosis of deep veins of lower extremity**

Use additional code, if applicable, for associated long-term (current) use of anticoagulants (Z79.01)

EXCLUDES 1   *personal history of venous embolism and thrombosis (Z86.718)*

AHA: 2020,2Q,20

√6ᵗʰ **I82.50** **Chronic embolism and thrombosis of unspecified deep veins of lower extremity**

EXCLUDES 1   *chronic embolism and thrombosis of unspecified deep veins of distal lower extremity (I82.5Z-)*

chronic embolism and thrombosis of unspecified deep veins of proximal lower extremity (I82.5Y-)

I82.501 **Chronic embolism and thrombosis of unspecified deep veins of right lower extremity** `CC` `HCC`

I82.502 **Chronic embolism and thrombosis of unspecified deep veins of left lower extremity** `CC` `HCC`

I82.503 **Chronic embolism and thrombosis of unspecified deep veins of lower extremity, bilateral** `CC` `HCC`

I82.509 **Chronic embolism and thrombosis of unspecified deep veins of unspecified lower extremity** `CC` `HCC`

√6ᵗʰ **I82.51** **Chronic embolism and thrombosis of femoral vein**

Chronic embolism and thrombosis of common femoral vein

Chronic embolism and thrombosis of deep femoral vein

I82.511 **Chronic embolism and thrombosis of right femoral vein** `CC` `HCC`

I82.512 **Chronic embolism and thrombosis of left femoral vein** `CC` `HCC`

I82.513 **Chronic embolism and thrombosis of femoral vein, bilateral** `CC` `HCC`

I82.519 **Chronic embolism and thrombosis of unspecified femoral vein** `CC` `HCC`

√6ᵗʰ **I82.52** **Chronic embolism and thrombosis of iliac vein**

Chronic embolism and thrombosis of common iliac vein

Chronic embolism and thrombosis of external iliac vein

Chronic embolism and thrombosis of internal iliac vein

I82.521 **Chronic embolism and thrombosis of right iliac vein** `CC` `HCC`

I82.522 **Chronic embolism and thrombosis of left iliac vein** `CC` `HCC`

I82.523 **Chronic embolism and thrombosis of iliac vein, bilateral** `CC` `HCC`

I82.529 **Chronic embolism and thrombosis of unspecified iliac vein** `CC` `HCC`

√6ᵗʰ **I82.53** **Chronic embolism and thrombosis of popliteal vein**

I82.531 **Chronic embolism and thrombosis of right popliteal vein** `CC` `HCC`

I82.532 **Chronic embolism and thrombosis of left popliteal vein** `CC` `HCC`

I82.533 **Chronic embolism and thrombosis of popliteal vein, bilateral** `CC` `HCC`

I82.539 **Chronic embolism and thrombosis of unspecified popliteal vein** `CC` `HCC`

√6ᵗʰ **I82.54** **Chronic embolism and thrombosis of tibial vein**

Chronic embolism and thrombosis of anterior tibial vein

Chronic embolism and thrombosis of posterior tibial vein

I82.541 **Chronic embolism and thrombosis of right tibial vein** `CC` `HCC`

I82.542 **Chronic embolism and thrombosis of left tibial vein** `CC` `HCC`

I82.543 **Chronic embolism and thrombosis of tibial vein, bilateral** `CC` `HCC`

I82.549 **Chronic embolism and thrombosis of unspecified tibial vein** `CC` `HCC`

N Newborn: 0   P Pediatric: 0-17   M Maternity: 9-64   A Adult: 15-124   MCC Major Complication/Comorbidity   CC Complication/Comorbidity   SW Severe Wound Dx

680   ICD-10-CM 2021

√6ᵗʰ **I82.55** **Chronic embolism and thrombosis of** peroneal vein
  AHA: 2019,4Q,8-10

     I82.551 **Chronic embolism and thrombosis of** right **peroneal vein**   CC HCC

     I82.552 **Chronic embolism and thrombosis of** left **peroneal vein**   CC HCC

     I82.553 **Chronic embolism and thrombosis of peroneal vein,** bilateral   CC HCC

     I82.559 **Chronic embolism and thrombosis of unspecified peroneal vein**   CC HCC

√6ᵗʰ **I82.56** **Chronic embolism and thrombosis of** calf muscular vein
  Chronic embolism and thrombosis of calf muscular vein NOS
  Chronic embolism and thrombosis of gastrocnemial vein
  Chronic embolism and thrombosis of soleal vein
  AHA: 2019,4Q,8-10

     I82.561 **Chronic embolism and thrombosis of** right **calf muscular vein**   HCC

     I82.562 **Chronic embolism and thrombosis of** left **calf muscular vein**   HCC

     I82.563 **Chronic embolism and thrombosis of calf muscular vein,** bilateral   HCC

     I82.569 **Chronic embolism and thrombosis of unspecified calf muscular vein**   HCC

√6ᵗʰ **I82.59** **Chronic embolism and thrombosis of other specified deep vein of lower extremity**

     I82.591 **Chronic embolism and thrombosis of other specified deep vein of** right **lower extremity**   CC HCC

     I82.592 **Chronic embolism and thrombosis of other specified deep vein of** left **lower extremity**   CC HCC

     I82.593 **Chronic embolism and thrombosis of other specified deep vein of lower extremity,** bilateral   CC HCC

     I82.599 **Chronic embolism and thrombosis of other specified deep vein of unspecified lower extremity**   CC HCC

√6ᵗʰ **I82.5Y** **Chronic embolism and thrombosis of unspecified deep veins of** proximal **lower extremity**
  Chronic embolism and thrombosis of deep veins of thigh NOS
  Chronic embolism and thrombosis of deep veins of upper leg NOS

     I82.5Y1 **Chronic embolism and thrombosis of unspecified deep veins of** right **proximal lower extremity**   CC HCC

     I82.5Y2 **Chronic embolism and thrombosis of unspecified deep veins of** left **proximal lower extremity**   CC HCC

     I82.5Y3 **Chronic embolism and thrombosis of unspecified deep veins of proximal lower extremity,** bilateral   CC HCC

     I82.5Y9 **Chronic embolism and thrombosis of unspecified deep veins of unspecified proximal lower extremity**   CC HCC

√6ᵗʰ **I82.5Z** **Chronic embolism and thrombosis of unspecified deep veins of** distal **lower extremity**
  Chronic embolism and thrombosis of deep veins of calf NOS
  Chronic embolism and thrombosis of deep veins of lower leg NOS

     I82.5Z1 **Chronic embolism and thrombosis of unspecified deep veins of** right **distal lower extremity**   CC HCC

     I82.5Z2 **Chronic embolism and thrombosis of unspecified deep veins of** left **distal lower extremity**   CC HCC

     I82.5Z3 **Chronic embolism and thrombosis of unspecified deep veins of distal lower extremity,** bilateral   CC HCC

     I82.5Z9 **Chronic embolism and thrombosis of unspecified deep veins of unspecified distal lower extremity**   CC HCC

√5ᵗʰ **I82.6** Acute **embolism and thrombosis of veins of** upper extremity

√6ᵗʰ **I82.60** **Acute embolism and thrombosis of unspecified veins of upper extremity**

     I82.601 **Acute embolism and thrombosis of unspecified veins of** right **upper extremity**   CC

     I82.602 **Acute embolism and thrombosis of unspecified veins of** left **upper extremity**   CC

     I82.603 **Acute embolism and thrombosis of unspecified veins of upper extremity,** bilateral   CC

     I82.609 **Acute embolism and thrombosis of unspecified veins of unspecified upper extremity**   CC

√6ᵗʰ **I82.61** **Acute embolism and thrombosis of** superficial veins **of upper extremity**
  Acute embolism and thrombosis of antecubital vein
  Acute embolism and thrombosis of basilic vein
  Acute embolism and thrombosis of cephalic vein

     I82.611 **Acute embolism and thrombosis of superficial veins of** right **upper extremity**   CC

     I82.612 **Acute embolism and thrombosis of superficial veins of** left **upper extremity**   CC

     I82.613 **Acute embolism and thrombosis of superficial veins of upper extremity,** bilateral   CC

     I82.619 **Acute embolism and thrombosis of superficial veins of unspecified upper extremity**   CC

√6ᵗʰ **I82.62** **Acute embolism and thrombosis of** deep veins **of upper extremity**
  Acute embolism and thrombosis of brachial vein
  Acute embolism and thrombosis of radial vein
  Acute embolism and thrombosis of ulnar vein

     I82.621 **Acute embolism and thrombosis of deep veins of** right **upper extremity**   CC HCC

     I82.622 **Acute embolism and thrombosis of deep veins of** left **upper extremity**   CC HCC

     I82.623 **Acute embolism and thrombosis of deep veins of upper extremity,** bilateral   CC HCC

     I82.629 **Acute embolism and thrombosis of deep veins of unspecified upper extremity**   CC HCC

√5ᵗʰ **I82.7** Chronic **embolism and thrombosis of veins of** upper extremity
  Use additional code, if applicable, for associated long-term (current) use of anticoagulants (Z79.01)
  EXCLUDES 1   *personal history of venous embolism and thrombosis (Z86.718)*

√6ᵗʰ **I82.70** **Chronic embolism and thrombosis of unspecified veins of upper extremity**

     I82.701 **Chronic embolism and thrombosis of unspecified veins of** right **upper extremity**   CC

     I82.702 **Chronic embolism and thrombosis of unspecified veins of** left **upper extremity**   CC

     I82.703 **Chronic embolism and thrombosis of unspecified veins of upper extremity,** bilateral   CC

     I82.709 **Chronic embolism and thrombosis of unspecified veins of unspecified upper extremity**   CC

√6ᵗʰ **I82.71** **Chronic embolism and thrombosis of** superficial veins **of upper extremity**
  Chronic embolism and thrombosis of antecubital vein
  Chronic embolism and thrombosis of basilic vein
  Chronic embolism and thrombosis of cephalic vein

     I82.711 **Chronic embolism and thrombosis of superficial veins of** right **upper extremity**   CC

     I82.712 **Chronic embolism and thrombosis of superficial veins of** left **upper extremity**   CC

     I82.713 **Chronic embolism and thrombosis of superficial veins of upper extremity,** bilateral   CC

✔ Additional Character Required   ✔x7ᵗʰ Placeholder   Unacceptable PDx   Questionable PDx   Manifestation   Unspecified Dx   H1-H14 HAC   HCC CMS-HCC Dx   HIV HIV Dx

ICD-10-CM 2021   681

I82.719 Chronic embolism and thrombosis of superficial veins of unspecified upper extremity `CC`

√6ᵗʰ **I82.72** Chronic embolism and thrombosis of deep veins of upper extremity
Chronic embolism and thrombosis of brachial vein
Chronic embolism and thrombosis of radial vein
Chronic embolism and thrombosis of ulnar vein

I82.721 Chronic embolism and thrombosis of deep veins of right upper extremity `CC` `HCC`

I82.722 Chronic embolism and thrombosis of deep veins of left upper extremity `CC` `HCC`

I82.723 Chronic embolism and thrombosis of deep veins of upper extremity, bilateral `CC` `HCC`

I82.729 Chronic embolism and thrombosis of deep veins of unspecified upper extremity `CC` `HCC`

√5ᵗʰ **I82.A** Embolism and thrombosis of axillary vein

√6ᵗʰ **I82.A1** Acute embolism and thrombosis of axillary vein

I82.A11 Acute embolism and thrombosis of right axillary vein `CC` `HCC`

I82.A12 Acute embolism and thrombosis of left axillary vein `CC` `HCC`

I82.A13 Acute embolism and thrombosis of axillary vein, bilateral `CC` `HCC`

I82.A19 Acute embolism and thrombosis of unspecified axillary vein `CC` `HCC`

√6ᵗʰ **I82.A2** Chronic embolism and thrombosis of axillary vein

I82.A21 Chronic embolism and thrombosis of right axillary vein `CC` `HCC`

I82.A22 Chronic embolism and thrombosis of left axillary vein `CC` `HCC`

I82.A23 Chronic embolism and thrombosis of axillary vein, bilateral `CC` `HCC`

I82.A29 Chronic embolism and thrombosis of unspecified axillary vein `CC` `HCC`

√5ᵗʰ **I82.B** Embolism and thrombosis of subclavian vein

√6ᵗʰ **I82.B1** Acute embolism and thrombosis of subclavian vein

I82.B11 Acute embolism and thrombosis of right subclavian vein `CC` `HCC`

I82.B12 Acute embolism and thrombosis of left subclavian vein `CC` `HCC`

I82.B13 Acute embolism and thrombosis of subclavian vein, bilateral `CC` `HCC`

I82.B19 Acute embolism and thrombosis of unspecified subclavian vein `CC` `HCC`

√6ᵗʰ **I82.B2** Chronic embolism and thrombosis of subclavian vein

I82.B21 Chronic embolism and thrombosis of right subclavian vein `CC` `HCC`

I82.B22 Chronic embolism and thrombosis of left subclavian vein `CC` `HCC`

I82.B23 Chronic embolism and thrombosis of subclavian vein, bilateral `CC` `HCC`

I82.B29 Chronic embolism and thrombosis of unspecified subclavian vein `CC` `HCC`

√5ᵗʰ **I82.C** Embolism and thrombosis of internal jugular vein

√6ᵗʰ **I82.C1** Acute embolism and thrombosis of internal jugular vein

I82.C11 Acute embolism and thrombosis of right internal jugular vein `CC` `HCC`

I82.C12 Acute embolism and thrombosis of left internal jugular vein `CC` `HCC`

I82.C13 Acute embolism and thrombosis of internal jugular vein, bilateral `CC` `HCC`

I82.C19 Acute embolism and thrombosis of unspecified internal jugular vein `CC` `HCC`

√6ᵗʰ **I82.C2** Chronic embolism and thrombosis of internal jugular vein

I82.C21 Chronic embolism and thrombosis of right internal jugular vein `CC` `HCC`

I82.C22 Chronic embolism and thrombosis of left internal jugular vein `CC` `HCC`

I82.C23 Chronic embolism and thrombosis of internal jugular vein, bilateral `CC` `HCC`

I82.C29 Chronic embolism and thrombosis of unspecified internal jugular vein `CC` `HCC`

√5ᵗʰ **I82.8** Embolism and thrombosis of other specified veins
Use additional code, if applicable, for associated long-term (current) use of anticoagulants (Z79.Ø1)

√6ᵗʰ **I82.81** Embolism and thrombosis of superficial veins of lower extremities
Embolism and thrombosis of saphenous vein (greater) (lesser)

I82.811 Embolism and thrombosis of superficial veins of right lower extremity `CC`

I82.812 Embolism and thrombosis of superficial veins of left lower extremity `CC`

I82.813 Embolism and thrombosis of superficial veins of lower extremities, bilateral `CC`

I82.819 Embolism and thrombosis of superficial veins of unspecified lower extremity `CC`

√6ᵗʰ **I82.89** Embolism and thrombosis of other specified veins

I82.89Ø Acute embolism and thrombosis of other specified veins `CC`

I82.891 Chronic embolism and thrombosis of other specified veins `CC`

√5ᵗʰ **I82.9** Embolism and thrombosis of unspecified vein

I82.9Ø Acute embolism and thrombosis of unspecified vein `CC`
Embolism of vein NOS
Thrombosis (vein) NOS

I82.91 Chronic embolism and thrombosis of unspecified vein `CC`

√4ᵗʰ **I83** Varicose veins of lower extremities

EXCLUDES 1   varicose veins complicating pregnancy (O22.Ø-)
varicose veins complicating the puerperium (O87.4)

√5ᵗʰ **I83.Ø** Varicose veins of lower extremities with ulcer
Use additional code to identify severity of ulcer (L97.-)

√6ᵗʰ **I83.ØØ** Varicose veins of unspecified lower extremity with ulcer

I83.ØØ1 Varicose veins of unspecified lower extremity with ulcer of thigh `HCC` `A`

I83.ØØ2 Varicose veins of unspecified lower extremity with ulcer of calf `HCC` `A`

I83.ØØ3 Varicose veins of unspecified lower extremity with ulcer of ankle `HCC` `A`

I83.ØØ4 Varicose veins of unspecified lower extremity with ulcer of heel and midfoot `HCC` `A`
Varicose veins of unspecified lower extremity with ulcer of plantar surface of midfoot

I83.ØØ5 Varicose veins of unspecified lower extremity with ulcer other part of foot `HCC` `A`
Varicose veins of unspecified lower extremity with ulcer of toe

I83.ØØ8 Varicose veins of unspecified lower extremity with ulcer other part of lower leg `HCC` `A`

I83.ØØ9 Varicose veins of unspecified lower extremity with ulcer of unspecified site `HCC` `A`

√6ᵗʰ **I83.Ø1** Varicose veins of right lower extremity with ulcer

I83.Ø11 Varicose veins of right lower extremity with ulcer of thigh `HCC` `A`

I83.Ø12 Varicose veins of right lower extremity with ulcer of calf `HCC` `A`

I83.Ø13 Varicose veins of right lower extremity with ulcer of ankle `HCC` `A`

I83.Ø14 Varicose veins of right lower extremity with ulcer of heel and midfoot `HCC` `A`
Varicose veins of right lower extremity with ulcer of plantar surface of midfoot

I83.Ø15 Varicose veins of right lower extremity with ulcer other part of foot `HCC` `A`
Varicose veins of right lower extremity with ulcer of toe

N Newborn: 0   P Pediatric: 0-17   M Maternity: 9-64   A Adult: 15-124   MCC Major Complication/Comorbidity   CC Complication/Comorbidity   SW Severe Wound Dx

682   ICD-10-CM 2021

        I83.018   **Varicose veins of right lower extremity with ulcer other part of lower leg** `HCC` `A`

        I83.019   **Varicose veins of right lower extremity with ulcer of unspecified site** `HCC` `A`

✓6ᵗʰ   I83.02   **Varicose veins of left lower extremity with ulcer**

        I83.021   **Varicose veins of left lower extremity with ulcer of thigh** `HCC` `A`

        I83.022   **Varicose veins of left lower extremity with ulcer of calf** `HCC` `A`

        I83.023   **Varicose veins of left lower extremity with ulcer of ankle** `HCC` `A`

        I83.024   **Varicose veins of left lower extremity with ulcer of heel and midfoot** `HCC` `A`
            Varicose veins of left lower extremity with ulcer of plantar surface of midfoot

        I83.025   **Varicose veins of left lower extremity with ulcer other part of foot** `HCC` `A`
            Varicose veins of left lower extremity with ulcer of toe

        I83.028   **Varicose veins of left lower extremity with ulcer other part of lower leg** `HCC` `A`

        I83.029   **Varicose veins of left lower extremity with ulcer of unspecified site** `HCC` `A`

✓5ᵗʰ   I83.1   **Varicose veins of lower extremities with inflammation**

        I83.10   **Varicose veins of unspecified lower extremity with inflammation** `A`

        I83.11   **Varicose veins of right lower extremity with inflammation** `A`

        I83.12   **Varicose veins of left lower extremity with inflammation** `A`

✓5ᵗʰ   I83.2   **Varicose veins of lower extremities with both ulcer and inflammation**
       Use additional code to identify severity of ulcer (L97.-)

✓6ᵗʰ   I83.20   **Varicose veins of unspecified lower extremity with both ulcer and inflammation**

        I83.201   **Varicose veins of unspecified lower extremity with both ulcer of thigh and inflammation** `CC` `HCC` `A`

        I83.202   **Varicose veins of unspecified lower extremity with both ulcer of calf and inflammation** `CC` `HCC` `A`

        I83.203   **Varicose veins of unspecified lower extremity with both ulcer of ankle and inflammation** `CC` `HCC` `A`

        I83.204   **Varicose veins of unspecified lower extremity with both ulcer of heel and midfoot and inflammation** `CC` `HCC` `A`
            Varicose veins of unspecified lower extremity with both ulcer of plantar surface of midfoot and inflammation

        I83.205   **Varicose veins of unspecified lower extremity with both ulcer of other part of foot and inflammation** `CC` `HCC` `A`
            Varicose veins of unspecified lower extremity with both ulcer of toe and inflammation

        I83.208   **Varicose veins of unspecified lower extremity with both ulcer of other part of lower extremity and inflammation** `CC` `HCC` `A`

        I83.209   **Varicose veins of unspecified lower extremity with both ulcer of unspecified site and inflammation** `CC` `HCC` `A`

✓6ᵗʰ   I83.21   **Varicose veins of right lower extremity with both ulcer and inflammation**

        I83.211   **Varicose veins of right lower extremity with both ulcer of thigh and inflammation** `CC` `HCC` `A`

        I83.212   **Varicose veins of right lower extremity with both ulcer of calf and inflammation** `CC` `HCC` `A`

        I83.213   **Varicose veins of right lower extremity with both ulcer of ankle and inflammation** `CC` `HCC` `A`

        I83.214   **Varicose veins of right lower extremity with both ulcer of heel and midfoot and inflammation** `CC` `HCC` `A`
            Varicose veins of right lower extremity with both ulcer of plantar surface of midfoot and inflammation

        I83.215   **Varicose veins of right lower extremity with both ulcer other part of foot and inflammation** `CC` `HCC` `A`
            Varicose veins of right lower extremity with both ulcer of toe and inflammation

        I83.218   **Varicose veins of right lower extremity with both ulcer of other part of lower extremity and inflammation** `CC` `HCC` `A`

        I83.219   **Varicose veins of right lower extremity with both ulcer of unspecified site and inflammation** `CC` `HCC` `A`

✓6ᵗʰ   I83.22   **Varicose veins of left lower extremity with both ulcer and inflammation**

        I83.221   **Varicose veins of left lower extremity with both ulcer of thigh and inflammation** `CC` `HCC` `A`

        I83.222   **Varicose veins of left lower extremity with both ulcer of calf and inflammation** `CC` `HCC` `A`

        I83.223   **Varicose veins of left lower extremity with both ulcer of ankle and inflammation** `CC` `HCC` `A`

        I83.224   **Varicose veins of left lower extremity with both ulcer of heel and midfoot and inflammation** `CC` `HCC` `A`
            Varicose veins of left lower extremity with both ulcer of plantar surface of midfoot and inflammation

        I83.225   **Varicose veins of left lower extremity with both ulcer other part of foot and inflammation** `CC` `HCC` `A`
            Varicose veins of left lower extremity with both ulcer of toe and inflammation

        I83.228   **Varicose veins of left lower extremity with both ulcer of other part of lower extremity and inflammation** `CC` `HCC` `A`

        I83.229   **Varicose veins of left lower extremity with both ulcer of unspecified site and inflammation** `CC` `HCC` `A`

✓5ᵗʰ   I83.8   **Varicose veins of lower extremities with other complications**

✓6ᵗʰ   I83.81   **Varicose veins of lower extremities with pain**

        I83.811   **Varicose veins of right lower extremity with pain** `A`

        I83.812   **Varicose veins of left lower extremity with pain** `A`

        I83.813   **Varicose veins of bilateral lower extremities with pain** `A`

        I83.819   **Varicose veins of unspecified lower extremity with pain** `A`

✓6ᵗʰ   I83.89   **Varicose veins of lower extremities with other complications**
       Varicose veins of lower extremities with edema
       Varicose veins of lower extremities with swelling

        I83.891   **Varicose veins of right lower extremity with other complications** `A`

        I83.892   **Varicose veins of left lower extremity with other complications** `A`

        I83.893   **Varicose veins of bilateral lower extremities with other complications** `A`

        I83.899   **Varicose veins of unspecified lower extremity with other complications** `A`

✓5ᵗʰ   I83.9   **Asymptomatic varicose veins of lower extremities**
       Phlebectasia of lower extremities
       Varicose veins of lower extremities
       Varix of lower extremities

        I83.90   **Asymptomatic varicose veins of unspecified lower extremity** `A`
            Varicose veins NOS

        I83.91   **Asymptomatic varicose veins of right lower extremity** `A`

        I83.92   **Asymptomatic varicose veins of left lower extremity** `A`

        I83.93   **Asymptomatic varicose veins of bilateral lower extremities** `A`

✓ Additional Character Required   ✓x7ᵗʰ Placeholder   Unacceptable PDx   Questionable PDx   Manifestation   Unspecified Dx   H1-H14 HAC   HCC CMS-HCC Dx   HIV HIV Dx

ICD-10-CM 2021   683

✓4th **I85 Esophageal varices**
Use additional code to identify:
  alcohol abuse and dependence (F10.-)

✓5th **I85.0 Esophageal varices**
Idiopathic esophageal varices
Primary esophageal varices

I85.00 Esophageal varices without bleeding   CC HCC
Esophageal varices NOS

I85.01 Esophageal varices with bleeding   MCC HCC

✓5th **I85.1 Secondary esophageal varices**
Esophageal varices secondary to alcoholic liver disease
Esophageal varices secondary to cirrhosis of liver
Esophageal varices secondary to schistosomiasis
Esophageal varices secondary to toxic liver disease
Code first underlying disease

I85.10 Secondary esophageal varices without bleeding   CC HCC

I85.11 Secondary esophageal varices with bleeding   MCC HCC

✓4th **I86 Varicose veins of other sites**
EXCLUDES 1 varicose veins of unspecified site (I83.9-)
EXCLUDES 2 retinal varices (H35.0-)

I86.0 Sublingual varices
DEF: Distended, tortuous veins beneath the tongue.

I86.1 Scrotal varices   ♂
Varicocele

I86.2 Pelvic varices

I86.3 Vulval varices   ♀
EXCLUDES 1 vulval varices complicating childbirth and the puerperium (O87.8)
  vulval varices complicating pregnancy (O22.1-)

I86.4 Gastric varices

I86.8 Varicose veins of other specified sites   A
Varicose ulcer of nasal septum

✓4th **I87 Other disorders of veins**

✓5th **I87.0 Postthrombotic syndrome**
Chronic venous hypertension due to deep vein thrombosis
Postphlebitic syndrome
EXCLUDES 1 chronic venous hypertension without deep vein thrombosis (I87.3-)

✓6th **I87.00 Postthrombotic syndrome** without complications
Asymptomatic postthrombotic syndrome

I87.001 Postthrombotic syndrome without complications of right lower **extremity**

I87.002 Postthrombotic syndrome without complications of left lower **extremity**

I87.003 Postthrombotic syndrome without complications of bilateral lower **extremity**

I87.009 Postthrombotic syndrome without complications of unspecified extremity
Postthrombotic syndrome NOS

✓6th **I87.01 Postthrombotic syndrome** with ulcer
Use additional code to specify site and severity of ulcer (L97.-)

I87.011 Postthrombotic syndrome with ulcer of right lower **extremity**   CC HCC

I87.012 Postthrombotic syndrome with ulcer of left lower **extremity**   CC HCC

I87.013 Postthrombotic syndrome with ulcer of bilateral lower **extremity**   CC HCC

I87.019 Postthrombotic syndrome with ulcer of unspecified lower extremity   CC HCC

✓6th **I87.02 Postthrombotic syndrome** with inflammation

I87.021 Postthrombotic syndrome with inflammation of right lower **extremity**

I87.022 Postthrombotic syndrome with inflammation of left lower **extremity**

I87.023 Postthrombotic syndrome with inflammation of bilateral lower **extremity**

I87.029 Postthrombotic syndrome with inflammation of unspecified lower extremity

✓6th **I87.03 Postthrombotic syndrome with** ulcer and inflammation
Use additional code to specify site and severity of ulcer (L97.-)

I87.031 Postthrombotic syndrome with ulcer and inflammation of right lower **extremity**   CC HCC

I87.032 Postthrombotic syndrome with ulcer and inflammation of left lower **extremity**   CC HCC

I87.033 Postthrombotic syndrome with ulcer and inflammation of bilateral lower **extremity**   CC HCC

I87.039 Postthrombotic syndrome with ulcer and inflammation of unspecified lower extremity   CC HCC

✓6th **I87.09 Postthrombotic syndrome with other complications**

I87.091 Postthrombotic syndrome with other complications of right lower **extremity**

I87.092 Postthrombotic syndrome with other complications of left lower **extremity**

I87.093 Postthrombotic syndrome with other complications of bilateral lower **extremity**

I87.099 Postthrombotic syndrome with other complications of unspecified lower extremity

I87.1 Compression of vein   CC
Stricture of vein
Vena cava syndrome (inferior) (superior)
EXCLUDES 2 compression of pulmonary vein (I28.8)

I87.2 Venous insufficiency (chronic) (peripheral)
Stasis dermatitis
EXCLUDES 1 stasis dermatitis with varicose veins of lower extremities (I83.1-, I83.2-)
DEF: Insufficient drainage of venous blood in any part of the body that results in edema or dermatosis.

✓5th **I87.3 Chronic venous hypertension (idiopathic)**
Stasis edema
EXCLUDES 1 chronic venous hypertension due to deep vein thrombosis (I87.0-)
  varicose veins of lower extremities (I83.-)

✓6th **I87.30 Chronic venous hypertension (idiopathic)** without complications
Asymptomatic chronic venous hypertension (idiopathic)

I87.301 Chronic venous hypertension (idiopathic) without complications of right lower **extremity**

I87.302 Chronic venous hypertension (idiopathic) without complications of left lower **extremity**

I87.303 Chronic venous hypertension (idiopathic) without complications of bilateral lower **extremity**

I87.309 Chronic venous hypertension (idiopathic) without complications of unspecified lower extremity
Chronic venous hypertension NOS

✓6th **I87.31 Chronic venous hypertension (idiopathic)** with ulcer
Use additional code to specify site and severity of ulcer (L97.-)

I87.311 Chronic venous hypertension (idiopathic) with ulcer of right lower **extremity**   CC HCC

I87.312 Chronic venous hypertension (idiopathic) with ulcer of left lower **extremity**   CC HCC

I87.313 Chronic venous hypertension (idiopathic) with ulcer of bilateral lower **extremity**   CC HCC

I87.319 Chronic venous hypertension (idiopathic) with ulcer of unspecified lower extremity   CC HCC

✓6th **I87.32 Chronic venous hypertension (idiopathic) with inflammation**

I87.321 Chronic venous hypertension (idiopathic) with inflammation of right lower **extremity**

I87.322 Chronic venous hypertension (idiopathic) with inflammation of left lower **extremity**

I87.323 Chronic venous hypertension (idiopathic) with inflammation of bilateral lower extremity

I87.329 Chronic venous hypertension (idiopathic) with inflammation of unspecified lower extremity

√6th **I87.33** Chronic venous hypertension (idiopathic) with ulcer and inflammation

Use additional code to specify site and severity of ulcer (L97.-)

I87.331 Chronic venous hypertension (idiopathic) with ulcer and inflammation of right lower extremity `CC` `HCC`

I87.332 Chronic venous hypertension (idiopathic) with ulcer and inflammation of left lower extremity `CC` `HCC`

I87.333 Chronic venous hypertension (idiopathic) with ulcer and inflammation of bilateral lower extremity `CC` `HCC`

I87.339 Chronic venous hypertension (idiopathic) with ulcer and inflammation of unspecified lower extremity `CC` `HCC`

√6th **I87.39** Chronic venous hypertension (idiopathic) with other complications

I87.391 Chronic venous hypertension (idiopathic) with other complications of right lower extremity

I87.392 Chronic venous hypertension (idiopathic) with other complications of left lower extremity

I87.393 Chronic venous hypertension (idiopathic) with other complications of bilateral lower extremity

I87.399 Chronic venous hypertension (idiopathic) with other complications of unspecified lower extremity

I87.8 Other specified disorders of veins
Phlebosclerosis
Venofibrosis

I87.9 Disorder of vein, unspecified

√4th **I88** Nonspecific lymphadenitis
EXCLUDES 1 acute lymphadenitis, except mesenteric (L04.-)
enlarged lymph nodes NOS (R59.-)
human immunodeficiency virus [HIV] disease resulting in generalized lymphadenopathy (B20)

I88.0 Nonspecific mesenteric lymphadenitis
Mesenteric lymphadenitis (acute)(chronic)

I88.1 Chronic lymphadenitis, except mesenteric
Adenitis
Lymphadenitis

I88.8 Other nonspecific lymphadenitis

I88.9 Nonspecific lymphadenitis, unspecified
Lymphadenitis NOS

√4th **I89** Other noninfective disorders of lymphatic vessels and lymph nodes
EXCLUDES 1 chylocele, tunica vaginalis (nonfilarial) NOS (N50.89)
enlarged lymph nodes NOS (R59.-)
filarial chylocele (B74.-)
hereditary lymphedema (Q82.0)

I89.0 Lymphedema, not elsewhere classified
Elephantiasis (nonfilarial) NOS
Lymphangiectasis
Obliteration, lymphatic vessel
Praecox lymphedema
Secondary lymphedema
EXCLUDES 1 postmastectomy lymphedema (I97.2)

I89.1 Lymphangitis
Chronic lymphangitis
Lymphangitis NOS
Subacute lymphangitis
EXCLUDES 1 acute lymphangitis (L03.-)

I89.8 Other specified noninfective disorders of lymphatic vessels and lymph nodes
Chylocele (nonfilarial)
Chylous ascites
Chylous cyst
Lipomelanotic reticulosis
Lymph node or vessel fistula
Lymph node or vessel infarction
Lymph node or vessel rupture

I89.9 Noninfective disorder of lymphatic vessels and lymph nodes, unspecified
Disease of lymphatic vessels NOS

Other and unspecified disorders of the circulatory system (I95-I99)

√4th **I95** Hypotension
EXCLUDES 1 cardiovascular collapse (R57.9) (~R57.9)
maternal hypotension syndrome (O26.5-)
nonspecific low blood pressure reading NOS (R03.1)

I95.0 Idiopathic hypotension

I95.1 Orthostatic hypotension
Hypotension, postural
EXCLUDES 1 neurogenic orthostatic hypotension [Shy-Drager] (G90.3)
orthostatic hypotension due to drugs (I95.2)

I95.2 Hypotension due to drugs
Orthostatic hypotension due to drugs
Use additional code for adverse effect, if applicable, to identify drug (T36-T50 with fifth or sixth character 5)

I95.3 Hypotension of hemodialysis
Intra-dialytic hypotension

√5th **I95.8** Other hypotension

I95.81 Postprocedural hypotension

I95.89 Other hypotension
Chronic hypotension

I95.9 Hypotension, unspecified

I96 Gangrene, not elsewhere classified `CC` `HCC`
Gangrenous cellulitis
EXCLUDES 1 gangrene in atherosclerosis of native arteries of the extremities (I70.26)
gangrene in hernia (K40.1, K40.4, K41.1, K41.4, K42.1, K43.1-, K44.1, K45.1, K46.1)
gangrene in other peripheral vascular diseases (I73.-)
gangrene of certain specified sites — see Alphabetical Index
gas gangrene (A48.0)
pyoderma gangrenosum (L88)
EXCLUDES 2 gangrene in diabetes mellitus (E08-E13 with .52)
AHA: 2018,4Q,87; 2018,3Q,3; 2017,3Q,6; 2013,2Q,34

√4th **I97** Intraoperative and postprocedural complications and disorders of circulatory system, not elsewhere classified
EXCLUDES 2 postprocedural shock (T81.1-)
AHA: 2019,2Q,21

I97.0 Postcardiotomy syndrome

√5th **I97.1** Other postprocedural cardiac functional disturbances
EXCLUDES 2 acute pulmonary insufficiency following thoracic surgery (J95.1)
intraoperative cardiac functional disturbances (I97.7-)

√6th **I97.11** Postprocedural cardiac insufficiency

I97.110 Postprocedural cardiac insufficiency following cardiac surgery `CC`

I97.111 Postprocedural cardiac insufficiency following other surgery `CC`

√6th **I97.12** Postprocedural cardiac arrest

I97.120 Postprocedural cardiac arrest following cardiac surgery `CC`

I97.121 Postprocedural cardiac arrest following other surgery `CC`

√6th **I97.13** Postprocedural heart failure
Use additional code to identify the heart failure (I50.-)

I97.130 Postprocedural heart failure following cardiac surgery `CC`

I97.131 Postprocedural heart failure following other surgery `CC`

I97.19   **Other postprocedural cardiac functional disturbances**
> Use additional code, if applicable, to further specify disorder

I97.190   **Other postprocedural cardiac functional disturbances following cardiac surgery** `cc`
> Use additional code, if applicable, for type 4 or type 5 myocardial infarction, to further specify disorder
> **AHA:** 2019,2Q,33

I97.191   **Other postprocedural cardiac functional disturbances following other surgery** `cc`

I97.2   **Postmastectomy lymphedema syndrome** `A`
> Elephantiasis due to mastectomy
> Obliteration of lymphatic vessels

I97.3   **Postprocedural hypertension**

I97.4   **Intraoperative hemorrhage and hematoma of a circulatory system organ or structure complicating a procedure**
> EXCLUDES 1: intraoperative hemorrhage and hematoma of a circulatory system organ or structure due to accidental puncture and laceration during a procedure (I97.5-)
> EXCLUDES 2: intraoperative cerebrovascular hemorrhage complicating a procedure (G97.3-)

I97.41   **Intraoperative hemorrhage and hematoma of a circulatory system organ or structure complicating a circulatory system procedure**

I97.410   **Intraoperative hemorrhage and hematoma of a circulatory system organ or structure complicating a cardiac catheterization** `cc`

I97.411   **Intraoperative hemorrhage and hematoma of a circulatory system organ or structure complicating a cardiac bypass** `cc`

I97.418   **Intraoperative hemorrhage and hematoma of a circulatory system organ or structure complicating other circulatory system procedure** `cc`

I97.42   **Intraoperative hemorrhage and hematoma of a circulatory system organ or structure complicating other procedure** `cc`
> **AHA:** 2020,1Q,19

I97.5   **Accidental puncture and laceration of a circulatory system organ or structure during a procedure**
> EXCLUDES 2: accidental puncture and laceration of brain during a procedure (G97.4-)

I97.51   **Accidental puncture and laceration of a circulatory system organ or structure during a circulatory system procedure** `cc`
> **AHA:** 2019,2Q,24

I97.52   **Accidental puncture and laceration of a circulatory system organ or structure during other procedure** `cc`

I97.6   **Postprocedural hemorrhage, hematoma and seroma of a circulatory system organ or structure following a procedure**
> EXCLUDES 2: postprocedural cerebrovascular hemorrhage complicating a procedure (G97.5-)
> **AHA:** 2016,4Q,9-10

I97.61   **Postprocedural hemorrhage of a circulatory system organ or structure following a circulatory system procedure**

I97.610   **Postprocedural hemorrhage of a circulatory system organ or structure following a cardiac catheterization** `cc`

I97.611   **Postprocedural hemorrhage of a circulatory system organ or structure following cardiac bypass** `cc`

I97.618   **Postprocedural hemorrhage of a circulatory system organ or structure following other circulatory system procedure** `cc`

I97.62   **Postprocedural hemorrhage, hematoma and seroma of a circulatory system organ or structure following other procedure**

I97.620   **Postprocedural hemorrhage of a circulatory system organ or structure following other procedure** `cc`

I97.621   **Postprocedural hematoma of a circulatory system organ or structure following other procedure** `cc`

I97.622   **Postprocedural seroma of a circulatory system organ or structure following other procedure** `cc`

I97.63   **Postprocedural hematoma of a circulatory system organ or structure following a circulatory system procedure**

I97.630   **Postprocedural hematoma of a circulatory system organ or structure following a cardiac catheterization** `cc`

I97.631   **Postprocedural hematoma of a circulatory system organ or structure following cardiac bypass** `cc`

I97.638   **Postprocedural hematoma of a circulatory system organ or structure following other circulatory system procedure** `cc`

I97.64   **Postprocedural seroma of a circulatory system organ or structure following a circulatory system procedure**

I97.640   **Postprocedural seroma of a circulatory system organ or structure following a cardiac catheterization** `cc`

I97.641   **Postprocedural seroma of a circulatory system organ or structure following cardiac bypass** `cc`

I97.648   **Postprocedural seroma of a circulatory system organ or structure following other circulatory system procedure** `cc`

I97.7   **Intraoperative cardiac functional disturbances**
> EXCLUDES 2: acute pulmonary insufficiency following thoracic surgery (J95.1)
> postprocedural cardiac functional disturbances (I97.1-)

I97.71   **Intraoperative cardiac arrest**

I97.710   **Intraoperative cardiac arrest during cardiac surgery** `cc`

I97.711   **Intraoperative cardiac arrest during other surgery** `cc`

I97.79   **Other intraoperative cardiac functional disturbances**
> Use additional code, if applicable, to further specify disorder

I97.790   **Other intraoperative cardiac functional disturbances during cardiac surgery** `cc`

I97.791   **Other intraoperative cardiac functional disturbances during other surgery** `cc`

I97.8   **Other intraoperative and postprocedural complications and disorders of the circulatory system, not elsewhere classified**
> Use additional code, if applicable, to further specify disorder

I97.81   **Intraoperative cerebrovascular infarction**

I97.810   **Intraoperative cerebrovascular infarction during cardiac surgery** `cc` `HCC`

I97.811   **Intraoperative cerebrovascular infarction during other surgery** `cc` `HCC`

I97.82   **Postprocedural cerebrovascular infarction**

I97.820   **Postprocedural cerebrovascular infarction following cardiac surgery** `cc` `HCC`

I97.821   **Postprocedural cerebrovascular infarction following other surgery** `cc` `HCC`

I97.88   **Other intraoperative complications of the circulatory system, not elsewhere classified** `cc`

I97.89   **Other postprocedural complications and disorders of the circulatory system, not elsewhere classified** `cc`
> **AHA:** 2019,2Q,33

I99   **Other and unspecified disorders of circulatory system**

I99.8   **Other disorder of circulatory system**

I99.9   **Unspecified disorder of circulatory system**

Chapter 10. Diseases of the Respiratory System (J00–J99), U07.0

Chapter-specific Guidelines with Coding Examples

The chapter-specific guidelines from the ICD-10-CM Official Guidelines for Coding and Reporting have been provided below. Along with these guidelines are coding examples, contained in the shaded boxes, that have been developed to help illustrate the coding and/or sequencing guidance found in these guidelines.

a. Chronic obstructive pulmonary disease [COPD] and asthma

1) Acute exacerbation of chronic obstructive bronchitis and asthma

The codes in categories J44 and J45 distinguish between uncomplicated cases and those in acute exacerbation. An acute exacerbation is a worsening or a decompensation of a chronic condition. An acute exacerbation is not equivalent to an infection superimposed on a chronic condition, though an exacerbation may be triggered by an infection.

Vancomycin IV was started to treat a patient with acute pneumonia due to *Streptococcus pneumoniae*. Patient also with acute exacerbation of COPD continued on home meds.

J13	**Pneumonia due to Streptococcus pneumoniae**
J44.0	**Chronic obstructive pulmonary disease with (acute) lower respiratory infection**
J44.1	**Chronic obstructive pulmonary disease with (acute) exacerbation**

Explanation: ICD-10-CM uses combination codes to create organism-specific classifications for acute pneumonia. Category J44 codes include combination codes with severity components, which differentiate between COPD with acute lower respiratory infection (acute pneumonia), COPD with acute exacerbation, and COPD without mention of a complication (unspecified).

An acute exacerbation is a worsening or a decompensation of a chronic condition. An acute exacerbation is not equivalent to an infection superimposed on a chronic condition, though an exacerbation may be triggered by an infection, as in this example. Treatment of the pneumonia necessitated the inpatient admission. Instructional notes at J44.0 say to "code also to identify the infection," which informs the coder that another code must be assigned if applicable. Sequencing of the pneumonia and COPD exacerbation are governed by the Section II, "Selection of Principal Diagnosis," guidelines. In this case it was the pneumonia that was "chiefly responsible for occasioning the admission" with the IV vancomycin treatment.

Exacerbation of moderate persistent asthma with status asthmaticus

J45.42	**Moderate persistent asthma with status asthmaticus**

Explanation: Category J45 Asthma includes severity-specific subcategories and fifth-character codes to distinguish between uncomplicated cases, those in acute exacerbation, and those with status asthmaticus.

b. Acute respiratory failure

1) Acute respiratory failure as principal diagnosis

A code from subcategory J96.0, Acute respiratory failure, or subcategory J96.2, Acute and chronic respiratory failure, may be assigned as a principal diagnosis when it is the condition established after study to be chiefly responsible for occasioning the admission to the hospital, and the selection is supported by the Alphabetic Index and Tabular List. However, chapter-specific coding guidelines (such as obstetrics, poisoning, HIV, newborn) that provide sequencing direction take precedence.

Acute hypoxic respiratory failure due to COPD exacerbation

J96.01	**Acute respiratory failure with hypoxia**
J44.1	**Chronic obstructive pulmonary disease with (acute) exacerbation**

Explanation: Category J96 classifies respiratory failure with combination codes that designate the severity and the presence of hypoxia and hypercapnia. Code J96.01 is sequenced as the first-listed diagnosis, as the reason for the admission. Respiratory failure may be assigned as a principal diagnosis when it is the condition established after study to be chiefly responsible for occasioning the admission to the hospital and the selection is supported by the Alphabetic Index and Tabular List.

2) Acute respiratory failure as secondary diagnosis

Respiratory failure may be listed as a secondary diagnosis if it occurs after admission, or if it is present on admission, but does not meet the definition of principal diagnosis.

Acute respiratory failure due to accidental oxycodone overdose

T40.2X1A	**Poisoning by other opioids, accidental (unintentional), initial encounter**
J96.00	**Acute respiratory failure, unspecified whether with hypoxia or hypercapnia**

Explanation: Respiratory failure may be assigned as a principal diagnosis when it is the condition established after study to be chiefly responsible for occasioning the admission to the hospital, and the selection is supported by the Alphabetic Index and Tabular List. However, chapter-specific coding guidelines, such as poisoning, that provide sequencing direction take precedence. When coding a poisoning or reaction to the improper use of a medication (e.g. overdose, wrong substance given or taken in error, wrong route of administration), first assign the appropriate code from categories T36–T50. Use additional code(s) for all manifestations of the poisoning. In this instance, the respiratory failure is a manifestation of the poisoning and is sequenced as a secondary diagnosis.

Acute pneumococcal pneumonia with subsequent development of acute respiratory failure

J13	**Pneumonia due to Streptococcus pneumoniae**
J96.00	**Acute respiratory failure, unspecified whether with hypoxia or hypercapnia**

Explanation: Acute respiratory failure may be listed as a secondary diagnosis if it occurs after admission, or if it is present on admission but does not meet the definition of principal diagnosis.

3) Sequencing of acute respiratory failure and another acute condition

When a patient is admitted with respiratory failure and another acute condition, (e.g., myocardial infarction, cerebrovascular accident, aspiration pneumonia), the principal diagnosis will not be the same in every situation. This applies whether the other acute condition is a respiratory or nonrespiratory condition. Selection of the principal diagnosis will be dependent on the circumstances of admission. If both the respiratory failure and the other acute condition are equally responsible for occasioning the admission to the hospital, and there are no chapter-specific sequencing rules, the guideline regarding two or more diagnoses that equally meet the definition for principal diagnosis (*Section II, C.*) may be applied in these situations.

If the documentation is not clear as to whether acute respiratory failure and another condition are equally responsible for occasioning the admission, query the provider for clarification.

Acute pneumococcal pneumonia and acute respiratory failure, both present on admission

J96.00	**Acute respiratory failure, unspecified whether with hypoxia or hypercapnia**
J13	**Pneumonia due to Streptococcus pneumoniae**

Explanation: When a patient is admitted with respiratory failure and another acute condition, such as a bacterial pneumonia, the principal diagnosis is not the same in every situation. This applies whether the other acute condition is a respiratory or nonrespiratory condition. The principal diagnosis depends on the circumstances of admission.

c. Influenza due to certain identified influenza viruses

Code only confirmed cases of influenza due to certain identified influenza viruses (category J09), and due to other identified influenza virus (category J10). This is an exception to the hospital inpatient guideline Section II, H. (Uncertain Diagnosis).

In this context, "confirmation" does not require documentation of positive laboratory testing specific for avian or other novel influenza A or other identified influenza virus. However, coding should be based on the provider's diagnostic statement that the patient has avian influenza, or other novel influenza A, for category J09, or has another particular identified strain of influenza, such as H1N1 or H3N2, but not identified as novel or variant, for category J10.

If the provider records "suspected" or "possible" or "probable" avian influenza, or novel influenza, or other identified influenza, then the appropriate influenza code from category J11, Influenza due to unidentified influenza virus, should be assigned. A code from category J09, Influenza due to certain identified influenza viruses, should not be assigned nor should a code from category J10, Influenza due to other identified influenza virus.

Influenza due to avian influenza virus with pneumonia

J09.X1   Influenza due to identified novel influenza A virus with pneumonia

Explanation: Codes in category J09 Influenza due to certain identified influenza viruses should be assigned only for confirmed cases. "Confirmation" does not require positive laboratory testing of a specific influenza virus but does need to be based on the provider's diagnostic statement, which should not include terms such as "possible," "probable," or "suspected."

d. Ventilator associated pneumonia

1) Documentation of ventilator associated pneumonia

As with all procedural or postprocedural complications, code assignment is based on the provider's documentation of the relationship between the condition and the procedure.

Code J95.851, Ventilator associated pneumonia, should be assigned only when the provider has documented ventilator associated pneumonia (VAP). An additional code to identify the organism (e.g., Pseudomonas aeruginosa, code B96.5) should also be assigned. Do not assign an additional code from categories J12-J18 to identify the type of pneumonia.

Code J95.851 should not be assigned for cases where the patient has pneumonia and is on a mechanical ventilator and the provider has not specifically stated that the pneumonia is ventilator-associated pneumonia. If the documentation is unclear as to whether the patient has a pneumonia that is a complication attributable to the mechanical ventilator, query the provider.

2) Ventilator associated pneumonia develops after admission

A patient may be admitted with one type of pneumonia (e.g., code J13, Pneumonia due to Streptococcus pneumonia) and subsequently develop VAP. In this instance, the principal diagnosis would be the appropriate code from categories J12-J18 for the pneumonia diagnosed at the time of admission. Code J95.851, Ventilator associated pneumonia, would be assigned as an additional diagnosis when the provider has also documented the presence of ventilator associated pneumonia.

Patient with pneumonia due to *Klebsiella pneumoniae* develops superimposed MRSA ventilator-associated pneumonia

J15.0   Pneumonia due to Klebsiella pneumoniae

J95.851   Ventilator associated pneumonia

B95.62   Methicillin resistant Staphylococcus aureus infection as the cause of diseases classified elsewhere

Explanation: Code assignment for ventilator-associated pneumonia is based on the provider's documentation of the relationship between the condition and the procedure and is reported only when the provider has documented ventilator-associated pneumonia (VAP).

A patient may be admitted with one type of pneumonia and subsequently develop VAP. In this example, the principal diagnosis code describes the pneumonia diagnosed at the time of admission, with code J95.851 Ventilator associated pneumonia, assigned as secondary.

e. Vaping-related disorders

For patients presenting with condition(s) related to vaping, assign code U07.0, Vaping-related disorder, as the principal diagnosis. For lung injury due to vaping, assign only code U07.0. Assign additional codes for other manifestations, such as acute respiratory failure (subcategory J96.0-) or pneumonitis (code J68.0).

Associated respiratory signs and symptoms due to vaping, such as cough, shortness of breath, etc., are not coded separately, when a definitive diagnosis has been established. However, it would be appropriate to code separately any gastrointestinal symptoms, such as diarrhea and abdominal pain.

23-year-old patient with history of anxiety disorder admitted with fever, dyspnea and nonproductive cough. Patient's respiratory function continued to clinically worsen, requiring intubation for suspected ARDS and required OGT suction for coffee ground hematemesis. Following extubating, patient confirmed the use of THC vaping cartridge preceding development of symptoms. Discharge diagnosis is ARDS due to EVALI and anxiety disorder.

U07.0   Vaping related disorder

J80   Acute respiratory distress syndrome

K92.0   Hematemesis

F41.9   Anxiety disorder, unspecified

Explanation: Codes U07.0 and J80 represent the vaping-related disorder and its associated manifestation, the acute respiratory distress syndrome (ARDS). The symptoms that brought the patient in are not coded separately because these are integral to the vaping disorder and the ARDS, unlike the hematemesis (vomiting blood) a gastrointestinal symptom that is not integral to either of these conditions.

Chapter 1Ø. Diseases of the Respiratory System (J0Ø-J99)

NOTE   When a respiratory condition is described as occurring in more than one site and is not specifically indexed, it should be classified to the lower anatomic site (e.g., tracheobronchitis to bronchitis in J4Ø).

Use additional code, where applicable, to identify:
exposure to environmental tobacco smoke (Z77.22)
exposure to tobacco smoke in the perinatal period (P96.81)
history of tobacco dependence (Z87.891)
occupational exposure to environmental tobacco smoke (Z57.31)
tobacco dependence (F17.-)
tobacco use (Z72.Ø)

EXCLUDES 2   *certain conditions originating in the perinatal period (PØ4-P96)*
certain infectious and parasitic diseases (AØØ-B99)
complications of pregnancy, childbirth and the puerperium (OØØ-O9A)
congenital malformations, deformations and chromosomal abnormalities (QØØ-Q99)
endocrine, nutritional and metabolic diseases (EØØ-E88)
injury, poisoning and certain other consequences of external causes (SØØ-T88)
neoplasms (CØØ-D49)
smoke inhalation (T59.81-)
symptoms, signs and abnormal clinical and laboratory findings, not elsewhere classified (RØØ-R94)

This chapter contains the following blocks:
JØØ-JØ6   Acute upper respiratory infections
JØ9-J18   Influenza and pneumonia
J2Ø-J22   Other acute lower respiratory infections
J3Ø-J39   Other diseases of upper respiratory tract
J4Ø-J47   Chronic lower respiratory diseases
J6Ø-J7Ø   Lung diseases due to external agents
J8Ø-J84   Other respiratory diseases principally affecting the interstitium
J85-J86   Suppurative and necrotic conditions of the lower respiratory tract
J9Ø-J94   Other diseases of the pleura
J95   Intraoperative and postprocedural complications and disorders of respiratory system, not elsewhere classified
J96-J99   Other diseases of the respiratory system

Acute upper respiratory infections (JØØ-JØ6)

EXCLUDES 1   *chronic obstructive pulmonary disease with acute lower respiratory infection (J44.Ø)*
~~influenza virus with other respiratory manifestations (JØ9.X2, J1Ø.1, J11.1)~~

JØØ   Acute nasopharyngitis [common cold]
Acute rhinitis
Coryza (acute)
Infective nasopharyngitis NOS
Infective rhinitis
Nasal catarrh, acute
Nasopharyngitis NOS

EXCLUDES 1   *acute pharyngitis (JØ2.-)*
acute sore throat NOS (JØ2.9)
▶*influenza virus with other respiratory manifestations (JØ9.X2, J1Ø.1, J11.1)*◀
pharyngitis NOS (JØ2.9)
rhinitis NOS (J31.Ø)
sore throat NOS (JØ2.9)

EXCLUDES 2   *allergic rhinitis (J3Ø.1-J3Ø.9)*
chronic pharyngitis (J31.2)
chronic rhinitis (J31.Ø)
chronic sore throat (J31.2)
nasopharyngitis, chronic (J31.1)
vasomotor rhinitis (J3Ø.Ø)

DEF: Acute inflammation of the mucous membranes that extends from the nares to the pharynx. It is characterized by nasal obstruction, sneezing, runny nose, and sore throat.

✓4ᵗʰ JØ1   Acute sinusitis
INCLUDES   acute abscess of sinus
acute empyema of sinus
acute infection of sinus
acute inflammation of sinus
acute suppuration of sinus
Use additional code (B95-B97) to identify infectious agent
EXCLUDES 1   *sinusitis NOS (J32.9)*
EXCLUDES 2   *chronic sinusitis (J32.Ø-J32.8)*

✓5ᵗʰ JØ1.Ø   Acute maxillary sinusitis
Acute antritis
JØ1.ØØ   Acute maxillary sinusitis, unspecified

JØ1.Ø1   Acute recurrent maxillary sinusitis

✓5ᵗʰ JØ1.1   Acute frontal sinusitis
JØ1.1Ø   Acute frontal sinusitis, unspecified
JØ1.11   Acute recurrent frontal sinusitis

✓5ᵗʰ JØ1.2   Acute ethmoidal sinusitis
JØ1.2Ø   Acute ethmoidal sinusitis, unspecified
JØ1.21   Acute recurrent ethmoidal sinusitis

✓5ᵗʰ JØ1.3   Acute sphenoidal sinusitis
JØ1.3Ø   Acute sphenoidal sinusitis, unspecified
JØ1.31   Acute recurrent sphenoidal sinusitis

✓5ᵗʰ JØ1.4   Acute pansinusitis
JØ1.4Ø   Acute pansinusitis, unspecified
JØ1.41   Acute recurrent pansinusitis

✓5ᵗʰ JØ1.8   Other acute sinusitis
JØ1.8Ø   Other acute sinusitis
Acute sinusitis involving more than one sinus but not pansinusitis
JØ1.81   Other acute recurrent sinusitis
Acute recurrent sinusitis involving more than one sinus but not pansinusitis

✓5ᵗʰ JØ1.9   Acute sinusitis, unspecified
JØ1.9Ø   Acute sinusitis, unspecified
JØ1.91   Acute recurrent sinusitis, unspecified

✓4ᵗʰ JØ2   Acute pharyngitis
INCLUDES   acute sore throat
EXCLUDES 1   *acute laryngopharyngitis (JØ6.Ø)*
peritonsillar abscess (J36)
pharyngeal abscess (J39.1)
retropharyngeal abscess (J39.Ø)
EXCLUDES 2   *chronic pharyngitis (J31.2)*

JØ2.Ø   Streptococcal pharyngitis
Septic pharyngitis
Streptococcal sore throat
EXCLUDES 2   *scarlet fever (A38.-)*

JØ2.8   Acute pharyngitis due to other specified organisms
Use additional code (B95-B97) to identify infectious agent
EXCLUDES 1   *acute pharyngitis due to coxsackie virus (BØ8.5)*
acute pharyngitis due to gonococcus (A54.5)
acute pharyngitis due to herpes [simplex] virus (BØØ.2)
acute pharyngitis due to infectious mononucleosis (B27.-)
enteroviral vesicular pharyngitis (BØ8.5)

JØ2.9   Acute pharyngitis, unspecified
Gangrenous pharyngitis (acute)
Infective pharyngitis (acute) NOS
Pharyngitis (acute) NOS
Sore throat (acute) NOS
Suppurative pharyngitis (acute)
Ulcerative pharyngitis (acute)
EXCLUDES 1   ▶*influenza virus with other respiratory manifestations (JØ9.X2, J1Ø.1, J11.1)*◀

✓4ᵗʰ JØ3   Acute tonsillitis
EXCLUDES 1   *acute sore throat (JØ2.-)*
hypertrophy of tonsils (J35.1)
peritonsillar abscess (J36)
sore throat NOS (JØ2.9)
streptococcal sore throat (JØ2.Ø)
EXCLUDES 2   *chronic tonsillitis (J35.Ø)*

✓5ᵗʰ JØ3.Ø   Streptococcal tonsillitis
JØ3.ØØ   Acute streptococcal tonsillitis, unspecified
JØ3.Ø1   Acute recurrent streptococcal tonsillitis

✓5ᵗʰ JØ3.8   Acute tonsillitis due to other specified organisms
Use additional code (B95-B97) to identify infectious agent
EXCLUDES 1   *diphtheritic tonsillitis (A36.Ø)*
herpesviral pharyngotonsillitis (BØØ.2)
streptococcal tonsillitis (JØ3.Ø)
tuberculous tonsillitis (A15.8)
Vincent's tonsillitis (A69.1)
JØ3.8Ø   Acute tonsillitis due to other specified organisms
JØ3.81   Acute recurrent tonsillitis due to other specified organisms

✓5ᵗʰ J03.9 Acute tonsillitis, unspecified
Follicular tonsillitis (acute)
Gangrenous tonsillitis (acute)
Infective tonsillitis (acute)
Tonsillitis (acute) NOS
Ulcerative tonsillitis (acute)
  EXCLUDES 1 ▶*influenza virus with other respiratory manifestations (J09.X2, J10.1, J11.1)*◀
J03.90 Acute tonsillitis, unspecified
J03.91 Acute recurrent tonsillitis, unspecified

✓4ᵗʰ J04 Acute laryngitis and tracheitis
▶Code also influenza, if present, such as:◀
  ▶influenza due to identified novel influenza A virus with other respiratory manifestations (J09.X2)◀
  ▶influenza due to other identified influenza virus with other respiratory manifestations (J10.1)◀
  ▶influenza due to unidentified influenza virus with other respiratory manifestations (J11.1)◀
Use additional code (B95-B97) to identify infectious agent
  EXCLUDES 1 acute obstructive laryngitis [croup] and epiglottitis (J05.-)
  EXCLUDES 2 laryngismus (stridulus) (J38.5)

J04.0 Acute laryngitis
Edematous laryngitis (acute)
Laryngitis (acute) NOS
Subglottic laryngitis (acute)
Suppurative laryngitis (acute)
Ulcerative laryngitis (acute)
  EXCLUDES 1 acute obstructive laryngitis (J05.0)
  EXCLUDES 2 chronic laryngitis (J37.0)

✓5ᵗʰ J04.1 Acute tracheitis
Acute viral tracheitis
Catarrhal tracheitis (acute)
Tracheitis (acute) NOS
  EXCLUDES 2 chronic tracheitis (J42)
J04.10 Acute tracheitis without obstruction
J04.11 Acute tracheitis with obstruction   MCC

J04.2 Acute laryngotracheitis
Laryngotracheitis NOS
Tracheitis (acute) with laryngitis (acute)
  EXCLUDES 1 acute obstructive laryngotracheitis (J05.0)
  EXCLUDES 2 chronic laryngotracheitis (J37.1)

✓5ᵗʰ J04.3 Supraglottitis, unspecified
J04.30 Supraglottitis, unspecified, without obstruction
J04.31 Supraglottitis, unspecified, with obstruction   MCC

✓4ᵗʰ J05 Acute obstructive laryngitis [croup] and epiglottitis
▶Code also, if present, such as:◀
  ▶influenza due to identified novel influenza A virus with other respiratory manifestations (J09.X2)◀
  ▶influenza due to other identified influenza virus with other respiratory manifestations (J10.1)◀
  ▶influenza due to unidentified influenza virus with other respiratory manifestations (J11.1)◀
Use additional code (B95-B97) to identify infectious agent

J05.0 Acute obstructive laryngitis [croup]
Obstructive laryngitis (acute) NOS
Obstructive laryngotracheitis NOS
DEF: Acute laryngeal obstruction due to allergies, foreign bodies, or in the majority of cases a viral infection. Symptoms include a harsh, barking cough, hoarseness, and a persistent, high-pitched respiratory sound (stridor).

✓5ᵗʰ J05.1 Acute epiglottitis
  EXCLUDES 2 epiglottitis, chronic (J37.0)
J05.10 Acute epiglottitis without obstruction   CC
Epiglottitis NOS
J05.11 Acute epiglottitis with obstruction   MCC

✓4ᵗʰ J06 Acute upper respiratory infections of multiple and unspecified sites
  EXCLUDES 1 acute respiratory infection NOS (J22)
  ▶*influenza virus with other respiratory manifestations (J09.X2, J10.1, J11.1)*◀
  streptococcal pharyngitis (J02.0)

J06.0 Acute laryngopharyngitis

J06.9 Acute upper respiratory infection, unspecified
Upper respiratory disease, acute
Upper respiratory infection NOS
Use additional code (B95-B97) to identify infectious agent, if known, such as:
  respiratory syncytial virus (RSV) (B97.4)
AHA: 2020,1Q,22

Influenza and pneumonia (J09-J18)

  EXCLUDES 2 allergic or eosinophilic pneumonia (J82)
  aspiration pneumonia NOS (J69.0)
  meconium pneumonia (P24.01)
  neonatal aspiration pneumonia (P24.-)
  pneumonia due to solids and liquids (J69.-)
  congenital pneumonia (P23.9)
  lipid pneumonia (J69.1)
  rheumatic pneumonia (I00)
  ventilator associated pneumonia (J95.851)
AHA: 2017,4Q,96
TIP: Assign J18.1 only when the provider specifically documents "lobar pneumonia" without specifying a causal organism. Lobar pneumonia may not be assumed based on an imaging report that identifies pneumonia in a specific lobe.
TIP: Documentation of lobar pneumonia or multilobar pneumonia should be coded to J18.1 when the specific organism causing the pneumonia is not identified. When the organism is documented, lobar pneumonia or multilobar pneumonia should be coded using categories J12-J16, depending on the organism that is present.
TIP: Hemoptysis (R04.2) is not customarily associated with pneumonia and may be reported separately.

✓4ᵗʰ J09 Influenza due to certain identified influenza viruses
  EXCLUDES 1 influenza A/H1N1 (J10.-)
  influenza due to other identified influenza virus (J10.-)
  influenza due to unidentified influenza virus (J11.-)
  seasonal influenza due to other identified influenza virus (J10.-)
  seasonal influenza due to unidentified influenza virus (J11.-)

✓5ᵗʰ J09.X Influenza due to identified novel influenza A virus
Avian influenza
Bird influenza
Influenza A/H5N1
Influenza of other animal origin, not bird or swine
Swine influenza virus (viruses that normally cause infections in pigs)
AHA: 2016,3Q,10
J09.X1 Influenza due to identified novel influenza A virus with pneumonia   HIV MCC
Code also, if applicable, associated:
  lung abscess (J85.1)
  other specified type of pneumonia

J09.X2 Influenza due to identified novel influenza A virus with other respiratory manifestations
Influenza due to identified novel influenza A virus NOS
Influenza due to identified novel influenza A virus with laryngitis
Influenza due to identified novel influenza A virus with pharyngitis
Influenza due to identified novel influenza A virus with upper respiratory symptoms
Use additional code, if applicable, for associated:
  pleural effusion (J91.8)
  sinusitis (J01.-)

J09.X3 Influenza due to identified novel influenza A virus with gastrointestinal manifestations
Influenza due to identified novel influenza A virus gastroenteritis
  EXCLUDES 1 'intestinal flu' [viral gastroenteritis] (A08.-)

J09.X9 Influenza due to identified novel influenza A virus with other manifestations
Influenza due to identified novel influenza A virus with encephalopathy
Influenza due to identified novel influenza A virus with myocarditis
Influenza due to identified novel influenza A virus with otitis media
Use additional code to identify manifestation

☑4ᵗʰ **J10 Influenza due to other identified influenza virus**

> INCLUDES ▶influenza A (non-novel)◄
> ▶influenza B◄
> ▶influenza C◄
>
> EXCLUDES 1 *influenza due to avian influenza virus (J09.X-)*
> *influenza due to swine flu (J09.X-)*
> *influenza due to unidentifed influenza virus (J11.-)*

☑5ᵗʰ **J10.0 Influenza due to other identified influenza virus with pneumonia**

> Code also associated lung abscess, if applicable (J85.1)

> **J10.00 Influenza due to other identified influenza virus with unspecified type of pneumonia**   MCC

> **J10.01 Influenza due to other identified influenza virus with the same other identified influenza virus pneumonia**   MCC

> **J10.08 Influenza due to other identified influenza virus with other specified pneumonia**   HIV MCC
>> Code also other specified type of pneumonia

J10.1 Influenza due to other identified influenza virus with other respiratory manifestations

> Influenza due to other identified influenza virus NOS
> Influenza due to other identified influenza virus with laryngitis
> Influenza due to other identified influenza virus with pharyngitis
> Influenza due to other identified influenza virus with upper respiratory symptoms
> Use additional code for associated pleural effusion, if applicable (J91.8)
> Use additional code for associated sinusitis, if applicable (J01.-)
> AHA: 2016,3Q,10-11

J10.2 Influenza due to other identified influenza virus with gastrointestinal manifestations

> Influenza due to other identified influenza virus gastroenteritis
> EXCLUDES 1 *"intestinal flu" [viral gastroenteritis] (A08.-)*

☑5ᵗʰ **J10.8 Influenza due to other identified influenza virus with other manifestations**

> **J10.81 Influenza due to other identified influenza virus with encephalopathy**

> **J10.82 Influenza due to other identified influenza virus with myocarditis**

> **J10.83 Influenza due to other identified influenza virus with otitis media**
>> Use additional code for any associated perforated tympanic membrane (H72.-)

> **J10.89 Influenza due to other identified influenza virus with other manifestations**
>> Use additional codes to identify the manifestations

☑4ᵗʰ **J11 Influenza due to unidentified influenza virus**

☑5ᵗʰ **J11.0 Influenza due to unidentified influenza virus with pneumonia**

> Code also associated lung abscess, if applicable (J85.1)
> AHA: 2016,3Q,11

> **J11.00 Influenza due to unidentified influenza virus with unspecified type of pneumonia**   MCC
>> Influenza with pneumonia NOS

> **J11.08 Influenza due to unidentified influenza virus with specified pneumonia**   MCC
>> Code also other specified type of pneumonia

J11.1 Influenza due to unidentified influenza virus with other respiratory manifestations

> Influenza NOS
> Influenzal laryngitis NOS
> Influenzal pharyngitis NOS
> Influenza with upper respiratory symptoms NOS
> Use additional code for associated pleural effusion, if applicable (J91.8)
> Use additional code for associated sinusitis, if applicable (J01.-)

J11.2 Influenza due to unidentified influenza virus with gastrointestinal manifestations

> Influenza gastroenteritis NOS
> EXCLUDES 1 *"intestinal flu" [viral gastroenteritis] (A08.-)*

☑5ᵗʰ **J11.8 Influenza due to unidentified influenza virus with other manifestations**

> **J11.81 Influenza due to unidentified influenza virus with encephalopathy**
>> Influenzal encephalopathy NOS

> **J11.82 Influenza due to unidentified influenza virus with myocarditis**
>> Influenzal myocarditis NOS

> **J11.83 Influenza due to unidentified influenza virus with otitis media**
>> Influenzal otitis media NOS
>> Use additional code for any associated perforated tympanic membrane (H72.-)

> **J11.89 Influenza due to unidentified influenza virus with other manifestations**
>> Use additional codes to identify the manifestations

☑4ᵗʰ **J12 Viral pneumonia, not elsewhere classified**

> INCLUDES bronchopneumonia due to viruses other than influenza viruses
> Code first associated influenza, if applicable (J09.X1, J10.0-, J11.0-)
> Code also associated abscess, if applicable (J85.1)
> EXCLUDES 1 *aspiration pneumonia due to anesthesia during labor and delivery (O74.0)*
> *aspiration pneumonia due to anesthesia during pregnancy (O29)*
> *aspiration pneumonia due to anesthesia during puerperium (O89.0)*
> *aspiration pneumonia due to solids and liquids (J69.-)*
> *aspiration pneumonia NOS (J69.0)*
> *congenital pneumonia (P23.0)*
> *congenital rubella pneumonitis (P35.0)*
> *interstitial pneumonia NOS (J84.9)*
> *lipid pneumonia (J69.1)*
> *neonatal aspiration pneumonia (P24.-)*
> AHA: 2020,2Q,28; 2019,1Q,35; 2018,3Q,24; 2016,3Q,15; 2013,4Q,118

J12.0 Adenoviral pneumonia   MCC

J12.1 Respiratory syncytial virus pneumonia   MCC
> RSV pneumonia

J12.2 Parainfluenza virus pneumonia   MCC

J12.3 Human metapneumovirus pneumonia   HIV MCC

☑5ᵗʰ **J12.8 Other viral pneumonia**

> **J12.81 Pneumonia due to SARS-associated coronavirus**   HIV MCC
>> Severe acute respiratory syndrome NOS
>> DEF: Severe adult respiratory syndrome caused by the coronavirus, specified as inflammation of the lungs with consolidation.

> **J12.89 Other viral pneumonia**   HIV MCC
>> AHA: 2020,2Q,8,11; 2020,1Q,34-36
>> TIP: For pneumonia confirmed as due to COVID-19, assign code U07.1 as the primary or first-listed diagnosis and J12.89 as a secondary diagnosis.

J12.9 Viral pneumonia, unspecified   HIV MCC

J13 Pneumonia due to Streptococcus pneumoniae   HIV MCC HCC
> Bronchopneumonia due to S. pneumoniae
> Code first associated influenza, if applicable (J09.X1, J10.0-, J11.0-)
> Code also associated abscess, if applicable (J85.1)
> EXCLUDES 1 *congenital pneumonia due to S. pneumoniae (P23.6)*
> *lobar pneumonia, unspecified organism (J18.1)*
> *pneumonia due to other streptococci (J15.3-J15.4)*
> AHA: 2020,2Q,28; 2019,1Q,35; 2018,3Q,24; 2016,3Q,15; 2013,4Q,118

J14 Pneumonia due to Hemophilus influenzae   HIV MCC HCC
> Bronchopneumonia due to H. influenzae
> Code first associated influenza, if applicable (J09.X1, J10.0-, J11.0-)
> Code also associated abscess, if applicable (J85.1)
> EXCLUDES 1 *congenital pneumonia due to H. influenzae (P23.6)*
> AHA: 2020,2Q,28; 2019,1Q,35; 2018,3Q,24; 2016,3Q,15; 2013,4Q,118

☑4ᵗʰ **J15 Bacterial pneumonia, not elsewhere classified**

> INCLUDES Bronchopneumonia due to bacteria other than S. pneumoniae and H. influenzae
> Code first associated influenza, if applicable (J09.X1, J10.0-, -J11.0-)
> Code also associated abscess, if applicable (J85.1)
> EXCLUDES 1 *chlamydial pneumonia (J16.0)*
> *congenital pneumonia (P23.-)*
> *Legionnaires' disease (A48.1)*
> *spirochetal pneumonia (A69.8)*
> AHA: 2020,2Q,28; 2019,1Q,35; 2018,3Q,24; 2016,3Q,15; 2013,4Q,118

J15.0 Pneumonia due to Klebsiella pneumoniae   HIV MCC HCC

J15.1 Pneumonia due to Pseudomonas   HIV MCC HCC

☑5ᵗʰ **J15.2 Pneumonia due to staphylococcus**

> **J15.20 Pneumonia due to staphylococcus, unspecified**   HIV MCC HCC

☑ Additional Character Required   ☑×7ᵗʰ Placeholder   Unacceptable PDx   Questionable PDx   Manifestation   Unspecified Dx   H1-H14 HAC   HCC CMS-HCC Dx   HIV HIV Dx

√6ᵗʰ **J15.21 Pneumonia due to Staphylococcus aureus**

    J15.211 Pneumonia due to methicillin susceptible Staphylococcus aureus `HIV` `MCC` `HCC`
      MSSA pneumonia
      Pneumonia due to Staphylococcus aureus NOS

    J15.212 Pneumonia due to methicillin resistant Staphylococcus aureus `HIV` `MCC` `HCC`

J15.29 Pneumonia due to other staphylococcus `HIV` `MCC` `HCC`

J15.3 Pneumonia due to streptococcus, group B `HIV` `MCC` `HCC`

J15.4 Pneumonia due to other streptococci `HIV` `MCC` `HCC`
    `EXCLUDES 1`   pneumonia due to streptococcus, group B (J15.3)
                        pneumonia due to Streptococcus pneumoniae (J13)

J15.5 Pneumonia due to Escherichia coli `HIV` `MCC` `HCC`

J15.6 Pneumonia due to other Gram-negative bacteria `HIV` `MCC` `HCC`
    Pneumonia due to other aerobic Gram-negative bacteria
    Pneumonia due to Serratia marcescens
    AHA: 2020,2Q,28

J15.7 Pneumonia due to Mycoplasma pneumoniae `MCC`

J15.8 Pneumonia due to other specified bacteria `HIV` `MCC` `HCC`

J15.9 Unspecified bacterial pneumonia `HIV` `MCC`
    Pneumonia due to gram-positive bacteria

√4ᵗʰ **J16 Pneumonia due to other infectious organisms, not elsewhere classified**
    Code first associated influenza, if applicable (J09.X1, J10.0-, J11.0-)
    Code also associated abscess, if applicable (J85.1)
    `EXCLUDES 1`   congenital pneumonia (P23.-)
                        ornithosis (A70)
                        pneumocystosis (B59)
                        pneumonia NOS (J18.9)
    AHA: 2020,2Q,28; 2019,1Q,35; 2018,3Q,24; 2016,3Q,15; 2013,4Q,118

J16.0 Chlamydial pneumonia `MCC`

J16.8 Pneumonia due to other specified infectious organisms `MCC`

J17 Pneumonia in diseases classified elsewhere `MCC`
    Code first underlying disease, such as:
      Q fever (A78)
      rheumatic fever (I00)
      schistosomiasis (B65.0-B65.9)
    `EXCLUDES 1`   candidial pneumonia (B37.1)
                        chlamydial pneumonia (J16.0)
                        gonorrheal pneumonia (A54.84)
                        histoplasmosis pneumonia (B39.0-B39.2)
                        measles pneumonia (B05.2)
                        nocardiosis pneumonia (A43.0)
                        pneumocystosis (B59)
                        pneumonia due to Pneumocystis carinii (B59)
                        pneumonia due to Pneumocystis jiroveci (B59)
                        pneumonia in actinomycosis (A42.0)
                        pneumonia in anthrax (A22.1)
                        pneumonia in ascariasis (B77.81)
                        pneumonia in aspergillosis (B44.0-B44.1)
                        pneumonia in coccidioidomycosis (B38.0-B38.2)
                        pneumonia in cytomegalovirus disease (B25.0)
                        pneumonia in toxoplasmosis (B58.3)
                        rubella pneumonia (B06.81)
                        salmonella pneumonia (A02.22)
                        spirochetal infection NEC with pneumonia (A69.8)
                        tularemia pneumonia (A21.2)
                        typhoid fever with pneumonia (A01.03)
                        varicella pneumonia (B01.2)
                        whooping cough with pneumonia (A37 with fifth character 1)
    AHA: 2020,2Q,28; 2019,1Q,35; 2016,3Q,15; 2013,4Q,118

J18 Pneumonia, unspecified organism √4ᵗʰ
    Code first associated influenza, if applicable (J09.X1, J10.0-, J11.0-)
    `EXCLUDES 1`   abscess of lung with pneumonia (J85.1)
                        aspiration pneumonia due to anesthesia during labor and delivery (O74.0)
                        aspiration pneumonia due to anesthesia during pregnancy (O29)
                        aspiration pneumonia due to anesthesia during puerperium (O89.0)
                        aspiration pneumonia due to solids and liquids (J69.-)
                        aspiration pneumonia NOS (J69.0)
                        congenital pneumonia (P23.0)
                        drug-induced interstitial lung disorder (J70.2-J70.4)
                        interstitial pneumonia NOS (J84.9)
                        lipid pneumonia (J69.1)
                        neonatal aspiration pneumonia (P24.-)
                        pneumonitis due to external agents (J67-J70)
                        pneumonitis due to fumes and vapors (J68.0)
                        usual interstitial pneumonia ▶(J84.178)◀
    AHA: 2020,2Q,28; 2019,1Q,35; 2016,3Q,15; 2013,4Q,118

J18.0 Bronchopneumonia, unspecified organism `MCC`
    `EXCLUDES 1`   hypostatic bronchopneumonia (J18.2)
                        lipid pneumonia (J69.1)
    `EXCLUDES 2`   acute bronchiolitis (J21.-)
                        chronic bronchiolitis (J44.9)

J18.1 Lobar pneumonia, unspecified organism `HIV` `MCC` `HCC`
    AHA: 2019,3Q,37; 2018,3Q,24
    TIP: Assign J18.1 only when the provider specifically documents "lobar pneumonia" without specifying a causal organism. Lobar pneumonia may not be assumed based on an imaging report that identifies pneumonia in a specific lobe.
    TIP: Use this code for documented lobar pneumonia or multilobar pneumonia when the causal organism is not identified. If the causal organism is identified, codes from categories J12-J16 should be used, depending on the organism that is present.

J18.2 Hypostatic pneumonia, unspecified organism `CC`
    Hypostatic bronchopneumonia
    Passive pneumonia

J18.8 Other pneumonia, unspecified organism `HIV` `MCC`

J18.9 Pneumonia, unspecified organism `HIV` `MCC`
    AHA: 2020,2Q,28; 2019,3Q,15; 2019,2Q,28; 2014,3Q,4; 2013,4Q,119; 2012,4Q,94

Other acute lower respiratory infections (J20-J22)

`EXCLUDES 2`   chronic obstructive pulmonary disease with acute lower respiratory infection (J44.0)

√4ᵗʰ **J20 Acute bronchitis**
    `INCLUDES`   acute and subacute bronchitis (with) bronchospasm
                     acute and subacute bronchitis (with) tracheitis
                     acute and subacute bronchitis (with) tracheobronchitis, acute
                     acute and subacute fibrinous bronchitis
                     acute and subacute membranous bronchitis
                     acute and subacute purulent bronchitis
                     acute and subacute septic bronchitis
    `EXCLUDES 1`   bronchitis NOS (J40)
                        tracheobronchitis NOS (J40)
    `EXCLUDES 2`   acute bronchitis with bronchiectasis (J47.0)
                        acute bronchitis with chronic obstructive asthma (J44.0)
                        acute bronchitis with chronic obstructive pulmonary disease (J44.0)
                        allergic bronchitis NOS (J45.909-)
                        bronchitis due to chemicals, fumes and vapors (J68.0)
                        chronic bronchitis NOS (J42)
                        chronic mucopurulent bronchitis (J41.1)
                        chronic obstructive bronchitis (J44.-)
                        chronic obstructive tracheobronchitis (J44.-)
                        chronic simple bronchitis (J41.0)
                        chronic tracheobronchitis (J42)
    AHA: 2019,1Q,35; 2016,3Q,10,16
    DEF: Acute inflammation of the main branches of the bronchial tree due to infectious or irritant agents. Symptoms include cough with a varied production of sputum, fever, substernal soreness, and lung rales. Bronchitis usually lasts three to 10 days.

J20.0 Acute bronchitis due to Mycoplasma pneumoniae

J20.1 Acute bronchitis due to Hemophilus influenzae

`N` Newborn: 0   `P` Pediatric: 0-17   `M` Maternity: 9-64   `A` Adult: 15-124   `MCC` Major Complication/Comorbidity   `CC` Complication/Comorbidity   `SW` Severe Wound Dx

692   ICD-10-CM 2021

J20.2   **Acute bronchitis due to** streptococcus

J20.3   **Acute bronchitis due to** coxsackievirus

J20.4   **Acute bronchitis due to** parainfluenza virus

J20.5   **Acute bronchitis due to** respiratory syncytial virus
     Acute bronchitis due to RSV

J20.6   **Acute bronchitis due to** rhinovirus

J20.7   **Acute bronchitis due to** echovirus

J20.8   **Acute bronchitis due to other specified organisms**
     AHA: 2020,1Q,34-36
     TIP: Assign as a secondary code for a patient with acute bronchitis confirmed as due to COVID-19; assign U07.1 as the principal or first-listed code.

J20.9   **Acute bronchitis, unspecified**

✓4ᵗʰ **J21**   **Acute bronchiolitis**

   INCLUDES   acute bronchiolitis with bronchospasm
   EXCLUDES 2   respiratory bronchiolitis interstitial lung disease (J84.115)

J21.0   **Acute bronchiolitis due to** respiratory syncytial virus   CC
     Acute bronchiolitis due to RSV

J21.1   **Acute bronchiolitis due to** human metapneumovirus   CC

J21.8   **Acute bronchiolitis due to other specified organisms**   CC

J21.9   **Acute bronchiolitis, unspecified**   CC
     Bronchiolitis (acute)
     EXCLUDES 1   chronic bronchiolitis (J44.-)

J22   **Unspecified acute lower respiratory infection**
     Acute (lower) respiratory (tract) infection NOS
     EXCLUDES 1   upper respiratory infection (acute) (J06.9)
     AHA: 2020,1Q,22,34-36
     TIP: Assign as a secondary code for a patient with a respiratory infection specified as acute or lower that is documented as being associated with COVID-19; assign U07.1 as the principal or first-listed code. If the respiratory infection documentation does not specify acute or lower, assign J98.8.

Other diseases of upper respiratory tract (J30-J39)

✓4ᵗʰ **J30**   **Vasomotor and allergic rhinitis**

   INCLUDES   spasmodic rhinorrhea
   EXCLUDES 1   allergic rhinitis with asthma (bronchial) (J45.909)
           rhinitis NOS (J31.0)

J30.0   **Vasomotor rhinitis**
     DEF: Noninfectious and nonallergic type of rhinitis for which the cause is often unknown. Symptoms often mimic those of allergic rhinitis with a diagnosis of vasomotor rhinitis typically made after ruling out allergens as the cause.

J30.1   **Allergic rhinitis due to** pollen
     Allergy NOS due to pollen
     Hay fever
     Pollinosis

J30.2   **Other** seasonal allergic **rhinitis**

J30.5   **Allergic rhinitis due to** food

✓5ᵗʰ **J30.8**   **Other allergic rhinitis**

     J30.81   **Allergic rhinitis due to** animal (cat) (dog) hair and dander

     J30.89   **Other allergic rhinitis**
           Perennial allergic rhinitis

J30.9   **Allergic rhinitis, unspecified**

✓4ᵗʰ **J31**   **Chronic rhinitis, nasopharyngitis and pharyngitis**
     Use additional code to identify:
       exposure to environmental tobacco smoke (Z77.22)
       exposure to tobacco smoke in the perinatal period (P96.81)
       history of tobacco dependence (Z87.891)
       occupational exposure to environmental tobacco smoke (Z57.31)
       tobacco dependence (F17.-)
       tobacco use (Z72.0)

   J31.0   **Chronic rhinitis**
     Atrophic rhinitis (chronic)
     Granulomatous rhinitis (chronic)
     Hypertrophic rhinitis (chronic)
     Obstructive rhinitis (chronic)
     Ozena
     Purulent rhinitis (chronic)
     Rhinitis (chronic) NOS
     Ulcerative rhinitis (chronic)
     EXCLUDES 1   allergic rhinitis (J30.1-J30.9)
           vasomotor rhinitis (J30.0)
     DEF: Persistent inflammation of the mucous membranes of the nose, characterized by a postnasal drip.

J31.1   **Chronic nasopharyngitis**
     EXCLUDES 2   acute nasopharyngitis (J00)
     DEF: Persistent inflammation of the mucous membranes extending from the nares to the pharynx. It is characterized by constant irritation in the nasopharynx and postnasal drip.

J31.2   **Chronic pharyngitis**
     Atrophic pharyngitis (chronic)
     Chronic sore throat
     Granular pharyngitis (chronic)
     Hypertrophic pharyngitis (chronic)
     EXCLUDES 2   acute pharyngitis (J02.9)

✓4ᵗʰ **J32**   **Chronic sinusitis**

   INCLUDES   sinus abscess
           sinus empyema
           sinus infection
           sinus suppuration
     Use additional code to identify:
       exposure to environmental tobacco smoke (Z77.22)
       exposure to tobacco smoke in the perinatal period (P96.81)
       history of tobacco dependence (Z87.891)
       infectious agent (B95-B97)
       occupational exposure to environmental tobacco smoke (Z57.31)
       tobacco dependence (F17.-),
       tobacco use (Z72.0)
     EXCLUDES 2   acute sinusitis (J01.-)

J32.0   **Chronic** maxillary **sinusitis**
     Antritis (chronic)
     Maxillary sinusitis NOS

J32.1   **Chronic** frontal **sinusitis**
     Frontal sinusitis NOS

J32.2   **Chronic** ethmoidal **sinusitis**
     Ethmoidal sinusitis NOS
     EXCLUDES 1   Woakes' ethmoiditis (J33.1)

J32.3   **Chronic** sphenoidal **sinusitis**
     Sphenoidal sinusitis NOS

J32.4   **Chronic** pansinusitis
     Pansinusitis NOS

J32.8   **Other chronic sinusitis**
     Sinusitis (chronic) involving more than one sinus but not pansinusitis

J32.9   **Chronic sinusitis, unspecified**
     Sinusitis (chronic) NOS

✓4ᵗʰ **J33**   **Nasal polyp**
     Use additional code to identify:
       exposure to environmental tobacco smoke (Z77.22)
       exposure to tobacco smoke in the perinatal period (P96.81)
       history of tobacco dependence (Z87.891)
       occupational exposure to environmental tobacco smoke (Z57.31)
       tobacco dependence (F17.-)
       tobacco use (Z72.0)
     EXCLUDES 1   adenomatous polyps (D14.0)

J33.0   **Polyp of nasal cavity**
     Choanal polyp
     Nasopharyngeal polyp

J33.1   **Polypoid sinus degeneration**
     Woakes' syndrome or ethmoiditis

J33.8   **Other polyp of sinus**
     Accessory polyp of sinus
     Ethmoidal polyp of sinus
     Maxillary polyp of sinus
     Sphenoidal polyp of sinus

J33.9   **Nasal polyp, unspecified**

✓4ᵗʰ **J34**   **Other and unspecified disorders of nose and nasal sinuses**
     EXCLUDES 2   varicose ulcer of nasal septum (I86.8)

J34.0   **Abscess, furuncle and carbuncle of nose**
     Cellulitis of nose
     Necrosis of nose
     Ulceration of nose

J34.1   **Cyst and mucocele of nose and nasal sinus**

J34.2   **Deviated nasal septum**
     Deflection or deviation of septum (nasal) (acquired)
     EXCLUDES 1   congenital deviated nasal septum (Q67.4)
     DEF: Condition in which the nasal septum, a thin wall composed of cartilage and bone that separates the two nostrils, is crooked or displaced from the midline.

☑ Additional Character Required   ✓x7ᵗʰ Placeholder   Unacceptable PDx   Questionable PDx   Manifestation   Unspecified Dx   H1-H14 HAC   HCC CMS-HCC Dx   HIV HIV Dx

ICD-10-CM 2021   693

Chapter 10. Diseases of the Respiratory System

J34.3 **Hypertrophy of nasal turbinates**
DEF: Overgrowth of bones within the nasal turbinate, which are ridges of bone and soft tissue that project from the sidewalls of the nasal passages. Hypertrophy can cause obstruction of the nasal passages.

√5ᵗʰ **J34.8** **Other specified disorders of nose and nasal sinuses**

J34.81 **Nasal mucositis (ulcerative)**
Code also type of associated therapy, such as:
antineoplastic and immunosuppressive drugs (T45.1X-)
radiological procedure and radiotherapy (Y84.2)
EXCLUDES 2   *gastrointestinal mucositis (ulcerative) (K92.81)*
mucositis (ulcerative) of vagina and vulva (N76.81)
oral mucositis (ulcerative) (K12.3-)

J34.89 **Other specified disorders of nose and nasal sinuses**
Perforation of nasal septum NOS
Rhinolith

J34.9 **Unspecified disorder of nose and nasal sinuses**

√4ᵗʰ **J35** **Chronic diseases of tonsils and adenoids**
Use additional code to identify:
exposure to environmental tobacco smoke (Z77.22)
exposure to tobacco smoke in the perinatal period (P96.81)
history of tobacco dependence (Z87.891)
occupational exposure to environmental tobacco smoke (Z57.31)
tobacco dependence (F17.-)
tobacco use (Z72.0)

√5ᵗʰ **J35.0** **Chronic tonsillitis and adenoiditis**
EXCLUDES 2   *acute tonsillitis (J03.-)*

J35.01 **Chronic tonsillitis**
J35.02 **Chronic adenoiditis**
J35.03 **Chronic tonsillitis and adenoiditis**

J35.1 **Hypertrophy of tonsils**
Enlargement of tonsils
EXCLUDES 1   *hypertrophy of tonsils with tonsillitis (J35.0-)*

J35.2 **Hypertrophy of adenoids**
Enlargement of adenoids
EXCLUDES 1   *hypertrophy of adenoids with adenoiditis (J35.0-)*

J35.3 **Hypertrophy of tonsils with hypertrophy of adenoids**
EXCLUDES 1   *hypertrophy of tonsils and adenoids with tonsillitis and adenoiditis (J35.03)*

J35.8 **Other chronic diseases of tonsils and adenoids**
Adenoid vegetations
Amygdalolith
Calculus, tonsil
Cicatrix of tonsil (and adenoid)
Tonsillar tag
Ulcer of tonsil

J35.9 **Chronic disease of tonsils and adenoids, unspecified**
Disease (chronic) of tonsils and adenoids NOS

J36 **Peritonsillar abscess**   CC
INCLUDES   abscess of tonsil
peritonsillar cellulitis
quinsy
Use additional code (B95-B97) to identify infectious agent
EXCLUDES 1   *acute tonsillitis (J03.-)*
chronic tonsillitis (J35.0)
retropharyngeal abscess (J39.0)
tonsillitis NOS (J03.9-)

√4ᵗʰ **J37** **Chronic laryngitis and laryngotracheitis**
Use additional code to identify:
exposure to environmental tobacco smoke (Z77.22)
exposure to tobacco smoke in the perinatal period (P96.81)
history of tobacco dependence (Z87.891)
infectious agent (B95-B97)
occupational exposure to environmental tobacco smoke (Z57.31)
tobacco dependence (F17.-)
tobacco use (Z72.0)

J37.0 **Chronic laryngitis**
Catarrhal laryngitis
Hypertrophic laryngitis
Sicca laryngitis
EXCLUDES 2   *acute laryngitis (J04.0)*
obstructive (acute) laryngitis (J05.0)

J37.1 **Chronic laryngotracheitis**
Laryngitis, chronic, with tracheitis (chronic)
Tracheitis, chronic, with laryngitis
EXCLUDES 1   *chronic tracheitis (J42)*
EXCLUDES 2   *acute laryngotracheitis (J04.2)*
acute tracheitis (J04.1)

√4ᵗʰ **J38** **Diseases of vocal cords and larynx, not elsewhere classified**
Use additional code to identify:
exposure to environmental tobacco smoke (Z77.22)
exposure to tobacco smoke in the perinatal period (P96.81)
history of tobacco dependence (Z87.891)
occupational exposure to environmental tobacco smoke (Z57.31)
tobacco dependence (F17.-)
tobacco use (Z72.0)
EXCLUDES 1   *congenital laryngeal stridor (P28.89)*
obstructive laryngitis (acute) (J05.0)
postprocedural subglottic stenosis (J95.5)
stridor (R06.1)
ulcerative laryngitis (J04.0)

√5ᵗʰ **J38.0** **Paralysis of vocal cords and larynx**
Laryngoplegia
Paralysis of glottis

J38.00 **Paralysis of vocal cords and larynx, unspecified**
J38.01 **Paralysis of vocal cords and larynx, unilateral**
J38.02 **Paralysis of vocal cords and larynx, bilateral**

J38.1 **Polyp of vocal cord and larynx**
EXCLUDES 1   *adenomatous polyps (D14.1)*

J38.2 **Nodules of vocal cords**
Chorditis (fibrinous)(nodosa)(tuberosa)
Singer's nodes
Teacher's nodes

J38.3 **Other diseases of vocal cords**
Abscess of vocal cords
Cellulitis of vocal cords
Granuloma of vocal cords
Leukokeratosis of vocal cords
Leukoplakia of vocal cords

J38.4 **Edema of larynx**
Edema (of) glottis
Subglottic edema
Supraglottic edema
EXCLUDES 1   *acute obstructive laryngitis [croup] (J05.0)*
edematous laryngitis (J04.0)

J38.5 **Laryngeal spasm**
Laryngismus (stridulus)

J38.6 **Stenosis of larynx**

J38.7 **Other diseases of larynx**
Abscess of larynx
Cellulitis of larynx
Disease of larynx NOS
Necrosis of larynx
Pachyderma of larynx
Perichondritis of larynx
Ulcer of larynx

√4ᵗʰ **J39** **Other diseases of upper respiratory tract**
EXCLUDES 1   *acute respiratory infection NOS (J22)*
acute upper respiratory infection (J06.9)
upper respiratory inflammation due to chemicals, gases, fumes or vapors (J68.2)

J39.0 **Retropharyngeal and parapharyngeal abscess**   CC
Peripharyngeal abscess
EXCLUDES 1   *peritonsillar abscess (J36)*
DEF: Purulent infection behind the pharynx and the front of the precerebral fascia, characterized by neck stiffness, cervical lymphadenopathy, sore throat, fever, and stridor.

J39.1 **Other abscess of pharynx**   CC
Cellulitis of pharynx
Nasopharyngeal abscess

J39.2 **Other diseases of pharynx**
Cyst of pharynx
Edema of pharynx
EXCLUDES 2   *chronic pharyngitis (J31.2)*
ulcerative pharyngitis (J02.9)

J39.3 **Upper respiratory tract hypersensitivity reaction, site unspecified**
> EXCLUDES 1   *hypersensitivity reaction of upper respiratory tract, such as:*
> *extrinsic allergic alveolitis (J67.9)*
> *pneumoconiosis (J60-J67.9)*

J39.8 **Other specified diseases of upper respiratory tract**

J39.9 **Disease of upper respiratory tract, unspecified**

Chronic lower respiratory diseases (J40-J47)

> EXCLUDES 1   *bronchitis due to chemicals, gases, fumes and vapors (J68.0)*
> EXCLUDES 2   *cystic fibrosis (E84.-)*

J40 **Bronchitis, not specified as acute or chronic**
Bronchitis NOS
Bronchitis with tracheitis NOS
Catarrhal bronchitis
Tracheobronchitis NOS
Use additional code to identify:
  exposure to environmental tobacco smoke (Z77.22)
  exposure to tobacco smoke in the perinatal period (P96.81)
  history of tobacco dependence (Z87.891)
  occupational exposure to environmental tobacco smoke (Z57.31)
  tobacco dependence (F17.-)
  tobacco use (Z72.0)
> EXCLUDES 1   *acute bronchitis (J20.-)*
> *allergic bronchitis NOS (J45.909-)*
> *asthmatic bronchitis NOS (J45.9-)*
> *bronchitis due to chemicals, gases, fumes and vapors (J68.0)*

AHA: 2020,1Q,34-36
TIP: Assign as a secondary code for a patient with bronchitis of unspecified acuity due to COVID-19; assign U07.1 as the principal or first-listed code.

✓4ᵗʰ J41 **Simple and mucopurulent chronic bronchitis**
Use additional code to identify:
  exposure to environmental tobacco smoke (Z77.22)
  exposure to tobacco smoke in the perinatal period (P96.81)
  history of tobacco dependence (Z87.891)
  occupational exposure to environmental tobacco smoke (Z57.31)
  tobacco dependence (F17.-)
  tobacco use (Z72.0)
> EXCLUDES 1   *chronic bronchitis NOS (J42)*
> *chronic obstructive bronchitis (J44.-)*

J41.0 **Simple chronic bronchitis**   HCC

J41.1 **Mucopurulent chronic bronchitis**   HCC

J41.8 **Mixed simple and mucopurulent chronic bronchitis**   HCC

J42 **Unspecified chronic bronchitis**   HCC
Chronic bronchitis NOS
Chronic tracheitis
Chronic tracheobronchitis
Use additional code to identify:
  exposure to environmental tobacco smoke (Z77.22)
  exposure to tobacco smoke in the perinatal period (P96.81)
  history of tobacco dependence (Z87.891)
  occupational exposure to environmental tobacco smoke (Z57.31)
  tobacco dependence (F17.-)
  tobacco use (Z72.0)
> EXCLUDES 1   *chronic asthmatic bronchitis (J44.-)*
> *chronic bronchitis with airways obstruction (J44.-)*
> *chronic emphysematous bronchitis (J44.-)*
> *chronic obstructive pulmonary disease NOS (J44.9)*
> *simple and mucopurulent chronic bronchitis (J41.-)*

✓4ᵗʰ J43 **Emphysema**
Use additional code to identify:
  exposure to environmental tobacco smoke (Z77.22)
  history of tobacco dependence (Z87.891)
  occupational exposure to environmental tobacco smoke (Z57.31)
  tobacco dependence (F17.-)
  tobacco use (Z72.0)
> EXCLUDES 1   *compensatory emphysema (J98.3)*
> *emphysema due to inhalation of chemicals, gases, fumes or vapors (J68.4)*
> *emphysema with chronic (obstructive) bronchitis (J44.-)*
> *emphysematous (obstructive) bronchitis (J44.-)*
> *interstitial emphysema (J98.2)*
> *mediastinal emphysema (J98.2)*
> *neonatal interstitial emphysema (P25.0)*
> *surgical (subcutaneous) emphysema (T81.82)*
> *traumatic subcutaneous emphysema (T79.7)*
> EXCLUDES 2   ▶*traumatic subcutaneous emphysema (T79.7)*◀

DEF: Pathological condition in which there is destructive enlargement of the air sacs in the lungs resulting in damage and lack of elasticity to the alveolar walls, commonly seen in long-term smokers.

Emphysema

Healthy alveoli — Patent bronchiole — Well-vascularized — Dilated alveoli — Excess mucus

Alveoli w/ Emphysema — Collapsed bronchiole — Enlarged alveoli — Broken/fewer capillaries — Alveolar membranes break down

J43.0 **Unilateral pulmonary emphysema [MacLeod's syndrome]**   HCC
Swyer-James syndrome
Unilateral emphysema
Unilateral hyperlucent lung
Unilateral pulmonary artery functional hypoplasia
Unilateral transparency of lung

J43.1 **Panlobular emphysema**   HCC
Panacinar emphysema

J43.2 **Centrilobular emphysema**   HCC

J43.8 **Other emphysema**   HCC

J43.9 **Emphysema, unspecified**   HCC
Bullous emphysema (lung)(pulmonary)
Emphysema (lung)(pulmonary) NOS
Emphysematous bleb
Vesicular emphysema (lung)(pulmonary)
AHA: 2019,1Q,34-36; 2017,4Q,97-98

☑ Additional Character Required   ✓x7ᵗʰ Placeholder   Unacceptable PDx   Questionable PDx   Manifestation   Unspecified Dx   H1 - H14 HAC   HCC CMS-HCC Dx   HIV HIV Dx
ICD-10-CM 2021   695

Chapter 10. Diseases of the Respiratory System

J39.3–J43.9

✓4ᵗʰ J44 Other chronic obstructive pulmonary disease

INCLUDES asthma with chronic obstructive pulmonary disease
chronic asthmatic (obstructive) bronchitis
chronic bronchitis with airways obstruction
chronic bronchitis with emphysema
chronic emphysematous bronchitis
chronic obstructive asthma
chronic obstructive bronchitis
chronic obstructive tracheobronchitis

Code also type of asthma, if applicable (J45.-)
Use additional code to identify:
exposure to environmental tobacco smoke (Z77.22)
history of tobacco dependence (Z87.891)
occupational exposure to environmental tobacco smoke (Z57.31)
tobacco dependence (F17.-)
tobacco use (Z72.0)

EXCLUDES 1 bronchiectasis (J47.-)
chronic bronchitis NOS (J42)
chronic simple and mucopurulent bronchitis (J41.-)
chronic tracheitis (J42)
chronic tracheobronchitis (J42)
emphysema without chronic bronchitis (J43.-)

AHA: 2019,1Q,34-36; 2017,4Q,97-98; 2017,1Q,25-26; 2016,3Q,15-16; 2013,4Q,109

J44.0 Chronic obstructive pulmonary disease with (acute) lower respiratory infection CC HCC

Code also to identify the infection
AHA: 2019,1Q,35; 2017,4Q,96; 2017,1Q,24-25
TIP: Do not assign when only aspiration pneumonia is present. Aspiration pneumonia is not classified as a respiratory infection.

J44.1 Chronic obstructive pulmonary disease with (acute) exacerbation CC HCC

Decompensated COPD
Decompensated COPD with (acute) exacerbation
EXCLUDES 2 chronic obstructive pulmonary disease [COPD] with acute bronchitis (J44.0)
lung diseases due to external agents (J60-J70)
AHA: 2019,1Q,34; 2017,4Q,96; 2017,1Q,26; 2016,1Q,36
TIP: Exacerbation of COPD should not be assumed based upon worsening of a concomitant respiratory disease or when COPD is described as end-stage.

J44.9 Chronic obstructive pulmonary disease, unspecified HCC

Chronic obstructive airway disease NOS
Chronic obstructive lung disease NOS
EXCLUDES 2 lung diseases due to external agents (J60-J70)
AHA: 2019,1Q,36; 2017,4Q,96-97; 2016,1Q,36; 2014,4Q,21; 2013,4Q,109

✓4ᵗʰ J45 Asthma

INCLUDES allergic (predominantly) asthma
allergic bronchitis NOS
allergic rhinitis with asthma
atopic asthma
extrinsic allergic asthma
hay fever with asthma
idiosyncratic asthma
intrinsic nonallergic asthma
nonallergic asthma

Use additional code to identify:
▶eosinophilic asthma (J82.83) ◀
exposure to environmental tobacco smoke (Z77.22)
exposure to tobacco smoke in the perinatal period (P96.81)
history of tobacco dependence (Z87.891)
occupational exposure to environmental tobacco smoke (Z57.31)
tobacco dependence (F17.-)
tobacco use (Z72.0)

EXCLUDES 1 detergent asthma (J69.8)
eosinophilic asthma (J82)
miner's asthma (J60)
wheezing NOS (R06.2)
wood asthma (J67.8)

EXCLUDES 2 asthma with chronic obstructive pulmonary disease (J44.9)
chronic asthmatic (obstructive) bronchitis (J44.9)
chronic obstructive asthma (J44.9)

AHA: 2019,1Q,36; 2017,1Q,25-26; 2012,4Q,99
DEF: Status asthmaticus: Severe, intractable episode of asthma that is unresponsive to normal therapeutic measures.

Asthma

Respiratory bronchiole
Smooth muscle fibers
Contraction of smooth muscle fibers
Mucus lining bronchial tubes
Alveoli
Extra mucus secretion in inflamed bronchial tubes
Air trapped within alveoli

Normal alveoli   Asthmatic alveoli

✓5ᵗʰ J45.2 Mild intermittent asthma

J45.20 Mild intermittent asthma, uncomplicated
Mild intermittent asthma NOS

J45.21 Mild intermittent asthma with (acute) exacerbation CC

J45.22 Mild intermittent asthma with status asthmaticus CC

✓5ᵗʰ J45.3 Mild persistent asthma

J45.30 Mild persistent asthma, uncomplicated
Mild persistent asthma NOS

J45.31 Mild persistent asthma with (acute) exacerbation CC
AHA: 2016,1Q,35

J45.32 Mild persistent asthma with status asthmaticus CC

✓5ᵗʰ J45.4 Moderate persistent asthma

J45.40 Moderate persistent asthma, uncomplicated
Moderate persistent asthma NOS

J45.41 Moderate persistent asthma with (acute) exacerbation CC
AHA: 2017,1Q,26

J45.42 Moderate persistent asthma with status asthmaticus CC

N Newborn: 0   P Pediatric: 0-17   M Maternity: 9-64   A Adult: 15-124   MCC Major Complication/Comorbidity   CC Complication/Comorbidity   SW Severe Wound Dx

696   ICD-10-CM 2021

✓5ᵗʰ **J45.5** Severe persistent **asthma**

    J45.50 **Severe persistent asthma,** uncomplicated
        Severe persistent asthma NOS

    J45.51 **Severe persistent asthma with (acute) exacerbation** `CC`

    J45.52 **Severe persistent asthma with** status **asthmaticus** `CC`

✓5ᵗʰ **J45.9** **Other and unspecified asthma**

    ✓6ᵗʰ **J45.90** **Unspecified asthma**
        Asthmatic bronchitis NOS
        Childhood asthma NOS
        Late onset asthma
        AHA: 2017,4Q,96; 2017,1Q,25

        J45.901 **Unspecified asthma with (acute) exacerbation** `CC`

        J45.902 **Unspecified asthma with** status **asthmaticus** `CC`

        J45.909 **Unspecified asthma,** uncomplicated
            Asthma NOS
            EXCLUDES 2 *lung diseases due to external agents (J60-J70)*
            AHA: 2017,1Q,25

    ✓6ᵗʰ **J45.99** **Other asthma**

        J45.990 **Exercise induced bronchospasm**
        J45.991 **Cough variant asthma**
        J45.998 **Other asthma**

✓4ᵗʰ **J47** **Bronchiectasis**

    INCLUDES bronchiolectasis
    Use additional code to identify:
      exposure to environmental tobacco smoke (Z77.22)
      exposure to tobacco smoke in the perinatal period (P96.81)
      history of tobacco dependence (Z87.891)
      occupational exposure to environmental tobacco smoke (Z57.31)
      tobacco dependence (F17.-)
      tobacco use (Z72.0)
    EXCLUDES 1 *congenital bronchiectasis (Q33.4)*
            tuberculous bronchiectasis (current disease) (A15.0)
    DEF: Dilation of the bronchi with mucus production and persistent cough due to infection or chronic conditions that causes diminished lung capacity and frequent infections of the lung.

    J47.0 **Bronchiectasis with acute lower respiratory infection** `CC` `HCC`
        Bronchiectasis with acute bronchitis
        Use additional code to identify the infection

    J47.1 **Bronchiectasis with (acute) exacerbation** `CC` `HCC`

    J47.9 **Bronchiectasis,** uncomplicated `HCC`
        Bronchiectasis NOS

Lung diseases due to external agents (J60-J70)

    EXCLUDES 2 *asthma (J45.-)*
            malignant neoplasm of bronchus and lung (C34.-)
    DEF: Pneumoconiosis: Condition caused by inhaling inorganic dust particles, typically associated with occupations that require regular exposure to mineral dusts. A form of interstitial lung disease that contributes to the inflammation of the air sacs, causing the lung tissue to harden.

J60 **Coalworker's pneumoconiosis** `HCC` `A`
    Anthracosilicosis
    Anthracosis
    Black lung disease
    Coalworker's lung
    EXCLUDES 1 *coalworker pneumoconiosis with tuberculosis, any type in A15 (J65)*

J61 **Pneumoconiosis due to asbestos and other mineral fibers** `HCC` `A`
    Asbestosis
    EXCLUDES 1 *pleural plaque with asbestosis (J92.0)*
            pneumoconiosis with tuberculosis, any type in A15 (J65)

✓4ᵗʰ **J62** **Pneumoconiosis due to dust containing silica**
    INCLUDES silicotic fibrosis (massive) of lung
    EXCLUDES 1 *pneumoconiosis with tuberculosis, any type in A15 (J65)*

    J62.0 **Pneumoconiosis due to talc dust** `HCC`

    J62.8 **Pneumoconiosis due to other dust containing silica** `HCC`
        Silicosis NOS

✓4ᵗʰ **J63** **Pneumoconiosis due to other inorganic dusts**
    EXCLUDES 1 *pneumoconiosis with tuberculosis, any type in A15 (J65)*

    J63.0 **Aluminosis (of lung)** `HCC`

    J63.1 **Bauxite fibrosis (of lung)** `HCC`
    J63.2 **Berylliosis** `HCC`
    J63.3 **Graphite fibrosis (of lung)** `HCC`
    J63.4 **Siderosis** `HCC`
        AHA: 2019,3Q,8
    J63.5 **Stannosis** `HCC`
    J63.6 **Pneumoconiosis due to other specified inorganic dusts** `HCC`

J64 **Unspecified pneumoconiosis** `HCC`
    EXCLUDES 1 *pneumonoconiosis with tuberculosis, any type in A15 (J65)*

J65 **Pneumoconiosis associated with tuberculosis** `HCC`
    Any condition in J60-J64 with tuberculosis, any type in A15
    Silicotuberculosis

✓4ᵗʰ **J66** **Airway disease due to specific organic dust**
    EXCLUDES 2 *allergic alveolitis (J67.-)*
            asbestosis (J61)
            bagassosis (J67.1)
            farmer's lung (J67.0)
            hypersensitivity pneumonitis due to organic dust (J67.-)
            reactive airways dysfunction syndrome (J68.3)

    J66.0 **Byssinosis** `HCC`
        Airway disease due to cotton dust

    J66.1 **Flax-dressers' disease** `HCC`
    J66.2 **Cannabinosis** `HCC`
    J66.8 **Airway disease due to other specific organic dusts** `HCC`

✓4ᵗʰ **J67** **Hypersensitivity pneumonitis due to organic dust**
    INCLUDES allergic alveolitis and pneumonitis due to inhaled organic dust and particles of fungal, actinomycetic or other origin
    EXCLUDES 1 *pneumonitis due to inhalation of chemicals, gases, fumes or vapors (J68.0)*

    J67.0 **Farmer's lung** `HCC`
        Harvester's lung
        Haymaker's lung
        Moldy hay disease

    J67.1 **Bagassosis** `HCC`
        Bagasse disease
        Bagasse pneumonitis

    J67.2 **Bird fancier's lung** `HCC`
        Budgerigar fancier's disease or lung
        Pigeon fancier's disease or lung

    J67.3 **Suberosis** `HCC`
        Corkhandler's disease or lung
        Corkworker's disease or lung

    J67.4 **Maltworker's lung** `HCC`
        Alveolitis due to Aspergillus clavatus

    J67.5 **Mushroom-worker's lung** `HCC`

    J67.6 **Maple-bark-stripper's lung** `HCC`
        Alveolitis due to Cryptostroma corticale
        Cryptostromosis

    J67.7 **Air conditioner and humidifier lung** `CC` `HCC`
        Allergic alveolitis due to fungal, thermophilic actinomycetes and other organisms growing in ventilation [air conditioning] systems

    J67.8 **Hypersensitivity pneumonitis due to other organic dusts** `CC` `HCC`
        Cheese-washer's lung
        Coffee-worker's lung
        Fish-meal worker's lung
        Furrier's lung
        Sequoiosis

    J67.9 **Hypersensitivity pneumonitis due to unspecified organic dust** `CC` `HCC`
        Allergic alveolitis (extrinsic) NOS
        Hypersensitivity pneumonitis NOS

Chapter 10. Diseases of the Respiratory System

✓4ᵗʰ **J68 Respiratory conditions due to inhalation of chemicals, gases, fumes and vapors**
    Code first (T51-T65) to identify cause
    Use additional code to identify associated respiratory conditions, such as:
    acute respiratory failure (J96.0-)

  J68.0 Bronchitis and pneumonitis due to chemicals, gases, fumes and vapors `CC` `HCC`
    Chemical bronchitis (acute)
    AHA: 2019,2Q,31

  J68.1 Pulmonary edema due to chemicals, gases, fumes and vapors `MCC` `HCC`
    Chemical pulmonary edema (acute) (chronic)
    EXCLUDES 1   *pulmonary edema (acute) (chronic) NOS (J81.-)*

  J68.2 Upper respiratory inflammation due to chemicals, gases, fumes and vapors, not elsewhere classified `HCC`

  J68.3 Other acute and subacute respiratory conditions due to chemicals, gases, fumes and vapors `HCC`
    Reactive airways dysfunction syndrome

  J68.4 Chronic respiratory conditions due to chemicals, gases, fumes and vapors `HCC`
    Emphysema (diffuse) (chronic) due to inhalation of chemicals, gases, fumes and vapors
    Obliterative bronchiolitis (chronic) (subacute) due to inhalation of chemicals, gases, fumes and vapors
    Pulmonary fibrosis (chronic) due to inhalation of chemicals, gases, fumes and vapors
    EXCLUDES 1   *chronic pulmonary edema due to chemicals, gases, fumes and vapors (J68.1)*

  J68.8 Other respiratory conditions due to chemicals, gases, fumes and vapors `HCC`

  J68.9 Unspecified respiratory condition due to chemicals, gases, fumes and vapors `HCC`

✓4ᵗʰ **J69 Pneumonitis due to solids and liquids**
    EXCLUDES 1   *neonatal aspiration syndromes (P24.-)*
        postprocedural pneumonitis (J95.4)
    AHA: 2017,1Q,24
    DEF: Pneumonitis: Noninfectious inflammation of the walls of the alveoli in the lung tissue due to inhalation of food, vomit, oils, essences, or other solids or liquids.

  J69.0 Pneumonitis due to inhalation of food and vomit `MCC` `HCC`
    Aspiration pneumonia NOS
    Aspiration pneumonia (due to) food (regurgitated)
    Aspiration pneumonia (due to) gastric secretions
    Aspiration pneumonia (due to) milk
    Aspiration pneumonia (due to) vomit
    Code also any associated foreign body in respiratory tract (T17.-)
    EXCLUDES 1   *chemical pneumonitis due to anesthesia (J95.4)*
        obstetric aspiration pneumonitis (O74.0)
    AHA: 2020,2Q,11,28; 2019,3Q,17; 2019,2Q,6,31

  J69.1 Pneumonitis due to inhalation of oils and essences `MCC` `HCC`
    Exogenous lipoid pneumonia
    Lipid pneumonia NOS
    Code first (T51-T65) to identify substance
    EXCLUDES 1   *endogenous lipoid pneumonia (J84.89)*

  J69.8 Pneumonitis due to inhalation of other solids and liquids `MCC` `HCC`
    Pneumonitis due to aspiration of blood
    Pneumonitis due to aspiration of detergent
    Code first (T51-T65) to identify substance

✓4ᵗʰ **J70 Respiratory conditions due to other external agents**

  J70.0 Acute pulmonary manifestations due to radiation `CC` `HCC`
    Radiation pneumonitis
    Use additional code (W88-W90, X39.0-) to identify the external cause

  J70.1 Chronic and other pulmonary manifestations due to radiation `CC` `HCC`
    Fibrosis of lung following radiation
    Use additional code (W88-W90, X39.0-) to identify the external cause

  J70.2 Acute drug-induced interstitial lung disorders `HCC`
    Use additional code for adverse effect, if applicable, to identify drug (T36-T50 with fifth or sixth character 5)
    EXCLUDES 1   *interstitial pneumonia NOS (J84.9)*
        lymphoid interstitial pneumonia (J84.2)
    AHA: 2019,2Q,28

  J70.3 Chronic drug-induced interstitial lung disorders `HCC`
    Use additional code for adverse effect, if applicable, to identify drug (T36-T50 with fifth or sixth character 5)
    EXCLUDES 1   *interstitial pneumonia NOS (J84.9)*
        lymphoid interstitial pneumonia (J84.2)

  J70.4 Drug-induced interstitial lung disorders, unspecified `HCC`
    Use additional code for adverse effect, if applicable, to identify drug (T36-T50 with fifth or sixth character 5)
    EXCLUDES 1   *interstitial pneumonia NOS (J84.9)*
        lymphoid interstitial pneumonia (J84.2)
    AHA: 2019,2Q,28

  J70.5 Respiratory conditions due to smoke inhalation `HCC`
    ~~Smoke inhalation NOS~~
    ▶Code first smoke inhalation (T59.81-)◀
    EXCLUDES 1   ~~*smoke inhalation due to chemicals, gases, fumes and vapors (J68.9)*~~
    EXCLUDES 2   ▶*smoke inhalation (J68.9)* ◀
        vapors (J68.9) ◀
    AHA: 2013,4Q,121

  J70.8 Respiratory conditions due to other specified external agents `HCC`
    Code first (T51-T65) to identify the external agent

  J70.9 Respiratory conditions due to unspecified external agent `HCC`
    Code first (T51-T65) to identify the external agent

Other respiratory diseases principally affecting the interstitium (J80-J84)

J80 Acute respiratory distress syndrome `MCC` `HCC`
    Acute respiratory distress syndrome in adult or child
    Adult hyaline membrane disease
    EXCLUDES 1   *respiratory distress syndrome in newborn (perinatal) (P22.0)*
    AHA: 2020,1Q,34-36; 2017,1Q,26
    DEF: Lung inflammation or injury resulting in a build-up of fluid in the air sacs, preventing the passage of oxygen from the air into the bloodstream.
    TIP: Assign as a secondary code for a patient with acute respiratory distress syndrome (ARDS) due to COVID-19; assign code U07.1 as the principal or first-listed code.

✓4ᵗʰ **J81 Pulmonary edema**
    Use additional code to identify:
    exposure to environmental tobacco smoke (Z77.22)
    history of tobacco dependence (Z87.891)
    occupational exposure to environmental tobacco smoke (Z57.31)
    tobacco dependence (F17.-)
    tobacco use (Z72.0)
    EXCLUDES 1   *chemical (acute) pulmonary edema (J68.1)*
        hypostatic pneumonia (J18.2)
        passive pneumonia (J18.2)
        pulmonary edema due to external agents (J60-J70)
        pulmonary edema with heart disease NOS (I50.1)
        pulmonary edema with heart failure (I50.1)
    DEF: Accumulation of fluid in the air sacs of the lungs, making it difficult to breathe.

  J81.0 Acute pulmonary edema `MCC` `HCC`
    Acute edema of lung

  J81.1 Chronic pulmonary edema `CC`
    Pulmonary congestion (chronic) (passive)
    Pulmonary edema NOS

▲ √4ᵗʰ **J82 Pulmonary eosinophilia, not elsewhere classified**
~~Allergic pneumonia~~
~~Eosinophilic asthma~~
~~Eosinophilic pneumonia~~
~~Löffler's pneumonia~~
~~Tropical (pulmonary) eosinophilia NOS~~
    EXCLUDES 1   ~~pulmonary eosinophilia due to aspergillosis (B44.-)~~
            ~~pulmonary eosinophilia due to drugs (J70.2-J70.4)~~
            ~~pulmonary eosinophilia due to specified parasitic infection~~
               ~~(B50-B83)~~
            ~~pulmonary eosinophilia due to systemic connective tissue~~
               ~~disorders (M30-M36)~~
            ~~pulmonary infiltrate NOS (R91.8)~~
    EXCLUDES 2   ▶pulmonary eosinophilia due to aspergillosis (B44.-) ◀
            ▶pulmonary eosinophilia due to drugs (J70.2-J70.4) ◀
            ▶pulmonary eosinophilia due to specified parasitic infection
               (B50-B83) ◀
            ▶pulmonary eosinophilia due to systemic connective tissue
               disorders (M30-M36) ◀
            ▶pulmonary infiltrate NOS (R91.8) ◀
    DEF: Infiltration of eosinophils (white blood cells of the immune system) into the parenchyma of the lungs, resulting in cough, fever, and dyspnea.

● √5ᵗʰ **J82.8 Pulmonary eosinophilia, not elsewhere classified**
●   **J82.81 Chronic eosinophilic pneumonia**   CC
             Eosinophilic pneumonia, NOS
●   **J82.82 Acute eosinophilic pneumonia**   CC
●   **J82.83 Eosinophilic asthma**   CC
             Code first asthma, by type, such as:
                mild intermittent asthma (J45.2-)
                mild persistent asthma (J45.3-)
                moderate persistent asthma (J45.4-)
                severe persistent asthma (J45.5-)
●   **J82.89 Other pulmonary eosinophilia, not elsewhere classified**   CC
             Allergic pneumonia
             Löffler's pneumonia
             Tropical (pulmonary) eosinophilia NOS

√4ᵗʰ **J84 Other interstitial pulmonary diseases**
    EXCLUDES 1   drug-induced interstitial lung disorders (J70.2-J70.4)
            interstitial emphysema (J98.2)
    EXCLUDES 2   lung diseases due to external agents (J60-J70)
    DEF: Interstitial: Within the small spaces or gaps occurring in tissue or organs.

√5ᵗʰ **J84.0 Alveolar and parieto-alveolar conditions**
      J84.01 Alveolar proteinosis   CC HCC
             DEF: Reduced ventilation due to proteinaceous deposits on alveoli. Symptoms include dyspnea, cough, chest pain, weakness, weight loss, and hemoptysis.
      J84.02 Pulmonary alveolar microlithiasis   CC HCC
      J84.03 *Idiopathic pulmonary hemosiderosis*   CC HCC
             Essential brown induration of lung
             Code first underlying disease, such as:
                disorders of iron metabolism (E83.1-)
             EXCLUDES 1   acute idiopathic pulmonary hemorrhage in infants [AIPHI] (R04.81)
             DEF: Fibrosis of the alveolar walls marked by abnormal accumulation of iron as hemosiderin in the lungs. It primarily affects children and symptoms include anemia, fluid in the lungs, and blood in the sputum. Etiology is unknown.
      J84.09 Other alveolar and parieto-alveolar conditions   CC HCC

√5ᵗʰ **J84.1 Other interstitial pulmonary diseases with fibrosis**
    EXCLUDES 1   pulmonary fibrosis (chronic) due to inhalation of chemicals, gases, fumes or vapors (J68.4)
            pulmonary fibrosis (chronic) following radiation (J70.1)
      J84.10 Pulmonary fibrosis, unspecified   HCC
             Capillary fibrosis of lung
             Cirrhosis of lung (chronic) NOS
             Fibrosis of lung (atrophic) (chronic) (confluent) (massive) (perialveolar) (peribronchial) NOS
             Induration of lung (chronic) NOS
             Postinflammatory pulmonary fibrosis

√6ᵗʰ **J84.11 Idiopathic interstitial pneumonia**
    EXCLUDES 1   lymphoid interstitial pneumonia (J84.2)
            pneumocystis pneumonia (B59)
      J84.111 Idiopathic interstitial pneumonia, not otherwise specified   HCC
      J84.112 Idiopathic pulmonary fibrosis   HCC
             Cryptogenic fibrosing alveolitis
             Idiopathic fibrosing alveolitis
      J84.113 Idiopathic non-specific interstitial pneumonitis   HCC
             EXCLUDES 1   non-specific interstitial pneumonia NOS, or due to known underlying cause (J84.89)
      J84.114 Acute interstitial pneumonitis   CC HCC
             Hamman-Rich syndrome
             EXCLUDES 1   pneumocystis pneumonia (B59)
      J84.115 Respiratory bronchiolitis interstitial lung disease   HCC
      J84.116 Cryptogenic organizing pneumonia   CC HCC
             EXCLUDES 1   organizing pneumonia NOS, or due to known underlying cause (J84.89)
      J84.117 Desquamative interstitial pneumonia   CC HCC

▲ √6ᵗʰ **J84.17 Other interstitial pulmonary diseases with fibrosis in diseases classified elsewhere**
             ~~Interstitial pneumonia (nonspecific) (usual) due to collagen vascular disease~~
             ~~Interstitial pneumonia (nonspecific) (usual) in diseases classified elsewhere~~
             ~~Organizing pneumonia due to collagen vascular disease~~
             ~~Organizing pneumonia in diseases classified elsewhere~~
             ~~Code first underlying disease, such as:~~
                ~~progressive systemic sclerosis (M34.0)~~
                ~~rheumatoid arthritis (M05.00-M06.9)~~
                ~~systemic lupus erythematosis (M32.0-M32.9)~~
●   **J84.170 *Interstitial lung disease with progressive fibrotic phenotype in diseases classified elsewhere***
             Progressive fibrotic interstitial lung disease
             Code first underlying disease, such as:
                lung diseases due to external agents (J60-J70)
                rheumatoid arthritis (M05.00-M06.9)
                sarcoidosis (D86)
                systemic connective tissue disorders (M30-M36)
●   **J84.178 *Other interstitial pulmonary diseases with fibrosis in diseases classified elsewhere***
             Interstitial pneumonia (nonspecific) (usual) due to collagen vascular disease
             Interstitial pneumonia (nonspecific) (usual) in diseases classified elsewhere
             Organizing pneumonia due to collagen vascular disease
             Organizing pneumonia in diseases classified elsewhere
             Code first underlying disease, such as:
                progressive systemic sclerosis (M34.0)
                rheumatoid arthritis (M05.00-M06.9)
                systemic lupus erythematosis (M32.0-M32.9)

J84.2 Lymphoid interstitial pneumonia   CC HCC
        Lymphoid interstitial pneumonitis

√5ᵗʰ **J84.8 Other specified interstitial pulmonary diseases**
    EXCLUDES 1   exogenous lipoid pneumonia (J69.1)
            unspecified lipoid pneumonia (J69.1)
      J84.81 Lymphangioleiomyomatosis   MCC HCC
             Lymphangiomyomatosis
      J84.82 Adult pulmonary Langerhans cell histiocytosis   CC HCC A
             Adult PLCH

J84.83 **Surfactant mutations of the lung** `MCC` `HCC`

DEF: Genetic disorder resulting in insufficient secretion of a complex mixture of phospholipids and proteins that reduce surface tension in the alveoli following the onset of breathing to facilitate lung expansion in the newborn. It is the leading indication for pediatric lung transplantation.

✓6th **J84.84** **Other interstitial lung diseases of** childhood

J84.841 **Neuroendocrine cell hyperplasia of infancy** `MCC` `HCC`

J84.842 **Pulmonary interstitial glycogenosis** `MCC` `HCC`

J84.843 **Alveolar capillary dysplasia with vein misalignment** `MCC` `HCC`

J84.848 **Other interstitial lung diseases of childhood** `MCC` `HCC`

J84.89 **Other specified interstitial pulmonary diseases** `HCC`

Endogenous lipoid pneumonia
Interstitial pneumonitis
Non-specific interstitial pneumonitis NOS
Organizing pneumonia NOS

Code first, if applicable:

poisoning due to drug or toxin (T51-T65 with fifth or sixth character to indicate intent), for toxic pneumonopathy

underlying cause of pneumonopathy, if known

Use additional code, for adverse effect, to identify drug (T36-T50 with fifth or sixth character 5), if drug-induced

EXCLUDES 1 *cryptogenic organizing pneumonia (J84.116)*

idiopathic non-specific interstitial pneumonitis (J84.113)

lymphoid interstitial pneumonia (J84.2)

lipoid pneumonia, exogenous or unspecified (J69.1)

AHA: 2019,2Q,28

J84.9 **Interstitial pulmonary disease, unspecified** `CC` `HCC`

Interstitial pneumonia NOS

Suppurative and necrotic conditions of the lower respiratory tract (J85-J86)

✓4th **J85** **Abscess of lung and mediastinum**

Use additional code (B95-B97) to identify infectious agent

J85.0 **Gangrene and necrosis of lung** `MCC` `HCC`

J85.1 **Abscess of lung with pneumonia** `MCC` `HCC`

Code also the type of pneumonia

J85.2 **Abscess of lung without pneumonia** `MCC` `HCC`

Abscess of lung NOS

J85.3 **Abscess of mediastinum** `MCC` `HCC`

✓4th **J86** **Pyothorax**

Use additional code (B95-B97) to identify infectious agent

EXCLUDES 1 *abscess of lung (J85.-)*

pyothorax due to tuberculosis (A15.6)

DEF: Collection of pus in the pleural space that is commonly caused by an infection that spreads from the lung, such as bacterial pneumonia or a lung abscess.

J86.0 **Pyothorax with fistula** `MCC` `HCC` `SW`

Bronchocutaneous fistula
Bronchopleural fistula
Hepatopleural fistula
Mediastinal fistula
Pleural fistula
Thoracic fistula
Any condition classifiable to J86.9 with fistula

DEF: Purulent infection of the respiratory cavity, with communication from a cavity to another structure.

J86.9 **Pyothorax without fistula** `MCC` `HCC`

Abscess of pleura
Abscess of thorax
Empyema (chest) (lung) (pleura)
Fibrinopurulent pleurisy
Purulent pleurisy
Pyopneumothorax
Septic pleurisy
Seropurulent pleurisy
Suppurative pleurisy

Other diseases of the pleura (J90-J94)

J90 **Pleural effusion, not elsewhere classified** `CC`

Encysted pleurisy
Pleural effusion NOS
Pleurisy with effusion (exudative) (serous)

EXCLUDES 1 *chylous (pleural) effusion (J94.0)*

malignant pleural effusion (J91.0))

pleurisy NOS (R09.1)

tuberculous pleural effusion (A15.6)

DEF: Collection of lymph and other fluid within the pleural space.

✓4th **J91** **Pleural effusion in conditions classified elsewhere**

EXCLUDES 2 *pleural effusion in heart failure (I50.-)*

pleural effusion in systemic lupus erythematosus (M32.13)

DEF: Collection of lymph and other fluid within the pleural space.

J91.0 *Malignant pleural effusion* `CC`

Code first underlying neoplasm

J91.8 *Pleural effusion in other conditions classified elsewhere* `CC`

Code first underlying disease, such as:

filariasis (B74.0-B74.9)
influenza (J09.X2, J10.1, J11.1)

AHA: 2015,2Q,15

TIP: Assign this code as a secondary diagnosis to congestive heart failure (I50.-) only if pleural effusion is specifically evaluated or treated.

Pleural Effusion

✓4th **J92** **Pleural plaque**

`INCLUDES` pleural thickening

DEF: Areas of fibrous thickening that form on the parietal or visceral pleura, the membranes that line the ribs and lungs.

J92.0 **Pleural plaque with presence of asbestos**

J92.9 **Pleural plaque without asbestos**

Pleural plaque NOS

`N` Newborn: 0   `P` Pediatric: 0-17   `M` Maternity: 9-64   `A` Adult: 15-124   `MCC` Major Complication/Comorbidity   `CC` Complication/Comorbidity   `SW` Severe Wound Dx

700   ICD-10-CM 2021

✓4th **J93 Pneumothorax and air leak**

> EXCLUDES 1   congenital or perinatal pneumothorax (P25.1)
> postprocedural air leak (J95.812)
> postprocedural pneumothorax (J95.811)
> pyopneumothorax (J86.-)
> traumatic pneumothorax (S27.0)
> tuberculous (current disease) pneumothorax (A15.-)

> **DEF:** Pneumothorax: Lung displacement due to abnormal leakage of air or gas that is trapped in the pleural space formed by the membrane that encloses the lungs and lines the thoracic cavity.

J93.0 Spontaneous tension pneumothorax   MCC

> **DEF:** Leaking air from the lung into the lining, causing collapse.

✓5th **J93.1 Other spontaneous pneumothorax**

     J93.11 Primary spontaneous pneumothorax   CC

     J93.12 Secondary spontaneous pneumothorax   CC

> Code first underlying condition, such as:
> catamenial pneumothorax due to endometriosis (N80.8)
> cystic fibrosis (E84.-)
> eosinophilic pneumonia (J82)
> lymphangioleiomyomatosis (J84.81)
> malignant neoplasm of bronchus and lung (C34.-)
> Marfan's syndrome (Q87.4)
> pneumonia due to Pneumocystis carinii (B59)
> secondary malignant neoplasm of lung (C78.0-)
> spontaneous rupture of the esophagus (K22.3)

✓5th **J93.8 Other pneumothorax and air leak**

     J93.81 Chronic pneumothorax   CC

     J93.82 Other air leak   CC
> Persistent air leak

     J93.83 Other pneumothorax   CC
> Acute pneumothorax
> Spontaneous pneumothorax NOS

J93.9 Pneumothorax, unspecified   CC
> Pneumothorax NOS

✓4th **J94 Other pleural conditions**

> EXCLUDES 1   pleurisy NOS (R09.1)
> traumatic hemopneumothorax (S27.2)
> traumatic hemothorax (S27.1)
> tuberculous pleural conditions (current disease) (A15.-)

J94.0 Chylous effusion   CC
> Chyliform effusion
> **DEF:** Fluid within the pleural space due to the leaking of lymph contents into the space, usually as a result of thoracic duct damage or injury or mediastinal lymphoma.

J94.1 Fibrothorax
> **DEF:** Fibrosis within the pleural lining of the lungs commonly seen as a stiff layer surrounding the lung typically attributed to traumatic hemothorax or pleural effusion.

J94.2 Hemothorax   CC
> Hemopneumothorax

J94.8 Other specified pleural conditions   CC
> Hydropneumothorax
> Hydrothorax

J94.9 Pleural condition, unspecified

Intraoperative and postprocedural complications and disorders of respiratory system, not elsewhere classified (J95)

✓4th **J95 Intraoperative and postprocedural complications and disorders of respiratory system, not elsewhere classified**

> EXCLUDES 2   aspiration pneumonia (J69.-)
> emphysema (subcutaneous) resulting from a procedure (T81.82)
> hypostatic pneumonia (J18.2)
> pulmonary manifestations due to radiation (J70.0-J70.1)

✓5th **J95.0 Tracheostomy complications**

> **DEF:** Tracheostomy: Formation of a tracheal opening on the neck surface with tube insertion to allow for respiration in cases of obstruction or decreased patency. A tracheostomy may be planned or performed on an emergency basis for temporary or long-term use.

Tracheostomy

Tracheostomy in place

Incision in trachea

Trachea

Tracheostomy tube

     J95.00 Unspecified tracheostomy complication   CC HCC

     J95.01 Hemorrhage from tracheostomy stoma   CC HCC

     J95.02 Infection of tracheostomy stoma   CC HCC
> Use additional code to identify type of infection, such as:
> cellulitis of neck (L03.221)
> sepsis (A40, A41.-)

     J95.03 Malfunction of tracheostomy stoma   CC HCC
> Mechanical complication of tracheostomy stoma
> Obstruction of tracheostomy airway
> Tracheal stenosis due to tracheostomy

     J95.04 Tracheo-esophageal fistula following tracheostomy   CC HCC

     J95.09 Other tracheostomy complication   CC HCC

J95.1 Acute pulmonary insufficiency following thoracic surgery   MCC HCC

> EXCLUDES 2   functional disturbances following cardiac surgery (I97.0, I97.1-)

J95.2 Acute pulmonary insufficiency following nonthoracic surgery   MCC HCC

> EXCLUDES 2   functional disturbances following cardiac surgery (I97.0, I97.1-)

J95.3 Chronic pulmonary insufficiency following surgery   MCC HCC

> EXCLUDES 2   functional disturbances following cardiac surgery (I97.0, I97.1-)

✓ Additional Character Required   ✓7th Placeholder   Unacceptable PDx   Questionable PDx   Manifestation   Unspecified Dx   H1-H14 HAC   HCC CMS-HCC Dx   HIV HIV Dx

ICD-10-CM 2021   701

J95.4　Chemical pneumonitis due to anesthesia　`CC`
　Mendelson's syndrome
　Postprocedural aspiration pneumonia
　Use additional code for adverse effect, if applicable, to identify drug (T41.- with fifth or sixth character 5)
　EXCLUDES 1　aspiration pneumonitis due to anesthesia complicating labor and delivery (O74.0)
　　　　aspiration pneumonitis due to anesthesia complicating pregnancy (O29)
　　　　aspiration pneumonitis due to anesthesia complicating the puerperium (O89.01)

J95.5　Postprocedural subglottic stenosis　`CC`

√5ᵗʰ **J95.6　Intraoperative hemorrhage and hematoma of a respiratory system organ or structure complicating a procedure**
　EXCLUDES 1　intraoperative hemorrhage and hematoma of a respiratory system organ or structure due to accidental puncture and laceration during procedure (J95.7-)

　J95.61　Intraoperative hemorrhage and hematoma of a respiratory system organ or structure complicating a respiratory system procedure　`CC`

　J95.62　Intraoperative hemorrhage and hematoma of a respiratory system organ or structure complicating other procedure　`CC`

√5ᵗʰ **J95.7　Accidental puncture and laceration of a respiratory system organ or structure during a procedure**
　EXCLUDES 2　postprocedural pneumothorax (J95.811)

　J95.71　Accidental puncture and laceration of a respiratory system organ or structure during a respiratory system procedure　`CC`

　J95.72　Accidental puncture and laceration of a respiratory system organ or structure during other procedure　`CC`

√5ᵗʰ **J95.8　Other intraoperative and postprocedural complications and disorders of respiratory system, not elsewhere classified**
　AHA: 2016,4Q,9-10

　√6ᵗʰ **J95.81　Postprocedural pneumothorax and air leak**
　　J95.811　Postprocedural pneumothorax　`CC` `H14`
　　J95.812　Postprocedural air leak　`CC`

　√6ᵗʰ **J95.82　Postprocedural respiratory failure**
　　EXCLUDES 1　respiratory failure in other conditions (J96.-)
　　J95.821　Acute postprocedural respiratory failure　`MCC` `HCC`
　　　Postprocedural respiratory failure NOS
　　J95.822　Acute and chronic postprocedural respiratory failure　`MCC` `HCC`

　√6ᵗʰ **J95.83　Postprocedural hemorrhage of a respiratory system organ or structure following a procedure**
　　J95.830　Postprocedural hemorrhage of a respiratory system organ or structure following a respiratory system procedure　`CC`
　　J95.831　Postprocedural hemorrhage of a respiratory system organ or structure following other procedure　`CC`

　J95.84　Transfusion-related acute lung injury (TRALI)　`CC`
　　DEF: Relatively rare, but serious, pulmonary complication of blood transfusion, with acute respiratory distress, noncardiogenic pulmonary edema, cyanosis, hypoxemia, hypotension, fever, and chills.

　√6ᵗʰ **J95.85　Complication of respirator [ventilator]**
　　J95.850　Mechanical complication of respirator　`CC` `HCC`
　　　EXCLUDES 1　encounter for respirator [ventilator] dependence during power failure (Z99.12)
　　J95.851　Ventilator associated pneumonia　`CC` `HCC`
　　　Ventilator associated pneumonitis
　　　Use additional code to identify the organism, if known (B95.-, B96.-, B97.-)
　　　EXCLUDES 1　ventilator lung in newborn (P27.8)
　　　AHA: 2020,2Q,17; 2017,1Q,25
　　J95.859　Other complication of respirator [ventilator]　`CC` `HCC`

√6ᵗʰ **J95.86　Postprocedural hematoma and seroma of a respiratory system organ or structure following a procedure**
　J95.860　Postprocedural hematoma of a respiratory system organ or structure following a respiratory system procedure　`CC`
　J95.861　Postprocedural hematoma of a respiratory system organ or structure following other procedure　`CC`
　J95.862　Postprocedural seroma of a respiratory system organ or structure following a respiratory system procedure　`CC`
　J95.863　Postprocedural seroma of a respiratory system organ or structure following other procedure　`CC`

J95.88　Other intraoperative complications of respiratory system, not elsewhere classified　`CC`

J95.89　Other postprocedural complications and disorders of respiratory system, not elsewhere classified　`CC`
　Use additional code to identify disorder, such as:
　　aspiration pneumonia (J69.-)
　　bacterial or viral pneumonia (J12-J18)
　EXCLUDES 2　acute pulmonary insufficiency following thoracic surgery (J95.1)
　　　　postprocedural subglottic stenosis (J95.5)

Other diseases of the respiratory system (J96-J99)

√4ᵗʰ **J96　Respiratory failure, not elsewhere classified**
　EXCLUDES 1　acute respiratory distress syndrome (J80)
　　　　cardiorespiratory failure (R09.2)
　　　　newborn respiratory distress syndrome (P22.0)
　　　　postprocedural respiratory failure (J95.82-)
　　　　respiratory arrest (R09.2)
　　　　respiratory arrest of newborn (P28.81)
　　　　respiratory failure of newborn (P28.5)

　√5ᵗʰ **J96.0　Acute respiratory failure**
　　J96.00　Acute respiratory failure, unspecified whether with hypoxia or hypercapnia　`MCC` `HCC`
　　　AHA: 2016,3Q,14; 2013,4Q,121
　　J96.01　Acute respiratory failure with hypoxia　`MCC` `HCC`
　　J96.02　Acute respiratory failure with hypercapnia　`MCC` `HCC`

　√5ᵗʰ **J96.1　Chronic respiratory failure**
　　J96.10　Chronic respiratory failure, unspecified whether with hypoxia or hypercapnia　`CC` `HCC`
　　　AHA: 2016,1Q,38; 2015,1Q,21
　　J96.11　Chronic respiratory failure with hypoxia　`CC` `HCC`
　　　AHA: 2013,4Q,129
　　J96.12　Chronic respiratory failure with hypercapnia　`CC` `HCC`

　√5ᵗʰ **J96.2　Acute and chronic respiratory failure**
　　Acute on chronic respiratory failure
　　J96.20　Acute and chronic respiratory failure, unspecified whether with hypoxia or hypercapnia　`MCC` `HCC`
　　J96.21　Acute and chronic respiratory failure with hypoxia　`MCC` `HCC`
　　J96.22　Acute and chronic respiratory failure with hypercapnia　`MCC` `HCC`

　√5ᵗʰ **J96.9　Respiratory failure, unspecified**
　　J96.90　Respiratory failure, unspecified, unspecified whether with hypoxia or hypercapnia　`MCC` `HCC`
　　J96.91　Respiratory failure, unspecified with hypoxia　`MCC` `HCC`
　　J96.92　Respiratory failure, unspecified with hypercapnia　`MCC` `HCC`

☑4ᵗʰ **J98 Other respiratory disorders**

Use additional code to identify:

exposure to environmental tobacco smoke (Z77.22)

exposure to tobacco smoke in the perinatal period (P96.81)

history of tobacco dependence (Z87.891)

occupational exposure to environmental tobacco smoke (Z57.31)

tobacco dependence (F17.-)

tobacco use (Z72.0)

     EXCLUDES 1   newborn apnea (P28.4)

                 newborn sleep apnea (P28.3)

     EXCLUDES 2   apnea NOS (R06.81)

                 sleep apnea (G47.3-)

☑5ᵗʰ **J98.0 Diseases of bronchus, not elsewhere classified**

     J98.01 Acute bronchospasm

         EXCLUDES 1   acute bronchiolitis with bronchospasm
                       (J21.-)

                       acute bronchitis with bronchospasm
                       (J20.-)

                       asthma (J45.-)

                       exercise induced bronchospasm (J45.990)

     J98.09 Other diseases of bronchus, not elsewhere classified

Broncholithiasis

Calcification of bronchus

Stenosis of bronchus

Tracheobronchial collapse

Tracheobronchial dyskinesia

Ulcer of bronchus

☑5ᵗʰ **J98.1 Pulmonary collapse**

     EXCLUDES 1   therapeutic collapse of lung status (Z98.3)

     J98.11 Atelectasis   CC

         EXCLUDES 1   newborn atelectasis

                       tuberculous atelectasis (current disease)
                       (A15)

         DEF: Collapse of lung tissue affecting part or all of one lung, preventing normal oxygen absorption to healthy tissues.

     J98.19 Other pulmonary collapse   CC

J98.2 Interstitial emphysema   HCC

Mediastinal emphysema

     EXCLUDES 1   emphysema NOS (J43.9)

                 emphysema in newborn (P25.0)

                 surgical emphysema (subcutaneous) (T81.82)

                 traumatic subcutaneous emphysema (T79.7)

J98.3 Compensatory emphysema   HCC

     DEF: Distention of all or part of the lung caused by disease processes or surgical intervention that decreased volume in another part of the lung, causing an overcompensation reaction. Compensatory emphysema occurs in association with pneumonias, pleural effusions, atelectasis, empyema, and pneumothorax.

J98.4 Other disorders of lung

Calcification of lung

Cystic lung disease (acquired)

Lung disease NOS

Pulmolithiasis

     EXCLUDES 1   acute interstitial pneumonitis (J84.114)

                 pulmonary insufficiency following surgery
                 (J95.1-J95.2)

☑5ᵗʰ **J98.5 Diseases of mediastinum, not elsewhere classified**

     EXCLUDES 2   abscess of mediastinum (J85.3)

     AHA: 2016,4Q,29

     J98.51 Mediastinitis   MCC   H8

         Code first underlying condition, if applicable, such as postoperative mediastinitis (T81.-)

     J98.59 Other diseases of mediastinum, not elsewhere classified   MCC   H8

Fibrosis of mediastinum

Hernia of mediastinum

Retraction of mediastinum

J98.6 Disorders of diaphragm

Diaphragmatitis

Paralysis of diaphragm

Relaxation of diaphragm

     EXCLUDES 1   congenital malformation of diaphragm NEC (Q79.1)

                 congenital diaphragmatic hernia (Q79.0)

     EXCLUDES 2   diaphragmatic hernia (K44.-)

J98.8 Other specified respiratory disorders

     AHA: 2020,1Q,34-36

     TIP: Assign as a secondary code for a patient with a respiratory infection that is not further specified but is documented as being associated with COVID-19; assign U07.1 as the principal or first-listed code. If the respiratory infection documentation specifies acute or lower respiratory infection (NOS), assign J22 instead.

J98.9 Respiratory disorder, unspecified

Respiratory disease (chronic) NOS

J99   *Respiratory disorders in diseases classified elsewhere*   HCC

Code first underlying disease, such as:

amyloidosis (E85.-)

ankylosing spondylitis (M45)

congenital syphilis (A50.5)

cryoglobulinemia (D89.1)

early congenital syphilis (A50.0)

plasminogen deficiency (E88.02)

schistosomiasis (B65.0-B65.9)

     EXCLUDES 1   respiratory disorders in:

                 amebiasis (A06.5)

                 blastomycosis (B40.0-B40.2)

                 candidiasis (B37.1)

                 coccidioidomycosis (B38.0-B38.2)

                 cystic fibrosis with pulmonary manifestations (E84.0)

                 dermatomyositis (M33.01, M33.11)

                 histoplasmosis (B39.0-B39.2)

                 late syphilis (A52.72, A52.73)

                 polymyositis (M33.21)

                 sicca syndrome (M35.02)

                 systemic lupus erythematosus (M32.13)

                 systemic sclerosis (M34.81)

                 Wegener's granulomatosis (M31.30-M31.31)

☑ Additional Character Required   x7ᵗʰ Placeholder   Unacceptable PDx   Questionable PDx   Manifestation   Unspecified Dx   H1-H14 HAC   HCC CMS-HCC Dx   HIV HIV Dx

ICD-10-CM 2021   703

Chapter 11. Diseases of the Digestive System (KØØ–K95)

Chapter-specific Guidelines with Coding Examples
Reserved for future guideline expansion.

Chapter 11. Diseases of the Digestive System

Chapter 11. Diseases of the Digestive System (K00-K95)

> EXCLUDES 2   certain conditions originating in the perinatal period (P04-P96)
> certain infectious and parasitic diseases (A00-B99)
> complications of pregnancy, childbirth and the puerperium (O00-O9A)
> congenital malformations, deformations and chromosomal abnormalities (Q00-Q99)
> endocrine, nutritional and metabolic diseases (E00-E88)
> injury, poisoning and certain other consequences of external causes (S00-T88)
> neoplasms (C00-D49)
> symptoms, signs and abnormal clinical and laboratory findings, not elsewhere classified (R00-R94)

This chapter contains the following blocks:

K00-K14   Diseases of oral cavity and salivary glands
K20-K31   Diseases of esophagus, stomach and duodenum
K35-K38   Diseases of appendix
K40-K46   Hernia
K50-K52   Noninfective enteritis and colitis
K55-K64   Other diseases of intestines
K65-K68   Diseases of peritoneum and retroperitoneum
K70-K77   Diseases of liver
K80-K87   Disorders of gallbladder, biliary tract and pancreas
K90-K95   Other diseases of the digestive system

Diseases of oral cavity and salivary glands (K00-K14)

✓4ᵗʰ **K00   Disorders of tooth development and eruption**

> EXCLUDES 2   embedded and impacted teeth (K01.-)

K00.0   Anodontia
Hypodontia
Oligodontia
> EXCLUDES 1   acquired absence of teeth (K08.1-)

DEF: Partial or complete absence of teeth due to a congenital defect involving the tooth bud.

K00.1   Supernumerary teeth
Distomolar
Fourth molar
Mesiodens
Paramolar
Supplementary teeth
> EXCLUDES 2   supernumerary roots (K00.2)

K00.2   Abnormalities of size and form of teeth
Concrescence of teeth
Fusion of teeth
Gemination of teeth
Dens evaginatus
Dens in dente
Dens invaginatus
Enamel pearls
Macrodontia
Microdontia
Peg-shaped [conical] teeth
Supernumerary roots
Taurodontism
Tuberculum paramolare
> EXCLUDES 1   abnormalities of teeth due to congenital syphilis (A50.5)
> tuberculum Carabelli, which is regarded as a normal variation and should not be coded

K00.3   Mottled teeth
Dental fluorosis
Mottling of enamel
Nonfluoride enamel opacities
> EXCLUDES 2   deposits [accretions] on teeth (K03.6)

K00.4   Disturbances in tooth formation
Aplasia and hypoplasia of cementum
Dilaceration of tooth
Enamel hypoplasia (neonatal) (postnatal) (prenatal)
Regional odontodysplasia
Turner's tooth
> EXCLUDES 1   Hutchinson's teeth and mulberry molars in congenital syphilis (A50.5)
> EXCLUDES 2   mottled teeth (K00.3)

K00.5   Hereditary disturbances in tooth structure, not elsewhere classified
Amelogenesis imperfecta
Dentinogenesis imperfecta
Odontogenesis imperfecta
Dentinal dysplasia
Shell teeth

K00.6   Disturbances in tooth eruption
Dentia praecox
Natal tooth
Neonatal tooth
Premature eruption of tooth
Premature shedding of primary [deciduous] tooth
Prenatal teeth
Retained [persistent] primary tooth
> EXCLUDES 2   embedded and impacted teeth (K01.-)

K00.7   Teething syndrome

K00.8   Other disorders of tooth development
Color changes during tooth formation
Intrinsic staining of teeth NOS
> EXCLUDES 2   posteruptive color changes (K03.7)

K00.9   Disorder of tooth development, unspecified
Disorder of odontogenesis NOS

✓4ᵗʰ **K01   Embedded and impacted teeth**
> EXCLUDES 1   abnormal position of fully erupted teeth (M26.3-)

K01.0   Embedded teeth

K01.1   Impacted teeth

✓4ᵗʰ **K02   Dental caries**
> INCLUDES   caries of dentine
> dental cavities
> early childhood caries
> pre-eruptive caries
> recurrent caries (dentino enamel junction) (enamel) (to the pulp)
> tooth decay

DEF: Localized section of tooth decay that begins on the tooth surface with destruction of the calcified enamel, allowing bacterial destruction to continue and form cavities and may extend to the dentin and pulp.

Tooth Anatomy

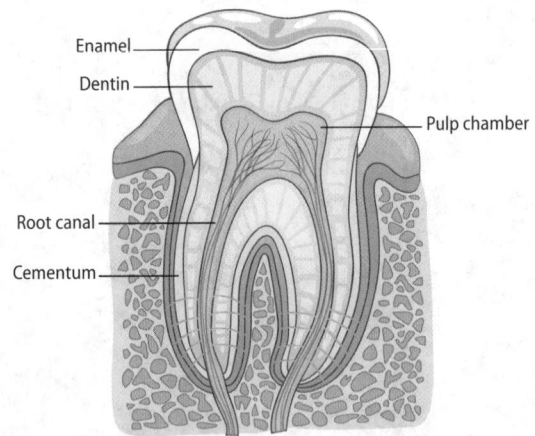

Enamel
Dentin
Pulp chamber
Root canal
Cementum

K02.3   Arrested dental caries
Arrested coronal and root caries

✓5ᵗʰ **K02.5   Dental caries on pit and fissure surface**
Dental caries on chewing surface of tooth

K02.51   Dental caries on pit and fissure surface limited to enamel
White spot lesions [initial caries] on pit and fissure surface of tooth

K02.52   Dental caries on pit and fissure surface penetrating into dentin
Primary dental caries, cervical origin

K02.53   Dental caries on pit and fissure surface penetrating into pulp

Ⓝ Newborn: 0   Ⓟ Pediatric: 0-17   Ⓜ Maternity: 9-64   Ⓐ Adult: 15-124   ᴹᶜᶜ Major Complication/Comorbidity   ᶜᶜ Complication/Comorbidity   ˢʷ Severe Wound Dx

706   ICD-10-CM 2021

K00–K02.53

✓5ᵗʰ **K02.6 Dental caries on** smooth surface

     K02.61 Dental caries on smooth surface limited to enamel
        White spot lesions [initial caries] on smooth surface of tooth

     K02.62 Dental caries on smooth surface penetrating into dentin

     K02.63 Dental caries on smooth surface penetrating into pulp

K02.7 Dental root **caries**

K02.9 Dental caries, unspecified

✓4ᵗʰ **K03 Other diseases of hard tissues of teeth**

     EXCLUDES 2   *bruxism (F45.8)*
                 dental caries (K02.-)
                 teeth-grinding NOS (F45.8)

K03.0 Excessive attrition of teeth
     Approximal wear of teeth
     Occlusal wear of teeth
     DEF: Attrition: In dentistry, wearing away or erosion of tooth surface from abrasive food or grinding teeth.

K03.1 Abrasion of teeth
     Dentifrice abrasion of teeth
     Habitual abrasion of teeth
     Occupational abrasion of teeth
     Ritual abrasion of teeth
     Traditional abrasion of teeth
     Wedge defect NOS

K03.2 Erosion of teeth
     Erosion of teeth due to diet
     Erosion of teeth due to drugs and medicaments
     Erosion of teeth due to persistent vomiting
     Erosion of teeth NOS
     Idiopathic erosion of teeth
     Occupational erosion of teeth

K03.3 Pathological resorption of teeth
     Internal granuloma of pulp
     Resorption of teeth (external)

K03.4 Hypercementosis
     Cementation hyperplasia

K03.5 Ankylosis of teeth

K03.6 Deposits [accretions] on teeth
     Betel deposits [accretions] on teeth
     Black deposits [accretions] on teeth
     Extrinsic staining of teeth NOS
     Green deposits [accretions] on teeth
     Materia alba deposits [accretions] on teeth
     Orange deposits [accretions] on teeth
     Staining of teeth NOS
     Subgingival dental calculus
     Supragingival dental calculus
     Tobacco deposits [accretions] on teeth

K03.7 Posteruptive color changes of dental hard tissues
     EXCLUDES 2   *deposits [accretions] on teeth (K03.6)*

✓5ᵗʰ **K03.8 Other specified diseases of hard tissues of teeth**

     K03.81 Cracked tooth
        EXCLUDES 1   *asymptomatic craze lines in enamel - omit code*
                broken or fractured tooth due to trauma (S02.5)

     K03.89 Other specified diseases of hard tissues of teeth

K03.9 Disease of hard tissues of teeth, unspecified

✓4ᵗʰ **K04 Diseases of pulp and periapical tissues**
     AHA: 2016,4Q,29-30

✓5ᵗʰ **K04.0 Pulpitis**
     Acute pulpitis
     Chronic (hyperplastic) (ulcerative) pulpitis

     K04.01 Reversible pulpitis   cc

     K04.02 Irreversible pulpitis   cc

K04.1 Necrosis of pulp
     Pulpal gangrene

K04.2 Pulp degeneration
     Denticles
     Pulpal calcifications
     Pulpal stones

K04.3 Abnormal hard tissue formation in pulp
     Secondary or irregular dentine

K04.4 Acute apical periodontitis of pulpal origin   cc
     Acute apical periodontitis NOS
     EXCLUDES 1   *acute periodontitis (K05.2-)*
     DEF: Severe inflammation of the area surrounding the tip of a tooth's root that is often secondary to infection or trauma.

K04.5 Chronic apical periodontitis
     Apical or periapical granuloma
     Apical periodontitis NOS
     EXCLUDES 1   *chronic periodontitis (K05.3-)*

K04.6 Periapical abscess with sinus   sw
     Dental abscess with sinus
     Dentoalveolar abscess with sinus

K04.7 Periapical abscess without sinus
     Dental abscess without sinus
     Dentoalveolar abscess without sinus

K04.8 Radicular cyst
     Apical (periodontal) cyst
     Periapical cyst
     Residual radicular cyst
     EXCLUDES 2   *lateral periodontal cyst (K09.0)*
     DEF: Most common odontogenic cyst in tissue around the tooth apex due to chronic inflammation of dental pulp.

✓5ᵗʰ **K04.9 Other and unspecified diseases of pulp and periapical tissues**

     K04.90 Unspecified diseases of pulp and periapical tissues
     K04.99 Other diseases of pulp and periapical tissues

✓4ᵗʰ **K05 Gingivitis and periodontal diseases**
     Use additional code to identify:
     alcohol abuse and dependence (F10.-)
     exposure to environmental tobacco smoke (Z77.22)
     exposure to tobacco smoke in the perinatal period (P96.81)
     history of tobacco dependence (Z87.891)
     occupational exposure to environmental tobacco smoke (Z57.31)
     tobacco dependence (F17.-)
     tobacco use (Z72.0)
     AHA: 2016,4Q,29-30

✓5ᵗʰ **K05.0 Acute gingivitis**
     EXCLUDES 1   *acute necrotizing ulcerative gingivitis (A69.1)*
                 herpesviral [herpes simplex] gingivostomatitis (B00.2)

     K05.00 Acute gingivitis, plaque induced
        Acute gingivitis NOS
        Plaque induced gingival disease

     K05.01 Acute gingivitis, non-plaque induced

✓5ᵗʰ **K05.1 Chronic gingivitis**

     Desquamative gingivitis (chronic)
     Gingivitis (chronic) NOS
     Hyperplastic gingivitis (chronic)
     Pregnancy associated gingivitis
     Simple marginal gingivitis (chronic)
     Ulcerative gingivitis (chronic)
     Code first, if applicable, diseases of the digestive system complicating pregnacy (O99.61-)

     K05.10 Chronic gingivitis, plaque induced
        Chronic gingivitis NOS
        Gingivitis NOS

     K05.11 Chronic gingivitis, non-plaque induced

✓5ᵗʰ **K05.2 Aggressive periodontitis**

     Acute pericoronitis
     EXCLUDES 1   *acute apical periodontitis (K04.4)*
                 periapical abscess (K04.7)
                 periapical abscess with sinus (K04.6)

     K05.20 Aggressive periodontitis, unspecified

✓6ᵗʰ **K05.21 Aggressive periodontitis,** localized
        Periodontal abscess

        K05.211 Aggressive periodontitis, localized, slight
        K05.212 Aggressive periodontitis, localized, moderate
        K05.213 Aggressive periodontitis, localized, severe
        K05.219 Aggressive periodontitis, localized, unspecified severity

✓6ᵗʰ **K05.22 Aggressive periodontitis,** generalized
        K05.221 Aggressive periodontitis, generalized, slight
        K05.222 Aggressive periodontitis, generalized, moderate
        K05.223 Aggressive periodontitis, generalized, severe

K05.229 Aggressive periodontitis, generalized, unspecified severity

√5ᵗʰ **K05.3 Chronic periodontitis**

Chronic pericoronitis
Complex periodontitis
Periodontitis NOS
Simplex periodontitis
EXCLUDES 1   chronic apical periodontitis (K04.5)

K05.30 Chronic periodontitis, unspecified

√6ᵗʰ **K05.31 Chronic periodontitis, localized**

K05.311 Chronic periodontitis, localized, slight
K05.312 Chronic periodontitis, localized, moderate
K05.313 Chronic periodontitis, localized, severe
K05.319 Chronic periodontitis, localized, unspecified severity

√6ᵗʰ **K05.32 Chronic periodontitis, generalized**

K05.321 Chronic periodontitis, generalized, slight
K05.322 Chronic periodontitis, generalized, moderate
K05.323 Chronic periodontitis, generalized, severe
K05.329 Chronic periodontitis, generalized, unspecified

K05.4 Periodontosis

Juvenile periodontosis

K05.5 Other periodontal diseases

Combined periodontic-endodontic lesion
Narrow gingival width (of periodontal soft tissue)
EXCLUDES 2   leukoplakia of gingiva (K13.21)

K05.6 Periodontal disease, unspecified

√4ᵗʰ **K06 Other disorders of gingiva and edentulous alveolar ridge**

EXCLUDES 2   acute gingivitis (K05.0)
atrophy of edentulous alveolar ridge (K08.2)
chronic gingivitis (K05.1)
gingivitis NOS (K05.1)
AHA: 2016,4Q,29-30

√5ᵗʰ **K06.0 Gingival recession**

Gingival recession (postinfective) (postprocedural)
AHA: 2017,4Q,16

√6ᵗʰ **K06.01 Gingival recession, localized**

K06.010 Localized gingival recession, unspecified
Localized gingival recession, NOS
K06.011 Localized gingival recession, minimal
K06.012 Localized gingival recession, moderate
K06.013 Localized gingival recession, severe

√6ᵗʰ **K06.02 Gingival recession, generalized**

K06.020 Generalized gingival recession, unspecified
Generalized gingival recession, NOS
K06.021 Generalized gingival recession, minimal
K06.022 Generalized gingival recession, moderate
K06.023 Generalized gingival recession, severe

K06.1 Gingival enlargement

Gingival fibromatosis

K06.2 Gingival and edentulous alveolar ridge lesions associated with trauma

Irritative hyperplasia of edentulous ridge [denture hyperplasia]
Use additional code (Chapter 20) to identify external cause or denture status (Z97.2)

K06.3 Horizontal alveolar bone loss

K06.8 Other specified disorders of gingiva and edentulous alveolar ridge

Fibrous epulis
Flabby alveolar ridge
Giant cell epulis
Peripheral giant cell granuloma of gingiva
Pyogenic granuloma of gingiva
Vertical ridge deficiency
EXCLUDES 2   gingival cyst (K09.0)

K06.9 Disorder of gingiva and edentulous alveolar ridge, unspecified

√4ᵗʰ **K08 Other disorders of teeth and supporting structures**

EXCLUDES 2   dentofacial anomalies [including malocclusion] (M26.-)
disorders of jaw (M27.-)
AHA: 2016,4Q,29-30

K08.0 Exfoliation of teeth due to systemic causes

Code also underlying systemic condition

√5ᵗʰ **K08.1 Complete loss of teeth**

Acquired loss of teeth, complete
EXCLUDES 1   congenital absence of teeth (K00.0)
exfoliation of teeth due to systemic causes (K08.0)
partial loss of teeth (K08.4-)
DEF: Loss of all teeth as a result of caries, trauma, extraction, periodontal disease, or other specified or unspecified causes.
Synonym(s): complete edentulism

√6ᵗʰ **K08.10 Complete loss of teeth, unspecified cause**

K08.101 Complete loss of teeth, unspecified cause, class I
K08.102 Complete loss of teeth, unspecified cause, class II
K08.103 Complete loss of teeth, unspecified cause, class III
K08.104 Complete loss of teeth, unspecified cause, class IV
K08.109 Complete loss of teeth, unspecified cause, unspecified class
Edentulism NOS

√6ᵗʰ **K08.11 Complete loss of teeth due to trauma**

K08.111 Complete loss of teeth due to trauma, class I
K08.112 Complete loss of teeth due to trauma, class II
K08.113 Complete loss of teeth due to trauma, class III
K08.114 Complete loss of teeth due to trauma, class IV
K08.119 Complete loss of teeth due to trauma, unspecified class

√6ᵗʰ **K08.12 Complete loss of teeth due to periodontal diseases**

K08.121 Complete loss of teeth due to periodontal diseases, class I
K08.122 Complete loss of teeth due to periodontal diseases, class II
K08.123 Complete loss of teeth due to periodontal diseases, class III
K08.124 Complete loss of teeth due to periodontal diseases, class IV
K08.129 Complete loss of teeth due to periodontal diseases, unspecified class

√6ᵗʰ **K08.13 Complete loss of teeth due to caries**

K08.131 Complete loss of teeth due to caries, class I
K08.132 Complete loss of teeth due to caries, class II
K08.133 Complete loss of teeth due to caries, class III
K08.134 Complete loss of teeth due to caries, class IV
K08.139 Complete loss of teeth due to caries, unspecified class

√6ᵗʰ **K08.19 Complete loss of teeth due to other specified cause**

K08.191 Complete loss of teeth due to other specified cause, class I
K08.192 Complete loss of teeth due to other specified cause, class II
K08.193 Complete loss of teeth due to other specified cause, class III
K08.194 Complete loss of teeth due to other specified cause, class IV
K08.199 Complete loss of teeth due to other specified cause, unspecified class

√5ᵗʰ **K08.2 Atrophy of edentulous alveolar ridge**

K08.20 Unspecified atrophy of edentulous alveolar ridge
Atrophy of the mandible NOS
Atrophy of the maxilla NOS
K08.21 Minimal atrophy of the mandible
Minimal atrophy of the edentulous mandible
K08.22 Moderate atrophy of the mandible
Moderate atrophy of the edentulous mandible

K08.23   Severe **atrophy of the** mandible
Severe atrophy of the edentulous mandible

K08.24   Minimal **atrophy of** maxilla
Minimal atrophy of the edentulous maxilla

K08.25   Moderate **atrophy of the** maxilla
Moderate atrophy of the edentulous maxilla

K08.26   Severe **atrophy of the** maxilla
Severe atrophy of the edentulous maxilla

K08.3   **Retained dental root**

✓5ᵗʰ **K08.4**   **Partial loss of teeth**
Acquired loss of teeth, partial
EXCLUDES 1   *complete loss of teeth (K08.1-)*
congenital absence of teeth (K00.0)
EXCLUDES 2   *exfoliation of teeth due to systemic causes (K08.0)*

✓6ᵗʰ **K08.40**   **Partial loss of teeth, unspecified cause**

K08.401   **Partial loss of teeth, unspecified cause, class I**

K08.402   **Partial loss of teeth, unspecified cause, class II**

K08.403   **Partial loss of teeth, unspecified cause, class III**

K08.404   **Partial loss of teeth, unspecified cause, class IV**

K08.409   **Partial loss of teeth, unspecified cause, unspecified class**
Tooth extraction status NOS

✓6ᵗʰ **K08.41**   **Partial loss of teeth due to** trauma

K08.411   **Partial loss of teeth due to trauma, class I**

K08.412   **Partial loss of teeth due to trauma, class II**

K08.413   **Partial loss of teeth due to trauma, class III**

K08.414   **Partial loss of teeth due to trauma, class IV**

K08.419   **Partial loss of teeth due to trauma, unspecified class**

✓6ᵗʰ **K08.42**   **Partial loss of teeth due to** periodontal diseases

K08.421   **Partial loss of teeth due to periodontal diseases, class I**

K08.422   **Partial loss of teeth due to periodontal diseases, class II**

K08.423   **Partial loss of teeth due to periodontal diseases, class III**

K08.424   **Partial loss of teeth due to periodontal diseases, class IV**

K08.429   **Partial loss of teeth due to periodontal diseases, unspecified class**

✓6ᵗʰ **K08.43**   **Partial loss of teeth due to** caries

K08.431   **Partial loss of teeth due to caries, class I**
K08.432   **Partial loss of teeth due to caries, class II**
K08.433   **Partial loss of teeth due to caries, class III**
K08.434   **Partial loss of teeth due to caries, class IV**
K08.439   **Partial loss of teeth due to caries, unspecified class**

✓6ᵗʰ **K08.49**   **Partial loss of teeth due to other specified cause**

K08.491   **Partial loss of teeth due to other specified cause, class I**

K08.492   **Partial loss of teeth due to other specified cause, class II**

K08.493   **Partial loss of teeth due to other specified cause, class III**

K08.494   **Partial loss of teeth due to other specified cause, class IV**

K08.499   **Partial loss of teeth due to other specified cause, unspecified class**

✓5ᵗʰ **K08.5**   **Unsatisfactory restoration of tooth**
Defective bridge, crown, filling
Defective dental restoration
EXCLUDES 1   *dental restoration status (Z98.811)*
EXCLUDES 2   *endosseous dental implant failure (M27.6-)*
unsatisfactory endodontic treatment (M27.5-)

K08.50   **Unsatisfactory restoration of tooth, unspecified**
Defective dental restoration NOS

K08.51   Open **restoration margins of tooth**
Dental restoration failure of marginal integrity
Open margin on tooth restoration
Poor gingival margin to tooth restoration

K08.52   **Unrepairable overhanging of dental restorative materials**
Overhanging of tooth restoration

✓6ᵗʰ **K08.53**   **Fractured dental restorative material**
EXCLUDES 1   *cracked tooth (K03.81)*
traumatic fracture of tooth (S02.5)

K08.530   **Fractured dental restorative material without loss of material**

K08.531   **Fractured dental restorative material with loss of material**

K08.539   **Fractured dental restorative material, unspecified**

K08.54   **Contour of existing restoration of tooth biologically incompatible with oral health**
Dental restoration failure of periodontal anatomical integrity
Unacceptable contours of existing restoration of tooth
Unacceptable morphology of existing restoration of tooth

K08.55   **Allergy to existing dental restorative material**
Use additional code to identify the specific type of allergy

K08.56   **Poor aesthetic of existing restoration of tooth**
Dental restoration aesthetically inadequate or displeasing

K08.59   **Other unsatisfactory restoration of tooth**
Other defective dental restoration

✓5ᵗʰ **K08.8**   **Other specified disorders of teeth and supporting structures**

K08.81   **Primary occlusal trauma**
K08.82   **Secondary occlusal trauma**
K08.89   **Other specified disorders of teeth and supporting structures**
Enlargement of alveolar ridge NOS
Insufficient anatomic crown height
Insufficient clinical crown length
Irregular alveolar process
Toothache NOS

K08.9   **Disorder of teeth and supporting structures, unspecified**

✓4ᵗʰ **K09**   **Cysts of oral region, not elsewhere classified**
INCLUDES   lesions showing histological features both of aneurysmal cyst and of another fibro-osseous lesion
EXCLUDES 2   *cysts of jaw (M27.0-, M27.4-)*
radicular cyst (K04.8)

K09.0   **Developmental odontogenic cysts**
Dentigerous cyst
Eruption cyst
Follicular cyst
Gingival cyst
Lateral periodontal cyst
Primordial cyst
EXCLUDES 2   *keratocysts (D16.4, D16.5)*
odontogenic keratocystic tumors (D16.4, D16.5)

K09.1   **Developmental (nonodontogenic) cysts of oral region**
Cyst (of) incisive canal
Cyst (of) palatine of papilla
Globulomaxillary cyst
Median palatal cyst
Nasoalveolar cyst
Nasolabial cyst
Nasopalatine duct cyst

K09.8   **Other cysts of oral region, not elsewhere classified**
Dermoid cyst
Epidermoid cyst
Lymphoepithelial cyst
Epstein's pearl

K09.9   **Cyst of oral region, unspecified**

✓4ᵗʰ **K11**   **Diseases of salivary glands**
Use additional code to identify:
alcohol abuse and dependence (F10.-)
exposure to environmental tobacco smoke (Z77.22)
exposure to tobacco smoke in the perinatal period (P96.81)
history of tobacco dependence (Z87.891)
occupational exposure to environmental tobacco smoke (Z57.31)
tobacco dependence (F17.-)
tobacco use (Z72.0)

K11.0   **Atrophy of salivary gland**

K11.1 **Hypertrophy** of salivary gland
  DEF: Overgrowth of or enlarged salivary gland tissue caused by infection, salivary duct blockage, autoimmune diseases, and benign and malignant tumors.

√5ᵗʰ **K11.2** **Sialoadenitis**
  Parotitis
    EXCLUDES 1   *epidemic parotitis (B26.-)*
          mumps (B26.-)
          uveoparotid fever [Heerfordt] (D86.89)
  DEF: Inflammation of the salivary gland.
  K11.20 **Sialoadenitis, unspecified**
  K11.21 **Acute sialoadenitis**
        EXCLUDES 1   *acute recurrent sialoadenitis (K11.22)*
  K11.22 **Acute recurrent sialoadenitis**
  K11.23 **Chronic sialoadenitis**

K11.3 **Abscess** of salivary gland   CC

K11.4 **Fistula** of salivary gland   CC SW
    EXCLUDES 1   *congenital fistula of salivary gland (Q38.4)*

K11.5 **Sialolithiasis**
  Calculus of salivary gland or duct
  Stone of salivary gland or duct

K11.6 **Mucocele** of salivary gland
  Mucous extravasation cyst of salivary gland
  Mucous retention cyst of salivary gland
  Ranula

K11.7 **Disturbances of salivary** secretion
  Hypoptyalism
  Ptyalism
  Xerostomia
    EXCLUDES 2   *dry mouth NOS (R68.2)*

K11.8 **Other diseases of salivary glands**
  Benign lymphoepithelial lesion of salivary gland
  Mikulicz' disease
  Necrotizing sialometaplasia
  Sialectasia
  Stenosis of salivary duct
  Stricture of salivary duct
    EXCLUDES 1   *sicca syndrome [Sjögren] (M35.0-)*

K11.9 **Disease of salivary gland, unspecified**
  Sialoadenopathy NOS

√4ᵗʰ **K12** **Stomatitis and related lesions**
  Use additional code to identify:
    alcohol abuse and dependence (F10.-)
    exposure to environmental tobacco smoke (Z77.22)
    exposure to tobacco smoke in the perinatal period (P96.81)
    history of tobacco dependence (Z87.891)
    occupational exposure to environmental tobacco smoke (Z57.31)
    tobacco dependence (F17.-)
    tobacco use (Z72.0)
    EXCLUDES 1   *cancrum oris (A69.0)*
          cheilitis (K13.0)
          gangrenous stomatitis (A69.0)
          herpesviral [herpes simplex] gingivostomatitis (B00.2)
          noma (A69.0)

K12.0 **Recurrent oral aphthae**
  Aphthous stomatitis (major) (minor)
  Bednar's aphthae
  Periadenitis mucosa necrotica recurrens
  Recurrent aphthous ulcer
  Stomatitis herpetiformis
  DEF: Disorder of unknown etiology with small oval or round painful ulcers of the mouth marked by a grayish exudate and a red halo effect.

K12.1 **Other forms of stomatitis**
  Stomatitis NOS
  Denture stomatitis
  Ulcerative stomatitis
  Vesicular stomatitis
    EXCLUDES 1   *acute necrotizing ulcerative stomatitis (A69.1)*
          Vincent's stomatitis (A69.1)

K12.2 **Cellulitis and abscess of mouth**   CC
  Cellulitis of mouth (floor)
  Submandibular abscess
    EXCLUDES 2   *abscess of salivary gland (K11.3)*
          abscess of tongue (K14.0)
          periapical abscess (K04.6-K04.7)
          periodontal abscess (K05.21)
          peritonsillar abscess (J36)

√5ᵗʰ **K12.3** **Oral mucositis (ulcerative)**
  Mucositis (oral) (oropharyneal)
    EXCLUDES 2   *gastrointestinal mucositis (ulcerative) (K92.81)*
          mucositis (ulcerative) of vagina and vulva (N76.81)
          nasal mucositis (ulcerative) (J34.81)
  K12.30 **Oral mucositis (ulcerative), unspecified**
  K12.31 **Oral mucositis (ulcerative) due to antineoplastic therapy**
      Use additional code for adverse effect, if applicable, to identify antineoplastic and immunosuppressive drugs (T45.1X5)
      Use additional code for other antineoplastic therapy, such as:
        radiological procedure and radiotherapy (Y84.2)
  K12.32 **Oral mucositis (ulcerative) due to other drugs**
      Use additional code for adverse effect, if applicable, to identify drug (T36-T50 with fifth or sixth character 5)
  K12.33 **Oral mucositis (ulcerative) due to radiation**
      Use additional external cause code (W88-W90, X39.0-) to identify cause
  K12.39 **Other oral mucositis (ulcerative)**
      Viral oral mucositis (ulcerative)

√4ᵗʰ **K13** **Other diseases of lip and oral mucosa**
  INCLUDES   epithelial disturbances of tongue
  Use additional code to identify:
    alcohol abuse and dependence (F10.-)
    exposure to environmental tobacco smoke (Z77.22)
    exposure to tobacco smoke in the perinatal period (P96.81)
    history of tobacco dependence (Z87.891)
    occupational exposure to environmental tobacco smoke (Z57.31)
    tobacco dependence (F17.-)
    tobacco use (Z72.0)
    EXCLUDES 2   *certain disorders of gingiva and edentulous alveolar ridge (K05-K06)*
          cysts of oral region (K09.-)
          diseases of tongue (K14.-)
          stomatitis and related lesions (K12.-)

K13.0 **Diseases of lips**
  Abscess of lips
  Angular cheilitis
  Cellulitis of lips
  Cheilitis NOS
  Cheilodynia
  Cheilosis
  Exfoliative cheilitis
  Fistula of lips
  Glandular cheilitis
  Hypertrophy of lips
  Perlèche NEC
    EXCLUDES 1   *ariboflavinosis (E53.0)*
          cheilitis due to radiation-related disorders (L55-L59)
          congenital fistula of lips (Q38.0)
          congenital hypertrophy of lips (Q18.6)
          perlèche due to candidiasis (B37.83)
          perlèche due to riboflavin deficiency (E53.0)

K13.1 **Cheek and lip biting**

√5ᵗʰ **K13.2** **Leukoplakia and other disturbances of oral epithelium, including tongue**

> EXCLUDES 1   *carcinoma in situ of oral epithelium (D00.0-)*
>   *hairy leukoplakia (K13.3)*

> **DEF:** Leukoplakia: Thickened white patches or lesions appearing on a mucous membrane, such as oral mucosa or tongue.

     K13.21 **Leukoplakia of oral mucosa, including tongue**
         Leukokeratosis of oral mucosa
         Leukoplakia of gingiva, lips, tongue

>   EXCLUDES 1   *hairy leukoplakia (K13.3)*
>   *leukokeratosis nicotina palati (K13.24)*

     K13.22 **Minimal keratinized residual ridge mucosa**
         Minimal keratinization of alveolar ridge mucosa

     K13.23 **Excessive keratinized residual ridge mucosa**
         Excessive keratinization of alveolar ridge mucosa

     K13.24 **Leukokeratosis nicotina palati**
         Smoker's palate

     K13.29 **Other disturbances of oral epithelium, including tongue**
         Erythroplakia of mouth or tongue
         Focal epithelial hyperplasia of mouth or tongue
         Leukoedema of mouth or tongue
         Other oral epithelium disturbances

K13.3 **Hairy leukoplakia**

K13.4 **Granuloma and granuloma-like lesions of oral mucosa**
     Eosinophilic granuloma
     Granuloma pyogenicum
     Verrucous xanthoma

K13.5 **Oral submucous fibrosis**
     Submucous fibrosis of tongue

K13.6 **Irritative hyperplasia of oral mucosa**

> EXCLUDES 2   *irritative hyperplasia of edentulous ridge [denture hyperplasia] (K06.2)*

√5ᵗʰ **K13.7** **Other and unspecified lesions of oral mucosa**

     K13.70 **Unspecified lesions of oral mucosa**
     K13.79 **Other lesions of oral mucosa**
         Focal oral mucinosis

√4ᵗʰ **K14** **Diseases of tongue**
     Use additional code to identify:
       alcohol abuse and dependence (F10.-)
       exposure to environmental tobacco smoke (Z77.22)
       history of tobacco dependence (Z87.891)
       occupational exposure to environmental tobacco smoke (Z57.31)
       tobacco dependence (F17.-)
       tobacco use (Z72.0)

> EXCLUDES 2   *erythroplakia (K13.29)*
>   *focal epithelial hyperplasia (K13.29)*
>   *leukedema of tongue (K13.29)*
>   *leukoplakia of tongue (K13.21)*
>   *hairy leukoplakia (K13.3)*
>   *macroglossia (congenital) (Q38.2)*
>   *submucous fibrosis of tongue (K13.5)*

K14.0 **Glossitis**
     Abscess of tongue
     Ulceration (traumatic) of tongue

> EXCLUDES 1   *atrophic glossitis (K14.4)*

> **DEF:** Inflammation and swelling of the tongue that may be associated with infection, adverse drug reactions, smoking, or injury.

K14.1 **Geographic tongue**
     Benign migratory glossitis
     Glossitis areata exfoliativa

K14.2 **Median rhomboid glossitis**

K14.3 **Hypertrophy of tongue papillae**
     Black hairy tongue
     Coated tongue
     Hypertrophy of foliate papillae
     Lingua villosa nigra

K14.4 **Atrophy of tongue papillae**
     Atrophic glossitis

K14.5 **Plicated tongue**
     Fissured tongue
     Furrowed tongue
     Scrotal tongue

> EXCLUDES 1   *fissured tongue, congenital (Q38.3)*

K14.6 **Glossodynia**
     Glossopyrosis
     Painful tongue

K14.8 **Other diseases of tongue**
     Atrophy of tongue
     Crenated tongue
     Enlargement of tongue
     Glossocele
     Glossoptosis
     Hypertrophy of tongue

K14.9 **Disease of tongue, unspecified**
     Glossopathy NOS

Diseases of esophagus, stomach and duodenum (K20-K31)

> EXCLUDES 2   *hiatus hernia (K44.-)*

√4ᵗʰ **K20** **Esophagitis**
     Use additional code to identify:
       alcohol abuse and dependence (F10.-)

> EXCLUDES 1   *erosion of esophagus (K22.1-)*
>   *esophagitis with gastro-esophageal reflux disease ▶(K21.0-)◀*
>   *reflux esophagitis ▶(K21.0-)◀*
>   *ulcerative esophagitis (K22.1-)*

> EXCLUDES 2   *eosinophilic gastritis or gastroenteritis (K52.81)*

     K20.0 **Eosinophilic esophagitis**

▲ √5ᵗʰ **K20.8** **Other esophagitis**
         ~~Abscess of esophagus~~

●   **K20.80** **Other esophagitis without bleeding**
           Abscess of esophagus
           Other esophagitis NOS

●   **K20.81** **Other esophagitis with bleeding**   MCC

▲ √5ᵗʰ **K20.9** **Esophagitis, unspecified**
         ~~Esophagitis NOS~~

●   **K20.90** **Esophagitis, unspecified without bleeding**
           Esophagitis NOS

●   **K20.91** **Esophagitis, unspecified with bleeding**   MCC

√4ᵗʰ **K21** **Gastro-esophageal reflux disease**

> EXCLUDES 1   *newborn esophageal reflux (P78.83)*

▲ √5ᵗʰ **K21.0** **Gastro-esophageal reflux disease with esophagitis**
         ~~Reflux esophagitis~~

●   **K21.00** **Gastro-esophageal reflux disease with esophagitis, without bleeding**
           Reflux esophagitis

●   **K21.01** **Gastro-esophageal reflux disease with esophagitis, with bleeding**   MCC

     K21.9 **Gastro-esophageal reflux disease without esophagitis**
         Esophageal reflux NOS
         AHA: 2016,1Q,18

√4ᵗʰ **K22** **Other diseases of esophagus**

> EXCLUDES 2   *esophageal varices (I85.-)*

     K22.0 **Achalasia of cardia**
         Achalasia NOS
         Cardiospasm

> EXCLUDES 1   *congenital cardiospasm (Q39.5)*

> **DEF:** Esophageal motility disorder that is caused by absence of the esophageal peristalsis and impaired relaxation of the lower esophageal sphincter. It is characterized by dysphagia, regurgitation, and heartburn.

☑ Additional Character Required   √x7ᵗʰ Placeholder   Unacceptable PDx   Questionable PDx   Manifestation   Unspecified Dx   H1-H14 HAC   HCC CMS-HCC Dx   HIV HIV Dx

ICD-10-CM 2021   711

✓5th **K22.1 Ulcer of esophagus**

Barrett's ulcer
Erosion of esophagus
Fungal ulcer of esophagus
Peptic ulcer of esophagus
Ulcer of esophagus due to ingestion of chemicals
Ulcer of esophagus due to ingestion of drugs and medicaments
Ulcerative esophagitis
Code first poisoning due to drug or toxin, if applicable (T36-T65 with fifth or sixth character 1-4 or 6)
Use additional code for adverse effect, if applicable, to identify drug (T36-T50 with fifth or sixth character 5)

EXCLUDES 1   Barrett's esophagus (K22.7-)

AHA: 2018,3Q,22; 2017,3Q,27
TIP: Assign a code for "with bleeding" when an esophageal ulcer and bleeding (hematemesis) are documented. The ICD-10-CM classification assumes the two are related without the provider linking the two conditions. Evidence of bleeding during a procedure is not required.
TIP: For bleeding ulcers resulting from anticoagulant therapy, code D68.32 Hemorrhagic disorder due to extrinsic circulating anticoagulant, and an adverse-effect code from subcategory T45.5- should also be assigned. Either the bleeding ulcer code or code D68.32 may be sequenced first, depending on the circumstances of admission.

K22.10 Ulcer of esophagus without bleeding   CC
Ulcer of esophagus NOS

K22.11 Ulcer of esophagus with bleeding   MCC
EXCLUDES 2   bleeding esophageal varices (I85.01, I85.11)

K22.2 Esophageal obstruction
Compression of esophagus
Constriction of esophagus
Stenosis of esophagus
Stricture of esophagus
EXCLUDES 1   congenital stenosis or stricture of esophagus (Q39.3)

K22.3 Perforation of esophagus   MCC
Rupture of esophagus
EXCLUDES 1   traumatic perforation of (thoracic) esophagus (S27.8-)

K22.4 Dyskinesia of esophagus
Corkscrew esophagus
Diffuse esophageal spasm
Spasm of esophagus
EXCLUDES 1   cardiospasm (K22.0)

K22.5 Diverticulum of esophagus, acquired
Esophageal pouch, acquired
EXCLUDES 1   diverticulum of esophagus (congenital) (Q39.6)

K22.6 Gastro-esophageal laceration-hemorrhage syndrome   MCC
Mallory-Weiss syndrome

✓5th **K22.7 Barrett's esophagus**

Barrett's disease
Barrett's syndrome
EXCLUDES 1   Barrett's ulcer (K22.1)
                 malignant neoplasm of esophagus (C15.-)

DEF: Metaplastic disorder in which specialized columnar epithelial cells replace the normal squamous epithelial cells. Secondary to chronic gastroesophageal reflux damage to the mucosa, this disorder increases the risk of developing adenocarcinoma.

K22.70 Barrett's esophagus without dysplasia
Barrett's esophagus NOS

✓6th **K22.71 Barrett's esophagus with dysplasia**

K22.710 Barrett's esophagus with low grade dysplasia

K22.711 Barrett's esophagus with high grade dysplasia

K22.719 Barrett's esophagus with dysplasia, unspecified

K22.8 Other specified diseases of esophagus
Hemorrhage of esophagus NOS
EXCLUDES 2   esophageal varices (I85.-)
                 Paterson-Kelly syndrome (D50.1)

AHA: 2020,1Q,16

K22.9 Disease of esophagus, unspecified

K23 Disorders of esophagus in diseases classified elsewhere
Code first underlying disease, such as:
congenital syphilis (A50.5)
EXCLUDES 1   late syphilis (A52.79)
                 megaesophagus due to Chagas' disease (B57.31)
                 tuberculosis (A18.83)

✓4th **K25 Gastric ulcer**

INCLUDES   erosion (acute) of stomach
              pylorus ulcer (peptic)
              stomach ulcer (peptic)
Use additional code to identify:
alcohol abuse and dependence (F10.-)
EXCLUDES 1   acute gastritis (K29.0-)
                 peptic ulcer NOS (K27.-)

AHA: 2017,3Q,27
TIP: Assign a code for "with hemorrhage" when a gastric ulcer and GI bleeding are documented. The ICD-10-CM classification assumes the two are related without the provider linking the two conditions. Evidence of bleeding during a procedure is not required.
TIP: For bleeding ulcers resulting from anticoagulant therapy, code D68.32 Hemorrhagic disorder due to extrinsic circulating anticoagulant, and an adverse-effect code from subcategory T45.5- should also be assigned. Either the bleeding ulcer code or code D68.32 may be sequenced first, depending on the circumstances of admission.

K25.0 Acute gastric ulcer with hemorrhage   MCC
K25.1 Acute gastric ulcer with perforation   MCC HCC
K25.2 Acute gastric ulcer with both hemorrhage and perforation   MCC HCC
K25.3 Acute gastric ulcer without hemorrhage or perforation   CC
K25.4 Chronic or unspecified gastric ulcer with hemorrhage   MCC
K25.5 Chronic or unspecified gastric ulcer with perforation   MCC HCC
K25.6 Chronic or unspecified gastric ulcer with both hemorrhage and perforation   MCC HCC
K25.7 Chronic gastric ulcer without hemorrhage or perforation
K25.9 Gastric ulcer, unspecified as acute or chronic, without hemorrhage or perforation

Gastrointestinal Ulcers

Esophagus
Esophageal ulcer
Stomach
Duodenal ulcer
Gastric ulcer
Small intestine

✓4th **K26 Duodenal ulcer**

INCLUDES   erosion (acute) of duodenum
              duodenum ulcer (peptic)
              postpyloric ulcer (peptic)
Use additional code to identify:
alcohol abuse and dependence (F10.-)
EXCLUDES 1   peptic ulcer NOS (K27.-)

AHA: 2017,3Q,27
TIP: Assign a code for "with hemorrhage" when a duodenal ulcer and GI bleeding are documented. The ICD-10-CM classification assumes the two are related without the provider linking the two conditions. Evidence of bleeding during a procedure is not required.
TIP: For bleeding ulcers resulting from anticoagulant therapy, code D68.32 Hemorrhagic disorder due to extrinsic circulating anticoagulant, and an adverse-effect code from subcategory T45.5- should also be assigned. Either the bleeding ulcer code or code D68.32 may be sequenced first, depending on the circumstances of admission.

K26.0 Acute duodenal ulcer with hemorrhage   MCC
K26.1 Acute duodenal ulcer with perforation   MCC HCC
K26.2 Acute duodenal ulcer with both hemorrhage and perforation   MCC HCC

K26.3   Acute duodenal ulcer without hemorrhage or perforation   `CC`

K26.4   Chronic or unspecified duodenal ulcer with hemorrhage   `MCC`
     AHA: 2016,1Q,14

K26.5   Chronic or unspecified duodenal ulcer with perforation   `MCC` `HCC`

K26.6   Chronic or unspecified duodenal ulcer with both hemorrhage and perforation   `MCC` `HCC`

K26.7   Chronic duodenal ulcer without hemorrhage or perforation

K26.9   Duodenal ulcer, unspecified as acute or chronic, without hemorrhage or perforation

✓4ᵗʰ **K27**   Peptic ulcer, site unspecified

    `INCLUDES`   gastroduodenal ulcer NOS
                 peptic ulcer NOS

   Use additional code to identify:
     alcohol abuse and dependence (F10.-)
    `EXCLUDES 1`   peptic ulcer of newborn (P78.82)

   AHA: 2017,3Q,27

   TIP: Assign a code for "with hemorrhage" when a peptic ulcer and GI bleeding are documented. The ICD-10-CM classification assumes the two are related without the provider linking the two conditions. Evidence of bleeding during a procedure is not required.

   TIP: For bleeding ulcers resulting from anticoagulant therapy, code D68.32 Hemorrhagic disorder due to extrinsic circulating anticoagulant, and an adverse-effect code from subcategory T45.5- should also be assigned. Either the bleeding ulcer code or code D68.32 may be sequenced first, depending on the circumstances of admission.

K27.0   Acute peptic ulcer, site unspecified, with hemorrhage   `MCC`

K27.1   Acute peptic ulcer, site unspecified, with perforation   `MCC` `HCC`

K27.2   Acute peptic ulcer, site unspecified, with both hemorrhage and perforation   `MCC` `HCC`

K27.3   Acute peptic ulcer, site unspecified, without hemorrhage or perforation   `CC`

K27.4   Chronic or unspecified peptic ulcer, site unspecified, with hemorrhage   `MCC`

K27.5   Chronic or unspecified peptic ulcer, site unspecified, with perforation   `MCC` `HCC`

K27.6   Chronic or unspecified peptic ulcer, site unspecified, with both hemorrhage and perforation   `MCC` `HCC`

K27.7   Chronic peptic ulcer, site unspecified, without hemorrhage or perforation

K27.9   Peptic ulcer, site unspecified, unspecified as acute or chronic, without hemorrhage or perforation

✓4ᵗʰ **K28**   Gastrojejunal ulcer

    `INCLUDES`   anastomotic ulcer (peptic) or erosion
                 gastrocolic ulcer (peptic) or erosion
                 gastrointestinal ulcer (peptic) or erosion
                 gastrojejunal ulcer (peptic) or erosion
                 jejunal ulcer (peptic) or erosion
                 marginal ulcer (peptic) or erosion
                 stomal ulcer (peptic) or erosion

   Use additional code to identify:
     alcohol abuse and dependence (F10.-)
    `EXCLUDES 1`   primary ulcer of small intestine (K63.3)

   AHA: 2017,3Q,27

   TIP: Assign a code for "with hemorrhage" when a gastrojejunal ulcer and GI bleeding are documented. The ICD-10-CM classification assumes the two are related without the provider linking the two conditions. Evidence of bleeding during a procedure is not required.

   TIP: For bleeding ulcers resulting from anticoagulant therapy, code D68.32 Hemorrhagic disorder due to extrinsic circulating anticoagulant, and an adverse-effect code from subcategory T45.5- should also be assigned. Either the bleeding ulcer code or code D68.32 may be sequenced first, depending on the circumstances of admission.

K28.0   Acute gastrojejunal ulcer with hemorrhage   `MCC`

K28.1   Acute gastrojejunal ulcer with perforation   `MCC` `HCC`

K28.2   Acute gastrojejunal ulcer with both hemorrhage and perforation   `MCC` `HCC`

K28.3   Acute gastrojejunal ulcer without hemorrhage or perforation   `CC`

K28.4   Chronic or unspecified gastrojejunal ulcer with hemorrhage   `MCC`

K28.5   Chronic or unspecified gastrojejunal ulcer with perforation   `MCC` `HCC`

K28.6   Chronic or unspecified gastrojejunal ulcer with both hemorrhage and perforation   `MCC` `HCC`

K28.7   Chronic gastrojejunal ulcer without hemorrhage or perforation

K28.9   Gastrojejunal ulcer, unspecified as acute or chronic, without hemorrhage or perforation

✓4ᵗʰ **K29**   Gastritis and duodenitis

    `EXCLUDES 1`   eosinophilic gastritis or gastroenteritis (K52.81)
                 Zollinger-Ellison syndrome (E16.4)

   AHA: 2018,3Q,22

   TIP: Assign a code for "with bleeding" when gastritis or duodenitis and GI bleeding are documented. The ICD-10-CM classification assumes the two are related without the provider linking the two conditions. Evidence of bleeding during a procedure is not required.

   TIP: For bleeding resulting from anticoagulant therapy, code D68.32 Hemorrhagic disorder due to extrinsic circulating anticoagulant, and an adverse-effect code from subcategory T45.5- should also be assigned. Either code K29 or code D68.32 may be sequenced first, depending on the circumstances of admission.

✓5ᵗʰ **K29.0**   Acute gastritis

   Use additional code to identify:
     alcohol abuse and dependence (F10.-)
    `EXCLUDES 1`   erosion (acute) of stomach (K25.-)

   K29.00   Acute gastritis without bleeding

   K29.01   Acute gastritis with bleeding   `MCC`

✓5ᵗʰ **K29.2**   Alcoholic gastritis

   Use additional code to identify:
     alcohol abuse and dependence (F10.-)

   K29.20   Alcoholic gastritis without bleeding

   K29.21   Alcoholic gastritis with bleeding   `MCC`

✓5ᵗʰ **K29.3**   Chronic superficial gastritis

   K29.30   Chronic superficial gastritis without bleeding

   K29.31   Chronic superficial gastritis with bleeding   `MCC`

✓5ᵗʰ **K29.4**   Chronic atrophic gastritis

   Gastric atrophy

   K29.40   Chronic atrophic gastritis without bleeding

   K29.41   Chronic atrophic gastritis with bleeding   `MCC`

✓5ᵗʰ **K29.5**   Unspecified chronic gastritis

   Chronic antral gastritis
   Chronic fundal gastritis

   K29.50   Unspecified chronic gastritis without bleeding

   K29.51   Unspecified chronic gastritis with bleeding   `MCC`

✓5ᵗʰ **K29.6**   Other gastritis

   Giant hypertrophic gastritis
   Granulomatous gastritis
   Ménétrier's disease

   K29.60   Other gastritis without bleeding

   K29.61   Other gastritis with bleeding   `MCC`

✓5ᵗʰ **K29.7**   Gastritis, unspecified

   K29.70   Gastritis, unspecified, without bleeding

   K29.71   Gastritis, unspecified, with bleeding   `MCC`

✓5ᵗʰ **K29.8**   Duodenitis

   K29.80   Duodenitis without bleeding

   K29.81   Duodenitis with bleeding   `MCC`

✓5ᵗʰ **K29.9**   Gastroduodenitis, unspecified

   K29.90   Gastroduodenitis, unspecified, without bleeding

   K29.91   Gastroduodenitis, unspecified, with bleeding   `MCC`

K30   Functional dyspepsia

   Indigestion

    `EXCLUDES 1`   dyspepsia NOS (R10.13)
                 heartburn (R12)
                 nervous dyspepsia (F45.8)
                 neurotic dyspepsia (F45.8)
                 psychogenic dyspepsia (F45.8)

✓4ᵗʰ **K31**   Other diseases of stomach and duodenum

    `INCLUDES`   functional disorders of stomach
    `EXCLUDES 2`   diabetic gastroparesis (E08.43, E09.43, E10.43, E11.43, E13.43)
                 diverticulum of duodenum (K57.00-K57.13)

   K31.0   Acute dilatation of stomach   `CC`

     Acute distention of stomach

   K31.1   Adult hypertrophic pyloric stenosis   `CC` `A`

     Pyloric stenosis NOS

      `EXCLUDES 1`   congenital or infantile pyloric stenosis (Q40.0)

✓ Additional Character Required   ✓×7ᵗʰ Placeholder   Unacceptable PDx   Questionable PDx   Manifestation   Unspecified Dx   `H1`-`H14` HAC   `HCC` CMS-HCC Dx   `HIV` HIV Dx

ICD-10-CM 2021   713

K31.2 Hourglass stricture and stenosis of stomach
> EXCLUDES 1   congenital hourglass stomach (Q40.2)
>   hourglass contraction of stomach (K31.89)

K31.3 Pylorospasm, not elsewhere classified
> EXCLUDES 1   congenital or infantile pylorospasm (Q40.0)
>   neurotic pylorospasm (F45.8)
>   psychogenic pylorospasm (F45.8)

K31.4 Gastric diverticulum
> EXCLUDES 1   congenital diverticulum of stomach (Q40.2)

K31.5 Obstruction of duodenum   CC
Constriction of duodenum
Duodenal ileus (chronic)
Stenosis of duodenum
Stricture of duodenum
Volvulus of duodenum
> EXCLUDES 1   congenital stenosis of duodenum (Q41.0)

K31.6 Fistula of stomach and duodenum   CC SW
Gastrocolic fistula
Gastrojejunocolic fistula

K31.7 Polyp of stomach and duodenum
> EXCLUDES 1   adenomatous polyp of stomach (D13.1)

AHA: 2020,1Q,16

✓5ᵗʰ **K31.8 Other specified diseases of stomach and duodenum**

  ✓6ᵗʰ **K31.81 Angiodysplasia of stomach and duodenum**
  > TIP: Assign a code for "with bleeding" when
  > angiodysplasia of the stomach or the duodenum and
  > GI bleeding are documented. The ICD-10-CM
  > classification assumes the two are related without the
  > provider linking the two conditions. Evidence of
  > bleeding during a procedure is not required.

    **K31.811 Angiodysplasia of stomach and
    duodenum with bleeding**   MCC

    **K31.819 Angiodysplasia of stomach and
    duodenum without bleeding**
    Angiodysplasia of stomach and duodenum
    NOS

  **K31.82 Dieulafoy lesion (hemorrhagic) of stomach and
  duodenum**   MCC
  > EXCLUDES 2   Dieulafoy lesion of intestine (K63.81)
  > DEF: Abnormally large submucosal artery protruding
  > through a defect in the stomach mucosa or intestines
  > that can cause massive and life-threatening
  > hemorrhaging.

  K31.83 Achlorhydria
  > DEF: Absence of hydrochloric acid in gastric secretions
  > due to gastric mucosa atrophy. Achlorhydria is
  > unresponsive to histamines.

  K31.84 Gastroparesis
  Gastroparalysis
  Code first underlying disease, if known, such as:
    anorexia nervosa (F50.0-)
    diabetes mellitus (E08.43, E09.43, E10.43, E11.43,
      E13.43)
    scleroderma (M34,-)
  AHA: 2013,4Q,114

  K31.89 Other diseases of stomach and duodenum
  AHA: 2020,1Q,15; 2017,1Q,28

  K31.9 Disease of stomach and duodenum, unspecified

Diseases of appendix (K35-K38)

✓4ᵗʰ **K35 Acute appendicitis**
AHA: 2018,4Q,17-18

  ✓5ᵗʰ **K35.2 Acute appendicitis with generalized peritonitis**
  Appendicitis (acute) with generalized (diffuse) peritonitis
  following rupture or perforation of appendix

    **K35.20 Acute appendicitis with generalized peritonitis,
    without abscess**   CC
    (Acute) appendicitis with generalized peritonitis NOS

    **K35.21 Acute appendicitis with generalized peritonitis,
    with abscess**   MCC

  ✓5ᵗʰ **K35.3 Acute appendicitis with localized peritonitis**

    **K35.30 Acute appendicitis with localized peritonitis,
    without perforation or gangrene**   CC
    Acute appendicitis with localized peritonitis NOS

    **K35.31 Acute appendicitis with localized peritonitis and
    gangrene, without perforation**   CC

**K35.32 Acute appendicitis with perforation and localized
peritonitis, without abscess**   MCC
(Acute) appendicitis with perforation NOS
Perforated appendix NOS
Ruptured appendix (with localized peritonitis) NOS
AHA: 2020,1Q,16

**K35.33 Acute appendicitis with perforation and localized
peritonitis, with abscess**   MCC
(Acute) appendicitis with (peritoneal) abscess NOS
Ruptured appendix with localized peritonitis and
abscess

✓5ᵗʰ **K35.8 Other and unspecified acute appendicitis**

  K35.80 Unspecified acute appendicitis   CC
  Acute appendicitis NOS
  Acute appendicitis without (localized) (generalized)
  peritonitis

  ✓6ᵗʰ **K35.89 Other acute appendicitis**
  AHA: 2020,1Q,16

    **K35.890 Other acute appendicitis without
    perforation or gangrene**   CC

    **K35.891 Other acute appendicitis without
    perforation, with gangrene**   CC
    (Acute) appendicitis with gangrene NOS

K36 Other appendicitis
Chronic appendicitis
Recurrent appendicitis

K37 Unspecified appendicitis
> EXCLUDES 1   unspecified appendicitis with peritonitis (K35.2-, K35.3-)

✓4ᵗʰ **K38 Other diseases of appendix**

  K38.0 Hyperplasia of appendix

  K38.1 Appendicular concretions
  Fecalith of appendix
  Stercolith of appendix

  K38.2 Diverticulum of appendix

  K38.3 Fistula of appendix

  K38.8 Other specified diseases of appendix
  Intussusception of appendix

  K38.9 Disease of appendix, unspecified

Hernia (K40-K46)

NOTE   Hernia with both gangrene and obstruction is classified to hernia
with gangrene.

INCLUDES   acquired hernia
            congenital [except diaphragmatic or hiatus] hernia
            recurrent hernia

✓4ᵗʰ **K40 Inguinal hernia**

  INCLUDES   bubonocele
              direct inguinal hernia
              double inguinal hernia
              indirect inguinal hernia
              inguinal hernia NOS
              oblique inguinal hernia
              scrotal hernia
  DEF: Within the groin region.

  ✓5ᵗʰ **K40.0 Bilateral inguinal hernia, with obstruction, without gangrene**
  Inguinal hernia (bilateral) causing obstruction without gangrene
  Incarcerated inguinal hernia (bilateral) without gangrene
  Irreducible inguinal hernia (bilateral) without gangrene
  Strangulated inguinal hernia (bilateral) without gangrene

    **K40.00 Bilateral inguinal hernia, with obstruction, without
    gangrene, not specified as recurrent**   CC
    Bilateral inguinal hernia, with obstruction, without
    gangrene NOS

    **K40.01 Bilateral inguinal hernia, with obstruction, without
    gangrene, recurrent**   CC

  ✓5ᵗʰ **K40.1 Bilateral inguinal hernia, with gangrene**

    **K40.10 Bilateral inguinal hernia, with gangrene, not
    specified as recurrent**   MCC
    Bilateral inguinal hernia, with gangrene NOS

    **K40.11 Bilateral inguinal hernia, with gangrene,
    recurrent**   MCC

✓5ᵗʰ K40.2 Bilateral **inguinal hernia, without obstruction or gangrene**

    K40.20 **Bilateral inguinal hernia, without obstruction or gangrene, not specified as recurrent**
        Bilateral inguinal hernia NOS

    K40.21 **Bilateral inguinal hernia, without obstruction or gangrene, recurrent**

✓5ᵗʰ K40.3 Unilateral **inguinal hernia, with obstruction, without gangrene**

    Inguinal hernia (unilateral) causing obstruction without gangrene
    Incarcerated inguinal hernia (unilateral) without gangrene
    Irreducible inguinal hernia (unilateral) without gangrene
    Strangulated inguinal hernia (unilateral) without gangrene

    K40.30 **Unilateral inguinal hernia, with obstruction, without gangrene, not specified as recurrent** `CC`
        Inguinal hernia, with obstruction NOS
        Unilateral inguinal hernia, with obstruction, without gangrene NOS

    K40.31 **Unilateral inguinal hernia, with obstruction, without gangrene, recurrent** `CC`

✓5ᵗʰ K40.4 Unilateral **inguinal hernia, with gangrene**

    K40.40 **Unilateral inguinal hernia, with gangrene, not specified as recurrent** `MCC`
        Inguinal hernia with gangrene NOS
        Unilateral inguinal hernia with gangrene NOS

    K40.41 **Unilateral inguinal hernia, with gangrene, recurrent** `MCC`

✓5ᵗʰ K40.9 Unilateral **inguinal hernia, without obstruction or gangrene**

    K40.90 **Unilateral inguinal hernia, without obstruction or gangrene, not specified as recurrent**
        Inguinal hernia NOS
        Unilateral inguinal hernia NOS

    K40.91 **Unilateral inguinal hernia, without obstruction or gangrene, recurrent**

Hernia Sites

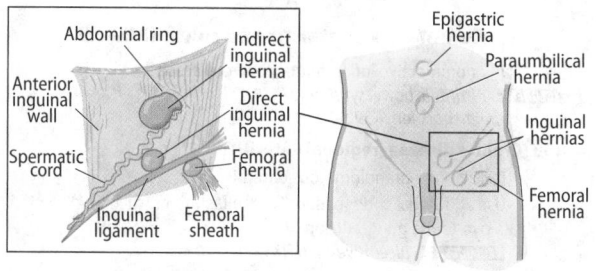

✓4ᵗʰ K41 **Femoral** hernia

✓5ᵗʰ K41.0 Bilateral **femoral hernia, with obstruction, without gangrene**

    Femoral hernia (bilateral) causing obstruction, without gangrene
    Incarcerated femoral hernia (bilateral), without gangrene
    Irreducible femoral hernia (bilateral), without gangrene
    Strangulated femoral hernia (bilateral), without gangrene

    K41.00 **Bilateral femoral hernia, with obstruction, without gangrene, not specified as recurrent** `CC`
        Bilateral femoral hernia, with obstruction, without gangrene NOS

    K41.01 **Bilateral femoral hernia, with obstruction, without gangrene, recurrent** `CC`

✓5ᵗʰ K41.1 Bilateral **femoral hernia, with gangrene**

    K41.10 **Bilateral femoral hernia, with gangrene, not specified as recurrent** `MCC`
        Bilateral femoral hernia, with gangrene NOS

    K41.11 **Bilateral femoral hernia, with gangrene, recurrent** `MCC`

✓5ᵗʰ K41.2 Bilateral **femoral hernia, without obstruction or gangrene**

    K41.20 **Bilateral femoral hernia, without obstruction or gangrene, not specified as recurrent**
        Bilateral femoral hernia NOS

    K41.21 **Bilateral femoral hernia, without obstruction or gangrene, recurrent**

✓5ᵗʰ K41.3 Unilateral **femoral hernia, with obstruction, without gangrene**

    Femoral hernia (unilateral) causing obstruction, without gangrene
    Incarcerated femoral hernia (unilateral), without gangrene
    Irreducible femoral hernia (unilateral), without gangrene
    Strangulated femoral hernia (unilateral), without gangrene

    K41.30 **Unilateral femoral hernia, with obstruction, without gangrene, not specified as recurrent** `CC`
        Femoral hernia, with obstruction NOS
        Unilateral femoral hernia, with obstruction NOS

    K41.31 **Unilateral femoral hernia, with obstruction, without gangrene, recurrent** `CC`

✓5ᵗʰ K41.4 Unilateral **femoral hernia, with gangrene**

    K41.40 **Unilateral femoral hernia, with gangrene, not specified as recurrent** `MCC`
        Femoral hernia, with gangrene NOS
        Unilateral femoral hernia, with gangrene NOS

    K41.41 **Unilateral femoral hernia, with gangrene, recurrent** `MCC`

✓5ᵗʰ K41.9 Unilateral **femoral hernia, without obstruction or gangrene**

    K41.90 **Unilateral femoral hernia, without obstruction or gangrene, not specified as recurrent**
        Femoral hernia NOS
        Unilateral femoral hernia NOS

    K41.91 **Unilateral femoral hernia, without obstruction or gangrene, recurrent**

✓4ᵗʰ K42 Umbilical **hernia**

    `INCLUDES` paraumbilical hernia
    `EXCLUDES 1` omphalocele (Q79.2)

    K42.0 **Umbilical hernia with obstruction, without gangrene** `CC`
        Umbilical hernia causing obstruction, without gangrene
        Incarcerated umbilical hernia, without gangrene
        Irreducible umbilical hernia, without gangrene
        Strangulated umbilical hernia, without gangrene

    K42.1 **Umbilical hernia with gangrene** `MCC`
        Gangrenous umbilical hernia

    K42.9 **Umbilical hernia without obstruction or gangrene**
        Umbilical hernia NOS

✓4ᵗʰ K43 Ventral **hernia**

    DEF: Condition in which a loop of bowel protrudes through a weakness in the abdominal wall muscles that may occur as a birth defect, past surgical site (incisional), or form at a stomal site (parastomal).

    K43.0 **Incisional hernia with obstruction, without gangrene** `CC`
        Incisional hernia causing obstruction, without gangrene
        Incarcerated incisional hernia, without gangrene
        Irreducible incisional hernia, without gangrene
        Strangulated incisional hernia, without gangrene

    K43.1 **Incisional hernia with gangrene** `MCC`
        Gangrenous incisional hernia
        AHA: 2020,2Q,22

    K43.2 **Incisional hernia without obstruction or gangrene**
        Incisional hernia NOS

    K43.3 **Parastomal hernia with obstruction, without gangrene** `CC`
        Incarcerated parastomal hernia, without gangrene
        Irreducible parastomal hernia, without gangrene
        Parastomal hernia causing obstruction, without gangrene
        Strangulated parastomal hernia, without gangrene

    K43.4 **Parastomal hernia with gangrene** `MCC`
        Gangrenous parastomal hernia

    K43.5 **Parastomal hernia without obstruction or gangrene**
        Parastomal hernia NOS

☑ Additional Character Required   ✓x7ᵗʰ Placeholder   Unacceptable PDx   Questionable PDx   Manifestation   Unspecified Dx   H1-H1d HAC   HCC CMS-HCC Dx   HIV HIV Dx

ICD-10-CM 2021   715

Chapter 11. Diseases of the Digestive System

K43.6 Other and unspecified ventral hernia with obstruction, without gangrene `CC`
Epigastric hernia causing obstruction, without gangrene
Hypogastric hernia causing obstruction, without gangrene
Incarcerated epigastric hernia without gangrene
Incarcerated hypogastric hernia without gangrene
Incarcerated midline hernia without gangrene
Incarcerated spigelian hernia without gangrene
Incarcerated subxiphoid hernia without gangrene
Irreducible epigastric hernia without gangrene
Irreducible hypogastric hernia without gangrene
Irreducible midline hernia without gangrene
Irreducible spigelian hernia without gangrene
Irreducible subxiphoid hernia without gangrene
Midline hernia causing obstruction, without gangrene
Spigelian hernia causing obstruction, without gangrene
Strangulated epigastric hernia without gangrene
Strangulated hypogastric hernia without gangrene
Strangulated midline hernia without gangrene
Strangulated spigelian hernia without gangrene
Strangulated subxiphoid hernia without gangrene
Subxiphoid hernia causing obstruction, without gangrene

K43.7 Other and unspecified ventral hernia with gangrene `MCC`
Any condition listed under K43.6 specified as gangrenous

K43.9 Ventral hernia without obstruction or gangrene
Epigastric hernia
Ventral hernia NOS

✓4ᵗʰ **K44 Diaphragmatic hernia**
INCLUDES   hiatus hernia (esophageal) (sliding)
paraesophageal hernia
EXCLUDES 1   *congenital diaphragmatic hernia (Q79.0)*
congenital hiatus hernia (Q40.1)
DEF: Protrusion of an abdominal organ, usually the stomach, through the esophageal opening within the diaphragm and occurring in two types: the sliding hiatal hernia and the paraesophageal hernia.

Hiatal Hernia

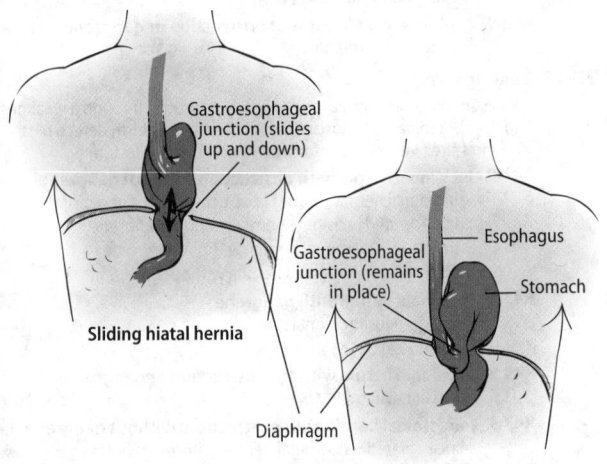

Gastroesophageal junction (slides up and down)

Sliding hiatal hernia

Gastroesophageal junction (remains in place)
Esophagus
Stomach
Diaphragm

Paraesophageal hiatal hernia

K44.0 Diaphragmatic hernia with obstruction, without gangrene `CC`
Diaphragmatic hernia causing obstruction
Incarcerated diaphragmatic hernia
Irreducible diaphragmatic hernia
Strangulated diaphragmatic hernia

K44.1 Diaphragmatic hernia with gangrene `MCC`
Gangrenous diaphragmatic hernia

K44.9 Diaphragmatic hernia without obstruction or gangrene
Diaphragmatic hernia NOS

✓4ᵗʰ **K45 Other abdominal hernia**
INCLUDES   abdominal hernia, specified site NEC
lumbar hernia
obturator hernia
pudendal hernia
retroperitoneal hernia
sciatic hernia

K45.0 Other specified abdominal hernia with obstruction, without gangrene `CC`
Other specified abdominal hernia causing obstruction
Other specified incarcerated abdominal hernia
Other specified irreducible abdominal hernia
Other specified strangulated abdominal hernia

K45.1 Other specified abdominal hernia with gangrene `MCC`
Any condition listed under K45 specified as gangrenous

K45.8 Other specified abdominal hernia without obstruction or gangrene

✓4ᵗʰ **K46 Unspecified abdominal hernia**
INCLUDES   enterocele
epiplocele
hernia NOS
interstitial hernia
intestinal hernia
intra-abdominal hernia
EXCLUDES 1   *vaginal enterocele (N81.5)*

K46.0 Unspecified abdominal hernia with obstruction, without gangrene `CC`
Unspecified abdominal hernia causing obstruction
Unspecified incarcerated abdominal hernia
Unspecified irreducible abdominal hernia
Unspecified strangulated abdominal hernia

K46.1 Unspecified abdominal hernia with gangrene `MCC`
Any condition listed under K46 specified as gangrenous

K46.9 Unspecified abdominal hernia without obstruction or gangrene
Abdominal hernia NOS

Noninfective enteritis and colitis (K50-K52)

INCLUDES   noninfective inflammatory bowel disease
EXCLUDES 1   *irritable bowel syndrome (K58.-)*
megacolon (K59.3-)

✓4ᵗʰ **K50 Crohn's disease [regional enteritis]**
INCLUDES   granulomatous enteritis
Use additional code to identify manifestations, such as:
pyoderma gangrenosum (L88)
EXCLUDES 1   *ulcerative colitis (K51.-)*
AHA: 2019,3Q,5; 2012,4Q,104
DEF: Chronic inflammation of the gastrointestinal tract characterized by chronic granulomatous disease, most commonly affecting the intestines and the terminal ileum.

✓5ᵗʰ **K50.0 Crohn's disease of small intestine**
Crohn's disease [regional enteritis] of duodenum
Crohn's disease [regional enteritis] of ileum
Crohn's disease [regional enteritis] of jejunum
Regional ileitis
Terminal ileitis
EXCLUDES 1   *Crohn's disease of both small and large intestine (K50.8-)*

K50.00 Crohn's disease of small intestine without complications `CC` `HCC`

✓6ᵗʰ **K50.01 Crohn's disease of small intestine with complications**

K50.011 Crohn's disease of small intestine with rectal bleeding `CC` `HCC`

K50.012 Crohn's disease of small intestine with intestinal obstruction `CC` `HCC`

K50.013 Crohn's disease of small intestine with fistula `CC` `HCC` `SW`

K50.014 Crohn's disease of small intestine with abscess `CC` `HCC`
AHA: 2012,4Q,104

K50.018 Crohn's disease of small intestine with other complication `CC` `HCC`

K50.019 Crohn's disease of small intestine with unspecified complications `CC` `HCC`

Chapter 11. Diseases of the Digestive System

√5ᵗʰ **K50.1 Crohn's disease of large intestine**
Crohn's disease [regional enteritis] of colon
Crohn's disease [regional enteritis] of large bowel
Crohn's disease [regional enteritis] of rectum
Granulomatous colitis
Regional colitis
EXCLUDES 1   *Crohn's disease of both small and large intestine (K50.8)*

     K50.10 Crohn's disease of large intestine without complications   CC HCC

√6ᵗʰ **K50.11 Crohn's disease of large intestine** with complications

        K50.111 Crohn's disease of large intestine with rectal bleeding   CC HCC

        K50.112 Crohn's disease of large intestine with intestinal obstruction   CC HCC

        K50.113 Crohn's disease of large intestine with fistula   CC HCC SW

        K50.114 Crohn's disease of large intestine with abscess   CC HCC

        K50.118 Crohn's disease of large intestine with other complication   CC HCC

        K50.119 Crohn's disease of large intestine with unspecified complications   CC HCC

√5ᵗʰ **K50.8 Crohn's disease of both small and large intestine**

     K50.80 Crohn's disease of both small and large intestine without complications   CC HCC

√6ᵗʰ **K50.81 Crohn's disease of both small and large intestine** with complications

        K50.811 Crohn's disease of both small and large intestine with rectal bleeding   CC HCC

        K50.812 Crohn's disease of both small and large intestine with intestinal obstruction   CC HCC

        K50.813 Crohn's disease of both small and large intestine with fistula   CC HCC SW

        K50.814 Crohn's disease of both small and large intestine with abscess   CC HCC

        K50.818 Crohn's disease of both small and large intestine with other complication   CC HCC

        K50.819 Crohn's disease of both small and large intestine with unspecified complications   CC HCC

√5ᵗʰ **K50.9 Crohn's disease, unspecified**

     K50.90 Crohn's disease, unspecified, without complications   CC HCC
Crohn's disease NOS
Regional enteritis NOS

√6ᵗʰ **K50.91 Crohn's disease, unspecified,** with complications

        K50.911 Crohn's disease, unspecified, with rectal bleeding   CC HCC

        K50.912 Crohn's disease, unspecified, with intestinal obstruction   CC HCC

        K50.913 Crohn's disease, unspecified, with fistula   CC HCC SW

        K50.914 Crohn's disease, unspecified, with abscess   CC HCC

        K50.918 Crohn's disease, unspecified, with other complication   CC HCC

        K50.919 Crohn's disease, unspecified, with unspecified complications   CC HCC

√4ᵗʰ **K51 Ulcerative colitis**
Use additional code to identify manifestations, such as:
   pyoderma gangrenosum (L88)
EXCLUDES 1   *Crohn's disease [regional enteritis] (K50.-)*

√5ᵗʰ **K51.0 Ulcerative (chronic) pancolitis**
Backwash ileitis

     K51.00 Ulcerative (chronic) pancolitis without complications   CC HCC
Ulcerative (chronic) pancolitis NOS

√6ᵗʰ **K51.01 Ulcerative (chronic) pancolitis** with complications

        K51.011 Ulcerative (chronic) pancolitis with rectal bleeding   CC HCC

        K51.012 Ulcerative (chronic) pancolitis with intestinal obstruction   CC HCC

        K51.013 Ulcerative (chronic) pancolitis with fistula   CC HCC SW

        K51.014 Ulcerative (chronic) pancolitis with abscess   CC HCC

        K51.018 Ulcerative (chronic) pancolitis with other complication   CC HCC

        K51.019 Ulcerative (chronic) pancolitis with unspecified complications   CC HCC

√5ᵗʰ **K51.2 Ulcerative (chronic) proctitis**

     K51.20 Ulcerative (chronic) proctitis without complications   CC HCC
Ulcerative (chronic) proctitis NOS

√6ᵗʰ **K51.21 Ulcerative (chronic) proctitis** with complications

        K51.211 Ulcerative (chronic) proctitis with rectal bleeding   CC HCC

        K51.212 Ulcerative (chronic) proctitis with intestinal obstruction   CC HCC

        K51.213 Ulcerative (chronic) proctitis with fistula   CC HCC SW

        K51.214 Ulcerative (chronic) proctitis with abscess   CC HCC

        K51.218 Ulcerative (chronic) proctitis with other complication   CC HCC

        K51.219 Ulcerative (chronic) proctitis with unspecified complications   CC HCC

√5ᵗʰ **K51.3 Ulcerative (chronic) rectosigmoiditis**

     K51.30 Ulcerative (chronic) rectosigmoiditis without complications   CC HCC
Ulcerative (chronic) rectosigmoiditis NOS

√6ᵗʰ **K51.31 Ulcerative (chronic) rectosigmoiditis** with complications

        K51.311 Ulcerative (chronic) rectosigmoiditis with rectal bleeding   CC HCC

        K51.312 Ulcerative (chronic) rectosigmoiditis with intestinal obstruction   CC HCC

        K51.313 Ulcerative (chronic) rectosigmoiditis with fistula   CC HCC SW

        K51.314 Ulcerative (chronic) rectosigmoiditis with abscess   CC HCC

        K51.318 Ulcerative (chronic) rectosigmoiditis with other complication   CC HCC

        K51.319 Ulcerative (chronic) rectosigmoiditis with unspecified complications   CC HCC

√5ᵗʰ **K51.4 Inflammatory polyps of colon**
EXCLUDES 1   *adenomatous polyp of colon (D12.6)*
         polyposis of colon (D12.6)
         polyps of colon NOS (K63.5)

     K51.40 Inflammatory polyps of colon without complications   CC HCC
Inflammatory polyps of colon NOS

√6ᵗʰ **K51.41 Inflammatory polyps of colon** with complications

        K51.411 Inflammatory polyps of colon with rectal bleeding   CC HCC

        K51.412 Inflammatory polyps of colon with intestinal obstruction   CC HCC

        K51.413 Inflammatory polyps of colon with fistula   CC HCC SW

        K51.414 Inflammatory polyps of colon with abscess   CC HCC

        K51.418 Inflammatory polyps of colon with other complication   CC HCC

        K51.419 Inflammatory polyps of colon with unspecified complications   CC HCC

√5ᵗʰ **K51.5 Left sided colitis**
Left hemicolitis

     K51.50 Left sided colitis without complications   CC HCC
Left sided colitis NOS

√6ᵗʰ **K51.51 Left sided colitis** with complications

        K51.511 Left sided colitis with rectal bleeding   CC HCC

        K51.512 Left sided colitis with intestinal obstruction   CC HCC

        K51.513 Left sided colitis with fistula   CC HCC SW

        K51.514 Left sided colitis with abscess   CC HCC

        K51.518 Left sided colitis with other complication   CC HCC

        K51.519 Left sided colitis with unspecified complications   CC HCC

✓5ᵗʰ **K51.8** **Other ulcerative colitis**

K51.80 **Other ulcerative colitis** without complications `CC` `HCC`

✓6ᵗʰ **K51.81** **Other ulcerative colitis** with complications

K51.811 **Other ulcerative colitis with** rectal bleeding `CC` `HCC`

K51.812 **Other ulcerative colitis with** intestinal obstruction `CC` `HCC`

K51.813 **Other ulcerative colitis with** fistula `CC` `HCC` `SW`

K51.814 **Other ulcerative colitis with** abscess `CC` `HCC`

K51.818 **Other ulcerative colitis with other** complication `CC` `HCC`

K51.819 **Other ulcerative colitis with unspecified** complications `CC` `HCC`

✓5ᵗʰ **K51.9** **Ulcerative colitis, unspecified**

K51.90 **Ulcerative colitis, unspecified,** without complications `CC` `HCC`

✓6ᵗʰ **K51.91** **Ulcerative colitis, unspecified,** with complications

K51.911 **Ulcerative colitis, unspecified with** rectal bleeding `CC` `HCC`

K51.912 **Ulcerative colitis, unspecified with** intestinal obstruction `CC` `HCC`

K51.913 **Ulcerative colitis, unspecified with** fistula `CC` `HCC` `SW`

K51.914 **Ulcerative colitis, unspecified with** abscess `CC` `HCC`

K51.918 **Ulcerative colitis, unspecified with other** complication `CC` `HCC`

K51.919 **Ulcerative colitis, unspecified with** unspecified complications `CC` `HCC`

✓4ᵗʰ **K52** **Other and unspecified noninfective gastroenteritis and colitis**

AHA: 2016,4Q,30-31

K52.0 **Gastroenteritis and colitis due to** radiation `CC`

K52.1 **Toxic** gastroenteritis and colitis `CC`

Drug-induced gastroenteritis and colitis

Code first (T51-T65) to identify toxic agent

Use additional code for adverse effect, if applicable, to identify drug (T36-T50 with fifth or sixth character 5)

AHA: 2019,1Q,17

✓5ᵗʰ **K52.2** **Allergic and dietetic** gastroenteritis and colitis

Food hypersensitivity gastroenteritis or colitis

Use additional code to identify type of food allergy (Z91.01-, Z91.02-)

`EXCLUDES 2` allergic eosinophilic colitis (K52.82)

allergic eosinophilic esophagitis (K20.0)

allergic eosinophilic gastritis (K52.81)

allergic eosinophilic gastroenteritis (K52.81)

food protein-induced proctocolitis (K52.82)

DEF: True immunoglobulin E (IgE)-mediated allergic reaction of the lining of the stomach, intestines, or colon to food proteins. It causes nausea, vomiting, diarrhea, and abdominal cramping.

TIP: Assign a code for "with hemorrhage" when angiodysplasia and GI bleeding are documented. The ICD-10-CM classification assumes the two are related without the provider linking the two conditions. Evidence of bleeding during a procedure is not required.

K52.21 **Food protein-induced** enterocolitis syndrome

FPIES

Use additional code for hypovolemic shock, if present (R57.1)

K52.22 **Food protein-induced** enteropathy

K52.29 **Other allergic and dietetic gastroenteritis and colitis**

Food hypersensitivity gastroenteritis or colitis

Immediate gastrointestinal hypersensitivity

K52.3 **Indeterminate** colitis

Colonic inflammatory bowel disease unclassified (IBDU)

`EXCLUDES 1` unspecified colitis (K52.9)

✓5ᵗʰ **K52.8** **Other specified noninfective gastroenteritis and colitis**

K52.81 **Eosinophilic gastritis or gastroenteritis**

Eosinophilic enteritis

`EXCLUDES 2` eosinophilic esophagitis (K20.0)

DEF: Disorder involving the accumulation of eosinophil in the lining of the stomach or multiple levels of the gastrointestinal tract, but without a known cause such as connective tissue disease, drug reaction, malignancy, or parasitic infection.

K52.82 **Eosinophilic colitis**

Allergic proctocolitis

Food-induced eosinophilic proctocolitis

Food protein-induced proctocolitis

Milk protein-induced proctocolitis

DEF: Disorder involving the accumulation of eosinophil in the tissues lining the colon, but without a known cause such as connective tissue disease, drug reaction, malignancy, or parasitic infection. The resultant inflammation may cause extreme abdominal pain, diarrhea, or bloody stool.

✓6ᵗʰ **K52.83** **Microscopic colitis**

K52.831 **Collagenous** colitis

K52.832 **Lymphocytic** colitis

K52.838 **Other microscopic colitis**

K52.839 **Microscopic colitis, unspecified**

K52.89 **Other specified noninfective gastroenteritis and colitis**

AHA: 2019,1Q,20

K52.9 **Noninfective gastroenteritis and colitis, unspecified**

Colitis NOS

Enteritis NOS

Gastroenteritis NOS

Ileitis NOS

Jejunitis NOS

Sigmoiditis NOS

`EXCLUDES 1` diarrhea NOS (R19.7)

functional diarrhea (K59.1)

infectious gastroenteritis and colitis NOS (A09)

neonatal diarrhea (noninfective) (P78.3)

psychogenic diarrhea (F45.8)

Other diseases of intestines (K55-K64)

✓4ᵗʰ **K55** **Vascular disorders of intestine**

`EXCLUDES 1` necrotizing enterocolitis of newborn (P77.-)

AHA: 2016,4Q,32

✓5ᵗʰ **K55.0** **Acute vascular disorders of intestine**

Infarction of appendices epiploicae

Mesenteric (artery) (vein) embolism

Mesenteric (artery) (vein) infarction

Mesenteric (artery) (vein) thrombosis

AHA: 2019,4Q,68

✓6ᵗʰ **K55.01** **Acute (reversible)** ischemia of small intestine

K55.011 **Focal (segmental) acute (reversible)** ischemia of small intestine `MCC` `HCC`

K55.012 **Diffuse acute (reversible) ischemia of** small intestine `MCC` `HCC`

K55.019 **Acute (reversible) ischemia of small** intestine, extent unspecified `MCC` `HCC`

✓6ᵗʰ **K55.02** **Acute infarction of small intestine**

Gangrene of small intestine

Necrosis of small intestine

K55.021 **Focal (segmental) acute infarction of** small intestine `MCC` `HCC`

K55.022 **Diffuse acute infarction of small** intestine `MCC` `HCC`

K55.029 **Acute infarction of small intestine, extent** unspecified `MCC` `HCC`

✓6ᵗʰ **K55.03** **Acute (reversible)** ischemia of large intestine

Acute fulminant ischemic colitis

Subacute ischemic colitis

K55.031 **Focal (segmental) acute (reversible)** ischemia of large intestine `MCC` `HCC`

K55.032 **Diffuse acute (reversible) ischemia of** large intestine `MCC` `HCC`

K55.039   **Acute (reversible) ischemia of large intestine, extent unspecified** `MCC` `HCC`
AHA: 2019,4Q,68

✓6ᵗʰ   **K55.04**   **Acute infarction of large intestine**
Gangrene of large intestine
Necrosis of large intestine

     K55.041   **Focal (segmental) acute infarction of large intestine** `MCC` `HCC`

     K55.042   **Diffuse acute infarction of large intestine** `MCC` `HCC`

     K55.049   **Acute infarction of large intestine, extent unspecified** `MCC` `HCC`

✓6ᵗʰ   **K55.05**   **Acute (reversible) ischemia of intestine, part unspecified**

     K55.051   **Focal (segmental) acute (reversible) ischemia of intestine, part unspecified** `MCC` `HCC`

     K55.052   **Diffuse acute (reversible) ischemia of intestine, part unspecified** `MCC` `HCC`

     K55.059   **Acute (reversible) ischemia of intestine, part and extent unspecified** `MCC` `HCC`

✓6ᵗʰ   **K55.06**   **Acute infarction of intestine, part unspecified**
Acute intestinal infarction
Gangrene of intestine
Necrosis of intestine

     K55.061   **Focal (segmental) acute infarction of intestine, part unspecified** `MCC` `HCC`

     K55.062   **Diffuse acute infarction of intestine, part unspecified** `MCC` `HCC`

     K55.069   **Acute infarction of intestine, part and extent unspecified** `MCC` `HCC`

K55.1   **Chronic vascular disorders of intestine** `CC` `HCC`
Chronic ischemic colitis
Chronic ischemic enteritis
Chronic ischemic enterocolitis
Ischemic stricture of intestine
Mesenteric atherosclerosis
Mesenteric vascular insufficiency

✓5ᵗʰ   **K55.2**   **Angiodysplasia of colon**

AHA: 2018,3Q,21
TIP: Assign a code for "with hemorrhage" when angiodysplasia and GI bleeding are documented. The ICD-10-CM classification assumes the two are related without the provider linking the two conditions. Evidence of bleeding during a procedure is not required.

     K55.20   **Angiodysplasia of colon without hemorrhage**

     K55.21   **Angiodysplasia of colon with hemorrhage** `MCC`
DEF: Small vascular abnormalities due to fragile blood vessels in the colon, resulting in blood loss from the gastrointestinal (GI) tract.

✓5ᵗʰ   **K55.3**   **Necrotizing enterocolitis**

     EXCLUDES 1   *necrotizing enterocolitis of newborn (P77.-)*
     EXCLUDES 2   *necrotizing enterocolitis due to Clostridium difficile (A04.7-)*

     K55.30   **Necrotizing enterocolitis, unspecified** `MCC` `HCC`
Necrotizing enterocolitis, NOS

     K55.31   **Stage 1 necrotizing enterocolitis** `MCC` `HCC`
Necrotizing enterocolitis without pneumatosis, without perforation

     K55.32   **Stage 2 necrotizing enterocolitis** `MCC` `HCC`
Necrotizing enterocolitis with pneumatosis, without perforation

     K55.33   **Stage 3 necrotizing enterocolitis** `MCC` `HCC`
Necrotizing enterocolitis with perforation
Necrotizing enterocolitis with pneumatosis and perforation

K55.8   **Other vascular disorders of intestine** `CC` `HCC`

K55.9   **Vascular disorder of intestine, unspecified** `CC` `HCC`
Ischemic colitis
Ischemic enteritis
Ischemic enterocolitis

✓4ᵗʰ   **K56**   **Paralytic ileus and intestinal obstruction without hernia**

     EXCLUDES 1   *congenital stricture or stenosis of intestine (Q41-Q42)*
         cystic fibrosis with meconium ileus (E84.11)
         ischemic stricture of intestine (K55.1)
         meconium ileus NOS (P76.0)
         neonatal intestinal obstructions classifiable to P76.-
         obstruction of duodenum (K31.5)
         postprocedural intestinal obstruction (K91.3-)
         ~~*stenosis of anus or rectum (K62.4)*~~

     EXCLUDES 2   ▶*stenosis of anus or rectum (K62.4)*◄

K56.0   **Paralytic ileus** `CC` `HCC`
Paralysis of bowel
Paralysis of colon
Paralysis of intestine

     EXCLUDES 1   *gallstone ileus (K56.3)*
         ileus NOS (K56.7)
         obstructive ileus NOS (K56.69-)

DEF: Intestinal obstruction due to paralysis of bowel motility or peristalsis.

K56.1   **Intussusception** `CC` `HCC`
Intussusception or invagination of bowel
Intussusception or invagination of colon
Intussusception or invagination of intestine
Intussusception or invagination of rectum

     EXCLUDES 2   *intussusception of appendix (K38.8)*

DEF: Intestinal obstruction due to prolapse of a bowel section into an adjacent section. It occurs primarily in children and symptoms include acute abdominal pain, vomiting, and passage of blood and mucus from the rectum.

K56.2   **Volvulus** `MCC` `HCC`
Strangulation of colon or intestine
Torsion of colon or intestine
Twist of colon or intestine

     EXCLUDES 2   *volvulus of duodenum (K31.5)*

DEF: Twisting, knotting, or entanglement of the bowel on itself that may quickly compromise oxygen supply to the intestinal tissues. A volvulus usually occurs at the sigmoid and ileocecal areas of the intestines.

Volvulus

Knotted intestine (volvulus)

K56.3   **Gallstone ileus** `CC` `HCC`
Obstruction of intestine by gallstone

✓5ᵗʰ   **K56.4**   **Other impaction of intestine**

     K56.41   **Fecal impaction** `HCC`
         EXCLUDES 1   *constipation (K59.0-)*
                 incomplete defecation (R15.0)

     K56.49   **Other impaction of intestine** `CC` `HCC`

✓ Additional Character Required   ✓x7ᵗʰ Placeholder   Unacceptable PDx   Questionable PDx   Manifestation   Unspecified Dx   `H1`-`H14` HAC   `HCC` CMS-HCC Dx   `HIV` HIV Dx

√5ᵗʰ **K56.5** Intestinal adhesions [bands] with obstruction (postinfection)
Abdominal hernia due to adhesions with obstruction
Peritoneal adhesions [bands] with intestinal obstruction (postinfection)
AHA: 2017,4Q,16-17

    K56.50 Intestinal adhesions [bands], unspecified as to partial versus complete obstruction CC HCC
Intestinal adhesions with obstruction NOS

    K56.51 Intestinal adhesions [bands], with partial obstruction CC HCC
Intestinal adhesions with incomplete obstruction

    K56.52 Intestinal adhesions [bands] with complete obstruction CC HCC

√5ᵗʰ **K56.6** Other and unspecified intestinal obstruction
AHA: 2017,4Q,16-17; 2017,2Q,12

   √6ᵗʰ **K56.60** Unspecified intestinal obstruction
     EXCLUDES 1   *intestinal obstruction due to specified condition - code to condition*

     K56.600 Partial intestinal obstruction, unspecified as to cause CC HCC
Incomplete intestinal obstruction, NOS

     K56.601 Complete intestinal obstruction, unspecified as to cause CC HCC

     K56.609 Unspecified intestinal obstruction, unspecified as to partial versus complete obstruction CC HCC
Intestinal obstruction NOS

   √6ᵗʰ **K56.69** Other intestinal obstruction
Enterostenosis NOS
Obstructive ileus NOS
Occlusion of colon or intestine NOS
Stenosis of colon or intestine NOS
Stricture of colon or intestine NOS
     EXCLUDES 1   *intestinal obstruction due to specified condition - code to condition*

     K56.690 Other partial intestinal obstruction CC HCC
Other incomplete intestinal obstruction

     K56.691 Other complete intestinal obstruction CC HCC

     K56.699 Other intestinal obstruction unspecified as to partial versus complete obstruction CC HCC
Other intestinal obstruction, NEC

   K56.7 Ileus, unspecified CC HCC
     EXCLUDES 1   *obstructive ileus (K56.69-)*
     EXCLUDES 2   *intestinal obstruction with hernia (K40-K46)*
     AHA: 2017,1Q,40

√4ᵗʰ **K57** Diverticular disease of intestine
Code also if applicable peritonitis K65.-
     EXCLUDES 1   *congenital diverticulum of intestine (Q43.8)*
         Meckel's diverticulum (Q43.0)
     EXCLUDES 2   *diverticulum of appendix (K38.2)*
     AHA: 2018,3Q,21
     TIP: Assign a code for "with bleeding" when diverticular disease of the intestine and GI bleeding are documented. The ICD-10-CM classification assumes the two are related without the provider linking the two conditions. Evidence of bleeding during a procedure is not required.

   √5ᵗʰ **K57.0** Diverticulitis of small intestine with perforation and abscess
Diverticulitis of small intestine with peritonitis
     EXCLUDES 1   *diverticulitis of both small and large intestine with perforation and abscess (K57.4-)*

    K57.00 Diverticulitis of small intestine with perforation and abscess without bleeding CC

    K57.01 Diverticulitis of small intestine with perforation and abscess with bleeding MCC

   √5ᵗʰ **K57.1** Diverticular disease of small intestine without perforation or abscess
     EXCLUDES 1   *diverticular disease of both small and large intestine without perforation or abscess (K57.5-)*

    K57.10 Diverticulosis of small intestine without perforation or abscess without bleeding
Diverticular disease of small intestine NOS

    K57.11 Diverticulosis of small intestine without perforation or abscess with bleeding MCC

    K57.12 Diverticulitis of small intestine without perforation or abscess without bleeding CC

    K57.13 Diverticulitis of small intestine without perforation or abscess with bleeding MCC

   √5ᵗʰ **K57.2** Diverticulitis of large intestine with perforation and abscess
Diverticulitis of colon with peritonitis
     EXCLUDES 1   *diverticulitis of both small and large intestine with perforation and abscess (K57.4-)*

    K57.20 Diverticulitis of large intestine with perforation and abscess without bleeding CC

    K57.21 Diverticulitis of large intestine with perforation and abscess with bleeding MCC

   √5ᵗʰ **K57.3** Diverticular disease of large intestine without perforation or abscess
     EXCLUDES 1   *diverticular disease of both small and large intestine without perforation or abscess (K57.5-)*

    K57.30 Diverticulosis of large intestine without perforation or abscess without bleeding
Diverticular disease of colon NOS

    K57.31 Diverticulosis of large intestine without perforation or abscess with bleeding MCC

    K57.32 Diverticulitis of large intestine without perforation or abscess without bleeding CC

    K57.33 Diverticulitis of large intestine without perforation or abscess with bleeding MCC

   √5ᵗʰ **K57.4** Diverticulitis of both small and large intestine with perforation and abscess
Diverticulitis of both small and large intestine with peritonitis

    K57.40 Diverticulitis of both small and large intestine with perforation and abscess without bleeding CC

    K57.41 Diverticulitis of both small and large intestine with perforation and abscess with bleeding MCC

   √5ᵗʰ **K57.5** Diverticular disease of both small and large intestine without perforation or abscess

    K57.50 Diverticulosis of both small and large intestine without perforation or abscess without bleeding
Diverticular disease of both small and large intestine NOS

    K57.51 Diverticulosis of both small and large intestine without perforation or abscess with bleeding MCC

    K57.52 Diverticulitis of both small and large intestine without perforation or abscess without bleeding CC

    K57.53 Diverticulitis of both small and large intestine without perforation or abscess with bleeding MCC

   √5ᵗʰ **K57.8** Diverticulitis of intestine, part unspecified, with perforation and abscess
Diverticulitis of intestine NOS with peritonitis

    K57.80 Diverticulitis of intestine, part unspecified, with perforation and abscess without bleeding CC

    K57.81 Diverticulitis of intestine, part unspecified, with perforation and abscess with bleeding MCC

   √5ᵗʰ **K57.9** Diverticular disease of intestine, part unspecified, without perforation or abscess

    K57.90 Diverticulosis of intestine, part unspecified, without perforation or abscess without bleeding
Diverticular disease of intestine NOS

    K57.91 Diverticulosis of intestine, part unspecified, without perforation or abscess with bleeding MCC

    K57.92 Diverticulitis of intestine, part unspecified, without perforation or abscess without bleeding CC

    K57.93 Diverticulitis of intestine, part unspecified, without perforation or abscess with bleeding MCC

√4ᵗʰ **K58** Irritable bowel syndrome
     INCLUDES   irritable colon
         spastic colon
     AHA: 2016,4Q,32-33

   K58.0 Irritable bowel syndrome with diarrhea

   K58.1 Irritable bowel syndrome with constipation

   K58.2 Mixed irritable bowel syndrome

   K58.8 Other irritable bowel syndrome

   K58.9 Irritable bowel syndrome without diarrhea
Irritable bowel syndrome NOS

✔4ᵗʰ K59 Other functional intestinal disorders

EXCLUDES 1   change in bowel habit NOS (R19.4)
           intestinal malabsorption (K90.-)
           psychogenic intestinal disorders (F45.8)

EXCLUDES 2   functional disorders of stomach (K31.-)

✔5ᵗʰ K59.0 Constipation

EXCLUDES 1   fecal impaction (K56.41)
           incomplete defecation (R15.0)

AHA: 2016,4Q,33

K59.00 Constipation, unspecified

K59.01 Slow transit constipation
   DEF: Delay in the transit of fecal material through the colon secondary to smooth muscle dysfunction or decreased peristaltic contractions along the colon.

K59.02 Outlet dysfunction constipation

K59.03 Drug induced constipation
   Use additional code for adverse effect, if applicable, to identify drug (T36-T50 with fifth or sixth character 5)

K59.04 Chronic idiopathic constipation
   Functional constipation

K59.09 Other constipation
   Chronic constipation

K59.1 Functional diarrhea

EXCLUDES 1   diarrhea NOS (R19.7)
           irritable bowel syndrome with diarrhea (K58.0)

K59.2 Neurogenic bowel, not elsewhere classified   cc
   DEF: Disorder of bowel due to a spinal cord lesion due to injury or as a complication of conditions such as multiple sclerosis (MS) or spina bifida. Loss of bowel control is the primary symptom, manifested as constipation or bowel incontinence.

✔5ᵗʰ K59.3 Megacolon, not elsewhere classified

Dilatation of colon

Code first, if applicable (T51-T65) to identify toxic agent

EXCLUDES 1   congenital megacolon (aganglionic) (Q43.1)
           megacolon (due to) (in) Chagas' disease (B57.32)
           megacolon (due to) (in) Clostridium difficile (A04.7-)
           megacolon (due to) (in) Hirschsprung's disease (Q43.1)

AHA: 2016,4Q,33-34

K59.31 Toxic megacolon   cc HCC

K59.39 Other megacolon   cc
   Megacolon NOS

K59.4 Anal spasm
Proctalgia fugax

▲ ✔5ᵗʰ K59.8 Other specified functional intestinal disorders

~~Atony of colon~~

~~Pseudo-obstruction (acute) (chronic) of intestine~~

● **K59.81 Ogilvie syndrome**
   Acute colonic pseudo-obstruction (ACPO)

● **K59.89 Other specified functional intestinal disorders**
   Atony of colon
   Pseudo-obstruction (acute) (chronic) of intestine

K59.9 Functional intestinal disorder, unspecified

✔4ᵗʰ K60 Fissure and fistula of anal and rectal regions

EXCLUDES 1   fissure and fistula of anal and rectal regions with abscess or cellulitis (K61.-)

EXCLUDES 2   anal sphincter tear (healed) (nontraumatic) (old) (K62.81)

K60.0 Acute anal fissure

K60.1 Chronic anal fissure

K60.2 Anal fissure, unspecified

K60.3 Anal fistula   SW

K60.4 Rectal fistula   SW
Fistula of rectum to skin

EXCLUDES 1   rectovaginal fistula (N82.3)
           vesicorectal fistual (N32.1)

K60.5 Anorectal fistula   SW

✔4ᵗʰ K61 Abscess of anal and rectal regions

INCLUDES   abscess of anal and rectal regions
           cellulitis of anal and rectal regions

K61.0 Anal abscess   cc
Perianal abscess

EXCLUDES 2   intrasphincteric abscess (K61.4)

K61.1 Rectal abscess   cc
Perirectal abscess

EXCLUDES 1   ischiorectal abscess (K61.39)

AHA: 2012,4Q,104

K61.2 Anorectal abscess   cc

✔5ᵗʰ K61.3 Ischiorectal abscess

AHA: 2018,4Q,19

K61.31 Horseshoe abscess

K61.39 Other ischiorectal abscess
   Abscess of ischiorectal fossa
   Ischiorectal abscess, NOS

K61.4 Intrasphincteric abscess   cc
Intersphincteric abscess

K61.5 Supralevator abscess
AHA: 2018,4Q,19

✔4ᵗʰ K62 Other diseases of anus and rectum

INCLUDES   anal canal

EXCLUDES 2   colostomy and enterostomy malfunction (K94.0-, K94.1-)
           fecal incontinence (R15.-)
           hemorrhoids (K64.-)

K62.0 Anal polyp

K62.1 Rectal polyp

EXCLUDES 1   adenomatous polyp (D12.8)

AHA: 2018,1Q,6

K62.2 Anal prolapse
Prolapse of anal canal

K62.3 Rectal prolapse
Prolapse of rectal mucosa

K62.4 Stenosis of anus and rectum
Stricture of anus (sphincter)

AHA: 2019,2Q,13

K62.5 Hemorrhage of anus and rectum   cc

EXCLUDES 1   gastrointestinal bleeding NOS (K92.2)
           melena (K92.1)
           neonatal rectal hemorrhage (P54.2)

AHA: 2019,1Q,21

K62.6 Ulcer of anus and rectum   cc
Solitary ulcer of anus and rectum
Stercoral ulcer of anus and rectum

EXCLUDES 1   fissure and fistula of anus and rectum (K60.-)
           ulcerative colitis (K51.-)

K62.7 Radiation proctitis
▶Use additional code to identify the type of radiation (W88.-) or radiation therapy (Y84.2)◀

AHA: 2019,1Q,21

✔5ᵗʰ K62.8 Other specified diseases of anus and rectum

EXCLUDES 2   ulcerative proctitis (K51.2)

K62.81 Anal sphincter tear (healed) (nontraumatic) (old)
   Tear of anus, nontraumatic
   Use additional code for any associated fecal incontinence (R15.-)

   EXCLUDES 2   anal fissure (K60.-)
                anal sphincter tear (healed) (old) complicating delivery (O34.7-)
                traumatic tear of anal sphincter (S31.831)

K62.82 Dysplasia of anus
   Anal intraepithelial neoplasia I and II (AIN I and II) (histologically confirmed)
   Dysplasia of anus NOS
   Mild and moderate dysplasia of anus (histologically confirmed)

   EXCLUDES 1   abnormal results from anal cytologic examination without histologic confirmation (R85.61-)
                anal intraepithelial neoplasia III (D01.3)
                carcinoma in situ of anus (D01.3)
                HGSIL of anus (R85.613)
                severe dysplasia of anus (D01.3)

K62.89 Other specified diseases of anus and rectum
   Proctitis NOS
   Use additional code for any associated fecal incontinence (R15.-)

K62.9 Disease of anus and rectum, unspecified

☑ Additional Character Required   ✔x7ᵗʰ Placeholder   Unacceptable PDx   Questionable PDx   Manifestation   Unspecified Dx   H1-H14 HAC   HCC CMS-HCC Dx   HIV HIV Dx

ICD-10-CM 2021   721

✓4th K63 Other diseases of intestine

K63.Ø Abscess of intestine `CC`
EXCLUDES 1   abscess of intestine with Crohn's disease (K50.014,
K50.114, K50.814, K50.914)
abscess of intestine with diverticular disease (K57.0,
K57.2, K57.4, K57.8)
abscess of intestine with ulcerative colitis (K51.014,
K51.214, K51.314, K51.414, K51.514, K51.814,
K51.914)
EXCLUDES 2   abscess of anal and rectal regions (K61.-)
abscess of appendix (K35.3-)

K63.1 Perforation of intestine (nontraumatic) `MCC` `HCC`
Perforation (nontraumatic) of rectum
EXCLUDES 1   perforation (nontraumatic) of duodenum (K26.-)
perforation (nontraumatic) of intestine with
diverticular disease (K57.0, K57.2, K57.4, K57.8)
EXCLUDES 2   perforation (nontraumatic) of appendix (K35.2-,
K35.3-)
AHA: 2020,2Q,22

K63.2 Fistula of intestine `CC` `SW`
EXCLUDES 1   fistula of duodenum (K31.6)
fistula of intestine with Crohn's disease (K50.013,
K50.113, K50.813, K50.913)
fistula of intestine with ulcerative colitis (K51.013,
K51.213, K51.313, K51.413, K51.513, K51.813,
K51.913)
EXCLUDES 2   fistula of anal and rectal regions (K60.-)
fistula of appendix (K38.3)
intestinal-genital fistula, female (N82.2-N82.4)
vesicointestinal fistula (N32.1)
AHA: 2017,3Q,4

K63.3 Ulcer of intestine `CC`
Primary ulcer of small intestine
EXCLUDES 1   duodenal ulcer (K26.-)
gastrointestinal ulcer (K28.-)
gastrojejunal ulcer (K28.-)
jejunal ulcer (K28.-)
peptic ulcer, site unspecified (K27.-)
ulcer of intestine with perforation (K63.1)
ulcer of anus or rectum (K62.6)
ulcerative colitis (K51.-)

K63.4 Enteroptosis

K63.5 Polyp of colon
EXCLUDES 1   adenomatous polyp of colon (D12.-)
inflammatory polyp of colon (K51.4-)
polyposis of colon (D12.6)
AHA: 2019,1Q,33; 2018,2Q,14; 2017,1Q,15; 2015,2Q,14
TIP: Assign this code when documentation states hyperplastic
colon polyp regardless of the site in the colon. Slow-growing,
hyperplastic polyps are not precancerous and are classified
differently from benign or adenomatous polyps.

✓5th K63.8 Other specified diseases of intestine

K63.81 Dieulafoy lesion of intestine `MCC`
EXCLUDES 2   Dieulafoy lesion of stomach and
duodenum (K31.82)
DEF: Abnormally large submucosal artery protruding
through a defect in the stomach mucosa or intestines
that can cause massive and life-threatening
hemorrhaging.

K63.89 Other specified diseases of intestine
AHA: 2013,2Q,31

K63.9 Disease of intestine, unspecified

✓4th K64 Hemorrhoids and perianal venous thrombosis
INCLUDES   piles
EXCLUDES 1   hemorrhoids complicating childbirth and the puerperium
(O87.2)
hemorrhoids complicating pregnancy (O22.4)

Hemorrhoids

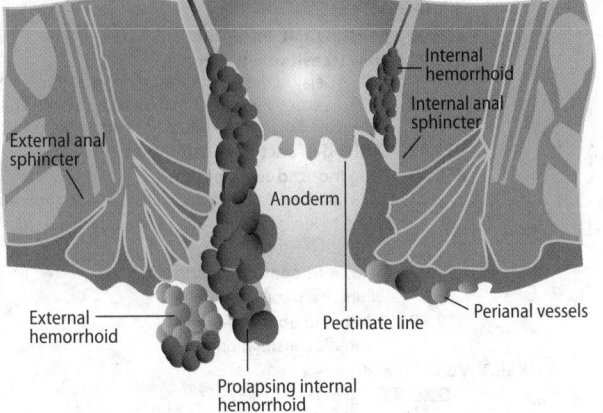

Internal hemorrhoid
Internal anal sphincter
External anal sphincter
Anoderm
External hemorrhoid
Pectinate line
Perianal vessels
Prolapsing internal hemorrhoid

K64.Ø First degree hemorrhoids
Grade/stage I hemorrhoids
Hemorrhoids (bleeding) without prolapse outside of anal canal

K64.1 Second degree hemorrhoids
Grade/stage II hemorrhoids
Hemorrhoids (bleeding) that prolapse with straining, but retract
spontaneously

K64.2 Third degree hemorrhoids
Grade/stage III hemorrhoids
Hemorrhoids (bleeding) that prolapse with straining and require
manual replacement back inside anal canal

K64.3 Fourth degree hemorrhoids
Grade/stage IV hemorrhoids
Hemorrhoids (bleeding) with prolapsed tissue that cannot be
manually replaced

K64.4 Residual hemorrhoidal skin tags
External hemorrhoids, NOS
Skin tags of anus

K64.5 Perianal venous thrombosis
External hemorrhoids with thrombosis
Perianal hematoma
Thrombosed hemorrhoids NOS

K64.8 Other hemorrhoids
Internal hemorrhoids, without mention of degree
Prolapsed hemorrhoids, degree not specified

K64.9 Unspecified hemorrhoids
Hemorrhoids (bleeding) NOS
Hemorrhoids (bleeding) without mention of degree

Diseases of peritoneum and retroperitoneum (K65-K68)

✓4ᵗʰ K65 Peritonitis

Use additional code (B95-B97), to identify infectious agent, if known
Code also if applicable diverticular disease of intestine (K57.-)

EXCLUDES 1   acute appendicitis with generalized peritonitis (K35.2-)
     aseptic peritonitis (T81.6)
     benign paroxysmal peritonitis (E85.0)
     chemical peritonitis (T81.6)
     gonococcal peritonitis (A54.85)
     neonatal peritonitis (P78.0-P78.1)
     pelvic peritonitis, female (N73.3-N73.5)
     periodic familial peritonitis (E85.0)
     peritonitis due to talc or other foreign substance (T81.6)
     peritonitis in chlamydia (A74.81)
     peritonitis in diphtheria (A36.89)
     peritonitis in syphilis (late) (A52.74)
     peritonitis in tuberculosis (A18.31)
     peritonitis with or following abortion or ectopic or molar
       pregnancy (O00-O07, O08.0)
     peritonitis with or following appendicitis (K35.-)
     puerperal peritonitis (O85)
     retroperitoneal infections (K68.-)

K65.0 Generalized (acute) peritonitis   `MCC` `HCC`
Pelvic peritonitis (acute), male
Subphrenic peritonitis (acute)
Suppurative peritonitis (acute)

K65.1 Peritoneal abscess   `MCC` `HCC`
Abdominopelvic abscess
Abscess (of) omentum
Abscess (of) peritoneum
Mesenteric abscess
Retrocecal abscess
Subdiaphragmatic abscess
Subhepatic abscess
Subphrenic abscess
AHA: 2019,1Q,15

K65.2 Spontaneous bacterial peritonitis   `MCC` `HCC`
EXCLUDES 1   bacterial peritonitis NOS (K65.9)

K65.3 Choleperitonitis   `MCC` `HCC`
Peritonitis due to bile
DEF: Inflammation of the peritoneum due to leakage of bile into
the peritoneal cavity resulting from rupture of the bile passages
or gallbladder.

K65.4 Sclerosing mesenteritis   `CC` `HCC`
Fat necrosis of peritoneum
(Idiopathic) sclerosing mesenteric fibrosis
Mesenteric lipodystrophy
Mesenteric panniculitis
Retractile mesenteritis

K65.8 Other peritonitis   `MCC` `HCC`
Chronic proliferative peritonitis
Peritonitis due to urine

K65.9 Peritonitis, unspecified   `MCC` `HCC`
Bacterial peritonitis NOS
AHA: 2013,2Q,31

✓4ᵗʰ K66 Other disorders of peritoneum

EXCLUDES 2   ascites (R18.-)
     peritoneal effusion (chronic) (R18.8)

K66.0 Peritoneal adhesions (postprocedural) (postinfection)
Adhesions (of) abdominal (wall)
Adhesions (of) diaphragm
Adhesions (of) intestine
Adhesions (of) male pelvis
Adhesions (of) omentum
Adhesions (of) stomach
Adhesive bands
Mesenteric adhesions
EXCLUDES 1   female pelvic adhesions [bands] (N73.6)
     peritoneal adhesions with intestinal obstruction
       (K56.5-)

K66.1 Hemoperitoneum   `MCC`
EXCLUDES 1   traumatic hemoperitoneum (S36.8-)

K66.8 Other specified disorders of peritoneum

K66.9 Disorder of peritoneum, unspecified

K67 Disorders of peritoneum in infectious diseases classified elsewhere   `MCC` `HCC`

Code first underlying disease, such as:
congenital syphilis (A50.0)
helminthiasis (B65.0-B83.9)

EXCLUDES 1   peritonitis in chlamydia (A74.81)
     peritonitis in diphtheria (A36.89)
     peritonitis in gonococcal (A54.85)
     peritonitis in syphilis (late) (A52.74)
     peritonitis in tuberculosis (A18.31)

✓4ᵗʰ K68 Disorders of retroperitoneum

✓5ᵗʰ K68.1 Retroperitoneal abscess

K68.11 Postprocedural retroperitoneal abscess   `CC` `H11` `H12` `H13`
EXCLUDES 2   infection following procedure (T81.4-)

K68.12 Psoas muscle abscess   `MCC` `HCC`

K68.19 Other retroperitoneal abscess   `MCC` `HCC`
AHA: 2019,1Q,15
TIP: This code should be used for a diagnosis of internal
presacral abscess. If an intra-abdominal abscess is also
present, code K65.1 can also be assigned; sequencing
depends on the circumstances of admission.

K68.9 Other disorders of retroperitoneum   `MCC`

Diseases of liver (K70-K77)

EXCLUDES 1   jaundice NOS (R17)
EXCLUDES 2   hemochromatosis (E83.11-)
     Reye's syndrome (G93.7)
     viral hepatitis (B15-B19)
     Wilson's disease (E83.0)

✓4ᵗʰ K70 Alcoholic liver disease

Use additional code to identify:
alcohol abuse and dependence (F10.-)

K70.0 Alcoholic fatty liver   `A`

✓5ᵗʰ K70.1 Alcoholic hepatitis

K70.10 Alcoholic hepatitis without ascites   `A`
K70.11 Alcoholic hepatitis with ascites   `A`

K70.2 Alcoholic fibrosis and sclerosis of liver   `A`

✓5ᵗʰ K70.3 Alcoholic cirrhosis of liver

Alcoholic cirrhosis NOS

K70.30 Alcoholic cirrhosis of liver without ascites   `HCC` `A`
K70.31 Alcoholic cirrhosis of liver with ascites   `HCC` `A`
AHA: 2018,1Q,4

✓5ᵗʰ K70.4 Alcoholic hepatic failure

Acute alcoholic hepatic failure
Alcoholic hepatic failure NOS
Chronic alcoholic hepatic failure
Subacute alcoholic hepatic failure

K70.40 Alcoholic hepatic failure without coma   `HCC` `A`
K70.41 Alcoholic hepatic failure with coma   `MCC` `HCC` `A`

K70.9 Alcoholic liver disease, unspecified   `HCC` `A`

✓4ᵗʰ K71 Toxic liver disease

INCLUDES   drug-induced idiosyncratic (unpredictable) liver disease
     drug-induced toxic (predictable) liver disease

Code first poisoning due to drug or toxin, if applicable (T36-T65 with
fifth or sixth character 1-4 or 6)
Use additional code for adverse effect, if applicable, to identify drug
(T36-T50 with fifth or sixth character 5)

EXCLUDES 2   alcoholic liver disease (K70.-)
     Budd-Chiari syndrome (I82.0)

K71.0 Toxic liver disease with cholestasis
Cholestasis with hepatocyte injury
"Pure" cholestasis

✓5ᵗʰ K71.1 Toxic liver disease with hepatic necrosis

Hepatic failure (acute) (chronic) due to drugs

K71.10 Toxic liver disease with hepatic necrosis, without coma
K71.11 Toxic liver disease with hepatic necrosis, with coma   `MCC` `HCC`

K71.2 Toxic liver disease with acute hepatitis
K71.3 Toxic liver disease with chronic persistent hepatitis
K71.4 Toxic liver disease with chronic lobular hepatitis

K71.5 **Toxic liver disease with** chronic active hepatitis
Toxic liver disease with lupoid hepatitis

K71.50 **Toxic liver disease with chronic active hepatitis** without ascites

K71.51 **Toxic liver disease with chronic active hepatitis** with ascites
AHA: 2018,1Q,4

K71.6 **Toxic liver disease with** hepatitis, not elsewhere classified

K71.7 **Toxic liver disease with** fibrosis and cirrhosis of liver

K71.8 **Toxic liver disease with other disorders of liver**
Toxic liver disease with focal nodular hyperplasia
Toxic liver disease with hepatic granulomas
Toxic liver disease with peliosis hepatis
Toxic liver disease with veno-occlusive disease of liver

K71.9 **Toxic liver disease, unspecified**

K72 **Hepatic failure, not elsewhere classified**

INCLUDES fulminant hepatitis NEC, with hepatic failure
hepatic encephalopathy NOS
liver (cell) necrosis with hepatic failure
malignant hepatitis NEC, with hepatic failure
yellow liver atrophy or dystrophy

EXCLUDES 1 *alcoholic hepatic failure (K70.4)*
hepatic failure with toxic liver disease (K71.1-)
icterus of newborn (P55-P59)
postprocedural hepatic failure (K91.82)

EXCLUDES 2 *hepatic failure complicating abortion or ectopic or molar pregnancy (O00-O07, O08.8)*
hepatic failure complicating pregnancy, childbirth and the puerperium (O26.6-)
viral hepatitis with hepatic coma (B15-B19)

AHA: 2017,1Q,41

K72.0 **Acute and subacute hepatic failure**
Acute non-viral hepatitis NOS
AHA: 2015,2Q,17; 2014,2Q,13

K72.00 **Acute and subacute hepatic failure** without coma MCC

K72.01 **Acute and subacute hepatic failure** with coma MCC HCC

K72.1 **Chronic hepatic failure**

K72.10 **Chronic hepatic failure** without coma HCC
K72.11 **Chronic hepatic failure** with coma MCC HCC

K72.9 **Hepatic failure, unspecified**

K72.90 **Hepatic failure, unspecified** without coma HCC
AHA: 2018,4Q,20; 2016,2Q,35

K72.91 **Hepatic failure, unspecified** with coma MCC HCC
Hepatic coma NOS

K73 **Chronic hepatitis, not elsewhere classified**

EXCLUDES 1 *alcoholic hepatitis (chronic) (K70.1-)*
drug-induced hepatitis (chronic) (K71.-)
granulomatous hepatitis (chronic) NEC (K75.3)
reactive, nonspecific hepatitis (chronic) (K75.2)
viral hepatitis (chronic) (B15-B19)

K73.0 **Chronic** persistent **hepatitis, not elsewhere classified** HCC
K73.1 **Chronic** lobular **hepatitis, not elsewhere classified** HCC
K73.2 **Chronic** active **hepatitis, not elsewhere classified** HCC
K73.8 **Other chronic hepatitis, not elsewhere classified** HCC
K73.9 **Chronic hepatitis, unspecified** HCC

K74 **Fibrosis and cirrhosis of liver**
Code also, if applicable, viral hepatitis (acute) (chronic) (B15-B19)

EXCLUDES 1 *alcoholic cirrhosis (of liver) (K70.3)*
alcoholic fibrosis of liver (K70.2)
cardiac sclerosis of liver (K76.1)
cirrhosis (of liver) with toxic liver disease (K71.7)
congenital cirrhosis (of liver) (P78.81)
pigmentary cirrhosis (of liver) (E83.110)

▲ **K74.0** **Hepatic** fibrosis
►Code first underlying liver disease, such as:◄
►nonalcoholic steatohepatitis (NASH) (K75.81)◄

● **K74.00** **Hepatic fibrosis, unspecified**

● **K74.01** **Hepatic fibrosis,** early fibrosis
Hepatic fibrosis, stage F1 or stage F2

● **K74.02** **Hepatic fibrosis,** advanced fibrosis
Hepatic fibrosis, stage F3
EXCLUDES 1 *cirrhosis of liver (K74.6-)*
hepatic fibrosis, stage F4 (K74.6-)

K74.1 **Hepatic** sclerosis
K74.2 **Hepatic** fibrosis with hepatic sclerosis
K74.3 **Primary biliary cirrhosis** HCC
Chronic nonsuppurative destructive cholangitis
Primary biliary cholangitis
EXCLUDES 2 *primary sclerosing cholangitis (K83.01)*

K74.4 **Secondary biliary cirrhosis** HCC
K74.5 **Biliary cirrhosis, unspecified** HCC

K74.6 **Other and unspecified cirrhosis of liver**

K74.60 **Unspecified cirrhosis of liver** HCC
Cirrhosis (of liver) NOS
AHA: 2018,1Q,4

K74.69 **Other cirrhosis of liver** HCC
Cryptogenic cirrhosis (of liver)
Macronodular cirrhosis (of liver)
Micronodular cirrhosis (of liver)
Mixed type cirrhosis (of liver)
Portal cirrhosis (of liver)
Postnecrotic cirrhosis (of liver)

K75 **Other inflammatory liver diseases**
EXCLUDES 2 *toxic liver disease (K71.-)*

K75.0 **Abscess of liver** MCC
Cholangitic hepatic abscess
Hematogenic hepatic abscess
Hepatic abscess NOS
Lymphogenic hepatic abscess
Pylephlebitic hepatic abscess
EXCLUDES 1 *amebic liver abscess (A06.4)*
cholangitis without liver abscess (K83.09)
pylephlebitis without liver abscess (K75.1)
EXCLUDES 2 *acute or subacute hepatitis NOS (B17.9)*
acute or subacute non-viral hepatitis (K72.0)
chronic hepatitis NEC (K73.8)

K75.1 **Phlebitis of portal vein** MCC
Pylephlebitis
EXCLUDES 1 *pylephlebitic liver abscess (K75.0)*
DEF: Inflammation of the portal vein or branches due to diverticulitis, perforated appendicitis, or peritonitis. Symptoms include fever, chills, jaundice, sweating, and abscess in various body parts.

K75.2 **Nonspecific reactive hepatitis**
EXCLUDES 1 *acute or subacute hepatitis (K72.0-)*
chronic hepatitis NEC (K73.-)
viral hepatitis (B15-B19)

K75.3 **Granulomatous hepatitis, not elsewhere classified**
EXCLUDES 1 *acute or subacute hepatitis (K72.0-)*
chronic hepatitis NEC (K73.-)
viral hepatitis (B15-B19)

K75.4 **Autoimmune hepatitis** HCC
Lupoid hepatitis NEC

K75.8 **Other specified inflammatory liver diseases**

K75.81 **Nonalcoholic steatohepatitis (NASH)**
►Use additional code, if applicable, hepatic fibrosis (K74.0-)◄

K75.89 **Other specified inflammatory liver diseases**

K75.9 **Inflammatory liver disease, unspecified**
Hepatitis NOS
EXCLUDES 1 *acute or subacute hepatitis (K72.0-)*
chronic hepatitis NEC (K73.-)
viral hepatitis (B15-B19)

AHA: 2015,2Q,17

N Newborn: 0 | P Pediatric: 0-17 | M Maternity: 9-64 | A Adult: 15-124 | MCC Major Complication/Comorbidity | CC Complication/Comorbidity | SW Severe Wound Dx

724 | ICD-10-CM 2021

☑4ᵗʰ **K76 Other diseases of liver**

EXCLUDES 2 *alcoholic liver disease (K70.-)*
amyloid degeneration of liver (E85.-)
cystic disease of liver (congenital) (Q44.6)
hepatic vein thrombosis (I82.0)
hepatomegaly NOS (R16.0)
pigmentary cirrhosis (of liver) (E83.110)
portal vein thrombosis (I81)
toxic liver disease (K71.-)

K76.0 Fatty (change of) liver, not elsewhere classified
Nonalcoholic fatty liver disease (NAFLD)
EXCLUDES 1 *nonalcoholic steatohepatitis (NASH) (K75.81)*

K76.1 Chronic passive congestion of liver
Cardiac cirrhosis
Cardiac sclerosis

K76.2 Central hemorrhagic necrosis of liver MCC
EXCLUDES 1 *liver necrosis with hepatic failure (K72.-)*

K76.3 Infarction of liver MCC

K76.4 Peliosis hepatis
Hepatic angiomatosis

K76.5 Hepatic veno-occlusive disease
EXCLUDES 1 *Budd-Chiari syndrome (I82.0)*

K76.6 Portal hypertension CC HCC
Use additional code for any associated complications, such as:
portal hypertensive gastropathy (K31.89)
AHA: 2020,1Q,15

K76.7 Hepatorenal syndrome MCC HCC
EXCLUDES 1 *hepatorenal syndrome following labor and delivery (O90.4)*
postprocedural hepatorenal syndrome (K91.83)

☑5ᵗʰ **K76.8 Other specified diseases of liver**

K76.81 Hepatopulmonary syndrome HCC
Code first underlying liver disease, such as:
alcoholic cirrhosis of liver (K70.3-)
cirrhosis of liver without mention of alcohol (K74.6-)

K76.89 Other specified diseases of liver
Cyst (simple) of liver
Focal nodular hyperplasia of liver
Hepatoptosis

K76.9 Liver disease, unspecified

K77 Liver disorders in diseases classified elsewhere CC
Code first underlying disease, such as:
amyloidosis (E85.-)
congenital syphilis (A50.0, A50.5)
congenital toxoplasmosis (P37.1)
schistosomiasis (B65.0-B65.9)
EXCLUDES 1 *alcoholic hepatitis (K70.1-)*
alcoholic liver disease (K70.-)
cytomegaloviral hepatitis (B25.1)
herpesviral [herpes simplex] hepatitis (B00.81)
infectious mononucleosis with liver disease (B27.0-B27.9 with .9)
mumps hepatitis (B26.81)
sarcoidosis with liver disease (D86.89)
secondary syphilis with liver disease (A51.45)
syphilis (late) with liver disease (A52.74)
toxoplasmosis (acquired) hepatitis (B58.1)
tuberculosis with liver disease (A18.83)

Disorders of gallbladder, biliary tract and pancreas (K80-K87)

☑4ᵗʰ **K80 Cholelithiasis**
EXCLUDES 1 *retained cholelithiasis following cholecystectomy (K91.86)*
AHA: 2018,4Q,20
DEF: Presence or formation of concretions (calculi or "gallstones") in the gallbladder. The stones contain cholesterol, calcium carbonate, or calcium bilirubinate in pure forms or in various combinations.

Cholelithiasis

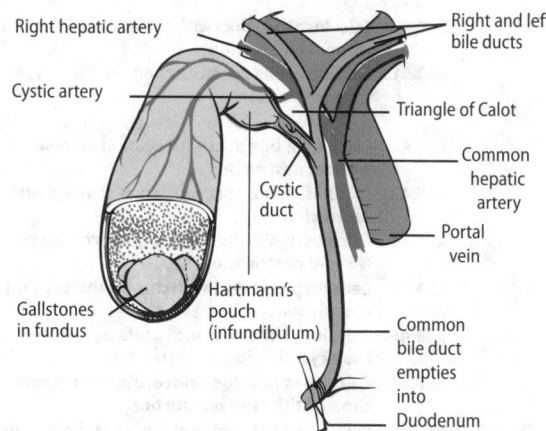

Right hepatic artery — Cystic artery — Cystic duct — Gallstones in fundus — Hartmann's pouch (infundibulum) — Right and left bile ducts — Triangle of Calot — Common hepatic artery — Portal vein — Common bile duct empties into Duodenum

☑5ᵗʰ **K80.0 Calculus of gallbladder with acute cholecystitis**
Any condition listed in K80.2 with acute cholecystitis
Use additional code if applicable for associated gangrene of gallbladder (K82.A1), or perforation of gallbladder (K82.A2)

K80.00 Calculus of gallbladder with acute cholecystitis without obstruction CC

K80.01 Calculus of gallbladder with acute cholecystitis with obstruction CC

☑5ᵗʰ **K80.1 Calculus of gallbladder with other cholecystitis**
Use additional code if applicable for associated gangrene of gallbladder (K82.A1), or perforation of gallbladder (K82.A2)

K80.10 Calculus of gallbladder with chronic cholecystitis without obstruction CC
Cholelithiasis with cholecystitis NOS

K80.11 Calculus of gallbladder with chronic cholecystitis with obstruction CC

K80.12 Calculus of gallbladder with acute and chronic cholecystitis without obstruction CC

K80.13 Calculus of gallbladder with acute and chronic cholecystitis with obstruction CC

K80.18 Calculus of gallbladder with other cholecystitis without obstruction CC

K80.19 Calculus of gallbladder with other cholecystitis with obstruction CC

☑5ᵗʰ **K80.2 Calculus of gallbladder without cholecystitis**
Cholecystolithiasis without cholecystitis
Cholelithiasis (without cholecystitis)
Colic (recurrent) of gallbladder (without cholecystitis)
Gallstone (impacted) of cystic duct (without cholecystitis)
Gallstone (impacted) of gallbladder (without cholecystitis)

K80.20 Calculus of gallbladder without cholecystitis without obstruction

K80.21 Calculus of gallbladder without cholecystitis with obstruction CC

☑5ᵗʰ **K80.3 Calculus of bile duct with cholangitis**
Any condition listed in K80.5 with cholangitis
DEF: Cholangitis: Inflammation of the bile ducts.

K80.30 Calculus of bile duct with cholangitis, unspecified, without obstruction CC

K80.31 Calculus of bile duct with cholangitis, unspecified, with obstruction CC

K80.32 Calculus of bile duct with acute cholangitis without obstruction CC

K80.33 Calculus of bile duct with acute cholangitis with obstruction CC

K80.34 Calculus of bile duct with chronic cholangitis without obstruction CC

☑ Additional Character Required   ✓x7ᵗʰ Placeholder   Unacceptable PDx   Questionable PDx   Manifestation   Unspecified Dx   H1-H14 HAC   HCC CMS-HCC Dx   HIV HIV Dx

ICD-10-CM 2021

725

K76–K80.34

K80.35 Calculus of bile duct with chronic cholangitis with obstruction `CC`

K80.36 Calculus of bile duct with acute and chronic cholangitis without obstruction `CC`

K80.37 Calculus of bile duct with acute and chronic cholangitis with obstruction `CC`

√5ᵗʰ **K80.4** **Calculus of bile duct with cholecystitis**

Any condition listed in K80.5 with cholecystitis (with cholangitis)

▶Codes also fistula of bile duct (K83.3)◀

Use additional code if applicable for associated gangrene of gallbladder (K82.A1), or perforation of gallbladder (K82.A2)

AHA: 2019,1Q,17

K80.40 Calculus of bile duct with cholecystitis, unspecified, without obstruction `CC`

K80.41 Calculus of bile duct with cholecystitis, unspecified, with obstruction `CC`

AHA: 2019,1Q,17

K80.42 Calculus of bile duct with acute cholecystitis without obstruction `CC`

K80.43 Calculus of bile duct with acute cholecystitis with obstruction `CC`

K80.44 Calculus of bile duct with chronic cholecystitis without obstruction `CC`

K80.45 Calculus of bile duct with chronic cholecystitis with obstruction `CC`

K80.46 Calculus of bile duct with acute and chronic cholecystitis without obstruction `CC`

K80.47 Calculus of bile duct with acute and chronic cholecystitis with obstruction `CC`

√5ᵗʰ **K80.5** **Calculus of bile duct without cholangitis or cholecystitis**

Choledocholithiasis (without cholangitis or cholecystitis)

Gallstone (impacted) of bile duct NOS (without cholangitis or cholecystitis)

Gallstone (impacted) of common duct (without cholangitis or cholecystitis)

Gallstone (impacted) of hepatic duct (without cholangitis or cholecystitis)

Hepatic cholelithiasis (without cholangitis or cholecystitis)

Hepatic colic (recurrent) (without cholangitis or cholecystitis)

DEF: Cholangitis: Inflammation of the bile ducts.

K80.50 Calculus of bile duct without cholangitis or cholecystitis without obstruction

K80.51 Calculus of bile duct without cholangitis or cholecystitis with obstruction `CC`

√5ᵗʰ **K80.6** **Calculus of gallbladder and bile duct with cholecystitis**

Use additional code if applicable for associated gangrene of gallbladder (K82.A1), or perforation of gallbladder (K82.A2)

K80.60 Calculus of gallbladder and bile duct with cholecystitis, unspecified, without obstruction `CC`

K80.61 Calculus of gallbladder and bile duct with cholecystitis, unspecified, with obstruction `CC`

K80.62 Calculus of gallbladder and bile duct with acute cholecystitis without obstruction `CC`

K80.63 Calculus of gallbladder and bile duct with acute cholecystitis with obstruction `CC`

K80.64 Calculus of gallbladder and bile duct with chronic cholecystitis without obstruction `CC`

K80.65 Calculus of gallbladder and bile duct with chronic cholecystitis with obstruction `CC`

K80.66 Calculus of gallbladder and bile duct with acute and chronic cholecystitis without obstruction `CC`

K80.67 Calculus of gallbladder and bile duct with acute and chronic cholecystitis with obstruction `MCC`

√5ᵗʰ **K80.7** **Calculus of gallbladder and bile duct without cholecystitis**

K80.70 Calculus of gallbladder and bile duct without cholecystitis without obstruction

K80.71 Calculus of gallbladder and bile duct without cholecystitis with obstruction `CC`

√5ᵗʰ **K80.8** **Other cholelithiasis**

K80.80 Other cholelithiasis without obstruction

K80.81 Other cholelithiasis with obstruction `CC`

√4ᵗʰ **K81** **Cholecystitis**

Use additional code if applicable for associated gangrene of gallbladder (K82.A1), or perforation of gallbladder (K82.A2)

EXCLUDES 1 cholecystitis with cholelithiasis (K80.-)

AHA: 2018,4Q,20

K81.0 **Acute cholecystitis** `CC`

Abscess of gallbladder

Angiocholecystitis

Emphysematous (acute) cholecystitis

Empyema of gallbladder

Gangrene of gallbladder

Gangrenous cholecystitis

Suppurative cholecystitis

K81.1 **Chronic cholecystitis**

K81.2 **Acute cholecystitis with chronic cholecystitis** `CC`

K81.9 **Cholecystitis, unspecified**

√4ᵗʰ **K82** **Other diseases of gallbladder**

EXCLUDES 1 nonvisualization of gallbladder (R93.2)

postcholecystectomy syndrome (K91.5)

K82.0 **Obstruction of gallbladder** `CC`

Occlusion of cystic duct or gallbladder without cholelithiasis

Stenosis of cystic duct or gallbladder without cholelithiasis

Stricture of cystic duct or gallbladder without cholelithiasis

EXCLUDES 1 obstruction of gallbladder with cholelithiasis (K80.-)

K82.1 **Hydrops of gallbladder** `CC`

Mucocele of gallbladder

K82.2 **Perforation of gallbladder** `MCC`

Rupture of cystic duct or gallbladder

EXCLUDES 1 perforation of gallbladder in cholecystitis (K82.A2)

K82.3 **Fistula of gallbladder** `CC`

Cholecystocolic fistula

Cholecystoduodenal fistula

K82.4 **Cholesterolosis of gallbladder**

Strawberry gallbladder

EXCLUDES 1 cholesterolosis of gallbladder with cholecystitis (K81.-)

cholesterolosis of gallbladder with cholelithiasis (K80.-)

K82.8 **Other specified diseases of gallbladder**

Adhesions of cystic duct or gallbladder

Atrophy of cystic duct or gallbladder

Cyst of cystic duct or gallbladder

Dyskinesia of cystic duct or gallbladder

Hypertrophy of cystic duct or gallbladder

Nonfunctioning of cystic duct or gallbladder

Ulcer of cystic duct or gallbladder

K82.9 **Disease of gallbladder, unspecified**

√5ᵗʰ **K82.A** **Disorders of gallbladder in diseases classified elsewhere**

Code first the type of cholecystitis (K81.-), or cholelithiasis with cholecystitis (K80.00-K80.19, K80.40-K80.47, K80.60-K80.67)

AHA: 2018,4Q,19-20

K82.A1 *Gangrene of gallbladder in cholecystitis*

K82.A2 *Perforation of gallbladder in cholecystitis* `CC`

√4ᵗʰ **K83** **Other diseases of biliary tract**

EXCLUDES 1 postcholecystectomy syndrome (K91.5)

EXCLUDES 2 conditions involving the gallbladder (K81-K82)

conditions involving the cystic duct (K81-K82)

√5ᵗʰ **K83.0** **Cholangitis**

EXCLUDES 1 cholangitic liver abscess (K75.0)

cholangitis with choledocholithiasis (K80.3-, K80.4-)

EXCLUDES 2 chronic nonsuppurative destructive cholangitis (K74.3)

primary biliary cholangitis (K74.3)

primary biliary cirrhosis (K74.3)

AHA: 2018,4Q,20

K83.01 **Primary sclerosing cholangitis** `CC`

`N` Newborn: 0   `P` Pediatric: 0-17   `M` Maternity: 9-64   `A` Adult: 15-124   `MCC` Major Complication/Comorbidity   `CC` Complication/Comorbidity   `SW` Severe Wound Dx

726 ICD-10-CM 2021

K83.09 **Other cholangitis** `CC`
Ascending cholangitis
Cholangitis NOS
Primary cholangitis
Recurrent cholangitis
Sclerosing cholangitis
Secondary cholangitis
Stenosing cholangitis
Suppurative cholangitis

K83.1 **Obstruction of bile duct** `MCC`
Occlusion of bile duct without cholelithiasis
Stenosis of bile duct without cholelithiasis
Stricture of bile duct without cholelithiasis
    EXCLUDES 1   *congenital obstruction of bile duct (Q44.3)*
          obstruction of bile duct with cholelithiasis (K80.-)
AHA: 2016,1Q,18

K83.2 **Perforation of bile duct** `MCC`
Rupture of bile duct

K83.3 **Fistula of bile duct** `CC`
Choledochoduodenal fistula
AHA: 2019,1Q,17

K83.4 **Spasm of sphincter of Oddi**

K83.5 **Biliary cyst**

K83.8 **Other specified diseases of biliary tract**
Adhesions of biliary tract
Atrophy of biliary tract
Hypertrophy of biliary tract
Ulcer of biliary tract

K83.9 **Disease of biliary tract, unspecified**

✓4ᵗʰ K85 Acute pancreatitis
    INCLUDES   acute (recurrent) pancreatitis
            subacute pancreatitis
AHA: 2016,4Q,34

✓5ᵗʰ **K85.0** **Idiopathic acute pancreatitis**
    K85.00 **Idiopathic acute pancreatitis without necrosis or infection** `MCC`
    K85.01 **Idiopathic acute pancreatitis with uninfected necrosis** `MCC`
    K85.02 **Idiopathic acute pancreatitis with infected necrosis** `MCC`

✓5ᵗʰ **K85.1** **Biliary acute pancreatitis**
Gallstone pancreatitis
    K85.10 **Biliary acute pancreatitis without necrosis or infection** `MCC`
    K85.11 **Biliary acute pancreatitis with uninfected necrosis** `MCC`
    K85.12 **Biliary acute pancreatitis with infected necrosis** `MCC`

✓5ᵗʰ **K85.2** **Alcohol induced acute pancreatitis**
    EXCLUDES 2   *alcohol induced chronic pancreatitis (K86.0)*
    K85.20 **Alcohol induced acute pancreatitis without necrosis or infection** `MCC`
        AHA: 2020,1Q,9
    K85.21 **Alcohol induced acute pancreatitis with uninfected necrosis** `MCC`
    K85.22 **Alcohol induced acute pancreatitis with infected necrosis** `MCC`

✓5ᵗʰ **K85.3** **Drug induced acute pancreatitis**
Use additional code for adverse effect, if applicable, to identify drug (T36-T50 with fifth or sixth character 5)
Use additional code to identify drug abuse and dependence (F11.- F17.-)
    K85.30 **Drug induced acute pancreatitis without necrosis or infection** `MCC`
    K85.31 **Drug induced acute pancreatitis with uninfected necrosis** `MCC`
    K85.32 **Drug induced acute pancreatitis with infected necrosis** `MCC`

✓5ᵗʰ **K85.8** **Other acute pancreatitis**
    K85.80 **Other acute pancreatitis without necrosis or infection** `MCC`
    K85.81 **Other acute pancreatitis with uninfected necrosis** `MCC`
    K85.82 **Other acute pancreatitis with infected necrosis** `MCC`

✓5ᵗʰ **K85.9** **Acute pancreatitis, unspecified**
Pancreatitis NOS
    K85.90 **Acute pancreatitis without necrosis or infection, unspecified** `MCC`
    K85.91 **Acute pancreatitis with uninfected necrosis, unspecified** `MCC`
    K85.92 **Acute pancreatitis with infected necrosis, unspecified** `MCC`

✓4ᵗʰ K86 Other diseases of pancreas
    EXCLUDES 2   *fibrocystic disease of pancreas (E84.-)*
            islet cell tumor (of pancreas) (D13.7)
            pancreatic steatorrhea (K90.3)

K86.0 **Alcohol-induced chronic pancreatitis** `CC` `HCC`
Use additional code to identify:
  alcohol abuse and dependence (F10.-)
Code also exocrine pancreatic insufficiency (K86.81)
    EXCLUDES 2   *alcohol induced acute pancreatitis (K85.2-)*

K86.1 **Other chronic pancreatitis** `CC` `HCC`
Chronic pancreatitis NOS
Infectious chronic pancreatitis
Recurrent chronic pancreatitis
Relapsing chronic pancreatitis
Code also exocrine pancreatic insufficiency (K86.81)

K86.2 **Cyst of pancreas** `CC`

K86.3 **Pseudocyst of pancreas** `CC`

✓5ᵗʰ **K86.8** **Other specified diseases of pancreas**
AHA: 2016,4Q,34-35
    K86.81 **Exocrine pancreatic insufficiency**
    K86.89 **Other specified diseases of pancreas**
        Aseptic pancreatic necrosis, unrelated to acute pancreatitis
        Atrophy of pancreas
        Calculus of pancreas
        Cirrhosis of pancreas
        Fibrosis of pancreas
        Pancreatic fat necrosis, unrelated to acute pancreatitis
        Pancreatic infantilism
        Pancreatic necrosis NOS, unrelated to acute pancreatitis

K86.9 **Disease of pancreas, unspecified**

K87 Disorders of gallbladder, biliary tract and pancreas in diseases classified elsewhere
Code first underlying disease
    EXCLUDES 1   *cytomegaloviral pancreatitis (B25.2)*
            mumps pancreatitis (B26.3)
            syphilitic gallbladder (A52.74)
            syphilitic pancreas (A52.74)
            tuberculosis of gallbladder (A18.83)
            tuberculosis of pancreas (A18.83)

Other diseases of the digestive system (K90-K95)

✓4ᵗʰ K90 Intestinal malabsorption
    EXCLUDES 1   *intestinal malabsorption following gastrointestinal surgery (K91.2)*
AHA: 2017,4Q,108

K90.0 **Celiac disease**
Celiac disease with steatorrhea
Celiac gluten-sensitive enteropathy
Nontropical sprue
Use additional code for associated disorders including:
  dermatitis herpetiformis (L13.0)
  gluten ataxia (G32.81)
Code also exocrine pancreatic insufficiency (K86.81)
DEF: Malabsorption syndrome due to gluten consumption. Symptoms include fetid, bulky, frothy, oily stools; a distended abdomen; gas; asthenia; electrolyte depletion; and vitamin B, D, and K deficiency.

K90.1 **Tropical sprue** `CC`
Sprue NOS
Tropical steatorrhea

K90.2 **Blind loop syndrome, not elsewhere classified** `CC`
Blind loop syndrome NOS
    EXCLUDES 1   *congenital blind loop syndrome (Q43.8)*
            postsurgical blind loop syndrome (K91.2)

K90.3 **Pancreatic steatorrhea** `CC`

✔ Additional Character Required   ✓x7ᵗʰ Placeholder   Unacceptable PDx   Questionable PDx   Manifestation   Unspecified Dx   H1-H14 HAC   HCC CMS-HCC Dx   HIV HIV Dx

Chapter 11. Diseases of the Digestive System

K90.4–K94.01

✓5ᵗʰ **K90.4** **Other malabsorption due to intolerance**
> EXCLUDES 2   *celiac gluten-sensitive enteropathy (K90.0)*
> *lactose intolerance (E73.-)*
> **AHA:** 2016,4Q,35-36

     K90.41 **Non-celiac gluten sensitivity**   CC
> Gluten sensitivity NOS
> Non-celiac gluten sensitive enteropathy

     K90.49 **Malabsorption due to intolerance, not elsewhere classified**
> Malabsorption due to intolerance to carbohydrate
> Malabsorption due to intolerance to fat
> Malabsorption due to intolerance to protein
> Malabsorption due to intolerance to starch

✓5ᵗʰ **K90.8** **Other intestinal malabsorption**

     K90.81 **Whipple's disease**   CC

     K90.89 **Other intestinal malabsorption**   CC

   K90.9 **Intestinal malabsorption, unspecified**   CC

✓4ᵗʰ **K91** **Intraoperative and postprocedural complications and disorders of digestive system, not elsewhere classified**
> EXCLUDES 2   *complications of artificial opening of digestive system (K94.-)*
> *complications of bariatric procedures (K95.-)*
> *gastrojejunal ulcer (K28.-)*
> *postprocedural (radiation) retroperitoneal abscess (K68.11)*
> *radiation colitis (K52.0)*
> *radiation gastroenteritis (K52.0)*
> *radiation proctitis (K62.7)*
> **AHA:** 2016,4Q,9-10

   K91.0 **Vomiting following gastrointestinal surgery**

   K91.1 **Postgastric surgery syndromes**
> Dumping syndrome
> Postgastrectomy syndrome
> Postvagotomy syndrome

   K91.2 **Postsurgical malabsorption, not elsewhere classified**   CC
> Postsurgical blind loop syndrome
> EXCLUDES 1   *malabsorption osteomalacia in adults (M83.2)*
> *malabsorption osteoporosis, postsurgical (M80.8-, M81.8)*

✓5ᵗʰ **K91.3** **Postprocedural intestinal obstruction**
> **AHA:** 2017,4Q,16-17; 2017,1Q,40

     K91.30 **Postprocedural intestinal obstruction, unspecified as to partial versus complete**   CC
> Postprocedural intestinal obstruction NOS

     K91.31 **Postprocedural partial intestinal obstruction**   CC
> Postprocedural incomplete intestinal obstruction

     K91.32 **Postprocedural complete intestinal obstruction**   CC

   K91.5 **Postcholecystectomy syndrome**

✓5ᵗʰ **K91.6** **Intraoperative hemorrhage and hematoma of a digestive system organ or structure complicating a procedure**
> EXCLUDES 1   *intraoperative hemorrhage and hematoma of a digestive system organ or structure due to accidental puncture and laceration during a procedure (K91.7-)*

     K91.61 **Intraoperative hemorrhage and hematoma of a digestive system organ or structure complicating a digestive system procedure**   CC
> **AHA:** 2020,1Q,19

     K91.62 **Intraoperative hemorrhage and hematoma of a digestive system organ or structure complicating other procedure**   CC

✓5ᵗʰ **K91.7** **Accidental puncture and laceration of a digestive system organ or structure during a procedure**

     K91.71 **Accidental puncture and laceration of a digestive system organ or structure during a digestive system procedure**   CC

     K91.72 **Accidental puncture and laceration of a digestive system organ or structure during other procedure**   CC
> **AHA:** 2019,2Q,23

✓5ᵗʰ **K91.8** **Other intraoperative and postprocedural complications and disorders of digestive system**

     K91.81 **Other intraoperative complications of digestive system**   CC

     K91.82 **Postprocedural hepatic failure**   CC

     K91.83 **Postprocedural hepatorenal syndrome**   CC

✓6ᵗʰ **K91.84** **Postprocedural hemorrhage of a digestive system organ or structure following a procedure**

     K91.840 **Postprocedural hemorrhage of a digestive system organ or structure following a digestive system procedure**   CC
> **AHA:** 2016,1Q,15

     K91.841 **Postprocedural hemorrhage of a digestive system organ or structure following other procedure**   CC

✓6ᵗʰ **K91.85** **Complications of intestinal pouch**

     K91.850 **Pouchitis**   CC HCC
> Inflammation of internal ileoanal pouch
> **DEF:** Inflammatory complication of an existing surgically created ileoanal pouch, resulting in multiple GI complaints, including diarrhea, abdominal pain, rectal bleeding, fecal urgency, or incontinence.

     K91.858 **Other complications of intestinal pouch**   CC HCC
> **AHA:** 2019,2Q,13

     K91.86 **Retained cholelithiasis following cholecystectomy**   CC

✓6ᵗʰ **K91.87** **Postprocedural hematoma and seroma of a digestive system organ or structure following a procedure**

     K91.870 **Postprocedural hematoma of a digestive system organ or structure following a digestive system procedure**   CC

     K91.871 **Postprocedural hematoma of a digestive system organ or structure following other procedure**   CC

     K91.872 **Postprocedural seroma of a digestive system organ or structure following a digestive system procedure**   CC

     K91.873 **Postprocedural seroma of a digestive system organ or structure following other procedure**   CC

     K91.89 **Other postprocedural complications and disorders of digestive system**   CC
> Use additional code, if applicable, to further specify disorder
> EXCLUDES 2   *postprocedural retroperitoneal abscess (K68.11)*
> **AHA:** 2020,2Q,22; 2017,1Q,40

✓4ᵗʰ **K92** **Other diseases of digestive system**
> EXCLUDES 1   *neonatal gastrointestinal hemorrhage (P54.0-P54.3)*

   K92.0 **Hematemesis**   CC

   K92.1 **Melena**   CC
> EXCLUDES 1   *occult blood in feces (R19.5)*

   K92.2 **Gastrointestinal hemorrhage, unspecified**   CC
> Gastric hemorrhage NOS
> Intestinal hemorrhage NOS
> EXCLUDES 1   *acute hemorrhagic gastritis (K29.01)*
> *hemorrhage of anus and rectum (K62.5)*
> *angiodysplasia of stomach with hemorrhage (K31.811)*
> *diverticular disease with hemorrhage (K57.-)*
> *gastritis and duodenitis with hemorrhage (K29.-)*
> *peptic ulcer with hemorrhage (K25-K28)*

✓5ᵗʰ **K92.8** **Other specified diseases of the digestive system**

     K92.81 **Gastrointestinal mucositis (ulcerative)**   CC
> Code also type of associated therapy, such as:
> antineoplastic and immunosuppressive drugs (T45.1X-)
> radiological procedure and radiotherapy (Y84.2)
> EXCLUDES 2   *mucositis (ulcerative) of vagina and vulva (N76.81)*
> *nasal mucositis (ulcerative) (J34.81)*
> *oral mucositis (ulcerative) (K12.3-)*

     K92.89 **Other specified diseases of the digestive system**

   K92.9 **Disease of digestive system, unspecified**

✓4ᵗʰ **K94** **Complications of artificial openings of the digestive system**

✓5ᵗʰ **K94.0** **Colostomy complications**

     K94.00 **Colostomy complication, unspecified**   HCC

     K94.01 **Colostomy hemorrhage**   CC HCC

N Newborn: 0   P Pediatric: 0-17   M Maternity: 9-64   A Adult: 15-124   MCC Major Complication/Comorbidity   CC Complication/Comorbidity   SW Severe Wound Dx

728   ICD-10-CM 2021

	K94.02	**Colostomy** infection `CC` `HCC`	

Use additional code to specify type of infection, such as:

cellulitis of abdominal wall (L03.311)
sepsis (A40.-, A41.-)

K94.03   **Colostomy** malfunction   `CC` `HCC`
Mechanical complication of colostomy

K94.09   **Other complications of colostomy**   `CC` `HCC`

✓5ᵗʰ **K94.1** **Enterostomy** complications

K94.10   **Enterostomy complication, unspecified**   `HCC`

K94.11   **Enterostomy** hemorrhage   `CC` `HCC`

K94.12   **Enterostomy** infection   `CC` `HCC`
Use additional code to specify type of infection, such as:

cellulitis of abdominal wall (L03.311)
sepsis (A40.-, A41.-)

K94.13   **Enterostomy** malfunction   `CC` `HCC`
Mechanical complication of enterostomy

K94.19   **Other complications of enterostomy**   `CC` `HCC`

✓5ᵗʰ **K94.2** **Gastrostomy** complications

K94.20   **Gastrostomy complication, unspecified**   `HCC`

K94.21   **Gastrostomy** hemorrhage   `HCC`

K94.22   **Gastrostomy** infection   `CC` `HCC`
Use additional code to specify type of infection, such as:

cellulitis of abdominal wall (L03.311)
sepsis (A40.-, A41.-)

K94.23   **Gastrostomy** malfunction   `CC` `HCC`
Mechanical complication of gastrostomy
AHA: 2019,1Q,26

K94.29   **Other complications of gastrostomy**   `HCC`

✓5ᵗʰ **K94.3** **Esophagostomy** complications

K94.30   **Esophagostomy complications, unspecified**   `CC` `HCC`

K94.31   **Esophagostomy** hemorrhage   `CC` `HCC`

K94.32   **Esophagostomy** infection   `CC` `HCC`
Use additional code to identify the infection

K94.33   **Esophagostomy** malfunction   `CC` `HCC`
Mechanical complication of esophagostomy

K94.39   **Other complications of esophagostomy**   `CC` `HCC`

✓4ᵗʰ **K95** **Complications of bariatric procedures**

✓5ᵗʰ **K95.0** **Complications of** gastric band procedure

K95.01   **Infection** due to gastric band procedure   `CC` `H11`
Use additional code to specify type of infection or organism, such as:
bacterial and viral infectious agents (B95.-, B96.-)
cellulitis of abdominal wall (L03.311)
sepsis (A40.-, A41.-)

K95.09   **Other complications of gastric band procedure**   `CC`
Use additional code, if applicable, to further specify complication

✓5ᵗʰ **K95.8** **Complications of other bariatric procedure**
`EXCLUDES 1`   complications of gastric band surgery (K95.0-)

K95.81   **Infection** due to other bariatric procedure   `CC` `H11`
Use additional code to specify type of infection or organism, such as:
bacterial and viral infectious agents (B95.-, B96.-)
cellulitis of abdominal wall (L03.311)
sepsis (A40.-, A41.-)

K95.89   **Other complications of other bariatric procedure**   `CC`
Use additional code, if applicable, to further specify complication

Chapter 12. Diseases of the Skin and Subcutaneous Tissue (L00–L99)

Chapter-specific Guidelines with Coding Examples

The chapter-specific guidelines from the ICD-10-CM Official Guidelines for Coding and Reporting have been provided below. Along with these guidelines are coding examples, contained in the shaded boxes, that have been developed to help illustrate the coding and/or sequencing guidance found in these guidelines.

a. Pressure ulcer stage codes

1) Pressure ulcer stages

Codes in category L89, Pressure ulcer, identify the site and stage of the pressure ulcer.

The ICD-10-CM classifies pressure ulcer stages based on severity, which is designated by stages 1-4, deep tissue pressure injury, unspecified stage, and unstageable.

Assign as many codes from category L89 as needed to identify all the pressure ulcers the patient has, if applicable.

See Section I.B.14 for pressure ulcer stage documentation by clinicians other than patient's provider

> Nursing notes: Dressings changed daily on stage 4 ulcer on heel and stage 2 ulcer on elbow
>
> Discharge summary: Pressure ulcers on right heel and left elbow
>
> **L89.614   Pressure ulcer of right heel, stage 4**
>
> **L89.022   Pressure ulcer of left elbow, stage 2**
>
> *Explanation:* Right heel and left elbow pressure ulcers were documented by the patient's provider in the discharge summary. Although the stage of these ulcers was not included in the provider's diagnostic statement, it is appropriate to code the stage from documentation from other clinicians involved in the patient's care, such as the nurse's notes, according to section I.B.14. Combination codes from category L89 Pressure ulcer, identify the site of the pressure ulcer as well as the stage. Assign as many codes from category L89 as needed to identify all the pressure ulcers the patient has.

2) Unstageable pressure ulcers

Assignment of the code for unstageable pressure ulcer (L89.--0) should be based on the clinical documentation. These codes are used for pressure ulcers whose stage cannot be clinically determined (e.g., the ulcer is covered by eschar or has been treated with a skin or muscle graft). This code should not be confused with the codes for unspecified stage (L89.--9). When there is no documentation regarding the stage of the pressure ulcer, assign the appropriate code for unspecified stage (L89.--9).

> Pressure ulcer of the right lower back documented as unstageable due to the presence of thick eschar covering the ulcer
>
> **L89.130   Pressure ulcer of right lower back, unstageable**
>
> *Explanation:* Codes for unstageable pressure ulcers are assigned when the stage cannot be clinically determined (e.g., the ulcer is covered by eschar or has been treated with a skin or muscle graft).

3) Documented pressure ulcer stage

Assignment of the pressure ulcer stage code should be guided by clinical documentation of the stage or documentation of the terms found in the Alphabetic Index. For clinical terms describing the stage that are not found in the Alphabetic Index, and there is no documentation of the stage, the provider should be queried.

> Left heel pressure ulcer with partial thickness skin loss involving the dermis
>
> **L89.622   Pressure ulcer of left heel, stage 2**
>
> *Explanation:* Code assignment for the pressure ulcer stage should be guided by either the clinical documentation of the stage or the documentation of terms found in the Alphabetic Index. The clinical documentation describing the left heel pressure ulcer "partial thickness skin loss involving the dermis" matches the ICD-10-CM index parenthetical description for stage 2 "(abrasion, blister, partial thickness skin loss involving epidermis and/or dermis)."

4) Patients admitted with pressure ulcers documented as healed

No code is assigned if the documentation states that the pressure ulcer is completely healed at the time of admission.

5) Pressure ulcers documented as healing

Pressure ulcers described as healing should be assigned the appropriate pressure ulcer stage code based on the documentation in the medical record. If the documentation does not provide information about the stage of the healing pressure ulcer, assign the appropriate code for unspecified stage.

If the documentation is unclear as to whether the patient has a current (new) pressure ulcer or if the patient is being treated for a healing pressure ulcer, query the provider.

For ulcers that were present on admission but healed at the time of discharge, assign the code for the site and stage of the pressure ulcer at the time of admission.

> H & P noted healing stage 2 sacral pressure ulcer. Resolved at time of discharge summary.
>
> **L89.152   Pressure ulcer of sacral region, stage 2**
>
> *Explanation:* Although completely healed upon discharge, the pressure ulcer required observation and/or treatment and should be coded based on the site and stage upon admission.

6) Patient admitted with pressure ulcer evolving into another stage during the admission

If a patient is admitted to an inpatient hospital with a pressure ulcer at one stage and it progresses to a higher stage, two separate codes should be assigned: one code for the site and stage of the ulcer on admission and a second code for the same ulcer site and the highest stage reported during the stay.

> Stage 3 right hip pressure ulcer worsened during admission to a stage 4
>
> **L89.213   Pressure ulcer of right hip, stage 3**
>
> **L89.214   Pressure ulcer of right hip, stage 4**
>
> *Explanation:* A pressure ulcer that progresses from a lower stage to a higher stage is assigned two codes, one for the documented stage upon admission and one for the documented stage at discharge.

7) Pressure-induced deep tissue damage

For pressure-induced deep tissue damage or deep tissue pressure injury, assign only the appropriate code for pressure-induced deep tissue damage (L89.--6).

b. Non-pressure chronic ulcers

1) Patients admitted with non-pressure ulcers documented as healed

No code is assigned if the documentation states that the non-pressure ulcer is completely healed at the time of admission.

2) Non-pressure ulcers documented as healing

Non-pressure ulcers described as healing should be assigned the appropriate non-pressure ulcer code based on the documentation in the medical record. If the documentation does not provide information about the severity of the healing non-pressure ulcer, assign the appropriate code for unspecified severity.

If the documentation is unclear as to whether the patient has a current (new) non-pressure ulcer or if the patient is being treated for a healing non-pressure ulcer, query the provider.

For ulcers that were present on admission but healed at the time of discharge, assign the code for the site and severity of the non-pressure ulcer at the time of admission.

> Admission diagnosis: Chronic ulcer, fat layer exposed, on left ankle
>
> Discharge diagnosis: Resolution of ulcer on the left ankle
>
> **L97.322   Non-pressure chronic ulcer of left ankle with fat layer exposed**
>
> *Explanation:* Although the ulcer was documented as resolved (healed) at discharge, a code representing the site and severity of the ulcer upon admission should be appended.

3) Patient admitted with non-pressure ulcer that progresses to another severity level during the admission

If a patient is admitted to an inpatient hospital with a non-pressure ulcer at one severity level and it progresses to a higher severity level, two separate codes should be assigned: one code for the site and severity level of the ulcer on admission and a second code for the same ulcer site and the highest severity level reported during the stay.

See Section I.B.14 for pressure ulcer stage documentation by clinicians other than patient's provider

Chapter 12. Diseases of the Skin and Subcutaneous Tissue (L00-L99)

EXCLUDES 2   *certain conditions originating in the perinatal period (P04-P96)*
certain infectious and parasitic diseases (A00-B99)
complications of pregnancy, childbirth and the puerperium (O00-O9A)
congenital malformations, deformations, and chromosomal abnormalities (Q00-Q99)
endocrine, nutritional and metabolic diseases (E00-E88)
lipomelanotic reticulosis (I89.8)
neoplasms (C00-D49)
symptoms, signs and abnormal clinical and laboratory findings, not elsewhere classified (R00-R94)
systemic connective tissue disorders (M30-M36)
viral warts (B07.-)

This chapter contains the following blocks:

L00-L08   Infections of the skin and subcutaneous tissue
L10-L14   Bullous disorders
L20-L30   Dermatitis and eczema
L40-L45   Papulosquamous disorders
L49-L54   Urticaria and erythema
L55-L59   Radiation-related disorders of the skin and subcutaneous tissue
L60-L75   Disorders of skin appendages
L76   Intraoperative and postprocedural complications of skin and subcutaneous tissue
L80-L99   Other disorders of the skin and subcutaneous tissue

Infections of the skin and subcutaneous tissue (L00-L08)

Use additional code (B95-B97) to identify infectious agent

EXCLUDES 2   *hordeolum (H00.0)*
infective dermatitis (L30.3)
local infections of skin classified in Chapter 1
lupus panniculitis (L93.2)
panniculitis NOS (M79.3)
panniculitis of neck and back (M54.0-)
perlèche NOS (K13.0)
perlèche due to candidiasis (B37.0)
perlèche due to riboflavin deficiency (E53.0)
pyogenic granuloma (L98.0)
relapsing panniculitis [Weber-Christian] (M35.6)
viral warts (B07.-)
zoster (B02.-)

L00 Staphylococcal scalded skin syndrome
Ritter's disease
· Use additional code to identify percentage of skin exfoliation (L49.-)

EXCLUDES 1   *bullous impetigo (L01.03)*
pemphigus neonatorum (L01.03)
toxic epidermal necrolysis [Lyell] (L51.2)

DEF: Infectious skin disease of children younger than 5 years marked by eruptions ranging from a few localized blisters to widespread, easily ruptured, fine vesicles and bullae affecting almost the entire body. It results in exfoliation of large planes of skin and leaves raw areas.

✓4ᵗʰ **L01 Impetigo**

EXCLUDES 1   *impetigo herpetiformis (L40.1)*

DEF: Acute, superficial, highly contagious skin infection commonly occurring in children. Skin lesions usually appear on the face and consist of vesicles and bullae that burst and form yellow crusts.

✓5ᵗʰ **L01.0 Impetigo**
Impetigo contagiosa
Impetigo vulgaris

L01.00 Impetigo, unspecified
Impetigo NOS

L01.01 Non-bullous impetigo

L01.02 Bockhart's impetigo
Impetigo follicularis
Perifolliculitis NOS
Superficial pustular perifolliculitis
DEF: Superficial inflammation of the hair follicles most commonly caused by staph aureus that manifests as rounded, sphere-shaped, pustular eruptions in the areas of the scalp, beard, underarms, extremities, and buttocks.

L01.03 Bullous impetigo
Impetigo neonatorum
Pemphigus neonatorum

L01.09 Other impetigo
Ulcerative impetigo

L01.1 Impetiginization of other dermatoses

✓4ᵗʰ **L02 Cutaneous abscess, furuncle and carbuncle**
Use additional code to identify organism (B95-B96)

EXCLUDES 2   *abscess of anus and rectal regions (K61.-)*
abscess of female genital organs (external) (N76.4)
abscess of male genital organs (external) (N48.2, N49.-)

DEF: Carbuncle: Infection of the skin that arises from a collection of interconnected infected boils or furuncles, usually from hair follicles infected by *Staphylococcus*. This condition can produce pus and form drainage cavities.
DEF: Furuncle: Inflamed, painful abscess, cyst, or nodule on the skin caused by bacteria, often *Staphylococcus*, entering along the hair follicle.

✓5ᵗʰ **L02.0 Cutaneous abscess, furuncle and carbuncle of face**

EXCLUDES 2   *abscess of ear, external (H60.0)*
abscess of eyelid (H00.0)
abscess of head [any part, except face] (L02.8)
abscess of lacrimal gland (H04.0)
abscess of lacrimal passages (H04.3)
abscess of mouth (K12.2)
abscess of nose (J34.0)
abscess of orbit (H05.0)
submandibular abscess (K12.2)

L02.01 Cutaneous abscess of face CC

L02.02 Furuncle of face
Boil of face
Folliculitis of face

L02.03 Carbuncle of face

✓5ᵗʰ **L02.1 Cutaneous abscess, furuncle and carbuncle of neck**

L02.11 Cutaneous abscess of neck CC

L02.12 Furuncle of neck
Boil of neck
Folliculitis of neck

L02.13 Carbuncle of neck

✓5ᵗʰ **L02.2 Cutaneous abscess, furuncle and carbuncle of trunk**

EXCLUDES 1   *non-newborn omphalitis (L08.82)*
omphalitis of newborn (P38.-)

EXCLUDES 2   *abscess of breast (N61.1)*
abscess of buttocks (L02.3)
abscess of female external genital organs (N76.4)
abscess of hip (L02.4)
abscess of male external genital organs (N48.2, N49.-)

✓6ᵗʰ **L02.21 Cutaneous abscess of trunk**

L02.211 Cutaneous abscess of abdominal wall CC

L02.212 Cutaneous abscess of back [any part, except buttock] CC

L02.213 Cutaneous abscess of chest wall CC

L02.214 Cutaneous abscess of groin CC

L02.215 Cutaneous abscess of perineum CC

L02.216 Cutaneous abscess of umbilicus CC

L02.219 Cutaneous abscess of trunk, unspecified CC

✓6ᵗʰ **L02.22 Furuncle of trunk**
Boil of trunk
Folliculitis of trunk

L02.221 Furuncle of abdominal wall

L02.222 Furuncle of back [any part, except buttock]

L02.223 Furuncle of chest wall

L02.224 Furuncle of groin

L02.225 Furuncle of perineum

L02.226 Furuncle of umbilicus

L02.229 Furuncle of trunk, unspecified

✓6ᵗʰ **L02.23 Carbuncle of trunk**

L02.231 Carbuncle of abdominal wall

L02.232 Carbuncle of back [any part, except buttock]

L02.233 Carbuncle of chest wall

L02.234 Carbuncle of groin

L02.235 Carbuncle of perineum

L02.236 Carbuncle of umbilicus

L02.239 Carbuncle of trunk, unspecified

✓5ᵗʰ **L02.3 Cutaneous abscess, furuncle and carbuncle of buttock**

EXCLUDES 1   *pilonidal cyst with abscess (L05.01)*

L02.31 Cutaneous abscess of buttock CC
Cutaneous abscess of gluteal region

Chapter 12. Diseases of the Skin and Subcutaneous Tissue

L02.32   **Furuncle** of buttock
Boil of buttock
Folliculitis of buttock
Furuncle of gluteal region

L02.33   **Carbuncle** of buttock
Carbuncle of gluteal region

✓5ᵗʰ **L02.4**   **Cutaneous abscess, furuncle and carbuncle of limb**
> EXCLUDES 2   *cutaneous abscess, furuncle and carbuncle of groin (L02.214, L02.224, L02.234)*
> *cutaneous abscess, furuncle and carbuncle of hand (L02.5-)*
> *cutaneous abscess, furuncle and carbuncle of foot (L02.6-)*

✓6ᵗʰ **L02.41**   **Cutaneous abscess** of limb

L02.411   **Cutaneous abscess** of right axilla   CC
L02.412   **Cutaneous abscess** of left axilla   CC
L02.413   **Cutaneous abscess** of right upper limb   CC
L02.414   **Cutaneous abscess** of left upper limb   CC
L02.415   **Cutaneous abscess** of right lower limb   CC
L02.416   **Cutaneous abscess** of left lower limb   CC
L02.419   **Cutaneous abscess** of limb, unspecified   CC

✓6ᵗʰ **L02.42**   **Furuncle** of limb
Boil of limb
Folliculitis of limb

L02.421   **Furuncle** of right axilla
L02.422   **Furuncle** of left axilla
L02.423   **Furuncle** of right upper limb
L02.424   **Furuncle** of left upper limb
L02.425   **Furuncle** of right lower limb
L02.426   **Furuncle** of left lower limb
L02.429   **Furuncle** of limb, unspecified

✓6ᵗʰ **L02.43**   **Carbuncle** of limb

L02.431   **Carbuncle** of right axilla
L02.432   **Carbuncle** of left axilla
L02.433   **Carbuncle** of right upper limb
L02.434   **Carbuncle** of left upper limb
L02.435   **Carbuncle** of right lower limb
L02.436   **Carbuncle** of left lower limb
L02.439   **Carbuncle** of limb, unspecified

✓5ᵗʰ **L02.5**   **Cutaneous abscess, furuncle and carbuncle of hand**

✓6ᵗʰ **L02.51**   **Cutaneous abscess** of hand

L02.511   **Cutaneous abscess** of right hand   CC
L02.512   **Cutaneous abscess** of left hand   CC
L02.519   **Cutaneous abscess** of unspecified hand   CC

✓6ᵗʰ **L02.52**   **Furuncle** hand
Boil of hand
Folliculitis of hand

L02.521   **Furuncle** right hand
L02.522   **Furuncle** left hand
L02.529   **Furuncle** unspecified hand

✓6ᵗʰ **L02.53**   **Carbuncle** of hand

L02.531   **Carbuncle** of right hand
L02.532   **Carbuncle** of left hand
L02.539   **Carbuncle** of unspecified hand

✓5ᵗʰ **L02.6**   **Cutaneous abscess, furuncle and carbuncle of foot**

✓6ᵗʰ **L02.61**   **Cutaneous abscess** of foot

L02.611   **Cutaneous abscess** of right foot   CC
L02.612   **Cutaneous abscess** of left foot   CC
L02.619   **Cutaneous abscess** of unspecified foot   CC

✓6ᵗʰ **L02.62**   **Furuncle** of foot
Boil of foot
Folliculitis of foot

L02.621   **Furuncle** of right foot
L02.622   **Furuncle** of left foot
L02.629   **Furuncle** of unspecified foot

✓6ᵗʰ **L02.63**   **Carbuncle** of foot

L02.631   **Carbuncle** of right foot
L02.632   **Carbuncle** of left foot
L02.639   **Carbuncle** of unspecified foot

✓5ᵗʰ **L02.8**   **Cutaneous abscess, furuncle and carbuncle of other sites**

✓6ᵗʰ **L02.81**   **Cutaneous abscess** of other sites

L02.811   **Cutaneous abscess** of head [any part, except face]   CC
L02.818   **Cutaneous abscess** of other sites   CC

✓6ᵗʰ **L02.82**   **Furuncle** of other sites
Boil of other sites
Folliculitis of other sites

L02.821   **Furuncle** of head [any part, except face]
L02.828   **Furuncle** of other sites

✓6ᵗʰ **L02.83**   **Carbuncle** of other sites

L02.831   **Carbuncle** of head [any part, except face]
L02.838   **Carbuncle** of other sites

✓5ᵗʰ **L02.9**   **Cutaneous abscess, furuncle and carbuncle, unspecified**

L02.91   **Cutaneous abscess, unspecified**   CC
L02.92   **Furuncle, unspecified**
Boil NOS
Furunculosis NOS
L02.93   **Carbuncle, unspecified**

✓4ᵗʰ **L03**   **Cellulitis and acute lymphangitis**
> EXCLUDES 2   *cellulitis of anal and rectal region (K61.-)*
> *cellulitis of external auditory canal (H60.1)*
> *cellulitis of eyelid (H00.0)*
> *cellulitis of female external genital organs (N76.4)*
> *cellulitis of lacrimal apparatus (H04.3)*
> *cellulitis of male external genital organs (N48.2, N49.-)*
> *cellulitis of mouth (K12.2)*
> *cellulitis of nose (J34.0)*
> *eosinophilic cellulitis [Wells] (L98.3)*
> *febrile neutrophilic dermatosis [Sweet] (L98.2)*
> *lymphangitis (chronic) (subacute) (I89.1)*

AHA: 2017,4Q,100
DEF: Cellulitis: Infection of the skin and subcutaneous tissues, most often caused by *Staphylococcus* or *Streptococcus* bacteria secondary to a cutaneous lesion. Progression of the inflammation may lead to abscess and tissue death, or even systemic infection-like bacteremia.
DEF: Lymphangitis: Inflammation of the lymph channels most often caused by *Streptococcus*.

✓5ᵗʰ **L03.0**   **Cellulitis and acute lymphangitis of finger and toe**
Infection of nail
Onychia
Paronychia
Perionychia

✓6ᵗʰ **L03.01**   **Cellulitis** of finger
Felon
Whitlow
> EXCLUDES 1   *herpetic whitlow (B00.89)*

DEF: Felon: Superficial bacterial skin infection at the tip of the finger.

L03.011   **Cellulitis** of right finger
L03.012   **Cellulitis** of left finger
L03.019   **Cellulitis** of unspecified finger

✓6ᵗʰ **L03.02**   **Acute lymphangitis** of finger
Hangnail with lymphangitis of finger

L03.021   **Acute lymphangitis** of right finger
L03.022   **Acute lymphangitis** of left finger
L03.029   **Acute lymphangitis** of unspecified finger

✓6ᵗʰ **L03.03**   **Cellulitis** of toe

L03.031   **Cellulitis** of right toe
L03.032   **Cellulitis** of left toe
L03.039   **Cellulitis** of unspecified toe

✓6ᵗʰ **L03.04**   **Acute lymphangitis** of toe
Hangnail with lymphangitis of toe

L03.041   **Acute lymphangitis** of right toe
L03.042   **Acute lymphangitis** of left toe
L03.049   **Acute lymphangitis** of unspecified toe

✓5ᵗʰ **L03.1**   **Cellulitis and acute lymphangitis of other parts of limb**

✓6ᵗʰ **L03.11**   **Cellulitis** of other parts of limb
> EXCLUDES 2   *cellulitis of fingers (L03.01-)*
> *cellulitis of toes (L03.03-)*
> *groin (L03.314)*

L03.111   **Cellulitis** of right axilla   CC
L03.112   **Cellulitis** of left axilla   CC
L03.113   **Cellulitis** of right upper limb   CC
L03.114   **Cellulitis** of left upper limb   CC

L03.115 Cellulitis of right lower limb `CC`
L03.116 Cellulitis of left lower limb `CC`
L03.119 Cellulitis of unspecified part of limb `CC`
√6ᵗʰ **L03.12** Acute lymphangitis of other parts of limb
　　　EXCLUDES 2 *acute lymphangitis of fingers (L03.2-)*
　　　　acute lymphangitis of groin (L03.324)
　　　　acute lymphangitis of toes (L03.04-)
L03.121 Acute lymphangitis of right axilla `CC`
L03.122 Acute lymphangitis of left axilla `CC`
L03.123 Acute lymphangitis of right upper limb `CC`
L03.124 Acute lymphangitis of left upper limb `CC`
L03.125 Acute lymphangitis of right lower limb `CC`
L03.126 Acute lymphangitis of left lower limb `CC`
L03.129 Acute lymphangitis of unspecified part of limb `CC`
√5ᵗʰ **L03.2** Cellulitis and acute lymphangitis of face and neck
√6ᵗʰ **L03.21** Cellulitis and acute lymphangitis of face
L03.211 Cellulitis of face `CC`
　　　EXCLUDES 2 *abscess of orbit (H05.01-)*
　　　　cellulitis of ear (H60.1-)
　　　　cellulitis of eyelid (H00.0-)
　　　　cellulitis of head (L03.81)
　　　　cellulitis of lacrimal apparatus (H04.3)
　　　　cellulitis of lip (K13.0)
　　　　cellulitis of mouth (K12.2)
　　　　cellulitis of nose (internal) (J34.0)
　　　　cellulitis of orbit (H05.01-)
　　　　cellulitis of scalp (L03.81)
　　　AHA: 2013,4Q,123
L03.212 Acute lymphangitis of face `CC`
L03.213 Periorbital cellulitis `CC`
　　　Preseptal cellulitis
　　　AHA: 2016,4Q,36
√6ᵗʰ **L03.22** Cellulitis and acute lymphangitis of neck
L03.221 Cellulitis of neck `CC`
L03.222 Acute lymphangitis of neck `CC`
√5ᵗʰ **L03.3** Cellulitis and acute lymphangitis of trunk
√6ᵗʰ **L03.31** Cellulitis of trunk
　　　EXCLUDES 2 *cellulitis of anal and rectal regions (K61.-)*
　　　　cellulitis of breast NOS (N61.0)
　　　　cellulitis of female external genital organs (N76.4)
　　　　cellulitis of male external genital organs (N48.2, N49.-)
　　　　omphalitis of newborn (P38.-)
　　　　puerperal cellulitis of breast (O91.2)
L03.311 Cellulitis of abdominal wall `CC`
　　　EXCLUDES 2 *cellulitis of umbilicus (L03.316)*
　　　　cellulitis of groin (L03.314)
L03.312 Cellulitis of back [any part except buttock] `CC`
L03.313 Cellulitis of chest wall `CC`
L03.314 Cellulitis of groin `CC`
L03.315 Cellulitis of perineum `CC`
L03.316 Cellulitis of umbilicus `CC`
L03.317 Cellulitis of buttock `CC`
L03.319 Cellulitis of trunk, unspecified `CC`
√6ᵗʰ **L03.32** Acute lymphangitis of trunk
L03.321 Acute lymphangitis of abdominal wall `CC`
L03.322 Acute lymphangitis of back [any part except buttock] `CC`
L03.323 Acute lymphangitis of chest wall `CC`
L03.324 Acute lymphangitis of groin `CC`
L03.325 Acute lymphangitis of perineum `CC`
L03.326 Acute lymphangitis of umbilicus `CC`
L03.327 Acute lymphangitis of buttock `CC`

L03.329 Acute lymphangitis of trunk, unspecified `CC`
√5ᵗʰ **L03.8** Cellulitis and acute lymphangitis of other sites
√6ᵗʰ **L03.81** Cellulitis of other sites
L03.811 Cellulitis of head [any part, except face] `CC`
　　　Cellulitis of scalp
　　　EXCLUDES 2 *cellulitis of face (L03.211)*
L03.818 Cellulitis of other sites `CC`
√6ᵗʰ **L03.89** Acute lymphangitis of other sites
L03.891 Acute lymphangitis of head [any part, except face] `CC`
L03.898 Acute lymphangitis of other sites `CC`
√5ᵗʰ **L03.9** Cellulitis and acute lymphangitis, unspecified
L03.90 Cellulitis, unspecified `CC`
L03.91 Acute lymphangitis, unspecified `CC`
　　　EXCLUDES 1 *lymphangitis NOS (I89.1)*
√4ᵗʰ **L04** Acute lymphadenitis
　　　INCLUDES abscess (acute) of lymph nodes, except mesenteric
　　　　acute lymphadenitis, except mesenteric
　　　EXCLUDES 1 *chronic or subacute lymphadenitis, except mesenteric (I88.1)*
　　　　enlarged lymph nodes (R59.-)
　　　　human immunodeficiency virus [HIV] disease resulting in generalized lymphadenopathy (B20)
　　　　lymphadenitis NOS (I88.9)
　　　　nonspecific mesenteric lymphadenitis (I88.0)
　　　DEF: Inflammation or enlargement of the lymph nodes.
L04.0 Acute lymphadenitis of face, head and neck
L04.1 Acute lymphadenitis of trunk
L04.2 Acute lymphadenitis of upper limb
　　　Acute lymphadenitis of axilla
　　　Acute lymphadenitis of shoulder
L04.3 Acute lymphadenitis of lower limb
　　　Acute lymphadenitis of hip
　　　EXCLUDES 2 *acute lymphadenitis of groin (L04.1)*
L04.8 Acute lymphadenitis of other sites
L04.9 Acute lymphadenitis, unspecified
√4ᵗʰ **L05** Pilonidal cyst and sinus
　　　DEF: Pilonidal cyst: Sac or sinus cavity of trapped epithelial tissues in the sacrococcygeal region, usually associated with ingrown hair.
　　　DEF: Pilonidal sinus: Fistula, tract, or channel that extends from an infected area of ingrown hair to another site within the skin or out to the skin surface.

Pilonidal Cyst

- Skin
- Fistula
- Pilonidal cyst
- Fat
- Bone

√5ᵗʰ **L05.0** Pilonidal cyst and sinus with abscess
L05.01 Pilonidal cyst with abscess `CC` `SW`
　　　Pilonidal abscess
　　　Pilonidal dimple with abscess
　　　Postanal dimple with abscess
　　　EXCLUDES 2 *congenital sacral dimple (Q82.6)*
　　　　parasacral dimple (Q82.6)

       L05.02   **Pilonidal sinus with abscess**   `CC` `SW`
Coccygeal fistula with abscess
Coccygeal sinus with abscess
Pilonidal fistula with abscess

√5ᵗʰ **L05.9**   **Pilonidal cyst and sinus without abscess**

       L05.91   **Pilonidal cyst without abscess**
Pilonidal dimple
Postanal dimple
Pilonidal cyst NOS
EXCLUDES 2   congenital sacral dimple (Q82.6)
          parasacral dimple (Q82.6)

       L05.92   **Pilonidal sinus without abscess**   `SW`
Coccygeal fistula
Coccygeal sinus without abscess
Pilonidal fistula

√4ᵗʰ **L08**   **Other local infections of skin and subcutaneous tissue**

     L08.0   **Pyoderma**
Dermatitis gangrenosa
Purulent dermatitis
Septic dermatitis
Suppurative dermatitis
EXCLUDES 1   pyoderma gangrenosum (L88)
          pyoderma vegetans (L08.81)
DEF: Any superficial skin disease commonly characterized by the discharging of pus not attributed to another condition.

     L08.1   **Erythrasma**   `HIV` `CC`
DEF: Chronic, superficial skin infection of brown scaly patches, commonly found in skin folds most prevalent in the overweight or diabetic population.

√5ᵗʰ **L08.8**   **Other specified local infections of the skin and subcutaneous tissue**

       L08.81   **Pyoderma vegetans**
EXCLUDES 1   pyoderma gangrenosum (L88)
          pyoderma NOS (L08.0)

       L08.82   **Omphalitis not of newborn**
EXCLUDES 1   omphalitis of newborn (P38.-)

       L08.89   **Other specified local infections of the skin and subcutaneous tissue**

     L08.9   **Local infection of the skin and subcutaneous tissue, unspecified**

Bullous disorders (L10-L14)

EXCLUDES 1   benign familial pemphigus [Hailey-Hailey] (Q82.8)
          staphylococcal scalded skin syndrome (L00)
          toxic epidermal necrolysis [Lyell] (L51.2)

√4ᵗʰ **L10**   **Pemphigus**
EXCLUDES 1   pemphigus neonatorum (L01.03)

     L10.0   **Pemphigus vulgaris**   `CC`
     L10.1   **Pemphigus vegetans**   `CC`
     L10.2   **Pemphigus foliaceous**   `CC`
     L10.3   **Brazilian pemphigus [fogo selvagem]**   `CC`
     L10.4   **Pemphigus erythematosus**   `CC`
Senear-Usher syndrome
     L10.5   **Drug-induced pemphigus**   `CC`
Use additional code for adverse effect, if applicable, to identify drug (T36-T50 with fifth or sixth character 5)

√5ᵗʰ **L10.8**   **Other pemphigus**
       L10.81   **Paraneoplastic pemphigus**   `CC`
       L10.89   **Other pemphigus**   `CC`
     L10.9   **Pemphigus, unspecified**   `CC`

√4ᵗʰ **L11**   **Other acantholytic disorders**

     L11.0   **Acquired keratosis follicularis**
EXCLUDES 1   keratosis follicularis (congenital) [Darier-White] (Q82.8)
     L11.1   **Transient acantholytic dermatosis [Grover]**
     L11.8   **Other specified acantholytic disorders**
     L11.9   **Acantholytic disorder, unspecified**

√4ᵗʰ **L12**   **Pemphigoid**
EXCLUDES 1   herpes gestationis (O26.4-)
          impetigo herpetiformis (L40.1)
     L12.0   **Bullous pemphigoid**   `CC`

     L12.1   **Cicatricial pemphigoid**
Benign mucous membrane pemphigoid
DEF: Chronic autoimmune disease characterized by subepidermal blistering lesions of the mucosa, including the conjunctiva. It is seen predominantly in the elderly and produces adhesions and scarring.

     L12.2   **Chronic bullous disease of childhood**   `P`
Juvenile dermatitis herpetiformis

√5ᵗʰ **L12.3**   **Acquired epidermolysis bullosa**
EXCLUDES 1   epidermolysis bullosa (congenital) (Q81.-)
       L12.30   **Acquired epidermolysis bullosa, unspecified**   `CC` `HCC`
       L12.31   **Epidermolysis bullosa due to drug**   `CC` `HCC`
Use additional code for adverse effect, if applicable, to identify drug (T36-T50 with fifth or sixth character 5)
       L12.35   **Other acquired epidermolysis bullosa**   `CC` `HCC`

     L12.8   **Other pemphigoid**   `CC`
     L12.9   **Pemphigoid, unspecified**   `CC`

√4ᵗʰ **L13**   **Other bullous disorders**

     L13.0   **Dermatitis herpetiformis**
Duhring's disease
Hydroa herpetiformis
EXCLUDES 1   juvenile dermatitis herpetiformis (L12.2)
          senile dermatitis herpetiformis (L12.0)
DEF: Skin disease to which people are genetically predisposed resulting from an immunological response to gluten. Dermatitis herpetiformis is an extremely pruritic eruption of various lesions that frequently heal, leaving hyperpigmentation or hypopigmentation and occasionally scarring. It is usually associated with asymptomatic gluten-sensitive enteropathy.

     L13.1   **Subcorneal pustular dermatitis**
Sneddon-Wilkinson disease
     L13.8   **Other specified bullous disorders**
     L13.9   **Bullous disorder, unspecified**

L14   *Bullous disorders in diseases classified elsewhere*
Code first underlying disease

Dermatitis and eczema (L20-L30)

`NOTE`   In this block the terms dermatitis and eczema are used synonymously and interchangeably.

EXCLUDES 2   chronic (childhood) granulomatous disease (D71)
          dermatitis gangrenosa (L08.0)
          dermatitis herpetiformis (L13.0)
          dry skin dermatitis (L85.3)
          factitial dermatitis (L98.1)
          perioral dermatitis (L71.0)
          radiation-related disorders of the skin and subcutaneous tissue (L55-L59)
          stasis dermatitis (I87.2)

√4ᵗʰ **L20**   **Atopic dermatitis**

     L20.0   **Besnier's prurigo**

√5ᵗʰ **L20.8**   **Other atopic dermatitis**
EXCLUDES 2   circumscribed neurodermatitis (L28.0)
       L20.81   **Atopic neurodermatitis**
Diffuse neurodermatitis
       L20.82   **Flexural eczema**
       L20.83   **Infantile (acute) (chronic) eczema**   `P`
       L20.84   **Intrinsic (allergic) eczema**
       L20.89   **Other atopic dermatitis**
     L20.9   **Atopic dermatitis, unspecified**

√4ᵗʰ **L21**   **Seborrheic dermatitis**
EXCLUDES 2   infective dermatitis (L30.3)
          seborrheic keratosis (L82.-)

     L21.0   **Seborrhea capitis**
Cradle cap
AHA: 2018,1Q,6
TIP: Assign for dandruff in an adult patient.
     L21.1   **Seborrheic infantile dermatitis**   `P`
     L21.8   **Other seborrheic dermatitis**
     L21.9   **Seborrheic dermatitis, unspecified**
Seborrhea NOS

Chapter 12. Diseases of the Skin and Subcutaneous Tissue

L22–L27.9

L22 Diaper dermatitis
Diaper erythema
Diaper rash
Psoriasiform diaper rash

✓4ᵗʰ **L23 Allergic contact dermatitis**
     EXCLUDES 1   *allergy NOS (T78.40)*
                   contact dermatitis NOS (L25.9)
                   dermatitis NOS (L30.9)
     EXCLUDES 2   *dermatitis due to substances taken internally (L27.-)*
                   dermatitis of eyelid (H01.1-)
                   diaper dermatitis (L22)
                   eczema of external ear (H60.5-)
                   irritant contact dermatitis (L24.-)
                   perioral dermatitis (L71.0)
                   radiation-related disorders of the skin and subcutaneous tissue (L55-L59)

L23.0 Allergic contact dermatitis due to metals
Allergic contact dermatitis due to chromium
Allergic contact dermatitis due to nickel

L23.1 Allergic contact dermatitis due to adhesives

L23.2 Allergic contact dermatitis due to cosmetics

L23.3 Allergic contact dermatitis due to drugs in contact with skin
Use additional code for adverse effect, if applicable, to identify drug (T36-T50 with fifth or sixth character 5)
     EXCLUDES 2   *dermatitis due to ingested drugs and medicaments (L27.0-L27.1)*

L23.4 Allergic contact dermatitis due to dyes

L23.5 Allergic contact dermatitis due to other chemical products
Allergic contact dermatitis due to cement
Allergic contact dermatitis due to insecticide
Allergic contact dermatitis due to plastic
Allergic contact dermatitis due to rubber

L23.6 Allergic contact dermatitis due to food in contact with the skin
     EXCLUDES 2   *dermatitis due to ingested food (L27.2)*

L23.7 Allergic contact dermatitis due to plants, except food
     EXCLUDES 2   *allergy NOS due to pollen (J30.1)*

✓5ᵗʰ **L23.8 Allergic contact dermatitis due to other agents**

     L23.81 Allergic contact dermatitis due to animal (cat) (dog) dander
         Allergic contact dermatitis due to animal (cat) (dog) hair

     L23.89 Allergic contact dermatitis due to other agents

L23.9 Allergic contact dermatitis, unspecified cause
Allergic contact eczema NOS

✓4ᵗʰ **L24 Irritant contact dermatitis**
     EXCLUDES 1   *allergy NOS (T78.40)*
                   contact dermatitis NOS (L25.9)
                   dermatitis NOS (L30.9)
     EXCLUDES 2   *allergic contact dermatitis (L23.-)*
                   dermatitis due to substances taken internally (L27.-)
                   dermatitis of eyelid (H01.1-)
                   diaper dermatitis (L22)
                   eczema of external ear (H60.5-)
                   perioral dermatitis (L71.0)
                   radiation-related disorders of the skin and subcutaneous tissue (L55-L59)

L24.0 Irritant contact dermatitis due to detergents

L24.1 Irritant contact dermatitis due to oils and greases

L24.2 Irritant contact dermatitis due to solvents
Irritant contact dermatitis due to chlorocompound
Irritant contact dermatitis due to cyclohexane
Irritant contact dermatitis due to ester
Irritant contact dermatitis due to glycol
Irritant contact dermatitis due to hydrocarbon
Irritant contact dermatitis due to ketone

L24.3 Irritant contact dermatitis due to cosmetics

L24.4 Irritant contact dermatitis due to drugs in contact with skin
Use additional code for adverse effect, if applicable, to identify drug (T36-T50 with fifth or sixth character 5)

L24.5 Irritant contact dermatitis due to other chemical products
Irritant contact dermatitis due to cement
Irritant contact dermatitis due to insecticide
Irritant contact dermatitis due to plastic
Irritant contact dermatitis due to rubber

L24.6 Irritant contact dermatitis due to food in contact with skin
     EXCLUDES 2   *dermatitis due to ingested food (L27.2)*

L24.7 Irritant contact dermatitis due to plants, except food
     EXCLUDES 2   *allergy NOS to pollen (J30.1)*

✓5ᵗʰ **L24.8 Irritant contact dermatitis due to other agents**

     L24.81 Irritant contact dermatitis due to metals
         Irritant contact dermatitis due to chromium
         Irritant contact dermatitis due to nickel

     L24.89 Irritant contact dermatitis due to other agents
         Irritant contact dermatitis due to dyes

L24.9 Irritant contact dermatitis, unspecified cause
Irritant contact eczema NOS

✓4ᵗʰ **L25 Unspecified contact dermatitis**
     EXCLUDES 1   *allergic contact dermatitis (L23.-)*
                   allergy NOS (T78.40)
                   dermatitis NOS (L30.9)
                   irritant contact dermatitis (L24.-)
     EXCLUDES 2   *dermatitis due to ingested substances (L27.-)*
                   dermatitis of eyelid (H01.1-)
                   eczema of external ear (H60.5-)
                   perioral dermatitis (L71.0)
                   radiation-related disorders of the skin and subcutaneous tissue (L55-L59)

L25.0 Unspecified contact dermatitis due to cosmetics

L25.1 Unspecified contact dermatitis due to drugs in contact with skin
Use additional code for adverse effect, if applicable, to identify drug (T36-T50 with fifth or sixth character 5)
     EXCLUDES 2   *dermatitis due to ingested drugs and medicaments (L27.0-L27.1)*

L25.2 Unspecified contact dermatitis due to dyes

L25.3 Unspecified contact dermatitis due to other chemical products
Unspecified contact dermatitis due to cement
Unspecified contact dermatitis due to insecticide

L25.4 Unspecified contact dermatitis due to food in contact with skin
     EXCLUDES 2   *dermatitis due to ingested food (L27.2)*

L25.5 Unspecified contact dermatitis due to plants, except food
     EXCLUDES 1   *nettle rash (L50.9)*
     EXCLUDES 2   *allergy NOS due to pollen (J30.1)*

L25.8 Unspecified contact dermatitis due to other agents

L25.9 Unspecified contact dermatitis, unspecified cause
Contact dermatitis (occupational) NOS
Contact eczema (occupational) NOS

L26 Exfoliative dermatitis
Hebra's pityriasis
     EXCLUDES 1   *Ritter's disease (L00)*

✓4ᵗʰ **L27 Dermatitis due to substances taken internally**
     EXCLUDES 1   *allergy NOS (T78.40)*
     EXCLUDES 2   *adverse food reaction, except dermatitis (T78.0-T78.1)*
                   contact dermatitis (L23-L25)
                   drug photoallergic response (L56.1)
                   drug phototoxic response (L56.0)
                   urticaria (L50.-)

L27.0 Generalized skin eruption due to drugs and medicaments taken internally
Use additional code for adverse effect, if applicable, to identify drug (T36-T50 with fifth or sixth character 5)

L27.1 Localized skin eruption due to drugs and medicaments taken internally
Use additional code for adverse effect, if applicable, to identify drug (T36-T50 with fifth or sixth character 5)

L27.2 Dermatitis due to ingested food
     EXCLUDES 2   *dermatitis due to food in contact with skin (L23.6, L24.6, L25.4)*

L27.8 Dermatitis due to other substances taken internally

L27.9 Dermatitis due to unspecified substance taken internally

---

Ⓝ Newborn: 0   Ⓟ Pediatric: 0-17   Ⓜ Maternity: 9-64   Ⓐ Adult: 15-124   **MCC** Major Complication/Comorbidity   **CC** Complication/Comorbidity   **SW** Severe Wound Dx

736   ICD-10-CM 2021

√4th **L28 Lichen simplex chronicus and prurigo**

    L28.0 Lichen simplex chronicus
        Circumscribed neurodermatitis
        Lichen NOS

    L28.1 Prurigo nodularis

    L28.2 Other prurigo
        Prurigo NOS
        Prurigo Hebra
        Prurigo mitis
        Urticaria papulosa

√4th **L29 Pruritus**

    EXCLUDES1   neurotic excoriation (L98.1)
                psychogenic pruritus (F45.8)

    L29.0 Pruritus ani

    L29.1 Pruritus scroti   ♂

    L29.2 Pruritus vulvae   ♀

    L29.3 Anogenital pruritus, unspecified

    L29.8 Other pruritus

    L29.9 Pruritus, unspecified
        Itch NOS

√4th **L30 Other and unspecified dermatitis**

    EXCLUDES2   contact dermatitis (L23-L25)
                dry skin dermatitis (L85.3)
                small plaque parapsoriasis (L41.3)
                stasis dermatitis (I87.2)

    L30.0 Nummular dermatitis

    L30.1 Dyshidrosis [pompholyx]

    L30.2 Cutaneous autosensitization
        Candidid [levurid]
        Dermatophytid
        Eczematid

    L30.3 Infective dermatitis
        Infectious eczematoid dermatitis

    L30.4 Erythema intertrigo

    L30.5 Pityriasis alba
        AHA: 2018,1Q,6

    L30.8 Other specified dermatitis

    L30.9 Dermatitis, unspecified
        Eczema NOS

Papulosquamous disorders (L40-L45)

√4th **L40 Psoriasis**

    DEF: Chronic autoimmune condition that speeds up skin cell growth, causing excessive immature skin cells to form raised, rounded erythematous lesions covered by dry, silvery scaling patches. Most commonly found on the scalp, elbows, knees, hands, feet, and genitals, it can also affect the joints with stiffness and swelling.

    L40.0 Psoriasis vulgaris
        Nummular psoriasis
        Plaque psoriasis

    L40.1 Generalized pustular psoriasis
        Impetigo herpetiformis
        Von Zumbusch's disease

    L40.2 Acrodermatitis continua

    L40.3 Pustulosis palmaris et plantaris

    L40.4 Guttate psoriasis

√6th   **L40.5 Arthropathic psoriasis**

        L40.50 Arthropathic psoriasis, unspecified   HCC
        L40.51 Distal interphalangeal psoriatic arthropathy   HCC
        L40.52 Psoriatic arthritis mutilans   HCC
        L40.53 Psoriatic spondylitis   HCC
        L40.54 Psoriatic juvenile arthropathy   HCC
        L40.59 Other psoriatic arthropathy   HCC

    L40.8 Other psoriasis
        Flexural psoriasis

    L40.9 Psoriasis, unspecified

√4th **L41 Parapsoriasis**

    EXCLUDES1   poikiloderma vasculare atrophicans (L94.5)

    L41.0 Pityriasis lichenoides et varioliformis acuta
        Mucha-Habermann disease

    L41.1 Pityriasis lichenoides chronica

    L41.3 Small plaque parapsoriasis

    L41.4 Large plaque parapsoriasis

    L41.5 Retiform parapsoriasis

    L41.8 Other parapsoriasis

    L41.9 Parapsoriasis, unspecified

L42 Pityriasis rosea

√4th **L43 Lichen planus**

    EXCLUDES1   lichen planopilaris (L66.1)

    L43.0 Hypertrophic lichen planus

    L43.1 Bullous lichen planus

    L43.2 Lichenoid drug reaction
        Use additional code for adverse effect, if applicable, to identify drug (T36-T50 with fifth or sixth character 5)

    L43.3 Subacute (active) lichen planus
        Lichen planus tropicus

    L43.8 Other lichen planus

    L43.9 Lichen planus, unspecified

√4th **L44 Other papulosquamous disorders**

    L44.0 Pityriasis rubra pilaris

    L44.1 Lichen nitidus
        DEF: Chronic, inflammatory, asymptomatic skin disorder, characterized by numerous glistening, flat-topped, discrete, skin-colored micropapules, most often on the penis, lower abdomen, inner thighs, wrists, forearms, breasts, and buttocks.

    L44.2 Lichen striatus

    L44.3 Lichen ruber moniliformis

    L44.4 Infantile papular acrodermatitis [Gianotti-Crosti]   P

    L44.8 Other specified papulosquamous disorders

    L44.9 Papulosquamous disorder, unspecified

L45 Papulosquamous disorders in diseases classified elsewhere
    Code first underlying disease

Urticaria and erythema (L49-L54)

    EXCLUDES1   Lyme disease (A69.2-)
                rosacea (L71.-)

√4th **L49 Exfoliation due to erythematous conditions according to extent of body surface involved**

    Code first erythematous condition causing exfoliation, such as:
        Ritter's disease (L00)
        (Staphylococcal) scalded skin syndrome (L00)
        Stevens-Johnson syndrome (L51.1)
        Stevens-Johnson syndrome-toxic epidermal necrolysis overlap syndrome (L51.3)
        toxic epidermal necrolysis (L51.2)
    DEF: Exfoliation: Falling or sloughing off skin in layers.

    L49.0 Exfoliation due to erythematous condition involving less than 10 percent of body surface
        Exfoliation due to erythematous condition NOS

    L49.1 Exfoliation due to erythematous condition involving 10-19 percent of body surface

    L49.2 Exfoliation due to erythematous condition involving 20-29 percent of body surface

    L49.3 Exfoliation due to erythematous condition involving 30-39 percent of body surface   CC

    L49.4 Exfoliation due to erythematous condition involving 40-49 percent of body surface   CC

    L49.5 Exfoliation due to erythematous condition involving 50-59 percent of body surface   CC

    L49.6 Exfoliation due to erythematous condition involving 60-69 percent of body surface   CC

    L49.7 Exfoliation due to erythematous condition involving 70-79 percent of body surface   CC

    L49.8 Exfoliation due to erythematous condition involving 80-89 percent of body surface   CC

    L49.9 Exfoliation due to erythematous condition involving 90 or more percent of body surface   CC

☑ Additional Character Required   √x7th Placeholder   Unacceptable PDx   Questionable PDx   Manifestation   Unspecified Dx   H1-H14 HAC   HCC CMS-HCC Dx   HIV HIV Dx

ICD-10-CM 2021   737

Chapter 12. Diseases of the Skin and Subcutaneous Tissue

L50–L58.9

✓4ᵗʰ L50 Urticaria

> EXCLUDES 1   allergic contact dermatitis (L23.-)
> angioneurotic edema (T78.3)
> giant urticaria (T78.3)
> hereditary angio-edema (D84.1)
> Quincke's edema (T78.3)
> serum urticaria (T80.6-)
> solar urticaria (L56.3)
> urticaria neonatorum (P83.8)
> urticaria papulosa (L28.2)
> urticaria pigmentosa (D47.01)

> **DEF:** Eruption of itching edema of the skin. **Synonym(s):** hives.

L50.0 Allergic urticaria

L50.1 Idiopathic urticaria

L50.2 Urticaria due to cold and heat
> EXCLUDES 2   familial cold urticaria (M04.2)

L50.3 Dermatographic urticaria

L50.4 Vibratory urticaria

L50.5 Cholinergic urticaria

L50.6 Contact urticaria

L50.8 Other urticaria
> Chronic urticaria
> Recurrent periodic urticaria

L50.9 Urticaria, unspecified

✓4ᵗʰ L51 Erythema multiforme

> Use additional code for adverse effect, if applicable, to identify drug (T36-T50 with fifth or sixth character 5)
> Use additional code to identify associated manifestations, such as:
> arthropathy associated with dermatological disorders (M14.8-)
> conjunctival edema (H11.42)
> conjunctivitis (H10.22-)
> corneal scars and opacities (H17.-)
> corneal ulcer (H16.0-)
> edema of eyelid (H02.84-)
> inflammation of eyelid (H01.8)
> keratoconjunctivitis sicca (H16.22-)
> mechanical lagophthalmos (H02.22-)
> stomatitis (K12.-)
> symblepharon (H11.23-)
> Use additional code to identify percentage of skin exfoliation (L49.-)

> EXCLUDES 1   staphylococcal scalded skin syndrome (L00)
> Ritter's disease (L00)

> **DEF:** Acute complex of symptoms with a varied pattern of skin eruptions, such as macular, bullous, popular, nodose, or vesicular lesions on the neck, face, and legs. Erythema (redness of skin and mucous membranes) multiforme (multiple forms) is a hypersensitivity (allergic) reaction that can occur at any age but primarily affects children or young adults.

L51.0 Nonbullous erythema multiforme

L51.1 Stevens-Johnson syndrome   CC HCC

L51.2 Toxic epidermal necrolysis [Lyell]   CC HCC

L51.3 Stevens-Johnson syndrome-toxic epidermal necrolysis overlap syndrome   CC HCC
> SJS-TEN overlap syndrome

L51.8 Other erythema multiforme

L51.9 Erythema multiforme, unspecified
> Erythema iris
> Erythema multiforme major NOS
> Erythema multiforme minor NOS
> Herpes iris

L52 Erythema nodosum

> EXCLUDES 1   tuberculous erythema nodosum (A18.4)

> **DEF:** Form of panniculitis (inflammation of the fat layer beneath the skin) most often occurring in women. Commonly seen as a hypersensitivity reaction to infections, drugs, sarcoidosis, and specific enteropathies. The acute stage is associated with fever, malaise, and arthralgia. The lesions are pink to blue in color as tender nodules and are found on the front of the legs below the knees.

✓4ᵗʰ L53 Other erythematous conditions

> EXCLUDES 1   erythema ab igne (L59.0)
> erythema due to external agents in contact with skin (L23-L25)
> erythema intertrigo (L30.4)

L53.0 Toxic erythema   CC
> Code first poisoning due to drug or toxin, if applicable (T36-T65 with fifth or sixth character 1-4 or 6)
> Use additional code for adverse effect, if applicable, to identify drug (T36-T50 with fifth or sixth character 5)
> EXCLUDES 1   neonatal erythema toxicum (P83.1)

L53.1 Erythema annulare centrifugum   CC

L53.2 Erythema marginatum   CC

L53.3 Other chronic figurate erythema   CC

L53.8 Other specified erythematous conditions

L53.9 Erythematous condition, unspecified
> Erythema NOS
> Erythroderma NOS

L54 Erythema in diseases classified elsewhere
> Code first underlying disease

Radiation-related disorders of the skin and subcutaneous tissue (L55-L59)

✓4ᵗʰ L55 Sunburn

L55.0 Sunburn of first degree

L55.1 Sunburn of second degree

L55.2 Sunburn of third degree

L55.9 Sunburn, unspecified

✓4ᵗʰ L56 Other acute skin changes due to ultraviolet radiation

> Use additional code to identify the source of the ultraviolet radiation (W89, X32)

L56.0 Drug phototoxic response
> Use additional code for adverse effect, if applicable, to identify drug (T36-T50 with fifth or sixth character 5)

L56.1 Drug photoallergic response
> Use additional code for adverse effect, if applicable, to identify drug (T36-T50 with fifth or sixth character 5)

L56.2 Photocontact dermatitis [berloque dermatitis]

L56.3 Solar urticaria

L56.4 Polymorphous light eruption

L56.5 Disseminated superficial actinic porokeratosis (DSAP)
> **DEF:** Autosomal dominant skin condition occurring in sun-exposed areas of the skin (particularly the arms and legs), characterized by superficial annular, keratotic, brownish-red spots or thickenings with depressed centers and sharp, ridged borders. It may evolve into squamous cell carcinoma.

L56.8 Other specified acute skin changes due to ultraviolet radiation

L56.9 Acute skin change due to ultraviolet radiation, unspecified

✓4ᵗʰ L57 Skin changes due to chronic exposure to nonionizing radiation

> ▶Use additional code to identify the source of the ultraviolet radiation (W89), or other nonionizing radiation (W90)◀

L57.0 Actinic keratosis
> Keratosis NOS
> Senile keratosis
> Solar keratosis

L57.1 Actinic reticuloid

L57.2 Cutis rhomboidalis nuchae

L57.3 Poikiloderma of Civatte

L57.4 Cutis laxa senilis
> Elastosis senilis

L57.5 Actinic granuloma

L57.8 Other skin changes due to chronic exposure to nonionizing radiation
> Farmer's skin
> Sailor's skin
> Solar dermatitis

L57.9 Skin changes due to chronic exposure to nonionizing radiation, unspecified

✓4ᵗʰ L58 Radiodermatitis

> Use additional code to identify the source of the radiation (W88, W90)

L58.0 Acute radiodermatitis

L58.1 Chronic radiodermatitis

L58.9 Radiodermatitis, unspecified

√4ᵗʰ **L59 Other disorders of skin and subcutaneous tissue related to radiation**

L59.0 Erythema ab igne [dermatitis ab igne]

L59.8 Other specified disorders of the skin and subcutaneous tissue related to radiation
AHA: 2017,1Q,33

L59.9 Disorder of the skin and subcutaneous tissue related to radiation, unspecified

Disorders of skin appendages (L60-L75)

EXCLUDES 1   *congenital malformations of integument (Q84.-)*

√4ᵗʰ **L60 Nail disorders**

EXCLUDES 2   *clubbing of nails (R68.3)*
          onychia and paronychia (L03.0-)

Nail Disorders

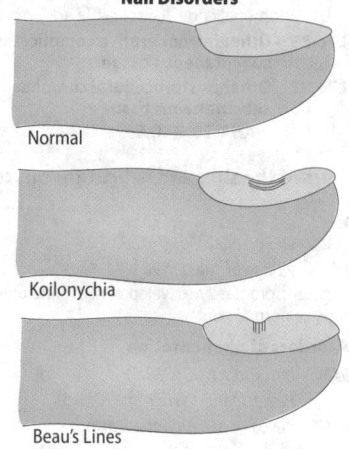

Normal

Koilonychia

Beau's Lines

L60.0 Ingrowing nail
L60.1 Onycholysis
L60.2 Onychogryphosis
L60.3 Nail dystrophy
L60.4 Beau's lines
L60.5 Yellow nail syndrome
L60.8 Other nail disorders
L60.9 Nail disorder, unspecified

L62 Nail disorders in diseases classified elsewhere
Code first underlying disease, such as:
pachydermoperiostosis (M89.4-)

√4ᵗʰ **L63 Alopecia areata**

L63.0 Alopecia (capitis) totalis
L63.1 Alopecia universalis
L63.2 Ophiasis
L63.8 Other alopecia areata
L63.9 Alopecia areata, unspecified

√4ᵗʰ **L64 Androgenic alopecia**

INCLUDES   male-pattern baldness

L64.0 Drug-induced androgenic alopecia
Use additional code for adverse effect, if applicable, to identify drug (T36-T50 with fifth or sixth character 5)

L64.8 Other androgenic alopecia
L64.9 Androgenic alopecia, unspecified

√4ᵗʰ **L65 Other nonscarring hair loss**

Use additional code for adverse effect, if applicable, to identify drug (T36-T50 with fifth or sixth character 5)

EXCLUDES 1   *trichotillomania (F63.3)*

L65.0 Telogen effluvium
DEF: Form of nonscarring alopecia characterized by shedding of hair from premature telogen development in follicles due to stress, including shock, childbirth, surgery, drugs, or weight loss.

L65.1 Anagen effluvium
L65.2 Alopecia mucinosa
L65.8 Other specified nonscarring hair loss
L65.9 Nonscarring hair loss, unspecified
Alopecia NOS

√4ᵗʰ **L66 Cicatricial alopecia [scarring hair loss]**

L66.0 Pseudopelade

L66.1 Lichen planopilaris
Follicular lichen planus

L66.2 Folliculitis decalvans
L66.3 Perifolliculitis capitis abscedens
L66.4 Folliculitis ulerythematosa reticulata
L66.8 Other cicatricial alopecia
AHA: 2015,1Q,19

L66.9 Cicatricial alopecia, unspecified

√4ᵗʰ **L67 Hair color and hair shaft abnormalities**

EXCLUDES 1   *monilethrix (Q84.1)*
          pili annulati (Q84.1)
          telogen effluvium (L65.0)

L67.0 Trichorrhexis nodosa
L67.1 Variations in hair color
Canities
Greyness, hair (premature)
Heterochromia of hair
Poliosis circumscripta, acquired
Poliosis NOS

L67.8 Other hair color and hair shaft abnormalities
Fragilitas crinium

L67.9 Hair color and hair shaft abnormality, unspecified

√4ᵗʰ **L68 Hypertrichosis**

INCLUDES   excess hair
EXCLUDES 1   *congenital hypertrichosis (Q84.2)*
          persistent lanugo (Q84.2)

L68.0 Hirsutism
L68.1 Acquired hypertrichosis lanuginosa
L68.2 Localized hypertrichosis
L68.3 Polytrichia
L68.8 Other hypertrichosis
L68.9 Hypertrichosis, unspecified

√4ᵗʰ **L70 Acne**

EXCLUDES 2   *acne keloid (L73.0)*

L70.0 Acne vulgaris
L70.1 Acne conglobata
L70.2 Acne varioliformis
Acne necrotica miliaris
DEF: Rare form of acne characterized by development of persistent brown papulopustules followed by scar formation. This type of acne usually presents on the brow and temporoparietal part of the scalp.

L70.3 Acne tropica
L70.4 Infantile acne   P
L70.5 Acné excoriée
Acné excoriée des jeunes filles
Picker's acne

L70.8 Other acne
L70.9 Acne, unspecified

√4ᵗʰ **L71 Rosacea**

Use additional code for adverse effect, if applicable, to identify drug (T36-T50 with fifth or sixth character 5)

L71.0 Perioral dermatitis
L71.1 Rhinophyma
L71.8 Other rosacea
AHA: 2018,4Q,15

L71.9 Rosacea, unspecified

√4ᵗʰ **L72 Follicular cysts of skin and subcutaneous tissue**

L72.0 Epidermal cyst
√5ᵗʰ **L72.1 Pilar and trichodermal cyst**

L72.11 Pilar cyst
L72.12 Trichodermal cyst
Trichilemmal (proliferating) cyst

L72.2 Steatocystoma multiplex
L72.3 Sebaceous cyst
EXCLUDES 2   *pilar cyst (L72.11)*
          trichilemmal (proliferating) cyst (L72.12)

L72.8 Other follicular cysts of the skin and subcutaneous tissue
L72.9 Follicular cyst of the skin and subcutaneous tissue, unspecified

√4ᵗʰ **L73 Other follicular disorders**

L73.0 Acne keloid
L73.1 Pseudofolliculitis barbae

✔ Additional Character Required   √x7ᵗʰ Placeholder   Unacceptable PDx   Questionable PDx   Manifestation   Unspecified Dx   H1-H14 HAC   HCC CMS-HCC Dx   HIV HIV Dx

ICD-10-CM 2021   739

Chapter 12. Diseases of the Skin and Subcutaneous Tissue

L73.2–L85.2

L73.2 Hidradenitis suppurativa

L73.8 Other specified follicular disorders
Sycosis barbae

L73.9 Follicular disorder, unspecified

√4ᵗʰ **L74 Eccrine sweat disorders**

EXCLUDES 2   *generalized hyperhidrosis (R61)*

DEF: Eccrine sweat glands: Glands found in the dermal and hypodermal layer of the skin throughout the body, particularly on the forehead, scalp, axillae, palms, and soles. These glands produce watery and neutral or slightly acidic sweat.

L74.0 Miliaria rubra

L74.1 Miliaria crystallina

L74.2 Miliaria profunda
Miliaria tropicalis

L74.3 Miliaria, unspecified

L74.4 Anhidrosis
Hypohidrosis
DEF: Inability to sweat normally. When the body can't cool itself through perspiration it can lead to heatstroke, a life-threatening condition.

√5ᵗʰ **L74.5 Focal hyperhidrosis**

√6ᵗʰ **L74.51 Primary focal hyperhidrosis**

L74.510 Primary focal hyperhidrosis, axilla

L74.511 Primary focal hyperhidrosis, face

L74.512 Primary focal hyperhidrosis, palms

L74.513 Primary focal hyperhidrosis, soles

L74.519 Primary focal hyperhidrosis, unspecified

L74.52 Secondary focal hyperhidrosis
Frey's syndrome

L74.8 Other eccrine sweat disorders

L74.9 Eccrine sweat disorder, unspecified
Sweat gland disorder NOS

√4ᵗʰ **L75 Apocrine sweat disorders**

EXCLUDES 1   *dyshidrosis (L30.1)*
               hidradenitis suppurativa (L73.2)

DEF: Apocrine sweat glands: Found in the axilla, areola, and circumanal region, these glands begin to function in puberty and produce viscid milky secretions in response to external stimuli.

L75.0 Bromhidrosis

L75.1 Chromhidrosis

L75.2 Apocrine miliaria
Fox-Fordyce disease
DEF: Chronic, usually pruritic disease evidenced by small follicular papular eruptions, especially in the axillary and pubic areas. Apocrine miliaria develops from the closure and rupture of the affected apocrine glands' intraepidermal portion of the ducts.

L75.8 Other apocrine sweat disorders

L75.9 Apocrine sweat disorder, unspecified

Intraoperative and postprocedural complications of skin and subcutaneous tissue (L76)

√4ᵗʰ **L76 Intraoperative and postprocedural complications of skin and subcutaneous tissue**
AHA: 2016,4Q,9-10

√5ᵗʰ **L76.0 Intraoperative hemorrhage and hematoma of skin and subcutaneous tissue complicating a procedure**

EXCLUDES 1   *intraoperative hemorrhage and hematoma of skin and subcutaneous tissue due to accidental puncture and laceration during a procedure (L76.1-)*

L76.01 Intraoperative hemorrhage and hematoma of skin and subcutaneous tissue complicating a dermatologic procedure CC

L76.02 Intraoperative hemorrhage and hematoma of skin and subcutaneous tissue complicating other procedure CC

√5ᵗʰ **L76.1 Accidental puncture and laceration of skin and subcutaneous tissue during a procedure**

L76.11 Accidental puncture and laceration of skin and subcutaneous tissue during a dermatologic procedure CC

L76.12 Accidental puncture and laceration of skin and subcutaneous tissue during other procedure CC

√5ᵗʰ **L76.2 Postprocedural hemorrhage of skin and subcutaneous tissue following a procedure**

L76.21 Postprocedural hemorrhage of skin and subcutaneous tissue following a dermatologic procedure CC

L76.22 Postprocedural hemorrhage of skin and subcutaneous tissue following other procedure CC

√5ᵗʰ **L76.3 Postprocedural hematoma and seroma of skin and subcutaneous tissue following a procedure**

L76.31 Postprocedural hematoma of skin and subcutaneous tissue following a dermatologic procedure CC

L76.32 Postprocedural hematoma of skin and subcutaneous tissue following other procedure CC

L76.33 Postprocedural seroma of skin and subcutaneous tissue following a dermatologic procedure CC

L76.34 Postprocedural seroma of skin and subcutaneous tissue following other procedure CC

√5ᵗʰ **L76.8 Other intraoperative and postprocedural complications of skin and subcutaneous tissue**
Use additional code, if applicable, to further specify disorder

L76.81 Other intraoperative complications of skin and subcutaneous tissue

L76.82 Other postprocedural complications of skin and subcutaneous tissue
AHA: 2017,3Q,6

Other disorders of the skin and subcutaneous tissue (L80-L99)

L80 Vitiligo

EXCLUDES 2   *vitiligo of eyelids (H02.73-)*
               vitiligo of vulva (N90.89)

DEF: Persistent, progressive development of nonpigmented white patches on otherwise normal skin.

√4ᵗʰ **L81 Other disorders of pigmentation**

EXCLUDES 1   *birthmark NOS (Q82.5)*
               Peutz-Jeghers syndrome (Q85.8)

EXCLUDES 2   *nevus — see Alphabetical Index*

L81.0 Postinflammatory hyperpigmentation

L81.1 Chloasma

L81.2 Freckles

L81.3 Café au lait spots

L81.4 Other melanin hyperpigmentation
Lentigo

L81.5 Leukoderma, not elsewhere classified

L81.6 Other disorders of diminished melanin formation

L81.7 Pigmented purpuric dermatosis
Angioma serpiginosum

L81.8 Other specified disorders of pigmentation
Iron pigmentation
Tattoo pigmentation

L81.9 Disorder of pigmentation, unspecified

√4ᵗʰ **L82 Seborrheic keratosis**

INCLUDES   basal cell papilloma
              dermatosis papulosa nigra
              Leser-Trélat disease

EXCLUDES 2   *seborrheic dermatitis (L21.-)*

DEF: Common, benign, noninvasive, lightly pigmented, warty growth composed of basaloid cells that usually appear at middle age as soft, easily crumbling plaques on the face, trunk, and extremities.

L82.0 Inflamed seborrheic keratosis

L82.1 Other seborrheic keratosis
Seborrheic keratosis NOS

L83 Acanthosis nigricans
Confluent and reticulated papillomatosis
DEF: Diffuse, velvety hyperplasia of the spinous skin layer of the axilla and other body folds marked by gray, brown, or black pigmentation. In adult form, it is often associated with malignant acanthosis nigricans in a benign, nevoid form relatively generalized.

L84 Corns and callosities
Callus
Clavus

√4ᵗʰ **L85 Other epidermal thickening**

EXCLUDES 2   *hypertrophic disorders of the skin (L91.-)*

L85.0 Acquired ichthyosis
EXCLUDES 1   *congenital ichthyosis (Q80.-)*

L85.1 Acquired keratosis [keratoderma] palmaris et plantaris
EXCLUDES 1   *inherited keratosis palmaris et plantaris (Q82.8)*

L85.2 Keratosis punctata (palmaris et plantaris)

N Newborn: 0   P Pediatric: 0-17   M Maternity: 9-64   A Adult: 15-124   MCC Major Complication/Comorbidity   CC Complication/Comorbidity   SW Severe Wound Dx

740   ICD-10-CM 2021

Chapter 12. Diseases of the Skin and Subcutaneous Tissue

L85.3 **Xerosis cutis**
Dry skin dermatitis

L85.8 **Other specified epidermal thickening**
Cutaneous horn

L85.9 **Epidermal thickening, unspecified**

L86 *Keratoderma in diseases classified elsewhere*
Code first underlying disease, such as:
Reiter's disease (M02.3-)

   EXCLUDES 1   gonococcal keratoderma (A54.89)
gonococcal keratosis (A54.89)
keratoderma due to vitamin A deficiency (E50.8)
keratosis due to vitamin A deficiency (E50.8)
xeroderma due to vitamin A deficiency (E50.8)

☑4ᵗʰ **L87 Transepidermal elimination disorders**

   EXCLUDES 1   granuloma annulare (perforating) (L92.0)

L87.0 **Keratosis follicularis et parafollicularis in cutem penetrans**
Hyperkeratosis follicularis penetrans
Kyrle disease

L87.1 **Reactive perforating collagenosis**

L87.2 **Elastosis perforans serpiginosa**

L87.8 **Other transepidermal elimination disorders**

L87.9 **Transepidermal elimination disorder, unspecified**

L88 Pyoderma gangrenosum   CC
Phagedenic pyoderma

   EXCLUDES 1   dermatitis gangrenosa (L08.0)

DEF: Persistent debilitating skin disease characterized by irregular, boggy, blue-red ulcerations, with central healing and undermined edges.

☑4ᵗʰ **L89 Pressure ulcer**

   INCLUDES   bed sore
decubitus ulcer
plaster ulcer
pressure area
pressure sore

Code first any associated gangrene (I96)

   EXCLUDES 2   decubitus (trophic) ulcer of cervix (uteri) (N86)
diabetic ulcers (E08.621, E08.622, E09.621, E09.622, E10.621, E10.622, E11.621, E11.622, E13.621, E13.622)
non-pressure chronic ulcer of skin (L97.-)
skin infections (L00-L08)
varicose ulcer (I83.0, I83.2)

AHA: 2019,4Q,10-11,54; 2018,4Q,69; 2018,3Q,3; 2018,2Q,21; 2017,4Q,109; 2017,1Q,49; 2016,4Q,143

TIP: The stage of a diagnosed pressure ulcer can be based on documentation from clinicians who are not the patient's provider.

Four Stages of Pressure Ulcer

Stage 1
Persistent focal edema

Stage 2
Abrasion, blister, partial thickness skin loss involving epidermis and/or dermis

Stage 3
Full thickness skin loss involving damage or necrosis of subcutaneous tissue

Stage 4
Necrosis of soft tissues through to underlying muscle, tendon, or bone

☑5ᵗʰ **L89.0 Pressure ulcer of elbow**

☑6ᵗʰ **L89.00 Pressure ulcer of unspecified elbow**

L89.000 Pressure ulcer of unspecified elbow, unstageable   HCC SW

L89.001 Pressure ulcer of unspecified elbow, stage 1
Healing pressure ulcer of unspecified elbow, stage 1
Pressure pre-ulcer skin changes limited to persistent focal edema, unspecified elbow

L89.002 Pressure ulcer of unspecified elbow, stage 2   HCC
Healing pressure ulcer of unspecified elbow, stage 2
Pressure ulcer with abrasion, blister, partial thickness skin loss involving epidermis and/or dermis, unspecified elbow

L89.003 Pressure ulcer of unspecified elbow, stage 3   MCC H4 HCC SW
Healing pressure ulcer of unspecified elbow, stage 3
Pressure ulcer with full thickness skin loss involving damage or necrosis of subcutaneous tissue, unspecified elbow

L89.004 Pressure ulcer of unspecified elbow, stage 4   MCC H4 HCC SW
Healing pressure ulcer of unspecified elbow, stage 4
Pressure ulcer with necrosis of soft tissues through to underlying muscle, tendon, or bone, unspecified elbow

L89.006 Pressure-induced deep tissue damage of unspecified elbow

L89.009 Pressure ulcer of unspecified elbow, unspecified stage
Healing pressure ulcer of elbow NOS
Healing pressure ulcer of unspecified elbow, unspecified stage

☑6ᵗʰ **L89.01 Pressure ulcer of right elbow**

L89.010 Pressure ulcer of right elbow, unstageable   HCC SW

L89.011 Pressure ulcer of right elbow, stage 1
Healing pressure ulcer of right elbow, stage 1
Pressure pre-ulcer skin changes limited to persistent focal edema, right elbow

L89.012 Pressure ulcer of right elbow, stage 2   HCC
Healing pressure ulcer of right elbow, stage 2
Pressure ulcer with abrasion, blister, partial thickness skin loss involving epidermis and/or dermis, right elbow

L89.013 Pressure ulcer of right elbow, stage 3   MCC H4 HCC SW
Healing pressure ulcer of right elbow, stage 3
Pressure ulcer with full thickness skin loss involving damage or necrosis of subcutaneous tissue, right elbow

L89.014 Pressure ulcer of right elbow, stage 4   MCC H4 HCC SW
Healing pressure ulcer of right elbow, stage 4
Pressure ulcer with necrosis of soft tissues through to underlying muscle, tendon, or bone, right elbow

L89.016 Pressure-induced deep tissue damage of right elbow

L89.019 Pressure ulcer of right elbow, unspecified stage
Healing pressure right of elbow NOS
Healing pressure ulcer of right elbow, unspecified stage

☑6ᵗʰ **L89.02 Pressure ulcer of left elbow**

L89.020 Pressure ulcer of left elbow, unstageable   HCC SW

☑ Additional Character Required   ☑x7ᵗʰ Placeholder   Unacceptable PDx   Questionable PDx   Manifestation   Unspecified Dx   H1–H14 HAC   HCC CMS-HCC Dx   HIV HIV Dx

ICD-10-CM 2021   741

L89.021 Pressure ulcer of left elbow, stage 1
Healing pressure ulcer of left elbow, stage 1
Pressure pre-ulcer skin changes limited to persistent focal edema, left elbow

L89.022 Pressure ulcer of left elbow, stage 2 `HCC`
Healing pressure ulcer of left elbow, stage 2
Pressure ulcer with abrasion, blister, partial thickness skin loss involving epidermis and/or dermis, left elbow

L89.023 Pressure ulcer of left elbow, stage 3 `MCC` `H4` `HCC` `SW`
Healing pressure ulcer of left elbow, stage 3
Pressure ulcer with full thickness skin loss involving damage or necrosis of subcutaneous tissue, left elbow

L89.024 Pressure ulcer of left elbow, stage 4 `MCC` `H4` `HCC` `SW`
Healing pressure ulcer of left elbow, stage 4
Pressure ulcer with necrosis of soft tissues through to underlying muscle, tendon, or bone, left elbow

L89.026 Pressure-induced deep tissue damage of left elbow

L89.029 Pressure ulcer of left elbow, unspecified stage
Healing pressure ulcer of left of elbow NOS
Healing pressure ulcer of left elbow, unspecified stage

√5ᵗʰ **L89.1 Pressure ulcer of back**

√6ᵗʰ **L89.10 Pressure ulcer of unspecified part of back**

L89.100 Pressure ulcer of unspecified part of back, unstageable `HCC` `SW`

L89.101 Pressure ulcer of unspecified part of back, stage 1
Healing pressure ulcer of unspecified part of back, stage 1
Pressure pre-ulcer skin changes limited to persistent focal edema, unspecified part of back

L89.102 Pressure ulcer of unspecified part of back, stage 2 `HCC`
Healing pressure ulcer of unspecified part of back, stage 2
Pressure ulcer with abrasion, blister, partial thickness skin loss involving epidermis and/or dermis, unspecified part of back

L89.103 Pressure ulcer of unspecified part of back, stage 3 `MCC` `H4` `HCC` `SW`
Healing pressure ulcer of unspecified part of back, stage 3
Pressure ulcer with full thickness skin loss involving damage or necrosis of subcutaneous tissue, unspecified part of back

L89.104 Pressure ulcer of unspecified part of back, stage 4 `MCC` `H4` `HCC` `SW`
Healing pressure ulcer of unspecified part of back, stage 4
Pressure ulcer with necrosis of soft tissues through to underlying muscle, tendon, or bone, unspecified part of back

L89.106 Pressure-induced deep tissue damage of unspecified part of back

L89.109 Pressure ulcer of unspecified part of back, unspecified stage
Healing pressure ulcer of unspecified part of back NOS
Healing pressure ulcer of unspecified part of back, unspecified stage

√6ᵗʰ **L89.11 Pressure ulcer of right upper back**
Pressure ulcer of right shoulder blade

L89.110 Pressure ulcer of right upper back, unstageable `HCC` `SW`

L89.111 Pressure ulcer of right upper back, stage 1
Healing pressure ulcer of right upper back, stage 1
Pressure pre-ulcer skin changes limited to persistent focal edema, right upper back

L89.112 Pressure ulcer of right upper back, stage 2 `HCC`
Healing pressure ulcer of right upper back, stage 2
Pressure ulcer with abrasion, blister, partial thickness skin loss involving epidermis and/or dermis, right upper back

L89.113 Pressure ulcer of right upper back, stage 3 `MCC` `H4` `HCC` `SW`
Healing pressure ulcer of right upper back, stage 3
Pressure ulcer with full thickness skin loss involving damage or necrosis of subcutaneous tissue, right upper back

L89.114 Pressure ulcer of right upper back, stage 4 `MCC` `H4` `HCC` `SW`
Healing pressure ulcer of right upper back, stage 4
Pressure ulcer with necrosis of soft tissues through to underlying muscle, tendon, or bone, right upper back

L89.116 Pressure-induced deep tissue damage of right upper back

L89.119 Pressure ulcer of right upper back, unspecified stage
Healing pressure ulcer of right upper back NOS
Healing pressure ulcer of right upper back, unspecified stage

√6ᵗʰ **L89.12 Pressure ulcer of left upper back**
Pressure ulcer of left shoulder blade

L89.120 Pressure ulcer of left upper back, unstageable `HCC` `SW`

L89.121 Pressure ulcer of left upper back, stage 1
Healing pressure ulcer of left upper back, stage 1
Pressure pre-ulcer skin changes limited to persistent focal edema, left upper back

L89.122 Pressure ulcer of left upper back, stage 2 `HCC`
Healing pressure ulcer of left upper back, stage 2
Pressure ulcer with abrasion, blister, partial thickness skin loss involving epidermis and/or dermis, left upper back

L89.123 Pressure ulcer of left upper back, stage 3 `MCC` `H4` `HCC` `SW`
Healing pressure ulcer of left upper back, stage 3
Pressure ulcer with full thickness skin loss involving damage or necrosis of subcutaneous tissue, left upper back

L89.124 Pressure ulcer of left upper back, stage 4 `MCC` `H4` `HCC` `SW`
Healing pressure ulcer of left upper back, stage 4
Pressure ulcer with necrosis of soft tissues through to underlying muscle, tendon, or bone, left upper back

L89.126 Pressure-induced deep tissue damage of left upper back

L89.129 **Pressure ulcer of left upper back, unspecified stage**
     Healing pressure ulcer of left upper back NOS
     Healing pressure ulcer of left upper back, unspecified stage

✓6ᵗʰ **L89.13** **Pressure ulcer of right lower back**

   L89.130 **Pressure ulcer of right lower back, unstageable** `HCC` `SW`

   L89.131 **Pressure ulcer of right lower back, stage 1**
     Healing pressure ulcer of right lower back, stage 1
     Pressure pre-ulcer skin changes limited to persistent focal edema, right lower back

   L89.132 **Pressure ulcer of right lower back, stage 2** `HCC`
     Healing pressure ulcer of right lower back, stage 2
     Pressure ulcer with abrasion, blister, partial thickness skin loss involving epidermis and/or dermis, right lower back

   L89.133 **Pressure ulcer of right lower back, stage 3** `MCC` `H4` `HCC` `SW`
     Healing pressure ulcer of right lower back, stage 3
     Pressure ulcer with full thickness skin loss involving damage or necrosis of subcutaneous tissue, right lower back

   L89.134 **Pressure ulcer of right lower back, stage 4** `MCC` `H4` `HCC` `SW`
     Healing pressure ulcer of right lower back, stage 4
     Pressure ulcer with necrosis of soft tissues through to underlying muscle, tendon, or bone, right lower back

   L89.136 **Pressure-induced deep tissue damage of right lower back**

   L89.139 **Pressure ulcer of right lower back, unspecified stage**
     Healing pressure ulcer of right lower back NOS
     Healing pressure ulcer of right lower back, unspecified stage

✓6ᵗʰ **L89.14** **Pressure ulcer of left lower back**

   L89.140 **Pressure ulcer of left lower back, unstageable** `HCC` `SW`

   L89.141 **Pressure ulcer of left lower back, stage 1**
     Healing pressure ulcer of left lower back, stage 1
     Pressure pre-ulcer skin changes limited to persistent focal edema, left lower back

   L89.142 **Pressure ulcer of left lower back, stage 2** `HCC`
     Healing pressure ulcer of left lower back, stage 2
     Pressure ulcer with abrasion, blister, partial thickness skin loss involving epidermis and/or dermis, left lower back

   L89.143 **Pressure ulcer of left lower back, stage 3** `MCC` `H4` `HCC` `SW`
     Healing pressure ulcer of left lower back, stage 3
     Pressure ulcer with full thickness skin loss involving damage or necrosis of subcutaneous tissue, left lower back

   L89.144 **Pressure ulcer of left lower back, stage 4** `MCC` `H4` `HCC` `SW`
     Healing pressure ulcer of left lower back, stage 4
     Pressure ulcer with necrosis of soft tissues through to underlying muscle, tendon, or bone, left lower back

   L89.146 **Pressure-induced deep tissue damage of left lower back**

L89.149 **Pressure ulcer of left lower back, unspecified stage**
     Healing pressure ulcer of left lower back NOS
     Healing pressure ulcer of left lower back, unspecified stage

✓6ᵗʰ **L89.15** **Pressure ulcer of sacral region**
   Pressure ulcer of coccyx
   Pressure ulcer of tailbone

   L89.150 **Pressure ulcer of sacral region, unstageable** `HCC` `SW`

   L89.151 **Pressure ulcer of sacral region, stage 1**
     Healing pressure ulcer of sacral region, stage 1
     Pressure pre-ulcer skin changes limited to persistent focal edema, sacral region

   L89.152 **Pressure ulcer of sacral region, stage 2** `HCC`
     Healing pressure ulcer of sacral region, stage 2
     Pressure ulcer with abrasion, blister, partial thickness skin loss involving epidermis and/or dermis, sacral region

   L89.153 **Pressure ulcer of sacral region, stage 3** `MCC` `H4` `HCC` `SW`
     Healing pressure ulcer of sacral region, stage 3
     Pressure ulcer with full thickness skin loss involving damage or necrosis of subcutaneous tissue, sacral region

   L89.154 **Pressure ulcer of sacral region, stage 4** `MCC` `H4` `HCC` `SW`
     Healing pressure ulcer of sacral region, stage 4
     Pressure ulcer with necrosis of soft tissues through to underlying muscle, tendon, or bone, sacral region

   L89.156 **Pressure-induced deep tissue damage of sacral region**

   L89.159 **Pressure ulcer of sacral region, unspecified stage**
     Healing pressure ulcer of sacral region NOS
     Healing pressure ulcer of sacral region, unspecified stage

✓5ᵗʰ **L89.2** **Pressure ulcer of hip**

   ✓6ᵗʰ **L89.20** **Pressure ulcer of unspecified hip**

     L89.200 **Pressure ulcer of unspecified hip, unstageable** `HCC` `SW`

     L89.201 **Pressure ulcer of unspecified hip, stage 1**
       Healing pressure ulcer of unspecified hip back, stage 1
       Pressure pre-ulcer skin changes limited to persistent focal edema, unspecified hip

     L89.202 **Pressure ulcer of unspecified hip, stage 2** `HCC`
       Healing pressure ulcer of unspecified hip, stage 2
       Pressure ulcer with abrasion, blister, partial thickness skin loss involving epidermis and/or dermis, unspecified hip

     L89.203 **Pressure ulcer of unspecified hip, stage 3** `MCC` `H4` `HCC` `SW`
       Healing pressure ulcer of unspecified hip, stage 3
       Pressure ulcer with full thickness skin loss involving damage or necrosis of subcutaneous tissue, unspecified hip

     L89.204 **Pressure ulcer of unspecified hip, stage 4** `MCC` `H4` `HCC` `SW`
       Healing pressure ulcer of unspecified hip, stage 4
       Pressure ulcer with necrosis of soft tissues through to underlying muscle, tendon, or bone, unspecified hip

☑ Additional Character Required   ✓x7ᵗʰ Placeholder   Unacceptable PDx   Questionable PDx   Manifestation   Unspecified Dx   `H1`-`H14` HAC   `HCC` CMS-HCC Dx   `HIV` HIV Dx

ICD-10-CM 2021   **743**

L89.206 Pressure-induced deep tissue damage of unspecified hip

L89.209 Pressure ulcer of unspecified hip, unspecified stage
     Healing pressure ulcer of unspecified hip NOS
     Healing pressure ulcer of unspecified hip, unspecified stage

√6ᵗʰ **L89.21 Pressure ulcer of right hip**

L89.210 Pressure ulcer of right hip, unstageable   HCC SW

L89.211 Pressure ulcer of right hip, stage 1
     Healing pressure ulcer of right hip back, stage 1
     Pressure pre-ulcer skin changes limited to persistent focal edema, right hip

L89.212 Pressure ulcer of right hip, stage 2   HCC
     Healing pressure ulcer of right hip, stage 2
     Pressure ulcer with abrasion, blister, partial thickness skin loss involving epidermis and/or dermis, right hip

L89.213 Pressure ulcer of right hip, stage 3   MCC H4 HCC SW
     Healing pressure ulcer of right hip, stage 3
     Pressure ulcer with full thickness skin loss involving damage or necrosis of subcutaneous tissue, right hip

L89.214 Pressure ulcer of right hip, stage 4   MCC H4 HCC SW
     Healing pressure ulcer of right hip, stage 4
     Pressure ulcer with necrosis of soft tissues through to underlying muscle, tendon, or bone, right hip

L89.216 Pressure-induced deep tissue damage of right hip

L89.219 Pressure ulcer of right hip, unspecified stage
     Healing pressure ulcer of right hip NOS
     Healing pressure ulcer of right hip, unspecified stage

√6ᵗʰ **L89.22 Pressure ulcer of left hip**

L89.220 Pressure ulcer of left hip, unstageable   HCC SW

L89.221 Pressure ulcer of left hip, stage 1
     Healing pressure ulcer of left hip back, stage 1
     Pressure pre-ulcer skin changes limited to persistent focal edema, left hip

L89.222 Pressure ulcer of left hip, stage 2   HCC
     Healing pressure ulcer of left hip, stage 2
     Pressure ulcer with abrasion, blister, partial thickness skin loss involving epidermis and/or dermis, left hip

L89.223 Pressure ulcer of left hip, stage 3   MCC H4 HCC SW
     Healing pressure ulcer of left hip, stage 3
     Pressure ulcer with full thickness skin loss involving damage or necrosis of subcutaneous tissue, left hip

L89.224 Pressure ulcer of left hip, stage 4   MCC H4 HCC SW
     Healing pressure ulcer of left hip, stage 4
     Pressure ulcer with necrosis of soft tissues through to underlying muscle, tendon, or bone, left hip

L89.226 Pressure-induced deep tissue damage of left hip

L89.229 Pressure ulcer of left hip, unspecified stage
     Healing pressure ulcer of left hip NOS
     Healing pressure ulcer of left hip, unspecified stage

√5ᵗʰ **L89.3 Pressure ulcer of buttock**

√6ᵗʰ **L89.30 Pressure ulcer of unspecified buttock**

L89.300 Pressure ulcer of unspecified buttock, unstageable   HCC SW

L89.301 Pressure ulcer of unspecified buttock, stage 1
     Healing pressure ulcer of unspecified buttock, stage 1
     Pressure pre-ulcer skin changes limited to persistent focal edema, unspecified buttock

L89.302 Pressure ulcer of unspecified buttock, stage 2   HCC
     Healing pressure ulcer of unspecified buttock, stage 2
     Pressure ulcer with abrasion, blister, partial thickness skin loss involving epidermis and/or dermis, unspecified buttock

L89.303 Pressure ulcer of unspecified buttock, stage 3   MCC H4 HCC SW
     Healing pressure ulcer of unspecified buttock, stage 3
     Pressure ulcer with full thickness skin loss involving damage or necrosis of subcutaneous tissue, unspecified buttock

L89.304 Pressure ulcer of unspecified buttock, stage 4   MCC H4 HCC SW
     Healing pressure ulcer of unspecified buttock, stage 4
     Pressure ulcer with necrosis of soft tissues through to underlying muscle, tendon, or bone, unspecified buttock

L89.306 Pressure-induced deep tissue damage of unspecified buttock

L89.309 Pressure ulcer of unspecified buttock, unspecified stage
     Healing pressure ulcer of unspecified buttock NOS
     Healing pressure ulcer of unspecified buttock, unspecified stage

√6ᵗʰ **L89.31 Pressure ulcer of right buttock**

L89.310 Pressure ulcer of right buttock, unstageable   HCC SW

L89.311 Pressure ulcer of right buttock, stage 1
     Healing pressure ulcer of right buttock, stage 1
     Pressure pre-ulcer skin changes limited to persistent focal edema, right buttock

L89.312 Pressure ulcer of right buttock, stage 2   HCC
     Healing pressure ulcer of right buttock, stage 2
     Pressure ulcer with abrasion, blister, partial thickness skin loss involving epidermis and/or dermis, right buttock

L89.313 Pressure ulcer of right buttock, stage 3   MCC H4 HCC SW
     Healing pressure ulcer of right buttock, stage 3
     Pressure ulcer with full thickness skin loss involving damage or necrosis of subcutaneous tissue, right buttock

L89.314 Pressure ulcer of right buttock, stage 4   MCC H4 HCC SW
     Healing pressure ulcer of right buttock, stage 4
     Pressure ulcer with necrosis of soft tissues through to underlying muscle, tendon, or bone, right buttock

L89.316 Pressure-induced deep tissue damage of right buttock

L89.319 Pressure ulcer of right buttock, unspecified stage
     Healing pressure ulcer of right buttock NOS
     Healing pressure ulcer of right buttock, unspecified stage

√6ᵗʰ **L89.32 Pressure ulcer of left buttock**

L89.320 Pressure ulcer of left buttock, unstageable   HCC SW

N Newborn: 0   P Pediatric: 0-17   M Maternity: 9-64   A Adult: 15-124   MCC Major Complication/Comorbidity   CC Complication/Comorbidity   SW Severe Wound Dx

744

ICD-10-CM 2021

L89.321 Pressure ulcer of left buttock, stage 1
Healing pressure ulcer of left buttock, stage 1
Pressure pre-ulcer skin changes limited to persistent focal edema, left buttock

L89.322 Pressure ulcer of left buttock, stage 2 `HCC`
Healing pressure ulcer of left buttock, stage 2
Pressure ulcer with abrasion, blister, partial thickness skin loss involving epidermis and/or dermis, left buttock

L89.323 Pressure ulcer of left buttock, stage 3 `MCC` `H4` `HCC` `SW`
Healing pressure ulcer of left buttock, stage 3
Pressure ulcer with full thickness skin loss involving damage or necrosis of subcutaneous tissue, left buttock

L89.324 Pressure ulcer of left buttock, stage 4 `MCC` `H4` `HCC` `SW`
Healing pressure ulcer of left buttock, stage 4
Pressure ulcer with necrosis of soft tissues through to underlying muscle, tendon, or bone, left buttock

L89.326 Pressure-induced deep tissue damage of left buttock

L89.329 Pressure ulcer of left buttock, unspecified stage
Healing pressure ulcer of left buttock NOS
Healing pressure ulcer of left buttock, unspecified stage

✓5ᵗʰ **L89.4 Pressure ulcer of contiguous site of back, buttock and hip**

L89.40 Pressure ulcer of contiguous site of back, buttock and hip, unspecified stage
Healing pressure ulcer of contiguous site of back, buttock and hip NOS
Healing pressure ulcer of contiguous site of back, buttock and hip, unspecified stage

L89.41 Pressure ulcer of contiguous site of back, buttock and hip, stage 1
Healing pressure ulcer of contiguous site of back, buttock and hip, stage 1
Pressure pre-ulcer skin changes limited to persistent focal edema, contiguous site of back, buttock and hip

L89.42 Pressure ulcer of contiguous site of back, buttock and hip, stage 2 `HCC`
Healing pressure ulcer of contiguous site of back, buttock and hip, stage 2
Pressure ulcer with abrasion, blister, partial thickness skin loss involving epidermis and/or dermis, contiguous site of back, buttock and hip

L89.43 Pressure ulcer of contiguous site of back, buttock and hip, stage 3 `MCC` `H4` `HCC` `SW`
Healing pressure ulcer of contiguous site of back, buttock and hip, stage 3
Pressure ulcer with full thickness skin loss involving damage or necrosis of subcutaneous tissue, contiguous site of back, buttock and hip

L89.44 Pressure ulcer of contiguous site of back, buttock and hip, stage 4 `MCC` `H4` `HCC` `SW`
Healing pressure ulcer of contiguous site of back, buttock and hip, stage 4
Pressure ulcer with necrosis of soft tissues through to underlying muscle, tendon, or bone, contiguous site of back, buttock and hip

L89.45 Pressure ulcer of contiguous site of back, buttock and hip, unstageable `HCC` `SW`

L89.46 Pressure-induced deep tissue damage of contiguous site of back, buttock and hip

✓5ᵗʰ **L89.5 Pressure ulcer of ankle**

✓6ᵗʰ **L89.50 Pressure ulcer of unspecified ankle**

L89.500 Pressure ulcer of unspecified ankle, unstageable `HCC` `SW`

L89.501 Pressure ulcer of unspecified ankle, stage 1
Healing pressure ulcer of unspecified ankle, stage 1
Pressure pre-ulcer skin changes limited to persistent focal edema, unspecified ankle

L89.502 Pressure ulcer of unspecified ankle, stage 2 `HCC`
Healing pressure ulcer of unspecified ankle, stage 2
Pressure ulcer with abrasion, blister, partial thickness skin loss involving epidermis and/or dermis, unspecified ankle

L89.503 Pressure ulcer of unspecified ankle, stage 3 `MCC` `H4` `HCC` `SW`
Healing pressure ulcer of unspecified ankle, stage 3
Pressure ulcer with full thickness skin loss involving damage or necrosis of subcutaneous tissue, unspecified ankle

L89.504 Pressure ulcer of unspecified ankle, stage 4 `MCC` `H4` `HCC` `SW`
Healing pressure ulcer of unspecified ankle, stage 4
Pressure ulcer with necrosis of soft tissues through to underlying muscle, tendon, or bone, unspecified ankle

L89.506 Pressure-induced deep tissue damage of unspecified ankle

L89.509 Pressure ulcer of unspecified ankle, unspecified stage
Healing pressure ulcer of unspecified ankle NOS
Healing pressure ulcer of unspecified ankle, unspecified stage

✓6ᵗʰ **L89.51 Pressure ulcer of right ankle**

L89.510 Pressure ulcer of right ankle, unstageable `HCC` `SW`

L89.511 Pressure ulcer of right ankle, stage 1
Healing pressure ulcer of right ankle, stage 1
Pressure pre-ulcer skin changes limited to persistent focal edema, right ankle

L89.512 Pressure ulcer of right ankle, stage 2 `HCC`
Healing pressure ulcer of right ankle, stage 2
Pressure ulcer with abrasion, blister, partial thickness skin loss involving epidermis and/or dermis, right ankle

L89.513 Pressure ulcer of right ankle, stage 3 `MCC` `H4` `HCC` `SW`
Healing pressure ulcer of right ankle, stage 3
Pressure ulcer with full thickness skin loss involving damage or necrosis of subcutaneous tissue, right ankle

L89.514 Pressure ulcer of right ankle, stage 4 `MCC` `H4` `HCC` `SW`
Healing pressure ulcer of right ankle, stage 4
Pressure ulcer with necrosis of soft tissues through to underlying muscle, tendon, or bone, right ankle

L89.516 Pressure-induced deep tissue damage of right ankle

L89.519 Pressure ulcer of right ankle, unspecified stage
Healing pressure ulcer of right ankle NOS
Healing pressure ulcer of right ankle, unspecified stage

✓6ᵗʰ **L89.52 Pressure ulcer of left ankle**

L89.520 Pressure ulcer of left ankle, unstageable `HCC` `SW`

✓ Additional Character Required   ✓x7ᵗʰ Placeholder   Unacceptable PDx   Questionable PDx   Manifestation   Unspecified Dx   H1-H14 HAC   HCC CMS-HCC Dx   HIV HIV Dx

ICD-10-CM 2021   745

L89.521 **Pressure ulcer of left ankle, stage 1**
Healing pressure ulcer of left ankle, stage 1
Pressure pre-ulcer skin changes limited to persistent focal edema, left ankle

L89.522 **Pressure ulcer of left ankle, stage 2** HCC
Healing pressure ulcer of left ankle, stage 2
Pressure ulcer with abrasion, blister, partial thickness skin loss involving epidermis and/or dermis, left ankle

L89.523 **Pressure ulcer of left ankle, stage 3** MCC H4 HCC SW
Healing pressure ulcer of left ankle, stage 3
Pressure ulcer with full thickness skin loss involving damage or necrosis of subcutaneous tissue, left ankle

L89.524 **Pressure ulcer of left ankle, stage 4** MCC H4 HCC SW
Healing pressure ulcer of left ankle, stage 4
Pressure ulcer with necrosis of soft tissues through to underlying muscle, tendon, or bone, left ankle

L89.526 **Pressure-induced deep tissue damage of left ankle**

L89.529 **Pressure ulcer of left ankle, unspecified stage**
Healing pressure ulcer of left ankle NOS
Healing pressure ulcer of left ankle, unspecified stage

√5ᵗʰ **L89.6** **Pressure ulcer of heel**

√6ᵗʰ **L89.60** **Pressure ulcer of unspecified heel**

L89.600 **Pressure ulcer of unspecified heel, unstageable** HCC SW

L89.601 **Pressure ulcer of unspecified heel, stage 1**
Healing pressure ulcer of unspecified heel, stage 1
Pressure pre-ulcer skin changes limited to persistent focal edema, unspecified heel

L89.602 **Pressure ulcer of unspecified heel, stage 2** HCC
Healing pressure ulcer of unspecified heel, stage 2
Pressure ulcer with abrasion, blister, partial thickness skin loss involving epidermis and/or dermis, unspecified heel

L89.603 **Pressure ulcer of unspecified heel, stage 3** MCC H4 HCC SW
Healing pressure ulcer of unspecified heel, stage 3
Pressure ulcer with full thickness skin loss involving damage or necrosis of subcutaneous tissue, unspecified heel

L89.604 **Pressure ulcer of unspecified heel, stage 4** MCC H4 HCC SW
Healing pressure ulcer of unspecified heel, stage 4
Pressure ulcer with necrosis of soft tissues through to underlying muscle, tendon, or bone, unspecified heel

L89.606 **Pressure-induced deep tissue damage of unspecified heel**

L89.609 **Pressure ulcer of unspecified heel, unspecified stage**
Healing pressure ulcer of unspecified heel NOS
Healing pressure ulcer of unspecified heel, unspecified stage

√6ᵗʰ **L89.61** **Pressure ulcer of right heel**

L89.610 **Pressure ulcer of right heel, unstageable** HCC SW

L89.611 **Pressure ulcer of right heel, stage 1**
Healing pressure ulcer of right heel, stage 1
Pressure pre-ulcer skin changes limited to persistent focal edema, right heel

L89.612 **Pressure ulcer of right heel, stage 2** HCC
Healing pressure ulcer of right heel, stage 2
Pressure ulcer with abrasion, blister, partial thickness skin loss involving epidermis and/or dermis, right heel

L89.613 **Pressure ulcer of right heel, stage 3** MCC H4 HCC SW
Healing pressure ulcer of right heel, stage 3
Pressure ulcer with full thickness skin loss involving damage or necrosis of subcutaneous tissue, right heel

L89.614 **Pressure ulcer of right heel, stage 4** MCC H4 HCC SW
Healing pressure ulcer of right heel, stage 4
Pressure ulcer with necrosis of soft tissues through to underlying muscle, tendon, or bone, right heel

L89.616 **Pressure-induced deep tissue damage of right heel**

L89.619 **Pressure ulcer of right heel, unspecified stage**
Healing pressure ulcer of right heel NOS
Healing pressure ulcer of right heel, unspecified stage

√6ᵗʰ **L89.62** **Pressure ulcer of left heel**

L89.620 **Pressure ulcer of left heel, unstageable** HCC SW

L89.621 **Pressure ulcer of left heel, stage 1**
Healing pressure ulcer of left heel, stage 1
Pressure pre-ulcer skin changes limited to persistent focal edema, left heel

L89.622 **Pressure ulcer of left heel, stage 2** HCC
Healing pressure ulcer of left heel, stage 2
Pressure ulcer with abrasion, blister, partial thickness skin loss involving epidermis and/or dermis, left heel

L89.623 **Pressure ulcer of left heel, stage 3** MCC H4 HCC SW
Healing pressure ulcer of left heel, stage 3
Pressure ulcer with full thickness skin loss involving damage or necrosis of subcutaneous tissue, left heel

L89.624 **Pressure ulcer of left heel, stage 4** MCC H4 HCC SW
Healing pressure ulcer of left heel, stage 4
Pressure ulcer with necrosis of soft tissues through to underlying muscle, tendon, or bone, left heel

L89.626 **Pressure-induced deep tissue damage of left heel**

L89.629 **Pressure ulcer of left heel, unspecified stage**
Healing pressure ulcer of left heel NOS
Healing pressure ulcer of left heel, unspecified stage

√5ᵗʰ **L89.8** **Pressure ulcer of other site**

√6ᵗʰ **L89.81** **Pressure ulcer of head**
Pressure ulcer of face

L89.810 **Pressure ulcer of head, unstageable** HCC SW

L89.811 **Pressure ulcer of head, stage 1**
Healing pressure ulcer of head, stage 1
Pressure pre-ulcer skin changes limited to persistent focal edema, head

L89.812 **Pressure ulcer of head, stage 2** HCC
Healing pressure ulcer of head, stage 2
Pressure ulcer with abrasion, blister, partial thickness skin loss involving epidermis and/or dermis, head

L89.813 **Pressure ulcer of head, stage 3** MCC H4 HCC SW
Healing pressure ulcer of head, stage 3
Pressure ulcer with full thickness skin loss involving damage or necrosis of subcutaneous tissue, head

L89.814 **Pressure ulcer of head, stage 4** `MCC` `H4` `HCC` `SW`
Healing pressure ulcer of head, stage 4
Pressure ulcer with necrosis of soft tissues through to underlying muscle, tendon, or bone, head

L89.816 **Pressure-induced deep tissue damage of head**

L89.819 **Pressure ulcer of head, unspecified stage**
Healing pressure ulcer of head NOS
Healing pressure ulcer of head, unspecified stage

√6th **L89.89 Pressure ulcer of other site**

L89.890 **Pressure ulcer of other site, unstageable** `HCC` `SW`

L89.891 **Pressure ulcer of other site, stage 1**
Healing pressure ulcer of other site, stage 1
Pressure pre-ulcer skin changes limited to persistent focal edema, other site

L89.892 **Pressure ulcer of other site, stage 2** `HCC`
Healing pressure ulcer of other site, stage 2
Pressure ulcer with abrasion, blister, partial thickness skin loss involving epidermis and/or dermis, other site

L89.893 **Pressure ulcer of other site, stage 3** `MCC` `H4` `HCC` `SW`
Healing pressure ulcer of other site, stage 3
Pressure ulcer with full thickness skin loss involving damage or necrosis of subcutaneous tissue, other site

L89.894 **Pressure ulcer of other site, stage 4** `MCC` `H4` `HCC` `SW`
Healing pressure ulcer of other site, stage 4
Pressure ulcer with necrosis of soft tissues through to underlying muscle, tendon, or bone, other site

L89.896 **Pressure-induced deep tissue damage of other site**

L89.899 **Pressure ulcer of other site, unspecified stage**
Healing pressure ulcer of other site NOS
Healing pressure ulcer of other site, unspecified stage

√5th **L89.9 Pressure ulcer of unspecified site**

L89.90 **Pressure ulcer of unspecified site, unspecified stage**
Healing pressure ulcer of unspecified site NOS
Healing pressure ulcer of unspecified site, unspecified stage

L89.91 **Pressure ulcer of unspecified site, stage 1**
Healing pressure ulcer of unspecified site, stage 1
Pressure pre-ulcer skin changes limited to persistent focal edema, unspecified site

L89.92 **Pressure ulcer of unspecified site, stage 2** `HCC`
Healing pressure ulcer of unspecified site, stage 2
Pressure ulcer with abrasion, blister, partial thickness skin loss involving epidermis and/or dermis, unspecified site

L89.93 **Pressure ulcer of unspecified site, stage 3** `MCC` `H4` `HCC` `SW`
Healing pressure ulcer of unspecified site, stage 3
Pressure ulcer with full thickness skin loss involving damage or necrosis of subcutaneous tissue, unspecified site

L89.94 **Pressure ulcer of unspecified site, stage 4** `MCC` `H4` `HCC` `SW`
Healing pressure ulcer of unspecified site, stage 4
Pressure ulcer with necrosis of soft tissues through to underlying muscle, tendon, or bone, unspecified site

L89.95 **Pressure ulcer of unspecified site, unstageable** `HCC` `SW`

L89.96 **Pressure-induced deep tissue damage of unspecified site**

√4th **L90 Atrophic disorders of skin**

L90.0 **Lichen sclerosus et atrophicus**
EXCLUDES 2   *lichen sclerosus of external female genital organs (N90.4)*
lichen sclerosus of external male genital organs (N48.0)

L90.1 **Anetoderma of Schweninger-Buzzi**

L90.2 **Anetoderma of Jadassohn-Pellizzari**

L90.3 **Atrophoderma of Pasini and Pierini**

L90.4 **Acrodermatitis chronica atrophicans**

L90.5 **Scar conditions and fibrosis of skin**
Adherent scar (skin)
Cicatrix
Disfigurement of skin due to scar
Fibrosis of skin NOS
Scar NOS
EXCLUDES 2   *hypertrophic scar (L91.0)*
keloid scar (L91.0)
AHA: 2016,2Q,5; 2015,1Q,19

L90.6 **Striae atrophicae**

L90.8 **Other atrophic disorders of skin**

L90.9 **Atrophic disorder of skin, unspecified**

√4th **L91 Hypertrophic disorders of skin**

L91.0 **Hypertrophic scar**
Keloid
Keloid scar
EXCLUDES 2   *acne keloid (L73.0)*
scar NOS (L90.5)
DEF: Overgrowth of scar tissue due to excess amounts of collagen during connective tissue repair, occurring mainly on the upper trunk and face.

L91.8 **Other hypertrophic disorders of the skin**

L91.9 **Hypertrophic disorder of the skin, unspecified**

√4th **L92 Granulomatous disorders of skin and subcutaneous tissue**
EXCLUDES 2   *actinic granuloma (L57.5)*

L92.0 **Granuloma annulare**
Perforating granuloma annulare

L92.1 **Necrobiosis lipoidica, not elsewhere classified**
EXCLUDES 1   *necrobiosis lipoidica associated with diabetes mellitus (E08-E13 with .620)*

L92.2 **Granuloma faciale [eosinophilic granuloma of skin]**

L92.3 **Foreign body granuloma of the skin and subcutaneous tissue**
Use additional code to identify the type of retained foreign body (Z18.-)

L92.8 **Other granulomatous disorders of the skin and subcutaneous tissue**

L92.9 **Granulomatous disorder of the skin and subcutaneous tissue, unspecified**
EXCLUDES 2   *umbilical granuloma (P83.81)*
AHA: 2017,4Q,21-22

√4th **L93 Lupus erythematosus**
Use additional code for adverse effect, if applicable, to identify drug (T36-T50 with fifth or sixth character 5)
EXCLUDES 1   *lupus exedens (A18.4)*
lupus vulgaris (A18.4)
scleroderma (M34.-)
systemic lupus erythematosus (M32.-)
DEF: Inflammatory, autoimmune skin condition in which the body's autoimmune system attacks healthy tissue of the integumentary system.

L93.0 **Discoid lupus erythematosus**
Lupus erythematosus NOS

L93.1 **Subacute cutaneous lupus erythematosus**

L93.2 **Other local lupus erythematosus**
Lupus erythematosus profundus
Lupus panniculitis

√4th **L94 Other localized connective tissue disorders**
EXCLUDES 1   *systemic connective tissue disorders (M30-M36)*

L94.0 **Localized scleroderma [morphea]**
Circumscribed scleroderma

L94.1 **Linear scleroderma**
En coup de sabre lesion

L94.2 **Calcinosis cutis**

L94.3 **Sclerodactyly**

L94.4 **Gottron's papules**

L94.5 **Poikiloderma vasculare atrophicans**

L94.6 **Ainhum**

L94.8 **Other specified localized connective tissue disorders**

L94.9 **Localized connective tissue disorder, unspecified**

√4ᵗʰ L95 **Vasculitis limited to skin, not elsewhere classified**

> EXCLUDES 1   angioma serpiginosum (L81.7)
> Henoch(-Schönlein) purpura (D69.0)
> hypersensitivity angiitis (M31.0)
> lupus panniculitis (L93.2)
> panniculitis NOS (M79.3)
> panniculitis of neck and back (M54.0-)
> polyarteritis nodosa (M30.0)
> relapsing panniculitis (M35.6)
> rheumatoid vasculitis (M05.2)
> serum sickness (T80.6-)
> urticaria (L50.-)
> Wegener's granulomatosis (M31.3-)

L95.0 **Livedoid vasculitis**

Atrophie blanche (en plaque)

L95.1 **Erythema elevatum diutinum**

L95.8 **Other vasculitis limited to the skin**

L95.9 **Vasculitis limited to the skin, unspecified**

√4ᵗʰ L97 **Non-pressure chronic ulcer of lower limb, not elsewhere classified**

> INCLUDES   chronic ulcer of skin of lower limb NOS
> non-healing ulcer of skin
> non-infected sinus of skin
> trophic ulcer NOS
> tropical ulcer NOS
> ulcer of skin of lower limb NOS

Code first any associated underlying condition, such as:
any associated gangrene (I96)
atherosclerosis of the lower extremities (I70.23-, I70.24-, I70.33-, I70.34-, I70.43-, I70.44-, I70.53-, I70.54-, I70.63-, I70.64-, I70.73-, I70.74-)
chronic venous hypertension (I87.31-, I87.33-)
diabetic ulcers (E08.621, E08.622, E09.621, E09.622, E10.621, E10.622, E11.621, E11.622, E13.621, E13.622)
postphlebitic syndrome (I87.01-, I87.03-)
postthrombotic syndrome (I87.01-, I87.03-)
varicose ulcer (I83.0-, I83.2-)

> EXCLUDES 2   pressure ulcer (pressure area) (L89.-)
> skin infections (L00-L08)
> specific infections classified to A00-B99

AHA: 2020,2Q,19; 2018,4Q,69; 2017,4Q,17

TIP: The depth and/or severity of a diagnosed nonpressure ulcer can be determined based on medical record documentation from clinicians who are not the patient's provider.

TIP: Assign a code from this category/subcategory for nonpressure ulcers documented as acute.

√5ᵗʰ L97.1 **Non-pressure chronic ulcer of** thigh

√6ᵗʰ L97.10 **Non-pressure chronic ulcer of unspecified thigh**

L97.101 **Non-pressure chronic ulcer of unspecified thigh** limited to breakdown of skin CC HCC

L97.102 **Non-pressure chronic ulcer of unspecified thigh** with fat layer exposed CC HCC SW

L97.103 **Non-pressure chronic ulcer of unspecified thigh** with necrosis of muscle CC HCC SW

L97.104 **Non-pressure chronic ulcer of unspecified thigh** with necrosis of bone CC HCC SW

L97.105 **Non-pressure chronic ulcer of unspecified thigh** with muscle involvement without evidence of necrosis CC HCC

L97.106 **Non-pressure chronic ulcer of unspecified thigh** with bone involvement without evidence of necrosis CC HCC

L97.108 **Non-pressure chronic ulcer of unspecified thigh** with other specified severity CC HCC

L97.109 **Non-pressure chronic ulcer of unspecified thigh** with unspecified severity CC HCC

√6ᵗʰ L97.11 **Non-pressure chronic ulcer of** right **thigh**

L97.111 **Non-pressure chronic ulcer of right thigh** limited to breakdown of skin CC HCC

L97.112 **Non-pressure chronic ulcer of right thigh** with fat layer exposed CC HCC SW

L97.113 **Non-pressure chronic ulcer of right thigh** with necrosis of muscle CC HCC SW

L97.114 **Non-pressure chronic ulcer of right thigh** with necrosis of bone CC HCC SW

L97.115 **Non-pressure chronic ulcer of right thigh** with muscle involvement without evidence of necrosis CC HCC

L97.116 **Non-pressure chronic ulcer of right thigh** with bone involvement without evidence of necrosis CC HCC

L97.118 **Non-pressure chronic ulcer of right thigh** with other specified severity CC HCC

L97.119 **Non-pressure chronic ulcer of right thigh** with unspecified severity CC HCC

√6ᵗʰ L97.12 **Non-pressure chronic ulcer of** left **thigh**

L97.121 **Non-pressure chronic ulcer of left thigh** limited to breakdown of skin CC HCC

L97.122 **Non-pressure chronic ulcer of left thigh** with fat layer exposed CC HCC SW

L97.123 **Non-pressure chronic ulcer of left thigh** with necrosis of muscle CC HCC SW

L97.124 **Non-pressure chronic ulcer of left thigh** with necrosis of bone CC HCC SW

L97.125 **Non-pressure chronic ulcer of left thigh** with muscle involvement without evidence of necrosis CC HCC

L97.126 **Non-pressure chronic ulcer of left thigh** with bone involvement without evidence of necrosis CC HCC

L97.128 **Non-pressure chronic ulcer of left thigh** with other specified severity CC HCC

L97.129 **Non-pressure chronic ulcer of left thigh** with unspecified severity CC HCC

√5ᵗʰ L97.2 **Non-pressure chronic ulcer of** calf

√6ᵗʰ L97.20 **Non-pressure chronic ulcer of unspecified calf**

L97.201 **Non-pressure chronic ulcer of unspecified calf** limited to breakdown of skin CC HCC

L97.202 **Non-pressure chronic ulcer of unspecified calf** with fat layer exposed CC HCC SW

L97.203 **Non-pressure chronic ulcer of unspecified calf** with necrosis of muscle CC HCC SW

L97.204 **Non-pressure chronic ulcer of unspecified calf** with necrosis of bone CC HCC SW

L97.205 **Non-pressure chronic ulcer of unspecified calf** with muscle involvement without evidence of necrosis CC HCC

L97.206 **Non-pressure chronic ulcer of unspecified calf** with bone involvement without evidence of necrosis CC HCC

L97.208 **Non-pressure chronic ulcer of unspecified calf** with other specified severity CC HCC

L97.209 **Non-pressure chronic ulcer of unspecified calf** with unspecified severity CC HCC

√6ᵗʰ L97.21 **Non-pressure chronic ulcer of** right **calf**

L97.211 **Non-pressure chronic ulcer of right calf** limited to breakdown of skin CC HCC

L97.212 **Non-pressure chronic ulcer of right calf** with fat layer exposed CC HCC SW

L97.213 **Non-pressure chronic ulcer of right calf** with necrosis of muscle CC HCC SW

L97.214 **Non-pressure chronic ulcer of right calf** with necrosis of bone CC HCC SW

L97.215 **Non-pressure chronic ulcer of right calf** with muscle involvement without evidence of necrosis CC HCC

L97.216 **Non-pressure chronic ulcer of right calf** with bone involvement without evidence of necrosis CC HCC

L97.218 **Non-pressure chronic ulcer of right calf** with other specified severity CC HCC

L97.219 **Non-pressure chronic ulcer of right calf** with unspecified severity CC HCC

√6ᵗʰ L97.22 **Non-pressure chronic ulcer of** left **calf**

L97.221 **Non-pressure chronic ulcer of left calf** limited to breakdown of skin CC HCC

L97.222 **Non-pressure chronic ulcer of left calf** with fat layer exposed CC HCC SW

N Newborn: 0   P Pediatric: 0-17   M Maternity: 9-64   A Adult: 15-124   MCC Major Complication/Comorbidity   CC Complication/Comorbidity   SW Severe Wound Dx

748   ICD-10-CM 2021

    L97.223 **Non-pressure chronic ulcer of left calf with necrosis of muscle** `CC` `HCC` `SW`

    L97.224 **Non-pressure chronic ulcer of left calf with necrosis of bone** `CC` `HCC` `SW`

    L97.225 **Non-pressure chronic ulcer of left calf with muscle involvement without evidence of necrosis** `CC` `HCC`

    L97.226 **Non-pressure chronic ulcer of left calf with bone involvement without evidence of necrosis** `CC` `HCC`

    L97.228 **Non-pressure chronic ulcer of left calf with other specified severity** `CC` `HCC`

    L97.229 **Non-pressure chronic ulcer of left calf with unspecified severity** `CC` `HCC`

✓5ᵗʰ **L97.3 Non-pressure chronic ulcer of ankle**

  ✓6ᵗʰ **L97.30 Non-pressure chronic ulcer of unspecified ankle**

    L97.301 **Non-pressure chronic ulcer of unspecified ankle limited to breakdown of skin** `CC` `HCC`

    L97.302 **Non-pressure chronic ulcer of unspecified ankle with fat layer exposed** `CC` `HCC` `SW`

    L97.303 **Non-pressure chronic ulcer of unspecified ankle with necrosis of muscle** `CC` `HCC` `SW`

    L97.304 **Non-pressure chronic ulcer of unspecified ankle with necrosis of bone** `CC` `HCC` `SW`

    L97.305 **Non-pressure chronic ulcer of unspecified ankle with muscle involvement without evidence of necrosis** `CC` `HCC`

    L97.306 **Non-pressure chronic ulcer of unspecified ankle with bone involvement without evidence of necrosis** `CC` `HCC`

    L97.308 **Non-pressure chronic ulcer of unspecified ankle with other specified severity** `CC` `HCC`

    L97.309 **Non-pressure chronic ulcer of unspecified ankle with unspecified severity** `CC` `HCC`

  ✓6ᵗʰ **L97.31 Non-pressure chronic ulcer of right ankle**

    L97.311 **Non-pressure chronic ulcer of right ankle limited to breakdown of skin** `CC` `HCC`

    L97.312 **Non-pressure chronic ulcer of right ankle with fat layer exposed** `CC` `HCC` `SW`

    L97.313 **Non-pressure chronic ulcer of right ankle with necrosis of muscle** `CC` `HCC` `SW`

    L97.314 **Non-pressure chronic ulcer of right ankle with necrosis of bone** `CC` `HCC` `SW`

    L97.315 **Non-pressure chronic ulcer of right ankle with muscle involvement without evidence of necrosis** `CC` `HCC`

    L97.316 **Non-pressure chronic ulcer of right ankle with bone involvement without evidence of necrosis** `CC` `HCC`

    L97.318 **Non-pressure chronic ulcer of right ankle with other specified severity** `CC` `HCC`

    L97.319 **Non-pressure chronic ulcer of right ankle with unspecified severity** `CC` `HCC`

  ✓6ᵗʰ **L97.32 Non-pressure chronic ulcer of left ankle**

    L97.321 **Non-pressure chronic ulcer of left ankle limited to breakdown of skin** `CC` `HCC`

    L97.322 **Non-pressure chronic ulcer of left ankle with fat layer exposed** `CC` `HCC` `SW`

    L97.323 **Non-pressure chronic ulcer of left ankle with necrosis of muscle** `CC` `HCC` `SW`

    L97.324 **Non-pressure chronic ulcer of left ankle with necrosis of bone** `CC` `HCC` `SW`

    L97.325 **Non-pressure chronic ulcer of left ankle with muscle involvement without evidence of necrosis** `CC` `HCC`

    L97.326 **Non-pressure chronic ulcer of left ankle with bone involvement without evidence of necrosis** `CC` `HCC`

    L97.328 **Non-pressure chronic ulcer of left ankle with other specified severity** `CC` `HCC`

    L97.329 **Non-pressure chronic ulcer of left ankle with unspecified severity** `CC` `HCC`

✓5ᵗʰ **L97.4 Non-pressure chronic ulcer of heel and midfoot**

Non-pressure chronic ulcer of plantar surface of midfoot

  ✓6ᵗʰ **L97.40 Non-pressure chronic ulcer of unspecified heel and midfoot**

    L97.401 **Non-pressure chronic ulcer of unspecified heel and midfoot limited to breakdown of skin** `CC` `HCC`

    L97.402 **Non-pressure chronic ulcer of unspecified heel and midfoot with fat layer exposed** `CC` `HCC` `SW`

    L97.403 **Non-pressure chronic ulcer of unspecified heel and midfoot with necrosis of muscle** `CC` `HCC` `SW`

    L97.404 **Non-pressure chronic ulcer of unspecified heel and midfoot with necrosis of bone** `CC` `HCC` `SW`

    L97.405 **Non-pressure chronic ulcer of unspecified heel and midfoot with muscle involvement without evidence of necrosis** `CC` `HCC`

    L97.406 **Non-pressure chronic ulcer of unspecified heel and midfoot with bone involvement without evidence of necrosis** `CC` `HCC`

    L97.408 **Non-pressure chronic ulcer of unspecified heel and midfoot with other specified severity** `CC` `HCC`

    L97.409 **Non-pressure chronic ulcer of unspecified heel and midfoot with unspecified severity** `CC` `HCC`

  ✓6ᵗʰ **L97.41 Non-pressure chronic ulcer of right heel and midfoot**

    L97.411 **Non-pressure chronic ulcer of right heel and midfoot limited to breakdown of skin** `CC` `HCC`

    L97.412 **Non-pressure chronic ulcer of right heel and midfoot with fat layer exposed** `CC` `HCC` `SW`

      AHA: 2020,2Q,19

    L97.413 **Non-pressure chronic ulcer of right heel and midfoot with necrosis of muscle** `CC` `HCC` `SW`

    L97.414 **Non-pressure chronic ulcer of right heel and midfoot with necrosis of bone** `CC` `HCC` `SW`

    L97.415 **Non-pressure chronic ulcer of right heel and midfoot with muscle involvement without evidence of necrosis** `CC` `HCC`

    L97.416 **Non-pressure chronic ulcer of right heel and midfoot with bone involvement without evidence of necrosis** `CC` `HCC`

    L97.418 **Non-pressure chronic ulcer of right heel and midfoot with other specified severity** `CC` `HCC`

    L97.419 **Non-pressure chronic ulcer of right heel and midfoot with unspecified severity** `CC` `HCC`

  ✓6ᵗʰ **L97.42 Non-pressure chronic ulcer of left heel and midfoot**

    L97.421 **Non-pressure chronic ulcer of left heel and midfoot limited to breakdown of skin** `CC` `HCC`

      AHA: 2016,1Q,12

    L97.422 **Non-pressure chronic ulcer of left heel and midfoot with fat layer exposed** `CC` `HCC` `SW`

      AHA: 2020,2Q,19

    L97.423 **Non-pressure chronic ulcer of left heel and midfoot with necrosis of muscle** `CC` `HCC` `SW`

    L97.424 **Non-pressure chronic ulcer of left heel and midfoot with necrosis of bone** `CC` `HCC` `SW`

    L97.425 **Non-pressure chronic ulcer of left heel and midfoot with muscle involvement without evidence of necrosis** `CC` `HCC`

    L97.426 **Non-pressure chronic ulcer of left heel and midfoot with bone involvement without evidence of necrosis** `CC` `HCC`

    L97.428 **Non-pressure chronic ulcer of left heel and midfoot with other specified severity** `CC` `HCC`

L97.429 Non-pressure chronic ulcer of left heel and midfoot with unspecified severity CC HCC

✓5th L97.5 Non-pressure chronic ulcer of other part of foot
Non-pressure chronic ulcer of toe

✓6th L97.50 Non-pressure chronic ulcer of other part of unspecified foot

L97.501 Non-pressure chronic ulcer of other part of unspecified foot limited to breakdown of skin HCC

L97.502 Non-pressure chronic ulcer of other part of unspecified foot with fat layer exposed HCC SW

L97.503 Non-pressure chronic ulcer of other part of unspecified foot with necrosis of muscle HCC SW

L97.504 Non-pressure chronic ulcer of other part of unspecified foot with necrosis of bone HCC SW

L97.505 Non-pressure chronic ulcer of other part of unspecified foot with muscle involvement without evidence of necrosis CC HCC

L97.506 Non-pressure chronic ulcer of other part of unspecified foot with bone involvement without evidence of necrosis CC HCC

L97.508 Non-pressure chronic ulcer of other part of unspecified foot with other specified severity CC HCC

L97.509 Non-pressure chronic ulcer of other part of unspecified foot with unspecified severity HCC

✓6th L97.51 Non-pressure chronic ulcer of other part of right foot
AHA: 2020,1Q,12

L97.511 Non-pressure chronic ulcer of other part of right foot limited to breakdown of skin HCC

L97.512 Non-pressure chronic ulcer of other part of right foot with fat layer exposed HCC SW
AHA: 2020,2Q,19

L97.513 Non-pressure chronic ulcer of other part of right foot with necrosis of muscle HCC SW

L97.514 Non-pressure chronic ulcer of other part of right foot with necrosis of bone HCC SW

L97.515 Non-pressure chronic ulcer of other part of right foot with muscle involvement without evidence of necrosis CC HCC

L97.516 Non-pressure chronic ulcer of other part of right foot with bone involvement without evidence of necrosis CC HCC

L97.518 Non-pressure chronic ulcer of other part of right foot with other specified severity CC HCC

L97.519 Non-pressure chronic ulcer of other part of right foot with unspecified severity HCC

✓6th L97.52 Non-pressure chronic ulcer of other part of left foot
AHA: 2020,1Q,12

L97.521 Non-pressure chronic ulcer of other part of left foot limited to breakdown of skin HCC

L97.522 Non-pressure chronic ulcer of other part of left foot with fat layer exposed HCC SW
AHA: 2020,2Q,19

L97.523 Non-pressure chronic ulcer of other part of left foot with necrosis of muscle HCC SW

L97.524 Non-pressure chronic ulcer of other part of left foot with necrosis of bone HCC SW

L97.525 Non-pressure chronic ulcer of other part of left foot with muscle involvement without evidence of necrosis CC HCC

L97.526 Non-pressure chronic ulcer of other part of left foot with bone involvement without evidence of necrosis CC HCC

L97.528 Non-pressure chronic ulcer of other part of left foot with other specified severity CC HCC

L97.529 Non-pressure chronic ulcer of other part of left foot with unspecified severity HCC

✓5th L97.8 Non-pressure chronic ulcer of other part of lower leg

✓6th L97.80 Non-pressure chronic ulcer of other part of unspecified lower leg

L97.801 Non-pressure chronic ulcer of other part of unspecified lower leg limited to breakdown of skin CC HCC

L97.802 Non-pressure chronic ulcer of other part of unspecified lower leg with fat layer exposed CC HCC SW

L97.803 Non-pressure chronic ulcer of other part of unspecified lower leg with necrosis of muscle CC HCC SW

L97.804 Non-pressure chronic ulcer of other part of unspecified lower leg with necrosis of bone CC HCC SW

L97.805 Non-pressure chronic ulcer of other part of unspecified lower leg with muscle involvement without evidence of necrosis CC HCC

L97.806 Non-pressure chronic ulcer of other part of unspecified lower leg with bone involvement without evidence of necrosis CC HCC

L97.808 Non-pressure chronic ulcer of other part of unspecified lower leg with other specified severity CC HCC

L97.809 Non-pressure chronic ulcer of other part of unspecified lower leg with unspecified severity CC HCC

✓6th L97.81 Non-pressure chronic ulcer of other part of right lower leg

L97.811 Non-pressure chronic ulcer of other part of right lower leg limited to breakdown of skin CC HCC

L97.812 Non-pressure chronic ulcer of other part of right lower leg with fat layer exposed CC HCC SW

L97.813 Non-pressure chronic ulcer of other part of right lower leg with necrosis of muscle CC HCC SW

L97.814 Non-pressure chronic ulcer of other part of right lower leg with necrosis of bone CC HCC SW

L97.815 Non-pressure chronic ulcer of other part of right lower leg with muscle involvement without evidence of necrosis CC HCC

L97.816 Non-pressure chronic ulcer of other part of right lower leg with bone involvement without evidence of necrosis CC HCC

L97.818 Non-pressure chronic ulcer of other part of right lower leg with other specified severity CC HCC

L97.819 Non-pressure chronic ulcer of other part of right lower leg with unspecified severity CC HCC

✓6th L97.82 Non-pressure chronic ulcer of other part of left lower leg

L97.821 Non-pressure chronic ulcer of other part of left lower leg limited to breakdown of skin CC HCC

L97.822 Non-pressure chronic ulcer of other part of left lower leg with fat layer exposed CC HCC SW

L97.823 Non-pressure chronic ulcer of other part of left lower leg with necrosis of muscle CC HCC SW

L97.824 Non-pressure chronic ulcer of other part of left lower leg with necrosis of bone CC HCC SW

L97.825 Non-pressure chronic ulcer of other part of left lower leg with muscle involvement without evidence of necrosis CC HCC

L97.826 Non-pressure chronic ulcer of other part of left lower leg with bone involvement without evidence of necrosis CC HCC

    L97.828   Non-pressure chronic ulcer of other part of left lower leg with other specified severity   `CC` `HCC`

    L97.829   Non-pressure chronic ulcer of other part of left lower leg with unspecified severity   `CC` `HCC`

✓5th **L97.9**   Non-pressure chronic ulcer of unspecified part of lower leg

  ✓6th **L97.90**   Non-pressure chronic ulcer of unspecified part of unspecified lower leg

    L97.901   Non-pressure chronic ulcer of unspecified part of unspecified lower leg limited to breakdown of skin   `CC` `HCC`

    L97.902   Non-pressure chronic ulcer of unspecified part of unspecified lower leg with fat layer exposed   `CC` `HCC` `SW`

    L97.903   Non-pressure chronic ulcer of unspecified part of unspecified lower leg with necrosis of muscle   `CC` `HCC` `SW`

    L97.904   Non-pressure chronic ulcer of unspecified part of unspecified lower leg with necrosis of bone   `CC` `HCC` `SW`

    L97.905   Non-pressure chronic ulcer of unspecified part of unspecified lower leg with muscle involvement without evidence of necrosis   `CC` `HCC`

    L97.906   Non-pressure chronic ulcer of unspecified part of unspecified lower leg with bone involvement without evidence of necrosis   `CC` `HCC`

    L97.908   Non-pressure chronic ulcer of unspecified part of unspecified lower leg with other specified severity   `CC` `HCC`

    L97.909   Non-pressure chronic ulcer of unspecified part of unspecified lower leg with unspecified severity   `CC` `HCC`

  ✓6th **L97.91**   Non-pressure chronic ulcer of unspecified part of right lower leg

    L97.911   Non-pressure chronic ulcer of unspecified part of right lower leg limited to breakdown of skin   `CC` `HCC`

    L97.912   Non-pressure chronic ulcer of unspecified part of right lower leg with fat layer exposed   `CC` `HCC` `SW`

    L97.913   Non-pressure chronic ulcer of unspecified part of right lower leg with necrosis of muscle   `CC` `HCC` `SW`

    L97.914   Non-pressure chronic ulcer of unspecified part of right lower leg with necrosis of bone   `CC` `HCC` `SW`

    L97.915   Non-pressure chronic ulcer of unspecified part of right lower leg with muscle involvement without evidence of necrosis   `CC` `HCC`

    L97.916   Non-pressure chronic ulcer of unspecified part of right lower leg with bone involvement without evidence of necrosis   `CC` `HCC`

    L97.918   Non-pressure chronic ulcer of unspecified part of right lower leg with other specified severity   `CC` `HCC`

    L97.919   Non-pressure chronic ulcer of unspecified part of right lower leg with unspecified severity   `CC` `HCC`

  ✓6th **L97.92**   Non-pressure chronic ulcer of unspecified part of left lower leg

    L97.921   Non-pressure chronic ulcer of unspecified part of left lower leg limited to breakdown of skin   `CC` `HCC` `SW`

    L97.922   Non-pressure chronic ulcer of unspecified part of left lower leg with fat layer exposed   `CC` `HCC` `SW`

    L97.923   Non-pressure chronic ulcer of unspecified part of left lower leg with necrosis of muscle   `CC` `HCC` `SW`

    L97.924   Non-pressure chronic ulcer of unspecified part of left lower leg with necrosis of bone   `CC` `HCC` `SW`

    L97.925   Non-pressure chronic ulcer of unspecified part of left lower leg with muscle involvement without evidence of necrosis   `CC` `HCC`

    L97.926   Non-pressure chronic ulcer of unspecified part of left lower leg with bone involvement without evidence of necrosis   `CC` `HCC`

    L97.928   Non-pressure chronic ulcer of unspecified part of left lower leg with other specified severity   `CC` `HCC`

    L97.929   Non-pressure chronic ulcer of unspecified part of left lower leg with unspecified severity   `CC` `HCC`

✓4th **L98**   **Other disorders of skin and subcutaneous tissue, not elsewhere classified**

  L98.0   **Pyogenic granuloma**

    EXCLUDES 2   pyogenic granuloma of gingiva (K06.8)

         pyogenic granuloma of maxillary alveolar ridge (K04.5)

         pyogenic granuloma of oral mucosa (K13.4)

    DEF: Solitary polypoid capillary hemangioma often associated with local irritation, trauma, and superimposed inflammation. Located on the skin and gingival or oral mucosa, they bleed easily and may ulcerate and form crusted sores.

  L98.1   **Factitial dermatitis**

    Neurotic excoriation

    EXCLUDES 1   excoriation (skin-picking) disorder (F42.4)

    AHA: 2016,4Q,15

    DEF: Self-inflicted skin lesions to satisfy an unconscious psychological or emotional need. Methods used to injure the skin include deep excoriations with a sharp instrument, scarification with a knife, or the application of caustic chemicals and burning, sometimes with a cigarette.

  L98.2   **Febrile neutrophilic dermatosis [Sweet]**

  L98.3   **Eosinophilic cellulitis [Wells]**   `CC`

✓5th **L98.4**   **Non-pressure chronic ulcer of skin, not elsewhere classified**

    Chronic ulcer of skin NOS

    Tropical ulcer NOS

    Ulcer of skin NOS

    EXCLUDES 2   gangrene (I96)

         pressure ulcer (pressure area) (L89.-)

         skin infections (L00-L08)

         specific infections classified to A00-B99

         ulcer of lower limb NEC (L97.-)

         varicose ulcer ▶(I83.0-I83.93)◀

    AHA: 2017,4Q,17

    TIP: The depth and/or severity of a diagnosed nonpressure ulcer can be determined based on medical record documentation from clinicians who are not the patient's provider.

    TIP: Assign a code from this category/subcategory for nonpressure ulcers documented as acute.

  ✓6th **L98.41**   **Non-pressure chronic ulcer of buttock**

    L98.411   Non-pressure chronic ulcer of buttock limited to breakdown of skin   `HCC`

    L98.412   Non-pressure chronic ulcer of buttock with fat layer exposed   `HCC` `SW`

    L98.413   Non-pressure chronic ulcer of buttock with necrosis of muscle   `HCC` `SW`

    L98.414   Non-pressure chronic ulcer of buttock with necrosis of bone   `HCC` `SW`

    L98.415   Non-pressure chronic ulcer of buttock with muscle involvement without evidence of necrosis   `CC` `HCC`

    L98.416   Non-pressure chronic ulcer of buttock with bone involvement without evidence of necrosis   `CC` `HCC`

    L98.418   Non-pressure chronic ulcer of buttock with other specified severity   `CC` `HCC`

    L98.419   Non-pressure chronic ulcer of buttock with unspecified severity   `HCC`

  ✓6th **L98.42**   **Non-pressure chronic ulcer of back**

    L98.421   Non-pressure chronic ulcer of back limited to breakdown of skin   `HCC`

    L98.422   Non-pressure chronic ulcer of back with fat layer exposed   `HCC` `SW`

    L98.423   Non-pressure chronic ulcer of back with necrosis of muscle   `HCC` `SW`

    L98.424   Non-pressure chronic ulcer of back with necrosis of bone   `HCC` `SW`

    L98.425   Non-pressure chronic ulcer of back with muscle involvement without evidence of necrosis   `CC` `HCC`

☑ Additional Character Required   ✓x7th Placeholder   Unacceptable PDx   Questionable PDx   Manifestation   Unspecified Dx   `H1`-`H14` HAC   `HCC` CMS-HCC Dx   `HIV` HIV Dx

ICD-10-CM 2021   751

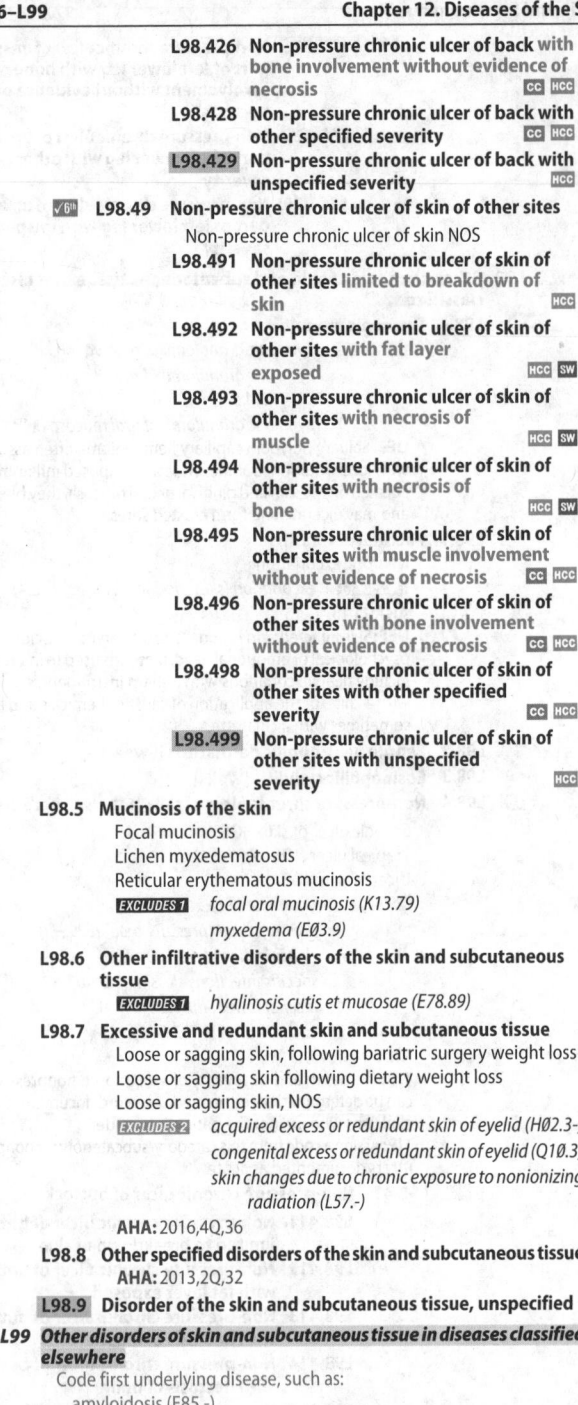

L98.426 **Non-pressure chronic ulcer of back** with bone involvement without evidence of necrosis `CC` `HCC`

L98.428 **Non-pressure chronic ulcer of back** with other specified severity `CC` `HCC`

L98.429 **Non-pressure chronic ulcer of back** with unspecified severity `HCC`

√6ᵗʰ **L98.49** **Non-pressure chronic ulcer of skin of other sites**
  Non-pressure chronic ulcer of skin NOS

L98.491 **Non-pressure chronic ulcer of skin of other sites** limited to breakdown of skin `HCC`

L98.492 **Non-pressure chronic ulcer of skin of other sites** with fat layer exposed `HCC` `SW`

L98.493 **Non-pressure chronic ulcer of skin of other sites** with necrosis of muscle `HCC` `SW`

L98.494 **Non-pressure chronic ulcer of skin of other sites** with necrosis of bone `HCC` `SW`

L98.495 **Non-pressure chronic ulcer of skin of other sites** with muscle involvement without evidence of necrosis `CC` `HCC`

L98.496 **Non-pressure chronic ulcer of skin of other sites** with bone involvement without evidence of necrosis `CC` `HCC`

L98.498 **Non-pressure chronic ulcer of skin of other sites** with other specified severity `CC` `HCC`

L98.499 **Non-pressure chronic ulcer of skin of other sites** with unspecified severity `HCC`

L98.5 **Mucinosis of the skin**
  Focal mucinosis
  Lichen myxedematosus
  Reticular erythematous mucinosis
  EXCLUDES 1   *focal oral mucinosis (K13.79)*
           myxedema (E03.9)

L98.6 **Other infiltrative disorders of the skin and subcutaneous tissue**
  EXCLUDES 1   *hyalinosis cutis et mucosae (E78.89)*

L98.7 **Excessive and redundant skin and subcutaneous tissue**
  Loose or sagging skin, following bariatric surgery weight loss
  Loose or sagging skin following dietary weight loss
  Loose or sagging skin, NOS
  EXCLUDES 2   *acquired excess or redundant skin of eyelid (H02.3-)*
           congenital excess or redundant skin of eyelid (Q10.3)
           skin changes due to chronic exposure to nonionizing radiation (L57.-)
  AHA: 2016,4Q,36

L98.8 **Other specified disorders of the skin and subcutaneous tissue**
  AHA: 2013,2Q,32

L98.9 **Disorder of the skin and subcutaneous tissue, unspecified**

L99 *Other disorders of skin and subcutaneous tissue in diseases classified elsewhere*
  Code first underlying disease, such as:
  amyloidosis (E85.-)
  EXCLUDES 1   *skin disorders in diabetes (E08-E13 with .62)*
           skin disorders in gonorrhea (A54.89)
           skin disorders in syphilis (A51.31, A52.79)

N Newborn: 0   P Pediatric: 0-17   M Maternity: 9-64   A Adult: 15-124   MCC Major Complication/Comorbidity   CC Complication/Comorbidity   SW Severe Wound Dx

752   ICD-10-CM 2021

Chapter 13. Diseases of the Musculoskeletal System and Connective Tissue (M00–M99)

Chapter-specific Guidelines with Coding Examples

The chapter-specific guidelines from the ICD-10-CM Official Guidelines for Coding and Reporting have been provided below. Along with these guidelines are coding examples, contained in the shaded boxes, that have been developed to help illustrate the coding and/or sequencing guidance found in these guidelines.

a. Site and laterality

Most of the codes within Chapter 13 have site and laterality designations. The site represents the bone, joint or the muscle involved. For some conditions where more than one bone, joint or muscle is usually involved, such as osteoarthritis, there is a "multiple sites" code available. For categories where no multiple site code is provided and more than one bone, joint or muscle is involved, multiple codes should be used to indicate the different sites involved.

Rheumatoid arthritis of multiple sites without rheumatoid factor

M06.09   **Rheumatoid arthritis without rheumatoid factor, multiple sites**

Explanation: For some conditions where more than one bone, joint or muscle is usually involved, such as rheumatoid arthritis, there is a "multiple sites" code available.

Osteomyelitis of the fourth thoracic and second lumbar vertebrae

M46.24   **Osteomyelitis of vertebra, thoracic region**

M46.26   **Osteomyelitis of vertebra, lumbar region**

Explanation: For categories without a multiple site code and more than one bone, joint, or muscle is involved, multiple codes should be used to indicate the different sites involved.

---

1) Bone versus joint

For certain conditions, the bone may be affected at the upper or lower end, (e.g., avascular necrosis of bone, M87, Osteoporosis, M80, M81). Though the portion of the bone affected may be at the joint, the site designation will be the bone, not the joint.

Idiopathic avascular necrosis of the femoral head of the left hip joint

M87.052   **Idiopathic aseptic necrosis of left femur**

Explanation: For certain conditions such as avascular necrosis, the bone may be affected at the joint, but the site designation is the bone, not the joint.

---

b. Acute traumatic versus chronic or recurrent musculoskeletal conditions

Many musculoskeletal conditions are a result of previous injury or trauma to a site, or are recurrent conditions. Bone, joint or muscle conditions that are the result of a healed injury are usually found in chapter 13. Recurrent bone, joint or muscle conditions are also usually found in chapter 13. Any current, acute injury should be coded to the appropriate injury code from chapter 19. Chronic or recurrent conditions should generally be coded with a code from chapter 13. If it is difficult to determine from the documentation in the record which code is best to describe a condition, query the provider.

Acute traumatic bucket-handle tear of right medial meniscus

S83.211A   **Bucket-handle tear of medial meniscus, current injury, right knee, initial encounter**

Explanation: Any current, acute injury is not coded in chapter 13. It should instead be coded to the appropriate injury code from chapter 19.

Old bucket-handle tear of right medial meniscus

M23.203   **Derangement of unspecified medial meniscus due to old tear or injury, right knee**

Explanation: Chronic or recurrent conditions should generally be coded with a code from chapter 13.

---

c. Coding of pathologic fractures

7th character A is for use as long as the patient is receiving active treatment for the fracture. Examples of active treatment are: surgical treatment, emergency department encounter, evaluation and continuing treatment by the same or a different physician. While the patient may be seen by a new or different provider over the course of treatment for a pathological fracture,

assignment of the 7th character is based on whether the patient is undergoing active treatment and not whether the provider is seeing the patient for the first time.

Patient admitted for repair of pathologic fracture of left foot, unknown cause. The surgery will be performed by his orthopedic specialist who he has been seeing for this fracture for the past month.

M84.475A   **Pathological fracture, left foot, initial encounter for fracture**

Explanation: Seventh character A is for use as long as the patient is receiving active treatment for a pathologic fracture. Examples of active treatment are surgical treatment, emergency department encounter, evaluation, and continuing treatment by the same or a different physician.

The seventh character is based on whether the patient is undergoing active treatment such as surgery, and not whether the provider is seeing the patient for the first time.

7th character D is to be used for encounters after the patient has completed active treatment for the fracture and is receiving routine care for the fracture during the healing or recovery phase. The other 7th characters, listed under each subcategory in the Tabular List, are to be used for subsequent encounters for treatment of problems associated with the healing, such as malunions, nonunions, and sequelae.

Care for complications of surgical treatment for fracture repairs during the healing or recovery phase should be coded with the appropriate complication codes.

See Section I.C.19. Coding of traumatic fractures.

d. Osteoporosis

Osteoporosis is a systemic condition, meaning that all bones of the musculoskeletal system are affected. Therefore, site is not a component of the codes under category M81, Osteoporosis without current pathological fracture. The site codes under category M80, Osteoporosis with current pathological fracture, identify the site of the fracture, not the osteoporosis.

1) Osteoporosis without pathological fracture

Category M81, Osteoporosis without current pathological fracture, is for use for patients with osteoporosis who do not currently have a pathologic fracture due to the osteoporosis, even if they have had a fracture in the past. For patients with a history of osteoporosis fractures, status code Z87.310, Personal history of (healed) osteoporosis fracture, should follow the code from M81.

Age-related osteoporosis with healed osteoporotic fracture of the lumbar vertebra

M81.0   **Age-related osteoporosis without current pathological fracture**

Z87.310   **Personal history of (healed) osteoporosis fracture**

Explanation: Category M81 is used for patients with osteoporosis who do not currently have a pathologic fracture due to the osteoporosis. To report a previous (healed) fracture, status code Z87.310 Personal history of (healed) osteoporosis fracture, should follow the code from M81.

---

2) Osteoporosis with current pathological fracture

Category M80, Osteoporosis with current pathological fracture, is for patients who have a current pathologic fracture at the time of an encounter. The codes under M80 identify the site of the fracture. A code from category M80, not a traumatic fracture code, should be used for any patient with known osteoporosis who suffers a fracture, even if the patient had a minor fall or trauma, if that fall or trauma would not usually break a normal, healthy bone.

Disuse osteoporosis with current fracture of right shoulder sustained lifting a grocery bag, initial encounter

M80.811A   **Other osteoporosis with current pathological fracture, right shoulder, initial encounter for fracture**

Explanation: A code from category M80, not a traumatic fracture code, should be used for any patient with known osteoporosis who suffers a fracture, even if the patient had a minor fall or trauma, if that fall or trauma would not usually break a normal, healthy bone.

Chapter 13. Diseases of the Musculoskeletal System and Connective Tissue

Muscle/Tendon Table

ICD-10-CM categorizes certain muscles and tendons in the upper and lower extremities by their action (e.g., extension, flexion), their anatomical location (e.g., posterior, anterior), and/or whether they are intrinsic or extrinsic to a certain anatomical area. The Muscle/Tendon Table is provided at the beginning of chapters 13 and 19 as a resource to help users when code selection depends on one or more of these characteristics. Please note that this table is not all-inclusive, and proper code assignment should be based on the provider's documentation.

Body Region	Muscle	Extensor Tendon	Flexor Tendon	Other Tendon
Shoulder				
	Deltoid	Posterior deltoid	Anterior deltoid	
	Rotator cuff			
	Infraspinatus			Infraspinatus
	Subscapularis			Subscapularis
	Supraspinatus			Supraspinatus
	Teres minor			Teres minor
	Teres major	Teres major		
Upper arm				
	Anterior muscles			
	Biceps brachii — long head		Biceps brachii — long head	
	Biceps brachii — short head		Biceps brachii — short head	
	Brachialis		Brachialis	
	Coracobrachialis		Coracobrachialis	
	Posterior muscles			
	Triceps brachii	Triceps brachii		
Forearm				
	Anterior muscles			
	Flexors			
	Deep			
	Flexor digitorum profundus		Flexor digitorum profundus	
	Flexor pollicis longus		Flexor pollicis longus	
	Intermediate			
	Flexor digitorum superficialis		Flexor digitorum superficialis	
	Superficial			
	Flexor carpi radialis		Flexor carpi radialis	
	Flexor carpi ulnaris		Flexor carpi ulnaris	
	Palmaris longus		Palmaris longus	
	Pronators			
	Pronator quadratus			Pronator quadratus
	Pronator teres			Pronator teres
	Posterior muscles			
	Extensors			
	Deep			
	Abductor pollicis longus			Abductor pollicis longus
	Extensor indicis	Extensor indicis		
	Extensor pollicis brevis	Extensor pollicis brevis		
	Extensor pollicis longus	Extensor pollicis longus		
	Superficial			
	Brachioradialis			Brachioradialis
	Extensor carpi radialis brevis	Extensor carpi radialis brevis		
	Extensor carpi radialis longus	Extensor carpi radialis longus		
	Extensor carpi ulnaris	Extensor carpi ulnaris		
	Extensor digiti minimi	Extensor digiti minimi		
	Extensor digitorum	Extensor digitorum		
	Anconeus	Anconeus		
	Supinator			Supinator

Body Region	Muscle	Extensor Tendon	Flexor Tendon	Other Tendon
Hand				
Extrinsic — attach to a site in the forearm as well as a site in the hand with action related to hand movement at the wrist				
	Extensor carpi radialis brevis	Extensor carpi radialis brevis		
	Extensor carpi radialis longus	Extensor carpi radialis longus		
	Extensor carpi ulnaris	Extensor carpi ulnaris		
	Flexor carpi radialis		Flexor carpi radialis	
	Flexor carpi ulnaris		Flexor carpi ulnaris	
	Flexor digitorum superficialis		Flexor digitorum superficialis	
	Palmaris longus		Palmaris longus	
Extrinsic — attach to a site in the forearm as well as a site in the hand with action in the hand related to finger movement				
	Adductor pollicis longus			Adductor pollicis longus
	Extensor digiti minimi	Extensor digiti minimi		
	Extensor digitorum	Extensor digitorum		
	Extensor indicis	Extensor indicis		
	Flexor digitorum profundus		Flexor digitorum profundus	
	Flexor digitorum superficialis		Flexor digitorum superficialis	
Extrinsic — attach to a site in the forearm as well as a site in the hand with action in the hand related to thumb movement				
	Extensor pollicis brevis	Extensor pollicis brevis		
	Extensor pollicis longus	Extensor pollicis longus		
	Flexor pollicis longus		Flexor pollicis longus	
Intrinsic — found within the hand only				
	Adductor pollicis			Adductor pollicis
	Dorsal interossei	Dorsal interossei	Dorsal interossei	
	Lumbricals	Lumbricals	Lumbricals	
	Palmaris brevis			Palmaris brevis
	Palmar interossei	Palmar interossei	Palmar interossei	
	Hypothenar muscles			
	Abductor digiti minimi			Abductor digiti minimi
	Flexor digiti minimi brevis		Flexor digiti minimi brevis	
	Opponens digiti minimi		Opponens digiti minimi	
	Thenar muscles			
	Abductor pollicis brevis			Abductor pollicis brevis
	Flexor pollicis brevis		Flexor pollicis brevis	
	Opponens pollicis		Opponens pollicis	
Thigh				
	Anterior muscles			
	Iliopsoas		Iliopsoas	
	Pectineus		Pectineus	
	Quadriceps	Quadriceps		
	Rectus femoris	Rectus femoris — Extends knee	Rectus femoris — Flexes hip	
	Vastus intermedius	Vastus intermedius		
	Vastus lateralis	Vastus lateralis		
	Vastus medialis	Vastus medialis		
	Sartorius		Sartorius	
	Medial muscles			
	Adductor brevis			Adductor brevis
	Adductor longus			Adductor longus
	Adductor magnus			Adductor magnus
	Gracilis			Gracilis
	Obturator externus			Obturator externus
	Posterior muscles			
	Hamstring	Hamstring — Extends hip	Hamstring — Flexes knee	
	Biceps femoris	Biceps femoris	Biceps femoris	
	Semimembranosus	Semimembranosus	Semimembranosus	
	Semitendinosus	Semitendinosus	Semitendinosus	

Chapter 13. Diseases of the Musculoskeletal System and Connective Tissue

Body Region	Muscle	Extensor Tendon	Flexor Tendon	Other Tendon
Lower leg				
	Anterior muscles			
	Extensor digitorum longus	Extensor digitorum longus		
	Extensor hallucis longus	Extensor hallucis longus		
	Fibularis (peroneus) tertius	Fibularis (peroneus) tertius		
	Tibialis anterior	Tibialis anterior		Tibialis anterior
	Lateral muscles			
	Fibularis (peroneus) brevis		Fibularis (peroneus) brevis	
	Fibularis (peroneus) longus		Fibularis (peroneus) longus	
	Posterior muscles			
	Deep			
	Flexor digitorum longus		Flexor digitorum longus	
	Flexor hallucis longus		Flexor hallucis longus	
	Popliteus		Popliteus	
	Tibialis posterior		Tibialis posterior	
	Superficial			
	Gastrocnemius		Gastrocnemius	
	Plantaris		Plantaris	
	Soleus		Soleus	
				Calcaneal (Achilles)
Ankle/Foot				
Extrinsic — attach to a site in the lower leg as well as a site in the foot with action related to foot movement at the ankle				
	Plantaris		Plantaris	
	Soleus		Soleus	
	Tibialis anterior	Tibialis anterior		
	Tibialis posterior		Tibialis posterior	
Extrinsic — attach to a site in the lower leg as well as a site in the foot with action in the foot related to toe movement				
	Extensor digitorum longus	Extensor digitorum longus		
	Extensor hallucis longus	Extensor hallucis longus		
	Flexor digitorum longus		Flexor digitorum longus	
	Flexor hallucis longus		Flexor hallucis longus	
Intrinsic — found within the ankle/foot only				
	Dorsal muscles			
	Extensor digitorum brevis	Extensor digitorum brevis		
	Extensor hallucis brevis	Extensor hallucis brevis		
	Plantar muscles			
	Abductor digiti minimi		Abductor digiti minimi	
	Abductor hallucis		Abductor hallucis	
	Dorsal interossei	Dorsal interossei	Dorsal interossei	
	Flexor digiti minimi brevis		Flexor digiti minimi brevis	
	Flexor digitorum brevis		Flexor digitorum brevis	
	Flexor hallucis brevis		Flexor hallucis brevis	
	Lumbricals	Lumbricals	Lumbricals	
	Quadratus plantae		Quadratus plantae	
	Plantar interossei	Plantar interossei	Plantar interossei	

Chapter 13. Diseases of the Musculoskeletal System and Connective Tissue (M00-M99)

NOTE   Use an external cause code following the code for the musculoskeletal condition, if applicable, to identify the cause of the musculoskeletal condition

EXCLUDES 2   arthropathic psoriasis (L40.5-)
certain conditions originating in the perinatal period (P04-P96)
certain infectious and parasitic diseases (A00-B99)
compartment syndrome (traumatic) (T79.A-)
complications of pregnancy, childbirth and the puerperium (O00-O9A)
congenital malformations, deformations, and chromosomal abnormalities (Q00-Q99)
endocrine, nutritional and metabolic diseases (E00-E88)
injury, poisoning and certain other consequences of external causes (S00-T88)
neoplasms (C00-D49)
symptoms, signs and abnormal clinical and laboratory findings, not elsewhere classified (R00-R94)

This chapter contains the following blocks:

M00-M02	Infectious arthropathies
M04	Autoinflammatory syndromes
M05-M14	Inflammatory polyarthropathies
M15-M19	Osteoarthritis
M20-M25	Other joint disorders
M26-M27	Dentofacial anomalies [including malocclusion] and other disorders of jaw
M30-M36	Systemic connective tissue disorders
M40-M43	Deforming dorsopathies
M45-M49	Spondylopathies
M50-M54	Other dorsopathies
M60-M63	Disorders of muscles
M65-M67	Disorders of synovium and tendon
M70-M79	Other soft tissue disorders
M80-M85	Disorders of bone density and structure
M86-M90	Other osteopathies
M91-M94	Chondropathies
M95	Other disorders of the musculoskeletal system and connective tissue
M96	Intraoperative and postprocedural complications and disorders of musculoskeletal system, not elsewhere classified
M97	Periprosthetic fracture around internal prosthetic joint
M99	Biomechanical lesions, not elsewhere classified

ARTHROPATHIES (M00-M25)

INCLUDES   disorders affecting predominantly peripheral (limb) joints

Infectious arthropathies (M00-M02)

NOTE   This block comprises arthropathies due to microbiological agents. Distinction is made between the following types of etiological relationship:

a) direct infection of joint, where organisms invade synovial tissue and microbial antigen is present in the joint;

b) indirect infection, which may be of two types: a reactive arthropathy, where microbial infection of the body is established but neither organisms nor antigens can be identified in the joint, and a postinfective arthropathy, where microbial antigen is present but recovery of an organism is inconstant and evidence of local multiplication is lacking.

AHA: 2019,3Q,16

✓4ᵗʰ **M00 Pyogenic arthritis**

   EXCLUDES 2   ▶infection and inflammatory reaction due to internal joint prosthesis (T84.5-)◀

   DEF: Pyogenic: Relating to or involving pus production, often referred to as suppurative or purulent.

   ✓5ᵗʰ **M00.0 Staphylococcal arthritis and polyarthritis**

     Use additional code (B95.61-B95.8) to identify bacterial agent

     EXCLUDES 2   infection and inflammatory reaction due to internal joint prosthesis (T84.5-)

     M00.00 Staphylococcal arthritis, unspecified joint cc HCC

     ✓6ᵗʰ **M00.01 Staphylococcal arthritis, shoulder**

       M00.011 Staphylococcal arthritis, right shoulder cc HCC

       M00.012 Staphylococcal arthritis, left shoulder cc HCC

       M00.019 Staphylococcal arthritis, unspecified shoulder cc HCC

     ✓6ᵗʰ **M00.02 Staphylococcal arthritis, elbow**

       M00.021 Staphylococcal arthritis, right elbow cc HCC

       M00.022 Staphylococcal arthritis, left elbow cc HCC

       M00.029 Staphylococcal arthritis, unspecified elbow cc HCC

     ✓6ᵗʰ **M00.03 Staphylococcal arthritis, wrist**

       Staphylococcal arthritis of carpal bones

       M00.031 Staphylococcal arthritis, right wrist cc HCC

       M00.032 Staphylococcal arthritis, left wrist cc HCC

       M00.039 Staphylococcal arthritis, unspecified wrist cc HCC

     ✓6ᵗʰ **M00.04 Staphylococcal arthritis, hand**

       Staphylococcal arthritis of metacarpus and phalanges

       M00.041 Staphylococcal arthritis, right hand cc HCC

       M00.042 Staphylococcal arthritis, left hand cc HCC

       M00.049 Staphylococcal arthritis, unspecified hand cc HCC

     ✓6ᵗʰ **M00.05 Staphylococcal arthritis, hip**

       M00.051 Staphylococcal arthritis, right hip cc HCC

       M00.052 Staphylococcal arthritis, left hip cc HCC

       M00.059 Staphylococcal arthritis, unspecified hip cc HCC

     ✓6ᵗʰ **M00.06 Staphylococcal arthritis, knee**

       M00.061 Staphylococcal arthritis, right knee cc HCC

       M00.062 Staphylococcal arthritis, left knee cc HCC

       M00.069 Staphylococcal arthritis, unspecified knee cc HCC

     ✓6ᵗʰ **M00.07 Staphylococcal arthritis, ankle and foot**

       Staphylococcal arthritis, tarsus, metatarsus and phalanges

       M00.071 Staphylococcal arthritis, right ankle and foot cc HCC

       M00.072 Staphylococcal arthritis, left ankle and foot cc HCC

       M00.079 Staphylococcal arthritis, unspecified ankle and foot cc HCC

     M00.08 Staphylococcal arthritis, vertebrae cc HCC

     M00.09 Staphylococcal polyarthritis cc HCC

   ✓5ᵗʰ **M00.1 Pneumococcal arthritis and polyarthritis**

     M00.10 Pneumococcal arthritis, unspecified joint cc HCC

     ✓6ᵗʰ **M00.11 Pneumococcal arthritis, shoulder**

       M00.111 Pneumococcal arthritis, right shoulder cc HCC

       M00.112 Pneumococcal arthritis, left shoulder cc HCC

       M00.119 Pneumococcal arthritis, unspecified shoulder cc HCC

     ✓6ᵗʰ **M00.12 Pneumococcal arthritis, elbow**

       M00.121 Pneumococcal arthritis, right elbow cc HCC

       M00.122 Pneumococcal arthritis, left elbow cc HCC

       M00.129 Pneumococcal arthritis, unspecified elbow cc HCC

     ✓6ᵗʰ **M00.13 Pneumococcal arthritis, wrist**

       Pneumococcal arthritis of carpal bones

       M00.131 Pneumococcal arthritis, right wrist cc HCC

       M00.132 Pneumococcal arthritis, left wrist cc HCC

       M00.139 Pneumococcal arthritis, unspecified wrist cc HCC

     ✓6ᵗʰ **M00.14 Pneumococcal arthritis, hand**

       Pneumococcal arthritis of metacarpus and phalanges

       M00.141 Pneumococcal arthritis, right hand cc HCC

       M00.142 Pneumococcal arthritis, left hand cc HCC

       M00.149 Pneumococcal arthritis, unspecified hand cc HCC

✓ Additional Character Required   ✓x7ᵗʰ Placeholder   Unacceptable PDx   Questionable PDx   Manifestation   Unspecified Dx   H1-H14 HAC   HCC CMS-HCC Dx   HIV HIV Dx

ICD-10-CM 2021   757

Chapter 13. Diseases of the Musculoskeletal System and Connective Tissue

M00.15–M00.9

✓6ᵗʰ **M00.15 Pneumococcal arthritis,** hip

    M00.151 Pneumococcal arthritis, right hip `CC` `HCC`

    M00.152 Pneumococcal arthritis, left hip `CC` `HCC`

    M00.159 Pneumococcal arthritis, unspecified hip `CC` `HCC`

✓6ᵗʰ **M00.16 Pneumococcal arthritis,** knee

    M00.161 Pneumococcal arthritis, right knee `CC` `HCC`

    M00.162 Pneumococcal arthritis, left knee `CC` `HCC`

    M00.169 Pneumococcal arthritis, unspecified knee `CC` `HCC`

✓6ᵗʰ **M00.17 Pneumococcal arthritis,** ankle and foot

    Pneumococcal arthritis, tarsus, metatarsus and phalanges

    M00.171 Pneumococcal arthritis, right ankle and foot `CC` `HCC`

    M00.172 Pneumococcal arthritis, left ankle and foot `CC` `HCC`

    M00.179 Pneumococcal arthritis, unspecified ankle and foot `CC` `HCC`

  M00.18 Pneumococcal arthritis, vertebrae `CC` `HCC`

  M00.19 Pneumococcal polyarthritis `CC` `HCC`

✓5ᵗʰ **M00.2 Other streptococcal arthritis and polyarthritis**

    Use additional code (B95.0-B95.2, B95.4-B95.5) to identify bacterial agent

  M00.20 Other streptococcal arthritis, unspecified joint `CC` `HCC`

✓6ᵗʰ **M00.21 Other streptococcal arthritis,** shoulder

    M00.211 Other streptococcal arthritis, right shoulder `CC` `HCC`

    M00.212 Other streptococcal arthritis, left shoulder `CC` `HCC`

    M00.219 Other streptococcal arthritis, unspecified shoulder `CC` `HCC`

✓6ᵗʰ **M00.22 Other streptococcal arthritis,** elbow

    M00.221 Other streptococcal arthritis, right elbow `CC` `HCC`

    M00.222 Other streptococcal arthritis, left elbow `CC` `HCC`

    M00.229 Other streptococcal arthritis, unspecified elbow `CC` `HCC`

✓6ᵗʰ **M00.23 Other streptococcal arthritis,** wrist

    Other streptococcal arthritis of carpal bones

    M00.231 Other streptococcal arthritis, right wrist `CC` `HCC`

    M00.232 Other streptococcal arthritis, left wrist `CC` `HCC`

    M00.239 Other streptococcal arthritis, unspecified wrist `CC` `HCC`

✓6ᵗʰ **M00.24 Other streptococcal arthritis,** hand

    Other streptococcal arthritis metacarpus and phalanges

    M00.241 Other streptococcal arthritis, right hand `CC` `HCC`

    M00.242 Other streptococcal arthritis, left hand `CC` `HCC`

    M00.249 Other streptococcal arthritis, unspecified hand `CC` `HCC`

✓6ᵗʰ **M00.25 Other streptococcal arthritis,** hip

    M00.251 Other streptococcal arthritis, right hip `CC` `HCC`

    M00.252 Other streptococcal arthritis, left hip `CC` `HCC`

    M00.259 Other streptococcal arthritis, unspecified hip `CC` `HCC`

✓6ᵗʰ **M00.26 Other streptococcal arthritis,** knee

    M00.261 Other streptococcal arthritis, right knee `CC` `HCC`

    M00.262 Other streptococcal arthritis, left knee `CC` `HCC`

    M00.269 Other streptococcal arthritis, unspecified knee `CC` `HCC`

✓6ᵗʰ **M00.27 Other streptococcal arthritis,** ankle and foot

    Other streptococcal arthritis, tarsus, metatarsus and phalanges

    M00.271 Other streptococcal arthritis, right ankle and foot `CC` `HCC`

    M00.272 Other streptococcal arthritis, left ankle and foot `CC` `HCC`

    M00.279 Other streptococcal arthritis, unspecified ankle and foot `CC` `HCC`

  M00.28 Other streptococcal arthritis, vertebrae `CC` `HCC`

  M00.29 Other streptococcal polyarthritis `CC` `HCC`

✓5ᵗʰ **M00.8 Arthritis and polyarthritis due to other bacteria**

    Use additional code (B96) to identify bacteria

  M00.80 Arthritis due to other bacteria, unspecified joint `CC` `HCC`

✓6ᵗʰ **M00.81 Arthritis due to other bacteria,** shoulder

    M00.811 Arthritis due to other bacteria, right shoulder `CC` `HCC`

    M00.812 Arthritis due to other bacteria, left shoulder `CC` `HCC`

    M00.819 Arthritis due to other bacteria, unspecified shoulder `CC` `HCC`

✓6ᵗʰ **M00.82 Arthritis due to other bacteria,** elbow

    M00.821 Arthritis due to other bacteria, right elbow `CC` `HCC`

    M00.822 Arthritis due to other bacteria, left elbow `CC` `HCC`

    M00.829 Arthritis due to other bacteria, unspecified elbow `CC` `HCC`

✓6ᵗʰ **M00.83 Arthritis due to other bacteria,** wrist

    Arthritis due to other bacteria, carpal bones

    M00.831 Arthritis due to other bacteria, right wrist `CC` `HCC`

    M00.832 Arthritis due to other bacteria, left wrist `CC` `HCC`

    M00.839 Arthritis due to other bacteria, unspecified wrist `CC` `HCC`

✓6ᵗʰ **M00.84 Arthritis due to other bacteria,** hand

    Arthritis due to other bacteria, metacarpus and phalanges

    M00.841 Arthritis due to other bacteria, right hand `CC` `HCC`

    M00.842 Arthritis due to other bacteria, left hand `CC` `HCC`

    M00.849 Arthritis due to other bacteria, unspecified hand `CC` `HCC`

✓6ᵗʰ **M00.85 Arthritis due to other bacteria,** hip

    M00.851 Arthritis due to other bacteria, right hip `CC` `HCC`

    M00.852 Arthritis due to other bacteria, left hip `CC` `HCC`

    M00.859 Arthritis due to other bacteria, unspecified hip `CC` `HCC`

✓6ᵗʰ **M00.86 Arthritis due to other bacteria,** knee

    AHA: 2019,3Q,16

    M00.861 Arthritis due to other bacteria, right knee `CC` `HCC`

    M00.862 Arthritis due to other bacteria, left knee `CC` `HCC`

    M00.869 Arthritis due to other bacteria, unspecified knee `CC` `HCC`

✓6ᵗʰ **M00.87 Arthritis due to other bacteria,** ankle and foot

    Arthritis due to other bacteria, tarsus, metatarsus, and phalanges

    M00.871 Arthritis due to other bacteria, right ankle and foot `CC` `HCC`

    M00.872 Arthritis due to other bacteria, left ankle and foot `CC` `HCC`

    M00.879 Arthritis due to other bacteria, unspecified ankle and foot `CC` `HCC`

  M00.88 Arthritis due to other bacteria, vertebrae `CC` `HCC`

  M00.89 Polyarthritis due to other bacteria `CC` `HCC`

M00.9 Pyogenic arthritis, unspecified

    Infective arthritis NOS

`N` Newborn: 0   `P` Pediatric: 0-17   `M` Maternity: 9-64   `A` Adult: 15-124   `MCC` Major Complication/Comorbidity   `CC` Complication/Comorbidity   `SW` Severe Wound Dx

758   ICD-10-CM 2021

M01   **Direct infections of joint in infectious and parasitic diseases classified elsewhere**

Code first underlying disease, such as:
leprosy [Hansen's disease] (A30.-)
mycoses (B35-B49)
O'nyong-nyong fever (A92.1)
paratyphoid fever (A01.1-A01.4)

EXCLUDES 1   *arthropathy in Lyme disease (A69.23)*
gonococcal arthritis (A54.42)
meningococcal arthritis (A39.83)
mumps arthritis (B26.85)
postinfective arthropathy (M02.-)
postmeningococcal arthritis (A39.84)
reactive arthritis (M02.3)
rubella arthritis (B06.82)
sarcoidosis arthritis (D86.86)
typhoid fever arthritis (A01.04)
tuberculosis arthritis (A18.01-A18.02)

M01.X   **Direct infection of joint in infectious and parasitic diseases classified elsewhere**

M01.X0   **Direct infection of unspecified joint in infectious and parasitic diseases classified elsewhere** `CC` `HCC`

M01.X1   **Direct infection of shoulder joint in infectious and parasitic diseases classified elsewhere**

  M01.X11   Direct infection of *right* shoulder in infectious and parasitic diseases classified elsewhere `CC` `HCC`

  M01.X12   Direct infection of *left* shoulder in infectious and parasitic diseases classified elsewhere `CC` `HCC`

  M01.X19   Direct infection of unspecified shoulder in infectious and parasitic diseases classified elsewhere `CC` `HCC`

M01.X2   **Direct infection of elbow in infectious and parasitic diseases classified elsewhere**

  M01.X21   Direct infection of *right* elbow in infectious and parasitic diseases classified elsewhere `CC` `HCC`

  M01.X22   Direct infection of *left* elbow in infectious and parasitic diseases classified elsewhere `CC` `HCC`

  M01.X29   Direct infection of unspecified elbow in infectious and parasitic diseases classified elsewhere `CC` `HCC`

M01.X3   **Direct infection of wrist in infectious and parasitic diseases classified elsewhere**

Direct infection of carpal bones in infectious and parasitic diseases classified elsewhere

  M01.X31   Direct infection of *right* wrist in infectious and parasitic diseases classified elsewhere `CC` `HCC`

  M01.X32   Direct infection of *left* wrist in infectious and parasitic diseases classified elsewhere `CC` `HCC`

  M01.X39   Direct infection of unspecified wrist in infectious and parasitic diseases classified elsewhere `CC` `HCC`

M01.X4   **Direct infection of hand in infectious and parasitic diseases classified elsewhere**

Direct infection of metacarpus and phalanges in infectious and parasitic diseases classified elsewhere

  M01.X41   Direct infection of *right* hand in infectious and parasitic diseases classified elsewhere `CC` `HCC`

  M01.X42   Direct infection of *left* hand in infectious and parasitic diseases classified elsewhere `CC` `HCC`

  M01.X49   Direct infection of unspecified hand in infectious and parasitic diseases classified elsewhere `CC` `HCC`

M01.X5   **Direct infection of hip in infectious and parasitic diseases classified elsewhere**

  M01.X51   Direct infection of *right* hip in infectious and parasitic diseases classified elsewhere `CC` `HCC`

  M01.X52   Direct infection of *left* hip in infectious and parasitic diseases classified elsewhere `CC` `HCC`

  M01.X59   Direct infection of unspecified hip in infectious and parasitic diseases classified elsewhere `CC` `HCC`

M01.X6   **Direct infection of knee in infectious and parasitic diseases classified elsewhere**

  M01.X61   Direct infection of *right* knee in infectious and parasitic diseases classified elsewhere `CC` `HCC`

  M01.X62   Direct infection of *left* knee in infectious and parasitic diseases classified elsewhere `CC` `HCC`

  M01.X69   Direct infection of unspecified knee in infectious and parasitic diseases classified elsewhere `CC` `HCC`

M01.X7   **Direct infection of ankle and foot in infectious and parasitic diseases classified elsewhere**

Direct infection of tarsus, metatarsus and phalanges in infectious and parasitic diseases classified elsewhere

  M01.X71   Direct infection of *right* ankle and foot in infectious and parasitic diseases classified elsewhere `CC` `HCC`

  M01.X72   Direct infection of *left* ankle and foot in infectious and parasitic diseases classified elsewhere `CC` `HCC`

  M01.X79   Direct infection of unspecified ankle and foot in infectious and parasitic diseases classified elsewhere `CC` `HCC`

M01.X8   **Direct infection of vertebrae in infectious and parasitic diseases classified elsewhere** `CC` `HCC`

M01.X9   **Direct infection of multiple joints in infectious and parasitic diseases classified elsewhere** `CC` `HCC`

M02   **Postinfective and reactive arthropathies**

Code first underlying disease, such as:
congenital syphilis [Clutton's joints] (A50.5)
enteritis due to Yersinia enterocolitica (A04.6)
infective endocarditis (I33.0)
viral hepatitis (B15-B19)

EXCLUDES 1   *Behçet's disease (M35.2)*
direct infections of joint in infectious and parasitic diseases classified elsewhere (M01.-)
mumps arthritis (B26.85)
postmeningococcal arthritis (A39.84)
rheumatic fever (I00)
rubella arthritis (B06.82)
syphilis arthritis (late) (A52.77)
tabetic arthropathy [Charcôt's] (A52.16)

M02.0   **Arthropathy following intestinal bypass**

M02.00   **Arthropathy following intestinal bypass, unspecified site**

M02.01   **Arthropathy following intestinal bypass, shoulder**

  M02.011   Arthropathy following intestinal bypass, right shoulder

  M02.012   Arthropathy following intestinal bypass, left shoulder

  M02.019   Arthropathy following intestinal bypass, unspecified shoulder

M02.02   **Arthropathy following intestinal bypass, elbow**

  M02.021   Arthropathy following intestinal bypass, right elbow

  M02.022   Arthropathy following intestinal bypass, left elbow

  M02.029   Arthropathy following intestinal bypass, unspecified elbow

M02.03   **Arthropathy following intestinal bypass, wrist**

Arthropathy following intestinal bypass, carpal bones

  M02.031   Arthropathy following intestinal bypass, right wrist

  M02.032   Arthropathy following intestinal bypass, left wrist

  M02.039   Arthropathy following intestinal bypass, unspecified wrist

M02.04   **Arthropathy following intestinal bypass, hand**

Arthropathy following intestinal bypass, metacarpals and phalanges

  M02.041   Arthropathy following intestinal bypass, right hand

  M02.042   Arthropathy following intestinal bypass, left hand

✔ Additional Character Required   ✔x7ᵗʰ Placeholder   Unacceptable PDx   Questionable PDx   Manifestation   Unspecified Dx   `H1`-`H4` HAC   `HCC` CMS-HCC Dx   `HIV` HIV Dx

ICD-10-CM 2021   759

      M02.049 Arthropathy following intestinal bypass, unspecified hand

√6th **M02.05** Arthropathy following intestinal bypass, hip

      M02.051 Arthropathy following intestinal bypass, right hip

      M02.052 Arthropathy following intestinal bypass, left hip

      M02.059 Arthropathy following intestinal bypass, unspecified hip

√6th **M02.06** Arthropathy following intestinal bypass, knee

      M02.061 Arthropathy following intestinal bypass, right knee

      M02.062 Arthropathy following intestinal bypass, left knee

      M02.069 Arthropathy following intestinal bypass, unspecified knee

√6th **M02.07** Arthropathy following intestinal bypass, ankle and foot

      Arthropathy following intestinal bypass, tarsus, metatarsus and phalanges

      M02.071 Arthropathy following intestinal bypass, right ankle and foot

      M02.072 Arthropathy following intestinal bypass, left ankle and foot

      M02.079 Arthropathy following intestinal bypass, unspecified ankle and foot

      M02.08 Arthropathy following intestinal bypass, vertebrae

      M02.09 Arthropathy following intestinal bypass, multiple sites

√5th **M02.1** Postdysenteric arthropathy

      M02.10 Postdysenteric arthropathy, unspecified site   CC HCC

√6th **M02.11** Postdysenteric arthropathy, shoulder

      M02.111 Postdysenteric arthropathy, right shoulder   CC HCC

      M02.112 Postdysenteric arthropathy, left shoulder   CC HCC

      M02.119 Postdysenteric arthropathy, unspecified shoulder   CC HCC

√6th **M02.12** Postdysenteric arthropathy, elbow

      M02.121 Postdysenteric arthropathy, right elbow   CC HCC

      M02.122 Postdysenteric arthropathy, left elbow   CC HCC

      M02.129 Postdysenteric arthropathy, unspecified elbow   CC HCC

√6th **M02.13** Postdysenteric arthropathy, wrist

      Postdysenteric arthropathy, carpal bones

      M02.131 Postdysenteric arthropathy, right wrist   CC HCC

      M02.132 Postdysenteric arthropathy, left wrist   CC HCC

      M02.139 Postdysenteric arthropathy, unspecified wrist   CC HCC

√6th **M02.14** Postdysenteric arthropathy, hand

      Postdysenteric arthropathy, metacarpus and phalanges

      M02.141 Postdysenteric arthropathy, right hand   CC HCC

      M02.142 Postdysenteric arthropathy, left hand   CC HCC

      M02.149 Postdysenteric arthropathy, unspecified hand   CC HCC

√6th **M02.15** Postdysenteric arthropathy, hip

      M02.151 Postdysenteric arthropathy, right hip   CC HCC

      M02.152 Postdysenteric arthropathy, left hip   CC HCC

      M02.159 Postdysenteric arthropathy, unspecified hip   CC HCC

√6th **M02.16** Postdysenteric arthropathy, knee

      M02.161 Postdysenteric arthropathy, right knee   CC HCC

      M02.162 Postdysenteric arthropathy, left knee   CC HCC

      M02.169 Postdysenteric arthropathy, unspecified knee   CC HCC

√6th **M02.17** Postdysenteric arthropathy, ankle and foot

      Postdysenteric arthropathy, tarsus, metatarsus and phalanges

      M02.171 Postdysenteric arthropathy, right ankle and foot   CC HCC

      M02.172 Postdysenteric arthropathy, left ankle and foot   CC HCC

      M02.179 Postdysenteric arthropathy, unspecified ankle and foot   CC HCC

      M02.18 Postdysenteric arthropathy, vertebrae   CC HCC

      M02.19 Postdysenteric arthropathy, multiple sites   CC HCC

√5th **M02.2** Postimmunization arthropathy

      M02.20 Postimmunization arthropathy, unspecified site

√6th **M02.21** Postimmunization arthropathy, shoulder

      M02.211 Postimmunization arthropathy, right shoulder

      M02.212 Postimmunization arthropathy, left shoulder

      M02.219 Postimmunization arthropathy, unspecified shoulder

√6th **M02.22** Postimmunization arthropathy, elbow

      M02.221 Postimmunization arthropathy, right elbow

      M02.222 Postimmunization arthropathy, left elbow

      M02.229 Postimmunization arthropathy, unspecified elbow

√6th **M02.23** Postimmunization arthropathy, wrist

      Postimmunization arthropathy, carpal bones

      M02.231 Postimmunization arthropathy, right wrist

      M02.232 Postimmunization arthropathy, left wrist

      M02.239 Postimmunization arthropathy, unspecified wrist

√6th **M02.24** Postimmunization arthropathy, hand

      Postimmunization arthropathy, metacarpus and phalanges

      M02.241 Postimmunization arthropathy, right hand

      M02.242 Postimmunization arthropathy, left hand

      M02.249 Postimmunization arthropathy, unspecified hand

√6th **M02.25** Postimmunization arthropathy, hip

      M02.251 Postimmunization arthropathy, right hip

      M02.252 Postimmunization arthropathy, left hip

      M02.259 Postimmunization arthropathy, unspecified hip

√6th **M02.26** Postimmunization arthropathy, knee

      M02.261 Postimmunization arthropathy, right knee

      M02.262 Postimmunization arthropathy, left knee

      M02.269 Postimmunization arthropathy, unspecified knee

√6th **M02.27** Postimmunization arthropathy, ankle and foot

      Postimmunization arthropathy, tarsus, metatarsus and phalanges

      M02.271 Postimmunization arthropathy, right ankle and foot

      M02.272 Postimmunization arthropathy, left ankle and foot

      M02.279 Postimmunization arthropathy, unspecified ankle and foot

      M02.28 Postimmunization arthropathy, vertebrae

      M02.29 Postimmunization arthropathy, multiple sites

√5th **M02.3** Reiter's disease

      Reactive arthritis

      DEF: Arthritis, iridocyclitis, and urethritis, sometimes with diarrhea. While symptoms may recur, arthritis is constant.

      M02.30 Reiter's disease, unspecified site   CC HCC

√6th **M02.31** Reiter's disease, shoulder

      M02.311 Reiter's disease, right shoulder   CC HCC

      M02.312 Reiter's disease, left shoulder   CC HCC

      M02.319 Reiter's disease, unspecified shoulder   CC HCC

√6th **M02.32** Reiter's disease, elbow

      M02.321 Reiter's disease, right elbow   CC HCC

      M02.322 Reiter's disease, left elbow   CC HCC

N Newborn: 0   P Pediatric: 0-17   M Maternity: 9-64   A Adult: 15-124   MCC Major Complication/Comorbidity   CC Complication/Comorbidity   SW Severe Wound Dx

760   ICD-10-CM 2021

✓6ᵗʰ   **M02.329**   Reiter's disease, unspecified elbow   `CC` `HCC`

✓6ᵗʰ   **M02.33**   Reiter's disease, wrist

     Reiter's disease, carpal bones

     M02.331   Reiter's disease, right wrist   `CC` `HCC`

     M02.332   Reiter's disease, left wrist   `CC` `HCC`

     M02.339   Reiter's disease, unspecified wrist   `CC` `HCC`

✓6ᵗʰ   **M02.34**   Reiter's disease, hand

     Reiter's disease, metacarpus and phalanges

     M02.341   Reiter's disease, right hand   `CC` `HCC`

     M02.342   Reiter's disease, left hand   `CC` `HCC`

     M02.349   Reiter's disease, unspecified hand   `CC` `HCC`

✓6ᵗʰ   **M02.35**   Reiter's disease, hip

     M02.351   Reiter's disease, right hip   `CC` `HCC`

     M02.352   Reiter's disease, left hip   `CC` `HCC`

     M02.359   Reiter's disease, unspecified hip   `CC` `HCC`

✓6ᵗʰ   **M02.36**   Reiter's disease, knee

     M02.361   Reiter's disease, right knee   `CC` `HCC`

     M02.362   Reiter's disease, left knee   `CC` `HCC`

     M02.369   Reiter's disease, unspecified knee   `CC` `HCC`

✓6ᵗʰ   **M02.37**   Reiter's disease, ankle and foot

     Reiter's disease, tarsus, metatarsus and phalanges

     M02.371   Reiter's disease, right ankle and foot   `CC` `HCC`

     M02.372   Reiter's disease, left ankle and foot   `CC` `HCC`

     M02.379   Reiter's disease, unspecified ankle and foot   `CC` `HCC`

     M02.38   Reiter's disease, vertebrae   `CC` `HCC`

     M02.39   Reiter's disease, multiple sites   `CC` `HCC`

✓5ᵗʰ   **M02.8**   Other reactive arthropathies

     M02.80   *Other reactive arthropathies, unspecified site*   `CC` `HCC`

✓6ᵗʰ   **M02.81**   Other reactive arthropathies, shoulder

     M02.811   *Other reactive arthropathies, right shoulder*   `CC` `HCC`

     M02.812   *Other reactive arthropathies, left shoulder*   `CC` `HCC`

     M02.819   *Other reactive arthropathies, unspecified shoulder*   `CC` `HCC`

✓6ᵗʰ   **M02.82**   Other reactive arthropathies, elbow

     M02.821   *Other reactive arthropathies, right elbow*   `CC` `HCC`

     M02.822   *Other reactive arthropathies, left elbow*   `CC` `HCC`

     M02.829   *Other reactive arthropathies, unspecified elbow*   `CC` `HCC`

✓6ᵗʰ   **M02.83**   Other reactive arthropathies, wrist

     Other reactive arthropathies, carpal bones

     M02.831   *Other reactive arthropathies, right wrist*   `CC` `HCC`

     M02.832   *Other reactive arthropathies, left wrist*   `CC` `HCC`

     M02.839   *Other reactive arthropathies, unspecified wrist*   `CC` `HCC`

✓6ᵗʰ   **M02.84**   Other reactive arthropathies, hand

     Other reactive arthropathies, metacarpus and phalanges

     M02.841   *Other reactive arthropathies, right hand*   `CC` `HCC`

     M02.842   *Other reactive arthropathies, left hand*   `CC` `HCC`

     M02.849   *Other reactive arthropathies, unspecified hand*   `CC` `HCC`

✓6ᵗʰ   **M02.85**   Other reactive arthropathies, hip

     M02.851   *Other reactive arthropathies, right hip*   `CC` `HCC`

     M02.852   *Other reactive arthropathies, left hip*   `CC` `HCC`

     M02.859   *Other reactive arthropathies, unspecified hip*   `CC` `HCC`

✓6ᵗʰ   **M02.86**   Other reactive arthropathies, knee

     M02.861   *Other reactive arthropathies, right knee*   `CC` `HCC`

     M02.862   *Other reactive arthropathies, left knee*   `CC` `HCC`

     M02.869   *Other reactive arthropathies, unspecified knee*   `CC` `HCC`

✓6ᵗʰ   **M02.87**   Other reactive arthropathies, ankle and foot

     Other reactive arthropathies, tarsus, metatarsus and phalanges

     M02.871   *Other reactive arthropathies, right ankle and foot*   `CC` `HCC`

     M02.872   *Other reactive arthropathies, left ankle and foot*   `CC` `HCC`

     M02.879   *Other reactive arthropathies, unspecified ankle and foot*   `CC` `HCC`

     M02.88   *Other reactive arthropathies, vertebrae*   `CC` `HCC`

     M02.89   *Other reactive arthropathies, multiple sites*   `CC` `HCC`

  M02.9   *Reactive arthropathy, unspecified*   `HCC`

Autoinflammatory syndromes (M04)

✓4ᵗʰ   **M04**   Autoinflammatory syndromes

     `EXCLUDES 2`   Crohn's disease (K50.-)

     AHA: 2016,4Q,37

   M04.1   **Periodic fever syndromes**   `HCC`

     Familial Mediterranean fever

     Hyperimmunoglobin D syndrome

     Mevalonate kinase deficiency

     Tumor necrosis factor receptor associated periodic syndrome [TRAPS]

   M04.2   **Cryopyrin-associated periodic syndromes**   `HCC`

     Chronic infantile neurological, cutaneous and articular syndrome [CINCA]

     Familial cold autoinflammatory syndrome

     Familial cold urticaria

     Muckle-Wells syndrome

     Neonatal onset multisystemic inflammatory disorder [NOMID]

   M04.8   **Other autoinflammatory syndromes**   `HCC`

     Blau syndrome

     Deficiency of interleukin 1 receptor antagonist [DIRA]

     Majeed syndrome

     Periodic fever, aphthous stomatitis, pharyngitis, and adenopathy syndrome [PFAPA]

     Pyogenic arthritis, pyoderma gangrenosum, and acne syndrome [PAPA]

   M04.9   **Autoinflammatory syndrome, unspecified**   `HCC`

Inflammatory polyarthropathies (M05-M14)

✓4ᵗʰ   **M05**   Rheumatoid arthritis with rheumatoid factor

     `EXCLUDES 1`   rheumatic fever (I00)

                  juvenile rheumatoid arthritis (M08.-)

                   rheumatoid arthritis of spine (M45.-)

     DEF: Rheumatoid arthritis: Autoimmune systemic disease that causes chronic inflammation of the joints and other areas of the body, manifested by inflammatory changes in articular structures and synovial membranes, atrophy, and loss in bone density.

✓5ᵗʰ   **M05.0**   Felty's syndrome

     Rheumatoid arthritis with splenoadenomegaly and leukopenia

     M05.00   Felty's syndrome, unspecified site   `HCC`

✓6ᵗʰ   **M05.01**   Felty's syndrome, shoulder

     M05.011   Felty's syndrome, right shoulder   `HCC`

     M05.012   Felty's syndrome, left shoulder   `HCC`

     M05.019   Felty's syndrome, unspecified shoulder   `HCC`

✓6ᵗʰ   **M05.02**   Felty's syndrome, elbow

     M05.021   Felty's syndrome, right elbow   `HCC`

     M05.022   Felty's syndrome, left elbow   `HCC`

     M05.029   Felty's syndrome, unspecified elbow   `HCC`

✓6ᵗʰ   **M05.03**   Felty's syndrome, wrist

     Felty's syndrome, carpal bones

     M05.031   Felty's syndrome, right wrist   `HCC`

     M05.032   Felty's syndrome, left wrist   `HCC`

✓ Additional Character Required   ✓x7ᵗʰ Placeholder   Unacceptable PDx   Questionable PDx   Manifestation   Unspecified Dx   `H1`-`H14` HAC   `HCC` CMS-HCC Dx   `HIV` HIV Dx

ICD-10-CM 2021   761

M05.039   Felty's syndrome, unspecified wrist   `HCC`

✓6ᵗʰ   M05.04   Felty's syndrome, hand

    Felty's syndrome, metacarpus and phalanges

   M05.041   Felty's syndrome, right hand   `HCC`

   M05.042   Felty's syndrome, left hand   `HCC`

   M05.049   Felty's syndrome, unspecified hand   `HCC`

✓6ᵗʰ   M05.05   Felty's syndrome, hip

   M05.051   Felty's syndrome, right hip   `HCC`

   M05.052   Felty's syndrome, left hip   `HCC`

   M05.059   Felty's syndrome, unspecified hip   `HCC`

✓6ᵗʰ   M05.06   Felty's syndrome, knee

   M05.061   Felty's syndrome, right knee   `HCC`

   M05.062   Felty's syndrome, left knee   `HCC`

   M05.069   Felty's syndrome, unspecified knee   `HCC`

✓6ᵗʰ   M05.07   Felty's syndrome, ankle and foot

    Felty's syndrome, tarsus, metatarsus and phalanges

   M05.071   Felty's syndrome, right ankle and foot   `HCC`

   M05.072   Felty's syndrome, left ankle and foot   `HCC`

   M05.079   Felty's syndrome, unspecified ankle and foot   `HCC`

   M05.09   Felty's syndrome, multiple sites   `HCC`

✓5ᵗʰ   M05.1   Rheumatoid lung disease with rheumatoid arthritis

    DEF: Lung disorders associated with rheumatoid arthritis.

   M05.10   Rheumatoid lung disease with rheumatoid arthritis of unspecified site   `HCC`

✓6ᵗʰ   M05.11   Rheumatoid lung disease with rheumatoid arthritis of shoulder

   M05.111   Rheumatoid lung disease with rheumatoid arthritis of right shoulder   `HCC`

   M05.112   Rheumatoid lung disease with rheumatoid arthritis of left shoulder   `HCC`

   M05.119   Rheumatoid lung disease with rheumatoid arthritis of unspecified shoulder   `HCC`

✓6ᵗʰ   M05.12   Rheumatoid lung disease with rheumatoid arthritis of elbow

   M05.121   Rheumatoid lung disease with rheumatoid arthritis of right elbow   `HCC`

   M05.122   Rheumatoid lung disease with rheumatoid arthritis of left elbow   `HCC`

   M05.129   Rheumatoid lung disease with rheumatoid arthritis of unspecified elbow   `HCC`

✓6ᵗʰ   M05.13   Rheumatoid lung disease with rheumatoid arthritis of wrist

    Rheumatoid lung disease with rheumatoid arthritis, carpal bones

   M05.131   Rheumatoid lung disease with rheumatoid arthritis of right wrist   `HCC`

   M05.132   Rheumatoid lung disease with rheumatoid arthritis of left wrist   `HCC`

   M05.139   Rheumatoid lung disease with rheumatoid arthritis of unspecified wrist   `HCC`

✓6ᵗʰ   M05.14   Rheumatoid lung disease with rheumatoid arthritis of hand

    Rheumatoid lung disease with rheumatoid arthritis, metacarpus and phalanges

   M05.141   Rheumatoid lung disease with rheumatoid arthritis of right hand   `HCC`

   M05.142   Rheumatoid lung disease with rheumatoid arthritis of left hand   `HCC`

   M05.149   Rheumatoid lung disease with rheumatoid arthritis of unspecified hand   `HCC`

✓6ᵗʰ   M05.15   Rheumatoid lung disease with rheumatoid arthritis of hip

   M05.151   Rheumatoid lung disease with rheumatoid arthritis of right hip   `HCC`

   M05.152   Rheumatoid lung disease with rheumatoid arthritis of left hip   `HCC`

   M05.159   Rheumatoid lung disease with rheumatoid arthritis of unspecified hip   `HCC`

✓6ᵗʰ   M05.16   Rheumatoid lung disease with rheumatoid arthritis of knee

   M05.161   Rheumatoid lung disease with rheumatoid arthritis of right knee   `HCC`

   M05.162   Rheumatoid lung disease with rheumatoid arthritis of left knee   `HCC`

   M05.169   Rheumatoid lung disease with rheumatoid arthritis of unspecified knee   `HCC`

✓6ᵗʰ   M05.17   Rheumatoid lung disease with rheumatoid arthritis of ankle and foot

    Rheumatoid lung disease with rheumatoid arthritis, tarsus, metatarsus and phalanges

   M05.171   Rheumatoid lung disease with rheumatoid arthritis of right ankle and foot   `HCC`

   M05.172   Rheumatoid lung disease with rheumatoid arthritis of left ankle and foot   `HCC`

   M05.179   Rheumatoid lung disease with rheumatoid arthritis of unspecified ankle and foot   `HCC`

   M05.19   Rheumatoid lung disease with rheumatoid arthritis of multiple sites   `HCC`

✓5ᵗʰ   M05.2   Rheumatoid vasculitis with rheumatoid arthritis

   M05.20   Rheumatoid vasculitis with rheumatoid arthritis of unspecified site   `HCC`

✓6ᵗʰ   M05.21   Rheumatoid vasculitis with rheumatoid arthritis of shoulder

   M05.211   Rheumatoid vasculitis with rheumatoid arthritis of right shoulder   `HCC`

   M05.212   Rheumatoid vasculitis with rheumatoid arthritis of left shoulder   `HCC`

   M05.219   Rheumatoid vasculitis with rheumatoid arthritis of unspecified shoulder   `HCC`

✓6ᵗʰ   M05.22   Rheumatoid vasculitis with rheumatoid arthritis of elbow

   M05.221   Rheumatoid vasculitis with rheumatoid arthritis of right elbow   `HCC`

   M05.222   Rheumatoid vasculitis with rheumatoid arthritis of left elbow   `HCC`

   M05.229   Rheumatoid vasculitis with rheumatoid arthritis of unspecified elbow   `HCC`

✓6ᵗʰ   M05.23   Rheumatoid vasculitis with rheumatoid arthritis of wrist

    Rheumatoid vasculitis with rheumatoid arthritis, carpal bones

   M05.231   Rheumatoid vasculitis with rheumatoid arthritis of right wrist   `HCC`

   M05.232   Rheumatoid vasculitis with rheumatoid arthritis of left wrist   `HCC`

   M05.239   Rheumatoid vasculitis with rheumatoid arthritis of unspecified wrist   `HCC`

✓6ᵗʰ   M05.24   Rheumatoid vasculitis with rheumatoid arthritis of hand

    Rheumatoid vasculitis with rheumatoid arthritis, metacarpus and phalanges

   M05.241   Rheumatoid vasculitis with rheumatoid arthritis of right hand   `HCC`

   M05.242   Rheumatoid vasculitis with rheumatoid arthritis of left hand   `HCC`

   M05.249   Rheumatoid vasculitis with rheumatoid arthritis of unspecified hand   `HCC`

✓6ᵗʰ   M05.25   Rheumatoid vasculitis with rheumatoid arthritis of hip

   M05.251   Rheumatoid vasculitis with rheumatoid arthritis of right hip   `HCC`

   M05.252   Rheumatoid vasculitis with rheumatoid arthritis of left hip   `HCC`

   M05.259   Rheumatoid vasculitis with rheumatoid arthritis of unspecified hip   `HCC`

✓6ᵗʰ   M05.26   Rheumatoid vasculitis with rheumatoid arthritis of knee

   M05.261   Rheumatoid vasculitis with rheumatoid arthritis of right knee   `HCC`

   M05.262   Rheumatoid vasculitis with rheumatoid arthritis of left knee   `HCC`

Ⓝ Newborn: 0   Ⓟ Pediatric: 0-17   Ⓜ Maternity: 9-64   Ⓐ Adult: 15-124   `MCC` Major Complication/Comorbidity   `CC` Complication/Comorbidity   `SW` Severe Wound Dx

762   ICD-10-CM 2021

M05.269 **Rheumatoid vasculitis with rheumatoid arthritis of unspecified knee** HCC

✓6ᵗʰ M05.27 **Rheumatoid vasculitis with rheumatoid arthritis of ankle and foot**

Rheumatoid vasculitis with rheumatoid arthritis, tarsus, metatarsus and phalanges

M05.271 **Rheumatoid vasculitis with rheumatoid arthritis of right ankle and foot** HCC

M05.272 **Rheumatoid vasculitis with rheumatoid arthritis of left ankle and foot** HCC

M05.279 **Rheumatoid vasculitis with rheumatoid arthritis of unspecified ankle and foot** HCC

M05.29 **Rheumatoid vasculitis with rheumatoid arthritis of multiple sites** HCC

✓5ᵗʰ M05.3 **Rheumatoid heart disease with rheumatoid arthritis**

Rheumatoid carditis
Rheumatoid endocarditis
Rheumatoid myocarditis
Rheumatoid pericarditis

M05.30 **Rheumatoid heart disease with rheumatoid arthritis of unspecified site** HCC

✓6ᵗʰ M05.31 **Rheumatoid heart disease with rheumatoid arthritis of shoulder**

M05.311 **Rheumatoid heart disease with rheumatoid arthritis of right shoulder** HCC

M05.312 **Rheumatoid heart disease with rheumatoid arthritis of left shoulder** HCC

M05.319 **Rheumatoid heart disease with rheumatoid arthritis of unspecified shoulder** HCC

✓6ᵗʰ M05.32 **Rheumatoid heart disease with rheumatoid arthritis of elbow**

M05.321 **Rheumatoid heart disease with rheumatoid arthritis of right elbow** HCC

M05.322 **Rheumatoid heart disease with rheumatoid arthritis of left elbow** HCC

M05.329 **Rheumatoid heart disease with rheumatoid arthritis of unspecified elbow** HCC

✓6ᵗʰ M05.33 **Rheumatoid heart disease with rheumatoid arthritis of wrist**

Rheumatoid heart disease with rheumatoid arthritis, carpal bones

M05.331 **Rheumatoid heart disease with rheumatoid arthritis of right wrist** HCC

M05.332 **Rheumatoid heart disease with rheumatoid arthritis of left wrist** HCC

M05.339 **Rheumatoid heart disease with rheumatoid arthritis of unspecified wrist** HCC

✓6ᵗʰ M05.34 **Rheumatoid heart disease with rheumatoid arthritis of hand**

Rheumatoid heart disease with rheumatoid arthritis, metacarpus and phalanges

M05.341 **Rheumatoid heart disease with rheumatoid arthritis of right hand** HCC

M05.342 **Rheumatoid heart disease with rheumatoid arthritis of left hand** HCC

M05.349 **Rheumatoid heart disease with rheumatoid arthritis of unspecified hand** HCC

✓6ᵗʰ M05.35 **Rheumatoid heart disease with rheumatoid arthritis of hip**

M05.351 **Rheumatoid heart disease with rheumatoid arthritis of right hip** HCC

M05.352 **Rheumatoid heart disease with rheumatoid arthritis of left hip** HCC

M05.359 **Rheumatoid heart disease with rheumatoid arthritis of unspecified hip** HCC

✓6ᵗʰ M05.36 **Rheumatoid heart disease with rheumatoid arthritis of knee**

M05.361 **Rheumatoid heart disease with rheumatoid arthritis of right knee** HCC

M05.362 **Rheumatoid heart disease with rheumatoid arthritis of left knee** HCC

M05.369 **Rheumatoid heart disease with rheumatoid arthritis of unspecified knee** HCC

✓6ᵗʰ M05.37 **Rheumatoid heart disease with rheumatoid arthritis of ankle and foot**

Rheumatoid heart disease with rheumatoid arthritis, tarsus, metatarsus and phalanges

M05.371 **Rheumatoid heart disease with rheumatoid arthritis of right ankle and foot** HCC

M05.372 **Rheumatoid heart disease with rheumatoid arthritis of left ankle and foot** HCC

M05.379 **Rheumatoid heart disease with rheumatoid arthritis of unspecified ankle and foot** HCC

M05.39 **Rheumatoid heart disease with rheumatoid arthritis of multiple sites** HCC

✓5ᵗʰ M05.4 **Rheumatoid myopathy with rheumatoid arthritis**

M05.40 **Rheumatoid myopathy with rheumatoid arthritis of unspecified site** CC HCC

✓6ᵗʰ M05.41 **Rheumatoid myopathy with rheumatoid arthritis of shoulder**

M05.411 **Rheumatoid myopathy with rheumatoid arthritis of right shoulder** CC HCC

M05.412 **Rheumatoid myopathy with rheumatoid arthritis of left shoulder** CC HCC

M05.419 **Rheumatoid myopathy with rheumatoid arthritis of unspecified shoulder** CC HCC

✓6ᵗʰ M05.42 **Rheumatoid myopathy with rheumatoid arthritis of elbow**

M05.421 **Rheumatoid myopathy with rheumatoid arthritis of right elbow** CC HCC

M05.422 **Rheumatoid myopathy with rheumatoid arthritis of left elbow** CC HCC

M05.429 **Rheumatoid myopathy with rheumatoid arthritis of unspecified elbow** CC HCC

✓6ᵗʰ M05.43 **Rheumatoid myopathy with rheumatoid arthritis of wrist**

Rheumatoid myopathy with rheumatoid arthritis, carpal bones

M05.431 **Rheumatoid myopathy with rheumatoid arthritis of right wrist** CC HCC

M05.432 **Rheumatoid myopathy with rheumatoid arthritis of left wrist** CC HCC

M05.439 **Rheumatoid myopathy with rheumatoid arthritis of unspecified wrist** CC HCC

✓6ᵗʰ M05.44 **Rheumatoid myopathy with rheumatoid arthritis of hand**

Rheumatoid myopathy with rheumatoid arthritis, metacarpus and phalanges

M05.441 **Rheumatoid myopathy with rheumatoid arthritis of right hand** CC HCC

M05.442 **Rheumatoid myopathy with rheumatoid arthritis of left hand** CC HCC

M05.449 **Rheumatoid myopathy with rheumatoid arthritis of unspecified hand** CC HCC

✓6ᵗʰ M05.45 **Rheumatoid myopathy with rheumatoid arthritis of hip**

M05.451 **Rheumatoid myopathy with rheumatoid arthritis of right hip** CC HCC

M05.452 **Rheumatoid myopathy with rheumatoid arthritis of left hip** CC HCC

M05.459 **Rheumatoid myopathy with rheumatoid arthritis of unspecified hip** CC HCC

✓6ᵗʰ M05.46 **Rheumatoid myopathy with rheumatoid arthritis of knee**

M05.461 **Rheumatoid myopathy with rheumatoid arthritis of right knee** CC HCC

M05.462 **Rheumatoid myopathy with rheumatoid arthritis of left knee** CC HCC

M05.469 **Rheumatoid myopathy with rheumatoid arthritis of unspecified knee** CC HCC

✓6ᵗʰ M05.47 **Rheumatoid myopathy with rheumatoid arthritis of ankle and foot**

Rheumatoid myopathy with rheumatoid arthritis, tarsus, metatarsus and phalanges

M05.471 **Rheumatoid myopathy with rheumatoid arthritis of right ankle and foot** CC HCC

☑ Additional Character Required   ✓x7ᵗʰ Placeholder   Unacceptable PDx   Questionable PDx   Manifestation   Unspecified Dx   H1-H14 HAC   HCC CMS-HCC Dx   HIV HIV Dx

ICD-10-CM 2021   **763**

M05.472   Rheumatoid myopathy with rheumatoid arthritis of left ankle and foot   CC HCC

M05.479   Rheumatoid myopathy with rheumatoid arthritis of unspecified ankle and foot   CC HCC

M05.49   Rheumatoid myopathy with rheumatoid arthritis of multiple sites   CC HCC

√5th **M05.5**   Rheumatoid polyneuropathy with rheumatoid arthritis

M05.50   Rheumatoid polyneuropathy with rheumatoid arthritis of unspecified site   HCC

√6th **M05.51**   Rheumatoid polyneuropathy with rheumatoid arthritis of shoulder

M05.511   Rheumatoid polyneuropathy with rheumatoid arthritis of right shoulder   HCC

M05.512   Rheumatoid polyneuropathy with rheumatoid arthritis of left shoulder   HCC

M05.519   Rheumatoid polyneuropathy with rheumatoid arthritis of unspecified shoulder   HCC

√6th **M05.52**   Rheumatoid polyneuropathy with rheumatoid arthritis of elbow

M05.521   Rheumatoid polyneuropathy with rheumatoid arthritis of right elbow   HCC

M05.522   Rheumatoid polyneuropathy with rheumatoid arthritis of left elbow   HCC

M05.529   Rheumatoid polyneuropathy with rheumatoid arthritis of unspecified elbow   HCC

√6th **M05.53**   Rheumatoid polyneuropathy with rheumatoid arthritis of wrist

   Rheumatoid polyneuropathy with rheumatoid arthritis, carpal bones

M05.531   Rheumatoid polyneuropathy with rheumatoid arthritis of right wrist   HCC

M05.532   Rheumatoid polyneuropathy with rheumatoid arthritis of left wrist   HCC

M05.539   Rheumatoid polyneuropathy with rheumatoid arthritis of unspecified wrist   HCC

√6th **M05.54**   Rheumatoid polyneuropathy with rheumatoid arthritis of hand

   Rheumatoid polyneuropathy with rheumatoid arthritis, metacarpus and phalanges

M05.541   Rheumatoid polyneuropathy with rheumatoid arthritis of right hand   HCC

M05.542   Rheumatoid polyneuropathy with rheumatoid arthritis of left hand   HCC

M05.549   Rheumatoid polyneuropathy with rheumatoid arthritis of unspecified hand   HCC

√6th **M05.55**   Rheumatoid polyneuropathy with rheumatoid arthritis of hip

M05.551   Rheumatoid polyneuropathy with rheumatoid arthritis of right hip   HCC

M05.552   Rheumatoid polyneuropathy with rheumatoid arthritis of left hip   HCC

M05.559   Rheumatoid polyneuropathy with rheumatoid arthritis of unspecified hip   HCC

√6th **M05.56**   Rheumatoid polyneuropathy with rheumatoid arthritis of knee

M05.561   Rheumatoid polyneuropathy with rheumatoid arthritis of right knee   HCC

M05.562   Rheumatoid polyneuropathy with rheumatoid arthritis of left knee   HCC

M05.569   Rheumatoid polyneuropathy with rheumatoid arthritis of unspecified knee   HCC

√6th **M05.57**   Rheumatoid polyneuropathy with rheumatoid arthritis of ankle and foot

   Rheumatoid polyneuropathy with rheumatoid arthritis, tarsus, metatarsus and phalanges

M05.571   Rheumatoid polyneuropathy with rheumatoid arthritis of right ankle and foot   HCC

M05.572   Rheumatoid polyneuropathy with rheumatoid arthritis of left ankle and foot   HCC

M05.579   Rheumatoid polyneuropathy with rheumatoid arthritis of unspecified ankle and foot   HCC

M05.59   Rheumatoid polyneuropathy with rheumatoid arthritis of multiple sites   HCC

√5th **M05.6**   Rheumatoid arthritis with involvement of other organs and systems

M05.60   Rheumatoid arthritis of unspecified site with involvement of other organs and systems   HCC

√6th **M05.61**   Rheumatoid arthritis of shoulder with involvement of other organs and systems

M05.611   Rheumatoid arthritis of right shoulder with involvement of other organs and systems   HCC

M05.612   Rheumatoid arthritis of left shoulder with involvement of other organs and systems   HCC

M05.619   Rheumatoid arthritis of unspecified shoulder with involvement of other organs and systems   HCC

√6th **M05.62**   Rheumatoid arthritis of elbow with involvement of other organs and systems

M05.621   Rheumatoid arthritis of right elbow with involvement of other organs and systems   HCC

M05.622   Rheumatoid arthritis of left elbow with involvement of other organs and systems   HCC

M05.629   Rheumatoid arthritis of unspecified elbow with involvement of other organs and systems   HCC

√6th **M05.63**   Rheumatoid arthritis of wrist with involvement of other organs and systems

   Rheumatoid arthritis of carpal bones with involvement of other organs and systems

M05.631   Rheumatoid arthritis of right wrist with involvement of other organs and systems   HCC

M05.632   Rheumatoid arthritis of left wrist with involvement of other organs and systems   HCC

M05.639   Rheumatoid arthritis of unspecified wrist with involvement of other organs and systems   HCC

√6th **M05.64**   Rheumatoid arthritis of hand with involvement of other organs and systems

   Rheumatoid arthritis of metacarpus and phalanges with involvement of other organs and systems

M05.641   Rheumatoid arthritis of right hand with involvement of other organs and systems   HCC

M05.642   Rheumatoid arthritis of left hand with involvement of other organs and systems   HCC

M05.649   Rheumatoid arthritis of unspecified hand with involvement of other organs and systems   HCC

√6th **M05.65**   Rheumatoid arthritis of hip with involvement of other organs and systems

M05.651   Rheumatoid arthritis of right hip with involvement of other organs and systems   HCC

M05.652   Rheumatoid arthritis of left hip with involvement of other organs and systems   HCC

M05.659   Rheumatoid arthritis of unspecified hip with involvement of other organs and systems   HCC

√6th **M05.66**   Rheumatoid arthritis of knee with involvement of other organs and systems

M05.661   Rheumatoid arthritis of right knee with involvement of other organs and systems   HCC

M05.662   Rheumatoid arthritis of left knee with involvement of other organs and systems   HCC

M05.669   Rheumatoid arthritis of unspecified knee with involvement of other organs and systems   HCC

N Newborn: 0   P Pediatric: 0-17   M Maternity: 9-64   A Adult: 15-124   MCC Major Complication/Comorbidity   CC Complication/Comorbidity   SW Severe Wound Dx

764   ICD-10-CM 2021

√6ᵗʰ **M05.67 Rheumatoid arthritis of ankle and foot with involvement of other organs and systems**
Rheumatoid arthritis of tarsus, metatarsus and phalanges with involvement of other organs and systems

> **M05.671 Rheumatoid arthritis of right ankle and foot with involvement of other organs and systems** HCC
>
> **M05.672 Rheumatoid arthritis of left ankle and foot with involvement of other organs and systems** HCC
>
> **M05.679 Rheumatoid arthritis of unspecified ankle and foot with involvement of other organs and systems** HCC

M05.69 Rheumatoid arthritis of multiple sites with involvement of other organs and systems HCC

√5ᵗʰ **M05.7 Rheumatoid arthritis with rheumatoid factor without organ or systems involvement**

> **M05.70 Rheumatoid arthritis with rheumatoid factor of unspecified site without organ or systems involvement** HCC

√6ᵗʰ **M05.71 Rheumatoid arthritis with rheumatoid factor of shoulder without organ or systems involvement**

> **M05.711 Rheumatoid arthritis with rheumatoid factor of right shoulder without organ or systems involvement** HCC
>
> **M05.712 Rheumatoid arthritis with rheumatoid factor of left shoulder without organ or systems involvement** HCC
>
> **M05.719 Rheumatoid arthritis with rheumatoid factor of unspecified shoulder without organ or systems involvement** HCC

√6ᵗʰ **M05.72 Rheumatoid arthritis with rheumatoid factor of elbow without organ or systems involvement**

> **M05.721 Rheumatoid arthritis with rheumatoid factor of right elbow without organ or systems involvement** HCC
>
> **M05.722 Rheumatoid arthritis with rheumatoid factor of left elbow without organ or systems involvement** HCC
>
> **M05.729 Rheumatoid arthritis with rheumatoid factor of unspecified elbow without organ or systems involvement** HCC

√6ᵗʰ **M05.73 Rheumatoid arthritis with rheumatoid factor of wrist without organ or systems involvement**

> **M05.731 Rheumatoid arthritis with rheumatoid factor of right wrist without organ or systems involvement** HCC
>
> **M05.732 Rheumatoid arthritis with rheumatoid factor of left wrist without organ or systems involvement** HCC
>
> **M05.739 Rheumatoid arthritis with rheumatoid factor of unspecified wrist without organ or systems involvement** HCC

√6ᵗʰ **M05.74 Rheumatoid arthritis with rheumatoid factor of hand without organ or systems involvement**

> **M05.741 Rheumatoid arthritis with rheumatoid factor of right hand without organ or systems involvement** HCC
>
> **M05.742 Rheumatoid arthritis with rheumatoid factor of left hand without organ or systems involvement** HCC
>
> **M05.749 Rheumatoid arthritis with rheumatoid factor of unspecified hand without organ or systems involvement** HCC

√6ᵗʰ **M05.75 Rheumatoid arthritis with rheumatoid factor of hip without organ or systems involvement**

> **M05.751 Rheumatoid arthritis with rheumatoid factor of right hip without organ or systems involvement** HCC
>
> **M05.752 Rheumatoid arthritis with rheumatoid factor of left hip without organ or systems involvement** HCC
>
> **M05.759 Rheumatoid arthritis with rheumatoid factor of unspecified hip without organ or systems involvement** HCC

√6ᵗʰ **M05.76 Rheumatoid arthritis with rheumatoid factor of knee without organ or systems involvement**

> **M05.761 Rheumatoid arthritis with rheumatoid factor of right knee without organ or systems involvement** HCC
>
> **M05.762 Rheumatoid arthritis with rheumatoid factor of left knee without organ or systems involvement** HCC
>
> **M05.769 Rheumatoid arthritis with rheumatoid factor of unspecified knee without organ or systems involvement** HCC

√6ᵗʰ **M05.77 Rheumatoid arthritis with rheumatoid factor of ankle and foot without organ or systems involvement**

> **M05.771 Rheumatoid arthritis with rheumatoid factor of right ankle and foot without organ or systems involvement** HCC
>
> **M05.772 Rheumatoid arthritis with rheumatoid factor of left ankle and foot without organ or systems involvement** HCC
>
> **M05.779 Rheumatoid arthritis with rheumatoid factor of unspecified ankle and foot without organ or systems involvement** HCC

M05.79 Rheumatoid arthritis with rheumatoid factor of multiple sites without organ or systems involvement HCC

• **M05.7A Rheumatoid arthritis with rheumatoid factor of other specified site without organ or systems involvement**

√5ᵗʰ **M05.8 Other rheumatoid arthritis with rheumatoid factor**

> **M05.80 Other rheumatoid arthritis with rheumatoid factor of unspecified site** HCC

√6ᵗʰ **M05.81 Other rheumatoid arthritis with rheumatoid factor of shoulder**

> **M05.811 Other rheumatoid arthritis with rheumatoid factor of right shoulder** HCC
>
> **M05.812 Other rheumatoid arthritis with rheumatoid factor of left shoulder** HCC
>
> **M05.819 Other rheumatoid arthritis with rheumatoid factor of unspecified shoulder** HCC

√6ᵗʰ **M05.82 Other rheumatoid arthritis with rheumatoid factor of elbow**

> **M05.821 Other rheumatoid arthritis with rheumatoid factor of right elbow** HCC
>
> **M05.822 Other rheumatoid arthritis with rheumatoid factor of left elbow** HCC
>
> **M05.829 Other rheumatoid arthritis with rheumatoid factor of unspecified elbow** HCC

√6ᵗʰ **M05.83 Other rheumatoid arthritis with rheumatoid factor of wrist**

> **M05.831 Other rheumatoid arthritis with rheumatoid factor of right wrist** HCC
>
> **M05.832 Other rheumatoid arthritis with rheumatoid factor of left wrist** HCC
>
> **M05.839 Other rheumatoid arthritis with rheumatoid factor of unspecified wrist** HCC

√6ᵗʰ **M05.84 Other rheumatoid arthritis with rheumatoid factor of hand**

> **M05.841 Other rheumatoid arthritis with rheumatoid factor of right hand** HCC
>
> **M05.842 Other rheumatoid arthritis with rheumatoid factor of left hand** HCC
>
> **M05.849 Other rheumatoid arthritis with rheumatoid factor of unspecified hand** HCC

√6ᵗʰ **M05.85 Other rheumatoid arthritis with rheumatoid factor of hip**

> **M05.851 Other rheumatoid arthritis with rheumatoid factor of right hip** HCC
>
> **M05.852 Other rheumatoid arthritis with rheumatoid factor of left hip** HCC
>
> **M05.859 Other rheumatoid arthritis with rheumatoid factor of unspecified hip** HCC

√6ᵗʰ **M05.86 Other rheumatoid arthritis with rheumatoid factor of knee**

> **M05.861 Other rheumatoid arthritis with rheumatoid factor of right knee** HCC
>
> **M05.862 Other rheumatoid arthritis with rheumatoid factor of left knee** HCC

☑ Additional Character Required   √x7ᵗʰ Placeholder   Unacceptable PDx   Questionable PDx   Manifestation   Unspecified Dx   H1-H14 HAC   HCC CMS-HCC Dx   HIV HIV Dx

        M05.869   Other rheumatoid arthritis with rheumatoid factor of unspecified knee   HCC

✓6th   M05.87   Other rheumatoid arthritis with rheumatoid factor of ankle and foot

        M05.871   Other rheumatoid arthritis with rheumatoid factor of right ankle and foot   HCC

        M05.872   Other rheumatoid arthritis with rheumatoid factor of left ankle and foot   HCC

        M05.879   Other rheumatoid arthritis with rheumatoid factor of unspecified ankle and foot   HCC

    M05.89   Other rheumatoid arthritis with rheumatoid factor of multiple sites   HCC

    M05.8A   Other rheumatoid arthritis with rheumatoid factor of other specified site

  M05.9   Rheumatoid arthritis with rheumatoid factor, unspecified   HCC

✓4th   **M06**   **Other rheumatoid arthritis**

DEF: Rheumatoid arthritis: Autoimmune systemic disease that causes chronic inflammation of the joints and other areas of the body, manifested by inflammatory changes in articular structures and synovial membranes, atrophy, and loss in bone density.

✓5th   M06.0   Rheumatoid arthritis without rheumatoid factor

    M06.00   Rheumatoid arthritis without rheumatoid factor, unspecified site   HCC

✓6th   M06.01   Rheumatoid arthritis without rheumatoid factor, shoulder

        M06.011   Rheumatoid arthritis without rheumatoid factor, right shoulder   HCC

        M06.012   Rheumatoid arthritis without rheumatoid factor, left shoulder   HCC

        M06.019   Rheumatoid arthritis without rheumatoid factor, unspecified shoulder   HCC

✓6th   M06.02   Rheumatoid arthritis without rheumatoid factor, elbow

        M06.021   Rheumatoid arthritis without rheumatoid factor, right elbow   HCC

        M06.022   Rheumatoid arthritis without rheumatoid factor, left elbow   HCC

        M06.029   Rheumatoid arthritis without rheumatoid factor, unspecified elbow   HCC

✓6th   M06.03   Rheumatoid arthritis without rheumatoid factor, wrist

        M06.031   Rheumatoid arthritis without rheumatoid factor, right wrist   HCC

        M06.032   Rheumatoid arthritis without rheumatoid factor, left wrist   HCC

        M06.039   Rheumatoid arthritis without rheumatoid factor, unspecified wrist   HCC

✓6th   M06.04   Rheumatoid arthritis without rheumatoid factor, hand

        M06.041   Rheumatoid arthritis without rheumatoid factor, right hand   HCC

        M06.042   Rheumatoid arthritis without rheumatoid factor, left hand   HCC

        M06.049   Rheumatoid arthritis without rheumatoid factor, unspecified hand   HCC

✓6th   M06.05   Rheumatoid arthritis without rheumatoid factor, hip

        M06.051   Rheumatoid arthritis without rheumatoid factor, right hip   HCC

        M06.052   Rheumatoid arthritis without rheumatoid factor, left hip   HCC

        M06.059   Rheumatoid arthritis without rheumatoid factor, unspecified hip   HCC

✓6th   M06.06   Rheumatoid arthritis without rheumatoid factor, knee

        M06.061   Rheumatoid arthritis without rheumatoid factor, right knee   HCC

        M06.062   Rheumatoid arthritis without rheumatoid factor, left knee   HCC

        M06.069   Rheumatoid arthritis without rheumatoid factor, unspecified knee   HCC

✓6th   M06.07   Rheumatoid arthritis without rheumatoid factor, ankle and foot

        M06.071   Rheumatoid arthritis without rheumatoid factor, right ankle and foot   HCC

        M06.072   Rheumatoid arthritis without rheumatoid factor, left ankle and foot   HCC

        M06.079   Rheumatoid arthritis without rheumatoid factor, unspecified ankle and foot   HCC

    M06.08   Rheumatoid arthritis without rheumatoid factor, vertebrae   HCC

    M06.09   Rheumatoid arthritis without rheumatoid factor, multiple sites   HCC

    M06.0A   Rheumatoid arthritis without rheumatoid factor, other specified site

  M06.1   Adult-onset Still's disease   HCC A

    EXCLUDES 1   Still's disease NOS (M08.2-)

    DEF: Type of systemic arthritis characterized by a transient rash and spiking fevers. This condition may resolve or develop into a chronic condition and may affect internal organs, as well as joints. *Synonym(s): AOSD*

✓5th   M06.2   Rheumatoid bursitis

    M06.20   Rheumatoid bursitis, unspecified site   HCC

✓6th   M06.21   Rheumatoid bursitis, shoulder

        M06.211   Rheumatoid bursitis, right shoulder   HCC

        M06.212   Rheumatoid bursitis, left shoulder   HCC

        M06.219   Rheumatoid bursitis, unspecified shoulder   HCC

✓6th   M06.22   Rheumatoid bursitis, elbow

        M06.221   Rheumatoid bursitis, right elbow   HCC

        M06.222   Rheumatoid bursitis, left elbow   HCC

        M06.229   Rheumatoid bursitis, unspecified elbow   HCC

✓6th   M06.23   Rheumatoid bursitis, wrist

        M06.231   Rheumatoid bursitis, right wrist   HCC

        M06.232   Rheumatoid bursitis, left wrist   HCC

        M06.239   Rheumatoid bursitis, unspecified wrist   HCC

✓6th   M06.24   Rheumatoid bursitis, hand

        M06.241   Rheumatoid bursitis, right hand   HCC

        M06.242   Rheumatoid bursitis, left hand   HCC

        M06.249   Rheumatoid bursitis, unspecified hand   HCC

✓6th   M06.25   Rheumatoid bursitis, hip

        M06.251   Rheumatoid bursitis, right hip   HCC

        M06.252   Rheumatoid bursitis, left hip   HCC

        M06.259   Rheumatoid bursitis, unspecified hip   HCC

✓6th   M06.26   Rheumatoid bursitis, knee

        M06.261   Rheumatoid bursitis, right knee   HCC

        M06.262   Rheumatoid bursitis, left knee   HCC

        M06.269   Rheumatoid bursitis, unspecified knee   HCC

✓6th   M06.27   Rheumatoid bursitis, ankle and foot

        M06.271   Rheumatoid bursitis, right ankle and foot   HCC

        M06.272   Rheumatoid bursitis, left ankle and foot   HCC

        M06.279   Rheumatoid bursitis, unspecified ankle and foot   HCC

    M06.28   Rheumatoid bursitis, vertebrae   HCC

    M06.29   Rheumatoid bursitis, multiple sites   HCC

✓5th   M06.3   Rheumatoid nodule

    M06.30   Rheumatoid nodule, unspecified site   HCC

✓6th   M06.31   Rheumatoid nodule, shoulder

        M06.311   Rheumatoid nodule, right shoulder   HCC

        M06.312   Rheumatoid nodule, left shoulder   HCC

        M06.319   Rheumatoid nodule, unspecified shoulder   HCC

✓6th   M06.32   Rheumatoid nodule, elbow

        M06.321   Rheumatoid nodule, right elbow   HCC

        M06.322   Rheumatoid nodule, left elbow   HCC

        M06.329   Rheumatoid nodule, unspecified elbow   HCC

✓6th   M06.33   Rheumatoid nodule, wrist

        M06.331   Rheumatoid nodule, right wrist   HCC

        M06.332   Rheumatoid nodule, left wrist   HCC

        M06.339   Rheumatoid nodule, unspecified wrist   HCC

N Newborn: 0   P Pediatric: 0-17   M Maternity: 9-64   A Adult: 15-124   MCC Major Complication/Comorbidity   CC Complication/Comorbidity   SW Severe Wound Dx

766   ICD-10-CM 2021

√6th **M06.34 Rheumatoid nodule,** hand

    M06.341 **Rheumatoid nodule,** right **hand** HCC

    M06.342 **Rheumatoid nodule,** left **hand** HCC

    M06.349 **Rheumatoid nodule, unspecified hand** HCC

√6th **M06.35 Rheumatoid nodule,** hip

    M06.351 **Rheumatoid nodule,** right **hip** HCC

    M06.352 **Rheumatoid nodule,** left **hip** HCC

    M06.359 **Rheumatoid nodule, unspecified hip** HCC

√6th **M06.36 Rheumatoid nodule,** knee

    M06.361 **Rheumatoid nodule,** right **knee** HCC

    M06.362 **Rheumatoid nodule,** left **knee** HCC

    M06.369 **Rheumatoid nodule, unspecified knee** HCC

√6th **M06.37 Rheumatoid nodule,** ankle and foot

    M06.371 **Rheumatoid nodule,** right **ankle and foot** HCC

    M06.372 **Rheumatoid nodule,** left **ankle and foot** HCC

    M06.379 **Rheumatoid nodule, unspecified ankle and foot** HCC

    M06.38 Rheumatoid nodule, vertebrae HCC

    M06.39 Rheumatoid nodule, multiple sites HCC

M06.4 Inflammatory polyarthropathy HCC

    EXCLUDES 1   *polyarthritis NOS (M13.0)*

√5th **M06.8 Other specified rheumatoid arthritis**

    M06.80 **Other specified rheumatoid arthritis, unspecified site** HCC

√6th **M06.81 Other specified rheumatoid arthritis,** shoulder

    M06.811 **Other specified rheumatoid arthritis, right shoulder** HCC

    M06.812 **Other specified rheumatoid arthritis,** left **shoulder** HCC

    M06.819 **Other specified rheumatoid arthritis, unspecified shoulder** HCC

√6th **M06.82 Other specified rheumatoid arthritis,** elbow

    M06.821 **Other specified rheumatoid arthritis, right elbow** HCC

    M06.822 **Other specified rheumatoid arthritis,** left **elbow** HCC

    M06.829 **Other specified rheumatoid arthritis, unspecified elbow** HCC

√6th **M06.83 Other specified rheumatoid arthritis,** wrist

    M06.831 **Other specified rheumatoid arthritis, right wrist** HCC

    M06.832 **Other specified rheumatoid arthritis,** left **wrist** HCC

    M06.839 **Other specified rheumatoid arthritis, unspecified wrist** HCC

√6th **M06.84 Other specified rheumatoid arthritis,** hand

    M06.841 **Other specified rheumatoid arthritis, right hand** HCC

    M06.842 **Other specified rheumatoid arthritis,** left **hand** HCC

    M06.849 **Other specified rheumatoid arthritis, unspecified hand** HCC

√6th **M06.85 Other specified rheumatoid arthritis,** hip

    M06.851 **Other specified rheumatoid arthritis, right hip** HCC

    M06.852 **Other specified rheumatoid arthritis,** left **hip** HCC

    M06.859 **Other specified rheumatoid arthritis, unspecified hip** HCC

√6th **M06.86 Other specified rheumatoid arthritis,** knee

    M06.861 **Other specified rheumatoid arthritis, right knee** HCC

    M06.862 **Other specified rheumatoid arthritis,** left **knee** HCC

    M06.869 **Other specified rheumatoid arthritis, unspecified knee** HCC

√6th **M06.87 Other specified rheumatoid arthritis,** ankle and foot

    M06.871 **Other specified rheumatoid arthritis, right ankle and foot** HCC

    M06.872 **Other specified rheumatoid arthritis,** left **ankle and foot** HCC

    M06.879 **Other specified rheumatoid arthritis, unspecified ankle and foot** HCC

    M06.88 Other specified rheumatoid arthritis, vertebrae HCC

    M06.89 Other specified rheumatoid arthritis, multiple sites HCC

    ● **M06.8A Other specified rheumatoid arthritis, other specified site**

    M06.9 Rheumatoid arthritis, unspecified HCC

√4th **M07 Enteropathic arthropathies**

Code also associated enteropathy, such as:
    regional enteritis [Crohn's disease] (K50.-)
    ulcerative colitis (K51.-)

    EXCLUDES 1   *psoriatic arthropathies (L40.5-)*

√5th **M07.6 Enteropathic arthropathies**

    M07.60 **Enteropathic arthropathies, unspecified site**

√6th **M07.61 Enteropathic arthropathies,** shoulder

    M07.611 **Enteropathic arthropathies, right shoulder**

    M07.612 **Enteropathic arthropathies,** left **shoulder**

    M07.619 **Enteropathic arthropathies, unspecified shoulder**

√6th **M07.62 Enteropathic arthropathies,** elbow

    M07.621 **Enteropathic arthropathies,** right **elbow**

    M07.622 **Enteropathic arthropathies,** left **elbow**

    M07.629 **Enteropathic arthropathies, unspecified elbow**

√6th **M07.63 Enteropathic arthropathies,** wrist

    M07.631 **Enteropathic arthropathies,** right **wrist**

    M07.632 **Enteropathic arthropathies,** left **wrist**

    M07.639 **Enteropathic arthropathies, unspecified wrist**

√6th **M07.64 Enteropathic arthropathies,** hand

    M07.641 **Enteropathic arthropathies,** right **hand**

    M07.642 **Enteropathic arthropathies,** left **hand**

    M07.649 **Enteropathic arthropathies, unspecified hand**

√6th **M07.65 Enteropathic arthropathies,** hip

    M07.651 **Enteropathic arthropathies,** right **hip**

    M07.652 **Enteropathic arthropathies,** left **hip**

    M07.659 **Enteropathic arthropathies, unspecified hip**

√6th **M07.66 Enteropathic arthropathies,** knee

    M07.661 **Enteropathic arthropathies,** right **knee**

    M07.662 **Enteropathic arthropathies,** left **knee**

    M07.669 **Enteropathic arthropathies, unspecified knee**

√6th **M07.67 Enteropathic arthropathies,** ankle and foot

    M07.671 **Enteropathic arthropathies,** right **ankle and foot**

    M07.672 **Enteropathic arthropathies,** left **ankle and foot**

    M07.679 **Enteropathic arthropathies, unspecified ankle and foot**

    M07.68 Enteropathic arthropathies, vertebrae

    M07.69 Enteropathic arthropathies, multiple sites

√4th **M08 Juvenile arthritis**

Code also any associated underlying condition, such as:
    regional enteritis [Crohn's disease] (K50.-)
    ulcerative colitis (K51.-)

    EXCLUDES 1   *arthropathy in Whipple's disease (M14.8)*

            Felty's syndrome (M05.0)

            juvenile dermatomyositis (M33.0-)

            psoriatic juvenile arthropathy (L40.54)

√5th **M08.0 Unspecified juvenile rheumatoid arthritis**

Juvenile rheumatoid arthritis with or without rheumatoid factor

    M08.00 **Unspecified juvenile rheumatoid arthritis of unspecified site** HCC

√6th **M08.01 Unspecified juvenile rheumatoid arthritis,** shoulder

    M08.011 **Unspecified juvenile rheumatoid arthritis, right shoulder** HCC

    M08.012 **Unspecified juvenile rheumatoid arthritis, left shoulder** HCC

    M08.019 **Unspecified juvenile rheumatoid arthritis, unspecified shoulder** HCC

☑ Additional Character Required   √x7th Placeholder   Unacceptable PDx   Questionable PDx   Manifestation   Unspecified Dx   H1 - H14 HAC   HCC CMS-HCC Dx   HIV HIV Dx

ICD-10-CM 2021   767

Chapter 13. Diseases of the Musculoskeletal System and Connective Tissue

✓6ᵗʰ **M08.02** Unspecified juvenile rheumatoid arthritis of elbow

    M08.021 Unspecified juvenile rheumatoid arthritis, right elbow   HCC

    M08.022 Unspecified juvenile rheumatoid arthritis, left elbow   HCC

    M08.029 Unspecified juvenile rheumatoid arthritis, unspecified elbow   HCC

✓6ᵗʰ **M08.03** Unspecified juvenile rheumatoid arthritis, wrist

    M08.031 Unspecified juvenile rheumatoid arthritis, right wrist   HCC

    M08.032 Unspecified juvenile rheumatoid arthritis, left wrist   HCC

    M08.039 Unspecified juvenile rheumatoid arthritis, unspecified wrist   HCC

✓6ᵗʰ **M08.04** Unspecified juvenile rheumatoid arthritis, hand

    M08.041 Unspecified juvenile rheumatoid arthritis, right hand   HCC

    M08.042 Unspecified juvenile rheumatoid arthritis, left hand   HCC

    M08.049 Unspecified juvenile rheumatoid arthritis, unspecified hand   HCC

✓6ᵗʰ **M08.05** Unspecified juvenile rheumatoid arthritis, hip

    M08.051 Unspecified juvenile rheumatoid arthritis, right hip   HCC

    M08.052 Unspecified juvenile rheumatoid arthritis, left hip   HCC

    M08.059 Unspecified juvenile rheumatoid arthritis, unspecified hip   HCC

✓6ᵗʰ **M08.06** Unspecified juvenile rheumatoid arthritis, knee

    M08.061 Unspecified juvenile rheumatoid arthritis, right knee   HCC

    M08.062 Unspecified juvenile rheumatoid arthritis, left knee   HCC

    M08.069 Unspecified juvenile rheumatoid arthritis, unspecified knee   HCC

✓6ᵗʰ **M08.07** Unspecified juvenile rheumatoid arthritis, ankle and foot

    M08.071 Unspecified juvenile rheumatoid arthritis, right ankle and foot   HCC

    M08.072 Unspecified juvenile rheumatoid arthritis, left ankle and foot   HCC

    M08.079 Unspecified juvenile rheumatoid arthritis, unspecified ankle and foot   HCC

M08.08 Unspecified juvenile rheumatoid arthritis, vertebrae   HCC

M08.09 Unspecified juvenile rheumatoid arthritis, multiple sites   HCC

M08.0A Unspecified juvenile rheumatoid arthritis, other specified site

M08.1 Juvenile ankylosing spondylitis   HCC

    EXCLUDES 1   ankylosing spondylitis in adults (M45.0-)

✓5ᵗʰ **M08.2** Juvenile rheumatoid arthritis with systemic onset

    Still's disease NOS

    EXCLUDES 1   adult-onset Still's disease (M06.1-)

    DEF: Systemic juvenile rheumatoid arthritis characterized by a transient rash and spiking fevers that may affect internal organs, as well as joints.

    M08.20 Juvenile rheumatoid arthritis with systemic onset, unspecified site   HCC

✓6ᵗʰ **M08.21** Juvenile rheumatoid arthritis with systemic onset, shoulder

    M08.211 Juvenile rheumatoid arthritis with systemic onset, right shoulder   HCC

    M08.212 Juvenile rheumatoid arthritis with systemic onset, left shoulder   HCC

    M08.219 Juvenile rheumatoid arthritis with systemic onset, unspecified shoulder   HCC

✓6ᵗʰ **M08.22** Juvenile rheumatoid arthritis with systemic onset, elbow

    M08.221 Juvenile rheumatoid arthritis with systemic onset, right elbow   HCC

    M08.222 Juvenile rheumatoid arthritis with systemic onset, left elbow   HCC

    M08.229 Juvenile rheumatoid arthritis with systemic onset, unspecified elbow   HCC

✓6ᵗʰ **M08.23** Juvenile rheumatoid arthritis with systemic onset, wrist

    M08.231 Juvenile rheumatoid arthritis with systemic onset, right wrist   HCC

    M08.232 Juvenile rheumatoid arthritis with systemic onset, left wrist   HCC

    M08.239 Juvenile rheumatoid arthritis with systemic onset, unspecified wrist   HCC

✓6ᵗʰ **M08.24** Juvenile rheumatoid arthritis with systemic onset, hand

    M08.241 Juvenile rheumatoid arthritis with systemic onset, right hand   HCC

    M08.242 Juvenile rheumatoid arthritis with systemic onset, left hand   HCC

    M08.249 Juvenile rheumatoid arthritis with systemic onset, unspecified hand   HCC

✓6ᵗʰ **M08.25** Juvenile rheumatoid arthritis with systemic onset, hip

    M08.251 Juvenile rheumatoid arthritis with systemic onset, right hip   HCC

    M08.252 Juvenile rheumatoid arthritis with systemic onset, left hip   HCC

    M08.259 Juvenile rheumatoid arthritis with systemic onset, unspecified hip   HCC

✓6ᵗʰ **M08.26** Juvenile rheumatoid arthritis with systemic onset, knee

    M08.261 Juvenile rheumatoid arthritis with systemic onset, right knee   HCC

    M08.262 Juvenile rheumatoid arthritis with systemic onset, left knee   HCC

    M08.269 Juvenile rheumatoid arthritis with systemic onset, unspecified knee   HCC

✓6ᵗʰ **M08.27** Juvenile rheumatoid arthritis with systemic onset, ankle and foot

    M08.271 Juvenile rheumatoid arthritis with systemic onset, right ankle and foot   HCC

    M08.272 Juvenile rheumatoid arthritis with systemic onset, left ankle and foot   HCC

    M08.279 Juvenile rheumatoid arthritis with systemic onset, unspecified ankle and foot   HCC

M08.28 Juvenile rheumatoid arthritis with systemic onset, vertebrae   HCC

M08.29 Juvenile rheumatoid arthritis with systemic onset, multiple sites   HCC

M08.2A Juvenile rheumatoid arthritis with systemic onset, other specified site

M08.3 Juvenile rheumatoid polyarthritis (seronegative)   HCC

✓5ᵗʰ **M08.4** Pauciarticular juvenile rheumatoid arthritis

    M08.40 Pauciarticular juvenile rheumatoid arthritis, unspecified site   HCC

✓6ᵗʰ **M08.41** Pauciarticular juvenile rheumatoid arthritis, shoulder

    M08.411 Pauciarticular juvenile rheumatoid arthritis, right shoulder   HCC

    M08.412 Pauciarticular juvenile rheumatoid arthritis, left shoulder   HCC

    M08.419 Pauciarticular juvenile rheumatoid arthritis, unspecified shoulder   HCC

✓6ᵗʰ **M08.42** Pauciarticular juvenile rheumatoid arthritis, elbow

    M08.421 Pauciarticular juvenile rheumatoid arthritis, right elbow   HCC

    M08.422 Pauciarticular juvenile rheumatoid arthritis, left elbow   HCC

    M08.429 Pauciarticular juvenile rheumatoid arthritis, unspecified elbow   HCC

✓6ᵗʰ **M08.43** Pauciarticular juvenile rheumatoid arthritis, wrist

    M08.431 Pauciarticular juvenile rheumatoid arthritis, right wrist   HCC

    M08.432 Pauciarticular juvenile rheumatoid arthritis, left wrist   HCC

    M08.439 Pauciarticular juvenile rheumatoid arthritis, unspecified wrist   HCC

✓6ᵗʰ **M08.44** Pauciarticular juvenile rheumatoid arthritis, hand

    M08.441 Pauciarticular juvenile rheumatoid arthritis, right hand   HCC

    M08.442 Pauciarticular juvenile rheumatoid arthritis, left hand   HCC

    M08.449 Pauciarticular juvenile rheumatoid arthritis, unspecified hand   HCC

✓6ᵗʰ **M08.45** Pauciarticular juvenile rheumatoid arthritis, hip

    M08.451 Pauciarticular juvenile rheumatoid arthritis, right hip   HCC

N Newborn: 0   P Pediatric: 0-17   M Maternity: 9-64   A Adult: 15-124   MCC Major Complication/Comorbidity   CC Complication/Comorbidity   SW Severe Wound Dx

768   ICD-10-CM 2021

M08.452 Pauciarticular juvenile rheumatoid arthritis, left hip   HCC

M08.459 Pauciarticular juvenile rheumatoid arthritis, unspecified hip   HCC

√6ᵗʰ M08.46 Pauciarticular juvenile rheumatoid arthritis, knee

M08.461 Pauciarticular juvenile rheumatoid arthritis, right knee   HCC

M08.462 Pauciarticular juvenile rheumatoid arthritis, left knee   HCC

M08.469 Pauciarticular juvenile rheumatoid arthritis, unspecified knee   HCC

√6ᵗʰ M08.47 Pauciarticular juvenile rheumatoid arthritis, ankle and foot

M08.471 Pauciarticular juvenile rheumatoid arthritis, right ankle and foot   HCC

M08.472 Pauciarticular juvenile rheumatoid arthritis, left ankle and foot   HCC

M08.479 Pauciarticular juvenile rheumatoid arthritis, unspecified ankle and foot   HCC

M08.48 Pauciarticular juvenile rheumatoid arthritis, vertebrae   HCC

M08.4A Pauciarticular juvenile rheumatoid arthritis, other specified site

√5ᵗʰ M08.8 Other juvenile arthritis

M08.80 Other juvenile arthritis, unspecified site   HCC

√6ᵗʰ M08.81 Other juvenile arthritis, shoulder

M08.811 Other juvenile arthritis, right shoulder   HCC

M08.812 Other juvenile arthritis, left shoulder   HCC

M08.819 Other juvenile arthritis, unspecified shoulder   HCC

√6ᵗʰ M08.82 Other juvenile arthritis, elbow

M08.821 Other juvenile arthritis, right elbow   HCC

M08.822 Other juvenile arthritis, left elbow   HCC

M08.829 Other juvenile arthritis, unspecified elbow   HCC

√6ᵗʰ M08.83 Other juvenile arthritis, wrist

M08.831 Other juvenile arthritis, right wrist   HCC

M08.832 Other juvenile arthritis, left wrist   HCC

M08.839 Other juvenile arthritis, unspecified wrist   HCC

√6ᵗʰ M08.84 Other juvenile arthritis, hand

M08.841 Other juvenile arthritis, right hand   HCC

M08.842 Other juvenile arthritis, left hand   HCC

M08.849 Other juvenile arthritis, unspecified hand   HCC

√6ᵗʰ M08.85 Other juvenile arthritis, hip

M08.851 Other juvenile arthritis, right hip   HCC

M08.852 Other juvenile arthritis, left hip   HCC

M08.859 Other juvenile arthritis, unspecified hip   HCC

√6ᵗʰ M08.86 Other juvenile arthritis, knee

M08.861 Other juvenile arthritis, right knee   HCC

M08.862 Other juvenile arthritis, left knee   HCC

M08.869 Other juvenile arthritis, unspecified knee   HCC

√6ᵗʰ M08.87 Other juvenile arthritis, ankle and foot

M08.871 Other juvenile arthritis, right ankle and foot   HCC

M08.872 Other juvenile arthritis, left ankle and foot   HCC

M08.879 Other juvenile arthritis, unspecified ankle and foot   HCC

M08.88 Other juvenile arthritis, other specified site   HCC
    Other juvenile arthritis, vertebrae

M08.89 Other juvenile arthritis, multiple sites   HCC

√5ᵗʰ M08.9 Juvenile arthritis, unspecified

    EXCLUDES 1   juvenile rheumatoid arthritis, unspecified (M08.0-)

M08.90 Juvenile arthritis, unspecified, unspecified site   HCC

√6ᵗʰ M08.91 Juvenile arthritis, unspecified, shoulder

M08.911 Juvenile arthritis, unspecified, right shoulder   HCC

M08.912 Juvenile arthritis, unspecified, left shoulder   HCC

M08.919 Juvenile arthritis, unspecified, unspecified shoulder   HCC

√6ᵗʰ M08.92 Juvenile arthritis, unspecified, elbow

M08.921 Juvenile arthritis, unspecified, right elbow   HCC

M08.922 Juvenile arthritis, unspecified, left elbow   HCC

M08.929 Juvenile arthritis, unspecified, unspecified elbow   HCC

√6ᵗʰ M08.93 Juvenile arthritis, unspecified, wrist

M08.931 Juvenile arthritis, unspecified, right wrist   HCC

M08.932 Juvenile arthritis, unspecified, left wrist   HCC

M08.939 Juvenile arthritis, unspecified, unspecified wrist   HCC

√6ᵗʰ M08.94 Juvenile arthritis, unspecified, hand

M08.941 Juvenile arthritis, unspecified, right hand   HCC

M08.942 Juvenile arthritis, unspecified, left hand   HCC

M08.949 Juvenile arthritis, unspecified, unspecified hand   HCC

√6ᵗʰ M08.95 Juvenile arthritis, unspecified, hip

M08.951 Juvenile arthritis, unspecified, right hip   HCC

M08.952 Juvenile arthritis, unspecified, left hip   HCC

M08.959 Juvenile arthritis, unspecified, unspecified hip   HCC

√6ᵗʰ M08.96 Juvenile arthritis, unspecified, knee

M08.961 Juvenile arthritis, unspecified, right knee   HCC

M08.962 Juvenile arthritis, unspecified, left knee   HCC

M08.969 Juvenile arthritis, unspecified, unspecified knee   HCC

√6ᵗʰ M08.97 Juvenile arthritis, unspecified, ankle and foot

M08.971 Juvenile arthritis, unspecified, right ankle and foot   HCC

M08.972 Juvenile arthritis, unspecified, left ankle and foot   HCC

M08.979 Juvenile arthritis, unspecified, unspecified ankle and foot   HCC

M08.98 Juvenile arthritis, unspecified, vertebrae   HCC

M08.99 Juvenile arthritis, unspecified, multiple sites   HCC

M08.9A Juvenile arthritis, unspecified, other specified site

√4ᵗʰ **M1A Chronic gout**

Use additional code to identify:
    autonomic neuropathy in diseases classified elsewhere (G99.0)
    calculus of urinary tract in diseases classified elsewhere (N22)
    cardiomyopathy in diseases classified elsewhere (I43)
    disorders of external ear in diseases classified elsewhere (H61.1-, H62.8-)
    disorders of iris and ciliary body in diseases classified elsewhere (H22)
    glomerular disorders in diseases classified elsewhere (N08)

EXCLUDES 1   gout NOS (M10.-)

EXCLUDES 2   acute gout (M10.-)

The appropriate 7th character is to be added to each code from category M1A.
0   without tophus (tophi)
1   with tophus (tophi)

√5ᵗʰ M1A.0 Idiopathic chronic gout

    Chronic gouty bursitis
    Primary chronic gout

√x7ᵗʰ M1A.00 Idiopathic chronic gout, unspecified site

√6ᵗʰ M1A.01 Idiopathic chronic gout, shoulder

√7ᵗʰ M1A.011 Idiopathic chronic gout, right shoulder

√7ᵗʰ M1A.012 Idiopathic chronic gout, left shoulder

√7ᵗʰ M1A.019 Idiopathic chronic gout, unspecified shoulder

√6ᵗʰ M1A.02 Idiopathic chronic gout, elbow

√7ᵗʰ M1A.021 Idiopathic chronic gout, right elbow

☑ Additional Character Required   √x7ᵗʰ Placeholder   Unacceptable PDx   Questionable PDx   Manifestation   Unspecified Dx   H1-H14 HAC   HCC CMS-HCC Dx   HIV HIV Dx

ICD-10-CM 2021   769

✓7ᵗʰ **M1A.Ø22** Idiopathic chronic gout, left elbow

✓7ᵗʰ **M1A.Ø29** Idiopathic chronic gout, unspecified elbow

✓6ᵗʰ **M1A.Ø3** Idiopathic chronic gout, wrist

  ✓7ᵗʰ **M1A.Ø31** Idiopathic chronic gout, right wrist

  ✓7ᵗʰ **M1A.Ø32** Idiopathic chronic gout, left wrist

  ✓7ᵗʰ **M1A.Ø39** Idiopathic chronic gout, unspecified wrist

✓6ᵗʰ **M1A.Ø4** Idiopathic chronic gout, hand

  ✓7ᵗʰ **M1A.Ø41** Idiopathic chronic gout, right hand

  ✓7ᵗʰ **M1A.Ø42** Idiopathic chronic gout, left hand

  ✓7ᵗʰ **M1A.Ø49** Idiopathic chronic gout, unspecified hand

✓6ᵗʰ **M1A.Ø5** Idiopathic chronic gout, hip

  ✓7ᵗʰ **M1A.Ø51** Idiopathic chronic gout, right hip

  ✓7ᵗʰ **M1A.Ø52** Idiopathic chronic gout, left hip

  ✓7ᵗʰ **M1A.Ø59** Idiopathic chronic gout, unspecified hip

✓6ᵗʰ **M1A.Ø6** Idiopathic chronic gout, knee

  ✓7ᵗʰ **M1A.Ø61** Idiopathic chronic gout, right knee

  ✓7ᵗʰ **M1A.Ø62** Idiopathic chronic gout, left knee

  ✓7ᵗʰ **M1A.Ø69** Idiopathic chronic gout, unspecified knee

✓6ᵗʰ **M1A.Ø7** Idiopathic chronic gout, ankle and foot

  ✓7ᵗʰ **M1A.Ø71** Idiopathic chronic gout, right ankle and foot

  ✓7ᵗʰ **M1A.Ø72** Idiopathic chronic gout, left ankle and foot

  ✓7ᵗʰ **M1A.Ø79** Idiopathic chronic gout, unspecified ankle and foot

✓x7ᵗʰ **M1A.Ø8** Idiopathic chronic gout, vertebrae

✓x7ᵗʰ **M1A.Ø9** Idiopathic chronic gout, multiple sites

✓5ᵗʰ **M1A.1** Lead-induced chronic gout

  Code first toxic effects of lead and its compounds (T56.Ø-)

✓x7ᵗʰ **M1A.1Ø** Lead-induced chronic gout, unspecified site

✓6ᵗʰ **M1A.11** Lead-induced chronic gout, shoulder

  ✓7ᵗʰ **M1A.111** Lead-induced chronic gout, right shoulder

  ✓7ᵗʰ **M1A.112** Lead-induced chronic gout, left shoulder

  ✓7ᵗʰ **M1A.119** Lead-induced chronic gout, unspecified shoulder

✓6ᵗʰ **M1A.12** Lead-induced chronic gout, elbow

  ✓7ᵗʰ **M1A.121** Lead-induced chronic gout, right elbow

  ✓7ᵗʰ **M1A.122** Lead-induced chronic gout, left elbow

  ✓7ᵗʰ **M1A.129** Lead-induced chronic gout, unspecified elbow

✓6ᵗʰ **M1A.13** Lead-induced chronic gout, wrist

  ✓7ᵗʰ **M1A.131** Lead-induced chronic gout, right wrist

  ✓7ᵗʰ **M1A.132** Lead-induced chronic gout, left wrist

  ✓7ᵗʰ **M1A.139** Lead-induced chronic gout, unspecified wrist

✓6ᵗʰ **M1A.14** Lead-induced chronic gout, hand

  ✓7ᵗʰ **M1A.141** Lead-induced chronic gout, right hand

  ✓7ᵗʰ **M1A.142** Lead-induced chronic gout, left hand

  ✓7ᵗʰ **M1A.149** Lead-induced chronic gout, unspecified hand

✓6ᵗʰ **M1A.15** Lead-induced chronic gout, hip

  ✓7ᵗʰ **M1A.151** Lead-induced chronic gout, right hip

  ✓7ᵗʰ **M1A.152** Lead-induced chronic gout, left hip

  ✓7ᵗʰ **M1A.159** Lead-induced chronic gout, unspecified hip

✓6ᵗʰ **M1A.16** Lead-induced chronic gout, knee

  ✓7ᵗʰ **M1A.161** Lead-induced chronic gout, right knee

  ✓7ᵗʰ **M1A.162** Lead-induced chronic gout, left knee

  ✓7ᵗʰ **M1A.169** Lead-induced chronic gout, unspecified knee

✓6ᵗʰ **M1A.17** Lead-induced chronic gout, ankle and foot

  ✓7ᵗʰ **M1A.171** Lead-induced chronic gout, right ankle and foot

  ✓7ᵗʰ **M1A.172** Lead-induced chronic gout, left ankle and foot

  ✓7ᵗʰ **M1A.179** Lead-induced chronic gout, unspecified ankle and foot

✓x7ᵗʰ **M1A.18** Lead-induced chronic gout, vertebrae

✓x7ᵗʰ **M1A.19** Lead-induced chronic gout, multiple sites

✓5ᵗʰ **M1A.2** Drug-induced chronic gout

  Use additional code for adverse effect, if applicable, to identify drug (T36-T5Ø with fifth or sixth character 5)

✓x7ᵗʰ **M1A.2Ø** Drug-induced chronic gout, unspecified site

✓6ᵗʰ **M1A.21** Drug-induced chronic gout, shoulder

  ✓7ᵗʰ **M1A.211** Drug-induced chronic gout, right shoulder

  ✓7ᵗʰ **M1A.212** Drug-induced chronic gout, left shoulder

  ✓7ᵗʰ **M1A.219** Drug-induced chronic gout, unspecified shoulder

✓6ᵗʰ **M1A.22** Drug-induced chronic gout, elbow

  ✓7ᵗʰ **M1A.221** Drug-induced chronic gout, right elbow

  ✓7ᵗʰ **M1A.222** Drug-induced chronic gout, left elbow

  ✓7ᵗʰ **M1A.229** Drug-induced chronic gout, unspecified elbow

✓6ᵗʰ **M1A.23** Drug-induced chronic gout, wrist

  ✓7ᵗʰ **M1A.231** Drug-induced chronic gout, right wrist

  ✓7ᵗʰ **M1A.232** Drug-induced chronic gout, left wrist

  ✓7ᵗʰ **M1A.239** Drug-induced chronic gout, unspecified wrist

✓6ᵗʰ **M1A.24** Drug-induced chronic gout, hand

  ✓7ᵗʰ **M1A.241** Drug-induced chronic gout, right hand

  ✓7ᵗʰ **M1A.242** Drug-induced chronic gout, left hand

  ✓7ᵗʰ **M1A.249** Drug-induced chronic gout, unspecified hand

✓6ᵗʰ **M1A.25** Drug-induced chronic gout, hip

  ✓7ᵗʰ **M1A.251** Drug-induced chronic gout, right hip

  ✓7ᵗʰ **M1A.252** Drug-induced chronic gout, left hip

  ✓7ᵗʰ **M1A.259** Drug-induced chronic gout, unspecified hip

✓6ᵗʰ **M1A.26** Drug-induced chronic gout, knee

  ✓7ᵗʰ **M1A.261** Drug-induced chronic gout, right knee

  ✓7ᵗʰ **M1A.262** Drug-induced chronic gout, left knee

  ✓7ᵗʰ **M1A.269** Drug-induced chronic gout, unspecified knee

✓6ᵗʰ **M1A.27** Drug-induced chronic gout, ankle and foot

  ✓7ᵗʰ **M1A.271** Drug-induced chronic gout, right ankle and foot

  ✓7ᵗʰ **M1A.272** Drug-induced chronic gout, left ankle and foot

  ✓7ᵗʰ **M1A.279** Drug-induced chronic gout, unspecified ankle and foot

✓x7ᵗʰ **M1A.28** Drug-induced chronic gout, vertebrae

✓x7ᵗʰ **M1A.29** Drug-induced chronic gout, multiple sites

✓5ᵗʰ **M1A.3** Chronic gout due to renal impairment

  Code first associated renal disease

✓x7ᵗʰ **M1A.3Ø** Chronic gout due to renal impairment, unspecified site

✓6ᵗʰ **M1A.31** Chronic gout due to renal impairment, shoulder

  ✓7ᵗʰ **M1A.311** Chronic gout due to renal impairment, right shoulder

  ✓7ᵗʰ **M1A.312** Chronic gout due to renal impairment, left shoulder

  ✓7ᵗʰ **M1A.319** Chronic gout due to renal impairment, unspecified shoulder

✓6ᵗʰ **M1A.32** Chronic gout due to renal impairment, elbow

  ✓7ᵗʰ **M1A.321** Chronic gout due to renal impairment, right elbow

  ✓7ᵗʰ **M1A.322** Chronic gout due to renal impairment, left elbow

  ✓7ᵗʰ **M1A.329** Chronic gout due to renal impairment, unspecified elbow

✓6ᵗʰ **M1A.33** Chronic gout due to renal impairment, wrist

  ✓7ᵗʰ **M1A.331** Chronic gout due to renal impairment, right wrist

  ✓7ᵗʰ **M1A.332** Chronic gout due to renal impairment, left wrist

  ✓7ᵗʰ **M1A.339** Chronic gout due to renal impairment, unspecified wrist

✓6ᵗʰ **M1A.34** Chronic gout due to renal impairment, hand

  ✓7ᵗʰ **M1A.341** Chronic gout due to renal impairment, right hand

  ✓7ᵗʰ **M1A.342** Chronic gout due to renal impairment, left hand

  ✓7ᵗʰ **M1A.349** Chronic gout due to renal impairment, unspecified hand

√6ᵗʰ **M1A.35** Chronic gout due to renal impairment, hip

     √7ᵗʰ **M1A.351** Chronic gout due to renal impairment, right hip

     √7ᵗʰ **M1A.352** Chronic gout due to renal impairment, left hip

     √7ᵗʰ **M1A.359** Chronic gout due to renal impairment, unspecified hip

√6ᵗʰ **M1A.36** Chronic gout due to renal impairment, knee

     √7ᵗʰ **M1A.361** Chronic gout due to renal impairment, right knee

     √7ᵗʰ **M1A.362** Chronic gout due to renal impairment, left knee

     √7ᵗʰ **M1A.369** Chronic gout due to renal impairment, unspecified knee

√6ᵗʰ **M1A.37** Chronic gout due to renal impairment, ankle and foot

     √7ᵗʰ **M1A.371** Chronic gout due to renal impairment, right ankle and foot

     √7ᵗʰ **M1A.372** Chronic gout due to renal impairment, left ankle and foot

     √7ᵗʰ **M1A.379** Chronic gout due to renal impairment, unspecified ankle and foot

√x7ᵗʰ **M1A.38** Chronic gout due to renal impairment, vertebrae

√x7ᵗʰ **M1A.39** Chronic gout due to renal impairment, multiple sites

√5ᵗʰ **M1A.4** Other secondary chronic gout

     Code first associated condition

√x7ᵗʰ **M1A.40** Other secondary chronic gout, unspecified site

√6ᵗʰ **M1A.41** Other secondary chronic gout, shoulder

     √7ᵗʰ **M1A.411** Other secondary chronic gout, right shoulder

     √7ᵗʰ **M1A.412** Other secondary chronic gout, left shoulder

     √7ᵗʰ **M1A.419** Other secondary chronic gout, unspecified shoulder

√6ᵗʰ **M1A.42** Other secondary chronic gout, elbow

     √7ᵗʰ **M1A.421** Other secondary chronic gout, right elbow

     √7ᵗʰ **M1A.422** Other secondary chronic gout, left elbow

     √7ᵗʰ **M1A.429** Other secondary chronic gout, unspecified elbow

√6ᵗʰ **M1A.43** Other secondary chronic gout, wrist

     √7ᵗʰ **M1A.431** Other secondary chronic gout, right wrist

     √7ᵗʰ **M1A.432** Other secondary chronic gout, left wrist

     √7ᵗʰ **M1A.439** Other secondary chronic gout, unspecified wrist

√6ᵗʰ **M1A.44** Other secondary chronic gout, hand

     √7ᵗʰ **M1A.441** Other secondary chronic gout, right hand

     √7ᵗʰ **M1A.442** Other secondary chronic gout, left hand

     √7ᵗʰ **M1A.449** Other secondary chronic gout, unspecified hand

√6ᵗʰ **M1A.45** Other secondary chronic gout, hip

     √7ᵗʰ **M1A.451** Other secondary chronic gout, right hip

     √7ᵗʰ **M1A.452** Other secondary chronic gout, left hip

     √7ᵗʰ **M1A.459** Other secondary chronic gout, unspecified hip

√6ᵗʰ **M1A.46** Other secondary chronic gout, knee

     √7ᵗʰ **M1A.461** Other secondary chronic gout, right knee

     √7ᵗʰ **M1A.462** Other secondary chronic gout, left knee

     √7ᵗʰ **M1A.469** Other secondary chronic gout, unspecified knee

√6ᵗʰ **M1A.47** Other secondary chronic gout, ankle and foot

     √7ᵗʰ **M1A.471** Other secondary chronic gout, right ankle and foot

     √7ᵗʰ **M1A.472** Other secondary chronic gout, left ankle and foot

     √7ᵗʰ **M1A.479** Other secondary chronic gout, unspecified ankle and foot

√x7ᵗʰ **M1A.48** Other secondary chronic gout, vertebrae

√x7ᵗʰ **M1A.49** Other secondary chronic gout, multiple sites

√x7ᵗʰ **M1A.9** Chronic gout, unspecified

√4ᵗʰ **M10** Gout

     Acute gout
     Gout attack
     Gout flare
     Podagra
     Use additional code to identify:
         autonomic neuropathy in diseases classified elsewhere (G99.0)
         calculus of urinary tract in diseases classified elsewhere (N22)
         cardiomyopathy in diseases classified elsewhere (I43)
         disorders of external ear in diseases classified elsewhere (H61.1-, H62.8-)
         disorders of iris and ciliary body in diseases classified elsewhere (H22)
         glomerular disorders in diseases classified elsewhere (N08)

     EXCLUDES 2   chronic gout (M1A.-)

     DEF: Purine and pyrimidine metabolic disorders, manifested by hyperuricemia and recurrent acute inflammatory arthritis. Monosodium urate or monohydrate crystals may be deposited in and around the joints, leading to joint destruction and severe crippling.

√5ᵗʰ **M10.0** Idiopathic gout

     Gouty bursitis
     Primary gout

     M10.00 Idiopathic gout, unspecified site

√6ᵗʰ **M10.01** Idiopathic gout, shoulder

     M10.011 Idiopathic gout, right shoulder
     M10.012 Idiopathic gout, left shoulder
     M10.019 Idiopathic gout, unspecified shoulder

√6ᵗʰ **M10.02** Idiopathic gout, elbow

     M10.021 Idiopathic gout, right elbow
     M10.022 Idiopathic gout, left elbow
     M10.029 Idiopathic gout, unspecified elbow

√6ᵗʰ **M10.03** Idiopathic gout, wrist

     M10.031 Idiopathic gout, right wrist
     M10.032 Idiopathic gout, left wrist
     M10.039 Idiopathic gout, unspecified wrist

√6ᵗʰ **M10.04** Idiopathic gout, hand

     M10.041 Idiopathic gout, right hand
     M10.042 Idiopathic gout, left hand
     M10.049 Idiopathic gout, unspecified hand

√6ᵗʰ **M10.05** Idiopathic gout, hip

     M10.051 Idiopathic gout, right hip
     M10.052 Idiopathic gout, left hip
     M10.059 Idiopathic gout, unspecified hip

√6ᵗʰ **M10.06** Idiopathic gout, knee

     M10.061 Idiopathic gout, right knee
     M10.062 Idiopathic gout, left knee
     M10.069 Idiopathic gout, unspecified knee

√6ᵗʰ **M10.07** Idiopathic gout, ankle and foot

     M10.071 Idiopathic gout, right ankle and foot
     M10.072 Idiopathic gout, left ankle and foot
     M10.079 Idiopathic gout, unspecified ankle and foot

     M10.08 Idiopathic gout, vertebrae

     M10.09 Idiopathic gout, multiple sites

√5ᵗʰ **M10.1** Lead-induced gout

     Code first toxic effects of lead and its compounds (T56.0-)

     M10.10 Lead-induced gout, unspecified site

√6ᵗʰ **M10.11** Lead-induced gout, shoulder

     M10.111 Lead-induced gout, right shoulder
     M10.112 Lead-induced gout, left shoulder
     M10.119 Lead-induced gout, unspecified shoulder

√6ᵗʰ **M10.12** Lead-induced gout, elbow

     M10.121 Lead-induced gout, right elbow
     M10.122 Lead-induced gout, left elbow
     M10.129 Lead-induced gout, unspecified elbow

√6ᵗʰ **M10.13** Lead-induced gout, wrist

     M10.131 Lead-induced gout, right wrist
     M10.132 Lead-induced gout, left wrist
     M10.139 Lead-induced gout, unspecified wrist

√6ᵗʰ **M10.14** Lead-induced gout, hand

     M10.141 Lead-induced gout, right hand
     M10.142 Lead-induced gout, left hand
     M10.149 Lead-induced gout, unspecified hand

√6ᵗʰ **M10.15** Lead-induced gout, hip

     M10.151 Lead-induced gout, right hip
     M10.152 Lead-induced gout, left hip
     M10.159 Lead-induced gout, unspecified hip

☑ Additional Character Required   √x7ᵗʰ Placeholder   Unacceptable PDx   Questionable PDx   Manifestation   Unspecified Dx   H1-H14 HAC   HCC CMS-HCC Dx   HIV HIV Dx

ICD-10-CM 2021   771

✓6ᵗʰ **M10.16** Lead-induced gout, knee

     M10.161 Lead-induced gout, right knee
     M10.162 Lead-induced gout, left knee
     M10.169 Lead-induced gout, unspecified knee

✓6ᵗʰ **M10.17** Lead-induced gout, ankle and foot

     M10.171 Lead-induced gout, right ankle and foot
     M10.172 Lead-induced gout, left ankle and foot
     M10.179 Lead-induced gout, unspecified ankle and foot

M10.18 Lead-induced gout, vertebrae
M10.19 Lead-induced gout, multiple sites

✓5ᵗʰ **M10.2** Drug-induced gout

Use additional code for adverse effect, if applicable, to identify drug (T36-T50 with fifth or sixth character 5)

     M10.20 Drug-induced gout, unspecified site

✓6ᵗʰ **M10.21** Drug-induced gout, shoulder

     M10.211 Drug-induced gout, right shoulder
     M10.212 Drug-induced gout, left shoulder
     M10.219 Drug-induced gout, unspecified shoulder

✓6ᵗʰ **M10.22** Drug-induced gout, elbow

     M10.221 Drug-induced gout, right elbow
     M10.222 Drug-induced gout, left elbow
     M10.229 Drug-induced gout, unspecified elbow

✓6ᵗʰ **M10.23** Drug-induced gout, wrist

     M10.231 Drug-induced gout, right wrist
     M10.232 Drug-induced gout, left wrist
     M10.239 Drug-induced gout, unspecified wrist

✓6ᵗʰ **M10.24** Drug-induced gout, hand

     M10.241 Drug-induced gout, right hand
     M10.242 Drug-induced gout, left hand
     M10.249 Drug-induced gout, unspecified hand

✓6ᵗʰ **M10.25** Drug-induced gout, hip

     M10.251 Drug-induced gout, right hip
     M10.252 Drug-induced gout, left hip
     M10.259 Drug-induced gout, unspecified hip

✓6ᵗʰ **M10.26** Drug-induced gout, knee

     M10.261 Drug-induced gout, right knee
     M10.262 Drug-induced gout, left knee
     M10.269 Drug-induced gout, unspecified knee

✓6ᵗʰ **M10.27** Drug-induced gout, ankle and foot

     M10.271 Drug-induced gout, right ankle and foot
     M10.272 Drug-induced gout, left ankle and foot
     M10.279 Drug-induced gout, unspecified ankle and foot

M10.28 Drug-induced gout, vertebrae
M10.29 Drug-induced gout, multiple sites

✓5ᵗʰ **M10.3** Gout due to renal impairment

Code first associated renal disease

     M10.30 Gout due to renal impairment, unspecified site

✓6ᵗʰ **M10.31** Gout due to renal impairment, shoulder

     M10.311 Gout due to renal impairment, right shoulder
     M10.312 Gout due to renal impairment, left shoulder
     M10.319 Gout due to renal impairment, unspecified shoulder

✓6ᵗʰ **M10.32** Gout due to renal impairment, elbow

     M10.321 Gout due to renal impairment, right elbow
     M10.322 Gout due to renal impairment, left elbow
     M10.329 Gout due to renal impairment, unspecified elbow

✓6ᵗʰ **M10.33** Gout due to renal impairment, wrist

     M10.331 Gout due to renal impairment, right wrist
     M10.332 Gout due to renal impairment, left wrist
     M10.339 Gout due to renal impairment, unspecified wrist

✓6ᵗʰ **M10.34** Gout due to renal impairment, hand

     M10.341 Gout due to renal impairment, right hand
     M10.342 Gout due to renal impairment, left hand
     M10.349 Gout due to renal impairment, unspecified hand

✓6ᵗʰ **M10.35** Gout due to renal impairment, hip

     M10.351 Gout due to renal impairment, right hip
     M10.352 Gout due to renal impairment, left hip

     M10.359 Gout due to renal impairment, unspecified hip

✓6ᵗʰ **M10.36** Gout due to renal impairment, knee

     M10.361 Gout due to renal impairment, right knee
     M10.362 Gout due to renal impairment, left knee
     M10.369 Gout due to renal impairment, unspecified knee

✓6ᵗʰ **M10.37** Gout due to renal impairment, ankle and foot

     M10.371 Gout due to renal impairment, right ankle and foot
     M10.372 Gout due to renal impairment, left ankle and foot
     M10.379 Gout due to renal impairment, unspecified ankle and foot

M10.38 Gout due to renal impairment, vertebrae
M10.39 Gout due to renal impairment, multiple sites

✓5ᵗʰ **M10.4** Other secondary gout

Code first associated condition

     M10.40 Other secondary gout, unspecified site

✓6ᵗʰ **M10.41** Other secondary gout, shoulder

     M10.411 Other secondary gout, right shoulder
     M10.412 Other secondary gout, left shoulder
     M10.419 Other secondary gout, unspecified shoulder

✓6ᵗʰ **M10.42** Other secondary gout, elbow

     M10.421 Other secondary gout, right elbow
     M10.422 Other secondary gout, left elbow
     M10.429 Other secondary gout, unspecified elbow

✓6ᵗʰ **M10.43** Other secondary gout, wrist

     M10.431 Other secondary gout, right wrist
     M10.432 Other secondary gout, left wrist
     M10.439 Other secondary gout, unspecified wrist

✓6ᵗʰ **M10.44** Other secondary gout, hand

     M10.441 Other secondary gout, right hand
     M10.442 Other secondary gout, left hand
     M10.449 Other secondary gout, unspecified hand

✓6ᵗʰ **M10.45** Other secondary gout, hip

     M10.451 Other secondary gout, right hip
     M10.452 Other secondary gout, left hip
     M10.459 Other secondary gout, unspecified hip

✓6ᵗʰ **M10.46** Other secondary gout, knee

     M10.461 Other secondary gout, right knee
     M10.462 Other secondary gout, left knee
     M10.469 Other secondary gout, unspecified knee

✓6ᵗʰ **M10.47** Other secondary gout, ankle and foot

     M10.471 Other secondary gout, right ankle and foot
     M10.472 Other secondary gout, left ankle and foot
     M10.479 Other secondary gout, unspecified ankle and foot

M10.48 Other secondary gout, vertebrae
M10.49 Other secondary gout, multiple sites

M10.9 Gout, unspecified
Gout NOS

✓4ᵗʰ **M11** Other crystal arthropathies

✓5ᵗʰ **M11.0** Hydroxyapatite deposition disease

DEF: Disease caused by deposits of calcium phosphate crystals in the soft tissues close to the joint (especially tendons) or in the joints. These calcifications can be mono or polyarticular and can cause destruction of the joint involved.

     M11.00 Hydroxyapatite deposition disease, unspecified site

✓6ᵗʰ **M11.01** Hydroxyapatite deposition disease, shoulder

     M11.011 Hydroxyapatite deposition disease, right shoulder
     M11.012 Hydroxyapatite deposition disease, left shoulder
     M11.019 Hydroxyapatite deposition disease, unspecified shoulder

✓6ᵗʰ **M11.02** Hydroxyapatite deposition disease, elbow

     M11.021 Hydroxyapatite deposition disease, right elbow
     M11.022 Hydroxyapatite deposition disease, left elbow
     M11.029 Hydroxyapatite deposition disease, unspecified elbow

√6ᵗʰ **M11.03** Hydroxyapatite deposition disease, wrist

    M11.031 Hydroxyapatite deposition disease, right wrist

    M11.032 Hydroxyapatite deposition disease, left wrist

    M11.039 Hydroxyapatite deposition disease, unspecified wrist

√6ᵗʰ **M11.04** Hydroxyapatite deposition disease, hand

    M11.041 Hydroxyapatite deposition disease, right hand

    M11.042 Hydroxyapatite deposition disease, left hand

    M11.049 Hydroxyapatite deposition disease, unspecified hand

√6ᵗʰ **M11.05** Hydroxyapatite deposition disease, hip

    M11.051 Hydroxyapatite deposition disease, right hip

    M11.052 Hydroxyapatite deposition disease, left hip

    M11.059 Hydroxyapatite deposition disease, unspecified hip

√6ᵗʰ **M11.06** Hydroxyapatite deposition disease, knee

    M11.061 Hydroxyapatite deposition disease, right knee

    M11.062 Hydroxyapatite deposition disease, left knee

    M11.069 Hydroxyapatite deposition disease, unspecified knee

√6ᵗʰ **M11.07** Hydroxyapatite deposition disease, ankle and foot

    M11.071 Hydroxyapatite deposition disease, right ankle and foot

    M11.072 Hydroxyapatite deposition disease, left ankle and foot

    M11.079 Hydroxyapatite deposition disease, unspecified ankle and foot

  M11.08 Hydroxyapatite deposition disease, vertebrae

  M11.09 Hydroxyapatite deposition disease, multiple sites

√5ᵗʰ **M11.1** Familial chondrocalcinosis

  M11.10 Familial chondrocalcinosis, unspecified site

√6ᵗʰ **M11.11** Familial chondrocalcinosis, shoulder

    M11.111 Familial chondrocalcinosis, right shoulder

    M11.112 Familial chondrocalcinosis, left shoulder

    M11.119 Familial chondrocalcinosis, unspecified shoulder

√6ᵗʰ **M11.12** Familial chondrocalcinosis, elbow

    M11.121 Familial chondrocalcinosis, right elbow

    M11.122 Familial chondrocalcinosis, left elbow

    M11.129 Familial chondrocalcinosis, unspecified elbow

√6ᵗʰ **M11.13** Familial chondrocalcinosis, wrist

    M11.131 Familial chondrocalcinosis, right wrist

    M11.132 Familial chondrocalcinosis, left wrist

    M11.139 Familial chondrocalcinosis, unspecified wrist

√6ᵗʰ **M11.14** Familial chondrocalcinosis, hand

    M11.141 Familial chondrocalcinosis, right hand

    M11.142 Familial chondrocalcinosis, left hand

    M11.149 Familial chondrocalcinosis, unspecified hand

√6ᵗʰ **M11.15** Familial chondrocalcinosis, hip

    M11.151 Familial chondrocalcinosis, right hip

    M11.152 Familial chondrocalcinosis, left hip

    M11.159 Familial chondrocalcinosis, unspecified hip

√6ᵗʰ **M11.16** Familial chondrocalcinosis, knee

    M11.161 Familial chondrocalcinosis, right knee

    M11.162 Familial chondrocalcinosis, left knee

    M11.169 Familial chondrocalcinosis, unspecified knee

√6ᵗʰ **M11.17** Familial chondrocalcinosis, ankle and foot

    M11.171 Familial chondrocalcinosis, right ankle and foot

    M11.172 Familial chondrocalcinosis, left ankle and foot

    M11.179 Familial chondrocalcinosis, unspecified ankle and foot

  M11.18 Familial chondrocalcinosis, vertebrae

  M11.19 Familial chondrocalcinosis, multiple sites

√5ᵗʰ **M11.2** Other chondrocalcinosis

Chondrocalcinosis NOS

AHA: 2018,3Q,20

TIP: Pseudogout is captured with codes in this subcategory.

  M11.20 Other chondrocalcinosis, unspecified site

√6ᵗʰ **M11.21** Other chondrocalcinosis, shoulder

    M11.211 Other chondrocalcinosis, right shoulder

    M11.212 Other chondrocalcinosis, left shoulder

    M11.219 Other chondrocalcinosis, unspecified shoulder

√6ᵗʰ **M11.22** Other chondrocalcinosis, elbow

    M11.221 Other chondrocalcinosis, right elbow

    M11.222 Other chondrocalcinosis, left elbow

    M11.229 Other chondrocalcinosis, unspecified elbow

√6ᵗʰ **M11.23** Other chondrocalcinosis, wrist

    M11.231 Other chondrocalcinosis, right wrist

    M11.232 Other chondrocalcinosis, left wrist

    M11.239 Other chondrocalcinosis, unspecified wrist

√6ᵗʰ **M11.24** Other chondrocalcinosis, hand

    M11.241 Other chondrocalcinosis, right hand

    M11.242 Other chondrocalcinosis, left hand

    M11.249 Other chondrocalcinosis, unspecified hand

√6ᵗʰ **M11.25** Other chondrocalcinosis, hip

    M11.251 Other chondrocalcinosis, right hip

    M11.252 Other chondrocalcinosis, left hip

    M11.259 Other chondrocalcinosis, unspecified hip

√6ᵗʰ **M11.26** Other chondrocalcinosis, knee

    M11.261 Other chondrocalcinosis, right knee

    M11.262 Other chondrocalcinosis, left knee

    M11.269 Other chondrocalcinosis, unspecified knee

√6ᵗʰ **M11.27** Other chondrocalcinosis, ankle and foot

    M11.271 Other chondrocalcinosis, right ankle and foot

    M11.272 Other chondrocalcinosis, left ankle and foot

    M11.279 Other chondrocalcinosis, unspecified ankle and foot

  M11.28 Other chondrocalcinosis, vertebrae

  M11.29 Other chondrocalcinosis, multiple sites

√5ᵗʰ **M11.8** Other specified crystal arthropathies

  M11.80 Other specified crystal arthropathies, unspecified site

√6ᵗʰ **M11.81** Other specified crystal arthropathies, shoulder

    M11.811 Other specified crystal arthropathies, right shoulder

    M11.812 Other specified crystal arthropathies, left shoulder

    M11.819 Other specified crystal arthropathies, unspecified shoulder

√6ᵗʰ **M11.82** Other specified crystal arthropathies, elbow

    M11.821 Other specified crystal arthropathies, right elbow

    M11.822 Other specified crystal arthropathies, left elbow

    M11.829 Other specified crystal arthropathies, unspecified elbow

√6ᵗʰ **M11.83** Other specified crystal arthropathies, wrist

    M11.831 Other specified crystal arthropathies, right wrist

    M11.832 Other specified crystal arthropathies, left wrist

    M11.839 Other specified crystal arthropathies, unspecified wrist

√6ᵗʰ **M11.84** Other specified crystal arthropathies, hand

    M11.841 Other specified crystal arthropathies, right hand

    M11.842 Other specified crystal arthropathies, left hand

    M11.849 Other specified crystal arthropathies, unspecified hand

√6ᵗʰ **M11.85** Other specified crystal arthropathies, hip

    M11.851 Other specified crystal arthropathies, right hip

☑ Additional Character Required   √x7ᵗʰ Placeholder   Unacceptable PDx   Questionable PDx   Manifestation   Unspecified Dx   H1-H14 HAC   HCC CMS-HCC Dx   HIV HIV Dx

ICD-10-CM 2021   773

     M11.852 Other specified crystal arthropathies, left hip
     M11.859 Other specified crystal arthropathies, unspecified hip
   ✓6ᵗʰ **M11.86** Other specified crystal arthropathies, knee
     M11.861 Other specified crystal arthropathies, right knee
     M11.862 Other specified crystal arthropathies, left knee
     M11.869 Other specified crystal arthropathies, unspecified knee
   ✓6ᵗʰ **M11.87** Other specified crystal arthropathies, ankle and foot
     M11.871 Other specified crystal arthropathies, right ankle and foot
     M11.872 Other specified crystal arthropathies, left ankle and foot
     M11.879 Other specified crystal arthropathies, unspecified ankle and foot
    M11.88 Other specified crystal arthropathies, vertebrae
    M11.89 Other specified crystal arthropathies, multiple sites
   M11.9 Crystal arthropathy, unspecified
✓4ᵗʰ **M12** Other and unspecified arthropathy
   EXCLUDES 1   arthrosis (M15-M19)
          cricoarytenoid arthropathy (J38.7)
   ✓5ᵗʰ **M12.0** Chronic postrheumatic arthropathy [Jaccoud]
     M12.00 Chronic postrheumatic arthropathy [Jaccoud], unspecified site   HCC
    ✓6ᵗʰ **M12.01** Chronic postrheumatic arthropathy [Jaccoud], shoulder
     M12.011 Chronic postrheumatic arthropathy [Jaccoud], right shoulder   HCC
     M12.012 Chronic postrheumatic arthropathy [Jaccoud], left shoulder   HCC
     M12.019 Chronic postrheumatic arthropathy [Jaccoud], unspecified shoulder   HCC
    ✓6ᵗʰ **M12.02** Chronic postrheumatic arthropathy [Jaccoud], elbow
     M12.021 Chronic postrheumatic arthropathy [Jaccoud], right elbow   HCC
     M12.022 Chronic postrheumatic arthropathy [Jaccoud], left elbow   HCC
     M12.029 Chronic postrheumatic arthropathy [Jaccoud], unspecified elbow   HCC
    ✓6ᵗʰ **M12.03** Chronic postrheumatic arthropathy [Jaccoud], wrist
     M12.031 Chronic postrheumatic arthropathy [Jaccoud], right wrist   HCC
     M12.032 Chronic postrheumatic arthropathy [Jaccoud], left wrist   HCC
     M12.039 Chronic postrheumatic arthropathy [Jaccoud], unspecified wrist   HCC
    ✓6ᵗʰ **M12.04** Chronic postrheumatic arthropathy [Jaccoud], hand
     M12.041 Chronic postrheumatic arthropathy [Jaccoud], right hand   HCC
     M12.042 Chronic postrheumatic arthropathy [Jaccoud], left hand   HCC
     M12.049 Chronic postrheumatic arthropathy [Jaccoud], unspecified hand   HCC
    ✓6ᵗʰ **M12.05** Chronic postrheumatic arthropathy [Jaccoud], hip
     M12.051 Chronic postrheumatic arthropathy [Jaccoud], right hip   HCC
     M12.052 Chronic postrheumatic arthropathy [Jaccoud], left hip   HCC
     M12.059 Chronic postrheumatic arthropathy [Jaccoud], unspecified hip   HCC
    ✓6ᵗʰ **M12.06** Chronic postrheumatic arthropathy [Jaccoud], knee
     M12.061 Chronic postrheumatic arthropathy [Jaccoud], right knee   HCC
     M12.062 Chronic postrheumatic arthropathy [Jaccoud], left knee   HCC
     M12.069 Chronic postrheumatic arthropathy [Jaccoud], unspecified knee   HCC
    ✓6ᵗʰ **M12.07** Chronic postrheumatic arthropathy [Jaccoud], ankle and foot
     M12.071 Chronic postrheumatic arthropathy [Jaccoud], right ankle and foot   HCC
     M12.072 Chronic postrheumatic arthropathy [Jaccoud], left ankle and foot   HCC

     M12.079 Chronic postrheumatic arthropathy [Jaccoud], unspecified ankle and foot   HCC
    M12.08 Chronic postrheumatic arthropathy [Jaccoud], other specified site   HCC
       Chronic postrheumatic arthropathy [Jaccoud], vertebrae
    M12.09 Chronic postrheumatic arthropathy [Jaccoud], multiple sites   HCC
   ✓5ᵗʰ **M12.1** Kaschin-Beck disease
     Osteochondroarthrosis deformans endemica
     M12.10 Kaschin-Beck disease, unspecified site
    ✓6ᵗʰ **M12.11** Kaschin-Beck disease, shoulder
     M12.111 Kaschin-Beck disease, right shoulder
     M12.112 Kaschin-Beck disease, left shoulder
     M12.119 Kaschin-Beck disease, unspecified shoulder
    ✓6ᵗʰ **M12.12** Kaschin-Beck disease, elbow
     M12.121 Kaschin-Beck disease, right elbow
     M12.122 Kaschin-Beck disease, left elbow
     M12.129 Kaschin-Beck disease, unspecified elbow
    ✓6ᵗʰ **M12.13** Kaschin-Beck disease, wrist
     M12.131 Kaschin-Beck disease, right wrist
     M12.132 Kaschin-Beck disease, left wrist
     M12.139 Kaschin-Beck disease, unspecified wrist
    ✓6ᵗʰ **M12.14** Kaschin-Beck disease, hand
     M12.141 Kaschin-Beck disease, right hand
     M12.142 Kaschin-Beck disease, left hand
     M12.149 Kaschin-Beck disease, unspecified hand
    ✓6ᵗʰ **M12.15** Kaschin-Beck disease, hip
     M12.151 Kaschin-Beck disease, right hip
     M12.152 Kaschin-Beck disease, left hip
     M12.159 Kaschin-Beck disease, unspecified hip
    ✓6ᵗʰ **M12.16** Kaschin-Beck disease, knee
     M12.161 Kaschin-Beck disease, right knee
     M12.162 Kaschin-Beck disease, left knee
     M12.169 Kaschin-Beck disease, unspecified knee
    ✓6ᵗʰ **M12.17** Kaschin-Beck disease, ankle and foot
     M12.171 Kaschin-Beck disease, right ankle and foot
     M12.172 Kaschin-Beck disease, left ankle and foot
     M12.179 Kaschin-Beck disease, unspecified ankle and foot
    M12.18 Kaschin-Beck disease, vertebrae
    M12.19 Kaschin-Beck disease, multiple sites
   ✓5ᵗʰ **M12.2** Villonodular synovitis (pigmented)
     M12.20 Villonodular synovitis (pigmented), unspecified site
    ✓6ᵗʰ **M12.21** Villonodular synovitis (pigmented), shoulder
     M12.211 Villonodular synovitis (pigmented), right shoulder
     M12.212 Villonodular synovitis (pigmented), left shoulder
     M12.219 Villonodular synovitis (pigmented), unspecified shoulder
    ✓6ᵗʰ **M12.22** Villonodular synovitis (pigmented), elbow
     M12.221 Villonodular synovitis (pigmented), right elbow
     M12.222 Villonodular synovitis (pigmented), left elbow
     M12.229 Villonodular synovitis (pigmented), unspecified elbow
    ✓6ᵗʰ **M12.23** Villonodular synovitis (pigmented), wrist
     M12.231 Villonodular synovitis (pigmented), right wrist
     M12.232 Villonodular synovitis (pigmented), left wrist
     M12.239 Villonodular synovitis (pigmented), unspecified wrist
    ✓6ᵗʰ **M12.24** Villonodular synovitis (pigmented), hand
     M12.241 Villonodular synovitis (pigmented), right hand
     M12.242 Villonodular synovitis (pigmented), left hand
     M12.249 Villonodular synovitis (pigmented), unspecified hand

N Newborn: 0   P Pediatric: 0-17   M Maternity: 9-64   A Adult: 15-124   MCC Major Complication/Comorbidity   CC Complication/Comorbidity   SW Severe Wound Dx

774   ICD-10-CM 2021

☑6ᵗʰ **M12.25** Villonodular synovitis (pigmented), hip

     M12.251 Villonodular synovitis (pigmented), right hip

     M12.252 Villonodular synovitis (pigmented), left hip

     M12.259 Villonodular synovitis (pigmented), unspecified hip

☑6ᵗʰ **M12.26** Villonodular synovitis (pigmented), knee

     M12.261 Villonodular synovitis (pigmented), right knee

     M12.262 Villonodular synovitis (pigmented), left knee

     M12.269 Villonodular synovitis (pigmented), unspecified knee

☑6ᵗʰ **M12.27** Villonodular synovitis (pigmented), ankle and foot

     M12.271 Villonodular synovitis (pigmented), right ankle and foot

     M12.272 Villonodular synovitis (pigmented), left ankle and foot

     M12.279 Villonodular synovitis (pigmented), unspecified ankle and foot

     M12.28 Villonodular synovitis (pigmented), other specified site

         Villonodular synovitis (pigmented), vertebrae

     M12.29 Villonodular synovitis (pigmented), multiple sites

☑5ᵗʰ **M12.3** Palindromic rheumatism

     DEF: Sudden and recurring attacks of moderate to severe joint pain and swelling generally occurring in the hands or feet of unknown etiology. After the attack subsides, the joints appear normal again.

     M12.30 Palindromic rheumatism, unspecified site

☑6ᵗʰ **M12.31** Palindromic rheumatism, shoulder

     M12.311 Palindromic rheumatism, right shoulder

     M12.312 Palindromic rheumatism, left shoulder

     M12.319 Palindromic rheumatism, unspecified shoulder

☑6ᵗʰ **M12.32** Palindromic rheumatism, elbow

     M12.321 Palindromic rheumatism, right elbow

     M12.322 Palindromic rheumatism, left elbow

     M12.329 Palindromic rheumatism, unspecified elbow

☑6ᵗʰ **M12.33** Palindromic rheumatism, wrist

     M12.331 Palindromic rheumatism, right wrist

     M12.332 Palindromic rheumatism, left wrist

     M12.339 Palindromic rheumatism, unspecified wrist

☑6ᵗʰ **M12.34** Palindromic rheumatism, hand

     M12.341 Palindromic rheumatism, right hand

     M12.342 Palindromic rheumatism, left hand

     M12.349 Palindromic rheumatism, unspecified hand

☑6ᵗʰ **M12.35** Palindromic rheumatism, hip

     M12.351 Palindromic rheumatism, right hip

     M12.352 Palindromic rheumatism, left hip

     M12.359 Palindromic rheumatism, unspecified hip

☑6ᵗʰ **M12.36** Palindromic rheumatism, knee

     M12.361 Palindromic rheumatism, right knee

     M12.362 Palindromic rheumatism, left knee

     M12.369 Palindromic rheumatism, unspecified knee

☑6ᵗʰ **M12.37** Palindromic rheumatism, ankle and foot

     M12.371 Palindromic rheumatism, right ankle and foot

     M12.372 Palindromic rheumatism, left ankle and foot

     M12.379 Palindromic rheumatism, unspecified ankle and foot

     M12.38 Palindromic rheumatism, other specified site

         Palindromic rheumatism, vertebrae

     M12.39 Palindromic rheumatism, multiple sites

☑5ᵗʰ **M12.4** Intermittent hydrarthrosis

     M12.40 Intermittent hydrarthrosis, unspecified site

☑6ᵗʰ **M12.41** Intermittent hydrarthrosis, shoulder

     M12.411 Intermittent hydrarthrosis, right shoulder

     M12.412 Intermittent hydrarthrosis, left shoulder

     M12.419 Intermittent hydrarthrosis, unspecified shoulder

☑6ᵗʰ **M12.42** Intermittent hydrarthrosis, elbow

     M12.421 Intermittent hydrarthrosis, right elbow

     M12.422 Intermittent hydrarthrosis, left elbow

     M12.429 Intermittent hydrarthrosis, unspecified elbow

☑6ᵗʰ **M12.43** Intermittent hydrarthrosis, wrist

     M12.431 Intermittent hydrarthrosis, right wrist

     M12.432 Intermittent hydrarthrosis, left wrist

     M12.439 Intermittent hydrarthrosis, unspecified wrist

☑6ᵗʰ **M12.44** Intermittent hydrarthrosis, hand

     M12.441 Intermittent hydrarthrosis, right hand

     M12.442 Intermittent hydrarthrosis, left hand

     M12.449 Intermittent hydrarthrosis, unspecified hand

☑6ᵗʰ **M12.45** Intermittent hydrarthrosis, hip

     M12.451 Intermittent hydrarthrosis, right hip

     M12.452 Intermittent hydrarthrosis, left hip

     M12.459 Intermittent hydrarthrosis, unspecified hip

☑6ᵗʰ **M12.46** Intermittent hydrarthrosis, knee

     M12.461 Intermittent hydrarthrosis, right knee

     M12.462 Intermittent hydrarthrosis, left knee

     M12.469 Intermittent hydrarthrosis, unspecified knee

☑6ᵗʰ **M12.47** Intermittent hydrarthrosis, ankle and foot

     M12.471 Intermittent hydrarthrosis, right ankle and foot

     M12.472 Intermittent hydrarthrosis, left ankle and foot

     M12.479 Intermittent hydrarthrosis, unspecified ankle and foot

     M12.48 Intermittent hydrarthrosis, other site

     M12.49 Intermittent hydrarthrosis, multiple sites

☑5ᵗʰ **M12.5** Traumatic arthropathy

     EXCLUDES 1   *current injury—see Alphabetic Index*

         post-traumatic osteoarthritis of first carpometacarpal joint (M18.2-M18.3)

         post-traumatic osteoarthritis of hip (M16.4-M16.5)

         post-traumatic osteoarthritis of knee (M17.2-M17.3)

         post-traumatic osteoarthritis NOS (M19.1-)

         post-traumatic osteoarthritis of other single joints (M19.1-)

     AHA: 2015,1Q,17

     M12.50 Traumatic arthropathy, unspecified site

☑6ᵗʰ **M12.51** Traumatic arthropathy, shoulder

     M12.511 Traumatic arthropathy, right shoulder

     M12.512 Traumatic arthropathy, left shoulder

     M12.519 Traumatic arthropathy, unspecified shoulder

☑6ᵗʰ **M12.52** Traumatic arthropathy, elbow

     M12.521 Traumatic arthropathy, right elbow

     M12.522 Traumatic arthropathy, left elbow

     M12.529 Traumatic arthropathy, unspecified elbow

☑6ᵗʰ **M12.53** Traumatic arthropathy, wrist

     M12.531 Traumatic arthropathy, right wrist

     M12.532 Traumatic arthropathy, left wrist

     M12.539 Traumatic arthropathy, unspecified wrist

☑6ᵗʰ **M12.54** Traumatic arthropathy, hand

     M12.541 Traumatic arthropathy, right hand

     M12.542 Traumatic arthropathy, left hand

     M12.549 Traumatic arthropathy, unspecified hand

☑6ᵗʰ **M12.55** Traumatic arthropathy, hip

     M12.551 Traumatic arthropathy, right hip

     M12.552 Traumatic arthropathy, left hip

     M12.559 Traumatic arthropathy, unspecified hip

☑6ᵗʰ **M12.56** Traumatic arthropathy, knee

     M12.561 Traumatic arthropathy, right knee

     M12.562 Traumatic arthropathy, left knee

     M12.569 Traumatic arthropathy, unspecified knee

☑6ᵗʰ **M12.57** Traumatic arthropathy, ankle and foot

     M12.571 Traumatic arthropathy, right ankle and foot

     M12.572 Traumatic arthropathy, left ankle and foot

☑ Additional Character Required   ☑x7ᵗʰ Placeholder   Unacceptable PDx   Questionable PDx   Manifestation   Unspecified Dx   H1-H14 HAC   HCC CMS-HCC Dx   HIV HIV Dx

ICD-10-CM 2021   **775**

M12.579 Traumatic arthropathy, unspecified ankle and foot

M12.58 Traumatic arthropathy, other specified site
Traumatic arthropathy, vertebrae

M12.59 Traumatic arthropathy, multiple sites

√5ᵗʰ **M12.8** Other specific arthropathies, not elsewhere classified
Transient arthropathy

M12.80 Other specific arthropathies, not elsewhere classified, unspecified site

√6ᵗʰ **M12.81** Other specific arthropathies, not elsewhere classified, shoulder

M12.811 Other specific arthropathies, not elsewhere classified, right shoulder

M12.812 Other specific arthropathies, not elsewhere classified, left shoulder

M12.819 Other specific arthropathies, not elsewhere classified, unspecified shoulder

√6ᵗʰ **M12.82** Other specific arthropathies, not elsewhere classified, elbow

M12.821 Other specific arthropathies, not elsewhere classified, right elbow

M12.822 Other specific arthropathies, not elsewhere classified, left elbow

M12.829 Other specific arthropathies, not elsewhere classified, unspecified elbow

√6ᵗʰ **M12.83** Other specific arthropathies, not elsewhere classified, wrist

M12.831 Other specific arthropathies, not elsewhere classified, right wrist

M12.832 Other specific arthropathies, not elsewhere classified, left wrist

M12.839 Other specific arthropathies, not elsewhere classified, unspecified wrist

√6ᵗʰ **M12.84** Other specific arthropathies, not elsewhere classified, hand

M12.841 Other specific arthropathies, not elsewhere classified, right hand

M12.842 Other specific arthropathies, not elsewhere classified, left hand

M12.849 Other specific arthropathies, not elsewhere classified, unspecified hand

√6ᵗʰ **M12.85** Other specific arthropathies, not elsewhere classified, hip

M12.851 Other specific arthropathies, not elsewhere classified, right hip

M12.852 Other specific arthropathies, not elsewhere classified, left hip

M12.859 Other specific arthropathies, not elsewhere classified, unspecified hip

√6ᵗʰ **M12.86** Other specific arthropathies, not elsewhere classified, knee

M12.861 Other specific arthropathies, not elsewhere classified, right knee

M12.862 Other specific arthropathies, not elsewhere classified, left knee

M12.869 Other specific arthropathies, not elsewhere classified, unspecified knee

√6ᵗʰ **M12.87** Other specific arthropathies, not elsewhere classified, ankle and foot

M12.871 Other specific arthropathies, not elsewhere classified, right ankle and foot

M12.872 Other specific arthropathies, not elsewhere classified, left ankle and foot

M12.879 Other specific arthropathies, not elsewhere classified, unspecified ankle and foot

M12.88 Other specific arthropathies, not elsewhere classified, other specified site
Other specific arthropathies, not elsewhere classified, vertebrae

M12.89 Other specific arthropathies, not elsewhere classified, multiple sites

M12.9 Arthropathy, unspecified

√4ᵗʰ **M13** Other arthritis
EXCLUDES 1   arthrosis (M15-M19)
             osteoarthritis (M15-M19)

M13.0 Polyarthritis, unspecified

√5ᵗʰ **M13.1** Monoarthritis, not elsewhere classified

M13.10 Monoarthritis, not elsewhere classified, unspecified site

√6ᵗʰ **M13.11** Monoarthritis, not elsewhere classified, shoulder

M13.111 Monoarthritis, not elsewhere classified, right shoulder

M13.112 Monoarthritis, not elsewhere classified, left shoulder

M13.119 Monoarthritis, not elsewhere classified, unspecified shoulder

√6ᵗʰ **M13.12** Monoarthritis, not elsewhere classified, elbow

M13.121 Monoarthritis, not elsewhere classified, right elbow

M13.122 Monoarthritis, not elsewhere classified, left elbow

M13.129 Monoarthritis, not elsewhere classified, unspecified elbow

√6ᵗʰ **M13.13** Monoarthritis, not elsewhere classified, wrist

M13.131 Monoarthritis, not elsewhere classified, right wrist

M13.132 Monoarthritis, not elsewhere classified, left wrist

M13.139 Monoarthritis, not elsewhere classified, unspecified wrist

√6ᵗʰ **M13.14** Monoarthritis, not elsewhere classified, hand

M13.141 Monoarthritis, not elsewhere classified, right hand

M13.142 Monoarthritis, not elsewhere classified, left hand

M13.149 Monoarthritis, not elsewhere classified, unspecified hand

√6ᵗʰ **M13.15** Monoarthritis, not elsewhere classified, hip

M13.151 Monoarthritis, not elsewhere classified, right hip

M13.152 Monoarthritis, not elsewhere classified, left hip

M13.159 Monoarthritis, not elsewhere classified, unspecified hip

√6ᵗʰ **M13.16** Monoarthritis, not elsewhere classified, knee

M13.161 Monoarthritis, not elsewhere classified, right knee

M13.162 Monoarthritis, not elsewhere classified, left knee

M13.169 Monoarthritis, not elsewhere classified, unspecified knee

√6ᵗʰ **M13.17** Monoarthritis, not elsewhere classified, ankle and foot

M13.171 Monoarthritis, not elsewhere classified, right ankle and foot

M13.172 Monoarthritis, not elsewhere classified, left ankle and foot

M13.179 Monoarthritis, not elsewhere classified, unspecified ankle and foot

√5ᵗʰ **M13.8** Other specified arthritis
Allergic arthritis
EXCLUDES 1   osteoarthritis (M15-M19)

M13.80 Other specified arthritis, unspecified site

√6ᵗʰ **M13.81** Other specified arthritis, shoulder

M13.811 Other specified arthritis, right shoulder
M13.812 Other specified arthritis, left shoulder
M13.819 Other specified arthritis, unspecified shoulder

√6ᵗʰ **M13.82** Other specified arthritis, elbow

M13.821 Other specified arthritis, right elbow
M13.822 Other specified arthritis, left elbow
M13.829 Other specified arthritis, unspecified elbow

√6ᵗʰ **M13.83** Other specified arthritis, wrist

M13.831 Other specified arthritis, right wrist
M13.832 Other specified arthritis, left wrist
M13.839 Other specified arthritis, unspecified wrist

√6ᵗʰ **M13.84** Other specified arthritis, hand

M13.841 Other specified arthritis, right hand
M13.842 Other specified arthritis, left hand
M13.849 Other specified arthritis, unspecified hand

√6ᵗʰ **M13.85** Other specified arthritis, hip

M13.851 Other specified arthritis, right hip
M13.852 Other specified arthritis, left hip
M13.859 Other specified arthritis, unspecified hip

☑6ᵗʰ **M13.86** **Other specified arthritis,** knee

   M13.861 **Other specified arthritis,** right **knee**
   M13.862 **Other specified arthritis,** left **knee**
   M13.869 **Other specified arthritis, unspecified knee**

☑6ᵗʰ **M13.87** **Other specified arthritis,** ankle and foot

   M13.871 **Other specified arthritis,** right **ankle and foot**
   M13.872 **Other specified arthritis,** left **ankle and foot**
   M13.879 **Other specified arthritis, unspecified ankle and foot**

   M13.88 **Other specified arthritis, other site**
   M13.89 **Other specified arthritis,** multiple sites

☑4ᵗʰ **M14** **Arthropathies in other diseases classified elsewhere**

   EXCLUDES 1   *arthropathy in:*
     diabetes mellitus (E08-E13 with .61-)
     hematological disorders (M36.2-M36.3)
     hypersensitivity reactions (M36.4)
     neoplastic disease (M36.1)
     neurosyphillis (A52.16)
     sarcoidosis (D86.86)
    enteropathic arthropathies (M07.-)
    juvenile psoriatic arthropathy (L40.54)
    lipoid dermatoarthritis (E78.81)

☑5ᵗʰ **M14.6** **Charcôt's joint**

   Neuropathic arthropathy
   EXCLUDES 1   *Charcôt's joint in diabetes mellitus (E08-E13 with .610)*
      Charcôt's joint in tabes dorsalis (A52.16)
   DEF: Progressive neurologic arthropathy in which chronic degeneration of joints in the weight-bearing areas with peripheral hypertrophy occurs as a complication of a neuropathy disorder. Supporting structures relax from a loss of sensation resulting in chronic joint instability.

   M14.60 **Charcôt's joint, unspecified site**

☑6ᵗʰ **M14.61** **Charcôt's joint,** shoulder

   M14.611 **Charcôt's joint,** right **shoulder**
   M14.612 **Charcôt's joint,** left **shoulder**
   M14.619 **Charcôt's joint, unspecified shoulder**

☑6ᵗʰ **M14.62** **Charcôt's joint,** elbow

   M14.621 **Charcôt's joint,** right **elbow**
   M14.622 **Charcôt's joint,** left **elbow**
   M14.629 **Charcôt's joint, unspecified elbow**

☑6ᵗʰ **M14.63** **Charcôt's joint,** wrist

   M14.631 **Charcôt's joint,** right **wrist**
   M14.632 **Charcôt's joint,** left **wrist**
   M14.639 **Charcôt's joint, unspecified wrist**

☑6ᵗʰ **M14.64** **Charcôt's joint,** hand

   M14.641 **Charcôt's joint,** right **hand**
   M14.642 **Charcôt's joint,** left **hand**
   M14.649 **Charcôt's joint, unspecified hand**

☑6ᵗʰ **M14.65** **Charcôt's joint,** hip

   M14.651 **Charcôt's joint,** right **hip**
   M14.652 **Charcôt's joint,** left **hip**
   M14.659 **Charcôt's joint, unspecified hip**

☑6ᵗʰ **M14.66** **Charcôt's joint,** knee

   M14.661 **Charcôt's joint,** right **knee**
   M14.662 **Charcôt's joint,** left **knee**
   M14.669 **Charcôt's joint, unspecified knee**

☑6ᵗʰ **M14.67** **Charcôt's joint,** ankle and foot

   M14.671 **Charcôt's joint,** right **ankle and foot**
   M14.672 **Charcôt's joint,** left **ankle and foot**
   M14.679 **Charcôt's joint, unspecified ankle and foot**

   M14.68 **Charcôt's joint,** vertebrae
   M14.69 **Charcôt's joint,** multiple sites

☑5ᵗʰ **M14.8** **Arthropathies in other specified diseases classified elsewhere**

   Code first underlying disease, such as:
     amyloidosis (E85.-)
     erythema multiforme (L51.-)
     erythema nodosum (L52)
     hemochromatosis (E83.11-)
     hyperparathyroidism (E21.-)
     hypothyroidism (E00-E03)
     sickle-cell disorders (D57.-)
     thyrotoxicosis [hyperthyroidism] (E05.-)
     Whipple's disease (K90.81)

   M14.80 *Arthropathies in other specified diseases classified elsewhere, unspecified site*

☑6ᵗʰ **M14.81** **Arthropathies in other specified diseases classified elsewhere,** shoulder

   M14.811 *Arthropathies in other specified diseases classified elsewhere,* right *shoulder*
   M14.812 *Arthropathies in other specified diseases classified elsewhere,* left *shoulder*
   M14.819 *Arthropathies in other specified diseases classified elsewhere, unspecified shoulder*

☑6ᵗʰ **M14.82** **Arthropathies in other specified diseases classified elsewhere,** elbow

   M14.821 *Arthropathies in other specified diseases classified elsewhere,* right *elbow*
   M14.822 *Arthropathies in other specified diseases classified elsewhere,* left *elbow*
   M14.829 *Arthropathies in other specified diseases classified elsewhere, unspecified elbow*

☑6ᵗʰ **M14.83** **Arthropathies in other specified diseases classified elsewhere,** wrist

   M14.831 *Arthropathies in other specified diseases classified elsewhere,* right *wrist*
   M14.832 *Arthropathies in other specified diseases classified elsewhere,* left *wrist*
   M14.839 *Arthropathies in other specified diseases classified elsewhere, unspecified wrist*

☑6ᵗʰ **M14.84** **Arthropathies in other specified diseases classified elsewhere,** hand

   M14.841 *Arthropathies in other specified diseases classified elsewhere,* right *hand*
   M14.842 *Arthropathies in other specified diseases classified elsewhere,* left *hand*
   M14.849 *Arthropathies in other specified diseases classified elsewhere, unspecified hand*

☑6ᵗʰ **M14.85** **Arthropathies in other specified diseases classified elsewhere,** hip

   M14.851 *Arthropathies in other specified diseases classified elsewhere,* right *hip*
   M14.852 *Arthropathies in other specified diseases classified elsewhere,* left *hip*
   M14.859 *Arthropathies in other specified diseases classified elsewhere, unspecified hip*

☑6ᵗʰ **M14.86** **Arthropathies in other specified diseases classified elsewhere,** knee

   M14.861 *Arthropathies in other specified diseases classified elsewhere,* right *knee*
   M14.862 *Arthropathies in other specified diseases classified elsewhere,* left *knee*
   M14.869 *Arthropathies in other specified diseases classified elsewhere, unspecified knee*

☑6ᵗʰ **M14.87** **Arthropathies in other specified diseases classified elsewhere,** ankle and foot

   M14.871 *Arthropathies in other specified diseases classified elsewhere,* right *ankle and foot*
   M14.872 *Arthropathies in other specified diseases classified elsewhere,* left *ankle and foot*
   M14.879 *Arthropathies in other specified diseases classified elsewhere, unspecified ankle and foot*

   M14.88 *Arthropathies in other specified diseases classified elsewhere,* vertebrae
   M14.89 *Arthropathies in other specified diseases classified elsewhere,* multiple sites

☑ Additional Character Required   ☑x7ᵗʰ Placeholder   Unacceptable PDx   Questionable PDx   Manifestation   Unspecified Dx   H1-H14 HAC   HCC CMS-HCC Dx   HIV HIV Dx

ICD-10-CM 2021   777

Osteoarthritis (M15-M19)

EXCLUDES 2 *osteoarthritis of spine (M47.-)*
AHA: 2020,2Q,14; 2016,4Q,147
TIP: Assign a primary osteoarthritis code when the site of the osteoarthritis is documented but the type of osteoarthritis — primary, secondary, generalized, or post-traumatic — is not documented. Primary is considered the default.

✓4ᵗʰ **M15 Polyosteoarthritis**
     INCLUDES arthritis of multiple sites
     EXCLUDES 1 *bilateral involvement of single joint (M16-M19)*

     M15.0 Primary generalized (osteo)arthritis
     M15.1 Heberden's nodes (with arthropathy)
         Interphalangeal distal osteoarthritis
     M15.2 Bouchard's nodes (with arthropathy)
         Juxtaphalangeal distal osteoarthritis
     M15.3 Secondary multiple arthritis
         Post-traumatic polyosteoarthritis
     M15.4 Erosive (osteo)arthritis
     M15.8 Other polyosteoarthritis
     M15.9 Polyosteoarthritis, unspecified
         Generalized osteoarthritis NOS

✓4ᵗʰ **M16 Osteoarthritis of hip**
     AHA: 2016,4Q,146

     M16.0 Bilateral primary osteoarthritis of hip
         AHA: 2018,2Q,15
    ✓5ᵗʰ **M16.1 Unilateral primary osteoarthritis of hip**
         Primary osteoarthritis of hip NOS
         AHA: 2018,2Q,15
        M16.10 Unilateral primary osteoarthritis, unspecified hip
        M16.11 Unilateral primary osteoarthritis, right hip
        M16.12 Unilateral primary osteoarthritis, left hip
     M16.2 Bilateral osteoarthritis resulting from hip dysplasia
    ✓5ᵗʰ **M16.3 Unilateral osteoarthritis resulting from hip dysplasia**
         Dysplastic osteoarthritis of hip NOS
        M16.30 Unilateral osteoarthritis resulting from hip dysplasia, unspecified hip
        M16.31 Unilateral osteoarthritis resulting from hip dysplasia, right hip
        M16.32 Unilateral osteoarthritis resulting from hip dysplasia, left hip
     M16.4 Bilateral post-traumatic osteoarthritis of hip
    ✓5ᵗʰ **M16.5 Unilateral post-traumatic osteoarthritis of hip**
         Post-traumatic osteoarthritis of hip NOS
        M16.50 Unilateral post-traumatic osteoarthritis, unspecified hip
        M16.51 Unilateral post-traumatic osteoarthritis, right hip
        M16.52 Unilateral post-traumatic osteoarthritis, left hip
     M16.6 Other bilateral secondary osteoarthritis of hip
     M16.7 Other unilateral secondary osteoarthritis of hip
         Secondary osteoarthritis of hip NOS
     M16.9 Osteoarthritis of hip, unspecified

✓4ᵗʰ **M17 Osteoarthritis of knee**
     AHA: 2016,4Q,146-147

     M17.0 Bilateral primary osteoarthritis of knee
         AHA: 2018,2Q,15
    ✓5ᵗʰ **M17.1 Unilateral primary osteoarthritis of knee**
         Primary osteoarthritis of knee NOS
         AHA: 2018,2Q,15
        M17.10 Unilateral primary osteoarthritis, unspecified knee
        M17.11 Unilateral primary osteoarthritis, right knee
        M17.12 Unilateral primary osteoarthritis, left knee
     M17.2 Bilateral post-traumatic osteoarthritis of knee
    ✓5ᵗʰ **M17.3 Unilateral post-traumatic osteoarthritis of knee**
         Post-traumatic osteoarthritis of knee NOS
        M17.30 Unilateral post-traumatic osteoarthritis, unspecified knee
        M17.31 Unilateral post-traumatic osteoarthritis, right knee
        M17.32 Unilateral post-traumatic osteoarthritis, left knee
     M17.4 Other bilateral secondary osteoarthritis of knee
     M17.5 Other unilateral secondary osteoarthritis of knee
         Secondary osteoarthritis of knee NOS
     M17.9 Osteoarthritis of knee, unspecified

✓4ᵗʰ **M18 Osteoarthritis of first carpometacarpal joint**

     M18.0 Bilateral primary osteoarthritis of first carpometacarpal joints

✓5ᵗʰ **M18.1 Unilateral primary osteoarthritis of first carpometacarpal joint**
     Primary osteoarthritis of first carpometacarpal joint NOS
     M18.10 Unilateral primary osteoarthritis of first carpometacarpal joint, unspecified hand
     M18.11 Unilateral primary osteoarthritis of first carpometacarpal joint, right hand
     M18.12 Unilateral primary osteoarthritis of first carpometacarpal joint, left hand
     M18.2 Bilateral post-traumatic osteoarthritis of first carpometacarpal joints
✓5ᵗʰ **M18.3 Unilateral post-traumatic osteoarthritis of first carpometacarpal joint**
     Post-traumatic osteoarthritis of first carpometacarpal joint NOS
     M18.30 Unilateral post-traumatic osteoarthritis of first carpometacarpal joint, unspecified hand
     M18.31 Unilateral post-traumatic osteoarthritis of first carpometacarpal joint, right hand
     M18.32 Unilateral post-traumatic osteoarthritis of first carpometacarpal joint, left hand
     M18.4 Other bilateral secondary osteoarthritis of first carpometacarpal joints
✓5ᵗʰ **M18.5 Other unilateral secondary osteoarthritis of first carpometacarpal joint**
     Secondary osteoarthritis of first carpometacarpal joint NOS
     M18.50 Other unilateral secondary osteoarthritis of first carpometacarpal joint, unspecified hand
     M18.51 Other unilateral secondary osteoarthritis of first carpometacarpal joint, right hand
     M18.52 Other unilateral secondary osteoarthritis of first carpometacarpal joint, left hand
     M18.9 Osteoarthritis of first carpometacarpal joint, unspecified

✓4ᵗʰ **M19 Other and unspecified osteoarthritis**
     EXCLUDES 1 *polyarthritis (M15.-)*
     EXCLUDES 2 *arthrosis of spine (M47.-)*
              hallux rigidus (M20.2)
              osteoarthritis of spine (M47.-)

✓5ᵗʰ **M19.0 Primary osteoarthritis of other joints**
     AHA: 2018,2Q,15; 2016,4Q,145
    ✓6ᵗʰ **M19.01 Primary osteoarthritis, shoulder**
         M19.011 Primary osteoarthritis, right shoulder
         M19.012 Primary osteoarthritis, left shoulder
         M19.019 Primary osteoarthritis, unspecified shoulder
    ✓6ᵗʰ **M19.02 Primary osteoarthritis, elbow**
         M19.021 Primary osteoarthritis, right elbow
         M19.022 Primary osteoarthritis, left elbow
         M19.029 Primary osteoarthritis, unspecified elbow
    ✓6ᵗʰ **M19.03 Primary osteoarthritis, wrist**
         M19.031 Primary osteoarthritis, right wrist
         M19.032 Primary osteoarthritis, left wrist
         M19.039 Primary osteoarthritis, unspecified wrist
    ✓6ᵗʰ **M19.04 Primary osteoarthritis, hand**
         EXCLUDES 2 *primary osteoarthritis of first carpometacarpal joint (M18.0-, M18.1-)*
         M19.041 Primary osteoarthritis, right hand
         M19.042 Primary osteoarthritis, left hand
         M19.049 Primary osteoarthritis, unspecified hand
    ✓6ᵗʰ **M19.07 Primary osteoarthritis ankle and foot**
         M19.071 Primary osteoarthritis, right ankle and foot
         M19.072 Primary osteoarthritis, left ankle and foot
         M19.079 Primary osteoarthritis, unspecified ankle and foot
         M19.09 Primary osteoarthritis, other specified site
    ✓5ᵗʰ **M19.1 Post-traumatic osteoarthritis of other joints**
    ✓6ᵗʰ **M19.11 Post-traumatic osteoarthritis, shoulder**
         M19.111 Post-traumatic osteoarthritis, right shoulder
         M19.112 Post-traumatic osteoarthritis, left shoulder
         M19.119 Post-traumatic osteoarthritis, unspecified shoulder
    ✓6ᵗʰ **M19.12 Post-traumatic osteoarthritis, elbow**
         M19.121 Post-traumatic osteoarthritis, right elbow
         M19.122 Post-traumatic osteoarthritis, left elbow

N Newborn: 0   P Pediatric: 0-17   M Maternity: 9-64   A Adult: 15-124   MCC Major Complication/Comorbidity   CC Complication/Comorbidity   SW Severe Wound Dx

778   ICD-10-CM 2021

M19.129   Post-traumatic osteoarthritis, unspecified elbow

✓6ᵗʰ   **M19.13**   **Post-traumatic osteoarthritis, wrist**

M19.131   Post-traumatic osteoarthritis, right wrist

M19.132   Post-traumatic osteoarthritis, left wrist

M19.139   Post-traumatic osteoarthritis, unspecified wrist

✓6ᵗʰ   **M19.14**   **Post-traumatic osteoarthritis, hand**

EXCLUDES 2   post-traumatic osteoarthritis of first carpometacarpal joint (M18.2-, M18.3-)

M19.141   Post-traumatic osteoarthritis, right hand

M19.142   Post-traumatic osteoarthritis, left hand

M19.149   Post-traumatic osteoarthritis, unspecified hand

✓6ᵗʰ   **M19.17**   **Post-traumatic osteoarthritis, ankle and foot**

M19.171   Post-traumatic osteoarthritis, right ankle and foot

M19.172   Post-traumatic osteoarthritis, left ankle and foot

M19.179   Post-traumatic osteoarthritis, unspecified ankle and foot

M19.19   Post-traumatic osteoarthritis, other specified site

✓5ᵗʰ   **M19.2**   **Secondary osteoarthritis of other joints**

✓6ᵗʰ   **M19.21**   **Secondary osteoarthritis, shoulder**

M19.211   Secondary osteoarthritis, right shoulder

M19.212   Secondary osteoarthritis, left shoulder

M19.219   Secondary osteoarthritis, unspecified shoulder

✓6ᵗʰ   **M19.22**   **Secondary osteoarthritis, elbow**

M19.221   Secondary osteoarthritis, right elbow

M19.222   Secondary osteoarthritis, left elbow

M19.229   Secondary osteoarthritis, unspecified elbow

✓6ᵗʰ   **M19.23**   **Secondary osteoarthritis, wrist**

M19.231   Secondary osteoarthritis, right wrist

M19.232   Secondary osteoarthritis, left wrist

M19.239   Secondary osteoarthritis, unspecified wrist

✓6ᵗʰ   **M19.24**   **Secondary osteoarthritis, hand**

M19.241   Secondary osteoarthritis, right hand

M19.242   Secondary osteoarthritis, left hand

M19.249   Secondary osteoarthritis, unspecified hand

✓6ᵗʰ   **M19.27**   **Secondary osteoarthritis, ankle and foot**

M19.271   Secondary osteoarthritis, right ankle and foot

M19.272   Secondary osteoarthritis, left ankle and foot

M19.279   Secondary osteoarthritis, unspecified ankle and foot

M19.29   Secondary osteoarthritis, other specified site

✓5ᵗʰ   **M19.9**   **Osteoarthritis, unspecified site**

TIP: Assign M19.90 when neither the site nor the type of osteoarthritis — primary, secondary, or post-traumatic — is documented.

M19.90   **Unspecified osteoarthritis, unspecified site**
Arthrosis NOS
Arthritis NOS
Osteoarthritis NOS
AHA: 2016,4Q,145-147

M19.91   **Primary osteoarthritis, unspecified site**
Primary osteoarthritis NOS

M19.92   **Post-traumatic osteoarthritis, unspecified site**
Post-traumatic osteoarthritis NOS

M19.93   **Secondary osteoarthritis, unspecified site**
Secondary osteoarthritis NOS

Other joint disorders (M20-M25)

EXCLUDES 2   joints of the spine (M40-M54)

✓4ᵗʰ   **M20**   **Acquired deformities of fingers and toes**

EXCLUDES 1   acquired absence of fingers and toes (Z89.-)
congenital absence of fingers and toes (Q71.3-, Q72.3-)
congenital deformities and malformations of fingers and toes (Q66.-, Q68-Q70, Q74.-)

✓5ᵗʰ   **M20.0**   **Deformity of finger(s)**

EXCLUDES 1   clubbing of fingers (R68.3)
palmar fascial fibromatosis [Dupuytren] (M72.0)
trigger finger (M65.3)

✓6ᵗʰ   **M20.00**   **Unspecified deformity of finger(s)**

M20.001   Unspecified deformity of right finger(s)

M20.002   Unspecified deformity of left finger(s)

M20.009   Unspecified deformity of unspecified finger(s)

✓6ᵗʰ   **M20.01**   **Mallet finger**

M20.011   Mallet finger of right finger(s)

M20.012   Mallet finger of left finger(s)

M20.019   Mallet finger of unspecified finger(s)

✓6ᵗʰ   **M20.02**   **Boutonnière deformity**

DEF: Deformity of the finger caused by flexion of the proximal interphalangeal joint and hyperextension of the distal joint. The deformity results from rheumatoid arthritis, osteoarthritis, or injury.

M20.021   Boutonnière deformity of right finger(s)

M20.022   Boutonnière deformity of left finger(s)

M20.029   Boutonnière deformity of unspecified finger(s)

✓6ᵗʰ   **M20.03**   **Swan-neck deformity**

DEF: Flexed distal and hyperextended proximal interphalangeal joint most commonly caused by rheumatoid arthritis.

M20.031   Swan-neck deformity of right finger(s)

M20.032   Swan-neck deformity of left finger(s)

M20.039   Swan-neck deformity of unspecified finger(s)

✓6ᵗʰ   **M20.09**   **Other deformity of finger(s)**

M20.091   Other deformity of right finger(s)

M20.092   Other deformity of left finger(s)

M20.099   Other deformity of finger(s), unspecified finger(s)

✓5ᵗʰ   **M20.1**   **Hallux valgus (acquired)**

EXCLUDES 2   bunion (M21.6-)

AHA: 2016,4Q,38

DEF: Deformity in which the great toe deviates toward the other toes and may even be positioned over or under the second toe.

Hallux Valgus

Hallux valgus

Medial eminence of metatarsal bone

Right foot

M20.10   Hallux valgus (acquired), unspecified foot

M20.11   Hallux valgus (acquired), right foot

M20.12   Hallux valgus (acquired), left foot

☑ Additional Character Required   ✓x7ᵗʰ Placeholder   Unacceptable PDx   Questionable PDx   Manifestation   Unspecified Dx   H1-H14 HAC   HCC CMS-HCC Dx   HIV HIV Dx

ICD-10-CM 2021   779

√5ᵗʰ **M20.2** Hallux rigidus
- **M20.20** Hallux rigidus, unspecified foot
- **M20.21** Hallux rigidus, **right** foot
- **M20.22** Hallux rigidus, **left** foot

√5ᵗʰ **M20.3** Hallux varus (acquired)
> **DEF:** Deformity in which the great toe deviates away from the other toes.
- **M20.30** Hallux varus (acquired), unspecified foot
- **M20.31** Hallux varus (acquired), **right** foot
- **M20.32** Hallux varus (acquired), **left** foot

√5ᵗʰ **M20.4** Other hammer toe(s) (acquired)
- **M20.40** Other hammer toe(s) (acquired), unspecified foot
- **M20.41** Other hammer toe(s) (acquired), **right** foot
- **M20.42** Other hammer toe(s) (acquired), **left** foot

√5ᵗʰ **M20.5** Other deformities of toe(s) (acquired)
- √6ᵗʰ **M20.5X** Other deformities of **toe(s)** (acquired)
  - **M20.5X1** Other deformities of toe(s) (acquired), **right** foot
  - **M20.5X2** Other deformities of toe(s) (acquired), **left** foot
  - **M20.5X9** Other deformities of toe(s) (acquired), unspecified foot

√5ᵗʰ **M20.6** Acquired deformities of **toe(s)**, unspecified
- **M20.60** Acquired deformities of toe(s), unspecified, unspecified foot
- **M20.61** Acquired deformities of toe(s), unspecified, **right** foot
- **M20.62** Acquired deformities of toe(s), unspecified, **left** foot

√4ᵗʰ **M21** **Other acquired deformities of limbs**
> **EXCLUDES 1**   acquired absence of limb (Z89.-)
> congenital absence of limbs (Q71-Q73)
> congenital deformities and malformations of limbs (Q65-Q66, Q68-Q74)
> **EXCLUDES 2**   acquired deformities of fingers or toes (M20.-)
> coxa plana (M91.2)

√5ᵗʰ **M21.0** Valgus deformity, not elsewhere classified
> **EXCLUDES 1**   metatarsus valgus (Q66.6)
> talipes calcaneovalgus (Q66.4-)
- **M21.00** Valgus deformity, not elsewhere classified, unspecified site
- √6ᵗʰ **M21.02** Valgus deformity, not elsewhere classified, **elbow**
  > Cubitus valgus
  - **M21.021** Valgus deformity, not elsewhere classified, **right** elbow
  - **M21.022** Valgus deformity, not elsewhere classified, **left** elbow
  - **M21.029** Valgus deformity, not elsewhere classified, unspecified elbow
- √6ᵗʰ **M21.05** Valgus deformity, not elsewhere classified, **hip**
  - **M21.051** Valgus deformity, not elsewhere classified, **right** hip
  - **M21.052** Valgus deformity, not elsewhere classified, **left** hip
  - **M21.059** Valgus deformity, not elsewhere classified, unspecified hip

√6ᵗʰ **M21.06** Valgus deformity, not elsewhere classified, **knee**
> Genu valgum
> Knock knee
> **DEF:** Genu valga/valgum: Condition in which the thighs slant inward, causing the knees to be angled abnormally close together, leaving the space between the ankles wider than normal.

Genu Valga (knock-knee)

- **M21.061** Valgus deformity, not elsewhere classified, **right** knee
- **M21.062** Valgus deformity, not elsewhere classified, **left** knee
- **M21.069** Valgus deformity, not elsewhere classified, unspecified knee

√6ᵗʰ **M21.07** Valgus deformity, not elsewhere classified, **ankle**
- **M21.071** Valgus deformity, not elsewhere classified, **right** ankle
- **M21.072** Valgus deformity, not elsewhere classified, **left** ankle
- **M21.079** Valgus deformity, not elsewhere classified, unspecified ankle

√5ᵗʰ **M21.1** Varus deformity, not elsewhere classified
> **EXCLUDES 1**   metatarsus varus (Q66.22-)
> tibia vara ▶(M92.51-)◀
- **M21.10** Varus deformity, not elsewhere classified, unspecified site
- √6ᵗʰ **M21.12** Varus deformity, not elsewhere classified, **elbow**
  > Cubitus varus, elbow
  - **M21.121** Varus deformity, not elsewhere classified, **right** elbow
  - **M21.122** Varus deformity, not elsewhere classified, **left** elbow
  - **M21.129** Varus deformity, not elsewhere classified, unspecified elbow
- √6ᵗʰ **M21.15** Varus deformity, not elsewhere classified, **hip**
  - **M21.151** Varus deformity, not elsewhere classified, **right** hip
  - **M21.152** Varus deformity, not elsewhere classified, **left** hip
  - **M21.159** Varus deformity, not elsewhere classified, unspecified

✓6ᵗʰ **M21.16 Varus deformity, not elsewhere classified, knee**
Bow leg
Genu varum
DEF: Genu varus/varum: Condition in which the thighs and/or legs are bowed in an outward curve with an abnormally increased space between the knees.

Genu Varus (bowleg)

M21.161 Varus deformity, not elsewhere classified, right knee
M21.162 Varus deformity, not elsewhere classified, left knee
M21.169 Varus deformity, not elsewhere classified, unspecified knee

✓6ᵗʰ **M21.17 Varus deformity, not elsewhere classified, ankle**
M21.171 Varus deformity, not elsewhere classified, right ankle
M21.172 Varus deformity, not elsewhere classified, left ankle
M21.179 Varus deformity, not elsewhere classified, unspecified ankle

✓5ᵗʰ **M21.2 Flexion deformity**
M21.20 Flexion deformity, unspecified site
✓6ᵗʰ **M21.21 Flexion deformity, shoulder**
M21.211 Flexion deformity, right shoulder
M21.212 Flexion deformity, left shoulder
M21.219 Flexion deformity, unspecified shoulder
✓6ᵗʰ **M21.22 Flexion deformity, elbow**
M21.221 Flexion deformity, right elbow
M21.222 Flexion deformity, left elbow
M21.229 Flexion deformity, unspecified elbow
✓6ᵗʰ **M21.23 Flexion deformity, wrist**
M21.231 Flexion deformity, right wrist
M21.232 Flexion deformity, left wrist
M21.239 Flexion deformity, unspecified wrist
✓6ᵗʰ **M21.24 Flexion deformity, finger joints**
M21.241 Flexion deformity, right finger joints
M21.242 Flexion deformity, left finger joints
M21.249 Flexion deformity, unspecified finger joints
✓6ᵗʰ **M21.25 Flexion deformity, hip**
M21.251 Flexion deformity, right hip
M21.252 Flexion deformity, left hip
M21.259 Flexion deformity, unspecified hip
✓6ᵗʰ **M21.26 Flexion deformity, knee**
M21.261 Flexion deformity, right knee
M21.262 Flexion deformity, left knee
M21.269 Flexion deformity, unspecified knee
✓6ᵗʰ **M21.27 Flexion deformity, ankle and toes**
M21.271 Flexion deformity, right ankle and toes
M21.272 Flexion deformity, left ankle and toes
M21.279 Flexion deformity, unspecified ankle and toes

✓5ᵗʰ **M21.3 Wrist or foot drop (acquired)**
✓6ᵗʰ **M21.33 Wrist drop (acquired)**
M21.331 Wrist drop, right wrist
M21.332 Wrist drop, left wrist
M21.339 Wrist drop, unspecified wrist
✓6ᵗʰ **M21.37 Foot drop (acquired)**
M21.371 Foot drop, right foot
M21.372 Foot drop, left foot
M21.379 Foot drop, unspecified foot

✓5ᵗʰ **M21.4 Flat foot [pes planus] (acquired)**
EXCLUDES 1   congenital pes planus (Q66.5-)
M21.40 Flat foot [pes planus] (acquired), unspecified foot
M21.41 Flat foot [pes planus] (acquired), right foot
M21.42 Flat foot [pes planus] (acquired), left foot

✓5ᵗʰ **M21.5 Acquired clawhand, clubhand, clawfoot and clubfoot**
EXCLUDES 1   clubfoot, not specified as acquired (Q66.89)
✓6ᵗʰ **M21.51 Acquired clawhand**
M21.511 Acquired clawhand, right hand
M21.512 Acquired clawhand, left hand
M21.519 Acquired clawhand, unspecified hand
✓6ᵗʰ **M21.52 Acquired clubhand**
M21.521 Acquired clubhand, right hand
M21.522 Acquired clubhand, left hand
M21.529 Acquired clubhand, unspecified hand
✓6ᵗʰ **M21.53 Acquired clawfoot**
DEF: High foot arch with hyperextended toes at the metatarsophalangeal joint and flexed toes at the distal joints.
M21.531 Acquired clawfoot, right foot
M21.532 Acquired clawfoot, left foot
M21.539 Acquired clawfoot, unspecified foot
✓6ᵗʰ **M21.54 Acquired clubfoot**
DEF: Acquired anomaly of the foot with the heel elevated and rotated outward and the toes pointing inward.
M21.541 Acquired clubfoot, right foot
M21.542 Acquired clubfoot, left foot
M21.549 Acquired clubfoot, unspecified foot

✓5ᵗʰ **M21.6 Other acquired deformities of foot**
EXCLUDES 2   deformities of toe (acquired) (M20.1-M20.6-)
AHA: 2016,4Q,38
✓6ᵗʰ **M21.61 Bunion**
M21.611 Bunion of right foot
M21.612 Bunion of left foot
M21.619 Bunion of unspecified foot
✓6ᵗʰ **M21.62 Bunionette**
M21.621 Bunionette of right foot
M21.622 Bunionette of left foot
M21.629 Bunionette of unspecified foot
✓6ᵗʰ **M21.6X Other acquired deformities of foot**
M21.6X1 Other acquired deformities of right foot
M21.6X2 Other acquired deformities of left foot
M21.6X9 Other acquired deformities of unspecified foot

✓5ᵗʰ **M21.7 Unequal limb length (acquired)**
NOTE   The site used should correspond to the shorter limb
M21.70 Unequal limb length (acquired), unspecified site
✓6ᵗʰ **M21.72 Unequal limb length (acquired), humerus**
M21.721 Unequal limb length (acquired), right humerus
M21.722 Unequal limb length (acquired), left humerus
M21.729 Unequal limb length (acquired), unspecified humerus
✓6ᵗʰ **M21.73 Unequal limb length (acquired), ulna and radius**
M21.731 Unequal limb length (acquired), right ulna
M21.732 Unequal limb length (acquired), left ulna
M21.733 Unequal limb length (acquired), right radius
M21.734 Unequal limb length (acquired), left radius
M21.739 Unequal limb length (acquired), unspecified ulna and radius

√6ᵗʰ **M21.75** Unequal limb length (acquired), femur

     M21.751 Unequal limb length (acquired), right femur

     M21.752 Unequal limb length (acquired), left femur

     M21.759 Unequal limb length (acquired), unspecified femur

√6ᵗʰ **M21.76** Unequal limb length (acquired), tibia and fibula

     M21.761 Unequal limb length (acquired), right tibia

     M21.762 Unequal limb length (acquired), left tibia

     M21.763 Unequal limb length (acquired), right fibula

     M21.764 Unequal limb length (acquired), left fibula

     M21.769 Unequal limb length (acquired), unspecified tibia and fibula

√5ᵗʰ **M21.8** Other specified acquired deformities of limbs

     EXCLUDES 2   *coxa plana (M91.2)*

     M21.80 Other specified acquired deformities of unspecified limb

√6ᵗʰ **M21.82** Other specified acquired deformities of upper arm

     M21.821 Other specified acquired deformities of right upper arm

     M21.822 Other specified acquired deformities of left upper arm

     M21.829 Other specified acquired deformities of unspecified upper arm

√6ᵗʰ **M21.83** Other specified acquired deformities of forearm

     M21.831 Other specified acquired deformities of right forearm

     M21.832 Other specified acquired deformities of left forearm

     M21.839 Other specified acquired deformities of unspecified forearm

√6ᵗʰ **M21.85** Other specified acquired deformities of thigh

     M21.851 Other specified acquired deformities of right thigh

     M21.852 Other specified acquired deformities of left thigh

     M21.859 Other specified acquired deformities of unspecified thigh

√6ᵗʰ **M21.86** Other specified acquired deformities of lower leg

     M21.861 Other specified acquired deformities of right lower leg

     M21.862 Other specified acquired deformities of left lower leg

     M21.869 Other specified acquired deformities of unspecified lower leg

√5ᵗʰ **M21.9** Unspecified acquired deformity of limb and hand

     M21.90 Unspecified acquired deformity of unspecified limb

√6ᵗʰ **M21.92** Unspecified acquired deformity of upper arm

     M21.921 Unspecified acquired deformity of right upper arm

     M21.922 Unspecified acquired deformity of left upper arm

     M21.929 Unspecified acquired deformity of unspecified upper arm

√6ᵗʰ **M21.93** Unspecified acquired deformity of forearm

     M21.931 Unspecified acquired deformity of right forearm

     M21.932 Unspecified acquired deformity of left forearm

     M21.939 Unspecified acquired deformity of unspecified forearm

√6ᵗʰ **M21.94** Unspecified acquired deformity of hand

     M21.941 Unspecified acquired deformity of hand, right hand

     M21.942 Unspecified acquired deformity of hand, left hand

     M21.949 Unspecified acquired deformity of hand, unspecified hand

√6ᵗʰ **M21.95** Unspecified acquired deformity of thigh

     M21.951 Unspecified acquired deformity of right thigh

     M21.952 Unspecified acquired deformity of left thigh

     M21.959 Unspecified acquired deformity of unspecified thigh

√6ᵗʰ **M21.96** Unspecified acquired deformity of lower leg

     M21.961 Unspecified acquired deformity of right lower leg

     M21.962 Unspecified acquired deformity of left lower leg

     M21.969 Unspecified acquired deformity of unspecified lower leg

√4ᵗʰ **M22** Disorder of patella

     EXCLUDES 1   *traumatic dislocation of patella (S83.0-)*

     EXCLUDES 2   ▶*traumatic dislocation of patella (S83.0-)*◀

√5ᵗʰ **M22.0** Recurrent dislocation of patella

     M22.00 Recurrent dislocation of patella, unspecified knee

     M22.01 Recurrent dislocation of patella, right knee

     M22.02 Recurrent dislocation of patella, left knee

√5ᵗʰ **M22.1** Recurrent subluxation of patella

     Incomplete dislocation of patella

     M22.10 Recurrent subluxation of patella, unspecified knee

     M22.11 Recurrent subluxation of patella, right knee

     M22.12 Recurrent subluxation of patella, left knee

√5ᵗʰ **M22.2** Patellofemoral disorders

     √6ᵗʰ **M22.2X** Patellofemoral disorders

         M22.2X1 Patellofemoral disorders, right knee

         M22.2X2 Patellofemoral disorders, left knee

         M22.2X9 Patellofemoral disorders, unspecified knee

√5ᵗʰ **M22.3** Other derangements of patella

     √6ᵗʰ **M22.3X** Other derangements of patella

         M22.3X1 Other derangements of patella, right knee

         M22.3X2 Other derangements of patella, left knee

         M22.3X9 Other derangements of patella, unspecified knee

√5ᵗʰ **M22.4** Chondromalacia patellae

     M22.40 Chondromalacia patellae, unspecified knee

     M22.41 Chondromalacia patellae, right knee

     M22.42 Chondromalacia patellae, left knee

√5ᵗʰ **M22.8** Other disorders of patella

     √6ᵗʰ **M22.8X** Other disorders of patella

         M22.8X1 Other disorders of patella, right knee

         M22.8X2 Other disorders of patella, left knee

         M22.8X9 Other disorders of patella, unspecified knee

√5ᵗʰ **M22.9** Unspecified disorder of patella

     M22.90 Unspecified disorder of patella, unspecified knee

     M22.91 Unspecified disorder of patella, right knee

     M22.92 Unspecified disorder of patella, left knee

√4ᵗʰ **M23** Internal derangement of knee

     EXCLUDES 1   *ankylosis (M24.66)*

         current injury — see injury of knee and lower leg (S80-S89)

         deformity of knee (M21.-)

         osteochondritis dissecans (M93.2)

         recurrent dislocation or subluxation of joints (M24.4)

         recurrent dislocation or subluxation of patella (M22.0-M22.1)

     EXCLUDES 2   ▶*current injury — see injury of knee and lower leg (S80-S89)*◀

         ▶*recurrent dislocation or subluxation of joints (M24.4)*◀

         ▶*recurrent dislocation or subluxation of patella (M22.0-M22.1)*◀

√5ᵗʰ **M23.0** Cystic meniscus

     √6ᵗʰ **M23.00** Cystic meniscus, unspecified meniscus

         Cystic meniscus, unspecified lateral meniscus

         Cystic meniscus, unspecified medial meniscus

         M23.000 Cystic meniscus, unspecified lateral meniscus, right knee

         M23.001 Cystic meniscus, unspecified lateral meniscus, left knee

         M23.002 Cystic meniscus, unspecified lateral meniscus, unspecified knee

         M23.003 Cystic meniscus, unspecified medial meniscus, right knee

         M23.004 Cystic meniscus, unspecified medial meniscus, left knee

         M23.005 Cystic meniscus, unspecified medial meniscus, unspecified knee

         M23.006 Cystic meniscus, unspecified meniscus, right knee

N Newborn: 0   P Pediatric: 0-17   M Maternity: 9-64   A Adult: 15-124   MCC Major Complication/Comorbidity   CC Complication/Comorbidity   SW Severe Wound Dx

782   ICD-10-CM 2021

M23.007 Cystic meniscus, unspecified meniscus, left knee

M23.009 Cystic meniscus, unspecified meniscus, unspecified knee

√6ᵗʰ **M23.01** Cystic meniscus, anterior horn of medial meniscus

   M23.011 Cystic meniscus, anterior horn of medial meniscus, right knee

   M23.012 Cystic meniscus, anterior horn of medial meniscus, left knee

   M23.019 Cystic meniscus, anterior horn of medial meniscus, unspecified knee

√6ᵗʰ **M23.02** Cystic meniscus, posterior horn of medial meniscus

   M23.021 Cystic meniscus, posterior horn of medial meniscus, right knee

   M23.022 Cystic meniscus, posterior horn of medial meniscus, left knee

   M23.029 Cystic meniscus, posterior horn of medial meniscus, unspecified knee

√6ᵗʰ **M23.03** Cystic meniscus, other medial meniscus

   M23.031 Cystic meniscus, other medial meniscus, right knee

   M23.032 Cystic meniscus, other medial meniscus, left knee

   M23.039 Cystic meniscus, other medial meniscus, unspecified knee

√6ᵗʰ **M23.04** Cystic meniscus, anterior horn of lateral meniscus

   M23.041 Cystic meniscus, anterior horn of lateral meniscus, right knee

   M23.042 Cystic meniscus, anterior horn of lateral meniscus, left knee

   M23.049 Cystic meniscus, anterior horn of lateral meniscus, unspecified knee

√6ᵗʰ **M23.05** Cystic meniscus, posterior horn of lateral meniscus

   M23.051 Cystic meniscus, posterior horn of lateral meniscus, right knee

   M23.052 Cystic meniscus, posterior horn of lateral meniscus, left knee

   M23.059 Cystic meniscus, posterior horn of lateral meniscus, unspecified knee

√6ᵗʰ **M23.06** Cystic meniscus, other lateral meniscus

   M23.061 Cystic meniscus, other lateral meniscus, right knee

   M23.062 Cystic meniscus, other lateral meniscus, left knee

   M23.069 Cystic meniscus, other lateral meniscus, unspecified knee

√5ᵗʰ **M23.2** Derangement of meniscus due to old tear or injury

Old bucket-handle tear

AHA: 2019,2Q,26

Derangement of Meniscus

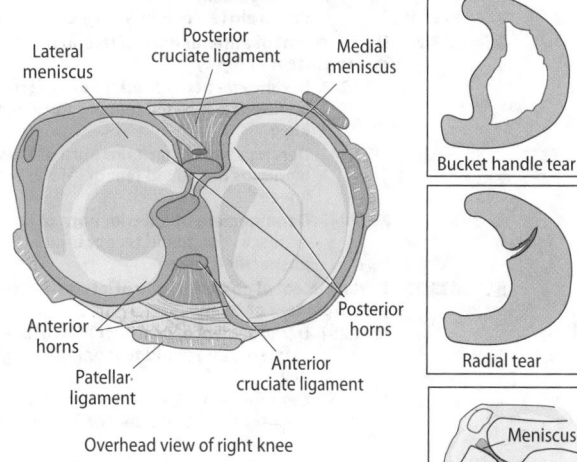

Overhead view of right knee

Bucket handle tear

Radial tear

Meniscus

√6ᵗʰ **M23.20** Derangement of unspecified meniscus due to old tear or injury

Derangement of unspecified lateral meniscus due to old tear or injury

Derangement of unspecified medial meniscus due to old tear or injury

   M23.200 Derangement of unspecified lateral meniscus due to old tear or injury, right knee

   M23.201 Derangement of unspecified lateral meniscus due to old tear or injury, left knee

   M23.202 Derangement of unspecified lateral meniscus due to old tear or injury, unspecified knee

   M23.203 Derangement of unspecified medial meniscus due to old tear or injury, right knee

   M23.204 Derangement of unspecified medial meniscus due to old tear or injury, left knee

   M23.205 Derangement of unspecified medial meniscus due to old tear or injury, unspecified knee

   M23.206 Derangement of unspecified meniscus due to old tear or injury, right knee

   M23.207 Derangement of unspecified meniscus due to old tear or injury, left knee

   M23.209 Derangement of unspecified meniscus due to old tear or injury, unspecified knee

√6ᵗʰ **M23.21** Derangement of anterior horn of medial meniscus due to old tear or injury

   M23.211 Derangement of anterior horn of medial meniscus due to old tear or injury, right knee

   M23.212 Derangement of anterior horn of medial meniscus due to old tear or injury, left knee

   M23.219 Derangement of anterior horn of medial meniscus due to old tear or injury, unspecified knee

√6ᵗʰ **M23.22** Derangement of posterior horn of medial meniscus due to old tear or injury

   M23.221 Derangement of posterior horn of medial meniscus due to old tear or injury, right knee

   M23.222 Derangement of posterior horn of medial meniscus due to old tear or injury, left knee

   M23.229 Derangement of posterior horn of medial meniscus due to old tear or injury, unspecified knee

✓ Additional Character Required   √x7ᵗʰ Placeholder   Unacceptable PDx   Questionable PDx   Manifestation   Unspecified Dx   H1-H14 HAC   HCC CMS-HCC Dx   HIV HIV Dx

ICD-10-CM 2021   783

✓6ᵗʰ **M23.23 Derangement of** other medial **meniscus due to old tear or injury**

    M23.231 Derangement of other medial meniscus due to old tear or injury, right knee

    M23.232 Derangement of other medial meniscus due to old tear or injury, left knee

    M23.239 Derangement of other medial meniscus due to old tear or injury, unspecified knee

✓6ᵗʰ **M23.24 Derangement of** anterior horn of lateral **meniscus due to old tear or injury**

    M23.241 Derangement of anterior horn of lateral meniscus due to old tear or injury, right knee

    M23.242 Derangement of anterior horn of lateral meniscus due to old tear or injury, left knee

    M23.249 Derangement of anterior horn of lateral meniscus due to old tear or injury, unspecified knee

✓6ᵗʰ **M23.25 Derangement of** posterior horn of lateral **meniscus due to old tear or injury**

    M23.251 Derangement of posterior horn of lateral meniscus due to old tear or injury, right knee

    M23.252 Derangement of posterior horn of lateral meniscus due to old tear or injury, left knee

    M23.259 Derangement of posterior horn of lateral meniscus due to old tear or injury, unspecified knee

✓6ᵗʰ **M23.26 Derangement of** other lateral **meniscus due to old tear or injury**

    M23.261 Derangement of other lateral meniscus due to old tear or injury, right knee

    M23.262 Derangement of other lateral meniscus due to old tear or injury, left knee

    M23.269 Derangement of other lateral meniscus due to old tear or injury, unspecified knee

✓5ᵗʰ **M23.3 Other meniscus derangements**

    Degenerate meniscus

    Detached meniscus

    Retained meniscus

✓6ᵗʰ **M23.30 Other meniscus derangements, unspecified meniscus**

    Other meniscus derangements, unspecified lateral meniscus

    Other meniscus derangements, unspecified medial meniscus

    M23.300 Other meniscus derangements, unspecified lateral meniscus, right knee

    M23.301 Other meniscus derangements, unspecified lateral meniscus, left knee

    M23.302 Other meniscus derangements, unspecified lateral meniscus, unspecified knee

    M23.303 Other meniscus derangements, unspecified medial meniscus, right knee

    M23.304 Other meniscus derangements, unspecified medial meniscus, left knee

    M23.305 Other meniscus derangements, unspecified medial meniscus, unspecified knee

    M23.306 Other meniscus derangements, unspecified meniscus, right knee

    M23.307 Other meniscus derangements, unspecified meniscus, left knee

    M23.309 Other meniscus derangements, unspecified meniscus, unspecified knee

✓6ᵗʰ **M23.31 Other meniscus derangements,** anterior horn of medial **meniscus**

    M23.311 Other meniscus derangements, anterior horn of medial meniscus, right knee

    M23.312 Other meniscus derangements, anterior horn of medial meniscus, left knee

    M23.319 Other meniscus derangements, anterior horn of medial meniscus, unspecified knee

✓6ᵗʰ **M23.32 Other meniscus derangements,** posterior horn of medial **meniscus**

    M23.321 Other meniscus derangements, posterior horn of medial meniscus, right knee

    M23.322 Other meniscus derangements, posterior horn of medial meniscus, left knee

    M23.329 Other meniscus derangements, posterior horn of medial meniscus, unspecified knee

✓6ᵗʰ **M23.33 Other meniscus derangements,** other medial **meniscus**

    M23.331 Other meniscus derangements, other medial meniscus, right knee

    M23.332 Other meniscus derangements, other medial meniscus, left knee

    M23.339 Other meniscus derangements, other medial meniscus, unspecified knee

✓6ᵗʰ **M23.34 Other meniscus derangements,** anterior horn of lateral **meniscus**

    M23.341 Other meniscus derangements, anterior horn of lateral meniscus, right knee

    M23.342 Other meniscus derangements, anterior horn of lateral meniscus, left knee

    M23.349 Other meniscus derangements, anterior horn of lateral meniscus, unspecified knee

✓6ᵗʰ **M23.35 Other meniscus derangements,** posterior horn of lateral **meniscus**

    M23.351 Other meniscus derangements, posterior horn of lateral meniscus, right knee

    M23.352 Other meniscus derangements, posterior horn of lateral meniscus, left knee

    M23.359 Other meniscus derangements, posterior horn of lateral meniscus, unspecified knee

✓6ᵗʰ **M23.36 Other meniscus derangements,** other lateral **meniscus**

    M23.361 Other meniscus derangements, other lateral meniscus, right knee

    M23.362 Other meniscus derangements, other lateral meniscus, left knee

    M23.369 Other meniscus derangements, other lateral meniscus, unspecified knee

✓5ᵗʰ **M23.4 Loose body in knee**

    M23.40 Loose body in knee, unspecified knee

    M23.41 Loose body in knee, right knee

    M23.42 Loose body in knee, left knee

✓5ᵗʰ **M23.5 Chronic instability of knee**

    M23.50 Chronic instability of knee, unspecified knee

    M23.51 Chronic instability of knee, right knee

    M23.52 Chronic instability of knee, left knee

✓5ᵗʰ **M23.6 Other spontaneous disruption of ligament(s) of knee**

✓6ᵗʰ **M23.60 Other spontaneous disruption of unspecified ligament of knee**

    M23.601 Other spontaneous disruption of unspecified ligament of right knee

    M23.602 Other spontaneous disruption of unspecified ligament of left knee

    M23.609 Other spontaneous disruption of unspecified ligament of unspecified knee

✓6ᵗʰ **M23.61 Other spontaneous disruption of** anterior cruciate **ligament of knee**

    M23.611 Other spontaneous disruption of anterior cruciate ligament of right knee

    M23.612 Other spontaneous disruption of anterior cruciate ligament of left knee

    M23.619 Other spontaneous disruption of anterior cruciate ligament of unspecified knee

✓6ᵗʰ **M23.62 Other spontaneous disruption of** posterior cruciate **ligament of knee**

    M23.621 Other spontaneous disruption of posterior cruciate ligament of right knee

    M23.622 Other spontaneous disruption of posterior cruciate ligament of left knee

    M23.629 Other spontaneous disruption of posterior cruciate ligament of unspecified knee

✓6ᵗʰ **M23.63 Other spontaneous disruption of** medial collateral **ligament of knee**

    M23.631 Other spontaneous disruption of medial collateral ligament of right knee

    M23.632 Other spontaneous disruption of medial collateral ligament of left knee

    M23.639 Other spontaneous disruption of medial collateral ligament of unspecified knee

N Newborn: 0   P Pediatric: 0-17   M Maternity: 9-64   A Adult: 15-124   MCC Major Complication/Comorbidity   CC Complication/Comorbidity   SW Severe Wound Dx

784   ICD-10-CM 2021

✓6ᵗʰ **M23.64** Other spontaneous disruption of lateral collateral ligament of knee

     M23.641 Other spontaneous disruption of lateral collateral ligament of right knee

     M23.642 Other spontaneous disruption of lateral collateral ligament of left knee

     M23.649 Other spontaneous disruption of lateral collateral ligament of unspecified knee

✓6ᵗʰ **M23.67** Other spontaneous disruption of capsular ligament of knee

     M23.671 Other spontaneous disruption of capsular ligament of right knee

     M23.672 Other spontaneous disruption of capsular ligament of left knee

     M23.679 Other spontaneous disruption of capsular ligament of unspecified knee

✓5ᵗʰ **M23.8** Other internal derangements of knee

     Laxity of ligament of knee

     Snapping knee

     ✓6ᵗʰ **M23.8X** Other internal derangements of knee

        M23.8X1 Other internal derangements of right knee

        M23.8X2 Other internal derangements of left knee

        M23.8X9 Other internal derangements of unspecified knee

✓5ᵗʰ **M23.9** Unspecified internal derangement of knee

     M23.90 Unspecified internal derangement of unspecified knee

     M23.91 Unspecified internal derangement of right knee

     M23.92 Unspecified internal derangement of left knee

✓4ᵗʰ **M24** **Other specific joint derangements**

     EXCLUDES 1   current injury — see injury of joint by body region

     EXCLUDES 2   ganglion (M67.4)

                 snapping knee (M23.8-)

                 temporomandibular joint disorders (M26.6-)

✓5ᵗʰ **M24.0** Loose body in joint

     EXCLUDES 2   loose body in knee (M23.4)

     M24.00 Loose body in unspecified joint

     ✓6ᵗʰ **M24.01** Loose body in shoulder

        M24.011 Loose body in right shoulder

        M24.012 Loose body in left shoulder

        M24.019 Loose body in unspecified shoulder

     ✓6ᵗʰ **M24.02** Loose body in elbow

        M24.021 Loose body in right elbow

        M24.022 Loose body in left elbow

        M24.029 Loose body in unspecified elbow

     ✓6ᵗʰ **M24.03** Loose body in wrist

        M24.031 Loose body in right wrist

        M24.032 Loose body in left wrist

        M24.039 Loose body in unspecified wrist

     ✓6ᵗʰ **M24.04** Loose body in finger joints

        M24.041 Loose body in right finger joint(s)

        M24.042 Loose body in left finger joint(s)

        M24.049 Loose body in unspecified finger joint(s)

     ✓6ᵗʰ **M24.05** Loose body in hip

        M24.051 Loose body in right hip

        M24.052 Loose body in left hip

        M24.059 Loose body in unspecified hip

     ✓6ᵗʰ **M24.07** Loose body in ankle and toe joints

        M24.071 Loose body in right ankle

        M24.072 Loose body in left ankle

        M24.073 Loose body in unspecified ankle

        M24.074 Loose body in right toe joint(s)

        M24.075 Loose body in left toe joint(s)

        M24.076 Loose body in unspecified toe joints

     M24.08 Loose body, other site

✓5ᵗʰ **M24.1** Other articular cartilage disorders

     EXCLUDES 2   chondrocalcinosis (M11.1, M11.2-)

                 internal derangement of knee (M23.-)

                 metastatic calcification (E83.5)

                 ochronosis (E70.2)

     M24.10 Other articular cartilage disorders, unspecified site

     ✓6ᵗʰ **M24.11** Other articular cartilage disorders, shoulder

        M24.111 Other articular cartilage disorders, right shoulder

        M24.112 Other articular cartilage disorders, left shoulder

        M24.119 Other articular cartilage disorders, unspecified shoulder

     ✓6ᵗʰ **M24.12** Other articular cartilage disorders, elbow

        M24.121 Other articular cartilage disorders, right elbow

        M24.122 Other articular cartilage disorders, left elbow

        M24.129 Other articular cartilage disorders, unspecified elbow

     ✓6ᵗʰ **M24.13** Other articular cartilage disorders, wrist

        M24.131 Other articular cartilage disorders, right wrist

        M24.132 Other articular cartilage disorders, left wrist

        M24.139 Other articular cartilage disorders, unspecified wrist

     ✓6ᵗʰ **M24.14** Other articular cartilage disorders, hand

        M24.141 Other articular cartilage disorders, right hand

        M24.142 Other articular cartilage disorders, left hand

        M24.149 Other articular cartilage disorders, unspecified hand

     ✓6ᵗʰ **M24.15** Other articular cartilage disorders, hip

        M24.151 Other articular cartilage disorders, right hip

        M24.152 Other articular cartilage disorders, left hip

        M24.159 Other articular cartilage disorders, unspecified hip

     ✓6ᵗʰ **M24.17** Other articular cartilage disorders, ankle and foot

        M24.171 Other articular cartilage disorders, right ankle

        M24.172 Other articular cartilage disorders, left ankle

        M24.173 Other articular cartilage disorders, unspecified ankle

        M24.174 Other articular cartilage disorders, right foot

        M24.175 Other articular cartilage disorders, left foot

        M24.176 Other articular cartilage disorders, unspecified foot

     M24.19 Other articular cartilage disorders, other specified site

✓5ᵗʰ **M24.2** Disorder of ligament

     Instability secondary to old ligament injury

     Ligamentous laxity NOS

     EXCLUDES 1   familial ligamentous laxity (M35.7)

     EXCLUDES 2   internal derangement of knee (M23.5-M23.8X9)

     M24.20 Disorder of ligament, unspecified site

     ✓6ᵗʰ **M24.21** Disorder of ligament, shoulder

        M24.211 Disorder of ligament, right shoulder

        M24.212 Disorder of ligament, left shoulder

        M24.219 Disorder of ligament, unspecified shoulder

     ✓6ᵗʰ **M24.22** Disorder of ligament, elbow

        M24.221 Disorder of ligament, right elbow

        M24.222 Disorder of ligament, left elbow

        M24.229 Disorder of ligament, unspecified elbow

     ✓6ᵗʰ **M24.23** Disorder of ligament, wrist

        M24.231 Disorder of ligament, right wrist

        M24.232 Disorder of ligament, left wrist

        M24.239 Disorder of ligament, unspecified wrist

     ✓6ᵗʰ **M24.24** Disorder of ligament, hand

        M24.241 Disorder of ligament, right hand

        M24.242 Disorder of ligament, left hand

        M24.249 Disorder of ligament, unspecified hand

     ✓6ᵗʰ **M24.25** Disorder of ligament, hip

        M24.251 Disorder of ligament, right hip

        M24.252 Disorder of ligament, left hip

        M24.259 Disorder of ligament, unspecified hip

     ✓6ᵗʰ **M24.27** Disorder of ligament, ankle and foot

        M24.271 Disorder of ligament, right ankle

        M24.272 Disorder of ligament, left ankle

        M24.273 Disorder of ligament, unspecified ankle

☑ Additional Character Required   ✓x7ᵗʰ Placeholder   Unacceptable PDx   Questionable PDx   Manifestation   Unspecified Dx   H1 - H14 HAC   HCC CMS-HCC Dx   HIV HIV Dx

ICD-10-CM 2021   785

M24.274 Disorder of ligament, right foot
M24.275 Disorder of ligament, left foot
M24.276 Disorder of ligament, unspecified foot
M24.28 Disorder of ligament, vertebrae
● M24.29 Disorder of ligament, other specified site

√5ᵗʰ M24.3 Pathological dislocation of joint, not elsewhere classified

EXCLUDES 1   congenital dislocation or displacement of joint —
see congenital malformations and deformations
of the musculoskeletal system (Q65-Q79)
current injury — see injury of joints and ligaments
by body region
recurrent dislocation of joint (M24.4-)

M24.30 Pathological dislocation of unspecified joint, not
elsewhere classified
√6ᵗʰ M24.31 Pathological dislocation of shoulder, not elsewhere
classified
M24.311 Pathological dislocation of right
shoulder, not elsewhere classified
M24.312 Pathological dislocation of left shoulder,
not elsewhere classified
M24.319 Pathological dislocation of unspecified
shoulder, not elsewhere classified
√6ᵗʰ M24.32 Pathological dislocation of elbow, not elsewhere
classified
M24.321 Pathological dislocation of right elbow,
not elsewhere classified
M24.322 Pathological dislocation of left elbow, not
elsewhere classified
M24.329 Pathological dislocation of unspecified
elbow, not elsewhere classified
√6ᵗʰ M24.33 Pathological dislocation of wrist, not elsewhere
classified
M24.331 Pathological dislocation of right wrist,
not elsewhere classified
M24.332 Pathological dislocation of left wrist, not
elsewhere classified
M24.339 Pathological dislocation of unspecified
wrist, not elsewhere classified
√6ᵗʰ M24.34 Pathological dislocation of hand, not elsewhere
classified
M24.341 Pathological dislocation of right hand,
not elsewhere classified
M24.342 Pathological dislocation of left hand, not
elsewhere classified
M24.349 Pathological dislocation of unspecified
hand, not elsewhere classified
√6ᵗʰ M24.35 Pathological dislocation of hip, not elsewhere
classified
M24.351 Pathological dislocation of right hip, not
elsewhere classified
M24.352 Pathological dislocation of left hip, not
elsewhere classified
M24.359 Pathological dislocation of unspecified
hip, not elsewhere classified
√6ᵗʰ M24.36 Pathological dislocation of knee, not elsewhere
classified
M24.361 Pathological dislocation of right knee,
not elsewhere classified
M24.362 Pathological dislocation of left knee, not
elsewhere classified
M24.369 Pathological dislocation of unspecified
knee, not elsewhere classified
√6ᵗʰ M24.37 Pathological dislocation of ankle and foot, not
elsewhere classified
M24.371 Pathological dislocation of right ankle,
not elsewhere classified
M24.372 Pathological dislocation of left ankle, not
elsewhere classified
M24.373 Pathological dislocation of unspecified
ankle, not elsewhere classified
M24.374 Pathological dislocation of right foot, not
elsewhere classified
M24.375 Pathological dislocation of left foot, not
elsewhere classified
M24.376 Pathological dislocation of unspecified
foot, not elsewhere classified
● M24.39 Pathological dislocation of other specified joint,
not elsewhere classified

√5ᵗʰ M24.4 Recurrent dislocation of joint
Recurrent subluxation of joint
EXCLUDES 2   recurrent dislocation of patella (M22.0-M22.1)
recurrent vertebral dislocation (M43.3-, M43.4,
M43.5-)
M24.40 Recurrent dislocation, unspecified joint
√6ᵗʰ M24.41 Recurrent dislocation, shoulder
M24.411 Recurrent dislocation, right shoulder
M24.412 Recurrent dislocation, left shoulder
M24.419 Recurrent dislocation, unspecified
shoulder
√6ᵗʰ M24.42 Recurrent dislocation, elbow
M24.421 Recurrent dislocation, right elbow
M24.422 Recurrent dislocation, left elbow
M24.429 Recurrent dislocation, unspecified elbow
√6ᵗʰ M24.43 Recurrent dislocation, wrist
M24.431 Recurrent dislocation, right wrist
M24.432 Recurrent dislocation, left wrist
M24.439 Recurrent dislocation, unspecified wrist
√6ᵗʰ M24.44 Recurrent dislocation, hand and finger(s)
M24.441 Recurrent dislocation, right hand
M24.442 Recurrent dislocation, left hand
M24.443 Recurrent dislocation, unspecified hand
M24.444 Recurrent dislocation, right finger
M24.445 Recurrent dislocation, left finger
M24.446 Recurrent dislocation, unspecified finger
√6ᵗʰ M24.45 Recurrent dislocation, hip
M24.451 Recurrent dislocation, right hip
M24.452 Recurrent dislocation, left hip
M24.459 Recurrent dislocation, unspecified hip
√6ᵗʰ M24.46 Recurrent dislocation, knee
M24.461 Recurrent dislocation, right knee
M24.462 Recurrent dislocation, left knee
M24.469 Recurrent dislocation, unspecified knee
√6ᵗʰ M24.47 Recurrent dislocation, ankle, foot and toes
M24.471 Recurrent dislocation, right ankle
M24.472 Recurrent dislocation, left ankle
M24.473 Recurrent dislocation, unspecified ankle
M24.474 Recurrent dislocation, right foot
M24.475 Recurrent dislocation, left foot
M24.476 Recurrent dislocation, unspecified foot
M24.477 Recurrent dislocation, right toe(s)
M24.478 Recurrent dislocation, left toe(s)
M24.479 Recurrent dislocation, unspecified toe(s)
● M24.49 Recurrent dislocation, other specified joint

√5ᵗʰ M24.5 Contracture of joint
EXCLUDES 1   contracture of muscle without contracture of joint
(M62.4-)
contracture of tendon (sheath) without contracture
of joint (M62.4-)
Dupuytren's contracture (M72.0)
EXCLUDES 2   acquired deformities of limbs (M20-M21)
AHA: 2016,2Q,6
M24.50 Contracture, unspecified joint
√6ᵗʰ M24.51 Contracture, shoulder
M24.511 Contracture, right shoulder
M24.512 Contracture, left shoulder
M24.519 Contracture, unspecified shoulder
√6ᵗʰ M24.52 Contracture, elbow
M24.521 Contracture, right elbow
M24.522 Contracture, left elbow
M24.529 Contracture, unspecified elbow
√6ᵗʰ M24.53 Contracture, wrist
M24.531 Contracture, right wrist
M24.532 Contracture, left wrist
M24.539 Contracture, unspecified wrist
√6ᵗʰ M24.54 Contracture, hand
M24.541 Contracture, right hand
M24.542 Contracture, left hand
M24.549 Contracture, unspecified hand
√6ᵗʰ M24.55 Contracture, hip
M24.551 Contracture, right hip
M24.552 Contracture, left hip
M24.559 Contracture, unspecified hip

√6ᵗʰ **M24.56 Contracture, knee**

M24.561 Contracture, right knee
M24.562 Contracture, left knee
M24.569 Contracture, unspecified knee

√6ᵗʰ **M24.57 Contracture, ankle and foot**

M24.571 Contracture, right ankle
M24.572 Contracture, left ankle
M24.573 Contracture, unspecified ankle
M24.574 Contracture, right foot
M24.575 Contracture, left foot
M24.576 Contracture, unspecified foot

● **M24.59 Contracture, other specified joint**

√5ᵗʰ **M24.6 Ankylosis of joint**

> **EXCLUDES 1** *stiffness of joint without ankylosis (M25.6-)*
> **EXCLUDES 2** *spine (M43.2-)*
> **DEF:** Ankylosis: Abnormal union or fusion of bones in a joint, which is normally moveable.

M24.60 Ankylosis, unspecified joint

√6ᵗʰ **M24.61 Ankylosis, shoulder**

M24.611 Ankylosis, right shoulder
M24.612 Ankylosis, left shoulder
M24.619 Ankylosis, unspecified shoulder

√6ᵗʰ **M24.62 Ankylosis, elbow**

M24.621 Ankylosis, right elbow
M24.622 Ankylosis, left elbow
M24.629 Ankylosis, unspecified elbow

√6ᵗʰ **M24.63 Ankylosis, wrist**

M24.631 Ankylosis, right wrist
M24.632 Ankylosis, left wrist
M24.639 Ankylosis, unspecified wrist

√6ᵗʰ **M24.64 Ankylosis, hand**

M24.641 Ankylosis, right hand
M24.642 Ankylosis, left hand
M24.649 Ankylosis, unspecified hand

√6ᵗʰ **M24.65 Ankylosis, hip**

M24.651 Ankylosis, right hip
M24.652 Ankylosis, left hip
M24.659 Ankylosis, unspecified hip

√6ᵗʰ **M24.66 Ankylosis, knee**

M24.661 Ankylosis, right knee
M24.662 Ankylosis, left knee
M24.669 Ankylosis, unspecified knee

√6ᵗʰ **M24.67 Ankylosis, ankle and foot**

M24.671 Ankylosis, right ankle
M24.672 Ankylosis, left ankle
M24.673 Ankylosis, unspecified ankle
M24.674 Ankylosis, right foot
M24.675 Ankylosis, left foot
M24.676 Ankylosis, unspecified foot

● **M24.69 Ankylosis, other specified joint**

M24.7 Protrusio acetabuli

> **DEF:** Intrapelvic protrusion of the acetabulum characterized by the sinking of the floor of the acetabulum, causing the femoral head to protrude. It limits hip movement and is of unknown etiology. ***Synonym(s):*** *Otto's pelvis.*

√5ᵗʰ **M24.8 Other specific joint derangements, not elsewhere classified**

> **EXCLUDES 2** *iliotibial band syndrome (M76.3)*

M24.80 Other specific joint derangements of unspecified joint, not elsewhere classified

√6ᵗʰ **M24.81 Other specific joint derangements of shoulder, not elsewhere classified**

M24.811 Other specific joint derangements of right shoulder, not elsewhere classified
M24.812 Other specific joint derangements of left shoulder, not elsewhere classified
M24.819 Other specific joint derangements of unspecified shoulder, not elsewhere classified

√6ᵗʰ **M24.82 Other specific joint derangements of elbow, not elsewhere classified**

M24.821 Other specific joint derangements of right elbow, not elsewhere classified
M24.822 Other specific joint derangements of left elbow, not elsewhere classified
M24.829 Other specific joint derangements of unspecified elbow, not elsewhere classified

√6ᵗʰ **M24.83 Other specific joint derangements of wrist, not elsewhere classified**

M24.831 Other specific joint derangements of right wrist, not elsewhere classified
M24.832 Other specific joint derangements of left wrist, not elsewhere classified
M24.839 Other specific joint derangements of unspecified wrist, not elsewhere classified

√6ᵗʰ **M24.84 Other specific joint derangements of hand, not elsewhere classified**

M24.841 Other specific joint derangements of right hand, not elsewhere classified
M24.842 Other specific joint derangements of left hand, not elsewhere classified
M24.849 Other specific joint derangements of unspecified hand, not elsewhere classified

√6ᵗʰ **M24.85 Other specific joint derangements of hip, not elsewhere classified**

Irritable hip

M24.851 Other specific joint derangements of right hip, not elsewhere classified
M24.852 Other specific joint derangements of left hip, not elsewhere classified
M24.859 Other specific joint derangements of unspecified hip, not elsewhere classified

√6ᵗʰ **M24.87 Other specific joint derangements of ankle and foot, not elsewhere classified**

M24.871 Other specific joint derangements of right ankle, not elsewhere classified
M24.872 Other specific joint derangements of left ankle, not elsewhere classified
M24.873 Other specific joint derangements of unspecified ankle, not elsewhere classified
M24.874 Other specific joint derangements of right foot, not elsewhere classified
M24.875 Other specific joint derangements of left foot, not elsewhere classified
M24.876 Other specific joint derangements of unspecified foot, not elsewhere classified

● **M24.89 Other specific joint derangement of other specified joint, not elsewhere classified**

M24.9 Joint derangement, unspecified

√4ᵗʰ **M25 Other joint disorder, not elsewhere classified**

> **EXCLUDES 2** *abnormality of gait and mobility (R26.-)*
> *acquired deformities of limb (M20-M21)*
> *calcification of bursa (M71.4-)*
> *calcification of shoulder (joint) (M75.3)*
> *calcification of tendon (M65.2-)*
> *difficulty in walking (R26.2)*
> *temporomandibular joint disorder (M26.6-)*

√5ᵗʰ **M25.0 Hemarthrosis**

> **EXCLUDES 1** *current injury — see injury of joint by body region*
> *hemophilic arthropathy (M36.2)*

M25.00 Hemarthrosis, unspecified joint `CC`

√6ᵗʰ **M25.01 Hemarthrosis, shoulder**

M25.011 Hemarthrosis, right shoulder `CC`
M25.012 Hemarthrosis, left shoulder `CC`
M25.019 Hemarthrosis, unspecified shoulder `CC`

√6ᵗʰ **M25.02 Hemarthrosis, elbow**

M25.021 Hemarthrosis, right elbow `CC`
M25.022 Hemarthrosis, left elbow `CC`
M25.029 Hemarthrosis, unspecified elbow `CC`

√6ᵗʰ **M25.03 Hemarthrosis, wrist**

M25.031 Hemarthrosis, right wrist `CC`
M25.032 Hemarthrosis, left wrist `CC`
M25.039 Hemarthrosis, unspecified wrist `CC`

√6ᵗʰ **M25.04 Hemarthrosis, hand**

M25.041 Hemarthrosis, right hand `CC`
M25.042 Hemarthrosis, left hand `CC`
M25.049 Hemarthrosis, unspecified hand `CC`

√6ᵗʰ **M25.05 Hemarthrosis, hip**

M25.051 Hemarthrosis, right hip `CC`
M25.052 Hemarthrosis, left hip `CC`
M25.059 Hemarthrosis, unspecified hip `CC`

Chapter 13. Diseases of the Musculoskeletal System and Connective Tissue

M25.06–M25.459

√6ᵗʰ **M25.06** **Hemarthrosis,** knee
- **M25.061** **Hemarthrosis,** right knee   `CC`
- **M25.062** **Hemarthrosis,** left knee   `CC`
- **M25.069** **Hemarthrosis,** unspecified knee   `CC`

√6ᵗʰ **M25.07** **Hemarthrosis,** ankle and foot
- **M25.071** **Hemarthrosis,** right ankle   `CC`
- **M25.072** **Hemarthrosis,** left ankle   `CC`
- **M25.073** **Hemarthrosis,** unspecified ankle   `CC`
- **M25.074** **Hemarthrosis,** right foot   `CC`
- **M25.075** **Hemarthrosis,** left foot   `CC`
- **M25.076** **Hemarthrosis,** unspecified foot   `CC`

M25.08 **Hemarthrosis,** other specified site   `CC`
Hemarthrosis, vertebrae

√5ᵗʰ **M25.1** **Fistula of joint**

M25.10 **Fistula,** unspecified joint   `SW`

√6ᵗʰ **M25.11** **Fistula,** shoulder
- **M25.111** **Fistula,** right shoulder   `SW`
- **M25.112** **Fistula,** left shoulder   `SW`
- **M25.119** **Fistula,** unspecified shoulder   `SW`

√6ᵗʰ **M25.12** **Fistula,** elbow
- **M25.121** **Fistula,** right elbow   `SW`
- **M25.122** **Fistula,** left elbow   `SW`
- **M25.129** **Fistula,** unspecified elbow   `SW`

√6ᵗʰ **M25.13** **Fistula,** wrist
- **M25.131** **Fistula,** right wrist   `SW`
- **M25.132** **Fistula,** left wrist   `SW`
- **M25.139** **Fistula,** unspecified wrist   `SW`

√6ᵗʰ **M25.14** **Fistula,** hand
- **M25.141** **Fistula,** right hand   `SW`
- **M25.142** **Fistula,** left hand   `SW`
- **M25.149** **Fistula,** unspecified hand   `SW`

√6ᵗʰ **M25.15** **Fistula,** hip
- **M25.151** **Fistula,** right hip   `SW`
- **M25.152** **Fistula,** left hip   `SW`
- **M25.159** **Fistula,** unspecified hip   `SW`

√6ᵗʰ **M25.16** **Fistula,** knee
- **M25.161** **Fistula,** right knee   `SW`
- **M25.162** **Fistula,** left knee   `SW`
- **M25.169** **Fistula,** unspecified knee   `SW`

√6ᵗʰ **M25.17** **Fistula,** ankle and foot
- **M25.171** **Fistula,** right ankle   `SW`
- **M25.172** **Fistula,** left ankle   `SW`
- **M25.173** **Fistula,** unspecified ankle   `SW`
- **M25.174** **Fistula,** right foot   `SW`
- **M25.175** **Fistula,** left foot   `SW`
- **M25.176** **Fistula,** unspecified foot   `SW`

M25.18 **Fistula,** other specified site   `SW`
Fistula, vertebrae

√5ᵗʰ **M25.2** **Flail joint**

DEF: Hinged joint that exhibits an abnormal or excessive degree of range and mobility.

M25.20 **Flail joint,** unspecified joint

√6ᵗʰ **M25.21** **Flail joint,** shoulder
- **M25.211** **Flail joint,** right shoulder
- **M25.212** **Flail joint,** left shoulder
- **M25.219** **Flail joint,** unspecified shoulder

√6ᵗʰ **M25.22** **Flail joint,** elbow
- **M25.221** **Flail joint,** right elbow
- **M25.222** **Flail joint,** left elbow
- **M25.229** **Flail joint,** unspecified elbow

√6ᵗʰ **M25.23** **Flail joint,** wrist
- **M25.231** **Flail joint,** right wrist
- **M25.232** **Flail joint,** left wrist
- **M25.239** **Flail joint,** unspecified wrist

√6ᵗʰ **M25.24** **Flail joint,** hand
- **M25.241** **Flail joint,** right hand
- **M25.242** **Flail joint,** left hand
- **M25.249** **Flail joint,** unspecified hand

√6ᵗʰ **M25.25** **Flail joint,** hip
- **M25.251** **Flail joint,** right hip
- **M25.252** **Flail joint,** left hip
- **M25.259** **Flail joint,** unspecified hip

√6ᵗʰ **M25.26** **Flail joint,** knee
- **M25.261** **Flail joint,** right knee
- **M25.262** **Flail joint,** left knee
- **M25.269** **Flail joint,** unspecified knee

√6ᵗʰ **M25.27** **Flail joint,** ankle and foot
- **M25.271** **Flail joint,** right ankle and foot
- **M25.272** **Flail joint,** left ankle and foot
- **M25.279** **Flail joint,** unspecified ankle and foot

M25.28 **Flail joint,** other site

√5ᵗʰ **M25.3** **Other instability of joint**

EXCLUDES 1   instability of joint secondary to old ligament injury (M24.2-)

instability of joint secondary to removal of joint prosthesis (M96.8-)

EXCLUDES 2   spinal instabilities (M53.2-)

M25.30 **Other instability,** unspecified joint

√6ᵗʰ **M25.31** **Other instability,** shoulder
- **M25.311** **Other instability,** right shoulder
- **M25.312** **Other instability,** left shoulder
- **M25.319** **Other instability,** unspecified shoulder

√6ᵗʰ **M25.32** **Other instability,** elbow
- **M25.321** **Other instability,** right elbow
- **M25.322** **Other instability,** left elbow
- **M25.329** **Other instability,** unspecified elbow

√6ᵗʰ **M25.33** **Other instability,** wrist
- **M25.331** **Other instability,** right wrist
- **M25.332** **Other instability,** left wrist
- **M25.339** **Other instability,** unspecified wrist

√6ᵗʰ **M25.34** **Other instability,** hand
- **M25.341** **Other instability,** right hand
- **M25.342** **Other instability,** left hand
- **M25.349** **Other instability,** unspecified hand

√6ᵗʰ **M25.35** **Other instability,** hip
- **M25.351** **Other instability,** right hip
- **M25.352** **Other instability,** left hip
- **M25.359** **Other instability,** unspecified hip

√6ᵗʰ **M25.36** **Other instability,** knee
- **M25.361** **Other instability,** right knee
- **M25.362** **Other instability,** left knee
- **M25.369** **Other instability,** unspecified knee

√6ᵗʰ **M25.37** **Other instability,** ankle and foot
- **M25.371** **Other instability,** right ankle
- **M25.372** **Other instability,** left ankle
- **M25.373** **Other instability,** unspecified ankle
- **M25.374** **Other instability,** right foot
- **M25.375** **Other instability,** left foot
- **M25.376** **Other instability,** unspecified foot

M25.39 **Other instability,** other specified joint

√5ᵗʰ **M25.4** **Effusion of joint**

EXCLUDES 1   hydrarthrosis in yaws (A66.6)

intermittent hydrarthrosis (M12.4-)

other infective (teno)synovitis (M65.1-)

M25.40 **Effusion,** unspecified joint

√6ᵗʰ **M25.41** **Effusion,** shoulder
- **M25.411** **Effusion,** right shoulder
- **M25.412** **Effusion,** left shoulder
- **M25.419** **Effusion,** unspecified shoulder

√6ᵗʰ **M25.42** **Effusion,** elbow
- **M25.421** **Effusion,** right elbow
- **M25.422** **Effusion,** left elbow
- **M25.429** **Effusion,** unspecified elbow

√6ᵗʰ **M25.43** **Effusion,** wrist
- **M25.431** **Effusion,** right wrist
- **M25.432** **Effusion,** left wrist
- **M25.439** **Effusion,** unspecified wrist

√6ᵗʰ **M25.44** **Effusion,** hand
- **M25.441** **Effusion,** right hand
- **M25.442** **Effusion,** left hand
- **M25.449** **Effusion,** unspecified hand

√6ᵗʰ **M25.45** **Effusion,** hip
- **M25.451** **Effusion,** right hip
- **M25.452** **Effusion,** left hip
- **M25.459** **Effusion,** unspecified hip

Ⓝ Newborn: 0   Ⓟ Pediatric: 0-17   Ⓜ Maternity: 9-64   Ⓐ Adult: 15-124   `MCC` Major Complication/Comorbidity   `CC` Complication/Comorbidity   `SW` Severe Wound Dx

788

ICD-10-CM 2021

√6ᵗʰ **M25.46** **Effusion,** knee

M25.461 **Effusion,** right knee
M25.462 **Effusion,** left knee
M25.469 **Effusion,** unspecified knee

√6ᵗʰ **M25.47** **Effusion,** ankle and foot

M25.471 **Effusion,** right ankle
M25.472 **Effusion,** left ankle
M25.473 **Effusion,** unspecified ankle
M25.474 **Effusion,** right foot
M25.475 **Effusion,** left foot
M25.476 **Effusion,** unspecified foot

M25.48 **Effusion,** other site

√5ᵗʰ **M25.5** **Pain in joint**

EXCLUDES 2   pain in hand (M79.64-)
pain in fingers (M79.64-)
pain in foot (M79.67-)
pain in limb (M79.6-)
pain in toes (M79.67-)

M25.50 **Pain in unspecified joint**

√6ᵗʰ **M25.51** **Pain in** shoulder

M25.511 **Pain in** right shoulder
M25.512 **Pain in** left shoulder
M25.519 **Pain in** unspecified shoulder

√6ᵗʰ **M25.52** **Pain in** elbow

M25.521 **Pain in** right elbow
M25.522 **Pain in** left elbow
M25.529 **Pain in** unspecified elbow

√6ᵗʰ **M25.53** **Pain in** wrist

M25.531 **Pain in** right wrist
M25.532 **Pain in** left wrist
M25.539 **Pain in** unspecified wrist

√6ᵗʰ **M25.54** **Pain in** joints of hand

AHA: 2016,4Q,38

M25.541 **Pain in joints of** right hand
M25.542 **Pain in joints of** left hand
M25.549 **Pain in joints of** unspecified hand
Pain in joints of hand NOS

√6ᵗʰ **M25.55** **Pain in** hip

M25.551 **Pain in** right hip
M25.552 **Pain in** left hip
M25.559 **Pain in** unspecified hip

√6ᵗʰ **M25.56** **Pain in** knee

M25.561 **Pain in** right knee
M25.562 **Pain in** left knee
M25.569 **Pain in** unspecified knee

√6ᵗʰ **M25.57** **Pain in** ankle and joints of foot

M25.571 **Pain in** right ankle and joints of right foot
M25.572 **Pain in** left ankle and joints of left foot
M25.579 **Pain in** unspecified ankle and joints of unspecified foot

M25.59 **Pain in other specified joint**

√5ᵗʰ **M25.6** **Stiffness of joint, not elsewhere classified**

EXCLUDES 1   ankylosis of joint (M24.6-)
contracture of joint (M24.5-)

M25.60 **Stiffness of unspecified joint, not elsewhere classified**

√6ᵗʰ **M25.61** **Stiffness of** shoulder, not elsewhere classified

M25.611 **Stiffness of** right shoulder, not elsewhere classified
M25.612 **Stiffness of** left shoulder, not elsewhere classified
M25.619 **Stiffness of** unspecified shoulder, not elsewhere classified

√6ᵗʰ **M25.62** **Stiffness of** elbow, not elsewhere classified

M25.621 **Stiffness of** right elbow, not elsewhere classified
M25.622 **Stiffness of** left elbow, not elsewhere classified
M25.629 **Stiffness of** unspecified elbow, not elsewhere classified

√6ᵗʰ **M25.63** **Stiffness of** wrist, not elsewhere classified

M25.631 **Stiffness of** right wrist, not elsewhere classified
M25.632 **Stiffness of** left wrist, not elsewhere classified

M25.639 **Stiffness of unspecified wrist, not elsewhere classified**

√6ᵗʰ **M25.64** **Stiffness of** hand, not elsewhere classified

M25.641 **Stiffness of** right hand, not elsewhere classified
M25.642 **Stiffness of** left hand, not elsewhere classified
M25.649 **Stiffness of unspecified hand, not elsewhere classified**

√6ᵗʰ **M25.65** **Stiffness of** hip, not elsewhere classified

M25.651 **Stiffness of** right hip, not elsewhere classified
M25.652 **Stiffness of** left hip, not elsewhere classified
M25.659 **Stiffness of unspecified hip, not elsewhere classified**

√6ᵗʰ **M25.66** **Stiffness of** knee, not elsewhere classified

M25.661 **Stiffness of** right knee, not elsewhere classified
M25.662 **Stiffness of** left knee, not elsewhere classified
M25.669 **Stiffness of unspecified knee, not elsewhere classified**

√6ᵗʰ **M25.67** **Stiffness of** ankle and foot, not elsewhere classified

M25.671 **Stiffness of** right ankle, not elsewhere classified
M25.672 **Stiffness of** left ankle, not elsewhere classified
M25.673 **Stiffness of unspecified ankle, not elsewhere classified**
M25.674 **Stiffness of** right foot, not elsewhere classified
M25.675 **Stiffness of** left foot, not elsewhere classified
M25.676 **Stiffness of unspecified foot, not elsewhere classified**

M25.69 **Stiffness of other specified joint, not elsewhere classified**

√5ᵗʰ **M25.7** **Osteophyte**

M25.70 **Osteophyte, unspecified joint**

√6ᵗʰ **M25.71** **Osteophyte,** shoulder

M25.711 **Osteophyte,** right shoulder
M25.712 **Osteophyte,** left shoulder
M25.719 **Osteophyte, unspecified shoulder**

√6ᵗʰ **M25.72** **Osteophyte,** elbow

M25.721 **Osteophyte,** right elbow
M25.722 **Osteophyte,** left elbow
M25.729 **Osteophyte, unspecified elbow**

√6ᵗʰ **M25.73** **Osteophyte,** wrist

M25.731 **Osteophyte,** right wrist
M25.732 **Osteophyte,** left wrist
M25.739 **Osteophyte, unspecified wrist**

√6ᵗʰ **M25.74** **Osteophyte,** hand

M25.741 **Osteophyte,** right hand
M25.742 **Osteophyte,** left hand
M25.749 **Osteophyte, unspecified hand**

√6ᵗʰ **M25.75** **Osteophyte,** hip

M25.751 **Osteophyte,** right hip
M25.752 **Osteophyte,** left hip
M25.759 **Osteophyte, unspecified hip**

√6ᵗʰ **M25.76** **Osteophyte,** knee

M25.761 **Osteophyte,** right knee
M25.762 **Osteophyte,** left knee
M25.769 **Osteophyte, unspecified knee**

√6ᵗʰ **M25.77** **Osteophyte,** ankle and foot

M25.771 **Osteophyte,** right ankle
M25.772 **Osteophyte,** left ankle
M25.773 **Osteophyte, unspecified ankle**
M25.774 **Osteophyte,** right foot
M25.775 **Osteophyte,** left foot
M25.776 **Osteophyte, unspecified foot**

M25.78 **Osteophyte,** vertebrae

√5ᵗʰ **M25.8** **Other specified joint disorders**

M25.80 **Other specified joint disorders, unspecified joint**

√6ᵗʰ **M25.81** **Other specified joint disorders,** shoulder

M25.811 **Other specified joint disorders,** right shoulder

☑ Additional Character Required   √x7ᵗʰ Placeholder   Unacceptable PDx   Questionable PDx   Manifestation   Unspecified Dx   H1-H4 HAC   HCC CMS-HCC Dx   HIV HIV Dx

ICD-10-CM 2021   789

M25.812 **Other specified joint disorders, left shoulder**

M25.819 **Other specified joint disorders, unspecified shoulder**

√6ᵗʰ M25.82 **Other specified joint disorders, elbow**

M25.821 **Other specified joint disorders, right elbow**

M25.822 **Other specified joint disorders, left elbow**

M25.829 **Other specified joint disorders, unspecified elbow**

√6ᵗʰ M25.83 **Other specified joint disorders, wrist**

M25.831 **Other specified joint disorders, right wrist**

M25.832 **Other specified joint disorders, left wrist**

M25.839 **Other specified joint disorders, unspecified wrist**

√6ᵗʰ M25.84 **Other specified joint disorders, hand**

M25.841 **Other specified joint disorders, right hand**

M25.842 **Other specified joint disorders, left hand**

M25.849 **Other specified joint disorders, unspecified hand**

√6ᵗʰ M25.85 **Other specified joint disorders, hip**

AHA: 2014,4Q,25

M25.851 **Other specified joint disorders, right hip**

M25.852 **Other specified joint disorders, left hip**

M25.859 **Other specified joint disorders, unspecified hip**

√6ᵗʰ M25.86 **Other specified joint disorders, knee**

M25.861 **Other specified joint disorders, right knee**

M25.862 **Other specified joint disorders, left knee**

M25.869 **Other specified joint disorders, unspecified knee**

√6ᵗʰ M25.87 **Other specified joint disorders, ankle and foot**

M25.871 **Other specified joint disorders, right ankle and foot**

M25.872 **Other specified joint disorders, left ankle and foot**

M25.879 **Other specified joint disorders, unspecified ankle and foot**

M25.9 **Joint disorder, unspecified**

Dentofacial anomalies [including malocclusion] and other disorders of jaw (M26-M27)

EXCLUDES 1 *hemifacial atrophy or hypertrophy (Q67.4)*
unilateral condylar hyperplasia or hypoplasia (M27.8)

√4ᵗʰ **M26 Dentofacial anomalies [including malocclusion]**

√5ᵗʰ M26.0 **Major anomalies of jaw size**

EXCLUDES 1 *acromegaly (E22.0)*
Robin's syndrome (Q87.0)

M26.00 **Unspecified anomaly of jaw size**

M26.01 **Maxillary hyperplasia**

M26.02 **Maxillary hypoplasia**

AHA: 2014,3Q,23

M26.03 **Mandibular hyperplasia**

M26.04 **Mandibular hypoplasia**

M26.05 **Macrogenia**

M26.06 **Microgenia**

M26.07 **Excessive tuberosity of jaw**
Entire maxillary tuberosity

M26.09 **Other specified anomalies of jaw size**

√5ᵗʰ M26.1 **Anomalies of jaw-cranial base relationship**

M26.10 **Unspecified anomaly of jaw-cranial base relationship**

M26.11 **Maxillary asymmetry**

M26.12 **Other jaw asymmetry**

M26.19 **Other specified anomalies of jaw-cranial base relationship**

AHA: 2020,1Q,21

√5ᵗʰ M26.2 **Anomalies of dental arch relationship**

M26.20 **Unspecified anomaly of dental arch relationship**

√6ᵗʰ M26.21 **Malocclusion, Angle's class**

M26.211 **Malocclusion, Angle's class I**
Neutro-occlusion

M26.212 **Malocclusion, Angle's class II**
Disto-occlusion Division I
Disto-occlusion Division II

M26.213 **Malocclusion, Angle's class III**
Mesio-occlusion

M26.219 **Malocclusion, Angle's class, unspecified**

√6ᵗʰ M26.22 **Open occlusal relationship**

M26.220 **Open anterior occlusal relationship**
Anterior open bite

M26.221 **Open posterior occlusal relationship**
Posterior open bite

M26.23 **Excessive horizontal overlap**
Excessive horizontal overjet

M26.24 **Reverse articulation**
Crossbite (anterior) (posterior)

M26.25 **Anomalies of interarch distance**

M26.29 **Other anomalies of dental arch relationship**
Midline deviation of dental arch
Overbite (excessive) deep
Overbite (excessive) horizontal
Overbite (excessive) vertical
Posterior lingual occlusion of mandibular teeth

√5ᵗʰ M26.3 **Anomalies of tooth position of fully erupted tooth or teeth**

EXCLUDES 2 *embedded and impacted teeth (K01.-)*

M26.30 **Unspecified anomaly of tooth position of fully erupted tooth or teeth**
Abnormal spacing of fully erupted tooth or teeth NOS
Displacement of fully erupted tooth or teeth NOS
Transposition of fully erupted tooth or teeth NOS

M26.31 **Crowding of fully erupted teeth**

M26.32 **Excessive spacing of fully erupted teeth**
Diastema of fully erupted tooth or teeth NOS

M26.33 **Horizontal displacement of fully erupted tooth or teeth**
Tipped tooth or teeth
Tipping of fully erupted tooth

M26.34 **Vertical displacement of fully erupted tooth or teeth**
Extruded tooth
Infraeruption of tooth or teeth
Supraeruption of tooth or teeth

M26.35 **Rotation of fully erupted tooth or teeth**

M26.36 **Insufficient interocclusal distance of fully erupted teeth (ridge)**
Lack of adequate intermaxillary vertical dimension of fully erupted teeth

M26.37 **Excessive interocclusal distance of fully erupted teeth**
Excessive intermaxillary vertical dimension of fully erupted teeth
Loss of occlusal vertical dimension of fully erupted teeth

M26.39 **Other anomalies of tooth position of fully erupted tooth or teeth**

M26.4 **Malocclusion, unspecified**

√5ᵗʰ M26.5 **Dentofacial functional abnormalities**

EXCLUDES 1 *bruxism (F45.8)*
teeth-grinding NOS (F45.8)

M26.50 **Dentofacial functional abnormalities, unspecified**

M26.51 **Abnormal jaw closure**

M26.52 **Limited mandibular range of motion**

M26.53 **Deviation in opening and closing of the mandible**

M26.54 **Insufficient anterior guidance**
Insufficient anterior occlusal guidance

M26.55 **Centric occlusion maximum intercuspation discrepancy**
EXCLUDES 1 *centric occlusion NOS (M26.59)*

M26.56 **Non-working side interference**
Balancing side interference

M26.57 **Lack of posterior occlusal support**

M26.59 **Other dentofacial functional abnormalities**
Centric occlusion (of teeth) NOS
Malocclusion due to abnormal swallowing
Malocclusion due to mouth breathing
Malocclusion due to tongue, lip or finger habits

N Newborn: 0   P Pediatric: 0-17   M Maternity: 9-64   A Adult: 15-124   MCC Major Complication/Comorbidity   CC Complication/Comorbidity   SW Severe Wound Dx

790   ICD-10-CM 2021

✓5th **M26.6 Temporomandibular joint disorders**

    EXCLUDES 2   current temporomandibular joint dislocation (S03.0)
                  current temporomandibular joint sprain (S03.4)

    AHA: 2016,4Q,38-39

Temporomandibular Joint

Cutaway detail

Upper joint space

Articular disc (meniscus)

Lower joint space

Condyle

Mandible   Cutaway view of temporomandibular joint (TMJ)

✓6th **M26.60 Temporomandibular joint disorder, unspecified**

    M26.601 Right temporomandibular joint disorder, unspecified

    M26.602 Left temporomandibular joint disorder, unspecified

    M26.603 Bilateral temporomandibular joint disorder, unspecified

    M26.609 Unspecified temporomandibular joint disorder, unspecified side
           Temporomandibular joint disorder NOS

✓6th **M26.61 Adhesions and ankylosis of temporomandibular joint**

    M26.611 Adhesions and ankylosis of right temporomandibular joint

    M26.612 Adhesions and ankylosis of left temporomandibular joint

    M26.613 Adhesions and ankylosis of bilateral temporomandibular joint

    M26.619 Adhesions and ankylosis of temporomandibular joint, unspecified side

✓6th **M26.62 Arthralgia of temporomandibular joint**

    M26.621 Arthralgia of right temporomandibular joint

    M26.622 Arthralgia of left temporomandibular joint

    M26.623 Arthralgia of bilateral temporomandibular joint

    M26.629 Arthralgia of temporomandibular joint, unspecified side

✓6th **M26.63 Articular disc disorder of temporomandibular joint**

    M26.631 Articular disc disorder of right temporomandibular joint

    M26.632 Articular disc disorder of left temporomandibular joint

    M26.633 Articular disc disorder of bilateral temporomandibular joint

    M26.639 Articular disc disorder of temporomandibular joint, unspecified side

✓6th **M26.64 Arthritis of temporomandibular joint**

    M26.641 Arthritis of right temporomandibular joint

    M26.642 Arthritis of left temporomandibular joint

    M26.643 Arthritis of bilateral temporomandibular joint

    M26.649 Arthritis of unspecified temporomandibular joint

✓6th **M26.65 Arthropathy of temporomandibular joint**

    M26.651 Arthropathy of right temporomandibular joint

    M26.652 Arthropathy of left temporomandibular joint

    M26.653 Arthropathy of bilateral temporomandibular joint

    M26.659 Arthropathy of unspecified temporomandibular joint

    M26.69 Other specified disorders of temporomandibular joint

✓5th **M26.7 Dental alveolar anomalies**

    M26.70 Unspecified alveolar anomaly

    M26.71 Alveolar maxillary hyperplasia

    M26.72 Alveolar mandibular hyperplasia

    M26.73 Alveolar maxillary hypoplasia

    M26.74 Alveolar mandibular hypoplasia

    M26.79 Other specified alveolar anomalies

✓5th **M26.8 Other dentofacial anomalies**

    M26.81 Anterior soft tissue impingement
           Anterior soft tissue impingement on teeth

    M26.82 Posterior soft tissue impingement
           Posterior soft tissue impingement on teeth

    M26.89 Other dentofacial anomalies

    M26.9 Dentofacial anomaly, unspecified

✓4th **M27 Other diseases of jaws**

    M27.0 Developmental disorders of jaws
           Latent bone cyst of jaw
           Stafne's cyst
           Torus mandibularis
           Torus palatinus

    M27.1 Giant cell granuloma, central
           Giant cell granuloma NOS
        EXCLUDES 1   peripheral giant cell granuloma (K06.8)

    M27.2 Inflammatory conditions of jaws
           Osteitis of jaw(s)
           Osteomyelitis (neonatal) jaw(s)
           Osteoradionecrosis jaw(s)
           Periostitis jaw(s)
           Sequestrum of jaw bone
           Use additional code (W88-W90, X39.0) to identify radiation, if radiation-induced
        EXCLUDES 2   osteonecrosis of jaw due to drug (M87.180)

    M27.3 Alveolitis of jaws
           Alveolar osteitis
           Dry socket

✓5th **M27.4 Other and unspecified cysts of jaw**
        EXCLUDES 1   cysts of oral region (K09.-)
                   latent bone cyst of jaw (M27.0)
                   Stafne's cyst (M27.0)

    M27.40 Unspecified cyst of jaw
           Cyst of jaw NOS

    M27.49 Other cysts of jaw
           Aneurysmal cyst of jaw
           Hemorrhagic cyst of jaw
           Traumatic cyst of jaw

✓5th **M27.5 Periradicular pathology associated with previous endodontic treatment**

    M27.51 Perforation of root canal space due to endodontic treatment

    M27.52 Endodontic overfill

    M27.53 Endodontic underfill

    M27.59 Other periradicular pathology associated with previous endodontic treatment

✓5th **M27.6 Endosseous dental implant failure**

    M27.61 Osseointegration failure of dental implant
           Hemorrhagic complications of dental implant placement
           Iatrogenic osseointegration failure of dental implant
           Osseointegration failure of dental implant due to complications of systemic disease
           Osseointegration failure of dental implant due to poor bone quality
           Pre-integration failure of dental implant NOS
           Pre-osseointegration failure of dental implant

☑ Additional Character Required   ✓x7th Placeholder   Unacceptable PDx   Questionable PDx   Manifestation   Unspecified Dx   H1-H4 HAC   HCC CMS-HCC Dx   HIV HIV Dx

ICD-10-CM 2021   791

Chapter 13. Diseases of the Musculoskeletal System and Connective Tissue

M27.62–M33.91

M27.62   **Post-osseointegration biological failure of dental implant**
Failure of dental implant due to lack of attached gingiva
Failure of dental implant due to occlusal trauma (caused by poor prosthetic design)
Failure of dental implant due to parafunctional habits
Failure of dental implant due to periodontal infection (peri-implantitis)
Failure of dental implant due to poor oral hygiene
Iatrogenic post-osseointegration failure of dental implant
Post-osseointegration failure of dental implant due to complications of systemic disease

M27.63   **Post-osseointegration mechanical failure of dental implant**
Failure of dental prosthesis causing loss of dental implant
Fracture of dental implant
   EXCLUDES 2   *cracked tooth (K03.81)*
     fractured dental restorative material with loss of material (K08.531)
     fractured dental restorative material without loss of material (K08.530)
     fractured tooth (S02.5)

M27.69   **Other endosseous dental implant failure**
Dental implant failure NOS

M27.8   **Other specified diseases of jaws**
Cherubism
Exostosis
Fibrous dysplasia
Unilateral condylar hyperplasia
Unilateral condylar hypoplasia
   EXCLUDES 1   *jaw pain (R68.84)*

M27.9   **Disease of jaws, unspecified**

Systemic connective tissue disorders (M30-M36)

INCLUDES   autoimmune disease NOS
collagen (vascular) disease NOS
systemic autoimmune disease
systemic collagen (vascular) disease
EXCLUDES 1   *autoimmune disease, single organ or single cell-type-code to relevant condition category*

✓4ᵗʰ **M30**   **Polyarteritis nodosa and related conditions**
   EXCLUDES 1   *microscopic polyarteritis (M31.7)*

M30.0   **Polyarteritis nodosa**   CC HCC

M30.1   **Polyarteritis with lung involvement [Churg-Strauss]**   CC HCC
Allergic granulomatous angiitis
▶Eosinophilic granulomatosis with polyangiitis [EGPA] ◀

M30.2   **Juvenile polyarteritis**   CC HCC

M30.3   **Mucocutaneous lymph node syndrome [Kawasaki]**   CC HCC

M30.8   **Other conditions related to polyarteritis nodosa**   CC HCC
Polyangiitis overlap syndrome

✓4ᵗʰ **M31**   **Other necrotizing vasculopathies**

M31.0   **Hypersensitivity angiitis**   CC HCC
Goodpasture's syndrome

M31.1   **Thrombotic microangiopathy**   MCC HCC
Thrombotic thrombocytopenic purpura

M31.2   **Lethal midline granuloma**   CC HCC

✓5ᵗʰ **M31.3**   **Wegener's granulomatosis**
▶Granulomatosis with polyangiitis◀
Necrotizing respiratory granulomatosis

M31.30   **Wegener's granulomatosis without renal involvement**   CC HCC
Wegener's granulomatosis NOS

M31.31   **Wegener's granulomatosis with renal involvement**   CC HCC

M31.4   **Aortic arch syndrome [Takayasu]**   CC HCC

M31.5   **Giant cell arteritis with polymyalgia rheumatica**   HCC

M31.6   **Other giant cell arteritis**   HCC

M31.7   **Microscopic polyangiitis**   CC HCC
Microscopic polyarteritis
   EXCLUDES 1   *polyarteritis nodosa (M30.0)*

M31.8   **Other specified necrotizing vasculopathies**   CC HCC
Hypocomplementemic vasculitis
Septic vasculitis

M31.9   **Necrotizing vasculopathy, unspecified**   CC HCC

✓4ᵗʰ **M32**   **Systemic lupus erythematosus (SLE)**
   EXCLUDES 1   *lupus erythematosus (discoid) (NOS) (L93.0)*
   AHA: 2018,3Q,14
   TIP: There is no default code for "lupus NOS." Query the provider for the specific type of lupus in order to assign the appropriate code.

M32.0   **Drug-induced systemic lupus erythematosus**   HCC
Use additional code for adverse effect, if applicable, to identify drug (T36-T50 with fifth or sixth character 5)

✓5ᵗʰ **M32.1**   **Systemic lupus erythematosus with organ or system involvement**

M32.10   **Systemic lupus erythematosus, organ or system involvement unspecified**   HCC

M32.11   **Endocarditis in systemic lupus erythematosus**   CC HCC
Libman-Sacks disease

M32.12   **Pericarditis in systemic lupus erythematosus**   CC HCC
Lupus pericarditis

M32.13   **Lung involvement in systemic lupus erythematosus**   HCC
Pleural effusion due to systemic lupus erythematosus

M32.14   **Glomerular disease in systemic lupus erythematosus**   HCC
Lupus renal disease NOS
   AHA: 2013,4Q,125

M32.15   **Tubulo-interstitial nephropathy in systemic lupus erythematosus**   HCC

M32.19   **Other organ or system involvement in systemic lupus erythematosus**   HCC

M32.8   **Other forms of systemic lupus erythematosus**   HCC

M32.9   **Systemic lupus erythematosus, unspecified**   HCC
SLE NOS
Systemic lupus erythematosus NOS
Systemic lupus erythematosus without organ involvement

✓4ᵗʰ **M33**   **Dermatopolymyositis**
   AHA: 2017,4Q,18

✓5ᵗʰ **M33.0**   **Juvenile dermatomyositis**

M33.00   **Juvenile dermatomyositis, organ involvement unspecified**   CC HCC

M33.01   **Juvenile dermatomyositis with respiratory involvement**   CC HCC

M33.02   **Juvenile dermatomyositis with myopathy**   CC HCC

M33.03   **Juvenile dermatomyositis without myopathy**   CC HCC

M33.09   **Juvenile dermatomyositis with other organ involvement**   CC HCC

✓5ᵗʰ **M33.1**   **Other dermatomyositis**
Adult dermatomyositis

M33.10   **Other dermatomyositis, organ involvement unspecified**   CC HCC

M33.11   **Other dermatomyositis with respiratory involvement**   CC HCC

M33.12   **Other dermatomyositis with myopathy**   CC HCC

M33.13   **Other dermatomyositis without myopathy**   CC HCC
Dermatomyositis NOS

M33.19   **Other dermatomyositis with other organ involvement**   CC HCC

✓5ᵗʰ **M33.2**   **Polymyositis**

M33.20   **Polymyositis, organ involvement unspecified**   CC HCC

M33.21   **Polymyositis with respiratory involvement**   CC HCC

M33.22   **Polymyositis with myopathy**   CC HCC

M33.29   **Polymyositis with other organ involvement**   CC HCC

✓5ᵗʰ **M33.9**   **Dermatopolymyositis, unspecified**

M33.90   **Dermatopolymyositis, unspecified, organ involvement unspecified**   CC HCC

M33.91   **Dermatopolymyositis, unspecified with respiratory involvement**   CC HCC

M33.92 Dermatopolymyositis, unspecified with myopathy `CC` `HCC`

M33.93 Dermatopolymyositis, unspecified without myopathy `CC` `HCC`

M33.99 Dermatopolymyositis, unspecified with other organ involvement `CC` `HCC`

✓4ᵗʰ **M34** Systemic sclerosis [scleroderma]

     EXCLUDES 1   *circumscribed scleroderma (L94.0)*
                   neonatal scleroderma (P83.88)

M34.0 Progressive systemic sclerosis `HCC`

M34.1 CR(E)ST syndrome `HCC`
     Combination of calcinosis, Raynaud's phenomenon, esophageal dysfunction, sclerodactyly, telangiectasia

M34.2 Systemic sclerosis induced by drug and chemical `HCC`
     Code first poisoning due to drug or toxin, if applicable (T36-T65 with fifth or sixth character 1-4 or 6)
     Use additional code for adverse effect, if applicable, to identify drug (T36-T50 with fifth or sixth character 5)

✓5ᵗʰ **M34.8** Other forms of systemic sclerosis

     M34.81 Systemic sclerosis with lung involvement `CC` `HCC`
     M34.82 Systemic sclerosis with myopathy `CC` `HCC`
     M34.83 Systemic sclerosis with polyneuropathy `HCC`
     M34.89 Other systemic sclerosis `HCC`

M34.9 Systemic sclerosis, unspecified `HCC`

✓4ᵗʰ **M35** Other systemic involvement of connective tissue

     EXCLUDES 1   *reactive perforating collagenosis (L87.1)*

✓5ᵗʰ **M35.0** Sicca syndrome [Sjögren]

     DEF: Autoimmune disease associated with keratoconjunctivitis, laryngopharyngitis, rhinitis, dry mouth, enlarged parotid gland, and chronic polyarthritis.

     M35.00 Sicca syndrome, unspecified `HCC`
     M35.01 Sicca syndrome with keratoconjunctivitis `HCC`
     M35.02 Sicca syndrome with lung involvement `HCC`
     M35.03 Sicca syndrome with myopathy `CC` `HCC`
     M35.04 Sicca syndrome with tubulo-interstitial nephropathy `HCC`
             Renal tubular acidosis in sicca syndrome
     M35.09 Sicca syndrome with other organ involvement `HCC`

M35.1 Other overlap syndromes `CC` `HCC`
     Mixed connective tissue disease
     EXCLUDES 1   *polyangiitis overlap syndrome (M30.8)*

M35.2 Behçet's disease `CC` `HCC`

M35.3 Polymyalgia rheumatica `HCC`
     EXCLUDES 1   *polymyalgia rheumatica with giant cell arteritis (M31.5)*

M35.4 Diffuse (eosinophilic) fasciitis

M35.5 Multifocal fibrosclerosis `CC` `HCC`

M35.6 Relapsing panniculitis [Weber-Christian]
     EXCLUDES 1   *lupus panniculitis (L93.2)*
                   panniculitis NOS (M79.3-)

M35.7 Hypermobility syndrome
     Familial ligamentous laxity
     EXCLUDES 1   ►*Ehlers-Danlos syndromes*◄ *(Q79.6-)*
                   ligamentous laxity, NOS (M24.2-)

M35.8 Other specified systemic involvement of connective tissue `CC` `HCC`

M35.9 Systemic involvement of connective tissue, unspecified `HCC`
     Autoimmune disease (systemic) NOS
     Collagen (vascular) disease NOS

✓4ᵗʰ **M36** Systemic disorders of connective tissue in diseases classified elsewhere

     EXCLUDES 2   *arthropathies in diseases classified elsewhere (M14.-)*

M36.0 *Dermato(poly)myositis in neoplastic disease* `CC` `HCC`
     Code first underlying neoplasm (C00-D49)

M36.1 *Arthropathy in neoplastic disease*
     Code first underlying neoplasm, such as:
         leukemia (C91-C95)
         malignant histiocytosis (C96.A)
         multiple myeloma (C90.0)

M36.2 *Hemophilic arthropathy*
     Hemarthrosis in hemophilic arthropathy
     Code first underlying disease, such as:
         factor VIII deficiency (D66)
             with vascular defect (D68.0)
         factor IX deficiency (D67)
         hemophilia (classical) (D66)
         hemophilia B (D67)
         hemophilia C (D68.1)

M36.3 *Arthropathy in other blood disorders*

M36.4 *Arthropathy in hypersensitivity reactions classified elsewhere*
     Code first underlying disease, such as:
         Henoch (-Schönlein) purpura (D69.0)
         serum sickness (T80.6-)

M36.8 *Systemic disorders of connective tissue in other diseases classified elsewhere* `HCC`
     Code first underlying disease, such as:
         alkaptonuria (E70.2)
         hypogammaglobulinemia (D80.-)
         ochronosis (E70.2)

DORSOPATHIES (M40-M54)

Deforming dorsopathies (M40-M43)

✓4ᵗʰ **M40** Kyphosis and lordosis

     EXCLUDES 1   *congenital kyphosis and lordosis (Q76.4)*
                   kyphoscoliosis (M41.-)
                   postprocedural kyphosis and lordosis (M96.-)

Kyphosis and Lordosis

Kyphosis: Excessive convexity in the thoracic region

Lordosis: Excessive concavity in the lumbar region

✓5ᵗʰ **M40.0** Postural kyphosis

     EXCLUDES 1   *osteochondrosis of spine (M42.-)*

     M40.00 Postural kyphosis, site unspecified
     M40.03 Postural kyphosis, cervicothoracic region
     M40.04 Postural kyphosis, thoracic region
     M40.05 Postural kyphosis, thoracolumbar region

✓5ᵗʰ **M40.1** Other secondary kyphosis

     M40.10 Other secondary kyphosis, site unspecified
     M40.12 Other secondary kyphosis, cervical region
     M40.13 Other secondary kyphosis, cervicothoracic region
     M40.14 Other secondary kyphosis, thoracic region
     M40.15 Other secondary kyphosis, thoracolumbar region

✓5ᵗʰ **M40.2** Other and unspecified kyphosis

     ✓6ᵗʰ **M40.20** Unspecified kyphosis

         M40.202 Unspecified kyphosis, cervical region
         M40.203 Unspecified kyphosis, cervicothoracic region
         M40.204 Unspecified kyphosis, thoracic region
         M40.205 Unspecified kyphosis, thoracolumbar region
         M40.209 Unspecified kyphosis, site unspecified

     ✓6ᵗʰ **M40.29** Other kyphosis

         M40.292 Other kyphosis, cervical region
         M40.293 Other kyphosis, cervicothoracic region
         M40.294 Other kyphosis, thoracic region
         M40.295 Other kyphosis, thoracolumbar region

☑ Additional Character Required   ✓x7ᵗʰ Placeholder   Unacceptable PDx   Questionable PDx   Manifestation   Unspecified Dx   H1-H16 HAC   HCC CMS-HCC Dx   HIV HIV Dx

ICD-10-CM 2021   793

M40.299 Other kyphosis, site unspecified

✓5ᵗʰ **M40.3** Flatback syndrome

M40.30 Flatback syndrome, site unspecified
M40.35 Flatback syndrome, thoracolumbar region
M40.36 Flatback syndrome, lumbar region
M40.37 Flatback syndrome, lumbosacral region

✓5ᵗʰ **M40.4** Postural lordosis

Acquired lordosis

M40.40 Postural lordosis, site unspecified
M40.45 Postural lordosis, thoracolumbar region
M40.46 Postural lordosis, lumbar region
M40.47 Postural lordosis, lumbosacral region

✓5ᵗʰ **M40.5** Lordosis, unspecified

M40.50 Lordosis, unspecified, site unspecified
M40.55 Lordosis, unspecified, thoracolumbar region
M40.56 Lordosis, unspecified, lumbar region
M40.57 Lordosis, unspecified, lumbosacral region

✓4ᵗʰ **M41** Scoliosis

INCLUDES　kyphoscoliosis
EXCLUDES 1　congenital scoliosis due to bony malformation (Q76.3)
　　　　　congenital scoliosis NOS (Q67.5)
　　　　　kyphoscoliotic heart disease (I27.1)
　　　　　postprocedural scoliosis (M96.-)
　　　　　postural congenital scoliosis (Q67.5)

Scoliosis

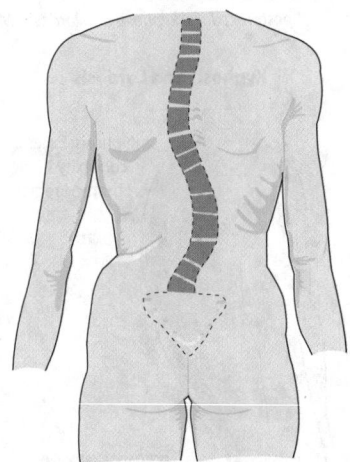

Lateral curvature of spine

✓5ᵗʰ **M41.0** Infantile idiopathic scoliosis

AHA: 2014,4Q,26

M41.00 Infantile idiopathic scoliosis, site unspecified
M41.02 Infantile idiopathic scoliosis, cervical region
M41.03 Infantile idiopathic scoliosis, cervicothoracic region
M41.04 Infantile idiopathic scoliosis, thoracic region
M41.05 Infantile idiopathic scoliosis, thoracolumbar region
M41.06 Infantile idiopathic scoliosis, lumbar region
M41.07 Infantile idiopathic scoliosis, lumbosacral region
M41.08 Infantile idiopathic scoliosis, sacral and sacrococcygeal region

✓5ᵗʰ **M41.1** Juvenile and adolescent idiopathic scoliosis

✓6ᵗʰ **M41.11** Juvenile idiopathic scoliosis

AHA: 2014,4Q,28

M41.112 Juvenile idiopathic scoliosis, cervical region
M41.113 Juvenile idiopathic scoliosis, cervicothoracic region
M41.114 Juvenile idiopathic scoliosis, thoracic region
M41.115 Juvenile idiopathic scoliosis, thoracolumbar region
M41.116 Juvenile idiopathic scoliosis, lumbar region
M41.117 Juvenile idiopathic scoliosis, lumbosacral region
M41.119 Juvenile idiopathic scoliosis, site unspecified

✓6ᵗʰ **M41.12** Adolescent scoliosis

M41.122 Adolescent idiopathic scoliosis, cervical region
M41.123 Adolescent idiopathic scoliosis, cervicothoracic region
M41.124 Adolescent idiopathic scoliosis, thoracic region
M41.125 Adolescent idiopathic scoliosis, thoracolumbar region
M41.126 Adolescent idiopathic scoliosis, lumbar region
M41.127 Adolescent idiopathic scoliosis, lumbosacral region
M41.129 Adolescent idiopathic scoliosis, site unspecified

✓5ᵗʰ **M41.2** Other idiopathic scoliosis

M41.20 Other idiopathic scoliosis, site unspecified
M41.22 Other idiopathic scoliosis, cervical region
M41.23 Other idiopathic scoliosis, cervicothoracic region
M41.24 Other idiopathic scoliosis, thoracic region
M41.25 Other idiopathic scoliosis, thoracolumbar region
M41.26 Other idiopathic scoliosis, lumbar region
M41.27 Other idiopathic scoliosis, lumbosacral region

✓5ᵗʰ **M41.3** Thoracogenic scoliosis

M41.30 Thoracogenic scoliosis, site unspecified
M41.34 Thoracogenic scoliosis, thoracic region
M41.35 Thoracogenic scoliosis, thoracolumbar region

✓5ᵗʰ **M41.4** Neuromuscular scoliosis

Scoliosis secondary to cerebral palsy, Friedreich's ataxia, poliomyelitis and other neuromuscular disorders
Code also underlying condition
AHA: 2014,4Q,27

M41.40 Neuromuscular scoliosis, site unspecified
M41.41 Neuromuscular scoliosis, occipito-atlanto-axial region
M41.42 Neuromuscular scoliosis, cervical region
M41.43 Neuromuscular scoliosis, cervicothoracic region
M41.44 Neuromuscular scoliosis, thoracic region
M41.45 Neuromuscular scoliosis, thoracolumbar region
M41.46 Neuromuscular scoliosis, lumbar region
M41.47 Neuromuscular scoliosis, lumbosacral region

✓5ᵗʰ **M41.5** Other secondary scoliosis

AHA: 2019,1Q,19

M41.50 Other secondary scoliosis, site unspecified
M41.52 Other secondary scoliosis, cervical region
M41.53 Other secondary scoliosis, cervicothoracic region
M41.54 Other secondary scoliosis, thoracic region
M41.55 Other secondary scoliosis, thoracolumbar region
M41.56 Other secondary scoliosis, lumbar region
M41.57 Other secondary scoliosis, lumbosacral region

✓5ᵗʰ **M41.8** Other forms of scoliosis

M41.80 Other forms of scoliosis, site unspecified
M41.82 Other forms of scoliosis, cervical region
M41.83 Other forms of scoliosis, cervicothoracic region
M41.84 Other forms of scoliosis, thoracic region
M41.85 Other forms of scoliosis, thoracolumbar region
M41.86 Other forms of scoliosis, lumbar region
M41.87 Other forms of scoliosis, lumbosacral region

M41.9 Scoliosis, unspecified

✓4ᵗʰ **M42** Spinal osteochondrosis

✓5ᵗʰ **M42.0** Juvenile osteochondrosis of spine

Calvé's disease
Scheuermann's disease
EXCLUDES 1　postural kyphosis (M40.0)

M42.00 Juvenile osteochondrosis of spine, site unspecified
M42.01 Juvenile osteochondrosis of spine, occipito-atlanto-axial region
M42.02 Juvenile osteochondrosis of spine, cervical region
M42.03 Juvenile osteochondrosis of spine, cervicothoracic region
M42.04 Juvenile osteochondrosis of spine, thoracic region
M42.05 Juvenile osteochondrosis of spine, thoracolumbar region
M42.06 Juvenile osteochondrosis of spine, lumbar region
M42.07 Juvenile osteochondrosis of spine, lumbosacral region

M42.08   **Juvenile osteochondrosis of spine,** sacral and sacrococcygeal region

M42.09   **Juvenile osteochondrosis of spine,** multiple sites in spine

√5ᵗʰ **M42.1   Adult osteochondrosis of spine**

    M42.10   Adult osteochondrosis of spine, site unspecified   A

    M42.11   **Adult osteochondrosis of spine,** occipito-atlanto-axial region   A

    M42.12   **Adult osteochondrosis of spine,** cervical region   A

    M42.13   **Adult osteochondrosis of spine,** cervicothoracic region   A

    M42.14   **Adult osteochondrosis of spine,** thoracic region   A

    M42.15   **Adult osteochondrosis of spine,** thoracolumbar region   A

    M42.16   **Adult osteochondrosis of spine,** lumbar region   A

    M42.17   **Adult osteochondrosis of spine,** lumbosacral region   A

    M42.18   **Adult osteochondrosis of** spine, sacral and sacrococcygeal region   A

    M42.19   **Adult osteochondrosis of spine,** multiple sites in spine   A

    M42.9   Spinal osteochondrosis, unspecified

√4ᵗʰ **M43   Other deforming dorsopathies**

    EXCLUDES 1   *congenital spondylolysis and spondylolisthesis (Q76.2)*
        hemivertebra (Q76.3-Q76.4)
        Klippel-Feil syndrome (Q76.1)
        lumbarization and sacralization (Q76.4)
        platyspondylisis (Q76.4)
        spina bifida occulta (Q76.0)
        spinal curvature in osteoporosis (M80.-)
        spinal curvature in Paget's disease of bone [osteitis deformans] (M88.-)

√5ᵗʰ **M43.0   Spondylolysis**

    EXCLUDES 1   *congenital spondylolysis (Q76.2)*
        spondylolisthesis (M43.1)

    M43.00   Spondylolysis, site unspecified

    M43.01   **Spondylolysis,** occipito-atlanto-axial region

    M43.02   **Spondylolysis,** cervical region

    M43.03   **Spondylolysis,** cervicothoracic region

    M43.04   **Spondylolysis,** thoracic region

    M43.05   **Spondylolysis,** thoracolumbar region

    M43.06   **Spondylolysis,** lumbar region

    M43.07   **Spondylolysis,** lumbosacral region

    M43.08   **Spondylolysis,** sacral and sacrococcygeal region

    M43.09   **Spondylolysis,** multiple sites in spine

√5ᵗʰ **M43.1   Spondylolisthesis**

    EXCLUDES 1   *acute traumatic of lumbosacral region (S33.1)*
        acute traumatic of sites other than lumbosacral — code to Fracture, vertebra, by region
        congenital spondylolisthesis (Q76.2)

    AHA: 2020,2Q,21; 2018,3Q,18
    TIP: Code also any associated radiculopathy (M54.1-) and/or myelopathy (G99.2).

    M43.10   Spondylolisthesis, site unspecified

    M43.11   **Spondylolisthesis,** occipito-atlanto-axial region

    M43.12   **Spondylolisthesis,** cervical region

    M43.13   **Spondylolisthesis,** cervicothoracic region

    M43.14   **Spondylolisthesis,** thoracic region

    M43.15   **Spondylolisthesis,** thoracolumbar region

    M43.16   **Spondylolisthesis,** lumbar region

    M43.17   **Spondylolisthesis,** lumbosacral region

    M43.18   **Spondylolisthesis,** sacral and sacrococcygeal region

    M43.19   **Spondylolisthesis,** multiple sites in spine

√5ᵗʰ **M43.2   Fusion of spine**

    Ankylosis of spinal joint

    EXCLUDES 1   *ankylosing spondylitis (M45.0-)*
        congenital fusion of spine (Q76.4)

    EXCLUDES 2   *arthrodesis status (Z98.1)*
        pseudoarthrosis after fusion or arthrodesis (M96.0)

    M43.20   Fusion of spine, site unspecified

    M43.21   **Fusion of spine,** occipito-atlanto-axial region

    M43.22   **Fusion of spine,** cervical region

    M43.23   **Fusion of spine,** cervicothoracic region

    M43.24   **Fusion of spine,** thoracic region

    M43.25   **Fusion of spine,** thoracolumbar region

    M43.26   **Fusion of spine,** lumbar region

    M43.27   **Fusion of spine,** lumbosacral region

    M43.28   **Fusion of spine,** sacral and sacrococcygeal region

    M43.3   Recurrent atlantoaxial dislocation with myelopathy

    M43.4   Other recurrent atlantoaxial dislocation

√5ᵗʰ **M43.5   Other recurrent vertebral dislocation**

    EXCLUDES 1   *biomechanical lesions NEC (M99.-)*

    √6ᵗʰ **M43.5X   Other recurrent vertebral dislocation**

        M43.5X2   **Other recurrent vertebral dislocation,** cervical region

        M43.5X3   **Other recurrent vertebral dislocation,** cervicothoracic region

        M43.5X4   **Other recurrent vertebral dislocation,** thoracic region

        M43.5X5   **Other recurrent vertebral dislocation,** thoracolumbar region

        M43.5X6   **Other recurrent vertebral dislocation,** lumbar region

        M43.5X7   **Other recurrent vertebral dislocation,** lumbosacral region

        M43.5X8   **Other recurrent vertebral dislocation,** sacral and sacrococcygeal region

        M43.5X9   Other recurrent vertebral dislocation, site unspecified

    M43.6   Torticollis

    EXCLUDES 1   *congenital (sternomastoid) torticollis (Q68.0)*
        current injury — see Injury, of spine, by body region
        ocular torticollis (R29.891)
        psychogenic torticollis (F45.8)
        spasmodic torticollis (G24.3)
        torticollis due to birth injury (P15.2)

    DEF: Twisted, unnatural position of the neck due to contracted cervical muscles that pull the head to one side.

√5ᵗʰ **M43.8   Other specified deforming dorsopathies**

    EXCLUDES 2   *kyphosis and lordosis (M40.-)*
        scoliosis (M41.-)

    √6ᵗʰ **M43.8X   Other specified deforming dorsopathies**

        M43.8X1   **Other specified deforming dorsopathies,** occipito-atlanto-axial region

        M43.8X2   **Other specified deforming dorsopathies,** cervical region

        M43.8X3   **Other specified deforming dorsopathies,** cervicothoracic region

        M43.8X4   **Other specified deforming dorsopathies,** thoracic region

        M43.8X5   **Other specified deforming dorsopathies,** thoracolumbar region

        M43.8X6   **Other specified deforming dorsopathies,** lumbar region

        M43.8X7   **Other specified deforming dorsopathies,** lumbosacral region

        M43.8X8   **Other specified deforming dorsopathies,** sacral and sacrococcygeal region

        M43.8X9   Other specified deforming dorsopathies, site unspecified

    M43.9   Deforming dorsopathy, unspecified
        Curvature of spine NOS

Spondylopathies (M45-M49)

√4ᵗʰ **M45   Ankylosing spondylitis**

    Rheumatoid arthritis of spine

    EXCLUDES 1   *arthropathy in Reiter's disease (M02.3-)*
        juvenile (ankylosing) spondylitis (M08.1)

    EXCLUDES 2   *Behçet's disease (M35.2)*

    M45.0   Ankylosing spondylitis of multiple sites in spine   HCC

    M45.1   Ankylosing spondylitis of occipito-atlanto-axial region   HCC

    M45.2   Ankylosing spondylitis of cervical region   HCC

    M45.3   Ankylosing spondylitis of cervicothoracic region   HCC

    M45.4   Ankylosing spondylitis of thoracic region   HCC

    M45.5   Ankylosing spondylitis of thoracolumbar region   HCC

    M45.6   Ankylosing spondylitis lumbar region   HCC

    M45.7   Ankylosing spondylitis of lumbosacral region   HCC

M45.8 Ankylosing spondylitis sacral and sacrococcygeal region `HCC`

M45.9 Ankylosing spondylitis of unspecified sites in spine `HCC`

✓4ᵗʰ **M46 Other inflammatory spondylopathies**

  ✓5ᵗʰ **M46.0 Spinal enthesopathy**

    Disorder of ligamentous or muscular attachments of spine

    M46.00 Spinal enthesopathy, site unspecified `HCC`

    M46.01 Spinal enthesopathy, occipito-atlanto-axial region `HCC`

    M46.02 Spinal enthesopathy, cervical region `HCC`

    M46.03 Spinal enthesopathy, cervicothoracic region `HCC`

    M46.04 Spinal enthesopathy, thoracic region `HCC`

    M46.05 Spinal enthesopathy, thoracolumbar region `HCC`

    M46.06 Spinal enthesopathy, lumbar region `HCC`

    M46.07 Spinal enthesopathy, lumbosacral region `HCC`

    M46.08 Spinal enthesopathy, sacral and sacrococcygeal region `HCC`

    M46.09 Spinal enthesopathy, multiple sites in spine `HCC`

  M46.1 Sacroiliitis, not elsewhere classified `HCC`

    AHA: 2020,2Q,14

    DEF: Inflammation of the sacroiliac joint (situated at the juncture of the sacrum and hip). Symptoms include pain in the buttocks or lower back that can extend down one or both legs.

  ✓5ᵗʰ **M46.2 Osteomyelitis of vertebra**

    M46.20 Osteomyelitis of vertebra, site unspecified `CC` `HCC`

    M46.21 Osteomyelitis of vertebra, occipito-atlanto-axial region `CC` `HCC`

    M46.22 Osteomyelitis of vertebra, cervical region `CC` `HCC`

    M46.23 Osteomyelitis of vertebra, cervicothoracic region `CC` `HCC`

    M46.24 Osteomyelitis of vertebra, thoracic region `CC` `HCC`

    M46.25 Osteomyelitis of vertebra, thoracolumbar region `CC` `HCC`

    M46.26 Osteomyelitis of vertebra, lumbar region `CC` `HCC`

    M46.27 Osteomyelitis of vertebra, lumbosacral region `CC` `HCC`

    M46.28 Osteomyelitis of vertebra, sacral and sacrococcygeal region `CC` `HCC`

  ✓5ᵗʰ **M46.3 Infection of intervertebral disc (pyogenic)**

    Use additional code (B95-B97) to identify infectious agent

    M46.30 Infection of intervertebral disc (pyogenic), site unspecified `CC` `HCC`

    M46.31 Infection of intervertebral disc (pyogenic), occipito-atlanto-axial region `CC` `HCC`

    M46.32 Infection of intervertebral disc (pyogenic), cervical region `CC` `HCC`

    M46.33 Infection of intervertebral disc (pyogenic), cervicothoracic region `CC` `HCC`

    M46.34 Infection of intervertebral disc (pyogenic), thoracic region `CC` `HCC`

    M46.35 Infection of intervertebral disc (pyogenic), thoracolumbar region `CC` `HCC`

    M46.36 Infection of intervertebral disc (pyogenic), lumbar region `CC` `HCC`

    M46.37 Infection of intervertebral disc (pyogenic), lumbosacral region `CC` `HCC`

    M46.38 Infection of intervertebral disc (pyogenic), sacral and sacrococcygeal region `CC` `HCC`

    M46.39 Infection of intervertebral disc (pyogenic), multiple sites in spine `CC` `HCC`

  ✓5ᵗʰ **M46.4 Discitis, unspecified**

    M46.40 Discitis, unspecified, site unspecified

    M46.41 Discitis, unspecified, occipito-atlanto-axial region

    M46.42 Discitis, unspecified, cervical region

    M46.43 Discitis, unspecified, cervicothoracic region

    M46.44 Discitis, unspecified, thoracic region

    M46.45 Discitis, unspecified, thoracolumbar region

    M46.46 Discitis, unspecified, lumbar region

    M46.47 Discitis, unspecified, lumbosacral region

    M46.48 Discitis, unspecified, sacral and sacrococcygeal region

    M46.49 Discitis, unspecified, multiple sites in spine

  ✓5ᵗʰ **M46.5 Other infective spondylopathies**

    M46.50 Other infective spondylopathies, site unspecified `HCC`

    M46.51 Other infective spondylopathies, occipito-atlanto-axial region `HCC`

    M46.52 Other infective spondylopathies, cervical region `HCC`

    M46.53 Other infective spondylopathies, cervicothoracic region `HCC`

    M46.54 Other infective spondylopathies, thoracic region `HCC`

    M46.55 Other infective spondylopathies, thoracolumbar region `HCC`

    M46.56 Other infective spondylopathies, lumbar region `HCC`

    M46.57 Other infective spondylopathies, lumbosacral region `HCC`

    M46.58 Other infective spondylopathies, sacral and sacrococcygeal region `HCC`

    M46.59 Other infective spondylopathies, multiple sites in spine `HCC`

  ✓5ᵗʰ **M46.8 Other specified inflammatory spondylopathies**

    M46.80 Other specified inflammatory spondylopathies, site unspecified `HCC`

    M46.81 Other specified inflammatory spondylopathies, occipito-atlanto-axial region `HCC`

    M46.82 Other specified inflammatory spondylopathies, cervical region `HCC`

    M46.83 Other specified inflammatory spondylopathies, cervicothoracic region `HCC`

    M46.84 Other specified inflammatory spondylopathies, thoracic region `HCC`

    M46.85 Other specified inflammatory spondylopathies, thoracolumbar region `HCC`

    M46.86 Other specified inflammatory spondylopathies, lumbar region `HCC`

    M46.87 Other specified inflammatory spondylopathies, lumbosacral region `HCC`

    M46.88 Other specified inflammatory spondylopathies, sacral and sacrococcygeal region `HCC`

    M46.89 Other specified inflammatory spondylopathies, multiple sites in spine `HCC`

  ✓5ᵗʰ **M46.9 Unspecified inflammatory spondylopathy**

    M46.90 Unspecified inflammatory spondylopathy, site unspecified `HCC`

    M46.91 Unspecified inflammatory spondylopathy, occipito-atlanto-axial region `HCC`

    M46.92 Unspecified inflammatory spondylopathy, cervical region `HCC`

      AHA: 2019,3Q,10

    M46.93 Unspecified inflammatory spondylopathy, cervicothoracic region `HCC`

    M46.94 Unspecified inflammatory spondylopathy, thoracic region `HCC`

    M46.95 Unspecified inflammatory spondylopathy, thoracolumbar region `HCC`

    M46.96 Unspecified inflammatory spondylopathy, lumbar region `HCC`

    M46.97 Unspecified inflammatory spondylopathy, lumbosacral region `HCC`

    M46.98 Unspecified inflammatory spondylopathy, sacral and sacrococcygeal region `HCC`

    M46.99 Unspecified inflammatory spondylopathy, multiple sites in spine `HCC`

✓4ᵗʰ **M47 Spondylosis**

  `INCLUDES` arthrosis or osteoarthritis of spine

     degeneration of facet joints

  AHA: 2020,1Q,17; 2019,3Q,10-11; 2016,4Q,147

  ✓5ᵗʰ **M47.0 Anterior spinal and vertebral artery compression syndromes**

    ✓6ᵗʰ **M47.01 Anterior spinal artery compression syndromes**

      M47.011 Anterior spinal artery compression syndromes, occipito-atlanto-axial region `CC`

      M47.012 Anterior spinal artery compression syndromes, cervical region `CC`

      M47.013 Anterior spinal artery compression syndromes, cervicothoracic region `CC`

      M47.014 Anterior spinal artery compression syndromes, thoracic region `CC`

      M47.015 Anterior spinal artery compression syndromes, thoracolumbar region `CC`

`N` Newborn: 0   `P` Pediatric: 0-17   `M` Maternity: 9-64   `A` Adult: 15-124   `MCC` Major Complication/Comorbidity   `CC` Complication/Comorbidity   `SW` Severe Wound Dx

796   ICD-10-CM 2021

M47.Ø16 **Anterior spinal artery compression syndromes, lumbar region** `cc`

M47.Ø19 **Anterior spinal artery compression syndromes, site unspecified** `cc`

√6ᵗʰ M47.Ø2 Vertebral artery compression syndromes

M47.Ø21 **Vertebral artery compression syndromes, occipito-atlanto-axial region** `cc`

M47.Ø22 **Vertebral artery compression syndromes, cervical region** `cc`

M47.Ø29 **Vertebral artery compression syndromes, site unspecified** `cc`

√5ᵗʰ M47.1 **Other spondylosis** with myelopathy

Spondylogenic compression of spinal cord

EXCLUDES 1   vertebral subluxation (M43.3-M43.5X9)

AHA: 2020,1Q,17

M47.1Ø **Other spondylosis with myelopathy, site unspecified** `cc`

M47.11 **Other spondylosis with myelopathy, occipito-atlanto-axial region** `cc`

M47.12 **Other spondylosis with myelopathy, cervical region** `cc`

M47.13 **Other spondylosis with myelopathy, cervicothoracic region** `cc`

M47.14 **Other spondylosis with myelopathy, thoracic region** `cc`

M47.15 **Other spondylosis with myelopathy, thoracolumbar region** `cc`

M47.16 **Other spondylosis with myelopathy, lumbar region** `cc`

√5ᵗʰ M47.2 **Other spondylosis** with radiculopathy

AHA: 2020,1Q,17

M47.2Ø **Other spondylosis with radiculopathy, site unspecified**

M47.21 **Other spondylosis with radiculopathy, occipito-atlanto-axial region**

M47.22 **Other spondylosis with radiculopathy, cervical region**

M47.23 **Other spondylosis with radiculopathy, cervicothoracic region**

M47.24 **Other spondylosis with radiculopathy, thoracic region**

M47.25 **Other spondylosis with radiculopathy, thoracolumbar region**

M47.26 **Other spondylosis with radiculopathy, lumbar region**

M47.27 **Other spondylosis with radiculopathy, lumbosacral region**

M47.28 **Other spondylosis with radiculopathy, sacral and sacrococcygeal region**

√5ᵗʰ M47.8 **Other spondylosis**

√6ᵗʰ M47.81 **Spondylosis** without myelopathy or radiculopathy

AHA: 2019,3Q,10-11; 2018,2Q,14

M47.811 **Spondylosis without myelopathy or radiculopathy, occipito-atlanto-axial region**

M47.812 **Spondylosis without myelopathy or radiculopathy, cervical region**

M47.813 **Spondylosis without myelopathy or radiculopathy, cervicothoracic region**

M47.814 **Spondylosis without myelopathy or radiculopathy, thoracic region**

M47.815 **Spondylosis without myelopathy or radiculopathy, thoracolumbar region**

M47.816 **Spondylosis without myelopathy or radiculopathy, lumbar region**

M47.817 **Spondylosis without myelopathy or radiculopathy, lumbosacral region**

M47.818 **Spondylosis without myelopathy or radiculopathy, sacral and sacrococcygeal region**

M47.819 **Spondylosis without myelopathy or radiculopathy, site unspecified**

√6ᵗʰ M47.89 **Other spondylosis**

M47.891 **Other spondylosis,** occipito-atlanto-axial region

M47.892 **Other spondylosis,** cervical region

M47.893 **Other spondylosis,** cervicothoracic region

M47.894 **Other spondylosis,** thoracic region

M47.895 **Other spondylosis,** thoracolumbar region

M47.896 **Other spondylosis,** lumbar region

M47.897 **Other spondylosis,** lumbosacral region

M47.898 **Other spondylosis,** sacral and sacrococcygeal region

M47.899 **Other spondylosis, site unspecified**

M47.9 **Spondylosis, unspecified**

√4ᵗʰ M48 **Other spondylopathies**

√5ᵗʰ M48.Ø **Spinal stenosis**

Caudal stenosis

AHA: 2020,1Q,17; 2018,3Q,18-19

TIP: Code also any associated radiculopathy (M54.1-) and/or myelopathy (G99.2).

M48.ØØ **Spinal stenosis, site unspecified**

M48.Ø1 **Spinal stenosis,** occipito-atlanto-axial region

M48.Ø2 **Spinal stenosis,** cervical region

M48.Ø3 **Spinal stenosis,** cervicothoracic region

M48.Ø4 **Spinal stenosis,** thoracic region

M48.Ø5 **Spinal stenosis,** thoracolumbar region

√6ᵗʰ M48.Ø6 **Spinal stenosis,** lumbar region

AHA: 2018,3Q,19; 2017,4Q,18-19

DEF: Spinal canal narrowing in the lumbar area with nerve root compression, causing muscle pain, fatigue, and weakness during extension of the lumbar spine. Pain is relieved by sitting or bending.

M48.Ø61 **Spinal stenosis, lumbar region** without neurogenic claudication

Spinal stenosis, lumbar region NOS

M48.Ø62 **Spinal stenosis, lumbar region** with neurogenic claudication

M48.Ø7 **Spinal stenosis,** lumbosacral region

M48.Ø8 **Spinal stenosis,** sacral and sacrococcygeal region

√5ᵗʰ M48.1 **Ankylosing hyperostosis [Forestier]**

Diffuse idiopathic skeletal hyperostosis [DISH]

M48.1Ø **Ankylosing hyperostosis [Forestier], site unspecified**

M48.11 **Ankylosing hyperostosis [Forestier],** occipito-atlanto-axial region

M48.12 **Ankylosing hyperostosis [Forestier],** cervical region

M48.13 **Ankylosing hyperostosis [Forestier],** cervicothoracic region

M48.14 **Ankylosing hyperostosis [Forestier],** thoracic region

M48.15 **Ankylosing hyperostosis [Forestier],** thoracolumbar region

M48.16 **Ankylosing hyperostosis [Forestier],** lumbar region

M48.17 **Ankylosing hyperostosis [Forestier],** lumbosacral region

M48.18 **Ankylosing hyperostosis [Forestier],** sacral and sacrococcygeal region

M48.19 **Ankylosing hyperostosis [Forestier],** multiple sites in spine

√5ᵗʰ M48.2 **Kissing spine**

M48.2Ø **Kissing spine, site unspecified**

M48.21 **Kissing spine,** occipito-atlanto-axial region

M48.22 **Kissing spine,** cervical region

M48.23 **Kissing spine,** cervicothoracic region

M48.24 **Kissing spine,** thoracic region

M48.25 **Kissing spine,** thoracolumbar region

M48.26 **Kissing spine,** lumbar region

M48.27 **Kissing spine,** lumbosacral region

√5ᵗʰ M48.3 **Traumatic spondylopathy**

M48.3Ø **Traumatic spondylopathy, site unspecified** `cc`

M48.31 **Traumatic spondylopathy,** occipito-atlanto-axial region `cc`

M48.32 **Traumatic spondylopathy,** cervical region `cc`

M48.33 **Traumatic spondylopathy,** cervicothoracic region `cc`

M48.34 **Traumatic spondylopathy,** thoracic region `cc`

M48.35 **Traumatic spondylopathy,** thoracolumbar region `cc`

M48.36 **Traumatic spondylopathy,** lumbar region `cc`

M48.37 **Traumatic spondylopathy,** lumbosacral region `cc`

M48.38 **Traumatic spondylopathy,** sacral and sacrococcygeal region `cc`

✔ Additional Character Required   √x7ᵗʰ Placeholder   Unacceptable PDx   Questionable PDx   Manifestation   Unspecified Dx   H1 -H14 HAC   HCC CMS-HCC Dx   HIV HIV Dx

ICD-10-CM 2021   797

Chapter 13. Diseases of the Musculoskeletal System and Connective Tissue

M48.4–M50.01

✓5ᵗʰ **M48.4** **Fatigue fracture of vertebra**
Stress fracture of vertebra
EXCLUDES 1   *pathological fracture NOS (M84.4-)*
pathological fracture of vertebra due to neoplasm (M84.58)
pathological fracture of vertebra due to osteoporosis (M80.-)
pathological fracture of vertebra due to other diagnosis (M84.68)
traumatic fracture of vertebrae (S12.0-S12.3-, S22.0-, S32.0-)

The appropriate 7th character is to be added to each code from subcategory M48.4.
A   initial encounter for fracture
D   subsequent encounter for fracture with routine healing
G   subsequent encounter for fracture with delayed healing
S   sequela of fracture

✓x7ᵗʰ **M48.40** **Fatigue fracture of vertebra, site unspecified**
✓x7ᵗʰ **M48.41** **Fatigue fracture of vertebra, occipito-atlanto-axial region**
✓x7ᵗʰ **M48.42** **Fatigue fracture of vertebra, cervical region**
✓x7ᵗʰ **M48.43** **Fatigue fracture of vertebra, cervicothoracic region**
✓x7ᵗʰ **M48.44** **Fatigue fracture of vertebra, thoracic region**
✓x7ᵗʰ **M48.45** **Fatigue fracture of vertebra, thoracolumbar region**
✓x7ᵗʰ **M48.46** **Fatigue fracture of vertebra, lumbar region**
✓x7ᵗʰ **M48.47** **Fatigue fracture of vertebra, lumbosacral region**
✓x7ᵗʰ **M48.48** **Fatigue fracture of vertebra, sacral and sacrococcygeal region**

✓5ᵗʰ **M48.5** **Collapsed vertebra, not elsewhere classified**
Collapsed vertebra NOS
Compression fracture of vertebra NOS
Wedging of vertebra NOS
EXCLUDES 1   *current injury — see Injury of spine, by body region*
fatigue fracture of vertebra (M48.4)
pathological fracture NOS (M84.4-)
pathological fracture of vertebra due to neoplasm (M84.58)
pathological fracture of vertebra due to osteoporosis (M80.-)
pathological fracture of vertebra due to other diagnosis (M84.68)
stress fracture of vertebra (M48.4-)
traumatic fracture of vertebra (S12.-, S22.-, S32.-)

The appropriate 7th character is to be added to each code from subcategory M48.5.
A   initial encounter for fracture
D   subsequent encounter for fracture with routine healing
G   subsequent encounter for fracture with delayed healing
S   sequela of fracture

6 ✓x7ᵗʰ **M48.50** **Collapsed vertebra, not elsewhere classified, site unspecified**   CC HCC
6 ✓x7ᵗʰ **M48.51** **Collapsed vertebra, not elsewhere classified, occipito-atlanto-axial region**   CC HCC
6 ✓x7ᵗʰ **M48.52** **Collapsed vertebra, not elsewhere classified, cervical region**   CC HCC
6 ✓x7ᵗʰ **M48.53** **Collapsed vertebra, not elsewhere classified, cervicothoracic region**   CC HCC
6 ✓x7ᵗʰ **M48.54** **Collapsed vertebra, not elsewhere classified, thoracic region**   CC HCC
6 ✓x7ᵗʰ **M48.55** **Collapsed vertebra, not elsewhere classified, thoracolumbar region**   CC HCC
6 ✓x7ᵗʰ **M48.56** **Collapsed vertebra, not elsewhere classified, lumbar region**   CC HCC
6 ✓x7ᵗʰ **M48.57** **Collapsed vertebra, not elsewhere classified, lumbosacral region**   CC HCC
6 ✓x7ᵗʰ **M48.58** **Collapsed vertebra, not elsewhere classified, sacral and sacrococcygeal region**   CC HCC

✓5ᵗʰ **M48.8** **Other specified spondylopathies**
Ossification of posterior longitudinal ligament
✓6ᵗʰ **M48.8X** **Other specified spondylopathies**
M48.8X1 **Other specified spondylopathies, occipito-atlanto-axial region**   HCC
M48.8X2 **Other specified spondylopathies, cervical region**   HCC

M48.8X3 **Other specified spondylopathies, cervicothoracic region**   HCC
M48.8X4 **Other specified spondylopathies, thoracic region**   HCC
M48.8X5 **Other specified spondylopathies, thoracolumbar region**   HCC
M48.8X6 **Other specified spondylopathies, lumbar region**   HCC
M48.8X7 **Other specified spondylopathies, lumbosacral region**   HCC
M48.8X8 **Other specified spondylopathies, sacral and sacrococcygeal region**   HCC
M48.8X9 **Other specified spondylopathies, site unspecified**   HCC

M48.9 **Spondylopathy, unspecified**

✓4ᵗʰ **M49** **Spondylopathies in diseases classified elsewhere**
INCLUDES   curvature of spine in diseases classified elsewhere
deformity of spine in diseases classified elsewhere
kyphosis in diseases classified elsewhere
scoliosis in diseases classified elsewhere
spondylopathy in diseases classified elsewhere
Code first underlying disease, such as:
brucellosis (A23.-)
Charcôt-Marie-Tooth disease (G60.0)
enterobacterial infections (A01-A04)
osteitis fibrosa cystica (E21.0)
EXCLUDES 1   *curvature of spine in tuberculosis [Pott's] (A18.01)*
enteropathic arthropathies (M07.-)
gonococcal spondylitis (A54.41)
neuropathic spondylopathy in syringomyelia (G95.0)
neuropathic spondylopathy in tabes dorsalis (A52.11)
neuropathic [tabes dorsalis] spondylitis (A52.11)
nonsyphilitic neuropathic spondylopathy NEC (G98.0)
spondylitis in syphilis (acquired) (A52.77)
tuberculous spondylitis (A18.01)
typhoid fever spondylitis (A01.05)

✓5ᵗʰ **M49.8** **Spondylopathy in diseases classified elsewhere**
M49.80 *Spondylopathy in diseases classified elsewhere, site unspecified*   HCC
M49.81 *Spondylopathy in diseases classified elsewhere, occipito-atlanto-axial region*   HCC
M49.82 *Spondylopathy in diseases classified elsewhere, cervical region*   HCC
M49.83 *Spondylopathy in diseases classified elsewhere, cervicothoracic region*   HCC
M49.84 *Spondylopathy in diseases classified elsewhere, thoracic region*   HCC
M49.85 *Spondylopathy in diseases classified elsewhere, thoracolumbar region*   HCC
M49.86 *Spondylopathy in diseases classified elsewhere, lumbar region*   HCC
M49.87 *Spondylopathy in diseases classified elsewhere, lumbosacral region*   HCC
M49.88 *Spondylopathy in diseases classified elsewhere, sacral and sacrococcygeal region*   HCC
M49.89 *Spondylopathy in diseases classified elsewhere, multiple sites in spine*   HCC

Other dorsopathies (M50-M54)

EXCLUDES 1   *current injury — see injury of spine by body region*
discitis NOS (M46.4-)

✓4ᵗʰ **M50** **Cervical disc disorders**
NOTE   Code to the most superior level of disorder
INCLUDES   cervicothoracic disc disorders
cervicothoracic disc disorders with cervicalgia
AHA: 2016,4Q,39-40; 2016,1Q,17
✓5ᵗʰ **M50.0** **Cervical disc disorder with myelopathy**
AHA: 2018,3Q,19
M50.00 **Cervical disc disorder with myelopathy, unspecified cervical region**   CC
M50.01 **Cervical disc disorder with myelopathy, high cervical region**   CC
C2-C3 disc disorder with myelopathy
C3-C4 disc disorder with myelopathy

√6ᵗʰ **M50.02 Cervical disc disorder with myelopathy, mid-cervical region**

    M50.020 Cervical disc disorder with myelopathy, mid-cervical region, unspecified level `cc`

    M50.021 **Cervical disc disorder at C4-C5 level with myelopathy** `cc`

      C4-C5 disc disorder with myelopathy

    M50.022 **Cervical disc disorder at C5-C6 level with myelopathy** `cc`

      C5-C6 disc disorder with myelopathy

    M50.023 **Cervical disc disorder at C6-C7 level with myelopathy** `cc`

      C6-C7 disc disorder with myelopathy

M50.03 Cervical disc disorder with myelopathy, cervicothoracic region `cc`

   C7-T1 disc disorder with myelopathy

√5ᵗʰ **M50.1 Cervical disc disorder with radiculopathy**

   EXCLUDES 2   brachial radiculitis NOS (M54.13)

   AHA: 2018,3Q,19

   M50.10 Cervical disc disorder with radiculopathy, unspecified cervical region

   M50.11 **Cervical disc disorder with radiculopathy, high cervical region**

     C2-C3 disc disorder with radiculopathy

     C3 radiculopathy due to disc disorder

     C3-C4 disc disorder with radiculopathy

     C4 radiculopathy due to disc disorder

√6ᵗʰ **M50.12 Cervical disc disorder with radiculopathy, mid-cervical region**

    M50.120 Mid-cervical disc disorder, unspecified level

    M50.121 **Cervical disc disorder at C4-C5 level with radiculopathy**

      C4-C5 disc disorder with radiculopathy

      C5 radiculopathy due to disc disorder

    M50.122 **Cervical disc disorder at C5-C6 level with radiculopathy**

      C5-C6 disc disorder with radiculopathy

      C6 radiculopathy due to disc disorder

    M50.123 **Cervical disc disorder at C6-C7 level with radiculopathy**

      C6-C7 disc disorder with radiculopathy

      C7 radiculopathy due to disc disorder

M50.13 Cervical disc disorder with radiculopathy, cervicothoracic region

   C7-T1 disc disorder with radiculopathy

   C8 radiculopathy due to disc disorder

√5ᵗʰ **M50.2 Other cervical disc displacement**

   M50.20 Other cervical disc displacement, unspecified cervical region

   M50.21 **Other cervical disc displacement, high cervical region**

     Other C2-C3 cervical disc displacement

     Other C3-C4 cervical disc displacement

√6ᵗʰ **M50.22 Other cervical disc displacement, mid-cervical region**

    M50.220 Other cervical disc displacement, mid-cervical region, unspecified level

    M50.221 **Other cervical disc displacement at C4-C5 level**

      Other C4-C5 cervical disc displacement

    M50.222 **Other cervical disc displacement at C5-C6 level**

      Other C5-C6 cervical disc displacement

    M50.223 **Other cervical disc displacement at C6-C7 level**

      Other C6-C7 cervical disc displacement

M50.23 Other cervical disc displacement, cervicothoracic region

   Other C7-T1 cervical disc displacement

√5ᵗʰ **M50.3 Other cervical disc degeneration**

   M50.30 Other cervical disc degeneration, unspecified cervical region

   M50.31 **Other cervical disc degeneration, high cervical region**

     Other C2-C3 cervical disc degeneration

     Other C3-C4 cervical disc degeneration

√6ᵗʰ **M50.32 Other cervical disc degeneration, mid-cervical region**

    M50.320 Other cervical disc degeneration, mid-cervical region, unspecified level

    M50.321 **Other cervical disc degeneration at C4-C5 level**

      Other C4-C5 cervical disc degeneration

    M50.322 **Other cervical disc degeneration at C5-C6 level**

      Other C5-C6 cervical disc degeneration

    M50.323 **Other cervical disc degeneration at C6-C7 level**

      Other C6-C7 cervical disc degeneration

M50.33 Other cervical disc degeneration, cervicothoracic region

   Other C7-T1 cervical disc degeneration

√5ᵗʰ **M50.8 Other cervical disc disorders**

   M50.80 Other cervical disc disorders, unspecified cervical region

   M50.81 **Other cervical disc disorders, high cervical region**

     Other C2-C3 cervical disc disorders

     Other C3-C4 cervical disc disorders

√6ᵗʰ **M50.82 Other cervical disc disorders, mid-cervical region**

    M50.820 Other cervical disc disorders, mid-cervical region, unspecified level

    M50.821 **Other cervical disc disorders at C4-C5 level**

      Other C4-C5 cervical disc disorders

    M50.822 **Other cervical disc disorders at C5-C6 level**

      Other C5-C6 cervical disc disorders

    M50.823 **Other cervical disc disorders at C6-C7 level**

      Other C6-C7 cervical disc disorders

M50.83 Other cervical disc disorders, cervicothoracic region

   Other C7-T1 cervical disc disorders

√5ᵗʰ **M50.9 Cervical disc disorder, unspecified**

   M50.90 Cervical disc disorder, unspecified, unspecified cervical region

   M50.91 Cervical disc disorder, unspecified, high cervical region

     C2-C3 cervical disc disorder, unspecified

     C3-C4 cervical disc disorder, unspecified

√6ᵗʰ **M50.92 Cervical disc disorder, unspecified, mid-cervical region**

    M50.920 Unspecified cervical disc disorder, mid-cervical region, unspecified level

    M50.921 Unspecified cervical disc disorder at C4-C5 level

      Unspecified C4-C5 cervical disc disorder

    M50.922 Unspecified cervical disc disorder at C5-C6 level

      Unspecified C5-C6 cervical disc disorder

    M50.923 Unspecified cervical disc disorder at C6-C7 level

      Unspecified C6-C7 cervical disc disorder

M50.93 Cervical disc disorder, unspecified, cervicothoracic region

   C7-T1 cervical disc disorder, unspecified

√4ᵗʰ **M51 Thoracic, thoracolumbar, and lumbosacral intervertebral disc disorders**

   EXCLUDES 2   cervical and cervicothoracic disc disorders (M50.-)

              sacral and sacrococcygeal disorders (M53.3)

√5ᵗʰ **M51.0 Thoracic, thoracolumbar and lumbosacral intervertebral disc disorders with myelopathy**

   M51.04 **Intervertebral disc disorders with myelopathy, thoracic region** `cc`

   M51.05 **Intervertebral disc disorders with myelopathy, thoracolumbar region** `cc`

   M51.06 **Intervertebral disc disorders with myelopathy, lumbar region** `cc`

√5ᵗʰ **M51.1 Thoracic, thoracolumbar and lumbosacral intervertebral disc disorders with radiculopathy**

   Sciatica due to intervertebral disc disorder

   EXCLUDES 1   lumbar radiculitis NOS (M54.16)

              sciatica NOS (M54.3)

   AHA: 2018,3Q,18

   M51.14 **Intervertebral disc disorders with radiculopathy, thoracic region**

✔ Additional Character Required   √x7ᵗʰ Placeholder   Unacceptable PDx   Questionable PDx   Manifestation   Unspecified Dx   H1-H4 HAC   HCC CMS-HCC Dx   HIV HIV Dx

ICD-10-CM 2021   799

M51.15   **Intervertebral disc disorders with radiculopathy, thoracolumbar region**

M51.16   **Intervertebral disc disorders with radiculopathy, lumbar region**

M51.17   **Intervertebral disc disorders with radiculopathy, lumbosacral region**

√5ᵗʰ **M51.2**   **Other thoracic, thoracolumbar and lumbosacral intervertebral disc** displacement

     Lumbago due to displacement of intervertebral disc

Displacement Intervertebral Disc

Normal Top View   Herniated Top View

Lamina

Nucleus pulposus

Ligamentum flavum

Disc annulus

Nucleus pulposus

Spinal cord

Herniates through annulus

Spinal nerve

M51.24   **Other intervertebral disc displacement, thoracic region**

M51.25   **Other intervertebral disc displacement, thoracolumbar region**

M51.26   **Other intervertebral disc displacement, lumbar region**

M51.27   **Other intervertebral disc displacement, lumbosacral region**

√5ᵗʰ **M51.3**   **Other thoracic, thoracolumbar and lumbosacral intervertebral disc** degeneration

     AHA: 2018,2Q,15; 2013,3Q,22

M51.34   **Other intervertebral disc degeneration, thoracic region**

M51.35   **Other intervertebral disc degeneration, thoracolumbar region**

M51.36   **Other intervertebral disc degeneration, lumbar region**

M51.37   **Other intervertebral disc degeneration, lumbosacral region**

√5ᵗʰ **M51.4**   **Schmorl's nodes**

     DEF: Irregular bone defect in the margin of the vertebral body that causes herniation into the end plate of the vertebral body.

M51.44   **Schmorl's nodes, thoracic region**

M51.45   **Schmorl's nodes, thoracolumbar region**

M51.46   **Schmorl's nodes, lumbar region**

M51.47   **Schmorl's nodes, lumbosacral region**

√5ᵗʰ **M51.8**   **Other thoracic, thoracolumbar and lumbosacral intervertebral** disc disorders

M51.84   **Other intervertebral disc disorders, thoracic region**

M51.85   **Other intervertebral disc disorders, thoracolumbar region**

M51.86   **Other intervertebral disc disorders, lumbar region**

M51.87   **Other intervertebral disc disorders, lumbosacral region**

M51.9   **Unspecified thoracic, thoracolumbar and lumbosacral intervertebral disc disorder**

√4ᵗʰ **M53**   **Other and unspecified dorsopathies, not elsewhere classified**

M53.0   **Cervicocranial syndrome**

     Posterior cervical sympathetic syndrome

M53.1   **Cervicobrachial syndrome**

     EXCLUDES 2   *cervical disc disorder (M50.-)*

             thoracic outlet syndrome (G54.0)

√5ᵗʰ **M53.2**   **Spinal instabilities**

√6ᵗʰ **M53.2X**   **Spinal** instabilities

M53.2X1   **Spinal instabilities, occipito-atlanto-axial region**

M53.2X2   **Spinal instabilities, cervical region**

M53.2X3   **Spinal instabilities, cervicothoracic region**

M53.2X4   **Spinal instabilities, thoracic region**

M53.2X5   **Spinal instabilities, thoracolumbar region**

M53.2X6   **Spinal instabilities, lumbar region**

M53.2X7   **Spinal instabilities, lumbosacral region**

M53.2X8   **Spinal instabilities, sacral and sacrococcygeal region**

M53.2X9   **Spinal instabilities, site unspecified**

M53.3   **Sacrococcygeal disorders, not elsewhere classified**

     Coccygodynia

√5ᵗʰ **M53.8**   **Other specified** dorsopathies

M53.80   **Other specified dorsopathies, site unspecified**

M53.81   **Other specified dorsopathies, occipito-atlanto-axial region**

M53.82   **Other specified dorsopathies, cervical region**

M53.83   **Other specified dorsopathies, cervicothoracic region**

M53.84   **Other specified dorsopathies, thoracic region**

M53.85   **Other specified dorsopathies, thoracolumbar region**

M53.86   **Other specified dorsopathies, lumbar region**

M53.87   **Other specified dorsopathies, lumbosacral region**

M53.88   **Other specified dorsopathies, sacral and sacrococcygeal region**

M53.9   **Dorsopathy, unspecified**

√4ᵗʰ **M54**   **Dorsalgia**

     EXCLUDES 1   *psychogenic dorsalgia (F45.41)*

√5ᵗʰ **M54.0**   **Panniculitis affecting regions of neck and back**

     EXCLUDES 1   *lupus panniculitis (L93.2)*

             panniculitis NOS (M79.3)

             relapsing [Weber-Christian] panniculitis (M35.6)

M54.00   **Panniculitis affecting regions of neck and back, site unspecified**

M54.01   **Panniculitis affecting regions of neck and back, occipito-atlanto-axial region**

M54.02   **Panniculitis affecting regions of neck and back, cervical region**

M54.03   **Panniculitis affecting regions of neck and back, cervicothoracic region**

M54.04   **Panniculitis affecting regions of neck and back, thoracic region**

M54.05   **Panniculitis affecting regions of neck and back, thoracolumbar region**

M54.06   **Panniculitis affecting regions of neck and back, lumbar region**

M54.07   **Panniculitis affecting regions of neck and back, lumbosacral region**

M54.08   **Panniculitis affecting regions of neck and back, sacral and sacrococcygeal region**

M54.09   **Panniculitis affecting regions, neck and back, multiple sites in spine**

√5ᵗʰ **M54.1**   **Radiculopathy**

     Brachial neuritis or radiculitis NOS

     Lumbar neuritis or radiculitis NOS

     Lumbosacral neuritis or radiculitis NOS

     Thoracic neuritis or radiculitis NOS

     Radiculitis NOS

     EXCLUDES 1   *neuralgia and neuritis NOS (M79.2)*

             radiculopathy with cervical disc disorder (M50.1)

             radiculopathy with lumbar and other intervertebral disc disorder (M51.1-)

             radiculopathy with spondylosis (M47.2-)

     AHA: 2018,3Q,18

     TIP: A code from this subcategory can be used in addition to a spondylolisthesis code (M43.1-) or a spinal stenosis code (M48.0-) when either condition is documented as the cause of the radiculopathy.

M54.10   **Radiculopathy, site unspecified**

M54.11   **Radiculopathy, occipito-atlanto-axial region**

M54.12   **Radiculopathy, cervical region**

M54.13   **Radiculopathy, cervicothoracic region**

M54.14   **Radiculopathy, thoracic region**

M54.15   **Radiculopathy, thoracolumbar region**

M54.16   **Radiculopathy, lumbar region**

M54.17   **Radiculopathy, lumbosacral region**

M54.18   **Radiculopathy, sacral and sacrococcygeal region**

M54.2   **Cervicalgia**

     EXCLUDES 1   *cervicalgia due to intervertebral cervical disc disorder (M50.-)*

✓5ᵗʰ **M54.3 Sciatica**

> EXCLUDES 1   lesion of sciatic nerve (G57.0)
>
> sciatica due to intervertebral disc disorder (M51.1-)
>
> sciatica with lumbago (M54.4-)

    M54.30   Sciatica, unspecified side

    M54.31   Sciatica, right side

    M54.32   Sciatica, left side

✓5ᵗʰ **M54.4 Lumbago with sciatica**

> EXCLUDES 1   lumbago with sciatica due to intervertebral disc disorder (M51.1-)

    AHA: 2016,2Q,7

    M54.40   Lumbago with sciatica, unspecified side

    M54.41   Lumbago with sciatica, right side

    M54.42   Lumbago with sciatica, left side

M54.5 Low back pain

    Loin pain

    Lumbago NOS

> EXCLUDES 1   low back strain (S39.012)
>
> lumbago due to intervertebral disc displacement (M51.2-)
>
> lumbago with sciatica (M54.4-)

M54.6 Pain in thoracic spine

> EXCLUDES 1   pain in thoracic spine due to intervertebral disc disorder (M51.-)

✓5ᵗʰ **M54.8 Other dorsalgia**

> EXCLUDES 1   dorsalgia in thoracic region (M54.6)
>
> low back pain (M54.5)

    M54.81   Occipital neuralgia

    M54.89   Other dorsalgia

M54.9 Dorsalgia, unspecified

    Backache NOS

    Back pain NOS

SOFT TISSUE DISORDERS (M60-M79)

Disorders of muscles (M60-M63)

> EXCLUDES 1   dermatopolymyositis (M33.-)
>
> muscular dystrophies and myopathies (G71-G72)
>
> myopathy in amyloidosis (E85.-)
>
> myopathy in polyarteritis nodosa (M30.0)
>
> myopathy in rheumatoid arthritis (M05.32)
>
> myopathy in scleroderma (M34.-)
>
> myopathy in Sjögren's syndrome (M35.03)
>
> myopathy in systemic lupus erythematosus (M32.-)

✓4ᵗʰ **M60 Myositis**

> EXCLUDES 2   inclusion body myositis [IBM] (G72.41)

✓5ᵗʰ **M60.0 Infective myositis**

    Tropical pyomyositis

    Use additional code (B95-B97) to identify infectious agent

✓6ᵗʰ   **M60.00**   Infective myositis, unspecified site

     M60.000   Infective myositis, unspecified right arm   cc

       Infective myositis, right upper limb NOS

     M60.001   Infective myositis, unspecified left arm   cc

       Infective myositis, left upper limb NOS

     M60.002   Infective myositis, unspecified arm   cc

       Infective myositis, upper limb NOS

     M60.003   Infective myositis, unspecified right leg   cc

       Infective myositis, right lower limb NOS

     M60.004   Infective myositis, unspecified left leg   cc

       Infective myositis, left lower limb NOS

     M60.005   Infective myositis, unspecified leg   cc

       Infective myositis, lower limb NOS

     M60.009   Infective myositis, unspecified site   cc

✓6ᵗʰ   **M60.01**   Infective myositis, shoulder

     M60.011   Infective myositis, right shoulder   cc

     M60.012   Infective myositis, left shoulder   cc

     M60.019   Infective myositis, unspecified shoulder   cc

✓6ᵗʰ   **M60.02**   Infective myositis, upper arm

     M60.021   Infective myositis, right upper arm   cc

     M60.022   Infective myositis, left upper arm   cc

     M60.029   Infective myositis, unspecified upper arm   cc

✓6ᵗʰ   **M60.03**   Infective myositis, forearm

     M60.031   Infective myositis, right forearm   cc

     M60.032   Infective myositis, left forearm   cc

     M60.039   Infective myositis, unspecified forearm   cc

✓6ᵗʰ   **M60.04**   Infective myositis, hand and fingers

     M60.041   Infective myositis, right hand   cc

     M60.042   Infective myositis, left hand   cc

     M60.043   Infective myositis, unspecified hand   cc

     M60.044   Infective myositis, right finger(s)   cc

     M60.045   Infective myositis, left finger(s)   cc

     M60.046   Infective myositis, unspecified finger(s)   cc

✓6ᵗʰ   **M60.05**   Infective myositis, thigh

     M60.051   Infective myositis, right thigh   cc

     M60.052   Infective myositis, left thigh   cc

     M60.059   Infective myositis, unspecified thigh   cc

✓6ᵗʰ   **M60.06**   Infective myositis, lower leg

     M60.061   Infective myositis, right lower leg   cc

     M60.062   Infective myositis, left lower leg   cc

     M60.069   Infective myositis, unspecified lower leg   cc

✓6ᵗʰ   **M60.07**   Infective myositis, ankle, foot and toes

     M60.070   Infective myositis, right ankle   cc

     M60.071   Infective myositis, left ankle   cc

     M60.072   Infective myositis, unspecified ankle   cc

     M60.073   Infective myositis, right foot   cc

     M60.074   Infective myositis, left foot   cc

     M60.075   Infective myositis, unspecified foot   cc

     M60.076   Infective myositis, right toe(s)   cc

     M60.077   Infective myositis, left toe(s)   cc

     M60.078   Infective myositis, unspecified toe(s)   cc

    M60.08   Infective myositis, other site   cc

    M60.09   Infective myositis, multiple sites   cc

✓5ᵗʰ **M60.1 Interstitial myositis**

    M60.10   Interstitial myositis of unspecified site

✓6ᵗʰ   **M60.11**   Interstitial myositis, shoulder

     M60.111   Interstitial myositis, right shoulder

     M60.112   Interstitial myositis, left shoulder

     M60.119   Interstitial myositis, unspecified shoulder

✓6ᵗʰ   **M60.12**   Interstitial myositis, upper arm

     M60.121   Interstitial myositis, right upper arm

     M60.122   Interstitial myositis, left upper arm

     M60.129   Interstitial myositis, unspecified upper arm

✓6ᵗʰ   **M60.13**   Interstitial myositis, forearm

     M60.131   Interstitial myositis, right forearm

     M60.132   Interstitial myositis, left forearm

     M60.139   Interstitial myositis, unspecified forearm

✓6ᵗʰ   **M60.14**   Interstitial myositis, hand

     M60.141   Interstitial myositis, right hand

     M60.142   Interstitial myositis, left hand

     M60.149   Interstitial myositis, unspecified hand

✓6ᵗʰ   **M60.15**   Interstitial myositis, thigh

     M60.151   Interstitial myositis, right thigh

     M60.152   Interstitial myositis, left thigh

     M60.159   Interstitial myositis, unspecified thigh

✓6ᵗʰ   **M60.16**   Interstitial myositis, lower leg

     M60.161   Interstitial myositis, right lower leg

     M60.162   Interstitial myositis, left lower leg

     M60.169   Interstitial myositis, unspecified lower leg

✓6ᵗʰ   **M60.17**   Interstitial myositis, ankle and foot

     M60.171   Interstitial myositis, right ankle and foot

     M60.172   Interstitial myositis, left ankle and foot

     M60.179   Interstitial myositis, unspecified ankle and foot

    M60.18   Interstitial myositis, other site

    M60.19   Interstitial myositis, multiple sites

☑ Additional Character Required   ✓×7ᵗʰ Placeholder   Unacceptable PDx   Questionable PDx   Manifestation   Unspecified Dx   H1-H14 HAC   HCC CMS-HCC Dx   HIV HIV Dx

ICD-10-CM 2021   801

√5ᵗʰ **M60.2** **Foreign body granuloma of soft tissue, not elsewhere classified**

   Use additional code to identify the type of retained foreign body (Z18.-)

     EXCLUDES 1 *foreign body granuloma of skin and subcutaneous tissue (L92.3)*

   M60.20 Foreign body granuloma of soft tissue, not elsewhere classified, unspecified site

√6ᵗʰ **M60.21** Foreign body granuloma of soft tissue, not elsewhere classified, shoulder

   M60.211 Foreign body granuloma of soft tissue, not elsewhere classified, right shoulder

   M60.212 Foreign body granuloma of soft tissue, not elsewhere classified, left shoulder

   M60.219 Foreign body granuloma of soft tissue, not elsewhere classified, unspecified shoulder

√6ᵗʰ **M60.22** Foreign body granuloma of soft tissue, not elsewhere classified, upper arm

   M60.221 Foreign body granuloma of soft tissue, not elsewhere classified, right upper arm

   M60.222 Foreign body granuloma of soft tissue, not elsewhere classified, left upper arm

   M60.229 Foreign body granuloma of soft tissue, not elsewhere classified, unspecified upper arm

√6ᵗʰ **M60.23** Foreign body granuloma of soft tissue, not elsewhere classified, forearm

   M60.231 Foreign body granuloma of soft tissue, not elsewhere classified, right forearm

   M60.232 Foreign body granuloma of soft tissue, not elsewhere classified, left forearm

   M60.239 Foreign body granuloma of soft tissue, not elsewhere classified, unspecified forearm

√6ᵗʰ **M60.24** Foreign body granuloma of soft tissue, not elsewhere classified, hand

   M60.241 Foreign body granuloma of soft tissue, not elsewhere classified, right hand

   M60.242 Foreign body granuloma of soft tissue, not elsewhere classified, left hand

   M60.249 Foreign body granuloma of soft tissue, not elsewhere classified, unspecified hand

√6ᵗʰ **M60.25** Foreign body granuloma of soft tissue, not elsewhere classified, thigh

   M60.251 Foreign body granuloma of soft tissue, not elsewhere classified, right thigh

   M60.252 Foreign body granuloma of soft tissue, not elsewhere classified, left thigh

   M60.259 Foreign body granuloma of soft tissue, not elsewhere classified, unspecified thigh

√6ᵗʰ **M60.26** Foreign body granuloma of soft tissue, not elsewhere classified, lower leg

   M60.261 Foreign body granuloma of soft tissue, not elsewhere classified, right lower leg

   M60.262 Foreign body granuloma of soft tissue, not elsewhere classified, left lower leg

   M60.269 Foreign body granuloma of soft tissue, not elsewhere classified, unspecified lower leg

√6ᵗʰ **M60.27** Foreign body granuloma of soft tissue, not elsewhere classified, ankle and foot

   M60.271 Foreign body granuloma of soft tissue, not elsewhere classified, right ankle and foot

   M60.272 Foreign body granuloma of soft tissue, not elsewhere classified, left ankle and foot

   M60.279 Foreign body granuloma of soft tissue, not elsewhere classified, unspecified ankle and foot

   M60.28 Foreign body granuloma of soft tissue, not elsewhere classified, other site

√5ᵗʰ **M60.8** **Other myositis**

   M60.80 Other myositis, unspecified site

√6ᵗʰ **M60.81** Other myositis shoulder

   M60.811 Other myositis, right shoulder

   M60.812 Other myositis, left shoulder

   M60.819 Other myositis, unspecified shoulder

√6ᵗʰ **M60.82** Other myositis, upper arm

   M60.821 Other myositis, right upper arm

   M60.822 Other myositis, left upper arm

   M60.829 Other myositis, unspecified upper arm

√6ᵗʰ **M60.83** Other myositis, forearm

   M60.831 Other myositis, right forearm

   M60.832 Other myositis, left forearm

   M60.839 Other myositis, unspecified forearm

√6ᵗʰ **M60.84** Other myositis, hand

   M60.841 Other myositis, right hand

   M60.842 Other myositis, left hand

   M60.849 Other myositis, unspecified hand

√6ᵗʰ **M60.85** Other myositis, thigh

   M60.851 Other myositis, right thigh

   M60.852 Other myositis, left thigh

   M60.859 Other myositis, unspecified thigh

√6ᵗʰ **M60.86** Other myositis, lower leg

   M60.861 Other myositis, right lower leg

   M60.862 Other myositis, left lower leg

   M60.869 Other myositis, unspecified lower leg

√6ᵗʰ **M60.87** Other myositis, ankle and foot

   M60.871 Other myositis, right ankle and foot

   M60.872 Other myositis, left ankle and foot

   M60.879 Other myositis, unspecified ankle and foot

   M60.88 Other myositis, other site

   M60.89 Other myositis, multiple sites

M60.9 Myositis, unspecified

√4ᵗʰ **M61** **Calcification and ossification of muscle**

√5ᵗʰ **M61.0** **Myositis ossificans traumatica**

   M61.00 Myositis ossificans traumatica, unspecified site

√6ᵗʰ **M61.01** Myositis ossificans traumatica, shoulder

   M61.011 Myositis ossificans traumatica, right shoulder

   M61.012 Myositis ossificans traumatica, left shoulder

   M61.019 Myositis ossificans traumatica, unspecified shoulder

√6ᵗʰ **M61.02** Myositis ossificans traumatica, upper arm

   M61.021 Myositis ossificans traumatica, right upper arm

   M61.022 Myositis ossificans traumatica, left upper arm

   M61.029 Myositis ossificans traumatica, unspecified upper arm

√6ᵗʰ **M61.03** Myositis ossificans traumatica, forearm

   M61.031 Myositis ossificans traumatica, right forearm

   M61.032 Myositis ossificans traumatica, left forearm

   M61.039 Myositis ossificans traumatica, unspecified forearm

√6ᵗʰ **M61.04** Myositis ossificans traumatica, hand

   M61.041 Myositis ossificans traumatica, right hand

   M61.042 Myositis ossificans traumatica, left hand

   M61.049 Myositis ossificans traumatica, unspecified hand

√6ᵗʰ **M61.05** Myositis ossificans traumatica, thigh

   M61.051 Myositis ossificans traumatica, right thigh

   M61.052 Myositis ossificans traumatica, left thigh

   M61.059 Myositis ossificans traumatica, unspecified thigh

√6ᵗʰ **M61.06** Myositis ossificans traumatica, lower leg

   M61.061 Myositis ossificans traumatica, right lower leg

   M61.062 Myositis ossificans traumatica, left lower leg

   M61.069 Myositis ossificans traumatica, unspecified lower leg

√6ᵗʰ **M61.07** Myositis ossificans traumatica, ankle and foot

   M61.071 Myositis ossificans traumatica, right ankle and foot

   M61.072 Myositis ossificans traumatica, left ankle and foot

   M61.079 Myositis ossificans traumatica, unspecified ankle and foot

   M61.08 Myositis ossificans traumatica, other site

N Newborn: 0 P Pediatric: 0-17 M Maternity: 9-64 A Adult: 15-124 MCC Major Complication/Comorbidity CC Complication/Comorbidity SW Severe Wound Dx

802   ICD-10-CM 2021

M61.Ø9 **Myositis ossificans traumatica,** multiple sites

✓5ᵗʰ M61.1 **Myositis ossificans** progressiva

Fibrodysplasia ossificans progressiva

M61.1Ø **Myositis ossificans progressiva, unspecified site**

✓6ᵗʰ M61.11 **Myositis ossificans progressiva,** shoulder

M61.111 **Myositis ossificans progressiva,** right shoulder

M61.112 **Myositis ossificans progressiva,** left shoulder

M61.119 **Myositis ossificans progressiva, unspecified shoulder**

✓6ᵗʰ M61.12 **Myositis ossificans progressiva,** upper arm

M61.121 **Myositis ossificans progressiva,** right upper arm

M61.122 **Myositis ossificans progressiva,** left upper arm

M61.129 **Myositis ossificans progressiva, unspecified arm**

✓6ᵗʰ M61.13 **Myositis ossificans progressiva,** forearm

M61.131 **Myositis ossificans progressiva,** right forearm

M61.132 **Myositis ossificans progressiva,** left forearm

M61.139 **Myositis ossificans progressiva, unspecified forearm**

✓6ᵗʰ M61.14 **Myositis ossificans progressiva,** hand and finger(s)

M61.141 **Myositis ossificans progressiva,** right hand

M61.142 **Myositis ossificans progressiva,** left hand

M61.143 **Myositis ossificans progressiva, unspecified hand**

M61.144 **Myositis ossificans progressiva,** right finger(s)

M61.145 **Myositis ossificans progressiva,** left finger(s)

M61.146 **Myositis ossificans progressiva, unspecified finger(s)**

✓6ᵗʰ M61.15 **Myositis ossificans progressiva,** thigh

M61.151 **Myositis ossificans progressiva,** right thigh

M61.152 **Myositis ossificans progressiva,** left thigh

M61.159 **Myositis ossificans progressiva, unspecified thigh**

✓6ᵗʰ M61.16 **Myositis ossificans progressiva,** lower leg

M61.161 **Myositis ossificans progressiva,** right lower leg

M61.162 **Myositis ossificans progressiva,** left lower leg

M61.169 **Myositis ossificans progressiva, unspecified lower leg**

✓6ᵗʰ M61.17 **Myositis ossificans progressiva,** ankle, foot and toe(s)

M61.171 **Myositis ossificans progressiva,** right ankle

M61.172 **Myositis ossificans progressiva,** left ankle

M61.173 **Myositis ossificans progressiva, unspecified ankle**

M61.174 **Myositis ossificans progressiva,** right foot

M61.175 **Myositis ossificans progressiva,** left foot

M61.176 **Myositis ossificans progressiva, unspecified foot**

M61.177 **Myositis ossificans progressiva,** right toe(s)

M61.178 **Myositis ossificans progressiva,** left toe(s)

M61.179 **Myositis ossificans progressiva, unspecified toe(s)**

M61.18 **Myositis ossificans progressiva, other site**

M61.19 **Myositis ossificans progressiva,** multiple sites

✓5ᵗʰ M61.2 **Paralytic** calcification and ossification of muscle

Myositis ossificans associated with quadriplegia or paraplegia

M61.2Ø **Paralytic calcification and ossification of muscle, unspecified site**

✓6ᵗʰ M61.21 **Paralytic calcification and ossification of muscle,** shoulder

M61.211 **Paralytic calcification and ossification of muscle,** right shoulder

M61.212 **Paralytic calcification and ossification of muscle,** left shoulder

M61.219 **Paralytic calcification and ossification of muscle, unspecified shoulder**

✓6ᵗʰ M61.22 **Paralytic calcification and ossification of muscle,** upper arm

M61.221 **Paralytic calcification and ossification of muscle,** right upper arm

M61.222 **Paralytic calcification and ossification of muscle,** left upper arm

M61.229 **Paralytic calcification and ossification of muscle, unspecified upper arm**

✓6ᵗʰ M61.23 **Paralytic calcification and ossification of muscle,** forearm

M61.231 **Paralytic calcification and ossification of muscle,** right forearm

M61.232 **Paralytic calcification and ossification of muscle,** left forearm

M61.239 **Paralytic calcification and ossification of muscle, unspecified forearm**

✓6ᵗʰ M61.24 **Paralytic calcification and ossification of muscle,** hand

M61.241 **Paralytic calcification and ossification of muscle,** right hand

M61.242 **Paralytic calcification and ossification of muscle,** left hand

M61.249 **Paralytic calcification and ossification of muscle, unspecified hand**

✓6ᵗʰ M61.25 **Paralytic calcification and ossification of muscle,** thigh

M61.251 **Paralytic calcification and ossification of muscle,** right thigh

M61.252 **Paralytic calcification and ossification of muscle,** left thigh

M61.259 **Paralytic calcification and ossification of muscle, unspecified thigh**

✓6ᵗʰ M61.26 **Paralytic calcification and ossification of muscle,** lower leg

M61.261 **Paralytic calcification and ossification of muscle,** right lower leg

M61.262 **Paralytic calcification and ossification of muscle,** left lower leg

M61.269 **Paralytic calcification and ossification of muscle, unspecified lower leg**

✓6ᵗʰ M61.27 **Paralytic calcification and ossification of muscle,** ankle and foot

M61.271 **Paralytic calcification and ossification of muscle,** right ankle and foot

M61.272 **Paralytic calcification and ossification of muscle,** left ankle and foot

M61.279 **Paralytic calcification and ossification of muscle, unspecified ankle and foot**

M61.28 **Paralytic calcification and ossification of muscle, other site**

M61.29 **Paralytic calcification and ossification of muscle,** multiple sites

✓5ᵗʰ M61.3 **Calcification and ossification of muscles** associated with burns

Myositis ossificans associated with burns

M61.3Ø **Calcification and ossification of muscles associated with burns, unspecified site**

✓6ᵗʰ M61.31 **Calcification and ossification of muscles associated with burns,** shoulder

M61.311 **Calcification and ossification of muscles associated with burns,** right shoulder

M61.312 **Calcification and ossification of muscles associated with burns,** left shoulder

M61.319 **Calcification and ossification of muscles associated with burns, unspecified shoulder**

✓6ᵗʰ M61.32 **Calcification and ossification of muscles associated with burns,** upper arm

M61.321 **Calcification and ossification of muscles associated with burns,** right upper arm

M61.322 **Calcification and ossification of muscles associated with burns,** left upper arm

M61.329 **Calcification and ossification of muscles associated with burns, unspecified upper arm**

✓6ᵗʰ M61.33 **Calcification and ossification of muscles associated with burns,** forearm

M61.331 **Calcification and ossification of muscles associated with burns,** right forearm

M61.332 **Calcification and ossification of muscles associated with burns,** left forearm

☑ Additional Character Required ✓x7ᵗʰ Placeholder Unacceptable PDx Questionable PDx Manifestation Unspecified Dx H1-H14 HAC HCC CMS-HCC Dx HIV HIV Dx

ICD-10-CM 2021

803

M61.339 Calcification and ossification of muscles associated with burns, unspecified forearm

☑6ᵗʰ M61.34 Calcification and ossification of muscles associated with burns, hand

M61.341 Calcification and ossification of muscles associated with burns, right hand

M61.342 Calcification and ossification of muscles associated with burns, left hand

M61.349 Calcification and ossification of muscles associated with burns, unspecified hand

☑6ᵗʰ M61.35 Calcification and ossification of muscles associated with burns, thigh

M61.351 Calcification and ossification of muscles associated with burns, right thigh

M61.352 Calcification and ossification of muscles associated with burns, left thigh

M61.359 Calcification and ossification of muscles associated with burns, unspecified thigh

☑6ᵗʰ M61.36 Calcification and ossification of muscles associated with burns, lower leg

M61.361 Calcification and ossification of muscles associated with burns, right lower leg

M61.362 Calcification and ossification of muscles associated with burns, left lower leg

M61.369 Calcification and ossification of muscles associated with burns, unspecified lower leg

☑6ᵗʰ M61.37 Calcification and ossification of muscles associated with burns, ankle and foot

M61.371 Calcification and ossification of muscles associated with burns, right ankle and foot

M61.372 Calcification and ossification of muscles associated with burns, left ankle and foot

M61.379 Calcification and ossification of muscles associated with burns, unspecified ankle and foot

M61.38 Calcification and ossification of muscles associated with burns, other site

M61.39 Calcification and ossification of muscles associated with burns, multiple sites

☑5ᵗʰ M61.4 Other calcification of muscle

> **EXCLUDES 1**   calcific tendinitis NOS (M65.2-)
> calcific tendinitis of shoulder (M75.3)

M61.40 Other calcification of muscle, unspecified site

☑6ᵗʰ M61.41 Other calcification of muscle, shoulder

M61.411 Other calcification of muscle, right shoulder

M61.412 Other calcification of muscle, left shoulder

M61.419 Other calcification of muscle, unspecified shoulder

☑6ᵗʰ M61.42 Other calcification of muscle, upper arm

M61.421 Other calcification of muscle, right upper arm

M61.422 Other calcification of muscle, left upper arm

M61.429 Other calcification of muscle, unspecified upper arm

☑6ᵗʰ M61.43 Other calcification of muscle, forearm

M61.431 Other calcification of muscle, right forearm

M61.432 Other calcification of muscle, left forearm

M61.439 Other calcification of muscle, unspecified forearm

☑6ᵗʰ M61.44 Other calcification of muscle, hand

M61.441 Other calcification of muscle, right hand

M61.442 Other calcification of muscle, left hand

M61.449 Other calcification of muscle, unspecified hand

☑6ᵗʰ M61.45 Other calcification of muscle, thigh

M61.451 Other calcification of muscle, right thigh

M61.452 Other calcification of muscle, left thigh

M61.459 Other calcification of muscle, unspecified thigh

☑6ᵗʰ M61.46 Other calcification of muscle, lower leg

M61.461 Other calcification of muscle, right lower leg

M61.462 Other calcification of muscle, left lower leg

M61.469 Other calcification of muscle, unspecified lower leg

☑6ᵗʰ M61.47 Other calcification of muscle, ankle and foot

M61.471 Other calcification of muscle, right ankle and foot

M61.472 Other calcification of muscle, left ankle and foot

M61.479 Other calcification of muscle, unspecified ankle and foot

M61.48 Other calcification of muscle, other site

M61.49 Other calcification of muscle, multiple sites

☑5ᵗʰ M61.5 Other ossification of muscle

M61.50 Other ossification of muscle, unspecified site

☑6ᵗʰ M61.51 Other ossification of muscle, shoulder

M61.511 Other ossification of muscle, right shoulder

M61.512 Other ossification of muscle, left shoulder

M61.519 Other ossification of muscle, unspecified shoulder

☑6ᵗʰ M61.52 Other ossification of muscle, upper arm

M61.521 Other ossification of muscle, right upper arm

M61.522 Other ossification of muscle, left upper arm

M61.529 Other ossification of muscle, unspecified upper arm

☑6ᵗʰ M61.53 Other ossification of muscle, forearm

M61.531 Other ossification of muscle, right forearm

M61.532 Other ossification of muscle, left forearm

M61.539 Other ossification of muscle, unspecified forearm

☑6ᵗʰ M61.54 Other ossification of muscle, hand

M61.541 Other ossification of muscle, right hand

M61.542 Other ossification of muscle, left hand

M61.549 Other ossification of muscle, unspecified hand

☑6ᵗʰ M61.55 Other ossification of muscle, thigh

M61.551 Other ossification of muscle, right thigh

M61.552 Other ossification of muscle, left thigh

M61.559 Other ossification of muscle, unspecified thigh

☑6ᵗʰ M61.56 Other ossification of muscle, lower leg

M61.561 Other ossification of muscle, right lower leg

M61.562 Other ossification of muscle, left lower leg

M61.569 Other ossification of muscle, unspecified lower leg

☑6ᵗʰ M61.57 Other ossification of muscle, ankle and foot

M61.571 Other ossification of muscle, right ankle and foot

M61.572 Other ossification of muscle, left ankle and foot

M61.579 Other ossification of muscle, unspecified ankle and foot

M61.58 Other ossification of muscle, other site

M61.59 Other ossification of muscle, multiple sites

M61.9 Calcification and ossification of muscle, unspecified

☑4ᵗʰ **M62 Other disorders of muscle**

> **EXCLUDES 1**   alcoholic myopathy (G72.1)
> cramp and spasm (R25.2)
> drug-induced myopathy (G72.0)
> myalgia (M79.1-)
> stiff-man syndrome (G25.82)
>
> **EXCLUDES 2**   nontraumatic hematoma of muscle (M79.81)

☑5ᵗʰ M62.0 Separation of muscle (nontraumatic)

Diastasis of muscle

> **EXCLUDES 1**   diastasis recti complicating pregnancy, labor and delivery (O71.8)
> traumatic separation of muscle — see strain of muscle by body region

M62.00 Separation of muscle (nontraumatic), unspecified site

☑6ᵗʰ M62.01 Separation of muscle (nontraumatic), shoulder

M62.011 Separation of muscle (nontraumatic), right shoulder

Ⓝ Newborn: 0   Ⓟ Pediatric: 0-17   Ⓜ Maternity: 9-64   Ⓐ Adult: 15-124   ᴹᶜᶜ Major Complication/Comorbidity   ᶜᶜ Complication/Comorbidity   ˢʷ Severe Wound Dx

804   ICD-10-CM 2021

M62.012 Separation of muscle (nontraumatic), left shoulder

M62.019 Separation of muscle (nontraumatic), unspecified shoulder

√6ᵗʰ **M62.02 Separation of muscle (nontraumatic), upper arm**

M62.021 Separation of muscle (nontraumatic), right upper arm

M62.022 Separation of muscle (nontraumatic), left upper arm

M62.029 Separation of muscle (nontraumatic), unspecified upper arm

√6ᵗʰ **M62.03 Separation of muscle (nontraumatic), forearm**

M62.031 Separation of muscle (nontraumatic), right forearm

M62.032 Separation of muscle (nontraumatic), left forearm

M62.039 Separation of muscle (nontraumatic), unspecified forearm

√6ᵗʰ **M62.04 Separation of muscle (nontraumatic), hand**

M62.041 Separation of muscle (nontraumatic), right hand

M62.042 Separation of muscle (nontraumatic), left hand

M62.049 Separation of muscle (nontraumatic), unspecified hand

√6ᵗʰ **M62.05 Separation of muscle (nontraumatic), thigh**

M62.051 Separation of muscle (nontraumatic), right thigh

M62.052 Separation of muscle (nontraumatic), left thigh

M62.059 Separation of muscle (nontraumatic), unspecified thigh

√6ᵗʰ **M62.06 Separation of muscle (nontraumatic), lower leg**

M62.061 Separation of muscle (nontraumatic), right lower leg

M62.062 Separation of muscle (nontraumatic), left lower leg

M62.069 Separation of muscle (nontraumatic), unspecified lower leg

√6ᵗʰ **M62.07 Separation of muscle (nontraumatic), ankle and foot**

M62.071 Separation of muscle (nontraumatic), right ankle and foot

M62.072 Separation of muscle (nontraumatic), left ankle and foot

M62.079 Separation of muscle (nontraumatic), unspecified ankle and foot

M62.08 Separation of muscle (nontraumatic), other site

√5ᵗʰ **M62.1 Other rupture of muscle (nontraumatic)**

EXCLUDES 1 traumatic rupture of muscle — see strain of muscle by body region

EXCLUDES 2 rupture of tendon (M66.-)

M62.10 Other rupture of muscle (nontraumatic), unspecified site

√6ᵗʰ **M62.11 Other rupture of muscle (nontraumatic), shoulder**

M62.111 Other rupture of muscle (nontraumatic), right shoulder

M62.112 Other rupture of muscle (nontraumatic), left shoulder

M62.119 Other rupture of muscle (nontraumatic), unspecified shoulder

√6ᵗʰ **M62.12 Other rupture of muscle (nontraumatic), upper arm**

M62.121 Other rupture of muscle (nontraumatic), right upper arm

M62.122 Other rupture of muscle (nontraumatic), left upper arm

M62.129 Other rupture of muscle (nontraumatic), unspecified upper arm

√6ᵗʰ **M62.13 Other rupture of muscle (nontraumatic), forearm**

M62.131 Other rupture of muscle (nontraumatic), right forearm

M62.132 Other rupture of muscle (nontraumatic), left forearm

M62.139 Other rupture of muscle (nontraumatic), unspecified forearm

√6ᵗʰ **M62.14 Other rupture of muscle (nontraumatic), hand**

M62.141 Other rupture of muscle (nontraumatic), right hand

M62.142 Other rupture of muscle (nontraumatic), left hand

M62.149 Other rupture of muscle (nontraumatic), unspecified hand

√6ᵗʰ **M62.15 Other rupture of muscle (nontraumatic), thigh**

M62.151 Other rupture of muscle (nontraumatic), right thigh

M62.152 Other rupture of muscle (nontraumatic), left thigh

M62.159 Other rupture of muscle (nontraumatic), unspecified thigh

√6ᵗʰ **M62.16 Other rupture of muscle (nontraumatic), lower leg**

M62.161 Other rupture of muscle (nontraumatic), right lower leg

M62.162 Other rupture of muscle (nontraumatic), left lower leg

M62.169 Other rupture of muscle (nontraumatic), unspecified lower leg

√6ᵗʰ **M62.17 Other rupture of muscle (nontraumatic), ankle and foot**

M62.171 Other rupture of muscle (nontraumatic), right ankle and foot

M62.172 Other rupture of muscle (nontraumatic), left ankle and foot

M62.179 Other rupture of muscle (nontraumatic), unspecified ankle and foot

M62.18 Other rupture of muscle (nontraumatic), other site

√5ᵗʰ **M62.2 Nontraumatic ischemic infarction of muscle**

EXCLUDES 1 compartment syndrome (traumatic) (T79.A-)
nontraumatic compartment syndrome (M79.A-)
rhabdomyolysis (M62.82)
traumatic ischemia of muscle (T79.6)
Volkmann's ischemic contracture (T79.6)

M62.20 Nontraumatic ischemic infarction of muscle, unspecified site

√6ᵗʰ **M62.21 Nontraumatic ischemic infarction of muscle, shoulder**

M62.211 Nontraumatic ischemic infarction of muscle, right shoulder

M62.212 Nontraumatic ischemic infarction of muscle, left shoulder

M62.219 Nontraumatic ischemic infarction of muscle, unspecified shoulder

√6ᵗʰ **M62.22 Nontraumatic ischemic infarction of muscle, upper arm**

M62.221 Nontraumatic ischemic infarction of muscle, right upper arm

M62.222 Nontraumatic ischemic infarction of muscle, left upper arm

M62.229 Nontraumatic ischemic infarction of muscle, unspecified upper arm

√6ᵗʰ **M62.23 Nontraumatic ischemic infarction of muscle, forearm**

M62.231 Nontraumatic ischemic infarction of muscle, right forearm

M62.232 Nontraumatic ischemic infarction of muscle, left forearm

M62.239 Nontraumatic ischemic infarction of muscle, unspecified forearm

√6ᵗʰ **M62.24 Nontraumatic ischemic infarction of muscle, hand**

M62.241 Nontraumatic ischemic infarction of muscle, right hand

M62.242 Nontraumatic ischemic infarction of muscle, left hand

M62.249 Nontraumatic ischemic infarction of muscle, unspecified hand

√6ᵗʰ **M62.25 Nontraumatic ischemic infarction of muscle, thigh**

M62.251 Nontraumatic ischemic infarction of muscle, right thigh

M62.252 Nontraumatic ischemic infarction of muscle, left thigh

M62.259 Nontraumatic ischemic infarction of muscle, unspecified thigh

√6ᵗʰ **M62.26 Nontraumatic ischemic infarction of muscle, lower leg**

M62.261 Nontraumatic ischemic infarction of muscle, right lower leg

M62.262 Nontraumatic ischemic infarction of muscle, left lower leg

M62.269 Nontraumatic ischemic infarction of muscle, unspecified lower leg

✓6th **M62.27 Nontraumatic ischemic infarction of muscle, ankle and foot**
     M62.271 Nontraumatic ischemic infarction of muscle, right ankle and foot
     M62.272 Nontraumatic ischemic infarction of muscle, left ankle and foot
     M62.279 Nontraumatic ischemic infarction of muscle, unspecified ankle and foot
     M62.28 Nontraumatic ischemic infarction of muscle, other site

M62.3 Immobility syndrome (paraplegic)

✓5th **M62.4 Contracture of muscle**
     Contracture of tendon (sheath)
     EXCLUDES 1   contracture of joint (M24.5-)
     M62.40 Contracture of muscle, unspecified site
✓6th **M62.41 Contracture of muscle, shoulder**
     M62.411 Contracture of muscle, right shoulder
     M62.412 Contracture of muscle, left shoulder
     M62.419 Contracture of muscle, unspecified shoulder
✓6th **M62.42 Contracture of muscle, upper arm**
     M62.421 Contracture of muscle, right upper arm
     M62.422 Contracture of muscle, left upper arm
     M62.429 Contracture of muscle, unspecified upper arm
✓6th **M62.43 Contracture of muscle, forearm**
     M62.431 Contracture of muscle, right forearm
     M62.432 Contracture of muscle, left forearm
     M62.439 Contracture of muscle, unspecified forearm
✓6th **M62.44 Contracture of muscle, hand**
     M62.441 Contracture of muscle, right hand
     M62.442 Contracture of muscle, left hand
     M62.449 Contracture of muscle, unspecified hand
✓6th **M62.45 Contracture of muscle, thigh**
     M62.451 Contracture of muscle, right thigh
     M62.452 Contracture of muscle, left thigh
     M62.459 Contracture of muscle, unspecified thigh
✓6th **M62.46 Contracture of muscle, lower leg**
     M62.461 Contracture of muscle, right lower leg
     M62.462 Contracture of muscle, left lower leg
     M62.469 Contracture of muscle, unspecified lower leg
✓6th **M62.47 Contracture of muscle, ankle and foot**
     M62.471 Contracture of muscle, right ankle and foot
     M62.472 Contracture of muscle, left ankle and foot
     M62.479 Contracture of muscle, unspecified ankle and foot
     M62.48 Contracture of muscle, other site
     M62.49 Contracture of muscle, multiple sites

✓5th **M62.5 Muscle wasting and atrophy, not elsewhere classified**
     Disuse atrophy NEC
     EXCLUDES 1   neuralgic amyotrophy (G54.5)
                 progressive muscular atrophy (G12.21)
                 sarcopenia (M62.84)
     EXCLUDES 2   pelvic muscle wasting (N81.84)
     M62.50 Muscle wasting and atrophy, not elsewhere classified, unspecified site
✓6th **M62.51 Muscle wasting and atrophy, not elsewhere classified, shoulder**
     M62.511 Muscle wasting and atrophy, not elsewhere classified, right shoulder
     M62.512 Muscle wasting and atrophy, not elsewhere classified, left shoulder
     M62.519 Muscle wasting and atrophy, not elsewhere classified, unspecified shoulder
✓6th **M62.52 Muscle wasting and atrophy, not elsewhere classified, upper arm**
     M62.521 Muscle wasting and atrophy, not elsewhere classified, right upper arm
     M62.522 Muscle wasting and atrophy, not elsewhere classified, left upper arm
     M62.529 Muscle wasting and atrophy, not elsewhere classified, unspecified upper arm

✓6th **M62.53 Muscle wasting and atrophy, not elsewhere classified, forearm**
     M62.531 Muscle wasting and atrophy, not elsewhere classified, right forearm
     M62.532 Muscle wasting and atrophy, not elsewhere classified, left forearm
     M62.539 Muscle wasting and atrophy, not elsewhere classified, unspecified forearm
✓6th **M62.54 Muscle wasting and atrophy, not elsewhere classified, hand**
     M62.541 Muscle wasting and atrophy, not elsewhere classified, right hand
     M62.542 Muscle wasting and atrophy, not elsewhere classified, left hand
     M62.549 Muscle wasting and atrophy, not elsewhere classified, unspecified hand
✓6th **M62.55 Muscle wasting and atrophy, not elsewhere classified, thigh**
     M62.551 Muscle wasting and atrophy, not elsewhere classified, right thigh
     M62.552 Muscle wasting and atrophy, not elsewhere classified, left thigh
     M62.559 Muscle wasting and atrophy, not elsewhere classified, unspecified thigh
✓6th **M62.56 Muscle wasting and atrophy, not elsewhere classified, lower leg**
     M62.561 Muscle wasting and atrophy, not elsewhere classified, right lower leg
     M62.562 Muscle wasting and atrophy, not elsewhere classified, left lower leg
     M62.569 Muscle wasting and atrophy, not elsewhere classified, unspecified lower leg
✓6th **M62.57 Muscle wasting and atrophy, not elsewhere classified, ankle and foot**
     M62.571 Muscle wasting and atrophy, not elsewhere classified, right ankle and foot
     M62.572 Muscle wasting and atrophy, not elsewhere classified, left ankle and foot
     M62.579 Muscle wasting and atrophy, not elsewhere classified, unspecified ankle and foot
     M62.58 Muscle wasting and atrophy, not elsewhere classified, other site
     M62.59 Muscle wasting and atrophy, not elsewhere classified, multiple sites

✓5th **M62.8 Other specified disorders of muscle**
     EXCLUDES 2   nontraumatic hematoma of muscle (M79.81)
     M62.81 Muscle weakness (generalized)
         EXCLUDES 1   muscle weakness in sarcopenia (M62.84)
     M62.82 Rhabdomyolysis   CC
         EXCLUDES 1   traumatic rhabdomyolysis (T79.6)
         AHA: 2019,2Q,12
         DEF: Rapid disintegration or destruction of skeletal muscle caused by direct or indirect injury, resulting in the excretion of muscle protein myoglobin into the urine.
✓6th **M62.83 Muscle spasm**
     M62.830 Muscle spasm of back
     M62.831 Muscle spasm of calf
         Charley-horse
     M62.838 Other muscle spasm
     M62.84 Sarcopenia
         Age-related sarcopenia
         Code first underlying disease, if applicable, such as:
            disorders of myoneural junction and muscle disease in diseases classified elsewhere (G73.-)
            other and unspecified myopathies (G72.-)
            primary disorders of muscles (G71.-)
         AHA: 2016,4Q,41
     M62.89 Other specified disorders of muscle
         Muscle (sheath) hernia

M62.9 Disorder of muscle, unspecified

N Newborn: 0   P Pediatric: 0-17   M Maternity: 9-64   A Adult: 15-124   MCC Major Complication/Comorbidity   CC Complication/Comorbidity   SW Severe Wound Dx

806   ICD-10-CM 2021

✓4ᵗʰ **M63 Disorders of muscle in diseases classified elsewhere**

Code first underlying disease, such as:
leprosy (A3Ø.-)
neoplasm (C49.-, C79.89, D21.-, D48.1)
schistosomiasis (B65.-)
trichinellosis (B75)

EXCLUDES 1   myopathy in cysticercosis (B69.81)
myopathy in endocrine diseases (G73.7)
myopathy in metabolic diseases (G73.7)
myopathy in sarcoidosis (D86.87)
myopathy in secondary syphilis (A51.49)
myopathy in syphilis (late) (A52.78)
myopathy in toxoplasmosis (B58.82)
myopathy in tuberculosis (A18.Ø9)

✓5ᵗʰ **M63.8 Disorders of muscle in diseases classified elsewhere**

    M63.8Ø Disorders of muscle in diseases classified elsewhere, unspecified site

✓6ᵗʰ **M63.81 Disorders of muscle in diseases classified elsewhere, shoulder**

    M63.811 Disorders of muscle in diseases classified elsewhere, right shoulder
    M63.812 Disorders of muscle in diseases classified elsewhere, left shoulder
    M63.819 Disorders of muscle in diseases classified elsewhere, unspecified shoulder

✓6ᵗʰ **M63.82 Disorders of muscle in diseases classified elsewhere, upper arm**

    M63.821 Disorders of muscle in diseases classified elsewhere, right upper arm
    M63.822 Disorders of muscle in diseases classified elsewhere, left upper arm
    M63.829 Disorders of muscle in diseases classified elsewhere, unspecified upper arm

✓6ᵗʰ **M63.83 Disorders of muscle in diseases classified elsewhere, forearm**

    M63.831 Disorders of muscle in diseases classified elsewhere, right forearm
    M63.832 Disorders of muscle in diseases classified elsewhere, left forearm
    M63.839 Disorders of muscle in diseases classified elsewhere, unspecified forearm

✓6ᵗʰ **M63.84 Disorders of muscle in diseases classified elsewhere, hand**

    M63.841 Disorders of muscle in diseases classified elsewhere, right hand
    M63.842 Disorders of muscle in diseases classified elsewhere, left hand
    M63.849 Disorders of muscle in diseases classified elsewhere, unspecified hand

✓6ᵗʰ **M63.85 Disorders of muscle in diseases classified elsewhere, thigh**

    M63.851 Disorders of muscle in diseases classified elsewhere, right thigh
    M63.852 Disorders of muscle in diseases classified elsewhere, left thigh
    M63.859 Disorders of muscle in diseases classified elsewhere, unspecified thigh

✓6ᵗʰ **M63.86 Disorders of muscle in diseases classified elsewhere, lower leg**

    M63.861 Disorders of muscle in diseases classified elsewhere, right lower leg
    M63.862 Disorders of muscle in diseases classified elsewhere, left lower leg
    M63.869 Disorders of muscle in diseases classified elsewhere, unspecified lower leg

✓6ᵗʰ **M63.87 Disorders of muscle in diseases classified elsewhere, ankle and foot**

    M63.871 Disorders of muscle in diseases classified elsewhere, right ankle and foot
    M63.872 Disorders of muscle in diseases classified elsewhere, left ankle and foot
    M63.879 Disorders of muscle in diseases classified elsewhere, unspecified ankle and foot

    M63.88 Disorders of muscle in diseases classified elsewhere, other site

    M63.89 Disorders of muscle in diseases classified elsewhere, multiple sites

Disorders of synovium and tendon (M65-M67)

✓4ᵗʰ **M65 Synovitis and tenosynovitis**

EXCLUDES 1   chronic crepitant synovitis of hand and wrist (M7Ø.Ø-)
current injury — see injury of ligament or tendon by body region
soft tissue disorders related to use, overuse and pressure (M7Ø.-)

✓5ᵗʰ **M65.Ø Abscess of tendon sheath**

Use additional code (B95-B96) to identify bacterial agent.

    M65.ØØ Abscess of tendon sheath, unspecified site

✓6ᵗʰ **M65.Ø1 Abscess of tendon sheath, shoulder**

    M65.Ø11 Abscess of tendon sheath, right shoulder
    M65.Ø12 Abscess of tendon sheath, left shoulder
    M65.Ø19 Abscess of tendon sheath, unspecified shoulder

✓6ᵗʰ **M65.Ø2 Abscess of tendon sheath, upper arm**

    M65.Ø21 Abscess of tendon sheath, right upper arm
    M65.Ø22 Abscess of tendon sheath, left upper arm
    M65.Ø29 Abscess of tendon sheath, unspecified upper arm

✓6ᵗʰ **M65.Ø3 Abscess of tendon sheath, forearm**

    M65.Ø31 Abscess of tendon sheath, right forearm
    M65.Ø32 Abscess of tendon sheath, left forearm
    M65.Ø39 Abscess of tendon sheath, unspecified forearm

✓6ᵗʰ **M65.Ø4 Abscess of tendon sheath, hand**

    M65.Ø41 Abscess of tendon sheath, right hand
    M65.Ø42 Abscess of tendon sheath, left hand
    M65.Ø49 Abscess of tendon sheath, unspecified hand

✓6ᵗʰ **M65.Ø5 Abscess of tendon sheath, thigh**

    M65.Ø51 Abscess of tendon sheath, right thigh
    M65.Ø52 Abscess of tendon sheath, left thigh
    M65.Ø59 Abscess of tendon sheath, unspecified thigh

✓6ᵗʰ **M65.Ø6 Abscess of tendon sheath, lower leg**

    M65.Ø61 Abscess of tendon sheath, right lower leg
    M65.Ø62 Abscess of tendon sheath, left lower leg
    M65.Ø69 Abscess of tendon sheath, unspecified lower leg

✓6ᵗʰ **M65.Ø7 Abscess of tendon sheath, ankle and foot**

    M65.Ø71 Abscess of tendon sheath, right ankle and foot
    M65.Ø72 Abscess of tendon sheath, left ankle and foot
    M65.Ø79 Abscess of tendon sheath, unspecified ankle and foot

    M65.Ø8 Abscess of tendon sheath, other site

✓5ᵗʰ **M65.1 Other infective (teno)synovitis**

    M65.1Ø Other infective (teno)synovitis, unspecified site

✓6ᵗʰ **M65.11 Other infective (teno)synovitis, shoulder**

    M65.111 Other infective (teno)synovitis, right shoulder
    M65.112 Other infective (teno)synovitis, left shoulder
    M65.119 Other infective (teno)synovitis, unspecified shoulder

✓6ᵗʰ **M65.12 Other infective (teno)synovitis, elbow**

    M65.121 Other infective (teno)synovitis, right elbow
    M65.122 Other infective (teno)synovitis, left elbow
    M65.129 Other infective (teno)synovitis, unspecified elbow

✓6ᵗʰ **M65.13 Other infective (teno)synovitis, wrist**

    M65.131 Other infective (teno)synovitis, right wrist
    M65.132 Other infective (teno)synovitis, left wrist
    M65.139 Other infective (teno)synovitis, unspecified wrist

✓6ᵗʰ **M65.14 Other infective (teno)synovitis, hand**

    M65.141 Other infective (teno)synovitis, right hand
    M65.142 Other infective (teno)synovitis, left hand
    M65.149 Other infective (teno)synovitis, unspecified hand

✓6ᵗʰ **M65.15 Other infective (teno)synovitis, hip**

    M65.151 Other infective (teno)synovitis, right hip

    M65.152 Other infective (teno)synovitis, left hip

    M65.159 Other infective (teno)synovitis, unspecified hip

✓6ᵗʰ **M65.16 Other infective (teno)synovitis, knee**

    M65.161 Other infective (teno)synovitis, right knee

    M65.162 Other infective (teno)synovitis, left knee

    M65.169 Other infective (teno)synovitis, unspecified knee

✓6ᵗʰ **M65.17 Other infective (teno)synovitis, ankle and foot**

    M65.171 Other infective (teno)synovitis, right ankle and foot

    M65.172 Other infective (teno)synovitis, left ankle and foot

    M65.179 Other infective (teno)synovitis, unspecified ankle and foot

    M65.18 Other infective (teno)synovitis, other site

    M65.19 Other infective (teno)synovitis, multiple sites

✓5ᵗʰ **M65.2 Calcific tendinitis**

    EXCLUDES 1   *tendinitis as classified in M75-M77*

                calcified tendinitis of shoulder (M75.3)

    M65.20 Calcific tendinitis, unspecified site

✓6ᵗʰ **M65.22 Calcific tendinitis, upper arm**

    M65.221 Calcific tendinitis, right upper arm

    M65.222 Calcific tendinitis, left upper arm

    M65.229 Calcific tendinitis, unspecified upper arm

✓6ᵗʰ **M65.23 Calcific tendinitis, forearm**

    M65.231 Calcific tendinitis, right forearm

    M65.232 Calcific tendinitis, left forearm

    M65.239 Calcific tendinitis, unspecified forearm

✓6ᵗʰ **M65.24 Calcific tendinitis, hand**

    M65.241 Calcific tendinitis, right hand

    M65.242 Calcific tendinitis, left hand

    M65.249 Calcific tendinitis, unspecified hand

✓6ᵗʰ **M65.25 Calcific tendinitis, thigh**

    M65.251 Calcific tendinitis, right thigh

    M65.252 Calcific tendinitis, left thigh

    M65.259 Calcific tendinitis, unspecified thigh

✓6ᵗʰ **M65.26 Calcific tendinitis, lower leg**

    M65.261 Calcific tendinitis, right lower leg

    M65.262 Calcific tendinitis, left lower leg

    M65.269 Calcific tendinitis, unspecified lower leg

✓6ᵗʰ **M65.27 Calcific tendinitis, ankle and foot**

    M65.271 Calcific tendinitis, right ankle and foot

    M65.272 Calcific tendinitis, left ankle and foot

    M65.279 Calcific tendinitis, unspecified ankle and foot

    M65.28 Calcific tendinitis, other site

    M65.29 Calcific tendinitis, multiple sites

✓5ᵗʰ **M65.3 Trigger finger**

    Nodular tendinous disease

    M65.30 Trigger finger, unspecified finger

✓6ᵗʰ **M65.31 Trigger thumb**

    M65.311 Trigger thumb, right thumb

    M65.312 Trigger thumb, left thumb

    M65.319 Trigger thumb, unspecified thumb

✓6ᵗʰ **M65.32 Trigger finger, index finger**

    M65.321 Trigger finger, right index finger

    M65.322 Trigger finger, left index finger

    M65.329 Trigger finger, unspecified index finger

✓6ᵗʰ **M65.33 Trigger finger, middle finger**

    M65.331 Trigger finger, right middle finger

    M65.332 Trigger finger, left middle finger

    M65.339 Trigger finger, unspecified middle finger

✓6ᵗʰ **M65.34 Trigger finger, ring finger**

    M65.341 Trigger finger, right ring finger

    M65.342 Trigger finger, left ring finger

    M65.349 Trigger finger, unspecified ring finger

✓6ᵗʰ **M65.35 Trigger finger, little finger**

    M65.351 Trigger finger, right little finger

    M65.352 Trigger finger, left little finger

    M65.359 Trigger finger, unspecified little finger

    M65.4 Radial styloid tenosynovitis [de Quervain]

✓5ᵗʰ **M65.8 Other synovitis and tenosynovitis**

    M65.80 Other synovitis and tenosynovitis, unspecified site

✓6ᵗʰ **M65.81 Other synovitis and tenosynovitis, shoulder**

    M65.811 Other synovitis and tenosynovitis, right shoulder

    M65.812 Other synovitis and tenosynovitis, left shoulder

    M65.819 Other synovitis and tenosynovitis, unspecified shoulder

✓6ᵗʰ **M65.82 Other synovitis and tenosynovitis, upper arm**

    M65.821 Other synovitis and tenosynovitis, right upper arm

    M65.822 Other synovitis and tenosynovitis, left upper arm

    M65.829 Other synovitis and tenosynovitis, unspecified upper arm

✓6ᵗʰ **M65.83 Other synovitis and tenosynovitis, forearm**

    M65.831 Other synovitis and tenosynovitis, right forearm

    M65.832 Other synovitis and tenosynovitis, left forearm

    M65.839 Other synovitis and tenosynovitis, unspecified forearm

✓6ᵗʰ **M65.84 Other synovitis and tenosynovitis, hand**

    M65.841 Other synovitis and tenosynovitis, right hand

    M65.842 Other synovitis and tenosynovitis, left hand

    M65.849 Other synovitis and tenosynovitis, unspecified hand

✓6ᵗʰ **M65.85 Other synovitis and tenosynovitis, thigh**

    M65.851 Other synovitis and tenosynovitis, right thigh

    M65.852 Other synovitis and tenosynovitis, left thigh

    M65.859 Other synovitis and tenosynovitis, unspecified thigh

✓6ᵗʰ **M65.86 Other synovitis and tenosynovitis, lower leg**

    M65.861 Other synovitis and tenosynovitis, right lower leg

    M65.862 Other synovitis and tenosynovitis, left lower leg

    M65.869 Other synovitis and tenosynovitis, unspecified lower leg

✓6ᵗʰ **M65.87 Other synovitis and tenosynovitis, ankle and foot**

    M65.871 Other synovitis and tenosynovitis, right ankle and foot

    M65.872 Other synovitis and tenosynovitis, left ankle and foot

    M65.879 Other synovitis and tenosynovitis, unspecified ankle and foot

    M65.88 Other synovitis and tenosynovitis, other site

    M65.89 Other synovitis and tenosynovitis, multiple sites

    M65.9 Synovitis and tenosynovitis, unspecified

✓4ᵗʰ **M66 Spontaneous rupture of synovium and tendon**

    INCLUDES   rupture that occurs when a normal force is applied to tissues that are inferred to have less than normal strength

    EXCLUDES 2   *rotator cuff syndrome (M75.1-)*

                rupture where an abnormal force is applied to normal tissue — see injury of tendon by body region

    M66.0 Rupture of popliteal cyst

✓5ᵗʰ **M66.1 Rupture of synovium**

    Rupture of synovial cyst

    EXCLUDES 2   *rupture of popliteal cyst (M66.0)*

    M66.10 Rupture of synovium, unspecified joint

✓6ᵗʰ **M66.11 Rupture of synovium, shoulder**

    M66.111 Rupture of synovium, right shoulder

    M66.112 Rupture of synovium, left shoulder

    M66.119 Rupture of synovium, unspecified shoulder

✓6ᵗʰ **M66.12 Rupture of synovium, elbow**

    M66.121 Rupture of synovium, right elbow

    M66.122 Rupture of synovium, left elbow

    M66.129 Rupture of synovium, unspecified elbow

✓6ᵗʰ **M66.13 Rupture of synovium, wrist**

    M66.131 Rupture of synovium, right wrist

    M66.132 Rupture of synovium, left wrist

N Newborn: 0   P Pediatric: 0-17   M Maternity: 9-64   A Adult: 15-124   MCC Major Complication/Comorbidity   CC Complication/Comorbidity   SW Severe Wound Dx

808   ICD-10-CM 2021

M66.139 Rupture of synovium, unspecified wrist

√6ᵗʰ M66.14 Rupture of synovium, hand and fingers

M66.141 Rupture of synovium, right hand
M66.142 Rupture of synovium, left hand
M66.143 Rupture of synovium, unspecified hand
M66.144 Rupture of synovium, right finger(s)
M66.145 Rupture of synovium, left finger(s)
M66.146 Rupture of synovium, unspecified finger(s)

√6ᵗʰ M66.15 Rupture of synovium, hip

M66.151 Rupture of synovium, right hip
M66.152 Rupture of synovium, left hip
M66.159 Rupture of synovium, unspecified hip

√6ᵗʰ M66.17 Rupture of synovium, ankle, foot and toes

M66.171 Rupture of synovium, right ankle
M66.172 Rupture of synovium, left ankle
M66.173 Rupture of synovium, unspecified ankle
M66.174 Rupture of synovium, right foot
M66.175 Rupture of synovium, left foot
M66.176 Rupture of synovium, unspecified foot
M66.177 Rupture of synovium, right toe(s)
M66.178 Rupture of synovium, left toe(s)
M66.179 Rupture of synovium, unspecified toe(s)

M66.18 Rupture of synovium, other site

√5ᵗʰ M66.2 Spontaneous rupture of extensor tendons

TIP: Refer to the Muscle/Tendon table at the beginning of this chapter.

M66.20 Spontaneous rupture of extensor tendons, unspecified site

√6ᵗʰ M66.21 Spontaneous rupture of extensor tendons, shoulder

M66.211 Spontaneous rupture of extensor tendons, right shoulder
M66.212 Spontaneous rupture of extensor tendons, left shoulder
M66.219 Spontaneous rupture of extensor tendons, unspecified shoulder

√6ᵗʰ M66.22 Spontaneous rupture of extensor tendons, upper arm

M66.221 Spontaneous rupture of extensor tendons, right upper arm
M66.222 Spontaneous rupture of extensor tendons, left upper arm
M66.229 Spontaneous rupture of extensor tendons, unspecified upper arm

√6ᵗʰ M66.23 Spontaneous rupture of extensor tendons, forearm

M66.231 Spontaneous rupture of extensor tendons, right forearm
M66.232 Spontaneous rupture of extensor tendons, left forearm
M66.239 Spontaneous rupture of extensor tendons, unspecified forearm

√6ᵗʰ M66.24 Spontaneous rupture of extensor tendons, hand

M66.241 Spontaneous rupture of extensor tendons, right hand
M66.242 Spontaneous rupture of extensor tendons, left hand
M66.249 Spontaneous rupture of extensor tendons, unspecified hand

√6ᵗʰ M66.25 Spontaneous rupture of extensor tendons, thigh

M66.251 Spontaneous rupture of extensor tendons, right thigh
M66.252 Spontaneous rupture of extensor tendons, left thigh
M66.259 Spontaneous rupture of extensor tendons, unspecified thigh

√6ᵗʰ M66.26 Spontaneous rupture of extensor tendons, lower leg

M66.261 Spontaneous rupture of extensor tendons, right lower leg
M66.262 Spontaneous rupture of extensor tendons, left lower leg
M66.269 Spontaneous rupture of extensor tendons, unspecified lower leg

√6ᵗʰ M66.27 Spontaneous rupture of extensor tendons, ankle and foot

M66.271 Spontaneous rupture of extensor tendons, right ankle and foot
M66.272 Spontaneous rupture of extensor tendons, left ankle and foot

M66.279 Spontaneous rupture of extensor tendons, unspecified ankle and foot

M66.28 Spontaneous rupture of extensor tendons, other site

M66.29 Spontaneous rupture of extensor tendons, multiple sites

√5ᵗʰ M66.3 Spontaneous rupture of flexor tendons

TIP: Refer to the Muscle/Tendon table at the beginning of this chapter.

M66.30 Spontaneous rupture of flexor tendons, unspecified site

√6ᵗʰ M66.31 Spontaneous rupture of flexor tendons, shoulder

M66.311 Spontaneous rupture of flexor tendons, right shoulder
M66.312 Spontaneous rupture of flexor tendons, left shoulder
M66.319 Spontaneous rupture of flexor tendons, unspecified shoulder

√6ᵗʰ M66.32 Spontaneous rupture of flexor tendons, upper arm

M66.321 Spontaneous rupture of flexor tendons, right upper arm
M66.322 Spontaneous rupture of flexor tendons, left upper arm
M66.329 Spontaneous rupture of flexor tendons, unspecified upper arm

√6ᵗʰ M66.33 Spontaneous rupture of flexor tendons, forearm

M66.331 Spontaneous rupture of flexor tendons, right forearm
M66.332 Spontaneous rupture of flexor tendons, left forearm
M66.339 Spontaneous rupture of flexor tendons, unspecified forearm

√6ᵗʰ M66.34 Spontaneous rupture of flexor tendons, hand

M66.341 Spontaneous rupture of flexor tendons, right hand
M66.342 Spontaneous rupture of flexor tendons, left hand
M66.349 Spontaneous rupture of flexor tendons, unspecified hand

√6ᵗʰ M66.35 Spontaneous rupture of flexor tendons, thigh

M66.351 Spontaneous rupture of flexor tendons, right thigh
M66.352 Spontaneous rupture of flexor tendons, left thigh
M66.359 Spontaneous rupture of flexor tendons, unspecified thigh

√6ᵗʰ M66.36 Spontaneous rupture of flexor tendons, lower leg

M66.361 Spontaneous rupture of flexor tendons, right lower leg
M66.362 Spontaneous rupture of flexor tendons, left lower leg
M66.369 Spontaneous rupture of flexor tendons, unspecified lower leg

√6ᵗʰ M66.37 Spontaneous rupture of flexor tendons, ankle and foot

M66.371 Spontaneous rupture of flexor tendons, right ankle and foot
M66.372 Spontaneous rupture of flexor tendons, left ankle and foot
M66.379 Spontaneous rupture of flexor tendons, unspecified ankle and foot

M66.38 Spontaneous rupture of flexor tendons, other site

M66.39 Spontaneous rupture of flexor tendons, multiple sites

√5ᵗʰ M66.8 Spontaneous rupture of other tendons

TIP: Refer to the Muscle/Tendon table at the beginning of this chapter.

M66.80 Spontaneous rupture of other tendons, unspecified site

√6ᵗʰ M66.81 Spontaneous rupture of other tendons, shoulder

M66.811 Spontaneous rupture of other tendons, right shoulder
M66.812 Spontaneous rupture of other tendons, left shoulder
M66.819 Spontaneous rupture of other tendons, unspecified shoulder

√6ᵗʰ M66.82 Spontaneous rupture of other tendons, upper arm

M66.821 Spontaneous rupture of other tendons, right upper arm

M66.822   Spontaneous rupture of other tendons, left upper arm

M66.829   Spontaneous rupture of other tendons, unspecified upper arm

√6th   M66.83   Spontaneous rupture of other tendons, forearm

M66.831   Spontaneous rupture of other tendons, right forearm

M66.832   Spontaneous rupture of other tendons, left forearm

M66.839   Spontaneous rupture of other tendons, unspecified forearm

√6th   M66.84   Spontaneous rupture of other tendons, hand

M66.841   Spontaneous rupture of other tendons, right hand

M66.842   Spontaneous rupture of other tendons, left hand

M66.849   Spontaneous rupture of other tendons, unspecified hand

√6th   M66.85   Spontaneous rupture of other tendons, thigh

M66.851   Spontaneous rupture of other tendons, right thigh

M66.852   Spontaneous rupture of other tendons, left thigh

M66.859   Spontaneous rupture of other tendons, unspecified thigh

√6th   M66.86   Spontaneous rupture of other tendons, lower leg

M66.861   Spontaneous rupture of other tendons, right lower leg

M66.862   Spontaneous rupture of other tendons, left lower leg

M66.869   Spontaneous rupture of other tendons, unspecified lower leg

√6th   M66.87   Spontaneous rupture of other tendons, ankle and foot

M66.871   Spontaneous rupture of other tendons, right ankle and foot

M66.872   Spontaneous rupture of other tendons, left ankle and foot

M66.879   Spontaneous rupture of other tendons, unspecified ankle and foot

M66.88   Spontaneous rupture of other tendons, other sites

M66.89   Spontaneous rupture of other tendons, multiple sites

M66.9   Spontaneous rupture of unspecified tendon

Rupture at musculotendinous junction, nontraumatic

√4th   **M67   Other disorders of synovium and tendon**

EXCLUDES 1   palmar fascial fibromatosis [Dupuytren] (M72.0)

tendinitis NOS (M77.9-)

xanthomatosis localized to tendons (E78.2)

√5th   M67.0   Short Achilles tendon (acquired)

M67.00   Short Achilles tendon (acquired), unspecified ankle

M67.01   Short Achilles tendon (acquired), right ankle

M67.02   Short Achilles tendon (acquired), left ankle

√5th   M67.2   Synovial hypertrophy, not elsewhere classified

EXCLUDES 1   villonodular synovitis (pigmented) (M12.2-)

M67.20   Synovial hypertrophy, not elsewhere classified, unspecified site

√6th   M67.21   Synovial hypertrophy, not elsewhere classified, shoulder

M67.211   Synovial hypertrophy, not elsewhere classified, right shoulder

M67.212   Synovial hypertrophy, not elsewhere classified, left shoulder

M67.219   Synovial hypertrophy, not elsewhere classified, unspecified shoulder

√6th   M67.22   Synovial hypertrophy, not elsewhere classified, upper arm

M67.221   Synovial hypertrophy, not elsewhere classified, right upper arm

M67.222   Synovial hypertrophy, not elsewhere classified, left upper arm

M67.229   Synovial hypertrophy, not elsewhere classified, unspecified upper arm

√6th   M67.23   Synovial hypertrophy, not elsewhere classified, forearm

M67.231   Synovial hypertrophy, not elsewhere classified, right forearm

M67.232   Synovial hypertrophy, not elsewhere classified, left forearm

M67.239   Synovial hypertrophy, not elsewhere classified, unspecified forearm

√6th   M67.24   Synovial hypertrophy, not elsewhere classified, hand

M67.241   Synovial hypertrophy, not elsewhere classified, right hand

M67.242   Synovial hypertrophy, not elsewhere classified, left hand

M67.249   Synovial hypertrophy, not elsewhere classified, unspecified hand

√6th   M67.25   Synovial hypertrophy, not elsewhere classified, thigh

M67.251   Synovial hypertrophy, not elsewhere classified, right thigh

M67.252   Synovial hypertrophy, not elsewhere classified, left thigh

M67.259   Synovial hypertrophy, not elsewhere classified, unspecified thigh

√6th   M67.26   Synovial hypertrophy, not elsewhere classified, lower leg

M67.261   Synovial hypertrophy, not elsewhere classified, right lower leg

M67.262   Synovial hypertrophy, not elsewhere classified, left lower leg

M67.269   Synovial hypertrophy, not elsewhere classified, unspecified lower leg

√6th   M67.27   Synovial hypertrophy, not elsewhere classified, ankle and foot

M67.271   Synovial hypertrophy, not elsewhere classified, right ankle and foot

M67.272   Synovial hypertrophy, not elsewhere classified, left ankle and foot

M67.279   Synovial hypertrophy, not elsewhere classified, unspecified ankle and foot

M67.28   Synovial hypertrophy, not elsewhere classified, other site

M67.29   Synovial hypertrophy, not elsewhere classified, multiple sites

√5th   M67.3   Transient synovitis

Toxic synovitis

EXCLUDES 1   palindromic rheumatism (M12.3-)

M67.30   Transient synovitis, unspecified site

√6th   M67.31   Transient synovitis, shoulder

M67.311   Transient synovitis, right shoulder

M67.312   Transient synovitis, left shoulder

M67.319   Transient synovitis, unspecified shoulder

√6th   M67.32   Transient synovitis, elbow

M67.321   Transient synovitis, right elbow

M67.322   Transient synovitis, left elbow

M67.329   Transient synovitis, unspecified elbow

√6th   M67.33   Transient synovitis, wrist

M67.331   Transient synovitis, right wrist

M67.332   Transient synovitis, left wrist

M67.339   Transient synovitis, unspecified wrist

√6th   M67.34   Transient synovitis, hand

M67.341   Transient synovitis, right hand

M67.342   Transient synovitis, left hand

M67.349   Transient synovitis, unspecified hand

√6th   M67.35   Transient synovitis, hip

M67.351   Transient synovitis, right hip

M67.352   Transient synovitis, left hip

M67.359   Transient synovitis, unspecified hip

√6th   M67.36   Transient synovitis, knee

M67.361   Transient synovitis, right knee

M67.362   Transient synovitis, left knee

M67.369   Transient synovitis, unspecified knee

√6th   M67.37   Transient synovitis, ankle and foot

M67.371   Transient synovitis, right ankle and foot

M67.372   Transient synovitis, left ankle and foot

M67.379   Transient synovitis, unspecified ankle and foot

M67.38   Transient synovitis, other site

M67.39   Transient synovitis, multiple sites

N Newborn: 0   P Pediatric: 0-17   M Maternity: 9-64   A Adult: 15-124   MCC Major Complication/Comorbidity   CC Complication/Comorbidity   SW Severe Wound Dx

810   ICD-10-CM 2021

√5ᵗʰ **M67.4 Ganglion**

Ganglion of joint or tendon (sheath)

    EXCLUDES 1   *ganglion in yaws (A66.6)*

    EXCLUDES 2   *cyst of bursa (M71.2-M71.3)*

                cyst of synovium (M71.2-M71.3)

DEF: Fluid-filled, benign cyst appearing on a tendon sheath or aponeurosis, frequently connecting to an underlying joint.

    M67.40   Ganglion, unspecified site

√6ᵗʰ   **M67.41**   Ganglion, shoulder

         M67.411   Ganglion, right shoulder

         M67.412   Ganglion, left shoulder

         M67.419   Ganglion, unspecified shoulder

√6ᵗʰ   **M67.42**   Ganglion, elbow

         M67.421   Ganglion, right elbow

         M67.422   Ganglion, left elbow

         M67.429   Ganglion, unspecified elbow

√6ᵗʰ   **M67.43**   Ganglion, wrist

Ganglion of Wrist

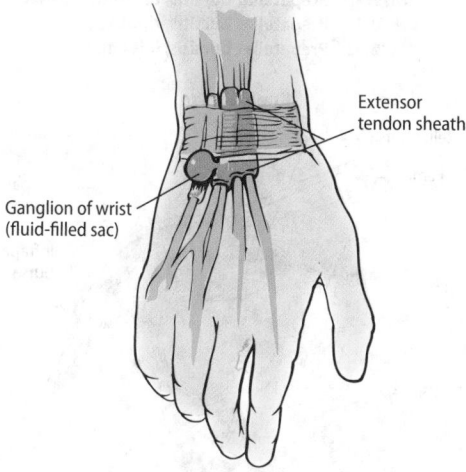

Ganglion of wrist
(fluid-filled sac)

Extensor
tendon sheaths

         M67.431   Ganglion, right wrist

         M67.432   Ganglion, left wrist

         M67.439   Ganglion, unspecified wrist

√6ᵗʰ   **M67.44**   Ganglion, hand

         M67.441   Ganglion, right hand

         M67.442   Ganglion, left hand

         M67.449   Ganglion, unspecified hand

√6ᵗʰ   **M67.45**   Ganglion, hip

         M67.451   Ganglion, right hip

         M67.452   Ganglion, left hip

         M67.459   Ganglion, unspecified hip

√6ᵗʰ   **M67.46**   Ganglion, knee

         M67.461   Ganglion, right knee

         M67.462   Ganglion, left knee

         M67.469   Ganglion, unspecified knee

√6ᵗʰ   **M67.47**   Ganglion, ankle and foot

         M67.471   Ganglion, right ankle and foot

         M67.472   Ganglion, left ankle and foot

         M67.479   Ganglion, unspecified ankle and foot

    M67.48   Ganglion, other site

    M67.49   Ganglion, multiple sites

√5ᵗʰ **M67.5 Plica syndrome**

Plica knee

    M67.50   Plica syndrome, unspecified knee

    M67.51   Plica syndrome, right knee

    M67.52   Plica syndrome, left knee

√5ᵗʰ **M67.8 Other specified disorders of synovium and tendon**

    M67.80   Other specified disorders of synovium and tendon, unspecified site

√6ᵗʰ   **M67.81**   Other specified disorders of synovium and tendon, shoulder

         M67.811   Other specified disorders of synovium, right shoulder

         M67.812   Other specified disorders of synovium, left shoulder

         M67.813   Other specified disorders of tendon, right shoulder

         M67.814   Other specified disorders of tendon, left shoulder

         M67.819   Other specified disorders of synovium and tendon, unspecified shoulder

√6ᵗʰ   **M67.82**   Other specified disorders of synovium and tendon, elbow

         M67.821   Other specified disorders of synovium, right elbow

         M67.822   Other specified disorders of synovium, left elbow

         M67.823   Other specified disorders of tendon, right elbow

         M67.824   Other specified disorders of tendon, left elbow

         M67.829   Other specified disorders of synovium and tendon, unspecified elbow

√6ᵗʰ   **M67.83**   Other specified disorders of synovium and tendon, wrist

         M67.831   Other specified disorders of synovium, right wrist

         M67.832   Other specified disorders of synovium, left wrist

         M67.833   Other specified disorders of tendon, right wrist

         M67.834   Other specified disorders of tendon, left wrist

         M67.839   Other specified disorders of synovium and tendon, unspecified wrist

√6ᵗʰ   **M67.84**   Other specified disorders of synovium and tendon, hand

         M67.841   Other specified disorders of synovium, right hand

         M67.842   Other specified disorders of synovium, left hand

         M67.843   Other specified disorders of tendon, right hand

         M67.844   Other specified disorders of tendon, left hand

         M67.849   Other specified disorders of synovium and tendon, unspecified hand

√6ᵗʰ   **M67.85**   Other specified disorders of synovium and tendon, hip

         M67.851   Other specified disorders of synovium, right hip

         M67.852   Other specified disorders of synovium, left hip

         M67.853   Other specified disorders of tendon, right hip

         M67.854   Other specified disorders of tendon, left hip

         M67.859   Other specified disorders of synovium and tendon, unspecified hip

√6ᵗʰ   **M67.86**   Other specified disorders of synovium and tendon, knee

         M67.861   Other specified disorders of synovium, right knee

         M67.862   Other specified disorders of synovium, left knee

         M67.863   Other specified disorders of tendon, right knee

         M67.864   Other specified disorders of tendon, left knee

         M67.869   Other specified disorders of synovium and tendon, unspecified knee

√6ᵗʰ   **M67.87**   Other specified disorders of synovium and tendon, ankle and foot

         M67.871   Other specified disorders of synovium, right ankle and foot

         M67.872   Other specified disorders of synovium, left ankle and foot

         M67.873   Other specified disorders of tendon, right ankle and foot

         M67.874   Other specified disorders of tendon, left ankle and foot

         M67.879   Other specified disorders of synovium and tendon, unspecified ankle and foot

    M67.88   Other specified disorders of synovium and tendon, other site

    M67.89   Other specified disorders of synovium and tendon, multiple sites

✔ Additional Character Required   √x7ᵗʰ Placeholder   Unacceptable PDx   Questionable PDx   Manifestation   Unspecified Dx   H1–H14 HAC   HCC CMS-HCC Dx   HIV HIV Dx

ICD-10-CM 2021   811

✓5ᵗʰ **M67.9** Unspecified disorder of synovium and tendon

    M67.90 Unspecified disorder of synovium and tendon, unspecified site

    ✓6ᵗʰ **M67.91** Unspecified disorder of synovium and tendon, shoulder

      M67.911 Unspecified disorder of synovium and tendon, right shoulder

      M67.912 Unspecified disorder of synovium and tendon, left shoulder

      M67.919 Unspecified disorder of synovium and tendon, unspecified shoulder

    ✓6ᵗʰ **M67.92** Unspecified disorder of synovium and tendon, upper arm

      M67.921 Unspecified disorder of synovium and tendon, right upper arm

      M67.922 Unspecified disorder of synovium and tendon, left upper arm

      M67.929 Unspecified disorder of synovium and tendon, unspecified upper arm

    ✓6ᵗʰ **M67.93** Unspecified disorder of synovium and tendon, forearm

      M67.931 Unspecified disorder of synovium and tendon, right forearm

      M67.932 Unspecified disorder of synovium and tendon, left forearm

      M67.939 Unspecified disorder of synovium and tendon, unspecified forearm

    ✓6ᵗʰ **M67.94** Unspecified disorder of synovium and tendon, hand

      M67.941 Unspecified disorder of synovium and tendon, right hand

      M67.942 Unspecified disorder of synovium and tendon, left hand

      M67.949 Unspecified disorder of synovium and tendon, unspecified hand

    ✓6ᵗʰ **M67.95** Unspecified disorder of synovium and tendon, thigh

      M67.951 Unspecified disorder of synovium and tendon, right thigh

      M67.952 Unspecified disorder of synovium and tendon, left thigh

      M67.959 Unspecified disorder of synovium and tendon, unspecified thigh

    ✓6ᵗʰ **M67.96** Unspecified disorder of synovium and tendon, lower leg

      M67.961 Unspecified disorder of synovium and tendon, right lower leg

      M67.962 Unspecified disorder of synovium and tendon, left lower leg

      M67.969 Unspecified disorder of synovium and tendon, unspecified lower leg

    ✓6ᵗʰ **M67.97** Unspecified disorder of synovium and tendon, ankle and foot

      M67.971 Unspecified disorder of synovium and tendon, right ankle and foot

      M67.972 Unspecified disorder of synovium and tendon, left ankle and foot

      M67.979 Unspecified disorder of synovium and tendon, unspecified ankle and foot

    M67.98 Unspecified disorder of synovium and tendon, other site

    M67.99 Unspecified disorder of synovium and tendon, multiple sites

Other soft tissue disorders (M70-M79)

✓4ᵗʰ **M70 Soft tissue disorders related to use, overuse and pressure**

    INCLUDES   soft tissue disorders of occupational origin

    Use additional external cause code to identify activity causing disorder (Y93.-)

    EXCLUDES 1   bursitis NOS (M71.9-)

    EXCLUDES 2   bursitis of shoulder (M75.5)

      enthesopathies (M76-M77)

      pressure ulcer (pressure area) (L89.-)

    ✓5ᵗʰ **M70.0** Crepitant synovitis (acute) (chronic) of hand and wrist

      ✓6ᵗʰ **M70.03** Crepitant synovitis (acute) (chronic), wrist

        M70.031 Crepitant synovitis (acute) (chronic), right wrist

        M70.032 Crepitant synovitis (acute) (chronic), left wrist

        M70.039 Crepitant synovitis (acute) (chronic), unspecified wrist

    ✓6ᵗʰ **M70.04** Crepitant synovitis (acute) (chronic), hand

      M70.041 Crepitant synovitis (acute) (chronic), right hand

      M70.042 Crepitant synovitis (acute) (chronic), left hand

      M70.049 Crepitant synovitis (acute) (chronic), unspecified hand

    ✓5ᵗʰ **M70.1** Bursitis of hand

      M70.10 Bursitis, unspecified hand

      M70.11 Bursitis, right hand

      M70.12 Bursitis, left hand

    ✓5ᵗʰ **M70.2** Olecranon bursitis

      M70.20 Olecranon bursitis, unspecified elbow

      M70.21 Olecranon bursitis, right elbow

      M70.22 Olecranon bursitis, left elbow

    ✓5ᵗʰ **M70.3** Other bursitis of elbow

      M70.30 Other bursitis of elbow, unspecified elbow

      M70.31 Other bursitis of elbow, right elbow

      M70.32 Other bursitis of elbow, left elbow

    ✓5ᵗʰ **M70.4** Prepatellar bursitis

      M70.40 Prepatellar bursitis, unspecified knee

      M70.41 Prepatellar bursitis, right knee

      M70.42 Prepatellar bursitis, left knee

Knee Bursae

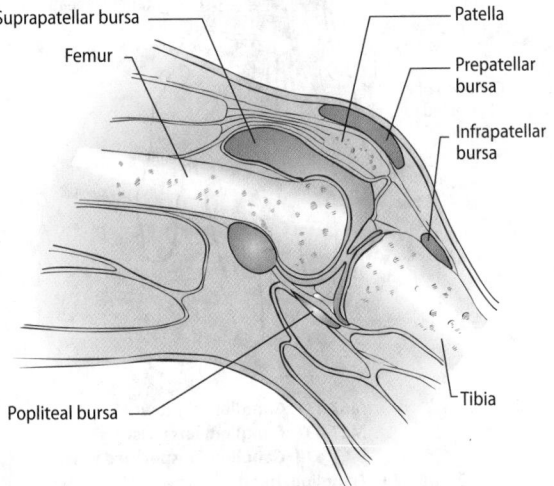

✓5ᵗʰ **M70.5** Other bursitis of knee

      M70.50 Other bursitis of knee, unspecified knee

      M70.51 Other bursitis of knee, right knee

      M70.52 Other bursitis of knee, left knee

✓5ᵗʰ **M70.6** Trochanteric bursitis

    Trochanteric tendinitis

      M70.60 Trochanteric bursitis, unspecified hip

      M70.61 Trochanteric bursitis, right hip

      M70.62 Trochanteric bursitis, left hip

✓5ᵗʰ **M70.7** Other bursitis of hip

    Ischial bursitis

      M70.70 Other bursitis of hip, unspecified hip

      M70.71 Other bursitis of hip, right hip

      M70.72 Other bursitis of hip, left hip

✓5ᵗʰ **M70.8** Other soft tissue disorders related to use, overuse and pressure

      M70.80 Other soft tissue disorders related to use, overuse and pressure of unspecified site

    ✓6ᵗʰ **M70.81** Other soft tissue disorders related to use, overuse and pressure of shoulder

      M70.811 Other soft tissue disorders related to use, overuse and pressure, right shoulder

      M70.812 Other soft tissue disorders related to use, overuse and pressure, left shoulder

      M70.819 Other soft tissue disorders related to use, overuse and pressure, unspecified shoulder

    ✓6ᵗʰ **M70.82** Other soft tissue disorders related to use, overuse and pressure of upper arm

      M70.821 Other soft tissue disorders related to use, overuse and pressure, right upper arm

M70.822   Other soft tissue disorders related to use, overuse and pressure, left upper arm

M70.829   Other soft tissue disorders related to use, overuse and pressure, unspecified upper arms

✓6th **M70.83**   Other soft tissue disorders related to use, overuse and pressure of forearm

     M70.831   Other soft tissue disorders related to use, overuse and pressure, right forearm

     M70.832   Other soft tissue disorders related to use, overuse and pressure, left forearm

     M70.839   Other soft tissue disorders related to use, overuse and pressure, unspecified forearm

✓6th **M70.84**   Other soft tissue disorders related to use, overuse and pressure of hand

     M70.841   Other soft tissue disorders related to use, overuse and pressure, right hand

     M70.842   Other soft tissue disorders related to use, overuse and pressure, left hand

     M70.849   Other soft tissue disorders related to use, overuse and pressure, unspecified hand

✓6th **M70.85**   Other soft tissue disorders related to use, overuse and pressure of thigh

     M70.851   Other soft tissue disorders related to use, overuse and pressure, right thigh

     M70.852   Other soft tissue disorders related to use, overuse and pressure, left thigh

     M70.859   Other soft tissue disorders related to use, overuse and pressure, unspecified thigh

✓6th **M70.86**   Other soft tissue disorders related to use, overuse and pressure lower leg

     M70.861   Other soft tissue disorders related to use, overuse and pressure, right lower leg

     M70.862   Other soft tissue disorders related to use, overuse and pressure, left lower leg

     M70.869   Other soft tissue disorders related to use, overuse and pressure, unspecified leg

✓6th **M70.87**   Other soft tissue disorders related to use, overuse and pressure of ankle and foot

     M70.871   Other soft tissue disorders related to use, overuse and pressure, right ankle and foot

     M70.872   Other soft tissue disorders related to use, overuse and pressure, left ankle and foot

     M70.879   Other soft tissue disorders related to use, overuse and pressure, unspecified ankle and foot

     M70.88   Other soft tissue disorders related to use, overuse and pressure other site

     M70.89   Other soft tissue disorders related to use, overuse and pressure multiple sites

✓5th **M70.9**   Unspecified soft tissue disorder related to use, overuse and pressure

     M70.90   Unspecified soft tissue disorder related to use, overuse and pressure of unspecified site

✓6th **M70.91**   Unspecified soft tissue disorder related to use, overuse and pressure of shoulder

     M70.911   Unspecified soft tissue disorder related to use, overuse and pressure, right shoulder

     M70.912   Unspecified soft tissue disorder related to use, overuse and pressure, left shoulder

     M70.919   Unspecified soft tissue disorder related to use, overuse and pressure, unspecified shoulder

✓6th **M70.92**   Unspecified soft tissue disorder related to use, overuse and pressure of upper arm

     M70.921   Unspecified soft tissue disorder related to use, overuse and pressure, right upper arm

     M70.922   Unspecified soft tissue disorder related to use, overuse and pressure, left upper arm

     M70.929   Unspecified soft tissue disorder related to use, overuse and pressure, unspecified upper arm

✓6th **M70.93**   Unspecified soft tissue disorder related to use, overuse and pressure of forearm

     M70.931   Unspecified soft tissue disorder related to use, overuse and pressure, right forearm

M70.932   Unspecified soft tissue disorder related to use, overuse and pressure, left forearm

M70.939   Unspecified soft tissue disorder related to use, overuse and pressure, unspecified forearm

✓6th **M70.94**   Unspecified soft tissue disorder related to use, overuse and pressure of hand

     M70.941   Unspecified soft tissue disorder related to use, overuse and pressure, right hand

     M70.942   Unspecified soft tissue disorder related to use, overuse and pressure, left hand

     M70.949   Unspecified soft tissue disorder related to use, overuse and pressure, unspecified hand

✓6th **M70.95**   Unspecified soft tissue disorder related to use, overuse and pressure of thigh

     M70.951   Unspecified soft tissue disorder related to use, overuse and pressure, right thigh

     M70.952   Unspecified soft tissue disorder related to use, overuse and pressure, left thigh

     M70.959   Unspecified soft tissue disorder related to use, overuse and pressure, unspecified thigh

✓6th **M70.96**   Unspecified soft tissue disorder related to use, overuse and pressure lower leg

     M70.961   Unspecified soft tissue disorder related to use, overuse and pressure, right lower leg

     M70.962   Unspecified soft tissue disorder related to use, overuse and pressure, left lower leg

     M70.969   Unspecified soft tissue disorder related to use, overuse and pressure, unspecified lower leg

✓6th **M70.97**   Unspecified soft tissue disorder related to use, overuse and pressure of ankle and foot

     M70.971   Unspecified soft tissue disorder related to use, overuse and pressure, right ankle and foot

     M70.972   Unspecified soft tissue disorder related to use, overuse and pressure, left ankle and foot

     M70.979   Unspecified soft tissue disorder related to use, overuse and pressure, unspecified ankle and foot

     M70.98   Unspecified soft tissue disorder related to use, overuse and pressure other

     M70.99   Unspecified soft tissue disorder related to use, overuse and pressure multiple sites

✓4th **M71**   **Other bursopathies**

     EXCLUDES 1   bunion (M20.1)

                 bursitis related to use, overuse or pressure (M70.-)

                 enthesopathies (M76-M77)

✓5th **M71.0**   **Abscess of bursa**

     Use additional code (B95.-, B96.-) to identify causative organism

     M71.00   Abscess of bursa, unspecified site

✓6th **M71.01**   Abscess of bursa, shoulder

     M71.011   Abscess of bursa, right shoulder

     M71.012   Abscess of bursa, left shoulder

     M71.019   Abscess of bursa, unspecified shoulder

✓6th **M71.02**   Abscess of bursa, elbow

     M71.021   Abscess of bursa, right elbow

     M71.022   Abscess of bursa, left elbow

     M71.029   Abscess of bursa, unspecified elbow

✓6th **M71.03**   Abscess of bursa, wrist

     M71.031   Abscess of bursa, right wrist

     M71.032   Abscess of bursa, left wrist

     M71.039   Abscess of bursa, unspecified wrist

✓6th **M71.04**   Abscess of bursa, hand

     M71.041   Abscess of bursa, right hand

     M71.042   Abscess of bursa, left hand

     M71.049   Abscess of bursa, unspecified hand

✓6th **M71.05**   Abscess of bursa, hip

     M71.051   Abscess of bursa, right hip

     M71.052   Abscess of bursa, left hip

     M71.059   Abscess of bursa, unspecified hip

✓6th **M71.06**   Abscess of bursa, knee

     M71.061   Abscess of bursa, right knee

     M71.062   Abscess of bursa, left knee

     M71.069   Abscess of bursa, unspecified knee

✓6ᵗʰ **M71.07** **Abscess of bursa,** ankle and foot
    M71.071 **Abscess of bursa,** right ankle and foot
    M71.072 **Abscess of bursa,** left ankle and foot
    M71.079 **Abscess of bursa,** unspecified ankle and foot
  M71.08 **Abscess of bursa,** other site
  M71.09 **Abscess of bursa,** multiple sites
✓5ᵗʰ **M71.1** **Other infective bursitis**
    Use additional code (B95.-, B96.-) to identify causative organism
  M71.10 **Other infective bursitis,** unspecified site
✓6ᵗʰ **M71.11** **Other infective bursitis,** shoulder
    M71.111 **Other infective bursitis,** right shoulder
    M71.112 **Other infective bursitis,** left shoulder
    M71.119 **Other infective bursitis,** unspecified shoulder
✓6ᵗʰ **M71.12** **Other infective bursitis,** elbow
    M71.121 **Other infective bursitis,** right elbow
    M71.122 **Other infective bursitis,** left elbow
    M71.129 **Other infective bursitis,** unspecified elbow
✓6ᵗʰ **M71.13** **Other infective bursitis,** wrist
    M71.131 **Other infective bursitis,** right wrist
    M71.132 **Other infective bursitis,** left wrist
    M71.139 **Other infective bursitis,** unspecified wrist
✓6ᵗʰ **M71.14** **Other infective bursitis,** hand
    M71.141 **Other infective bursitis,** right hand
    M71.142 **Other infective bursitis,** left hand
    M71.149 **Other infective bursitis,** unspecified hand
✓6ᵗʰ **M71.15** **Other infective bursitis,** hip
    M71.151 **Other infective bursitis,** right hip
    M71.152 **Other infective bursitis,** left hip
    M71.159 **Other infective bursitis,** unspecified hip
✓6ᵗʰ **M71.16** **Other infective bursitis,** knee
    M71.161 **Other infective bursitis,** right knee
    M71.162 **Other infective bursitis,** left knee
    M71.169 **Other infective bursitis,** unspecified knee
✓6ᵗʰ **M71.17** **Other infective bursitis,** ankle and foot
    M71.171 **Other infective bursitis,** right ankle and foot
    M71.172 **Other infective bursitis,** left ankle and foot
    M71.179 **Other infective bursitis,** unspecified ankle and foot
  M71.18 **Other infective bursitis,** other site
  M71.19 **Other infective bursitis,** multiple sites
✓5ᵗʰ **M71.2** **Synovial cyst of popliteal space [Baker]**
    EXCLUDES 1 *synovial cyst of popliteal space with rupture (M66.0)*
    DEF: Sac filled with clear synovial fluid in adults, usually secondary to disease inside the joint, located on the back of the knee in the popliteal fossa area. In children, the cyst usually represents a ganglion of one of the tendons in the knee.

Baker's Cyst

Baker's cyst connected to knee joint synovial cavity

  M71.20 **Synovial cyst of popliteal space [Baker],** unspecified knee

  M71.21 **Synovial cyst of popliteal space [Baker],** right knee
  M71.22 **Synovial cyst of popliteal space [Baker],** left knee
✓5ᵗʰ **M71.3** **Other bursal cyst**
    Synovial cyst NOS
    EXCLUDES 1 *synovial cyst with rupture (M66.1-)*
  M71.30 **Other bursal cyst,** unspecified site
✓6ᵗʰ **M71.31** **Other bursal cyst,** shoulder
    M71.311 **Other bursal cyst,** right shoulder
    M71.312 **Other bursal cyst,** left shoulder
    M71.319 **Other bursal cyst,** unspecified shoulder
✓6ᵗʰ **M71.32** **Other bursal cyst,** elbow
    M71.321 **Other bursal cyst,** right elbow
    M71.322 **Other bursal cyst,** left elbow
    M71.329 **Other bursal cyst,** unspecified elbow
✓6ᵗʰ **M71.33** **Other bursal cyst,** wrist
    M71.331 **Other bursal cyst,** right wrist
    M71.332 **Other bursal cyst,** left wrist
    M71.339 **Other bursal cyst,** unspecified wrist
✓6ᵗʰ **M71.34** **Other bursal cyst,** hand
    M71.341 **Other bursal cyst,** right hand
    M71.342 **Other bursal cyst,** left hand
    M71.349 **Other bursal cyst,** unspecified hand
✓6ᵗʰ **M71.35** **Other bursal cyst,** hip
    M71.351 **Other bursal cyst,** right hip
    M71.352 **Other bursal cyst,** left hip
    M71.359 **Other bursal cyst,** unspecified hip
✓6ᵗʰ **M71.37** **Other bursal cyst,** ankle and foot
    M71.371 **Other bursal cyst,** right ankle and foot
    M71.372 **Other bursal cyst,** left ankle and foot
    M71.379 **Other bursal cyst,** unspecified ankle and foot
  M71.38 **Other bursal cyst,** other site
  M71.39 **Other bursal cyst,** multiple sites
✓5ᵗʰ **M71.4** **Calcium deposit in bursa**
    EXCLUDES 2 *calcium deposit in bursa of shoulder (M75.3)*
  M71.40 **Calcium deposit in bursa,** unspecified site
✓6ᵗʰ **M71.42** **Calcium deposit in bursa,** elbow
    M71.421 **Calcium deposit in bursa,** right elbow
    M71.422 **Calcium deposit in bursa,** left elbow
    M71.429 **Calcium deposit in bursa,** unspecified elbow
✓6ᵗʰ **M71.43** **Calcium deposit in bursa,** wrist
    M71.431 **Calcium deposit in bursa,** right wrist
    M71.432 **Calcium deposit in bursa,** left wrist
    M71.439 **Calcium deposit in bursa,** unspecified wrist
✓6ᵗʰ **M71.44** **Calcium deposit in bursa,** hand
    M71.441 **Calcium deposit in bursa,** right hand
    M71.442 **Calcium deposit in bursa,** left hand
    M71.449 **Calcium deposit in bursa,** unspecified hand
✓6ᵗʰ **M71.45** **Calcium deposit in bursa,** hip
    M71.451 **Calcium deposit in bursa,** right hip
    M71.452 **Calcium deposit in bursa,** left hip
    M71.459 **Calcium deposit in bursa,** unspecified hip
✓6ᵗʰ **M71.46** **Calcium deposit in bursa,** knee
    M71.461 **Calcium deposit in bursa,** right knee
    M71.462 **Calcium deposit in bursa,** left knee
    M71.469 **Calcium deposit in bursa,** unspecified knee
✓6ᵗʰ **M71.47** **Calcium deposit in bursa,** ankle and foot
    M71.471 **Calcium deposit in bursa,** right ankle and foot
    M71.472 **Calcium deposit in bursa,** left ankle and foot
    M71.479 **Calcium deposit in bursa,** unspecified ankle and foot
  M71.48 **Calcium deposit in bursa,** other site
  M71.49 **Calcium deposit in bursa,** multiple sites
✓5ᵗʰ **M71.5** **Other bursitis, not elsewhere classified**
    EXCLUDES 1 *bursitis NOS (M71.9-)*
    EXCLUDES 2 *bursitis of shoulder (M75.5)*
          bursitis of tibial collateral [Pellegrini-Stieda] (M76.4-)
  M71.50 **Other bursitis, not elsewhere classified,** unspecified site

✓6ᵗʰ **M71.52 Other bursitis, not elsewhere classified, elbow**

    M71.521 Other bursitis, not elsewhere classified, right elbow

    M71.522 Other bursitis, not elsewhere classified, left elbow

    M71.529 Other bursitis, not elsewhere classified, unspecified elbow

✓6ᵗʰ **M71.53 Other bursitis, not elsewhere classified, wrist**

    M71.531 Other bursitis, not elsewhere classified, right wrist

    M71.532 Other bursitis, not elsewhere classified, left wrist

    M71.539 Other bursitis, not elsewhere classified, unspecified wrist

✓6ᵗʰ **M71.54 Other bursitis, not elsewhere classified, hand**

    M71.541 Other bursitis, not elsewhere classified, right hand

    M71.542 Other bursitis, not elsewhere classified, left hand

    M71.549 Other bursitis, not elsewhere classified, unspecified hand

✓6ᵗʰ **M71.55 Other bursitis, not elsewhere classified, hip**

    M71.551 Other bursitis, not elsewhere classified, right hip

    M71.552 Other bursitis, not elsewhere classified, left hip

    M71.559 Other bursitis, not elsewhere classified, unspecified hip

✓6ᵗʰ **M71.56 Other bursitis, not elsewhere classified, knee**

    M71.561 Other bursitis, not elsewhere classified, right knee

    M71.562 Other bursitis, not elsewhere classified, left knee

    M71.569 Other bursitis, not elsewhere classified, unspecified knee

✓6ᵗʰ **M71.57 Other bursitis, not elsewhere classified, ankle and foot**

    M71.571 Other bursitis, not elsewhere classified, right ankle and foot

    M71.572 Other bursitis, not elsewhere classified, left ankle and foot

    M71.579 Other bursitis, not elsewhere classified, unspecified ankle and foot

    M71.58 Other bursitis, not elsewhere classified, other site

✓5ᵗʰ **M71.8 Other specified bursopathies**

    M71.80 Other specified bursopathies, unspecified site

✓6ᵗʰ **M71.81 Other specified bursopathies, shoulder**

    M71.811 Other specified bursopathies, right shoulder

    M71.812 Other specified bursopathies, left shoulder

    M71.819 Other specified bursopathies, unspecified shoulder

✓6ᵗʰ **M71.82 Other specified bursopathies, elbow**

    M71.821 Other specified bursopathies, right elbow

    M71.822 Other specified bursopathies, left elbow

    M71.829 Other specified bursopathies, unspecified elbow

✓6ᵗʰ **M71.83 Other specified bursopathies, wrist**

    M71.831 Other specified bursopathies, right wrist

    M71.832 Other specified bursopathies, left wrist

    M71.839 Other specified bursopathies, unspecified wrist

✓6ᵗʰ **M71.84 Other specified bursopathies, hand**

    M71.841 Other specified bursopathies, right hand

    M71.842 Other specified bursopathies, left hand

    M71.849 Other specified bursopathies, unspecified hand

✓6ᵗʰ **M71.85 Other specified bursopathies, hip**

    M71.851 Other specified bursopathies, right hip

    M71.852 Other specified bursopathies, left hip

    M71.859 Other specified bursopathies, unspecified hip

✓6ᵗʰ **M71.86 Other specified bursopathies, knee**

    M71.861 Other specified bursopathies, right knee

    M71.862 Other specified bursopathies, left knee

    M71.869 Other specified bursopathies, unspecified knee

✓6ᵗʰ **M71.87 Other specified bursopathies, ankle and foot**

    M71.871 Other specified bursopathies, right ankle and foot

    M71.872 Other specified bursopathies, left ankle and foot

    M71.879 Other specified bursopathies, unspecified ankle and foot

    M71.88 Other specified bursopathies, other site

    M71.89 Other specified bursopathies, multiple sites

M71.9 Bursopathy, unspecified
Bursitis NOS

✓4ᵗʰ **M72 Fibroblastic disorders**

    EXCLUDES 2   *retroperitoneal fibromatosis (D48.3)*

    M72.0 Palmar fascial fibromatosis [Dupuytren]   A

        DEF: Dupuytren's contracture: Flexion deformity of a finger, due to shortened, thickened fibrosing of palmar fascia. The cause is unknown, but it is associated with long-standing epilepsy.

    M72.1 Knuckle pads

    M72.2 Plantar fascial fibromatosis
        Plantar fasciitis
        DEF: Rapid-growing and multiplanar nodular swellings and pain in the foot that is not associated with contractures.

    M72.4 Pseudosarcomatous fibromatosis
        Nodular fasciitis

    M72.6 Necrotizing fasciitis   MCC HCC
        Use additional code (B95.-, B96.-) to identify causative organism

    M72.8 Other fibroblastic disorders
        Abscess of fascia
        Fasciitis NEC
        Other infective fasciitis
        Use additional code to (B95.-, B96.-) identify causative organism

        EXCLUDES 1   *diffuse (eosinophilic) fasciitis (M35.4)*
                 necrotizing fasciitis (M72.6)
                 nodular fasciitis (M72.4)
                 perirenal fasciitis NOS (N13.5)
                 perirenal fasciitis with infection (N13.6)
                 plantar fasciitis (M72.2)

    M72.9 Fibroblastic disorder, unspecified
        Fasciitis NOS
        Fibromatosis NOS

✓4ᵗʰ **M75 Shoulder lesions**

    EXCLUDES 2   *shoulder-hand syndrome (M89.0-)*

✓5ᵗʰ **M75.0 Adhesive capsulitis of shoulder**

        Frozen shoulder
        Periarthritis of shoulder
        AHA: 2015,2Q,23

    M75.00 Adhesive capsulitis of unspecified shoulder

    M75.01 Adhesive capsulitis of right shoulder

    M75.02 Adhesive capsulitis of left shoulder

✓5ᵗʰ **M75.1 Rotator cuff tear or rupture, not specified as traumatic**

        Rotator cuff syndrome
        Supraspinatus syndrome
        Supraspinatus tear or rupture, not specified as traumatic

        EXCLUDES 1   *tear of rotator cuff, traumatic (S46.01-)*

    ✓6ᵗʰ **M75.10 Unspecified rotator cuff tear or rupture, not specified as traumatic**

        M75.100 Unspecified rotator cuff tear or rupture of unspecified shoulder, not specified as traumatic

        M75.101 Unspecified rotator cuff tear or rupture of right shoulder, not specified as traumatic

        M75.102 Unspecified rotator cuff tear or rupture of left shoulder, not specified as traumatic

    ✓6ᵗʰ **M75.11 Incomplete rotator cuff tear or rupture not specified as traumatic**

        M75.110 Incomplete rotator cuff tear or rupture of unspecified shoulder, not specified as traumatic

        M75.111 Incomplete rotator cuff tear or rupture of right shoulder, not specified as traumatic

        M75.112 Incomplete rotator cuff tear or rupture of left shoulder, not specified as traumatic

☑ Additional Character Required   ✓x7ᵗʰ Placeholder   Unacceptable PDx   Questionable PDx   Manifestation   Unspecified Dx   H1-H14 HAC   HCC CMS-HCC Dx   HIV HIV Dx

ICD-10-CM 2021   815

√6ᵗʰ **M75.12** Complete rotator cuff tear or rupture not specified as traumatic

     M75.120 Complete rotator cuff tear or rupture of unspecified shoulder, not specified as traumatic

     M75.121 Complete rotator cuff tear or rupture of right shoulder, not specified as traumatic

     M75.122 Complete rotator cuff tear or rupture of left shoulder, not specified as traumatic

√5ᵗʰ **M75.2** Bicipital tendinitis

     M75.20 Bicipital tendinitis, unspecified shoulder

     M75.21 Bicipital tendinitis, right shoulder

     M75.22 Bicipital tendinitis, left shoulder

√5ᵗʰ **M75.3** Calcific tendinitis of shoulder

     Calcified bursa of shoulder

     M75.30 Calcific tendinitis of unspecified shoulder

     M75.31 Calcific tendinitis of right shoulder

     M75.32 Calcific tendinitis of left shoulder

√5ᵗʰ **M75.4** Impingement syndrome of shoulder

     M75.40 Impingement syndrome of unspecified shoulder

     M75.41 Impingement syndrome of right shoulder

     M75.42 Impingement syndrome of left shoulder

√5ᵗʰ **M75.5** Bursitis of shoulder

     M75.50 Bursitis of unspecified shoulder

     M75.51 Bursitis of right shoulder

     M75.52 Bursitis of left shoulder

√5ᵗʰ **M75.8** Other shoulder lesions

     M75.80 Other shoulder lesions, unspecified shoulder

     M75.81 Other shoulder lesions, right shoulder

     M75.82 Other shoulder lesions, left shoulder

√5ᵗʰ **M75.9** Shoulder lesion, unspecified

     M75.90 Shoulder lesion, unspecified, unspecified shoulder

     M75.91 Shoulder lesion, unspecified, right shoulder

     M75.92 Shoulder lesion, unspecified, left shoulder

√4ᵗʰ **M76** Enthesopathies, lower limb, excluding foot

     EXCLUDES 2   *bursitis due to use, overuse and pressure (M70.-)*

                enthesopathies of ankle and foot (M77.5-)

√5ᵗʰ **M76.0** Gluteal tendinitis

     M76.00 Gluteal tendinitis, unspecified hip

     M76.01 Gluteal tendinitis, right hip

     M76.02 Gluteal tendinitis, left hip

√5ᵗʰ **M76.1** Psoas tendinitis

     M76.10 Psoas tendinitis, unspecified hip

     M76.11 Psoas tendinitis, right hip

     M76.12 Psoas tendinitis, left hip

√5ᵗʰ **M76.2** Iliac crest spur

     M76.20 Iliac crest spur, unspecified hip

     M76.21 Iliac crest spur, right hip

     M76.22 Iliac crest spur, left hip

√5ᵗʰ **M76.3** Iliotibial band syndrome

     M76.30 Iliotibial band syndrome, unspecified leg

     M76.31 Iliotibial band syndrome, right leg

     M76.32 Iliotibial band syndrome, left leg

√5ᵗʰ **M76.4** Tibial collateral bursitis [Pellegrini-Stieda]

     M76.40 Tibial collateral bursitis [Pellegrini-Stieda], unspecified leg

     M76.41 Tibial collateral bursitis [Pellegrini-Stieda], right leg

     M76.42 Tibial collateral bursitis [Pellegrini-Stieda], left leg

√5ᵗʰ **M76.5** Patellar tendinitis

     M76.50 Patellar tendinitis, unspecified knee

     M76.51 Patellar tendinitis, right knee

     M76.52 Patellar tendinitis, left knee

√5ᵗʰ **M76.6** Achilles tendinitis

     Achilles bursitis

     M76.60 Achilles tendinitis, unspecified leg

     M76.61 Achilles tendinitis, right leg

     M76.62 Achilles tendinitis, left leg

√5ᵗʰ **M76.7** Peroneal tendinitis

     M76.70 Peroneal tendinitis, unspecified leg

     M76.71 Peroneal tendinitis, right leg

     M76.72 Peroneal tendinitis, left leg

√5ᵗʰ **M76.8** Other specified enthesopathies of lower limb, excluding foot

     √6ᵗʰ **M76.81** Anterior tibial syndrome

         M76.811 Anterior tibial syndrome, right leg

         M76.812 Anterior tibial syndrome, left leg

         M76.819 Anterior tibial syndrome, unspecified leg

     √6ᵗʰ **M76.82** Posterior tibial tendinitis

         M76.821 Posterior tibial tendinitis, right leg

         M76.822 Posterior tibial tendinitis, left leg

         M76.829 Posterior tibial tendinitis, unspecified leg

     √6ᵗʰ **M76.89** Other specified enthesopathies of lower limb, excluding foot

         M76.891 Other specified enthesopathies of right lower limb, excluding foot

         M76.892 Other specified enthesopathies of left lower limb, excluding foot

         M76.899 Other specified enthesopathies of unspecified lower limb, excluding foot

     M76.9 Unspecified enthesopathy, lower limb, excluding foot

√4ᵗʰ **M77** Other enthesopathies

     EXCLUDES 1   *bursitis NOS (M71.9-)*

     EXCLUDES 2   *bursitis due to use, overuse and pressure (M70.-)*

                osteophyte (M25.7)

                spinal enthesopathy (M46.0-)

√5ᵗʰ **M77.0** Medial epicondylitis

     M77.00 Medial epicondylitis, unspecified elbow

     M77.01 Medial epicondylitis, right elbow

     M77.02 Medial epicondylitis, left elbow

√5ᵗʰ **M77.1** Lateral epicondylitis

     Tennis elbow

     M77.10 Lateral epicondylitis, unspecified elbow

     M77.11 Lateral epicondylitis, right elbow

     M77.12 Lateral epicondylitis, left elbow

√5ᵗʰ **M77.2** Periarthritis of wrist

     M77.20 Periarthritis, unspecified wrist

     M77.21 Periarthritis, right wrist

     M77.22 Periarthritis, left wrist

√5ᵗʰ **M77.3** Calcaneal spur

     DEF: Overgrowth of calcaneus bone on the underside of the heel that causes pain on walking. Calcaneal spur is due to a chronic avulsion injury of the plantar fascia from the calcaneus.

     M77.30 Calcaneal spur, unspecified foot

     M77.31 Calcaneal spur, right foot

     M77.32 Calcaneal spur, left foot

√5ᵗʰ **M77.4** Metatarsalgia

     EXCLUDES 1   *Morton's metatarsalgia (G57.6)*

     M77.40 Metatarsalgia, unspecified foot

     M77.41 Metatarsalgia, right foot

     M77.42 Metatarsalgia, left foot

√5ᵗʰ **M77.5** Other enthesopathy of foot and ankle

     M77.50 Other enthesopathy of unspecified foot and ankle

     M77.51 Other enthesopathy of right foot and ankle

     M77.52 Other enthesopathy of left foot and ankle

     M77.8 Other enthesopathies, not elsewhere classified

     M77.9 Enthesopathy, unspecified

     Bone spur NOS

     Capsulitis NOS

     Periarthritis NOS

     Tendinitis NOS

√4ᵗʰ **M79** Other and unspecified soft tissue disorders, not elsewhere classified

     EXCLUDES 1   *psychogenic rheumatism (F45.8)*

                soft tissue pain, psychogenic (F45.41)

     M79.0 Rheumatism, unspecified

         EXCLUDES 1   *fibromyalgia (M79.7)*

                    palindromic rheumatism (M12.3-)

√5ᵗʰ **M79.1** Myalgia

     Myofascial pain syndrome

     EXCLUDES 1   *fibromyalgia (M79.7)*

                myositis (M60.-)

     AHA: 2018,4Q,21

     M79.10 Myalgia, unspecified site

     M79.11 Myalgia of mastication muscle

     M79.12 Myalgia of auxiliary muscles, head and neck

     M79.18 Myalgia, other site

Ⓝ Newborn: 0   Ⓟ Pediatric: 0-17   Ⓜ Maternity: 9-64   Ⓐ Adult: 15-124   **MCC** Major Complication/Comorbidity   **CC** Complication/Comorbidity   **SW** Severe Wound Dx

816   ICD-10-CM 2021

M79.2 **Neuralgia and neuritis, unspecified**
    EXCLUDES 1   *brachial radiculitis NOS (M54.1)*
                 lumbosacral radiculitis NOS (M54.1)
                 mononeuropathies (G56-G58)
                 radiculitis NOS (M54.1)
                 sciatica (M54.3-M54.4)
    TIP: Assign for documented neuropathic pain.

M79.3 **Panniculitis, unspecified**
    EXCLUDES 1   *lupus panniculitis (L93.2)*
                 neck and back panniculitis (M54.0-)
                 relapsing [Weber-Christian] panniculitis (M35.6)

M79.4 **Hypertrophy of (infrapatellar) fat pad**

M79.5 **Residual foreign body in soft tissue**
    EXCLUDES 1   *foreign body granuloma of skin and subcutaneous*
                 tissue (L92.3)
                 foreign body granuloma of soft tissue (M60.2-)

√5ᵗʰ **M79.6** **Pain in limb, hand, foot, fingers and toes**
    EXCLUDES 2   *pain in joint (M25.5-)*

  √6ᵗʰ **M79.60** **Pain in limb, unspecified**
      M79.601 Pain in **right arm**
          Pain in right upper limb NOS
      M79.602 Pain in **left arm**
          Pain in left upper limb NOS
      M79.603 Pain in **arm, unspecified**
          Pain in upper limb NOS
      M79.604 Pain in **right leg**
          Pain in right lower limb NOS
      M79.605 Pain in **left leg**
          Pain in left lower limb NOS
      M79.606 Pain in **leg, unspecified**
          Pain in lower limb NOS
      M79.609 Pain in **unspecified limb**
          Pain in limb NOS

  √6ᵗʰ **M79.62** **Pain in upper arm**
       Pain in axillary region
      M79.621 **Pain in right upper arm**
      M79.622 **Pain in left upper arm**
      M79.629 **Pain in unspecified upper arm**

  √6ᵗʰ **M79.63** **Pain in forearm**
      M79.631 **Pain in right forearm**
      M79.632 **Pain in left forearm**
      M79.639 **Pain in unspecified forearm**

  √6ᵗʰ **M79.64** **Pain in hand and fingers**
      M79.641 **Pain in right hand**
      M79.642 **Pain in left hand**
      M79.643 **Pain in unspecified hand**
      M79.644 **Pain in right finger(s)**
      M79.645 **Pain in left finger(s)**
      M79.646 **Pain in unspecified finger(s)**

  √6ᵗʰ **M79.65** **Pain in thigh**
      M79.651 **Pain in right thigh**
      M79.652 **Pain in left thigh**
      M79.659 **Pain in unspecified thigh**

  √6ᵗʰ **M79.66** **Pain in lower leg**
      M79.661 **Pain in right lower leg**
      M79.662 **Pain in left lower leg**
      M79.669 **Pain in unspecified lower leg**

  √6ᵗʰ **M79.67** **Pain in foot and toes**
      M79.671 **Pain in right foot**
      M79.672 **Pain in left foot**
      M79.673 **Pain in unspecified foot**
      M79.674 **Pain in right toe(s)**
      M79.675 **Pain in left toe(s)**
      M79.676 **Pain in unspecified toe(s)**

M79.7 **Fibromyalgia**
    Fibromyositis
    Fibrositis
    Myofibrositis

√5ᵗʰ **M79.A** **Nontraumatic compartment syndrome**
    Code first, if applicable, associated postprocedural complication
    EXCLUDES 1   *compartment syndrome NOS (T79.A-)*
                 fibromyalgia (M79.7)
                 nontraumatic ischemic infarction of muscle (M62.2-)
                 traumatic compartment syndrome (T79.A-)

  √6ᵗʰ **M79.A1** **Nontraumatic compartment syndrome of upper extremity**
       Nontraumatic compartment syndrome of shoulder, arm, forearm, wrist, hand, and fingers
      M79.A11 **Nontraumatic compartment syndrome of right upper extremity**   cc
      M79.A12 **Nontraumatic compartment syndrome of left upper extremity**   cc
      M79.A19 **Nontraumatic compartment syndrome of unspecified upper extremity**   cc

  √6ᵗʰ **M79.A2** **Nontraumatic compartment syndrome of lower extremity**
       Nontraumatic compartment syndrome of hip, buttock, thigh, leg, foot, and toes
      M79.A21 **Nontraumatic compartment syndrome of right lower extremity**   cc
      M79.A22 **Nontraumatic compartment syndrome of left lower extremity**   cc
      M79.A29 **Nontraumatic compartment syndrome of unspecified lower extremity**   cc

    M79.A3 **Nontraumatic compartment syndrome of abdomen**   cc
    M79.A9 **Nontraumatic compartment syndrome of other sites**   cc

√5ᵗʰ **M79.8** **Other specified soft tissue disorders**
    M79.81 **Nontraumatic hematoma of soft tissue**
       Nontraumatic hematoma of muscle
       Nontraumatic seroma of muscle and soft tissue
    M79.89 **Other specified soft tissue disorders**
       Polyalgia

M79.9 **Soft tissue disorder, unspecified**

OSTEOPATHIES AND CHONDROPATHIES (M80-M94)

Disorders of bone density and structure (M80-M85)

√4ᵗʰ **M80** **Osteoporosis with current pathological fracture**
    INCLUDES   osteoporosis with current fragility fracture
    Use additional code to identify major osseous defect, if applicable (M89.7-)
    EXCLUDES 1   *collapsed vertebra NOS (M48.5)*
                 pathological fracture NOS (M84.4)
                 wedging of vertebra NOS (M48.5)
    EXCLUDES 2   *personal history of (healed) osteoporosis fracture (Z87.310)*
    AHA: 2018,2Q,12
    TIP: The site codes in this category identify the site of the fracture, not the site of the osteoporosis.

    > The appropriate 7th character is to be added to each code from category M80:
    > A   initial encounter for fracture
    > D   subsequent encounter for fracture with routine healing
    > G   subsequent encounter for fracture with delayed healing
    > K   subsequent encounter for fracture with nonunion
    > P   subsequent encounter for fracture with malunion
    > S   sequela

√5ᵗʰ **M80.0** **Age-related osteoporosis with current pathological fracture**
     Involutional osteoporosis with current pathological fracture
     Osteoporosis NOS with current pathological fracture
     Postmenopausal osteoporosis with current pathological fracture
     Senile osteoporosis with current pathological fracture

  ³ √×7ᵗʰ **M80.00** **Age-related osteoporosis with current pathological fracture, unspecified site**   cc A

  √6ᵗʰ **M80.01** **Age-related osteoporosis with current pathological fracture, shoulder**
    ³ √7ᵗʰ **M80.011** **Age-related osteoporosis with current pathological fracture, right shoulder**   cc A
    ³ √7ᵗʰ **M80.012** **Age-related osteoporosis with current pathological fracture, left shoulder**   cc A

☑ Additional Character Required   √×7ᵗʰ Placeholder   Unacceptable PDx   Questionable PDx   Manifestation   Unspecified Dx   H1-H14 HAC   HCC CMS-HCC Dx   HIV HIV Dx

ICD-10-CM 2021   817

3 √7ᵗʰ **M80.019** Age-related osteoporosis with current pathological fracture, unspecified shoulder   cc A

√6ᵗʰ **M80.02** Age-related osteoporosis with current pathological fracture, humerus

   3 √7ᵗʰ **M80.021** Age-related osteoporosis with current pathological fracture, right humerus   cc A

   3 √7ᵗʰ **M80.022** Age-related osteoporosis with current pathological fracture, left humerus   cc A

   3 √7ᵗʰ **M80.029** Age-related osteoporosis with current pathological fracture, unspecified humerus   cc A

√6ᵗʰ **M80.03** Age-related osteoporosis with current pathological fracture, forearm
> Age-related osteoporosis with current pathological fracture of wrist

   3 √7ᵗʰ **M80.031** Age-related osteoporosis with current pathological fracture, right forearm   cc A

   3 √7ᵗʰ **M80.032** Age-related osteoporosis with current pathological fracture, left forearm   cc A

   3 √7ᵗʰ **M80.039** Age-related osteoporosis with current pathological fracture, unspecified forearm   cc A

√6ᵗʰ **M80.04** Age-related osteoporosis with current pathological fracture, hand

   3 √7ᵗʰ **M80.041** Age-related osteoporosis with current pathological fracture, right hand   cc A

   3 √7ᵗʰ **M80.042** Age-related osteoporosis with current pathological fracture, left hand   cc A

   3 √7ᵗʰ **M80.049** Age-related osteoporosis with current pathological fracture, unspecified hand   cc A

√6ᵗʰ **M80.05** Age-related osteoporosis with current pathological fracture, femur
> Age-related osteoporosis with current pathological fracture of hip

   3,6 √7ᵗʰ **M80.051** Age-related osteoporosis with current pathological fracture, right femur   cc HCC A

   3,6 √7ᵗʰ **M80.052** Age-related osteoporosis with current pathological fracture, left femur   cc HCC A

   3,6 √7ᵗʰ **M80.059** Age-related osteoporosis with current pathological fracture, unspecified femur   cc HCC A

√6ᵗʰ **M80.06** Age-related osteoporosis with current pathological fracture, lower leg

   3 √7ᵗʰ **M80.061** Age-related osteoporosis with current pathological fracture, right lower leg   cc A

   3 √7ᵗʰ **M80.062** Age-related osteoporosis with current pathological fracture, left lower leg   cc A

   3 √7ᵗʰ **M80.069** Age-related osteoporosis with current pathological fracture, unspecified lower leg   cc A

√6ᵗʰ **M80.07** Age-related osteoporosis with current pathological fracture, ankle and foot

   3 √7ᵗʰ **M80.071** Age-related osteoporosis with current pathological fracture, right ankle and foot   cc A

   3 √7ᵗʰ **M80.072** Age-related osteoporosis with current pathological fracture, left ankle and foot   cc A

   3 √7ᵗʰ **M80.079** Age-related osteoporosis with current pathological fracture, unspecified ankle and foot   cc A

3,6 √x7ᵗʰ **M80.08** Age-related osteoporosis with current pathological fracture, vertebra(e)   cc HCC A

● 3 √x7ᵗʰ **M80.0A** Age-related osteoporosis with current pathological fracture, other site   cc A

√5ᵗʰ **M80.8** Other osteoporosis with current pathological fracture
> Drug-induced osteoporosis with current pathological fracture
> Idiopathic osteoporosis with current pathological fracture
> Osteoporosis of disuse with current pathological fracture
> Postoophorectomy osteoporosis with current pathological fracture
> Postsurgical malabsorption osteoporosis with current pathological fracture
> Post-traumatic osteoporosis with current pathological fracture
> Use additional code for adverse effect, if applicable, to identify drug (T36-T50 with fifth or sixth character 5)

3 √x7ᵗʰ **M80.80** Other osteoporosis with current pathological fracture, unspecified site   cc

√6ᵗʰ **M80.81** Other osteoporosis with pathological fracture, shoulder

   3 √7ᵗʰ **M80.811** Other osteoporosis with current pathological fracture, right shoulder   cc

   3 √7ᵗʰ **M80.812** Other osteoporosis with current pathological fracture, left shoulder   cc

   3 √7ᵗʰ **M80.819** Other osteoporosis with current pathological fracture, unspecified shoulder   cc

√6ᵗʰ **M80.82** Other osteoporosis with current pathological fracture, humerus

   3 √7ᵗʰ **M80.821** Other osteoporosis with current pathological fracture, right humerus   cc

   3 √7ᵗʰ **M80.822** Other osteoporosis with current pathological fracture, left humerus   cc

   3 √7ᵗʰ **M80.829** Other osteoporosis with current pathological fracture, unspecified humerus   cc

√6ᵗʰ **M80.83** Other osteoporosis with current pathological fracture, forearm
> Other osteoporosis with current pathological fracture of wrist

   3 √7ᵗʰ **M80.831** Other osteoporosis with current pathological fracture, right forearm   cc

   3 √7ᵗʰ **M80.832** Other osteoporosis with current pathological fracture, left forearm   cc

   3 √7ᵗʰ **M80.839** Other osteoporosis with current pathological fracture, unspecified forearm   cc

√6ᵗʰ **M80.84** Other osteoporosis with current pathological fracture, hand

   3 √7ᵗʰ **M80.841** Other osteoporosis with current pathological fracture, right hand   cc

   3 √7ᵗʰ **M80.842** Other osteoporosis with current pathological fracture, left hand   cc

   3 √7ᵗʰ **M80.849** Other osteoporosis with current pathological fracture, unspecified hand   cc

√6ᵗʰ **M80.85** Other osteoporosis with current pathological fracture, femur
> Other osteoporosis with current pathological fracture of hip

   3,6 √7ᵗʰ **M80.851** Other osteoporosis with current pathological fracture, right femur   cc HCC

   3,6 √7ᵗʰ **M80.852** Other osteoporosis with current pathological fracture, left femur   cc HCC

   3,6 √7ᵗʰ **M80.859** Other osteoporosis with current pathological fracture, unspecified femur   cc HCC

√6ᵗʰ **M80.86** Other osteoporosis with current pathological fracture, lower leg

   3 √7ᵗʰ **M80.861** Other osteoporosis with current pathological fracture, right lower leg   cc

   3 √7ᵗʰ **M80.862** Other osteoporosis with current pathological fracture, left lower leg   cc

   3 √7ᵗʰ **M80.869** Other osteoporosis with current pathological fracture, unspecified lower leg   cc

N Newborn: 0   P Pediatric: 0-17   M Maternity: 9-64   A Adult: 15-124   MCC Major Complication/Comorbidity   CC Complication/Comorbidity   SW Severe Wound Dx

818   ICD-10-CM 2021

√6ᵗʰ **M80.87** **Other osteoporosis with current pathological fracture**, ankle and foot

   ³ √7ᵗʰ **M80.871** **Other osteoporosis with current pathological fracture**, right ankle and foot   CC

   ³ √7ᵗʰ **M80.872** **Other osteoporosis with current pathological fracture**, left ankle and foot   CC

   ³ √7ᵗʰ **M80.879** **Other osteoporosis with current pathological fracture**, unspecified ankle and foot   CC

³,⁶ √7ᵗʰ **M80.88** **Other osteoporosis with current pathological fracture**, vertebra(e)   CC HCC

● ³ √x7ᵗʰ **M80.8A** **Other osteoporosis with current pathological fracture**, other site   CC

√4ᵗʰ **M81** **Osteoporosis** without current pathological fracture

   Use additional code to identify:

     major osseous defect, if applicable (M89.7-)

     personal history of (healed) osteoporosis fracture, if applicable (Z87.310)

   EXCLUDES 1   osteoporosis with current pathological fracture (M80.-)

            Sudeck's atrophy (M89.0)

M81.0 **Age-related** osteoporosis without current pathological fracture   A

   Involutional osteoporosis without current pathological fracture

   Osteoporosis NOS

   Postmenopausal osteoporosis without current pathological fracture

   Senile osteoporosis without current pathological fracture

M81.6 **Localized** osteoporosis [Lequesne]

   EXCLUDES 1   Sudeck's atrophy (M89.0)

M81.8 **Other osteoporosis** without current pathological fracture

   Drug-induced osteoporosis without current pathological fracture

   Idiopathic osteoporosis without current pathological fracture

   Osteoporosis of disuse without current pathological fracture

   Postoophorectomy osteoporosis without current pathological fracture

   Postsurgical malabsorption osteoporosis without current pathological fracture

   Post-traumatic osteoporosis without current pathological fracture

   Use additional code for adverse effect, if applicable, to identify drug (T36-T50 with fifth or sixth character 5)

√4ᵗʰ **M83** **Adult osteomalacia**

   EXCLUDES 1   infantile and juvenile osteomalacia (E55.0)

            renal osteodystrophy (N25.0)

            rickets (active) (E55.0)

            rickets (active) sequelae (E64.3)

            vitamin D-resistant osteomalacia (E83.3)

            vitamin D-resistant rickets (active) (E83.3)

M83.0 **Puerperal** osteomalacia   M ♀

M83.1 **Senile** osteomalacia   A

M83.2 **Adult osteomalacia** due to malabsorption   A

   Postsurgical malabsorption osteomalacia in adults

M83.3 **Adult osteomalacia** due to malnutrition   A

M83.4 **Aluminum bone disease**

M83.5 **Other drug-induced** osteomalacia in adults   A

   Use additional code for adverse effect, if applicable, to identify drug (T36-T50 with fifth or sixth character 5)

M83.8 **Other adult osteomalacia**   A

M83.9 **Adult osteomalacia, unspecified**   A

√4ᵗʰ **M84** **Disorder of continuity of bone**

   EXCLUDES 2   traumatic fracture of bone-see fracture, by site

√5ᵗʰ **M84.3** **Stress fracture**

   Fatigue fracture

   March fracture

   Stress fracture NOS

   Stress reaction

   Use additional external cause code(s) to identify the cause of the stress fracture

   EXCLUDES 1   pathological fracture due to osteoporosis (M80.-)

            pathological fracture NOS (M84.4.-)

            traumatic fracture (S12.-, S22.-, S32.-, S42.-, S52.-, S62.-, S72.-, S82.-, S92.-)

   EXCLUDES 2   personal history of (healed) stress (fatigue) fracture (Z87.312)

            stress fracture of vertebra (M48.4-)

The appropriate 7th character is to be added to each code from subcategory M84.3.
A   initial encounter for fracture
D   subsequent encounter for fracture with routine healing
G   subsequent encounter for fracture with delayed healing
K   subsequent encounter for fracture with nonunion
P   subsequent encounter for fracture with malunion
S   sequela

⁴ √x7ᵗʰ **M84.30** **Stress fracture, unspecified site**   CC

√6ᵗʰ **M84.31** **Stress fracture,** shoulder

   ⁴ √7ᵗʰ **M84.311** **Stress fracture,** right shoulder   CC

   ⁴ √7ᵗʰ **M84.312** **Stress fracture,** left shoulder   CC

   ⁴ √7ᵗʰ **M84.319** **Stress fracture, unspecified shoulder**   CC

√6ᵗʰ **M84.32** **Stress fracture,** humerus

   ⁴ √7ᵗʰ **M84.321** **Stress fracture,** right humerus   CC

   ⁴ √7ᵗʰ **M84.322** **Stress fracture,** left humerus   CC

   ⁴ √7ᵗʰ **M84.329** **Stress fracture, unspecified humerus**   CC

√6ᵗʰ **M84.33** **Stress fracture,** ulna and radius

   ⁴ √7ᵗʰ **M84.331** **Stress fracture,** right ulna   CC

   ⁴ √7ᵗʰ **M84.332** **Stress fracture,** left ulna   CC

   ⁴ √7ᵗʰ **M84.333** **Stress fracture,** right radius   CC

   ⁴ √7ᵗʰ **M84.334** **Stress fracture,** left radius   CC

   ⁴ √7ᵗʰ **M84.339** **Stress fracture, unspecified ulna and radius**   CC

√6ᵗʰ **M84.34** **Stress fracture,** hand and fingers

   ⁴ √7ᵗʰ **M84.341** **Stress fracture,** right hand   CC

   ⁴ √7ᵗʰ **M84.342** **Stress fracture,** left hand   CC

   ⁴ √7ᵗʰ **M84.343** **Stress fracture, unspecified hand**   CC

   ⁴ √7ᵗʰ **M84.344** **Stress fracture,** right finger(s)   CC

   ⁴ √7ᵗʰ **M84.345** **Stress fracture,** left finger(s)   CC

   ⁴ √7ᵗʰ **M84.346** **Stress fracture, unspecified finger(s)**   CC

√6ᵗʰ **M84.35** **Stress fracture,** pelvis and femur

   Stress fracture, hip

   ⁴ √7ᵗʰ **M84.350** **Stress fracture,** pelvis   CC

   ⁴ √7ᵗʰ **M84.351** **Stress fracture,** right femur   CC

   ⁴ √7ᵗʰ **M84.352** **Stress fracture,** left femur   CC

   ⁴ √7ᵗʰ **M84.353** **Stress fracture, unspecified femur**   CC

   ⁴ √7ᵗʰ **M84.359** **Stress fracture, hip, unspecified**   CC

√6ᵗʰ **M84.36** **Stress fracture,** tibia and fibula

   ⁴ √7ᵗʰ **M84.361** **Stress fracture,** right tibia   CC

   ⁴ √7ᵗʰ **M84.362** **Stress fracture,** left tibia   CC

   ⁴ √7ᵗʰ **M84.363** **Stress fracture,** right fibula   CC

   ⁴ √7ᵗʰ **M84.364** **Stress fracture,** left fibula   CC

   ⁴ √7ᵗʰ **M84.369** **Stress fracture, unspecified tibia and fibula**   CC

√6ᵗʰ **M84.37** **Stress fracture,** ankle, foot and toes

   ⁴ √7ᵗʰ **M84.371** **Stress fracture,** right ankle   CC

   ⁴ √7ᵗʰ **M84.372** **Stress fracture,** left ankle   CC

   ⁴ √7ᵗʰ **M84.373** **Stress fracture, unspecified ankle**   CC

   ⁴ √7ᵗʰ **M84.374** **Stress fracture,** right foot   CC

   ⁴ √7ᵗʰ **M84.375** **Stress fracture,** left foot   CC

☑ Additional Character Required   √x7ᵗʰ Placeholder   Unacceptable PDx   Questionable PDx   Manifestation   Unspecified Dx   H1-H14 HAC   HCC CMS-HCC Dx   HIV HIV Dx

ICD-10-CM 2021   819

4 √7th **M84.376** Stress fracture, unspecified foot `CC`

4 √7th **M84.377** Stress fracture, right toe(s) `CC`

4 √7th **M84.378** Stress fracture, left toe(s) `CC`

4 √7th **M84.379** Stress fracture, unspecified toe(s) `CC`

4 √x7th **M84.38** Stress fracture, other site `CC`

> *EXCLUDES 2*   stress fracture of vertebra (M48.4-)

√5th **M84.4** Pathological fracture, not elsewhere classified

Chronic fracture

Pathological fracture NOS

> *EXCLUDES 1*   collapsed vertebra NEC (M48.5)
> pathological fracture in neoplastic disease (M84.5-)
> pathological fracture in osteoporosis (M8Ø.-)
> pathological fracture in other disease (M84.6-)
> stress fracture (M84.3-)
> traumatic fracture (S12.-, S22.-, S32.-, S42.-, S52.-, S62.-, S72.-, S82.-, S92.-)

> *EXCLUDES 2*   personal history of (healed) pathological fracture (Z87.311)

The appropriate 7th character is to be added to each code from subcategory M84.4.
A   initial encounter for fracture
D   subsequent encounter for fracture with routine healing
G   subsequent encounter for fracture with delayed healing
K   subsequent encounter for fracture with nonunion
P   subsequent encounter for fracture with malunion
S   sequela

3 √x7th **M84.4Ø** Pathological fracture, unspecified site `CC`

√6th **M84.41** Pathological fracture, shoulder

3 √7th **M84.411** Pathological fracture, right shoulder `CC`

3 √7th **M84.412** Pathological fracture, left shoulder `CC`

3 √7th **M84.419** Pathological fracture, unspecified shoulder `CC`

√6th **M84.42** Pathological fracture, humerus

3 √7th **M84.421** Pathological fracture, right humerus `CC`

3 √7th **M84.422** Pathological fracture, left humerus `CC`

3 √7th **M84.429** Pathological fracture, unspecified humerus `CC`

√6th **M84.43** Pathological fracture, ulna and radius

3 √7th **M84.431** Pathological fracture, right ulna `CC`

3 √7th **M84.432** Pathological fracture, left ulna `CC`

3 √7th **M84.433** Pathological fracture, right radius `CC`

3 √7th **M84.434** Pathological fracture, left radius `CC`

3 √7th **M84.439** Pathological fracture, unspecified ulna and radius `CC`

√6th **M84.44** Pathological fracture, hand and fingers

3 √7th **M84.441** Pathological fracture, right hand `CC`

3 √7th **M84.442** Pathological fracture, left hand `CC`

3 √7th **M84.443** Pathological fracture, unspecified hand `CC`

3 √7th **M84.444** Pathological fracture, right finger(s) `CC`

3 √7th **M84.445** Pathological fracture, left finger(s) `CC`

3 √7th **M84.446** Pathological fracture, unspecified finger(s) `CC`

√6th **M84.45** Pathological fracture, femur and pelvis

AHA: 2016,4Q,43

3,6 √7th **M84.451** Pathological fracture, right femur `CC` `HCC`

3,6 √7th **M84.452** Pathological fracture, left femur `CC` `HCC`

3,6 √7th **M84.453** Pathological fracture, unspecified femur `CC` `HCC`

3 √7th **M84.454** Pathological fracture, pelvis `CC`

3,6 √7th **M84.459** Pathological fracture, hip, unspecified `CC` `HCC`

√6th **M84.46** Pathological fracture, tibia and fibula

3 √7th **M84.461** Pathological fracture, right tibia `CC`

3 √7th **M84.462** Pathological fracture, left tibia `CC`

3 √7th **M84.463** Pathological fracture, right fibula `CC`

3 √7th **M84.464** Pathological fracture, left fibula `CC`

3 √7th **M84.469** Pathological fracture, unspecified tibia and fibula `CC`

√6th **M84.47** Pathological fracture, ankle, foot and toes

3 √7th **M84.471** Pathological fracture, right ankle `CC`

3 √7th **M84.472** Pathological fracture, left ankle `CC`

3 √7th **M84.473** Pathological fracture, unspecified ankle `CC`

3 √7th **M84.474** Pathological fracture, right foot `CC`

3 √7th **M84.475** Pathological fracture, left foot `CC`

3 √7th **M84.476** Pathological fracture, unspecified foot `CC`

3 √7th **M84.477** Pathological fracture, right toe(s) `CC`

3 √7th **M84.478** Pathological fracture, left toe(s) `CC`

3 √7th **M84.479** Pathological fracture, unspecified toe(s) `CC`

3 √x7th **M84.48** Pathological fracture, other site `CC`

√5th **M84.5** Pathological fracture in neoplastic disease

Code also underlying neoplasm

The appropriate 7th character is to be added to each code from subcategory M84.5.
A   initial encounter for fracture
D   subsequent encounter for fracture with routine healing
G   subsequent encounter for fracture with delayed healing
K   subsequent encounter for fracture with nonunion
P   subsequent encounter for fracture with malunion
S   sequela

3 √x7th **M84.5Ø** Pathological fracture in neoplastic disease, unspecified site `CC`

√6th **M84.51** Pathological fracture in neoplastic disease, shoulder

3 √7th **M84.511** Pathological fracture in neoplastic disease, right shoulder `CC`

3 √7th **M84.512** Pathological fracture in neoplastic disease, left shoulder `CC`

3 √7th **M84.519** Pathological fracture in neoplastic disease, unspecified shoulder `CC`

√6th **M84.52** Pathological fracture in neoplastic disease, humerus

3 √7th **M84.521** Pathological fracture in neoplastic disease, right humerus `CC`

3 √7th **M84.522** Pathological fracture in neoplastic disease, left humerus `CC`

3 √7th **M84.529** Pathological fracture in neoplastic disease, unspecified humerus `CC`

√6th **M84.53** Pathological fracture in neoplastic disease, ulna and radius

3 √7th **M84.531** Pathological fracture in neoplastic disease, right ulna `CC`

3 √7th **M84.532** Pathological fracture in neoplastic disease, left ulna `CC`

3 √7th **M84.533** Pathological fracture in neoplastic disease, right radius `CC`

3 √7th **M84.534** Pathological fracture in neoplastic disease, left radius `CC`

3 √7th **M84.539** Pathological fracture in neoplastic disease, unspecified ulna and radius `CC`

√6th **M84.54** Pathological fracture in neoplastic disease, hand

3 √7th **M84.541** Pathological fracture in neoplastic disease, right hand `CC`

3 √7th **M84.542** Pathological fracture in neoplastic disease, left hand `CC`

3 √7th **M84.549** Pathological fracture in neoplastic disease, unspecified hand `CC`

√6th **M84.55** Pathological fracture in neoplastic disease, pelvis and femur

3 √7th **M84.55Ø** Pathological fracture in neoplastic disease, pelvis `CC`

3,6 √7th **M84.551** Pathological fracture in neoplastic disease, right femur `CC` `HCC`

3,6 √7th **M84.552** Pathological fracture in neoplastic disease, left femur `CC` `HCC`

3,6 √7th **M84.553** Pathological fracture in neoplastic disease, unspecified femur `CC` `HCC`

3,6 √7th **M84.559** Pathological fracture in neoplastic disease, hip, unspecified `CC` `HCC`

N Newborn: 0   P Pediatric: 0-17   M Maternity: 9-64   A Adult: 15-124   MCC Major Complication/Comorbidity   CC Complication/Comorbidity   SW Severe Wound Dx

820   ICD-10-CM 2021

√6ᵗʰ **M84.56 Pathological fracture in neoplastic disease, tibia and fibula**

- ³ √7ᵗʰ **M84.561 Pathological fracture in neoplastic disease, right tibia** `CC`
- ³ √7ᵗʰ **M84.562 Pathological fracture in neoplastic disease, left tibia** `CC`
- ³ √7ᵗʰ **M84.563 Pathological fracture in neoplastic disease, right fibula** `CC`
- ³ √7ᵗʰ **M84.564 Pathological fracture in neoplastic disease, left fibula** `CC`
- ³ √7ᵗʰ **M84.569 Pathological fracture in neoplastic disease, unspecified tibia and fibula** `CC`

√6ᵗʰ **M84.57 Pathological fracture in neoplastic disease, ankle and foot**

- ³ √7ᵗʰ **M84.571 Pathological fracture in neoplastic disease, right ankle** `CC`
- ³ √7ᵗʰ **M84.572 Pathological fracture in neoplastic disease, left ankle** `CC`
- ³ √7ᵗʰ **M84.573 Pathological fracture in neoplastic disease, unspecified ankle** `CC`
- ³ √7ᵗʰ **M84.574 Pathological fracture in neoplastic disease, right foot** `CC`
- ³ √7ᵗʰ **M84.575 Pathological fracture in neoplastic disease, left foot** `CC`
- ³ √7ᵗʰ **M84.576 Pathological fracture in neoplastic disease, unspecified foot** `CC`

³ √x7ᵗʰ **M84.58 Pathological fracture in neoplastic disease, other specified site** `CC`

Pathological fracture in neoplastic disease, vertebrae

√5ᵗʰ **M84.6 Pathological fracture in other disease**

Code also underlying condition

EXCLUDES 1 *pathological fracture in osteoporosis (M80.-)*

The appropriate 7th character is to be added to each code from subcategory M84.6.
A   initial encounter for fracture
D   subsequent encounter for fracture with routine healing
G   subsequent encounter for fracture with delayed healing
K   subsequent encounter for fracture with nonunion
P   subsequent encounter for fracture with malunion
S   sequela

³ √x7ᵗʰ **M84.60 Pathological fracture in other disease, unspecified site** `CC`

√6ᵗʰ **M84.61 Pathological fracture in other disease, shoulder**

- ³ √7ᵗʰ **M84.611 Pathological fracture in other disease, right shoulder** `CC`
- ³ √7ᵗʰ **M84.612 Pathological fracture in other disease, left shoulder** `CC`
- ³ √7ᵗʰ **M84.619 Pathological fracture in other disease, unspecified shoulder** `CC`

√6ᵗʰ **M84.62 Pathological fracture in other disease, humerus**

- ³ √7ᵗʰ **M84.621 Pathological fracture in other disease, right humerus** `CC`
- ³ √7ᵗʰ **M84.622 Pathological fracture in other disease, left humerus** `CC`
- ³ √7ᵗʰ **M84.629 Pathological fracture in other disease, unspecified humerus** `CC`

√6ᵗʰ **M84.63 Pathological fracture in other disease, ulna and radius**

- ³ √7ᵗʰ **M84.631 Pathological fracture in other disease, right ulna** `CC`
- ³ √7ᵗʰ **M84.632 Pathological fracture in other disease, left ulna** `CC`
- ³ √7ᵗʰ **M84.633 Pathological fracture in other disease, right radius** `CC`
- ³ √7ᵗʰ **M84.634 Pathological fracture in other disease, left radius** `CC`
- ³ √7ᵗʰ **M84.639 Pathological fracture in other disease, unspecified ulna and radius** `CC`

√6ᵗʰ **M84.64 Pathological fracture in other disease, hand**

- ³ √7ᵗʰ **M84.641 Pathological fracture in other disease, right hand** `CC`
- ³ √7ᵗʰ **M84.642 Pathological fracture in other disease, left hand** `CC`
- ³ √7ᵗʰ **M84.649 Pathological fracture in other disease, unspecified hand** `CC`

√6ᵗʰ **M84.65 Pathological fracture in other disease, pelvis and femur**

- ³ √7ᵗʰ **M84.650 Pathological fracture in other disease, pelvis** `CC`
- ³,⁶ √7ᵗʰ **M84.651 Pathological fracture in other disease, right femur** `CC` `HCC`
- ³,⁶ √7ᵗʰ **M84.652 Pathological fracture in other disease, left femur** `CC` `HCC`
- ³,⁶ √7ᵗʰ **M84.653 Pathological fracture in other disease, unspecified femur** `CC` `HCC`
- ³,⁶ √7ᵗʰ **M84.659 Pathological fracture in other disease, hip, unspecified** `CC` `HCC`

√6ᵗʰ **M84.66 Pathological fracture in other disease, tibia and fibula**

- ³ √7ᵗʰ **M84.661 Pathological fracture in other disease, right tibia** `CC`
- ³ √7ᵗʰ **M84.662 Pathological fracture in other disease, left tibia** `CC`
- ³ √7ᵗʰ **M84.663 Pathological fracture in other disease, right fibula** `CC`
- ³ √7ᵗʰ **M84.664 Pathological fracture in other disease, left fibula** `CC`
- ³ √7ᵗʰ **M84.669 Pathological fracture in other disease, unspecified tibia and fibula** `CC`

√6ᵗʰ **M84.67 Pathological fracture in other disease, ankle and foot**

- ³ √7ᵗʰ **M84.671 Pathological fracture in other disease, right ankle** `CC`
- ³ √7ᵗʰ **M84.672 Pathological fracture in other disease, left ankle** `CC`
- ³ √7ᵗʰ **M84.673 Pathological fracture in other disease, unspecified ankle** `CC`
- ³ √7ᵗʰ **M84.674 Pathological fracture in other disease, right foot** `CC`
- ³ √7ᵗʰ **M84.675 Pathological fracture in other disease, left foot** `CC`
- ³ √7ᵗʰ **M84.676 Pathological fracture in other disease, unspecified foot** `CC`

³ √x7ᵗʰ **M84.68 Pathological fracture in other disease, other site** `CC`

√5ᵗʰ **M84.7 Nontraumatic fracture, not elsewhere classified**

√6ᵗʰ **M84.75 Atypical femoral fracture**

AHA: 2016,4Q,41-42

The appropriate 7th character is to be added to each code from M84.75.
A   initial encounter for fracture
D   subsequent encounter for fracture with routine healing
G   subsequent encounter for fracture with delayed healing
K   subsequent encounter for fracture with nonunion
P   subsequent encounter for fracture with malunion
S   sequela

- ³ √7ᵗʰ **M84.750 Atypical femoral fracture, unspecified** `CC`
- ³ √7ᵗʰ **M84.751 Incomplete atypical femoral fracture, right leg** `CC`
- ³ √7ᵗʰ **M84.752 Incomplete atypical femoral fracture, left leg** `CC`
- ³ √7ᵗʰ **M84.753 Incomplete atypical femoral fracture, unspecified leg** `CC`
- ³,⁶ √7ᵗʰ **M84.754 Complete transverse atypical femoral fracture, right leg** `CC` `HCC`
- ³,⁶ √7ᵗʰ **M84.755 Complete transverse atypical femoral fracture, left leg** `CC` `HCC`
- ³,⁶ √7ᵗʰ **M84.756 Complete transverse atypical femoral fracture, unspecified leg** `CC` `HCC`
- ³,⁶ √7ᵗʰ **M84.757 Complete oblique atypical femoral fracture, right leg** `CC` `HCC`
- ³,⁶ √7ᵗʰ **M84.758 Complete oblique atypical femoral fracture, left leg** `CC` `HCC`
- ³,⁶ √7ᵗʰ **M84.759 Complete oblique atypical femoral fracture, unspecified leg** `CC` `HCC`

√5ᵗʰ **M84.8 Other disorders of continuity of bone**

M84.80 Other disorders of continuity of bone, unspecified site

---

☑ Additional Character Required   √x7ᵗʰ Placeholder   Unacceptable PDx   Questionable PDx   Manifestation   Unspecified Dx   H1-H14 HAC   HCC CMS-HCC Dx   HIV HIV Dx

ICD-10-CM 2021   821

✓6ᵗʰ **M84.81** **Other disorders of continuity of bone,** shoulder

     M84.811 Other disorders of continuity of bone, right shoulder

     M84.812 Other disorders of continuity of bone, left shoulder

     M84.819 Other disorders of continuity of bone, unspecified shoulder

✓6ᵗʰ **M84.82** **Other disorders of continuity of bone,** humerus

     M84.821 Other disorders of continuity of bone, right humerus

     M84.822 Other disorders of continuity of bone, left humerus

     M84.829 Other disorders of continuity of bone, unspecified humerus

✓6ᵗʰ **M84.83** **Other disorders of continuity of bone,** ulna and radius

     M84.831 Other disorders of continuity of bone, right ulna

     M84.832 Other disorders of continuity of bone, left ulna

     M84.833 Other disorders of continuity of bone, right radius

     M84.834 Other disorders of continuity of bone, left radius

     M84.839 Other disorders of continuity of bone, unspecified ulna and radius

✓6ᵗʰ **M84.84** **Other disorders of continuity of bone,** hand

     M84.841 Other disorders of continuity of bone, right hand

     M84.842 Other disorders of continuity of bone, left hand

     M84.849 Other disorders of continuity of bone, unspecified hand

✓6ᵗʰ **M84.85** **Other disorders of continuity of bone,** pelvic region and thigh

     M84.851 Other disorders of continuity of bone, right pelvic region and thigh

     M84.852 Other disorders of continuity of bone, left pelvic region and thigh

     M84.859 Other disorders of continuity of bone, unspecified pelvic region and thigh

✓6ᵗʰ **M84.86** **Other disorders of continuity of bone,** tibia and fibula

     M84.861 Other disorders of continuity of bone, right tibia

     M84.862 Other disorders of continuity of bone, left tibia

     M84.863 Other disorders of continuity of bone, right fibula

     M84.864 Other disorders of continuity of bone, left fibula

     M84.869 Other disorders of continuity of bone, unspecified tibia and fibula

✓6ᵗʰ **M84.87** **Other disorders of continuity of bone,** ankle and foot

     M84.871 Other disorders of continuity of bone, right ankle and foot

     M84.872 Other disorders of continuity of bone, left ankle and foot

     M84.879 Other disorders of continuity of bone, unspecified ankle and foot

   M84.88 Other disorders of continuity of bone, other site

   M84.9 **Disorder of continuity of bone, unspecified**

✓4ᵗʰ **M85** **Other disorders of bone density and structure**

     EXCLUDES 1   osteogenesis imperfecta (Q78.0)
              osteopetrosis (Q78.2)
              osteopoikilosis (Q78.8)
              polyostotic fibrous dysplasia (Q78.1)

✓5ᵗʰ **M85.0** **Fibrous dysplasia (monostotic)**

     EXCLUDES 2   fibrous dysplasia of jaw (M27.8)

   M85.00 **Fibrous dysplasia (monostotic), unspecified site**

✓6ᵗʰ **M85.01** **Fibrous dysplasia (monostotic),** shoulder

     M85.011 Fibrous dysplasia (monostotic), right shoulder

     M85.012 Fibrous dysplasia (monostotic), left shoulder

     M85.019 Fibrous dysplasia (monostotic), unspecified shoulder

✓6ᵗʰ **M85.02** **Fibrous dysplasia (monostotic),** upper arm

     M85.021 Fibrous dysplasia (monostotic), right upper arm

     M85.022 Fibrous dysplasia (monostotic), left upper arm

     M85.029 Fibrous dysplasia (monostotic), unspecified upper arm

✓6ᵗʰ **M85.03** **Fibrous dysplasia (monostotic),** forearm

     M85.031 Fibrous dysplasia (monostotic), right forearm

     M85.032 Fibrous dysplasia (monostotic), left forearm

     M85.039 Fibrous dysplasia (monostotic), unspecified forearm

✓6ᵗʰ **M85.04** **Fibrous dysplasia (monostotic),** hand

     M85.041 Fibrous dysplasia (monostotic), right hand

     M85.042 Fibrous dysplasia (monostotic), left hand

     M85.049 Fibrous dysplasia (monostotic), unspecified hand

✓6ᵗʰ **M85.05** **Fibrous dysplasia (monostotic),** thigh

     M85.051 Fibrous dysplasia (monostotic), right thigh

     M85.052 Fibrous dysplasia (monostotic), left thigh

     M85.059 Fibrous dysplasia (monostotic), unspecified thigh

✓6ᵗʰ **M85.06** **Fibrous dysplasia (monostotic),** lower leg

     M85.061 Fibrous dysplasia (monostotic), right lower leg

     M85.062 Fibrous dysplasia (monostotic), left lower leg

     M85.069 Fibrous dysplasia (monostotic), unspecified lower leg

✓6ᵗʰ **M85.07** **Fibrous dysplasia (monostotic),** ankle and foot

     M85.071 Fibrous dysplasia (monostotic), right ankle and foot

     M85.072 Fibrous dysplasia (monostotic), left ankle and foot

     M85.079 Fibrous dysplasia (monostotic), unspecified ankle and foot

   M85.08 Fibrous dysplasia (monostotic), other site

   M85.09 Fibrous dysplasia (monostotic), multiple sites

✓5ᵗʰ **M85.1** **Skeletal fluorosis**

   M85.10 Skeletal fluorosis, unspecified site

✓6ᵗʰ **M85.11** **Skeletal fluorosis,** shoulder

     M85.111 Skeletal fluorosis, right shoulder

     M85.112 Skeletal fluorosis, left shoulder

     M85.119 Skeletal fluorosis, unspecified shoulder

✓6ᵗʰ **M85.12** **Skeletal fluorosis,** upper arm

     M85.121 Skeletal fluorosis, right upper arm

     M85.122 Skeletal fluorosis, left upper arm

     M85.129 Skeletal fluorosis, unspecified upper arm

✓6ᵗʰ **M85.13** **Skeletal fluorosis,** forearm

     M85.131 Skeletal fluorosis, right forearm

     M85.132 Skeletal fluorosis, left forearm

     M85.139 Skeletal fluorosis, unspecified forearm

✓6ᵗʰ **M85.14** **Skeletal fluorosis,** hand

     M85.141 Skeletal fluorosis, right hand

     M85.142 Skeletal fluorosis, left hand

     M85.149 Skeletal fluorosis, unspecified hand

✓6ᵗʰ **M85.15** **Skeletal fluorosis,** thigh

     M85.151 Skeletal fluorosis, right thigh

     M85.152 Skeletal fluorosis, left thigh

     M85.159 Skeletal fluorosis, unspecified thigh

✓6ᵗʰ **M85.16** **Skeletal fluorosis,** lower leg

     M85.161 Skeletal fluorosis, right lower leg

     M85.162 Skeletal fluorosis, left lower leg

     M85.169 Skeletal fluorosis, unspecified lower leg

✓6ᵗʰ **M85.17** **Skeletal fluorosis,** ankle and foot

     M85.171 Skeletal fluorosis, right ankle and foot

     M85.172 Skeletal fluorosis, left ankle and foot

     M85.179 Skeletal fluorosis, unspecified ankle and foot

   M85.18 Skeletal fluorosis, other site

   M85.19 Skeletal fluorosis, multiple sites

N Newborn: 0   P Pediatric: 0-17   M Maternity: 9-64   A Adult: 15-124   MCC Major Complication/Comorbidity   CC Complication/Comorbidity   SW Severe Wound Dx

822   ICD-10-CM 2021

M85.2 Hyperostosis of skull
> **DEF:** Abnormal bone growth on the inner aspect of the cranial bones.

√5ᵗʰ **M85.3 Osteitis condensans**

    M85.30 Osteitis condensans, unspecified site

√6ᵗʰ   **M85.31** Osteitis condensans, **shoulder**

     M85.311 Osteitis condensans, **right** shoulder
     M85.312 Osteitis condensans, **left** shoulder
     M85.319 Osteitis condensans, **unspecified** shoulder

√6ᵗʰ   **M85.32** Osteitis condensans, **upper arm**

     M85.321 Osteitis condensans, **right** upper arm
     M85.322 Osteitis condensans, **left** upper arm
     M85.329 Osteitis condensans, **unspecified** upper arm

√6ᵗʰ   **M85.33** Osteitis condensans, **forearm**

     M85.331 Osteitis condensans, **right** forearm
     M85.332 Osteitis condensans, **left** forearm
     M85.339 Osteitis condensans, **unspecified** forearm

√6ᵗʰ   **M85.34** Osteitis condensans, **hand**

     M85.341 Osteitis condensans, **right** hand
     M85.342 Osteitis condensans, **left** hand
     M85.349 Osteitis condensans, **unspecified** hand

√6ᵗʰ   **M85.35** Osteitis condensans, **thigh**

     M85.351 Osteitis condensans, **right** thigh
     M85.352 Osteitis condensans, **left** thigh
     M85.359 Osteitis condensans, **unspecified** thigh

√6ᵗʰ   **M85.36** Osteitis condensans, **lower leg**

     M85.361 Osteitis condensans, **right** lower leg
     M85.362 Osteitis condensans, **left** lower leg
     M85.369 Osteitis condensans, **unspecified** lower leg

√6ᵗʰ   **M85.37** Osteitis condensans, **ankle and foot**

     M85.371 Osteitis condensans, **right** ankle and foot
     M85.372 Osteitis condensans, **left** ankle and foot
     M85.379 Osteitis condensans, **unspecified** ankle and foot

    M85.38 Osteitis condensans, other site
    M85.39 Osteitis condensans, **multiple sites**

√5ᵗʰ **M85.4 Solitary bone cyst**

> EXCLUDES 2   *solitary cyst of jaw (M27.4)*

    M85.40 Solitary bone cyst, unspecified site

√6ᵗʰ   **M85.41** Solitary bone cyst, **shoulder**

     M85.411 Solitary bone cyst, **right** shoulder
     M85.412 Solitary bone cyst, **left** shoulder
     M85.419 Solitary bone cyst, **unspecified** shoulder

√6ᵗʰ   **M85.42** Solitary bone cyst, **humerus**

     M85.421 Solitary bone cyst, **right** humerus
     M85.422 Solitary bone cyst, **left** humerus
     M85.429 Solitary bone cyst, **unspecified** humerus

√6ᵗʰ   **M85.43** Solitary bone cyst, **ulna and radius**

     M85.431 Solitary bone cyst, **right** ulna and radius
     M85.432 Solitary bone cyst, **left** ulna and radius
     M85.439 Solitary bone cyst, **unspecified** ulna and radius

√6ᵗʰ   **M85.44** Solitary bone cyst, **hand**

     M85.441 Solitary bone cyst, **right** hand
     M85.442 Solitary bone cyst, **left** hand
     M85.449 Solitary bone cyst, **unspecified** hand

√6ᵗʰ   **M85.45** Solitary bone cyst, **pelvis**

     M85.451 Solitary bone cyst, **right** pelvis
     M85.452 Solitary bone cyst, **left** pelvis
     M85.459 Solitary bone cyst, **unspecified** pelvis

√6ᵗʰ   **M85.46** Solitary bone cyst, **tibia and fibula**

     M85.461 Solitary bone cyst, **right** tibia and fibula
     M85.462 Solitary bone cyst, **left** tibia and fibula
     M85.469 Solitary bone cyst, **unspecified** tibia and fibula

√6ᵗʰ   **M85.47** Solitary bone cyst, **ankle and foot**

     M85.471 Solitary bone cyst, **right** ankle and foot
     M85.472 Solitary bone cyst, **left** ankle and foot
     M85.479 Solitary bone cyst, **unspecified** ankle and foot

    M85.48 Solitary bone cyst, other site

√5ᵗʰ **M85.5 Aneurysmal bone cyst**

> EXCLUDES 2   *aneurysmal cyst of jaw (M27.4)*
> **DEF:** Solitary bone lesion that bulges into the periosteum and is marked by a calcified rim.

    M85.50 Aneurysmal bone cyst, unspecified site

√6ᵗʰ   **M85.51** Aneurysmal bone cyst, **shoulder**

     M85.511 Aneurysmal bone cyst, **right** shoulder
     M85.512 Aneurysmal bone cyst, **left** shoulder
     M85.519 Aneurysmal bone cyst, **unspecified** shoulder

√6ᵗʰ   **M85.52** Aneurysmal bone cyst, **upper arm**

     M85.521 Aneurysmal bone cyst, **right** upper arm
     M85.522 Aneurysmal bone cyst, **left** upper arm
     M85.529 Aneurysmal bone cyst, **unspecified** upper arm

√6ᵗʰ   **M85.53** Aneurysmal bone cyst, **forearm**

     M85.531 Aneurysmal bone cyst, **right** forearm
     M85.532 Aneurysmal bone cyst, **left** forearm
     M85.539 Aneurysmal bone cyst, **unspecified** forearm

√6ᵗʰ   **M85.54** Aneurysmal bone cyst, **hand**

     M85.541 Aneurysmal bone cyst, **right** hand
     M85.542 Aneurysmal bone cyst, **left** hand
     M85.549 Aneurysmal bone cyst, **unspecified** hand

√6ᵗʰ   **M85.55** Aneurysmal bone cyst, **thigh**

     M85.551 Aneurysmal bone cyst, **right** thigh
     M85.552 Aneurysmal bone cyst, **left** thigh
     M85.559 Aneurysmal bone cyst, **unspecified** thigh

√6ᵗʰ   **M85.56** Aneurysmal bone cyst, **lower leg**

     M85.561 Aneurysmal bone cyst, **right** lower leg
     M85.562 Aneurysmal bone cyst, **left** lower leg
     M85.569 Aneurysmal bone cyst, **unspecified** lower leg

√6ᵗʰ   **M85.57** Aneurysmal bone cyst, **ankle and foot**

     M85.571 Aneurysmal bone cyst, **right** ankle and foot
     M85.572 Aneurysmal bone cyst, **left** ankle and foot
     M85.579 Aneurysmal bone cyst, **unspecified** ankle and foot

    M85.58 Aneurysmal bone cyst, other site
    M85.59 Aneurysmal bone cyst, **multiple sites**

√5ᵗʰ **M85.6 Other cyst of bone**

> EXCLUDES 1   *cyst of jaw NEC (M27.4)*
> *osteitis fibrosa cystica generalisata [von Recklinghausen's disease of bone] (E21.0)*

    M85.60 Other cyst of bone, unspecified site

√6ᵗʰ   **M85.61** Other cyst of bone, **shoulder**

     M85.611 Other cyst of bone, **right** shoulder
     M85.612 Other cyst of bone, **left** shoulder
     M85.619 Other cyst of bone, **unspecified** shoulder

√6ᵗʰ   **M85.62** Other cyst of bone, **upper arm**

     M85.621 Other cyst of bone, **right** upper arm
     M85.622 Other cyst of bone, **left** upper arm
     M85.629 Other cyst of bone, **unspecified** upper arm

√6ᵗʰ   **M85.63** Other cyst of bone, **forearm**

     M85.631 Other cyst of bone, **right** forearm
     M85.632 Other cyst of bone, **left** forearm
     M85.639 Other cyst of bone, **unspecified** forearm

√6ᵗʰ   **M85.64** Other cyst of bone, **hand**

     M85.641 Other cyst of bone, **right** hand
     M85.642 Other cyst of bone, **left** hand
     M85.649 Other cyst of bone, **unspecified** hand

√6ᵗʰ   **M85.65** Other cyst of bone, **thigh**

     M85.651 Other cyst of bone, **right** thigh
     M85.652 Other cyst of bone, **left** thigh
     M85.659 Other cyst of bone, **unspecified** thigh

√6ᵗʰ   **M85.66** Other cyst of bone, **lower leg**

     M85.661 Other cyst of bone, **right** lower leg
     M85.662 Other cyst of bone, **left** lower leg
     M85.669 Other cyst of bone, **unspecified** lower leg

√6ᵗʰ   **M85.67** Other cyst of bone, **ankle and foot**

     M85.671 Other cyst of bone, **right** ankle and foot
     M85.672 Other cyst of bone, **left** ankle and foot
     M85.679 Other cyst of bone, **unspecified** ankle and foot

    M85.68 Other cyst of bone, other site

☑ Additional Character Required   √x7ᵗʰ Placeholder   Unacceptable PDx   Questionable PDx   Manifestation   Unspecified Dx   H1–H14 HAC   HCC CMS-HCC Dx   HIV HIV Dx

ICD-10-CM 2021   823

     M85.69   Other cyst of bone, multiple sites

✓5ᵗʰ **M85.8**   Other specified disorders of bone density and structure

     Hyperostosis of bones, except skull

     Osteosclerosis, acquired

     EXCLUDES 1   diffuse idiopathic skeletal hyperostosis [DISH] (M48.1)

                osteosclerosis congenita (Q77.4)

                osteosclerosis fragilitas (generalista) (Q78.2)

                osteosclerosis myelofibrosis (D75.81)

     M85.80   Other specified disorders of bone density and structure, unspecified site

     ✓6ᵗʰ **M85.81**   Other specified disorders of bone density and structure, shoulder

         M85.811   Other specified disorders of bone density and structure, right shoulder

         M85.812   Other specified disorders of bone density and structure, left shoulder

         M85.819   Other specified disorders of bone density and structure, unspecified shoulder

     ✓6ᵗʰ **M85.82**   Other specified disorders of bone density and structure, upper arm

         M85.821   Other specified disorders of bone density and structure, right upper arm

         M85.822   Other specified disorders of bone density and structure, left upper arm

         M85.829   Other specified disorders of bone density and structure, unspecified upper arm

     ✓6ᵗʰ **M85.83**   Other specified disorders of bone density and structure, forearm

         M85.831   Other specified disorders of bone density and structure, right forearm

         M85.832   Other specified disorders of bone density and structure, left forearm

         M85.839   Other specified disorders of bone density and structure, unspecified forearm

     ✓6ᵗʰ **M85.84**   Other specified disorders of bone density and structure, hand

         M85.841   Other specified disorders of bone density and structure, right hand

         M85.842   Other specified disorders of bone density and structure, left hand

         M85.849   Other specified disorders of bone density and structure, unspecified hand

     ✓6ᵗʰ **M85.85**   Other specified disorders of bone density and structure, thigh

         M85.851   Other specified disorders of bone density and structure, right thigh

         M85.852   Other specified disorders of bone density and structure, left thigh

         M85.859   Other specified disorders of bone density and structure, unspecified thigh

     ✓6ᵗʰ **M85.86**   Other specified disorders of bone density and structure, lower leg

         M85.861   Other specified disorders of bone density and structure, right lower leg

         M85.862   Other specified disorders of bone density and structure, left lower leg

         M85.869   Other specified disorders of bone density and structure, unspecified lower leg

     ✓6ᵗʰ **M85.87**   Other specified disorders of bone density and structure, ankle and foot

         M85.871   Other specified disorders of bone density and structure, right ankle and foot

         M85.872   Other specified disorders of bone density and structure, left ankle and foot

         M85.879   Other specified disorders of bone density and structure, unspecified ankle and foot

     M85.88   Other specified disorders of bone density and structure, other site

     M85.89   Other specified disorders of bone density and structure, multiple sites

M85.9   Disorder of bone density and structure, unspecified

Other osteopathies (M86-M90)

     EXCLUDES 1   postprocedural osteopathies (M96.-)

✓4ᵗʰ **M86**   Osteomyelitis

     Use additional code (B95-B97) to identify infectious agent

     Use additional code to identify major osseous defect, if applicable (M89.7-)

     EXCLUDES 1   osteomyelitis due to:

                echinococcus (B67.2)

                gonococcus (A54.43)

                salmonella (A02.24)

     EXCLUDES 2   ostemyelitis of:

                orbit (H05.0-)

                petrous bone (H70.2-)

                vertebra (M46.2-)

     ✓5ᵗʰ **M86.0**   Acute hematogenous osteomyelitis

         M86.00   Acute hematogenous osteomyelitis, unspecified site   CC HCC

         ✓6ᵗʰ **M86.01**   Acute hematogenous osteomyelitis, shoulder

             M86.011   Acute hematogenous osteomyelitis, right shoulder   CC HCC

             M86.012   Acute hematogenous osteomyelitis, left shoulder   CC HCC

             M86.019   Acute hematogenous osteomyelitis, unspecified shoulder

         ✓6ᵗʰ **M86.02**   Acute hematogenous osteomyelitis, humerus

             M86.021   Acute hematogenous osteomyelitis, right humerus   CC HCC

             M86.022   Acute hematogenous osteomyelitis, left humerus   CC HCC

             M86.029   Acute hematogenous osteomyelitis, unspecified humerus   CC HCC

         ✓6ᵗʰ **M86.03**   Acute hematogenous osteomyelitis, radius and ulna

             M86.031   Acute hematogenous osteomyelitis, right radius and ulna   CC HCC

             M86.032   Acute hematogenous osteomyelitis, left radius and ulna   CC HCC

             M86.039   Acute hematogenous osteomyelitis, unspecified radius and ulna   CC HCC

         ✓6ᵗʰ **M86.04**   Acute hematogenous osteomyelitis, hand

             M86.041   Acute hematogenous osteomyelitis, right hand   CC HCC

             M86.042   Acute hematogenous osteomyelitis, left hand   CC HCC

             M86.049   Acute hematogenous osteomyelitis, unspecified hand

         ✓6ᵗʰ **M86.05**   Acute hematogenous osteomyelitis, femur

             M86.051   Acute hematogenous osteomyelitis, right femur   CC HCC

             M86.052   Acute hematogenous osteomyelitis, left femur   CC HCC

             M86.059   Acute hematogenous osteomyelitis, unspecified femur   CC HCC

         ✓6ᵗʰ **M86.06**   Acute hematogenous osteomyelitis, tibia and fibula

             M86.061   Acute hematogenous osteomyelitis, right tibia and fibula   CC HCC

             M86.062   Acute hematogenous osteomyelitis, left tibia and fibula   CC HCC

             M86.069   Acute hematogenous osteomyelitis, unspecified tibia and fibula   CC HCC

         ✓6ᵗʰ **M86.07**   Acute hematogenous osteomyelitis, ankle and foot

             M86.071   Acute hematogenous osteomyelitis, right ankle and foot   CC HCC

             M86.072   Acute hematogenous osteomyelitis, left ankle and foot   CC HCC

             M86.079   Acute hematogenous osteomyelitis, unspecified ankle and foot   CC HCC

         M86.08   Acute hematogenous osteomyelitis, other sites   CC HCC

         M86.09   Acute hematogenous osteomyelitis, multiple sites   CC HCC

     ✓5ᵗʰ **M86.1**   Other acute osteomyelitis

         M86.10   Other acute osteomyelitis, unspecified site   CC HCC

N Newborn: 0   P Pediatric: 0-17   M Maternity: 9-64   A Adult: 15-124   MCC Major Complication/Comorbidity   CC Complication/Comorbidity   SW Severe Wound Dx

824   ICD-10-CM 2021

✓6ᵗʰ **M86.11** Other acute osteomyelitis, shoulder

    M86.111 Other acute osteomyelitis, right shoulder   CC HCC

    M86.112 Other acute osteomyelitis, left shoulder   CC HCC

    M86.119 Other acute osteomyelitis, unspecified shoulder   CC HCC

✓6ᵗʰ **M86.12** Other acute osteomyelitis, humerus

    M86.121 Other acute osteomyelitis, right humerus   CC HCC

    M86.122 Other acute osteomyelitis, left humerus   CC HCC

    M86.129 Other acute osteomyelitis, unspecified humerus   CC HCC

✓6ᵗʰ **M86.13** Other acute osteomyelitis, radius and ulna

    M86.131 Other acute osteomyelitis, right radius and ulna   CC HCC

    M86.132 Other acute osteomyelitis, left radius and ulna   CC HCC

    M86.139 Other acute osteomyelitis, unspecified radius and ulna   CC HCC

✓6ᵗʰ **M86.14** Other acute osteomyelitis, hand

    M86.141 Other acute osteomyelitis, right hand   CC HCC

    M86.142 Other acute osteomyelitis, left hand   CC HCC

    M86.149 Other acute osteomyelitis, unspecified hand   CC HCC

✓6ᵗʰ **M86.15** Other acute osteomyelitis, femur

    M86.151 Other acute osteomyelitis, right femur   CC HCC

    M86.152 Other acute osteomyelitis, left femur   CC HCC

    M86.159 Other acute osteomyelitis, unspecified femur   CC HCC

✓6ᵗʰ **M86.16** Other acute osteomyelitis, tibia and fibula

    M86.161 Other acute osteomyelitis, right tibia and fibula   CC HCC

    M86.162 Other acute osteomyelitis, left tibia and fibula   CC HCC

    M86.169 Other acute osteomyelitis, unspecified tibia and fibula   CC HCC

✓6ᵗʰ **M86.17** Other acute osteomyelitis, ankle and foot

    AHA: 2020,1Q,12

    M86.171 Other acute osteomyelitis, right ankle and foot   CC HCC

    M86.172 Other acute osteomyelitis, left ankle and foot   CC HCC

    M86.179 Other acute osteomyelitis, unspecified ankle and foot   CC HCC

M86.18 Other acute osteomyelitis, other site   CC HCC

M86.19 Other acute osteomyelitis, multiple sites   CC HCC

✓5ᵗʰ **M86.2** Subacute osteomyelitis

    M86.20 Subacute osteomyelitis, unspecified site   CC HCC

✓6ᵗʰ **M86.21** Subacute osteomyelitis, shoulder

    M86.211 Subacute osteomyelitis, right shoulder   CC HCC

    M86.212 Subacute osteomyelitis, left shoulder   CC HCC

    M86.219 Subacute osteomyelitis, unspecified shoulder   CC HCC

✓6ᵗʰ **M86.22** Subacute osteomyelitis, humerus

    M86.221 Subacute osteomyelitis, right humerus   CC HCC

    M86.222 Subacute osteomyelitis, left humerus   CC HCC

    M86.229 Subacute osteomyelitis, unspecified humerus   CC HCC

✓6ᵗʰ **M86.23** Subacute osteomyelitis, radius and ulna

    M86.231 Subacute osteomyelitis, right radius and ulna   CC HCC

    M86.232 Subacute osteomyelitis, left radius and ulna   CC HCC

    M86.239 Subacute osteomyelitis, unspecified radius and ulna   CC HCC

✓6ᵗʰ **M86.24** Subacute osteomyelitis, hand

    M86.241 Subacute osteomyelitis, right hand   CC HCC

    M86.242 Subacute osteomyelitis, left hand   CC HCC

    M86.249 Subacute osteomyelitis, unspecified hand   CC HCC

✓6ᵗʰ **M86.25** Subacute osteomyelitis, femur

    M86.251 Subacute osteomyelitis, right femur   CC HCC

    M86.252 Subacute osteomyelitis, left femur   CC HCC

    M86.259 Subacute osteomyelitis, unspecified femur   CC HCC

✓6ᵗʰ **M86.26** Subacute osteomyelitis, tibia and fibula

    M86.261 Subacute osteomyelitis, right tibia and fibula   CC HCC

    M86.262 Subacute osteomyelitis, left tibia and fibula   CC HCC

    M86.269 Subacute osteomyelitis, unspecified tibia and fibula   CC HCC

✓6ᵗʰ **M86.27** Subacute osteomyelitis, ankle and foot

    M86.271 Subacute osteomyelitis, right ankle and foot   CC HCC

    M86.272 Subacute osteomyelitis, left ankle and foot   CC HCC

    M86.279 Subacute osteomyelitis, unspecified ankle and foot   CC HCC

M86.28 Subacute osteomyelitis, other site   CC HCC

M86.29 Subacute osteomyelitis, multiple sites   CC HCC

✓5ᵗʰ **M86.3** Chronic multifocal osteomyelitis

    M86.30 Chronic multifocal osteomyelitis, unspecified site   CC HCC

✓6ᵗʰ **M86.31** Chronic multifocal osteomyelitis, shoulder

    M86.311 Chronic multifocal osteomyelitis, right shoulder   CC HCC

    M86.312 Chronic multifocal osteomyelitis, left shoulder   CC HCC

    M86.319 Chronic multifocal osteomyelitis, unspecified shoulder   CC HCC

✓6ᵗʰ **M86.32** Chronic multifocal osteomyelitis, humerus

    M86.321 Chronic multifocal osteomyelitis, right humerus   CC HCC

    M86.322 Chronic multifocal osteomyelitis, left humerus   CC HCC

    M86.329 Chronic multifocal osteomyelitis, unspecified humerus   CC HCC

✓6ᵗʰ **M86.33** Chronic multifocal osteomyelitis, radius and ulna

    M86.331 Chronic multifocal osteomyelitis, right radius and ulna   CC HCC

    M86.332 Chronic multifocal osteomyelitis, left radius and ulna   CC HCC

    M86.339 Chronic multifocal osteomyelitis, unspecified radius and ulna   CC HCC

✓6ᵗʰ **M86.34** Chronic multifocal osteomyelitis, hand

    M86.341 Chronic multifocal osteomyelitis, right hand   CC HCC

    M86.342 Chronic multifocal osteomyelitis, left hand   CC HCC

    M86.349 Chronic multifocal osteomyelitis, unspecified hand   CC HCC

✓6ᵗʰ **M86.35** Chronic multifocal osteomyelitis, femur

    M86.351 Chronic multifocal osteomyelitis, right femur   CC HCC

    M86.352 Chronic multifocal osteomyelitis, left femur   CC HCC

    M86.359 Chronic multifocal osteomyelitis, unspecified femur   CC HCC

✓6ᵗʰ **M86.36** Chronic multifocal osteomyelitis, tibia and fibula

    M86.361 Chronic multifocal osteomyelitis, right tibia and fibula   CC HCC

    M86.362 Chronic multifocal osteomyelitis, left tibia and fibula   CC HCC

    M86.369 Chronic multifocal osteomyelitis, unspecified tibia and fibula   CC HCC

✓6ᵗʰ **M86.37** Chronic multifocal osteomyelitis, ankle and foot

    M86.371 Chronic multifocal osteomyelitis, right ankle and foot   CC HCC

    M86.372 Chronic multifocal osteomyelitis, left ankle and foot   CC HCC

✓ Additional Character Required   ✓x7ᵗʰ Placeholder   Unacceptable PDx   Questionable PDx   Manifestation   Unspecified Dx   H1-H14 HAC   HCC CMS-HCC Dx   HIV HIV Dx

ICD-10-CM 2021   825

        M86.379 Chronic multifocal osteomyelitis, unspecified ankle and foot `cc` `HCC`

     M86.38 Chronic multifocal osteomyelitis, other site `cc` `HCC`

     M86.39 Chronic multifocal osteomyelitis, multiple sites `cc` `HCC`

✓5th **M86.4** Chronic osteomyelitis with draining sinus

      M86.40 Chronic osteomyelitis with draining sinus, unspecified site `cc` `HCC`

  ✓6th **M86.41** Chronic osteomyelitis with draining sinus, shoulder

        M86.411 Chronic osteomyelitis with draining sinus, right shoulder `cc` `HCC`

        M86.412 Chronic osteomyelitis with draining sinus, left shoulder `cc` `HCC`

        M86.419 Chronic osteomyelitis with draining sinus, unspecified shoulder `cc` `HCC`

  ✓6th **M86.42** Chronic osteomyelitis with draining sinus, humerus

        M86.421 Chronic osteomyelitis with draining sinus, right humerus `cc` `HCC`

        M86.422 Chronic osteomyelitis with draining sinus, left humerus `cc` `HCC`

        M86.429 Chronic osteomyelitis with draining sinus, unspecified humerus `cc` `HCC`

  ✓6th **M86.43** Chronic osteomyelitis with draining sinus, radius and ulna

        M86.431 Chronic osteomyelitis with draining sinus, right radius and ulna `cc` `HCC`

        M86.432 Chronic osteomyelitis with draining sinus, left radius and ulna `cc` `HCC`

        M86.439 Chronic osteomyelitis with draining sinus, unspecified radius and ulna `cc` `HCC`

  ✓6th **M86.44** Chronic osteomyelitis with draining sinus, hand

        M86.441 Chronic osteomyelitis with draining sinus, right hand `cc` `HCC`

        M86.442 Chronic osteomyelitis with draining sinus, left hand `cc` `HCC`

        M86.449 Chronic osteomyelitis with draining sinus, unspecified hand `cc` `HCC`

  ✓6th **M86.45** Chronic osteomyelitis with draining sinus, femur

        M86.451 Chronic osteomyelitis with draining sinus, right femur `cc` `HCC`

        M86.452 Chronic osteomyelitis with draining sinus, left femur `cc` `HCC`

        M86.459 Chronic osteomyelitis with draining sinus, unspecified femur `cc` `HCC`

  ✓6th **M86.46** Chronic osteomyelitis with draining sinus, tibia and fibula

        M86.461 Chronic osteomyelitis with draining sinus, right tibia and fibula `cc` `HCC`

        M86.462 Chronic osteomyelitis with draining sinus, left tibia and fibula `cc` `HCC`

        M86.469 Chronic osteomyelitis with draining sinus, unspecified tibia and fibula `cc` `HCC`

  ✓6th **M86.47** Chronic osteomyelitis with draining sinus, ankle and foot

        M86.471 Chronic osteomyelitis with draining sinus, right ankle and foot `cc` `HCC`

        M86.472 Chronic osteomyelitis with draining sinus, left ankle and foot `cc` `HCC`

        M86.479 Chronic osteomyelitis with draining sinus, unspecified ankle and foot `cc` `HCC`

     M86.48 Chronic osteomyelitis with draining sinus, other site `cc` `HCC`

     M86.49 Chronic osteomyelitis with draining sinus, multiple sites `cc` `HCC`

✓5th **M86.5** Other chronic hematogenous osteomyelitis

      M86.50 Other chronic hematogenous osteomyelitis, unspecified site `cc` `HCC`

  ✓6th **M86.51** Other chronic hematogenous osteomyelitis, shoulder

        M86.511 Other chronic hematogenous osteomyelitis, right shoulder `cc` `HCC`

        M86.512 Other chronic hematogenous osteomyelitis, left shoulder `cc` `HCC`

        M86.519 Other chronic hematogenous osteomyelitis, unspecified shoulder `cc` `HCC`

✓6th **M86.52** Other chronic hematogenous osteomyelitis, humerus

        M86.521 Other chronic hematogenous osteomyelitis, right humerus `cc` `HCC`

        M86.522 Other chronic hematogenous osteomyelitis, left humerus `cc` `HCC`

        M86.529 Other chronic hematogenous osteomyelitis, unspecified humerus `cc` `HCC`

✓6th **M86.53** Other chronic hematogenous osteomyelitis, radius and ulna

        M86.531 Other chronic hematogenous osteomyelitis, right radius and ulna `cc` `HCC`

        M86.532 Other chronic hematogenous osteomyelitis, left radius and ulna `cc` `HCC`

        M86.539 Other chronic hematogenous osteomyelitis, unspecified radius and ulna `cc` `HCC`

✓6th **M86.54** Other chronic hematogenous osteomyelitis, hand

        M86.541 Other chronic hematogenous osteomyelitis, right hand `cc` `HCC`

        M86.542 Other chronic hematogenous osteomyelitis, left hand `cc` `HCC`

        M86.549 Other chronic hematogenous osteomyelitis, unspecified hand `cc` `HCC`

✓6th **M86.55** Other chronic hematogenous osteomyelitis, femur

        M86.551 Other chronic hematogenous osteomyelitis, right femur `cc` `HCC`

        M86.552 Other chronic hematogenous osteomyelitis, left femur `cc` `HCC`

        M86.559 Other chronic hematogenous osteomyelitis, unspecified femur `cc` `HCC`

✓6th **M86.56** Other chronic hematogenous osteomyelitis, tibia and fibula

        M86.561 Other chronic hematogenous osteomyelitis, right tibia and fibula `cc` `HCC`

        M86.562 Other chronic hematogenous osteomyelitis, left tibia and fibula `cc` `HCC`

        M86.569 Other chronic hematogenous osteomyelitis, unspecified tibia and fibula `cc` `HCC`

✓6th **M86.57** Other chronic hematogenous osteomyelitis, ankle and foot

        M86.571 Other chronic hematogenous osteomyelitis, right ankle and foot `cc` `HCC`

        M86.572 Other chronic hematogenous osteomyelitis, left ankle and foot `cc` `HCC`

        M86.579 Other chronic hematogenous osteomyelitis, unspecified ankle and foot `cc` `HCC`

     M86.58 Other chronic hematogenous osteomyelitis, other site `cc` `HCC`

     M86.59 Other chronic hematogenous osteomyelitis, multiple sites `cc` `HCC`

✓5th **M86.6** Other chronic osteomyelitis

      M86.60 Other chronic osteomyelitis, unspecified site `cc` `HCC`

✓6th **M86.61** Other chronic osteomyelitis, shoulder

        M86.611 Other chronic osteomyelitis, right shoulder `cc` `HCC`

        M86.612 Other chronic osteomyelitis, left shoulder `cc` `HCC`

        M86.619 Other chronic osteomyelitis, unspecified shoulder `cc` `HCC`

✓6th **M86.62** Other chronic osteomyelitis, humerus

        M86.621 Other chronic osteomyelitis, right humerus `cc` `HCC`

        M86.622 Other chronic osteomyelitis, left humerus `cc` `HCC`

        M86.629 Other chronic osteomyelitis, unspecified humerus `cc` `HCC`

Ⓝ Newborn: 0   Ⓟ Pediatric: 0-17   Ⓜ Maternity: 9-64   Ⓐ Adult: 15-124   `MCC` Major Complication/Comorbidity   `CC` Complication/Comorbidity   `SW` Severe Wound Dx

826   ICD-10-CM 2021

√6ᵗʰ **M86.63** Other chronic osteomyelitis, radius and ulna

M86.631 Other chronic osteomyelitis, right radius and ulna `CC` `HCC`

M86.632 Other chronic osteomyelitis, left radius and ulna `CC` `HCC`

M86.639 Other chronic osteomyelitis, unspecified radius and ulna `CC` `HCC`

√6ᵗʰ **M86.64** Other chronic osteomyelitis, hand

M86.641 Other chronic osteomyelitis, right hand `CC` `HCC`

M86.642 Other chronic osteomyelitis, left hand `CC` `HCC`

M86.649 Other chronic osteomyelitis, unspecified hand `CC` `HCC`

√6ᵗʰ **M86.65** Other chronic osteomyelitis, thigh

M86.651 Other chronic osteomyelitis, right thigh `CC` `HCC`

M86.652 Other chronic osteomyelitis, left thigh `CC` `HCC`

M86.659 Other chronic osteomyelitis, unspecified thigh `CC` `HCC`

√6ᵗʰ **M86.66** Other chronic osteomyelitis, tibia and fibula

M86.661 Other chronic osteomyelitis, right tibia and fibula `CC` `HCC`

M86.662 Other chronic osteomyelitis, left tibia and fibula `CC` `HCC`

M86.669 Other chronic osteomyelitis, unspecified tibia and fibula `CC` `HCC`

√6ᵗʰ **M86.67** Other chronic osteomyelitis, ankle and foot

M86.671 Other chronic osteomyelitis, right ankle and foot `CC` `HCC`
  AHA: 2016,1Q,13

M86.672 Other chronic osteomyelitis, left ankle and foot `CC` `HCC`

M86.679 Other chronic osteomyelitis, unspecified ankle and foot `CC` `HCC`

M86.68 Other chronic osteomyelitis, other site `CC` `HCC`

M86.69 Other chronic osteomyelitis, multiple sites `CC` `HCC`

√5ᵗʰ **M86.8** Other osteomyelitis
  Brodie's abscess

√6ᵗʰ **M86.8X** Other osteomyelitis

M86.8X0 Other osteomyelitis, multiple sites `CC` `HCC`

M86.8X1 Other osteomyelitis, shoulder `CC` `HCC`

M86.8X2 Other osteomyelitis, upper arm `CC` `HCC`

M86.8X3 Other osteomyelitis, forearm `CC` `HCC`

M86.8X4 Other osteomyelitis, hand `CC` `HCC`

M86.8X5 Other osteomyelitis, thigh `CC` `HCC`

M86.8X6 Other osteomyelitis, lower leg `CC` `HCC`

M86.8X7 Other osteomyelitis, ankle and foot `CC` `HCC`

M86.8X8 Other osteomyelitis, other site `CC` `HCC`

M86.8X9 Other osteomyelitis, unspecified sites `CC` `HCC`

M86.9 Osteomyelitis, unspecified `CC` `HCC`
  Infection of bone NOS
  Periostitis without osteomyelitis

√4ᵗʰ **M87 Osteonecrosis**

`INCLUDES`   avascular necrosis of bone
  Use additional code to identify major osseous defect, if applicable (M89.7-)

`EXCLUDES 1`   juvenile osteonecrosis (M91-M92)
  osteochondropathies (M90-M93)

√5ᵗʰ **M87.0** Idiopathic aseptic necrosis of bone

M87.00 Idiopathic aseptic necrosis of unspecified bone `CC` `HCC`

√6ᵗʰ **M87.01** Idiopathic aseptic necrosis of shoulder
  Idiopathic aseptic necrosis of clavicle and scapula

M87.011 Idiopathic aseptic necrosis of right shoulder `CC` `HCC`

M87.012 Idiopathic aseptic necrosis of left shoulder `CC` `HCC`

M87.019 Idiopathic aseptic necrosis of unspecified shoulder `CC` `HCC`

√6ᵗʰ **M87.02** Idiopathic aseptic necrosis of humerus

M87.021 Idiopathic aseptic necrosis of right humerus `CC` `HCC`

M87.022 Idiopathic aseptic necrosis of left humerus `CC` `HCC`

M87.029 Idiopathic aseptic necrosis of unspecified humerus `CC` `HCC`

√6ᵗʰ **M87.03** Idiopathic aseptic necrosis of radius, ulna and carpus

M87.031 Idiopathic aseptic necrosis of right radius `CC` `HCC`

M87.032 Idiopathic aseptic necrosis of left radius `CC` `HCC`

M87.033 Idiopathic aseptic necrosis of unspecified radius `CC` `HCC`

M87.034 Idiopathic aseptic necrosis of right ulna `CC` `HCC`

M87.035 Idiopathic aseptic necrosis of left ulna `CC` `HCC`

M87.036 Idiopathic aseptic necrosis of unspecified ulna `CC` `HCC`

M87.037 Idiopathic aseptic necrosis of right carpus `CC` `HCC`

M87.038 Idiopathic aseptic necrosis of left carpus `CC` `HCC`

M87.039 Idiopathic aseptic necrosis of unspecified carpus `CC` `HCC`

√6ᵗʰ **M87.04** Idiopathic aseptic necrosis of hand and fingers
  Idiopathic aseptic necrosis of metacarpals and phalanges of hands

M87.041 Idiopathic aseptic necrosis of right hand `CC` `HCC`

M87.042 Idiopathic aseptic necrosis of left hand `CC` `HCC`

M87.043 Idiopathic aseptic necrosis of unspecified hand `CC` `HCC`

M87.044 Idiopathic aseptic necrosis of right finger(s) `CC` `HCC`

M87.045 Idiopathic aseptic necrosis of left finger(s) `CC` `HCC`

M87.046 Idiopathic aseptic necrosis of unspecified finger(s) `CC` `HCC`

√6ᵗʰ **M87.05** Idiopathic aseptic necrosis of pelvis and femur

M87.050 Idiopathic aseptic necrosis of pelvis `CC` `HCC`

M87.051 Idiopathic aseptic necrosis of right femur `CC` `HCC`

M87.052 Idiopathic aseptic necrosis of left femur `CC` `HCC`

M87.059 Idiopathic aseptic necrosis of unspecified femur `CC` `HCC`

√6ᵗʰ **M87.06** Idiopathic aseptic necrosis of tibia and fibula

M87.061 Idiopathic aseptic necrosis of right tibia `CC` `HCC`

M87.062 Idiopathic aseptic necrosis of left tibia `CC` `HCC`

M87.063 Idiopathic aseptic necrosis of unspecified tibia `CC` `HCC`

M87.064 Idiopathic aseptic necrosis of right fibula `CC` `HCC`

M87.065 Idiopathic aseptic necrosis of left fibula `CC` `HCC`

M87.066 Idiopathic aseptic necrosis of unspecified fibula `CC` `HCC`

√6ᵗʰ **M87.07** Idiopathic aseptic necrosis of ankle, foot and toes
  Idiopathic aseptic necrosis of metatarsus, tarsus, and phalanges of toes

M87.071 Idiopathic aseptic necrosis of right ankle `CC` `HCC`

M87.072 Idiopathic aseptic necrosis of left ankle `CC` `HCC`

M87.073 Idiopathic aseptic necrosis of unspecified ankle `CC` `HCC`

M87.074 Idiopathic aseptic necrosis of right foot `CC` `HCC`

M87.075 Idiopathic aseptic necrosis of left foot `CC` `HCC`

M87.076 Idiopathic aseptic necrosis of unspecified foot `CC` `HCC`

M87.077   Idiopathic aseptic necrosis of right toe(s)   `CC` `HCC`

M87.078   Idiopathic aseptic necrosis of left toe(s)   `CC` `HCC`

M87.079   Idiopathic aseptic necrosis of unspecified toe(s)   `CC` `HCC`

M87.08   Idiopathic aseptic necrosis of bone, other site   `CC` `HCC`

M87.09   Idiopathic aseptic necrosis of bone, multiple sites   `CC` `HCC`

√5ᵗʰ **M87.1**   Osteonecrosis due to drugs

> Use additional code for adverse effect, if applicable, to identify drug (T36-T50 with fifth or sixth character 5)

M87.10   Osteonecrosis due to drugs, unspecified bone   `CC` `HCC`

√6ᵗʰ **M87.11**   Osteonecrosis due to drugs, shoulder

M87.111   Osteonecrosis due to drugs, right shoulder   `CC` `HCC`

M87.112   Osteonecrosis due to drugs, left shoulder   `CC` `HCC`

M87.119   Osteonecrosis due to drugs, unspecified shoulder   `CC` `HCC`

√6ᵗʰ **M87.12**   Osteonecrosis due to drugs, humerus

M87.121   Osteonecrosis due to drugs, right humerus   `CC` `HCC`

M87.122   Osteonecrosis due to drugs, left humerus   `CC` `HCC`

M87.129   Osteonecrosis due to drugs, unspecified humerus   `CC` `HCC`

√6ᵗʰ **M87.13**   Osteonecrosis due to drugs of radius, ulna and carpus

M87.131   Osteonecrosis due to drugs of right radius   `CC` `HCC`

M87.132   Osteonecrosis due to drugs of left radius   `CC` `HCC`

M87.133   Osteonecrosis due to drugs of unspecified radius   `CC` `HCC`

M87.134   Osteonecrosis due to drugs of right ulna   `CC` `HCC`

M87.135   Osteonecrosis due to drugs of left ulna   `CC` `HCC`

M87.136   Osteonecrosis due to drugs of unspecified ulna   `CC` `HCC`

M87.137   Osteonecrosis due to drugs of right carpus   `CC` `HCC`

M87.138   Osteonecrosis due to drugs of left carpus   `CC` `HCC`

M87.139   Osteonecrosis due to drugs of unspecified carpus   `CC` `HCC`

√6ᵗʰ **M87.14**   Osteonecrosis due to drugs, hand and fingers

M87.141   Osteonecrosis due to drugs, right hand   `CC` `HCC`

M87.142   Osteonecrosis due to drugs, left hand   `CC` `HCC`

M87.143   Osteonecrosis due to drugs, unspecified hand   `CC` `HCC`

M87.144   Osteonecrosis due to drugs, right finger(s)   `CC` `HCC`

M87.145   Osteonecrosis due to drugs, left finger(s)   `CC` `HCC`

M87.146   Osteonecrosis due to drugs, unspecified finger(s)   `CC` `HCC`

√6ᵗʰ **M87.15**   Osteonecrosis due to drugs, pelvis and femur

M87.150   Osteonecrosis due to drugs, pelvis   `CC` `HCC`

M87.151   Osteonecrosis due to drugs, right femur   `CC` `HCC`

M87.152   Osteonecrosis due to drugs, left femur   `CC` `HCC`

M87.159   Osteonecrosis due to drugs, unspecified femur   `CC` `HCC`

√6ᵗʰ **M87.16**   Osteonecrosis due to drugs, tibia and fibula

M87.161   Osteonecrosis due to drugs, right tibia   `CC` `HCC`

M87.162   Osteonecrosis due to drugs, left tibia   `CC` `HCC`

M87.163   Osteonecrosis due to drugs, unspecified tibia   `CC` `HCC`

M87.164   Osteonecrosis due to drugs, right fibula   `CC` `HCC`

M87.165   Osteonecrosis due to drugs, left fibula   `CC` `HCC`

M87.166   Osteonecrosis due to drugs, unspecified fibula   `CC` `HCC`

√6ᵗʰ **M87.17**   Osteonecrosis due to drugs, ankle, foot and toes

M87.171   Osteonecrosis due to drugs, right ankle   `CC` `HCC`

M87.172   Osteonecrosis due to drugs, left ankle   `CC` `HCC`

M87.173   Osteonecrosis due to drugs, unspecified ankle   `CC` `HCC`

M87.174   Osteonecrosis due to drugs, right foot   `CC` `HCC`

M87.175   Osteonecrosis due to drugs, left foot   `CC` `HCC`

M87.176   Osteonecrosis due to drugs, unspecified foot   `CC` `HCC`

M87.177   Osteonecrosis due to drugs, right toe(s)   `CC` `HCC`

M87.178   Osteonecrosis due to drugs, left toe(s)   `CC` `HCC`

M87.179   Osteonecrosis due to drugs, unspecified toe(s)   `CC` `HCC`

√6ᵗʰ **M87.18**   Osteonecrosis due to drugs, other site

M87.180   Osteonecrosis due to drugs, jaw   `CC` `HCC`

M87.188   Osteonecrosis due to drugs, other site   `CC` `HCC`

M87.19   Osteonecrosis due to drugs, multiple sites   `CC` `HCC`

√5ᵗʰ **M87.2**   Osteonecrosis due to previous trauma

M87.20   Osteonecrosis due to previous trauma, unspecified bone   `CC` `HCC`

√6ᵗʰ **M87.21**   Osteonecrosis due to previous trauma, shoulder

M87.211   Osteonecrosis due to previous trauma, right shoulder   `CC` `HCC`

M87.212   Osteonecrosis due to previous trauma, left shoulder   `CC` `HCC`

M87.219   Osteonecrosis due to previous trauma, unspecified shoulder   `CC` `HCC`

√6ᵗʰ **M87.22**   Osteonecrosis due to previous trauma, humerus

M87.221   Osteonecrosis due to previous trauma, right humerus   `CC` `HCC`

M87.222   Osteonecrosis due to previous trauma, left humerus   `CC` `HCC`

M87.229   Osteonecrosis due to previous trauma, unspecified humerus   `CC` `HCC`

√6ᵗʰ **M87.23**   Osteonecrosis due to previous trauma of radius, ulna and carpus

M87.231   Osteonecrosis due to previous trauma of right radius   `CC` `HCC`

M87.232   Osteonecrosis due to previous trauma of left radius   `CC` `HCC`

M87.233   Osteonecrosis due to previous trauma of unspecified radius   `CC` `HCC`

M87.234   Osteonecrosis due to previous trauma of right ulna   `CC` `HCC`

M87.235   Osteonecrosis due to previous trauma of left ulna   `CC` `HCC`

M87.236   Osteonecrosis due to previous trauma of unspecified ulna   `CC` `HCC`

M87.237   Osteonecrosis due to previous trauma of right carpus   `CC` `HCC`

M87.238   Osteonecrosis due to previous trauma of left carpus   `CC` `HCC`

M87.239   Osteonecrosis due to previous trauma of unspecified carpus   `CC` `HCC`

√6ᵗʰ **M87.24**   Osteonecrosis due to previous trauma, hand and fingers

M87.241   Osteonecrosis due to previous trauma, right hand   `CC` `HCC`

M87.242   Osteonecrosis due to previous trauma, left hand   `CC` `HCC`

M87.243   Osteonecrosis due to previous trauma, unspecified hand   `CC` `HCC`

M87.244   Osteonecrosis due to previous trauma, right finger(s)   `CC` `HCC`

N Newborn: 0   P Pediatric: 0-17   M Maternity: 9-64   A Adult: 15-124   `MCC` Major Complication/Comorbidity   `CC` Complication/Comorbidity   `SW` Severe Wound Dx

828   ICD-10-CM 2021

M87.245   Osteonecrosis due to previous trauma, left finger(s)   `CC` `HCC`

M87.246   Osteonecrosis due to previous trauma, unspecified finger(s)   `CC` `HCC`

√6th   **M87.25**   Osteonecrosis due to previous trauma, pelvis and femur

M87.250   Osteonecrosis due to previous trauma, pelvis   `CC` `HCC`

M87.251   Osteonecrosis due to previous trauma, right femur   `CC` `HCC`

M87.252   Osteonecrosis due to previous trauma, left femur   `CC` `HCC`

M87.256   Osteonecrosis due to previous trauma, unspecified femur   `CC` `HCC`

√6th   **M87.26**   Osteonecrosis due to previous trauma, tibia and fibula

M87.261   Osteonecrosis due to previous trauma, right tibia   `CC` `HCC`

M87.262   Osteonecrosis due to previous trauma, left tibia   `CC` `HCC`

M87.263   Osteonecrosis due to previous trauma, unspecified tibia   `CC` `HCC`

M87.264   Osteonecrosis due to previous trauma, right fibula   `CC` `HCC`

M87.265   Osteonecrosis due to previous trauma, left fibula   `CC` `HCC`

M87.266   Osteonecrosis due to previous trauma, unspecified fibula   `CC` `HCC`

√6th   **M87.27**   Osteonecrosis due to previous trauma, ankle, foot and toes

M87.271   Osteonecrosis due to previous trauma, right ankle   `CC` `HCC`

M87.272   Osteonecrosis due to previous trauma, left ankle   `CC` `HCC`

M87.273   Osteonecrosis due to previous trauma, unspecified ankle   `CC` `HCC`

M87.274   Osteonecrosis due to previous trauma, right foot   `CC` `HCC`

M87.275   Osteonecrosis due to previous trauma, left foot   `CC` `HCC`

M87.276   Osteonecrosis due to previous trauma, unspecified foot   `CC` `HCC`

M87.277   Osteonecrosis due to previous trauma, right toe(s)   `CC` `HCC`

M87.278   Osteonecrosis due to previous trauma, left toe(s)   `CC` `HCC`

M87.279   Osteonecrosis due to previous trauma, unspecified toe(s)   `CC` `HCC`

M87.28   Osteonecrosis due to previous trauma, other site   `CC` `HCC`

M87.29   Osteonecrosis due to previous trauma, multiple sites   `CC` `HCC`

√5th   **M87.3**   Other secondary osteonecrosis

M87.30   Other secondary osteonecrosis, unspecified bone   `CC` `HCC`

√6th   **M87.31**   Other secondary osteonecrosis, shoulder

M87.311   Other secondary osteonecrosis, right shoulder   `CC` `HCC`

M87.312   Other secondary osteonecrosis, left shoulder   `CC` `HCC`

M87.319   Other secondary osteonecrosis, unspecified shoulder   `CC` `HCC`

√6th   **M87.32**   Other secondary osteonecrosis, humerus

M87.321   Other secondary osteonecrosis, right humerus   `CC` `HCC`

M87.322   Other secondary osteonecrosis, left humerus   `CC` `HCC`

M87.329   Other secondary osteonecrosis, unspecified humerus   `CC` `HCC`

√6th   **M87.33**   Other secondary osteonecrosis of radius, ulna and carpus

M87.331   Other secondary osteonecrosis of right radius   `CC` `HCC`

M87.332   Other secondary osteonecrosis of left radius   `CC` `HCC`

M87.333   Other secondary osteonecrosis of unspecified radius   `CC` `HCC`

M87.334   Other secondary osteonecrosis of right ulna   `CC` `HCC`

M87.335   Other secondary osteonecrosis of left ulna   `CC` `HCC`

M87.336   Other secondary osteonecrosis of unspecified ulna   `CC` `HCC`

M87.337   Other secondary osteonecrosis of right carpus   `CC` `HCC`

M87.338   Other secondary osteonecrosis of left carpus   `CC` `HCC`

M87.339   Other secondary osteonecrosis of unspecified carpus   `CC` `HCC`

√6th   **M87.34**   Other secondary osteonecrosis, hand and fingers

M87.341   Other secondary osteonecrosis, right hand   `CC` `HCC`

M87.342   Other secondary osteonecrosis, left hand   `CC` `HCC`

M87.343   Other secondary osteonecrosis, unspecified hand   `CC` `HCC`

M87.344   Other secondary osteonecrosis, right finger(s)   `CC` `HCC`

M87.345   Other secondary osteonecrosis, left finger(s)   `CC` `HCC`

M87.346   Other secondary osteonecrosis, unspecified finger(s)   `CC` `HCC`

√6th   **M87.35**   Other secondary osteonecrosis, pelvis and femur

M87.350   Other secondary osteonecrosis, pelvis   `CC` `HCC`

M87.351   Other secondary osteonecrosis, right femur   `CC` `HCC`

M87.352   Other secondary osteonecrosis, left femur   `CC` `HCC`

M87.353   Other secondary osteonecrosis, unspecified femur   `CC` `HCC`

√6th   **M87.36**   Other secondary osteonecrosis, tibia and fibula

M87.361   Other secondary osteonecrosis, right tibia   `CC` `HCC`

M87.362   Other secondary osteonecrosis, left tibia   `CC` `HCC`

M87.363   Other secondary osteonecrosis, unspecified tibia   `CC` `HCC`

M87.364   Other secondary osteonecrosis, right fibula   `CC` `HCC`

M87.365   Other secondary osteonecrosis, left fibula   `CC` `HCC`

M87.366   Other secondary osteonecrosis, unspecified fibula   `CC` `HCC`

√6th   **M87.37**   Other secondary osteonecrosis, ankle and foot

M87.371   Other secondary osteonecrosis, right ankle   `CC` `HCC`

M87.372   Other secondary osteonecrosis, left ankle   `CC` `HCC`

M87.373   Other secondary osteonecrosis, unspecified ankle   `CC` `HCC`

M87.374   Other secondary osteonecrosis, right foot   `CC` `HCC`

M87.375   Other secondary osteonecrosis, left foot   `CC` `HCC`

M87.376   Other secondary osteonecrosis, unspecified foot   `CC` `HCC`

M87.377   Other secondary osteonecrosis, right toe(s)   `CC` `HCC`

M87.378   Other secondary osteonecrosis, left toe(s)   `CC` `HCC`

M87.379   Other secondary osteonecrosis, unspecified toe(s)   `CC` `HCC`

M87.38   Other secondary osteonecrosis, other site   `CC` `HCC`

M87.39   Other secondary osteonecrosis, multiple sites   `CC` `HCC`

√5th   **M87.8**   Other osteonecrosis

M87.80   Other osteonecrosis, unspecified bone   `CC` `HCC`

√6th   **M87.81**   Other osteonecrosis, shoulder

M87.811   Other osteonecrosis, right shoulder   `CC` `HCC`

M87.812   Other osteonecrosis, left shoulder   `CC` `HCC`

M87.819   Other osteonecrosis, unspecified shoulder   `CC` `HCC`

√6th   **M87.82**   Other osteonecrosis, humerus

M87.821   Other osteonecrosis, right humerus   `CC` `HCC`

✓ Additional Character Required   ✓x7th Placeholder   Unacceptable PDx   Questionable PDx   Manifestation   Unspecified Dx   H1-H14 HAC   HCC CMS-HCC Dx   HIV HIV Dx

ICD-10-CM 2021   829

M87.822 Other osteonecrosis, left humerus CC HCC
M87.829 Other osteonecrosis, unspecified humerus CC HCC
✓6th **M87.83** Other osteonecrosis of radius, ulna and carpus
M87.831 Other osteonecrosis of right radius CC HCC
M87.832 Other osteonecrosis of left radius CC HCC
M87.833 Other osteonecrosis of unspecified radius CC HCC
M87.834 Other osteonecrosis of right ulna CC HCC
M87.835 Other osteonecrosis of left ulna CC HCC
M87.836 Other osteonecrosis of unspecified ulna CC HCC
M87.837 Other osteonecrosis of right carpus CC HCC
M87.838 Other osteonecrosis of left carpus CC HCC
M87.839 Other osteonecrosis of unspecified carpus CC HCC
✓6th **M87.84** Other osteonecrosis, hand and fingers
M87.841 Other osteonecrosis, right hand CC HCC
M87.842 Other osteonecrosis, left hand CC HCC
M87.843 Other osteonecrosis, unspecified hand CC HCC
M87.844 Other osteonecrosis, right finger(s) CC HCC
M87.845 Other osteonecrosis, left finger(s) CC HCC
M87.849 Other osteonecrosis, unspecified finger(s) CC HCC
✓6th **M87.85** Other osteonecrosis, pelvis and femur
M87.850 Other osteonecrosis, pelvis CC HCC
M87.851 Other osteonecrosis, right femur CC HCC
M87.852 Other osteonecrosis, left femur CC HCC
M87.859 Other osteonecrosis, unspecified femur CC HCC
✓6th **M87.86** Other osteonecrosis, tibia and fibula
M87.861 Other osteonecrosis, right tibia CC HCC
M87.862 Other osteonecrosis, left tibia CC HCC
M87.863 Other osteonecrosis, unspecified tibia CC HCC
M87.864 Other osteonecrosis, right fibula CC HCC
M87.865 Other osteonecrosis, left fibula CC HCC
M87.869 Other osteonecrosis, unspecified fibula CC HCC
✓6th **M87.87** Other osteonecrosis, ankle, foot and toes
M87.871 Other osteonecrosis, right ankle CC HCC
M87.872 Other osteonecrosis, left ankle CC HCC
M87.873 Other osteonecrosis, unspecified ankle CC HCC
M87.874 Other osteonecrosis, right foot CC HCC
M87.875 Other osteonecrosis, left foot CC HCC
M87.876 Other osteonecrosis, unspecified foot CC HCC
M87.877 Other osteonecrosis, right toe(s) CC HCC
M87.878 Other osteonecrosis, left toe(s) CC HCC
M87.879 Other osteonecrosis, unspecified toe(s) CC HCC
M87.88 Other osteonecrosis, other site CC HCC
M87.89 Other osteonecrosis, multiple sites CC HCC
M87.9 Osteonecrosis, unspecified CC HCC
Necrosis of bone NOS

✓4th **M88** Osteitis deformans [Paget's disease of bone]
EXCLUDES 1 osteitis deformans in neoplastic disease (M90.6)
DEF: Bone disease characterized by numerous cycles of bone resorption by the body. Resorption is followed by accelerated repair attempts, causing bone deformities and bowing, with associated fractures and pain.
M88.0 Osteitis deformans of skull
M88.1 Osteitis deformans of vertebrae

✓5th **M88.8** Osteitis deformans of other bones
✓6th **M88.81** Osteitis deformans of shoulder
M88.811 Osteitis deformans of right shoulder
M88.812 Osteitis deformans of left shoulder
M88.819 Osteitis deformans of unspecified shoulder
✓6th **M88.82** Osteitis deformans of upper arm
M88.821 Osteitis deformans of right upper arm
M88.822 Osteitis deformans of left upper arm
M88.829 Osteitis deformans of unspecified upper arm
✓6th **M88.83** Osteitis deformans of forearm
M88.831 Osteitis deformans of right forearm
M88.832 Osteitis deformans of left forearm
M88.839 Osteitis deformans of unspecified forearm
✓6th **M88.84** Osteitis deformans of hand
M88.841 Osteitis deformans of right hand
M88.842 Osteitis deformans of left hand
M88.849 Osteitis deformans of unspecified hand
✓6th **M88.85** Osteitis deformans of thigh
M88.851 Osteitis deformans of right thigh
M88.852 Osteitis deformans of left thigh
M88.859 Osteitis deformans of unspecified thigh
✓6th **M88.86** Osteitis deformans of lower leg
M88.861 Osteitis deformans of right lower leg
M88.862 Osteitis deformans of left lower leg
M88.869 Osteitis deformans of unspecified lower leg
✓6th **M88.87** Osteitis deformans of ankle and foot
M88.871 Osteitis deformans of right ankle and foot
M88.872 Osteitis deformans of left ankle and foot
M88.879 Osteitis deformans of unspecified ankle and foot
M88.88 Osteitis deformans of other bones
EXCLUDES 2 osteitis deformans of skull (M88.0)
osteitis deformans of vertebrae (M88.1)
M88.89 Osteitis deformans of multiple sites
M88.9 Osteitis deformans of unspecified bone

✓4th **M89** Other disorders of bone
✓5th **M89.0** Algoneurodystrophy
Shoulder-hand syndrome
Sudeck's atrophy
EXCLUDES 1 causalgia, lower limb (G57.7-)
causalgia, upper limb (G56.4-)
complex regional pain syndrome II, lower limb (G57.7-)
complex regional pain syndrome II, upper limb (G56.4-)
reflex sympathetic dystrophy (G90.5-)
M89.00 Algoneurodystrophy, unspecified site
✓6th **M89.01** Algoneurodystrophy, shoulder
M89.011 Algoneurodystrophy, right shoulder
M89.012 Algoneurodystrophy, left shoulder
M89.019 Algoneurodystrophy, unspecified shoulder
✓6th **M89.02** Algoneurodystrophy, upper arm
M89.021 Algoneurodystrophy, right upper arm
M89.022 Algoneurodystrophy, left upper arm
M89.029 Algoneurodystrophy, unspecified upper arm
✓6th **M89.03** Algoneurodystrophy, forearm
M89.031 Algoneurodystrophy, right forearm
M89.032 Algoneurodystrophy, left forearm
M89.039 Algoneurodystrophy, unspecified forearm
✓6th **M89.04** Algoneurodystrophy, hand
M89.041 Algoneurodystrophy, right hand
M89.042 Algoneurodystrophy, left hand
M89.049 Algoneurodystrophy, unspecified hand
✓6th **M89.05** Algoneurodystrophy, thigh
M89.051 Algoneurodystrophy, right thigh
M89.052 Algoneurodystrophy, left thigh
M89.059 Algoneurodystrophy, unspecified thigh

✓6ᵗʰ **M89.06 Algoneurodystrophy, lower leg**

     M89.061 Algoneurodystrophy, right lower leg

     M89.062 Algoneurodystrophy, left lower leg

     M89.069 Algoneurodystrophy, unspecified lower leg

✓6ᵗʰ **M89.07 Algoneurodystrophy, ankle and foot**

     M89.071 Algoneurodystrophy, right ankle and foot

     M89.072 Algoneurodystrophy, left ankle and foot

     M89.079 Algoneurodystrophy, unspecified ankle and foot

     M89.08 Algoneurodystrophy, other site

     M89.09 Algoneurodystrophy, multiple sites

✓5ᵗʰ **M89.1 Physeal arrest**

     Arrest of growth plate

     Epiphyseal arrest

     Growth plate arrest

✓6ᵗʰ **M89.12 Physeal arrest, humerus**

     M89.121 Complete physeal arrest, right proximal humerus

     M89.122 Complete physeal arrest, left proximal humerus

     M89.123 Partial physeal arrest, right proximal humerus

     M89.124 Partial physeal arrest, left proximal humerus

     M89.125 Complete physeal arrest, right distal humerus

     M89.126 Complete physeal arrest, left distal humerus

     M89.127 Partial physeal arrest, right distal humerus

     M89.128 Partial physeal arrest, left distal humerus

     M89.129 Physeal arrest, humerus, unspecified

✓6ᵗʰ **M89.13 Physeal arrest, forearm**

     M89.131 Complete physeal arrest, right distal radius

     M89.132 Complete physeal arrest, left distal radius

     M89.133 Partial physeal arrest, right distal radius

     M89.134 Partial physeal arrest, left distal radius

     M89.138 Other physeal arrest of forearm

     M89.139 Physeal arrest, forearm, unspecified

✓6ᵗʰ **M89.15 Physeal arrest, femur**

     M89.151 Complete physeal arrest, right proximal femur

     M89.152 Complete physeal arrest, left proximal femur

     M89.153 Partial physeal arrest, right proximal femur

     M89.154 Partial physeal arrest, left proximal femur

     M89.155 Complete physeal arrest, right distal femur

     M89.156 Complete physeal arrest, left distal femur

     M89.157 Partial physeal arrest, right distal femur

     M89.158 Partial physeal arrest, left distal femur

     M89.159 Physeal arrest, femur, unspecified

✓6ᵗʰ **M89.16 Physeal arrest, lower leg**

     M89.160 Complete physeal arrest, right proximal tibia

     M89.161 Complete physeal arrest, left proximal tibia

     M89.162 Partial physeal arrest, right proximal tibia

     M89.163 Partial physeal arrest, left proximal tibia

     M89.164 Complete physeal arrest, right distal tibia

     M89.165 Complete physeal arrest, left distal tibia

     M89.166 Partial physeal arrest, right distal tibia

     M89.167 Partial physeal arrest, left distal tibia

     M89.168 Other physeal arrest of lower leg

     M89.169 Physeal arrest, lower leg, unspecified

     M89.18 Physeal arrest, other site

✓5ᵗʰ **M89.2 Other disorders of bone development and growth**

     M89.20 Other disorders of bone development and growth, unspecified site

✓6ᵗʰ **M89.21 Other disorders of bone development and growth, shoulder**

     M89.211 Other disorders of bone development and growth, right shoulder

     M89.212 Other disorders of bone development and growth, left shoulder

     M89.219 Other disorders of bone development and growth, unspecified shoulder

✓6ᵗʰ **M89.22 Other disorders of bone development and growth, humerus**

     M89.221 Other disorders of bone development and growth, right humerus

     M89.222 Other disorders of bone development and growth, left humerus

     M89.229 Other disorders of bone development and growth, unspecified humerus

✓6ᵗʰ **M89.23 Other disorders of bone development and growth, ulna and radius**

     M89.231 Other disorders of bone development and growth, right ulna

     M89.232 Other disorders of bone development and growth, left ulna

     M89.233 Other disorders of bone development and growth, right radius

     M89.234 Other disorders of bone development and growth, left radius

     M89.239 Other disorders of bone development and growth, unspecified ulna and radius

✓6ᵗʰ **M89.24 Other disorders of bone development and growth, hand**

     M89.241 Other disorders of bone development and growth, right hand

     M89.242 Other disorders of bone development and growth, left hand

     M89.249 Other disorders of bone development and growth, unspecified hand

✓6ᵗʰ **M89.25 Other disorders of bone development and growth, femur**

     M89.251 Other disorders of bone development and growth, right femur

     M89.252 Other disorders of bone development and growth, left femur

     M89.259 Other disorders of bone development and growth, unspecified femur

✓6ᵗʰ **M89.26 Other disorders of bone development and growth, tibia and fibula**

     M89.261 Other disorders of bone development and growth, right tibia

     M89.262 Other disorders of bone development and growth, left tibia

     M89.263 Other disorders of bone development and growth, right fibula

     M89.264 Other disorders of bone development and growth, left fibula

     M89.269 Other disorders of bone development and growth, unspecified lower leg

✓6ᵗʰ **M89.27 Other disorders of bone development and growth, ankle and foot**

     M89.271 Other disorders of bone development and growth, right ankle and foot

     M89.272 Other disorders of bone development and growth, left ankle and foot

     M89.279 Other disorders of bone development and growth, unspecified ankle and foot

     M89.28 Other disorders of bone development and growth, other site

     M89.29 Other disorders of bone development and growth, multiple sites

✓5ᵗʰ **M89.3 Hypertrophy of bone**

     M89.30 Hypertrophy of bone, unspecified site

✓6ᵗʰ **M89.31 Hypertrophy of bone, shoulder**

     M89.311 Hypertrophy of bone, right shoulder

     M89.312 Hypertrophy of bone, left shoulder

     M89.319 Hypertrophy of bone, unspecified shoulder

✓6ᵗʰ **M89.32 Hypertrophy of bone, humerus**

     M89.321 Hypertrophy of bone, right humerus

     M89.322 Hypertrophy of bone, left humerus

     M89.329 Hypertrophy of bone, unspecified humerus

✓6ᵗʰ **M89.33 Hypertrophy of bone, ulna and radius**

     M89.331 Hypertrophy of bone, right ulna

     M89.332 Hypertrophy of bone, left ulna

     M89.333 Hypertrophy of bone, right radius

     M89.334 Hypertrophy of bone, left radius

     M89.339 Hypertrophy of bone, unspecified ulna and radius

✔ Additional Character Required   ✓x7ᵗʰ Placeholder   Unacceptable PDx   Questionable PDx   Manifestation   Unspecified Dx   H1–H14 HAC   HCC CMS-HCC Dx   HIV HIV Dx

ICD-10-CM 2021   831

√6ᵗʰ **M89.34** **Hypertrophy of bone,** hand

     M89.341 **Hypertrophy of bone, right** hand
     M89.342 **Hypertrophy of bone, left** hand
     M89.349 **Hypertrophy of bone, unspecified hand**

√6ᵗʰ **M89.35** **Hypertrophy of bone,** femur

     M89.351 **Hypertrophy of bone, right** femur
     M89.352 **Hypertrophy of bone, left** femur
     M89.359 **Hypertrophy of bone, unspecified femur**

√6ᵗʰ **M89.36** **Hypertrophy of bone,** tibia and fibula

     M89.361 **Hypertrophy of bone, right** tibia
     M89.362 **Hypertrophy of bone, left** tibia
     M89.363 **Hypertrophy of bone, right** fibula
     M89.364 **Hypertrophy of bone, left** fibula
     M89.369 **Hypertrophy of bone, unspecified tibia and fibula**

√6ᵗʰ **M89.37** **Hypertrophy of bone,** ankle and foot

     M89.371 **Hypertrophy of bone, right** ankle and foot
     M89.372 **Hypertrophy of bone, left** ankle and foot
     M89.379 **Hypertrophy of bone, unspecified ankle and foot**

     M89.38 **Hypertrophy of bone, other site**

     M89.39 **Hypertrophy of bone,** multiple sites

√5ᵗʰ **M89.4** **Other hypertrophic osteoarthropathy**

     Marie-Bamberger disease
     Pachydermoperiostosis

     M89.40 **Other hypertrophic osteoarthropathy, unspecified site**

√6ᵗʰ **M89.41** **Other hypertrophic osteoarthropathy,** shoulder

     M89.411 **Other hypertrophic osteoarthropathy, right shoulder**
     M89.412 **Other hypertrophic osteoarthropathy, left shoulder**
     M89.419 **Other hypertrophic osteoarthropathy, unspecified shoulder**

√6ᵗʰ **M89.42** **Other hypertrophic osteoarthropathy,** upper arm

     M89.421 **Other hypertrophic osteoarthropathy, right upper arm**
     M89.422 **Other hypertrophic osteoarthropathy, left upper arm**
     M89.429 **Other hypertrophic osteoarthropathy, unspecified upper arm**

√6ᵗʰ **M89.43** **Other hypertrophic osteoarthropathy,** forearm

     M89.431 **Other hypertrophic osteoarthropathy, right forearm**
     M89.432 **Other hypertrophic osteoarthropathy, left forearm**
     M89.439 **Other hypertrophic osteoarthropathy, unspecified forearm**

√6ᵗʰ **M89.44** **Other hypertrophic osteoarthropathy,** hand

     M89.441 **Other hypertrophic osteoarthropathy, right hand**
     M89.442 **Other hypertrophic osteoarthropathy, left hand**
     M89.449 **Other hypertrophic osteoarthropathy, unspecified hand**

√6ᵗʰ **M89.45** **Other hypertrophic osteoarthropathy,** thigh

     M89.451 **Other hypertrophic osteoarthropathy, right thigh**
     M89.452 **Other hypertrophic osteoarthropathy, left thigh**
     M89.459 **Other hypertrophic osteoarthropathy, unspecified thigh**

√6ᵗʰ **M89.46** **Other hypertrophic osteoarthropathy,** lower leg

     M89.461 **Other hypertrophic osteoarthropathy, right lower leg**
     M89.462 **Other hypertrophic osteoarthropathy, left lower leg**
     M89.469 **Other hypertrophic osteoarthropathy, unspecified lower leg**

√6ᵗʰ **M89.47** **Other hypertrophic osteoarthropathy,** ankle and foot

     M89.471 **Other hypertrophic osteoarthropathy, right ankle and foot**
     M89.472 **Other hypertrophic osteoarthropathy, left ankle and foot**
     M89.479 **Other hypertrophic osteoarthropathy, unspecified ankle and foot**

     M89.48 **Other hypertrophic osteoarthropathy, other site**

     M89.49 **Other hypertrophic osteoarthropathy,** multiple sites

√5ᵗʰ **M89.5** **Osteolysis**

     Use additional code to identify major osseous defect, if applicable (M89.7-)

     EXCLUDES 2   *periprosthetic osteolysis of internal prosthetic joint (T84.Ø5-)*

     M89.50 **Osteolysis, unspecified site**

√6ᵗʰ **M89.51** **Osteolysis,** shoulder

     M89.511 **Osteolysis, right shoulder**
     M89.512 **Osteolysis, left shoulder**
     M89.519 **Osteolysis, unspecified shoulder**

√6ᵗʰ **M89.52** **Osteolysis,** upper arm

     M89.521 **Osteolysis, right upper arm**
     M89.522 **Osteolysis, left upper arm**
     M89.529 **Osteolysis, unspecified upper arm**

√6ᵗʰ **M89.53** **Osteolysis,** forearm

     M89.531 **Osteolysis, right forearm**
     M89.532 **Osteolysis, left forearm**
     M89.539 **Osteolysis, unspecified forearm**

√6ᵗʰ **M89.54** **Osteolysis,** hand

     M89.541 **Osteolysis, right hand**
     M89.542 **Osteolysis, left hand**
     M89.549 **Osteolysis, unspecified hand**

√6ᵗʰ **M89.55** **Osteolysis,** thigh

     M89.551 **Osteolysis, right thigh**
     M89.552 **Osteolysis, left thigh**
     M89.559 **Osteolysis, unspecified thigh**

√6ᵗʰ **M89.56** **Osteolysis,** lower leg

     M89.561 **Osteolysis, right lower leg**
     M89.562 **Osteolysis, left lower leg**
     M89.569 **Osteolysis, unspecified lower leg**

√6ᵗʰ **M89.57** **Osteolysis,** ankle and foot

     M89.571 **Osteolysis, right ankle and foot**
     M89.572 **Osteolysis, left ankle and foot**
     M89.579 **Osteolysis, unspecified ankle and foot**

     M89.58 **Osteolysis, other site**

     M89.59 **Osteolysis,** multiple sites

√5ᵗʰ **M89.6** **Osteopathy after poliomyelitis**

     Use additional code (B91) to identify previous poliomyelitis

     EXCLUDES 1   *postpolio syndrome (G14)*

     M89.60 **Osteopathy after poliomyelitis, unspecified site** HCC

√6ᵗʰ **M89.61** **Osteopathy after poliomyelitis,** shoulder

     M89.611 **Osteopathy after poliomyelitis, right shoulder** HCC
     M89.612 **Osteopathy after poliomyelitis, left shoulder** HCC
     M89.619 **Osteopathy after poliomyelitis, unspecified shoulder** HCC

√6ᵗʰ **M89.62** **Osteopathy after poliomyelitis,** upper arm

     M89.621 **Osteopathy after poliomyelitis, right upper arm** HCC
     M89.622 **Osteopathy after poliomyelitis, left upper arm** HCC
     M89.629 **Osteopathy after poliomyelitis, unspecified upper arm** HCC

√6ᵗʰ **M89.63** **Osteopathy after poliomyelitis,** forearm

     M89.631 **Osteopathy after poliomyelitis, right forearm** HCC
     M89.632 **Osteopathy after poliomyelitis, left forearm** HCC
     M89.639 **Osteopathy after poliomyelitis, unspecified forearm** HCC

√6ᵗʰ **M89.64** **Osteopathy after poliomyelitis,** hand

     M89.641 **Osteopathy after poliomyelitis, right hand** HCC
     M89.642 **Osteopathy after poliomyelitis, left hand** HCC
     M89.649 **Osteopathy after poliomyelitis, unspecified hand** HCC

√6ᵗʰ **M89.65** **Osteopathy after poliomyelitis,** thigh

     M89.651 **Osteopathy after poliomyelitis, right thigh** HCC
     M89.652 **Osteopathy after poliomyelitis, left thigh** HCC

M89.659 Osteopathy after poliomyelitis, unspecified thigh **HCC**

✓6th M89.66 Osteopathy after poliomyelitis, lower leg

M89.661 Osteopathy after poliomyelitis, right lower leg **HCC**

M89.662 Osteopathy after poliomyelitis, left lower leg **HCC**

M89.669 Osteopathy after poliomyelitis, unspecified lower leg **HCC**

✓6th M89.67 Osteopathy after poliomyelitis, ankle and foot

M89.671 Osteopathy after poliomyelitis, right ankle and foot **HCC**

M89.672 Osteopathy after poliomyelitis, left ankle and foot **HCC**

M89.679 Osteopathy after poliomyelitis, unspecified ankle and foot **HCC**

M89.68 Osteopathy after poliomyelitis, other site **HCC**

M89.69 Osteopathy after poliomyelitis, multiple sites **HCC**

✓5th M89.7 Major osseous defect

Code first underlying disease, if known, such as:
aseptic necrosis of bone (M87.-)
malignant neoplasm of bone (C40.-)
osteolysis (M89.5)
osteomyelitis (M86.-)
osteonecrosis (M87.-)
osteoporosis (M80.-, M81.-)
periprosthetic osteolysis (T84.05-)

M89.70 Major osseous defect, unspecified site

✓6th M89.71 Major osseous defect, shoulder region

Major osseous defect clavicle or scapula

M89.711 Major osseous defect, right shoulder region

M89.712 Major osseous defect, left shoulder region

M89.719 Major osseous defect, unspecified shoulder region

✓6th M89.72 Major osseous defect, humerus

M89.721 Major osseous defect, right humerus

M89.722 Major osseous defect, left humerus

M89.729 Major osseous defect, unspecified humerus

✓6th M89.73 Major osseous defect, forearm

Major osseous defect of radius and ulna

M89.731 Major osseous defect, right forearm

M89.732 Major osseous defect, left forearm

M89.739 Major osseous defect, unspecified forearm

✓6th M89.74 Major osseous defect, hand

Major osseous defect of carpus, fingers, metacarpus

M89.741 Major osseous defect, right hand

M89.742 Major osseous defect, left hand

M89.749 Major osseous defect, unspecified hand

✓6th M89.75 Major osseous defect, pelvic region and thigh

Major osseous defect of femur and pelvis

M89.751 Major osseous defect, right pelvic region and thigh

M89.752 Major osseous defect, left pelvic region and thigh

M89.759 Major osseous defect, unspecified pelvic region and thigh

✓6th M89.76 Major osseous defect, lower leg

Major osseous defect of fibula and tibia

M89.761 Major osseous defect, right lower leg

M89.762 Major osseous defect, left lower leg

M89.769 Major osseous defect, unspecified lower leg

✓6th M89.77 Major osseous defect, ankle and foot

Major osseous defect of metatarsus, tarsus, toes

M89.771 Major osseous defect, right ankle and foot

M89.772 Major osseous defect, left ankle and foot

M89.779 Major osseous defect, unspecified ankle and foot

M89.78 Major osseous defect, other site

M89.79 Major osseous defect, multiple sites

✓5th M89.8 Other specified disorders of bone

Infantile cortical hyperostoses
Post-traumatic subperiosteal ossification

✓6th M89.8X Other specified disorders of bone

M89.8X0 Other specified disorders of bone, multiple sites

M89.8X1 Other specified disorders of bone, shoulder

M89.8X2 Other specified disorders of bone, upper arm

M89.8X3 Other specified disorders of bone, forearm
    AHA: 2019,3Q,9

M89.8X4 Other specified disorders of bone, hand

M89.8X5 Other specified disorders of bone, thigh

M89.8X6 Other specified disorders of bone, lower leg

M89.8X7 Other specified disorders of bone, ankle and foot

M89.8X8 Other specified disorders of bone, other site

M89.8X9 Other specified disorders of bone, unspecified site

M89.9 Disorder of bone, unspecified

✓4th **M90** Osteopathies in diseases classified elsewhere

EXCLUDES 1   osteochondritis, osteomyelitis, and osteopathy (in):
cryptococcosis (B45.3)
diabetes mellitus (E08-E13 with .69-)
gonococcal (A54.43)
neurogenic syphilis (A52.11)
renal osteodystrophy (N25.0)
salmonellosis (A02.24)
secondary syphilis (A51.46)
syphilis (late) (A52.77)

✓5th M90.5 Osteonecrosis in diseases classified elsewhere

Code first underlying disease, such as:
caisson disease (T70.3)
hemoglobinopathy (D50-D64)

M90.50 Osteonecrosis in diseases classified elsewhere, unspecified site **CC** **HCC**

✓6th M90.51 Osteonecrosis in diseases classified elsewhere, shoulder

M90.511 Osteonecrosis in diseases classified elsewhere, right shoulder **CC** **HCC**

M90.512 Osteonecrosis in diseases classified elsewhere, left shoulder **CC** **HCC**

M90.519 Osteonecrosis in diseases classified elsewhere, unspecified shoulder **CC** **HCC**

✓6th M90.52 Osteonecrosis in diseases classified elsewhere, upper arm

M90.521 Osteonecrosis in diseases classified elsewhere, right upper arm **CC** **HCC**

M90.522 Osteonecrosis in diseases classified elsewhere, left upper arm **CC** **HCC**

M90.529 Osteonecrosis in diseases classified elsewhere, unspecified upper arm **CC** **HCC**

✓6th M90.53 Osteonecrosis in diseases classified elsewhere, forearm

M90.531 Osteonecrosis in diseases classified elsewhere, right forearm **CC** **HCC**

M90.532 Osteonecrosis in diseases classified elsewhere, left forearm **CC** **HCC**

M90.539 Osteonecrosis in diseases classified elsewhere, unspecified forearm **CC** **HCC**

✓6th M90.54 Osteonecrosis in diseases classified elsewhere, hand

M90.541 Osteonecrosis in diseases classified elsewhere, right hand **CC** **HCC**

M90.542 Osteonecrosis in diseases classified elsewhere, left hand **CC** **HCC**

M90.549 Osteonecrosis in diseases classified elsewhere, unspecified hand **CC** **HCC**

✓6th M90.55 Osteonecrosis in diseases classified elsewhere, thigh

M90.551 Osteonecrosis in diseases classified elsewhere, right thigh **CC** **HCC**

M90.552 Osteonecrosis in diseases classified elsewhere, left thigh **CC** **HCC**

✅ Additional Character Required   ✓x7th Placeholder   Unacceptable PDx   Questionable PDx   Manifestation   Unspecified Dx   **H1**-**H4** HAC   **HCC** CMS-HCC Dx   **HIV** HIV Dx

ICD-10-CM 2021   833

M90.559 Osteonecrosis in diseases classified elsewhere, unspecified thigh `CC` `HCC`

✓6ᵗʰ M90.56 Osteonecrosis in diseases classified elsewhere, lower leg

    M90.561 Osteonecrosis in diseases classified elsewhere, right lower leg `CC` `HCC`

    M90.562 Osteonecrosis in diseases classified elsewhere, left lower leg `CC` `HCC`

    M90.569 Osteonecrosis in diseases classified elsewhere, unspecified lower leg `CC` `HCC`

✓6ᵗʰ M90.57 Osteonecrosis in diseases classified elsewhere, ankle and foot

    M90.571 Osteonecrosis in diseases classified elsewhere, right ankle and foot `CC` `HCC`

    M90.572 Osteonecrosis in diseases classified elsewhere, left ankle and foot `CC` `HCC`

    M90.579 Osteonecrosis in diseases classified elsewhere, unspecified ankle and foot `CC` `HCC`

M90.58 Osteonecrosis in diseases classified elsewhere, other site `CC` `HCC`

M90.59 Osteonecrosis in diseases classified elsewhere, multiple sites `CC` `HCC`

✓5ᵗʰ M90.6 Osteitis deformans in neoplastic diseases

Osteitis deformans in malignant neoplasm of bone
Code first the neoplasm (C40.-, C41.-)

EXCLUDES 1   osteitis deformans [Paget's disease of bone] (M88.-)

M90.60 Osteitis deformans in neoplastic diseases, unspecified site

✓6ᵗʰ M90.61 Osteitis deformans in neoplastic diseases, shoulder

    M90.611 Osteitis deformans in neoplastic diseases, right shoulder

    M90.612 Osteitis deformans in neoplastic diseases, left shoulder

    M90.619 Osteitis deformans in neoplastic diseases, unspecified shoulder

✓6ᵗʰ M90.62 Osteitis deformans in neoplastic diseases, upper arm

    M90.621 Osteitis deformans in neoplastic diseases, right upper arm

    M90.622 Osteitis deformans in neoplastic diseases, left upper arm

    M90.629 Osteitis deformans in neoplastic diseases, unspecified upper arm

✓6ᵗʰ M90.63 Osteitis deformans in neoplastic diseases, forearm

    M90.631 Osteitis deformans in neoplastic diseases, right forearm

    M90.632 Osteitis deformans in neoplastic diseases, left forearm

    M90.639 Osteitis deformans in neoplastic diseases, unspecified forearm

✓6ᵗʰ M90.64 Osteitis deformans in neoplastic diseases, hand

    M90.641 Osteitis deformans in neoplastic diseases, right hand

    M90.642 Osteitis deformans in neoplastic diseases, left hand

    M90.649 Osteitis deformans in neoplastic diseases, unspecified hand

✓6ᵗʰ M90.65 Osteitis deformans in neoplastic diseases, thigh

    M90.651 Osteitis deformans in neoplastic diseases, right thigh

    M90.652 Osteitis deformans in neoplastic diseases, left thigh

    M90.659 Osteitis deformans in neoplastic diseases, unspecified thigh

✓6ᵗʰ M90.66 Osteitis deformans in neoplastic diseases, lower leg

    M90.661 Osteitis deformans in neoplastic diseases, right lower leg

    M90.662 Osteitis deformans in neoplastic diseases, left lower leg

    M90.669 Osteitis deformans in neoplastic diseases, unspecified lower leg

✓6ᵗʰ M90.67 Osteitis deformans in neoplastic diseases, ankle and foot

    M90.671 Osteitis deformans in neoplastic diseases, right ankle and foot

    M90.672 Osteitis deformans in neoplastic diseases, left ankle and foot

    M90.679 Osteitis deformans in neoplastic diseases, unspecified ankle and foot

M90.68 Osteitis deformans in neoplastic diseases, other site

M90.69 Osteitis deformans in neoplastic diseases, multiple sites

✓5ᵗʰ M90.8 Osteopathy in diseases classified elsewhere

Code first underlying disease, such as:
   rickets (E55.0)
   vitamin-D-resistant rickets (E83.3)

M90.80 Osteopathy in diseases classified elsewhere, unspecified site

✓6ᵗʰ M90.81 Osteopathy in diseases classified elsewhere, shoulder

    M90.811 Osteopathy in diseases classified elsewhere, right shoulder

    M90.812 Osteopathy in diseases classified elsewhere, left shoulder

    M90.819 Osteopathy in diseases classified elsewhere, unspecified shoulder

✓6ᵗʰ M90.82 Osteopathy in diseases classified elsewhere, upper arm

    M90.821 Osteopathy in diseases classified elsewhere, right upper arm

    M90.822 Osteopathy in diseases classified elsewhere, left upper arm

    M90.829 Osteopathy in diseases classified elsewhere, unspecified upper arm

✓6ᵗʰ M90.83 Osteopathy in diseases classified elsewhere, forearm

    M90.831 Osteopathy in diseases classified elsewhere, right forearm

    M90.832 Osteopathy in diseases classified elsewhere, left forearm

    M90.839 Osteopathy in diseases classified elsewhere, unspecified forearm

✓6ᵗʰ M90.84 Osteopathy in diseases classified elsewhere, hand

    M90.841 Osteopathy in diseases classified elsewhere, right hand

    M90.842 Osteopathy in diseases classified elsewhere, left hand

    M90.849 Osteopathy in diseases classified elsewhere, unspecified hand

✓6ᵗʰ M90.85 Osteopathy in diseases classified elsewhere, thigh

    M90.851 Osteopathy in diseases classified elsewhere, right thigh

    M90.852 Osteopathy in diseases classified elsewhere, left thigh

    M90.859 Osteopathy in diseases classified elsewhere, unspecified thigh

✓6ᵗʰ M90.86 Osteopathy in diseases classified elsewhere, lower leg

    M90.861 Osteopathy in diseases classified elsewhere, right lower leg

    M90.862 Osteopathy in diseases classified elsewhere, left lower leg

    M90.869 Osteopathy in diseases classified elsewhere, unspecified lower leg

✓6ᵗʰ M90.87 Osteopathy in diseases classified elsewhere, ankle and foot

    M90.871 Osteopathy in diseases classified elsewhere, right ankle and foot

    M90.872 Osteopathy in diseases classified elsewhere, left ankle and foot

    M90.879 Osteopathy in diseases classified elsewhere, unspecified ankle and foot

M90.88 Osteopathy in diseases classified elsewhere, other site

M90.89 Osteopathy in diseases classified elsewhere, multiple sites

Chondropathies (M91-M94)

EXCLUDES 1   postprocedural chondropathies (M96.-)

✓4ᵗʰ M91 Juvenile osteochondrosis of hip and pelvis

EXCLUDES 1   slipped upper femoral epiphysis (nontraumatic) (M93.0)

M91.0 Juvenile osteochondrosis of pelvis

Osteochondrosis (juvenile) of acetabulum
Osteochondrosis (juvenile) of iliac crest [Buchanan]
Osteochondrosis (juvenile) of ischiopubic synchondrosis [van Neck]
Osteochondrosis (juvenile) of symphysis pubis [Pierson]

N Newborn: 0   P Pediatric: 0-17   M Maternity: 9-64   A Adult: 15-124   MCC Major Complication/Comorbidity   CC Complication/Comorbidity   SW Severe Wound Dx

834   ICD-10-CM 2021

√5ᵗʰ **M91.1** Juvenile osteochondrosis of **head of femur [Legg-Calvé-Perthes]**
- **M91.10** Juvenile osteochondrosis of head of femur [Legg-Calvé-Perthes], unspecified leg
- **M91.11** Juvenile osteochondrosis of head of femur [Legg-Calvé-Perthes], right leg
- **M91.12** Juvenile osteochondrosis of head of femur [Legg-Calvé-Perthes], left leg

√5ᵗʰ **M91.2** **Coxa plana**

Hip deformity due to previous juvenile osteochondrosis
- **M91.20** Coxa plana, unspecified hip
- **M91.21** Coxa plana, right hip
- **M91.22** Coxa plana, left hip

√5ᵗʰ **M91.3** **Pseudocoxalgia**
- **M91.30** Pseudocoxalgia, unspecified hip
- **M91.31** Pseudocoxalgia, right hip
- **M91.32** Pseudocoxalgia, left hip

√5ᵗʰ **M91.4** **Coxa magna**
- **M91.40** Coxa magna, unspecified hip
- **M91.41** Coxa magna, right hip
- **M91.42** Coxa magna, left hip

√5ᵗʰ **M91.8** Other juvenile osteochondrosis of hip and pelvis

Juvenile osteochondrosis after reduction of congenital dislocation of hip
- **M91.80** Other juvenile osteochondrosis of hip and pelvis, unspecified leg
- **M91.81** Other juvenile osteochondrosis of hip and pelvis, right leg
- **M91.82** Other juvenile osteochondrosis of hip and pelvis, left leg

√5ᵗʰ **M91.9** Juvenile osteochondrosis of hip and pelvis, unspecified
- **M91.90** Juvenile osteochondrosis of hip and pelvis, unspecified, unspecified leg
- **M91.91** Juvenile osteochondrosis of hip and pelvis, unspecified, right leg
- **M91.92** Juvenile osteochondrosis of hip and pelvis, unspecified, left leg

√4ᵗʰ **M92** **Other juvenile osteochondrosis**

√5ᵗʰ **M92.0** Juvenile osteochondrosis of **humerus**

Osteochondrosis (juvenile) of capitulum of humerus [Panner]
Osteochondrosis (juvenile) of head of humerus [Haas]
- **M92.00** Juvenile osteochondrosis of humerus, unspecified arm
- **M92.01** Juvenile osteochondrosis of humerus, right arm
- **M92.02** Juvenile osteochondrosis of humerus, left arm

√5ᵗʰ **M92.1** Juvenile osteochondrosis of **radius and ulna**

Osteochondrosis (juvenile) of lower ulna [Burns]
Osteochondrosis (juvenile) of radial head [Brailsford]
- **M92.10** Juvenile osteochondrosis of radius and ulna, unspecified arm
- **M92.11** Juvenile osteochondrosis of radius and ulna, right arm
- **M92.12** Juvenile osteochondrosis of radius and ulna, left arm

√5ᵗʰ **M92.2** Juvenile osteochondrosis, **hand**

√6ᵗʰ **M92.20** Unspecified juvenile osteochondrosis, **hand**
- **M92.201** Unspecified juvenile osteochondrosis, right hand
- **M92.202** Unspecified juvenile osteochondrosis, left hand
- **M92.209** Unspecified juvenile osteochondrosis, unspecified hand

√6ᵗʰ **M92.21** Osteochondrosis (juvenile) of **carpal lunate [Kienböck]**
- **M92.211** Osteochondrosis (juvenile) of carpal lunate [Kienböck], right hand
- **M92.212** Osteochondrosis (juvenile) of carpal lunate [Kienböck], left hand
- **M92.219** Osteochondrosis (juvenile) of carpal lunate [Kienböck], unspecified hand

√6ᵗʰ **M92.22** Osteochondrosis (juvenile) of **metacarpal heads [Mauclaire]**
- **M92.221** Osteochondrosis (juvenile) of metacarpal heads [Mauclaire], right hand
- **M92.222** Osteochondrosis (juvenile) of metacarpal heads [Mauclaire], left hand
- **M92.229** Osteochondrosis (juvenile) of metacarpal heads [Mauclaire], unspecified hand

√6ᵗʰ **M92.29** Other juvenile osteochondrosis, **hand**
- **M92.291** Other juvenile osteochondrosis, right hand
- **M92.292** Other juvenile osteochondrosis, left hand
- **M92.299** Other juvenile osteochondrosis, unspecified hand

√5ᵗʰ **M92.3** Other juvenile osteochondrosis, **upper limb**
- **M92.30** Other juvenile osteochondrosis, unspecified upper limb
- **M92.31** Other juvenile osteochondrosis, right upper limb
- **M92.32** Other juvenile osteochondrosis, left upper limb

√5ᵗʰ **M92.4** Juvenile osteochondrosis of **patella**

Osteochondrosis (juvenile) of primary patellar center [Köhler]
Osteochondrosis (juvenile) of secondary patellar centre [Sinding Larsen]
- **M92.40** Juvenile osteochondrosis of patella, unspecified knee
- **M92.41** Juvenile osteochondrosis of patella, right knee
- **M92.42** Juvenile osteochondrosis of patella, left knee

√5ᵗʰ **M92.5** Juvenile osteochondrosis of **tibia and fibula**

~~Osteochondrosis (juvenile) of proximal tibia [Blount]~~
~~Osteochondrosis (juvenile) of tibial tubercle [Osgood-Schlatter]~~
~~Tibia vara~~

▲ √6ᵗʰ **M92.50** Unspecified juvenile osteochondrosis of tibia and fibula
- ● **M92.501** Unspecified juvenile osteochondrosis, right leg
- ● **M92.502** Unspecified juvenile osteochondrosis, left leg
- ● **M92.503** Unspecified juvenile osteochondrosis, bilateral leg
- ● **M92.509** Unspecified juvenile osteochondrosis, unspecified leg

▲ √6ᵗʰ **M92.51** Juvenile osteochondrosis of **proximal tibia**

▶Blount disease◀
▶Tibia vara◀
- **M92.511** Juvenile osteochondrosis of proximal tibia, right leg
- **M92.512** Juvenile osteochondrosis of proximal tibia, left leg
- **M92.513** Juvenile osteochondrosis of proximal tibia, bilateral
- **M92.519** Juvenile osteochondrosis of proximal tibia, unspecified leg

▲ √6ᵗʰ **M92.52** Juvenile osteochondrosis of **tibia tubercle**

▶Osgood-Schlatter disease◀
- **M92.521** Juvenile osteochondrosis of tibia tubercle, right leg
- **M92.522** Juvenile osteochondrosis of tibia tubercle, left leg
- **M92.523** Juvenile osteochondrosis of tibia tubercle, bilateral
- **M92.529** Juvenile osteochondrosis of tibia tubercle, unspecified leg

√6ᵗʰ **M92.59** Other juvenile osteochondrosis of tibia and fibula
- **M92.591** Other juvenile osteochondrosis of tibia and fibula, right leg
- **M92.592** Other juvenile osteochondrosis of tibia and fibula, left leg
- **M92.593** Other juvenile osteochondrosis of tibia and fibula, bilateral
- **M92.599** Other juvenile osteochondrosis of tibia and fibula, unspecified leg

√5ᵗʰ **M92.6** Juvenile osteochondrosis of **tarsus**

Osteochondrosis (juvenile) of calcaneum [Sever]
Osteochondrosis (juvenile) of os tibiale externum [Haglund]
Osteochondrosis (juvenile) of talus [Diaz]
Osteochondrosis (juvenile) of tarsal navicular [Köhler]
- **M92.60** Juvenile osteochondrosis of tarsus, unspecified ankle
- **M92.61** Juvenile osteochondrosis of tarsus, right ankle
- **M92.62** Juvenile osteochondrosis of tarsus, left ankle

√5ᵗʰ **M92.7** Juvenile osteochondrosis of **metatarsus**

Osteochondrosis (juvenile) of fifth metatarsus [Iselin]
Osteochondrosis (juvenile) of second metatarsus [Freiberg]
- **M92.70** Juvenile osteochondrosis of metatarsus, unspecified foot
- **M92.71** Juvenile osteochondrosis of metatarsus, right foot
- **M92.72** Juvenile osteochondrosis of metatarsus, left foot

---

☑ Additional Character Required √x7ᵗʰ Placeholder Unacceptable PDx Questionable PDx Manifestation Unspecified Dx **H1**-**H14** HAC **HCC** CMS-HCC Dx **HIV** HIV Dx

M92.8 Other specified juvenile osteochondrosis
Calcaneal apophysitis
DEF: Calcaneal apophysitis: Inflammation of the calcaneus at the point of Achilles tendon insertion usually occurring in boys ages 8 to 14. Pain, tenderness, and localized swelling are present.

M92.9 Juvenile osteochondrosis, unspecified
Juvenile apophysitis NOS
Juvenile epiphysitis NOS
Juvenile osteochondritis NOS
Juvenile osteochondrosis NOS

✓4th **M93 Other osteochondropathies**
EXCLUDES 2 osteochondrosis of spine (M42.-)

✓5th **M93.0 Slipped upper femoral epiphysis (nontraumatic)**
Use additional code for associated chondrolysis (M94.3)

✓6th **M93.00 Unspecified slipped upper femoral epiphysis (nontraumatic)**
M93.001 Unspecified slipped upper femoral epiphysis (nontraumatic), right hip
M93.002 Unspecified slipped upper femoral epiphysis (nontraumatic), left hip
M93.003 Unspecified slipped upper femoral epiphysis (nontraumatic), unspecified hip

✓6th **M93.01 Acute slipped upper femoral epiphysis (nontraumatic)**
M93.011 Acute slipped upper femoral epiphysis (nontraumatic), right hip
M93.012 Acute slipped upper femoral epiphysis (nontraumatic), left hip
M93.013 Acute slipped upper femoral epiphysis (nontraumatic), unspecified hip

✓6th **M93.02 Chronic slipped upper femoral epiphysis (nontraumatic)**
M93.021 Chronic slipped upper femoral epiphysis (nontraumatic), right hip
M93.022 Chronic slipped upper femoral epiphysis (nontraumatic), left hip
M93.023 Chronic slipped upper femoral epiphysis (nontraumatic), unspecified hip

✓6th **M93.03 Acute on chronic slipped upper femoral epiphysis (nontraumatic)**
M93.031 Acute on chronic slipped upper femoral epiphysis (nontraumatic), right hip
M93.032 Acute on chronic slipped upper femoral epiphysis (nontraumatic), left hip
M93.033 Acute on chronic slipped upper femoral epiphysis (nontraumatic), unspecified hip

M93.1 Kienböck's disease of adults A
Adult osteochondrosis of carpal lunates

✓5th **M93.2 Osteochondritis dissecans**
DEF: Avascular necrosis caused by lack of blood flow to the bone and cartilage of a joint causing the bone to die. This can result in splinters or pieces of cartilage breaking off in the joint.

M93.20 Osteochondritis dissecans of unspecified site

✓6th **M93.21 Osteochondritis dissecans of shoulder**
M93.211 Osteochondritis dissecans, right shoulder
M93.212 Osteochondritis dissecans, left shoulder
M93.219 Osteochondritis dissecans, unspecified shoulder

✓6th **M93.22 Osteochondritis dissecans of elbow**
M93.221 Osteochondritis dissecans, right elbow
M93.222 Osteochondritis dissecans, left elbow
M93.229 Osteochondritis dissecans, unspecified elbow

✓6th **M93.23 Osteochondritis dissecans of wrist**
M93.231 Osteochondritis dissecans, right wrist
M93.232 Osteochondritis dissecans, left wrist
M93.239 Osteochondritis dissecans, unspecified wrist

✓6th **M93.24 Osteochondritis dissecans of joints of hand**
M93.241 Osteochondritis dissecans, joints of right hand
M93.242 Osteochondritis dissecans, joints of left hand
M93.249 Osteochondritis dissecans, joints of unspecified hand

✓6th **M93.25 Osteochondritis dissecans of hip**
M93.251 Osteochondritis dissecans, right hip
M93.252 Osteochondritis dissecans, left hip
M93.259 Osteochondritis dissecans, unspecified hip

✓6th **M93.26 Osteochondritis dissecans knee**
M93.261 Osteochondritis dissecans, right knee
M93.262 Osteochondritis dissecans, left knee
M93.269 Osteochondritis dissecans, unspecified knee

✓6th **M93.27 Osteochondritis dissecans of ankle and joints of foot**
M93.271 Osteochondritis dissecans, right ankle and joints of right foot
M93.272 Osteochondritis dissecans, left ankle and joints of left foot
M93.279 Osteochondritis dissecans, unspecified ankle and joints of foot

M93.28 Osteochondritis dissecans other site
M93.29 Osteochondritis dissecans multiple sites

✓5th **M93.8 Other specified osteochondropathies**

M93.80 Other specified osteochondropathies of unspecified site

✓6th **M93.81 Other specified osteochondropathies of shoulder**
M93.811 Other specified osteochondropathies, right shoulder
M93.812 Other specified osteochondropathies, left shoulder
M93.819 Other specified osteochondropathies, unspecified shoulder

✓6th **M93.82 Other specified osteochondropathies of upper arm**
M93.821 Other specified osteochondropathies, right upper arm
M93.822 Other specified osteochondropathies, left upper arm
M93.829 Other specified osteochondropathies, unspecified upper arm

✓6th **M93.83 Other specified osteochondropathies of forearm**
M93.831 Other specified osteochondropathies, right forearm
M93.832 Other specified osteochondropathies, left forearm
M93.839 Other specified osteochondropathies, unspecified forearm

✓6th **M93.84 Other specified osteochondropathies of hand**
M93.841 Other specified osteochondropathies, right hand
M93.842 Other specified osteochondropathies, left hand
M93.849 Other specified osteochondropathies, unspecified hand

✓6th **M93.85 Other specified osteochondropathies of thigh**
M93.851 Other specified osteochondropathies, right thigh
M93.852 Other specified osteochondropathies, left thigh
M93.859 Other specified osteochondropathies, unspecified thigh

✓6th **M93.86 Other specified osteochondropathies lower leg**
M93.861 Other specified osteochondropathies, right lower leg
M93.862 Other specified osteochondropathies, left lower leg
M93.869 Other specified osteochondropathies, unspecified lower leg

✓6th **M93.87 Other specified osteochondropathies of ankle and foot**
M93.871 Other specified osteochondropathies, right ankle and foot
M93.872 Other specified osteochondropathies, left ankle and foot
M93.879 Other specified osteochondropathies, unspecified ankle and foot

M93.88 Other specified osteochondropathies other site
M93.89 Other specified osteochondropathies multiple sites

✓5th **M93.9 Osteochondropathy, unspecified**
Apophysitis NOS
Epiphysitis NOS
Osteochondritis NOS
Osteochondrosis NOS
M93.90 Osteochondropathy, unspecified of unspecified site

✓6ᵗʰ **M93.91** Osteochondropathy, unspecified of shoulder

     M93.911 Osteochondropathy, unspecified, right shoulder

     M93.912 Osteochondropathy, unspecified, left shoulder

     M93.919 Osteochondropathy, unspecified, unspecified shoulder

✓6ᵗʰ **M93.92** Osteochondropathy, unspecified of upper arm

     M93.921 Osteochondropathy, unspecified, right upper arm

     M93.922 Osteochondropathy, unspecified, left upper arm

     M93.929 Osteochondropathy, unspecified, unspecified upper arm

✓6ᵗʰ **M93.93** Osteochondropathy, unspecified of forearm

     M93.931 Osteochondropathy, unspecified, right forearm

     M93.932 Osteochondropathy, unspecified, left forearm

     M93.939 Osteochondropathy, unspecified, unspecified forearm

✓6ᵗʰ **M93.94** Osteochondropathy, unspecified of hand

     M93.941 Osteochondropathy, unspecified, right hand

     M93.942 Osteochondropathy, unspecified, left hand

     M93.949 Osteochondropathy, unspecified, unspecified hand

✓6ᵗʰ **M93.95** Osteochondropathy, unspecified of thigh

     M93.951 Osteochondropathy, unspecified, right thigh

     M93.952 Osteochondropathy, unspecified, left thigh

     M93.959 Osteochondropathy, unspecified, unspecified thigh

✓6ᵗʰ **M93.96** Osteochondropathy, unspecified lower leg

     M93.961 Osteochondropathy, unspecified, right lower leg

     M93.962 Osteochondropathy, unspecified, left lower leg

     M93.969 Osteochondropathy, unspecified, unspecified lower leg

✓6ᵗʰ **M93.97** Osteochondropathy, unspecified of ankle and foot

     M93.971 Osteochondropathy, unspecified, right ankle and foot

     M93.972 Osteochondropathy, unspecified, left ankle and foot

     M93.979 Osteochondropathy, unspecified, unspecified ankle and foot

M93.98 Osteochondropathy, unspecified other site

M93.99 Osteochondropathy, unspecified multiple sites

✓4ᵗʰ **M94** **Other disorders of cartilage**

M94.0 **Chondrocostal junction syndrome [Tietze]**
Costochondritis

M94.1 **Relapsing polychondritis**

✓5ᵗʰ **M94.2** **Chondromalacia**

     EXCLUDES 1   chondromalacia patellae (M22.4)

     M94.20 Chondromalacia, unspecified site

✓6ᵗʰ **M94.21** Chondromalacia, shoulder

     M94.211 Chondromalacia, right shoulder

     M94.212 Chondromalacia, left shoulder

     M94.219 Chondromalacia, unspecified shoulder

✓6ᵗʰ **M94.22** Chondromalacia, elbow

     M94.221 Chondromalacia, right elbow

     M94.222 Chondromalacia, left elbow

     M94.229 Chondromalacia, unspecified elbow

✓6ᵗʰ **M94.23** Chondromalacia, wrist

     M94.231 Chondromalacia, right wrist

     M94.232 Chondromalacia, left wrist

     M94.239 Chondromalacia, unspecified wrist

✓6ᵗʰ **M94.24** Chondromalacia, joints of hand

     M94.241 Chondromalacia, joints of right hand

     M94.242 Chondromalacia, joints of left hand

     M94.249 Chondromalacia, joints of unspecified hand

✓6ᵗʰ **M94.25** Chondromalacia, hip

     M94.251 Chondromalacia, right hip

     M94.252 Chondromalacia, left hip

     M94.259 Chondromalacia, unspecified hip

✓6ᵗʰ **M94.26** Chondromalacia, knee

     M94.261 Chondromalacia, right knee

     M94.262 Chondromalacia, left knee

     M94.269 Chondromalacia, unspecified knee

✓6ᵗʰ **M94.27** Chondromalacia, ankle and joints of foot

     M94.271 Chondromalacia, right ankle and joints of right foot

     M94.272 Chondromalacia, left ankle and joints of left foot

     M94.279 Chondromalacia, unspecified ankle and joints of foot

     M94.28 Chondromalacia, other site

     M94.29 Chondromalacia, multiple sites

✓5ᵗʰ **M94.3** **Chondrolysis**

     Code first any associated slipped upper femoral epiphysis (nontraumatic) (M93.0-)

✓6ᵗʰ **M94.35** Chondrolysis, hip

     M94.351 Chondrolysis, right hip

     M94.352 Chondrolysis, left hip

     M94.359 Chondrolysis, unspecified hip

✓5ᵗʰ **M94.8** **Other specified disorders of cartilage**

✓6ᵗʰ **M94.8X** Other specified disorders of cartilage

     M94.8X0 Other specified disorders of cartilage, multiple sites

     M94.8X1 Other specified disorders of cartilage, shoulder

     M94.8X2 Other specified disorders of cartilage, upper arm

     M94.8X3 Other specified disorders of cartilage, forearm

     M94.8X4 Other specified disorders of cartilage, hand

     M94.8X5 Other specified disorders of cartilage, thigh

     M94.8X6 Other specified disorders of cartilage, lower leg

     M94.8X7 Other specified disorders of cartilage, ankle and foot

     M94.8X8 Other specified disorders of cartilage, other site

     M94.8X9 Other specified disorders of cartilage, unspecified sites

M94.9 **Disorder of cartilage, unspecified**

Other disorders of the musculoskeletal system and connective tissue (M95)

✓4ᵗʰ **M95** **Other acquired deformities of musculoskeletal system and connective tissue**

     EXCLUDES 2   acquired absence of limbs and organs (Z89-Z90)
            acquired deformities of limbs (M20-M21)
            congenital malformations and deformations of the musculoskeletal system (Q65-Q79)
            deforming dorsopathies (M40-M43)
            dentofacial anomalies [including malocclusion] (M26.-)
            postprocedural musculoskeletal disorders (M96.-)

M95.0 **Acquired deformity of nose**

     EXCLUDES 2   deviated nasal septum (J34.2)

✓5ᵗʰ **M95.1** **Cauliflower ear**

     EXCLUDES 2   other acquired deformities of ear (H61.1)

     DEF: Acquired deformity of the external ear due to injury or subsequent perichondritis.

     M95.10 Cauliflower ear, unspecified ear

     M95.11 Cauliflower ear, right ear

     M95.12 Cauliflower ear, left ear

M95.2 **Other acquired deformity of head**

M95.3 **Acquired deformity of neck**

M95.4 **Acquired deformity of chest and rib**
     AHA: 2014,4Q,26-27

M95.5 **Acquired deformity of pelvis**

     EXCLUDES 1   maternal care for known or suspected disproportion (O33.-)

M95.8 **Other specified acquired deformities of musculoskeletal system**

M95.9 **Acquired deformity of musculoskeletal system, unspecified**

Chapter 13. Diseases of the Musculoskeletal System and Connective Tissue

M96–M97.12

Intraoperative and postprocedural complications and disorders of musculoskeletal system, not elsewhere classified (M96)

✓4th **M96**   **Intraoperative and postprocedural complications and disorders of musculoskeletal system, not elsewhere classified**
   EXCLUDES 2   *arthropathy following intestinal bypass (M02.0-)*
     complications of internal orthopedic prosthetic devices, implants and grafts (T84.-)
     disorders associated with osteoporosis (M80)
     periprosthetic fracture around internal prosthetic joint (M97.-)
     presence of functional implants and other devices (Z96-Z97)

M96.0   **Pseudarthrosis after fusion or arthrodesis**   CC

M96.1   **Postlaminectomy syndrome, not elsewhere classified**

M96.2   **Postradiation kyphosis**

M96.3   **Postlaminectomy kyphosis**

M96.4   **Postsurgical lordosis**

M96.5   **Postradiation scoliosis**

✓5th **M96.6**   **Fracture of bone following insertion of orthopedic implant, joint prosthesis, or bone plate**
     Intraoperative fracture of bone during insertion of orthopedic implant, joint prosthesis, or bone plate
     EXCLUDES 2   *complication of internal orthopedic devices, implants or grafts (T84.-)*

   ✓6th **M96.62**   Fracture of **humerus** following insertion of orthopedic implant, joint prosthesis, or bone plate
     M96.621   Fracture of humerus following insertion of orthopedic implant, joint prosthesis, or bone plate, **right** arm   CC HCC
     M96.622   Fracture of humerus following insertion of orthopedic implant, joint prosthesis, or bone plate, **left** arm   CC HCC
     M96.629   Fracture of humerus following insertion of orthopedic implant, joint prosthesis, or bone plate, **unspecified** arm   CC HCC

   ✓6th **M96.63**   Fracture of **radius or ulna** following insertion of orthopedic implant, joint prosthesis, or bone plate
     M96.631   Fracture of radius or ulna following insertion of orthopedic implant, joint prosthesis, or bone plate, **right** arm   CC HCC
     M96.632   Fracture of radius or ulna following insertion of orthopedic implant, joint prosthesis, or bone plate, **left** arm   CC HCC
     M96.639   Fracture of radius or ulna following insertion of orthopedic implant, joint prosthesis, or bone plate, **unspecified** arm   CC HCC

   M96.65   Fracture of **pelvis** following insertion of orthopedic implant, joint prosthesis, or bone plate   CC HCC

   ✓6th **M96.66**   Fracture of **femur** following insertion of orthopedic implant, joint prosthesis, or bone plate
     M96.661   Fracture of femur following insertion of orthopedic implant, joint prosthesis, or bone plate, **right** leg   CC HCC
     M96.662   Fracture of femur following insertion of orthopedic implant, joint prosthesis, or bone plate, **left** leg   CC HCC
     M96.669   Fracture of femur following insertion of orthopedic implant, joint prosthesis, or bone plate, **unspecified** leg   CC HCC

   ✓6th **M96.67**   Fracture of **tibia** or **fibula** following insertion of orthopedic implant, joint prosthesis, or bone plate
     M96.671   Fracture of tibia or fibula following insertion of orthopedic implant, joint prosthesis, or bone plate, **right** leg   CC HCC
     M96.672   Fracture of tibia or fibula following insertion of orthopedic implant, joint prosthesis, or bone plate, **left** leg   CC HCC
     M96.679   Fracture of tibia or fibula following insertion of orthopedic implant, joint prosthesis, or bone plate, **unspecified** leg   CC HCC

   M96.69   Fracture of other bone following insertion of orthopedic implant, joint prosthesis, or bone plate   CC HCC

✓5th **M96.8**   **Other intraoperative and postprocedural complications and disorders of musculoskeletal system, not elsewhere classified**
     AHA: 2016,4Q,9-10

   ✓6th **M96.81**   **Intraoperative hemorrhage and hematoma** of a musculoskeletal structure complicating a procedure
     EXCLUDES 1   *intraoperative hemorrhage and hematoma of a musculoskeletal structure due to accidental puncture and laceration during a procedure (M96.82-)*
     M96.810   Intraoperative hemorrhage and hematoma of a musculoskeletal structure complicating a **musculoskeletal system procedure**   CC
     M96.811   Intraoperative hemorrhage and hematoma of a musculoskeletal structure complicating **other procedure**   CC

   ✓6th **M96.82**   **Accidental puncture and laceration** of a musculoskeletal structure during a procedure
     M96.820   Accidental puncture and laceration of a musculoskeletal structure during a **musculoskeletal system procedure**   CC
     M96.821   Accidental puncture and laceration of a musculoskeletal structure during **other procedure**   CC

   ✓6th **M96.83**   **Postprocedural hemorrhage** of a musculoskeletal structure following a procedure
     M96.830   Postprocedural hemorrhage of a musculoskeletal structure following a **musculoskeletal system procedure**   CC
     M96.831   Postprocedural hemorrhage of a musculoskeletal structure following **other procedure**   CC

   ✓6th **M96.84**   **Postprocedural hematoma and seroma** of a musculoskeletal structure following a procedure
     M96.840   Postprocedural **hematoma** of a musculoskeletal structure following a **musculoskeletal system procedure**   CC
     M96.841   Postprocedural **hematoma** of a musculoskeletal structure following **other procedure**   CC
       AHA: 2016,4Q,10
     M96.842   Postprocedural **seroma** of a musculoskeletal structure following a **musculoskeletal system procedure**   CC
     M96.843   Postprocedural **seroma** of a musculoskeletal structure following **other procedure**   CC
       AHA: 2018,3Q,6

   M96.89   **Other intraoperative and postprocedural complications and disorders of the musculoskeletal system**   CC
     Instability of joint secondary to removal of joint prosthesis
     Use additional code, if applicable, to further specify disorder

Periprosthetic fractures around internal prosthetic joint (M97)

✓4th **M97**   **Periprosthetic fracture around internal prosthetic joint**
   EXCLUDES 2   *breakage (fracture) of prosthetic joint (T84.01-)*
     fracture of bone following insertion of orthopedic implant, joint prosthesis or bone plate (M96.6-)
   AHA: 2016,4Q,42-43

> The appropriate 7th character is to be added to each code from category M97.
> A   initial encounter
> D   subsequent encounter
> S   sequela

✓5th **M97.0**   **Periprosthetic fracture around internal prosthetic hip joint**
     AHA: 2018,1Q,21; 2016,4Q,42

   ✓x7th **M97.01**   **Periprosthetic fracture around internal prosthetic right hip joint**   CC HCC

   ✓x7th **M97.02**   **Periprosthetic fracture around internal prosthetic left hip joint**   CC HCC

✓5th **M97.1**   **Periprosthetic fracture around internal prosthetic knee joint**

   ✓x7th **M97.11**   **Periprosthetic fracture around internal prosthetic right knee joint**   CC

   ✓x7th **M97.12**   **Periprosthetic fracture around internal prosthetic left knee joint**   CC

N Newborn: 0   P Pediatric: 0-17   M Maternity: 9-64   A Adult: 15-124   MCC Major Complication/Comorbidity   CC Complication/Comorbidity   SW Severe Wound Dx

838   ICD-10-CM 2021

√5ᵗʰ **M97.2 Periprosthetic fracture around internal prosthetic ankle joint**

   √x7ᵗʰ **M97.21 Periprosthetic fracture around internal prosthetic right ankle joint** `cc`

   √x7ᵗʰ **M97.22 Periprosthetic fracture around internal prosthetic left ankle joint** `cc`

√5ᵗʰ **M97.3 Periprosthetic fracture around internal prosthetic shoulder joint**

   √x7ᵗʰ **M97.31 Periprosthetic fracture around internal prosthetic right shoulder joint** `cc`

   √x7ᵗʰ **M97.32 Periprosthetic fracture around internal prosthetic left shoulder joint** `cc`

√5ᵗʰ **M97.4 Periprosthetic fracture around internal prosthetic elbow joint**

   √x7ᵗʰ **M97.41 Periprosthetic fracture around internal prosthetic right elbow joint** `cc`

   √x7ᵗʰ **M97.42 Periprosthetic fracture around internal prosthetic left elbow joint** `cc`

√x7ᵗʰ **M97.8 Periprosthetic fracture around other internal prosthetic joint** `cc`

Periprosthetic fracture around internal prosthetic finger joint
Periprosthetic fracture around internal prosthetic spinal joint
Periprosthetic fracture around internal prosthetic toe joint
Periprosthetic fracture around internal prosthetic wrist joint
Use additional code to identify the joint (Z96.6-)

√x7ᵗʰ **M97.9 Periprosthetic fracture around unspecified internal prosthetic joint** `cc`

Biomechanical lesions, not elsewhere classified (M99)

√4ᵗʰ **M99 Biomechanical lesions, not elsewhere classified**

   NOTE This category should not be used if the condition can be classified elsewhere.

   DEF: Biomechanical lesion: Term used by osteopathic and chiropractic physicians to describe musculoskeletal conditions treated that are not more appropriately classified elsewhere.

√5ᵗʰ **M99.0 Segmental and somatic dysfunction**

   M99.00 Segmental and somatic dysfunction of head region
   M99.01 Segmental and somatic dysfunction of cervical region
   M99.02 Segmental and somatic dysfunction of thoracic region
   M99.03 Segmental and somatic dysfunction of lumbar region
   M99.04 Segmental and somatic dysfunction of sacral region
   M99.05 Segmental and somatic dysfunction of pelvic region
   M99.06 Segmental and somatic dysfunction of lower extremity
   M99.07 Segmental and somatic dysfunction of upper extremity
   M99.08 Segmental and somatic dysfunction of rib cage
   M99.09 Segmental and somatic dysfunction of abdomen and other regions

√5ᵗʰ **M99.1 Subluxation complex (vertebral)**

   M99.10 Subluxation complex (vertebral) of head region `cc` `H5`
   M99.11 Subluxation complex (vertebral) of cervical region `cc` `H5`
   M99.12 Subluxation complex (vertebral) of thoracic region
   M99.13 Subluxation complex (vertebral) of lumbar region
   M99.14 Subluxation complex (vertebral) of sacral region
   M99.15 Subluxation complex (vertebral) of pelvic region
   M99.16 Subluxation complex (vertebral) of lower extremity
   M99.17 Subluxation complex (vertebral) of upper extremity
   M99.18 Subluxation complex (vertebral) of rib cage `cc` `H5`
   M99.19 Subluxation complex (vertebral) of abdomen and other regions

√5ᵗʰ **M99.2 Subluxation stenosis of neural canal**

   M99.20 Subluxation stenosis of neural canal of head region
   M99.21 Subluxation stenosis of neural canal of cervical region
   M99.22 Subluxation stenosis of neural canal of thoracic region
   M99.23 Subluxation stenosis of neural canal of lumbar region
   M99.24 Subluxation stenosis of neural canal of sacral region
   M99.25 Subluxation stenosis of neural canal of pelvic region
   M99.26 Subluxation stenosis of neural canal of lower extremity

   M99.27 Subluxation stenosis of neural canal of upper extremity
   M99.28 Subluxation stenosis of neural canal of rib cage
   M99.29 Subluxation stenosis of neural canal of abdomen and other regions

√5ᵗʰ **M99.3 Osseous stenosis of neural canal**

   M99.30 Osseous stenosis of neural canal of head region
   M99.31 Osseous stenosis of neural canal of cervical region
   M99.32 Osseous stenosis of neural canal of thoracic region
   M99.33 Osseous stenosis of neural canal of lumbar region
   M99.34 Osseous stenosis of neural canal of sacral region
   M99.35 Osseous stenosis of neural canal of pelvic region
   M99.36 Osseous stenosis of neural canal of lower extremity
   M99.37 Osseous stenosis of neural canal of upper extremity
   M99.38 Osseous stenosis of neural canal of rib cage
   M99.39 Osseous stenosis of neural canal of abdomen and other regions

√5ᵗʰ **M99.4 Connective tissue stenosis of neural canal**

   M99.40 Connective tissue stenosis of neural canal of head region
   M99.41 Connective tissue stenosis of neural canal of cervical region
   M99.42 Connective tissue stenosis of neural canal of thoracic region
   M99.43 Connective tissue stenosis of neural canal of lumbar region
   M99.44 Connective tissue stenosis of neural canal of sacral region
   M99.45 Connective tissue stenosis of neural canal of pelvic region
   M99.46 Connective tissue stenosis of neural canal of lower extremity
   M99.47 Connective tissue stenosis of neural canal of upper extremity
   M99.48 Connective tissue stenosis of neural canal of rib cage
   M99.49 Connective tissue stenosis of neural canal of abdomen and other regions

√5ᵗʰ **M99.5 Intervertebral disc stenosis of neural canal**

   M99.50 Intervertebral disc stenosis of neural canal of head region
   M99.51 Intervertebral disc stenosis of neural canal of cervical region
   M99.52 Intervertebral disc stenosis of neural canal of thoracic region
   M99.53 Intervertebral disc stenosis of neural canal of lumbar region
   M99.54 Intervertebral disc stenosis of neural canal of sacral region
   M99.55 Intervertebral disc stenosis of neural canal of pelvic region
   M99.56 Intervertebral disc stenosis of neural canal of lower extremity
   M99.57 Intervertebral disc stenosis of neural canal of upper extremity
   M99.58 Intervertebral disc stenosis of neural canal of rib cage
   M99.59 Intervertebral disc stenosis of neural canal of abdomen and other regions

√5ᵗʰ **M99.6 Osseous and subluxation stenosis of intervertebral foramina**

   M99.60 Osseous and subluxation stenosis of intervertebral foramina of head region
   M99.61 Osseous and subluxation stenosis of intervertebral foramina of cervical region
   M99.62 Osseous and subluxation stenosis of intervertebral foramina of thoracic region
   M99.63 Osseous and subluxation stenosis of intervertebral foramina of lumbar region
   M99.64 Osseous and subluxation stenosis of intervertebral foramina of sacral region
   M99.65 Osseous and subluxation stenosis of intervertebral foramina of pelvic region
   M99.66 Osseous and subluxation stenosis of intervertebral foramina of lower extremity
   M99.67 Osseous and subluxation stenosis of intervertebral foramina of upper extremity
   M99.68 Osseous and subluxation stenosis of intervertebral foramina of rib cage
   M99.69 Osseous and subluxation stenosis of intervertebral foramina of abdomen and other regions

☑5ᵗʰ **M99.7**   **Connective tissue and disc stenosis of intervertebral foramina**

     M99.70   **Connective tissue and disc stenosis of intervertebral foramina of head region**

     M99.71   **Connective tissue and disc stenosis of intervertebral foramina of cervical region**

     M99.72   **Connective tissue and disc stenosis of intervertebral foramina of thoracic region**

     M99.73   **Connective tissue and disc stenosis of intervertebral foramina of lumbar region**

     M99.74   **Connective tissue and disc stenosis of intervertebral foramina of sacral region**

     M99.75   **Connective tissue and disc stenosis of intervertebral foramina of pelvic region**

     M99.76   **Connective tissue and disc stenosis of intervertebral foramina of lower extremity**

     M99.77   **Connective tissue and disc stenosis of intervertebral foramina of upper extremity**

     M99.78   **Connective tissue and disc stenosis of intervertebral foramina of rib cage**

     M99.79   **Connective tissue and disc stenosis of intervertebral foramina of abdomen and other regions**

☑5ᵗʰ **M99.8**   **Other biomechanical lesions**

     M99.80   **Other biomechanical lesions of head region**

     M99.81   **Other biomechanical lesions of cervical region**

     M99.82   **Other biomechanical lesions of thoracic region**

     M99.83   **Other biomechanical lesions of lumbar region**

     M99.84   **Other biomechanical lesions of sacral region**

     M99.85   **Other biomechanical lesions of pelvic region**

     M99.86   **Other biomechanical lesions of lower extremity**

     M99.87   **Other biomechanical lesions of upper extremity**

     M99.88   **Other biomechanical lesions of rib cage**

     M99.89   **Other biomechanical lesions of abdomen and other regions**

     M99.9   **Biomechanical lesion, unspecified**

Ⓝ Newborn: 0   Ⓟ Pediatric: 0-17   Ⓜ Maternity: 9-64   Ⓐ Adult: 15-124   **MCC** Major Complication/Comorbidity   **CC** Complication/Comorbidity   **SW** Severe Wound Dx

840   ICD-10-CM 2021

Chapter 14. Diseases of Genitourinary System (NØØ–N99)

Chapter-specific Guidelines with Coding Examples

The chapter-specific guidelines from the ICD-10-CM Official Guidelines for Coding and Reporting have been provided below. Along with these guidelines are coding examples, contained in the shaded boxes, that have been developed to help illustrate the coding and/or sequencing guidance found in these guidelines.

a. Chronic kidney disease

1) Stages of chronic kidney disease (CKD)

The ICD-10-CM classifies CKD based on severity. The severity of CKD is designated by stages 1-5. Stage 2, code N18.2, equates to mild CKD; stage 3, **codes N18.3Ø-N18.32,** equate to moderate CKD; and stage 4, code N18.4, equates to severe CKD. Code N18.6, End stage renal disease (ESRD), is assigned when the provider has documented end-stage renal disease (ESRD).

If both a stage of CKD and ESRD are documented, assign code N18.6 only.

Stage 5 chronic kidney disease with ESRD requiring chronic dialysis

N18.6	**End stage renal disease**
Z99.2	**Dependence on renal dialysis**

Explanation: The diagnostic statement indicates the patient has chronic kidney disease, documented both as stage 5 and as ESRD requiring chronic dialysis. Code N18.6 End stage renal disease (ESRD), is assigned when the provider has documented end-stage-renal disease (ESRD). If both a stage of CKD and ESRD are documented, assign code N18.6 only.

2) Chronic kidney disease and kidney transplant status

Patients who have undergone kidney transplant may still have some form of chronic kidney disease (CKD) because the kidney transplant may not fully restore kidney function. Therefore, the presence of CKD alone does not constitute a transplant complication. Assign the appropriate N18 code for the patient's stage of CKD and code Z94.Ø, Kidney transplant status. If a transplant complication such as failure or rejection or other transplant complication is documented, see section I.C.19.g for information on coding complications of a kidney transplant. If the documentation is unclear as to whether the patient has a complication of the transplant, query the provider.

Patient with residual chronic kidney disease stage 1 after kidney transplant

N18.1	**Chronic kidney disease, stage 1**
Z94.Ø	**Kidney transplant status**

Explanation: Patients who have undergone kidney transplant may still have some form of chronic kidney disease (CKD) because the kidney transplant may not fully restore kidney function. The presence of CKD alone does not constitute a transplant complication. Assign the appropriate N18 code for the patient's stage of CKD and code Z94.Ø Kidney transplant status.

3) Chronic kidney disease with other conditions

Patients with CKD may also suffer from other serious conditions, most commonly diabetes mellitus and hypertension. The sequencing of the CKD code in relationship to codes for other contributing conditions is based on the conventions in the Tabular List.

See I.C.9. Hypertensive chronic kidney disease.

See I.C.19. Chronic kidney disease and kidney transplant complications.

Type 1 diabetic chronic kidney disease, stage 2

E1Ø.22	**Type 1 diabetes mellitus with diabetic chronic kidney disease**
N18.2	**Chronic kidney disease, stage 2 (mild)**

Explanation: Patients with CKD may also suffer from other serious conditions such as diabetes mellitus. The sequencing of the CKD code in relationship to codes for other contributing conditions is based on the conventions in the Tabular List. Diabetic CKD code E1Ø.22 includes an instructional note to "Use additional code to identify stage of chronic kidney disease (N18.1–N18.6)," thus providing sequencing direction.

Chapter 14. Diseases of the Genitourinary System (N00-N99)

EXCLUDES 2   *certain conditions originating in the perinatal period (P04-P96)*
certain infectious and parasitic diseases (A00-B99)
complications of pregnancy, childbirth and the puerperium (O00-O9A)
congenital malformations, deformations and chromosomal abnormalities (Q00-Q99)
endocrine, nutritional and metabolic diseases (E00-E88)
injury, poisoning and certain other consequences of external causes (S00-T88)
neoplasms (C00-D49)
symptoms, signs and abnormal clinical and laboratory findings, not elsewhere classified (R00-R94)

This chapter contains the following blocks:

N00-N08	Glomerular diseases
N10-N16	Renal tubulo-interstitial diseases
N17-N19	Acute kidney failure and chronic kidney disease
N20-N23	Urolithiasis
N25-N29	Other disorders of kidney and ureter
N30-N39	Other diseases of the urinary system
N40-N53	Diseases of male genital organs
N60-N65	Disorders of breast
N70-N77	Inflammatory diseases of female pelvic organs
N80-N98	Noninflammatory disorders of female genital tract
N99	Intraoperative and postprocedural complications and disorders of genitourinary system, not elsewhere classified

Glomerular diseases (N00-N08)

Code also any associated kidney failure (N17-N19).

EXCLUDES 1   *hypertensive chronic kidney disease (I12.-)*

DEF: Glomeruli: Clusters of microscopic blood vessels located within the kidneys containing small pores through which waste products are filtered from the blood and urine is formed.

DEF: Glomerulonephritis: Disease of the kidney with diffuse inflammation of the capillary loops of the glomeruli.

✓4ᵗʰ **N00**   **Acute nephritic syndrome**

INCLUDES   acute glomerular disease
acute glomerulonephritis
acute nephritis

EXCLUDES 1   *acute tubulo-interstitial nephritis (N10)*
nephritic syndrome NOS (N05.-)

N00.0   **Acute nephritic syndrome with minor glomerular abnormality**   MCC
Acute nephritic syndrome with minimal change lesion

N00.1   **Acute nephritic syndrome with focal and segmental glomerular lesions**   MCC
Acute nephritic syndrome with focal and segmental hyalinosis
Acute nephritic syndrome with focal and segmental sclerosis
Acute nephritic syndrome with focal glomerulonephritis

N00.2   **Acute nephritic syndrome with diffuse membranous glomerulonephritis**   MCC

N00.3   **Acute nephritic syndrome with diffuse mesangial proliferative glomerulonephritis**   MCC

N00.4   **Acute nephritic syndrome with diffuse endocapillary proliferative glomerulonephritis**   MCC

N00.5   **Acute nephritic syndrome with diffuse mesangiocapillary glomerulonephritis**   MCC
Acute nephritic syndrome with membranoproliferative glomerulonephritis, types 1 and 3, or NOS
EXCLUDES 1   ▶*acute nephritic syndrome with C3 glomerulonephritis (N00.A)*◀
▶*acute nephritic syndrome with C3 glomerulopathy (N00.A)*◀

N00.6   **Acute nephritic syndrome with dense deposit disease**   MCC
▶Acute nephritic syndrome with C3 glomerulopathy with dense deposit disease◀
Acute nephritic syndrome with membranoproliferative glomerulonephritis, type 2

N00.7   **Acute nephritic syndrome with diffuse crescentic glomerulonephritis**   MCC
Acute nephritic syndrome with extracapillary glomerulonephritis

N00.8   **Acute nephritic syndrome with other morphologic changes**   MCC
Acute nephritic syndrome with proliferative glomerulonephritis NOS

N00.9   **Acute nephritic syndrome with unspecified morphologic changes**   MCC

● **N00.A**   **Acute nephritic syndrome with C3 glomerulonephritis**   MCC
Acute nephritic syndrome with C3 glomerulopathy, NOS
EXCLUDES 1   *acute nephritic syndrome (with C3 glomerulopathy) with dense deposit disease (N00.6)*

✓4ᵗʰ **N01**   **Rapidly progressive nephritic syndrome**

INCLUDES   rapidly progressive glomerular disease
rapidly progressive glomerulonephritis
rapidly progressive nephritis

EXCLUDES 1   *nephritic syndrome NOS (N05.-)*

N01.0   **Rapidly progressive nephritic syndrome with minor glomerular abnormality**   MCC
Rapidly progressive nephritic syndrome with minimal change lesion

N01.1   **Rapidly progressive nephritic syndrome with focal and segmental glomerular lesions**   MCC
Rapidly progressive nephritic syndrome with focal and segmental hyalinosis
Rapidly progressive nephritic syndrome with focal and segmental sclerosis
Rapidly progressive nephritic syndrome with focal glomerulonephritis

N01.2   **Rapidly progressive nephritic syndrome with diffuse membranous glomerulonephritis**   MCC

N01.3   **Rapidly progressive nephritic syndrome with diffuse mesangial proliferative glomerulonephritis**   MCC

N01.4   **Rapidly progressive nephritic syndrome with diffuse endocapillary proliferative glomerulonephritis**   MCC

N01.5   **Rapidly progressive nephritic syndrome with diffuse mesangiocapillary glomerulonephritis**   MCC
Rapidly progressive nephritic syndrome with membranoproliferative glomerulonephritis, types 1 and 3, or NOS
EXCLUDES 1   ▶*rapidly progressive nephritic syndrome with C3 glomerulonephritis (N01.A)*◀
▶*rapidly progressive nephritic syndrome with C3 glomerulopathy (N01.A)*◀

N01.6   **Rapidly progressive nephritic syndrome with dense deposit disease**   MCC
▶Rapidly progressive nephritic syndrome with C3 glomerulopathy with dense deposit disease◀
Rapidly progressive nephritic syndrome with membranoproliferative glomerulonephritis, type 2

N01.7   **Rapidly progressive nephritic syndrome with diffuse crescentic glomerulonephritis**   MCC
Rapidly progressive nephritic syndrome with extracapillary glomerulonephritis

N01.8   **Rapidly progressive nephritic syndrome with other morphologic changes**   MCC
Rapidly progressive nephritic syndrome with proliferative glomerulonephritis NOS

N01.9   **Rapidly progressive nephritic syndrome with unspecified morphologic changes**   MCC

● **N01.A**   **Rapidly progressive nephritic syndrome with C3 glomerulonephritis**   MCC
Rapidly progressive nephritic syndrome with C3 glomerulopathy, NOS
EXCLUDES 1   *rapidly progressive nephritic syndrome (with C3 glomerulopathy) with dense deposit disease (N01.6)*

✓4ᵗʰ **N02**   **Recurrent and persistent hematuria**

EXCLUDES 1   *acute cystitis with hematuria (N30.01)*
hematuria NOS (R31.9)
hematuria not associated with specified morphologic lesions (R31.-)

N02.0   **Recurrent and persistent hematuria with minor glomerular abnormality**   CC
Recurrent and persistent hematuria with minimal change lesion

N02.1   **Recurrent and persistent hematuria with focal and segmental glomerular lesions**   CC
Recurrent and persistent hematuria with focal and segmental hyalinosis
Recurrent and persistent hematuria with focal and segmental sclerosis
Recurrent and persistent hematuria with focal glomerulonephritis

N02.2   **Recurrent and persistent hematuria with diffuse membranous glomerulonephritis**   CC

N Newborn: 0   P Pediatric: 0-17   M Maternity: 9-64   A Adult: 15-124   MCC Major Complication/Comorbidity   CC Complication/Comorbidity   SW Severe Wound Dx

N02.3 **Recurrent and persistent hematuria with** diffuse mesangial proliferative glomerulonephritis `cc`

N02.4 **Recurrent and persistent hematuria with** diffuse endocapillary proliferative glomerulonephritis `cc`

N02.5 **Recurrent and persistent hematuria with** diffuse mesangiocapillary glomerulonephritis `cc`

Recurrent and persistent hematuria with membranoproliferative glomerulonephritis, types 1 and 3, or NOS

EXCLUDES 1 ▶recurrent and persistent hematuria with C3 glomerulonephritis (N02.A)◀
▶recurrent and persistent hematuria with C3 glomerulopathy (N02.A)◀

N02.6 **Recurrent and persistent hematuria with** dense deposit disease `cc`

▶Recurrent and persistent hematuria with C3 glomerulopathy with dense deposit disease◀
Recurrent and persistent hematuria with membranoproliferative glomerulonephritis, type 2

N02.7 **Recurrent and persistent hematuria with** diffuse crescentic glomerulonephritis `cc`

Recurrent and persistent hematuria with extracapillary glomerulonephritis

N02.8 **Recurrent and persistent hematuria with other morphologic changes** `cc`

Recurrent and persistent hematuria with proliferative glomerulonephritis NOS

N02.9 **Recurrent and persistent hematuria with unspecified morphologic changes** `cc`

AHA: 2017,2Q,5

● **N02.A** **Recurrent and persistent hematuria with** C3 glomerulonephritis `cc`

Recurrent and persistent hematuria with C3 glomerulopathy

EXCLUDES 1 recurrent and persistent hematuria (with C3 glomerulopathy) with dense deposit disease (N02.6)

✓4ᵗʰ **N03** **Chronic nephritic syndrome**

INCLUDES chronic glomerular disease
chronic glomerulonephritis
chronic nephritis

EXCLUDES 1 chronic tubulo-interstitial nephritis (N11.-)
diffuse sclerosing glomerulonephritis (N05.8-)
nephritic syndrome NOS (N05.-)

DEF: Slow, progressive type of nephritis characterized by inflammation of the capillary loops in the glomeruli of the kidney, which leads to renal failure.

N03.0 **Chronic nephritic syndrome with** minor glomerular abnormality `cc`

Chronic nephritic syndrome with minimal change lesion

N03.1 **Chronic nephritic syndrome with** focal and segmental glomerular lesions

Chronic nephritic syndrome with focal and segmental hyalinosis
Chronic nephritic syndrome with focal and segmental sclerosis
Chronic nephritic syndrome with focal glomerulonephritis

N03.2 **Chronic nephritic syndrome with** diffuse membranous glomerulonephritis `cc`

N03.3 **Chronic nephritic syndrome with** diffuse mesangial proliferative glomerulonephritis `cc`

N03.4 **Chronic nephritic syndrome with** diffuse endocapillary proliferative glomerulonephritis `cc`

N03.5 **Chronic nephritic syndrome with diffuse** mesangiocapillary glomerulonephritis `cc`

Chronic nephritic syndrome with membranoproliferative glomerulonephritis, types 1 and 3, or NOS

EXCLUDES 1 ▶chronic nephritic syndrome with C3 glomerulonephritis (N03.A)◀
▶chronic nephritic syndrome with C3 glomerulopathy (N03.A)◀

N03.6 **Chronic nephritic syndrome with** dense deposit disease `cc`

▶Chronic nephritic syndrome with C3 glomerulopathy with dense deposit disease◀
Chronic nephritic syndrome with membranoproliferative glomerulonephritis, type 2

N03.7 **Chronic nephritic syndrome with** diffuse crescentic glomerulonephritis `cc`

Chronic nephritic syndrome with extracapillary glomerulonephritis

N03.8 **Chronic nephritic syndrome with other morphologic changes** `cc`

Chronic nephritic syndrome with proliferative glomerulonephritis NOS

N03.9 **Chronic nephritic syndrome with unspecified morphologic changes** `cc`

● **N03.A** **Chronic nephritic syndrome with** C3 glomerulonephritis `cc`

Chronic nephritic syndrome with C3 glomerulopathy

EXCLUDES 1 chronic nephritic syndrome (with C3 glomerulopathy) with dense deposit disease (N03.6)

✓4ᵗʰ **N04** **Nephrotic syndrome**

INCLUDES congenital nephrotic syndrome
lipoid nephrosis

N04.0 **Nephrotic syndrome with** minor glomerular abnormality `cc`

Nephrotic syndrome with minimal change lesion

N04.1 **Nephrotic syndrome with** focal and segmental glomerular lesions `cc`

Nephrotic syndrome with focal and segmental hyalinosis
Nephrotic syndrome with focal and segmental sclerosis
Nephrotic syndrome with focal glomerulonephritis

N04.2 **Nephrotic syndrome with** diffuse membranous glomerulonephritis `cc`

N04.3 **Nephrotic syndrome with** diffuse mesangial proliferative glomerulonephritis `cc`

N04.4 **Nephrotic syndrome with** diffuse endocapillary proliferative glomerulonephritis `cc`

N04.5 **Nephrotic syndrome with** diffuse mesangiocapillary glomerulonephritis `cc`

Nephrotic syndrome with membranoproliferative glomerulonephritis, types 1 and 3, or NOS

EXCLUDES 1 ▶nephrotic syndrome with C3 glomerulonephritis (N04.A)◀
▶nephrotic syndrome with C3 glomerulopathy (N04.A)◀

N04.6 **Nephrotic syndrome with** dense deposit disease `cc`

▶Nephrotic syndrome with C3 glomerulopathy with dense deposit disease◀
Nephrotic syndrome with membranoproliferative glomerulonephritis, type 2

N04.7 **Nephrotic syndrome with** diffuse crescentic glomerulonephritis `cc`

Nephrotic syndrome with extracapillary glomerulonephritis

N04.8 **Nephrotic syndrome with other morphologic changes** `cc`

Nephrotic syndrome with proliferative glomerulonephritis NOS

N04.9 **Nephrotic syndrome with unspecified morphologic changes** `cc`

● **N04.A** **Nephrotic syndrome with** C3 glomerulonephritis `cc`

Nephrotic syndrome with C3 glomerulopathy

EXCLUDES 1 nephrotic syndrome (with C3 glomerulopathy) with dense deposit disease (N04.6)

✓4ᵗʰ **N05** **Unspecified nephritic syndrome**

INCLUDES glomerular disease NOS
glomerulonephritis NOS
nephritis NOS
nephropathy NOS and renal disease NOS with morphological lesion specified in .0-.8

EXCLUDES 1 nephropathy NOS with no stated morphological lesion (N28.9)
renal disease NOS with no stated morphological lesion (N28.9)
tubulo-interstitial nephritis NOS (N12)

N05.0 **Unspecified nephritic syndrome with** minor glomerular abnormality

Unspecified nephritic syndrome with minimal change lesion

N05.1 **Unspecified nephritic syndrome with** focal and segmental glomerular lesions

Unspecified nephritic syndrome with focal and segmental hyalinosis
Unspecified nephritic syndrome with focal and segmental sclerosis
Unspecified nephritic syndrome with focal glomerulonephritis

N05.2 **Unspecified nephritic syndrome with** diffuse membranous glomerulonephritis `cc`

N05.3 **Unspecified nephritic syndrome with** diffuse mesangial proliferative glomerulonephritis `cc`

N05.4 **Unspecified nephritic syndrome with** diffuse endocapillary proliferative glomerulonephritis `cc`

N05.5 **Unspecified nephritic syndrome with diffuse mesangiocapillary glomerulonephritis** `CC`

Unspecified nephritic syndrome with membranoproliferative glomerulonephritis, types 1 and 3, or NOS

EXCLUDES 1 ▶unspecified nephritic syndrome with C3 glomerulonephritis (N05.A)◀

▶unspecified nephritic syndrome with C3 glomerulopathy (N05.A)◀

N05.6 **Unspecified nephritic syndrome with dense deposit disease**

▶Unspecified nephritic syndrome with C3 glomerulopathy with dense deposit disease◀

Unspecified nephritic syndrome with membranoproliferative glomerulonephritis, type 2

N05.7 **Unspecified nephritic syndrome with diffuse crescentic glomerulonephritis**

Unspecified nephritic syndrome with extracapillary glomerulonephritis

N05.8 **Unspecified nephritic syndrome with other morphologic changes**

Unspecified nephritic syndrome with proliferative glomerulonephritis NOS

N05.9 **Unspecified nephritic syndrome with unspecified morphologic changes**

● **N05.A** **Unspecified nephritic syndrome with C3 glomerulonephritis** `CC`

Unspecified nephritic syndrome with C3 glomerulopathy

EXCLUDES 1 unspecified nephritic syndrome (with C3 glomerulopathy) with dense deposit disease (N05.6)

✓4ᵗʰ **N06** **Isolated proteinuria with specified morphological lesion**

EXCLUDES 1 proteinuria not associated with specific morphologic lesions (R80.0)

N06.0 **Isolated proteinuria with minor glomerular abnormality**

Isolated proteinuria with minimal change lesion

N06.1 **Isolated proteinuria with focal and segmental glomerular lesions**

Isolated proteinuria with focal and segmental hyalinosis

Isolated proteinuria with focal and segmental sclerosis

Isolated proteinuria with focal glomerulonephritis

N06.2 **Isolated proteinuria with diffuse membranous glomerulonephritis** `CC`

N06.3 **Isolated proteinuria with diffuse mesangial proliferative glomerulonephritis** `CC`

N06.4 **Isolated proteinuria with diffuse endocapillary proliferative glomerulonephritis** `CC`

N06.5 **Isolated proteinuria with diffuse mesangiocapillary glomerulonephritis** `CC`

Isolated proteinuria with membranoproliferative glomerulonephritis, types 1 and 3, or NOS

EXCLUDES 1 ▶isolated proteinuria with C3 glomerulonephritis (N06.A)◀

▶isolated proteinuria with C3 glomerulopathy (N06.A)◀

N06.6 **Isolated proteinuria with dense deposit disease**

▶Isolated proteinuria with C3 glomerulopathy with dense deposit disease◀

Isolated proteinuria with membranoproliferative glomerulonephritis, type 2

N06.7 **Isolated proteinuria with diffuse crescentic glomerulonephritis**

Isolated proteinuria with extracapillary glomerulonephritis

N06.8 **Isolated proteinuria with other morphologic lesion**

Isolated proteinuria with proliferative glomerulonephritis NOS

N06.9 **Isolated proteinuria with unspecified morphologic lesion**

● **N06.A** **Isolated proteinuria with C3 glomerulonephritis** `CC`

Isolated proteinuria with C3 glomerulopathy

EXCLUDES 1 isolated proteinuria (with C3 glomerulopathy) with dense deposit disease (N06.6)

✓4ᵗʰ **N07** **Hereditary nephropathy, not elsewhere classified**

EXCLUDES 2 Alport's syndrome (Q87.81-)

hereditary amyloid nephropathy (E85.-)

nail patella syndrome (Q87.2)

non-neuropathic heredofamilial amyloidosis (E85.-)

N07.0 **Hereditary nephropathy, not elsewhere classified with minor glomerular abnormality**

Hereditary nephropathy, not elsewhere classified with minimal change lesion

N07.1 **Hereditary nephropathy, not elsewhere classified with focal and segmental glomerular lesions**

Hereditary nephropathy, not elsewhere classified with focal and segmental hyalinosis

Hereditary nephropathy, not elsewhere classified with focal and segmental sclerosis

Hereditary nephropathy, not elsewhere classified with focal glomerulonephritis

N07.2 **Hereditary nephropathy, not elsewhere classified with diffuse membranous glomerulonephritis** `CC`

N07.3 **Hereditary nephropathy, not elsewhere classified with diffuse mesangial proliferative glomerulonephritis** `CC`

N07.4 **Hereditary nephropathy, not elsewhere classified with diffuse endocapillary proliferative glomerulonephritis** `CC`

N07.5 **Hereditary nephropathy, not elsewhere classified with diffuse mesangiocapillary glomerulonephritis** `CC`

Hereditary nephropathy, not elsewhere classified with membranoproliferative glomerulonephritis, types 1 and 3, or NOS

EXCLUDES 1 ▶hereditary nephropathy, not elsewhere classified with C3 glomerulonephritis (N07.A)◀

▶hereditary nephropathy, not elsewhere classified with C3 glomerulopathy (N07.A)◀

N07.6 **Hereditary nephropathy, not elsewhere classified with dense deposit disease**

▶Hereditary nephropathy, not elsewhere classified with C3 glomerulopathy with dense deposit disease◀

Hereditary nephropathy, not elsewhere classified with membranoproliferative glomerulonephritis, type 2

N07.7 **Hereditary nephropathy, not elsewhere classified with diffuse crescentic glomerulonephritis**

Hereditary nephropathy, not elsewhere classified with extracapillary glomerulonephritis

N07.8 **Hereditary nephropathy, not elsewhere classified with other morphologic lesions**

Hereditary nephropathy, not elsewhere classified with proliferative glomerulonephritis NOS

N07.9 **Hereditary nephropathy, not elsewhere classified with unspecified morphologic lesions**

● **N07.A** **Hereditary nephropathy, not elsewhere classified with C3 glomerulonephritis** `CC`

Hereditary nephropathy, not elsewhere classified with C3 glomerulopathy

EXCLUDES 1 hereditary nephropathy, not elsewhere classified (with C3 glomerulopathy) with dense deposit disease (N07.6)

`N` Newborn: 0　`P` Pediatric: 0-17　`M` Maternity: 9-64　`A` Adult: 15-124　`MCC` Major Complication/Comorbidity　`CC` Complication/Comorbidity　`SW` Severe Wound Dx

N08 Glomerular disorders in diseases classified elsewhere
    Glomerulonephritis
    Nephritis
    Nephropathy
    Code first underlying disease, such as:
      amyloidosis (E85.-)
      congenital syphilis (A50.5)
      cryoglobulinemia (D89.1)
      disseminated intravascular coagulation (D65)
      gout (M1A.-, M10.-)
      microscopic polyangiitis (M31.7)
      multiple myeloma (C90.0-)
      sepsis (A40.0-A41.9)
      sickle-cell disease (D57.0-D57.8)
      EXCLUDES 1   *glomerulonephritis, nephritis and nephropathy (in):*
        antiglomerular basement membrane disease (M31.0)
        diabetes (E08-E13 with .21)
        gonococcal (A54.21)
        Goodpasture's syndrome (M31.0)
        hemolytic-uremic syndrome (D59.3)
        lupus (M32.14)
        mumps (B26.83)
        syphilis (A52.75)
        systemic lupus erythematosus (M32.14)
        Wegener's granulomatosis (M31.31)
      pyelonephritis in diseases classified elsewhere (N16)
      renal tubulo-interstitial disorders classified elsewhere (N16)

Renal tubulo-interstitial diseases (N10-N16)

  INCLUDES   pyelonephritis
  EXCLUDES 1   *pyeloureteritis cystica (N28.85)*

N10 Acute pyelonephritis   `CC` `H6`
    Acute infectious interstitial nephritis
    Acute pyelitis
    Acute tubulo-interstitial nephritis
    Hemoglobin nephrosis
    Myoglobin nephrosis
    Use additional code (B95-B97), to identify infectious agent
    AHA: 2019,3Q,13

N11 Chronic tubulo-interstitial nephritis   ✓4th
    INCLUDES   chronic infectious interstitial nephritis
             chronic pyelitis
             chronic pyelonephritis
    Use additional code (B95-B97), to identify infectious agent

  N11.0 Nonobstructive reflux-associated chronic pyelonephritis
    Pyelonephritis (chronic) associated with (vesicoureteral) reflux
    EXCLUDES 1   *vesicoureteral reflux NOS (N13.70)*

  N11.1 Chronic obstructive pyelonephritis   `CC`
    Pyelonephritis (chronic) associated with anomaly of
      pelviureteric junction
    Pyelonephritis (chronic) associated with anomaly of
      pyeloureteric junction
    Pyelonephritis (chronic) associated with crossing of vessel
    Pyelonephritis (chronic) associated with kinking of ureter
    Pyelonephritis (chronic) associated with obstruction of ureter
    Pyelonephritis (chronic) associated with stricture of pelviureteric
      junction
    Pyelonephritis (chronic) associated with stricture of ureter
    EXCLUDES 1   *calculous pyelonephritis (N20.9)*
           obstructive uropathy (N13.-)

  N11.8 Other chronic tubulo-interstitial nephritis   `CC`
    Nonobstructive chronic pyelonephritis NOS

  N11.9 Chronic tubulo-interstitial nephritis, unspecified   `CC` `H6`
    Chronic interstitial nephritis NOS
    Chronic pyelitis NOS
    Chronic pyelonephritis NOS

N12 Tubulo-interstitial nephritis, not specified as acute or chronic   `CC` `H6`
    Interstitial nephritis NOS
    Pyelitis NOS
    Pyelonephritis NOS
    EXCLUDES 1   *calculous pyelonephritis (N20.9)*

N13 Obstructive and reflux uropathy   ✓4th
    EXCLUDES 2   *calculus of kidney and ureter without hydronephrosis (N20.-)*
      congenital obstructive defects of renal pelvis and ureter
        (Q62.0-Q62.3)
      hydronephrosis with ureteropelvic junction obstruction
        (Q62.11)
      obstructive pyelonephritis (N11.1)
    DEF: Hydronephrosis: Distension of the kidney caused by an accumulation of urine that cannot flow out due to an obstruction that may be caused by conditions such as kidney stones or vesicoureteral reflux.

  N13.0 Hydronephrosis with ureteropelvic junction obstruction   `CC`
    Hydronephrosis due to acquired occlusion of ureteropelvic junction
    EXCLUDES 2   *hydronephrosis with ureteropelvic junction obstruction due to calculus (N13.2)*
    AHA: 2016,4Q,43

Hydronephrosis/UPJ Obstruction

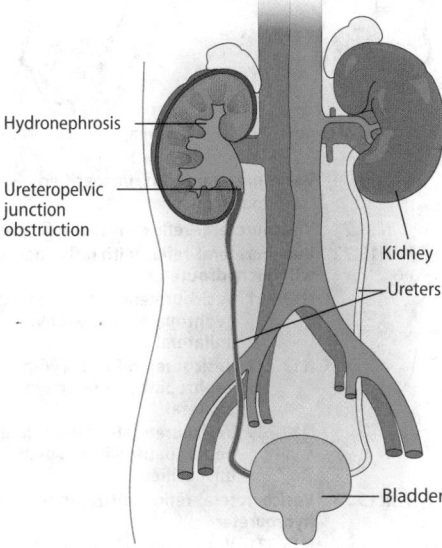

  N13.1 Hydronephrosis with ureteral stricture, not elsewhere classified   `CC`
    EXCLUDES 1   *hydronephrosis with ureteral stricture with infection (N13.6)*

  N13.2 Hydronephrosis with renal and ureteral calculous obstruction   `CC`
    EXCLUDES 1   *hydronephrosis with renal and ureteral calculous obstruction with infection (N13.6)*

  N13.3 Other and unspecified hydronephrosis   ✓5th
    EXCLUDES 1   *hydronephrosis with infection (N13.6)*
    N13.30 Unspecified hydronephrosis   `CC`
    N13.39 Other hydronephrosis   `CC`

  N13.4 Hydroureter   `CC`
    EXCLUDES 1   *congenital hydroureter (Q62.3-)*
           hydroureter with infection (N13.6)
           vesicoureteral-reflux with hydroureter (N13.73-)
    DEF: Abnormal enlargement or distension of the ureter with water or urine caused by an obstruction.

  N13.5 Crossing vessel and stricture of ureter without hydronephrosis
    Kinking and stricture of ureter without hydronephrosis
    EXCLUDES 1   *crossing vessel and stricture of ureter without hydronephrosis with infection (N13.6)*

  N13.6 Pyonephrosis   `CC` `H6`
    Conditions in N13.0-N13.5 with infection
    Obstructive uropathy with infection
    Use additional code (B95-B97), to identify infectious agent
    AHA: 2018,2Q,21

☑ Additional Character Required   ✓x7th Placeholder   Unacceptable PDx   Questionable PDx   Manifestation   Unspecified Dx   H1-H14 HAC   HCC CMS-HCC Dx   HIV HIV Dx

ICD-10-CM 2021   845

Chapter 14. Diseases of the Genitourinary System

N13.7–N18.2

✓6ᵗʰ N13.7 Vesicoureteral-reflux

> **EXCLUDES 1**   reflux-associated pyelonephritis (N11.Ø)
>
> **DEF:** Urine passage from the bladder flows backward up into the ureter and kidneys that can lead to bacterial infection and an increase in hydrostatic pressure, causing kidney damage.

Vesicoureteral Reflux

Kidneys

Ureters

Bladder

Normal flow of urine   Urine flowing the wrong way (VUR)

N13.70 Vesicoureteral-reflux, unspecified
Vesicoureteral-reflux NOS

N13.71 Vesicoureteral-reflux without reflux nephropathy

✓6ᵗʰ **N13.72 Vesicoureteral-reflux with reflux nephropathy without hydroureter**

     N13.721 Vesicoureteral-reflux with reflux nephropathy without hydroureter, unilateral

     N13.722 Vesicoureteral-reflux with reflux nephropathy without hydroureter, bilateral

     N13.729 Vesicoureteral-reflux with reflux nephropathy without hydroureter, unspecified

✓6ᵗʰ **N13.73 Vesicoureteral-reflux with reflux nephropathy with hydroureter**

     N13.731 Vesicoureteral-reflux with reflux nephropathy with hydroureter, unilateral

     N13.732 Vesicoureteral-reflux with reflux nephropathy with hydroureter, bilateral

     N13.739 Vesicoureteral-reflux with reflux nephropathy with hydroureter, unspecified

N13.8 Other obstructive and reflux uropathy   CC
Urinary tract obstruction due to specified cause
Code first, if applicable, any causal condition, such as:
     enlarged prostate (N40.1)

N13.9 Obstructive and reflux uropathy, unspecified
Urinary tract obstruction NOS

✓4ᵗʰ N14 Drug- and heavy-metal-induced tubulo-interstitial and tubular conditions

Code first poisoning due to drug or toxin, if applicable (T36-T65 with fifth or sixth character 1-4 or 6)
Use additional code for adverse effect, if applicable, to identify drug (T36-T50 with fifth or sixth character 5)

N14.Ø Analgesic nephropathy

N14.1 Nephropathy induced by other drugs, medicaments and biological substances

N14.2 Nephropathy induced by unspecified drug, medicament or biological substance

N14.3 Nephropathy induced by heavy metals

N14.4 Toxic nephropathy, not elsewhere classified

✓4ᵗʰ N15 Other renal tubulo-interstitial diseases

N15.Ø Balkan nephropathy
Balkan endemic nephropathy

N15.1 Renal and perinephric abscess   MCC H6

N15.8 Other specified renal tubulo-interstitial diseases

N15.9 Renal tubulo-interstitial disease, unspecified
Infection of kidney NOS
> **EXCLUDES 1**   urinary tract infection NOS (N39.Ø)

N16 Renal tubulo-interstitial disorders in diseases classified elsewhere

Pyelonephritis
Tubulo-interstitial nephritis
Code first underlying disease, such as:
     brucellosis (A23.Ø-A23.9)
     cryoglobulinemia (D89.1)
     glycogen storage disease (E74.Ø)
     leukemia (C91-C95)
     lymphoma (C81.Ø-C85.9, C96.Ø-C96.9)
     multiple myeloma (C9Ø.Ø-)
     sepsis (A4Ø.Ø-A41.9)
     Wilson's disease (E83.Ø)

> **EXCLUDES 1**   diphtheritic pyelonephritis and tubulo-interstitial nephritis (A36.84)
>
> pyelonephritis and tubulo-interstitial nephritis in candidiasis (B37.49)
>
> pyelonephritis and tubulo-interstitial nephritis in cystinosis (E72.Ø4)
>
> pyelonephritis and tubulo-interstitial nephritis in salmonella infection (AØ2.25)
>
> pyelonephritis and tubulo-interstitial nephritis in sarcoidosis (D86.84)
>
> pyelonephritis and tubulo-interstitial nephritis in sicca syndrome [Sjogren's] (M35.Ø4)
>
> pyelonephritis and tubulo-interstitial nephritis in systemic lupus erythematosus (M32.15)
>
> pyelonephritis and tubulo-interstitial nephritis in toxoplasmosis (B58.83)
>
> renal tubular degeneration in diabetes (EØ8-E13 with .29)
>
> syphilitic pyelonephritis and tubulo-interstitial nephritis (A52.75)

Acute kidney failure and chronic kidney disease (N17-N19)

> **EXCLUDES 2**   congenital renal failure (P96.Ø)
>
> drug- and heavy-metal-induced tubulo-interstitial and tubular conditions (N14.-)
>
> extrarenal uremia (R39.2)
>
> hemolytic-uremic syndrome (D59.3)
>
> hepatorenal syndrome (K76.7)
>
> postpartum hepatorenal syndrome (O9Ø.4)
>
> posttraumatic renal failure (T79.5)
>
> prerenal uremia (R39.2)
>
> renal failure complicating abortion or ectopic or molar pregnancy (OØØ-OØ7, OØ8.4)
>
> renal failure following labor and delivery (O9Ø.4)
>
> renal failure postprocedural (N99.Ø)

✓4ᵗʰ N17 Acute kidney failure

Code also associated underlying condition
> **EXCLUDES 1**   posttraumatic renal failure (T79.5)

AHA: 2019,2Q,7; 2019,1Q,12; 2013,4Q,124

N17.Ø Acute kidney failure with tubular necrosis   MCC HCC
Acute tubular necrosis
Renal tubular necrosis
Tubular necrosis NOS

N17.1 Acute kidney failure with acute cortical necrosis   MCC HCC
Acute cortical necrosis
Cortical necrosis NOS
Renal cortical necrosis

N17.2 Acute kidney failure with medullary necrosis   MCC HCC
Medullary [papillary] necrosis NOS
Acute medullary [papillary] necrosis
Renal medullary [papillary] necrosis

N17.8 Other acute kidney failure   CC HCC

N17.9 Acute kidney failure, unspecified   CC HCC
Acute kidney injury (nontraumatic)
> **EXCLUDES 2**   traumatic kidney injury (S37.Ø-)

✓4ᵗʰ N18 Chronic kidney disease (CKD)

Code first any associated:
     diabetic chronic kidney disease (EØ8.22, EØ9.22, E1Ø.22, E11.22, E13.22)
     hypertensive chronic kidney disease (I12.-, I13.-)
Use additional code to identify kidney transplant status, if applicable, (Z94.Ø)

AHA: 2019,3Q,3; 2018,4Q,88; 2013,1Q,24

N18.1 Chronic kidney disease, stage 1

N18.2 Chronic kidney disease, stage 2 (mild)

N Newborn: 0   P Pediatric: 0-17   M Maternity: 9-64   A Adult: 15-124   MCC Major Complication/Comorbidity   CC Complication/Comorbidity   SW Severe Wound Dx

846   ICD-10-CM 2021

▲   ✓5ᵗʰ   **N18.3**   **Chronic kidney disease, stage 3 (moderate)**

●   **N18.30**   **Chronic kidney disease, stage 3 unspecified**

●   **N18.31**   **Chronic kidney disease,** stage 3a

●   **N18.32**   **Chronic kidney disease,** stage 3b

    N18.4   **Chronic kidney disease,** stage 4 (severe)   `CC` `HCC`

    N18.5   **Chronic kidney disease,** stage 5   `CC` `HCC`
       EXCLUDES 1   chronic kidney disease, stage 5 requiring chronic dialysis (N18.6)
       DEF: End-stage renal disease (ESRD) with a GFR value of 15 ml/min or less not yet requiring chronic dialysis.
       TIP: When both ESRD and CKD 5 are documented, code only for ESRD.

    N18.6   **End stage renal disease**   `MCC` `HCC`
       Chronic kidney disease requiring chronic dialysis
       Use additional code to identify dialysis status (Z99.2)
       AHA: 2016,3Q,22; 2016,1Q,12; 2013,4Q,124-125
       TIP: When both ESRD and CKD 5 are documented, code only for ESRD.

    N18.9   **Chronic kidney disease, unspecified**
       Chronic renal disease
       Chronic renal failure NOS
       Chronic renal insufficiency
       Chronic uremia NOS
       Diffuse sclerosing glomerulonephritis NOS

N19   **Unspecified kidney failure**
    Uremia NOS
    EXCLUDES 1   acute kidney failure (N17.-)
         chronic kidney disease (N18.-)
         chronic uremia (N18.9)
         extrarenal uremia (R39.2)
         prerenal uremia (R39.2)
         renal insufficiency (acute) (N28.9)
         uremia of newborn (P96.0)

Urolithiasis (N20-N23)

AHA: 2017,1Q,5; 2015,2Q,8
TIP: Codes from this code block can be assigned based on the diagnosis listed in a radiology report when authenticated by a radiologist and available at the time of code assignment.

✓4ᵗʰ   **N20**   **Calculus of kidney and ureter**
    Calculous pyelonephritis
    EXCLUDES 1   nephrocalcinosis (E83.5)
         that with hydronephrosis (N13.2)
    AHA: 2019,3Q,13

    N20.0   **Calculus of kidney**
       Nephrolithiasis NOS
       Renal calculus
       Renal stone
       Staghorn calculus
       Stone in kidney
       AHA: 2019,3Q,13

    N20.1   **Calculus of ureter**   `CC`
       ▶Calculus of the ureteropelvic junction◀
       Ureteric stone
       AHA: 2016,3Q,22

    N20.2   **Calculus of kidney with calculus of ureter**   `CC`
    N20.9   **Urinary calculus, unspecified**

✓4ᵗʰ   **N21**   **Calculus of lower urinary tract**
    INCLUDES   calculus of lower urinary tract with cystitis and urethritis

    N21.0   **Calculus in bladder**
       Calculus in diverticulum of bladder
       Urinary bladder stone
       EXCLUDES 2   staghorn calculus (N20.0)

    N21.1   **Calculus in urethra**
       EXCLUDES 2   calculus of prostate (N42.0)

    N21.8   **Other lower urinary tract calculus**
    N21.9   **Calculus of lower urinary tract, unspecified**
       EXCLUDES 1   calculus of urinary tract NOS (N20.9)

N22   *Calculus of urinary tract in diseases classified elsewhere*
    Code first underlying disease, such as:
       gout (M1A.-, M10.-)
       schistosomiasis (B65.0-B65.9)

N23   **Unspecified renal colic**

Other disorders of kidney and ureter (N25-N29)

    EXCLUDES 2   disorders of kidney and ureter with urolithiasis (N20-N23)

✓4ᵗʰ   **N25**   **Disorders resulting from impaired renal tubular function**

    N25.0   **Renal osteodystrophy**
       Azotemic osteodystrophy
       Phosphate-losing tubular disorders
       Renal rickets
       Renal short stature
       EXCLUDES 2   metabolic disorders classifiable to E70-E88
       DEF: Various bone diseases occurring when kidney function is impaired or fails. Abnormal levels of phosphorous and calcium can lead to osteomalacia, osteoporosis, or osteosclerosis.

    N25.1   **Nephrogenic diabetes insipidus**   `CC` `HCC`
       EXCLUDES 1   diabetes insipidus NOS (E23.2)
       DEF: Type of diabetes due to the inability of renal tubules to reabsorb water back into the body. It is not responsive to vasopressin (antidiuretic hormone) and it is characterized by excessive thirst and excessive urine production. It may develop into chronic renal insufficiency.

✓5ᵗʰ   **N25.8**   **Other disorders resulting from impaired renal tubular function**

       N25.81   **Secondary hyperparathyroidism of renal origin**   `CC` `HCC`
          EXCLUDES 1   secondary hyperparathyroidism, non-renal (E21.1)
          EXCLUDES 2   metabolic disorders classifiable to E70-E88
          DEF: Parathyroid dysfunction caused by chronic renal failure. Phosphate clearance and vitamin D production is impaired resulting in lowered calcium blood levels and an excessive production of parathyroid hormone.

       N25.89   **Other disorders resulting from impaired renal tubular function**
          Hypokalemic nephropathy
          Lightwood-Albright syndrome
          Renal tubular acidosis NOS

    N25.9   **Disorder resulting from impaired renal tubular function, unspecified**

✓4ᵗʰ   **N26**   **Unspecified contracted kidney**
    EXCLUDES 1   contracted kidney due to hypertension (I12.-)
         diffuse sclerosing glomerulonephritis (N05.8.-)
         hypertensive nephrosclerosis (arteriolar) (arteriosclerotic) (I12.-)
         small kidney of unknown cause (N27.-)

    N26.1   **Atrophy of kidney (terminal)**
    N26.2   **Page kidney**
    N26.9   **Renal sclerosis, unspecified**

✓4ᵗʰ   **N27**   **Small kidney of unknown cause**
    INCLUDES   oligonephronia

    N27.0   **Small kidney, unilateral**
    N27.1   **Small kidney, bilateral**
    N27.9   **Small kidney, unspecified**

✓4ᵗʰ   **N28**   **Other disorders of kidney and ureter, not elsewhere classified**

    N28.0   **Ischemia and infarction of kidney**   `CC` `HCC`
       Renal artery embolism
       Renal artery obstruction
       Renal artery occlusion
       Renal artery thrombosis
       Renal infarct
       EXCLUDES 1   atherosclerosis of renal artery (extrarenal part) (I70.1)
          congenital stenosis of renal artery (Q27.1)
          Goldblatt's kidney (I70.1)

    N28.1   **Cyst of kidney, acquired**
       Cyst (multiple) (solitary) of kidney (acquired)
       EXCLUDES 1   cystic kidney disease (congenital) (Q61.-)

✓5ᵗʰ   **N28.8**   **Other specified disorders of kidney and ureter**
       EXCLUDES 1   hydroureter (N13.4)
         ureteric stricture with hydronephrosis (N13.1)
         ureteric stricture without hydronephrosis (N13.5)

       N28.81   **Hypertrophy of kidney**
       N28.82   **Megaloureter**
       N28.83   **Nephroptosis**
       N28.84   **Pyelitis cystica**   `CC` `H6`
       N28.85   **Pyeloureteritis cystica**   `CC` `H6`
       N28.86   **Ureteritis cystica**   `CC` `H6`

☑ Additional Character Required   ✓x7ᵗʰ Placeholder   Unacceptable PDx   Questionable PDx   Manifestation   Unspecified Dx   `H1`-`H14` HAC   `HCC` CMS-HCC Dx   `HIV` HIV Dx

ICD-10-CM 2021   **847**

N28.89　**Other specified disorders of kidney and ureter**

N28.9　**Disorder of kidney and ureter, unspecified**
Nephropathy NOS
Renal disease (acute) NOS
Renal insufficiency (acute)
　EXCLUDES 1　*chronic renal insufficiency (N18.9)*
　　　　　　unspecified nephritic syndrome (N05.-)
AHA: 2016,1Q,13

N29　***Other disorders of kidney and ureter in diseases classified elsewhere***
Code first underlying disease, such as:
　amyloidosis (E85.-)
　nephrocalcinosis (E83.5)
　schistosomiasis (B65.0-B65.9)
　EXCLUDES 1　*disorders of kidney and ureter in:*
　　　　　　cystinosis (E72.0)
　　　　　　gonorrhea (A54.21)
　　　　　　syphilis (A52.75)
　　　　　　tuberculosis (A18.11)

Other diseases of the urinary system (N30-N39)

EXCLUDES 1　*urinary infection (complicating):*
　　　abortion or ectopic or molar pregnancy (O00-O07, O08.8)
　　　pregnancy, childbirth and the puerperium (O23.-, O75.3, O86.2-)

✓4ᵗʰ **N30**　**Cystitis**
Use additional code to identify infectious agent (B95-B97)
　EXCLUDES 1　*prostatocystitis (N41.3)*
AHA: 2017,1Q,6
DEF: Inflammation of the urinary bladder. Symptoms include dysuria, frequency of urination, urgency, and hematuria.

✓5ᵗʰ **N30.0**　**Acute cystitis**
　　　EXCLUDES 1　*irradiation cystitis (N30.4-)*
　　　　　　　trigonitis (N30.3-)
　　N30.00　**Acute cystitis without hematuria**　CC H6
　　N30.01　**Acute cystitis with hematuria**　CC H6

✓5ᵗʰ **N30.1**　**Interstitial cystitis (chronic)**
　　N30.10　**Interstitial cystitis (chronic) without hematuria**
　　N30.11　**Interstitial cystitis (chronic) with hematuria**

✓5ᵗʰ **N30.2**　**Other chronic cystitis**
　　N30.20　**Other chronic cystitis without hematuria**
　　N30.21　**Other chronic cystitis with hematuria**

✓5ᵗʰ **N30.3**　**Trigonitis**
　Urethrotrigonitis
　　N30.30　**Trigonitis without hematuria**
　　N30.31　**Trigonitis with hematuria**

✓5ᵗʰ **N30.4**　**Irradiation cystitis**
　　N30.40　**Irradiation cystitis without hematuria**　CC
　　N30.41　**Irradiation cystitis with hematuria**　CC

✓5ᵗʰ **N30.8**　**Other cystitis**
　Abscess of bladder
　　N30.80　**Other cystitis without hematuria**
　　N30.81　**Other cystitis with hematuria**

✓5ᵗʰ **N30.9**　**Cystitis, unspecified**
　　N30.90　**Cystitis, unspecified without hematuria**
　　N30.91　**Cystitis, unspecified with hematuria**

✓4ᵗʰ **N31**　**Neuromuscular dysfunction of bladder, not elsewhere classified**
Use additional code to identify any associated urinary incontinence (N39.3-N39.4-)
　EXCLUDES 1　*cord bladder NOS (G95.89)*
　　　　　　neurogenic bladder due to cauda equina syndrome (G83.4)
　　　　　　neuromuscular dysfunction due to spinal cord lesion (G95.89)

N31.0　**Uninhibited neuropathic bladder, not elsewhere classified**
N31.1　**Reflex neuropathic bladder, not elsewhere classified**
N31.2　**Flaccid neuropathic bladder, not elsewhere classified**
　Atonic (motor) (sensory) neuropathic bladder
　Autonomous neuropathic bladder
　Nonreflex neuropathic bladder
N31.8　**Other neuromuscular dysfunction of bladder**
N31.9　**Neuromuscular dysfunction of bladder, unspecified**
　Neurogenic bladder dysfunction NOS

✓4ᵗʰ **N32**　**Other disorders of bladder**
　EXCLUDES 2　*calculus of bladder (N21.0)*
　　　　　　cystocele (N81.1-)
　　　　　　hernia or prolapse of bladder, female (N81.1-)

N32.0　**Bladder-neck obstruction**
　Bladder-neck stenosis (acquired)
　EXCLUDES 1　*congenital bladder-neck obstruction (Q64.3-)*
　DEF: Bladder outlet and vesicourethral obstruction that occurs as a consequence of benign prostatic hypertrophy or prostatic cancer. It may also occur in either sex due to strictures, radiation, cystoscopy, catheterization, injury, infection, blood clots, bladder cancer, impaction, or other disease that compresses the bladder neck.

N32.1　**Vesicointestinal fistula**　CC
　Vesicorectal fistula

N32.2　**Vesical fistula, not elsewhere classified**　CC
　EXCLUDES 1　*fistula between bladder and female genital tract (N82.0-N82.1)*

N32.3　**Diverticulum of bladder**
　EXCLUDES 1　*congenital diverticulum of bladder (Q64.6)*
　　　　　　diverticulitis of bladder (N30.8-)

✓5ᵗʰ **N32.8**　**Other specified disorders of bladder**
　N32.81　**Overactive bladder**
　　Detrusor muscle hyperactivity
　　EXCLUDES 1　*frequent urination due to specified bladder condition — code to condition*
　　DEF: Sudden involuntary contractions of the muscular wall of the bladder that results in a sudden, strong urge to urinate.
　N32.89　**Other specified disorders of bladder**
　　Bladder hemorrhage
　　Bladder hypertrophy
　　Calcified bladder
　　Contracted bladder

N32.9　**Bladder disorder, unspecified**

N33　***Bladder disorders in diseases classified elsewhere***
Code first underlying disease, such as:
　schistosomiasis (B65.0-B65.9)
　EXCLUDES 1　*bladder disorder in syphilis (A52.76)*
　　　　　　bladder disorder in tuberculosis (A18.12)
　　　　　　candidal cystitis (B37.41)
　　　　　　chlamydial cystitis (A56.01)
　　　　　　cystitis in gonorrhea (A54.01)
　　　　　　cystitis in neurogenic bladder (N31.-)
　　　　　　diphtheritic cystitis (A36.85)
　　　　　　neurogenic bladder (N31.-)
　　　　　　syphilitic cystitis (A52.76)
　　　　　　trichomonal cystitis (A59.03)

✓4ᵗʰ **N34**　**Urethritis and urethral syndrome**
Use additional code (B95-B97), to identify infectious agent
　EXCLUDES 2　*Reiter's disease (M02.3-)*
　　　　　　urethritis in diseases with a predominantly sexual mode of transmission (A50-A64)
　　　　　　urethrotrigonitis (N30.3-)
AHA: 2017,1Q,6

N34.0　**Urethral abscess**　CC H6
　Abscess (of) Cowper's gland
　Abscess (of) Littré's gland
　Abscess (of) urethral (gland)
　Periurethral abscess
　EXCLUDES 1　*urethral caruncle (N36.2)*

N34.1　**Nonspecific urethritis**
　Nongonococcal urethritis
　Nonvenereal urethritis

N34.2　**Other urethritis**
　Meatitis, urethral
　Postmenopausal urethritis
　Ulcer of urethra (meatus)
　Urethritis NOS

N34.3　**Urethral syndrome, unspecified**

☑4ᵗʰ **N35 Urethral stricture**
> *EXCLUDES 1*   congenital urethral stricture (Q64.3-)
>   postprocedural urethral stricture (N99.1-)
> **AHA:** 2018,4Q,21-22

   ☑5ᵗʰ **N35.0 Post-traumatic urethral stricture**
>   Urethral stricture due to injury
>   *EXCLUDES 1*   postprocedural urethral stricture (N99.1-)

     ☑6ᵗʰ **N35.01 Post-traumatic urethral stricture, male**
>   **N35.010 Post-traumatic urethral stricture, male, meatal** ♂
>   **N35.011 Post-traumatic bulbous urethral stricture** ♂
>   **N35.012 Post-traumatic membranous urethral stricture** ♂
>   **N35.013 Post-traumatic anterior urethral stricture** ♂
>   **N35.014 Post-traumatic urethral stricture, male, unspecified** ♂
>   **N35.016 Post-traumatic urethral stricture, male, overlapping sites** ♂

     ☑6ᵗʰ **N35.02 Post-traumatic urethral stricture, female**
>   **N35.021 Urethral stricture due to childbirth** ♀
>   **N35.028 Other post-traumatic urethral stricture, female** ♀

   ☑5ᵗʰ **N35.1 Postinfective urethral stricture, not elsewhere classified**
>   *EXCLUDES 1*   gonococcal urethral stricture (A54.01)
>   syphilitic urethral stricture (A52.76)
>   urethral stricture associated with schistosomiasis (B65.-, N29)

     ☑6ᵗʰ **N35.11 Postinfective urethral stricture, not elsewhere classified, male**
>   **N35.111 Postinfective urethral stricture, not elsewhere classified, male, meatal** ♂
>   **N35.112 Postinfective bulbous urethral stricture, not elsewhere classified, male** ♂
>   **N35.113 Postinfective membranous urethral stricture, not elsewhere classified, male** ♂
>   **N35.114 Postinfective anterior urethral stricture, not elsewhere classified, male** ♂
>   **N35.116 Postinfective urethral stricture, not elsewhere classified, male, overlapping sites** ♂
>   **N35.119 Postinfective urethral stricture, not elsewhere classified, male, unspecified** ♂

     N35.12 Postinfective urethral stricture, not elsewhere classified, female ♀

   ☑5ᵗʰ **N35.8 Other urethral stricture**
>   *EXCLUDES 1*   postprocedural urethral stricture (N99.1-)

     ☑6ᵗʰ **N35.81 Other urethral stricture, male**
>   **N35.811 Other urethral stricture, male, meatal** ♂
>   **N35.812 Other urethral bulbous stricture, male** ♂
>   **N35.813 Other membranous urethral stricture, male** ♂
>   **N35.814 Other anterior urethral stricture, male** ♂
>   **N35.816 Other urethral stricture, male, overlapping sites** ♂
>   **N35.819 Other urethral stricture, male, unspecified site** ♂

     N35.82 Other urethral stricture, female ♀

   ☑5ᵗʰ **N35.9 Urethral stricture, unspecified**

     ☑6ᵗʰ **N35.91 Urethral stricture, unspecified, male**
>   **N35.911 Unspecified urethral stricture, male, meatal** ♂
>   **N35.912 Unspecified bulbous urethral stricture, male** ♂
>   **N35.913 Unspecified membranous urethral stricture, male** ♂
>   **N35.914 Unspecified anterior urethral stricture, male** ♂
>   **N35.916 Unspecified urethral stricture, male, overlapping sites** ♂

   N35.919 Unspecified urethral stricture, male, unspecified site ♂
>   Pinhole meatus NOS
>   Urethral stricture NOS

     N35.92 Unspecified urethral stricture, female ♀

☑4ᵗʰ **N36 Other disorders of urethra**

   N36.0 Urethral fistula   CC
>   Urethroperineal fistula
>   Urethrorectal fistula
>   Urinary fistula NOS
>   *EXCLUDES 1*   urethroscrotal fistula (N50.89)
>   urethrovaginal fistula (N82.1)
>   urethrovesicovaginal fistula (N82.1)

   N36.1 Urethral diverticulum
   N36.2 Urethral caruncle

   ☑5ᵗʰ **N36.4 Urethral functional and muscular disorders**
>   Use additional code to identify associated urinary stress incontinence (N39.3)
>   **N36.41 Hypermobility of urethra**
>   **N36.42 Intrinsic sphincter deficiency (ISD)**
>   **N36.43 Combined hypermobility of urethra and intrinsic sphincter deficiency**
>   **N36.44 Muscular disorders of urethra**
>   Bladder sphincter dyssynergy

   N36.5 Urethral false passage

   N36.8 Other specified disorders of urethra
>   *EXCLUDES 1*   congenital urethrocele (Q64.7)
>   female urethrocele (N81.0)

   N36.9 Urethral disorder, unspecified

N37 Urethral disorders in diseases classified elsewhere
> Code first underlying disease
> *EXCLUDES 1*   urethritis (in):
>   candidal infection (B37.41)
>   chlamydial (A56.01)
>   gonorrhea (A54.01)
>   syphilis (A52.76)
>   trichomonal infection (A59.03)
>   tuberculosis (A18.13)

☑4ᵗʰ **N39 Other disorders of urinary system**
> *EXCLUDES 2*   hematuria NOS (R31.-)
>   recurrent or persistent hematuria (N02.-)
>   recurrent or persistent hematuria with specified morphological lesion (N02.-)
>   proteinuria NOS (R80.-)

   N39.0 Urinary tract infection, site not specified   CC   H6
>   Use additional code (B95-B97), to identify infectious agent
>   *EXCLUDES 1*   candidiasis of urinary tract (B37.4-)
>   neonatal urinary tract infection (P39.3)
>   pyuria (R82.81)
>   urinary tract infection of specified site, such as:
>   cystitis (N30.-)
>   urethritis (N34.-)
>   **AHA:** 2019,3Q,17; 2018,2Q,21,22; 2018,1Q,16; 2017,1Q,6; 2012,4Q,94

   N39.3 Stress incontinence (female) (male)
>   Code also any associated overactive bladder (N32.81)
>   *EXCLUDES 1*   mixed incontinence (N39.46)

   ☑5ᵗʰ **N39.4 Other specified urinary incontinence**
>   Code also any associated overactive bladder (N32.81)
>   *EXCLUDES 1*   enuresis NOS (R32)
>   functional urinary incontinence (R39.81)
>   urinary incontinence associated with cognitive impairment (R39.81)
>   urinary incontinence NOS (R32)
>   urinary incontinence of nonorganic origin (F98.0)

   N39.41 Urge incontinence
>   *EXCLUDES 1*   mixed incontinence (N39.46)

   N39.42 Incontinence without sensory awareness
>   Insensible (urinary) incontinence

   N39.43 Post-void dribbling
   N39.44 Nocturnal enuresis
   N39.45 Continuous leakage

Chapter 14. Diseases of the Genitourinary System

    N39.46   **Mixed incontinence**
         Urge and stress incontinence

☑6ᵗʰ   **N39.49**   **Other specified urinary incontinence**

         AHA: 2016,4Q,44

         N39.490   **Overflow incontinence**
         N39.491   **Coital incontinence**
         N39.492   **Postural (urinary) incontinence**
         N39.498   **Other specified urinary incontinence**
            Reflex incontinence
            Total incontinence

  N39.8   **Other specified disorders of urinary system**

  N39.9   **Disorder of urinary system, unspecified**

Diseases of male genital organs (N40-N53)

☑4ᵗʰ **N40** **Benign prostatic hyperplasia**

     INCLUDES   adenofibromatous hypertrophy of prostate
                  benign hypertrophy of the prostate
                  benign prostatic hypertrophy
                  BPH
                  enlarged prostate
                  nodular prostate
                  polyp of prostate

     EXCLUDES 1   *benign neoplasms of prostate (adenoma, benign)*
                  (fibroadenoma) (fibroma) (myoma) (D29.1)

     EXCLUDES 2   *malignant neoplasm of prostate (C61)*

     DEF: Enlargement of the prostate gland due to an abnormal proliferation of fibrostromal tissue in the paraurethral glands. This condition causes impingement of the urethra resulting in obstructed urinary flow.

  N40.0   **Benign prostatic hyperplasia** without lower urinary tract symptoms   A ♂
       Enlarged prostate NOS
       Enlarged prostate without LUTS

  N40.1   **Benign prostatic hyperplasia** with lower urinary tract symptoms   A ♂
       Enlarged prostate with LUTS
       Use additional code for associated symptoms, when specified:
         incomplete bladder emptying (R39.14)
         nocturia (R35.1)
         straining on urination (R39.16)
         urinary frequency (R35.0)
         urinary hesitancy (R39.11)
         urinary incontinence (N39.4-)
         urinary obstruction (N13.8)
         urinary retention (R33.8)
         urinary urgency (R39.15)
         weak urinary stream (R39.12)
       AHA: 2018,4Q,55

  N40.2   **Nodular prostate** without lower urinary tract symptoms   A ♂
       Nodular prostate without LUTS

  N40.3   **Nodular prostate** with lower urinary tract symptoms   A ♂
       Use additional code for associated symptoms, when specified:
         incomplete bladder emptying (R39.14)
         nocturia (R35.1)
         straining on urination (R39.16)
         urinary frequency (R35.0)
         urinary hesitancy (R39.11)
         urinary incontinence (N39.4-)
         urinary obstruction (N13.8)
         urinary retention (R33.8)
         urinary urgency (R39.15)
         weak urinary stream (R39.12)

☑4ᵗʰ **N41** **Inflammatory diseases of prostate**
       Use additional code (B95-B97), to identify infectious agent

  N41.0   **Acute prostatitis**   CC A ♂
  N41.1   **Chronic prostatitis**   A ♂
  N41.2   **Abscess of prostate**   CC A ♂
  N41.3   **Prostatocystitis**   A ♂
  N41.4   **Granulomatous prostatitis**   A ♂
  N41.8   **Other inflammatory diseases of prostate**   A ♂
  N41.9   **Inflammatory disease of prostate, unspecified**   A ♂
       Prostatitis NOS

☑4ᵗʰ **N42** **Other and unspecified disorders of prostate**

  N42.0   **Calculus of prostate**   A ♂
       Prostatic stone
       DEF: Formation of a small, solid stone often composed of calcium carbonate or calcium phosphate in the prostate gland.

  N42.1   **Congestion and hemorrhage of prostate**   A ♂
     EXCLUDES 1   *enlarged prostate (N40.-)*
                 hematuria (R31.-)
                 hyperplasia of prostate (N40.-)
                 inflammatory diseases of prostate (N41.-)

☑5ᵗʰ **N42.3**   **Dysplasia of prostate**
       AHA: 2016,4Q,44

     N42.30   **Unspecified dysplasia of prostate**   ♂
     N42.31   **Prostatic intraepithelial neoplasia**   ♂
         PIN
         Prostatic intraepithelial neoplasia I (PIN I)
         Prostatic intraepithelial neoplasia II (PIN II)
       EXCLUDES 1   *prostatic intraepithelial neoplasia III (PIN III) (D07.5)*
         DEF: Abnormality of shape and size of the intraepithelial tissues of the prostate. It is a premalignant condition characterized by stalks and absence of a basilar cell layer.

     N42.32   **Atypical small acinar proliferation of prostate**   ♂
     N42.39   **Other dysplasia of prostate**   ♂

☑5ᵗʰ **N42.8**   **Other specified disorders of prostate**
     N42.81   **Prostatodynia syndrome**   A ♂
         Painful prostate syndrome
     N42.82   **Prostatosis syndrome**   A ♂
     N42.83   **Cyst of prostate**   A ♂
     N42.89   **Other specified disorders of prostate**   A ♂

  N42.9   **Disorder of prostate, unspecified**   A ♂

☑4ᵗʰ **N43** **Hydrocele and spermatocele**
     INCLUDES   hydrocele of spermatic cord, testis or tunica vaginalis
     EXCLUDES 1   *congenital hydrocele (P83.5)*
     DEF: Hydrocele: Serous fluid that collects in the tunica vaginalis of the scrotum along the spermatic cord in males.

  N43.0   **Encysted hydrocele**   ♂
  N43.1   **Infected hydrocele**   CC ♂
       Use additional code (B95-B97), to identify infectious agent
  N43.2   **Other hydrocele**   ♂

Hydrocele

Normal   Noncommunicating hydrocele   Communicating hydrocele   Hydrocele of the cord

  N43.3   **Hydrocele, unspecified**   ♂
☑5ᵗʰ **N43.4**   **Spermatocele of epididymis**
       Spermatic cyst
       DEF: Spermatocele: Noncancerous accumulation of fluid and dead sperm cells normally located at the head of the epididymis that exhibits itself as a hard, smooth scrotal mass and do not normally require treatment unless they become enlarged or cause pain.

     N43.40   **Spermatocele of epididymis, unspecified**   ♂
     N43.41   **Spermatocele of epididymis, single**   ♂
     N43.42   **Spermatocele of epididymis, multiple**   ♂

☑4ᵗʰ **N44** **Noninflammatory disorders of testis**
☑5ᵗʰ **N44.0**   **Torsion of testis**
     N44.00   **Torsion of testis, unspecified**   CC ♂

N Newborn: 0   P Pediatric: 0-17   M Maternity: 9-64   A Adult: 15-124   MCC Major Complication/Comorbidity   CC Complication/Comorbidity   SW Severe Wound Dx

850   ICD-10-CM 2021

N44.01   **Extravaginal torsion of spermatic cord**   CC ♂
     DEF: Torsion of the spermatic cord just below the tunica vaginalis attachments.

N44.02   **Intravaginal torsion of spermatic cord**   CC ♂
     Torsion of spermatic cord NOS

N44.03   **Torsion of appendix testis**   CC ♂

N44.04   **Torsion of appendix epididymis**   CC ♂

N44.1   **Cyst of tunica albuginea testis**   ♂

N44.2   **Benign cyst of testis**   ♂

N44.8   **Other noninflammatory disorders of the testis**   ♂

✓4th **N45**   **Orchitis and epididymitis**
     Use additional code (B95-B97), to identify infectious agent

N45.1   **Epididymitis**   ♂

N45.2   **Orchitis**   ♂

N45.3   **Epididymo-orchitis**   ♂

N45.4   **Abscess of epididymis or testis**   CC ♂

✓4th **N46**   **Male infertility**
     EXCLUDES 1   vasectomy status (Z98.52)

✓5th **N46.0**   **Azoospermia**
     Absolute male infertility
     Male infertility due to germinal (cell) aplasia
     Male infertility due to spermatogenic arrest (complete)
     DEF: Failure of the development of sperm or the absence of sperm in semen.

N46.01   **Organic azoospermia**   A ♂
     Azoospermia NOS

✓6th **N46.02**   **Azoospermia due to extratesticular causes**
     Code also associated cause

N46.021   **Azoospermia due to drug therapy**   A ♂

N46.022   **Azoospermia due to infection**   A ♂

N46.023   **Azoospermia due to obstruction of efferent ducts**   ♂

N46.024   **Azoospermia due to radiation**   A ♂

N46.025   **Azoospermia due to systemic disease**   A ♂

N46.029   **Azoospermia due to other extratesticular causes**   A ♂

✓5th **N46.1**   **Oligospermia**
     Male infertility due to germinal cell desquamation
     Male infertility due to hypospermatogenesis
     Male infertility due to incomplete spermatogenic arrest
     DEF: Insufficient production of sperm in semen.

N46.11   **Organic oligospermia**   A ♂
     Oligospermia NOS

✓6th **N46.12**   **Oligospermia due to extratesticular causes**
     Code also associated cause

N46.121   **Oligospermia due to drug therapy**   A ♂

N46.122   **Oligospermia due to infection**   A ♂

N46.123   **Oligospermia due to obstruction of efferent ducts**   A ♂

N46.124   **Oligospermia due to radiation**   A ♂

N46.125   **Oligospermia due to systemic disease**   A ♂

N46.129   **Oligospermia due to other extratesticular causes**   A ♂

N46.8   **Other male infertility**   A ♂

N46.9   **Male infertility, unspecified**   A ♂

✓4th **N47**   **Disorders of prepuce**

N47.0   **Adherent prepuce, newborn**   N ♂

N47.1   **Phimosis**
     DEF: Condition in which the foreskin is contracted and cannot be drawn back behind the glans penis.

N47.2   **Paraphimosis**   ♂

N47.3   **Deficient foreskin**   ♂

N47.4   **Benign cyst of prepuce**   ♂

N47.5   **Adhesions of prepuce and glans penis**   ♂

N47.6   **Balanoposthitis**   ♂
     Use additional code (B95-B97), to identify infectious agent
     EXCLUDES 1   balanitis (N48.1)

N47.7   **Other inflammatory diseases of prepuce**   ♂
     Use additional code (B95-B97), to identify infectious agent

N47.8   **Other disorders of prepuce**   ♂

✓4th **N48**   **Other disorders of penis**

N48.0   **Leukoplakia of penis**   ♂
     Balanitis xerotica obliterans
     Kraurosis of penis
     Lichen sclerosus of external male genital organs
     EXCLUDES 1   carcinoma in situ of penis (D07.4)

N48.1   **Balanitis**   ♂
     Use additional code (B95-B97), to identify infectious agent
     EXCLUDES 1   amebic balanitis (A06.8)
         balanitis xerotica obliterans (N48.0)
         candidal balanitis (B37.42)
         gonococcal balanitis (A54.23)
         herpesviral [herpes simplex] balanitis (A60.01)
     DEF: Inflammation of the glans penis, most often affecting uncircumcised males.

✓5th **N48.2**   **Other inflammatory disorders of penis**
     Use additional code (B95-B97), to identify infectious agent
     EXCLUDES 1   balanitis (N48.1)
         balanitis xerotica obliterans (N48.0)
         balanoposthitis (N47.6)

N48.21   **Abscess of corpus cavernosum and penis**   ♂

N48.22   **Cellulitis of corpus cavernosum and penis**   ♂

N48.29   **Other inflammatory disorders of penis**   ♂

✓5th **N48.3**   **Priapism**
     Painful erection
     Code first underlying cause

N48.30   **Priapism, unspecified**   CC ♂

N48.31   **Priapism due to trauma**   CC ♂

N48.32   *Priapism due to disease classified elsewhere*   CC ♂

N48.33   **Priapism, drug-induced**   CC ♂

N48.39   **Other priapism**   CC ♂

N48.5   **Ulcer of penis**   ♂

N48.6   **Induration penis plastica**   ♂
     Peyronie's disease
     Plastic induration of penis

✓5th **N48.8**   **Other specified disorders of penis**

N48.81   **Thrombosis of superficial vein of penis**   ♂

N48.82   **Acquired torsion of penis**   ♂
     Acquired torsion of penis NOS
     EXCLUDES 1   congenital torsion of penis (Q55.63)

N48.83   **Acquired buried penis**   ♂
     EXCLUDES 1   congenital hidden penis (Q55.64)

N48.89   **Other specified disorders of penis**   ♂

N48.9   **Disorder of penis, unspecified**   ♂

✓4th **N49**   **Inflammatory disorders of male genital organs, not elsewhere classified**
     Use additional code (B95-B97), to identify infectious agent
     EXCLUDES 1   inflammation of penis (N48.1, N48.2-)
         orchitis and epididymitis (N45.-)

N49.0   **Inflammatory disorders of seminal vesicle**   ♂
     Vesiculitis NOS

N49.1   **Inflammatory disorders of spermatic cord, tunica vaginalis and vas deferens**   ♂
     Vasitis

N49.2   **Inflammatory disorders of scrotum**   ♂

N49.3   **Fournier gangrene**   ♂
     AHA: 2020,2Q,18

N49.8   **Inflammatory disorders of other specified male genital organs**   ♂
     Inflammation of multiple sites in male genital organs

N49.9   **Inflammatory disorder of unspecified male genital organ**   ♂
     Abscess of unspecified male genital organ
     Boil of unspecified male genital organ
     Carbuncle of unspecified male genital organ
     Cellulitis of unspecified male genital organ

✓4th **N50**   **Other and unspecified disorders of male genital organs**
     EXCLUDES 2   torsion of testis (N44.0-)

N50.0   **Atrophy of testis**   ♂

N50.1   **Vascular disorders of male genital organs**   ♂
     Hematocele, NOS, of male genital organs
     Hemorrhage of male genital organs
     Thrombosis of male genital organs

N50.3   **Cyst of epididymis**   ♂

☑ Additional Character Required   ✓x7th Placeholder   Unacceptable PDx   Questionable PDx   Manifestation   Unspecified Dx   H1-H14 HAC   HCC CMS-HCC Dx   HIV HIV Dx

Chapter 14. Diseases of the Genitourinary System

N50.8–N61.0

✓5ᵗʰ **N50.8 Other specified disorders of male genital organs**

    AHA: 2016,4Q,45

    ✓6ᵗʰ **N50.81 Testicular pain**

        N50.811 Right testicular pain ♂

        N50.812 Left testicular pain ♂

        N50.819 Testicular pain, unspecified ♂

    N50.82 Scrotal pain ♂

    N50.89 Other specified disorders of the male genital organs ♂

        Atrophy of scrotum, seminal vesicle, spermatic cord, tunica vaginalis and vas deferens

        Chylocele, tunica vaginalis (nonfilarial) NOS

        Edema of scrotum, seminal vesicle, spermatic cord, tunica vaginalis and vas deferens

        Hypertrophy of scrotum, seminal vesicle, spermatic cord, tunica vaginalis and vas deferens

        Stricture of spermatic cord, tunica vaginalis, and vas deferens

        Ulcer of scrotum, seminal vesicle, spermatic cord, testis, tunica vaginalis and vas deferens

        Urethroscrotal fistula

    N50.9 Disorder of male genital organs, unspecified ♂

N51 Disorders of male genital organs in diseases classified elsewhere ♂

    Code first underlying disease, such as:

        filariasis (B74.0-B74.9)

    EXCLUDES 1   amebic balanitis (A06.8)

        candidal balanitis (B37.42)

        gonococcal balanitis (A54.23)

        gonococcal prostatitis (A54.22)

        herpesviral [herpes simplex] balanitis (A60.01)

        trichomonal prostatitis (A59.02)

        tuberculous prostatitis (A18.14)

✓4ᵗʰ **N52 Male erectile dysfunction**

    EXCLUDES 1   psychogenic impotence (F52.21)

    ✓5ᵗʰ **N52.0 Vasculogenic erectile dysfunction**

        N52.01 Erectile dysfunction due to arterial insufficiency A ♂

        N52.02 Corporo-venous occlusive erectile dysfunction A ♂

        N52.03 Combined arterial insufficiency and corporo-venous occlusive erectile dysfunction A ♂

    N52.1 Erectile dysfunction due to diseases classified elsewhere A ♂

        Code first underlying disease

    N52.2 Drug-induced erectile dysfunction A ♂

    ✓5ᵗʰ **N52.3 Postprocedural erectile dysfunction**

        AHA: 2016,4Q,45

        N52.31 Erectile dysfunction following radical prostatectomy A ♂

        N52.32 Erectile dysfunction following radical cystectomy A ♂

        N52.33 Erectile dysfunction following urethral surgery A ♂

        N52.34 Erectile dysfunction following simple prostatectomy A ♂

        N52.35 Erectile dysfunction following radiation therapy A ♂

        N52.36 Erectile dysfunction following interstitial seed therapy A ♂

        N52.37 Erectile dysfunction following prostate ablative therapy A ♂

        Erectile dysfunction following cryotherapy

        Erectile dysfunction following other prostate ablative therapies

        Erectile dysfunction following ultrasound ablative therapies

        N52.39 Other and unspecified postprocedural erectile dysfunction A ♂

    N52.8 Other male erectile dysfunction A ♂

    N52.9 Male erectile dysfunction, unspecified A ♂

        Impotence NOS

✓4ᵗʰ **N53 Other male sexual dysfunction**

    EXCLUDES 1   psychogenic sexual dysfunction (F52.-)

    ✓5ᵗʰ **N53.1 Ejaculatory dysfunction**

        EXCLUDES 1   premature ejaculation (F52.4)

        N53.11 Retarded ejaculation ♂

        N53.12 Painful ejaculation ♂

        N53.13 Anejaculatory orgasm ♂

        N53.14 Retrograde ejaculation ♂

        DEF: Form of male sexual dysfunction in which the semen enters the bladder instead of going out through the urethra during ejaculation.

        N53.19 Other ejaculatory dysfunction ♂

        Ejaculatory dysfunction NOS

    N53.8 Other male sexual dysfunction ♂

    N53.9 Unspecified male sexual dysfunction ♂

Disorders of breast (N60-N65)

EXCLUDES 1   disorders of breast associated with childbirth (O91-O92)

✓4ᵗʰ **N60 Benign mammary dysplasia**

    INCLUDES   fibrocystic mastopathy

    ✓5ᵗʰ **N60.0 Solitary cyst of breast**

        Cyst of breast

        N60.01 Solitary cyst of right breast

        N60.02 Solitary cyst of left breast

        N60.09 Solitary cyst of unspecified breast

    ✓5ᵗʰ **N60.1 Diffuse cystic mastopathy**

        Cystic breast

        Fibrocystic disease of breast

        EXCLUDES 1   diffuse cystic mastopathy with epithelial proliferation (N60.3-)

        N60.11 Diffuse cystic mastopathy of right breast A

        N60.12 Diffuse cystic mastopathy of left breast A

        N60.19 Diffuse cystic mastopathy of unspecified breast A

    ✓5ᵗʰ **N60.2 Fibroadenosis of breast**

        Adenofibrosis of breast

        EXCLUDES 2   fibroadenoma of breast (D24.-)

        N60.21 Fibroadenosis of right breast

        N60.22 Fibroadenosis of left breast

        N60.29 Fibroadenosis of unspecified breast

    ✓5ᵗʰ **N60.3 Fibrosclerosis of breast**

        Cystic mastopathy with epithelial proliferation

        N60.31 Fibrosclerosis of right breast

        N60.32 Fibrosclerosis of left breast

        N60.39 Fibrosclerosis of unspecified breast

    ✓5ᵗʰ **N60.4 Mammary duct ectasia**

        N60.41 Mammary duct ectasia of right breast

        N60.42 Mammary duct ectasia of left breast

        N60.49 Mammary duct ectasia of unspecified breast

    ✓5ᵗʰ **N60.8 Other benign mammary dysplasias**

        N60.81 Other benign mammary dysplasias of right breast

        N60.82 Other benign mammary dysplasias of left breast

        N60.89 Other benign mammary dysplasias of unspecified breast

    ✓5ᵗʰ **N60.9 Unspecified benign mammary dysplasia**

        N60.91 Unspecified benign mammary dysplasia of right breast

        N60.92 Unspecified benign mammary dysplasia of left breast

        N60.99 Unspecified benign mammary dysplasia of unspecified breast

✓4ᵗʰ **N61 Inflammatory disorders of breast**

    EXCLUDES 1   inflammatory carcinoma of breast (C50.9)

        inflammatory disorder of breast associated with childbirth (O91.-)

        neonatal infective mastitis (P39.0)

        thrombophlebitis of breast [Mondor's disease] (I80.8)

    N61.0 Mastitis without abscess

        Infective mastitis (acute) (nonpuerperal) (subacute)

        Mastitis (acute) (nonpuerperal) (subacute) NOS

        Cellulitis (acute) (nonpuerperal) (subacute) of breast NOS

        Cellulitis (acute) (nonpuerperal) (subacute) of nipple NOS

N Newborn: 0   P Pediatric: 0-17   M Maternity: 9-64   A Adult: 15-124   MCC Major Complication/Comorbidity   CC Complication/Comorbidity   SW Severe Wound Dx

852

ICD-10-CM 2021

N61.1   **Abscess of the breast and nipple**
Abscess (acute) (chronic) (nonpuerperal) of areola
Abscess (acute) (chronic) (nonpuerperal) of breast
Carbuncle of breast
Mastitis with abscess

●   ✓5ᵗʰ   **N61.2**   **Granulomatous mastitis**

●   **N61.20**   **Granulomatous mastitis, unspecified breast**

●   **N61.21**   **Granulomatous mastitis, right breast**

●   **N61.22**   **Granulomatous mastitis, left breast**

●   **N61.23**   **Granulomatous mastitis, bilateral breast**

N62   **Hypertrophy of breast**
Gynecomastia
Hypertrophy of breast NOS
Massive pubertal hypertrophy of breast
   EXCLUDES 1   *breast engorgement of newborn (P83.4)*
            disproportion of reconstructed breast (N65.1)

✓4ᵗʰ   **N63**   **Unspecified lump in breast**
Nodule(s) NOS in breast
AHA: 2019,4Q,12; 2017,4Q,19

   N63.0   **Unspecified lump in unspecified breast**

✓5ᵗʰ   **N63.1**   **Unspecified lump in the right breast**

     N63.10   **Unspecified lump in the right breast, unspecified quadrant**

     N63.11   **Unspecified lump in the right breast, upper outer quadrant**

     N63.12   **Unspecified lump in the right breast, upper inner quadrant**

     N63.13   **Unspecified lump in the right breast, lower outer quadrant**

     N63.14   **Unspecified lump in the right breast, lower inner quadrant**

     N63.15   **Unspecified lump in the right breast, overlapping quadrants**

✓5ᵗʰ   **N63.2**   **Unspecified lump in the left breast**

     N63.20   **Unspecified lump in the left breast, unspecified quadrant**

     N63.21   **Unspecified lump in the left breast, upper outer quadrant**

     N63.22   **Unspecified lump in the left breast, upper inner quadrant**

     N63.23   **Unspecified lump in the left breast, lower outer quadrant**

     N63.24   **Unspecified lump in the left breast, lower inner quadrant**

     N63.25   **Unspecified lump in the left breast, overlapping quadrants**

✓5ᵗʰ   **N63.3**   **Unspecified lump in axillary tail**

     N63.31   **Unspecified lump in axillary tail of the right breast**
     N63.32   **Unspecified lump in axillary tail of the left breast**

✓5ᵗʰ   **N63.4**   **Unspecified lump in breast, subareolar**

     N63.41   **Unspecified lump in right breast, subareolar**

     N63.42   **Unspecified lump in left breast, subareolar**

✓4ᵗʰ   **N64**   **Other disorders of breast**
   EXCLUDES 2   *mechanical complication of breast prosthesis and implant (T85.4-)*

   N64.0   **Fissure and fistula of nipple**

   N64.1   **Fat necrosis of breast**
Fat necrosis (segmental) of breast
Code first breast necrosis due to breast graft (T85.898)

   N64.2   **Atrophy of breast**

   N64.3   **Galactorrhea not associated with childbirth**

   N64.4   **Mastodynia**

✓5ᵗʰ   **N64.5**   **Other signs and symptoms in breast**
     EXCLUDES 2   *abnormal findings on diagnostic imaging of breast (R92.-)*

     N64.51   **Induration of breast**

     N64.52   **Nipple discharge**
       EXCLUDES 1   *abnormal findings in nipple discharge (R89.-)*

     N64.53   **Retraction of nipple**

     N64.59   **Other signs and symptoms in breast**

✓5ᵗʰ   **N64.8**   **Other specified disorders of breast**

   N64.81   **Ptosis of breast**   A
     EXCLUDES 1   *ptosis of native breast in relation to reconstructed breast (N65.1)*

   N64.82   **Hypoplasia of breast**   A
Micromastia
     EXCLUDES 1   *congenital absence of breast (Q83.0)*
            hypoplasia of native breast in relation to reconstructed breast (N65.1)

   N64.89   **Other specified disorders of breast**
Galactocele
Subinvolution of breast (postlactational)
AHA: 2019,1Q,32; 2018,1Q,3

   N64.9   **Disorder of breast, unspecified**

✓4ᵗʰ   **N65**   **Deformity and disproportion of reconstructed breast**

   N65.0   **Deformity of reconstructed breast**   A
Contour irregularity in reconstructed breast
Excess tissue in reconstructed breast
Misshapen reconstructed breast

   N65.1   **Disproportion of reconstructed breast**   A
Breast asymmetry between native breast and reconstructed breast
Disproportion between native breast and reconstructed breast

Inflammatory diseases of female pelvic organs (N70-N77)

   EXCLUDES 1   *inflammatory diseases of female pelvic organs complicating:*
     abortion or ectopic or molar pregnancy (O00-O07, O08.0)
     pregnancy, childbirth and the puerperium (O23.-, O75.3, O85, O86.-)

✓4ᵗʰ   **N70**   **Salpingitis and oophoritis**
   INCLUDES   abscess (of) fallopian tube
           abscess (of) ovary
           pyosalpinx
           salpingo-oophoritis
           tubo-ovarian abscess
           tubo-ovarian inflammatory disease
Use additional code (B95-B97), to identify infectious agent
   EXCLUDES 1   *gonococcal infection (A54.24)*
           tuberculous infection (A18.17)

✓5ᵗʰ   **N70.0**   **Acute salpingitis and oophoritis**

     N70.01   **Acute salpingitis**   CC ♀

     N70.02   **Acute oophoritis**   CC ♀

     N70.03   **Acute salpingitis and oophoritis**   CC ♀

✓5ᵗʰ   **N70.1**   **Chronic salpingitis and oophoritis**
Hydrosalpinx

     N70.11   **Chronic salpingitis**   ♀

     N70.12   **Chronic oophoritis**   ♀

     N70.13   **Chronic salpingitis and oophoritis**   ♀

✓5ᵗʰ   **N70.9**   **Salpingitis and oophoritis, unspecified**

     N70.91   **Salpingitis, unspecified**   ♀

     N70.92   **Oophoritis, unspecified**   ♀

     N70.93   **Salpingitis and oophoritis, unspecified**   ♀

✓4ᵗʰ   **N71**   **Inflammatory disease of uterus, except cervix**
   INCLUDES   endo (myo) metritis
           metritis
           myometritis
           pyometra
           uterine abscess
Use additional code (B95-B97), to identify infectious agent
   EXCLUDES 1   *hyperplastic endometritis (N85.0-)*
           infection of uterus following delivery (O85, O86.-)

   N71.0   **Acute inflammatory disease of uterus**   CC ♀

   N71.1   **Chronic inflammatory disease of uterus**   ♀

   N71.9   **Inflammatory disease of uterus, unspecified**   ♀

N72   **Inflammatory disease of cervix uteri**   ♀
   INCLUDES   cervicitis (with or without erosion or ectropion)
           endocervicitis (with or without erosion or ectropion)
           exocervicitis (with or without erosion or ectropion)
Use additional code (B95-B97), to identify infectious agent
   EXCLUDES 1   *erosion and ectropion of cervix without cervicitis (N86)*

☑ Additional Character Required   ✓x7ᵗʰ Placeholder   Unacceptable PDx   Questionable PDx   Manifestation   Unspecified Dx   H1-H14 HAC   HCC CMS-HCC Dx   HIV HIV Dx

Chapter 14. Diseases of the Genitourinary System

✓4ᵗʰ **N73 Other female pelvic inflammatory diseases**

Use additional code (B95-B97), to identify infectious agent

N73.0 Acute parametritis and pelvic cellulitis   CC ♀

Abscess of broad ligament

Abscess of parametrium

Pelvic cellulitis, female

DEF: Parametritis: Inflammation of the parametrium.

N73.1 Chronic parametritis and pelvic cellulitis   ♀

Any condition in N73.0 specified as chronic

EXCLUDES 1   *tuberculous parametritis and pelvic cellulitis (A18.17)*

N73.2 Unspecified parametritis and pelvic cellulitis   ♀

Any condition in N73.0 unspecified whether acute or chronic

N73.3 Female acute pelvic peritonitis   MCC ♀

N73.4 Female chronic pelvic peritonitis   CC ♀

EXCLUDES 1   *tuberculous pelvic (female) peritonitis (A18.17)*

N73.5 Female pelvic peritonitis, unspecified   ♀

N73.6 Female pelvic peritoneal adhesions (postinfective)   ♀

EXCLUDES 2   *postprocedural pelvic peritoneal adhesions (N99.4)*

AHA: 2014,1Q,6

N73.8 Other specified female pelvic inflammatory diseases   ♀

N73.9 Female pelvic inflammatory disease, unspecified   ♀

Female pelvic infection or inflammation NOS

N74 *Female pelvic inflammatory disorders in diseases classified elsewhere*   ♀

Code first underlying disease

EXCLUDES 1   *chlamydial cervicitis (A56.02)*

chlamydial pelvic inflammatory disease (A56.11)

gonococcal cervicitis (A54.03)

gonococcal pelvic inflammatory disease (A54.24)

herpesviral [herpes simplex] cervicitis (A60.03)

herpesviral [herpes simplex] pelvic inflammatory disease (A60.09)

syphilitic cervicitis (A52.76)

syphilitic pelvic inflammatory disease (A52.76)

trichomonal cervicitis (A59.09)

tuberculous cervicitis (A18.16)

tuberculous pelvic inflammatory disease (A18.17)

✓4ᵗʰ **N75 Diseases of Bartholin's gland**

DEF: Bartholin's gland: Mucous-producing gland found in the vestibular bulbs on either side of the vaginal orifice and connected to the mucosal membrane at the opening by a duct.

N75.0 Cyst of Bartholin's gland   ♀

N75.1 Abscess of Bartholin's gland   CC ♀

N75.8 Other diseases of Bartholin's gland   ♀

Bartholinitis

N75.9 Disease of Bartholin's gland, unspecified   ♀

✓4ᵗʰ **N76 Other inflammation of vagina and vulva**

Use additional code (B95-B97), to identify infectious agent

EXCLUDES 2   *senile (atrophic) vaginitis (N95.2)*

vulvar vestibulitis (N94.810)

N76.0 Acute vaginitis   ♀

Acute vulvovaginitis

Vaginitis NOS

Vulvovaginitis NOS

N76.1 Subacute and chronic vaginitis   ♀

Chronic vulvovaginitis

Subacute vulvovaginitis

N76.2 Acute vulvitis   ♀

Vulvitis NOS

N76.3 Subacute and chronic vulvitis   ♀

N76.4 Abscess of vulva   CC ♀

Furuncle of vulva

N76.5 Ulceration of vagina   ♀

N76.6 Ulceration of vulva   ♀

✓5ᵗʰ **N76.8 Other specified inflammation of vagina and vulva**

N76.81 Mucositis (ulcerative) of vagina and vulva   CC ♀

Code also type of associated therapy, such as:

antineoplastic and immunosuppressive drugs (T45.1X-)

radiological procedure and radiotherapy (Y84.2)

EXCLUDES 2   *gastrointestinal mucositis (ulcerative) (K92.81)*

nasal mucositis (ulcerative) (J34.81)

oral mucositis (ulcerative) (K12.3-)

N76.89 Other specified inflammation of vagina and vulva   ♀

✓4ᵗʰ **N77 Vulvovaginal ulceration and inflammation in diseases classified elsewhere**

N77.0 *Ulceration of vulva in diseases classified elsewhere*   ♀

Code first underlying disease, such as:

Behçet's disease (M35.2)

EXCLUDES 1   *ulceration of vulva in gonococcal infection (A54.02)*

ulceration of vulva in herpesviral [herpes simplex] infection (A60.04)

ulceration of vulva in syphilis (A51.0)

ulceration of vulva in tuberculosis (A18.18)

N77.1 *Vaginitis, vulvitis and vulvovaginitis in diseases classified elsewhere*   ♀

Code first underlying disease, such as:

pinworm (B80)

EXCLUDES 1   *candidal vulvovaginitis (B37.3)*

chlamydial vulvovaginitis (A56.02)

gonococcal vulvovaginitis (A54.02)

herpesviral [herpes simplex] vulvovaginitis (A60.04)

trichomonal vulvovaginitis (A59.01)

tuberculous vulvovaginitis (A18.18)

vulvovaginitis in early syphilis (A51.0)

vulvovaginitis in late syphilis (A52.76)

Noninflammatory disorders of female genital tract (N80-N98)

✓4ᵗʰ **N80 Endometriosis**

DEF: Aberrant uterine mucosal tissue appearing in areas of the pelvic cavity outside of its normal location, lining the uterus, and inflaming surrounding tissues often resulting in infertility or spontaneous abortion.

N80.0 Endometriosis of uterus   ♀

Adenomyosis

EXCLUDES 1   *stromal endometriosis (D39.0)*

N80.1 Endometriosis of ovary   ♀

N80.2 Endometriosis of fallopian tube   ♀

N80.3 Endometriosis of pelvic peritoneum   ♀

N80.4 Endometriosis of rectovaginal septum and vagina   ♀

N80.5 Endometriosis of intestine   ♀

N80.6 Endometriosis in cutaneous scar   ♀

N80.8 Other endometriosis

Endometriosis of thorax

N80.9 Endometriosis, unspecified   ♀

N Newborn: 0   P Pediatric: 0-17   M Maternity: 9-64   A Adult: 15-124   MCC Major Complication/Comorbidity   CC Complication/Comorbidity   SW Severe Wound Dx

854   ICD-10-CM 2021

✓4ᵗʰ N81 Female genital prolapse

    EXCLUDES 1   *genital prolapse complicating pregnancy, labor or delivery (O34.5-)*
                  prolapse and hernia of ovary and fallopian tube (N83.4-)
                  prolapse of vaginal vault after hysterectomy (N99.3)

Types of Pelvic Organ Prolapse

Urethrocele

Cystocele

Rectocele

Enterocele

N81.0 Urethrocele ♀
    EXCLUDES 1   *urethrocele with cystocele (N81.1-)*
                  urethrocele with prolapse of uterus (N81.2-N81.4)

✓5ᵗʰ N81.1 Cystocele
    Cystocele with urethrocele
    Cystourethrocele
    EXCLUDES 1   *cystocele with prolapse of uterus (N81.2-N81.4)*

    N81.10 Cystocele, unspecified ♀
        Prolapse of (anterior) vaginal wall NOS

    N81.11 Cystocele, midline ♀
    N81.12 Cystocele, lateral ♀
        Paravaginal cystocele
        DEF: Detachment of the lateral support connections of the vagina at the arcus tendineus fasciae pelvis (ATFP) that results in bladder drop. The bladder herniates into the vagina laterally.

N81.2 Incomplete uterovaginal prolapse ♀
    First degree uterine prolapse
    Prolapse of cervix NOS
    Second degree uterine prolapse
    EXCLUDES 1   *cervical stump prolapse (N81.85)*

N81.3 Complete uterovaginal prolapse ♀
    Procidentia (uteri) NOS
    Third degree uterine prolapse

N81.4 Uterovaginal prolapse, unspecified ♀
    Prolapse of uterus NOS

N81.5 Vaginal enterocele ♀
    EXCLUDES 1   *enterocele with prolapse of uterus (N81.2-N81.4)*

N81.6 Rectocele ♀
    Prolapse of posterior vaginal wall
    Use additional code for any associated fecal incontinence, if applicable (R15.-)
    EXCLUDES 2   *perineocele (N81.81)*
                  rectal prolapse (K62.3)
                  rectocele with prolapse of uterus (N81.2-N81.4)

✓5ᵗʰ N81.8 Other female genital prolapse
    N81.81 Perineocele ♀
    N81.82 Incompetence or weakening of pubocervical tissue ♀
    N81.83 Incompetence or weakening of rectovaginal tissue ♀
    N81.84 Pelvic muscle wasting ♀
        Disuse atrophy of pelvic muscles and anal sphincter
    N81.85 Cervical stump prolapse ♀

    N81.89 Other female genital prolapse ♀
        Deficient perineum
        Old laceration of muscles of pelvic floor

N81.9 Female genital prolapse, unspecified ♀

✓4ᵗʰ N82 Fistulae involving female genital tract
    EXCLUDES 1   *vesicointestinal fistulae (N32.1)*

N82.0 Vesicovaginal fistula   CC SW ♀

N82.1 Other female urinary-genital tract fistulae   CC ♀
    Cervicovesical fistula
    Ureterovaginal fistula
    Urethrovaginal fistula
    Uteroureteric fistula
    Uterovesical fistula
    AHA: 2017,3Q,3

N82.2 Fistula of vagina to small intestine   CC SW ♀

N82.3 Fistula of vagina to large intestine   CC SW ♀
    Rectovaginal fistula

N82.4 Other female intestinal-genital tract fistulae   CC SW ♀
    Intestinouterine fistula

N82.5 Female genital tract-skin fistulae   CC SW ♀
    Uterus to abdominal wall fistula
    Vaginoperineal fistula

N82.8 Other female genital tract fistulae   CC ♀

N82.9 Female genital tract fistula, unspecified   CC ♀

✓4ᵗʰ N83 Noninflammatory disorders of ovary, fallopian tube and broad ligament
    EXCLUDES 2   *hydrosalpinx (N70.1-)*
    AHA: 2016,4Q,46

✓5ᵗʰ N83.0 Follicular cyst of ovary
    Cyst of graafian follicle
    Hemorrhagic follicular cyst (of ovary)

    N83.00 Follicular cyst of ovary, unspecified side ♀
    N83.01 Follicular cyst of right ovary ♀
    N83.02 Follicular cyst of left ovary ♀

✓5ᵗʰ N83.1 Corpus luteum cyst
    Hemorrhagic corpus luteum cyst

    N83.10 Corpus luteum cyst of ovary, unspecified side ♀
    N83.11 Corpus luteum cyst of right ovary ♀
    N83.12 Corpus luteum cyst of left ovary ♀

✓5ᵗʰ N83.2 Other and unspecified ovarian cysts
    EXCLUDES 1   *developmental ovarian cyst (Q50.1)*
                  neoplastic ovarian cyst (D27.-)
                  polycystic ovarian syndrome (E28.2)
                  Stein-Leventhal syndrome (E28.2)

    ✓6ᵗʰ N83.20 Unspecified ovarian cysts
        N83.201 Unspecified ovarian cyst, right side ♀
        N83.202 Unspecified ovarian cyst, left side ♀
        N83.209 Unspecified ovarian cyst, unspecified side ♀
            Ovarian cyst, NOS

    ✓6ᵗʰ N83.29 Other ovarian cysts
        Retention cyst of ovary
        Simple cyst of ovary
        N83.291 Other ovarian cyst, right side ♀
        N83.292 Other ovarian cyst, left side ♀
        N83.299 Other ovarian cyst, unspecified side ♀

✓5ᵗʰ N83.3 Acquired atrophy of ovary and fallopian tube
    ✓6ᵗʰ N83.31 Acquired atrophy of ovary
        N83.311 Acquired atrophy of right ovary ♀
        N83.312 Acquired atrophy of left ovary ♀
        N83.319 Acquired atrophy of ovary, unspecified side ♀
            Acquired atrophy of ovary, NOS

    ✓6ᵗʰ N83.32 Acquired atrophy of fallopian tube
        N83.321 Acquired atrophy of right fallopian tube ♀
        N83.322 Acquired atrophy of left fallopian tube ♀
        N83.329 Acquired atrophy of fallopian tube, unspecified side ♀
            Acquired atrophy of fallopian tube, NOS

    ✓6ᵗʰ N83.33 Acquired atrophy of ovary and fallopian tube
        N83.331 Acquired atrophy of right ovary and fallopian tube ♀

N83.332   **Acquired atrophy of left ovary and fallopian tube** ♀

N83.339   **Acquired atrophy of ovary and fallopian tube, unspecified side** ♀
Acquired atrophy of ovary and fallopian tube, NOS

✓5ᵗʰ **N83.4**   **Prolapse and hernia of ovary and fallopian tube**

N83.40   **Prolapse and hernia of ovary and fallopian tube, unspecified side** ♀
Prolapse and hernia of ovary and fallopian tube, NOS

N83.41   **Prolapse and hernia of right ovary and fallopian tube** ♀

N83.42   **Prolapse and hernia of left ovary and fallopian tube** ♀

✓5ᵗʰ **N83.5**   **Torsion of ovary, ovarian pedicle and fallopian tube**
Torsion of accessory tube

✓6ᵗʰ **N83.51**   **Torsion of ovary and ovarian pedicle**

N83.511   **Torsion of right ovary and ovarian pedicle** CC ♀

N83.512   **Torsion of left ovary and ovarian pedicle** CC ♀

N83.519   **Torsion of ovary and ovarian pedicle, unspecified side** CC ♀
Torsion of ovary and ovarian pedicle, NOS

✓6ᵗʰ **N83.52**   **Torsion of fallopian tube**
Torsion of hydatid of Morgagni

N83.521   **Torsion of right fallopian tube** CC ♀

N83.522   **Torsion of left fallopian tube** CC ♀

N83.529   **Torsion of fallopian tube, unspecified side** CC ♀
Torsion of fallopian tube, NOS

N83.53   **Torsion of ovary, ovarian pedicle and fallopian tube** CC ♀

N83.6   **Hematosalpinx** ♀
   EXCLUDES 1   *hematosalpinx (with) (in):*
     hematocolpos (N89.7)
     hematometra (N85.7)
     tubal pregnancy (O00.1-)

N83.7   **Hematoma of broad ligament** ♀

N83.8   **Other noninflammatory disorders of ovary, fallopian tube and broad ligament** ♀
Broad ligament laceration syndrome [Allen-Masters]

N83.9   **Noninflammatory disorder of ovary, fallopian tube and broad ligament, unspecified** ♀

✓4ᵗʰ **N84**   **Polyp of female genital tract**
   EXCLUDES 1   *adenomatous polyp (D28.-)*
     placental polyp (O90.89)

N84.0   **Polyp of corpus uteri** ♀
Polyp of endometrium
Polyp of uterus NOS
   EXCLUDES 1   *polypoid endometrial hyperplasia (N85.0-)*

N84.1   **Polyp of cervix uteri** ♀
Mucous polyp of cervix

N84.2   **Polyp of vagina** ♀

N84.3   **Polyp of vulva** ♀
Polyp of labia

N84.8   **Polyp of other parts of female genital tract** ♀

N84.9   **Polyp of female genital tract, unspecified** ♀

✓4ᵗʰ **N85**   **Other noninflammatory disorders of uterus, except cervix**
   EXCLUDES 1   *endometriosis (N80.-)*
     inflammatory diseases of uterus (N71.-)
     noninflammatory disorders of cervix, except malposition (N86-N88)
     polyp of corpus uteri (N84.0)
     uterine prolapse (N81.-)

✓5ᵗʰ **N85.0**   **Endometrial hyperplasia**

N85.00   **Endometrial hyperplasia, unspecified** ♀
Hyperplasia (adenomatous) (cystic) (glandular) of endometrium
Hyperplastic endometritis

N85.01   **Benign endometrial hyperplasia** ♀
Endometrial hyperplasia (complex) (simple) without atypia

N85.02   **Endometrial intraepithelial neoplasia [EIN]** ♀
Endometrial hyperplasia with atypia
   EXCLUDES 1   *malignant neoplasm of endometrium (with endometrial intraepithelial neoplasia [EIN]) (C54.1)*

N85.2   **Hypertrophy of uterus** ♀
Bulky or enlarged uterus
   EXCLUDES 1   *puerperal hypertrophy of uterus (O90.89)*

N85.3   **Subinvolution of uterus** ♀
   EXCLUDES 1   *puerperal subinvolution of uterus (O90.89)*

N85.4   **Malposition of uterus** ♀
Anteversion of uterus
Retroflexion of uterus
Retroversion of uterus
   EXCLUDES 1   *malposition of uterus complicating pregnancy, labor or delivery (O34.5-, O65.5)*

N85.5   **Inversion of uterus** ♀
   EXCLUDES 1   *current obstetric trauma (O71.2)*
     postpartum inversion of uterus (O71.2)
   DEF: Abnormality in which the uterus turns inside out.

Inversion of Uterus

Uterus

N85.6   **Intrauterine synechiae** ♀

N85.7   **Hematometra** ♀
Hematosalpinx with hematometra
   EXCLUDES 1   *hematometra with hematocolpos (N89.7)*
   DEF: Accumulation of blood within the uterus.

N85.8   **Other specified noninflammatory disorders of uterus** ♀
Atrophy of uterus, acquired
Fibrosis of uterus NOS

N85.9   **Noninflammatory disorder of uterus, unspecified** ♀
Disorder of uterus NOS

N86   **Erosion and ectropion of cervix uteri** ♀
Decubitus (trophic) ulcer of cervix
Eversion of cervix
   EXCLUDES 1   *erosion and ectropion of cervix with cervicitis (N72)*

✓4ᵗʰ **N87**   **Dysplasia of cervix uteri**
   EXCLUDES 1   *abnormal results from cervical cytologic examination without histologic confirmation (R87.61-)*
     carcinoma in situ of cervix uteri (D06.-)
     cervical intraepithelial neoplasia III [CIN III] (D06.-)
     HGSIL of cervix (R87.613)
     severe dysplasia of cervix uteri (D06.-)

N87.0   **Mild cervical dysplasia** ♀
Cervical intraepithelial neoplasia I [CIN I]

N87.1   **Moderate cervical dysplasia** ♀
Cervical intraepithelial neoplasia II [CIN II]

N87.9   **Dysplasia of cervix uteri, unspecified** ♀
Anaplasia of cervix
Cervical atypism
Cervical dysplasia NOS

✓4ᵗʰ **N88**   **Other noninflammatory disorders of cervix uteri**
   EXCLUDES 2   *inflammatory disease of cervix (N72)*
     polyp of cervix (N84.1)

N88.0   **Leukoplakia of cervix uteri** ♀

Ⓝ Newborn: 0   Ⓟ Pediatric: 0-17   Ⓜ Maternity: 9-64   Ⓐ Adult: 15-124   MCC Major Complication/Comorbidity   CC Complication/Comorbidity   SW Severe Wound Dx

856   ICD-10-CM 2021

N88.1 **Old laceration of cervix uteri** ♀
Adhesions of cervix
EXCLUDES 1　*current obstetric trauma (O71.3)*

N88.2 **Stricture and stenosis of cervix uteri** ♀
EXCLUDES 1　*stricture and stenosis of cervix uteri complicating labor (O65.5)*

N88.3 **Incompetence of cervix uteri** ♀
Investigation and management of (suspected) cervical incompetence in a nonpregnant woman
EXCLUDES 1　*cervical incompetence complicating pregnancy (O34.3-)*
DEF: Inadequate functioning of the cervix marked by abnormal widening during pregnancy and causing premature birth or miscarriage.

N88.4 **Hypertrophic elongation of cervix uteri** ♀

N88.8 **Other specified noninflammatory disorders of cervix uteri** ♀
EXCLUDES 1　*current obstetric trauma (O71.3)*

N88.9 **Noninflammatory disorder of cervix uteri, unspecified** ♀

✓4ᵗʰ **N89** **Other noninflammatory disorders of vagina**
EXCLUDES 1　*abnormal results from vaginal cytologic examination without histologic confirmation (R87.62-)*
carcinoma in situ of vagina (D07.2)
HGSIL of vagina (R87.623)
inflammation of vagina (N76.-)
senile (atrophic) vaginitis (N95.2)
severe dysplasia of vagina (D07.2)
trichomonal leukorrhea (A59.00)
vaginal intraepithelial neoplasia [VAIN], grade III (D07.2)

N89.0 **Mild vaginal dysplasia** ♀
Vaginal intraepithelial neoplasia [VAIN], grade I

N89.1 **Moderate vaginal dysplasia** ♀
Vaginal intraepithelial neoplasia [VAIN], grade II

N89.3 **Dysplasia of vagina, unspecified** ♀

N89.4 **Leukoplakia of vagina** ♀

N89.5 **Stricture and atresia of vagina** ♀
Vaginal adhesions
Vaginal stenosis
EXCLUDES 1　*congenital atresia or stricture (Q52.4)*
postprocedural adhesions of vagina (N99.2)

N89.6 **Tight hymenal ring** ♀
Rigid hymen
Tight introitus
EXCLUDES 1　*imperforate hymen (Q52.3)*

N89.7 **Hematocolpos** ♀
Hematocolpos with hematometra or hematosalpinx
AHA: 2016,4Q,58

N89.8 **Other specified noninflammatory disorders of vagina** ♀
Leukorrhea NOS
Old vaginal laceration
Pessary ulcer of vagina
EXCLUDES 1　*current obstetric trauma (O70.-, O71.4, O71.7-O71.8)*
old laceration involving muscles of pelvic floor (N81.8)

N89.9 **Noninflammatory disorder of vagina, unspecified** ♀

✓4ᵗʰ **N90** **Other noninflammatory disorders of vulva and perineum**
EXCLUDES 1　*anogenital (venereal) warts (A63.0)*
carcinoma in situ of vulva (D07.1)
condyloma acuminatum (A63.0)
current obstetric trauma (O70.-, O71.7-O71.8)
inflammation of vulva (N76.-)
severe dysplasia of vulva (D07.1)
vulvar intraepithelial neoplasm III [VIN III] (D07.1)

N90.0 **Mild vulvar dysplasia** ♀
Vulvar intraepithelial neoplasia [VIN], grade I

N90.1 **Moderate vulvar dysplasia** ♀
Vulvar intraepithelial neoplasia [VIN], grade II

N90.3 **Dysplasia of vulva, unspecified** ♀

N90.4 **Leukoplakia of vulva** ♀
Dystrophy of vulva
Kraurosis of vulva
Lichen sclerosus of external female genital organs

N90.5 **Atrophy of vulva** ♀
Stenosis of vulva

✓5ᵗʰ **N90.6** **Hypertrophy of vulva**
AHA: 2016,4Q,46

N90.60 **Unspecified hypertrophy of vulva** ♀
Unspecified hypertrophy of labia

N90.61 **Childhood asymmetric labium majus enlargement** ♀
CALME

N90.69 **Other specified hypertrophy of vulva** ♀
Other specified hypertrophy of labia

N90.7 **Vulvar cyst** ♀

✓5ᵗʰ **N90.8** **Other specified noninflammatory disorders of vulva and perineum**

✓6ᵗʰ **N90.81** **Female genital mutilation status**
Female genital cutting status

N90.810 **Female genital mutilation status, unspecified** ♀
Female genital cutting status, unspecified
Female genital mutilation status NOS

N90.811 **Female genital mutilation Type I status** ♀
Clitorectomy status
Female genital cutting Type I status

N90.812 **Female genital mutilation Type II status** ♀
Clitorectomy with excision of labia minora status
Female genital cutting Type II status

N90.813 **Female genital mutilation Type III status** ♀
Female genital cutting Type III status
Infibulation status

N90.818 **Other female genital mutilation status** ♀
Female genital cutting Type IV status
Female genital mutilation Type IV status
Other female genital cutting status

N90.89 **Other specified noninflammatory disorders of vulva and perineum** ♀
Adhesions of vulva
Hypertrophy of clitoris

N90.9 **Noninflammatory disorder of vulva and perineum, unspecified** ♀

✓4ᵗʰ **N91** **Absent, scanty and rare menstruation**
EXCLUDES 1　*ovarian dysfunction (E28.-)*

N91.0 **Primary amenorrhea** ♀
N91.1 **Secondary amenorrhea** ♀
N91.2 **Amenorrhea, unspecified** ♀
N91.3 **Primary oligomenorrhea** ♀
N91.4 **Secondary oligomenorrhea** ♀
N91.5 **Oligomenorrhea, unspecified** ♀
Hypomenorrhea NOS

✓4ᵗʰ **N92** **Excessive, frequent and irregular menstruation**
EXCLUDES 1　*postmenopausal bleeding (N95.0)*
precocious puberty (menstruation) (E30.1)

N92.0 **Excessive and frequent menstruation with regular cycle** ♀
Heavy periods NOS
Menorrhagia NOS
Polymenorrhea

N92.1 **Excessive and frequent menstruation with irregular cycle** ♀
Irregular intermenstrual bleeding
Irregular, shortened intervals between menstrual bleeding
Menometrorrhagia
Metrorrhagia

N92.2 **Excessive menstruation at puberty** P ♀
Excessive bleeding associated with onset of menstrual periods
Pubertal menorrhagia
Puberty bleeding

N92.3 **Ovulation bleeding** ♀
Regular intermenstrual bleeding

N92.4 Excessive bleeding in the premenopausal period   ♀
    Climacteric menorrhagia or metrorrhagia
    Menopausal menorrhagia or metrorrhagia
    Perimenopausal bleeding
    Perimenopausal menorrhagia or metrorrhagia
    Preclimacteric menorrhagia or metrorrhagia
    Premenopausal menorrhagia or metrorrhagia

N92.5 Other specified irregular menstruation   ♀

N92.6 Irregular menstruation, unspecified   ♀
    Irregular bleeding NOS
    Irregular periods NOS
        EXCLUDES 1 irregular menstruation with:
            lengthened intervals or scanty bleeding
                (N91.3-N91.5)
            shortened intervals or excessive bleeding (N92.1)

✓4ᵗʰ **N93 Other abnormal uterine and vaginal bleeding**
    EXCLUDES 1 neonatal vaginal hemorrhage (P54.6)
        precocious puberty (menstruation) (E30.1)
        pseudomenses (P54.6)

N93.0 Postcoital and contact bleeding   ♀

N93.1 Pre-pubertal vaginal bleeding   ♀
    AHA: 2016,4Q,47

N93.8 Other specified abnormal uterine and vaginal bleeding ♀
    Dysfunctional or functional uterine or vaginal bleeding NOS

N93.9 Abnormal uterine and vaginal bleeding, unspecified   ♀

✓4ᵗʰ **N94 Pain and other conditions associated with female genital organs and menstrual cycle**

N94.0 Mittelschmerz   ♀
    DEF: One-sided, lower abdominal pain occurring between
        menstrual periods that is associated with ovulation.

✓5ᵗʰ **N94.1 Dyspareunia**
    EXCLUDES 1 psychogenic dyspareunia (F52.6)
    AHA: 2016,4Q,47
        N94.10 Unspecified dyspareunia   ♀
        N94.11 Superficial (introital) dyspareunia   ♀
        N94.12 Deep dyspareunia   ♀
        N94.19 Other specified dyspareunia   ♀

N94.2 Vaginismus   ♀
    EXCLUDES 1 psychogenic vaginismus (F52.5)
    DEF: Spontaneous contractions of the muscles surrounding the
        vagina, causing it to constrict or close.

N94.3 Premenstrual tension syndrome   ♀
    Code also associated menstrual migraine (G43.82-, G43.83-)
    EXCLUDES 1 premenstrual dysphoric disorder (F32.81)

N94.4 Primary dysmenorrhea   ♀

N94.5 Secondary dysmenorrhea   ♀

N94.6 Dysmenorrhea, unspecified   ♀
    EXCLUDES 1 psychogenic dysmenorrhea (F45.8)

✓5ᵗʰ **N94.8 Other specified conditions associated with female genital organs and menstrual cycle**
    ✓6ᵗʰ **N94.81 Vulvodynia**
        N94.810 Vulvar vestibulitis   ♀
        N94.818 Other vulvodynia   ♀
        N94.819 Vulvodynia, unspecified   ♀
            Vulvodynia NOS
    N94.89 Other specified conditions associated with female genital organs and menstrual cycle   ♀
        DEF: Hydrocele: Serous fluid that collects in the canal
            of Nuck in females.

N94.9 Unspecified condition associated with female genital organs and menstrual cycle   ♀

✓4ᵗʰ **N95 Menopausal and other perimenopausal disorders**
    Menopausal and other perimenopausal disorders due to naturally
        occurring (age-related) menopause and perimenopause
    EXCLUDES 1 excessive bleeding in the premenopausal period (N92.4)
        menopausal and perimenopausal disorders due to artificial
            or premature menopause (E89.4-, E28.31-)
        premature menopause (E28.31-)
    EXCLUDES 2 postmenopausal osteoporosis (M81.0-)
        postmenopausal osteoporosis with current pathological
            fracture (M80.0-)
        postmenopausal urethritis (N34.2)

N95.0 Postmenopausal bleeding   ♀

N95.1 Menopausal and female climacteric states   ♀
    Symptoms such as flushing, sleeplessness, headache, lack of
        concentration, associated with natural (age-related)
        menopause
    Use additional code for associated symptoms
        EXCLUDES 1 asymptomatic menopausal state (Z78.0)
            symptoms associated with artificial menopause
                (E89.41)
            symptoms associated with premature menopause
                (E28.310)

N95.2 Postmenopausal atrophic vaginitis   ♀
    Senile (atrophic) vaginitis

N95.8 Other specified menopausal and perimenopausal disorders   ♀

N95.9 Unspecified menopausal and perimenopausal disorder   ♀

N96 Recurrent pregnancy loss   ♀
    Investigation or care in a nonpregnant woman with history of recurrent
        pregnancy loss
    EXCLUDES 1 recurrent pregnancy loss with current pregnancy (O26.2-)

✓4ᵗʰ **N97 Female infertility**
    INCLUDES inability to achieve a pregnancy
        sterility, female NOS
    EXCLUDES 1 female infertility associated with:
        hypopituitarism (E23.0)
        Stein-Leventhal syndrome (E28.2)
    EXCLUDES 2 incompetence of cervix uteri (N88.3)
    DEF: Infertility: Inability to conceive for at least one year with regular
        intercourse.
    DEF: Primary infertility: Infertility occurring in patients who have never
        conceived.
    DEF: Secondary infertility: Infertility occurring in patients who have
        previously conceived.

N97.0 Female infertility associated with anovulation   ♀

N97.1 Female infertility of tubal origin   ♀
    Female infertility associated with congenital anomaly of tube
    Female infertility due to tubal block
    Female infertility due to tubal occlusion
    Female infertility due to tubal stenosis

N97.2 Female infertility of uterine origin   ♀
    Female infertility associated with congenital anomaly of uterus
    Female infertility due to nonimplantation of ovum

N97.8 Female infertility of other origin   ♀

N97.9 Female infertility, unspecified   ♀

✓4ᵗʰ **N98 Complications associated with artificial fertilization**

N98.0 Infection associated with artificial insemination   CC ♀

N98.1 Hyperstimulation of ovaries   CC ♀
    Hyperstimulation of ovaries NOS
    Hyperstimulation of ovaries associated with induced ovulation

N98.2 Complications of attempted introduction of fertilized ovum following in vitro fertilization   CC ♀

N98.3 Complications of attempted introduction of embryo in embryo transfer   CC ♀

N98.8 Other complications associated with artificial fertilization   CC ♀

N98.9 Complication associated with artificial fertilization, unspecified   CC ♀

Intraoperative and postprocedural complications and disorders of genitourinary system, not elsewhere classified (N99)

✓4ᵗʰ **N99 Intraoperative and postprocedural complications and disorders of genitourinary system, not elsewhere classified**
    EXCLUDES 2 irradiation cystitis (N30.4-)
        postoophorectomy osteoporosis with current pathological
            fracture (M80.8-)
        postoophorectomy osteoporosis without current pathological
            fracture (M81.8)

N99.0 Postprocedural (acute) (chronic) kidney failure
    Use additional code to type of kidney disease

✓5ᵗʰ **N99.1 Postprocedural urethral stricture**
    Postcatheterization urethral stricture
    ✓6ᵗʰ **N99.11 Postprocedural urethral stricture, male**
        AHA: 2016,4Q,47-48
        N99.110 Postprocedural urethral stricture, male, meatal   ♂

Ⓝ Newborn: 0   Ⓟ Pediatric: 0-17   Ⓜ Maternity: 9-64   Ⓐ Adult: 15-124   MCC Major Complication/Comorbidity   CC Complication/Comorbidity   SW Severe Wound Dx

858   ICD-10-CM 2021

       N99.111   Postprocedural bulbous urethral stricture, male ♂

       N99.112   Postprocedural membranous urethral stricture, male ♂

       N99.113   Postprocedural anterior bulbous urethral stricture, male ♂

       N99.114   Postprocedural urethral stricture, male, unspecified ♂

       N99.115   Postprocedural fossa navicularis urethral stricture ♂

       N99.116   Postprocedural urethral stricture, male, overlapping sites ♂

    N99.12   Postprocedural urethral stricture, female ♀

N99.2   Postprocedural adhesions of vagina ♀

N99.3   Prolapse of vaginal vault after hysterectomy ♀

N99.4   Postprocedural pelvic peritoneal adhesions

    EXCLUDES 2   pelvic peritoneal adhesions NOS (N73.6)

              postinfective pelvic peritoneal adhesions (N73.6)

✓5ᵗʰ **N99.5**   Complications of stoma of urinary tract

    EXCLUDES 2   mechanical complication of urinary catheter (T83.0-)

    AHA: 2016,4Q,48

  ✓6ᵗʰ **N99.51**   Complication of cystostomy

       N99.510   Cystostomy hemorrhage   CC HCC

       N99.511   Cystostomy infection   CC HCC

       N99.512   Cystostomy malfunction   CC HCC

       N99.518   Other cystostomy complication   CC HCC

  ✓6ᵗʰ **N99.52**   Complication of incontinent external stoma of urinary tract

       N99.520   Hemorrhage of incontinent external stoma of urinary tract   HCC

       N99.521   Infection of incontinent external stoma of urinary tract   HCC

       N99.522   Malfunction of incontinent external stoma of urinary tract   HCC

       N99.523   Herniation of incontinent stoma of urinary tract   HCC

       N99.524   Stenosis of incontinent stoma of urinary tract   HCC

       N99.528   Other complication of incontinent external stoma of urinary tract   HCC

  ✓6ᵗʰ **N99.53**   Complication of continent stoma of urinary tract

       N99.530   Hemorrhage of continent stoma of urinary tract   HCC

       N99.531   Infection of continent stoma of urinary tract   HCC

       N99.532   Malfunction of continent stoma of urinary tract   HCC

       N99.533   Herniation of continent stoma of urinary tract   HCC

       N99.534   Stenosis of continent stoma of urinary tract   HCC

       N99.538   Other complication of continent stoma of urinary tract   HCC

✓5ᵗʰ **N99.6**   Intraoperative hemorrhage and hematoma of a genitourinary system organ or structure complicating a procedure

    EXCLUDES 1   intraoperative hemorrhage and hematoma of a genitourinary system organ or structure due to accidental puncture or laceration during a procedure (N99.7-)

    N99.61   Intraoperative hemorrhage and hematoma of a genitourinary system organ or structure complicating a genitourinary system procedure   CC

    N99.62   Intraoperative hemorrhage and hematoma of a genitourinary system organ or structure complicating other procedure   CC

✓5ᵗʰ **N99.7**   Accidental puncture and laceration of a genitourinary system organ or structure during a procedure

    N99.71   Accidental puncture and laceration of a genitourinary system organ or structure during a genitourinary system procedure   CC

    N99.72   Accidental puncture and laceration of a genitourinary system organ or structure during other procedure   CC

✓5ᵗʰ **N99.8**   Other intraoperative and postprocedural complications and disorders of genitourinary system

    AHA: 2016,4Q,9-10

    N99.81   Other intraoperative complications of genitourinary system

  ✓6ᵗʰ **N99.82**   Postprocedural hemorrhage of a genitourinary system organ or structure following a procedure

       N99.820   Postprocedural hemorrhage of a genitourinary system organ or structure following a genitourinary system procedure   CC

       N99.821   Postprocedural hemorrhage of a genitourinary system organ or structure following other procedure   CC

    N99.83   Residual ovary syndrome ♀

  ✓6ᵗʰ **N99.84**   Postprocedural hematoma and seroma of a genitourinary system organ or structure following a procedure

       N99.840   Postprocedural hematoma of a genitourinary system organ or structure following a genitourinary system procedure   CC

       N99.841   Postprocedural hematoma of a genitourinary system organ or structure following other procedure   CC

       N99.842   Postprocedural seroma of a genitourinary system organ or structure following a genitourinary system procedure   CC

       N99.843   Postprocedural seroma of a genitourinary system organ or structure following other procedure   CC

    N99.85   Post endometrial ablation syndrome ♀

       AHA: 2019,4Q,12

    N99.89   Other postprocedural complications and disorders of genitourinary system

☑ Additional Character Required   ✓x7ᵗʰ Placeholder   Unacceptable PDx   Questionable PDx   Manifestation   Unspecified Dx   H1-H14 HAC   HCC CMS-HCC Dx   HIV HIV Dx

ICD-10-CM 2021   859

Chapter 15. Pregnancy, Childbirth and the Puerperium (O00–O9A)

Chapter-specific Guidelines with Coding Examples

The chapter-specific guidelines from the ICD-10-CM Official Guidelines for Coding and Reporting have been provided below. Along with these guidelines are coding examples, contained in the shaded boxes, that have been developed to help illustrate the coding and/or sequencing guidance found in these guidelines.

a. General rules for obstetric cases

1) Codes from Chapter 15 and sequencing priority

Obstetric cases require codes from chapter 15, codes in the range O00-O9A, Pregnancy, Childbirth, and the Puerperium. Chapter 15 codes have sequencing priority over codes from other chapters. Additional codes from other chapters may be used in conjunction with chapter 15 codes to further specify conditions. Should the provider document that the pregnancy is incidental to the encounter, then code Z33.1, Pregnant state, incidental, should be used in place of any chapter 15 codes. It is the provider's responsibility to state that the condition being treated is not affecting the pregnancy.

> Pregnant patient at 25 weeks' gestation admitted for bladder abscess
>
> **O23.12** **Infections of bladder in pregnancy, second trimester**
>
> **N30.80** **Other cystitis without hematuria**
>
> **Z3A.25** **25 weeks gestation of pregnancy**
>
> *Explanation:* The documentation does not indicate that the pregnancy is incidental or in any way unaffected by the bladder abscess; therefore, an obstetrics code should be sequenced first. An additional code was provided to identify the specific bladder condition as this information is not called out specifically in the obstetrics code.

2) Chapter 15 codes used only on the maternal record

Chapter 15 codes are to be used only on the maternal record, never on the record of the newborn.

3) Final character for trimester

The majority of codes in Chapter 15 have a final character indicating the trimester of pregnancy. The timeframes for the trimesters are indicated at the beginning of the chapter. If trimester is not a component of a code, it is because the condition always occurs in a specific trimester, or the concept of trimester of pregnancy is not applicable. Certain codes have characters for only certain trimesters because the condition does not occur in all trimesters, but it may occur in more than just one.

Assignment of the final character for trimester should be based on the provider's documentation of the trimester (or number of weeks) for the current admission/encounter. This applies to the assignment of trimester for pre-existing conditions as well as those that develop during or are due to the pregnancy. The provider's documentation of the number of weeks may be used to assign the appropriate code identifying the trimester.

Whenever delivery occurs during the current admission, and there is an "in childbirth" option for the obstetric complication being coded, the "in childbirth" code should be assigned.

> Pregnant patient at 21 weeks' gestation admitted with excessive vomiting
>
> **O21.2** **Late vomiting of pregnancy**
>
> **Z3A.21** **21 weeks gestation of pregnancy**
>
> *Explanation:* Category O21 classifies vomiting in pregnancy. Although code selection is based on whether the vomiting is before or after 20 completed weeks, these codes are not further classified by trimester. If vomiting only in the second trimester was documented, the provider should be queried for the specific week of gestation, as this will affect code selection.

4) Selection of trimester for inpatient admissions that encompass more than one trimester

In instances when a patient is admitted to a hospital for complications of pregnancy during one trimester and remains in the hospital into a subsequent trimester, the trimester character for the antepartum complication code should be assigned on the basis of the trimester when the complication developed, not the trimester of the discharge. If the condition developed prior to the current admission/encounter or represents a pre-existing condition, the trimester character for the trimester at the time of the admission/encounter should be assigned.

> Patient admitted at 27 6/7 weeks' gestation for hemorrhaging from partial placenta previa; three days after admission at 28 1/7 weeks' gestation, she developed gestational hypertension
>
> **O44.32** **Partial placenta previa with hemorrhage, second trimester**
>
> **O13.3** **Gestational [pregnancy-induced] hypertension without significant proteinuria, third trimester**
>
> **Z3A.27** **27 weeks gestation of pregnancy**
>
> *Explanation:* The patient presented with hemorrhaging from partial placenta previa while still in her 27th week, which falls within the second trimester. The gestational hypertension did not occur until three days after admission, putting the patient in her 28th week of pregnancy or what is considered to be the third trimester. The weeks of gestation captured by a code from category Z3A should represent only the gestational weeks upon admission.

5) Unspecified trimester

Each category that includes codes for trimester has a code for "unspecified trimester." The "unspecified trimester" code should rarely be used, such as when the documentation in the record is insufficient to determine the trimester and it is not possible to obtain clarification.

6) 7th character for fetus identification

Where applicable, a 7th character is to be assigned for certain categories (O31, O32, O33.3 - O33.6, O35, O36, O40, O41, O60.1, O60.2, O64, and O69) to identify the fetus for which the complication code applies.

Assign 7th character "0":

- For single gestations
- When the documentation in the record is insufficient to determine the fetus affected and it is not possible to obtain clarification.
- When it is not possible to clinically determine which fetus is affected.

> Maternal patient with twin gestations is seen after ultrasound identifies fetus B to be in breech presentation
>
> **O32.1XX2** **Maternal care for breech presentation, fetus 2**
>
> *Explanation:* The documentation indicates that although there are two fetuses, only one fetus is determined to be in breech presentation. Whether fetus 2 or fetus B is used, the coder can assign the seventh character of 2 to identify the second fetus as the one in breech.

b. Selection of OB principal or first-listed diagnosis

1) Routine outpatient prenatal visits

For routine outpatient prenatal visits when no complications are present, a code from category Z34, Encounter for supervision of normal pregnancy, should be used as the first-listed diagnosis. These codes should not be used in conjunction with chapter 15 codes.

2) Supervision of high-risk pregnancy

Codes from category O09, Supervision of high-risk pregnancy, are intended for use only during the prenatal period. For complications during the labor or delivery episode as a result of a high-risk pregnancy, assign the applicable complication codes from Chapter 15. If there are no complications during the labor or delivery episode, assign code O80, Encounter for full-term uncomplicated delivery.

For routine prenatal outpatient visits for patients with high-risk pregnancies, a code from category O09, Supervision of high-risk pregnancy, should be used as the first-listed diagnosis. Secondary chapter 15 codes may be used in conjunction with these codes if appropriate.

> 36-year-old with history of preterm labor admitted in labor with second child at 39 weeks' gestation, delivered healthy baby without complications
>
> **O80** **Encounter for full-term uncomplicated delivery**
>
> **Z3A.39** **39 weeks gestation of pregnancy**
>
> **Z37.0** **Single live birth**
>
> *Explanation:* Although this patient is over 35 and having her second child (elderly multigravida) and has a history of preterm labor with her first child, no codes from category O09.- should be appended. In the absence of any other complications noted during the encounter, code O80 is the most appropriate code to describe the principal diagnosis.

3) Episodes when no delivery occurs

In episodes when no delivery occurs, the principal diagnosis should correspond to the principal complication of the pregnancy which necessitated the encounter. Should more than one complication exist, all of which are treated or monitored, any of the complication codes may be sequenced first.

4) When a delivery occurs

When an obstetric patient is admitted and delivers during that admission, the condition that prompted the admission should be sequenced as the principal diagnosis. If multiple conditions prompted the admission, sequence the one most related to the delivery as the principal diagnosis. A code for any complication of the delivery should be assigned as an additional diagnosis. In cases of cesarean delivery, if the patient was admitted with a condition that resulted in the performance of a cesarean procedure, that condition should be selected as the principal diagnosis. If the reason for the admission was unrelated to the condition resulting in the cesarean delivery, the condition related to the reason for the admission should be selected as the principal diagnosis.

Maternal patient with diet-controlled gestational diabetes was admitted at 38 weeks' gestation in obstructed labor due to footling presentation; cesarean performed for the malpresentation

O64.8XX0	Obstructed labor due to other malposition and malpresentation, not applicable or unspecified
O24.420	Gestational diabetes mellitus in childbirth, diet controlled
Z3A.38	38 weeks gestation of pregnancy
Z37.0	Single live birth

Explanation: The obstructed labor necessitated the cesarean procedure.

At 39 weeks' gestation, a maternal patient presents with hemorrhage with coagulation defect; the next day the patient goes into labor and eventually delivers via cesarean section due to arrested active phase of labor

O46.003	Antepartum hemorrhage with coagulation defect, unspecified, third trimester
O62.1	Secondary uterine inertia
Z3A.39	39 weeks gestation of pregnancy
Z37.0	Single live birth

Explanation: The patient was admitted because of the antepartum hemorrhage with coagulation defect. The arrested active phase, although the reason for the cesarean delivery, did not develop until later into the stay.

5) Outcome of delivery

A code from category Z37, Outcome of delivery, should be included on every maternal record when a delivery has occurred. These codes are not to be used on subsequent records or on the newborn record.

c. Pre-existing conditions versus conditions due to the pregnancy

Certain categories in Chapter 15 distinguish between conditions of the mother that existed prior to pregnancy (pre-existing) and those that are a direct result of pregnancy. When assigning codes from Chapter 15, it is important to assess if a condition was pre-existing prior to pregnancy or developed during or due to the pregnancy in order to assign the correct code.

Categories that do not distinguish between pre-existing and pregnancy-related conditions may be used for either. It is acceptable to use codes specifically for the puerperium with codes complicating pregnancy and childbirth if a condition arises postpartum during the delivery encounter.

d. Pre-existing hypertension in pregnancy

Category O10, Pre-existing hypertension complicating pregnancy, childbirth and the puerperium, includes codes for hypertensive heart and hypertensive chronic kidney disease. When assigning one of the O10 codes that includes hypertensive heart disease or hypertensive chronic kidney disease, it is necessary to add a secondary code from the appropriate hypertension category to specify the type of heart failure or chronic kidney disease.

See Section I.C.9. Hypertension.

e. Fetal conditions affecting the management of the mother

1) Codes from categories O35 and O36

Codes from categories O35, Maternal care for known or suspected fetal abnormality and damage, and O36, Maternal care for other fetal problems, are assigned only when the fetal condition is actually responsible for modifying the management of the mother, i.e., by requiring diagnostic studies, additional observation, special care, or termination of pregnancy. The fact that the fetal condition exists does not justify assigning a code from this series to the mother's record.

A patient is seen in ED for spotting 15 weeks into her pregnancy; the doctors also suspect fetal hydrocephalus.

| O26.852 | Spotting complicating pregnancy, second trimester |
| Z3A.15 | 15 weeks gestation of pregnancy |

Explanation: Whether the fetal hydrocephalus was suspected or confirmed, an additional code is not warranted for this condition as the documentation does not indicate that this fetal condition is in any way altering the management of the mother or complicating her pregnancy.

2) In utero surgery

In cases when surgery is performed on the fetus, a diagnosis code from category O35, Maternal care for known or suspected fetal abnormality and damage, should be assigned identifying the fetal condition. Assign the appropriate procedure code for the procedure performed.

No code from Chapter 16, the perinatal codes, should be used on the mother's record to identify fetal conditions. Surgery performed in utero on a fetus is still to be coded as an obstetric encounter.

f. HIV infection in pregnancy, childbirth and the puerperium

During pregnancy, childbirth or the puerperium, a patient admitted because of an HIV-related illness should receive a principal diagnosis from subcategory O98.7-, Human immunodeficiency [HIV] disease complicating pregnancy, childbirth and the puerperium, followed by the code(s) for the HIV-related illness(es).

Patients with asymptomatic HIV infection status admitted during pregnancy, childbirth, or the puerperium should receive codes of O98.7- and Z21, Asymptomatic human immunodeficiency virus [HIV] infection status.

A previously asymptomatic HIV patient who is 13 weeks pregnant is admitted with oral thrush.

O98.711	Human immunodeficiency virus [HIV] disease complicating pregnancy, first trimester
B20	Human immunodeficiency virus [HIV] disease
B37.0	Candidal stomatitis
Z3A.13	13 weeks gestation of pregnancy

Explanation: Because oral thrush is an HIV-related condition, this patient is now considered to have HIV disease. An obstetrics code indicating that HIV is complicating the pregnancy is coded first, followed by B20 for HIV disease as well as a code for the oral thrush.

g. Diabetes mellitus in pregnancy

Diabetes mellitus is a significant complicating factor in pregnancy. Pregnant women who are diabetic should be assigned a code from category O24, Diabetes mellitus in pregnancy, childbirth, and the puerperium, first, followed by the appropriate diabetes code(s) (E08-E13) from Chapter 4.

h. Long term use of insulin and oral hypoglycemics

See section I.C.4.a.3 for information on the long-term use of insulin and oral hypoglycemics.

i. Gestational (pregnancy induced) diabetes

Gestational (pregnancy induced) diabetes can occur during the second and third trimester of pregnancy in women who were not diabetic prior to pregnancy. Gestational diabetes can cause complications in the pregnancy similar to those of pre-existing diabetes mellitus. It also puts the woman at greater risk of developing diabetes after the pregnancy. Codes for gestational diabetes are in subcategory O24.4, Gestational diabetes mellitus. No other code from category O24, Diabetes mellitus in pregnancy, childbirth, and the puerperium, should be used with a code from O24.4.

The codes under subcategory O24.4 include diet controlled, insulin controlled, and controlled by oral hypoglycemic drugs. If a patient with gestational diabetes is treated with both diet and insulin, only the code for insulin-controlled is required. If a patient with gestational diabetes is treated with both diet and oral hypoglycemic medications, only the code for "controlled by oral hypoglycemic drugs" is required. Code Z79.4, Long-term (current) use of insulin or code Z79.84, Long-term (current) use of oral hypoglycemic drugs, should not be assigned with codes from subcategory O24.4.

An abnormal glucose tolerance in pregnancy is assigned a code from subcategory O99.81, Abnormal glucose complicating pregnancy, childbirth, and the puerperium.

> Patient at 39 weeks term pregnancy with gestational diabetes was admitted in labor and delivered a healthy newborn. Patient is on a diabetic diet with daily metformin.
>
> **O24.425**   **Gestational diabetes mellitus in childbirth, controlled by oral hypoglycemic drugs**
>
> **Z3A.39**   **39 weeks gestation of pregnancy**
>
> **Z37.0**   **Single live birth**
>
> *Explanation:* When the patient is admitted for delivery and the patient's gestational diabetes is controlled by both diet and oral hypoglycemic medications, only the combination code in subcategory O24.4- Gestational diabetes mellitus, is reported. No code is added for diet controlled diabetes, and no Z code for long-term use of oral hypoglycemics is reported with the O24.4 combination codes.

j. Sepsis and septic shock complicating abortion, pregnancy, childbirth and the puerperium

When assigning a chapter 15 code for sepsis complicating abortion, pregnancy, childbirth, and the puerperium, a code for the specific type of infection should be assigned as an additional diagnosis. If severe sepsis is present, a code from subcategory R65.2, Severe sepsis, and code(s) for associated organ dysfunction(s) should also be assigned as additional diagnoses.

> Patient is seen several days after a miscarriage with sepsis; cultures return MSSA
>
> **O03.87**   **Sepsis following complete or unspecified spontaneous abortion**
>
> **B95.61**   **Methicillin susceptible Staphylococcus aureus infection as the cause of diseases classified elsewhere**
>
> *Explanation:* The type of infection that caused this patient to become septic was methicillin susceptible *Staphylococcus aureus* (MSSA), which as a secondary code helps capture all aspects related to this patient's septic condition.

k. Puerperal sepsis

Code O85, Puerperal sepsis, should be assigned with a secondary code to identify the causal organism (e.g., for a bacterial infection, assign a code from category B95-B96, Bacterial infections in conditions classified elsewhere). A code from category A40, Streptococcal sepsis, or A41, Other sepsis, should not be used for puerperal sepsis. If applicable, use additional codes to identify severe sepsis (R65.2-) and any associated acute organ dysfunction.

Code O85 should not be assigned for sepsis following an obstetrical procedure (See Section I.C.1.d.5.b., Sepsis due to a postprocedural infection).

l. Alcohol, tobacco and drug use during pregnancy, childbirth and the puerperium

1) Alcohol use during pregnancy, childbirth and the puerperium

Codes under subcategory O99.31, Alcohol use complicating pregnancy, childbirth, and the puerperium, should be assigned for any pregnancy case when a mother uses alcohol during the pregnancy or postpartum. A secondary code from category F10, Alcohol related disorders, should also be assigned to identify manifestations of the alcohol use.

2) Tobacco use during pregnancy, childbirth and the puerperium

Codes under subcategory O99.33, Smoking (tobacco) complicating pregnancy, childbirth, and the puerperium, should be assigned for any pregnancy case when a mother uses any type of tobacco product during the pregnancy or postpartum. A secondary code from category F17, Nicotine dependence, should also be assigned to identify the type of nicotine dependence.

3) Drug use during pregnancy, childbirth and the puerperium

Codes under subcategory O99.32, Drug use complicating pregnancy, childbirth, and the puerperium, should be assigned for any pregnancy case when a mother uses drugs during the pregnancy or postpartum. This can involve illegal drugs, or inappropriate use or abuse of prescription drugs. Secondary code(s) from categories F11-F16 and F18-F19 should also be assigned to identify manifestations of the drug use.

m. Poisoning, toxic effects, adverse effects and underdosing in a pregnant patient

A code from subcategory O9A.2, Injury, poisoning and certain other consequences of external causes complicating pregnancy, childbirth, and the puerperium, should be sequenced first, followed by the appropriate injury, poisoning, toxic effect, adverse effect or underdosing code, and then the additional code(s) that specifies the condition caused by the poisoning, toxic effect, adverse effect or underdosing.

See Section I.C.19. Adverse effects, poisoning, underdosing and toxic effects.

> Patient admitted with accidental carbon monoxide poisoning from a gas heating implement; the patient is 18 weeks' pregnant
>
> **O9A.212**   **Injury, poisoning and certain other consequences of external causes complicating pregnancy, second trimester**
>
> **T58.11XA**   **Toxic effect of carbon monoxide from utility gas, accidental (unintentional), initial encounter**
>
> **Z3A.18**   **18 weeks gestation of pregnancy**
>
> *Explanation:* Although the carbon monoxide poisoning is the reason the patient was admitted, a code from the obstetrics chapter must be sequenced first. Chapter 15 codes have sequencing priority over codes from other chapters.

n. Normal delivery, code O80

1) Encounter for full term uncomplicated delivery

Code O80 should be assigned when a woman is admitted for a full-term normal delivery and delivers a single, healthy infant without any complications antepartum, during the delivery, or postpartum during the delivery episode. Code O80 is always a principal diagnosis. It is not to be used if any other code from chapter 15 is needed to describe a current complication of the antenatal, delivery, or postnatal period. Additional codes from other chapters may be used with code O80 if they are not related to or are in any way complicating the pregnancy.

2) Uncomplicated delivery with resolved antepartum complication

Code O80 may be used if the patient had a complication at some point during the pregnancy, but the complication is not present at the time of the admission for delivery.

> Patient presents in labor at 39 weeks' gestation and delivers a healthy newborn; patient had abnormal glucose levels in her first trimester, which have since resolved
>
> **O80**   **Encounter for full-term uncomplicated delivery**
>
> **Z37.0**   **Single live birth**
>
> *Explanation:* The abnormal glucose levels during the first trimester cannot be coded if they are not affecting the patient's current trimester. Without additional complications associated with the pregnancy, fetus, or mother, code O80 is appropriate.

3) Outcome of delivery for O80

Z37.0, Single live birth, is the only outcome of delivery code appropriate for use with O80.

o. The peripartum and postpartum periods

1) Peripartum and postpartum periods

The postpartum period begins immediately after delivery and continues for six weeks following delivery. The peripartum period is defined as the last month of pregnancy to five months postpartum.

2) Peripartum and postpartum complication

A postpartum complication is any complication occurring within the six-week period.

Chapter 15. Pregnancy, Childbirth and the Puerperium

3) Pregnancy-related complications after 6-week period

Chapter 15 codes may also be used to describe pregnancy-related complications after the peripartum or postpartum period if the provider documents that a condition is pregnancy related.

> Patient admitted for varicose veins. She had a baby boy three months ago; the varicose veins started to appear one month ago. The doctor attributes the patient's pregnancy as the cause of the varicose veins, which continue to be painful and bother the patient. She is seeking surgical relief.
>
> **O87.4   Varicose veins of the lower extremity in the puerperium**
>
> *Explanation:* Although the varicose veins occurred several months after the delivery of the newborn, the doctor attributed the varicose veins to pregnancy and therefore a code from chapter 15 is appropriate.

4) Admission for routine postpartum care following delivery outside hospital

When the mother delivers outside the hospital prior to admission and is admitted for routine postpartum care and no complications are noted, code Z39.0, Encounter for care and examination of mother immediately after delivery, should be assigned as the principal diagnosis.

5) Pregnancy associated cardiomyopathy

Pregnancy associated cardiomyopathy, code O90.3, is unique in that it may be diagnosed in the third trimester of pregnancy but may continue to progress months after delivery. For this reason, it is referred to as peripartum cardiomyopathy. Code O90.3 is only for use when the cardiomyopathy develops as a result of pregnancy in a woman who did not have pre-existing heart disease.

p. Code O94, Sequelae of complication of pregnancy, childbirth, and the puerperium

1) Code O94

Code O94, Sequelae of complication of pregnancy, childbirth, and the puerperium, is for use in those cases when an initial complication of a pregnancy develops a sequelae requiring care or treatment at a future date.

2) After the initial postpartum period

This code may be used at any time after the initial postpartum period.

3) Sequencing of code O94

This code, like all sequela codes, is to be sequenced following the code describing the sequelae of the complication.

q. Termination of pregnancy and spontaneous abortions

1) Abortion with liveborn fetus

When an attempted termination of pregnancy results in a liveborn fetus, assign code Z33.2, Encounter for elective termination of pregnancy and a code from category Z37, Outcome of Delivery.

2) Retained products of conception following an abortion

Subsequent encounters for retained products of conception following a spontaneous abortion or elective termination of pregnancy, without complications are assigned O03.4, Incomplete spontaneous, abortion without complication, or code O07.4, Failed attempted termination of pregnancy without complication. This advice is appropriate even when the patient was discharged previously with a discharge diagnosis of complete abortion. If the patient has a specific complication associated with the spontaneous abortion or elective termination of pregnancy in addition to retained products of conception, assign the appropriate complication code (e.g., O03.-, O04.-, O07.-) instead of code O03.4 or O07.4.

> Patient was seen two days ago for complete spontaneous abortion but returns today for urinary tract infection (UTI) with ultrasound showing retained products of conception
>
> **O03.38   Urinary tract infection following incomplete spontaneous abortion**
>
> *Explanation:* Although the diagnosis from the patient's previous stay indicated that the patient had a complete abortion, it is now determined that there were actually retained products of conception (POC). An abortion with retained POC is considered incomplete and in this case resulted in the patient developing a UTI.

3) Complications leading to abortion

Codes from Chapter 15 may be used as additional codes to identify any documented complications of the pregnancy in conjunction with codes in categories in O04, O07 and O08.

r. Abuse in a pregnant patient

For suspected or confirmed cases of abuse of a pregnant patient, a code(s) from subcategories O9A.3, Physical abuse complicating pregnancy, childbirth, and the puerperium, O9A.4, Sexual abuse complicating pregnancy, childbirth, and the puerperium, and O9A.5, Psychological abuse complicating pregnancy, childbirth, and the puerperium, should be sequenced first, followed by the appropriate codes (if applicable) to identify any associated current injury due to physical abuse, sexual abuse, and the perpetrator of abuse.

See Section I.C.19. Adult and child abuse, neglect and other maltreatment.

s. COVID-19 infection in pregnancy, childbirth, and the puerperium

During pregnancy, childbirth or the puerperium, when COVID-19 is the reason for admission/encounter , code O98.5-, Other viral diseases complicating pregnancy, childbirth and the puerperium, should be sequenced as the principal/first-listed diagnosis, and code U07.1, COVID-19, and the appropriate codes for associated manifestation(s) should be assigned as additional diagnoses. Codes from Chapter 15 always take sequencing priority.

If the reason for admission/encounter is unrelated to COVID-19 but the patient tests positive for COVID-19 during the admission/encounter, the appropriate code for the reason for admission/encounter should be sequenced as the principal/first-listed diagnosis, and codes O98.5- and U07.1, as well as the appropriate codes for associated COVID-19 manifestations, should be assigned as additional diagnoses.

> Patient admitted in labor at 39 weeks' gestation and delivered a healthy newborn. Prenatal care consisted of some hyperemesis early in the pregnancy that has since resolved. No complications encountered during or following delivery. As per hospital protocol, during the pandemic, all patients are to be screened for COVID-19, and the patient tested positive. She remains asymptomatic, will be sent home to quarantine for 14 days.
>
> **O98.52   Other viral diseases complicating childbirth**
>
> **U07.1   COVID-19**
>
> **Z3A.39   39 weeks gestation of pregnancy**
>
> **Z37.0   Single live birth**
>
> *Explanation:* No code is assigned for the hyperemesis as it resolved prior to this admission. Per guideline I.C.1.g.1.f, a screening code is generally not appropriate during the pandemic phase of COVID-19. Most hospitals screen their patients upon admission to the hospital to ensure proper protocols are in place for monitoring and treating those patients who do test positive for the disease. A positive test result alone is confirmation of the disease, according to guideline I.C.1.g.1.a, and code U07.1 should be assigned. A claim for any patient admitted during pregnancy, childbirth, or the puerperium and who tests positive or is treated for COVID-19 should have a code from subcategory O98.5- sequenced first, followed by code U07.1. As the patient was asymptomatic, no additional codes are assigned to represent any manifestation of the COVID-19 infection.

Chapter 15. Pregnancy, Childbirth and the Puerperium (O00-O9A)

NOTE   CODES FROM THIS CHAPTER ARE FOR USE ONLY ON MATERNAL RECORDS, NEVER ON NEWBORN RECORDS

Codes from this chapter are for use for conditions related to or aggravated by the pregnancy, childbirth, or by the puerperium (maternal causes or obstetric causes)

NOTE   Trimesters are counted from the first day of the last menstrual period. They are defined as follows:

1st trimester- less than 14 weeks 0 days

2nd trimester- 14 weeks 0 days to less than 28 weeks 0 days

3rd trimester- 28 weeks 0 days until delivery

Use additional code from category Z3A, Weeks of gestation, to identify the specific week of the pregnancy, if known.

EXCLUDES 1   supervision of normal pregnancy (Z34.-)

EXCLUDES 2   mental and behavioral disorders associated with the puerperium (F53.-)
obstetrical tetanus (A34)
postpartum necrosis of pituitary gland (E23.0)
puerperal osteomalacia (M83.0)

AHA: 2016,1Q,3-5; 2014,3Q,17

This chapter contains the following blocks:

O00-O08	Pregnancy with abortive outcome
O09	Supervision of high risk pregnancy
O10-O16	Edema, proteinuria and hypertensive disorders in pregnancy, childbirth and the puerperium
O20-O29	Other maternal disorders predominantly related to pregnancy
O30-O48	Maternal care related to the fetus and amniotic cavity and possible delivery problems
O60-O77	Complications of labor and delivery
O80-O82	Encounter for delivery
O85-O92	Complications predominantly related to the puerperium
O94-O9A	Other obstetric conditions, not elsewhere classified

Pregnancy with abortive outcome (O00-O08)

EXCLUDES 1   continuing pregnancy in multiple gestation after abortion of one fetus or more (O31.1-, O31.3-)

TIP: Do not assign a code from category Z3A with codes in this code block.

✓4ᵗʰ O00 Ectopic pregnancy

INCLUDES   ruptured ectopic pregnancy

Use additional code from category O08 to identify any associated complication

AHA: 2016,4Q,48-50; 2014,3Q,17

DEF: Implantation of a fertilized egg outside the uterus, usually in the fallopian tube or abdomen that requires emergency treatment.

Ectopic Pregnancy

Cornual/interstitial
Isthmic
Ampullar
Tubal (fallopian)
Infundibular
Ovarian
Intraligamentous
Abdominal
Cervical
Intramural/mural

✓5ᵗʰ O00.0 Abdominal pregnancy

EXCLUDES 1   maternal care for viable fetus in abdominal pregnancy (O36.7-)

O00.00 Abdominal pregnancy without intrauterine pregnancy   cc M ♀
Abdominal pregnancy NOS

O00.01 Abdominal pregnancy with intrauterine pregnancy   cc M ♀

✓5ᵗʰ O00.1 Tubal pregnancy
Fallopian pregnancy
Rupture of (fallopian) tube due to pregnancy
Tubal abortion
AHA: 2017,4Q,20

✓6ᵗʰ O00.10 Tubal pregnancy without intrauterine pregnancy
Tubal pregnancy NOS

O00.101 Right tubal pregnancy without intrauterine pregnancy   cc M ♀

O00.102 Left tubal pregnancy without intrauterine pregnancy   cc M ♀

O00.109 Unspecified tubal pregnancy without intrauterine pregnancy   cc M ♀

✓6ᵗʰ O00.11 Tubal pregnancy with intrauterine pregnancy

O00.111 Right tubal pregnancy with intrauterine pregnancy   cc M ♀

O00.112 Left tubal pregnancy with intrauterine pregnancy   cc M ♀

O00.119 Unspecified tubal pregnancy with intrauterine pregnancy   cc M ♀

✓5ᵗʰ O00.2 Ovarian pregnancy
AHA: 2017,4Q,20

✓6ᵗʰ O00.20 Ovarian pregnancy without intrauterine pregnancy
Ovarian pregnancy NOS

O00.201 Right ovarian pregnancy without intrauterine pregnancy   cc M ♀

O00.202 Left ovarian pregnancy without intrauterine pregnancy   cc M ♀

O00.209 Unspecified ovarian pregnancy without intrauterine pregnancy   cc M ♀

✓6ᵗʰ O00.21 Ovarian pregnancy with intrauterine pregnancy

O00.211 Right ovarian pregnancy with intrauterine pregnancy   cc M ♀

O00.212 Left ovarian pregnancy with intrauterine pregnancy   cc M ♀

O00.219 Unspecified ovarian pregnancy with intrauterine pregnancy   cc M ♀

✓5ᵗʰ O00.8 Other ectopic pregnancy
Cervical pregnancy
Cornual pregnancy
Intraligamentous pregnancy
Mural pregnancy

O00.80 Other ectopic pregnancy without intrauterine pregnancy   cc M ♀
Other ectopic pregnancy NOS

O00.81 Other ectopic pregnancy with intrauterine pregnancy   cc M ♀

✓5ᵗʰ O00.9 Ectopic pregnancy, unspecified

O00.90 Unspecified ectopic pregnancy without intrauterine pregnancy   cc M ♀
Ectopic pregnancy NOS

O00.91 Unspecified ectopic pregnancy with intrauterine pregnancy   cc M ♀

✓4ᵗʰ O01 Hydatidiform mole

Use additional code from category O08 to identify any associated complication

EXCLUDES 1   chorioadenoma (destruens) (D39.2)
malignant hydatidiform mole (D39.2)

AHA: 2014,3Q,17

DEF: Abnormal product of pregnancy, marked by a mass of cysts resembling a bunch of grapes due to chorionic villi proliferation and dissolution. It must be surgically removed.

O01.0 Classical hydatidiform mole   M ♀
Complete hydatidiform mole

O01.1 Incomplete and partial hydatidiform mole   M ♀

O01.9 Hydatidiform mole, unspecified   M ♀
Trophoblastic disease NOS
Vesicular mole NOS

☑ Additional Character Required   ✓x7ᵗʰ Placeholder   Unacceptable PDx   Questionable PDx   Manifestation   Unspecified Dx   H1-H4 HAC   HCC CMS-HCC Dx   HIV HIV Dx

ICD-10-CM 2021   **865**

✓4ᵗʰ O02 Other abnormal products of conception

Use additional code from category O08 to identify any associated complication

EXCLUDES 1   *papyraceous fetus (O31.0-)*

AHA: 2014,3Q,17

O02.0 Blighted ovum and nonhydatidiform mole   M ♀

Carneous mole
Fleshy mole
Intrauterine mole NOS
Molar pregnancy NEC
Pathological ovum

O02.1 Missed abortion   M ♀

Early fetal death, before completion of 20 weeks of gestation, with retention of dead fetus

EXCLUDES 1   *failed induced abortion (O07.-)*
fetal death (intrauterine) (late) (O36.4)
missed abortion with blighted ovum (O02.0)
missed abortion with hydatidiform mole (O01.-)
missed abortion with nonhydatidiform (O02.0)
missed abortion with other abnormal products of conception (O02.8-)
missed delivery (O36.4)
stillbirth (P95)

AHA: 2019,3Q,11

✓5ᵗʰ O02.8 Other specified abnormal products of conception

EXCLUDES 1   *abnormal products of conception with blighted ovum (O02.0)*
abnormal products of conception with hydatidiform mole (O01.-)
abnormal products of conception with nonhydatidiform mole (O02.0)

O02.81 Inappropriate change in quantitative human chorionic gonadotropin (hCG) in early pregnancy   M ♀

Biochemical pregnancy
Chemical pregnancy
Inappropriate level of quantitative human chorionic gonadotropin (hCG) for gestational age in early pregnancy

O02.89 Other abnormal products of conception   M ♀

O02.9 Abnormal product of conception, unspecified   M ♀

✓4ᵗʰ O03 Spontaneous abortion

NOTE   Incomplete abortion includes retained products of conception following spontaneous abortion

INCLUDES   miscarriage

O03.0 Genital tract and pelvic infection following incomplete spontaneous abortion   CC M ♀

Endometritis following incomplete spontaneous abortion
Oophoritis following incomplete spontaneous abortion
Parametritis following incomplete spontaneous abortion
Pelvic peritonitis following incomplete spontaneous abortion
Salpingitis following incomplete spontaneous abortion
Salpingo-oophoritis following incomplete spontaneous abortion

EXCLUDES 1   *sepsis following incomplete spontaneous abortion (O03.37)*
urinary tract infection following incomplete spontaneous abortion (O03.38)

O03.1 Delayed or excessive hemorrhage following incomplete spontaneous abortion   M ♀

Afibrinogenemia following incomplete spontaneous abortion
Defibrination syndrome following incomplete spontaneous abortion
Hemolysis following incomplete spontaneous abortion
Intravascular coagulation following incomplete spontaneous abortion

O03.2 Embolism following incomplete spontaneous abortion   MCC M ♀

Air embolism following incomplete spontaneous abortion
Amniotic fluid embolism following incomplete spontaneous abortion
Blood-clot embolism following incomplete spontaneous abortion
Embolism NOS following incomplete spontaneous abortion
Fat embolism following incomplete spontaneous abortion
Pulmonary embolism following incomplete spontaneous abortion
Pyemic embolism following incomplete spontaneous abortion
Septic or septicopyemic embolism following incomplete spontaneous abortion
Soap embolism following incomplete spontaneous abortion

✓5ᵗʰ O03.3 Other and unspecified complications following incomplete spontaneous abortion

O03.30 Unspecified complication following incomplete spontaneous abortion   CC M ♀

O03.31 Shock following incomplete spontaneous abortion   MCC M ♀

Circulatory collapse following incomplete spontaneous abortion
Shock (postprocedural) following incomplete spontaneous abortion

EXCLUDES 1   *shock due to infection following incomplete spontaneous abortion (O03.37)*

O03.32 Renal failure following incomplete spontaneous abortion   MCC M ♀

Kidney failure (acute) following incomplete spontaneous abortion
Oliguria following incomplete spontaneous abortion
Renal shutdown following incomplete spontaneous abortion
Renal tubular necrosis following incomplete spontaneous abortion
Uremia following incomplete spontaneous abortion

O03.33 Metabolic disorder following incomplete spontaneous abortion   CC M ♀

O03.34 Damage to pelvic organs following incomplete spontaneous abortion   CC M ♀

Laceration, perforation, tear or chemical damage of bladder following incomplete spontaneous abortion
Laceration, perforation, tear or chemical damage of bowel following incomplete spontaneous abortion
Laceration, perforation, tear or chemical damage of broad ligament following incomplete spontaneous abortion
Laceration, perforation, tear or chemical damage of cervix following incomplete spontaneous abortion
Laceration, perforation, tear or chemical damage of periurethral tissue following incomplete spontaneous abortion
Laceration, perforation, tear or chemical damage of uterus following incomplete spontaneous abortion
Laceration, perforation, tear or chemical damage of vagina following incomplete spontaneous abortion

O03.35 Other venous complications following incomplete spontaneous abortion   CC M ♀

O03.36 Cardiac arrest following incomplete spontaneous abortion   CC M ♀

O03.37 Sepsis following incomplete spontaneous abortion   CC M ♀

Use additional code to identify infectious agent (B95-B97)
Use additional code to identify severe sepsis, if applicable (R65.2-)

EXCLUDES 1   *septic or septicopyemic embolism following incomplete spontaneous abortion (O03.2)*

O03.38 **Urinary tract infection following incomplete spontaneous abortion** `CC` `M` ♀
Cystitis following incomplete spontaneous abortion

O03.39 **Incomplete spontaneous abortion with other complications** `CC` `M` ♀

O03.4 **Incomplete spontaneous abortion without complication** `M` ♀

O03.5 **Genital tract and pelvic infection following complete or unspecified spontaneous abortion** `CC` `M` ♀
Endometritis following complete or unspecified spontaneous abortion
Oophoritis following complete or unspecified spontaneous abortion
Parametritis following complete or unspecified spontaneous abortion
Pelvic peritonitis following complete or unspecified spontaneous abortion
Salpingitis following complete or unspecified spontaneous abortion
Salpingo-oophoritis following complete or unspecified spontaneous abortion
> **EXCLUDES 1** *sepsis following complete or unspecified spontaneous abortion (O03.87)*
> *urinary tract infection following complete or unspecified spontaneous abortion (O03.88)*

O03.6 **Delayed or excessive hemorrhage following complete or unspecified spontaneous abortion** `M` ♀
Afibrinogenemia following complete or unspecified spontaneous abortion
Defibrination syndrome following complete or unspecified spontaneous abortion
Hemolysis following complete or unspecified spontaneous abortion
Intravascular coagulation following complete or unspecified spontaneous abortion

O03.7 **Embolism following complete or unspecified spontaneous abortion** `CC` `M` ♀
Air embolism following complete or unspecified spontaneous abortion
Amniotic fluid embolism following complete or unspecified spontaneous abortion
Blood-clot embolism following complete or unspecified spontaneous abortion
Embolism NOS following complete or unspecified spontaneous abortion
Fat embolism following complete or unspecified spontaneous abortion
Pulmonary embolism following complete or unspecified spontaneous abortion
Pyemic embolism following complete or unspecified spontaneous abortion
Septic or septicopyemic embolism following complete or unspecified spontaneous abortion
Soap embolism following complete or unspecified spontaneous abortion

√5ᵗʰ **O03.8** **Other and unspecified complications following complete or unspecified spontaneous abortion**

O03.80 **Unspecified complication following complete or unspecified spontaneous abortion** `CC` `M` ♀

O03.81 **Shock following complete or unspecified spontaneous abortion** `MCC` `M` ♀
Circulatory collapse following complete or unspecified spontaneous abortion
Shock (postprocedural) following complete or unspecified spontaneous abortion
> **EXCLUDES 1** *shock due to infection following complete or unspecified spontaneous abortion (O03.87)*

O03.82 **Renal failure following complete or unspecified spontaneous abortion** `MCC` `M` ♀
Kidney failure (acute) following complete or unspecified spontaneous abortion
Oliguria following complete or unspecified spontaneous abortion
Renal shutdown following complete or unspecified spontaneous abortion
Renal tubular necrosis following complete or unspecified spontaneous abortion
Uremia following complete or unspecified spontaneous abortion

O03.83 **Metabolic disorder following complete or unspecified spontaneous abortion** `CC` `M` ♀

O03.84 **Damage to pelvic organs following complete or unspecified spontaneous abortion** `CC` `M` ♀
Laceration, perforation, tear or chemical damage of bladder following complete or unspecified spontaneous abortion
Laceration, perforation, tear or chemical damage of bowel following complete or unspecified spontaneous abortion
Laceration, perforation, tear or chemical damage of broad ligament following complete or unspecified spontaneous abortion
Laceration, perforation, tear or chemical damage of cervix following complete or unspecified spontaneous abortion
Laceration, perforation, tear or chemical damage of periurethral tissue following complete or unspecified spontaneous abortion
Laceration, perforation, tear or chemical damage of uterus following complete or unspecified spontaneous abortion
Laceration, perforation, tear or chemical damage of vagina following complete or unspecified spontaneous abortion

O03.85 **Other venous complications following complete or unspecified spontaneous abortion** `CC` `M` ♀

O03.86 **Cardiac arrest following complete or unspecified spontaneous abortion** `CC` `M` ♀

O03.87 **Sepsis following complete or unspecified spontaneous abortion** `CC` `M` ♀
Use additional code to identify infectious agent (B95-B97)
Use additional code to identify severe sepsis, if applicable (R65.2-)
> **EXCLUDES 1** *septic or septicopyemic embolism following complete or unspecified spontaneous abortion (O03.7)*

O03.88 **Urinary tract infection following complete or unspecified spontaneous abortion** `CC` `M` ♀
Cystitis following complete or unspecified spontaneous abortion

O03.89 **Complete or unspecified spontaneous abortion with other complications** `CC` `M` ♀

O03.9 **Complete or unspecified spontaneous abortion without complication** `M` ♀
Miscarriage NOS
Spontaneous abortion NOS

Chapter 15. Pregnancy, Childbirth and the Puerperium

O03.38–O03.9

Chapter 15. Pregnancy, Childbirth and the Puerperium (side tab)

☑4ᵗʰ **O04 Complications following (induced) termination of pregnancy**

INCLUDES   complications following (induced) termination of pregnancy

EXCLUDES 1   *encounter for elective termination of pregnancy, uncomplicated (Z33.2)*
failed attempted termination of pregnancy (O07.-)

O04.5 Genital tract and pelvic infection following (induced) termination of pregnancy   CC M ♀

Endometritis following (induced) termination of pregnancy
Oophoritis following (induced) termination of pregnancy
Parametritis following (induced) termination of pregnancy
Pelvic peritonitis following (induced) termination of pregnancy
Salpingitis following (induced) termination of pregnancy
Salpingo-oophoritis following (induced) termination of pregnancy

EXCLUDES 1   *sepsis following (induced) termination of pregnancy (O04.87)*
urinary tract infection following (induced) termination of pregnancy (O04.88)

O04.6 Delayed or excessive hemorrhage following (induced) termination of pregnancy   M ♀

Afibrinogenemia following (induced) termination of pregnancy
Defibrination syndrome following (induced) termination of pregnancy
Hemolysis following (induced) termination of pregnancy
Intravascular coagulation following (induced) termination of pregnancy

AHA: 2019,3Q,11

O04.7 Embolism following (induced) termination of pregnancy   MCC M ♀

Air embolism following (induced) termination of pregnancy
Amniotic fluid embolism following (induced) termination of pregnancy
Blood-clot embolism following (induced) termination of pregnancy
Embolism NOS following (induced) termination of pregnancy
Fat embolism following (induced) termination of pregnancy
Pulmonary embolism following (induced) termination of pregnancy
Pyemic embolism following (induced) termination of pregnancy
Septic or septicopyemic embolism following (induced) termination of pregnancy
Soap embolism following (induced) termination of pregnancy

☑5ᵗʰ **O04.8 (Induced) termination of pregnancy with other and unspecified complications**

O04.80 (Induced) termination of pregnancy with unspecified complications   CC M ♀

O04.81 Shock following (induced) termination of pregnancy   MCC M ♀

Circulatory collapse following (induced) termination of pregnancy
Shock (postprocedural) following (induced) termination of pregnancy

EXCLUDES 1   *shock due to infection following (induced) termination of pregnancy (O04.87)*

O04.82 Renal failure following (induced) termination of pregnancy   MCC M ♀

Kidney failure (acute) following (induced) termination of pregnancy
Oliguria following (induced) termination of pregnancy
Renal shutdown following (induced) termination of pregnancy
Renal tubular necrosis following (induced) termination of pregnancy
Uremia following (induced) termination of pregnancy

O04.83 Metabolic disorder following (induced) termination of pregnancy   CC M ♀

O04.84 Damage to pelvic organs following (induced) termination of pregnancy   CC M ♀

Laceration, perforation, tear or chemical damage of bladder following (induced) termination of pregnancy
Laceration, perforation, tear or chemical damage of bowel following (induced) termination of pregnancy
Laceration, perforation, tear or chemical damage of broad ligament following (induced) termination of pregnancy
Laceration, perforation, tear or chemical damage of cervix following (induced) termination of pregnancy
Laceration, perforation, tear or chemical damage of periurethral tissue following (induced) termination of pregnancy
Laceration, perforation, tear or chemical damage of uterus following (induced) termination of pregnancy
Laceration, perforation, tear or chemical damage of vagina following (induced) termination of pregnancy

O04.85 Other venous complications following (induced) termination of pregnancy   CC M ♀

O04.86 Cardiac arrest following (induced) termination of pregnancy   CC M ♀

O04.87 Sepsis following (induced) termination of pregnancy   MCC M ♀

Use additional code to identify infectious agent (B95-B97)
Use additional code to identify severe sepsis, if applicable (R65.2-)

EXCLUDES 1   *septic or septicopyemic embolism following (induced) termination of pregnancy (O04.7)*

O04.88 Urinary tract infection following (induced) termination of pregnancy   CC M ♀

Cystitis following (induced) termination of pregnancy

O04.89 (Induced) termination of pregnancy with other complications   CC M ♀

☑4ᵗʰ **O07 Failed attempted termination of pregnancy**

INCLUDES   failure of attempted induction of termination of pregnancy
incomplete elective abortion

EXCLUDES 1   *incomplete spontaneous abortion (O03.0-)*

O07.0 Genital tract and pelvic infection following failed attempted termination of pregnancy   CC M ♀

Endometritis following failed attempted termination of pregnancy
Oophoritis following failed attempted termination of pregnancy
Parametritis following failed attempted termination of pregnancy
Pelvic peritonitis following failed attempted termination of pregnancy
Salpingitis following failed attempted termination of pregnancy
Salpingo-oophoritis following failed attempted termination of pregnancy

EXCLUDES 1   *sepsis following failed attempted termination of pregnancy (O07.37)*
urinary tract infection following failed attempted termination of pregnancy (O07.38)

O07.1 Delayed or excessive hemorrhage following failed attempted termination of pregnancy   CC M ♀

Afibrinogenemia following failed attempted termination of pregnancy
Defibrination syndrome following failed attempted termination of pregnancy
Hemolysis following failed attempted termination of pregnancy
Intravascular coagulation following failed attempted termination of pregnancy

N Newborn: 0   P Pediatric: 0-17   M Maternity: 9-64   A Adult: 15-124   MCC Major Complication/Comorbidity   CC Complication/Comorbidity   SW Severe Wound Dx

868   ICD-10-CM 2021

O07.2 Embolism following failed attempted termination of pregnancy   `MCC` `M` ♀

Air embolism following failed attempted termination of pregnancy

Amniotic fluid embolism following failed attempted termination of pregnancy

Blood-clot embolism following failed attempted termination of pregnancy

Embolism NOS following failed attempted termination of pregnancy

Fat embolism following failed attempted termination of pregnancy

Pulmonary embolism following failed attempted termination of pregnancy

Pyemic embolism following failed attempted termination of pregnancy

Septic or septicopyemic embolism following failed attempted termination of pregnancy

Soap embolism following failed attempted termination of pregnancy

✓5ᵗʰ O07.3 Failed attempted termination of pregnancy with other and unspecified complications

O07.30 Failed attempted termination of pregnancy with unspecified complications   `CC` `M` ♀

O07.31 Shock following failed attempted termination of pregnancy   `MCC` `M` ♀

Circulatory collapse following failed attempted termination of pregnancy

Shock (postprocedural) following failed attempted termination of pregnancy

   `EXCLUDES 1`   *shock due to infection following failed attempted termination of pregnancy (O07.37)*

O07.32 Renal failure following failed attempted termination of pregnancy   `MCC` `M` ♀

Kidney failure (acute) following failed attempted termination of pregnancy

Oliguria following failed attempted termination of pregnancy

Renal shutdown following failed attempted termination of pregnancy

Renal tubular necrosis following failed attempted termination of pregnancy

Uremia following failed attempted termination of pregnancy

O07.33 Metabolic disorder following failed attempted termination of pregnancy   `CC` `M` ♀

O07.34 Damage to pelvic organs following failed attempted termination of pregnancy   `CC` `M` ♀

Laceration, perforation, tear or chemical damage of bladder following failed attempted termination of pregnancy

Laceration, perforation, tear or chemical damage of bowel following failed attempted termination of pregnancy

Laceration, perforation, tear or chemical damage of broad ligament following failed attempted termination of pregnancy

Laceration, perforation, tear or chemical damage of cervix following failed attempted termination of pregnancy

Laceration, perforation, tear or chemical damage of periurethral tissue following failed attempted termination of pregnancy

Laceration, perforation, tear or chemical damage of uterus following failed attempted termination of pregnancy

Laceration, perforation, tear or chemical damage of vagina following failed attempted termination of pregnancy

O07.35 Other venous complications following failed attempted termination of pregnancy   `CC` `M` ♀

O07.36 Cardiac arrest following failed attempted termination of pregnancy   `CC` `M` ♀

O07.37 Sepsis following failed attempted termination of pregnancy   `CC` `M` ♀

Use additional code (B95-B97), to identify infectious agent

Use additional code (R65.2-) to identify severe sepsis, if applicable

   `EXCLUDES 1`   *septic or septicopyemic embolism following failed attempted termination of pregnancy (O07.2)*

O07.38 Urinary tract infection following failed attempted termination of pregnancy   `CC` `M` ♀

Cystitis following failed attempted termination of pregnancy

O07.39 Failed attempted termination of pregnancy with other complications   `CC` `M` ♀

O07.4 Failed attempted termination of pregnancy without complication   `M` ♀

✓4ᵗʰ O08 Complications following ectopic and molar pregnancy

This category is for use with categories O00-O02 to identify any associated complications

O08.0 Genital tract and pelvic infection following ectopic and molar pregnancy   `CC` `M` ♀

Endometritis following ectopic and molar pregnancy

Oophoritis following ectopic and molar pregnancy

Parametritis following ectopic and molar pregnancy

Pelvic peritonitis following ectopic and molar pregnancy

Salpingitis following ectopic and molar pregnancy

Salpingo-oophoritis following ectopic and molar pregnancy

   `EXCLUDES 1`   *sepsis following ectopic and molar pregnancy (O08.82)*
       urinary tract infection (O08.83)

O08.1 Delayed or excessive hemorrhage following ectopic and molar pregnancy   `CC` `M` ♀

Afibrinogenemia following ectopic and molar pregnancy

Defibrination syndrome following ectopic and molar pregnancy

Hemolysis following ectopic and molar pregnancy

Intravascular coagulation following ectopic and molar pregnancy

   `EXCLUDES 1`   *delayed or excessive hemorrhage due to incomplete abortion (O03.1)*

O08.2 Embolism following ectopic and molar pregnancy   `MCC` `M` ♀

Air embolism following ectopic and molar pregnancy

Amniotic fluid embolism following ectopic and molar pregnancy

Blood-clot embolism following ectopic and molar pregnancy

Embolism NOS following ectopic and molar pregnancy

Fat embolism following ectopic and molar pregnancy

Pulmonary embolism following ectopic and molar pregnancy

Pyemic embolism following ectopic and molar pregnancy

Septic or septicopyemic embolism following ectopic and molar pregnancy

Soap embolism following ectopic and molar pregnancy

O08.3 Shock following ectopic and molar pregnancy   `MCC` `M` ♀

Circulatory collapse following ectopic and molar pregnancy

Shock (postprocedural) following ectopic and molar pregnancy

   `EXCLUDES 1`   *shock due to infection following ectopic and molar pregnancy (O08.82)*

O08.4 Renal failure following ectopic and molar pregnancy   `MCC` `M` ♀

Kidney failure (acute) following ectopic and molar pregnancy

Oliguria following ectopic and molar pregnancy

Renal shutdown following ectopic and molar pregnancy

Renal tubular necrosis following ectopic and molar pregnancy

Uremia following ectopic and molar pregnancy

O08.5 Metabolic disorders following an ectopic and molar pregnancy   `CC` `M` ♀

✓ Additional Character Required   `✓x7ᵗʰ` Placeholder   <u>Unacceptable PDx</u>   Questionable PDx   Manifestation   <u>Unspecified Dx</u>   `H1`-`H14` HAC   `HCC` CMS-HCC Dx   `HIV` HIV Dx

ICD-10-CM 2021   **869**

Chapter 15. Pregnancy, Childbirth and the Puerperium

O08.6 Damage to pelvic organs and tissues following an ectopic and molar pregnancy CC M ♀
Laceration, perforation, tear or chemical damage of bladder following an ectopic and molar pregnancy
Laceration, perforation, tear or chemical damage of bowel following an ectopic and molar pregnancy
Laceration, perforation, tear or chemical damage of broad ligament following an ectopic and molar pregnancy
Laceration, perforation, tear or chemical damage of cervix following an ectopic and molar pregnancy
Laceration, perforation, tear or chemical damage of periurethral tissue following an ectopic and molar pregnancy
Laceration, perforation, tear or chemical damage of uterus following an ectopic and molar pregnancy
Laceration, perforation, tear or chemical damage of vagina following an ectopic and molar pregnancy

O08.7 Other venous complications following an ectopic and molar pregnancy CC M ♀

✓5ᵗʰ **O08.8 Other complications following an ectopic and molar pregnancy**

O08.81 Cardiac arrest following an ectopic and molar pregnancy CC M ♀

O08.82 Sepsis following ectopic and molar pregnancy CC M ♀
Use additional code (B95-B97), to identify infectious agent
Use additional code (R65.2-) to identify severe sepsis, if applicable
EXCLUDES 1   septic or septicopyemic embolism following ectopic and molar pregnancy (O08.2)

O08.83 Urinary tract infection following an ectopic and molar pregnancy CC M ♀
Cystitis following an ectopic and molar pregnancy

O08.89 Other complications following an ectopic and molar pregnancy CC M ♀

O08.9 Unspecified complication following an ectopic and molar pregnancy CC M ♀

Supervision of high risk pregnancy (O09)

✓4ᵗʰ **O09 Supervision of high risk pregnancy**
AHA: 2019,3Q,5; 2016,4Q,48-50,150

✓5ᵗʰ **O09.0 Supervision of pregnancy with history of infertility**
DEF: Infertility: Inability to conceive for at least one year with regular intercourse.

O09.00 Supervision of pregnancy with history of infertility, unspecified trimester M ♀

O09.01 Supervision of pregnancy with history of infertility, first trimester M ♀

O09.02 Supervision of pregnancy with history of infertility, second trimester M ♀

O09.03 Supervision of pregnancy with history of infertility, third trimester M ♀

✓5ᵗʰ **O09.1 Supervision of pregnancy with history of ectopic pregnancy**
DEF: Ectopic pregnancy: Implantation of a fertilized egg outside the uterus, usually in the fallopian tube or abdomen that requires emergency treatment.

O09.10 Supervision of pregnancy with history of ectopic pregnancy, unspecified trimester M ♀

O09.11 Supervision of pregnancy with history of ectopic pregnancy, first trimester M ♀

O09.12 Supervision of pregnancy with history of ectopic pregnancy, second trimester M ♀

O09.13 Supervision of pregnancy with history of ectopic pregnancy, third trimester M ♀

✓5ᵗʰ **O09.A Supervision of pregnancy with history of molar pregnancy**
DEF: Molar pregnancy: Trophoblastic neoplasm that mimics pregnancy by proliferating from a pathologic ovum and resulting only in a mass of cysts resembling grapes, 80 percent of which are benign, but require surgical removal.

O09.A0 Supervision of pregnancy with history of molar pregnancy, unspecified trimester M ♀

O09.A1 Supervision of pregnancy with history of molar pregnancy, first trimester M ♀

O09.A2 Supervision of pregnancy with history of molar pregnancy, second trimester M ♀

O09.A3 Supervision of pregnancy with history of molar pregnancy, third trimester M ♀

✓5ᵗʰ **O09.2 Supervision of pregnancy with other poor reproductive or obstetric history**
EXCLUDES 2   pregnancy care for patient with history of recurrent pregnancy loss (O26.2-)

✓6ᵗʰ **O09.21 Supervision of pregnancy with history of pre-term labor**

O09.211 Supervision of pregnancy with history of pre-term labor, first trimester M ♀

O09.212 Supervision of pregnancy with history of pre-term labor, second trimester M ♀

O09.213 Supervision of pregnancy with history of pre-term labor, third trimester M ♀

O09.219 Supervision of pregnancy with history of pre-term labor, unspecified trimester M ♀

✓6ᵗʰ **O09.29 Supervision of pregnancy with other poor reproductive or obstetric history**
Supervision of pregnancy with history of neonatal death
Supervision of pregnancy with history of stillbirth

O09.291 Supervision of pregnancy with other poor reproductive or obstetric history, first trimester M ♀

O09.292 Supervision of pregnancy with other poor reproductive or obstetric history, second trimester M ♀

O09.293 Supervision of pregnancy with other poor reproductive or obstetric history, third trimester M ♀

O09.299 Supervision of pregnancy with other poor reproductive or obstetric history, unspecified trimester M ♀

✓5ᵗʰ **O09.3 Supervision of pregnancy with insufficient antenatal care**
Supervision of concealed pregnancy
Supervision of hidden pregnancy

O09.30 Supervision of pregnancy with insufficient antenatal care, unspecified trimester M ♀

O09.31 Supervision of pregnancy with insufficient antenatal care, first trimester M ♀

O09.32 Supervision of pregnancy with insufficient antenatal care, second trimester M ♀

O09.33 Supervision of pregnancy with insufficient antenatal care, third trimester M ♀

✓5ᵗʰ **O09.4 Supervision of pregnancy with grand multiparity**

O09.40 Supervision of pregnancy with grand multiparity, unspecified trimester M ♀

O09.41 Supervision of pregnancy with grand multiparity, first trimester M ♀

O09.42 Supervision of pregnancy with grand multiparity, second trimester M ♀

O09.43 Supervision of pregnancy with grand multiparity, third trimester M ♀

✓5ᵗʰ **O09.5 Supervision of elderly primigravida and multigravida**
Pregnancy for a female 35 years and older at expected date of delivery

✓6ᵗʰ **O09.51 Supervision of elderly primigravida**

O09.511 Supervision of elderly primigravida, first trimester M ♀

O09.512 Supervision of elderly primigravida, second trimester M ♀

O09.513 Supervision of elderly primigravida, third trimester M ♀

O09.519 Supervision of elderly primigravida, unspecified trimester M ♀

✓6ᵗʰ **O09.52 Supervision of elderly multigravida**

O09.521 Supervision of elderly multigravida, first trimester M ♀

O09.522 Supervision of elderly multigravida, second trimester M ♀

O09.523 Supervision of elderly multigravida, third trimester M ♀

O09.529 Supervision of elderly multigravida, unspecified trimester M ♀

✓5ᵗʰ **O09.6 Supervision of young primigravida and multigravida**
Supervision of pregnancy for a female less than 16 years old at expected date of delivery

✓6ᵗʰ **O09.61 Supervision of young primigravida**

O09.611 Supervision of young primigravida, first trimester M ♀

            O09.612   **Supervision of young primigravida, second trimester**   M ♀

            O09.613   **Supervision of young primigravida, third trimester**   M ♀

            O09.619   **Supervision of young primigravida, unspecified trimester**   M ♀

√6th   **O09.62**   **Supervision of young multigravida**

            O09.621   **Supervision of young multigravida, first trimester**   M ♀

            O09.622   **Supervision of young multigravida, second trimester**   M ♀

            O09.623   **Supervision of young multigravida, third trimester**   M ♀

            O09.629   **Supervision of young multigravida, unspecified trimester**   M ♀

√5th   **O09.7**   **Supervision of high risk pregnancy due to social problems**

       O09.70   **Supervision of high risk pregnancy due to social problems, unspecified trimester**   M ♀

       O09.71   **Supervision of high risk pregnancy due to social problems, first trimester**   M ♀

       O09.72   **Supervision of high risk pregnancy due to social problems, second trimester**   M ♀

       O09.73   **Supervision of high risk pregnancy due to social problems, third trimester**   M ♀

√5th   **O09.8**   **Supervision of other high risk pregnancies**

√6th   **O09.81**   **Supervision of pregnancy resulting from assisted reproductive technology**

       Supervision of pregnancy resulting from in-vitro fertilization

       EXCLUDES 2   *gestational carrier status (Z33.3)*

            O09.811   **Supervision of pregnancy resulting from assisted reproductive technology, first trimester**   M ♀

            O09.812   **Supervision of pregnancy resulting from assisted reproductive technology, second trimester**   M ♀

            O09.813   **Supervision of pregnancy resulting from assisted reproductive technology, third trimester**   M ♀

            O09.819   **Supervision of pregnancy resulting from assisted reproductive technology, unspecified trimester**   M ♀

√6th   **O09.82**   **Supervision of pregnancy with history of in utero procedure during previous pregnancy**

            O09.821   **Supervision of pregnancy with history of in utero procedure during previous pregnancy, first trimester**   M ♀

            O09.822   **Supervision of pregnancy with history of in utero procedure during previous pregnancy, second trimester**   M ♀

            O09.823   **Supervision of pregnancy with history of in utero procedure during previous pregnancy, third trimester**   M ♀

            O09.829   **Supervision of pregnancy with history of in utero procedure during previous pregnancy, unspecified trimester**   M ♀

                  EXCLUDES 1   *supervision of pregnancy affected by in utero procedure during current pregnancy (O35.7)*

√6th   **O09.89**   **Supervision of other high risk pregnancies**

            O09.891   **Supervision of other high risk pregnancies, first trimester**   M ♀

            O09.892   **Supervision of other high risk pregnancies, second trimester**   M ♀

            O09.893   **Supervision of other high risk pregnancies, third trimester**   M ♀

            O09.899   **Supervision of other high risk pregnancies, unspecified trimester**   M ♀

√5th   **O09.9**   **Supervision of high risk pregnancy, unspecified**

       O09.90   **Supervision of high risk pregnancy, unspecified, unspecified trimester**   M ♀

       O09.91   **Supervision of high risk pregnancy, unspecified, first trimester**   M ♀

       O09.92   **Supervision of high risk pregnancy, unspecified, second trimester**   M ♀

       O09.93   **Supervision of high risk pregnancy, unspecified, third trimester**   M ♀

Edema, proteinuria and hypertensive disorders in pregnancy, childbirth and the puerperium (O10-O16)

AHA: 2016,4Q,50

√4th   **O10**   **Pre-existing hypertension complicating pregnancy, childbirth and the puerperium**

     INCLUDES   pre-existing hypertension with pre-existing proteinuria complicating pregnancy, childbirth and the puerperium

     EXCLUDES 2   *pre-existing hypertension with superimposed pre-eclampsia complicating pregnancy, childbirth and the puerperium (O11.-)*

√5th   **O10.0**   **Pre-existing essential hypertension complicating pregnancy, childbirth and the puerperium**

       Any condition in I10 specified as a reason for obstetric care during pregnancy, childbirth or the puerperium

√6th   **O10.01**   **Pre-existing essential hypertension complicating pregnancy**

            O10.011   **Pre-existing essential hypertension complicating pregnancy, first trimester**   CC M ♀

            O10.012   **Pre-existing essential hypertension complicating pregnancy, second trimester**   CC M ♀

            O10.013   **Pre-existing essential hypertension complicating pregnancy, third trimester**   CC ♀

            O10.019   **Pre-existing essential hypertension complicating pregnancy, unspecified trimester**   M ♀

       O10.02   **Pre-existing essential hypertension complicating childbirth**   CC M ♀

       O10.03   **Pre-existing essential hypertension complicating the puerperium**   M ♀

√5th   **O10.1**   **Pre-existing hypertensive heart disease complicating pregnancy, childbirth and the puerperium**

       Any condition in I11 specified as a reason for obstetric care during pregnancy, childbirth or the puerperium

       Use additional code from I11 to identify the type of hypertensive heart disease

√6th   **O10.11**   **Pre-existing hypertensive heart disease complicating pregnancy**

            O10.111   **Pre-existing hypertensive heart disease complicating pregnancy, first trimester**   M ♀

            O10.112   **Pre-existing hypertensive heart disease complicating pregnancy, second trimester**   M ♀

            O10.113   **Pre-existing hypertensive heart disease complicating pregnancy, third trimester**   M ♀

            O10.119   **Pre-existing hypertensive heart disease complicating pregnancy, unspecified trimester**   M ♀

       O10.12   **Pre-existing hypertensive heart disease complicating childbirth**   M ♀

       O10.13   **Pre-existing hypertensive heart disease complicating the puerperium**   M ♀

√5th   **O10.2**   **Pre-existing hypertensive chronic kidney disease complicating pregnancy, childbirth and the puerperium**

       Any condition in I12 specified as a reason for obstetric care during pregnancy, childbirth or the puerperium

       Use additional code from I12 to identify the type of hypertensive chronic kidney disease

√6th   **O10.21**   **Pre-existing hypertensive chronic kidney disease complicating pregnancy**

            O10.211   **Pre-existing hypertensive chronic kidney disease complicating pregnancy, first trimester**   M ♀

            O10.212   **Pre-existing hypertensive chronic kidney disease complicating pregnancy, second trimester**   M ♀

            O10.213   **Pre-existing hypertensive chronic kidney disease complicating pregnancy, third trimester**   M ♀

            O10.219   **Pre-existing hypertensive chronic kidney disease complicating pregnancy, unspecified trimester**   M ♀

       O10.22   **Pre-existing hypertensive chronic kidney disease complicating childbirth**   M ♀

☑ Additional Character Required   √x7th Placeholder   Unacceptable PDx   Questionable PDx   Manifestation   Unspecified Dx   H1 -H14 HAC   HCC CMS-HCC Dx   HIV HIV Dx

ICD-10-CM 2021   **871**

Chapter 15. Pregnancy, Childbirth and the Puerperium

O10.23   **Pre-existing hypertensive chronic kidney disease complicating the** puerperium   M♀

✓5th O10.3   **Pre-existing hypertensive heart and chronic kidney disease complicating pregnancy, childbirth and the puerperium**
Any condition in I13 specified as a reason for obstetric care during pregnancy, childbirth or the puerperium
Use additional code from I13 to identify the type of hypertensive heart and chronic kidney disease

   ✓6th O10.31   **Pre-existing hypertensive heart and chronic kidney disease complicating** pregnancy

     O10.311   **Pre-existing hypertensive heart and chronic kidney disease complicating pregnancy, first trimester**   M♀

     O10.312   **Pre-existing hypertensive heart and chronic kidney disease complicating pregnancy, second trimester**   M♀

     O10.313   **Pre-existing hypertensive heart and chronic kidney disease complicating pregnancy, third trimester**   M♀

     O10.319   **Pre-existing hypertensive heart and chronic kidney disease complicating pregnancy, unspecified trimester**   M♀

   O10.32   **Pre-existing hypertensive heart and chronic kidney disease complicating** childbirth   M♀

   O10.33   **Pre-existing hypertensive heart and chronic kidney disease complicating the** puerperium   M♀

✓5th O10.4   **Pre-existing secondary hypertension complicating pregnancy, childbirth and the puerperium**
Any condition in I15 specified as a reason for obstetric care during pregnancy, childbirth or the puerperium
Use additional code from I15 to identify the type of secondary hypertension

   ✓6th O10.41   **Pre-existing secondary hypertension complicating** pregnancy

     O10.411   **Pre-existing secondary hypertension complicating pregnancy, first trimester**   CC M♀

     O10.412   **Pre-existing secondary hypertension complicating pregnancy, second trimester**   CC M♀

     O10.413   **Pre-existing secondary hypertension complicating pregnancy, third trimester**   CC M♀

     O10.419   **Pre-existing secondary hypertension complicating pregnancy, unspecified trimester**   M♀

   O10.42   **Pre-existing secondary hypertension complicating** childbirth   MCC M♀

   O10.43   **Pre-existing secondary hypertension complicating the** puerperium   CC M♀

✓5th O10.9   **Unspecified pre-existing hypertension complicating pregnancy, childbirth and the puerperium**

   ✓6th O10.91   **Unspecified pre-existing hypertension complicating** pregnancy

     O10.911   **Unspecified pre-existing hypertension complicating pregnancy, first trimester**   CC M♀

     O10.912   **Unspecified pre-existing hypertension complicating pregnancy, second trimester**   CC M♀

     O10.913   **Unspecified pre-existing hypertension complicating pregnancy, third trimester**   CC M♀

     O10.919   **Unspecified pre-existing hypertension complicating pregnancy, unspecified trimester**   M♀

   O10.92   **Unspecified pre-existing hypertension complicating** childbirth   CC M♀

   O10.93   **Unspecified pre-existing hypertension complicating the** puerperium   M♀

✓4th O11   **Pre-existing hypertension with pre-eclampsia**
INCLUDES   conditions in O10 complicated by pre-eclampsia
pre-eclampsia superimposed pre-existing in hypertension
Use additional code from O10 to identify the type of hypertension
DEF: Complication of pregnancy manifesting in the development of borderline hypertension, protein in the urine, and unresponsive swelling between the 20th week of pregnancy and the end of the first week following birth in mild to moderate cases. Severe preeclampsia presents with hypertension, associated with marked swelling, proteinuria, abdominal pain, and/or visual changes.

O11.1   **Pre-existing hypertension with pre-eclampsia, first trimester**   MCC M♀

O11.2   **Pre-existing hypertension with pre-eclampsia, second trimester**   MCC M♀

O11.3   **Pre-existing hypertension with pre-eclampsia, third trimester**   MCC M♀

O11.4   **Pre-existing hypertension with pre-eclampsia, complicating childbirth**   M♀

O11.5   **Pre-existing hypertension with pre-eclampsia, complicating the** puerperium   M♀

O11.9   **Pre-existing hypertension with pre-eclampsia, unspecified trimester**   M♀

✓4th O12   **Gestational [pregnancy-induced] edema and proteinuria** without hypertension

   ✓5th O12.0   **Gestational** edema

     O12.00   **Gestational edema, unspecified trimester**   M♀

     O12.01   **Gestational edema, first trimester**   M♀

     O12.02   **Gestational edema, second trimester**   M♀

     O12.03   **Gestational edema, third trimester**   M♀

     O12.04   **Gestational edema, complicating childbirth**   M♀

     O12.05   **Gestational edema, complicating the puerperium**   M♀

   ✓5th O12.1   **Gestational** proteinuria

     O12.10   **Gestational proteinuria, unspecified trimester**   M♀

     O12.11   **Gestational proteinuria, first trimester**   CC M♀

     O12.12   **Gestational proteinuria, second trimester**   CC M♀

     O12.13   **Gestational proteinuria, third trimester**   CC M♀

     O12.14   **Gestational proteinuria, complicating childbirth**   M♀

     O12.15   **Gestational proteinuria, complicating the puerperium**   M♀

   ✓5th O12.2   **Gestational** edema with proteinuria

     O12.20   **Gestational edema with proteinuria, unspecified trimester**   M♀

     O12.21   **Gestational edema with proteinuria, first trimester**   CC M♀

     O12.22   **Gestational edema with proteinuria, second trimester**   CC M♀

     O12.23   **Gestational edema with proteinuria, third trimester**   CC M♀

     O12.24   **Gestational edema with proteinuria, complicating childbirth**   M♀

     O12.25   **Gestational edema with proteinuria, complicating the** puerperium   M♀

✓4th O13   **Gestational [pregnancy-induced] hypertension without significant proteinuria**
INCLUDES   gestational hypertension NOS
transient hypertension of pregnancy
AHA: 2016,1Q,5

O13.1   **Gestational [pregnancy-induced] hypertension without significant proteinuria, first trimester**   M♀

O13.2   **Gestational [pregnancy-induced] hypertension without significant proteinuria, second trimester**   M♀

O13.3   **Gestational [pregnancy-induced] hypertension without significant proteinuria, third trimester**   M♀

O13.4   **Gestational [pregnancy-induced] hypertension without significant proteinuria, complicating childbirth**   M♀

O13.5   **Gestational [pregnancy-induced] hypertension without significant proteinuria, complicating the** puerperium   M♀

O13.9   **Gestational [pregnancy-induced] hypertension without significant proteinuria, unspecified trimester**   M♀

N Newborn: 0   P Pediatric: 0-17   M Maternity: 9-64   A Adult: 15-124   MCC Major Complication/Comorbidity   CC Complication/Comorbidity   SW Severe Wound Dx

872   ICD-10-CM 2021

☑4ᵗʰ O14 Pre-eclampsia

> **EXCLUDES 1**   *pre-existing hypertension with pre-eclampsia (O11)*
> **DEF:** Complication of pregnancy manifesting in the development of borderline hypertension, protein in the urine, and unresponsive swelling between the 20th week of pregnancy and the end of the first week following birth in mild to moderate cases. Severe preeclampsia presents with hypertension, associated with marked swelling, proteinuria, abdominal pain, and/or visual changes.

√5ᵗʰ O14.0   Mild to moderate pre-eclampsia

> **AHA:** 2019,3Q,12; 2019,2Q,8

     O14.00   Mild to moderate pre-eclampsia, unspecified trimester   M ♀

     O14.02   Mild to moderate pre-eclampsia, second trimester   CC M ♀

     O14.03   Mild to moderate pre-eclampsia, third trimester   CC M ♀

     O14.04   Mild to moderate pre-eclampsia, complicating childbirth   M ♀
> **AHA:** 2019,2Q,8

     O14.05   Mild to moderate pre-eclampsia, complicating the puerperium   M ♀

√5ᵗʰ O14.1   Severe pre-eclampsia

> **EXCLUDES 1**   *HELLP syndrome (O14.2-)*
> **AHA:** 2019,3Q,12

     O14.10   Severe pre-eclampsia, unspecified trimester   M ♀

     O14.12   Severe pre-eclampsia, second trimester   MCC M ♀

     O14.13   Severe pre-eclampsia, third trimester   MCC M ♀

     O14.14   Severe pre-eclampsia complicating childbirth   M ♀

     O14.15   Severe pre-eclampsia, complicating the puerperium   M ♀

√5ᵗʰ O14.2   HELLP syndrome

> Severe pre-eclampsia with hemolysis, elevated liver enzymes and low platelet count (HELLP)
> **AHA:** 2019,3Q,12

     O14.20   HELLP syndrome (HELLP), unspecified trimester   M ♀

     O14.22   HELLP syndrome (HELLP), second trimester   MCC M ♀

     O14.23   HELLP syndrome (HELLP), third trimester   MCC M ♀

     O14.24   HELLP syndrome, complicating childbirth   M ♀

     O14.25   HELLP syndrome, complicating the puerperium   M ♀

√5ᵗʰ O14.9   Unspecified pre-eclampsia

     O14.90   Unspecified pre-eclampsia, unspecified trimester   M ♀

     O14.92   Unspecified pre-eclampsia, second trimester   CC M ♀

     O14.93   Unspecified pre-eclampsia, third trimester   CC M ♀

     O14.94   Unspecified pre-eclampsia, complicating childbirth   M ♀

     O14.95   Unspecified pre-eclampsia, complicating the puerperium   M ♀

√4ᵗʰ O15   Eclampsia

> **INCLUDES**   convulsions following conditions in O10–O14 and O16
> **DEF:** Tetany and toxemia producing seizure activity or coma in a pregnant patient who most often has presented with prior preeclampsia (i.e., hypertension, albuminuria, and edema).

√5ᵗʰ O15.0   Eclampsia complicating pregnancy

     O15.00   Eclampsia complicating pregnancy, unspecified trimester   M ♀

     O15.02   Eclampsia complicating pregnancy, second trimester   MCC M ♀

     O15.03   Eclampsia complicating pregnancy, third trimester   MCC M ♀

     O15.1   Eclampsia complicating labor   MCC M ♀

     O15.2   Eclampsia complicating the puerperium   MCC M ♀

     O15.9   Eclampsia, unspecified as to time period   M ♀
> Eclampsia NOS

√4ᵗʰ O16   Unspecified maternal hypertension

     O16.1   Unspecified maternal hypertension, first trimester   CC M ♀

     O16.2   Unspecified maternal hypertension, second trimester   CC M ♀

     O16.3   Unspecified maternal hypertension, third trimester   CC M ♀

     O16.4   Unspecified maternal hypertension, complicating childbirth   M ♀

     O16.5   Unspecified maternal hypertension, complicating the puerperium   M ♀

     O16.9   Unspecified maternal hypertension, unspecified trimester   M ♀

Other maternal disorders predominantly related to pregnancy (O20-O29)

> **EXCLUDES 2**   *maternal care related to the fetus and amniotic cavity and possible delivery problems (O30–O48)*
> *maternal diseases classifiable elsewhere but complicating pregnancy, labor and delivery, and the puerperium (O98-O99)*

√4ᵗʰ O20   Hemorrhage in early pregnancy

> **INCLUDES**   hemorrhage before completion of 20 weeks gestation
> **EXCLUDES 1**   *pregnancy with abortive outcome (O00-O08)*

     O20.0   Threatened abortion   CC M ♀
> Hemorrhage specified as due to threatened abortion
> **DEF:** Bloody discharge during pregnancy. The cervix may be dilated and pregnancy threatened, but the pregnancy is not terminated.

     O20.8   Other hemorrhage in early pregnancy   M ♀

     O20.9   Hemorrhage in early pregnancy, unspecified   CC M ♀

√4ᵗʰ O21   Excessive vomiting in pregnancy

     O21.0   Mild hyperemesis gravidarum   M ♀
> Hyperemesis gravidarum, mild or unspecified, starting before the end of the 20th week of gestation

     O21.1   Hyperemesis gravidarum with metabolic disturbance   M ♀
> Hyperemesis gravidarum, starting before the end of the 20th week of gestation, with metabolic disturbance such as carbohydrate depletion
> Hyperemesis gravidarum, starting before the end of the 20th week of gestation, with metabolic disturbance such as dehydration
> Hyperemesis gravidarum, starting before the end of the 20th week of gestation, with metabolic disturbance such as electrolyte imbalance

     O21.2   Late vomiting of pregnancy   M ♀
> Excessive vomiting starting after 20 completed weeks of gestation

     O21.8   Other vomiting complicating pregnancy   M ♀
> Vomiting due to diseases classified elsewhere, complicating pregnancy
> Use additional code, to identify cause

     O21.9   Vomiting of pregnancy, unspecified   M ♀

√4ᵗʰ O22   Venous complications and hemorrhoids in pregnancy

> **EXCLUDES 1**   *venous complications of:*
>   *abortion NOS (O03.9)*
>   *ectopic or molar pregnancy (O08.7)*
>   *failed attempted abortion (O07.35)*
>   *induced abortion (O04.85)*
>   *spontaneous abortion (O03.89)*
> **EXCLUDES 2**   *obstetric pulmonary embolism (O88.-)*
>   *venous complications and hemorrhoids of childbirth and the puerperium (O87.-)*

√5ᵗʰ O22.0   Varicose veins of lower extremity in pregnancy

> Varicose veins NOS in pregnancy
> **DEF:** Distended, tortuous veins of the lower extremities associated with pregnancy.

     O22.00   Varicose veins of lower extremity in pregnancy, unspecified trimester   M ♀

     O22.01   Varicose veins of lower extremity in pregnancy, first trimester   M ♀

     O22.02   Varicose veins of lower extremity in pregnancy, second trimester   M ♀

     O22.03   Varicose veins of lower extremity in pregnancy, third trimester   M ♀

√5ᵗʰ O22.1   Genital varices in pregnancy

> Perineal varices in pregnancy
> Vaginal varices in pregnancy
> Vulval varices in pregnancy

     O22.10   Genital varices in pregnancy, unspecified trimester   M ♀

     O22.11   Genital varices in pregnancy, first trimester   M ♀

     O22.12   Genital varices in pregnancy, second trimester   M ♀

O22.13   **Genital varices in pregnancy, third trimester**   M ♀

✓5ᵗʰ   **O22.2   Superficial thrombophlebitis in pregnancy**

Phlebitis in pregnancy NOS
Thrombophlebitis of legs in pregnancy
Thrombosis in pregnancy NOS
Use additional code to identify the superficial thrombophlebitis (I80.0-)

O22.20   **Superficial thrombophlebitis in pregnancy, unspecified trimester**   cc M ♀

O22.21   **Superficial thrombophlebitis in pregnancy, first trimester**   cc M ♀

O22.22   **Superficial thrombophlebitis in pregnancy, second trimester**   cc M ♀

O22.23   **Superficial thrombophlebitis in pregnancy, third trimester**   cc M ♀

✓5ᵗʰ   **O22.3   Deep phlebothrombosis in pregnancy**

Deep vein thrombosis, antepartum
Use additional code to identify the deep vein thrombosis (I82.4-, I82.5-, I82.62-. I82.72-)
Use additional code, if applicable, for associated long-term (current) use of anticoagulants (Z79.01)

O22.30   **Deep phlebothrombosis in pregnancy, unspecified trimester**   cc M ♀

O22.31   **Deep phlebothrombosis in pregnancy, first trimester**   MCC M ♀

O22.32   **Deep phlebothrombosis in pregnancy, second trimester**   MCC M ♀

O22.33   **Deep phlebothrombosis in pregnancy, third trimester**   MCC M ♀

✓5ᵗʰ   **O22.4   Hemorrhoids in pregnancy**

O22.40   **Hemorrhoids in pregnancy, unspecified trimester**   cc M ♀

O22.41   **Hemorrhoids in pregnancy, first trimester**   cc M ♀

O22.42   **Hemorrhoids in pregnancy, second trimester**   cc M ♀

O22.43   **Hemorrhoids in pregnancy, third trimester**   cc M ♀

✓5ᵗʰ   **O22.5   Cerebral venous thrombosis in pregnancy**

Cerebrovenous sinus thrombosis in pregnancy

O22.50   **Cerebral venous thrombosis in pregnancy, unspecified trimester**   cc M ♀

O22.51   **Cerebral venous thrombosis in pregnancy, first trimester**   cc M ♀

O22.52   **Cerebral venous thrombosis in pregnancy, second trimester**   cc M ♀

O22.53   **Cerebral venous thrombosis in pregnancy, third trimester**   cc M ♀

✓5ᵗʰ   **O22.8   Other venous complications in pregnancy**

✓6ᵗʰ   **O22.8X   Other venous complications in pregnancy**

O22.8X1   **Other venous complications in pregnancy, first trimester**   cc M ♀

O22.8X2   **Other venous complications in pregnancy, second trimester**   cc M ♀

O22.8X3   **Other venous complications in pregnancy, third trimester**   cc M ♀

O22.8X9   **Other venous complications in pregnancy, unspecified trimester**   cc M ♀

✓5ᵗʰ   **O22.9   Venous complication in pregnancy, unspecified**

Gestational phlebitis NOS
Gestational phlebopathy NOS
Gestational thrombosis NOS

O22.90   **Venous complication in pregnancy, unspecified, unspecified trimester**   cc M ♀

O22.91   **Venous complication in pregnancy, unspecified, first trimester**   M ♀

O22.92   **Venous complication in pregnancy, unspecified, second trimester**   M ♀

O22.93   **Venous complication in pregnancy, unspecified, third trimester**   M ♀

✓4ᵗʰ   **O23   Infections of genitourinary tract in pregnancy**

Use additional code to identify organism (B95.-, B96.-)

EXCLUDES 2   gonococcal infections complicating pregnancy, childbirth and the puerperium (O98.2)
infections with a predominantly sexual mode of transmission NOS complicating pregnancy, childbirth and the puerperium (O98.3)
syphilis complicating pregnancy, childbirth and the puerperium (O98.1)
tuberculosis of genitourinary system complicating pregnancy, childbirth and the puerperium (O98.0)
venereal disease NOS complicating pregnancy, childbirth and the puerperium (O98.3)

AHA: 2018,2Q,20

✓5ᵗʰ   **O23.0   Infections of kidney in pregnancy**

Pyelonephritis in pregnancy

O23.00   **Infections of kidney in pregnancy, unspecified trimester**   M ♀

O23.01   **Infections of kidney in pregnancy, first trimester**   cc M ♀

O23.02   **Infections of kidney in pregnancy, second trimester**   cc M ♀

O23.03   **Infections of kidney in pregnancy, third trimester**   cc M ♀

✓5ᵗʰ   **O23.1   Infections of bladder in pregnancy**

O23.10   **Infections of bladder in pregnancy, unspecified trimester**   M ♀

O23.11   **Infections of bladder in pregnancy, first trimester**   cc M ♀

O23.12   **Infections of bladder in pregnancy, second trimester**   cc M ♀

O23.13   **Infections of bladder in pregnancy, third trimester**   cc M ♀

✓5ᵗʰ   **O23.2   Infections of urethra in pregnancy**

O23.20   **Infections of urethra in pregnancy, unspecified trimester**   M ♀

O23.21   **Infections of urethra in pregnancy, first trimester**   cc M ♀

O23.22   **Infections of urethra in pregnancy, second trimester**   cc M ♀

O23.23   **Infections of urethra in pregnancy, third trimester**   cc M ♀

✓5ᵗʰ   **O23.3   Infections of other parts of urinary tract in pregnancy**

O23.30   **Infections of other parts of urinary tract in pregnancy, unspecified trimester**   M ♀

O23.31   **Infections of other parts of urinary tract in pregnancy, first trimester**   cc M ♀

O23.32   **Infections of other parts of urinary tract in pregnancy, second trimester**   cc M ♀

O23.33   **Infections of other parts of urinary tract in pregnancy, third trimester**   cc M ♀

✓5ᵗʰ   **O23.4   Unspecified infection of urinary tract in pregnancy**

O23.40   **Unspecified infection of urinary tract in pregnancy, unspecified trimester**   M ♀

O23.41   **Unspecified infection of urinary tract in pregnancy, first trimester**   cc M ♀

O23.42   **Unspecified infection of urinary tract in pregnancy, second trimester**   cc M ♀

O23.43   **Unspecified infection of urinary tract in pregnancy, third trimester**   cc M ♀

✓5ᵗʰ   **O23.5   Infections of the genital tract in pregnancy**

✓6ᵗʰ   **O23.51   Infection of cervix in pregnancy**

O23.511   **Infections of cervix in pregnancy, first trimester**   cc M ♀

O23.512   **Infections of cervix in pregnancy, second trimester**   cc M ♀

O23.513   **Infections of cervix in pregnancy, third trimester**   cc M ♀

O23.519   **Infections of cervix in pregnancy, unspecified trimester**   M ♀

✓6ᵗʰ   **O23.52   Salpingo-oophoritis in pregnancy**

Oophoritis in pregnancy
Salpingitis in pregnancy

O23.521   **Salpingo-oophoritis in pregnancy, first trimester**   cc M ♀

O23.522   **Salpingo-oophoritis in pregnancy, second trimester**   cc M ♀

N Newborn: 0   P Pediatric: 0-17   M Maternity: 9-64   A Adult: 15-124   MCC Major Complication/Comorbidity   cc Complication/Comorbidity   SW Severe Wound Dx

874   ICD-10-CM 2021

O23.523 **Salpingo-oophoritis in pregnancy, third trimester** CC M ♀

O23.529 **Salpingo-oophoritis in pregnancy, unspecified trimester** M ♀

√6ᵗʰ O23.59 **Infection of other part of genital tract in pregnancy**

O23.591 **Infection of other part of genital tract in pregnancy, first trimester** CC M ♀

O23.592 **Infection of other part of genital tract in pregnancy, second trimester** CC M ♀

O23.593 **Infection of other part of genital tract in pregnancy, third trimester** CC M ♀

O23.599 **Infection of other part of genital tract in pregnancy, unspecified trimester** M ♀

√5ᵗʰ O23.9 **Unspecified genitourinary tract infection in pregnancy**

Genitourinary tract infection in pregnancy NOS

O23.90 **Unspecified genitourinary tract infection in pregnancy, unspecified trimester** M ♀

O23.91 **Unspecified genitourinary tract infection in pregnancy, first trimester** CC M ♀

O23.92 **Unspecified genitourinary tract infection in pregnancy, second trimester** CC M ♀

O23.93 **Unspecified genitourinary tract infection in pregnancy, third trimester** CC M ♀

√4ᵗʰ **O24** Diabetes mellitus **in pregnancy, childbirth and the puerperium**

√5ᵗʰ O24.0 **Pre-existing type 1 diabetes mellitus, in pregnancy, childbirth and the puerperium**

Juvenile onset diabetes mellitus, in pregnancy, childbirth and the puerperium

Ketosis-prone diabetes mellitus in pregnancy, childbirth and the puerperium

Use additional code from category E10 to further identify any manifestations

√6ᵗʰ O24.01 **Pre-existing type 1 diabetes mellitus, in pregnancy**

O24.011 **Pre-existing type 1 diabetes mellitus, in pregnancy, first trimester** CC M ♀

O24.012 **Pre-existing type 1 diabetes mellitus, in pregnancy, second trimester** CC M ♀

O24.013 **Pre-existing type 1 diabetes mellitus, in pregnancy, third trimester** CC M ♀

O24.019 **Pre-existing type 1 diabetes mellitus, in pregnancy, unspecified trimester** CC M ♀

O24.02 **Pre-existing type 1 diabetes mellitus, in childbirth** MCC M ♀

O24.03 **Pre-existing type 1 diabetes mellitus, in the puerperium** CC M ♀

√5ᵗʰ O24.1 **Pre-existing type 2 diabetes mellitus, in pregnancy, childbirth and the puerperium**

Insulin-resistant diabetes mellitus in pregnancy, childbirth and the puerperium

Use additional code (for):

from category E11 to further identify any manifestations

long-term (current) use of insulin (Z79.4)

√6ᵗʰ O24.11 **Pre-existing type 2 diabetes mellitus, in pregnancy**

O24.111 **Pre-existing type 2 diabetes mellitus, in pregnancy, first trimester** CC M ♀

O24.112 **Pre-existing type 2 diabetes mellitus, in pregnancy, second trimester** CC M ♀

O24.113 **Pre-existing type 2 diabetes mellitus, in pregnancy, third trimester** CC M ♀

O24.119 **Pre-existing type 2 diabetes mellitus, in pregnancy, unspecified trimester** CC M ♀

O24.12 **Pre-existing type 2 diabetes mellitus, in childbirth** MCC M ♀

O24.13 **Pre-existing type 2 diabetes mellitus, in the puerperium** CC M ♀

√5ᵗʰ O24.3 **Unspecified pre-existing diabetes mellitus in pregnancy, childbirth and the puerperium**

Use additional code (for):

from category E11 to further identify any manifestation

long-term (current) use of insulin (Z79.4)

√6ᵗʰ O24.31 **Unspecified pre-existing diabetes mellitus in pregnancy**

O24.311 **Unspecified pre-existing diabetes mellitus in pregnancy, first trimester** CC M ♀

O24.312 **Unspecified pre-existing diabetes mellitus in pregnancy, second trimester** CC M ♀

O24.313 **Unspecified pre-existing diabetes mellitus in pregnancy, third trimester** CC M ♀

O24.319 **Unspecified pre-existing diabetes mellitus in pregnancy, unspecified trimester** CC M ♀

O24.32 **Unspecified pre-existing diabetes mellitus in childbirth** MCC M ♀

O24.33 **Unspecified pre-existing diabetes mellitus in the puerperium** CC M ♀

√5ᵗʰ O24.4 **Gestational diabetes mellitus**

Diabetes mellitus arising in pregnancy

Gestational diabetes mellitus NOS

AHA: 2016,4Q,50; 2015,4Q,34

√6ᵗʰ O24.41 **Gestational diabetes mellitus in pregnancy**

O24.410 **Gestational diabetes mellitus in pregnancy, diet controlled** M ♀

O24.414 **Gestational diabetes mellitus in pregnancy, insulin controlled** M ♀

O24.415 **Gestational diabetes mellitus in pregnancy, controlled by oral hypoglycemic drugs** M ♀

Gestational diabetes mellitus in pregnancy, controlled by oral antidiabetic drugs

O24.419 **Gestational diabetes mellitus in pregnancy, unspecified control** M ♀

√6ᵗʰ O24.42 **Gestational diabetes mellitus in childbirth**

AHA: 2016,1Q,5

O24.420 **Gestational diabetes mellitus in childbirth, diet controlled** M ♀

O24.424 **Gestational diabetes mellitus in childbirth, insulin controlled** M ♀

O24.425 **Gestational diabetes mellitus in childbirth, controlled by oral hypoglycemic drugs** M ♀

Gestational diabetes mellitus in childbirth, controlled by oral antidiabetic drugs

O24.429 **Gestational diabetes mellitus in childbirth, unspecified control** M ♀

√6ᵗʰ O24.43 **Gestational diabetes mellitus in the puerperium**

O24.430 **Gestational diabetes mellitus in the puerperium, diet controlled** M ♀

O24.434 **Gestational diabetes mellitus in the puerperium, insulin controlled** M ♀

O24.435 **Gestational diabetes mellitus in puerperium, controlled by oral hypoglycemic drugs** M ♀

Gestational diabetes mellitus in puerperium, controlled by oral antidiabetic drugs

O24.439 **Gestational diabetes mellitus in the puerperium, unspecified control** M ♀

√5ᵗʰ O24.8 **Other pre-existing diabetes mellitus in pregnancy, childbirth, and the puerperium**

Use additional code (for):

from categories E08, E09 and E13 to further identify any manifestation

long-term (current) use of insulin (Z79.4)

√6ᵗʰ O24.81 **Other pre-existing diabetes mellitus in pregnancy**

O24.811 **Other pre-existing diabetes mellitus in pregnancy, first trimester** CC M ♀

O24.812 **Other pre-existing diabetes mellitus in pregnancy, second trimester** CC M ♀

O24.813 **Other pre-existing diabetes mellitus in pregnancy, third trimester** CC M ♀

O24.819 **Other pre-existing diabetes mellitus in pregnancy, unspecified trimester** CC M ♀

O24.82 **Other pre-existing diabetes mellitus in childbirth** MCC M ♀

O24.83 **Other pre-existing diabetes mellitus in the puerperium** CC M ♀

☑ Additional Character Required   √x7ᵗʰ Placeholder   Unacceptable PDx   Questionable PDx   Manifestation   Unspecified Dx   H1-H14 HAC   HCC CMS-HCC Dx   HIV HIV Dx

ICD-10-CM 2021   **875**

√5ᵗʰ **O24.9 Unspecified diabetes mellitus in pregnancy, childbirth and the puerperium**
Use additional code for long-term (current) use of insulin (Z79.4)

    √6ᵗʰ **O24.91 Unspecified diabetes mellitus in** pregnancy

        O24.911 Unspecified diabetes mellitus in pregnancy, first trimester   CC M ♀

        O24.912 Unspecified diabetes mellitus in pregnancy, second trimester   CC M ♀

        O24.913 Unspecified diabetes mellitus in pregnancy, third trimester   CC M ♀

        O24.919 Unspecified diabetes mellitus in pregnancy, unspecified trimester   CC M ♀

    O24.92 Unspecified diabetes mellitus in childbirth   M ♀

    O24.93 Unspecified diabetes mellitus in the puerperium   CC M ♀

√4ᵗʰ **O25 Malnutrition in pregnancy, childbirth and the puerperium**

    √5ᵗʰ **O25.1 Malnutrition in** pregnancy

        O25.10 Malnutrition in pregnancy, unspecified trimester   M ♀

        O25.11 Malnutrition in pregnancy, first trimester   M ♀

        O25.12 Malnutrition in pregnancy, second trimester   M ♀

        O25.13 Malnutrition in pregnancy, third trimester   M ♀

    O25.2 Malnutrition in childbirth   M ♀

    O25.3 Malnutrition in the puerperium   M ♀

√4ᵗʰ **O26 Maternal care for other conditions predominantly related to pregnancy**

    √5ᵗʰ **O26.0 Excessive weight gain in pregnancy**

        EXCLUDES 2   gestational edema (O12.0, O12.2)

        O26.00 Excessive weight gain in pregnancy, unspecified trimester   M ♀

        O26.01 Excessive weight gain in pregnancy, first trimester   M ♀

        O26.02 Excessive weight gain in pregnancy, second trimester   M ♀

        O26.03 Excessive weight gain in pregnancy, third trimester   M ♀

    √5ᵗʰ **O26.1 Low weight gain in pregnancy**

        O26.10 Low weight gain in pregnancy, unspecified trimester   M ♀

        O26.11 Low weight gain in pregnancy, first trimester   M ♀

        O26.12 Low weight gain in pregnancy, second trimester   M ♀

        O26.13 Low weight gain in pregnancy, third trimester   M ♀

    √5ᵗʰ **O26.2 Pregnancy care for patient with recurrent pregnancy loss**

        O26.20 Pregnancy care for patient with recurrent pregnancy loss, unspecified trimester   ♀

        O26.21 Pregnancy care for patient with recurrent pregnancy loss, first trimester   M ♀

        O26.22 Pregnancy care for patient with recurrent pregnancy loss, second trimester   M ♀

        O26.23 Pregnancy care for patient with recurrent pregnancy loss, third trimester   M ♀

    √5ᵗʰ **O26.3 Retained intrauterine contraceptive device in pregnancy**

        O26.30 Retained intrauterine contraceptive device in pregnancy, unspecified trimester   M ♀

        O26.31 Retained intrauterine contraceptive device in pregnancy, first trimester   M ♀

        O26.32 Retained intrauterine contraceptive device in pregnancy, second trimester   M ♀

        O26.33 Retained intrauterine contraceptive device in pregnancy, third trimester   M ♀

    √5ᵗʰ **O26.4 Herpes gestationis**

        DEF: Rare skin disorder of unknown origin that appears on the abdomen in the second and third trimester as intensely itchy blisters that spread to other sites.

        O26.40 Herpes gestationis, unspecified trimester   M ♀

        O26.41 Herpes gestationis, first trimester   M ♀

        O26.42 Herpes gestationis, second trimester   M ♀

        O26.43 Herpes gestationis, third trimester   M ♀

    √5ᵗʰ **O26.5 Maternal hypotension syndrome**

        Supine hypotensive syndrome

        O26.50 Maternal hypotension syndrome, unspecified trimester   M ♀

        O26.51 Maternal hypotension syndrome, first trimester   M ♀

        O26.52 Maternal hypotension syndrome, second trimester   M ♀

        O26.53 Maternal hypotension syndrome, third trimester   M ♀

√5ᵗʰ **O26.6 Liver and biliary tract disorders in pregnancy, childbirth and the puerperium**
Use additional code to identify the specific disorder

    EXCLUDES 2   hepatorenal syndrome following labor and delivery (O90.4)

    √6ᵗʰ **O26.61 Liver and biliary tract disorders in** pregnancy

        O26.611 Liver and biliary tract disorders in pregnancy, first trimester   CC M ♀

        O26.612 Liver and biliary tract disorders in pregnancy, second trimester   CC M ♀

        O26.613 Liver and biliary tract disorders in pregnancy, third trimester   CC M ♀

        O26.619 Liver and biliary tract disorders in pregnancy, unspecified trimester   M ♀

    O26.62 Liver and biliary tract disorders in childbirth   CC M ♀

    O26.63 Liver and biliary tract disorders in the puerperium   M ♀

√5ᵗʰ **O26.7 Subluxation of symphysis (pubis) in pregnancy, childbirth and the puerperium**

    EXCLUDES 1   traumatic separation of symphysis (pubis) during childbirth (O71.6)

    √6ᵗʰ **O26.71 Subluxation of symphysis (pubis) in** pregnancy

        O26.711 Subluxation of symphysis (pubis) in pregnancy, first trimester   M ♀

        O26.712 Subluxation of symphysis (pubis) in pregnancy, second trimester   M ♀

        O26.713 Subluxation of symphysis (pubis) in pregnancy, third trimester   M ♀

        O26.719 Subluxation of symphysis (pubis) in pregnancy, unspecified trimester   M ♀

    O26.72 Subluxation of symphysis (pubis) in childbirth   M ♀

    O26.73 Subluxation of symphysis (pubis) in the puerperium   M ♀

√5ᵗʰ **O26.8 Other specified pregnancy related conditions**

    √6ᵗʰ **O26.81 Pregnancy related exhaustion and fatigue**

        O26.811 Pregnancy related exhaustion and fatigue, first trimester   M ♀

        O26.812 Pregnancy related exhaustion and fatigue, second trimester   M ♀

        O26.813 Pregnancy related exhaustion and fatigue, third trimester   M ♀

        O26.819 Pregnancy related exhaustion and fatigue, unspecified trimester   M ♀

    √6ᵗʰ **O26.82 Pregnancy related peripheral neuritis**

        O26.821 Pregnancy related peripheral neuritis, first trimester   M ♀

        O26.822 Pregnancy related peripheral neuritis, second trimester   M ♀

        O26.823 Pregnancy related peripheral neuritis, third trimester   M ♀

        O26.829 Pregnancy related peripheral neuritis, unspecified trimester   M ♀

    √6ᵗʰ **O26.83 Pregnancy related renal disease**
Use additional code to identify the specific disorder

        O26.831 Pregnancy related renal disease, first trimester   CC M ♀

        O26.832 Pregnancy related renal disease, second trimester   CC M ♀

        O26.833 Pregnancy related renal disease, third trimester   CC M ♀

        O26.839 Pregnancy related renal disease, unspecified trimester   M ♀

    √6ᵗʰ **O26.84 Uterine size-date discrepancy complicating pregnancy**

        EXCLUDES 1   encounter for suspected problem with fetal growth ruled out (Z03.74)

        O26.841 Uterine size-date discrepancy, first trimester   M ♀

        O26.842 Uterine size-date discrepancy, second trimester   M ♀

N Newborn: 0   P Pediatric: 0-17   M Maternity: 9-64   A Adult: 15-124   MCC Major Complication/Comorbidity   CC Complication/Comorbidity   SW Severe Wound Dx

876   ICD-10-CM 2021

O26.843 Uterine size-date discrepancy, third trimester ⓜ♀

O26.849 Uterine size-date discrepancy, unspecified trimester ⓜ♀

✓6ᵗʰ **O26.85** Spotting complicating pregnancy

O26.851 Spotting complicating pregnancy, first trimester ⓜ♀

O26.852 Spotting complicating pregnancy, second trimester ⓜ♀

O26.853 Spotting complicating pregnancy, third trimester ⓜ♀

O26.859 Spotting complicating pregnancy, unspecified trimester ⓜ♀

O26.86 Pruritic urticarial papules and plaques of pregnancy (PUPPP) ⓜ♀

Polymorphic eruption of pregnancy

✓6ᵗʰ **O26.87** Cervical shortening

EXCLUDES 1 encounter for suspected cervical shortening ruled out (Z03.75)

DEF: Cervix that has shortened to less than 25 mm before the 24th week of pregnancy. A shortened cervix is a warning sign for impending premature delivery and is treated by cervical cerclage placement or progesterone.

O26.872 Cervical shortening, second trimester CC ⓜ♀

O26.873 Cervical shortening, third trimester CC ⓜ♀

O26.879 Cervical shortening, unspecified trimester CC ⓜ♀

✓6ᵗʰ **O26.89** Other specified pregnancy related conditions

AHA: 2015,3Q,40

O26.891 Other specified pregnancy related conditions, first trimester ⓜ♀

O26.892 Other specified pregnancy related conditions, second trimester ⓜ♀

O26.893 Other specified pregnancy related conditions, third trimester ⓜ♀

O26.899 Other specified pregnancy related conditions, unspecified trimester ⓜ♀

✓5ᵗʰ **O26.9** Pregnancy related conditions, unspecified

O26.90 Pregnancy related conditions, unspecified, unspecified trimester ⓜ♀

O26.91 Pregnancy related conditions, unspecified, first trimester ⓜ♀

O26.92 Pregnancy related conditions, unspecified, second trimester ⓜ♀

O26.93 Pregnancy related conditions, unspecified, third trimester ⓜ♀

✓4ᵗʰ **O28 Abnormal findings on antenatal screening of mother**

EXCLUDES 1 diagnostic findings classified elsewhere — see Alphabetical Index

O28.0 Abnormal hematological finding on antenatal screening of mother ⓜ♀

O28.1 Abnormal biochemical finding on antenatal screening of mother ⓜ♀

O28.2 Abnormal cytological finding on antenatal screening of mother ⓜ♀

O28.3 Abnormal ultrasonic finding on antenatal screening of mother ⓜ♀

O28.4 Abnormal radiological finding on antenatal screening of mother ⓜ♀

O28.5 Abnormal chromosomal and genetic finding on antenatal screening of mother ⓜ♀

O28.8 Other abnormal findings on antenatal screening of mother ⓜ♀

O28.9 Unspecified abnormal findings on antenatal screening of mother ⓜ♀

✓4ᵗʰ **O29 Complications of anesthesia during pregnancy**

INCLUDES maternal complications arising from the administration of a general, regional or local anesthetic, analgesic or other sedation during pregnancy

Use additional code, if necessary, to identify the complication

EXCLUDES 2 complications of anesthesia during labor and delivery (O74.-)
complications of anesthesia during the puerperium (O89.-)

✓5ᵗʰ **O29.0** Pulmonary complications of anesthesia during pregnancy

✓6ᵗʰ **O29.01** Aspiration pneumonitis due to anesthesia during pregnancy

Inhalation of stomach contents or secretions NOS due to anesthesia during pregnancy
Mendelson's syndrome due to anesthesia during pregnancy

O29.011 Aspiration pneumonitis due to anesthesia during pregnancy, first trimester ⓜ♀

O29.012 Aspiration pneumonitis due to anesthesia during pregnancy, second trimester ⓜ♀

O29.013 Aspiration pneumonitis due to anesthesia during pregnancy, third trimester ⓜ♀

O29.019 Aspiration pneumonitis due to anesthesia during pregnancy, unspecified trimester ⓜ♀

✓6ᵗʰ **O29.02** Pressure collapse of lung due to anesthesia during pregnancy

O29.021 Pressure collapse of lung due to anesthesia during pregnancy, first trimester ⓜ♀

O29.022 Pressure collapse of lung due to anesthesia during pregnancy, second trimester ⓜ♀

O29.023 Pressure collapse of lung due to anesthesia during pregnancy, third trimester ⓜ♀

O29.029 Pressure collapse of lung due to anesthesia during pregnancy, unspecified trimester ⓜ♀

✓6ᵗʰ **O29.09** Other pulmonary complications of anesthesia during pregnancy

O29.091 Other pulmonary complications of anesthesia during pregnancy, first trimester ⓜ♀

O29.092 Other pulmonary complications of anesthesia during pregnancy, second trimester ⓜ♀

O29.093 Other pulmonary complications of anesthesia during pregnancy, third trimester ⓜ♀

O29.099 Other pulmonary complications of anesthesia during pregnancy, unspecified trimester ⓜ♀

✓5ᵗʰ **O29.1** Cardiac complications of anesthesia during pregnancy

✓6ᵗʰ **O29.11** Cardiac arrest due to anesthesia during pregnancy

O29.111 Cardiac arrest due to anesthesia during pregnancy, first trimester ⓜ♀

O29.112 Cardiac arrest due to anesthesia during pregnancy, second trimester ⓜ♀

O29.113 Cardiac arrest due to anesthesia during pregnancy, third trimester ⓜ♀

O29.119 Cardiac arrest due to anesthesia during pregnancy, unspecified trimester ⓜ♀

✓6ᵗʰ **O29.12** Cardiac failure due to anesthesia during pregnancy

O29.121 Cardiac failure due to anesthesia during pregnancy, first trimester ⓜ♀

O29.122 Cardiac failure due to anesthesia during pregnancy, second trimester ⓜ♀

O29.123 Cardiac failure due to anesthesia during pregnancy, third trimester ⓜ♀

O29.129 Cardiac failure due to anesthesia during pregnancy, unspecified trimester ⓜ♀

✓6ᵗʰ **O29.19** Other cardiac complications of anesthesia during pregnancy

O29.191 Other cardiac complications of anesthesia during pregnancy, first trimester ⓜ♀

O29.192 Other cardiac complications of anesthesia during pregnancy, second trimester ⓜ♀

O29.193 Other cardiac complications of anesthesia during pregnancy, third trimester ⓜ♀

☑ Additional Character Required · ✓x7ᵗʰ Placeholder · Unacceptable PDx · Questionable PDx · Manifestation · Unspecified Dx · H1-H14 HAC · HCC CMS-HCC Dx · HIV HIV Dx

ICD-10-CM 2021 · 877

O29.199 Other cardiac complications of anesthesia during pregnancy, unspecified trimester   M ♀

√5ᵗʰ **O29.2** **Central nervous system** complications of anesthesia during pregnancy

   √6ᵗʰ **O29.21** **Cerebral anoxia** due to anesthesia during pregnancy

     O29.211 Cerebral anoxia due to anesthesia during pregnancy, **first trimester**   M ♀

     O29.212 Cerebral anoxia due to anesthesia during pregnancy, **second trimester**   M ♀

     O29.213 Cerebral anoxia due to anesthesia during pregnancy, **third trimester**   M ♀

     O29.219 Cerebral anoxia due to anesthesia during pregnancy, **unspecified trimester**   M ♀

   √6ᵗʰ **O29.29** Other central nervous system complications of anesthesia during pregnancy

     O29.291 Other central nervous system complications of anesthesia during pregnancy, **first trimester**   M ♀

     O29.292 Other central nervous system complications of anesthesia during pregnancy, **second trimester**   M ♀

     O29.293 Other central nervous system complications of anesthesia during pregnancy, **third trimester**   M ♀

     O29.299 Other central nervous system complications of anesthesia during pregnancy, **unspecified trimester**   M ♀

√5ᵗʰ **O29.3** **Toxic reaction** to local anesthesia during pregnancy

   √6ᵗʰ **O29.3X** Toxic reaction to local anesthesia during pregnancy

     O29.3X1 Toxic reaction to local anesthesia during pregnancy, **first trimester**   M ♀

     O29.3X2 Toxic reaction to local anesthesia during pregnancy, **second trimester**   M ♀

     O29.3X3 Toxic reaction to local anesthesia during pregnancy, **third trimester**   M ♀

     O29.3X9 Toxic reaction to local anesthesia during pregnancy, **unspecified trimester**   M ♀

√5ᵗʰ **O29.4** **Spinal and epidural anesthesia induced headache** during pregnancy

     O29.40 Spinal and epidural anesthesia induced headache during pregnancy, **unspecified trimester**   M ♀

     O29.41 Spinal and epidural anesthesia induced headache during pregnancy, **first trimester**   M ♀

     O29.42 Spinal and epidural anesthesia induced headache during pregnancy, **second trimester**   M ♀

     O29.43 Spinal and epidural anesthesia induced headache during pregnancy, **third trimester**   M ♀

√5ᵗʰ **O29.5** **Other complications of** spinal and epidural anesthesia during pregnancy

   √6ᵗʰ **O29.5X** Other complications of spinal and epidural anesthesia during pregnancy

     O29.5X1 Other complications of spinal and epidural anesthesia during pregnancy, **first trimester**   M ♀

     O29.5X2 Other complications of spinal and epidural anesthesia during pregnancy, **second trimester**   M ♀

     O29.5X3 Other complications of spinal and epidural anesthesia during pregnancy, **third trimester**   M ♀

     O29.5X9 Other complications of spinal and epidural anesthesia during pregnancy, **unspecified trimester**   M ♀

   √6ᵗʰ **O29.6** **Failed or difficult intubation** for anesthesia during pregnancy

     O29.60 Failed or difficult intubation for anesthesia during pregnancy, **unspecified trimester**   M ♀

     O29.61 Failed or difficult intubation for anesthesia during pregnancy, **first trimester**   M ♀

     O29.62 Failed or difficult intubation for anesthesia during pregnancy, **second trimester**   M ♀

     O29.63 Failed or difficult intubation for anesthesia during pregnancy, **third trimester**   M ♀

√5ᵗʰ **O29.8** **Other complications** of anesthesia during pregnancy

   √6ᵗʰ **O29.8X** Other complications of anesthesia during pregnancy

     O29.8X1 Other complications of anesthesia during pregnancy, **first trimester**   M ♀

     O29.8X2 Other complications of anesthesia during pregnancy, **second trimester**   M ♀

O29.8X3 Other complications of anesthesia during pregnancy, **third trimester**   M ♀

O29.8X9 Other complications of anesthesia during pregnancy, **unspecified trimester**   M ♀

√5ᵗʰ **O29.9** **Unspecified complication** of anesthesia during pregnancy

   O29.90 Unspecified complication of anesthesia during pregnancy, **unspecified trimester**   M ♀

   O29.91 Unspecified complication of anesthesia during pregnancy, **first trimester**   M ♀

   O29.92 Unspecified complication of anesthesia during pregnancy, **second trimester**   M ♀

   O29.93 Unspecified complication of anesthesia during pregnancy, **third trimester**   M ♀

Maternal care related to the fetus and amniotic cavity and possible delivery problems (O30-O48)

√4ᵗʰ **O30** **Multiple gestation**

Code also any complications specific to multiple gestation
AHA: 2016,4Q,51

√5ᵗʰ **O30.0** **Twin** pregnancy

   √6ᵗʰ **O30.00** Twin pregnancy, unspecified number of placenta and unspecified number of amniotic sacs

     O30.001 Twin pregnancy, unspecified number of placenta and unspecified number of amniotic sacs, **first trimester**   M ♀

     O30.002 Twin pregnancy, unspecified number of placenta and unspecified number of amniotic sacs, **second trimester**   M ♀

     O30.003 Twin pregnancy, unspecified number of placenta and unspecified number of amniotic sacs, **third trimester**   M ♀

     O30.009 Twin pregnancy, unspecified number of placenta and unspecified number of amniotic sacs, **unspecified trimester**   M ♀

   √6ᵗʰ **O30.01** Twin pregnancy, **monochorionic/monoamniotic**

Twin pregnancy, one placenta, one amniotic sac
EXCLUDES 1   conjoined twins (O30.02-)

Twin Gestation – Monochorionic/Monoamniotic

- 1 Chorionic sac
- 1 Amniotic sac
- 2 Fetuses
- 2 Umbilical cords
- 1 Placenta

     O30.011 Twin pregnancy, monochorionic/monoamniotic, **first trimester**   M ♀

     O30.012 Twin pregnancy, monochorionic/monoamniotic, **second trimester**   M ♀

     O30.013 Twin pregnancy, monochorionic/monoamniotic, **third trimester**   M ♀

     O30.019 Twin pregnancy, monochorionic/monoamniotic, **unspecified trimester**   M ♀

   √6ᵗʰ **O30.02** **Conjoined** twin pregnancy

     O30.021 Conjoined twin pregnancy, **first trimester**   M ♀

     O30.022 Conjoined twin pregnancy, **second trimester**   M ♀

     O30.023 Conjoined twin pregnancy, **third trimester**   M ♀

     O30.029 Conjoined twin pregnancy, **unspecified trimester**   M ♀

N Newborn: 0   P Pediatric: 0-17   M Maternity: 9-64   A Adult: 15-124   MCC Major Complication/Comorbidity   CC Complication/Comorbidity   SW Severe Wound Dx

878   ICD-10-CM 2021

√6ᵗʰ **O30.03**   **Twin pregnancy, monochorionic/diamniotic**
Twin pregnancy, one placenta, two amniotic sacs

Twin Gestation – Monochorionic/Diamniotic

- 1 Chorionic sac
- 2 Amniotic sacs
- 2 Fetuses
- 2 Umbilical cords
- 1 Placenta

O30.031   **Twin pregnancy, monochorionic/diamniotic, first trimester**   M ♀

O30.032   **Twin pregnancy, monochorionic/diamniotic, second trimester**   M ♀

O30.033   **Twin pregnancy, monochorionic/diamniotic, third trimester**   M ♀

O30.039   **Twin pregnancy, monochorionic/diamniotic, unspecified trimester**   M ♀

√6ᵗʰ **O30.04**   **Twin pregnancy, dichorionic/diamniotic**
Twin pregnancy, two placentae, two amniotic sacs

Twin Gestation – Dichorionic/Diamniotic

- 2 Chorionic sacs
- 2 Amniotic sacs
- 2 Fetuses
- 2 Umbilical cords
- 2 Placentas

O30.041   **Twin pregnancy, dichorionic/diamniotic, first trimester**   M ♀

O30.042   **Twin pregnancy, dichorionic/diamniotic, second trimester**   M ♀

O30.043   **Twin pregnancy, dichorionic/diamniotic, third trimester**   M ♀

O30.049   **Twin pregnancy, dichorionic/diamniotic, unspecified trimester**   M ♀

√6ᵗʰ **O30.09**   **Twin pregnancy, unable to determine number of placenta and number of amniotic sacs**

O30.091   **Twin pregnancy, unable to determine number of placenta and number of amniotic sacs, first trimester**   M ♀

O30.092   **Twin pregnancy, unable to determine number of placenta and number of amniotic sacs, second trimester**   M ♀

O30.093   **Twin pregnancy, unable to determine number of placenta and number of amniotic sacs, third trimester**   M ♀

O30.099   **Twin pregnancy, unable to determine number of placenta and number of amniotic sacs, unspecified trimester**   M ♀

√5ᵗʰ **O30.1**   **Triplet pregnancy**

√6ᵗʰ **O30.10**   **Triplet pregnancy, unspecified number of placenta and unspecified number of amniotic sacs**
AHA: 2016,2Q,8

O30.101   **Triplet pregnancy, unspecified number of placenta and unspecified number of amniotic sacs, first trimester**   CC M ♀

O30.102   **Triplet pregnancy, unspecified number of placenta and unspecified number of amniotic sacs, second trimester**   CC M ♀

O30.103   **Triplet pregnancy, unspecified number of placenta and unspecified number of amniotic sacs, third trimester**   CC M ♀

O30.109   **Triplet pregnancy, unspecified number of placenta and unspecified number of amniotic sacs, unspecified trimester**   M ♀

√6ᵗʰ **O30.11**   **Triplet pregnancy with two or more monochorionic fetuses**

O30.111   **Triplet pregnancy with two or more monochorionic fetuses, first trimester**   CC M ♀

O30.112   **Triplet pregnancy with two or more monochorionic fetuses, second trimester**   CC M ♀

O30.113   **Triplet pregnancy with two or more monochorionic fetuses, third trimester**   CC M ♀

O30.119   **Triplet pregnancy with two or more monochorionic fetuses, unspecified trimester**   M ♀

√6ᵗʰ **O30.12**   **Triplet pregnancy with two or more monoamniotic fetuses**

O30.121   **Triplet pregnancy with two or more monoamniotic fetuses, first trimester**   CC M ♀

O30.122   **Triplet pregnancy with two or more monoamniotic fetuses, second trimester**   CC M ♀

O30.123   **Triplet pregnancy with two or more monoamniotic fetuses, third trimester**   CC M ♀

O30.129   **Triplet pregnancy with two or more monoamniotic fetuses, unspecified trimester**   M ♀

√6ᵗʰ **O30.13**   **Triplet pregnancy, trichorionic/triamniotic**
AHA: 2018,4Q,22

O30.131   **Triplet pregnancy, trichorionic/triamniotic, first trimester**   CC M ♀

O30.132   **Triplet pregnancy, trichorionic/triamniotic, second trimester**   CC M ♀

O30.133   **Triplet pregnancy, trichorionic/triamniotic, third trimester**   CC M ♀

O30.139   **Triplet pregnancy, trichorionic/triamniotic, unspecified trimester**   M ♀

√6ᵗʰ **O30.19**   **Triplet pregnancy, unable to determine number of placenta and number of amniotic sacs**

O30.191   **Triplet pregnancy, unable to determine number of placenta and number of amniotic sacs, first trimester**   CC M ♀

O30.192   **Triplet pregnancy, unable to determine number of placenta and number of amniotic sacs, second trimester**   CC M ♀

O30.193   **Triplet pregnancy, unable to determine number of placenta and number of amniotic sacs, third trimester**   CC M ♀

O30.199   **Triplet pregnancy, unable to determine number of placenta and number of amniotic sacs, unspecified trimester**   M ♀

√5ᵗʰ **O30.2**   **Quadruplet pregnancy**

√6ᵗʰ **O30.20**   **Quadruplet pregnancy, unspecified number of placenta and unspecified number of amniotic sacs**

O30.201   **Quadruplet pregnancy, unspecified number of placenta and unspecified number of amniotic sacs, first trimester**   CC M ♀

O30.202   Quadruplet pregnancy, unspecified number of placenta and unspecified number of amniotic sacs, second trimester   cc M ♀

O30.203   Quadruplet pregnancy, unspecified number of placenta and unspecified number of amniotic sacs, third trimester   cc M ♀

O30.209   Quadruplet pregnancy, unspecified number of placenta and unspecified number of amniotic sacs, unspecified trimester   M ♀

√6ᵗʰ   **O30.21**   **Quadruplet pregnancy with** two or more monochorionic fetuses

O30.211   Quadruplet pregnancy with two or more monochorionic fetuses, first trimester   cc M ♀

O30.212   Quadruplet pregnancy with two or more monochorionic fetuses, second trimester   cc M ♀

O30.213   Quadruplet pregnancy with two or more monochorionic fetuses, third trimester   cc M ♀

O30.219   Quadruplet pregnancy with two or more monochorionic fetuses, unspecified trimester   M ♀

√6ᵗʰ   **O30.22**   **Quadruplet pregnancy with** two or more monoamniotic fetuses

O30.221   Quadruplet pregnancy with two or more monoamniotic fetuses, first trimester   cc M ♀

O30.222   Quadruplet pregnancy with two or more monoamniotic fetuses, second trimester   cc M ♀

O30.223   Quadruplet pregnancy with two or more monoamniotic fetuses, third trimester   cc M ♀

O30.229   Quadruplet pregnancy with two or more monoamniotic fetuses, unspecified trimester   M ♀

√6ᵗʰ   **O30.23**   **Quadruplet pregnancy, quadrachorionic/quadra-amniotic**
    AHA: 2018,4Q,22

O30.231   Quadruplet pregnancy, quadrachorionic/quadra-amniotic, first trimester   cc M ♀

O30.232   Quadruplet pregnancy, quadrachorionic/quadra-amniotic, second trimester   cc M ♀

O30.233   Quadruplet pregnancy, quadrachorionic/quadra-amniotic, third trimester   cc M ♀

O30.239   Quadruplet pregnancy, quadrachorionic/quadra-amniotic, unspecified trimester   M ♀

√6ᵗʰ   **O30.29**   **Quadruplet pregnancy,** unable to determine number **of placenta and number of amniotic sacs**

O30.291   Quadruplet pregnancy, unable to determine number of placenta and number of amniotic sacs, first trimester   cc M ♀

O30.292   Quadruplet pregnancy, unable to determine number of placenta and number of amniotic sacs, second trimester   cc M ♀

O30.293   Quadruplet pregnancy, unable to determine number of placenta and number of amniotic sacs, third trimester   cc M ♀

O30.299   Quadruplet pregnancy, unable to determine number of placenta and number of amniotic sacs, unspecified trimester   M ♀

√5ᵗʰ   **O30.8**   **Other specified multiple gestation**
    Multiple gestation pregnancy greater then quadruplets

√6ᵗʰ   **O30.80**   **Other specified multiple gestation, unspecified number of placenta and unspecified number of amniotic sacs**

O30.801   Other specified multiple gestation, unspecified number of placenta and unspecified number of amniotic sacs, first trimester   cc M ♀

O30.802   Other specified multiple gestation, unspecified number of placenta and unspecified number of amniotic sacs, second trimester   cc M ♀

O30.803   Other specified multiple gestation, unspecified number of placenta and unspecified number of amniotic sacs, third trimester   cc M ♀

O30.809   Other specified multiple gestation, unspecified number of placenta and unspecified number of amniotic sacs, unspecified trimester   M ♀

√6ᵗʰ   **O30.81**   **Other specified multiple gestation with** two or more monochorionic fetuses

O30.811   Other specified multiple gestation with two or more monochorionic fetuses, first trimester   cc M ♀

O30.812   Other specified multiple gestation with two or more monochorionic fetuses, second trimester   cc M ♀

O30.813   Other specified multiple gestation with two or more monochorionic fetuses, third trimester   cc M ♀

O30.819   Other specified multiple gestation with two or more monochorionic fetuses, unspecified trimester   M ♀

√6ᵗʰ   **O30.82**   **Other specified multiple gestation with** two or more monoamniotic fetuses

O30.821   Other specified multiple gestation with two or more monoamniotic fetuses, first trimester   cc M ♀

O30.822   Other specified multiple gestation with two or more monoamniotic fetuses, second trimester   cc M ♀

O30.823   Other specified multiple gestation with two or more monoamniotic fetuses, third trimester   cc M ♀

O30.829   Other specified multiple gestation with two or more monoamniotic fetuses, unspecified trimester   M ♀

√6ᵗʰ   **O30.83**   **Other specified multiple gestation,** number of chorions and amnions are both equal to the number of fetuses
    Pentachorionic, penta-amniotic pregnancy (quintuplets)
    Hexachorionic, hexa-amniotic pregnancy (sextuplets)
    Heptachorionic, hepta-amniotic pregnancy (septuplets)
    AHA: 2018,4Q,22

O30.831   Other specified multiple gestation, number of chorions and amnions are both equal to the number of fetuses, first trimester   cc M ♀

O30.832   Other specified multiple gestation, number of chorions and amnions are both equal to the number of fetuses, second trimester   cc M ♀

O30.833   Other specified multiple gestation, number of chorions and amnions are both equal to the number of fetuses, third trimester   cc M ♀

O30.839   Other specified multiple gestation, number of chorions and amnions are both equal to the number of fetuses, unspecified trimester   M ♀

√6ᵗʰ   **O30.89**   **Other specified multiple gestation,** unable to determine number **of placenta and number of amniotic sacs**

O30.891   Other specified multiple gestation, unable to determine number of placenta and number of amniotic sacs, first trimester   cc M ♀

O30.892   Other specified multiple gestation, unable to determine number of placenta and number of amniotic sacs, second trimester   cc M ♀

O30.893   Other specified multiple gestation, unable to determine number of placenta and number of amniotic sacs, third trimester   cc M ♀

O30.899   Other specified multiple gestation, unable to determine number of placenta and number of amniotic sacs, unspecified trimester   M ♀

N Newborn: 0   P Pediatric: 0-17   M Maternity: 9-64   A Adult: 15-124   MCC Major Complication/Comorbidity   CC Complication/Comorbidity   SW Severe Wound Dx

880   ICD-10-CM 2021

√5ᵗʰ **O30.9 Multiple gestation, unspecified**

Multiple pregnancy NOS

O30.90 Multiple gestation, unspecified, unspecified trimester Ⓜ ♀

O30.91 Multiple gestation, unspecified, first trimester Ⓜ ♀

O30.92 Multiple gestation, unspecified, second trimester Ⓜ ♀

O30.93 Multiple gestation, unspecified, third trimester Ⓜ ♀

√4ᵗʰ **O31 Complications specific to multiple gestation**

EXCLUDES 2   *delayed delivery of second twin, triplet, etc. (O63.2)*
malpresentation of one fetus or more (O32.9)
placental transfusion syndromes (O43.0-)

AHA: 2012,4Q,107

One of the following 7th characters is to be assigned to each code under category O31. 7th character 0 is for single gestations and multiple gestations where the fetus is unspecified. 7th characters 1 through 9 are for cases of multiple gestations to identify the fetus for which the code applies. The appropriate code from category O30, Multiple gestation, must also be assigned when assigning a code from category O31 that has a 7th character of 1 through 9.

0   not applicable or unspecified
1   fetus 1
2   fetus 2
3   fetus 3
4   fetus 4
5   fetus 5
9   other fetus

√5ᵗʰ **O31.0 Papyraceous fetus**

Fetus compressus
DEF: Fetus that has died, but remains in utero for weeks before delivery, becoming compacted and mummified in appearance, with skin resembling parchment. Occurs most commonly in multigestational pregnancies. *Synonym(s): paper doll fetus.*

√x7ᵗʰ **O31.00 Papyraceous fetus, unspecified trimester** Ⓜ ♀

√x7ᵗʰ **O31.01 Papyraceous fetus, first trimester** Ⓜ ♀

√x7ᵗʰ **O31.02 Papyraceous fetus, second trimester** Ⓜ ♀

√x7ᵗʰ **O31.03 Papyraceous fetus, third trimester** Ⓜ ♀

√5ᵗʰ **O31.1 Continuing pregnancy after spontaneous abortion of one fetus or more**

√x7ᵗʰ **O31.10 Continuing pregnancy after spontaneous abortion of one fetus or more, unspecified trimester** Ⓜ ♀

√x7ᵗʰ **O31.11 Continuing pregnancy after spontaneous abortion of one fetus or more, first trimester** Ⓜ ♀

√x7ᵗʰ **O31.12 Continuing pregnancy after spontaneous abortion of one fetus or more, second trimester** Ⓜ ♀

√x7ᵗʰ **O31.13 Continuing pregnancy after spontaneous abortion of one fetus or more, third trimester** Ⓜ ♀

√5ᵗʰ **O31.2 Continuing pregnancy after intrauterine death of one fetus or more**

√x7ᵗʰ **O31.20 Continuing pregnancy after intrauterine death of one fetus or more, unspecified trimester** Ⓜ ♀

√x7ᵗʰ **O31.21 Continuing pregnancy after intrauterine death of one fetus or more, first trimester** Ⓜ ♀

√x7ᵗʰ **O31.22 Continuing pregnancy after intrauterine death of one fetus or more, second trimester** Ⓜ ♀

√x7ᵗʰ **O31.23 Continuing pregnancy after intrauterine death of one fetus or more, third trimester** Ⓜ ♀

√5ᵗʰ **O31.3 Continuing pregnancy after elective fetal reduction of one fetus or more**

Continuing pregnancy after selective termination of one fetus or more

√x7ᵗʰ **O31.30 Continuing pregnancy after elective fetal reduction of one fetus or more, unspecified trimester** Ⓜ ♀

√x7ᵗʰ **O31.31 Continuing pregnancy after elective fetal reduction of one fetus or more, first trimester** Ⓜ ♀

√x7ᵗʰ **O31.32 Continuing pregnancy after elective fetal reduction of one fetus or more, second trimester** Ⓜ ♀

√x7ᵗʰ **O31.33 Continuing pregnancy after elective fetal reduction of one fetus or more, third trimester** Ⓜ ♀

√5ᵗʰ **O31.8 Other complications specific to multiple gestation**

√6ᵗʰ **O31.8X Other complications specific to multiple gestation**

√7ᵗʰ **O31.8X1 Other complications specific to multiple gestation, first trimester** CC Ⓜ ♀

√7ᵗʰ **O31.8X2 Other complications specific to multiple gestation, second trimester** CC Ⓜ ♀

√7ᵗʰ **O31.8X3 Other complications specific to multiple gestation, third trimester** CC Ⓜ ♀

√7ᵗʰ **O31.8X9 Other complications specific to multiple gestation, unspecified trimester** CC Ⓜ ♀

√4ᵗʰ **O32 Maternal care for malpresentation of fetus**

INCLUDES   the listed conditions as a reason for observation, hospitalization or other obstetric care of the mother, or for cesarean delivery before onset of labor

EXCLUDES 1   *malpresentation of fetus with obstructed labor (O64.-)*

AHA: 2012,4Q,107

One of the following 7th characters is to be assigned to each code under category O32. 7th character 0 is for single gestations and multiple gestations where the fetus is unspecified. 7th characters 1 through 9 are for cases of multiple gestations to identify the fetus for which the code applies. The appropriate code from category O30, Multiple gestation, must also be assigned when assigning a code from category O32 that has a 7th character of 1 through 9.

0   not applicable or unspecified
1   fetus 1
2   fetus 2
3   fetus 3
4   fetus 4
5   fetus 5
9   other fetus

√x7ᵗʰ **O32.0 Maternal care for unstable lie** Ⓜ ♀

√x7ᵗʰ **O32.1 Maternal care for breech presentation** Ⓜ ♀

Maternal care for buttocks presentation
Maternal care for complete breech
Maternal care for frank breech
EXCLUDES 1   *footling presentation (O32.8)*
incomplete breech (O32.8)
DEF: Fetus presentation in a longitudinal lie with the buttocks or feet closest to birth canal that may require external cephalic version or cesarean delivery.

√x7ᵗʰ **O32.2 Maternal care for transverse and oblique lie** Ⓜ ♀

Maternal care for oblique presentation
Maternal care for transverse presentation

√x7ᵗʰ **O32.3 Maternal care for face, brow and chin presentation** Ⓜ ♀

√x7ᵗʰ **O32.4 Maternal care for high head at term** Ⓜ ♀

Maternal care for failure of head to enter pelvic brim

√x7ᵗʰ **O32.6 Maternal care for compound presentation** Ⓜ ♀

√x7ᵗʰ **O32.8 Maternal care for other malpresentation of fetus** Ⓜ ♀

Maternal care for footling presentation
Maternal care for incomplete breech

√x7ᵗʰ **O32.9 Maternal care for malpresentation of fetus, unspecified** Ⓜ ♀

Fetal Malpresentation

Breech

Shoulder (arm prolapse)

Mother's pelvis

Compound (extremity together with head)

Face (mentum)

Oblique

☑ Additional Character Required   √x7ᵗʰ Placeholder   Unacceptable PDx   Questionable PDx   Manifestation   Unspecified Dx   H1-H14 HAC   HCC CMS-HCC Dx   HIV HIV Dx

ICD-10-CM 2021   881

√4ᵗʰ **O33 Maternal care for disproportion**

INCLUDES   the listed conditions as a reason for observation, hospitalization or other obstetric care of the mother, or for cesarean delivery before onset of labor

EXCLUDES 1   *disproportion with obstructed labor (O65-O66)*

O33.0 Maternal care for disproportion due to deformity of maternal pelvic bones   CC M ♀

Maternal care for disproportion due to pelvic deformity causing disproportion NOS

O33.1 Maternal care for disproportion due to generally contracted pelvis   M ♀

Maternal care for disproportion due to contracted pelvis NOS causing disproportion

O33.2 Maternal care for disproportion due to inlet contraction of pelvis   M ♀

Maternal care for disproportion due to inlet contraction (pelvis) causing disproportion

√7ᵗʰ **O33.3 Maternal care for disproportion due to outlet contraction of pelvis**   M ♀

Maternal care for disproportion due to mid-cavity contraction (pelvis)

Maternal care for disproportion due to outlet contraction (pelvis)

One of the following 7th characters is to be assigned to code O33.3. 7th character Ø is for single gestations and multiple gestations where the fetus is unspecified. 7th characters 1 through 9 are for cases of multiple gestations to identify the fetus for which the code applies. The appropriate code from category O30, Multiple gestation, must also be assigned when assigning code O33.3 with a 7th character of 1 through 9.

Ø   not applicable or unspecified
1   fetus 1
2   fetus 2
3   fetus 3
4   fetus 4
5   fetus 5
9   other fetus

√7ᵗʰ **O33.4 Maternal care for disproportion of mixed maternal and fetal origin**   M ♀

One of the following 7th characters is to be assigned to code O33.4. 7th character Ø is for single gestations and multiple gestations where the fetus is unspecified. 7th characters 1 through 9 are for cases of multiple gestations to identify the fetus for which the code applies. The appropriate code from category O30, Multiple gestation, must also be assigned when assigning code O33.4 with a 7th character of 1 through 9.

Ø   not applicable or unspecified
1   fetus 1
2   fetus 2
3   fetus 3
4   fetus 4
5   fetus 5
9   other fetus

√7ᵗʰ **O33.5 Maternal care for disproportion due to unusually large fetus**   M ♀

Maternal care for disproportion due to disproportion of fetal origin with normally formed fetus

Maternal care for disproportion due to fetal disproportion NOS

One of the following 7th characters is to be assigned to code O33.5. 7th character Ø is for single gestations and multiple gestations where the fetus is unspecified. 7th characters 1 through 9 are for cases of multiple gestations to identify the fetus for which the code applies. The appropriate code from category O30, Multiple gestation, must also be assigned when assigning code O33.5 with a 7th character of 1 through 9.

Ø   not applicable or unspecified
1   fetus 1
2   fetus 2
3   fetus 3
4   fetus 4
5   fetus 5
9   other fetus

√x7ᵗʰ **O33.6 Maternal care for disproportion due to hydrocephalic fetus**   M ♀

One of the following 7th characters is to be assigned to code O33.6. 7th character Ø is for single gestations and multiple gestations where the fetus is unspecified. 7th characters 1 through 9 are for cases of multiple gestations to identify the fetus for which the code applies. The appropriate code from category O30, Multiple gestation, must also be assigned when assigning code O33.6 with a 7th character of 1 through 9.

Ø   not applicable or unspecified
1   fetus 1
2   fetus 2
3   fetus 3
4   fetus 4
5   fetus 5
9   other fetus

√x7ᵗʰ **O33.7 Maternal care for disproportion due to other fetal deformities**   M ♀

Maternal care for disproportion due to fetal ascites

Maternal care for disproportion due to fetal hydrops

Maternal care for disproportion due to fetal meningomyelocele

Maternal care for disproportion due to fetal sacral teratoma

Maternal care for disproportion due to fetal tumor

EXCLUDES 1   *obstructed labor due to other fetal deformities (O66.3)*

AHA: 2016,4Q,51

One of the following 7th characters is to be assigned to code O33.7. 7th character Ø is for single gestations and multiple gestations where the fetus is unspecified. 7th characters 1 through 9 are for cases of multiple gestations to identify the fetus for which the code applies. The appropriate code from category O30, Multiple gestation, must also be assigned when assigning code O33.7 with a 7th character of 1 through 9.

Ø   not applicable or unspecified
1   fetus 1
2   fetus 2
3   fetus 3
4   fetus 4
5   fetus 5
9   other fetus

O33.8 Maternal care for disproportion of other origin   M ♀

O33.9 Maternal care for disproportion, unspecified   M ♀

Maternal care for disproportion due to cephalopelvic disproportion NOS

Maternal care for disproportion due to fetopelvic disproportion NOS

√4ᵗʰ **O34 Maternal care for abnormality of pelvic organs**

INCLUDES   the listed conditions as a reason for hospitalization or other obstetric care of the mother, or for cesarean delivery before onset of labor

Code first any associated obstructed labor (O65.5)

Use additional code for specific condition

√5ᵗʰ **O34.0 Maternal care for congenital malformation of uterus**

Maternal care for double uterus

Maternal care for uterus bicornis

O34.00 Maternal care for unspecified congenital malformation of uterus, unspecified trimester   M ♀

O34.01 Maternal care for unspecified congenital malformation of uterus, first trimester   M ♀

O34.02 Maternal care for unspecified congenital malformation of uterus, second trimester   M ♀

O34.03 Maternal care for unspecified congenital malformation of uterus, third trimester   M ♀

√5ᵗʰ **O34.1 Maternal care for benign tumor of corpus uteri**

EXCLUDES 2   *maternal care for benign tumor of cervix (O34.4-)*

maternal care for malignant neoplasm of uterus (O9A.1-)

O34.10 Maternal care for benign tumor of corpus uteri, unspecified trimester   M ♀

O34.11 Maternal care for benign tumor of corpus uteri, first trimester   M ♀

O34.12 Maternal care for benign tumor of corpus uteri, second trimester   M ♀

O34.13 Maternal care for benign tumor of corpus uteri, third trimester   M ♀

N Newborn: 0   P Pediatric: 0-17   M Maternity: 9-64   A Adult: 15-124   MCC Major Complication/Comorbidity   CC Complication/Comorbidity   SW Severe Wound Dx

882   ICD-10-CM 2021

✓5ᵗʰ O34.2 Maternal care due to uterine scar from previous surgery
    AHA: 2016,4Q,76

   ✓6ᵗʰ O34.21 Maternal care for scar from previous cesarean delivery
      AHA: 2018,3Q,23; 2016,4Q,51-52

    O34.211 Maternal care for low transverse scar from previous cesarean delivery   M ♀

    O34.212 Maternal care for vertical scar from previous cesarean delivery   M ♀
      Maternal care for classical scar from previous cesarean delivery

    O34.218 Maternal care for other type scar from previous cesarean delivery   M ♀
      Mid-transverse T incision

    O34.219 Maternal care for unspecified type scar from previous cesarean delivery   M ♀

   O34.22 Maternal care for cesarean scar defect (isthmocele)   M ♀

   O34.29 Maternal care due to uterine scar from other previous surgery   M ♀
    Maternal care due to uterine scar from other transmural uterine incision

✓5ᵗʰ O34.3 Maternal care for cervical incompetence
   Maternal care for cerclage with or without cervical incompetence
   Maternal care for Shirodkar suture with or without cervical incompetence
   DEF: Inadequate functioning of the cervix marked by abnormal widening during pregnancy and causing premature birth or miscarriage.

   O34.30 Maternal care for cervical incompetence, unspecified trimester   M ♀

   O34.31 Maternal care for cervical incompetence, first trimester   MCC M ♀

   O34.32 Maternal care for cervical incompetence, second trimester   MCC M ♀

   O34.33 Maternal care for cervical incompetence, third trimester   MCC M ♀

✓5ᵗʰ O34.4 Maternal care for other abnormalities of cervix

   O34.40 Maternal care for other abnormalities of cervix, unspecified trimester   M ♀

   O34.41 Maternal care for other abnormalities of cervix, first trimester   M ♀

   O34.42 Maternal care for other abnormalities of cervix, second trimester   M ♀

   O34.43 Maternal care for other abnormalities of cervix, third trimester   M ♀

✓5ᵗʰ O34.5 Maternal care for other abnormalities of gravid uterus

   ✓6ᵗʰ O34.51 Maternal care for incarceration of gravid uterus

    O34.511 Maternal care for incarceration of gravid uterus, first trimester   M ♀

    O34.512 Maternal care for incarceration of gravid uterus, second trimester   M ♀

    O34.513 Maternal care for incarceration of gravid uterus, third trimester   M ♀

    O34.519 Maternal care for incarceration of gravid uterus, unspecified trimester   M ♀

   ✓6ᵗʰ O34.52 Maternal care for prolapse of gravid uterus

    O34.521 Maternal care for prolapse of gravid uterus, first trimester   M ♀

    O34.522 Maternal care for prolapse of gravid uterus, second trimester   M ♀

    O34.523 Maternal care for prolapse of gravid uterus, third trimester   M ♀

    O34.529 Maternal care for prolapse of gravid uterus, unspecified trimester   M ♀

   ✓6ᵗʰ O34.53 Maternal care for retroversion of gravid uterus

    O34.531 Maternal care for retroversion of gravid uterus, first trimester   M ♀

    O34.532 Maternal care for retroversion of gravid uterus, second trimester   M ♀

    O34.533 Maternal care for retroversion of gravid uterus, third trimester   M ♀

    O34.539 Maternal care for retroversion of gravid uterus, unspecified trimester   M ♀

   ✓6ᵗʰ O34.59 Maternal care for other abnormalities of gravid uterus

    O34.591 Maternal care for other abnormalities of gravid uterus, first trimester   M ♀

    O34.592 Maternal care for other abnormalities of gravid uterus, second trimester   M ♀

    O34.593 Maternal care for other abnormalities of gravid uterus, third trimester   M ♀

    O34.599 Maternal care for other abnormalities of gravid uterus, unspecified trimester   M ♀

✓5ᵗʰ O34.6 Maternal care for abnormality of vagina
   EXCLUDES 2   maternal care for vaginal varices in pregnancy (O22.1-)

   O34.60 Maternal care for abnormality of vagina, unspecified trimester   M ♀

   O34.61 Maternal care for abnormality of vagina, first trimester   M ♀

   O34.62 Maternal care for abnormality of vagina, second trimester   M ♀

   O34.63 Maternal care for abnormality of vagina, third trimester   M ♀

✓5ᵗʰ O34.7 Maternal care for abnormality of vulva and perineum
   EXCLUDES 2   maternal care for perineal and vulval varices in pregnancy (O22.1-)

   O34.70 Maternal care for abnormality of vulva and perineum, unspecified trimester   M ♀

   O34.71 Maternal care for abnormality of vulva and perineum, first trimester   M ♀

   O34.72 Maternal care for abnormality of vulva and perineum, second trimester   M ♀

   O34.73 Maternal care for abnormality of vulva and perineum, third trimester   M ♀

✓5ᵗʰ O34.8 Maternal care for other abnormalities of pelvic organs

   O34.80 Maternal care for other abnormalities of pelvic organs, unspecified trimester   M ♀

   O34.81 Maternal care for other abnormalities of pelvic organs, first trimester   M ♀

   O34.82 Maternal care for other abnormalities of pelvic organs, second trimester   M ♀

   O34.83 Maternal care for other abnormalities of pelvic organs, third trimester   M ♀

✓5ᵗʰ O34.9 Maternal care for abnormality of pelvic organ, unspecified

   O34.90 Maternal care for abnormality of pelvic organ, unspecified, unspecified trimester   M ♀

   O34.91 Maternal care for abnormality of pelvic organ, unspecified, first trimester   M ♀

   O34.92 Maternal care for abnormality of pelvic organ, unspecified, second trimester   M ♀

   O34.93 Maternal care for abnormality of pelvic organ, unspecified, third trimester   M ♀

✓4ᵗʰ O35 Maternal care for known or suspected fetal abnormality and damage
   INCLUDES   the listed conditions in the fetus as a reason for hospitalization or other obstetric care to the mother, or for termination of pregnancy
   Code also any associated maternal condition
   EXCLUDES 1   encounter for suspected maternal and fetal conditions ruled out (Z03.7-)

   One of the following 7th characters is to be assigned to each code under category O35. 7th character Ø is for single gestations and multiple gestations where the fetus is unspecified. 7th characters 1 through 9 are for cases of multiple gestations to identify the fetus for which the code applies. The appropriate code from category O30, Multiple gestation, must also be assigned when assigning a code from category O35 that has a 7th character of 1 through 9.
   Ø   not applicable or unspecified
   1   fetus 1
   2   fetus 2
   3   fetus 3
   4   fetus 4
   5   fetus 5
   9   other fetus

   ✓x7ᵗʰ O35.Ø Maternal care for (suspected) central nervous system malformation in fetus   M ♀
    Maternal care for fetal anencephaly
    Maternal care for fetal hydrocephalus
    Maternal care for fetal spina bifida
    EXCLUDES 2   chromosomal abnormality in fetus (O35.1)

   ✓x7ᵗʰ O35.1 Maternal care for (suspected) chromosomal abnormality in fetus   M ♀

☑ Additional Character Required   ✓x7ᵗʰ Placeholder   Unacceptable PDx   Questionable PDx   Manifestation   Unspecified Dx   H1-H14 HAC   HCC CMS-HCC Dx   HIV HIV Dx

ICD-10-CM 2021   **883**

✓x7ᵗʰ O35.2 Maternal care for (suspected) hereditary disease in fetus M ♀
> EXCLUDES 2   chromosomal abnormality in fetus (O35.1)

✓x7ᵗʰ O35.3 Maternal care for (suspected) damage to fetus from viral disease in mother M ♀
Maternal care for damage to fetus from maternal cytomegalovirus infection
Maternal care for damage to fetus from maternal rubella

✓x7ᵗʰ O35.4 Maternal care for (suspected) damage to fetus from alcohol M ♀

✓x7ᵗʰ O35.5 Maternal care for (suspected) damage to fetus by drugs M ♀
Maternal care for damage to fetus from drug addiction

✓x7ᵗʰ O35.6 Maternal care for (suspected) damage to fetus by radiation M ♀

✓x7ᵗʰ O35.7 Maternal care for (suspected) damage to fetus by other medical procedures M ♀
Maternal care for damage to fetus by amniocentesis
Maternal care for damage to fetus by biopsy procedures
Maternal care for damage to fetus by hematological investigation
Maternal care for damage to fetus by intrauterine contraceptive device
Maternal care for damage to fetus by intrauterine surgery

✓x7ᵗʰ O35.8 Maternal care for other (suspected) fetal abnormality and damage M ♀
Maternal care for damage to fetus from maternal listeriosis
Maternal care for damage to fetus from maternal toxoplasmosis

✓x7ᵗʰ O35.9 Maternal care for (suspected) fetal abnormality and damage, unspecified M ♀

✓4ᵗʰ O36 Maternal care for other fetal problems
> INCLUDES   the listed conditions in the fetus as a reason for hospitalization or other obstetric care of the mother, or for termination of pregnancy
> EXCLUDES 1   encounter for suspected maternal and fetal conditions ruled out (Z03.7-)
>   placental transfusion syndromes (O43.0-)
> EXCLUDES 2   labor and delivery complicated by fetal stress (O77.-)
> AHA: 2015,3Q,40

One of the following 7th characters is to be assigned to each code under category O36. 7th character 0 is for single gestations and multiple gestations where the fetus is unspecified. 7th characters 1 through 9 are for cases of multiple gestations to identify the fetus for which the code applies. The appropriate code from category O30, Multiple gestation, must also be assigned when assigning a code from category O36 that has a 7th character of 1 through 9.
0   not applicable or unspecified
1   fetus 1
2   fetus 2
3   fetus 3
4   fetus 4
5   fetus 5
9   other fetus

✓5ᵗʰ O36.0 Maternal care for rhesus isoimmunization
Maternal care for Rh incompatibility (with hydrops fetalis)

✓6ᵗʰ O36.01 Maternal care for anti-D [Rh] antibodies
> AHA: 2014,4Q,17

✓7ᵗʰ O36.011 Maternal care for anti-D [Rh] antibodies, first trimester CC M ♀

✓7ᵗʰ O36.012 Maternal care for anti-D [Rh] antibodies, second trimester CC M ♀

✓7ᵗʰ O36.013 Maternal care for anti-D [Rh] antibodies, third trimester CC M ♀

✓7ᵗʰ O36.019 Maternal care for anti-D [Rh] antibodies, unspecified trimester M ♀

✓6ᵗʰ O36.09 Maternal care for other rhesus isoimmunization

✓7ᵗʰ O36.091 Maternal care for other rhesus isoimmunization, first trimester CC M ♀

✓7ᵗʰ O36.092 Maternal care for other rhesus isoimmunization, second trimester CC M ♀

✓7ᵗʰ O36.093 Maternal care for other rhesus isoimmunization, third trimester CC M ♀

✓7ᵗʰ O36.099 Maternal care for other rhesus isoimmunization, unspecified trimester M ♀

✓5ᵗʰ O36.1 Maternal care for other isoimmunization
Maternal care for ABO isoimmunization

✓6ᵗʰ O36.11 Maternal care for Anti-A sensitization
Maternal care for isoimmunization NOS (with hydrops fetalis)

✓7ᵗʰ O36.111 Maternal care for Anti-A sensitization, first trimester M ♀

✓7ᵗʰ O36.112 Maternal care for Anti-A sensitization, second trimester M ♀

✓7ᵗʰ O36.113 Maternal care for Anti-A sensitization, third trimester M ♀

✓7ᵗʰ O36.119 Maternal care for Anti-A sensitization, unspecified trimester M ♀

✓6ᵗʰ O36.19 Maternal care for other isoimmunization
Maternal care for Anti-B sensitization

✓7ᵗʰ O36.191 Maternal care for other isoimmunization, first trimester M ♀

✓7ᵗʰ O36.192 Maternal care for other isoimmunization, second trimester M ♀

✓7ᵗʰ O36.193 Maternal care for other isoimmunization, third trimester M ♀

✓7ᵗʰ O36.199 Maternal care for other isoimmunization, unspecified trimester M ♀

✓5ᵗʰ O36.2 Maternal care for hydrops fetalis
Maternal care for hydrops fetalis NOS
Maternal care for hydrops fetalis not associated with isoimmunization
> EXCLUDES 1   hydrops fetalis associated with ABO isoimmunization (O36.1-)
>   hydrops fetalis associated with rhesus isoimmunization (O36.0-)
> DEF: Hydrops fetalis: Abnormal fluid buildup in at least two of the following fetal organ spaces: the skin (edema), abdomen (ascites), around the heart (pericardia effusion), and around the lung (pleural effusion). Fluid accumulation may also occur in the mother as polyhydramnios and edema of the placenta.

✓x7ᵗʰ O36.20 Maternal care for hydrops fetalis, unspecified trimester M ♀

✓x7ᵗʰ O36.21 Maternal care for hydrops fetalis, first trimester M ♀

✓x7ᵗʰ O36.22 Maternal care for hydrops fetalis, second trimester M ♀

✓x7ᵗʰ O36.23 Maternal care for hydrops fetalis, third trimester M ♀

✓x7ᵗʰ O36.4 Maternal care for intrauterine death CC M ♀
Maternal care for intrauterine fetal death NOS
Maternal care for intrauterine fetal death after completion of 20 weeks of gestation
Maternal care for late fetal death
Maternal care for missed delivery
> EXCLUDES 1   missed abortion (O02.1)
>   stillbirth (P95)

✓5ᵗʰ O36.5 Maternal care for known or suspected poor fetal growth

✓6ᵗʰ O36.51 Maternal care for known or suspected placental insufficiency

✓7ᵗʰ O36.511 Maternal care for known or suspected placental insufficiency, first trimester M ♀

✓7ᵗʰ O36.512 Maternal care for known or suspected placental insufficiency, second trimester M ♀

✓7ᵗʰ O36.513 Maternal care for known or suspected placental insufficiency, third trimester M ♀

✓7ᵗʰ O36.519 Maternal care for known or suspected placental insufficiency, unspecified trimester M ♀

✓6ᵗʰ O36.59 Maternal care for other known or suspected poor fetal growth
Maternal care for known or suspected light-for-dates NOS
Maternal care for known or suspected small-for-dates NOS

✓7ᵗʰ O36.591 Maternal care for other known or suspected poor fetal growth, first trimester M ♀

✓7ᵗʰ O36.592 Maternal care for other known or suspected poor fetal growth, second trimester M ♀

N Newborn: 0   P Pediatric: 0-17   M Maternity: 9-64   A Adult: 15-124   MCC Major Complication/Comorbidity   CC Complication/Comorbidity   SW Severe Wound Dx

884   ICD-10-CM 2021

√7ᵗʰ O36.593 Maternal care for other known or suspected poor fetal growth, third trimester Ⓜ ♀

√7ᵗʰ O36.599 Maternal care for other known or suspected poor fetal growth, unspecified trimester Ⓜ ♀

√5ᵗʰ O36.6 Maternal care for excessive fetal growth
Maternal care for known or suspected large-for-dates

√x7ᵗʰ O36.60 Maternal care for excessive fetal growth, unspecified trimester Ⓜ ♀

O36.61 Maternal care for excessive fetal growth, first trimester Ⓜ ♀

√x7ᵗʰ O36.62 Maternal care for excessive fetal growth, second trimester Ⓜ ♀

√x7ᵗʰ O36.63 Maternal care for excessive fetal growth, third trimester Ⓜ ♀

√5ᵗʰ O36.7 Maternal care for viable fetus in abdominal pregnancy

√x7ᵗʰ O36.70 Maternal care for viable fetus in abdominal pregnancy, unspecified trimester Ⓜ ♀

√x7ᵗʰ O36.71 Maternal care for viable fetus in abdominal pregnancy, first trimester Ⓜ ♀

√x7ᵗʰ O36.72 Maternal care for viable fetus in abdominal pregnancy, second trimester Ⓜ ♀

√x7ᵗʰ O36.73 Maternal care for viable fetus in abdominal pregnancy, third trimester Ⓜ ♀

√5ᵗʰ O36.8 Maternal care for other specified fetal problems

√x7ᵗʰ O36.80 Pregnancy with inconclusive fetal viability Ⓜ ♀
Encounter to determine fetal viability of pregnancy
AHA: 2019,2Q,29

√6ᵗʰ O36.81 Decreased fetal movements

√7ᵗʰ O36.812 Decreased fetal movements, second trimester Ⓜ ♀

√7ᵗʰ O36.813 Decreased fetal movements, third trimester Ⓜ ♀

√7ᵗʰ O36.819 Decreased fetal movements, unspecified trimester Ⓜ ♀

√6ᵗʰ O36.82 Fetal anemia and thrombocytopenia

√7ᵗʰ O36.821 Fetal anemia and thrombocytopenia, first trimester Ⓜ ♀

√7ᵗʰ O36.822 Fetal anemia and thrombocytopenia, second trimester Ⓜ ♀

√7ᵗʰ O36.823 Fetal anemia and thrombocytopenia, third trimester Ⓜ ♀

√7ᵗʰ O36.829 Fetal anemia and thrombocytopenia, unspecified trimester Ⓜ ♀

√6ᵗʰ O36.83 Maternal care for abnormalities of the fetal heart rate or rhythm
Maternal care for depressed fetal heart rate tones
Maternal care for fetal bradycardia
Maternal care for fetal heart rate abnormal variability
Maternal care for fetal heart rate decelerations
Maternal care for fetal heart rate irregularity
Maternal care for fetal tachycardia
Maternal care for non-reassuring fetal heart rate or rhythm
AHA: 2017,4Q,20
TIP: Assign for documented fetal tachycardia, bradycardia, decelerations, or loss of variability detected during antenatal testing.

√7ᵗʰ O36.831 Maternal care for abnormalities of the fetal heart rate or rhythm, first trimester Ⓜ ♀

√7ᵗʰ O36.832 Maternal care for abnormalities of the fetal heart rate or rhythm, second trimester Ⓜ ♀

√7ᵗʰ O36.833 Maternal care for abnormalities of the fetal heart rate or rhythm, third trimester Ⓜ ♀

√7ᵗʰ O36.839 Maternal care for abnormalities of the fetal heart rate or rhythm, unspecified trimester Ⓜ ♀

√6ᵗʰ O36.89 Maternal care for other specified fetal problems

√7ᵗʰ O36.891 Maternal care for other specified fetal problems, first trimester Ⓜ ♀

√7ᵗʰ O36.892 Maternal care for other specified fetal problems, second trimester Ⓜ ♀

√7ᵗʰ O36.893 Maternal care for other specified fetal problems, third trimester Ⓜ ♀

√7ᵗʰ O36.899 Maternal care for other specified fetal problems, unspecified trimester Ⓜ ♀

√5ᵗʰ O36.9 Maternal care for fetal problem, unspecified

√x7ᵗʰ O36.90 Maternal care for fetal problem, unspecified, unspecified trimester Ⓜ ♀

√x7ᵗʰ O36.91 Maternal care for fetal problem, unspecified, first trimester Ⓜ ♀

√x7ᵗʰ O36.92 Maternal care for fetal problem, unspecified, second trimester Ⓜ ♀

√x7ᵗʰ O36.93 Maternal care for fetal problem, unspecified, third trimester Ⓜ ♀

√4ᵗʰ O40 Polyhydramnios
INCLUDES   hydramnios
EXCLUDES 1   encounter for suspected maternal and fetal conditions ruled out (Z03.7-)
AHA: 2016,1Q,4
DEF: Excess amniotic fluid surrounding the fetus, typically defined as a total fluid volume of greater than 24.0 cc.

One of the following 7th characters is to be assigned to each code under category O40. 7th character Ø is for single gestations and multiple gestations where the fetus is unspecified. 7th characters 1 through 9 are for cases of multiple gestations to identify the fetus for which the code applies. The appropriate code from category O30, Multiple gestation, must be assigned when assigning a code from category O40 that has a 7th character of 1 through 9.
Ø   not applicable or unspecified
1   fetus 1
2   fetus 2
3   fetus 3
4   fetus 4
5   fetus 5
9   other fetus

√x7ᵗʰ O40.1 Polyhydramnios, first trimester Ⓜ ♀

√x7ᵗʰ O40.2 Polyhydramnios, second trimester Ⓜ ♀

√x7ᵗʰ O40.3 Polyhydramnios, third trimester Ⓜ ♀

√x7ᵗʰ O40.9 Polyhydramnios, unspecified trimester Ⓜ ♀

√4ᵗʰ O41 Other disorders of amniotic fluid and membranes
EXCLUDES 1   encounter for suspected maternal and fetal conditions ruled out (Z03.7-)

One of the following 7th characters is to be assigned to each code under category O41. 7th character Ø is for single gestations and multiple gestations where the fetus is unspecified. 7th characters 1 through 9 are for cases of multiple gestations to identify the fetus for which the code applies. The appropriate code from category O30, Multiple gestation, must also be assigned when assigning a code from category O41 that has a 7th character of 1 through 9.
Ø   not applicable or unspecified
1   fetus 1
2   fetus 2
3   fetus 3
4   fetus 4
5   fetus 5
9   other fetus

√5ᵗʰ O41.0 Oligohydramnios
Oligohydramnios without rupture of membranes
DEF: Low amniotic fluid, occurring most frequently in the last trimester.

√x7ᵗʰ O41.00 Oligohydramnios, unspecified trimester Ⓜ ♀

√x7ᵗʰ O41.01 Oligohydramnios, first trimester CC Ⓜ ♀

√x7ᵗʰ O41.02 Oligohydramnios, second trimester CC Ⓜ ♀

√x7ᵗʰ O41.03 Oligohydramnios, third trimester CC Ⓜ ♀

√5ᵗʰ O41.1 Infection of amniotic sac and membranes

√6ᵗʰ O41.10 Infection of amniotic sac and membranes, unspecified

√7ᵗʰ O41.101 Infection of amniotic sac and membranes, unspecified, first trimester MCC Ⓜ ♀

√7ᵗʰ O41.102 Infection of amniotic sac and membranes, unspecified, second trimester MCC Ⓜ ♀

√7ᵗʰ O41.103 Infection of amniotic sac and membranes, unspecified, third trimester MCC Ⓜ ♀

√7ᵗʰ O41.109 Infection of amniotic sac and membranes, unspecified, unspecified trimester Ⓜ ♀

√6ᵗʰ **O41.12 Chorioamnionitis**
AHA: 2019,2Q,34

√7ᵗʰ **O41.121 Chorioamnionitis, first trimester** MCC M ♀

√7ᵗʰ **O41.122 Chorioamnionitis, second trimester** MCC M ♀

√7ᵗʰ **O41.123 Chorioamnionitis, third trimester** MCC M ♀

√7ᵗʰ **O41.129 Chorioamnionitis, unspecified trimester** M ♀

√6ᵗʰ **O41.14 Placentitis**

√7ᵗʰ **O41.141 Placentitis, first trimester** MCC M ♀

√7ᵗʰ **O41.142 Placentitis, second trimester** MCC M ♀

√7ᵗʰ **O41.143 Placentitis, third trimester** MCC M ♀

√7ᵗʰ **O41.149 Placentitis, unspecified trimester** M ♀

√5ᵗʰ **O41.8 Other specified disorders of amniotic fluid and membranes**

√6ᵗʰ **O41.8X Other specified disorders of amniotic fluid and membranes**

√7ᵗʰ **O41.8X1 Other specified disorders of amniotic fluid and membranes, first trimester** M ♀

√7ᵗʰ **O41.8X2 Other specified disorders of amniotic fluid and membranes, second trimester** M ♀

√7ᵗʰ **O41.8X3 Other specified disorders of amniotic fluid and membranes, third trimester** M ♀

√7ᵗʰ **O41.8X9 Other specified disorders of amniotic fluid and membranes, unspecified trimester** M ♀

√5ᵗʰ **O41.9 Disorder of amniotic fluid and membranes, unspecified**

√x7ᵗʰ **O41.90 Disorder of amniotic fluid and membranes, unspecified, unspecified trimester** M ♀

√x7ᵗʰ **O41.91 Disorder of amniotic fluid and membranes, unspecified, first trimester** M ♀

√x7ᵗʰ **O41.92 Disorder of amniotic fluid and membranes, unspecified, second trimester** M ♀

√x7ᵗʰ **O41.93 Disorder of amniotic fluid and membranes, unspecified, third trimester** M ♀

√4ᵗʰ **O42 Premature rupture of membranes**
AHA: 2016,1Q,3

√5ᵗʰ **O42.0 Premature rupture of membranes, onset of labor within 24 hours of rupture**

O42.00 Premature rupture of membranes, onset of labor within 24 hours of rupture, unspecified weeks of gestation M ♀

√6ᵗʰ **O42.01 Preterm premature rupture of membranes, onset of labor within 24 hours of rupture**
Premature rupture of membranes before 37 completed weeks of gestation

O42.011 Preterm premature rupture of membranes, onset of labor within 24 hours of rupture, first trimester M ♀

O42.012 Preterm premature rupture of membranes, onset of labor within 24 hours of rupture, second trimester M ♀

O42.013 Preterm premature rupture of membranes, onset of labor within 24 hours of rupture, third trimester M ♀

O42.019 Preterm premature rupture of membranes, onset of labor within 24 hours of rupture, unspecified trimester M ♀

O42.02 Full-term premature rupture of membranes, onset of labor within 24 hours of rupture M ♀
Premature rupture of membranes at or after 37 completed weeks of gestation, onset of labor within 24 hours of rupture

√5ᵗʰ **O42.1 Premature rupture of membranes, onset of labor more than 24 hours following rupture**
AHA: 2016,1Q,5

O42.10 Premature rupture of membranes, onset of labor more than 24 hours following rupture, unspecified weeks of gestation M ♀

√6ᵗʰ **O42.11 Preterm premature rupture of membranes, onset of labor more than 24 hours following rupture**
Premature rupture of membranes before 37 completed weeks of gestation

O42.111 Preterm premature rupture of membranes, onset of labor more than 24 hours following rupture, first trimester M ♀

O42.112 Preterm premature rupture of membranes, onset of labor more than 24 hours following rupture, second trimester M ♀

O42.113 Preterm premature rupture of membranes, onset of labor more than 24 hours following rupture, third trimester M ♀

O42.119 Preterm premature rupture of membranes, onset of labor more than 24 hours following rupture, unspecified trimester M ♀

O42.12 Full-term premature rupture of membranes, onset of labor more than 24 hours following rupture M ♀
Premature rupture of membranes at or after 37 completed weeks of gestation, onset of labor more than 24 hours following rupture

√5ᵗʰ **O42.9 Premature rupture of membranes, unspecified as to length of time between rupture and onset of labor**

O42.90 Premature rupture of membranes, unspecified as to length of time between rupture and onset of labor, unspecified weeks of gestation M ♀

√6ᵗʰ **O42.91 Preterm premature rupture of membranes, unspecified as to length of time between rupture and onset of labor**
Premature rupture of membranes before 37 completed weeks of gestation

O42.911 Preterm premature rupture of membranes, unspecified as to length of time between rupture and onset of labor, first trimester M ♀

O42.912 Preterm premature rupture of membranes, unspecified as to length of time between rupture and onset of labor, second trimester M ♀

O42.913 Preterm premature rupture of membranes, unspecified as to length of time between rupture and onset of labor, third trimester M ♀

O42.919 Preterm premature rupture of membranes, unspecified as to length of time between rupture and onset of labor, unspecified trimester M ♀

O42.92 Full-term premature rupture of membranes, unspecified as to length of time between rupture and onset of labor M ♀
Premature rupture of membranes at or after 37 completed weeks of gestation, unspecified as to length of time between rupture and onset of labor

√4ᵗʰ **O43 Placental disorders**

EXCLUDES 2 maternal care for poor fetal growth due to placental insufficiency (O36.5-)
placenta previa (O44.-)
placental polyp (O90.89)
placentitis (O41.14-)
premature separation of placenta [abruptio placentae] (O45.-)

√5ᵗʰ **O43.0 Placental transfusion syndromes**

√6ᵗʰ **O43.01 Fetomaternal placental transfusion syndrome**
Maternofetal placental transfusion syndrome

O43.011 Fetomaternal placental transfusion syndrome, first trimester M ♀

O43.012 Fetomaternal placental transfusion syndrome, second trimester M ♀

O43.013 Fetomaternal placental transfusion syndrome, third trimester M ♀

O43.019 Fetomaternal placental transfusion syndrome, unspecified trimester M ♀

N Newborn: 0   P Pediatric: 0-17   M Maternity: 9-64   A Adult: 15-124   MCC Major Complication/Comorbidity   CC Complication/Comorbidity   SW Severe Wound Dx

886   ICD-10-CM 2021

√6ᵗʰ **O43.02 Fetus-to-fetus** placental transfusion syndrome

DEF: Condition in which an imbalance in amniotic fluid occurs due to uneven blood flow between twins sharing a placenta.

Twin to Twin Transfusion Syndrome (TTTS)

Healthy twins   Twins with TTTS

O43.021 Fetus-to-fetus placental transfusion syndrome, **first trimester** Ⓜ♀

O43.022 Fetus-to-fetus placental transfusion syndrome, **second trimester** Ⓜ♀

O43.023 Fetus-to-fetus placental transfusion syndrome, **third trimester** Ⓜ♀

O43.029 Fetus-to-fetus placental transfusion syndrome, unspecified trimester Ⓜ♀

√5ᵗʰ **O43.1 Malformation of placenta**

√6ᵗʰ **O43.10 Malformation of placenta, unspecified**

Abnormal placenta NOS

O43.101 Malformation of placenta, unspecified, first trimester Ⓜ♀

O43.102 Malformation of placenta, unspecified, second trimester Ⓜ♀

O43.103 Malformation of placenta, unspecified, third trimester Ⓜ♀

O43.109 Malformation of placenta, unspecified, unspecified trimester Ⓜ♀

√6ᵗʰ **O43.11 Circumvallate** placenta

O43.111 Circumvallate placenta, first trimester Ⓜ♀

O43.112 Circumvallate placenta, second trimester Ⓜ♀

O43.113 Circumvallate placenta, third trimester Ⓜ♀

O43.119 Circumvallate placenta, unspecified trimester Ⓜ♀

√6ᵗʰ **O43.12 Velamentous insertion of umbilical cord**

O43.121 Velamentous insertion of umbilical cord, first trimester Ⓜ♀

O43.122 Velamentous insertion of umbilical cord, second trimester Ⓜ♀

O43.123 Velamentous insertion of umbilical cord, third trimester Ⓜ♀

O43.129 Velamentous insertion of umbilical cord, unspecified trimester Ⓜ♀

√6ᵗʰ **O43.19 Other malformation of placenta**

O43.191 Other malformation of placenta, first trimester Ⓜ♀

O43.192 Other malformation of placenta, second trimester Ⓜ♀

O43.193 Other malformation of placenta, third trimester Ⓜ♀

O43.199 Other malformation of placenta, unspecified trimester Ⓜ♀

√5ᵗʰ **O43.2 Morbidly adherent placenta**

Code also associated third stage postpartum hemorrhage, if applicable (O72.0)

EXCLUDES 1   retained placenta (O73.-)

√6ᵗʰ **O43.21 Placenta accreta**

DEF: Condition where the placenta adheres too deeply to the uterine wall; often associated with placenta previa.

O43.211 Placenta accreta, first trimester Ⓜ♀

O43.212 Placenta accreta, second trimester Ⓜ♀

O43.213 Placenta accreta, third trimester Ⓜ♀

O43.219 Placenta accreta, unspecified trimester Ⓜ♀

√6ᵗʰ **O43.22 Placenta increta**

DEF: Condition where the placenta adheres too deeply to the uterine wall and penetrates the muscle; often associated with placenta previa.

O43.221 Placenta increta, first trimester Ⓜ♀

O43.222 Placenta increta, second trimester Ⓜ♀

O43.223 Placenta increta, third trimester Ⓜ♀

O43.229 Placenta increta, unspecified trimester Ⓜ♀

√6ᵗʰ **O43.23 Placenta percreta**

DEF: Condition where the placenta attaches through the uterine muscle and may invade other organs, resulting in antenatal complications, premature delivery, retention of all or a portion of the placenta, or postpartum bleeding.

O43.231 Placenta percreta, first trimester Ⓜ♀

O43.232 Placenta percreta, second trimester Ⓜ♀

O43.233 Placenta percreta, third trimester Ⓜ♀

O43.239 Placenta percreta, unspecified trimester Ⓜ♀

√5ᵗʰ **O43.8 Other placental disorders**

√6ᵗʰ **O43.81 Placental infarction**

O43.811 Placental infarction, first trimester Ⓜ♀

O43.812 Placental infarction, second trimester Ⓜ♀

O43.813 Placental infarction, third trimester Ⓜ♀

O43.819 Placental infarction, unspecified trimester Ⓜ♀

√6ᵗʰ **O43.89 Other placental disorders**

Placental dysfunction

O43.891 Other placental disorders, first trimester Ⓜ♀

O43.892 Other placental disorders, second trimester Ⓜ♀

O43.893 Other placental disorders, third trimester Ⓜ♀

O43.899 Other placental disorders, unspecified trimester Ⓜ♀

√5ᵗʰ **O43.9 Unspecified placental disorder**

O43.90 Unspecified placental disorder, unspecified trimester Ⓜ♀

O43.91 Unspecified placental disorder, first trimester Ⓜ♀

O43.92 Unspecified placental disorder, second trimester Ⓜ♀

O43.93 Unspecified placental disorder, third trimester Ⓜ♀

√4ᵗʰ **O44 Placenta previa**

AHA: 2016,4Q,52-53

DEF: Placenta implanted in the lower segment of the uterus, which commonly causes hemorrhage in the last trimester of pregnancy.

√5ᵗʰ **O44.0 Complete placenta previa NOS or without hemorrhage**

Placenta previa NOS

O44.00 Complete placenta previa NOS or without hemorrhage, unspecified trimester Ⓜ♀

O44.01 Complete placenta previa NOS or without hemorrhage, first trimester 𝖢𝖢 Ⓜ♀

O44.02 Complete placenta previa NOS or without hemorrhage, second trimester 𝖢𝖢 Ⓜ♀

☑ Additional Character Required   √x7ᵗʰ Placeholder   Unacceptable PDx   Questionable PDx   Manifestation   Unspecified Dx   𝐇𝟏-𝐇𝟒 HAC   𝐇𝐂𝐂 CMS-HCC Dx   𝐇𝐈𝐕 HIV Dx

ICD-10-CM 2021   887

     O44.Ø3   **Complete placenta previa NOS or without hemorrhage,** third trimester   CC M ♀

√5ᵗʰ **O44.1**   Complete **placenta previa** with hemorrhage

      EXCLUDES 1   *labor and delivery complicated by hemorrhage from vasa previa (O69.4)*

     O44.1Ø   **Complete placenta previa with hemorrhage, unspecified trimester**   M ♀

     O44.11   **Complete placenta previa with hemorrhage,** first trimester   MCC M ♀

     O44.12   **Complete placenta previa with hemorrhage,** second trimester   MCC M ♀

     O44.13   **Complete placenta previa with hemorrhage,** third trimester   MCC M ♀

√5ᵗʰ **O44.2**   Partial **placenta previa** without hemorrhage

     Marginal placenta previa, NOS or without hemorrhage

     O44.2Ø   **Partial placenta previa NOS or without hemorrhage, unspecified trimester**   M ♀

     O44.21   **Partial placenta previa NOS or without hemorrhage, first trimester**   CC M ♀

     O44.22   **Partial placenta previa NOS or without hemorrhage, second trimester**   CC M ♀

     O44.23   **Partial placenta previa NOS or without hemorrhage, third trimester**   CC ♀

√5ᵗʰ **O44.3**   Partial **placenta previa** with hemorrhage

     Marginal placenta previa with hemorrhage

     O44.3Ø   **Partial placenta previa with hemorrhage, unspecified trimester**   M ♀

     O44.31   **Partial placenta previa with hemorrhage,** first trimester   MCC M ♀

     O44.32   **Partial placenta previa with hemorrhage,** second trimester   MCC M ♀

     O44.33   **Partial placenta previa with hemorrhage,** third trimester   MCC ♀

√5ᵗʰ **O44.4**   Low lying **placenta NOS or** without hemorrhage

     Low implantation of placenta NOS or without hemorrhage

     O44.4Ø   **Low lying placenta NOS or without hemorrhage, unspecified trimester**   M ♀

     O44.41   **Low lying placenta NOS or without hemorrhage, first trimester**   CC M ♀

     O44.42   **Low lying placenta NOS or without hemorrhage,** second trimester   CC M ♀

     O44.43   **Low lying placenta NOS or without hemorrhage,** third trimester   CC M ♀

√5ᵗʰ **O44.5**   Low lying **placenta** with hemorrhage

     Low implantation of placenta with hemorrhage

     O44.5Ø   **Low lying placenta with hemorrhage, unspecified trimester**   M ♀

     O44.51   **Low lying placenta with hemorrhage,** first trimester   MCC M ♀

     O44.52   **Low lying placenta with hemorrhage,** second trimester   MCC M ♀

     O44.53   **Low lying placenta with hemorrhage,** third trimester   MCC M ♀

√4ᵗʰ **O45**   **Premature separation of placenta [abruptio placentae]**

√5ᵗʰ **O45.Ø**   **Premature separation of placenta** with coagulation defect

√6ᵗʰ   **O45.ØØ**   **Premature separation of placenta with coagulation defect, unspecified**

     O45.ØØ1   **Premature separation of placenta with coagulation defect, unspecified,** first trimester   MCC M ♀

     O45.ØØ2   **Premature separation of placenta with coagulation defect, unspecified,** second trimester   MCC ♀

     O45.ØØ3   **Premature separation of placenta with coagulation defect, unspecified,** third trimester   MCC M ♀

     O45.ØØ9   **Premature separation of placenta with coagulation defect, unspecified, unspecified trimester**   M ♀

√6ᵗʰ   **O45.Ø1**   **Premature separation of placenta** with afibrinogenemia

     Premature separation of placenta with hypofibrinogenemia

     O45.Ø11   **Premature separation of placenta with afibrinogenemia,** first trimester   MCC M ♀

     O45.Ø12   **Premature separation of placenta with afibrinogenemia,** second trimester   MCC M ♀

     O45.Ø13   **Premature separation of placenta with afibrinogenemia,** third trimester   MCC M ♀

     O45.Ø19   **Premature separation of placenta with afibrinogenemia, unspecified trimester**   M ♀

√6ᵗʰ   **O45.Ø2**   **Premature separation of placenta** with disseminated intravascular coagulation

     O45.Ø21   **Premature separation of placenta with disseminated intravascular coagulation, first trimester**   MCC M ♀

     O45.Ø22   **Premature separation of placenta with disseminated intravascular coagulation, second trimester**   MCC M ♀

     O45.Ø23   **Premature separation of placenta with disseminated intravascular coagulation, third trimester**   MCC M ♀

     O45.Ø29   **Premature separation of placenta with disseminated intravascular coagulation, unspecified trimester**   M ♀

√6ᵗʰ   **O45.Ø9**   **Premature separation of placenta with other coagulation defect**

     O45.Ø91   **Premature separation of placenta with other coagulation defect,** first trimester   MCC M ♀

     O45.Ø92   **Premature separation of placenta with other coagulation defect,** second trimester   MCC M ♀

     O45.Ø93   **Premature separation of placenta with other coagulation defect,** third trimester   MCC M ♀

     O45.Ø99   **Premature separation of placenta with other coagulation defect, unspecified trimester**   M ♀

√5ᵗʰ **O45.8**   **Other premature separation of placenta**

√6ᵗʰ   **O45.8X**   **Other premature separation of placenta**

     O45.8X1   **Other premature separation of placenta,** first trimester   MCC M ♀

     O45.8X2   **Other premature separation of placenta,** second trimester   MCC M ♀

     O45.8X3   **Other premature separation of placenta,** third trimester   MCC M ♀

     O45.8X9   **Other premature separation of placenta, unspecified trimester**   M ♀

√5ᵗʰ **O45.9**   **Premature separation of placenta, unspecified**

     Abruptio placentae NOS

     O45.9Ø   **Premature separation of placenta, unspecified, unspecified trimester**   M ♀

     O45.91   **Premature separation of placenta, unspecified,** first trimester   MCC M ♀

     O45.92   **Premature separation of placenta, unspecified,** second trimester   MCC M ♀

     O45.93   **Premature separation of placenta, unspecified,** third trimester   MCC M ♀

√4ᵗʰ **O46**   **Antepartum hemorrhage, not elsewhere classified**

      EXCLUDES 1   *hemorrhage in early pregnancy (O2Ø.-)*

                intrapartum hemorrhage NEC (O67.-)

                placenta previa (O44.-)

                premature separation of placenta [abruptio placentae] (O45.-)

     DEF: Uterine hemorrhage prior to delivery that is not related to placenta previa or abruptio placentae.

√5ᵗʰ **O46.Ø**   **Antepartum hemorrhage** with coagulation defect

√6ᵗʰ   **O46.ØØ**   **Antepartum hemorrhage with coagulation defect, unspecified**

     O46.ØØ1   **Antepartum hemorrhage with coagulation defect, unspecified,** first trimester   MCC M ♀

     O46.ØØ2   **Antepartum hemorrhage with coagulation defect, unspecified,** second trimester   MCC M ♀

     O46.ØØ3   **Antepartum hemorrhage with coagulation defect, unspecified,** third trimester   MCC M ♀

     O46.ØØ9   **Antepartum hemorrhage with coagulation defect, unspecified, unspecified trimester**   M ♀

N Newborn: 0   P Pediatric: 0-17   M Maternity: 9-64   A Adult: 15-124   MCC Major Complication/Comorbidity   CC Complication/Comorbidity   SW Severe Wound Dx

888   ICD-10-CM 2021

√6ᵗʰ **O46.Ø1 Antepartum hemorrhage** with afibrinogenemia
Antepartum hemorrhage with hypofibrinogenemia

O46.Ø11 Antepartum hemorrhage with afibrinogenemia, first trimester MCC M ♀

O46.Ø12 Antepartum hemorrhage with afibrinogenemia, second trimester MCC M ♀

O46.Ø13 Antepartum hemorrhage with afibrinogenemia, third trimester MCC M ♀

O46.Ø19 Antepartum hemorrhage with afibrinogenemia, unspecified trimester M ♀

√6ᵗʰ **O46.Ø2 Antepartum hemorrhage** with disseminated intravascular coagulation

O46.Ø21 Antepartum hemorrhage with disseminated intravascular coagulation, first trimester MCC M ♀

O46.Ø22 Antepartum hemorrhage with disseminated intravascular coagulation, second trimester MCC M ♀

O46.Ø23 Antepartum hemorrhage with disseminated intravascular coagulation, third trimester MCC M ♀

O46.Ø29 Antepartum hemorrhage with disseminated intravascular coagulation, unspecified trimester M ♀

√6ᵗʰ **O46.Ø9 Antepartum hemorrhage with** other **coagulation defect**

O46.Ø91 Antepartum hemorrhage with other coagulation defect, first trimester MCC M ♀

O46.Ø92 Antepartum hemorrhage with other coagulation defect, second trimester MCC M ♀

O46.Ø93 Antepartum hemorrhage with other coagulation defect, third trimester MCC M ♀

O46.Ø99 Antepartum hemorrhage with other coagulation defect, unspecified trimester M ♀

√5ᵗʰ **O46.8 Other antepartum hemorrhage**

√6ᵗʰ **O46.8X Other antepartum hemorrhage**

O46.8X1 Other antepartum hemorrhage, first **trimester** M ♀

O46.8X2 Other antepartum hemorrhage, second **trimester** M ♀

O46.8X3 Other antepartum hemorrhage, third **trimester** M ♀

O46.8X9 Other antepartum hemorrhage, unspecified trimester M ♀

√5ᵗʰ **O46.9 Antepartum hemorrhage, unspecified**

O46.9Ø Antepartum hemorrhage, unspecified, unspecified trimester M ♀

O46.91 Antepartum hemorrhage, unspecified, first trimester M ♀

O46.92 Antepartum hemorrhage, unspecified, second trimester M ♀

O46.93 Antepartum hemorrhage, unspecified, third trimester M ♀

√4ᵗʰ **O47 False labor**

INCLUDES   Braxton Hicks contractions
threatened labor
EXCLUDES 1   *preterm labor (O6Ø.-)*

√5ᵗʰ **O47.Ø False labor** before 37 completed weeks of gestation

O47.ØØ False labor before 37 completed weeks of gestation, unspecified trimester M ♀

O47.Ø2 False labor before 37 completed weeks of gestation, second trimester CC M ♀

O47.Ø3 False labor before 37 completed weeks of gestation, third trimester CC M ♀

O47.1 False labor at or after 37 completed weeks of gestation CC M ♀

O47.9 False labor, unspecified M ♀

√4ᵗʰ **O48 Late pregnancy**

O48.Ø Post-term pregnancy M ♀
Pregnancy over 4Ø completed weeks to 42 completed weeks gestation

O48.1 Prolonged pregnancy M ♀
Pregnancy which has advanced beyond 42 completed weeks gestation
AHA: 2016,1Q,5

Complications of labor and delivery (O6Ø-O77)

√4ᵗʰ **O6Ø Preterm labor**

INCLUDES   onset (spontaneous) of labor before 37 completed weeks of gestation
EXCLUDES 1   *false labor (O47.Ø-)*
threatened labor NOS (O47.Ø-)

√5ᵗʰ **O6Ø.Ø Preterm labor** without delivery

O6Ø.ØØ Preterm labor without delivery, unspecified trimester M ♀

O6Ø.Ø2 Preterm labor without delivery, second trimester MCC M ♀

O6Ø.Ø3 Preterm labor without delivery, third trimester MCC M ♀

√5ᵗʰ **O6Ø.1 Preterm labor** with preterm delivery
AHA: 2016,2Q,10

One of the following 7th characters is to be assigned to each code under subcategory O6Ø.1. 7th character Ø is for single gestations and multiple gestations where the fetus is unspecified. 7th characters 1 through 9 are for cases of multiple gestations to identify the fetus for which the code applies. The appropriate code from category O3Ø, Multiple gestation, must also be assigned when assigning a code from subcategory O6Ø.1 that has a 7th character of 1 through 9.
Ø   not applicable or unspecified
1   fetus 1
2   fetus 2
3   fetus 3
4   fetus 4
5   fetus 5
9   other fetus

√x7ᵗʰ **O6Ø.1Ø Preterm labor with preterm delivery, unspecified trimester** CC M ♀
Preterm labor with delivery NOS

√x7ᵗʰ **O6Ø.12 Preterm labor** second trimester **with preterm delivery** second trimester MCC M ♀

√x7ᵗʰ **O6Ø.13 Preterm labor** second trimester **with preterm delivery** third trimester MCC M ♀

√x7ᵗʰ **O6Ø.14 Preterm labor** third trimester **with preterm delivery** third trimester MCC M ♀

√5ᵗʰ **O6Ø.2 Term delivery with preterm labor**

One of the following 7th characters is to be assigned to each code under subcategory O6Ø.2. 7th character Ø is for single gestations and multiple gestations where the fetus is unspecified. 7th characters 1 through 9 are for cases of multiple gestations to identify the fetus for which the code applies. The appropriate code from category O3Ø, Multiple gestation, must also be assigned when assigning a code from subcategory O6Ø.2 that has a 7th character of 1 through 9.
Ø   not applicable or unspecified
1   fetus 1
2   fetus 2
3   fetus 3
4   fetus 4
5   fetus 5
9   other fetus

√x7ᵗʰ **O6Ø.2Ø Term delivery with preterm labor, unspecified trimester** CC M ♀

√x7ᵗʰ **O6Ø.22 Term delivery with preterm labor,** second trimester MCC M ♀

√x7ᵗʰ **O6Ø.23 Term delivery with preterm labor,** third trimester MCC M ♀

√4ᵗʰ **O61 Failed induction of labor**

O61.Ø Failed medical **induction of labor** M ♀
Failed induction (of labor) by oxytocin
Failed induction (of labor) by prostaglandins

Chapter 15. Pregnancy, Childbirth and the Puerperium

O46.Ø1–O61.Ø

O61.1 Failed instrumental induction of labor Ⓜ ♀
Failed mechanical induction (of labor)
Failed surgical induction (of labor)

O61.8 Other failed induction of labor Ⓜ ♀

O61.9 Failed induction of labor, unspecified Ⓜ ♀

✓4ᵗʰ **O62 Abnormalities of forces of labor**
DEF: Uterine inertia: Weak or poorly coordinated contractions of the uterus during labor.

O62.0 Primary inadequate contractions Ⓜ ♀
Failure of cervical dilatation
Primary hypotonic uterine dysfunction
Uterine inertia during latent phase of labor

O62.1 Secondary uterine inertia Ⓜ ♀
Arrested active phase of labor
Secondary hypotonic uterine dysfunction

O62.2 Other uterine inertia Ⓜ ♀
Atony of uterus without hemorrhage
Atony of uterus NOS
Desultory labor
Hypotonic uterine dysfunction NOS
Irregular labor
Poor contractions
Slow slope active phase of labor
Uterine inertia NOS
> EXCLUDES 1   *atony of uterus with hemorrhage (postpartum) (O72.1)*
> *postpartum atony of uterus without hemorrhage (O75.89)*

DEF: Uterine atony: Failure of the uterine muscles to contract after the fetus and placenta are delivered.

O62.3 Precipitate labor Ⓜ ♀
DEF: Rapid labor with delivery occurring in three hours or less from the onset of contractions.

O62.4 Hypertonic, incoordinate, and prolonged uterine contractions Ⓜ ♀
Cervical spasm
Contraction ring dystocia
Dyscoordinate labor
Hour-glass contraction of uterus
Hypertonic uterine dysfunction
Incoordinate uterine action
Tetanic contractions
Uterine dystocia NOS
Uterine spasm
> EXCLUDES 1   *dystocia (fetal) (maternal) NOS (O66.9)*

O62.8 Other abnormalities of forces of labor Ⓜ ♀

O62.9 Abnormality of forces of labor, unspecified Ⓜ ♀

✓4ᵗʰ **O63 Long labor**

O63.0 Prolonged first stage (of labor) Ⓜ ♀

O63.1 Prolonged second stage (of labor) Ⓜ ♀

O63.2 Delayed delivery of second twin, triplet, etc. Ⓜ ♀

O63.9 Long labor, unspecified cc Ⓜ ♀
Prolonged labor NOS

✓4ᵗʰ **O64 Obstructed labor due to malposition and malpresentation of fetus**

One of the following 7th characters is to be assigned to each code under category O64. 7th character 0 is for single gestations and multiple gestations where the fetus is unspecified. 7th characters 1 through 9 are for cases of multiple gestations to identify the fetus for which the code applies. The appropriate code from category O30, Multiple gestation, must also be assigned when assigning a code from category O64 that has a 7th character of 1 through 9.
0   not applicable or unspecified
1   fetus 1
2   fetus 2
3   fetus 3
4   fetus 4
5   fetus 5
9   other fetus

Fetal Malposition

Breech

Shoulder
(arm prolapse)

Mother's pelvis

Compound
(extremity together with head)

Oblique

Face
(mentum)

✓x7ᵗʰ **O64.0 Obstructed labor due to incomplete rotation of fetal head** Ⓜ ♀
Deep transverse arrest
Obstructed labor due to persistent occipitoiliac (position)
Obstructed labor due to persistent occipitoposterior (position)
Obstructed labor due to persistent occipitosacral (position)
Obstructed labor due to persistent occipitotransverse (position)

✓x7ᵗʰ **O64.1 Obstructed labor due to breech presentation** Ⓜ ♀
Obstructed labor due to buttocks presentation
Obstructed labor due to complete breech presentation
Obstructed labor due to frank breech presentation

✓x7ᵗʰ **O64.2 Obstructed labor due to face presentation** Ⓜ ♀
Obstructed labor due to chin presentation

✓x7ᵗʰ **O64.3 Obstructed labor due to brow presentation** Ⓜ ♀

✓x7ᵗʰ **O64.4 Obstructed labor due to shoulder presentation** Ⓜ ♀
Prolapsed arm
> EXCLUDES 1   *impacted shoulders (O66.0)*
> *shoulder dystocia (O66.0)*

✓x7ᵗʰ **O64.5 Obstructed labor due to compound presentation** Ⓜ ♀

✓x7ᵗʰ **O64.8 Obstructed labor due to other malposition and malpresentation** Ⓜ ♀
Obstructed labor due to footling presentation
Obstructed labor due to incomplete breech presentation

✓x7ᵗʰ **O64.9 Obstructed labor due to malposition and malpresentation, unspecified** Ⓜ ♀

✓4ᵗʰ **O65 Obstructed labor due to maternal pelvic abnormality**

O65.0 Obstructed labor due to deformed pelvis Ⓜ ♀
O65.1 Obstructed labor due to generally contracted pelvis Ⓜ ♀
O65.2 Obstructed labor due to pelvic inlet contraction Ⓜ ♀
O65.3 Obstructed labor due to pelvic outlet and mid-cavity contraction Ⓜ ♀
O65.4 Obstructed labor due to fetopelvic disproportion, unspecified Ⓜ ♀
> EXCLUDES 1   *dystocia due to abnormality of fetus (O66.2-O66.3)*

O65.5 **Obstructed labor due to** abnormality of maternal pelvic organs   M ♀
    Obstructed labor due to conditions listed in O34.-
    Use additional code to identify abnormality of pelvic organs O34.-

O65.8 **Obstructed labor due to other maternal pelvic abnormalities**   M ♀

O65.9 **Obstructed labor due to maternal pelvic abnormality, unspecified**   M ♀

✓4ᵗʰ **O66** **Other obstructed labor**

O66.0 **Obstructed labor due to** shoulder dystocia   M ♀
    Impacted shoulders
    DEF: Obstructed labor due to impacted fetal shoulders. It is an emergency condition that may require cesarean section, forceps delivery, vacuum extraction, or symphysiotomy.

O66.1 **Obstructed labor due to** locked twins   M ♀

O66.2 **Obstructed labor due to** unusually large fetus   M ♀

O66.3 **Obstructed labor due to other abnormalities of fetus**   M ♀
    Dystocia due to fetal ascites
    Dystocia due to fetal hydrops
    Dystocia due to fetal meningomyelocele
    Dystocia due to fetal sacral teratoma
    Dystocia due to fetal tumor
    Dystocia due to hydrocephalic fetus
    Use additional code to identify cause of obstruction

✓5ᵗʰ **O66.4** **Failed trial of labor**

    O66.40 **Failed trial of labor, unspecified**   M ♀

    O66.41 **Failed** attempted vaginal birth after previous cesarean delivery   M ♀
       Code first rupture of uterus, if applicable (O71.0-, O71.1)

O66.5 **Attempted application of** vacuum extractor and forceps   M ♀
    Attempted application of vacuum or forceps, with subsequent delivery by forceps or cesarean delivery

O66.6 **Obstructed labor due to other multiple fetuses**   M ♀

O66.8 **Other specified obstructed labor**   M ♀
    Use additional code to identify cause of obstruction

O66.9 **Obstructed labor, unspecified**   M ♀
    Dystocia NOS
    Fetal dystocia NOS
    Maternal dystocia NOS

✓4ᵗʰ **O67** **Labor and delivery complicated by intrapartum hemorrhage, not elsewhere classified**
    EXCLUDES 1   *antepartum hemorrhage NEC (O46.-)*
       placenta previa (O44.-)
       premature separation of placenta [abruptio placentae] (O45.-)
    EXCLUDES 2   *postpartum hemorrhage (O72.-)*

O67.0 **Intrapartum hemorrhage with coagulation defect**   MCC M ♀
    Intrapartum hemorrhage (excessive) associated with afibrinogenemia
    Intrapartum hemorrhage (excessive) associated with disseminated intravascular coagulation
    Intrapartum hemorrhage (excessive) associated with hyperfibrinolysis
    Intrapartum hemorrhage (excessive) associated with hypofibrinogenemia

O67.8 **Other intrapartum hemorrhage**   M ♀
    Excessive intrapartum hemorrhage

O67.9 **Intrapartum hemorrhage, unspecified**   M ♀

O68 **Labor and delivery complicated by abnormality of fetal acid-base balance**   CC M ♀
    Fetal acidemia complicating labor and delivery
    Fetal acidosis complicating labor and delivery
    Fetal alkalosis complicating labor and delivery
    Fetal metabolic acidemia complicating labor and delivery
    EXCLUDES 1   *fetal stress NOS (O77.9)*
       labor and delivery complicated by electrocardiographic evidence of fetal stress (O77.8)
       labor and delivery complicated by ultrasonic evidence of fetal stress (O77.8)
    EXCLUDES 2   *abnormality in fetal heart rate or rhythm (O76)*
       labor and delivery complicated by meconium in amniotic fluid (O77.0)

✓4ᵗʰ **O69** **Labor and delivery complicated by umbilical cord complications**
    AHA: 2016,1Q,5

    One of the following 7th characters is to be assigned to each code under category O69. 7th character Ø is for single gestations and multiple gestations where the fetus is unspecified. 7th characters 1 through 9 are for cases of multiple gestations to identify the fetus for which the code applies. The appropriate code from category O30, Multiple gestation, must also be assigned when assigning a code from category O69 that has a 7th character of 1 through 9.
    Ø   not applicable or unspecified
    1   fetus 1
    2   fetus 2
    3   fetus 3
    4   fetus 4
    5   fetus 5
    9   other fetus

✓x 7ᵗʰ **O69.0** **Labor and delivery complicated by** prolapse of cord   M ♀
    DEF: Abnormal presentation of the fetus marked by a protruding umbilical cord during labor. It can cause fetal death.

✓x 7ᵗʰ **O69.1** **Labor and delivery complicated by** cord around neck, with compression   M ♀
    EXCLUDES 1   *labor and delivery complicated by cord around neck, without compression (O69.81)*

✓x 7ᵗʰ **O69.2** **Labor and delivery complicated by** other cord entanglement, with compression   M ♀
    Labor and delivery complicated by compression of cord NOS
    Labor and delivery complicated by entanglement of cords of twins in monoamniotic sac
    Labor and delivery complicated by knot in cord
    EXCLUDES 1   *labor and delivery complicated by other cord entanglement, without compression (O69.82)*

✓x 7ᵗʰ **O69.3** **Labor and delivery complicated by** short cord   M ♀

✓x 7ᵗʰ **O69.4** **Labor and delivery complicated by** vasa previa   M ♀
    Labor and delivery complicated by hemorrhage from vasa previa

✓x 7ᵗʰ **O69.5** **Labor and delivery complicated by** vascular lesion of cord   M ♀
    Labor and delivery complicated by cord bruising
    Labor and delivery complicated by cord hematoma
    Labor and delivery complicated by thrombosis of umbilical vessels

✓5ᵗʰ **O69.8** **Labor and delivery complicated by other cord complications**

    ✓x 7ᵗʰ **O69.81** **Labor and delivery complicated by** cord around neck, without compression   M ♀
       AHA: 2016,1Q,5

    ✓x 7ᵗʰ **O69.82** **Labor and delivery complicated by** other cord entanglement, without compression   M ♀

    ✓x 7ᵗʰ **O69.89** **Labor and delivery complicated by other cord complications**   M ♀

✓x 7ᵗʰ **O69.9** **Labor and delivery complicated by cord complication, unspecified**   M ♀

✓4ᵗʰ **O70** **Perineal laceration during delivery**
    INCLUDES   episiotomy extended by laceration
    EXCLUDES 1   *obstetric high vaginal laceration alone (O71.4)*
    AHA: 2016,2Q,34; 2016,1Q,3-4,5

O70.0 **First degree** perineal laceration during delivery   M ♀
    Perineal laceration, rupture or tear involving fourchette during delivery
    Perineal laceration, rupture or tear involving labia during delivery
    Perineal laceration, rupture or tear involving skin during delivery
    Perineal laceration, rupture or tear involving vagina during delivery
    Perineal laceration, rupture or tear involving vulva during delivery
    Slight perineal laceration, rupture or tear during delivery

O70.1 **Second degree** perineal laceration during delivery   M ♀
    Perineal laceration, rupture or tear during delivery as in O70.0, also involving pelvic floor
    Perineal laceration, rupture or tear during delivery as in O70.0, also involving perineal muscles
    Perineal laceration, rupture or tear during delivery as in O70.0, also involving vaginal muscles
    EXCLUDES 1   *perineal laceration involving anal sphincter (O70.2)*

✓ Additional Character Required   ✓x7ᵗʰ Placeholder   Unacceptable PDx   Questionable PDx   Manifestation   Unspecified Dx   H1-H14 HAC   HCC CMS-HCC Dx   HIV HIV Dx

O70.2 ✓5ᵗʰ **Third degree perineal laceration during delivery**
Perineal laceration, rupture or tear during delivery as in O70.1, also involving anal sphincter
Perineal laceration, rupture or tear during delivery as in O70.1, also involving rectovaginal septum
Perineal laceration, rupture or tear during delivery as in O70.1, also involving sphincter NOS
> EXCLUDES 1 *anal sphincter tear during delivery without third degree perineal laceration (O70.4)*
> *perineal laceration involving anal or rectal mucosa (O70.3)*

AHA: 2016,4Q,53-54

O70.20 **Third degree perineal laceration during delivery, unspecified** CC M ♀

O70.21 **Third degree perineal laceration during delivery, IIIa** CC M ♀
Third degree perineal laceration during delivery with less than 50% of external anal sphincter (EAS) thickness torn

O70.22 **Third degree perineal laceration during delivery, IIIb** CC M ♀
Third degree perineal laceration during delivery with more than 50% external anal sphincter (EAS) thickness torn

O70.23 **Third degree perineal laceration during delivery, IIIc** CC M ♀
Third degree perineal laceration during delivery with both external anal sphincter (EAS) and internal anal sphincter (IAS) torn

O70.3 **Fourth degree perineal laceration during delivery** CC M ♀
Perineal laceration, rupture or tear during delivery as in O70.2, also involving anal mucosa
Perineal laceration, rupture or tear during delivery as in O70.2, also involving rectal mucosa

O70.4 **Anal sphincter tear complicating delivery, not associated with third degree laceration** CC M ♀
> EXCLUDES 1 *anal sphincter tear with third degree perineal laceration (O70.2)*

O70.9 **Perineal laceration during delivery, unspecified** M ♀

O71 ✓4ᵗʰ **Other obstetric trauma**
> INCLUDES obstetric damage from instruments

O71.0 ✓5ᵗʰ **Rupture of uterus (spontaneous) before onset of labor**
> EXCLUDES 1 *disruption of (current) cesarean delivery wound (O90.0)*
> *laceration of uterus, NEC (O71.81)*

O71.00 **Rupture of uterus before onset of labor, unspecified trimester** M ♀

O71.02 **Rupture of uterus before onset of labor, second trimester** MCC M ♀

O71.03 **Rupture of uterus before onset of labor, third trimester** MCC M ♀

O71.1 **Rupture of uterus during labor** MCC M ♀
Rupture of uterus not stated as occurring before onset of labor
> EXCLUDES 1 *disruption of cesarean delivery wound (O90.0)*
> *laceration of uterus, NEC (O71.81)*

O71.2 **Postpartum inversion of uterus** CC M ♀

O71.3 **Obstetric laceration of cervix** CC M ♀
Annular detachment of cervix

O71.4 **Obstetric high vaginal laceration alone** CC M ♀
Laceration of vaginal wall without perineal laceration
> EXCLUDES 1 *obstetric high vaginal laceration with perineal laceration (O70.-)*

AHA: 2016,1Q,5

O71.5 **Other obstetric injury to pelvic organs** CC M ♀
Obstetric injury to bladder
Obstetric injury to urethra
> EXCLUDES 2 *obstetric periurethral trauma (O71.82)*

AHA: 2014,4Q,18

O71.6 **Obstetric damage to pelvic joints and ligaments** CC M ♀
Obstetric avulsion of inner symphyseal cartilage
Obstetric damage to coccyx
Obstetric traumatic separation of symphysis (pubis)

O71.7 **Obstetric hematoma of pelvis** CC M ♀
Obstetric hematoma of perineum
Obstetric hematoma of vagina
Obstetric hematoma of vulva

O71.8 ✓5ᵗʰ **Other specified obstetric trauma**

O71.81 **Laceration of uterus, not elsewhere classified** M ♀

O71.82 **Other specified trauma to perineum and vulva** M ♀
Obstetric periurethral trauma
AHA: 2016,1Q,4; 2014,4Q,18

O71.89 **Other specified obstetric trauma** M ♀

O71.9 **Obstetric trauma, unspecified** M ♀

O72 ✓4ᵗʰ **Postpartum hemorrhage**
> INCLUDES hemorrhage after delivery of fetus or infant

O72.0 **Third-stage hemorrhage** CC M ♀
Hemorrhage associated with retained, trapped or adherent placenta
Retained placenta NOS
Code also type of adherent placenta (O43.2-)
AHA: 2019,3Q,11

O72.1 **Other immediate postpartum hemorrhage** CC M ♀
Hemorrhage following delivery of placenta
Postpartum hemorrhage (atonic) NOS
Uterine atony with hemorrhage
> EXCLUDES 1 *uterine atony NOS (O62.2)*
> *uterine atony without hemorrhage (O62.2)*
> *postpartum atony of uterus without hemorrhage (O75.89)*

AHA: 2016,1Q,4
DEF: Uterine atony: Failure of the uterine muscles to contract after the fetus and placenta are delivered.

O72.2 **Delayed and secondary postpartum hemorrhage** CC M ♀
Hemorrhage associated with retained portions of placenta or membranes after the first 24 hours following delivery of placenta
Retained products of conception NOS, following delivery

O72.3 **Postpartum coagulation defects** M ♀
Postpartum afibrinogenemia
Postpartum fibrinolysis

O73 ✓4ᵗʰ **Retained placenta and membranes, without hemorrhage**
> EXCLUDES 1 *placenta accreta (O43.21-)*
> *placenta increta (O43.22-)*
> *placenta percreta (O43.23-)*

DEF: Postpartum condition resulting from failure to expel placental membrane tissues due to failed contractions of the uterine wall.

O73.0 **Retained placenta without hemorrhage** M ♀
Adherent placenta, without hemorrhage
Trapped placenta without hemorrhage

O73.1 **Retained portions of placenta and membranes, without hemorrhage** M ♀
Retained products of conception following delivery, without hemorrhage

O74 ✓4ᵗʰ **Complications of anesthesia during labor and delivery**
> INCLUDES maternal complications arising from the administration of a general, regional or local anesthetic, analgesic or other sedation during labor and delivery

Use additional code, if applicable, to identify specific complication

O74.0 **Aspiration pneumonitis due to anesthesia during labor and delivery** M ♀
Inhalation of stomach contents or secretions NOS due to anesthesia during labor and delivery
Mendelson's syndrome due to anesthesia during labor and delivery

O74.1 **Other pulmonary complications of anesthesia during labor and delivery** M ♀

O74.2 **Cardiac complications of anesthesia during labor and delivery** M ♀

O74.3 **Central nervous system complications of anesthesia during labor and delivery** M ♀

O74.4 **Toxic reaction to local anesthesia during labor and delivery** M ♀

O74.5 **Spinal and epidural anesthesia-induced headache during labor and delivery** M ♀

O74.6 **Other complications of spinal and epidural anesthesia during labor and delivery** M ♀

N Newborn: 0   P Pediatric: 0-17   M Maternity: 9-64   A Adult: 15-124   MCC Major Complication/Comorbidity   CC Complication/Comorbidity   SW Severe Wound Dx

892   ICD-10-CM 2021

O74.7 **Failed or difficult intubation** for anesthesia during labor and delivery   Ⓜ ♀

O74.8 Other complications of anesthesia during labor and delivery   Ⓜ ♀

O74.9 Complication of anesthesia during labor and delivery, unspecified   Ⓜ ♀

✓4ᵗʰ **O75** **Other complications of labor and delivery, not elsewhere classified**

   EXCLUDES 2   *puerperal (postpartum) infection (O86.-)*
          puerperal (postpartum) sepsis (O85)

O75.0 **Maternal distress during labor and delivery**   Ⓜ ♀

O75.1 **Shock during or following labor and delivery**   MCC Ⓜ ♀
    Obstetric shock following labor and delivery

O75.2 **Pyrexia during labor, not elsewhere classified**   CC Ⓜ ♀

O75.3 **Other infection during labor**   MCC Ⓜ ♀
    Sepsis during labor
    Use additional code (B95-B97), to identify infectious agent

O75.4 **Other complications of obstetric surgery and procedures**   Ⓜ ♀
    Cardiac arrest following obstetric surgery or procedures
    Cardiac failure following obstetric surgery or procedures
    Cerebral anoxia following obstetric surgery or procedures
    Pulmonary edema following obstetric surgery or procedures
    Use additional code to identify specific complication
    EXCLUDES 2   *complications of anesthesia during labor and delivery (O74.-)*
          disruption of obstetrical (surgical) wound (O90.0-O90.1)
          hematoma of obstetrical (surgical) wound (O90.2)
          infection of obstetrical (surgical) wound (O86.0-)

O75.5 **Delayed delivery after artificial rupture of membranes**   Ⓜ ♀

✓5ᵗʰ **O75.8** **Other specified complications of labor and delivery**

   O75.81 **Maternal exhaustion complicating labor and delivery**   Ⓜ ♀

   O75.82 **Onset (spontaneous) of labor after 37 completed weeks of gestation but before 39 completed weeks gestation, with delivery by (planned) cesarean section**   Ⓜ ♀
      Delivery by (planned) cesarean section occurring after 37 completed weeks of gestation but before 39 completed weeks gestation due to (spontaneous) onset of labor
      Code first to specify reason for planned cesarean section such as:
        cephalopelvic disproportion (normally formed fetus) (O33.9)
        previous cesarean delivery (O34.21)

   O75.89 **Other specified complications of labor and delivery**   Ⓜ ♀

O75.9 Complication of labor and delivery, unspecified   Ⓜ ♀

O76 **Abnormality in fetal heart rate and rhythm complicating labor and delivery**   Ⓜ ♀
    Depressed fetal heart rate tones complicating labor and delivery
    Fetal bradycardia complicating labor and delivery
    Fetal heart rate decelerations complicating labor and delivery
    Fetal heart rate irregularity complicating labor and delivery
    Fetal heart rate abnormal variability complicating labor and delivery
    Fetal tachycardia complicating labor and delivery
    Non-reassuring fetal heart rate or rhythm complicating labor and delivery
    EXCLUDES 1   *fetal stress NOS (O77.9)*
          labor and delivery complicated by electrocardiographic evidence of fetal stress (O77.8)
          labor and delivery complicated by ultrasonic evidence of fetal stress (O77.8)
    EXCLUDES 2   *fetal metabolic acidemia (O68)*
          other fetal stress (O77.0-O77.1)
    AHA: 2013,4Q,118

✓4ᵗʰ **O77** **Other fetal stress complicating labor and delivery**

O77.0 **Labor and delivery complicated by meconium in amniotic fluid**   Ⓜ ♀
    AHA: 2013,4Q,117-118

O77.1 **Fetal stress in labor or delivery due to drug administration**   Ⓜ ♀

O77.8 **Labor and delivery complicated by other evidence of fetal stress**   Ⓜ ♀
    Labor and delivery complicated by electrocardiographic evidence of fetal stress
    Labor and delivery complicated by ultrasonic evidence of fetal stress
    EXCLUDES 1   *abnormality of fetal acid-base balance (O68)*
          abnormality in fetal heart rate or rhythm (O76)
          fetal metabolic acidemia (O68)

O77.9 **Labor and delivery complicated by fetal stress, unspecified**   Ⓜ ♀
    EXCLUDES 1   *abnormality of fetal acid-base balance (O68)*
          abnormality in fetal heart rate or rhythm (O76)
          fetal metabolic acidemia (O68)

Encounter for delivery (O80-O82)

O80 **Encounter for full-term uncomplicated delivery**   Ⓜ ♀
    NOTE   Delivery requiring minimal or no assistance, with or without episiotomy, without fetal manipulation [e.g., rotation version] or instrumentation [forceps] of a spontaneous, cephalic, vaginal, full-term, single, live-born infant. This code is for use as a single diagnosis code and is not to be used with any other code from chapter 15.
    Use additional code to indicate outcome of delivery (Z37.0)
    AHA: 2016,4Q,150; 2014,2Q,9

O82 **Encounter for cesarean delivery without indication**   Ⓜ ♀
    Use additional code to indicate outcome of delivery (Z37.0)

Complications predominantly related to the puerperium (O85-O92)

EXCLUDES 2   *mental and behavioral disorders associated with the puerperium (F53.-)*
        obstetrical tetanus (A34)
        puerperal osteomalacia (M83.0)

O85 **Puerperal sepsis**   MCC Ⓜ ♀
    Postpartum sepsis
    Puerperal peritonitis
    Puerperal pyemia
    Use additional code (B95-B97), to identify infectious agent
    Use additional code (R65.2-) to identify severe sepsis, if applicable
    EXCLUDES 1   *fever of unknown origin following delivery (O86.4)*
          genital tract infection following delivery (O86.1-)
          obstetric pyemic and septic embolism (O88.3-)
          puerperal septic thrombophlebitis (O86.81)
          urinary tract infection following delivery (O86.2-)
    EXCLUDES 2   *sepsis during labor (O75.3)*
    AHA: 2020,2Q,32; 2019,2Q,39; 2018,4Q,23

✓4ᵗʰ **O86** **Other puerperal infections**
    Use additional code (B95-B97), to identify infectious agent
    EXCLUDES 2   *infection during labor (O75.3)*
          obstetrical tetanus (A34)

✓5ᵗʰ **O86.0** **Infection of obstetric surgical wound**
    Infected cesarean delivery wound following delivery
    Infected perineal repair following delivery
    EXCLUDES 1   *complications of procedures, not elsewhere classified (T81.4-)*
          postprocedural fever NOS (R50.82)
          postprocedural retroperitoneal abscess (K68.11)
    AHA: 2020,2Q,32; 2018,4Q,22-23,62

   O86.00 **Infection of obstetric surgical wound, unspecified**   Ⓜ ♀

   O86.01 **Infection of obstetric surgical wound, superficial incisional site**   Ⓜ ♀
      Subcutaneous abscess following an obstetrical procedure
      Stitch abscess following an obstetrical procedure

   O86.02 **Infection of obstetric surgical wound, deep incisional site**   Ⓜ ♀
      Intramuscular abscess following an obstetrical procedure
      Sub-fascial abscess following an obstetrical procedure
      AHA: 2020,2Q,32

☑ Additional Character Required   ✓x7ᵗʰ Placeholder   Unacceptable PDx   Questionable PDx   Manifestation   Unspecified Dx   H1-H4ᵗʰ HAC   HCC CMS-HCC Dx   HIV HIV Dx

ICD-10-CM 2021   **893**

Chapter 15. Pregnancy, Childbirth and the Puerperium

O86.03   **Infection of obstetric surgical wound, organ and space site**   M ♀
> Intraabdominal abscess following an obstetrical procedure
> Subphrenic abscess following an obstetrical procedure

O86.04   **Sepsis following an obstetrical procedure**   MCC M ♀
> Use additional code to identify the sepsis
> AHA: 2020,2Q,32; 2019,2Q,39

O86.09   **Infection of obstetric surgical wound, other surgical site**   M ♀

√5ᵗʰ **O86.1**   **Other infection of genital tract following delivery**

O86.11   **Cervicitis following delivery**   CC M ♀

O86.12   **Endometritis following delivery**   CC M ♀

O86.13   **Vaginitis following delivery**   CC M ♀

O86.19   **Other infection of genital tract following delivery**   CC M ♀

√5ᵗʰ **O86.2**   **Urinary tract infection following delivery**

O86.20   **Urinary tract infection following delivery, unspecified**   CC M ♀
> Puerperal urinary tract infection NOS

O86.21   **Infection of kidney following delivery**   CC M ♀

O86.22   **Infection of bladder following delivery**   CC M ♀
> Infection of urethra following delivery

O86.29   **Other urinary tract infection following delivery**   CC M ♀

O86.4   **Pyrexia of unknown origin following delivery**   CC ♀
> Puerperal infection NOS following delivery
> Puerperal pyrexia NOS following delivery
> EXCLUDES 2   pyrexia during labor (O75.2)
> **DEF:** Fever of unknown origin experienced by the mother after childbirth.

√5ᵗʰ **O86.8**   **Other specified puerperal infections**

O86.81   **Puerperal septic thrombophlebitis**   MCC M ♀

O86.89   **Other specified puerperal infections**   MCC M ♀

√4ᵗʰ **O87**   **Venous complications and hemorrhoids in the puerperium**
> INCLUDES   venous complications in labor, delivery and the puerperium
> EXCLUDES 2   obstetric embolism (O88.-)
>   puerperal septic thrombophlebitis (O86.81)
>   venous complications in pregnancy (O22.-)

O87.0   **Superficial thrombophlebitis in the puerperium**   CC M ♀
> Puerperal phlebitis NOS
> Puerperal thrombosis NOS

O87.1   **Deep phlebothrombosis in the puerperium**   MCC M ♀
> Deep vein thrombosis, postpartum
> Pelvic thrombophlebitis, postpartum
> Use additional code to identify the deep vein thrombosis (I82.4-, I82.5-, I82.62-, I82.72-)
> Use additional code, if applicable, for associated long-term (current) use of anticoagulants (Z79.01)

O87.2   **Hemorrhoids in the puerperium**   CC M ♀

O87.3   **Cerebral venous thrombosis in the puerperium**   CC M ♀
> Cerebrovenous sinus thrombosis in the puerperium

O87.4   **Varicose veins of lower extremity in the puerperium**   M ♀

O87.8   **Other venous complications in the puerperium**   CC M ♀
> Genital varices in the puerperium

O87.9   **Venous complication in the puerperium, unspecified**   M ♀
> Puerperal phlebopathy NOS

√4ᵗʰ **O88**   **Obstetric embolism**
> EXCLUDES 1   embolism complicating abortion NOS (O03.2)
>   embolism complicating ectopic or molar pregnancy (O08.2)
>   embolism complicating failed attempted abortion (O07.2)
>   embolism complicating induced abortion (O04.7)
>   embolism complicating spontaneous abortion (O03.2, O03.7)

√5ᵗʰ **O88.0**   **Obstetric air embolism**
> **DEF:** Sudden blocking of the pulmonary artery or right ventricle with air or nitrogen bubbles.

√6ᵗʰ **O88.01**   **Obstetric air embolism in pregnancy**

O88.011   **Air embolism in pregnancy, first trimester**   MCC M ♀

O88.012   **Air embolism in pregnancy, second trimester**   MCC M ♀

O88.013   **Air embolism in pregnancy, third trimester**   MCC M ♀

O88.019   **Air embolism in pregnancy, unspecified trimester**   M ♀

O88.02   **Air embolism in childbirth**   MCC M ♀

O88.03   **Air embolism in the puerperium**   MCC M ♀

√5ᵗʰ **O88.1**   **Amniotic fluid embolism**
> Anaphylactoid syndrome in pregnancy

√6ᵗʰ **O88.11**   **Amniotic fluid embolism in pregnancy**

O88.111   **Amniotic fluid embolism in pregnancy, first trimester**   MCC M ♀

O88.112   **Amniotic fluid embolism in pregnancy, second trimester**   MCC M ♀

O88.113   **Amniotic fluid embolism in pregnancy, third trimester**   MCC M ♀

O88.119   **Amniotic fluid embolism in pregnancy, unspecified trimester**   M ♀

O88.12   **Amniotic fluid embolism in childbirth**   MCC M ♀

O88.13   **Amniotic fluid embolism in the puerperium**   MCC M ♀

√5ᵗʰ **O88.2**   **Obstetric thromboembolism**

√6ᵗʰ **O88.21**   **Thromboembolism in pregnancy**
> Obstetric (pulmonary) embolism NOS

O88.211   **Thromboembolism in pregnancy, first trimester**   MCC M ♀

O88.212   **Thromboembolism in pregnancy, second trimester**   MCC M ♀

O88.213   **Thromboembolism in pregnancy, third trimester**   MCC M ♀

O88.219   **Thromboembolism in pregnancy, unspecified trimester**   M ♀

O88.22   **Thromboembolism in childbirth**   MCC M ♀

O88.23   **Thromboembolism in the puerperium**   MCC M ♀
> Puerperal (pulmonary) embolism NOS

√5ᵗʰ **O88.3**   **Obstetric pyemic and septic embolism**

√6ᵗʰ **O88.31**   **Pyemic and septic embolism in pregnancy**

O88.311   **Pyemic and septic embolism in pregnancy, first trimester**   MCC M ♀

O88.312   **Pyemic and septic embolism in pregnancy, second trimester**   MCC M ♀

O88.313   **Pyemic and septic embolism in pregnancy, third trimester**   MCC M ♀

O88.319   **Pyemic and septic embolism in pregnancy, unspecified trimester**   CC M ♀

O88.32   **Pyemic and septic embolism in childbirth**   MCC M ♀

O88.33   **Pyemic and septic embolism in the puerperium**   MCC M ♀

√5ᵗʰ **O88.8**   **Other obstetric embolism**
> Obstetric fat embolism

√6ᵗʰ **O88.81**   **Other embolism in pregnancy**

O88.811   **Other embolism in pregnancy, first trimester**   MCC M ♀

O88.812   **Other embolism in pregnancy, second trimester**   MCC M ♀

O88.813   **Other embolism in pregnancy, third trimester**   MCC M ♀

O88.819   **Other embolism in pregnancy, unspecified trimester**   M ♀

O88.82   **Other embolism in childbirth**   MCC M ♀

O88.83   **Other embolism in the puerperium**   MCC M ♀

√4ᵗʰ **O89**   **Complications of anesthesia during the puerperium**
> INCLUDES   maternal complications arising from the administration of a general, regional or local anesthetic, analgesic or other sedation during the puerperium
> Use additional code, if applicable, to identify specific complication

√5ᵗʰ **O89.0**   **Pulmonary complications of anesthesia during the puerperium**

O89.01   **Aspiration pneumonitis due to anesthesia during the puerperium**   M ♀
> Inhalation of stomach contents or secretions NOS due to anesthesia during the puerperium
> Mendelson's syndrome due to anesthesia during the puerperium

O89.09   **Other pulmonary complications of anesthesia during the puerperium**   M ♀

O89.1   **Cardiac complications of anesthesia during the puerperium**   M ♀

O89.2 **Central nervous system complications of anesthesia during the puerperium**   M ♀

O89.3 **Toxic reaction to local anesthesia during the puerperium**   M ♀

O89.4 **Spinal and epidural anesthesia-induced headache during the puerperium**   M ♀

O89.5 **Other complications of spinal and epidural anesthesia during the puerperium**   M ♀

O89.6 **Failed or difficult intubation for anesthesia during the puerperium**   M ♀

O89.8 **Other complications of anesthesia during the puerperium**   M ♀

O89.9 **Complication of anesthesia during the puerperium, unspecified**   M ♀

✓4ᵗʰ O90 **Complications of the puerperium, not elsewhere classified**

     O90.0 **Disruption of cesarean delivery wound**   M ♀
Dehiscence of cesarean delivery wound
EXCLUDES 1   *rupture of uterus (spontaneous) before onset of labor (O71.0-)*
     rupture of uterus during labor (O71.1)

     O90.1 **Disruption of perineal obstetric wound**   M ♀
Disruption of wound of episiotomy
Disruption of wound of perineal laceration
Secondary perineal tear

     O90.2 **Hematoma of obstetric wound**   M ♀

     O90.3 **Peripartum cardiomyopathy**   MCC M ♀
Conditions in I42- arising during pregnancy and the puerperium
EXCLUDES 1   *pre-existing heart disease complicating pregnancy and the puerperium (O99.4-)*
DEF: Any structural or functional abnormality of the ventricular myocardium. It is a noninflammatory disease of obscure or unknown etiology with onset during the postpartum period.

     O90.4 **Postpartum acute kidney failure**   MCC M ♀
Hepatorenal syndrome following labor and delivery

     O90.5 **Postpartum thyroiditis**   M ♀

     O90.6 **Postpartum mood disturbance**   M ♀
Postpartum blues
Postpartum dysphoria
Postpartum sadness
EXCLUDES 1   *postpartum depression (F53.0)*
     puerperal psychosis (F53.1)

✓5ᵗʰ O90.8 **Other complications of the puerperium, not elsewhere classified**

     O90.81 **Anemia of the puerperium**   M ♀
Postpartum anemia NOS
EXCLUDES 1   *pre-existing anemia complicating the puerperium (O99.03)*
AHA: 2019,3Q,11

     O90.89 **Other complications of the puerperium, not elsewhere classified**   M ♀
Placental polyp

     O90.9 **Complication of the puerperium, unspecified**   M ♀

✓4ᵗʰ O91 **Infections of breast associated with pregnancy, the puerperium and lactation**
Use additional code to identify infection

✓5ᵗʰ O91.0 **Infection of nipple associated with pregnancy, the puerperium and lactation**

     ✓6ᵗʰ O91.01 **Infection of nipple associated with pregnancy**
Gestational abscess of nipple

       O91.011 **Infection of nipple associated with pregnancy, first trimester**   M ♀

       O91.012 **Infection of nipple associated with pregnancy, second trimester**   M ♀

       O91.013 **Infection of nipple associated with pregnancy, third trimester**   M ♀

       O91.019 **Infection of nipple associated with pregnancy, unspecified trimester**   M ♀

     O91.02 **Infection of nipple associated with the puerperium**   M ♀
Puerperal abscess of nipple

     O91.03 **Infection of nipple associated with lactation**   M ♀
Abscess of nipple associated with lactation

✓5ᵗʰ O91.1 **Abscess of breast associated with pregnancy, the puerperium and lactation**

     ✓6ᵗʰ O91.11 **Abscess of breast associated with pregnancy**
Gestational mammary abscess
Gestational purulent mastitis
Gestational subareolar abscess

       O91.111 **Abscess of breast associated with pregnancy, first trimester**   M ♀

       O91.112 **Abscess of breast associated with pregnancy, second trimester**   M ♀

       O91.113 **Abscess of breast associated with pregnancy, third trimester**   M ♀

       O91.119 **Abscess of breast associated with pregnancy, unspecified trimester**   M ♀

     O91.12 **Abscess of breast associated with the puerperium**   M ♀
Puerperal mammary abscess
Puerperal purulent mastitis
Puerperal subareolar abscess

     O91.13 **Abscess of breast associated with lactation**   M ♀
Mammary abscess associated with lactation
Purulent mastitis associated with lactation
Subareolar abscess associated with lactation

✓5ᵗʰ O91.2 **Nonpurulent mastitis associated with pregnancy, the puerperium and lactation**

     ✓6ᵗʰ O91.21 **Nonpurulent mastitis associated with pregnancy**
Gestational interstitial mastitis
Gestational lymphangitis of breast
Gestational mastitis NOS
Gestational parenchymatous mastitis

       O91.211 **Nonpurulent mastitis associated with pregnancy, first trimester**   M ♀

       O91.212 **Nonpurulent mastitis associated with pregnancy, second trimester**   M ♀

       O91.213 **Nonpurulent mastitis associated with pregnancy, third trimester**   M ♀

       O91.219 **Nonpurulent mastitis associated with pregnancy, unspecified trimester**   M ♀

     O91.22 **Nonpurulent mastitis associated with the puerperium**   M ♀
Puerperal interstitial mastitis
Puerperal lymphangitis of breast
Puerperal mastitis NOS
Puerperal parenchymatous mastitis

     O91.23 **Nonpurulent mastitis associated with lactation**   M ♀
Interstitial mastitis associated with lactation
Lymphangitis of breast associated with lactation
Mastitis NOS associated with lactation
Parenchymatous mastitis associated with lactation

✓4ᵗʰ O92 **Other disorders of breast and disorders of lactation associated with pregnancy and the puerperium**

✓5ᵗʰ O92.0 **Retracted nipple associated with pregnancy, the puerperium, and lactation**

     ✓6ᵗʰ O92.01 **Retracted nipple associated with pregnancy**

       O92.011 **Retracted nipple associated with pregnancy, first trimester**   M ♀

       O92.012 **Retracted nipple associated with pregnancy, second trimester**   M ♀

       O92.013 **Retracted nipple associated with pregnancy, third trimester**   M ♀

       O92.019 **Retracted nipple associated with pregnancy, unspecified trimester**   M ♀

     O92.02 **Retracted nipple associated with the puerperium**   M ♀

     O92.03 **Retracted nipple associated with lactation**   M ♀

✓5ᵗʰ O92.1 **Cracked nipple associated with pregnancy, the puerperium, and lactation**
Fissure of nipple, gestational or puerperal

     ✓6ᵗʰ O92.11 **Cracked nipple associated with pregnancy**

       O92.111 **Cracked nipple associated with pregnancy, first trimester**   M ♀

       O92.112 **Cracked nipple associated with pregnancy, second trimester**   M ♀

       O92.113 **Cracked nipple associated with pregnancy, third trimester**   M ♀

       O92.119 **Cracked nipple associated with pregnancy, unspecified trimester**   M ♀

O92.12   **Cracked nipple associated with the puerperium**   M ♀

O92.13   **Cracked nipple associated with** lactation   M ♀

✓5ᵗʰ   O92.2   **Other and unspecified disorders of breast associated with pregnancy and the puerperium**

O92.20   **Unspecified disorder of breast associated with pregnancy and the puerperium**   M ♀

O92.29   **Other disorders of breast associated with pregnancy and the puerperium**   M ♀

O92.3   **Agalactia**   M ♀

Primary agalactia

EXCLUDES 1   *elective agalactia (O92.5)*

secondary agalactia (O92.5)

therapeutic agalactia (O92.5)

DEF: Absence of milk secretion in a female after delivery.

O92.4   **Hypogalactia**   M ♀

O92.5   **Suppressed lactation**   M ♀

Elective agalactia

Secondary agalactia

Therapeutic agalactia

EXCLUDES 1   *primary agalactia (O92.3)*

O92.6   **Galactorrhea**   M ♀

DEF: Excessive or persistent milk secretion by the breast that may occur in the absence of nursing.

✓5ᵗʰ   O92.7   **Other and unspecified disorders of lactation**

O92.70   **Unspecified disorders of lactation**   M ♀

O92.79   **Other disorders of lactation**   M ♀

Puerperal galactocele

Other obstetric conditions, not elsewhere classified (O94-O9A)

O94   **Sequelae of complication of pregnancy, childbirth, and the puerperium**   M ♀

NOTE   This category is to be used to indicate conditions in O00-O77.-, O85-O94 and O98-O9A.- as the cause of late effects. The sequelae include conditions specified as such, or as late effects, which may occur at any time after the puerperium

Code first condition resulting from (sequela) of complication of pregnancy, childbirth, and the puerperium

✓4ᵗʰ   O98   **Maternal infectious and parasitic diseases classifiable elsewhere but complicating pregnancy, childbirth and the puerperium**

INCLUDES   the listed conditions when complicating the pregnant state, when aggravated by the pregnancy, or as a reason for obstetric care

Use additional code (Chapter 1), to identify specific infectious or parasitic disease

EXCLUDES 2   *herpes gestationis (O26.4-)*

infectious carrier state (O99.82-, O99.83-)

obstetrical tetanus (A34)

puerperal infection (O86.-)

puerperal sepsis (O85)

when the reason for maternal care is that the disease is known or suspected to have affected the fetus (O35-O36)

✓5ᵗʰ   O98.0   **Tuberculosis complicating pregnancy, childbirth and the puerperium**

Conditions in A15-A19

✓6ᵗʰ   O98.01   **Tuberculosis complicating** pregnancy

O98.011   **Tuberculosis complicating pregnancy, first trimester**   CC M ♀

O98.012   **Tuberculosis complicating pregnancy, second trimester**   CC M ♀

O98.013   **Tuberculosis complicating pregnancy, third trimester**   CC M ♀

O98.019   **Tuberculosis complicating pregnancy, unspecified trimester**   M ♀

O98.02   **Tuberculosis complicating** childbirth   CC M ♀

O98.03   **Tuberculosis complicating the puerperium**   CC M ♀

✓5ᵗʰ   O98.1   **Syphilis complicating pregnancy, childbirth and the puerperium**

Conditions in A50-A53

✓6ᵗʰ   O98.11   **Syphilis complicating** pregnancy

O98.111   **Syphilis complicating pregnancy, first trimester**   CC M ♀

O98.112   **Syphilis complicating pregnancy, second trimester**   CC M ♀

O98.113   **Syphilis complicating pregnancy, third trimester**   CC M ♀

O98.119   **Syphilis complicating pregnancy, unspecified trimester**   M ♀

O98.12   **Syphilis complicating** childbirth   CC M ♀

O98.13   **Syphilis complicating the** puerperium   CC M ♀

✓5ᵗʰ   O98.2   **Gonorrhea complicating pregnancy, childbirth and the puerperium**

Conditions in A54.-

✓6ᵗʰ   O98.21   **Gonorrhea complicating** pregnancy

O98.211   **Gonorrhea complicating pregnancy, first trimester**   CC M ♀

O98.212   **Gonorrhea complicating pregnancy, second trimester**   CC M ♀

O98.213   **Gonorrhea complicating pregnancy, third trimester**   CC M ♀

O98.219   **Gonorrhea complicating pregnancy, unspecified trimester**   M ♀

O98.22   **Gonorrhea complicating** childbirth   CC M ♀

O98.23   **Gonorrhea complicating the** puerperium   CC M ♀

✓5ᵗʰ   O98.3   **Other infections with a predominantly sexual mode of transmission complicating pregnancy, childbirth and the puerperium**

Conditions in A55-A64

AHA: 2020,1Q,20

✓6ᵗʰ   O98.31   **Other infections with a predominantly sexual mode of transmission complicating** pregnancy

O98.311   **Other infections with a predominantly sexual mode of transmission complicating pregnancy, first trimester**   CC M ♀

O98.312   **Other infections with a predominantly sexual mode of transmission complicating pregnancy, second trimester**   CC M ♀

O98.313   **Other infections with a predominantly sexual mode of transmission complicating pregnancy, third trimester**   CC M ♀

O98.319   **Other infections with a predominantly sexual mode of transmission complicating pregnancy, unspecified trimester**   M ♀

O98.32   **Other infections with a predominantly sexual mode of transmission complicating** childbirth   CC M ♀

O98.33   **Other infections with a predominantly sexual mode of transmission complicating the** puerperium   CC M ♀

✓5ᵗʰ   O98.4   **Viral hepatitis complicating pregnancy, childbirth and the puerperium**

Conditions in B15-B19

✓6ᵗʰ   O98.41   **Viral hepatitis complicating** pregnancy

O98.411   **Viral hepatitis complicating pregnancy, first trimester**   CC M ♀

O98.412   **Viral hepatitis complicating pregnancy, second trimester**   CC M ♀

O98.413   **Viral hepatitis complicating pregnancy, third trimester**   CC M ♀

O98.419   **Viral hepatitis complicating pregnancy, unspecified trimester**   M ♀

O98.42   **Viral hepatitis complicating** childbirth   CC M ♀

O98.43   **Viral hepatitis complicating the puerperium**   CC M ♀

✓5ᵗʰ   O98.5   **Other viral diseases complicating pregnancy, childbirth and the puerperium**

Conditions in A80-B09, B25-B34, R87.81-, R87.82-

EXCLUDES 1   *human immunodeficiency virus [HIV] disease complicating pregnancy, childbirth and the puerperium (O98.7-)*

TIP: Assign a code from this subcategory as the principal or first-listed diagnosis for a patient admitted/presenting during pregnancy, childbirth, or the puerperium because of COVID-19; assign U07.1 and codes for associated manifestations as secondary codes.

✓6ᵗʰ   O98.51   **Other viral diseases complicating** pregnancy

O98.511   **Other viral diseases complicating pregnancy, first trimester**   CC M ♀

O98.512   **Other viral diseases complicating pregnancy, second trimester**   CC M ♀

O98.513   **Other viral diseases complicating pregnancy, third trimester**   CC M ♀

N Newborn: 0   P Pediatric: 0-17   M Maternity: 9-64   A Adult: 15-124   MCC Major Complication/Comorbidity   CC Complication/Comorbidity   SW Severe Wound Dx

896   ICD-10-CM 2021

O98.519   **Other viral diseases complicating pregnancy, unspecified trimester**   M ♀

O98.52   **Other viral diseases complicating** childbirth   CC M ♀

O98.53   **Other viral diseases complicating the** puerperium   CC M ♀

√5ᵗʰ **O98.6**   Protozoal diseases **complicating pregnancy, childbirth and the puerperium**
Conditions in B50-B64

    √6ᵗʰ **O98.61**   **Protozoal diseases complicating** pregnancy

       O98.611   **Protozoal diseases complicating pregnancy, first trimester**   CC M ♀

       O98.612   **Protozoal diseases complicating pregnancy, second trimester**   CC M ♀

       O98.613   **Protozoal diseases complicating pregnancy, third trimester**   CC M ♀

       O98.619   **Protozoal diseases complicating pregnancy, unspecified trimester**   M ♀

    O98.62   **Protozoal diseases complicating** childbirth   CC M ♀

    O98.63   **Protozoal diseases complicating the** puerperium   CC M ♀

√5ᵗʰ **O98.7**   Human immunodeficiency virus [HIV] disease **complicating pregnancy, childbirth and the puerperium**
Use additional code to identify the type of HIV disease:
acquired immune deficiency syndrome (AIDS) (B20)
asymptomatic HIV status (Z21)
HIV positive NOS (Z21)
symptomatic HIV disease (B20)

    √6ᵗʰ **O98.71**   **Human immunodeficiency virus [HIV] disease complicating** pregnancy

       O98.711   **Human immunodeficiency virus [HIV] disease complicating pregnancy, first trimester**   CC M ♀

       O98.712   **Human immunodeficiency virus [HIV] disease complicating pregnancy, second trimester**   CC M ♀

       O98.713   **Human immunodeficiency virus [HIV] disease complicating pregnancy, third trimester**   CC M ♀

       O98.719   **Human immunodeficiency virus [HIV] disease complicating pregnancy, unspecified trimester**   M ♀

    O98.72   **Human immunodeficiency virus [HIV] disease complicating** childbirth   CC ♀

    O98.73   **Human immunodeficiency virus [HIV] disease complicating the** puerperium   CC ♀

√5ᵗʰ **O98.8**   **Other maternal infectious and parasitic diseases complicating pregnancy, childbirth and the puerperium**
AHA: 2020,1Q,10

    √6ᵗʰ **O98.81**   **Other maternal infectious and parasitic diseases complicating** pregnancy

       O98.811   **Other maternal infectious and parasitic diseases complicating pregnancy, first trimester**   CC M ♀

       O98.812   **Other maternal infectious and parasitic diseases complicating pregnancy, second trimester**   CC M ♀

       O98.813   **Other maternal infectious and parasitic diseases complicating pregnancy, third trimester**   CC M ♀

       O98.819   **Other maternal infectious and parasitic diseases complicating pregnancy, unspecified trimester**   M ♀

    O98.82   **Other maternal infectious and parasitic diseases complicating** childbirth   CC M ♀

    O98.83   **Other maternal infectious and parasitic diseases complicating the** puerperium   CC M ♀

√5ᵗʰ **O98.9**   **Unspecified maternal infectious and parasitic disease complicating pregnancy, childbirth and the puerperium**

    √6ᵗʰ **O98.91**   **Unspecified maternal infectious and parasitic disease complicating** pregnancy

       O98.911   **Unspecified maternal infectious and parasitic disease complicating pregnancy, first trimester**   CC M ♀

       O98.912   **Unspecified maternal infectious and parasitic disease complicating pregnancy, second trimester**   CC M ♀

       O98.913   **Unspecified maternal infectious and parasitic disease complicating pregnancy, third trimester**   CC M ♀

       O98.919   **Unspecified maternal infectious and parasitic disease complicating pregnancy, unspecified trimester**   M ♀

    O98.92   **Unspecified maternal infectious and parasitic disease complicating** childbirth   CC M ♀

    O98.93   **Unspecified maternal infectious and parasitic disease complicating the** puerperium   CC M ♀

√4ᵗʰ **O99**   **Other maternal diseases classifiable elsewhere but complicating pregnancy, childbirth and the puerperium**
INCLUDES   conditions which complicate the pregnant state, are aggravated by the pregnancy or are a main reason for obstetric care
Use additional code to identify specific condition
EXCLUDES 2   *when the reason for maternal care is that the condition is known or suspected to have affected the fetus (O35-O36)*

√5ᵗʰ **O99.0**   Anemia **complicating pregnancy, childbirth and the puerperium**
Conditions in D50-D64
EXCLUDES 1   *anemia arising in the puerperium (O90.81)*
postpartum anemia NOS (O90.81)
AHA: 2019,3Q,11

    √6ᵗʰ **O99.01**   **Anemia complicating** pregnancy
AHA: 2016,1Q,4

       O99.011   **Anemia complicating pregnancy, first trimester**   M ♀

       O99.012   **Anemia complicating pregnancy, second trimester**   M ♀

       O99.013   **Anemia complicating pregnancy, third trimester**   M ♀

       O99.019   **Anemia complicating pregnancy, unspecified trimester**   M ♀

    O99.02   **Anemia complicating** childbirth   M ♀

    O99.03   **Anemia complicating the** puerperium   M ♀
EXCLUDES 1   *postpartum anemia not pre-existing prior to delivery (O90.81)*

√5ᵗʰ **O99.1**   **Other diseases of the** blood and blood-forming organs and certain disorders involving the immune mechanism **complicating pregnancy, childbirth and the puerperium**
Conditions in D65-D89
EXCLUDES 1   *hemorrhage with coagulation defects (O45.-, O46.0-, O67.0, O72.3)*

    √6ᵗʰ **O99.11**   **Other diseases of the blood and blood-forming organs and certain disorders involving the immune mechanism complicating** pregnancy

       O99.111   **Other diseases of the blood and blood-forming organs and certain disorders involving the immune mechanism complicating pregnancy,** first trimester   CC M ♀

       O99.112   **Other diseases of the blood and blood-forming organs and certain disorders involving the immune mechanism complicating pregnancy,** second trimester   CC M ♀

       O99.113   **Other diseases of the blood and blood-forming organs and certain disorders involving the immune mechanism complicating pregnancy,** third trimester   CC M ♀

       O99.119   **Other diseases of the blood and blood-forming organs and certain disorders involving the immune mechanism complicating pregnancy, unspecified trimester**   CC M ♀

    O99.12   **Other diseases of the blood and blood-forming organs and certain disorders involving the immune mechanism complicating** childbirth   CC M ♀

    O99.13   **Other diseases of the blood and blood-forming organs and certain disorders involving the immune mechanism complicating the** puerperium   CC M ♀

Chapter 15. Pregnancy, Childbirth and the Puerperium

O99.2–O99.355

√5ᵗʰ **O99.2 Endocrine, nutritional and metabolic diseases complicating pregnancy, childbirth and the puerperium**
►Conditions in E00-E89◄

EXCLUDES 2   *diabetes mellitus (O24.-)*
     malnutrition (O25.-)
     postpartum thyroiditis (O90.5)

√6ᵗʰ **O99.21 Obesity complicating pregnancy, childbirth, and the puerperium**
Use additional code to identify the type of obesity (E66.-)
AHA: 2018,4Q,80
TIP: Do not assign a BMI code (Z68.-) for obese or overweight patients who are pregnant.

O99.210 Obesity complicating pregnancy, unspecified trimester Ⓜ♀

O99.211 Obesity complicating pregnancy, first trimester Ⓜ♀

O99.212 Obesity complicating pregnancy, second trimester Ⓜ♀

O99.213 Obesity complicating pregnancy, third trimester Ⓜ♀

O99.214 Obesity complicating childbirth Ⓜ♀

O99.215 Obesity complicating the puerperium Ⓜ♀

√6ᵗʰ **O99.28 Other endocrine, nutritional and metabolic diseases complicating pregnancy, childbirth and the puerperium**

O99.280 Endocrine, nutritional and metabolic diseases complicating pregnancy, unspecified trimester Ⓜ♀

O99.281 Endocrine, nutritional and metabolic diseases complicating pregnancy, first trimester Ⓜ♀

O99.282 Endocrine, nutritional and metabolic diseases complicating pregnancy, second trimester Ⓜ♀

O99.283 Endocrine, nutritional and metabolic diseases complicating pregnancy, third trimester Ⓜ♀

O99.284 Endocrine, nutritional and metabolic diseases complicating childbirth Ⓜ♀

O99.285 Endocrine, nutritional and metabolic diseases complicating the puerperium Ⓜ♀

√5ᵗʰ **O99.3 Mental disorders and diseases of the nervous system complicating pregnancy, childbirth and the puerperium**

√6ᵗʰ **O99.31 Alcohol use complicating pregnancy, childbirth, and the puerperium**
Use additional code(s) from F10 to identify manifestations of the alcohol use

O99.310 Alcohol use complicating pregnancy, unspecified trimester Ⓜ♀

O99.311 Alcohol use complicating pregnancy, first trimester Ⓜ♀

O99.312 Alcohol use complicating pregnancy, second trimester Ⓜ♀

O99.313 Alcohol use complicating pregnancy, third trimester Ⓜ♀

O99.314 Alcohol use complicating childbirth Ⓜ♀

O99.315 Alcohol use complicating the puerperium Ⓜ♀

√6ᵗʰ **O99.32 Drug use complicating pregnancy, childbirth, and the puerperium**
Use additional code(s) from F11-F16 and F18-F19 to identify manifestations of the drug use
AHA: 2018,4Q,69-70; 2018,2Q,10
TIP: When drug use is documented during pregnancy, assign first a code from this subcategory followed by an additional code from F11-F16 and F18-F19 identifying the specific drug use even if not documented as associated with a physical, mental, or behavioral disorder. According to chapter 15 guidelines, it is the provider's responsibility to state that the condition being treated is *not* affecting the pregnancy.

O99.320 Drug use complicating pregnancy, unspecified trimester Ⓜ♀

O99.321 Drug use complicating pregnancy, first trimester cc Ⓜ♀

O99.322 Drug use complicating pregnancy, second trimester cc Ⓜ♀

O99.323 Drug use complicating pregnancy, third trimester cc Ⓜ♀

O99.324 Drug use complicating childbirth cc Ⓜ♀

O99.325 Drug use complicating the puerperium cc Ⓜ♀

√6ᵗʰ **O99.33 Tobacco use disorder complicating pregnancy, childbirth, and the puerperium**
Smoking complicating pregnancy, childbirth, and the puerperium
Use additional code from category F17 to identify type of tobacco nicotine dependence

O99.330 Smoking (tobacco) complicating pregnancy, unspecified trimester Ⓜ♀

O99.331 Smoking (tobacco) complicating pregnancy, first trimester Ⓜ♀

O99.332 Smoking (tobacco) complicating pregnancy, second trimester Ⓜ♀

O99.333 Smoking (tobacco) complicating pregnancy, third trimester Ⓜ♀

O99.334 Smoking (tobacco) complicating childbirth Ⓜ♀

O99.335 Smoking (tobacco) complicating the puerperium Ⓜ♀

√6ᵗʰ **O99.34 Other mental disorders complicating pregnancy, childbirth, and the puerperium**
►Conditions in F01-F09, F20-F52 and F54-F99◄

EXCLUDES 2   *postpartum mood disturbance (O90.6)*
     postnatal psychosis (F53.1)
     puerperal psychosis (F53.1)

O99.340 Other mental disorders complicating pregnancy, unspecified trimester Ⓜ♀

O99.341 Other mental disorders complicating pregnancy, first trimester Ⓜ♀

O99.342 Other mental disorders complicating pregnancy, second trimester Ⓜ♀

O99.343 Other mental disorders complicating pregnancy, third trimester Ⓜ♀

O99.344 Other mental disorders complicating childbirth Ⓜ♀

O99.345 Other mental disorders complicating the puerperium Ⓜ♀
AHA: 2018,4Q,8

√6ᵗʰ **O99.35 Diseases of the nervous system complicating pregnancy, childbirth, and the puerperium**
Conditions in G00-G99

EXCLUDES 2   *pregnancy related peripheral neuritis (O26.8-)*

O99.350 Diseases of the nervous system complicating pregnancy, unspecified trimester Ⓜ♀

O99.351 Diseases of the nervous system complicating pregnancy, first trimester Ⓜ♀

O99.352 Diseases of the nervous system complicating pregnancy, second trimester Ⓜ♀

O99.353 Diseases of the nervous system complicating pregnancy, third trimester Ⓜ♀

O99.354 Diseases of the nervous system complicating childbirth cc Ⓜ♀

O99.355 Diseases of the nervous system complicating the puerperium cc Ⓜ♀

☑5ᵗʰ **O99.4 Diseases of the** circulatory system **complicating pregnancy, childbirth and the puerperium**
     Conditions in I00-I99
     EXCLUDES 1   *peripartum cardiomyopathy (O90.3)*
     EXCLUDES 2   *hypertensive disorders (O10-O16)*
         obstetric embolism (O88.-)
         venous complications and cerebrovenous sinus thrombosis in labor, childbirth and the puerperium (O87.-)
         venous complications and cerebrovenous sinus thrombosis in pregnancy (O22.-)
     AHA: 2016,2Q,8

   ☑6ᵗʰ **O99.41 Diseases of the circulatory system complicating** pregnancy
     O99.411 Diseases of the circulatory system complicating pregnancy, first trimester CC M ♀
     O99.412 Diseases of the circulatory system complicating pregnancy, second trimester CC M ♀
     O99.413 Diseases of the circulatory system complicating pregnancy, third trimester CC M ♀
     O99.419 Diseases of the circulatory system complicating pregnancy, unspecified trimester M ♀
   O99.42 Diseases of the circulatory system complicating childbirth MCC M ♀
   O99.43 Diseases of the circulatory system complicating the puerperium CC M ♀

☑5ᵗʰ **O99.5 Diseases of the** respiratory system **complicating pregnancy, childbirth and the puerperium**
     Conditions in J00-J99
   ☑6ᵗʰ **O99.51 Diseases of the respiratory system complicating** pregnancy
     O99.511 Diseases of the respiratory system complicating pregnancy, first trimester M ♀
     O99.512 Diseases of the respiratory system complicating pregnancy, second trimester M ♀
     O99.513 Diseases of the respiratory system complicating pregnancy, third trimester M ♀
     O99.519 Diseases of the respiratory system complicating pregnancy, unspecified trimester M ♀
   O99.52 Diseases of the respiratory system complicating childbirth M ♀
   O99.53 Diseases of the respiratory system complicating the puerperium M ♀

☑5ᵗʰ **O99.6 Diseases of the** digestive system **complicating pregnancy, childbirth and the puerperium**
     Conditions in K00-K93
     EXCLUDES 2   *hemorrhoids in pregnancy (O22.4-)*
         liver and biliary tract disorders in pregnancy, childbirth and the puerperium (O26.6-)
   ☑6ᵗʰ **O99.61 Diseases of the digestive system complicating** pregnancy
     AHA: 2016,1Q,4
     O99.611 Diseases of the digestive system complicating pregnancy, first trimester M ♀
     O99.612 Diseases of the digestive system complicating pregnancy, second trimester M ♀
     O99.613 Diseases of the digestive system complicating pregnancy, third trimester M ♀
     O99.619 Diseases of the digestive system complicating pregnancy, unspecified trimester M ♀
   O99.62 Diseases of the digestive system complicating childbirth M ♀
   O99.63 Diseases of the digestive system complicating the puerperium M ♀

☑5ᵗʰ **O99.7 Diseases of the** skin and subcutaneous **tissue complicating pregnancy, childbirth and the puerperium**
     Conditions in L00-L99
     EXCLUDES 2   *herpes gestationis (O26.4)*
         pruritic urticarial papules and plaques of pregnancy (PUPPP) (O26.86)
   ☑6ᵗʰ **O99.71 Diseases of the skin and subcutaneous tissue complicating** pregnancy
     O99.711 Diseases of the skin and subcutaneous tissue complicating pregnancy, first trimester M ♀
     O99.712 Diseases of the skin and subcutaneous tissue complicating pregnancy, second trimester M ♀
     O99.713 Diseases of the skin and subcutaneous tissue complicating pregnancy, third trimester M ♀
     O99.719 Diseases of the skin and subcutaneous tissue complicating pregnancy, unspecified trimester M ♀
   O99.72 Diseases of the skin and subcutaneous tissue complicating childbirth M ♀
   O99.73 Diseases of the skin and subcutaneous tissue complicating the puerperium M ♀

☑5ᵗʰ **O99.8 Other specified diseases and conditions complicating pregnancy, childbirth and the puerperium**
     Conditions in D00-D48, H00-H95, M00-N99, and Q00-Q99
     Use additional code to identify condition
     EXCLUDES 2   *genitourinary infections in pregnancy (O23.-)*
         infection of genitourinary tract following delivery (O86.1-O86.4)
         malignant neoplasm complicating pregnancy, childbirth and the puerperium (O9A.1-)
         maternal care for known or suspected abnormality of maternal pelvic organs (O34.-)
         postpartum acute kidney failure (O90.4)
         traumatic injuries in pregnancy (O9A.2-)
   ☑6ᵗʰ **O99.81 Abnormal glucose complicating pregnancy, childbirth and the puerperium**
     EXCLUDES 1   *gestational diabetes (O24.4-)*
     O99.810 Abnormal glucose complicating pregnancy M ♀
     O99.814 Abnormal glucose complicating childbirth M ♀
     O99.815 Abnormal glucose complicating the puerperium M ♀
   ☑6ᵗʰ **O99.82 Streptococcus B carrier state complicating pregnancy, childbirth and the puerperium**
     EXCLUDES 1   *carrier of streptococcus group B (GBS) in a nonpregnant woman (Z22.330)*
     DEF: *Streptococcus* group B colonization: Bacteria normally found in the vagina or lower intestine of many healthy adult women that may infect the fetus during childbirth, causing mental or physical handicaps or death. Women who test positive for *streptococcus* Group B during pregnancy are considered a "colonized" status and are treated with IV antibiotics at the time of delivery and may also be treated with oral antibiotics during the pregnancy.
     O99.820 Streptococcus B carrier state complicating pregnancy M ♀
     O99.824 Streptococcus B carrier state complicating childbirth M ♀
         AHA: 2019,2Q,8
     O99.825 Streptococcus B carrier state complicating the puerperium M ♀
   ☑6ᵗʰ **O99.83 Other infection carrier state complicating pregnancy, childbirth and the puerperium**
     Use additional code to identify the carrier state (Z22.-)
     O99.830 Other infection carrier state complicating pregnancy CC M ♀
     O99.834 Other infection carrier state complicating childbirth CC M ♀
     O99.835 Other infection carrier state complicating the puerperium CC M ♀

Chapter 15. Pregnancy, Childbirth and the Puerperium

✓6ᵗʰ **O99.84** **Bariatric surgery status complicating pregnancy, childbirth and the puerperium**
Gastric banding status complicating pregnancy, childbirth and the puerperium
Gastric bypass status for obesity complicating pregnancy, childbirth and the puerperium
Obesity surgery status complicating pregnancy, childbirth and the puerperium

     O99.840 **Bariatric surgery status complicating pregnancy, unspecified trimester** Ⓜ ♀

     O99.841 **Bariatric surgery status complicating pregnancy, first trimester** Ⓜ ♀

     O99.842 **Bariatric surgery status complicating pregnancy, second trimester** Ⓜ ♀

     O99.843 **Bariatric surgery status complicating pregnancy, third trimester** Ⓜ ♀

     O99.844 **Bariatric surgery status complicating childbirth** Ⓜ ♀

     O99.845 **Bariatric surgery status complicating the puerperium** Ⓜ ♀

▲ ✓6ᵗʰ **O99.89** **Other specified diseases and conditions complicating pregnancy, childbirth and the puerperium**

●   **O99.891** **Other specified diseases and conditions complicating pregnancy** Ⓜ ♀

●   **O99.892** **Other specified diseases and conditions complicating childbirth** Ⓜ ♀

●   **O99.893** **Other specified diseases and conditions complicating puerperium** Ⓜ ♀

✓4ᵗʰ **O9A** **Maternal malignant neoplasms, traumatic injuries and abuse classifiable elsewhere but complicating pregnancy, childbirth and the puerperium**

✓5ᵗʰ **O9A.1** **Malignant neoplasm complicating pregnancy, childbirth and the puerperium**
Conditions in C00-C96
Use additional code to identify neoplasm
EXCLUDES 2 *maternal care for benign tumor of corpus uteri (O34.1-)*
maternal care for benign tumor of cervix (O34.4-)
AHA: 2015,3Q,19

     ✓6ᵗʰ **O9A.11** **Malignant neoplasm complicating pregnancy**

     O9A.111 **Malignant neoplasm complicating pregnancy, first trimester** Ⓜ ♀

     O9A.112 **Malignant neoplasm complicating pregnancy, second trimester** Ⓜ ♀

     O9A.113 **Malignant neoplasm complicating pregnancy, third trimester** Ⓜ ♀

     O9A.119 **Malignant neoplasm complicating pregnancy, unspecified trimester** Ⓜ ♀

     O9A.12 **Malignant neoplasm complicating childbirth** Ⓜ ♀

     O9A.13 **Malignant neoplasm complicating the puerperium** Ⓜ ♀

✓5ᵗʰ **O9A.2** **Injury, poisoning and certain other consequences of external causes complicating pregnancy, childbirth and the puerperium**
Conditions in S00-T88, except T74 and T76
Use additional code(s) to identify the injury or poisoning
EXCLUDES 2 *physical, sexual and psychological abuse complicating pregnancy, childbirth and the puerperium (O9A.3-, O9A.4-, O9A.5-)*

     ✓6ᵗʰ **O9A.21** **Injury, poisoning and certain other consequences of external causes complicating pregnancy**

     O9A.211 **Injury, poisoning and certain other consequences of external causes complicating pregnancy, first trimester** Ⓜ ♀

     O9A.212 **Injury, poisoning and certain other consequences of external causes complicating pregnancy, second trimester** Ⓜ ♀

     O9A.213 **Injury, poisoning and certain other consequences of external causes complicating pregnancy, third trimester** Ⓜ ♀

     O9A.219 **Injury, poisoning and certain other consequences of external causes complicating pregnancy, unspecified trimester** Ⓜ ♀

     O9A.22 **Injury, poisoning and certain other consequences of external causes complicating childbirth** Ⓜ ♀

     O9A.23 **Injury, poisoning and certain other consequences of external causes complicating the puerperium** Ⓜ ♀

✓5ᵗʰ **O9A.3** **Physical abuse complicating pregnancy, childbirth and the puerperium**
Conditions in T74.11 or T76.11
Use additional code (if applicable):
to identify any associated current injury due to physical abuse
to identify the perpetrator of abuse (Y07.-)
EXCLUDES 2 *sexual abuse complicating pregnancy, childbirth and the puerperium (O9A.4)*

     ✓6ᵗʰ **O9A.31** **Physical abuse complicating pregnancy**

     O9A.311 **Physical abuse complicating pregnancy, first trimester** Ⓜ ♀

     O9A.312 **Physical abuse complicating pregnancy, second trimester** Ⓜ ♀

     O9A.313 **Physical abuse complicating pregnancy, third trimester** Ⓜ ♀

     O9A.319 **Physical abuse complicating pregnancy, unspecified trimester** Ⓜ ♀

     O9A.32 **Physical abuse complicating childbirth** Ⓜ ♀

     O9A.33 **Physical abuse complicating the puerperium** Ⓜ ♀

✓5ᵗʰ **O9A.4** **Sexual abuse complicating pregnancy, childbirth and the puerperium**
Conditions in T74.21 or T76.21
Use additional code (if applicable):
to identify any associated current injury due to sexual abuse
to identify the perpetrator of abuse (Y07.-)

     ✓6ᵗʰ **O9A.41** **Sexual abuse complicating pregnancy**

     O9A.411 **Sexual abuse complicating pregnancy, first trimester** Ⓜ ♀

     O9A.412 **Sexual abuse complicating pregnancy, second trimester** Ⓜ ♀

     O9A.413 **Sexual abuse complicating pregnancy, third trimester** Ⓜ ♀

     O9A.419 **Sexual abuse complicating pregnancy, unspecified trimester** Ⓜ ♀

     O9A.42 **Sexual abuse complicating childbirth** Ⓜ ♀

     O9A.43 **Sexual abuse complicating the puerperium** Ⓜ ♀

✓5ᵗʰ **O9A.5** **Psychological abuse complicating pregnancy, childbirth and the puerperium**
Conditions in T74.31 or T76.31
Use additional code to identify the perpetrator of abuse (Y07.-)

     ✓6ᵗʰ **O9A.51** **Psychological abuse complicating pregnancy**

     O9A.511 **Psychological abuse complicating pregnancy, first trimester** Ⓜ ♀

     O9A.512 **Psychological abuse complicating pregnancy, second trimester** Ⓜ ♀

     O9A.513 **Psychological abuse complicating pregnancy, third trimester** Ⓜ ♀

     O9A.519 **Psychological abuse complicating pregnancy, unspecified trimester** Ⓜ ♀

     O9A.52 **Psychological abuse complicating childbirth** Ⓜ ♀

     O9A.53 **Psychological abuse complicating the puerperium** Ⓜ ♀

Ⓝ Newborn: 0   Ⓟ Pediatric: 0-17   Ⓜ Maternity: 9-64   Ⓐ Adult: 15-124   ᴹᶜᶜ Major Complication/Comorbidity   ᶜᶜ Complication/Comorbidity   ˢᵂ Severe Wound Dx

900   ICD-10-CM 2021

Chapter 16. Certain Conditions Originating in the Perinatal Period (PØØ–P96)

Chapter-specific Guidelines with Coding Examples

The chapter-specific guidelines from the ICD-10-CM Official Guidelines for Coding and Reporting have been provided below. Along with these guidelines are coding examples, contained in the shaded boxes, that have been developed to help illustrate the coding and/or sequencing guidance found in these guidelines.

For coding and reporting purposes the perinatal period is defined as before birth through the 28th day following birth. The following guidelines are provided for reporting purposes

a. General perinatal rules

1) Use of Chapter 16 codes

Codes in this chapter are <u>never</u> for use on the maternal record. Codes from Chapter 15, the obstetric chapter, are never permitted on the newborn record. Chapter 16 codes may be used throughout the life of the patient if the condition is still present.

2) Principal diagnosis for birth record

When coding the birth episode in a newborn record, assign a code from category Z38, Liveborn infants according to place of birth and type of delivery, as the principal diagnosis. A code from category Z38 is assigned only once, to a newborn at the time of birth. If a newborn is transferred to another institution, a code from category Z38 should not be used at the receiving hospital.

A code from category Z38 is used only on the newborn record, not on the mother's record.

> Newborn delivered via vaginal delivery in Rural Hospital A, experienced meconium aspiration resulting in pneumonia. Rural Hospital A is not equipped to handle the extensive respiratory therapy this baby needs and transfers the patient to Metropolis Hospital B, where the pneumonia resolves and the newborn is eventually discharged.
>
> *Rural Hospital A*
>
> **Z38.ØØ**   **Single liveborn infant, delivered vaginally**
>
> **P24.Ø1**   **Meconium aspiration with respiratory symptoms**
>
> *Metropolis Hospital B*
>
> **P24.Ø1**   **Meconium aspiration with respiratory symptoms**
>
> *Explanation:* A code from category Z38 is a one-time use only code. The hospital that actually delivered the newborn, in this case Rural Hospital A, can append a code from category Z38 but for the delivery admission only. Once the patient is transferred or discharged, the Z38 category no longer applies for that patient.
>
> The reason for the transfer to Metropolis Hospital B was for the respiratory symptoms (pneumonia) the newborn was exhibiting secondary to aspirating meconium.

3) Use of codes from other chapters with codes from Chapter 16

Codes from other chapters may be used with codes from chapter 16 if the codes from the other chapters provide more specific detail. Codes for signs and symptoms may be assigned when a definitive diagnosis has not been established. If the reason for the encounter is a perinatal condition, the code from chapter 16 should be sequenced first.

4) Use of Chapter 16 codes after the perinatal period

Should a condition originate in the perinatal period, and continue throughout the life of the patient, the perinatal code should continue to be used regardless of the patient's age.

> A 7-year-old patient with history of birth injury that resulted in Erb's palsy is seen for subscapularis release
>
> **P14.Ø**   **Erb's paralysis due to birth injury**
>
> *Explanation:* Although in this instance Erb's palsy is specifically related to a birth injury, it has not resolved and continues to be a health concern. A perinatal code is appropriate even though this patient is beyond the perinatal period.

5) Birth process or community acquired conditions

If a newborn has a condition that may be either due to the birth process or community acquired and the documentation does not indicate which it is, the default is due to the birth process and the code from Chapter 16 should be used. If the condition is community-acquired, a code from Chapter 16 should not be assigned.

<u>For COVID-19 infection in a newborn, see guideline I.C.16.h.</u>

6) Code all clinically significant conditions

All clinically significant conditions noted on routine newborn examination should be coded. A condition is clinically significant if it requires:

clinical evaluation; or

therapeutic treatment; or

diagnostic procedures; or

extended length of hospital stay; or

increased nursing care and/or monitoring; or

has implications for future health care needs

Note: The perinatal guidelines listed above are the same as the general coding guidelines for "additional diagnoses", except for the final point regarding implications for future health care needs. Codes should be assigned for conditions that have been specified by the provider as having implications for future health care needs.

b. Observation and evaluation of newborns for suspected conditions not found

1) Use of Z05 codes

Assign a code from category Z05, Observation and evaluation of newborns and infants for suspected conditions ruled out, to identify those instances when a healthy newborn is evaluated for a suspected condition that is determined after study not to be present. Do not use a code from category Z05 when the patient has identified signs or symptoms of a suspected problem; in such cases code the sign or symptom.

2) Z05 on Other than the birth record

A code from category Z05 may also be assigned as a principal or first-listed code for readmissions or encounters when the code from category Z38 code no longer applies. Codes from category Z05 are for use only for healthy newborns and infants for which no condition after study is found to be present.

3) Z05 on a birth record

A code from category Z05 is to be used as a secondary code after the code from category Z38, Liveborn infants according to place of birth and type of delivery.

> Newborn delivered via vaginal delivery; previous ultrasounds showed what appeared to be an abnormality of the right kidney. Kidney function tests were performed and ultrasounds taken and any genitourinary conditions ruled out.
>
> **Z38.ØØ**   **Single liveborn infant, delivered vaginally**
>
> **Z05.6**   **Observation and evaluation of newborn for suspected genitourinary condition ruled out**
>
> Explanation: The newborn had no signs or symptoms of kidney or other genitourinary condition but was evaluated after delivery due to the abnormal prenatal ultrasound findings. A Z code describing the type and place of birth should be coded first, followed by a Z05 category code for the work performed to rule out a suspected genitourinary condition.

c. Coding additional perinatal diagnoses

1) Assigning codes for conditions that require treatment

Assign codes for conditions that require treatment or further investigation, prolong the length of stay, or require resource utilization.

2) Codes for conditions specified as having implications for future health care needs

Assign codes for conditions that have been specified by the provider as having implications for future health care needs.

Note: This guideline should not be used for adult patients.

An abnormal noise was heard in the left hip of a post-term newborn during a physical examination. The pediatrician would like to follow the patient after discharge as a hip click can be an early sign of hip dysplasia. The newborn was delivered via cesarean at 41 weeks.

Z38.01	Single liveborn infant, delivered by cesarean
P08.21	Post-term newborn
R29.4	Clicking hip

Explanation: The abnormal hip noise or click is appended as a secondary diagnosis not only because it is an abnormal finding upon examination, but also due to its potential to be part of a bigger health issue. The hip dysplasia has not yet been diagnosed and does not warrant a code at this time.

d. Prematurity and fetal growth retardation

Providers utilize different criteria in determining prematurity. A code for prematurity should not be assigned unless it is documented. Assignment of codes in categories P05, Disorders of newborn related to slow fetal growth and fetal malnutrition, and P07, Disorders of newborn related to short gestation and low birth weight, not elsewhere classified, should be based on the recorded birth weight and estimated gestational age.

When both birth weight and gestational age are available, two codes from category P07 should be assigned, with the code for birth weight sequenced before the code for gestational age.

e. Low birth weight and immaturity status

Codes from category P07, Disorders of newborn related to short gestation and low birth weight, not elsewhere classified, are for use for a child or adult who was premature or had a low birth weight as a newborn and this is affecting the patient's current health status.

See Section I.C.21. Factors influencing health status and contact with health services, Status.

A 35-year-old patient, who weighed 659 grams at birth, is seen for heart disease documented as being a consequence of the low birth weight

I51.9	Heart disease, unspecified
P07.02	Extremely low birth weight newborn, 500–749 grams

Explanation: A code from subcategories P07.0- and P07.1- is appropriate, regardless of the age of the patient, as long as the documentation provides a clear link between the patient's current illness and the low birth weight.

f. Bacterial sepsis of newborn

Category P36, Bacterial sepsis of newborn, includes congenital sepsis. If a perinate is documented as having sepsis without documentation of congenital or community acquired, the default is congenital and a code from category P36 should be assigned. If the P36 code includes the causal organism, an additional code from category B95, Streptococcus, Staphylococcus, and Enterococcus as the cause of diseases classified elsewhere, or B96, Other bacterial agents as the cause of diseases classified elsewhere, should not be assigned. If the P36 code does not include the causal organism, assign an additional code from category B96. If applicable, use additional codes to identify severe sepsis (R65.2-) and any associated acute organ dysfunction.

A full-term infant develops severe sepsis 24 hours after discharge from the hospital and is readmitted; cultures identified *E. coli* as the infective agent

P36.4	Sepsis of newborn due to Escherichia coli
R65.20	Severe sepsis without septic shock

Explanation: Even though this newborn was discharged and could have acquired *E. coli* from his/her external environment, due to the lack of documentation specifying specifically how this pathogen was acquired, the default is to code the *E. coli* sepsis as congenital. A code from chapter 1, "Certain Infectious and Parasitic Diseases," is not required because the perinatal sepsis code identifies both the sepsis and the bacteria causing the sepsis.

g. Stillbirth

Code P95, Stillbirth, is only for use in institutions that maintain separate records for stillbirths. No other code should be used with P95. Code P95 should not be used on the mother's record.

h. COVID-19 Infection in Newborn

For a newborn that tests positive for COVID-19, assign code U07.1, COVID-19, and the appropriate codes for associated manifestation(s) in neonates/newborns in the absence of documentation indicating a specific type of transmission. For a newborn that tests positive for COVID-19 and the provider documents the condition was contracted in utero or during the birth process, assign codes P35.8, Other congenital viral diseases, and U07.1, COVID-19. When coding the birth episode in a newborn record, the appropriate code from category Z38, Liveborn infants according to place of birth and type of delivery, should be assigned as the principal diagnosis.

Chapter 16. Certain Conditions Originating in the Perinatal Period (P00–P96)

NOTE   Codes from this chapter are for use on newborn records only, never on maternal records

INCLUDES   conditions that have their origin in the fetal or perinatal period (before birth through the first 28 days after birth) even if morbidity occurs later

EXCLUDES 2   congenital malformations, deformations and chromosomal abnormalities (Q00-Q99)

endocrine, nutritional and metabolic diseases (E00-E88)

injury, poisoning and certain other consequences of external causes (S00-T88)

neoplasms (C00-D49)

tetanus neonatorum (A33)

This chapter contains the following blocks:

P00-P04	Newborn affected by maternal factors and by complications of pregnancy, labor, and delivery
P05-P08	Disorders of newborn related to length of gestation and fetal growth
P09	Abnormal findings on neonatal screening
P10-P15	Birth trauma
P19-P29	Respiratory and cardiovascular disorders specific to the perinatal period
P35-P39	Infections specific to the perinatal period
P50-P61	Hemorrhagic and hematological disorders of newborn
P70-P74	Transitory endocrine and metabolic disorders specific to newborn
P76-P78	Digestive system disorders of newborn
P80-P83	Conditions involving the integument and temperature regulation of newborn
P84	Other problems with newborn
P90-P96	Other disorders originating in the perinatal period

Newborn affected by maternal factors and by complications of pregnancy, labor, and delivery (P00-P04)

NOTE   These codes are for use when the listed maternal conditions are specified as the cause of confirmed morbidity or potential morbidity which have their origin in the perinatal period (before birth through the first 28 days after birth).

AHA: 2016,4Q,54-55

√4ᵗʰ P00 Newborn affected by maternal conditions that may be unrelated to present pregnancy

Code first any current condition in newborn

     EXCLUDES 2   encounter for observation of newborn for suspected diseases and conditions ruled out (Z05.-)

newborn affected by maternal complications of pregnancy (P01.-)

newborn affected by maternal endocrine and metabolic disorders (P70-P74)

newborn affected by noxious substances transmitted via placenta or breast milk (P04.-)

P00.0 Newborn affected by maternal hypertensive disorders
Newborn affected by maternal conditions classifiable to O10-O11, O13-O16

P00.1 Newborn affected by maternal renal and urinary tract diseases
Newborn affected by maternal conditions classifiable to N00-N39

P00.2 Newborn affected by maternal infectious and parasitic diseases
Newborn affected by maternal infectious disease classifiable to A00-B99, J09 and J10

     EXCLUDES 1   maternal genital tract or other localized infections (P00.8)

     EXCLUDES 2   infections specific to the perinatal period (P35-P39)

     AHA: 2019,2Q,10; 2015,3Q,20

P00.3 Newborn affected by other maternal circulatory and respiratory diseases
Newborn affected by maternal conditions classifiable to I00-I99, J00-J99, Q20-Q34 and not included in P00.0, P00.2

P00.4 Newborn affected by maternal nutritional disorders
Newborn affected by maternal disorders classifiable to E40-E64
Maternal malnutrition NOS

P00.5 Newborn affected by maternal injury
Newborn affected by maternal conditions classifiable to O9A.2-

P00.6 Newborn affected by surgical procedure on mother
Newborn affected by amniocentesis

     EXCLUDES 1   Cesarean delivery for present delivery (P03.4)

damage to placenta from amniocentesis, Cesarean delivery or surgical induction (P02.1)

previous surgery to uterus or pelvic organs (P03.89)

     EXCLUDES 2   newborn affected by complication of (fetal) intrauterine procedure (P96.5)

P00.7 Newborn affected by other medical procedures on mother, not elsewhere classified
Newborn affected by radiation to mother

     EXCLUDES 1   damage to placenta from amniocentesis, cesarean delivery or surgical induction (P02.1)

newborn affected by other complications of labor and delivery (P03.-)

√5ᵗʰ P00.8 Newborn affected by other maternal conditions

     P00.81 Newborn affected by periodontal disease in mother

     P00.89 Newborn affected by other maternal conditions
Newborn affected by conditions classifiable to T80-T88

Newborn affected by maternal genital tract or other localized infections

Newborn affected by maternal systemic lupus erythematosus

▶Use additional code to identify infectious agent, if known◀

     AHA: 2019,2Q,9

P00.9 Newborn affected by unspecified maternal condition

√4ᵗʰ P01 Newborn affected by maternal complications of pregnancy

Code first any current condition in newborn

     EXCLUDES 2   encounter for observation of newborn for suspected diseases and conditions ruled out (Z05.-)

P01.0 Newborn affected by incompetent cervix

P01.1 Newborn affected by premature rupture of membranes

P01.2 Newborn affected by oligohydramnios

     EXCLUDES 1   oligohydramnios due to premature rupture of membranes (P01.1)

DEF: Oligohydramnios: Low amniotic fluid level, resulting in underdeveloped organs in the fetus.

P01.3 Newborn affected by polyhydramnios
Newborn affected by hydramnios
DEF: Polyhydramnios: Excess amniotic fluid surrounding the fetus, typically defined as a total fluid volume of greater than 24.0 cc.

P01.4 Newborn affected by ectopic pregnancy
Newborn affected by abdominal pregnancy

P01.5 Newborn affected by multiple pregnancy
Newborn affected by triplet (pregnancy)
Newborn affected by twin (pregnancy)

P01.6 Newborn affected by maternal death

P01.7 Newborn affected by malpresentation before labor
Newborn affected by breech presentation before labor
Newborn affected by external version before labor
Newborn affected by face presentation before labor
Newborn affected by transverse lie before labor
Newborn affected by unstable lie before labor

P01.8 Newborn affected by other maternal complications of pregnancy

P01.9 Newborn affected by maternal complication of pregnancy, unspecified

√4ᵗʰ P02 Newborn affected by complications of placenta, cord and membranes

Code first any current condition in newborn

     EXCLUDES 2   encounter for observation of newborn for suspected diseases and conditions ruled out (Z05.-)

P02.0 Newborn affected by placenta previa
DEF: Placenta developed in the lower segment of the uterus that can cause hemorrhaging leading to preterm delivery.

P02.1 Newborn affected by other forms of placental separation and hemorrhage
Newborn affected by abruptio placenta
Newborn affected by accidental hemorrhage
Newborn affected by antepartum hemorrhage
Newborn affected by damage to placenta from amniocentesis, cesarean delivery or surgical induction
Newborn affected by maternal blood loss
Newborn affected by premature separation of placenta

✅ Additional Character Required   √x7ᵗʰ Placeholder   Unacceptable PDx   Questionable PDx   Manifestation   Unspecified Dx   H1-H14 HAC   HCC CMS-HCC Dx   HIV HIV Dx

Chapter 16. Certain Conditions Originating in the Perinatal Period

P02.2–P04.0

✓5th   **P02.2   Newborn affected by other and unspecified morphological and functional abnormalities of placenta**

    P02.20   Newborn affected by unspecified morphological and functional abnormalities of placenta

    P02.29   Newborn affected by other morphological and functional abnormalities of placenta
       Newborn affected by placental dysfunction
       Newborn affected by placental infarction
       Newborn affected by placental insufficiency

P02.3   Newborn affected by placental transfusion syndromes
     Newborn affected by placental and cord abnormalities resulting in twin-to-twin or other transplacental transfusion

P02.4   Newborn affected by prolapsed cord

P02.5   Newborn affected by other compression of umbilical cord
     Newborn affected by umbilical cord (tightly) around neck
     Newborn affected by entanglement of umbilical cord
     Newborn affected by knot in umbilical cord

✓5th   **P02.6   Newborn affected by other and unspecified conditions of umbilical cord**

    P02.60   Newborn affected by unspecified conditions of umbilical cord

    P02.69   Newborn affected by other conditions of umbilical cord
       Newborn affected by short umbilical cord
       Newborn affected by vasa previa
       EXCLUDES 1   newborn affected by single umbilical artery (Q27.0)

✓5th   **P02.7   Newborn affected by chorioamnionitis**
     AHA: 2018,4Q,23-24
     DEF: Inflammation of the fetal membranes due to maternal infection characterized by fetal tachycardia, respiratory distress, apnea, weak cries, and poor sucking.

    P02.70   Newborn affected by fetal inflammatory response syndrome   **MCC**
       Newborn affected by FIRS

    P02.78   Newborn affected by other conditions from chorioamnionitis
       Newborn affected by amnionitis
       Newborn affected by membranitis
       Newborn affected by placentitis

P02.8   Newborn affected by other abnormalities of membranes

P02.9   Newborn affected by abnormality of membranes, unspecified

✓4th   **P03   Newborn affected by other complications of labor and delivery**
     Code first any current condition in newborn
     EXCLUDES 2   encounter for observation of newborn for suspected diseases and conditions ruled out (Z05.-)

P03.0   Newborn affected by breech delivery and extraction

P03.1   Newborn affected by other malpresentation, malposition and disproportion during labor and delivery
     Newborn affected by contracted pelvis
     Newborn affected by conditions classifiable to O64-O66
     Newborn affected by persistent occipitoposterior
     Newborn affected by transverse lie

P03.2   Newborn affected by forceps delivery

Forceps Assisted Birth

Forceps extractor

P03.3   Newborn affected by delivery by vacuum extractor [ventouse]

Vacuum Assisted Birth

Vacuum extractor

P03.4   Newborn affected by Cesarean delivery

P03.5   Newborn affected by precipitate delivery
     Newborn affected by rapid second stage

P03.6   Newborn affected by abnormal uterine contractions
     Newborn affected by conditions classifiable to O62.-, except O62.3
     Newborn affected by hypertonic labor
     Newborn affected by uterine inertia

✓5th   **P03.8   Newborn affected by other specified complications of labor and delivery**

    ✓6th   **P03.81   Newborn affected by abnormality in fetal (intrauterine) heart rate or rhythm**
       EXCLUDES 1   neonatal cardiac dysrhythmia (P29.1-)

       P03.810   Newborn affected by abnormality in fetal (intrauterine) heart rate or rhythm before the onset of labor

       P03.811   Newborn affected by abnormality in fetal (intrauterine) heart rate or rhythm during labor

       P03.819   Newborn affected by abnormality in fetal (intrauterine) heart rate or rhythm, unspecified as to time of onset

    P03.82   Meconium passage during delivery
       EXCLUDES 1   meconium aspiration (P24.00, P24.01)
                 meconium staining (P96.83)
       DEF: Fetal intestinal activity that increases in response to a fetomaternal distressed state during delivery. The anal sphincter relaxes and meconium is passed into the amniotic fluid.

    P03.89   Newborn affected by other specified complications of labor and delivery
       Newborn affected by abnormality of maternal soft tissues
       Newborn affected by conditions classifiable to O60-O75 and by procedures used in labor and delivery not included in P02.- and P03.0-P03.6
       Newborn affected by induction of labor

P03.9   Newborn affected by complication of labor and delivery, unspecified

✓4th   **P04   Newborn affected by noxious substances transmitted via placenta or breast milk**
     INCLUDES   nonteratogenic effects of substances transmitted via placenta
     EXCLUDES 2   congenital malformations (Q00-Q99)
           encounter for observation of newborn for suspected diseases and conditions ruled out (Z05.-)
           neonatal jaundice from excessive hemolysis due to drugs or toxins transmitted from mother (P58.4)
           newborn in contact with and (suspected) exposures hazardous to health not transmitted via placenta or breast milk (Z77.-)

P04.0   Newborn affected by maternal anesthesia and analgesia in pregnancy, labor and delivery
     Newborn affected by reactions and intoxications from maternal opiates and tranquilizers administered for procedures during pregnancy or labor and delivery
     EXCLUDES 2   newborn affected by other maternal medication (P04.1-)

N Newborn: 0   P Pediatric: 0-17   M Maternity: 9-64   A Adult: 15-124   MCC Major Complication/Comorbidity   CC Complication/Comorbidity   SW Severe Wound Dx

904   ICD-10-CM 2021

✓5ᵗʰ P04.1 Newborn affected by other maternal medication

Code first withdrawal symptoms from maternal use of drugs of addiction, if applicable (P96.1)

EXCLUDES 1 *dysmorphism due to warfarin (Q86.2)*
  fetal hydantoin syndrome (Q86.1)

EXCLUDES 2 *maternal anesthesia and analgesia in pregnancy, labor and delivery (P04.0)*
  maternal use of drugs of addiction (P04.4-)

AHA: 2018,4Q,24-25

P04.11 Newborn affected by maternal antineoplastic chemotherapy

P04.12 Newborn affected by maternal cytotoxic drugs

P04.13 Newborn affected by maternal use of anticonvulsants

P04.14 Newborn affected by maternal use of opiates

P04.15 Newborn affected by maternal use of antidepressants

P04.16 Newborn affected by maternal use of amphetamines

P04.17 Newborn affected by maternal use of sedative-hypnotics

P04.1A Newborn affected by maternal use of anxiolytics

P04.18 Newborn affected by other maternal medication

P04.19 Newborn affected by maternal use of unspecified medication

P04.2 Newborn affected by maternal use of tobacco

Newborn affected by exposure in utero to tobacco smoke

EXCLUDES 2 *newborn exposure to environmental tobacco smoke (P96.81)*

P04.3 Newborn affected by maternal use of alcohol

EXCLUDES 1 *fetal alcohol syndrome (Q86.0)*

✓5ᵗʰ P04.4 Newborn affected by maternal use of drugs of addiction

AHA: 2018,4Q,25

P04.40 Newborn affected by maternal use of unspecified drugs of addiction

P04.41 Newborn affected by maternal use of cocaine

P04.42 Newborn affected by maternal use of hallucinogens

EXCLUDES 2 *newborn affected by other maternal medication (P04.1-)*

P04.49 Newborn affected by maternal use of other drugs of addiction

EXCLUDES 2 *newborn affected by maternal anesthesia and analgesia (P04.0)*
  withdrawal symptoms from maternal use of drugs of addiction (P96.1)

P04.5 Newborn affected by maternal use of nutritional chemical substances

P04.6 Newborn affected by maternal exposure to environmental chemical substances

✓5ᵗʰ P04.8 Newborn affected by other maternal noxious substances

AHA: 2018,4Q,25

P04.81 Newborn affected by maternal use of cannabis

P04.89 Newborn affected by other maternal noxious substances

P04.9 Newborn affected by maternal noxious substance, unspecified

Disorders of newborn related to length of gestation and fetal growth (P05-P08)

✓4ᵗʰ P05 Disorders of newborn related to slow fetal growth and fetal malnutrition

AHA: 2016,4Q,55-56

✓5ᵗʰ P05.0 Newborn light for gestational age

Newborn light-for-dates

Weight below but length above 10th percentile for gestational age

P05.00 Newborn light for gestational age, unspecified weight

P05.01 Newborn light for gestational age, less than 500 grams

P05.02 Newborn light for gestational age, 500-749 grams

P05.03 Newborn light for gestational age, 750-999 grams

P05.04 Newborn light for gestational age, 1000-1249 grams

P05.05 Newborn light for gestational age, 1250-1499 grams

P05.06 Newborn light for gestational age, 1500-1749 grams

P05.07 Newborn light for gestational age, 1750-1999 grams

P05.08 Newborn light for gestational age, 2000-2499 grams

P05.09 Newborn light for gestational age, 2500 grams and over

Newborn light for gestational age, other

✓5ᵗʰ P05.1 Newborn small for gestational age

Newborn small-and-light-for-dates

Newborn small-for-dates

Weight and length below 10th percentile for gestational age

P05.10 Newborn small for gestational age, unspecified weight

P05.11 Newborn small for gestational age, less than 500 grams

P05.12 Newborn small for gestational age, 500-749 grams

P05.13 Newborn small for gestational age, 750-999 grams

P05.14 Newborn small for gestational age, 1000-1249 grams

P05.15 Newborn small for gestational age, 1250-1499 grams

P05.16 Newborn small for gestational age, 1500-1749 grams

P05.17 Newborn small for gestational age, 1750-1999 grams

P05.18 Newborn small for gestational age, 2000-2499 grams

P05.19 Newborn small for gestational age, other

Newborn small for gestational age, 2500 grams and over

P05.2 Newborn affected by fetal (intrauterine) malnutrition not light or small for gestational age

Infant, not light or small for gestational age, showing signs of fetal malnutrition, such as dry, peeling skin and loss of subcutaneous tissue

EXCLUDES 1 *newborn affected by fetal malnutrition with light for gestational age (P05.0-)*
  newborn affected by fetal malnutrition with small for gestational age (P05.1-)

P05.9 Newborn affected by slow intrauterine growth, unspecified

Newborn affected by fetal growth retardation NOS

✓4ᵗʰ P07 Disorders of newborn related to short gestation and low birth weight, not elsewhere classified

NOTE When both birth weight and gestational age of the newborn are available, both should be coded with birth weight sequenced before gestational age

INCLUDES the listed conditions, without further specification, as the cause of morbidity or additional care, in newborn

✓5ᵗʰ P07.0 Extremely low birth weight newborn

Newborn birth weight 999 g. or less

EXCLUDES 1 *low birth weight due to slow fetal growth and fetal malnutrition (P05.-)*

P07.00 Extremely low birth weight newborn, unspecified weight

P07.01 Extremely low birth weight newborn, less than 500 grams

P07.02 Extremely low birth weight newborn, 500-749 grams

P07.03 Extremely low birth weight newborn, 750-999 grams

✓5ᵗʰ P07.1 Other low birth weight newborn

Newborn birth weight 1000-2499 g.

EXCLUDES 1 *low birth weight due to slow fetal growth and fetal malnutrition (P05.-)*

P07.10 Other low birth weight newborn, unspecified weight

P07.14 Other low birth weight newborn, 1000-1249 grams

P07.15 Other low birth weight newborn, 1250-1499 grams

P07.16 Other low birth weight newborn, 1500-1749 grams

P07.17 Other low birth weight newborn, 1750-1999 grams

P07.18 Other low birth weight newborn, 2000-2499 grams

✓5ᵗʰ P07.2 Extreme immaturity of newborn

Less than 28 completed weeks (less than 196 completed days) of gestation

P07.20 Extreme immaturity of newborn, unspecified weeks of gestation

Gestational age less than 28 completed weeks NOS

✓ Additional Character Required ✓x7ᵗʰ Placeholder Unacceptable PDx Questionable PDx Manifestation Unspecified Dx H1 - H14 HAC HCC CMS-HCC Dx HIV HIV Dx

Chapter 16. Certain Conditions Originating in the Perinatal Period

P07.21   **Extreme immaturity of newborn, gestational age less than 23 completed weeks**
     Extreme immaturity of newborn, gestational age less than 23 weeks, Ø days

P07.22   **Extreme immaturity of newborn, gestational age 23 completed weeks**
     Extreme immaturity of newborn, gestational age 23 weeks, Ø days through 23 weeks, 6 days

P07.23   **Extreme immaturity of newborn, gestational age 24 completed weeks**
     Extreme immaturity of newborn, gestational age 24 weeks, Ø days through 24 weeks, 6 days

P07.24   **Extreme immaturity of newborn, gestational age 25 completed weeks**
     Extreme immaturity of newborn, gestational age 25 weeks, Ø days through 25 weeks, 6 days

P07.25   **Extreme immaturity of newborn, gestational age 26 completed weeks**
     Extreme immaturity of newborn, gestational age 26 weeks, Ø days through 26 weeks, 6 days

P07.26   **Extreme immaturity of newborn, gestational age 27 completed weeks**
     Extreme immaturity of newborn, gestational age 27 weeks, Ø days through 27 weeks, 6 days

√5ᵗʰ **P07.3**   **Preterm [premature] newborn [other]**
     28 completed weeks or more but less than 37 completed weeks (196 completed days but less than 259 completed days) of gestation
     Prematurity NOS
     AHA: 2017,3Q,26

     P07.30   **Preterm newborn, unspecified weeks of gestation**

     P07.31   **Preterm newborn, gestational age 28 completed weeks**
         Preterm newborn, gestational age 28 weeks, Ø days through 28 weeks, 6 days

     P07.32   **Preterm newborn, gestational age 29 completed weeks**
         Preterm newborn, gestational age 29 weeks, Ø days through 29 weeks, 6 days

     P07.33   **Preterm newborn, gestational age 30 completed weeks**
         Preterm newborn, gestational age 30 weeks, Ø days through 30 weeks, 6 days

     P07.34   **Preterm newborn, gestational age 31 completed weeks**
         Preterm newborn, gestational age 31 weeks, Ø days through 31 weeks, 6 days

     P07.35   **Preterm newborn, gestational age 32 completed weeks**
         Preterm newborn, gestational age 32 weeks, Ø days through 32 weeks, 6 days

     P07.36   **Preterm newborn, gestational age 33 completed weeks**
         Preterm newborn, gestational age 33 weeks, Ø days through 33 weeks, 6 days

     P07.37   **Preterm newborn, gestational age 34 completed weeks**
         Preterm newborn, gestational age 34 weeks, Ø days through 34 weeks, 6 days

     P07.38   **Preterm newborn, gestational age 35 completed weeks**
         Preterm newborn, gestational age 35 weeks, Ø days through 35 weeks, 6 days

     P07.39   **Preterm newborn, gestational age 36 completed weeks**
         Preterm newborn, gestational age 36 weeks, Ø days through 36 weeks, 6 days

√4ᵗʰ **P08**   **Disorders of newborn related to long gestation and high birth weight**

     NOTE   When both birth weight and gestational age of the newborn are available, priority of assignment should be given to birth weight

     INCLUDES   the listed conditions, without further specification, as causes of morbidity or additional care, in newborn

     P08.0   **Exceptionally large newborn baby**
         Usually implies a birth weight of 4500 g. or more
         EXCLUDES 1   *syndrome of infant of diabetic mother (P70.1)*
            syndrome of infant of mother with gestational diabetes (P70.0)

     P08.1   **Other heavy for gestational age newborn**
         Other newborn heavy- or large-for-dates regardless of period of gestation
         Usually implies a birth weight of 4000 g. to 4499 g.
         EXCLUDES 1   *newborn with a birth weight of 4500 or more (P08.0)*
            syndrome of infant of diabetic mother (P70.1)
            syndrome of infant of mother with gestational diabetes (P70.0).

√5ᵗʰ **P08.2**   **Late newborn, not heavy for gestational age**
     AHA: 2014,1Q,14

     P08.21   **Post-term newborn**
         Newborn with gestation period over 40 completed weeks to 42 completed weeks

     P08.22   **Prolonged gestation of newborn**
         Newborn with gestation period over 42 completed weeks (294 days or more), not heavy- or large-for-dates.
         Postmaturity NOS

Abnormal findings on neonatal screening (P09)

P09   **Abnormal findings on neonatal screening**
     Use additional code to identify signs, symptoms and conditions associated with the screening
     EXCLUDES 2   *nonspecific serologic evidence of human immunodeficiency virus [HIV] (R75)*

Birth trauma (P10-P15)

√4ᵗʰ **P10**   **Intracranial laceration and hemorrhage due to birth injury**
     EXCLUDES 1   *intracranial hemorrhage of newborn NOS (P52.9)*
         intracranial hemorrhage of newborn due to anoxia or hypoxia (P52.-)
         nontraumatic intracranial hemorrhage of newborn (P52.-)

     P10.0   **Subdural hemorrhage due to birth injury**   `MCC`
         Subdural hematoma (localized) due to birth injury
         EXCLUDES 1   *subdural hemorrhage accompanying tentorial tear (P10.4)*

     P10.1   **Cerebral hemorrhage due to birth injury**   `MCC`

     P10.2   **Intraventricular hemorrhage due to birth injury**   `CC`

     P10.3   **Subarachnoid hemorrhage due to birth injury**   `MCC`

     P10.4   **Tentorial tear due to birth injury**   `MCC`

     P10.8   **Other intracranial lacerations and hemorrhages due to birth injury**   `MCC`

     P10.9   **Unspecified intracranial laceration and hemorrhage due to birth injury**   `MCC`

√4ᵗʰ **P11**   **Other birth injuries to central nervous system**

     P11.0   **Cerebral edema due to birth injury**   `MCC`

     P11.1   **Other specified brain damage due to birth injury**

     P11.2   **Unspecified brain damage due to birth injury**   `MCC`

     P11.3   **Birth injury to facial nerve**
         Facial palsy due to birth injury

     P11.4   **Birth injury to other cranial nerves**

     P11.5   **Birth injury to spine and spinal cord**
         Fracture of spine due to birth injury

     P11.9   **Birth injury to central nervous system, unspecified**   `MCC`

N Newborn: 0   P Pediatric: 0-17   M Maternity: 9-64   A Adult: 15-124   MCC Major Complication/Comorbidity   CC Complication/Comorbidity   SW Severe Wound Dx

906   ICD-10-CM 2021

☑4th P12 Birth injury to scalp

Birth Injuries to Scalp

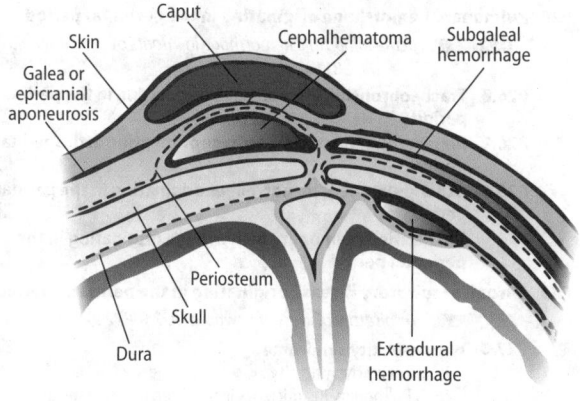

P12.0 Cephalhematoma due to birth injury
> **DEF:** Condition that occurs in a neonate when blood vessels between the skull and periosteum rupture and blood collects in the subperiosteal space (below the periosteum). It is typically caused by prolonged labor or trauma due to instrument-assisted delivery (e.g., forceps, vacuum extraction), although in rare circumstances, it may indicate a linear skull fracture with intracranial hemorrhage.

P12.1 Chignon (from vacuum extraction) due to birth injury
> **DEF:** Artificial swelling of the scalp that occurs when a collection of interstitial fluid and blood forms in the area of the scalp where the suction cup was applied during a vacuum-assisted delivery.

P12.2 Epicranial subaponeurotic hemorrhage due to birth injury `CC`
> Subgaleal hemorrhage

P12.3 Bruising of scalp due to birth injury

P12.4 Injury of scalp of newborn due to monitoring equipment
> Sampling incision of scalp of newborn
> Scalp clip (electrode) injury of newborn

☑5th P12.8 Other birth injuries to scalp

P12.81 Caput succedaneum
> **DEF:** Swelling of the scalp as a result of pressure being exerted on the head from the vaginal walls, uterus, or instrumentation used in assisting a delivery (e.g., vacuum).

P12.89 Other birth injuries to scalp

P12.9 Birth injury to scalp, unspecified

☑4th P13 Birth injury to skeleton

> **EXCLUDES 2** birth injury to spine (P11.5)

P13.0 Fracture of skull due to birth injury

P13.1 Other birth injuries to skull
> **EXCLUDES 1** cephalhematoma (P12.0)

P13.2 Birth injury to femur

P13.3 Birth injury to other long bones

P13.4 Fracture of clavicle due to birth injury

P13.8 Birth injuries to other parts of skeleton

P13.9 Birth injury to skeleton, unspecified

☑4th P14 Birth injury to peripheral nervous system

P14.0 Erb's paralysis due to birth injury
> **DEF:** Erb's paralysis: Most common type of brachial plexus (peripheral nerve) injury in a neonate that involves nerve damage at the level of C5-C6. **Synonym(s):** Erb's palsy

P14.1 Klumpke's paralysis due to birth injury

P14.2 Phrenic nerve paralysis due to birth injury

P14.3 Other brachial plexus birth injuries

P14.8 Birth injuries to other parts of peripheral nervous system

P14.9 Birth injury to peripheral nervous system, unspecified

☑4th P15 Other birth injuries

P15.0 Birth injury to liver
> Rupture of liver due to birth injury

P15.1 Birth injury to spleen
> Rupture of spleen due to birth injury

P15.2 Sternomastoid injury due to birth injury

P15.3 Birth injury to eye
> Subconjunctival hemorrhage due to birth injury
> Traumatic glaucoma due to birth injury

P15.4 Birth injury to face
> Facial congestion due to birth injury

P15.5 Birth injury to external genitalia

P15.6 Subcutaneous fat necrosis due to birth injury

P15.8 Other specified birth injuries

P15.9 Birth injury, unspecified

Respiratory and cardiovascular disorders specific to the perinatal period (P19-P29)

☑4th P19 Metabolic acidemia in newborn

> **INCLUDES** metabolic acidemia in newborn

P19.0 Metabolic acidemia in newborn first noted before onset of labor

P19.1 Metabolic acidemia in newborn first noted during labor

P19.2 Metabolic acidemia noted at birth

P19.9 Metabolic acidemia, unspecified

☑4th P22 Respiratory distress of newborn

> **AHA:** 2019,2Q,29

P22.0 Respiratory distress syndrome of newborn `MCC`
> Cardiorespiratory distress syndrome of newborn
> Hyaline membrane disease
> Idiopathic respiratory distress syndrome [IRDS or RDS] of newborn
> Pulmonary hypoperfusion syndrome
> Respiratory distress syndrome, type I
> **EXCLUDES 2** respiratory arrest of newborn (P28.81)
> respiratory failure of newborn NOS (P28.5)
>
> **AHA:** 2019,2Q,29
> **DEF:** Severe chest contractions upon air intake and expiratory grunting. The infant appears blue due to oxygen deficiency and has a rapid respiratory rate, formerly called hyaline membrane disease.

P22.1 Transient tachypnea of newborn
> Idiopathic tachypnea of newborn
> Respiratory distress syndrome, type II
> Wet lung syndrome
> **DEF:** Rapid, labored breathing of a newborn. It is a short-term problem that begins after birth and lasts about three days.

P22.8 Other respiratory distress of newborn
> **EXCLUDES 1** respiratory arrest of newborn (P28.81)
> respiratory failure of newborn NOS (P28.5)

P22.9 Respiratory distress of newborn, unspecified
> **EXCLUDES 1** respiratory arrest of newborn (P28.81)
> respiratory failure of newborn NOS (P28.5)

☑4th P23 Congenital pneumonia

> **INCLUDES** infective pneumonia acquired in utero or during birth
> **EXCLUDES 1** neonatal pneumonia resulting from aspiration (P24.-)

P23.0 Congenital pneumonia due to viral agent `MCC`
> Use additional code (B97) to identify organism
> **EXCLUDES 1** congenital rubella pneumonitis (P35.0)

P23.1 Congenital pneumonia due to Chlamydia `MCC`

P23.2 Congenital pneumonia due to staphylococcus `MCC`

P23.3 Congenital pneumonia due to streptococcus, group B `MCC`

P23.4 Congenital pneumonia due to Escherichia coli `MCC`

P23.5 Congenital pneumonia due to Pseudomonas `MCC`

P23.6 Congenital pneumonia due to other bacterial agents `MCC`
> Congenital pneumonia due to Hemophilus influenzae
> Congenital pneumonia due to Klebsiella pneumoniae
> Congenital pneumonia due to Mycoplasma
> Congenital pneumonia due to Streptococcus, except group B
> Use additional code (B95-B96) to identify organism

P23.8 Congenital pneumonia due to other organisms `MCC`

P23.9 Congenital pneumonia, unspecified `MCC`

✓4ᵗʰ P24 Neonatal aspiration

INCLUDES aspiration in utero and during delivery

✓5ᵗʰ P24.0 Meconium aspiration

EXCLUDES 1 meconium passage (without aspiration) during delivery (P03.82)

meconium staining (P96.83)

DEF: Meconium in the trachea or seen on chest x-ray after birth.

P24.00 Meconium aspiration without respiratory symptoms

Meconium aspiration NOS

P24.01 Meconium aspiration with respiratory symptoms MCC

Meconium aspiration pneumonia

Meconium aspiration pneumonitis

Meconium aspiration syndrome NOS

Use additional code to identify any secondary pulmonary hypertension, if applicable (I27.2-)

DEF: Aspiration of fetal gastrointestinal material during or prior to delivery. If is usually a complication of placental insufficiency, causing pneumonitis and bronchial obstruction (inflammatory reaction of lungs).

✓5ᵗʰ P24.1 Neonatal aspiration of (clear) amniotic fluid and mucus

Neonatal aspiration of liquor (amnii)

P24.10 Neonatal aspiration of (clear) amniotic fluid and mucus without respiratory symptoms

Neonatal aspiration of amniotic fluid and mucus NOS

P24.11 Neonatal aspiration of (clear) amniotic fluid and mucus with respiratory symptoms MCC

Neonatal aspiration of amniotic fluid and mucus with pneumonia

Neonatal aspiration of amniotic fluid and mucus with pneumonitis

Use additional code to identify any secondary pulmonary hypertension, if applicable (I27.2-)

✓5ᵗʰ P24.2 Neonatal aspiration of blood

P24.20 Neonatal aspiration of blood without respiratory symptoms

Neonatal aspiration of blood NOS

P24.21 Neonatal aspiration of blood with respiratory symptoms MCC

Neonatal aspiration of blood with pneumonia

Neonatal aspiration of blood with pneumonitis

Use additional code to identify any secondary pulmonary hypertension, if applicable (I27.2-)

✓5ᵗʰ P24.3 Neonatal aspiration of milk and regurgitated food

Neonatal aspiration of stomach contents

P24.30 Neonatal aspiration of milk and regurgitated food without respiratory symptoms

Neonatal aspiration of milk and regurgitated food NOS

P24.31 Neonatal aspiration of milk and regurgitated food with respiratory symptoms MCC

Neonatal aspiration of milk and regurgitated food with pneumonia

Neonatal aspiration of milk and regurgitated food with pneumonitis

Use additional code to identify any secondary pulmonary hypertension, if applicable (I27.2-)

✓5ᵗʰ P24.8 Other neonatal aspiration

P24.80 Other neonatal aspiration without respiratory symptoms

Neonatal aspiration NEC

P24.81 Other neonatal aspiration with respiratory symptoms MCC

Neonatal aspiration pneumonia NEC

Neonatal aspiration with pneumonitis NEC

Neonatal aspiration with pneumonia NOS

Neonatal aspiration with pneumonitis NOS

Use additional code to identify any secondary pulmonary hypertension, if applicable (I27.2-)

P24.9 Neonatal aspiration, unspecified

✓4ᵗʰ P25 Interstitial emphysema and related conditions originating in the perinatal period

P25.0 Interstitial emphysema originating in the perinatal period MCC

P25.1 Pneumothorax originating in the perinatal period MCC

P25.2 Pneumomediastinum originating in the perinatal period MCC

P25.3 Pneumopericardium originating in the perinatal period MCC

P25.8 Other conditions related to interstitial emphysema originating in the perinatal period MCC

✓4ᵗʰ P26 Pulmonary hemorrhage originating in the perinatal period

EXCLUDES 1 acute idiopathic hemorrhage in infants over 28 days old (R04.81)

P26.0 Tracheobronchial hemorrhage originating in the perinatal period

P26.1 Massive pulmonary hemorrhage originating in the perinatal period MCC

P26.8 Other pulmonary hemorrhages originating in the perinatal period MCC

P26.9 Unspecified pulmonary hemorrhage originating in the perinatal period MCC

✓4ᵗʰ P27 Chronic respiratory disease originating in the perinatal period

EXCLUDES 2 respiratory distress of newborn (P22.0-P22.9)

P27.0 Wilson-Mikity syndrome MCC

Pulmonary dysmaturity

DEF: Pulmonary insufficiency in newborn babies, especially those with low birth weight. Rapid onset of hypercapnia and cyanosis occur during the first month of life frequently resulting in death.

P27.1 Bronchopulmonary dysplasia originating in the perinatal period MCC

P27.8 Other chronic respiratory diseases originating in the perinatal period MCC

Congenital pulmonary fibrosis

Ventilator lung in newborn

P27.9 Unspecified chronic respiratory disease originating in the perinatal period MCC

✓4ᵗʰ P28 Other respiratory conditions originating in the perinatal period

EXCLUDES 1 congenital malformations of the respiratory system (Q30-Q34)

P28.0 Primary atelectasis of newborn CC

Primary failure to expand terminal respiratory units

Pulmonary hypoplasia associated with short gestation

Pulmonary immaturity NOS

✓5ᵗʰ P28.1 Other and unspecified atelectasis of newborn

P28.10 Unspecified atelectasis of newborn CC

Atelectasis of newborn NOS

P28.11 Resorption atelectasis without respiratory distress syndrome CC

EXCLUDES 1 resorption atelectasis with respiratory distress syndrome (P22.0)

P28.19 Other atelectasis of newborn CC

Partial atelectasis of newborn

Secondary atelectasis of newborn

P28.2 Cyanotic attacks of newborn CC

EXCLUDES 1 apnea of newborn (P28.3-P28.4)

P28.3 Primary sleep apnea of newborn CC

Central sleep apnea of newborn

Obstructive sleep apnea of newborn

Sleep apnea of newborn NOS

DEF: Unexplained cessation of breathing when a neonate makes no respiratory effort for 20 seconds or longer or when a neonate's breathing cessation is accompanied by cyanosis, bradycardia, or hypotonia.

P28.4 Other apnea of newborn CC

Apnea of prematurity

Obstructive apnea of newborn

EXCLUDES 1 obstructive sleep apnea of newborn (P28.3)

P28.5 Respiratory failure of newborn MCC

EXCLUDES 1 respiratory arrest of newborn (P28.81)

respiratory distress of newborn (P22.0-)

AHA: 2019,2Q,29

✓5ᵗʰ P28.8 Other specified respiratory conditions of newborn

P28.81 Respiratory arrest of newborn MCC

P28.89 Other specified respiratory conditions of newborn

Congenital laryngeal stridor

Sniffles in newborn

Snuffles in newborn

EXCLUDES 1 early congenital syphilitic rhinitis (A50.05)

P28.9 Respiratory condition of newborn, unspecified

Respiratory depression in newborn

N Newborn: 0 | P Pediatric: 0-17 | M Maternity: 9-64 | A Adult: 15-124 | MCC Major Complication/Comorbidity | CC Complication/Comorbidity | SW Severe Wound Dx

908 | ICD-10-CM 2021

✓4ᵗʰ **P29 Cardiovascular disorders originating in the perinatal period**

    EXCLUDES 1   *congenital malformations of the circulatory system (Q20-Q28)*

  P29.0 Neonatal cardiac failure

✓5ᵗʰ **P29.1 Neonatal cardiac dysrhythmia**

    P29.11 Neonatal tachycardia

    P29.12 Neonatal bradycardia

  P29.2 Neonatal hypertension

✓5ᵗʰ **P29.3 Persistent fetal circulation**

    AHA: 2017,4Q,20-21

    P29.30 Pulmonary hypertension of newborn   MCC

      Persistent pulmonary hypertension of newborn

      DEF: Condition that occurs when pressure within the pulmonary artery is elevated and vascular resistance is observed in the lungs.

    P29.38 Other persistent fetal circulation   MCC

      Delayed closure of ductus arteriosus

  P29.4 Transient myocardial ischemia in newborn

✓5ᵗʰ **P29.8 Other cardiovascular disorders originating in the perinatal period**

    P29.81 Cardiac arrest of newborn   MCC

    P29.89 Other cardiovascular disorders originating in the perinatal period

      AHA: 2014,4Q,23

  P29.9 Cardiovascular disorder originating in the perinatal period, unspecified

Infections specific to the perinatal period (P35-P39)

Infections acquired in utero, during birth via the umbilicus, or during the first 28 days after birth

  EXCLUDES 2   *asymptomatic human immunodeficiency virus [HIV] infection status (Z21)*

    congenital gonococcal infection (A54.-)

    congenital pneumonia (P23.-)

    congenital syphilis (A50.-)

    human immunodeficiency virus [HIV] disease (B20)

    infant botulism (A48.51)

    infectious diseases not specific to the perinatal period (A00-B99, J09, J10.-)

    intestinal infectious disease (A00-A09)

    laboratory evidence of human immunodeficiency virus [HIV] (R75)

    tetanus neonatorum (A33)

✓4ᵗʰ **P35 Congenital viral diseases**

  INCLUDES   infections acquired in utero or during birth

  P35.0 Congenital rubella syndrome   CC

    Congenital rubella pneumonitis

  P35.1 Congenital cytomegalovirus infection   MCC

  P35.2 Congenital herpesviral [herpes simplex] infection   MCC

  P35.3 Congenital viral hepatitis   MCC

  P35.4 Congenital Zika virus disease   MCC

    Use additional code to identify manifestations of congenital Zika virus disease

    AHA: 2018,4Q,25-26

  P35.8 Other congenital viral diseases   MCC

    Congenital varicella [chickenpox]

    AHA: 2020,2Q,13

  P35.9 Congenital viral disease, unspecified   MCC

✓4ᵗʰ **P36 Bacterial sepsis of newborn**

  INCLUDES   congenital sepsis

  Use additional code(s), if applicable, to identify severe sepsis (R65.2-) and associated acute organ dysfunction(s)

  P36.0 Sepsis of newborn due to streptococcus, group B   MCC HCC

✓5ᵗʰ **P36.1 Sepsis of newborn due to other and unspecified streptococci**

    P36.10 Sepsis of newborn due to unspecified streptococci   MCC HCC

    P36.19 Sepsis of newborn due to other streptococci   MCC HCC

  P36.2 Sepsis of newborn due to Staphylococcus aureus   MCC HCC

✓5ᵗʰ **P36.3 Sepsis of newborn due to other and unspecified staphylococci**

    P36.30 Sepsis of newborn due to unspecified staphylococci   MCC HCC

    P36.39 Sepsis of newborn due to other staphylococci   MCC HCC

  P36.4 Sepsis of newborn due to Escherichia coli   MCC HCC

  P36.5 Sepsis of newborn due to anaerobes   MCC HCC

  P36.8 Other bacterial sepsis of newborn   MCC HCC

    Use additional code from category B96 to identify organism

  P36.9 Bacterial sepsis of newborn, unspecified   MCC HCC

✓4ᵗʰ **P37 Other congenital infectious and parasitic diseases**

  EXCLUDES 2   *congenital syphilis (A50.-)*

    infectious neonatal diarrhea (A00-A09)

    necrotizing enterocolitis in newborn (P77.-)

    noninfectious neonatal diarrhea (P78.3)

    ophthalmia neonatorum due to gonococcus (A54.31)

    tetanus neonatorum (A33)

  P37.0 Congenital tuberculosis   MCC

  P37.1 Congenital toxoplasmosis   MCC

    Hydrocephalus due to congenital toxoplasmosis

  P37.2 Neonatal (disseminated) listeriosis   MCC

  P37.3 Congenital falciparum malaria   MCC

  P37.4 Other congenital malaria   MCC

  P37.5 Neonatal candidiasis

  P37.8 Other specified congenital infectious and parasitic diseases   MCC

  P37.9 Congenital infectious or parasitic disease, unspecified   MCC

✓4ᵗʰ **P38 Omphalitis of newborn**

  EXCLUDES 1   *omphalitis not of newborn (L08.82)*

    tetanus omphalitis (A33)

    umbilical hemorrhage of newborn (P51.-)

  DEF: Omphalitis: Infection and inflammation of the umbilical stump, often due to bacteria that can spread beyond the umbilical stump to the fascia, muscle, or even the umbilical vessels.

  P38.1 Omphalitis with mild hemorrhage   CC

  P38.9 Omphalitis without hemorrhage   CC

    Omphalitis of newborn NOS

✓4ᵗʰ **P39 Other infections specific to the perinatal period**

  Use additional code to identify organism or specific infection

  P39.0 Neonatal infective mastitis   CC

    EXCLUDES 1   *breast engorgement of newborn (P83.4)*

      noninfective mastitis of newborn (P83.4)

  P39.1 Neonatal conjunctivitis and dacryocystitis

    Neonatal chlamydial conjunctivitis

    Ophthalmia neonatorum NOS

    EXCLUDES 1   *gonococcal conjunctivitis (A54.31)*

  P39.2 Intra-amniotic infection affecting newborn, not elsewhere classified   CC

  P39.3 Neonatal urinary tract infection   CC

  P39.4 Neonatal skin infection   CC

    Neonatal pyoderma

    EXCLUDES 1   *pemphigus neonatorum (L00)*

      staphylococcal scalded skin syndrome (L00)

  P39.8 Other specified infections specific to the perinatal period   CC

  P39.9 Infection specific to the perinatal period, unspecified   CC

Hemorrhagic and hematological disorders of newborn (P50-P61)

  EXCLUDES 1   *congenital stenosis and stricture of bile ducts (Q44.3)*

    Crigler-Najjar syndrome (E80.5)

    Dubin-Johnson syndrome (E80.6)

    Gilbert syndrome (E80.4)

    hereditary hemolytic anemias (D55-D58)

✓4ᵗʰ **P50 Newborn affected by intrauterine (fetal) blood loss**

  EXCLUDES 1   *congenital anemia from intrauterine (fetal) blood loss (P61.3)*

  P50.0 Newborn affected by intrauterine (fetal) blood loss from vasa previa

  P50.1 Newborn affected by intrauterine (fetal) blood loss from ruptured cord

  P50.2 Newborn affected by intrauterine (fetal) blood loss from placenta

  P50.3 Newborn affected by hemorrhage into co-twin

  P50.4 Newborn affected by hemorrhage into maternal circulation

  P50.5 Newborn affected by intrauterine (fetal) blood loss from cut end of co-twin's cord

  P50.8 Newborn affected by other intrauterine (fetal) blood loss

  P50.9 Newborn affected by intrauterine (fetal) blood loss, unspecified

    Newborn affected by fetal hemorrhage NOS

☑ Additional Character Required   ✓x7ᵗʰ Placeholder   Unacceptable PDx   Questionable PDx   Manifestation   Unspecified Dx   H1-H14 HAC   HCC CMS-HCC Dx   HIV HIV Dx

ICD-10-CM 2021   **909**

Chapter 16. Certain Conditions Originating in the Perinatal Period

P51-P59.9

✓4ᵗʰ **P51** Umbilical hemorrhage of newborn
> EXCLUDES 1   *omphalitis with mild hemorrhage (P38.1)*
> *umbilical hemorrhage from cut end of co-twins cord (P50.5)*

P51.0 Massive umbilical hemorrhage of newborn

P51.8 Other umbilical hemorrhages of newborn
> Slipped umbilical ligature NOS

P51.9 Umbilical hemorrhage of newborn, unspecified

✓4ᵗʰ **P52** Intracranial nontraumatic hemorrhage of newborn
> INCLUDES   intracranial hemorrhage due to anoxia or hypoxia
> EXCLUDES 1   *intracranial hemorrhage due to birth injury (P10.-)*
> *intracranial hemorrhage due to other injury (S06.-)*

P52.0 Intraventricular (nontraumatic) hemorrhage, grade 1, of newborn   CC
> Subependymal hemorrhage (without intraventricular extension)
> Bleeding into germinal matrix

P52.1 Intraventricular (nontraumatic) hemorrhage, grade 2, of newborn   CC
> Subependymal hemorrhage with intraventricular extension
> Bleeding into ventricle

✓5ᵗʰ **P52.2** Intraventricular (nontraumatic) hemorrhage, grade 3 and grade 4, of newborn

    P52.21 Intraventricular (nontraumatic) hemorrhage, grade 3, of newborn   MCC
> Subependymal hemorrhage with intraventricular extension with enlargement of ventricle

    P52.22 Intraventricular (nontraumatic) hemorrhage, grade 4, of newborn   MCC
> Bleeding into cerebral cortex
> Subependymal hemorrhage with intracerebral extension

P52.3 Unspecified intraventricular (nontraumatic) hemorrhage of newborn   CC

P52.4 Intracerebral (nontraumatic) hemorrhage of newborn   MCC

P52.5 Subarachnoid (nontraumatic) hemorrhage of newborn   MCC

P52.6 Cerebellar (nontraumatic) and posterior fossa hemorrhage of newborn   MCC

P52.8 Other intracranial (nontraumatic) hemorrhages of newborn   MCC

P52.9 Intracranial (nontraumatic) hemorrhage of newborn, unspecified   MCC

P53 Hemorrhagic disease of newborn   CC
> Vitamin K deficiency of newborn

✓4ᵗʰ **P54** Other neonatal hemorrhages
> EXCLUDES 1   *newborn affected by (intrauterine) blood loss (P50.-)*
> *pulmonary hemorrhage originating in the perinatal period (P26.-)*

P54.0 Neonatal hematemesis
> EXCLUDES 1   *neonatal hematemesis due to swallowed maternal blood (P78.2)*

P54.1 Neonatal melena   MCC
> EXCLUDES 1   *neonatal melena due to swallowed maternal blood (P78.2)*

P54.2 Neonatal rectal hemorrhage   MCC

P54.3 Other neonatal gastrointestinal hemorrhage   MCC

P54.4 Neonatal adrenal hemorrhage   CC

P54.5 Neonatal cutaneous hemorrhage
> Neonatal bruising
> Neonatal ecchymoses
> Neonatal petechiae
> Neonatal superficial hematomata
> EXCLUDES 2   *bruising of scalp due to birth injury (P12.3)*
> *cephalhematoma due to birth injury (P12.0)*

P54.6 Neonatal vaginal hemorrhage   ♀
> Neonatal pseudomenses

P54.8 Other specified neonatal hemorrhages

P54.9 Neonatal hemorrhage, unspecified

✓4ᵗʰ **P55** Hemolytic disease of newborn

P55.0 Rh isoimmunization of newborn
> **DEF:** Incompatible Rh fetal-maternal blood grouping that prematurely destroys red blood cells. Symptoms include jaundice, asphyxia, pulmonary hypertension, edema, respiratory distress, kernicterus, and coagulopathies. It is detected by a Coombs test.
> **TIP:** A positive Coombs test without documentation of associated Rh isoimmunization should be coded to R79.89 Other specified abnormal findings of blood chemistry.

P55.1 ABO isoimmunization of newborn
> AHA: 2015,3Q,20

P55.8 Other hemolytic diseases of newborn
> AHA: 2018,3Q,24

P55.9 Hemolytic disease of newborn, unspecified

✓4ᵗʰ **P56** Hydrops fetalis due to hemolytic disease
> EXCLUDES 1   *hydrops fetalis NOS (P83.2)*

P56.0 Hydrops fetalis due to isoimmunization   MCC

✓5ᵗʰ **P56.9** Hydrops fetalis due to other and unspecified hemolytic disease

    P56.90 Hydrops fetalis due to unspecified hemolytic disease   MCC

    P56.99 Hydrops fetalis due to other hemolytic disease   MCC

✓4ᵗʰ **P57** Kernicterus

P57.0 Kernicterus due to isoimmunization   MCC
> **DEF:** Complication of erythroblastosis fetalis associated with severe neural symptoms, high blood bilirubin levels, and nerve cell destruction. It results in bilirubin-pigmented gray matter of the central nervous system.

P57.8 Other specified kernicterus   MCC
> EXCLUDES 1   *Crigler-Najjar syndrome (E80.5)*

P57.9 Kernicterus, unspecified   MCC

✓4ᵗʰ **P58** Neonatal jaundice due to other excessive hemolysis
> EXCLUDES 1   *jaundice due to isoimmunization (P55-P57)*

P58.0 Neonatal jaundice due to bruising

P58.1 Neonatal jaundice due to bleeding

P58.2 Neonatal jaundice due to infection

P58.3 Neonatal jaundice due to polycythemia

✓5ᵗʰ **P58.4** Neonatal jaundice due to drugs or toxins transmitted from mother or given to newborn
> Code first poisoning due to drug or toxin, if applicable (T36-T65 with fifth or sixth character 1-4 or 6)
> Use additional code for adverse effect, if applicable, to identify drug (T36-T50 with fifth or sixth character 5)

    P58.41 Neonatal jaundice due to drugs or toxins transmitted from mother

    P58.42 Neonatal jaundice due to drugs or toxins given to newborn

P58.5 Neonatal jaundice due to swallowed maternal blood

P58.8 Neonatal jaundice due to other specified excessive hemolysis

P58.9 Neonatal jaundice due to excessive hemolysis, unspecified

✓4ᵗʰ **P59** Neonatal jaundice from other and unspecified causes
> EXCLUDES 1   *jaundice due to inborn errors of metabolism (E70-E88)*
> *kernicterus (P57.-)*

P59.0 Neonatal jaundice associated with preterm delivery
> Hyperbilirubinemia of prematurity
> Jaundice due to delayed conjugation associated with preterm delivery

P59.1 Inspissated bile syndrome   MCC
> **DEF:** Biliary obstruction in newborn resulting from obstruction of outflow tract.

✓5ᵗʰ **P59.2** Neonatal jaundice from other and unspecified hepatocellular damage
> EXCLUDES 1   *congenital viral hepatitis (P35.3)*

    P59.20 Neonatal jaundice from unspecified hepatocellular damage   MCC

    P59.29 Neonatal jaundice from other hepatocellular damage   MCC
> Neonatal giant cell hepatitis
> Neonatal (idiopathic) hepatitis

P59.3 Neonatal jaundice from breast milk inhibitor

P59.8 Neonatal jaundice from other specified causes

P59.9 Neonatal jaundice, unspecified
> Neonatal physiological jaundice (intense)(prolonged) NOS
> AHA: 2015,3Q,20

N Newborn: 0   P Pediatric: 0-17   M Maternity: 9-64   A Adult: 15-124   MCC Major Complication/Comorbidity   CC Complication/Comorbidity   SW Severe Wound Dx

910   ICD-10-CM 2021

P60   **Disseminated intravascular coagulation of newborn**   `MCC`
Defibrination syndrome of newborn

`√4ᵗʰ` **P61**   **Other perinatal hematological disorders**
    `EXCLUDES 1`   *transient hypogammaglobulinemia of infancy (D80.7)*

    P61.0   **Transient neonatal thrombocytopenia**   `MCC`
       Neonatal thrombocytopenia due to exchange transfusion
       Neonatal thrombocytopenia due to idiopathic maternal thrombocytopenia
       Neonatal thrombocytopenia due to isoimmunization
       DEF: Temporary decrease in blood platelets of a newborn that is secondary to placental insufficiency.

    P61.1   **Polycythemia neonatorum**
       DEF: Abnormal increase of total red blood cells of a newborn that results in hyperviscosity, which slows the flow of blood through small blood vessels.

    P61.2   **Anemia of prematurity**   `CC`
    P61.3   **Congenital anemia from fetal blood loss**   `CC`
    P61.4   **Other congenital anemias, not elsewhere classified**   `CC`
       Congenital anemia NOS

    P61.5   **Transient neonatal neutropenia**   `MCC`
       `EXCLUDES 1`   *congenital neutropenia (nontransient) (D70.0)*
       DEF: Low blood neutrophil counts of newborn that occurs due to maternal hypertension, sepsis, twin-twin transfusion, alloimmunization, and hemolytic disease.

    P61.6   **Other transient neonatal disorders of coagulation**   `CC`
    P61.8   **Other specified perinatal hematological disorders**
    P61.9   **Perinatal hematological disorder, unspecified**

Transitory endocrine and metabolic disorders specific to newborn (P70-P74)

    `INCLUDES`   transitory endocrine and metabolic disturbances caused by the infant's response to maternal endocrine and metabolic factors, or its adjustment to extrauterine environment

AHA: 2018,2Q,6

`√4ᵗʰ` **P70**   **Transitory disorders of carbohydrate metabolism specific to newborn**

    P70.0   **Syndrome of infant of mother with gestational diabetes**
       Newborn (with hypoglycemia) affected by maternal gestational diabetes
       `EXCLUDES 1`   *newborn (with hypoglycemia) affected by maternal (pre-existing) diabetes mellitus (P70.1)*
              syndrome of infant of a diabetic mother (P70.1)

    P70.1   **Syndrome of infant of a diabetic mother**
       Newborn (with hypoglycemia) affected by maternal (pre-existing) diabetes mellitus
       `EXCLUDES 1`   *newborn (with hypoglycemia) affected by maternal gestational diabetes (P70.0)*
              syndrome of infant of mother with gestational diabetes (P70.0)

    P70.2   **Neonatal diabetes mellitus**   `CC`
    P70.3   **Iatrogenic neonatal hypoglycemia**
    P70.4   **Other neonatal hypoglycemia**
       Transitory neonatal hypoglycemia
    P70.8   **Other transitory disorders of carbohydrate metabolism of newborn**   `CC`
    P70.9   **Transitory disorder of carbohydrate metabolism of newborn, unspecified**

`√4ᵗʰ` **P71**   **Transitory neonatal disorders of calcium and magnesium metabolism**
    P71.0   **Cow's milk hypocalcemia in newborn**   `CC`
    P71.1   **Other neonatal hypocalcemia**   `CC`
       `EXCLUDES 1`   *neonatal hypoparathyroidism (P71.4)*
    P71.2   **Neonatal hypomagnesemia**   `CC`
    P71.3   **Neonatal tetany without calcium or magnesium deficiency**   `CC`
       Neonatal tetany NOS
    P71.4   **Transitory neonatal hypoparathyroidism**   `CC`
    P71.8   **Other transitory neonatal disorders of calcium and magnesium metabolism**   `CC`
       AHA: 2016,4Q,54
    P71.9   **Transitory neonatal disorder of calcium and magnesium metabolism, unspecified**   `CC`

`√4ᵗʰ` **P72**   **Other transitory neonatal endocrine disorders**
    `EXCLUDES 1`   *congenital hypothyroidism with or without goiter (E03.0-E03.1)*
           dyshormogenetic goiter (E07.1)
           Pendred's syndrome (E07.1)

    P72.0   **Neonatal goiter, not elsewhere classified**   `CC`
       Transitory congenital goiter with normal functioning
    P72.1   **Transitory neonatal hyperthyroidism**   `CC`
       Neonatal thyrotoxicosis
    P72.2   **Other transitory neonatal disorders of thyroid function, not elsewhere classified**   `CC`
       Transitory neonatal hypothyroidism
    P72.8   **Other specified transitory neonatal endocrine disorders**   `CC`
    P72.9   **Transitory neonatal endocrine disorder, unspecified**

`√4ᵗʰ` **P74**   **Other transitory neonatal electrolyte and metabolic disturbances**
    AHA: 2018,4Q,26-27

    P74.0   **Late metabolic acidosis of newborn**   `MCC`
       `EXCLUDES 1`   *(fetal) metabolic acidosis of newborn (P19)*
    P74.1   **Dehydration of newborn**
   `√5ᵗʰ` **P74.2**   **Disturbances of sodium balance of newborn**
       P74.21   **Hypernatremia of newborn**
       P74.22   **Hyponatremia of newborn**
   `√5ᵗʰ` **P74.3**   **Disturbances of potassium balance of newborn**
       P74.31   **Hyperkalemia of newborn**
       P74.32   **Hypokalemia of newborn**
   `√5ᵗʰ` **P74.4**   **Other transitory electrolyte disturbances of newborn**
       P74.41   **Alkalosis of newborn**   `CC`
           Hyperbicarbonatemia
     `√6ᵗʰ` **P74.42**   **Disturbances of chlorine balance of newborn**
          P74.421   **Hyperchloremia of newborn**
             Hyperchloremic metabolic acidosis
             `EXCLUDES 2`   *late metabolic acidosis of the newborn (P74.0)*
          P74.422   **Hypochloremia of newborn**
       P74.49   **Other transitory electrolyte disturbance of newborn**
    P74.5   **Transitory tyrosinemia of newborn**   `CC`
    P74.6   **Transitory hyperammonemia of newborn**   `CC`
    P74.8   **Other transitory metabolic disturbances of newborn**   `CC`
       Amino-acid metabolic disorders described as transitory
    P74.9   **Transitory metabolic disturbance of newborn, unspecified**

Digestive system disorders of newborn (P76-P78)

`√4ᵗʰ` **P76**   **Other intestinal obstruction of newborn**

    P76.0   **Meconium plug syndrome**
       Meconium ileus NOS
       `EXCLUDES 1`   *meconium ileus in cystic fibrosis (E84.11)*
       DEF: Meconium obstruction of a newborn's intestines, resulting from unusually thick or hard meconium.

    P76.1   **Transitory ileus of newborn**   `CC`
       `EXCLUDES 1`   *Hirschsprung's disease (Q43.1)*
    P76.2   **Intestinal obstruction due to inspissated milk**
    P76.8   **Other specified intestinal obstruction of newborn**
       `EXCLUDES 1`   *intestinal obstruction classifiable to K56.-*
    P76.9   **Intestinal obstruction of newborn, unspecified**

`√4ᵗʰ` **P77**   **Necrotizing enterocolitis of newborn**
    DEF: Serious intestinal infection and inflammation in preterm infants. Severity is measured by stages and may progress to life-threatening perforation or peritonitis. Resection surgical treatment may be necessary.

    P77.1   **Stage 1 necrotizing enterocolitis in newborn**   `MCC`
       Necrotizing enterocolitis without pneumatosis, without perforation
       DEF: Broad-spectrum symptoms with nonspecific signs, including feeding intolerance, abdominal distention, bradycardia, and metabolic abnormalities.

    P77.2   **Stage 2 necrotizing enterocolitis in newborn**   `MCC`
       Necrotizing enterocolitis with pneumatosis, without perforation
       DEF: Radiographic confirmation of necrotizing enterocolitis showing intestinal dilatation, fixed loops of bowels, pneumatosis intestinalis, metabolic acidosis, and thrombocytopenia.

☑ Additional Character Required   `√x7ᵗʰ` Placeholder   Unacceptable PDx   Questionable PDx   Manifestation   Unspecified Dx   `H1`-`H14` HAC   `HCC` CMS-HCC Dx   `HIV` HIV Dx

ICD-10-CM 2021   **911**

P77.3 Stage 3 **necrotizing enterocolitis in newborn** MCC
Necrotizing enterocolitis with perforation
Necrotizing enterocolitis with pneumatosis and perforation
DEF: Advanced stage in which an infant demonstrates signs of bowel perforation, septic shock, metabolic acidosis, ascites, disseminated intravascular coagulopathy, and neutropenia.

P77.9 Necrotizing enterocolitis in newborn, unspecified MCC
Necrotizing enterocolitis in newborn, NOS

✓4ᵗʰ **P78** **Other perinatal digestive system disorders**
EXCLUDES 1 cystic fibrosis (E84.0-E84.9)
neonatal gastrointestinal hemorrhages (P54.0-P54.3)

P78.0 **Perinatal intestinal perforation** MCC
Meconium peritonitis

P78.1 **Other neonatal peritonitis**
Neonatal peritonitis NOS

P78.2 **Neonatal hematemesis and melena due to swallowed maternal blood**

P78.3 **Noninfective neonatal diarrhea**
Neonatal diarrhea NOS

✓5ᵗʰ **P78.8** **Other specified perinatal digestive system disorders**

P78.81 **Congenital cirrhosis (of liver)**

P78.82 **Peptic ulcer of newborn**

P78.83 **Newborn esophageal reflux**
Neonatal esophageal reflux

P78.84 **Gestational alloimmune liver disease**
GALD
Neonatal hemochromatosis
EXCLUDES 1 hemochromatosis (E83.11-)
AHA: 2017,4Q,21
DEF: Severe hepatic injury with onset during fetal development with manifestations beginning during fetal life. It is due to maternal antibodies to fetal hepatic cells (hepatocytes) that cross the placenta into the fetal circulation, causing hepatic cell necrosis.

P78.89 **Other specified perinatal digestive system disorders**

P78.9 **Perinatal digestive system disorder, unspecified**

Conditions involving the integument and temperature regulation of newborn (P80-P83)

✓4ᵗʰ **P80** **Hypothermia of newborn**
DEF: Decrease in newborn body temperature due to their larger ratio of surface area to body weight, thin skin with blood vessels close to the surface, and a limited amount of subcutaneous fat.

P80.0 **Cold injury syndrome**
Severe and usually chronic hypothermia associated with a pink flushed appearance, edema and neurological and biochemical abnormalities.
EXCLUDES 1 mild hypothermia of newborn (P80.8)

P80.8 **Other hypothermia of newborn**
Mild hypothermia of newborn

P80.9 **Hypothermia of newborn, unspecified**

✓4ᵗʰ **P81** **Other disturbances of temperature regulation of newborn**

P81.0 **Environmental hyperthermia of newborn**

P81.8 **Other specified disturbances of temperature regulation of newborn**

P81.9 **Disturbance of temperature regulation of newborn, unspecified**
Fever of newborn NOS

✓4ᵗʰ **P83** **Other conditions of integument specific to newborn**
EXCLUDES 1 congenital malformations of skin and integument (Q80-Q84)
hydrops fetalis due to hemolytic disease (P56.-)
neonatal skin infection (P39.4)
staphylococcal scalded skin syndrome (L00)
EXCLUDES 2 cradle cap (L21.0)
diaper [napkin] dermatitis (L22)

P83.0 **Sclerema neonatorum** CC
DEF: Diffuse, rapidly progressing white, waxy, nonpitting hardening of tissue, usually of legs and feet that is life-threatening. It is found in preterm or debilitated infants. Etiology is unknown.

P83.1 **Neonatal erythema toxicum**

P83.2 **Hydrops fetalis not due to hemolytic disease** MCC
Hydrops fetalis NOS
DEF: Severe, life-threatening problem of a newborn characterized by severe edema of the entire body. It is unrelated to immune response.

✓5ᵗʰ **P83.3** **Other and unspecified edema specific to newborn**

P83.30 **Unspecified edema specific to newborn** CC

P83.39 **Other edema specific to newborn** CC

P83.4 **Breast engorgement of newborn**
Noninfective mastitis of newborn

P83.5 **Congenital hydrocele** ♂
DEF: Hydrocele: Serous fluid that collects in the tunica vaginalis of the scrotum along the spermatic cord in males.

P83.6 **Umbilical polyp of newborn**

✓5ᵗʰ **P83.8** **Other specified conditions of integument specific to newborn**
AHA: 2017,4Q,21-22

P83.81 **Umbilical granuloma**
EXCLUDES 2 granulomatous disorder of the skin and subcutaneous tissue, unspecified (L92.9)

P83.88 **Other specified conditions of integument specific to newborn**
Bronze baby syndrome
Neonatal scleroderma
Urticaria neonatorum

P83.9 **Condition of the integument specific to newborn, unspecified**

Other problems with newborn (P84)

P84 **Other problems with newborn**
Acidemia of newborn
Acidosis of newborn
Anoxia of newborn NOS
Asphyxia of newborn NOS
Hypercapnia of newborn
Hypoxemia of newborn
Hypoxia of newborn NOS
Mixed metabolic and respiratory acidosis of newborn
EXCLUDES 1 intracranial hemorrhage due to anoxia or hypoxia (P52.-)
hypoxic ischemic encephalopathy [HIE] (P91.6-)
late metabolic acidosis of newborn (P74.0)

Other disorders originating in the perinatal period (P90-P96)

P90 **Convulsions of newborn** MCC
EXCLUDES 1 benign myoclonic epilepsy in infancy (G40.3-)
benign neonatal convulsions (familial) (G40.3-)

✓4ᵗʰ **P91** **Other disturbances of cerebral status of newborn**

P91.0 **Neonatal cerebral ischemia** MCC
EXCLUDES 1 ▶neonatal cerebral infarction (P91.82-)◀

P91.1 **Acquired periventricular cysts of newborn** MCC

P91.2 **Neonatal cerebral leukomalacia** MCC
Periventricular leukomalacia

P91.3 **Neonatal cerebral irritability** MCC

P91.4 **Neonatal cerebral depression** MCC

P91.5 **Neonatal coma** MCC

✓5ᵗʰ **P91.6** **Hypoxic ischemic encephalopathy [HIE]**
EXCLUDES 1 neonatal cerebral depression (P91.4)
neonatal cerebral irritability (P91.3)
neonatal coma (P91.5)
AHA: 2017,4Q,22

P91.60 **Hypoxic ischemic encephalopathy [HIE], unspecified** CC

P91.61 **Mild hypoxic ischemic encephalopathy [HIE]** CC

P91.62 **Moderate hypoxic ischemic encephalopathy [HIE]** CC

P91.63 **Severe hypoxic ischemic encephalopathy [HIE]** MCC

✓5ᵗʰ **P91.8** **Other specified disturbances of cerebral status of newborn**
AHA: 2017,4Q,22

✓6ᵗʰ **P91.81** **Neonatal encephalopathy**

P91.811 **Neonatal encephalopathy in diseases classified elsewhere**
Code first underlying condition, if known, such as:
congenital cirrhosis (of liver) (P78.81)
intracranial nontraumatic hemorrhage of newborn (P52.-)
kernicterus (P57.-)

P91.819 **Neonatal encephalopathy, unspecified**

N Newborn: 0 P Pediatric: 0-17 M Maternity: 9-64 A Adult: 15-124 MCC Major Complication/Comorbidity CC Complication/Comorbidity SW Severe Wound Dx

912 ICD-10-CM 2021

- ✓6ᵗʰ **P91.82** **Neonatal** cerebral infarction
  Neonatal stroke
  Perinatal arterial ischemic stroke
  Perinatal cerebral infarction
  EXCLUDES 1 *cerebral infarction (I63.-)*
  EXCLUDES 2 *intracranial hemorrhage of newborn (P52.-)*

- **P91.821** **Neonatal cerebral infarction, right side of brain** MCC
- **P91.822** **Neonatal cerebral infarction, left side of brain** MCC
- **P91.823** **Neonatal cerebral infarction, bilateral** MCC
- **P91.829** **Neonatal cerebral infarction, unspecified side** MCC

  P91.88 **Other specified disturbances of cerebral status of newborn**
  P91.9 **Disturbance of cerebral status of newborn, unspecified**

✓4ᵗʰ **P92 Feeding problems of newborn**
  EXCLUDES 1 *eating disorders (F50.-)*
  feeding problems in child over 28 days old (R63.3)
  AHA: 2016,3Q,19
  TIP: Continue to assign a code from this category for feeding problems in a patient greater than 28 days old when that feeding problem was initially diagnosed between day 0 and day 28. Do not assign code R63.3.

✓5ᵗʰ **P92.0** **Vomiting of newborn**
    EXCLUDES 1 *vomiting of child over 28 days old (R11.-)*
  P92.01 **Bilious vomiting of newborn** MCC
    EXCLUDES 1 *bilious vomiting in child over 28 days old (R11.14)*
  P92.09 **Other vomiting of newborn**
    EXCLUDES 1 *regurgitation of food in newborn (P92.1)*

P92.1 **Regurgitation and rumination of newborn**
P92.2 **Slow feeding of newborn**
P92.3 **Underfeeding of newborn**
P92.4 **Overfeeding of newborn**
P92.5 **Neonatal difficulty in feeding at breast**
    AHA: 2017,1Q,28
P92.6 **Failure to thrive in newborn**
    EXCLUDES 1 *failure to thrive in child over 28 days old (R62.51)*
P92.8 **Other feeding problems of newborn**
P92.9 **Feeding problem of newborn, unspecified**

✓4ᵗʰ **P93 Reactions and intoxications due to drugs administered to newborn**
  INCLUDES reactions and intoxications due to drugs administered to fetus affecting newborn
  EXCLUDES 1 *jaundice due to drugs or toxins transmitted from mother or given to newborn (P58.4-)*
  reactions and intoxications from maternal opiates, tranquilizers and other medication (P04.0-P04.1, P04.4-)
  withdrawal symptoms from maternal use of drugs of addiction (P96.1)
  withdrawal symptoms from therapeutic use of drugs in newborn (P96.2)

P93.0 **Grey baby syndrome** CC
  Grey syndrome from chloramphenicol administration in newborn
P93.8 **Other reactions and intoxications due to drugs administered to newborn** CC
  Use additional code for adverse effect, if applicable, to identify drug (T36-T50 with fifth or sixth character 5)

✓4ᵗʰ **P94 Disorders of muscle tone of newborn**
  P94.0 **Transient neonatal myasthenia gravis** CC
    EXCLUDES 1 *myasthenia gravis (G70.0)*
  P94.1 **Congenital hypertonia**
  P94.2 **Congenital hypotonia**
    Floppy baby syndrome, unspecified
  P94.8 **Other disorders of muscle tone of newborn**
  P94.9 **Disorder of muscle tone of newborn, unspecified**

P95 Stillbirth
  Deadborn fetus NOS
  Fetal death of unspecified cause
  Stillbirth NOS
  EXCLUDES 1 *maternal care for intrauterine death (O36.4)*
  missed abortion (O02.1)
  outcome of delivery, stillbirth (Z37.1, Z37.3, Z37.4, Z37.7)

✓4ᵗʰ **P96 Other conditions originating in the perinatal period**
  P96.0 **Congenital renal failure**
    Uremia of newborn
  P96.1 **Neonatal withdrawal symptoms from maternal use of drugs of addiction** CC
    Drug withdrawal syndrome in infant of dependent mother
    Neonatal abstinence syndrome
    EXCLUDES 1 *reactions and intoxications from maternal opiates and tranquilizers administered during labor and delivery (P04.0)*
    AHA: 2018,4Q,24-25
  P96.2 **Withdrawal symptoms from therapeutic use of drugs in newborn** CC
  P96.3 **Wide cranial sutures of newborn**
    Neonatal craniotabes
  P96.5 **Complication to newborn due to (fetal) intrauterine procedure**
    EXCLUDES 2 *newborn affected by amniocentesis (P00.6)*

✓5ᵗʰ **P96.8** **Other specified conditions originating in the perinatal period**
  P96.81 **Exposure to (parental) (environmental) tobacco smoke in the perinatal period**
    EXCLUDES 2 *newborn affected by in utero exposure to tobacco (P04.2)*
    exposure to environmental tobacco smoke after the perinatal period (Z77.22)
  P96.82 **Delayed separation of umbilical cord**
  P96.83 **Meconium staining**
    EXCLUDES 1 *meconium aspiration (P24.00, P24.01)*
    meconium passage during delivery (P03.82)
    DEF: Meconium passed in utero causing discoloration on the fetal skin and nails or on the umbilicus. This staining may be incidental or may be an indicator of significant fetal stress that could affect outcomes.
  P96.89 **Other specified conditions originating in the perinatal period**
    Use additional code to specify condition

P96.9 **Condition originating in the perinatal period, unspecified**
  Congenital debility NOS

Chapter 17. Congenital Malformations, Deformations and Chromosomal Abnormalities (Q00–Q99)

Chapter-specific Guidelines with Coding Examples

The chapter-specific guidelines from the ICD-10-CM Official Guidelines for Coding and Reporting have been provided below. Along with these guidelines are coding examples, contained in the shaded boxes, that have been developed to help illustrate the coding and/or sequencing guidance found in these guidelines.

Assign an appropriate code(s) from categories Q00-Q99, Congenital malformations, deformations, and chromosomal abnormalities when a malformation/deformation or chromosomal abnormality is documented. A malformation/deformation/or chromosomal abnormality may be the principal/first-listed diagnosis on a record or a secondary diagnosis.

When a malformation/deformation/or chromosomal abnormality does not have a unique code assignment, assign additional code(s) for any manifestations that may be present.

When the code assignment specifically identifies the malformation/deformation/or chromosomal abnormality, manifestations that are an inherent component of the anomaly should not be coded separately. Additional codes should be assigned for manifestations that are not an inherent component.

8-day-old infant with tetralogy of Fallot and pulmonary stenosis

Q21.3   **Tetralogy of Fallot**

Explanation: Pulmonary stenosis is inherent in the disease process of tetralogy of Fallot. When the code assignment specifically identifies the malformation/deformation/or chromosomal abnormality, manifestations that are inherent components of the anomaly should not be coded separately.

7-month-old infant with Down syndrome and common atrioventricular canal

Q90.9   **Down syndrome, unspecified**

Q21.2   **Atrioventricular septal defect**

Explanation: While a common atrioventricular canal is often associated with patients with Down syndrome, this manifestation is not an inherent component and may be reported separately. When the code assignment specifically identifies the anomaly, manifestations that are inherent components of the condition should not be coded separately. Additional codes should be assigned for manifestations that are not inherent components.

Codes from Chapter 17 may be used throughout the life of the patient. If a congenital malformation or deformity has been corrected, a personal history code should be used to identify the history of the malformation or deformity. Although present at birth, a malformation/deformation/or chromosomal abnormality may not be identified until later in life. Whenever the condition is diagnosed by the provider, it is appropriate to assign a code from codes Q00-Q99. For the birth admission, the appropriate code from category Z38, Liveborn infants, according to place of birth and type of delivery, should be sequenced as the principal diagnosis, followed by any congenital anomaly codes, Q00- Q99.

Three-year-old with history of corrected ventricular septal defect

Z87.74   **Personal history of (corrected) congenital malformations of heart and circulatory system**

Explanation: If a congenital malformation or deformity has been corrected, a personal history code should be used to identify the history of the malformation or deformity.

Forty-year-old man with headaches diagnosed with congenital arteriovenous malformation of cerebral vessels by brain scan

Q28.2   **Arteriovenous malformation of cerebral vessels**

Explanation: Although present at birth, malformations may not be identified until later in life. Whenever a congenital condition is diagnosed by the physician, it is appropriate to assign a code from the range Q00–Q99.

Newborn with anencephaly delivered vaginally in hospital

Z38.00   **Single liveborn infant, delivered vaginally**

Q00.0   **Anencephaly**

Explanation: For the birth admission, the appropriate code from category Z38 Liveborn infants, according to place of birth and type of delivery, should be sequenced as the principal diagnosis, followed by any congenital anomaly codes, Q00–Q99.

Chapter 17. Congenital Malformations, Deformations and Chromosomal Abnormalities (Q00-Q99)

NOTE   Codes from this chapter are not for use on maternal records

EXCLUDES 2   *inborn errors of metabolism (E70-E88)*

This chapter contains the following blocks:

Q00-Q07   Congenital malformations of the nervous system
Q10-Q18   Congenital malformations of eye, ear, face and neck
Q20-Q28   Congenital malformations of the circulatory system
Q30-Q34   Congenital malformations of the respiratory system
Q35-Q37   Cleft lip and cleft palate
Q38-Q45   Other congenital malformations of the digestive system
Q50-Q56   Congenital malformations of genital organs
Q60-Q64   Congenital malformations of the urinary system
Q65-Q79   Congenital malformations and deformations of the musculoskeletal system
Q80-Q89   Other congenital malformations
Q90-Q99   Chromosomal abnormalities, not elsewhere classified

Congenital malformations of the nervous system (Q00-Q07)

☑4ᵗʰ Q00 Anencephaly and similar malformations

   Q00.0 Anencephaly   `MCC` `HCC`
     Acephaly
     Acrania
     Amyelencephaly
     Hemianencephaly
     Hemicephaly

   Q00.1 Craniorachischisis   `MCC` `HCC`

   Q00.2 Iniencephaly   `MCC` `HCC`

☑4ᵗʰ Q01 Encephalocele

   INCLUDES   Arnold-Chiari syndrome, type III
     encephalocystocele
     encephalomyelocele
     hydroencephalocele
     hydromeningocele, cranial
     meningocele, cerebral
     meningoencephalocele

   EXCLUDES 1   *Meckel-Gruber syndrome (Q61.9)*

   DEF: Congenital protrusion of brain tissue through a defect in the skull.

   Q01.0 Frontal encephalocele   `CC` `HCC`

   Q01.1 Nasofrontal encephalocele   `CC` `HCC`

   Q01.2 Occipital encephalocele   `CC` `HCC`

   Q01.8 Encephalocele of other sites   `CC` `HCC`

   Q01.9 Encephalocele, unspecified   `CC` `HCC`

Q02 Microcephaly   `HCC`

   INCLUDES   hydromicrocephaly
     micrencephalon

   Code first, if applicable, congenital Zika virus disease

   EXCLUDES 1   *Meckel-Gruber syndrome (Q61.9)*

   AHA: 2018,4Q,26

   DEF: Congenital disorder in which the head circumference is more than two standard deviations below the mean for age, sex, race, and gestation and associated with a decreased life expectancy.

☑4ᵗʰ Q03 Congenital hydrocephalus

   INCLUDES   hydrocephalus in newborn

   EXCLUDES 1   *Arnold-Chiari syndrome, type II (Q07.0-)*
     acquired hydrocephalus (G91.-)
     hydrocephalus due to congenital toxoplasmosis (P37.1)
     hydrocephalus with spina bifida (Q05.0-Q05.4)

   DEF: Hydrocephalus: Abnormal buildup of cerebrospinal fluid in the brain causing dilation of the ventricles.

Congenital Hydrocephalus

Pressure

Normal ventricles   Hydrocephalic ventricles

   Q03.0 Malformations of aqueduct of Sylvius   `HCC`
     Anomaly of aqueduct of Sylvius
     Obstruction of aqueduct of Sylvius, congenital
     Stenosis of aqueduct of Sylvius

   Q03.1 Atresia of foramina of Magendie and Luschka   `HCC`
     Dandy-Walker syndrome

   Q03.8 Other congenital hydrocephalus   `HCC`

   Q03.9 Congenital hydrocephalus, unspecified   `HCC`

☑4ᵗʰ Q04 Other congenital malformations of brain

   EXCLUDES 1   *cyclopia (Q87.0)*
     macrocephaly (Q75.3)

   Q04.0 Congenital malformations of corpus callosum   `MCC` `HCC`
     Agenesis of corpus callosum

   Q04.1 Arhinencephaly   `MCC` `HCC`

   Q04.2 Holoprosencephaly   `MCC` `HCC`

   Q04.3 Other reduction deformities of brain   `MCC` `HCC`
     Absence of part of brain
     Agenesis of part of brain
     Agyria
     Aplasia of part of brain
     Hydranencephaly
     Hypoplasia of part of brain
     Lissencephaly
     Microgyria
     Pachygyria

     EXCLUDES 1   *congenital malformations of corpus callosum (Q04.0)*

   Q04.4 Septo-optic dysplasia of brain   `CC` `HCC`

   Q04.5 Megalencephaly   `CC` `HCC`

   Q04.6 Congenital cerebral cysts   `CC` `HCC`
     Porencephaly
     Schizencephaly

     EXCLUDES 1   *acquired porencephalic cyst (G93.0)*

   Q04.8 Other specified congenital malformations of brain   `CC` `HCC`
     Arnold-Chiari syndrome, type IV
     Macrogyria

   Q04.9 Congenital malformation of brain, unspecified   `HCC`
     Congenital anomaly NOS of brain
     Congenital deformity NOS of brain
     Congenital disease or lesion NOS of brain
     Multiple anomalies NOS of brain, congenital

N Newborn: 0   **P** Pediatric: 0-17   **M** Maternity: 9-64   **A** Adult: 15-124   **MCC** Major Complication/Comorbidity   **CC** Complication/Comorbidity   **SW** Severe Wound Dx

916   ICD-10-CM 2021

☑4ᵗʰ **Q05　Spina bifida**

INCLUDES　hydromeningocele (spinal)
　　　　　meningocele (spinal)
　　　　　meningomyelocele
　　　　　myelocele
　　　　　myelomeningocele
　　　　　rachischisis
　　　　　spina bifida (aperta)(cystica)
　　　　　syringomyelocele

Use additional code for any associated paraplegia (paraparesis) (G82.2-)

EXCLUDES 1　Arnold-Chiari syndrome, type II (Q07.0-)
　　　　　spina bifida occulta (Q76.0)

DEF: Lack of closure in the vertebral column with protrusion of the spinal cord through the defect, often in the lumbosacral area. This condition can be recognized by the presence of alpha-fetoproteins in the amniotic fluid.

Spina Bifida

Spina bifida occulta　　Meningocele　　Myelomeningocele

Q05.0　Cervical **spina bifida with hydrocephalus**	CC HCC
Q05.1　Thoracic **spina bifida with hydrocephalus**	CC HCC
Dorsal spina bifida with hydrocephalus	
Thoracolumbar spina bifida with hydrocephalus	
Q05.2　Lumbar **spina bifida with hydrocephalus**	CC HCC
Lumbosacral spina bifida with hydrocephalus	
Q05.3　Sacral **spina bifida with hydrocephalus**	CC HCC
Q05.4　Unspecified spina bifida with hydrocephalus	CC HCC
Q05.5　Cervical **spina bifida without hydrocephalus**	HCC
Q05.6　Thoracic **spina bifida without hydrocephalus**	HCC
Dorsal spina bifida NOS	
Thoracolumbar spina bifida NOS	
Q05.7　Lumbar **spina bifida without hydrocephalus**	HCC
Lumbosacral spina bifida NOS	
Q05.8　Sacral **spina bifida without hydrocephalus**	HCC
Q05.9　Spina bifida, unspecified	HCC

☑4ᵗʰ **Q06　Other congenital malformations of spinal cord**

Q06.0　**Amyelia**	HCC
Q06.1　**Hypoplasia and dysplasia of spinal cord**	HCC
Atelomyelia	
Myelatelia	
Myelodysplasia of spinal cord	

Q06.2　**Diastematomyelia**　　HCC
　　　　DEF: Rare congenital anomaly often associated with spina bifida. The spinal cord is separated into longitudinal halves by a bony, cartilaginous or fibrous septum, each half surrounded by a dural sac.

Q06.3　**Other congenital cauda equina malformations**	HCC
Q06.4　**Hydromyelia**	HCC
Hydrorachis	
Q06.8　**Other specified congenital malformations of spinal cord**	HCC
Q06.9　**Congenital malformation of spinal cord, unspecified**	HCC
Congenital anomaly NOS of spinal cord	
Congenital deformity NOS of spinal cord	
Congenital disease or lesion NOS of spinal cord	

☑4ᵗʰ **Q07　Other congenital malformations of nervous system**

EXCLUDES 2　*congenital central alveolar hypoventilation syndrome (G47.35)*
　　　　　familial dysautonomia [Riley-Day] (G90.1)
　　　　　neurofibromatosis (nonmalignant) (Q85.0-)

☑5ᵗʰ **Q07.0　Arnold-Chiari syndrome**
　　　Arnold-Chiari syndrome, type II

EXCLUDES 1　*Arnold-Chiari syndrome, type III (Q01.-)*
　　　　　Arnold-Chiari syndrome, type IV (Q04.8)

DEF: Congenital malformation of the brain in which the cerebellum protrudes through the foramen magnum into the spinal canal.

Q07.00　**Arnold-Chiari syndrome** without spina bifida or hydrocephalus	HCC
Q07.01　**Arnold-Chiari syndrome** with spina bifida	HCC
Q07.02　**Arnold-Chiari syndrome** with hydrocephalus	CC HCC
Q07.03　**Arnold-Chiari syndrome** with spina bifida and hydrocephalus	CC HCC

Q07.8　**Other specified congenital malformations of nervous system**　　HCC
　　　Agenesis of nerve
　　　Displacement of brachial plexus
　　　Jaw-winking syndrome
　　　Marcus Gunn's syndrome

Q07.9　**Congenital malformation of nervous system, unspecified**　　HCC
　　　Congenital anomaly NOS of nervous system
　　　Congenital deformity NOS of nervous system
　　　Congenital disease or lesion NOS of nervous system

Congenital malformations of eye, ear, face and neck (Q10-Q18)

EXCLUDES 2　*cleft lip and cleft palate (Q35-Q37)*
　　　　　congenital malformation of cervical spine (Q05.0, Q05.5, Q67.5, Q76.0-Q76.4)
　　　　　congenital malformation of larynx (Q31.-)
　　　　　congenital malformation of lip NEC (Q38.0)
　　　　　congenital malformation of nose (Q30.-)
　　　　　congenital malformation of parathyroid gland (Q89.2)
　　　　　congenital malformation of thyroid gland (Q89.2)

☑4ᵗʰ **Q10　Congenital malformations of eyelid, lacrimal apparatus and orbit**

EXCLUDES 1　*cryptophthalmos NOS (Q11.2)*
　　　　　cryptophthalmos syndrome (Q87.0)

Q10.0　**Congenital ptosis**
　　　　DEF: Congenital drooping of the eyelid. Ptosis is mostly idiopathic, but may occur genetically.

Q10.1　**Congenital ectropion**

Q10.2　**Congenital entropion**

Q10.3　**Other congenital malformations of eyelid**
　　　Ablepharon
　　　Blepharophimosis, congenital
　　　Coloboma of eyelid
　　　Congenital absence or agenesis of cilia
　　　Congenital absence or agenesis of eyelid
　　　Congenital accessory eyelid
　　　Congenital accessory eye muscle
　　　Congenital malformation of eyelid NOS

Q10.4　**Absence and agenesis of lacrimal apparatus**
　　　Congenital absence of punctum lacrimale

Q10.5　**Congenital stenosis and stricture of lacrimal duct**

Q10.6　**Other congenital malformations of lacrimal apparatus**
　　　Congenital malformation of lacrimal apparatus NOS

Q10.7　**Congenital malformation of orbit**

☑4ᵗʰ **Q11　Anophthalmos, microphthalmos and macrophthalmos**

Q11.0　**Cystic eyeball**

Q11.1　**Other anophthalmos**
　　　Anophthalmos NOS
　　　Agenesis of eye
　　　Aplasia of eye

Q11.2　**Microphthalmos**
　　　Cryptophthalmos NOS
　　　Dysplasia of eye
　　　Hypoplasia of eye
　　　Rudimentary eye

EXCLUDES 1　*cryptophthalmos syndrome (Q87.0)*

Q11.3 Macrophthalmos
    EXCLUDES 1   *macrophthalmos in congenital glaucoma (Q15.0)*

✓4ᵗʰ **Q12 Congenital lens malformations**

   Q12.0 Congenital cataract

   Q12.1 Congenital displaced lens

   Q12.2 Coloboma of lens

Coloboma of Lens

Coloboma

   Q12.3 Congenital aphakia

   Q12.4 Spherophakia

   Q12.8 Other congenital lens malformations
     Microphakia

   Q12.9 Congenital lens malformation, unspecified

✓4ᵗʰ **Q13 Congenital malformations of anterior segment of eye**

   Q13.0 Coloboma of iris
     Coloboma NOS
     DEF: Defective or absent section of ocular tissue that may present as mild cupping or a small pit in the ocular disc due to extensive defects in the iris, ciliary body, choroids, and retina.

   Q13.1 Absence of iris
     Aniridia
     Use additional code for associated glaucoma (H42)
     DEF: Incompletely formed or absent iris. It affects both eyes and is a dominant trait.

   Q13.2 Other congenital malformations of iris
     Anisocoria, congenital
     Atresia of pupil
     Congenital malformation of iris NOS
     Corectopia

   Q13.3 Congenital corneal opacity

   Q13.4 Other congenital corneal malformations
     Congenital malformation of cornea NOS
     Microcornea
     Peter's anomaly

   Q13.5 Blue sclera

✓5ᵗʰ **Q13.8 Other congenital malformations of anterior segment of eye**

     Q13.81 Rieger's anomaly
       Use additional code for associated glaucoma (H42)

     Q13.89 Other congenital malformations of anterior segment of eye

   Q13.9 Congenital malformation of anterior segment of eye, unspecified

✓4ᵗʰ **Q14 Congenital malformations of posterior segment of eye**
    EXCLUDES 2   *optic nerve hypoplasia (H47.03-)*

   Q14.0 Congenital malformation of vitreous humor
     Congenital vitreous opacity

   Q14.1 Congenital malformation of retina
     Congenital retinal aneurysm

   Q14.2 Congenital malformation of optic disc
     Coloboma of optic disc

   Q14.3 Congenital malformation of choroid

   Q14.8 Other congenital malformations of posterior segment of eye
     Coloboma of the fundus

   Q14.9 Congenital malformation of posterior segment of eye, unspecified

✓4ᵗʰ **Q15 Other congenital malformations of eye**
    EXCLUDES 1   *congenital nystagmus (H55.01)*
                ocular albinism (E70.31-)
                optic nerve hypoplasia (H47.03-)
                retinitis pigmentosa (H35.52)

   Q15.0 Congenital glaucoma
     Axenfeld's anomaly
     Buphthalmos
     Glaucoma of childhood
     Glaucoma of newborn
     Hydrophthalmos
     Keratoglobus, congenital, with glaucoma
     Macrocornea with glaucoma
     Macrophthalmos in congenital glaucoma
     Megalocornea with glaucoma

   Q15.8 Other specified congenital malformations of eye

   Q15.9 Congenital malformation of eye, unspecified
     Congenital anomaly of eye
     Congenital deformity of eye

✓4ᵗʰ **Q16 Congenital malformations of ear causing impairment of hearing**
    EXCLUDES 1   *congenital deafness (H90.-)*

   Q16.0 Congenital absence of (ear) auricle

   Q16.1 Congenital absence, atresia and stricture of auditory canal (external)
     Congenital atresia or stricture of osseous meatus

   Q16.2 Absence of eustachian tube

   Q16.3 Congenital malformation of ear ossicles
     Congenital fusion of ear ossicles

   Q16.4 Other congenital malformations of middle ear
     Congenital malformation of middle ear NOS

   Q16.5 Congenital malformation of inner ear
     Congenital anomaly of membranous labyrinth
     Congenital anomaly of organ of Corti

   Q16.9 Congenital malformation of ear causing impairment of hearing, unspecified
     Congenital absence of ear NOS

✓4ᵗʰ **Q17 Other congenital malformations of ear**
    EXCLUDES 1   *congenital malformations of ear with impairment of hearing (Q16.0-Q16.9)*
                preauricular sinus (Q18.1)

   Q17.0 Accessory auricle
     Accessory tragus
     Polyotia
     Preauricular appendage or tag
     Supernumerary ear
     Supernumerary lobule

   Q17.1 Macrotia
     DEF: Birth defect characterized by abnormal enlargement of the pinna of the ear.

   Q17.2 Microtia

   Q17.3 Other misshapen ear
     Pointed ear

   Q17.4 Misplaced ear
     Low-set ears
     EXCLUDES 1   *cervical auricle (Q18.2)*

   Q17.5 Prominent ear
     Bat ear

   Q17.8 Other specified congenital malformations of ear
     Congenital absence of lobe of ear

   Q17.9 Congenital malformation of ear, unspecified
     Congenital anomaly of ear NOS

✓4ᵗʰ **Q18 Other congenital malformations of face and neck**
    EXCLUDES 1   *cleft lip and cleft palate (Q35-Q37)*
                conditions classified to Q67.0-Q67.4
                congenital malformations of skull and face bones (Q75.-)
                cyclopia (Q87.0)
                dentofacial anomalies [including malocclusion] (M26.-)
                malformation syndromes affecting facial appearance (Q87.0)
                persistent thyroglossal duct (Q89.2)

   Q18.0 Sinus, fistula and cyst of branchial cleft
     Branchial vestige

   Q18.1 Preauricular sinus and cyst   SW
     Fistula of auricle, congenital
     Cervicoaural fistula

N Newborn: 0   P Pediatric: 0-17   M Maternity: 9-64   A Adult: 15-124   MCC Major Complication/Comorbidity   CC Complication/Comorbidity   SW Severe Wound Dx

918   ICD-10-CM 2021

Q18.2 Other branchial cleft malformations
Branchial cleft malformation NOS
Cervical auricle
Otocephaly

Q18.3 Webbing of neck
Pterygium colli
DEF: Congenital malformation characterized by a thick, triangular skinfold that stretches from the lateral side of the neck across the shoulder. It is associated with genetic conditions such as Turner's and Noonan's syndromes.

Q18.4 Macrostomia
DEF: Rare congenital craniofacial bilateral or unilateral anomaly of the mouth due to malformed maxillary and mandibular processes. It results in an abnormally large mouth extending toward the ear.

Q18.5 Microstomia

Q18.6 Macrocheilia
Hypertrophy of lip, congenital

Q18.7 Microcheilia

Q18.8 Other specified congenital malformations of face and neck
Medial cyst of face and neck
Medial fistula of face and neck
Medial sinus of face and neck

Q18.9 Congenital malformation of face and neck, unspecified
Congenital anomaly NOS of face and neck

Congenital malformations of the circulatory system (Q20-Q28)

☑️4ᵗʰ Q20 Congenital malformations of cardiac chambers and connections
EXCLUDES 1   dextrocardia with situs inversus (Q89.3)
mirror-image atrial arrangement with situs inversus (Q89.3)

Q20.0 Common arterial trunk   MCC
Persistent truncus arteriosus
EXCLUDES 1   aortic septal defect (Q21.4)

Q20.1 Double outlet right ventricle   MCC
Taussig-Bing syndrome

Q20.2 Double outlet left ventricle   MCC

Q20.3 Discordant ventriculoarterial connection   MCC
Dextrotransposition of aorta
Transposition of great vessels (complete)

Q20.4 Double inlet ventricle   MCC
Common ventricle
Cor triloculare biatriatum
Single ventricle

Q20.5 Discordant atrioventricular connection   CC
Corrected transposition
Levotransposition
Ventricular inversion

Q20.6 Isomerism of atrial appendages
Isomerism of atrial appendages with asplenia or polysplenia

Q20.8 Other congenital malformations of cardiac chambers and connections
Cor binoculare

Q20.9 Congenital malformation of cardiac chambers and connections, unspecified

☑️4ᵗʰ Q21 Congenital malformations of cardiac septa
EXCLUDES 1   acquired cardiac septal defect (I51.0)

Q21.0 Ventricular septal defect   CC
Roger's disease

Ventricular Septal Defect

Q21.1 Atrial septal defect   CC
Coronary sinus defect
Patent or persistent foramen ovale
Patent or persistent ostium secundum defect (type II)
Patent or persistent sinus venosus defect

Atrial Septal Defect

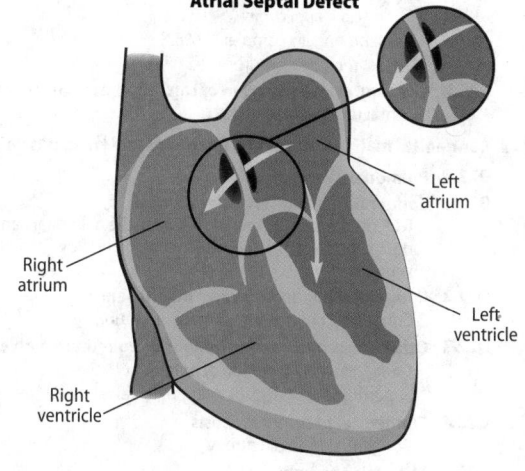

Left atrium

Right atrium

Left ventricle

Right ventricle

☑️ Additional Character Required   **✓ₓ7ᵗʰ** Placeholder   Unacceptable PDx   Questionable PDx   Manifestation   Unspecified Dx   **H1**-**H14** HAC   **HCC** CMS-HCC Dx   **HIV** HIV Dx

ICD-10-CM 2021   919

Q21.2 Atrioventricular **septal defect** `CC`
Common atrioventricular canal
Endocardial cushion defect
Ostium primum atrial septal defect (type I)

Atrioventricular Septal Defect

Aorta
Pulmonary artery
Left atrium
Common valve
Right atrium
Left ventricle
Right ventricle

Q21.3 **Tetralogy of Fallot** `MCC`
Ventricular septal defect with pulmonary stenosis or atresia, dextroposition of aorta and hypertrophy of right ventricle.
AHA: 2014,3Q,16

Q21.4 Aortopulmonary septal **defect**
Aortic septal defect
Aortopulmonary window

Q21.8 **Other congenital malformations of cardiac septa**
Eisenmenger's defect
Pentalogy of Fallot
Code also if applicable:
Eisenmenger's complex (I27.83)
Eisenmenger's syndrome (I27.83)

Q21.9 **Congenital malformation of cardiac septum, unspecified**
Septal (heart) defect NOS

☑4ᵗʰ **Q22** **Congenital malformations of pulmonary and tricuspid valves**

Q22.0 Pulmonary **valve atresia** `MCC`

Q22.1 Congenital pulmonary **valve stenosis** `CC`
DEF: Stenosis of the opening between the pulmonary artery and right ventricle, causing obstructed blood outflow from the right ventricle.

Q22.2 Congenital pulmonary **valve insufficiency** `CC`
Congenital pulmonary valve regurgitation

Q22.3 **Other congenital malformations of pulmonary valve** `CC`
Congenital malformation of pulmonary valve NOS
Supernumerary cusps of pulmonary valve

Q22.4 Congenital tricuspid **stenosis** `MCC`
Congenital tricuspid atresia

Q22.5 **Ebstein's anomaly** `MCC`
DEF: Malformation of the tricuspid valve characterized by septal and posterior leaflets attaching to the wall of the right ventricle. Ebstein's anomaly causes the right ventricle to fuse with the atrium into a large right atrium and a small ventricle and leads to heart failure and abnormal cardiac rhythm.

Q22.6 **Hypoplastic right heart syndrome** `MCC`

Q22.8 **Other congenital malformations of tricuspid valve** `MCC`

Q22.9 **Congenital malformation of tricuspid valve, unspecified** `MCC`

☑4ᵗʰ **Q23** **Congenital malformations of aortic and mitral valves**

Q23.0 **Congenital stenosis of aortic valve** `CC`
Congenital aortic atresia
Congenital aortic stenosis NOS
EXCLUDES 1   *congenital stenosis of aortic valve in hypoplastic left heart syndrome (Q23.4)*
     congenital subaortic stenosis (Q24.4)
     supravalvular aortic stenosis (congenital) (Q25.3)

Q23.1 **Congenital insufficiency of aortic valve** `CC`
Bicuspid aortic valve
Congenital aortic insufficiency

Q23.2 **Congenital mitral stenosis** `CC`
Congenital mitral atresia
DEF: Congenital stenosis of the mitral valve orifice between the left atrium and ventricle, at the supravalvular, valvular, or subvalvular levels, causing obstruction to left ventricular filling.

Q23.3 **Congenital mitral insufficiency** `CC`

Q23.4 **Hypoplastic left heart syndrome** `MCC`

Q23.8 **Other congenital malformations of aortic and mitral valves**

Q23.9 **Congenital malformation of aortic and mitral valves, unspecified**

☑4ᵗʰ **Q24** **Other congenital malformations of heart**
EXCLUDES 1   *endocardial fibroelastosis (I42.4)*

Q24.0 **Dextrocardia** `CC`
EXCLUDES 1   *dextrocardia with situs inversus (Q89.3)*
     isomerism of atrial appendages (with asplenia or polysplenia) (Q20.6)
     mirror-image atrial arrangement with situs inversus (Q89.3)
DEF: Congenital condition in which the heart is located on the right side of the chest rather than in its normal position on the left.

Q24.1 **Levocardia** `CC`

Q24.2 **Cor triatriatum** `MCC`

Q24.3 **Pulmonary infundibular stenosis** `CC`
Subvalvular pulmonic stenosis

Q24.4 **Congenital subaortic stenosis** `MCC`
DEF: Congenital heart defect characterized by stenosis of the left ventricular outflow tract due to a fibrous tissue ring or septal hypertrophy below the aortic valve.

Q24.5 **Malformation of coronary vessels** `CC`
Congenital coronary (artery) aneurysm

Q24.6 **Congenital heart block** `MCC`

Q24.8 **Other specified congenital malformations of heart**
Congenital diverticulum of left ventricle
Congenital malformation of myocardium
Congenital malformation of pericardium
Malposition of heart
Uhl's disease

Q24.9 **Congenital malformation of heart, unspecified**
Congenital anomaly of heart
Congenital disease of heart

☑4ᵗʰ **Q25** **Congenital malformations of great arteries**

Q25.0 Patent ductus arteriosus `CC`
Patent ductus Botallo
Persistent ductus arteriosus
DEF: Condition in which the normal channel between the pulmonary artery and the aorta fails to close at birth, causing arterial blood to recirculate in the lungs and inhibiting the blood supply to the aorta. **Synonym(s):** *PDA*.

Patent Ductus Arteriosus

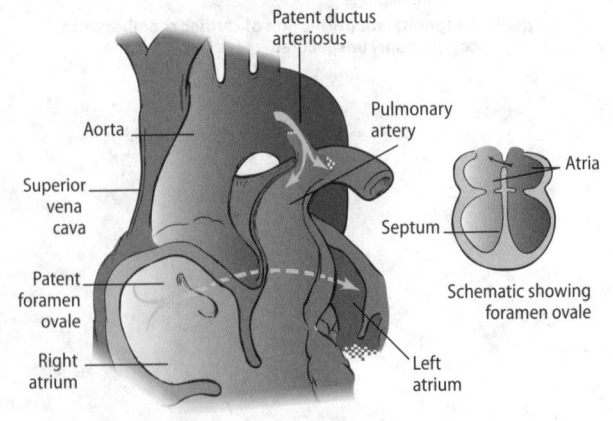

Patent ductus arteriosus
Pulmonary artery
Aorta
Superior vena cava
Atria
Septum
Patent foramen ovale
Right atrium
Schematic showing foramen ovale
Left atrium

Q25.1 Coarctation **of aorta** `CC`
Coarctation of aorta (preductal) (postductal)
Stenosis of aorta
AHA: 2016,4Q,56-57

N Newborn: 0   **P** Pediatric: 0-17   **M** Maternity: 9-64   **A** Adult: 15-124   **MCC** Major Complication/Comorbidity   **CC** Complication/Comorbidity   **SW** Severe Wound Dx

920   ICD-10-CM 2021

✓5th **Q25.2** Atresia of aorta
> **AHA:** 2016,4Q,56-57

     Q25.21 **Interruption of aortic arch** `CC`
> Atresia of aortic arch

     Q25.29 **Other atresia of aorta** `CC`
> Atresia of aorta

Q25.3 Supravalvular aortic stenosis `CC`
> **EXCLUDES 1**   *congenital aortic stenosis NOS (Q23.0)*
> *congenital stenosis of aortic valve (Q23.0)*

✓5th **Q25.4** Other congenital malformations of aorta
> **EXCLUDES 1**   *hypoplasia of aorta in hypoplastic left heart syndrome (Q23.4)*
>
> **AHA:** 2016,4Q,57

     Q25.40 **Congenital malformation of aorta unspecified** `CC`

     Q25.41 **Absence and aplasia of aorta** `CC`

     Q25.42 **Hypoplasia of aorta** `CC`

     Q25.43 **Congenital aneurysm of aorta** `CC`
> Congenital aneurysm of aortic root
> Congenital aneurysm of aortic sinus

     Q25.44 **Congenital dilation of aorta** `CC`

     Q25.45 **Double aortic arch** `CC`
> Vascular ring of aorta

Aortic Arch Anomalies

Normal aortic arch

Double aortic arch   Right aortic arch

     Q25.46 **Tortuous aortic arch** `CC`
> Persistent convolutions of aortic arch

     Q25.47 **Right aortic arch** `CC`
> Persistent right aortic arch

     Q25.48 **Anomalous origin of subclavian artery** `CC`

     Q25.49 **Other congenital malformations of aorta** `CC`
> Aortic arch
> Bovine arch

Q25.5 Atresia of pulmonary artery `MCC`

Q25.6 Stenosis of pulmonary artery `MCC`
> Supravalvular pulmonary stenosis

✓5th **Q25.7** Other congenital malformations of pulmonary artery

     Q25.71 **Coarctation of pulmonary artery** `MCC`

     Q25.72 **Congenital pulmonary arteriovenous malformation** `MCC`
> Congenital pulmonary arteriovenous aneurysm

     Q25.79 **Other congenital malformations of pulmonary artery** `MCC`
> Aberrant pulmonary artery
> Agenesis of pulmonary artery
> Congenital aneurysm of pulmonary artery
> Congenital anomaly of pulmonary artery
> Hypoplasia of pulmonary artery

Q25.8 Other congenital malformations of other great arteries `CC`

Q25.9 Congenital malformation of great arteries, unspecified `CC`

✓4th **Q26** Congenital malformations of great veins

     Q26.0 **Congenital stenosis of vena cava** `CC`
> Congenital stenosis of vena cava (inferior)(superior)

     Q26.1 **Persistent left superior vena cava** `CC`

     Q26.2 **Total anomalous pulmonary venous connection** `CC`
> Total anomalous pulmonary venous return [TAPVR], subdiaphragmatic
> Total anomalous pulmonary venous return [TAPVR], supradiaphragmatic

     Q26.3 **Partial anomalous pulmonary venous connection** `CC`
> Partial anomalous pulmonary venous return

     Q26.4 **Anomalous pulmonary venous connection, unspecified** `CC`

     Q26.5 **Anomalous portal venous connection**

     Q26.6 **Portal vein-hepatic artery fistula**

     Q26.8 **Other congenital malformations of great veins** `CC`
> Absence of vena cava (inferior) (superior)
> Azygos continuation of inferior vena cava
> Persistent left posterior cardinal vein
> Scimitar syndrome

     Q26.9 **Congenital malformation of great vein, unspecified** `CC`
> Congenital anomaly of vena cava (inferior) (superior) NOS

✓4th **Q27** Other congenital malformations of peripheral vascular system
> **EXCLUDES 2**   *anomalies of cerebral and precerebral vessels (Q28.0-Q28.3)*
> *anomalies of coronary vessels (Q24.5)*
> *anomalies of pulmonary artery (Q25.5-Q25.7)*
> *congenital retinal aneurysm (Q14.1)*
> *hemangioma and lymphangioma (D18.-)*

     Q27.0 **Congenital absence and hypoplasia of umbilical artery**
> Single umbilical artery

     Q27.1 **Congenital renal artery stenosis**

     Q27.2 **Other congenital malformations of renal artery**
> Congenital malformation of renal artery NOS
> Multiple renal arteries

✓5th **Q27.3** **Arteriovenous malformation (peripheral)**
> Arteriovenous aneurysm
> **EXCLUDES 1**   *acquired arteriovenous aneurysm (I77.0)*
> **EXCLUDES 2**   *arteriovenous malformation of cerebral vessels (Q28.2)*
> *arteriovenous malformation of precerebral vessels (Q28.0)*
>
> **DEF:** Arteriovenous malformation: Connecting passage between an artery and a vein.

     Q27.30 **Arteriovenous malformation, site unspecified** `CC`

     Q27.31 **Arteriovenous malformation of vessel of upper limb**

     Q27.32 **Arteriovenous malformation of vessel of lower limb**

     Q27.33 **Arteriovenous malformation of digestive system vessel**
> **AHA:** 2018,3Q,21

     Q27.34 **Arteriovenous malformation of renal vessel**

     Q27.39 **Arteriovenous malformation, other site**

     Q27.4 **Congenital phlebectasia** `CC`

     Q27.8 **Other specified congenital malformations of peripheral vascular system**
> Absence of peripheral vascular system
> Atresia of peripheral vascular system
> Congenital aneurysm (peripheral)
> Congenital stricture, artery
> Congenital varix
> **EXCLUDES 1**   *arteriovenous malformation (Q27.3-)*

     Q27.9 **Congenital malformation of peripheral vascular system, unspecified**
> Anomaly of artery or vein NOS

✓4th **Q28** Other congenital malformations of circulatory system
> **EXCLUDES 1**   *congenital aneurysm NOS (Q27.8)*
> *congenital coronary aneurysm (Q24.5)*
> *ruptured cerebral arteriovenous malformation (I60.8)*
> *ruptured malformation of precerebral vessels (I72.0)*
> **EXCLUDES 2**   *congenital peripheral aneurysm (Q27.8)*
> *congenital pulmonary aneurysm (Q25.79)*
> *congenital retinal aneurysm (Q14.1)*

     Q28.0 **Arteriovenous malformation of precerebral vessels** `CC`
> Congenital arteriovenous precerebral aneurysm (nonruptured)

☑ Additional Character Required   vx7th Placeholder   Unacceptable PDx   Questionable PDx   Manifestation   Unspecified Dx   H1-H14 HAC   HCC CMS-HCC Dx   HIV HIV Dx

ICD-10-CM 2021   **921**

Chapter 17. Congenital Malformations, Deformations and Chromosomal Abnormalities

Q28.1   **Other malformations of precerebral vessels**   `CC`
Congenital malformation of precerebral vessels NOS
Congenital precerebral aneurysm (nonruptured)

Q28.2   **Arteriovenous malformation of cerebral vessels**   `MCC`
Arteriovenous malformation of brain NOS
Congenital arteriovenous cerebral aneurysm (nonruptured)

Q28.3   **Other malformations of cerebral vessels**   `MCC`
Congenital cerebral aneurysm (nonruptured)
Congenital malformation of cerebral vessels NOS
Developmental venous anomaly

Q28.8   **Other specified congenital malformations of circulatory system**   `CC`
Congenital aneurysm, specified site NEC
Spinal vessel anomaly

Q28.9   **Congenital malformation of circulatory system, unspecified**   `CC`

Congenital malformations of the respiratory system (Q30-Q34)

✓4ᵗʰ **Q30**   **Congenital malformations of nose**
> EXCLUDES 1   *congenital deviation of nasal septum (Q67.4)*

Q30.0   **Choanal atresia**
Atresia of nares (anterior) (posterior)
Congenital stenosis of nares (anterior) (posterior)

Q30.1   **Agenesis and underdevelopment of nose**
Congenital absent of nose

Q30.2   **Fissured, notched and cleft nose**

Q30.3   **Congenital perforated nasal septum**

Q30.8   **Other congenital malformations of nose**
Accessory nose
Congenital anomaly of nasal sinus wall

Q30.9   **Congenital malformation of nose, unspecified**

✓4ᵗʰ **Q31**   **Congenital malformations of larynx**
> EXCLUDES 1   *congenital laryngeal stridor NOS (P28.89)*

Q31.0   **Web of larynx**
Glottic web of larynx
Subglottic web of larynx
Web of larynx NOS
DEF: Congenital malformation of the larynx marked by thin, translucent, or thick fibrotic membrane-like structure between the vocal folds. It is characterized by shortness of breath and stridor.

Q31.1   **Congenital subglottic stenosis**   `CC`

Q31.2   **Laryngeal hypoplasia**   `CC`

Q31.3   **Laryngocele**   `CC`

Q31.5   **Congenital laryngomalacia**   `CC`

Q31.8   **Other congenital malformations of larynx**   `CC`
Absence of larynx
Agenesis of larynx
Atresia of larynx
Congenital cleft thyroid cartilage
Congenital fissure of epiglottis
Congenital stenosis of larynx NEC
Posterior cleft of cricoid cartilage

Q31.9   **Congenital malformation of larynx, unspecified**   `CC`

✓4ᵗʰ **Q32**   **Congenital malformations of trachea and bronchus**
> EXCLUDES 1   *congenital bronchiectasis (Q33.4)*

Q32.0   **Congenital tracheomalacia**   `CC`

Q32.1   **Other congenital malformations of trachea**   `CC`
Atresia of trachea
Congenital anomaly of tracheal cartilage
Congenital dilatation of trachea
Congenital malformation of trachea
Congenital stenosis of trachea
Congenital tracheocele

Q32.2   **Congenital bronchomalacia**   `CC`

Q32.3   **Congenital stenosis of bronchus**   `CC`

Q32.4   **Other congenital malformations of bronchus**   `CC`
Absence of bronchus
Agenesis of bronchus
Atresia of bronchus
Congenital diverticulum of bronchus
Congenital malformation of bronchus NOS

✓4ᵗʰ **Q33**   **Congenital malformations of lung**

Q33.0   **Congenital cystic lung**   `CC`
Congenital cystic lung disease
Congenital honeycomb lung
Congenital polycystic lung disease
> EXCLUDES 1   cystic fibrosis (E84.0)
> cystic lung disease, acquired or unspecified (J98.4)

Q33.1   **Accessory lobe of lung**
Azygos lobe (fissured), lung

Q33.2   **Sequestration of lung**   `MCC`

Q33.3   **Agenesis of lung**   `MCC`
Congenital absence of lung (lobe)

Q33.4   **Congenital bronchiectasis**   `CC`

Q33.5   **Ectopic tissue in lung**

Q33.6   **Congenital hypoplasia and dysplasia of lung**   `MCC`
> EXCLUDES 1   pulmonary hypoplasia associated with short gestation (P28.0)

Q33.8   **Other congenital malformations of lung**

Q33.9   **Congenital malformation of lung, unspecified**

✓4ᵗʰ **Q34**   **Other congenital malformations of respiratory system**
> EXCLUDES 2   congenital central alveolar hypoventilation syndrome (G47.35)

Q34.0   **Anomaly of pleura**

Q34.1   **Congenital cyst of mediastinum**

Q34.8   **Other specified congenital malformations of respiratory system**
Atresia of nasopharynx

Q34.9   **Congenital malformation of respiratory system, unspecified**
Congenital absence of respiratory system
Congenital anomaly of respiratory system NOS

Cleft lip and cleft palate (Q35-Q37)

Use additional code to identify associated malformation of the nose (Q30.2)
> EXCLUDES 1   ▶Robin's syndrome (Q87.0)
> EXCLUDES 2   ▶Robin's syndrome (Q87.0)◀

✓4ᵗʰ **Q35**   **Cleft palate**
> INCLUDES   fissure of palate
> palatoschisis
> EXCLUDES 1   cleft palate with cleft lip (Q37.-)

DEF: Congenital fissure or defect of the roof of the mouth opening to the nasal cavity due to failure of embryonic cells to fuse completely.

Cleft Palate

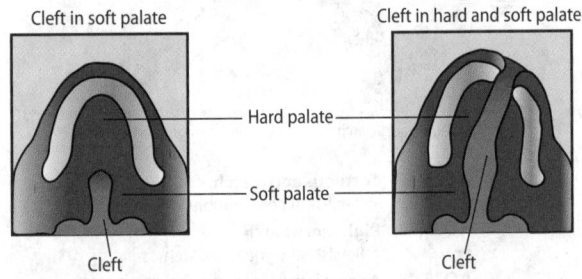

Cleft in soft palate   Cleft in hard and soft palate

Hard palate — Soft palate

Cleft   Cleft

Q35.1   **Cleft hard palate**

Q35.3   **Cleft soft palate**

Q35.5   **Cleft hard palate with cleft soft palate**

Q35.7   **Cleft uvula**

Q35.9   **Cleft palate, unspecified**
Cleft palate NOS

N Newborn: 0   P Pediatric: 0-17   M Maternity: 9-64   A Adult: 15-124   `MCC` Major Complication/Comorbidity   `CC` Complication/Comorbidity   `SW` Severe Wound Dx

922   ICD-10-CM 2021

☑4ᵗʰ **Q36 Cleft lip**

     [INCLUDES]   cheiloschisis
                    congenital fissure of lip
                    harelip
                    labium leporinum

     [EXCLUDES 1]   *cleft lip with cleft palate (Q37.-)*

     DEF: Congenital fissure or opening in the upper lip due to failure of embryonic cells to fuse completely.

Cleft Lip

Unilateral incomplete   Unilateral complete   Bilateral complete

    Q36.0 Cleft lip, bilateral
    Q36.1 Cleft lip, median
    Q36.9 Cleft lip, unilateral
            Cleft lip NOS

☑4ᵗʰ **Q37 Cleft palate with cleft lip**

     [INCLUDES]   cheilopalatoschisis

    Q37.0 Cleft hard palate with bilateral cleft lip
    Q37.1 Cleft hard palate with unilateral cleft lip
            Cleft hard palate with cleft lip NOS
    Q37.2 Cleft soft palate with bilateral cleft lip
    Q37.3 Cleft soft palate with unilateral cleft lip
            Cleft soft palate with cleft lip NOS
    Q37.4 Cleft hard and soft palate with bilateral cleft lip
    Q37.5 Cleft hard and soft palate with unilateral cleft lip
            Cleft hard and soft palate with cleft lip NOS
    Q37.8 Unspecified cleft palate with bilateral cleft lip
    Q37.9 Unspecified cleft palate with unilateral cleft lip
            Cleft palate with cleft lip NOS

Other congenital malformations of the digestive system (Q38-Q45)

☑4ᵗʰ **Q38 Other congenital malformations of tongue, mouth and pharynx**

     [EXCLUDES 1]   *dentofacial anomalies (M26.-)*
                    macrostomia (Q18.4)
                    microstomia (Q18.5)

    Q38.0 Congenital malformations of lips, not elsewhere classified
            Congenital fistula of lip
            Congenital malformation of lip NOS
            Van der Woude's syndrome
            [EXCLUDES 1]   *cleft lip (Q36.-)*
                          cleft lip with cleft palate (Q37.-)
                          macrocheilia (Q18.6)
                          microcheilia (Q18.7)
    Q38.1 Ankyloglossia
            Tongue tie
    Q38.2 Macroglossia
            Congenital hypertrophy of tongue
    Q38.3 Other congenital malformations of tongue
            Aglossia
            Bifid tongue
            Congenital adhesion of tongue
            Congenital fissure of tongue
            Congenital malformation of tongue NOS
            Double tongue
            Hypoglossia
            Hypoplasia of tongue
            Microglossia
    Q38.4 Congenital malformations of salivary glands and ducts
            Atresia of salivary glands and ducts
            Congenital absence of salivary glands and ducts
            Congenital accessory salivary glands and ducts
            Congenital fistula of salivary gland

    Q38.5 Congenital malformations of palate, not elsewhere classified
            Congenital absence of uvula
            Congenital malformation of palate NOS
            Congenital high arched palate
            [EXCLUDES 1]   *cleft palate (Q35.-)*
                          cleft palate with cleft lip (Q37.-)
    Q38.6 Other congenital malformations of mouth
            Congenital malformation of mouth NOS
    Q38.7 Congenital pharyngeal pouch
            Congenital diverticulum of pharynx
            [EXCLUDES 1]   *pharyngeal pouch syndrome (D82.1)*
    Q38.8 Other congenital malformations of pharynx
            Congenital malformation of pharynx NOS
            Imperforate pharynx

☑4ᵗʰ **Q39 Congenital malformations of esophagus**

    Q39.0 Atresia of esophagus without fistula   MCC
            Atresia of esophagus NOS
    Q39.1 Atresia of esophagus with tracheo-esophageal fistula   MCC
            Atresia of esophagus with broncho-esophageal fistula
    Q39.2 Congenital tracheo-esophageal fistula without atresia   MCC
            Congenital tracheo-esophageal fistula NOS
    Q39.3 Congenital stenosis and stricture of esophagus   MCC
    Q39.4 Esophageal web   MCC
    Q39.5 Congenital dilatation of esophagus   CC
            Congenital cardiospasm
    Q39.6 Congenital diverticulum of esophagus   CC
            Congenital esophageal pouch
    Q39.8 Other congenital malformations of esophagus   CC
            Congenital absence of esophagus
            Congenital displacement of esophagus
            Congenital duplication of esophagus
    Q39.9 Congenital malformation of esophagus, unspecified   CC

☑4ᵗʰ **Q40 Other congenital malformations of upper alimentary tract**

    Q40.0 Congenital hypertrophic pyloric stenosis
            Congenital or infantile constriction
            Congenital or infantile hypertrophy
            Congenital or infantile spasm
            Congenital or infantile stenosis
            Congenital or infantile stricture
    Q40.1 Congenital hiatus hernia
            Congenital displacement of cardia through esophageal hiatus
            [EXCLUDES 1]   *congenital diaphragmatic hernia (Q79.0)*
    Q40.2 Other specified congenital malformations of stomach
            Congenital displacement of stomach
            Congenital diverticulum of stomach
            Congenital hourglass stomach
            Congenital duplication of stomach
            Megalogastria
            Microgastria
    Q40.3 Congenital malformation of stomach, unspecified
    Q40.8 Other specified congenital malformations of upper alimentary tract
    Q40.9 Congenital malformation of upper alimentary tract, unspecified
            Congenital anomaly of upper alimentary tract
            Congenital deformity of upper alimentary tract

☑4ᵗʰ **Q41 Congenital absence, atresia and stenosis of small intestine**

     [INCLUDES]   congenital obstruction, occlusion or stricture of small intestine or intestine NOS
     [EXCLUDES 1]   *cystic fibrosis with intestinal manifestation (E84.11)*
                    meconium ileus NOS (without cystic fibrosis) (P76.0)

    Q41.0 Congenital absence, atresia and stenosis of duodenum   CC
    Q41.1 Congenital absence, atresia and stenosis of jejunum   CC
            Apple peel syndrome
            Imperforate jejunum
    Q41.2 Congenital absence, atresia and stenosis of ileum   CC
    Q41.8 Congenital absence, atresia and stenosis of other specified parts of small intestine   CC
    Q41.9 Congenital absence, atresia and stenosis of small intestine, part unspecified   CC
            Congenital absence, atresia and stenosis of intestine NOS

☑ Additional Character Required   ☑x7ᵗʰ Placeholder   Unacceptable PDx   Questionable PDx   Manifestation   Unspecified Dx   H1-H14 HAC   HCC CMS-HCC Dx   HIV HIV Dx

✓4ᵗʰ **Q42 Congenital absence, atresia and stenosis of large intestine**

INCLUDES congenital obstruction, occlusion and stricture of large intestine

Q42.Ø Congenital absence, atresia and stenosis of rectum with fistula CC

Q42.1 Congenital absence, atresia and stenosis of rectum without fistula CC
Imperforate rectum

Q42.2 Congenital absence, atresia and stenosis of anus with fistula CC

Q42.3 Congenital absence, atresia and stenosis of anus without fistula CC
Imperforate anus

Q42.8 Congenital absence, atresia and stenosis of other parts of large intestine

Q42.9 Congenital absence, atresia and stenosis of large intestine, part unspecified CC

✓4ᵗʰ **Q43 Other congenital malformations of intestine**

Q43.Ø Meckel's diverticulum (displaced) (hypertrophic)
Persistent omphalomesenteric duct
Persistent vitelline duct
DEF: Congenital, abnormal remnant of embryonic digestive system development that leaves a sacculation or outpouching from the wall of the small intestine near the terminal part of the ileum made of acid-secreting tissue as in the stomach.

Q43.1 Hirschsprung's disease CC
Aganglionosis
Congenital (aganglionic) megacolon
DEF: Congenital enlargement or dilation of the colon, with the absence of nerve cells in a segment of colon distally that causes the inability to defecate.

Q43.2 Other congenital functional disorders of colon CC
Congenital dilatation of colon

Q43.3 Congenital malformations of intestinal fixation CC
Congenital omental, anomalous adhesions [bands]
Congenital peritoneal adhesions [bands]
Incomplete rotation of cecum and colon
Insufficient rotation of cecum and colon
Jackson's membrane
Malrotation of colon
Rotation failure of cecum and colon
Universal mesentery

Q43.4 Duplication of intestine CC

Q43.5 Ectopic anus CC

Q43.6 Congenital fistula of rectum and anus CC
EXCLUDES 1 congenital fistula of anus with absence, atresia and stenosis (Q42.2)
congenital fistula of rectum with absence, atresia and stenosis (Q42.Ø)
congenital rectovaginal fistula (Q52.2)
congenital urethrorectal fistula (Q64.73)
pilonidal fistula or sinus (LØ5.-)

Q43.7 Persistent cloaca CC
Cloaca NOS

Q43.8 Other specified congenital malformations of intestine CC
Congenital blind loop syndrome
Congenital diverticulitis, colon
Congenital diverticulum, intestine
Dolichocolon
Megaloappendix
Megaloduodenum
Microcolon
Transposition of appendix
Transposition of colon
Transposition of intestine
AHA: 2013,2Q,31

Q43.9 Congenital malformation of intestine, unspecified CC

✓4ᵗʰ **Q44 Congenital malformations of gallbladder, bile ducts and liver**

Q44.Ø Agenesis, aplasia and hypoplasia of gallbladder CC
Congenital absence of gallbladder

Q44.1 Other congenital malformations of gallbladder CC
Congenital malformation of gallbladder NOS
Intrahepatic gallbladder

Q44.2 Atresia of bile ducts MCC

Q44.3 Congenital stenosis and stricture of bile ducts MCC

Q44.4 Choledochal cyst CC

Q44.5 Other congenital malformations of bile ducts CC
Accessory hepatic duct
Biliary duct duplication
Congenital malformation of bile duct NOS
Cystic duct duplication

Q44.6 Cystic disease of liver CC
Fibrocystic disease of liver

Q44.7 Other congenital malformations of liver CC
Accessory liver
Alagille's syndrome
Congenital absence of liver
Congenital hepatomegaly
Congenital malformation of liver NOS

✓4ᵗʰ **Q45 Other congenital malformations of digestive system**

EXCLUDES 2 congenital diaphragmatic hernia (Q79.Ø)
congenital hiatus hernia (Q4Ø.1)

Q45.Ø Agenesis, aplasia and hypoplasia of pancreas CC
Congenital absence of pancreas

Q45.1 Annular pancreas CC

Q45.2 Congenital pancreatic cyst CC

Q45.3 Other congenital malformations of pancreas and pancreatic duct CC
Accessory pancreas
Congenital malformation of pancreas or pancreatic duct NOS
EXCLUDES 1 congenital diabetes mellitus (E1Ø.-)
cystic fibrosis (E84.Ø-E84.9)
fibrocystic disease of pancreas (E84.-)
neonatal diabetes mellitus (P7Ø.2)

Q45.8 Other specified congenital malformations of digestive system
Absence (complete) (partial) of alimentary tract NOS
Duplication of digestive system
Malposition, congenital of digestive system

Q45.9 Congenital malformation of digestive system, unspecified
Congenital anomaly of digestive system
Congenital deformity of digestive system

Congenital malformations of genital organs (Q5Ø-Q56)

EXCLUDES 1 androgen insensitivity syndrome (E34.5-)
syndromes associated with anomalies in the number and form of chromosomes (Q9Ø-Q99)

✓4ᵗʰ **Q5Ø Congenital malformations of ovaries, fallopian tubes and broad ligaments**

✓5ᵗʰ **Q5Ø.Ø Congenital absence of ovary**
EXCLUDES 1 Turner's syndrome (Q96.-)

Q5Ø.Ø1 Congenital absence of ovary, unilateral ♀

Q5Ø.Ø2 Congenital absence of ovary, bilateral ♀

Q5Ø.1 Developmental ovarian cyst ♀

Q5Ø.2 Congenital torsion of ovary ♀

✓5ᵗʰ **Q5Ø.3 Other congenital malformations of ovary**

Q5Ø.31 Accessory ovary ♀

Q5Ø.32 Ovarian streak ♀
46, XX with streak gonads

Q5Ø.39 Other congenital malformation of ovary ♀
Congenital malformation of ovary NOS

Q5Ø.4 Embryonic cyst of fallopian tube ♀
Fimbrial cyst

Q5Ø.5 Embryonic cyst of broad ligament ♀
Epoophoron cyst
Parovarian cyst

Q5Ø.6 Other congenital malformations of fallopian tube and broad ligament ♀
Absence of fallopian tube and broad ligament
Accessory fallopian tube and broad ligament
Atresia of fallopian tube and broad ligament
Congenital malformation of fallopian tube or broad ligament NOS

✓4ᵗʰ **Q51 Congenital malformations of uterus and cervix**

Q51.Ø Agenesis and aplasia of uterus ♀
Congenital absence of uterus

N Newborn: 0   P Pediatric: 0-17   M Maternity: 9-64   A Adult: 15-124   MCC Major Complication/Comorbidity   CC Complication/Comorbidity   SW Severe Wound Dx

924   ICD-10-CM 2021

√5ᵗʰ **Q51.1 Doubling of uterus with doubling of cervix and vagina**

   Q51.10 Doubling of uterus with doubling of cervix and vagina without obstruction ♀
      Doubling of uterus with doubling of cervix and vagina NOS

   Q51.11 Doubling of uterus with doubling of cervix and vagina with obstruction ♀

√5ᵗʰ **Q51.2 Other doubling of uterus**
   Doubling of uterus NOS
   Septate uterus
   AHA: 2018,4Q,27

   Q51.20 Other doubling of uterus, unspecified

▲   **Q51.21 Complete doubling of uterus** ♀
      Complete septate uterus

▲   **Q51.22 Partial doubling of uterus** ♀
      Partial septate uterus

▲   **Q51.28 Other and unspecified doubling of uterus** ♀
      ▶Septate uterus NOS◀

Q51.3 Bicornate uterus ♀
   Bicornate uterus, complete or partial

Q51.4 Unicornate uterus ♀
   Unicornate uterus with or without a separate uterine horn
   Uterus with only one functioning horn

Q51.5 Agenesis and aplasia of cervix ♀
   Congenital absence of cervix

Q51.6 Embryonic cyst of cervix ♀

Q51.7 Congenital fistulae between uterus and digestive and urinary tracts ♀

√5ᵗʰ **Q51.8 Other congenital malformations of uterus and cervix**

  √6ᵗʰ **Q51.81 Other congenital malformations of uterus**
    Q51.810 Arcuate uterus ♀
      Arcuatus uterus
    Q51.811 Hypoplasia of uterus ♀
    Q51.818 Other congenital malformations of uterus ♀
      Müllerian anomaly of uterus NEC

  √6ᵗʰ **Q51.82 Other congenital malformations of cervix**
    Q51.820 Cervical duplication ♀
    Q51.821 Hypoplasia of cervix ♀
    Q51.828 Other congenital malformations of cervix ♀

Q51.9 Congenital malformation of uterus and cervix, unspecified ♀

√4ᵗʰ **Q52 Other congenital malformations of female genitalia**

Q52.0 Congenital absence of vagina ♀
   Vaginal agenesis, total or partial

√5ᵗʰ **Q52.1 Doubling of vagina**
   EXCLUDES 1 doubling of vagina with doubling of uterus and cervix (Q51.1-)

  Q52.10 Doubling of vagina, unspecified ♀
    Septate vagina NOS

  Q52.11 Transverse vaginal septum ♀

  √6ᵗʰ **Q52.12 Longitudinal vaginal septum**
    AHA: 2016,4Q,58-59
    Q52.120 Longitudinal vaginal septum, nonobstructing ♀
    Q52.121 Longitudinal vaginal septum, obstructing, right side ♀
    Q52.122 Longitudinal vaginal septum, obstructing, left side ♀
    Q52.123 Longitudinal vaginal septum, microperforate, right side ♀
    Q52.124 Longitudinal vaginal septum, microperforate, left side ♀
    Q52.129 Other and unspecified longitudinal vaginal septum ♀

Q52.2 Congenital rectovaginal fistula ♀
   EXCLUDES 1 cloaca (Q43.7)

Q52.3 Imperforate hymen ♀
   DEF: Obstructive anomaly of vagina, characterized by complete closure of the membranous fold around the external opening of the vagina, obstructing the vaginal introitus.

Q52.4 Other congenital malformations of vagina ♀
   Canal of Nuck cyst, congenital
   Congenital malformation of vagina NOS
   Embryonic vaginal cyst
   Gartner's duct cyst

Q52.5 Fusion of labia ♀

Q52.6 Congenital malformation of clitoris ♀

√5ᵗʰ **Q52.7 Other and unspecified congenital malformations of vulva**
  Q52.70 Unspecified congenital malformations of vulva ♀
    Congenital malformation of vulva NOS
  Q52.71 Congenital absence of vulva ♀
  Q52.79 Other congenital malformations of vulva ♀
    Congenital cyst of vulva

Q52.8 Other specified congenital malformations of female genitalia ♀

Q52.9 Congenital malformation of female genitalia, unspecified ♀

√4ᵗʰ **Q53 Undescended and ectopic testicle**

√5ᵗʰ **Q53.0 Ectopic testis**
  Q53.00 Ectopic testis, unspecified ♂
  Q53.01 Ectopic testis, unilateral ♂
  Q53.02 Ectopic testes, bilateral ♂

√5ᵗʰ **Q53.1 Undescended testicle, unilateral**
  AHA: 2017,4Q,22-23
  Q53.10 Unspecified undescended testicle, unilateral ♂
  √6ᵗʰ **Q53.11 Abdominal testis, unilateral**
    Q53.111 Unilateral intraabdominal testis ♂
    Q53.112 Unilateral inguinal testis ♂
  Q53.12 Ectopic perineal testis, unilateral ♂
  Q53.13 Unilateral high scrotal testis ♂

√5ᵗʰ **Q53.2 Undescended testicle, bilateral**
  AHA: 2017,4Q,22-23
  Q53.20 Undescended testicle, unspecified, bilateral ♂
  √6ᵗʰ **Q53.21 Abdominal testis, bilateral**
    Q53.211 Bilateral intraabdominal testes ♂
    Q53.212 Bilateral inguinal testes ♂
  Q53.22 Ectopic perineal testis, bilateral ♂
  Q53.23 Bilateral high scrotal testes ♂

Q53.9 Undescended testicle, unspecified ♂
   Cryptorchism NOS

√4ᵗʰ **Q54 Hypospadias**
   EXCLUDES 1 epispadias (Q64.0)
   DEF: Abnormal opening of the urethra on the ventral (underside) surface of the penis.

Hypospadias

Balanic (glanular, coronal) hypospadias
Subcoronal hypospadias
Penile hypospadias
Penile raphe
Scrotal hypospadias
Penoscrotal hypospadias
Scrotum
Scrotal raphe
Hypospadias (ventral view)
Perineal hypospadias

Q54.0 Hypospadias, balanic ♂
   Hypospadias, coronal
   Hypospadias, glandular

Q54.1 Hypospadias, penile ♂

Q54.2 Hypospadias, penoscrotal ♂

Q54.3 Hypospadias, perineal ♂

Q54.4 Congenital chordee ♂
   Chordee without hypospadias

Q54.8 Other hypospadias ♂
   Hypospadias with intersex state

Q54.9 Hypospadias, unspecified ♂

✓4ᵗʰ Q55 Other congenital malformations of male genital organs
> **EXCLUDES 1** *congenital hydrocele (P83.5)*
> *hypospadias (Q54.-)*

Q55.0 Absence and aplasia of testis ♂
> Monorchism

Q55.1 Hypoplasia of testis and scrotum ♂
> Fusion of testes

✓5ᵗʰ Q55.2 Other and unspecified congenital malformations of testis and scrotum

> **Q55.20 Unspecified congenital malformations of testis and scrotum**
> > Congenital malformation of testis or scrotum NOS

> **Q55.21 Polyorchism** ♂
> > **DEF:** Congenital anomaly in which there are more than two testes.

> **Q55.22 Retractile testis** ♂

> **Q55.23 Scrotal transposition** ♂

> **Q55.29 Other congenital malformations of testis and scrotum** ♂

Q55.3 Atresia of vas deferens ♂
> Code first any associated cystic fibrosis (E84.-)

Q55.4 Other congenital malformations of vas deferens, epididymis, seminal vesicles and prostate ♂
> Absence or aplasia of prostate
> Absence or aplasia of spermatic cord
> Congenital malformation of vas deferens, epididymis, seminal vesicles or prostate NOS

Q55.5 Congenital absence and aplasia of penis ♂

✓5ᵗʰ Q55.6 Other congenital malformations of penis

> **Q55.61 Curvature of penis (lateral)** ♂

> **Q55.62 Hypoplasia of penis** ♂
> > Micropenis

> **Q55.63 Congenital torsion of penis** ♂
> > **EXCLUDES 1** *acquired torsion of penis (N48.82)*

> **Q55.64 Hidden penis** ♂
> > Buried penis
> > Concealed penis
> > **EXCLUDES 1** *acquired buried penis (N48.83)*

> **Q55.69 Other congenital malformation of penis** ♂
> > Congenital malformation of penis NOS

Q55.7 Congenital vasocutaneous fistula ♂

Q55.8 Other specified congenital malformations of male genital organs ♂

Q55.9 Congenital malformation of male genital organ, unspecified ♂
> Congenital anomaly of male genital organ
> Congenital deformity of male genital organ

✓4ᵗʰ Q56 Indeterminate sex and pseudohermaphroditism
> **EXCLUDES 1** *46, XX true hermaphrodite (Q99.1)*
> *androgen insensitivity syndrome (E34.5-)*
> *chimera 46, XX/46, XY true hermaphrodite (Q99.0)*
> *female pseudohermaphroditism with adrenocortical disorder (E25.-)*
> *pseudohermaphroditism with specified chromosomal anomaly (Q96-Q99)*
> *pure gonadal dysgenesis (Q99.1)*

DEF: Indeterminate sex: External genitalia that is nondescript, lacking the physical appearance specific to either sex.
DEF: Pseudohermaphroditism: Presence of gonads of one sex and external genitalia of another sex.

Q56.0 Hermaphroditism, not elsewhere classified
> Ovotestis

Q56.1 Male pseudohermaphroditism, not elsewhere classified ♂
> 46, XY with streak gonads
> Male pseudohermaphroditism NOS

Q56.2 Female pseudohermaphroditism, not elsewhere classified ♀
> Female pseudohermaphroditism NOS

Q56.3 Pseudohermaphroditism, unspecified

Q56.4 Indeterminate sex, unspecified
> Ambiguous genitalia

Congenital malformations of the urinary system (Q60-Q64)

✓4ᵗʰ Q60 Renal agenesis and other reduction defects of kidney
> **INCLUDES** congenital absence of kidney
> congenital atrophy of kidney
> infantile atrophy of kidney

Q60.0 Renal agenesis, unilateral `cc`
Q60.1 Renal agenesis, bilateral `cc`
Q60.2 Renal agenesis, unspecified `cc`
Q60.3 Renal hypoplasia, unilateral `cc`
Q60.4 Renal hypoplasia, bilateral `cc`
Q60.5 Renal hypoplasia, unspecified `cc`
Q60.6 Potter's syndrome `cc`

✓4ᵗʰ Q61 Cystic kidney disease
> **EXCLUDES 1** *acquired cyst of kidney (N28.1)*
> *Potter's syndrome (Q60.6)*

✓5ᵗʰ Q61.0 Congenital renal cyst

> **Q61.00 Congenital renal cyst, unspecified** `cc`
> > Cyst of kidney NOS (congenital)

> **Q61.01 Congenital single renal cyst** `cc`

> **Q61.02 Congenital multiple renal cysts** `cc`

✓5ᵗʰ Q61.1 Polycystic kidney, infantile type
> Polycystic kidney, autosomal recessive

> **Q61.11 Cystic dilatation of collecting ducts** `cc`

> **Q61.19 Other polycystic kidney, infantile type** `cc`

Q61.2 Polycystic kidney, adult type
> Polycystic kidney, autosomal dominant

Q61.3 Polycystic kidney, unspecified `cc`
> **AHA:** 2016,3Q,22

Q61.4 Renal dysplasia `cc`
> Multicystic dysplastic kidney
> Multicystic kidney (development)
> Multicystic kidney disease
> Multicystic renal dysplasia
> **EXCLUDES 1** *polycystic kidney disease (Q61.11-Q61.3)*

Q61.5 Medullary cystic kidney `cc`
> Nephronopthisis
> Sponge kidney NOS
> **DEF:** Sponge kidney: Dilated collecting tubules that are usually asymptomatic. Calcinosis in tubules may cause renal insufficiency.

Q61.8 Other cystic kidney diseases `cc`
> Fibrocystic kidney
> Fibrocystic renal degeneration or disease

Q61.9 Cystic kidney disease, unspecified `cc`
> Meckel-Gruber syndrome

✓4ᵗʰ Q62 Congenital obstructive defects of renal pelvis **and congenital malformations of** ureter

Q62.0 Congenital hydronephrosis `cc`

✓5ᵗʰ Q62.1 Congenital occlusion of ureter
> Atresia and stenosis of ureter

> **Q62.10 Congenital occlusion of ureter, unspecified** `cc`

> **Q62.11 Congenital occlusion of ureteropelvic junction** `cc`

> **Q62.12 Congenital occlusion of ureterovesical orifice** `cc`

Q62.2 Congenital megaureter `cc`
> Congenital dilatation of ureter

✓5ᵗʰ Q62.3 Other obstructive defects of renal pelvis and ureter

> **Q62.31 Congenital ureterocele, orthotopic** `cc`

> **Q62.32 Cecoureterocele** `cc`
> > Ectopic ureterocele

> **Q62.39 Other obstructive defects of renal pelvis and ureter** `cc`
> > Ureteropelvic junction obstruction NOS

Q62.4 Agenesis of ureter
> Congenital absence ureter

Q62.5 Duplication of ureter
> Accessory ureter
> Double ureter

✓5ᵗʰ Q62.6 Malposition of ureter

> **Q62.60 Malposition of ureter, unspecified**

> **Q62.61 Deviation of ureter**

> **Q62.62 Displacement of ureter**

N Newborn: 0   **P** Pediatric: 0-17   **M** Maternity: 9-64   **A** Adult: 15-124   **MCC** Major Complication/Comorbidity   **CC** Complication/Comorbidity   **SW** Severe Wound Dx

926   ICD-10-CM 2021

Q62.63   Anomalous implantation of ureter
　　　　Ectopia of ureter
　　　　Ectopic ureter
Q62.69   **Other malposition of ureter**
Q62.7   **Congenital vesico-uretero-renal reflux**
Q62.8   **Other congenital malformations of ureter**
　　　　Anomaly of ureter NOS

☑4ᵗʰ **Q63   Other congenital malformations of kidney**
　　EXCLUDES 1   congenital nephrotic syndrome (N04.-)
Q63.0   **Accessory kidney**
Q63.1   **Lobulated, fused and horseshoe kidney**
Q63.2   **Ectopic kidney**
　　　　Congenital displaced kidney
　　　　Malrotation of kidney
Q63.3   **Hyperplastic and giant kidney**
　　　　Compensatory hypertrophy of kidney
Q63.8   **Other specified congenital malformations of kidney**
　　　　Congenital renal calculi
Q63.9   **Congenital malformation of kidney, unspecified**

☑4ᵗʰ **Q64   Other congenital malformations of urinary system**
Q64.0   **Epispadias**
　　EXCLUDES 1   hypospadias (Q54.-)

Epispadias

Normal external urethral orifice
Glans penis
Foreskin (retracted)
Epispadias

Epispadias (dorsal view)

☑5ᵗʰ Q64.1   **Exstrophy of urinary bladder**
　　Q64.10   **Exstrophy of urinary bladder, unspecified**   CC
　　　　　Ectopia vesicae
　　Q64.11   **Supravesical fissure of urinary bladder**   CC
　　Q64.12   **Cloacal exstrophy of urinary bladder**   CC
　　Q64.19   **Other exstrophy of urinary bladder**   CC
　　　　　Extroversion of bladder
Q64.2   **Congenital posterior urethral valves**   CC
☑5ᵗʰ Q64.3   **Other atresia and stenosis of urethra and bladder neck**
　　Q64.31   **Congenital bladder neck obstruction**   CC
　　　　　Congenital obstruction of vesicourethral orifice
　　Q64.32   **Congenital stricture of urethra**   CC
　　Q64.33   **Congenital stricture of urinary meatus**   CC
　　Q64.39   **Other atresia and stenosis of urethra and bladder neck**   CC
　　　　　Atresia and stenosis of urethra and bladder neck NOS
Q64.4   **Malformation of urachus**
　　　　Cyst of urachus
　　　　Patent urachus
　　　　Prolapse of urachus
Q64.5   **Congenital absence of bladder and urethra**
Q64.6   **Congenital diverticulum of bladder**
☑5ᵗʰ Q64.7   **Other and unspecified congenital malformations of bladder and urethra**
　　EXCLUDES 1   congenital prolapse of bladder (mucosa) (Q79.4)
　　Q64.70   **Unspecified congenital malformation of bladder and urethra**
　　　　　Malformation of bladder or urethra NOS
　　Q64.71   **Congenital prolapse of urethra**
　　Q64.72   **Congenital prolapse of urinary meatus**
　　Q64.73   **Congenital urethrorectal fistula**
　　Q64.74   **Double urethra**
　　Q64.75   **Double urinary meatus**
　　Q64.79   **Other congenital malformations of bladder and urethra**
Q64.8   **Other specified congenital malformations of urinary system**

Q64.9   **Congenital malformation of urinary system, unspecified**
　　　　Congenital anomaly NOS of urinary system
　　　　Congenital deformity NOS of urinary system

Congenital malformations and deformations of the musculoskeletal system (Q65-Q79)

☑4ᵗʰ **Q65   Congenital deformities of hip**
　　EXCLUDES 1   clicking hip (R29.4)
☑5ᵗʰ Q65.0   **Congenital dislocation of hip, unilateral**
　　Q65.00   **Congenital dislocation of unspecified hip, unilateral**
　　Q65.01   **Congenital dislocation of right hip, unilateral**
　　Q65.02   **Congenital dislocation of left hip, unilateral**
Q65.1   **Congenital dislocation of hip, bilateral**
Q65.2   **Congenital dislocation of hip, unspecified**
☑5ᵗʰ Q65.3   **Congenital partial dislocation of hip, unilateral**
　　Q65.30   **Congenital partial dislocation of unspecified hip, unilateral**
　　Q65.31   **Congenital partial dislocation of right hip, unilateral**
　　Q65.32   **Congenital partial dislocation of left hip, unilateral**
Q65.4   **Congenital partial dislocation of hip, bilateral**
Q65.5   **Congenital partial dislocation of hip, unspecified**
Q65.6   **Congenital unstable hip**
　　　　Congenital dislocatable hip
☑5ᵗʰ Q65.8   **Other congenital deformities of hip**
　　Q65.81   **Congenital coxa valga**
　　Q65.82   **Congenital coxa vara**
　　Q65.89   **Other specified congenital deformities of hip**
　　　　　Anteversion of femoral neck
　　　　　Congenital acetabular dysplasia
Q65.9   **Congenital deformity of hip, unspecified**

☑4ᵗʰ **Q66   Congenital deformities of feet**
　　EXCLUDES 1   reduction defects of feet (Q72.-)
　　　　　　valgus deformities (acquired) (M21.0-)
　　　　　　varus deformities (acquired) (M21.1-)
　　AHA: 2019,4Q,13
☑5ᵗʰ Q66.0   **Congenital talipes equinovarus**
　　Q66.00   **Congenital talipes equinovarus, unspecified foot**
　　Q66.01   **Congenital talipes equinovarus, right foot**
　　Q66.02   **Congenital talipes equinovarus, left foot**
☑5ᵗʰ Q66.1   **Congenital talipes calcaneovarus**
　　Q66.10   **Congenital talipes calcaneovarus, unspecified foot**
　　Q66.11   **Congenital talipes calcaneovarus, right foot**
　　Q66.12   **Congenital talipes calcaneovarus, left foot**
☑5ᵗʰ Q66.2   **Congenital metatarsus (primus) varus**
　　AHA: 2016,4Q,59
　　☑6ᵗʰ Q66.21   **Congenital metatarsus primus varus**
　　　　Q66.211   **Congenital metatarsus primus varus, right foot**
　　　　Q66.212   **Congenital metatarsus primus varus, left foot**
　　　　Q66.219   **Congenital metatarsus primus varus, unspecified foot**
　　☑6ᵗʰ Q66.22   **Congenital metatarsus adductus**
　　　　Congenital metatarsus varus
　　　　Q66.221   **Congenital metatarsus adductus, right foot**
　　　　Q66.222   **Congenital metatarsus adductus, left foot**
　　　　Q66.229   **Congenital metatarsus adductus, unspecified foot**
☑5ᵗʰ Q66.3   **Other congenital varus deformities of feet**
　　　　Hallux varus, congenital
　　Q66.30   **Other congenital varus deformities of feet, unspecified foot**
　　Q66.31   **Other congenital varus deformities of feet, right foot**
　　Q66.32   **Other congenital varus deformities of feet, left foot**
☑6ᵗʰ Q66.4   **Congenital talipes calcaneovalgus**
　　Q66.40   **Congenital talipes calcaneovalgus, unspecified foot**
　　Q66.41   **Congenital talipes calcaneovalgus, right foot**
　　Q66.42   **Congenital talipes calcaneovalgus, left foot**

Chapter 17. Congenital Malformations, Deformations and Chromosomal Abnormalities

Q66.5–Q71.13

√5ᵗʰ **Q66.5 Congenital pes planus**
- Congenital flat foot
- Congenital rigid flat foot
- Congenital spastic (everted) flat foot
  - *EXCLUDES 1*   pes planus, acquired (M21.4)

   Q66.50 Congenital pes planus, unspecified foot
   Q66.51 Congenital pes planus, right foot
   Q66.52 Congenital pes planus, left foot

Q66.6 Other congenital valgus deformities of feet
- Congenital metatarsus valgus

√5ᵗʰ **Q66.7 Congenital pes cavus**
   Q66.70 Congenital pes cavus, unspecified foot
   Q66.71 Congenital pes cavus, right foot
   Q66.72 Congenital pes cavus, left foot

√5ᵗʰ **Q66.8 Other congenital deformities of feet**
   Q66.80 Congenital vertical talus deformity, unspecified foot
   Q66.81 Congenital vertical talus deformity, right foot
   Q66.82 Congenital vertical talus deformity, left foot
   Q66.89 Other specified congenital deformities of feet
- Congenital asymmetric talipes
- Congenital clubfoot NOS
- Congenital talipes NOS
- Congenital tarsal coalition
- Hammer toe, congenital
  - **DEF:** Clubfoot: Congenital anomaly of the foot with the heel elevated and rotated outward and the toes pointing inward.

√5ᵗʰ **Q66.9 Congenital deformity of feet, unspecified**
   Q66.90 Congenital deformity of feet, unspecified, unspecified foot
   Q66.91 Congenital deformity of feet, unspecified, right foot
   Q66.92 Congenital deformity of feet, unspecified, left foot

√4ᵗʰ **Q67 Congenital musculoskeletal deformities of head, face, spine and chest**
- *EXCLUDES 1*   congenital malformation syndromes classified to Q87.-
  - Potter's syndrome (Q60.6)

Q67.0 Congenital facial asymmetry
Q67.1 Congenital compression facies
Q67.2 Dolichocephaly
Q67.3 Plagiocephaly
Q67.4 Other congenital deformities of skull, face and jaw
- Congenital depressions in skull
- Congenital hemifacial atrophy or hypertrophy
- Deviation of nasal septum, congenital
- Squashed or bent nose, congenital
  - *EXCLUDES 1*   dentofacial anomalies [including malocclusion] (M26.-)
    - syphilitic saddle nose (A50.5)
  - **DEF:** Deviated septum: Condition in which the nasal septum, a thin wall composed of cartilage and bone that separates the two nostrils, is crooked or displaced from the midline.

Q67.5 Congenital deformity of spine   `CC`
- Congenital postural scoliosis
- Congenital scoliosis NOS
  - *EXCLUDES 1*   infantile idiopathic scoliosis (M41.0)
    - scoliosis due to congenital bony malformation (Q76.3)
  - **AHA:** 2014,4Q,26

Q67.6 Pectus excavatum
- Congenital funnel chest
Q67.7 Pectus carinatum
- Congenital pigeon chest
Q67.8 Other congenital deformities of chest   `CC`
- Congenital deformity of chest wall NOS

√4ᵗʰ **Q68 Other congenital musculoskeletal deformities**
- *EXCLUDES 1*   reduction defects of limb(s) (Q71-Q73)
- *EXCLUDES 2*   congenital myotonic chondrodystrophy (G71.13)

Q68.0 Congenital deformity of sternocleidomastoid muscle
- Congenital contracture of sternocleidomastoid (muscle)
- Congenital (sternomastoid) torticollis
- Sternomastoid tumor (congenital)

Q68.1 Congenital deformity of finger(s) and hand   `CC`
- Congenital clubfinger
- Spade-like hand (congenital)
Q68.2 Congenital deformity of knee
- Congenital dislocation of knee
- Congenital genu recurvatum
Q68.3 Congenital bowing of femur
- *EXCLUDES 1*   anteversion of femur (neck) (Q65.89)
Q68.4 Congenital bowing of tibia and fibula
Q68.5 Congenital bowing of long bones of leg, unspecified
Q68.6 Discoid meniscus
Q68.8 Other specified congenital musculoskeletal deformities
- Congenital deformity of clavicle
- Congenital deformity of elbow
- Congenital deformity of forearm
- Congenital deformity of scapula
- Congenital deformity of wrist
- Congenital dislocation of elbow
- Congenital dislocation of shoulder
- Congenital dislocation of wrist

√4ᵗʰ **Q69 Polydactyly**
Q69.0 Accessory finger(s)
Q69.1 Accessory thumb(s)
Q69.2 Accessory toe(s)
- Accessory hallux
Q69.9 Polydactyly, unspecified
- Supernumerary digit(s) NOS

√4ᵗʰ **Q70 Syndactyly**
√5ᵗʰ **Q70.0 Fused fingers**
- Complex syndactyly of fingers with synostosis
   Q70.00 Fused fingers, unspecified hand
   Q70.01 Fused fingers, right hand
   Q70.02 Fused fingers, left hand
   Q70.03 Fused fingers, bilateral
√5ᵗʰ **Q70.1 Webbed fingers**
- Simple syndactyly of fingers without synostosis
   Q70.10 Webbed fingers, unspecified hand
   Q70.11 Webbed fingers, right hand
   Q70.12 Webbed fingers, left hand
   Q70.13 Webbed fingers, bilateral
√5ᵗʰ **Q70.2 Fused toes**
- Complex syndactyly of toes with synostosis
   Q70.20 Fused toes, unspecified foot
   Q70.21 Fused toes, right foot
   Q70.22 Fused toes, left foot
   Q70.23 Fused toes, bilateral
√5ᵗʰ **Q70.3 Webbed toes**
- Simple syndactyly of toes without synostosis
   Q70.30 Webbed toes, unspecified foot
   Q70.31 Webbed toes, right foot
   Q70.32 Webbed toes, left foot
   Q70.33 Webbed toes, bilateral
Q70.4 Polysyndactyly, unspecified
- *EXCLUDES 1*   specified syndactyly of hand and feet — code to specified conditions (Q70.0-Q70.3-)
Q70.9 Syndactyly, unspecified
- Symphalangy NOS

√4ᵗʰ **Q71 Reduction defects of upper limb**
√5ᵗʰ **Q71.0 Congenital complete absence of upper limb**
   Q71.00 Congenital complete absence of unspecified upper limb
   Q71.01 Congenital complete absence of right upper limb
   Q71.02 Congenital complete absence of left upper limb
   Q71.03 Congenital complete absence of upper limb, bilateral
√5ᵗʰ **Q71.1 Congenital absence of upper arm and forearm with hand present**
   Q71.10 Congenital absence of unspecified upper arm and forearm with hand present
   Q71.11 Congenital absence of right upper arm and forearm with hand present
   Q71.12 Congenital absence of left upper arm and forearm with hand present
   Q71.13 Congenital absence of upper arm and forearm with hand present, bilateral

N Newborn: 0   P Pediatric: 0-17   M Maternity: 9-64   A Adult: 15-124   MCC Major Complication/Comorbidity   CC Complication/Comorbidity   SW Severe Wound Dx

928   ICD-10-CM 2021

✓5ᵗʰ **Q71.2 Congenital** absence of both forearm and hand

     Q71.20 Congenital absence of both forearm and hand, unspecified upper limb

     Q71.21 Congenital absence of both forearm and hand, right **upper limb**

     Q71.22 Congenital absence of both forearm and hand, left **upper limb**

     Q71.23 Congenital absence of both forearm and hand, bilateral

✓5ᵗʰ **Q71.3 Congenital** absence of hand and finger

     Q71.30 Congenital absence of unspecified hand and finger

     Q71.31 Congenital absence of right **hand and finger**

     Q71.32 Congenital absence of left **hand and finger**

     Q71.33 Congenital absence of hand and finger, bilateral

✓5ᵗʰ **Q71.4 Longitudinal reduction defect of** radius

     Clubhand (congenital)

     Radial clubhand

     Q71.40 Longitudinal reduction defect of unspecified radius

     Q71.41 Longitudinal reduction defect of right **radius**

     Q71.42 Longitudinal reduction defect of left **radius**

     Q71.43 Longitudinal reduction defect of radius, bilateral

✓5ᵗʰ **Q71.5 Longitudinal reduction defect of** ulna

     Q71.50 Longitudinal reduction defect of unspecified ulna

     Q71.51 Longitudinal reduction defect of right **ulna**

     Q71.52 Longitudinal reduction defect of left **ulna**

     Q71.53 Longitudinal reduction defect of ulna, bilateral

✓5ᵗʰ **Q71.6** Lobster-claw hand

     Q71.60 Lobster-claw hand, unspecified hand

     Q71.61 Lobster-claw right **hand**

     Q71.62 Lobster-claw left **hand**

     Q71.63 Lobster-claw hand, bilateral

✓5ᵗʰ **Q71.8 Other reduction defects of** upper limb

     ✓6ᵗʰ **Q71.81 Congenital** shortening **of upper limb**

         Q71.811 Congenital shortening of right **upper limb**

         Q71.812 Congenital shortening of left **upper limb**

         Q71.813 Congenital shortening of upper limb, bilateral

         Q71.819 Congenital shortening of unspecified upper limb

     ✓6ᵗʰ **Q71.89 Other reduction defects of upper limb**

         Q71.891 Other reduction defects of right **upper limb**

         Q71.892 Other reduction defects of left **upper limb**

         Q71.893 Other reduction defects of upper limb, bilateral

         Q71.899 Other reduction defects of unspecified upper limb

✓5ᵗʰ **Q71.9 Unspecified reduction defect of upper limb**

     Q71.90 Unspecified reduction defect of unspecified upper limb

     Q71.91 Unspecified reduction defect of right **upper limb**

     Q71.92 Unspecified reduction defect of left **upper limb**

     Q71.93 Unspecified reduction defect of upper limb, bilateral

✓4ᵗʰ **Q72 Reduction defects of** lower limb

     ✓5ᵗʰ **Q72.0 Congenital** complete absence of lower limb

         Q72.00 Congenital complete absence of unspecified lower limb

         Q72.01 Congenital complete absence of right **lower limb**

         Q72.02 Congenital complete absence of left **lower limb**

         Q72.03 Congenital complete absence of lower limb, bilateral

     ✓5ᵗʰ **Q72.1 Congenital** absence of thigh and lower leg with foot present

         Q72.10 Congenital absence of unspecified thigh and lower leg with foot present

         Q72.11 Congenital absence of right **thigh and lower leg with foot present**

         Q72.12 Congenital absence of left **thigh and lower leg with foot present**

         Q72.13 Congenital absence of thigh and lower leg with foot present, bilateral

     ✓5ᵗʰ **Q72.2 Congenital** absence of both lower leg and foot

         Q72.20 Congenital absence of both lower leg and foot, unspecified lower limb

         Q72.21 Congenital absence of both lower leg and foot, right **lower limb**

         Q72.22 Congenital absence of both lower leg and foot, left **lower limb**

         Q72.23 Congenital absence of both lower leg and foot, bilateral

     ✓5ᵗʰ **Q72.3 Congenital** absence of foot and toe(s)

         Q72.30 Congenital absence of unspecified foot and toe(s)

         Q72.31 Congenital absence of right **foot and toe(s)**

         Q72.32 Congenital absence of left **foot and toe(s)**

         Q72.33 Congenital absence of foot and toe(s), bilateral

     ✓5ᵗʰ **Q72.4 Longitudinal reduction defect of femur**

         Proximal femoral focal deficiency

         Q72.40 Longitudinal reduction defect of unspecified femur

         Q72.41 Longitudinal reduction defect of right **femur**

         Q72.42 Longitudinal reduction defect of left **femur**

         Q72.43 Longitudinal reduction defect of femur, bilateral

     ✓5ᵗʰ **Q72.5 Longitudinal reduction defect of tibia**

         Q72.50 Longitudinal reduction defect of unspecified tibia

         Q72.51 Longitudinal reduction defect of right **tibia**

         Q72.52 Longitudinal reduction defect of left **tibia**

         Q72.53 Longitudinal reduction defect of tibia, bilateral

     ✓5ᵗʰ **Q72.6 Longitudinal reduction defect of** fibula

         Q72.60 Longitudinal reduction defect of unspecified fibula

         Q72.61 Longitudinal reduction defect of right **fibula**

         Q72.62 Longitudinal reduction defect of left **fibula**

         Q72.63 Longitudinal reduction defect of fibula, bilateral

     ✓5ᵗʰ **Q72.7 Split foot**

         Q72.70 Split foot, unspecified lower limb

         Q72.71 Split foot, right **lower limb**

         Q72.72 Split foot, left **lower limb**

         Q72.73 Split foot, bilateral

     ✓5ᵗʰ **Q72.8 Other reduction defects of lower limb**

         ✓6ᵗʰ **Q72.81 Congenital** shortening **of lower limb**

             Q72.811 Congenital shortening of right **lower limb**

             Q72.812 Congenital shortening of left **lower limb**

             Q72.813 Congenital shortening of lower limb, bilateral

             Q72.819 Congenital shortening of unspecified lower limb

         ✓6ᵗʰ **Q72.89 Other reduction defects of lower limb**

             Q72.891 Other reduction defects of right **lower limb**

             Q72.892 Other reduction defects of left **lower limb**

             Q72.893 Other reduction defects of lower limb, bilateral

             Q72.899 Other reduction defects of unspecified lower limb

     ✓5ᵗʰ **Q72.9 Unspecified reduction defect of lower limb**

         Q72.90 Unspecified reduction defect of unspecified lower limb

         Q72.91 Unspecified reduction defect of right **lower limb**

         Q72.92 Unspecified reduction defect of left **lower limb**

         Q72.93 Unspecified reduction defect of lower limb, bilateral

✓4ᵗʰ **Q73 Reduction defects of unspecified limb**

     Q73.0 Congenital absence **of unspecified limb(s)**

         Amelia NOS

     Q73.1 Phocomelia, **unspecified limb(s)**

         Phocomelia NOS

     Q73.8 Other reduction defects of unspecified limb(s)

         Longitudinal reduction deformity of unspecified limb(s)

         Ectromelia of limb NOS

         Hemimelia of limb NOS

         Reduction defect of limb NOS

✔ Additional Character Required   ✔x7ᵗʰ Placeholder   Unacceptable PDx   Questionable PDx   Manifestation   Unspecified Dx   H1 - H14 HAC   HCC CMS-HCC Dx   HIV HIV Dx

ICD-10-CM 2021

929

Chapter 17. Congenital Malformations, Deformations and Chromosomal Abnormalities

✓4ᵗʰ **Q74 Other congenital malformations of limb(s)**
     EXCLUDES 1   *polydactyly (Q69.-)*
                reduction defect of limb (Q71-Q73)
                syndactyly (Q70.-)

Q74.0 Other congenital malformations of upper limb(s), including shoulder girdle
     Accessory carpal bones
     Cleidocranial dysostosis
     Congenital pseudarthrosis of clavicle
     Macrodactylia (fingers)
     Madelung's deformity
     Radioulnar synostosis
     Sprengel's deformity
     Triphalangeal thumb

Q74.1 Congenital malformation of knee
     Congenital absence of patella
     Congenital dislocation of patella
     Congenital genu valgum
     Congenital genu varum
     Rudimentary patella
     EXCLUDES 1   *congenital dislocation of knee (Q68.2)*
                congenital genu recurvatum (Q68.2)
                nail patella syndrome (Q87.2)

Q74.2 Other congenital malformations of lower limb(s), including pelvic girdle
     Congenital fusion of sacroiliac joint
     Congenital malformation of ankle joint
     Congenital malformation of sacroiliac joint
     EXCLUDES 1   *anteversion of femur (neck) (Q65.89)*

Q74.3 Arthrogryposis multiplex congenita   CC
Q74.8 Other specified congenital malformations of limb(s)
Q74.9 Unspecified congenital malformation of limb(s)
     Congenital anomaly of limb(s) NOS

✓4ᵗʰ **Q75 Other congenital malformations of skull and face bones**
     EXCLUDES 1   *congenital malformation of face NOS (Q18.-)*
                congenital malformation syndromes classified to Q87.-
                dentofacial anomalies [including malocclusion] (M26.-)
                musculoskeletal deformities of head and face (Q67.0-Q67.4)
                skull defects associated with congenital anomalies of brain such as:
                anencephaly (Q00.0)
                encephalocele (Q01.-)
                hydrocephalus (Q03.-)
                microcephaly (Q02)

Q75.0 Craniosynostosis
     Acrocephaly
     Imperfect fusion of skull
     Oxycephaly
     Trigonocephaly
     DEF: Congenital condition in which one or more of the cranial sutures fuse prematurely, creating a deformed or aberrant head shape.

Q75.1 Craniofacial dysostosis
     Crouzon's disease

Q75.2 Hypertelorism
Q75.3 Macrocephaly
Q75.4 Mandibulofacial dysostosis
     Franceschetti syndrome
     Treacher Collins syndrome

Q75.5 Oculomandibular dysostosis
Q75.8 Other specified congenital malformations of skull and face bones
     Absence of skull bone, congenital
     Congenital deformity of forehead
     Platybasia

Q75.9 Congenital malformation of skull and face bones, unspecified
     Congenital anomaly of face bones NOS
     Congenital anomaly of skull NOS

✓4ᵗʰ **Q76 Congenital malformations of spine and bony thorax**
     EXCLUDES 1   *congenital musculoskeletal deformities of spine and chest (Q67.5-Q67.8)*

Q76.0 Spina bifida occulta
     EXCLUDES 1   *meningocele (spinal) (Q05.-)*
                spina bifida (aperta) (cystica) (Q05.-)

Q76.1 Klippel-Feil syndrome
     Cervical fusion syndrome

Q76.2 Congenital spondylolisthesis
     Congenital spondylolysis
     EXCLUDES 1   *spondylolisthesis (acquired) (M43.1-)*
                spondylolysis (acquired) (M43.0-)

Q76.3 Congenital scoliosis due to congenital bony malformation   CC
     Hemivertebra fusion or failure of segmentation with scoliosis

✓5ᵗʰ **Q76.4 Other congenital malformations of spine, not associated with scoliosis**

     ✓6ᵗʰ **Q76.41 Congenital kyphosis**

         Q76.411 Congenital kyphosis, occipito-atlanto-axial region
         Q76.412 Congenital kyphosis, cervical region
         Q76.413 Congenital kyphosis, cervicothoracic region
         Q76.414 Congenital kyphosis, thoracic region
         Q76.415 Congenital kyphosis, thoracolumbar region
         Q76.419 Congenital kyphosis, unspecified region

     ✓6ᵗʰ **Q76.42 Congenital lordosis**

         Q76.425 Congenital lordosis, thoracolumbar region   CC
         Q76.426 Congenital lordosis, lumbar region   CC
         Q76.427 Congenital lordosis, lumbosacral region   CC
         Q76.428 Congenital lordosis, sacral and sacrococcygeal region   CC
         Q76.429 Congenital lordosis, unspecified region   CC

     Q76.49 Other congenital malformations of spine, not associated with scoliosis
         Congenital absence of vertebra NOS
         Congenital fusion of spine NOS
         Congenital malformation of lumbosacral (joint) (region) NOS
         Congenital malformation of spine NOS
         Hemivertebra NOS
         Malformation of spine NOS
         Platyspondylisis NOS
         Supernumerary vertebra NOS

Q76.5 Cervical rib
     Supernumerary rib in cervical region

Q76.6 Other congenital malformations of ribs   CC
     Accessory rib
     Congenital absence of rib
     Congenital fusion of ribs
     Congenital malformation of ribs NOS
     EXCLUDES 1   *short rib syndrome (Q77.2)*

Q76.7 Congenital malformation of sternum   CC
     Congenital absence of sternum
     Sternum bifidum

Q76.8 Other congenital malformations of bony thorax   CC
Q76.9 Congenital malformation of bony thorax, unspecified   CC

✓4ᵗʰ **Q77 Osteochondrodysplasia with defects of growth of tubular bones and spine**
     EXCLUDES 1   *mucopolysaccharidosis (E76.0-E76.3)*
     EXCLUDES 2   *congenital myotonic chondrodystrophy (G71.13)*

Q77.0 Achondrogenesis
     Hypochondrogenesis

Q77.1 Thanatophoric short stature
Q77.2 Short rib syndrome   CC
     Asphyxiating thoracic dysplasia [Jeune]

Q77.3 Chondrodysplasia punctata
     EXCLUDES 1   *Rhizomelic chondrodysplasia punctata (E71.43)*

Q77.4 Achondroplasia
     Hypochondroplasia
     Osteosclerosis congenita

Q77.5 Diastrophic dysplasia
Q77.6 Chondroectodermal dysplasia
     Ellis-van Creveld syndrome

Q77.7 Spondyloepiphyseal dysplasia
Q77.8 Other osteochondrodysplasia with defects of growth of tubular bones and spine
Q77.9 Osteochondrodysplasia with defects of growth of tubular bones and spine, unspecified

---

N Newborn: 0   P Pediatric: 0-17   M Maternity: 9-64   A Adult: 15-124   MCC Major Complication/Comorbidity   CC Complication/Comorbidity   SW Severe Wound Dx

930   ICD-10-CM 2021

Q74–Q77.9

✓4ᵗʰ **Q78 Other osteochondrodysplasias**

    EXCLUDES 2   congenital myotonic chondrodystrophy (G71.13)

Q78.0 Osteogenesis imperfecta   CC
     Fragilitas ossium
     Osteopsathyrosis

Q78.1 Polyostotic fibrous dysplasia
     Albright(-McCune)(-Sternberg) syndrome

Q78.2 Osteopetrosis   CC
     Albers-Schönberg syndrome
     Osteosclerosis NOS
     DEF: Rare congenital condition in which the bones are excessively dense, resulting from a discrepancy in the formation and breakdown of bone.

Q78.3 Progressive diaphyseal dysplasia
     Camurati-Engelmann syndrome

Q78.4 Enchondromatosis
     Maffucci's syndrome
     Ollier's disease

Q78.5 Metaphyseal dysplasia
     Pyle's syndrome

Q78.6 Multiple congenital exostoses
     Diaphyseal aclasis

Q78.8 Other specified osteochondrodysplasias
     Osteopoikilosis

Q78.9 Osteochondrodysplasia, unspecified
     Chondrodystrophy NOS
     Osteodystrophy NOS

✓4ᵗʰ **Q79 Congenital malformations of musculoskeletal system, not elsewhere classified**

    EXCLUDES 2   congenital (sternomastoid) torticollis (Q68.0)

Q79.0 Congenital diaphragmatic hernia   MCC
    EXCLUDES 1   congenital hiatus hernia (Q40.1)

Q79.1 Other congenital malformations of diaphragm   MCC
     Absence of diaphragm
     Congenital malformation of diaphragm NOS
     Eventration of diaphragm

Q79.2 Exomphalos   MCC
     Omphalocele
    EXCLUDES 1   umbilical hernia (K42.-)

Q79.3 Gastroschisis   MCC

Gastroschisis

Herniated small bowel (gastroschisis)

Rectus abdominus m.

Umbilicus

skin

distal

proximal

Defect

Q79.4 Prune belly syndrome   MCC
     Congenital prolapse of bladder mucosa
     Eagle-Barrett syndrome

✓5ᵗʰ **Q79.5 Other congenital malformations of abdominal wall**

    EXCLUDES 1   umbilical hernia (K42.-)

Q79.51 Congenital hernia of bladder   MCC

Q79.59 Other congenital malformations of abdominal wall   MCC

✓5ᵗʰ **Q79.6 Ehlers-Danlos syndromes**

     AHA: 2019,4Q,13-14
     DEF: Connective tissue disorder that causes hyperextended skin and joints and results in fragile blood vessels with bleeding, poor wound healing, and subcutaneous pseudotumors.

Q79.60 Ehlers-Danlos syndrome, unspecified   CC

Q79.61 Classical Ehlers-Danlos syndrome   CC
     Classical EDS (cEDS)

Q79.62 Hypermobile Ehlers-Danlos syndrome   CC
     Hypermobile EDS (hEDS)

Q79.63 Vascular Ehlers-Danlos syndrome   CC
     Vascular EDS (vEDS)

Q79.69 Other Ehlers-Danlos syndromes   CC

Q79.8 Other congenital malformations of musculoskeletal system
     Absence of muscle
     Absence of tendon
     Accessory muscle
     Amyotrophia congenita
     Congenital constricting bands
     Congenital shortening of tendon
     Poland syndrome

Q79.9 Congenital malformation of musculoskeletal system, unspecified
     Congenital anomaly of musculoskeletal system NOS
     Congenital deformity of musculoskeletal system NOS

Other congenital malformations (Q80-Q89)

✓4ᵗʰ **Q80 Congenital ichthyosis**

    EXCLUDES 1   Refsum's disease (G60.1)
     DEF: Excessive production of skin cells resulting in red, dry, scaly skin.

Q80.0 Ichthyosis vulgaris

Q80.1 X-linked ichthyosis

Q80.2 Lamellar ichthyosis
     Collodion baby

Q80.3 Congenital bullous ichthyosiform erythroderma

Q80.4 Harlequin fetus

Q80.8 Other congenital ichthyosis

Q80.9 Congenital ichthyosis, unspecified

✓4ᵗʰ **Q81 Epidermolysis bullosa**

Q81.0 Epidermolysis bullosa simplex
    EXCLUDES 1   Cockayne's syndrome (Q87.19)

Q81.1 Epidermolysis bullosa letalis
     Herlitz' syndrome

Q81.2 Epidermolysis bullosa dystrophica

Q81.8 Other epidermolysis bullosa

Q81.9 Epidermolysis bullosa, unspecified

✓4ᵗʰ **Q82 Other congenital malformations of skin**

    EXCLUDES 1   acrodermatitis enteropathica (E83.2)
                congenital erythropoietic porphyria (E80.0)
                pilonidal cyst or sinus (L05.-)
                Sturge-Weber (-Dimitri) syndrome (Q85.8)

Q82.0 Hereditary lymphedema

Q82.1 Xeroderma pigmentosum

Q82.2 Congenital cutaneous mastocytosis
     Congenital diffuse cutaneous mastocytosis
     Congenital maculopapular cutaneous mastocytosis
     Congenital urticaria pigmentosa
    EXCLUDES 1   cutaneous mastocytosis NOS (D47.01)
                diffuse cutaneous mastocytosis (with onset after newborn period) (D47.01)
                malignant mastocytosis (C96.2-)
                systemic mastocytosis (D47.02)
                urticaria pigmentosa (non-congenital) (with onset after newborn period) (D47.01)

     AHA: 2017,4Q,5

Q82.3 Incontinentia pigmenti

Q82.4 Ectodermal dysplasia (anhidrotic)
    EXCLUDES 1   Ellis-van Creveld syndrome (Q77.6)

✓ Additional Character Required   ✓x7ᵗʰ Placeholder   Unacceptable PDx   Questionable PDx   Manifestation   Unspecified Dx   H1-H14 HAC   HCC CMS-HCC Dx   HIV HIV Dx

Q82.5   Congenital non-neoplastic nevus
Birthmark NOS
Flammeus Nevus
Portwine Nevus
Sanguineous Nevus
Strawberry Nevus
Vascular Nevus NOS
Verrucous Nevus
EXCLUDES 2   *araneus nevus (I78.1)*
Café au lait spots (L81.3)
lentigo (L81.4)
melanocytic nevus (D22.-)
nevus NOS (D22.-)
pigmented nevus (D22.-)
spider nevus (I78.1)
stellar nevus (I78.1)

Q82.6   Congenital sacral dimple
Parasacral dimple
EXCLUDES 2   *pilonidal cyst with abscess (L05.01)*
pilonidal cyst without abscess (L05.91)
AHA: 2016,4Q,60

Q82.8   Other specified congenital malformations of skin
Abnormal palmar creases
Accessory skin tags
Benign familial pemphigus [Hailey-Hailey]
Congenital poikiloderma
Cutis laxa (hyperelastica)
Dermatoglyphic anomalies
Inherited keratosis palmaris et plantaris
Keratosis follicularis [Darier-White]
EXCLUDES 1   ►*Ehlers-Danlos syndromes*◄ *(Q79.6-)*
AHA: 2016,1Q,17

Q82.9   Congenital malformation of skin, unspecified

✓4ᵗʰ **Q83   Congenital malformations of breast**
EXCLUDES 2   *absence of pectoral muscle (Q79.8)*
hypoplasia of breast (N64.82)
micromastia (N64.82)

Q83.0   Congenital absence of breast with absent nipple

Q83.1   Accessory breast
Supernumerary breast

Q83.2   Absent nipple

Q83.3   Accessory nipple
Supernumerary nipple

Q83.8   Other congenital malformations of breast

Q83.9   Congenital malformation of breast, unspecified

✓4ᵗʰ **Q84   Other congenital malformations of integument**

Q84.0   Congenital alopecia
Congenital atrichosis

Q84.1   Congenital morphological disturbances of hair, not elsewhere classified
Beaded hair
Monilethrix
Pili annulati
EXCLUDES 1   *Menkes' kinky hair syndrome (E83.0)*

Q84.2   Other congenital malformations of hair
Congenital hypertrichosis
Congenital malformation of hair NOS
Persistent lanugo

Q84.3   Anonychia
EXCLUDES 1   *nail patella syndrome (Q87.2)*

Q84.4   Congenital leukonychia

Q84.5   Enlarged and hypertrophic nails
Congenital onychauxis
Pachyonychia

Q84.6   Other congenital malformations of nails
Congenital clubnail
Congenital koilonychia
Congenital malformation of nail NOS

Q84.8   Other specified congenital malformations of integument
Aplasia cutis congenita

Q84.9   Congenital malformation of integument, unspecified
Congenital anomaly of integument NOS
Congenital deformity of integument NOS

✓4ᵗʰ **Q85   Phakomatoses, not elsewhere classified**
EXCLUDES 1   *ataxia telangiectasia [Louis-Bar] (G11.3)*
familial dysautonomia [Riley-Day] (G90.1)

✓5ᵗʰ **Q85.0   Neurofibromatosis (nonmalignant)**

Q85.00   Neurofibromatosis, unspecified   HCC

Q85.01   Neurofibromatosis, type 1   HCC
Von Recklinghausen disease

Q85.02   Neurofibromatosis, type 2   HCC
Acoustic neurofibromatosis
DEF: Inherited condition with cutaneous lesions, benign tumors of peripheral nerves, and bilateral 8th nerve masses.

Q85.03   Schwannomatosis   HCC
DEF: Genetic mutation (SMARCB1/INI1) causing multiple benign tumors along the nerve pathways, except on the 8th cranial (vestibular) nerve.

Q85.09   Other neurofibromatosis   HCC

Q85.1   Tuberous sclerosis   CC   HCC
Bourneville's disease
Epiloia

Q85.8   Other phakomatoses, not elsewhere classified   CC   HCC
Peutz-Jeghers Syndrome
Sturge-Weber(-Dimitri) syndrome
von Hippel-Lindau syndrome
EXCLUDES 1   *Meckel-Gruber syndrome (Q61.9)*

Q85.9   Phakomatosis, unspecified   CC   HCC
Hamartosis NOS

✓4ᵗʰ **Q86   Congenital malformation syndromes due to known exogenous causes, not elsewhere classified**
EXCLUDES 2   *iodine-deficiency-related hypothyroidism (E00-E02)*
nonteratogenic effects of substances transmitted via placenta or breast milk (P04.-)

Q86.0   Fetal alcohol syndrome (dysmorphic)

Q86.1   Fetal hydantoin syndrome
Meadow's syndrome

Q86.2   Dysmorphism due to warfarin

Q86.8   Other congenital malformation syndromes due to known exogenous causes

✓4ᵗʰ **Q87   Other specified congenital malformation syndromes affecting multiple systems**
Use additional code(s) to identify all associated manifestations

Q87.0   Congenital malformation syndromes predominantly affecting facial appearance
Acrocephalopolysyndactyly
Acrocephalosyndactyly [Apert]
Cryptophthalmos syndrome
Cyclopia
Goldenhar syndrome
Moebius syndrome
Oro-facial-digital syndrome
Robin syndrome
Whistling face

✓5ᵗʰ **Q87.1   Congenital malformation syndromes predominantly associated with short stature**
EXCLUDES 1   *Ellis-van Creveld syndrome (Q77.6)*
Smith-Lemli-Opitz syndrome (E78.72)
AHA: 2019,4Q,14-15

Q87.11   Prader-Willi syndrome   CC

Q87.19   Other congenital malformation syndromes predominantly associated with short stature   CC
Aarskog syndrome
Cockayne syndrome
De Lange syndrome
Dubowitz syndrome
Noonan syndrome
Robinow-Silverman-Smith syndrome
Russell-Silver syndrome
Seckel syndrome

Q87.2 **Congenital malformation syndromes predominantly involving limbs** `cc`
> Holt-Oram syndrome
> Klippel-Trenaunay-Weber syndrome
> Nail patella syndrome
> Rubinstein-Taybi syndrome
> Sirenomelia syndrome
> Thrombocytopenia with absent radius [TAR] syndrome
> VATER syndrome

Q87.3 **Congenital malformation syndromes involving early overgrowth** `cc`
> Beckwith-Wiedemann syndrome
> Sotos syndrome
> Weaver syndrome

√6ᵗʰ **Q87.4** **Marfan's syndrome**
> **DEF:** Disorder that affects the connective tissue of multiple systems, including disproportionally long or abnormal bone structure and eye and cardiovascular complications.

     Q87.40 **Marfan's syndrome, unspecified** `cc`

     √6ᵗʰ **Q87.41** **Marfan's syndrome with cardiovascular manifestations**

       Q87.410 **Marfan's syndrome with aortic dilation** `cc`

       Q87.418 **Marfan's syndrome with other cardiovascular manifestations** `cc`

     Q87.42 **Marfan's syndrome with ocular manifestations** `cc`

     Q87.43 **Marfan's syndrome with skeletal manifestation** `cc`

Q87.5 **Other congenital malformation syndromes with other skeletal changes** `cc`

√5ᵗʰ **Q87.8** **Other specified congenital malformation syndromes, not elsewhere classified**
> EXCLUDES 1   Zellweger syndrome (E71.510)

     Q87.81 **Alport syndrome** `cc`
> Use additional code to identify stage of chronic kidney disease (N18.1-N18.6)

     Q87.82 **Arterial tortuosity syndrome** `cc`
> **AHA:** 2016,4Q,60-61

     Q87.89 **Other specified congenital malformation syndromes, not elsewhere classified** `cc`
> Laurence-Moon (-Bardet)-Biedl syndrome

√4ᵗʰ **Q89** **Other congenital malformations, not elsewhere classified**

√5ᵗʰ **Q89.0** **Congenital absence and malformations of spleen**
> EXCLUDES 1   isomerism of atrial appendages (with asplenia or polysplenia) (Q20.6)

     Q89.01 **Asplenia (congenital)** `cc`

     Q89.09 **Congenital malformations of spleen** `cc`
> Congenital splenomegaly

Q89.1 **Congenital malformations of adrenal gland**
> EXCLUDES 1   adrenogenital disorders (E25.-)
>   congenital adrenal hyperplasia (E25.0)

Q89.2 **Congenital malformations of other endocrine glands**
> Congenital malformation of parathyroid or thyroid gland
> Persistent thyroglossal duct
> Thyroglossal cyst
> EXCLUDES 1   congenital goiter (E03.0)
>   congenital hypothyroidism (E03.1)

Q89.3 **Situs inversus** `cc`
> Dextrocardia with situs inversus
> Mirror-image atrial arrangement with situs inversus
> Situs inversus or transversus abdominalis
> Situs inversus or transversus thoracis
> Transposition of abdominal viscera
> Transposition of thoracic viscera
> EXCLUDES 1   dextrocardia NOS (Q24.0)
> **DEF:** Congenital anomaly in which the internal thoracic and abdominal organs are transposed laterally and found on the opposite side from the normal position.

Q89.4 **Conjoined twins** `MCC`
> Craniopagus
> Dicephaly
> Pygopagus
> Thoracopagus

Q89.7 **Multiple congenital malformations, not elsewhere classified** `cc`
> Multiple congenital anomalies NOS
> Multiple congenital deformities NOS
> EXCLUDES 1   congenital malformation syndromes affecting multiple systems (Q87.-)

Q89.8 **Other specified congenital malformations** `cc`
> Use additional code(s) to identify all associated manifestations

Q89.9 **Congenital malformation, unspecified**
> Congenital anomaly NOS
> Congenital deformity NOS

Chromosomal abnormalities, not elsewhere classified (Q90-Q99)

> EXCLUDES 2   mitochondrial metabolic disorders (E88.4-)

√4ᵗʰ **Q90** **Down syndrome**
> Use additional code(s) to identify any associated physical conditions and degree of intellectual disabilities (F70-F79)

     Q90.0 **Trisomy 21, nonmosaicism (meiotic nondisjunction)**

     Q90.1 **Trisomy 21, mosaicism (mitotic nondisjunction)**

     Q90.2 **Trisomy 21, translocation**

     Q90.9 **Down syndrome, unspecified**
> Trisomy 21 NOS

√4ᵗʰ **Q91** **Trisomy 18 and Trisomy 13**

     Q91.0 **Trisomy 18, nonmosaicism (meiotic nondisjunction)** `cc`

     Q91.1 **Trisomy 18, mosaicism (mitotic nondisjunction)** `cc`

     Q91.2 **Trisomy 18, translocation** `cc`

     Q91.3 **Trisomy 18, unspecified** `cc`

     Q91.4 **Trisomy 13, nonmosaicism (meiotic nondisjunction)** `cc`

     Q91.5 **Trisomy 13, mosaicism (mitotic nondisjunction)** `cc`

     Q91.6 **Trisomy 13, translocation** `cc`

     Q91.7 **Trisomy 13, unspecified** `cc`

√4ᵗʰ **Q92** **Other trisomies and partial trisomies of the autosomes, not elsewhere classified**
> INCLUDES   unbalanced translocations and insertions
> EXCLUDES 1   trisomies of chromosomes 13, 18, 21 (Q90-Q91)

     Q92.0 **Whole chromosome trisomy, nonmosaicism (meiotic nondisjunction)**

     Q92.1 **Whole chromosome trisomy, mosaicism (mitotic nondisjunction)**

     Q92.2 **Partial trisomy**
> Less than whole arm duplicated
> Whole arm or more duplicated
> EXCLUDES 1   partial trisomy due to unbalanced translocation (Q92.5)

     Q92.5 **Duplications with other complex rearrangements**
> Partial trisomy due to unbalanced translocations
> Code also any associated deletions due to unbalanced translocations, inversions and insertions (Q93.7)

     √5ᵗʰ **Q92.6** **Marker chromosomes**
> Trisomies due to dicentrics
> Trisomies due to extra rings
> Trisomies due to isochromosomes
> Individual with marker heterochromatin

       Q92.61 **Marker chromosomes in normal individual**

       Q92.62 **Marker chromosomes in abnormal individual**

     Q92.7 **Triploidy and polyploidy**

     Q92.8 **Other specified trisomies and partial trisomies of autosomes**
> Duplications identified by fluorescence in situ hybridization (FISH)
> Duplications identified by in situ hybridization (ISH)
> Duplications seen only at prometaphase

     Q92.9 **Trisomy and partial trisomy of autosomes, unspecified**

√4ᵗʰ **Q93** **Monosomies and deletions from the autosomes, not elsewhere classified**

     Q93.0 **Whole chromosome monosomy, nonmosaicism (meiotic nondisjunction)**

     Q93.1 **Whole chromosome monosomy, mosaicism (mitotic nondisjunction)**

     Q93.2 **Chromosome replaced with ring, dicentric or isochromosome**

     Q93.3 **Deletion of short arm of chromosome 4** `cc`
> Wolff-Hirschorn syndrome

     Q93.4 **Deletion of short arm of chromosome 5** `cc`
> Cri-du-chat syndrome

✔ Additional Character Required   ✔x7ᵗʰ Placeholder   Unacceptable PDx   Questionable PDx   Manifestation   Unspecified Dx   H1-H14 HAC   HCC CMS-HCC Dx   HIV HIV Dx

ICD-10-CM 2021   **933**

✓5ᵗʰ **Q93.5 Other deletions of** part of a chromosome
     AHA: 2018,4Q,28

  Q93.51 Angelman syndrome   CC

  Q93.59 Other deletions of part of a chromosome   CC

Q93.7 Deletions with other complex rearrangements   CC
     Deletions due to unbalanced translocations, inversions and insertions
     Code also any associated duplications due to unbalanced translocations, inversions and insertions (Q92.5)

✓5ᵗʰ **Q93.8 Other deletions from the autosomes**

  Q93.81 Velo-cardio-facial syndrome   MCC
     Deletion 22q11.2
     AHA: 2019,3Q,14
     DEF: Microdeletion syndrome affecting multiple organs characterized by a cleft palate, heart defects, an elongated face with almond-shaped eyes, wide nose, small ears, weak immune system, weak musculature, hypothyroidism, short stature, and scoliosis. The deletion occurs at q11.2 on the long arm of the chromosome 22.

  Q93.82 Williams syndrome   CC
     AHA: 2018,4Q,28-29

  Q93.88 Other microdeletions   CC
     Miller-Dieker syndrome
     Smith-Magenis syndrome

  Q93.89 Other deletions from the autosomes   CC
     Deletions identified by fluorescence in situ hybridization (FISH)
     Deletions identified by in situ hybridization (ISH)
     Deletions seen only at prometaphase

Q93.9 Deletion from autosomes, unspecified   CC

✓4ᵗʰ **Q95 Balanced rearrangements and structural markers, not elsewhere classified**
     INCLUDES   Robertsonian and balanced reciprocal translocations and insertions

Q95.0 Balanced translocation and insertion in normal individual

Q95.1 Chromosome inversion in normal individual

Q95.2 Balanced autosomal rearrangement in abnormal individual

Q95.3 Balanced sex/autosomal rearrangement in abnormal individual

Q95.5 Individual with autosomal fragile site

Q95.8 Other balanced rearrangements and structural markers

Q95.9 Balanced rearrangement and structural marker, unspecified

✓4ᵗʰ **Q96 Turner's syndrome**
     EXCLUDES 1   Noonan syndrome (Q87.19)

Q96.0 Karyotype 45, X   ♀

Q96.1 Karyotype 46, X iso (Xq)   ♀
     Karyotype 46, isochromosome Xq

Q96.2 Karyotype 46, X with abnormal sex chromosome, except iso (Xq)   ♀
     Karyotype 46, X with abnormal sex chromosome, except isochromosome Xq

Q96.3 Mosaicism, 45, X/46, XX or XY   ♀

Q96.4 Mosaicism, 45, X/other cell line(s) with abnormal sex chromosome   ♀

Q96.8 Other variants of Turner's syndrome   ♀

Q96.9 Turner's syndrome, unspecified   ♀

✓4ᵗʰ **Q97 Other sex chromosome abnormalities, female phenotype, not elsewhere classified**
     EXCLUDES 1   Turner's syndrome (Q96.-)

Q97.0 Karyotype 47, XXX   ♀

Q97.1 Female with more than three X chromosomes   ♀

Q97.2 Mosaicism, lines with various numbers of X chromosomes   ♀

Q97.3 Female with 46, XY karyotype   ♀

Q97.8 Other specified sex chromosome abnormalities, female phenotype   ♀

Q97.9 Sex chromosome abnormality, female phenotype, unspecified   ♀

✓4ᵗʰ **Q98 Other sex chromosome abnormalities, male phenotype, not elsewhere classified**

Q98.0 Klinefelter syndrome karyotype 47, XXY   ♂

Q98.1 Klinefelter syndrome, male with more than two X chromosomes   ♂

Q98.3 Other male with 46, XX karyotype   ♂

Q98.4 Klinefelter syndrome, unspecified   ♂

Q98.5 Karyotype 47, XYY

Q98.6 Male with structurally abnormal sex chromosome   ♂

Q98.7 Male with sex chromosome mosaicism   ♂

Q98.8 Other specified sex chromosome abnormalities, male phenotype   ♂

Q98.9 Sex chromosome abnormality, male phenotype, unspecified   ♂

✓4ᵗʰ **Q99 Other chromosome abnormalities, not elsewhere classified**

Q99.0 Chimera 46, XX/46, XY
     Chimera 46, XX/46, XY true hermaphrodite

Q99.1 46, XX true hermaphrodite
     46, XX with streak gonads
     46, XY with streak gonads
     Pure gonadal dysgenesis

Q99.2 Fragile X chromosome
     Fragile X syndrome

Q99.8 Other specified chromosome abnormalities

Q99.9 Chromosomal abnormality, unspecified

N Newborn: 0   P Pediatric: 0-17   M Maternity: 9-64   A Adult: 15-124   MCC Major Complication/Comorbidity   CC Complication/Comorbidity   SW Severe Wound Dx

934   ICD-10-CM 2021

Chapter 18. Symptoms, Signs and Abnormal Clinical and Laboratory Findings (R00–R99)

Chapter-specific Guidelines with Coding Examples

The chapter-specific guidelines from the ICD-10-CM Official Guidelines for Coding and Reporting have been provided below. Along with these guidelines are coding examples, contained in the shaded boxes, that have been developed to help illustrate the coding and/or sequencing guidance found in these guidelines.

Chapter 18 includes symptoms, signs, abnormal results of clinical or other investigative procedures, and ill-defined conditions regarding which no diagnosis classifiable elsewhere is recorded. Signs and symptoms that point to a specific diagnosis have been assigned to a category in other chapters of the classification.

a. Use of symptom codes

Codes that describe symptoms and signs are acceptable for reporting purposes when a related definitive diagnosis has not been established (confirmed) by the provider.

> Chest pain of unknown origin
>
> **R07.9**   **Chest pain, unspecified**
>
> *Explanation:* Codes that describe symptoms such as chest pain are acceptable for reporting purposes when the provider has not established (confirmed) a related definitive diagnosis.

b. Use of a symptom code with a definitive diagnosis code

Codes for signs and symptoms may be reported in addition to a related definitive diagnosis when the sign or symptom is not routinely associated with that diagnosis, such as the various signs and symptoms associated with complex syndromes. The definitive diagnosis code should be sequenced before the symptom code.

Signs or symptoms that are associated routinely with a disease process should not be assigned as additional codes, unless otherwise instructed by the classification.

> Pneumonia with hemoptysis
>
> **J18.9**   **Pneumonia, unspecified organism**
>
> **R04.2**   **Hemoptysis**
>
> *Explanation:* Codes for signs and symptoms may be reported in addition to a related definitive diagnosis when the sign or symptom is not routinely associated with that diagnosis.

> Abdominal pain due to acute appendicitis
>
> **K35.80**   **Unspecified acute appendicitis**
>
> *Explanation:* Codes for signs or symptoms routinely associated with a disease process should not be assigned unless the classification instructs otherwise.

c. Combination codes that include symptoms

ICD-10-CM contains a number of combination codes that identify both the definitive diagnosis and common symptoms of that diagnosis. When using one of these combination codes, an additional code should not be assigned for the symptom.

> Acute gastritis with hemorrhage
>
> **K29.01**   **Acute gastritis with bleeding**
>
> *Explanation:* When a combination code identifies both the definitive diagnosis and the symptom, an additional code should not be assigned for the symptom.

d. Repeated falls

Code R29.6, Repeated falls, is for use for encounters when a patient has recently fallen and the reason for the fall is being investigated.

Code Z91.81, History of falling, is for use when a patient has fallen in the past and is at risk for future falls. When appropriate, both codes R29.6 and Z91.81 may be assigned together.

e. Coma scale

The coma scale codes (R40.2-) can be used in conjunction with traumatic brain injury codes. These codes are primarily for use by trauma registries, but they may be used in any setting where this information is collected. The coma scale codes should be sequenced after the diagnosis code(s).

These codes, one from each subcategory, are needed to complete the scale. The 7th character indicates when the scale was recorded. The 7th character should match for all three codes.

At a minimum, report the initial score documented on presentation at your facility. This may be a score from the emergency medicine technician (EMT) or in the emergency department. If desired, a facility may choose to capture multiple coma scale scores.

Assign code R40.24, Glasgow coma scale, total score, when only the total score is documented in the medical record and not the individual score(s).

Do not report codes for individual or total Glasgow coma scale scores for a patient with a medically induced coma or a sedated patient.

See Section I.B.14 for coma scale documentation by clinicians other than patient's provider

> 23-year-old man found down after unknown injury with skull fracture and with concussion and loss of consciousness of unknown duration. EMS evaluated the patient in the field and reported the individual Glasgow coma scores:
>
> Eye opening response—3: eyes open to speech
>
> Verbal response—4: confused but coherent speech
>
> Motor response—6: obeys commands fully
>
> **S02.0XXA**   **Fracture of vault of skull, initial encounter for closed fracture**
>
> **S06.0X9A**   **Concussion with loss of consciousness of unspecified duration, initial encounter**
>
> **R40.2131**   **Coma scale, eyes open, to sound, in the field [EMT or ambulance]**
>
> **R40.2241**   **Coma scale, best verbal response, confused conversation, in the field [EMT or ambulance]**
>
> **R40.2361**   **Coma scale, best motor response, obeys commands, in the field [EMT or ambulance]**
>
> *Explanation:* When individual scores for the Glasgow coma scale are documented, one code from each category is needed to complete the scale. The seventh character indicates when the scale was recorded and should match for all three codes. Assign a code from subcategory R40.24- Glasgow coma scale, total score, when only the total and not the individual score(s) is documented.

> Patient with intractable epilepsy with status epilepticus arrives to ED with alteration of consciousness. Coma scale performed en route by EMT documented total coma score as 11. Another coma score was performed upon hospital admission that was documented as 14.
>
> **G40.911**   **Epilepsy, unspecified, intractable, with status epilepticus**
>
> **R40.2421**   **Glasgow coma scale score 9-12, in the field [EMT or ambulance]**
>
> **R40.2413**   **Glasgow coma scale score 13-15, at hospital admission**
>
> *Explanation:* Coma scores may be used to assess mental status in non-trauma conditions. Use only code R40.24- Glasgow coma scale, total scores when individual scores are unavailable. Multiple scores may be reported with the seventh character representing where or when the assessment was made.

f. Functional quadriplegia

GUIDELINE HAS BEEN DELETED EFFECTIVE OCTOBER 1, 2017

g. SIRS due to non-infectious process

The systemic inflammatory response syndrome (SIRS) can develop as a result of certain non-infectious disease processes, such as trauma, malignant neoplasm, or pancreatitis. When SIRS is documented with a noninfectious condition, and no subsequent infection is documented, the code for the underlying condition, such as an injury, should be assigned, followed by code R65.10, Systemic inflammatory response syndrome (SIRS) of non-infectious origin without acute organ dysfunction, or code R65.11, Systemic inflammatory response syndrome (SIRS) of non-infectious origin with acute organ dysfunction. If an associated acute organ dysfunction is documented, the appropriate code(s) for the specific type of organ dysfunction(s) should be assigned in addition to code R65.11. If acute organ dysfunction is documented, but it cannot be determined if the acute organ dysfunction is associated with SIRS or due to another condition (e.g., directly due to the trauma), the provider should be queried.

Systemic inflammatory response syndrome (SIRS) due to acute gallstone pancreatitis

K85.10   Biliary acute pancreatitis without necrosis or infection

R65.10   Systemic inflammatory response syndrome [SIRS] of non-infectious origin without acute organ dysfunction

Explanation: When SIRS is documented with a non-infectious condition without subsequent infection documented, the code for the underlying condition such as pancreatitis should be assigned followed by the appropriate code for SIRS of noninfectious origin, either with or without associated organ dysfunction.

h. Death NOS

Code R99, Ill-defined and unknown cause of mortality, is only for use in the very limited circumstance when a patient who has already died is brought into an emergency department or other healthcare facility and is pronounced dead upon arrival. It does not represent the discharge disposition of death.

i. NIHSS stroke scale

The NIH stroke scale (NIHSS) codes (R29.7- -) can be used in conjunction with acute stroke codes (I63) to identify the patient's neurological status and the severity of the stroke. The stroke scale codes should be sequenced after the acute stroke diagnosis code(s).

At a minimum, report the initial score documented. If desired, a facility may choose to capture multiple stroke scale scores.

See Section I.B.14 for NIHSS stroke scale documentation by clinicians other than patient's provider

Patient admitted with CVA seen by neurology consult who documents moderate to severe stroke, 17 on NIHSS stroke scale.

I63.9   Cerebral infarction, unspecified

R29.717   NIHSS score 17

Explanation: Unspecified cerebral vascular accident (CVA) is sequenced before the NIHSS stroke scale score code. The stroke scale is an assessment tool to help measure stroke-related neurological deficits. Fifteen items are evaluated by trained observers and include such conditions as levels of consciousness, language, dysarthria, ataxia, and sensory loss. A facility may report multiple stroke scale scores if it wants to.

Chapter 18. Symptoms, Signs and Abnormal Clinical and Laboratory Findings, Not Elsewhere Classified (R00-R99)

NOTE This chapter includes symptoms, signs, abnormal results of clinical or other investigative procedures, and ill-defined conditions regarding which no diagnosis classifiable elsewhere is recorded.

Signs and symptoms that point rather definitely to a given diagnosis have been assigned to a category in other chapters of the classification. In general, categories in this chapter include the less well-defined conditions and symptoms that, without the necessary study of the case to establish a final diagnosis, point perhaps equally to two or more diseases or to two or more systems of the body. Practically all categories in the chapter could be designated 'not otherwise specified', 'unknown etiology' or 'transient'. The Alphabetical Index should be consulted to determine which symptoms and signs are to be allocated here and which to other chapters. The residual subcategories, numbered .8, are generally provided for other relevant symptoms that cannot be allocated elsewhere in the classification.

The conditions and signs or symptoms included in categories R00-R94 consist of:

(a) cases for which no more specific diagnosis can be made even after all the facts bearing on the case have been investigated;

(b) signs or symptoms existing at the time of initial encounter that proved to be transient and whose causes could not be determined;

(c) provisional diagnosis in a patient who failed to return for further investigation or care;

(d) cases referred elsewhere for investigation or treatment before the diagnosis was made;

(e) cases in which a more precise diagnosis was not available for any other reason;

(f) certain symptoms, for which supplementary information is provided, that represent important problems in medical care in their own right.

EXCLUDES 2   *abnormal findings on antenatal screening of mother (O28.-)*
certain conditions originating in the perinatal period (P04-P96)
signs and symptoms classified in the body system chapters
signs and symptoms of breast (N63, N64.5)

AHA: 2017,1Q,6,7

This chapter contains the following blocks:

R00-R09   Symptoms and signs involving the circulatory and respiratory systems
R10-R19   Symptoms and signs involving the digestive system and abdomen
R20-R23   Symptoms and signs involving the skin and subcutaneous tissue
R25-R29   Symptoms and signs involving the nervous and musculoskeletal systems
R30-R39   Symptoms and signs involving the genitourinary system
R40-R46   Symptoms and signs involving cognition, perception, emotional state and behavior
R47-R49   Symptoms and signs involving speech and voice
R50-R69   General symptoms and signs
R70-R79   Abnormal findings on examination of blood, without diagnosis
R80-R82   Abnormal findings on examination of urine, without diagnosis
R83-R89   Abnormal findings on examination of other body fluids, substances and tissues, without diagnosis
R90-R94   Abnormal findings on diagnostic imaging and in function studies, without diagnosis
R97   Abnormal tumor markers
R99   Ill-defined and unknown cause of mortality

Symptoms and signs involving the circulatory and respiratory systems (R00-R09)

✓4ᵗʰ R00 Abnormalities of heart beat

     EXCLUDES 1   *abnormalities originating in the perinatal period (P29.1-)*
     EXCLUDES 2   *specified arrhythmias (I47-I49)*

     R00.0 Tachycardia, unspecified
         Rapid heart beat
         Sinoauricular tachycardia NOS
         Sinus [sinusal] tachycardia NOS
         EXCLUDES 1   *neonatal tachycardia (P29.11)*
                 paroxysmal tachycardia (I47.-)
         DEF: Excessively rapid heart rate of more than 100 beats per minute.

     R00.1 Bradycardia, unspecified
         Sinoatrial bradycardia
         Sinus bradycardia
         Slow heart beat
         Vagal bradycardia
         Use additional code for adverse effect, if applicable, to identify drug (T36-T50 with fifth or sixth character 5)
         EXCLUDES 1   *neonatal bradycardia (P29.12)*
         AHA: 2020,2Q,23
         DEF: Slowed heartbeat, usually defined as a rate fewer than 60 beats per minute. Heart rhythm may be slow as a result of a congenital defect or an acquired problem.

     R00.2 Palpitations
         Awareness of heart beat

     R00.8 Other abnormalities of heart beat

     R00.9 Unspecified abnormalities of heart beat

✓4ᵗʰ R01 Cardiac murmurs and other cardiac sounds

     EXCLUDES 1   *cardiac murmurs and sounds originating in the perinatal period (P29.8)*

     R01.0 Benign and innocent cardiac murmurs
         Functional cardiac murmur

     R01.1 Cardiac murmur, unspecified
         Cardiac bruit NOS
         Heart murmur NOS
         Systolic murmur NOS

     R01.2 Other cardiac sounds
         Cardiac dullness, increased or decreased
         Precordial friction

✓4ᵗʰ R03 Abnormal blood-pressure reading, without diagnosis

     R03.0 Elevated blood-pressure reading, without diagnosis of hypertension
         NOTE   This category is to be used to record an episode of elevated blood pressure in a patient in whom no formal diagnosis of hypertension has been made, or as an isolated incidental finding.

     R03.1 Nonspecific low blood-pressure reading
         EXCLUDES 1   *hypotension (I95.-)*
                 maternal hypotension syndrome (O26.5-)
                 neurogenic orthostatic hypotension (G90.3)

✓4ᵗʰ R04 Hemorrhage from respiratory passages

     R04.0 Epistaxis
         Hemorrhage from nose
         Nosebleed

     R04.1 Hemorrhage from throat
         EXCLUDES 2   *hemoptysis (R04.2)*

     R04.2 Hemoptysis   CC
         Blood-stained sputum
         Cough with hemorrhage
         AHA: 2013,4Q,118

     ✓5ᵗʰ R04.8 Hemorrhage from other sites in respiratory passages

         R04.81 Acute idiopathic pulmonary hemorrhage in infants   CC P
             AIPHI
             Acute idiopathic hemorrhage in infants over 28 days old
             EXCLUDES 1   *perinatal pulmonary hemorrhage (P26.-)*
                         von Willebrand's disease (D68.0)

         R04.89 Hemorrhage from other sites in respiratory passages   CC
             Pulmonary hemorrhage NOS

     R04.9 Hemorrhage from respiratory passages, unspecified   CC

R05 Cough
     EXCLUDES 1   *cough with hemorrhage (R04.2)*
                 smoker's cough (J41.0)
     AHA: 2016,2Q,33

☑ Additional Character Required   ✓x7ᵗʰ Placeholder   Unacceptable PDx   Questionable PDx   Manifestation   Unspecified Dx   H1-H14 HAC   HCC CMS-HCC Dx   HIV HIV Dx

ICD-10-CM 2021   937

✓4ᵗʰ **R06 Abnormalities of breathing**
> *EXCLUDES 1*   *acute respiratory distress syndrome (J80)*
> *respiratory arrest (R09.2)*
> *respiratory arrest of newborn (P28.81)*
> *respiratory distress syndrome of newborn (P22.-)*
> *respiratory failure (J96.-)*
> *respiratory failure of newborn (P28.5)*

✓5ᵗʰ **R06.0 Dyspnea**
> *EXCLUDES 1*   *tachypnea NOS (R06.82)*
> *transient tachypnea of newborn (P22.1)*

R06.00 Dyspnea, unspecified
   AHA: 2017,1Q,26
R06.01 Orthopnea
R06.02 Shortness of breath
R06.03 Acute respiratory distress
   AHA: 2017,4Q,23
R06.09 Other forms of dyspnea

R06.1 Stridor
> *EXCLUDES 1*   *congenital laryngeal stridor (P28.89)*
> *laryngismus (stridulus) (J38.5)*

DEF: Certain type of wheezing described as a loud, constant, musical sound produced when breathing with an obstructed airway, like the inspiratory sound heard when laryngeal or esophageal obstruction is present.

R06.2 Wheezing
> *EXCLUDES 1*   *asthma (J45.-)*

AHA: 2016,2Q,33
DEF: High-pitched whistling sound during breathing due to stenosis of the respiratory passageway. Wheezing is associated with asthma, sleep apnea, bronchiectasis, bronchiolitis, COPD, and pleural effusion.

R06.3 Periodic breathing   CC
   Cheyne-Stokes breathing
R06.4 Hyperventilation
> *EXCLUDES 1*   *psychogenic hyperventilation (F45.8)*

R06.5 Mouth breathing
> *EXCLUDES 2*   *dry mouth NOS (R68.2)*

R06.6 Hiccough
> *EXCLUDES 1*   *psychogenic hiccough (F45.8)*

R06.7 Sneezing
✓5ᵗʰ **R06.8 Other abnormalities of breathing**

R06.81 Apnea, not elsewhere classified
   Apnea NOS
> *EXCLUDES 1*   *apnea (of) newborn (P28.4)*
> *sleep apnea (G47.3-)*
> *sleep apnea of newborn (primary) (P28.3)*

R06.82 Tachypnea, not elsewhere classified
   Tachypnea NOS
> *EXCLUDES 1*   *transitory tachypnea of newborn (P22.1)*

R06.83 Snoring
R06.89 Other abnormalities of breathing
   Breath-holding (spells)
   Sighing

R06.9 Unspecified abnormalities of breathing

✓4ᵗʰ **R07 Pain in throat and chest**
> *EXCLUDES 1*   *epidemic myalgia (B33.0)*
> *EXCLUDES 2*   *jaw pain R68.84*
> *pain in breast (N64.4)*

R07.0 Pain in throat
> *EXCLUDES 1*   *chronic sore throat (J31.2)*
> *sore throat (acute) NOS (J02.9)*
> *EXCLUDES 2*   *dysphagia (R13.1-)*
> *pain in neck (M54.2)*

R07.1 Chest pain on breathing
   Painful respiration
R07.2 Precordial pain
   DEF: Pain felt in the anterior (front) chest wall over the region of the heart. This type of pain is generally felt slightly to the left of the sternum, but may also extend into the surrounding chest wall region.

✓5ᵗʰ **R07.8 Other chest pain**

R07.81 Pleurodynia
   Pleurodynia NOS
> *EXCLUDES 1*   *epidemic pleurodynia (B33.0)*

R07.82 Intercostal pain

R07.89 Other chest pain
   Anterior chest-wall pain NOS
R07.9 Chest pain, unspecified

✓4ᵗʰ **R09 Other symptoms and signs involving the circulatory and respiratory system**
> *EXCLUDES 1*   *acute respiratory distress syndrome (J80)*
> *respiratory arrest of newborn (P28.81)*
> *respiratory distress syndrome of newborn (P22.0)*
> *respiratory failure (J96.-)*
> *respiratory failure of newborn (P28.5)*

✓5ᵗʰ **R09.0 Asphyxia and hypoxemia**
> *EXCLUDES 1*   *asphyxia due to carbon monoxide (T58.-)*
> *asphyxia due to foreign body in respiratory tract (T17.-)*
> *birth (intrauterine) asphyxia (P84)*
> *hyperventilation (R06.4)*
> *traumatic asphyxia (T71.-)*
> *EXCLUDES 2*   *hypercapnia (R06.89)*

R09.01 Asphyxia   CC
   DEF: Interference of oxygen intake due to obstruction or injury of airways resulting in a lack of oxygen perfusion to the tissues or excessive carbon dioxide in the blood. Can cause unconsciousness or death.

R09.02 Hypoxemia
   AHA: 2019,3Q,15
   DEF: Insufficient oxygen in the arterial blood resulting in inadequate delivery of oxygen to the body tissues.

R09.1 Pleurisy
> *EXCLUDES 1*   *pleurisy with effusion (J90)*

¹ **R09.2 Respiratory arrest**   MCC HCC
   Cardiorespiratory failure
> *EXCLUDES 1*   *cardiac arrest (I46.-)*
> *respiratory arrest of newborn (P28.81)*
> *respiratory distress of newborn (P22.0)*
> *respiratory failure (J96.-)*
> *respiratory failure of newborn (P28.5)*
> *respiratory insufficiency (R06.89)*
> *respiratory insufficiency of newborn (P28.5)*

R09.3 Abnormal sputum
   Abnormal amount of sputum
   Abnormal color of sputum
   Abnormal odor of sputum
   Excessive sputum
> *EXCLUDES 1*   *blood-stained sputum (R04.2)*

✓5ᵗʰ **R09.8 Other specified symptoms and signs involving the circulatory and respiratory systems**
R09.81 Nasal congestion
R09.82 Postnasal drip
R09.89 Other specified symptoms and signs involving the circulatory and respiratory systems
   Abnormal chest percussion
   Bruit (arterial)
   Chest tympany
   Choking sensation
   Feeling of foreign body in throat
   Friction sounds in chest
   Rales
   Weak pulse
> *EXCLUDES 2*   *foreign body in throat (T17.2-)*
> *wheezing (R06.2)*

Symptoms and signs involving the digestive system and abdomen (R10-R19)

EXCLUDES 2   congenital or infantile pylorospasm (Q40.0)
gastrointestinal hemorrhage (K92.0-K92.2)
intestinal obstruction (K56.-)
newborn gastrointestinal hemorrhage (P54.0-P54.3)
newborn intestinal obstruction (P76.-)
pylorospasm (K31.3)
signs and symptoms involving the urinary system (R30-R39)
symptoms referable to female genital organs (N94.-)
symptoms referable to male genital organs (N48-N50)

✓4th **R10   Abdominal and pelvic pain**

    EXCLUDES 1   renal colic (N23)
    EXCLUDES 2   dorsalgia (M54.-)
       flatulence and related conditions (R14.-)

   R10.0   Acute abdomen
      Severe abdominal pain (generalized) (with abdominal rigidity)
      EXCLUDES 1   abdominal rigidity NOS (R19.3)
        generalized abdominal pain NOS (R10.84)
        localized abdominal pain (R10.1-R10.3-)

✓5th **R10.1   Pain localized to upper abdomen**
     R10.10   Upper abdominal pain, unspecified
     R10.11   Right upper quadrant pain
     R10.12   Left upper quadrant pain
     R10.13   Epigastric pain
       Dyspepsia
       EXCLUDES 1   functional dyspepsia (K30)

Abdominal Pain

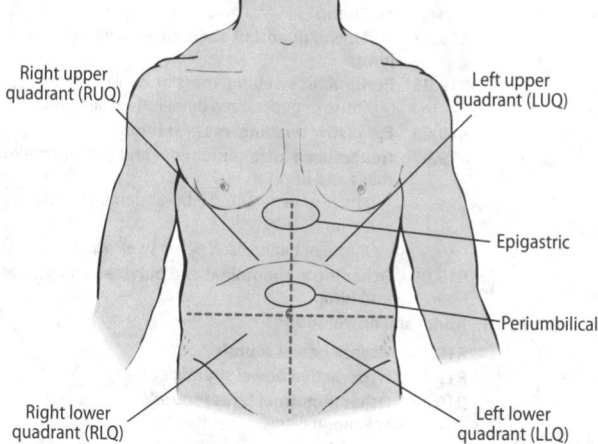

Right upper quadrant (RUQ)
Left upper quadrant (LUQ)
Epigastric
Periumbilical
Right lower quadrant (RLQ)
Left lower quadrant (LLQ)

   R10.2   Pelvic and perineal pain
      EXCLUDES 1   vulvodynia (N94.81)

✓5th **R10.3   Pain localized to other parts of lower abdomen**
     R10.30   Lower abdominal pain, unspecified
     R10.31   Right lower quadrant pain
     R10.32   Left lower quadrant pain
     R10.33   Periumbilical pain

✓5th **R10.8   Other abdominal pain**
   ✓6th **R10.81   Abdominal tenderness**
       Abdominal tenderness NOS
     R10.811   Right upper quadrant abdominal tenderness
     R10.812   Left upper quadrant abdominal tenderness
     R10.813   Right lower quadrant abdominal tenderness
     R10.814   Left lower quadrant abdominal tenderness
     R10.815   Periumbilic abdominal tenderness
     R10.816   Epigastric abdominal tenderness
     R10.817   Generalized abdominal tenderness
     R10.819   Abdominal tenderness, unspecified site
   ✓6th **R10.82   Rebound abdominal tenderness**
     R10.821   Right upper quadrant rebound abdominal tenderness

     R10.822   Left upper quadrant rebound abdominal tenderness
     R10.823   Right lower quadrant rebound abdominal tenderness
     R10.824   Left lower quadrant rebound abdominal tenderness
     R10.825   Periumbilic rebound abdominal tenderness
     R10.826   Epigastric rebound abdominal tenderness
     R10.827   Generalized rebound abdominal tenderness
     R10.829   Rebound abdominal tenderness, unspecified site

   R10.83   Colic   P
      Colic NOS
      Infantile colic
      EXCLUDES 1   colic in adult and child over 12 months old (R10.84)
      DEF: Inconsolable crying in an otherwise well-fed and healthy infant for more than three hours a day, three days a week, for more than three weeks.

   R10.84   Generalized abdominal pain
      EXCLUDES 1   generalized abdominal pain associated with acute abdomen (R10.0)

   R10.9   Unspecified abdominal pain

✓4th **R11   Nausea and vomiting**
    EXCLUDES 1   cyclical vomiting associated with migraine (G43.A-)
       excessive vomiting in pregnancy (O21.-)
       hematemesis (K92.0)
       neonatal hematemesis (P54.0)
       newborn vomiting (P92.0-)
       psychogenic vomiting (F50.89)
       vomiting associated with bulimia nervosa (F50.2)
       vomiting following gastrointestinal surgery (K91.0)

   AHA: 2017,1Q,28
   TIP: Assign a code from this category along with K31.89 Other diseases of stomach and duodenum, to describe cyclical vomiting not due to migraine.

   R11.0   Nausea
      Nausea NOS
      Nausea without vomiting

✓5th **R11.1   Vomiting**
     R11.10   Vomiting, unspecified
       Vomiting NOS
     R11.11   Vomiting without nausea
     R11.12   Projectile vomiting
     R11.13   Vomiting of fecal matter
     R11.14   Bilious vomiting
       Bilious emesis
     R11.15   Cyclical vomiting syndrome unrelated to migraine
       Cyclic vomiting syndrome NOS
       Persistent vomiting
       EXCLUDES 1   cyclical vomiting in migraine (G43.A-)
       EXCLUDES 2   bulimia nervosa (F50.2)
        diabetes mellitus due to underlying condition (E08.-)
      AHA: 2019,4Q,15

   R11.2   Nausea with vomiting, unspecified
      Persistent nausea with vomiting NOS
      AHA: 2020,1Q,8

R12   Heartburn
    EXCLUDES 1   dyspepsia NOS (R10.13)
       functional dyspepsia (K30)

✓4th **R13   Aphagia and dysphagia**
   R13.0   Aphagia
      Inability to swallow
      EXCLUDES 1   psychogenic aphagia (F50.9)

Chapter 18. Symptoms, Signs and Abnormal Clinical and Laboratory Findings

R13.1–R19.4

✓5ᵗʰ **R13.1 Dysphagia**

Code first, if applicable, dysphagia following cerebrovascular disease (I69. with final characters -91)

EXCLUDES 1 *psychogenic dysphagia (F45.8)*

Swallowing Function

Oral phase

Oropharyngeal phase

Pharyngeal phase

Pharyngoesophageal phase

R13.10 Dysphagia, unspecified
Difficulty in swallowing NOS

R13.11 Dysphagia, oral phase

R13.12 Dysphagia, oropharyngeal phase

R13.13 Dysphagia, pharyngeal phase

R13.14 Dysphagia, pharyngoesophageal phase

R13.19 Other dysphagia
Cervical dysphagia
Neurogenic dysphagia

✓4ᵗʰ **R14 Flatulence and related conditions**

EXCLUDES 1 *psychogenic aerophagy (F45.8)*

R14.0 Abdominal distension (gaseous)
Bloating
Tympanites (abdominal) (intestinal)

R14.1 Gas pain

R14.2 Eructation

R14.3 Flatulence

✓4ᵗʰ **R15 Fecal incontinence**

INCLUDES encopresis NOS

EXCLUDES 1 *fecal incontinence of nonorganic origin (F98.1)*

R15.0 Incomplete defecation

EXCLUDES 1 *constipation (K59.0-)*
fecal impaction (K56.41)

R15.1 Fecal smearing
Fecal soiling

R15.2 Fecal urgency

R15.9 Full incontinence of feces
Fecal incontinence NOS

✓4ᵗʰ **R16 Hepatomegaly and splenomegaly, not elsewhere classified**

R16.0 Hepatomegaly, not elsewhere classified
Hepatomegaly NOS

R16.1 Splenomegaly, not elsewhere classified
Splenomegaly NOS

R16.2 Hepatomegaly with splenomegaly, not elsewhere classified
Hepatosplenomegaly NOS

R17 Unspecified jaundice CC

EXCLUDES 1 *neonatal jaundice (P55, P57-P59)*

✓4ᵗʰ **R18 Ascites**

INCLUDES fluid in peritoneal cavity

EXCLUDES 1 *ascites in alcoholic cirrhosis (K70.31)*
ascites in alcoholic hepatitis (K70.11)
ascites in toxic liver disease with chronic active hepatitis (K71.51)

DEF: Abnormal accumulation of free fluid in the abdominal cavity, causing distention and tightness in addition to shortness of breath as the fluid accumulates. Ascites is usually an underlying disorder and can be a manifestation of any number of diseases.

R18.0 Malignant ascites CC
Code first malignancy, such as:
malignant neoplasm of ovary (C56.-)
secondary malignant neoplasm of retroperitoneum and peritoneum (C78.6)

R18.8 Other ascites CC
Ascites NOS
Peritoneal effusion (chronic)
AHA: 2018,1Q,4

✓4ᵗʰ **R19 Other symptoms and signs involving the digestive system and abdomen**

EXCLUDES 1 *acute abdomen (R10.0)*

✓5ᵗʰ **R19.0 Intra-abdominal and pelvic swelling, mass and lump**

EXCLUDES 1 *abdominal distension (gaseous) (R14.-)*
ascites (R18.-)

R19.00 Intra-abdominal and pelvic swelling, mass and lump, unspecified site

R19.01 Right upper quadrant abdominal swelling, mass and lump

R19.02 Left upper quadrant abdominal swelling, mass and lump

R19.03 Right lower quadrant abdominal swelling, mass and lump

R19.04 Left lower quadrant abdominal swelling, mass and lump

R19.05 Periumbilic swelling, mass or lump
Diffuse or generalized umbilical swelling or mass

R19.06 Epigastric swelling, mass or lump

R19.07 Generalized intra-abdominal and pelvic swelling, mass and lump
Diffuse or generalized intra-abdominal swelling or mass NOS
Diffuse or generalized pelvic swelling or mass NOS

R19.09 Other intra-abdominal and pelvic swelling, mass and lump

✓5ᵗʰ **R19.1 Abnormal bowel sounds**

R19.11 Absent bowel sounds

R19.12 Hyperactive bowel sounds

R19.15 Other abnormal bowel sounds
Abnormal bowel sounds NOS

R19.2 Visible peristalsis
Hyperperistalsis
DEF: Visible movements of muscular attempts to move food through the digestive tract due to pyloric obstruction, stomach obstruction, or intestinal obstruction.

✓5ᵗʰ **R19.3 Abdominal rigidity**

EXCLUDES 1 *abdominal rigidity with severe abdominal pain (R10.0)*

R19.30 Abdominal rigidity, unspecified site

R19.31 Right upper quadrant abdominal rigidity

R19.32 Left upper quadrant abdominal rigidity

R19.33 Right lower quadrant abdominal rigidity

R19.34 Left lower quadrant abdominal rigidity

R19.35 Periumbilic abdominal rigidity

R19.36 Epigastric abdominal rigidity

R19.37 Generalized abdominal rigidity

R19.4 Change in bowel habit

EXCLUDES 1 *constipation (K59.0-)*
functional diarrhea (K59.1)

R19.5 Other fecal abnormalities
Abnormal stool color
Bulky stools
Mucus in stools
Occult blood in feces
Occult blood in stools
EXCLUDES 1   melena (K92.1)
neonatal melena (P54.1)
AHA: 2019,1Q,32

R19.6 Halitosis

R19.7 Diarrhea, unspecified
Diarrhea NOS
EXCLUDES 1   functional diarrhea (K59.1)
neonatal diarrhea (P78.3)
psychogenic diarrhea (F45.8)

R19.8 Other specified symptoms and signs involving the digestive system and abdomen

Symptoms and signs involving the skin and subcutaneous tissue (R20-R23)

EXCLUDES 2   symptoms relating to breast (N64.4-N64.5)

✓4ᵗʰ **R20 Disturbances of skin sensation**
EXCLUDES 1   dissociative anesthesia and sensory loss (F44.6)
psychogenic disturbances (F45.8)

R20.0 Anesthesia of skin

R20.1 Hypoesthesia of skin

R20.2 Paresthesia of skin
Formication
Pins and needles
Tingling skin
EXCLUDES 1   acroparesthesia (I73.8)

R20.3 Hyperesthesia

R20.8 Other disturbances of skin sensation

R20.9 Unspecified disturbances of skin sensation

R21 Rash and other nonspecific skin eruption
INCLUDES   rash NOS
EXCLUDES 1   specified type of rash — code to condition
vesicular eruption (R23.8)

✓4ᵗʰ **R22 Localized swelling, mass and lump of skin and subcutaneous tissue**
INCLUDES   subcutaneous nodules (localized)(superficial)
EXCLUDES 1   abnormal findings on diagnostic imaging (R90-R93)
edema (R60.-)
enlarged lymph nodes (R59.-)
localized adiposity (E65)
swelling of joint (M25.4-)

R22.0 Localized swelling, mass and lump, head

R22.1 Localized swelling, mass and lump, neck

R22.2 Localized swelling, mass and lump, trunk
EXCLUDES 1   intra-abdominal or pelvic mass and lump (R19.0-)
intra-abdominal or pelvic swelling (R19.0-)
EXCLUDES 2   breast mass and lump (N63)

✓5ᵗʰ **R22.3 Localized swelling, mass and lump, upper limb**

R22.30 Localized swelling, mass and lump, unspecified upper limb

R22.31 Localized swelling, mass and lump, right upper limb

R22.32 Localized swelling, mass and lump, left upper limb

R22.33 Localized swelling, mass and lump, upper limb, bilateral

✓5ᵗʰ **R22.4 Localized swelling, mass and lump, lower limb**

R22.40 Localized swelling, mass and lump, unspecified lower limb

R22.41 Localized swelling, mass and lump, right lower limb

R22.42 Localized swelling, mass and lump, left lower limb

R22.43 Localized swelling, mass and lump, lower limb, bilateral

R22.9 Localized swelling, mass and lump, unspecified

✓4ᵗʰ **R23 Other skin changes**

R23.0 Cyanosis
EXCLUDES 1   acrocyanosis (I73.8)
cyanotic attacks of newborn (P28.2)
DEF: Bluish or purplish discoloration of the skin due to an inadequate oxygen blood level.

R23.1 Pallor
Clammy skin

R23.2 Flushing
Excessive blushing
Code first, if applicable, menopausal and female climacteric states (N95.1)

R23.3 Spontaneous ecchymoses
Petechiae
EXCLUDES 1   ecchymoses of newborn (P54.5)
purpura (D69.-)

R23.4 Changes in skin texture
Desquamation of skin
Induration of skin
Scaling of skin
EXCLUDES 1   epidermal thickening NOS (L85.9)

R23.8 Other skin changes

R23.9 Unspecified skin changes

Symptoms and signs involving the nervous and musculoskeletal systems (R25-R29)

✓4ᵗʰ **R25 Abnormal involuntary movements**
EXCLUDES 1   specific movement disorders (G20-G26)
stereotyped movement disorders (F98.4)
tic disorders (F95.-)

R25.0 Abnormal head movements

R25.1 Tremor, unspecified
EXCLUDES 1   chorea NOS (G25.5)
essential tremor (G25.0)
hysterical tremor (F44.4)
intention tremor (G25.2)

R25.2 Cramp and spasm
EXCLUDES 2   carpopedal spasm (R29.0)
charley-horse (M62.831)
infantile spasms (G40.4-)
muscle spasm of back (M62.830)
muscle spasm of calf (M62.831)

R25.3 Fasciculation
Twitching NOS

R25.8 Other abnormal involuntary movements

R25.9 Unspecified abnormal involuntary movements

✓4ᵗʰ **R26 Abnormalities of gait and mobility**
EXCLUDES 1   ataxia NOS (R27.0)
hereditary ataxia (G11.-)
locomotor (syphilitic) ataxia (A52.11)
immobility syndrome (paraplegic) (M62.3)

R26.0 Ataxic gait
Staggering gait

R26.1 Paralytic gait
Spastic gait

R26.2 Difficulty in walking, not elsewhere classified
EXCLUDES 1   falling (R29.6)
unsteadiness on feet (R26.81)
AHA: 2016,2Q,7

✓5ᵗʰ **R26.8 Other abnormalities of gait and mobility**

R26.81 Unsteadiness on feet

R26.89 Other abnormalities of gait and mobility
AHA: 2020,2Q,29

R26.9 Unspecified abnormalities of gait and mobility

✓4ᵗʰ **R27 Other lack of coordination**
EXCLUDES 1   ataxic gait (R26.0)
hereditary ataxia (G11.-)
vertigo NOS (R42)

R27.0 Ataxia, unspecified
EXCLUDES 1   ataxia following cerebrovascular disease (I69. with final characters -93)

R27.8 Other lack of coordination

R27.9 Unspecified lack of coordination

✓4th R29 Other symptoms and signs involving the nervous and musculoskeletal systems

R29.0 Tetany   **CC**

Carpopedal spasm

EXCLUDES 1   *hysterical tetany (F44.5)*
neonatal tetany (P71.3)
parathyroid tetany (E20.9)
post-thyroidectomy tetany (E89.2)

DEF: Calcium or other mineral imbalance causing voluntary muscles such as, hands, feet, or larynx to spasm rhythmically.

R29.1 Meningismus   **CC**

R29.2 Abnormal reflex

EXCLUDES 2   *abnormal pupillary reflex (H57.0)*
hyperactive gag reflex (J39.2)
vasovagal reaction or syncope (R55)

R29.3 Abnormal posture

R29.4 Clicking hip

EXCLUDES 1   *congenital deformities of hip (Q65.-)*

R29.5 Transient paralysis   **CC**

Code first any associated spinal cord injury (S14.0, S14.1-, S24.0, S24.1-, S34.0-, S34.1-)

EXCLUDES 1   *transient ischemic attack (G45.9)*

R29.6 Repeated falls

Falling

Tendency to fall

EXCLUDES 2   *at risk for falling (Z91.81)*
history of falling (Z91.81)

AHA: 2016,2Q,6

TIP: Code in addition to Parkinson's disease (G20), when documented.

✓5th R29.7 National Institutes of Health Stroke Scale (NIHSS) score

Code first the type of cerebral infarction ▶(I63.-)◀

AHA: 2016,4Q,61-62

TIP: Codes from this subcategory may be assigned based on medical record documentation from clinicians who are not the patient's provider.

✓6th R29.70 NIHSS score 0-9

R29.700 NIHSS score 0
R29.701 NIHSS score 1
R29.702 NIHSS score 2
R29.703 NIHSS score 3
R29.704 NIHSS score 4
R29.705 NIHSS score 5
R29.706 NIHSS score 6
R29.707 NIHSS score 7
R29.708 NIHSS score 8
R29.709 NIHSS score 9

✓6th R29.71 NIHSS score 10-19

R29.710 NIHSS score 10
R29.711 NIHSS score 11
R29.712 NIHSS score 12
R29.713 NIHSS score 13
R29.714 NIHSS score 14
R29.715 NIHSS score 15
R29.716 NIHSS score 16
R29.717 NIHSS score 17
R29.718 NIHSS score 18
R29.719 NIHSS score 19

✓6th R29.72 NIHSS score 20-29

R29.720 NIHSS score 20
R29.721 NIHSS score 21
R29.722 NIHSS score 22
R29.723 NIHSS score 23
R29.724 NIHSS score 24
R29.725 NIHSS score 25
R29.726 NIHSS score 26
R29.727 NIHSS score 27
R29.728 NIHSS score 28
R29.729 NIHSS score 29

✓6th R29.73 NIHSS score 30-39

R29.730 NIHSS score 30
R29.731 NIHSS score 31
R29.732 NIHSS score 32
R29.733 NIHSS score 33
R29.734 NIHSS score 34
R29.735 NIHSS score 35
R29.736 NIHSS score 36
R29.737 NIHSS score 37
R29.738 NIHSS score 38
R29.739 NIHSS score 39

✓6th R29.74 NIHSS score 40-42

R29.740 NIHSS score 40
R29.741 NIHSS score 41
R29.742 NIHSS score 42

✓5th R29.8 Other symptoms and signs involving the nervous and musculoskeletal systems

✓6th R29.81 Other symptoms and signs involving the nervous system

R29.810 Facial weakness

Facial droop

EXCLUDES 1   *Bell's palsy (G51.0)*
facial weakness following cerebrovascular disease (I69. with final characters -92)

R29.818 Other symptoms and signs involving the nervous system

✓6th R29.89 Other symptoms and signs involving the musculoskeletal system

EXCLUDES 2   *pain in limb (M79.6-)*

R29.890 Loss of height

EXCLUDES 1   *osteoporosis (M80-M81)*

R29.891 Ocular torticollis

EXCLUDES 1   *congenital (sternomastoid) torticollis Q68.0*
psychogenic torticollis (F45.8)
spasmodic torticollis (G24.3)
torticollis due to birth injury (P15.8)
torticollis NOS M43.6

DEF: Abnormal head posture as a result of a contracted state of cervical muscles to correct a visual disturbance, either double vision or a visual field defect.

R29.898 Other symptoms and signs involving the musculoskeletal system

✓5th R29.9 Unspecified symptoms and signs involving the nervous and musculoskeletal systems

R29.90 Unspecified symptoms and signs involving the nervous system

R29.91 Unspecified symptoms and signs involving the musculoskeletal system

Symptoms and signs involving the genitourinary system (R30-R39)

✓4th R30 Pain associated with micturition

EXCLUDES 1   *psychogenic pain associated with micturition (F45.8)*

R30.0 Dysuria

Strangury

R30.1 Vesical tenesmus

DEF: Feeling of a full bladder even when there is little or no urine in the bladder.

R30.9 Painful micturition, unspecified

Painful urination NOS

✓4th R31 Hematuria

EXCLUDES 1   *hematuria included with underlying conditions, such as:*
acute cystitis with hematuria (N30.01)
recurrent and persistent hematuria in glomerular diseases (N02.-)

AHA: 2017,1Q,17

R31.0 Gross hematuria

R31.1 Benign essential microscopic hematuria

✓5th R31.2 Other microscopic hematuria

AHA: 2016,4Q,62

R31.21 Asymptomatic microscopic hematuria

AMH

R31.29 Other microscopic hematuria

R31.9 Hematuria, unspecified

N Newborn: 0   P Pediatric: 0-17   M Maternity: 9-64   A Adult: 15-124   MCC Major Complication/Comorbidity   CC Complication/Comorbidity   SW Severe Wound Dx

R29–R31.9

942   ICD-10-CM 2021

R32   Unspecified urinary incontinence
     Enuresis NOS
     EXCLUDES 1   *functional urinary incontinence (R39.81)*
           nonorganic enuresis (F98.0)
           stress incontinence and other specified urinary incontinence (N39.3-N39.4-)
           urinary incontinence associated with cognitive impairment (R39.81)

✓4ᵗʰ **R33   Retention of urine**
     EXCLUDES 1   *psychogenic retention of urine (F45.8)*

     R33.0   Drug induced retention of urine
           Use additional code for adverse effect, if applicable, to identify drug (T36-T50 with fifth or sixth character 5)

     R33.8   Other retention of urine
           Code first, if applicable, any causal condition, such as:
           enlarged prostate (N40.1)
           AHA: 2018,4Q,55

     R33.9   Retention of urine, unspecified

R34   Anuria and oliguria
     EXCLUDES 1   *anuria and oliguria complicating abortion or ectopic or molar pregnancy (O00-O07, O08.4)*
           anuria and oliguria complicating pregnancy (O26.83-)
           anuria and oliguria complicating the puerperium (O90.4)

✓4ᵗʰ **R35   Polyuria**
     Code first, if applicable, any causal condition, such as:
           enlarged prostate (N40.1)
     EXCLUDES 1   *psychogenic polyuria (F45.8)*

     R35.0   Frequency of micturition
     R35.1   Nocturia
     R35.8   Other polyuria
           Polyuria NOS

✓4ᵗʰ **R36   Urethral discharge**
     R36.0   Urethral discharge without blood
     R36.1   Hematospermia   ♂
     R36.9   Urethral discharge, unspecified
           Penile discharge NOS
           Urethrorrhea

R37   Sexual dysfunction, unspecified

✓4ᵗʰ **R39   Other and unspecified symptoms and signs involving the genitourinary system**
     R39.0   Extravasation of urine   CC
✓5ᵗʰ   **R39.1   Other difficulties with micturition**
           Code first, if applicable, any causal condition, such as:
           enlarged prostate (N40.1)
         R39.11   Hesitancy of micturition
         R39.12   Poor urinary stream
           Weak urinary steam
         R39.13   Splitting of urinary stream
         R39.14   Feeling of incomplete bladder emptying
         R39.15   Urgency of urination
           EXCLUDES 1   *urge incontinence (N39.41, N39.46)*
         R39.16   Straining to void
✓6ᵗʰ   **R39.19   Other difficulties with micturition**
           AHA: 2016,4Q;63
           R39.191   Need to immediately re-void
           R39.192   Position dependent micturition
           R39.198   Other difficulties with micturition
     R39.2   Extrarenal uremia
           Prerenal uremia
           EXCLUDES 1   *uremia NOS (N19)*
✓5ᵗʰ   **R39.8   Other symptoms and signs involving the genitourinary system**
           AHA: 2017,4Q,22-23
         R39.81   Functional urinary incontinence
           Urinary incontinence due to cognitive impairment, or severe physical disability or immobility
           EXCLUDES 1   *stress incontinence and other specified urinary incontinence (N39.3-N39.4-)*
                   urinary incontinence NOS (R32)
         R39.82   Chronic bladder pain
           AHA: 2016,4Q,64
         R39.83   Unilateral non-palpable testicle   ♂
         R39.84   Bilateral non-palpable testicles   ♂

         R39.89   Other symptoms and signs involving the genitourinary system
     R39.9   Unspecified symptoms and signs involving the genitourinary system

Symptoms and signs involving cognition, perception, emotional state and behavior (R40-R46)

     EXCLUDES 2   *symptoms and signs constituting part of a pattern of mental disorder (F01-F99)*

✓4ᵗʰ **R40   Somnolence, stupor and coma**
     EXCLUDES 1   *neonatal coma (P91.5)*
           somnolence, stupor and coma in diabetes (E08-E13)
           somnolence, stupor and coma in hepatic failure (K72.-)
           somnolence, stupor and coma in hypoglycemia (nondiabetic) (E15)

     R40.0   Somnolence
           Drowsiness
           EXCLUDES 1   *coma (R40.2-)*

     R40.1   Stupor
           Catatonic stupor
           Semicoma
           EXCLUDES 1   *catatonic schizophrenia (F20.2)*
                   coma (R40.2-)
                   depressive stupor (F31-F33)
                   dissociative stupor (F44.2)
                   manic stupor (F30.2)

✓5ᵗʰ   **R40.2   Coma**
           Code first any associated:
           fracture of skull (S02.-)
           intracranial injury (S06.-)

           NOTE   One code from each subcategory, R40.21-R40.23, is required to complete the coma scale

           AHA: 2019,2Q,12; 2018,4Q,70; 2017,4Q,23-25,95; 2015,2Q,17; 2014,1Q,19
           TIP: Codes for individual (R40.21-, R40.22, R40.23-) or total (R40.24-) coma scale scores may be assigned based on medical record documentation from clinicians who are not the patient's provider.
           TIP: It is not appropriate to assign individual (R40.21-, R40.22-, R40.23-) or total (R40.24-) coma scale score codes for patients who are sedated or in medically induced comas.

         R40.20   Unspecified coma   MCC HCC
           Coma NOS
           Unconsciousness NOS
✓6ᵗʰ   **R40.21   Coma scale, eyes open**

           The following appropriate 7th character is to be added to subcategory R40.21-, R40.22-, R40.23-, and R40.24-.
           0   unspecified time
           1   in the field [EMT or ambulance]
           2   at arrival to emergency department
           3   at hospital admission
           4   24 hours or more after hospital admission

        ✓7ᵗʰ   **R40.211   Coma scale, eyes open, never**   MCC HCC
           Coma scale eye opening score of 1
        ✓7ᵗʰ   **R40.212   Coma scale, eyes open, to pain**   MCC HCC
           Coma scale eye opening score of 2
        ✓7ᵗʰ   **R40.213   Coma scale, eyes open, to sound**
           Coma scale eye opening score of 3
        ✓7ᵗʰ   **R40.214   Coma scale, eyes open, spontaneous**
           Coma scale eye opening score of 4
✓6ᵗʰ   **R40.22   Coma scale, best verbal response**
        ✓7ᵗʰ   **R40.221   Coma scale, best verbal response, none**   MCC HCC
           Coma scale verbal score of 1
        ✓7ᵗʰ   **R40.222   Coma scale, best verbal response, incomprehensible words**   MCC HCC
           Coma scale verbal score of 2
           Incomprehensible sounds (2-5 years of age)
           Moans/grunts to pain; restless (< 2 years old)

√7ᵗʰ **R40.223** **Coma scale, best verbal response, inappropriate words**
Coma scale verbal score of 3
Inappropriate crying or screaming (< 2 years of age)
Screaming (2-5 years of age)

√7ᵗʰ **R40.224** **Coma scale, best verbal response, confused conversation**
Coma scale verbal score of 4
Inappropriate words (2-5 years of age)
Irritable cries (< 2 years of age)

√7ᵗʰ **R40.225** **Coma scale, best verbal response, oriented**
Coma scale verbal score of 5
Cooing or babbling or crying appropriately (< 2 years of age)
Uses appropriate words (2-5 years of age)

√6ᵗʰ **R40.23** **Coma scale, best motor response**

√7ᵗʰ **R40.231** **Coma scale, best motor response, none** MCC HCC
Coma scale motor score of 1

√7ᵗʰ **R40.232** **Coma scale, best motor response, extension** MCC HCC
Abnormal extensor posturing to pain or noxious stimuli (< 2 years of age)
Coma scale motor score of 2
Extensor posturing to pain or noxious stimuli (2-5 years of age)

√7ᵗʰ **R40.233** **Coma scale, best motor response, abnormal flexion**
Abnormal flexure posturing to pain or noxious stimuli (2-5 years of age)
Coma scale motor score of 3
Flexion/decorticate posturing (< 2 years of age)

√7ᵗʰ **R40.234** **Coma scale, best motor response, flexion withdrawal** MCC HCC
Coma scale motor score of 4
Withdraws from pain or noxious stimuli (2-5 years of age)

√7ᵗʰ **R40.235** **Coma scale, best motor response, localizes pain**
Coma scale motor score of 5
Localizes pain (2-5 years of age)
Withdraws to touch (< 2 years of age)

√7ᵗʰ **R40.236** **Coma scale, best motor response, obeys commands**
Coma scale motor score of 6
Normal or spontaneous movement (< 2 years of age)
Obeys commands (2-5 years of age)

√6ᵗʰ **R40.24** **Glasgow coma scale, total score**
NOTE Assign a code from subcategory R40.24, when only the total coma score is documented
AHA: 2016,4Q,64-65

√7ᵗʰ **R40.241** **Glasgow coma scale score 13-15**

√7ᵗʰ **R40.242** **Glasgow coma scale score 9-12**

√7ᵗʰ **R40.243** **Glasgow coma scale score 3-8** HCC

√7ᵗʰ **R40.244** **Other coma, without documented Glasgow coma scale score, or with partial score reported** HCC

R40.3 **Persistent vegetative state** CC HCC
DEF: Persistent wakefulness without consciousness due to a nonfunctioning cerebral cortex.

R40.4 **Transient alteration of awareness**
AHA: 2020,2Q,24

√4ᵗʰ **R41** **Other symptoms and signs involving cognitive functions and awareness**
EXCLUDES 1 dissociative [conversion] disorders (F44.-)
mild cognitive impairment, so stated (G31.84)

R41.0 **Disorientation, unspecified**
Confusion NOS
Delirium NOS
AHA: 2019,2Q,34

R41.1 **Anterograde amnesia**

R41.2 **Retrograde amnesia**

R41.3 **Other amnesia**
Amnesia NOS
Memory loss NOS
EXCLUDES 1 amnestic disorder due to known physiologic condition (F04)
amnestic syndrome due to psychoactive substance use (F10-F19 with 5th character .6)
mild memory disturbance due to known physiological condition (F06.8)
transient global amnesia (G45.4)

R41.4 **Neurologic neglect syndrome** CC
Asomatognosia
Hemi-akinesia
Hemi-inattention
Hemispatial neglect
Left-sided neglect
Sensory neglect
Visuospatial neglect
EXCLUDES 1 visuospatial deficit (R41.842)

√5ᵗʰ **R41.8** **Other symptoms and signs involving cognitive functions and awareness**

R41.81 **Age-related cognitive decline** A
Senility NOS

R41.82 **Altered mental status, unspecified**
Change in mental status NOS
EXCLUDES 1 altered level of consciousness (R40.-)
altered mental status due to known condition — code to condition
delirium NOS (R41.0)
AHA: 2012,4Q,97

R41.83 **Borderline intellectual functioning**
IQ level 71 to 84
EXCLUDES 1 intellectual disabilities (F70-F79)

√6ᵗʰ **R41.84** **Other specified cognitive deficit**
EXCLUDES 1 cognitive deficits as sequelae of cerebrovascular disease (I69.01-, I69.11-, I69.21-, I69.31-, I69.81-, I69.91-)

R41.840 **Attention and concentration deficit**
EXCLUDES 1 attention-deficit hyperactivity disorders (F90.-)

R41.841 **Cognitive communication deficit**

R41.842 **Visuospatial deficit**

R41.843 **Psychomotor deficit**

R41.844 **Frontal lobe and executive function deficit**

R41.89 **Other symptoms and signs involving cognitive functions and awareness**
Anosognosia

R41.9 **Unspecified symptoms and signs involving cognitive functions and awareness**
Unspecified neurocognitive disorder

R42 **Dizziness and giddiness**
Light-headedness
Vertigo NOS
EXCLUDES 1 vertiginous syndromes (H81.-)
vertigo from infrasound (T75.23)

√4ᵗʰ **R43** **Disturbances of smell and taste**

R43.0 **Anosmia**
DEF: Permanent or transient absence of smell that may be congenital or acquired.

R43.1 **Parosmia**
DEF: Abnormal perception of smell usually triggered by environmental odors.

R43.2 **Parageusia**
DEF: Abnormal perception of taste.

R43.8 **Other disturbances of smell and taste**
Mixed disturbance of smell and taste

R43.9 **Unspecified disturbances of smell and taste**

N Newborn: 0   P Pediatric: 0-17   M Maternity: 9-64   A Adult: 15-124   MCC Major Complication/Comorbidity   CC Complication/Comorbidity   SW Severe Wound Dx

✓4th **R44** **Other symptoms and signs involving general sensations and perceptions**

> EXCLUDES 1   alcoholic hallucinations ▶(F10.151, F10.251, F10.951)◄
> hallucinations in drug psychosis ▶(F11-F19 with fifth to sixth characters 51)◄
> hallucinations in mood disorders with psychotic symptoms (F30.2, F31.5, F32.3, F33.3)
> hallucinations in schizophrenia, schizotypal and delusional disorders (F20-F29)
>
> EXCLUDES 2   disturbances of skin sensation (R20.-)

    R44.0   **Auditory** hallucinations   `cc`

    R44.1   **Visual** hallucinations

    R44.2   **Other hallucinations**   `cc`

    R44.3   **Hallucinations, unspecified**   `cc`

    R44.8   **Other symptoms and signs involving general sensations and perceptions**

    R44.9   **Unspecified symptoms and signs involving general sensations and perceptions**

✓4th **R45** **Symptoms and signs involving emotional state**

    R45.0   **Nervousness**
                Nervous tension

    R45.1   **Restlessness and agitation**

    R45.2   **Unhappiness**

    R45.3   **Demoralization and apathy**
          EXCLUDES 1   anhedonia (R45.84)

    R45.4   **Irritability and anger**

    R45.5   **Hostility**

    R45.6   **Violent behavior**

    R45.7   **State of emotional shock and stress, unspecified**

✓5th **R45.8**   **Other symptoms and signs involving emotional state**

        R45.81   **Low self-esteem**

        R45.82   **Worries**

        R45.83   **Excessive crying of child, adolescent or adult**
              EXCLUDES 1   excessive crying of infant (baby) R68.11

        R45.84   **Anhedonia**

        ✓6th **R45.85**   **Homicidal and suicidal ideations**
              EXCLUDES 1   suicide attempt (T14.91)

            R45.850   **Homicidal ideations**

            R45.851   **Suicidal ideations**   `cc`
                DEF: Thoughts of committing suicide but no actual attempt of suicide has been made.

        R45.86   **Emotional lability**

        R45.87   **Impulsiveness**

        R45.89   **Other symptoms and signs involving emotional state**

✓4th **R46** **Symptoms and signs involving appearance and behavior**

> EXCLUDES 1   appearance and behavior in schizophrenia, schizotypal and delusional disorders (F20-F29)
> mental and behavioral disorders (F01-F99)

    R46.0   **Very low level of personal hygiene**

    R46.1   **Bizarre personal appearance**

    R46.2   **Strange and inexplicable behavior**

    R46.3   **Overactivity**

    R46.4   **Slowness and poor responsiveness**
          EXCLUDES 1   stupor (R40.1)

    R46.5   **Suspiciousness and marked evasiveness**

    R46.6   **Undue concern and preoccupation with stressful events**

    R46.7   **Verbosity and circumstantial detail obscuring reason for contact**

✓5th **R46.8**   **Other symptoms and signs involving appearance and behavior**

        R46.81   **Obsessive-compulsive behavior**
              EXCLUDES 1   obsessive-compulsive disorder ▶(F42.-)◄

        R46.89   **Other symptoms and signs involving appearance and behavior**

Symptoms and signs involving speech and voice (R47-R49)

✓4th **R47** **Speech disturbances, not elsewhere classified**

> EXCLUDES 1   autism (F84.0)
> cluttering (F80.81)
> specific developmental disorders of speech and language (F80.-)
> stuttering (F80.81)

✓5th **R47.0**   **Dysphasia and aphasia**

        R47.01   **Aphasia**   `cc`
              EXCLUDES 1   aphasia following cerebrovascular disease (I69. with final characters -20)
                      progressive isolated aphasia (G31.01)

        R47.02   **Dysphasia**
              EXCLUDES 1   dysphasia following cerebrovascular disease (I69. with final characters -21)

    R47.1   **Dysarthria and anarthria**
          EXCLUDES 1   dysarthria following cerebrovascular disease (I69. with final characters -22)

✓5th **R47.8**   **Other speech disturbances**
          EXCLUDES 1   dysarthria following cerebrovascular disease (I69. with final characters -28)

        R47.81   **Slurred speech**

        R47.82   ***Fluency disorder in conditions classified elsewhere***
              Stuttering in conditions classified elsewhere
              Code first underlying disease or condition, such as:
                Parkinson's disease (G20)
              EXCLUDES 1   adult onset fluency disorder (F98.5)
                      childhood onset fluency disorder (F80.81)
                      fluency disorder (stuttering) following cerebrovascular disease (I69. with final characters -23)

        R47.89   **Other speech disturbances**

    R47.9   **Unspecified speech disturbances**

✓4th **R48** **Dyslexia and other symbolic dysfunctions, not elsewhere classified**

> EXCLUDES 1   specific developmental disorders of scholastic skills (F81.-)

    R48.0   **Dyslexia and alexia**

    R48.1   **Agnosia**
          Astereognosia (astereognosis)
          Autotopagnosia
          EXCLUDES 1   visual object agnosia (R48.3)
          DEF: Inability to recognize common things such as faces, objects, smells, or voices.

    R48.2   **Apraxia**
          EXCLUDES 1   apraxia following cerebrovascular disease (I69. with final characters -90)

    R48.3   **Visual agnosia**
          Prosopagnosia
          Simultanagnosia (asimultagnosia)

    R48.8   **Other symbolic dysfunctions**
          Acalculia
          Agraphia
          AHA: 2017,1Q,27

    R48.9   **Unspecified symbolic dysfunctions**

✓4th **R49** **Voice and resonance disorders**

> EXCLUDES 1   psychogenic voice and resonance disorders (F44.4)

    R49.0   **Dysphonia**
          Hoarseness

    R49.1   **Aphonia**
          Loss of voice

✓5th **R49.2**   **Hypernasality and hyponasality**

        R49.21   **Hypernasality**

        R49.22   **Hyponasality**

    R49.8   **Other voice and resonance disorders**

    R49.9   **Unspecified voice and resonance disorder**
          Change in voice NOS
          Resonance disorder NOS

✓ Additional Character Required   ✓x7th Placeholder   Unacceptable PDx   Questionable PDx   Manifestation   Unspecified Dx   H1-H14 HAC   HCC CMS-HCC Dx   HIV HIV Dx

ICD-10-CM 2021   **945**

General symptoms and signs (R50-R69)

✓4ᵗʰ R50 Fever of other and unknown origin

EXCLUDES 1 chills without fever (R68.83)
febrile convulsions (R56.0-)
fever of unknown origin during labor (O75.2)
fever of unknown origin in newborn (P81.9)
hypothermia due to illness (R68.0)
malignant hyperthermia due to anesthesia (T88.3)
puerperal pyrexia NOS (O86.4)

R50.2 Drug induced fever
Use additional code for adverse effect, if applicable, to identify drug (T36-T50 with fifth or sixth character 5)
EXCLUDES 1 postvaccination (postimmunization) fever (R50.83)

✓5ᵗʰ R50.8 Other specified fever

R50.81 Fever presenting with conditions classified elsewhere
Code first underlying condition when associated fever is present, such as with:
leukemia (C91-C95)
neutropenia (D70.-)
sickle-cell disease (D57.-)
AHA: 2014,4Q,22

R50.82 Postprocedural fever
EXCLUDES 1 postprocedural infection (T81.4-)
posttransfusion fever (R50.84)
postvaccination (postimmunization) fever (R50.83)

R50.83 Postvaccination fever
Postimmunization fever

R50.84 Febrile nonhemolytic transfusion reaction
FNHTR
Posttransfusion fever

R50.9 Fever, unspecified
Fever NOS
Fever of unknown origin [FUO]
Fever with chills
Fever with rigors
Hyperpyrexia NOS
Persistent fever
Pyrexia NOS

▲ ✓4ᵗʰ R51 Headache

Facial pain NOS
EXCLUDES 1 ~~atypical face pain (G50.1)~~
~~migraine and other headache syndromes (G43-G44)~~
~~trigeminal neuralgia (G50.0)~~
EXCLUDES 2 ▶atypical face pain (G50.1)◀
▶migraine and other headache syndromes (G43-G44)◀
▶trigeminal neuralgia (G50.0)◀

● **R51.0 Headache with orthostatic component, not elsewhere classified**
Headache with positional component, not elsewhere classified

● **R51.9 Headache, unspecified**
Facial pain NOS

R52 Pain, unspecified

Acute pain NOS
Generalized pain NOS
Pain NOS
EXCLUDES 1 acute and chronic pain, not elsewhere classified (G89.-)
localized pain, unspecified type — code to pain by site, such as:
abdomen pain (R10.-)
back pain (M54.9)
breast pain (N64.4)
chest pain (R07.1-R07.9)
ear pain (H92.0-)
eye pain (H57.1)
headache ▶(R51.9)◀
joint pain (M25.5-)
limb pain (M79.6-)
lumbar region pain (M54.5)
pelvic and perineal pain (R10.2)
renal colic (N23)
shoulder pain (M25.51-)
spine pain (M54.-)
throat pain (R07.0)
tongue pain (K14.6)
tooth pain (K08.8)
pain disorders exclusively related to psychological factors (F45.41)

✓4ᵗʰ R53 Malaise and fatigue

R53.0 Neoplastic (malignant) related fatigue
Code first associated neoplasm

R53.1 Weakness
Asthenia NOS
EXCLUDES 1 age-related weakness (R54)
▶muscle weakness (generalized) (M62.81)◀
sarcopenia (M62.84)
senile asthenia (R54)
AHA: 2017,1Q,7; 2015,1Q,25

R53.2 Functional quadriplegia MCC HCC
Complete immobility due to severe physical disability or frailty
EXCLUDES 1 frailty NOS (R54)
hysterical paralysis (F44.4)
immobility syndrome (M62.3)
neurologic quadriplegia (G82.5-)
quadriplegia (G82.50)
AHA: 2016,2Q,6
DEF: Inability to move due to a nonphysiological condition, such as dementia. The patient has no mental ability to move independently.

✓5ᵗʰ R53.8 Other malaise and fatigue

EXCLUDES 1 combat exhaustion and fatigue (F43.0)
congenital debility (P96.9)
exhaustion and fatigue due to excessive exertion (T73.3)
exhaustion and fatigue due to exposure (T73.2)
exhaustion and fatigue due to heat (T67.-)
exhaustion and fatigue due to pregnancy (O26.8-)
exhaustion and fatigue due to recurrent depressive episode (F33)
exhaustion and fatigue due to senile debility (R54)

R53.81 Other malaise
Chronic debility
Debility NOS
General physical deterioration
Malaise NOS
Nervous debility
EXCLUDES 1 age-related physical debility (R54)

R53.82 Chronic fatigue, unspecified
Chronic fatigue syndrome NOS
EXCLUDES 1 postviral fatigue syndrome (G93.3)

N Newborn: 0 | P Pediatric: 0-17 | M Maternity: 9-64 | A Adult: 15-124 | MCC Major Complication/Comorbidity | CC Complication/Comorbidity | SW Severe Wound Dx

946

R53.83 Other fatigue
Fatigue NOS
Lack of energy
Lethargy
Tiredness
EXCLUDES 2   exhaustion and fatigue due to depressive episode (F32.-)

R54 Age-related physical debility   A
Frailty
Old age
Senescence
Senile asthenia
Senile debility
EXCLUDES 1   age-related cognitive decline (R41.81)
sarcopenia (M62.84)
senile psychosis (F03)
senility NOS (R41.81)

R55 Syncope and collapse
Blackout
Fainting
Vasovagal attack
EXCLUDES 1   cardiogenic shock (R57.0)
carotid sinus syncope (G90.01)
heat syncope (T67.1)
neurocirculatory asthenia (F45.8)
neurogenic orthostatic hypotension (G90.3)
orthostatic hypotension (I95.1)
postprocedural shock (T81.1-)
psychogenic syncope (F48.8)
shock NOS (R57.9)
shock complicating or following abortion or ectopic or molar pregnancy (O00-O07, O08.3)
shock complicating or following labor and delivery (O75.1)
Stokes-Adams attack (I45.9)
unconsciousness NOS (R40.2-)

✓4ᵗʰ R56 Convulsions, not elsewhere classified
EXCLUDES 1   dissociative convulsions and seizures (F44.5)
epileptic convulsions and seizures (G40.-)
newborn convulsions and seizures (P90)

✓5ᵗʰ R56.0 Febrile convulsions

R56.00 Simple febrile convulsions   CC HCC
Febrile convulsion NOS
Febrile seizure NOS

R56.01 Complex febrile convulsions   CC HCC
Atypical febrile seizure
Complex febrile seizure
Complicated febrile seizure
EXCLUDES 1   status epilepticus (G40.901)

R56.1 Post traumatic seizures   CC HCC
EXCLUDES 1   post traumatic epilepsy (G40.-)

R56.9 Unspecified convulsions   HCC
Convulsion disorder
Fit NOS
Recurrent convulsions
Seizure(s) (convulsive) NOS
AHA: 2019,1Q,19

✓4ᵗʰ R57 Shock, not elsewhere classified
EXCLUDES 1   anaphylactic shock NOS (T78.2)
anaphylactic reaction or shock due to adverse food reaction (T78.0-)
anaphylactic shock due to adverse effect of correct drug or medicament properly administered (T88.6)
anaphylactic shock due to serum (T80.5-)
anesthetic shock (T88.3)
electric shock (T75.4)
obstetric shock (O75.1)
postprocedural shock (T81.1-)
psychic shock (F43.0)
shock complicating or following ectopic or molar pregnancy (O00-O07, O08.3)
shock due to lightning (T75.01)
traumatic shock (T79.4)
toxic shock syndrome (A48.3)

¹ R57.0 Cardiogenic shock   MCC HCC
EXCLUDES 2   septic shock (R65.21)
DEF: Associated with myocardial infarction, cardiac tamponade, and massive pulmonary embolism. Symptoms include mental confusion, reduced blood pressure, tachycardia, pallor, and cold, clammy skin.

¹ R57.1 Hypovolemic shock   MCC HCC
AHA: 2019,2Q,7

¹ R57.8 Other shock   MCC HCC

R57.9 Shock, unspecified   CC HCC
Failure of peripheral circulation NOS

R58 Hemorrhage, not elsewhere classified
Hemorrhage NOS
EXCLUDES 1   hemorrhage included with underlying conditions, such as:
acute duodenal ulcer with hemorrhage (K26.0)
acute gastritis with bleeding (K29.01)
ulcerative enterocolitis with rectal bleeding (K51.01)

✓4ᵗʰ R59 Enlarged lymph nodes
INCLUDES   swollen glands
EXCLUDES 1   acute lymphadenitis (L04.-)
chronic lymphadenitis (I88.1)
lymphadenitis NOS (I88.9)
mesenteric (acute) (chronic) lymphadenitis (I88.0)

R59.0 Localized enlarged lymph nodes

R59.1 Generalized enlarged lymph nodes
Lymphadenopathy NOS

R59.9 Enlarged lymph nodes, unspecified

✓4ᵗʰ R60 Edema, not elsewhere classified
EXCLUDES 1   angioneurotic edema (T78.3)
ascites (R18.-)
cerebral edema (G93.6)
cerebral edema due to birth injury (P11.0)
edema of larynx (J38.4)
edema of nasopharynx (J39.2)
edema of pharynx (J39.2)
gestational edema (O12.0-)
hereditary edema (Q82.0)
hydrops fetalis NOS (P83.2)
hydrothorax (J94.8)
hydrops fetalis NOS (P83.2)
newborn edema (P83.3)
pulmonary edema (J81.-)

R60.0 Localized edema

R60.1 Generalized edema
EXCLUDES 2   nutritional edema (E40-E46)

R60.9 Edema, unspecified
Fluid retention NOS

R61 Generalized hyperhidrosis
Excessive sweating
Night sweats
Secondary hyperhidrosis
Code first, if applicable, menopausal and female climacteric states (N95.1)
EXCLUDES 1   focal (primary) (secondary) hyperhidrosis (L74.5-)
Frey's syndrome (L74.52)
localized (primary) (secondary) hyperhidrosis (L74.5-)

✓4ᵗʰ R62 Lack of expected normal physiological development in childhood and adults

   EXCLUDES 1   *delayed puberty (E30.0)*

        gonadal dysgenesis (Q99.1)

        hypopituitarism (E23.0)

R62.0 Delayed milestone in childhood   P

  Delayed attainment of expected physiological developmental stage

  Late talker

  Late walker

✓5ᵗʰ R62.5 Other and unspecified lack of expected normal physiological development in childhood

   EXCLUDES 1   *HIV disease resulting in failure to thrive (B20)*

        physical retardation due to malnutrition (E45)

R62.50 Unspecified lack of expected normal physiological development in childhood

  Infantilism NOS

R62.51 Failure to thrive (child)   P

  Failure to gain weight

   EXCLUDES 1   *failure to thrive in child under 28 days old (P92.6)*

  AHA: 2018,4Q,82

  DEF: Organic failure to thrive (FTT): Acute or chronic illness that interferes with nutritional intake, absorption, metabolism excretion, and energy requirements.

  DEF: Nonorganic failure to thrive (FTT): Symptom of neglect or abuse.

R62.52 Short stature (child)

  Lack of growth

  Physical retardation

  Short stature NOS

   EXCLUDES 1   *short stature due to endocrine disorder (E34.3)*

R62.59 Other lack of expected normal physiological development in childhood

R62.7 Adult failure to thrive   A

✓4ᵗʰ R63 Symptoms and signs concerning food and fluid intake

   EXCLUDES 1   *bulimia NOS (F50.2)*

R63.0 Anorexia

  Loss of appetite

   EXCLUDES 1   *anorexia nervosa (F50.0-)*

        loss of appetite of nonorganic origin (F50.89)

  AHA: 2018,4Q,82

  TIP: Assign an additional code from category Z68 when BMI is documented. BMI can be based on documentation from clinicians who are not the patient's provider.

R63.1 Polydipsia

  Excessive thirst

R63.2 Polyphagia

  Excessive eating

  Hyperalimentation NOS

R63.3 Feeding difficulties

  Feeding problem (elderly) (infant) NOS

  Picky eater

   EXCLUDES 1   *eating disorders (F50.-)*

        feeding problems of newborn (P92.-)

        infant feeding disorder of nonorganic origin (F98.2-)

  AHA: 2017,1Q,28; 2016,3Q,19

  TIP: Do not assign for feeding problems in a patient greater than 28 days old if the feeding problem was initially diagnosed between day 0 and day 28; use a code from category P92 instead.

R63.4 Abnormal weight loss

  AHA: 2018,4Q,82

  TIP: Assign an additional code from category Z68 when BMI is documented. BMI can be based on documentation from clinicians who are not the patient's provider.

R63.5 Abnormal weight gain

   EXCLUDES 1   *excessive weight gain in pregnancy (O26.0-)*

        obesity (E66.-)

  AHA: 2018,4Q,82

  TIP: Assign an additional code from category Z68 when BMI is documented. BMI can be based on documentation from clinicians who are not the patient's provider.

R63.6 Underweight

  Use additional code to identify body mass index (BMI), if known (Z68.-)

   EXCLUDES 1   *abnormal weight loss (R63.4)*

        anorexia nervosa (F50.0-)

        malnutrition (E40-E46)

  AHA: 2018,4Q,82

R63.8 Other symptoms and signs concerning food and fluid intake

R64 Cachexia   CC HCC

  Wasting syndrome

  Code first underlying condition, if known

   EXCLUDES 1   *abnormal weight loss (R63.4)*

        nutritional marasmus (E41)

  AHA: 2018,4Q,82; 2017,3Q,24

✓4ᵗʰ R65 Symptoms and signs specifically associated with systemic inflammation and infection

  AHA: 2019,2Q,38

  TIP: When documentation states SIRS with an infection, assign only a code for the infection. ICD-10-CM does not offer a code for SIRS due to infectious process. If sepsis is suspected, query the provider.

✓5ᵗʰ R65.1 Systemic inflammatory response syndrome [SIRS] of non-infectious origin

  Code first underlying condition, such as:

    heatstroke (T67.0-)

    injury and trauma (S00-T88)

   EXCLUDES 1   *sepsis — code to infection*

        severe sepsis (R65.2)

R65.10 Systemic inflammatory response syndrome [SIRS] of non-infectious origin without acute organ dysfunction   CC HCC

  Systemic inflammatory response syndrome (SIRS) NOS

  AHA: 2019,2Q,24

R65.11 Systemic inflammatory response syndrome [SIRS] of non-infectious origin with acute organ dysfunction   MCC HCC

  Use additional code to identify specific acute organ dysfunction, such as:

    acute kidney failure (N17.-)

    acute respiratory failure (J96.0-)

    critical illness myopathy (G72.81)

    critical illness polyneuropathy (G62.81)

    disseminated intravascular coagulopathy [DIC] (D65)

    encephalopathy (metabolic) (septic) (G93.41)

    hepatic failure (K72.0-)

✓5ᵗʰ R65.2 Severe sepsis

  Infection with associated acute organ dysfunction

  Sepsis with acute organ dysfunction

  Sepsis with multiple organ dysfunction

  Systemic inflammatory response syndrome due to infectious process with acute organ dysfunction

  Code first underlying infection, such as:

    infection following a procedure (T81.4-)

    infections following infusion, transfusion and therapeutic injection (T80.2-)

    puerperal sepsis (O85)

    sepsis following complete or unspecified spontaneous abortion (O03.87)

    sepsis following ectopic and molar pregnancy (O08.82)

    sepsis following incomplete spontaneous abortion (O03.37)

    sepsis following (induced) termination of pregnancy (O04.87)

    sepsis NOS (A41.9)

  Use additional code to identify specific acute organ dysfunction, such as:

    acute kidney failure (N17.-)

    acute respiratory failure (J96.0-)

    critical illness myopathy (G72.81)

    critical illness polyneuropathy (G62.81)

    disseminated intravascular coagulopathy [DIC] (D65)

    encephalopathy (metabolic) (septic) (G93.41)

    hepatic failure (K72.0-)

  AHA: 2020,2Q,17; 2018,4Q,62-63; 2017,4Q,98-99; 2016,3Q,8

R65.20 Severe sepsis without septic shock   MCC HCC

  Severe sepsis NOS

  AHA: 2020,2Q,17; 2016,3Q,14; 2013,4Q,119

N Newborn: 0   P Pediatric: 0-17   M Maternity: 9-64   A Adult: 15-124   MCC Major Complication/Comorbidity   CC Complication/Comorbidity   SW Severe Wound Dx

948   ICD-10-CM 2021

R65.21   **Severe sepsis** with septic shock   MCC HCC
       AHA: 2018,4Q,63

✓4ᵗʰ R68   Other general symptoms and signs

R68.0   **Hypothermia, not associated with low environmental temperature**
     EXCLUDES 1   *hypothermia NOS (accidental) (T68)*
          hypothermia due to anesthesia (T88.51)
          hypothermia due to low environmental temperature (T68)
          newborn hypothermia (P80.-)

✓5ᵗʰ **R68.1**   **Nonspecific symptoms peculiar to infancy**
     EXCLUDES 1   *colic, infantile (R10.83)*
          neonatal cerebral irritability (P91.3)
          teething syndrome (K00.7)

R68.11   **Excessive crying of infant (baby)**   P
     EXCLUDES 1   *excessive crying of child, adolescent, or adult (R45.83)*

R68.12   **Fussy infant (baby)**   P
     Irritable infant

R68.13   **Apparent life threatening event in infant (ALTE)**   P
     Apparent life threatening event in newborn
     Brief resolved unexplained event (BRUE)
     Code first confirmed diagnosis, if known
     Use additional code(s) for associated signs and symptoms if no confirmed diagnosis established, or if signs and symptoms are not associated routinely with confirmed diagnosis, or provide additional information for cause of ALTE

R68.19   **Other nonspecific symptoms peculiar to infancy**   P

R68.2   **Dry mouth, unspecified**
     EXCLUDES 1   *dry mouth due to dehydration (E86.0)*
          dry mouth due to sicca syndrome [Sjögren] (M35.0-)
          salivary gland hyposecretion (K11.7)

R68.3   **Clubbing of fingers**
     Clubbing of nails
     EXCLUDES 1   *congenital clubfinger (Q68.1)*
     DEF: Enlarged soft tissue of the distal fingers that usually occurs in heart and lung diseases.

✓5ᵗʰ **R68.8**   **Other general symptoms and signs**

R68.81   **Early satiety**
     DEF: Premature feeling of being full after eating only a small amount of food. The mechanism of satiety is multifactorial.

R68.82   **Decreased libido**   A
     Decreased sexual desire

R68.83   **Chills (without fever)**
     Chills NOS
     EXCLUDES 1   *chills with fever (R50.9)*

R68.84   **Jaw pain**
     Mandibular pain
     Maxilla pain
     EXCLUDES 1   *temporomandibular joint arthralgia (M26.62-)*

R68.89   **Other general symptoms and signs**

R69   **Illness, unspecified**
     Unknown and unspecified cases of morbidity

Abnormal findings on examination of blood, without diagnosis (R70-R79)

EXCLUDES 2   *abnormal findings on antenatal screening of mother (O28.-)*
     abnormalities of lipids (E78.-)
     abnormalities of platelets and thrombocytes (D69.-)
     abnormalities of white blood cells classified elsewhere (D70-D72)
     coagulation hemorrhagic disorders (D65-D68)
     diagnostic abnormal findings classified elsewhere — see Alphabetical Index
     hemorrhagic and hematological disorders of newborn (P50-P61)

✓4ᵗʰ R70   Elevated erythrocyte sedimentation rate and abnormality of plasma viscosity

R70.0   **Elevated erythrocyte sedimentation rate**

R70.1   **Abnormal plasma viscosity**

✓4ᵗʰ R71   Abnormality of red blood cells

     EXCLUDES 1   *anemias (D50-D64)*
          anemia of premature infant (P61.2)
          benign (familial) polycythemia (D75.0)
          congenital anemias (P61.2-P61.4)
          newborn anemia due to isoimmunization (P55.-)
          polycythemia neonatorum (P61.1)
          polycythemia NOS (D75.1)
          polycythemia vera (D45)
          secondary polycythemia (D75.1)

R71.0   **Precipitous drop in hematocrit**   CC
     Drop (precipitous) in hemoglobin
     Drop in hematocrit

R71.8   **Other abnormality of red blood cells**
     Abnormal red-cell morphology NOS
     Abnormal red-cell volume NOS
     Anisocytosis
     Poikilocytosis

✓4ᵗʰ R73   Elevated blood glucose level

     EXCLUDES 1   *diabetes mellitus (E08-E13)*
          diabetes mellitus in pregnancy, childbirth and the puerperium (O24.-)
          neonatal disorders (P70.0-P70.2)
          postsurgical hypoinsulinemia (E89.1)

✓5ᵗʰ **R73.0**   **Abnormal glucose**
     EXCLUDES 1   *abnormal glucose in pregnancy (O99.81-)*
          diabetes mellitus (E08-E13)
          dysmetabolic syndrome X (E88.81)
          gestational diabetes (O24.4-)
          glycosuria (R81)
          hypoglycemia (E16.2)

R73.01   **Impaired fasting glucose**
     Elevated fasting glucose

R73.02   **Impaired glucose tolerance (oral)**
     Elevated glucose tolerance

R73.03   **Prediabetes**
     Latent diabetes
     AHA: 2016,4Q,65

R73.09   **Other abnormal glucose**
     Abnormal glucose NOS
     Abnormal non-fasting glucose tolerance

R73.9   **Hyperglycemia, unspecified**

✓4ᵗʰ R74   Abnormal serum enzyme levels

▲ ✓5ᵗʰ **R74.0**   **Nonspecific elevation of levels of transaminase and lactic acid dehydrogenase [LDH]**

●   **R74.01**   **Elevation of levels of liver transaminase levels**
     Elevation of levels of alanine transaminase (ALT)
     Elevation of levels of aspartate transaminase (AST)

●   **R74.02**   **Elevation of levels of lactic acid dehydrogenase [LDH]**

R74.8   **Abnormal levels of other serum enzymes**
     Abnormal level of acid phosphatase
     Abnormal level of alkaline phosphatase
     Abnormal level of amylase
     Abnormal level of lipase [triacylglycerol lipase]
     AHA: 2019,2Q,6

R74.9   **Abnormal serum enzyme level, unspecified**

R75   **Inconclusive laboratory evidence of human immunodeficiency virus [HIV]**
     Nonconclusive HIV-test finding in infants
     EXCLUDES 1   *asymptomatic human immunodeficiency virus [HIV] infection status (Z21)*
          human immunodeficiency virus [HIV] disease (B20)
     TIP: Do not assign for patients previously diagnosed with an HIV-related illness; assign code B20 instead.

✓4ᵗʰ R76   Other abnormal immunological findings in serum

R76.0   **Raised antibody titer**
     EXCLUDES 1   *isoimmunization in pregnancy (O36.0-O36.1)*
          isoimmunization affecting newborn (P55.-)

✔ Additional Character Required   ✓x7ᵗʰ Placeholder   Unacceptable PDx   Questionable PDx   Manifestation   Unspecified Dx   H1-H14 HAC   HCC CMS-HCC Dx   HIV HIV Dx

ICD-10-CM 2021   **949**

R65.21–R76.0

✓5ᵗʰ **R76.1 Nonspecific reaction to test for tuberculosis**

R76.11 Nonspecific reaction to tuberculin skin test without active tuberculosis

Abnormal result of Mantoux test

PPD positive

Tuberculin (skin test) positive

Tuberculin (skin test) reactor

> **EXCLUDES 1** nonspecific reaction to cell mediated immunity measurement of gamma interferon antigen response without active tuberculosis (R76.12)

R76.12 Nonspecific reaction to cell mediated immunity measurement of gamma interferon antigen response without active tuberculosis

Nonspecific reaction to QuantiFERON-TB test (QFT) without active tuberculosis

> **EXCLUDES 1** nonspecific reaction to tuberculin skin test without active tuberculosis (R76.11)
> positive tuberculin skin test (R76.11)

R76.8 Other specified abnormal immunological findings in serum

Raised level of immunoglobulins NOS

R76.9 Abnormal immunological finding in serum, unspecified

✓4ᵗʰ **R77 Other abnormalities of plasma proteins**

> **EXCLUDES 1** disorders of plasma-protein metabolism (E88.0-)

R77.0 Abnormality of albumin

R77.1 Abnormality of globulin

Hyperglobulinemia NOS

R77.2 Abnormality of alphafetoprotein

R77.8 Other specified abnormalities of plasma proteins

R77.9 Abnormality of plasma protein, unspecified

AHA: 2019,2Q,6

✓4ᵗʰ **R78 Findings of drugs and other substances, not normally found in blood**

Use additional code to identify the any retained foreign body, if applicable (Z18.-)

> **EXCLUDES 1** mental or behavioral disorders due to psychoactive substance use (F10-F19)

R78.0 Finding of alcohol **in blood**

Use additional external cause code (Y90.-), for detail regarding alcohol level

R78.1 Finding of opiate **drug in blood**

R78.2 Finding of cocaine **in blood**

R78.3 Finding of hallucinogen **in blood**

R78.4 Finding of other drugs of addictive potential in blood

R78.5 Finding of other psychotropic drug in blood

R78.6 Finding of steroid **agent in blood**

✓5ᵗʰ **R78.7 Finding of abnormal level of** heavy metals **in blood**

R78.71 Abnormal lead **level in blood**

> **EXCLUDES 1** lead poisoning (T56.0-)

R78.79 Finding of abnormal level of heavy metals **in blood**

✓5ᵗʰ **R78.8 Finding of other specified substances, not normally found in blood**

R78.81 Bacteremia CC

> **EXCLUDES 1** sepsis — code to specified infection

DEF: Laboratory finding of bacteria in the blood in the absence of two or more signs of sepsis. Transient in nature, it can progress to septicemia with a severe infectious process.

R78.89 Finding of other specified substances, not normally found in blood

Finding of abnormal level of lithium in blood

R78.9 Finding of unspecified substance, not normally found in blood

✓4ᵗʰ **R79 Other abnormal findings of blood chemistry**

Use additional code to identify any retained foreign body, if applicable (Z18.-)

> **EXCLUDES 1** asymptomatic hyperuricemia (E79.0)
> hyperglycemia NOS (R73.9)
> hypoglycemia NOS (E16.2)
> neonatal hypoglycemia (P70.3-P70.4)
> specific findings indicating disorder of amino-acid metabolism (E70-E72)
> specific findings indicating disorder of carbohydrate metabolism (E73-E74)
> specific findings indicating disorder of lipid metabolism (E75.-)

R79.0 Abnormal level of blood mineral

Abnormal blood level of cobalt

Abnormal blood level of copper

Abnormal blood level of iron

Abnormal blood level of magnesium

Abnormal blood level of mineral NEC

Abnormal blood level of zinc

> **EXCLUDES 1** abnormal level of lithium (R78.89)
> disorders of mineral metabolism (E83.-)
> neonatal hypomagnesemia (P71.2)
> nutritional mineral deficiency (E58-E61)

R79.1 Abnormal coagulation profile

Abnormal or prolonged bleeding time

Abnormal or prolonged coagulation time

Abnormal or prolonged partial thromboplastin time [PTT]

Abnormal or prolonged prothrombin time [PT]

> **EXCLUDES 1** coagulation defects (D68.-)

> **EXCLUDES 2** abnormality of fluid, electrolyte or acid-base balance (E86-E87)

✓5ᵗʰ **R79.8 Other specified abnormal findings of blood chemistry**

R79.81 Abnormal blood-gas **level**

R79.82 Elevated C-reactive protein [CRP]

R79.89 Other specified abnormal findings of blood chemistry

AHA: 2019,2Q,6

TIP: Assign for documented abnormal or elevated troponin level when a definitive diagnosis has not been established.

TIP: Assign for positive Coombs test when not further clarified in the documentation.

R79.9 Abnormal finding of blood chemistry, unspecified

Abnormal findings on examination of urine, without diagnosis (R80-R82)

> **EXCLUDES 1** abnormal findings on antenatal screening of mother (O28.-)
> diagnostic abnormal findings classified elsewhere — see Alphabetical Index
> specific findings indicating disorder of amino-acid metabolism (E70-E72)
> specific findings indicating disorder of carbohydrate metabolism (E73-E74)

✓4ᵗʰ **R80 Proteinuria**

> **EXCLUDES 1** gestational proteinuria (O12.1-)

R80.0 Isolated proteinuria

Idiopathic proteinuria

> **EXCLUDES 1** isolated proteinuria with specific morphological lesion (N06.-)

R80.1 Persistent proteinuria, unspecified

R80.2 Orthostatic proteinuria, unspecified

Postural proteinuria

R80.3 Bence Jones proteinuria

R80.8 Other proteinuria

R80.9 Proteinuria, unspecified

Albuminuria NOS

R81 Glycosuria

> **EXCLUDES 1** renal glycosuria ▶(E74.818)◀

✓4ᵗʰ **R82 Other and unspecified abnormal findings in urine**

> **INCLUDES** chromoabnormalities in urine

Use additional code to identify any retained foreign body, if applicable (Z18.-)

> **EXCLUDES 2** hematuria (R31.-)

R82.0 Chyluria CC

> **EXCLUDES 1** filarial chyluria (B74.-)

R82.1 Myoglobinuria CC

N Newborn: 0   **P** Pediatric: 0-17   **M** Maternity: 9-64   **A** Adult: 15-124   **MCC** Major Complication/Comorbidity   **CC** Complication/Comorbidity   **SW** Severe Wound Dx

950   ICD-10-CM 2021

R82.2 Biliuria

R82.3 Hemoglobinuria

> **EXCLUDES 1** *hemoglobinuria due to hemolysis from external causes NEC (D59.6)*
>
> *hemoglobinuria due to paroxysmal nocturnal [Marchiafava-Micheli] (D59.5)*
>
> **DEF:** Free hemoglobin in blood due to rapid hemolysis of red blood cells. Causes include burns, crushed injury, sickle cell anemia, thalassemia, parasitic infections, or kidney infections.

R82.4 Acetonuria

> Ketonuria
>
> **DEF:** Excessive excretion of acetone in urine that commonly occurs in diabetic acidosis.

R82.5 Elevated urine levels of drugs, medicaments and biological substances

> Elevated urine levels of catecholamines
>
> Elevated urine levels of indoleacetic acid
>
> Elevated urine levels of 17-ketosteroids
>
> Elevated urine levels of steroids

R82.6 Abnormal urine levels of substances chiefly nonmedicinal as to source

> Abnormal urine level of heavy metals

✓5ᵗʰ **R82.7** Abnormal findings on microbiological examination of urine

> **EXCLUDES 1** *colonization status (Z22.-)*
>
> **AHA:** 2016,4Q,65

R82.71 Bacteriuria

R82.79 Other abnormal findings on microbiological examination of urine

> Positive culture findings of urine

✓5ᵗʰ **R82.8** Abnormal findings on cytological and histological examination of urine

> **AHA:** 2019,4Q,16

R82.81 Pyuria

> Sterile pyuria

R82.89 Other abnormal findings on cytological and histological examination of urine

✓5ᵗʰ **R82.9** Other and unspecified abnormal findings in urine

R82.90 Unspecified abnormal findings in urine

R82.91 Other chromoabnormalities of urine

> Chromoconversion (dipstick)
>
> Idiopathic dipstick converts positive for blood with no cellular forms in sediment
>
> > **EXCLUDES 1** *hemoglobinuria (R82.3)*
> >
> > *myoglobinuria (R82.1)*

✓6ᵗʰ **R82.99** Other abnormal findings in urine

> **AHA:** 2018,4Q,29-30

R82.991 Hypocitraturia

R82.992 Hyperoxaluria

> **EXCLUDES 1** *primary hyperoxaluria (E72.53)*

R82.993 Hyperuricosuria

R82.994 Hypercalciuria

> Idiopathic hypercalciuria

R82.998 Other abnormal findings in urine

> Cells and casts in urine
>
> Crystalluria
>
> Melanuria

Abnormal findings on examination of other body fluids, substances and tissues, without diagnosis (R83-R89)

> **EXCLUDES 1** *abnormal findings on antenatal screening of mother (O28.-)*
>
> *diagnostic abnormal findings classified elsewhere — see Alphabetical Index*
>
> **EXCLUDES 2** *abnormal findings on examination of blood, without diagnosis (R70-R79)*
>
> *abnormal findings on examination of urine, without diagnosis (R80-R82)*
>
> *abnormal tumor markers (R97.-)*

✓4ᵗʰ **R83** Abnormal findings in cerebrospinal fluid

Cerebrospinal Fluid

Ventricles

Cerebrospinal fluid

Spinal cord

R83.0 Abnormal level of enzymes in cerebrospinal fluid

R83.1 Abnormal level of hormones in cerebrospinal fluid

R83.2 Abnormal level of other drugs, medicaments and biological substances in cerebrospinal fluid

R83.3 Abnormal level of substances chiefly nonmedicinal as to source in cerebrospinal fluid

R83.4 Abnormal immunological findings in cerebrospinal fluid

R83.5 Abnormal microbiological findings in cerebrospinal fluid

> Positive culture findings in cerebrospinal fluid
>
> **EXCLUDES 1** *colonization status (Z22.-)*

R83.6 Abnormal cytological findings in cerebrospinal fluid

R83.8 Other abnormal findings in cerebrospinal fluid

> Abnormal chromosomal findings in cerebrospinal fluid

R83.9 Unspecified abnormal finding in cerebrospinal fluid

✓4ᵗʰ **R84** Abnormal findings in specimens from respiratory organs and thorax

> **INCLUDES** abnormal findings in bronchial washings
>
> abnormal findings in nasal secretions
>
> abnormal findings in pleural fluid
>
> abnormal findings in sputum
>
> abnormal findings in throat scrapings
>
> **EXCLUDES 1** *blood-stained sputum (R04.2)*

R84.0 Abnormal level of enzymes in specimens from respiratory organs and thorax

R84.1 Abnormal level of hormones in specimens from respiratory organs and thorax

R84.2 Abnormal level of other drugs, medicaments and biological substances in specimens from respiratory organs and thorax

R84.3 Abnormal level of substances chiefly nonmedicinal as to source in specimens from respiratory organs and thorax

R84.4 Abnormal immunological findings in specimens from respiratory organs and thorax

☑ Additional Character Required   ✓x7ᵗʰ Placeholder   Unacceptable PDx   Questionable PDx   Manifestation   Unspecified Dx   H1-H14 HAC   HCC CMS-HCC Dx   HIV HIV Dx

ICD-10-CM 2021

951

R84.5   Abnormal microbiological findings in specimens from respiratory organs and thorax

> Positive culture findings in specimens from respiratory organs and thorax
>> EXCLUDES 1   colonization status (Z22.-)

R84.6   Abnormal cytological findings in specimens from respiratory organs and thorax

R84.7   Abnormal histological findings in specimens from respiratory organs and thorax

R84.8   Other abnormal findings in specimens from respiratory organs and thorax

> Abnormal chromosomal findings in specimens from respiratory organs and thorax

R84.9   Unspecified abnormal finding in specimens from respiratory organs and thorax

✓4ᵗʰ **R85**   Abnormal findings in specimens from digestive organs and abdominal cavity

> INCLUDES   abnormal findings in peritoneal fluid
> abnormal findings in saliva
>> EXCLUDES 1   cloudy peritoneal dialysis effluent (R88.0)
>> fecal abnormalities (R19.5)

R85.0   Abnormal level of enzymes in specimens from digestive organs and abdominal cavity

R85.1   Abnormal level of hormones in specimens from digestive organs and abdominal cavity

R85.2   Abnormal level of other drugs, medicaments and biological substances in specimens from digestive organs and abdominal cavity

R85.3   Abnormal level of substances chiefly nonmedicinal as to source in specimens from digestive organs and abdominal cavity

R85.4   Abnormal immunological findings in specimens from digestive organs and abdominal cavity

R85.5   Abnormal microbiological findings in specimens from digestive organs and abdominal cavity

> Positive culture findings in specimens from digestive organs and abdominal cavity
>> EXCLUDES 1   colonization status (Z22.-)

✓5ᵗʰ **R85.6**   Abnormal cytological findings in specimens from digestive organs and abdominal cavity

    ✓6ᵗʰ **R85.61**   Abnormal cytologic smear of anus

>> EXCLUDES 1   abnormal cytological findings in specimens from other digestive organs and abdominal cavity (R85.69)
>> anal intraepithelial neoplasia I [AIN I] (K62.82)
>> anal intraepithelial neoplasia II [AIN II] (K62.82)
>> anal intraepithelial neoplasia III [AIN III] (D01.3)
>> carcinoma in situ of anus (histologically confirmed) (D01.3)
>> dysplasia (mild) (moderate) of anus (histologically confirmed) (K62.82)
>> severe dysplasia of anus (histologically confirmed) (D01.3)
>>> EXCLUDES 2   anal high risk human papillomavirus (HPV) DNA test positive (R85.81)
>>> anal low risk human papillomavirus (HPV) DNA test positive (R85.82)

       R85.610   Atypical squamous cells of undetermined significance on cytologic smear of anus [ASC-US]

       R85.611   Atypical squamous cells cannot exclude high grade squamous intraepithelial lesion on cytologic smear of anus [ASC-H]

       R85.612   Low grade squamous intraepithelial lesion on cytologic smear of anus [LGSIL]

       R85.613   High grade squamous intraepithelial lesion on cytologic smear of anus [HGSIL]

       R85.614   Cytologic evidence of malignancy on smear of anus

       R85.615   Unsatisfactory cytologic smear of anus
>> Inadequate sample of cytologic smear of anus

       R85.616   Satisfactory anal smear but lacking transformation zone

       R85.618   Other abnormal cytological findings on specimens from anus

       R85.619   Unspecified abnormal cytological findings in specimens from anus
>> Abnormal anal cytology NOS
>> Atypical glandular cells of anus NOS

    R85.69   Abnormal cytological findings in specimens from other digestive organs and abdominal cavity

R85.7   Abnormal histological findings in specimens from digestive organs and abdominal cavity

✓5ᵗʰ **R85.8**   Other abnormal findings in specimens from digestive organs and abdominal cavity

    R85.81   Anal high risk human papillomavirus [HPV] DNA test positive

>> EXCLUDES 1   anogenital warts due to human papillomavirus (HPV) (A63.0)
>> condyloma acuminatum (A63.0)

    R85.82   Anal low risk human papillomavirus [HPV] DNA test positive

> Use additional code for associated human papillomavirus (B97.7)

    R85.89   Other abnormal findings in specimens from digestive organs and abdominal cavity

> Abnormal chromosomal findings in specimens from digestive organs and abdominal cavity

R85.9   Unspecified abnormal finding in specimens from digestive organs and abdominal cavity

✓4ᵗʰ **R86**   Abnormal findings in specimens from male genital organs

> INCLUDES   abnormal findings in prostatic secretions
> abnormal findings in semen, seminal fluid
> abnormal spermatozoa
>> EXCLUDES 1   azoospermia (N46.0-)
>> oligospermia (N46.1-)

R86.0   Abnormal level of enzymes in specimens from male genital organs ♂

R86.1   Abnormal level of hormones in specimens from male genital organs ♂

R86.2   Abnormal level of other drugs, medicaments and biological substances in specimens from male genital organs ♂

R86.3   Abnormal level of substances chiefly nonmedicinal as to source in specimens from male genital organs ♂

R86.4   Abnormal immunological findings in specimens from male genital organs ♂

R86.5   Abnormal microbiological findings in specimens from male genital organs ♂

> Positive culture findings in specimens from male genital organs
>> EXCLUDES 1   colonization status (Z22.-)

R86.6   Abnormal cytological findings in specimens from male genital organs ♂

R86.7   Abnormal histological findings in specimens from male genital organs ♂

R86.8   Other abnormal findings in specimens from male genital organs ♂

> Abnormal chromosomal findings in specimens from male genital organs

R86.9   Unspecified abnormal finding in specimens from male genital organs ♂

✓4ᵗʰ **R87**   Abnormal findings in specimens from female genital organs

> INCLUDES   abnormal findings in secretion and smears from cervix uteri
> abnormal findings in secretion and smears from vagina
> abnormal findings in secretion and smears from vulva

R87.0   Abnormal level of enzymes in specimens from female genital organs ♀

R87.1   Abnormal level of hormones in specimens from female genital organs ♀

R87.2   Abnormal level of other drugs, medicaments and biological substances in specimens from female genital organs ♀

R87.3   Abnormal level of substances chiefly nonmedicinal as to source in specimens from female genital organs ♀

R87.4   Abnormal immunological findings in specimens from female genital organs ♀

R87.5   Abnormal microbiological findings in specimens from female genital organs ♀

> Positive culture findings in specimens from female genital organs
>> EXCLUDES 1   colonization status (Z22.-)

N Newborn: 0   P Pediatric: 0-17   M Maternity: 9-64   A Adult: 15-124   MCC Major Complication/Comorbidity   CC Complication/Comorbidity   SW Severe Wound Dx

952   ICD-10-CM 2021

☑6ᵗʰ **R87.6** **Abnormal cytological findings in specimens from female genital organs**

☑6ᵗʰ **R87.61** **Abnormal cytological findings in specimens from cervix uteri**

EXCLUDES 1 *abnormal cytological findings in specimens from other female genital organs (R87.69)*

abnormal cytological findings in specimens from vagina (R87.62-)

carcinoma in situ of cervix uteri (histologically confirmed) (D06.-)

cervical intraepithelial neoplasia I [CIN I] (N87.0)

cervical intraepithelial neoplasia II [CIN II] (N87.1)

cervical intraepithelial neoplasia III [CIN III] (D06.-)

dysplasia (mild) (moderate) of cervix uteri (histologically confirmed) (N87.-)

severe dysplasia of cervix uteri (histologically confirmed) (D06.-)

EXCLUDES 2 *cervical high risk human papillomavirus (HPV) DNA test positive (R87.810)*

cervical low risk human papillomavirus (HPV) DNA test positive (R87.820)

R87.610 **Atypical squamous cells of undetermined significance on cytologic smear of cervix [ASC-US]** ♀

R87.611 **Atypical squamous cells cannot exclude high grade squamous intraepithelial lesion on cytologic smear of cervix [ASC-H]** ♀

R87.612 **Low grade squamous intraepithelial lesion on cytologic smear of cervix [LGSIL]** ♀

R87.613 **High grade squamous intraepithelial lesion on cytologic smear of cervix [HGSIL]** ♀

R87.614 **Cytologic evidence of malignancy on smear of cervix** ♀

R87.615 **Unsatisfactory cytologic smear of cervix** ♀

Inadequate sample of cytologic smear of cervix

R87.616 **Satisfactory cervical smear but lacking transformation zone** ♀

R87.618 **Other abnormal cytological findings on specimens from cervix uteri** ♀

R87.619 **Unspecified abnormal cytological findings in specimens from cervix uteri** ♀

Abnormal cervical cytology NOS
Abnormal Papanicolaou smear of cervix NOS
Abnormal thin preparation smear of cervix NOS
Atypical endocervial cells of cervix NOS
Atypical endometrial cells of cervix NOS
Atypical glandular cells of cervix NOS

☑6ᵗʰ **R87.62** **Abnormal cytological findings in specimens from vagina**

Use additional code to identify acquired absence of uterus and cervix, if applicable (Z90.71-)

EXCLUDES 1 *abnormal cytological findings in specimens from cervix uteri (R87.61-)*

abnormal cytological findings in specimens from other female genital organs (R87.69)

carcinoma in situ of vagina (histologically confirmed) (D07.2)

dysplasia (mild) (moderate) of vagina (histologically confirmed) (N89.-)

severe dysplasia of vagina (histologically confirmed) (D07.2)

vaginal intraepithelial neoplasia I [VAIN I] (N89.0)

vaginal intraepithelial neoplasia II [VAIN II] (N89.1)

vaginal intraepithelial neoplasia III [VAIN III] (D07.2)

EXCLUDES 2 *vaginal high risk human papillomavirus (HPV) DNA test positive (R87.811)*

vaginal low risk human papillomavirus (HPV) DNA test positive (R87.821)

R87.620 **Atypical squamous cells of undetermined significance on cytologic smear of vagina [ASC-US]** ♀

R87.621 **Atypical squamous cells cannot exclude high grade squamous intraepithelial lesion on cytologic smear of vagina [ASC-H]** ♀

R87.622 **Low grade squamous intraepithelial lesion on cytologic smear of vagina [LGSIL]** ♀

R87.623 **High grade squamous intraepithelial lesion on cytologic smear of vagina [HGSIL]** ♀

R87.624 **Cytologic evidence of malignancy on smear of vagina** ♀

R87.625 **Unsatisfactory cytologic smear of vagina** ♀

Inadequate sample of cytologic smear of vagina

R87.628 **Other abnormal cytological findings on specimens from vagina** ♀

R87.629 **Unspecified abnormal cytological findings in specimens from vagina** ♀

Abnormal Papanicolaou smear of vagina NOS
Abnormal thin preparation smear of vagina NOS
Abnormal vaginal cytology NOS
Atypical endocervical cells of vagina NOS
Atypical endometrial cells of vagina NOS
Atypical glandular cells of vagina NOS

R87.69 **Abnormal cytological findings in specimens from other female genital organs** ♀

Abnormal cytological findings in specimens from female genital organs NOS

EXCLUDES 1 *dysplasia of vulva (histologically confirmed) (N90.0-N90.3)*

☑ Additional Character Required   ☑x7ᵗʰ Placeholder   Unacceptable PDx   Questionable PDx   Manifestation   Unspecified Dx   H1-H4 HAC   HCC CMS-HCC Dx   HIV HIV Dx

ICD-10-CM 2021

953

R87.7 Abnormal histological findings in specimens from female genital organs ♀
> EXCLUDES 1   *carcinoma in situ (histologically confirmed) of female genital organs (D06-D07.3)*
> *cervical intraepithelial neoplasia I [CIN I] (N87.0)*
> *cervical intraepithelial neoplasia II [CIN II] (N87.1)*
> *cervical intraepithelial neoplasia III [CIN III] (D06.-)*
> *dysplasia (mild) (moderate) of cervix uteri (histologically confirmed) (N87.-)*
> *dysplasia (mild) (moderate) of vagina (histologically confirmed) (N89.-)*
> *severe dysplasia of cervix uteri (histologically confirmed) (D06.-)*
> *severe dysplasia of vagina (histologically confirmed) (D07.2)*
> *vaginal intraepithelial neoplasia I [VAIN I] (N89.0)*
> *vaginal intraepithelial neoplasia II [VAIN II] (N89.1)*
> *vaginal intraepithelial neoplasia III [VAIN III] (D07.2)*

✓5ᵗʰ **R87.8 Other abnormal findings in specimens from female genital organs**

✓6ᵗʰ **R87.81 High risk human papillomavirus [HPV] DNA test positive from female genital organs**
> EXCLUDES 1   *anogenital warts due to human papillomavirus (HPV) (A63.0)*
> *condyloma acuminatum (A63.0)*

R87.810 Cervical high risk human papillomavirus [HPV] DNA test positive ♀

R87.811 Vaginal high risk human papillomavirus [HPV] DNA test positive ♀

✓6ᵗʰ **R87.82 Low risk human papillomavirus [HPV] DNA test positive from female genital organs**
Use additional code for associated human papillomavirus (B97.7)

R87.820 Cervical low risk human papillomavirus [HPV] DNA test positive ♀

R87.821 Vaginal low risk human papillomavirus [HPV] DNA test positive ♀

R87.89 Other abnormal findings in specimens from female genital organs ♀
Abnormal chromosomal findings in specimens from female genital organs

R87.9 Unspecified abnormal finding in specimens from female genital organs ♀

✓4ᵗʰ **R88 Abnormal findings in other body fluids and substances**

R88.0 Cloudy (hemodialysis) (peritoneal) dialysis effluent

R88.8 Abnormal findings in other body fluids and substances

✓4ᵗʰ **R89 Abnormal findings in specimens from other organs, systems and tissues**
> INCLUDES   abnormal findings in nipple discharge
> abnormal findings in synovial fluid
> abnormal findings in wound secretions

R89.0 Abnormal level of enzymes in specimens from other organs, systems and tissues

R89.1 Abnormal level of hormones in specimens from other organs, systems and tissues

R89.2 Abnormal level of other drugs, medicaments and biological substances in specimens from other organs, systems and tissues

R89.3 Abnormal level of substances chiefly nonmedicinal as to source in specimens from other organs, systems and tissues

R89.4 Abnormal immunological findings in specimens from other organs, systems and tissues

R89.5 Abnormal microbiological findings in specimens from other organs, systems and tissues
Positive culture findings in specimens from other organs, systems and tissues
> EXCLUDES 1   *colonization status (Z22.-)*

R89.6 Abnormal cytological findings in specimens from other organs, systems and tissues

R89.7 Abnormal histological findings in specimens from other organs, systems and tissues

R89.8 Other abnormal findings in specimens from other organs, systems and tissues
Abnormal chromosomal findings in specimens from other organs, systems and tissues

R89.9 Unspecified abnormal finding in specimens from other organs, systems and tissues

Abnormal findings on diagnostic imaging and in function studies, without diagnosis (R90-R94)

> INCLUDES   nonspecific abnormal findings on diagnostic imaging by computerized axial tomography [CAT scan]
> nonspecific abnormal findings on diagnostic imaging by magnetic resonance imaging [MRI][NMR]
> nonspecific abnormal findings on diagnostic imaging by positron emission tomography [PET scan]
> nonspecific abnormal findings on diagnostic imaging by thermography
> nonspecific abnormal findings on diagnostic imaging by ultrasound [echogram]
> nonspecific abnormal findings on diagnostic imaging by X-ray examination

> EXCLUDES 1   *abnormal findings on antenatal screening of mother (O28.-)*
> *diagnostic abnormal findings classified elsewhere — see Alphabetical Index*

✓4ᵗʰ **R90 Abnormal findings on diagnostic imaging of central nervous system**

R90.0 Intracranial space-occupying lesion found on diagnostic imaging of central nervous system

✓5ᵗʰ **R90.8 Other abnormal findings on diagnostic imaging of central nervous system**

R90.81 Abnormal echoencephalogram

R90.82 White matter disease, unspecified

R90.89 Other abnormal findings on diagnostic imaging of central nervous system
Other cerebrovascular abnormality found on diagnostic imaging of central nervous system

✓4ᵗʰ **R91 Abnormal findings on diagnostic imaging of lung**

R91.1 Solitary pulmonary nodule
Coin lesion lung
Solitary pulmonary nodule, subsegmental branch of the bronchial tree

R91.8 Other nonspecific abnormal finding of lung field
Lung mass NOS found on diagnostic imaging of lung
Pulmonary infiltrate NOS
Shadow, lung

✓4ᵗʰ **R92 Abnormal and inconclusive findings on diagnostic imaging of breast**

R92.0 Mammographic microcalcification found on diagnostic imaging of breast
> EXCLUDES 2   *mammographic calcification (calculus) found on diagnostic imaging of breast (R92.1)*

DEF: Calcium and cellular debris deposits in the breast that cannot be felt but can be detected on a mammogram. The deposits can be a sign of cancer, benign conditions, or changes in the breast tissue as a result of inflammation, injury, or an obstructed duct.

R92.1 Mammographic calcification found on diagnostic imaging of breast
Mammographic calculus found on diagnostic imaging of breast

R92.2 Inconclusive mammogram
Dense breasts NOS
Inconclusive mammogram NEC
Inconclusive mammography due to dense breasts
Inconclusive mammography NEC
AHA: 2015,1Q,24

R92.8 Other abnormal and inconclusive findings on diagnostic imaging of breast

✓4ᵗʰ **R93 Abnormal findings on diagnostic imaging of other body structures**

R93.0 Abnormal findings on diagnostic imaging of skull and head, not elsewhere classified
> EXCLUDES 1   *intracranial space-occupying lesion found on diagnostic imaging (R90.0)*

R93.1 Abnormal findings on diagnostic imaging of heart and coronary circulation
Abnormal echocardiogram NOS
Abnormal heart shadow

R93.2 Abnormal findings on diagnostic imaging of liver and biliary tract
Nonvisualization of gallbladder

R93.3 Abnormal findings on diagnostic imaging of other parts of digestive tract

---

✓5ᵗʰ **R93.4** **Abnormal findings on diagnostic imaging of** urinary organs
  EXCLUDES 2 hypertrophy of kidney (N28.81)
  AHA: 2016,4Q,66

R93.41 **Abnormal radiologic findings on diagnostic imaging of** renal pelvis, ureter, or bladder
  Filling defect of bladder found on diagnostic imaging
  Filling defect of renal pelvis found on diagnostic imaging
  Filling defect of ureter found on diagnostic imaging

✓6ᵗʰ **R93.42** **Abnormal radiologic findings on diagnostic imaging of kidney**
  R93.421 **Abnormal radiologic findings on diagnostic imaging of** right **kidney**
  R93.422 **Abnormal radiologic findings on diagnostic imaging of** left **kidney**
  R93.429 **Abnormal radiologic findings on diagnostic imaging of unspecified kidney**

R93.49 **Abnormal radiologic findings on diagnostic imaging of other urinary organs**

R93.5 **Abnormal findings on diagnostic imaging of other abdominal regions, including retroperitoneum**

R93.6 **Abnormal findings on diagnostic imaging of** limbs
  EXCLUDES 2 abnormal finding in skin and subcutaneous tissue (R93.8-)
  AHA: 2020,1Q,14

R93.7 **Abnormal findings on diagnostic imaging of other parts of musculoskeletal system**
  EXCLUDES 2 abnormal findings on diagnostic imaging of skull (R93.0)

✓5ᵗʰ **R93.8** **Abnormal findings on diagnostic imaging of other specified body structures**
  AHA: 2018,4Q,30

✓6ᵗʰ **R93.81** **Abnormal radiologic findings on diagnostic imaging of** testis
  R93.811 **Abnormal radiologic findings on diagnostic imaging of** right **testicle** ♂
  R93.812 **Abnormal radiologic findings on diagnostic imaging of** left **testicle** ♂
  R93.813 **Abnormal radiologic findings on diagnostic imaging of testicles, bilateral** ♂
  R93.819 **Abnormal radiologic findings on diagnostic imaging of unspecified testicle** ♂

R93.89 **Abnormal findings on diagnostic imaging of other specified body structures**
  Abnormal finding by radioisotope localization of placenta
  Abnormal radiological finding in skin and subcutaneous tissue
  Mediastinal shift

R93.9 **Diagnostic imaging inconclusive due to** excess body fat of **patient**

✓4ᵗʰ **R94** **Abnormal results of function studies**
  INCLUDES abnormal results of radionuclide [radioisotope] uptake studies
  abnormal results of scintigraphy

✓5ᵗʰ **R94.0** **Abnormal results of function studies of** central nervous system
  R94.01 **Abnormal** electroencephalogram [EEG]
  R94.02 **Abnormal** brain scan
  R94.09 **Abnormal results of other function studies of central nervous system**

✓5ᵗʰ **R94.1** **Abnormal results of function studies of** peripheral nervous system and special senses
  ✓6ᵗʰ **R94.11** **Abnormal results of function studies of** eye
    R94.110 **Abnormal** electro-oculogram [EOG]
    R94.111 **Abnormal** electroretinogram [ERG]
      Abnormal retinal function study
    R94.112 **Abnormal** visually evoked potential [VEP]
    R94.113 **Abnormal** oculomotor **study**
    R94.118 **Abnormal results of other function studies of eye**
  ✓6ᵗʰ **R94.12** **Abnormal results of function studies of** ear and **other special senses**
    AHA: 2016,3Q,17
    R94.120 **Abnormal** auditory **function study**
    R94.121 **Abnormal** vestibular **function study**
    R94.128 **Abnormal results of other function studies of ear and other special senses**

✓6ᵗʰ **R94.13** **Abnormal results of function studies of** peripheral nervous system
  R94.130 **Abnormal response to nerve stimulation, unspecified**
  R94.131 **Abnormal** electromyogram [EMG]
    EXCLUDES 1 electromyogram of eye (R94.113)
  R94.138 **Abnormal results of other function studies of peripheral nervous system**

R94.2 **Abnormal results of** pulmonary function **studies**
  Reduced ventilatory capacity
  Reduced vital capacity

✓5ᵗʰ **R94.3** **Abnormal results of** cardiovascular function **studies**
  R94.30 **Abnormal result of cardiovascular function study, unspecified**
  R94.31 **Abnormal** electrocardiogram [ECG] [EKG]
    EXCLUDES 1 long QT syndrome (I45.81)
  R94.39 **Abnormal result of other cardiovascular function study**
    Abnormal electrophysiological intracardiac studies
    Abnormal phonocardiogram
    Abnormal vectorcardiogram

R94.4 **Abnormal results of** kidney function **studies**
  Abnormal renal function test

R94.5 **Abnormal results of** liver function **studies**

R94.6 **Abnormal results of** thyroid function **studies**

R94.7 **Abnormal results of other endocrine function studies**
  EXCLUDES 2 abnormal glucose (R73.0-)

R94.8 **Abnormal results of function studies of other organs and systems**
  Abnormal basal metabolic rate [BMR]
  Abnormal bladder function test
  Abnormal splenic function test

Abnormal tumor markers (R97)

✓4ᵗʰ **R97** **Abnormal tumor markers**
  Elevated tumor associated antigens [TAA]
  Elevated tumor specific antigens [TSA]
  R97.0 **Elevated carcinoembryonic antigen [CEA]**
  R97.1 **Elevated cancer antigen 125 [CA 125]**
  ✓5ᵗʰ **R97.2** **Elevated prostate specific antigen [PSA]**
    AHA: 2016,4Q,66
    R97.20 **Elevated prostate specific antigen [PSA]** A ♂
    R97.21 **Rising PSA following treatment for malignant neoplasm of prostate** A ♂
  R97.8 **Other abnormal tumor markers**

Ill-defined and unknown cause of mortality (R99)

R99 **Ill-defined and unknown cause of mortality**
  Death (unexplained) NOS
  Unspecified cause of mortality

Chapter 19. Injury, Poisoning and Certain Other Consequences of External Causes (SØØ–T88)

Chapter-specific Guidelines with Coding Examples

The chapter-specific guidelines from the ICD-10-CM Official Guidelines for Coding and Reporting have been provided below. Along with these guidelines are coding examples, contained in the shaded boxes, that have been developed to help illustrate the coding and/or sequencing guidance found in these guidelines.

a. Application of 7th characters in Chapter 19

Most categories in chapter 19 have a 7th character requirement for each applicable code. Most categories in this chapter have three 7th character values (with the exception of fractures): A, initial encounter, D, subsequent encounter and S, sequela. Categories for traumatic fractures have additional 7th character values. While the patient may be seen by a new or different provider over the course of treatment for an injury, assignment of the 7th character is based on whether the patient is undergoing active treatment and not whether the provider is seeing the patient for the first time.

For complication codes, active treatment refers to treatment for the condition described by the code, even though it may be related to an earlier precipitating problem. For example, code T84.50XA, Infection and inflammatory reaction due to unspecified internal joint prosthesis, initial encounter, is used when active treatment is provided for the infection, even though the condition relates to the prosthetic device, implant or graft that was placed at a previous encounter.

7th character "A", initial encounter is used for each encounter where the patient is receiving active treatment for the condition.

> Patient admitted after fall from a skateboard onto the sidewalk, x-rays identify a nondisplaced fracture to the distal pole of the right scaphoid bone. The patient is placed in a cast.
>
> | S62.014A | Nondisplaced fracture of distal pole of navicular [scaphoid] bone of right wrist, initial encounter for closed fracture |
> |---|---|
> | V00.131A | Fall from skateboard, initial encounter |
> | Y92.48Ø | Sidewalk as the place of occurrence of the external cause |
> | Y93.51 | Activity, roller skating (inline) and skateboarding |
> | Y99.8 | Other external cause status |
>
> *Explanation:* This fracture would be coded with a seventh character A for initial encounter because the patient received x-rays to identify the site of the fracture and treatment was rendered; this would be considered active treatment.

7th character "D" subsequent encounter is used for encounters after the patient has completed active treatment of the condition and is receiving routine care for the condition during the healing or recovery phase.

> Patient admitted after fall from a skateboard onto the sidewalk resulted in casting of the right arm. X-rays are taken to evaluate how well the nondisplaced fracture to the distal pole of the right scaphoid bone is healing. The physician feels the fracture is healing appropriately; no adjustments to the cast are made.
>
> | S62.014D | Nondisplaced fracture of distal pole of navicular [scaphoid] bone of right wrist, subsequent encounter for fracture with routine healing |
> |---|---|
> | V00.131D | Fall from skateboard, subsequent encounter |
>
> *Explanation:* This fracture would be coded with a seventh character D for subsequent encounter, whether the same physician who provided the initial cast application or a different physician is now seeing the patient. Although the patient received x-rays, the intent of the x-rays was to assess how the fracture was healing. There was no active treatment rendered and the visit is therefore considered a subsequent encounter.

The aftercare Z codes should not be used for aftercare for conditions such as injuries or poisonings, where 7th characters are provided to identify subsequent care. For example, for aftercare of an injury, assign the acute injury code with the 7th character "D" (subsequent encounter).

7th character "S", sequela, is for use for complications or conditions that arise as a direct result of a condition, such as scar formation after a burn. The scars are sequelae of the burn. When using 7th character "S", it is

necessary to use both the injury code that precipitated the sequela and the code for the sequela itself. The "S" is added only to the injury code, not the sequela code. The 7th character "S" identifies the injury responsible for the sequela. The specific type of sequela (e.g. scar) is sequenced first, followed by the injury code.

See Section I.B.1Ø Sequelae, (Late Effects)

> Patient with a history of a nondisplaced fracture to the distal pole of the right scaphoid bone due to a fall from a skateboard is admitted for evaluation of arthritis to the right wrist that has developed as a consequence of the traumatic fracture.
>
> | M12.531 | Traumatic arthropathy, right wrist |
> |---|---|
> | S62.014S | Nondisplaced fracture of distal pole of navicular [scaphoid] bone of right wrist, sequela |
> | V00.131S | Fall from skateboard, sequela |
>
> *Explanation:* The code identifying the specific sequela condition (traumatic arthritis) should be coded first followed by the injury that instigated the development of the sequela (fracture). The scaphoid fracture injury code is given a 7th character S for sequela to represent its role as the inciting injury. The fracture has healed and is not being managed or treated on this admit and therefore is not applicable as a first listed or principal diagnosis. However, it is directly related to the development of the arthritis and should be appended as a secondary code to signify this cause and effect relationship.

b. Coding of injuries

When coding injuries, assign separate codes for each injury unless a combination code is provided, in which case the combination code is assigned. Codes from category T07, Unspecified multiple injuries should not be assigned in the inpatient setting unless information for a more specific code is not available. Traumatic injury codes (SØØ-T14.9) are not to be used for normal, healing surgical wounds or to identify complications of surgical wounds.

The code for the most serious injury, as determined by the provider and the focus of treatment, is sequenced first.

1) Superficial injuries

Superficial injuries such as abrasions or contusions are not coded when associated with more severe injuries of the same site.

2) Primary injury with damage to nerves/blood vessels

When a primary injury results in minor damage to peripheral nerves or blood vessels, the primary injury is sequenced first with additional code(s) for injuries to nerves and spinal cord (such as category SØ4), and/or injury to blood vessels (such as category S15). When the primary injury is to the blood vessels or nerves, that injury should be sequenced first.

3) Iatrogenic injuries

Injury codes from Chapter 19 should not be assigned for injuries that occur during, or as a result of, a medical intervention. Assign the appropriate complication code(s).

c. Coding of traumatic fractures

The principles of multiple coding of injuries should be followed in coding fractures. Fractures of specified sites are coded individually by site in accordance with both the provisions within categories SØ2, S12, S22, S32, S42, S49, S52, S59, S62, S72, S79, S82, S89, S92 and the level of detail furnished by medical record content.

A fracture not indicated as open or closed should be coded to closed. A fracture not indicated whether displaced or not displaced should be coded to displaced.

More specific guidelines are as follows:

1) Initial vs. subsequent encounter for fractures

Traumatic fractures are coded using the appropriate 7th character for initial encounter (A, B, C) for each encounter where the patient is receiving active treatment for the fracture. The appropriate 7th character for initial encounter should also be assigned for a patient who delayed seeking treatment for the fracture or nonunion.

Fractures are coded using the appropriate 7th character for subsequent care for encounters after the patient has completed active treatment of the fracture and is receiving routine care for the fracture during the healing or recovery phase.

Care for complications of surgical treatment for fracture repairs during the healing or recovery phase should be coded with the appropriate complication codes.

Care of complications of fractures, such as malunion and nonunion, should be reported with the appropriate 7th character for subsequent care with nonunion (K, M, N,) or subsequent care with malunion (P, Q, R).

Malunion/nonunion: The appropriate 7th character for initial encounter should also be assigned for a patient who delayed seeking treatment for the fracture or nonunion.

Female patient fell during a forest hiking excursion almost six months ago and until recently did not feel she needed to seek medical attention for her left ankle pain; x-rays show nonunion of lateral malleolus and surgery has been scheduled

S82.62XA	**Displaced fracture of lateral malleolus of left fibula, initial encounter for closed fracture**
W01.0XXA	**Fall on same level from slipping, tripping and stumbling without subsequent striking against object, initial encounter**
Y92.821	**Forest as place of occurrence of the external cause**
Y93.01	**Activity, walking, marching and hiking**
Y99.8	**Other external cause status**

Explanation: A seventh character of A is used for the lateral malleolus nonunion fracture to signify that the fracture is receiving active treatment. The delayed care for the fracture has resulted in a nonunion, but capturing the nonunion in the seventh character is trumped by the provision of active care.

The open fracture designations in the assignment of the 7th character for fractures of the forearm, femur and lower leg, including ankle are based on the Gustilo open fracture classification. When the Gustilo classification type is not specified for an open fracture, the 7th character for open fracture type I or II should be assigned (B, E, H, M, Q).

A 17-year-old arrives at the trauma center with open, displaced right forearm fracture with extensive soft tissue damage. He fell while being tackled playing football for his high school team. On-call orthopaedic specialist documents segmental type IIIA fracture of radial shaft with no need for plastic consult.

S52.361C	**Displaced segmental fracture of shaft of radius, right arm, initial encounter for open fracture type IIIA, IIIB, or IIIC**
W03.XXXA	**Other fall on same level due to collision with another person, initial encounter**
Y92.321	**Football field as the place of occurrence of the external cause**
Y93.61	**Activity, American tackle football**

Explanation: The seventh character for forearm fractures capture the type of encounter and whether the fracture is open or closed; open fractures are broken down further by the type of fracture based on the Gustilo classification. The Gustilo classification describes the severity of open fracture and soft tissue injury. Type IIIA describes an open fracture with extensive soft tissue injury but adequate soft tissue remaining for wound coverage. A segmental fracture means that the bone is broken in two places, leaving at least one segment unattached to the bone. There is no need to report an additional code for the soft tissue injury as it is captured in the fracture code.

A code from category M80, not a traumatic fracture code, should be used for any patient with known osteoporosis who suffers a fracture, even if the patient had a minor fall or trauma, if that fall or trauma would not usually break a normal, healthy bone.

See Section I.C.13. Osteoporosis.

The aftercare Z codes should not be used for aftercare for traumatic fractures. For aftercare of a traumatic fracture, assign the acute fracture code with the appropriate 7th character.

2) Multiple fractures sequencing

Multiple fractures are sequenced in accordance with the severity of the fracture.

3) Physeal fractures

For physeal fractures, assign only the code identifying the type of physeal fracture. Do not assign a separate code to identify the specific bone that is fractured.

d. Coding of burns and corrosions

The ICD-10-CM makes a distinction between burns and corrosions. The burn codes are for thermal burns, except sunburns, that come from a heat source, such as a fire or hot appliance. The burn codes are also for burns resulting from electricity and radiation. Corrosions are burns due to chemicals. The guidelines are the same for burns and corrosions.

Current burns (T20-T25) are classified by depth, extent and by agent (X code). Burns are classified by depth as first degree (erythema), second degree (blistering), and third degree (full-thickness involvement). Burns of the eye and internal organs (T26-T28) are classified by site, but not by degree.

1) Sequencing of burn and related condition codes

Sequence first the code that reflects the highest degree of burn when more than one burn is present.

   a. When the reason for the admission or encounter is for treatment of external multiple burns, sequence first the code that reflects the burn of the highest degree.

   b. When a patient has both internal and external burns, the circumstances of admission govern the selection of the principal diagnosis or first-listed diagnosis.

   c. When a patient is admitted for burn injuries and other related conditions such as smoke inhalation and/or respiratory failure, the circumstances of admission govern the selection of the principal or first-listed diagnosis.

Patient admitted with minor first-degree burns to multiple sites of her right and left hands as well as severe smoke inhalation. While she was sleeping at home, a candle on her dresser lit the bedroom curtains on fire.

T59.811A	**Toxic effect of smoke, accidental (unintentional), initial encounter**
J70.5	**Respiratory conditions due to smoke inhalation**
T23.191A	**Burn of first degree of multiple sites of right wrist and hand, initial encounter**
T23.192A	**Burn of first degree of multiple sites of left wrist and hand, initial encounter**
X08.8XXA	**Exposure to other specified smoke, fire and flames, initial encounter**
Y92.003	**Bedroom of unspecified non-institutional (private) residence as the place of occurrence of the external cause**
Y93.84	**Activity, sleeping**

Explanation: Based on the documentation, the inhalation injury is more severe than the first-degree burns and is sequenced first. The burns to the hands are appended as secondary diagnoses.

2) Burns of the same anatomic site

Classify burns of the same anatomic site and on the same side but of different degrees to the subcategory identifying the highest degree recorded in the diagnosis (e.g., for second and third degree burns of right thigh, assign only code T24.311-).

3) Non-healing burns

Non-healing burns are coded as acute burns.

Necrosis of burned skin should be coded as a non-healed burn.

4) Infected burn

For any documented infected burn site, use an additional code for the infection.

5) Assign separate codes for each burn site

When coding burns, assign separate codes for each burn site. Category T30, Burn and corrosion, body region unspecified is extremely vague and should rarely be used.

Codes for burns of "multiple sites" should only be assigned when the medical record documentation does not specify the individual sites.

> Patient is admitted with third-degree burns of the scalp as well as second-degree burns to the back of the right hand
>
> **T20.35XA**   **Burn of third degree of scalp [any part], initial encounter**
>
> **T23.261A**   **Burn of second degree of back of right hand, initial encounter**
>
> *Explanation:* Two codes may be reported as the hand and face represent distinct burn sites.

6) **Burns and corrosions classified according to extent of body surface involved**

Assign codes from category T31, Burns classified according to extent of body surface involved, or T32, Corrosions classified according to extent of body surface involved, when the site of the burn is not specified or when there is a need for additional data. It is advisable to use category T31 as additional coding when needed to provide data for evaluating burn mortality, such as that needed by burn units. It is also advisable to use category T31 as an additional code for reporting purposes when there is mention of a third-degree burn involving 20 percent or more of the body surface.

Categories T31 and T32 are based on the classic "rule of nines" in estimating body surface involved: head and neck are assigned nine percent, each arm nine percent, each leg 18 percent, the anterior trunk 18 percent, posterior trunk 18 percent, and genitalia one percent. Providers may change these percentage assignments where necessary to accommodate infants and children who have proportionately larger heads than adults, and patients who have large buttocks, thighs, or abdomen that involve burns.

> Patient seen in burn unit for dressing change after he accidentally spilled acetic acid on himself two days ago. The second-degree burns to his right thigh, covering about 3 percent of his body surface, are healing appropriately.
>
> **T54.2X1D**   **Toxic effect of corrosive acids and acid-like substances, accidental (unintentional), subsequent encounter**
>
> **T24.611D**   **Corrosion of second degree of right thigh, subsequent encounter**
>
> **T32.0**   **Corrosions involving less than 10% of body surface**
>
> *Explanation:* Code T32.0 provides additional information as to how much of the patient's body was affected by the corrosive substance.

7) **Encounters for treatment of sequela of burns**

Encounters for the treatment of the late effects of burns or corrosions (i.e., scars or joint contractures) should be coded with a burn or corrosion code with the 7th character "S" for sequela.

8) **Sequelae with a late effect code and current burn**

When appropriate, both a code for a current burn or corrosion with 7th character "A" or "D" and a burn or corrosion code with 7th character "S" may be assigned on the same record (when both a current burn and sequelae of an old burn exist). Burns and corrosions do not heal at the same rate and a current healing wound may still exist with sequela of a healed burn or corrosion.

See Section I.B.10 Sequela (Late Effects)

> Female patient seen in ED for second-degree burn to the left ear; she also has significant scarring on her left elbow from a third-degree burn from childhood
>
> **T20.212A**   **Burn of second degree of left ear [any part, except ear drum], initial encounter**
>
> **L90.5**   **Scar conditions and fibrosis of skin**
>
> **T22.322S**   **Burn of third degree of left elbow, sequela**
>
> *Explanation:* The patient is being seen for management of a current second-degree burn, which is reflected in the code by appending the seventh character of A, indicating active treatment or management of this burn. The elbow scarring is a sequela of a previous third-degree burn. The sequela condition precedes the original burn injury, which is appended with a seventh character of S.

9) **Use of an external cause code with burns and corrosions**

An external cause code should be used with burns and corrosions to identify the source and intent of the burn, as well as the place where it occurred.

e. **Adverse effects, poisoning, underdosing and toxic effects**

Codes in categories T36-T65 are combination codes that include the substance that was taken as well as the intent. No additional external cause code is required for poisonings, toxic effects, adverse effects and underdosing codes.

1) **Do not code directly from the Table of Drugs**

Do not code directly from the Table of Drugs and Chemicals. Always refer back to the Tabular List.

2) **Use as many codes as necessary to describe**

Use as many codes as necessary to describe completely all drugs, medicinal or biological substances.

3) **If the same code would describe the causative agent**

If the same code would describe the causative agent for more than one adverse reaction, poisoning, toxic effect or underdosing, assign the code only once.

4) **If two or more drugs, medicinal or biological substances**

If two or more drugs, medicinal or biological substances are taken, code each individually unless a combination code is listed in the Table of Drugs and Chemicals.

If multiple unspecified drugs, medicinal or biological substances were taken, assign the appropriate code from subcategory T50.91, Poisoning by, adverse effect of and underdosing of multiple unspecified drugs, medicaments and biological substances.

5) **The occurrence of drug toxicity is classified in ICD-10-CM as follows:**
(a) **Adverse effect**

When coding an adverse effect of a drug that has been correctly prescribed and properly administered, assign the appropriate code for the nature of the adverse effect followed by the appropriate code for the adverse effect of the drug (T36-T50). The code for the drug should have a 5th or 6th character "5" (for example T36.0X5-) Examples of the nature of an adverse effect are tachycardia, delirium, gastrointestinal hemorrhaging, vomiting, hypokalemia, hepatitis, renal failure, or respiratory failure.

> Patient admitted for stomach pain and jaundice, indicated by physician as possible side-effects of Inderal, recently started for hypertension. Inderal was discontinued and the patient switched to Atenolol instead.
>
> **R10.9**   **Unspecified abdominal pain**
>
> **R17**   **Unspecified jaundice**
>
> **T44.7X5A**   **Adverse effect of beta-adrenoreceptor antagonists, initial encounter**
>
> **I10**   **Essential (primary) hypertension**
>
> *Explanation:* The side-effects caused by the drug are listed first, followed by the code for the adverse effect of the drug to capture the specific drug that was used.

(b) **Poisoning**

When coding a poisoning or reaction to the improper use of a medication (e.g., overdose, wrong substance given or taken in error, wrong route of administration), first assign the appropriate code from categories T36-T50. The poisoning codes have an associated intent as their 5th or 6th character (accidental, intentional self-harm, assault and undetermined. If the intent of the poisoning is unknown or unspecified, code the intent as accidental intent. The undetermined intent is only for use if the documentation in the record specifies that the intent cannot be determined. Use additional code(s) for all manifestations of poisonings.

A 55-year-old female status post recent left knee replacement is admitted due to confusion, dizziness, and nausea. Her spouse brought in her prescribed Xanax, Ambien, and Percocet bottles but has no idea how many she took. It is suspected that her symptoms are due to an overdose of these medications.

T42.4X1A	Poisoning by benzodiazepines, accidental (unintentional), initial encounter
T42.6X1A	Poisoning by other antiepileptic and sedative-hypnotic drugs, accidental (unintentional), initial encounter
T40.2X1A	Poisoning by other opioids, accidental (unintentional), initial encounter
R41.0	Disorientation, unspecified
R42	Dizziness and giddiness
R11.0	Nausea

Explanation: It was not documented whether the overdose of the drugs was accidental or intentional; therefore the correct reporting of the poisoning codes is accidental intent. The poisoning codes are sequenced first, followed by manifestations of the poisoning.

If there is also a diagnosis of abuse or dependence of the substance, the abuse or dependence is assigned as an additional code.

Examples of poisoning include:

(i)   Error was made in drug prescription

Errors made in drug prescription or in the administration of the drug by provider, nurse, patient, or other person.

(ii   Overdose of a drug intentionally taken

If an overdose of a drug was intentionally taken or administered and resulted in drug toxicity, it would be coded as a poisoning.

(iii)   Nonprescribed drug taken with correctly prescribed and properly administered drug

If a nonprescribed drug or medicinal agent was taken in combination with a correctly prescribed and properly administered drug, any drug toxicity or other reaction resulting from the interaction of the two drugs would be classified as a poisoning.

(iv)   Interaction of drug(s) and alcohol

When a reaction results from the interaction of a drug(s) and alcohol, this would be classified as poisoning.

See Section I.C.4. if poisoning is the result of insulin pump malfunctions.

(c) Underdosing

Underdosing refers to taking less of a medication than is prescribed by a provider or a manufacturer's instruction. Discontinuing the use of a prescribed medication on the patient's own initiative (not directed by the patient's provider) is also classified as an underdosing. For underdosing, assign the code from categories T36-T50 (fifth or sixth character "6").

Codes for underdosing should never be assigned as principal or first-listed codes. If a patient has a relapse or exacerbation of the medical condition for which the drug is prescribed because of the reduction in dose, then the medical condition itself should be coded.

Noncompliance (Z91.12-, Z91.13- and Z91.14-) or complication of care (Y63.6-Y63.9) codes are to be used with an underdosing code to indicate intent, if known.

Patient admitted for atrial fibrillation with history of chronic atrial fibrillation for which she is prescribed amiodarone. Financial concerns have left the patient unable to pay for her prescriptions and she has been skipping her amiodarone dose every other day to offset the cost.

I48.20	Chronic atrial fibrillation, unspecified
T46.2X6A	Underdosing of other antidysrhythmic drugs, initial encounter
Z91.120	Patient's intentional underdosing of medication regimen due to financial hardship

Explanation: By skipping her amiodarone pill every other day, the patient's atrial fibrillation returned. The condition for which the drug was being taken is reported first, followed by an underdosing code to show that the patient was not adhering to her prescription regimen. The Z code helps elaborate on the patient's social and/or economic circumstances that led to the patient taking less then what she was prescribed.

(d) Toxic effects

When a harmful substance is ingested or comes in contact with a person, this is classified as a toxic effect. The toxic effect codes are in categories T51-T65.

Toxic effect codes have an associated intent: accidental, intentional self-harm, assault and undetermined.

f.   Adult and child abuse, neglect and other maltreatment

Sequence first the appropriate code from categories T74.- (Adult and child abuse, neglect and other maltreatment, confirmed) or T76.- (Adult and child abuse, neglect and other maltreatment, suspected) for abuse, neglect and other maltreatment, followed by any accompanying mental health or injury code(s).

If the documentation in the medical record states abuse or neglect it is coded as confirmed (T74.-). It is coded as suspected if it is documented as suspected (T76.-).

For cases of confirmed abuse or neglect an external cause code from the assault section (X92-Y09) should be added to identify the cause of any physical injuries. A perpetrator code (Y07) should be added when the perpetrator of the abuse is known. For suspected cases of abuse or neglect, do not report external cause or perpetrator code.

If a suspected case of abuse, neglect or mistreatment is ruled out during an encounter code Z04.71, Encounter for examination and observation following alleged physical adult abuse, ruled out, or code Z04.72, Encounter for examination and observation following alleged child physical abuse, ruled out, should be used, not a code from T76.

If a suspected case of alleged rape or sexual abuse is ruled out during an encounter code Z04.41, Encounter for examination and observation following alleged adult rape or code Z04.42, Encounter for examination and observation following alleged child rape, should be used, not a code from T76.

If a suspected case of forced sexual exploitation or forced labor exploitation is ruled out during an encounter, code Z04.81, Encounter for examination and observation of victim following forced sexual exploitation, or code Z04.82, Encounter for examination and observation of victim following forced labor exploitation, should be used, not a code from T76.

See Section I.C.15. Abuse in a pregnant patient.

g.   Complications of care

1)   General guidelines for complications of care

(a) Documentation of complications of care

See Section I.B.16. for information on documentation of complications of care.

2)   Pain due to medical devices

Pain associated with devices, implants or grafts left in a surgical site (for example painful hip prosthesis) is assigned to the appropriate code(s) found in Chapter 19, Injury, poisoning, and certain other consequences of external causes. Specific codes for pain due to medical devices are found in the T code section of the ICD-10-CM. Use additional code(s) from category G89 to identify acute or chronic pain due to presence of the device, implant or graft (G89.18 or G89.28).

Chronic left breast pain secondary to breast implant

T85.848A	**Pain due to other internal prosthetic devices, implants and grafts, initial encounter**
N64.4	**Mastodynia**
G89.28	**Other chronic postprocedural pain**

Explanation: As the pain is a complication related to the breast implant, the complication code is sequenced first. The T code does not describe the site or type of pain, so additional codes may be appended to indicate that the patient is experiencing chronic pain in the breast.

3) Transplant complications

(a) Transplant complications other than kidney

Codes under category T86, Complications of transplanted organs and tissues, are for use for both complications and rejection of transplanted organs. A transplant complication code is only assigned if the complication affects the function of the transplanted organ. Two codes are required to fully describe a transplant complication: the appropriate code from category T86 and a secondary code that identifies the complication.

Pre-existing conditions or conditions that develop after the transplant are not coded as complications unless they affect the function of the transplanted organs.

See I.C.21. for transplant organ removal status

See I.C.2. for malignant neoplasm associated with transplanted organ.

(b) Kidney transplant complications

Patients who have undergone kidney transplant may still have some form of chronic kidney disease (CKD) because the kidney transplant may not fully restore kidney function. Code T86.1- should be assigned for documented complications of a kidney transplant, such as transplant failure or rejection or other transplant complication. Code T86.1- should not be assigned for post kidney transplant patients who have chronic kidney (CKD) unless a transplant complication such as transplant failure or rejection is documented. If the documentation is unclear as to whether the patient has a complication of the transplant, query the provider.

Conditions that affect the function of the transplanted kidney, other than CKD, should be assigned a code from subcategory T86.1, Complications of transplanted organ, Kidney, and a secondary code that identifies the complication.

For patients with CKD following a kidney transplant, but who do not have a complication such as failure or rejection, *see section I.C.14. Chronic kidney disease and kidney transplant status.*

Patient with chronic kidney disease stage 2; history of successful kidney transplant with no complications identified

N18.2	**Chronic kidney disease, stage 2 (mild)**
Z94.0	**Kidney transplant status**

Explanation: This patient's stage 2 CKD is not indicated as being due to the transplanted kidney but instead is just the residual disease the patient had prior to the transplant.

4) Complication codes that include the external cause

As with certain other T codes, some of the complications of care codes have the external cause included in the code. The code includes the nature of the complication as well as the type of procedure that caused the complication. No external cause code indicating the type of procedure is necessary for these codes.

5) Complications of care codes within the body system chapters

Intraoperative and postprocedural complication codes are found within the body system chapters with codes specific to the organs and structures of that body system. These codes should be sequenced first, followed by a code(s) for the specific complication, if applicable.

Complication codes from the body system chapters should be assigned for intraoperative and postprocedural complications (e.g., the appropriate complication code from chapter 9 would be assigned for a vascular intraoperative or postprocedural complication) unless the complication is specifically indexed to a T code in chapter 19.

During a spinal fusion procedure, the surgeon inadvertently punctured the dura. The midline durotomy was repaired, and the fusion procedure was completed.

G97.41	**Accidental puncture or laceration of dura during a procedure**

Explanation: The accidental durotomy is not coded to an injury code in chapter 19 but instead is categorized to the nervous system chapter.

Muscle/Tendon Table

ICD-10-CM categorizes certain muscles and tendons in the upper and lower extremities by their action (e.g., extension, flexion), their anatomical location (e.g., posterior, anterior), and/or whether they are intrinsic or extrinsic to a certain anatomical area. The Muscle/Tendon Table is provided at the beginning of chapters 13 and 19 as a resource to help users when code selection depends on one or more of these characteristics. Please note that this table is not all-inclusive, and proper code assignment should be based on the provider's documentation.

Body Region	Muscle	Extensor Tendon	Flexor Tendon	Other Tendon
Shoulder				
	Deltoid	Posterior deltoid	Anterior deltoid	
	Rotator cuff			
	Infraspinatus			Infraspinatus
	Subscapularis			Subscapularis
	Supraspinatus			Supraspinatus
	Teres minor			Teres minor
	Teres major	Teres major		
Upper arm				
	Anterior muscles			
	Biceps brachii — long head		Biceps brachii — long head	
	Biceps brachii — short head		Biceps brachii — short head	
	Brachialis		Brachialis	
	Coracobrachialis		Coracobrachialis	
	Posterior muscles			
	Triceps brachii	Triceps brachii		
Forearm				
	Anterior muscles			
	Flexors			
	Deep			
	Flexor digitorum profundus		Flexor digitorum profundus	
	Flexor pollicis longus		Flexor pollicis longus	
	Intermediate			
	Flexor digitorum superficialis		Flexor digitorum superficialis	
	Superficial			
	Flexor carpi radialis		Flexor carpi radialis	
	Flexor carpi ulnaris		Flexor carpi ulnaris	
	Palmaris longus		Palmaris longus	
	Pronators			
	Pronator quadratus			Pronator quadratus
	Pronator teres			Pronator teres
	Posterior muscles			
	Extensors			
	Deep			
	Abductor pollicis longus			Abductor pollicis longus
	Extensor indicis	Extensor indicis		
	Extensor pollicis brevis	Extensor pollicis brevis		
	Extensor pollicis longus	Extensor pollicis longus		
	Superficial			
	Brachioradialis			Brachioradialis
	Extensor carpi radialis brevis	Extensor carpi radialis brevis		
	Extensor carpi radialis longus	Extensor carpi radialis longus		
	Extensor carpi ulnaris	Extensor carpi ulnaris		
	Extensor digiti minimi	Extensor digiti minimi		
	Extensor digitorum	Extensor digitorum		
	Anconeus	Anconeus		
	Supinator			Supinator

Body Region	Muscle	Extensor Tendon	Flexor Tendon	Other Tendon
Hand				
Extrinsic — attach to a site in the forearm as well as a site in the hand with action related to hand movement at the wrist				
	Extensor carpi radialis brevis	Extensor carpi radialis brevis		
	Extensor carpi radialis longus	Extensor carpi radialis longus		
	Extensor carpi ulnaris	Extensor carpi ulnaris		
	Flexor carpi radialis		Flexor carpi radialis	
	Flexor carpi ulnaris		Flexor carpi ulnaris	
	Flexor digitorum superficialis		Flexor digitorum superficialis	
	Palmaris longus		Palmaris longus	
Extrinsic — attach to a site in the forearm as well as a site in the hand with action in the hand related to finger movement				
	Adductor pollicis longus			Adductor pollicis longus
	Extensor digiti minimi	Extensor digiti minimi		
	Extensor digitorum	Extensor digitorum		
	Extensor indicis	Extensor indicis		
	Flexor digitorum profundus		Flexor digitorum profundus	
	Flexor digitorum superficialis		Flexor digitorum superficialis	
Extrinsic — attach to a site in the forearm as well as a site in the hand with action in the hand related to thumb movement				
	Extensor pollicis brevis	Extensor pollicis brevis		
	Extensor pollicis longus	Extensor pollicis longus		
	Flexor pollicis longus		Flexor pollicis longus	
Intrinsic — found within the hand only				
	Adductor pollicis			Adductor pollicis
	Dorsal interossei	Dorsal interossei	Dorsal interossei	
	Lumbricals	Lumbricals	Lumbricals	
	Palmaris brevis			Palmaris brevis
	Palmar interossei	Palmar interossei	Palmar interossei	
	Hypothenar muscles			
	Abductor digiti minimi			Abductor digiti minimi
	Flexor digiti minimi brevis		Flexor digiti minimi brevis	
	Opponens digiti minimi		Opponens digiti minimi	
	Thenar muscles			
	Abductor pollicis brevis			Abductor pollicis brevis
	Flexor pollicis brevis		Flexor pollicis brevis	
	Opponens pollicis		Opponens pollicis	
Thigh				
	Anterior muscles			
	Iliopsoas		Iliopsoas	
	Pectineus		Pectineus	
	Quadriceps	Quadriceps		
	Rectus femoris	Rectus femoris — Extends knee	Rectus femoris — Flexes hip	
	Vastus intermedius	Vastus intermedius		
	Vastus lateralis	Vastus lateralis		
	Vastus medialis	Vastus medialis		
	Sartorius		Sartorius	
	Medial muscles			
	Adductor brevis			Adductor brevis
	Adductor longus			Adductor longus
	Adductor magnus			Adductor magnus
	Gracilis			Gracilis
	Obturator externus			Obturator externus
	Posterior muscles			
	Hamstring	Hamstring — Extends hip	Hamstring — Flexes knee	
	Biceps femoris	Biceps femoris	Biceps femoris	
	Semimembranosus	Semimembranosus	Semimembranosus	
	Semitendinosus	Semitendinosus	Semitendinosus	

Body Region	Muscle	Extensor Tendon	Flexor Tendon	Other Tendon
Lower leg				
	Anterior muscles			
	Extensor digitorum longus	Extensor digitorum longus		
	Extensor hallucis longus	Extensor hallucis longus		
	Fibularis (peroneus) tertius	Fibularis (peroneus) tertius		
	Tibialis anterior	Tibialis anterior		Tibialis anterior
	Lateral muscles			
	Fibularis (peroneus) brevis		Fibularis (peroneus) brevis	
	Fibularis (peroneus) longus		Fibularis (peroneus) longus	
	Posterior muscles			
	Deep			
	Flexor digitorum longus		Flexor digitorum longus	
	Flexor hallucis longus		Flexor hallucis longus	
	Popliteus		Popliteus	
	Tibialis posterior		Tibialis posterior	
	Superficial			
	Gastrocnemius		Gastrocnemius	
	Plantaris		Plantaris	
	Soleus		Soleus	
				Calcaneal (Achilles)
Ankle/Foot				
Extrinsic — attach to a site in the lower leg as well as a site in the foot with action related to foot movement at the ankle				
	Plantaris		Plantaris	
	Soleus		Soleus	
	Tibialis anterior	Tibialis anterior		
	Tibialis posterior		Tibialis posterior	
Extrinsic — attach to a site in the lower leg as well as a site in the foot with action in the foot related to toe movement				
	Extensor digitorum longus	Extensor digitorum longus		
	Extensor hallucis longus	Extensor hallucis longus		
	Flexor digitorum longus		Flexor digitorum longus	
	Flexor hallucis longus		Flexor hallucis longus	
Intrinsic — found within the ankle/foot only				
	Dorsal muscles			
	Extensor digitorum brevis	Extensor digitorum brevis		
	Extensor hallucis brevis	Extensor hallucis brevis		
	Plantar muscles			
	Abductor digiti minimi		Abductor digiti minimi	
	Abductor hallucis		Abductor hallucis	
	Dorsal interossei	Dorsal interossei	Dorsal interossei	
	Flexor digiti minimi brevis		Flexor digiti minimi brevis	
	Flexor digitorum brevis		Flexor digitorum brevis	
	Flexor hallucis brevis		Flexor hallucis brevis	
	Lumbricals	Lumbricals	Lumbricals	
	Quadratus plantae		Quadratus plantae	
	Plantar interossei	Plantar interossei	Plantar interossei	

Chapter 19. Injury, Poisoning and Certain Other Consequences of External Causes (S00-T88)

NOTE   Use secondary code(s) from Chapter 20, External causes of morbidity, to indicate cause of injury. Codes within the T section that include the external cause do not require an additional external cause code.

Use additional code to identify any retained foreign body, if applicable (Z18.-)

EXCLUDES 1   birth trauma (P10-P15)
       obstetric trauma (O70-O71)

NOTE   The chapter uses the S-section for coding different types of injuries related to single body regions and the T-section to cover injuries to unspecified body regions as well as poisoning and certain other consequences of external causes.

AHA: 2016,2Q,3-7; 2015,4Q,35-38; 2015,3Q,37-39,40; 2015,2Q,6; 2015,1Q,3-21

TIP: The specific site of an injury can be determined from the radiology report when authenticated by a radiologist and available at the time of code assignment.

This chapter contains the following blocks:

S00-S09	Injuries to the head
S10-S19	Injuries to the neck
S20-S29	Injuries to the thorax
S30-S39	Injuries to the abdomen, lower back, lumbar spine, pelvis and external genitals
S40-S49	Injuries to the shoulder and upper arm
S50-S59	Injuries to the elbow and forearm
S60-S69	Injuries to the wrist, hand and fingers
S70-S79	Injuries to the hip and thigh
S80-S89	Injuries to the knee and lower leg
S90-S99	Injuries to the ankle and foot
T07	Injuries involving multiple body regions
T14	Injury of unspecified body region
T15-T19	Effects of foreign body entering through natural orifice
T20-T25	Burns and corrosions of external body surface, specified by site
T26-T28	Burns and corrosions confined to eye and internal organs
T30-T32	Burns and corrosions of multiple and unspecified body regions
T33-T34	Frostbite
T36-T50	Poisoning by, adverse effect of and underdosing of drugs, medicaments and biological substances
T51-T65	Toxic effects of substances chiefly nonmedicinal as to source
T66-T78	Other and unspecified effects of external causes
T79	Certain early complications of trauma
T80-T88	Complications of surgical and medical care, not elsewhere classified

Injuries to the head (S00-S09)

INCLUDES   injuries of ear
       injuries of eye
       injuries of face [any part]
       injuries of gum
       injuries of jaw
       injuries of oral cavity
       injuries of palate
       injuries of periocular area
       injuries of scalp
       injuries of temporomandibular joint area
       injuries of tongue
       injuries of tooth

Code also for any associated infection

EXCLUDES 2   burns and corrosions (T20-T32)
       effects of foreign body in ear (T16)
       effects of foreign body in larynx (T17.3)
       effects of foreign body in mouth NOS (T18.0)
       effects of foreign body in nose (T17.0-T17.1)
       effects of foreign body in pharynx (T17.2)
       effects of foreign body on external eye (T15.-)
       frostbite (T33-T34)
       insect bite or sting, venomous (T63.4)

✓4th **S00**   **Superficial injury of head**

   EXCLUDES 1   diffuse cerebral contusion (S06.2-)
           focal cerebral contusion (S06.3-)
           injury of eye and orbit (S05.-)
           open wound of head (S01.-)

The appropriate 7th character is to be added to each code from category S00.
A   initial encounter
D   subsequent encounter
S   sequela

✓5th **S00.0**   **Superficial injury of scalp**

   ✓x7th **S00.00**   Unspecified superficial injury of scalp

   ✓x7th **S00.01**   **Abrasion** of scalp

   ✓x7th **S00.02**   **Blister (nonthermal)** of scalp

   ✓x7th **S00.03**   **Contusion** of scalp
       Bruise of scalp
       Hematoma of scalp

   ✓x7th **S00.04**   **External constriction** of part of scalp

   ✓x7th **S00.05**   **Superficial foreign body** of scalp
       Splinter in the scalp

   ✓x7th **S00.06**   **Insect bite (nonvenomous)** of scalp

   ✓x7th **S00.07**   **Other superficial** bite of scalp
       EXCLUDES 1   open bite of scalp (S01.05)

✓5th **S00.1**   **Contusion of eyelid and periocular area**
    Black eye
   EXCLUDES 2   contusion of eyeball and orbital tissues (S05.1)

   ✓x7th **S00.10**   Contusion of unspecified eyelid and periocular area

   ✓x7th **S00.11**   Contusion of **right** eyelid and periocular area

   ✓x7th **S00.12**   Contusion of **left** eyelid and periocular area

✓5th **S00.2**   **Other and unspecified superficial injuries of eyelid and periocular area**
   EXCLUDES 2   superficial injury of conjunctiva and cornea (S05.0-)

   ✓6th **S00.20**   **Unspecified superficial injury of eyelid and periocular area**

     ✓7th **S00.201**   Unspecified superficial injury of **right** eyelid and periocular area

     ✓7th **S00.202**   Unspecified superficial injury of **left** eyelid and periocular area

     ✓7th **S00.209**   Unspecified superficial injury of unspecified eyelid and periocular area

   ✓6th **S00.21**   **Abrasion** of eyelid and periocular area

     ✓7th **S00.211**   Abrasion of **right** eyelid and periocular area

     ✓7th **S00.212**   Abrasion of **left** eyelid and periocular area

     ✓7th **S00.219**   Abrasion of unspecified eyelid and periocular area

   ✓6th **S00.22**   **Blister (nonthermal)** of eyelid and periocular area

     ✓7th **S00.221**   Blister (nonthermal) of **right** eyelid and periocular area

     ✓7th **S00.222**   Blister (nonthermal) of **left** eyelid and periocular area

     ✓7th **S00.229**   Blister (nonthermal) of unspecified eyelid and periocular area

   ✓6th **S00.24**   **External constriction** of eyelid and periocular area

     ✓7th **S00.241**   External constriction of **right** eyelid and periocular area

     ✓7th **S00.242**   External constriction of **left** eyelid and periocular area

     ✓7th **S00.249**   External constriction of unspecified eyelid and periocular area

   ✓6th **S00.25**   **Superficial foreign body** of eyelid and periocular area
     Splinter of eyelid and periocular area
     EXCLUDES 2   retained foreign body in eyelid (H02.81-)

     ✓7th **S00.251**   Superficial foreign body of **right** eyelid and periocular area

     ✓7th **S00.252**   Superficial foreign body of **left** eyelid and periocular area

     ✓7th **S00.259**   Superficial foreign body of unspecified eyelid and periocular area

   ✓6th **S00.26**   **Insect bite (nonvenomous)** of eyelid and periocular area

     ✓7th **S00.261**   Insect bite (nonvenomous) of **right** eyelid and periocular area

     ✓7th **S00.262**   Insect bite (nonvenomous) of **left** eyelid and periocular area

     ✓7th **S00.269**   Insect bite (nonvenomous) of unspecified eyelid and periocular area

   ✓6th **S00.27**   **Other superficial** bite of eyelid and periocular area
     EXCLUDES 1   open bite of eyelid and periocular area (S01.15)

     ✓7th **S00.271**   Other superficial bite of **right** eyelid and periocular area

     ✓7th **S00.272**   Other superficial bite of **left** eyelid and periocular area

     ✓7th **S00.279**   Other superficial bite of unspecified eyelid and periocular area

✓5th **S00.3**   **Superficial injury of nose**

   ✓x7th **S00.30**   Unspecified superficial injury of nose

   ✓x7th **S00.31**   **Abrasion** of nose

   ✓x7th **S00.32**   **Blister (nonthermal)** of nose

✓ Additional Character Required   ✓x7th Placeholder   Unacceptable PDx   Questionable PDx   Manifestation   Unspecified Dx   H1-H14 HAC   HCC CMS-HCC Dx   HIV HIV Dx

ICD-10-CM 2021   965

√x7th **S00.33** **Contusion** of nose
> Bruise of nose
> Hematoma of nose

√x7th **S00.34** **External constriction** of nose

√x7th **S00.35** **Superficial** foreign body of nose
> Splinter in the nose

√x7th **S00.36** **Insect bite** (nonvenomous) of nose

√x7th **S00.37** **Other superficial** bite of nose
> EXCLUDES 1   open bite of nose (S01.25)

√5th **S00.4** **Superficial injury** of ear

  √6th **S00.40** **Unspecified superficial injury** of ear

    √7th **S00.401** Unspecified superficial injury of right ear

    √7th **S00.402** Unspecified superficial injury of left ear

    √7th **S00.409** Unspecified superficial injury of unspecified ear

  √6th **S00.41** **Abrasion** of ear

    √7th **S00.411** Abrasion of right ear

    √7th **S00.412** Abrasion of left ear

    √7th **S00.419** Abrasion of unspecified ear

  √6th **S00.42** **Blister** (nonthermal) of ear

    √7th **S00.421** Blister (nonthermal) of right ear

    √7th **S00.422** Blister (nonthermal) of left ear

    √7th **S00.429** Blister (nonthermal) of unspecified ear

  √6th **S00.43** **Contusion** of ear
> Bruise of ear
> Hematoma of ear

    √7th **S00.431** Contusion of right ear

    √7th **S00.432** Contusion of left ear

    √7th **S00.439** Contusion of unspecified ear

  √6th **S00.44** **External constriction** of ear

    √7th **S00.441** External constriction of right ear

    √7th **S00.442** External constriction of left ear

    √7th **S00.449** External constriction of unspecified ear

  √6th **S00.45** **Superficial** foreign body of ear
> Splinter in the ear

    √7th **S00.451** Superficial foreign body of right ear

    √7th **S00.452** Superficial foreign body of left ear

    √7th **S00.459** Superficial foreign body of unspecified ear

  √6th **S00.46** **Insect bite** (nonvenomous) of ear

    √7th **S00.461** Insect bite (nonvenomous) of right ear

    √7th **S00.462** Insect bite (nonvenomous) of left ear

    √7th **S00.469** Insect bite (nonvenomous) of unspecified ear

  √6th **S00.47** **Other superficial** bite of ear
> EXCLUDES 1   open bite of ear (S01.35)

    √7th **S00.471** Other superficial bite of right ear

    √7th **S00.472** Other superficial bite of left ear

    √7th **S00.479** Other superficial bite of unspecified ear

√5th **S00.5** **Superficial injury** of lip and oral cavity

  √6th **S00.50** **Unspecified superficial injury** of lip and oral cavity

    √7th **S00.501** Unspecified superficial injury of lip

    √7th **S00.502** Unspecified superficial injury of oral cavity

  √6th **S00.51** **Abrasion** of lip and oral cavity

    √7th **S00.511** Abrasion of lip

    √7th **S00.512** Abrasion of oral cavity

  √6th **S00.52** **Blister** (nonthermal) of lip and oral cavity

    √7th **S00.521** Blister (nonthermal) of lip

    √7th **S00.522** Blister (nonthermal) of oral cavity

  √6th **S00.53** **Contusion** of lip and oral cavity

    √7th **S00.531** Contusion of lip
> Bruise of lip
> Hematoma of lip

    √7th **S00.532** Contusion of oral cavity
> Bruise of oral cavity
> Hematoma of oral cavity

  √6th **S00.54** **External constriction** of lip and oral cavity

    √7th **S00.541** External constriction of lip

    √7th **S00.542** External constriction of oral cavity

  √6th **S00.55** **Superficial** foreign body of lip and oral cavity

    √7th **S00.551** Superficial foreign body of lip
> Splinter of lip and oral cavity

    √7th **S00.552** Superficial foreign body of oral cavity
> Splinter of lip and oral cavity

  √6th **S00.56** **Insect bite** (nonvenomous) of lip and oral cavity

    √7th **S00.561** Insect bite (nonvenomous) of lip

    √7th **S00.562** Insect bite (nonvenomous) of oral cavity

  √6th **S00.57** **Other superficial** bite of lip and oral cavity

    √7th **S00.571** Other superficial bite of lip
> EXCLUDES 1   open bite of lip (S01.551)

    √7th **S00.572** Other superficial bite of oral cavity
> EXCLUDES 1   open bite of oral cavity (S01.552)

√5th **S00.8** **Superficial injury** of other parts of head
> Superficial injuries of face [any part]

√x7th **S00.80** **Unspecified superficial injury** of other part of head

√x7th **S00.81** **Abrasion** of other part of head

√x7th **S00.82** **Blister** (nonthermal) of other part of head

√x7th **S00.83** **Contusion** of other part of head
> Bruise of other part of head
> Hematoma of other part of head

√x7th **S00.84** **External constriction** of other part of head

√x7th **S00.85** **Superficial** foreign body of other part of head
> Splinter in other part of head

√x7th **S00.86** **Insect bite** (nonvenomous) of other part of head

√x7th **S00.87** **Other superficial** bite of other part of head
> EXCLUDES 1   open bite of other part of head (S01.85)

√5th **S00.9** **Superficial injury** of unspecified part of head

√x7th **S00.90** **Unspecified superficial injury** of unspecified part of head

√x7th **S00.91** **Abrasion** of unspecified part of head

√x7th **S00.92** **Blister** (nonthermal) of unspecified part of head

√x7th **S00.93** **Contusion** of unspecified part of head
> Bruise of head
> Hematoma of head

√x7th **S00.94** **External constriction** of unspecified part of head

√x7th **S00.95** **Superficial** foreign body of unspecified part of head
> Splinter of head

√x7th **S00.96** **Insect bite** (nonvenomous) of unspecified part of head

√x7th **S00.97** **Other superficial** bite of unspecified part of head
> EXCLUDES 1   open bite of head (S01.95)

√4th **S01** **Open wound of head**
> Code also any associated:
>   injury of cranial nerve (S04.-)
>   injury of muscle and tendon of head (S09.1-)
>   intracranial injury (S06.-)
>   wound infection
> EXCLUDES 1   open skull fracture (S02.- with 7th character B)
> EXCLUDES 2   injury of eye and orbit (S05.-)
>   traumatic amputation of part of head (S08.-)

> The appropriate 7th character is to be added to each code from category S01.
> A   initial encounter
> D   subsequent encounter
> S   sequela

√6th **S01.0** **Open wound of scalp**
> EXCLUDES 1   avulsion of scalp (S08.0)

√x7th **S01.00** **Unspecified open wound of scalp**

√x7th **S01.01** **Laceration without foreign body** of scalp

√x7th **S01.02** **Laceration with foreign body** of scalp

√x7th **S01.03** **Puncture wound without foreign body** of scalp

√x7th **S01.04** **Puncture wound with foreign body** of scalp

√x7th **S01.05** **Open bite** of scalp
> Bite of scalp NOS
> EXCLUDES 1   superficial bite of scalp (S00.06, S00.07-)

√5ᵗʰ **S01.1** **Open wound of** eyelid and periocular area

Open wound of eyelid and periocular area with or without involvement of lacrimal passages

√6ᵗʰ **S01.10** **Unspecified open wound of eyelid and periocular area**

√7ᵗʰ **S01.101** **Unspecified open wound of** right **eyelid and periocular area** cc

√7ᵗʰ **S01.102** **Unspecified open wound of** left **eyelid and periocular area** cc

√7ᵗʰ **S01.109** **Unspecified open wound of unspecified eyelid and periocular area** cc

√6ᵗʰ **S01.11** **Laceration without foreign body of eyelid and periocular area**

√7ᵗʰ **S01.111** **Laceration without foreign body of** right **eyelid and periocular area**

√7ᵗʰ **S01.112** **Laceration without foreign body of** left **eyelid and periocular area**

√7ᵗʰ **S01.119** **Laceration without foreign body of unspecified eyelid and periocular area**

√6ᵗʰ **S01.12** **Laceration with foreign body of eyelid and periocular area**

√7ᵗʰ **S01.121** **Laceration with foreign body of** right **eyelid and periocular area**

√7ᵗʰ **S01.122** **Laceration with foreign body of** left **eyelid and periocular area**

√7ᵗʰ **S01.129** **Laceration with foreign body of unspecified eyelid and periocular area**

√6ᵗʰ **S01.13** **Puncture wound without foreign body of eyelid and periocular area**

√7ᵗʰ **S01.131** **Puncture wound without foreign body of** right **eyelid and periocular area**

√7ᵗʰ **S01.132** **Puncture wound without foreign body of** left **eyelid and periocular area**

√7ᵗʰ **S01.139** **Puncture wound without foreign body of unspecified eyelid and periocular area**

√6ᵗʰ **S01.14** **Puncture wound with foreign body of eyelid and periocular area**

√7ᵗʰ **S01.141** **Puncture wound with foreign body of** right **eyelid and periocular area**

√7ᵗʰ **S01.142** **Puncture wound with foreign body of** left **eyelid and periocular area**

√7ᵗʰ **S01.149** **Puncture wound with foreign body of unspecified eyelid and periocular area**

√6ᵗʰ **S01.15** **Open bite of eyelid and periocular area**

Bite of eyelid and periocular area NOS

EXCLUDES 1   *superficial bite of eyelid and periocular area (S00.26, S00.27)*

√7ᵗʰ **S01.151** **Open bite of** right **eyelid and periocular area**

√7ᵗʰ **S01.152** **Open bite of** left **eyelid and periocular area**

√7ᵗʰ **S01.159** **Open bite of unspecified eyelid and periocular area**

√5ᵗʰ **S01.2** **Open wound of** nose

√x7ᵗʰ **S01.20** **Unspecified open wound of nose**

√x7ᵗʰ **S01.21** **Laceration without foreign body of nose**

√x7ᵗʰ **S01.22** **Laceration with foreign body of nose**

√x7ᵗʰ **S01.23** **Puncture wound without foreign body of nose**

√x7ᵗʰ **S01.24** **Puncture wound with foreign body of nose**

√x7ᵗʰ **S01.25** **Open bite of nose**

Bite of nose NOS

EXCLUDES 1   *superficial bite of nose (S00.36, S00.37)*

√5ᵗʰ **S01.3** **Open wound of** ear

√6ᵗʰ **S01.30** **Unspecified open wound of ear**

√7ᵗʰ **S01.301** **Unspecified open wound of** right **ear**

√7ᵗʰ **S01.302** **Unspecified open wound of** left **ear**

√7ᵗʰ **S01.309** **Unspecified open wound of unspecified ear**

√6ᵗʰ **S01.31** **Laceration without foreign body of ear**

√7ᵗʰ **S01.311** **Laceration without foreign body of** right **ear**

√7ᵗʰ **S01.312** **Laceration without foreign body of** left **ear**

√7ᵗʰ **S01.319** **Laceration without foreign body of unspecified ear**

√6ᵗʰ **S01.32** **Laceration with foreign body of ear**

√7ᵗʰ **S01.321** **Laceration with foreign body of** right **ear**

√7ᵗʰ **S01.322** **Laceration with foreign body of** left **ear**

√7ᵗʰ **S01.329** **Laceration with foreign body of unspecified ear**

√6ᵗʰ **S01.33** **Puncture wound without foreign body of ear**

√7ᵗʰ **S01.331** **Puncture wound without foreign body of** right **ear**

√7ᵗʰ **S01.332** **Puncture wound without foreign body of** left **ear**

√7ᵗʰ **S01.339** **Puncture wound without foreign body of unspecified ear**

√6ᵗʰ **S01.34** **Puncture wound with foreign body of ear**

√7ᵗʰ **S01.341** **Puncture wound with foreign body of** right **ear**

√7ᵗʰ **S01.342** **Puncture wound with foreign body of** left **ear**

√7ᵗʰ **S01.349** **Puncture wound with foreign body of unspecified ear**

√6ᵗʰ **S01.35** **Open bite of ear**

Bite of ear NOS

EXCLUDES 1   *superficial bite of ear (S00.46, S00.47)*

√7ᵗʰ **S01.351** **Open bite of** right **ear**

√7ᵗʰ **S01.352** **Open bite of** left **ear**

√7ᵗʰ **S01.359** **Open bite of unspecified ear**

√5ᵗʰ **S01.4** **Open wound of** cheek and temporomandibular area

√6ᵗʰ **S01.40** **Unspecified open wound of cheek and temporomandibular area**

√7ᵗʰ **S01.401** **Unspecified open wound of** right **cheek and temporomandibular area**

√7ᵗʰ **S01.402** **Unspecified open wound of** left **cheek and temporomandibular area**

√7ᵗʰ **S01.409** **Unspecified open wound of unspecified cheek and temporomandibular area**

√6ᵗʰ **S01.41** **Laceration without foreign body of cheek and temporomandibular area**

√7ᵗʰ **S01.411** **Laceration without foreign body of** right **cheek and temporomandibular area**

√7ᵗʰ **S01.412** **Laceration without foreign body of** left **cheek and temporomandibular area**

√7ᵗʰ **S01.419** **Laceration without foreign body of unspecified cheek and temporomandibular area**

√6ᵗʰ **S01.42** **Laceration with foreign body of cheek and temporomandibular area**

√7ᵗʰ **S01.421** **Laceration with foreign body of** right **cheek and temporomandibular area**

√7ᵗʰ **S01.422** **Laceration with foreign body of** left **cheek and temporomandibular area**

√7ᵗʰ **S01.429** **Laceration with foreign body of unspecified cheek and temporomandibular area**

√6ᵗʰ **S01.43** **Puncture wound without foreign body of cheek and temporomandibular area**

√7ᵗʰ **S01.431** **Puncture wound without foreign body of** right **cheek and temporomandibular area**

√7ᵗʰ **S01.432** **Puncture wound without foreign body of** left **cheek and temporomandibular area**

√7ᵗʰ **S01.439** **Puncture wound without foreign body of unspecified cheek and temporomandibular area**

√6ᵗʰ **S01.44** **Puncture wound with foreign body of cheek and temporomandibular area**

√7ᵗʰ **S01.441** **Puncture wound with foreign body of** right **cheek and temporomandibular area**

√7ᵗʰ **S01.442** **Puncture wound with foreign body of** left **cheek and temporomandibular area**

√7ᵗʰ **S01.449** **Puncture wound with foreign body of unspecified cheek and temporomandibular area**

√6ᵗʰ **S01.45** **Open bite of cheek and temporomandibular area**

Bite of cheek and temporomandibular area NOS

EXCLUDES 2   *superficial bite of cheek and temporomandibular area (S00.86, S00.87)*

√7ᵗʰ **S01.451** **Open bite of** right **cheek and temporomandibular area**

√7ᵗʰ **S01.452** **Open bite of** left **cheek and temporomandibular area**

√7ᵗʰ **S01.459** **Open bite of unspecified cheek and temporomandibular area**

✔ Additional Character Required   √x7ᵗʰ Placeholder   Unacceptable PDx   Questionable PDx   Manifestation   Unspecified Dx   H1-H4 HAC   HCC CMS-HCC Dx   HIV HIV Dx

ICD-10-CM 2021   967

√5ᵗʰ **S01.5 Open wound of lip and oral cavity**

EXCLUDES 2 *tooth dislocation (S03.2)*
tooth fracture (S02.5)

√6ᵗʰ **S01.50 Unspecified open wound of lip and oral cavity**

√7ᵗʰ **S01.501 Unspecified open wound of lip**

√7ᵗʰ **S01.502 Unspecified open wound of oral cavity**

√6ᵗʰ **S01.51 Laceration of lip and oral cavity without foreign body**

√7ᵗʰ **S01.511 Laceration without foreign body of lip**

√7ᵗʰ **S01.512 Laceration without foreign body of oral cavity**

√6ᵗʰ **S01.52 Laceration of lip and oral cavity with foreign body**

√7ᵗʰ **S01.521 Laceration with foreign body of lip**

√7ᵗʰ **S01.522 Laceration with foreign body of oral cavity**

√6ᵗʰ **S01.53 Puncture wound of lip and oral cavity without foreign body**

√7ᵗʰ **S01.531 Puncture wound without foreign body of lip**

√7ᵗʰ **S01.532 Puncture wound without foreign body of oral cavity**

√6ᵗʰ **S01.54 Puncture wound of lip and oral cavity with foreign body**

√7ᵗʰ **S01.541 Puncture wound with foreign body of lip**

√7ᵗʰ **S01.542 Puncture wound with foreign body of oral cavity**

√6ᵗʰ **S01.55 Open bite of lip and oral cavity**

√7ᵗʰ **S01.551 Open bite of lip**

Bite of lip NOS

EXCLUDES 1 *superficial bite of lip (S00.571)*

√7ᵗʰ **S01.552 Open bite of oral cavity**

Bite of oral cavity NOS

EXCLUDES 1 *superficial bite of oral cavity (S00.572)*

√5ᵗʰ **S01.8 Open wound of other parts of head**

√x7ᵗʰ **S01.80 Unspecified open wound of other part of head**

√x7ᵗʰ **S01.81 Laceration without foreign body of other part of head**

√x7ᵗʰ **S01.82 Laceration with foreign body of other part of head**

√x7ᵗʰ **S01.83 Puncture wound without foreign body of other part of head**

√x7ᵗʰ **S01.84 Puncture wound with foreign body of other part of head**

√x7ᵗʰ **S01.85 Open bite of other part of head**

Bite of other part of head NOS

EXCLUDES 1 *superficial bite of other part of head (S00.87)*

√5ᵗʰ **S01.9 Open wound of unspecified part of head**

√x7ᵗʰ **S01.90 Unspecified open wound of unspecified part of head**

√x7ᵗʰ **S01.91 Laceration without foreign body of unspecified part of head**

√x7ᵗʰ **S01.92 Laceration with foreign body of unspecified part of head**

√x7ᵗʰ **S01.93 Puncture wound without foreign body of unspecified part of head**

√x7ᵗʰ **S01.94 Puncture wound with foreign body of unspecified part of head**

√x7ᵗʰ **S01.95 Open bite of unspecified part of head**

Bite of head NOS

EXCLUDES 1 *superficial bite of head NOS (S00.97)*

√4ᵗʰ **S02 Fracture of skull and facial bones**

NOTE A fracture not indicated as open or closed should be coded to closed.

Code also any associated intracranial injury (S06.-)
AHA: 2017,1Q,42; 2016,4Q,66-67

The appropriate 7th character is to be added to each code from category S02.
A initial encounter for closed fracture
B initial encounter for open fracture
D subsequent encounter for fracture with routine healing
G subsequent encounter for fracture with delayed healing
K subsequent encounter for fracture with nonunion
S sequela

2,3,7 √x7ᵗʰ **S02.0 Fracture of vault of skull** MCC CC H5 HCC

Fracture of frontal bone
Fracture of parietal bone

√5ᵗʰ **S02.1 Fracture of base of skull**

EXCLUDES 2 *lateral orbital wall (S02.84-)*
medial orbital wall (S02.83-)
orbital floor (S02.3-)

AHA: 2019,4Q,16-17

√6ᵗʰ **S02.10 Unspecified fracture of base of skull**

2,3,7 √7ᵗʰ **S02.101 Fracture of base of skull, right side** MCC CC H5 HCC

2,3,7 √7ᵗʰ **S02.102 Fracture of base of skull, left side** MCC CC H5 HCC

2,3,7 √7ᵗʰ **S02.109 Fracture of base of skull, unspecified side** MCC CC H5 HCC

√6ᵗʰ **S02.11 Fracture of occiput**

2,3,7 √7ᵗʰ **S02.110 Type I occipital condyle fracture, unspecified side** MCC CC H5 HCC

2,3,7 √7ᵗʰ **S02.111 Type II occipital condyle fracture, unspecified side** MCC CC H5 HCC

2,3,7 √7ᵗʰ **S02.112 Type III occipital condyle fracture, unspecified side** MCC CC H5 HCC

2,3,7 √7ᵗʰ **S02.113 Unspecified occipital condyle fracture** MCC CC H5 HCC

2,3,7 √7ᵗʰ **S02.118 Other fracture of occiput, unspecified side** MCC CC H5 HCC

2,3,7 √7ᵗʰ **S02.119 Unspecified fracture of occiput** MCC CC H5 HCC

2,3,7 √7ᵗʰ **S02.11A Type I occipital condyle fracture, right side** MCC CC H5 HCC

2,3,7 √7ᵗʰ **S02.11B Type I occipital condyle fracture, left side** MCC CC H5 HCC

2,3,7 √7ᵗʰ **S02.11C Type II occipital condyle fracture, right side** MCC CC H5 HCC

2,3,7 √7ᵗʰ **S02.11D Type II occipital condyle fracture, left side** MCC CC H5 HCC

2,3,7 √7ᵗʰ **S02.11E Type III occipital condyle fracture, right side** MCC CC H5 HCC

2,3,7 √7ᵗʰ **S02.11F Type III occipital condyle fracture, left side** MCC CC H5 HCC

2,3,7 √7ᵗʰ **S02.11G Other fracture of occiput, right side** MCC CC H5 HCC

2,3,7 √7ᵗʰ **S02.11H Other fracture of occiput, left side** MCC CC H5 HCC

√6ᵗʰ **S02.12 Fracture of orbital roof**

AHA: 2019,4Q,16-17

2,3,7 √7ᵗʰ **S02.121 Fracture of orbital roof, right side** MCC CC H5 HCC

2,3,7 √7ᵗʰ **S02.122 Fracture of orbital roof, left side** MCC CC H5 HCC

2,3,7 √7ᵗʰ **S02.129 Fracture of orbital roof, unspecified side** MCC CC H5 HCC

2,3,7 √x7ᵗʰ **S02.19 Other fracture of base of skull** MCC CC H5 HCC

Fracture of anterior fossa of base of skull
Fracture of ethmoid sinus
Fracture of frontal sinus
Fracture of middle fossa of base of skull
Fracture of posterior fossa of base of skull
Fracture of sphenoid
Fracture of temporal bone

3 √x7ᵗʰ **S02.2 Fracture of nasal bones** CC H5

√5ᵗʰ S02.3   Fracture of orbital floor

Fracture of inferior orbital wall

EXCLUDES 1   orbit NOS (S02.85)

EXCLUDES 2   lateral orbital wall (S02.84-)

medial orbital wall (S02.83-)

orbital roof (S02.1-)

3,7 √x7ᵗʰ S02.30   Fracture of orbital floor, unspecified side   `CC` `H5` `HCC`

3,7 √x7ᵗʰ S02.31   Fracture of orbital floor, right side   `CC` `H5` `HCC`

3,7 √x7ᵗʰ S02.32   Fracture of orbital floor, left side   `CC` `H5` `HCC`

√5ᵗʰ S02.4   Fracture of malar, maxillary and zygoma bones

Fracture of superior maxilla

Fracture of upper jaw (bone)

Fracture of zygomatic process of temporal bone

√6ᵗʰ S02.40   Fracture of malar, maxillary and zygoma bones, unspecified

3,7 √7ᵗʰ S02.400   Malar fracture, unspecified side   `CC` `H5` `HCC`

3,7 √7ᵗʰ S02.401   Maxillary fracture, unspecified side   `CC` `H5` `HCC`

3,7 √7ᵗʰ S02.402   Zygomatic fracture, unspecified side   `CC` `H5` `HCC`

3,7 √7ᵗʰ S02.40A   Malar fracture, right side   `CC` `H5` `HCC`

3,7 √7ᵗʰ S02.40B   Malar fracture, left side   `CC` `H5` `HCC`

3,7 √7ᵗʰ S02.40C   Maxillary fracture, right side   `CC` `H5` `HCC`

3,7 √7ᵗʰ S02.40D   Maxillary fracture, left side   `CC` `H5` `HCC`

3,7 √7ᵗʰ S02.40E   Zygomatic fracture, right side   `CC` `H5` `HCC`

3,7 √7ᵗʰ S02.40F   Zygomatic fracture, left side   `CC` `H5` `HCC`

√6ᵗʰ S02.41   LeFort fracture

DEF: Named for Rene Le Fort, these fractures describe different combinations of multiple fractures that occur from significant force to the midface. A common denominator in all three types of LeFort fractures is fracture of the pterygoid processes, which are two bony plates resembling wings that extend downward from the sphenoid bone.

LeFort Fracture Types

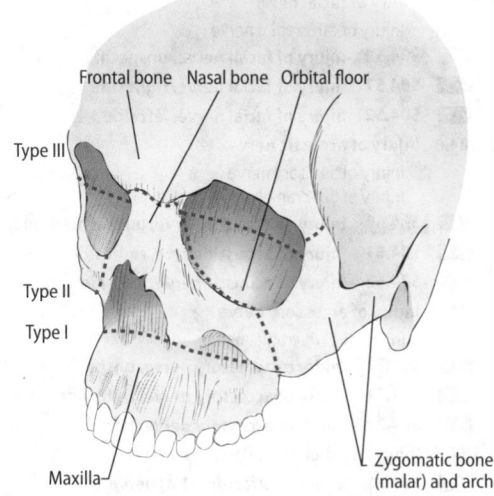

Frontal bone   Nasal bone   Orbital floor

Type III

Type II

Type I

Maxilla

Zygomatic bone (malar) and arch

3,7 √7ᵗʰ S02.411   LeFort I fracture   `CC` `H5` `HCC`

3,7 √7ᵗʰ S02.412   LeFort II fracture   `CC` `H5` `HCC`

3,7 √7ᵗʰ S02.413   LeFort III fracture   `CC` `H5` `HCC`

3,7 √x7ᵗʰ S02.42   Fracture of alveolus of maxilla   `CC` `H5` `HCC`

4 √x7ᵗʰ S02.5   Fracture of tooth (traumatic)   `CC`

Broken tooth

EXCLUDES 1   cracked tooth (nontraumatic) (K03.81)

√5ᵗʰ S02.6   Fracture of mandible

Fracture of lower jaw (bone)

√6ᵗʰ S02.60   Fracture of mandible, unspecified

3,7 √7ᵗʰ S02.600   Fracture of unspecified part of body of mandible, unspecified side   `CC` `H5` `HCC`

3,7 √7ᵗʰ S02.601   Fracture of unspecified part of body of right mandible   `CC` `H5` `HCC`

3,7 √7ᵗʰ S02.602   Fracture of unspecified part of body of left mandible   `CC` `H5` `HCC`

3,7 √7ᵗʰ S02.609   Fracture of mandible, unspecified   `CC` `H5` `HCC`

√6ᵗʰ S02.61   Fracture of condylar process of mandible

3,7 √7ᵗʰ S02.610   Fracture of condylar process of mandible, unspecified side   `CC` `H5` `HCC`

3,7 √7ᵗʰ S02.611   Fracture of condylar process of right mandible   `CC` `H5` `HCC`

3,7 √7ᵗʰ S02.612   Fracture of condylar process of left mandible   `CC` `H5` `HCC`

√6ᵗʰ S02.62   Fracture of subcondylar process of mandible

3,7 √7ᵗʰ S02.620   Fracture of subcondylar process of mandible, unspecified side   `CC` `H5` `HCC`

3,7 √7ᵗʰ S02.621   Fracture of subcondylar process of right mandible   `CC` `H5` `HCC`

3,7 √7ᵗʰ S02.622   Fracture of subcondylar process of left mandible   `CC` `H5` `HCC`

√6ᵗʰ S02.63   Fracture of coronoid process of mandible

3,7 √7ᵗʰ S02.630   Fracture of coronoid process of mandible, unspecified side   `CC` `H5` `HCC`

3,7 √7ᵗʰ S02.631   Fracture of coronoid process of right mandible   `CC` `H5` `HCC`

3,7 √7ᵗʰ S02.632   Fracture of coronoid process of left mandible   `CC` `H5` `HCC`

√6ᵗʰ S02.64   Fracture of ramus of mandible

3,7 √7ᵗʰ S02.640   Fracture of ramus of mandible, unspecified side   `CC` `H5` `HCC`

3,7 √7ᵗʰ S02.641   Fracture of ramus of right mandible   `CC` `H5` `HCC`

3,7 √7ᵗʰ S02.642   Fracture of ramus of left mandible   `CC` `H5` `HCC`

√6ᵗʰ S02.65   Fracture of angle of mandible

3,7 √7ᵗʰ S02.650   Fracture of angle of mandible, unspecified side   `CC` `H5` `HCC`

3,7 √7ᵗʰ S02.651   Fracture of angle of right mandible   `CC` `H5` `HCC`

3,7 √7ᵗʰ S02.652   Fracture of angle of left mandible   `CC` `H5` `HCC`

3,7 √x7ᵗʰ S02.66   Fracture of symphysis of mandible   `CC` `H5` `HCC`

√6ᵗʰ S02.67   Fracture of alveolus of mandible

3,7 √7ᵗʰ S02.670   Fracture of alveolus of mandible, unspecified side   `CC` `H5` `HCC`

3,7 √7ᵗʰ S02.671   Fracture of alveolus of right mandible   `CC` `H5` `HCC`

3,7 √7ᵗʰ S02.672   Fracture of alveolus of left mandible   `CC` `H5` `HCC`

3,7 √x7ᵗʰ S02.69   Fracture of mandible of other specified site   `CC` `H5` `HCC`

√5ᵗʰ S02.8   Fractures of other specified skull and facial bones

Fracture of palate

EXCLUDES 2   fracture of orbital floor (S02.3-)

fracture of orbital roof (S02.12-)

3,7 √x7ᵗʰ S02.80   Fracture of other specified skull and facial bones, unspecified side   `CC` `H5` `HCC`

3,7 √x7ᵗʰ S02.81   Fracture of other specified skull and facial bones, right side   `CC` `H5` `HCC`

3,7 √x7ᵗʰ S02.82   Fracture of other specified skull and facial bones, left side   `CC` `H5` `HCC`

√6ᵗʰ S02.83   Fracture of medial orbital wall

EXCLUDES 2   orbital floor (S02.3-)

orbital roof (S02.12-)

AHA: 2019,4Q,16-17

3,7 √7ᵗʰ S02.831   Fracture of medial orbital wall, right side   `CC` `H5` `HCC`

3,7 √7ᵗʰ S02.832   Fracture of medial orbital wall, left side   `CC` `H5` `HCC`

3,7 √7ᵗʰ S02.839   Fracture of medial orbital wall, unspecified side   `CC` `H5` `HCC`

√6ᵗʰ S02.84   Fracture of lateral orbital wall

EXCLUDES 2   orbital floor (S02.3-)

orbital roof (S02.12-)

AHA: 2019,4Q,16-17

3,7 √7ᵗʰ S02.841   Fracture of lateral orbital wall, right side   `CC` `H5` `HCC`

☑ Additional Character Required   √x7ᵗʰ Placeholder   Unacceptable PDx   Questionable PDx   Manifestation   Unspecified Dx   H1 - H14 HAC   HCC CMS-HCC Dx   HIV HIV Dx

ICD-10-CM 2021   969

3,7 √7th S02.842 Fracture of lateral orbital wall, left side CC H5 HCC

3,7 √7th S02.849 Fracture of lateral orbital wall, unspecified side CC H5 HCC

3,7 √x7th S02.85 Fracture of orbit, unspecified CC H5 HCC

    Fracture of orbit NOS
    Fracture of orbit wall NOS
    EXCLUDES 1   lateral orbital wall (S02.84-)
            medial orbital wall (S02.83-)
            orbital floor (S02.3-)
            orbital roof (S02.12-)

√5th S02.9 Fracture of unspecified skull and facial bones

2,3,7 √x7th S02.91 Unspecified fracture of skull MCC CC H5 HCC
    AHA: 2020,2Q,24

3,7 √x7th S02.92 Unspecified fracture of facial bones CC H5 HCC

√4th S03 Dislocation and sprain of joints and ligaments of head

    INCLUDES   avulsion of joint (capsule) or ligament of head
           laceration of cartilage, joint (capsule) or ligament of head
           sprain of cartilage, joint (capsule) or ligament of head
           traumatic hemarthrosis of joint or ligament of head
           traumatic rupture of joint or ligament of head
           traumatic subluxation of joint or ligament of head
           traumatic tear of joint or ligament of head
    Code also any associated open wound
    EXCLUDES 2   strain of muscle or tendon of head (S09.1)

    The appropriate 7th character is to be added to each code from category S03.
    A   initial encounter
    D   subsequent encounter
    S   sequela

√5th S03.0 Dislocation of jaw
    Dislocation of jaw (cartilage) (meniscus)
    Dislocation of mandible
    Dislocation of temporomandibular (joint)
    AHA: 2016,4Q,67

√x7th S03.00 Dislocation of jaw, unspecified side
√x7th S03.01 Dislocation of jaw, right side
√x7th S03.02 Dislocation of jaw, left side
√x7th S03.03 Dislocation of jaw, bilateral

√x7th S03.1 Dislocation of septal cartilage of nose
√x7th S03.2 Dislocation of tooth

√5th S03.4 Sprain of jaw
    Sprain of temporomandibular (joint) (ligament)
    AHA: 2016,4Q,67

√x7th S03.40 Sprain of jaw, unspecified side
√x7th S03.41 Sprain of jaw, right side
√x7th S03.42 Sprain of jaw, left side
√x7th S03.43 Sprain of jaw, bilateral

√x7th S03.8 Sprain of joints and ligaments of other parts of head
√x7th S03.9 Sprain of joints and ligaments of unspecified parts of head

√4th S04 Injury of cranial nerve

    The selection of side should be based on the side of the body being affected
    Code first any associated intracranial injury (S06.-)
    Code also any associated:
       open wound of head (S01.-)
       skull fracture (S02.-)

    The appropriate 7th character is to be added to each code from category S04.
    A   initial encounter
    D   subsequent encounter
    S   sequela

√5th S04.0 Injury of optic nerve and pathways
    Use additional code to identify any visual field defect or blindness (H53.4-, H54.-)

√6th S04.01 Injury of optic nerve
    Injury of 2nd cranial nerve

√7th S04.011 Injury of optic nerve, right eye CC
√7th S04.012 Injury of optic nerve, left eye CC

√7th S04.019 Injury of optic nerve, unspecified eye CC
    Injury of optic nerve NOS

√x7th S04.02 Injury of optic chiasm CC

√6th S04.03 Injury of optic tract and pathways CC
    Injury of optic radiation

√7th S04.031 Injury of optic tract and pathways, right side CC
√7th S04.032 Injury of optic tract and pathways, left side CC
√7th S04.039 Injury of optic tract and pathways, unspecified side CC
    Injury of optic tract and pathways NOS

√6th S04.04 Injury of visual cortex
√7th S04.041 Injury of visual cortex, right side CC
√7th S04.042 Injury of visual cortex, left side CC
√7th S04.049 Injury of visual cortex, unspecified side CC
    Injury of visual cortex NOS

√5th S04.1 Injury of oculomotor nerve
    Injury of 3rd cranial nerve
√x7th S04.10 Injury of oculomotor nerve, unspecified side CC
√x7th S04.11 Injury of oculomotor nerve, right side CC
√x7th S04.12 Injury of oculomotor nerve, left side CC

√5th S04.2 Injury of trochlear nerve
    Injury of 4th cranial nerve
√x7th S04.20 Injury of trochlear nerve, unspecified side CC
√x7th S04.21 Injury of trochlear nerve, right side CC
√x7th S04.22 Injury of trochlear nerve, left side CC

√5th S04.3 Injury of trigeminal nerve
    Injury of 5th cranial nerve
√x7th S04.30 Injury of trigeminal nerve, unspecified side CC
√x7th S04.31 Injury of trigeminal nerve, right side CC
√x7th S04.32 Injury of trigeminal nerve, left side CC

√5th S04.4 Injury of abducent nerve
    Injury of 6th cranial nerve
√x7th S04.40 Injury of abducent nerve, unspecified side CC
√x7th S04.41 Injury of abducent nerve, right side CC
√x7th S04.42 Injury of abducent nerve, left side CC

√5th S04.5 Injury of facial nerve
    Injury of 7th cranial nerve
√x7th S04.50 Injury of facial nerve, unspecified side CC
√x7th S04.51 Injury of facial nerve, right side CC
√x7th S04.52 Injury of facial nerve, left side CC

√5th S04.6 Injury of acoustic nerve
    Injury of auditory nerve
    Injury of 8th cranial nerve
√x7th S04.60 Injury of acoustic nerve, unspecified side CC
√x7th S04.61 Injury of acoustic nerve, right side CC
√x7th S04.62 Injury of acoustic nerve, left side CC

√5th S04.7 Injury of accessory nerve
    Injury of 11th cranial nerve
√x7th S04.70 Injury of accessory nerve, unspecified side CC
√x7th S04.71 Injury of accessory nerve, right side CC
√x7th S04.72 Injury of accessory nerve, left side CC

√5th S04.8 Injury of other cranial nerves
√6th S04.81 Injury of olfactory [1st] nerve
√7th S04.811 Injury of olfactory [1st] nerve, right side CC
√7th S04.812 Injury of olfactory [1st] nerve, left side CC
√7th S04.819 Injury of olfactory [1st] nerve, unspecified side CC

√6th S04.89 Injury of other cranial nerves
    Injury of vagus [10th] nerve
√7th S04.891 Injury of other cranial nerves, right side CC
√7th S04.892 Injury of other cranial nerves, left side CC
√7th S04.899 Injury of other cranial nerves, unspecified side CC

N Newborn: 0   P Pediatric: 0-17   M Maternity: 9-64   A Adult: 15-124   MCC Major Complication/Comorbidity   CC Complication/Comorbidity   SW Severe Wound Dx

970   ICD-10-CM 2021

√x7ᵗʰ **S04.9 Injury of unspecified cranial nerve** `CC`

√4ᵗʰ **S05 Injury of eye and orbit**

> `INCLUDES` open wound of eye and orbit
> `EXCLUDES 2` 2nd cranial [optic] nerve injury (S04.0-)
> 3rd cranial [oculomotor] nerve injury (S04.1-)
> open wound of eyelid and periocular area (S01.1-)
> orbital bone fracture (S02.1-, S02.3-, S02.8-)
> superficial injury of eyelid (S00.1-S00.2)

> The appropriate 7th character is to be added to each code from category S05.
> A initial encounter
> D subsequent encounter
> S sequela

√5ᵗʰ **S05.0 Injury of conjunctiva and corneal abrasion** without foreign body

> `EXCLUDES 1` foreign body in conjunctival sac (T15.1)
> foreign body in cornea (T15.0)

√x7ᵗʰ **S05.00 Injury of conjunctiva and corneal abrasion without foreign body, unspecified eye**

√x7ᵗʰ **S05.01 Injury of conjunctiva and corneal abrasion without foreign body, right eye**

√x7ᵗʰ **S05.02 Injury of conjunctiva and corneal abrasion without foreign body, left eye**

√5ᵗʰ **S05.1 Contusion of eyeball and orbital tissues**

> Traumatic hyphema
> `EXCLUDES 2` black eye NOS (S00.1)
> contusion of eyelid and periocular area (S00.1)

√x7ᵗʰ **S05.10 Contusion of eyeball and orbital tissues, unspecified eye**

√x7ᵗʰ **S05.11 Contusion of eyeball and orbital tissues, right eye**

√x7ᵗʰ **S05.12 Contusion of eyeball and orbital tissues, left eye**

√5ᵗʰ **S05.2 Ocular laceration and rupture** with prolapse or loss of intraocular tissue

√x7ᵗʰ **S05.20 Ocular laceration and rupture with prolapse or loss of intraocular tissue, unspecified eye** `CC`

√x7ᵗʰ **S05.21 Ocular laceration and rupture with prolapse or loss of intraocular tissue, right eye** `CC`

√x7ᵗʰ **S05.22 Ocular laceration and rupture with prolapse or loss of intraocular tissue, left eye** `CC`

√5ᵗʰ **S05.3 Ocular laceration** without prolapse or loss of intraocular tissue

> Laceration of eye NOS
> **DEF:** Tear in ocular tissue without displacing structures that is due to blunt trauma. It is characterized by pain, redness, and decreased vision.

√x7ᵗʰ **S05.30 Ocular laceration without prolapse or loss of intraocular tissue, unspecified eye** `CC`

√x7ᵗʰ **S05.31 Ocular laceration without prolapse or loss of intraocular tissue, right eye** `CC`

√x7ᵗʰ **S05.32 Ocular laceration without prolapse or loss of intraocular tissue, left eye** `CC`

√5ᵗʰ **S05.4 Penetrating wound of orbit** with or without foreign body

> `EXCLUDES 2` retained (old) foreign body following penetrating wound in orbit (H05.5-)

√x7ᵗʰ **S05.40 Penetrating wound of orbit with or without foreign body, unspecified eye** `CC`

√x7ᵗʰ **S05.41 Penetrating wound of orbit with or without foreign body, right eye** `CC`

√x7ᵗʰ **S05.42 Penetrating wound of orbit with or without foreign body, left eye** `CC`

√5ᵗʰ **S05.5 Penetrating wound with foreign body** of eyeball

> `EXCLUDES 2` retained (old) intraocular foreign body (H44.6-, H44.7)

√x7ᵗʰ **S05.50 Penetrating wound with foreign body of unspecified eyeball** `CC`

√x7ᵗʰ **S05.51 Penetrating wound with foreign body of right eyeball** `CC`

√x7ᵗʰ **S05.52 Penetrating wound with foreign body of left eyeball** `CC`

√5ᵗʰ **S05.6 Penetrating wound without foreign body** of eyeball

> Ocular penetration NOS

√x7ᵗʰ **S05.60 Penetrating wound without foreign body of unspecified eyeball**

√x7ᵗʰ **S05.61 Penetrating wound without foreign body of right eyeball**

√x7ᵗʰ **S05.62 Penetrating wound without foreign body of left eyeball**

√5ᵗʰ **S05.7 Avulsion of eye**

> Traumatic enucleation

√x7ᵗʰ **S05.70 Avulsion of unspecified eye** `CC`

√x7ᵗʰ **S05.71 Avulsion of right eye** `CC`

√x7ᵗʰ **S05.72 Avulsion of left eye** `CC`

√5ᵗʰ **S05.8 Other injuries of eye and orbit**

> Lacrimal duct injury

√6ᵗʰ **S05.8X Other injuries of eye and orbit**

√7ᵗʰ **S05.8X1 Other injuries of right eye and orbit** `CC`

√7ᵗʰ **S05.8X2 Other injuries of left eye and orbit** `CC`

√7ᵗʰ **S05.8X9 Other injuries of unspecified eye and orbit** `CC`

√5ᵗʰ **S05.9 Unspecified injury of eye and orbit**

> Injury of eye NOS

√x7ᵗʰ **S05.90 Unspecified injury of unspecified eye and orbit**

√x7ᵗʰ **S05.91 Unspecified injury of right eye and orbit** `CC`

√x7ᵗʰ **S05.92 Unspecified injury of left eye and orbit** `CC`

√4ᵗʰ **S06 Intracranial injury**

> `NOTE` 7th characters D and S do not apply to codes in category S06 with 6th character 7 – death due to brain injury prior to regaining consciousness, or 8 – death due to other cause prior to regaining consciousness.

> `INCLUDES` traumatic brain injury
> Code also any associated:
> open wound of head (S01.-)
> skull fracture (S02.-)
> `EXCLUDES 1` head injury NOS (S09.90)
> **AHA:** 2017,4Q,25; 2017,1Q,42; 2015,3Q,37
> **TIP:** Do not assign Z87.820 Personal history of traumatic brain injury, when residual conditions persist after an intracranial injury. The codes for the residual conditions should be first listed, followed by a code from category S06 using seventh character S to identify sequelae.

> The appropriate 7th character is to be added to each code from category S06.
> A initial encounter
> D subsequent encounter
> S sequela

√5ᵗʰ **S06.0 Concussion**

> Commotio cerebri
> `EXCLUDES 1` concussion with other intracranial injuries classified in subcategories S06.1- to S06.6- , S06.81- and S06.82- — code to specified intracranial injury
> **AHA:** 2016,4Q,67-68

√6ᵗʰ **S06.0X Concussion**

8 √7ᵗʰ **S06.0X0 Concussion** without loss of consciousness `CC` `HCC`

8 √7ᵗʰ **S06.0X1 Concussion with loss of consciousness of 30 minutes or less** `CC` `H5` `HCC`

8 √7ᵗʰ **S06.0X9 Concussion with loss of consciousness of unspecified duration** `CC` `H5` `HCC`

> Concussion NOS

√5ᵗʰ **S06.1 Traumatic cerebral edema**

> Diffuse traumatic cerebral edema
> Focal traumatic cerebral edema
> **AHA:** 2019,3Q,35; 2015,1Q,12-13

√6ᵗʰ **S06.1X Traumatic cerebral edema**

7 √7ᵗʰ **S06.1X0 Traumatic cerebral edema** without loss of consciousness `MCC` `HCC`

7 √7ᵗʰ **S06.1X1 Traumatic cerebral edema with loss of consciousness of 30 minutes or less** `MCC` `H5` `HCC`

7 √7ᵗʰ **S06.1X2 Traumatic cerebral edema with loss of consciousness of 31 minutes to 59 minutes** `MCC` `H5` `HCC`

7 √7ᵗʰ **S06.1X3 Traumatic cerebral edema with loss of consciousness of 1 hour to 5 hours 59 minutes** `MCC` `H5` `HCC`

7 √7ᵗʰ **S06.1X4 Traumatic cerebral edema with loss of consciousness of 6 hours to 24 hours** `MCC` `H5` `HCC`

7 √7ᵗʰ **S06.1X5 Traumatic cerebral edema with loss of consciousness greater than 24 hours with return to pre-existing conscious level** `MCC` `H5` `HCC`

☑ Additional Character Required   √x7ᵗʰ Placeholder   Unacceptable PDx   Questionable PDx   Manifestation   Unspecified Dx   H1 - H14 HAC   HCC CMS-HCC Dx   HIV HIV Dx

ICD-10-CM 2021   971

7 √7ᵗʰ **S06.1X6** **Traumatic cerebral edema with loss of consciousness** greater than 24 hours without return to pre-existing conscious level with patient surviving `MCC` `H5` `HCC`

√7ᵗʰ **S06.1X7** **Traumatic cerebral edema with loss of consciousness of** any duration with death due to brain injury prior to regaining consciousness `MCC` `H5`

√7ᵗʰ **S06.1X8** **Traumatic cerebral edema with loss of consciousness of** any duration with death due to **other** cause prior to regaining consciousness `MCC` `H5`

7 √7ᵗʰ **S06.1X9** **Traumatic cerebral edema with loss of consciousness of unspecified duration** `MCC` `H5` `HCC`
　　　Traumatic cerebral edema NOS

√5ᵗʰ **S06.2** **Diffuse traumatic brain injury**
　　Diffuse axonal brain injury
　　　EXCLUDES 1　traumatic diffuse cerebral edema (S06.1X-)

　　√6ᵗʰ **S06.2X** **Diffuse traumatic brain injury**

7 √7ᵗʰ **S06.2X0** **Diffuse traumatic brain injury without loss of consciousness** `HCC`

7 √7ᵗʰ **S06.2X1** **Diffuse traumatic brain injury with loss of consciousness of** 30 minutes or less `CC` `H5` `HCC`

7 √7ᵗʰ **S06.2X2** **Diffuse traumatic brain injury with loss of consciousness of** 31 minutes to 59 minutes `CC` `H5` `HCC`

7 √7ᵗʰ **S06.2X3** **Diffuse traumatic brain injury with loss of consciousness of** 1 hour to 5 hours 59 minutes `CC` `H5` `HCC`

7 √7ᵗʰ **S06.2X4** **Diffuse traumatic brain injury with loss of consciousness of** 6 hours to 24 hours `CC` `H5` `HCC`

7 √7ᵗʰ **S06.2X5** **Diffuse traumatic brain injury with loss of consciousness** greater than 24 hours with return to pre-existing conscious levels `CC` `H5` `HCC`

7 √7ᵗʰ **S06.2X6** **Diffuse traumatic brain injury with loss of consciousness** greater than 24 hours without return to pre-existing conscious level with patient surviving `MCC` `H5` `HCC`

√7ᵗʰ **S06.2X7** **Diffuse traumatic brain injury with loss of consciousness of** any duration with death due to brain injury prior to regaining consciousness `MCC` `H5`

√7ᵗʰ **S06.2X8** **Diffuse traumatic brain injury with loss of consciousness of** any duration with death due to **other** cause prior to regaining consciousness `MCC` `H5`

7 √7ᵗʰ **S06.2X9** **Diffuse traumatic brain injury with loss of consciousness of unspecified duration** `CC` `H5` `HCC`
　　　Diffuse traumatic brain injury NOS

√5ᵗʰ **S06.3** **Focal traumatic brain injury**
　　　EXCLUDES 1　any condition classifiable to S06.4-S06.6
　　　　　　　　　focal cerebral edema (S06.1)
　　　EXCLUDES 2　▶focal cerebral edema (S06.1)◀
　　AHA: 2019,3Q,35; 2015,1Q,12-13

　√6ᵗʰ **S06.30** **Unspecified focal traumatic brain injury**

7 √7ᵗʰ **S06.300** **Unspecified focal traumatic brain injury without loss of consciousness** `HCC`

7 √7ᵗʰ **S06.301** **Unspecified focal traumatic brain injury with loss of consciousness of** 30 minutes or less `CC` `H5` `HCC`

7 √7ᵗʰ **S06.302** **Unspecified focal traumatic brain injury with loss of consciousness of** 31 minutes to 59 minutes `CC` `H5` `HCC`

7 √7ᵗʰ **S06.303** **Unspecified focal traumatic brain injury with loss of consciousness of** 1 hour to 5 hours 59 minutes `CC` `H5` `HCC`

7 √7ᵗʰ **S06.304** **Unspecified focal traumatic brain injury with loss of consciousness of** 6 hours to 24 hours `CC` `H5` `HCC`

7 √7ᵗʰ **S06.305** **Unspecified focal traumatic brain injury with loss of consciousness** greater than 24 hours with return to pre-existing conscious level `CC` `H5` `HCC`

7 √7ᵗʰ **S06.306** **Unspecified focal traumatic brain injury with loss of consciousness** greater than 24 hours without return to pre-existing conscious level with patient surviving `MCC` `H5` `HCC`

√7ᵗʰ **S06.307** **Unspecified focal traumatic brain injury with loss of consciousness of** any duration with death due to brain injury prior to regaining consciousness `MCC` `H5`

√7ᵗʰ **S06.308** **Unspecified focal traumatic brain injury with loss of consciousness of** any duration with death due to **other** cause prior to regaining consciousness `MCC` `H5`

7 √7ᵗʰ **S06.309** **Unspecified focal traumatic brain injury with loss of consciousness of unspecified duration** `CC` `H5` `HCC`
　　　Unspecified focal traumatic brain injury NOS

√6ᵗʰ **S06.31** **Contusion and laceration of** right cerebrum

7 √7ᵗʰ **S06.310** **Contusion and laceration of right cerebrum without loss of consciousness** `MCC` `H5` `HCC`

7 √7ᵗʰ **S06.311** **Contusion and laceration of right cerebrum with loss of consciousness of** 30 minutes or less `MCC` `H5` `HCC`

7 √7ᵗʰ **S06.312** **Contusion and laceration of right cerebrum with loss of consciousness of** 31 minutes to 59 minutes `MCC` `H5` `HCC`

7 √7ᵗʰ **S06.313** **Contusion and laceration of right cerebrum with loss of consciousness of** 1 hour to 5 hours 59 minutes `MCC` `H5` `HCC`

7 √7ᵗʰ **S06.314** **Contusion and laceration of right cerebrum with loss of consciousness of** 6 hours to 24 hours `MCC` `H5` `HCC`

7 √7ᵗʰ **S06.315** **Contusion and laceration of right cerebrum with loss of consciousness** greater than 24 hours with return to pre-existing conscious level `MCC` `H5` `HCC`

7 √7ᵗʰ **S06.316** **Contusion and laceration of right cerebrum with loss of consciousness** greater than 24 hours without return to pre-existing conscious level with patient surviving `MCC` `H5` `HCC`

√7ᵗʰ **S06.317** **Contusion and laceration of right cerebrum with loss of consciousness of** any duration with death due to brain injury prior to regaining consciousness `MCC` `H5`

√7ᵗʰ **S06.318** **Contusion and laceration of right cerebrum with loss of consciousness of** any duration with death due to **other** cause prior to regaining consciousness `MCC` `H5`

7 √7ᵗʰ **S06.319** **Contusion and laceration of right cerebrum with loss of consciousness of unspecified duration** `MCC` `H5` `HCC`
　　　Contusion and laceration of right cerebrum NOS

√6ᵗʰ **S06.32** **Contusion and laceration of** left cerebrum

7 √7ᵗʰ **S06.320** **Contusion and laceration of left cerebrum without loss of consciousness** `MCC` `H5` `HCC`

7 √7ᵗʰ **S06.321** **Contusion and laceration of left cerebrum with loss of consciousness of** 30 minutes or less `MCC` `H5` `HCC`

7 √7ᵗʰ **S06.322** **Contusion and laceration of left cerebrum with loss of consciousness of** 31 minutes to 59 minutes `MCC` `H5` `HCC`

7 √7ᵗʰ **S06.323** **Contusion and laceration of left cerebrum with loss of consciousness of** 1 hour to 5 hours 59 minutes `MCC` `H5` `HCC`

7 √7ᵗʰ **S06.324** **Contusion and laceration of left cerebrum with loss of consciousness of** 6 hours to 24 hours `MCC` `H5` `HCC`

7 √7ᵗʰ **S06.325** **Contusion and laceration of left cerebrum with loss of consciousness** greater than 24 hours with return to pre-existing conscious level `MCC` `H5` `HCC`

`N` Newborn: 0　`P` Pediatric: 0-17　`M` Maternity: 9-64　`A` Adult: 15-124　`MCC` Major Complication/Comorbidity　`CC` Complication/Comorbidity　`SW` Severe Wound Dx

972　　ICD-10-CM 2021

⁷ ✓7ᵗʰ **S06.326** **Contusion and laceration of left cerebrum with loss of consciousness** greater than 24 hours without return to pre-existing conscious level with patient surviving   MCC H5 HCC

✓7ᵗʰ **S06.327** **Contusion and laceration of left cerebrum with loss of consciousness of** any duration with death due to brain injury prior to regaining consciousness   MCC H5

✓7ᵗʰ **S06.328** **Contusion and laceration of left cerebrum with loss of consciousness of** any duration with death due to **other** cause prior to regaining consciousness   MCC H5

⁷ ✓7ᵗʰ **S06.329** **Contusion and laceration of left cerebrum with loss of consciousness of unspecified duration**   MCC H5 HCC

Contusion and laceration of left cerebrum NOS

✓6ᵗʰ **S06.33** **Contusion and laceration of cerebrum, unspecified**

⁷ ✓7ᵗʰ **S06.330** **Contusion and laceration of cerebrum, unspecified,** without loss of consciousness   MCC H5 HCC

⁷ ✓7ᵗʰ **S06.331** **Contusion and laceration of cerebrum, unspecified, with loss of consciousness of** 30 minutes or less   MCC H5 HCC

⁷ ✓7ᵗʰ **S06.332** **Contusion and laceration of cerebrum, unspecified, with loss of consciousness of** 31 minutes to 59 minutes   MCC H5 HCC

⁷ ✓7ᵗʰ **S06.333** **Contusion and laceration of cerebrum, unspecified, with loss of consciousness of** 1 hour to 5 hours 59 minutes   MCC H5 HCC

⁷ ✓7ᵗʰ **S06.334** **Contusion and laceration of cerebrum, unspecified, with loss of consciousness of** 6 hours to 24 hours   MCC H5 HCC

⁷ ✓7ᵗʰ **S06.335** **Contusion and laceration of cerebrum, unspecified, with loss of consciousness** greater than 24 hours with return to pre-existing conscious level   MCC H5 HCC

⁷ ✓7ᵗʰ **S06.336** **Contusion and laceration of cerebrum, unspecified, with loss of consciousness** greater than 24 hours without return to pre-existing conscious level with patient surviving   MCC H5 HCC

✓7ᵗʰ **S06.337** **Contusion and laceration of cerebrum, unspecified, with loss of consciousness of** any duration with death due to brain injury prior to regaining consciousness   MCC H5

✓7ᵗʰ **S06.338** **Contusion and laceration of cerebrum, unspecified, with loss of consciousness of** any duration with death due to **other** cause prior to regaining consciousness   MCC H5

⁷ ✓7ᵗʰ **S06.339** **Contusion and laceration of cerebrum, unspecified, with loss of consciousness of unspecified duration**   MCC H5 HCC

Contusion and laceration of cerebrum NOS

✓6ᵗʰ **S06.34** **Traumatic hemorrhage of** right cerebrum

Traumatic intracerebral hemorrhage and hematoma of right cerebrum

⁷ ✓7ᵗʰ **S06.340** **Traumatic hemorrhage of right cerebrum** without loss of consciousness   MCC H5 HCC

⁷ ✓7ᵗʰ **S06.341** **Traumatic hemorrhage of right cerebrum with loss of consciousness of** 30 minutes or less   MCC H5 HCC

⁷ ✓7ᵗʰ **S06.342** **Traumatic hemorrhage of right cerebrum with loss of consciousness of** 31 minutes to 59 minutes   MCC H5 HCC

⁷ ✓7ᵗʰ **S06.343** **Traumatic hemorrhage of right cerebrum with loss of consciousness of** 1 hours to 5 hours 59 minutes   MCC H5 HCC

⁷ ✓7ᵗʰ **S06.344** **Traumatic hemorrhage of right cerebrum with loss of consciousness of** 6 hours to 24 hours   MCC H5 HCC

⁷ ✓7ᵗʰ **S06.345** **Traumatic hemorrhage of right cerebrum with loss of consciousness** greater than 24 hours with return to pre-existing conscious level   MCC H5 HCC

⁷ ✓7ᵗʰ **S06.346** **Traumatic hemorrhage of right cerebrum with loss of consciousness** greater than 24 hours without return to pre-existing conscious level with patient surviving   MCC H5 HCC

✓7ᵗʰ **S06.347** **Traumatic hemorrhage of right cerebrum with loss of consciousness of** any duration with death due to brain injury prior to regaining consciousness   MCC H5

✓7ᵗʰ **S06.348** **Traumatic hemorrhage of right cerebrum with loss of consciousness of** any duration with death due to **other** cause prior to regaining consciousness   MCC H5

⁷ ✓7ᵗʰ **S06.349** **Traumatic hemorrhage of right cerebrum with loss of consciousness of unspecified duration**   MCC H5 HCC

Traumatic hemorrhage of right cerebrum NOS

✓6ᵗʰ **S06.35** **Traumatic hemorrhage of** left cerebrum

Traumatic intracerebral hemorrhage and hematoma of left cerebrum

⁷ ✓7ᵗʰ **S06.350** **Traumatic hemorrhage of left cerebrum** without loss of consciousness   MCC H5 HCC

⁷ ✓7ᵗʰ **S06.351** **Traumatic hemorrhage of left cerebrum with loss of consciousness of** 30 minutes or less   MCC H5 HCC

⁷ ✓7ᵗʰ **S06.352** **Traumatic hemorrhage of left cerebrum with loss of consciousness of** 31 minutes to 59 minutes   MCC H5 HCC

⁷ ✓7ᵗʰ **S06.353** **Traumatic hemorrhage of left cerebrum with loss of consciousness of** 1 hours to 5 hours 59 minutes   MCC H5 HCC

⁷ ✓7ᵗʰ **S06.354** **Traumatic hemorrhage of left cerebrum with loss of consciousness of** 6 hours to 24 hours   MCC H5 HCC

⁷ ✓7ᵗʰ **S06.355** **Traumatic hemorrhage of left cerebrum with loss of consciousness** greater than 24 hours with return to pre-existing conscious level   MCC H5 HCC

⁷ ✓7ᵗʰ **S06.356** **Traumatic hemorrhage of left cerebrum with loss of consciousness** greater than 24 hours without return to pre-existing conscious level with patient surviving   MCC H5 HCC

✓7ᵗʰ **S06.357** **Traumatic hemorrhage of left cerebrum with loss of consciousness of** any duration with death due to brain injury prior to regaining consciousness   MCC H5

✓7ᵗʰ **S06.358** **Traumatic hemorrhage of left cerebrum with loss of consciousness of** any duration with death due to **other** cause prior to regaining consciousness   MCC H5

⁷ ✓7ᵗʰ **S06.359** **Traumatic hemorrhage of left cerebrum with loss of consciousness of unspecified duration**   MCC H5 HCC

Traumatic hemorrhage of left cerebrum NOS

✓6ᵗʰ **S06.36** **Traumatic hemorrhage of cerebrum, unspecified**

Traumatic intracerebral hemorrhage and hematoma, unspecified

⁷ ✓7ᵗʰ **S06.360** **Traumatic hemorrhage of cerebrum, unspecified,** without loss of consciousness   MCC H5 HCC

⁷ ✓7ᵗʰ **S06.361** **Traumatic hemorrhage of cerebrum, unspecified, with loss of consciousness of** 30 minutes or less   MCC H5 HCC

⁷ ✓7ᵗʰ **S06.362** **Traumatic hemorrhage of cerebrum, unspecified, with loss of consciousness of** 31 minutes to 59 minutes   MCC H5 HCC

⁷ ✓7ᵗʰ **S06.363** **Traumatic hemorrhage of cerebrum, unspecified, with loss of consciousness of** 1 hours to 5 hours 59 minutes   MCC H5 HCC

⁷ ✓7ᵗʰ **S06.364** **Traumatic hemorrhage of cerebrum, unspecified, with loss of consciousness of** 6 hours to 24 hours   MCC H5 HCC

⁷ ✓7ᵗʰ **S06.365** **Traumatic hemorrhage of cerebrum, unspecified, with loss of consciousness** greater than 24 hours with return to pre-existing conscious level   MCC H5 HCC

✓ Additional Character Required   ✓x7ᵗʰ Placeholder   Unacceptable PDx   Questionable PDx   Manifestation   Unspecified Dx   H1-H14 HAC   HCC CMS-HCC Dx   HIV HIV Dx

ICD-10-CM 2021   **973**

7 √7ᵗʰ **S06.366 Traumatic hemorrhage of cerebrum, unspecified, with loss of consciousness** greater than 24 hours without return to pre-existing conscious level with patient surviving   MCC H5

√7ᵗʰ **S06.367 Traumatic hemorrhage of cerebrum, unspecified, with loss of consciousness** of any duration with death due to brain injury prior to regaining consciousness   MCC H5

√7ᵗʰ **S06.368 Traumatic hemorrhage of cerebrum, unspecified, with loss of consciousness** of any duration with death due to other cause prior to regaining consciousness   MCC H5

7 √7ᵗʰ **S06.369 Traumatic hemorrhage of cerebrum, unspecified, with loss of consciousness** of unspecified duration   MCC H5 HCC
Traumatic hemorrhage of cerebrum NOS

√6ᵗʰ **S06.37 Contusion, laceration, and hemorrhage of cerebellum**

7 √7ᵗʰ **S06.370 Contusion, laceration, and hemorrhage of cerebellum** without loss of consciousness   MCC H5 HCC

7 √7ᵗʰ **S06.371 Contusion, laceration, and hemorrhage of cerebellum with loss of consciousness** of 30 minutes or less   CC H5 HCC

7 √7ᵗʰ **S06.372 Contusion, laceration, and hemorrhage of cerebellum with loss of consciousness** of 31 minutes to 59 minutes   CC H5 HCC

7 √7ᵗʰ **S06.373 Contusion, laceration, and hemorrhage of cerebellum with loss of consciousness** of 1 hour to 5 hours 59 minutes   CC H5 HCC

7 √7ᵗʰ **S06.374 Contusion, laceration, and hemorrhage of cerebellum with loss of consciousness** of 6 hours to 24 hours   CC H5 HCC

7 √7ᵗʰ **S06.375 Contusion, laceration, and hemorrhage of cerebellum with loss of consciousness** greater than 24 hours with return to pre-existing conscious level   CC H5 HCC

7 √7ᵗʰ **S06.376 Contusion, laceration, and hemorrhage of cerebellum with loss of consciousness** greater than 24 hours without return to pre-existing conscious level with patient surviving   MCC H5 HCC

7 √7ᵗʰ **S06.377 Contusion, laceration, and hemorrhage of cerebellum with loss of consciousness** of any duration with death due to brain injury prior to regaining consciousness   MCC H5

√7ᵗʰ **S06.378 Contusion, laceration, and hemorrhage of cerebellum with loss of consciousness** of any duration with death due to other cause prior to regaining consciousness   MCC H5

7 √7ᵗʰ **S06.379 Contusion, laceration, and hemorrhage of cerebellum with loss of consciousness** of unspecified duration   CC H5 HCC
Contusion, laceration, and hemorrhage of cerebellum NOS

√6ᵗʰ **S06.38 Contusion, laceration, and hemorrhage of brainstem**

7 √7ᵗʰ **S06.380 Contusion, laceration, and hemorrhage of brainstem** without loss of consciousness   MCC H5 HCC

7 √7ᵗʰ **S06.381 Contusion, laceration, and hemorrhage of brainstem with loss of consciousness** of 30 minutes or less   CC H5 HCC

7 √7ᵗʰ **S06.382 Contusion, laceration, and hemorrhage of brainstem with loss of consciousness** of 31 minutes to 59 minutes   CC H5 HCC

7 √7ᵗʰ **S06.383 Contusion, laceration, and hemorrhage of brainstem with loss of consciousness** of 1 hour to 5 hours 59 minutes   CC H5 HCC

7 √7ᵗʰ **S06.384 Contusion, laceration, and hemorrhage of brainstem with loss of consciousness** of 6 hours to 24 hours   CC H5 HCC

7 √7ᵗʰ **S06.385 Contusion, laceration, and hemorrhage of brainstem with loss of consciousness** greater than 24 hours with return to pre-existing conscious level   CC H5 HCC

7 √7ᵗʰ **S06.386 Contusion, laceration, and hemorrhage of brainstem with loss of consciousness** greater than 24 hours without return to pre-existing conscious level with patient surviving   MCC H5 HCC

√7ᵗʰ **S06.387 Contusion, laceration, and hemorrhage of brainstem with loss of consciousness** of any duration with death due to brain injury prior to regaining consciousness   MCC H5

√7ᵗʰ **S06.388 Contusion, laceration, and hemorrhage of brainstem with loss of consciousness** of any duration with death due to other cause prior to regaining consciousness   MCC H5

7 √7ᵗʰ **S06.389 Contusion, laceration, and hemorrhage of brainstem with loss of consciousness** of unspecified duration   CC H5 HCC
Contusion, laceration, and hemorrhage of brainstem NOS

√5ᵗʰ **S06.4 Epidural hemorrhage**
Extradural hemorrhage NOS
Extradural hemorrhage (traumatic)
DEF: Epidural space: Space between the endosteum of the cranium (skull) and the dura mater, the outermost layer of a three-layer membrane that covers the brain.

√6ᵗʰ **S06.4X Epidural hemorrhage**

7 √7ᵗʰ **S06.4X0 Epidural hemorrhage** without loss of consciousness   MCC H5 HCC

7 √7ᵗʰ **S06.4X1 Epidural hemorrhage with loss of consciousness** of 30 minutes or less   MCC H5 HCC

7 √7ᵗʰ **S06.4X2 Epidural hemorrhage with loss of consciousness** of 31 minutes to 59 minutes   MCC H5 HCC

7 √7ᵗʰ **S06.4X3 Epidural hemorrhage with loss of consciousness** of 1 hour to 5 hours 59 minutes   MCC H5 HCC

7 √7ᵗʰ **S06.4X4 Epidural hemorrhage with loss of consciousness** of 6 hours to 24 hours   MCC H5 HCC

7 √7ᵗʰ **S06.4X5 Epidural hemorrhage with loss of consciousness** greater than 24 hours with return to pre-existing conscious level   MCC H5 HCC

7 √7ᵗʰ **S06.4X6 Epidural hemorrhage with loss of consciousness** greater than 24 hours without return to pre-existing conscious level with patient surviving   MCC H5 HCC

√7ᵗʰ **S06.4X7 Epidural hemorrhage with loss of consciousness** of any duration with death due to brain injury prior to regaining consciousness   MCC H5

√7ᵗʰ **S06.4X8 Epidural hemorrhage with loss of consciousness** of any duration with death due to other causes prior to regaining consciousness   MCC H5

7 √7ᵗʰ **S06.4X9 Epidural hemorrhage with loss of consciousness** of unspecified duration   MCC H5 HCC
Epidural hemorrhage NOS

√5ᵗʰ **S06.5 Traumatic subdural hemorrhage**
DEF: Subdural: Potential space between the dura mater and arachnoid membrane around the brain.

√6ᵗʰ **S06.5X Traumatic subdural hemorrhage**

7 √7ᵗʰ **S06.5X0 Traumatic subdural hemorrhage** without loss of consciousness   MCC H5 HCC

7 √7ᵗʰ **S06.5X1 Traumatic subdural hemorrhage with loss of consciousness** of 30 minutes or less   MCC H5 HCC

7 √7ᵗʰ **S06.5X2 Traumatic subdural hemorrhage with loss of consciousness** of 31 minutes to 59 minutes   MCC H5 HCC

7 √7ᵗʰ **S06.5X3 Traumatic subdural hemorrhage with loss of consciousness** of 1 hour to 5 hours 59 minutes   MCC H5 HCC

7 √7ᵗʰ **S06.5X4 Traumatic subdural hemorrhage with loss of consciousness** of 6 hours to 24 hours   MCC H5 HCC

7 √7ᵗʰ **S06.5X5** Traumatic subdural hemorrhage with loss of consciousness greater than 24 hours with return to pre-existing conscious level   MCC H5 HCC

7 √7ᵗʰ **S06.5X6** Traumatic subdural hemorrhage with loss of consciousness greater than 24 hours without return to pre-existing conscious level with patient surviving   MCC H5 HCC

√7ᵗʰ **S06.5X7** Traumatic subdural hemorrhage with loss of consciousness of any duration with death due to brain injury before regaining consciousness   MCC H5

√7ᵗʰ **S06.5X8** Traumatic subdural hemorrhage with loss of consciousness of any duration with death due to other cause before regaining consciousness   MCC H5

7 √7ᵗʰ **S06.5X9** Traumatic subdural hemorrhage with loss of consciousness of unspecified duration   MCC H5 HCC
    Traumatic subdural hemorrhage NOS

√5ᵗʰ **S06.6** Traumatic subarachnoid hemorrhage
   DEF: Subarachnoid: Space located between the arachnoid membrane and the pia mater that contains cerebrospinal fluid.

√6ᵗʰ **S06.6X** Traumatic subarachnoid hemorrhage

7 √7ᵗʰ **S06.6X0** Traumatic subarachnoid hemorrhage without loss of consciousness   MCC H5 HCC

7 √7ᵗʰ **S06.6X1** Traumatic subarachnoid hemorrhage with loss of consciousness of 30 minutes or less   MCC H5 HCC

7 √7ᵗʰ **S06.6X2** Traumatic subarachnoid hemorrhage with loss of consciousness of 31 minutes to 59 minutes   MCC H5 HCC

7 √7ᵗʰ **S06.6X3** Traumatic subarachnoid hemorrhage with loss of consciousness of 1 hour to 5 hours 59 minutes   MCC H5 HCC

7 √7ᵗʰ **S06.6X4** Traumatic subarachnoid hemorrhage with loss of consciousness of 6 hours to 24 hours   MCC H5 HCC

7 √7ᵗʰ **S06.6X5** Traumatic subarachnoid hemorrhage with loss of consciousness greater than 24 hours with return to pre-existing conscious level   MCC H5 HCC

7 √7ᵗʰ **S06.6X6** Traumatic subarachnoid hemorrhage with loss of consciousness greater than 24 hours without return to pre-existing conscious level with patient surviving   MCC H5 HCC

√7ᵗʰ **S06.6X7** Traumatic subarachnoid hemorrhage with loss of consciousness of any duration with death due to brain injury prior to regaining consciousness   MCC H5

√7ᵗʰ **S06.6X8** Traumatic subarachnoid hemorrhage with loss of consciousness of any duration with death due to other cause prior to regaining consciousness   MCC H5

7 √7ᵗʰ **S06.6X9** Traumatic subarachnoid hemorrhage with loss of consciousness of unspecified duration   MCC H5 HCC
    Traumatic subarachnoid hemorrhage NOS

√5ᵗʰ **S06.8** Other specified intracranial injuries

√6ᵗʰ **S06.81** Injury of right internal carotid artery, intracranial portion, not elsewhere classified

7 √7ᵗʰ **S06.810** Injury of right internal carotid artery, intracranial portion, not elsewhere classified without loss of consciousness   HCC

7 √7ᵗʰ **S06.811** Injury of right internal carotid artery, intracranial portion, not elsewhere classified with loss of consciousness of 30 minutes or less   CC H5 HCC

7 √7ᵗʰ **S06.812** Injury of right internal carotid artery, intracranial portion, not elsewhere classified with loss of consciousness of 31 minutes to 59 minutes   CC H5 HCC

7 √7ᵗʰ **S06.813** Injury of right internal carotid artery, intracranial portion, not elsewhere classified with loss of consciousness of 1 hour to 5 hours 59 minutes   CC H5 HCC

7 √7ᵗʰ **S06.814** Injury of right internal carotid artery, intracranial portion, not elsewhere classified with loss of consciousness of 6 hours to 24 hours   CC H5 HCC

7 √7ᵗʰ **S06.815** Injury of right internal carotid artery, intracranial portion, not elsewhere classified with loss of consciousness greater than 24 hours with return to pre-existing conscious level   CC H5 HCC

7 √7ᵗʰ **S06.816** Injury of right internal carotid artery, intracranial portion, not elsewhere classified with loss of consciousness greater than 24 hours without return to pre-existing conscious level with patient surviving   MCC H5 HCC

√7ᵗʰ **S06.817** Injury of right internal carotid artery, intracranial portion, not elsewhere classified with loss of consciousness of any duration with death due to brain injury prior to regaining consciousness   MCC H5

√7ᵗʰ **S06.818** Injury of right internal carotid artery, intracranial portion, not elsewhere classified with loss of consciousness of any duration with death due to other cause prior to regaining consciousness   MCC H5

7 √7ᵗʰ **S06.819** Injury of right internal carotid artery, intracranial portion, not elsewhere classified with loss of consciousness of unspecified duration   CC H5 HCC
    Injury of right internal carotid artery, intracranial portion, not elsewhere classified NOS

√6ᵗʰ **S06.82** Injury of left internal carotid artery, intracranial portion, not elsewhere classified

7 √7ᵗʰ **S06.820** Injury of left internal carotid artery, intracranial portion, not elsewhere classified without loss of consciousness   HCC

7 √7ᵗʰ **S06.821** Injury of left internal carotid artery, intracranial portion, not elsewhere classified with loss of consciousness of 30 minutes or less   CC H5 HCC

7 √7ᵗʰ **S06.822** Injury of left internal carotid artery, intracranial portion, not elsewhere classified with loss of consciousness of 31 minutes to 59 minutes   CC H5 HCC

7 √7ᵗʰ **S06.823** Injury of left internal carotid artery, intracranial portion, not elsewhere classified with loss of consciousness of 1 hour to 5 hours 59 minutes   CC H5 HCC

7 √7ᵗʰ **S06.824** Injury of left internal carotid artery, intracranial portion, not elsewhere classified with loss of consciousness of 6 hours to 24 hours   CC H5 HCC

7 √7ᵗʰ **S06.825** Injury of left internal carotid artery, intracranial portion, not elsewhere classified with loss of consciousness greater than 24 hours with return to pre-existing conscious level   CC H5 HCC

7 √7ᵗʰ **S06.826** Injury of left internal carotid artery, intracranial portion, not elsewhere classified with loss of consciousness greater than 24 hours without return to pre-existing conscious level with patient surviving   MCC H5 HCC

√7ᵗʰ **S06.827** Injury of left internal carotid artery, intracranial portion, not elsewhere classified with loss of consciousness of any duration with death due to brain injury prior to regaining consciousness   MCC H5

√7ᵗʰ **S06.828** Injury of left internal carotid artery, intracranial portion, not elsewhere classified with loss of consciousness of any duration with death due to other cause prior to regaining consciousness   MCC H5

7 ✓7ᵗʰ **S06.829** **Injury of left internal carotid artery, intracranial portion, not elsewhere classified with loss of consciousness of unspecified duration** CC H5 HCC

Injury of left internal carotid artery, intracranial portion, not elsewhere classified NOS

✓6ᵗʰ **S06.89** **Other specified intracranial injury**

EXCLUDES 1   concussion (S06.0X-)

7 ✓7ᵗʰ **S06.890** **Other specified intracranial injury without loss of consciousness** HCC

7 ✓7ᵗʰ **S06.891** **Other specified intracranial injury with loss of consciousness of 30 minutes or less** CC H5 HCC

7 ✓7ᵗʰ **S06.892** **Other specified intracranial injury with loss of consciousness of 31 minutes to 59 minutes** CC H5 HCC

7 ✓7ᵗʰ **S06.893** **Other specified intracranial injury with loss of consciousness of 1 hour to 5 hours 59 minutes** CC H5 HCC

7 ✓7ᵗʰ **S06.894** **Other specified intracranial injury with loss of consciousness of 6 hours to 24 hours** CC H5 HCC

7 ✓7ᵗʰ **S06.895** **Other specified intracranial injury with loss of consciousness greater than 24 hours with return to pre-existing conscious level** CC H5 HCC

7 ✓7ᵗʰ **S06.896** **Other specified intracranial injury with loss of consciousness greater than 24 hours without return to pre-existing conscious level with patient surviving** MCC H5 HCC

✓7ᵗʰ **S06.897** **Other specified intracranial injury with loss of consciousness of any duration with death due to brain injury prior to regaining consciousness** MCC H5

✓7ᵗʰ **S06.898** **Other specified intracranial injury with loss of consciousness of any duration with death due to other cause prior to regaining consciousness** MCC H5

7 ✓7ᵗʰ **S06.899** **Other specified intracranial injury with loss of consciousness of unspecified duration** CC H5 HCC

✓5ᵗʰ **S06.9** **Unspecified intracranial injury**

Brain injury NOS
Head injury NOS with loss of consciousness
Traumatic brain injury NOS

EXCLUDES 1   conditions classifiable to S06.0- to S06.8- code to specified intracranial injury
head injury NOS (S09.90)

AHA: 2020,2Q,31

✓6ᵗʰ **S06.9X** **Unspecified intracranial injury**

7 ✓7ᵗʰ **S06.9X0** **Unspecified intracranial injury without loss of consciousness** HCC

7 ✓7ᵗʰ **S06.9X1** **Unspecified intracranial injury with loss of consciousness of 30 minutes or less** CC H5 HCC

7 ✓7ᵗʰ **S06.9X2** **Unspecified intracranial injury with loss of consciousness of 31 minutes to 59 minutes** CC H5 HCC

7 ✓7ᵗʰ **S06.9X3** **Unspecified intracranial injury with loss of consciousness of 1 hour to 5 hours 59 minutes** CC H5 HCC

7 ✓7ᵗʰ **S06.9X4** **Unspecified intracranial injury with loss of consciousness of 6 hours to 24 hours** CC H5 HCC

7 ✓7ᵗʰ **S06.9X5** **Unspecified intracranial injury with loss of consciousness greater than 24 hours with return to pre-existing conscious level** CC H5 HCC

7 ✓7ᵗʰ **S06.9X6** **Unspecified intracranial injury with loss of consciousness greater than 24 hours without return to pre-existing conscious level with patient surviving** MCC H5 HCC

✓7ᵗʰ **S06.9X7** **Unspecified intracranial injury with loss of consciousness of any duration with death due to brain injury prior to regaining consciousness** MCC H5

✓7ᵗʰ **S06.9X8** **Unspecified intracranial injury with loss of consciousness of any duration with death due to other cause prior to regaining consciousness** MCC H5

7 ✓7ᵗʰ **S06.9X9** **Unspecified intracranial injury with loss of consciousness of unspecified duration** CC H5 HCC

✓4ᵗʰ **S07** **Crushing injury of head**

Use additional code for all associated injuries, such as:
intracranial injuries (S06.-)
skull fractures (S02.-)

The appropriate 7th character is to be added to each code from category S07.
A   initial encounter
D   subsequent encounter
S   sequela

✓x7ᵗʰ **S07.0** **Crushing injury of face** CC H5

✓x7ᵗʰ **S07.1** **Crushing injury of skull** CC H5

✓x7ᵗʰ **S07.8** **Crushing injury of other parts of head** CC H5

✓x7ᵗʰ **S07.9** **Crushing injury of head, part unspecified** CC H5

✓4ᵗʰ **S08** **Avulsion and traumatic amputation of part of head**

An amputation not identified as partial or complete should be coded to complete

The appropriate 7th character is to be added to each code from category S08.
A   initial encounter
D   subsequent encounter
S   sequela

✓x7ᵗʰ **S08.0** **Avulsion of scalp**

✓5ᵗʰ **S08.1** **Traumatic amputation of ear**

✓6ᵗʰ **S08.11** **Complete traumatic amputation of ear**

✓7ᵗʰ **S08.111** **Complete traumatic amputation of right ear**

✓7ᵗʰ **S08.112** **Complete traumatic amputation of left ear**

✓7ᵗʰ **S08.119** **Complete traumatic amputation of unspecified ear**

✓6ᵗʰ **S08.12** **Partial traumatic amputation of ear**

✓7ᵗʰ **S08.121** **Partial traumatic amputation of right ear**

✓7ᵗʰ **S08.122** **Partial traumatic amputation of left ear**

✓7ᵗʰ **S08.129** **Partial traumatic amputation of unspecified ear**

✓5ᵗʰ **S08.8** **Traumatic amputation of other parts of head**

✓6ᵗʰ **S08.81** **Traumatic amputation of nose**

✓7ᵗʰ **S08.811** **Complete traumatic amputation of nose**

✓7ᵗʰ **S08.812** **Partial traumatic amputation of nose**

✓x7ᵗʰ **S08.89** **Traumatic amputation of other parts of head**

✓4ᵗʰ **S09** **Other and unspecified injuries of head**

The appropriate 7th character is to be added to each code from category S09.
A   initial encounter
D   subsequent encounter
S   sequela

✓x7ᵗʰ **S09.0** **Injury of blood vessels of head, not elsewhere classified** CC

EXCLUDES 1   injury of cerebral blood vessels (S06.-)
injury of precerebral blood vessels (S15.-)

✓5ᵗʰ **S09.1** **Injury of muscle and tendon of head**

Code also any associated open wound (S01.-)

EXCLUDES 2   sprain to joints and ligament of head (S03.9)

✓x7ᵗʰ **S09.10** **Unspecified injury of muscle and tendon of head**

Injury of muscle and tendon of head NOS

✓x7ᵗʰ **S09.11** **Strain of muscle and tendon of head**

✓x7ᵗʰ **S09.12** **Laceration of muscle and tendon of head**

✓x7ᵗʰ **S09.19** **Other specified injury of muscle and tendon of head**

✓5ᵗʰ **S09.2** **Traumatic rupture of ear drum**

EXCLUDES 1   traumatic rupture of ear drum due to blast injury (S09.31-)

✓x7ᵗʰ **S09.20** **Traumatic rupture of unspecified ear drum** CC

✓x7ᵗʰ **S09.21** **Traumatic rupture of right ear drum** CC

✓x7ᵗʰ **S09.22** **Traumatic rupture of left ear drum** CC

N Newborn: 0   P Pediatric: 0-17   M Maternity: 9-64   A Adult: 15-124   MCC Major Complication/Comorbidity   CC Complication/Comorbidity   SW Severe Wound Dx

976   ICD-10-CM 2021

√5ᵗʰ S09.3 Other specified and unspecified injury of middle and inner ear

> EXCLUDES 1   injury to ear NOS (S09.91-)
> EXCLUDES 2   injury to external ear (S00.4-, S01.3-, S08.1-)

  √6ᵗʰ **S09.30 Unspecified injury of middle and inner ear**

    √7ᵗʰ **S09.301 Unspecified injury of right middle and inner ear**   cc

    √7ᵗʰ **S09.302 Unspecified injury of left middle and inner ear**   cc

    √7ᵗʰ **S09.309 Unspecified injury of unspecified middle and inner ear**   cc

  √6ᵗʰ **S09.31 Primary blast injury of ear**

    Blast injury of ear NOS

    √7ᵗʰ **S09.311 Primary blast injury of right ear**   cc

    √7ᵗʰ **S09.312 Primary blast injury of left ear**   cc

    √7ᵗʰ **S09.313 Primary blast injury of ear, bilateral**   cc

    √7ᵗʰ **S09.319 Primary blast injury of unspecified ear**   cc

  √6ᵗʰ **S09.39 Other specified injury of middle and inner ear**

    Secondary blast injury to ear

    √7ᵗʰ **S09.391 Other specified injury of right middle and inner ear**   cc

    √7ᵗʰ **S09.392 Other specified injury of left middle and inner ear**   cc

    √7ᵗʰ **S09.399 Other specified injury of unspecified middle and inner ear**   cc

√x7ᵗʰ S09.8 Other specified injuries of head

√5ᵗʰ S09.9 Unspecified injury of face and head

  √x7ᵗʰ **S09.90 Unspecified injury of head**

    Head injury NOS

> EXCLUDES 1   brain injury NOS (S06.9-)
>   head injury NOS with loss of consciousness (S06.9-)
>   intracranial injury NOS (S06.9-)

  √x7ᵗʰ **S09.91 Unspecified injury of ear**

    Injury of ear NOS

  √x7ᵗʰ **S09.92 Unspecified injury of nose**

    Injury of nose NOS

  √x7ᵗʰ **S09.93 Unspecified injury of face**

    Injury of face NOS

    AHA: 2019,2Q,23

Injuries to the neck (S10-S19)

> INCLUDES   injuries of nape
>   injuries of supraclavicular region
>   injuries of throat
> EXCLUDES 2   burns and corrosions (T20-T32)
>   effects of foreign body in esophagus (T18.1)
>   effects of foreign body in larynx (T17.3)
>   effects of foreign body in pharynx (T17.2)
>   effects of foreign body in trachea (T17.4)
>   frostbite (T33-T34)
>   insect bite or sting, venomous (T63.4)

√4ᵗʰ S10 Superficial injury of neck

> The appropriate 7th character is to be added to each code from category S10.
> A   initial encounter
> D   subsequent encounter
> S   sequela

√x7ᵗʰ S10.0 Contusion of throat

  Contusion of cervical esophagus
  Contusion of larynx
  Contusion of pharynx
  Contusion of trachea

√5ᵗʰ S10.1 Other and unspecified superficial injuries of throat

  √x7ᵗʰ **S10.10 Unspecified superficial injuries of throat**

  √x7ᵗʰ **S10.11 Abrasion of throat**

  √x7ᵗʰ **S10.12 Blister (nonthermal) of throat**

  √x7ᵗʰ **S10.14 External constriction of part of throat**

  √x7ᵗʰ **S10.15 Superficial foreign body of throat**

    Splinter in the throat

  √x7ᵗʰ **S10.16 Insect bite (nonvenomous) of throat**

  √x7ᵗʰ **S10.17 Other superficial bite of throat**

> EXCLUDES 1   open bite of throat (S11.85)

√5ᵗʰ S10.8 Superficial injury of other specified parts of neck

  √x7ᵗʰ **S10.80 Unspecified superficial injury of other specified part of neck**

  √x7ᵗʰ **S10.81 Abrasion of other specified part of neck**

  √x7ᵗʰ **S10.82 Blister (nonthermal) of other specified part of neck**

  √x7ᵗʰ **S10.83 Contusion of other specified part of neck**

  √x7ᵗʰ **S10.84 External constriction of other specified part of neck**

  √x7ᵗʰ **S10.85 Superficial foreign body of other specified part of neck**

    Splinter in other specified part of neck

  √x7ᵗʰ **S10.86 Insect bite of other specified part of neck**

  √x7ᵗʰ **S10.87 Other superficial bite of other specified part of neck**

> EXCLUDES 1   open bite of other specified parts of neck (S11.85)

√5ᵗʰ S10.9 Superficial injury of unspecified part of neck

  √x7ᵗʰ **S10.90 Unspecified superficial injury of unspecified part of neck**

  √x7ᵗʰ **S10.91 Abrasion of unspecified part of neck**

  √x7ᵗʰ **S10.92 Blister (nonthermal) of unspecified part of neck**

  √x7ᵗʰ **S10.93 Contusion of unspecified part of neck**

  √x7ᵗʰ **S10.94 External constriction of unspecified part of neck**

  √x7ᵗʰ **S10.95 Superficial foreign body of unspecified part of neck**

  √x7ᵗʰ **S10.96 Insect bite of unspecified part of neck**

  √x7ᵗʰ **S10.97 Other superficial bite of unspecified part of neck**

√4ᵗʰ S11 Open wound of neck

> Code also any associated:
>   spinal cord injury (S14.0, S14.1-)
>   wound infection
> EXCLUDES 2   open fracture of vertebra (S12.- with 7th character B)

> The appropriate 7th character is to be added to each code from category S11.
> A   initial encounter
> D   subsequent encounter
> S   sequela

√5ᵗʰ S11.0 Open wound of larynx and trachea

  √6ᵗʰ **S11.01 Open wound of larynx**

> EXCLUDES 2   open wound of vocal cord (S11.03)

    √7ᵗʰ **S11.011 Laceration without foreign body of larynx**   MCC

    √7ᵗʰ **S11.012 Laceration with foreign body of larynx**   MCC

    √7ᵗʰ **S11.013 Puncture wound without foreign body of larynx**   MCC

    √7ᵗʰ **S11.014 Puncture wound with foreign body of larynx**   MCC

    √7ᵗʰ **S11.015 Open bite of larynx**   MCC

    Bite of larynx NOS

    √7ᵗʰ **S11.019 Unspecified open wound of larynx**   MCC

  √6ᵗʰ **S11.02 Open wound of trachea**

    Open wound of cervical trachea
    Open wound of trachea NOS

> EXCLUDES 2   open wound of thoracic trachea (S27.5-)

    √7ᵗʰ **S11.021 Laceration without foreign body of trachea**   MCC

    √7ᵗʰ **S11.022 Laceration with foreign body of trachea**   MCC

    √7ᵗʰ **S11.023 Puncture wound without foreign body of trachea**   MCC

    √7ᵗʰ **S11.024 Puncture wound with foreign body of trachea**   MCC

    √7ᵗʰ **S11.025 Open bite of trachea**   MCC

    Bite of trachea NOS

    √7ᵗʰ **S11.029 Unspecified open wound of trachea**   MCC

  √6ᵗʰ **S11.03 Open wound of vocal cord**

    √7ᵗʰ **S11.031 Laceration without foreign body of vocal cord**   MCC

    √7ᵗʰ **S11.032 Laceration with foreign body of vocal cord**   MCC

    √7ᵗʰ **S11.033 Puncture wound without foreign body of vocal cord**   MCC

☑ Additional Character Required   √x7ᵗʰ Placeholder   Unacceptable PDx   Questionable PDx   Manifestation   Unspecified Dx   H1-H14 HAC   HCC CMS-HCC Dx   HIV HIV Dx

ICD-10-CM 2021   977

✓7ᵗʰ **S11.034** Puncture wound with foreign body of vocal cord   MCC

✓7ᵗʰ **S11.035** Open bite of vocal cord   MCC
Bite of vocal cord NOS

✓7ᵗʰ **S11.039** Unspecified open wound of vocal cord   MCC

✓5ᵗʰ **S11.1** Open wound of thyroid gland

✓x7ᵗʰ **S11.10** Unspecified open wound of thyroid gland   CC

✓x7ᵗʰ **S11.11** Laceration without foreign body of thyroid gland   CC

✓x7ᵗʰ **S11.12** Laceration with foreign body of thyroid gland   CC

✓x7ᵗʰ **S11.13** Puncture wound without foreign body of thyroid gland   CC

✓x7ᵗʰ **S11.14** Puncture wound with foreign body of thyroid gland   CC

✓x7ᵗʰ **S11.15** Open bite of thyroid gland   CC
Bite of thyroid gland NOS

✓5ᵗʰ **S11.2** Open wound of pharynx and cervical esophagus
EXCLUDES 1   open wound of esophagus NOS (S27.8-)

✓x7ᵗʰ **S11.20** Unspecified open wound of pharynx and cervical esophagus   CC

✓x7ᵗʰ **S11.21** Laceration without foreign body of pharynx and cervical esophagus   CC

✓x7ᵗʰ **S11.22** Laceration with foreign body of pharynx and cervical esophagus   CC

✓x7ᵗʰ **S11.23** Puncture wound without foreign body of pharynx and cervical esophagus   CC

✓x7ᵗʰ **S11.24** Puncture wound with foreign body of pharynx and cervical esophagus   CC

✓x7ᵗʰ **S11.25** Open bite of pharynx and cervical esophagus   CC
Bite of pharynx and cervical esophagus NOS

✓5ᵗʰ **S11.8** Open wound of other specified parts of neck

✓x7ᵗʰ **S11.80** Unspecified open wound of other specified part of neck

✓x7ᵗʰ **S11.81** Laceration without foreign body of other specified part of neck

✓x7ᵗʰ **S11.82** Laceration with foreign body of other specified part of neck

✓x7ᵗʰ **S11.83** Puncture wound without foreign body of other specified part of neck

✓x7ᵗʰ **S11.84** Puncture wound with foreign body of other specified part of neck

✓x7ᵗʰ **S11.85** Open bite of other specified part of neck
Bite of other specified part of neck NOS
EXCLUDES 1   superficial bite of other specified part of neck (S10.87)

✓x7ᵗʰ **S11.89** Other open wound of other specified part of neck

✓5ᵗʰ **S11.9** Open wound of unspecified part of neck

✓x7ᵗʰ **S11.90** Unspecified open wound of unspecified part of neck

✓x7ᵗʰ **S11.91** Laceration without foreign body of unspecified part of neck

✓x7ᵗʰ **S11.92** Laceration with foreign body of unspecified part of neck

✓x7ᵗʰ **S11.93** Puncture wound without foreign body of unspecified part of neck

✓x7ᵗʰ **S11.94** Puncture wound with foreign body of unspecified part of neck

✓x7ᵗʰ **S11.95** Open bite of unspecified part of neck
Bite of neck NOS
EXCLUDES 1   superficial bite of neck (S10.97)

✓4ᵗʰ **S12** Fracture of cervical vertebra and other parts of neck

NOTE   A fracture not indicated as displaced or nondisplaced should be coded to displaced.

A fracture not indicated as open or closed should be coded to closed.

INCLUDES   fracture of cervical neural arch
fracture of cervical spine
fracture of cervical spinous process
fracture of cervical transverse process
fracture of cervical vertebral arch
fracture of neck

Code first any associated cervical spinal cord injury (S14.0, S14.1-)
AHA: 2018,2Q,12; 2015,3Q,37-39

The appropriate 7th character is to be added to all codes from subcategories S12.0-S12.6.
A   initial encounter for closed fracture
B   initial encounter for open fracture
D   subsequent encounter for fracture with routine healing
G   subsequent encounter for fracture with delayed healing
K   subsequent encounter for fracture with nonunion
S   sequela

✓5ᵗʰ **S12.0** Fracture of first cervical vertebra
Atlas

✓6ᵗʰ **S12.00** Unspecified fracture of first cervical vertebra

2,3,6 ✓7ᵗʰ **S12.000** Unspecified displaced fracture of first cervical vertebra   MCC CC H5 HCC

2,3,6 ✓7ᵗʰ **S12.001** Unspecified nondisplaced fracture of first cervical vertebra   MCC CC H5 HCC

2,3,6 ✓x7ᵗʰ **S12.01** Stable burst fracture of first cervical vertebra   MCC CC H5 HCC

2,3,6 ✓x7ᵗʰ **S12.02** Unstable burst fracture of first cervical vertebra   MCC CC H5 HCC

✓6ᵗʰ **S12.03** Posterior arch fracture of first cervical vertebra

2,3,6 ✓7ᵗʰ **S12.030** Displaced posterior arch fracture of first cervical vertebra   MCC CC H5 HCC

2,3,6 ✓7ᵗʰ **S12.031** Nondisplaced posterior arch fracture of first cervical vertebra   MCC CC H5 HCC

✓6ᵗʰ **S12.04** Lateral mass fracture of first cervical vertebra

2,3,6 ✓7ᵗʰ **S12.040** Displaced lateral mass fracture of first cervical vertebra   MCC CC H5 HCC

2,3,6 ✓7ᵗʰ **S12.041** Nondisplaced lateral mass fracture of first cervical vertebra   MCC CC H5 HCC

✓6ᵗʰ **S12.09** Other fracture of first cervical vertebra

2,3,6 ✓7ᵗʰ **S12.090** Other displaced fracture of first cervical vertebra   MCC CC H5 HCC

2,3,6 ✓7ᵗʰ **S12.091** Other nondisplaced fracture of first cervical vertebra   MCC CC H5 HCC

✓5ᵗʰ **S12.1** Fracture of second cervical vertebra
Axis

✓6ᵗʰ **S12.10** Unspecified fracture of second cervical vertebra

2,3,6 ✓7ᵗʰ **S12.100** Unspecified displaced fracture of second cervical vertebra   MCC CC H5 HCC

2,3,6 ✓7ᵗʰ **S12.101** Unspecified nondisplaced fracture of second cervical vertebra   MCC CC H5 HCC

✓6ᵗʰ **S12.11** Type II dens fracture

2,3,6 ✓7ᵗʰ **S12.110** Anterior displaced Type II dens fracture   MCC CC H5 HCC

2,3,6 ✓7ᵗʰ **S12.111** Posterior displaced Type II dens fracture   MCC CC H5 HCC

2,3,6 ✓7ᵗʰ **S12.112** Nondisplaced Type II dens fracture   MCC CC H5 HCC

✓6ᵗʰ **S12.12** Other dens fracture

2,3,6 ✓7ᵗʰ **S12.120** Other displaced dens fracture   MCC CC H5 HCC

2,3,6 ✓7ᵗʰ **S12.121** Other nondisplaced dens fracture   MCC CC H5 HCC

✓6ᵗʰ **S12.13** Unspecified traumatic spondylolisthesis of second cervical vertebra

2,3,6 ✓7ᵗʰ **S12.130** Unspecified traumatic displaced spondylolisthesis of second cervical vertebra   MCC CC H5 HCC

2,3,6 ✓7ᵗʰ **S12.131** Unspecified traumatic nondisplaced spondylolisthesis of second cervical vertebra   MCC CC H5 HCC

2,3,6 √x7ᵗʰ **S12.14** Type III traumatic spondylolisthesis of second cervical vertebra   MCC CC H5 HCC

√6ᵗʰ **S12.15** Other traumatic spondylolisthesis of second cervical vertebra

    2,3,6 √7ᵗʰ **S12.150** Other traumatic displaced spondylolisthesis of second cervical vertebra   MCC CC H5 HCC

    2,3,6 √7ᵗʰ **S12.151** Other traumatic nondisplaced spondylolisthesis of second cervical vertebra   MCC CC H5 HCC

√6ᵗʰ **S12.19** Other fracture of second cervical vertebra

    2,3,6 √7ᵗʰ **S12.190** Other displaced fracture of second cervical vertebra   MCC CC H5 HCC

    2,3,6 √7ᵗʰ **S12.191** Other nondisplaced fracture of second cervical vertebra   MCC CC H5 HCC

√5ᵗʰ **S12.2** Fracture of third cervical vertebra

   √6ᵗʰ **S12.20** Unspecified fracture of third cervical vertebra

    2,3,6 √7ᵗʰ **S12.200** Unspecified displaced fracture of third cervical vertebra   MCC CC H5 HCC

    2,3,6 √7ᵗʰ **S12.201** Unspecified nondisplaced fracture of third cervical vertebra   MCC CC H5 HCC

   √6ᵗʰ **S12.23** Unspecified traumatic spondylolisthesis of third cervical vertebra

    2,3,6 √7ᵗʰ **S12.230** Unspecified traumatic displaced spondylolisthesis of third cervical vertebra   MCC CC H5 HCC

    2,3,6 √7ᵗʰ **S12.231** Unspecified traumatic nondisplaced spondylolisthesis of third cervical vertebra   MCC CC H5 HCC

2,3,6 √x7ᵗʰ **S12.24** Type III traumatic spondylolisthesis of third cervical vertebra   MCC CC H5 HCC

   √6ᵗʰ **S12.25** Other traumatic spondylolisthesis of third cervical vertebra

    2,3,6 √7ᵗʰ **S12.250** Other traumatic displaced spondylolisthesis of third cervical vertebra   MCC CC H5 HCC

    2,3,6 √7ᵗʰ **S12.251** Other traumatic nondisplaced spondylolisthesis of third cervical vertebra   MCC CC H5 HCC

   √6ᵗʰ **S12.29** Other fracture of third cervical vertebra

    2,3,6 √7ᵗʰ **S12.290** Other displaced fracture of third cervical vertebra   MCC CC H5 HCC

    2,3,6 √7ᵗʰ **S12.291** Other nondisplaced fracture of third cervical vertebra   MCC CC H5 HCC

√5ᵗʰ **S12.3** Fracture of fourth cervical vertebra

   √6ᵗʰ **S12.30** Unspecified fracture of fourth cervical vertebra

    2,3,6 √7ᵗʰ **S12.300** Unspecified displaced fracture of fourth cervical vertebra   MCC CC H5 HCC

    2,3,6 √7ᵗʰ **S12.301** Unspecified nondisplaced fracture of fourth cervical vertebra   MCC CC H5 HCC

   √6ᵗʰ **S12.33** Unspecified traumatic spondylolisthesis of fourth cervical vertebra

    2,3,6 √7ᵗʰ **S12.330** Unspecified traumatic displaced spondylolisthesis of fourth cervical vertebra   MCC CC H5 HCC

    2,3,6 √7ᵗʰ **S12.331** Unspecified traumatic nondisplaced spondylolisthesis of fourth cervical vertebra   MCC CC H5 HCC

2,3,6 √x7ᵗʰ **S12.34** Type III traumatic spondylolisthesis of fourth cervical vertebra   MCC CC H5 HCC

   √6ᵗʰ **S12.35** Other traumatic spondylolisthesis of fourth cervical vertebra

    2,3,6 √7ᵗʰ **S12.350** Other traumatic displaced spondylolisthesis of fourth cervical vertebra   MCC CC H5 HCC

    2,3,6 √7ᵗʰ **S12.351** Other traumatic nondisplaced spondylolisthesis of fourth cervical vertebra   MCC CC H5 HCC

   √6ᵗʰ **S12.39** Other fracture of fourth cervical vertebra

    2,3,6 √7ᵗʰ **S12.390** Other displaced fracture of fourth cervical vertebra   MCC CC H5 HCC

    2,3,6 √7ᵗʰ **S12.391** Other nondisplaced fracture of fourth cervical vertebra   MCC CC H5 HCC

√5ᵗʰ **S12.4** Fracture of fifth cervical vertebra

   √6ᵗʰ **S12.40** Unspecified fracture of fifth cervical vertebra

    2,3,6 √7ᵗʰ **S12.400** Unspecified displaced fracture of fifth cervical vertebra   MCC CC H5 HCC

    2,3,6 √7ᵗʰ **S12.401** Unspecified nondisplaced fracture of fifth cervical vertebra   MCC CC H5 HCC

√6ᵗʰ **S12.43** Unspecified traumatic spondylolisthesis of fifth cervical vertebra

    2,3,6 √7ᵗʰ **S12.430** Unspecified traumatic displaced spondylolisthesis of fifth cervical vertebra   MCC CC H5 HCC

    2,3,6 √7ᵗʰ **S12.431** Unspecified traumatic nondisplaced spondylolisthesis of fifth cervical vertebra   MCC CC H5 HCC

2,3,6 √x7ᵗʰ **S12.44** Type III traumatic spondylolisthesis of fifth cervical vertebra   MCC CC H5 HCC

   √6ᵗʰ **S12.45** Other traumatic spondylolisthesis of fifth cervical vertebra

    2,3,6 √7ᵗʰ **S12.450** Other traumatic displaced spondylolisthesis of fifth cervical vertebra   MCC CC H5 HCC

    2,3,6 √7ᵗʰ **S12.451** Other traumatic nondisplaced spondylolisthesis of fifth cervical vertebra   MCC CC H5 HCC

   √6ᵗʰ **S12.49** Other fracture of fifth cervical vertebra

    2,3,6 √7ᵗʰ **S12.490** Other displaced fracture of fifth cervical vertebra   MCC CC H5 HCC

    2,3,6 √7ᵗʰ **S12.491** Other nondisplaced fracture of fifth cervical vertebra   MCC CC H5 HCC

√5ᵗʰ **S12.5** Fracture of sixth cervical vertebra

   √6ᵗʰ **S12.50** Unspecified fracture of sixth cervical vertebra

    2,3,6 √7ᵗʰ **S12.500** Unspecified displaced fracture of sixth cervical vertebra   MCC CC H5 HCC

    2,3,6 √7ᵗʰ **S12.501** Unspecified nondisplaced fracture of sixth cervical vertebra   MCC CC H5 HCC

   √6ᵗʰ **S12.53** Unspecified traumatic spondylolisthesis of sixth cervical vertebra

    2,3,6 √7ᵗʰ **S12.530** Unspecified traumatic displaced spondylolisthesis of sixth cervical vertebra   MCC CC H5 HCC

    2,3,6 √7ᵗʰ **S12.531** Unspecified traumatic nondisplaced spondylolisthesis of sixth cervical vertebra   MCC CC H5 HCC

2,3,6 √x7ᵗʰ **S12.54** Type III traumatic spondylolisthesis of sixth cervical vertebra   MCC CC H5 HCC

   √6ᵗʰ **S12.55** Other traumatic spondylolisthesis of sixth cervical vertebra

    2,3,6 √7ᵗʰ **S12.550** Other traumatic displaced spondylolisthesis of sixth cervical vertebra   MCC CC H5 HCC

    2,3,6 √7ᵗʰ **S12.551** Other traumatic nondisplaced spondylolisthesis of sixth cervical vertebra   MCC CC H5 HCC

   √6ᵗʰ **S12.59** Other fracture of sixth cervical vertebra

    2,3,6 √7ᵗʰ **S12.590** Other displaced fracture of sixth cervical vertebra   MCC CC H5 HCC

    2,3,6 √7ᵗʰ **S12.591** Other nondisplaced fracture of sixth cervical vertebra   MCC CC H5 HCC

√5ᵗʰ **S12.6** Fracture of seventh cervical vertebra

   √6ᵗʰ **S12.60** Unspecified fracture of seventh cervical vertebra

    2,3,6 √7ᵗʰ **S12.600** Unspecified displaced fracture of seventh cervical vertebra   MCC CC H5 HCC

    2,3,6 √7ᵗʰ **S12.601** Unspecified nondisplaced fracture of seventh cervical vertebra   MCC CC H5 HCC

   √6ᵗʰ **S12.63** Unspecified traumatic spondylolisthesis of seventh cervical vertebra

    2,3,6 √7ᵗʰ **S12.630** Unspecified traumatic displaced spondylolisthesis of seventh cervical vertebra   MCC CC H5 HCC

    2,3,6 √7ᵗʰ **S12.631** Unspecified traumatic nondisplaced spondylolisthesis of seventh cervical vertebra   MCC CC H5 HCC

2,3,6 √x7ᵗʰ **S12.64** Type III traumatic spondylolisthesis of seventh cervical vertebra   MCC CC H5 HCC

   √6ᵗʰ **S12.65** Other traumatic spondylolisthesis of seventh cervical vertebra

    2,3,6 √7ᵗʰ **S12.650** Other traumatic displaced spondylolisthesis of seventh cervical vertebra   MCC CC H5 HCC

    2,3,6 √7ᵗʰ **S12.651** Other traumatic nondisplaced spondylolisthesis of seventh cervical vertebra   MCC CC H5 HCC

   √6ᵗʰ **S12.69** Other fracture of seventh cervical vertebra

    2,3,6 √7ᵗʰ **S12.690** Other displaced fracture of seventh cervical vertebra   MCC CC H5 HCC

☑ Additional Character Required   √x7ᵗʰ Placeholder   Unacceptable PDx   Questionable PDx   Manifestation   Unspecified Dx   H1-H14 HAC   HCC CMS-HCC Dx   HIV HIV Dx

ICD-10-CM 2021   **979**

2,3,6 √7th **S12.691** **Other nondisplaced fracture of seventh cervical vertebra** `MCC` `CC` `H5` `HCC`

6 √x7th **S12.8** **Fracture of other parts of neck** `MCC` `H5` `HCC`

Hyoid bone
Larynx
Thyroid cartilage
Trachea

The appropriate 7th character is to be added to code S12.8.
A initial encounter
D subsequent encounter
S sequela

6 √x7th **S12.9** **Fracture of neck, unspecified** `CC` `H5` `HCC`

Fracture of neck NOS
Fracture of cervical spine NOS
Fracture of cervical vertebra NOS

The appropriate 7th character is to be added to code S12.9.
A initial encounter
D subsequent encounter
S sequela

√4th **S13** **Dislocation and sprain of joints and ligaments at neck level**

`INCLUDES` avulsion of joint or ligament at neck level
laceration of cartilage, joint or ligament at neck level
sprain of cartilage, joint or ligament at neck level
traumatic hemarthrosis of joint or ligament at neck level
traumatic rupture of joint or ligament at neck level
traumatic subluxation of joint or ligament at neck level
traumatic tear of joint or ligament at neck level

Code also any associated open wound
`EXCLUDES 2` strain of muscle or tendon at neck level (S16.1)

The appropriate 7th character is to be added to each code from category S13.
A initial encounter
D subsequent encounter
S sequela

√x7th **S13.0** **Traumatic rupture of cervical intervertebral disc** `CC` `H5`

`EXCLUDES 1` rupture or displacement (nontraumatic) of cervical intervertebral disc NOS (M50.-)

√5th **S13.1** **Subluxation and dislocation of cervical vertebrae**

Code also any associated:
open wound of neck (S11.-)
spinal cord injury (S14.1-)
`EXCLUDES 2` fracture of cervical vertebrae (S12.0-S12.3-)

√6th **S13.10** **Subluxation and dislocation of unspecified cervical vertebrae**

√7th **S13.100** **Subluxation of unspecified cervical vertebrae** `CC` `H5`

√7th **S13.101** **Dislocation of unspecified cervical vertebrae** `CC` `H5`

√6th **S13.11** **Subluxation and dislocation of C0/C1 cervical vertebrae**

Subluxation and dislocation of atlantooccipital joint
Subluxation and dislocation of atloidooccipital joint
Subluxation and dislocation of occipitoatloid joint

√7th **S13.110** **Subluxation of C0/C1 cervical vertebrae** `CC` `H5`

√7th **S13.111** **Dislocation of C0/C1 cervical vertebrae** `CC` `H5`

√6th **S13.12** **Subluxation and dislocation of C1/C2 cervical vertebrae**

Subluxation and dislocation of atlantoaxial joint

√7th **S13.120** **Subluxation of C1/C2 cervical vertebrae** `CC` `H5`

√7th **S13.121** **Dislocation of C1/C2 cervical vertebrae** `CC` `H5`

√6th **S13.13** **Subluxation and dislocation of C2/C3 cervical vertebrae**

√7th **S13.130** **Subluxation of C2/C3 cervical vertebrae** `CC` `H5`

√7th **S13.131** **Dislocation of C2/C3 cervical vertebrae** `CC` `H5`

√6th **S13.14** **Subluxation and dislocation of C3/C4 cervical vertebrae**

√7th **S13.140** **Subluxation of C3/C4 cervical vertebrae** `CC` `H5`

√7th **S13.141** **Dislocation of C3/C4 cervical vertebrae** `CC` `H5`

√6th **S13.15** **Subluxation and dislocation of C4/C5 cervical vertebrae**

√7th **S13.150** **Subluxation of C4/C5 cervical vertebrae** `CC` `H5`

√7th **S13.151** **Dislocation of C4/C5 cervical vertebrae** `CC` `H5`

√6th **S13.16** **Subluxation and dislocation of C5/C6 cervical vertebrae**

√7th **S13.160** **Subluxation of C5/C6 cervical vertebrae** `CC` `H5`

√7th **S13.161** **Dislocation of C5/C6 cervical vertebrae** `CC` `H5`

√6th **S13.17** **Subluxation and dislocation of C6/C7 cervical vertebrae**

√7th **S13.170** **Subluxation of C6/C7 cervical vertebrae** `CC` `H5`

√7th **S13.171** **Dislocation of C6/C7 cervical vertebrae** `CC` `H5`

√6th **S13.18** **Subluxation and dislocation of C7/T1 cervical vertebrae**

√7th **S13.180** **Subluxation of C7/T1 cervical vertebrae** `CC` `H5`

√7th **S13.181** **Dislocation of C7/T1 cervical vertebrae** `CC` `H5`

√5th **S13.2** **Dislocation of other and unspecified parts of neck**

√x7th **S13.20** **Dislocation of unspecified parts of neck** `CC` `H5`

√x7th **S13.29** **Dislocation of other parts of neck** `CC` `H5`

√x7th **S13.4** **Sprain of ligaments of cervical spine**

Sprain of anterior longitudinal (ligament), cervical
Sprain of atlanto-axial (joints)
Sprain of atlanto-occipital (joints)
Whiplash injury of cervical spine

√x7th **S13.5** **Sprain of thyroid region**

Sprain of cricoarytenoid (joint) (ligament)
Sprain of cricothyroid (joint) (ligament)
Sprain of thyroid cartilage

√x7th **S13.8** **Sprain of joints and ligaments of other parts of neck**

√x7th **S13.9** **Sprain of joints and ligaments of unspecified parts of neck**

√4th **S14** **Injury of nerves and spinal cord at neck level**

`NOTE`   Code to highest level of cervical cord injury

Code also any associated:
fracture of cervical vertebra (S12.0- — S12.6.-)
open wound of neck (S11.-)
transient paralysis (R29.5)

The appropriate 7th character is to be added to each code from category S14.
A initial encounter
D subsequent encounter
S sequela

√x7th **S14.0** **Concussion and edema of cervical spinal cord** `MCC` `HCC`

√5th **S14.1** **Other and unspecified injuries of cervical spinal cord**

√6th **S14.10** **Unspecified injury of cervical spinal cord**

√7th **S14.101** **Unspecified injury at C1 level of cervical spinal cord** `MCC` `H5` `HCC`

√7th **S14.102** **Unspecified injury at C2 level of cervical spinal cord** `MCC` `H5` `HCC`

√7th **S14.103** **Unspecified injury at C3 level of cervical spinal cord** `MCC` `H5` `HCC`

√7th **S14.104** **Unspecified injury at C4 level of cervical spinal cord** `MCC` `H5` `HCC`

√7th **S14.105** **Unspecified injury at C5 level of cervical spinal cord** `MCC` `H5` `HCC`

√7th **S14.106** **Unspecified injury at C6 level of cervical spinal cord** `MCC` `H5` `HCC`

√7th **S14.107** **Unspecified injury at C7 level of cervical spinal cord** `MCC` `H5` `HCC`

√7th **S14.108** **Unspecified injury at C8 level of cervical spinal cord** `MCC` `HCC`

√7th **S14.109** **Unspecified injury at unspecified level of cervical spinal cord** `HCC`

Injury of cervical spinal cord NOS

√6th **S14.11** **Complete lesion of cervical spinal cord**

√7th **S14.111** **Complete lesion at C1 level of cervical spinal cord** `MCC` `H5` `HCC`

√7th **S14.112** **Complete lesion at C2 level of cervical spinal cord** `MCC` `H5` `HCC`

√7th **S14.113** **Complete lesion at** C3 **level of**
spinal cord `MCC` `H5` `HCC`

√7th **S14.114** **Complete lesion at** C4 **level of cervical**
spinal cord `MCC` `H5` `HCC`

√7th **S14.115** **Complete lesion at** C5 **level of cervical**
spinal cord `MCC` `H5` `HCC`

√7th **S14.116** **Complete lesion at** C6 **level of cervical**
spinal cord `MCC` `H5` `HCC`

√7th **S14.117** **Complete lesion at** C7 **level of cervical**
spinal cord `MCC` `H5` `HCC`

√7th **S14.118** **Complete lesion at** C8 **level of cervical**
spinal cord `MCC` `HCC`

√7th **S14.119** **Complete lesion at unspecified level of**
cervical spinal cord `HCC`

√6th **S14.12** Central cord syndrome **of cervical spinal cord**

√7th **S14.121** **Central cord syndrome at** C1 **level of**
cervical spinal cord `MCC` `H5` `HCC`

√7th **S14.122** **Central cord syndrome at** C2 **level of**
cervical spinal cord `MCC` `H5` `HCC`

√7th **S14.123** **Central cord syndrome at** C3 **level of**
cervical spinal cord `MCC` `H5` `HCC`

√7th **S14.124** **Central cord syndrome at** C4 **level of**
cervical spinal cord `MCC` `H5` `HCC`

√7th **S14.125** **Central cord syndrome at** C5 **level of**
cervical spinal cord `MCC` `H5` `HCC`

√7th **S14.126** **Central cord syndrome at** C6 **level of**
cervical spinal cord `MCC` `H5` `HCC`

√7th **S14.127** **Central cord syndrome at** C7 **level of**
cervical spinal cord `MCC` `H5` `HCC`

√7th **S14.128** **Central cord syndrome at** C8 **level of**
cervical spinal cord `MCC` `HCC`

√7th **S14.129** **Central cord syndrome at unspecified**
level of cervical spinal cord `HCC`

√6th **S14.13** Anterior cord syndrome **of cervical spinal cord**

√7th **S14.131** **Anterior cord syndrome at** C1 **level of**
cervical spinal cord `MCC` `H5` `HCC`

√7th **S14.132** **Anterior cord syndrome at** C2 **level of**
cervical spinal cord `MCC` `H5` `HCC`

√7th **S14.133** **Anterior cord syndrome at** C3 **level of**
cervical spinal cord `MCC` `H5` `HCC`

√7th **S14.134** **Anterior cord syndrome at** C4 **level of**
cervical spinal cord `MCC` `H5` `HCC`

√7th **S14.135** **Anterior cord syndrome at** C5 **level of**
cervical spinal cord `MCC` `H5` `HCC`

√7th **S14.136** **Anterior cord syndrome at** C6 **level of**
cervical spinal cord `MCC` `H5` `HCC`

√7th **S14.137** **Anterior cord syndrome at** C7 **level of**
cervical spinal cord `MCC` `H5` `HCC`

√7th **S14.138** **Anterior cord syndrome at** C8 **level of**
cervical spinal cord `MCC` `HCC`

√7th **S14.139** **Anterior cord syndrome at unspecified**
level of cervical spinal cord `HCC`

√6th **S14.14** Brown-Séquard syndrome **of cervical spinal cord**

√7th **S14.141** **Brown-Séquard syndrome at** C1 **level of**
cervical spinal cord `MCC` `HCC`

√7th **S14.142** **Brown-Séquard syndrome at** C2 **level of**
cervical spinal cord `MCC` `HCC`

√7th **S14.143** **Brown-Séquard syndrome at** C3 **level of**
cervical spinal cord `MCC` `HCC`

√7th **S14.144** **Brown-Séquard syndrome at** C4 **level of**
cervical spinal cord `MCC` `HCC`

√7th **S14.145** **Brown-Séquard syndrome at** C5 **level of**
cervical spinal cord `MCC` `HCC`

√7th **S14.146** **Brown-Séquard syndrome at** C6 **level of**
cervical spinal cord `MCC` `HCC`

√7th **S14.147** **Brown-Séquard syndrome at** C7 **level of**
cervical spinal cord `MCC` `HCC`

√7th **S14.148** **Brown-Séquard syndrome at** C8 **level of**
cervical spinal cord `MCC` `HCC`

√7th **S14.149** **Brown-Séquard syndrome at unspecified**
level of cervical spinal cord `HCC`

√6th **S14.15** **Other** incomplete lesions **of cervical spinal cord**

Incomplete lesion of cervical spinal cord NOS
Posterior cord syndrome of cervical spinal cord

√7th **S14.151** **Other incomplete lesion at** C1 **level of**
cervical spinal cord `MCC` `H5` `HCC`

√7th **S14.152** **Other incomplete lesion at** C2 **level of**
cervical spinal cord `MCC` `H5` `HCC`

√7th **S14.153** **Other incomplete lesion at** C3 **level of**
cervical spinal cord `MCC` `H5` `HCC`

√7th **S14.154** **Other incomplete lesion at** C4 **level of**
cervical spinal cord `MCC` `H5` `HCC`

√7th **S14.155** **Other incomplete lesion at** C5 **level of**
cervical spinal cord `MCC` `H5` `HCC`

√7th **S14.156** **Other incomplete lesion at** C6 **level of**
cervical spinal cord `MCC` `H5` `HCC`

√7th **S14.157** **Other incomplete lesion at** C7 **level of**
cervical spinal cord `MCC` `H5` `HCC`

√7th **S14.158** **Other incomplete lesion at** C8 **level of**
cervical spinal cord `MCC` `HCC`

√7th **S14.159** **Other incomplete lesion at unspecified**
level of cervical spinal cord `HCC`

√x7th **S14.2** **Injury of** nerve root of cervical spine

√x7th **S14.3** **Injury of** brachial plexus

√x7th **S14.4** **Injury of** peripheral nerves of neck

√x7th **S14.5** **Injury of** cervical sympathetic nerves

√x7th **S14.8** **Injury of other specified nerves of neck**

√x7th **S14.9** **Injury of unspecified nerves of neck**

√4th **S15** **Injury of blood vessels at neck level**

Code also any associated open wound (S11.-)

The appropriate 7th character is to be added to each code from
category S15.
A   initial encounter
D   subsequent encounter
S   sequela

√5th **S15.0** **Injury of** carotid artery **of neck**

Injury of carotid artery (common) (external) (internal,
extracranial portion)
Injury of carotid artery NOS

EXCLUDES 1   *injury of internal carotid artery, intracranial portion*
(S06.8)

√6th **S15.00** **Unspecified injury of carotid artery**

√7th **S15.001** **Unspecified injury of** right **carotid**
artery `CC`

√7th **S15.002** **Unspecified injury of** left **carotid**
artery `CC`

√7th **S15.009** **Unspecified injury of unspecified carotid**
artery `CC`

√6th **S15.01** **Minor laceration of carotid artery**

Incomplete transection of carotid artery
Laceration of carotid artery NOS
Superficial laceration of carotid artery

√7th **S15.011** **Minor laceration of** right **carotid**
artery `CC`

√7th **S15.012** **Minor laceration of** left **carotid**
artery `CC`

√7th **S15.019** **Minor laceration of unspecified carotid**
artery `CC`

√6th **S15.02** **Major laceration of carotid artery**

Complete transection of carotid artery
Traumatic rupture of carotid artery

√7th **S15.021** **Major laceration of** right **carotid**
artery `CC`

√7th **S15.022** **Major laceration of** left **carotid**
artery `CC`

√7th **S15.029** **Major laceration of unspecified carotid**
artery `CC`

√6th **S15.09** **Other specified injury of carotid artery**

√7th **S15.091** **Other specified injury of** right **carotid**
artery `CC`

√7th **S15.092** **Other specified injury of** left **carotid**
artery `CC`

√7th **S15.099** **Other specified injury of unspecified**
carotid artery `CC`

√5th **S15.1** **Injury of** vertebral artery

√6th **S15.10** **Unspecified injury of vertebral artery**

√7th **S15.101** **Unspecified injury of** right **vertebral**
artery `CC`

√7th **S15.102** **Unspecified injury of** left **vertebral**
artery `CC`

√7th **S15.109** **Unspecified injury of unspecified**
vertebral artery `CC`

☑ Additional Character Required   √x7th Placeholder   Unacceptable PDx   Questionable PDx   Manifestation   Unspecified Dx   `H1`-`H14` HAC   `HCC` CMS-HCC Dx   `HIV` HIV Dx

ICD-10-CM 2021   **981**

√6ᵗʰ **S15.11** **Minor laceration** of vertebral artery
Incomplete transection of vertebral artery
Laceration of vertebral artery NOS
Superficial laceration of vertebral artery
  √7ᵗʰ **S15.111** **Minor laceration of** right vertebral artery **cc**
  √7ᵗʰ **S15.112** **Minor laceration of** left vertebral artery **cc**
  √7ᵗʰ **S15.119** **Minor laceration of unspecified** vertebral artery **cc**

√6ᵗʰ **S15.12** **Major laceration** of vertebral artery
Complete transection of vertebral artery
Traumatic rupture of vertebral artery
  √7ᵗʰ **S15.121** **Major laceration of** right vertebral artery **cc**
  √7ᵗʰ **S15.122** **Major laceration of** left vertebral artery **cc**
  √7ᵗʰ **S15.129** **Major laceration of unspecified** vertebral artery **cc**

√6ᵗʰ **S15.19** **Other specified injury** of vertebral artery
  √7ᵗʰ **S15.191** **Other specified injury of** right vertebral artery **cc**
  √7ᵗʰ **S15.192** **Other specified injury of** left vertebral artery **cc**
  √7ᵗʰ **S15.199** **Other specified injury of unspecified** vertebral artery **cc**

√5ᵗʰ **S15.2** **Injury of** external jugular vein
  √6ᵗʰ **S15.20** **Unspecified injury of external jugular vein**
    √7ᵗʰ **S15.201** **Unspecified injury of** right external jugular vein **cc**
    √7ᵗʰ **S15.202** **Unspecified injury of** left external jugular vein **cc**
    √7ᵗʰ **S15.209** **Unspecified injury of unspecified** external jugular vein **cc**

  √6ᵗʰ **S15.21** **Minor laceration** of external jugular vein
Incomplete transection of external jugular vein
Laceration of external jugular vein NOS
Superficial laceration of external jugular vein
    √7ᵗʰ **S15.211** **Minor laceration of** right external jugular vein **cc**
    √7ᵗʰ **S15.212** **Minor laceration of** left external jugular vein **cc**
    √7ᵗʰ **S15.219** **Minor laceration of unspecified** external jugular vein **cc**

  √6ᵗʰ **S15.22** **Major laceration** of external jugular vein
Complete transection of external jugular vein
Traumatic rupture of external jugular vein
    √7ᵗʰ **S15.221** **Major laceration of** right external jugular vein **cc**
    √7ᵗʰ **S15.222** **Major laceration of** left external jugular vein **cc**
    √7ᵗʰ **S15.229** **Major laceration of unspecified** external jugular vein **cc**

  √6ᵗʰ **S15.29** **Other specified injury** of external jugular vein
    √7ᵗʰ **S15.291** **Other specified injury of** right external jugular vein **cc**
    √7ᵗʰ **S15.292** **Other specified injury of** left external jugular vein **cc**
    √7ᵗʰ **S15.299** **Other specified injury of unspecified** external jugular vein **cc**

√5ᵗʰ **S15.3** **Injury of** internal jugular vein
  √6ᵗʰ **S15.30** **Unspecified injury of internal jugular vein**
    √7ᵗʰ **S15.301** **Unspecified injury of** right internal jugular vein **cc**
    √7ᵗʰ **S15.302** **Unspecified injury of** left internal jugular vein **cc**
    √7ᵗʰ **S15.309** **Unspecified injury of unspecified** internal jugular vein **cc**

  √6ᵗʰ **S15.31** **Minor laceration** of internal jugular vein
Incomplete transection of internal jugular vein
Laceration of internal jugular vein NOS
Superficial laceration of internal jugular vein
    √7ᵗʰ **S15.311** **Minor laceration of** right internal jugular vein **cc**
    √7ᵗʰ **S15.312** **Minor laceration of** left internal jugular vein **cc**
    √7ᵗʰ **S15.319** **Minor laceration of unspecified** internal jugular vein **cc**

√6ᵗʰ **S15.32** **Major laceration** of internal jugular vein
Complete transection of internal jugular vein
Traumatic rupture of internal jugular vein
  √7ᵗʰ **S15.321** **Major laceration of** right internal jugular vein **cc**
  √7ᵗʰ **S15.322** **Major laceration of** left internal jugular vein **cc**
  √7ᵗʰ **S15.329** **Major laceration of unspecified** internal jugular vein **cc**

√6ᵗʰ **S15.39** **Other specified injury** of internal jugular vein
  √7ᵗʰ **S15.391** **Other specified injury of** right internal jugular vein **cc**
  √7ᵗʰ **S15.392** **Other specified injury of** left internal jugular vein **cc**
  √7ᵗʰ **S15.399** **Other specified injury of unspecified** internal jugular vein **cc**

√x7ᵗʰ **S15.8** **Injury of other specified blood vessels at neck level** **cc**
√x7ᵗʰ **S15.9** **Injury of unspecified blood vessel at neck level** **cc**

√4ᵗʰ **S16** **Injury of muscle, fascia and tendon at neck level**
Code also any associated open wound (S11.-)
EXCLUDES 2 sprain of joint or ligament at neck level (S13.9)

The appropriate 7th character is to be added to each code from category S16.
A initial encounter
D subsequent encounter
S sequela

√x7ᵗʰ **S16.1** **Strain of muscle, fascia and tendon at neck level**
√x7ᵗʰ **S16.2** **Laceration of muscle, fascia and tendon at neck level**
√x7ᵗʰ **S16.8** **Other specified injury of muscle, fascia and tendon at neck level**
√x7ᵗʰ **S16.9** **Unspecified injury of muscle, fascia and tendon at neck level**

√4ᵗʰ **S17** **Crushing injury of neck**
Use additional code for all associated injuries, such as:
injury of blood vessels (S15.-)
open wound of neck (S11.-)
spinal cord injury (S14.0, S14.1)
vertebral fracture (S12.0- — S12.3-)

The appropriate 7th character is to be added to each code from category S17.
A initial encounter
D subsequent encounter
S sequela

√x7ᵗʰ **S17.0** **Crushing injury of larynx and trachea** **cc** **H5**
√x7ᵗʰ **S17.8** **Crushing injury of other specified parts of neck** **cc** **H5**
√x7ᵗʰ **S17.9** **Crushing injury of neck, part unspecified** **cc** **H5**

√4ᵗʰ **S19** **Other specified and unspecified injuries of neck**

The appropriate 7th character is to be added to each code from category S19.
A initial encounter
D subsequent encounter
S sequela

√5ᵗʰ **S19.8** **Other specified injuries of neck**
  √x7ᵗʰ **S19.80** **Other specified injuries of unspecified part of neck**
  √x7ᵗʰ **S19.81** **Other specified injuries of larynx**
  √x7ᵗʰ **S19.82** **Other specified injuries of cervical trachea**
EXCLUDES 2 other specified injury of thoracic trachea (S27.5-)
  √x7ᵗʰ **S19.83** **Other specified injuries of vocal cord**
  √x7ᵗʰ **S19.84** **Other specified injuries of thyroid gland**
  √x7ᵗʰ **S19.85** **Other specified injuries of pharynx and cervical esophagus**
  √x7ᵗʰ **S19.89** **Other specified injuries of other specified part of neck**
√x7ᵗʰ **S19.9** **Unspecified injury of neck**

Injuries to the thorax (S20-S29)

INCLUDES   injuries of breast
injuries of chest (wall)
injuries of interscapular area

EXCLUDES 2   *burns and corrosions (T20-T32)*
effects of foreign body in bronchus (T17.5)
effects of foreign body in esophagus (T18.1)
effects of foreign body in lung (T17.8)
effects of foreign body in trachea (T17.4)
frostbite (T33-T34)
injuries of axilla
injuries of clavicle
injuries of scapular region
injuries of shoulder
insect bite or sting, venomous (T63.4)

√4th **S20**   **Superficial injury of thorax**

> The appropriate 7th character is to be added to each code from category S20.
> A   initial encounter
> D   subsequent encounter
> S   sequela

√5th   **S20.0**   **Contusion of breast**

    √x7th   **S20.00**   **Contusion of breast, unspecified breast**

    √x7th   **S20.01**   **Contusion of right breast**

    √x7th   **S20.02**   **Contusion of left breast**

√5th   **S20.1**   **Other and unspecified superficial injuries of breast**

    √6th   **S20.10**   **Unspecified superficial injuries of breast**

       √7th   **S20.101**   **Unspecified superficial injuries of breast, right breast**

       √7th   **S20.102**   **Unspecified superficial injuries of breast, left breast**

       √7th   **S20.109**   **Unspecified superficial injuries of breast, unspecified breast**

    √6th   **S20.11**   **Abrasion of breast**

       √7th   **S20.111**   **Abrasion of breast, right breast**

       √7th   **S20.112**   **Abrasion of breast, left breast**

       √7th   **S20.119**   **Abrasion of breast, unspecified breast**

    √6th   **S20.12**   **Blister (nonthermal) of breast**

       √7th   **S20.121**   **Blister (nonthermal) of breast, right breast**

       √7th   **S20.122**   **Blister (nonthermal) of breast, left breast**

       √7th   **S20.129**   **Blister (nonthermal) of breast, unspecified breast**

    √6th   **S20.14**   **External constriction of part of breast**

       √7th   **S20.141**   **External constriction of part of breast, right breast**

       √7th   **S20.142**   **External constriction of part of breast, left breast**

       √7th   **S20.149**   **External constriction of part of breast, unspecified breast**

    √6th   **S20.15**   **Superficial foreign body of breast**

       Splinter in the breast

       √7th   **S20.151**   **Superficial foreign body of breast, right breast**

       √7th   **S20.152**   **Superficial foreign body of breast, left breast**

       √7th   **S20.159**   **Superficial foreign body of breast, unspecified breast**

    √6th   **S20.16**   **Insect bite (nonvenomous) of breast**

       √7th   **S20.161**   **Insect bite (nonvenomous) of breast, right breast**

       √7th   **S20.162**   **Insect bite (nonvenomous) of breast, left breast**

       √7th   **S20.169**   **Insect bite (nonvenomous) of breast, unspecified breast**

    √6th   **S20.17**   **Other superficial bite of breast**

       EXCLUDES 1   *open bite of breast (S21.05-)*

       √7th   **S20.171**   **Other superficial bite of breast, right breast**

       √7th   **S20.172**   **Other superficial bite of breast, left breast**

       √7th   **S20.179**   **Other superficial bite of breast, unspecified breast**

√5th   **S20.2**   **Contusion of thorax**

    √x7th   **S20.20**   **Contusion of thorax, unspecified**

    √6th   **S20.21**   **Contusion of front wall of thorax**

       √7th   **S20.211**   **Contusion of right front wall of thorax**

       √7th   **S20.212**   **Contusion of left front wall of thorax**

       √7th   **S20.213**   **Contusion of bilateral front wall of thorax**

       √7th   **S20.214**   **Contusion of middle front wall of thorax**

       √7th   **S20.219**   **Contusion of unspecified front wall of thorax**

    √6th   **S20.22**   **Contusion of back wall of thorax**

       √7th   **S20.221**   **Contusion of right back wall of thorax**

       √7th   **S20.222**   **Contusion of left back wall of thorax**

       √7th   **S20.223**   **Contusion of bilateral back wall of thorax**

       √7th   **S20.224**   **Contusion of middle back wall of thorax**

       √7th   **S20.229**   **Contusion of unspecified back wall of thorax**

√5th   **S20.3**   **Other and unspecified superficial injuries of front wall of thorax**

    √6th   **S20.30**   **Unspecified superficial injuries of front wall of thorax**

       √7th   **S20.301**   **Unspecified superficial injuries of right front wall of thorax**

       √7th   **S20.302**   **Unspecified superficial injuries of left front wall of thorax**

       √7th   **S20.303**   **Unspecified superficial injuries of bilateral front wall of thorax**

       √7th   **S20.304**   **Unspecified superficial injuries of middle front wall of thorax**

       √7th   **S20.309**   **Unspecified superficial injuries of unspecified front wall of thorax**

    √6th   **S20.31**   **Abrasion of front wall of thorax**

       √7th   **S20.311**   **Abrasion of right front wall of thorax**

       √7th   **S20.312**   **Abrasion of left front wall of thorax**

       √7th   **S20.313**   **Abrasion of bilateral front wall of thorax**

       √7th   **S20.314**   **Abrasion of middle front wall of thorax**

       √7th   **S20.319**   **Abrasion of unspecified front wall of thorax**

    √6th   **S20.32**   **Blister (nonthermal) of front wall of thorax**

       √7th   **S20.321**   **Blister (nonthermal) of right front wall of thorax**

       √7th   **S20.322**   **Blister (nonthermal) of left front wall of thorax**

       √7th   **S20.323**   **Blister (nonthermal) of bilateral front wall of thorax**

       √7th   **S20.324**   **Blister (nonthermal) of middle front wall of thorax**

       √7th   **S20.329**   **Blister (nonthermal) of unspecified front wall of thorax**

    √6th   **S20.34**   **External constriction of front wall of thorax**

       √7th   **S20.341**   **External constriction of right front wall of thorax**

       √7th   **S20.342**   **External constriction of left front wall of thorax**

       √7th   **S20.343**   **External constriction of bilateral front wall of thorax**

       √7th   **S20.344**   **External constriction of middle front wall of thorax**

       √7th   **S20.349**   **External constriction of unspecified front wall of thorax**

    √6th   **S20.35**   **Superficial foreign body of front wall of thorax**

       Splinter in front wall of thorax

       √7th   **S20.351**   **Superficial foreign body of right front wall of thorax**

       √7th   **S20.352**   **Superficial foreign body of left front wall of thorax**

       √7th   **S20.353**   **Superficial foreign body of bilateral front wall of thorax**

       √7th   **S20.354**   **Superficial foreign body of middle front wall of thorax**

       √7th   **S20.359**   **Superficial foreign body of unspecified front wall of thorax**

    √6th   **S20.36**   **Insect bite (nonvenomous) of front wall of thorax**

       √7th   **S20.361**   **Insect bite (nonvenomous) of right front wall of thorax**

       √7th   **S20.362**   **Insect bite (nonvenomous) of left front wall of thorax**

       √7th   **S20.363**   **Insect bite (nonvenomous) of bilateral front wall of thorax**

       √7th   **S20.364**   **Insect bite (nonvenomous) of middle front wall of thorax**

☑ Additional Character Required   √x7th Placeholder   Unacceptable PDx   Questionable PDx   Manifestation   Unspecified Dx   H1-H14 HAC   HCC CMS-HCC Dx   HIV HIV Dx

ICD-10-CM 2021   983

√7ᵗʰ **S20.369** **Insect bite** (nonvenomous) of unspecified front wall of thorax

√6ᵗʰ **S20.37** Other superficial bite of front wall of thorax

> EXCLUDES 1   *open bite of front wall of thorax (S21.15)*

√7ᵗʰ **S20.371** Other superficial bite of right front wall of thorax

√7ᵗʰ **S20.372** Other superficial bite of left front wall of thorax

√7ᵗʰ **S20.373** Other superficial bite of bilateral front wall of thorax

√7ᵗʰ **S20.374** Other superficial bite of middle front wall of thorax

√7ᵗʰ **S20.379** Other superficial bite of unspecified front wall of thorax

√5ᵗʰ **S20.4** Other and unspecified superficial injuries of back wall of thorax

√6ᵗʰ **S20.40** Unspecified superficial injuries of back wall of thorax

√7ᵗʰ **S20.401** Unspecified superficial injuries of right back wall of thorax

√7ᵗʰ **S20.402** Unspecified superficial injuries of left back wall of thorax

√7ᵗʰ **S20.409** Unspecified superficial injuries of unspecified back wall of thorax

√6ᵗʰ **S20.41** Abrasion of back wall of thorax

√7ᵗʰ **S20.411** Abrasion of right back wall of thorax

√7ᵗʰ **S20.412** Abrasion of left back wall of thorax

√7ᵗʰ **S20.419** Abrasion of unspecified back wall of thorax

√6ᵗʰ **S20.42** Blister (nonthermal) of back wall of thorax

√7ᵗʰ **S20.421** Blister (nonthermal) of right back wall of thorax

√7ᵗʰ **S20.422** Blister (nonthermal) of left back wall of thorax

√7ᵗʰ **S20.429** Blister (nonthermal) of unspecified back wall of thorax

√6ᵗʰ **S20.44** External constriction of back wall of thorax

√7ᵗʰ **S20.441** External constriction of right back wall of thorax

√7ᵗʰ **S20.442** External constriction of left back wall of thorax

√7ᵗʰ **S20.449** External constriction of unspecified back wall of thorax

√6ᵗʰ **S20.45** Superficial foreign body of back wall of thorax

> Splinter of back wall of thorax

√7ᵗʰ **S20.451** Superficial foreign body of right back wall of thorax

√7ᵗʰ **S20.452** Superficial foreign body of left back wall of thorax

√7ᵗʰ **S20.459** Superficial foreign body of unspecified back wall of thorax

√6ᵗʰ **S20.46** Insect bite (nonvenomous) of back wall of thorax

√7ᵗʰ **S20.461** Insect bite (nonvenomous) of right back wall of thorax

√7ᵗʰ **S20.462** Insect bite (nonvenomous) of left back wall of thorax

√7ᵗʰ **S20.469** Insect bite (nonvenomous) of unspecified back wall of thorax

√6ᵗʰ **S20.47** Other superficial bite of back wall of thorax

> EXCLUDES 1   *open bite of back wall of thorax (S21.25)*

√7ᵗʰ **S20.471** Other superficial bite of right back wall of thorax

√7ᵗʰ **S20.472** Other superficial bite of left back wall of thorax

√7ᵗʰ **S20.479** Other superficial bite of unspecified back wall of thorax

√5ᵗʰ **S20.9** Superficial injury of unspecified parts of thorax

> EXCLUDES 1   *contusion of thorax NOS (S20.20)*

√x7ᵗʰ **S20.90** Unspecified superficial injury of unspecified parts of thorax

> Superficial injury of thoracic wall NOS

√x7ᵗʰ **S20.91** Abrasion of unspecified parts of thorax

√x7ᵗʰ **S20.92** Blister (nonthermal) of unspecified parts of thorax

√x7ᵗʰ **S20.94** External constriction of unspecified parts of thorax

√x7ᵗʰ **S20.95** Superficial foreign body of unspecified parts of thorax

> Splinter in thorax NOS

√x7ᵗʰ **S20.96** Insect bite (nonvenomous) of unspecified parts of thorax

√x7ᵗʰ **S20.97** Other superficial bite of unspecified parts of thorax

> EXCLUDES 1   *open bite of thorax NOS (S21.95)*

√4ᵗʰ **S21** **Open wound of thorax**

> Code also any associated injury, such as:
> injury of heart (S26.-)
> injury of intrathoracic organs (S27.-)
> rib fracture (S22.3-, S22.4-)
> spinal cord injury (S24.0-, S24.1-)
> traumatic hemopneumothorax (S27.3)
> traumatic hemothorax (S27.1)
> traumatic pneumothorax (S27.0)
> wound infection

> EXCLUDES 1   *traumatic amputation (partial) of thorax (S28.1)*

> The appropriate 7th character is to be added to each code from category S21.
> A   initial encounter
> D   subsequent encounter
> S   sequela

√5ᵗʰ **S21.0** Open wound of breast

√6ᵗʰ **S21.00** Unspecified open wound of breast

√7ᵗʰ **S21.001** Unspecified open wound of right breast

√7ᵗʰ **S21.002** Unspecified open wound of left breast

√7ᵗʰ **S21.009** Unspecified open wound of unspecified breast

√6ᵗʰ **S21.01** Laceration without foreign body of breast

√7ᵗʰ **S21.011** Laceration without foreign body of right breast

√7ᵗʰ **S21.012** Laceration without foreign body of left breast

√7ᵗʰ **S21.019** Laceration without foreign body of unspecified breast

√6ᵗʰ **S21.02** Laceration with foreign body of breast

√7ᵗʰ **S21.021** Laceration with foreign body of right breast

√7ᵗʰ **S21.022** Laceration with foreign body of left breast

√7ᵗʰ **S21.029** Laceration with foreign body of unspecified breast

√6ᵗʰ **S21.03** Puncture wound without foreign body of breast

√7ᵗʰ **S21.031** Puncture wound without foreign body of right breast

√7ᵗʰ **S21.032** Puncture wound without foreign body of left breast

√7ᵗʰ **S21.039** Puncture wound without foreign body of unspecified breast

√6ᵗʰ **S21.04** Puncture wound with foreign body of breast

√7ᵗʰ **S21.041** Puncture wound with foreign body of right breast

√7ᵗʰ **S21.042** Puncture wound with foreign body of left breast

√7ᵗʰ **S21.049** Puncture wound with foreign body of unspecified breast

√6ᵗʰ **S21.05** Open bite of breast

> Bite of breast NOS

> EXCLUDES 1   *superficial bite of breast (S20.17)*

√7ᵗʰ **S21.051** Open bite of right breast

√7ᵗʰ **S21.052** Open bite of left breast

√7ᵗʰ **S21.059** Open bite of unspecified breast

√5ᵗʰ **S21.1** Open wound of front wall of thorax without penetration into thoracic cavity

> Open wound of chest without penetration into thoracic cavity

√6ᵗʰ **S21.10** Unspecified open wound of front wall of thorax without penetration into thoracic cavity

√7ᵗʰ **S21.101** Unspecified open wound of right front wall of thorax without penetration into thoracic cavity   CC

√7ᵗʰ **S21.102** Unspecified open wound of left front wall of thorax without penetration into thoracic cavity   CC

√7ᵗʰ **S21.109** Unspecified open wound of unspecified front wall of thorax without penetration into thoracic cavity   CC

√6ᵗʰ **S21.11** Laceration without foreign body of front wall of thorax without penetration into thoracic cavity

√7ᵗʰ **S21.111** Laceration without foreign body of right front wall of thorax without penetration into thoracic cavity   CC

N Newborn: 0   P Pediatric: 0-17   M Maternity: 9-64   A Adult: 15-124   MCC Major Complication/Comorbidity   CC Complication/Comorbidity   SW Severe Wound Dx

984   ICD-10-CM 2021

   √7ᵗʰ **S21.112** Laceration without foreign body of left front wall of thorax without penetration into thoracic cavity   cc

   √7ᵗʰ **S21.119** Laceration without foreign body of unspecified front wall of thorax without penetration into thoracic cavity   cc

√6ᵗʰ **S21.12** Laceration with foreign body of front wall of thorax without penetration into thoracic cavity

   √7ᵗʰ **S21.121** Laceration with foreign body of right front wall of thorax without penetration into thoracic cavity   cc

   √7ᵗʰ **S21.122** Laceration with foreign body of left front wall of thorax without penetration into thoracic cavity   cc

   √7ᵗʰ **S21.129** Laceration with foreign body of unspecified front wall of thorax without penetration into thoracic cavity   cc

√6ᵗʰ **S21.13** Puncture wound without foreign body of front wall of thorax without penetration into thoracic cavity

   √7ᵗʰ **S21.131** Puncture wound without foreign body of right front wall of thorax without penetration into thoracic cavity   cc

   √7ᵗʰ **S21.132** Puncture wound without foreign body of left front wall of thorax without penetration into thoracic cavity   cc

   √7ᵗʰ **S21.139** Puncture wound without foreign body of unspecified front wall of thorax without penetration into thoracic cavity   cc

√6ᵗʰ **S21.14** Puncture wound with foreign body of front wall of thorax without penetration into thoracic cavity

   √7ᵗʰ **S21.141** Puncture wound with foreign body of right front wall of thorax without penetration into thoracic cavity   cc

   √7ᵗʰ **S21.142** Puncture wound with foreign body of left front wall of thorax without penetration into thoracic cavity   cc

   √7ᵗʰ **S21.149** Puncture wound with foreign body of unspecified front wall of thorax without penetration into thoracic cavity   cc

√6ᵗʰ **S21.15** Open bite of front wall of thorax without penetration into thoracic cavity

Bite of front wall of thorax NOS

    EXCLUDES 1   superficial bite of front wall of thorax (S20.37)

   √7ᵗʰ **S21.151** Open bite of right front wall of thorax without penetration into thoracic cavity   cc

   √7ᵗʰ **S21.152** Open bite of left front wall of thorax without penetration into thoracic cavity   cc

   √7ᵗʰ **S21.159** Open bite of unspecified front wall of thorax without penetration into thoracic cavity   cc

√5ᵗʰ **S21.2** Open wound of back wall of thorax without penetration into thoracic cavity

√6ᵗʰ **S21.20** Unspecified open wound of back wall of thorax without penetration into thoracic cavity

   √7ᵗʰ **S21.201** Unspecified open wound of right back wall of thorax without penetration into thoracic cavity

   √7ᵗʰ **S21.202** Unspecified open wound of left back wall of thorax without penetration into thoracic cavity

   √7ᵗʰ **S21.209** Unspecified open wound of unspecified back wall of thorax without penetration into thoracic cavity

√6ᵗʰ **S21.21** Laceration without foreign body of back wall of thorax without penetration into thoracic cavity

   √7ᵗʰ **S21.211** Laceration without foreign body of right back wall of thorax without penetration into thoracic cavity

   √7ᵗʰ **S21.212** Laceration without foreign body of left back wall of thorax without penetration into thoracic cavity

   √7ᵗʰ **S21.219** Laceration without foreign body of unspecified back wall of thorax without penetration into thoracic cavity

√6ᵗʰ **S21.22** Laceration with foreign body of back wall of thorax without penetration into thoracic cavity

   √7ᵗʰ **S21.221** Laceration with foreign body of right back wall of thorax without penetration into thoracic cavity

   √7ᵗʰ **S21.222** Laceration with foreign body of left back wall of thorax without penetration into thoracic cavity

   √7ᵗʰ **S21.229** Laceration with foreign body of unspecified back wall of thorax without penetration into thoracic cavity

√6ᵗʰ **S21.23** Puncture wound without foreign body of back wall of thorax without penetration into thoracic cavity

   √7ᵗʰ **S21.231** Puncture wound without foreign body of right back wall of thorax without penetration into thoracic cavity

   √7ᵗʰ **S21.232** Puncture wound without foreign body of left back wall of thorax without penetration into thoracic cavity

   √7ᵗʰ **S21.239** Puncture wound without foreign body of unspecified back wall of thorax without penetration into thoracic cavity

√6ᵗʰ **S21.24** Puncture wound with foreign body of back wall of thorax without penetration into thoracic cavity

   √7ᵗʰ **S21.241** Puncture wound with foreign body of right back wall of thorax without penetration into thoracic cavity

   √7ᵗʰ **S21.242** Puncture wound with foreign body of left back wall of thorax without penetration into thoracic cavity

   √7ᵗʰ **S21.249** Puncture wound with foreign body of unspecified back wall of thorax without penetration into thoracic cavity

√6ᵗʰ **S21.25** Open bite of back wall of thorax without penetration into thoracic cavity

Bite of back wall of thorax NOS

    EXCLUDES 1   superficial bite of back wall of thorax (S20.47)

   √7ᵗʰ **S21.251** Open bite of right back wall of thorax without penetration into thoracic cavity

   √7ᵗʰ **S21.252** Open bite of left back wall of thorax without penetration into thoracic cavity

   √7ᵗʰ **S21.259** Open bite of unspecified back wall of thorax without penetration into thoracic cavity

√5ᵗʰ **S21.3** Open wound of front wall of thorax with penetration into thoracic cavity

Open wound of chest with penetration into thoracic cavity

√6ᵗʰ **S21.30** Unspecified open wound of front wall of thorax with penetration into thoracic cavity

   √7ᵗʰ **S21.301** Unspecified open wound of right front wall of thorax with penetration into thoracic cavity   MCC

   √7ᵗʰ **S21.302** Unspecified open wound of left front wall of thorax with penetration into thoracic cavity   MCC

   √7ᵗʰ **S21.309** Unspecified open wound of unspecified front wall of thorax with penetration into thoracic cavity   MCC

√6ᵗʰ **S21.31** Laceration without foreign body of front wall of thorax with penetration into thoracic cavity

   √7ᵗʰ **S21.311** Laceration without foreign body of right front wall of thorax with penetration into thoracic cavity   MCC

   √7ᵗʰ **S21.312** Laceration without foreign body of left front wall of thorax with penetration into thoracic cavity   MCC

   √7ᵗʰ **S21.319** Laceration without foreign body of unspecified front wall of thorax with penetration into thoracic cavity   MCC

√6ᵗʰ **S21.32** Laceration with foreign body of front wall of thorax with penetration into thoracic cavity

   √7ᵗʰ **S21.321** Laceration with foreign body of right front wall of thorax with penetration into thoracic cavity   MCC

   √7ᵗʰ **S21.322** Laceration with foreign body of left front wall of thorax with penetration into thoracic cavity   MCC

   √7ᵗʰ **S21.329** Laceration with foreign body of unspecified front wall of thorax with penetration into thoracic cavity   MCC

√6ᵗʰ **S21.33** Puncture wound without foreign body of front wall of thorax with penetration into thoracic cavity

   √7ᵗʰ **S21.331** Puncture wound without foreign body of right front wall of thorax with penetration into thoracic cavity   MCC

   √7ᵗʰ **S21.332** Puncture wound without foreign body of left front wall of thorax with penetration into thoracic cavity   MCC

☑ Additional Character Required   √x7ᵗʰ Placeholder   Unacceptable PDx   Questionable PDx   Manifestation   Unspecified Dx   H1 - H4 HAC   HCC CMS-HCC Dx   HIV HIV Dx

√7ᵗʰ **S21.339** Puncture wound without foreign body of unspecified front wall of thorax with penetration into thoracic cavity **MCC**

√6ᵗʰ **S21.34** Puncture wound with foreign body of front wall of thorax with penetration into thoracic cavity

√7ᵗʰ **S21.341** Puncture wound with foreign body of right front wall of thorax with penetration into thoracic cavity **MCC**

√7ᵗʰ **S21.342** Puncture wound with foreign body of left front wall of thorax with penetration into thoracic cavity **MCC**

√7ᵗʰ **S21.349** Puncture wound with foreign body of unspecified front wall of thorax with penetration into thoracic cavity **MCC**

√6ᵗʰ **S21.35** Open bite of front wall of thorax with penetration into thoracic cavity

EXCLUDES 1 superficial bite of front wall of thorax (S20.37)

√7ᵗʰ **S21.351** Open bite of right front wall of thorax with penetration into thoracic cavity **MCC**

√7ᵗʰ **S21.352** Open bite of left front wall of thorax with penetration into thoracic cavity **MCC**

√7ᵗʰ **S21.359** Open bite of unspecified front wall of thorax with penetration into thoracic cavity **MCC**

√5ᵗʰ **S21.4** Open wound of back wall of thorax with penetration into thoracic cavity

√6ᵗʰ **S21.40** Unspecified open wound of back wall of thorax with penetration into thoracic cavity

√7ᵗʰ **S21.401** Unspecified open wound of right back wall of thorax with penetration into thoracic cavity **MCC**

√7ᵗʰ **S21.402** Unspecified open wound of left back wall of thorax with penetration into thoracic cavity **MCC**

√7ᵗʰ **S21.409** Unspecified open wound of unspecified back wall of thorax with penetration into thoracic cavity **MCC**

√6ᵗʰ **S21.41** Laceration without foreign body of back wall of thorax with penetration into thoracic cavity

√7ᵗʰ **S21.411** Laceration without foreign body of right back wall of thorax with penetration into thoracic cavity **MCC**

√7ᵗʰ **S21.412** Laceration without foreign body of left back wall of thorax with penetration into thoracic cavity **MCC**

√7ᵗʰ **S21.419** Laceration without foreign body of unspecified back wall of thorax with penetration into thoracic cavity **MCC**

√6ᵗʰ **S21.42** Laceration with foreign body of back wall of thorax with penetration into thoracic cavity

√7ᵗʰ **S21.421** Laceration with foreign body of right back wall of thorax with penetration into thoracic cavity **MCC**

√7ᵗʰ **S21.422** Laceration with foreign body of left back wall of thorax with penetration into thoracic cavity **MCC**

√7ᵗʰ **S21.429** Laceration with foreign body of unspecified back wall of thorax with penetration into thoracic cavity **MCC**

√6ᵗʰ **S21.43** Puncture wound without foreign body of back wall of thorax with penetration into thoracic cavity

√7ᵗʰ **S21.431** Puncture wound without foreign body of right back wall of thorax with penetration into thoracic cavity **MCC**

√7ᵗʰ **S21.432** Puncture wound without foreign body of left back wall of thorax with penetration into thoracic cavity **MCC**

√7ᵗʰ **S21.439** Puncture wound without foreign body of unspecified back wall of thorax with penetration into thoracic cavity **MCC**

√6ᵗʰ **S21.44** Puncture wound with foreign body of back wall of thorax with penetration into thoracic cavity

√7ᵗʰ **S21.441** Puncture wound with foreign body of right back wall of thorax with penetration into thoracic cavity **MCC**

√7ᵗʰ **S21.442** Puncture wound with foreign body of left back wall of thorax with penetration into thoracic cavity **MCC**

√7ᵗʰ **S21.449** Puncture wound with foreign body of unspecified back wall of thorax with penetration into thoracic cavity **MCC**

√6ᵗʰ **S21.45** Open bite of back wall of thorax with penetration into thoracic cavity

Bite of back wall of thorax NOS

EXCLUDES 1 superficial bite of back wall of thorax (S20.47)

√7ᵗʰ **S21.451** Open bite of right back wall of thorax with penetration into thoracic cavity **MCC**

√7ᵗʰ **S21.452** Open bite of left back wall of thorax with penetration into thoracic cavity **MCC**

√7ᵗʰ **S21.459** Open bite of unspecified back wall of thorax with penetration into thoracic cavity **MCC**

√5ᵗʰ **S21.9** Open wound of unspecified part of thorax

Open wound of thoracic wall NOS

√x7ᵗʰ **S21.90** Unspecified open wound of unspecified part of thorax **CC**

√x7ᵗʰ **S21.91** Laceration without foreign body of unspecified part of thorax **CC**

√x7ᵗʰ **S21.92** Laceration with foreign body of unspecified part of thorax **CC**

√x7ᵗʰ **S21.93** Puncture wound without foreign body of unspecified part of thorax **CC**

√x7ᵗʰ **S21.94** Puncture wound with foreign body of unspecified part of thorax **CC**

√x7ᵗʰ **S21.95** Open bite of unspecified part of thorax **CC**

EXCLUDES 1 superficial bite of thorax (S20.97)

√4ᵗʰ **S22** Fracture of rib(s), sternum and thoracic spine

NOTE A fracture not indicated as displaced or nondisplaced should be coded to displaced

A fracture not indicated as open or closed should be coded to closed

INCLUDES fracture of thoracic neural arch

fracture of thoracic spinous process

fracture of thoracic transverse process

fracture of thoracic vertebra

fracture of thoracic vertebral arch

Code first any associated:

injury of intrathoracic organ (S27.-)

spinal cord injury (S24.0-, S24.1-)

EXCLUDES 1 transection of thorax (S28.1)

EXCLUDES 2 fracture of clavicle (S42.0-)

fracture of scapula (S42.1-)

AHA: 2018,2Q,12; 2015,3Q,37-39

The appropriate 7th character is to be added to each code from category S22.

A initial encounter for closed fracture

B initial encounter for open fracture

D subsequent encounter for fracture with routine healing

G subsequent encounter for fracture with delayed healing

K subsequent encounter for fracture with nonunion

S sequela

√5ᵗʰ **S22.0** Fracture of thoracic vertebra

√6ᵗʰ **S22.00** Fracture of unspecified thoracic vertebra

2,3,6 √7ᵗʰ **S22.000** Wedge compression fracture of unspecified thoracic vertebra **MCC CC HS HCC**

2,3,6 √7ᵗʰ **S22.001** Stable burst fracture of unspecified thoracic vertebra **MCC CC HS HCC**

2,3,6 √7ᵗʰ **S22.002** Unstable burst fracture of unspecified thoracic vertebra **MCC CC HS HCC**

2,3,6 √7ᵗʰ **S22.008** Other fracture of unspecified thoracic vertebra **MCC CC HS HCC**

2,3,6 √7ᵗʰ **S22.009** Unspecified fracture of unspecified thoracic vertebra **MCC CC HS HCC**

√6ᵗʰ **S22.01** Fracture of first thoracic vertebra

2,3,6 √7ᵗʰ **S22.010** Wedge compression fracture of first thoracic vertebra **MCC CC HS HCC**

2,3,6 √7ᵗʰ **S22.011** Stable burst fracture of first thoracic vertebra **MCC CC HS HCC**

2,3,6 √7ᵗʰ **S22.012** Unstable burst fracture of first thoracic vertebra **MCC CC HS HCC**

2,3,6 √7ᵗʰ **S22.018** Other fracture of first thoracic vertebra **MCC CC HS HCC**

2,3,6 √7ᵗʰ **S22.019** Unspecified fracture of first thoracic vertebra **MCC CC HS HCC**

N Newborn: 0   **P** Pediatric: 0-17   **M** Maternity: 9-64   **A** Adult: 15-124   **MCC** Major Complication/Comorbidity   **CC** Complication/Comorbidity   **SW** Severe Wound Dx

986 ICD-10-CM 2021

√6ᵗʰ **S22.02** Fracture of second thoracic vertebra

2,3,6 √7ᵗʰ **S22.020** Wedge compression fracture of second thoracic vertebra MCC CC H5 HCC

2,3,6 √7ᵗʰ **S22.021** Stable burst fracture of second thoracic vertebra MCC CC H5 HCC

2,3,6 √7ᵗʰ **S22.022** Unstable burst fracture of second thoracic vertebra MCC CC H5 HCC

2,3,6 √7ᵗʰ **S22.028** Other fracture of second thoracic vertebra MCC CC H5 HCC

2,3,6 √7ᵗʰ **S22.029** Unspecified fracture of second thoracic vertebra MCC CC H5 HCC

√6ᵗʰ **S22.03** Fracture of third thoracic vertebra

2,3,6 √7ᵗʰ **S22.030** Wedge compression fracture of third thoracic vertebra MCC CC H5 HCC

2,3,6 √7ᵗʰ **S22.031** Stable burst fracture of third thoracic vertebra MCC CC H5 HCC

2,3,6 √7ᵗʰ **S22.032** Unstable burst fracture of third thoracic vertebra MCC CC H5 HCC

2,3,6 √7ᵗʰ **S22.038** Other fracture of third thoracic vertebra MCC CC H5 HCC

2,3,6 √7ᵗʰ **S22.039** Unspecified fracture of third thoracic vertebra MCC CC H5 HCC

√6ᵗʰ **S22.04** Fracture of fourth thoracic vertebra

2,3,6 √7ᵗʰ **S22.040** Wedge compression fracture of fourth thoracic vertebra MCC CC H5 HCC

2,3,6 √7ᵗʰ **S22.041** Stable burst fracture of fourth thoracic vertebra MCC CC H5 HCC

2,3,6 √7ᵗʰ **S22.042** Unstable burst fracture of fourth thoracic vertebra MCC CC H5 HCC

2,3,6 √7ᵗʰ **S22.048** Other fracture of fourth thoracic vertebra MCC CC H5 HCC

2,3,6 √7ᵗʰ **S22.049** Unspecified fracture of fourth thoracic vertebra MCC CC H5 HCC

√6ᵗʰ **S22.05** Fracture of T5-T6 vertebra

2,3,6 √7ᵗʰ **S22.050** Wedge compression fracture of T5-T6 vertebra MCC CC H5 HCC

2,3,6 √7ᵗʰ **S22.051** Stable burst fracture of T5-T6 vertebra MCC CC H5 HCC

2,3,6 √7ᵗʰ **S22.052** Unstable burst fracture of T5-T6 vertebra MCC CC H5 HCC

2,3,6 √7ᵗʰ **S22.058** Other fracture of T5-T6 vertebra MCC CC H5 HCC

2,3,6 √7ᵗʰ **S22.059** Unspecified fracture of T5-T6 vertebra MCC CC H5 HCC

√6ᵗʰ **S22.06** Fracture of T7-T8 vertebra

2,3,6 √7ᵗʰ **S22.060** Wedge compression fracture of T7-T8 vertebra MCC CC H5 HCC

2,3,6 √7ᵗʰ **S22.061** Stable burst fracture of T7-T8 vertebra MCC CC H5 HCC

2,3,6 √7ᵗʰ **S22.062** Unstable burst fracture of T7-T8 vertebra MCC CC H5 HCC

2,3,6 √7ᵗʰ **S22.068** Other fracture of T7-T8 thoracic vertebra MCC CC H5 HCC

2,3,6 √7ᵗʰ **S22.069** Unspecified fracture of T7-T8 vertebra MCC CC H5 HCC

√6ᵗʰ **S22.07** Fracture of T9-T10 vertebra

2,3,6 √7ᵗʰ **S22.070** Wedge compression fracture of T9-T10 vertebra MCC CC H5 HCC

2,3,6 √7ᵗʰ **S22.071** Stable burst fracture of T9-T10 vertebra MCC CC H5 HCC

2,3,6 √7ᵗʰ **S22.072** Unstable burst fracture of T9-T10 vertebra MCC CC H5 HCC

2,3,6 √7ᵗʰ **S22.078** Other fracture of T9-T10 vertebra MCC CC H5 HCC

2,3,6 √7ᵗʰ **S22.079** Unspecified fracture of T9-T10 vertebra MCC CC H5 HCC

√6ᵗʰ **S22.08** Fracture of T11-T12 vertebra

2,3,6 √7ᵗʰ **S22.080** Wedge compression fracture of T11-T12 vertebra MCC CC H5 HCC

2,3,6 √7ᵗʰ **S22.081** Stable burst fracture of T11-T12 vertebra MCC CC H5 HCC

2,3,6 √7ᵗʰ **S22.082** Unstable burst fracture of T11-T12 vertebra MCC CC H5 HCC

2,3,6 √7ᵗʰ **S22.088** Other fracture of T11-T12 vertebra MCC CC H5 HCC

2,3,6 √7ᵗʰ **S22.089** Unspecified fracture of T11-T12 vertebra MCC CC H5 HCC

√5ᵗʰ **S22.2** Fracture of sternum

DEF: Break in flat bone (breast bone) in the anterior thorax caused by blunt trauma to the anterior chest.

2,3 √x7ᵗʰ **S22.20** Unspecified fracture of sternum MCC CC H5

2,3 √x7ᵗʰ **S22.21** Fracture of manubrium MCC CC H5

2,3 √x7ᵗʰ **S22.22** Fracture of body of sternum MCC CC H5

2,3 √x7ᵗʰ **S22.23** Sternal manubrial dissociation MCC CC H5

2,3 √x7ᵗʰ **S22.24** Fracture of xiphoid process MCC CC H5

√5ᵗʰ **S22.3** Fracture of one rib

2,3 √x7ᵗʰ **S22.31** Fracture of one rib, right side MCC CC H5

2,3 √x7ᵗʰ **S22.32** Fracture of one rib, left side MCC CC H5

2,3 √x7ᵗʰ **S22.39** Fracture of one rib, unspecified side MCC CC H5

√5ᵗʰ **S22.4** Multiple fractures of ribs

Fractures of two or more ribs
EXCLUDES 1 flail chest (S22.5-)

2,3 √x7ᵗʰ **S22.41** Multiple fractures of ribs, right side MCC CC H5

2,3 √x7ᵗʰ **S22.42** Multiple fractures of ribs, left side MCC CC H5

2,3 √x7ᵗʰ **S22.43** Multiple fractures of ribs, bilateral MCC CC H5

2,3 √x7ᵗʰ **S22.49** Multiple fractures of ribs, unspecified side MCC CC H5

4 √x7ᵗʰ **S22.5** Flail chest MCC CC H5

2,3 √x7ᵗʰ **S22.9** Fracture of bony thorax, part unspecified MCC CC H5

√4ᵗʰ **S23** Dislocation and sprain of joints and ligaments of thorax

INCLUDES avulsion of joint or ligament of thorax
laceration of cartilage, joint or ligament of thorax
sprain of cartilage, joint or ligament of thorax
traumatic hemarthrosis of joint or ligament of thorax
traumatic rupture of joint or ligament of thorax
traumatic subluxation of joint or ligament of thorax
traumatic tear of joint or ligament of thorax

Code also any associated open wound
EXCLUDES 2 dislocation, sprain of sternoclavicular joint (S43.2, S43.6)
strain of muscle or tendon of thorax (S29.01-)

The appropriate 7th character is to be added to each code from category S23.
A initial encounter
D subsequent encounter
S sequela

√x7ᵗʰ **S23.0** Traumatic rupture of thoracic intervertebral disc

EXCLUDES 1 rupture or displacement (nontraumatic) of thoracic intervertebral disc NOS (M51.- with fifth character 4)

√5ᵗʰ **S23.1** Subluxation and dislocation of thoracic vertebra

Code also any associated:
open wound of thorax (S21.-)
spinal cord injury (S24.0-, S24.1-)
EXCLUDES 2 fracture of thoracic vertebrae (S22.0-)

√6ᵗʰ **S23.10** Subluxation and dislocation of unspecified thoracic vertebra

√7ᵗʰ **S23.100** Subluxation of unspecified thoracic vertebra

√7ᵗʰ **S23.101** Dislocation of unspecified thoracic vertebra

√6ᵗʰ **S23.11** Subluxation and dislocation of T1/T2 thoracic vertebra

√7ᵗʰ **S23.110** Subluxation of T1/T2 thoracic vertebra

√7ᵗʰ **S23.111** Dislocation of T1/T2 thoracic vertebra

√6ᵗʰ **S23.12** Subluxation and dislocation of T2/T3-T3/T4 thoracic vertebra

√7ᵗʰ **S23.120** Subluxation of T2/T3 thoracic vertebra

√7ᵗʰ **S23.121** Dislocation of T2/T3 thoracic vertebra

√7ᵗʰ **S23.122** Subluxation of T3/T4 thoracic vertebra

√7ᵗʰ **S23.123** Dislocation of T3/T4 thoracic vertebra

√6ᵗʰ **S23.13** Subluxation and dislocation of T4/T5-T5/T6 thoracic vertebra

√7ᵗʰ **S23.130** Subluxation of T4/T5 thoracic vertebra

√7ᵗʰ **S23.131** Dislocation of T4/T5 thoracic vertebra

√7ᵗʰ **S23.132** Subluxation of T5/T6 thoracic vertebra

√7ᵗʰ **S23.133** Dislocation of T5/T6 thoracic vertebra

√6ᵗʰ **S23.14** Subluxation and dislocation of T6/T7-T7/T8 thoracic vertebra

√7ᵗʰ **S23.140** Subluxation of T6/T7 thoracic vertebra

✓ Additional Character Required √x7ᵗʰ Placeholder Unacceptable PDx Questionable PDx Manifestation Unspecified Dx H1-H14 HAC HCC CMS-HCC Dx HIV HIV Dx

√7ᵗʰ **S23.141** Dislocation of T6/T7 thoracic vertebra

√7ᵗʰ **S23.142** Subluxation of T7/T8 thoracic vertebra

√7ᵗʰ **S23.143** Dislocation of T7/T8 thoracic vertebra

√6ᵗʰ **S23.15** Subluxation and dislocation of T8/T9-T9/T10 thoracic vertebra

√7ᵗʰ **S23.150** Subluxation of T8/T9 thoracic vertebra

√7ᵗʰ **S23.151** Dislocation of T8/T9 thoracic vertebra

√7ᵗʰ **S23.152** Subluxation of T9/T10 thoracic vertebra

√7ᵗʰ **S23.153** Dislocation of T9/T10 thoracic vertebra

√6ᵗʰ **S23.16** Subluxation and dislocation of T10/T11-T11/T12 thoracic vertebra

√7ᵗʰ **S23.160** Subluxation of T10/T11 thoracic vertebra

√7ᵗʰ **S23.161** Dislocation of T10/T11 thoracic vertebra

√7ᵗʰ **S23.162** Subluxation of T11/T12 thoracic vertebra

√7ᵗʰ **S23.163** Dislocation of T11/T12 thoracic vertebra

√6ᵗʰ **S23.17** Subluxation and dislocation of T12/L1 thoracic vertebra

√7ᵗʰ **S23.170** Subluxation of T12/L1 thoracic vertebra

√7ᵗʰ **S23.171** Dislocation of T12/L1 thoracic vertebra

√5ᵗʰ **S23.2** Dislocation of other and unspecified parts of thorax

√x7ᵗʰ **S23.20** Dislocation of unspecified part of thorax

√x7ᵗʰ **S23.29** Dislocation of other parts of thorax

√x7ᵗʰ **S23.3** Sprain of ligaments of thoracic spine

√5ᵗʰ **S23.4** Sprain of ribs and sternum

√x7ᵗʰ **S23.41** Sprain of ribs

√6ᵗʰ **S23.42** Sprain of sternum

√7ᵗʰ **S23.420** Sprain of sternoclavicular (joint) (ligament)

√7ᵗʰ **S23.421** Sprain of chondrosternal joint

√7ᵗʰ **S23.428** Other sprain of sternum

√7ᵗʰ **S23.429** Unspecified sprain of sternum

√x7ᵗʰ **S23.8** Sprain of other specified parts of thorax

√x7ᵗʰ **S23.9** Sprain of unspecified parts of thorax

√4ᵗʰ **S24** Injury of nerves and spinal cord at thorax level

NOTE   Code to highest level of thoracic spinal cord injury.

Injuries to the spinal cord (S24.0 and S24.1) refer to the cord level and not bone level injury, and can affect nerve roots at and below the level given.

Code also any associated:

fracture of thoracic vertebra (S22.0-)

open wound of thorax (S21.-)

transient paralysis (R29.5)

EXCLUDES 2   injury of brachial plexus (S14.3)

The appropriate 7th character is to be added to each code from category S24.
A   initial encounter
D   subsequent encounter
S   sequela

√x7ᵗʰ **S24.0** Concussion and edema of thoracic spinal cord   MCC HCC

√5ᵗʰ **S24.1** Other and unspecified injuries of thoracic spinal cord

√6ᵗʰ **S24.10** Unspecified injury of thoracic spinal cord

√7ᵗʰ **S24.101** Unspecified injury at T1 level of thoracic spinal cord   MCC H5 HCC

√7ᵗʰ **S24.102** Unspecified injury at T2-T6 level of thoracic spinal cord   MCC H5 HCC

√7ᵗʰ **S24.103** Unspecified injury at T7-T10 level of thoracic spinal cord   MCC H5 HCC

√7ᵗʰ **S24.104** Unspecified injury at T11-T12 level of thoracic spinal cord   MCC H5 HCC

√7ᵗʰ **S24.109** Unspecified injury at unspecified level of thoracic spinal cord   HCC

Injury of thoracic spinal cord NOS

√6ᵗʰ **S24.11** Complete lesion of thoracic spinal cord

√7ᵗʰ **S24.111** Complete lesion at T1 level of thoracic spinal cord   MCC H5 HCC

√7ᵗʰ **S24.112** Complete lesion at T2-T6 level of thoracic spinal cord   MCC H5 HCC

√7ᵗʰ **S24.113** Complete lesion at T7-T10 level of thoracic spinal cord   MCC H5 HCC

√7ᵗʰ **S24.114** Complete lesion at T11-T12 level of thoracic spinal cord   MCC H5 HCC

√7ᵗʰ **S24.119** Complete lesion at unspecified level of thoracic spinal cord   HCC

√6ᵗʰ **S24.13** Anterior cord syndrome of thoracic spinal cord

√7ᵗʰ **S24.131** Anterior cord syndrome at T1 level of thoracic spinal cord   MCC H5 HCC

√7ᵗʰ **S24.132** Anterior cord syndrome at T2-T6 level of thoracic spinal cord   MCC H5 HCC

√7ᵗʰ **S24.133** Anterior cord syndrome at T7-T10 level of thoracic spinal cord   MCC H5 HCC

√7ᵗʰ **S24.134** Anterior cord syndrome at T11-T12 level of thoracic spinal cord   MCC H5 HCC

√7ᵗʰ **S24.139** Anterior cord syndrome at unspecified level of thoracic spinal cord   HCC

√6ᵗʰ **S24.14** Brown-Séquard syndrome of thoracic spinal cord

√7ᵗʰ **S24.141** Brown-Séquard syndrome at T1 level of thoracic spinal cord   MCC HCC

√7ᵗʰ **S24.142** Brown-Séquard syndrome at T2-T6 level of thoracic spinal cord   MCC HCC

√7ᵗʰ **S24.143** Brown-Séquard syndrome at T7-T10 level of thoracic spinal cord   MCC HCC

√7ᵗʰ **S24.144** Brown-Séquard syndrome at T11-T12 level of thoracic spinal cord   MCC HCC

√7ᵗʰ **S24.149** Brown-Séquard syndrome at unspecified level of thoracic spinal cord   HCC

√6ᵗʰ **S24.15** Other incomplete lesions of thoracic spinal cord

Incomplete lesion of thoracic spinal cord NOS
Posterior cord syndrome of thoracic spinal cord

√7ᵗʰ **S24.151** Other incomplete lesion at T1 level of thoracic spinal cord   MCC H5 HCC

√7ᵗʰ **S24.152** Other incomplete lesion at T2-T6 level of thoracic spinal cord   MCC H5 HCC

√7ᵗʰ **S24.153** Other incomplete lesion at T7-T10 level of thoracic spinal cord   MCC H5 HCC

√7ᵗʰ **S24.154** Other incomplete lesion at T11-T12 level of thoracic spinal cord   MCC H5 HCC

√7ᵗʰ **S24.159** Other incomplete lesion at unspecified level of thoracic spinal cord   HCC

√x7ᵗʰ **S24.2** Injury of nerve root of thoracic spine

√x7ᵗʰ **S24.3** Injury of peripheral nerves of thorax

√x7ᵗʰ **S24.4** Injury of thoracic sympathetic nervous system

Injury of cardiac plexus
Injury of esophageal plexus
Injury of pulmonary plexus
Injury of stellate ganglion
Injury of thoracic sympathetic ganglion

√x7ᵗʰ **S24.8** Injury of other specified nerves of thorax

√x7ᵗʰ **S24.9** Injury of unspecified nerve of thorax

√4ᵗʰ **S25** Injury of blood vessels of thorax

Code also any associated open wound (S21.-)

The appropriate 7th character is to be added to each code from category S25.
A   initial encounter
D   subsequent encounter
S   sequela

√5ᵗʰ **S25.0** Injury of thoracic aorta

Injury of aorta NOS

√x7ᵗʰ **S25.00** Unspecified injury of thoracic aorta   MCC

√x7ᵗʰ **S25.01** Minor laceration of thoracic aorta   MCC

Incomplete transection of thoracic aorta
Laceration of thoracic aorta NOS
Superficial laceration of thoracic aorta

√x7ᵗʰ **S25.02** Major laceration of thoracic aorta   MCC

Complete transection of thoracic aorta
Traumatic rupture of thoracic aorta

√x7ᵗʰ **S25.09** Other specified injury of thoracic aorta   MCC

√5ᵗʰ **S25.1** Injury of innominate or subclavian artery

√6ᵗʰ **S25.10** Unspecified injury of innominate or subclavian artery

√7ᵗʰ **S25.101** Unspecified injury of right innominate or subclavian artery   MCC

√7ᵗʰ **S25.102** Unspecified injury of left innominate or subclavian artery   MCC

√7ᵗʰ **S25.109** Unspecified injury of unspecified innominate or subclavian artery   MCC

N Newborn: 0   P Pediatric: 0-17   M Maternity: 9-64   A Adult: 15-124   MCC Major Complication/Comorbidity   CC Complication/Comorbidity   SW Severe Wound Dx

988   ICD-10-CM 2021

√6ᵗʰ **S25.11** Minor laceration of innominate or subclavian artery

    Incomplete transection of innominate or subclavian artery

    Laceration of innominate or subclavian artery NOS

    Superficial laceration of innominate or subclavian artery

    √7ᵗʰ **S25.111** Minor laceration of right innominate or subclavian artery   MCC

    √7ᵗʰ **S25.112** Minor laceration of left innominate or subclavian artery   MCC

    √7ᵗʰ **S25.119** Minor laceration of unspecified innominate or subclavian artery   MCC

√6ᵗʰ **S25.12** Major laceration of innominate or subclavian artery

    Complete transection of innominate or subclavian artery

    Traumatic rupture of innominate or subclavian artery

    √7ᵗʰ **S25.121** Major laceration of right innominate or subclavian artery   MCC

    √7ᵗʰ **S25.122** Major laceration of left innominate or subclavian artery   MCC

    √7ᵗʰ **S25.129** Major laceration of unspecified innominate or subclavian artery   MCC

√6ᵗʰ **S25.19** Other specified injury of innominate or subclavian artery

    √7ᵗʰ **S25.191** Other specified injury of right innominate or subclavian artery   MCC

    √7ᵗʰ **S25.192** Other specified injury of left innominate or subclavian artery   MCC

    √7ᵗʰ **S25.199** Other specified injury of unspecified innominate or subclavian artery   MCC

√5ᵗʰ **S25.2** Injury of superior vena cava

    Injury of vena cava NOS

  √×7ᵗʰ **S25.20** Unspecified injury of superior vena cava   MCC

  √×7ᵗʰ **S25.21** Minor laceration of superior vena cava   MCC

    Incomplete transection of superior vena cava

    Laceration of superior vena cava NOS

    Superficial laceration of superior vena cava

  √×7ᵗʰ **S25.22** Major laceration of superior vena cava   MCC

    Complete transection of superior vena cava

    Traumatic rupture of superior vena cava

  √×7ᵗʰ **S25.29** Other specified injury of superior vena cava   MCC

√5ᵗʰ **S25.3** Injury of innominate or subclavian vein

  √6ᵗʰ **S25.30** Unspecified injury of innominate or subclavian vein

    √7ᵗʰ **S25.301** Unspecified injury of right innominate or subclavian vein   MCC

    √7ᵗʰ **S25.302** Unspecified injury of left innominate or subclavian vein   MCC

    √7ᵗʰ **S25.309** Unspecified injury of unspecified innominate or subclavian vein   MCC

  √6ᵗʰ **S25.31** Minor laceration of innominate or subclavian vein

    Incomplete transection of innominate or subclavian vein

    Laceration of innominate or subclavian vein NOS

    Superficial laceration of innominate or subclavian vein

    √7ᵗʰ **S25.311** Minor laceration of right innominate or subclavian vein   MCC

    √7ᵗʰ **S25.312** Minor laceration of left innominate or subclavian vein   MCC

    √7ᵗʰ **S25.319** Minor laceration of unspecified innominate or subclavian vein   MCC

  √6ᵗʰ **S25.32** Major laceration of innominate or subclavian vein

    Complete transection of innominate or subclavian vein

    Traumatic rupture of innominate or subclavian vein

    √7ᵗʰ **S25.321** Major laceration of right innominate or subclavian vein   MCC

    √7ᵗʰ **S25.322** Major laceration of left innominate or subclavian vein   MCC

    √7ᵗʰ **S25.329** Major laceration of unspecified innominate or subclavian vein   MCC

  √6ᵗʰ **S25.39** Other specified injury of innominate or subclavian vein

    √7ᵗʰ **S25.391** Other specified injury of right innominate or subclavian vein   MCC

    √7ᵗʰ **S25.392** Other specified injury of left innominate or subclavian vein   MCC

    √7ᵗʰ **S25.399** Other specified injury of unspecified innominate or subclavian vein   MCC

√5ᵗʰ **S25.4** Injury of pulmonary blood vessels

  √6ᵗʰ **S25.40** Unspecified injury of pulmonary blood vessels

    √7ᵗʰ **S25.401** Unspecified injury of right pulmonary blood vessels   MCC

    √7ᵗʰ **S25.402** Unspecified injury of left pulmonary blood vessels   MCC

    √7ᵗʰ **S25.409** Unspecified injury of unspecified pulmonary blood vessels   MCC

  √6ᵗʰ **S25.41** Minor laceration of pulmonary blood vessels

    Incomplete transection of pulmonary blood vessels

    Laceration of pulmonary blood vessels NOS

    Superficial laceration of pulmonary blood vessels

    √7ᵗʰ **S25.411** Minor laceration of right pulmonary blood vessels   MCC

    √7ᵗʰ **S25.412** Minor laceration of left pulmonary blood vessels   MCC

    √7ᵗʰ **S25.419** Minor laceration of unspecified pulmonary blood vessels   MCC

  √6ᵗʰ **S25.42** Major laceration of pulmonary blood vessels

    Complete transection of pulmonary blood vessels

    Traumatic rupture of pulmonary blood vessels

    √7ᵗʰ **S25.421** Major laceration of right pulmonary blood vessels   MCC

    √7ᵗʰ **S25.422** Major laceration of left pulmonary blood vessels   MCC

    √7ᵗʰ **S25.429** Major laceration of unspecified pulmonary blood vessels   MCC

  √6ᵗʰ **S25.49** Other specified injury of pulmonary blood vessels

    √7ᵗʰ **S25.491** Other specified injury of right pulmonary blood vessels   MCC

    √7ᵗʰ **S25.492** Other specified injury of left pulmonary blood vessels   MCC

    √7ᵗʰ **S25.499** Other specified injury of unspecified pulmonary blood vessels   MCC

√5ᵗʰ **S25.5** Injury of intercostal blood vessels

  √6ᵗʰ **S25.50** Unspecified injury of intercostal blood vessels

    √7ᵗʰ **S25.501** Unspecified injury of intercostal blood vessels, right side   CC

    √7ᵗʰ **S25.502** Unspecified injury of intercostal blood vessels, left side   CC

    √7ᵗʰ **S25.509** Unspecified injury of intercostal blood vessels, unspecified side   CC

  √6ᵗʰ **S25.51** Laceration of intercostal blood vessels

    √7ᵗʰ **S25.511** Laceration of intercostal blood vessels, right side   CC

    √7ᵗʰ **S25.512** Laceration of intercostal blood vessels, left side   CC

    √7ᵗʰ **S25.519** Laceration of intercostal blood vessels, unspecified side   CC

  √6ᵗʰ **S25.59** Other specified injury of intercostal blood vessels

    √7ᵗʰ **S25.591** Other specified injury of intercostal blood vessels, right side   CC

    √7ᵗʰ **S25.592** Other specified injury of intercostal blood vessels, left side   CC

    √7ᵗʰ **S25.599** Other specified injury of intercostal blood vessels, unspecified side   CC

√5ᵗʰ **S25.8** Injury of other blood vessels of thorax

    Injury of azygos vein

    Injury of mammary artery or vein

  √6ᵗʰ **S25.80** Unspecified injury of other blood vessels of thorax

    √7ᵗʰ **S25.801** Unspecified injury of other blood vessels of thorax, right side   CC

    √7ᵗʰ **S25.802** Unspecified injury of other blood vessels of thorax, left side   CC

    √7ᵗʰ **S25.809** Unspecified injury of other blood vessels of thorax, unspecified side   CC

  √6ᵗʰ **S25.81** Laceration of other blood vessels of thorax

    √7ᵗʰ **S25.811** Laceration of other blood vessels of thorax, right side   CC

    √7ᵗʰ **S25.812** Laceration of other blood vessels of thorax, left side   CC

    √7ᵗʰ **S25.819** Laceration of other blood vessels of thorax, unspecified side   CC

✔ Additional Character Required   √×7ᵗʰ Placeholder   Unacceptable PDx   Questionable PDx   Manifestation   Unspecified Dx   H1-H14 HAC   HCC CMS-HCC Dx   HIV HIV Dx

ICD-10-CM 2021   **989**

Chapter 19. Injury, Poisoning and Certain Other Consequences of External Causes

☑6th **S25.89** Other specified injury of other blood vessels of thorax

    ☑7th **S25.891** Other specified injury of other blood vessels of thorax, **right** side   `CC`

    ☑7th **S25.892** Other specified injury of other blood vessels of thorax, **left** side   `CC`

    ☑7th **S25.899** Other specified injury of other blood vessels of thorax, unspecified side   `CC`

☑5th **S25.9** Injury of unspecified blood vessel of thorax

  ☑x7th **S25.90** Unspecified injury of unspecified blood vessel of thorax   `CC`

  ☑x7th **S25.91** **Laceration** of unspecified blood vessel of thorax   `CC`

  ☑x7th **S25.99** Other specified injury of unspecified blood vessel of thorax   `CC`

☑4th **S26** **Injury of heart**

Code also any associated:
  open wound of thorax (S21.-)
  traumatic hemopneumothorax (S27.2)
  traumatic hemothorax (S27.1)
  traumatic pneumothorax (S27.0)

> The appropriate 7th character is to be added to each code from category S26.
> A   initial encounter
> D   subsequent encounter
> S   sequela

☑5th **S26.0** **Injury of heart** with hemopericardium

  ☑x7th **S26.00** Unspecified injury of heart with hemopericardium   `CC`

  ☑x7th **S26.01** **Contusion** of heart with hemopericardium   `CC`

  ☑6th **S26.02** **Laceration** of heart with hemopericardium

    ☑7th **S26.020** **Mild** laceration of heart with hemopericardium   `MCC`
      Laceration of heart without penetration of heart chamber

    ☑7th **S26.021** **Moderate** laceration of heart with hemopericardium   `MCC`
      Laceration of heart with penetration of heart chamber

    ☑7th **S26.022** **Major** laceration of heart with hemopericardium   `MCC`
      Laceration of heart with penetration of multiple heart chambers

  ☑x7th **S26.09** Other injury of heart with hemopericardium   `CC`

☑5th **S26.1** **Injury of heart** without hemopericardium

  ☑x7th **S26.10** Unspecified injury of heart without hemopericardium   `CC`

  ☑x7th **S26.11** **Contusion** of heart without hemopericardium   `CC`

  ☑x7th **S26.12** **Laceration** of heart without hemopericardium   `MCC`

  ☑x7th **S26.19** Other injury of heart without hemopericardium   `CC`

☑5th **S26.9** Injury of heart, unspecified with or without hemopericardium

  ☑x7th **S26.90** Unspecified injury of heart, unspecified with or without hemopericardium   `CC`

  ☑x7th **S26.91** **Contusion** of heart, unspecified with or without hemopericardium   `CC`
    DEF: Bruising within the heart muscle, with no mention of an open wound, usually caused by blunt chest trauma in motor vehicle accidents, falling from great heights, or receiving CPR.

  ☑x7th **S26.92** **Laceration** of heart, unspecified with or without hemopericardium   `MCC`
    Laceration of heart NOS
    AHA: 2019,2Q,24

  ☑x7th **S26.99** Other injury of heart, unspecified with or without hemopericardium   `CC`

☑4th **S27** **Injury of other and unspecified intrathoracic organs**

Code also any associated open wound of thorax (S21.-)

EXCLUDES 2   injury of cervical esophagus (S10–S19)
                injury of trachea (cervical) (S10–S19)

> The appropriate 7th character is to be added to each code from category S27.
> A   initial encounter
> D   subsequent encounter
> S   sequela

☑x7th **S27.0** **Traumatic pneumothorax**   `CC`
    EXCLUDES 1   spontaneous pneumothorax (J93.-)

☑x7th **S27.1** **Traumatic hemothorax**   `MCC`

☑x7th **S27.2** **Traumatic hemopneumothorax**   `MCC`

☑5th **S27.3** Other and unspecified injuries of **lung**

  ☑6th **S27.30** Unspecified injury of lung

    ☑7th **S27.301** Unspecified injury of lung, **unilateral**   `CC`

    ☑7th **S27.302** Unspecified injury of lung, **bilateral**   `CC`

    ☑7th **S27.309** Unspecified injury of lung, unspecified   `CC`

  ☑6th **S27.31** **Primary blast** injury of lung
    Blast injury of lung NOS

    ☑7th **S27.311** Primary blast injury of lung, **unilateral**   `CC`

    ☑7th **S27.312** Primary blast injury of lung, **bilateral**   `CC`

    ☑7th **S27.319** Primary blast injury of lung, unspecified   `CC`

  ☑6th **S27.32** **Contusion** of lung
    DEF: Bruising of the lung without mention of an open wound.

    ☑7th **S27.321** Contusion of lung, **unilateral**   `CC`

    ☑7th **S27.322** Contusion of lung, **bilateral**   `CC`

    ☑7th **S27.329** Contusion of lung, unspecified   `CC`

  ☑6th **S27.33** **Laceration** of lung

    ☑7th **S27.331** Laceration of lung, **unilateral**   `MCC`

    ☑7th **S27.332** Laceration of lung, **bilateral**   `MCC`

    ☑7th **S27.339** Laceration of lung, unspecified   `MCC`

  ☑6th **S27.39** **Other injuries of lung**
    Secondary blast injury of lung

    ☑7th **S27.391** Other injuries of lung, **unilateral**   `CC`

    ☑7th **S27.392** Other injuries of lung, **bilateral**   `CC`

    ☑7th **S27.399** Other injuries of lung, unspecified   `CC`

☑5th **S27.4** Injury of **bronchus**

  ☑6th **S27.40** Unspecified injury of bronchus

    ☑7th **S27.401** Unspecified injury of bronchus, **unilateral**   `MCC`

    ☑7th **S27.402** Unspecified injury of bronchus, **bilateral**   `MCC`

    ☑7th **S27.409** Unspecified injury of bronchus, unspecified   `MCC`

  ☑6th **S27.41** **Primary blast** injury of bronchus
    Blast injury of bronchus NOS

    ☑7th **S27.411** Primary blast injury of bronchus, **unilateral**   `MCC`

    ☑7th **S27.412** Primary blast injury of bronchus, **bilateral**   `MCC`

    ☑7th **S27.419** Primary blast injury of bronchus, unspecified   `MCC`

  ☑6th **S27.42** **Contusion** of bronchus

    ☑7th **S27.421** Contusion of bronchus, **unilateral**   `MCC`

    ☑7th **S27.422** Contusion of bronchus, **bilateral**   `MCC`

    ☑7th **S27.429** Contusion of bronchus, unspecified   `MCC`

  ☑6th **S27.43** **Laceration** of bronchus

    ☑7th **S27.431** Laceration of bronchus, **unilateral**   `MCC`

    ☑7th **S27.432** Laceration of bronchus, **bilateral**   `MCC`

    ☑7th **S27.439** Laceration of bronchus, unspecified   `MCC`

`N` Newborn: 0   `P` Pediatric: 0-17   `M` Maternity: 9-64   `A` Adult: 15-124   `MCC` Major Complication/Comorbidity   `CC` Complication/Comorbidity   `SW` Severe Wound Dx

990   ICD-10-CM 2021

√6ᵗʰ **S27.49**   **Other injury of bronchus**
Secondary blast injury of bronchus

    √7ᵗʰ **S27.491**   **Other injury of bronchus, unilateral**   `MCC`

    √7ᵗʰ **S27.492**   **Other injury of bronchus, bilateral**   `MCC`

    √7ᵗʰ **S27.499**   **Other injury of bronchus, unspecified**   `MCC`

√5ᵗʰ **S27.5**   **Injury of thoracic trachea**

   √x7ᵗʰ **S27.50**   **Unspecified injury of thoracic trachea**   `CC`

   √x7ᵗʰ **S27.51**   **Primary blast injury of thoracic trachea**   `CC`
Blast injury of thoracic trachea NOS

   √x7ᵗʰ **S27.52**   **Contusion of thoracic trachea**   `CC`

   √x7ᵗʰ **S27.53**   **Laceration of thoracic trachea**   `CC`

   √x7ᵗʰ **S27.59**   **Other injury of thoracic trachea**   `CC`
Secondary blast injury of thoracic trachea

√5ᵗʰ **S27.6**   **Injury of pleura**

   √x7ᵗʰ **S27.60**   **Unspecified injury of pleura**   `CC`

   √x7ᵗʰ **S27.63**   **Laceration of pleura**   `CC`

   √x7ᵗʰ **S27.69**   **Other injury of pleura**   `CC`

√5ᵗʰ **S27.8**   **Injury of other specified intrathoracic organs**

   √6ᵗʰ **S27.80**   **Injury of diaphragm**

    √7ᵗʰ **S27.802**   **Contusion of diaphragm**   `CC`

    √7ᵗʰ **S27.803**   **Laceration of diaphragm**   `CC`

    √7ᵗʰ **S27.808**   **Other injury of diaphragm**   `CC`

    √7ᵗʰ **S27.809**   **Unspecified injury of diaphragm**   `CC`

   √6ᵗʰ **S27.81**   **Injury of esophagus (thoracic part)**

    √7ᵗʰ **S27.812**   **Contusion of esophagus (thoracic part)**   `MCC`

    √7ᵗʰ **S27.813**   **Laceration of esophagus (thoracic part)**   `MCC`

    √7ᵗʰ **S27.818**   **Other injury of esophagus (thoracic part)**   `MCC`

    √7ᵗʰ **S27.819**   **Unspecified injury of esophagus (thoracic part)**   `MCC`

   √6ᵗʰ **S27.89**   **Injury of other specified intrathoracic organs**
Injury of lymphatic thoracic duct
Injury of thymus gland

    √7ᵗʰ **S27.892**   **Contusion of other specified intrathoracic organs**   `CC`

    √7ᵗʰ **S27.893**   **Laceration of other specified intrathoracic organs**   `CC`

    √7ᵗʰ **S27.898**   **Other injury of other specified intrathoracic organs**   `CC`

    √7ᵗʰ **S27.899**   **Unspecified injury of other specified intrathoracic organs**   `CC`

   √x7ᵗʰ **S27.9**   **Injury of unspecified intrathoracic organ**   `CC`

√4ᵗʰ **S28**   **Crushing injury of thorax, and traumatic amputation of part of thorax**

> The appropriate 7th character is to be added to each code from category S28.
> A   initial encounter
> D   subsequent encounter
> S   sequela

   √x7ᵗʰ **S28.0**   **Crushed chest**
Use additional code for all associated injuries
   EXCLUDES 1   flail chest (S22.5)

   √x7ᵗʰ **S28.1**   **Traumatic amputation (partial) of part of thorax, except breast**   `CC`

   √5ᵗʰ **S28.2**   **Traumatic amputation of breast**

   √6ᵗʰ **S28.21**   **Complete traumatic amputation of breast**
Traumatic amputation of breast NOS

    √7ᵗʰ **S28.211**   **Complete traumatic amputation of right breast**

    √7ᵗʰ **S28.212**   **Complete traumatic amputation of left breast**

    √7ᵗʰ **S28.219**   **Complete traumatic amputation of unspecified breast**

   √6ᵗʰ **S28.22**   **Partial traumatic amputation of breast**

    √7ᵗʰ **S28.221**   **Partial traumatic amputation of right breast**

    √7ᵗʰ **S28.222**   **Partial traumatic amputation of left breast**

    √7ᵗʰ **S28.229**   **Partial traumatic amputation of unspecified breast**

√4ᵗʰ **S29**   **Other and unspecified injuries of thorax**
Code also any associated open wound (S21.-)

> The appropriate 7th character is to be added to each code from category S29.
> A   initial encounter
> D   subsequent encounter
> S   sequela

   √5ᵗʰ **S29.0**   **Injury of muscle and tendon at thorax level**

   √6ᵗʰ **S29.00**   **Unspecified injury of muscle and tendon of thorax**

    √7ᵗʰ **S29.001**   **Unspecified injury of muscle and tendon of front wall of thorax**

    √7ᵗʰ **S29.002**   **Unspecified injury of muscle and tendon of back wall of thorax**

    √7ᵗʰ **S29.009**   **Unspecified injury of muscle and tendon of unspecified wall of thorax**

   √6ᵗʰ **S29.01**   **Strain of muscle and tendon of thorax**

    √7ᵗʰ **S29.011**   **Strain of muscle and tendon of front wall of thorax**

    √7ᵗʰ **S29.012**   **Strain of muscle and tendon of back wall of thorax**

    √7ᵗʰ **S29.019**   **Strain of muscle and tendon of unspecified wall of thorax**

   √6ᵗʰ **S29.02**   **Laceration of muscle and tendon of thorax**

    √7ᵗʰ **S29.021**   **Laceration of muscle and tendon of front wall of thorax**   `CC`

    √7ᵗʰ **S29.022**   **Laceration of muscle and tendon of back wall of thorax**

    √7ᵗʰ **S29.029**   **Laceration of muscle and tendon of unspecified wall of thorax**   `CC`

   √6ᵗʰ **S29.09**   **Other injury of muscle and tendon of thorax**

    √7ᵗʰ **S29.091**   **Other injury of muscle and tendon of front wall of thorax**

    √7ᵗʰ **S29.092**   **Other injury of muscle and tendon of back wall of thorax**

    √7ᵗʰ **S29.099**   **Other injury of muscle and tendon of unspecified wall of thorax**

   √x7ᵗʰ **S29.8**   **Other specified injuries of thorax**

   √x7ᵗʰ **S29.9**   **Unspecified injury of thorax**

Injuries to the abdomen, lower back, lumbar spine, pelvis and external genitals (S30-S39)

`INCLUDES`   injuries to the abdominal wall
injuries to the anus
injuries to the buttock
injuries to the external genitalia
injuries to the flank
injuries to the groin

EXCLUDES 2   burns and corrosions (T20-T32)
effects of foreign body in anus and rectum (T18.5)
effects of foreign body in genitourinary tract (T19.-)
effects of foreign body in stomach, small intestine and colon (T18.2-T18.4)
frostbite (T33-T34)
insect bite or sting, venomous (T63.4)

√4ᵗʰ **S30**   **Superficial injury of abdomen, lower back, pelvis and external genitals**
   EXCLUDES 2   superficial injury of hip (S70.-)

> The appropriate 7th character is to be added to each code from category S30.
> A   initial encounter
> D   subsequent encounter
> S   sequela

   √x7ᵗʰ **S30.0**   **Contusion of lower back and pelvis**
Contusion of buttock

   √x7ᵗʰ **S30.1**   **Contusion of abdominal wall**
Contusion of flank
Contusion of groin

   √5ᵗʰ **S30.2**   **Contusion of external genital organs**

   √6ᵗʰ **S30.20**   **Contusion of unspecified external genital organ**

    √7ᵗʰ **S30.201**   **Contusion of unspecified external genital organ, male**   ♂

    √7ᵗʰ **S30.202**   **Contusion of unspecified external genital organ, female**   ♀

   √x7ᵗʰ **S30.21**   **Contusion of penis**   ♂

✅ Additional Character Required   √x7ᵗʰ Placeholder   Unacceptable PDx   Questionable PDx   Manifestation   Unspecified Dx   `HI`-`HI` HAC   `HCC` CMS-HCC Dx   `HIV` HIV Dx

√x7ᵗʰ **S30.22**   **Contusion of** scrotum and testes   ♂

√x7ᵗʰ **S30.23**   **Contusion of** vagina and vulva   ♀

√x7ᵗʰ **S30.3**   **Contusion of** anus

√5ᵗʰ **S30.8**   **Other superficial injuries of abdomen, lower back, pelvis and external genitals**

  √6ᵗʰ **S30.81**   **Abrasion of abdomen, lower back, pelvis and external genitals**

    √7ᵗʰ **S30.810**   **Abrasion of** lower back and pelvis

    √7ᵗʰ **S30.811**   **Abrasion of** abdominal wall

    √7ᵗʰ **S30.812**   **Abrasion of** penis   ♂

    √7ᵗʰ **S30.813**   **Abrasion of** scrotum and testes   ♂

    √7ᵗʰ **S30.814**   **Abrasion of** vagina and vulva   ♀

    √7ᵗʰ **S30.815**   **Abrasion of unspecified** external genital organs, male   ♂

    √7ᵗʰ **S30.816**   **Abrasion of unspecified** external genital organs, female   ♀

    √7ᵗʰ **S30.817**   **Abrasion of** anus

  √6ᵗʰ **S30.82**   **Blister (nonthermal) of abdomen, lower back, pelvis and external genitals**

    √7ᵗʰ **S30.820**   **Blister (nonthermal) of** lower back and pelvis

    √7ᵗʰ **S30.821**   **Blister (nonthermal) of** abdominal wall

    √7ᵗʰ **S30.822**   **Blister (nonthermal) of** penis   ♂

    √7ᵗʰ **S30.823**   **Blister (nonthermal) of** scrotum and testes   ♂

    √7ᵗʰ **S30.824**   **Blister (nonthermal) of** vagina and vulva   ♀

    √7ᵗʰ **S30.825**   **Blister (nonthermal) of unspecified** external genital organs, male   ♂

    √7ᵗʰ **S30.826**   **Blister (nonthermal) of unspecified** external genital organs, female   ♀

    √7ᵗʰ **S30.827**   **Blister (nonthermal) of** anus

  √6ᵗʰ **S30.84**   **External constriction of abdomen, lower back, pelvis and external genitals**

    √7ᵗʰ **S30.840**   **External constriction of** lower back and pelvis

    √7ᵗʰ **S30.841**   **External constriction of** abdominal wall

    √7ᵗʰ **S30.842**   **External constriction of** penis   ♂

      Hair tourniquet syndrome of penis

      Use additional cause code to identify the constricting item (W49.0-)

    √7ᵗʰ **S30.843**   **External constriction of** scrotum and testes   ♂

    √7ᵗʰ **S30.844**   **External constriction of** vagina and vulva   ♀

    √7ᵗʰ **S30.845**   **External constriction of unspecified** external genital organs, male   ♂

    √7ᵗʰ **S30.846**   **External constriction of unspecified** external genital organs, female   ♀

  √6ᵗʰ **S30.85**   **Superficial foreign body of abdomen, lower back, pelvis and external genitals**

      Splinter in the abdomen, lower back, pelvis and external genitals

    √7ᵗʰ **S30.850**   **Superficial foreign body of** lower back and pelvis

    √7ᵗʰ **S30.851**   **Superficial foreign body of** abdominal wall

    √7ᵗʰ **S30.852**   **Superficial foreign body of** penis   ♂

    √7ᵗʰ **S30.853**   **Superficial foreign body of** scrotum and testes   ♂

    √7ᵗʰ **S30.854**   **Superficial foreign body of** vagina and vulva   ♀

    √7ᵗʰ **S30.855**   **Superficial foreign body of unspecified** external genital organs, male   ♂

    √7ᵗʰ **S30.856**   **Superficial foreign body of unspecified** external genital organs, female   ♀

    √7ᵗʰ **S30.857**   **Superficial foreign body of** anus

  √6ᵗʰ **S30.86**   **Insect bite (nonvenomous) of abdomen, lower back, pelvis and external genitals**

    √7ᵗʰ **S30.860**   **Insect bite (nonvenomous) of** lower back and pelvis

    √7ᵗʰ **S30.861**   **Insect bite (nonvenomous) of** abdominal wall

    √7ᵗʰ **S30.862**   **Insect bite (nonvenomous) of** penis   ♂

    √7ᵗʰ **S30.863**   **Insect bite (nonvenomous) of** scrotum and testes   ♂

    √7ᵗʰ **S30.864**   **Insect bite (nonvenomous) of** vagina and vulva   ♀

    √7ᵗʰ **S30.865**   **Insect bite (nonvenomous) of unspecified** external genital organs, male   ♂

    √7ᵗʰ **S30.866**   **Insect bite (nonvenomous) of unspecified** external genital organs, female   ♀

    √7ᵗʰ **S30.867**   **Insect bite (nonvenomous) of** anus

  √6ᵗʰ **S30.87**   **Other superficial bite of abdomen, lower back, pelvis and external genitals**

    EXCLUDES 1   open bite of abdomen, lower back, pelvis and external genitals (S31.05, S31.15, S31.25, S31.35, S31.45, S31.55)

    √7ᵗʰ **S30.870**   **Other superficial bite of** lower back and pelvis

    √7ᵗʰ **S30.871**   **Other superficial bite of** abdominal wall

    √7ᵗʰ **S30.872**   **Other superficial bite of** penis   ♂

    √7ᵗʰ **S30.873**   **Other superficial bite of** scrotum and testes   ♂

    √7ᵗʰ **S30.874**   **Other superficial bite of** vagina and vulva   ♀

    √7ᵗʰ **S30.875**   **Other superficial bite of unspecified** external genital organs, male   ♂

    √7ᵗʰ **S30.876**   **Other superficial bite of unspecified** external genital organs, female   ♀

    √7ᵗʰ **S30.877**   **Other superficial bite of** anus

√5ᵗʰ **S30.9**   **Unspecified superficial injury of abdomen, lower back, pelvis and external genitals**

  √x7ᵗʰ **S30.91**   **Unspecified superficial injury of** lower back and pelvis

  √x7ᵗʰ **S30.92**   **Unspecified superficial injury of** abdominal wall

  √x7ᵗʰ **S30.93**   **Unspecified superficial injury of** penis   ♂

  √x7ᵗʰ **S30.94**   **Unspecified superficial injury of** scrotum and testes   ♂

  √x7ᵗʰ **S30.95**   **Unspecified superficial injury of** vagina and vulva   ♀

  √x7ᵗʰ **S30.96**   **Unspecified superficial injury of unspecified** external genital organs, male   ♂

  √x7ᵗʰ **S30.97**   **Unspecified superficial injury of unspecified** external genital organs, female   ♀

  √x7ᵗʰ **S30.98**   **Unspecified superficial injury of** anus

√4ᵗʰ **S31**   **Open wound of abdomen, lower back, pelvis and external genitals**

  Code also any associated:

    spinal cord injury (S24.0, S24.1-, S34.0-, S34.1-)

    wound infection

  EXCLUDES 1   traumatic amputation of part of abdomen, lower back and pelvis (S38.2-, S38.3)

  EXCLUDES 2   open wound of hip (S71.00-S71.02)

    open fracture of pelvis (S32.1- – S32.9 with 7th character B)

> The appropriate 7th character is to be added to each code from category S31.
> A   initial encounter
> D   subsequent encounter
> S   sequela

  √5ᵗʰ **S31.0**   **Open wound of** lower back and pelvis

    √6ᵗʰ **S31.00**   **Unspecified open wound of lower back and pelvis**

      √7ᵗʰ **S31.000**   **Unspecified open wound of lower back and pelvis** without penetration into retroperitoneum

        Unspecified open wound of lower back and pelvis NOS

      √7ᵗʰ **S31.001**   **Unspecified open wound of lower back and pelvis** with penetration into retroperitoneum   MCC

    √6ᵗʰ **S31.01**   **Laceration without foreign body of** lower back and pelvis

      √7ᵗʰ **S31.010**   **Laceration without foreign body of lower back and pelvis** without penetration into retroperitoneum

        Laceration without foreign body of lower back and pelvis NOS

      √7ᵗʰ **S31.011**   **Laceration without foreign body of lower back and pelvis** with penetration into retroperitoneum   MCC

✓6ᵗʰ **S31.02** Laceration with foreign body of lower back and pelvis

     ✓7ᵗʰ **S31.020** **Laceration with foreign body of lower back and pelvis** without penetration into retroperitoneum

         Laceration with foreign body of lower back and pelvis NOS

     ✓7ᵗʰ **S31.021** **Laceration with foreign body of lower back and pelvis** with penetration into retroperitoneum   **MCC**

✓6ᵗʰ **S31.03** Puncture wound without foreign body of lower back and pelvis

     ✓7ᵗʰ **S31.030** **Puncture wound without foreign body of lower back and pelvis** without penetration into retroperitoneum

         Puncture wound without foreign body of lower back and pelvis NOS

     ✓7ᵗʰ **S31.031** **Puncture wound without foreign body of lower back and pelvis** with penetration into retroperitoneum   **MCC**

✓6ᵗʰ **S31.04** Puncture wound with foreign body of lower back and pelvis

     ✓7ᵗʰ **S31.040** **Puncture wound with foreign body of lower back and pelvis** without penetration into retroperitoneum

         Puncture wound with foreign body of lower back and pelvis NOS

     ✓7ᵗʰ **S31.041** **Puncture wound with foreign body of lower back and pelvis** with penetration into retroperitoneum   **MCC**

✓6ᵗʰ **S31.05** Open bite of lower back and pelvis

     Bite of lower back and pelvis NOS

         EXCLUDES 1   superficial bite of lower back and pelvis (S30.860, S30.870)

     ✓7ᵗʰ **S31.050** **Open bite of lower back and pelvis** without penetration into retroperitoneum

         Open bite of lower back and pelvis NOS

     ✓7ᵗʰ **S31.051** **Open bite of lower back and pelvis** with penetration into retroperitoneum   **MCC**

✓5ᵗʰ **S31.1** **Open wound of** abdominal wall without penetration into peritoneal cavity

     Open wound of abdominal wall NOS

     EXCLUDES 2   open wound of abdominal wall with penetration into peritoneal cavity (S31.6-)

✓6ᵗʰ **S31.10** Unspecified open wound of abdominal wall without penetration into peritoneal cavity

     ✓7ᵗʰ **S31.100** **Unspecified open wound of abdominal wall, right upper quadrant** without penetration into peritoneal cavity

     ✓7ᵗʰ **S31.101** **Unspecified open wound of abdominal wall, left upper quadrant** without penetration into peritoneal cavity

     ✓7ᵗʰ **S31.102** **Unspecified open wound of abdominal wall, epigastric region** without penetration into peritoneal cavity

     ✓7ᵗʰ **S31.103** **Unspecified open wound of abdominal wall, right lower quadrant** without penetration into peritoneal cavity

     ✓7ᵗʰ **S31.104** **Unspecified open wound of abdominal wall, left lower quadrant** without penetration into peritoneal cavity

     ✓7ᵗʰ **S31.105** **Unspecified open wound of abdominal wall, periumbilic region** without penetration into peritoneal cavity

     ✓7ᵗʰ **S31.109** **Unspecified open wound of abdominal wall, unspecified quadrant** without penetration into peritoneal cavity

         Unspecified open wound of abdominal wall NOS

✓6ᵗʰ **S31.11** Laceration without foreign body of abdominal wall without penetration into peritoneal cavity

     ✓7ᵗʰ **S31.110** **Laceration without foreign body of abdominal wall, right upper quadrant** without penetration into peritoneal cavity

     ✓7ᵗʰ **S31.111** **Laceration without foreign body of abdominal wall, left upper quadrant** without penetration into peritoneal cavity

     ✓7ᵗʰ **S31.112** **Laceration without foreign body of abdominal wall, epigastric region** without penetration into peritoneal cavity

     ✓7ᵗʰ **S31.113** **Laceration without foreign body of abdominal wall, right lower quadrant** without penetration into peritoneal cavity

     ✓7ᵗʰ **S31.114** **Laceration without foreign body of abdominal wall, left lower quadrant** without penetration into peritoneal cavity

     ✓7ᵗʰ **S31.115** **Laceration without foreign body of abdominal wall, periumbilic region** without penetration into peritoneal cavity

     ✓7ᵗʰ **S31.119** **Laceration without foreign body of abdominal wall, unspecified quadrant** without penetration into peritoneal cavity

✓6ᵗʰ **S31.12** Laceration with foreign body of abdominal wall without penetration into peritoneal cavity

     ✓7ᵗʰ **S31.120** **Laceration of abdominal wall with foreign body, right upper quadrant** without penetration into peritoneal cavity

     ✓7ᵗʰ **S31.121** **Laceration of abdominal wall with foreign body, left upper quadrant** without penetration into peritoneal cavity

     ✓7ᵗʰ **S31.122** **Laceration of abdominal wall with foreign body, epigastric region** without penetration into peritoneal cavity

     ✓7ᵗʰ **S31.123** **Laceration of abdominal wall with foreign body, right lower quadrant** without penetration into peritoneal cavity

     ✓7ᵗʰ **S31.124** **Laceration of abdominal wall with foreign body, left lower quadrant** without penetration into peritoneal cavity

     ✓7ᵗʰ **S31.125** **Laceration of abdominal wall with foreign body, periumbilic region** without penetration into peritoneal cavity

     ✓7ᵗʰ **S31.129** **Laceration of abdominal wall with foreign body, unspecified quadrant** without penetration into peritoneal cavity

✓6ᵗʰ **S31.13** Puncture wound of abdominal wall without foreign body without penetration into peritoneal cavity

     ✓7ᵗʰ **S31.130** **Puncture wound of abdominal wall without foreign body, right upper quadrant** without penetration into peritoneal cavity

     ✓7ᵗʰ **S31.131** **Puncture wound of abdominal wall without foreign body, left upper quadrant** without penetration into peritoneal cavity

     ✓7ᵗʰ **S31.132** **Puncture wound of abdominal wall without foreign body, epigastric region** without penetration into peritoneal cavity

     ✓7ᵗʰ **S31.133** **Puncture wound of abdominal wall without foreign body, right lower quadrant** without penetration into peritoneal cavity

     ✓7ᵗʰ **S31.134** **Puncture wound of abdominal wall without foreign body, left lower quadrant** without penetration into peritoneal cavity

     ✓7ᵗʰ **S31.135** **Puncture wound of abdominal wall without foreign body, periumbilic region** without penetration into peritoneal cavity

     ✓7ᵗʰ **S31.139** **Puncture wound of abdominal wall without foreign body, unspecified quadrant** without penetration into peritoneal cavity

✓6ᵗʰ **S31.14** Puncture wound of abdominal wall with foreign body without penetration into peritoneal cavity

     ✓7ᵗʰ **S31.140** **Puncture wound of abdominal wall with foreign body, right upper quadrant** without penetration into peritoneal cavity

     ✓7ᵗʰ **S31.141** **Puncture wound of abdominal wall with foreign body, left upper quadrant** without penetration into peritoneal cavity

     ✓7ᵗʰ **S31.142** **Puncture wound of abdominal wall with foreign body, epigastric region** without penetration into peritoneal cavity

     ✓7ᵗʰ **S31.143** **Puncture wound of abdominal wall with foreign body, right lower quadrant** without penetration into peritoneal cavity

✓ Additional Character Required   ✓x7ᵗʰ Placeholder   Unacceptable PDx   Questionable PDx   Manifestation   Unspecified Dx   **H1**-**H14** HAC   **HCC** CMS-HCC Dx   **HIV** HIV Dx

ICD-10-CM 2021   **993**

√7ᵗʰ **S31.144** Puncture wound of abdominal wall with foreign body, left lower quadrant without penetration into peritoneal cavity

√7ᵗʰ **S31.145** Puncture wound of abdominal wall with foreign body, periumbilic region without penetration into peritoneal cavity

√7ᵗʰ **S31.149** Puncture wound of abdominal wall with foreign body, unspecified quadrant without penetration into peritoneal cavity

√6ᵗʰ **S31.15** Open bite of abdominal wall without penetration into peritoneal cavity

Bite of abdominal wall NOS

EXCLUDES 1   superficial bite of abdominal wall (S30.871)

√7ᵗʰ **S31.150** Open bite of abdominal wall, right upper quadrant without penetration into peritoneal cavity

√7ᵗʰ **S31.151** Open bite of abdominal wall, left upper quadrant without penetration into peritoneal cavity

√7ᵗʰ **S31.152** Open bite of abdominal wall, epigastric region without penetration into peritoneal cavity

√7ᵗʰ **S31.153** Open bite of abdominal wall, right lower quadrant without penetration into peritoneal cavity

√7ᵗʰ **S31.154** Open bite of abdominal wall, left lower quadrant without penetration into peritoneal cavity

√7ᵗʰ **S31.155** Open bite of abdominal wall, periumbilic region without penetration into peritoneal cavity

√7ᵗʰ **S31.159** Open bite of abdominal wall, unspecified quadrant without penetration into peritoneal cavity

√5ᵗʰ **S31.2** Open wound of penis

√x7ᵗʰ **S31.20** Unspecified open wound of penis   ♂

√x7ᵗʰ **S31.21** Laceration without foreign body of penis   ♂

√x7ᵗʰ **S31.22** Laceration with foreign body of penis   ♂

√x7ᵗʰ **S31.23** Puncture wound without foreign body of penis   ♂

√x7ᵗʰ **S31.24** Puncture wound with foreign body of penis   ♂

√x7ᵗʰ **S31.25** Open bite of penis   ♂

Bite of penis NOS

EXCLUDES 1   superficial bite of penis (S30.862, S30.872)

√5ᵗʰ **S31.3** Open wound of scrotum and testes

√x7ᵗʰ **S31.30** Unspecified open wound of scrotum and testes   ♂

√x7ᵗʰ **S31.31** Laceration without foreign body of scrotum and testes   ♂

√x7ᵗʰ **S31.32** Laceration with foreign body of scrotum and testes   ♂

√x7ᵗʰ **S31.33** Puncture wound without foreign body of scrotum and testes   ♂

√x7ᵗʰ **S31.34** Puncture wound with foreign body of scrotum and testes   ♂

√x7ᵗʰ **S31.35** Open bite of scrotum and testes   ♂

Bite of scrotum and testes NOS

EXCLUDES 1   superficial bite of scrotum and testes (S30.863, S30.873)

√5ᵗʰ **S31.4** Open wound of vagina and vulva

EXCLUDES 1   injury to vagina and vulva during delivery (O70.-, O71.4)

√x7ᵗʰ **S31.40** Unspecified open wound of vagina and vulva   ♀

√x7ᵗʰ **S31.41** Laceration without foreign body of vagina and vulva   ♀

√x7ᵗʰ **S31.42** Laceration with foreign body of vagina and vulva   ♀

√x7ᵗʰ **S31.43** Puncture wound without foreign body of vagina and vulva   ♀

√x7ᵗʰ **S31.44** Puncture wound with foreign body of vagina and vulva   ♀

√x7ᵗʰ **S31.45** Open bite of vagina and vulva   ♀

Bite of vagina and vulva NOS

EXCLUDES 1   superficial bite of vagina and vulva (S30.864, S30.874)

√5ᵗʰ **S31.5** Open wound of unspecified external genital organs

EXCLUDES 1   traumatic amputation of external genital organs (S38.21, S38.22)

√6ᵗʰ **S31.50** Unspecified open wound of unspecified external genital organs

√7ᵗʰ **S31.501** Unspecified open wound of unspecified external genital organs, male   ♂

√7ᵗʰ **S31.502** Unspecified open wound of unspecified external genital organs, female   ♀

√6ᵗʰ **S31.51** Laceration without foreign body of unspecified external genital organs

√7ᵗʰ **S31.511** Laceration without foreign body of unspecified external genital organs, male   ♂

√7ᵗʰ **S31.512** Laceration without foreign body of unspecified external genital organs, female   ♀

√6ᵗʰ **S31.52** Laceration with foreign body of unspecified external genital organs

√7ᵗʰ **S31.521** Laceration with foreign body of unspecified external genital organs, male   ♂

√7ᵗʰ **S31.522** Laceration with foreign body of unspecified external genital organs, female   ♀

√6ᵗʰ **S31.53** Puncture wound without foreign body of unspecified external genital organs

√7ᵗʰ **S31.531** Puncture wound without foreign body of unspecified external genital organs, male   ♂

√7ᵗʰ **S31.532** Puncture wound without foreign body of unspecified external genital organs, female   ♀

√6ᵗʰ **S31.54** Puncture wound with foreign body of unspecified external genital organs

√7ᵗʰ **S31.541** Puncture wound with foreign body of unspecified external genital organs, male   ♂

√7ᵗʰ **S31.542** Puncture wound with foreign body of unspecified external genital organs, female   ♀

√6ᵗʰ **S31.55** Open bite of unspecified external genital organs

Bite of unspecified external genital organs NOS

EXCLUDES 1   superficial bite of unspecified external genital organs (S30.865, S30.866, S30.875, S30.876)

√7ᵗʰ **S31.551** Open bite of unspecified external genital organs, male   ♂

√7ᵗʰ **S31.552** Open bite of unspecified external genital organs, female   ♀

√5ᵗʰ **S31.6** Open wound of abdominal wall with penetration into peritoneal cavity

√6ᵗʰ **S31.60** Unspecified open wound of abdominal wall with penetration into peritoneal cavity

√7ᵗʰ **S31.600** Unspecified open wound of abdominal wall, right upper quadrant with penetration into peritoneal cavity   MCC

√7ᵗʰ **S31.601** Unspecified open wound of abdominal wall, left upper quadrant with penetration into peritoneal cavity   MCC

√7ᵗʰ **S31.602** Unspecified open wound of abdominal wall, epigastric region with penetration into peritoneal cavity   MCC

√7ᵗʰ **S31.603** Unspecified open wound of abdominal wall, right lower quadrant with penetration into peritoneal cavity   MCC

√7ᵗʰ **S31.604** Unspecified open wound of abdominal wall, left lower quadrant with penetration into peritoneal cavity   MCC

√7ᵗʰ **S31.605** Unspecified open wound of abdominal wall, periumbilic region with penetration into peritoneal cavity   MCC

√7ᵗʰ **S31.609** Unspecified open wound of abdominal wall, unspecified quadrant with penetration into peritoneal cavity   MCC

√6ᵗʰ **S31.61** Laceration without foreign body of abdominal wall with penetration into peritoneal cavity

√7ᵗʰ **S31.610** Laceration without foreign body of abdominal wall, right upper quadrant with penetration into peritoneal cavity   MCC

N Newborn: 0   P Pediatric: 0-17   M Maternity: 9-64   A Adult: 15-124   MCC Major Complication/Comorbidity   CC Complication/Comorbidity   SW Severe Wound Dx

994   ICD-10-CM 2021

√7ᵗʰ **S31.611** **Laceration without foreign body of abdominal wall, left upper quadrant with penetration into peritoneal cavity** `MCC`

√7ᵗʰ **S31.612** **Laceration without foreign body of abdominal wall, epigastric region with penetration into peritoneal cavity** `MCC`

√7ᵗʰ **S31.613** **Laceration without foreign body of abdominal wall, right lower quadrant with penetration into peritoneal cavity** `MCC`

√7ᵗʰ **S31.614** **Laceration without foreign body of abdominal wall, left lower quadrant with penetration into peritoneal cavity** `MCC`

√7ᵗʰ **S31.615** **Laceration without foreign body of abdominal wall, periumbilic region with penetration into peritoneal cavity** `MCC`

√7ᵗʰ **S31.619** **Laceration without foreign body of abdominal wall, unspecified quadrant with penetration into peritoneal cavity** `MCC`

√6ᵗʰ **S31.62** Laceration with foreign body of abdominal wall with penetration into peritoneal cavity

√7ᵗʰ **S31.620** **Laceration with foreign body of abdominal wall, right upper quadrant with penetration into peritoneal cavity** `MCC`

√7ᵗʰ **S31.621** **Laceration with foreign body of abdominal wall, left upper quadrant with penetration into peritoneal cavity** `MCC`

√7ᵗʰ **S31.622** **Laceration with foreign body of abdominal wall, epigastric region with penetration into peritoneal cavity** `MCC`

√7ᵗʰ **S31.623** **Laceration with foreign body of abdominal wall, right lower quadrant with penetration into peritoneal cavity** `MCC`

√7ᵗʰ **S31.624** **Laceration with foreign body of abdominal wall, left lower quadrant with penetration into peritoneal cavity** `MCC`

√7ᵗʰ **S31.625** **Laceration with foreign body of abdominal wall, periumbilic region with penetration into peritoneal cavity** `MCC`

√7ᵗʰ **S31.629** **Laceration with foreign body of abdominal wall, unspecified quadrant with penetration into peritoneal cavity** `MCC`

√6ᵗʰ **S31.63** Puncture wound without foreign body of abdominal wall with penetration into peritoneal cavity

√7ᵗʰ **S31.630** **Puncture wound without foreign body of abdominal wall, right upper quadrant with penetration into peritoneal cavity** `MCC`

√7ᵗʰ **S31.631** **Puncture wound without foreign body of abdominal wall, left upper quadrant with penetration into peritoneal cavity** `MCC`

√7ᵗʰ **S31.632** **Puncture wound without foreign body of abdominal wall, epigastric region with penetration into peritoneal cavity** `MCC`

√7ᵗʰ **S31.633** **Puncture wound without foreign body of abdominal wall, right lower quadrant with penetration into peritoneal cavity** `MCC`

√7ᵗʰ **S31.634** **Puncture wound without foreign body of abdominal wall, left lower quadrant with penetration into peritoneal cavity** `MCC`

√7ᵗʰ **S31.635** **Puncture wound without foreign body of abdominal wall, periumbilic region with penetration into peritoneal cavity** `MCC`

√7ᵗʰ **S31.639** **Puncture wound without foreign body of abdominal wall, unspecified quadrant with penetration into peritoneal cavity** `MCC`

√6ᵗʰ **S31.64** Puncture wound with foreign body of abdominal wall with penetration into peritoneal cavity

√7ᵗʰ **S31.640** **Puncture wound with foreign body of abdominal wall, right upper quadrant with penetration into peritoneal cavity** `MCC`

√7ᵗʰ **S31.641** **Puncture wound with foreign body of abdominal wall, left upper quadrant with penetration into peritoneal cavity** `MCC`

√7ᵗʰ **S31.642** **Puncture wound with foreign body of abdominal wall, epigastric region with penetration into peritoneal cavity** `MCC`

√7ᵗʰ **S31.643** **Puncture wound with foreign body of abdominal wall, right lower quadrant with penetration into peritoneal cavity** `MCC`

√7ᵗʰ **S31.644** **Puncture wound with foreign body of abdominal wall, left lower quadrant with penetration into peritoneal cavity** `MCC`

√7ᵗʰ **S31.645** **Puncture wound with foreign body of abdominal wall, periumbilic region with penetration into peritoneal cavity** `MCC`

√7ᵗʰ **S31.649** **Puncture wound with foreign body of abdominal wall, unspecified quadrant with penetration into peritoneal cavity** `MCC`

√6ᵗʰ **S31.65** Open bite of abdominal wall with penetration into peritoneal cavity

    EXCLUDES 1   superficial bite of abdominal wall (S30.861, S30.871)

√7ᵗʰ **S31.650** **Open bite of abdominal wall, right upper quadrant with penetration into peritoneal cavity** `MCC`

√7ᵗʰ **S31.651** **Open bite of abdominal wall, left upper quadrant with penetration into peritoneal cavity** `MCC`

√7ᵗʰ **S31.652** **Open bite of abdominal wall, epigastric region with penetration into peritoneal cavity** `MCC`

√7ᵗʰ **S31.653** **Open bite of abdominal wall, right lower quadrant with penetration into peritoneal cavity** `MCC`

√7ᵗʰ **S31.654** **Open bite of abdominal wall, left lower quadrant with penetration into peritoneal cavity** `MCC`

√7ᵗʰ **S31.655** **Open bite of abdominal wall, periumbilic region with penetration into peritoneal cavity** `MCC`

√7ᵗʰ **S31.659** **Open bite of abdominal wall, unspecified quadrant with penetration into peritoneal cavity** `MCC`

√5ᵗʰ **S31.8** **Open wound of other parts of abdomen, lower back and pelvis**

√6ᵗʰ **S31.80** **Open wound of unspecified buttock**

√7ᵗʰ **S31.801** Laceration without foreign body of unspecified buttock

√7ᵗʰ **S31.802** Laceration with foreign body of unspecified buttock

√7ᵗʰ **S31.803** Puncture wound without foreign body of unspecified buttock

√7ᵗʰ **S31.804** Puncture wound with foreign body of unspecified buttock

√7ᵗʰ **S31.805** Open bite of unspecified buttock

    Bite of buttock NOS

    EXCLUDES 1   superficial bite of buttock (S30.870)

√7ᵗʰ **S31.809** Unspecified open wound of unspecified buttock

√6ᵗʰ **S31.81** **Open wound of right buttock**

√7ᵗʰ **S31.811** Laceration without foreign body of right buttock

√7ᵗʰ **S31.812** Laceration with foreign body of right buttock

√7ᵗʰ **S31.813** Puncture wound without foreign body of right buttock

√7ᵗʰ **S31.814** Puncture wound with foreign body of right buttock

√7ᵗʰ **S31.815** Open bite of right buttock

    Bite of right buttock NOS

    EXCLUDES 1   superficial bite of buttock (S30.870)

√7ᵗʰ **S31.819** Unspecified open wound of right buttock

√6ᵗʰ **S31.82** **Open wound of left buttock**

√7ᵗʰ **S31.821** Laceration without foreign body of left buttock

√7ᵗʰ **S31.822** Laceration with foreign body of left buttock

√7ᵗʰ **S31.823** Puncture wound without foreign body of left buttock

√7ᵗʰ **S31.824** Puncture wound with foreign body of left buttock

---

☑ Additional Character Required   √x7ᵗʰ Placeholder   Unacceptable PDx   Questionable PDx   Manifestation   Unspecified Dx   `H1`-`H14` HAC   `HCC` CMS-HCC Dx   `HIV` HIV Dx

√7ᵗʰ **S31.825** Open bite of left buttock
Bite of left buttock NOS
EXCLUDES 1 *superficial bite of buttock (S30.870)*

√7ᵗʰ **S31.829** Unspecified open wound of left buttock

√6ᵗʰ **S31.83** Open wound of anus

√7ᵗʰ **S31.831** Laceration without foreign body of anus

√7ᵗʰ **S31.832** Laceration with foreign body of anus

√7ᵗʰ **S31.833** Puncture wound without foreign body of anus

√7ᵗʰ **S31.834** Puncture wound with foreign body of anus

√7ᵗʰ **S31.835** Open bite of anus
Bite of anus NOS
EXCLUDES 1 *superficial bite of anus (S30.877)*

√7ᵗʰ **S31.839** Unspecified open wound of anus

√4ᵗʰ **S32** Fracture of lumbar spine and pelvis

NOTE A fracture not indicated as displaced or nondisplaced should be coded to displaced.

A fracture not indicated as opened or closed should be coded to closed.

INCLUDES fracture of lumbosacral neural arch
fracture of lumbosacral spinous process
fracture of lumbosacral transverse process
fracture of lumbosacral vertebra
fracture of lumbosacral vertebral arch

Code first any associated spinal cord and spinal nerve injury (S34.-)

EXCLUDES 1 *transection of abdomen (S38.3)*

EXCLUDES 2 *fracture of hip NOS (S72.0-)*

AHA: 2018,2Q,12; 2015,3Q,37-39; 2012,4Q,93

The appropriate 7th character is to be added to each code from category S32.
A initial encounter for closed fracture
B initial encounter for open fracture
D subsequent encounter for fracture with routine healing
G subsequent encounter for fracture with delayed healing
K subsequent encounter for fracture with nonunion
S sequela

√5ᵗʰ **S32.0** Fracture of lumbar vertebra
Fracture of lumbar spine NOS

√6ᵗʰ **S32.00** Fracture of unspecified lumbar vertebra

2,3,6 √7ᵗʰ **S32.000** Wedge compression fracture of unspecified lumbar vertebra `MCC` `CC` `H5` `HCC`

2,3,6 √7ᵗʰ **S32.001** Stable burst fracture of unspecified lumbar vertebra `MCC` `CC` `H5` `HCC`

2,3,6 √7ᵗʰ **S32.002** Unstable burst fracture of unspecified lumbar vertebra `MCC` `CC` `H5` `HCC`

2,3,6 √7ᵗʰ **S32.008** Other fracture of unspecified lumbar vertebra `MCC` `CC` `H5` `HCC`

2,3,6 √7ᵗʰ **S32.009** Unspecified fracture of unspecified lumbar vertebra `MCC` `CC` `H5` `HCC`

√6ᵗʰ **S32.01** Fracture of first lumbar vertebra

2,3,6 √7ᵗʰ **S32.010** Wedge compression fracture of first lumbar vertebra `MCC` `CC` `H5` `HCC`

2,3,6 √7ᵗʰ **S32.011** Stable burst fracture of first lumbar vertebra `MCC` `CC` `H5` `HCC`

2,3,6 √7ᵗʰ **S32.012** Unstable burst fracture of first lumbar vertebra `MCC` `CC` `H5` `HCC`

2,3,6 √7ᵗʰ **S32.018** Other fracture of first lumbar vertebra `MCC` `CC` `H5` `HCC`

2,3,6 √7ᵗʰ **S32.019** Unspecified fracture of first lumbar vertebra `MCC` `CC` `H5` `HCC`

√6ᵗʰ **S32.02** Fracture of second lumbar vertebra

2,3,6 √7ᵗʰ **S32.020** Wedge compression fracture of second lumbar vertebra `MCC` `CC` `H5` `HCC`

2,3,6 √7ᵗʰ **S32.021** Stable burst fracture of second lumbar vertebra `MCC` `CC` `H5` `HCC`

2,3,6 √7ᵗʰ **S32.022** Unstable burst fracture of second lumbar vertebra `MCC` `CC` `H5` `HCC`

2,3,6 √7ᵗʰ **S32.028** Other fracture of second lumbar vertebra `MCC` `CC` `H5` `HCC`

2,3,6 √7ᵗʰ **S32.029** Unspecified fracture of second lumbar vertebra `MCC` `CC` `H5` `HCC`

√6ᵗʰ **S32.03** Fracture of third lumbar vertebra

2,3,6 √7ᵗʰ **S32.030** Wedge compression fracture of third lumbar vertebra `MCC` `CC` `H5` `HCC`

2,3,6 √7ᵗʰ **S32.031** Stable burst fracture of third lumbar vertebra `MCC` `CC` `H5` `HCC`

2,3,6 √7ᵗʰ **S32.032** Unstable burst fracture of third lumbar vertebra `MCC` `CC` `H5` `HCC`

2,3,6 √7ᵗʰ **S32.038** Other fracture of third lumbar vertebra `MCC` `CC` `H5` `HCC`

2,3,6 √7ᵗʰ **S32.039** Unspecified fracture of third lumbar vertebra `MCC` `CC` `H5` `HCC`

√6ᵗʰ **S32.04** Fracture of fourth lumbar vertebra

2,3,6 √7ᵗʰ **S32.040** Wedge compression fracture of fourth lumbar vertebra `MCC` `CC` `H5` `HCC`

2,3,6 √7ᵗʰ **S32.041** Stable burst fracture of fourth lumbar vertebra `MCC` `CC` `H5` `HCC`

2,3,6 √7ᵗʰ **S32.042** Unstable burst fracture of fourth lumbar vertebra `MCC` `CC` `H5` `HCC`

2,3,6 √7ᵗʰ **S32.048** Other fracture of fourth lumbar vertebra `MCC` `CC` `H5` `HCC`

2,3,6 √7ᵗʰ **S32.049** Unspecified fracture of fourth lumbar vertebra `MCC` `CC` `H5` `HCC`

√6ᵗʰ **S32.05** Fracture of fifth lumbar vertebra

2,3,6 √7ᵗʰ **S32.050** Wedge compression fracture of fifth lumbar vertebra `MCC` `CC` `H5` `HCC`

2,3,6 √7ᵗʰ **S32.051** Stable burst fracture of fifth lumbar vertebra `MCC` `CC` `H5` `HCC`

2,3,6 √7ᵗʰ **S32.052** Unstable burst fracture of fifth lumbar vertebra `MCC` `CC` `H5` `HCC`

2,3,6 √7ᵗʰ **S32.058** Other fracture of fifth lumbar vertebra `MCC` `CC` `H5` `HCC`

2,3,6 √7ᵗʰ **S32.059** Unspecified fracture of fifth lumbar vertebra `MCC` `CC` `H5` `HCC`

√5ᵗʰ **S32.1** Fracture of sacrum

NOTE For vertical fractures, code to most medial fracture extension

Use two codes if both a vertical and transverse fracture are present

Code also any associated fracture of pelvic ring (S32.8-)

2,3,6 √x7ᵗʰ **S32.10** Unspecified fracture of sacrum `MCC` `CC` `H5` `HCC`

√6ᵗʰ **S32.11** Zone I fracture of sacrum
Vertical sacral ala fracture of sacrum

Vertical Sacral Fracture Zones

Zones: ① ② ③

2,3,6 √7ᵗʰ **S32.110** Nondisplaced Zone I fracture of sacrum `MCC` `CC` `H5` `HCC`

2,3,6 √7ᵗʰ **S32.111** Minimally displaced Zone I fracture of sacrum `MCC` `CC` `H5` `HCC`

2,3,6 √7ᵗʰ **S32.112** Severely displaced Zone I fracture of sacrum `MCC` `CC` `H5` `HCC`

2,3,6 √7ᵗʰ **S32.119** Unspecified Zone I fracture of sacrum `MCC` `CC` `H5` `HCC`

√6ᵗʰ **S32.12** Zone II fracture of sacrum
Vertical foraminal region fracture of sacrum

2,3,6 √7ᵗʰ **S32.120** Nondisplaced Zone II fracture of sacrum `MCC` `CC` `H5` `HCC`

2,3,6 √7ᵗʰ **S32.121** Minimally displaced Zone II fracture of sacrum `MCC` `CC` `H5` `HCC`

2,3,6 √7ᵗʰ **S32.122** Severely displaced Zone II fracture of sacrum `MCC` `CC` `H5` `HCC`

N Newborn: 0   **P** Pediatric: 0-17   **M** Maternity: 9-64   **A** Adult: 15-124   `MCC` Major Complication/Comorbidity   `CC` Complication/Comorbidity   `SW` Severe Wound Dx

996   ICD-10-CM 2021

2,3,6 ✓7ᵗʰ **S32.129** Unspecified Zone II fracture of sacrum   `MCC` `CC` `H5` `HCC`

✓6ᵗʰ **S32.13** Zone III fracture of sacrum

Vertical fracture into spinal canal region of sacrum

2,3,6 ✓7ᵗʰ **S32.130** Nondisplaced Zone III fracture of sacrum   `MCC` `CC` `H5` `HCC`

2,3,6 ✓7ᵗʰ **S32.131** Minimally displaced Zone III fracture of sacrum   `MCC` `CC` `H5` `HCC`

2,3,6 ✓7ᵗʰ **S32.132** Severely displaced Zone III fracture of sacrum   `MCC` `CC` `H5` `HCC`

2,3,6 ✓7ᵗʰ **S32.139** Unspecified Zone III fracture of sacrum   `MCC` `CC` `H5` `HCC`

Transverse Sacral Fracture Types

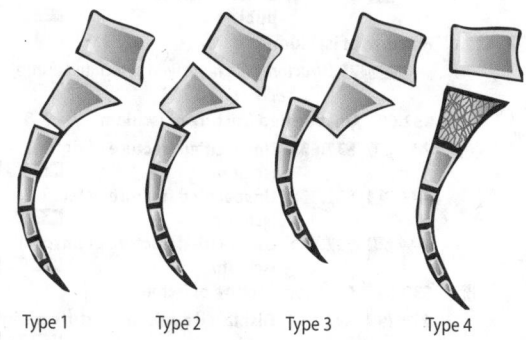

Type 1   Type 2   Type 3   Type 4

2,3,6 ✓x7ᵗʰ **S32.14** Type 1 fracture of sacrum   `MCC` `CC` `H5` `HCC`

Transverse flexion fracture of sacrum without displacement

2,3,6 ✓x7ᵗʰ **S32.15** Type 2 fracture of sacrum   `MCC` `CC` `H5` `HCC`

Transverse flexion fracture of sacrum with posterior displacement

2,3,6 ✓x7ᵗʰ **S32.16** Type 3 fracture of sacrum   `MCC` `CC` `H5` `HCC`

Transverse extension fracture of sacrum with anterior displacement

2,3,6 ✓x7ᵗʰ **S32.17** Type 4 fracture of sacrum   `MCC` `CC` `H5` `HCC`

Transverse segmental comminution of upper sacrum

2,3,6 ✓x7ᵗʰ **S32.19** Other fracture of sacrum   `MCC` `CC` `H5` `HCC`

2,3,6 ✓x7ᵗʰ **S32.2** Fracture of coccyx   `MCC` `CC` `H5` `HCC`

✓5ᵗʰ **S32.3** Fracture of ilium

EXCLUDES 1   *fracture of ilium with associated disruption of pelvic ring (S32.8-)*

✓6ᵗʰ **S32.30** Unspecified fracture of ilium

2,3,6 ✓7ᵗʰ **S32.301** Unspecified fracture of right ilium   `MCC` `CC` `H5` `HCC`

2,3,6 ✓7ᵗʰ **S32.302** Unspecified fracture of left ilium   `MCC` `CC` `H5` `HCC`

2,3,6 ✓7ᵗʰ **S32.309** Unspecified fracture of unspecified ilium   `MCC` `CC` `H5` `HCC`

✓6ᵗʰ **S32.31** Avulsion fracture of ilium

2,3,6 ✓7ᵗʰ **S32.311** Displaced avulsion fracture of right ilium   `MCC` `CC` `H5` `HCC`

2,3,6 ✓7ᵗʰ **S32.312** Displaced avulsion fracture of left ilium   `MCC` `CC` `H5` `HCC`

2,3,6 ✓7ᵗʰ **S32.313** Displaced avulsion fracture of unspecified ilium   `MCC` `CC` `H5` `HCC`

2,3,6 ✓7ᵗʰ **S32.314** Nondisplaced avulsion fracture of right ilium   `MCC` `CC` `H5` `HCC`

2,3,6 ✓7ᵗʰ **S32.315** Nondisplaced avulsion fracture of left ilium   `MCC` `CC` `H5` `HCC`

2,3,6 ✓7ᵗʰ **S32.316** Nondisplaced avulsion fracture of unspecified ilium   `MCC` `CC` `H5` `HCC`

✓6ᵗʰ **S32.39** Other fracture of ilium

2,3,6 ✓7ᵗʰ **S32.391** Other fracture of right ilium   `MCC` `CC` `H5` `HCC`

2,3,6 ✓7ᵗʰ **S32.392** Other fracture of left ilium   `MCC` `CC` `H5` `HCC`

2,3,6 ✓7ᵗʰ **S32.399** Other fracture of unspecified ilium   `MCC` `CC` `H5` `HCC`

✓5ᵗʰ **S32.4** Fracture of acetabulum

Code also any associated fracture of pelvic ring (S32.8-)

AHA: 2016,3Q,16

✓6ᵗʰ **S32.40** Unspecified fracture of acetabulum

4,6 ✓7ᵗʰ **S32.401** Unspecified fracture of right acetabulum   `MCC` `CC` `H5` `HCC`

4,6 ✓7ᵗʰ **S32.402** Unspecified fracture of left acetabulum   `MCC` `CC` `H5` `HCC`

4,6 ✓7ᵗʰ **S32.409** Unspecified fracture of unspecified acetabulum   `MCC` `CC` `H5` `HCC`

✓6ᵗʰ **S32.41** Fracture of anterior wall of acetabulum

4,6 ✓7ᵗʰ **S32.411** Displaced fracture of anterior wall of right acetabulum   `MCC` `CC` `H5` `HCC`

4,6 ✓7ᵗʰ **S32.412** Displaced fracture of anterior wall of left acetabulum   `MCC` `CC` `H5` `HCC`

4,6 ✓7ᵗʰ **S32.413** Displaced fracture of anterior wall of unspecified acetabulum   `MCC` `CC` `H5` `HCC`

4,6 ✓7ᵗʰ **S32.414** Nondisplaced fracture of anterior wall of right acetabulum   `MCC` `CC` `H5` `HCC`

4,6 ✓7ᵗʰ **S32.415** Nondisplaced fracture of anterior wall of left acetabulum   `MCC` `CC` `H5` `HCC`

4,6 ✓7ᵗʰ **S32.416** Nondisplaced fracture of anterior wall of unspecified acetabulum   `MCC` `CC` `H5` `HCC`

✓6ᵗʰ **S32.42** Fracture of posterior wall of acetabulum

4,6 ✓7ᵗʰ **S32.421** Displaced fracture of posterior wall of right acetabulum   `MCC` `CC` `H5` `HCC`

4,6 ✓7ᵗʰ **S32.422** Displaced fracture of posterior wall of left acetabulum   `MCC` `CC` `H5` `HCC`

4,6 ✓7ᵗʰ **S32.423** Displaced fracture of posterior wall of unspecified acetabulum   `MCC` `CC` `H5` `HCC`

4,6 ✓7ᵗʰ **S32.424** Nondisplaced fracture of posterior wall of right acetabulum   `MCC` `CC` `H5` `HCC`

4,6 ✓7ᵗʰ **S32.425** Nondisplaced fracture of posterior wall of left acetabulum   `MCC` `CC` `H5` `HCC`

4,6 ✓7ᵗʰ **S32.426** Nondisplaced fracture of posterior wall of unspecified acetabulum   `MCC` `CC` `H5` `HCC`

✓6ᵗʰ **S32.43** Fracture of anterior column [iliopubic] of acetabulum

4,6 ✓7ᵗʰ **S32.431** Displaced fracture of anterior column [iliopubic] of right acetabulum   `MCC` `CC` `H5` `HCC`

4,6 ✓7ᵗʰ **S32.432** Displaced fracture of anterior column [iliopubic] of left acetabulum   `MCC` `CC` `H5` `HCC`

4,6 ✓7ᵗʰ **S32.433** Displaced fracture of anterior column [iliopubic] of unspecified acetabulum   `MCC` `CC` `H5` `HCC`

4,6 ✓7ᵗʰ **S32.434** Nondisplaced fracture of anterior column [iliopubic] of right acetabulum   `MCC` `CC` `H5` `HCC`

4,6 ✓7ᵗʰ **S32.435** Nondisplaced fracture of anterior column [iliopubic] of left acetabulum   `MCC` `CC` `H5` `HCC`

4,6 ✓7ᵗʰ **S32.436** Nondisplaced fracture of anterior column [iliopubic] of unspecified acetabulum   `MCC` `CC` `H5` `HCC`

✓6ᵗʰ **S32.44** Fracture of posterior column [ilioischial] of acetabulum

4,6 ✓7ᵗʰ **S32.441** Displaced fracture of posterior column [ilioischial] of right acetabulum   `MCC` `CC` `H5` `HCC`

4,6 ✓7ᵗʰ **S32.442** Displaced fracture of posterior column [ilioischial] of left acetabulum   `MCC` `CC` `H5` `HCC`

4,6 ✓7ᵗʰ **S32.443** Displaced fracture of posterior column [ilioischial] of unspecified acetabulum   `MCC` `CC` `H5` `HCC`

4,6 ✓7ᵗʰ **S32.444** Nondisplaced fracture of posterior column [ilioischial] of right acetabulum   `MCC` `CC` `H5` `HCC`

4,6 ✓7ᵗʰ **S32.445** Nondisplaced fracture of posterior column [ilioischial] of left acetabulum   `MCC` `CC` `H5` `HCC`

4,6 ✓7ᵗʰ **S32.446** Nondisplaced fracture of posterior column [ilioischial] of unspecified acetabulum   `MCC` `CC` `H5` `HCC`

√6ᵗʰ **S32.45** Transverse fracture of acetabulum

    4,6 √7ᵗʰ **S32.451** Displaced transverse fracture of **right** acetabulum `MCC` `CC` `H5` `HCC`

    4,6 √7ᵗʰ **S32.452** Displaced transverse fracture of **left** acetabulum `MCC` `CC` `H5` `HCC`

    4,6 √7ᵗʰ **S32.453** Displaced transverse fracture of unspecified acetabulum `MCC` `CC` `H5` `HCC`

    4,6 √7ᵗʰ **S32.454** Nondisplaced transverse fracture of **right** acetabulum `MCC` `CC` `H5` `HCC`

    4,6 √7ᵗʰ **S32.455** Nondisplaced transverse fracture of **left** acetabulum `MCC` `CC` `H5` `HCC`

    4,6 √7ᵗʰ **S32.456** Nondisplaced transverse fracture of unspecified acetabulum `MCC` `CC` `H5` `HCC`

√6ᵗʰ **S32.46** Associated transverse-posterior fracture of acetabulum

    4,6 √7ᵗʰ **S32.461** Displaced associated transverse-posterior fracture of **right** acetabulum `MCC` `CC` `H5` `HCC`

    4,6 √7ᵗʰ **S32.462** Displaced associated transverse-posterior fracture of **left** acetabulum `MCC` `CC` `H5` `HCC`

    4,6 √7ᵗʰ **S32.463** Displaced associated transverse-posterior fracture of unspecified acetabulum `MCC` `CC` `H5` `HCC`

    4,6 √7ᵗʰ **S32.464** Nondisplaced associated transverse-posterior fracture of **right** acetabulum `MCC` `CC` `H5` `HCC`

    4,6 √7ᵗʰ **S32.465** Nondisplaced associated transverse-posterior fracture of **left** acetabulum `MCC` `CC` `H5` `HCC`

    4,6 √7ᵗʰ **S32.466** Nondisplaced associated transverse-posterior fracture of unspecified acetabulum `MCC` `CC` `H5` `HCC`

√6ᵗʰ **S32.47** Fracture of medial wall of acetabulum

    4,6 √7ᵗʰ **S32.471** Displaced fracture of medial wall of **right** acetabulum `MCC` `CC` `H5` `HCC`

    4,6 √7ᵗʰ **S32.472** Displaced fracture of medial wall of **left** acetabulum `MCC` `CC` `H5` `HCC`

    4,6 √7ᵗʰ **S32.473** Displaced fracture of medial wall of unspecified acetabulum `MCC` `CC` `H5` `HCC`

    4,6 √7ᵗʰ **S32.474** Nondisplaced fracture of medial wall of **right** acetabulum `MCC` `CC` `H5` `HCC`

    4,6 √7ᵗʰ **S32.475** Nondisplaced fracture of medial wall of **left** acetabulum `MCC` `CC` `H5` `HCC`

    4,6 √7ᵗʰ **S32.476** Nondisplaced fracture of medial wall of unspecified acetabulum `MCC` `CC` `H5` `HCC`

√6ᵗʰ **S32.48** Dome fracture of acetabulum

    4,6 √7ᵗʰ **S32.481** Displaced dome fracture of **right** acetabulum `MCC` `CC` `H5` `HCC`

    4,6 √7ᵗʰ **S32.482** Displaced dome fracture of **left** acetabulum `MCC` `CC` `H5` `HCC`

    4,6 √7ᵗʰ **S32.483** Displaced dome fracture of unspecified acetabulum `MCC` `CC` `H5` `HCC`

    4,6 √7ᵗʰ **S32.484** Nondisplaced dome fracture of **right** acetabulum `MCC` `CC` `H5` `HCC`

    4,6 √7ᵗʰ **S32.485** Nondisplaced dome fracture of **left** acetabulum `MCC` `CC` `H5` `HCC`

    4,6 √7ᵗʰ **S32.486** Nondisplaced dome fracture of unspecified acetabulum `MCC` `CC` `H5` `HCC`

√6ᵗʰ **S32.49** Other specified fracture of acetabulum

    4,6 √7ᵗʰ **S32.491** Other specified fracture of **right** acetabulum `MCC` `CC` `H5` `HCC`

    4,6 √7ᵗʰ **S32.492** Other specified fracture of **left** acetabulum `MCC` `CC` `H5` `HCC`

    4,6 √7ᵗʰ **S32.499** Other specified fracture of unspecified acetabulum `MCC` `CC` `H5` `HCC`

√5ᵗʰ **S32.5** Fracture of pubis

> *EXCLUDES 1*   fracture of pubis with associated disruption of pelvic ring (S32.8-)

√6ᵗʰ **S32.50** Unspecified fracture of pubis

    2,3,6 √7ᵗʰ **S32.501** Unspecified fracture of **right** pubis `MCC` `CC` `H5` `HCC`

    2,3,6 √7ᵗʰ **S32.502** Unspecified fracture of **left** pubis `MCC` `CC` `H5` `HCC`

    2,3,6 √7ᵗʰ **S32.509** Unspecified fracture of unspecified pubis `MCC` `CC` `H5` `HCC`

√6ᵗʰ **S32.51** Fracture of superior rim of pubis

    2,3,6 √7ᵗʰ **S32.511** Fracture of superior rim of **right** pubis `MCC` `CC` `H5` `HCC`

    2,3,6 √7ᵗʰ **S32.512** Fracture of superior rim of **left** pubis `MCC` `CC` `H5` `HCC`

    2,3,6 √7ᵗʰ **S32.519** Fracture of superior rim of unspecified pubis `MCC` `CC` `H5` `HCC`

√6ᵗʰ **S32.59** Other specified fracture of pubis

    2,3,6 √7ᵗʰ **S32.591** Other specified fracture of **right** pubis `MCC` `CC` `H5` `HCC`

    2,3,6 √7ᵗʰ **S32.592** Other specified fracture of **left** pubis `MCC` `CC` `H5` `HCC`

    2,3,6 √7ᵗʰ **S32.599** Other specified fracture of unspecified pubis `MCC` `CC` `H5` `HCC`

√5ᵗʰ **S32.6** Fracture of ischium

> *EXCLUDES 1*   fracture of ischium with associated disruption of pelvic ring (S32.8-)

√6ᵗʰ **S32.60** Unspecified fracture of ischium

    2,3,6 √7ᵗʰ **S32.601** Unspecified fracture of **right** ischium `MCC` `CC` `H5` `HCC`

    2,3,6 √7ᵗʰ **S32.602** Unspecified fracture of **left** ischium `MCC` `CC` `H5` `HCC`

    2,3,6 √7ᵗʰ **S32.609** Unspecified fracture of unspecified ischium `MCC` `CC` `H5` `HCC`

√6ᵗʰ **S32.61** Avulsion fracture of ischium

    2,3,6 √7ᵗʰ **S32.611** Displaced avulsion fracture of **right** ischium `MCC` `CC` `H5` `HCC`

    2,3,6 √7ᵗʰ **S32.612** Displaced avulsion fracture of **left** ischium `MCC` `CC` `H5` `HCC`

    2,3,6 √7ᵗʰ **S32.613** Displaced avulsion fracture of unspecified ischium `MCC` `CC` `H5` `HCC`

    2,3,6 √7ᵗʰ **S32.614** Nondisplaced avulsion fracture of **right** ischium `MCC` `CC` `H5` `HCC`

    2,3,6 √7ᵗʰ **S32.615** Nondisplaced avulsion fracture of **left** ischium `MCC` `CC` `H5` `HCC`

    2,3,6 √7ᵗʰ **S32.616** Nondisplaced avulsion fracture of unspecified ischium `MCC` `CC` `H5` `HCC`

√6ᵗʰ **S32.69** Other specified fracture of ischium

    2,3,6 √7ᵗʰ **S32.691** Other specified fracture of **right** ischium `MCC` `CC` `H5` `HCC`

    2,3,6 √7ᵗʰ **S32.692** Other specified fracture of **left** ischium `MCC` `CC` `H5` `HCC`

    2,3,6 √7ᵗʰ **S32.699** Other specified fracture of unspecified ischium `MCC` `CC` `H5` `HCC`

√5ᵗʰ **S32.8** Fracture of other parts of pelvis

> Code also any associated:
> fracture of acetabulum (S32.4-)
> sacral fracture (S32.1-)

Fractures Disrupting Pelvic Circle

√6ᵗʰ **S32.81** Multiple fractures of pelvis with disruption of pelvic ring

> Multiple pelvic fractures with disruption of pelvic circle

    2,3,6 √7ᵗʰ **S32.810** Multiple fractures of pelvis with stable disruption of pelvic ring `MCC` `CC` `H5` `HCC`

Ⓝ Newborn: 0   Ⓟ Pediatric: 0-17   Ⓜ Maternity: 9-64   Ⓐ Adult: 15-124   **MCC** Major Complication/Comorbidity   **CC** Complication/Comorbidity   **SW** Severe Wound Dx

998   ICD-10-CM 2021

2,3,6 ✓7th **S32.811** **Multiple fractures of pelvis with** unstable disruption of pelvic ring   `MCC` `CC` `H5` `HCC`

2,3,6 ✓x7th **S32.82** **Multiple fractures of pelvis** without disruption of pelvic ring   `MCC` `CC` `H5` `HCC`

> Multiple pelvic fractures without disruption of pelvic circle

2,3,6 ✓x7th **S32.89** **Fracture of other parts of pelvis**   `MCC` `CC` `H5` `HCC`

2,3,6 ✓x7th **S32.9** **Fracture of unspecified parts of lumbosacral spine and pelvis**   `MCC` `CC` `H5` `HCC`

> Fracture of lumbosacral spine NOS
> Fracture of pelvis NOS
> **AHA:** 2012,4Q,93

✓4th **S33** **Dislocation and sprain of joints and ligaments of lumbar spine and pelvis**

> `INCLUDES`   avulsion of joint or ligament of lumbar spine and pelvis
> laceration of cartilage, joint or ligament of lumbar spine and pelvis
> sprain of cartilage, joint or ligament of lumbar spine and pelvis
> traumatic hemarthrosis of joint or ligament of lumbar spine and pelvis
> traumatic rupture of joint or ligament of lumbar spine and pelvis
> traumatic subluxation of joint or ligament of lumbar spine and pelvis
> traumatic tear of joint or ligament of lumbar spine and pelvis

Code also any associated open wound

> `EXCLUDES 1`   nontraumatic rupture or displacement of lumbar intervertebral disc NOS (M51.-)
> obstetric damage to pelvic joints and ligaments (O71.6)
> `EXCLUDES 2`   dislocation and sprain of joints and ligaments of hip (S73.-)
> strain of muscle of lower back and pelvis (S39.01-)

The appropriate 7th character is to be added to each code from category S33.
A   initial encounter
D   subsequent encounter
S   sequela

✓x7th **S33.0** **Traumatic rupture of lumbar intervertebral disc**

> `EXCLUDES 1`   rupture or displacement (nontraumatic) of lumbar intervertebral disc NOS (M51.- with fifth character 6)

✓5th **S33.1** **Subluxation and dislocation of** lumbar vertebra

> Code also any associated:
> open wound of abdomen, lower back and pelvis (S31)
> spinal cord injury (S24.0, S24.1-, S34.0-, S34.1-)
> `EXCLUDES 2`   fracture of lumbar vertebrae (S32.0-)

   ✓6th **S33.10** **Subluxation and dislocation of unspecified lumbar vertebra**

     ✓7th **S33.100** **Subluxation of unspecified lumbar vertebra**

     ✓7th **S33.101** **Dislocation of unspecified lumbar vertebra**

   ✓6th **S33.11** **Subluxation and dislocation of** L1/L2 **lumbar vertebra**

     ✓7th **S33.110** **Subluxation of L1/L2 lumbar vertebra**

     ✓7th **S33.111** **Dislocation of L1/L2 lumbar vertebra**

   ✓6th **S33.12** **Subluxation and dislocation of** L2/L3 **lumbar vertebra**

     ✓7th **S33.120** **Subluxation of L2/L3 lumbar vertebra**

     ✓7th **S33.121** **Dislocation of L2/L3 lumbar vertebra**

   ✓6th **S33.13** **Subluxation and dislocation of** L3/L4 **lumbar vertebra**

     ✓7th **S33.130** **Subluxation of L3/L4 lumbar vertebra**

     ✓7th **S33.131** **Dislocation of L3/L4 lumbar vertebra**

   ✓6th **S33.14** **Subluxation and dislocation of** L4/L5 **lumbar vertebra**

     ✓7th **S33.140** **Subluxation of L4/L5 lumbar vertebra**

     ✓7th **S33.141** **Dislocation of L4/L5 lumbar vertebra**

✓x7th **S33.2** **Dislocation of** sacroiliac and sacrococcygeal **joint**

✓5th **S33.3** **Dislocation of other and unspecified parts of lumbar spine and pelvis**

   ✓x7th **S33.30** **Dislocation of unspecified parts of lumbar spine and pelvis**

✓x7th **S33.39** **Dislocation of other parts of lumbar spine and pelvis**

✓x7th **S33.4** **Traumatic rupture of** symphysis pubis

✓x7th **S33.5** **Sprain of ligaments of** lumbar spine

✓x7th **S33.6** **Sprain of** sacroiliac joint

✓x7th **S33.8** **Sprain of other parts of lumbar spine and pelvis**

✓x7th **S33.9** **Sprain of unspecified parts of lumbar spine and pelvis**

✓4th **S34** **Injury of lumbar and sacral spinal cord and nerves at abdomen, lower back and pelvis level**

> `NOTE`   Code to highest level of lumbar cord injury.
> Injuries to the spinal cord (S34.0 and S34.1) refer to the cord level and not bone level injury, and can affect nerve roots at and below the level given.

Code also any associated:
fracture of vertebra (S22.0-, S32.0-)
open wound of abdomen, lower back and pelvis (S31.-)
transient paralysis (R29.5)

The appropriate 7th character is to be added to each code from category S34.
A   initial encounter
D   subsequent encounter
S   sequela

✓5th **S34.0** **Concussion and edema of lumbar and sacral spinal cord**

   ✓x7th **S34.01** **Concussion and edema of** lumbar **spinal cord**   `MCC` `HCC`

   ✓x7th **S34.02** **Concussion and edema of** sacral **spinal cord**   `MCC` `HCC`

> Concussion and edema of conus medullaris

✓5th **S34.1** **Other and unspecified injury of lumbar and sacral spinal cord**

   ✓6th **S34.10** **Unspecified injury to lumbar spinal cord**

     ✓7th **S34.101** **Unspecified injury to** L1 **level of lumbar spinal cord**   `MCC` `H5` `HCC`

> Unspecified injury to lumbar spinal cord level 1

     ✓7th **S34.102** **Unspecified injury to** L2 **level of lumbar spinal cord**   `MCC` `H5` `HCC`

> Unspecified injury to lumbar spinal cord level 2

     ✓7th **S34.103** **Unspecified injury to** L3 **level of lumbar spinal cord**   `MCC` `H5` `HCC`

> Unspecified injury to lumbar spinal cord level 3

     ✓7th **S34.104** **Unspecified injury to** L4 **level of lumbar spinal cord**   `MCC` `H5` `HCC`

> Unspecified injury to lumbar spinal cord level 4

     ✓7th **S34.105** **Unspecified injury to** L5 **level of lumbar spinal cord**   `MCC` `H5` `HCC`

> Unspecified injury to lumbar spinal cord level 5

     ✓7th **S34.109** **Unspecified injury to unspecified level of lumbar spinal cord**   `MCC` `H5` `HCC`

   ✓6th **S34.11** **Complete lesion of lumbar spinal cord**

     ✓7th **S34.111** **Complete lesion of** L1 **level of lumbar spinal cord**   `MCC` `H5` `HCC`

> Complete lesion of lumbar spinal cord level 1

     ✓7th **S34.112** **Complete lesion of** L2 **level of lumbar spinal cord**   `MCC` `H5` `HCC`

> Complete lesion of lumbar spinal cord level 2

     ✓7th **S34.113** **Complete lesion of** L3 **level of lumbar spinal cord**   `MCC` `H5` `HCC`

> Complete lesion of lumbar spinal cord level 3

     ✓7th **S34.114** **Complete lesion of** L4 **level of lumbar spinal cord**   `MCC` `H5` `HCC`

> Complete lesion of lumbar spinal cord level 4

     ✓7th **S34.115** **Complete lesion of** L5 **level of lumbar spinal cord**   `MCC` `H5` `HCC`

> Complete lesion of lumbar spinal cord level 5

     ✓7th **S34.119** **Complete lesion of unspecified level of lumbar spinal cord**   `MCC` `H5` `HCC`

✓ Additional Character Required   ✓x7th Placeholder   Unacceptable PDx   Questionable PDx   Manifestation   Unspecified Dx   H1 - H14 HAC   HCC CMS-HCC Dx   HIV HIV Dx

ICD-10-CM 2021   999

Chapter 19. Injury, Poisoning and Certain Other Consequences of External Causes

S32.811–S34.119

√6ᵗʰ **S34.12** **Incomplete lesion** of lumbar spinal cord

√7ᵗʰ   **S34.121** **Incomplete lesion of** L1 level **of lumbar spinal cord**   MCC H5 HCC

Incomplete lesion of lumbar spinal cord level 1

√7ᵗʰ   **S34.122** **Incomplete lesion of** L2 level **of lumbar spinal cord**   MCC H5 HCC

Incomplete lesion of lumbar spinal cord level 2

√7ᵗʰ   **S34.123** **Incomplete lesion of** L3 level **of lumbar spinal cord**   MCC H5 HCC

Incomplete lesion of lumbar spinal cord level 3

√7ᵗʰ   **S34.124** **Incomplete lesion of** L4 level **of lumbar spinal cord**   MCC H5 HCC

Incomplete lesion of lumbar spinal cord level 4

√7ᵗʰ   **S34.125** **Incomplete lesion of** L5 level **of lumbar spinal cord**   MCC H5 HCC

Incomplete lesion of lumbar spinal cord level 5

√7ᵗʰ   **S34.129** **Incomplete lesion of unspecified level of lumbar spinal cord**   MCC H5 HCC

√6ᵗʰ **S34.13** **Other and unspecified injury to sacral spinal cord**

Other injury to conus medullaris

√7ᵗʰ   **S34.131** **Complete lesion of sacral spinal cord**   MCC H5 HCC

Complete lesion of conus medullaris

√7ᵗʰ   **S34.132** **Incomplete lesion of sacral spinal cord**   MCC H5 HCC

Incomplete lesion of conus medullaris

√7ᵗʰ   **S34.139** **Unspecified injury to sacral spinal cord**   MCC H5 HCC

Unspecified injury of conus medullaris

√5ᵗʰ **S34.2** **Injury of nerve root of lumbar and sacral spine**

√x7ᵗʰ **S34.21** **Injury of nerve root of** lumbar spine

√x7ᵗʰ **S34.22** **Injury of nerve root of** sacral spine

6 √x7ᵗʰ **S34.3** **Injury of cauda equina**   MCC H5 HCC

√x7ᵗʰ **S34.4** **Injury of lumbosacral plexus**

√x7ᵗʰ **S34.5** **Injury of lumbar, sacral and pelvic sympathetic nerves**

Injury of celiac ganglion or plexus

Injury of hypogastric plexus

Injury of mesenteric plexus (inferior) (superior)

Injury of splanchnic nerve

√x7ᵗʰ **S34.6** **Injury of peripheral nerve(s) at abdomen, lower back and pelvis level**

√x7ᵗʰ **S34.8** **Injury of other nerves at abdomen, lower back and pelvis level**

√x7ᵗʰ **S34.9** **Injury of unspecified nerves at abdomen, lower back and pelvis level**

√4ᵗʰ **S35** **Injury of blood vessels at abdomen, lower back and pelvis level**

Code also any associated open wound (S31.-)

The appropriate 7th character is to be added to each code from category S35.

A   initial encounter

D   subsequent encounter

S   sequela

√5ᵗʰ **S35.0** **Injury of** abdominal aorta

EXCLUDES 1   injury of aorta NOS (S25.0)

√x7ᵗʰ **S35.00** **Unspecified injury of abdominal aorta**   MCC

√x7ᵗʰ **S35.01** **Minor laceration of abdominal aorta**   MCC

Incomplete transection of abdominal aorta

Laceration of abdominal aorta NOS

Superficial laceration of abdominal aorta

√x7ᵗʰ **S35.02** **Major laceration of abdominal aorta**   MCC

Complete transection of abdominal aorta

Traumatic rupture of abdominal aorta

√x7ᵗʰ **S35.09** **Other injury of abdominal aorta**   MCC

√5ᵗʰ **S35.1** **Injury of** inferior vena cava

Injury of hepatic vein

EXCLUDES 1   injury of vena cava NOS (S25.2)

√x7ᵗʰ **S35.10** **Unspecified injury of inferior vena cava**   MCC

√x7ᵗʰ **S35.11** **Minor laceration of inferior vena cava**   MCC

Incomplete transection of inferior vena cava

Laceration of inferior vena cava NOS

Superficial laceration of inferior vena cava

√x7ᵗʰ **S35.12** **Major laceration of inferior vena cava**   MCC

Complete transection of inferior vena cava

Traumatic rupture of inferior vena cava

√x7ᵗʰ **S35.19** **Other injury of inferior vena cava**   MCC

√5ᵗʰ **S35.2** **Injury of celiac or mesenteric artery and branches**

√6ᵗʰ **S35.21** **Injury of** celiac artery

√7ᵗʰ   **S35.211** **Minor laceration of celiac artery**   MCC

Incomplete transection of celiac artery

Laceration of celiac artery NOS

Superficial laceration of celiac artery

√7ᵗʰ   **S35.212** **Major laceration of celiac artery**   MCC

Complete transection of celiac artery

Traumatic rupture of celiac artery

√7ᵗʰ   **S35.218** **Other injury of celiac artery**   MCC

√7ᵗʰ   **S35.219** **Unspecified injury of celiac artery**   MCC

√6ᵗʰ **S35.22** **Injury of** superior mesenteric artery

√7ᵗʰ   **S35.221** **Minor laceration of superior mesenteric artery**   MCC

Incomplete transection of superior mesenteric artery

Laceration of superior mesenteric artery NOS

Superficial laceration of superior mesenteric artery

√7ᵗʰ   **S35.222** **Major laceration of superior mesenteric artery**   MCC

Complete transection of superior mesenteric artery

Traumatic rupture of superior mesenteric artery

√7ᵗʰ   **S35.228** **Other injury of superior mesenteric artery**   MCC

√7ᵗʰ   **S35.229** **Unspecified injury of superior mesenteric artery**   MCC

√6ᵗʰ **S35.23** **Injury of** inferior mesenteric artery

√7ᵗʰ   **S35.231** **Minor laceration of inferior mesenteric artery**   MCC

Incomplete transection of inferior mesenteric artery

Laceration of inferior mesenteric artery NOS

Superficial laceration of inferior mesenteric artery

√7ᵗʰ   **S35.232** **Major laceration of inferior mesenteric artery**   MCC

Complete transection of inferior mesenteric artery

Traumatic rupture of inferior mesenteric artery

√7ᵗʰ   **S35.238** **Other injury of inferior mesenteric artery**   MCC

√7ᵗʰ   **S35.239** **Unspecified injury of inferior mesenteric artery**   MCC

√6ᵗʰ **S35.29** **Injury of** branches of celiac and mesenteric artery

Injury of gastric artery

Injury of gastroduodenal artery

Injury of hepatic artery

Injury of splenic artery

√7ᵗʰ   **S35.291** **Minor laceration of branches of celiac and mesenteric artery**   MCC

Incomplete transection of branches of celiac and mesenteric artery

Laceration of branches of celiac and mesenteric artery NOS

Superficial laceration of branches of celiac and mesenteric artery

√7ᵗʰ   **S35.292** **Major laceration of branches of celiac and mesenteric artery**   MCC

Complete transection of branches of celiac and mesenteric artery

Traumatic rupture of branches of celiac and mesenteric artery

N Newborn: 0   P Pediatric: 0-17   M Maternity: 9-64   A Adult: 15-124   MCC Major Complication/Comorbidity   CC Complication/Comorbidity   SW Severe Wound Dx

1000   ICD-10-CM 2021

√7ᵗʰ **S35.298** Other injury of branches of celiac and mesenteric artery   `MCC`

√7ᵗʰ **S35.299** Unspecified injury of branches of celiac and mesenteric artery   `MCC`

√5ᵗʰ **S35.3** Injury of portal or splenic vein and branches

√6ᵗʰ **S35.31** Injury of portal vein

√7ᵗʰ **S35.311** Laceration of portal vein   `MCC`

√7ᵗʰ **S35.318** Other specified injury of portal vein   `MCC`

√7ᵗʰ **S35.319** Unspecified injury of portal vein   `MCC`

√6ᵗʰ **S35.32** Injury of splenic vein

√7ᵗʰ **S35.321** Laceration of splenic vein   `MCC`

√7ᵗʰ **S35.328** Other specified injury of splenic vein   `MCC`

√7ᵗʰ **S35.329** Unspecified injury of splenic vein   `MCC`

√6ᵗʰ **S35.33** Injury of superior mesenteric vein

√7ᵗʰ **S35.331** Laceration of superior mesenteric vein   `MCC`

√7ᵗʰ **S35.338** Other specified injury of superior mesenteric vein   `MCC`

√7ᵗʰ **S35.339** Unspecified injury of superior mesenteric vein   `MCC`

√6ᵗʰ **S35.34** Injury of inferior mesenteric vein

√7ᵗʰ **S35.341** Laceration of inferior mesenteric vein   `MCC`

√7ᵗʰ **S35.348** Other specified injury of inferior mesenteric vein   `MCC`

√7ᵗʰ **S35.349** Unspecified injury of inferior mesenteric vein   `MCC`

√5ᵗʰ **S35.4** Injury of renal blood vessels

√6ᵗʰ **S35.40** Unspecified injury of renal blood vessel

√7ᵗʰ **S35.401** Unspecified injury of right renal artery   `MCC`

√7ᵗʰ **S35.402** Unspecified injury of left renal artery   `MCC`

√7ᵗʰ **S35.403** Unspecified injury of unspecified renal artery   `MCC`

√7ᵗʰ **S35.404** Unspecified injury of right renal vein   `MCC`

√7ᵗʰ **S35.405** Unspecified injury of left renal vein   `MCC`

√7ᵗʰ **S35.406** Unspecified injury of unspecified renal vein   `MCC`

√6ᵗʰ **S35.41** Laceration of renal blood vessel

√7ᵗʰ **S35.411** Laceration of right renal artery   `MCC`

√7ᵗʰ **S35.412** Laceration of left renal artery   `MCC`

√7ᵗʰ **S35.413** Laceration of unspecified renal artery   `MCC`

√7ᵗʰ **S35.414** Laceration of right renal vein   `MCC`

√7ᵗʰ **S35.415** Laceration of left renal vein   `MCC`

√7ᵗʰ **S35.416** Laceration of unspecified renal vein   `MCC`

√6ᵗʰ **S35.49** Other specified injury of renal blood vessel

√7ᵗʰ **S35.491** Other specified injury of right renal artery   `MCC`

√7ᵗʰ **S35.492** Other specified injury of left renal artery   `MCC`

√7ᵗʰ **S35.493** Other specified injury of unspecified renal artery   `MCC`

√7ᵗʰ **S35.494** Other specified injury of right renal vein   `MCC`

√7ᵗʰ **S35.495** Other specified injury of left renal vein   `MCC`

√7ᵗʰ **S35.496** Other specified injury of unspecified renal vein   `MCC`

√5ᵗʰ **S35.5** Injury of iliac blood vessels

√x7ᵗʰ **S35.50** Injury of unspecified iliac blood vessel(s)   `MCC`

√6ᵗʰ **S35.51** Injury of iliac artery or vein

Injury of hypogastric artery or vein

√7ᵗʰ **S35.511** Injury of right iliac artery   `MCC`

√7ᵗʰ **S35.512** Injury of left iliac artery   `MCC`

√7ᵗʰ **S35.513** Injury of unspecified iliac artery   `MCC`

√7ᵗʰ **S35.514** Injury of right iliac vein   `MCC`

√7ᵗʰ **S35.515** Injury of left iliac vein   `MCC`

√7ᵗʰ **S35.516** Injury of unspecified iliac vein   `MCC`

√6ᵗʰ **S35.53** Injury of uterine artery or vein

√7ᵗʰ **S35.531** Injury of right uterine artery   `CC` ♀

√7ᵗʰ **S35.532** Injury of left uterine artery   `CC` ♀

√7ᵗʰ **S35.533** Injury of unspecified uterine artery   `CC` ♀

√7ᵗʰ **S35.534** Injury of right uterine vein   `CC` ♀

√7ᵗʰ **S35.535** Injury of left uterine vein   `CC` ♀

√7ᵗʰ **S35.536** Injury of unspecified uterine vein   `CC` ♀

√x7ᵗʰ **S35.59** Injury of other iliac blood vessels   `MCC`

√5ᵗʰ **S35.8** Injury of other blood vessels at abdomen, lower back and pelvis level

Injury of ovarian artery or vein

√6ᵗʰ **S35.8X** Injury of other blood vessels at abdomen, lower back and pelvis level

√7ᵗʰ **S35.8X1** Laceration of other blood vessels at abdomen, lower back and pelvis level   `CC`

√7ᵗʰ **S35.8X8** Other specified injury of other blood vessels at abdomen, lower back and pelvis level   `CC`

√7ᵗʰ **S35.8X9** Unspecified injury of other blood vessels at abdomen, lower back and pelvis level   `CC`

√5ᵗʰ **S35.9** Injury of unspecified blood vessel at abdomen, lower back and pelvis level

√x7ᵗʰ **S35.90** Unspecified injury of unspecified blood vessel at abdomen, lower back and pelvis level   `CC`

√x7ᵗʰ **S35.91** Laceration of unspecified blood vessel at abdomen, lower back and pelvis level   `CC`

√x7ᵗʰ **S35.99** Other specified injury of unspecified blood vessel at abdomen, lower back and pelvis level   `CC`

√4ᵗʰ **S36 Injury of intra-abdominal organs**

Code also any associated open wound (S31.-)

The appropriate 7th character is to be added to each code from category S36.
A   initial encounter
D   subsequent encounter
S   sequela

√5ᵗʰ **S36.0** Injury of spleen

AHA: 2015,2Q,36; 2015,1Q,10

√x7ᵗʰ **S36.00** Unspecified injury of spleen   `CC`

√6ᵗʰ **S36.02** Contusion of spleen

TIP: When both traumatic splenic laceration and contusion are documented in the same encounter, code only the laceration, as contusions are not coded when they occur with a more severe injury in the same body site.

√7ᵗʰ **S36.020** Minor contusion of spleen   `CC`
Contusion of spleen less than 2 cm

√7ᵗʰ **S36.021** Major contusion of spleen   `CC`
Contusion of spleen greater than 2 cm

√7ᵗʰ **S36.029** Unspecified contusion of spleen   `CC`

√6ᵗʰ **S36.03** Laceration of spleen

TIP: When both traumatic splenic laceration and contusion are documented in the same encounter, code only the laceration, as contusions are not coded when they occur with a more severe injury in the same body site.

√7ᵗʰ **S36.030** Superficial (capsular) laceration of spleen   `CC`
Laceration of spleen less than 1 cm
Minor laceration of spleen

√7ᵗʰ **S36.031** Moderate laceration of spleen   `MCC`
Laceration of spleen 1 to 3 cm

√7ᵗʰ **S36.032** Major laceration of spleen   `MCC`
Avulsion of spleen
Laceration of spleen greater than 3 cm
Massive laceration of spleen
Multiple moderate lacerations of spleen
Stellate laceration of spleen

√7ᵗʰ **S36.039** Unspecified laceration of spleen   `CC`

√x7ᵗʰ **S36.09** Other injury of spleen   `CC`

✔ Additional Character Required   √x7ᵗʰ Placeholder   Unacceptable PDx   Questionable PDx   Manifestation   Unspecified Dx   `H1`-`H14` HAC   `HCC` CMS-HCC Dx   `HIV` HIV Dx

ICD-10-CM 2021   1001

√5ᵗʰ **S36.1**   **Injury of liver and gallbladder and bile duct**

   √6ᵗʰ **S36.11**   **Injury of liver**

     √7ᵗʰ **S36.112**   Contusion of liver   `CC`

     √7ᵗʰ **S36.113**   Laceration of liver, unspecified degree   `CC`

     √7ᵗʰ **S36.114**   Minor laceration of liver   `CC`

       Laceration involving capsule only, or, without significant involvement of hepatic parenchyma [i.e., less than 1 cm deep]

     √7ᵗʰ **S36.115**   Moderate laceration of liver   `MCC`

       Laceration involving parenchyma but without major disruption of parenchyma [i.e., less than 10 cm long and less than 3 cm deep]

     √7ᵗʰ **S36.116**   Major laceration of liver   `MCC`

       Laceration with significant disruption of hepatic parenchyma [i.e., greater than 10 cm long and 3 cm deep]

       Multiple moderate lacerations, with or without hematoma

       Stellate laceration of liver

     √7ᵗʰ **S36.118**   Other injury of liver   `CC`

     √7ᵗʰ **S36.119**   Unspecified injury of liver   `CC`

   √6ᵗʰ **S36.12**   **Injury of gallbladder**

     √7ᵗʰ **S36.122**   Contusion of gallbladder   `CC`

     √7ᵗʰ **S36.123**   Laceration of gallbladder   `CC`

     √7ᵗʰ **S36.128**   Other injury of gallbladder   `CC`

     √7ᵗʰ **S36.129**   Unspecified injury of gallbladder   `CC`

   √x7ᵗʰ **S36.13**   **Injury of bile duct**   `CC`

√5ᵗʰ **S36.2**   **Injury of pancreas**

   √6ᵗʰ **S36.20**   **Unspecified injury of pancreas**

     √7ᵗʰ **S36.200**   Unspecified injury of head of pancreas   `CC`

     √7ᵗʰ **S36.201**   Unspecified injury of body of pancreas   `CC`

     √7ᵗʰ **S36.202**   Unspecified injury of tail of pancreas   `CC`

     √7ᵗʰ **S36.209**   Unspecified injury of unspecified part of pancreas   `CC`

   √6ᵗʰ **S36.22**   **Contusion of pancreas**

     √7ᵗʰ **S36.220**   Contusion of head of pancreas   `CC`

     √7ᵗʰ **S36.221**   Contusion of body of pancreas   `CC`

     √7ᵗʰ **S36.222**   Contusion of tail of pancreas   `CC`

     √7ᵗʰ **S36.229**   Contusion of unspecified part of pancreas   `CC`

   √6ᵗʰ **S36.23**   **Laceration of pancreas, unspecified degree**

     √7ᵗʰ **S36.230**   Laceration of head of pancreas, unspecified degree   `CC`

     √7ᵗʰ **S36.231**   Laceration of body of pancreas, unspecified degree   `CC`

     √7ᵗʰ **S36.232**   Laceration of tail of pancreas, unspecified degree   `CC`

     √7ᵗʰ **S36.239**   Laceration of unspecified part of pancreas, unspecified degree   `CC`

   √6ᵗʰ **S36.24**   **Minor laceration of pancreas**

     √7ᵗʰ **S36.240**   Minor laceration of head of pancreas   `CC`

     √7ᵗʰ **S36.241**   Minor laceration of body of pancreas   `CC`

     √7ᵗʰ **S36.242**   Minor laceration of tail of pancreas   `CC`

     √7ᵗʰ **S36.249**   Minor laceration of unspecified part of pancreas   `CC`

   √6ᵗʰ **S36.25**   **Moderate laceration of pancreas**

     √7ᵗʰ **S36.250**   Moderate laceration of head of pancreas   `CC`

     √7ᵗʰ **S36.251**   Moderate laceration of body of pancreas   `CC`

     √7ᵗʰ **S36.252**   Moderate laceration of tail of pancreas   `CC`

     √7ᵗʰ **S36.259**   Moderate laceration of unspecified part of pancreas   `CC`

   √6ᵗʰ **S36.26**   **Major laceration of pancreas**

     √7ᵗʰ **S36.260**   Major laceration of head of pancreas   `CC`

     √7ᵗʰ **S36.261**   Major laceration of body of pancreas   `CC`

     √7ᵗʰ **S36.262**   Major laceration of tail of pancreas   `CC`

     √7ᵗʰ **S36.269**   Major laceration of unspecified part of pancreas   `CC`

   √6ᵗʰ **S36.29**   **Other injury of pancreas**

     √7ᵗʰ **S36.290**   Other injury of head of pancreas   `CC`

     √7ᵗʰ **S36.291**   Other injury of body of pancreas   `CC`

     √7ᵗʰ **S36.292**   Other injury of tail of pancreas   `CC`

     √7ᵗʰ **S36.299**   Other injury of unspecified part of pancreas   `CC`

√5ᵗʰ **S36.3**   **Injury of stomach**

   √x7ᵗʰ **S36.30**   **Unspecified injury of stomach**   `CC`

   √x7ᵗʰ **S36.32**   **Contusion of stomach**   `CC`

   √x7ᵗʰ **S36.33**   **Laceration of stomach**   `CC`

   √x7ᵗʰ **S36.39**   **Other injury of stomach**   `CC`

√5ᵗʰ **S36.4**   **Injury of small intestine**

   √6ᵗʰ **S36.40**   **Unspecified injury of small intestine**

     √7ᵗʰ **S36.400**   Unspecified injury of duodenum   `CC`

     √7ᵗʰ **S36.408**   Unspecified injury of other part of small intestine   `CC`

     √7ᵗʰ **S36.409**   Unspecified injury of unspecified part of small intestine   `CC`

   √6ᵗʰ **S36.41**   **Primary blast injury of small intestine**

       Blast injury of small intestine NOS

     √7ᵗʰ **S36.410**   Primary blast injury of duodenum   `CC`

     √7ᵗʰ **S36.418**   Primary blast injury of other part of small intestine   `CC`

     √7ᵗʰ **S36.419**   Primary blast injury of unspecified part of small intestine   `CC`

   √6ᵗʰ **S36.42**   **Contusion of small intestine**

     √7ᵗʰ **S36.420**   Contusion of duodenum   `CC`

     √7ᵗʰ **S36.428**   Contusion of other part of small intestine   `CC`

     √7ᵗʰ **S36.429**   Contusion of unspecified part of small intestine   `CC`

   √6ᵗʰ **S36.43**   **Laceration of small intestine**

     √7ᵗʰ **S36.430**   Laceration of duodenum   `CC`

     √7ᵗʰ **S36.438**   Laceration of other part of small intestine   `CC`

     √7ᵗʰ **S36.439**   Laceration of unspecified part of small intestine   `CC`

   √6ᵗʰ **S36.49**   **Other injury of small intestine**

     √7ᵗʰ **S36.490**   Other injury of duodenum   `CC`

     √7ᵗʰ **S36.498**   Other injury of other part of small intestine   `CC`

     √7ᵗʰ **S36.499**   Other injury of unspecified part of small intestine   `CC`

√5ᵗʰ **S36.5**   **Injury of colon**

     `EXCLUDES 2`   injury of rectum (S36.6-)

   √6ᵗʰ **S36.50**   **Unspecified injury of colon**

     √7ᵗʰ **S36.500**   Unspecified injury of ascending [right] colon   `CC`

     √7ᵗʰ **S36.501**   Unspecified injury of transverse colon   `CC`

     √7ᵗʰ **S36.502**   Unspecified injury of descending [left] colon   `CC`

     √7ᵗʰ **S36.503**   Unspecified injury of sigmoid colon   `CC`

     √7ᵗʰ **S36.508**   Unspecified injury of other part of colon   `CC`

     √7ᵗʰ **S36.509**   Unspecified injury of unspecified part of colon   `CC`

   √6ᵗʰ **S36.51**   **Primary blast injury of colon**

       Blast injury of colon NOS

     √7ᵗʰ **S36.510**   Primary blast injury of ascending [right] colon   `CC`

     √7ᵗʰ **S36.511**   Primary blast injury of transverse colon   `CC`

     √7ᵗʰ **S36.512**   Primary blast injury of descending [left] colon   `CC`

     √7ᵗʰ **S36.513**   Primary blast injury of sigmoid colon   `CC`

     √7ᵗʰ **S36.518**   Primary blast injury of other part of colon   `CC`

N Newborn: 0   P Pediatric: 0-17   M Maternity: 9-64   A Adult: 15-124   `MCC` Major Complication/Comorbidity   `CC` Complication/Comorbidity   `SW` Severe Wound Dx

1002   ICD-10-CM 2021

√7ᵗʰ **S36.519**   Primary blast injury of unspecified part of colon   CC

√6ᵗʰ **S36.52**   Contusion of colon

    √7ᵗʰ **S36.520**   Contusion of ascending [right] colon   CC

    √7ᵗʰ **S36.521**   Contusion of transverse colon   CC

    √7ᵗʰ **S36.522**   Contusion of descending [left] colon   CC

    √7ᵗʰ **S36.523**   Contusion of sigmoid colon   CC

    √7ᵗʰ **S36.528**   Contusion of other part of colon   CC

    √7ᵗʰ **S36.529**   Contusion of unspecified part of colon   CC

√6ᵗʰ **S36.53**   Laceration of colon

    √7ᵗʰ **S36.530**   Laceration of ascending [right] colon   CC

    √7ᵗʰ **S36.531**   Laceration of transverse colon   CC

    √7ᵗʰ **S36.532**   Laceration of descending [left] colon   CC

    √7ᵗʰ **S36.533**   Laceration of sigmoid colon   CC

    √7ᵗʰ **S36.538**   Laceration of other part of colon   CC

    √7ᵗʰ **S36.539**   Laceration of unspecified part of colon   CC

√6ᵗʰ **S36.59**   Other injury of colon

    Secondary blast injury of colon

    √7ᵗʰ **S36.590**   Other injury of ascending [right] colon   CC

    √7ᵗʰ **S36.591**   Other injury of transverse colon   CC

    √7ᵗʰ **S36.592**   Other injury of descending [left] colon   CC

    √7ᵗʰ **S36.593**   Other injury of sigmoid colon   CC

    √7ᵗʰ **S36.598**   Other injury of other part of colon   CC

    √7ᵗʰ **S36.599**   Other injury of unspecified part of colon   CC

√5ᵗʰ **S36.6**   Injury of rectum

  √x7ᵗʰ **S36.60**   Unspecified injury of rectum   CC

  √x7ᵗʰ **S36.61**   Primary blast injury of rectum   CC

    Blast injury of rectum NOS

  √x7ᵗʰ **S36.62**   Contusion of rectum   CC

  √x7ᵗʰ **S36.63**   Laceration of rectum   CC

  √x7ᵗʰ **S36.69**   Other injury of rectum   CC

    Secondary blast injury of rectum

√5ᵗʰ **S36.8**   Injury of other intra-abdominal organs

  √x7ᵗʰ **S36.81**   Injury of peritoneum   CC

  √6ᵗʰ **S36.89**   Injury of other intra-abdominal organs

    Injury of retroperitoneum

    √7ᵗʰ **S36.892**   Contusion of other intra-abdominal organs   CC

    √7ᵗʰ **S36.893**   Laceration of other intra-abdominal organs   CC

    √7ᵗʰ **S36.898**   Other injury of other intra-abdominal organs   CC

    √7ᵗʰ **S36.899**   Unspecified injury of other intra-abdominal organs   CC

√5ᵗʰ **S36.9**   Injury of unspecified intra-abdominal organ

  √x7ᵗʰ **S36.90**   Unspecified injury of unspecified intra-abdominal organ   CC

  √x7ᵗʰ **S36.92**   Contusion of unspecified intra-abdominal organ   CC

  √x7ᵗʰ **S36.93**   Laceration of unspecified intra-abdominal organ   CC

  √x7ᵗʰ **S36.99**   Other injury of unspecified intra-abdominal organ   CC

√4ᵗʰ **S37**   Injury of urinary and pelvic organs

    Code also any associated open wound (S31.-)

    EXCLUDES 1   obstetric trauma to pelvic organs (O71.-)

    EXCLUDES 2   injury of peritoneum (S36.81)

       injury of retroperitoneum (S36.89-)

    The appropriate 7th character is to be added to each code from category S37.
    A   initial encounter
    D   subsequent encounter
    S   sequela

√5ᵗʰ **S37.0**   Injury of kidney

    EXCLUDES 2   acute kidney injury (nontraumatic) (N17.9)

  √6ᵗʰ **S37.00**   Unspecified injury of kidney

    √7ᵗʰ **S37.001**   Unspecified injury of right kidney   CC

    √7ᵗʰ **S37.002**   Unspecified injury of left kidney   CC

    √7ᵗʰ **S37.009**   Unspecified injury of unspecified kidney   CC

  √6ᵗʰ **S37.01**   Minor contusion of kidney

    Contusion of kidney less than 2 cm
    Contusion of kidney NOS

    √7ᵗʰ **S37.011**   Minor contusion of right kidney   CC

    √7ᵗʰ **S37.012**   Minor contusion of left kidney   CC

    √7ᵗʰ **S37.019**   Minor contusion of unspecified kidney   CC

  √6ᵗʰ **S37.02**   Major contusion of kidney

    Contusion of kidney greater than 2 cm

    √7ᵗʰ **S37.021**   Major contusion of right kidney   CC

    √7ᵗʰ **S37.022**   Major contusion of left kidney   CC

    √7ᵗʰ **S37.029**   Major contusion of unspecified kidney   CC

  √6ᵗʰ **S37.03**   Laceration of kidney, unspecified degree

    √7ᵗʰ **S37.031**   Laceration of right kidney, unspecified degree   CC

    √7ᵗʰ **S37.032**   Laceration of left kidney, unspecified degree   CC

    √7ᵗʰ **S37.039**   Laceration of unspecified kidney, unspecified degree   CC

  √6ᵗʰ **S37.04**   Minor laceration of kidney

    Laceration of kidney less than 1 cm

    √7ᵗʰ **S37.041**   Minor laceration of right kidney   CC

    √7ᵗʰ **S37.042**   Minor laceration of left kidney   CC

    √7ᵗʰ **S37.049**   Minor laceration of unspecified kidney   CC

  √6ᵗʰ **S37.05**   Moderate laceration of kidney

    Laceration of kidney 1 to 3 cm

    √7ᵗʰ **S37.051**   Moderate laceration of right kidney   CC

    √7ᵗʰ **S37.052**   Moderate laceration of left kidney   CC

    √7ᵗʰ **S37.059**   Moderate laceration of unspecified kidney   CC

  √6ᵗʰ **S37.06**   Major laceration of kidney

    Avulsion of kidney
    Laceration of kidney greater than 3 cm
    Massive laceration of kidney
    Multiple moderate lacerations of kidney
    Stellate laceration of kidney

    √7ᵗʰ **S37.061**   Major laceration of right kidney   MCC

    √7ᵗʰ **S37.062**   Major laceration of left kidney   MCC

    √7ᵗʰ **S37.069**   Major laceration of unspecified kidney   MCC

  √6ᵗʰ **S37.09**   Other injury of kidney

    √7ᵗʰ **S37.091**   Other injury of right kidney   MCC

    √7ᵗʰ **S37.092**   Other injury of left kidney   MCC

    √7ᵗʰ **S37.099**   Other injury of unspecified kidney   MCC

√5ᵗʰ **S37.1**   Injury of ureter

  √x7ᵗʰ **S37.10**   Unspecified injury of ureter   CC

  √x7ᵗʰ **S37.12**   Contusion of ureter   CC

  √x7ᵗʰ **S37.13**   Laceration of ureter   CC

  √x7ᵗʰ **S37.19**   Other injury of ureter   CC

√5ᵗʰ **S37.2**   Injury of bladder

  √x7ᵗʰ **S37.20**   Unspecified injury of bladder   CC

√ Additional Character Required   √x7ᵗʰ Placeholder   Unacceptable PDx   Questionable PDx   Manifestation   Unspecified Dx   H1-H14 HAC   HCC CMS-HCC Dx   HIV HIV Dx

√x7th S37.22 **Contusion** of bladder `CC`

√x7th S37.23 **Laceration** of bladder `CC`

√x7th S37.29 Other injury of bladder `CC`

√5th **S37.3 Injury of urethra**

√x7th S37.30 Unspecified injury of urethra `CC`

√x7th S37.32 **Contusion** of urethra `CC`

√x7th S37.33 **Laceration** of urethra `CC`

√x7th S37.39 Other injury of urethra `CC`

√5th **S37.4 Injury of ovary**

√6th S37.40 Unspecified injury of ovary

  √7th S37.401 Unspecified injury of ovary, unilateral ♀

  √7th S37.402 Unspecified injury of ovary, bilateral ♀

  √7th S37.409 Unspecified injury of ovary, unspecified ♀

√6th S37.42 **Contusion** of ovary

  √7th S37.421 Contusion of ovary, unilateral ♀

  √7th S37.422 Contusion of ovary, bilateral ♀

  √7th S37.429 Contusion of ovary, unspecified ♀

√6th S37.43 **Laceration** of ovary

  √7th S37.431 Laceration of ovary, unilateral ♀

  √7th S37.432 Laceration of ovary, bilateral ♀

  √7th S37.439 Laceration of ovary, unspecified ♀

√6th S37.49 Other injury of ovary

  √7th S37.491 Other injury of ovary, unilateral ♀

  √7th S37.492 Other injury of ovary, bilateral ♀

  √7th S37.499 Other injury of ovary, unspecified ♀

√5th **S37.5 Injury of fallopian tube**

√6th S37.50 Unspecified injury of fallopian tube

  √7th S37.501 Unspecified injury of fallopian tube, unilateral ♀

  √7th S37.502 Unspecified injury of fallopian tube, bilateral ♀

  √7th S37.509 Unspecified injury of fallopian tube, unspecified ♀

√6th S37.51 **Primary blast** injury of fallopian tube

  Blast injury of fallopian tube NOS

  √7th S37.511 Primary blast injury of fallopian tube, unilateral ♀

  √7th S37.512 Primary blast injury of fallopian tube, bilateral ♀

  √7th S37.519 Primary blast injury of fallopian tube, unspecified ♀

√6th S37.52 **Contusion** of fallopian tube

  √7th S37.521 Contusion of fallopian tube, unilateral ♀

  √7th S37.522 Contusion of fallopian tube, bilateral ♀

  √7th S37.529 Contusion of fallopian tube, unspecified ♀

√6th S37.53 **Laceration** of fallopian tube

  √7th S37.531 Laceration of fallopian tube, unilateral ♀

  √7th S37.532 Laceration of fallopian tube, bilateral ♀

  √7th S37.539 Laceration of fallopian tube, unspecified ♀

√6th S37.59 Other injury of fallopian tube

  Secondary blast injury of fallopian tube

  √7th S37.591 Other injury of fallopian tube, unilateral ♀

  √7th S37.592 Other injury of fallopian tube, bilateral ♀

  √7th S37.599 Other injury of fallopian tube, unspecified ♀

√5th **S37.6 Injury of uterus**

  EXCLUDES 1 *injury to gravid uterus (O9A.2-)*
  injury to uterus during delivery (O71.-)

√x7th S37.60 Unspecified injury of uterus `CC` ♀

√x7th S37.62 **Contusion** of uterus `CC` ♀

√x7th S37.63 **Laceration** of uterus `CC` ♀

√x7th S37.69 Other injury of uterus `CC` ♀

√5th **S37.8 Injury of other urinary and pelvic organs**

√6th S37.81 Injury of adrenal gland

  √7th S37.812 **Contusion** of adrenal gland `CC`

  √7th S37.813 **Laceration** of adrenal gland `CC`

  √7th S37.818 Other injury of adrenal gland `CC`

  √7th S37.819 Unspecified injury of adrenal gland `CC`

√6th S37.82 Injury of prostate

  √7th S37.822 **Contusion** of prostate ♂

  √7th S37.823 **Laceration** of prostate ♂

  √7th S37.828 Other injury of prostate ♂

  √7th S37.829 Unspecified injury of prostate ♂

√6th S37.89 Injury of other urinary and pelvic organ

  √7th S37.892 **Contusion** of other urinary and pelvic organ `CC`

  √7th S37.893 **Laceration** of other urinary and pelvic organ `CC`

  √7th S37.898 Other injury of other urinary and pelvic organ

  √7th S37.899 Unspecified injury of other urinary and pelvic organ `CC`

√5th **S37.9 Injury of unspecified urinary and pelvic organ**

√x7th S37.90 Unspecified injury of unspecified urinary and pelvic organ `CC`

√x7th S37.92 **Contusion** of unspecified urinary and pelvic organ `CC`

√x7th S37.93 **Laceration** of unspecified urinary and pelvic organ `CC`

√x7th S37.99 Other injury of unspecified urinary and pelvic organ `CC`

√4th **S38 Crushing injury and traumatic amputation of abdomen, lower back, pelvis and external genitals**

  NOTE An amputation not identified as partial or complete should be coded to complete

  The appropriate 7th character is to be added to each code from category S38.
  A initial encounter
  D subsequent encounter
  S sequela

√5th **S38.0 Crushing injury of external genital organs**

  Use additional code for any associated injuries

√6th S38.00 Crushing injury of unspecified external genital organs

  √7th S38.001 Crushing injury of unspecified external genital organs, male ♂

  √7th S38.002 Crushing injury of unspecified external genital organs, female ♀

√x7th S38.01 Crushing injury of penis ♂

√x7th S38.02 Crushing injury of scrotum and testis ♂

√x7th S38.03 Crushing injury of vulva ♀

√x7th **S38.1 Crushing injury of abdomen, lower back, and pelvis**

  Use additional code for all associated injuries, such as:
  fracture of thoracic or lumbar spine and pelvis (S22.0-, S32.-)
  injury to intra-abdominal organs (S36.-)
  injury to urinary and pelvic organs (S37.-)
  open wound of abdominal wall (S31.-)
  spinal cord injury (S34.0, S34.1-)

  EXCLUDES 2 *crushing injury of external genital organs (S38.0-)*

√5th **S38.2 Traumatic amputation of external genital organs**

√6th S38.21 Traumatic amputation of female external genital organs

  Traumatic amputation of clitoris
  Traumatic amputation of labium (majus) (minus)
  Traumatic amputation of vulva

  √7th S38.211 **Complete** traumatic amputation of female external genital organs ♀

  √7th S38.212 **Partial** traumatic amputation of female external genital organs ♀

√6th S38.22 Traumatic amputation of penis

  √7th S38.221 **Complete** traumatic amputation of penis ♂

  √7th S38.222 **Partial** traumatic amputation of penis ♂

√6ᵗʰ S38.23 Traumatic amputation of scrotum and testis

    √7ᵗʰ S38.231 Complete traumatic amputation of scrotum and testis ♂

    √7ᵗʰ S38.232 Partial traumatic amputation of scrotum and testis ♂

√x7ᵗʰ S38.3 Transection (partial) of abdomen

√4ᵗʰ S39 Other and unspecified injuries of abdomen, lower back, pelvis and external genitals

    Code also any associated open wound (S31.-)

    EXCLUDES 2   sprain of joints and ligaments of lumbar spine and pelvis (S33.-)

    The appropriate 7th character is to be added to each code from category S39.
    A   initial encounter
    D   subsequent encounter
    S   sequela

  √5ᵗʰ S39.0 Injury of muscle, fascia and tendon of abdomen, lower back and pelvis

    √6ᵗʰ S39.00 Unspecified injury of muscle, fascia and tendon of abdomen, lower back and pelvis

      √7ᵗʰ S39.001 Unspecified injury of muscle, fascia and tendon of abdomen

      √7ᵗʰ S39.002 Unspecified injury of muscle, fascia and tendon of lower back

      √7ᵗʰ S39.003 Unspecified injury of muscle, fascia and tendon of pelvis

    √6ᵗʰ S39.01 Strain of muscle, fascia and tendon of abdomen, lower back and pelvis

      √7ᵗʰ S39.011 Strain of muscle, fascia and tendon of abdomen

      √7ᵗʰ S39.012 Strain of muscle, fascia and tendon of lower back

      √7ᵗʰ S39.013 Strain of muscle, fascia and tendon of pelvis

    √6ᵗʰ S39.02 Laceration of muscle, fascia and tendon of abdomen, lower back and pelvis

      √7ᵗʰ S39.021 Laceration of muscle, fascia and tendon of abdomen

      √7ᵗʰ S39.022 Laceration of muscle, fascia and tendon of lower back

      √7ᵗʰ S39.023 Laceration of muscle, fascia and tendon of pelvis

    √6ᵗʰ S39.09 Other injury of muscle, fascia and tendon of abdomen, lower back and pelvis

      √7ᵗʰ S39.091 Other injury of muscle, fascia and tendon of abdomen

      √7ᵗʰ S39.092 Other injury of muscle, fascia and tendon of lower back

      √7ᵗʰ S39.093 Other injury of muscle, fascia and tendon of pelvis

  √5ᵗʰ S39.8 Other specified injuries of abdomen, lower back, pelvis and external genitals

    √x7ᵗʰ S39.81 Other specified injuries of abdomen

    √x7ᵗʰ S39.82 Other specified injuries of lower back

    √x7ᵗʰ S39.83 Other specified injuries of pelvis

    √6ᵗʰ S39.84 Other specified injuries of external genitals

      √7ᵗʰ S39.840 Fracture of corpus cavernosum penis ♂

      √7ᵗʰ S39.848 Other specified injuries of external genitals

          TIP: Assign for traumatic rupture of testis.

  √5ᵗʰ S39.9 Unspecified injury of abdomen, lower back, pelvis and external genitals

    √x7ᵗʰ S39.91 Unspecified injury of abdomen

    √x7ᵗʰ S39.92 Unspecified injury of lower back

    √x7ᵗʰ S39.93 Unspecified injury of pelvis

    √x7ᵗʰ S39.94 Unspecified injury of external genitals

Injuries to the shoulder and upper arm (S40-S49)

INCLUDES   injuries of axilla
          injuries of scapular region
EXCLUDES 2 *burns and corrosions (T20-T32)*
          frostbite (T33-T34)
          injuries of elbow (S50-S59)
          insect bite or sting, venomous (T63.4)

√4ᵗʰ S40 Superficial injury of shoulder and upper arm

    The appropriate 7th character is to be added to each code from category S40.
    A   initial encounter
    D   subsequent encounter
    S   sequela

  √5ᵗʰ S40.0 Contusion of shoulder and upper arm

    √6ᵗʰ S40.01 Contusion of shoulder

      √7ᵗʰ S40.011 Contusion of right shoulder

      √7ᵗʰ S40.012 Contusion of left shoulder

      √7ᵗʰ S40.019 Contusion of unspecified shoulder

    √6ᵗʰ S40.02 Contusion of upper arm

      √7ᵗʰ S40.021 Contusion of right upper arm

      √7ᵗʰ S40.022 Contusion of left upper arm

      √7ᵗʰ S40.029 Contusion of unspecified upper arm

  √5ᵗʰ S40.2 Other superficial injuries of shoulder

    √6ᵗʰ S40.21 Abrasion of shoulder

      √7ᵗʰ S40.211 Abrasion of right shoulder

      √7ᵗʰ S40.212 Abrasion of left shoulder

      √7ᵗʰ S40.219 Abrasion of unspecified shoulder

    √6ᵗʰ S40.22 Blister (nonthermal) of shoulder

      √7ᵗʰ S40.221 Blister (nonthermal) of right shoulder

      √7ᵗʰ S40.222 Blister (nonthermal) of left shoulder

      √7ᵗʰ S40.229 Blister (nonthermal) of unspecified shoulder

    √6ᵗʰ S40.24 External constriction of shoulder

      √7ᵗʰ S40.241 External constriction of right shoulder

      √7ᵗʰ S40.242 External constriction of left shoulder

      √7ᵗʰ S40.249 External constriction of unspecified shoulder

    √6ᵗʰ S40.25 Superficial foreign body of shoulder

      Splinter in the shoulder

      √7ᵗʰ S40.251 Superficial foreign body of right shoulder

      √7ᵗʰ S40.252 Superficial foreign body of left shoulder

      √7ᵗʰ S40.259 Superficial foreign body of unspecified shoulder

    √6ᵗʰ S40.26 Insect bite (nonvenomous) of shoulder

      √7ᵗʰ S40.261 Insect bite (nonvenomous) of right shoulder

      √7ᵗʰ S40.262 Insect bite (nonvenomous) of left shoulder

      √7ᵗʰ S40.269 Insect bite (nonvenomous) of unspecified shoulder

    √6ᵗʰ S40.27 Other superficial bite of shoulder

      EXCLUDES 1 *open bite of shoulder (S41.05)*

      √7ᵗʰ S40.271 Other superficial bite of right shoulder

      √7ᵗʰ S40.272 Other superficial bite of left shoulder

      √7ᵗʰ S40.279 Other superficial bite of unspecified shoulder

  √5ᵗʰ S40.8 Other superficial injuries of upper arm

    √6ᵗʰ S40.81 Abrasion of upper arm

      √7ᵗʰ S40.811 Abrasion of right upper arm

      √7ᵗʰ S40.812 Abrasion of left upper arm

      √7ᵗʰ S40.819 Abrasion of unspecified upper arm

    √6ᵗʰ S40.82 Blister (nonthermal) of upper arm

      √7ᵗʰ S40.821 Blister (nonthermal) of right upper arm

      √7ᵗʰ S40.822 Blister (nonthermal) of left upper arm

      √7ᵗʰ S40.829 Blister (nonthermal) of unspecified upper arm

    √6ᵗʰ S40.84 External constriction of upper arm

      √7ᵗʰ S40.841 External constriction of right upper arm

      √7ᵗʰ S40.842 External constriction of left upper arm

√7th **S40.849**　**External constriction of unspecified upper arm**

√6th **S40.85**　**Superficial foreign body of upper arm**

　Splinter in the upper arm

√7th **S40.851**　**Superficial foreign body of right upper arm**

√7th **S40.852**　**Superficial foreign body of left upper arm**

√7th **S40.859**　**Superficial foreign body of unspecified upper arm**

√6th **S40.86**　**Insect bite (nonvenomous) of upper arm**

√7th **S40.861**　**Insect bite (nonvenomous) of right upper arm**

√7th **S40.862**　**Insect bite (nonvenomous) of left upper arm**

√7th **S40.869**　**Insect bite (nonvenomous) of unspecified upper arm**

√6th **S40.87**　**Other superficial bite of upper arm**

　　EXCLUDES 1　open bite of upper arm (S41.14)

　　EXCLUDES 2　other superficial bite of shoulder (S40.27-)

√7th **S40.871**　**Other superficial bite of right upper arm**

√7th **S40.872**　**Other superficial bite of left upper arm**

√7th **S40.879**　**Other superficial bite of unspecified upper arm**

√5th **S40.9**　**Unspecified superficial injury of shoulder and upper arm**

√6th **S40.91**　**Unspecified superficial injury of shoulder**

√7th **S40.911**　**Unspecified superficial injury of right shoulder**

√7th **S40.912**　**Unspecified superficial injury of left shoulder**

√7th **S40.919**　**Unspecified superficial injury of unspecified shoulder**

√6th **S40.92**　**Unspecified superficial injury of upper arm**

√7th **S40.921**　**Unspecified superficial injury of right upper arm**

√7th **S40.922**　**Unspecified superficial injury of left upper arm**

√7th **S40.929**　**Unspecified superficial injury of unspecified upper arm**

√4th **S41**　**Open wound of shoulder and upper arm**

　Code also any associated wound infection

　EXCLUDES 1　traumatic amputation of shoulder and upper arm (S48.-)

　EXCLUDES 2　open fracture of shoulder and upper arm (S42.- with 7th character B or C)

> The appropriate 7th character is to be added to each code from category S41.
> A　initial encounter
> D　subsequent encounter
> S　sequela

√5th **S41.0**　**Open wound of shoulder**

√6th **S41.00**　**Unspecified open wound of shoulder**

√7th **S41.001**　**Unspecified open wound of right shoulder**

√7th **S41.002**　**Unspecified open wound of left shoulder**

√7th **S41.009**　**Unspecified open wound of unspecified shoulder**

√6th **S41.01**　**Laceration without foreign body of shoulder**

√7th **S41.011**　**Laceration without foreign body of right shoulder**

√7th **S41.012**　**Laceration without foreign body of left shoulder**

√7th **S41.019**　**Laceration without foreign body of unspecified shoulder**

√6th **S41.02**　**Laceration with foreign body of shoulder**

√7th **S41.021**　**Laceration with foreign body of right shoulder**

√7th **S41.022**　**Laceration with foreign body of left shoulder**

√7th **S41.029**　**Laceration with foreign body of unspecified shoulder**

√6th **S41.03**　**Puncture wound without foreign body of shoulder**

√7th **S41.031**　**Puncture wound without foreign body of right shoulder**

√7th **S41.032**　**Puncture wound without foreign body of left shoulder**

√7th **S41.039**　**Puncture wound without foreign body of unspecified shoulder**

√6th **S41.04**　**Puncture wound with foreign body of shoulder**

√7th **S41.041**　**Puncture wound with foreign body of right shoulder**

√7th **S41.042**　**Puncture wound with foreign body of left shoulder**

√7th **S41.049**　**Puncture wound with foreign body of unspecified shoulder**

√6th **S41.05**　**Open bite of shoulder**

　Bite of shoulder NOS

　　EXCLUDES 1　superficial bite of shoulder (S40.27)

√7th **S41.051**　**Open bite of right shoulder**

√7th **S41.052**　**Open bite of left shoulder**

√7th **S41.059**　**Open bite of unspecified shoulder**

√5th **S41.1**　**Open wound of upper arm**

√6th **S41.10**　**Unspecified open wound of upper arm**

　AHA: 2016,3Q,24

√7th **S41.101**　**Unspecified open wound of right upper arm**

√7th **S41.102**　**Unspecified open wound of left upper arm**

√7th **S41.109**　**Unspecified open wound of unspecified upper arm**

√6th **S41.11**　**Laceration without foreign body of upper arm**

√7th **S41.111**　**Laceration without foreign body of right upper arm**

√7th **S41.112**　**Laceration without foreign body of left upper arm**

√7th **S41.119**　**Laceration without foreign body of unspecified upper arm**

√6th **S41.12**　**Laceration with foreign body of upper arm**

√7th **S41.121**　**Laceration with foreign body of right upper arm**

√7th **S41.122**　**Laceration with foreign body of left upper arm**

√7th **S41.129**　**Laceration with foreign body of unspecified upper arm**

√6th **S41.13**　**Puncture wound without foreign body of upper arm**

　AHA: 2016,3Q,24

√7th **S41.131**　**Puncture wound without foreign body of right upper arm**

√7th **S41.132**　**Puncture wound without foreign body of left upper arm**

√7th **S41.139**　**Puncture wound without foreign body of unspecified upper arm**

√6th **S41.14**　**Puncture wound with foreign body of upper arm**

　AHA: 2016,3Q,24

√7th **S41.141**　**Puncture wound with foreign body of right upper arm**

√7th **S41.142**　**Puncture wound with foreign body of left upper arm**

√7th **S41.149**　**Puncture wound with foreign body of unspecified upper arm**

√6th **S41.15**　**Open bite of upper arm**

　Bite of upper arm NOS

　　EXCLUDES 1　superficial bite of upper arm (S40.87)

√7th **S41.151**　**Open bite of right upper arm**

√7th **S41.152**　**Open bite of left upper arm**

√7th **S41.159**　**Open bite of unspecified upper arm**

N Newborn: 0　　P Pediatric: 0-17　　M Maternity: 9-64　　A Adult: 15-124　　MCC Major Complication/Comorbidity　　CC Complication/Comorbidity　　SW Severe Wound Dx

1006　　ICD-10-CM 2021

√4ᵗʰ **S42 Fracture of shoulder and upper arm**

> **NOTE**   A fracture not indicated as displaced or nondisplaced should be coded to displaced
>
> A fracture not indicated as open or closed should be coded to closed

> **EXCLUDES 1**   *traumatic amputation of shoulder and upper arm (S48.-)*

AHA: 2018,2Q,12; 2015,3Q,37-39
DEF: Diaphysis: Central shaft of a long bone.
DEF: Epiphysis: Proximal and distal rounded ends of a long bone, communicates with the joint.
DEF: Metaphysis: Section of a long bone located between the epiphysis and diaphysis at the proximal and distal ends.
DEF: Physis (growth plate): Narrow zone of cartilaginous tissue between the epiphysis and metaphysis at each end of a long bone. In childhood, proliferation of cells in this zone lengthens the bone. As the bone matures, this area thins, ossification eventually fusing into solid bone and growth stops. *Synonyms: Epiphyseal plate.*

> The appropriate 7th character is to be added to all codes from category S42 [unless otherwise indicated].
> A   initial encounter for closed fracture
> B   initial encounter for open fracture
> D   subsequent encounter for fracture with routine healing
> G   subsequent encounter for fracture with delayed healing
> K   subsequent encounter for fracture with nonunion
> P   subsequent encounter for fracture with malunion
> S   sequela

√5ᵗʰ **S42.0 Fracture of clavicle**

  √6ᵗʰ **S42.00 Fracture of unspecified part of clavicle**

    3 √7ᵗʰ **S42.001 Fracture of unspecified part of right clavicle** CC H5

    3 √7ᵗʰ **S42.002 Fracture of unspecified part of left clavicle** CC H5

    3 √7ᵗʰ **S42.009 Fracture of unspecified part of unspecified clavicle** CC H5
             AHA: 2012,4Q,93

  √6ᵗʰ **S42.01 Fracture of sternal end of clavicle**

    3 √7ᵗʰ **S42.011 Anterior displaced fracture of sternal end of right clavicle** CC H5

    3 √7ᵗʰ **S42.012 Anterior displaced fracture of sternal end of left clavicle** CC H5

    3 √7ᵗʰ **S42.013 Anterior displaced fracture of sternal end of unspecified clavicle** CC H5
             Displaced fracture of sternal end of clavicle NOS

    3 √7ᵗʰ **S42.014 Posterior displaced fracture of sternal end of right clavicle** CC H5

    3 √7ᵗʰ **S42.015 Posterior displaced fracture of sternal end of left clavicle** CC H5

    3 √7ᵗʰ **S42.016 Posterior displaced fracture of sternal end of unspecified clavicle** CC H5

    3 √7ᵗʰ **S42.017 Nondisplaced fracture of sternal end of right clavicle** CC H5

    3 √7ᵗʰ **S42.018 Nondisplaced fracture of sternal end of left clavicle** CC H5

    3 √7ᵗʰ **S42.019 Nondisplaced fracture of sternal end of unspecified clavicle** CC H5

  √6ᵗʰ **S42.02 Fracture of shaft of clavicle**

    3 √7ᵗʰ **S42.021 Displaced fracture of shaft of right clavicle** CC H5

    3 √7ᵗʰ **S42.022 Displaced fracture of shaft of left clavicle** CC H5

    3 √7ᵗʰ **S42.023 Displaced fracture of shaft of unspecified clavicle** CC H5

    3 √7ᵗʰ **S42.024 Nondisplaced fracture of shaft of right clavicle** CC H5

    3 √7ᵗʰ **S42.025 Nondisplaced fracture of shaft of left clavicle** CC H5

    3 √7ᵗʰ **S42.026 Nondisplaced fracture of shaft of unspecified clavicle** CC H5

  √6ᵗʰ **S42.03 Fracture of lateral end of clavicle**
          Fracture of acromial end of clavicle

    3 √7ᵗʰ **S42.031 Displaced fracture of lateral end of right clavicle** CC H5

    3 √7ᵗʰ **S42.032 Displaced fracture of lateral end of left clavicle** CC H5

    3 √7ᵗʰ **S42.033 Displaced fracture of lateral end of unspecified clavicle** CC H5

    3 √7ᵗʰ **S42.034 Nondisplaced fracture of lateral end of right clavicle** CC H5

    3 √7ᵗʰ **S42.035 Nondisplaced fracture of lateral end of left clavicle** CC H5

    3 √7ᵗʰ **S42.036 Nondisplaced fracture of lateral end of unspecified clavicle** CC H5

√5ᵗʰ **S42.1 Fracture of scapula**

  √6ᵗʰ **S42.10 Fracture of unspecified part of scapula**

    3 √7ᵗʰ **S42.101 Fracture of unspecified part of scapula, right shoulder** CC H5

    3 √7ᵗʰ **S42.102 Fracture of unspecified part of scapula, left shoulder** CC H5

    3 √7ᵗʰ **S42.109 Fracture of unspecified part of scapula, unspecified shoulder** CC H5

  √6ᵗʰ **S42.11 Fracture of body of scapula**

    3 √7ᵗʰ **S42.111 Displaced fracture of body of scapula, right shoulder** CC H5

    3 √7ᵗʰ **S42.112 Displaced fracture of body of scapula, left shoulder** CC H5

    3 √7ᵗʰ **S42.113 Displaced fracture of body of scapula, unspecified shoulder** CC H5

    3 √7ᵗʰ **S42.114 Nondisplaced fracture of body of scapula, right shoulder** CC H5

    3 √7ᵗʰ **S42.115 Nondisplaced fracture of body of scapula, left shoulder** CC H5

    3 √7ᵗʰ **S42.116 Nondisplaced fracture of body of scapula, unspecified shoulder** CC H5

  √6ᵗʰ **S42.12 Fracture of acromial process**

    3 √7ᵗʰ **S42.121 Displaced fracture of acromial process, right shoulder** CC H5

    3 √7ᵗʰ **S42.122 Displaced fracture of acromial process, left shoulder** CC H5

    3 √7ᵗʰ **S42.123 Displaced fracture of acromial process, unspecified shoulder** CC H5

    3 √7ᵗʰ **S42.124 Nondisplaced fracture of acromial process, right shoulder** CC H5

    3 √7ᵗʰ **S42.125 Nondisplaced fracture of acromial process, left shoulder** CC H5

    3 √7ᵗʰ **S42.126 Nondisplaced fracture of acromial process, unspecified shoulder** CC H5

  √6ᵗʰ **S42.13 Fracture of coracoid process**

    3 √7ᵗʰ **S42.131 Displaced fracture of coracoid process, right shoulder** CC H5

    3 √7ᵗʰ **S42.132 Displaced fracture of coracoid process, left shoulder** CC H5

    3 √7ᵗʰ **S42.133 Displaced fracture of coracoid process, unspecified shoulder** CC H5

    3 √7ᵗʰ **S42.134 Nondisplaced fracture of coracoid process, right shoulder** CC H5

    3 √7ᵗʰ **S42.135 Nondisplaced fracture of coracoid process, left shoulder** CC H5

    3 √7ᵗʰ **S42.136 Nondisplaced fracture of coracoid process, unspecified shoulder** CC H5

  √6ᵗʰ **S42.14 Fracture of glenoid cavity of scapula**

    3 √7ᵗʰ **S42.141 Displaced fracture of glenoid cavity of scapula, right shoulder** CC H5

    3 √7ᵗʰ **S42.142 Displaced fracture of glenoid cavity of scapula, left shoulder** CC H5

    3 √7ᵗʰ **S42.143 Displaced fracture of glenoid cavity of scapula, unspecified shoulder** CC H5

    3 √7ᵗʰ **S42.144 Nondisplaced fracture of glenoid cavity of scapula, right shoulder** CC H5

    3 √7ᵗʰ **S42.145 Nondisplaced fracture of glenoid cavity of scapula, left shoulder** CC H5

    3 √7ᵗʰ **S42.146 Nondisplaced fracture of glenoid cavity of scapula, unspecified shoulder** CC H5

  √6ᵗʰ **S42.15 Fracture of neck of scapula**

    3 √7ᵗʰ **S42.151 Displaced fracture of neck of scapula, right shoulder** CC H5

    3 √7ᵗʰ **S42.152 Displaced fracture of neck of scapula, left shoulder** CC H5

    3 √7ᵗʰ **S42.153 Displaced fracture of neck of scapula, unspecified shoulder** CC H5

    3 √7ᵗʰ **S42.154 Nondisplaced fracture of neck of scapula, right shoulder** CC H5

    3 √7ᵗʰ **S42.155 Nondisplaced fracture of neck of scapula, left shoulder** CC H5

☑ Additional Character Required   √x7ᵗʰ Placeholder   Unacceptable PDx   Questionable PDx   Manifestation   Unspecified Dx   H1-H14 HAC   HCC CMS-HCC Dx   HIV HIV Dx

ICD-10-CM 2021   1007

Chapter 19. Injury, Poisoning and Certain Other Consequences of External Causes

S42.156–S42.309

³ √7ᵗʰ **S42.156** **Nondisplaced** fracture of neck of scapula, unspecified shoulder   CC H5

√6ᵗʰ **S42.19** **Fracture of other part of scapula**

³ √7ᵗʰ **S42.191** Fracture of other part of scapula, **right** shoulder   CC H5

³ √7ᵗʰ **S42.192** Fracture of other part of scapula, **left** shoulder   CC H5

³ √7ᵗʰ **S42.199** Fracture of other part of scapula, unspecified shoulder   CC H5

√5ᵗʰ **S42.2** **Fracture of upper end of humerus**

Fracture of proximal end of humerus

EXCLUDES 2   *fracture of shaft of humerus (S42.3-)*

physeal fracture of upper end of humerus (S49.0-)

√6ᵗʰ **S42.20** **Unspecified fracture of upper end of humerus**

²,³ √7ᵗʰ **S42.201** Unspecified fracture of upper end of **right** humerus   MCC CC H5

²,³ √7ᵗʰ **S42.202** Unspecified fracture of upper end of **left** humerus   MCC CC H5

²,³ √7ᵗʰ **S42.209** Unspecified fracture of upper end of unspecified humerus   MCC CC H5

√6ᵗʰ **S42.21** **Unspecified fracture of surgical neck of humerus**

Fracture of neck of humerus NOS

²,³ √7ᵗʰ **S42.211** Unspecified **displaced** fracture of surgical neck of **right** humerus   MCC CC H5

²,³ √7ᵗʰ **S42.212** Unspecified **displaced** fracture of surgical neck of **left** humerus   MCC CC H5

²,³ √7ᵗʰ **S42.213** Unspecified **displaced** fracture of surgical neck of unspecified humerus   MCC CC H5

²,³ √7ᵗʰ **S42.214** Unspecified **nondisplaced** fracture of surgical neck of **right** humerus   MCC CC H5

²,³ √7ᵗʰ **S42.215** Unspecified **nondisplaced** fracture of surgical neck of **left** humerus   MCC CC H5

²,³ √7ᵗʰ **S42.216** Unspecified **nondisplaced** fracture of surgical neck of unspecified humerus   MCC CC H5

√6ᵗʰ **S42.22** **2-part fracture of surgical neck of humerus**

²,³ √7ᵗʰ **S42.221** 2-part **displaced** fracture of surgical neck of **right** humerus   MCC CC H5

²,³ √7ᵗʰ **S42.222** 2-part **displaced** fracture of surgical neck of **left** humerus   MCC CC H5

²,³ √7ᵗʰ **S42.223** 2-part **displaced** fracture of surgical neck of unspecified humerus   MCC CC H5

²,³ √7ᵗʰ **S42.224** 2-part **nondisplaced** fracture of surgical neck of **right** humerus   MCC CC H5

²,³ √7ᵗʰ **S42.225** 2-part **nondisplaced** fracture of surgical neck of **left** humerus   MCC CC H5

²,³ √7ᵗʰ **S42.226** 2-part **nondisplaced** fracture of surgical neck of unspecified humerus   MCC CC H5

√6ᵗʰ **S42.23** **3-part fracture of surgical neck of humerus**

²,³ √7ᵗʰ **S42.231** 3-part fracture of surgical neck of **right** humerus   MCC CC H5

²,³ √7ᵗʰ **S42.232** 3-part fracture of surgical neck of **left** humerus   MCC CC H5

²,³ √7ᵗʰ **S42.239** 3-part fracture of surgical neck of unspecified humerus   MCC CC H5

√6ᵗʰ **S42.24** **4-part fracture of surgical neck of humerus**

²,³ √7ᵗʰ **S42.241** 4-part fracture of surgical neck of **right** humerus   MCC CC H5

²,³ √7ᵗʰ **S42.242** 4-part fracture of surgical neck of **left** humerus   MCC CC H5

²,³ √7ᵗʰ **S42.249** 4-part fracture of surgical neck of unspecified humerus   MCC CC H5

√6ᵗʰ **S42.25** **Fracture of greater tuberosity of humerus**

²,³ √7ᵗʰ **S42.251** **Displaced** fracture of greater tuberosity of **right** humerus   MCC CC H5

²,³ √7ᵗʰ **S42.252** **Displaced** fracture of greater tuberosity of **left** humerus   MCC CC H5

²,³ √7ᵗʰ **S42.253** **Displaced** fracture of greater tuberosity of unspecified humerus   MCC CC H5

²,³ √7ᵗʰ **S42.254** **Nondisplaced** fracture of greater tuberosity of **right** humerus   MCC CC H5

²,³ √7ᵗʰ **S42.255** **Nondisplaced** fracture of greater tuberosity of **left** humerus   MCC CC H5

²,³ √7ᵗʰ **S42.256** **Nondisplaced** fracture of greater tuberosity of unspecified humerus   MCC CC H5

√6ᵗʰ **S42.26** **Fracture of lesser tuberosity of humerus**

²,³ √7ᵗʰ **S42.261** **Displaced** fracture of lesser tuberosity of **right** humerus   MCC CC H5

²,³ √7ᵗʰ **S42.262** **Displaced** fracture of lesser tuberosity of **left** humerus   MCC CC H5

²,³ √7ᵗʰ **S42.263** **Displaced** fracture of lesser tuberosity of unspecified humerus   MCC CC H5

²,³ √7ᵗʰ **S42.264** **Nondisplaced** fracture of lesser tuberosity of **right** humerus   MCC CC H5

²,³ √7ᵗʰ **S42.265** **Nondisplaced** fracture of lesser tuberosity of **left** humerus   MCC CC H5

²,³ √7ᵗʰ **S42.266** **Nondisplaced** fracture of lesser tuberosity of unspecified humerus   MCC CC H5

√6ᵗʰ **S42.27** **Torus fracture of upper end of humerus**

The appropriate 7th character is to be added to all codes in subcategory S42.27

A   initial encounter for closed fracture

D   subsequent encounter for fracture with routine healing

G   subsequent encounter for fracture with delayed healing

K   subsequent encounter for fracture with nonunion

P   subsequent encounter for fracture with malunion

S   sequela

³ √7ᵗʰ **S42.271** Torus fracture of upper end of **right** humerus   CC H5

³ √7ᵗʰ **S42.272** Torus fracture of upper end of **left** humerus   CC H5

³ √7ᵗʰ **S42.279** Torus fracture of upper end of unspecified humerus   CC H5

√6ᵗʰ **S42.29** **Other fracture of upper end of humerus**

Fracture of anatomical neck of humerus

Fracture of articular head of humerus

AHA: 2019,1Q,18

²,³ √7ᵗʰ **S42.291** Other **displaced** fracture of upper end of **right** humerus   MCC CC H5

²,³ √7ᵗʰ **S42.292** Other **displaced** fracture of upper end of **left** humerus   MCC CC H5

²,³ √7ᵗʰ **S42.293** Other **displaced** fracture of upper end of unspecified humerus   MCC CC H5

²,³ √7ᵗʰ **S42.294** Other **nondisplaced** fracture of upper end of **right** humerus   MCC CC H5

²,³ √7ᵗʰ **S42.295** Other **nondisplaced** fracture of upper end of **left** humerus   MCC CC H5

²,³ √7ᵗʰ **S42.296** Other **nondisplaced** fracture of upper end of unspecified humerus   MCC CC H5

√5ᵗʰ **S42.3** **Fracture of shaft of humerus**

Fracture of humerus NOS

Fracture of upper arm NOS

EXCLUDES 2   *physeal fractures of upper end of humerus (S49.0-)*

physeal fractures of lower end of humerus (S49.1-)

√6ᵗʰ **S42.30** **Unspecified fracture of shaft of humerus**

²,³ √7ᵗʰ **S42.301** Unspecified fracture of shaft of humerus, **right arm**   MCC CC H5

²,³ √7ᵗʰ **S42.302** Unspecified fracture of shaft of humerus, **left arm**   MCC CC H5

²,³ √7ᵗʰ **S42.309** Unspecified fracture of shaft of humerus, unspecified arm   MCC CC H5

N Newborn: 0   P Pediatric: 0-17   M Maternity: 9-64   A Adult: 15-124   MCC Major Complication/Comorbidity   CC Complication/Comorbidity   SW Severe Wound Dx

1008   ICD-10-CM 2021

√6ᵗʰ **S42.31** **Greenstick** fracture of shaft of humerus

> The appropriate 7th character is to be added to all codes in subcategory S42.31
> A initial encounter for closed fracture
> D subsequent encounter for fracture with routine healing
> G subsequent encounter for fracture with delayed healing
> K subsequent encounter for fracture with nonunion
> P subsequent encounter for fracture with malunion
> S sequela

    ³ √7ᵗʰ **S42.311** **Greenstick** fracture of shaft of humerus, **right arm** `CC` `H5`

    ³ √7ᵗʰ **S42.312** **Greenstick** fracture of shaft of humerus, **left arm** `CC` `H5`

    ³ √7ᵗʰ **S42.319** **Greenstick** fracture of shaft of humerus, **unspecified arm** `CC` `H5`

√6ᵗʰ **S42.32** **Transverse** fracture of shaft of humerus

    ²,³ √7ᵗʰ **S42.321** Displaced **transverse** fracture of shaft of humerus, **right arm** `MCC` `CC` `H5`

    ²,³ √7ᵗʰ **S42.322** Displaced **transverse** fracture of shaft of humerus, **left arm** `MCC` `CC` `H5`

    ²,³ √7ᵗʰ **S42.323** Displaced **transverse** fracture of shaft of humerus, **unspecified arm** `MCC` `CC` `H5`

    ²,³ √7ᵗʰ **S42.324** Nondisplaced **transverse** fracture of shaft of humerus, **right arm** `MCC` `CC` `H5`

    ²,³ √7ᵗʰ **S42.325** Nondisplaced **transverse** fracture of shaft of humerus, **left arm** `MCC` `CC` `H5`

    ²,³ √7ᵗʰ **S42.326** Nondisplaced **transverse** fracture of shaft of humerus, **unspecified arm** `MCC` `CC` `H5`

√6ᵗʰ **S42.33** **Oblique** fracture of shaft of humerus

    ²,³ √7ᵗʰ **S42.331** Displaced **oblique** fracture of shaft of humerus, **right arm** `MCC` `CC` `H5`

    ²,³ √7ᵗʰ **S42.332** Displaced **oblique** fracture of shaft of humerus, **left arm** `MCC` `CC` `H5`

    ²,³ √7ᵗʰ **S42.333** Displaced **oblique** fracture of shaft of humerus, **unspecified arm** `MCC` `CC` `H5`

    ²,³ √7ᵗʰ **S42.334** Nondisplaced **oblique** fracture of shaft of humerus, **right arm** `MCC` `CC` `H5`

    ²,³ √7ᵗʰ **S42.335** Nondisplaced **oblique** fracture of shaft of humerus, **left arm** `MCC` `CC` `H5`

    ²,³ √7ᵗʰ **S42.336** Nondisplaced **oblique** fracture of shaft of humerus, **unspecified arm** `MCC` `CC` `H5`

√6ᵗʰ **S42.34** **Spiral** fracture of shaft of humerus

    ²,³ √7ᵗʰ **S42.341** Displaced **spiral** fracture of shaft of humerus, **right arm** `MCC` `CC` `H5`

    ²,³ √7ᵗʰ **S42.342** Displaced **spiral** fracture of shaft of humerus, **left arm** `MCC` `CC` `H5`

    ²,³ √7ᵗʰ **S42.343** Displaced **spiral** fracture of shaft of humerus, **unspecified arm** `MCC` `CC` `H5`

    ²,³ √7ᵗʰ **S42.344** Nondisplaced **spiral** fracture of shaft of humerus, **right arm** `MCC` `CC` `H5`

    ²,³ √7ᵗʰ **S42.345** Nondisplaced **spiral** fracture of shaft of humerus, **left arm** `MCC` `CC` `H5`

    ²,³ √7ᵗʰ **S42.346** Nondisplaced **spiral** fracture of shaft of humerus, **unspecified arm** `MCC` `CC` `H5`

√6ᵗʰ **S42.35** **Comminuted** fracture of shaft of humerus

    ²,³ √7ᵗʰ **S42.351** Displaced **comminuted** fracture of shaft of humerus, **right arm** `MCC` `CC` `H5`

    ²,³ √7ᵗʰ **S42.352** Displaced **comminuted** fracture of shaft of humerus, **left arm** `MCC` `CC` `H5`

    ²,³ √7ᵗʰ **S42.353** Displaced **comminuted** fracture of shaft of humerus, **unspecified arm** `MCC` `CC` `H5`

    ²,³ √7ᵗʰ **S42.354** Nondisplaced **comminuted** fracture of shaft of humerus, **right arm** `MCC` `CC` `H5`

    ²,³ √7ᵗʰ **S42.355** Nondisplaced **comminuted** fracture of shaft of humerus, **left arm** `MCC` `CC` `H5`

    ²,³ √7ᵗʰ **S42.356** Nondisplaced **comminuted** fracture of shaft of humerus, **unspecified arm** `MCC` `CC` `H5`

√6ᵗʰ **S42.36** **Segmental** fracture of shaft of humerus

    ²,³ √7ᵗʰ **S42.361** Displaced **segmental** fracture of shaft of humerus, **right arm** `MCC` `CC` `H5`

    ²,³ √7ᵗʰ **S42.362** Displaced **segmental** fracture of shaft of humerus, **left arm** `MCC` `CC` `H5`

    ²,³ √7ᵗʰ **S42.363** Displaced **segmental** fracture of shaft of humerus, **unspecified arm** `MCC` `CC` `H5`

    ²,³ √7ᵗʰ **S42.364** Nondisplaced **segmental** fracture of shaft of humerus, **right arm** `MCC` `CC` `H5`

    ²,³ √7ᵗʰ **S42.365** Nondisplaced **segmental** fracture of shaft of humerus, **left arm** `MCC` `CC` `H5`

    ²,³ √7ᵗʰ **S42.366** Nondisplaced **segmental** fracture of shaft of humerus, **unspecified arm** `MCC` `CC` `H5`

√6ᵗʰ **S42.39** **Other** fracture of shaft of humerus

    ²,³ √7ᵗʰ **S42.391** **Other** fracture of shaft of **right** humerus `MCC` `CC` `H5`

    ²,³ √7ᵗʰ **S42.392** **Other** fracture of shaft of **left** humerus `MCC` `CC` `H5`

    ²,³ √7ᵗʰ **S42.399** **Other** fracture of shaft of **unspecified** humerus `MCC` `CC` `H5`

√5ᵗʰ **S42.4** Fracture of **lower end** of humerus

Fracture of distal end of humerus

> *EXCLUDES 2*   *fracture of shaft of humerus (S42.3-)*
> *physeal fracture of lower end of humerus (S49.1-)*

√6ᵗʰ **S42.40** **Unspecified** fracture of lower end of humerus

Fracture of elbow NOS

    ²,³ √7ᵗʰ **S42.401** **Unspecified** fracture of lower end of **right** humerus `MCC` `CC` `H5`

    ²,³ √7ᵗʰ **S42.402** **Unspecified** fracture of lower end of **left** humerus `MCC` `CC` `H5`

    ²,³ √7ᵗʰ **S42.409** **Unspecified** fracture of lower end of **unspecified** humerus `MCC` `CC` `H5`

√6ᵗʰ **S42.41** **Simple supracondylar** fracture without **intercondylar** fracture of humerus

    ²,³ √7ᵗʰ **S42.411** Displaced **simple supracondylar** fracture without intercondylar fracture of **right** humerus `MCC` `CC` `H5`

    ²,³ √7ᵗʰ **S42.412** Displaced **simple supracondylar** fracture without intercondylar fracture of **left** humerus `MCC` `CC` `H5`

    ²,³ √7ᵗʰ **S42.413** Displaced **simple supracondylar** fracture without intercondylar fracture of **unspecified** humerus `MCC` `CC` `H5`

    ²,³ √7ᵗʰ **S42.414** Nondisplaced **simple supracondylar** fracture without intercondylar fracture of **right** humerus `MCC` `CC` `H5`

    ²,³ √7ᵗʰ **S42.415** Nondisplaced **simple supracondylar** fracture without intercondylar fracture of **left** humerus `MCC` `CC` `H5`

    ²,³ √7ᵗʰ **S42.416** Nondisplaced **simple supracondylar** fracture without intercondylar fracture of **unspecified** humerus `MCC` `CC` `H5`

√6ᵗʰ **S42.42** **Comminuted supracondylar** fracture without **intercondylar** fracture of humerus

    ²,³ √7ᵗʰ **S42.421** Displaced **comminuted supracondylar** fracture without intercondylar fracture of **right** humerus `MCC` `CC` `H5`

    ²,³ √7ᵗʰ **S42.422** Displaced **comminuted supracondylar** fracture without intercondylar fracture of **left** humerus `MCC` `CC` `H5`

    ²,³ √7ᵗʰ **S42.423** Displaced **comminuted supracondylar** fracture without intercondylar fracture of **unspecified** humerus `MCC` `CC` `H5`

    ²,³ √7ᵗʰ **S42.424** Nondisplaced **comminuted supracondylar** fracture without intercondylar fracture of **right** humerus `MCC` `CC` `H5`

    ²,³ √7ᵗʰ **S42.425** Nondisplaced **comminuted supracondylar** fracture without intercondylar fracture of **left** humerus `MCC` `CC` `H5`

    ²,³ √7ᵗʰ **S42.426** Nondisplaced **comminuted supracondylar** fracture without intercondylar fracture of **unspecified** humerus `MCC` `CC` `H5`

√6ᵗʰ **S42.43** Fracture (avulsion) of **lateral epicondyle** of humerus

    ²,³ √7ᵗʰ **S42.431** Displaced **fracture (avulsion)** of lateral epicondyle of **right** humerus `MCC` `CC` `H5`

    ²,³ √7ᵗʰ **S42.432** Displaced **fracture (avulsion)** of lateral epicondyle of **left** humerus `MCC` `CC` `H5`

    ²,³ √7ᵗʰ **S42.433** Displaced **fracture (avulsion)** of lateral epicondyle of **unspecified** humerus `MCC` `CC` `H5`

2,3 ✓7ᵗʰ **S42.434** Nondisplaced fracture (avulsion) of lateral epicondyle of right humerus `MCC` `CC` `H5`

2,3 ✓7ᵗʰ **S42.435** Nondisplaced fracture (avulsion) of lateral epicondyle of left humerus `MCC` `CC` `H5`

2,3 ✓7ᵗʰ **S42.436** Nondisplaced fracture (avulsion) of lateral epicondyle of unspecified humerus `MCC` `CC` `H5`

✓6ᵗʰ **S42.44** Fracture (avulsion) of medial epicondyle of humerus

    2,3 ✓7ᵗʰ **S42.441** Displaced fracture (avulsion) of medial epicondyle of right humerus `MCC` `CC` `H5`

    2,3 ✓7ᵗʰ **S42.442** Displaced fracture (avulsion) of medial epicondyle of left humerus `MCC` `CC` `H5`

    2,3 ✓7ᵗʰ **S42.443** Displaced fracture (avulsion) of medial epicondyle of unspecified humerus `MCC` `CC` `H5`

    2,3 ✓7ᵗʰ **S42.444** Nondisplaced fracture (avulsion) of medial epicondyle of right humerus `MCC` `CC` `H5`

    2,3 ✓7ᵗʰ **S42.445** Nondisplaced fracture (avulsion) of medial epicondyle of left humerus `MCC` `CC` `H5`

    2,3 ✓7ᵗʰ **S42.446** Nondisplaced fracture (avulsion) of medial epicondyle of unspecified humerus `MCC` `CC` `H5`

    2,3 ✓7ᵗʰ **S42.447** Incarcerated fracture (avulsion) of medial epicondyle of right humerus `MCC` `CC` `H5`

    2,3 ✓7ᵗʰ **S42.448** Incarcerated fracture (avulsion) of medial epicondyle of left humerus `MCC` `CC` `H5`

    2,3 ✓7ᵗʰ **S42.449** Incarcerated fracture (avulsion) of medial epicondyle of unspecified humerus `MCC` `CC` `H5`

✓6ᵗʰ **S42.45** Fracture of lateral condyle of humerus

    Fracture of capitellum of humerus

    2,3 ✓7ᵗʰ **S42.451** Displaced fracture of lateral condyle of right humerus `MCC` `CC` `H5`

    2,3 ✓7ᵗʰ **S42.452** Displaced fracture of lateral condyle of left humerus `MCC` `CC` `H5`

    2,3 ✓7ᵗʰ **S42.453** Displaced fracture of lateral condyle of unspecified humerus `MCC` `CC` `H5`

    2,3 ✓7ᵗʰ **S42.454** Nondisplaced fracture of lateral condyle of right humerus `MCC` `CC` `H5`

    2,3 ✓7ᵗʰ **S42.455** Nondisplaced fracture of lateral condyle of left humerus `MCC` `CC` `H5`

    2,3 ✓7ᵗʰ **S42.456** Nondisplaced fracture of lateral condyle of unspecified humerus `MCC` `CC` `H5`

✓6ᵗʰ **S42.46** Fracture of medial condyle of humerus

    Trochlea fracture of humerus

    2,3 ✓7ᵗʰ **S42.461** Displaced fracture of medial condyle of right humerus `MCC` `CC` `H5`

    2,3 ✓7ᵗʰ **S42.462** Displaced fracture of medial condyle of left humerus `MCC` `CC` `H5`

    2,3 ✓7ᵗʰ **S42.463** Displaced fracture of medial condyle of unspecified humerus `MCC` `CC` `H5`

    2,3 ✓7ᵗʰ **S42.464** Nondisplaced fracture of medial condyle of right humerus `MCC` `CC` `H5`

    2,3 ✓7ᵗʰ **S42.465** Nondisplaced fracture of medial condyle of left humerus `MCC` `CC` `H5`

    2,3 ✓7ᵗʰ **S42.466** Nondisplaced fracture of medial condyle of unspecified humerus `MCC` `CC` `H5`

✓6ᵗʰ **S42.47** Transcondylar fracture of humerus

    2,3 ✓7ᵗʰ **S42.471** Displaced transcondylar fracture of right humerus `MCC` `CC` `H5`

    2,3 ✓7ᵗʰ **S42.472** Displaced transcondylar fracture of left humerus `MCC` `CC` `H5`

    2,3 ✓7ᵗʰ **S42.473** Displaced transcondylar fracture of unspecified humerus `MCC` `CC` `H5`

    2,3 ✓7ᵗʰ **S42.474** Nondisplaced transcondylar fracture of right humerus `MCC` `CC` `H5`

    2,3 ✓7ᵗʰ **S42.475** Nondisplaced transcondylar fracture of left humerus `MCC` `CC` `H5`

    2,3 ✓7ᵗʰ **S42.476** Nondisplaced transcondylar fracture of unspecified humerus `MCC` `CC` `H5`

✓6ᵗʰ **S42.48** Torus fracture of lower end of humerus

> The appropriate 7th character is to be added to all codes in subcategory S42.48.
> A   initial encounter for closed fracture
> D   subsequent encounter for fracture with routine healing
> G   subsequent encounter for fracture with delayed healing
> K   subsequent encounter for fracture with nonunion
> P   subsequent encounter for fracture with malunion
> S   sequela

    3 ✓7ᵗʰ **S42.481** Torus fracture of lower end of right humerus `CC` `H5`

    3 ✓7ᵗʰ **S42.482** Torus fracture of lower end of left humerus `CC` `H5`

    3 ✓7ᵗʰ **S42.489** Torus fracture of lower end of unspecified humerus `CC` `H5`

✓6ᵗʰ **S42.49** Other fracture of lower end of humerus

    2,3 ✓7ᵗʰ **S42.491** Other displaced fracture of lower end of right humerus `MCC` `CC` `H5`

    2,3 ✓7ᵗʰ **S42.492** Other displaced fracture of lower end of left humerus `MCC` `CC` `H5`

    2,3 ✓7ᵗʰ **S42.493** Other displaced fracture of lower end of unspecified humerus `MCC` `CC` `H5`

    2,3 ✓7ᵗʰ **S42.494** Other nondisplaced fracture of lower end of right humerus `MCC` `CC` `H5`

    2,3 ✓7ᵗʰ **S42.495** Other nondisplaced fracture of lower end of left humerus `MCC` `CC` `H5`

    2,3 ✓7ᵗʰ **S42.496** Other nondisplaced fracture of lower end of unspecified humerus `MCC` `CC` `H5`

✓5ᵗʰ **S42.9** Fracture of shoulder girdle, part unspecified

    Fracture of shoulder NOS

    2,3 ✓x7ᵗʰ **S42.90** Fracture of unspecified shoulder girdle, part unspecified `MCC` `CC` `H5`

    2,3 ✓x7ᵗʰ **S42.91** Fracture of right shoulder girdle, part unspecified `MCC` `CC` `H5`

    2,3 ✓x7ᵗʰ **S42.92** Fracture of left shoulder girdle, part unspecified `MCC` `CC` `H5`

✓4ᵗʰ **S43** Dislocation and sprain of joints and ligaments of shoulder girdle

> `INCLUDES` avulsion of joint or ligament of shoulder girdle
> laceration of cartilage, joint or ligament of shoulder girdle
> sprain of cartilage, joint or ligament of shoulder girdle
> traumatic hemarthrosis of joint or ligament of shoulder girdle
> traumatic rupture of joint or ligament of shoulder girdle
> traumatic subluxation of joint or ligament of shoulder girdle
> traumatic tear of joint or ligament of shoulder girdle

Code also any associated open wound

> `EXCLUDES 2` strain of muscle, fascia and tendon of shoulder and upper arm (S46.-)

> The appropriate 7th character is to be added to each code from category S43.
> A   initial encounter
> D   subsequent encounter
> S   sequela

✓5ᵗʰ **S43.0** Subluxation and dislocation of shoulder joint

    Dislocation of glenohumeral joint
    Subluxation of glenohumeral joint

    ✓6ᵗʰ **S43.00** Unspecified subluxation and dislocation of shoulder joint

       Dislocation of humerus NOS
       Subluxation of humerus NOS

       ✓7ᵗʰ **S43.001** Unspecified subluxation of right shoulder joint

       ✓7ᵗʰ **S43.002** Unspecified subluxation of left shoulder joint

       ✓7ᵗʰ **S43.003** Unspecified subluxation of unspecified shoulder joint

       ✓7ᵗʰ **S43.004** Unspecified dislocation of right shoulder joint

       ✓7ᵗʰ **S43.005** Unspecified dislocation of left shoulder joint

       ✓7ᵗʰ **S43.006** Unspecified dislocation of unspecified shoulder joint

Ⓝ Newborn: 0   Ⓟ Pediatric: 0-17   Ⓜ Maternity: 9-64   Ⓐ Adult: 15-124   `MCC` Major Complication/Comorbidity   `CC` Complication/Comorbidity   `SW` Severe Wound Dx

1010   ICD-10-CM 2021

√6ᵗʰ **S43.01** Anterior subluxation and dislocation of humerus
- √7ᵗʰ **S43.011** Anterior subluxation of right humerus
- √7ᵗʰ **S43.012** Anterior subluxation of left humerus
- √7ᵗʰ **S43.013** Anterior subluxation of unspecified humerus
- √7ᵗʰ **S43.014** Anterior dislocation of right humerus
- √7ᵗʰ **S43.015** Anterior dislocation of left humerus
- √7ᵗʰ **S43.016** Anterior dislocation of unspecified humerus

√6ᵗʰ **S43.02** Posterior subluxation and dislocation of humerus
- √7ᵗʰ **S43.021** Posterior subluxation of right humerus
- √7ᵗʰ **S43.022** Posterior subluxation of left humerus
- √7ᵗʰ **S43.023** Posterior subluxation of unspecified humerus
- √7ᵗʰ **S43.024** Posterior dislocation of right humerus
- √7ᵗʰ **S43.025** Posterior dislocation of left humerus
- √7ᵗʰ **S43.026** Posterior dislocation of unspecified humerus

√6ᵗʰ **S43.03** Inferior subluxation and dislocation of humerus
- √7ᵗʰ **S43.031** Inferior subluxation of right humerus
- √7ᵗʰ **S43.032** Inferior subluxation of left humerus
- √7ᵗʰ **S43.033** Inferior subluxation of unspecified humerus
- √7ᵗʰ **S43.034** Inferior dislocation of right humerus
- √7ᵗʰ **S43.035** Inferior dislocation of left humerus
- √7ᵗʰ **S43.036** Inferior dislocation of unspecified humerus

√6ᵗʰ **S43.08** Other subluxation and dislocation of shoulder joint
- √7ᵗʰ **S43.081** Other subluxation of right shoulder joint
- √7ᵗʰ **S43.082** Other subluxation of left shoulder joint
- √7ᵗʰ **S43.083** Other subluxation of unspecified shoulder joint
- √7ᵗʰ **S43.084** Other dislocation of right shoulder joint
- √7ᵗʰ **S43.085** Other dislocation of left shoulder joint
- √7ᵗʰ **S43.086** Other dislocation of unspecified shoulder joint

√5ᵗʰ **S43.1** Subluxation and dislocation of acromioclavicular joint

√6ᵗʰ **S43.10** Unspecified dislocation of acromioclavicular joint
- √7ᵗʰ **S43.101** Unspecified dislocation of right acromioclavicular joint
- √7ᵗʰ **S43.102** Unspecified dislocation of left acromioclavicular joint
- √7ᵗʰ **S43.109** Unspecified dislocation of unspecified acromioclavicular joint

√6ᵗʰ **S43.11** Subluxation of acromioclavicular joint
- √7ᵗʰ **S43.111** Subluxation of right acromioclavicular joint
- √7ᵗʰ **S43.112** Subluxation of left acromioclavicular joint
- √7ᵗʰ **S43.119** Subluxation of unspecified acromioclavicular joint

√6ᵗʰ **S43.12** Dislocation of acromioclavicular joint, 100%-200% displacement
- √7ᵗʰ **S43.121** Dislocation of right acromioclavicular joint, 100%-200% displacement
- √7ᵗʰ **S43.122** Dislocation of left acromioclavicular joint, 100%-200% displacement
- √7ᵗʰ **S43.129** Dislocation of unspecified acromioclavicular joint, 100%-200% displacement

√6ᵗʰ **S43.13** Dislocation of acromioclavicular joint, greater than 200% displacement
- √7ᵗʰ **S43.131** Dislocation of right acromioclavicular joint, greater than 200% displacement
- √7ᵗʰ **S43.132** Dislocation of left acromioclavicular joint, greater than 200% displacement
- √7ᵗʰ **S43.139** Dislocation of unspecified acromioclavicular joint, greater than 200% displacement

√6ᵗʰ **S43.14** Inferior dislocation of acromioclavicular joint
- √7ᵗʰ **S43.141** Inferior dislocation of right acromioclavicular joint
- √7ᵗʰ **S43.142** Inferior dislocation of left acromioclavicular joint
- √7ᵗʰ **S43.149** Inferior dislocation of unspecified acromioclavicular joint

√6ᵗʰ **S43.15** Posterior dislocation of acromioclavicular joint
- √7ᵗʰ **S43.151** Posterior dislocation of right acromioclavicular joint
- √7ᵗʰ **S43.152** Posterior dislocation of left acromioclavicular joint
- √7ᵗʰ **S43.159** Posterior dislocation of unspecified acromioclavicular joint

√5ᵗʰ **S43.2** Subluxation and dislocation of sternoclavicular joint

√6ᵗʰ **S43.20** Unspecified subluxation and dislocation of sternoclavicular joint
- √7ᵗʰ **S43.201** Unspecified subluxation of right sternoclavicular joint   CC H5
- √7ᵗʰ **S43.202** Unspecified subluxation of left sternoclavicular joint   CC H5
- √7ᵗʰ **S43.203** Unspecified subluxation of unspecified sternoclavicular joint   CC H5
- √7ᵗʰ **S43.204** Unspecified dislocation of right sternoclavicular joint   CC H5
- √7ᵗʰ **S43.205** Unspecified dislocation of left sternoclavicular joint   CC H5
- √7ᵗʰ **S43.206** Unspecified dislocation of unspecified sternoclavicular joint   CC H5

√6ᵗʰ **S43.21** Anterior subluxation and dislocation of sternoclavicular joint
- √7ᵗʰ **S43.211** Anterior subluxation of right sternoclavicular joint   CC H5
- √7ᵗʰ **S43.212** Anterior subluxation of left sternoclavicular joint   CC H5
- √7ᵗʰ **S43.213** Anterior subluxation of unspecified sternoclavicular joint   CC H5
- √7ᵗʰ **S43.214** Anterior dislocation of right sternoclavicular joint   CC H5
- √7ᵗʰ **S43.215** Anterior dislocation of left sternoclavicular joint   CC H5
- √7ᵗʰ **S43.216** Anterior dislocation of unspecified sternoclavicular joint   CC H5

√6ᵗʰ **S43.22** Posterior subluxation and dislocation of sternoclavicular joint
- √7ᵗʰ **S43.221** Posterior subluxation of right sternoclavicular joint   CC H5
- √7ᵗʰ **S43.222** Posterior subluxation of left sternoclavicular joint   CC H5
- √7ᵗʰ **S43.223** Posterior subluxation of unspecified sternoclavicular joint   CC H5
- √7ᵗʰ **S43.224** Posterior dislocation of right sternoclavicular joint   CC H5
- √7ᵗʰ **S43.225** Posterior dislocation of left sternoclavicular joint   CC H5
- √7ᵗʰ **S43.226** Posterior dislocation of unspecified sternoclavicular joint   CC H5

√5ᵗʰ **S43.3** Subluxation and dislocation of other and unspecified parts of shoulder girdle

√6ᵗʰ **S43.30** Subluxation and dislocation of unspecified parts of shoulder girdle
- Dislocation of shoulder girdle NOS
- Subluxation of shoulder girdle NOS
- √7ᵗʰ **S43.301** Subluxation of unspecified parts of right shoulder girdle
- √7ᵗʰ **S43.302** Subluxation of unspecified parts of left shoulder girdle
- √7ᵗʰ **S43.303** Subluxation of unspecified parts of unspecified shoulder girdle
- √7ᵗʰ **S43.304** Dislocation of unspecified parts of right shoulder girdle
- √7ᵗʰ **S43.305** Dislocation of unspecified parts of left shoulder girdle
- √7ᵗʰ **S43.306** Dislocation of unspecified parts of unspecified shoulder girdle

√6ᵗʰ **S43.31** Subluxation and dislocation of scapula
- √7ᵗʰ **S43.311** Subluxation of right scapula
- √7ᵗʰ **S43.312** Subluxation of left scapula
- √7ᵗʰ **S43.313** Subluxation of unspecified scapula
- √7ᵗʰ **S43.314** Dislocation of right scapula
- √7ᵗʰ **S43.315** Dislocation of left scapula
- √7ᵗʰ **S43.316** Dislocation of unspecified scapula

√6ᵗʰ **S43.39** Subluxation and dislocation of other parts of shoulder girdle
- √7ᵗʰ **S43.391** Subluxation of other parts of right shoulder girdle

✓ Additional Character Required   ✓ₓ7ᵗʰ Placeholder   Unacceptable PDx   Questionable PDx   Manifestation   Unspecified Dx   H1-H14 HAC   HCC CMS-HCC Dx   HIV HIV Dx

ICD-10-CM 2021   1011

√7th **S43.392** Subluxation of other parts of left shoulder girdle

√7th **S43.393** Subluxation of other parts of unspecified shoulder girdle

√7th **S43.394** Dislocation of other parts of right shoulder girdle

√7th **S43.395** Dislocation of other parts of left shoulder girdle

√7th **S43.396** Dislocation of other parts of unspecified shoulder girdle

√5th **S43.4** Sprain of shoulder joint

√6th **S43.40** Unspecified sprain of shoulder joint

√7th **S43.401** Unspecified sprain of right shoulder joint

√7th **S43.402** Unspecified sprain of left shoulder joint

√7th **S43.409** Unspecified sprain of unspecified shoulder joint

√6th **S43.41** Sprain of coracohumeral (ligament)

√7th **S43.411** Sprain of right coracohumeral (ligament)

√7th **S43.412** Sprain of left coracohumeral (ligament)

√7th **S43.419** Sprain of unspecified coracohumeral (ligament)

√6th **S43.42** Sprain of rotator cuff capsule

EXCLUDES 1   rotator cuff syndrome (complete) (incomplete), not specified as traumatic (M75.1-)

EXCLUDES 2   injury of tendon of rotator cuff (S46.0-)

√7th **S43.421** Sprain of right rotator cuff capsule

√7th **S43.422** Sprain of left rotator cuff capsule

√7th **S43.429** Sprain of unspecified rotator cuff capsule

√6th **S43.43** Superior glenoid labrum lesion

SLAP lesion

AHA: 2019,2Q,26

DEF: Detachment injury of the superior aspect of the glenoid labrum, which is the ring of fibrocartilage attached to the rim of the glenoid cavity of the scapula.

√7th **S43.431** Superior glenoid labrum lesion of right shoulder

√7th **S43.432** Superior glenoid labrum lesion of left shoulder

√7th **S43.439** Superior glenoid labrum lesion of unspecified shoulder

√6th **S43.49** Other sprain of shoulder joint

√7th **S43.491** Other sprain of right shoulder joint

√7th **S43.492** Other sprain of left shoulder joint

√7th **S43.499** Other sprain of unspecified shoulder joint

√5th **S43.5** Sprain of acromioclavicular joint

Sprain of acromioclavicular ligament

√x7th **S43.50** Sprain of unspecified acromioclavicular joint

√x7th **S43.51** Sprain of right acromioclavicular joint

√x7th **S43.52** Sprain of left acromioclavicular joint

√5th **S43.6** Sprain of sternoclavicular joint

√x7th **S43.60** Sprain of unspecified sternoclavicular joint

√x7th **S43.61** Sprain of right sternoclavicular joint

√x7th **S43.62** Sprain of left sternoclavicular joint

√5th **S43.8** Sprain of other specified parts of shoulder girdle

√x7th **S43.80** Sprain of other specified parts of unspecified shoulder girdle

√x7th **S43.81** Sprain of other specified parts of right shoulder girdle

√x7th **S43.82** Sprain of other specified parts of left shoulder girdle

√5th **S43.9** Sprain of unspecified parts of shoulder girdle

√x7th **S43.90** Sprain of unspecified parts of unspecified shoulder girdle

Sprain of shoulder girdle NOS

√x7th **S43.91** Sprain of unspecified parts of right shoulder girdle

√x7th **S43.92** Sprain of unspecified parts of left shoulder girdle

√4th **S44** Injury of nerves at shoulder and upper arm level

Code also any associated open wound (S41.-)

EXCLUDES 2   injury of brachial plexus (S14.3-)

The appropriate 7th character is to be added to each code from category S44.

A   initial encounter
D   subsequent encounter
S   sequela

√5th **S44.0** Injury of ulnar nerve at upper arm level

EXCLUDES 1   ulnar nerve NOS (S54.0)

√x7th **S44.00** Injury of ulnar nerve at upper arm level, unspecified arm

√x7th **S44.01** Injury of ulnar nerve at upper arm level, right arm

√x7th **S44.02** Injury of ulnar nerve at upper arm level, left arm

√5th **S44.1** Injury of median nerve at upper arm level

EXCLUDES 1   median nerve NOS (S54.1)

√x7th **S44.10** Injury of median nerve at upper arm level, unspecified arm

√x7th **S44.11** Injury of median nerve at upper arm level, right arm

√x7th **S44.12** Injury of median nerve at upper arm level, left arm

√5th **S44.2** Injury of radial nerve at upper arm level

EXCLUDES 1   radial nerve NOS (S54.2)

√x7th **S44.20** Injury of radial nerve at upper arm level, unspecified arm

√x7th **S44.21** Injury of radial nerve at upper arm level, right arm

√x7th **S44.22** Injury of radial nerve at upper arm level, left arm

√5th **S44.3** Injury of axillary nerve

√x7th **S44.30** Injury of axillary nerve, unspecified arm

√x7th **S44.31** Injury of axillary nerve, right arm

√x7th **S44.32** Injury of axillary nerve, left arm

√5th **S44.4** Injury of musculocutaneous nerve

√x7th **S44.40** Injury of musculocutaneous nerve, unspecified arm

√x7th **S44.41** Injury of musculocutaneous nerve, right arm

√x7th **S44.42** Injury of musculocutaneous nerve, left arm

√5th **S44.5** Injury of cutaneous sensory nerve at shoulder and upper arm level

√x7th **S44.50** Injury of cutaneous sensory nerve at shoulder and upper arm level, unspecified arm

√x7th **S44.51** Injury of cutaneous sensory nerve at shoulder and upper arm level, right arm

√x7th **S44.52** Injury of cutaneous sensory nerve at shoulder and upper arm level, left arm

√5th **S44.8** Injury of other nerves at shoulder and upper arm level

√6th **S44.8X** Injury of other nerves at shoulder and upper arm level

√7th **S44.8X1** Injury of other nerves at shoulder and upper arm level, right arm

√7th **S44.8X2** Injury of other nerves at shoulder and upper arm level, left arm

√7th **S44.8X9** Injury of other nerves at shoulder and upper arm level, unspecified arm

√5th **S44.9** Injury of unspecified nerve at shoulder and upper arm level

√x7th **S44.90** Injury of unspecified nerve at shoulder and upper arm level, unspecified arm

√x7th **S44.91** Injury of unspecified nerve at shoulder and upper arm level, right arm

√x7th **S44.92** Injury of unspecified nerve at shoulder and upper arm level, left arm

√4th **S45** Injury of blood vessels at shoulder and upper arm level

Code also any associated open wound (S41.-)

EXCLUDES 2   injury of subclavian artery (S25.1)

injury of subclavian vein (S25.3)

The appropriate 7th character is to be added to each code from category S45.

A   initial encounter
D   subsequent encounter
S   sequela

√5th **S45.0** Injury of axillary artery

√6th **S45.00** Unspecified injury of axillary artery

√7th **S45.001** Unspecified injury of axillary artery, right side   MCC

N Newborn: 0   P Pediatric: 0-17   M Maternity: 9-64   A Adult: 15-124   MCC Major Complication/Comorbidity   CC Complication/Comorbidity   SW Severe Wound Dx

1012   ICD-10-CM 2021

√7ᵗʰ **S45.002** Unspecified injury of axillary artery, left side   MCC

√7ᵗʰ **S45.009** Unspecified injury of axillary artery, unspecified side   MCC

√6ᵗʰ **S45.01** Laceration of axillary artery

√7ᵗʰ **S45.011** Laceration of axillary artery, right side   MCC

√7ᵗʰ **S45.012** Laceration of axillary artery, left side   MCC

√7ᵗʰ **S45.019** Laceration of axillary artery, unspecified   MCC

√6ᵗʰ **S45.09** Other specified injury of axillary artery

√7ᵗʰ **S45.091** Other specified injury of axillary artery, right side   MCC

√7ᵗʰ **S45.092** Other specified injury of axillary artery, left side   MCC

√7ᵗʰ **S45.099** Other specified injury of axillary artery, unspecified side   MCC

√5ᵗʰ **S45.1** Injury of brachial artery

√6ᵗʰ **S45.10** Unspecified injury of brachial artery

√7ᵗʰ **S45.101** Unspecified injury of brachial artery, right side   CC

√7ᵗʰ **S45.102** Unspecified injury of brachial artery, left side   CC

√7ᵗʰ **S45.109** Unspecified injury of brachial artery, unspecified side   CC

√6ᵗʰ **S45.11** Laceration of brachial artery

√7ᵗʰ **S45.111** Laceration of brachial artery, right side   CC

√7ᵗʰ **S45.112** Laceration of brachial artery, left side   CC

√7ᵗʰ **S45.119** Laceration of brachial artery, unspecified side   CC

√6ᵗʰ **S45.19** Other specified injury of brachial artery

√7ᵗʰ **S45.191** Other specified injury of brachial artery, right side   CC

√7ᵗʰ **S45.192** Other specified injury of brachial artery, left side   CC

√7ᵗʰ **S45.199** Other specified injury of brachial artery, unspecified side   CC

√5ᵗʰ **S45.2** Injury of axillary or brachial vein

√6ᵗʰ **S45.20** Unspecified injury of axillary or brachial vein

√7ᵗʰ **S45.201** Unspecified injury of axillary or brachial vein, right side   CC

√7ᵗʰ **S45.202** Unspecified injury of axillary or brachial vein, left side   CC

√7ᵗʰ **S45.209** Unspecified injury of axillary or brachial vein, unspecified side   CC

√6ᵗʰ **S45.21** Laceration of axillary or brachial vein

√7ᵗʰ **S45.211** Laceration of axillary or brachial vein, right side   CC

√7ᵗʰ **S45.212** Laceration of axillary or brachial vein, left side   CC

√7ᵗʰ **S45.219** Laceration of axillary or brachial vein, unspecified side   CC

√6ᵗʰ **S45.29** Other specified injury of axillary or brachial vein

√7ᵗʰ **S45.291** Other specified injury of axillary or brachial vein, right side   CC

√7ᵗʰ **S45.292** Other specified injury of axillary or brachial vein, left side   CC

√7ᵗʰ **S45.299** Other specified injury of axillary or brachial vein, unspecified side   CC

√5ᵗʰ **S45.3** Injury of superficial vein at shoulder and upper arm level

√6ᵗʰ **S45.30** Unspecified injury of superficial vein at shoulder and upper arm level

√7ᵗʰ **S45.301** Unspecified injury of superficial vein at shoulder and upper arm level, right arm   CC

√7ᵗʰ **S45.302** Unspecified injury of superficial vein at shoulder and upper arm level, left arm   CC

√7ᵗʰ **S45.309** Unspecified injury of superficial vein at shoulder and upper arm level, unspecified arm   CC

√6ᵗʰ **S45.31** Laceration of superficial vein at shoulder and upper arm level

√7ᵗʰ **S45.311** Laceration of superficial vein at shoulder and upper arm level, right arm   CC

√7ᵗʰ **S45.312** Laceration of superficial vein at shoulder and upper arm level, left arm   CC

√7ᵗʰ **S45.319** Laceration of superficial vein at shoulder and upper arm level, unspecified   CC

√6ᵗʰ **S45.39** Other specified injury of superficial vein at shoulder and upper arm level

√7ᵗʰ **S45.391** Other specified injury of superficial vein at shoulder and upper arm level, right arm   CC

√7ᵗʰ **S45.392** Other specified injury of superficial vein at shoulder and upper arm level, left arm   CC

√7ᵗʰ **S45.399** Other specified injury of superficial vein at shoulder and upper arm level, unspecified arm   CC

√5ᵗʰ **S45.8** Injury of other specified blood vessels at shoulder and upper arm level

√6ᵗʰ **S45.80** Unspecified injury of other specified blood vessels at shoulder and upper arm level

√7ᵗʰ **S45.801** Unspecified injury of other specified blood vessels at shoulder and upper arm level, right arm   CC

√7ᵗʰ **S45.802** Unspecified injury of other specified blood vessels at shoulder and upper arm level, left arm   CC

√7ᵗʰ **S45.809** Unspecified injury of other specified blood vessels at shoulder and upper arm level, unspecified arm   CC

√6ᵗʰ **S45.81** Laceration of other specified blood vessels at shoulder and upper arm level

√7ᵗʰ **S45.811** Laceration of other specified blood vessels at shoulder and upper arm level, right arm   CC

√7ᵗʰ **S45.812** Laceration of other specified blood vessels at shoulder and upper arm level, left arm   CC

√7ᵗʰ **S45.819** Laceration of other specified blood vessels at shoulder and upper arm level, unspecified arm   CC

√6ᵗʰ **S45.89** Other specified injury of other specified blood vessels at shoulder and upper arm level

√7ᵗʰ **S45.891** Other specified injury of other specified blood vessels at shoulder and upper arm level, right arm   CC

√7ᵗʰ **S45.892** Other specified injury of other specified blood vessels at shoulder and upper arm level, left arm   CC

√7ᵗʰ **S45.899** Other specified injury of other specified blood vessels at shoulder and upper arm level, unspecified arm   CC

√5ᵗʰ **S45.9** Injury of unspecified blood vessel at shoulder and upper arm level

√6ᵗʰ **S45.90** Unspecified injury of unspecified blood vessel at shoulder and upper arm level

√7ᵗʰ **S45.901** Unspecified injury of unspecified blood vessel at shoulder and upper arm level, right arm   CC

√7ᵗʰ **S45.902** Unspecified injury of unspecified blood vessel at shoulder and upper arm level, left arm   CC

√7ᵗʰ **S45.909** Unspecified injury of unspecified blood vessel at shoulder and upper arm level, unspecified arm   CC

√6ᵗʰ **S45.91** Laceration of unspecified blood vessel at shoulder and upper arm level

√7ᵗʰ **S45.911** Laceration of unspecified blood vessel at shoulder and upper arm level, right arm   CC

√7ᵗʰ **S45.912** Laceration of unspecified blood vessel at shoulder and upper arm level, left arm   CC

√7ᵗʰ **S45.919** Laceration of unspecified blood vessel at shoulder and upper arm level, unspecified arm   CC

√6ᵗʰ **S45.99** Other specified injury of unspecified blood vessel at shoulder and upper arm level

√7ᵗʰ **S45.991** Other specified injury of unspecified blood vessel at shoulder and upper arm level, right arm   CC

√7ᵗʰ **S45.992** Other specified injury of unspecified blood vessel at shoulder and upper arm level, left arm   CC

✔ Additional Character Required   √x7ᵗʰ Placeholder   Unacceptable PDx   Questionable PDx   Manifestation   Unspecified Dx   H1-H14 HAC   HCC CMS-HCC Dx   HIV HIV Dx

ICD-10-CM 2021   **1013**

√7ᵗʰ **S45.999** Other specified injury of unspecified blood vessel at shoulder and upper arm level, unspecified arm   cc

√4ᵗʰ **S46 Injury of muscle, fascia and tendon at shoulder and upper arm level**

Code also any associated open wound (S41.-)

EXCLUDES 2   injury of muscle, fascia and tendon at elbow (S56.-)
sprain of joints and ligaments of shoulder girdle (S43.9)

TIP: Refer to the Muscle/Tendon table at the beginning of this chapter.

The appropriate 7th character is to be added to each code from category S46.
A   initial encounter
D   subsequent encounter
S   sequela

√5ᵗʰ **S46.0 Injury of muscle(s) and tendon(s) of the rotator cuff of shoulder**

√6ᵗʰ **S46.00** Unspecified injury of muscle(s) and tendon(s) of the rotator cuff of shoulder

√7ᵗʰ **S46.001** Unspecified injury of muscle(s) and tendon(s) of the rotator cuff of right shoulder

√7ᵗʰ **S46.002** Unspecified injury of muscle(s) and tendon(s) of the rotator cuff of left shoulder

√7ᵗʰ **S46.009** Unspecified injury of muscle(s) and tendon(s) of the rotator cuff of unspecified shoulder

√6ᵗʰ **S46.01** Strain of muscle(s) and tendon(s) of the rotator cuff of shoulder

√7ᵗʰ **S46.011** Strain of muscle(s) and tendon(s) of the rotator cuff of right shoulder

√7ᵗʰ **S46.012** Strain of muscle(s) and tendon(s) of the rotator cuff of left shoulder

√7ᵗʰ **S46.019** Strain of muscle(s) and tendon(s) of the rotator cuff of unspecified shoulder

√6ᵗʰ **S46.02** Laceration of muscle(s) and tendon(s) of the rotator cuff of shoulder

√7ᵗʰ **S46.021** Laceration of muscle(s) and tendon(s) of the rotator cuff of right shoulder   cc

√7ᵗʰ **S46.022** Laceration of muscle(s) and tendon(s) of the rotator cuff of left shoulder   cc

√7ᵗʰ **S46.029** Laceration of muscle(s) and tendon(s) of the rotator cuff of unspecified shoulder   cc

√6ᵗʰ **S46.09** Other injury of muscle(s) and tendon(s) of the rotator cuff of shoulder

√7ᵗʰ **S46.091** Other injury of muscle(s) and tendon(s) of the rotator cuff of right shoulder

√7ᵗʰ **S46.092** Other injury of muscle(s) and tendon(s) of the rotator cuff of left shoulder

√7ᵗʰ **S46.099** Other injury of muscle(s) and tendon(s) of the rotator cuff of unspecified shoulder

√5ᵗʰ **S46.1 Injury of muscle, fascia and tendon of long head of biceps**

√6ᵗʰ **S46.10** Unspecified injury of muscle, fascia and tendon of long head of biceps

√7ᵗʰ **S46.101** Unspecified injury of muscle, fascia and tendon of long head of biceps, right arm

√7ᵗʰ **S46.102** Unspecified injury of muscle, fascia and tendon of long head of biceps, left arm

√7ᵗʰ **S46.109** Unspecified injury of muscle, fascia and tendon of long head of biceps, unspecified arm

√6ᵗʰ **S46.11** Strain of muscle, fascia and tendon of long head of biceps

AHA: 2020,1Q,38; 2019,2Q,27

√7ᵗʰ **S46.111** Strain of muscle, fascia and tendon of long head of biceps, right arm

√7ᵗʰ **S46.112** Strain of muscle, fascia and tendon of long head of biceps, left arm

√7ᵗʰ **S46.119** Strain of muscle, fascia and tendon of long head of biceps, unspecified arm

√6ᵗʰ **S46.12** Laceration of muscle, fascia and tendon of long head of biceps

√7ᵗʰ **S46.121** Laceration of muscle, fascia and tendon of long head of biceps, right arm   cc

√7ᵗʰ **S46.122** Laceration of muscle, fascia and tendon of long head of biceps, left arm   cc

√7ᵗʰ **S46.129** Laceration of muscle, fascia and tendon of long head of biceps, unspecified arm   cc

√6ᵗʰ **S46.19** Other injury of muscle, fascia and tendon of long head of biceps

√7ᵗʰ **S46.191** Other injury of muscle, fascia and tendon of long head of biceps, right arm

√7ᵗʰ **S46.192** Other injury of muscle, fascia and tendon of long head of biceps, left arm

√7ᵗʰ **S46.199** Other injury of muscle, fascia and tendon of long head of biceps, unspecified arm

√5ᵗʰ **S46.2 Injury of muscle, fascia and tendon of other parts of biceps**

√6ᵗʰ **S46.20** Unspecified injury of muscle, fascia and tendon of other parts of biceps

√7ᵗʰ **S46.201** Unspecified injury of muscle, fascia and tendon of other parts of biceps, right arm

√7ᵗʰ **S46.202** Unspecified injury of muscle, fascia and tendon of other parts of biceps, left arm

√7ᵗʰ **S46.209** Unspecified injury of muscle, fascia and tendon of other parts of biceps, unspecified arm

√6ᵗʰ **S46.21** Strain of muscle, fascia and tendon of other parts of biceps

√7ᵗʰ **S46.211** Strain of muscle, fascia and tendon of other parts of biceps, right arm

√7ᵗʰ **S46.212** Strain of muscle, fascia and tendon of other parts of biceps, left arm

√7ᵗʰ **S46.219** Strain of muscle, fascia and tendon of other parts of biceps, unspecified arm

√6ᵗʰ **S46.22** Laceration of muscle, fascia and tendon of other parts of biceps

√7ᵗʰ **S46.221** Laceration of muscle, fascia and tendon of other parts of biceps, right arm   cc

√7ᵗʰ **S46.222** Laceration of muscle, fascia and tendon of other parts of biceps, left arm   cc

√7ᵗʰ **S46.229** Laceration of muscle, fascia and tendon of other parts of biceps, unspecified arm   cc

√6ᵗʰ **S46.29** Other injury of muscle, fascia and tendon of other parts of biceps

√7ᵗʰ **S46.291** Other injury of muscle, fascia and tendon of other parts of biceps, right arm

√7ᵗʰ **S46.292** Other injury of muscle, fascia and tendon of other parts of biceps, left arm

√7ᵗʰ **S46.299** Other injury of muscle, fascia and tendon of other parts of biceps, unspecified arm

√5ᵗʰ **S46.3 Injury of muscle, fascia and tendon of triceps**

√6ᵗʰ **S46.30** Unspecified injury of muscle, fascia and tendon of triceps

√7ᵗʰ **S46.301** Unspecified injury of muscle, fascia and tendon of triceps, right arm

√7ᵗʰ **S46.302** Unspecified injury of muscle, fascia and tendon of triceps, left arm

√7ᵗʰ **S46.309** Unspecified injury of muscle, fascia and tendon of triceps, unspecified arm

√6ᵗʰ **S46.31** Strain of muscle, fascia and tendon of triceps

√7ᵗʰ **S46.311** Strain of muscle, fascia and tendon of triceps, right arm

√7ᵗʰ **S46.312** Strain of muscle, fascia and tendon of triceps, left arm

√7ᵗʰ **S46.319** Strain of muscle, fascia and tendon of triceps, unspecified arm

√6ᵗʰ **S46.32** Laceration of muscle, fascia and tendon of triceps

√7ᵗʰ **S46.321** Laceration of muscle, fascia and tendon of triceps, right arm   cc

√7ᵗʰ **S46.322** Laceration of muscle, fascia and tendon of triceps, left arm   cc

√7ᵗʰ **S46.329** Laceration of muscle, fascia and tendon of triceps, unspecified arm   cc

√6ᵗʰ **S46.39** Other injury of muscle, fascia and tendon of triceps

√7ᵗʰ **S46.391** Other injury of muscle, fascia and tendon of triceps, right arm

√7ᵗʰ **S46.392** Other injury of muscle, fascia and tendon of triceps, left arm

√7ᵗʰ **S46.399** Other injury of muscle, fascia and tendon of triceps, unspecified arm

√5ᵗʰ **S46.8 Injury of other muscles, fascia and tendons at shoulder and upper arm level**

√6ᵗʰ **S46.80** Unspecified injury of other muscles, fascia and tendons at shoulder and upper arm level

√7ᵗʰ **S46.801** Unspecified injury of other muscles, fascia and tendons at shoulder and upper arm level, right arm

N Newborn: 0   P Pediatric: 0-17   M Maternity: 9-64   A Adult: 15-124   MCC Major Complication/Comorbidity   CC Complication/Comorbidity   SW Severe Wound Dx

1014   ICD-10-CM 2021

✓7th S46.802 Unspecified injury of other muscles, fascia and tendons at shoulder and upper arm level, **left arm**

✓7th S46.809 Unspecified injury of other muscles, fascia and tendons at shoulder and upper arm level, **unspecified arm**

✓6th S46.81 Strain of other muscles, fascia and tendons at shoulder and upper arm level

  ✓7th S46.811 Strain of other muscles, fascia and tendons at shoulder and upper arm level, **right arm**

  ✓7th S46.812 Strain of other muscles, fascia and tendons at shoulder and upper arm level, **left arm**

  ✓7th S46.819 Strain of other muscles, fascia and tendons at shoulder and upper arm level, **unspecified arm**

✓6th S46.82 Laceration of other muscles, fascia and tendons at shoulder and upper arm level

  S46.821 Laceration of other muscles, fascia and tendons at shoulder and upper arm level, **right arm** `cc`

  S46.822 Laceration of other muscles, fascia and tendons at shoulder and upper arm level, **left arm** `cc`

  ✓7th S46.829 Laceration of other muscles, fascia and tendons at shoulder and upper arm level, **unspecified arm** `cc`

✓6th S46.89 Other injury of other muscles, fascia and tendons at shoulder and upper arm level

  ✓7th S46.891 Other injury of other muscles, fascia and tendons at shoulder and upper arm level, **right arm**

  ✓7th S46.892 Other injury of other muscles, fascia and tendons at shoulder and upper arm level, **left arm**

  ✓7th S46.899 Other injury of other muscles, fascia and tendons at shoulder and upper arm level, **unspecified arm**

✓5th S46.9 Injury of unspecified muscle, fascia and tendon at shoulder and upper arm level

✓6th S46.90 Unspecified injury of unspecified muscle, fascia and tendon at shoulder and upper arm level

  ✓7th S46.901 Unspecified injury of unspecified muscle, fascia and tendon at shoulder and upper arm level, **right arm**

  ✓7th S46.902 Unspecified injury of unspecified muscle, fascia and tendon at shoulder and upper arm level, **left arm**

  ✓7th S46.909 Unspecified injury of unspecified muscle, fascia and tendon at shoulder and upper arm level, **unspecified arm**

✓6th S46.91 Strain of unspecified muscle, fascia and tendon at shoulder and upper arm level

  ✓7th S46.911 Strain of unspecified muscle, fascia and tendon at shoulder and upper arm level, **right arm**

  ✓7th S46.912 Strain of unspecified muscle, fascia and tendon at shoulder and upper arm level, **left arm**

  ✓7th S46.919 Strain of unspecified muscle, fascia and tendon at shoulder and upper arm level, **unspecified arm**

✓6th S46.92 Laceration of unspecified muscle, fascia and tendon at shoulder and upper arm level

  ✓7th S46.921 Laceration of unspecified muscle, fascia and tendon at shoulder and upper arm level, **right arm** `cc`

  ✓7th S46.922 Laceration of unspecified muscle, fascia and tendon at shoulder and upper arm level, **left arm** `cc`

  ✓7th S46.929 Laceration of unspecified muscle, fascia and tendon at shoulder and upper arm level, **unspecified arm** `cc`

✓6th S46.99 Other injury of unspecified muscle, fascia and tendon at shoulder and upper arm level

  ✓7th S46.991 Other injury of unspecified muscle, fascia and tendon at shoulder and upper arm level, **right arm**

  ✓7th S46.992 Other injury of unspecified muscle, fascia and tendon at shoulder and upper arm level, **left arm**

✓7th S46.999 Other injury of unspecified muscle, fascia and tendon at shoulder and upper arm level, **unspecified arm**

✓4th S47 Crushing injury of shoulder and upper arm

Use additional code for all associated injuries

EXCLUDES 2 crushing injury of elbow (S57.0-)

The appropriate 7th character is to be added to each code from category S47.
A initial encounter
D subsequent encounter
S sequela

✓x7th S47.1 Crushing injury of **right** shoulder and upper arm

✓x7th S47.2 Crushing injury of **left** shoulder and upper arm

✓x7th S47.9 Crushing injury of shoulder and upper arm, unspecified arm

✓4th S48 Traumatic amputation of shoulder and upper arm

An amputation not identified as partial or complete should be coded to complete

EXCLUDES 1 traumatic amputation at elbow level (S58.0)

The appropriate 7th character is to be added to each code from category S48.
A initial encounter
D subsequent encounter
S sequela

✓5th S48.0 Traumatic amputation at **shoulder joint**

✓6th S48.01 **Complete** traumatic amputation at shoulder joint

  7 ✓7th S48.011 Complete traumatic amputation at **right** shoulder joint `cc` `HCC`

  7 ✓7th S48.012 Complete traumatic amputation at **left** shoulder joint `cc` `HCC`

  7 ✓7th S48.019 Complete traumatic amputation at unspecified shoulder joint `cc` `HCC`

✓6th S48.02 **Partial** traumatic amputation at shoulder joint

  7 ✓7th S48.021 Partial traumatic amputation at **right** shoulder joint `cc` `HCC`

  7 ✓7th S48.022 Partial traumatic amputation at **left** shoulder joint `cc` `HCC`

  7 ✓7th S48.029 Partial traumatic amputation at unspecified shoulder joint `cc` `HCC`

✓5th S48.1 Traumatic amputation at **level between shoulder and elbow**

✓6th S48.11 **Complete** traumatic amputation at level between shoulder and elbow

  7 ✓7th S48.111 Complete traumatic amputation at level between **right** shoulder and elbow `cc` `HCC`

  7 ✓7th S48.112 Complete traumatic amputation at level between **left** shoulder and elbow `cc` `HCC`

  7 ✓7th S48.119 Complete traumatic amputation at level between unspecified shoulder and elbow `cc` `HCC`

✓6th S48.12 **Partial** traumatic amputation at level between shoulder and elbow

  7 ✓7th S48.121 Partial traumatic amputation at level between **right** shoulder and elbow `cc` `HCC`

  7 ✓7th S48.122 Partial traumatic amputation at level between **left** shoulder and elbow `cc` `HCC`

  7 ✓7th S48.129 Partial traumatic amputation at level between unspecified shoulder and elbow `cc` `HCC`

✓5th S48.9 Traumatic amputation of shoulder and upper arm, level unspecified

✓6th S48.91 **Complete** traumatic amputation of shoulder and upper arm, level unspecified

  7 ✓7th S48.911 Complete traumatic amputation of **right** shoulder and upper arm, level unspecified `cc` `HCC`

  7 ✓7th S48.912 Complete traumatic amputation of **left** shoulder and upper arm, level unspecified `cc` `HCC`

  7 ✓7th S48.919 Complete traumatic amputation of unspecified shoulder and upper arm, level unspecified `cc` `HCC`

Chapter 19. Injury, Poisoning and Certain Other Consequences of External Causes

√6ᵗʰ **S48.92** Partial traumatic amputation of shoulder and upper arm, level unspecified

    7 √7ᵗʰ **S48.921** Partial traumatic amputation of right shoulder and upper arm, level unspecified   `CC` `HCC`

    7 √7ᵗʰ **S48.922** Partial traumatic amputation of left shoulder and upper arm, level unspecified   `CC` `HCC`

    7 √7ᵗʰ **S48.929** Partial traumatic amputation of unspecified shoulder and upper arm, level unspecified   `CC` `HCC`

√4ᵗʰ **S49** Other and unspecified injuries of shoulder and upper arm

AHA: 2018,2Q,12; 2018,1Q,3

> The appropriate 7th character is to be added to each code from subcategories S49.0 and S49.1.
> A   initial encounter for closed fracture
> D   subsequent encounter for fracture with routine healing
> G   subsequent encounter for fracture with delayed healing
> K   subsequent encounter for fracture with nonunion
> P   subsequent encounter for fracture with malunion
> S   sequela

√5ᵗʰ **S49.0** Physeal fracture of upper end of humerus

AHA: 2019,4Q,56

√6ᵗʰ **S49.00** Unspecified physeal fracture of upper end of humerus

    3 √7ᵗʰ **S49.001** Unspecified physeal fracture of upper end of humerus, right arm   `CC` `H5`

    3 √7ᵗʰ **S49.002** Unspecified physeal fracture of upper end of humerus, left arm   `CC` `H5`

    3 √7ᵗʰ **S49.009** Unspecified physeal fracture of upper end of humerus, unspecified arm   `CC` `H5`

√6ᵗʰ **S49.01** Salter-Harris Type I physeal fracture of upper end of humerus

    3 √7ᵗʰ **S49.011** Salter-Harris Type I physeal fracture of upper end of humerus, right arm   `CC` `H5`

    3 √7ᵗʰ **S49.012** Salter-Harris Type I physeal fracture of upper end of humerus, left arm   `CC` `H5`

    3 √7ᵗʰ **S49.019** Salter-Harris Type I physeal fracture of upper end of humerus, unspecified arm   `CC` `H5`

√6ᵗʰ **S49.02** Salter-Harris Type II physeal fracture of upper end of humerus

    3 √7ᵗʰ **S49.021** Salter-Harris Type II physeal fracture of upper end of humerus, right arm   `CC` `H5`

    3 √7ᵗʰ **S49.022** Salter-Harris Type II physeal fracture of upper end of humerus, left arm   `CC` `H5`

    3 √7ᵗʰ **S49.029** Salter-Harris Type II physeal fracture of upper end of humerus, unspecified arm   `CC` `H5`

√6ᵗʰ **S49.03** Salter-Harris Type III physeal fracture of upper end of humerus

    3 √7ᵗʰ **S49.031** Salter-Harris Type III physeal fracture of upper end of humerus, right arm   `CC` `H5`

    3 √7ᵗʰ **S49.032** Salter-Harris Type III physeal fracture of upper end of humerus, left arm   `CC` `H5`

    3 √7ᵗʰ **S49.039** Salter-Harris Type III physeal fracture of upper end of humerus, unspecified arm   `CC` `H5`

√6ᵗʰ **S49.04** Salter-Harris Type IV physeal fracture of upper end of humerus

    3 √7ᵗʰ **S49.041** Salter-Harris Type IV physeal fracture of upper end of humerus, right arm   `CC` `H5`

    3 √7ᵗʰ **S49.042** Salter-Harris Type IV physeal fracture of upper end of humerus, left arm   `CC` `H5`

    3 √7ᵗʰ **S49.049** Salter-Harris Type IV physeal fracture of upper end of humerus, unspecified arm   `CC` `H5`

√6ᵗʰ **S49.09** Other physeal fracture of upper end of humerus

    3 √7ᵗʰ **S49.091** Other physeal fracture of upper end of humerus, right arm   `CC` `H5`

    3 √7ᵗʰ **S49.092** Other physeal fracture of upper end of humerus, left arm   `CC` `H5`

    3 √7ᵗʰ **S49.099** Other physeal fracture of upper end of humerus, unspecified arm   `CC` `H5`

√5ᵗʰ **S49.1** Physeal fracture of lower end of humerus

AHA: 2019,4Q,56

√6ᵗʰ **S49.10** Unspecified physeal fracture of lower end of humerus

    3 √7ᵗʰ **S49.101** Unspecified physeal fracture of lower end of humerus, right arm   `CC` `H5`

    3 √7ᵗʰ **S49.102** Unspecified physeal fracture of lower end of humerus, left arm   `CC` `H5`

    3 √7ᵗʰ **S49.109** Unspecified physeal fracture of lower end of humerus, unspecified arm   `CC` `H5`

√6ᵗʰ **S49.11** Salter-Harris Type I physeal fracture of lower end of humerus

    3 √7ᵗʰ **S49.111** Salter-Harris Type I physeal fracture of lower end of humerus, right arm   `CC` `H5`

    3 √7ᵗʰ **S49.112** Salter-Harris Type I physeal fracture of lower end of humerus, left arm   `CC` `H5`

    3 √7ᵗʰ **S49.119** Salter-Harris Type I physeal fracture of lower end of humerus, unspecified arm   `CC` `H5`

√6ᵗʰ **S49.12** Salter-Harris Type II physeal fracture of lower end of humerus

    3 √7ᵗʰ **S49.121** Salter-Harris Type II physeal fracture of lower end of humerus, right arm   `CC` `H5`

    3 √7ᵗʰ **S49.122** Salter-Harris Type II physeal fracture of lower end of humerus, left arm   `CC` `H5`

    3 √7ᵗʰ **S49.129** Salter-Harris Type II physeal fracture of lower end of humerus, unspecified arm   `CC` `H5`

√6ᵗʰ **S49.13** Salter-Harris Type III physeal fracture of lower end of humerus

    3 √7ᵗʰ **S49.131** Salter-Harris Type III physeal fracture of lower end of humerus, right arm   `CC` `H5`

    3 √7ᵗʰ **S49.132** Salter-Harris Type III physeal fracture of lower end of humerus, left arm   `CC` `H5`

    3 √7ᵗʰ **S49.139** Salter-Harris Type III physeal fracture of lower end of humerus, unspecified arm   `CC` `H5`

√6ᵗʰ **S49.14** Salter-Harris Type IV physeal fracture of lower end of humerus

    3 √7ᵗʰ **S49.141** Salter-Harris Type IV physeal fracture of lower end of humerus, right arm   `CC` `H5`

    3 √7ᵗʰ **S49.142** Salter-Harris Type IV physeal fracture of lower end of humerus, left arm   `CC` `H5`

    3 √7ᵗʰ **S49.149** Salter-Harris Type IV physeal fracture of lower end of humerus, unspecified arm   `CC` `H5`

√6ᵗʰ **S49.19** Other physeal fracture of lower end of humerus

    3 √7ᵗʰ **S49.191** Other physeal fracture of lower end of humerus, right arm   `CC` `H5`

    3 √7ᵗʰ **S49.192** Other physeal fracture of lower end of humerus, left arm   `CC` `H5`

    3 √7ᵗʰ **S49.199** Other physeal fracture of lower end of humerus, unspecified arm   `CC` `H5`

√5ᵗʰ **S49.8** Other specified injuries of shoulder and upper arm

> The appropriate 7th character is to be added to each code in subcategory S49.8.
> A   initial encounter
> D   subsequent encounter
> S   sequela

√x7ᵗʰ **S49.80** Other specified injuries of shoulder and upper arm, unspecified arm

√x7ᵗʰ **S49.81** Other specified injuries of right shoulder and upper arm

√x7ᵗʰ **S49.82** Other specified injuries of left shoulder and upper arm

√5ᵗʰ **S49.9** Unspecified injury of shoulder and upper arm

> The appropriate 7th character is to be added to each code in subcategory S49.9.
> A   initial encounter
> D   subsequent encounter
> S   sequela

√x7ᵗʰ **S49.90** Unspecified injury of shoulder and upper arm, unspecified arm

√x7ᵗʰ **S49.91** Unspecified injury of right shoulder and upper arm

√x7ᵗʰ **S49.92** Unspecified injury of left shoulder and upper arm

---

`N` Newborn: 0   `P` Pediatric: 0-17   `M` Maternity: 9-64   `A` Adult: 15-124   `MCC` Major Complication/Comorbidity   `CC` Complication/Comorbidity   `SW` Severe Wound Dx

1016   ICD-10-CM 2021

Injuries to the elbow and forearm (S50-S59)

EXCLUDES 2   burns and corrosions (T20-T32)
frostbite (T33-T34)
injuries of wrist and hand (S60-S69)
insect bite or sting, venomous (T63.4)

√4ᵗʰ **S50 Superficial injury of elbow and forearm**

EXCLUDES 2   superficial injury of wrist and hand (S60.-)

The appropriate 7th character is to be added to each code from category S50.
A   initial encounter
D   subsequent encounter
S   sequela

√5ᵗʰ **S50.0 Contusion of elbow**

√x7ᵗʰ **S50.00 Contusion of unspecified elbow**

√x7ᵗʰ **S50.01 Contusion of right elbow**

√x7ᵗʰ **S50.02 Contusion of left elbow**

√5ᵗʰ **S50.1 Contusion of forearm**

√x7ᵗʰ **S50.10 Contusion of unspecified forearm**

√x7ᵗʰ **S50.11 Contusion of right forearm**

√x7ᵗʰ **S50.12 Contusion of left forearm**

√5ᵗʰ **S50.3 Other superficial injuries of elbow**

√6ᵗʰ **S50.31 Abrasion of elbow**

√7ᵗʰ **S50.311 Abrasion of right elbow**

√7ᵗʰ **S50.312 Abrasion of left elbow**

√7ᵗʰ **S50.319 Abrasion of unspecified elbow**

√6ᵗʰ **S50.32 Blister (nonthermal) of elbow**

√7ᵗʰ **S50.321 Blister (nonthermal) of right elbow**

√7ᵗʰ **S50.322 Blister (nonthermal) of left elbow**

√7ᵗʰ **S50.329 Blister (nonthermal) of unspecified elbow**

√6ᵗʰ **S50.34 External constriction of elbow**

√7ᵗʰ **S50.341 External constriction of right elbow**

√7ᵗʰ **S50.342 External constriction of left elbow**

√7ᵗʰ **S50.349 External constriction of unspecified elbow**

√6ᵗʰ **S50.35 Superficial foreign body of elbow**

Splinter in the elbow

√7ᵗʰ **S50.351 Superficial foreign body of right elbow**

√7ᵗʰ **S50.352 Superficial foreign body of left elbow**

√7ᵗʰ **S50.359 Superficial foreign body of unspecified elbow**

√6ᵗʰ **S50.36 Insect bite (nonvenomous) of elbow**

√7ᵗʰ **S50.361 Insect bite (nonvenomous) of right elbow**

√7ᵗʰ **S50.362 Insect bite (nonvenomous) of left elbow**

√7ᵗʰ **S50.369 Insect bite (nonvenomous) of unspecified elbow**

√6ᵗʰ **S50.37 Other superficial bite of elbow**

EXCLUDES 1   open bite of elbow (S51.05)

√7ᵗʰ **S50.371 Other superficial bite of right elbow**

√7ᵗʰ **S50.372 Other superficial bite of left elbow**

√7ᵗʰ **S50.379 Other superficial bite of unspecified elbow**

√5ᵗʰ **S50.8 Other superficial injuries of forearm**

√6ᵗʰ **S50.81 Abrasion of forearm**

√7ᵗʰ **S50.811 Abrasion of right forearm**

√7ᵗʰ **S50.812 Abrasion of left forearm**

√7ᵗʰ **S50.819 Abrasion of unspecified forearm**

√6ᵗʰ **S50.82 Blister (nonthermal) of forearm**

√7ᵗʰ **S50.821 Blister (nonthermal) of right forearm**

√7ᵗʰ **S50.822 Blister (nonthermal) of left forearm**

√7ᵗʰ **S50.829 Blister (nonthermal) of unspecified forearm**

√6ᵗʰ **S50.84 External constriction of forearm**

√7ᵗʰ **S50.841 External constriction of right forearm**

√7ᵗʰ **S50.842 External constriction of left forearm**

√7ᵗʰ **S50.849 External constriction of unspecified forearm**

√6ᵗʰ **S50.85 Superficial foreign body of forearm**

Splinter in the forearm

√7ᵗʰ **S50.851 Superficial foreign body of right forearm**

√7ᵗʰ **S50.852 Superficial foreign body of left forearm**

√7ᵗʰ **S50.859 Superficial foreign body of unspecified forearm**

√6ᵗʰ **S50.86 Insect bite (nonvenomous) of forearm**

√7ᵗʰ **S50.861 Insect bite (nonvenomous) of right forearm**

√7ᵗʰ **S50.862 Insect bite (nonvenomous) of left forearm**

√7ᵗʰ **S50.869 Insect bite (nonvenomous) of unspecified forearm**

√6ᵗʰ **S50.87 Other superficial bite of forearm**

EXCLUDES 1   open bite of forearm (S51.85)

√7ᵗʰ **S50.871 Other superficial bite of right forearm**

√7ᵗʰ **S50.872 Other superficial bite of left forearm**

√7ᵗʰ **S50.879 Other superficial bite of unspecified forearm**

√5ᵗʰ **S50.9 Unspecified superficial injury of elbow and forearm**

√6ᵗʰ **S50.90 Unspecified superficial injury of elbow**

√7ᵗʰ **S50.901 Unspecified superficial injury of right elbow**

√7ᵗʰ **S50.902 Unspecified superficial injury of left elbow**

√7ᵗʰ **S50.909 Unspecified superficial injury of unspecified elbow**

√6ᵗʰ **S50.91 Unspecified superficial injury of forearm**

√7ᵗʰ **S50.911 Unspecified superficial injury of right forearm**

√7ᵗʰ **S50.912 Unspecified superficial injury of left forearm**

√7ᵗʰ **S50.919 Unspecified superficial injury of unspecified forearm**

√4ᵗʰ **S51 Open wound of elbow and forearm**

Code also any associated wound infection

EXCLUDES 1   open fracture of elbow and forearm (S52.- with open fracture 7th character)
traumatic amputation of elbow and forearm (S58.-)

EXCLUDES 2   open wound of wrist and hand (S61.-)

The appropriate 7th character is to be added to each code from category S51.
A   initial encounter
D   subsequent encounter
S   sequela

√5ᵗʰ **S51.0 Open wound of elbow**

√6ᵗʰ **S51.00 Unspecified open wound of elbow**

√7ᵗʰ **S51.001 Unspecified open wound of right elbow**

AHA: 2012,4Q,108

√7ᵗʰ **S51.002 Unspecified open wound of left elbow**

√7ᵗʰ **S51.009 Unspecified open wound of unspecified elbow**

Open wound of elbow NOS

√6ᵗʰ **S51.01 Laceration without foreign body of elbow**

√7ᵗʰ **S51.011 Laceration without foreign body of right elbow**

√7ᵗʰ **S51.012 Laceration without foreign body of left elbow**

√7ᵗʰ **S51.019 Laceration without foreign body of unspecified elbow**

√6ᵗʰ **S51.02 Laceration with foreign body of elbow**

√7ᵗʰ **S51.021 Laceration with foreign body of right elbow**

√7ᵗʰ **S51.022 Laceration with foreign body of left elbow**

√7ᵗʰ **S51.029 Laceration with foreign body of unspecified elbow**

√6ᵗʰ **S51.03 Puncture wound without foreign body of elbow**

√7ᵗʰ **S51.031 Puncture wound without foreign body of right elbow**

√7ᵗʰ **S51.032 Puncture wound without foreign body of left elbow**

√7ᵗʰ **S51.039 Puncture wound without foreign body of unspecified elbow**

√6ᵗʰ **S51.04 Puncture wound with foreign body of elbow**

√7ᵗʰ **S51.041 Puncture wound with foreign body of right elbow**

☑ Additional Character Required   √x7ᵗʰ Placeholder   Unacceptable PDx   Questionable PDx   Manifestation   Unspecified Dx   H1 -H14 HAC   HCC CMS-HCC Dx   HIV HIV Dx

ICD-10-CM 2021   1017

✓7ᵗʰ **S51.042** Puncture wound with foreign body of left elbow

✓7ᵗʰ **S51.049** Puncture wound with foreign body of unspecified elbow

✓6ᵗʰ **S51.05** **Open bite** of elbow

Bite of elbow NOS

EXCLUDES 1   *superficial bite of elbow (S50.36, S50.37)*

✓7ᵗʰ **S51.051** Open bite, right elbow

✓7ᵗʰ **S51.052** Open bite, left elbow

✓7ᵗʰ **S51.059** Open bite, unspecified elbow

✓5ᵗʰ **S51.8** **Open wound of** forearm

EXCLUDES 2   *open wound of elbow (S51.0-)*

✓6ᵗʰ **S51.80** **Unspecified open wound of forearm**

AHA: 2016,3Q,24

✓7ᵗʰ **S51.801** Unspecified open wound of right forearm

✓7ᵗʰ **S51.802** Unspecified open wound of left forearm

✓7ᵗʰ **S51.809** Unspecified open wound of unspecified forearm

Open wound of forearm NOS

✓6ᵗʰ **S51.81** **Laceration without foreign body** of forearm

✓7ᵗʰ **S51.811** Laceration without foreign body of right forearm

✓7ᵗʰ **S51.812** Laceration without foreign body of left forearm

✓7ᵗʰ **S51.819** Laceration without foreign body of unspecified forearm

✓6ᵗʰ **S51.82** **Laceration with foreign body** of forearm

✓7ᵗʰ **S51.821** Laceration with foreign body of right forearm

✓7ᵗʰ **S51.822** Laceration with foreign body of left forearm

✓7ᵗʰ **S51.829** Laceration with foreign body of unspecified forearm

✓6ᵗʰ **S51.83** **Puncture wound without foreign body** of forearm

AHA: 2016,3Q,24

✓7ᵗʰ **S51.831** Puncture wound without foreign body of right forearm

✓7ᵗʰ **S51.832** Puncture wound without foreign body of left forearm

✓7ᵗʰ **S51.839** Puncture wound without foreign body of unspecified forearm

✓6ᵗʰ **S51.84** **Puncture wound with foreign body** of forearm

AHA: 2016,3Q,24

✓7ᵗʰ **S51.841** Puncture wound with foreign body of right forearm

✓7ᵗʰ **S51.842** Puncture wound with foreign body of left forearm

✓7ᵗʰ **S51.849** Puncture wound with foreign body of unspecified forearm

✓6ᵗʰ **S51.85** **Open bite** of forearm

Bite of forearm NOS

EXCLUDES 1   *superficial bite of forearm (S50.86, S50.87)*

✓7ᵗʰ **S51.851** Open bite of right forearm

✓7ᵗʰ **S51.852** Open bite of left forearm

✓7ᵗʰ **S51.859** Open bite of unspecified forearm

✓4ᵗʰ **S52** **Fracture of forearm**

NOTE   A fracture not indicated as displaced or nondisplaced should be coded to displaced.

A fracture not indicated as open or closed should be coded to closed.

The open fracture designations are based on the Gustilo open fracture classification.

EXCLUDES 1   *traumatic amputation of forearm (S58.-)*

EXCLUDES 2   *fracture at wrist and hand level (S62.-)*

AHA: 2018,2Q,12; 2016,1Q,33; 2015,3Q,37-39

DEF: Diaphysis: Central shaft of a long bone.

DEF: Epiphysis: Proximal and distal rounded ends of a long bone, communicates with the joint.

DEF: Metaphysis: Section of a long bone located between the epiphysis and diaphysis at the proximal and distal ends.

DEF: Physis (growth plate): Narrow zone of cartilaginous tissue between the epiphysis and metaphysis at each end of a long bone. In childhood, proliferation of cells in this zone lengthens the bone. As the bone matures, this area thins, ossification eventually fusing into solid bone and growth stops. **Synonyms:** *Epiphyseal plate.*

The appropriate 7th character is to be added to all codes from category S52 [unless otherwise indicated].

A   initial encounter for closed fracture

B   initial encounter for open fracture type I or II

    initial encounter for open fracture NOS

C   initial encounter for open fracture type IIIA, IIIB, or IIIC

D   subsequent encounter for closed fracture with routine healing

E   subsequent encounter for open fracture type I or II with routine healing

F   subsequent encounter for open fracture type IIIA, IIIB, or IIIC with routine healing

G   subsequent encounter for closed fracture with delayed healing

H   subsequent encounter for open fracture type I or II with delayed healing

J   subsequent encounter for open fracture type IIIA, IIIB, or IIIC with delayed healing

K   subsequent encounter for closed fracture with nonunion

M   subsequent encounter for open fracture type I or II with nonunion

N   subsequent encounter for open fracture type IIIA, IIIB, or IIIC with nonunion

P   subsequent encounter for closed fracture with malunion

Q   subsequent encounter for open fracture type I or II with malunion

R   subsequent encounter for open fracture type IIIA, IIIB, or IIIC with malunion

S   sequela

✓5ᵗʰ **S52.0** **Fracture of** upper end of ulna

Fracture of proximal end of ulna

EXCLUDES 2   *fracture of elbow NOS (S42.40-)*

    fractures of shaft of ulna (S52.2-)

✓6ᵗʰ **S52.00** **Unspecified fracture of upper end of ulna**

2,4 ✓7ᵗʰ **S52.001** Unspecified fracture of upper end of right ulna   MCC CC H5

2,4 ✓7ᵗʰ **S52.002** Unspecified fracture of upper end of left ulna   MCC CC H5

2,4 ✓7ᵗʰ **S52.009** Unspecified fracture of upper end of unspecified ulna   MCC CC H5

✓6ᵗʰ **S52.01** **Torus** fracture of upper end of ulna

The appropriate 7th character is to be added to all codes in subcategory S52.01

A   initial encounter for closed fracture

D   subsequent encounter for fracture with routine healing

G   subsequent encounter for fracture with delayed healing

K   subsequent encounter for fracture with nonunion

P   subsequent encounter for fracture with malunion

S   sequela

3 ✓7ᵗʰ **S52.011** Torus fracture of upper end of right ulna   CC H5

3 ✓7ᵗʰ **S52.012** Torus fracture of upper end of left ulna   CC H5

3 ✓7ᵗʰ **S52.019** Torus fracture of upper end of unspecified ulna   CC H5

N Newborn: 0   P Pediatric: 0-17   M Maternity: 9-64   A Adult: 15-124   MCC Major Complication/Comorbidity   CC Complication/Comorbidity   SW Severe Wound Dx

1018   ICD-10-CM 2021

√6ᵗʰ **S52.02** Fracture of olecranon process without intraarticular extension of ulna

2,4 √7ᵗʰ **S52.021** Displaced fracture of olecranon process without intraarticular extension of right ulna   MCC CC H5

2,4 √7ᵗʰ **S52.022** Displaced fracture of olecranon process without intraarticular extension of left ulna   MCC CC H5

2,4 √7ᵗʰ **S52.023** Displaced fracture of olecranon process without intraarticular extension of unspecified ulna   MCC CC H5

2,4 √7ᵗʰ **S52.024** Nondisplaced fracture of olecranon process without intraarticular extension of right ulna   MCC CC H5

2,4 √7ᵗʰ **S52.025** Nondisplaced fracture of olecranon process without intraarticular extension of left ulna   MCC CC H5

2,4 √7ᵗʰ **S52.026** Nondisplaced fracture of olecranon process without intraarticular extension of unspecified ulna   MCC CC H5

√6ᵗʰ **S52.03** Fracture of olecranon process with intraarticular extension of ulna

2,4 √7ᵗʰ **S52.031** Displaced fracture of olecranon process with intraarticular extension of right ulna   MCC CC H5

2,4 √7ᵗʰ **S52.032** Displaced fracture of olecranon process with intraarticular extension of left ulna   MCC CC H5

2,4 √7ᵗʰ **S52.033** Displaced fracture of olecranon process with intraarticular extension of unspecified ulna   MCC CC H5

2,4 √7ᵗʰ **S52.034** Nondisplaced fracture of olecranon process with intraarticular extension of right ulna   MCC CC H5

2,4 √7ᵗʰ **S52.035** Nondisplaced fracture of olecranon process with intraarticular extension of left ulna   MCC CC H5

2,4 √7ᵗʰ **S52.036** Nondisplaced fracture of olecranon process with intraarticular extension of unspecified ulna   MCC CC H5

√6ᵗʰ **S52.04** Fracture of coronoid process of ulna

2,4 √7ᵗʰ **S52.041** Displaced fracture of coronoid process of right ulna   MCC CC H5

2,4 √7ᵗʰ **S52.042** Displaced fracture of coronoid process of left ulna   MCC CC H5

2,4 √7ᵗʰ **S52.043** Displaced fracture of coronoid process of unspecified ulna   MCC CC H5

2,4 √7ᵗʰ **S52.044** Nondisplaced fracture of coronoid process of right ulna   MCC CC H5

2,4 √7ᵗʰ **S52.045** Nondisplaced fracture of coronoid process of left ulna   MCC CC H5

2,4 √7ᵗʰ **S52.046** Nondisplaced fracture of coronoid process of unspecified ulna   MCC CC H5

√6ᵗʰ **S52.09** Other fracture of upper end of ulna

2,4 √7ᵗʰ **S52.091** Other fracture of upper end of right ulna   MCC CC H5

2,4 √7ᵗʰ **S52.092** Other fracture of upper end of left ulna   MCC CC H5

2,4 √7ᵗʰ **S52.099** Other fracture of upper end of unspecified ulna   MCC CC H5

√5ᵗʰ **S52.1** Fracture of upper end of radius

Fracture of proximal end of radius

EXCLUDES 2   physeal fractures of upper end of radius (S59.2-)
fracture of shaft of radius (S52.3-)

√6ᵗʰ **S52.10** Unspecified fracture of upper end of radius

2,4 √7ᵗʰ **S52.101** Unspecified fracture of upper end of right radius   MCC CC H5

2,4 √7ᵗʰ **S52.102** Unspecified fracture of upper end of left radius   MCC CC H5

2,4 √7ᵗʰ **S52.109** Unspecified fracture of upper end of unspecified radius   MCC CC H5

√6ᵗʰ **S52.11** Torus fracture of upper end of radius

The appropriate 7th character is to be added to all codes in subcategory S52.11
A   initial encounter for closed fracture
D   subsequent encounter for fracture with routine healing
G   subsequent encounter for fracture with delayed healing
K   subsequent encounter for fracture with nonunion
P   subsequent encounter for fracture with malunion
S   sequela

3 √7ᵗʰ **S52.111** Torus fracture of upper end of right radius   CC H5

3 √7ᵗʰ **S52.112** Torus fracture of upper end of left radius   CC H5

3 √7ᵗʰ **S52.119** Torus fracture of upper end of unspecified radius   CC H5

√6ᵗʰ **S52.12** Fracture of head of radius

2,4 √7ᵗʰ **S52.121** Displaced fracture of head of right radius   MCC CC H5

2,4 √7ᵗʰ **S52.122** Displaced fracture of head of left radius   MCC CC H5

2,4 √7ᵗʰ **S52.123** Displaced fracture of head of unspecified radius   MCC CC H5

2,4 √7ᵗʰ **S52.124** Nondisplaced fracture of head of right radius   MCC CC H5

2,4 √7ᵗʰ **S52.125** Nondisplaced fracture of head of left radius   MCC CC H5

2,4 √7ᵗʰ **S52.126** Nondisplaced fracture of head of unspecified radius   MCC CC H5

√6ᵗʰ **S52.13** Fracture of neck of radius

2,4 √7ᵗʰ **S52.131** Displaced fracture of neck of right radius   MCC CC H5

2,4 √7ᵗʰ **S52.132** Displaced fracture of neck of left radius   MCC CC H5

2,4 √7ᵗʰ **S52.133** Displaced fracture of neck of unspecified radius   MCC CC H5

2,4 √7ᵗʰ **S52.134** Nondisplaced fracture of neck of right radius   MCC CC H5

2,4 √7ᵗʰ **S52.135** Nondisplaced fracture of neck of left radius   MCC CC H5

2,4 √7ᵗʰ **S52.136** Nondisplaced fracture of neck of unspecified radius   MCC CC H5

√6ᵗʰ **S52.18** Other fracture of upper end of radius

2,4 √7ᵗʰ **S52.181** Other fracture of upper end of right radius   MCC CC H5

2,4 √7ᵗʰ **S52.182** Other fracture of upper end of left radius   MCC CC H5

2,4 √7ᵗʰ **S52.189** Other fracture of upper end of unspecified radius   MCC CC H5

√5ᵗʰ **S52.2** Fracture of shaft of ulna

√6ᵗʰ **S52.20** Unspecified fracture of shaft of ulna

Fracture of ulna NOS

2,3 √7ᵗʰ **S52.201** Unspecified fracture of shaft of right ulna   MCC CC H5

2,3 √7ᵗʰ **S52.202** Unspecified fracture of shaft of left ulna   MCC CC H5

2,3 √7ᵗʰ **S52.209** Unspecified fracture of shaft of unspecified ulna   MCC CC H5

√6ᵗʰ **S52.21** Greenstick fracture of shaft of ulna

The appropriate 7th character is to be added to all codes in subcategory S52.21
A   initial encounter for closed fracture
D   subsequent encounter for fracture with routine healing
G   subsequent encounter for fracture with delayed healing
K   subsequent encounter for fracture with nonunion
P   subsequent encounter for fracture with malunion
S   sequela

3 √7ᵗʰ **S52.211** Greenstick fracture of shaft of right ulna   CC H5

✔ Additional Character Required   √x7ᵗʰ Placeholder   Unacceptable PDx   Questionable PDx   Manifestation   Unspecified Dx   H1-H14 HAC   HCC CMS-HCC Dx   HIV HIV Dx

ICD-10-CM 2021   1019

³ √7ᵗʰ **S52.212** Greenstick fracture of shaft of left ulna   CC H5

³ √7ᵗʰ **S52.219** Greenstick fracture of shaft of unspecified ulna   CC H5

√6ᵗʰ **S52.22** Transverse fracture of shaft of ulna

2,3 √7ᵗʰ **S52.221** Displaced transverse fracture of shaft of right ulna   MCC CC H5

2,3 √7ᵗʰ **S52.222** Displaced transverse fracture of shaft of left ulna   MCC CC H5

2,3 √7ᵗʰ **S52.223** Displaced transverse fracture of shaft of unspecified ulna   MCC CC H5

2,3 √7ᵗʰ **S52.224** Nondisplaced transverse fracture of shaft of right ulna   MCC CC H5

2,3 √7ᵗʰ **S52.225** Nondisplaced transverse fracture of shaft of left ulna   MCC CC H5

2,3 √7ᵗʰ **S52.226** Nondisplaced transverse fracture of shaft of unspecified ulna   MCC CC H5

√6ᵗʰ **S52.23** Oblique fracture of shaft of ulna

2,3 √7ᵗʰ **S52.231** Displaced oblique fracture of shaft of right ulna   MCC CC H5

2,3 √7ᵗʰ **S52.232** Displaced oblique fracture of shaft of left ulna   MCC CC H5

2,3 √7ᵗʰ **S52.233** Displaced oblique fracture of shaft of unspecified ulna   MCC CC H5

2,3 √7ᵗʰ **S52.234** Nondisplaced oblique fracture of shaft of right ulna   MCC CC H5

2,3 √7ᵗʰ **S52.235** Nondisplaced oblique fracture of shaft of left ulna   MCC CC H5

2,3 √7ᵗʰ **S52.236** Nondisplaced oblique fracture of shaft of unspecified ulna   MCC CC H5

√6ᵗʰ **S52.24** Spiral fracture of shaft of ulna

2,3 √7ᵗʰ **S52.241** Displaced spiral fracture of shaft of ulna, right arm   MCC CC H5

2,3 √7ᵗʰ **S52.242** Displaced spiral fracture of shaft of ulna, left arm   MCC CC H5

2,3 √7ᵗʰ **S52.243** Displaced spiral fracture of shaft of ulna, unspecified arm   MCC CC H5

2,3 √7ᵗʰ **S52.244** Nondisplaced spiral fracture of shaft of ulna, right arm   MCC CC H5

2,3 √7ᵗʰ **S52.245** Nondisplaced spiral fracture of shaft of ulna, left arm   MCC CC H5

2,3 √7ᵗʰ **S52.246** Nondisplaced spiral fracture of shaft of ulna, unspecified arm   MCC CC H5

√6ᵗʰ **S52.25** Comminuted fracture of shaft of ulna

2,3 √7ᵗʰ **S52.251** Displaced comminuted fracture of shaft of ulna, right arm   MCC CC H5

2,3 √7ᵗʰ **S52.252** Displaced comminuted fracture of shaft of ulna, left arm   MCC CC H5

2,3 √7ᵗʰ **S52.253** Displaced comminuted fracture of shaft of ulna, unspecified arm   MCC CC H5

2,3 √7ᵗʰ **S52.254** Nondisplaced comminuted fracture of shaft of ulna, right arm   MCC CC H5

2,3 √7ᵗʰ **S52.255** Nondisplaced comminuted fracture of shaft of ulna, left arm   MCC CC H5

2,3 √7ᵗʰ **S52.256** Nondisplaced comminuted fracture of shaft of ulna, unspecified arm   MCC CC H5

√6ᵗʰ **S52.26** Segmental fracture of shaft of ulna

2,3 √7ᵗʰ **S52.261** Displaced segmental fracture of shaft of ulna, right arm   MCC CC H5

2,3 √7ᵗʰ **S52.262** Displaced segmental fracture of shaft of ulna, left arm   MCC CC H5

2,3 √7ᵗʰ **S52.263** Displaced segmental fracture of shaft of ulna, unspecified arm   MCC CC H5

2,3 √7ᵗʰ **S52.264** Nondisplaced segmental fracture of shaft of ulna, right arm   MCC CC H5

2,3 √7ᵗʰ **S52.265** Nondisplaced segmental fracture of shaft of ulna, left arm   MCC CC H5

2,3 √7ᵗʰ **S52.266** Nondisplaced segmental fracture of shaft of ulna, unspecified arm   MCC CC H5

√6ᵗʰ **S52.27** Monteggia's fracture of ulna

Fracture of upper shaft of ulna with dislocation of radial head

2,4 √7ᵗʰ **S52.271** Monteggia's fracture of right ulna   MCC CC H5

2,4 √7ᵗʰ **S52.272** Monteggia's fracture of left ulna   MCC CC H5

2,4 √7ᵗʰ **S52.279** Monteggia's fracture of unspecified ulna   MCC CC H5

√6ᵗʰ **S52.28** Bent bone of ulna

2,3 √7ᵗʰ **S52.281** Bent bone of right ulna   MCC CC H5

2,3 √7ᵗʰ **S52.282** Bent bone of left ulna   MCC CC H5

2,3 √7ᵗʰ **S52.283** Bent bone of unspecified ulna   MCC CC H5

√6ᵗʰ **S52.29** Other fracture of shaft of ulna

2,3 √7ᵗʰ **S52.291** Other fracture of shaft of right ulna   MCC CC H5

2,3 √7ᵗʰ **S52.292** Other fracture of shaft of left ulna   MCC CC H5

2,3 √7ᵗʰ **S52.299** Other fracture of shaft of unspecified ulna   MCC CC H5

√5ᵗʰ **S52.3** Fracture of shaft of radius

√6ᵗʰ **S52.30** Unspecified fracture of shaft of radius

2,3 √7ᵗʰ **S52.301** Unspecified fracture of shaft of right radius   MCC CC H5

2,3 √7ᵗʰ **S52.302** Unspecified fracture of shaft of left radius   MCC CC H5

2,3 √7ᵗʰ **S52.309** Unspecified fracture of shaft of unspecified radius   MCC CC H5

√6ᵗʰ **S52.31** Greenstick fracture of shaft of radius

> The appropriate 7th character is to be added to all codes in subcategory S52.31.
> A   initial encounter for closed fracture
> D   subsequent encounter for fracture with routine healing
> G   subsequent encounter for fracture with delayed healing
> K   subsequent encounter for fracture with nonunion
> P   subsequent encounter for fracture with malunion
> S   sequela

³ √7ᵗʰ **S52.311** Greenstick fracture of shaft of radius, right arm   CC H5

³ √7ᵗʰ **S52.312** Greenstick fracture of shaft of radius, left arm   CC H5

³ √7ᵗʰ **S52.319** Greenstick fracture of shaft of radius, unspecified arm   CC H5

√6ᵗʰ **S52.32** Transverse fracture of shaft of radius

2,3 √7ᵗʰ **S52.321** Displaced transverse fracture of shaft of right radius   MCC CC H5

2,3 √7ᵗʰ **S52.322** Displaced transverse fracture of shaft of left radius   MCC CC H5

2,3 √7ᵗʰ **S52.323** Displaced transverse fracture of shaft of unspecified radius   MCC CC H5

2,3 √7ᵗʰ **S52.324** Nondisplaced transverse fracture of shaft of right radius   MCC CC H5

2,3 √7ᵗʰ **S52.325** Nondisplaced transverse fracture of shaft of left radius   MCC CC H5

2,3 √7ᵗʰ **S52.326** Nondisplaced transverse fracture of shaft of unspecified radius   MCC CC H5

√6ᵗʰ **S52.33** Oblique fracture of shaft of radius

2,3 √7ᵗʰ **S52.331** Displaced oblique fracture of shaft of right radius   MCC CC H5

2,3 √7ᵗʰ **S52.332** Displaced oblique fracture of shaft of left radius   MCC CC H5

2,3 √7ᵗʰ **S52.333** Displaced oblique fracture of shaft of unspecified radius   MCC CC H5

2,3 √7ᵗʰ **S52.334** Nondisplaced oblique fracture of shaft of right radius   MCC CC H5

2,3 √7ᵗʰ **S52.335** Nondisplaced oblique fracture of shaft of left radius   MCC CC H5

2,3 √7ᵗʰ **S52.336** Nondisplaced oblique fracture of shaft of unspecified radius   MCC CC H5

√6ᵗʰ **S52.34** Spiral fracture of shaft of radius

2,3 √7ᵗʰ **S52.341** Displaced spiral fracture of shaft of radius, right arm   MCC CC H5

2,3 √7ᵗʰ **S52.342** Displaced spiral fracture of shaft of radius, left arm   MCC CC H5

2,3 √7ᵗʰ **S52.343** Displaced spiral fracture of shaft of radius, unspecified arm   MCC CC H5

2,3 √7ᵗʰ **S52.344** Nondisplaced spiral fracture of shaft of radius, right arm   MCC CC H5

2,3 √7ᵗʰ **S52.345** Nondisplaced spiral fracture of shaft of radius, left arm   MCC CC H5

N Newborn: 0   P Pediatric: 0-17   M Maternity: 9-64   A Adult: 15-124   MCC Major Complication/Comorbidity   CC Complication/Comorbidity   SW Severe Wound Dx

1020   ICD-10-CM 2021

2,3 √7ᵗʰ **S52.346** Nondisplaced spiral fracture of shaft of radius, unspecified arm `MCC` `CC` `H5`

√6ᵗʰ **S52.35** Comminuted fracture of shaft of radius

2,3 √7ᵗʰ **S52.351** Displaced comminuted fracture of shaft of radius, right arm `MCC` `CC` `H5`

2,3 √7ᵗʰ **S52.352** Displaced comminuted fracture of shaft of radius, left arm `MCC` `CC` `H5`

2,3 √7ᵗʰ **S52.353** Displaced comminuted fracture of shaft of radius, unspecified arm `MCC` `CC` `H5`

2,3 √7ᵗʰ **S52.354** Nondisplaced comminuted fracture of shaft of radius, right arm `MCC` `CC` `H5`

2,3 √7ᵗʰ **S52.355** Nondisplaced comminuted fracture of shaft of radius, left arm `MCC` `CC` `H5`

2,3 √7ᵗʰ **S52.356** Nondisplaced comminuted fracture of shaft of radius, unspecified arm `MCC` `CC` `H5`

√6ᵗʰ **S52.36** Segmental fracture of shaft of radius

2,3 √7ᵗʰ **S52.361** Displaced segmental fracture of shaft of radius, right arm `MCC` `CC` `H5`

2,3 √7ᵗʰ **S52.362** Displaced segmental fracture of shaft of radius, left arm `MCC` `CC` `H5`

2,3 √7ᵗʰ **S52.363** Displaced segmental fracture of shaft of radius, unspecified arm `MCC` `CC` `H5`

2,3 √7ᵗʰ **S52.364** Nondisplaced segmental fracture of shaft of radius, right arm `MCC` `CC` `H5`

2,3 √7ᵗʰ **S52.365** Nondisplaced segmental fracture of shaft of radius, left arm `MCC` `CC` `H5`

2,3 √7ᵗʰ **S52.366** Nondisplaced segmental fracture of shaft of radius, unspecified arm `MCC` `CC` `H5`

√6ᵗʰ **S52.37** Galeazzi's fracture

Fracture of lower shaft of radius with radioulnar joint dislocation

2,3 √7ᵗʰ **S52.371** Galeazzi's fracture of right radius `MCC` `CC` `H5`

2,3 √7ᵗʰ **S52.372** Galeazzi's fracture of left radius `MCC` `CC` `H5`

2,3 √7ᵗʰ **S52.379** Galeazzi's fracture of unspecified radius `MCC` `CC` `H5`

√6ᵗʰ **S52.38** Bent bone of radius

2,3 √7ᵗʰ **S52.381** Bent bone of right radius `MCC` `CC` `H5`

2,3 √7ᵗʰ **S52.382** Bent bone of left radius `MCC` `CC` `H5`

2,3 √7ᵗʰ **S52.389** Bent bone of unspecified radius `MCC` `CC` `H5`

√6ᵗʰ **S52.39** Other fracture of shaft of radius

2,3 √7ᵗʰ **S52.391** Other fracture of shaft of radius, right arm `MCC` `CC` `H5`

2,3 √7ᵗʰ **S52.392** Other fracture of shaft of radius, left arm `MCC` `CC` `H5`

2,3 √7ᵗʰ **S52.399** Other fracture of shaft of radius, unspecified arm `MCC` `CC` `H5`

√5ᵗʰ **S52.5** Fracture of lower end of radius

Fracture of distal end of radius

EXCLUDES 2   physeal fractures of lower end of radius (S59.2-)

DEF: Fracture of the distal end of the radius above the wrist, most commonly caused by a fall onto an outstretched hand.

√6ᵗʰ **S52.50** Unspecified fracture of the lower end of radius

2,3 √7ᵗʰ **S52.501** Unspecified fracture of the lower end of right radius `MCC` `CC` `H5`

2,3 √7ᵗʰ **S52.502** Unspecified fracture of the lower end of left radius `MCC` `CC` `H5`

2,3 √7ᵗʰ **S52.509** Unspecified fracture of the lower end of unspecified radius `MCC` `CC` `H5`

√6ᵗʰ **S52.51** Fracture of radial styloid process

2,3 √7ᵗʰ **S52.511** Displaced fracture of right radial styloid process `MCC` `CC` `H5`

2,3 √7ᵗʰ **S52.512** Displaced fracture of left radial styloid process `MCC` `CC` `H5`

2,3 √7ᵗʰ **S52.513** Displaced fracture of unspecified radial styloid process `MCC` `CC` `H5`

2,3 √7ᵗʰ **S52.514** Nondisplaced fracture of right radial styloid process `MCC` `CC` `H5`

2,3 √7ᵗʰ **S52.515** Nondisplaced fracture of left radial styloid process `MCC` `CC` `H5`

2,3 √7ᵗʰ **S52.516** Nondisplaced fracture of unspecified radial styloid process `MCC` `CC` `H5`

√6ᵗʰ **S52.52** Torus fracture of lower end of radius

The appropriate 7th character is to be added to all codes in subcategory S52.52.

A   initial encounter for closed fracture
D   subsequent encounter for fracture with routine healing
G   subsequent encounter for fracture with delayed healing
K   subsequent encounter for fracture with nonunion
P   subsequent encounter for fracture with malunion
S   sequela

3 √7ᵗʰ **S52.521** Torus fracture of lower end of right radius `CC` `H5`

3 √7ᵗʰ **S52.522** Torus fracture of lower end of left radius `CC` `H5`

3 √7ᵗʰ **S52.529** Torus fracture of lower end of unspecified radius `CC` `H5`

√6ᵗʰ **S52.53** Colles' fracture

AHA: 2016,2Q,4

DEF: Fracture of the radius at the wrist in which the distal fragment is pushed posteriorly. The dorsal angulation of the fragment results in the wrist cocking up.

2,3 √7ᵗʰ **S52.531** Colles' fracture of right radius `MCC` `CC` `H5`

2,3 √7ᵗʰ **S52.532** Colles' fracture of left radius `MCC` `CC` `H5`

2,3 √7ᵗʰ **S52.539** Colles' fracture of unspecified radius `MCC` `CC` `H5`

√6ᵗʰ **S52.54** Smith's fracture

2,3 √7ᵗʰ **S52.541** Smith's fracture of right radius `MCC` `CC` `H5`

2,3 √7ᵗʰ **S52.542** Smith's fracture of left radius `MCC` `CC` `H5`

2,3 √7ᵗʰ **S52.549** Smith's fracture of unspecified radius `MCC` `CC` `H5`

√6ᵗʰ **S52.55** Other extraarticular fracture of lower end of radius

2,3 √7ᵗʰ **S52.551** Other extraarticular fracture of lower end of right radius `MCC` `CC` `H5`

2,3 √7ᵗʰ **S52.552** Other extraarticular fracture of lower end of left radius `MCC` `CC` `H5`

2,3 √7ᵗʰ **S52.559** Other extraarticular fracture of lower end of unspecified radius `MCC` `CC` `H5`

√6ᵗʰ **S52.56** Barton's fracture

2,3 √7ᵗʰ **S52.561** Barton's fracture of right radius `MCC` `CC` `H5`

2,3 √7ᵗʰ **S52.562** Barton's fracture of left radius `MCC` `CC` `H5`

2,3 √7ᵗʰ **S52.569** Barton's fracture of unspecified radius `MCC` `CC` `H5`

√6ᵗʰ **S52.57** Other intraarticular fracture of lower end of radius

2,3 √7ᵗʰ **S52.571** Other intraarticular fracture of lower end of right radius `MCC` `CC` `H5`

2,3 √7ᵗʰ **S52.572** Other intraarticular fracture of lower end of left radius `MCC` `CC` `H5`

2,3 √7ᵗʰ **S52.579** Other intraarticular fracture of lower end of unspecified radius `MCC` `CC` `H5`

√6ᵗʰ **S52.59** Other fractures of lower end of radius

AHA: 2019,3Q,9

2,3 √7ᵗʰ **S52.591** Other fractures of lower end of right radius `MCC` `CC` `H5`

2,3 √7ᵗʰ **S52.592** Other fractures of lower end of left radius `MCC` `CC` `H5`

2,3 √7ᵗʰ **S52.599** Other fractures of lower end of unspecified radius `MCC` `CC` `H5`

√5ᵗʰ **S52.6** Fracture of lower end of ulna

√6ᵗʰ **S52.60** Unspecified fracture of lower end of ulna

2,3 √7ᵗʰ **S52.601** Unspecified fracture of lower end of right ulna `MCC` `CC` `H5`

2,3 √7ᵗʰ **S52.602** Unspecified fracture of lower end of left ulna `MCC` `CC` `H5`

2,3 √7ᵗʰ **S52.609** Unspecified fracture of lower end of unspecified ulna `MCC` `CC` `H5`

☑ Additional Character Required   √x7ᵗʰ Placeholder   Unacceptable PDx   Questionable PDx   Manifestation   Unspecified Dx   H1-H14 HAC   HCC CMS-HCC Dx   HIV HIV Dx

ICD-10-CM 2021   1021

√6ᵗʰ **S52.61** Fracture of ulna styloid process

2,3 √7ᵗʰ **S52.611** Displaced fracture of right ulna styloid process   MCC CC H5

2,3 √7ᵗʰ **S52.612** Displaced fracture of left ulna styloid process   MCC CC H5

2,3 √7ᵗʰ **S52.613** Displaced fracture of unspecified ulna styloid process   MCC CC H5

2,3 √7ᵗʰ **S52.614** Nondisplaced fracture of right ulna styloid process   MCC CC H5

2,3 √7ᵗʰ **S52.615** Nondisplaced fracture of left ulna styloid process   MCC CC H5

2,3 √7ᵗʰ **S52.616** Nondisplaced fracture of unspecified ulna styloid process   MCC CC H5

√6ᵗʰ **S52.62** Torus fracture of lower end of ulna

> The appropriate 7th character is to be added to all codes in subcategory S52.62.
> A   initial encounter for closed fracture
> D   subsequent encounter for fracture with routine healing
> G   subsequent encounter for fracture with delayed healing
> K   subsequent encounter for fracture with nonunion
> P   subsequent encounter for fracture with malunion
> S   sequela

3 √7ᵗʰ **S52.621** Torus fracture of lower end of right ulna   CC H5

3 √7ᵗʰ **S52.622** Torus fracture of lower end of left ulna   CC H5

3 √7ᵗʰ **S52.629** Torus fracture of lower end of unspecified ulna   CC H5

√6ᵗʰ **S52.69** Other fracture of lower end of ulna

AHA: 2019,3Q,9

2,3 √7ᵗʰ **S52.691** Other fracture of lower end of right ulna   MCC CC H5

2,3 √7ᵗʰ **S52.692** Other fracture of lower end of left ulna   MCC CC H5

2,3 √7ᵗʰ **S52.699** Other fracture of lower end of unspecified ulna   MCC CC H5

√5ᵗʰ **S52.9** Unspecified fracture of forearm

2,3 √x7ᵗʰ **S52.90** Unspecified fracture of unspecified forearm   MCC CC H5

2,3 √x7ᵗʰ **S52.91** Unspecified fracture of right forearm   MCC CC H5

2,3 √x7ᵗʰ **S52.92** Unspecified fracture of left forearm   MCC CC H5

√4ᵗʰ **S53** Dislocation and sprain of joints and ligaments of elbow

INCLUDES   avulsion of joint or ligament of elbow
laceration of cartilage, joint or ligament of elbow
sprain of cartilage, joint or ligament of elbow
traumatic hemarthrosis of joint or ligament of elbow
traumatic rupture of joint or ligament of elbow
traumatic subluxation of joint or ligament of elbow
traumatic tear of joint or ligament of elbow

Code also any associated open wound

EXCLUDES 2   *strain of muscle, fascia and tendon at forearm level (S56.-)*

> The appropriate 7th character is to be added to each code from category S53.
> A   initial encounter
> D   subsequent encounter
> S   sequela

√5ᵗʰ **S53.0** Subluxation and dislocation of radial head

Dislocation of radiohumeral joint
Subluxation of radiohumeral joint

EXCLUDES 1   *Monteggia's fracture-dislocation (S52.27-)*

√6ᵗʰ **S53.00** Unspecified subluxation and dislocation of radial head

√7ᵗʰ **S53.001** Unspecified subluxation of right radial head

√7ᵗʰ **S53.002** Unspecified subluxation of left radial head

√7ᵗʰ **S53.003** Unspecified subluxation of unspecified radial head

√7ᵗʰ **S53.004** Unspecified dislocation of right radial head

√7ᵗʰ **S53.005** Unspecified dislocation of left radial head

√7ᵗʰ **S53.006** Unspecified dislocation of unspecified radial head

√6ᵗʰ **S53.01** Anterior subluxation and dislocation of radial head

Anteriomedial subluxation and dislocation of radial head

√7ᵗʰ **S53.011** Anterior subluxation of right radial head

√7ᵗʰ **S53.012** Anterior subluxation of left radial head

√7ᵗʰ **S53.013** Anterior subluxation of unspecified radial head

√7ᵗʰ **S53.014** Anterior dislocation of right radial head

√7ᵗʰ **S53.015** Anterior dislocation of left radial head

√7ᵗʰ **S53.016** Anterior dislocation of unspecified radial head

√6ᵗʰ **S53.02** Posterior subluxation and dislocation of radial head

Posteriolateral subluxation and dislocation of radial head

√7ᵗʰ **S53.021** Posterior subluxation of right radial head

√7ᵗʰ **S53.022** Posterior subluxation of left radial head

√7ᵗʰ **S53.023** Posterior subluxation of unspecified radial head

√7ᵗʰ **S53.024** Posterior dislocation of right radial head

√7ᵗʰ **S53.025** Posterior dislocation of left radial head

√7ᵗʰ **S53.026** Posterior dislocation of unspecified radial head

√6ᵗʰ **S53.03** Nursemaid's elbow

√7ᵗʰ **S53.031** Nursemaid's elbow, right elbow

√7ᵗʰ **S53.032** Nursemaid's elbow, left elbow

√7ᵗʰ **S53.033** Nursemaid's elbow, unspecified elbow

√6ᵗʰ **S53.09** Other subluxation and dislocation of radial head

√7ᵗʰ **S53.091** Other subluxation of right radial head

√7ᵗʰ **S53.092** Other subluxation of left radial head

√7ᵗʰ **S53.093** Other subluxation of unspecified radial head

√7ᵗʰ **S53.094** Other dislocation of right radial head

√7ᵗʰ **S53.095** Other dislocation of left radial head

√7ᵗʰ **S53.096** Other dislocation of unspecified radial head

√5ᵗʰ **S53.1** Subluxation and dislocation of ulnohumeral joint

Subluxation and dislocation of elbow NOS

EXCLUDES 1   *dislocation of radial head alone (S53.0-)*

√6ᵗʰ **S53.10** Unspecified subluxation and dislocation of ulnohumeral joint

√7ᵗʰ **S53.101** Unspecified subluxation of right ulnohumeral joint

√7ᵗʰ **S53.102** Unspecified subluxation of left ulnohumeral joint

√7ᵗʰ **S53.103** Unspecified subluxation of unspecified ulnohumeral joint

√7ᵗʰ **S53.104** Unspecified dislocation of right ulnohumeral joint

√7ᵗʰ **S53.105** Unspecified dislocation of left ulnohumeral joint

√7ᵗʰ **S53.106** Unspecified dislocation of unspecified ulnohumeral joint

√6ᵗʰ **S53.11** Anterior subluxation and dislocation of ulnohumeral joint

√7ᵗʰ **S53.111** Anterior subluxation of right ulnohumeral joint

√7ᵗʰ **S53.112** Anterior subluxation of left ulnohumeral joint

√7ᵗʰ **S53.113** Anterior subluxation of unspecified ulnohumeral joint

√7ᵗʰ **S53.114** Anterior dislocation of right ulnohumeral joint

AHA: 2012,4Q,108

√7ᵗʰ **S53.115** Anterior dislocation of left ulnohumeral joint

√7ᵗʰ **S53.116** Anterior dislocation of unspecified ulnohumeral joint

√6ᵗʰ **S53.12** Posterior subluxation and dislocation of ulnohumeral joint

√7ᵗʰ **S53.121** Posterior subluxation of right ulnohumeral joint

√7ᵗʰ **S53.122** Posterior subluxation of left ulnohumeral joint

√7ᵗʰ **S53.123** Posterior subluxation of unspecified ulnohumeral joint

N Newborn: 0   P Pediatric: 0-17   M Maternity: 9-64   A Adult: 15-124   MCC Major Complication/Comorbidity   CC Complication/Comorbidity   SW Severe Wound Dx

1022   ICD-10-CM 2021

√7ᵗʰ **S53.124** Posterior dislocation of right ulnohumeral joint

√7ᵗʰ **S53.125** Posterior dislocation of left ulnohumeral joint

√7ᵗʰ **S53.126** Posterior dislocation of unspecified ulnohumeral joint

√6ᵗʰ **S53.13** Medial subluxation and dislocation of ulnohumeral joint

√7ᵗʰ **S53.131** Medial subluxation of right ulnohumeral joint

√7ᵗʰ **S53.132** Medial subluxation of left ulnohumeral joint

√7ᵗʰ **S53.133** Medial subluxation of unspecified ulnohumeral joint

√7ᵗʰ **S53.134** Medial dislocation of right ulnohumeral joint

√7ᵗʰ **S53.135** Medial dislocation of left ulnohumeral joint

√7ᵗʰ **S53.136** Medial dislocation of unspecified ulnohumeral joint

√6ᵗʰ **S53.14** Lateral subluxation and dislocation of ulnohumeral joint

√7ᵗʰ **S53.141** Lateral subluxation of right ulnohumeral joint

√7ᵗʰ **S53.142** Lateral subluxation of left ulnohumeral joint

√7ᵗʰ **S53.143** Lateral subluxation of unspecified ulnohumeral joint

√7ᵗʰ **S53.144** Lateral dislocation of right ulnohumeral joint

√7ᵗʰ **S53.145** Lateral dislocation of left ulnohumeral joint

√7ᵗʰ **S53.146** Lateral dislocation of unspecified ulnohumeral joint

√6ᵗʰ **S53.19** Other subluxation and dislocation of ulnohumeral joint

√7ᵗʰ **S53.191** Other subluxation of right ulnohumeral joint

√7ᵗʰ **S53.192** Other subluxation of left ulnohumeral joint

√7ᵗʰ **S53.193** Other subluxation of unspecified ulnohumeral joint

√7ᵗʰ **S53.194** Other dislocation of right ulnohumeral joint

√7ᵗʰ **S53.195** Other dislocation of left ulnohumeral joint

√7ᵗʰ **S53.196** Other dislocation of unspecified ulnohumeral joint

√5ᵗʰ **S53.2** Traumatic rupture of radial collateral ligament

> *EXCLUDES 1*   sprain of radial collateral ligament NOS (S53.43-)

√x7ᵗʰ **S53.20** Traumatic rupture of unspecified radial collateral ligament

√x7ᵗʰ **S53.21** Traumatic rupture of right radial collateral ligament

√x7ᵗʰ **S53.22** Traumatic rupture of left radial collateral ligament

√5ᵗʰ **S53.3** Traumatic rupture of ulnar collateral ligament

> *EXCLUDES 1*   sprain of ulnar collateral ligament (S53.44-)

√x7ᵗʰ **S53.30** Traumatic rupture of unspecified ulnar collateral ligament

√x7ᵗʰ **S53.31** Traumatic rupture of right ulnar collateral ligament

√x7ᵗʰ **S53.32** Traumatic rupture of left ulnar collateral ligament

√5ᵗʰ **S53.4** Sprain of elbow

> *EXCLUDES 2*   traumatic rupture of radial collateral ligament (S53.2-)
> traumatic rupture of ulnar collateral ligament (S53.3-)

√6ᵗʰ **S53.40** Unspecified sprain of elbow

√7ᵗʰ **S53.401** Unspecified sprain of right elbow

√7ᵗʰ **S53.402** Unspecified sprain of left elbow

√7ᵗʰ **S53.409** Unspecified sprain of unspecified elbow
Sprain of elbow NOS

√6ᵗʰ **S53.41** Radiohumeral (joint) sprain

√7ᵗʰ **S53.411** Radiohumeral (joint) sprain of right elbow

√7ᵗʰ **S53.412** Radiohumeral (joint) sprain of left elbow

√7ᵗʰ **S53.419** Radiohumeral (joint) sprain of unspecified elbow

√6ᵗʰ **S53.42** Ulnohumeral (joint) sprain

√7ᵗʰ **S53.421** Ulnohumeral (joint) sprain of right elbow

√7ᵗʰ **S53.422** Ulnohumeral (joint) sprain of left elbow

√7ᵗʰ **S53.429** Ulnohumeral (joint) sprain of unspecified elbow

√6ᵗʰ **S53.43** Radial collateral ligament sprain

√7ᵗʰ **S53.431** Radial collateral ligament sprain of right elbow

√7ᵗʰ **S53.432** Radial collateral ligament sprain of left elbow

√7ᵗʰ **S53.439** Radial collateral ligament sprain of unspecified elbow

√6ᵗʰ **S53.44** Ulnar collateral ligament sprain

√7ᵗʰ **S53.441** Ulnar collateral ligament sprain of right elbow

√7ᵗʰ **S53.442** Ulnar collateral ligament sprain of left elbow

√7ᵗʰ **S53.449** Ulnar collateral ligament sprain of unspecified elbow

√6ᵗʰ **S53.49** Other sprain of elbow

√7ᵗʰ **S53.491** Other sprain of right elbow

√7ᵗʰ **S53.492** Other sprain of left elbow

√7ᵗʰ **S53.499** Other sprain of unspecified elbow

√4ᵗʰ **S54** **Injury of nerves at forearm level**

Code also any associated open wound (S51.-)

> *EXCLUDES 2*   injury of nerves at wrist and hand level (S64.-)

> The appropriate 7th character is to be added to each code from category S54.
> A   initial encounter
> D   subsequent encounter
> S   sequela

√5ᵗʰ **S54.0** Injury of ulnar nerve at forearm level
Injury of ulnar nerve NOS

√x7ᵗʰ **S54.00** Injury of ulnar nerve at forearm level, unspecified arm

√x7ᵗʰ **S54.01** Injury of ulnar nerve at forearm level, right arm

√x7ᵗʰ **S54.02** Injury of ulnar nerve at forearm level, left arm

√5ᵗʰ **S54.1** Injury of median nerve at forearm level
Injury of median nerve NOS

√x7ᵗʰ **S54.10** Injury of median nerve at forearm level, unspecified arm

√x7ᵗʰ **S54.11** Injury of median nerve at forearm level, right arm

√x7ᵗʰ **S54.12** Injury of median nerve at forearm level, left arm

√5ᵗʰ **S54.2** Injury of radial nerve at forearm level
Injury of radial nerve NOS

√x7ᵗʰ **S54.20** Injury of radial nerve at forearm level, unspecified arm

√x7ᵗʰ **S54.21** Injury of radial nerve at forearm level, right arm

√x7ᵗʰ **S54.22** Injury of radial nerve at forearm level, left arm

√5ᵗʰ **S54.3** Injury of cutaneous sensory nerve at forearm level

√x7ᵗʰ **S54.30** Injury of cutaneous sensory nerve at forearm level, unspecified arm

√x7ᵗʰ **S54.31** Injury of cutaneous sensory nerve at forearm level, right arm

√x7ᵗʰ **S54.32** Injury of cutaneous sensory nerve at forearm level, left arm

√5ᵗʰ **S54.8** Injury of other nerves at forearm level

√6ᵗʰ **S54.8X** Injury of other nerves at forearm level

√7ᵗʰ **S54.8X1** Injury of other nerves at forearm level, right arm

√7ᵗʰ **S54.8X2** Injury of other nerves at forearm level, left arm

√7ᵗʰ **S54.8X9** Injury of other nerves at forearm level, unspecified arm

√5ᵗʰ **S54.9** Injury of unspecified nerve at forearm level

√x7ᵗʰ **S54.90** Injury of unspecified nerve at forearm level, unspecified arm

√x7ᵗʰ **S54.91** Injury of unspecified nerve at forearm level, right arm

√x7ᵗʰ **S54.92** Injury of unspecified nerve at forearm level, left arm

---

☑ Additional Character Required   √x7ᵗʰ Placeholder   Unacceptable PDx   Questionable PDx   Manifestation   Unspecified Dx   H1-H14 HAC   HCC CMS-HCC Dx   HIV HIV Dx

Chapter 19. Injury, Poisoning and Certain Other Consequences of External Causes

S55–S56.011

√4ᵗʰ **S55 Injury of blood vessels at forearm level**

Code also any associated open wound (S51.-)

EXCLUDES 2   injury of blood vessels at wrist and hand level (S65.-)
     injury of brachial vessels (S45.1-S45.2)

The appropriate 7th character is to be added to each code from category S55.
A   initial encounter
D   subsequent encounter
S   sequela

√5ᵗʰ **S55.0 Injury of ulnar artery at forearm level**

√6ᵗʰ **S55.00 Unspecified injury of ulnar artery at forearm level**

√7ᵗʰ **S55.001** Unspecified injury of ulnar artery at forearm level, right arm   CC

√7ᵗʰ **S55.002** Unspecified injury of ulnar artery at forearm level, left arm   CC

√7ᵗʰ **S55.009** Unspecified injury of ulnar artery at forearm level, unspecified arm   CC

√6ᵗʰ **S55.01 Laceration of ulnar artery at forearm level**

√7ᵗʰ **S55.011** Laceration of ulnar artery at forearm level, right arm   CC

√7ᵗʰ **S55.012** Laceration of ulnar artery at forearm level, left arm   CC

√7ᵗʰ **S55.019** Laceration of ulnar artery at forearm level, unspecified arm   CC

√6ᵗʰ **S55.09 Other specified injury of ulnar artery at forearm level**

√7ᵗʰ **S55.091** Other specified injury of ulnar artery at forearm level, right arm   CC

√7ᵗʰ **S55.092** Other specified injury of ulnar artery at forearm level, left arm   CC

√7ᵗʰ **S55.099** Other specified injury of ulnar artery at forearm level, unspecified arm   CC

√5ᵗʰ **S55.1 Injury of radial artery at forearm level**

√6ᵗʰ **S55.10 Unspecified injury of radial artery at forearm level**

√7ᵗʰ **S55.101** Unspecified injury of radial artery at forearm level, right arm   CC

√7ᵗʰ **S55.102** Unspecified injury of radial artery at forearm level, left arm   CC

√7ᵗʰ **S55.109** Unspecified injury of radial artery at forearm level, unspecified arm   CC

√6ᵗʰ **S55.11 Laceration of radial artery at forearm level**

√7ᵗʰ **S55.111** Laceration of radial artery at forearm level, right arm   CC

√7ᵗʰ **S55.112** Laceration of radial artery at forearm level, left arm   CC

√7ᵗʰ **S55.119** Laceration of radial artery at forearm level, unspecified arm   CC

√6ᵗʰ **S55.19 Other specified injury of radial artery at forearm level**

√7ᵗʰ **S55.191** Other specified injury of radial artery at forearm level, right arm   CC

√7ᵗʰ **S55.192** Other specified injury of radial artery at forearm level, left arm   CC

√7ᵗʰ **S55.199** Other specified injury of radial artery at forearm level, unspecified arm   CC

√5ᵗʰ **S55.2 Injury of vein at forearm level**

√6ᵗʰ **S55.20 Unspecified injury of vein at forearm level**

√7ᵗʰ **S55.201** Unspecified injury of vein at forearm level, right arm   CC

√7ᵗʰ **S55.202** Unspecified injury of vein at forearm level, left arm   CC

√7ᵗʰ **S55.209** Unspecified injury of vein at forearm level, unspecified arm   CC

√6ᵗʰ **S55.21 Laceration of vein at forearm level**

√7ᵗʰ **S55.211** Laceration of vein at forearm level, right arm   CC

√7ᵗʰ **S55.212** Laceration of vein at forearm level, left arm   CC

√7ᵗʰ **S55.219** Laceration of vein at forearm level, unspecified arm   CC

√6ᵗʰ **S55.29 Other specified injury of vein at forearm level**

√7ᵗʰ **S55.291** Other specified injury of vein at forearm level, right arm   CC

√7ᵗʰ **S55.292** Other specified injury of vein at forearm level, left arm   CC

√7ᵗʰ **S55.299** Other specified injury of vein at forearm level, unspecified arm   CC

√5ᵗʰ **S55.8 Injury of other blood vessels at forearm level**

√6ᵗʰ **S55.80 Unspecified injury of other blood vessels at forearm level**

√7ᵗʰ **S55.801** Unspecified injury of other blood vessels at forearm level, right arm   CC

√7ᵗʰ **S55.802** Unspecified injury of other blood vessels at forearm level, left arm   CC

√7ᵗʰ **S55.809** Unspecified injury of other blood vessels at forearm level, unspecified arm   CC

√6ᵗʰ **S55.81 Laceration of other blood vessels at forearm level**

√7ᵗʰ **S55.811** Laceration of other blood vessels at forearm level, right arm   CC

√7ᵗʰ **S55.812** Laceration of other blood vessels at forearm level, left arm   CC

√7ᵗʰ **S55.819** Laceration of other blood vessels at forearm level, unspecified arm   CC

√6ᵗʰ **S55.89 Other specified injury of other blood vessels at forearm level**

√7ᵗʰ **S55.891** Other specified injury of other blood vessels at forearm level, right arm   CC

√7ᵗʰ **S55.892** Other specified injury of other blood vessels at forearm level, left arm   CC

√7ᵗʰ **S55.899** Other specified injury of other blood vessels at forearm level, unspecified arm   CC

√5ᵗʰ **S55.9 Injury of unspecified blood vessel at forearm level**

√6ᵗʰ **S55.90 Unspecified injury of unspecified blood vessel at forearm level**

√7ᵗʰ **S55.901** Unspecified injury of unspecified blood vessel at forearm level, right arm   CC

√7ᵗʰ **S55.902** Unspecified injury of unspecified blood vessel at forearm level, left arm   CC

√7ᵗʰ **S55.909** Unspecified injury of unspecified blood vessel at forearm level, unspecified arm   CC

√6ᵗʰ **S55.91 Laceration of unspecified blood vessel at forearm level**

√7ᵗʰ **S55.911** Laceration of unspecified blood vessel at forearm level, right arm   CC

√7ᵗʰ **S55.912** Laceration of unspecified blood vessel at forearm level, left arm   CC

√7ᵗʰ **S55.919** Laceration of unspecified blood vessel at forearm level, unspecified arm   CC

√6ᵗʰ **S55.99 Other specified injury of unspecified blood vessel at forearm level**

√7ᵗʰ **S55.991** Other specified injury of unspecified blood vessel at forearm level, right arm   CC

√7ᵗʰ **S55.992** Other specified injury of unspecified blood vessel at forearm level, left arm   CC

√7ᵗʰ **S55.999** Other specified injury of unspecified blood vessel at forearm level, unspecified arm   CC

√4ᵗʰ **S56 Injury of muscle, fascia and tendon at forearm level**

Code also any associated open wound (S51.-)

EXCLUDES 2   injury of muscle, fascia and tendon at or below wrist (S66.-)
     sprain of joints and ligaments of elbow (S53.4-)

TIP: Refer to the Muscle/Tendon table at the beginning of this chapter

The appropriate 7th character is to be added to each code from category S56.
A   initial encounter
D   subsequent encounter
S   sequela

√5ᵗʰ **S56.0 Injury of flexor muscle, fascia and tendon of thumb at forearm level**

√6ᵗʰ **S56.00 Unspecified injury of flexor muscle, fascia and tendon of thumb at forearm level**

√7ᵗʰ **S56.001** Unspecified injury of flexor muscle, fascia and tendon of right thumb at forearm level

√7ᵗʰ **S56.002** Unspecified injury of flexor muscle, fascia and tendon of left thumb at forearm level

√7ᵗʰ **S56.009** Unspecified injury of flexor muscle, fascia and tendon of unspecified thumb at forearm level

√6ᵗʰ **S56.01 Strain of flexor muscle, fascia and tendon of thumb at forearm level**

√7ᵗʰ **S56.011** Strain of flexor muscle, fascia and tendon of right thumb at forearm level

N Newborn: 0   P Pediatric: 0-17   M Maternity: 9-64   A Adult: 15-124   MCC Major Complication/Comorbidity   CC Complication/Comorbidity   SW Severe Wound Dx

1024   ICD-10-CM 2021

√7ᵗʰ S56.012 Strain of flexor muscle, fascia and tendon of left thumb at forearm level

√7ᵗʰ **S56.019** Strain of flexor muscle, fascia and tendon of unspecified thumb at forearm level

√6ᵗʰ S56.02 Laceration of flexor muscle, fascia and tendon of thumb at forearm level

√7ᵗʰ S56.021 Laceration of flexor muscle, fascia and tendon of right thumb at forearm level **cc**

√7ᵗʰ S56.022 Laceration of flexor muscle, fascia and tendon of left thumb at forearm level **cc**

√7ᵗʰ **S56.029** Laceration of flexor muscle, fascia and tendon of unspecified thumb at forearm level **cc**

√6ᵗʰ S56.09 Other injury of flexor muscle, fascia and tendon of thumb at forearm level

√7ᵗʰ S56.091 Other injury of flexor muscle, fascia and tendon of right thumb at forearm level

√7ᵗʰ S56.092 Other injury of flexor muscle, fascia and tendon of left thumb at forearm level

√7ᵗʰ **S56.099** Other injury of flexor muscle, fascia and tendon of unspecified thumb at forearm level

√5ᵗʰ S56.1 Injury of flexor muscle, fascia and tendon of other and unspecified finger at forearm level

√6ᵗʰ S56.10 Unspecified injury of flexor muscle, fascia and tendon of other and unspecified finger at forearm level

√7ᵗʰ **S56.101** Unspecified injury of flexor muscle, fascia and tendon of right index finger at forearm level

√7ᵗʰ **S56.102** Unspecified injury of flexor muscle, fascia and tendon of left index finger at forearm level

√7ᵗʰ **S56.103** Unspecified injury of flexor muscle, fascia and tendon of right middle finger at forearm level

√7ᵗʰ **S56.104** Unspecified injury of flexor muscle, fascia and tendon of left middle finger at forearm level

√7ᵗʰ **S56.105** Unspecified injury of flexor muscle, fascia and tendon of right ring finger at forearm level

√7ᵗʰ **S56.106** Unspecified injury of flexor muscle, fascia and tendon of left ring finger at forearm level

√7ᵗʰ **S56.107** Unspecified injury of flexor muscle, fascia and tendon of right little finger at forearm level

√7ᵗʰ **S56.108** Unspecified injury of flexor muscle, fascia and tendon of left little finger at forearm level

√7ᵗʰ **S56.109** Unspecified injury of flexor muscle, fascia and tendon of unspecified finger at forearm level

√6ᵗʰ S56.11 Strain of flexor muscle, fascia and tendon of other and unspecified finger at forearm level

√7ᵗʰ S56.111 Strain of flexor muscle, fascia and tendon of right index finger at forearm level

√7ᵗʰ S56.112 Strain of flexor muscle, fascia and tendon of left index finger at forearm level

√7ᵗʰ S56.113 Strain of flexor muscle, fascia and tendon of right middle finger at forearm level

√7ᵗʰ S56.114 Strain of flexor muscle, fascia and tendon of left middle finger at forearm level

√7ᵗʰ S56.115 Strain of flexor muscle, fascia and tendon of right ring finger at forearm level

√7ᵗʰ S56.116 Strain of flexor muscle, fascia and tendon of left ring finger at forearm level

√7ᵗʰ S56.117 Strain of flexor muscle, fascia and tendon of right little finger at forearm level

√7ᵗʰ S56.118 Strain of flexor muscle, fascia and tendon of left little finger at forearm level

√7ᵗʰ **S56.119** Strain of flexor muscle, fascia and tendon of finger of unspecified finger at forearm level

√6ᵗʰ S56.12 Laceration of flexor muscle, fascia and tendon of other and unspecified finger at forearm level

√7ᵗʰ S56.121 Laceration of flexor muscle, fascia and tendon of right index finger at forearm level **cc**

√7ᵗʰ S56.122 Laceration of flexor muscle, fascia and tendon of left index finger at forearm level **cc**

√7ᵗʰ S56.123 Laceration of flexor muscle, fascia and tendon of right middle finger at forearm level **cc**

√7ᵗʰ S56.124 Laceration of flexor muscle, fascia and tendon of left middle finger at forearm level **cc**

√7ᵗʰ S56.125 Laceration of flexor muscle, fascia and tendon of right ring finger at forearm level **cc**

√7ᵗʰ S56.126 Laceration of flexor muscle, fascia and tendon of left ring finger at forearm level **cc**

√7ᵗʰ S56.127 Laceration of flexor muscle, fascia and tendon of right little finger at forearm level **cc**

√7ᵗʰ S56.128 Laceration of flexor muscle, fascia and tendon of left little finger at forearm level **cc**

√7ᵗʰ **S56.129** Laceration of flexor muscle, fascia and tendon of unspecified finger at forearm level **cc**

√6ᵗʰ S56.19 Other injury of flexor muscle, fascia and tendon of other and unspecified finger at forearm level

√7ᵗʰ S56.191 Other injury of flexor muscle, fascia and tendon of right index finger at forearm level

√7ᵗʰ S56.192 Other injury of flexor muscle, fascia and tendon of left index finger at forearm level

√7ᵗʰ S56.193 Other injury of flexor muscle, fascia and tendon of right middle finger at forearm level

√7ᵗʰ S56.194 Other injury of flexor muscle, fascia and tendon of left middle finger at forearm level

√7ᵗʰ S56.195 Other injury of flexor muscle, fascia and tendon of right ring finger at forearm level

√7ᵗʰ S56.196 Other injury of flexor muscle, fascia and tendon of left ring finger at forearm level

√7ᵗʰ S56.197 Other injury of flexor muscle, fascia and tendon of right little finger at forearm level

√7ᵗʰ S56.198 Other injury of flexor muscle, fascia and tendon of left little finger at forearm level

√7ᵗʰ **S56.199** Other injury of flexor muscle, fascia and tendon of unspecified finger at forearm level

√5ᵗʰ S56.2 Injury of other flexor muscle, fascia and tendon at forearm level

√6ᵗʰ S56.20 Unspecified injury of other flexor muscle, fascia and tendon at forearm level

√7ᵗʰ **S56.201** Unspecified injury of other flexor muscle, fascia and tendon at forearm level, right arm

√7ᵗʰ **S56.202** Unspecified injury of other flexor muscle, fascia and tendon at forearm level, left arm

√7ᵗʰ **S56.209** Unspecified injury of other flexor muscle, fascia and tendon at forearm level, unspecified arm

√6ᵗʰ S56.21 Strain of other flexor muscle, fascia and tendon at forearm level

√7ᵗʰ S56.211 Strain of other flexor muscle, fascia and tendon at forearm level, right arm

√7ᵗʰ S56.212 Strain of other flexor muscle, fascia and tendon at forearm level, left arm

√7ᵗʰ **S56.219** Strain of other flexor muscle, fascia and tendon at forearm level, unspecified arm

√6ᵗʰ S56.22 Laceration of other flexor muscle, fascia and tendon at forearm level

√7ᵗʰ S56.221 Laceration of other flexor muscle, fascia and tendon at forearm level, right arm **cc**

√7ᵗʰ S56.222 Laceration of other flexor muscle, fascia and tendon at forearm level, left arm **cc**

√7ᵗʰ **S56.229** Laceration of other flexor muscle, fascia and tendon at forearm level, unspecified arm **cc**

☑ Additional Character Required √x7ᵗʰ Placeholder   Unacceptable PDx   Questionable PDx   Manifestation   Unspecified Dx   H1 -H14 HAC   HCC CMS-HCC Dx   HIV HIV Dx

ICD-10-CM 2021   1025

✓6ᵗʰ **S56.29** Other injury of other flexor muscle, fascia and tendon at forearm level

    ✓7ᵗʰ **S56.291** Other injury of other flexor muscle, fascia and tendon at forearm level, right arm

    ✓7ᵗʰ **S56.292** Other injury of other flexor muscle, fascia and tendon at forearm level, left arm

    ✓7ᵗʰ **S56.299** Other injury of other flexor muscle, fascia and tendon at forearm level, unspecified arm

✓5ᵗʰ **S56.3** Injury of extensor or abductor muscles, fascia and tendons of thumb at forearm level

    ✓6ᵗʰ **S56.30** Unspecified injury of extensor or abductor muscles, fascia and tendons of thumb at forearm level

      ✓7ᵗʰ **S56.301** Unspecified injury of extensor or abductor muscles, fascia and tendons of right thumb at forearm level

      ✓7ᵗʰ **S56.302** Unspecified injury of extensor or abductor muscles, fascia and tendons of left thumb at forearm level

      ✓7ᵗʰ **S56.309** Unspecified injury of extensor or abductor muscles, fascia and tendons of unspecified thumb at forearm level

    ✓6ᵗʰ **S56.31** Strain of extensor or abductor muscles, fascia and tendons of thumb at forearm level

      ✓7ᵗʰ **S56.311** Strain of extensor or abductor muscles, fascia and tendons of right thumb at forearm level

      ✓7ᵗʰ **S56.312** Strain of extensor or abductor muscles, fascia and tendons of left thumb at forearm level

      ✓7ᵗʰ **S56.319** Strain of extensor or abductor muscles, fascia and tendons of unspecified thumb at forearm level

    ✓6ᵗʰ **S56.32** Laceration of extensor or abductor muscles, fascia and tendons of thumb at forearm level

      ✓7ᵗʰ **S56.321** Laceration of extensor or abductor muscles, fascia and tendons of right thumb at forearm level   cc

      ✓7ᵗʰ **S56.322** Laceration of extensor or abductor muscles, fascia and tendons of left thumb at forearm level   cc

      ✓7ᵗʰ **S56.329** Laceration of extensor or abductor muscles, fascia and tendons of unspecified thumb at forearm level   cc

    ✓6ᵗʰ **S56.39** Other injury of extensor or abductor muscles, fascia and tendons of thumb at forearm level

      ✓7ᵗʰ **S56.391** Other injury of extensor or abductor muscles, fascia and tendons of right thumb at forearm level

      ✓7ᵗʰ **S56.392** Other injury of extensor or abductor muscles, fascia and tendons of left thumb at forearm level

      ✓7ᵗʰ **S56.399** Other injury of extensor or abductor muscles, fascia and tendons of unspecified thumb at forearm level

✓5ᵗʰ **S56.4** Injury of extensor muscle, fascia and tendon of other and unspecified finger at forearm level

    ✓6ᵗʰ **S56.40** Unspecified injury of extensor muscle, fascia and tendon of other and unspecified finger at forearm level

      ✓7ᵗʰ **S56.401** Unspecified injury of extensor muscle, fascia and tendon of right index finger at forearm level

      ✓7ᵗʰ **S56.402** Unspecified injury of extensor muscle, fascia and tendon of left index finger at forearm level

      ✓7ᵗʰ **S56.403** Unspecified injury of extensor muscle, fascia and tendon of right middle finger at forearm level

      ✓7ᵗʰ **S56.404** Unspecified injury of extensor muscle, fascia and tendon of left middle finger at forearm level

      ✓7ᵗʰ **S56.405** Unspecified injury of extensor muscle, fascia and tendon of right ring finger at forearm level

      ✓7ᵗʰ **S56.406** Unspecified injury of extensor muscle, fascia and tendon of left ring finger at forearm level

      ✓7ᵗʰ **S56.407** Unspecified injury of extensor muscle, fascia and tendon of right little finger at forearm level

      ✓7ᵗʰ **S56.408** Unspecified injury of extensor muscle, fascia and tendon of left little finger at forearm level

      ✓7ᵗʰ **S56.409** Unspecified injury of extensor muscle, fascia and tendon of unspecified finger at forearm level

    ✓6ᵗʰ **S56.41** Strain of extensor muscle, fascia and tendon of other and unspecified finger at forearm level

      ✓7ᵗʰ **S56.411** Strain of extensor muscle, fascia and tendon of right index finger at forearm level

      ✓7ᵗʰ **S56.412** Strain of extensor muscle, fascia and tendon of left index finger at forearm level

      ✓7ᵗʰ **S56.413** Strain of extensor muscle, fascia and tendon of right middle finger at forearm level

      ✓7ᵗʰ **S56.414** Strain of extensor muscle, fascia and tendon of left middle finger at forearm level

      ✓7ᵗʰ **S56.415** Strain of extensor muscle, fascia and tendon of right ring finger at forearm level

      ✓7ᵗʰ **S56.416** Strain of extensor muscle, fascia and tendon of left ring finger at forearm level

      ✓7ᵗʰ **S56.417** Strain of extensor muscle, fascia and tendon of right little finger at forearm level

      ✓7ᵗʰ **S56.418** Strain of extensor muscle, fascia and tendon of left little finger at forearm level

      ✓7ᵗʰ **S56.419** Strain of extensor muscle, fascia and tendon of finger, unspecified finger at forearm level

    ✓6ᵗʰ **S56.42** Laceration of extensor muscle, fascia and tendon of other and unspecified finger at forearm level

      ✓7ᵗʰ **S56.421** Laceration of extensor muscle, fascia and tendon of right index finger at forearm level   cc

      ✓7ᵗʰ **S56.422** Laceration of extensor muscle, fascia and tendon of left index finger at forearm level   cc

      ✓7ᵗʰ **S56.423** Laceration of extensor muscle, fascia and tendon of right middle finger at forearm level   cc

      ✓7ᵗʰ **S56.424** Laceration of extensor muscle, fascia and tendon of left middle finger at forearm level   cc

      ✓7ᵗʰ **S56.425** Laceration of extensor muscle, fascia and tendon of right ring finger at forearm level   cc

      ✓7ᵗʰ **S56.426** Laceration of extensor muscle, fascia and tendon of left ring finger at forearm level   cc

      ✓7ᵗʰ **S56.427** Laceration of extensor muscle, fascia and tendon of right little finger at forearm level   cc

      ✓7ᵗʰ **S56.428** Laceration of extensor muscle, fascia and tendon of left little finger at forearm level   cc

      ✓7ᵗʰ **S56.429** Laceration of extensor muscle, fascia and tendon of unspecified finger at forearm level   cc

    ✓6ᵗʰ **S56.49** Other injury of extensor muscle, fascia and tendon of other and unspecified finger at forearm level

      ✓7ᵗʰ **S56.491** Other injury of extensor muscle, fascia and tendon of right index finger at forearm level

      ✓7ᵗʰ **S56.492** Other injury of extensor muscle, fascia and tendon of left index finger at forearm level

      ✓7ᵗʰ **S56.493** Other injury of extensor muscle, fascia and tendon of right middle finger at forearm level

      ✓7ᵗʰ **S56.494** Other injury of extensor muscle, fascia and tendon of left middle finger at forearm level

      ✓7ᵗʰ **S56.495** Other injury of extensor muscle, fascia and tendon of right ring finger at forearm level

      ✓7ᵗʰ **S56.496** Other injury of extensor muscle, fascia and tendon of left ring finger at forearm level

      ✓7ᵗʰ **S56.497** Other injury of extensor muscle, fascia and tendon of right little finger at forearm level

N Newborn: 0   P Pediatric: 0-17   M Maternity: 9-64   A Adult: 15-124   MCC Major Complication/Comorbidity   cc Complication/Comorbidity   SW Severe Wound Dx

1026   ICD-10-CM 2021

√7ᵗʰ **S56.498** Other injury of extensor muscle, fascia and tendon of left little finger at forearm level

√7ᵗʰ **S56.499** Other injury of extensor muscle, fascia and tendon of unspecified finger at forearm level

√5ᵗʰ **S56.5** Injury of other extensor muscle, fascia and tendon at forearm level

  √6ᵗʰ **S56.50** Unspecified injury of other extensor muscle, fascia and tendon at forearm level

    √7ᵗʰ **S56.501** Unspecified injury of other extensor muscle, fascia and tendon at forearm level, right arm

    √7ᵗʰ **S56.502** Unspecified injury of other extensor muscle, fascia and tendon at forearm level, left arm

    √7ᵗʰ **S56.509** Unspecified injury of other extensor muscle, fascia and tendon at forearm level, unspecified arm

  √6ᵗʰ **S56.51** Strain of other extensor muscle, fascia and tendon at forearm level

    √7ᵗʰ **S56.511** Strain of other extensor muscle, fascia and tendon at forearm level, right arm

    √7ᵗʰ **S56.512** Strain of other extensor muscle, fascia and tendon at forearm level, left arm

    √7ᵗʰ **S56.519** Strain of other extensor muscle, fascia and tendon at forearm level, unspecified arm

  √6ᵗʰ **S56.52** Laceration of other extensor muscle, fascia and tendon at forearm level

    √7ᵗʰ **S56.521** Laceration of other extensor muscle, fascia and tendon at forearm level, right arm CC

    √7ᵗʰ **S56.522** Laceration of other extensor muscle, fascia and tendon at forearm level, left arm CC

    √7ᵗʰ **S56.529** Laceration of other extensor muscle, fascia and tendon at forearm level, unspecified arm CC

  √6ᵗʰ **S56.59** Other injury of other extensor muscle, fascia and tendon at forearm level

    √7ᵗʰ **S56.591** Other injury of other extensor muscle, fascia and tendon at forearm level, right arm

    √7ᵗʰ **S56.592** Other injury of other extensor muscle, fascia and tendon at forearm level, left arm

    √7ᵗʰ **S56.599** Other injury of other extensor muscle, fascia and tendon at forearm level, unspecified arm

√5ᵗʰ **S56.8** Injury of other muscles, fascia and tendons at forearm level

  √6ᵗʰ **S56.80** Unspecified injury of other muscles, fascia and tendons at forearm level

    √7ᵗʰ **S56.801** Unspecified injury of other muscles, fascia and tendons at forearm level, right arm

    √7ᵗʰ **S56.802** Unspecified injury of other muscles, fascia and tendons at forearm level, left arm

    √7ᵗʰ **S56.809** Unspecified injury of other muscles, fascia and tendons at forearm level, unspecified arm

  √6ᵗʰ **S56.81** Strain of other muscles, fascia and tendons at forearm level

    √7ᵗʰ **S56.811** Strain of other muscles, fascia and tendons at forearm level, right arm

    √7ᵗʰ **S56.812** Strain of other muscles, fascia and tendons at forearm level, left arm

    √7ᵗʰ **S56.819** Strain of other muscles, fascia and tendons at forearm level, unspecified arm

  √6ᵗʰ **S56.82** Laceration of other muscles, fascia and tendons at forearm level

    √7ᵗʰ **S56.821** Laceration of other muscles, fascia and tendons at forearm level, right arm CC

    √7ᵗʰ **S56.822** Laceration of other muscles, fascia and tendons at forearm level, left arm CC

    √7ᵗʰ **S56.829** Laceration of other muscles, fascia and tendons at forearm level, unspecified arm CC

  √6ᵗʰ **S56.89** Other injury of other muscles, fascia and tendons at forearm level

    √7ᵗʰ **S56.891** Other injury of other muscles, fascia and tendons at forearm level, right arm

    √7ᵗʰ **S56.892** Other injury of other muscles, fascia and tendons at forearm level, left arm

    √7ᵗʰ **S56.899** Other injury of other muscles, fascia and tendons at forearm level, unspecified arm

√5ᵗʰ **S56.9** Injury of unspecified muscles, fascia and tendons at forearm level

  √6ᵗʰ **S56.90** Unspecified injury of unspecified muscles, fascia and tendons at forearm level

    √7ᵗʰ **S56.901** Unspecified injury of unspecified muscles, fascia and tendons at forearm level, right arm

    √7ᵗʰ **S56.902** Unspecified injury of unspecified muscles, fascia and tendons at forearm level, left arm

    √7ᵗʰ **S56.909** Unspecified injury of unspecified muscles, fascia and tendons at forearm level, unspecified arm

  √6ᵗʰ **S56.91** Strain of unspecified muscles, fascia and tendons at forearm level

    √7ᵗʰ **S56.911** Strain of unspecified muscles, fascia and tendons at forearm level, right arm

    √7ᵗʰ **S56.912** Strain of unspecified muscles, fascia and tendons at forearm level, left arm

    √7ᵗʰ **S56.919** Strain of unspecified muscles, fascia and tendons at forearm level, unspecified arm

  √6ᵗʰ **S56.92** Laceration of unspecified muscles, fascia and tendons at forearm level

    √7ᵗʰ **S56.921** Laceration of unspecified muscles, fascia and tendons at forearm level, right arm CC

    √7ᵗʰ **S56.922** Laceration of unspecified muscles, fascia and tendons at forearm level, left arm CC

    √7ᵗʰ **S56.929** Laceration of unspecified muscles, fascia and tendons at forearm level, unspecified arm CC

  √6ᵗʰ **S56.99** Other injury of unspecified muscles, fascia and tendons at forearm level

    √7ᵗʰ **S56.991** Other injury of unspecified muscles, fascia and tendons at forearm level, right arm

    √7ᵗʰ **S56.992** Other injury of unspecified muscles, fascia and tendons at forearm level, left arm

    √7ᵗʰ **S56.999** Other injury of unspecified muscles, fascia and tendons at forearm level, unspecified arm

√4ᵗʰ **S57** Crushing injury of elbow and forearm

  Use additional code(s) for all associated injuries

  EXCLUDES 2   crushing injury of wrist and hand (S67.-)

  The appropriate 7th character is to be added to each code from category S57.
  A initial encounter
  D subsequent encounter
  S sequela

  √5ᵗʰ **S57.0** Crushing injury of elbow

    √x7ᵗʰ **S57.00** Crushing injury of unspecified elbow

    √x7ᵗʰ **S57.01** Crushing injury of right elbow

    √x7ᵗʰ **S57.02** Crushing injury of left elbow

  √5ᵗʰ **S57.8** Crushing injury of forearm

    √x7ᵗʰ **S57.80** Crushing injury of unspecified forearm

    √x7ᵗʰ **S57.81** Crushing injury of right forearm

    √x7ᵗʰ **S57.82** Crushing injury of left forearm

√4ᵗʰ **S58** Traumatic amputation of elbow and forearm

  An amputation not identified as partial or complete should be coded to complete

  EXCLUDES 1   traumatic amputation of wrist and hand (S68.-)

  The appropriate 7th character is to be added to each code from category S58.
  A initial encounter
  D subsequent encounter
  S sequela

  √5ᵗʰ **S58.0** Traumatic amputation at elbow level

    √6ᵗʰ **S58.01** Complete traumatic amputation at elbow level

      7 √7ᵗʰ **S58.011** Complete traumatic amputation at elbow level, right arm CC HCC

      7 √7ᵗʰ **S58.012** Complete traumatic amputation at elbow level, left arm CC HCC

☑ Additional Character Required   √x7ᵗʰ Placeholder   Unacceptable PDx   Questionable PDx   Manifestation   Unspecified Dx   H1-H14 HAC   HCC CMS-HCC Dx   HIV HIV Dx

ICD-10-CM 2021   1027

7 √7ᵗʰ **S58.019** Complete traumatic amputation at elbow level, unspecified arm `CC` `HCC`

√6ᵗʰ **S58.02** Partial traumatic amputation at elbow level

7 √7ᵗʰ S58.021 Partial traumatic amputation at elbow level, right arm `CC` `HCC`

7 √7ᵗʰ S58.022 Partial traumatic amputation at elbow level, left arm `CC` `HCC`

7 √7ᵗʰ **S58.029** Partial traumatic amputation at elbow level, unspecified arm `CC` `HCC`

√5ᵗʰ **S58.1** Traumatic amputation at level between elbow and wrist

√6ᵗʰ **S58.11** Complete traumatic amputation at level between elbow and wrist

7 √7ᵗʰ S58.111 Complete traumatic amputation at level between elbow and wrist, right arm `CC` `HCC`

7 √7ᵗʰ S58.112 Complete traumatic amputation at level between elbow and wrist, left arm `CC` `HCC`

7 √7ᵗʰ **S58.119** Complete traumatic amputation at level between elbow and wrist, unspecified arm `CC` `HCC`

√6ᵗʰ **S58.12** Partial traumatic amputation at level between elbow and wrist

7 √7ᵗʰ S58.121 Partial traumatic amputation at level between elbow and wrist, right arm `CC` `HCC`

7 √7ᵗʰ S58.122 Partial traumatic amputation at level between elbow and wrist, left arm `CC` `HCC`

7 √7ᵗʰ **S58.129** Partial traumatic amputation at level between elbow and wrist, unspecified arm `CC` `HCC`

√5ᵗʰ **S58.9** Traumatic amputation of forearm, level unspecified

EXCLUDES 1   traumatic amputation of wrist (S68.-)

√6ᵗʰ **S58.91** Complete traumatic amputation of forearm, level unspecified

7 √7ᵗʰ **S58.911** Complete traumatic amputation of right forearm, level unspecified `CC` `HCC`

7 √7ᵗʰ **S58.912** Complete traumatic amputation of left forearm, level unspecified `CC` `HCC`

7 √7ᵗʰ **S58.919** Complete traumatic amputation of unspecified forearm, level unspecified `CC` `HCC`

√6ᵗʰ **S58.92** Partial traumatic amputation of forearm, level unspecified

7 √7ᵗʰ **S58.921** Partial traumatic amputation of right forearm, level unspecified `CC` `HCC`

7 √7ᵗʰ **S58.922** Partial traumatic amputation of left forearm, level unspecified `CC` `HCC`

7 √7ᵗʰ **S58.929** Partial traumatic amputation of unspecified forearm, level unspecified `CC` `HCC`

√4ᵗʰ **S59** Other and unspecified injuries of elbow and forearm

EXCLUDES 2   other and unspecified injuries of wrist and hand (S69.-)

AHA: 2018,2Q,12; 2018,1Q,3; 2015,3Q,37-39

The appropriate 7th character is to be added to each code from subcategories S59.0, S59.1, and S59.2.
A   initial encounter for closed fracture
D   subsequent encounter for fracture with routine healing
G   subsequent encounter for fracture with delayed healing
K   subsequent encounter for fracture with nonunion
P   subsequent encounter for fracture with malunion
S   sequela

√5ᵗʰ **S59.0** Physeal fracture of lower end of ulna

AHA: 2019,4Q,56

√6ᵗʰ **S59.00** Unspecified physeal fracture of lower end of ulna

3 √7ᵗʰ **S59.001** Unspecified physeal fracture of lower end of ulna, right arm `CC` `H5`

3 √7ᵗʰ **S59.002** Unspecified physeal fracture of lower end of ulna, left arm `CC` `H5`

3 √7ᵗʰ **S59.009** Unspecified physeal fracture of lower end of ulna, unspecified arm `CC` `H5`

√6ᵗʰ **S59.01** Salter-Harris Type I physeal fracture of lower end of ulna

3 √7ᵗʰ S59.011 Salter-Harris Type I physeal fracture of lower end of ulna, right arm `CC` `H5`

3 √7ᵗʰ S59.012 Salter-Harris Type I physeal fracture of lower end of ulna, left arm

3 √7ᵗʰ **S59.019** Salter-Harris Type I physeal fracture of lower end of ulna, unspecified arm `CC` `H5`

√6ᵗʰ **S59.02** Salter-Harris Type II physeal fracture of lower end of ulna

3 √7ᵗʰ S59.021 Salter-Harris Type II physeal fracture of lower end of ulna, right arm `CC` `H5`

3 √7ᵗʰ S59.022 Salter-Harris Type II physeal fracture of lower end of ulna, left arm `CC` `H5`

3 √7ᵗʰ **S59.029** Salter-Harris Type II physeal fracture of lower end of ulna, unspecified arm `CC` `H5`

√6ᵗʰ **S59.03** Salter-Harris Type III physeal fracture of lower end of ulna

3 √7ᵗʰ S59.031 Salter-Harris Type III physeal fracture of lower end of ulna, right arm `CC` `H5`

3 √7ᵗʰ S59.032 Salter-Harris Type III physeal fracture of lower end of ulna, left arm `CC` `H5`

3 √7ᵗʰ **S59.039** Salter-Harris Type III physeal fracture of lower end of ulna, unspecified arm `CC` `H5`

√6ᵗʰ **S59.04** Salter-Harris Type IV physeal fracture of lower end of ulna

3 √7ᵗʰ S59.041 Salter-Harris Type IV physeal fracture of lower end of ulna, right arm `CC` `H5`

3 √7ᵗʰ S59.042 Salter-Harris Type IV physeal fracture of lower end of ulna, left arm `CC` `H5`

3 √7ᵗʰ **S59.049** Salter-Harris Type IV physeal fracture of lower end of ulna, unspecified arm `CC` `H5`

√6ᵗʰ **S59.09** Other physeal fracture of lower end of ulna

3 √7ᵗʰ S59.091 Other physeal fracture of lower end of ulna, right arm `CC` `H5`

3 √7ᵗʰ S59.092 Other physeal fracture of lower end of ulna, left arm `CC` `H5`

3 √7ᵗʰ **S59.099** Other physeal fracture of lower end of ulna, unspecified arm `CC` `H5`

√5ᵗʰ **S59.1** Physeal fracture of upper end of radius

AHA: 2019,4Q,56

√6ᵗʰ **S59.10** Unspecified physeal fracture of upper end of radius

4 √7ᵗʰ **S59.101** Unspecified physeal fracture of upper end of radius, right arm `CC`

4 √7ᵗʰ **S59.102** Unspecified physeal fracture of upper end of radius, left arm `CC`

4 √7ᵗʰ **S59.109** Unspecified physeal fracture of upper end of radius, unspecified arm `CC`

√6ᵗʰ **S59.11** Salter-Harris Type I physeal fracture of upper end of radius

4 √7ᵗʰ S59.111 Salter-Harris Type I physeal fracture of upper end of radius, right arm `CC`

4 √7ᵗʰ S59.112 Salter-Harris Type I physeal fracture of upper end of radius, left arm `CC`

4 √7ᵗʰ **S59.119** Salter-Harris Type I physeal fracture of upper end of radius, unspecified arm `CC`

√6ᵗʰ **S59.12** Salter-Harris Type II physeal fracture of upper end of radius

4 √7ᵗʰ S59.121 Salter-Harris Type II physeal fracture of upper end of radius, right arm `CC`

4 √7ᵗʰ S59.122 Salter-Harris Type II physeal fracture of upper end of radius, left arm `CC`

4 √7ᵗʰ **S59.129** Salter-Harris Type II physeal fracture of upper end of radius, unspecified arm `CC`

√6ᵗʰ **S59.13** Salter-Harris Type III physeal fracture of upper end of radius

4 √7ᵗʰ S59.131 Salter-Harris Type III physeal fracture of upper end of radius, right arm `CC`

4 √7ᵗʰ S59.132 Salter-Harris Type III physeal fracture of upper end of radius, left arm `CC`

4 √7ᵗʰ **S59.139** Salter-Harris Type III physeal fracture of upper end of radius, unspecified arm `CC`

√6ᵗʰ **S59.14** Salter-Harris Type IV physeal fracture of upper end of radius

4 √7ᵗʰ **S59.141** Salter-Harris Type IV physeal fracture of upper end of radius, right arm `CC`

4 √7ᵗʰ **S59.142** Salter-Harris Type IV physeal fracture of upper end of radius, left arm `CC`

    ⁴ √7ᵗʰ **S59.149** Salter-Harris Type IV physeal fracture of upper end of radius, unspecified arm   **CC**

√6ᵗʰ **S59.19** Other physeal fracture of upper end of radius

    ⁴ √7ᵗʰ **S59.191** Other physeal fracture of upper end of radius, right arm   **CC**

    ⁴ √7ᵗʰ **S59.192** Other physeal fracture of upper end of radius, left arm   **CC**

    ⁴ √7ᵗʰ **S59.199** Other physeal fracture of upper end of radius, unspecified arm   **CC**

√5ᵗʰ **S59.2** Physeal fracture of lower end of radius

    AHA: 2019,4Q,56

√6ᵗʰ **S59.20** Unspecified physeal fracture of lower end of radius

    ³ √7ᵗʰ **S59.201** Unspecified physeal fracture of lower end of radius, right arm   **CC H5**

    ³ √7ᵗʰ **S59.202** Unspecified physeal fracture of lower end of radius, left arm   **CC H5**

    ³ √7ᵗʰ **S59.209** Unspecified physeal fracture of lower end of radius, unspecified arm   **CC H5**

√6ᵗʰ **S59.21** Salter-Harris Type I physeal fracture of lower end of radius

    ³ √7ᵗʰ **S59.211** Salter-Harris Type I physeal fracture of lower end of radius, right arm   **CC H5**

    ³ √7ᵗʰ **S59.212** Salter-Harris Type I physeal fracture of lower end of radius, left arm   **CC H5**

    ³ √7ᵗʰ **S59.219** Salter-Harris Type I physeal fracture of lower end of radius, unspecified arm   **CC H5**

√6ᵗʰ **S59.22** Salter-Harris Type II physeal fracture of lower end of radius

    ³ √7ᵗʰ **S59.221** Salter-Harris Type II physeal fracture of lower end of radius, right arm   **CC H5**

    ³ √7ᵗʰ **S59.222** Salter-Harris Type II physeal fracture of lower end of radius, left arm   **CC H5**

    ³ √7ᵗʰ **S59.229** Salter-Harris Type II physeal fracture of lower end of radius, unspecified arm   **CC H5**

√6ᵗʰ **S59.23** Salter-Harris Type III physeal fracture of lower end of radius

    ³ √7ᵗʰ **S59.231** Salter-Harris Type III physeal fracture of lower end of radius, right arm   **CC H5**

    ³ √7ᵗʰ **S59.232** Salter-Harris Type III physeal fracture of lower end of radius, left arm   **CC H5**

    ³ √7ᵗʰ **S59.239** Salter-Harris Type III physeal fracture of lower end of radius, unspecified arm   **CC H5**

√6ᵗʰ **S59.24** Salter-Harris Type IV physeal fracture of lower end of radius

    ³ √7ᵗʰ **S59.241** Salter-Harris Type IV physeal fracture of lower end of radius, right arm   **CC H5**

    ³ √7ᵗʰ **S59.242** Salter-Harris Type IV physeal fracture of lower end of radius, left arm   **CC H5**

    ³ √7ᵗʰ **S59.249** Salter-Harris Type IV physeal fracture of lower end of radius, unspecified arm   **CC H5**

√6ᵗʰ **S59.29** Other physeal fracture of lower end of radius

    ³ √7ᵗʰ **S59.291** Other physeal fracture of lower end of radius, right arm   **CC H5**

    ³ √7ᵗʰ **S59.292** Other physeal fracture of lower end of radius, left arm   **CC H5**

    ³ √7ᵗʰ **S59.299** Other physeal fracture of lower end of radius, unspecified arm   **CC H5**

√5ᵗʰ **S59.8** Other specified injuries of elbow and forearm

The appropriate 7th character is to be added to each code in subcategory S59.8.
A   initial encounter
D   subsequent encounter
S   sequela

√6ᵗʰ **S59.80** Other specified injuries of elbow

    √7ᵗʰ **S59.801** Other specified injuries of right elbow

    √7ᵗʰ **S59.802** Other specified injuries of left elbow

    √7ᵗʰ **S59.809** Other specified injuries of unspecified elbow

√6ᵗʰ **S59.81** Other specified injuries of forearm

    √7ᵗʰ **S59.811** Other specified injuries right forearm

    √7ᵗʰ **S59.812** Other specified injuries left forearm

    √7ᵗʰ **S59.819** Other specified injuries unspecified forearm

√5ᵗʰ **S59.9** Unspecified injury of elbow and forearm

The appropriate 7th character is to be added to each code in subcategory S59.9.
A   initial encounter
D   subsequent encounter
S   sequela

√6ᵗʰ **S59.90** Unspecified injury of elbow

    √7ᵗʰ **S59.901** Unspecified injury of right elbow

    √7ᵗʰ **S59.902** Unspecified injury of left elbow

    √7ᵗʰ **S59.909** Unspecified injury of unspecified elbow

√6ᵗʰ **S59.91** Unspecified injury of forearm

    √7ᵗʰ **S59.911** Unspecified injury of right forearm

    √7ᵗʰ **S59.912** Unspecified injury of left forearm

    √7ᵗʰ **S59.919** Unspecified injury of unspecified forearm

Injuries to the wrist, hand and fingers (S60-S69)

EXCLUDES 2   burns and corrosions (T20-T32)
frostbite (T33-T34)
insect bite or sting, venomous (T63.4)

√4ᵗʰ **S60** Superficial injury of wrist, hand and fingers

The appropriate 7th character is to be added to each code from category S60.
A   initial encounter
D   subsequent encounter
S   sequela

√5ᵗʰ **S60.0** Contusion of finger without damage to nail

    EXCLUDES 1   contusion involving nail (matrix) (S60.1)

√x7ᵗʰ **S60.00** Contusion of unspecified finger without damage to nail

Contusion of finger(s) NOS

√6ᵗʰ **S60.01** Contusion of thumb without damage to nail

    √7ᵗʰ **S60.011** Contusion of right thumb without damage to nail

    √7ᵗʰ **S60.012** Contusion of left thumb without damage to nail

    √7ᵗʰ **S60.019** Contusion of unspecified thumb without damage to nail

√6ᵗʰ **S60.02** Contusion of index finger without damage to nail

    √7ᵗʰ **S60.021** Contusion of right index finger without damage to nail

    √7ᵗʰ **S60.022** Contusion of left index finger without damage to nail

    √7ᵗʰ **S60.029** Contusion of unspecified index finger without damage to nail

√6ᵗʰ **S60.03** Contusion of middle finger without damage to nail

    √7ᵗʰ **S60.031** Contusion of right middle finger without damage to nail

    √7ᵗʰ **S60.032** Contusion of left middle finger without damage to nail

    √7ᵗʰ **S60.039** Contusion of unspecified middle finger without damage to nail

√6ᵗʰ **S60.04** Contusion of ring finger without damage to nail

    √7ᵗʰ **S60.041** Contusion of right ring finger without damage to nail

    √7ᵗʰ **S60.042** Contusion of left ring finger without damage to nail

    √7ᵗʰ **S60.049** Contusion of unspecified ring finger without damage to nail

√6ᵗʰ **S60.05** Contusion of little finger without damage to nail

    √7ᵗʰ **S60.051** Contusion of right little finger without damage to nail

    √7ᵗʰ **S60.052** Contusion of left little finger without damage to nail

    √7ᵗʰ **S60.059** Contusion of unspecified little finger without damage to nail

√5ᵗʰ **S60.1** Contusion of finger with damage to nail

√x7ᵗʰ **S60.10** Contusion of unspecified finger with damage to nail

√6ᵗʰ **S60.11** Contusion of thumb with damage to nail

    √7ᵗʰ **S60.111** Contusion of right thumb with damage to nail

    √7ᵗʰ **S60.112** Contusion of left thumb with damage to nail

    √7ᵗʰ **S60.119** Contusion of unspecified thumb with damage to nail

✔ Additional Character Required   √x7ᵗʰ Placeholder   Unacceptable PDx   Questionable PDx   Manifestation   Unspecified Dx   **H1**-**H14** HAC   **HCC** CMS-HCC Dx   **HIV** HIV Dx

ICD-10-CM 2021   1029

Chapter 19. Injury, Poisoning and Certain Other Consequences of External Causes

√6ᵗʰ **S60.12**   Contusion of index finger with damage to nail
- √7ᵗʰ **S60.121**   Contusion of right index finger with damage to nail
- √7ᵗʰ **S60.122**   Contusion of left index finger with damage to nail
- √7ᵗʰ **S60.129**   Contusion of unspecified index finger with damage to nail

√6ᵗʰ **S60.13**   Contusion of middle finger with damage to nail
- √7ᵗʰ **S60.131**   Contusion of right middle finger with damage to nail
- √7ᵗʰ **S60.132**   Contusion of left middle finger with damage to nail
- √7ᵗʰ **S60.139**   Contusion of unspecified middle finger with damage to nail

√6ᵗʰ **S60.14**   Contusion of ring finger with damage to nail
- √7ᵗʰ **S60.141**   Contusion of right ring finger with damage to nail
- √7ᵗʰ **S60.142**   Contusion of left ring finger with damage to nail
- √7ᵗʰ **S60.149**   Contusion of unspecified ring finger with damage to nail

√6ᵗʰ **S60.15**   Contusion of little finger with damage to nail
- √7ᵗʰ **S60.151**   Contusion of right little finger with damage to nail
- √7ᵗʰ **S60.152**   Contusion of left little finger with damage to nail
- √7ᵗʰ **S60.159**   Contusion of unspecified little finger with damage to nail

√5ᵗʰ **S60.2**   Contusion of wrist and hand
> EXCLUDES 2   contusion of fingers (S60.0-, S60.1-)

√6ᵗʰ **S60.21**   Contusion of wrist
- √7ᵗʰ **S60.211**   Contusion of right wrist
- √7ᵗʰ **S60.212**   Contusion of left wrist
- √7ᵗʰ **S60.219**   Contusion of unspecified wrist

√6ᵗʰ **S60.22**   Contusion of hand
- √7ᵗʰ **S60.221**   Contusion of right hand
- √7ᵗʰ **S60.222**   Contusion of left hand
- √7ᵗʰ **S60.229**   Contusion of unspecified hand

√5ᵗʰ **S60.3**   Other superficial injuries of thumb

√6ᵗʰ **S60.31**   Abrasion of thumb
- √7ᵗʰ **S60.311**   Abrasion of right thumb
- √7ᵗʰ **S60.312**   Abrasion of left thumb
- √7ᵗʰ **S60.319**   Abrasion of unspecified thumb

√6ᵗʰ **S60.32**   Blister (nonthermal) of thumb
- √7ᵗʰ **S60.321**   Blister (nonthermal) of right thumb
- √7ᵗʰ **S60.322**   Blister (nonthermal) of left thumb
- √7ᵗʰ **S60.329**   Blister (nonthermal) of unspecified thumb

√6ᵗʰ **S60.34**   External constriction of thumb
> Hair tourniquet syndrome of thumb
> Use additional cause code to identify the constricting item (W49.0-)
- √7ᵗʰ **S60.341**   External constriction of right thumb
- √7ᵗʰ **S60.342**   External constriction of left thumb
- √7ᵗʰ **S60.349**   External constriction of unspecified thumb

√6ᵗʰ **S60.35**   Superficial foreign body of thumb
> Splinter in the thumb
- √7ᵗʰ **S60.351**   Superficial foreign body of right thumb
- √7ᵗʰ **S60.352**   Superficial foreign body of left thumb
- √7ᵗʰ **S60.359**   Superficial foreign body of unspecified thumb

√6ᵗʰ **S60.36**   Insect bite (nonvenomous) of thumb
- √7ᵗʰ **S60.361**   Insect bite (nonvenomous) of right thumb
- √7ᵗʰ **S60.362**   Insect bite (nonvenomous) of left thumb
- √7ᵗʰ **S60.369**   Insect bite (nonvenomous) of unspecified thumb

√6ᵗʰ **S60.37**   Other superficial bite of thumb
> EXCLUDES 1   open bite of thumb (S61.05-, S61.15-)
- √7ᵗʰ **S60.371**   Other superficial bite of right thumb
- √7ᵗʰ **S60.372**   Other superficial bite of left thumb
- √7ᵗʰ **S60.379**   Other superficial bite of unspecified thumb

√6ᵗʰ **S60.39**   Other superficial injuries of thumb
- √7ᵗʰ **S60.391**   Other superficial injuries of right thumb
- √7ᵗʰ **S60.392**   Other superficial injuries of left thumb
- √7ᵗʰ **S60.399**   Other superficial injuries of unspecified thumb

√5ᵗʰ **S60.4**   Other superficial injuries of other fingers

√6ᵗʰ **S60.41**   Abrasion of fingers
- √7ᵗʰ **S60.410**   Abrasion of right index finger
- √7ᵗʰ **S60.411**   Abrasion of left index finger
- √7ᵗʰ **S60.412**   Abrasion of right middle finger
- √7ᵗʰ **S60.413**   Abrasion of left middle finger
- √7ᵗʰ **S60.414**   Abrasion of right ring finger
- √7ᵗʰ **S60.415**   Abrasion of left ring finger
- √7ᵗʰ **S60.416**   Abrasion of right little finger
- √7ᵗʰ **S60.417**   Abrasion of left little finger
- √7ᵗʰ **S60.418**   Abrasion of other finger
  > Abrasion of specified finger with unspecified laterality
- √7ᵗʰ **S60.419**   Abrasion of unspecified finger

√6ᵗʰ **S60.42**   Blister (nonthermal) of fingers
- √7ᵗʰ **S60.420**   Blister (nonthermal) of right index finger
- √7ᵗʰ **S60.421**   Blister (nonthermal) of left index finger
- √7ᵗʰ **S60.422**   Blister (nonthermal) of right middle finger
- √7ᵗʰ **S60.423**   Blister (nonthermal) of left middle finger
- √7ᵗʰ **S60.424**   Blister (nonthermal) of right ring finger
- √7ᵗʰ **S60.425**   Blister (nonthermal) of left ring finger
- √7ᵗʰ **S60.426**   Blister (nonthermal) of right little finger
- √7ᵗʰ **S60.427**   Blister (nonthermal) of left little finger
- √7ᵗʰ **S60.428**   Blister (nonthermal) of other finger
  > Blister (nonthermal) of specified finger with unspecified laterality
- √7ᵗʰ **S60.429**   Blister (nonthermal) of unspecified finger

√6ᵗʰ **S60.44**   External constriction of fingers
> Hair tourniquet syndrome of finger
> Use additional cause code to identify the constricting item (W49.0-)
- √7ᵗʰ **S60.440**   External constriction of right index finger
- √7ᵗʰ **S60.441**   External constriction of left index finger
- √7ᵗʰ **S60.442**   External constriction of right middle finger
- √7ᵗʰ **S60.443**   External constriction of left middle finger
- √7ᵗʰ **S60.444**   External constriction of right ring finger
- √7ᵗʰ **S60.445**   External constriction of left ring finger
- √7ᵗʰ **S60.446**   External constriction of right little finger
- √7ᵗʰ **S60.447**   External constriction of left little finger
- √7ᵗʰ **S60.448**   External constriction of other finger
  > External constriction of specified finger with unspecified laterality
- √7ᵗʰ **S60.449**   External constriction of unspecified finger

√6ᵗʰ **S60.45**   Superficial foreign body of fingers
> Splinter in the finger(s)
- √7ᵗʰ **S60.450**   Superficial foreign body of right index finger
- √7ᵗʰ **S60.451**   Superficial foreign body of left index finger
- √7ᵗʰ **S60.452**   Superficial foreign body of right middle finger
- √7ᵗʰ **S60.453**   Superficial foreign body of left middle finger
- √7ᵗʰ **S60.454**   Superficial foreign body of right ring finger
- √7ᵗʰ **S60.455**   Superficial foreign body of left ring finger
- √7ᵗʰ **S60.456**   Superficial foreign body of right little finger
- √7ᵗʰ **S60.457**   Superficial foreign body of left little finger
- √7ᵗʰ **S60.458**   Superficial foreign body of other finger
  > Superficial foreign body of specified finger with unspecified laterality
- √7ᵗʰ **S60.459**   Superficial foreign body of unspecified finger

Ⓝ Newborn: 0   Ⓟ Pediatric: 0-17   Ⓜ Maternity: 9-64   Ⓐ Adult: 15-124   **MCC** Major Complication/Comorbidity   **CC** Complication/Comorbidity   **SW** Severe Wound Dx

1030   ICD-10-CM 2021

√6ᵗʰ **S60.46** Insect bite (nonvenomous) of fingers

     √7ᵗʰ **S60.460** Insect bite (nonvenomous) of right index finger

     √7ᵗʰ **S60.461** Insect bite (nonvenomous) of left index finger

     √7ᵗʰ **S60.462** Insect bite (nonvenomous) of right middle finger

     √7ᵗʰ **S60.463** Insect bite (nonvenomous) of left middle finger

     √7ᵗʰ **S60.464** Insect bite (nonvenomous) of right ring finger

     √7ᵗʰ **S60.465** Insect bite (nonvenomous) of left ring finger

     √7ᵗʰ **S60.466** Insect bite (nonvenomous) of right little finger

     √7ᵗʰ **S60.467** Insect bite (nonvenomous) of left little finger

     √7ᵗʰ **S60.468** Insect bite (nonvenomous) of other finger

         Insect bite (nonvenomous) of specified finger with unspecified laterality

     √7ᵗʰ **S60.469** Insect bite (nonvenomous) of unspecified finger

√6ᵗʰ **S60.47** Other superficial bite of fingers

     EXCLUDES 1   open bite of fingers (S61.25-, S61.35-)

     √7ᵗʰ **S60.470** Other superficial bite of right index finger

     √7ᵗʰ **S60.471** Other superficial bite of left index finger

     √7ᵗʰ **S60.472** Other superficial bite of right middle finger

     √7ᵗʰ **S60.473** Other superficial bite of left middle finger

     √7ᵗʰ **S60.474** Other superficial bite of right ring finger

     √7ᵗʰ **S60.475** Other superficial bite of left ring finger

     √7ᵗʰ **S60.476** Other superficial bite of right little finger

     √7ᵗʰ **S60.477** Other superficial bite of left little finger

     √7ᵗʰ **S60.478** Other superficial bite of other finger

         Other superficial bite of specified finger with unspecified laterality

     √7ᵗʰ **S60.479** Other superficial bite of unspecified finger

√5ᵗʰ **S60.5** Other superficial injuries of hand

     EXCLUDES 2   superficial injuries of fingers (S60.3-, S60.4-)

√6ᵗʰ **S60.51** Abrasion of hand

     √7ᵗʰ **S60.511** Abrasion of right hand

     √7ᵗʰ **S60.512** Abrasion of left hand

     √7ᵗʰ **S60.519** Abrasion of unspecified hand

√6ᵗʰ **S60.52** Blister (nonthermal) of hand

     √7ᵗʰ **S60.521** Blister (nonthermal) of right hand

     √7ᵗʰ **S60.522** Blister (nonthermal) of left hand

     √7ᵗʰ **S60.529** Blister (nonthermal) of unspecified hand

√6ᵗʰ **S60.54** External constriction of hand

     √7ᵗʰ **S60.541** External constriction of right hand

     √7ᵗʰ **S60.542** External constriction of left hand

     √7ᵗʰ **S60.549** External constriction of unspecified hand

√6ᵗʰ **S60.55** Superficial foreign body of hand

     Splinter in the hand

     √7ᵗʰ **S60.551** Superficial foreign body of right hand

     √7ᵗʰ **S60.552** Superficial foreign body of left hand

     √7ᵗʰ **S60.559** Superficial foreign body of unspecified hand

√6ᵗʰ **S60.56** Insect bite (nonvenomous) of hand

     √7ᵗʰ **S60.561** Insect bite (nonvenomous) of right hand

     √7ᵗʰ **S60.562** Insect bite (nonvenomous) of left hand

     √7ᵗʰ **S60.569** Insect bite (nonvenomous) of unspecified hand

√6ᵗʰ **S60.57** Other superficial bite of hand

     EXCLUDES 1   open bite of hand (S61.45-)

     √7ᵗʰ **S60.571** Other superficial bite of hand of right hand

     √7ᵗʰ **S60.572** Other superficial bite of hand of left hand

     √7ᵗʰ **S60.579** Other superficial bite of hand of unspecified hand

√5ᵗʰ **S60.8** Other superficial injuries of wrist

√6ᵗʰ **S60.81** Abrasion of wrist

     √7ᵗʰ **S60.811** Abrasion of right wrist

     √7ᵗʰ **S60.812** Abrasion of left wrist

     √7ᵗʰ **S60.819** Abrasion of unspecified wrist

√6ᵗʰ **S60.82** Blister (nonthermal) of wrist

     √7ᵗʰ **S60.821** Blister (nonthermal) of right wrist

     √7ᵗʰ **S60.822** Blister (nonthermal) of left wrist

     √7ᵗʰ **S60.829** Blister (nonthermal) of unspecified wrist

√6ᵗʰ **S60.84** External constriction of wrist

     √7ᵗʰ **S60.841** External constriction of right wrist

     √7ᵗʰ **S60.842** External constriction of left wrist

     √7ᵗʰ **S60.849** External constriction of unspecified wrist

√6ᵗʰ **S60.85** Superficial foreign body of wrist

     Splinter in the wrist

     √7ᵗʰ **S60.851** Superficial foreign body of right wrist

     √7ᵗʰ **S60.852** Superficial foreign body of left wrist

     √7ᵗʰ **S60.859** Superficial foreign body of unspecified wrist

√6ᵗʰ **S60.86** Insect bite (nonvenomous) of wrist

     √7ᵗʰ **S60.861** Insect bite (nonvenomous) of right wrist

     √7ᵗʰ **S60.862** Insect bite (nonvenomous) of left wrist

     √7ᵗʰ **S60.869** Insect bite (nonvenomous) of unspecified wrist

√6ᵗʰ **S60.87** Other superficial bite of wrist

     EXCLUDES 1   open bite of wrist (S61.55)

     √7ᵗʰ **S60.871** Other superficial bite of right wrist

     √7ᵗʰ **S60.872** Other superficial bite of left wrist

     √7ᵗʰ **S60.879** Other superficial bite of unspecified wrist

√5ᵗʰ **S60.9** Unspecified superficial injury of wrist, hand and fingers

√6ᵗʰ **S60.91** Unspecified superficial injury of wrist

     √7ᵗʰ **S60.911** Unspecified superficial injury of right wrist

     √7ᵗʰ **S60.912** Unspecified superficial injury of left wrist

     √7ᵗʰ **S60.919** Unspecified superficial injury of unspecified wrist

√6ᵗʰ **S60.92** Unspecified superficial injury of hand

     √7ᵗʰ **S60.921** Unspecified superficial injury of right hand

     √7ᵗʰ **S60.922** Unspecified superficial injury of left hand

     √7ᵗʰ **S60.929** Unspecified superficial injury of unspecified hand

√6ᵗʰ **S60.93** Unspecified superficial injury of thumb

     √7ᵗʰ **S60.931** Unspecified superficial injury of right thumb

     √7ᵗʰ **S60.932** Unspecified superficial injury of left thumb

     √7ᵗʰ **S60.939** Unspecified superficial injury of unspecified thumb

√6ᵗʰ **S60.94** Unspecified superficial injury of other fingers

     √7ᵗʰ **S60.940** Unspecified superficial injury of right index finger

     √7ᵗʰ **S60.941** Unspecified superficial injury of left index finger

     √7ᵗʰ **S60.942** Unspecified superficial injury of right middle finger

     √7ᵗʰ **S60.943** Unspecified superficial injury of left middle finger

     √7ᵗʰ **S60.944** Unspecified superficial injury of right ring finger

     √7ᵗʰ **S60.945** Unspecified superficial injury of left ring finger

     √7ᵗʰ **S60.946** Unspecified superficial injury of right little finger

     √7ᵗʰ **S60.947** Unspecified superficial injury of left little finger

     √7ᵗʰ **S60.948** Unspecified superficial injury of other finger

         Unspecified superficial injury of specified finger with unspecified laterality

     √7ᵗʰ **S60.949** Unspecified superficial injury of unspecified finger

☑ Additional Character Required   √x7ᵗʰ Placeholder   Unacceptable PDx   Questionable PDx   Manifestation   Unspecified Dx   **H1**-**H14** HAC   **HCC** CMS-HCC Dx   **HIV** HIV Dx

ICD-10-CM 2021   1031

√4th **S61 Open wound of wrist, hand and fingers**

Code also any associated wound infection

EXCLUDES 1 *open fracture of wrist, hand and finger (S62.- with 7th character B)*

traumatic amputation of wrist and hand (S68.-)

The appropriate 7th character is to be added to each code from category S61.

A initial encounter

D subsequent encounter

S sequela

√5th **S61.0 Open wound of thumb without damage to nail**

EXCLUDES 1 *open wound of thumb with damage to nail (S61.1-)*

√6th **S61.00 Unspecified open wound of thumb without damage to nail**

√7th **S61.001 Unspecified open wound of right thumb without damage to nail**

√7th **S61.002 Unspecified open wound of left thumb without damage to nail**

√7th **S61.009 Unspecified open wound of unspecified thumb without damage to nail**

√6th **S61.01 Laceration without foreign body of thumb without damage to nail**

√7th **S61.011 Laceration without foreign body of right thumb without damage to nail**

√7th **S61.012 Laceration without foreign body of left thumb without damage to nail**

√7th **S61.019 Laceration without foreign body of unspecified thumb without damage to nail**

√6th **S61.02 Laceration with foreign body of thumb without damage to nail**

√7th **S61.021 Laceration with foreign body of right thumb without damage to nail**

√7th **S61.022 Laceration with foreign body of left thumb without damage to nail**

√7th **S61.029 Laceration with foreign body of unspecified thumb without damage to nail**

√6th **S61.03 Puncture wound without foreign body of thumb without damage to nail**

√7th **S61.031 Puncture wound without foreign body of right thumb without damage to nail**

√7th **S61.032 Puncture wound without foreign body of left thumb without damage to nail**

√7th **S61.039 Puncture wound without foreign body of unspecified thumb without damage to nail**

√6th **S61.04 Puncture wound with foreign body of thumb without damage to nail**

√7th **S61.041 Puncture wound with foreign body of right thumb without damage to nail**

√7th **S61.042 Puncture wound with foreign body of left thumb without damage to nail**

√7th **S61.049 Puncture wound with foreign body of unspecified thumb without damage to nail**

√6th **S61.05 Open bite of thumb without damage to nail**

Bite of thumb NOS

EXCLUDES 1 *superficial bite of thumb (S60.36-, S60.37-)*

√7th **S61.051 Open bite of right thumb without damage to nail**

√7th **S61.052 Open bite of left thumb without damage to nail**

√7th **S61.059 Open bite of unspecified thumb without damage to nail**

√5th **S61.1 Open wound of thumb with damage to nail**

√6th **S61.10 Unspecified open wound of thumb with damage to nail**

√7th **S61.101 Unspecified open wound of right thumb with damage to nail**

√7th **S61.102 Unspecified open wound of left thumb with damage to nail**

√7th **S61.109 Unspecified open wound of unspecified thumb with damage to nail**

√6th **S61.11 Laceration without foreign body of thumb with damage to nail**

√7th **S61.111 Laceration without foreign body of right thumb with damage to nail**

√7th **S61.112 Laceration without foreign body of left thumb with damage to nail**

√7th **S61.119 Laceration without foreign body of unspecified thumb with damage to nail**

√6th **S61.12 Laceration with foreign body of thumb with damage to nail**

√7th **S61.121 Laceration with foreign body of right thumb with damage to nail**

√7th **S61.122 Laceration with foreign body of left thumb with damage to nail**

√7th **S61.129 Laceration with foreign body of unspecified thumb with damage to nail**

√6th **S61.13 Puncture wound without foreign body of thumb with damage to nail**

√7th **S61.131 Puncture wound without foreign body of right thumb with damage to nail**

√7th **S61.132 Puncture wound without foreign body of left thumb with damage to nail**

√7th **S61.139 Puncture wound without foreign body of unspecified thumb with damage to nail**

√6th **S61.14 Puncture wound with foreign body of thumb with damage to nail**

√7th **S61.141 Puncture wound with foreign body of right thumb with damage to nail**

√7th **S61.142 Puncture wound with foreign body of left thumb with damage to nail**

√7th **S61.149 Puncture wound with foreign body of unspecified thumb with damage to nail**

√6th **S61.15 Open bite of thumb with damage to nail**

Bite of thumb with damage to nail NOS

EXCLUDES 1 *superficial bite of thumb (S60.36-, S60.37-)*

√7th **S61.151 Open bite of right thumb with damage to nail**

√7th **S61.152 Open bite of left thumb with damage to nail**

√7th **S61.159 Open bite of unspecified thumb with damage to nail**

√5th **S61.2 Open wound of other finger without damage to nail**

EXCLUDES 1 *open wound of finger involving nail (matrix) (S61.3-)*

EXCLUDES 2 *open wound of thumb without damage to nail (S61.0-)*

√6th **S61.20 Unspecified open wound of other finger without damage to nail**

√7th **S61.200 Unspecified open wound of right index finger without damage to nail**

√7th **S61.201 Unspecified open wound of left index finger without damage to nail**

√7th **S61.202 Unspecified open wound of right middle finger without damage to nail**

√7th **S61.203 Unspecified open wound of left middle finger without damage to nail**

√7th **S61.204 Unspecified open wound of right ring finger without damage to nail**

√7th **S61.205 Unspecified open wound of left ring finger without damage to nail**

√7th **S61.206 Unspecified open wound of right little finger without damage to nail**

√7th **S61.207 Unspecified open wound of left little finger without damage to nail**

√7th **S61.208 Unspecified open wound of other finger without damage to nail**

Unspecified open wound of specified finger with unspecified laterality without damage to nail

√7th **S61.209 Unspecified open wound of unspecified finger without damage to nail**

√6th **S61.21 Laceration without foreign body of finger without damage to nail**

√7th **S61.210 Laceration without foreign body of right index finger without damage to nail**

√7th **S61.211 Laceration without foreign body of left index finger without damage to nail**

√7th **S61.212 Laceration without foreign body of right middle finger without damage to nail**

√7th **S61.213 Laceration without foreign body of left middle finger without damage to nail**

√7th **S61.214 Laceration without foreign body of right ring finger without damage to nail**

√7th **S61.215 Laceration without foreign body of left ring finger without damage to nail**

√7th **S61.216 Laceration without foreign body of right little finger without damage to nail**

√7th **S61.217 Laceration without foreign body of left little finger without damage to nail**

N Newborn: 0　P Pediatric: 0-17　M Maternity: 9-64　A Adult: 15-124　MCC Major Complication/Comorbidity　CC Complication/Comorbidity　SW Severe Wound Dx

1032

ICD-10-CM 2021

√7ᵗʰ **S61.218** **Laceration without foreign body of other finger without damage to nail**
Laceration without foreign body of specified finger with unspecified laterality without damage to nail

√7ᵗʰ **S61.219** **Laceration without foreign body of unspecified finger without damage to nail**

√6ᵗʰ **S61.22** **Laceration with foreign body of finger without damage to nail**

√7ᵗʰ **S61.220** **Laceration with foreign body of right index finger without damage to nail**

√7ᵗʰ **S61.221** **Laceration with foreign body of left index finger without damage to nail**

√7ᵗʰ **S61.222** **Laceration with foreign body of right middle finger without damage to nail**

√7ᵗʰ **S61.223** **Laceration with foreign body of left middle finger without damage to nail**

√7ᵗʰ **S61.224** **Laceration with foreign body of right ring finger without damage to nail**

√7ᵗʰ **S61.225** **Laceration with foreign body of left ring finger without damage to nail**

√7ᵗʰ **S61.226** **Laceration with foreign body of right little finger without damage to nail**

√7ᵗʰ **S61.227** **Laceration with foreign body of left little finger without damage to nail**

√7ᵗʰ **S61.228** **Laceration with foreign body of other finger without damage to nail**
Laceration with foreign body of specified finger with unspecified laterality without damage to nail

√7ᵗʰ **S61.229** **Laceration with foreign body of unspecified finger without damage to nail**

√6ᵗʰ **S61.23** **Puncture wound without foreign body of finger without damage to nail**

√7ᵗʰ **S61.230** **Puncture wound without foreign body of right index finger without damage to nail**

√7ᵗʰ **S61.231** **Puncture wound without foreign body of left index finger without damage to nail**

√7ᵗʰ **S61.232** **Puncture wound without foreign body of right middle finger without damage to nail**

√7ᵗʰ **S61.233** **Puncture wound without foreign body of left middle finger without damage to nail**

√7ᵗʰ **S61.234** **Puncture wound without foreign body of right ring finger without damage to nail**

√7ᵗʰ **S61.235** **Puncture wound without foreign body of left ring finger without damage to nail**

√7ᵗʰ **S61.236** **Puncture wound without foreign body of right little finger without damage to nail**

√7ᵗʰ **S61.237** **Puncture wound without foreign body of left little finger without damage to nail**

√7ᵗʰ **S61.238** **Puncture wound without foreign body of other finger without damage to nail**
Puncture wound without foreign body of specified finger with unspecified laterality without damage to nail

√7ᵗʰ **S61.239** **Puncture wound without foreign body of unspecified finger without damage to nail**

√6ᵗʰ **S61.24** **Puncture wound with foreign body of finger without damage to nail**

√7ᵗʰ **S61.240** **Puncture wound with foreign body of right index finger without damage to nail**

√7ᵗʰ **S61.241** **Puncture wound with foreign body of left index finger without damage to nail**

√7ᵗʰ **S61.242** **Puncture wound with foreign body of right middle finger without damage to nail**

√7ᵗʰ **S61.243** **Puncture wound with foreign body of left middle finger without damage to nail**

√7ᵗʰ **S61.244** **Puncture wound with foreign body of right ring finger without damage to nail**

√7ᵗʰ **S61.245** **Puncture wound with foreign body of left ring finger without damage to nail**

√7ᵗʰ **S61.246** **Puncture wound with foreign body of right little finger without damage to nail**

√7ᵗʰ **S61.247** **Puncture wound with foreign body of left little finger without damage to nail**

√7ᵗʰ **S61.248** **Puncture wound with foreign body of other finger without damage to nail**
Puncture wound with foreign body of specified finger with unspecified laterality without damage to nail

√7ᵗʰ **S61.249** **Puncture wound with foreign body of unspecified finger without damage to nail**

√6ᵗʰ **S61.25** **Open bite of finger without damage to nail**
Bite of finger without damage to nail NOS
EXCLUDES 1   superficial bite of finger (S60.46-, S60.47-)

√7ᵗʰ **S61.250** **Open bite of right index finger without damage to nail**

√7ᵗʰ **S61.251** **Open bite of left index finger without damage to nail**

√7ᵗʰ **S61.252** **Open bite of right middle finger without damage to nail**

√7ᵗʰ **S61.253** **Open bite of left middle finger without damage to nail**

√7ᵗʰ **S61.254** **Open bite of right ring finger without damage to nail**

√7ᵗʰ **S61.255** **Open bite of left ring finger without damage to nail**

√7ᵗʰ **S61.256** **Open bite of right little finger without damage to nail**

√7ᵗʰ **S61.257** **Open bite of left little finger without damage to nail**

√7ᵗʰ **S61.258** **Open bite of other finger without damage to nail**
Open bite of specified finger with unspecified laterality without damage to nail

√7ᵗʰ **S61.259** **Open bite of unspecified finger without damage to nail**

√5ᵗʰ **S61.3** **Open wound of other finger with damage to nail**

√6ᵗʰ **S61.30** **Unspecified open wound of finger with damage to nail**

√7ᵗʰ **S61.300** **Unspecified open wound of right index finger with damage to nail**

√7ᵗʰ **S61.301** **Unspecified open wound of left index finger with damage to nail**

√7ᵗʰ **S61.302** **Unspecified open wound of right middle finger with damage to nail**

√7ᵗʰ **S61.303** **Unspecified open wound of left middle finger with damage to nail**

√7ᵗʰ **S61.304** **Unspecified open wound of right ring finger with damage to nail**

√7ᵗʰ **S61.305** **Unspecified open wound of left ring finger with damage to nail**

√7ᵗʰ **S61.306** **Unspecified open wound of right little finger with damage to nail**

√7ᵗʰ **S61.307** **Unspecified open wound of left little finger with damage to nail**

√7ᵗʰ **S61.308** **Unspecified open wound of other finger with damage to nail**
Unspecified open wound of specified finger with unspecified laterality with damage to nail

√7ᵗʰ **S61.309** **Unspecified open wound of unspecified finger with damage to nail**

√6ᵗʰ **S61.31** **Laceration without foreign body of finger with damage to nail**

√7ᵗʰ **S61.310** **Laceration without foreign body of right index finger with damage to nail**

√7ᵗʰ **S61.311** **Laceration without foreign body of left index finger with damage to nail**

√7ᵗʰ **S61.312** **Laceration without foreign body of right middle finger with damage to nail**

√7ᵗʰ **S61.313** **Laceration without foreign body of left middle finger with damage to nail**

√7ᵗʰ **S61.314** **Laceration without foreign body of right ring finger with damage to nail**

√7ᵗʰ **S61.315** **Laceration without foreign body of left ring finger with damage to nail**

√7ᵗʰ **S61.316** **Laceration without foreign body of right little finger with damage to nail**

√7ᵗʰ **S61.317** **Laceration without foreign body of left little finger with damage to nail**

✓ Additional Character Required   √x7ᵗʰ Placeholder   Unacceptable PDx   Questionable PDx   Manifestation   Unspecified Dx   H1-H16 HAC   HCC CMS-HCC Dx   HIV HIV Dx

ICD-10-CM 2021   1033

√7ᵗʰ **S61.318** **Laceration without foreign body of other finger with damage to nail**
Laceration without foreign body of specified finger with unspecified laterality with damage to nail

√7ᵗʰ **S61.319** **Laceration without foreign body of unspecified finger with damage to nail**

√6ᵗʰ **S61.32** Laceration with foreign body of finger with damage to nail

√7ᵗʰ **S61.320** **Laceration with foreign body of right index finger with damage to nail**

√7ᵗʰ **S61.321** **Laceration with foreign body of left index finger with damage to nail**

√7ᵗʰ **S61.322** **Laceration with foreign body of right middle finger with damage to nail**

√7ᵗʰ **S61.323** **Laceration with foreign body of left middle finger with damage to nail**

√7ᵗʰ **S61.324** **Laceration with foreign body of right ring finger with damage to nail**

√7ᵗʰ **S61.325** **Laceration with foreign body of left ring finger with damage to nail**

√7ᵗʰ **S61.326** **Laceration with foreign body of right little finger with damage to nail**

√7ᵗʰ **S61.327** **Laceration with foreign body of left little finger with damage to nail**

√7ᵗʰ **S61.328** **Laceration with foreign body of other finger with damage to nail**
Laceration with foreign body of specified finger with unspecified laterality with damage to nail

√7ᵗʰ **S61.329** **Laceration with foreign body of unspecified finger with damage to nail**

√6ᵗʰ **S61.33** Puncture wound without foreign body of finger with damage to nail

√7ᵗʰ **S61.330** **Puncture wound without foreign body of right index finger with damage to nail**

√7ᵗʰ **S61.331** **Puncture wound without foreign body of left index finger with damage to nail**

√7ᵗʰ **S61.332** **Puncture wound without foreign body of right middle finger with damage to nail**

√7ᵗʰ **S61.333** **Puncture wound without foreign body of left middle finger with damage to nail**

√7ᵗʰ **S61.334** **Puncture wound without foreign body of right ring finger with damage to nail**

√7ᵗʰ **S61.335** **Puncture wound without foreign body of left ring finger with damage to nail**

√7ᵗʰ **S61.336** **Puncture wound without foreign body of right little finger with damage to nail**

√7ᵗʰ **S61.337** **Puncture wound without foreign body of left little finger with damage to nail**

√7ᵗʰ **S61.338** **Puncture wound without foreign body of other finger with damage to nail**
Puncture wound without foreign body of specified finger with unspecified laterality with damage to nail

√7ᵗʰ **S61.339** **Puncture wound without foreign body of unspecified finger with damage to nail**

√6ᵗʰ **S61.34** Puncture wound with foreign body of finger with damage to nail

√7ᵗʰ **S61.340** **Puncture wound with foreign body of right index finger with damage to nail**

√7ᵗʰ **S61.341** **Puncture wound with foreign body of left index finger with damage to nail**

√7ᵗʰ **S61.342** **Puncture wound with foreign body of right middle finger with damage to nail**

√7ᵗʰ **S61.343** **Puncture wound with foreign body of left middle finger with damage to nail**

√7ᵗʰ **S61.344** **Puncture wound with foreign body of right ring finger with damage to nail**

√7ᵗʰ **S61.345** **Puncture wound with foreign body of left ring finger with damage to nail**

√7ᵗʰ **S61.346** **Puncture wound with foreign body of right little finger with damage to nail**

√7ᵗʰ **S61.347** **Puncture wound with foreign body of left little finger with damage to nail**

√7ᵗʰ **S61.348** **Puncture wound with foreign body of other finger with damage to nail**
Puncture wound with foreign body of specified finger with unspecified laterality with damage to nail

√7ᵗʰ **S61.349** **Puncture wound with foreign body of unspecified finger with damage to nail**

√6ᵗʰ **S61.35** Open bite of finger with damage to nail
Bite of finger with damage to nail NOS
EXCLUDES 1 *superficial bite of finger (S60.46-, S60.47-)*

√7ᵗʰ **S61.350** **Open bite of right index finger with damage to nail**

√7ᵗʰ **S61.351** **Open bite of left index finger with damage to nail**

√7ᵗʰ **S61.352** **Open bite of right middle finger with damage to nail**

√7ᵗʰ **S61.353** **Open bite of left middle finger with damage to nail**

√7ᵗʰ **S61.354** **Open bite of right ring finger with damage to nail**

√7ᵗʰ **S61.355** **Open bite of left ring finger with damage to nail**

√7ᵗʰ **S61.356** **Open bite of right little finger with damage to nail**

√7ᵗʰ **S61.357** **Open bite of left little finger with damage to nail**

√7ᵗʰ **S61.358** **Open bite of other finger with damage to nail**
Open bite of specified finger with unspecified laterality with damage to nail

√7ᵗʰ **S61.359** **Open bite of unspecified finger with damage to nail**

√5ᵗʰ **S61.4** **Open wound of hand**

√6ᵗʰ **S61.40** **Unspecified open wound of hand**

√7ᵗʰ **S61.401** **Unspecified open wound of right hand**

√7ᵗʰ **S61.402** **Unspecified open wound of left hand**

√7ᵗʰ **S61.409** **Unspecified open wound of unspecified hand**

√6ᵗʰ **S61.41** Laceration without foreign body of hand

√7ᵗʰ **S61.411** **Laceration without foreign body of right hand**

√7ᵗʰ **S61.412** **Laceration without foreign body of left hand**

√7ᵗʰ **S61.419** **Laceration without foreign body of unspecified hand**

√6ᵗʰ **S61.42** Laceration with foreign body of hand

√7ᵗʰ **S61.421** **Laceration with foreign body of right hand**

√7ᵗʰ **S61.422** **Laceration with foreign body of left hand**

√7ᵗʰ **S61.429** **Laceration with foreign body of unspecified hand**

√6ᵗʰ **S61.43** Puncture wound without foreign body of hand

√7ᵗʰ **S61.431** **Puncture wound without foreign body of right hand**

√7ᵗʰ **S61.432** **Puncture wound without foreign body of left hand**

√7ᵗʰ **S61.439** **Puncture wound without foreign body of unspecified hand**

√6ᵗʰ **S61.44** Puncture wound with foreign body of hand

√7ᵗʰ **S61.441** **Puncture wound with foreign body of right hand**

√7ᵗʰ **S61.442** **Puncture wound with foreign body of left hand**

√7ᵗʰ **S61.449** **Puncture wound with foreign body of unspecified hand**

√6ᵗʰ **S61.45** Open bite of hand
Bite of hand NOS
EXCLUDES 1 *superficial bite of hand (S60.56-, S60.57-)*

√7ᵗʰ **S61.451** **Open bite of right hand**

√7ᵗʰ **S61.452** **Open bite of left hand**

√7ᵗʰ **S61.459** **Open bite of unspecified hand**

√5ᵗʰ **S61.5** **Open wound of wrist**

√6ᵗʰ **S61.50** **Unspecified open wound of wrist**

√7ᵗʰ **S61.501** **Unspecified open wound of right wrist**

√7ᵗʰ **S61.502** **Unspecified open wound of left wrist**

√7ᵗʰ **S61.509** **Unspecified open wound of unspecified wrist**

√6ᵗʰ **S61.51** Laceration without foreign body of wrist

√7ᵗʰ **S61.511** **Laceration without foreign body of right wrist**

√7ᵗʰ **S61.512** **Laceration without foreign body of left wrist**

√7ᵗʰ **S61.519** Laceration without foreign body of unspecified wrist

√6ᵗʰ **S61.52** Laceration with foreign body of wrist

√7ᵗʰ **S61.521** Laceration with foreign body of right wrist

√7ᵗʰ **S61.522** Laceration with foreign body of left wrist

√7ᵗʰ **S61.529** Laceration with foreign body of unspecified wrist

√6ᵗʰ **S61.53** Puncture wound without foreign body of wrist

√7ᵗʰ **S61.531** Puncture wound without foreign body of right wrist

√7ᵗʰ **S61.532** Puncture wound without foreign body of left wrist

√7ᵗʰ **S61.539** Puncture wound without foreign body of unspecified wrist

√6ᵗʰ **S61.54** Puncture wound with foreign body of wrist

√7ᵗʰ **S61.541** Puncture wound with foreign body of right wrist

√7ᵗʰ **S61.542** Puncture wound with foreign body of left wrist

√7ᵗʰ **S61.549** Puncture wound with foreign body of unspecified wrist

√6ᵗʰ **S61.55** Open bite of wrist

Bite of wrist NOS

EXCLUDES 1   superficial bite of wrist (S60.86-, S60.87-)

√7ᵗʰ **S61.551** Open bite of right wrist

√7ᵗʰ **S61.552** Open bite of left wrist

√7ᵗʰ **S61.559** Open bite of unspecified wrist

√4ᵗʰ **S62 Fracture at wrist and hand level**

NOTE   A fracture not indicated as displaced or nondisplaced should be coded to displaced

A fracture not indicated as open or closed should be coded to closed

EXCLUDES 1   traumatic amputation of wrist and hand (S68.-)

EXCLUDES 2   fracture of distal parts of ulna and radius (S52.-)

AHA: 2018,2Q,12; 2015,3Q,37-39

The appropriate 7th character is to be added to each code from category S62.
A   initial encounter for closed fracture
B   initial encounter for open fracture
D   subsequent encounter for fracture with routine healing
G   subsequent encounter for fracture with delayed healing
K   subsequent encounter for fracture with nonunion
P   subsequent encounter for fracture with malunion
S   sequela

√5ᵗʰ **S62.0** Fracture of navicular [scaphoid] bone of wrist

√6ᵗʰ **S62.00** Unspecified fracture of navicular [scaphoid] bone of wrist

3 √7ᵗʰ **S62.001** Unspecified fracture of navicular [scaphoid] bone of right wrist   CC H5

3 √7ᵗʰ **S62.002** Unspecified fracture of navicular [scaphoid] bone of left wrist   CC H5

AHA: 2012,4Q,106

3 √7ᵗʰ **S62.009** Unspecified fracture of navicular [scaphoid] bone of unspecified wrist   CC H5

√6ᵗʰ **S62.01** Fracture of distal pole of navicular [scaphoid] bone of wrist

Fracture of volar tuberosity of navicular [scaphoid] bone of wrist

3 √7ᵗʰ **S62.011** Displaced fracture of distal pole of navicular [scaphoid] bone of right wrist   CC H5

3 √7ᵗʰ **S62.012** Displaced fracture of distal pole of navicular [scaphoid] bone of left wrist   CC H5

3 √7ᵗʰ **S62.013** Displaced fracture of distal pole of navicular [scaphoid] bone of unspecified wrist   CC H5

3 √7ᵗʰ **S62.014** Nondisplaced fracture of distal pole of navicular [scaphoid] bone of right wrist   CC H5

3 √7ᵗʰ **S62.015** Nondisplaced fracture of distal pole of navicular [scaphoid] bone of left wrist   CC H5

3 √7ᵗʰ **S62.016** Nondisplaced fracture of distal pole of navicular [scaphoid] bone of unspecified wrist   CC H5

√6ᵗʰ **S62.02** Fracture of middle third of navicular [scaphoid] bone of wrist

3 √7ᵗʰ **S62.021** Displaced fracture of middle third of navicular [scaphoid] bone of right wrist   CC H5

3 √7ᵗʰ **S62.022** Displaced fracture of middle third of navicular [scaphoid] bone of left wrist   CC H5

3 √7ᵗʰ **S62.023** Displaced fracture of middle third of navicular [scaphoid] bone of unspecified wrist   CC H5

3 √7ᵗʰ **S62.024** Nondisplaced fracture of middle third of navicular [scaphoid] bone of right wrist   CC H5

3 √7ᵗʰ **S62.025** Nondisplaced fracture of middle third of navicular [scaphoid] bone of left wrist   CC H5

3 √7ᵗʰ **S62.026** Nondisplaced fracture of middle third of navicular [scaphoid] bone of unspecified wrist   CC H5

√6ᵗʰ **S62.03** Fracture of proximal third of navicular [scaphoid] bone of wrist

3 √7ᵗʰ **S62.031** Displaced fracture of proximal third of navicular [scaphoid] bone of right wrist   CC H5

3 √7ᵗʰ **S62.032** Displaced fracture of proximal third of navicular [scaphoid] bone of left wrist   CC H5

3 √7ᵗʰ **S62.033** Displaced fracture of proximal third of navicular [scaphoid] bone of unspecified wrist   CC H5

3 √7ᵗʰ **S62.034** Nondisplaced fracture of proximal third of navicular [scaphoid] bone of right wrist   CC H5

3 √7ᵗʰ **S62.035** Nondisplaced fracture of proximal third of navicular [scaphoid] bone of left wrist   CC H5

3 √7ᵗʰ **S62.036** Nondisplaced fracture of proximal third of navicular [scaphoid] bone of unspecified wrist   CC H5

√5ᵗʰ **S62.1** Fracture of other and unspecified carpal bone(s)

EXCLUDES 2   fracture of scaphoid of wrist (S62.0-)

√6ᵗʰ **S62.10** Fracture of unspecified carpal bone

Fracture of wrist NOS

3 √7ᵗʰ **S62.101** Fracture of unspecified carpal bone, right wrist   CC H5

3 √7ᵗʰ **S62.102** Fracture of unspecified carpal bone, left wrist   CC H5

AHA: 2012,4Q,95

3 √7ᵗʰ **S62.109** Fracture of unspecified carpal bone, unspecified wrist   CC H5

√6ᵗʰ **S62.11** Fracture of triquetrum [cuneiform] bone of wrist

3 √7ᵗʰ **S62.111** Displaced fracture of triquetrum [cuneiform] bone, right wrist   CC H5

3 √7ᵗʰ **S62.112** Displaced fracture of triquetrum [cuneiform] bone, left wrist   CC H5

3 √7ᵗʰ **S62.113** Displaced fracture of triquetrum [cuneiform] bone, unspecified wrist   CC H5

3 √7ᵗʰ **S62.114** Nondisplaced fracture of triquetrum [cuneiform] bone, right wrist   CC H5

3 √7ᵗʰ **S62.115** Nondisplaced fracture of triquetrum [cuneiform] bone, left wrist   CC H5

3 √7ᵗʰ **S62.116** Nondisplaced fracture of triquetrum [cuneiform] bone, unspecified wrist   CC H5

√6ᵗʰ **S62.12** Fracture of lunate [semilunar]

3 √7ᵗʰ **S62.121** Displaced fracture of lunate [semilunar], right wrist   CC H5

3 √7ᵗʰ **S62.122** Displaced fracture of lunate [semilunar], left wrist   CC H5

3 √7ᵗʰ **S62.123** Displaced fracture of lunate [semilunar], unspecified wrist   CC H5

3 √7ᵗʰ **S62.124** Nondisplaced fracture of lunate [semilunar], right wrist   CC H5

3 √7ᵗʰ **S62.125** Nondisplaced fracture of lunate [semilunar], left wrist   CC H5

✔ Additional Character Required   √x7ᵗʰ Placeholder   Unacceptable PDx   Questionable PDx   Manifestation   Unspecified Dx   H1-H14 HAC   HCC CMS-HCC Dx   HIV HIV Dx

³ √7ᵗʰ **S62.126** **Nondisplaced** fracture of lunate [semilunar], unspecified wrist `CC` `H5`

√6ᵗʰ **S62.13** Fracture of capitate [os magnum] bone

³ √7ᵗʰ **S62.131** **Displaced** fracture of capitate [os magnum] bone, **right wrist** `CC` `H5`

³ √7ᵗʰ **S62.132** **Displaced** fracture of capitate [os magnum] bone, **left wrist** `CC` `H5`

³ √7ᵗʰ **S62.133** **Displaced** fracture of capitate [os magnum] bone, unspecified wrist `CC` `H5`

³ √7ᵗʰ **S62.134** **Nondisplaced** fracture of capitate [os magnum] bone, **right wrist** `CC` `H5`

³ √7ᵗʰ **S62.135** **Nondisplaced** fracture of capitate [os magnum] bone, **left wrist** `CC` `H5`

³ √7ᵗʰ **S62.136** **Nondisplaced** fracture of capitate [os magnum] bone, unspecified wrist `CC` `H5`

√6ᵗʰ **S62.14** Fracture of body of hamate [unciform] bone
Fracture of hamate [unciform] bone NOS

³ √7ᵗʰ **S62.141** **Displaced** fracture of body of hamate [unciform] bone, **right wrist** `CC` `H5`

³ √7ᵗʰ **S62.142** **Displaced** fracture of body of hamate [unciform] bone, **left wrist** `CC` `H5`

³ √7ᵗʰ **S62.143** **Displaced** fracture of body of hamate [unciform] bone, unspecified wrist `CC` `H5`

³ √7ᵗʰ **S62.144** **Nondisplaced** fracture of body of hamate [unciform] bone, **right wrist** `CC` `H5`

³ √7ᵗʰ **S62.145** **Nondisplaced** fracture of body of hamate [unciform] bone, **left wrist** `CC` `H5`

³ √7ᵗʰ **S62.146** **Nondisplaced** fracture of body of hamate [unciform] bone, unspecified wrist `CC` `H5`

√6ᵗʰ **S62.15** Fracture of hook process of hamate [unciform] bone
Fracture of unciform process of hamate [unciform] bone

³ √7ᵗʰ **S62.151** **Displaced** fracture of hook process of hamate [unciform] bone, **right wrist** `CC` `H5`

³ √7ᵗʰ **S62.152** **Displaced** fracture of hook process of hamate [unciform] bone, **left wrist** `CC` `H5`

³ √7ᵗʰ **S62.153** **Displaced** fracture of hook process of hamate [unciform] bone, unspecified wrist `CC` `H5`

³ √7ᵗʰ **S62.154** **Nondisplaced** fracture of hook process of hamate [unciform] bone, **right wrist** `CC` `H5`

³ √7ᵗʰ **S62.155** **Nondisplaced** fracture of hook process of hamate [unciform] bone, **left wrist** `CC` `H5`

³ √7ᵗʰ **S62.156** **Nondisplaced** fracture of hook process of hamate [unciform] bone, unspecified wrist `CC` `H5`

√6ᵗʰ **S62.16** Fracture of pisiform

³ √7ᵗʰ **S62.161** **Displaced** fracture of pisiform, **right wrist** `CC` `H5`

³ √7ᵗʰ **S62.162** **Displaced** fracture of pisiform, **left wrist** `CC` `H5`

³ √7ᵗʰ **S62.163** **Displaced** fracture of pisiform, unspecified wrist `CC` `H5`

³ √7ᵗʰ **S62.164** **Nondisplaced** fracture of pisiform, **right wrist** `CC` `H5`

³ √7ᵗʰ **S62.165** **Nondisplaced** fracture of pisiform, **left wrist** `CC` `H5`

³ √7ᵗʰ **S62.166** **Nondisplaced** fracture of pisiform, unspecified wrist `CC` `H5`

√6ᵗʰ **S62.17** Fracture of trapezium [larger multangular]

³ √7ᵗʰ **S62.171** **Displaced** fracture of trapezium [larger multangular], **right wrist** `CC` `H5`

³ √7ᵗʰ **S62.172** **Displaced** fracture of trapezium [larger multangular], **left wrist** `CC` `H5`

³ √7ᵗʰ **S62.173** **Displaced** fracture of trapezium [larger multangular], unspecified wrist `CC` `H5`

³ √7ᵗʰ **S62.174** **Nondisplaced** fracture of trapezium [larger multangular], **right wrist** `CC` `H5`

³ √7ᵗʰ **S62.175** **Nondisplaced** fracture of trapezium [larger multangular], **left wrist**

³ √7ᵗʰ **S62.176** **Nondisplaced** fracture of trapezium [larger multangular], unspecified wrist `CC` `H5`

√6ᵗʰ **S62.18** Fracture of trapezoid [smaller multangular]

³ √7ᵗʰ **S62.181** **Displaced** fracture of trapezoid [smaller multangular], **right wrist** `CC` `H5`

³ √7ᵗʰ **S62.182** **Displaced** fracture of trapezoid [smaller multangular], **left wrist** `CC` `H5`

³ √7ᵗʰ **S62.183** **Displaced** fracture of trapezoid [smaller multangular], unspecified wrist `CC` `H5`

³ √7ᵗʰ **S62.184** **Nondisplaced** fracture of trapezoid [smaller multangular], **right wrist** `CC` `H5`

³ √7ᵗʰ **S62.185** **Nondisplaced** fracture of trapezoid [smaller multangular], **left wrist** `CC` `H5`

³ √7ᵗʰ **S62.186** **Nondisplaced** fracture of trapezoid [smaller multangular], unspecified wrist `CC` `H5`

√5ᵗʰ **S62.2** Fracture of first metacarpal bone

√6ᵗʰ **S62.20** Unspecified fracture of first metacarpal bone

³ √7ᵗʰ **S62.201** Unspecified fracture of first metacarpal bone, **right hand** `CC` `H5`

³ √7ᵗʰ **S62.202** Unspecified fracture of first metacarpal bone, **left hand** `CC` `H5`

³ √7ᵗʰ **S62.209** Unspecified fracture of first metacarpal bone, unspecified hand `CC` `H5`

√6ᵗʰ **S62.21** Bennett's fracture
DEF: Intra-articular, two-part fracture at the base of the first metacarpal bone (thumb) on the ulnar side at the carpometacarpal (CMC) joint.

³ √7ᵗʰ **S62.211** Bennett's fracture, **right hand** `CC` `H5`

³ √7ᵗʰ **S62.212** Bennett's fracture, **left hand** `CC` `H5`

³ √7ᵗʰ **S62.213** Bennett's fracture, unspecified hand `CC` `H5`

√6ᵗʰ **S62.22** Rolando's fracture
DEF: Comminuted, three part intra-articular fracture at the base of the thumb metacarpal.

³ √7ᵗʰ **S62.221** **Displaced** Rolando's fracture, **right hand** `CC` `H5`

³ √7ᵗʰ **S62.222** **Displaced** Rolando's fracture, **left hand** `CC` `H5`

³ √7ᵗʰ **S62.223** **Displaced** Rolando's fracture, unspecified hand `CC` `H5`

³ √7ᵗʰ **S62.224** **Nondisplaced** Rolando's fracture, **right hand** `CC` `H5`

³ √7ᵗʰ **S62.225** **Nondisplaced** Rolando's fracture, **left hand** `CC` `H5`

³ √7ᵗʰ **S62.226** **Nondisplaced** Rolando's fracture, unspecified hand `CC` `H5`

√6ᵗʰ **S62.23** Other fracture of base of first metacarpal bone

³ √7ᵗʰ **S62.231** Other **displaced** fracture of base of first metacarpal bone, **right hand** `CC` `H5`

³ √7ᵗʰ **S62.232** Other **displaced** fracture of base of first metacarpal bone, **left hand** `CC` `H5`

³ √7ᵗʰ **S62.233** Other **displaced** fracture of base of first metacarpal bone, unspecified hand `CC` `H5`

³ √7ᵗʰ **S62.234** Other **nondisplaced** fracture of base of first metacarpal bone, **right hand** `CC` `H5`

³ √7ᵗʰ **S62.235** Other **nondisplaced** fracture of base of first metacarpal bone, **left hand** `CC` `H5`

³ √7ᵗʰ **S62.236** Other **nondisplaced** fracture of base of first metacarpal bone, unspecified hand `CC` `H5`

√6ᵗʰ **S62.24** Fracture of shaft of first metacarpal bone

³ √7ᵗʰ **S62.241** **Displaced** fracture of shaft of first metacarpal bone, **right hand** `CC` `H5`

³ √7ᵗʰ **S62.242** **Displaced** fracture of shaft of first metacarpal bone, **left hand** `CC` `H5`

³ √7ᵗʰ **S62.243** **Displaced** fracture of shaft of first metacarpal bone, unspecified hand `CC` `H5`

³ √7ᵗʰ **S62.244** **Nondisplaced** fracture of shaft of first metacarpal bone, **right hand** `CC` `H5`

³ √7ᵗʰ **S62.245** **Nondisplaced** fracture of shaft of first metacarpal bone, **left hand** `CC` `H5`

Ⓝ Newborn: 0   Ⓟ Pediatric: 0-17   Ⓜ Maternity: 9-64   Ⓐ Adult: 15-124   `MCC` Major Complication/Comorbidity   `CC` Complication/Comorbidity   `SW` Severe Wound Dx

1036   ICD-10-CM 2021

³ √7ᵗʰ **S62.246** Nondisplaced fracture of shaft of first metacarpal bone, unspecified hand   CC H5

√6ᵗʰ **S62.25** Fracture of neck of first metacarpal bone

³ √7ᵗʰ **S62.251** Displaced fracture of neck of first metacarpal bone, right hand   CC H5

³ √7ᵗʰ **S62.252** Displaced fracture of neck of first metacarpal bone, left hand   CC H5

³ √7ᵗʰ **S62.253** Displaced fracture of neck of first metacarpal bone, unspecified hand   CC H5

³ √7ᵗʰ **S62.254** Nondisplaced fracture of neck of first metacarpal bone, right hand   CC H5

³ √7ᵗʰ **S62.255** Nondisplaced fracture of neck of first metacarpal bone, left hand   CC H5

³ √7ᵗʰ **S62.256** Nondisplaced fracture of neck of first metacarpal bone, unspecified hand   CC H5

√6ᵗʰ **S62.29** Other fracture of first metacarpal bone

³ √7ᵗʰ **S62.291** Other fracture of first metacarpal bone, right hand   CC H5

³ √7ᵗʰ **S62.292** Other fracture of first metacarpal bone, left hand   CC H5

³ √7ᵗʰ **S62.299** Other fracture of first metacarpal bone, unspecified hand   CC H5

√5ᵗʰ **S62.3** Fracture of other and unspecified metacarpal bone

    EXCLUDES 2   *fracture of first metacarpal bone (S62.2-)*

√6ᵗʰ **S62.30** Unspecified fracture of other metacarpal bone

³ √7ᵗʰ **S62.300** Unspecified fracture of second metacarpal bone, right hand   CC H5

³ √7ᵗʰ **S62.301** Unspecified fracture of second metacarpal bone, left hand   CC H5

³ √7ᵗʰ **S62.302** Unspecified fracture of third metacarpal bone, right hand   CC H5

³ √7ᵗʰ **S62.303** Unspecified fracture of third metacarpal bone, left hand   CC H5

³ √7ᵗʰ **S62.304** Unspecified fracture of fourth metacarpal bone, right hand   CC H5

³ √7ᵗʰ **S62.305** Unspecified fracture of fourth metacarpal bone, left hand   CC H5

³ √7ᵗʰ **S62.306** Unspecified fracture of fifth metacarpal bone, right hand   CC H5

³ √7ᵗʰ **S62.307** Unspecified fracture of fifth metacarpal bone, left hand   CC H5

³ √7ᵗʰ **S62.308** Unspecified fracture of other metacarpal bone   CC H5

    Unspecified fracture of specified metacarpal bone with unspecified laterality

³ √7ᵗʰ **S62.309** Unspecified fracture of unspecified metacarpal bone   CC H5

√6ᵗʰ **S62.31** Displaced fracture of base of other metacarpal bone

³ √7ᵗʰ **S62.310** Displaced fracture of base of second metacarpal bone, right hand   CC H5

³ √7ᵗʰ **S62.311** Displaced fracture of base of second metacarpal bone, left hand   CC H5

³ √7ᵗʰ **S62.312** Displaced fracture of base of third metacarpal bone, right hand   CC H5

³ √7ᵗʰ **S62.313** Displaced fracture of base of third metacarpal bone, left hand   CC H5

³ √7ᵗʰ **S62.314** Displaced fracture of base of fourth metacarpal bone, right hand   CC H5

³ √7ᵗʰ **S62.315** Displaced fracture of base of fourth metacarpal bone, left hand   CC H5

³ √7ᵗʰ **S62.316** Displaced fracture of base of fifth metacarpal bone, right hand   CC H5

³ √7ᵗʰ **S62.317** Displaced fracture of base of fifth metacarpal bone, left hand   CC H5

³ √7ᵗʰ **S62.318** Displaced fracture of base of other metacarpal bone   CC H5

    Displaced fracture of base of specified metacarpal bone with unspecified laterality

³ √7ᵗʰ **S62.319** Displaced fracture of base of unspecified metacarpal bone   CC H5

√6ᵗʰ **S62.32** Displaced fracture of shaft of other metacarpal bone

³ √7ᵗʰ **S62.320** Displaced fracture of shaft of second metacarpal bone, right hand   CC H5

³ √7ᵗʰ **S62.321** Displaced fracture of shaft of second metacarpal bone, left hand   CC H5

³ √7ᵗʰ **S62.322** Displaced fracture of shaft of third metacarpal bone, right hand   CC H5

³ √7ᵗʰ **S62.323** Displaced fracture of shaft of third metacarpal bone, left hand   CC H5

³ √7ᵗʰ **S62.324** Displaced fracture of shaft of fourth metacarpal bone, right hand   CC H5

³ √7ᵗʰ **S62.325** Displaced fracture of shaft of fourth metacarpal bone, left hand   CC H5

³ √7ᵗʰ **S62.326** Displaced fracture of shaft of fifth metacarpal bone, right hand   CC H5

³ √7ᵗʰ **S62.327** Displaced fracture of shaft of fifth metacarpal bone, left hand   CC H5

³ √7ᵗʰ **S62.328** Displaced fracture of shaft of other metacarpal bone   CC H5

    Displaced fracture of shaft of specified metacarpal bone with unspecified laterality

³ √7ᵗʰ **S62.329** Displaced fracture of shaft of unspecified metacarpal bone   CC H5

√6ᵗʰ **S62.33** Displaced fracture of neck of other metacarpal bone

³ √7ᵗʰ **S62.330** Displaced fracture of neck of second metacarpal bone, right hand   CC H5

³ √7ᵗʰ **S62.331** Displaced fracture of neck of second metacarpal bone, left hand   CC H5

³ √7ᵗʰ **S62.332** Displaced fracture of neck of third metacarpal bone, right hand   CC H5

³ √7ᵗʰ **S62.333** Displaced fracture of neck of third metacarpal bone, left hand   CC H5

³ √7ᵗʰ **S62.334** Displaced fracture of neck of fourth metacarpal bone, right hand   CC H5

³ √7ᵗʰ **S62.335** Displaced fracture of neck of fourth metacarpal bone, left hand   CC H5

³ √7ᵗʰ **S62.336** Displaced fracture of neck of fifth metacarpal bone, right hand   CC H5

³ √7ᵗʰ **S62.337** Displaced fracture of neck of fifth metacarpal bone, left hand   CC H5

³ √7ᵗʰ **S62.338** Displaced fracture of neck of other metacarpal bone   CC H5

    Displaced fracture of neck of specified metacarpal bone with unspecified laterality

³ √7ᵗʰ **S62.339** Displaced fracture of neck of unspecified metacarpal bone   CC H5

√6ᵗʰ **S62.34** Nondisplaced fracture of base of other metacarpal bone

³ √7ᵗʰ **S62.340** Nondisplaced fracture of base of second metacarpal bone, right hand   CC H5

³ √7ᵗʰ **S62.341** Nondisplaced fracture of base of second metacarpal bone, left hand   CC H5

³ √7ᵗʰ **S62.342** Nondisplaced fracture of base of third metacarpal bone, right hand   CC H5

³ √7ᵗʰ **S62.343** Nondisplaced fracture of base of third metacarpal bone, left hand   CC H5

³ √7ᵗʰ **S62.344** Nondisplaced fracture of base of fourth metacarpal bone, right hand   CC H5

³ √7ᵗʰ **S62.345** Nondisplaced fracture of base of fourth metacarpal bone, left hand   CC H5

³ √7ᵗʰ **S62.346** Nondisplaced fracture of base of fifth metacarpal bone, right hand   CC H5

³ √7ᵗʰ **S62.347** Nondisplaced fracture of base of fifth metacarpal bone, left hand   CC H5

³ √7ᵗʰ **S62.348** Nondisplaced fracture of base of other metacarpal bone   CC H5

    Nondisplaced fracture of base of specified metacarpal bone with unspecified laterality

³ √7ᵗʰ **S62.349** Nondisplaced fracture of base of unspecified metacarpal bone   CC H5

√6ᵗʰ **S62.35** Nondisplaced fracture of shaft of other metacarpal bone

³ √7ᵗʰ **S62.350** Nondisplaced fracture of shaft of second metacarpal bone, right hand   CC H5

³ √7ᵗʰ **S62.351** Nondisplaced fracture of shaft of second metacarpal bone, left hand   CC H5

³ √7ᵗʰ **S62.352** Nondisplaced fracture of shaft of third metacarpal bone, right hand   CC H5

³ √7ᵗʰ **S62.353** Nondisplaced fracture of shaft of third metacarpal bone, left hand   CC H5

✔ Additional Character Required   √x7ᵗʰ Placeholder   Unacceptable PDx   Questionable PDx   Manifestation   Unspecified Dx   H1-H14 HAC   HCC CMS-HCC Dx   HIV HIV Dx

ICD-10-CM 2021   1037

³ √7ᵗʰ **S62.354** **Nondisplaced fracture of shaft of fourth metacarpal bone, right hand** CC H5

³ √7ᵗʰ **S62.355** **Nondisplaced fracture of shaft of fourth metacarpal bone, left hand** CC H5

³ √7ᵗʰ **S62.356** **Nondisplaced fracture of shaft of fifth metacarpal bone, right hand** CC H5

³ √7ᵗʰ **S62.357** **Nondisplaced fracture of shaft of fifth metacarpal bone, left hand** CC H5

³ √7ᵗʰ **S62.358** **Nondisplaced fracture of shaft of other metacarpal bone** CC H5
Nondisplaced fracture of shaft of specified metacarpal bone with unspecified laterality

³ √7ᵗʰ **S62.359** **Nondisplaced fracture of shaft of unspecified metacarpal bone** CC H5

√6ᵗʰ **S62.36** **Nondisplaced fracture of neck of other metacarpal bone**

³ √7ᵗʰ **S62.360** **Nondisplaced fracture of neck of second metacarpal bone, right hand** CC H5

³ √7ᵗʰ **S62.361** **Nondisplaced fracture of neck of second metacarpal bone, left hand** CC H5

³ √7ᵗʰ **S62.362** **Nondisplaced fracture of neck of third metacarpal bone, right hand** CC H5

³ √7ᵗʰ **S62.363** **Nondisplaced fracture of neck of third metacarpal bone, left hand** CC H5

³ √7ᵗʰ **S62.364** **Nondisplaced fracture of neck of fourth metacarpal bone, right hand** CC H5

³ √7ᵗʰ **S62.365** **Nondisplaced fracture of neck of fourth metacarpal bone, left hand** CC H5

³ √7ᵗʰ **S62.366** **Nondisplaced fracture of neck of fifth metacarpal bone, right hand** CC H5

³ √7ᵗʰ **S62.367** **Nondisplaced fracture of neck of fifth metacarpal bone, left hand** CC H5

³ √7ᵗʰ **S62.368** **Nondisplaced fracture of neck of other metacarpal bone** CC H5
Nondisplaced fracture of neck of specified metacarpal bone with unspecified laterality

³ √7ᵗʰ **S62.369** **Nondisplaced fracture of neck of unspecified metacarpal bone** CC H5

√6ᵗʰ **S62.39** **Other fracture of other metacarpal bone**

³ √7ᵗʰ **S62.390** **Other fracture of second metacarpal bone, right hand** CC H5

³ √7ᵗʰ **S62.391** **Other fracture of second metacarpal bone, left hand** CC H5

³ √7ᵗʰ **S62.392** **Other fracture of third metacarpal bone, right hand** CC H5

³ √7ᵗʰ **S62.393** **Other fracture of third metacarpal bone, left hand** CC H5

³ √7ᵗʰ **S62.394** **Other fracture of fourth metacarpal bone, right hand** CC H5

³ √7ᵗʰ **S62.395** **Other fracture of fourth metacarpal bone, left hand** CC H5

³ √7ᵗʰ **S62.396** **Other fracture of fifth metacarpal bone, right hand** CC H5

³ √7ᵗʰ **S62.397** **Other fracture of fifth metacarpal bone, left hand** CC H5

³ √7ᵗʰ **S62.398** **Other fracture of other metacarpal bone** CC H5
Other fracture of specified metacarpal bone with unspecified laterality

³ √7ᵗʰ **S62.399** **Other fracture of unspecified metacarpal bone** CC H5

√5ᵗʰ **S62.5** **Fracture of thumb**

√6ᵗʰ **S62.50** **Fracture of unspecified phalanx of thumb**

³ √7ᵗʰ **S62.501** **Fracture of unspecified phalanx of right thumb** CC H5

³ √7ᵗʰ **S62.502** **Fracture of unspecified phalanx of left thumb** CC H5

³ √7ᵗʰ **S62.509** **Fracture of unspecified phalanx of unspecified thumb** CC H5

√6ᵗʰ **S62.51** **Fracture of proximal phalanx of thumb**

³ √7ᵗʰ **S62.511** **Displaced fracture of proximal phalanx of right thumb** CC H5

³ √7ᵗʰ **S62.512** **Displaced fracture of proximal phalanx of left thumb** CC H5

³ √7ᵗʰ **S62.513** **Displaced fracture of proximal phalanx of unspecified thumb** CC H5

³ √7ᵗʰ **S62.514** **Nondisplaced fracture of proximal phalanx of right thumb** CC H5

³ √7ᵗʰ **S62.515** **Nondisplaced fracture of proximal phalanx of left thumb** CC H5

³ √7ᵗʰ **S62.516** **Nondisplaced fracture of proximal phalanx of unspecified thumb** CC H5

√6ᵗʰ **S62.52** **Fracture of distal phalanx of thumb**

³ √7ᵗʰ **S62.521** **Displaced fracture of distal phalanx of right thumb** CC H5

³ √7ᵗʰ **S62.522** **Displaced fracture of distal phalanx of left thumb** CC H5

³ √7ᵗʰ **S62.523** **Displaced fracture of distal phalanx of unspecified thumb** CC H5

³ √7ᵗʰ **S62.524** **Nondisplaced fracture of distal phalanx of right thumb** CC H5

³ √7ᵗʰ **S62.525** **Nondisplaced fracture of distal phalanx of left thumb** CC H5

³ √7ᵗʰ **S62.526** **Nondisplaced fracture of distal phalanx of unspecified thumb** CC H5

√5ᵗʰ **S62.6** **Fracture of other and unspecified finger(s)**

EXCLUDES 2   *fracture of thumb (S62.5-)*

√6ᵗʰ **S62.60** **Fracture of unspecified phalanx of finger**

³ √7ᵗʰ **S62.600** **Fracture of unspecified phalanx of right index finger** CC H5

³ √7ᵗʰ **S62.601** **Fracture of unspecified phalanx of left index finger** CC H5

³ √7ᵗʰ **S62.602** **Fracture of unspecified phalanx of right middle finger** CC H5

³ √7ᵗʰ **S62.603** **Fracture of unspecified phalanx of left middle finger** CC H5

³ √7ᵗʰ **S62.604** **Fracture of unspecified phalanx of right ring finger** CC H5

³ √7ᵗʰ **S62.605** **Fracture of unspecified phalanx of left ring finger** CC H5

³ √7ᵗʰ **S62.606** **Fracture of unspecified phalanx of right little finger** CC H5

³ √7ᵗʰ **S62.607** **Fracture of unspecified phalanx of left little finger** CC H5

³ √7ᵗʰ **S62.608** **Fracture of unspecified phalanx of other finger** CC H5
Fracture of unspecified phalanx of specified finger with unspecified laterality

³ √7ᵗʰ **S62.609** **Fracture of unspecified phalanx of unspecified finger** CC H5

√6ᵗʰ **S62.61** **Displaced fracture of proximal phalanx of finger**

³ √7ᵗʰ **S62.610** **Displaced fracture of proximal phalanx of right index finger** CC H5

³ √7ᵗʰ **S62.611** **Displaced fracture of proximal phalanx of left index finger** CC H5

³ √7ᵗʰ **S62.612** **Displaced fracture of proximal phalanx of right middle finger** CC H5

³ √7ᵗʰ **S62.613** **Displaced fracture of proximal phalanx of left middle finger** CC H5

³ √7ᵗʰ **S62.614** **Displaced fracture of proximal phalanx of right ring finger** CC H5

³ √7ᵗʰ **S62.615** **Displaced fracture of proximal phalanx of left ring finger** CC H5

³ √7ᵗʰ **S62.616** **Displaced fracture of proximal phalanx of right little finger** CC H5

³ √7ᵗʰ **S62.617** **Displaced fracture of proximal phalanx of left little finger** CC H5

³ √7ᵗʰ **S62.618** **Displaced fracture of proximal phalanx of other finger** CC H5
Displaced fracture of proximal phalanx of specified finger with unspecified laterality

³ √7ᵗʰ **S62.619** **Displaced fracture of proximal phalanx of unspecified finger** CC H5

√6ᵗʰ **S62.62** **Displaced fracture of middle phalanx of finger**

³ √7ᵗʰ **S62.620** **Displaced fracture of middle phalanx of right index finger** CC H5

³ √7ᵗʰ **S62.621** **Displaced fracture of middle phalanx of left index finger** CC H5

³ √7ᵗʰ **S62.622** **Displaced fracture of middle phalanx of right middle finger** CC H5

³ √7ᵗʰ **S62.623** **Displaced fracture of middle phalanx of left middle finger** CC H5

N Newborn: 0   P Pediatric: 0-17   M Maternity: 9-64   A Adult: 15-124   MCC Major Complication/Comorbidity   CC Complication/Comorbidity   SW Severe Wound Dx

1038   ICD-10-CM 2021

3 √7ᵗʰ **S62.624 Displaced fracture of middle phalanx of right ring finger** CC H5

3 √7ᵗʰ **S62.625 Displaced fracture of middle phalanx of left ring finger** CC H5

3 √7ᵗʰ **S62.626 Displaced fracture of middle phalanx of right little finger** CC H5

3 √7ᵗʰ **S62.627 Displaced fracture of middle phalanx of left little finger** CC H5

3 √7ᵗʰ **S62.628 Displaced fracture of middle phalanx of other finger** CC H5
    Displaced fracture of middle phalanx of specified finger with unspecified laterality

3 √7ᵗʰ **S62.629 Displaced fracture of middle phalanx of unspecified finger** CC H5

√6ᵗʰ **S62.63 Displaced fracture of distal phalanx of finger**

3 √7ᵗʰ **S62.630 Displaced fracture of distal phalanx of right index finger** CC H5

3 √7ᵗʰ **S62.631 Displaced fracture of distal phalanx of left index finger** CC H5

3 √7ᵗʰ **S62.632 Displaced fracture of distal phalanx of right middle finger** CC H5

3 √7ᵗʰ **S62.633 Displaced fracture of distal phalanx of left middle finger** CC H5

3 √7ᵗʰ **S62.634 Displaced fracture of distal phalanx of right ring finger** CC H5

3 √7ᵗʰ **S62.635 Displaced fracture of distal phalanx of left ring finger** CC H5

3 √7ᵗʰ **S62.636 Displaced fracture of distal phalanx of right little finger** CC H5

3 √7ᵗʰ **S62.637 Displaced fracture of distal phalanx of left little finger** CC H5

3 √7ᵗʰ **S62.638 Displaced fracture of distal phalanx of other finger** CC H5
    Displaced fracture of distal phalanx of specified finger with unspecified laterality

3 √7ᵗʰ **S62.639 Displaced fracture of distal phalanx of unspecified finger** CC H5

√6ᵗʰ **S62.64 Nondisplaced fracture of proximal phalanx of finger**

3 √7ᵗʰ **S62.640 Nondisplaced fracture of proximal phalanx of right index finger** CC H5

3 √7ᵗʰ **S62.641 Nondisplaced fracture of proximal phalanx of left index finger** CC H5

3 √7ᵗʰ **S62.642 Nondisplaced fracture of proximal phalanx of right middle finger** CC H5

3 √7ᵗʰ **S62.643 Nondisplaced fracture of proximal phalanx of left middle finger** CC H5

3 √7ᵗʰ **S62.644 Nondisplaced fracture of proximal phalanx of right ring finger** CC H5

3 √7ᵗʰ **S62.645 Nondisplaced fracture of proximal phalanx of left ring finger** CC H5

3 √7ᵗʰ **S62.646 Nondisplaced fracture of proximal phalanx of right little finger** CC H5

3 √7ᵗʰ **S62.647 Nondisplaced fracture of proximal phalanx of left little finger** CC H5

3 √7ᵗʰ **S62.648 Nondisplaced fracture of proximal phalanx of other finger** CC H5
    Nondisplaced fracture of proximal phalanx of specified finger with unspecified laterality

3 √7ᵗʰ **S62.649 Nondisplaced fracture of proximal phalanx of unspecified finger** CC H5

√6ᵗʰ **S62.65 Nondisplaced fracture of middle phalanx of finger**

3 √7ᵗʰ **S62.650 Nondisplaced fracture of middle phalanx of right index finger** CC H5

3 √7ᵗʰ **S62.651 Nondisplaced fracture of middle phalanx of left index finger** CC H5

3 √7ᵗʰ **S62.652 Nondisplaced fracture of middle phalanx of right middle finger** CC H5

3 √7ᵗʰ **S62.653 Nondisplaced fracture of middle phalanx of left middle finger** CC H5

3 √7ᵗʰ **S62.654 Nondisplaced fracture of middle phalanx of right ring finger** CC H5

3 √7ᵗʰ **S62.655 Nondisplaced fracture of middle phalanx of left ring finger** CC H5

3 √7ᵗʰ **S62.656 Nondisplaced fracture of middle phalanx of right little finger** CC H5

3 √7ᵗʰ **S62.657 Nondisplaced fracture of middle phalanx of left little finger** CC H5

3 √7ᵗʰ **S62.658 Nondisplaced fracture of middle phalanx of other finger** CC H5
    Nondisplaced fracture of middle phalanx of specified finger with unspecified laterality

3 √7ᵗʰ **S62.659 Nondisplaced fracture of middle phalanx of unspecified finger** CC H5

√6ᵗʰ **S62.66 Nondisplaced fracture of distal phalanx of finger**

3 √7ᵗʰ **S62.660 Nondisplaced fracture of distal phalanx of right index finger** CC H5

3 √7ᵗʰ **S62.661 Nondisplaced fracture of distal phalanx of left index finger** CC H5

3 √7ᵗʰ **S62.662 Nondisplaced fracture of distal phalanx of right middle finger** CC H5

3 √7ᵗʰ **S62.663 Nondisplaced fracture of distal phalanx of left middle finger** CC H5

3 √7ᵗʰ **S62.664 Nondisplaced fracture of distal phalanx of right ring finger** CC H5

3 √7ᵗʰ **S62.665 Nondisplaced fracture of distal phalanx of left ring finger** CC H5

3 √7ᵗʰ **S62.666 Nondisplaced fracture of distal phalanx of right little finger** CC H5

3 √7ᵗʰ **S62.667 Nondisplaced fracture of distal phalanx of left little finger** CC H5

3 √7ᵗʰ **S62.668 Nondisplaced fracture of distal phalanx of other finger** CC H5
    Nondisplaced fracture of distal phalanx of specified finger with unspecified laterality

3 √7ᵗʰ **S62.669 Nondisplaced fracture of distal phalanx of unspecified finger** CC H5

√5ᵗʰ **S62.9 Unspecified fracture of wrist and hand**

3 √x7ᵗʰ **S62.90 Unspecified fracture of unspecified wrist and hand** CC H5

3 √x7ᵗʰ **S62.91 Unspecified fracture of right wrist and hand** CC H5

3 √x7ᵗʰ **S62.92 Unspecified fracture of left wrist and hand** CC H5

√4ᵗʰ **S63 Dislocation and sprain of joints and ligaments at wrist and hand level**

   [INCLUDES]   avulsion of joint or ligament at wrist and hand level
       laceration of cartilage, joint or ligament at wrist and hand level
       sprain of cartilage, joint or ligament at wrist and hand level
       traumatic hemarthrosis of joint or ligament at wrist and hand level
       traumatic rupture of joint or ligament at wrist and hand level
       traumatic subluxation of joint or ligament at wrist and hand level
       traumatic tear of joint or ligament at wrist and hand level

Code also any associated open wound

EXCLUDES 2   strain of muscle, fascia and tendon of wrist and hand (S66.-)

The appropriate 7th character is to be added to each code from category S63.
A   initial encounter
D   subsequent encounter
S   sequela

√5ᵗʰ **S63.0 Subluxation and dislocation of wrist and hand joints**

√6ᵗʰ **S63.00 Unspecified subluxation and dislocation of wrist and hand**
    Dislocation of carpal bone NOS
    Dislocation of distal end of radius NOS
    Subluxation of carpal bone NOS
    Subluxation of distal end of radius NOS

√7ᵗʰ **S63.001 Unspecified subluxation of right wrist and hand**

√7ᵗʰ **S63.002 Unspecified subluxation of left wrist and hand**

√7ᵗʰ **S63.003 Unspecified subluxation of unspecified wrist and hand**

√7ᵗʰ **S63.004 Unspecified dislocation of right wrist and hand**

√7ᵗʰ **S63.005 Unspecified dislocation of left wrist and hand**

✔ Additional Character Required   √x7ᵗʰ Placeholder   Unacceptable PDx   Questionable PDx   Manifestation   Unspecified Dx   H1-H14 HAC   HCC CMS-HCC Dx   HIV HIV Dx

ICD-10-CM 2021   1039

√7ᵗʰ **S63.006** Unspecified dislocation of unspecified wrist and hand

√6ᵗʰ **S63.01** Subluxation and dislocation of distal radioulnar joint

    √7ᵗʰ **S63.011** Subluxation of distal radioulnar joint of right wrist

    √7ᵗʰ **S63.012** Subluxation of distal radioulnar joint of left wrist

    √7ᵗʰ **S63.013** Subluxation of distal radioulnar joint of unspecified wrist

    √7ᵗʰ **S63.014** Dislocation of distal radioulnar joint of right wrist

    √7ᵗʰ **S63.015** Dislocation of distal radioulnar joint of left wrist

    √7ᵗʰ **S63.016** Dislocation of distal radioulnar joint of unspecified wrist

√6ᵗʰ **S63.02** Subluxation and dislocation of radiocarpal joint

    √7ᵗʰ **S63.021** Subluxation of radiocarpal joint of right wrist

    √7ᵗʰ **S63.022** Subluxation of radiocarpal joint of left wrist

    √7ᵗʰ **S63.023** Subluxation of radiocarpal joint of unspecified wrist

    √7ᵗʰ **S63.024** Dislocation of radiocarpal joint of right wrist

    √7ᵗʰ **S63.025** Dislocation of radiocarpal joint of left wrist

    √7ᵗʰ **S63.026** Dislocation of radiocarpal joint of unspecified wrist

√6ᵗʰ **S63.03** Subluxation and dislocation of midcarpal joint

    √7ᵗʰ **S63.031** Subluxation of midcarpal joint of right wrist

    √7ᵗʰ **S63.032** Subluxation of midcarpal joint of left wrist

    √7ᵗʰ **S63.033** Subluxation of midcarpal joint of unspecified wrist

    √7ᵗʰ **S63.034** Dislocation of midcarpal joint of right wrist

    √7ᵗʰ **S63.035** Dislocation of midcarpal joint of left wrist

    √7ᵗʰ **S63.036** Dislocation of midcarpal joint of unspecified wrist

√6ᵗʰ **S63.04** Subluxation and dislocation of carpometacarpal joint of thumb

    EXCLUDES 2   interphalangeal subluxation and dislocation of thumb (S63.1-)

    √7ᵗʰ **S63.041** Subluxation of carpometacarpal joint of right thumb

    √7ᵗʰ **S63.042** Subluxation of carpometacarpal joint of left thumb

    √7ᵗʰ **S63.043** Subluxation of carpometacarpal joint of unspecified thumb

    √7ᵗʰ **S63.044** Dislocation of carpometacarpal joint of right thumb

    √7ᵗʰ **S63.045** Dislocation of carpometacarpal joint of left thumb

    √7ᵗʰ **S63.046** Dislocation of carpometacarpal joint of unspecified thumb

√6ᵗʰ **S63.05** Subluxation and dislocation of other carpometacarpal joint

    EXCLUDES 2   subluxation and dislocation of carpometacarpal joint of thumb (S63.04-)

    √7ᵗʰ **S63.051** Subluxation of other carpometacarpal joint of right hand

    √7ᵗʰ **S63.052** Subluxation of other carpometacarpal joint of left hand

    √7ᵗʰ **S63.053** Subluxation of other carpometacarpal joint of unspecified hand

    √7ᵗʰ **S63.054** Dislocation of other carpometacarpal joint of right hand

    √7ᵗʰ **S63.055** Dislocation of other carpometacarpal joint of left hand

    √7ᵗʰ **S63.056** Dislocation of other carpometacarpal joint of unspecified hand

√6ᵗʰ **S63.06** Subluxation and dislocation of metacarpal (bone), proximal end

    √7ᵗʰ **S63.061** Subluxation of metacarpal (bone), proximal end of right hand

    √7ᵗʰ **S63.062** Subluxation of metacarpal (bone), proximal end of left hand

    √7ᵗʰ **S63.063** Subluxation of metacarpal (bone), proximal end of unspecified hand

    √7ᵗʰ **S63.064** Dislocation of metacarpal (bone), proximal end of right hand

    √7ᵗʰ **S63.065** Dislocation of metacarpal (bone), proximal end of left hand

    √7ᵗʰ **S63.066** Dislocation of metacarpal (bone), proximal end of unspecified hand

√6ᵗʰ **S63.07** Subluxation and dislocation of distal end of ulna

    √7ᵗʰ **S63.071** Subluxation of distal end of right ulna

    √7ᵗʰ **S63.072** Subluxation of distal end of left ulna

    √7ᵗʰ **S63.073** Subluxation of distal end of unspecified ulna

    √7ᵗʰ **S63.074** Dislocation of distal end of right ulna

    √7ᵗʰ **S63.075** Dislocation of distal end of left ulna

    √7ᵗʰ **S63.076** Dislocation of distal end of unspecified ulna

√6ᵗʰ **S63.09** Other subluxation and dislocation of wrist and hand

    √7ᵗʰ **S63.091** Other subluxation of right wrist and hand

    √7ᵗʰ **S63.092** Other subluxation of left wrist and hand

    √7ᵗʰ **S63.093** Other subluxation of unspecified wrist and hand

    √7ᵗʰ **S63.094** Other dislocation of right wrist and hand

    √7ᵗʰ **S63.095** Other dislocation of left wrist and hand

    √7ᵗʰ **S63.096** Other dislocation of unspecified wrist and hand

√5ᵗʰ **S63.1** Subluxation and dislocation of thumb

√6ᵗʰ **S63.10** Unspecified subluxation and dislocation of thumb

    √7ᵗʰ **S63.101** Unspecified subluxation of right thumb

    √7ᵗʰ **S63.102** Unspecified subluxation of left thumb

    √7ᵗʰ **S63.103** Unspecified subluxation of unspecified thumb

    √7ᵗʰ **S63.104** Unspecified dislocation of right thumb

    √7ᵗʰ **S63.105** Unspecified dislocation of left thumb

    √7ᵗʰ **S63.106** Unspecified dislocation of unspecified thumb

√6ᵗʰ **S63.11** Subluxation and dislocation of metacarpophalangeal joint of thumb

    √7ᵗʰ **S63.111** Subluxation of metacarpophalangeal joint of right thumb

    √7ᵗʰ **S63.112** Subluxation of metacarpophalangeal joint of left thumb

    √7ᵗʰ **S63.113** Subluxation of metacarpophalangeal joint of unspecified thumb

    √7ᵗʰ **S63.114** Dislocation of metacarpophalangeal joint of right thumb

    √7ᵗʰ **S63.115** Dislocation of metacarpophalangeal joint of left thumb

    √7ᵗʰ **S63.116** Dislocation of metacarpophalangeal joint of unspecified thumb

√6ᵗʰ **S63.12** Subluxation and dislocation of interphalangeal joint of thumb

    √7ᵗʰ **S63.121** Subluxation of interphalangeal joint of right thumb

    √7ᵗʰ **S63.122** Subluxation of interphalangeal joint of left thumb

    √7ᵗʰ **S63.123** Subluxation of interphalangeal joint of unspecified thumb

    √7ᵗʰ **S63.124** Dislocation of interphalangeal joint of right thumb

    √7ᵗʰ **S63.125** Dislocation of interphalangeal joint of left thumb

    √7ᵗʰ **S63.126** Dislocation of interphalangeal joint of unspecified thumb

√5ᵗʰ **S63.2** Subluxation and dislocation of other finger(s)

    EXCLUDES 2   subluxation and dislocation of thumb (S63.1-)

√6ᵗʰ **S63.20** Unspecified subluxation of other finger

    √7ᵗʰ **S63.200** Unspecified subluxation of right index finger

    √7ᵗʰ **S63.201** Unspecified subluxation of left index finger

    √7ᵗʰ **S63.202** Unspecified subluxation of right middle finger

    √7ᵗʰ **S63.203** Unspecified subluxation of left middle finger

    √7ᵗʰ **S63.204** Unspecified subluxation of right ring finger

    √7ᵗʰ **S63.205** Unspecified subluxation of left ring finger

    √7ᵗʰ **S63.206** Unspecified subluxation of right little finger

N Newborn: 0   P Pediatric: 0-17   M Maternity: 9-64   A Adult: 15-124   MCC Major Complication/Comorbidity   CC Complication/Comorbidity   SW Severe Wound Dx

1040   ICD-10-CM 2021

√7ᵗʰ **S63.207** **Unspecified subluxation of** left little finger

√7ᵗʰ **S63.208** **Unspecified subluxation of other finger**
    Unspecified subluxation of specified finger with unspecified laterality

√7ᵗʰ **S63.209** **Unspecified subluxation of unspecified finger**

√6ᵗʰ **S63.21** **Subluxation of** metacarpophalangeal joint **of finger**

√7ᵗʰ **S63.210** **Subluxation of metacarpophalangeal joint of** right index **finger**

√7ᵗʰ **S63.211** **Subluxation of metacarpophalangeal joint of** left index **finger**

√7ᵗʰ **S63.212** **Subluxation of metacarpophalangeal joint of** right middle **finger**

√7ᵗʰ **S63.213** **Subluxation of metacarpophalangeal joint of** left middle **finger**

√7ᵗʰ **S63.214** **Subluxation of metacarpophalangeal joint of** right ring **finger**

√7ᵗʰ **S63.215** **Subluxation of metacarpophalangeal joint of** left ring **finger**

√7ᵗʰ **S63.216** **Subluxation of metacarpophalangeal joint of** right little **finger**

√7ᵗʰ **S63.217** **Subluxation of metacarpophalangeal joint of** left little **finger**

√7ᵗʰ **S63.218** **Subluxation of metacarpophalangeal joint of other finger**
    Subluxation of metacarpophalangeal joint of specified finger with unspecified laterality

√7ᵗʰ **S63.219** **Subluxation of metacarpophalangeal joint of unspecified finger**

√6ᵗʰ **S63.22** **Subluxation of unspecified** interphalangeal joint **of finger**

√7ᵗʰ **S63.220** **Subluxation of unspecified interphalangeal joint of** right index **finger**

√7ᵗʰ **S63.221** **Subluxation of unspecified interphalangeal joint of** left index **finger**

√7ᵗʰ **S63.222** **Subluxation of unspecified interphalangeal joint of** right middle **finger**

√7ᵗʰ **S63.223** **Subluxation of unspecified interphalangeal joint of** left middle **finger**

√7ᵗʰ **S63.224** **Subluxation of unspecified interphalangeal joint of** right ring **finger**

√7ᵗʰ **S63.225** **Subluxation of unspecified interphalangeal joint of** left ring **finger**

√7ᵗʰ **S63.226** **Subluxation of unspecified interphalangeal joint of** right little **finger**

√7ᵗʰ **S63.227** **Subluxation of unspecified interphalangeal joint of** left little **finger**

√7ᵗʰ **S63.228** **Subluxation of unspecified interphalangeal joint of other finger**
    Subluxation of unspecified interphalangeal joint of specified finger with unspecified laterality

√7ᵗʰ **S63.229** **Subluxation of unspecified interphalangeal joint of unspecified finger**

√6ᵗʰ **S63.23** **Subluxation of** proximal interphalangeal **joint of finger**

√7ᵗʰ **S63.230** **Subluxation of proximal interphalangeal joint of** right index **finger**

√7ᵗʰ **S63.231** **Subluxation of proximal interphalangeal joint of** left index **finger**

√7ᵗʰ **S63.232** **Subluxation of proximal interphalangeal joint of** right middle **finger**

√7ᵗʰ **S63.233** **Subluxation of proximal interphalangeal joint of** left middle **finger**

√7ᵗʰ **S63.234** **Subluxation of proximal interphalangeal joint of** right ring **finger**

√7ᵗʰ **S63.235** **Subluxation of proximal interphalangeal joint of** left ring **finger**

√7ᵗʰ **S63.236** **Subluxation of proximal interphalangeal joint of** right little **finger**

√7ᵗʰ **S63.237** **Subluxation of proximal interphalangeal joint of** left little **finger**

√7ᵗʰ **S63.238** **Subluxation of proximal interphalangeal joint of other finger**
    Subluxation of proximal interphalangeal joint of specified finger with unspecified laterality

√7ᵗʰ **S63.239** **Subluxation of proximal interphalangeal joint of unspecified finger**

√6ᵗʰ **S63.24** **Subluxation of** distal interphalangeal **joint of finger**

√7ᵗʰ **S63.240** **Subluxation of distal interphalangeal joint of** right index **finger**

√7ᵗʰ **S63.241** **Subluxation of distal interphalangeal joint of** left index **finger**

√7ᵗʰ **S63.242** **Subluxation of distal interphalangeal joint of** right middle **finger**

√7ᵗʰ **S63.243** **Subluxation of distal interphalangeal joint of** left middle **finger**

√7ᵗʰ **S63.244** **Subluxation of distal interphalangeal joint of** right ring **finger**

√7ᵗʰ **S63.245** **Subluxation of distal interphalangeal joint of** left ring **finger**

√7ᵗʰ **S63.246** **Subluxation of distal interphalangeal joint of** right little **finger**

√7ᵗʰ **S63.247** **Subluxation of distal interphalangeal joint of** left little **finger**

√7ᵗʰ **S63.248** **Subluxation of distal interphalangeal joint of other finger**
    Subluxation of distal interphalangeal joint of specified finger with unspecified laterality

√7ᵗʰ **S63.249** **Subluxation of distal interphalangeal joint of unspecified finger**

√6ᵗʰ **S63.25** **Unspecified dislocation of other finger**

√7ᵗʰ **S63.250** **Unspecified dislocation of** right index **finger**

√7ᵗʰ **S63.251** **Unspecified dislocation of** left index **finger**

√7ᵗʰ **S63.252** **Unspecified dislocation of** right middle **finger**

√7ᵗʰ **S63.253** **Unspecified dislocation of** left middle **finger**

√7ᵗʰ **S63.254** **Unspecified dislocation of** right ring **finger**

√7ᵗʰ **S63.255** **Unspecified dislocation of** left ring **finger**

√7ᵗʰ **S63.256** **Unspecified dislocation of** right little **finger**

√7ᵗʰ **S63.257** **Unspecified dislocation of** left little **finger**

√7ᵗʰ **S63.258** **Unspecified dislocation of other finger**
    Unspecified dislocation of specified finger with unspecified laterality

√7ᵗʰ **S63.259** **Unspecified dislocation of unspecified finger**
    Unspecified dislocation of unspecified finger with unspecified laterality

√6ᵗʰ **S63.26** **Dislocation of** metacarpophalangeal joint **of finger**

√7ᵗʰ **S63.260** **Dislocation of metacarpophalangeal joint of** right index **finger**

√7ᵗʰ **S63.261** **Dislocation of metacarpophalangeal joint of** left index **finger**

√7ᵗʰ **S63.262** **Dislocation of metacarpophalangeal joint of** right middle **finger**

√7ᵗʰ **S63.263** **Dislocation of metacarpophalangeal joint of** left middle **finger**

√7ᵗʰ **S63.264** **Dislocation of metacarpophalangeal joint of** right ring **finger**

√7ᵗʰ **S63.265** **Dislocation of metacarpophalangeal joint of** left ring **finger**

√7ᵗʰ **S63.266** **Dislocation of metacarpophalangeal joint of** right little **finger**

√7ᵗʰ **S63.267** **Dislocation of metacarpophalangeal joint of** left little **finger**

√7ᵗʰ **S63.268** **Dislocation of metacarpophalangeal joint of other finger**
    Dislocation of metacarpophalangeal joint of specified finger with unspecified laterality

√7ᵗʰ **S63.269** **Dislocation of metacarpophalangeal joint of unspecified finger**

√6ᵗʰ **S63.27** **Dislocation of unspecified interphalangeal joint of finger**

√7ᵗʰ **S63.270** **Dislocation of unspecified interphalangeal joint of** right index **finger**

√7ᵗʰ **S63.271** **Dislocation of unspecified interphalangeal joint of** left index **finger**

√7ᵗʰ **S63.272** **Dislocation of unspecified interphalangeal joint of** right middle **finger**

☑ Additional Character Required   √x7ᵗʰ Placeholder   Unacceptable PDx   Questionable PDx   Manifestation   Unspecified Dx   H1-H14 HAC   HCC CMS-HCC Dx   HIV HIV Dx

ICD-10-CM 2021   1041

√7ᵗʰ **S63.273** Dislocation of unspecified interphalangeal joint of left middle finger

√7ᵗʰ **S63.274** Dislocation of unspecified interphalangeal joint of right ring finger

√7ᵗʰ **S63.275** Dislocation of unspecified interphalangeal joint of left ring finger

√7ᵗʰ **S63.276** Dislocation of unspecified interphalangeal joint of right little finger

√7ᵗʰ **S63.277** Dislocation of unspecified interphalangeal joint of left little finger

√7ᵗʰ **S63.278** Dislocation of unspecified interphalangeal joint of other finger

Dislocation of unspecified interphalangeal joint of specified finger with unspecified laterality

√7ᵗʰ **S63.279** Dislocation of unspecified interphalangeal joint of unspecified finger

Dislocation of unspecified interphalangeal joint of unspecified finger without specified laterality

√6ᵗʰ **S63.28** Dislocation of proximal interphalangeal joint of finger

√7ᵗʰ **S63.280** Dislocation of proximal interphalangeal joint of right index finger

√7ᵗʰ **S63.281** Dislocation of proximal interphalangeal joint of left index finger

√7ᵗʰ **S63.282** Dislocation of proximal interphalangeal joint of right middle finger

√7ᵗʰ **S63.283** Dislocation of proximal interphalangeal joint of left middle finger

√7ᵗʰ **S63.284** Dislocation of proximal interphalangeal joint of right ring finger

√7ᵗʰ **S63.285** Dislocation of proximal interphalangeal joint of left ring finger

√7ᵗʰ **S63.286** Dislocation of proximal interphalangeal joint of right little finger

√7ᵗʰ **S63.287** Dislocation of proximal interphalangeal joint of left little finger

√7ᵗʰ **S63.288** Dislocation of proximal interphalangeal joint of other finger

Dislocation of proximal interphalangeal joint of specified finger with unspecified laterality

√7ᵗʰ **S63.289** Dislocation of proximal interphalangeal joint of unspecified finger

√6ᵗʰ **S63.29** Dislocation of distal interphalangeal joint of finger

√7ᵗʰ **S63.290** Dislocation of distal interphalangeal joint of right index finger

√7ᵗʰ **S63.291** Dislocation of distal interphalangeal joint of left index finger

√7ᵗʰ **S63.292** Dislocation of distal interphalangeal joint of right middle finger

√7ᵗʰ **S63.293** Dislocation of distal interphalangeal joint of left middle finger

√7ᵗʰ **S63.294** Dislocation of distal interphalangeal joint of right ring finger

√7ᵗʰ **S63.295** Dislocation of distal interphalangeal joint of left ring finger

√7ᵗʰ **S63.296** Dislocation of distal interphalangeal joint of right little finger

√7ᵗʰ **S63.297** Dislocation of distal interphalangeal joint of left little finger

√7ᵗʰ **S63.298** Dislocation of distal interphalangeal joint of other finger

Dislocation of distal interphalangeal joint of specified finger with unspecified laterality

√7ᵗʰ **S63.299** Dislocation of distal interphalangeal joint of unspecified finger

√5ᵗʰ **S63.3** Traumatic rupture of ligament of wrist

√6ᵗʰ **S63.30** Traumatic rupture of unspecified ligament of wrist

√7ᵗʰ **S63.301** Traumatic rupture of unspecified ligament of right wrist

√7ᵗʰ **S63.302** Traumatic rupture of unspecified ligament of left wrist

√7ᵗʰ **S63.309** Traumatic rupture of unspecified ligament of unspecified wrist

√6ᵗʰ **S63.31** Traumatic rupture of collateral ligament of wrist

√7ᵗʰ **S63.311** Traumatic rupture of collateral ligament of right wrist

√7ᵗʰ **S63.312** Traumatic rupture of collateral ligament of left wrist

√7ᵗʰ **S63.319** Traumatic rupture of collateral ligament of unspecified wrist

√6ᵗʰ **S63.32** Traumatic rupture of radiocarpal ligament

√7ᵗʰ **S63.321** Traumatic rupture of right radiocarpal ligament

√7ᵗʰ **S63.322** Traumatic rupture of left radiocarpal ligament

√7ᵗʰ **S63.329** Traumatic rupture of unspecified radiocarpal ligament

√6ᵗʰ **S63.33** Traumatic rupture of ulnocarpal (palmar) ligament

√7ᵗʰ **S63.331** Traumatic rupture of right ulnocarpal (palmar) ligament

√7ᵗʰ **S63.332** Traumatic rupture of left ulnocarpal (palmar) ligament

√7ᵗʰ **S63.339** Traumatic rupture of unspecified ulnocarpal (palmar) ligament

√6ᵗʰ **S63.39** Traumatic rupture of other ligament of wrist

√7ᵗʰ **S63.391** Traumatic rupture of other ligament of right wrist

√7ᵗʰ **S63.392** Traumatic rupture of other ligament of left wrist

√7ᵗʰ **S63.399** Traumatic rupture of other ligament of unspecified wrist

√5ᵗʰ **S63.4** Traumatic rupture of ligament of finger at metacarpophalangeal and interphalangeal joint(s)

√6ᵗʰ **S63.40** Traumatic rupture of unspecified ligament of finger at metacarpophalangeal and interphalangeal joint

√7ᵗʰ **S63.400** Traumatic rupture of unspecified ligament of right index finger at metacarpophalangeal and interphalangeal joint

√7ᵗʰ **S63.401** Traumatic rupture of unspecified ligament of left index finger at metacarpophalangeal and interphalangeal joint

√7ᵗʰ **S63.402** Traumatic rupture of unspecified ligament of right middle finger at metacarpophalangeal and interphalangeal joint

√7ᵗʰ **S63.403** Traumatic rupture of unspecified ligament of left middle finger at metacarpophalangeal and interphalangeal joint

√7ᵗʰ **S63.404** Traumatic rupture of unspecified ligament of right ring finger at metacarpophalangeal and interphalangeal joint

√7ᵗʰ **S63.405** Traumatic rupture of unspecified ligament of left ring finger at metacarpophalangeal and interphalangeal joint

√7ᵗʰ **S63.406** Traumatic rupture of unspecified ligament of right little finger at metacarpophalangeal and interphalangeal joint

√7ᵗʰ **S63.407** Traumatic rupture of unspecified ligament of left little finger at metacarpophalangeal and interphalangeal joint

√7ᵗʰ **S63.408** Traumatic rupture of unspecified ligament of other finger at metacarpophalangeal and interphalangeal joint

Traumatic rupture of unspecified ligament of specified finger with unspecified laterality at metacarpophalangeal and interphalangeal joint

√7ᵗʰ **S63.409** Traumatic rupture of unspecified ligament of unspecified finger at metacarpophalangeal and interphalangeal joint

√6ᵗʰ **S63.41** Traumatic rupture of collateral ligament of finger at metacarpophalangeal and interphalangeal joint

√7ᵗʰ **S63.410** Traumatic rupture of collateral ligament of right index finger at metacarpophalangeal and interphalangeal joint

√7ᵗʰ **S63.411** Traumatic rupture of collateral ligament of left index finger at metacarpophalangeal and interphalangeal joint

Ⓝ Newborn: 0   Ⓟ Pediatric: 0-17   Ⓜ Maternity: 9-64   Ⓐ Adult: 15-124   ᴹᶜᶜ Major Complication/Comorbidity   ᶜᶜ Complication/Comorbidity   ˢᵂ Severe Wound Dx

1042   ICD-10-CM 2021

√7ᵗʰ **S63.412** **Traumatic rupture of collateral ligament of** right middle **finger at metacarpophalangeal and interphalangeal joint**

√7ᵗʰ **S63.413** **Traumatic rupture of collateral ligament of** left middle **finger at metacarpophalangeal and interphalangeal joint**

√7ᵗʰ **S63.414** **Traumatic rupture of collateral ligament of** right ring **finger at metacarpophalangeal and interphalangeal joint**

√7ᵗʰ **S63.415** **Traumatic rupture of collateral ligament of** left ring **finger at metacarpophalangeal and interphalangeal joint**

√7ᵗʰ **S63.416** **Traumatic rupture of collateral ligament of** right little **finger at metacarpophalangeal and interphalangeal joint**

√7ᵗʰ **S63.417** **Traumatic rupture of collateral ligament of** left little **finger at metacarpophalangeal and interphalangeal joint**

√7ᵗʰ **S63.418** **Traumatic rupture of collateral ligament of other finger at metacarpophalangeal and interphalangeal joint**
Traumatic rupture of collateral ligament of specified finger with unspecified laterality at metacarpophalangeal and interphalangeal joint

√7ᵗʰ **S63.419** **Traumatic rupture of collateral ligament of unspecified finger at metacarpophalangeal and interphalangeal joint**

√6ᵗʰ **S63.42** **Traumatic rupture of** palmar ligament **of finger at metacarpophalangeal and interphalangeal joint**

√7ᵗʰ **S63.420** **Traumatic rupture of palmar ligament of** right index **finger at metacarpophalangeal and interphalangeal joint**

√7ᵗʰ **S63.421** **Traumatic rupture of palmar ligament of** left index **finger at metacarpophalangeal and interphalangeal joint**

√7ᵗʰ **S63.422** **Traumatic rupture of palmar ligament of** right middle **finger at metacarpophalangeal and interphalangeal joint**

√7ᵗʰ **S63.423** **Traumatic rupture of palmar ligament of** left middle **finger at metacarpophalangeal and interphalangeal joint**

√7ᵗʰ **S63.424** **Traumatic rupture of palmar ligament of** right ring **finger at metacarpophalangeal and interphalangeal joint**

√7ᵗʰ **S63.425** **Traumatic rupture of palmar ligament of** left ring **finger at metacarpophalangeal and interphalangeal joint**

√7ᵗʰ **S63.426** **Traumatic rupture of palmar ligament of** right little **finger at metacarpophalangeal and interphalangeal joint**

√7ᵗʰ **S63.427** **Traumatic rupture of palmar ligament of** left little **finger at metacarpophalangeal and interphalangeal joint**

√7ᵗʰ **S63.428** **Traumatic rupture of palmar ligament of other finger at metacarpophalangeal and interphalangeal joint**
Traumatic rupture of palmar ligament of specified finger with unspecified laterality at metacarpophalangeal and interphalangeal joint

√7ᵗʰ **S63.429** **Traumatic rupture of palmar ligament of unspecified finger at metacarpophalangeal and interphalangeal joint**

√6ᵗʰ **S63.43** **Traumatic rupture of** volar plate **of finger at metacarpophalangeal and interphalangeal joint**

√7ᵗʰ **S63.430** **Traumatic rupture of volar plate of** right index **finger at metacarpophalangeal and interphalangeal joint**

√7ᵗʰ **S63.431** **Traumatic rupture of volar plate of** left index **finger at metacarpophalangeal and interphalangeal joint**

√7ᵗʰ **S63.432** **Traumatic rupture of volar plate of** right middle **finger at metacarpophalangeal and interphalangeal joint**

√7ᵗʰ **S63.433** **Traumatic rupture of volar plate of** left middle **finger at metacarpophalangeal and interphalangeal joint**

√7ᵗʰ **S63.434** **Traumatic rupture of volar plate of** right ring **finger at metacarpophalangeal and interphalangeal joint**

√7ᵗʰ **S63.435** **Traumatic rupture of volar plate of** left ring **finger at metacarpophalangeal and interphalangeal joint**

√7ᵗʰ **S63.436** **Traumatic rupture of volar plate of** right little **finger at metacarpophalangeal and interphalangeal joint**

√7ᵗʰ **S63.437** **Traumatic rupture of volar plate of** left little **finger at metacarpophalangeal and interphalangeal joint**

√7ᵗʰ **S63.438** **Traumatic rupture of volar plate of other finger at metacarpophalangeal and interphalangeal joint**
Traumatic rupture of volar plate of specified finger with unspecified laterality at metacarpophalangeal and interphalangeal joint

√7ᵗʰ **S63.439** **Traumatic rupture of volar plate of unspecified finger at metacarpophalangeal and interphalangeal joint**

√6ᵗʰ **S63.49** **Traumatic rupture of other ligament of finger at metacarpophalangeal and interphalangeal joint**

√7ᵗʰ **S63.490** **Traumatic rupture of other ligament of** right index **finger at metacarpophalangeal and interphalangeal joint**

√7ᵗʰ **S63.491** **Traumatic rupture of other ligament of** left index **finger at metacarpophalangeal and interphalangeal joint**

√7ᵗʰ **S63.492** **Traumatic rupture of other ligament of** right middle **finger at metacarpophalangeal and interphalangeal joint**

√7ᵗʰ **S63.493** **Traumatic rupture of other ligament of** left middle **finger at metacarpophalangeal and interphalangeal joint**

√7ᵗʰ **S63.494** **Traumatic rupture of other ligament of** right ring **finger at metacarpophalangeal and interphalangeal joint**

√7ᵗʰ **S63.495** **Traumatic rupture of other ligament of** left ring **finger at metacarpophalangeal and interphalangeal joint**

√7ᵗʰ **S63.496** **Traumatic rupture of other ligament of** right little **finger at metacarpophalangeal and interphalangeal joint**

√7ᵗʰ **S63.497** **Traumatic rupture of other ligament of** left little **finger at metacarpophalangeal and interphalangeal joint**

√7ᵗʰ **S63.498** **Traumatic rupture of other ligament of other finger at metacarpophalangeal and interphalangeal joint**
Traumatic rupture of ligament of specified finger with unspecified laterality at metacarpophalangeal and interphalangeal joint

√7ᵗʰ **S63.499** **Traumatic rupture of other ligament of unspecified finger at metacarpophalangeal and interphalangeal joint**

√5ᵗʰ **S63.5** **Other and unspecified** sprain of wrist

√6ᵗʰ **S63.50** **Unspecified sprain of wrist**

√7ᵗʰ **S63.501** **Unspecified sprain of** right **wrist**

√7ᵗʰ **S63.502** **Unspecified sprain of** left **wrist**

√7ᵗʰ **S63.509** **Unspecified sprain of unspecified wrist**

√6ᵗʰ **S63.51** **Sprain of** carpal **(joint)**

√7ᵗʰ **S63.511** **Sprain of carpal joint of** right **wrist**

√7ᵗʰ **S63.512** **Sprain of carpal joint of** left **wrist**

√7ᵗʰ **S63.519** **Sprain of carpal joint of unspecified wrist**

☑ Additional Character Required   √ₓ7ᵗʰ Placeholder   Unacceptable PDx   Questionable PDx   Manifestation   Unspecified Dx   H1-H14 HAC   HCC CMS-HCC Dx   HIV HIV Dx

ICD-10-CM 2021   1043

Chapter 19. Injury, Poisoning and Certain Other Consequences of External Causes

S63.52–S64.21

√6ᵗʰ **S63.52**   **Sprain of radiocarpal joint**
> **EXCLUDES 1**   *traumatic rupture of radiocarpal ligament (S63.32-)*

    √7ᵗʰ **S63.521**   **Sprain of radiocarpal joint of right wrist**

    √7ᵗʰ **S63.522**   **Sprain of radiocarpal joint of left wrist**

    √7ᵗʰ **S63.529**   **Sprain of radiocarpal joint of unspecified wrist**

√6ᵗʰ **S63.59**   **Other specified sprain of wrist**

    √7ᵗʰ **S63.591**   **Other specified sprain of right wrist**

    √7ᵗʰ **S63.592**   **Other specified sprain of left wrist**

    √7ᵗʰ **S63.599**   **Other specified sprain of unspecified wrist**

√5ᵗʰ **S63.6**   **Other and unspecified sprain of finger(s)**
> **EXCLUDES 1**   *traumatic rupture of ligament of finger at metacarpophalangeal and interphalangeal joint(s) (S63.4-)*

√6ᵗʰ **S63.60**   **Unspecified sprain of thumb**

    √7ᵗʰ **S63.601**   **Unspecified sprain of right thumb**

    √7ᵗʰ **S63.602**   **Unspecified sprain of left thumb**

    √7ᵗʰ **S63.609**   **Unspecified sprain of unspecified thumb**

√6ᵗʰ **S63.61**   **Unspecified sprain of other and unspecified finger(s)**

    √7ᵗʰ **S63.610**   **Unspecified sprain of right index finger**

    √7ᵗʰ **S63.611**   **Unspecified sprain of left index finger**

    √7ᵗʰ **S63.612**   **Unspecified sprain of right middle finger**

    √7ᵗʰ **S63.613**   **Unspecified sprain of left middle finger**

    √7ᵗʰ **S63.614**   **Unspecified sprain of right ring finger**

    √7ᵗʰ **S63.615**   **Unspecified sprain of left ring finger**

    √7ᵗʰ **S63.616**   **Unspecified sprain of right little finger**

    √7ᵗʰ **S63.617**   **Unspecified sprain of left little finger**

    √7ᵗʰ **S63.618**   **Unspecified sprain of other finger**
> Unspecified sprain of specified finger with unspecified laterality

    √7ᵗʰ **S63.619**   **Unspecified sprain of unspecified finger**

√6ᵗʰ **S63.62**   **Sprain of interphalangeal joint of thumb**

    √7ᵗʰ **S63.621**   **Sprain of interphalangeal joint of right thumb**

    √7ᵗʰ **S63.622**   **Sprain of interphalangeal joint of left thumb**

    √7ᵗʰ **S63.629**   **Sprain of interphalangeal joint of unspecified thumb**

√6ᵗʰ **S63.63**   **Sprain of interphalangeal joint of other and unspecified finger(s)**

    √7ᵗʰ **S63.630**   **Sprain of interphalangeal joint of right index finger**

    √7ᵗʰ **S63.631**   **Sprain of interphalangeal joint of left index finger**

    √7ᵗʰ **S63.632**   **Sprain of interphalangeal joint of right middle finger**

    √7ᵗʰ **S63.633**   **Sprain of interphalangeal joint of left middle finger**

    √7ᵗʰ **S63.634**   **Sprain of interphalangeal joint of right ring finger**

    √7ᵗʰ **S63.635**   **Sprain of interphalangeal joint of left ring finger**

    √7ᵗʰ **S63.636**   **Sprain of interphalangeal joint of right little finger**

    √7ᵗʰ **S63.637**   **Sprain of interphalangeal joint of left little finger**

    √7ᵗʰ **S63.638**   **Sprain of interphalangeal joint of other finger**

    √7ᵗʰ **S63.639**   **Sprain of interphalangeal joint of unspecified finger**

√6ᵗʰ **S63.64**   **Sprain of metacarpophalangeal joint of thumb**

    √7ᵗʰ **S63.641**   **Sprain of metacarpophalangeal joint of right thumb**

    √7ᵗʰ **S63.642**   **Sprain of metacarpophalangeal joint of left thumb**

    √7ᵗʰ **S63.649**   **Sprain of metacarpophalangeal joint of unspecified thumb**

√6ᵗʰ **S63.65**   **Sprain of metacarpophalangeal joint of other and unspecified finger(s)**

    √7ᵗʰ **S63.650**   **Sprain of metacarpophalangeal joint of right index finger**

    √7ᵗʰ **S63.651**   **Sprain of metacarpophalangeal joint of left index finger**

    √7ᵗʰ **S63.652**   **Sprain of metacarpophalangeal joint of right middle finger**

    √7ᵗʰ **S63.653**   **Sprain of metacarpophalangeal joint of left middle finger**

    √7ᵗʰ **S63.654**   **Sprain of metacarpophalangeal joint of right ring finger**

    √7ᵗʰ **S63.655**   **Sprain of metacarpophalangeal joint of left ring finger**

    √7ᵗʰ **S63.656**   **Sprain of metacarpophalangeal joint of right little finger**

    √7ᵗʰ **S63.657**   **Sprain of metacarpophalangeal joint of left little finger**

    √7ᵗʰ **S63.658**   **Sprain of metacarpophalangeal joint of other finger**
> Sprain of metacarpophalangeal joint of specified finger with unspecified laterality

    √7ᵗʰ **S63.659**   **Sprain of metacarpophalangeal joint of unspecified finger**

√6ᵗʰ **S63.68**   **Other sprain of thumb**

    √7ᵗʰ **S63.681**   **Other sprain of right thumb**

    √7ᵗʰ **S63.682**   **Other sprain of left thumb**

    √7ᵗʰ **S63.689**   **Other sprain of unspecified thumb**

√6ᵗʰ **S63.69**   **Other sprain of other and unspecified finger(s)**

    √7ᵗʰ **S63.690**   **Other sprain of right index finger**

    √7ᵗʰ **S63.691**   **Other sprain of left index finger**

    √7ᵗʰ **S63.692**   **Other sprain of right middle finger**

    √7ᵗʰ **S63.693**   **Other sprain of left middle finger**

    √7ᵗʰ **S63.694**   **Other sprain of right ring finger**

    √7ᵗʰ **S63.695**   **Other sprain of left ring finger**

    √7ᵗʰ **S63.696**   **Other sprain of right little finger**

    √7ᵗʰ **S63.697**   **Other sprain of left little finger**

    √7ᵗʰ **S63.698**   **Other sprain of other finger**
> Other sprain of specified finger with unspecified laterality

    √7ᵗʰ **S63.699**   **Other sprain of unspecified finger**

√5ᵗʰ **S63.8**   **Sprain of other part of wrist and hand**

√6ᵗʰ **S63.8X**   **Sprain of other part of wrist and hand**

    √7ᵗʰ **S63.8X1**   **Sprain of other part of right wrist and hand**

    √7ᵗʰ **S63.8X2**   **Sprain of other part of left wrist and hand**

    √7ᵗʰ **S63.8X9**   **Sprain of other part of unspecified wrist and hand**

√5ᵗʰ **S63.9**   **Sprain of unspecified part of wrist and hand**

    √×7ᵗʰ **S63.90**   **Sprain of unspecified part of unspecified wrist and hand**

    √×7ᵗʰ **S63.91**   **Sprain of unspecified part of right wrist and hand**

    √×7ᵗʰ **S63.92**   **Sprain of unspecified part of left wrist and hand**

√4ᵗʰ **S64**   **Injury of nerves at wrist and hand level**
> Code also any associated open wound (S61.-)

> The appropriate 7th character is to be added to each code from category S64.
> A   initial encounter
> D   subsequent encounter
> S   sequela

√5ᵗʰ **S64.0**   **Injury of ulnar nerve at wrist and hand level**

    √×7ᵗʰ **S64.00**   **Injury of ulnar nerve at wrist and hand level of unspecified arm**

    √×7ᵗʰ **S64.01**   **Injury of ulnar nerve at wrist and hand level of right arm**

    √×7ᵗʰ **S64.02**   **Injury of ulnar nerve at wrist and hand level of left arm**

√5ᵗʰ **S64.1**   **Injury of median nerve at wrist and hand level**

    √×7ᵗʰ **S64.10**   **Injury of median nerve at wrist and hand level of unspecified arm**

    √×7ᵗʰ **S64.11**   **Injury of median nerve at wrist and hand level of right arm**

    √×7ᵗʰ **S64.12**   **Injury of median nerve at wrist and hand level of left arm**

√5ᵗʰ **S64.2**   **Injury of radial nerve at wrist and hand level**

    √×7ᵗʰ **S64.20**   **Injury of radial nerve at wrist and hand level of unspecified arm**

    √×7ᵗʰ **S64.21**   **Injury of radial nerve at wrist and hand level of right arm**

ℕ Newborn: 0   ℙ Pediatric: 0-17   Ⅿ Maternity: 9-64   Ⓐ Adult: 15-124   **MCC** Major Complication/Comorbidity   **CC** Complication/Comorbidity   **SW** Severe Wound Dx

1044   ICD-10-CM 2021

√x7ᵗʰ **S64.22** Injury of radial nerve at wrist and hand level of left arm

√5ᵗʰ **S64.3** Injury of digital nerve of thumb

    √x7ᵗʰ **S64.30** Injury of digital nerve of unspecified thumb

    √x7ᵗʰ **S64.31** Injury of digital nerve of right thumb

    √x7ᵗʰ **S64.32** Injury of digital nerve of left thumb

√5ᵗʰ **S64.4** Injury of digital nerve of other and unspecified finger

    √x7ᵗʰ **S64.40** Injury of digital nerve of unspecified finger

    √6ᵗʰ **S64.49** Injury of digital nerve of other finger

        7ᵗʰ **S64.490** Injury of digital nerve of right index finger

        7ᵗʰ **S64.491** Injury of digital nerve of left index finger

        7ᵗʰ **S64.492** Injury of digital nerve of right middle finger

        7ᵗʰ **S64.493** Injury of digital nerve of left middle finger

        7ᵗʰ **S64.494** Injury of digital nerve of right ring finger

        7ᵗʰ **S64.495** Injury of digital nerve of left ring finger

        7ᵗʰ **S64.496** Injury of digital nerve of right little finger

        7ᵗʰ **S64.497** Injury of digital nerve of left little finger

        7ᵗʰ **S64.498** Injury of digital nerve of other finger

          Injury of digital nerve of specified finger with unspecified laterality

√5ᵗʰ **S64.8** Injury of other nerves at wrist and hand level

    √6ᵗʰ **S64.8X** Injury of other nerves at wrist and hand level

        7ᵗʰ **S64.8X1** Injury of other nerves at wrist and hand level of right arm

        7ᵗʰ **S64.8X2** Injury of other nerves at wrist and hand level of left arm

        7ᵗʰ **S64.8X9** Injury of other nerves at wrist and hand level of unspecified arm

√5ᵗʰ **S64.9** Injury of unspecified nerve at wrist and hand level

    √x7ᵗʰ **S64.90** Injury of unspecified nerve at wrist and hand level of unspecified arm

    √x7ᵗʰ **S64.91** Injury of unspecified nerve at wrist and hand level of right arm

    √x7ᵗʰ **S64.92** Injury of unspecified nerve at wrist and hand level of left arm

√4ᵗʰ **S65** Injury of blood vessels at wrist and hand level

    Code also any associated open wound (S61.-)

> The appropriate 7th character is to be added to each code from category S65.
> A   initial encounter
> D subsequent encounter
> S   sequela

√5ᵗʰ **S65.0** Injury of ulnar artery at wrist and hand level

    √6ᵗʰ **S65.00** Unspecified injury of ulnar artery at wrist and hand level

        7ᵗʰ **S65.001** Unspecified injury of ulnar artery at wrist and hand level of right arm CC

        7ᵗʰ **S65.002** Unspecified injury of ulnar artery at wrist and hand level of left arm CC

        7ᵗʰ **S65.009** Unspecified injury of ulnar artery at wrist and hand level of unspecified arm CC

    √6ᵗʰ **S65.01** Laceration of ulnar artery at wrist and hand level

        7ᵗʰ **S65.011** Laceration of ulnar artery at wrist and hand level of right arm CC

        7ᵗʰ **S65.012** Laceration of ulnar artery at wrist and hand level of left arm CC

        7ᵗʰ **S65.019** Laceration of ulnar artery at wrist and hand level of unspecified arm CC

    √6ᵗʰ **S65.09** Other specified injury of ulnar artery at wrist and hand level

        7ᵗʰ **S65.091** Other specified injury of ulnar artery at wrist and hand level of right arm CC

        7ᵗʰ **S65.092** Other specified injury of ulnar artery at wrist and hand level of left arm CC

        7ᵗʰ **S65.099** Other specified injury of ulnar artery at wrist and hand level of unspecified arm CC

√5ᵗʰ **S65.1** Injury of radial artery at wrist and hand level

    √6ᵗʰ **S65.10** Unspecified injury of radial artery at wrist and hand level

        7ᵗʰ **S65.101** Unspecified injury of radial artery at wrist and hand level of right arm CC

        7ᵗʰ **S65.102** Unspecified injury of radial artery at wrist and hand level of left arm CC

        7ᵗʰ **S65.109** Unspecified injury of radial artery at wrist and hand level of unspecified arm CC

    √6ᵗʰ **S65.11** Laceration of radial artery at wrist and hand level

        7ᵗʰ **S65.111** Laceration of radial artery at wrist and hand level of right arm

        7ᵗʰ **S65.112** Laceration of radial artery at wrist and hand level of left arm

        7ᵗʰ **S65.119** Laceration of radial artery at wrist and hand level of unspecified arm

    √6ᵗʰ **S65.19** Other specified injury of radial artery at wrist and hand level

        7ᵗʰ **S65.191** Other specified injury of radial artery at wrist and hand level of right arm CC

        7ᵗʰ **S65.192** Other specified injury of radial artery at wrist and hand level of left arm CC

        7ᵗʰ **S65.199** Other specified injury of radial artery at wrist and hand level of unspecified arm CC

√5ᵗʰ **S65.2** Injury of superficial palmar arch

    √6ᵗʰ **S65.20** Unspecified injury of superficial palmar arch

        7ᵗʰ **S65.201** Unspecified injury of superficial palmar arch of right hand CC

        7ᵗʰ **S65.202** Unspecified injury of superficial palmar arch of left hand CC

        7ᵗʰ **S65.209** Unspecified injury of superficial palmar arch of unspecified hand CC

    √6ᵗʰ **S65.21** Laceration of superficial palmar arch

        7ᵗʰ **S65.211** Laceration of superficial palmar arch of right hand CC

        7ᵗʰ **S65.212** Laceration of superficial palmar arch of left hand CC

        7ᵗʰ **S65.219** Laceration of superficial palmar arch of unspecified hand CC

    √6ᵗʰ **S65.29** Other specified injury of superficial palmar arch

        7ᵗʰ **S65.291** Other specified injury of superficial palmar arch of right hand CC

        7ᵗʰ **S65.292** Other specified injury of superficial palmar arch of left hand CC

        7ᵗʰ **S65.299** Other specified injury of superficial palmar arch of unspecified hand CC

√5ᵗʰ **S65.3** Injury of deep palmar arch

    √6ᵗʰ **S65.30** Unspecified injury of deep palmar arch

        7ᵗʰ **S65.301** Unspecified injury of deep palmar arch of right hand CC

        7ᵗʰ **S65.302** Unspecified injury of deep palmar arch of left hand CC

        7ᵗʰ **S65.309** Unspecified injury of deep palmar arch of unspecified hand CC

    √6ᵗʰ **S65.31** Laceration of deep palmar arch

        7ᵗʰ **S65.311** Laceration of deep palmar arch of right hand CC

        7ᵗʰ **S65.312** Laceration of deep palmar arch of left hand CC

        7ᵗʰ **S65.319** Laceration of deep palmar arch of unspecified hand CC

    √6ᵗʰ **S65.39** Other specified injury of deep palmar arch

        7ᵗʰ **S65.391** Other specified injury of deep palmar arch of right hand CC

        7ᵗʰ **S65.392** Other specified injury of deep palmar arch of left hand CC

        7ᵗʰ **S65.399** Other specified injury of deep palmar arch of unspecified hand CC

√5ᵗʰ **S65.4** Injury of blood vessel of thumb

    √6ᵗʰ **S65.40** Unspecified injury of blood vessel of thumb

        7ᵗʰ **S65.401** Unspecified injury of blood vessel of right thumb CC

        7ᵗʰ **S65.402** Unspecified injury of blood vessel of left thumb CC

        7ᵗʰ **S65.409** Unspecified injury of blood vessel of unspecified thumb CC

    √6ᵗʰ **S65.41** Laceration of blood vessel of thumb

        7ᵗʰ **S65.411** Laceration of blood vessel of right thumb CC

        7ᵗʰ **S65.412** Laceration of blood vessel of left thumb CC

✔ Additional Character Required   √x7ᵗʰ Placeholder   Unacceptable PDx   Questionable PDx   Manifestation   Unspecified Dx   H1-H14 HAC   HCC CMS-HCC Dx   HIV HIV Dx

✓7ᵗʰ **S65.419** Laceration of blood vessel of unspecified thumb   cc

✓6ᵗʰ **S65.49** Other specified injury of blood vessel of thumb

     ✓7ᵗʰ **S65.491** Other specified injury of blood vessel of right thumb   cc

     ✓7ᵗʰ **S65.492** Other specified injury of blood vessel of left thumb   cc

     ✓7ᵗʰ **S65.499** Other specified injury of blood vessel of unspecified thumb   cc

✓5ᵗʰ **S65.5** Injury of blood vessel of other and unspecified finger

     ✓6ᵗʰ **S65.50** Unspecified injury of blood vessel of other and unspecified finger

         ✓7ᵗʰ **S65.500** Unspecified injury of blood vessel of right index finger   cc

         ✓7ᵗʰ **S65.501** Unspecified injury of blood vessel of left index finger   cc

         ✓7ᵗʰ **S65.502** Unspecified injury of blood vessel of right middle finger   cc

         ✓7ᵗʰ **S65.503** Unspecified injury of blood vessel of left middle finger   cc

         ✓7ᵗʰ **S65.504** Unspecified injury of blood vessel of right ring finger   cc

         ✓7ᵗʰ **S65.505** Unspecified injury of blood vessel of left ring finger   cc

         ✓7ᵗʰ **S65.506** Unspecified injury of blood vessel of right little finger   cc

         ✓7ᵗʰ **S65.507** Unspecified injury of blood vessel of left little finger   cc

         ✓7ᵗʰ **S65.508** Unspecified injury of blood vessel of other finger   cc
            Unspecified injury of blood vessel of specified finger with unspecified laterality

         ✓7ᵗʰ **S65.509** Unspecified injury of blood vessel of unspecified finger   cc

     ✓6ᵗʰ **S65.51** Laceration of blood vessel of other and unspecified finger

         ✓7ᵗʰ **S65.510** Laceration of blood vessel of right index finger   cc

         ✓7ᵗʰ **S65.511** Laceration of blood vessel of left index finger   cc

         ✓7ᵗʰ **S65.512** Laceration of blood vessel of right middle finger   cc

         ✓7ᵗʰ **S65.513** Laceration of blood vessel of left middle finger   cc

         ✓7ᵗʰ **S65.514** Laceration of blood vessel of right ring finger   cc

         ✓7ᵗʰ **S65.515** Laceration of blood vessel of left ring finger   cc

         ✓7ᵗʰ **S65.516** Laceration of blood vessel of right little finger   cc

         ✓7ᵗʰ **S65.517** Laceration of blood vessel of left little finger   cc

         ✓7ᵗʰ **S65.518** Laceration of blood vessel of other finger   cc
            Laceration of blood vessel of specified finger with unspecified laterality

         ✓7ᵗʰ **S65.519** Laceration of blood vessel of unspecified finger   cc

     ✓6ᵗʰ **S65.59** Other specified injury of blood vessel of other and unspecified finger

         ✓7ᵗʰ **S65.590** Other specified injury of blood vessel of right index finger   cc

         ✓7ᵗʰ **S65.591** Other specified injury of blood vessel of left index finger   cc

         ✓7ᵗʰ **S65.592** Other specified injury of blood vessel of right middle finger   cc

         ✓7ᵗʰ **S65.593** Other specified injury of blood vessel of left middle finger   cc

         ✓7ᵗʰ **S65.594** Other specified injury of blood vessel of right ring finger   cc

         ✓7ᵗʰ **S65.595** Other specified injury of blood vessel of left ring finger   cc

         ✓7ᵗʰ **S65.596** Other specified injury of blood vessel of right little finger   cc

         ✓7ᵗʰ **S65.597** Other specified injury of blood vessel of left little finger   cc

         ✓7ᵗʰ **S65.598** Other specified injury of blood vessel of other finger   cc
            Other specified injury of blood vessel of specified finger with unspecified laterality

         ✓7ᵗʰ **S65.599** Other specified injury of blood vessel of unspecified finger   cc

✓5ᵗʰ **S65.8** Injury of other blood vessels at wrist and hand level

     ✓6ᵗʰ **S65.80** Unspecified injury of other blood vessels at wrist and hand level

         ✓7ᵗʰ **S65.801** Unspecified injury of other blood vessels at wrist and hand level of right arm   cc

         ✓7ᵗʰ **S65.802** Unspecified injury of other blood vessels at wrist and hand level of left arm   cc

         ✓7ᵗʰ **S65.809** Unspecified injury of other blood vessels at wrist and hand level of unspecified arm   cc

     ✓6ᵗʰ **S65.81** Laceration of other blood vessels at wrist and hand level

         ✓7ᵗʰ **S65.811** Laceration of other blood vessels at wrist and hand level of right arm   cc

         ✓7ᵗʰ **S65.812** Laceration of other blood vessels at wrist and hand level of left arm   cc

         ✓7ᵗʰ **S65.819** Laceration of other blood vessels at wrist and hand level of unspecified arm   cc

     ✓6ᵗʰ **S65.89** Other specified injury of other blood vessels at wrist and hand level

         ✓7ᵗʰ **S65.891** Other specified injury of other blood vessels at wrist and hand level of right arm   cc

         ✓7ᵗʰ **S65.892** Other specified injury of other blood vessels at wrist and hand level of left arm   cc

         ✓7ᵗʰ **S65.899** Other specified injury of other blood vessels at wrist and hand level of unspecified arm   cc

✓5ᵗʰ **S65.9** Injury of unspecified blood vessel at wrist and hand level

     ✓6ᵗʰ **S65.90** Unspecified injury of unspecified blood vessel at wrist and hand level

         ✓7ᵗʰ **S65.901** Unspecified injury of unspecified blood vessel at wrist and hand level of right arm   cc

         ✓7ᵗʰ **S65.902** Unspecified injury of unspecified blood vessel at wrist and hand level of left arm   cc

         ✓7ᵗʰ **S65.909** Unspecified injury of unspecified blood vessel at wrist and hand level of unspecified arm   cc

     ✓6ᵗʰ **S65.91** Laceration of unspecified blood vessel at wrist and hand level

         ✓7ᵗʰ **S65.911** Laceration of unspecified blood vessel at wrist and hand level of right arm   cc

         ✓7ᵗʰ **S65.912** Laceration of unspecified blood vessel at wrist and hand level of left arm   cc

         ✓7ᵗʰ **S65.919** Laceration of unspecified blood vessel at wrist and hand level of unspecified arm   cc

     ✓6ᵗʰ **S65.99** Other specified injury of unspecified blood vessel at wrist and hand level

         ✓7ᵗʰ **S65.991** Other specified injury of unspecified blood vessel at wrist and hand of right arm   cc

         ✓7ᵗʰ **S65.992** Other specified injury of unspecified blood vessel at wrist and hand of left arm   cc

         ✓7ᵗʰ **S65.999** Other specified injury of unspecified blood vessel at wrist and hand of unspecified arm   cc

N Newborn: 0   **P** Pediatric: 0-17   **M** Maternity: 9-64   **A** Adult: 15-124   **MCC** Major Complication/Comorbidity   **CC** Complication/Comorbidity   **SW** Severe Wound Dx

1046   ICD-10-CM 2021

✓4ᵗʰ **S66** **Injury of muscle, fascia and tendon at wrist and hand level**

Code also any associated open wound (S61.-)

EXCLUDES 2   *sprain of joints and ligaments of wrist and hand (S63.-)*

TIP: Refer to the Muscle/Tendon table at the beginning of this chapter.

The appropriate 7th character is to be added to each code from category S66.
A   initial encounter
D   subsequent encounter
S   sequela

✓5ᵗʰ **S66.0** **Injury of long flexor muscle, fascia and tendon of thumb at wrist and hand level**

✓6ᵗʰ **S66.00** **Unspecified injury of long flexor muscle, fascia and tendon of thumb at wrist and hand level**

✓7ᵗʰ **S66.001** **Unspecified injury of long flexor muscle, fascia and tendon of right thumb at wrist and hand level**

✓7ᵗʰ **S66.002** **Unspecified injury of long flexor muscle, fascia and tendon of left thumb at wrist and hand level**

✓7ᵗʰ **S66.009** **Unspecified injury of long flexor muscle, fascia and tendon of unspecified thumb at wrist and hand level**

✓6ᵗʰ **S66.01** **Strain of long flexor muscle, fascia and tendon of thumb at wrist and hand level**

✓7ᵗʰ **S66.011** **Strain of long flexor muscle, fascia and tendon of right thumb at wrist and hand level**

✓7ᵗʰ **S66.012** **Strain of long flexor muscle, fascia and tendon of left thumb at wrist and hand level**

✓7ᵗʰ **S66.019** **Strain of long flexor muscle, fascia and tendon of unspecified thumb at wrist and hand level**

✓6ᵗʰ **S66.02** **Laceration of long flexor muscle, fascia and tendon of thumb at wrist and hand level**

✓7ᵗʰ **S66.021** **Laceration of long flexor muscle, fascia and tendon of right thumb at wrist and hand level**   CC

✓7ᵗʰ **S66.022** **Laceration of long flexor muscle, fascia and tendon of left thumb at wrist and hand level**   CC

✓7ᵗʰ **S66.029** **Laceration of long flexor muscle, fascia and tendon of unspecified thumb at wrist and hand level**   CC

✓6ᵗʰ **S66.09** **Other specified injury of long flexor muscle, fascia and tendon of thumb at wrist and hand level**

✓7ᵗʰ **S66.091** **Other specified injury of long flexor muscle, fascia and tendon of right thumb at wrist and hand level**

✓7ᵗʰ **S66.092** **Other specified injury of long flexor muscle, fascia and tendon of left thumb at wrist and hand level**

✓7ᵗʰ **S66.099** **Other specified injury of long flexor muscle, fascia and tendon of unspecified thumb at wrist and hand level**

✓5ᵗʰ **S66.1** **Injury of flexor muscle, fascia and tendon of other and unspecified finger at wrist and hand level**

EXCLUDES 2   *injury of long flexor muscle, fascia and tendon of thumb at wrist and hand level (S66.0-)*

✓6ᵗʰ **S66.10** **Unspecified injury of flexor muscle, fascia and tendon of other and unspecified finger at wrist and hand level**

✓7ᵗʰ **S66.100** **Unspecified injury of flexor muscle, fascia and tendon of right index finger at wrist and hand level**

✓7ᵗʰ **S66.101** **Unspecified injury of flexor muscle, fascia and tendon of left index finger at wrist and hand level**

✓7ᵗʰ **S66.102** **Unspecified injury of flexor muscle, fascia and tendon of right middle finger at wrist and hand level**

✓7ᵗʰ **S66.103** **Unspecified injury of flexor muscle, fascia and tendon of left middle finger at wrist and hand level**

✓7ᵗʰ **S66.104** **Unspecified injury of flexor muscle, fascia and tendon of right ring finger at wrist and hand level**

✓7ᵗʰ **S66.105** **Unspecified injury of flexor muscle, fascia and tendon of left ring finger at wrist and hand level**

✓7ᵗʰ **S66.106** **Unspecified injury of flexor muscle, fascia and tendon of right little finger at wrist and hand level**

✓7ᵗʰ **S66.107** **Unspecified injury of flexor muscle, fascia and tendon of left little finger at wrist and hand level**

✓7ᵗʰ **S66.108** **Unspecified injury of flexor muscle, fascia and tendon of other finger at wrist and hand level**

Unspecified injury of flexor muscle, fascia and tendon of specified finger with unspecified laterality at wrist and hand level

✓7ᵗʰ **S66.109** **Unspecified injury of flexor muscle, fascia and tendon of unspecified finger at wrist and hand level**

✓6ᵗʰ **S66.11** **Strain of flexor muscle, fascia and tendon of other and unspecified finger at wrist and hand level**

✓7ᵗʰ **S66.110** **Strain of flexor muscle, fascia and tendon of right index finger at wrist and hand level**

✓7ᵗʰ **S66.111** **Strain of flexor muscle, fascia and tendon of left index finger at wrist and hand level**

✓7ᵗʰ **S66.112** **Strain of flexor muscle, fascia and tendon of right middle finger at wrist and hand level**

✓7ᵗʰ **S66.113** **Strain of flexor muscle, fascia and tendon of left middle finger at wrist and hand level**

✓7ᵗʰ **S66.114** **Strain of flexor muscle, fascia and tendon of right ring finger at wrist and hand level**

✓7ᵗʰ **S66.115** **Strain of flexor muscle, fascia and tendon of left ring finger at wrist and hand level**

✓7ᵗʰ **S66.116** **Strain of flexor muscle, fascia and tendon of right little finger at wrist and hand level**

✓7ᵗʰ **S66.117** **Strain of flexor muscle, fascia and tendon of left little finger at wrist and hand level**

✓7ᵗʰ **S66.118** **Strain of flexor muscle, fascia and tendon of other finger at wrist and hand level**

Strain of flexor muscle, fascia and tendon of specified finger with unspecified laterality at wrist and hand level

✓7ᵗʰ **S66.119** **Strain of flexor muscle, fascia and tendon of unspecified finger at wrist and hand level**

✓6ᵗʰ **S66.12** **Laceration of flexor muscle, fascia and tendon of other and unspecified finger at wrist and hand level**

✓7ᵗʰ **S66.120** **Laceration of flexor muscle, fascia and tendon of right index finger at wrist and hand level**   CC

✓7ᵗʰ **S66.121** **Laceration of flexor muscle, fascia and tendon of left index finger at wrist and hand level**   CC

✓7ᵗʰ **S66.122** **Laceration of flexor muscle, fascia and tendon of right middle finger at wrist and hand level**   CC

✓7ᵗʰ **S66.123** **Laceration of flexor muscle, fascia and tendon of left middle finger at wrist and hand level**   CC

✓7ᵗʰ **S66.124** **Laceration of flexor muscle, fascia and tendon of right ring finger at wrist and hand level**   CC

✓7ᵗʰ **S66.125** **Laceration of flexor muscle, fascia and tendon of left ring finger at wrist and hand level**   CC

✓7ᵗʰ **S66.126** **Laceration of flexor muscle, fascia and tendon of right little finger at wrist and hand level**   CC

✓7ᵗʰ **S66.127** **Laceration of flexor muscle, fascia and tendon of left little finger at wrist and hand level**   CC

✓7ᵗʰ **S66.128** **Laceration of flexor muscle, fascia and tendon of other finger at wrist and hand level**   CC

Laceration of flexor muscle, fascia and tendon of specified finger with unspecified laterality at wrist and hand level

✓7ᵗʰ **S66.129** **Laceration of flexor muscle, fascia and tendon of unspecified finger at wrist and hand level**   CC

√6ᵗʰ **S66.19** **Other injury of flexor muscle, fascia and tendon of other and unspecified finger at wrist and hand level**

√7ᵗʰ **S66.190** Other injury of flexor muscle, fascia and tendon of right index finger at wrist and hand level

√7ᵗʰ **S66.191** Other injury of flexor muscle, fascia and tendon of left index finger at wrist and hand level

√7ᵗʰ **S66.192** Other injury of flexor muscle, fascia and tendon of right middle finger at wrist and hand level

√7ᵗʰ **S66.193** Other injury of flexor muscle, fascia and tendon of left middle finger at wrist and hand level

√7ᵗʰ **S66.194** Other injury of flexor muscle, fascia and tendon of right ring finger at wrist and hand level

√7ᵗʰ **S66.195** Other injury of flexor muscle, fascia and tendon of left ring finger at wrist and hand level

√7ᵗʰ **S66.196** Other injury of flexor muscle, fascia and tendon of right little finger at wrist and hand level

√7ᵗʰ **S66.197** Other injury of flexor muscle, fascia and tendon of left little finger at wrist and hand level

√7ᵗʰ **S66.198** Other injury of flexor muscle, fascia and tendon of other finger at wrist and hand level

Other injury of flexor muscle, fascia and tendon of specified finger with unspecified laterality at wrist and hand level

√7ᵗʰ **S66.199** Other injury of flexor muscle, fascia and tendon of unspecified finger at wrist and hand level

√5ᵗʰ **S66.2** **Injury of extensor muscle, fascia and tendon of thumb at wrist and hand level**

√6ᵗʰ **S66.20** **Unspecified injury of extensor muscle, fascia and tendon of thumb at wrist and hand level**

√7ᵗʰ **S66.201** Unspecified injury of extensor muscle, fascia and tendon of right thumb at wrist and hand level

√7ᵗʰ **S66.202** Unspecified injury of extensor muscle, fascia and tendon of left thumb at wrist and hand level

√7ᵗʰ **S66.209** Unspecified injury of extensor muscle, fascia and tendon of unspecified thumb at wrist and hand level

√6ᵗʰ **S66.21** **Strain of extensor muscle, fascia and tendon of thumb at wrist and hand level**

√7ᵗʰ **S66.211** Strain of extensor muscle, fascia and tendon of right thumb at wrist and hand level

√7ᵗʰ **S66.212** Strain of extensor muscle, fascia and tendon of left thumb at wrist and hand level

√7ᵗʰ **S66.219** Strain of extensor muscle, fascia and tendon of unspecified thumb at wrist and hand level

√6ᵗʰ **S66.22** **Laceration of extensor muscle, fascia and tendon of thumb at wrist and hand level**

√7ᵗʰ **S66.221** Laceration of extensor muscle, fascia and tendon of right thumb at wrist and hand level `cc`

√7ᵗʰ **S66.222** Laceration of extensor muscle, fascia and tendon of left thumb at wrist and hand level `cc`

√7ᵗʰ **S66.229** Laceration of extensor muscle, fascia and tendon of unspecified thumb at wrist and hand level `cc`

√6ᵗʰ **S66.29** **Other specified injury of extensor muscle, fascia and tendon of thumb at wrist and hand level**

√7ᵗʰ **S66.291** Other specified injury of extensor muscle, fascia and tendon of right thumb at wrist and hand level

√7ᵗʰ **S66.292** Other specified injury of extensor muscle, fascia and tendon of left thumb at wrist and hand level

√7ᵗʰ **S66.299** Other specified injury of extensor muscle, fascia and tendon of unspecified thumb at wrist and hand level

√5ᵗʰ **S66.3** **Injury of extensor muscle, fascia and tendon of other and unspecified finger at wrist and hand level**

EXCLUDES 2 *injury of extensor muscle, fascia and tendon of thumb at wrist and hand level (S66.2-)*

√6ᵗʰ **S66.30** **Unspecified injury of extensor muscle, fascia and tendon of other and unspecified finger at wrist and hand level**

√7ᵗʰ **S66.300** Unspecified injury of extensor muscle, fascia and tendon of right index finger at wrist and hand level

√7ᵗʰ **S66.301** Unspecified injury of extensor muscle, fascia and tendon of left index finger at wrist and hand level

√7ᵗʰ **S66.302** Unspecified injury of extensor muscle, fascia and tendon of right middle finger at wrist and hand level

√7ᵗʰ **S66.303** Unspecified injury of extensor muscle, fascia and tendon of left middle finger at wrist and hand level

√7ᵗʰ **S66.304** Unspecified injury of extensor muscle, fascia and tendon of right ring finger at wrist and hand level

√7ᵗʰ **S66.305** Unspecified injury of extensor muscle, fascia and tendon of left ring finger at wrist and hand level

√7ᵗʰ **S66.306** Unspecified injury of extensor muscle, fascia and tendon of right little finger at wrist and hand level

√7ᵗʰ **S66.307** Unspecified injury of extensor muscle, fascia and tendon of left little finger at wrist and hand level

√7ᵗʰ **S66.308** Unspecified injury of extensor muscle, fascia and tendon of other finger at wrist and hand level

Unspecified injury of extensor muscle, fascia and tendon of specified finger with unspecified laterality at wrist and hand level

√7ᵗʰ **S66.309** Unspecified injury of extensor muscle, fascia and tendon of unspecified finger at wrist and hand level

√6ᵗʰ **S66.31** **Strain of extensor muscle, fascia and tendon of other and unspecified finger at wrist and hand level**

√7ᵗʰ **S66.310** Strain of extensor muscle, fascia and tendon of right index finger at wrist and hand level

√7ᵗʰ **S66.311** Strain of extensor muscle, fascia and tendon of left index finger at wrist and hand level

√7ᵗʰ **S66.312** Strain of extensor muscle, fascia and tendon of right middle finger at wrist and hand level

√7ᵗʰ **S66.313** Strain of extensor muscle, fascia and tendon of left middle finger at wrist and hand level

√7ᵗʰ **S66.314** Strain of extensor muscle, fascia and tendon of right ring finger at wrist and hand level

√7ᵗʰ **S66.315** Strain of extensor muscle, fascia and tendon of left ring finger at wrist and hand level

√7ᵗʰ **S66.316** Strain of extensor muscle, fascia and tendon of right little finger at wrist and hand level

√7ᵗʰ **S66.317** Strain of extensor muscle, fascia and tendon of left little finger at wrist and hand level

√7ᵗʰ **S66.318** Strain of extensor muscle, fascia and tendon of other finger at wrist and hand level

Strain of extensor muscle, fascia and tendon of specified finger with unspecified laterality at wrist and hand level

√7ᵗʰ **S66.319** Strain of extensor muscle, fascia and tendon of unspecified finger at wrist and hand level

√6ᵗʰ **S66.32** **Laceration of extensor muscle, fascia and tendon of other and unspecified finger at wrist and hand level**

√7ᵗʰ **S66.320** Laceration of extensor muscle, fascia and tendon of right index finger at wrist and hand level `cc`

N Newborn: 0   P Pediatric: 0-17   M Maternity: 9-64   A Adult: 15-124   MCC Major Complication/Comorbidity   CC Complication/Comorbidity   SW Severe Wound Dx

1048   ICD-10-CM 2021

√7ᵗʰ **S66.321** Laceration of extensor muscle, fascia and tendon of left index finger at wrist and hand level   cc

√7ᵗʰ **S66.322** Laceration of extensor muscle, fascia and tendon of right middle finger at wrist and hand level   cc

√7ᵗʰ **S66.323** Laceration of extensor muscle, fascia and tendon of left middle finger at wrist and hand level   cc

√7ᵗʰ **S66.324** Laceration of extensor muscle, fascia and tendon of right ring finger at wrist and hand level   cc

√7ᵗʰ **S66.325** Laceration of extensor muscle, fascia and tendon of left ring finger at wrist and hand level   cc

√7ᵗʰ **S66.326** Laceration of extensor muscle, fascia and tendon of right little finger at wrist and hand level   cc

√7ᵗʰ **S66.327** Laceration of extensor muscle, fascia and tendon of left little finger at wrist and hand level   cc

√7ᵗʰ **S66.328** Laceration of extensor muscle, fascia and tendon of other finger at wrist and hand level   cc

Laceration of extensor muscle, fascia and tendon of specified finger with unspecified laterality at wrist and hand level

√7ᵗʰ **S66.329** Laceration of extensor muscle, fascia and tendon of unspecified finger at wrist and hand level   cc

√6ᵗʰ **S66.39** Other injury of extensor muscle, fascia and tendon of other and unspecified finger at wrist and hand level

√7ᵗʰ **S66.390** Other injury of extensor muscle, fascia and tendon of right index finger at wrist and hand level

√7ᵗʰ **S66.391** Other injury of extensor muscle, fascia and tendon of left index finger at wrist and hand level

√7ᵗʰ **S66.392** Other injury of extensor muscle, fascia and tendon of right middle finger at wrist and hand level

√7ᵗʰ **S66.393** Other injury of extensor muscle, fascia and tendon of left middle finger at wrist and hand level

√7ᵗʰ **S66.394** Other injury of extensor muscle, fascia and tendon of right ring finger at wrist and hand level

√7ᵗʰ **S66.395** Other injury of extensor muscle, fascia and tendon of left ring finger at wrist and hand level

√7ᵗʰ **S66.396** Other injury of extensor muscle, fascia and tendon of right little finger at wrist and hand level

√7ᵗʰ **S66.397** Other injury of extensor muscle, fascia and tendon of left little finger at wrist and hand level

√7ᵗʰ **S66.398** Other injury of extensor muscle, fascia and tendon of other finger at wrist and hand level

Other injury of extensor muscle, fascia and tendon of specified finger with unspecified laterality at wrist and hand level

√7ᵗʰ **S66.399** Other injury of extensor muscle, fascia and tendon of unspecified finger at wrist and hand level

√5ᵗʰ **S66.4** Injury of intrinsic muscle, fascia and tendon of thumb at wrist and hand level

√6ᵗʰ **S66.40** Unspecified injury of intrinsic muscle, fascia and tendon of thumb at wrist and hand level

√7ᵗʰ **S66.401** Unspecified injury of intrinsic muscle, fascia and tendon of right thumb at wrist and hand level

√7ᵗʰ **S66.402** Unspecified injury of intrinsic muscle, fascia and tendon of left thumb at wrist and hand level

√7ᵗʰ **S66.409** Unspecified injury of intrinsic muscle, fascia and tendon of unspecified thumb at wrist and hand level

√6ᵗʰ **S66.41** Strain of intrinsic muscle, fascia and tendon of thumb at wrist and hand level

√7ᵗʰ **S66.411** Strain of intrinsic muscle, fascia and tendon of right thumb at wrist and hand level

√7ᵗʰ **S66.412** Strain of intrinsic muscle, fascia and tendon of left thumb at wrist and hand level

√7ᵗʰ **S66.419** Strain of intrinsic muscle, fascia and tendon of unspecified thumb at wrist and hand level

√6ᵗʰ **S66.42** Laceration of intrinsic muscle, fascia and tendon of thumb at wrist and hand level

√7ᵗʰ **S66.421** Laceration of intrinsic muscle, fascia and tendon of right thumb at wrist and hand level   cc

√7ᵗʰ **S66.422** Laceration of intrinsic muscle, fascia and tendon of left thumb at wrist and hand level   cc

√7ᵗʰ **S66.429** Laceration of intrinsic muscle, fascia and tendon of unspecified thumb at wrist and hand level   cc

√6ᵗʰ **S66.49** Other specified injury of intrinsic muscle, fascia and tendon of thumb at wrist and hand level

√7ᵗʰ **S66.491** Other specified injury of intrinsic muscle, fascia and tendon of right thumb at wrist and hand level

√7ᵗʰ **S66.492** Other specified injury of intrinsic muscle, fascia and tendon of left thumb at wrist and hand level

√7ᵗʰ **S66.499** Other specified injury of intrinsic muscle, fascia and tendon of unspecified thumb at wrist and hand level

√5ᵗʰ **S66.5** Injury of intrinsic muscle, fascia and tendon of other and unspecified finger at wrist and hand level

EXCLUDES 2   injury of intrinsic muscle, fascia and tendon of thumb at wrist and hand level (S66.4-)

√6ᵗʰ **S66.50** Unspecified injury of intrinsic muscle, fascia and tendon of other and unspecified finger at wrist and hand level

√7ᵗʰ **S66.500** Unspecified injury of intrinsic muscle, fascia and tendon of right index finger at wrist and hand level

√7ᵗʰ **S66.501** Unspecified injury of intrinsic muscle, fascia and tendon of left index finger at wrist and hand level

√7ᵗʰ **S66.502** Unspecified injury of intrinsic muscle, fascia and tendon of right middle finger at wrist and hand level

√7ᵗʰ **S66.503** Unspecified injury of intrinsic muscle, fascia and tendon of left middle finger at wrist and hand level

√7ᵗʰ **S66.504** Unspecified injury of intrinsic muscle, fascia and tendon of right ring finger at wrist and hand level

√7ᵗʰ **S66.505** Unspecified injury of intrinsic muscle, fascia and tendon of left ring finger at wrist and hand level

√7ᵗʰ **S66.506** Unspecified injury of intrinsic muscle, fascia and tendon of right little finger at wrist and hand level

√7ᵗʰ **S66.507** Unspecified injury of intrinsic muscle, fascia and tendon of left little finger at wrist and hand level

√7ᵗʰ **S66.508** Unspecified injury of intrinsic muscle, fascia and tendon of other finger at wrist and hand level

Unspecified injury of intrinsic muscle, fascia and tendon of specified finger with unspecified laterality at wrist and hand level

√7ᵗʰ **S66.509** Unspecified injury of intrinsic muscle, fascia and tendon of unspecified finger at wrist and hand level

√6ᵗʰ **S66.51** Strain of intrinsic muscle, fascia and tendon of other and unspecified finger at wrist and hand level

√7ᵗʰ **S66.510** Strain of intrinsic muscle, fascia and tendon of right index finger at wrist and hand level

√7ᵗʰ **S66.511** Strain of intrinsic muscle, fascia and tendon of left index finger at wrist and hand level

√7ᵗʰ **S66.512** Strain of intrinsic muscle, fascia and tendon of right middle finger at wrist and hand level

√7ᵗʰ **S66.513** Strain of intrinsic muscle, fascia and tendon of left middle finger at wrist and hand level

√7ᵗʰ **S66.514** Strain of intrinsic muscle, fascia and tendon of right ring finger at wrist and hand level

√7ᵗʰ **S66.515** Strain of intrinsic muscle, fascia and tendon of left ring finger at wrist and hand level

√7ᵗʰ **S66.516** Strain of intrinsic muscle, fascia and tendon of right little finger at wrist and hand level

√7ᵗʰ **S66.517** Strain of intrinsic muscle, fascia and tendon of left little finger at wrist and hand level

√7ᵗʰ **S66.518** Strain of intrinsic muscle, fascia and tendon of other finger at wrist and hand level

Strain of intrinsic muscle, fascia and tendon of specified finger with unspecified laterality at wrist and hand level

√7ᵗʰ **S66.519** Strain of intrinsic muscle, fascia and tendon of unspecified finger at wrist and hand level

√6ᵗʰ **S66.52** Laceration of intrinsic muscle, fascia and tendon of other and unspecified finger at wrist and hand level

√7ᵗʰ **S66.520** Laceration of intrinsic muscle, fascia and tendon of right index finger at wrist and hand level   `CC`

√7ᵗʰ **S66.521** Laceration of intrinsic muscle, fascia and tendon of left index finger at wrist and hand level   `CC`

√7ᵗʰ **S66.522** Laceration of intrinsic muscle, fascia and tendon of right middle finger at wrist and hand level   `CC`

√7ᵗʰ **S66.523** Laceration of intrinsic muscle, fascia and tendon of left middle finger at wrist and hand level   `CC`

√7ᵗʰ **S66.524** Laceration of intrinsic muscle, fascia and tendon of right ring finger at wrist and hand level   `CC`

√7ᵗʰ **S66.525** Laceration of intrinsic muscle, fascia and tendon of left ring finger at wrist and hand level   `CC`

√7ᵗʰ **S66.526** Laceration of intrinsic muscle, fascia and tendon of right little finger at wrist and hand level   `CC`

√7ᵗʰ **S66.527** Laceration of intrinsic muscle, fascia and tendon of left little finger at wrist and hand level   `CC`

√7ᵗʰ **S66.528** Laceration of intrinsic muscle, fascia and tendon of other finger at wrist and hand level   `CC`

Laceration of intrinsic muscle, fascia and tendon of specified finger with unspecified laterality at wrist and hand level

√7ᵗʰ **S66.529** Laceration of intrinsic muscle, fascia and tendon of unspecified finger at wrist and hand level   `CC`

√6ᵗʰ **S66.59** Other injury of intrinsic muscle, fascia and tendon of other and unspecified finger at wrist and hand level

√7ᵗʰ **S66.590** Other injury of intrinsic muscle, fascia and tendon of right index finger at wrist and hand level

√7ᵗʰ **S66.591** Other injury of intrinsic muscle, fascia and tendon of left index finger at wrist and hand level

√7ᵗʰ **S66.592** Other injury of intrinsic muscle, fascia and tendon of right middle finger at wrist and hand level

√7ᵗʰ **S66.593** Other injury of intrinsic muscle, fascia and tendon of left middle finger at wrist and hand level

√7ᵗʰ **S66.594** Other injury of intrinsic muscle, fascia and tendon of right ring finger at wrist and hand level

√7ᵗʰ **S66.595** Other injury of intrinsic muscle, fascia and tendon of left ring finger at wrist and hand level

√7ᵗʰ **S66.596** Other injury of intrinsic muscle, fascia and tendon of right little finger at wrist and hand level

√7ᵗʰ **S66.597** Other injury of intrinsic muscle, fascia and tendon of left little finger at wrist and hand level

√7ᵗʰ **S66.598** Other injury of intrinsic muscle, fascia and tendon of other finger at wrist and hand level

Other injury of intrinsic muscle, fascia and tendon of specified finger with unspecified laterality at wrist and hand level

√7ᵗʰ **S66.599** Other injury of intrinsic muscle, fascia and tendon of unspecified finger at wrist and hand level

√5ᵗʰ **S66.8** Injury of other specified muscles, fascia and tendons at wrist and hand level

√6ᵗʰ **S66.80** Unspecified injury of other specified muscles, fascia and tendons at wrist and hand level

√7ᵗʰ **S66.801** Unspecified injury of other specified muscles, fascia and tendons at wrist and hand level, right hand

√7ᵗʰ **S66.802** Unspecified injury of other specified muscles, fascia and tendons at wrist and hand level, left hand

√7ᵗʰ **S66.809** Unspecified injury of other specified muscles, fascia and tendons at wrist and hand level, unspecified hand

√6ᵗʰ **S66.81** Strain of other specified muscles, fascia and tendons at wrist and hand level

√7ᵗʰ **S66.811** Strain of other specified muscles, fascia and tendons at wrist and hand level, right hand

√7ᵗʰ **S66.812** Strain of other specified muscles, fascia and tendons at wrist and hand level, left hand

√7ᵗʰ **S66.819** Strain of other specified muscles, fascia and tendons at wrist and hand level, unspecified hand

√6ᵗʰ **S66.82** Laceration of other specified muscles, fascia and tendons at wrist and hand level

√7ᵗʰ **S66.821** Laceration of other specified muscles, fascia and tendons at wrist and hand level, right hand   `CC`

√7ᵗʰ **S66.822** Laceration of other specified muscles, fascia and tendons at wrist and hand level, left hand   `CC`

√7ᵗʰ **S66.829** Laceration of other specified muscles, fascia and tendons at wrist and hand level, unspecified hand   `CC`

√6ᵗʰ **S66.89** Other injury of other specified muscles, fascia and tendons at wrist and hand level

√7ᵗʰ **S66.891** Other injury of other specified muscles, fascia and tendons at wrist and hand level, right hand

√7ᵗʰ **S66.892** Other injury of other specified muscles, fascia and tendons at wrist and hand level, left hand

√7ᵗʰ **S66.899** Other injury of other specified muscles, fascia and tendons at wrist and hand level, unspecified hand

√5ᵗʰ **S66.9** Injury of unspecified muscle, fascia and tendon at wrist and hand level

√6ᵗʰ **S66.90** Unspecified injury of unspecified muscle, fascia and tendon at wrist and hand level

√7ᵗʰ **S66.901** Unspecified injury of unspecified muscle, fascia and tendon at wrist and hand level, right hand

√7ᵗʰ **S66.902** Unspecified injury of unspecified muscle, fascia and tendon at wrist and hand level, left hand

√7ᵗʰ **S66.909** Unspecified injury of unspecified muscle, fascia and tendon at wrist and hand level, unspecified hand

√6ᵗʰ **S66.91** Strain of unspecified muscle, fascia and tendon at wrist and hand level

√7ᵗʰ **S66.911** Strain of unspecified muscle, fascia and tendon at wrist and hand level, right hand

√7ᵗʰ **S66.912** Strain of unspecified muscle, fascia and tendon at wrist and hand level, left hand

N Newborn: 0   **P** Pediatric: 0-17   **M** Maternity: 9-64   **A** Adult: 15-124   `MCC` Major Complication/Comorbidity   `CC` Complication/Comorbidity   `SW` Severe Wound Dx

1050   ICD-10-CM 2021

√7ᵗʰ **S66.919** Strain of unspecified muscle, fascia and tendon at wrist and hand level, unspecified hand

√6ᵗʰ **S66.92** Laceration of unspecified muscle, fascia and tendon at wrist and hand level

    √7ᵗʰ **S66.921** Laceration of unspecified muscle, fascia and tendon at wrist and hand level, right hand   CC

    √7ᵗʰ **S66.922** Laceration of unspecified muscle, fascia and tendon at wrist and hand level, left hand   CC

    √7ᵗʰ **S66.929** Laceration of unspecified muscle, fascia and tendon at wrist and hand level, unspecified hand   CC

√6ᵗʰ **S66.99** Other injury of unspecified muscle, fascia and tendon at wrist and hand level

    √7ᵗʰ **S66.991** Other injury of unspecified muscle, fascia and tendon at wrist and hand level, right hand

    √7ᵗʰ **S66.992** Other injury of unspecified muscle, fascia and tendon at wrist and hand level, left hand

    √7ᵗʰ **S66.999** Other injury of unspecified muscle, fascia and tendon at wrist and hand level, unspecified hand

√4ᵗʰ **S67** Crushing injury of wrist, hand and fingers

Use additional code for all associated injuries, such as:
  fracture of wrist and hand (S62.-)
  open wound of wrist and hand (S61.-)

The appropriate 7th character is to be added to each code from category S67.
  A   initial encounter
  D   subsequent encounter
  S   sequela

√5ᵗʰ **S67.0** Crushing injury of thumb

  √x7ᵗʰ **S67.00** Crushing injury of unspecified thumb

  √x7ᵗʰ **S67.01** Crushing injury of right thumb

  √x7ᵗʰ **S67.02** Crushing injury of left thumb

√5ᵗʰ **S67.1** Crushing injury of other and unspecified finger(s)

    EXCLUDES 2   crushing injury of thumb (S67.0-)

  √x7ᵗʰ **S67.10** Crushing injury of unspecified finger(s)

  √6ᵗʰ **S67.19** Crushing injury of other finger(s)

    √7ᵗʰ **S67.190** Crushing injury of right index finger

    √7ᵗʰ **S67.191** Crushing injury of left index finger

    √7ᵗʰ **S67.192** Crushing injury of right middle finger

    √7ᵗʰ **S67.193** Crushing injury of left middle finger

    √7ᵗʰ **S67.194** Crushing injury of right ring finger

    √7ᵗʰ **S67.195** Crushing injury of left ring finger

    √7ᵗʰ **S67.196** Crushing injury of right little finger

    √7ᵗʰ **S67.197** Crushing injury of left little finger

    √7ᵗʰ **S67.198** Crushing injury of other finger
      Crushing injury of specified finger with unspecified laterality

√5ᵗʰ **S67.2** Crushing injury of hand

    EXCLUDES 2   crushing injury of fingers (S67.1-)
        crushing injury of thumb (S67.0-)

  √x7ᵗʰ **S67.20** Crushing injury of unspecified hand

  √x7ᵗʰ **S67.21** Crushing injury of right hand

  √x7ᵗʰ **S67.22** Crushing injury of left hand

√5ᵗʰ **S67.3** Crushing injury of wrist

  √x7ᵗʰ **S67.30** Crushing injury of unspecified wrist

  √x7ᵗʰ **S67.31** Crushing injury of right wrist

  √x7ᵗʰ **S67.32** Crushing injury of left wrist

√5ᵗʰ **S67.4** Crushing injury of wrist and hand

    EXCLUDES 1   crushing injury of hand alone (S67.2-)
        crushing injury of wrist alone (S67.3-)
    EXCLUDES 2   crushing injury of fingers (S67.1-)
        crushing injury of thumb (S67.0-)

  √x7ᵗʰ **S67.40** Crushing injury of unspecified wrist and hand

  √x7ᵗʰ **S67.41** Crushing injury of right wrist and hand

  √x7ᵗʰ **S67.42** Crushing injury of left wrist and hand

√5ᵗʰ **S67.9** Crushing injury of unspecified part(s) of wrist, hand and fingers

  √x7ᵗʰ **S67.90** Crushing injury of unspecified part(s) of unspecified wrist, hand and fingers

  √x7ᵗʰ **S67.91** Crushing injury of unspecified part(s) of right wrist, hand and fingers

  √x7ᵗʰ **S67.92** Crushing injury of unspecified part(s) of left wrist, hand and fingers

√4ᵗʰ **S68** Traumatic amputation of wrist, hand and fingers

An amputation not identified as partial or complete should be coded to complete.

The appropriate 7th character is to be added to each code from category S68.
  A   initial encounter
  D   subsequent encounter
  S   sequela

√5ᵗʰ **S68.0** Traumatic metacarpophalangeal amputation of thumb
  Traumatic amputation of thumb NOS

  √6ᵗʰ **S68.01** Complete traumatic metacarpophalangeal amputation of thumb

    8 √7ᵗʰ **S68.011** Complete traumatic metacarpophalangeal amputation of right thumb   HCC

    8 √7ᵗʰ **S68.012** Complete traumatic metacarpophalangeal amputation of left thumb   HCC

    8 √7ᵗʰ **S68.019** Complete traumatic metacarpophalangeal amputation of unspecified thumb   HCC

  √6ᵗʰ **S68.02** Partial traumatic metacarpophalangeal amputation of thumb

    8 √7ᵗʰ **S68.021** Partial traumatic metacarpophalangeal amputation of right thumb   HCC

    8 √7ᵗʰ **S68.022** Partial traumatic metacarpophalangeal amputation of left thumb   HCC

    8 √7ᵗʰ **S68.029** Partial traumatic metacarpophalangeal amputation of unspecified thumb   HCC

√5ᵗʰ **S68.1** Traumatic metacarpophalangeal amputation of other and unspecified finger
  Traumatic amputation of finger NOS

    EXCLUDES 2   traumatic metacarpophalangeal amputation of thumb (S68.0-)

  √6ᵗʰ **S68.11** Complete traumatic metacarpophalangeal amputation of other and unspecified finger

    8 √7ᵗʰ **S68.110** Complete traumatic metacarpophalangeal amputation of right index finger   HCC

    8 √7ᵗʰ **S68.111** Complete traumatic metacarpophalangeal amputation of left index finger   HCC

    8 √7ᵗʰ **S68.112** Complete traumatic metacarpophalangeal amputation of right middle finger   HCC

    8 √7ᵗʰ **S68.113** Complete traumatic metacarpophalangeal amputation of left middle finger   HCC

    8 √7ᵗʰ **S68.114** Complete traumatic metacarpophalangeal amputation of right ring finger   HCC

    8 √7ᵗʰ **S68.115** Complete traumatic metacarpophalangeal amputation of left ring finger   HCC

    8 √7ᵗʰ **S68.116** Complete traumatic metacarpophalangeal amputation of right little finger   HCC

    8 √7ᵗʰ **S68.117** Complete traumatic metacarpophalangeal amputation of left little finger   HCC

    8 √7ᵗʰ **S68.118** Complete traumatic metacarpophalangeal amputation of other finger
      Complete traumatic metacarpophalangeal amputation of specified finger with unspecified laterality

    8 √7ᵗʰ **S68.119** Complete traumatic metacarpophalangeal amputation of unspecified finger   HCC

  √6ᵗʰ **S68.12** Partial traumatic metacarpophalangeal amputation of other and unspecified finger

    8 √7ᵗʰ **S68.120** Partial traumatic metacarpophalangeal amputation of right index finger   HCC

✔ Additional Character Required   √x7ᵗʰ Placeholder   Unacceptable PDx   Questionable PDx   Manifestation   Unspecified Dx   H1-H14 HAC   HCC CMS-HCC Dx   HIV HIV Dx

ICD-10-CM 2021   1051

Chapter 19. Injury, Poisoning and Certain Other Consequences of External Causes

S68.121–S69.92

8 √7ᵗʰ **S68.121 Partial traumatic metacarpophalangeal amputation of** left index **finger** HCC

8 √7ᵗʰ **S68.122 Partial traumatic metacarpophalangeal amputation of** right middle **finger** HCC

8 √7ᵗʰ **S68.123 Partial traumatic metacarpophalangeal amputation of** left middle **finger** HCC

8 √7ᵗʰ **S68.124 Partial traumatic metacarpophalangeal amputation of** right ring **finger** HCC

8 √7ᵗʰ **S68.125 Partial traumatic metacarpophalangeal amputation of** left ring **finger** HCC

8 √7ᵗʰ **S68.126 Partial traumatic metacarpophalangeal amputation of** right little **finger** HCC

8 √7ᵗʰ **S68.127 Partial traumatic metacarpophalangeal amputation of** left little **finger** HCC

8 √7ᵗʰ **S68.128 Partial traumatic metacarpophalangeal amputation of other finger** HCC

Partial traumatic metacarpophalangeal amputation of specified finger with unspecified laterality

8 √7ᵗʰ **S68.129 Partial traumatic metacarpophalangeal amputation of unspecified finger** HCC

√5ᵗʰ **S68.4 Traumatic amputation of** hand at wrist level

Traumatic amputation of hand NOS

Traumatic amputation of wrist

√6ᵗʰ **S68.41 Complete traumatic amputation of hand at wrist level**

7 √7ᵗʰ **S68.411 Complete traumatic amputation of** right **hand at wrist level** CC HCC

7 √7ᵗʰ **S68.412 Complete traumatic amputation of** left **hand at wrist level** CC HCC

7 √7ᵗʰ **S68.419 Complete traumatic amputation of unspecified hand at wrist level** CC HCC

√6ᵗʰ **S68.42 Partial traumatic amputation of hand at wrist level**

7 √7ᵗʰ **S68.421 Partial traumatic amputation of** right **hand at wrist level** CC HCC

7 √7ᵗʰ **S68.422 Partial traumatic amputation of** left **hand at wrist level** CC HCC

7 √7ᵗʰ **S68.429 Partial traumatic amputation of unspecified hand at wrist level** CC HCC

√5ᵗʰ **S68.5 Traumatic** transphalangeal **amputation of** thumb

Traumatic interphalangeal joint amputation of thumb

√6ᵗʰ **S68.51 Complete traumatic transphalangeal amputation of thumb**

8 √7ᵗʰ **S68.511 Complete traumatic transphalangeal amputation of** right **thumb** HCC

8 √7ᵗʰ **S68.512 Complete traumatic transphalangeal amputation of** left **thumb** HCC

8 √7ᵗʰ **S68.519 Complete traumatic transphalangeal amputation of unspecified thumb** HCC

√6ᵗʰ **S68.52 Partial traumatic transphalangeal amputation of thumb**

8 √7ᵗʰ **S68.521 Partial traumatic transphalangeal amputation of** right **thumb** HCC

8 √7ᵗʰ **S68.522 Partial traumatic transphalangeal amputation of** left **thumb** HCC

8 √7ᵗʰ **S68.529 Partial traumatic transphalangeal amputation of unspecified thumb** HCC

√5ᵗʰ **S68.6 Traumatic** transphalangeal **amputation of other and unspecified finger**

√6ᵗʰ **S68.61 Complete traumatic transphalangeal amputation of other and unspecified finger(s)**

8 √7ᵗʰ **S68.610 Complete traumatic transphalangeal amputation of** right index **finger** HCC

8 √7ᵗʰ **S68.611 Complete traumatic transphalangeal amputation of** left index **finger** HCC

8 √7ᵗʰ **S68.612 Complete traumatic transphalangeal amputation of** right middle **finger** HCC

8 √7ᵗʰ **S68.613 Complete traumatic transphalangeal amputation of** left middle **finger** HCC

8 √7ᵗʰ **S68.614 Complete traumatic transphalangeal amputation of** right ring **finger** HCC

8 √7ᵗʰ **S68.615 Complete traumatic transphalangeal amputation of** left ring **finger** HCC

8 √7ᵗʰ **S68.616 Complete traumatic transphalangeal amputation of** right little **finger** HCC

8 √7ᵗʰ **S68.617 Complete traumatic transphalangeal amputation of** left little **finger** HCC

8 √7ᵗʰ **S68.618 Complete traumatic transphalangeal amputation of other finger** HCC

Complete traumatic transphalangeal amputation of specified finger with unspecified laterality

8 √7ᵗʰ **S68.619 Complete traumatic transphalangeal amputation of unspecified finger** HCC

√6ᵗʰ **S68.62 Partial traumatic transphalangeal amputation of other and unspecified finger**

8 √7ᵗʰ **S68.620 Partial traumatic transphalangeal amputation of** right index **finger** HCC

8 √7ᵗʰ **S68.621 Partial traumatic transphalangeal amputation of** left index **finger** HCC

8 √7ᵗʰ **S68.622 Partial traumatic transphalangeal amputation of** right middle **finger** HCC

8 √7ᵗʰ **S68.623 Partial traumatic transphalangeal amputation of** left middle **finger** HCC

8 √7ᵗʰ **S68.624 Partial traumatic transphalangeal amputation of** right ring **finger** HCC

8 √7ᵗʰ **S68.625 Partial traumatic transphalangeal amputation of** left ring **finger** HCC

8 √7ᵗʰ **S68.626 Partial traumatic transphalangeal amputation of** right little **finger** HCC

8 √7ᵗʰ **S68.627 Partial traumatic transphalangeal amputation of** left little **finger** HCC

8 √7ᵗʰ **S68.628 Partial traumatic transphalangeal amputation of other finger** HCC

Partial traumatic transphalangeal amputation of specified finger with unspecified laterality

8 √7ᵗʰ **S68.629 Partial traumatic transphalangeal amputation of unspecified finger** HCC

√5ᵗʰ **S68.7 Traumatic** transmetacarpal **amputation of hand**

√6ᵗʰ **S68.71 Complete traumatic transmetacarpal amputation of hand**

7 √7ᵗʰ **S68.711 Complete traumatic transmetacarpal amputation of** right **hand** CC HCC

7 √7ᵗʰ **S68.712 Complete traumatic transmetacarpal amputation of** left **hand** CC HCC

7 √7ᵗʰ **S68.719 Complete traumatic transmetacarpal amputation of unspecified hand** CC HCC

√6ᵗʰ **S68.72 Partial traumatic transmetacarpal amputation of hand**

7 √7ᵗʰ **S68.721 Partial traumatic transmetacarpal amputation of** right **hand** CC HCC

7 √7ᵗʰ **S68.722 Partial traumatic transmetacarpal amputation of** left **hand** CC HCC

7 √7ᵗʰ **S68.729 Partial traumatic transmetacarpal amputation of unspecified hand** CC HCC

√4ᵗʰ **S69 Other and unspecified injuries of wrist, hand and finger(s)**

The appropriate 7th character is to be added to each code from category S69.

A   initial encounter

D   subsequent encounter

S   sequela

√5ᵗʰ **S69.8 Other specified injuries of wrist, hand and finger(s)**

√x7ᵗʰ **S69.80 Other specified injuries of unspecified wrist, hand and finger(s)**

√x7ᵗʰ **S69.81 Other specified injuries of** right **wrist, hand and finger(s)**

√x7ᵗʰ **S69.82 Other specified injuries of** left **wrist, hand and finger(s)**

√5ᵗʰ **S69.9 Unspecified injury of wrist, hand and finger(s)**

√x7ᵗʰ **S69.90 Unspecified injury of unspecified wrist, hand and finger(s)**

√x7ᵗʰ **S69.91 Unspecified injury of** right **wrist, hand and finger(s)**

√x7ᵗʰ **S69.92 Unspecified injury of** left **wrist, hand and finger(s)**

N Newborn: 0   P Pediatric: 0-17   M Maternity: 9-64   A Adult: 15-124   MCC Major Complication/Comorbidity   CC Complication/Comorbidity   SW Severe Wound Dx

1052   ICD-10-CM 2021

Injuries to the hip and thigh (S70-S79)

EXCLUDES 2   burns and corrosions (T20-T32)
     frostbite (T33-T34)
     snake bite (T63.0-)
     venomous insect bite or sting (T63.4-)

√4th **S70**   **Superficial injury of hip and thigh**

The appropriate 7th character is to be added to each code from category S70.
A   initial encounter
D   subsequent encounter
S   sequela

√5th **S70.0**   **Contusion of** hip
- √x7th **S70.00**   **Contusion of unspecified hip**
- √x7th **S70.01**   **Contusion of right hip**
- √x7th **S70.02**   **Contusion of left hip**

√5th **S70.1**   **Contusion of** thigh
- √x7th **S70.10**   **Contusion of unspecified thigh**
- √x7th **S70.11**   **Contusion of right thigh**
- √x7th **S70.12**   **Contusion of left thigh**

√5th **S70.2**   **Other superficial injuries of** hip
- √6th **S70.21**   Abrasion of hip
  - √7th **S70.211**   **Abrasion, right hip**
  - √7th **S70.212**   **Abrasion, left hip**
  - √7th **S70.219**   **Abrasion, unspecified hip**
- √6th **S70.22**   Blister (nonthermal) of hip
  - √7th **S70.221**   **Blister (nonthermal), right hip**
  - √7th **S70.222**   **Blister (nonthermal), left hip**
  - √7th **S70.229**   **Blister (nonthermal), unspecified hip**
- √6th **S70.24**   External constriction of hip
  - √7th **S70.241**   **External constriction, right hip**
  - √7th **S70.242**   **External constriction, left hip**
  - √7th **S70.249**   **External constriction, unspecified hip**
- √6th **S70.25**   **Superficial** foreign body **of hip**
  - Splinter in the hip
  - √7th **S70.251**   **Superficial foreign body, right hip**
  - √7th **S70.252**   **Superficial foreign body, left hip**
  - √7th **S70.259**   **Superficial foreign body, unspecified hip**
- √6th **S70.26**   Insect bite (nonvenomous) of hip
  - √7th **S70.261**   **Insect bite (nonvenomous), right hip**
  - √7th **S70.262**   **Insect bite (nonvenomous), left hip**
  - √7th **S70.269**   **Insect bite (nonvenomous), unspecified hip**
- √6th **S70.27**   **Other superficial** bite **of hip**
  - EXCLUDES 1   open bite of hip (S71.05-)
  - √7th **S70.271**   **Other superficial bite of hip, right hip**
  - √7th **S70.272**   **Other superficial bite of hip, left hip**
  - √7th **S70.279**   **Other superficial bite of hip, unspecified hip**

√5th **S70.3**   **Other superficial injuries of** thigh
- √6th **S70.31**   Abrasion of thigh
  - √7th **S70.311**   **Abrasion, right thigh**
  - √7th **S70.312**   **Abrasion, left thigh**
  - √7th **S70.319**   **Abrasion, unspecified thigh**
- √6th **S70.32**   Blister (nonthermal) of thigh
  - √7th **S70.321**   **Blister (nonthermal), right thigh**
  - √7th **S70.322**   **Blister (nonthermal), left thigh**
  - √7th **S70.329**   **Blister (nonthermal), unspecified thigh**
- √6th **S70.34**   External constriction of thigh
  - √7th **S70.341**   **External constriction, right thigh**
  - √7th **S70.342**   **External constriction, left thigh**
  - √7th **S70.349**   **External constriction, unspecified thigh**
- √6th **S70.35**   **Superficial** foreign body **of thigh**
  - Splinter in the thigh
  - √7th **S70.351**   **Superficial foreign body, right thigh**
  - √7th **S70.352**   **Superficial foreign body, left thigh**
  - √7th **S70.359**   **Superficial foreign body, unspecified thigh**

- √6th **S70.36**   Insect bite (nonvenomous) of thigh
  - √7th **S70.361**   **Insect bite (nonvenomous), right thigh**
  - √7th **S70.362**   **Insect bite (nonvenomous), left thigh**
  - √7th **S70.369**   **Insect bite (nonvenomous), unspecified thigh**
- √6th **S70.37**   **Other superficial** bite **of thigh**
  - EXCLUDES 1   open bite of thigh (S71.15)
  - √7th **S70.371**   **Other superficial bite of right thigh**
  - √7th **S70.372**   **Other superficial bite of left thigh**
  - √7th **S70.379**   **Other superficial bite of unspecified thigh**

√5th **S70.9**   **Unspecified superficial injury of** hip and thigh
- √6th **S70.91**   **Unspecified superficial injury of** hip
  - √7th **S70.911**   **Unspecified superficial injury of right hip**
  - √7th **S70.912**   **Unspecified superficial injury of left hip**
  - √7th **S70.919**   **Unspecified superficial injury of unspecified hip**
- √6th **S70.92**   **Unspecified superficial injury of** thigh
  - √7th **S70.921**   **Unspecified superficial injury of right thigh**
  - √7th **S70.922**   **Unspecified superficial injury of left thigh**
  - √7th **S70.929**   **Unspecified superficial injury of unspecified thigh**

√4th **S71**   **Open wound of hip and thigh**

Code also any associated wound infection
- EXCLUDES 1   open fracture of hip and thigh (S72.-)
  - traumatic amputation of hip and thigh (S78.-)
- EXCLUDES 2   bite of venomous animal (T63.-)
  - open wound of ankle, foot and toes (S91.-)
  - open wound of knee and lower leg (S81.-)

The appropriate 7th character is to be added to each code from category S71.
A   initial encounter
D   subsequent encounter
S   sequela

√5th **S71.0**   **Open wound of** hip
- √6th **S71.00**   Unspecified open wound of hip
  - √7th **S71.001**   **Unspecified open wound, right hip**
  - √7th **S71.002**   **Unspecified open wound, left hip**
  - √7th **S71.009**   **Unspecified open wound, unspecified hip**
- √6th **S71.01**   Laceration without foreign body of hip
  - √7th **S71.011**   **Laceration without foreign body, right hip**
  - √7th **S71.012**   **Laceration without foreign body, left hip**
  - √7th **S71.019**   **Laceration without foreign body, unspecified hip**
- √6th **S71.02**   Laceration with foreign body of hip
  - √7th **S71.021**   **Laceration with foreign body, right hip**
  - √7th **S71.022**   **Laceration with foreign body, left hip**
  - √7th **S71.029**   **Laceration with foreign body, unspecified hip**
- √6th **S71.03**   Puncture wound without foreign body of hip
  - √7th **S71.031**   **Puncture wound without foreign body, right hip**
  - √7th **S71.032**   **Puncture wound without foreign body, left hip**
  - √7th **S71.039**   **Puncture wound without foreign body, unspecified hip**
- √6th **S71.04**   Puncture wound with foreign body of hip
  - √7th **S71.041**   **Puncture wound with foreign body, right hip**
  - √7th **S71.042**   **Puncture wound with foreign body, left hip**
  - √7th **S71.049**   **Puncture wound with foreign body, unspecified hip**
- √6th **S71.05**   Open bite of hip
  - Bite of hip NOS
  - EXCLUDES 1   superficial bite of hip (S70.26, S70.27)
  - √7th **S71.051**   **Open bite, right hip**
  - √7th **S71.052**   **Open bite, left hip**
  - √7th **S71.059**   **Open bite, unspecified hip**

√5ᵗʰ **S71.1   Open wound of thigh**

√6ᵗʰ **S71.10   Unspecified open wound of thigh**
AHA: 2016,3Q,24

√7ᵗʰ **S71.101   Unspecified open wound, right thigh**

√7ᵗʰ **S71.102   Unspecified open wound, left thigh**

√7ᵗʰ **S71.109   Unspecified open wound, unspecified thigh**

√6ᵗʰ **S71.11   Laceration without foreign body of thigh**

√7ᵗʰ **S71.111   Laceration without foreign body, right thigh**

√7ᵗʰ **S71.112   Laceration without foreign body, left thigh**

√7ᵗʰ **S71.119   Laceration without foreign body, unspecified thigh**

√6ᵗʰ **S71.12   Laceration with foreign body of thigh**

√7ᵗʰ **S71.121   Laceration with foreign body, right thigh**

√7ᵗʰ **S71.122   Laceration with foreign body, left thigh**

√7ᵗʰ **S71.129   Laceration with foreign body, unspecified thigh**

√6ᵗʰ **S71.13   Puncture wound without foreign body of thigh**
AHA: 2016,3Q,24

√7ᵗʰ **S71.131   Puncture wound without foreign body, right thigh**

√7ᵗʰ **S71.132   Puncture wound without foreign body, left thigh**

√7ᵗʰ **S71.139   Puncture wound without foreign body, unspecified thigh**

√6ᵗʰ **S71.14   Puncture wound with foreign body of thigh**
AHA: 2016,3Q,24

√7ᵗʰ **S71.141   Puncture wound with foreign body, right thigh**

√7ᵗʰ **S71.142   Puncture wound with foreign body, left thigh**

√7ᵗʰ **S71.149   Puncture wound with foreign body, unspecified thigh**

√6ᵗʰ **S71.15   Open bite of thigh**
Bite of thigh NOS
EXCLUDES 1   superficial bite of thigh (S70.37-)

√7ᵗʰ **S71.151   Open bite, right thigh**

√7ᵗʰ **S71.152   Open bite, left thigh**

√7ᵗʰ **S71.159   Open bite, unspecified thigh**

√4ᵗʰ **S72   Fracture of femur**

NOTE   A fracture not indicated as displaced or nondisplaced should be coded to displaced.

A fracture not indicated as open or closed should be coded to closed.

The open fracture designations are based on the Gustilo open fracture classification.

EXCLUDES 1   traumatic amputation of hip and thigh (S78.-)

EXCLUDES 2   fracture of lower leg and ankle (S82.-)
fracture of foot (S92.-)
periprosthetic fracture of prosthetic implant of hip (M97.0-)

AHA: 2018,2Q,12; 2016,1Q,33; 2015,3Q,37-39; 2015,1Q,17; 2013,4Q,128
DEF: Diaphysis: Central shaft of a long bone.
DEF: Epiphysis: Proximal and distal rounded ends of a long bone communicates with the joint.
DEF: Metaphysis: Section of a long bone located between the epiphysis and diaphysis at the proximal and distal ends.
DEF: Physis (growth plate): Narrow zone of cartilaginous tissue between the epiphysis and metaphysis at each end of a long bone. In childhood, proliferation of cells in this zone lengthens the bone. As the bone matures, this area thins, ossification eventually fusing into solid bone and growth stops. *Synonyms: Epiphyseal plate.*

The appropriate 7th character is to be added to all codes from category S72 [unless otherwise indicated].
A   initial encounter for closed fracture
B   initial encounter for open fracture type I or II
      initial encounter for open fracture NOS
C   initial encounter for open fracture type IIIA, IIIB, or IIIC
D   subsequent encounter for closed fracture with routine healing
E   subsequent encounter for open fracture type I or II with routine healing
F   subsequent encounter for open fracture type IIIA, IIIB, or IIIC with routine healing
G   subsequent encounter for closed fracture with delayed healing
H   subsequent encounter for open fracture type I or II with delayed healing
J   subsequent encounter for open fracture type IIIA, IIIB, or IIIC with delayed healing
K   subsequent encounter for closed fracture with nonunion
M   subsequent encounter for open fracture type I or II with nonunion
N   subsequent encounter for open fracture type IIIA, IIIB, or IIIC with nonunion
P   subsequent encounter for closed fracture with malunion
Q   subsequent encounter for open fracture type I or II with malunion
R   subsequent encounter for open fracture type IIIA, IIIB, or IIIC with malunion
S   sequela

√5ᵗʰ **S72.0   Fracture of head and neck of femur**
EXCLUDES 2   physeal fracture of upper end of femur (S79.0-)
AHA: 2016,3Q,16

√6ᵗʰ **S72.00   Fracture of unspecified part of neck of femur**
Fracture of hip NOS
Fracture of neck of femur NOS

4,6 √7ᵗʰ **S72.001   Fracture of unspecified part of neck of right femur**   MCC CC H5 HCC

4,6 √7ᵗʰ **S72.002   Fracture of unspecified part of neck of left femur**   MCC CC H5 HCC

4,6 √7ᵗʰ **S72.009   Fracture of unspecified part of neck of unspecified femur**   MCC CC H5 HCC

√6ᵗʰ **S72.01   Unspecified intracapsular fracture of femur**
Subcapital fracture of femur

4,6 √7ᵗʰ **S72.011   Unspecified intracapsular fracture of right femur**   MCC CC H5 HCC

4,6 √7ᵗʰ **S72.012   Unspecified intracapsular fracture of left femur**   MCC CC H5 HCC

4,6 √7ᵗʰ **S72.019   Unspecified intracapsular fracture of unspecified femur**   MCC CC H5 HCC

√6ᵗʰ **S72.02   Fracture of epiphysis (separation) (upper) of femur**
Transepiphyseal fracture of femur
EXCLUDES 1   capital femoral epiphyseal fracture (pediatric) of femur (S79.01-)
Salter-Harris Type I physeal fracture of upper end of femur (S79.01-)

4,6 √7ᵗʰ **S72.021   Displaced fracture of epiphysis (separation) (upper) of right femur**   MCC CC H5 HCC

4,6 √7ᵗʰ **S72.022** Displaced fracture of epiphysis (separation) (upper) of left femur `MCC` `CC` `H5` `HCC`

4,6 √7ᵗʰ **S72.023** Displaced fracture of epiphysis (separation) (upper) of unspecified femur `MCC` `CC` `H5` `HCC`

4,6 √7ᵗʰ **S72.024** Nondisplaced fracture of epiphysis (separation) (upper) of right femur `MCC` `CC` `H5` `HCC`

4,6 √7ᵗʰ **S72.025** Nondisplaced fracture of epiphysis (separation) (upper) of left femur `MCC` `CC` `H5` `HCC`

4,6 √7ᵗʰ **S72.026** Nondisplaced fracture of epiphysis (separation) (upper) of unspecified femur `MCC` `CC` `H5` `HCC`

√6ᵗʰ **S72.03** Midcervical fracture of femur

    Transcervical fracture of femur NOS

4,6 √7ᵗʰ **S72.031** Displaced midcervical fracture of right femur `MCC` `CC` `H5` `HCC`

4,6 √7ᵗʰ **S72.032** Displaced midcervical fracture of left femur `MCC` `CC` `H5` `HCC`

4,6 √7ᵗʰ **S72.033** Displaced midcervical fracture of unspecified femur `MCC` `CC` `H5` `HCC`

4,6 √7ᵗʰ **S72.034** Nondisplaced midcervical fracture of right femur `MCC` `CC` `H5` `HCC`

4,6 √7ᵗʰ **S72.035** Nondisplaced midcervical fracture of left femur `MCC` `CC` `H5` `HCC`

4,6 √7ᵗʰ **S72.036** Nondisplaced midcervical fracture of unspecified femur `MCC` `CC` `H5` `HCC`

√6ᵗʰ **S72.04** Fracture of base of neck of femur

    Cervicotrochanteric fracture of femur

4,6 √7ᵗʰ **S72.041** Displaced fracture of base of neck of right femur `MCC` `CC` `H5` `HCC`

4,6 √7ᵗʰ **S72.042** Displaced fracture of base of neck of left femur `MCC` `CC` `H5` `HCC`

4,6 √7ᵗʰ **S72.043** Displaced fracture of base of neck of unspecified femur `MCC` `CC` `H5` `HCC`

4,6 √7ᵗʰ **S72.044** Nondisplaced fracture of base of neck of right femur `MCC` `CC` `H5` `HCC`

4,6 √7ᵗʰ **S72.045** Nondisplaced fracture of base of neck of left femur `MCC` `CC` `H5` `HCC`

4,6 √7ᵗʰ **S72.046** Nondisplaced fracture of base of neck of unspecified femur `MCC` `CC` `H5` `HCC`

√6ᵗʰ **S72.05** Unspecified fracture of head of femur

    Fracture of head of femur NOS

4,6 √7ᵗʰ **S72.051** Unspecified fracture of head of right femur `MCC` `CC` `H5` `HCC`

4,6 √7ᵗʰ **S72.052** Unspecified fracture of head of left femur `MCC` `CC` `H5` `HCC`

4,6 √7ᵗʰ **S72.059** Unspecified fracture of head of unspecified femur `MCC` `CC` `H5` `HCC`

√6ᵗʰ **S72.06** Articular fracture of head of femur

4,6 √7ᵗʰ **S72.061** Displaced articular fracture of head of right femur `MCC` `CC` `H5` `HCC`

4,6 √7ᵗʰ **S72.062** Displaced articular fracture of head of left femur `MCC` `CC` `H5` `HCC`

4,6 √7ᵗʰ **S72.063** Displaced articular fracture of head of unspecified femur `MCC` `CC` `H5` `HCC`

4,6 √7ᵗʰ **S72.064** Nondisplaced articular fracture of head of right femur `MCC` `CC` `H5` `HCC`

4,6 √7ᵗʰ **S72.065** Nondisplaced articular fracture of head of left femur `MCC` `CC` `H5` `HCC`

4,6 √7ᵗʰ **S72.066** Nondisplaced articular fracture of head of unspecified femur `MCC` `CC` `H5` `HCC`

√6ᵗʰ **S72.09** Other fracture of head and neck of femur

4,6 √7ᵗʰ **S72.091** Other fracture of head and neck of right femur `MCC` `CC` `H5` `HCC`

4,6 √7ᵗʰ **S72.092** Other fracture of head and neck of left femur `MCC` `CC` `H5` `HCC`

4,6 √7ᵗʰ **S72.099** Other fracture of head and neck of unspecified femur `MCC` `CC` `H5` `HCC`

√5ᵗʰ **S72.1** Pertrochanteric fracture

    AHA: 2016,3Q,16

√6ᵗʰ **S72.10** Unspecified trochanteric fracture of femur

    Fracture of trochanter NOS

4,6 √7ᵗʰ **S72.101** Unspecified trochanteric fracture of right femur `MCC` `CC` `H5` `HCC`

4,6 √7ᵗʰ **S72.102** Unspecified trochanteric fracture of left femur `MCC` `CC` `H5` `HCC`

4,6 √7ᵗʰ **S72.109** Unspecified trochanteric fracture of unspecified femur `MCC` `CC` `H5` `HCC`

√6ᵗʰ **S72.11** Fracture of greater trochanter of femur

4,6 √7ᵗʰ **S72.111** Displaced fracture of greater trochanter of right femur `MCC` `CC` `H5` `HCC`

4,6 √7ᵗʰ **S72.112** Displaced fracture of greater trochanter of left femur `MCC` `CC` `H5` `HCC`

4,6 √7ᵗʰ **S72.113** Displaced fracture of greater trochanter of unspecified femur `MCC` `CC` `H5` `HCC`

4,6 √7ᵗʰ **S72.114** Nondisplaced fracture of greater trochanter of right femur `MCC` `CC` `H5` `HCC`

4,6 √7ᵗʰ **S72.115** Nondisplaced fracture of greater trochanter of left femur `MCC` `CC` `H5` `HCC`

4,6 √7ᵗʰ **S72.116** Nondisplaced fracture of greater trochanter of unspecified femur `MCC` `CC` `H5` `HCC`

√6ᵗʰ **S72.12** Fracture of lesser trochanter of femur

4,6 √7ᵗʰ **S72.121** Displaced fracture of lesser trochanter of right femur `MCC` `CC` `H5` `HCC`

4,6 √7ᵗʰ **S72.122** Displaced fracture of lesser trochanter of left femur `MCC` `CC` `H5` `HCC`

4,6 √7ᵗʰ **S72.123** Displaced fracture of lesser trochanter of unspecified femur `MCC` `CC` `H5` `HCC`

4,6 √7ᵗʰ **S72.124** Nondisplaced fracture of lesser trochanter of right femur `MCC` `CC` `H5` `HCC`

4,6 √7ᵗʰ **S72.125** Nondisplaced fracture of lesser trochanter of left femur `MCC` `CC` `H5` `HCC`

4,6 √7ᵗʰ **S72.126** Nondisplaced fracture of lesser trochanter of unspecified femur `MCC` `CC` `H5` `HCC`

√6ᵗʰ **S72.13** Apophyseal fracture of femur

    EXCLUDES 1   chronic (nontraumatic) slipped upper femoral epiphysis (M93.0-)

4,6 √7ᵗʰ **S72.131** Displaced apophyseal fracture of right femur `MCC` `CC` `H5` `HCC`

4,6 √7ᵗʰ **S72.132** Displaced apophyseal fracture of left femur `MCC` `CC` `H5` `HCC`

4,6 √7ᵗʰ **S72.133** Displaced apophyseal fracture of unspecified femur `MCC` `CC` `H5` `HCC`

4,6 √7ᵗʰ **S72.134** Nondisplaced apophyseal fracture of right femur `MCC` `CC` `H5` `HCC`

4,6 √7ᵗʰ **S72.135** Nondisplaced apophyseal fracture of left femur `MCC` `CC` `H5` `HCC`

4,6 √7ᵗʰ **S72.136** Nondisplaced apophyseal fracture of unspecified femur `MCC` `CC` `H5` `HCC`

√6ᵗʰ **S72.14** Intertrochanteric fracture of femur

4,6 √7ᵗʰ **S72.141** Displaced intertrochanteric fracture of right femur `MCC` `CC` `H5` `HCC`

4,6 √7ᵗʰ **S72.142** Displaced intertrochanteric fracture of left femur `MCC` `CC` `H5` `HCC`

4,6 √7ᵗʰ **S72.143** Displaced intertrochanteric fracture of unspecified femur `MCC` `CC` `H5` `HCC`

4,6 √7ᵗʰ **S72.144** Nondisplaced intertrochanteric fracture of right femur `MCC` `CC` `H5` `HCC`

4,6 √7ᵗʰ **S72.145** Nondisplaced intertrochanteric fracture of left femur `MCC` `CC` `H5` `HCC`

4,6 √7ᵗʰ **S72.146** Nondisplaced intertrochanteric fracture of unspecified femur `MCC` `CC` `H5` `HCC`

√5ᵗʰ **S72.2** Subtrochanteric fracture of femur

4,6 √x7ᵗʰ **S72.21** Displaced subtrochanteric fracture of right femur `MCC` `CC` `H5` `HCC`

4,6 √x7ᵗʰ **S72.22** Displaced subtrochanteric fracture of left femur `MCC` `CC` `H5` `HCC`

4,6 √x7ᵗʰ **S72.23** Displaced subtrochanteric fracture of unspecified femur `MCC` `CC` `H5` `HCC`

4,6 √x7ᵗʰ **S72.24** Nondisplaced subtrochanteric fracture of right femur `MCC` `CC` `H5` `HCC`

4,6 √x7ᵗʰ **S72.25** Nondisplaced subtrochanteric fracture of left femur `MCC` `CC` `H5` `HCC`

4,6 √x7ᵗʰ **S72.26** Nondisplaced subtrochanteric fracture of unspecified femur `MCC` `CC` `H5` `HCC`

√5ᵗʰ **S72.3** Fracture of shaft of femur

√6ᵗʰ **S72.30** Unspecified fracture of shaft of femur

4,6 √7ᵗʰ **S72.301** Unspecified fracture of shaft of right femur `MCC` `CC` `H5` `HCC`

✅ Additional Character Required   √x7ᵗʰ Placeholder   Unacceptable PDx   Questionable PDx   Manifestation   Unspecified Dx   `H1`-`H14` HAC   `HCC` CMS-HCC Dx   `HIV` HIV Dx

ICD-10-CM 2021   1055

4,6 √7ᵗʰ **S72.302** Unspecified fracture of shaft of left femur `MCC` `CC` `H5` `HCC`

4,6 √7ᵗʰ **S72.309** Unspecified fracture of shaft of unspecified femur `MCC` `CC` `H5` `HCC`

√6ᵗʰ **S72.32** Transverse fracture of shaft of femur

4,6 √7ᵗʰ **S72.321** Displaced transverse fracture of shaft of right femur `MCC` `CC` `H5` `HCC`

4,6 √7ᵗʰ **S72.322** Displaced transverse fracture of shaft of left femur `MCC` `CC` `H5` `HCC`

4,6 √7ᵗʰ **S72.323** Displaced transverse fracture of shaft of unspecified femur `MCC` `CC` `H5` `HCC`

4,6 √7ᵗʰ **S72.324** Nondisplaced transverse fracture of shaft of right femur `MCC` `CC` `H5` `HCC`

4,6 √7ᵗʰ **S72.325** Nondisplaced transverse fracture of shaft of left femur `MCC` `CC` `H5` `HCC`

4,6 √7ᵗʰ **S72.326** Nondisplaced transverse fracture of shaft of unspecified femur `MCC` `CC` `H5` `HCC`

√6ᵗʰ **S72.33** Oblique fracture of shaft of femur

4,6 √7ᵗʰ **S72.331** Displaced oblique fracture of shaft of right femur `MCC` `CC` `H5` `HCC`

4,6 √7ᵗʰ **S72.332** Displaced oblique fracture of shaft of left femur `MCC` `CC` `H5` `HCC`

4,6 √7ᵗʰ **S72.333** Displaced oblique fracture of shaft of unspecified femur `MCC` `CC` `H5` `HCC`

4,6 √7ᵗʰ **S72.334** Nondisplaced oblique fracture of shaft of right femur `MCC` `CC` `H5` `HCC`

4,6 √7ᵗʰ **S72.335** Nondisplaced oblique fracture of shaft of left femur `MCC` `CC` `H5` `HCC`

4,6 √7ᵗʰ **S72.336** Nondisplaced oblique fracture of shaft of unspecified femur `MCC` `CC` `H5` `HCC`

√6ᵗʰ **S72.34** Spiral fracture of shaft of femur

4,6 √7ᵗʰ **S72.341** Displaced spiral fracture of shaft of right femur `MCC` `CC` `H5` `HCC`

4,6 √7ᵗʰ **S72.342** Displaced spiral fracture of shaft of left femur `MCC` `CC` `H5` `HCC`

4,6 √7ᵗʰ **S72.343** Displaced spiral fracture of shaft of unspecified femur `MCC` `CC` `H5` `HCC`

4,6 √7ᵗʰ **S72.344** Nondisplaced spiral fracture of shaft of right femur `MCC` `CC` `H5` `HCC`

4,6 √7ᵗʰ **S72.345** Nondisplaced spiral fracture of shaft of left femur `MCC` `CC` `H5` `HCC`

4,6 √7ᵗʰ **S72.346** Nondisplaced spiral fracture of shaft of unspecified femur `MCC` `CC` `H5` `HCC`

√6ᵗʰ **S72.35** Comminuted fracture of shaft of femur

4,6 √7ᵗʰ **S72.351** Displaced comminuted fracture of shaft of right femur `MCC` `CC` `H5` `HCC`

4,6 √7ᵗʰ **S72.352** Displaced comminuted fracture of shaft of left femur `MCC` `CC` `H5` `HCC`

4,6 √7ᵗʰ **S72.353** Displaced comminuted fracture of shaft of unspecified femur `MCC` `CC` `H5` `HCC`

4,6 √7ᵗʰ **S72.354** Nondisplaced comminuted fracture of shaft of right femur `MCC` `CC` `H5` `HCC`

4,6 √7ᵗʰ **S72.355** Nondisplaced comminuted fracture of shaft of left femur `MCC` `CC` `H5` `HCC`

4,6 √7ᵗʰ **S72.356** Nondisplaced comminuted fracture of shaft of unspecified femur `MCC` `CC` `H5` `HCC`

√6ᵗʰ **S72.36** Segmental fracture of shaft of femur

4,6 √7ᵗʰ **S72.361** Displaced segmental fracture of shaft of right femur `MCC` `CC` `H5` `HCC`

4,6 √7ᵗʰ **S72.362** Displaced segmental fracture of shaft of left femur `MCC` `CC` `H5` `HCC`

4,6 √7ᵗʰ **S72.363** Displaced segmental fracture of shaft of unspecified femur `MCC` `CC` `H5` `HCC`

4,6 √7ᵗʰ **S72.364** Nondisplaced segmental fracture of shaft of right femur `MCC` `CC` `H5` `HCC`

4,6 √7ᵗʰ **S72.365** Nondisplaced segmental fracture of shaft of left femur `MCC` `CC` `H5` `HCC`

4,6 √7ᵗʰ **S72.366** Nondisplaced segmental fracture of shaft of unspecified femur `MCC` `CC` `H5` `HCC`

√6ᵗʰ **S72.39** Other fracture of shaft of femur

4,6 √7ᵗʰ **S72.391** Other fracture of shaft of right femur `MCC` `CC` `H5` `HCC`

4,6 √7ᵗʰ **S72.392** Other fracture of shaft of left femur `MCC` `CC` `H5` `HCC`

4,6 √7ᵗʰ **S72.399** Other fracture of shaft of unspecified femur `MCC` `CC` `H5` `HCC`

√5ᵗʰ **S72.4** Fracture of lower end of femur

Fracture of distal end of femur

EXCLUDES 2   fracture of shaft of femur (S72.3-)

physeal fracture of lower end of femur (S79.1-)

AHA: 2016,4Q,42

√6ᵗʰ **S72.40** Unspecified fracture of lower end of femur

AHA: 2018,1Q,21; 2016,4Q,42

2,3,6 √7ᵗʰ **S72.401** Unspecified fracture of lower end of right femur `MCC` `CC` `H5` `HCC`

2,3,6 √7ᵗʰ **S72.402** Unspecified fracture of lower end of left femur `MCC` `CC` `H5` `HCC`

2,3,6 √7ᵗʰ **S72.409** Unspecified fracture of lower end of unspecified femur `MCC` `CC` `H5` `HCC`

√6ᵗʰ **S72.41** Unspecified condyle fracture of lower end of femur

Condyle fracture of femur NOS

2,3,6 √7ᵗʰ **S72.411** Displaced unspecified condyle fracture of lower end of right femur `MCC` `CC` `H5` `HCC`

2,3,6 √7ᵗʰ **S72.412** Displaced unspecified condyle fracture of lower end of left femur `MCC` `CC` `H5` `HCC`

2,3,6 √7ᵗʰ **S72.413** Displaced unspecified condyle fracture of lower end of unspecified femur `MCC` `CC` `H5` `HCC`

2,3,6 √7ᵗʰ **S72.414** Nondisplaced unspecified condyle fracture of lower end of right femur `MCC` `CC` `H5` `HCC`

2,3,6 √7ᵗʰ **S72.415** Nondisplaced unspecified condyle fracture of lower end of left femur `MCC` `CC` `H5` `HCC`

2,3,6 √7ᵗʰ **S72.416** Nondisplaced unspecified condyle fracture of lower end of unspecified femur `MCC` `CC` `H5` `HCC`

√6ᵗʰ **S72.42** Fracture of lateral condyle of femur

2,3,6 √7ᵗʰ **S72.421** Displaced fracture of lateral condyle of right femur `MCC` `CC` `H5` `HCC`

2,3,6 √7ᵗʰ **S72.422** Displaced fracture of lateral condyle of left femur `MCC` `CC` `H5` `HCC`

2,3,6 √7ᵗʰ **S72.423** Displaced fracture of lateral condyle of unspecified femur `MCC` `CC` `H5` `HCC`

2,3,6 √7ᵗʰ **S72.424** Nondisplaced fracture of lateral condyle of right femur `MCC` `CC` `H5` `HCC`

2,3,6 √7ᵗʰ **S72.425** Nondisplaced fracture of lateral condyle of left femur `MCC` `CC` `H5` `HCC`

2,3,6 √7ᵗʰ **S72.426** Nondisplaced fracture of lateral condyle of unspecified femur `MCC` `CC` `H5` `HCC`

√6ᵗʰ **S72.43** Fracture of medial condyle of femur

2,3,6 √7ᵗʰ **S72.431** Displaced fracture of medial condyle of right femur `MCC` `CC` `H5` `HCC`

2,3,6 √7ᵗʰ **S72.432** Displaced fracture of medial condyle of left femur `MCC` `CC` `H5` `HCC`

2,3,6 √7ᵗʰ **S72.433** Displaced fracture of medial condyle of unspecified femur `MCC` `CC` `H5` `HCC`

2,3,6 √7ᵗʰ **S72.434** Nondisplaced fracture of medial condyle of right femur `MCC` `CC` `H5` `HCC`

2,3,6 √7ᵗʰ **S72.435** Nondisplaced fracture of medial condyle of left femur `MCC` `CC` `H5` `HCC`

2,3,6 √7ᵗʰ **S72.436** Nondisplaced fracture of medial condyle of unspecified femur `MCC` `CC` `H5` `HCC`

√6ᵗʰ **S72.44** Fracture of lower epiphysis (separation) of femur

EXCLUDES 1   Salter-Harris Type I physeal fracture of lower end of femur (S79.11-)

2,3,6 √7ᵗʰ **S72.441** Displaced fracture of lower epiphysis (separation) of right femur `MCC` `CC` `H5` `HCC`

2,3,6 √7ᵗʰ **S72.442** Displaced fracture of lower epiphysis (separation) of left femur `MCC` `CC` `H5` `HCC`

2,3,6 √7ᵗʰ **S72.443** Displaced fracture of lower epiphysis (separation) of unspecified femur `MCC` `CC` `H5` `HCC`

2,3,6 √7ᵗʰ **S72.444** Nondisplaced fracture of lower epiphysis (separation) of right femur `MCC` `CC` `H5` `HCC`

2,3,6 √7ᵗʰ **S72.445** Nondisplaced fracture of lower epiphysis (separation) of left femur `MCC` `CC` `H5` `HCC`

N Newborn: 0   P Pediatric: 0-17   M Maternity: 9-64   A Adult: 15-124   MCC Major Complication/Comorbidity   CC Complication/Comorbidity   SW Severe Wound Dx

1056

ICD-10-CM 2021

2,3,6 √7ᵗʰ **S72.446** Nondisplaced **fracture of lower epiphysis (separation) of** unspecified **femur** `MCC` `CC` `H5` `HCC`

√6ᵗʰ **S72.45** Supracondylar **fracture without intracondylar extension of lower end of femur**
Supracondylar fracture of lower end of femur NOS
EXCLUDES 1 *supracondylar fracture with intracondylar extension of lower end of femur (S72.46-)*

2,3,6 √7ᵗʰ **S72.451** Displaced **supracondylar fracture without intracondylar extension of lower end of** right **femur** `MCC` `CC` `H5` `HCC`

2,3,6 √7ᵗʰ **S72.452** Displaced **supracondylar fracture without intracondylar extension of lower end of** left **femur** `MCC` `CC` `H5` `HCC`

2,3,6 √7ᵗʰ **S72.453** Displaced **supracondylar fracture without intracondylar extension of lower end of** unspecified **femur** `MCC` `CC` `H5` `HCC`

2,3,6 √7ᵗʰ **S72.454** Nondisplaced **supracondylar fracture without intracondylar extension of lower end of** right **femur** `MCC` `CC` `H5` `HCC`

2,3,6 √7ᵗʰ **S72.455** Nondisplaced **supracondylar fracture without intracondylar extension of lower end of** left **femur** `MCC` `CC` `H5` `HCC`

2,3,6 √7ᵗʰ **S72.456** Nondisplaced **supracondylar fracture without intracondylar extension of lower end of** femur `MCC` `CC` `H5` `HCC`

√6ᵗʰ **S72.46** Supracondylar **fracture with intracondylar extension of lower end of femur**
EXCLUDES 1 *supracondylar fracture without intracondylar extension of lower end of femur (S72.45-)*

2,3,6 √7ᵗʰ **S72.461** Displaced **supracondylar fracture with intracondylar extension of lower end of** right **femur** `MCC` `CC` `H5` `HCC`

2,3,6 √7ᵗʰ **S72.462** Displaced **supracondylar fracture with intracondylar extension of lower end of** left **femur** `MCC` `CC` `H5` `HCC`

2,3,6 √7ᵗʰ **S72.463** Displaced **supracondylar fracture with intracondylar extension of lower end of** unspecified **femur** `MCC` `CC` `H5` `HCC`

2,3,6 √7ᵗʰ **S72.464** Nondisplaced **supracondylar fracture with intracondylar extension of lower end of** right **femur** `MCC` `CC` `H5` `HCC`

2,3,6 √7ᵗʰ **S72.465** Nondisplaced **supracondylar fracture with intracondylar extension of lower end of** left **femur** `MCC` `CC` `H5` `HCC`

2,3,6 √7ᵗʰ **S72.466** Nondisplaced **supracondylar fracture with intracondylar extension of lower end of** unspecified **femur** `MCC` `CC` `H5` `HCC`

√6ᵗʰ **S72.47** Torus **fracture of lower end of femur**

> The appropriate 7th character is to be added to all codes in subcategory S72.47.
> A   initial encounter for closed fracture
> D   subsequent encounter for fracture with routine healing
> G   subsequent encounter for fracture with delayed healing
> K   subsequent encounter for fracture with nonunion
> P   subsequent encounter for fracture with malunion
> S   sequela

3,6 √7ᵗʰ **S72.471** Torus **fracture of lower end of** right **femur** `CC` `H5` `HCC`

3,6 √7ᵗʰ **S72.472** Torus **fracture of lower end of** left **femur** `CC` `H5` `HCC`

3,6 √7ᵗʰ **S72.479** Torus **fracture of lower end of** unspecified **femur** `CC` `H5` `HCC`

√6ᵗʰ **S72.49** Other fracture of lower end of femur

2,3,6 √7ᵗʰ **S72.491** Other fracture of lower end of right **femur** `MCC` `CC` `H5` `HCC`

2,3,6 √7ᵗʰ **S72.492** Other fracture of lower end of left **femur** `MCC` `CC` `H5` `HCC`

2,3,6 √7ᵗʰ **S72.499** Other fracture of lower end of unspecified **femur** `MCC` `CC` `H5` `HCC`

√5ᵗʰ **S72.8** Other fracture of femur

√6ᵗʰ **S72.8X** Other fracture of femur

4,6 √7ᵗʰ **S72.8X1** Other fracture of right **femur** `MCC` `CC` `H5` `HCC`

4,6 √7ᵗʰ **S72.8X2** Other fracture of left **femur** `MCC` `CC` `H5` `HCC`

4,6 √7ᵗʰ **S72.8X9** Other fracture of unspecified **femur** `MCC` `CC` `H5` `HCC`

√5ᵗʰ **S72.9** Unspecified fracture of femur
Fracture of thigh NOS
Fracture of upper leg NOS
EXCLUDES 1 *fracture of hip NOS (S72.00-, S72.01-)*

4,6 √x7ᵗʰ **S72.90** Unspecified fracture of unspecified **femur** `MCC` `CC` `H5` `HCC`
AHA: 2012,4Q,93

4,6 √x7ᵗʰ **S72.91** Unspecified fracture of right **femur** `MCC` `CC` `H5` `HCC`

4,6 √x7ᵗʰ **S72.92** Unspecified fracture of left **femur** `MCC` `CC` `H5` `HCC`

√4ᵗʰ **S73** Dislocation and sprain of joint and ligaments of hip

INCLUDES avulsion of joint or ligament of hip
laceration of cartilage, joint or ligament of hip
sprain of cartilage, joint or ligament of hip
traumatic hemarthrosis of joint or ligament of hip
traumatic rupture of joint or ligament of hip
traumatic subluxation of joint or ligament of hip
traumatic tear of joint or ligament of hip

Code also any associated open wound
EXCLUDES 2 *strain of muscle, fascia and tendon of hip and thigh (S76.-)*

> The appropriate 7th character is to be added to each code from category S73.
> A   initial encounter
> D   subsequent encounter
> S   sequela

√5ᵗʰ **S73.0** Subluxation and dislocation of hip
EXCLUDES 2 *dislocation and subluxation of hip prosthesis (T84.020, T84.021)*

√6ᵗʰ **S73.00** Unspecified subluxation and dislocation of hip
Dislocation of hip NOS
Subluxation of hip NOS

6 √7ᵗʰ **S73.001** Unspecified subluxation of right **hip** `CC` `H5` `HCC`

6 √7ᵗʰ **S73.002** Unspecified subluxation of left **hip** `CC` `H5` `HCC`

6 √7ᵗʰ **S73.003** Unspecified subluxation of unspecified **hip** `CC` `H5` `HCC`

6 √7ᵗʰ **S73.004** Unspecified dislocation of right **hip** `CC` `H5` `HCC`

6 √7ᵗʰ **S73.005** Unspecified dislocation of left **hip** `CC` `H5` `HCC`

6 √7ᵗʰ **S73.006** Unspecified dislocation of unspecified **hip** `CC` `H5` `HCC`

√6ᵗʰ **S73.01** Posterior subluxation and dislocation of hip

6 √7ᵗʰ **S73.011** Posterior subluxation of right **hip** `CC` `H5` `HCC`

6 √7ᵗʰ **S73.012** Posterior subluxation of left **hip** `CC` `H5` `HCC`

6 √7ᵗʰ **S73.013** Posterior subluxation of unspecified **hip** `CC` `H5` `HCC`

6 √7ᵗʰ **S73.014** Posterior dislocation of right **hip** `CC` `H5` `HCC`

6 √7ᵗʰ **S73.015** Posterior dislocation of left **hip** `CC` `H5` `HCC`

6 √7ᵗʰ **S73.016** Posterior dislocation of unspecified **hip** `CC` `H5` `HCC`

√6ᵗʰ **S73.02** Obturator subluxation and dislocation of hip

6 √7ᵗʰ **S73.021** Obturator subluxation of right **hip** `CC` `H5` `HCC`

6 √7ᵗʰ **S73.022** Obturator subluxation of left **hip** `CC` `H5` `HCC`

6 √7ᵗʰ **S73.023** Obturator subluxation of unspecified **hip** `CC` `H5` `HCC`

6 √7ᵗʰ **S73.024** Obturator dislocation of right **hip** `CC` `H5` `HCC`

6 √7ᵗʰ **S73.025** Obturator dislocation of left **hip** `CC` `H5` `HCC`

⁶ √7ᵗʰ **S73.026** **Obturator** dislocation **of unspecified hip** CC H5 HCC

√6ᵗʰ **S73.03** **Other** anterior **subluxation and dislocation of hip**

⁶ √7ᵗʰ **S73.031** **Other anterior** subluxation **of** right **hip** CC H5 HCC

⁶ √7ᵗʰ **S73.032** **Other anterior** subluxation **of** left **hip** CC H5 HCC

⁶ √7ᵗʰ **S73.033** **Other anterior** subluxation **of unspecified hip** CC H5 HCC

⁶ √7ᵗʰ **S73.034** **Other anterior** dislocation **of** right **hip** CC H5 HCC

⁶ √7ᵗʰ **S73.035** **Other anterior** dislocation **of** left **hip** CC H5 HCC

⁶ √7ᵗʰ **S73.036** **Other anterior** dislocation **of unspecified hip** CC H5 HCC

√6ᵗʰ **S73.04** **Central** subluxation **and dislocation of hip**

⁶ √7ᵗʰ **S73.041** **Central** subluxation **of** right **hip** CC H5 HCC

⁶ √7ᵗʰ **S73.042** **Central** subluxation **of** left **hip** CC H5 HCC

⁶ √7ᵗʰ **S73.043** **Central** subluxation **of unspecified hip** CC H5 HCC

⁶ √7ᵗʰ **S73.044** **Central** dislocation **of** right **hip** CC H5 HCC

⁶ √7ᵗʰ **S73.045** **Central** dislocation **of** left **hip** CC H5 HCC

⁶ √7ᵗʰ **S73.046** **Central** dislocation **of unspecified hip** CC H5 HCC

√5ᵗʰ **S73.1** **Sprain of hip**
AHA: 2014,4Q,25

√6ᵗʰ **S73.10** **Unspecified sprain of hip**

√7ᵗʰ **S73.101** **Unspecified sprain of** right **hip**

√7ᵗʰ **S73.102** **Unspecified sprain of** left **hip**

√7ᵗʰ **S73.109** **Unspecified sprain of unspecified hip**

√6ᵗʰ **S73.11** **Iliofemoral ligament sprain of hip**

√7ᵗʰ **S73.111** **Iliofemoral ligament sprain of** right **hip**

√7ᵗʰ **S73.112** **Iliofemoral ligament sprain of** left **hip**

√7ᵗʰ **S73.119** **Iliofemoral ligament sprain of unspecified hip**

√6ᵗʰ **S73.12** **Ischiocapsular (ligament) sprain of hip**

√7ᵗʰ **S73.121** **Ischiocapsular ligament sprain of** right **hip**

√7ᵗʰ **S73.122** **Ischiocapsular ligament sprain of** left **hip**

√7ᵗʰ **S73.129** **Ischiocapsular ligament sprain of unspecified hip**

√6ᵗʰ **S73.19** **Other sprain of hip**

√7ᵗʰ **S73.191** **Other sprain of** right **hip**

√7ᵗʰ **S73.192** **Other sprain of** left **hip**

√7ᵗʰ **S73.199** **Other sprain of unspecified hip**

√4ᵗʰ **S74** **Injury of nerves at hip and thigh level**
Code also any associated open wound (S71.-)
EXCLUDES 2 injury of nerves at ankle and foot level (S94.-)
injury of nerves at lower leg level (S84.-)

The appropriate 7th character is to be added to each code from category S74.
A initial encounter
D subsequent encounter
S sequela

√5ᵗʰ **S74.0** **Injury of** sciatic nerve **at hip and thigh level**

√x7ᵗʰ **S74.00** **Injury of sciatic nerve at hip and thigh level, unspecified leg**

√x7ᵗʰ **S74.01** **Injury of sciatic nerve at hip and thigh level,** right **leg**

√x7ᵗʰ **S74.02** **Injury of sciatic nerve at hip and thigh level,** left **leg**

√5ᵗʰ **S74.1** **Injury of** femoral nerve **at hip and thigh level**

√x7ᵗʰ **S74.10** **Injury of femoral nerve at hip and thigh level, unspecified leg**

√x7ᵗʰ **S74.11** **Injury of femoral nerve at hip and thigh level,** right **leg**

√x7ᵗʰ **S74.12** **Injury of femoral nerve at hip and thigh level,** left **leg**

√5ᵗʰ **S74.2** **Injury of** cutaneous sensory nerve **at hip and thigh level**

√x7ᵗʰ **S74.20** **Injury of cutaneous sensory nerve at hip and thigh level, unspecified leg**

√x7ᵗʰ **S74.21** **Injury of cutaneous sensory nerve at hip and high level,** right **leg**

√x7ᵗʰ **S74.22** **Injury of cutaneous sensory nerve at hip and thigh level,** left **leg**

√5ᵗʰ **S74.8** **Injury of other nerves at hip and thigh level**

√6ᵗʰ **S74.8X** **Injury of other nerves at hip and thigh level**

√7ᵗʰ **S74.8X1** **Injury of other nerves at hip and thigh level,** right **leg**

√7ᵗʰ **S74.8X2** **Injury of other nerves at hip and thigh level,** left **leg**

√7ᵗʰ **S74.8X9** **Injury of other nerves at hip and thigh level, unspecified leg**

√5ᵗʰ **S74.9** **Injury of unspecified nerve at hip and thigh level**

√x7ᵗʰ **S74.90** **Injury of unspecified nerve at hip and thigh level, unspecified leg**

√x7ᵗʰ **S74.91** **Injury of unspecified nerve at hip and thigh level,** right **leg**

√x7ᵗʰ **S74.92** **Injury of unspecified nerve at hip and thigh level,** left **leg**

√4ᵗʰ **S75** **Injury of blood vessels at hip and thigh level**
Code also any associated open wound (S71.-)
EXCLUDES 2 injury of blood vessels at lower leg level (S85.-)
injury of popliteal artery (S85.0)

The appropriate 7th character is to be added to each code from category S75.
A initial encounter
D subsequent encounter
S sequela

√5ᵗʰ **S75.0** **Injury of** femoral artery

√6ᵗʰ **S75.00** **Unspecified injury of femoral artery**

√7ᵗʰ **S75.001** **Unspecified injury of femoral artery,** right **leg** MCC

√7ᵗʰ **S75.002** **Unspecified injury of femoral artery,** left **leg** MCC

√7ᵗʰ **S75.009** **Unspecified injury of femoral artery, unspecified leg** MCC

√6ᵗʰ **S75.01** **Minor laceration of femoral artery**
Incomplete transection of femoral artery
Laceration of femoral artery NOS
Superficial laceration of femoral artery

√7ᵗʰ **S75.011** **Minor laceration of femoral artery,** right **leg** MCC

√7ᵗʰ **S75.012** **Minor laceration of femoral artery,** left **leg** MCC

√7ᵗʰ **S75.019** **Minor laceration of femoral artery, unspecified leg** MCC

√6ᵗʰ **S75.02** **Major laceration of femoral artery**
Complete transection of femoral artery
Traumatic rupture of femoral artery

√7ᵗʰ **S75.021** **Major laceration of femoral artery,** right **leg** MCC

√7ᵗʰ **S75.022** **Major laceration of femoral artery,** left **leg** MCC

√7ᵗʰ **S75.029** **Major laceration of femoral artery, unspecified leg** MCC

√6ᵗʰ **S75.09** **Other specified injury of femoral artery**

√7ᵗʰ **S75.091** **Other specified injury of femoral artery,** right **leg** MCC

√7ᵗʰ **S75.092** **Other specified injury of femoral artery,** left **leg** MCC

√7ᵗʰ **S75.099** **Other specified injury of femoral artery, unspecified leg** MCC

√5ᵗʰ **S75.1** **Injury of** femoral vein **at hip and thigh level**

√6ᵗʰ **S75.10** **Unspecified injury of femoral vein at hip and thigh level**

√7ᵗʰ **S75.101** **Unspecified injury of femoral vein at hip and thigh level,** right **leg** MCC

√7ᵗʰ **S75.102** **Unspecified injury of femoral vein at hip and thigh level,** left **leg** MCC

√7ᵗʰ **S75.109** **Unspecified injury of femoral vein at hip and thigh level, unspecified leg** MCC

√6ᵗʰ **S75.11** Minor laceration of femoral vein at hip and thigh level

    Incomplete transection of femoral vein at hip and thigh level

    Laceration of femoral vein at hip and thigh level NOS

    Superficial laceration of femoral vein at hip and thigh level

    √7ᵗʰ **S75.111** Minor laceration of femoral vein at hip and thigh level, right leg `MCC`

    √7ᵗʰ **S75.112** Minor laceration of femoral vein at hip and thigh level, left leg `MCC`

    √7ᵗʰ **S75.119** Minor laceration of femoral vein at hip and thigh level, unspecified leg `MCC`

√6ᵗʰ **S75.12** Major laceration of femoral vein at hip and thigh level

    Complete transection of femoral vein at hip and thigh level

    Traumatic rupture of femoral vein at hip and thigh level

    √7ᵗʰ **S75.121** Major laceration of femoral vein at hip and thigh level, right leg `MCC`

    √7ᵗʰ **S75.122** Major laceration of femoral vein at hip and thigh level, left leg `MCC`

    √7ᵗʰ **S75.129** Major laceration of femoral vein at hip and thigh level, unspecified leg `MCC`

√6ᵗʰ **S75.19** Other specified injury of femoral vein at hip and thigh level

    √7ᵗʰ **S75.191** Other specified injury of femoral vein at hip and thigh level, right leg `MCC`

    √7ᵗʰ **S75.192** Other specified injury of femoral vein at hip and thigh level, left leg `MCC`

    √7ᵗʰ **S75.199** Other specified injury of femoral vein at hip and thigh level, unspecified leg `MCC`

√5ᵗʰ **S75.2** Injury of greater saphenous vein at hip and thigh level

    EXCLUDES 1   greater saphenous vein NOS (S85.3)

    √6ᵗʰ **S75.20** Unspecified injury of greater saphenous vein at hip and thigh level

        √7ᵗʰ **S75.201** Unspecified injury of greater saphenous vein at hip and thigh level, right leg `CC`

        √7ᵗʰ **S75.202** Unspecified injury of greater saphenous vein at hip and thigh level, left leg `CC`

        √7ᵗʰ **S75.209** Unspecified injury of greater saphenous vein at hip and thigh level, unspecified leg `CC`

    √6ᵗʰ **S75.21** Minor laceration of greater saphenous vein at hip and thigh level

        Incomplete transection of greater saphenous vein at hip and thigh level

        Laceration of greater saphenous vein at hip and thigh level NOS

        Superficial laceration of greater saphenous vein at hip and thigh level

        √7ᵗʰ **S75.211** Minor laceration of greater saphenous vein at hip and thigh level, right leg `CC`

        √7ᵗʰ **S75.212** Minor laceration of greater saphenous vein at hip and thigh level, left leg `CC`

        √7ᵗʰ **S75.219** Minor laceration of greater saphenous vein at hip and thigh level, unspecified leg `CC`

    √6ᵗʰ **S75.22** Major laceration of greater saphenous vein at hip and thigh level

        Complete transection of greater saphenous vein at hip and thigh level

        Traumatic rupture of greater saphenous vein at hip and thigh level

        √7ᵗʰ **S75.221** Major laceration of greater saphenous vein at hip and thigh level, right leg `CC`

        √7ᵗʰ **S75.222** Major laceration of greater saphenous vein at hip and thigh level, left leg `CC`

        √7ᵗʰ **S75.229** Major laceration of greater saphenous vein at hip and thigh level, unspecified leg `CC`

    √6ᵗʰ **S75.29** Other specified injury of greater saphenous vein at hip and thigh level

        √7ᵗʰ **S75.291** Other specified injury of greater saphenous vein at hip and thigh level, right leg `CC`

        √7ᵗʰ **S75.292** Other specified injury of greater saphenous vein at hip and thigh level, left leg `CC`

        √7ᵗʰ **S75.299** Other specified injury of greater saphenous vein at hip and thigh level, unspecified leg `CC`

√5ᵗʰ **S75.8** Injury of other blood vessels at hip and thigh level

    √6ᵗʰ **S75.80** Unspecified injury of other blood vessels at hip and thigh level

        √7ᵗʰ **S75.801** Unspecified injury of other blood vessels at hip and thigh level, right leg `CC`

        √7ᵗʰ **S75.802** Unspecified injury of other blood vessels at hip and thigh level, left leg `CC`

        √7ᵗʰ **S75.809** Unspecified injury of other blood vessels at hip and thigh level, unspecified leg `CC`

    √6ᵗʰ **S75.81** Laceration of other blood vessels at hip and thigh level

        √7ᵗʰ **S75.811** Laceration of other blood vessels at hip and thigh level, right leg `CC`

        √7ᵗʰ **S75.812** Laceration of other blood vessels at hip and thigh level, left leg `CC`

        √7ᵗʰ **S75.819** Laceration of other blood vessels at hip and thigh level, unspecified leg `CC`

    √6ᵗʰ **S75.89** Other specified injury of other blood vessels at hip and thigh level

        √7ᵗʰ **S75.891** Other specified injury of other blood vessels at hip and thigh level, right leg `CC`

        √7ᵗʰ **S75.892** Other specified injury of other blood vessels at hip and thigh level, left leg `CC`

        √7ᵗʰ **S75.899** Other specified injury of other blood vessels at hip and thigh level, unspecified leg `CC`

√5ᵗʰ **S75.9** Injury of unspecified blood vessel at hip and thigh level

    √6ᵗʰ **S75.90** Unspecified injury of unspecified blood vessel at hip and thigh level

        √7ᵗʰ **S75.901** Unspecified injury of unspecified blood vessel at hip and thigh level, right leg `CC`

        √7ᵗʰ **S75.902** Unspecified injury of unspecified blood vessel at hip and thigh level, left leg `CC`

        √7ᵗʰ **S75.909** Unspecified injury of unspecified blood vessel at hip and thigh level, unspecified leg `CC`

    √6ᵗʰ **S75.91** Laceration of unspecified blood vessel at hip and thigh level

        √7ᵗʰ **S75.911** Laceration of unspecified blood vessel at hip and thigh level, right leg `CC`

        √7ᵗʰ **S75.912** Laceration of unspecified blood vessel at hip and thigh level, left leg `CC`

        √7ᵗʰ **S75.919** Laceration of unspecified blood vessel at hip and thigh level, unspecified leg `CC`

    √6ᵗʰ **S75.99** Other specified injury of unspecified blood vessel at hip and thigh level

        √7ᵗʰ **S75.991** Other specified injury of unspecified blood vessel at hip and thigh level, right leg `CC`

        √7ᵗʰ **S75.992** Other specified injury of unspecified blood vessel at hip and thigh level, left leg `CC`

        √7ᵗʰ **S75.999** Other specified injury of unspecified blood vessel at hip and thigh level, unspecified leg `CC`

☑ Additional Character Required   √x7ᵗʰ Placeholder   Unacceptable PDx   Questionable PDx   Manifestation   Unspecified Dx   H1-H14 HAC   HCC CMS-HCC Dx   HIV HIV Dx

ICD-10-CM 2021   1059

√4ᵗʰ S76 Injury of muscle, fascia and tendon at hip and thigh level

Code also any associated open wound (S71.-)

EXCLUDES 2 injury of muscle, fascia and tendon at lower leg level (S86)

sprain of joint and ligament of hip (S73.1)

TIP: Refer to the Muscle/Tendon table at the beginning of this chapter.

The appropriate 7th character is to be added to each code from category S76.

A   initial encounter

D   subsequent encounter

S   sequela

√5ᵗʰ S76.0 Injury of muscle, fascia and tendon of hip

√6ᵗʰ S76.00 Unspecified injury of muscle, fascia and tendon of hip

√7ᵗʰ **S76.001** Unspecified injury of muscle, fascia and tendon of right hip

√7ᵗʰ **S76.002** Unspecified injury of muscle, fascia and tendon of left hip

√7ᵗʰ **S76.009** Unspecified injury of muscle, fascia and tendon of unspecified hip

√6ᵗʰ S76.01 Strain of muscle, fascia and tendon of hip

√7ᵗʰ **S76.011** Strain of muscle, fascia and tendon of right hip

√7ᵗʰ S76.012 Strain of muscle, fascia and tendon of left hip

√7ᵗʰ **S76.019** Strain of muscle, fascia and tendon of unspecified hip

√6ᵗʰ S76.02 Laceration of muscle, fascia and tendon of hip

√7ᵗʰ **S76.021** Laceration of muscle, fascia and tendon of right hip `CC`

√7ᵗʰ **S76.022** Laceration of muscle, fascia and tendon of left hip `CC`

√7ᵗʰ **S76.029** Laceration of muscle, fascia and tendon of unspecified hip `CC`

√6ᵗʰ S76.09 Other specified injury of muscle, fascia and tendon of hip

√7ᵗʰ S76.091 Other specified injury of muscle, fascia and tendon of right hip

√7ᵗʰ S76.092 Other specified injury of muscle, fascia and tendon of left hip

√7ᵗʰ **S76.099** Other specified injury of muscle, fascia and tendon of unspecified hip

√5ᵗʰ S76.1 Injury of quadriceps muscle, fascia and tendon

Injury of patellar ligament (tendon)

√6ᵗʰ S76.10 Unspecified injury of quadriceps muscle, fascia and tendon

√7ᵗʰ **S76.101** Unspecified injury of right quadriceps muscle, fascia and tendon

√7ᵗʰ **S76.102** Unspecified injury of left quadriceps muscle, fascia and tendon

√7ᵗʰ **S76.109** Unspecified injury of unspecified quadriceps muscle, fascia and tendon

√6ᵗʰ S76.11 Strain of quadriceps muscle, fascia and tendon

√7ᵗʰ **S76.111** Strain of right quadriceps muscle, fascia and tendon

√7ᵗʰ **S76.112** Strain of left quadriceps muscle, fascia and tendon

√7ᵗʰ **S76.119** Strain of unspecified quadriceps muscle, fascia and tendon

√6ᵗʰ S76.12 Laceration of quadriceps muscle, fascia and tendon

√7ᵗʰ **S76.121** Laceration of right quadriceps muscle, fascia and tendon `CC`

√7ᵗʰ **S76.122** Laceration of left quadriceps muscle, fascia and tendon `CC`

√7ᵗʰ **S76.129** Laceration of unspecified quadriceps muscle, fascia and tendon `CC`

√6ᵗʰ S76.19 Other specified injury of quadriceps muscle, fascia and tendon

√7ᵗʰ **S76.191** Other specified injury of right quadriceps muscle, fascia and tendon

√7ᵗʰ S76.192 Other specified injury of left quadriceps muscle, fascia and tendon

√7ᵗʰ **S76.199** Other specified injury of unspecified quadriceps muscle, fascia and tendon

√5ᵗʰ S76.2 Injury of adductor muscle, fascia and tendon of thigh

√6ᵗʰ S76.20 Unspecified injury of adductor muscle, fascia and tendon of thigh

√7ᵗʰ **S76.201** Unspecified injury of adductor muscle, fascia and tendon of right thigh

√7ᵗʰ **S76.202** Unspecified injury of adductor muscle, fascia and tendon of left thigh

√7ᵗʰ **S76.209** Unspecified injury of adductor muscle, fascia and tendon of unspecified thigh

√6ᵗʰ S76.21 Strain of adductor muscle, fascia and tendon of thigh

√7ᵗʰ **S76.211** Strain of adductor muscle, fascia and tendon of right thigh

√7ᵗʰ **S76.212** Strain of adductor muscle, fascia and tendon of left thigh

√7ᵗʰ **S76.219** Strain of adductor muscle, fascia and tendon of unspecified thigh

√6ᵗʰ S76.22 Laceration of adductor muscle, fascia and tendon of thigh

√7ᵗʰ **S76.221** Laceration of adductor muscle, fascia and tendon of right thigh `CC`

√7ᵗʰ **S76.222** Laceration of adductor muscle, fascia and tendon of left thigh `CC`

√7ᵗʰ **S76.229** Laceration of adductor muscle, fascia and tendon of unspecified thigh `CC`

√6ᵗʰ S76.29 Other injury of adductor muscle, fascia and tendon of thigh

√7ᵗʰ **S76.291** Other injury of adductor muscle, fascia and tendon of right thigh

√7ᵗʰ **S76.292** Other injury of adductor muscle, fascia and tendon of left thigh

√7ᵗʰ **S76.299** Other injury of adductor muscle, fascia and tendon of unspecified thigh

√5ᵗʰ S76.3 Injury of muscle, fascia and tendon of the posterior muscle group at thigh level

√6ᵗʰ S76.30 Unspecified injury of muscle, fascia and tendon of the posterior muscle group at thigh level

√7ᵗʰ **S76.301** Unspecified injury of muscle, fascia and tendon of the posterior muscle group at thigh level, right thigh

√7ᵗʰ **S76.302** Unspecified injury of muscle, fascia and tendon of the posterior muscle group at thigh level, left thigh

√7ᵗʰ **S76.309** Unspecified injury of muscle, fascia and tendon of the posterior muscle group at thigh level, unspecified thigh

√6ᵗʰ S76.31 Strain of muscle, fascia and tendon of the posterior muscle group at thigh level

√7ᵗʰ **S76.311** Strain of muscle, fascia and tendon of the posterior muscle group at thigh level, right thigh

√7ᵗʰ **S76.312** Strain of muscle, fascia and tendon of the posterior muscle group at thigh level, left thigh

√7ᵗʰ **S76.319** Strain of muscle, fascia and tendon of the posterior muscle group at thigh level, unspecified thigh

√6ᵗʰ S76.32 Laceration of muscle, fascia and tendon of the posterior muscle group at thigh level

√7ᵗʰ **S76.321** Laceration of muscle, fascia and tendon of the posterior muscle group at thigh level, right thigh `CC`

√7ᵗʰ **S76.322** Laceration of muscle, fascia and tendon of the posterior muscle group at thigh level, left thigh `CC`

√7ᵗʰ **S76.329** Laceration of muscle, fascia and tendon of the posterior muscle group at thigh level, unspecified thigh `CC`

√6ᵗʰ S76.39 Other specified injury of muscle, fascia and tendon of the posterior muscle group at thigh level

√7ᵗʰ **S76.391** Other specified injury of muscle, fascia and tendon of the posterior muscle group at thigh level, right thigh

√7ᵗʰ **S76.392** Other specified injury of muscle, fascia and tendon of the posterior muscle group at thigh level, left thigh

√7ᵗʰ **S76.399** Other specified injury of muscle, fascia and tendon of the posterior muscle group at thigh level, unspecified thigh

√5ᵗʰ S76.8 Injury of other specified muscles, fascia and tendons at thigh level

√6ᵗʰ S76.80 Unspecified injury of other specified muscles, fascia and tendons at thigh level

√7ᵗʰ **S76.801** Unspecified injury of other specified muscles, fascia and tendons at thigh level, right thigh

√7ᵗʰ **S76.802** Unspecified injury of other specified muscles, fascia and tendons at thigh level, left thigh

N Newborn: 0 **P** Pediatric: 0-17 **M** Maternity: 9-64 **A** Adult: 15-124 **MCC** Major Complication/Comorbidity **CC** Complication/Comorbidity **SW** Severe Wound Dx

1060 ICD-10-CM 2021

✓7ᵗʰ S76.809 Unspecified injury of other specified muscles, fascia and tendons at thigh level, unspecified thigh

✓6ᵗʰ S76.81 Strain of other specified muscles, fascia and tendons at thigh level

    ✓7ᵗʰ S76.811 Strain of other specified muscles, fascia and tendons at thigh level, right thigh

    ✓7ᵗʰ S76.812 Strain of other specified muscles, fascia and tendons at thigh level, left thigh

    ✓7ᵗʰ S76.819 Strain of other specified muscles, fascia and tendons at thigh level, unspecified thigh

✓6ᵗʰ S76.82 Laceration of other specified muscles, fascia and tendons at thigh level

    ✓7ᵗʰ S76.821 Laceration of other specified muscles, fascia and tendons at thigh level, right thigh `CC`

    ✓7ᵗʰ S76.822 Laceration of other specified muscles, fascia and tendons at thigh level, left thigh `CC`

    ✓7ᵗʰ S76.829 Laceration of other specified muscles, fascia and tendons at thigh level, unspecified thigh `CC`

✓6ᵗʰ S76.89 Other injury of other specified muscles, fascia and tendons at thigh level

    ✓7ᵗʰ S76.891 Other injury of other specified muscles, fascia and tendons at thigh level, right thigh

    ✓7ᵗʰ S76.892 Other injury of other specified muscles, fascia and tendons at thigh level, left thigh

    ✓7ᵗʰ S76.899 Other injury of other specified muscles, fascia and tendons at thigh level, unspecified thigh

✓5ᵗʰ S76.9 Injury of unspecified muscles, fascia and tendons at thigh level

✓6ᵗʰ S76.90 Unspecified injury of unspecified muscles, fascia and tendons at thigh level

    ✓7ᵗʰ S76.901 Unspecified injury of unspecified muscles, fascia and tendons at thigh level, right thigh

    ✓7ᵗʰ S76.902 Unspecified injury of unspecified muscles, fascia and tendons at thigh level, left thigh

    ✓7ᵗʰ S76.909 Unspecified injury of unspecified muscles, fascia and tendons at thigh level, unspecified thigh

✓6ᵗʰ S76.91 Strain of unspecified muscles, fascia and tendons at thigh level

    ✓7ᵗʰ S76.911 Strain of unspecified muscles, fascia and tendons at thigh level, right thigh

    ✓7ᵗʰ S76.912 Strain of unspecified muscles, fascia and tendons at thigh level, left thigh

    ✓7ᵗʰ S76.919 Strain of unspecified muscles, fascia and tendons at thigh level, unspecified thigh

✓6ᵗʰ S76.92 Laceration of unspecified muscles, fascia and tendons at thigh level

    ✓7ᵗʰ S76.921 Laceration of unspecified muscles, fascia and tendons at thigh level, right thigh `CC`

    ✓7ᵗʰ S76.922 Laceration of unspecified muscles, fascia and tendons at thigh level, left thigh `CC`

    ✓7ᵗʰ S76.929 Laceration of unspecified muscles, fascia and tendons at thigh level, unspecified thigh `CC`

✓6ᵗʰ S76.99 Other specified injury of unspecified muscles, fascia and tendons at thigh level

    ✓7ᵗʰ S76.991 Other specified injury of unspecified muscles, fascia and tendons at thigh level, right thigh

    ✓7ᵗʰ S76.992 Other specified injury of unspecified muscles, fascia and tendons at thigh level, left thigh

    ✓7ᵗʰ S76.999 Other specified injury of unspecified muscles, fascia and tendons at thigh level, unspecified thigh

✓4ᵗʰ S77 Crushing injury of hip and thigh

Use additional code(s) for all associated injuries

EXCLUDES 2 crushing injury of ankle and foot (S97.-)

    crushing injury of lower leg (S87.-)

The appropriate 7th character is to be added to each code from category S77.
A initial encounter
D subsequent encounter
S sequela

✓5ᵗʰ S77.0 Crushing injury of hip

    ✓x7ᵗʰ S77.00 Crushing injury of unspecified hip `CC` `H5`

    ✓x7ᵗʰ S77.01 Crushing injury of right hip `CC` `H5`

    ✓x7ᵗʰ S77.02 Crushing injury of left hip `CC` `H5`

✓5ᵗʰ S77.1 Crushing injury of thigh

    ✓x7ᵗʰ S77.10 Crushing injury of unspecified thigh `CC` `H5`

    ✓x7ᵗʰ S77.11 Crushing injury of right thigh `CC` `H5`

    ✓x7ᵗʰ S77.12 Crushing injury of left thigh `CC` `H5`

✓5ᵗʰ S77.2 Crushing injury of hip with thigh

    ✓x7ᵗʰ S77.20 Crushing injury of unspecified hip with thigh

    ✓x7ᵗʰ S77.21 Crushing injury of right hip with thigh

    ✓x7ᵗʰ S77.22 Crushing injury of left hip with thigh

✓4ᵗʰ S78 Traumatic amputation of hip and thigh

An amputation not identified as partial or complete should be coded to complete

EXCLUDES 1 traumatic amputation of knee (S88.0-)

The appropriate 7th character is to be added to each code from category S78.
A initial encounter
D subsequent encounter
S sequela

✓5ᵗʰ S78.0 Traumatic amputation at hip joint

✓6ᵗʰ S78.01 Complete traumatic amputation at hip joint

    ✓7ᵗʰ S78.011 Complete traumatic amputation at right hip joint `CC` `HCC`

    ✓7ᵗʰ S78.012 Complete traumatic amputation at left hip joint `CC` `HCC`

    ✓7ᵗʰ S78.019 Complete traumatic amputation at unspecified hip joint `CC` `HCC`

✓6ᵗʰ S78.02 Partial traumatic amputation at hip joint

    ✓7ᵗʰ S78.021 Partial traumatic amputation at right hip joint `CC` `HCC`

    ✓7ᵗʰ S78.022 Partial traumatic amputation at left hip joint `CC` `HCC`

    ✓7ᵗʰ S78.029 Partial traumatic amputation at unspecified hip joint `CC` `HCC`

✓5ᵗʰ S78.1 Traumatic amputation at level between hip and knee

EXCLUDES 1 traumatic amputation of knee (S88.0-)

✓6ᵗʰ S78.11 Complete traumatic amputation at level between hip and knee

    ✓7ᵗʰ S78.111 Complete traumatic amputation at level between right hip and knee `CC` `HCC`

    ✓7ᵗʰ S78.112 Complete traumatic amputation at level between left hip and knee `CC` `HCC`

    ✓7ᵗʰ S78.119 Complete traumatic amputation at level between unspecified hip and knee `CC` `HCC`

✓6ᵗʰ S78.12 Partial traumatic amputation at level between hip and knee

    ✓7ᵗʰ S78.121 Partial traumatic amputation at level between right hip and knee `CC` `HCC`

    ✓7ᵗʰ S78.122 Partial traumatic amputation at level between left hip and knee `CC` `HCC`

    ✓7ᵗʰ S78.129 Partial traumatic amputation at level between unspecified hip and knee `CC` `HCC`

✓5ᵗʰ S78.9 Traumatic amputation of hip and thigh, level unspecified

✓6ᵗʰ S78.91 Complete traumatic amputation of hip and thigh, level unspecified

    ✓7ᵗʰ S78.911 Complete traumatic amputation of right hip and thigh, level unspecified `CC` `HCC`

    ✓7ᵗʰ S78.912 Complete traumatic amputation of left hip and thigh, level unspecified `CC` `HCC`

☑ Additional Character Required ✓x7ᵗʰ Placeholder Unacceptable PDx Questionable PDx Manifestation Unspecified Dx H1 - H14 HAC HCC CMS-HCC Dx HIV HIV Dx

ICD-10-CM 2021   1061

Chapter 19. Injury, Poisoning and Certain Other Consequences of External Causes

S78.919–S79.929

√7ᵗʰ **S78.919** Complete traumatic amputation of unspecified hip and thigh, level unspecified   CC HCC

√6ᵗʰ **S78.92** Partial traumatic amputation of hip and thigh, level unspecified

    √7ᵗʰ **S78.921** Partial traumatic amputation of right hip and thigh, level unspecified   CC HCC

    √7ᵗʰ **S78.922** Partial traumatic amputation of left hip and thigh, level unspecified   CC HCC

    √7ᵗʰ **S78.929** Partial traumatic amputation of unspecified hip and thigh, level unspecified   CC HCC

√4ᵗʰ **S79** **Other and unspecified injuries of hip and thigh**

> **NOTE** A fracture not indicated as open or closed should be coded to closed

AHA: 2018,2Q,12; 2018,1Q,3; 2015,3Q,37-39

> The appropriate 7th character is to be added to each code from subcategories S79.0 and S79.1.
> A   initial encounter for closed fracture
> D   subsequent encounter for fracture with routine healing
> G   subsequent encounter for fracture with delayed healing
> K   subsequent encounter for fracture with nonunion
> P   subsequent encounter for fracture with malunion
> S   sequela

√5ᵗʰ **S79.0** **Physeal fracture of upper end of femur**

> **EXCLUDES 1**   apophyseal fracture of upper end of femur (S72.13-)
> nontraumatic slipped upper femoral epiphysis (M93.0-)

AHA: 2019,4Q,56

√6ᵗʰ **S79.00** Unspecified physeal fracture of upper end of femur

    4,6 √7ᵗʰ **S79.001** Unspecified physeal fracture of upper end of right femur   MCC CC H5 HCC

    4,6 √7ᵗʰ **S79.002** Unspecified physeal fracture of upper end of left femur   MCC CC H5 HCC

    4,6 √7ᵗʰ **S79.009** Unspecified physeal fracture of upper end of unspecified femur   MCC CC H5 HCC

√6ᵗʰ **S79.01** Salter-Harris Type I physeal fracture of upper end of femur

    Acute on chronic slipped capital femoral epiphysis (traumatic)
    Acute slipped capital femoral epiphysis (traumatic)
    Capital femoral epiphyseal fracture

> **EXCLUDES 1**   chronic slipped upper femoral epiphysis (nontraumatic) (M93.02-)

    4,6 √7ᵗʰ **S79.011** Salter-Harris Type I physeal fracture of upper end of right femur   MCC CC H5 HCC

    4,6 √7ᵗʰ **S79.012** Salter-Harris Type I physeal fracture of upper end of left femur   MCC CC H5 HCC

    4,6 √7ᵗʰ **S79.019** Salter-Harris Type I physeal fracture of upper end of unspecified femur   MCC CC H5 HCC

√6ᵗʰ **S79.09** Other physeal fracture of upper end of femur

    4,6 √7ᵗʰ **S79.091** Other physeal fracture of upper end of right femur   MCC CC H5 HCC

    4,6 √7ᵗʰ **S79.092** Other physeal fracture of upper end of left femur   MCC CC H5 HCC

    4,6 √7ᵗʰ **S79.099** Other physeal fracture of upper end of unspecified femur   MCC CC H5 HCC

√5ᵗʰ **S79.1** **Physeal fracture of lower end of femur**

AHA: 2019,4Q,56

√6ᵗʰ **S79.10** Unspecified physeal fracture of lower end of femur

    3,6 √7ᵗʰ **S79.101** Unspecified physeal fracture of lower end of right femur   CC H5 HCC

    3,6 √7ᵗʰ **S79.102** Unspecified physeal fracture of lower end of left femur   CC H5 HCC

    3,6 √7ᵗʰ **S79.109** Unspecified physeal fracture of lower end of unspecified femur   CC H5 HCC

√6ᵗʰ **S79.11** Salter-Harris Type I physeal fracture of lower end of femur

    3,6 √7ᵗʰ **S79.111** Salter-Harris Type I physeal fracture of lower end of right femur   CC H5 HCC

    3,6 √7ᵗʰ **S79.112** Salter-Harris Type I physeal fracture of lower end of left femur   CC H5 HCC

    3,6 √7ᵗʰ **S79.119** Salter-Harris Type I physeal fracture of lower end of unspecified femur   CC H5 HCC

√6ᵗʰ **S79.12** Salter-Harris Type II physeal fracture of lower end of femur

    3,6 √7ᵗʰ **S79.121** Salter-Harris Type II physeal fracture of lower end of right femur   CC H5 HCC

    3,6 √7ᵗʰ **S79.122** Salter-Harris Type II physeal fracture of lower end of left femur   CC H5 HCC

    3,6 √7ᵗʰ **S79.129** Salter-Harris Type II physeal fracture of lower end of unspecified femur   CC H5 HCC

√6ᵗʰ **S79.13** Salter-Harris Type III physeal fracture of lower end of femur

    3,6 √7ᵗʰ **S79.131** Salter-Harris Type III physeal fracture of lower end of right femur   CC H5 HCC

    3,6 √7ᵗʰ **S79.132** Salter-Harris Type III physeal fracture of lower end of left femur   CC H5 HCC

    3,6 √7ᵗʰ **S79.139** Salter-Harris Type III physeal fracture of lower end of unspecified femur   CC H5 HCC

√6ᵗʰ **S79.14** Salter-Harris Type IV physeal fracture of lower end of femur

    3,6 √7ᵗʰ **S79.141** Salter-Harris Type IV physeal fracture of lower end of right femur   CC H5 HCC

    3,6 √7ᵗʰ **S79.142** Salter-Harris Type IV physeal fracture of lower end of left femur   CC H5 HCC

    3,6 √7ᵗʰ **S79.149** Salter-Harris Type IV physeal fracture of lower end of unspecified femur   CC H5 HCC

√6ᵗʰ **S79.19** Other physeal fracture of lower end of femur

    3,6 √7ᵗʰ **S79.191** Other physeal fracture of lower end of right femur   CC H5 HCC

    3,6 √7ᵗʰ **S79.192** Other physeal fracture of lower end of left femur   CC H5 HCC

    3,6 √7ᵗʰ **S79.199** Other physeal fracture of lower end of unspecified femur   CC H5 HCC

√5ᵗʰ **S79.8** **Other specified injuries of hip and thigh**

> The appropriate 7th character is to be added to each code in subcategory S79.8.
> A   initial encounter
> D   subsequent encounter
> S   sequela

√6ᵗʰ **S79.81** Other specified injuries of hip

    √7ᵗʰ **S79.811** Other specified injuries of right hip

    √7ᵗʰ **S79.812** Other specified injuries of left hip

    √7ᵗʰ **S79.819** Other specified injuries of unspecified hip

√6ᵗʰ **S79.82** Other specified injuries of thigh

    √7ᵗʰ **S79.821** Other specified injuries of right thigh

    √7ᵗʰ **S79.822** Other specified injuries of left thigh

    √7ᵗʰ **S79.829** Other specified injuries of unspecified thigh

√5ᵗʰ **S79.9** **Unspecified injury of hip and thigh**

> The appropriate 7th character is to be added to each code in subcategory S79.9.
> A   initial encounter
> D   subsequent encounter
> S   sequela

√6ᵗʰ **S79.91** Unspecified injury of hip

    √7ᵗʰ **S79.911** Unspecified injury of right hip

    √7ᵗʰ **S79.912** Unspecified injury of left hip

    √7ᵗʰ **S79.919** Unspecified injury of unspecified hip

√6ᵗʰ **S79.92** Unspecified injury of thigh

    √7ᵗʰ **S79.921** Unspecified injury of right thigh

    √7ᵗʰ **S79.922** Unspecified injury of left thigh

    √7ᵗʰ **S79.929** Unspecified injury of unspecified thigh

N Newborn: 0   P Pediatric: 0-17   M Maternity: 9-64   A Adult: 15-124   MCC Major Complication/Comorbidity   CC Complication/Comorbidity   SW Severe Wound Dx

1062   ICD-10-CM 2021

Injuries to the knee and lower leg (S80-S89)

EXCLUDES 2   burns and corrosions (T20-T32)
frostbite (T33-T34)
injuries of ankle and foot, except fracture of ankle and malleolus (S90-S99)
insect bite or sting, venomous (T63.4)

√4ᵗʰ **S80 Superficial injury of knee and lower leg**

EXCLUDES 2   superficial injury of ankle and foot (S90.-)

The appropriate 7th character is to be added to each code from category S80.
A   initial encounter
D   subsequent encounter
S   sequela

√5ᵗʰ **S80.0 Contusion of knee**
- √x7ᵗʰ **S80.00** Contusion of unspecified knee
- √x7ᵗʰ **S80.01** Contusion of right knee
- √x7ᵗʰ **S80.02** Contusion of left knee

√5ᵗʰ **S80.1 Contusion of lower leg**
- √x7ᵗʰ **S80.10** Contusion of unspecified lower leg
- √x7ᵗʰ **S80.11** Contusion of right lower leg
- √x7ᵗʰ **S80.12** Contusion of left lower leg

√5ᵗʰ **S80.2 Other superficial injuries of knee**
- √6ᵗʰ **S80.21 Abrasion of knee**
  - √7ᵗʰ **S80.211** Abrasion, right knee
  - √7ᵗʰ **S80.212** Abrasion, left knee
  - √7ᵗʰ **S80.219** Abrasion, unspecified knee
- √6ᵗʰ **S80.22 Blister (nonthermal) of knee**
  - √7ᵗʰ **S80.221** Blister (nonthermal), right knee
  - √7ᵗʰ **S80.222** Blister (nonthermal), left knee
  - √7ᵗʰ **S80.229** Blister (nonthermal), unspecified knee
- √6ᵗʰ **S80.24 External constriction of knee**
  - √7ᵗʰ **S80.241** External constriction, right knee
  - √7ᵗʰ **S80.242** External constriction, left knee
  - √7ᵗʰ **S80.249** External constriction, unspecified knee
- √6ᵗʰ **S80.25 Superficial foreign body of knee**
  Splinter in the knee
  - √7ᵗʰ **S80.251** Superficial foreign body, right knee
  - √7ᵗʰ **S80.252** Superficial foreign body, left knee
  - √7ᵗʰ **S80.259** Superficial foreign body, unspecified knee
- √6ᵗʰ **S80.26 Insect bite (nonvenomous) of knee**
  - √7ᵗʰ **S80.261** Insect bite (nonvenomous), right knee
  - √7ᵗʰ **S80.262** Insect bite (nonvenomous), left knee
  - √7ᵗʰ **S80.269** Insect bite (nonvenomous), unspecified knee
- √6ᵗʰ **S80.27 Other superficial bite of knee**
  EXCLUDES 1   open bite of knee (S81.05-)
  - √7ᵗʰ **S80.271** Other superficial bite of right knee
  - √7ᵗʰ **S80.272** Other superficial bite of left knee
  - √7ᵗʰ **S80.279** Other superficial bite of unspecified knee

√5ᵗʰ **S80.8 Other superficial injuries of lower leg**
- √6ᵗʰ **S80.81 Abrasion of lower leg**
  - √7ᵗʰ **S80.811** Abrasion, right lower leg
  - √7ᵗʰ **S80.812** Abrasion, left lower leg
  - √7ᵗʰ **S80.819** Abrasion, unspecified lower leg
- √6ᵗʰ **S80.82 Blister (nonthermal) of lower leg**
  - √7ᵗʰ **S80.821** Blister (nonthermal), right lower leg
  - √7ᵗʰ **S80.822** Blister (nonthermal), left lower leg
  - √7ᵗʰ **S80.829** Blister (nonthermal), unspecified lower leg
- √6ᵗʰ **S80.84 External constriction of lower leg**
  - √7ᵗʰ **S80.841** External constriction, right lower leg
  - √7ᵗʰ **S80.842** External constriction, left lower leg
  - √7ᵗʰ **S80.849** External constriction, unspecified lower leg
- √6ᵗʰ **S80.85 Superficial foreign body of lower leg**
  Splinter in the lower leg
  - √7ᵗʰ **S80.851** Superficial foreign body, right lower leg

- √7ᵗʰ **S80.852** Superficial foreign body, left lower leg
- √7ᵗʰ **S80.859** Superficial foreign body, unspecified lower leg
- √6ᵗʰ **S80.86 Insect bite (nonvenomous) of lower leg**
  - √7ᵗʰ **S80.861** Insect bite (nonvenomous), right lower leg
  - √7ᵗʰ **S80.862** Insect bite (nonvenomous), left lower leg
  - √7ᵗʰ **S80.869** Insect bite (nonvenomous), unspecified lower leg
- √6ᵗʰ **S80.87 Other superficial bite of lower leg**
  EXCLUDES 1   open bite of lower leg (S81.85-)
  - √7ᵗʰ **S80.871** Other superficial bite, right lower leg
  - √7ᵗʰ **S80.872** Other superficial bite, left lower leg
  - √7ᵗʰ **S80.879** Other superficial bite, unspecified lower leg

√5ᵗʰ **S80.9 Unspecified superficial injury of knee and lower leg**
- √6ᵗʰ **S80.91 Unspecified superficial injury of knee**
  - √7ᵗʰ **S80.911** Unspecified superficial injury of right knee
  - √7ᵗʰ **S80.912** Unspecified superficial injury of left knee
  - √7ᵗʰ **S80.919** Unspecified superficial injury of unspecified knee
- √6ᵗʰ **S80.92 Unspecified superficial injury of lower leg**
  - √7ᵗʰ **S80.921** Unspecified superficial injury of right lower leg
  - √7ᵗʰ **S80.922** Unspecified superficial injury of left lower leg
  - √7ᵗʰ **S80.929** Unspecified superficial injury of unspecified lower leg

√4ᵗʰ **S81 Open wound of knee and lower leg**
Code also any associated wound infection
EXCLUDES 1   open fracture of knee and lower leg (S82.-)
traumatic amputation of lower leg (S88.-)
EXCLUDES 2   open wound of ankle and foot (S91.-)

The appropriate 7th character is to be added to each code from category S81.
A   initial encounter
D   subsequent encounter
S   sequela

√5ᵗʰ **S81.0 Open wound of knee**
- √6ᵗʰ **S81.00 Unspecified open wound of knee**
  - √7ᵗʰ **S81.001** Unspecified open wound, right knee
  - √7ᵗʰ **S81.002** Unspecified open wound, left knee
  - √7ᵗʰ **S81.009** Unspecified open wound, unspecified knee
- √6ᵗʰ **S81.01 Laceration without foreign body of knee**
  - √7ᵗʰ **S81.011** Laceration without foreign body, right knee
  - √7ᵗʰ **S81.012** Laceration without foreign body, left knee
  - √7ᵗʰ **S81.019** Laceration without foreign body, unspecified knee
- √6ᵗʰ **S81.02 Laceration with foreign body of knee**
  - √7ᵗʰ **S81.021** Laceration with foreign body, right knee
  - √7ᵗʰ **S81.022** Laceration with foreign body, left knee
  - √7ᵗʰ **S81.029** Laceration with foreign body, unspecified knee
- √6ᵗʰ **S81.03 Puncture wound without foreign body of knee**
  - √7ᵗʰ **S81.031** Puncture wound without foreign body, right knee
  - √7ᵗʰ **S81.032** Puncture wound without foreign body, left knee
  - √7ᵗʰ **S81.039** Puncture wound without foreign body, unspecified knee
- √6ᵗʰ **S81.04 Puncture wound with foreign body of knee**
  - √7ᵗʰ **S81.041** Puncture wound with foreign body, right knee
  - √7ᵗʰ **S81.042** Puncture wound with foreign body, left knee
  - √7ᵗʰ **S81.049** Puncture wound with foreign body, unspecified knee
- √6ᵗʰ **S81.05 Open bite of knee**
  Bite of knee NOS
  EXCLUDES 1   superficial bite of knee (S80.27-)
  - √7ᵗʰ **S81.051** Open bite, right knee

☑ Additional Character Required   √x7ᵗʰ Placeholder   Unacceptable PDx   Questionable PDx   Manifestation   Unspecified Dx   H1-H14 HAC   HCC CMS-HCC Dx   HIV HIV Dx

ICD-10-CM 2021   1063

√7ᵗʰ **S81.052** Open bite, left knee

√7ᵗʰ **S81.059** Open bite, unspecified knee

√5ᵗʰ **S81.8** Open wound of lower leg

√6ᵗʰ **S81.80** Unspecified open wound of lower leg
AHA: 2016,3Q,24

√7ᵗʰ **S81.801** Unspecified open wound, right lower leg

√7ᵗʰ **S81.802** Unspecified open wound, left lower leg

√7ᵗʰ **S81.809** Unspecified open wound, unspecified lower leg

√6ᵗʰ **S81.81** Laceration without foreign body of lower leg

√7ᵗʰ **S81.811** Laceration without foreign body, right lower leg

√7ᵗʰ **S81.812** Laceration without foreign body, left lower leg

√7ᵗʰ **S81.819** Laceration without foreign body, unspecified lower leg

√6ᵗʰ **S81.82** Laceration with foreign body of lower leg

√7ᵗʰ **S81.821** Laceration with foreign body, right lower leg

√7ᵗʰ **S81.822** Laceration with foreign body, left lower leg

√7ᵗʰ **S81.829** Laceration with foreign body, unspecified lower leg

√6ᵗʰ **S81.83** Puncture wound without foreign body of lower leg
AHA: 2016,3Q,24

√7ᵗʰ **S81.831** Puncture wound without foreign body, right lower leg

√7ᵗʰ **S81.832** Puncture wound without foreign body, left lower leg

√7ᵗʰ **S81.839** Puncture wound without foreign body, unspecified lower leg

√6ᵗʰ **S81.84** Puncture wound with foreign body of lower leg
AHA: 2016,3Q,24

√7ᵗʰ **S81.841** Puncture wound with foreign body, right lower leg

√7ᵗʰ **S81.842** Puncture wound with foreign body, left lower leg

√7ᵗʰ **S81.849** Puncture wound with foreign body, unspecified lower leg

√6ᵗʰ **S81.85** Open bite of lower leg
Bite of lower leg NOS
EXCLUDES 1 superficial bite of lower leg (S80.86-, S80.87-)

√7ᵗʰ **S81.851** Open bite, right lower leg

√7ᵗʰ **S81.852** Open bite, left lower leg

√7ᵗʰ **S81.859** Open bite, unspecified lower leg

√4ᵗʰ **S82** Fracture of lower leg, including ankle

NOTE A fracture not indicated as displaced or nondisplaced should be coded to displaced

A fracture not indicated as open or closed should be coded to closed

The open fracture designations are based on the Gustilo open fracture classification.

INCLUDES fracture of malleolus

EXCLUDES 1 traumatic amputation of lower leg (S88.-)

EXCLUDES 2 fracture of foot, except ankle (S92.-)
periprosthetic fracture of prosthetic implant of knee (M97.0-)

AHA: 2018,2Q,12; 2016,1Q,33; 2015,3Q,37-39

DEF: Diaphysis: Central shaft of a long bone.

DEF: Epiphysis: Proximal and distal rounded ends of a long bone, communicates with the joint.

DEF: Metaphysis: Section of a long bone located between the epiphysis and diaphysis at the proximal and distal ends.

DEF: Physis (growth plate): Narrow zone of cartilaginous tissue between the epiphysis and metaphysis at each end of a long bone. In childhood, proliferation of cells in this zone lengthens the bone. As the bone matures, this area thins, ossification eventually fusing into solid bone and growth stops. **Synonyms:** Epiphyseal plate.

The appropriate 7th character is to be added to all codes from category S82 [unless otherwise indicated].
A   initial encounter for closed fracture
B   initial encounter for open fracture type I or II
     initial encounter for open fracture NOS
C   initial encounter for open fracture type IIIA, IIIB, or IIIC
D   subsequent encounter for closed fracture with routine healing
E   subsequent encounter for open fracture type I or II with routine healing
F   subsequent encounter for open fracture type IIIA, IIIB, or IIIC with routine healing
G   subsequent encounter for closed fracture with delayed healing
H   subsequent encounter for open fracture type I or II with delayed healing
J   subsequent encounter for open fracture type IIIA, IIIB, or IIIC with delayed healing
K   subsequent encounter for closed fracture with nonunion
M   subsequent encounter for open fracture type I or II with nonunion
N   subsequent encounter for open fracture type IIIA, IIIB, or IIIC with nonunion
P   subsequent encounter for closed fracture with malunion
Q   subsequent encounter for open fracture type I or II with malunion
R   subsequent encounter for open fracture type IIIA, IIIB, or IIIC with malunion
S   sequela

√5ᵗʰ **S82.0** Fracture of patella
Knee cap

√6ᵗʰ **S82.00** Unspecified fracture of patella

³ √7ᵗʰ **S82.001** Unspecified fracture of right patella — CC H5

³ √7ᵗʰ **S82.002** Unspecified fracture of left patella — CC H5

³ √7ᵗʰ **S82.009** Unspecified fracture of unspecified patella — CC H5

√6ᵗʰ **S82.01** Osteochondral fracture of patella

³ √7ᵗʰ **S82.011** Displaced osteochondral fracture of right patella — CC H5

³ √7ᵗʰ **S82.012** Displaced osteochondral fracture of left patella — CC H5

³ √7ᵗʰ **S82.013** Displaced osteochondral fracture of unspecified patella — CC H5

³ √7ᵗʰ **S82.014** Nondisplaced osteochondral fracture of right patella — CC H5

³ √7ᵗʰ **S82.015** Nondisplaced osteochondral fracture of left patella — CC H5

³ √7ᵗʰ **S82.016** Nondisplaced osteochondral fracture of unspecified patella — CC H5

√6ᵗʰ **S82.02** Longitudinal fracture of patella

³ √7ᵗʰ **S82.021** Displaced longitudinal fracture of right patella — CC H5

³ √7ᵗʰ **S82.022** Displaced longitudinal fracture of left patella — CC H5

³ √7ᵗʰ **S82.023** Displaced longitudinal fracture of unspecified patella — CC H5

³ ✓7ᵗʰ **S82.024** Nondisplaced longitudinal fracture of right patella   CC H5

³ ✓7ᵗʰ **S82.025** Nondisplaced longitudinal fracture of left patella   CC H5

³ ✓7ᵗʰ **S82.026** Nondisplaced longitudinal fracture of unspecified patella   CC H5

✓6ᵗʰ **S82.03** Transverse fracture of patella

  ³ ✓7ᵗʰ **S82.031** Displaced transverse fracture of right patella   CC H5

  ³ ✓7ᵗʰ **S82.032** Displaced transverse fracture of left patella   CC H5

  ³ ✓7ᵗʰ **S82.033** Displaced transverse fracture of unspecified patella   CC H5

  ³ ✓7ᵗʰ **S82.034** Nondisplaced transverse fracture of right patella   CC H5

  ³ ✓7ᵗʰ **S82.035** Nondisplaced transverse fracture of left patella   CC H5

  ³ ✓7ᵗʰ **S82.036** Nondisplaced transverse fracture of unspecified patella   CC H5

✓6ᵗʰ **S82.04** Comminuted fracture of patella

  ³ ✓7ᵗʰ **S82.041** Displaced comminuted fracture of right patella   CC H5

  ³ ✓7ᵗʰ **S82.042** Displaced comminuted fracture of left patella   CC H5

  ³ ✓7ᵗʰ **S82.043** Displaced comminuted fracture of unspecified patella   CC H5

  ³ ✓7ᵗʰ **S82.044** Nondisplaced comminuted fracture of right patella   CC H5

  ³ ✓7ᵗʰ **S82.045** Nondisplaced comminuted fracture of left patella   CC H5

  ³ ✓7ᵗʰ **S82.046** Nondisplaced comminuted fracture of unspecified patella   CC H5

✓6ᵗʰ **S82.09** Other fracture of patella

  ³ ✓7ᵗʰ **S82.091** Other fracture of right patella   CC H5

  ³ ✓7ᵗʰ **S82.092** Other fracture of left patella   CC H5

  ³ ✓7ᵗʰ **S82.099** Other fracture of unspecified patella   CC H5

✓5ᵗʰ **S82.1** Fracture of upper end of tibia

  Fracture of proximal end of tibia

  EXCLUDES 2   fracture of shaft of tibia (S82.2-)

              physeal fracture of upper end of tibia (S89.0-)

✓6ᵗʰ **S82.10** Unspecified fracture of upper end of tibia

  ²,³ ✓7ᵗʰ **S82.101** Unspecified fracture of upper end of right tibia   MCC CC H5

  ²,³ ✓7ᵗʰ **S82.102** Unspecified fracture of upper end of left tibia   MCC CC H5

  ²,³ ✓7ᵗʰ **S82.109** Unspecified fracture of upper end of unspecified tibia   MCC CC H5

✓6ᵗʰ **S82.11** Fracture of tibial spine

  ²,³ ✓7ᵗʰ **S82.111** Displaced fracture of right tibial spine   MCC CC H5

  ²,³ ✓7ᵗʰ **S82.112** Displaced fracture of left tibial spine   MCC CC H5

  ²,³ ✓7ᵗʰ **S82.113** Displaced fracture of unspecified tibial spine   MCC CC H5

  ²,³ ✓7ᵗʰ **S82.114** Nondisplaced fracture of right tibial spine   MCC CC H5

  ²,³ ✓7ᵗʰ **S82.115** Nondisplaced fracture of left tibial spine   MCC CC H5

  ²,³ ✓7ᵗʰ **S82.116** Nondisplaced fracture of unspecified tibial spine   MCC CC H5

✓6ᵗʰ **S82.12** Fracture of lateral condyle of tibia

  ²,³ ✓7ᵗʰ **S82.121** Displaced fracture of lateral condyle of right tibia   MCC CC H5

  ²,³ ✓7ᵗʰ **S82.122** Displaced fracture of lateral condyle of left tibia   MCC CC H5

  ²,³ ✓7ᵗʰ **S82.123** Displaced fracture of lateral condyle of unspecified tibia   MCC CC H5

  ²,³ ✓7ᵗʰ **S82.124** Nondisplaced fracture of lateral condyle of right tibia   MCC CC H5

  ²,³ ✓7ᵗʰ **S82.125** Nondisplaced fracture of lateral condyle of left tibia   MCC CC H5

  ²,³ ✓7ᵗʰ **S82.126** Nondisplaced fracture of lateral condyle of unspecified tibia   MCC CC H5

✓6ᵗʰ **S82.13** Fracture of medial condyle of tibia

  ²,³ ✓7ᵗʰ **S82.131** Displaced fracture of medial condyle of right tibia   MCC CC H5

  ²,³ ✓7ᵗʰ **S82.132** Displaced fracture of medial condyle of left tibia   MCC CC H5

  ²,³ ✓7ᵗʰ **S82.133** Displaced fracture of medial condyle of unspecified tibia   MCC CC H5

  ²,³ ✓7ᵗʰ **S82.134** Nondisplaced fracture of medial condyle of right tibia   MCC CC H5

  ²,³ ✓7ᵗʰ **S82.135** Nondisplaced fracture of medial condyle of left tibia   MCC CC H5

  ²,³ ✓7ᵗʰ **S82.136** Nondisplaced fracture of medial condyle of unspecified tibia   MCC CC H5

✓6ᵗʰ **S82.14** Bicondylar fracture of tibia

  Fracture of tibial plateau NOS

  ²,³ ✓7ᵗʰ **S82.141** Displaced bicondylar fracture of right tibia   MCC CC H5

  ²,³ ✓7ᵗʰ **S82.142** Displaced bicondylar fracture of left tibia   MCC CC H5

  ²,³ ✓7ᵗʰ **S82.143** Displaced bicondylar fracture of unspecified tibia   MCC CC H5

  ²,³ ✓7ᵗʰ **S82.144** Nondisplaced bicondylar fracture of right tibia   MCC CC H5

  ²,³ ✓7ᵗʰ **S82.145** Nondisplaced bicondylar fracture of left tibia   MCC CC H5

  ²,³ ✓7ᵗʰ **S82.146** Nondisplaced bicondylar fracture of unspecified tibia   MCC CC H5

✓6ᵗʰ **S82.15** Fracture of tibial tuberosity

  ²,³ ✓7ᵗʰ **S82.151** Displaced fracture of right tibial tuberosity   MCC CC H5

  ²,³ ✓7ᵗʰ **S82.152** Displaced fracture of left tibial tuberosity   MCC CC H5

  ²,³ ✓7ᵗʰ **S82.153** Displaced fracture of unspecified tibial tuberosity   MCC CC H5

  ²,³ ✓7ᵗʰ **S82.154** Nondisplaced fracture of right tibial tuberosity   MCC CC H5

  ²,³ ✓7ᵗʰ **S82.155** Nondisplaced fracture of left tibial tuberosity   MCC CC H5

  ²,³ ✓7ᵗʰ **S82.156** Nondisplaced fracture of unspecified tibial tuberosity   MCC CC H5

✓6ᵗʰ **S82.16** Torus fracture of upper end of tibia

> The appropriate 7th character is to be added to all codes in subcategory S82.16.
> A   initial encounter for closed fracture
> D   subsequent encounter for fracture with routine healing
> G   subsequent encounter for fracture with delayed healing
> K   subsequent encounter for fracture with nonunion
> P   subsequent encounter for fracture with malunion
> S   sequela

  ³ ✓7ᵗʰ **S82.161** Torus fracture of upper end of right tibia   CC H5

  ³ ✓7ᵗʰ **S82.162** Torus fracture of upper end of left tibia   CC H5

  ³ ✓7ᵗʰ **S82.169** Torus fracture of upper end of unspecified tibia   CC H5

✓6ᵗʰ **S82.19** Other fracture of upper end of tibia

  ²,³ ✓7ᵗʰ **S82.191** Other fracture of upper end of right tibia   MCC CC H5

  ²,³ ✓7ᵗʰ **S82.192** Other fracture of upper end of left tibia   MCC CC H5

  ²,³ ✓7ᵗʰ **S82.199** Other fracture of upper end of unspecified tibia   MCC CC H5

✓5ᵗʰ **S82.2** Fracture of shaft of tibia

✓6ᵗʰ **S82.20** Unspecified fracture of shaft of tibia

  Fracture of tibia NOS

  ²,³ ✓7ᵗʰ **S82.201** Unspecified fracture of shaft of right tibia   MCC CC H5

  ²,³ ✓7ᵗʰ **S82.202** Unspecified fracture of shaft of left tibia   MCC CC H5

  ²,³ ✓7ᵗʰ **S82.209** Unspecified fracture of shaft of unspecified tibia   MCC CC H5

✓6ᵗʰ **S82.22** Transverse fracture of shaft of tibia

  ²,³ ✓7ᵗʰ **S82.221** Displaced transverse fracture of shaft of right tibia   MCC CC H5

  ²,³ ✓7ᵗʰ **S82.222** Displaced transverse fracture of shaft of left tibia   MCC CC H5

✓ Additional Character Required   ✓x7ᵗʰ Placeholder   Unacceptable PDx   Questionable PDx   Manifestation   Unspecified Dx   H1-H14 HAC   HCC CMS-HCC Dx   HIV HIV Dx

2,3 √7th **S82.223** Displaced **transverse fracture of shaft of unspecified tibia** MCC CC H5

2,3 √7th **S82.224** Nondisplaced **transverse fracture of shaft of right tibia** MCC CC H5

2,3 √7th **S82.225** Nondisplaced **transverse fracture of shaft of left tibia** MCC CC H5

2,3 √7th **S82.226** Nondisplaced **transverse fracture of shaft of unspecified tibia** MCC CC H5

√6th **S82.23** Oblique **fracture of shaft of tibia**

2,3 √7th **S82.231** Displaced **oblique fracture of shaft of right tibia** MCC CC H5

2,3 √7th **S82.232** Displaced **oblique fracture of shaft of left tibia** MCC CC H5

2,3 √7th **S82.233** Displaced **oblique fracture of shaft of unspecified tibia** MCC CC H5

2,3 √7th **S82.234** Nondisplaced **oblique fracture of shaft of right tibia** MCC CC H5

2,3 √7th **S82.235** Nondisplaced **oblique fracture of shaft of left tibia** MCC CC H5

2,3 √7th **S82.236** Nondisplaced **oblique fracture of shaft of unspecified tibia** MCC CC H5

√6th **S82.24** Spiral **fracture of shaft of tibia**
　　　　Toddler fracture

2,3 √7th **S82.241** Displaced **spiral fracture of shaft of right tibia** MCC CC H5

2,3 √7th **S82.242** Displaced **spiral fracture of shaft of left tibia** MCC CC H5

2,3 √7th **S82.243** Displaced **spiral fracture of shaft of unspecified tibia** MCC CC H5

2,3 √7th **S82.244** Nondisplaced **spiral fracture of shaft of right tibia** MCC CC H5

2,3 √7th **S82.245** Nondisplaced **spiral fracture of shaft of left tibia** MCC CC H5

2,3 √7th **S82.246** Nondisplaced **spiral fracture of shaft of unspecified tibia** MCC CC H5

√6th **S82.25** Comminuted **fracture of shaft of tibia**

2,3 √7th **S82.251** Displaced **comminuted fracture of shaft of right tibia** MCC CC H5

2,3 √7th **S82.252** Displaced **comminuted fracture of shaft of left tibia** MCC CC H5

2,3 √7th **S82.253** Displaced **comminuted fracture of shaft of unspecified tibia** MCC CC H5

2,3 √7th **S82.254** Nondisplaced **comminuted fracture of shaft of right tibia** MCC CC H5

2,3 √7th **S82.255** Nondisplaced **comminuted fracture of shaft of left tibia** MCC CC H5

2,3 √7th **S82.256** Nondisplaced **comminuted fracture of shaft of unspecified tibia** MCC CC H5

√6th **S82.26** Segmental **fracture of shaft of tibia**

2,3 √7th **S82.261** Displaced **segmental fracture of shaft of right tibia** MCC CC H5

2,3 √7th **S82.262** Displaced **segmental fracture of shaft of left tibia** MCC CC H5

2,3 √7th **S82.263** Displaced **segmental fracture of shaft of unspecified tibia** MCC CC H5

2,3 √7th **S82.264** Nondisplaced **segmental fracture of shaft of right tibia** MCC CC H5

2,3 √7th **S82.265** Nondisplaced **segmental fracture of shaft of left tibia** MCC CC H5

2,3 √7th **S82.266** Nondisplaced **segmental fracture of shaft of unspecified tibia** MCC CC H5

√6th **S82.29** Other **fracture of shaft of tibia**

2,3 √7th **S82.291** Other **fracture of shaft of right tibia** MCC CC H5

2,3 √7th **S82.292** Other **fracture of shaft of left tibia** MCC CC H5

2,3 √7th **S82.299** Other **fracture of shaft of unspecified tibia** MCC CC H5

√5th **S82.3** Fracture of **lower end of tibia**

　　EXCLUDES 1　bimalleolar fracture of lower leg (S82.84-)
　　　　　fracture of medial malleolus alone (S82.5-)
　　　　　Maisonneuve's fracture (S82.86-)
　　　　　pilon fracture of distal tibia (S82.87-)
　　　　　trimalleolar fractures of lower leg (S82.85-)

√6th **S82.30** Unspecified **fracture of lower end of tibia**

3 √7th **S82.301** Unspecified **fracture of lower end of right tibia** CC H5

3 √7th **S82.302** Unspecified **fracture of lower end of tibia** CC H5

3 √7th **S82.309** Unspecified **fracture of lower end of unspecified tibia** CC H5

√6th **S82.31** Torus **fracture of lower end of tibia**

The appropriate 7th character is to be added to all codes in subcategory S82.31.
A　initial encounter for closed fracture
D　subsequent encounter for fracture with routine healing
G　subsequent encounter for fracture with delayed healing
K　subsequent encounter for fracture with nonunion
P　subsequent encounter for fracture with malunion
S　sequela

3 √7th **S82.311** Torus **fracture of lower end of right tibia** CC H5

3 √7th **S82.312** Torus **fracture of lower end of left tibia** CC H5

3 √7th **S82.319** Torus **fracture of lower end of unspecified tibia** CC H5

√6th **S82.39** Other **fracture of lower end of tibia**
　　　　AHA: 2015,1Q,25

3 √7th **S82.391** Other **fracture of lower end of right tibia** CC H5

3 √7th **S82.392** Other **fracture of lower end of left tibia** CC H5

3 √7th **S82.399** Other **fracture of lower end of unspecified tibia** CC H5

√5th **S82.4** Fracture of **shaft of fibula**

　　EXCLUDES 2　fracture of lateral malleolus alone (S82.6-)

√6th **S82.40** Unspecified **fracture of shaft of fibula**

2,4 √7th **S82.401** Unspecified **fracture of shaft of right fibula** MCC CC H5

2,4 √7th **S82.402** Unspecified **fracture of shaft of left fibula** MCC CC H5

2,4 √7th **S82.409** Unspecified **fracture of shaft of unspecified fibula** MCC CC H5

√6th **S82.42** Transverse **fracture of shaft of fibula**

2,4 √7th **S82.421** Displaced **transverse fracture of shaft of right fibula** MCC CC H5

2,4 √7th **S82.422** Displaced **transverse fracture of shaft of left fibula** MCC CC H5

2,4 √7th **S82.423** Displaced **transverse fracture of shaft of unspecified fibula** MCC CC H5

2,4 √7th **S82.424** Nondisplaced **transverse fracture of shaft of right fibula** MCC CC H5

2,4 √7th **S82.425** Nondisplaced **transverse fracture of shaft of left fibula** MCC CC H5

2,4 √7th **S82.426** Nondisplaced **transverse fracture of shaft of unspecified fibula** MCC CC H5

√6th **S82.43** Oblique **fracture of shaft of fibula**

2,4 √7th **S82.431** Displaced **oblique fracture of shaft of right fibula** MCC CC H5

2,4 √7th **S82.432** Displaced **oblique fracture of shaft of left fibula** MCC CC H5

2,4 √7th **S82.433** Displaced **oblique fracture of shaft of unspecified fibula** MCC CC H5

2,4 √7th **S82.434** Nondisplaced **oblique fracture of shaft of right fibula** MCC CC H5

2,4 √7th **S82.435** Nondisplaced **oblique fracture of shaft of left fibula** MCC CC H5

2,4 √7th **S82.436** Nondisplaced **oblique fracture of shaft of unspecified fibula** MCC CC H5

√6th **S82.44** Spiral **fracture of shaft of fibula**

2,4 √7th **S82.441** Displaced **spiral fracture of shaft of right fibula** MCC CC H5

2,4 √7th **S82.442** Displaced **spiral fracture of shaft of left fibula** MCC CC H5

2,4 √7th **S82.443** Displaced **spiral fracture of shaft of unspecified fibula** MCC CC H5

2,4 √7th **S82.444** Nondisplaced **spiral fracture of shaft of right fibula** MCC CC H5

2,4 √7th **S82.445** Nondisplaced **spiral fracture of shaft of left fibula** MCC CC H5

2,4 ✓7ᵗʰ **S82.446** Nondisplaced spiral fracture of shaft of unspecified fibula   MCC CC H5

✓6ᵗʰ **S82.45** Comminuted fracture of shaft of fibula

2,4 ✓7ᵗʰ **S82.451** Displaced comminuted fracture of shaft of right fibula   MCC CC H5

2,4 ✓7ᵗʰ **S82.452** Displaced comminuted fracture of shaft of left fibula   MCC CC H5

2,4 ✓7ᵗʰ **S82.453** Displaced comminuted fracture of shaft of unspecified fibula   MCC CC H5

2,4 ✓7ᵗʰ **S82.454** Nondisplaced comminuted fracture of shaft of right fibula   MCC CC H5

2,4 ✓7ᵗʰ **S82.455** Nondisplaced comminuted fracture of shaft of left fibula   MCC CC H5

2,4 ✓7ᵗʰ **S82.456** Nondisplaced comminuted fracture of shaft of unspecified fibula   MCC CC H5

✓6ᵗʰ **S82.46** Segmental fracture of shaft of fibula

2,4 ✓7ᵗʰ **S82.461** Displaced segmental fracture of shaft of right fibula   MCC CC H5

2,4 ✓7ᵗʰ **S82.462** Displaced segmental fracture of shaft of left fibula   MCC CC H5

2,4 ✓7ᵗʰ **S82.463** Displaced segmental fracture of shaft of unspecified fibula   MCC CC H5

2,4 ✓7ᵗʰ **S82.464** Nondisplaced segmental fracture of shaft of right fibula   MCC CC H5

2,4 ✓7ᵗʰ **S82.465** Nondisplaced segmental fracture of shaft of left fibula   MCC CC H5

2,4 ✓7ᵗʰ **S82.466** Nondisplaced segmental fracture of shaft of unspecified fibula   MCC CC H5

✓6ᵗʰ **S82.49** Other fracture of shaft of fibula

2,4 ✓7ᵗʰ **S82.491** Other fracture of shaft of right fibula   MCC CC H5

2,4 ✓7ᵗʰ **S82.492** Other fracture of shaft of left fibula   MCC CC H5

2,4 ✓7ᵗʰ **S82.499** Other fracture of shaft of unspecified fibula   MCC CC H5

✓5ᵗʰ **S82.5** Fracture of medial malleolus

EXCLUDES 1   pilon fracture of distal tibia (S82.87-)
Salter-Harris type III of lower end of tibia (S89.13-)
Salter-Harris type IV of lower end of tibia (S89.14-)

3 ✓x7ᵗʰ **S82.51** Displaced fracture of medial malleolus of right tibia   CC H5

3 ✓x7ᵗʰ **S82.52** Displaced fracture of medial malleolus of left tibia   CC H5

3 ✓x7ᵗʰ **S82.53** Displaced fracture of medial malleolus of unspecified tibia   CC H5

3 ✓x7ᵗʰ **S82.54** Nondisplaced fracture of medial malleolus of right tibia   CC H5

3 ✓x7ᵗʰ **S82.55** Nondisplaced fracture of medial malleolus of left tibia   CC H5

3 ✓x7ᵗʰ **S82.56** Nondisplaced fracture of medial malleolus of unspecified tibia   CC H5

✓5ᵗʰ **S82.6** Fracture of lateral malleolus

EXCLUDES 1   pilon fracture of distal tibia (S82.87-)

3 ✓x7ᵗʰ **S82.61** Displaced fracture of lateral malleolus of right fibula   CC H5

3 ✓x7ᵗʰ **S82.62** Displaced fracture of lateral malleolus of left fibula   CC H5

3 ✓x7ᵗʰ **S82.63** Displaced fracture of lateral malleolus of unspecified fibula   CC H5

3 ✓x7ᵗʰ **S82.64** Nondisplaced fracture of lateral malleolus of right fibula   CC H5

3 ✓x7ᵗʰ **S82.65** Nondisplaced fracture of lateral malleolus of left fibula   CC H5

3 ✓x7ᵗʰ **S82.66** Nondisplaced fracture of lateral malleolus of unspecified fibula   CC H5

✓5ᵗʰ **S82.8** Other fractures of lower leg

✓6ᵗʰ **S82.81** Torus fracture of upper end of fibula

The appropriate 7th character is to be added to all codes in subcategory S82.81
A   initial encounter for closed fracture
D   subsequent encounter for fracture with routine healing
G   subsequent encounter for fracture with delayed healing
K   subsequent encounter for fracture with nonunion
P   subsequent encounter for fracture with malunion
S   sequela

4 ✓7ᵗʰ **S82.811** Torus fracture of upper end of right fibula   CC

4 ✓7ᵗʰ **S82.812** Torus fracture of upper end of left fibula   CC

4 ✓7ᵗʰ **S82.819** Torus fracture of upper end of unspecified fibula   CC

✓6ᵗʰ **S82.82** Torus fracture of lower end of fibula

The appropriate 7th character is to be added to all codes in subcategory S82.82.
A   initial encounter for closed fracture
D   subsequent encounter for fracture with routine healing
G   subsequent encounter for fracture with delayed healing
K   subsequent encounter for fracture with nonunion
P   subsequent encounter for fracture with malunion
S   sequela

4 ✓7ᵗʰ **S82.821** Torus fracture of lower end of right fibula   CC

4 ✓7ᵗʰ **S82.822** Torus fracture of lower end of left fibula   CC

4 ✓7ᵗʰ **S82.829** Torus fracture of lower end of unspecified fibula   CC

✓6ᵗʰ **S82.83** Other fracture of upper and lower end of fibula
AHA: 2015,1Q,25

2,4 ✓7ᵗʰ **S82.831** Other fracture of upper and lower end of right fibula   MCC CC H5

2,4 ✓7ᵗʰ **S82.832** Other fracture of upper and lower end of left fibula   MCC CC H5

2,4 ✓7ᵗʰ **S82.839** Other fracture of upper and lower end of unspecified fibula   MCC CC H5

Chapter 19. Injury, Poisoning and Certain Other Consequences of External Causes

S82.446–S82.839

√6th **S82.84** **Bimalleolar** fracture of lower leg

Right Bimalleolar Fracture

- Patella
- Tibial plateau
- Tibial tubercle
- Fibula
- Tibia
- Fracture medial malleolus
- Fracture lateral malleolus
- Talus
- Medial (tibial) malleolus
- Lateral (fibular) malleolus

3 √7th **S82.841** Displaced **bimalleolar** fracture of **right** lower leg   CC H5

3 √7th **S82.842** Displaced **bimalleolar** fracture of **left** lower leg   CC H5

3 √7th **S82.843** Displaced **bimalleolar** fracture of **unspecified** lower leg   CC H5

3 √7th **S82.844** Nondisplaced **bimalleolar** fracture of **right** lower leg   CC H5

3 √7th **S82.845** Nondisplaced **bimalleolar** fracture of **left** lower leg   CC H5

3 √7th **S82.846** Nondisplaced **bimalleolar** fracture of **unspecified** lower leg   CC H5

√6th **S82.85** **Trimalleolar** fracture of lower leg

3 √7th **S82.851** Displaced **trimalleolar** fracture of **right** lower leg   CC H5

3 √7th **S82.852** Displaced **trimalleolar** fracture of **left** lower leg   CC H5

3 √7th **S82.853** Displaced **trimalleolar** fracture of **unspecified** lower leg   CC H5

3 √7th **S82.854** Nondisplaced **trimalleolar** fracture of **right** lower leg   CC H5

3 √7th **S82.855** Nondisplaced **trimalleolar** fracture of **left** lower leg   CC H5

3 √7th **S82.856** Nondisplaced **trimalleolar** fracture of **unspecified** lower leg   CC H5

√6th **S82.86** **Maisonneuve's** fracture

2,4 √7th **S82.861** Displaced **Maisonneuve's** fracture of **right** leg   MCC CC H5

2,4 √7th **S82.862** Displaced **Maisonneuve's** fracture of **left** leg   MCC CC H5

2,4 √7th **S82.863** Displaced **Maisonneuve's** fracture of **unspecified** leg   MCC CC H5

2,4 √7th **S82.864** Nondisplaced **Maisonneuve's** fracture of **right** leg   MCC CC H5

2,4 √7th **S82.865** Nondisplaced **Maisonneuve's** fracture of **left** leg   MCC CC H5

2,4 √7th **S82.866** Nondisplaced **Maisonneuve's** fracture of **unspecified** leg   MCC CC H5

√6th **S82.87** **Pilon** fracture of tibia

3 √7th **S82.871** Displaced **pilon** fracture of **right** tibia   CC H5

3 √7th **S82.872** Displaced **pilon** fracture of **left** tibia   CC H5

3 √7th **S82.873** Displaced **pilon** fracture of **unspecified** tibia   CC H5

3 √7th **S82.874** Nondisplaced **pilon** fracture of **right** tibia   CC H5

3 √7th **S82.875** Nondisplaced **pilon** fracture of **left** tibia   CC H5

3 √7th **S82.876** Nondisplaced **pilon** fracture of **unspecified** tibia   CC H5

√6th **S82.89** Other fractures of lower leg

Fracture of ankle NOS

3 √7th **S82.891** Other fracture of **right** lower leg   CC H5

3 √7th **S82.892** Other fracture of **left** lower leg   CC H5

3 √7th **S82.899** Other fracture of **unspecified** lower leg   CC H5

√5th **S82.9** **Unspecified** fracture of lower leg

3 √x7th **S82.90** **Unspecified** fracture of **unspecified** lower leg   CC H5

3 √x7th **S82.91** **Unspecified** fracture of **right** lower leg   CC H5

3 √x7th **S82.92** **Unspecified** fracture of **left** lower leg   CC H5

√4th **S83** **Dislocation and sprain of joints and ligaments of knee**

INCLUDES   avulsion of joint or ligament of knee
laceration of cartilage, joint or ligament of knee
sprain of cartilage, joint or ligament of knee
traumatic hemarthrosis of joint or ligament of knee
traumatic rupture of joint or ligament of knee
traumatic subluxation of joint or ligament of knee
traumatic tear of joint or ligament of knee

Code also any associated open wound

EXCLUDES 1   *derangement of patella (M22.0-M22.3)*
injury of patellar ligament (tendon) (S76.1-)
internal derangement of knee (M23.-)
old dislocation of knee (M23.8X)
pathological dislocation of knee (M24.36)
recurrent dislocation of knee (M22.0)

EXCLUDES 2   ▶*derangement of patella (M22.0-M22.3)*◀
▶*injury of patellar ligament (tendon) (S76.1-)*◀
▶*internal derangement of knee (M23.-)*◀
▶*old dislocation of knee (M24.36)*◀
▶*pathological dislocation of knee (M24.36)*◀
▶*recurrent dislocation of knee (M22.0)*◀
strain of muscle, fascia and tendon of lower leg (S86.-)

The appropriate 7th character is to be added to each code from category S83.
A   initial encounter
D   subsequent encounter
S   sequela

√5th **S83.0** **Subluxation and dislocation of patella**

√6th **S83.00** **Unspecified subluxation and dislocation of patella**

√7th **S83.001** **Unspecified subluxation of right patella**

√7th **S83.002** **Unspecified subluxation of left patella**

√7th **S83.003** **Unspecified subluxation of unspecified patella**

√7th **S83.004** **Unspecified dislocation of right patella**

√7th **S83.005** **Unspecified dislocation of left patella**

√7th **S83.006** **Unspecified dislocation of unspecified patella**

√6th **S83.01** **Lateral subluxation and dislocation of patella**

√7th **S83.011** **Lateral subluxation of right patella**

√7th **S83.012** **Lateral subluxation of left patella**

√7th **S83.013** **Lateral subluxation of unspecified patella**

√7th **S83.014** **Lateral dislocation of right patella**

√7th **S83.015** **Lateral dislocation of left patella**

√7th **S83.016** **Lateral dislocation of unspecified patella**

√6th **S83.09** **Other subluxation and dislocation of patella**

√7th **S83.091** **Other subluxation of right patella**

√7th **S83.092** **Other subluxation of left patella**

√7th **S83.093** **Other subluxation of unspecified patella**

√7th **S83.094** **Other dislocation of right patella**

√7th **S83.095** **Other dislocation of left patella**

√7th **S83.096** **Other dislocation of unspecified patella**

√5th **S83.1** **Subluxation and dislocation of knee**

EXCLUDES 2   *instability of knee prosthesis (T84.022, T84.023)*

√6th **S83.10** **Unspecified subluxation and dislocation of knee**

√7th **S83.101** **Unspecified subluxation of right knee**

√7th **S83.102** **Unspecified subluxation of left knee**

√7th **S83.103** **Unspecified subluxation of unspecified knee**

√7ᵗʰ **S83.104** Unspecified dislocation of right knee

√7ᵗʰ **S83.105** Unspecified dislocation of left knee

√7ᵗʰ **S83.106** Unspecified dislocation of unspecified knee

√6ᵗʰ **S83.11** Anterior subluxation and dislocation of proximal end of tibia

   Posterior subluxation and dislocation of distal end of femur

√7ᵗʰ **S83.111** Anterior subluxation of proximal end of tibia, right knee

√7ᵗʰ **S83.112** Anterior subluxation of proximal end of tibia, left knee

√7ᵗʰ **S83.113** Anterior subluxation of proximal end of tibia, unspecified knee

√7ᵗʰ **S83.114** Anterior dislocation of proximal end of tibia, right knee

√7ᵗʰ **S83.115** Anterior dislocation of proximal end of tibia, left knee

√7ᵗʰ **S83.116** Anterior dislocation of proximal end of tibia, unspecified knee

√6ᵗʰ **S83.12** Posterior subluxation and dislocation of proximal end of tibia

   Anterior dislocation of distal end of femur

√7ᵗʰ **S83.121** Posterior subluxation of proximal end of tibia, right knee

√7ᵗʰ **S83.122** Posterior subluxation of proximal end of tibia, left knee

√7ᵗʰ **S83.123** Posterior subluxation of proximal end of tibia, unspecified knee

√7ᵗʰ **S83.124** Posterior dislocation of proximal end of tibia, right knee

√7ᵗʰ **S83.125** Posterior dislocation of proximal end of tibia, left knee

√7ᵗʰ **S83.126** Posterior dislocation of proximal end of tibia, unspecified knee

√6ᵗʰ **S83.13** Medial subluxation and dislocation of proximal end of tibia

√7ᵗʰ **S83.131** Medial subluxation of proximal end of tibia, right knee

√7ᵗʰ **S83.132** Medial subluxation of proximal end of tibia, left knee

√7ᵗʰ **S83.133** Medial subluxation of proximal end of tibia, unspecified knee

√7ᵗʰ **S83.134** Medial dislocation of proximal end of tibia, right knee

√7ᵗʰ **S83.135** Medial dislocation of proximal end of tibia, left knee

√7ᵗʰ **S83.136** Medial dislocation of proximal end of tibia, unspecified knee

√6ᵗʰ **S83.14** Lateral subluxation and dislocation of proximal end of tibia

√7ᵗʰ **S83.141** Lateral subluxation of proximal end of tibia, right knee

√7ᵗʰ **S83.142** Lateral subluxation of proximal end of tibia, left knee

√7ᵗʰ **S83.143** Lateral subluxation of proximal end of tibia, unspecified knee

√7ᵗʰ **S83.144** Lateral dislocation of proximal end of tibia, right knee

√7ᵗʰ **S83.145** Lateral dislocation of proximal end of tibia, left knee

√7ᵗʰ **S83.146** Lateral dislocation of proximal end of tibia, unspecified knee

√6ᵗʰ **S83.19** Other subluxation and dislocation of knee

√7ᵗʰ **S83.191** Other subluxation of right knee

√7ᵗʰ **S83.192** Other subluxation of left knee

√7ᵗʰ **S83.193** Other subluxation of unspecified knee

√7ᵗʰ **S83.194** Other dislocation of right knee

√7ᵗʰ **S83.195** Other dislocation of left knee

√7ᵗʰ **S83.196** Other dislocation of unspecified knee

√5ᵗʰ **S83.2** Tear of meniscus, current injury

   EXCLUDES 1 old bucket-handle tear (M23.2)

   AHA: 2019,2Q,26

√6ᵗʰ **S83.20** Tear of unspecified meniscus, current injury

   Tear of meniscus of knee NOS

√7ᵗʰ **S83.200** Bucket-handle tear of unspecified meniscus, current injury, right knee

√7ᵗʰ **S83.201** Bucket-handle tear of unspecified meniscus, current injury, left knee

√7ᵗʰ **S83.202** Bucket-handle tear of unspecified meniscus, current injury, unspecified knee

√7ᵗʰ **S83.203** Other tear of unspecified meniscus, current injury, right knee

√7ᵗʰ **S83.204** Other tear of unspecified meniscus, current injury, left knee

√7ᵗʰ **S83.205** Other tear of unspecified meniscus, current injury, unspecified knee

√7ᵗʰ **S83.206** Unspecified tear of unspecified meniscus, current injury, right knee

√7ᵗʰ **S83.207** Unspecified tear of unspecified meniscus, current injury, left knee

√7ᵗʰ **S83.209** Unspecified tear of unspecified meniscus, current injury, unspecified knee

√6ᵗʰ **S83.21** Bucket-handle tear of medial meniscus, current injury

√7ᵗʰ **S83.211** Bucket-handle tear of medial meniscus, current injury, right knee

√7ᵗʰ **S83.212** Bucket-handle tear of medial meniscus, current injury, left knee

√7ᵗʰ **S83.219** Bucket-handle tear of medial meniscus, current injury, unspecified knee

√6ᵗʰ **S83.22** Peripheral tear of medial meniscus, current injury

√7ᵗʰ **S83.221** Peripheral tear of medial meniscus, current injury, right knee

√7ᵗʰ **S83.222** Peripheral tear of medial meniscus, current injury, left knee

√7ᵗʰ **S83.229** Peripheral tear of medial meniscus, current injury, unspecified knee

√6ᵗʰ **S83.23** Complex tear of medial meniscus, current injury

√7ᵗʰ **S83.231** Complex tear of medial meniscus, current injury, right knee

√7ᵗʰ **S83.232** Complex tear of medial meniscus, current injury, left knee

√7ᵗʰ **S83.239** Complex tear of medial meniscus, current injury, unspecified knee

√6ᵗʰ **S83.24** Other tear of medial meniscus, current injury

√7ᵗʰ **S83.241** Other tear of medial meniscus, current injury, right knee

√7ᵗʰ **S83.242** Other tear of medial meniscus, current injury, left knee

√7ᵗʰ **S83.249** Other tear of medial meniscus, current injury, unspecified knee

√6ᵗʰ **S83.25** Bucket-handle tear of lateral meniscus, current injury

√7ᵗʰ **S83.251** Bucket-handle tear of lateral meniscus, current injury, right knee

√7ᵗʰ **S83.252** Bucket-handle tear of lateral meniscus, current injury, left knee

√7ᵗʰ **S83.259** Bucket-handle tear of lateral meniscus, current injury, unspecified knee

√6ᵗʰ **S83.26** Peripheral tear of lateral meniscus, current injury

√7ᵗʰ **S83.261** Peripheral tear of lateral meniscus, current injury, right knee

√7ᵗʰ **S83.262** Peripheral tear of lateral meniscus, current injury, left knee

√7ᵗʰ **S83.269** Peripheral tear of lateral meniscus, current injury, unspecified knee

√6ᵗʰ **S83.27** Complex tear of lateral meniscus, current injury

√7ᵗʰ **S83.271** Complex tear of lateral meniscus, current injury, right knee

√7ᵗʰ **S83.272** Complex tear of lateral meniscus, current injury, left knee

√7ᵗʰ **S83.279** Complex tear of lateral meniscus, current injury, unspecified knee

√6ᵗʰ **S83.28** Other tear of lateral meniscus, current injury

√7ᵗʰ **S83.281** Other tear of lateral meniscus, current injury, right knee

√7ᵗʰ **S83.282** Other tear of lateral meniscus, current injury, left knee

√7ᵗʰ **S83.289** Other tear of lateral meniscus, current injury, unspecified knee

√5ᵗʰ **S83.3** Tear of articular cartilage of knee, current

√x7ᵗʰ **S83.30** Tear of articular cartilage of unspecified knee, current

√x7ᵗʰ **S83.31** Tear of articular cartilage of right knee, current

√x7ᵗʰ **S83.32** Tear of articular cartilage of left knee, current

✔ Additional Character Required   √x7ᵗʰ Placeholder   Unacceptable PDx   Questionable PDx   Manifestation   Unspecified Dx   H1–H14 HAC   HCC CMS-HCC Dx   HIV HIV Dx

ICD-10-CM 2021   1069

Chapter 19. Injury, Poisoning and Certain Other Consequences of External Causes

S83.4–S85.119

√5ᵗʰ **S83.4 Sprain of collateral ligament of knee**

√6ᵗʰ **S83.40 Sprain of unspecified collateral ligament of knee**

√7ᵗʰ **S83.401 Sprain of unspecified collateral ligament of right knee**

√7ᵗʰ **S83.402 Sprain of unspecified collateral ligament of left knee**

√7ᵗʰ **S83.409 Sprain of unspecified collateral ligament of unspecified knee**

√6ᵗʰ **S83.41 Sprain of medial collateral ligament of knee**

     Sprain of tibial collateral ligament

√7ᵗʰ **S83.411 Sprain of medial collateral ligament of right knee**

√7ᵗʰ **S83.412 Sprain of medial collateral ligament of left knee**

√7ᵗʰ **S83.419 Sprain of medial collateral ligament of unspecified knee**

√6ᵗʰ **S83.42 Sprain of lateral collateral ligament of knee**

     Sprain of fibular collateral ligament

√7ᵗʰ **S83.421 Sprain of lateral collateral ligament of right knee**

√7ᵗʰ **S83.422 Sprain of lateral collateral ligament of left knee**

√7ᵗʰ **S83.429 Sprain of lateral collateral ligament of unspecified knee**

√5ᵗʰ **S83.5 Sprain of cruciate ligament of knee**

     AHA: 2016,2Q,3

√6ᵗʰ **S83.50 Sprain of unspecified cruciate ligament of knee**

√7ᵗʰ **S83.501 Sprain of unspecified cruciate ligament of right knee**

√7ᵗʰ **S83.502 Sprain of unspecified cruciate ligament of left knee**

√7ᵗʰ **S83.509 Sprain of unspecified cruciate ligament of unspecified knee**

√6ᵗʰ **S83.51 Sprain of anterior cruciate ligament of knee**

√7ᵗʰ **S83.511 Sprain of anterior cruciate ligament of right knee**

√7ᵗʰ **S83.512 Sprain of anterior cruciate ligament of left knee**

√7ᵗʰ **S83.519 Sprain of anterior cruciate ligament of unspecified knee**

√6ᵗʰ **S83.52 Sprain of posterior cruciate ligament of knee**

√7ᵗʰ **S83.521 Sprain of posterior cruciate ligament of right knee**

√7ᵗʰ **S83.522 Sprain of posterior cruciate ligament of left knee**

√7ᵗʰ **S83.529 Sprain of posterior cruciate ligament of unspecified knee**

√5ᵗʰ **S83.6 Sprain of the superior tibiofibular joint and ligament**

√x7ᵗʰ **S83.60 Sprain of the superior tibiofibular joint and ligament, unspecified knee**

√x7ᵗʰ **S83.61 Sprain of the superior tibiofibular joint and ligament, right knee**

√x7ᵗʰ **S83.62 Sprain of the superior tibiofibular joint and ligament, left knee**

√5ᵗʰ **S83.8 Sprain of other specified parts of knee**

√6ᵗʰ **S83.8X Sprain of other specified parts of knee**

√7ᵗʰ **S83.8X1 Sprain of other specified parts of right knee**

√7ᵗʰ **S83.8X2 Sprain of other specified parts of left knee**

√7ᵗʰ **S83.8X9 Sprain of other specified parts of unspecified knee**

√5ᵗʰ **S83.9 Sprain of unspecified site of knee**

√x7ᵗʰ **S83.90 Sprain of unspecified site of unspecified knee**

√x7ᵗʰ **S83.91 Sprain of unspecified site of right knee**

√x7ᵗʰ **S83.92 Sprain of unspecified site of left knee**

√4ᵗʰ **S84 Injury of nerves at lower leg level**

     Code also any associated open wound (S81.-)

     EXCLUDES 2   *injury of nerves at ankle and foot level (S94.-)*

The appropriate 7th character is to be added to each code from category S84.
A   initial encounter
D   subsequent encounter
S   sequela

√5ᵗʰ **S84.0 Injury of tibial nerve at lower leg level**

√x7ᵗʰ **S84.00 Injury of tibial nerve at lower leg level, unspecified leg**

√x7ᵗʰ **S84.01 Injury of tibial nerve at lower leg level, right leg**

√x7ᵗʰ **S84.02 Injury of tibial nerve at lower leg level, left leg**

√5ᵗʰ **S84.1 Injury of peroneal nerve at lower leg level**

√x7ᵗʰ **S84.10 Injury of peroneal nerve at lower leg level, unspecified leg**

√x7ᵗʰ **S84.11 Injury of peroneal nerve at lower leg level, right leg**

√x7ᵗʰ **S84.12 Injury of peroneal nerve at lower leg level, left leg**

√5ᵗʰ **S84.2 Injury of cutaneous sensory nerve at lower leg level**

√x7ᵗʰ **S84.20 Injury of cutaneous sensory nerve at lower leg level, unspecified leg**

√x7ᵗʰ **S84.21 Injury of cutaneous sensory nerve at lower leg level, right leg**

√x7ᵗʰ **S84.22 Injury of cutaneous sensory nerve at lower leg level, left leg**

√5ᵗʰ **S84.8 Injury of other nerves at lower leg level**

√6ᵗʰ **S84.80 Injury of other nerves at lower leg level**

√7ᵗʰ **S84.801 Injury of other nerves at lower leg level, right leg**

√7ᵗʰ **S84.802 Injury of other nerves at lower leg level, left leg**

√7ᵗʰ **S84.809 Injury of other nerves at lower leg level, unspecified leg**

√5ᵗʰ **S84.9 Injury of unspecified nerve at lower leg level**

√x7ᵗʰ **S84.90 Injury of unspecified nerve at lower leg level, unspecified leg**

√x7ᵗʰ **S84.91 Injury of unspecified nerve at lower leg level, right leg**

√x7ᵗʰ **S84.92 Injury of unspecified nerve at lower leg level, left leg**

√4ᵗʰ **S85 Injury of blood vessels at lower leg level**

     Code also any associated open wound (S81.-)

     EXCLUDES 2   *injury of blood vessels at ankle and foot level (S95.-)*

The appropriate 7th character is to be added to each code from category S85.
A   initial encounter
D   subsequent encounter
S   sequela

√5ᵗʰ **S85.0 Injury of popliteal artery**

√6ᵗʰ **S85.00 Unspecified injury of popliteal artery**

√7ᵗʰ **S85.001 Unspecified injury of popliteal artery, right leg**   MCC

√7ᵗʰ **S85.002 Unspecified injury of popliteal artery, left leg**   MCC

√7ᵗʰ **S85.009 Unspecified injury of popliteal artery, unspecified leg**   MCC

√6ᵗʰ **S85.01 Laceration of popliteal artery**

√7ᵗʰ **S85.011 Laceration of popliteal artery, right leg**   MCC

√7ᵗʰ **S85.012 Laceration of popliteal artery, left leg**   MCC

√7ᵗʰ **S85.019 Laceration of popliteal artery, unspecified leg**   MCC

√6ᵗʰ **S85.09 Other specified injury of popliteal artery**

√7ᵗʰ **S85.091 Other specified injury of popliteal artery, right leg**   MCC

√7ᵗʰ **S85.092 Other specified injury of popliteal artery, left leg**   MCC

√7ᵗʰ **S85.099 Other specified injury of popliteal artery, unspecified leg**   MCC

√5ᵗʰ **S85.1 Injury of tibial artery**

√6ᵗʰ **S85.10 Unspecified injury of unspecified tibial artery**

     Injury of tibial artery NOS

√7ᵗʰ **S85.101 Unspecified injury of unspecified tibial artery, right leg**   CC

√7ᵗʰ **S85.102 Unspecified injury of unspecified tibial artery, left leg**   CC

√7ᵗʰ **S85.109 Unspecified injury of unspecified tibial artery, unspecified leg**   CC

√6ᵗʰ **S85.11 Laceration of unspecified tibial artery**

√7ᵗʰ **S85.111 Laceration of unspecified tibial artery, right leg**   CC

√7ᵗʰ **S85.112 Laceration of unspecified tibial artery, left leg**   CC

√7ᵗʰ **S85.119 Laceration of unspecified tibial artery, unspecified leg**   CC

√6ᵗʰ **S85.12 Other specified injury of unspecified tibial artery**

    √7ᵗʰ **S85.121 Other specified injury of unspecified tibial artery, right leg** `CC`

    √7ᵗʰ **S85.122 Other specified injury of unspecified tibial artery, left leg** `CC`

    √7ᵗʰ **S85.129 Other specified injury of unspecified tibial artery, unspecified leg** `CC`

√6ᵗʰ **S85.13 Unspecified injury of anterior tibial artery**

    √7ᵗʰ **S85.131 Unspecified injury of anterior tibial artery, right leg** `CC`

    √7ᵗʰ **S85.132 Unspecified injury of anterior tibial artery, left leg** `CC`

    √7ᵗʰ **S85.139 Unspecified injury of anterior tibial artery, unspecified leg** `CC`

√6ᵗʰ **S85.14 Laceration of anterior tibial artery**

    √7ᵗʰ **S85.141 Laceration of anterior tibial artery, right leg** `CC`

    √7ᵗʰ **S85.142 Laceration of anterior tibial artery, left leg** `CC`

    √7ᵗʰ **S85.149 Laceration of anterior tibial artery, unspecified leg** `CC`

√6ᵗʰ **S85.15 Other specified injury of anterior tibial artery**

    √7ᵗʰ **S85.151 Other specified injury of anterior tibial artery, right leg** `CC`

    √7ᵗʰ **S85.152 Other specified injury of anterior tibial artery, left leg** `CC`

    √7ᵗʰ **S85.159 Other specified injury of anterior tibial artery, unspecified leg** `CC`

√6ᵗʰ **S85.16 Unspecified injury of posterior tibial artery**

    √7ᵗʰ **S85.161 Unspecified injury of posterior tibial artery, right leg** `CC`

    √7ᵗʰ **S85.162 Unspecified injury of posterior tibial artery, left leg** `CC`

    √7ᵗʰ **S85.169 Unspecified injury of posterior tibial artery, unspecified leg** `CC`

√6ᵗʰ **S85.17 Laceration of posterior tibial artery**

    √7ᵗʰ **S85.171 Laceration of posterior tibial artery, right leg** `CC`

    √7ᵗʰ **S85.172 Laceration of posterior tibial artery, left leg** `CC`

    √7ᵗʰ **S85.179 Laceration of posterior tibial artery, unspecified leg** `CC`

√6ᵗʰ **S85.18 Other specified injury of posterior tibial artery**

    √7ᵗʰ **S85.181 Other specified injury of posterior tibial artery, right leg** `CC`

    √7ᵗʰ **S85.182 Other specified injury of posterior tibial artery, left leg** `CC`

    √7ᵗʰ **S85.189 Other specified injury of posterior tibial artery, unspecified leg** `CC`

√5ᵗʰ **S85.2 Injury of peroneal artery**

√6ᵗʰ **S85.20 Unspecified injury of peroneal artery**

    √7ᵗʰ **S85.201 Unspecified injury of peroneal artery, right leg** `CC`

    √7ᵗʰ **S85.202 Unspecified injury of peroneal artery, left leg** `CC`

    √7ᵗʰ **S85.209 Unspecified injury of peroneal artery, unspecified leg** `CC`

√6ᵗʰ **S85.21 Laceration of peroneal artery**

    √7ᵗʰ **S85.211 Laceration of peroneal artery, right leg** `CC`

    √7ᵗʰ **S85.212 Laceration of peroneal artery, left leg** `CC`

    √7ᵗʰ **S85.219 Laceration of peroneal artery, unspecified leg** `CC`

√6ᵗʰ **S85.29 Other specified injury of peroneal artery**

    √7ᵗʰ **S85.291 Other specified injury of peroneal artery, right leg** `CC`

    √7ᵗʰ **S85.292 Other specified injury of peroneal artery, left leg** `CC`

    √7ᵗʰ **S85.299 Other specified injury of peroneal artery, unspecified leg** `CC`

√6ᵗʰ **S85.3 Injury of greater saphenous vein at lower leg level**

    Injury of greater saphenous vein NOS
    Injury of saphenous vein NOS

√6ᵗʰ **S85.30 Unspecified injury of greater saphenous vein at lower leg level**

    √7ᵗʰ **S85.301 Unspecified injury of greater saphenous vein at lower leg level, right leg** `CC`

    √7ᵗʰ **S85.302 Unspecified injury of greater saphenous vein at lower leg level, left leg** `CC`

    √7ᵗʰ **S85.309 Unspecified injury of greater saphenous vein at lower leg level, unspecified leg** `CC`

√6ᵗʰ **S85.31 Laceration of greater saphenous vein at lower leg level**

    √7ᵗʰ **S85.311 Laceration of greater saphenous vein at lower leg level, right leg** `CC`

    √7ᵗʰ **S85.312 Laceration of greater saphenous vein at lower leg level, left leg** `CC`

    √7ᵗʰ **S85.319 Laceration of greater saphenous vein at lower leg level, unspecified leg** `CC`

√6ᵗʰ **S85.39 Other specified injury of greater saphenous vein at lower leg level**

    √7ᵗʰ **S85.391 Other specified injury of greater saphenous vein at lower leg level, right leg** `CC`

    √7ᵗʰ **S85.392 Other specified injury of greater saphenous vein at lower leg level, left leg** `CC`

    √7ᵗʰ **S85.399 Other specified injury of greater saphenous vein at lower leg level, unspecified leg** `CC`

√5ᵗʰ **S85.4 Injury of lesser saphenous vein at lower leg level**

√6ᵗʰ **S85.40 Unspecified injury of lesser saphenous vein at lower leg level**

    √7ᵗʰ **S85.401 Unspecified injury of lesser saphenous vein at lower leg level, right leg** `CC`

    √7ᵗʰ **S85.402 Unspecified injury of lesser saphenous vein at lower leg level, left leg** `CC`

    √7ᵗʰ **S85.409 Unspecified injury of lesser saphenous vein at lower leg level, unspecified leg** `CC`

√6ᵗʰ **S85.41 Laceration of lesser saphenous vein at lower leg level**

    √7ᵗʰ **S85.411 Laceration of lesser saphenous vein at lower leg level, right leg** `CC`

    √7ᵗʰ **S85.412 Laceration of lesser saphenous vein at lower leg level, left leg** `CC`

    √7ᵗʰ **S85.419 Laceration of lesser saphenous vein at lower leg level, unspecified leg** `CC`

√6ᵗʰ **S85.49 Other specified injury of lesser saphenous vein at lower leg level**

    √7ᵗʰ **S85.491 Other specified injury of lesser saphenous vein at lower leg level, right leg** `CC`

    √7ᵗʰ **S85.492 Other specified injury of lesser saphenous vein at lower leg level, left leg** `CC`

    √7ᵗʰ **S85.499 Other specified injury of lesser saphenous vein at lower leg level, unspecified leg** `CC`

√5ᵗʰ **S85.5 Injury of popliteal vein**

√6ᵗʰ **S85.50 Unspecified injury of popliteal vein**

    √7ᵗʰ **S85.501 Unspecified injury of popliteal vein, right leg** `MCC`

    √7ᵗʰ **S85.502 Unspecified injury of popliteal vein, left leg** `MCC`

    √7ᵗʰ **S85.509 Unspecified injury of popliteal vein, unspecified leg** `MCC`

√6ᵗʰ **S85.51 Laceration of popliteal vein**

    √7ᵗʰ **S85.511 Laceration of popliteal vein, right leg** `MCC`

    √7ᵗʰ **S85.512 Laceration of popliteal vein, left leg** `MCC`

    √7ᵗʰ **S85.519 Laceration of popliteal vein, unspecified leg** `MCC`

√6ᵗʰ **S85.59 Other specified injury of popliteal vein**

    √7ᵗʰ **S85.591 Other specified injury of popliteal vein, right leg** `MCC`

    √7ᵗʰ **S85.592 Other specified injury of popliteal vein, left leg** `MCC`

    √7ᵗʰ **S85.599 Other specified injury of popliteal vein, unspecified leg** `MCC`

√5ᵗʰ **S85.8 Injury of other blood vessels at lower leg level**

√6ᵗʰ **S85.80 Unspecified injury of other blood vessels at lower leg level**

    √7ᵗʰ **S85.801 Unspecified injury of other blood vessels at lower leg level, right leg** `CC`

    √7ᵗʰ **S85.802 Unspecified injury of other blood vessels at lower leg level, left leg** `CC`

☑ Additional Character Required √x7ᵗʰ Placeholder Unacceptable PDx Questionable PDx Manifestation Unspecified Dx H1 - H14 HAC HCC CMS-HCC Dx HIV HIV Dx

Chapter 19. Injury, Poisoning and Certain Other Consequences of External Causes

S85.809–S86.222

√7ᵗʰ **S85.809** Unspecified injury of other blood vessels at lower leg level, unspecified leg   cc

√6ᵗʰ **S85.81** Laceration of other blood vessels at lower leg level

√7ᵗʰ **S85.811** Laceration of other blood vessels at lower leg level, right leg   cc

√7ᵗʰ **S85.812** Laceration of other blood vessels at lower leg level, left leg   cc

√7ᵗʰ **S85.819** Laceration of other blood vessels at lower leg level, unspecified leg   cc

√6ᵗʰ **S85.89** Other specified injury of other blood vessels at lower leg level

√7ᵗʰ **S85.891** Other specified injury of other blood vessels at lower leg level, right leg   cc

√7ᵗʰ **S85.892** Other specified injury of other blood vessels at lower leg level, left leg   cc

√7ᵗʰ **S85.899** Other specified injury of other blood vessels at lower leg level, unspecified leg   cc

√5ᵗʰ **S85.9** Injury of unspecified blood vessel at lower leg level

√6ᵗʰ **S85.90** Unspecified injury of unspecified blood vessel at lower leg level

√7ᵗʰ **S85.901** Unspecified injury of unspecified blood vessel at lower leg level, right leg   cc

√7ᵗʰ **S85.902** Unspecified injury of unspecified blood vessel at lower leg level, left leg   cc

√7ᵗʰ **S85.909** Unspecified injury of unspecified blood vessel at lower leg level, unspecified leg   cc

√6ᵗʰ **S85.91** Laceration of unspecified blood vessel at lower leg level

√7ᵗʰ **S85.911** Laceration of unspecified blood vessel at lower leg level, right leg   cc

√7ᵗʰ **S85.912** Laceration of unspecified blood vessel at lower leg level, left leg   cc

√7ᵗʰ **S85.919** Laceration of unspecified blood vessel at lower leg level, unspecified leg   cc

√6ᵗʰ **S85.99** Other specified injury of unspecified blood vessel at lower leg level

√7ᵗʰ **S85.991** Other specified injury of unspecified blood vessel at lower leg level, right leg   cc

√7ᵗʰ **S85.992** Other specified injury of unspecified blood vessel at lower leg level, left leg   cc

√7ᵗʰ **S85.999** Other specified injury of unspecified blood vessel at lower leg level, unspecified leg   cc

√4ᵗʰ **S86** **Injury of muscle, fascia and tendon at lower leg level**

Code also any associated open wound (S81.-)

EXCLUDES 2   *injury of muscle, fascia and tendon at ankle (S96.-)*
injury of patellar ligament (tendon) (S76.1-)
sprain of joints and ligaments of knee (S83.-)

TIP: Refer to the Muscle/Tendon table at the beginning of this chapter.

The appropriate 7th character is to be added to each code from category S86.
A   initial encounter
D   subsequent encounter
S   sequela

√5ᵗʰ **S86.0** Injury of Achilles tendon

√6ᵗʰ **S86.00** Unspecified injury of Achilles tendon

√7ᵗʰ **S86.001** Unspecified injury of right Achilles tendon

√7ᵗʰ **S86.002** Unspecified injury of left Achilles tendon

√7ᵗʰ **S86.009** Unspecified injury of unspecified Achilles tendon

√6ᵗʰ **S86.01** Strain of Achilles tendon

√7ᵗʰ **S86.011** Strain of right Achilles tendon

√7ᵗʰ **S86.012** Strain of left Achilles tendon

√7ᵗʰ **S86.019** Strain of unspecified Achilles tendon

√6ᵗʰ **S86.02** Laceration of Achilles tendon

√7ᵗʰ **S86.021** Laceration of right Achilles tendon   cc

√7ᵗʰ **S86.022** Laceration of left Achilles tendon   cc

√7ᵗʰ **S86.029** Laceration of unspecified Achilles tendon   cc

√6ᵗʰ **S86.09** Other specified injury of Achilles tendon

√7ᵗʰ **S86.091** Other specified injury of right Achilles tendon

√7ᵗʰ **S86.092** Other specified injury of left Achilles tendon

√7ᵗʰ **S86.099** Other specified injury of unspecified Achilles tendon

√5ᵗʰ **S86.1** Injury of other muscle(s) and tendon(s) of posterior muscle group at lower leg level

√6ᵗʰ **S86.10** Unspecified injury of other muscle(s) and tendon(s) of posterior muscle group at lower leg level

√7ᵗʰ **S86.101** Unspecified injury of other muscle(s) and tendon(s) of posterior muscle group at lower leg level, right leg

√7ᵗʰ **S86.102** Unspecified injury of other muscle(s) and tendon(s) of posterior muscle group at lower leg level, left leg

√7ᵗʰ **S86.109** Unspecified injury of other muscle(s) and tendon(s) of posterior muscle group at lower leg level, unspecified leg

√6ᵗʰ **S86.11** Strain of other muscle(s) and tendon(s) of posterior muscle group at lower leg level

√7ᵗʰ **S86.111** Strain of other muscle(s) and tendon(s) of posterior muscle group at lower leg level, right leg

√7ᵗʰ **S86.112** Strain of other muscle(s) and tendon(s) of posterior muscle group at lower leg level, left leg

√7ᵗʰ **S86.119** Strain of other muscle(s) and tendon(s) of posterior muscle group at lower leg level, unspecified leg

√6ᵗʰ **S86.12** Laceration of other muscle(s) and tendon(s) of posterior muscle group at lower leg level

√7ᵗʰ **S86.121** Laceration of other muscle(s) and tendon(s) of posterior muscle group at lower leg level, right leg   cc

√7ᵗʰ **S86.122** Laceration of other muscle(s) and tendon(s) of posterior muscle group at lower leg level, left leg   cc

√7ᵗʰ **S86.129** Laceration of other muscle(s) and tendon(s) of posterior muscle group at lower leg level, unspecified leg   cc

√6ᵗʰ **S86.19** Other injury of other muscle(s) and tendon(s) of posterior muscle group at lower leg level

√7ᵗʰ **S86.191** Other injury of other muscle(s) and tendon(s) of posterior muscle group at lower leg level, right leg

√7ᵗʰ **S86.192** Other injury of other muscle(s) and tendon(s) of posterior muscle group at lower leg level, left leg

√7ᵗʰ **S86.199** Other injury of other muscle(s) and tendon(s) of posterior muscle group at lower leg level, unspecified leg

√5ᵗʰ **S86.2** Injury of muscle(s) and tendon(s) of anterior muscle group at lower leg level

√6ᵗʰ **S86.20** Unspecified injury of muscle(s) and tendon(s) of anterior muscle group at lower leg level

√7ᵗʰ **S86.201** Unspecified injury of muscle(s) and tendon(s) of anterior muscle group at lower leg level, right leg

√7ᵗʰ **S86.202** Unspecified injury of muscle(s) and tendon(s) of anterior muscle group at lower leg level, left leg

√7ᵗʰ **S86.209** Unspecified injury of muscle(s) and tendon(s) of anterior muscle group at lower leg level, unspecified leg

√6ᵗʰ **S86.21** Strain of muscle(s) and tendon(s) of anterior muscle group at lower leg level

√7ᵗʰ **S86.211** Strain of muscle(s) and tendon(s) of anterior muscle group at lower leg level, right leg

√7ᵗʰ **S86.212** Strain of muscle(s) and tendon(s) of anterior muscle group at lower leg level, left leg

√7ᵗʰ **S86.219** Strain of muscle(s) and tendon(s) of anterior muscle group at lower leg level, unspecified leg

√6ᵗʰ **S86.22** Laceration of muscle(s) and tendon(s) of anterior muscle group at lower leg level

√7ᵗʰ **S86.221** Laceration of muscle(s) and tendon(s) of anterior muscle group at lower leg level, right leg   cc

√7ᵗʰ **S86.222** Laceration of muscle(s) and tendon(s) of anterior muscle group at lower leg level, left leg   cc

N Newborn: 0   P Pediatric: 0-17   M Maternity: 9-64   A Adult: 15-124   MCC Major Complication/Comorbidity   CC Complication/Comorbidity   SW Severe Wound Dx

1072   ICD-10-CM 2021

√7ᵗʰ **S86.229** Laceration of muscle(s) and tendon(s) of anterior muscle group at lower leg level, unspecified leg   CC

√6ᵗʰ **S86.29** Other injury of muscle(s) and tendon(s) of anterior muscle group at lower leg level

√7ᵗʰ **S86.291** Other injury of muscle(s) and tendon(s) of anterior muscle group at lower leg level, right leg

√7ᵗʰ **S86.292** Other injury of muscle(s) and tendon(s) of anterior muscle group at lower leg level, left leg

√7ᵗʰ **S86.299** Other injury of muscle(s) and tendon(s) of anterior muscle group at lower leg level, unspecified leg

√5ᵗʰ **S86.3** Injury of muscle(s) and tendon(s) of peroneal muscle group at lower leg level

√6ᵗʰ **S86.30** Unspecified injury of muscle(s) and tendon(s) of peroneal muscle group at lower leg level

√7ᵗʰ **S86.301** Unspecified injury of muscle(s) and tendon(s) of peroneal muscle group at lower leg level, right leg

√7ᵗʰ **S86.302** Unspecified injury of muscle(s) and tendon(s) of peroneal muscle group at lower leg level, left leg

√7ᵗʰ **S86.309** Unspecified injury of muscle(s) and tendon(s) of peroneal muscle group at lower leg level, unspecified leg

√6ᵗʰ **S86.31** Strain of muscle(s) and tendon(s) of peroneal muscle group at lower leg level

√7ᵗʰ **S86.311** Strain of muscle(s) and tendon(s) of peroneal muscle group at lower leg level, right leg

√7ᵗʰ **S86.312** Strain of muscle(s) and tendon(s) of peroneal muscle group at lower leg level, left leg

√7ᵗʰ **S86.319** Strain of muscle(s) and tendon(s) of peroneal muscle group at lower leg level, unspecified leg

√6ᵗʰ **S86.32** Laceration of muscle(s) and tendon(s) of peroneal muscle group at lower leg level

√7ᵗʰ **S86.321** Laceration of muscle(s) and tendon(s) of peroneal muscle group at lower leg level, right leg   CC

√7ᵗʰ **S86.322** Laceration of muscle(s) and tendon(s) of peroneal muscle group at lower leg level, left leg   CC

√7ᵗʰ **S86.329** Laceration of muscle(s) and tendon(s) of peroneal muscle group at lower leg level, unspecified leg   CC

√6ᵗʰ **S86.39** Other injury of muscle(s) and tendon(s) of peroneal muscle group at lower leg level

√7ᵗʰ **S86.391** Other injury of muscle(s) and tendon(s) of peroneal muscle group at lower leg level, right leg

√7ᵗʰ **S86.392** Other injury of muscle(s) and tendon(s) of peroneal muscle group at lower leg level, left leg

√7ᵗʰ **S86.399** Other injury of muscle(s) and tendon(s) of peroneal muscle group at lower leg level, unspecified leg

√5ᵗʰ **S86.8** Injury of other muscles and tendons at lower leg level

√6ᵗʰ **S86.80** Unspecified injury of other muscles and tendons at lower leg level

√7ᵗʰ **S86.801** Unspecified injury of other muscle(s) and tendon(s) at lower leg level, right leg

√7ᵗʰ **S86.802** Unspecified injury of other muscle(s) and tendon(s) at lower leg level, left leg

√7ᵗʰ **S86.809** Unspecified injury of other muscle(s) and tendon(s) at lower leg level, unspecified leg

√6ᵗʰ **S86.81** Strain of other muscles and tendons at lower leg level

√7ᵗʰ **S86.811** Strain of other muscle(s) and tendon(s) at lower leg level, right leg

√7ᵗʰ **S86.812** Strain of other muscle(s) and tendon(s) at lower leg level, left leg

√7ᵗʰ **S86.819** Strain of other muscle(s) and tendon(s) at lower leg level, unspecified leg

√6ᵗʰ **S86.82** Laceration of other muscles and tendons at lower leg level

√7ᵗʰ **S86.821** Laceration of other muscle(s) and tendon(s) at lower leg level, right leg   CC

√7ᵗʰ **S86.822** Laceration of other muscle(s) and tendon(s) at lower leg level, left leg   CC

√7ᵗʰ **S86.829** Laceration of other muscle(s) and tendon(s) at lower leg level, unspecified leg   CC

√6ᵗʰ **S86.89** Other injury of other muscles and tendons at lower leg level

√7ᵗʰ **S86.891** Other injury of other muscle(s) and tendon(s) at lower leg level, right leg

√7ᵗʰ **S86.892** Other injury of other muscle(s) and tendon(s) at lower leg level, left leg

√7ᵗʰ **S86.899** Other injury of other muscle(s) and tendon(s) at lower leg level, unspecified leg

√5ᵗʰ **S86.9** Injury of unspecified muscle and tendon at lower leg level

√6ᵗʰ **S86.90** Unspecified injury of unspecified muscle and tendon at lower leg level

√7ᵗʰ **S86.901** Unspecified injury of unspecified muscle(s) and tendon(s) at lower leg level, right leg

√7ᵗʰ **S86.902** Unspecified injury of unspecified muscle(s) and tendon(s) at lower leg level, left leg

√7ᵗʰ **S86.909** Unspecified injury of unspecified muscle(s) and tendon(s) at lower leg level, unspecified leg

√6ᵗʰ **S86.91** Strain of unspecified muscle and tendon at lower leg level

√7ᵗʰ **S86.911** Strain of unspecified muscle(s) and tendon(s) at lower leg level, right leg

√7ᵗʰ **S86.912** Strain of unspecified muscle(s) and tendon(s) at lower leg level, left leg

√7ᵗʰ **S86.919** Strain of unspecified muscle(s) and tendon(s) at lower leg level, unspecified leg

√6ᵗʰ **S86.92** Laceration of unspecified muscle and tendon at lower leg level

√7ᵗʰ **S86.921** Laceration of unspecified muscle(s) and tendon(s) at lower leg level, right leg   CC

√7ᵗʰ **S86.922** Laceration of unspecified muscle(s) and tendon(s) at lower leg level, left leg   CC

√7ᵗʰ **S86.929** Laceration of unspecified muscle(s) and tendon(s) at lower leg level, unspecified leg   CC

√6ᵗʰ **S86.99** Other injury of unspecified muscle and tendon at lower leg level

√7ᵗʰ **S86.991** Other injury of unspecified muscle(s) and tendon(s) at lower leg level, right leg

√7ᵗʰ **S86.992** Other injury of unspecified muscle(s) and tendon(s) at lower leg level, left leg

√7ᵗʰ **S86.999** Other injury of unspecified muscle(s) and tendon(s) at lower leg level, unspecified leg

√4ᵗʰ **S87** **Crushing injury of lower leg**

Use additional code(s) for all associated injuries

EXCLUDES 2   crushing injury of ankle and foot (S97.-)

> The appropriate 7th character is to be added to each code from category S87.
> A   initial encounter
> D   subsequent encounter
> S   sequela

√5ᵗʰ **S87.0** Crushing injury of knee

√x7ᵗʰ **S87.00** Crushing injury of unspecified knee

√x7ᵗʰ **S87.01** Crushing injury of right knee

√x7ᵗʰ **S87.02** Crushing injury of left knee

√5ᵗʰ **S87.8** Crushing injury of lower leg

√x7ᵗʰ **S87.80** Crushing injury of unspecified lower leg

√x7ᵗʰ **S87.81** Crushing injury of right lower leg

√x7ᵗʰ **S87.82** Crushing injury of left lower leg

✓ Additional Character Required   √x7ᵗʰ Placeholder   Unacceptable PDx   Questionable PDx   Manifestation   Unspecified Dx   H1-H14 HAC   HCC CMS-HCC Dx   HIV HIV Dx

ICD-10-CM 2021   1073

√4ᵗʰ **S88 Traumatic amputation of lower leg**

> An amputation not identified as partial or complete should be coded to complete
>
> EXCLUDES 1   *traumatic amputation of ankle and foot (S98.-)*

> The appropriate 7th character is to be added to each code from category S88.
> A   initial encounter
> D   subsequent encounter
> S   sequela

√5ᵗʰ **S88.0 Traumatic amputation at knee level**

  √6ᵗʰ **S88.01 Complete traumatic amputation at knee level**

    √7ᵗʰ **S88.011** Complete traumatic amputation at knee level, **right** lower leg   CC HCC

    √7ᵗʰ **S88.012** Complete traumatic amputation at knee level, **left** lower leg   CC HCC

    √7ᵗʰ **S88.019** Complete traumatic amputation at knee level, unspecified lower leg   CC HCC

  √6ᵗʰ **S88.02 Partial traumatic amputation at knee level**

    √7ᵗʰ **S88.021** Partial traumatic amputation at knee level, **right** lower leg   CC HCC

    √7ᵗʰ **S88.022** Partial traumatic amputation at knee level, **left** lower leg   CC HCC

    √7ᵗʰ **S88.029** Partial traumatic amputation at knee level, unspecified lower leg   CC HCC

√5ᵗʰ **S88.1 Traumatic amputation at level between knee and ankle**

  √6ᵗʰ **S88.11 Complete traumatic amputation at level between knee and ankle**

    √7ᵗʰ **S88.111** Complete traumatic amputation at level between knee and ankle, **right** lower leg   CC HCC

    √7ᵗʰ **S88.112** Complete traumatic amputation at level between knee and ankle, **left** lower leg   CC HCC

    √7ᵗʰ **S88.119** Complete traumatic amputation at level between knee and ankle, unspecified lower leg   CC HCC

  √6ᵗʰ **S88.12 Partial traumatic amputation at level between knee and ankle**

    √7ᵗʰ **S88.121** Partial traumatic amputation at level between knee and ankle, **right** lower leg   CC HCC

    √7ᵗʰ **S88.122** Partial traumatic amputation at level between knee and ankle, **left** lower leg   CC HCC

    √7ᵗʰ **S88.129** Partial traumatic amputation at level between knee and ankle, unspecified lower leg   CC HCC

√5ᵗʰ **S88.9 Traumatic amputation of lower leg, level unspecified**

  √6ᵗʰ **S88.91 Complete traumatic amputation of lower leg, level unspecified**

    √7ᵗʰ **S88.911** Complete traumatic amputation of **right** lower leg, level unspecified   CC HCC

    √7ᵗʰ **S88.912** Complete traumatic amputation of **left** lower leg, level unspecified   CC HCC

    √7ᵗʰ **S88.919** Complete traumatic amputation of unspecified lower leg, level unspecified   CC HCC

  √6ᵗʰ **S88.92 Partial traumatic amputation of lower leg, level unspecified**

    √7ᵗʰ **S88.921** Partial traumatic amputation of **right** lower leg, level unspecified   CC HCC

    √7ᵗʰ **S88.922** Partial traumatic amputation of **left** lower leg, level unspecified   CC HCC

    √7ᵗʰ **S88.929** Partial traumatic amputation of unspecified lower leg, level unspecified   CC HCC

√4ᵗʰ **S89 Other and unspecified injuries of lower leg**

> NOTE   A fracture not indicated as open or closed should be coded to closed.
>
> EXCLUDES 2   *other and unspecified injuries of ankle and foot (S99.-)*

AHA: 2018,2Q,12; 2018,1Q,3; 2015,3Q,37-39

> The appropriate 7th character is to be added to each code from subcategories S89.0, S89.1, S89.2, and S89.3.
> A   initial encounter for closed fracture
> D   subsequent encounter for fracture with routine healing
> G   subsequent encounter for fracture with delayed healing
> K   subsequent encounter for fracture with nonunion
> P   subsequent encounter for fracture with malunion
> S   sequela

√5ᵗʰ **S89.0 Physeal fracture of upper end of tibia**

  AHA: 2019,4Q,56

  √6ᵗʰ **S89.00 Unspecified physeal fracture of upper end of tibia**

    ³ √7ᵗʰ **S89.001** Unspecified physeal fracture of upper end of **right** tibia   CC H5

    ³ √7ᵗʰ **S89.002** Unspecified physeal fracture of upper end of **left** tibia   CC H5

    ³ √7ᵗʰ **S89.009** Unspecified physeal fracture of upper end of **unspecified** tibia   CC H5

  √6ᵗʰ **S89.01 Salter-Harris Type I physeal fracture of upper end of tibia**

    ³ √7ᵗʰ **S89.011** Salter-Harris Type I physeal fracture of upper end of **right** tibia   CC H5

    ³ √7ᵗʰ **S89.012** Salter-Harris Type I physeal fracture of upper end of **left** tibia   CC H5

    ³ √7ᵗʰ **S89.019** Salter-Harris Type I physeal fracture of upper end of **unspecified** tibia   CC H5

  √6ᵗʰ **S89.02 Salter-Harris Type II physeal fracture of upper end of tibia**

    ³ √7ᵗʰ **S89.021** Salter-Harris Type II physeal fracture of upper end of **right** tibia   CC H5

    ³ √7ᵗʰ **S89.022** Salter-Harris Type II physeal fracture of upper end of **left** tibia   CC H5

    ³ √7ᵗʰ **S89.029** Salter-Harris Type II physeal fracture of upper end of **unspecified** tibia   CC H5

  √6ᵗʰ **S89.03 Salter-Harris Type III physeal fracture of upper end of tibia**

    ³ √7ᵗʰ **S89.031** Salter-Harris Type III physeal fracture of upper end of **right** tibia   CC H5

    ³ √7ᵗʰ **S89.032** Salter-Harris Type III physeal fracture of upper end of **left** tibia   CC H5

    ³ √7ᵗʰ **S89.039** Salter-Harris Type III physeal fracture of upper end of **unspecified** tibia   CC H5

  √6ᵗʰ **S89.04 Salter-Harris Type IV physeal fracture of upper end of tibia**

    ³ √7ᵗʰ **S89.041** Salter-Harris Type IV physeal fracture of upper end of **right** tibia   CC H5

    ³ √7ᵗʰ **S89.042** Salter-Harris Type IV physeal fracture of upper end of **left** tibia   CC H5

    ³ √7ᵗʰ **S89.049** Salter-Harris Type IV physeal fracture of upper end of **unspecified** tibia   CC H5

  √6ᵗʰ **S89.09 Other physeal fracture of upper end of tibia**

    ³ √7ᵗʰ **S89.091** Other physeal fracture of upper end of **right** tibia   CC H5

    ³ √7ᵗʰ **S89.092** Other physeal fracture of upper end of **left** tibia   CC H5

    ³ √7ᵗʰ **S89.099** Other physeal fracture of upper end of **unspecified** tibia   CC H5

√5ᵗʰ **S89.1 Physeal fracture of lower end of tibia**

  AHA: 2019,4Q,56

  √6ᵗʰ **S89.10 Unspecified physeal fracture of lower end of tibia**

    ⁴ √7ᵗʰ **S89.101** Unspecified physeal fracture of lower end of **right** tibia   CC

    ⁴ √7ᵗʰ **S89.102** Unspecified physeal fracture of lower end of **left** tibia   CC

    ⁴ √7ᵗʰ **S89.109** Unspecified physeal fracture of lower end of **unspecified** tibia   CC

  √6ᵗʰ **S89.11 Salter-Harris Type I physeal fracture of lower end of tibia**

    ⁴ √7ᵗʰ **S89.111** Salter-Harris Type I physeal fracture of lower end of **right** tibia   CC

    ⁴ √7ᵗʰ **S89.112** Salter-Harris Type I physeal fracture of lower end of **left** tibia   CC

    ⁴ √7ᵗʰ **S89.119** Salter-Harris Type I physeal fracture of lower end of **unspecified** tibia   CC

N Newborn: 0   P Pediatric: 0-17   M Maternity: 9-64   A Adult: 15-124   MCC Major Complication/Comorbidity   CC Complication/Comorbidity   SW Severe Wound Dx

1074   ICD-10-CM 2021

S89.12 Salter-Harris Type II physeal fracture of lower end of tibia

 S89.121 Salter-Harris Type II physeal fracture of lower end of right tibia　CC

 S89.122 Salter-Harris Type II physeal fracture of lower end of left tibia　CC

 S89.129 Salter-Harris Type II physeal fracture of lower end of unspecified tibia　CC

S89.13 Salter-Harris Type III physeal fracture of lower end of tibia

 EXCLUDES 1　fracture of medial malleolus (adult) (S82.5-)

 S89.131 Salter-Harris Type III physeal fracture of lower end of right tibia　CC

 S89.132 Salter-Harris Type III physeal fracture of lower end of left tibia　CC

 S89.139 Salter-Harris Type III physeal fracture of lower end of unspecified tibia　CC

S89.14 Salter-Harris Type IV physeal fracture of lower end of tibia

 EXCLUDES 1　fracture of medial malleolus (adult) (S82.5-)

 S89.141 Salter-Harris Type IV physeal fracture of lower end of right tibia　CC

 S89.142 Salter-Harris Type IV physeal fracture of lower end of left tibia　CC

 S89.149 Salter-Harris Type IV physeal fracture of lower end of unspecified tibia　CC

S89.19 Other physeal fracture of lower end of tibia

 S89.191 Other physeal fracture of lower end of right tibia　CC

 S89.192 Other physeal fracture of lower end of left tibia　CC

 S89.199 Other physeal fracture of lower end of unspecified tibia　CC

S89.2 Physeal fracture of upper end of fibula

 AHA: 2019,4Q,56

S89.20 Unspecified physeal fracture of upper end of fibula

 S89.201 Unspecified physeal fracture of upper end of right fibula　CC

 S89.202 Unspecified physeal fracture of upper end of left fibula　CC

 S89.209 Unspecified physeal fracture of upper end of unspecified fibula　CC

S89.21 Salter-Harris Type I physeal fracture of upper end of fibula

 S89.211 Salter-Harris Type I physeal fracture of upper end of right fibula　CC

 S89.212 Salter-Harris Type I physeal fracture of upper end of left fibula　CC

 S89.219 Salter-Harris Type I physeal fracture of upper end of unspecified fibula　CC

S89.22 Salter-Harris Type II physeal fracture of upper end of fibula

 S89.221 Salter-Harris Type II physeal fracture of upper end of right fibula　CC

 S89.222 Salter-Harris Type II physeal fracture of upper end of left fibula　CC

 S89.229 Salter-Harris Type II physeal fracture of upper end of unspecified fibula　CC

S89.29 Other physeal fracture of upper end of fibula

 S89.291 Other physeal fracture of upper end of right fibula　CC

 S89.292 Other physeal fracture of upper end of left fibula　CC

 S89.299 Other physeal fracture of upper end of unspecified fibula　CC

S89.3 Physeal fracture of lower end of fibula

 AHA: 2019,4Q,56

S89.30 Unspecified physeal fracture of lower end of fibula

 S89.301 Unspecified physeal fracture of lower end of right fibula　CC

 S89.302 Unspecified physeal fracture of lower end of left fibula　CC

 S89.309 Unspecified physeal fracture of lower end of unspecified fibula　CC

S89.31 Salter-Harris Type I physeal fracture of lower end of fibula

 S89.311 Salter-Harris Type I physeal fracture of lower end of right fibula　CC

 S89.312 Salter-Harris Type I physeal fracture of lower end of left fibula　CC

 S89.319 Salter-Harris Type I physeal fracture of lower end of unspecified fibula　CC

S89.32 Salter-Harris Type II physeal fracture of lower end of fibula

 S89.321 Salter-Harris Type II physeal fracture of lower end of right fibula　CC

 S89.322 Salter-Harris Type II physeal fracture of lower end of left fibula　CC

 S89.329 Salter-Harris Type II physeal fracture of lower end of unspecified fibula　CC

S89.39 Other physeal fracture of lower end of fibula

 S89.391 Other physeal fracture of lower end of right fibula　CC

 S89.392 Other physeal fracture of lower end of left fibula　CC

 S89.399 Other physeal fracture of lower end of unspecified fibula　CC

S89.8 Other specified injuries of lower leg

> The appropriate 7th character is to be added to each code in subcategory S89.8.
> A　initial encounter
> D　subsequent encounter
> S　sequela

S89.80 Other specified injuries of unspecified lower leg

S89.81 Other specified injuries of right lower leg

S89.82 Other specified injuries of left lower leg

S89.9 Unspecified injury of lower leg

> The appropriate 7th character is to be added to each code in subcategory S89.9.
> A　initial encounter
> D　subsequent encounter
> S　sequela

S89.90 Unspecified injury of unspecified lower leg

S89.91 Unspecified injury of right lower leg

S89.92 Unspecified injury of left lower leg

Injuries to the ankle and foot (S90-S99)

EXCLUDES 2　burns and corrosions (T20-T32)
fracture of ankle and malleolus (S82.-)
frostbite (T33-T34)
insect bite or sting, venomous (T63.4)

S90 Superficial injury of ankle, foot and toes

> The appropriate 7th character is to be added to each code from category S90.
> A　initial encounter
> D　subsequent encounter
> S　sequela

S90.0 Contusion of ankle

S90.00 Contusion of unspecified ankle

S90.01 Contusion of right ankle

S90.02 Contusion of left ankle

S90.1 Contusion of toe without damage to nail

S90.11 Contusion of great toe without damage to nail

 S90.111 Contusion of right great toe without damage to nail

 S90.112 Contusion of left great toe without damage to nail

 S90.119 Contusion of unspecified great toe without damage to nail

S90.12 Contusion of lesser toe without damage to nail

 S90.121 Contusion of right lesser toe(s) without damage to nail

 S90.122 Contusion of left lesser toe(s) without damage to nail

 S90.129 Contusion of unspecified lesser toe(s) without damage to nail
  Contusion of toe NOS

S90.2 Contusion of toe with damage to nail

S90.21 Contusion of great toe with damage to nail

 S90.211 Contusion of right great toe with damage to nail

√7ᵗʰ **S90.212** Contusion of left great toe with damage to nail

√7ᵗʰ **S90.219** Contusion of unspecified great toe with damage to nail

√6ᵗʰ **S90.22** Contusion of lesser toe with damage to nail

√7ᵗʰ **S90.221** Contusion of right lesser toe(s) with damage to nail

√7ᵗʰ **S90.222** Contusion of left lesser toe(s) with damage to nail

√7ᵗʰ **S90.229** Contusion of unspecified lesser toe(s) with damage to nail

√5ᵗʰ **S90.3** Contusion of foot

     EXCLUDES 2   contusion of toes (S90.1-, S90.2-)

√x7ᵗʰ **S90.30** Contusion of unspecified foot

     Contusion of foot NOS

√x7ᵗʰ **S90.31** Contusion of right foot

√x7ᵗʰ **S90.32** Contusion of left foot

√5ᵗʰ **S90.4** Other superficial injuries of toe

√6ᵗʰ **S90.41** Abrasion of toe

√7ᵗʰ **S90.411** Abrasion, right great toe

√7ᵗʰ **S90.412** Abrasion, left great toe

√7ᵗʰ **S90.413** Abrasion, unspecified great toe

√7ᵗʰ **S90.414** Abrasion, right lesser toe(s)

√7ᵗʰ **S90.415** Abrasion, left lesser toe(s)

√7ᵗʰ **S90.416** Abrasion, unspecified lesser toe(s)

√6ᵗʰ **S90.42** Blister (nonthermal) of toe

√7ᵗʰ **S90.421** Blister (nonthermal), right great toe

√7ᵗʰ **S90.422** Blister (nonthermal), left great toe

√7ᵗʰ **S90.423** Blister (nonthermal), unspecified great toe

√7ᵗʰ **S90.424** Blister (nonthermal), right lesser toe(s)

√7ᵗʰ **S90.425** Blister (nonthermal), left lesser toe(s)

√7ᵗʰ **S90.426** Blister (nonthermal), unspecified lesser toe(s)

√6ᵗʰ **S90.44** External constriction of toe

     Hair tourniquet syndrome of toe

√7ᵗʰ **S90.441** External constriction, right great toe

√7ᵗʰ **S90.442** External constriction, left great toe

√7ᵗʰ **S90.443** External constriction, unspecified great toe

√7ᵗʰ **S90.444** External constriction, right lesser toe(s)

√7ᵗʰ **S90.445** External constriction, left lesser toe(s)

√7ᵗʰ **S90.446** External constriction, unspecified lesser toe(s)

√6ᵗʰ **S90.45** Superficial foreign body of toe

     Splinter in the toe

√7ᵗʰ **S90.451** Superficial foreign body, right great toe

√7ᵗʰ **S90.452** Superficial foreign body, left great toe

√7ᵗʰ **S90.453** Superficial foreign body, unspecified great toe

√7ᵗʰ **S90.454** Superficial foreign body, right lesser toe(s)

√7ᵗʰ **S90.455** Superficial foreign body, left lesser toe(s)

√7ᵗʰ **S90.456** Superficial foreign body, unspecified lesser toe(s)

√6ᵗʰ **S90.46** Insect bite (nonvenomous) of toe

√7ᵗʰ **S90.461** Insect bite (nonvenomous), right great toe

√7ᵗʰ **S90.462** Insect bite (nonvenomous), left great toe

√7ᵗʰ **S90.463** Insect bite (nonvenomous), unspecified great toe

√7ᵗʰ **S90.464** Insect bite (nonvenomous), right lesser toe(s)

√7ᵗʰ **S90.465** Insect bite (nonvenomous), left lesser toe(s)

√7ᵗʰ **S90.466** Insect bite (nonvenomous), unspecified lesser toe(s)

√6ᵗʰ **S90.47** Other superficial bite of toe

     EXCLUDES 1   open bite of toe (S91.15-, S91.25-)

√7ᵗʰ **S90.471** Other superficial bite of right great toe

√7ᵗʰ **S90.472** Other superficial bite of left great toe

√7ᵗʰ **S90.473** Other superficial bite of unspecified great toe

√7ᵗʰ **S90.474** Other superficial bite of right lesser toe(s)

√7ᵗʰ **S90.475** Other superficial bite of left lesser toe(s)

√7ᵗʰ **S90.476** Other superficial bite of unspecified lesser toe(s)

√5ᵗʰ **S90.5** Other superficial injuries of ankle

√6ᵗʰ **S90.51** Abrasion of ankle

√7ᵗʰ **S90.511** Abrasion, right ankle

√7ᵗʰ **S90.512** Abrasion, left ankle

√7ᵗʰ **S90.519** Abrasion, unspecified ankle

√6ᵗʰ **S90.52** Blister (nonthermal) of ankle

√7ᵗʰ **S90.521** Blister (nonthermal), right ankle

√7ᵗʰ **S90.522** Blister (nonthermal), left ankle

√7ᵗʰ **S90.529** Blister (nonthermal), unspecified ankle

√6ᵗʰ **S90.54** External constriction of ankle

√7ᵗʰ **S90.541** External constriction, right ankle

√7ᵗʰ **S90.542** External constriction, left ankle

√7ᵗʰ **S90.549** External constriction, unspecified ankle

√6ᵗʰ **S90.55** Superficial foreign body of ankle

     Splinter in the ankle

√7ᵗʰ **S90.551** Superficial foreign body, right ankle

√7ᵗʰ **S90.552** Superficial foreign body, left ankle

√7ᵗʰ **S90.559** Superficial foreign body, unspecified ankle

√6ᵗʰ **S90.56** Insect bite (nonvenomous) of ankle

√7ᵗʰ **S90.561** Insect bite (nonvenomous), right ankle

√7ᵗʰ **S90.562** Insect bite (nonvenomous), left ankle

√7ᵗʰ **S90.569** Insect bite (nonvenomous), unspecified ankle

√6ᵗʰ **S90.57** Other superficial bite of ankle

     EXCLUDES 1   open bite of ankle (S91.05-)

√7ᵗʰ **S90.571** Other superficial bite of ankle, right ankle

√7ᵗʰ **S90.572** Other superficial bite of ankle, left ankle

√7ᵗʰ **S90.579** Other superficial bite of ankle, unspecified ankle

√5ᵗʰ **S90.8** Other superficial injuries of foot

√6ᵗʰ **S90.81** Abrasion of foot

√7ᵗʰ **S90.811** Abrasion, right foot

√7ᵗʰ **S90.812** Abrasion, left foot

√7ᵗʰ **S90.819** Abrasion, unspecified foot

√6ᵗʰ **S90.82** Blister (nonthermal) of foot

√7ᵗʰ **S90.821** Blister (nonthermal), right foot

√7ᵗʰ **S90.822** Blister (nonthermal), left foot

√7ᵗʰ **S90.829** Blister (nonthermal), unspecified foot

√6ᵗʰ **S90.84** External constriction of foot

√7ᵗʰ **S90.841** External constriction, right foot

√7ᵗʰ **S90.842** External constriction, left foot

√7ᵗʰ **S90.849** External constriction, unspecified foot

√6ᵗʰ **S90.85** Superficial foreign body of foot

     Splinter in the foot

√7ᵗʰ **S90.851** Superficial foreign body, right foot

√7ᵗʰ **S90.852** Superficial foreign body, left foot

√7ᵗʰ **S90.859** Superficial foreign body, unspecified foot

√6ᵗʰ **S90.86** Insect bite (nonvenomous) of foot

√7ᵗʰ **S90.861** Insect bite (nonvenomous), right foot

√7ᵗʰ **S90.862** Insect bite (nonvenomous), left foot

√7ᵗʰ **S90.869** Insect bite (nonvenomous), unspecified foot

√6ᵗʰ **S90.87** Other superficial bite of foot

     EXCLUDES 1   open bite of foot (S91.35-)

√7ᵗʰ **S90.871** Other superficial bite of right foot

√7ᵗʰ **S90.872** Other superficial bite of left foot

√7ᵗʰ **S90.879** Other superficial bite of unspecified foot

√5ᵗʰ **S90.9** Unspecified superficial injury of ankle, foot and toe

√6ᵗʰ **S90.91** Unspecified superficial injury of ankle

√7ᵗʰ **S90.911** Unspecified superficial injury of right ankle

√7ᵗʰ **S90.912** Unspecified superficial injury of left ankle

√7ᵗʰ **S90.919** Unspecified superficial injury of unspecified ankle

N Newborn: 0   P Pediatric: 0-17   M Maternity: 9-64   A Adult: 15-124   MCC Major Complication/Comorbidity   CC Complication/Comorbidity   SW Severe Wound Dx

1076   ICD-10-CM 2021

√6ᵗʰ **S90.92 Unspecified superficial injury of foot**

√7ᵗʰ **S90.921 Unspecified superficial injury of right foot**

√7ᵗʰ **S90.922 Unspecified superficial injury of left foot**

√7ᵗʰ **S90.929 Unspecified superficial injury of unspecified foot**

√6ᵗʰ **S90.93 Unspecified superficial injury of toes**

√7ᵗʰ **S90.931 Unspecified superficial injury of right great toe**

√7ᵗʰ **S90.932 Unspecified superficial injury of left great toe**

√7ᵗʰ **S90.933 Unspecified superficial injury of unspecified great toe**

√7ᵗʰ **S90.934 Unspecified superficial injury of right lesser toe(s)**

√7ᵗʰ **S90.935 Unspecified superficial injury of left lesser toe(s)**

√7ᵗʰ **S90.936 Unspecified superficial injury of unspecified lesser toe(s)**

√4ᵗʰ **S91 Open wound of ankle, foot and toes**

Code also any associated wound infection

EXCLUDES 1   open fracture of ankle, foot and toes (S92.- with 7th character B)

traumatic amputation of ankle and foot (S98.-)

The appropriate 7th character is to be added to each code from category S91.
A   initial encounter
D   subsequent encounter
S   sequela

√5ᵗʰ **S91.0 Open wound of ankle**

√6ᵗʰ **S91.00 Unspecified open wound of ankle**

√7ᵗʰ **S91.001 Unspecified open wound, right ankle**

√7ᵗʰ **S91.002 Unspecified open wound, left ankle**

√7ᵗʰ **S91.009 Unspecified open wound, unspecified ankle**

√6ᵗʰ **S91.01 Laceration without foreign body of ankle**

√7ᵗʰ **S91.011 Laceration without foreign body, right ankle**

√7ᵗʰ **S91.012 Laceration without foreign body, left ankle**

√7ᵗʰ **S91.019 Laceration without foreign body, unspecified ankle**

√6ᵗʰ **S91.02 Laceration with foreign body of ankle**

√7ᵗʰ **S91.021 Laceration with foreign body, right ankle**

√7ᵗʰ **S91.022 Laceration with foreign body, left ankle**

√7ᵗʰ **S91.029 Laceration with foreign body, unspecified ankle**

√6ᵗʰ **S91.03 Puncture wound without foreign body of ankle**

√7ᵗʰ **S91.031 Puncture wound without foreign body, right ankle**

√7ᵗʰ **S91.032 Puncture wound without foreign body, left ankle**

√7ᵗʰ **S91.039 Puncture wound without foreign body, unspecified ankle**

√6ᵗʰ **S91.04 Puncture wound with foreign body of ankle**

√7ᵗʰ **S91.041 Puncture wound with foreign body, right ankle**

√7ᵗʰ **S91.042 Puncture wound with foreign body, left ankle**

√7ᵗʰ **S91.049 Puncture wound with foreign body, unspecified ankle**

√6ᵗʰ **S91.05 Open bite of ankle**

EXCLUDES 1   superficial bite of ankle (S90.56-, S90.57-)

√7ᵗʰ **S91.051 Open bite, right ankle**

√7ᵗʰ **S91.052 Open bite, left ankle**

√7ᵗʰ **S91.059 Open bite, unspecified ankle**

√5ᵗʰ **S91.1 Open wound of toe without damage to nail**

√6ᵗʰ **S91.10 Unspecified open wound of toe without damage to nail**

√7ᵗʰ **S91.101 Unspecified open wound of right great toe without damage to nail**

√7ᵗʰ **S91.102 Unspecified open wound of left great toe without damage to nail**

√7ᵗʰ **S91.103 Unspecified open wound of unspecified great toe without damage to nail**

√7ᵗʰ **S91.104 Unspecified open wound of right lesser toe(s) without damage to nail**

√7ᵗʰ **S91.105 Unspecified open wound of left lesser toe(s) without damage to nail**

√7ᵗʰ **S91.106 Unspecified open wound of unspecified lesser toe(s) without damage to nail**

√7ᵗʰ **S91.109 Unspecified open wound of unspecified toe(s) without damage to nail**

√6ᵗʰ **S91.11 Laceration without foreign body of toe without damage to nail**

√7ᵗʰ **S91.111 Laceration without foreign body of right great toe without damage to nail**

√7ᵗʰ **S91.112 Laceration without foreign body of left great toe without damage to nail**

√7ᵗʰ **S91.113 Laceration without foreign body of unspecified great toe without damage to nail**

√7ᵗʰ **S91.114 Laceration without foreign body of right lesser toe(s) without damage to nail**

√7ᵗʰ **S91.115 Laceration without foreign body of left lesser toe(s) without damage to nail**

√7ᵗʰ **S91.116 Laceration without foreign body of unspecified lesser toe(s) without damage to nail**

√7ᵗʰ **S91.119 Laceration without foreign body of unspecified toe without damage to nail**

√6ᵗʰ **S91.12 Laceration with foreign body of toe without damage to nail**

√7ᵗʰ **S91.121 Laceration with foreign body of right great toe without damage to nail**

√7ᵗʰ **S91.122 Laceration with foreign body of left great toe without damage to nail**

√7ᵗʰ **S91.123 Laceration with foreign body of unspecified great toe without damage to nail**

√7ᵗʰ **S91.124 Laceration with foreign body of right lesser toe(s) without damage to nail**

√7ᵗʰ **S91.125 Laceration with foreign body of left lesser toe(s) without damage to nail**

√7ᵗʰ **S91.126 Laceration with foreign body of unspecified lesser toe(s) without damage to nail**

√7ᵗʰ **S91.129 Laceration with foreign body of unspecified toe(s) without damage to nail**

√6ᵗʰ **S91.13 Puncture wound without foreign body of toe without damage to nail**

√7ᵗʰ **S91.131 Puncture wound without foreign body of right great toe without damage to nail**

√7ᵗʰ **S91.132 Puncture wound without foreign body of left great toe without damage to nail**

√7ᵗʰ **S91.133 Puncture wound without foreign body of unspecified great toe without damage to nail**

√7ᵗʰ **S91.134 Puncture wound without foreign body of right lesser toe(s) without damage to nail**

√7ᵗʰ **S91.135 Puncture wound without foreign body of left lesser toe(s) without damage to nail**

√7ᵗʰ **S91.136 Puncture wound without foreign body of unspecified lesser toe(s) without damage to nail**

√7ᵗʰ **S91.139 Puncture wound without foreign body of unspecified toe(s) without damage to nail**

√6ᵗʰ **S91.14 Puncture wound with foreign body of toe without damage to nail**

√7ᵗʰ **S91.141 Puncture wound with foreign body of right great toe without damage to nail**

√7ᵗʰ **S91.142 Puncture wound with foreign body of left great toe without damage to nail**

√7ᵗʰ **S91.143 Puncture wound with foreign body of unspecified great toe without damage to nail**

√7ᵗʰ **S91.144 Puncture wound with foreign body of right lesser toe(s) without damage to nail**

√7ᵗʰ **S91.145 Puncture wound with foreign body of left lesser toe(s) without damage to nail**

√7ᵗʰ **S91.146 Puncture wound with foreign body of unspecified lesser toe(s) without damage to nail**

√7ᵗʰ **S91.149 Puncture wound with foreign body of unspecified toe(s) without damage to nail**

√6ᵗʰ **S91.15 Open bite of toe without damage to nail**

Bite of toe NOS

EXCLUDES 1   superficial bite of toe (S90.46-, S90.47-)

√7ᵗʰ **S91.151 Open bite of right great toe without damage to nail**

√7ᵗʰ **S91.152** Open bite of left great toe without damage to nail

√7ᵗʰ **S91.153** Open bite of unspecified great toe without damage to nail

√7ᵗʰ **S91.154** Open bite of right lesser toe(s) without damage to nail

√7ᵗʰ **S91.155** Open bite of left lesser toe(s) without damage to nail

√7ᵗʰ **S91.156** Open bite of unspecified lesser toe(s) without damage to nail

√7ᵗʰ **S91.159** Open bite of unspecified toe(s) without damage to nail

√5ᵗʰ **S91.2** Open wound of toe with damage to nail

√6ᵗʰ **S91.20** Unspecified open wound of toe with damage to nail

√7ᵗʰ **S91.201** Unspecified open wound of right great toe with damage to nail

√7ᵗʰ **S91.202** Unspecified open wound of left great toe with damage to nail

√7ᵗʰ **S91.203** Unspecified open wound of unspecified great toe with damage to nail

√7ᵗʰ **S91.204** Unspecified open wound of right lesser toe(s) with damage to nail

√7ᵗʰ **S91.205** Unspecified open wound of left lesser toe(s) with damage to nail

√7ᵗʰ **S91.206** Unspecified open wound of unspecified lesser toe(s) with damage to nail

√7ᵗʰ **S91.209** Unspecified open wound of unspecified toe(s) with damage to nail

√6ᵗʰ **S91.21** Laceration without foreign body of toe with damage to nail

√7ᵗʰ **S91.211** Laceration without foreign body of right great toe with damage to nail

√7ᵗʰ **S91.212** Laceration without foreign body of left great toe with damage to nail

√7ᵗʰ **S91.213** Laceration without foreign body of unspecified great toe with damage to nail

√7ᵗʰ **S91.214** Laceration without foreign body of right lesser toe(s) with damage to nail

√7ᵗʰ **S91.215** Laceration without foreign body of left lesser toe(s) with damage to nail

√7ᵗʰ **S91.216** Laceration without foreign body of unspecified lesser toe(s) with damage to nail

√7ᵗʰ **S91.219** Laceration without foreign body of unspecified toe(s) with damage to nail

√6ᵗʰ **S91.22** Laceration with foreign body of toe with damage to nail

√7ᵗʰ **S91.221** Laceration with foreign body of right great toe with damage to nail

√7ᵗʰ **S91.222** Laceration with foreign body of left great toe with damage to nail

√7ᵗʰ **S91.223** Laceration with foreign body of unspecified great toe with damage to nail

√7ᵗʰ **S91.224** Laceration with foreign body of right lesser toe(s) with damage to nail

√7ᵗʰ **S91.225** Laceration with foreign body of left lesser toe(s) with damage to nail

√7ᵗʰ **S91.226** Laceration with foreign body of unspecified lesser toe(s) with damage to nail

√7ᵗʰ **S91.229** Laceration with foreign body of unspecified toe(s) with damage to nail

√6ᵗʰ **S91.23** Puncture wound without foreign body of toe with damage to nail

√7ᵗʰ **S91.231** Puncture wound without foreign body of right great toe with damage to nail

√7ᵗʰ **S91.232** Puncture wound without foreign body of left great toe with damage to nail

√7ᵗʰ **S91.233** Puncture wound without foreign body of unspecified great toe with damage to nail

√7ᵗʰ **S91.234** Puncture wound without foreign body of right lesser toe(s) with damage to nail

√7ᵗʰ **S91.235** Puncture wound without foreign body of left lesser toe(s) with damage to nail

√7ᵗʰ **S91.236** Puncture wound without foreign body of unspecified lesser toe(s) with damage to nail

√7ᵗʰ **S91.239** Puncture wound without foreign body of unspecified toe(s) with damage to nail

√6ᵗʰ **S91.24** Puncture wound with foreign body of toe with damage to nail

√7ᵗʰ **S91.241** Puncture wound with foreign body of right great toe with damage to nail

√7ᵗʰ **S91.242** Puncture wound with foreign body of left great toe with damage to nail

√7ᵗʰ **S91.243** Puncture wound with foreign body of unspecified great toe with damage to nail

√7ᵗʰ **S91.244** Puncture wound with foreign body of right lesser toe(s) with damage to nail

√7ᵗʰ **S91.245** Puncture wound with foreign body of left lesser toe(s) with damage to nail

√7ᵗʰ **S91.246** Puncture wound with foreign body of unspecified lesser toe(s) with damage to nail

√7ᵗʰ **S91.249** Puncture wound with foreign body of unspecified toe(s) with damage to nail

√6ᵗʰ **S91.25** Open bite of toe with damage to nail

Bite of toe with damage to nail NOS

EXCLUDES 1 *superficial bite of toe (S90.46-, S90.47-)*

√7ᵗʰ **S91.251** Open bite of right great toe with damage to nail

√7ᵗʰ **S91.252** Open bite of left great toe with damage to nail

√7ᵗʰ **S91.253** Open bite of unspecified great toe with damage to nail

√7ᵗʰ **S91.254** Open bite of right lesser toe(s) with damage to nail

√7ᵗʰ **S91.255** Open bite of left lesser toe(s) with damage to nail

√7ᵗʰ **S91.256** Open bite of unspecified lesser toe(s) with damage to nail

√7ᵗʰ **S91.259** Open bite of unspecified toe(s) with damage to nail

√5ᵗʰ **S91.3** Open wound of foot

√6ᵗʰ **S91.30** Unspecified open wound of foot

√7ᵗʰ **S91.301** Unspecified open wound, right foot

√7ᵗʰ **S91.302** Unspecified open wound, left foot

√7ᵗʰ **S91.309** Unspecified open wound, unspecified foot

√6ᵗʰ **S91.31** Laceration without foreign body of foot

√7ᵗʰ **S91.311** Laceration without foreign body, right foot

√7ᵗʰ **S91.312** Laceration without foreign body, left foot

√7ᵗʰ **S91.319** Laceration without foreign body, unspecified foot

√6ᵗʰ **S91.32** Laceration with foreign body of foot

√7ᵗʰ **S91.321** Laceration with foreign body, right foot

√7ᵗʰ **S91.322** Laceration with foreign body, left foot

√7ᵗʰ **S91.329** Laceration with foreign body, unspecified foot

√6ᵗʰ **S91.33** Puncture wound without foreign body of foot

√7ᵗʰ **S91.331** Puncture wound without foreign body, right foot

√7ᵗʰ **S91.332** Puncture wound without foreign body, left foot

√7ᵗʰ **S91.339** Puncture wound without foreign body, unspecified foot

√6ᵗʰ **S91.34** Puncture wound with foreign body of foot

√7ᵗʰ **S91.341** Puncture wound with foreign body, right foot

√7ᵗʰ **S91.342** Puncture wound with foreign body, left foot

√7ᵗʰ **S91.349** Puncture wound with foreign body, unspecified foot

√6ᵗʰ **S91.35** Open bite of foot

EXCLUDES 1 *superficial bite of foot (S90.86-, S90.87-)*

√7ᵗʰ **S91.351** Open bite, right foot

√7ᵗʰ **S91.352** Open bite, left foot

√7ᵗʰ **S91.359** Open bite, unspecified foot

Ⓝ Newborn: 0   Ⓟ Pediatric: 0-17   Ⓜ Maternity: 9-64   Ⓐ Adult: 15-124   **MCC** Major Complication/Comorbidity   **CC** Complication/Comorbidity   **SW** Severe Wound Dx

✓4ᵗʰ S92 Fracture of foot and toe, except ankle

> **NOTE**   A fracture not indicated as displaced or nondisplaced should be coded to displaced
>
> A fracture not indicated as open or closed should be coded to closed.

EXCLUDES 1   traumatic amputation of ankle and foot (S98.-)
EXCLUDES 2   fracture of ankle (S82.-)
          fracture of malleolus (S82.-)

AHA: 2018,2Q,12; 2015,3Q,37-39

> The appropriate 7th character is to be added to each code from category S92.
> A   initial encounter for closed fracture
> B   initial encounter for open fracture
> D   subsequent encounter for fracture with routine healing
> G   subsequent encounter for fracture with delayed healing
> K   subsequent encounter for fracture with nonunion
> P   subsequent encounter for fracture with malunion
> S   sequela

✓5ᵗʰ S92.0 Fracture of calcaneus
Heel bone
Os calcis
EXCLUDES 2   physeal fracture of calcaneus (S99.0-)

✓6ᵗʰ S92.00 Unspecified fracture of calcaneus
- ³ ✓7ᵗʰ **S92.001** Unspecified fracture of right calcaneus   CC H5
- ³ ✓7ᵗʰ **S92.002** Unspecified fracture of left calcaneus   CC H5
- ³ ✓7ᵗʰ **S92.009** Unspecified fracture of unspecified calcaneus   CC H5

✓6ᵗʰ S92.01 Fracture of body of calcaneus
- ³ ✓7ᵗʰ **S92.011** Displaced fracture of body of right calcaneus   CC H5
- ³ ✓7ᵗʰ **S92.012** Displaced fracture of body of left calcaneus   CC H5
- ³ ✓7ᵗʰ **S92.013** Displaced fracture of body of unspecified calcaneus   CC H5
- ³ ✓7ᵗʰ **S92.014** Nondisplaced fracture of body of right calcaneus   CC H5
- ³ ✓7ᵗʰ **S92.015** Nondisplaced fracture of body of left calcaneus   CC H5
- ³ ✓7ᵗʰ **S92.016** Nondisplaced fracture of body of unspecified calcaneus   CC H5

✓6ᵗʰ S92.02 Fracture of anterior process of calcaneus
- ³ ✓7ᵗʰ **S92.021** Displaced fracture of anterior process of right calcaneus   CC H5
- ³ ✓7ᵗʰ **S92.022** Displaced fracture of anterior process of left calcaneus   CC H5
- ³ ✓7ᵗʰ **S92.023** Displaced fracture of anterior process of unspecified calcaneus   CC H5
- ³ ✓7ᵗʰ **S92.024** Nondisplaced fracture of anterior process of right calcaneus   CC H5
- ³ ✓7ᵗʰ **S92.025** Nondisplaced fracture of anterior process of left calcaneus   CC H5
- ³ ✓7ᵗʰ **S92.026** Nondisplaced fracture of anterior process of unspecified calcaneus   CC H5

✓6ᵗʰ S92.03 Avulsion fracture of tuberosity of calcaneus
- ³ ✓7ᵗʰ **S92.031** Displaced avulsion fracture of tuberosity of right calcaneus   CC H5
- ³ ✓7ᵗʰ **S92.032** Displaced avulsion fracture of tuberosity of left calcaneus   CC H5
- ³ ✓7ᵗʰ **S92.033** Displaced avulsion fracture of tuberosity of unspecified calcaneus   CC H5
- ³ ✓7ᵗʰ **S92.034** Nondisplaced avulsion fracture of tuberosity of right calcaneus   CC H5
- ³ ✓7ᵗʰ **S92.035** Nondisplaced avulsion fracture of tuberosity of left calcaneus   CC H5
- ³ ✓7ᵗʰ **S92.036** Nondisplaced avulsion fracture of tuberosity of unspecified calcaneus   CC H5

✓6ᵗʰ S92.04 Other fracture of tuberosity of calcaneus
- ³ ✓7ᵗʰ **S92.041** Displaced other fracture of tuberosity of right calcaneus   CC H5
- ³ ✓7ᵗʰ **S92.042** Displaced other fracture of tuberosity of left calcaneus   CC H5
- ³ ✓7ᵗʰ **S92.043** Displaced other fracture of tuberosity of unspecified calcaneus   CC H5
- ³ ✓7ᵗʰ **S92.044** Nondisplaced other fracture of tuberosity of right calcaneus   CC H5
- ³ ✓7ᵗʰ **S92.045** Nondisplaced other fracture of tuberosity of left calcaneus   CC H5
- ³ ✓7ᵗʰ **S92.046** Nondisplaced other fracture of tuberosity of unspecified calcaneus   CC H5

✓6ᵗʰ S92.05 Other extraarticular fracture of calcaneus
- ³ ✓7ᵗʰ **S92.051** Displaced other extraarticular fracture of right calcaneus   CC H5
- ³ ✓7ᵗʰ **S92.052** Displaced other extraarticular fracture of left calcaneus   CC H5
- ³ ✓7ᵗʰ **S92.053** Displaced other extraarticular fracture of unspecified calcaneus   CC H5
- ³ ✓7ᵗʰ **S92.054** Nondisplaced other extraarticular fracture of right calcaneus   CC H5
- ³ ✓7ᵗʰ **S92.055** Nondisplaced other extraarticular fracture of left calcaneus   CC H5
- ³ ✓7ᵗʰ **S92.056** Nondisplaced other extraarticular fracture of unspecified calcaneus   CC H5

✓6ᵗʰ S92.06 Intraarticular fracture of calcaneus
- ³ ✓7ᵗʰ **S92.061** Displaced intraarticular fracture of right calcaneus   CC H5
- ³ ✓7ᵗʰ **S92.062** Displaced intraarticular fracture of left calcaneus   CC H5
- ³ ✓7ᵗʰ **S92.063** Displaced intraarticular fracture of unspecified calcaneus   CC H5
- ³ ✓7ᵗʰ **S92.064** Nondisplaced intraarticular fracture of right calcaneus   CC H5
- ³ ✓7ᵗʰ **S92.065** Nondisplaced intraarticular fracture of left calcaneus   CC H5
- ³ ✓7ᵗʰ **S92.066** Nondisplaced intraarticular fracture of unspecified calcaneus   CC H5

✓5ᵗʰ S92.1 Fracture of talus
Astragalus

✓6ᵗʰ S92.10 Unspecified fracture of talus
- ³ ✓7ᵗʰ **S92.101** Unspecified fracture of right talus   CC H5
- ³ ✓7ᵗʰ **S92.102** Unspecified fracture of left talus   CC H5
- ³ ✓7ᵗʰ **S92.109** Unspecified fracture of unspecified talus   CC H5

✓6ᵗʰ S92.11 Fracture of neck of talus
- ³ ✓7ᵗʰ **S92.111** Displaced fracture of neck of right talus   CC H5
- ³ ✓7ᵗʰ **S92.112** Displaced fracture of neck of left talus   CC H5
- ³ ✓7ᵗʰ **S92.113** Displaced fracture of neck of unspecified talus   CC H5
- ³ ✓7ᵗʰ **S92.114** Nondisplaced fracture of neck of right talus   CC H5
- ³ ✓7ᵗʰ **S92.115** Nondisplaced fracture of neck of left talus   CC H5
- ³ ✓7ᵗʰ **S92.116** Nondisplaced fracture of neck of unspecified talus   CC H5

✓6ᵗʰ S92.12 Fracture of body of talus
- ³ ✓7ᵗʰ **S92.121** Displaced fracture of body of right talus   CC H5
- ³ ✓7ᵗʰ **S92.122** Displaced fracture of body of left talus   CC H5
- ³ ✓7ᵗʰ **S92.123** Displaced fracture of body of unspecified talus   CC H5
- ³ ✓7ᵗʰ **S92.124** Nondisplaced fracture of body of right talus   CC H5
- ³ ✓7ᵗʰ **S92.125** Nondisplaced fracture of body of left talus   CC H5
- ³ ✓7ᵗʰ **S92.126** Nondisplaced fracture of body of unspecified talus   CC H5

✓6ᵗʰ S92.13 Fracture of posterior process of talus
- ³ ✓7ᵗʰ **S92.131** Displaced fracture of posterior process of right talus   CC H5
- ³ ✓7ᵗʰ **S92.132** Displaced fracture of posterior process of left talus   CC H5
- ³ ✓7ᵗʰ **S92.133** Displaced fracture of posterior process of unspecified talus   CC H5
- ³ ✓7ᵗʰ **S92.134** Nondisplaced fracture of posterior process of right talus   CC H5

3 √7ᵗʰ **S92.135** Nondisplaced fracture of posterior process of left talus   CC H5

3 √7ᵗʰ **S92.136** Nondisplaced fracture of posterior process of unspecified talus   CC H5

√6ᵗʰ **S92.14** Dome fracture of talus

    EXCLUDES 1   osteochondritis dissecans (M93.2)

3 √7ᵗʰ **S92.141** Displaced dome fracture of right talus   CC H5

3 √7ᵗʰ **S92.142** Displaced dome fracture of left talus   CC H5

3 √7ᵗʰ **S92.143** Displaced dome fracture of unspecified talus   CC H5

3 √7ᵗʰ **S92.144** Nondisplaced dome fracture of right talus   CC H5

3 √7ᵗʰ **S92.145** Nondisplaced dome fracture of left talus   CC H5

3 √7ᵗʰ **S92.146** Nondisplaced dome fracture of unspecified talus   CC H5

√6ᵗʰ **S92.15** Avulsion fracture (chip fracture) of talus

3 √7ᵗʰ **S92.151** Displaced avulsion fracture (chip fracture) of right talus   CC H5

3 √7ᵗʰ **S92.152** Displaced avulsion fracture (chip fracture) of left talus   CC H5

3 √7ᵗʰ **S92.153** Displaced avulsion fracture (chip fracture) of unspecified talus   CC H5

3 √7ᵗʰ **S92.154** Nondisplaced avulsion fracture (chip fracture) of right talus   CC H5

3 √7ᵗʰ **S92.155** Nondisplaced avulsion fracture (chip fracture) of left talus   CC H5

3 √7ᵗʰ **S92.156** Nondisplaced avulsion fracture (chip fracture) of unspecified talus   CC H5

√6ᵗʰ **S92.19** Other fracture of talus

3 √7ᵗʰ **S92.191** Other fracture of right talus   CC H5

3 √7ᵗʰ **S92.192** Other fracture of left talus   CC H5

3 √7ᵗʰ **S92.199** Other fracture of unspecified talus   CC H5

√5ᵗʰ **S92.2** Fracture of other and unspecified tarsal bone(s)

√6ᵗʰ **S92.20** Fracture of unspecified tarsal bone(s)

3 √7ᵗʰ **S92.201** Fracture of unspecified tarsal bone(s) of right foot   CC H5

3 √7ᵗʰ **S92.202** Fracture of unspecified tarsal bone(s) of left foot   CC H5

3 √7ᵗʰ **S92.209** Fracture of unspecified tarsal bone(s) of unspecified foot   CC H5

√6ᵗʰ **S92.21** Fracture of cuboid bone

3 √7ᵗʰ **S92.211** Displaced fracture of cuboid bone of right foot   CC H5

3 √7ᵗʰ **S92.212** Displaced fracture of cuboid bone of left foot   CC H5

3 √7ᵗʰ **S92.213** Displaced fracture of cuboid bone of unspecified foot   CC H5

3 √7ᵗʰ **S92.214** Nondisplaced fracture of cuboid bone of right foot   CC H5

3 √7ᵗʰ **S92.215** Nondisplaced fracture of cuboid bone of left foot   CC H5

3 √7ᵗʰ **S92.216** Nondisplaced fracture of cuboid bone of unspecified foot   CC H5

√6ᵗʰ **S92.22** Fracture of lateral cuneiform

3 √7ᵗʰ **S92.221** Displaced fracture of lateral cuneiform of right foot   CC H5

3 √7ᵗʰ **S92.222** Displaced fracture of lateral cuneiform of left foot   CC H5

3 √7ᵗʰ **S92.223** Displaced fracture of lateral cuneiform of unspecified foot   CC H5

3 √7ᵗʰ **S92.224** Nondisplaced fracture of lateral cuneiform of right foot   CC H5

3 √7ᵗʰ **S92.225** Nondisplaced fracture of lateral cuneiform of left foot   CC H5

3 √7ᵗʰ **S92.226** Nondisplaced fracture of lateral cuneiform of unspecified foot   CC H5

√6ᵗʰ **S92.23** Fracture of intermediate cuneiform

3 √7ᵗʰ **S92.231** Displaced fracture of intermediate cuneiform of right foot   CC H5

3 √7ᵗʰ **S92.232** Displaced fracture of intermediate cuneiform of left foot   CC H5

3 √7ᵗʰ **S92.233** Displaced fracture of intermediate cuneiform of unspecified foot   CC H5

3 √7ᵗʰ **S92.234** Nondisplaced fracture of intermediate cuneiform of right foot   CC H5

3 √7ᵗʰ **S92.235** Nondisplaced fracture of intermediate cuneiform of left foot   CC H5

3 √7ᵗʰ **S92.236** Nondisplaced fracture of intermediate cuneiform of unspecified foot   CC H5

√6ᵗʰ **S92.24** Fracture of medial cuneiform

3 √7ᵗʰ **S92.241** Displaced fracture of medial cuneiform of right foot   CC H5

3 √7ᵗʰ **S92.242** Displaced fracture of medial cuneiform of left foot   CC H5

3 √7ᵗʰ **S92.243** Displaced fracture of medial cuneiform of unspecified foot   CC H5

3 √7ᵗʰ **S92.244** Nondisplaced fracture of medial cuneiform of right foot   CC H5

3 √7ᵗʰ **S92.245** Nondisplaced fracture of medial cuneiform of left foot   CC H5

3 √7ᵗʰ **S92.246** Nondisplaced fracture of medial cuneiform of unspecified foot   CC H5

√6ᵗʰ **S92.25** Fracture of navicular [scaphoid] of foot

3 √7ᵗʰ **S92.251** Displaced fracture of navicular [scaphoid] of right foot   CC H5

3 √7ᵗʰ **S92.252** Displaced fracture of navicular [scaphoid] of left foot   CC H5

3 √7ᵗʰ **S92.253** Displaced fracture of navicular [scaphoid] of unspecified foot   CC H5

3 √7ᵗʰ **S92.254** Nondisplaced fracture of navicular [scaphoid] of right foot   CC H5

3 √7ᵗʰ **S92.255** Nondisplaced fracture of navicular [scaphoid] of left foot   CC H5

3 √7ᵗʰ **S92.256** Nondisplaced fracture of navicular [scaphoid] of unspecified foot   CC H5

√5ᵗʰ **S92.3** Fracture of metatarsal bone(s)

    EXCLUDES 2   physeal fracture of metatarsal (S99.1-)

    AHA: 2018,1Q,3

√6ᵗʰ **S92.30** Fracture of unspecified metatarsal bone(s)

3 √7ᵗʰ **S92.301** Fracture of unspecified metatarsal bone(s), right foot   CC H5

3 √7ᵗʰ **S92.302** Fracture of unspecified metatarsal bone(s), left foot   CC H5

3 √7ᵗʰ **S92.309** Fracture of unspecified metatarsal bone(s), unspecified foot   CC H5

√6ᵗʰ **S92.31** Fracture of first metatarsal bone

3 √7ᵗʰ **S92.311** Displaced fracture of first metatarsal bone, right foot   CC H5

3 √7ᵗʰ **S92.312** Displaced fracture of first metatarsal bone, left foot   CC H5

3 √7ᵗʰ **S92.313** Displaced fracture of first metatarsal bone, unspecified foot   CC H5

3 √7ᵗʰ **S92.314** Nondisplaced fracture of first metatarsal bone, right foot   CC H5

3 √7ᵗʰ **S92.315** Nondisplaced fracture of first metatarsal bone, left foot   CC H5

3 √7ᵗʰ **S92.316** Nondisplaced fracture of first metatarsal bone, unspecified foot   CC H5

√6ᵗʰ **S92.32** Fracture of second metatarsal bone

3 √7ᵗʰ **S92.321** Displaced fracture of second metatarsal bone, right foot   CC H5

3 √7ᵗʰ **S92.322** Displaced fracture of second metatarsal bone, left foot   CC H5

3 √7ᵗʰ **S92.323** Displaced fracture of second metatarsal bone, unspecified foot   CC H5

3 √7ᵗʰ **S92.324** Nondisplaced fracture of second metatarsal bone, right foot   CC H5

3 √7ᵗʰ **S92.325** Nondisplaced fracture of second metatarsal bone, left foot   CC H5

3 √7ᵗʰ **S92.326** Nondisplaced fracture of second metatarsal bone, unspecified foot   CC H5

√6ᵗʰ **S92.33** Fracture of third metatarsal bone

3 √7ᵗʰ **S92.331** Displaced fracture of third metatarsal bone, right foot   CC H5

3 √7ᵗʰ **S92.332** Displaced fracture of third metatarsal bone, left foot   CC H5

3 √7ᵗʰ **S92.333** Displaced fracture of third metatarsal bone, unspecified foot   CC H5

3 √7ᵗʰ **S92.334** Nondisplaced fracture of third metatarsal bone, right foot   CC H5

N Newborn: 0   P Pediatric: 0-17   M Maternity: 9-64   A Adult: 15-124   MCC Major Complication/Comorbidity   CC Complication/Comorbidity   SW Severe Wound Dx

1080   ICD-10-CM 2021

³ √7ᵗʰ **S92.335** Nondisplaced fracture of third metatarsal bone, left foot `CC` `H5`

³ √7ᵗʰ **S92.336** Nondisplaced fracture of third metatarsal bone, unspecified foot `CC` `H5`

√6ᵗʰ **S92.34** Fracture of fourth metatarsal bone

³ √7ᵗʰ **S92.341** Displaced fracture of fourth metatarsal bone, right foot `CC` `H5`

³ √7ᵗʰ **S92.342** Displaced fracture of fourth metatarsal bone, left foot `CC` `H5`

³ √7ᵗʰ **S92.343** Displaced fracture of fourth metatarsal bone, unspecified foot `CC` `H5`

³ √7ᵗʰ **S92.344** Nondisplaced fracture of fourth metatarsal bone, right foot `CC` `H5`

³ √7ᵗʰ **S92.345** Nondisplaced fracture of fourth metatarsal bone, left foot `CC` `H5`

³ √7ᵗʰ **S92.346** Nondisplaced fracture of fourth metatarsal bone, unspecified foot `CC` `H5`

√6ᵗʰ **S92.35** Fracture of fifth metatarsal bone

³ √7ᵗʰ **S92.351** Displaced fracture of fifth metatarsal bone, right foot `CC` `H5`

³ √7ᵗʰ **S92.352** Displaced fracture of fifth metatarsal bone, left foot `CC` `H5`

³ √7ᵗʰ **S92.353** Displaced fracture of fifth metatarsal bone, unspecified foot `CC` `H5`

³ √7ᵗʰ **S92.354** Nondisplaced fracture of fifth metatarsal bone, right foot `CC` `H5`

³ √7ᵗʰ **S92.355** Nondisplaced fracture of fifth metatarsal bone, left foot `CC` `H5`

³ √7ᵗʰ **S92.356** Nondisplaced fracture of fifth metatarsal bone, unspecified foot `CC` `H5`

√5ᵗʰ **S92.4** Fracture of great toe

EXCLUDES 2   *physeal fracture of phalanx of toe (S99.2-)*

√6ᵗʰ **S92.40** Unspecified fracture of great toe

⁴ √7ᵗʰ **S92.401** Displaced unspecified fracture of right great toe `CC`

⁴ √7ᵗʰ **S92.402** Displaced unspecified fracture of left great toe `CC`

⁴ √7ᵗʰ **S92.403** Displaced unspecified fracture of unspecified great toe `CC`

⁴ √7ᵗʰ **S92.404** Nondisplaced unspecified fracture of right great toe `CC`

⁴ √7ᵗʰ **S92.405** Nondisplaced unspecified fracture of left great toe `CC`

⁴ √7ᵗʰ **S92.406** Nondisplaced unspecified fracture of unspecified great toe `CC`

√6ᵗʰ **S92.41** Fracture of proximal phalanx of great toe

⁴ √7ᵗʰ **S92.411** Displaced fracture of proximal phalanx of right great toe `CC`

⁴ √7ᵗʰ **S92.412** Displaced fracture of proximal phalanx of left great toe `CC`

⁴ √7ᵗʰ **S92.413** Displaced fracture of proximal phalanx of unspecified great toe `CC`

⁴ √7ᵗʰ **S92.414** Nondisplaced fracture of proximal phalanx of right great toe `CC`

⁴ √7ᵗʰ **S92.415** Nondisplaced fracture of proximal phalanx of left great toe `CC`

⁴ √7ᵗʰ **S92.416** Nondisplaced fracture of proximal phalanx of unspecified great toe `CC`

√6ᵗʰ **S92.42** Fracture of distal phalanx of great toe

⁴ √7ᵗʰ **S92.421** Displaced fracture of distal phalanx of right great toe `CC`

⁴ √7ᵗʰ **S92.422** Displaced fracture of distal phalanx of left great toe `CC`

⁴ √7ᵗʰ **S92.423** Displaced fracture of distal phalanx of unspecified great toe `CC`

⁴ √7ᵗʰ **S92.424** Nondisplaced fracture of distal phalanx of right great toe `CC`

⁴ √7ᵗʰ **S92.425** Nondisplaced fracture of distal phalanx of left great toe `CC`

⁴ √7ᵗʰ **S92.426** Nondisplaced fracture of distal phalanx of unspecified great toe `CC`

√6ᵗʰ **S92.49** Other fracture of great toe

⁴ √7ᵗʰ **S92.491** Other fracture of right great toe `CC`

⁴ √7ᵗʰ **S92.492** Other fracture of left great toe `CC`

⁴ √7ᵗʰ **S92.499** Other fracture of unspecified great toe `CC`

√5ᵗʰ **S92.5** Fracture of lesser toe(s)

EXCLUDES 2   *physeal fracture of phalanx of toe (S99.2-)*

√6ᵗʰ **S92.50** Unspecified fracture of lesser toe(s)

⁴ √7ᵗʰ **S92.501** Displaced unspecified fracture of right lesser toe(s) `CC`

⁴ √7ᵗʰ **S92.502** Displaced unspecified fracture of left lesser toe(s) `CC`

⁴ √7ᵗʰ **S92.503** Displaced unspecified fracture of unspecified lesser toe(s) `CC`

⁴ √7ᵗʰ **S92.504** Nondisplaced unspecified fracture of right lesser toe(s) `CC`

⁴ √7ᵗʰ **S92.505** Nondisplaced unspecified fracture of left lesser toe(s) `CC`

⁴ √7ᵗʰ **S92.506** Nondisplaced unspecified fracture of unspecified lesser toe(s) `CC`

√6ᵗʰ **S92.51** Fracture of proximal phalanx of lesser toe(s)

⁴ √7ᵗʰ **S92.511** Displaced fracture of proximal phalanx of right lesser toe(s) `CC`

⁴ √7ᵗʰ **S92.512** Displaced fracture of proximal phalanx of left lesser toe(s) `CC`

⁴ √7ᵗʰ **S92.513** Displaced fracture of proximal phalanx of unspecified lesser toe(s) `CC`

⁴ √7ᵗʰ **S92.514** Nondisplaced fracture of proximal phalanx of right lesser toe(s) `CC`

⁴ √7ᵗʰ **S92.515** Nondisplaced fracture of proximal phalanx of left lesser toe(s)) `CC`

⁴ √7ᵗʰ **S92.516** Nondisplaced fracture of proximal phalanx of unspecified lesser toe(s) `CC`

√6ᵗʰ **S92.52** Fracture of middle phalanx of lesser toe(s)

⁴ √7ᵗʰ **S92.521** Displaced fracture of middle phalanx of right lesser toe(s) `CC`

⁴ √7ᵗʰ **S92.522** Displaced fracture of middle phalanx of left lesser toe(s) `CC`

⁴ √7ᵗʰ **S92.523** Displaced fracture of middle phalanx of unspecified lesser toe(s) `CC`

⁴ √7ᵗʰ **S92.524** Nondisplaced fracture of middle phalanx of right lesser toe(s) `CC`

⁴ √7ᵗʰ **S92.525** Nondisplaced fracture of middle phalanx of left lesser toe(s) `CC`

⁴ √7ᵗʰ **S92.526** Nondisplaced fracture of middle phalanx of unspecified lesser toe(s) `CC`

√6ᵗʰ **S92.53** Fracture of distal phalanx of lesser toe(s)

⁴ √7ᵗʰ **S92.531** Displaced fracture of distal phalanx of right lesser toe(s) `CC`

⁴ √7ᵗʰ **S92.532** Displaced fracture of distal phalanx of left lesser toe(s) `CC`

⁴ √7ᵗʰ **S92.533** Displaced fracture of distal phalanx of unspecified lesser toe(s) `CC`

⁴ √7ᵗʰ **S92.534** Nondisplaced fracture of distal phalanx of right lesser toe(s) `CC`

⁴ √7ᵗʰ **S92.535** Nondisplaced fracture of distal phalanx of left lesser toe(s) `CC`

⁴ √7ᵗʰ **S92.536** Nondisplaced fracture of distal phalanx of unspecified lesser toe(s) `CC`

√6ᵗʰ **S92.59** Other fracture of lesser toe(s)

⁴ √7ᵗʰ **S92.591** Other fracture of right lesser toe(s) `CC`

⁴ √7ᵗʰ **S92.592** Other fracture of left lesser toe(s) `CC`

⁴ √7ᵗʰ **S92.599** Other fracture of unspecified lesser toe(s) `CC`

√5ᵗʰ **S92.8** Other fracture of foot, except ankle

√6ᵗʰ **S92.81** Other fracture of foot

Sesamoid fracture of foot

AHA: 2016,4Q,68

³ √7ᵗʰ **S92.811** Other fracture of right foot `CC` `H5`

³ √7ᵗʰ **S92.812** Other fracture of left foot `CC` `H5`

³ √7ᵗʰ **S92.819** Other fracture of unspecified foot `CC` `H5`

√5ᵗʰ **S92.9** Unspecified fracture of foot and toe

√6ᵗʰ **S92.90** Unspecified fracture of foot

³ √7ᵗʰ **S92.901** Unspecified fracture of right foot `CC` `H5`

³ √7ᵗʰ **S92.902** Unspecified fracture of left foot `CC` `H5`

³ √7ᵗʰ **S92.909** Unspecified fracture of unspecified foot `CC` `H5`

√6ᵗʰ **S92.91** Unspecified fracture of toe

⁴ √7ᵗʰ **S92.911** Unspecified fracture of right toe(s) `CC`

✔ Additional Character Required   √x7ᵗʰ Placeholder   Unacceptable PDx   Questionable PDx   Manifestation   Unspecified Dx   `H1`-`H4` HAC   `HCC` CMS-HCC Dx   `HIV` HIV Dx

ICD-10-CM 2021   1081

4 √7th **S92.912** **Unspecified fracture of** left **toe(s)** CC

4 √7th **S92.919** **Unspecified fracture of unspecified toe(s)** CC

√4th **S93** **Dislocation and sprain of joints and ligaments at ankle, foot and toe level**

INCLUDES   avulsion of joint or ligament of ankle, foot and toe
    laceration of cartilage, joint or ligament of ankle, foot and toe
    sprain of cartilage, joint or ligament of ankle, foot and toe
    traumatic hemarthrosis of joint or ligament of ankle, foot and toe
    traumatic rupture of joint or ligament of ankle, foot and toe
    traumatic subluxation of joint or ligament of ankle, foot and toe
    traumatic tear of joint or ligament of ankle, foot and toe

Code also any associated open wound

EXCLUDES 2   *strain of muscle and tendon of ankle and foot (S96.-)*

The appropriate 7th character is to be added to each code from category S93.
A   initial encounter
D   subsequent encounter
S   sequela

√5th **S93.0** **Subluxation and dislocation of** ankle joint

Subluxation and dislocation of astragalus
Subluxation and dislocation of fibula, lower end
Subluxation and dislocation of talus
Subluxation and dislocation of tibia, lower end

√x7th **S93.01** **Subluxation of** right **ankle joint**

√x7th **S93.02** **Subluxation of** left **ankle joint**

√x7th **S93.03** **Subluxation of unspecified ankle joint**

√x7th **S93.04** **Dislocation of** right **ankle joint**

√x7th **S93.05** **Dislocation of** left **ankle joint**

√x7th **S93.06** **Dislocation of unspecified ankle joint**

√5th **S93.1** **Subluxation and dislocation of** toe

√6th **S93.10** **Unspecified subluxation and dislocation of toe**

Dislocation of toe NOS
Subluxation of toe NOS

√7th **S93.101** **Unspecified** subluxation **of** right **toe(s)**

√7th **S93.102** **Unspecified** subluxation **of** left **toe(s)**

√7th **S93.103** **Unspecified** subluxation **of unspecified toe(s)**

√7th **S93.104** **Unspecified** dislocation **of** right **toe(s)**

√7th **S93.105** **Unspecified** dislocation **of** left **toe(s)**

√7th **S93.106** **Unspecified** dislocation **of unspecified toe(s)**

√6th **S93.11** **Dislocation of** interphalangeal joint

√7th **S93.111** **Dislocation of interphalangeal joint of** right great **toe**

√7th **S93.112** **Dislocation of interphalangeal joint of** left great **toe**

√7th **S93.113** **Dislocation of interphalangeal joint of unspecified great toe**

√7th **S93.114** **Dislocation of interphalangeal joint of** right lesser **toe(s)**

√7th **S93.115** **Dislocation of interphalangeal joint of** left lesser **toe(s)**

√7th **S93.116** **Dislocation of interphalangeal joint of unspecified lesser toe(s)**

√7th **S93.119** **Dislocation of interphalangeal joint of unspecified toe(s)**

√6th **S93.12** **Dislocation of** metatarsophalangeal joint

√7th **S93.121** **Dislocation of metatarsophalangeal joint of** right great **toe**

√7th **S93.122** **Dislocation of metatarsophalangeal joint of** left great **toe**

√7th **S93.123** **Dislocation of metatarsophalangeal joint of unspecified great toe**

√7th **S93.124** **Dislocation of metatarsophalangeal joint of** right lesser **toe(s)**

√7th **S93.125** **Dislocation of metatarsophalangeal joint of** left lesser **toe(s)**

√7th **S93.126** **Dislocation of metatarsophalangeal joint of unspecified lesser toe(s)**

√7th **S93.129** **Dislocation of metatarsophalangeal joint of unspecified toe(s)**

√6th **S93.13** **Subluxation of** interphalangeal joint

√7th **S93.131** **Subluxation of interphalangeal joint of** right great **toe**

√7th **S93.132** **Subluxation of interphalangeal joint of** left great **toe**

√7th **S93.133** **Subluxation of interphalangeal joint of unspecified great toe**

√7th **S93.134** **Subluxation of interphalangeal joint of** right lesser **toe(s)**

√7th **S93.135** **Subluxation of interphalangeal joint of** left lesser **toe(s)**

√7th **S93.136** **Subluxation of interphalangeal joint of unspecified lesser toe(s)**

√7th **S93.139** **Subluxation of interphalangeal joint of unspecified toe(s)**

√6th **S93.14** **Subluxation of** metatarsophalangeal joint

√7th **S93.141** **Subluxation of metatarsophalangeal joint of** right great **toe**

√7th **S93.142** **Subluxation of metatarsophalangeal joint of** left great **toe**

√7th **S93.143** **Subluxation of metatarsophalangeal joint of unspecified great toe**

√7th **S93.144** **Subluxation of metatarsophalangeal joint of** right lesser **toe(s)**

√7th **S93.145** **Subluxation of metatarsophalangeal joint of** left lesser **toe(s)**

√7th **S93.146** **Subluxation of metatarsophalangeal joint of unspecified lesser toe(s)**

√7th **S93.149** **Subluxation of metatarsophalangeal joint of unspecified toe(s)**

√5th **S93.3** **Subluxation and dislocation of** foot

EXCLUDES 2   *dislocation of toe (S93.1-)*

√6th **S93.30** **Unspecified subluxation and dislocation of foot**

Dislocation of foot NOS
Subluxation of foot NOS

√7th **S93.301** **Unspecified** subluxation **of** right **foot**

√7th **S93.302** **Unspecified** subluxation **of** left **foot**

√7th **S93.303** **Unspecified** subluxation **of unspecified foot**

√7th **S93.304** **Unspecified** dislocation **of** right **foot**

√7th **S93.305** **Unspecified** dislocation **of** left **foot**

√7th **S93.306** **Unspecified** dislocation **of unspecified foot**

√6th **S93.31** **Subluxation and dislocation of** tarsal joint

√7th **S93.311** **Subluxation of tarsal joint of** right **foot**

√7th **S93.312** **Subluxation of tarsal joint of** left **foot**

√7th **S93.313** **Subluxation of tarsal joint of unspecified foot**

√7th **S93.314** **Dislocation of tarsal joint of** right **foot**

√7th **S93.315** **Dislocation of tarsal joint of** left **foot**

√7th **S93.316** **Dislocation of tarsal joint of unspecified foot**

√6th **S93.32** **Subluxation and dislocation of** tarsometatarsal joint

√7th **S93.321** **Subluxation of tarsometatarsal joint of** right **foot**

√7th **S93.322** **Subluxation of tarsometatarsal joint of** left **foot**

√7th **S93.323** **Subluxation of tarsometatarsal joint of unspecified foot**

√7th **S93.324** **Dislocation of tarsometatarsal joint of** right **foot**

√7th **S93.325** **Dislocation of tarsometatarsal joint of** left **foot**

√7th **S93.326** **Dislocation of tarsometatarsal joint of unspecified foot**

√6th **S93.33** **Other subluxation and dislocation of foot**

√7th **S93.331** **Other** subluxation **of** right **foot**

√7th **S93.332** **Other** subluxation **of** left **foot**

√7th **S93.333** **Other** subluxation **of unspecified foot**

√7th **S93.334** **Other** dislocation **of** right **foot**

√7th **S93.335** **Other** dislocation **of** left **foot**

√7th **S93.336** **Other** dislocation **of unspecified foot**

√5ᵗʰ **S93.4 Sprain of ankle**

> EXCLUDES 2   *injury of Achilles tendon (S86.0-)*

> √6ᵗʰ **S93.40 Sprain of unspecified ligament of ankle**
>> Sprain of ankle NOS
>> Sprained ankle NOS
>>> √7ᵗʰ **S93.401** Sprain of unspecified ligament of right ankle
>>> √7ᵗʰ **S93.402** Sprain of unspecified ligament of left ankle
>>> √7ᵗʰ **S93.409** Sprain of unspecified ligament of unspecified ankle

> √6ᵗʰ **S93.41 Sprain of calcaneofibular ligament**
>>> √7ᵗʰ **S93.411** Sprain of calcaneofibular ligament of right ankle
>>> √7ᵗʰ **S93.412** Sprain of calcaneofibular ligament of left ankle
>>> √7ᵗʰ **S93.419** Sprain of calcaneofibular ligament of unspecified ankle

> √6ᵗʰ **S93.42 Sprain of deltoid ligament**
>>> √7ᵗʰ **S93.421** Sprain of deltoid ligament of right ankle
>>> √7ᵗʰ **S93.422** Sprain of deltoid ligament of left ankle
>>> √7ᵗʰ **S93.429** Sprain of deltoid ligament of unspecified ankle

> √6ᵗʰ **S93.43 Sprain of tibiofibular ligament**
>>> √7ᵗʰ **S93.431** Sprain of tibiofibular ligament of right ankle
>>> √7ᵗʰ **S93.432** Sprain of tibiofibular ligament of left ankle
>>> √7ᵗʰ **S93.439** Sprain of tibiofibular ligament of unspecified ankle

> √6ᵗʰ **S93.49 Sprain of other ligament of ankle**
>> Sprain of internal collateral ligament
>> Sprain of talofibular ligament
>>> √7ᵗʰ **S93.491** Sprain of other ligament of right ankle
>>> √7ᵗʰ **S93.492** Sprain of other ligament of left ankle
>>> √7ᵗʰ **S93.499** Sprain of other ligament of unspecified ankle

√5ᵗʰ **S93.5 Sprain of toe**

> √6ᵗʰ **S93.50 Unspecified sprain of toe**
>>> √7ᵗʰ **S93.501** Unspecified sprain of right great toe
>>> √7ᵗʰ **S93.502** Unspecified sprain of left great toe
>>> √7ᵗʰ **S93.503** Unspecified sprain of unspecified great toe
>>> √7ᵗʰ **S93.504** Unspecified sprain of right lesser toe(s)
>>> √7ᵗʰ **S93.505** Unspecified sprain of left lesser toe(s)
>>> √7ᵗʰ **S93.506** Unspecified sprain of unspecified lesser toe(s)
>>> √7ᵗʰ **S93.509** Unspecified sprain of unspecified toe(s)

> √6ᵗʰ **S93.51 Sprain of interphalangeal joint of toe**
>>> √7ᵗʰ **S93.511** Sprain of interphalangeal joint of right great toe
>>> √7ᵗʰ **S93.512** Sprain of interphalangeal joint of left great toe
>>> √7ᵗʰ **S93.513** Sprain of interphalangeal joint of unspecified great toe
>>> √7ᵗʰ **S93.514** Sprain of interphalangeal joint of right lesser toe(s)
>>> √7ᵗʰ **S93.515** Sprain of interphalangeal joint of left lesser toe(s)
>>> √7ᵗʰ **S93.516** Sprain of interphalangeal joint of unspecified lesser toe(s)
>>> √7ᵗʰ **S93.519** Sprain of interphalangeal joint of unspecified toe(s)

> √6ᵗʰ **S93.52 Sprain of metatarsophalangeal joint of toe**
>>> √7ᵗʰ **S93.521** Sprain of metatarsophalangeal joint of right great toe
>>> √7ᵗʰ **S93.522** Sprain of metatarsophalangeal joint of left great toe
>>> √7ᵗʰ **S93.523** Sprain of metatarsophalangeal joint of unspecified great toe
>>> √7ᵗʰ **S93.524** Sprain of metatarsophalangeal joint of right lesser toe(s)
>>> √7ᵗʰ **S93.525** Sprain of metatarsophalangeal joint of left lesser toe(s)
>>> √7ᵗʰ **S93.526** Sprain of metatarsophalangeal joint of unspecified lesser toe(s)
>>> √7ᵗʰ **S93.529** Sprain of metatarsophalangeal joint of unspecified toe(s)

√5ᵗʰ **S93.6 Sprain of foot**

> EXCLUDES 2   *sprain of metatarsophalangeal joint of toe (S93.52-)*
>> *sprain of toe (S93.5-)*

> √6ᵗʰ **S93.60 Unspecified sprain of foot**
>>> √7ᵗʰ **S93.601** Unspecified sprain of right foot
>>> √7ᵗʰ **S93.602** Unspecified sprain of left foot
>>> √7ᵗʰ **S93.609** Unspecified sprain of unspecified foot

> √6ᵗʰ **S93.61 Sprain of tarsal ligament of foot**
>>> √7ᵗʰ **S93.611** Sprain of tarsal ligament of right foot
>>> √7ᵗʰ **S93.612** Sprain of tarsal ligament of left foot
>>> √7ᵗʰ **S93.619** Sprain of tarsal ligament of unspecified foot

> √6ᵗʰ **S93.62 Sprain of tarsometatarsal ligament of foot**
>>> √7ᵗʰ **S93.621** Sprain of tarsometatarsal ligament of right foot
>>> √7ᵗʰ **S93.622** Sprain of tarsometatarsal ligament of left foot
>>> √7ᵗʰ **S93.629** Sprain of tarsometatarsal ligament of unspecified foot

> √6ᵗʰ **S93.69 Other sprain of foot**
>>> √7ᵗʰ **S93.691** Other sprain of right foot
>>> √7ᵗʰ **S93.692** Other sprain of left foot
>>> √7ᵗʰ **S93.699** Other sprain of unspecified foot

√4ᵗʰ **S94 Injury of nerves at ankle and foot level**

> Code also any associated open wound (S91.-)

> The appropriate 7th character is to be added to each code from category S94.
> A   initial encounter
> D   subsequent encounter
> S   sequela

√5ᵗʰ **S94.0 Injury of lateral plantar nerve**
> √x7ᵗʰ **S94.00** Injury of lateral plantar nerve, unspecified leg
> √x7ᵗʰ **S94.01** Injury of lateral plantar nerve, right leg
> √x7ᵗʰ **S94.02** Injury of lateral plantar nerve, left leg

√5ᵗʰ **S94.1 Injury of medial plantar nerve**
> √x7ᵗʰ **S94.10** Injury of medial plantar nerve, unspecified leg
> √x7ᵗʰ **S94.11** Injury of medial plantar nerve, right leg
> √x7ᵗʰ **S94.12** Injury of medial plantar nerve, left leg

√5ᵗʰ **S94.2 Injury of deep peroneal nerve at ankle and foot level**
>> Injury of terminal, lateral branch of deep peroneal nerve
> √x7ᵗʰ **S94.20** Injury of deep peroneal nerve at ankle and foot level, unspecified leg
> √x7ᵗʰ **S94.21** Injury of deep peroneal nerve at ankle and foot level, right leg
> √x7ᵗʰ **S94.22** Injury of deep peroneal nerve at ankle and foot level, left leg

√5ᵗʰ **S94.3 Injury of cutaneous sensory nerve at ankle and foot level**
> √x7ᵗʰ **S94.30** Injury of cutaneous sensory nerve at ankle and foot level, unspecified leg
> √x7ᵗʰ **S94.31** Injury of cutaneous sensory nerve at ankle and foot level, right leg
> √x7ᵗʰ **S94.32** Injury of cutaneous sensory nerve at ankle and foot level, left leg

√5ᵗʰ **S94.8 Injury of other nerves at ankle and foot level**
> √6ᵗʰ **S94.8X Injury of other nerves at ankle and foot level**
>>> √7ᵗʰ **S94.8X1** Injury of other nerves at ankle and foot level, right leg
>>> √7ᵗʰ **S94.8X2** Injury of other nerves at ankle and foot level, left leg
>>> √7ᵗʰ **S94.8X9** Injury of other nerves at ankle and foot level, unspecified leg

√5ᵗʰ **S94.9 Injury of unspecified nerve at ankle and foot level**
> √x7ᵗʰ **S94.90** Injury of unspecified nerve at ankle and foot level, unspecified leg
> √x7ᵗʰ **S94.91** Injury of unspecified nerve at ankle and foot level, right leg
> √x7ᵗʰ **S94.92** Injury of unspecified nerve at ankle and foot level, left leg

☑ Additional Character Required   √x7ᵗʰ Placeholder   Unacceptable PDx   Questionable PDx   Manifestation   Unspecified Dx   H1-H14 HAC   HCC CMS-HCC Dx   HIV HIV Dx

ICD-10-CM 2021   1083

✓4ᵗʰ **S95 Injury of blood vessels at ankle and foot level**

Code also any associated open wound (S91.-)

EXCLUDES 2   *injury of posterior tibial artery and vein (S85.1-, S85.8-)*

The appropriate 7th character is to be added to each code from category S95.
A   initial encounter
D   subsequent encounter
S   sequela

✓5ᵗʰ **S95.0 Injury of dorsal artery of foot**

    ✓6ᵗʰ **S95.00 Unspecified injury of dorsal artery of foot**

       ✓7ᵗʰ **S95.001** Unspecified injury of dorsal artery of right foot `CC`

       ✓7ᵗʰ **S95.002** Unspecified injury of dorsal artery of left foot `CC`

       ✓7ᵗʰ **S95.009** Unspecified injury of dorsal artery of unspecified foot `CC`

    ✓6ᵗʰ **S95.01 Laceration of dorsal artery of foot**

       ✓7ᵗʰ **S95.011** Laceration of dorsal artery of right foot `CC`

       ✓7ᵗʰ **S95.012** Laceration of dorsal artery of left foot `CC`

       ✓7ᵗʰ **S95.019** Laceration of dorsal artery of unspecified foot `CC`

    ✓6ᵗʰ **S95.09 Other specified injury of dorsal artery of foot**

       ✓7ᵗʰ **S95.091** Other specified injury of dorsal artery of right foot `CC`

       ✓7ᵗʰ **S95.092** Other specified injury of dorsal artery of left foot `CC`

       ✓7ᵗʰ **S95.099** Other specified injury of dorsal artery of unspecified foot `CC`

✓5ᵗʰ **S95.1 Injury of plantar artery of foot**

    ✓6ᵗʰ **S95.10 Unspecified injury of plantar artery of foot**

       ✓7ᵗʰ **S95.101** Unspecified injury of plantar artery of right foot `CC`

       ✓7ᵗʰ **S95.102** Unspecified injury of plantar artery of left foot `CC`

       ✓7ᵗʰ **S95.109** Unspecified injury of plantar artery of unspecified foot `CC`

    ✓6ᵗʰ **S95.11 Laceration of plantar artery of foot**

       ✓7ᵗʰ **S95.111** Laceration of plantar artery of right foot `CC`

       ✓7ᵗʰ **S95.112** Laceration of plantar artery of left foot `CC`

       ✓7ᵗʰ **S95.119** Laceration of plantar artery of unspecified foot `CC`

    ✓6ᵗʰ **S95.19 Other specified injury of plantar artery of foot**

       ✓7ᵗʰ **S95.191** Other specified injury of plantar artery of right foot `CC`

       ✓7ᵗʰ **S95.192** Other specified injury of plantar artery of left foot `CC`

       ✓7ᵗʰ **S95.199** Other specified injury of plantar artery of unspecified foot `CC`

✓5ᵗʰ **S95.2 Injury of dorsal vein of foot**

    ✓6ᵗʰ **S95.20 Unspecified injury of dorsal vein of foot**

       ✓7ᵗʰ **S95.201** Unspecified injury of dorsal vein of right foot `CC`

       ✓7ᵗʰ **S95.202** Unspecified injury of dorsal vein of left foot `CC`

       ✓7ᵗʰ **S95.209** Unspecified injury of dorsal vein of unspecified foot `CC`

    ✓6ᵗʰ **S95.21 Laceration of dorsal vein of foot**

       ✓7ᵗʰ **S95.211** Laceration of dorsal vein of right foot `CC`

       ✓7ᵗʰ **S95.212** Laceration of dorsal vein of left foot `CC`

       ✓7ᵗʰ **S95.219** Laceration of dorsal vein of unspecified foot `CC`

    ✓6ᵗʰ **S95.29 Other specified injury of dorsal vein of foot**

       ✓7ᵗʰ **S95.291** Other specified injury of dorsal vein of right foot `CC`

       ✓7ᵗʰ **S95.292** Other specified injury of dorsal vein of left foot `CC`

       ✓7ᵗʰ **S95.299** Other specified injury of dorsal vein of unspecified foot `CC`

✓5ᵗʰ **S95.8 Injury of other blood vessels at ankle and foot level**

    ✓6ᵗʰ **S95.80 Unspecified injury of other blood vessels at ankle and foot level**

       ✓7ᵗʰ **S95.801** Unspecified injury of other blood vessels at ankle and foot level, right leg `CC`

       ✓7ᵗʰ **S95.802** Unspecified injury of other blood vessels at ankle and foot level, left leg `CC`

       ✓7ᵗʰ **S95.809** Unspecified injury of other blood vessels at ankle and foot level, unspecified leg `CC`

    ✓6ᵗʰ **S95.81 Laceration of other blood vessels at ankle and foot level**

       ✓7ᵗʰ **S95.811** Laceration of other blood vessels at ankle and foot level, right leg `CC`

       ✓7ᵗʰ **S95.812** Laceration of other blood vessels at ankle and foot level, left leg `CC`

       ✓7ᵗʰ **S95.819** Laceration of other blood vessels at ankle and foot level, unspecified leg `CC`

    ✓6ᵗʰ **S95.89 Other specified injury of other blood vessels at ankle and foot level**

       ✓7ᵗʰ **S95.891** Other specified injury of other blood vessels at ankle and foot level, right leg `CC`

       ✓7ᵗʰ **S95.892** Other specified injury of other blood vessels at ankle and foot level, left leg `CC`

       ✓7ᵗʰ **S95.899** Other specified injury of other blood vessels at ankle and foot level, unspecified leg `CC`

✓5ᵗʰ **S95.9 Injury of unspecified blood vessel at ankle and foot level**

    ✓6ᵗʰ **S95.90 Unspecified injury of unspecified blood vessel at ankle and foot level**

       ✓7ᵗʰ **S95.901** Unspecified injury of unspecified blood vessel at ankle and foot level, right leg `CC`

       ✓7ᵗʰ **S95.902** Unspecified injury of unspecified blood vessel at ankle and foot level, left leg `CC`

       ✓7ᵗʰ **S95.909** Unspecified injury of unspecified blood vessel at ankle and foot level, unspecified leg `CC`

    ✓6ᵗʰ **S95.91 Laceration of unspecified blood vessel at ankle and foot level**

       ✓7ᵗʰ **S95.911** Laceration of unspecified blood vessel at ankle and foot level, right leg `CC`

       ✓7ᵗʰ **S95.912** Laceration of unspecified blood vessel at ankle and foot level, left leg `CC`

       ✓7ᵗʰ **S95.919** Laceration of unspecified blood vessel at ankle and foot level, unspecified leg `CC`

    ✓6ᵗʰ **S95.99 Other specified injury of unspecified blood vessel at ankle and foot level**

       ✓7ᵗʰ **S95.991** Other specified injury of unspecified blood vessel at ankle and foot level, right leg `CC`

       ✓7ᵗʰ **S95.992** Other specified injury of unspecified blood vessel at ankle and foot level, left leg `CC`

       ✓7ᵗʰ **S95.999** Other specified injury of unspecified blood vessel at ankle and foot level, unspecified leg `CC`

✓4ᵗʰ **S96 Injury of muscle and tendon at ankle and foot level**

Code also any associated open wound (S91.-)

EXCLUDES 2   *injury of Achilles tendon (S86.0-)*

          sprain of joints and ligaments of ankle and foot (S93.-)

TIP: Refer to the Muscle/Tendon table at the beginning of this chapter,

The appropriate 7th character is to be added to each code from category S96.
A   initial encounter
D   subsequent encounter
S   sequela

✓5ᵗʰ **S96.0 Injury of muscle and tendon of long flexor muscle of toe at ankle and foot level**

    ✓6ᵗʰ **S96.00 Unspecified injury of muscle and tendon of long flexor muscle of toe at ankle and foot level**

       ✓7ᵗʰ **S96.001** Unspecified injury of muscle and tendon of long flexor muscle of toe at ankle and foot level, right foot

       ✓7ᵗʰ **S96.002** Unspecified injury of muscle and tendon of long flexor muscle of toe at ankle and foot level, left foot

Ⓝ Newborn: 0   Ⓟ Pediatric: 0-17   Ⓜ Maternity: 9-64   Ⓐ Adult: 15-124   `MCC` Major Complication/Comorbidity   `CC` Complication/Comorbidity   `SW` Severe Wound Dx

1084   ICD-10-CM 2021

√7ᵗʰ **S96.009** Unspecified injury of muscle and tendon of long flexor muscle of toe at ankle and foot level, unspecified foot

√6ᵗʰ **S96.01** Strain of muscle and tendon of long flexor muscle of toe at ankle and foot level

    √7ᵗʰ **S96.011** Strain of muscle and tendon of long flexor muscle of toe at ankle and foot level, right foot

    √7ᵗʰ **S96.012** Strain of muscle and tendon of long flexor muscle of toe at ankle and foot level, left foot

    √7ᵗʰ **S96.019** Strain of muscle and tendon of long flexor muscle of toe at ankle and foot level, unspecified foot

√6ᵗʰ **S96.02** Laceration of muscle and tendon of long flexor muscle of toe at ankle and foot level

    √7ᵗʰ **S96.021** Laceration of muscle and tendon of long flexor muscle of toe at ankle and foot level, right foot   CC

    √7ᵗʰ **S96.022** Laceration of muscle and tendon of long flexor muscle of toe at ankle and foot level, left foot   CC

    √7ᵗʰ **S96.029** Laceration of muscle and tendon of long flexor muscle of toe at ankle and foot level, unspecified foot   CC

√6ᵗʰ **S96.09** Other injury of muscle and tendon of long flexor muscle of toe at ankle and foot level

    √7ᵗʰ **S96.091** Other injury of muscle and tendon of long flexor muscle of toe at ankle and foot level, right foot

    √7ᵗʰ **S96.092** Other injury of muscle and tendon of long flexor muscle of toe at ankle and foot level, left foot

    √7ᵗʰ **S96.099** Other injury of muscle and tendon of long flexor muscle of toe at ankle and foot level, unspecified foot

√5ᵗʰ **S96.1** Injury of muscle and tendon of long extensor muscle of toe at ankle and foot level

√6ᵗʰ **S96.10** Unspecified injury of muscle and tendon of long extensor muscle of toe at ankle and foot level

    √7ᵗʰ **S96.101** Unspecified injury of muscle and tendon of long extensor muscle of toe at ankle and foot level, right foot

    √7ᵗʰ **S96.102** Unspecified injury of muscle and tendon of long extensor muscle of toe at ankle and foot level, left foot

    √7ᵗʰ **S96.109** Unspecified injury of muscle and tendon of long extensor muscle of toe at ankle and foot level, unspecified foot

√6ᵗʰ **S96.11** Strain of muscle and tendon of long extensor muscle of toe at ankle and foot level

    √7ᵗʰ **S96.111** Strain of muscle and tendon of long extensor muscle of toe at ankle and foot level, right foot

    √7ᵗʰ **S96.112** Strain of muscle and tendon of long extensor muscle of toe at ankle and foot level, left foot

    √7ᵗʰ **S96.119** Strain of muscle and tendon of long extensor muscle of toe at ankle and foot level, unspecified foot

√6ᵗʰ **S96.12** Laceration of muscle and tendon of long extensor muscle of toe at ankle and foot level

    √7ᵗʰ **S96.121** Laceration of muscle and tendon of long extensor muscle of toe at ankle and foot level, right foot   CC

    √7ᵗʰ **S96.122** Laceration of muscle and tendon of long extensor muscle of toe at ankle and foot level, left foot   CC

    √7ᵗʰ **S96.129** Laceration of muscle and tendon of long extensor muscle of toe at ankle and foot level, unspecified foot   CC

√6ᵗʰ **S96.19** Other specified injury of muscle and tendon of long extensor muscle of toe at ankle and foot level

    √7ᵗʰ **S96.191** Other specified injury of muscle and tendon of long extensor muscle of toe at ankle and foot level, right foot

    √7ᵗʰ **S96.192** Other specified injury of muscle and tendon of long extensor muscle of toe at ankle and foot level, left foot

    √7ᵗʰ **S96.199** Other specified injury of muscle and tendon of long extensor muscle of toe at ankle and foot level, unspecified foot

√5ᵗʰ **S96.2** Injury of intrinsic muscle and tendon at ankle and foot level

√6ᵗʰ **S96.20** Unspecified injury of intrinsic muscle and tendon at ankle and foot level

    √7ᵗʰ **S96.201** Unspecified injury of intrinsic muscle and tendon at ankle and foot level, right foot

    √7ᵗʰ **S96.202** Unspecified injury of intrinsic muscle and tendon at ankle and foot level, left foot

    √7ᵗʰ **S96.209** Unspecified injury of intrinsic muscle and tendon at ankle and foot level, unspecified foot

√6ᵗʰ **S96.21** Strain of intrinsic muscle and tendon at ankle and foot level

    √7ᵗʰ **S96.211** Strain of intrinsic muscle and tendon at ankle and foot level, right foot

    √7ᵗʰ **S96.212** Strain of intrinsic muscle and tendon at ankle and foot level, left foot

    √7ᵗʰ **S96.219** Strain of intrinsic muscle and tendon at ankle and foot level, unspecified foot

√6ᵗʰ **S96.22** Laceration of intrinsic muscle and tendon at ankle and foot level

    √7ᵗʰ **S96.221** Laceration of intrinsic muscle and tendon at ankle and foot level, right foot   CC

    √7ᵗʰ **S96.222** Laceration of intrinsic muscle and tendon at ankle and foot level, left foot   CC

    √7ᵗʰ **S96.229** Laceration of intrinsic muscle and tendon at ankle and foot level, unspecified foot   CC

√6ᵗʰ **S96.29** Other specified injury of intrinsic muscle and tendon at ankle and foot level

    √7ᵗʰ **S96.291** Other specified injury of intrinsic muscle and tendon at ankle and foot level, right foot

    √7ᵗʰ **S96.292** Other specified injury of intrinsic muscle and tendon at ankle and foot level, left foot

    √7ᵗʰ **S96.299** Other specified injury of intrinsic muscle and tendon at ankle and foot level, unspecified foot

√5ᵗʰ **S96.8** Injury of other specified muscles and tendons at ankle and foot level

√6ᵗʰ **S96.80** Unspecified injury of other specified muscles and tendons at ankle and foot level

    √7ᵗʰ **S96.801** Unspecified injury of other specified muscles and tendons at ankle and foot level, right foot

    √7ᵗʰ **S96.802** Unspecified injury of other specified muscles and tendons at ankle and foot level, left foot

    √7ᵗʰ **S96.809** Unspecified injury of other specified muscles and tendons at ankle and foot level, unspecified foot

√6ᵗʰ **S96.81** Strain of other specified muscles and tendons at ankle and foot level

    √7ᵗʰ **S96.811** Strain of other specified muscles and tendons at ankle and foot level, right foot

    √7ᵗʰ **S96.812** Strain of other specified muscles and tendons at ankle and foot level, left foot

    √7ᵗʰ **S96.819** Strain of other specified muscles and tendons at ankle and foot level, unspecified foot

√6ᵗʰ **S96.82** Laceration of other specified muscles and tendons at ankle and foot level

    √7ᵗʰ **S96.821** Laceration of other specified muscles and tendons at ankle and foot level, right foot   CC

    √7ᵗʰ **S96.822** Laceration of other specified muscles and tendons at ankle and foot level, left foot   CC

    √7ᵗʰ **S96.829** Laceration of other specified muscles and tendons at ankle and foot level, unspecified foot   CC

√6ᵗʰ **S96.89** Other specified injury of other specified muscles and tendons at ankle and foot level

    √7ᵗʰ **S96.891** Other specified injury of other specified muscles and tendons at ankle and foot level, right foot

    √7ᵗʰ **S96.892** Other specified injury of other specified muscles and tendons at ankle and foot level, left foot

    √7ᵗʰ **S96.899** Other specified injury of other specified muscles and tendons at ankle and foot level, unspecified foot

☑ Additional Character Required   √xᵗʰ Placeholder   Unacceptable PDx   Questionable PDx   Manifestation   Unspecified Dx   H1-H16 HAC   HCC CMS-HCC Dx   HIV HIV Dx

ICD-10-CM 2021   1085

Chapter 19. Injury, Poisoning and Certain Other Consequences of External Causes

S96.9–S98.312

✓5ᵗʰ **S96.9** **Injury of unspecified muscle and tendon at ankle and foot level**

  ✓6ᵗʰ **S96.90** **Unspecified injury of unspecified muscle and tendon at ankle and foot level**

    ✓7ᵗʰ **S96.901** Unspecified injury of unspecified muscle and tendon at ankle and foot level, right foot

    ✓7ᵗʰ **S96.902** Unspecified injury of unspecified muscle and tendon at ankle and foot level, left foot

    ✓7ᵗʰ **S96.909** Unspecified injury of unspecified muscle and tendon at ankle and foot level, unspecified foot

  ✓6ᵗʰ **S96.91** **Strain of unspecified muscle and tendon at ankle and foot level**

    ✓7ᵗʰ **S96.911** Strain of unspecified muscle and tendon at ankle and foot level, right foot

    ✓7ᵗʰ **S96.912** Strain of unspecified muscle and tendon at ankle and foot level, left foot

    ✓7ᵗʰ **S96.919** Strain of unspecified muscle and tendon at ankle and foot level, unspecified foot

  ✓6ᵗʰ **S96.92** **Laceration of unspecified muscle and tendon at ankle and foot level**

    ✓7ᵗʰ **S96.921** Laceration of unspecified muscle and tendon at ankle and foot level, right foot   CC

    ✓7ᵗʰ **S96.922** Laceration of unspecified muscle and tendon at ankle and foot level, left foot   CC

    ✓7ᵗʰ **S96.929** Laceration of unspecified muscle and tendon at ankle and foot level, unspecified foot   CC

  ✓6ᵗʰ **S96.99** **Other specified injury of unspecified muscle and tendon at ankle and foot level**

    ✓7ᵗʰ **S96.991** Other specified injury of unspecified muscle and tendon at ankle and foot level, right foot

    ✓7ᵗʰ **S96.992** Other specified injury of unspecified muscle and tendon at ankle and foot level, left foot

    ✓7ᵗʰ **S96.999** Other specified injury of unspecified muscle and tendon at ankle and foot level, unspecified foot

✓4ᵗʰ **S97** **Crushing injury of ankle and foot**

Use additional code(s) for all associated injuries

The appropriate 7th character is to be added to each code from category S97.
A initial encounter
D subsequent encounter
S sequela

  ✓5ᵗʰ **S97.0** **Crushing injury of ankle**

    ✓×7ᵗʰ **S97.00** Crushing injury of unspecified ankle

    ✓×7ᵗʰ **S97.01** Crushing injury of right ankle

    ✓×7ᵗʰ **S97.02** Crushing injury of left ankle

  ✓5ᵗʰ **S97.1** **Crushing injury of toe**

    ✓6ᵗʰ **S97.10** **Crushing injury of unspecified toe(s)**

      ✓7ᵗʰ **S97.101** Crushing injury of unspecified right toe(s)

      ✓7ᵗʰ **S97.102** Crushing injury of unspecified left toe(s)

      ✓7ᵗʰ **S97.109** Crushing injury of unspecified toe(s)

        Crushing injury of toe NOS

    ✓6ᵗʰ **S97.11** **Crushing injury of great toe**

      ✓7ᵗʰ **S97.111** Crushing injury of right great toe

      ✓7ᵗʰ **S97.112** Crushing injury of left great toe

      ✓7ᵗʰ **S97.119** Crushing injury of unspecified great toe

    ✓6ᵗʰ **S97.12** **Crushing injury of lesser toe(s)**

      ✓7ᵗʰ **S97.121** Crushing injury of right lesser toe(s)

      ✓7ᵗʰ **S97.122** Crushing injury of left lesser toe(s)

      ✓7ᵗʰ **S97.129** Crushing injury of unspecified lesser toe(s)

  ✓5ᵗʰ **S97.8** **Crushing injury of foot**

    ✓×7ᵗʰ **S97.80** Crushing injury of unspecified foot

      Crushing injury of foot NOS

    ✓×7ᵗʰ **S97.81** Crushing injury of right foot

    ✓×7ᵗʰ **S97.82** Crushing injury of left foot

✓4ᵗʰ **S98** **Traumatic amputation of ankle and foot**

An amputation not identified as partial or complete should be coded to complete

The appropriate 7th character is to be added to each code from category S98.
A initial encounter
D subsequent encounter
S sequela

  ✓5ᵗʰ **S98.0** **Traumatic amputation of foot at ankle level**

    ✓6ᵗʰ **S98.01** **Complete traumatic amputation of foot at ankle level**

      ✓7ᵗʰ **S98.011** Complete traumatic amputation of right foot at ankle level   CC HCC

      ✓7ᵗʰ **S98.012** Complete traumatic amputation of left foot at ankle level   CC HCC

      ✓7ᵗʰ **S98.019** Complete traumatic amputation of unspecified foot at ankle level   CC HCC

    ✓6ᵗʰ **S98.02** **Partial traumatic amputation of foot at ankle level**

      ✓7ᵗʰ **S98.021** Partial traumatic amputation of right foot at ankle level   CC HCC

      ✓7ᵗʰ **S98.022** Partial traumatic amputation of left foot at ankle level   CC HCC

      ✓7ᵗʰ **S98.029** Partial traumatic amputation of unspecified foot at ankle level   CC HCC

  ✓5ᵗʰ **S98.1** **Traumatic amputation of one toe**

    ✓6ᵗʰ **S98.11** **Complete traumatic amputation of great toe**

      ✓7ᵗʰ **S98.111** Complete traumatic amputation of right great toe   HCC

      ✓7ᵗʰ **S98.112** Complete traumatic amputation of left great toe   HCC

      ✓7ᵗʰ **S98.119** Complete traumatic amputation of unspecified great toe   HCC

    ✓6ᵗʰ **S98.12** **Partial traumatic amputation of great toe**

      ✓7ᵗʰ **S98.121** Partial traumatic amputation of right great toe   HCC

      ✓7ᵗʰ **S98.122** Partial traumatic amputation of left great toe   HCC

      ✓7ᵗʰ **S98.129** Partial traumatic amputation of unspecified great toe   HCC

    ✓6ᵗʰ **S98.13** **Complete traumatic amputation of one lesser toe**

      Traumatic amputation of toe NOS

      ✓7ᵗʰ **S98.131** Complete traumatic amputation of one right lesser toe   HCC

      ✓7ᵗʰ **S98.132** Complete traumatic amputation of one left lesser toe   HCC

      ✓7ᵗʰ **S98.139** Complete traumatic amputation of one unspecified lesser toe   HCC

    ✓6ᵗʰ **S98.14** **Partial traumatic amputation of one lesser toe**

      ✓7ᵗʰ **S98.141** Partial traumatic amputation of one right lesser toe   HCC

      ✓7ᵗʰ **S98.142** Partial traumatic amputation of one left lesser toe   HCC

      ✓7ᵗʰ **S98.149** Partial traumatic amputation of one unspecified lesser toe   HCC

  ✓5ᵗʰ **S98.2** **Traumatic amputation of two or more lesser toes**

    ✓6ᵗʰ **S98.21** **Complete traumatic amputation of two or more lesser toes**

      ✓7ᵗʰ **S98.211** Complete traumatic amputation of two or more right lesser toes   HCC

      ✓7ᵗʰ **S98.212** Complete traumatic amputation of two or more left lesser toes   HCC

      ✓7ᵗʰ **S98.219** Complete traumatic amputation of two or more unspecified lesser toes   HCC

    ✓6ᵗʰ **S98.22** **Partial traumatic amputation of two or more lesser toes**

      ✓7ᵗʰ **S98.221** Partial traumatic amputation of two or more right lesser toes   HCC

      ✓7ᵗʰ **S98.222** Partial traumatic amputation of two or more left lesser toes   HCC

      ✓7ᵗʰ **S98.229** Partial traumatic amputation of two or more unspecified lesser toes   HCC

  ✓5ᵗʰ **S98.3** **Traumatic amputation of midfoot**

    ✓6ᵗʰ **S98.31** **Complete traumatic amputation of midfoot**

      ✓7ᵗʰ **S98.311** Complete traumatic amputation of right midfoot   CC HCC

      ✓7ᵗʰ **S98.312** Complete traumatic amputation of left midfoot   CC HCC

N Newborn: 0   P Pediatric: 0-17   M Maternity: 9-64   A Adult: 15-124   MCC Major Complication/Comorbidity   CC Complication/Comorbidity   SW Severe Wound Dx

1086   ICD-10-CM 2021

✓7ᵗʰ **S98.319** Complete traumatic amputation of unspecified midfoot   CC HCC

✓6ᵗʰ **S98.32** Partial traumatic amputation of midfoot

    ✓7ᵗʰ **S98.321** Partial traumatic amputation of right midfoot   CC HCC

    ✓7ᵗʰ **S98.322** Partial traumatic amputation of left midfoot   CC HCC

    ✓7ᵗʰ **S98.329** Partial traumatic amputation of unspecified midfoot   CC HCC

✓5ᵗʰ **S98.9** Traumatic amputation of foot, level unspecified

   ✓6ᵗʰ **S98.91** Complete traumatic amputation of foot, level unspecified

    ✓7ᵗʰ **S98.911** Complete traumatic amputation of right foot, level unspecified   CC HCC

    ✓7ᵗʰ **S98.912** Complete traumatic amputation of left foot, level unspecified   CC HCC

    ✓7ᵗʰ **S98.919** Complete traumatic amputation of unspecified foot, level unspecified   CC HCC

   ✓6ᵗʰ **S98.92** Partial traumatic amputation of foot, level unspecified

    ✓7ᵗʰ **S98.921** Partial traumatic amputation of right foot, level unspecified   CC HCC

    ✓7ᵗʰ **S98.922** Partial traumatic amputation of left foot, level unspecified   CC HCC

    ✓7ᵗʰ **S98.929** Partial traumatic amputation of unspecified foot, level unspecified   CC HCC

✓4ᵗʰ **S99 Other and unspecified injuries of ankle and foot**

   AHA: 2018,2Q,12; 2018,1Q,3; 2016,4Q,68-69

✓5ᵗʰ **S99.0** Physeal fracture of calcaneus

   AHA: 2019,4Q,56

> The appropriate 7th character is to be added to each code from subcategory S99.0.
> A   initial encounter for closed fracture
> B   initial encounter for open fracture
> D   subsequent encounter for fracture with routine healing
> G   subsequent encounter for fracture with delayed healing
> K   subsequent encounter for fracture with nonunion
> P   subsequent encounter for fracture with malunion
> S   sequela

   ✓6ᵗʰ **S99.00** Unspecified physeal fracture of calcaneus

    ✓7ᵗʰ **S99.001** Unspecified physeal fracture of right calcaneus

    ✓7ᵗʰ **S99.002** Unspecified physeal fracture of left calcaneus

    ✓7ᵗʰ **S99.009** Unspecified physeal fracture of unspecified calcaneus

   ✓6ᵗʰ **S99.01** Salter-Harris Type I physeal fracture of calcaneus

    ✓7ᵗʰ **S99.011** Salter-Harris Type I physeal fracture of right calcaneus

    ✓7ᵗʰ **S99.012** Salter-Harris Type I physeal fracture of left calcaneus

    ✓7ᵗʰ **S99.019** Salter-Harris Type I physeal fracture of unspecified calcaneus

   ✓6ᵗʰ **S99.02** Salter-Harris Type II physeal fracture of calcaneus

    ✓7ᵗʰ **S99.021** Salter-Harris Type II physeal fracture of right calcaneus

    ✓7ᵗʰ **S99.022** Salter-Harris Type II physeal fracture of left calcaneus

    ✓7ᵗʰ **S99.029** Salter-Harris Type II physeal fracture of unspecified calcaneus

   ✓6ᵗʰ **S99.03** Salter-Harris Type III physeal fracture of calcaneus

    ✓7ᵗʰ **S99.031** Salter-Harris Type III physeal fracture of right calcaneus

    ✓7ᵗʰ **S99.032** Salter-Harris Type III physeal fracture of left calcaneus

    ✓7ᵗʰ **S99.039** Salter-Harris Type III physeal fracture of unspecified calcaneus

   ✓6ᵗʰ **S99.04** Salter-Harris Type IV physeal fracture of calcaneus

    ✓7ᵗʰ **S99.041** Salter-Harris Type IV physeal fracture of right calcaneus

    ✓7ᵗʰ **S99.042** Salter-Harris Type IV physeal fracture of left calcaneus

    ✓7ᵗʰ **S99.049** Salter-Harris Type IV physeal fracture of unspecified calcaneus

   ✓6ᵗʰ **S99.09** Other physeal fracture of calcaneus

    ✓7ᵗʰ **S99.091** Other physeal fracture of right calcaneus

    ✓7ᵗʰ **S99.092** Other physeal fracture of left calcaneus

    ✓7ᵗʰ **S99.099** Other physeal fracture of unspecified calcaneus

✓5ᵗʰ **S99.1** Physeal fracture of metatarsal

   AHA: 2019,4Q,56

> The appropriate 7th character is to be added to each code from subcategory S99.1
> A   initial encounter for closed fracture
> B   initial encounter for open fracture
> D   subsequent encounter for fracture with routine healing
> G   subsequent encounter for fracture with delayed healing
> K   subsequent encounter for fracture with nonunion
> P   subsequent encounter for fracture with malunion
> S   sequela

   ✓6ᵗʰ **S99.10** Unspecified physeal fracture of metatarsal

    ✓7ᵗʰ **S99.101** Unspecified physeal fracture of right metatarsal

    ✓7ᵗʰ **S99.102** Unspecified physeal fracture of left metatarsal

    ✓7ᵗʰ **S99.109** Unspecified physeal fracture of unspecified metatarsal

   ✓6ᵗʰ **S99.11** Salter-Harris Type I physeal fracture of metatarsal

    ✓7ᵗʰ **S99.111** Salter-Harris Type I physeal fracture of right metatarsal

    ✓7ᵗʰ **S99.112** Salter-Harris Type I physeal fracture of left metatarsal

    ✓7ᵗʰ **S99.119** Salter-Harris Type I physeal fracture of unspecified metatarsal

   ✓6ᵗʰ **S99.12** Salter-Harris Type II physeal fracture of metatarsal

    ✓7ᵗʰ **S99.121** Salter-Harris Type II physeal fracture of right metatarsal

    ✓7ᵗʰ **S99.122** Salter-Harris Type II physeal fracture of left metatarsal

    ✓7ᵗʰ **S99.129** Salter-Harris Type II physeal fracture of unspecified metatarsal

   ✓6ᵗʰ **S99.13** Salter-Harris Type III physeal fracture of metatarsal

    ✓7ᵗʰ **S99.131** Salter-Harris Type III physeal fracture of right metatarsal

    ✓7ᵗʰ **S99.132** Salter-Harris Type III physeal fracture of left metatarsal

    ✓7ᵗʰ **S99.139** Salter-Harris Type III physeal fracture of unspecified metatarsal

   ✓6ᵗʰ **S99.14** Salter-Harris Type IV physeal fracture of metatarsal

    ✓7ᵗʰ **S99.141** Salter-Harris Type IV physeal fracture of right metatarsal

    ✓7ᵗʰ **S99.142** Salter-Harris Type IV physeal fracture of left metatarsal

    ✓7ᵗʰ **S99.149** Salter-Harris Type IV physeal fracture of unspecified metatarsal

   ✓6ᵗʰ **S99.19** Other physeal fracture of metatarsal

    ✓7ᵗʰ **S99.191** Other physeal fracture of right metatarsal

    ✓7ᵗʰ **S99.192** Other physeal fracture of left metatarsal

    ✓7ᵗʰ **S99.199** Other physeal fracture of unspecified metatarsal

✓5ᵗʰ **S99.2** Physeal fracture of phalanx of toe

   AHA: 2019,4Q,56

> The appropriate 7th character is to be added to each code from subcategories S99.2.
> A   initial encounter for closed fracture
> B   initial encounter for open fracture
> D   subsequent encounter for fracture with routine healing
> G   subsequent encounter for fracture with delayed healing
> K   subsequent encounter for fracture with nonunion
> P   subsequent encounter for fracture with malunion
> S   sequela

   ✓6ᵗʰ **S99.20** Unspecified physeal fracture of phalanx of toe

    ✓7ᵗʰ **S99.201** Unspecified physeal fracture of phalanx of right toe

    ✓7ᵗʰ **S99.202** Unspecified physeal fracture of phalanx of left toe

    ✓7ᵗʰ **S99.209** Unspecified physeal fracture of phalanx of unspecified toe

   ✓6ᵗʰ **S99.21** Salter-Harris Type I physeal fracture of phalanx of toe

    ✓7ᵗʰ **S99.211** Salter-Harris Type I physeal fracture of phalanx of right toe

    ✓7ᵗʰ **S99.212** Salter-Harris Type I physeal fracture of phalanx of left toe

✔ Additional Character Required   ✓x7ᵗʰ Placeholder   Unacceptable PDx   Questionable PDx   Manifestation   Unspecified Dx   H1-H14 HAC   HCC CMS-HCC Dx   HIV HIV Dx

ICD-10-CM 2021   1087

☑7ᵗʰ **S99.219** Salter-Harris Type I physeal fracture of phalanx of unspecified toe

☑6ᵗʰ **S99.22** Salter-Harris Type II physeal fracture of phalanx of toe

  ☑7ᵗʰ **S99.221** Salter-Harris Type II physeal fracture of phalanx of right toe

  ☑7ᵗʰ **S99.222** Salter-Harris Type II physeal fracture of phalanx of left toe

  ☑7ᵗʰ **S99.229** Salter-Harris Type II physeal fracture of phalanx of unspecified toe

☑6ᵗʰ **S99.23** Salter-Harris Type III physeal fracture of phalanx of toe

  ☑7ᵗʰ **S99.231** Salter-Harris Type III physeal fracture of phalanx of right toe

  ☑7ᵗʰ **S99.232** Salter-Harris Type III physeal fracture of phalanx of left toe

  ☑7ᵗʰ **S99.239** Salter-Harris Type III physeal fracture of phalanx of unspecified toe

☑6ᵗʰ **S99.24** Salter-Harris Type IV physeal fracture of phalanx of toe

  ☑7ᵗʰ **S99.241** Salter-Harris Type IV physeal fracture of phalanx of right toe

  ☑7ᵗʰ **S99.242** Salter-Harris Type IV physeal fracture of phalanx of left toe

  ☑7ᵗʰ **S99.249** Salter-Harris Type IV physeal fracture of phalanx of unspecified toe

☑6ᵗʰ **S99.29** Other physeal fracture of phalanx of toe

  ☑7ᵗʰ **S99.291** Other physeal fracture of phalanx of right toe

  ☑7ᵗʰ **S99.292** Other physeal fracture of phalanx of left toe

  ☑7ᵗʰ **S99.299** Other physeal fracture of phalanx of unspecified toe

☑5ᵗʰ **S99.8** Other specified injuries of ankle and foot

> The appropriate 7th character is to be added to each code from subcategory S99.8.
> A   initial encounter
> D   subsequent encounter
> S   sequela

☑6ᵗʰ **S99.81** Other specified injuries of ankle

  ☑7ᵗʰ **S99.811** Other specified injuries of right ankle

  ☑7ᵗʰ **S99.812** Other specified injuries of left ankle

  ☑7ᵗʰ **S99.819** Other specified injuries of unspecified ankle

☑6ᵗʰ **S99.82** Other specified injuries of foot

  ☑7ᵗʰ **S99.821** Other specified injuries of right foot

  ☑7ᵗʰ **S99.822** Other specified injuries of left foot

  ☑7ᵗʰ **S99.829** Other specified injuries of unspecified foot

☑5ᵗʰ **S99.9** Unspecified injury of ankle and foot

> The appropriate 7th character is to be added to each code from subcategory S99.9.
> A   initial encounter
> D   subsequent encounter
> S   sequela

☑6ᵗʰ **S99.91** Unspecified injury of ankle

  ☑7ᵗʰ **S99.911** Unspecified injury of right ankle

  ☑7ᵗʰ **S99.912** Unspecified injury of left ankle

  ☑7ᵗʰ **S99.919** Unspecified injury of unspecified ankle

☑6ᵗʰ **S99.92** Unspecified injury of foot

  ☑7ᵗʰ **S99.921** Unspecified injury of right foot

  ☑7ᵗʰ **S99.922** Unspecified injury of left foot

  ☑7ᵗʰ **S99.929** Unspecified injury of unspecified foot

INJURY, POISONING AND CERTAIN OTHER CONSEQUENCES OF EXTERNAL CAUSES (T07-T88)

Injuries involving multiple body regions (T07)

EXCLUDES 1   burns and corrosions (T20-T32)
     frostbite (T33-T34)
     insect bite or sting, venomous (T63.4)
     sunburn (L55.-)

☑x7ᵗʰ **T07** Unspecified multiple injuries

  EXCLUDES 1   injury NOS (T14.90)

  AHA: 2017,4Q,26

> The appropriate 7th character is to be added to code T07.
> A   initial encounter
> D   subsequent encounter
> S   sequela

Injury of unspecified body region (T14)

☑4ᵗʰ **T14** Injury of unspecified body region

  EXCLUDES 1   multiple unspecified injuries (T07)

  AHA: 2017,4Q,26

> The appropriate 7th character is to be added to each code from category T14.
> A   initial encounter
> D   subsequent encounter
> S   sequela

☑x7ᵗʰ **T14.8** Other injury of unspecified body region

  Abrasion NOS
  Contusion NOS
  Crush injury NOS
  Fracture NOS
  Skin injury NOS
  Vascular injury NOS
  Wound NOS

☑5ᵗʰ **T14.9** Unspecified injury

  ☑x7ᵗʰ **T14.90** Injury, unspecified

    Injury NOS

  ☑x7ᵗʰ **T14.91** Suicide attempt   `HCC`

    Attempted suicide NOS

Effects of foreign body entering through natural orifice (T15-T19)

EXCLUDES 2   foreign body accidentally left in operation wound (T81.5-)
     foreign body in penetrating wound — see open wound by body region
     residual foreign body in soft tissue (M79.5)
     splinter, without open wound — see superficial injury by body region

☑4ᵗʰ **T15** Foreign body on external eye

  EXCLUDES 2   foreign body in penetrating wound of orbit and eye ball (S05.4-, S05.5-)
     open wound of eyelid and periocular area (S01.1-)
     retained foreign body in eyelid (H02.8-)
     retained (old) foreign body in penetrating wound of orbit and eye ball (H05.5-, H44.6-, H44.7-)
     superficial foreign body of eyelid and periocular area (S00.25-)

> The appropriate 7th character is to be added to each code from category T15.
> A   initial encounter
> D   subsequent encounter
> S   sequela

☑5ᵗʰ **T15.0** Foreign body in cornea

  ☑x7ᵗʰ **T15.00** Foreign body in cornea, unspecified eye

  ☑x7ᵗʰ **T15.01** Foreign body in cornea, right eye

  ☑x7ᵗʰ **T15.02** Foreign body in cornea, left eye

☑5ᵗʰ **T15.1** Foreign body in conjunctival sac

  ☑x7ᵗʰ **T15.10** Foreign body in conjunctival sac, unspecified eye

  ☑x7ᵗʰ **T15.11** Foreign body in conjunctival sac, right eye

  ☑x7ᵗʰ **T15.12** Foreign body in conjunctival sac, left eye

☑5ᵗʰ **T15.8** Foreign body in other and multiple parts of external eye

  Foreign body in lacrimal punctum

  ☑x7ᵗʰ **T15.80** Foreign body in other and multiple parts of external eye, unspecified eye

N Newborn: 0   P Pediatric: 0-17   M Maternity: 9-64   A Adult: 15-124   **MCC** Major Complication/Comorbidity   **CC** Complication/Comorbidity   **SW** Severe Wound Dx

1088   ICD-10-CM 2021

√x7ᵗʰ **T15.81** **Foreign body in other and multiple parts of external eye, right eye**

√x7ᵗʰ **T15.82** **Foreign body in other and multiple parts of external eye, left eye**

√5ᵗʰ **T15.9** **Foreign body on external eye, part unspecified**

√x7ᵗʰ **T15.90** **Foreign body on external eye, part unspecified, unspecified eye**

√x7ᵗʰ **T15.91** **Foreign body on external eye, part unspecified, right eye**

√x7ᵗʰ **T15.92** **Foreign body on external eye, part unspecified, left eye**

√4ᵗʰ **T16** **Foreign body in ear**

INCLUDES   foreign body in auditory canal

The appropriate 7th character is to be added to each code from category T16.
A   initial encounter
D   subsequent encounter
S   sequela

√x7ᵗʰ **T16.1** **Foreign body in right ear**

√x7ᵗʰ **T16.2** **Foreign body in left ear**

√x7ᵗʰ **T16.9** **Foreign body in ear, unspecified ear**

√4ᵗʰ **T17** **Foreign body in respiratory tract**

The appropriate 7th character is to be added to each code from category T17.
A   initial encounter
D   subsequent encounter
S   sequela

√x7ᵗʰ **T17.0** **Foreign body in nasal sinus**

√x7ᵗʰ **T17.1** **Foreign body in nostril**

Foreign body in nose NOS

√5ᵗʰ **T17.2** **Foreign body in pharynx**

Foreign body in nasopharynx
Foreign body in throat NOS

√6ᵗʰ **T17.20** **Unspecified foreign body in pharynx**

√7ᵗʰ **T17.200** **Unspecified foreign body in pharynx causing asphyxiation**

√7ᵗʰ **T17.208** **Unspecified foreign body in pharynx causing other injury**

√6ᵗʰ **T17.21** **Gastric contents in pharynx**

Aspiration of gastric contents into pharynx
Vomitus in pharynx

√7ᵗʰ **T17.210** **Gastric contents in pharynx causing asphyxiation**

√7ᵗʰ **T17.218** **Gastric contents in pharynx causing other injury**

√6ᵗʰ **T17.22** **Food in pharynx**

Bones in pharynx
Seeds in pharynx

√7ᵗʰ **T17.220** **Food in pharynx causing asphyxiation**

√7ᵗʰ **T17.228** **Food in pharynx causing other injury**

√6ᵗʰ **T17.29** **Other foreign object in pharynx**

√7ᵗʰ **T17.290** **Other foreign object in pharynx causing asphyxiation**

√7ᵗʰ **T17.298** **Other foreign object in pharynx causing other injury**

√5ᵗʰ **T17.3** **Foreign body in larynx**

√6ᵗʰ **T17.30** **Unspecified foreign body in larynx**

√7ᵗʰ **T17.300** **Unspecified foreign body in larynx causing asphyxiation**

√7ᵗʰ **T17.308** **Unspecified foreign body in larynx causing other injury**

√6ᵗʰ **T17.31** **Gastric contents in larynx**

Aspiration of gastric contents into larynx
Vomitus in larynx

√7ᵗʰ **T17.310** **Gastric contents in larynx causing asphyxiation**

√7ᵗʰ **T17.318** **Gastric contents in larynx causing other injury**

√6ᵗʰ **T17.32** **Food in larynx**

Bones in larynx
Seeds in larynx

√7ᵗʰ **T17.320** **Food in larynx causing asphyxiation**

√7ᵗʰ **T17.328** **Food in larynx causing other injury**

√6ᵗʰ **T17.39** **Other foreign object in larynx**

√7ᵗʰ **T17.390** **Other foreign object in larynx causing asphyxiation**

√7ᵗʰ **T17.398** **Other foreign object in larynx causing other injury**

√5ᵗʰ **T17.4** **Foreign body in trachea**

√6ᵗʰ **T17.40** **Unspecified foreign body in trachea**

√7ᵗʰ **T17.400** **Unspecified foreign body in trachea causing asphyxiation** CC

√7ᵗʰ **T17.408** **Unspecified foreign body in trachea causing other injury** CC

√6ᵗʰ **T17.41** **Gastric contents in trachea**

Aspiration of gastric contents into trachea
Vomitus in trachea

√7ᵗʰ **T17.410** **Gastric contents in trachea causing asphyxiation** CC

√7ᵗʰ **T17.418** **Gastric contents in trachea causing other injury** CC

√6ᵗʰ **T17.42** **Food in trachea**

Bones in trachea
Seeds in trachea

√7ᵗʰ **T17.420** **Food in trachea causing asphyxiation** CC

√7ᵗʰ **T17.428** **Food in trachea causing other injury** CC

√6ᵗʰ **T17.49** **Other foreign object in trachea**

√7ᵗʰ **T17.490** **Other foreign object in trachea causing asphyxiation** CC

√7ᵗʰ **T17.498** **Other foreign object in trachea causing other injury** CC

√5ᵗʰ **T17.5** **Foreign body in bronchus**

√6ᵗʰ **T17.50** **Unspecified foreign body in bronchus**

√7ᵗʰ **T17.500** **Unspecified foreign body in bronchus causing asphyxiation** CC

√7ᵗʰ **T17.508** **Unspecified foreign body in bronchus causing other injury** CC

√6ᵗʰ **T17.51** **Gastric contents in bronchus**

Aspiration of gastric contents into bronchus
Vomitus in bronchus

√7ᵗʰ **T17.510** **Gastric contents in bronchus causing asphyxiation** CC

√7ᵗʰ **T17.518** **Gastric contents in bronchus causing other injury** CC

√6ᵗʰ **T17.52** **Food in bronchus**

Bones in bronchus
Seeds in bronchus

√7ᵗʰ **T17.520** **Food in bronchus causing asphyxiation** CC

√7ᵗʰ **T17.528** **Food in bronchus causing other injury** CC

√6ᵗʰ **T17.59** **Other foreign object in bronchus**

√7ᵗʰ **T17.590** **Other foreign object in bronchus causing asphyxiation** CC

√7ᵗʰ **T17.598** **Other foreign object in bronchus causing other injury** CC

√5ᵗʰ **T17.8** **Foreign body in other parts of respiratory tract**

Foreign body in bronchioles
Foreign body in lung

√6ᵗʰ **T17.80** **Unspecified foreign body in other parts of respiratory tract**

√7ᵗʰ **T17.800** **Unspecified foreign body in other parts of respiratory tract causing asphyxiation** CC

√7ᵗʰ **T17.808** **Unspecified foreign body in other parts of respiratory tract causing other injury** CC

√6ᵗʰ **T17.81** **Gastric contents in other parts of respiratory tract**

Aspiration of gastric contents into other parts of respiratory tract
Vomitus in other parts of respiratory tract

√7ᵗʰ **T17.810** **Gastric contents in other parts of respiratory tract causing asphyxiation** CC

√7ᵗʰ **T17.818** **Gastric contents in other parts of respiratory tract causing other injury** CC

√6ᵗʰ **T17.82** **Food** in other parts of respiratory tract

Bones in other parts of respiratory tract

Seeds in other parts of respiratory tract

√7ᵗʰ **T17.820** **Food in other parts of respiratory tract** causing asphyxiation   `CC`

√7ᵗʰ **T17.828** **Food in other parts of respiratory tract** causing other injury   `CC`

√6ᵗʰ **T17.89** **Other foreign object** in other parts of respiratory tract

√7ᵗʰ **T17.890** **Other foreign object in other parts of respiratory tract** causing asphyxiation   `CC`

√7ᵗʰ **T17.898** **Other foreign object in other parts of respiratory tract** causing other injury   `CC`

√5ᵗʰ **T17.9** **Foreign body** in respiratory tract, part unspecified

√6ᵗʰ **T17.90** **Unspecified foreign body** in respiratory tract, part unspecified

√7ᵗʰ **T17.900** **Unspecified foreign body in respiratory tract, part unspecified** causing asphyxiation

√7ᵗʰ **T17.908** **Unspecified foreign body in respiratory tract, part unspecified** causing other injury

√6ᵗʰ **T17.91** **Gastric contents** in respiratory tract, part unspecified

Aspiration of gastric contents into respiratory tract, part unspecified

Vomitus in trachea respiratory tract, part unspecified

√7ᵗʰ **T17.910** **Gastric contents in respiratory tract, part unspecified** causing asphyxiation

√7ᵗʰ **T17.918** **Gastric contents in respiratory tract, part unspecified** causing other injury

√6ᵗʰ **T17.92** **Food** in respiratory tract, part unspecified

Bones in respiratory tract, part unspecified

Seeds in respiratory tract, part unspecified

√7ᵗʰ **T17.920** **Food in respiratory tract, part unspecified** causing asphyxiation

√7ᵗʰ **T17.928** **Food in respiratory tract, part unspecified** causing other injury

√6ᵗʰ **T17.99** **Other foreign object** in respiratory tract, part unspecified

√7ᵗʰ **T17.990** **Other foreign object in respiratory tract, part unspecified** causing asphyxiation

AHA: 2019,3Q,15

√7ᵗʰ **T17.998** **Other foreign object in respiratory tract, part unspecified** causing other injury

√4ᵗʰ **T18** **Foreign body** in alimentary tract

`EXCLUDES 2`   foreign body in pharynx (T17.2-)

The appropriate 7th character is to be added to each code from category T18.

A   initial encounter

D   subsequent encounter

S   sequela

√x7ᵗʰ **T18.0** **Foreign body** in mouth

√5ᵗʰ **T18.1** **Foreign body** in esophagus

`EXCLUDES 2`   foreign body in respiratory tract (T17.-)

√6ᵗʰ **T18.10** **Unspecified foreign body** in esophagus

√7ᵗʰ **T18.100** **Unspecified foreign body in esophagus** causing compression of trachea

Unspecified foreign body in esophagus causing obstruction of respiration

√7ᵗʰ **T18.108** **Unspecified foreign body in esophagus** causing other injury

√6ᵗʰ **T18.11** **Gastric contents** in esophagus

Vomitus in esophagus

√7ᵗʰ **T18.110** **Gastric contents in esophagus** causing compression of trachea

Gastric contents in esophagus causing obstruction of respiration

√7ᵗʰ **T18.118** **Gastric contents in esophagus** causing other injury

√6ᵗʰ **T18.12** **Food** in esophagus

Bones in esophagus

Seeds in esophagus

√7ᵗʰ **T18.120** **Food in esophagus** causing compression of trachea

Food in esophagus causing obstruction of respiration

√7ᵗʰ **T18.128** **Food in esophagus** causing other injury

√6ᵗʰ **T18.19** **Other foreign object** in esophagus

AHA: 2015,1Q,23

√7ᵗʰ **T18.190** **Other foreign object in esophagus** causing compression of trachea

Other foreign body in esophagus causing obstruction of respiration

TIP: Any foreign object lodged in the esophagus requires immediate treatment and is considered an injury. Assign this code when there is respiratory compromise or compression.

√7ᵗʰ **T18.198** **Other foreign object in esophagus** causing other injury

TIP: Any foreign object lodged in the esophagus requires immediate treatment and is considered an injury. Assign this code when there is no respiratory compromise or compression.

√x7ᵗʰ **T18.2** **Foreign body** in stomach

√x7ᵗʰ **T18.3** **Foreign body** in small intestine

√x7ᵗʰ **T18.4** **Foreign body** in colon

√x7ᵗʰ **T18.5** **Foreign body** in anus and rectum

Foreign body in rectosigmoid (junction)

√x7ᵗʰ **T18.8** **Foreign body** in other parts of alimentary tract

√x7ᵗʰ **T18.9** **Foreign body** of alimentary tract, part unspecified

Foreign body in digestive system NOS

Swallowed foreign body NOS

√4ᵗʰ **T19** **Foreign body** in genitourinary tract

`EXCLUDES 2`   complications due to implanted mesh (T83.7-)

mechanical complications of contraceptive device (intrauterine) (vaginal) (T83.3-)

presence of contraceptive device (intrauterine) (vaginal) (Z97.5)

The appropriate 7th character is to be added to each code from category T19.

A   initial encounter

D   subsequent encounter

S   sequela

√x7ᵗʰ **T19.0** **Foreign body** in urethra

√x7ᵗʰ **T19.1** **Foreign body** in bladder

√x7ᵗʰ **T19.2** **Foreign body** in vulva and vagina   ♀

√x7ᵗʰ **T19.3** **Foreign body** in uterus   ♀

√x7ᵗʰ **T19.4** **Foreign body** in penis   ♂

√x7ᵗʰ **T19.8** **Foreign body** in other parts of genitourinary tract

√x7ᵗʰ **T19.9** **Foreign body** in genitourinary tract, part unspecified

N Newborn: 0   P Pediatric: 0-17   M Maternity: 9-64   A Adult: 15-124   MCC Major Complication/Comorbidity   CC Complication/Comorbidity   SW Severe Wound Dx

1090   ICD-10-CM 2021

BURNS AND CORROSIONS (T20-T32)

INCLUDES	burns (thermal) from electrical heating appliances
	burns (thermal) from electricity
	burns (thermal) from flame
	burns (thermal) from friction
	burns (thermal) from hot air and hot gases
	burns (thermal) from hot objects
	burns (thermal) from lightning
	burns (thermal) from radiation
	chemical burn [corrosion] (external) (internal)
	scalds
EXCLUDES 2	erythema [dermatitis] ab igne (L59.0)
	radiation-related disorders of the skin and subcutaneous tissue (L55-L59)
	sunburn (L55.-)

AHA: 2016,2Q,4

Burns and corrosions of external body surface, specified by site (T20-T25)

INCLUDES	burns and corrosions of first degree [erythema]
	burns and corrosions of second degree [blisters] [epidermal loss]
	burns and corrosions of third degree [deep necrosis of underlying tissue] [full-thickness skin loss]

Use additional code from category T31 or T32 to identify extent of body surface involved

√4ᵗʰ **T20 Burn and corrosion of head, face, and neck**

> EXCLUDES 2   *burn and corrosion of ear drum (T28.41, T28.91)*
> *burn and corrosion of eye and adnexa (T26.-)*
> *burn and corrosion of mouth and pharynx (T28.0)*

AHA: 2015,1Q,18-19

> The appropriate 7th character is to be added to each code from category T20.
> A   initial encounter
> D   subsequent encounter
> S   sequela

√5ᵗʰ **T20.0 Burn of unspecified degree of head, face, and neck**

> Use additional external cause code to identify the source, place and intent of the burn (X00-X19, X75-X77, X96-X98, Y92)

   √7ᵗʰ **T20.00 Burn of unspecified degree of head, face, and neck, unspecified site**

   √6ᵗʰ **T20.01 Burn of unspecified degree of ear [any part, except ear drum]**

> EXCLUDES 2   *burn of ear drum (T28.41-)*

     √7ᵗʰ **T20.011 Burn of unspecified degree of right ear [any part, except ear drum]**

     √7ᵗʰ **T20.012 Burn of unspecified degree of left ear [any part, except ear drum]**

     √7ᵗʰ **T20.019 Burn of unspecified degree of unspecified ear [any part, except ear drum]**

   √x7ᵗʰ **T20.02 Burn of unspecified degree of lip(s)**

   √x7ᵗʰ **T20.03 Burn of unspecified degree of chin**

   √x7ᵗʰ **T20.04 Burn of unspecified degree of nose (septum)**

   √x7ᵗʰ **T20.05 Burn of unspecified degree of scalp [any part]**

   √x7ᵗʰ **T20.06 Burn of unspecified degree of forehead and cheek**

   √x7ᵗʰ **T20.07 Burn of unspecified degree of neck**

   √x7ᵗʰ **T20.09 Burn of unspecified degree of multiple sites of head, face, and neck**

√5ᵗʰ **T20.1 Burn of first degree of head, face, and neck**

> Use additional external cause code to identify the source, place and intent of the burn (X00-X19, X75-X77, X96-X98, Y92)

   √x7ᵗʰ **T20.10 Burn of first degree of head, face, and neck, unspecified site**

   √6ᵗʰ **T20.11 Burn of first degree of ear [any part, except ear drum]**

> EXCLUDES 2   *burn of ear drum (T28.41-)*

     √7ᵗʰ **T20.111 Burn of first degree of right ear [any part, except ear drum]**

     √7ᵗʰ **T20.112 Burn of first degree of left ear [any part, except ear drum]**

     √7ᵗʰ **T20.119 Burn of first degree of unspecified ear [any part, except ear drum]**

   √x7ᵗʰ **T20.12 Burn of first degree of lip(s)**

   √x7ᵗʰ **T20.13 Burn of first degree of chin**

   √x7ᵗʰ **T20.14 Burn of first degree of nose (septum)**

   √x7ᵗʰ **T20.15 Burn of first degree of scalp [any part]**

   √x7ᵗʰ **T20.16 Burn of first degree of forehead and cheek**

   √x7ᵗʰ **T20.17 Burn of first degree of neck**

   √x7ᵗʰ **T20.19 Burn of first degree of multiple sites of head, face, and neck**

Degree of Burns

Epidermis — Dermis — Subcutaneous — Normal — First Degree Burn

Epidermis — Dermis — Subcutaneous — Second Degree Burn — Third Degree Burn

√5ᵗʰ **T20.2 Burn of second degree of head, face, and neck**

> Use additional external cause code to identify the source, place and intent of the burn (X00-X19, X75-X77, X96-X98, Y92)

   √x7ᵗʰ **T20.20 Burn of second degree of head, face, and neck, unspecified site**

   √6ᵗʰ **T20.21 Burn of second degree of ear [any part, except ear drum]**

> EXCLUDES 2   *burn of ear drum (T28.41-)*

     √7ᵗʰ **T20.211 Burn of second degree of right ear [any part, except ear drum]**

     √7ᵗʰ **T20.212 Burn of second degree of left ear [any part, except ear drum]**

     √7ᵗʰ **T20.219 Burn of second degree of unspecified ear [any part, except ear drum]**

   √x7ᵗʰ **T20.22 Burn of second degree of lip(s)**

   √x7ᵗʰ **T20.23 Burn of second degree of chin**

   √x7ᵗʰ **T20.24 Burn of second degree of nose (septum)**

   √x7ᵗʰ **T20.25 Burn of second degree of scalp [any part]**

   √x7ᵗʰ **T20.26 Burn of second degree of forehead and cheek**

   √x7ᵗʰ **T20.27 Burn of second degree of neck**

   √x7ᵗʰ **T20.29 Burn of second degree of multiple sites of head, face, and neck**

√5ᵗʰ **T20.3 Burn of third degree of head, face, and neck**

> Use additional external cause code to identify the source, place and intent of the burn (X00-X19, X75-X77, X96-X98, Y92)

   √x7ᵗʰ **T20.30 Burn of third degree of head, face, and neck, unspecified site**   CC H5 SW

   √6ᵗʰ **T20.31 Burn of third degree of ear [any part, except ear drum]**

> EXCLUDES 2   *burn of ear drum (T28.41-)*

> **AHA:** 2015,1Q,18

     √7ᵗʰ **T20.311 Burn of third degree of right ear [any part, except ear drum]**   CC H5 SW

     √7ᵗʰ **T20.312 Burn of third degree of left ear [any part, except ear drum]**   CC H5 SW

     √7ᵗʰ **T20.319 Burn of third degree of unspecified ear [any part, except ear drum]**   CC H5 SW

   √x7ᵗʰ **T20.32 Burn of third degree of lip(s)**   CC H5 SW

   √x7ᵗʰ **T20.33 Burn of third degree of chin**   CC H5 SW

   √x7ᵗʰ **T20.34 Burn of third degree of nose (septum)**   CC H5 SW

   √x7ᵗʰ **T20.35 Burn of third degree of scalp [any part]**   CC H5 SW

   √x7ᵗʰ **T20.36 Burn of third degree of forehead and cheek**   CC H5 SW

   √x7ᵗʰ **T20.37 Burn of third degree of neck**   CC H5 SW

   √x7ᵗʰ **T20.39 Burn of third degree of multiple sites of head, face, and neck**   CC H5 SW

✓ Additional Character Required   √x7ᵗʰ Placeholder   Unacceptable PDx   Questionable PDx   Manifestation   Unspecified Dx   H1-H15 HAC   HCC CMS-HCC Dx   HIV HIV Dx

ICD-10-CM 2021   1091

√5ᵗʰ **T20.4 Corrosion of unspecified degree of head, face, and neck**

Code first (T51-T65) to identify chemical and intent

Use additional external cause code to identify place (Y92)

√x7ᵗʰ **T20.40 Corrosion of unspecified degree of head, face, and neck, unspecified site**

√6ᵗʰ **T20.41 Corrosion of unspecified degree of ear [any part, except ear drum]**

EXCLUDES 2   corrosion of ear drum (T28.91-)

√7ᵗʰ **T20.411 Corrosion of unspecified degree of right ear [any part, except ear drum]**

√7ᵗʰ **T20.412 Corrosion of unspecified degree of left ear [any part, except ear drum]**

√7ᵗʰ **T20.419 Corrosion of unspecified degree of unspecified ear [any part, except ear drum]**

√x7ᵗʰ **T20.42 Corrosion of unspecified degree of lip(s)**

√x7ᵗʰ **T20.43 Corrosion of unspecified degree of chin**

√x7ᵗʰ **T20.44 Corrosion of unspecified degree of nose (septum)**

√x7ᵗʰ **T20.45 Corrosion of unspecified degree of scalp [any part]**

√x7ᵗʰ **T20.46 Corrosion of unspecified degree of forehead and cheek**

√x7ᵗʰ **T20.47 Corrosion of unspecified degree of neck**

√x7ᵗʰ **T20.49 Corrosion of unspecified degree of multiple sites of head, face, and neck**

√5ᵗʰ **T20.5 Corrosion of first degree of head, face, and neck**

Code first (T51-T65) to identify chemical and intent

Use additional external cause code to identify place (Y92)

√x7ᵗʰ **T20.50 Corrosion of first degree of head, face, and neck, unspecified site**

√6ᵗʰ **T20.51 Corrosion of first degree of ear [any part, except ear drum]**

EXCLUDES 2   corrosion of ear drum (T28.91-)

√7ᵗʰ **T20.511 Corrosion of first degree of right ear [any part, except ear drum]**

√7ᵗʰ **T20.512 Corrosion of first degree of left ear [any part, except ear drum]**

√7ᵗʰ **T20.519 Corrosion of first degree of unspecified ear [any part, except ear drum]**

√x7ᵗʰ **T20.52 Corrosion of first degree of lip(s)**

√x7ᵗʰ **T20.53 Corrosion of first degree of chin**

√x7ᵗʰ **T20.54 Corrosion of first degree of nose (septum)**

√x7ᵗʰ **T20.55 Corrosion of first degree of scalp [any part]**

√x7ᵗʰ **T20.56 Corrosion of first degree of forehead and cheek**

√x7ᵗʰ **T20.57 Corrosion of first degree of neck**

√x7ᵗʰ **T20.59 Corrosion of first degree of multiple sites of head, face, and neck**

√5ᵗʰ **T20.6 Corrosion of second degree of head, face, and neck**

Code first (T51-T65) to identify chemical and intent

Use additional external cause code to identify place (Y92)

√x7ᵗʰ **T20.60 Corrosion of second degree of head, face, and neck, unspecified site**

√6ᵗʰ **T20.61 Corrosion of second degree of ear [any part, except ear drum]**

EXCLUDES 2   corrosion of ear drum (T28.91-)

√7ᵗʰ **T20.611 Corrosion of second degree of right ear [any part, except ear drum]**

√7ᵗʰ **T20.612 Corrosion of second degree of left ear [any part, except ear drum]**

√7ᵗʰ **T20.619 Corrosion of second degree of unspecified ear [any part, except ear drum]**

√x7ᵗʰ **T20.62 Corrosion of second degree of lip(s)**

√x7ᵗʰ **T20.63 Corrosion of second degree of chin**

√x7ᵗʰ **T20.64 Corrosion of second degree of nose (septum)**

√x7ᵗʰ **T20.65 Corrosion of second degree of scalp [any part]**

√x7ᵗʰ **T20.66 Corrosion of second degree of forehead and cheek**

√x7ᵗʰ **T20.67 Corrosion of second degree of neck**

√x7ᵗʰ **T20.69 Corrosion of second degree of multiple sites of head, face, and neck**

√5ᵗʰ **T20.7 Corrosion of third degree of head, face, and neck**

Code first (T51-T65) to identify chemical and intent

Use additional external cause code to identify place (Y92)

√x7ᵗʰ **T20.70 Corrosion of third degree of head, face, and neck, unspecified site** `CC` `H5` `SW`

√6ᵗʰ **T20.71 Corrosion of third degree of ear [any part, except ear drum]**

EXCLUDES 2   corrosion of ear drum (T28.91-)

√7ᵗʰ **T20.711 Corrosion of third degree of right ear [any part, except ear drum]** `CC` `H5` `SW`

√7ᵗʰ **T20.712 Corrosion of third degree of left ear [any part, except ear drum]** `CC` `H5` `SW`

√7ᵗʰ **T20.719 Corrosion of third degree of unspecified ear [any part, except ear drum]** `CC` `H5` `SW`

√x7ᵗʰ **T20.72 Corrosion of third degree of lip(s)** `CC` `H5` `SW`

√x7ᵗʰ **T20.73 Corrosion of third degree of chin** `CC` `H5` `SW`

√x7ᵗʰ **T20.74 Corrosion of third degree of nose (septum)** `CC` `H5` `SW`

√x7ᵗʰ **T20.75 Corrosion of third degree of scalp [any part]** `CC` `H5` `SW`

√x7ᵗʰ **T20.76 Corrosion of third degree of forehead and cheek** `CC` `H5` `SW`

√x7ᵗʰ **T20.77 Corrosion of third degree of neck** `CC` `H5` `SW`

√x7ᵗʰ **T20.79 Corrosion of third degree of multiple sites of head, face, and neck** `CC` `H5` `SW`

√4ᵗʰ **T21 Burn and corrosion of trunk**

INCLUDES   burns and corrosion of hip region

EXCLUDES 2   burns and corrosion of axilla (T22.- with fifth character 4)

burns and corrosion of scapular region (T22.- with fifth character 6)

burns and corrosion of shoulder (T22.- with fifth character 5)

The appropriate 7th character is to be added to each code from category T21.

A   initial encounter

D   subsequent encounter

S   sequela

√5ᵗʰ **T21.0 Burn of unspecified degree of trunk**

Use additional external cause code to identify the source, place and intent of the burn (X00-X19, X75-X77, X96-X98, Y92)

√x7ᵗʰ **T21.00 Burn of unspecified degree of trunk, unspecified site**

√x7ᵗʰ **T21.01 Burn of unspecified degree of chest wall**

Burn of unspecified degree of breast

√x7ᵗʰ **T21.02 Burn of unspecified degree of abdominal wall**

Burn of unspecified degree of flank

Burn of unspecified degree of groin

√x7ᵗʰ **T21.03 Burn of unspecified degree of upper back**

Burn of unspecified degree of interscapular region

√x7ᵗʰ **T21.04 Burn of unspecified degree of lower back**

√x7ᵗʰ **T21.05 Burn of unspecified degree of buttock**

Burn of unspecified degree of anus

√x7ᵗʰ **T21.06 Burn of unspecified degree of male genital region** ♂

Burn of unspecified degree of penis

Burn of unspecified degree of scrotum

Burn of unspecified degree of testis

√x7ᵗʰ **T21.07 Burn of unspecified degree of female genital region** ♀

Burn of unspecified degree of labium (majus) (minus)

Burn of unspecified degree of perineum

Burn of unspecified degree of vulva

EXCLUDES 2   burn of vagina (T28.3)

√x7ᵗʰ **T21.09 Burn of unspecified degree of other site of trunk**

√5ᵗʰ **T21.1 Burn of first degree of trunk**

Use additional external cause code to identify the source, place and intent of the burn (X00-X19, X75-X77, X96-X98, Y92)

√x7ᵗʰ **T21.10 Burn of first degree of trunk, unspecified site**

√x7ᵗʰ **T21.11 Burn of first degree of chest wall**

Burn of first degree of breast

√x7ᵗʰ **T21.12 Burn of first degree of abdominal wall**

Burn of first degree of flank

Burn of first degree of groin

√x7ᵗʰ **T21.13 Burn of first degree of upper back**

Burn of first degree of interscapular region

√x7ᵗʰ **T21.14 Burn of first degree of lower back**

√x7ᵗʰ **T21.15 Burn of first degree of buttock**

Burn of first degree of anus

N Newborn: 0   P Pediatric: 0-17   M Maternity: 9-64   A Adult: 15-124   **MCC** Major Complication/Comorbidity   **CC** Complication/Comorbidity   **SW** Severe Wound Dx

1092   ICD-10-CM 2021

√x7ᵗʰ **T21.16 Burn of first degree of** male genital region ♂
Burn of first degree of penis
Burn of first degree of scrotum
Burn of first degree of testis

√x7ᵗʰ **T21.17 Burn of first degree of** female genital region ♀
Burn of first degree of labium (majus) (minus)
Burn of first degree of perineum
Burn of first degree of vulva
EXCLUDES 2   *burn of vagina (T28.3)*

√x7ᵗʰ **T21.19 Burn of first degree of other site of trunk**

√5ᵗʰ **T21.2   Burn of** second degree **of trunk**
Use additional external cause code to identify the source, place and intent of the burn (X00-X19, X75-X77, X96-X98, Y92)

√x7ᵗʰ **T21.20 Burn of second degree of trunk, unspecified site**

√x7ᵗʰ **T21.21 Burn of second degree of** chest wall
Burn of second degree of breast

√x7ᵗʰ **T21.22 Burn of second degree of** abdominal wall
Burn of second degree of flank
Burn of second degree of groin

√x7ᵗʰ **T21.23 Burn of second degree of** upper back
Burn of second degree of interscapular region

√x7ᵗʰ **T21.24 Burn of second degree of** lower back

√x7ᵗʰ **T21.25 Burn of second degree of** buttock
Burn of second degree of anus

√x7ᵗʰ **T21.26 Burn of second degree of** male genital region ♂
Burn of second degree of penis
Burn of second degree of scrotum
Burn of second degree of testis

√x7ᵗʰ **T21.27 Burn of second degree of** female genital region ♀
Burn of second degree of labium (majus) (minus)
Burn of second degree of perineum
Burn of second degree of vulva
EXCLUDES 2   *burn of vagina (T28.3)*

√x7ᵗʰ **T21.29 Burn of second degree of other site of trunk**

√5ᵗʰ **T21.3   Burn of** third degree **of trunk**
Use additional external cause code to identify the source, place and intent of the burn (X00-X19, X75-X77, X96-X98, Y92)

√x7ᵗʰ **T21.30 Burn of third degree of trunk, unspecified site**   CC H5 SW

√x7ᵗʰ **T21.31 Burn of third degree of** chest wall   CC H5 SW
Burn of third degree of breast
AHA: 2016,2Q,5

√x7ᵗʰ **T21.32 Burn of third degree of** abdominal wall   CC H5 SW
Burn of third degree of flank
Burn of third degree of groin

√x7ᵗʰ **T21.33 Burn of third degree of** upper back   CC H5 SW
Burn of third degree of interscapular region

√x7ᵗʰ **T21.34 Burn of third degree of** lower back   CC H5 SW

√x7ᵗʰ **T21.35 Burn of third degree of** buttock   CC H5 SW
Burn of third degree of anus

√x7ᵗʰ **T21.36 Burn of third degree of** male genital region   CC H5 SW ♂
Burn of third degree of penis
Burn of third degree of scrotum
Burn of third degree of testis

√x7ᵗʰ **T21.37 Burn of third degree of** female genital region   CC H5 SW ♀
Burn of third degree of labium (majus) (minus)
Burn of third degree of perineum
Burn of third degree of vulva
EXCLUDES 2   *burn of vagina (T28.3)*

√x7ᵗʰ **T21.39 Burn of third degree of other site of trunk**   CC H5 SW

√5ᵗʰ **T21.4   Corrosion of unspecified degree of trunk**
Code first (T51-T65) to identify chemical and intent
Use additional external cause code to identify place (Y92)

√x7ᵗʰ **T21.40 Corrosion of unspecified degree of trunk, unspecified site**

√x7ᵗʰ **T21.41 Corrosion of unspecified degree of** chest wall
Corrosion of unspecified degree of breast

√x7ᵗʰ **T21.42 Corrosion of unspecified degree of** abdominal wall
Corrosion of unspecified degree of flank
Corrosion of unspecified degree of groin

√x7ᵗʰ **T21.43 Corrosion of unspecified degree of** upper back
Corrosion of unspecified degree of interscapular region

√x7ᵗʰ **T21.44 Corrosion of unspecified degree of** lower back

√x7ᵗʰ **T21.45 Corrosion of unspecified degree of** buttock
Corrosion of unspecified degree of anus

√x7ᵗʰ **T21.46 Corrosion of unspecified degree of** male genital region ♂
Corrosion of unspecified degree of penis
Corrosion of unspecified degree of scrotum
Corrosion of unspecified degree of testis

√x7ᵗʰ **T21.47 Corrosion of unspecified degree of** female genital region ♀
Corrosion of unspecified degree of labium (majus) (minus)
Corrosion of unspecified degree of perineum
Corrosion of unspecified degree of vulva
EXCLUDES 2   *corrosion of vagina (T28.8)*

√x7ᵗʰ **T21.49 Corrosion of unspecified degree of other site of trunk**

√5ᵗʰ **T21.5   Corrosion of** first degree **of trunk**
Code first (T51-T65) to identify chemical and intent
Use additional external cause code to identify place (Y92)

√x7ᵗʰ **T21.50 Corrosion of first degree of trunk, unspecified site**

√x7ᵗʰ **T21.51 Corrosion of first degree of** chest wall
Corrosion of first degree of breast

√x7ᵗʰ **T21.52 Corrosion of first degree of** abdominal wall
Corrosion of first degree of flank
Corrosion of first degree of groin

√x7ᵗʰ **T21.53 Corrosion of first degree of** upper back
Corrosion of first degree of interscapular region

√x7ᵗʰ **T21.54 Corrosion of first degree of** lower back

√x7ᵗʰ **T21.55 Corrosion of first degree of** buttock
Corrosion of first degree of anus

√x7ᵗʰ **T21.56 Corrosion of first degree of** male genital region ♂
Corrosion of first degree of penis
Corrosion of first degree of scrotum
Corrosion of first degree of testis

√x7ᵗʰ **T21.57 Corrosion of first degree of** female genital region ♀
Corrosion of first degree of labium (majus) (minus)
Corrosion of first degree of perineum
Corrosion of first degree of vulva
EXCLUDES 2   *corrosion of vagina (T28.8)*

√x7ᵗʰ **T21.59 Corrosion of first degree of other site of trunk**

√5ᵗʰ **T21.6   Corrosion of** second degree **of trunk**
Code first (T51-T65) to identify chemical and intent
Use additional external cause code to identify place (Y92)

√x7ᵗʰ **T21.60 Corrosion of second degree of trunk, unspecified site**

√x7ᵗʰ **T21.61 Corrosion of second degree of** chest wall
Corrosion of second degree of breast

√x7ᵗʰ **T21.62 Corrosion of second degree of** abdominal wall
Corrosion of second degree of flank
Corrosion of second degree of groin

√x7ᵗʰ **T21.63 Corrosion of second degree of** upper back
Corrosion of second degree of interscapular region

√x7ᵗʰ **T21.64 Corrosion of second degree of** lower back

√x7ᵗʰ **T21.65 Corrosion of second degree of** buttock
Corrosion of second degree of anus

√x7ᵗʰ **T21.66 Corrosion of second degree of** male genital region ♂
Corrosion of second degree of penis
Corrosion of second degree of scrotum
Corrosion of second degree of testis

√x7ʰ **T21.67 Corrosion of second degree of** female genital region ♀
Corrosion of second degree of labium (majus) (minus)
Corrosion of second degree of perineum
Corrosion of second degree of vulva
EXCLUDES 2   corrosion of vagina (T28.8)

√x7ʰ **T21.69 Corrosion of second degree of other site of trunk**

√5ʰ **T21.7 Corrosion of** third degree **of trunk**
Code first (T51-T65) to identify chemical and intent
Use additional external cause code to identify place (Y92)

√x7ʰ **T21.70 Corrosion of third degree of trunk, unspecified site** `CC` `H5` `SW`

√x7ʰ **T21.71 Corrosion of third degree of** chest wall `CC` `H5` `SW`
Corrosion of third degree of breast

√x7ʰ **T21.72 Corrosion of third degree of** abdominal wall `CC` `H5` `SW`
Corrosion of third degree of flank
Corrosion of third degree of groin

√x7ʰ **T21.73 Corrosion of third degree of** upper back `CC` `H5` `SW`
Corrosion of third degree of interscapular region

√x7ʰ **T21.74 Corrosion of third degree of** lower back `CC` `H5` `SW`

√x7ʰ **T21.75 Corrosion of third degree of** buttock `CC` `H5` `SW`
Corrosion of third degree of anus

√x7ʰ **T21.76 Corrosion of third degree of** male genital region `CC` `H5` `SW` ♂
Corrosion of third degree of penis
Corrosion of third degree of scrotum
Corrosion of third degree of testis

√x7ʰ **T21.77 Corrosion of third degree of** female genital region `CC` `H5` `SW` ♀
Corrosion of third degree of labium (majus) (minus)
Corrosion of third degree of perineum
Corrosion of third degree of vulva
EXCLUDES 2   corrosion of vagina (T28.8)

√x7ʰ **T21.79 Corrosion of third degree of other site of trunk** `CC` `H5` `SW`

√4ʰ **T22 Burn and corrosion of shoulder and upper limb, except wrist and hand**
EXCLUDES 2   burn and corrosion of interscapular region (T21.-)
burn and corrosion of wrist and hand (T23.-)

The appropriate 7th character is to be added to each code from category T22.
A   initial encounter
D   subsequent encounter
S   sequela

√5ʰ **T22.0 Burn of unspecified degree of shoulder and upper limb, except wrist and hand**
Use additional external cause code to identify the source, place and intent of the burn (X00-X19, X75-X77, X96-X98, Y92)

√x7ʰ **T22.00 Burn of unspecified degree of shoulder and upper limb, except wrist and hand, unspecified site**

√6ʰ **T22.01 Burn of unspecified degree of** forearm

√7ʰ **T22.011 Burn of unspecified degree of** right forearm

√7ʰ **T22.012 Burn of unspecified degree of** left forearm

√7ʰ **T22.019 Burn of unspecified degree of unspecified forearm**

√6ʰ **T22.02 Burn of unspecified degree of** elbow

√7ʰ **T22.021 Burn of unspecified degree of** right elbow

√7ʰ **T22.022 Burn of unspecified degree of** left elbow

√7ʰ **T22.029 Burn of unspecified degree of unspecified elbow**

√6ʰ **T22.03 Burn of unspecified degree of** upper arm

√7ʰ **T22.031 Burn of unspecified degree of** right upper arm

√7ʰ **T22.032 Burn of unspecified degree of** left upper arm

√7ʰ **T22.039 Burn of unspecified degree of unspecified upper arm**

√6ʰ **T22.04 Burn of unspecified degree of** axilla

√7ʰ **T22.041 Burn of unspecified degree of** right axilla

√7ʰ **T22.042 Burn of unspecified degree of** left axilla

√7ʰ **T22.049 Burn of unspecified degree of unspecified axilla**

√6ʰ **T22.05 Burn of unspecified degree of** shoulder

√7ʰ **T22.051 Burn of unspecified degree of** right shoulder

√7ʰ **T22.052 Burn of unspecified degree of** left shoulder

√7ʰ **T22.059 Burn of unspecified degree of unspecified shoulder**

√6ʰ **T22.06 Burn of unspecified degree of** scapular region

√7ʰ **T22.061 Burn of unspecified degree of** right scapular region

√7ʰ **T22.062 Burn of unspecified degree of** left scapular region

√7ʰ **T22.069 Burn of unspecified degree of** unspecified scapular region

√6ʰ **T22.09 Burn of unspecified degree of** multiple sites **of shoulder and upper limb, except wrist and hand**

√7ʰ **T22.091 Burn of unspecified degree of multiple sites of** right **shoulder and upper limb, except wrist and hand**

√7ʰ **T22.092 Burn of unspecified degree of multiple sites of** left **shoulder and upper limb, except wrist and hand**

√7ʰ **T22.099 Burn of unspecified degree of multiple sites of unspecified shoulder and upper limb, except wrist and hand**

√5ʰ **T22.1 Burn of** first degree **of shoulder and upper limb, except wrist and hand**
Use additional external cause code to identify the source, place and intent of the burn (X00-X19, X75-X77, X96-X98, Y92)

√x7ʰ **T22.10 Burn of first degree of shoulder and upper limb, except wrist and hand, unspecified site**

√6ʰ **T22.11 Burn of first degree of** forearm

√7ʰ **T22.111 Burn of first degree of** right forearm

√7ʰ **T22.112 Burn of first degree of** left forearm

√7ʰ **T22.119 Burn of first degree of unspecified forearm**

√6ʰ **T22.12 Burn of first degree of** elbow

√7ʰ **T22.121 Burn of first degree of** right elbow

√7ʰ **T22.122 Burn of first degree of** left elbow

√7ʰ **T22.129 Burn of first degree of unspecified elbow**

√6ʰ **T22.13 Burn of first degree of** upper arm

√7ʰ **T22.131 Burn of first degree of** right upper arm

√7ʰ **T22.132 Burn of first degree of** left upper arm

√7ʰ **T22.139 Burn of first degree of unspecified upper arm**

√6ʰ **T22.14 Burn of first degree of** axilla

√7ʰ **T22.141 Burn of first degree of** right axilla

√7ʰ **T22.142 Burn of first degree of** left axilla

√7ʰ **T22.149 Burn of first degree of unspecified axilla**

√6ʰ **T22.15 Burn of first degree of** shoulder

√7ʰ **T22.151 Burn of first degree of** right shoulder

√7ʰ **T22.152 Burn of first degree of** left shoulder

√7ʰ **T22.159 Burn of first degree of unspecified shoulder**

√6ʰ **T22.16 Burn of first degree of** scapular region

√7ʰ **T22.161 Burn of first degree of** right scapular region

√7ʰ **T22.162 Burn of first degree of** left scapular region

√7ʰ **T22.169 Burn of first degree of unspecified scapular region**

√6ʰ **T22.19 Burn of first degree of** multiple sites **of shoulder and upper limb, except wrist and hand**

√7ʰ **T22.191 Burn of first degree of multiple sites of** right **shoulder and upper limb, except wrist and hand**

√7ʰ **T22.192 Burn of first degree of multiple sites of** left **shoulder and upper limb, except wrist and hand**

√7ʰ **T22.199 Burn of first degree of multiple sites of unspecified shoulder and upper limb, except wrist and hand**

√5ʰ **T22.2 Burn of** second degree **of shoulder and upper limb, except wrist and hand**
Use additional external cause code to identify the source, place and intent of the burn (X00-X19, X75-X77, X96-X98, Y92)

√x7ʰ **T22.20 Burn of second degree of shoulder and upper limb, except wrist and hand, unspecified site**

√6ᵗʰ **T22.21 Burn of second degree of forearm**
- √7ᵗʰ **T22.211** Burn of second degree of right forearm
- √7ᵗʰ **T22.212** Burn of second degree of left forearm
- √7ᵗʰ **T22.219** Burn of second degree of unspecified forearm

√6ᵗʰ **T22.22 Burn of second degree of elbow**
- √7ᵗʰ **T22.221** Burn of second degree of right elbow
- √7ᵗʰ **T22.222** Burn of second degree of left elbow
- √7ᵗʰ **T22.229** Burn of second degree of unspecified elbow

√6ᵗʰ **T22.23 Burn of second degree of upper arm**
- √7ᵗʰ **T22.231** Burn of second degree of right upper arm
- √7ᵗʰ **T22.232** Burn of second degree of left upper arm
- √7ᵗʰ **T22.239** Burn of second degree of unspecified upper arm

√6ᵗʰ **T22.24 Burn of second degree of axilla**
- √7ᵗʰ **T22.241** Burn of second degree of right axilla
- √7ᵗʰ **T22.242** Burn of second degree of left axilla
- √7ᵗʰ **T22.249** Burn of second degree of unspecified axilla

√6ᵗʰ **T22.25 Burn of second degree of shoulder**
- √7ᵗʰ **T22.251** Burn of second degree of right shoulder
- √7ᵗʰ **T22.252** Burn of second degree of left shoulder
- √7ᵗʰ **T22.259** Burn of second degree of unspecified shoulder

√6ᵗʰ **T22.26 Burn of second degree of scapular region**
- √7ᵗʰ **T22.261** Burn of second degree of right scapular region
- √7ᵗʰ **T22.262** Burn of second degree of left scapular region
- √7ᵗʰ **T22.269** Burn of second degree of unspecified scapular region

√6ᵗʰ **T22.29 Burn of second degree of multiple sites of shoulder and upper limb, except wrist and hand**
- √7ᵗʰ **T22.291** Burn of second degree of multiple sites of right shoulder and upper limb, except wrist and hand
- √7ᵗʰ **T22.292** Burn of second degree of multiple sites of left shoulder and upper limb, except wrist and hand
- √7ᵗʰ **T22.299** Burn of second degree of multiple sites of unspecified shoulder and upper limb, except wrist and hand

√5ᵗʰ **T22.3 Burn of third degree of shoulder and upper limb, except wrist and hand**
Use additional external cause code to identify the source, place and intent of the burn (X00-X19, X75-X77, X96-X98, Y92)

√x7ᵗʰ **T22.30** Burn of third degree of shoulder and upper limb, except wrist and hand, unspecified site   CC H5 SW

√6ᵗʰ **T22.31 Burn of third degree of forearm**
- √7ᵗʰ **T22.311** Burn of third degree of right forearm   CC H5 SW
- √7ᵗʰ **T22.312** Burn of third degree of left forearm   CC H5 SW
- √7ᵗʰ **T22.319** Burn of third degree of unspecified forearm   CC H5 SW

√6ᵗʰ **T22.32 Burn of third degree of elbow**
- √7ᵗʰ **T22.321** Burn of third degree of right elbow   CC H5 SW
- √7ᵗʰ **T22.322** Burn of third degree of left elbow   CC H5 SW
- √7ᵗʰ **T22.329** Burn of third degree of unspecified elbow   CC H5 SW

√6ᵗʰ **T22.33 Burn of third degree of upper arm**
- √7ᵗʰ **T22.331** Burn of third degree of right upper arm   CC H5 SW
- √7ᵗʰ **T22.332** Burn of third degree of left upper arm   CC H5 SW
- √7ᵗʰ **T22.339** Burn of third degree of unspecified upper arm   CC H5 SW

√6ᵗʰ **T22.34 Burn of third degree of axilla**
- √7ᵗʰ **T22.341** Burn of third degree of right axilla   CC H5 SW
- √7ᵗʰ **T22.342** Burn of third degree of left axilla   CC H5 SW
- √7ᵗʰ **T22.349** Burn of third degree of unspecified axilla   CC H5 SW

√6ᵗʰ **T22.35 Burn of third degree of shoulder**
- √7ᵗʰ **T22.351** Burn of third degree of right shoulder   CC H5 SW
- √7ᵗʰ **T22.352** Burn of third degree of left shoulder   CC H5 SW
- √7ᵗʰ **T22.359** Burn of third degree of unspecified shoulder   CC H5 SW

√6ᵗʰ **T22.36 Burn of third degree of scapular region**
- √7ᵗʰ **T22.361** Burn of third degree of right scapular region   CC H5 SW
- √7ᵗʰ **T22.362** Burn of third degree of left scapular region   CC H5 SW
- √7ᵗʰ **T22.369** Burn of third degree of unspecified scapular region   CC H5 SW

√6ᵗʰ **T22.39 Burn of third degree of multiple sites of shoulder and upper limb, except wrist and hand**
- √7ᵗʰ **T22.391** Burn of third degree of multiple sites of right shoulder and upper limb, except wrist and hand   CC H5 SW
- √7ᵗʰ **T22.392** Burn of third degree of multiple sites of left shoulder and upper limb, except wrist and hand   CC H5 SW
- √7ᵗʰ **T22.399** Burn of third degree of multiple sites of unspecified shoulder and upper limb, except wrist and hand   CC H5 SW

√5ᵗʰ **T22.4 Corrosion of unspecified degree of shoulder and upper limb, except wrist and hand**
Code first (T51-T65) to identify chemical and intent
Use additional external cause code to identify place (Y92)

√x7ᵗʰ **T22.40** Corrosion of unspecified degree of shoulder and upper limb, except wrist and hand, unspecified site

√6ᵗʰ **T22.41 Corrosion of unspecified degree of forearm**
- √7ᵗʰ **T22.411** Corrosion of unspecified degree of right forearm
- √7ᵗʰ **T22.412** Corrosion of unspecified degree of left forearm
- √7ᵗʰ **T22.419** Corrosion of unspecified degree of unspecified forearm

√6ᵗʰ **T22.42 Corrosion of unspecified degree of elbow**
- √7ᵗʰ **T22.421** Corrosion of unspecified degree of right elbow
- √7ᵗʰ **T22.422** Corrosion of unspecified degree of left elbow
- √7ᵗʰ **T22.429** Corrosion of unspecified degree of unspecified elbow

√6ᵗʰ **T22.43 Corrosion of unspecified degree of upper arm**
- √7ᵗʰ **T22.431** Corrosion of unspecified degree of right upper arm
- √7ᵗʰ **T22.432** Corrosion of unspecified degree of left upper arm
- √7ᵗʰ **T22.439** Corrosion of unspecified degree of unspecified upper arm

√6ᵗʰ **T22.44 Corrosion of unspecified degree of axilla**
- √7ᵗʰ **T22.441** Corrosion of unspecified degree of right axilla
- √7ᵗʰ **T22.442** Corrosion of unspecified degree of left axilla
- √7ᵗʰ **T22.449** Corrosion of unspecified degree of unspecified axilla

√6ᵗʰ **T22.45 Corrosion of unspecified degree of shoulder**
- √7ᵗʰ **T22.451** Corrosion of unspecified degree of right shoulder
- √7ᵗʰ **T22.452** Corrosion of unspecified degree of left shoulder
- √7ᵗʰ **T22.459** Corrosion of unspecified degree of unspecified shoulder

√6ᵗʰ **T22.46 Corrosion of unspecified degree of scapular region**
- √7ᵗʰ **T22.461** Corrosion of unspecified degree of right scapular region
- √7ᵗʰ **T22.462** Corrosion of unspecified degree of left scapular region
- √7ᵗʰ **T22.469** Corrosion of unspecified degree of unspecified scapular region

√6ᵗʰ **T22.49 Corrosion of unspecified degree of multiple sites of shoulder and upper limb, except wrist and hand**
- √7ᵗʰ **T22.491** Corrosion of unspecified degree of multiple sites of right shoulder and upper limb, except wrist and hand

---

√7ᵗʰ **T22.492** Corrosion of unspecified degree of multiple sites of left shoulder and upper limb, except wrist and hand

√7ᵗʰ **T22.499** Corrosion of unspecified degree of multiple sites of unspecified shoulder and upper limb, except wrist and hand

√5ᵗʰ **T22.5** Corrosion of first degree of shoulder and upper limb, except wrist and hand

Code first (T51-T65) to identify chemical and intent
Use additional external cause code to identify place (Y92)

√x7ᵗʰ **T22.50** Corrosion of first degree of shoulder and upper limb, except wrist and hand unspecified site

√6ᵗʰ **T22.51** Corrosion of first degree of forearm

√7ᵗʰ **T22.511** Corrosion of first degree of right forearm

√7ᵗʰ **T22.512** Corrosion of first degree of left forearm

√7ᵗʰ **T22.519** Corrosion of first degree of unspecified forearm

√6ᵗʰ **T22.52** Corrosion of first degree of elbow

√7ᵗʰ **T22.521** Corrosion of first degree of right elbow

√7ᵗʰ **T22.522** Corrosion of first degree of left elbow

√7ᵗʰ **T22.529** Corrosion of first degree of unspecified elbow

√6ᵗʰ **T22.53** Corrosion of first degree of upper arm

√7ᵗʰ **T22.531** Corrosion of first degree of right upper arm

√7ᵗʰ **T22.532** Corrosion of first degree of left upper arm

√7ᵗʰ **T22.539** Corrosion of first degree of unspecified upper arm

√6ᵗʰ **T22.54** Corrosion of first degree of axilla

√7ᵗʰ **T22.541** Corrosion of first degree of right axilla

√7ᵗʰ **T22.542** Corrosion of first degree of left axilla

√7ᵗʰ **T22.549** Corrosion of first degree of unspecified axilla

√6ᵗʰ **T22.55** Corrosion of first degree of shoulder

√7ᵗʰ **T22.551** Corrosion of first degree of right shoulder

√7ᵗʰ **T22.552** Corrosion of first degree of left shoulder

√7ᵗʰ **T22.559** Corrosion of first degree of unspecified shoulder

√6ᵗʰ **T22.56** Corrosion of first degree of scapular region

√7ᵗʰ **T22.561** Corrosion of first degree of right scapular region

√7ᵗʰ **T22.562** Corrosion of first degree of left scapular region

√7ᵗʰ **T22.569** Corrosion of first degree of unspecified scapular region

√6ᵗʰ **T22.59** Corrosion of first degree of multiple sites of shoulder and upper limb, except wrist and hand

√7ᵗʰ **T22.591** Corrosion of first degree of multiple sites of right shoulder and upper limb, except wrist and hand

√7ᵗʰ **T22.592** Corrosion of first degree of multiple sites of left shoulder and upper limb, except wrist and hand

√7ᵗʰ **T22.599** Corrosion of first degree of multiple sites of unspecified shoulder and upper limb, except wrist and hand

√5ᵗʰ **T22.6** Corrosion of second degree of shoulder and upper limb, except wrist and hand

Code first (T51-T65) to identify chemical and intent
Use additional external cause code to identify place (Y92)

√x7ᵗʰ **T22.60** Corrosion of second degree of shoulder and upper limb, except wrist and hand, unspecified site

√6ᵗʰ **T22.61** Corrosion of second degree of forearm

√7ᵗʰ **T22.611** Corrosion of second degree of right forearm

√7ᵗʰ **T22.612** Corrosion of second degree of left forearm

√7ᵗʰ **T22.619** Corrosion of second degree of unspecified forearm

√6ᵗʰ **T22.62** Corrosion of second degree of elbow

√7ᵗʰ **T22.621** Corrosion of second degree of right elbow

√7ᵗʰ **T22.622** Corrosion of second degree of left elbow

√7ᵗʰ **T22.629** Corrosion of second degree of unspecified elbow

√6ᵗʰ **T22.63** Corrosion of second degree of upper arm

√7ᵗʰ **T22.631** Corrosion of second degree of right upper arm

√7ᵗʰ **T22.632** Corrosion of second degree of left upper arm

√7ᵗʰ **T22.639** Corrosion of second degree of unspecified upper arm

√6ᵗʰ **T22.64** Corrosion of second degree of axilla

√7ᵗʰ **T22.641** Corrosion of second degree of right axilla

√7ᵗʰ **T22.642** Corrosion of second degree of left axilla

√7ᵗʰ **T22.649** Corrosion of second degree of unspecified axilla

√6ᵗʰ **T22.65** Corrosion of second degree of shoulder

√7ᵗʰ **T22.651** Corrosion of second degree of right shoulder

√7ᵗʰ **T22.652** Corrosion of second degree of left shoulder

√7ᵗʰ **T22.659** Corrosion of second degree of unspecified shoulder

√6ᵗʰ **T22.66** Corrosion of second degree of scapular region

√7ᵗʰ **T22.661** Corrosion of second degree of right scapular region

√7ᵗʰ **T22.662** Corrosion of second degree of left scapular region

√7ᵗʰ **T22.669** Corrosion of second degree of unspecified scapular region

√6ᵗʰ **T22.69** Corrosion of second degree of multiple sites of shoulder and upper limb, except wrist and hand

√7ᵗʰ **T22.691** Corrosion of second degree of multiple sites of right shoulder and upper limb, except wrist and hand

√7ᵗʰ **T22.692** Corrosion of second degree of multiple sites of left shoulder and upper limb, except wrist and hand

√7ᵗʰ **T22.699** Corrosion of second degree of multiple sites of unspecified shoulder and upper limb, except wrist and hand

√5ᵗʰ **T22.7** Corrosion of third degree of shoulder and upper limb, except wrist and hand

Code first (T51-T65) to identify chemical and intent
Use additional external cause code to identify place (Y92)

√x7ᵗʰ **T22.70** Corrosion of third degree of shoulder and upper limb, except wrist and hand, unspecified site **CC H5 SW**

√6ᵗʰ **T22.71** Corrosion of third degree of forearm

√7ᵗʰ **T22.711** Corrosion of third degree of right forearm **CC H5 SW**

√7ᵗʰ **T22.712** Corrosion of third degree of left forearm **CC H5 SW**

√7ᵗʰ **T22.719** Corrosion of third degree of unspecified forearm **CC H5 SW**

√6ᵗʰ **T22.72** Corrosion of third degree of elbow

√7ᵗʰ **T22.721** Corrosion of third degree of right elbow **CC H5 SW**

√7ᵗʰ **T22.722** Corrosion of third degree of left elbow **CC H5 SW**

√7ᵗʰ **T22.729** Corrosion of third degree of unspecified elbow **CC H5 SW**

√6ᵗʰ **T22.73** Corrosion of third degree of upper arm

√7ᵗʰ **T22.731** Corrosion of third degree of right upper arm **CC H5 SW**

√7ᵗʰ **T22.732** Corrosion of third degree of left upper arm **CC H5 SW**

√7ᵗʰ **T22.739** Corrosion of third degree of unspecified upper arm **CC H5 SW**

√6ᵗʰ **T22.74** Corrosion of third degree of axilla

√7ᵗʰ **T22.741** Corrosion of third degree of right axilla **CC H5 SW**

√7ᵗʰ **T22.742** Corrosion of third degree of left axilla **CC H5 SW**

√7ᵗʰ **T22.749** Corrosion of third degree of unspecified axilla **CC H5 SW**

√6ᵗʰ **T22.75** Corrosion of third degree of shoulder

√7ᵗʰ **T22.751** Corrosion of third degree of right shoulder **CC H5 SW**

√7ᵗʰ **T22.752** Corrosion of third degree of left shoulder **CC H5 SW**

√7ᵗʰ **T22.759** Corrosion of third degree of unspecified shoulder **CC H5 SW**

√6ᵗʰ **T22.76** Corrosion of third degree of scapular region

√7ᵗʰ **T22.761** Corrosion of third degree of right scapular region **CC H5 SW**

☑7ᵗʰ **T22.762** Corrosion of third degree of left scapular region `CC` `H5` `SW`

☑7ᵗʰ **T22.769** Corrosion of third degree of unspecified scapular region `CC` `H5` `SW`

☑6ᵗʰ **T22.79** Corrosion of third degree of multiple sites of shoulder and upper limb, except wrist and hand

☑7ᵗʰ **T22.791** Corrosion of third degree of multiple sites of right shoulder and upper limb, except wrist and hand `CC` `H5` `SW`

☑7ᵗʰ **T22.792** Corrosion of third degree of multiple sites of left shoulder and upper limb, except wrist and hand `CC` `H5` `SW`

☑7ᵗʰ **T22.799** Corrosion of third degree of multiple sites of unspecified shoulder and upper limb, except wrist and hand `CC` `H5` `SW`

☑4ᵗʰ **T23** **Burn and corrosion of wrist and hand**

AHA: 2015,1Q,19

The appropriate 7th character is to be added to each code from category T23.
A　initial encounter
D　subsequent encounter
S　sequela

☑5ᵗʰ **T23.0** **Burn of unspecified degree of wrist and hand**

Use additional external cause code to identify the source, place and intent of the burn (X00-X19, X75-X77, X96-X98, Y92)

☑6ᵗʰ **T23.00** Burn of unspecified degree of hand, unspecified site

☑7ᵗʰ **T23.001** Burn of unspecified degree of right hand, unspecified site

☑7ᵗʰ **T23.002** Burn of unspecified degree of left hand, unspecified site

☑7ᵗʰ **T23.009** Burn of unspecified degree of unspecified hand, unspecified site

☑6ᵗʰ **T23.01** Burn of unspecified degree of thumb (nail)

☑7ᵗʰ **T23.011** Burn of unspecified degree of right thumb (nail)

☑7ᵗʰ **T23.012** Burn of unspecified degree of left thumb (nail)

☑7ᵗʰ **T23.019** Burn of unspecified degree of unspecified thumb (nail)

☑6ᵗʰ **T23.02** Burn of unspecified degree of single finger (nail) except thumb

☑7ᵗʰ **T23.021** Burn of unspecified degree of single right finger (nail) except thumb

☑7ᵗʰ **T23.022** Burn of unspecified degree of single left finger (nail) except thumb

☑7ᵗʰ **T23.029** Burn of unspecified degree of unspecified single finger (nail) except thumb

☑6ᵗʰ **T23.03** Burn of unspecified degree of multiple fingers (nail), not including thumb

☑7ᵗʰ **T23.031** Burn of unspecified degree of multiple right fingers (nail), not including thumb

☑7ᵗʰ **T23.032** Burn of unspecified degree of multiple left fingers (nail), not including thumb

☑7ᵗʰ **T23.039** Burn of unspecified degree of unspecified multiple fingers (nail), not including thumb

☑6ᵗʰ **T23.04** Burn of unspecified degree of multiple fingers (nail), including thumb

☑7ᵗʰ **T23.041** Burn of unspecified degree of multiple right fingers (nail), including thumb

☑7ᵗʰ **T23.042** Burn of unspecified degree of multiple left fingers (nail), including thumb

☑7ᵗʰ **T23.049** Burn of unspecified degree of unspecified multiple fingers (nail), including thumb

☑6ᵗʰ **T23.05** Burn of unspecified degree of palm

☑7ᵗʰ **T23.051** Burn of unspecified degree of right palm

☑7ᵗʰ **T23.052** Burn of unspecified degree of left palm

☑7ᵗʰ **T23.059** Burn of unspecified degree of unspecified palm

☑6ᵗʰ **T23.06** Burn of unspecified degree of back of hand

☑7ᵗʰ **T23.061** Burn of unspecified degree of back of right hand

☑7ᵗʰ **T23.062** Burn of unspecified degree of back of left hand

☑7ᵗʰ **T23.069** Burn of unspecified degree of back of unspecified hand

☑6ᵗʰ **T23.07** Burn of unspecified degree of wrist

☑7ᵗʰ **T23.071** Burn of unspecified degree of right wrist

☑7ᵗʰ **T23.072** Burn of unspecified degree of left wrist

☑7ᵗʰ **T23.079** Burn of unspecified degree of unspecified wrist

☑6ᵗʰ **T23.09** Burn of unspecified degree of multiple sites of wrist and hand

☑7ᵗʰ **T23.091** Burn of unspecified degree of multiple sites of right wrist and hand

☑7ᵗʰ **T23.092** Burn of unspecified degree of multiple sites of left wrist and hand

☑7ᵗʰ **T23.099** Burn of unspecified degree of multiple sites of unspecified wrist and hand

☑5ᵗʰ **T23.1** **Burn of first degree of wrist and hand**

Use additional external cause code to identify the source, place and intent of the burn (X00-X19, X75-X77, X96-X98, Y92)

☑6ᵗʰ **T23.10** Burn of first degree of hand, unspecified site

☑7ᵗʰ **T23.101** Burn of first degree of right hand, unspecified site

☑7ᵗʰ **T23.102** Burn of first degree of left hand, unspecified site

☑7ᵗʰ **T23.109** Burn of first degree of unspecified hand, unspecified site

☑6ᵗʰ **T23.11** Burn of first degree of thumb (nail)

☑7ᵗʰ **T23.111** Burn of first degree of right thumb (nail)

☑7ᵗʰ **T23.112** Burn of first degree of left thumb (nail)

☑7ᵗʰ **T23.119** Burn of first degree of unspecified thumb (nail)

☑6ᵗʰ **T23.12** Burn of first degree of single finger (nail) except thumb

☑7ᵗʰ **T23.121** Burn of first degree of single right finger (nail) except thumb

☑7ᵗʰ **T23.122** Burn of first degree of single left finger (nail) except thumb

☑7ᵗʰ **T23.129** Burn of first degree of unspecified single finger (nail) except thumb

☑6ᵗʰ **T23.13** Burn of first degree of multiple fingers (nail), not including thumb

☑7ᵗʰ **T23.131** Burn of first degree of multiple right fingers (nail), not including thumb

☑7ᵗʰ **T23.132** Burn of first degree of multiple left fingers (nail), not including thumb

☑7ᵗʰ **T23.139** Burn of first degree of unspecified multiple fingers (nail), not including thumb

☑6ᵗʰ **T23.14** Burn of first degree of multiple fingers (nail), including thumb

☑7ᵗʰ **T23.141** Burn of first degree of multiple right fingers (nail), including thumb

☑7ᵗʰ **T23.142** Burn of first degree of multiple left fingers (nail), including thumb

☑7ᵗʰ **T23.149** Burn of first degree of unspecified multiple fingers (nail), including thumb

☑6ᵗʰ **T23.15** Burn of first degree of palm

☑7ᵗʰ **T23.151** Burn of first degree of right palm

☑7ᵗʰ **T23.152** Burn of first degree of left palm

☑7ᵗʰ **T23.159** Burn of first degree of unspecified palm

☑6ᵗʰ **T23.16** Burn of first degree of back of hand

☑7ᵗʰ **T23.161** Burn of first degree of back of right hand

☑7ᵗʰ **T23.162** Burn of first degree of back of left hand

☑7ᵗʰ **T23.169** Burn of first degree of back of unspecified hand

☑6ᵗʰ **T23.17** Burn of first degree of wrist

☑7ᵗʰ **T23.171** Burn of first degree of right wrist

☑7ᵗʰ **T23.172** Burn of first degree of left wrist

☑7ᵗʰ **T23.179** Burn of first degree of unspecified wrist

☑6ᵗʰ **T23.19** Burn of first degree of multiple sites of wrist and hand

☑7ᵗʰ **T23.191** Burn of first degree of multiple sites of right wrist and hand

☑7ᵗʰ **T23.192** Burn of first degree of multiple sites of left wrist and hand

☑7ᵗʰ **T23.199** Burn of first degree of multiple sites of unspecified wrist and hand

☑5ᵗʰ **T23.2** **Burn of second degree of wrist and hand**

Use additional external cause code to identify the source, place and intent of the burn (X00-X19, X75-X77, X96-X98, Y92)

☑6ᵗʰ **T23.20** Burn of second degree of hand, unspecified site

☑7ᵗʰ **T23.201** Burn of second degree of right hand, unspecified site

Chapter 19. Injury, Poisoning and Certain Other Consequences of External Causes

T23.202–T23.419

√7ᵗʰ **T23.202** Burn of second degree of left hand, unspecified site

√7ᵗʰ **T23.209** Burn of second degree of unspecified hand, unspecified site

√6ᵗʰ **T23.21** Burn of second degree of thumb (nail)

√7ᵗʰ **T23.211** Burn of second degree of right thumb (nail)

√7ᵗʰ **T23.212** Burn of second degree of left thumb (nail)

√7ᵗʰ **T23.219** Burn of second degree of unspecified thumb (nail)

√6ᵗʰ **T23.22** Burn of second degree of single finger (nail) except thumb

√7ᵗʰ **T23.221** Burn of second degree of single right finger (nail) except thumb

√7ᵗʰ **T23.222** Burn of second degree of single left finger (nail) except thumb

√7ᵗʰ **T23.229** Burn of second degree of unspecified single finger (nail) except thumb

√6ᵗʰ **T23.23** Burn of second degree of multiple fingers (nail), not including thumb

√7ᵗʰ **T23.231** Burn of second degree of multiple right fingers (nail), not including thumb

√7ᵗʰ **T23.232** Burn of second degree of multiple left fingers (nail), not including thumb

√7ᵗʰ **T23.239** Burn of second degree of unspecified multiple fingers (nail), not including thumb

√6ᵗʰ **T23.24** Burn of second degree of multiple fingers (nail), including thumb

√7ᵗʰ **T23.241** Burn of second degree of multiple right fingers (nail), including thumb

√7ᵗʰ **T23.242** Burn of second degree of multiple left fingers (nail), including thumb

√7ᵗʰ **T23.249** Burn of second degree of unspecified multiple fingers (nail), including thumb

√6ᵗʰ **T23.25** Burn of second degree of palm

√7ᵗʰ **T23.251** Burn of second degree of right palm

√7ᵗʰ **T23.252** Burn of second degree of left palm

√7ᵗʰ **T23.259** Burn of second degree of unspecified palm

√6ᵗʰ **T23.26** Burn of second degree of back of hand

√7ᵗʰ **T23.261** Burn of second degree of back of right hand

√7ᵗʰ **T23.262** Burn of second degree of back of left hand

√7ᵗʰ **T23.269** Burn of second degree of back of unspecified hand

√6ᵗʰ **T23.27** Burn of second degree of wrist

√7ᵗʰ **T23.271** Burn of second degree of right wrist

√7ᵗʰ **T23.272** Burn of second degree of left wrist

√7ᵗʰ **T23.279** Burn of second degree of unspecified wrist

√6ᵗʰ **T23.29** Burn of second degree of multiple sites of wrist and hand

√7ᵗʰ **T23.291** Burn of second degree of multiple sites of right wrist and hand

√7ᵗʰ **T23.292** Burn of second degree of multiple sites of left wrist and hand

√7ᵗʰ **T23.299** Burn of second degree of multiple sites of unspecified wrist and hand

√5ᵗʰ **T23.3** Burn of third degree of wrist and hand

Use additional external cause code to identify the source, place and intent of the burn (X00-X19, X75-X77, X96-X98, Y92)

√6ᵗʰ **T23.30** Burn of third degree of hand, unspecified site

AHA: 2016,2Q,5

√7ᵗʰ **T23.301** Burn of third degree of right hand, unspecified site   CC H5 SW

√7ᵗʰ **T23.302** Burn of third degree of left hand, unspecified site   CC H5 SW

√7ᵗʰ **T23.309** Burn of third degree of unspecified hand, unspecified site   CC H5 SW

√6ᵗʰ **T23.31** Burn of third degree of thumb (nail)

√7ᵗʰ **T23.311** Burn of third degree of right thumb (nail)   CC H5 SW

√7ᵗʰ **T23.312** Burn of third degree of left thumb (nail)   CC H5 SW

√7ᵗʰ **T23.319** Burn of third degree of unspecified thumb (nail)   CC H5 SW

√6ᵗʰ **T23.32** Burn of third degree of single finger (nail) except thumb

√7ᵗʰ **T23.321** Burn of third degree of single right finger (nail) except thumb   CC H5 SW

√7ᵗʰ **T23.322** Burn of third degree of single left finger (nail) except thumb   CC H5 SW

√7ᵗʰ **T23.329** Burn of third degree of unspecified single finger (nail) except thumb   CC H5 SW

√6ᵗʰ **T23.33** Burn of third degree of multiple fingers (nail), not including thumb

√7ᵗʰ **T23.331** Burn of third degree of multiple right fingers (nail), not including thumb   CC H5 SW

√7ᵗʰ **T23.332** Burn of third degree of multiple left fingers (nail), not including thumb   CC H5 SW

√7ᵗʰ **T23.339** Burn of third degree of unspecified multiple fingers (nail), not including thumb   CC H5 SW

√6ᵗʰ **T23.34** Burn of third degree of multiple fingers (nail), including thumb

√7ᵗʰ **T23.341** Burn of third degree of multiple right fingers (nail), including thumb   CC H5 SW

√7ᵗʰ **T23.342** Burn of third degree of multiple left fingers (nail), including thumb   CC H5 SW

√7ᵗʰ **T23.349** Burn of third degree of unspecified multiple fingers (nail), including thumb   CC H5 SW

√6ᵗʰ **T23.35** Burn of third degree of palm

√7ᵗʰ **T23.351** Burn of third degree of right palm   CC H5 SW

√7ᵗʰ **T23.352** Burn of third degree of left palm   CC H5 SW

√7ᵗʰ **T23.359** Burn of third degree of unspecified palm   CC H5 SW

√6ᵗʰ **T23.36** Burn of third degree of back of hand

√7ᵗʰ **T23.361** Burn of third degree of back of right hand   CC H5 SW

√7ᵗʰ **T23.362** Burn of third degree of back of left hand   CC H5 SW

√7ᵗʰ **T23.369** Burn of third degree of back of unspecified hand   CC H5 SW

√6ᵗʰ **T23.37** Burn of third degree of wrist

√7ᵗʰ **T23.371** Burn of third degree of right wrist   CC H5 SW

√7ᵗʰ **T23.372** Burn of third degree of left wrist   CC H5 SW

√7ᵗʰ **T23.379** Burn of third degree of unspecified wrist   CC H5 SW

√6ᵗʰ **T23.39** Burn of third degree of multiple sites of wrist and hand

√7ᵗʰ **T23.391** Burn of third degree of multiple sites of right wrist and hand   CC H5 SW

√7ᵗʰ **T23.392** Burn of third degree of multiple sites of left wrist and hand   CC H5 SW

√7ᵗʰ **T23.399** Burn of third degree of multiple sites of unspecified wrist and hand   CC H5 SW

√5ᵗʰ **T23.4** Corrosion of unspecified degree of wrist and hand

Code first (T51-T65) to identify chemical and intent
Use additional external cause code to identify place (Y92)

√6ᵗʰ **T23.40** Corrosion of unspecified degree of hand, unspecified site

√7ᵗʰ **T23.401** Corrosion of unspecified degree of right hand, unspecified site

√7ᵗʰ **T23.402** Corrosion of unspecified degree of left hand, unspecified site

√7ᵗʰ **T23.409** Corrosion of unspecified degree of unspecified hand, unspecified site

√6ᵗʰ **T23.41** Corrosion of unspecified degree of thumb (nail)

√7ᵗʰ **T23.411** Corrosion of unspecified degree of right thumb (nail)

√7ᵗʰ **T23.412** Corrosion of unspecified degree of left thumb (nail)

√7ᵗʰ **T23.419** Corrosion of unspecified degree of unspecified thumb (nail)

N Newborn: 0   P Pediatric: 0-17   M Maternity: 9-64   A Adult: 15-124   MCC Major Complication/Comorbidity   CC Complication/Comorbidity   SW Severe Wound Dx

1098

ICD-10-CM 2021

√6ᵗʰ **T23.42 Corrosion of unspecified degree of** single finger (nail) except thumb

    √7ᵗʰ **T23.421** Corrosion of unspecified degree of single right finger (nail) except thumb

    √7ᵗʰ **T23.422** Corrosion of unspecified degree of single left finger (nail) except thumb

    √7ᵗʰ **T23.429** Corrosion of unspecified degree of unspecified single finger (nail) except thumb

√6ᵗʰ **T23.43 Corrosion of unspecified degree of** multiple fingers (nail), not including thumb

    √7ᵗʰ **T23.431** Corrosion of unspecified degree of multiple right fingers (nail), not including thumb

    √7ᵗʰ **T23.432** Corrosion of unspecified degree of multiple left fingers (nail), not including thumb

    √7ᵗʰ **T23.439** Corrosion of unspecified degree of unspecified multiple fingers (nail), not including thumb

√6ᵗʰ **T23.44 Corrosion of unspecified degree of** multiple fingers (nail), including thumb

    √7ᵗʰ **T23.441** Corrosion of unspecified degree of multiple right fingers (nail), including thumb

    √7ᵗʰ **T23.442** Corrosion of unspecified degree of multiple left fingers (nail), including thumb

    √7ᵗʰ **T23.449** Corrosion of unspecified degree of unspecified multiple fingers (nail), including thumb

√6ᵗʰ **T23.45 Corrosion of unspecified degree of** palm

    √7ᵗʰ **T23.451** Corrosion of unspecified degree of right palm

    √7ᵗʰ **T23.452** Corrosion of unspecified degree of left palm

    √7ᵗʰ **T23.459** Corrosion of unspecified degree of unspecified palm

√6ᵗʰ **T23.46 Corrosion of unspecified degree of** back of hand

    √7ᵗʰ **T23.461** Corrosion of unspecified degree of back of right hand

    √7ᵗʰ **T23.462** Corrosion of unspecified degree of back of left hand

    √7ᵗʰ **T23.469** Corrosion of unspecified degree of back of unspecified hand

√6ᵗʰ **T23.47 Corrosion of unspecified degree of** wrist

    √7ᵗʰ **T23.471** Corrosion of unspecified degree of right wrist

    √7ᵗʰ **T23.472** Corrosion of unspecified degree of left wrist

    √7ᵗʰ **T23.479** Corrosion of unspecified degree of unspecified wrist

√6ᵗʰ **T23.49 Corrosion of unspecified degree of** multiple sites of wrist and hand

    √7ᵗʰ **T23.491** Corrosion of unspecified degree of multiple sites of right wrist and hand

    √7ᵗʰ **T23.492** Corrosion of unspecified degree of multiple sites of left wrist and hand

    √7ᵗʰ **T23.499** Corrosion of unspecified degree of multiple sites of unspecified wrist and hand

√5ᵗʰ **T23.5 Corrosion of** first degree **of wrist and hand**

    Code first (T51-T65) to identify chemical and intent
    Use additional external cause code to identify place (Y92)

√6ᵗʰ **T23.50 Corrosion of first degree of hand, unspecified site**

    √7ᵗʰ **T23.501** Corrosion of first degree of right hand, unspecified site

    √7ᵗʰ **T23.502** Corrosion of first degree of left hand, unspecified site

    √7ᵗʰ **T23.509** Corrosion of first degree of unspecified hand, unspecified site

√6ᵗʰ **T23.51 Corrosion of first degree of** thumb (nail)

    √7ᵗʰ **T23.511** Corrosion of first degree of right thumb (nail)

    √7ᵗʰ **T23.512** Corrosion of first degree of left thumb (nail)

    √7ᵗʰ **T23.519** Corrosion of first degree of unspecified thumb (nail)

√6ᵗʰ **T23.52 Corrosion of first degree of** single finger (nail) except thumb

    √7ᵗʰ **T23.521** Corrosion of first degree of single right finger (nail) except thumb

    √7ᵗʰ **T23.522** Corrosion of first degree of single left finger (nail) except thumb

    √7ᵗʰ **T23.529** Corrosion of first degree of unspecified single finger (nail) except thumb

√6ᵗʰ **T23.53 Corrosion of first degree of** multiple fingers (nail), not including thumb

    √7ᵗʰ **T23.531** Corrosion of first degree of multiple right fingers (nail), not including thumb

    √7ᵗʰ **T23.532** Corrosion of first degree of multiple left fingers (nail), not including thumb

    √7ᵗʰ **T23.539** Corrosion of first degree of unspecified multiple fingers (nail), not including thumb

√6ᵗʰ **T23.54 Corrosion of first degree of** multiple fingers (nail), including thumb

    √7ᵗʰ **T23.541** Corrosion of first degree of multiple right fingers (nail), including thumb

    √7ᵗʰ **T23.542** Corrosion of first degree of multiple left fingers (nail), including thumb

    √7ᵗʰ **T23.549** Corrosion of first degree of unspecified multiple fingers (nail), including thumb

√6ᵗʰ **T23.55 Corrosion of first degree of** palm

    √7ᵗʰ **T23.551** Corrosion of first degree of right palm

    √7ᵗʰ **T23.552** Corrosion of first degree of left palm

    √7ᵗʰ **T23.559** Corrosion of first degree of unspecified palm

√6ᵗʰ **T23.56 Corrosion of first degree of** back of hand

    √7ᵗʰ **T23.561** Corrosion of first degree of back of right hand

    √7ᵗʰ **T23.562** Corrosion of first degree of back of left hand

    √7ᵗʰ **T23.569** Corrosion of first degree of back of unspecified hand

√6ᵗʰ **T23.57 Corrosion of first degree of** wrist

    √7ᵗʰ **T23.571** Corrosion of first degree of right wrist

    √7ᵗʰ **T23.572** Corrosion of first degree of left wrist

    √7ᵗʰ **T23.579** Corrosion of first degree of unspecified wrist

√6ᵗʰ **T23.59 Corrosion of first degree of** multiple sites of wrist and hand

    √7ᵗʰ **T23.591** Corrosion of first degree of multiple sites of right wrist and hand

    √7ᵗʰ **T23.592** Corrosion of first degree of multiple sites of left wrist and hand

    √7ᵗʰ **T23.599** Corrosion of first degree of multiple sites of unspecified wrist and hand

√5ᵗʰ **T23.6 Corrosion of** second degree **of wrist and hand**

    Code first (T51-T65) to identify chemical and intent
    Use additional external cause code to identify place (Y92)

√6ᵗʰ **T23.60 Corrosion of second degree of hand, unspecified site**

    √7ᵗʰ **T23.601** Corrosion of second degree of right hand, unspecified site

    √7ᵗʰ **T23.602** Corrosion of second degree of left hand, unspecified site

    √7ᵗʰ **T23.609** Corrosion of second degree of unspecified hand, unspecified site

√6ᵗʰ **T23.61 Corrosion of second degree of** thumb (nail)

    √7ᵗʰ **T23.611** Corrosion of second degree of right thumb (nail)

    √7ᵗʰ **T23.612** Corrosion of second degree of left thumb (nail)

    √7ᵗʰ **T23.619** Corrosion of second degree of unspecified thumb (nail)

√6ᵗʰ **T23.62 Corrosion of second degree of** single finger (nail) except thumb

    √7ᵗʰ **T23.621** Corrosion of second degree of single right finger (nail) except thumb

    √7ᵗʰ **T23.622** Corrosion of second degree of single left finger (nail) except thumb

    √7ᵗʰ **T23.629** Corrosion of second degree of unspecified single finger (nail) except thumb

√6ᵗʰ **T23.63 Corrosion of second degree of** multiple fingers (nail), not including thumb

    √7ᵗʰ **T23.631** Corrosion of second degree of multiple right fingers (nail), not including thumb

    √7ᵗʰ **T23.632** Corrosion of second degree of multiple left fingers (nail), not including thumb

    √7ᵗʰ **T23.639** Corrosion of second degree of unspecified multiple fingers (nail), not including thumb

✔ Additional Character Required   √ₓ7ᵗʰ Placeholder   Unacceptable PDx   Questionable PDx   Manifestation   Unspecified Dx   H1-H14 HAC   HCC CMS-HCC Dx   HIV HIV Dx

ICD-10-CM 2021   1099

√6ᵗʰ **T23.64** **Corrosion of second degree of** multiple fingers (nail), including thumb

√7ᵗʰ **T23.641** **Corrosion of second degree of multiple** right **fingers (nail), including thumb**

√7ᵗʰ **T23.642** **Corrosion of second degree of multiple** left **fingers (nail), including thumb**

√7ᵗʰ **T23.649** **Corrosion of second degree of unspecified multiple fingers (nail), including thumb**

√6ᵗʰ **T23.65** **Corrosion of second degree of** palm

√7ᵗʰ **T23.651** **Corrosion of second degree of** right **palm**

√7ᵗʰ **T23.652** **Corrosion of second degree of** left **palm**

√7ᵗʰ **T23.659** **Corrosion of second degree of unspecified palm**

√6ᵗʰ **T23.66** **Corrosion of second degree of** back of hand

√7ᵗʰ **T23.661** **Corrosion of second degree back of** right **hand**

√7ᵗʰ **T23.662** **Corrosion of second degree back of** left **hand**

√7ᵗʰ **T23.669** **Corrosion of second degree back of unspecified hand**

√6ᵗʰ **T23.67** **Corrosion of second degree of** wrist

√7ᵗʰ **T23.671** **Corrosion of second degree of** right **wrist**

√7ᵗʰ **T23.672** **Corrosion of second degree of** left **wrist**

√7ᵗʰ **T23.679** **Corrosion of second degree of unspecified wrist**

√6ᵗʰ **T23.69** **Corrosion of second degree of** multiple sites **of wrist and hand**

√7ᵗʰ **T23.691** **Corrosion of second degree of multiple sites of** right **wrist and hand**

√7ᵗʰ **T23.692** **Corrosion of second degree of multiple sites of** left **wrist and hand**

√7ᵗʰ **T23.699** **Corrosion of second degree of multiple sites of unspecified wrist and hand**

√5ᵗʰ **T23.7** **Corrosion of** third degree **of wrist and hand**

Code first (T51-T65) to identify chemical and intent

Use additional external cause code to identify place (Y92)

√6ᵗʰ **T23.70** **Corrosion of third degree of hand, unspecified site**

√7ᵗʰ **T23.701** **Corrosion of third degree of** right **hand, unspecified site** `CC` `H5` `SW`

√7ᵗʰ **T23.702** **Corrosion of third degree of** left **hand, unspecified site** `CC` `H5` `SW`

√7ᵗʰ **T23.709** **Corrosion of third degree of unspecified hand, unspecified site** `CC` `H5` `SW`

√6ᵗʰ **T23.71** **Corrosion of third degree of** thumb (nail)

√7ᵗʰ **T23.711** **Corrosion of third degree of** right **thumb (nail)** `CC` `H5` `SW`

√7ᵗʰ **T23.712** **Corrosion of third degree of** left **thumb (nail)** `CC` `H5` `SW`

√7ᵗʰ **T23.719** **Corrosion of third degree of unspecified thumb (nail)** `CC` `H5` `SW`

√6ᵗʰ **T23.72** **Corrosion of third degree of** single finger (nail) **except thumb**

√7ᵗʰ **T23.721** **Corrosion of third degree of single** right **finger (nail) except thumb** `CC` `H5` `SW`

√7ᵗʰ **T23.722** **Corrosion of third degree of single** left **finger (nail) except thumb** `CC` `H5` `SW`

√7ᵗʰ **T23.729** **Corrosion of third degree of unspecified single finger (nail) except thumb** `CC` `H5` `SW`

√6ᵗʰ **T23.73** **Corrosion of third degree of** multiple fingers (nail), not including thumb

√7ᵗʰ **T23.731** **Corrosion of third degree of multiple** right **fingers (nail), not including thumb** `CC` `H5` `SW`

√7ᵗʰ **T23.732** **Corrosion of third degree of multiple** left **fingers (nail), not including thumb** `CC` `H5` `SW`

√7ᵗʰ **T23.739** **Corrosion of third degree of unspecified multiple fingers (nail), not including thumb** `CC` `H5` `SW`

√6ᵗʰ **T23.74** **Corrosion of third degree of** multiple fingers (nail), including thumb

√7ᵗʰ **T23.741** **Corrosion of third degree of multiple** right **fingers (nail), including thumb** `CC` `H5` `SW`

√7ᵗʰ **T23.742** **Corrosion of third degree of multiple** left **fingers (nail), including thumb** `CC` `H5` `SW`

√7ᵗʰ **T23.749** **Corrosion of third degree of unspecified multiple fingers (nail), including thumb** `CC` `H5` `SW`

√6ᵗʰ **T23.75** **Corrosion of third degree of** palm

√7ᵗʰ **T23.751** **Corrosion of third degree of** right **palm** `CC` `H5` `SW`

√7ᵗʰ **T23.752** **Corrosion of third degree of** left **palm** `CC` `H5` `SW`

√7ᵗʰ **T23.759** **Corrosion of third degree of unspecified palm** `CC` `H5` `SW`

√6ᵗʰ **T23.76** **Corrosion of third degree of** back of hand

√7ᵗʰ **T23.761** **Corrosion of third degree of back of** right **hand** `CC` `H5` `SW`

√7ᵗʰ **T23.762** **Corrosion of third degree of back of** left **hand** `CC` `H5` `SW`

√7ᵗʰ **T23.769** **Corrosion of third degree back of unspecified hand** `CC` `H5` `SW`

√6ᵗʰ **T23.77** **Corrosion of third degree of** wrist

√7ᵗʰ **T23.771** **Corrosion of third degree of** right **wrist** `CC` `H5` `SW`

√7ᵗʰ **T23.772** **Corrosion of third degree of** left **wrist** `CC` `H5` `SW`

√7ᵗʰ **T23.779** **Corrosion of third degree of unspecified wrist** `CC` `H5` `SW`

√6ᵗʰ **T23.79** **Corrosion of third degree of** multiple sites **of wrist and hand**

√7ᵗʰ **T23.791** **Corrosion of third degree of multiple sites of** right **wrist and hand** `CC` `H5` `SW`

√7ᵗʰ **T23.792** **Corrosion of third degree of multiple sites of** left **wrist and hand** `CC` `H5` `SW`

√7ᵗʰ **T23.799** **Corrosion of third degree of multiple sites of unspecified wrist and hand** `CC` `H5` `SW`

√4ᵗʰ **T24** **Burn and corrosion of lower limb, except ankle and foot**

EXCLUDES 2   *burn and corrosion of ankle and foot (T25.-)*

         burn and corrosion of hip region (T21.-)

The appropriate 7th character is to be added to each code from category T24.
A   initial encounter
D   subsequent encounter
S   sequela

√5ᵗʰ **T24.0** **Burn of unspecified degree of lower limb, except ankle and foot**

Use additional external cause code to identify the source, place and intent of the burn (X00-X19, X75-X77, X96-X98, Y92)

√6ᵗʰ **T24.00** **Burn of unspecified degree of unspecified site of lower limb, except ankle and foot**

√7ᵗʰ **T24.001** **Burn of unspecified degree of unspecified site of** right **lower limb, except ankle and foot**

√7ᵗʰ **T24.002** **Burn of unspecified degree of unspecified site of** left **lower limb, except ankle and foot**

√7ᵗʰ **T24.009** **Burn of unspecified degree of unspecified site of unspecified lower limb, except ankle and foot**

√6ᵗʰ **T24.01** **Burn of unspecified degree of** thigh

√7ᵗʰ **T24.011** **Burn of unspecified degree of** right **thigh**

√7ᵗʰ **T24.012** **Burn of unspecified degree of** left **thigh**

√7ᵗʰ **T24.019** **Burn of unspecified degree of unspecified thigh**

√6ᵗʰ **T24.02** **Burn of unspecified degree of** knee

√7ᵗʰ **T24.021** **Burn of unspecified degree of** right **knee**

√7ᵗʰ **T24.022** **Burn of unspecified degree of** left **knee**

√7ᵗʰ **T24.029** **Burn of unspecified degree of unspecified knee**

√6ᵗʰ **T24.03** **Burn of unspecified degree of** lower leg

√7ᵗʰ **T24.031** **Burn of unspecified degree of** right **lower leg**

√7ᵗʰ **T24.032** **Burn of unspecified degree of** left **lower leg**

√7ᵗʰ **T24.039** **Burn of unspecified degree of unspecified lower leg**

√6ᵗʰ **T24.09** **Burn of unspecified degree of** multiple sites **of lower limb, except ankle and foot**

√7ᵗʰ **T24.091** **Burn of unspecified degree of multiple sites of** right **lower limb, except ankle and foot**

Ⓝ Newborn: 0   Ⓟ Pediatric: 0-17   Ⓜ Maternity: 9-64   Ⓐ Adult: 15-124   `MCC` Major Complication/Comorbidity   `CC` Complication/Comorbidity   `SW` Severe Wound Dx

1100   ICD-10-CM 2021

√7ᵗʰ **T24.092** Burn of unspecified degree of multiple sites of **left** lower limb, except ankle and foot

√7ᵗʰ **T24.099** Burn of unspecified degree of multiple sites of unspecified lower limb, except ankle and foot

√5ᵗʰ **T24.1** Burn of **first degree** of lower limb, except ankle and foot
  Use additional external cause code to identify the source, place and intent of the burn (X00-X19, X75-X77, X96-X98, Y92)

√6ᵗʰ **T24.10** Burn of first degree of unspecified site of lower limb, except ankle and foot
  √7ᵗʰ **T24.101** Burn of first degree of unspecified site of **right** lower limb, except ankle and foot
  √7ᵗʰ **T24.102** Burn of first degree of unspecified site of **left** lower limb, except ankle and foot
  √7ᵗʰ **T24.109** Burn of first degree of unspecified site of unspecified lower limb, except ankle and foot

√6ᵗʰ **T24.11** Burn of first degree of **thigh**
  √7ᵗʰ **T24.111** Burn of first degree of **right** thigh
  √7ᵗʰ **T24.112** Burn of first degree of **left** thigh
  √7ᵗʰ **T24.119** Burn of first degree of unspecified thigh

√6ᵗʰ **T24.12** Burn of first degree of **knee**
  √7ᵗʰ **T24.121** Burn of first degree of **right** knee
  √7ᵗʰ **T24.122** Burn of first degree of **left** knee
  √7ᵗʰ **T24.129** Burn of first degree of unspecified knee

√6ᵗʰ **T24.13** Burn of first degree of **lower leg**
  √7ᵗʰ **T24.131** Burn of first degree of **right** lower leg
  √7ᵗʰ **T24.132** Burn of first degree of **left** lower leg
  √7ᵗʰ **T24.139** Burn of first degree of unspecified lower leg

√6ᵗʰ **T24.19** Burn of first degree of **multiple sites** of lower limb, except ankle and foot
  √7ᵗʰ **T24.191** Burn of first degree of multiple sites of **right** lower limb, except ankle and foot
  √7ᵗʰ **T24.192** Burn of first degree of multiple sites of **left** lower limb, except ankle and foot
  √7ᵗʰ **T24.199** Burn of first degree of multiple sites of unspecified lower limb, except ankle and foot

√5ᵗʰ **T24.2** Burn of **second degree** of lower limb, except ankle and foot
  Use additional external cause code to identify the source, place and intent of the burn (X00-X19, X75-X77, X96-X98, Y92)

√6ᵗʰ **T24.20** Burn of second degree of unspecified site of lower limb, except ankle and foot
  √7ᵗʰ **T24.201** Burn of second degree of unspecified site of **right** lower limb, except ankle and foot
  √7ᵗʰ **T24.202** Burn of second degree of unspecified site of **left** lower limb, except ankle and foot
  √7ᵗʰ **T24.209** Burn of second degree of unspecified site of unspecified lower limb, except ankle and foot

√6ᵗʰ **T24.21** Burn of second degree of **thigh**
  √7ᵗʰ **T24.211** Burn of second degree of **right** thigh
  √7ᵗʰ **T24.212** Burn of second degree of **left** thigh
  √7ᵗʰ **T24.219** Burn of second degree of unspecified thigh

√6ᵗʰ **T24.22** Burn of second degree of **knee**
  √7ᵗʰ **T24.221** Burn of second degree of **right** knee
  √7ᵗʰ **T24.222** Burn of second degree of **left** knee
  √7ᵗʰ **T24.229** Burn of second degree of unspecified knee

√6ᵗʰ **T24.23** Burn of second degree of **lower leg**
  √7ᵗʰ **T24.231** Burn of second degree of **right** lower leg
  √7ᵗʰ **T24.232** Burn of second degree of **left** lower leg
  √7ᵗʰ **T24.239** Burn of second degree of unspecified lower leg

√6ᵗʰ **T24.29** Burn of second degree of **multiple sites** of lower limb, except ankle and foot
  √7ᵗʰ **T24.291** Burn of second degree of multiple sites of **right** lower limb, except ankle and foot
  √7ᵗʰ **T24.292** Burn of second degree of multiple sites of **left** lower limb, except ankle and foot
  √7ᵗʰ **T24.299** Burn of second degree of multiple sites of unspecified lower limb, except ankle and foot

√5ᵗʰ **T24.3** Burn of **third degree** of lower limb, except ankle and foot
  Use additional external cause code to identify the source, place and intent of the burn (X00-X19, X75-X77, X96-X98, Y92)

√6ᵗʰ **T24.30** Burn of third degree of unspecified site of lower limb, except ankle and foot
  √7ᵗʰ **T24.301** Burn of third degree of unspecified site of **right** lower limb, except ankle and foot `CC` `H5` `SW`
  √7ᵗʰ **T24.302** Burn of third degree of unspecified site of **left** lower limb, except ankle and foot `CC` `H5` `SW`
  √7ᵗʰ **T24.309** Burn of third degree of unspecified site of unspecified lower limb, except ankle and foot `CC` `H5` `SW`

√6ᵗʰ **T24.31** Burn of third degree of **thigh**
  √7ᵗʰ **T24.311** Burn of third degree of **right** thigh `CC` `H5` `SW`
  √7ᵗʰ **T24.312** Burn of third degree of **left** thigh `CC` `H5` `SW`
  √7ᵗʰ **T24.319** Burn of third degree of unspecified thigh `CC` `H5` `SW`

√6ᵗʰ **T24.32** Burn of third degree of **knee**
  √7ᵗʰ **T24.321** Burn of third degree of **right** knee `CC` `H5` `SW`
  √7ᵗʰ **T24.322** Burn of third degree of **left** knee `CC` `H5` `SW`
  √7ᵗʰ **T24.329** Burn of third degree of unspecified knee `CC` `H5` `SW`

√6ᵗʰ **T24.33** Burn of third degree of **lower leg**
  √7ᵗʰ **T24.331** Burn of third degree of **right** lower leg `CC` `H5` `SW`
  √7ᵗʰ **T24.332** Burn of third degree of **left** lower leg `CC` `H5` `SW`
  √7ᵗʰ **T24.339** Burn of third degree of unspecified lower leg `CC` `H5` `SW`

√6ᵗʰ **T24.39** Burn of third degree of **multiple sites** of lower limb, except ankle and foot
  AHA: 2016,2Q,4
  √7ᵗʰ **T24.391** Burn of third degree of multiple sites of **right** lower limb, except ankle and foot `CC` `H5` `SW`
  √7ᵗʰ **T24.392** Burn of third degree of multiple sites of **left** lower limb, except ankle and foot `CC` `H5` `SW`
  √7ᵗʰ **T24.399** Burn of third degree of multiple sites of unspecified lower limb, except ankle and foot `CC` `H5` `SW`

√5ᵗʰ **T24.4** Corrosion of unspecified degree of lower limb, except ankle and foot
  Code first (T51-T65) to identify chemical and intent
  Use additional external cause code to identify place (Y92)

√6ᵗʰ **T24.40** Corrosion of unspecified degree of unspecified site of lower limb, except ankle and foot
  √7ᵗʰ **T24.401** Corrosion of unspecified degree of unspecified site of **right** lower limb, except ankle and foot
  √7ᵗʰ **T24.402** Corrosion of unspecified degree of unspecified site of **left** lower limb, except ankle and foot
  √7ᵗʰ **T24.409** Corrosion of unspecified degree of unspecified site of unspecified lower limb, except ankle and foot

√6ᵗʰ **T24.41** Corrosion of unspecified degree of **thigh**
  √7ᵗʰ **T24.411** Corrosion of unspecified degree of **right** thigh
  √7ᵗʰ **T24.412** Corrosion of unspecified degree of **left** thigh
  √7ᵗʰ **T24.419** Corrosion of unspecified degree of unspecified thigh

√6ᵗʰ **T24.42** Corrosion of unspecified degree of **knee**
  √7ᵗʰ **T24.421** Corrosion of unspecified degree of **right** knee
  √7ᵗʰ **T24.422** Corrosion of unspecified degree of **left** knee
  √7ᵗʰ **T24.429** Corrosion of unspecified degree of unspecified knee

√6ᵗʰ **T24.43** Corrosion of unspecified degree of **lower leg**
  √7ᵗʰ **T24.431** Corrosion of unspecified degree of **right** lower leg

☑ Additional Character Required   √₁₇ᵗʰ Placeholder   Unacceptable PDx   Questionable PDx   Manifestation   Unspecified Dx   **H1**-**H14** HAC   **HCC** CMS-HCC Dx   **HIV** HIV Dx

ICD-10-CM 2021   **1101**

√7ᵗʰ **T24.432** Corrosion of unspecified degree of left lower leg

√7ᵗʰ **T24.439** Corrosion of unspecified degree of unspecified lower leg

√6ᵗʰ **T24.49** Corrosion of unspecified degree of multiple sites of lower limb, except ankle and foot

√7ᵗʰ **T24.491** Corrosion of unspecified degree of multiple sites of right lower limb, except ankle and foot

√7ᵗʰ **T24.492** Corrosion of unspecified degree of multiple sites of left lower limb, except ankle and foot

√7ᵗʰ **T24.499** Corrosion of unspecified degree of multiple sites of unspecified lower limb, except ankle and foot

√5ᵗʰ **T24.5** Corrosion of first degree of lower limb, except ankle and foot

Code first (T51-T65) to identify chemical and intent
Use additional external cause code to identify place (Y92)

√6ᵗʰ **T24.50** Corrosion of first degree of unspecified site of lower limb, except ankle and foot

√7ᵗʰ **T24.501** Corrosion of first degree of unspecified site of right lower limb, except ankle and foot

√7ᵗʰ **T24.502** Corrosion of first degree of unspecified site of left lower limb, except ankle and foot

√7ᵗʰ **T24.509** Corrosion of first degree of unspecified site of unspecified lower limb, except ankle and foot

√6ᵗʰ **T24.51** Corrosion of first degree of thigh

√7ᵗʰ **T24.511** Corrosion of first degree of right thigh

√7ᵗʰ **T24.512** Corrosion of first degree of left thigh

√7ᵗʰ **T24.519** Corrosion of first degree of unspecified thigh

√6ᵗʰ **T24.52** Corrosion of first degree of knee

√7ᵗʰ **T24.521** Corrosion of first degree of right knee

√7ᵗʰ **T24.522** Corrosion of first degree of left knee

√7ᵗʰ **T24.529** Corrosion of first degree of unspecified knee

√6ᵗʰ **T24.53** Corrosion of first degree of lower leg

√7ᵗʰ **T24.531** Corrosion of first degree of right lower leg

√7ᵗʰ **T24.532** Corrosion of first degree of left lower leg

√7ᵗʰ **T24.539** Corrosion of first degree of unspecified lower leg

√6ᵗʰ **T24.59** Corrosion of first degree of multiple sites of lower limb, except ankle and foot

√7ᵗʰ **T24.591** Corrosion of first degree of multiple sites of right lower limb, except ankle and foot

√7ᵗʰ **T24.592** Corrosion of first degree of multiple sites of left lower limb, except ankle and foot

√7ᵗʰ **T24.599** Corrosion of first degree of multiple sites of unspecified lower limb, except ankle and foot

√5ᵗʰ **T24.6** Corrosion of second degree of lower limb, except ankle and foot

Code first (T51-T65) to identify chemical and intent
Use additional external cause code to identify place (Y92)

√6ᵗʰ **T24.60** Corrosion of second degree of unspecified site of lower limb, except ankle and foot

√7ᵗʰ **T24.601** Corrosion of second degree of unspecified site of right lower limb, except ankle and foot

√7ᵗʰ **T24.602** Corrosion of second degree of unspecified site of left lower limb, except ankle and foot

√7ᵗʰ **T24.609** Corrosion of second degree of unspecified site of unspecified lower limb, except ankle and foot

√6ᵗʰ **T24.61** Corrosion of second degree of thigh

√7ᵗʰ **T24.611** Corrosion of second degree of right thigh

√7ᵗʰ **T24.612** Corrosion of second degree of left thigh

√7ᵗʰ **T24.619** Corrosion of second degree of unspecified thigh

√6ᵗʰ **T24.62** Corrosion of second degree of knee

√7ᵗʰ **T24.621** Corrosion of second degree of right knee

√7ᵗʰ **T24.622** Corrosion of second degree of left knee

√7ᵗʰ **T24.629** Corrosion of second degree of unspecified knee

√6ᵗʰ **T24.63** Corrosion of second degree of lower leg

√7ᵗʰ **T24.631** Corrosion of second degree of right lower leg

√7ᵗʰ **T24.632** Corrosion of second degree of left lower leg

√7ᵗʰ **T24.639** Corrosion of second degree of unspecified lower leg

√6ᵗʰ **T24.69** Corrosion of second degree of multiple sites of lower limb, except ankle and foot

√7ᵗʰ **T24.691** Corrosion of second degree of multiple sites of right lower limb, except ankle and foot

√7ᵗʰ **T24.692** Corrosion of second degree of multiple sites of left lower limb, except ankle and foot

√7ᵗʰ **T24.699** Corrosion of second degree of multiple sites of unspecified lower limb, except ankle and foot

√5ᵗʰ **T24.7** Corrosion of third degree of lower limb, except ankle and foot

Code first (T51-T65) to identify chemical and intent
Use additional external cause code to identify place (Y92)

√6ᵗʰ **T24.70** Corrosion of third degree of unspecified site of lower limb, except ankle and foot

√7ᵗʰ **T24.701** Corrosion of third degree of unspecified site of right lower limb, except ankle and foot `CC` `H5` `SW`

√7ᵗʰ **T24.702** Corrosion of third degree of unspecified site of left lower limb, except ankle and foot `CC` `H5` `SW`

√7ᵗʰ **T24.709** Corrosion of third degree of unspecified site of unspecified lower limb, except ankle and foot `CC` `H5` `SW`

√6ᵗʰ **T24.71** Corrosion of third degree of thigh

√7ᵗʰ **T24.711** Corrosion of third degree of right thigh `CC` `H5` `SW`

√7ᵗʰ **T24.712** Corrosion of third degree of left thigh `CC` `H5` `SW`

√7ᵗʰ **T24.719** Corrosion of third degree of unspecified thigh `CC` `H5` `SW`

√6ᵗʰ **T24.72** Corrosion of third degree of knee

√7ᵗʰ **T24.721** Corrosion of third degree of right knee `CC` `H5` `SW`

√7ᵗʰ **T24.722** Corrosion of third degree of left knee `CC` `H5` `SW`

√7ᵗʰ **T24.729** Corrosion of third degree of unspecified knee `CC` `H5` `SW`

√6ᵗʰ **T24.73** Corrosion of third degree of lower leg

√7ᵗʰ **T24.731** Corrosion of third degree of right lower leg `CC` `H5` `SW`

√7ᵗʰ **T24.732** Corrosion of third degree of left lower leg `CC` `H5` `SW`

√7ᵗʰ **T24.739** Corrosion of third degree of unspecified lower leg `CC` `H5` `SW`

√6ᵗʰ **T24.79** Corrosion of third degree of multiple sites of lower limb, except ankle and foot

√7ᵗʰ **T24.791** Corrosion of third degree of multiple sites of right lower limb, except ankle and foot `CC` `H5` `SW`

√7ᵗʰ **T24.792** Corrosion of third degree of multiple sites of left lower limb, except ankle and foot `CC` `H5` `SW`

√7ᵗʰ **T24.799** Corrosion of third degree of multiple sites of unspecified lower limb, except ankle and foot `CC` `H5` `SW`

√4ᵗʰ **T25 Burn and corrosion of ankle and foot**

> The appropriate 7th character is to be added to each code from category T25.
> A   initial encounter
> D   subsequent encounter
> S   sequela

√5ᵗʰ **T25.0 Burn of unspecified degree of ankle and foot**

Use additional external cause code to identify the source, place and intent of the burn (X00-X19, X75-X77, X96-X98, Y92)

√6ᵗʰ **T25.01** Burn of unspecified degree of ankle

√7ᵗʰ **T25.011** Burn of unspecified degree of right ankle

√7ᵗʰ **T25.012** Burn of unspecified degree of left ankle

√7ᵗʰ **T25.019** Burn of unspecified degree of unspecified ankle

√6ᵗʰ **T25.02** **Burn of unspecified degree of** foot

    EXCLUDES 2   *burn of unspecified degree of toe(s) (nail) (T25.03-)*

    √7ᵗʰ **T25.021** Burn of unspecified degree of right foot

    √7ᵗʰ **T25.022** Burn of unspecified degree of left foot

    √7ᵗʰ **T25.029** Burn of unspecified degree of unspecified foot

√6ᵗʰ **T25.03** **Burn of unspecified degree of** toe(s) (nail)

    √7ᵗʰ **T25.031** Burn of unspecified degree of right toe(s) (nail)

    √7ᵗʰ **T25.032** Burn of unspecified degree of left toe(s) (nail)

    √7ᵗʰ **T25.039** Burn of unspecified degree of unspecified toe(s) (nail)

√6ᵗʰ **T25.09** **Burn of unspecified degree of** multiple sites **of ankle and foot**

    √7ᵗʰ **T25.091** Burn of unspecified degree of multiple sites of right ankle and foot

    √7ᵗʰ **T25.092** Burn of unspecified degree of multiple sites of left ankle and foot

    √7ᵗʰ **T25.099** Burn of unspecified degree of multiple sites of unspecified ankle and foot

√5ᵗʰ **T25.1** **Burn of** first degree **of ankle and foot**

    Use additional external cause code to identify the source, place and intent of the burn (X00-X19, X75-X77, X96-X98, Y92)

    √6ᵗʰ **T25.11** **Burn of first degree of** ankle

       √7ᵗʰ **T25.111** Burn of first degree of right ankle

       √7ᵗʰ **T25.112** Burn of first degree of left ankle

       √7ᵗʰ **T25.119** Burn of first degree of unspecified ankle

    √6ᵗʰ **T25.12** **Burn of first degree of** foot

       EXCLUDES 2   *burn of first degree of toe(s) (nail) (T25.13-)*

       √7ᵗʰ **T25.121** Burn of first degree of right foot

       √7ᵗʰ **T25.122** Burn of first degree of left foot

       √7ᵗʰ **T25.129** Burn of first degree of unspecified foot

    √6ᵗʰ **T25.13** **Burn of first degree of** toe(s) (nail)

       √7ᵗʰ **T25.131** Burn of first degree of right toe(s) (nail)

       √7ᵗʰ **T25.132** Burn of first degree of left toe(s) (nail)

       √7ᵗʰ **T25.139** Burn of first degree of unspecified toe(s) (nail)

    √6ᵗʰ **T25.19** **Burn of first degree of** multiple sites **of ankle and foot**

       √7ᵗʰ **T25.191** Burn of first degree of multiple sites of right ankle and foot

       √7ᵗʰ **T25.192** Burn of first degree of multiple sites of left ankle and foot

       √7ᵗʰ **T25.199** Burn of first degree of multiple sites of unspecified ankle and foot

√5ᵗʰ **T25.2** **Burn of** second degree **of ankle and foot**

    Use additional external cause code to identify the source, place and intent of the burn (X00-X19, X75-X77, X96-X98, Y92)

    √6ᵗʰ **T25.21** **Burn of second degree of** ankle

       √7ᵗʰ **T25.211** Burn of second degree of right ankle

       √7ᵗʰ **T25.212** Burn of second degree of left ankle

       √7ᵗʰ **T25.219** Burn of second degree of unspecified ankle

    √6ᵗʰ **T25.22** **Burn of second degree of** foot

       EXCLUDES 2   *burn of second degree of toe(s) (nail) (T25.23-)*

       √7ᵗʰ **T25.221** Burn of second degree of right foot

       √7ᵗʰ **T25.222** Burn of second degree of left foot

       √7ᵗʰ **T25.229** Burn of second degree of unspecified foot

    √6ᵗʰ **T25.23** **Burn of second degree of** toe(s) (nail)

       √7ᵗʰ **T25.231** Burn of second degree of right toe(s) (nail)

       √7ᵗʰ **T25.232** Burn of second degree of left toe(s) (nail)

       √7ᵗʰ **T25.239** Burn of second degree of unspecified toe(s) (nail)

    √6ᵗʰ **T25.29** **Burn of second degree of** multiple sites **of ankle and foot**

       √7ᵗʰ **T25.291** Burn of second degree of multiple sites of right ankle and foot

       √7ᵗʰ **T25.292** Burn of second degree of multiple sites of left ankle and foot

       √7ᵗʰ **T25.299** Burn of second degree of multiple sites of unspecified ankle and foot

√5ᵗʰ **T25.3** **Burn of** third degree **of ankle and foot**

    Use additional external cause code to identify the source, place and intent of the burn (X00-X19, X75-X77, X96-X98, Y92)

    √6ᵗʰ **T25.31** **Burn of third degree of** ankle

       √7ᵗʰ **T25.311** Burn of third degree of right ankle   CC H5 SW

       √7ᵗʰ **T25.312** Burn of third degree of left ankle   CC H5 SW

       √7ᵗʰ **T25.319** Burn of third degree of unspecified ankle   CC H5 SW

    √6ᵗʰ **T25.32** **Burn of third degree of** foot

       EXCLUDES 2   *burn of third degree of toe(s) (nail) (T25.33-)*

       √7ᵗʰ **T25.321** Burn of third degree of right foot   CC H5 SW

       √7ᵗʰ **T25.322** Burn of third degree of left foot   CC H5 SW

       √7ᵗʰ **T25.329** Burn of third degree of unspecified foot   CC H5 SW

    √6ᵗʰ **T25.33** **Burn of third degree of** toe(s) (nail)

       √7ᵗʰ **T25.331** Burn of third degree of right toe(s) (nail)   CC H5 SW

       √7ᵗʰ **T25.332** Burn of third degree of left toe(s) (nail)   CC H5 SW

       √7ᵗʰ **T25.339** Burn of third degree of unspecified toe(s) (nail)   CC H5 SW

    √6ᵗʰ **T25.39** **Burn of third degree of** multiple sites **of ankle and foot**

       √7ᵗʰ **T25.391** Burn of third degree of multiple sites of right ankle and foot   CC H5 SW

       √7ᵗʰ **T25.392** Burn of third degree of multiple sites of left ankle and foot   CC H5 SW

       √7ᵗʰ **T25.399** Burn of third degree of multiple sites of unspecified ankle and foot   CC H5 SW

√5ᵗʰ **T25.4** **Corrosion of unspecified degree of ankle and foot**

    Code first (T51-T65) to identify chemical and intent

    Use additional external cause code to identify place (Y92)

    √6ᵗʰ **T25.41** **Corrosion of unspecified degree of** ankle

       √7ᵗʰ **T25.411** Corrosion of unspecified degree of right ankle

       √7ᵗʰ **T25.412** Corrosion of unspecified degree of left ankle

       √7ᵗʰ **T25.419** Corrosion of unspecified degree of unspecified ankle

    √6ᵗʰ **T25.42** **Corrosion of unspecified degree of** foot

       EXCLUDES 2   *corrosion of unspecified degree of toe(s) (nail) (T25.43-)*

       √7ᵗʰ **T25.421** Corrosion of unspecified degree of right foot

       √7ᵗʰ **T25.422** Corrosion of unspecified degree of left foot

       √7ᵗʰ **T25.429** Corrosion of unspecified degree of unspecified foot

    √6ᵗʰ **T25.43** **Corrosion of unspecified degree of** toe(s) (nail)

       √7ᵗʰ **T25.431** Corrosion of unspecified degree of right toe(s) (nail)

       √7ᵗʰ **T25.432** Corrosion of unspecified degree of left toe(s) (nail)

       √7ᵗʰ **T25.439** Corrosion of unspecified degree of unspecified toe(s) (nail)

    √6ᵗʰ **T25.49** **Corrosion of unspecified degree of** multiple sites **of ankle and foot**

       √7ᵗʰ **T25.491** Corrosion of unspecified degree of multiple sites of right ankle and foot

       √7ᵗʰ **T25.492** Corrosion of unspecified degree of multiple sites of left ankle and foot

       √7ᵗʰ **T25.499** Corrosion of unspecified degree of multiple sites of unspecified ankle and foot

√5ᵗʰ **T25.5** **Corrosion of** first degree **of ankle and foot**

    Code first (T51-T65) to identify chemical and intent

    Use additional external cause code to identify place (Y92)

    √6ᵗʰ **T25.51** **Corrosion of first degree of** ankle

       √7ᵗʰ **T25.511** Corrosion of first degree of right ankle

       √7ᵗʰ **T25.512** Corrosion of first degree of left ankle

       √7ᵗʰ **T25.519** Corrosion of first degree of unspecified ankle

---

☑ Additional Character Required   √ˣ7ᵗʰ Placeholder   Unacceptable PDx   Questionable PDx   Manifestation   Unspecified Dx   H1-H14 HAC   HCC CMS-HCC Dx   HIV HIV Dx

√6ᵗʰ **T25.52 Corrosion of first degree of foot**

        EXCLUDES 2   corrosion of first degree of toe(s) (nail) (T25.53-)

   √7ᵗʰ **T25.521 Corrosion of first degree of right foot**

   √7ᵗʰ **T25.522 Corrosion of first degree of left foot**

   √7ᵗʰ **T25.529 Corrosion of first degree of unspecified foot**

√6ᵗʰ **T25.53 Corrosion of first degree of toe(s) (nail)**

   √7ᵗʰ **T25.531 Corrosion of first degree of right toe(s) (nail)**

   √7ᵗʰ **T25.532 Corrosion of first degree of left toe(s) (nail)**

   √7ᵗʰ **T25.539 Corrosion of first degree of unspecified toe(s) (nail)**

√6ᵗʰ **T25.59 Corrosion of first degree of multiple sites of ankle and foot**

   √7ᵗʰ **T25.591 Corrosion of first degree of multiple sites of right ankle and foot**

   √7ᵗʰ **T25.592 Corrosion of first degree of multiple sites of left ankle and foot**

   √7ᵗʰ **T25.599 Corrosion of first degree of multiple sites of unspecified ankle and foot**

√5ᵗʰ **T25.6 Corrosion of second degree of ankle and foot**

   Code first (T51-T65) to identify chemical and intent

   Use additional external cause code to identify place (Y92)

√6ᵗʰ **T25.61 Corrosion of second degree of ankle**

   √7ᵗʰ **T25.611 Corrosion of second degree of right ankle**

   √7ᵗʰ **T25.612 Corrosion of second degree of left ankle**

   √7ᵗʰ **T25.619 Corrosion of second degree of unspecified ankle**

√6ᵗʰ **T25.62 Corrosion of second degree of foot**

        EXCLUDES 2   corrosion of second degree of toe(s) (nail) (T25.63-)

   √7ᵗʰ **T25.621 Corrosion of second degree of right foot**

   √7ᵗʰ **T25.622 Corrosion of second degree of left foot**

   √7ᵗʰ **T25.629 Corrosion of second degree of unspecified foot**

√6ᵗʰ **T25.63 Corrosion of second degree of toe(s) (nail)**

   √7ᵗʰ **T25.631 Corrosion of second degree of right toe(s) (nail)**

   √7ᵗʰ **T25.632 Corrosion of second degree of left toe(s) (nail)**

   √7ᵗʰ **T25.639 Corrosion of second degree of unspecified toe(s) (nail)**

√6ᵗʰ **T25.69 Corrosion of second degree of multiple sites of ankle and foot**

   √7ᵗʰ **T25.691 Corrosion of second degree of right ankle and foot**

   √7ᵗʰ **T25.692 Corrosion of second degree of left ankle and foot**

   √7ᵗʰ **T25.699 Corrosion of second degree of unspecified ankle and foot**

√5ᵗʰ **T25.7 Corrosion of third degree of ankle and foot**

   Code first (T51-T65) to identify chemical and intent

   Use additional external cause code to identify place (Y92)

√6ᵗʰ **T25.71 Corrosion of third degree of ankle**

   √7ᵗʰ **T25.711 Corrosion of third degree of right ankle** CC H5 SW

   √7ᵗʰ **T25.712 Corrosion of third degree of left ankle** CC H5 SW

   √7ᵗʰ **T25.719 Corrosion of third degree of unspecified ankle** CC H5 SW

√6ᵗʰ **T25.72 Corrosion of third degree of foot**

        EXCLUDES 2   corrosion of third degree of toe(s) (nail) (T25.73-)

   √7ᵗʰ **T25.721 Corrosion of third degree of right foot** CC H5 SW

   √7ᵗʰ **T25.722 Corrosion of third degree of left foot** CC H5 SW

   √7ᵗʰ **T25.729 Corrosion of third degree of unspecified foot** CC H5 SW

√6ᵗʰ **T25.73 Corrosion of third degree of toe(s) (nail)**

   √7ᵗʰ **T25.731 Corrosion of third degree of right toe(s) (nail)** CC H5 SW

   √7ᵗʰ **T25.732 Corrosion of third degree of left toe(s) (nail)** CC H5 SW

√7ᵗʰ **T25.739 Corrosion of third degree of unspecified toe(s) (nail)** CC H5 SW

√6ᵗʰ **T25.79 Corrosion of third degree of multiple sites of ankle and foot**

   √7ᵗʰ **T25.791 Corrosion of third degree of multiple sites of right ankle and foot** CC H5 SW

   √7ᵗʰ **T25.792 Corrosion of third degree of multiple sites of left ankle and foot** CC H5 SW

   √7ᵗʰ **T25.799 Corrosion of third degree of multiple sites of unspecified ankle and foot** CC H5 SW

Burns and corrosions confined to eye and internal organs (T26-T28)

√4ᵗʰ **T26 Burn and corrosion confined to eye and adnexa**

   The appropriate 7th character is to be added to each code from category T26.

   A   initial encounter

   D   subsequent encounter

   S   sequela

√5ᵗʰ **T26.0 Burn of eyelid and periocular area**

   Use additional external cause code to identify the source, place and intent of the burn (X00-X19, X75-X77, X96-X98, Y92)

   √x7ᵗʰ **T26.00 Burn of unspecified eyelid and periocular area**

   √x7ᵗʰ **T26.01 Burn of right eyelid and periocular area**

   √x7ᵗʰ **T26.02 Burn of left eyelid and periocular area**

√5ᵗʰ **T26.1 Burn of cornea and conjunctival sac**

   Use additional external cause code to identify the source, place and intent of the burn (X00-X19, X75-X77, X96-X98, Y92)

   √x7ᵗʰ **T26.10 Burn of cornea and conjunctival sac, unspecified eye**

   √x7ᵗʰ **T26.11 Burn of cornea and conjunctival sac, right eye**

   √x7ᵗʰ **T26.12 Burn of cornea and conjunctival sac, left eye**

√5ᵗʰ **T26.2 Burn with resulting rupture and destruction of eyeball**

   Use additional external cause code to identify the source, place and intent of the burn (X00-X19, X75-X77, X96-X98, Y92)

   √x7ᵗʰ **T26.20 Burn with resulting rupture and destruction of unspecified eyeball** CC H5

   √x7ᵗʰ **T26.21 Burn with resulting rupture and destruction of right eyeball** CC H5

   √x7ᵗʰ **T26.22 Burn with resulting rupture and destruction of left eyeball** CC H5

√5ᵗʰ **T26.3 Burns of other specified parts of eye and adnexa**

   Use additional external cause code to identify the source, place and intent of the burn (X00-X19, X75-X77, X96-X98, Y92)

   √x7ᵗʰ **T26.30 Burns of other specified parts of unspecified eye and adnexa**

   √x7ᵗʰ **T26.31 Burns of other specified parts of right eye and adnexa**

   √x7ᵗʰ **T26.32 Burns of other specified parts of left eye and adnexa**

√5ᵗʰ **T26.4 Burn of eye and adnexa, part unspecified**

   Use additional external cause code to identify the source, place and intent of the burn (X00-X19, X75-X77, X96-X98, Y92)

   √x7ᵗʰ **T26.40 Burn of unspecified eye and adnexa, part unspecified**

   √x7ᵗʰ **T26.41 Burn of right eye and adnexa, part unspecified**

   √x7ᵗʰ **T26.42 Burn of left eye and adnexa, part unspecified**

√5ᵗʰ **T26.5 Corrosion of eyelid and periocular area**

   Code first (T51-T65) to identify chemical and intent

   Use additional external cause code to identify place (Y92)

   √x7ᵗʰ **T26.50 Corrosion of unspecified eyelid and periocular area**

   √x7ᵗʰ **T26.51 Corrosion of right eyelid and periocular area**

   √x7ᵗʰ **T26.52 Corrosion of left eyelid and periocular area**

√5ᵗʰ **T26.6 Corrosion of cornea and conjunctival sac**

   Code first (T51-T65) to identify chemical and intent

   Use additional external cause code to identify place (Y92)

   √x7ᵗʰ **T26.60 Corrosion of cornea and conjunctival sac, unspecified eye**

   √x7ᵗʰ **T26.61 Corrosion of cornea and conjunctival sac, right eye**

   √x7ᵗʰ **T26.62 Corrosion of cornea and conjunctival sac, left eye**

N Newborn: 0   P Pediatric: 0-17   M Maternity: 9-64   A Adult: 15-124   MCC Major Complication/Comorbidity   CC Complication/Comorbidity   SW Severe Wound Dx

1104   ICD-10-CM 2021

√5ᵗʰ **T26.7** Corrosion with resulting **rupture and destruction of eyeball**
Code first (T51-T65) to identify chemical and intent
Use additional external cause code to identify place (Y92)

  √x7ᵗʰ **T26.70** **Corrosion with resulting rupture and destruction of unspecified eyeball** CC H5

  √x7ᵗʰ **T26.71** **Corrosion with resulting rupture and destruction of right eyeball** CC H5

  √x7ᵗʰ **T26.72** **Corrosion with resulting rupture and destruction of left eyeball** CC H5

√5ᵗʰ **T26.8** Corrosions of other specified parts of eye and adnexa
Code first (T51-T65) to identify chemical and intent
Use additional external cause code to identify place (Y92)

  √x7ᵗʰ **T26.80** **Corrosions of other specified parts of unspecified eye and adnexa**

  √x7ᵗʰ **T26.81** **Corrosions of other specified parts of right eye and adnexa**

  √x7ᵗʰ **T26.82** **Corrosions of other specified parts of left eye and adnexa**

√5ᵗʰ **T26.9** Corrosion of eye and adnexa, part unspecified
Code first (T51-T65) to identify chemical and intent
Use additional external cause code to identify place (Y92)

  √x7ᵗʰ **T26.90** **Corrosion of unspecified eye and adnexa, part unspecified**

  √x7ᵗʰ **T26.91** **Corrosion of right eye and adnexa, part unspecified**

  √x7ᵗʰ **T26.92** **Corrosion of left eye and adnexa, part unspecified**

√4ᵗʰ **T27** Burn and corrosion of respiratory tract
Use additional external cause code to identify the source and intent of the burn (X00-X19, X75-X77, X96-X98)
Use additional external cause code to identify place (Y92)

The appropriate 7th character is to be added to each code from category T27.
A   initial encounter
D   subsequent encounter
S   sequela

√x7ᵗʰ **T27.0** Burn of **larynx and trachea** CC H5

√x7ᵗʰ **T27.1** Burn **involving larynx and trachea with lung** CC H5

√x7ᵗʰ **T27.2** Burn of **other parts of respiratory tract** CC H5
Burn of thoracic cavity

√x7ᵗʰ **T27.3** Burn of **respiratory tract, part unspecified** CC H5

√x7ᵗʰ **T27.4** Corrosion of **larynx and trachea** CC H5
Code first (T51-T65) to identify chemical and intent

√x7ᵗʰ **T27.5** Corrosion **involving larynx and trachea with lung** CC H5
Code first (T51-T65) to identify chemical and intent

√x7ᵗʰ **T27.6** Corrosion **of other parts of respiratory tract** CC H5
Code first (T51-T65) to identify chemical and intent

√x7ᵗʰ **T27.7** Corrosion **of respiratory tract, part unspecified** CC H5
Code first (T51-T65) to identify chemical and intent

√4ᵗʰ **T28** Burn and corrosion of other internal organs
Use additional external cause code to identify the source and intent of the burn (X00-X19, X75-X77, X96-X98)
Use additional external cause code to identify place (Y92)

The appropriate 7th character is to be added to each code from category T28.
A   initial encounter
D   subsequent encounter
S   sequela

√x7ᵗʰ **T28.0** Burn of **mouth and pharynx**

√x7ᵗʰ **T28.1** Burn of **esophagus** CC H5

√x7ᵗʰ **T28.2** Burn of **other parts of alimentary tract** CC H5

√x7ᵗʰ **T28.3** Burn of **internal genitourinary organs**

√5ᵗʰ **T28.4** Burns of other and unspecified internal organs

  √x7ᵗʰ **T28.40** **Burn of unspecified internal organ**

  √6ᵗʰ **T28.41** **Burn of ear drum**

    √7ᵗʰ **T28.411** **Burn of right ear drum**

    √7ᵗʰ **T28.412** **Burn of left ear drum**

    √7ᵗʰ **T28.419** **Burn of unspecified ear drum**

  √x7ᵗʰ **T28.49** **Burn of other internal organ**

√x7ᵗʰ **T28.5** Corrosion of **mouth and pharynx**
Code first (T51-T65) to identify chemical and intent

√x7ᵗʰ **T28.6** Corrosion of **esophagus** CC H5
Code first (T51-T65) to identify chemical and intent

√x7ᵗʰ **T28.7** Corrosion **of other parts of alimentary tract** CC H5
Code first (T51-T65) to identify chemical and intent

√x7ᵗʰ **T28.8** Corrosion of **internal genitourinary organs**
Code first (T51-T65) to identify chemical and intent

√5ᵗʰ **T28.9** Corrosions of other and unspecified internal organs
Code first (T51-T65) to identify chemical and intent

  √x7ᵗʰ **T28.90** **Corrosions of unspecified internal organs**

  √6ᵗʰ **T28.91** **Corrosions of ear drum**

    √7ᵗʰ **T28.911** **Corrosions of right ear drum**

    √7ᵗʰ **T28.912** **Corrosions of left ear drum**

    √7ᵗʰ **T28.919** **Corrosions of unspecified ear drum**

  √x7ᵗʰ **T28.99** **Corrosions of other internal organs**

Burns and corrosions of multiple and unspecified body regions (T30-T32)

√4ᵗʰ **T30** Burn and corrosion, body region unspecified

T30.0 Burn of unspecified body region, unspecified degree
This code is not for inpatient use. Code to specified site and degree of burns
Burn NOS
Multiple burns NOS

T30.4 Corrosion of unspecified body region, unspecified degree
This code is not for inpatient use. Code to specified site and degree of corrosion
Corrosion NOS
Multiple corrosion NOS

√4ᵗʰ **T31** Burns **classified according to extent of body surface involved**

NOTE   This category is to be used as the primary code only when the site of the burn is unspecified. It should be used as a supplementary code with categories T20-T25 when the site is specified.

T31.0 Burns involving **less than 10% of body surface**

√5ᵗʰ **T31.1** Burns involving **10-19% of body surface**

  T31.10 **Burns involving 10-19% of body surface with 0% to 9% third degree burns** CC H5
Burns involving 10-19% of body surface NOS

  T31.11 **Burns involving 10-19% of body surface with 10-19% third degree burns** CC H5 HCC

√5ᵗʰ **T31.2** Burns involving **20-29% of body surface**

  T31.20 **Burns involving 20-29% of body surface with 0% to 9% third degree burns** CC H5
Burns involving 20-29% of body surface NOS

  T31.21 **Burns involving 20-29% of body surface with 10-19% third degree burns** MCC H5 HCC

  T31.22 **Burns involving 20-29% of body surface with 20-29% third degree burns** MCC H5 HCC

√5ᵗʰ **T31.3** Burns involving **30-39% of body surface**

  T31.30 **Burns involving 30-39% of body surface with 0% to 9% third degree burns** CC H5
Burns involving 30-39% of body surface NOS

  T31.31 **Burns involving 30-39% of body surface with 10-19% third degree burns** MCC H5 HCC

  T31.32 **Burns involving 30-39% of body surface with 20-29% third degree burns** MCC H5 HCC

  T31.33 **Burns involving 30-39% of body surface with 30-39% third degree burns** MCC H5 HCC

√6ᵗʰ **T31.4** Burns involving **40-49% of body surface**

  T31.40 **Burns involving 40-49% of body surface with 0% to 9% third degree burns** CC H5
Burns involving 40-49% of body surface NOS

  T31.41 **Burns involving 40-49% of body surface with 10-19% third degree burns** MCC H5 HCC

  T31.42 **Burns involving 40-49% of body surface with 20-29% third degree burns** MCC H5 HCC

  T31.43 **Burns involving 40-49% of body surface with 30-39% third degree burns** MCC H5 HCC

  T31.44 **Burns involving 40-49% of body surface with 40-49% third degree burns** MCC H5 HCC

✓5ᵗʰ **T31.5** **Burns involving 50-59% of body surface**

T31.50 **Burns involving 50-59% of body surface with 0% to 9% third degree burns** `CC` `H5`
Burns involving 50-59% of body surface NOS

T31.51 **Burns involving 50-59% of body surface with 10-19% third degree burns** `MCC` `H5` `HCC`

T31.52 **Burns involving 50-59% of body surface with 20-29% third degree burns** `MCC` `H5` `HCC`

T31.53 **Burns involving 50-59% of body surface with 30-39% third degree burns** `MCC` `H5` `HCC`

T31.54 **Burns involving 50-59% of body surface with 40-49% third degree burns** `MCC` `H5` `HCC`

T31.55 **Burns involving 50-59% of body surface with 50-59% third degree burns** `MCC` `H5` `HCC`

✓5ᵗʰ **T31.6** **Burns involving 60-69% of body surface**

T31.60 **Burns involving 60-69% of body surface with 0% to 9% third degree burns** `CC` `H5`
Burns involving 60-69% of body surface NOS

T31.61 **Burns involving 60-69% of body surface with 10-19% third degree burns** `MCC` `H5` `HCC`

T31.62 **Burns involving 60-69% of body surface with 20-29% third degree burns** `MCC` `H5` `HCC`

T31.63 **Burns involving 60-69% of body surface with 30-39% third degree burns** `MCC` `H5` `HCC`

T31.64 **Burns involving 60-69% of body surface with 40-49% third degree burns** `MCC` `H5` `HCC`

T31.65 **Burns involving 60-69% of body surface with 50-59% third degree burns** `MCC` `H5` `HCC`

T31.66 **Burns involving 60-69% of body surface with 60-69% third degree burns** `MCC` `H5` `HCC`

✓5ᵗʰ **T31.7** **Burns involving 70-79% of body surface**

T31.70 **Burns involving 70-79% of body surface with 0% to 9% third degree burns** `CC` `H5`
Burns involving 70-79% of body surface NOS

T31.71 **Burns involving 70-79% of body surface with 10-19% third degree burns** `MCC` `H5` `HCC`

T31.72 **Burns involving 70-79% of body surface with 20-29% third degree burns** `MCC` `H5` `HCC`

T31.73 **Burns involving 70-79% of body surface with 30-39% third degree burns** `MCC` `H5` `HCC`

T31.74 **Burns involving 70-79% of body surface with 40-49% third degree burns** `MCC` `H5` `HCC`

T31.75 **Burns involving 70-79% of body surface with 50-59% third degree burns** `MCC` `H5` `HCC`

T31.76 **Burns involving 70-79% of body surface with 60-69% third degree burns** `MCC` `H5` `HCC`

T31.77 **Burns involving 70-79% of body surface with 70-79% third degree burns** `MCC` `H5` `HCC`

✓5ᵗʰ **T31.8** **Burns involving 80-89% of body surface**

T31.80 **Burns involving 80-89% of body surface with 0% to 9% third degree burns** `CC` `H5`
Burns involving 80-89% of body surface NOS

T31.81 **Burns involving 80-89% of body surface with 10-19% third degree burns** `MCC` `H5` `HCC`

T31.82 **Burns involving 80-89% of body surface with 20-29% third degree burns** `MCC` `H5` `HCC`

T31.83 **Burns involving 80-89% of body surface with 30-39% third degree burns** `MCC` `H5` `HCC`

T31.84 **Burns involving 80-89% of body surface with 40-49% third degree burns** `MCC` `H5` `HCC`

T31.85 **Burns involving 80-89% of body surface with 50-59% third degree burns** `MCC` `H5` `HCC`

T31.86 **Burns involving 80-89% of body surface with 60-69% third degree burns** `MCC` `H5` `HCC`

T31.87 **Burns involving 80-89% of body surface with 70-79% third degree burns** `MCC` `H5` `HCC`

T31.88 **Burns involving 80-89% of body surface with 80-89% third degree burns** `MCC` `H5` `HCC`

✓5ᵗʰ **T31.9** **Burns involving 90% or more of body surface**

T31.90 **Burns involving 90% or more of body surface with 0% to 9% third degree burns** `CC` `H5`
Burns involving 90% or more of body surface NOS

T31.91 **Burns involving 90% or more of body surface with 10-19% third degree burns** `MCC` `H5` `HCC`

T31.92 **Burns involving 90% or more of body surface with 20-29% third degree burns** `MCC` `H5` `HCC`

T31.93 **Burns involving 90% or more of body surface with 30-39% third degree burns** `MCC` `H5` `HCC`

T31.94 **Burns involving 90% or more of body surface with 40-49% third degree burns** `MCC` `H5` `HCC`

T31.95 **Burns involving 90% or more of body surface with 50-59% third degree burns** `MCC` `H5` `HCC`

T31.96 **Burns involving 90% or more of body surface with 60-69% third degree burns** `MCC` `H5` `HCC`

T31.97 **Burns involving 90% or more of body surface with 70-79% third degree burns** `MCC` `H5` `HCC`

T31.98 **Burns involving 90% or more of body surface with 80-89% third degree burns** `MCC` `H5` `HCC`

T31.99 **Burns involving 90% or more of body surface with 90% or more third degree burns** `MCC` `H5` `HCC`

Rule of Nines Estimation of Total Body Surface Burned

Head and neck 9%
Each arm 9%
Anterior trunk 18%
Genitalia 1%
Anterior leg 9%
Posterior trunk 18%
Posterior leg 9%

✓4ᵗʰ **T32** **Corrosions classified according to extent of body surface involved**

`NOTE` This category is to be used as the primary code only when the site of the corrosion is unspecified. It may be used as a supplementary code with categories T20-T25 when the site is specified.

T32.0 **Corrosions involving less than 10% of body surface**

✓5ᵗʰ **T32.1** **Corrosions involving 10-19% of body surface**

T32.10 **Corrosions involving 10-19% of body surface with 0% to 9% third degree corrosion** `CC` `H5`
Corrosions involving 10-19% of body surface NOS

T32.11 **Corrosions involving 10-19% of body surface with 10-19% third degree corrosion** `CC` `H5` `HCC`

✓5ᵗʰ **T32.2** **Corrosions involving 20-29% of body surface**

T32.20 **Corrosions involving 20-29% of body surface with 0% to 9% third degree corrosion** `CC` `H5`

T32.21 **Corrosions involving 20-29% of body surface with 10-19% third degree corrosion** `MCC` `H5` `HCC`

T32.22 **Corrosions involving 20-29% of body surface with 20-29% third degree corrosion** `MCC` `H5` `HCC`

✓5ᵗʰ **T32.3** **Corrosions involving 30-39% of body surface**

T32.30 **Corrosions involving 30-39% of body surface with 0% to 9% third degree corrosion** `CC` `H5`

T32.31 **Corrosions involving 30-39% of body surface with 10-19% third degree corrosion** `MCC` `H5` `HCC`

T32.32 **Corrosions involving 30-39% of body surface with 20-29% third degree corrosion** `MCC` `H5` `HCC`

T32.33 **Corrosions involving 30-39% of body surface with 30-39% third degree corrosion** `MCC` `H5` `HCC`

✓5ᵗʰ **T32.4** **Corrosions involving 40-49% of body surface**

T32.40 **Corrosions involving 40-49% of body surface with 0% to 9% third degree corrosion** `CC` `H5`

T32.41 **Corrosions involving 40-49% of body surface with 10-19% third degree corrosion** `MCC` `H5` `HCC`

T32.42 **Corrosions involving 40-49% of body surface with 20-29% third degree corrosion** `MCC` `H5` `HCC`

T32.43 **Corrosions involving 40-49% of body surface with 30-39% third degree corrosion** `MCC` `H5` `HCC`

T32.44 **Corrosions involving 40-49% of body surface with 40-49% third degree corrosion** `MCC` `H5` `HCC`

✓5ᵗʰ **T32.5** **Corrosions involving 50-59% of body surface**

T32.50 **Corrosions involving 50-59% of body surface with 0% to 9% third degree corrosion** `CC` `H5`

T32.51 **Corrosions involving 50-59% of body surface with 10-19% third degree corrosion** `MCC` `H5` `HCC`

T32.52   Corrosions involving 50-59% of body surface with 20-29% third degree **corrosion** `MCC` `H5` `HCC`

T32.53   Corrosions involving 50-59% of body surface with 30-39% third degree **corrosion** `MCC` `H5` `HCC`

T32.54   Corrosions involving 50-59% of body surface with 40-49% third degree **corrosion** `MCC` `H5` `HCC`

T32.55   Corrosions involving 50-59% of body surface with 50-59% third degree **corrosion** `MCC` `H5` `HCC`

√5ᵗʰ **T32.6**   Corrosions involving 60-69% of body surface

T32.60   Corrosions involving 60-69% of body surface with 0% to 9% third degree **corrosion** `CC` `H5`

T32.61   Corrosions involving 60-69% of body surface with 10-19% third degree **corrosion** `MCC` `H5` `HCC`

T32.62   Corrosions involving 60-69% of body surface with 20-29% third degree **corrosion** `MCC` `H5` `HCC`

T32.63   Corrosions involving 60-69% of body surface with 30-39% third degree **corrosion** `MCC` `H5` `HCC`

T32.64   Corrosions involving 60-69% of body surface with 40-49% third degree **corrosion** `MCC` `H5` `HCC`

T32.65   Corrosions involving 60-69% of body surface with 50-59% third degree **corrosion** `MCC` `H5` `HCC`

T32.66   Corrosions involving 60-69% of body surface with 60-69% third degree **corrosion** `MCC` `H5` `HCC`

√5ᵗʰ **T32.7**   Corrosions involving 70-79% of body surface

T32.70   Corrosions involving 70-79% of body surface with 0% to 9% third degree **corrosion** `CC` `H5`

T32.71   Corrosions involving 70-79% of body surface with 10-19% third degree **corrosion** `MCC` `H5` `HCC`

T32.72   Corrosions involving 70-79% of body surface with 20-29% third degree **corrosion** `MCC` `H5` `HCC`

T32.73   Corrosions involving 70-79% of body surface with 30-39% third degree **corrosion** `MCC` `H5` `HCC`

T32.74   Corrosions involving 70-79% of body surface with 40-49% third degree **corrosion** `MCC` `H5` `HCC`

T32.75   Corrosions involving 70-79% of body surface with 50-59% third degree **corrosion** `MCC` `H5` `HCC`

T32.76   Corrosions involving 70-79% of body surface with 60-69% third degree **corrosion** `MCC` `H5` `HCC`

T32.77   Corrosions involving 70-79% of body surface with 70-79% third degree **corrosion** `MCC` `H5` `HCC`

√5ᵗʰ **T32.8**   Corrosions involving 80-89% of body surface

T32.80   Corrosions involving 80-89% of body surface with 0% to 9% third degree **corrosion** `CC` `H5`

T32.81   Corrosions involving 80-89% of body surface with 10-19% third degree **corrosion** `MCC` `H5` `HCC`

T32.82   Corrosions involving 80-89% of body surface with 20-29% third degree **corrosion** `MCC` `H5` `HCC`

T32.83   Corrosions involving 80-89% of body surface with 30-39% third degree **corrosion** `MCC` `H5` `HCC`

T32.84   Corrosions involving 80-89% of body surface with 40-49% third degree **corrosion** `MCC` `H5` `HCC`

T32.85   Corrosions involving 80-89% of body surface with 50-59% third degree **corrosion** `MCC` `H5` `HCC`

T32.86   Corrosions involving 80-89% of body surface with 60-69% third degree **corrosion** `MCC` `H5` `HCC`

T32.87   Corrosions involving 80-89% of body surface with 70-79% third degree **corrosion** `MCC` `H5` `HCC`

T32.88   Corrosions involving 80-89% of body surface with 80-89% third degree **corrosion** `MCC` `H5` `HCC`

√5ᵗʰ **T32.9**   Corrosions involving 90% or more of body surface

T32.90   Corrosions involving 90% or more of body surface with 0% to 9% third degree **corrosion** `CC` `H5`

T32.91   Corrosions involving 90% or more of body surface with 10-19% third degree **corrosion** `MCC` `H5` `HCC`

T32.92   Corrosions involving 90% or more of body surface with 20-29% third degree **corrosion** `MCC` `H5` `HCC`

T32.93   Corrosions involving 90% or more of body surface with 30-39% third degree **corrosion** `MCC` `H5` `HCC`

T32.94   Corrosions involving 90% or more of body surface with 40-49% third degree **corrosion** `MCC` `H5` `HCC`

T32.95   Corrosions involving 90% or more of body surface with 50-59% third degree **corrosion** `MCC` `H5` `HCC`

T32.96   Corrosions involving 90% or more of body surface with 60-69% third degree **corrosion** `MCC` `H5` `HCC`

T32.97   Corrosions involving 90% or more of body surface with 70-79% third degree **corrosion** `MCC` `H5` `HCC`

T32.98   Corrosions involving 90% or more of body surface with 80-89% third degree **corrosion** `MCC` `H5` `HCC`

T32.99   Corrosions involving 90% or more of body surface with 90% or more third degree **corrosion** `MCC` `H5` `HCC`

Frostbite (T33-T34)

EXCLUDES 2   *hypothermia and other effects of reduced temperature (T68, T69.-)*

√4ᵗʰ **T33**   **Superficial frostbite**

INCLUDES   frostbite with partial thickness skin loss

> The appropriate 7th character is to be added to each code from category T33.
> A   initial encounter
> D   subsequent encounter
> S   sequela

√5ᵗʰ **T33.0**   **Superficial frostbite of** head

√6ᵗʰ   **T33.01**   **Superficial frostbite of** ear

√7ᵗʰ   T33.011   **Superficial frostbite of** right ear `CC` `H5`

√7ᵗʰ   T33.012   **Superficial frostbite of** left ear `CC` `H5`

√7ᵗʰ   T33.019   **Superficial frostbite of unspecified** ear `CC` `H5`

√x7ᵗʰ   **T33.02**   **Superficial frostbite of** nose `CC` `H5`

√x7ᵗʰ   **T33.09**   **Superficial frostbite of other part of head** `CC` `H5`

√x7ᵗʰ **T33.1**   **Superficial frostbite of** neck `CC` `H5`

√x7ᵗʰ **T33.2**   **Superficial frostbite of** thorax `CC` `H5`

√x7ᵗʰ **T33.3**   **Superficial frostbite of** abdominal wall, lower back and pelvis `CC` `H5`

√5ᵗʰ **T33.4**   **Superficial frostbite of** arm

EXCLUDES 2   *superficial frostbite of wrist and hand (T33.5-)*

√x7ᵗʰ   **T33.40**   **Superficial frostbite of unspecified arm** `CC` `H5`

√x7ᵗʰ   **T33.41**   **Superficial frostbite of** right arm `CC` `H5`

√x7ᵗʰ   **T33.42**   **Superficial frostbite of** left arm `CC` `H5`

√5ᵗʰ **T33.5**   **Superficial frostbite of** wrist, hand, and fingers

√6ᵗʰ   **T33.51**   **Superficial frostbite of** wrist

√7ᵗʰ   T33.511   **Superficial frostbite of** right wrist `CC` `H5`

√7ᵗʰ   T33.512   **Superficial frostbite of** left wrist `CC` `H5`

√7ᵗʰ   T33.519   **Superficial frostbite of unspecified** wrist `CC` `H5`

√6ᵗʰ   **T33.52**   **Superficial frostbite of** hand

EXCLUDES 2   *superficial frostbite of fingers (T33.53-)*

√7ᵗʰ   T33.521   **Superficial frostbite of** right hand `CC` `H5`

√7ᵗʰ   T33.522   **Superficial frostbite of** left hand `CC` `H5`

√7ᵗʰ   T33.529   **Superficial frostbite of unspecified** hand `CC` `H5`

√6ᵗʰ   **T33.53**   **Superficial frostbite of** finger(s)

√7ᵗʰ   T33.531   **Superficial frostbite of** right finger(s) `CC` `H5`

√7ᵗʰ   T33.532   **Superficial frostbite of** left finger(s) `CC` `H5`

√7ᵗʰ   T33.539   **Superficial frostbite of unspecified** finger(s) `CC` `H5`

√5ᵗʰ **T33.6**   **Superficial frostbite of** hip and thigh

√x7ᵗʰ   **T33.60**   **Superficial frostbite of unspecified hip and thigh** `CC` `H5`

√x7ᵗʰ   **T33.61**   **Superficial frostbite of** right hip and thigh `CC` `H5`

√x7ᵗʰ   **T33.62**   **Superficial frostbite of** left hip and thigh `CC` `H5`

√5ᵗʰ **T33.7**   **Superficial frostbite of** knee and lower leg

EXCLUDES 2   *superficial frostbite of ankle and foot (T33.8-)*

√x7ᵗʰ   **T33.70**   **Superficial frostbite of unspecified knee and lower leg** `CC` `H5`

√x7ᵗʰ   **T33.71**   **Superficial frostbite of** right knee and lower leg `CC` `H5`

√x7ᵗʰ   **T33.72**   **Superficial frostbite of** left knee and lower leg `CC` `H5`

√5ᵗʰ **T33.8**   **Superficial frostbite of** ankle, foot, and toe(s)

√6ᵗʰ   **T33.81**   **Superficial frostbite of** ankle

√7ᵗʰ   T33.811   **Superficial frostbite of** right ankle `CC` `H5`

√7ᵗʰ   T33.812   **Superficial frostbite of** left ankle `CC` `H5`

✓ Additional Character Required   √x7ᵗʰ Placeholder   Unacceptable PDx   Questionable PDx   Manifestation   Unspecified Dx   `H1`-`H4` HAC   `HCC` CMS-HCC Dx   `HIV` HIV Dx

ICD-10-CM 2021   1107

√7ᵗʰ **T33.819** **Superficial frostbite of unspecified ankle** `CC` `H5`

√6ᵗʰ **T33.82** **Superficial frostbite of** foot

    √7ᵗʰ **T33.821** **Superficial frostbite of** right **foot** `CC` `H5`

    √7ᵗʰ **T33.822** **Superficial frostbite of** left **foot** `CC` `H5`

    √7ᵗʰ **T33.829** **Superficial frostbite of unspecified foot** `CC` `H5`

√6ᵗʰ **T33.83** **Superficial frostbite of** toe(s)

    √7ᵗʰ **T33.831** **Superficial frostbite of** right **toe(s)** `CC` `H5`

    √7ᵗʰ **T33.832** **Superficial frostbite of** left **toe(s)** `CC` `H5`

    √7ᵗʰ **T33.839** **Superficial frostbite of unspecified toe(s)** `CC` `H5`

√5ᵗʰ **T33.9** **Superficial frostbite of other and unspecified sites**

    √x7ᵗʰ **T33.90** **Superficial frostbite of unspecified sites** `CC` `H5`
      Superficial frostbite NOS

    √x7ᵗʰ **T33.99** **Superficial frostbite of other sites** `CC` `H5`
      Superficial frostbite of leg NOS
      Superficial frostbite of trunk NOS

√4ᵗʰ **T34** **Frostbite** with tissue necrosis

> The appropriate 7th character is to be added to each code from category T34.
> A   initial encounter
> D   subsequent encounter
> S   sequela

√5ᵗʰ **T34.0** **Frostbite with tissue necrosis of** head

    √6ᵗʰ **T34.01** **Frostbite with tissue necrosis of** ear

      √7ᵗʰ **T34.011** **Frostbite with tissue necrosis of** right **ear** `CC` `H5`

      √7ᵗʰ **T34.012** **Frostbite with tissue necrosis of** left **ear** `CC` `H5`

      √7ᵗʰ **T34.019** **Frostbite with tissue necrosis of unspecified ear** `CC` `H5`

    √x7ᵗʰ **T34.02** **Frostbite with tissue necrosis of** nose `CC` `H5`

    √x7ᵗʰ **T34.09** **Frostbite with tissue necrosis of other part of head** `CC` `H5`

√x7ᵗʰ **T34.1** **Frostbite with tissue necrosis of** neck `CC` `H5`

√x7ᵗʰ **T34.2** **Frostbite with tissue necrosis of** thorax `CC` `H5`

√x7ᵗʰ **T34.3** **Frostbite with tissue necrosis of** abdominal wall, lower back and pelvis `CC` `H5`

√5ᵗʰ **T34.4** **Frostbite with tissue necrosis of** arm

   EXCLUDES 2   *frostbite with tissue necrosis of wrist and hand (T34.5-)*

    √x7ᵗʰ **T34.40** **Frostbite with tissue necrosis of unspecified arm** `CC` `H5`

    √x7ᵗʰ **T34.41** **Frostbite with tissue necrosis of** right **arm** `CC` `H5`

    √x7ᵗʰ **T34.42** **Frostbite with tissue necrosis of** left **arm** `CC` `H5`

√5ᵗʰ **T34.5** **Frostbite with tissue necrosis of** wrist, hand, and finger(s)

    √6ᵗʰ **T34.51** **Frostbite with tissue necrosis of** wrist

      √7ᵗʰ **T34.511** **Frostbite with tissue necrosis of** right **wrist** `CC` `H5`

      √7ᵗʰ **T34.512** **Frostbite with tissue necrosis of** left **wrist** `CC` `H5`

      √7ᵗʰ **T34.519** **Frostbite with tissue necrosis of unspecified wrist** `CC` `H5`

    √6ᵗʰ **T34.52** **Frostbite with tissue necrosis of** hand

      EXCLUDES 2   *frostbite with tissue necrosis of finger(s) (T34.53-)*

      √7ᵗʰ **T34.521** **Frostbite with tissue necrosis of** right **hand** `CC` `H5`

      √7ᵗʰ **T34.522** **Frostbite with tissue necrosis of** left **hand** `CC` `H5`

      √7ᵗʰ **T34.529** **Frostbite with tissue necrosis of unspecified hand** `CC` `H5`

    √6ᵗʰ **T34.53** **Frostbite with tissue necrosis of** finger(s)

      √7ᵗʰ **T34.531** **Frostbite with tissue necrosis of** right **finger(s)** `CC` `H5`

      √7ᵗʰ **T34.532** **Frostbite with tissue necrosis of** left **finger(s)** `CC` `H5`

      √7ᵗʰ **T34.539** **Frostbite with tissue necrosis of unspecified finger(s)** `CC` `H5`

√5ᵗʰ **T34.6** **Frostbite with tissue necrosis of** hip and thigh

    √x7ᵗʰ **T34.60** **Frostbite with tissue necrosis of unspecified hip and thigh** `CC` `H5`

    √x7ᵗʰ **T34.61** **Frostbite with tissue necrosis of** right **hip and thigh** `CC` `H5`

    √x7ᵗʰ **T34.62** **Frostbite with tissue necrosis of** left **hip and thigh** `CC` `H5`

√5ᵗʰ **T34.7** **Frostbite with tissue necrosis of** knee and lower leg

   EXCLUDES 2   *frostbite with tissue necrosis of ankle and foot (T34.8-)*

    √x7ᵗʰ **T34.70** **Frostbite with tissue necrosis of unspecified knee and lower leg** `CC` `H5`

    √x7ᵗʰ **T34.71** **Frostbite with tissue necrosis of** right **knee and lower leg** `CC` `H5`

    √x7ᵗʰ **T34.72** **Frostbite with tissue necrosis of** left **knee and lower leg** `CC` `H5`

√5ᵗʰ **T34.8** **Frostbite with tissue necrosis of** ankle, foot, and toe(s)

    √6ᵗʰ **T34.81** **Frostbite with tissue necrosis of** ankle

      √7ᵗʰ **T34.811** **Frostbite with tissue necrosis of** right **ankle** `CC` `H5`

      √7ᵗʰ **T34.812** **Frostbite with tissue necrosis of** left **ankle** `CC` `H5`

      √7ᵗʰ **T34.819** **Frostbite with tissue necrosis of unspecified ankle** `CC` `H5`

    √6ᵗʰ **T34.82** **Frostbite with tissue necrosis of** foot

      √7ᵗʰ **T34.821** **Frostbite with tissue necrosis of** right **foot** `CC` `H5`

      √7ᵗʰ **T34.822** **Frostbite with tissue necrosis of** left **foot** `CC` `H5`

      √7ᵗʰ **T34.829** **Frostbite with tissue necrosis of unspecified foot** `CC` `H5`

    √6ᵗʰ **T34.83** **Frostbite with tissue necrosis of** toe(s)

      √7ᵗʰ **T34.831** **Frostbite with tissue necrosis of** right **toe(s)** `CC` `H5`

      √7ᵗʰ **T34.832** **Frostbite with tissue necrosis of** left **toe(s)** `CC` `H5`

      √7ᵗʰ **T34.839** **Frostbite with tissue necrosis of unspecified toe(s)** `CC` `H5`

√5ᵗʰ **T34.9** **Frostbite with tissue necrosis of other and unspecified sites**

    √x7ᵗʰ **T34.90** **Frostbite with tissue necrosis of unspecified sites** `CC` `H5`
      Frostbite with tissue necrosis NOS

    √x7ᵗʰ **T34.99** **Frostbite with tissue necrosis of other sites** `CC` `H5`
      Frostbite with tissue necrosis of leg NOS
      Frostbite with tissue necrosis of trunk NOS

N Newborn: 0   P Pediatric: 0-17   M Maternity: 9-64   A Adult: 15-124   MCC Major Complication/Comorbidity   CC Complication/Comorbidity   SW Severe Wound Dx

1108   ICD-10-CM 2021

Poisoning by, adverse effects of and underdosing of drugs, medicaments and biological substances (T36–T50)

INCLUDES   adverse effect of correct substance properly administered
poisoning by overdose of substance
poisoning by wrong substance given or taken in error
underdosing by (inadvertently) (deliberately) taking less substance than prescribed or instructed

Code first, for adverse effects, the nature of the adverse effect, such as:
adverse effect NOS (T88.7)
aspirin gastritis (K29.-)
blood disorders (D56-D76)
contact dermatitis (L23-L25)
dermatitis due to substances taken internally (L27.-)
nephropathy (N14.0-N14.2)

NOTE   The drug giving rise to the adverse effect should be identified by use of codes from categories T36-T50 with fifth or sixth character 5.

Use additional code(s) to specify:
manifestations of poisoning
underdosing or failure in dosage during medical and surgical care (Y63.6, Y63.8-Y63.9)
underdosing of medication regimen (Z91.12-, Z91.13-)

EXCLUDES 1   *toxic reaction to local anesthesia in pregnancy (O29.3-)*
EXCLUDES 2   *abuse and dependence of psychoactive substances (F10-F19)*
abuse of non-dependence-producing substances (F55.-)
drug reaction and poisoning affecting newborn (P00-P96)
►*immunodeficiency due to drugs (D84.821)*◄
pathological drug intoxication (inebriation) (F10-F19)

AHA: 2018,4Q,71; 2016,2Q,8; 2015,3Q,22

☑4ᵗʰ **T36**   **Poisoning by, adverse effect of and underdosing of systemic antibiotics**

     EXCLUDES 1   *antineoplastic antibiotics (T45.1-)*
       locally applied antibiotic NEC (T49.0)
       topically used antibiotic for ear, nose and throat (T49.6)
       topically used antibiotic for eye (T49.5)

> The appropriate 7th character is to be added to each code from category T36.
> A   initial encounter
> D   subsequent encounter
> S   sequela

☑5ᵗʰ **T36.0**   **Poisoning by, adverse effect of and underdosing of penicillins**

   ☑6ᵗʰ **T36.0X**   **Poisoning by, adverse effect of and underdosing of penicillins**

     ☑7ᵗʰ **T36.0X1**   **Poisoning by penicillins, accidental (unintentional)**
         Poisoning by penicillins NOS

    7 ☑7ᵗʰ **T36.0X2**   **Poisoning by penicillins, intentional self-harm**   HCC

     ☑7ᵗʰ **T36.0X3**   **Poisoning by penicillins, assault**

     ☑7ᵗʰ **T36.0X4**   **Poisoning by penicillins, undetermined**

     ☑7ᵗʰ **T36.0X5**   Adverse effect of penicillins

     ☑7ᵗʰ **T36.0X6**   Underdosing of penicillins

☑5ᵗʰ **T36.1**   **Poisoning by, adverse effect of and underdosing of cephalosporins and other beta-lactam antibiotics**

   ☑6ᵗʰ **T36.1X**   **Poisoning by, adverse effect of and underdosing of cephalosporins and other beta-lactam antibiotics**

     ☑7ᵗʰ **T36.1X1**   **Poisoning by cephalosporins and other beta-lactam antibiotics, accidental (unintentional)**
         Poisoning by cephalosporins and other beta-lactam antibiotics NOS

    7 ☑7ᵗʰ **T36.1X2**   **Poisoning by cephalosporins and other beta-lactam antibiotics, intentional self-harm**   HCC

     ☑7ᵗʰ **T36.1X3**   **Poisoning by cephalosporins and other beta-lactam antibiotics, assault**

     ☑7ᵗʰ **T36.1X4**   **Poisoning by cephalosporins and other beta-lactam antibiotics, undetermined**

     ☑7ᵗʰ **T36.1X5**   Adverse effect of cephalosporins and other beta-lactam antibiotics

     ☑7ᵗʰ **T36.1X6**   Underdosing of cephalosporins and other beta-lactam antibiotics

☑5ᵗʰ **T36.2**   **Poisoning by, adverse effect of and underdosing of chloramphenicol group**

   ☑6ᵗʰ **T36.2X**   **Poisoning by, adverse effect of and underdosing of chloramphenicol group**

     ☑7ᵗʰ **T36.2X1**   **Poisoning by chloramphenicol group, accidental (unintentional)**
         Poisoning by chloramphenicol group NOS

    7 ☑7ᵗʰ **T36.2X2**   **Poisoning by chloramphenicol group, intentional self-harm**   HCC

     ☑7ᵗʰ **T36.2X3**   **Poisoning by chloramphenicol group, assault**

     ☑7ᵗʰ **T36.2X4**   **Poisoning by chloramphenicol group, undetermined**

     ☑7ᵗʰ **T36.2X5**   Adverse effect of chloramphenicol group

     ☑7ᵗʰ **T36.2X6**   Underdosing of chloramphenicol group

☑5ᵗʰ **T36.3**   **Poisoning by, adverse effect of and underdosing of macrolides**

   ☑6ᵗʰ **T36.3X**   **Poisoning by, adverse effect of and underdosing of macrolides**

     ☑7ᵗʰ **T36.3X1**   **Poisoning by macrolides, accidental (unintentional)**
         Poisoning by macrolides NOS

    7 ☑7ᵗʰ **T36.3X2**   **Poisoning by macrolides, intentional self-harm**   HCC

     ☑7ᵗʰ **T36.3X3**   **Poisoning by macrolides, assault**

     ☑7ᵗʰ **T36.3X4**   **Poisoning by macrolides, undetermined**

     ☑7ᵗʰ **T36.3X5**   Adverse effect of macrolides

     ☑7ᵗʰ **T36.3X6**   Underdosing of macrolides

☑5ᵗʰ **T36.4**   **Poisoning by, adverse effect of and underdosing of tetracyclines**

   ☑6ᵗʰ **T36.4X**   **Poisoning by, adverse effect of and underdosing of tetracyclines**

     ☑7ᵗʰ **T36.4X1**   **Poisoning by tetracyclines, accidental (unintentional)**
         Poisoning by tetracyclines NOS

    7 ☑7ᵗʰ **T36.4X2**   **Poisoning by tetracyclines, intentional self-harm**   HCC

     ☑7ᵗʰ **T36.4X3**   **Poisoning by tetracyclines, assault**

     ☑7ᵗʰ **T36.4X4**   **Poisoning by tetracyclines, undetermined**

     ☑7ᵗʰ **T36.4X5**   Adverse effect of tetracyclines

     ☑7ᵗʰ **T36.4X6**   Underdosing of tetracyclines

☑5ᵗʰ **T36.5**   **Poisoning by, adverse effect of and underdosing of aminoglycosides**
     Poisoning by, adverse effect of and underdosing of streptomycin

   ☑6ᵗʰ **T36.5X**   **Poisoning by, adverse effect of and underdosing of aminoglycosides**

     ☑7ᵗʰ **T36.5X1**   **Poisoning by aminoglycosides, accidental (unintentional)**
         Poisoning by aminoglycosides NOS

    7 ☑7ᵗʰ **T36.5X2**   **Poisoning by aminoglycosides, intentional self-harm**   HCC

     ☑7ᵗʰ **T36.5X3**   **Poisoning by aminoglycosides, assault**

     ☑7ᵗʰ **T36.5X4**   **Poisoning by aminoglycosides, undetermined**

     ☑7ᵗʰ **T36.5X5**   Adverse effect of aminoglycosides

     ☑7ᵗʰ **T36.5X6**   Underdosing of aminoglycosides

☑5ᵗʰ **T36.6**   **Poisoning by, adverse effect of and underdosing of rifampicins**

   ☑6ᵗʰ **T36.6X**   **Poisoning by, adverse effect of and underdosing of rifampicins**

     ☑7ᵗʰ **T36.6X1**   **Poisoning by rifampicins, accidental (unintentional)**
         Poisoning by rifampicins NOS

    7 ☑7ᵗʰ **T36.6X2**   **Poisoning by rifampicins, intentional self-harm**   HCC

     ☑7ᵗʰ **T36.6X3**   **Poisoning by rifampicins, assault**

     ☑7ᵗʰ **T36.6X4**   **Poisoning by rifampicins, undetermined**

     ☑7ᵗʰ **T36.6X5**   Adverse effect of rifampicins

     ☑7ᵗʰ **T36.6X6**   Underdosing of rifampicins

☑5ᵗʰ **T36.7**   **Poisoning by, adverse effect of and underdosing of antifungal antibiotics, systemically used**

   ☑6ᵗʰ **T36.7X**   **Poisoning by, adverse effect of and underdosing of antifungal antibiotics, systemically used**

     ☑7ᵗʰ **T36.7X1**   **Poisoning by antifungal antibiotics, systemically used, accidental (unintentional)**
         Poisoning by antifungal antibiotics, systemically used NOS

    7 ☑7ᵗʰ **T36.7X2**   **Poisoning by antifungal antibiotics, systemically used, intentional self-harm**   HCC

     ☑7ᵗʰ **T36.7X3**   **Poisoning by antifungal antibiotics, systemically used, assault**

     ☑7ᵗʰ **T36.7X4**   **Poisoning by antifungal antibiotics, systemically used, undetermined**

☑ Additional Character Required   ☑x7ᵗʰ Placeholder   Unacceptable PDx   Questionable PDx   Manifestation   Unspecified Dx   H1-H4 HAC   HCC CMS-HCC Dx   HIV HIV Dx

✓7th **T36.7X5** Adverse effect of antifungal antibiotics, systemically used

✓7th **T36.7X6** Underdosing of antifungal antibiotics, systemically used

✓5th **T36.8** Poisoning by, adverse effect of and underdosing of other systemic antibiotics

  ✓6th **T36.8X** Poisoning by, adverse effect of and underdosing of other systemic antibiotics
    AHA: 2017,1Q,39

    ✓7th **T36.8X1** Poisoning by other systemic antibiotics, accidental (unintentional)
        Poisoning by other systemic antibiotics NOS

    7 ✓7th **T36.8X2** Poisoning by other systemic antibiotics, intentional self-harm   HCC

    ✓7th **T36.8X3** Poisoning by other systemic antibiotics, assault

    ✓7th **T36.8X4** Poisoning by other systemic antibiotics, undetermined

    ✓7th **T36.8X5** Adverse effect of other systemic antibiotics

    ✓7th **T36.8X6** Underdosing of other systemic antibiotics

✓5th **T36.9** Poisoning by, adverse effect of and underdosing of unspecified systemic antibiotic

  ✓x7th **T36.91** Poisoning by unspecified systemic antibiotic, accidental (unintentional)
    Poisoning by systemic antibiotic NOS

  7 ✓x7th **T36.92** Poisoning by unspecified systemic antibiotic, intentional self-harm   HCC

  ✓x7th **T36.93** Poisoning by unspecified systemic antibiotic, assault

  ✓x7th **T36.94** Poisoning by unspecified systemic antibiotic, undetermined

  ✓x7th **T36.95** Adverse effect of unspecified systemic antibiotic

  ✓x7th **T36.96** Underdosing of unspecified systemic antibiotic

✓4th **T37** Poisoning by, adverse effect of and underdosing of other systemic anti-infectives and antiparasitics

  EXCLUDES 1   anti-infectives topically used for ear, nose and throat (T49.6-)
           anti-infectives topically used for eye (T49.5-)
           locally applied anti-infectives NEC (T49.Ø-)

The appropriate 7th character is to be added to each code from category T37.
A   initial encounter
D   subsequent encounter
S   sequela

✓5th **T37.Ø** Poisoning by, adverse effect of and underdosing of sulfonamides

  ✓6th **T37.ØX** Poisoning by, adverse effect of and underdosing of sulfonamides

    ✓7th **T37.ØX1** Poisoning by sulfonamides, accidental (unintentional)
        Poisoning by sulfonamides NOS

    7 ✓7th **T37.ØX2** Poisoning by sulfonamides, intentional self-harm   HCC

    ✓7th **T37.ØX3** Poisoning by sulfonamides, assault

    ✓7th **T37.ØX4** Poisoning by sulfonamides, undetermined

    ✓7th **T37.ØX5** Adverse effect of sulfonamides

    ✓7th **T37.ØX6** Underdosing of sulfonamides

✓5th **T37.1** Poisoning by, adverse effect of and underdosing of antimycobacterial drugs

  EXCLUDES 1   rifampicins (T36.6-)
           streptomycin (T36.5-)

  ✓6th **T37.1X** Poisoning by, adverse effect of and underdosing of antimycobacterial drugs

    ✓7th **T37.1X1** Poisoning by antimycobacterial drugs, accidental (unintentional)
        Poisoning by antimycobacterial drugs NOS

    7 ✓7th **T37.1X2** Poisoning by antimycobacterial drugs, intentional self-harm   HCC

    ✓7th **T37.1X3** Poisoning by antimycobacterial drugs, assault

    ✓7th **T37.1X4** Poisoning by antimycobacterial drugs, undetermined

    ✓7th **T37.1X5** Adverse effect of antimycobacterial drugs

    ✓7th **T37.1X6** Underdosing of antimycobacterial drugs

✓5th **T37.2** Poisoning by, adverse effect of and underdosing of antimalarials and drugs acting on other blood protozoa

  EXCLUDES 1   hydroxyquinoline derivatives (T37.8-)

  ✓6th **T37.2X** Poisoning by, adverse effect of and underdosing of antimalarials and drugs acting on other blood protozoa

    ✓7th **T37.2X1** Poisoning by antimalarials and drugs acting on other blood protozoa, accidental (unintentional)
        Poisoning by antimalarials and drugs acting on other blood protozoa NOS

    7 ✓7th **T37.2X2** Poisoning by antimalarials and drugs acting on other blood protozoa, intentional self-harm   HCC

    ✓7th **T37.2X3** Poisoning by antimalarials and drugs acting on other blood protozoa, assault

    ✓7th **T37.2X4** Poisoning by antimalarials and drugs acting on other blood protozoa, undetermined

    ✓7th **T37.2X5** Adverse effect of antimalarials and drugs acting on other blood protozoa

    ✓7th **T37.2X6** Underdosing of antimalarials and drugs acting on other blood protozoa

✓5th **T37.3** Poisoning by, adverse effect of and underdosing of other antiprotozoal drugs

  ✓6th **T37.3X** Poisoning by, adverse effect of and underdosing of other antiprotozoal drugs

    ✓7th **T37.3X1** Poisoning by other antiprotozoal drugs, accidental (unintentional)
        Poisoning by other antiprotozoal drugs NOS

    7 ✓7th **T37.3X2** Poisoning by other antiprotozoal drugs, intentional self-harm   HCC

    ✓7th **T37.3X3** Poisoning by other antiprotozoal drugs, assault

    ✓7th **T37.3X4** Poisoning by other antiprotozoal drugs, undetermined

    ✓7th **T37.3X5** Adverse effect of other antiprotozoal drugs

    ✓7th **T37.3X6** Underdosing of other antiprotozoal drugs

✓5th **T37.4** Poisoning by, adverse effect of and underdosing of anthelminthics

  ✓6th **T37.4X** Poisoning by, adverse effect of and underdosing of anthelminthics

    ✓7th **T37.4X1** Poisoning by anthelminthics, accidental (unintentional)
        Poisoning by anthelminthics NOS

    7 ✓7th **T37.4X2** Poisoning by anthelminthics, intentional self-harm   HCC

    ✓7th **T37.4X3** Poisoning by anthelminthics, assault

    ✓7th **T37.4X4** Poisoning by anthelminthics, undetermined

    ✓7th **T37.4X5** Adverse effect of anthelminthics

    ✓7th **T37.4X6** Underdosing of anthelminthics

✓5th **T37.5** Poisoning by, adverse effect of and underdosing of antiviral drugs

  EXCLUDES 1   amantadine (T42.8-)
           cytarabine (T45.1-)

  ✓6th **T37.5X** Poisoning by, adverse effect of and underdosing of antiviral drugs

    ✓7th **T37.5X1** Poisoning by antiviral drugs, accidental (unintentional)
        Poisoning by antiviral drugs NOS

    7 ✓7th **T37.5X2** Poisoning by antiviral drugs, intentional self-harm   HCC

    ✓7th **T37.5X3** Poisoning by antiviral drugs, assault

    ✓7th **T37.5X4** Poisoning by antiviral drugs, undetermined

    ✓7th **T37.5X5** Adverse effect of antiviral drugs

    ✓7th **T37.5X6** Underdosing of antiviral drugs

√5ᵗʰ **T37.8 Poisoning by, adverse effect of and underdosing of other specified systemic anti-infectives and antiparasitics**
Poisoning by, adverse effect of and underdosing of hydroxyquinoline derivatives
EXCLUDES 1   antimalarial drugs (T37.2-)

√6ᵗʰ **T37.8X Poisoning by, adverse effect of and underdosing of other specified systemic anti-infectives and antiparasitics**

√7ᵗʰ **T37.8X1 Poisoning by other specified systemic anti-infectives and antiparasitics, accidental (unintentional)**
Poisoning by other specified systemic anti-infectives and antiparasitics NOS

⁷ √7ᵗʰ **T37.8X2 Poisoning by other specified systemic anti-infectives and antiparasitics, intentional self-harm**   HCC

√7ᵗʰ **T37.8X3 Poisoning by other specified systemic anti-infectives and antiparasitics, assault**

√7ᵗʰ **T37.8X4 Poisoning by other specified systemic anti-infectives and antiparasitics, undetermined**

√7ᵗʰ **T37.8X5 Adverse effect of other specified systemic anti-infectives and antiparasitics**

√7ᵗʰ **T37.8X6 Underdosing of other specified systemic anti-infectives and antiparasitics**

√5ᵗʰ **T37.9 Poisoning by, adverse effect of and underdosing of unspecified systemic anti-infective and antiparasitics**

√x7ᵗʰ **T37.91 Poisoning by unspecified systemic anti-infective and antiparasitics, accidental (unintentional)**
Poisoning by, adverse effect of and underdosing of systemic anti-infective and antiparasitics NOS

⁷ √x7ᵗʰ **T37.92 Poisoning by unspecified systemic anti-infective and antiparasitics, intentional self-harm**   HCC

√x7ᵗʰ **T37.93 Poisoning by unspecified systemic anti-infective and antiparasitics, assault**

√x7ᵗʰ **T37.94 Poisoning by unspecified systemic anti-infective and antiparasitics, undetermined**

√x7ᵗʰ **T37.95 Adverse effect of unspecified systemic anti-infective and antiparasitic**

√x7ᵗʰ **T37.96 Underdosing of unspecified systemic anti-infectives and antiparasitics**

√4ᵗʰ **T38 Poisoning by, adverse effect of and underdosing of hormones and their synthetic substitutes and antagonists, not elsewhere classified**
EXCLUDES 1   mineralocorticoids and their antagonists (T50.0-)
     oxytocic hormones (T48.0-)
     parathyroid hormones and derivatives (T50.9-)

The appropriate 7th character is to be added to each code from category T38.
A   initial encounter
D   subsequent encounter
S   sequela

√5ᵗʰ **T38.0 Poisoning by, adverse effect of and underdosing of glucocorticoids and synthetic analogues**
EXCLUDES 1   glucocorticoids, topically used (T49.-)

√6ᵗʰ **T38.0X Poisoning by, adverse effect of and underdosing of glucocorticoids and synthetic analogues**

√7ᵗʰ **T38.0X1 Poisoning by glucocorticoids and synthetic analogues, accidental (unintentional)**
Poisoning by glucocorticoids and synthetic analogues NOS

⁷ √7ᵗʰ **T38.0X2 Poisoning by glucocorticoids and synthetic analogues, intentional self-harm**   HCC

√7ᵗʰ **T38.0X3 Poisoning by glucocorticoids and synthetic analogues, assault**

√7ᵗʰ **T38.0X4 Poisoning by glucocorticoids and synthetic analogues, undetermined**

√7ᵗʰ **T38.0X5 Adverse effect of glucocorticoids and synthetic analogues**

√7ᵗʰ **T38.0X6 Underdosing of glucocorticoids and synthetic analogues**

√5ᵗʰ **T38.1 Poisoning by, adverse effect of and underdosing of thyroid hormones and substitutes**

√6ᵗʰ **T38.1X Poisoning by, adverse effect of and underdosing of thyroid hormones and substitutes**

√7ᵗʰ **T38.1X1 Poisoning by thyroid hormones and substitutes, accidental (unintentional)**
Poisoning by thyroid hormones and substitutes NOS

⁷ √7ᵗʰ **T38.1X2 Poisoning by thyroid hormones and substitutes, intentional self-harm**   HCC

√7ᵗʰ **T38.1X3 Poisoning by thyroid hormones and substitutes, assault**

√7ᵗʰ **T38.1X4 Poisoning by thyroid hormones and substitutes, undetermined**

√7ᵗʰ **T38.1X5 Adverse effect of thyroid hormones and substitutes**

√7ᵗʰ **T38.1X6 Underdosing of thyroid hormones and substitutes**

√5ᵗʰ **T38.2 Poisoning by, adverse effect of and underdosing of antithyroid drugs**

√6ᵗʰ **T38.2X Poisoning by, adverse effect of and underdosing of antithyroid drugs**

√7ᵗʰ **T38.2X1 Poisoning by antithyroid drugs, accidental (unintentional)**
Poisoning by antithyroid drugs NOS

⁷ √7ᵗʰ **T38.2X2 Poisoning by antithyroid drugs, intentional self-harm**   HCC

√7ᵗʰ **T38.2X3 Poisoning by antithyroid drugs, assault**

√7ᵗʰ **T38.2X4 Poisoning by antithyroid drugs, undetermined**

√7ᵗʰ **T38.2X5 Adverse effect of antithyroid drugs**

√7ᵗʰ **T38.2X6 Underdosing of antithyroid drugs**

√5ᵗʰ **T38.3 Poisoning by, adverse effect of and underdosing of insulin and oral hypoglycemic [antidiabetic] drugs**

√6ᵗʰ **T38.3X Poisoning by, adverse effect of and underdosing of insulin and oral hypoglycemic [antidiabetic] drugs**

√7ᵗʰ **T38.3X1 Poisoning by insulin and oral hypoglycemic [antidiabetic] drugs, accidental (unintentional)**
Poisoning by insulin and oral hypoglycemic [antidiabetic] drugs NOS

⁷ √7ᵗʰ **T38.3X2 Poisoning by insulin and oral hypoglycemic [antidiabetic] drugs, intentional self-harm**   HCC

√7ᵗʰ **T38.3X3 Poisoning by insulin and oral hypoglycemic [antidiabetic] drugs, assault**

√7ᵗʰ **T38.3X4 Poisoning by insulin and oral hypoglycemic [antidiabetic] drugs, undetermined**

√7ᵗʰ **T38.3X5 Adverse effect of insulin and oral hypoglycemic [antidiabetic] drugs**

√7ᵗʰ **T38.3X6 Underdosing of insulin and oral hypoglycemic [antidiabetic] drugs**

√5ᵗʰ **T38.4 Poisoning by, adverse effect of and underdosing of oral contraceptives**
Poisoning by, adverse effect of and underdosing of multiple- and single-ingredient oral contraceptive preparations

√6ᵗʰ **T38.4X Poisoning by, adverse effect of and underdosing of oral contraceptives**

√7ᵗʰ **T38.4X1 Poisoning by oral contraceptives, accidental (unintentional)**
Poisoning by oral contraceptives NOS

⁷ √7ᵗʰ **T38.4X2 Poisoning by oral contraceptives, intentional self-harm**   HCC

√7ᵗʰ **T38.4X3 Poisoning by oral contraceptives, assault**

√7ᵗʰ **T38.4X4 Poisoning by oral contraceptives, undetermined**

√7ᵗʰ **T38.4X5 Adverse effect of oral contraceptives**

√7ᵗʰ **T38.4X6 Underdosing of oral contraceptives**

✓5ᵗʰ **T38.5** **Poisoning by, adverse effect of and underdosing of other estrogens and progestogens**
　　　Poisoning by, adverse effect of and underdosing of estrogens and progestogens mixtures and substitutes

　　✓6ᵗʰ **T38.5X** **Poisoning by, adverse effect of and underdosing of other estrogens and progestogens**

　　　　✓7ᵗʰ **T38.5X1** **Poisoning by other estrogens and progestogens, accidental (unintentional)**
　　　　　　Poisoning by other estrogens and progestogens NOS

　　　　7 ✓7ᵗʰ **T38.5X2** **Poisoning by other estrogens and progestogens, intentional self-harm**　　HCC

　　　　✓7ᵗʰ **T38.5X3** **Poisoning by other estrogens and progestogens, assault**

　　　　✓7ᵗʰ **T38.5X4** **Poisoning by other estrogens and progestogens, undetermined**

　　　　✓7ᵗʰ **T38.5X5** **Adverse effect of other estrogens and progestogens**

　　　　✓7ᵗʰ **T38.5X6** **Underdosing of other estrogens and progestogens**

✓5ᵗʰ **T38.6** **Poisoning by, adverse effect of and underdosing of antigonadotrophins, antiestrogens, antiandrogens, not elsewhere classified**
　　　Poisoning by, adverse effect of and underdosing of tamoxifen

　　✓6ᵗʰ **T38.6X** **Poisoning by, adverse effect of and underdosing of antigonadotrophins, antiestrogens, antiandrogens, not elsewhere classified**

　　　　✓7ᵗʰ **T38.6X1** **Poisoning by antigonadotrophins, antiestrogens, antiandrogens, not elsewhere classified, accidental (unintentional)**
　　　　　　Poisoning by antigonadotrophins, antiestrogens, antiandrogens, not elsewhere classified NOS

　　　　7 ✓7ᵗʰ **T38.6X2** **Poisoning by antigonadotrophins, antiestrogens, antiandrogens, not elsewhere classified, intentional self-harm**　　HCC

　　　　✓7ᵗʰ **T38.6X3** **Poisoning by antigonadotrophins, antiestrogens, antiandrogens, not elsewhere classified, assault**

　　　　✓7ᵗʰ **T38.6X4** **Poisoning by antigonadotrophins, antiestrogens, antiandrogens, not elsewhere classified, undetermined**

　　　　✓7ᵗʰ **T38.6X5** **Adverse effect of antigonadotrophins, antiestrogens, antiandrogens, not elsewhere classified**

　　　　✓7ᵗʰ **T38.6X6** **Underdosing of antigonadotrophins, antiestrogens, antiandrogens, not elsewhere classified**

✓5ᵗʰ **T38.7** **Poisoning by, adverse effect of and underdosing of androgens and anabolic congeners**

　　✓6ᵗʰ **T38.7X** **Poisoning by, adverse effect of and underdosing of androgens and anabolic congeners**

　　　　✓7ᵗʰ **T38.7X1** **Poisoning by androgens and anabolic congeners, accidental (unintentional)**
　　　　　　Poisoning by androgens and anabolic congeners NOS

　　　　7 ✓7ᵗʰ **T38.7X2** **Poisoning by androgens and anabolic congeners, intentional self-harm**　　HCC

　　　　✓7ᵗʰ **T38.7X3** **Poisoning by androgens and anabolic congeners, assault**

　　　　✓7ᵗʰ **T38.7X4** **Poisoning by androgens and anabolic congeners, undetermined**

　　　　✓7ᵗʰ **T38.7X5** **Adverse effect of androgens and anabolic congeners**

　　　　✓7ᵗʰ **T38.7X6** **Underdosing of androgens and anabolic congeners**

✓5ᵗʰ **T38.8** **Poisoning by, adverse effect of and underdosing of other and unspecified hormones and synthetic substitutes**

　　✓6ᵗʰ **T38.80** **Poisoning by, adverse effect of and underdosing of unspecified hormones and synthetic substitutes**

　　　　✓7ᵗʰ **T38.801** **Poisoning by unspecified hormones and synthetic substitutes, accidental (unintentional)**
　　　　　　Poisoning by unspecified hormones and synthetic substitutes NOS

　　　　7 ✓7ᵗʰ **T38.802** **Poisoning by unspecified hormones and synthetic substitutes, intentional self-harm**　　HCC

　　　　✓7ᵗʰ **T38.803** **Poisoning by unspecified hormones and synthetic substitutes, assault**

　　　　✓7ᵗʰ **T38.804** **Poisoning by unspecified hormones and synthetic substitutes, undetermined**

　　　　✓7ᵗʰ **T38.805** **Adverse effect of unspecified hormones and synthetic substitutes**

　　　　✓7ᵗʰ **T38.806** **Underdosing of unspecified hormones and synthetic substitutes**

　　✓6ᵗʰ **T38.81** **Poisoning by, adverse effect of and underdosing of anterior pituitary [adenohypophyseal] hormones**

　　　　✓7ᵗʰ **T38.811** **Poisoning by anterior pituitary [adenohypophyseal] hormones, accidental (unintentional)**
　　　　　　Poisoning by anterior pituitary [adenohypophyseal] hormones NOS

　　　　7 ✓7ᵗʰ **T38.812** **Poisoning by anterior pituitary [adenohypophyseal] hormones, intentional self-harm**　　HCC

　　　　✓7ᵗʰ **T38.813** **Poisoning by anterior pituitary [adenohypophyseal] hormones, assault**

　　　　✓7ᵗʰ **T38.814** **Poisoning by anterior pituitary [adenohypophyseal] hormones, undetermined**

　　　　✓7ᵗʰ **T38.815** **Adverse effect of anterior pituitary [adenohypophyseal] hormones**

　　　　✓7ᵗʰ **T38.816** **Underdosing of anterior pituitary [adenohypophyseal] hormones**

　　✓6ᵗʰ **T38.89** **Poisoning by, adverse effect of and underdosing of other hormones and synthetic substitutes**

　　　　✓7ᵗʰ **T38.891** **Poisoning by other hormones and synthetic substitutes, accidental (unintentional)**
　　　　　　Poisoning by other hormones and synthetic substitutes NOS

　　　　7 ✓7ᵗʰ **T38.892** **Poisoning by other hormones and synthetic substitutes, intentional self-harm**　　HCC

　　　　✓7ᵗʰ **T38.893** **Poisoning by other hormones and synthetic substitutes, assault**

　　　　✓7ᵗʰ **T38.894** **Poisoning by other hormones and synthetic substitutes, undetermined**

　　　　✓7ᵗʰ **T38.895** **Adverse effect of other hormones and synthetic substitutes**

　　　　✓7ᵗʰ **T38.896** **Underdosing of other hormones and synthetic substitutes**

✓5ᵗʰ **T38.9** **Poisoning by, adverse effect of and underdosing of other and unspecified hormone antagonists**

　　✓6ᵗʰ **T38.90** **Poisoning by, adverse effect of and underdosing of unspecified hormone antagonists**

　　　　✓7ᵗʰ **T38.901** **Poisoning by unspecified hormone antagonists, accidental (unintentional)**
　　　　　　Poisoning by unspecified hormone antagonists NOS

　　　　7 ✓7ᵗʰ **T38.902** **Poisoning by unspecified hormone antagonists, intentional self-harm**　　HCC

　　　　✓7ᵗʰ **T38.903** **Poisoning by unspecified hormone antagonists, assault**

　　　　✓7ᵗʰ **T38.904** **Poisoning by unspecified hormone antagonists, undetermined**

　　　　✓7ᵗʰ **T38.905** **Adverse effect of unspecified hormone antagonists**

　　　　✓7ᵗʰ **T38.906** **Underdosing of unspecified hormone antagonists**

　　✓6ᵗʰ **T38.99** **Poisoning by, adverse effect of and underdosing of other hormone antagonists**

　　　　✓7ᵗʰ **T38.991** **Poisoning by other hormone antagonists, accidental (unintentional)**
　　　　　　Poisoning by other hormone antagonists NOS

　　　　7 ✓7ᵗʰ **T38.992** **Poisoning by other hormone antagonists, intentional self-harm**　　HCC

　　　　✓7ᵗʰ **T38.993** **Poisoning by other hormone antagonists, assault**

　　　　✓7ᵗʰ **T38.994** **Poisoning by other hormone antagonists, undetermined**

　　　　✓7ᵗʰ **T38.995** **Adverse effect of other hormone antagonists**

　　　　✓7ᵗʰ **T38.996** **Underdosing of other hormone antagonists**

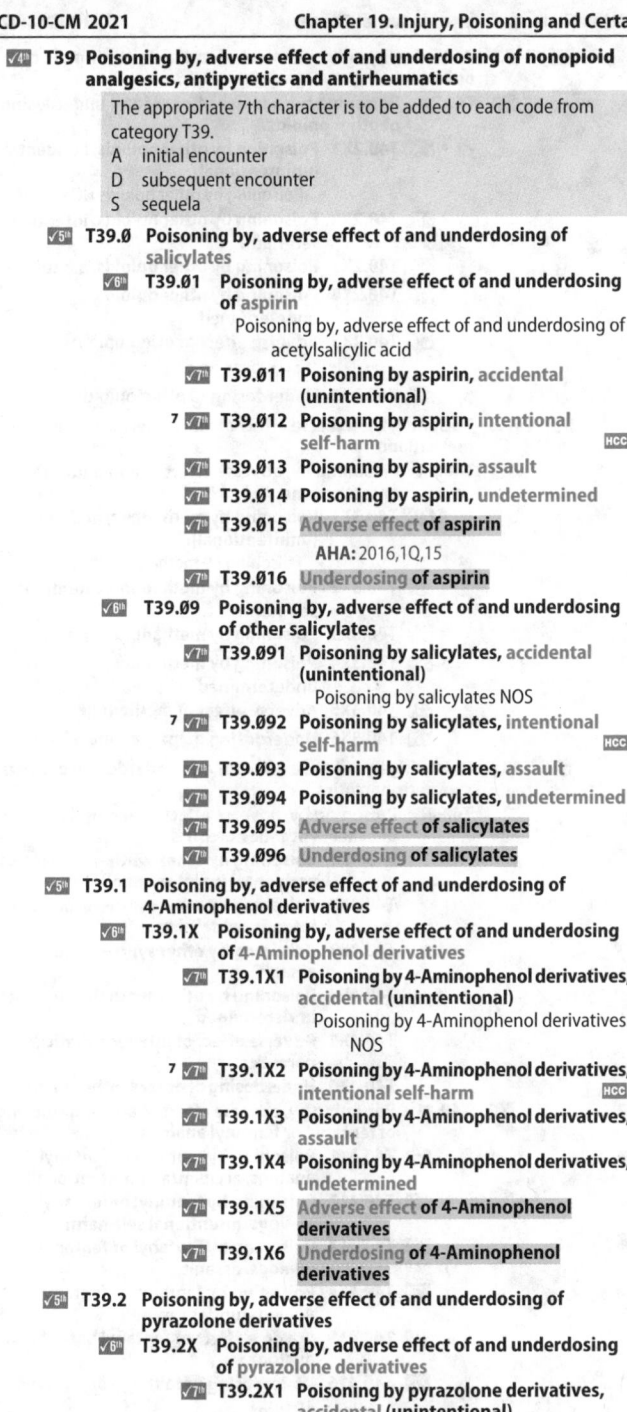

√4ᵗʰ **T39** **Poisoning by, adverse effect of and underdosing of nonopioid analgesics, antipyretics and antirheumatics**

> The appropriate 7th character is to be added to each code from category T39.
> A   initial encounter
> D   subsequent encounter
> S   sequela

√5ᵗʰ **T39.0** **Poisoning by, adverse effect of and underdosing of salicylates**

   √6ᵗʰ **T39.01** **Poisoning by, adverse effect of and underdosing of aspirin**

     Poisoning by, adverse effect of and underdosing of acetylsalicylic acid

     √7ᵗʰ **T39.011** **Poisoning by aspirin, accidental (unintentional)**

     7 √7ᵗʰ **T39.012** **Poisoning by aspirin, intentional self-harm** HCC

     √7ᵗʰ **T39.013** **Poisoning by aspirin, assault**

     √7ᵗʰ **T39.014** **Poisoning by aspirin, undetermined**

     √7ᵗʰ **T39.015** Adverse effect **of aspirin**

       AHA: 2016,1Q,15

     √7ᵗʰ **T39.016** Underdosing **of aspirin**

   √6ᵗʰ **T39.09** **Poisoning by, adverse effect of and underdosing of other salicylates**

     √7ᵗʰ **T39.091** **Poisoning by salicylates, accidental (unintentional)**

       Poisoning by salicylates NOS

     7 √7ᵗʰ **T39.092** **Poisoning by salicylates, intentional self-harm** HCC

     √7ᵗʰ **T39.093** **Poisoning by salicylates, assault**

     √7ᵗʰ **T39.094** **Poisoning by salicylates, undetermined**

     √7ᵗʰ **T39.095** Adverse effect **of salicylates**

     √7ᵗʰ **T39.096** Underdosing **of salicylates**

√5ᵗʰ **T39.1** **Poisoning by, adverse effect of and underdosing of 4-Aminophenol derivatives**

   √6ᵗʰ **T39.1X** **Poisoning by, adverse effect of and underdosing of 4-Aminophenol derivatives**

     √7ᵗʰ **T39.1X1** **Poisoning by 4-Aminophenol derivatives, accidental (unintentional)**

       Poisoning by 4-Aminophenol derivatives NOS

     7 √7ᵗʰ **T39.1X2** **Poisoning by 4-Aminophenol derivatives, intentional self-harm** HCC

     √7ᵗʰ **T39.1X3** **Poisoning by 4-Aminophenol derivatives, assault**

     √7ᵗʰ **T39.1X4** **Poisoning by 4-Aminophenol derivatives, undetermined**

     √7ᵗʰ **T39.1X5** Adverse effect **of 4-Aminophenol derivatives**

     √7ᵗʰ **T39.1X6** Underdosing **of 4-Aminophenol derivatives**

√5ᵗʰ **T39.2** **Poisoning by, adverse effect of and underdosing of pyrazolone derivatives**

   √6ᵗʰ **T39.2X** **Poisoning by, adverse effect of and underdosing of pyrazolone derivatives**

     √7ᵗʰ **T39.2X1** **Poisoning by pyrazolone derivatives, accidental (unintentional)**

       Poisoning by pyrazolone derivatives NOS

     7 √7ᵗʰ **T39.2X2** **Poisoning by pyrazolone derivatives, intentional self-harm** HCC

     √7ᵗʰ **T39.2X3** **Poisoning by pyrazolone derivatives, assault**

     √7ᵗʰ **T39.2X4** **Poisoning by pyrazolone derivatives, undetermined**

     √7ᵗʰ **T39.2X5** Adverse effect **of pyrazolone derivatives**

     √7ᵗʰ **T39.2X6** Underdosing **of pyrazolone derivatives**

√5ᵗʰ **T39.3** **Poisoning by, adverse effect of and underdosing of other nonsteroidal anti-inflammatory drugs [NSAID]**

   √6ᵗʰ **T39.31** **Poisoning by, adverse effect of and underdosing of propionic acid derivatives**

     Poisoning by, adverse effect of and underdosing of fenoprofen

     Poisoning by, adverse effect of and underdosing of flurbiprofen

     Poisoning by, adverse effect of and underdosing of ibuprofen

     Poisoning by, adverse effect of and underdosing of ketoprofen

     Poisoning by, adverse effect of and underdosing of naproxen

     Poisoning by, adverse effect of and underdosing of oxaprozin

     √7ᵗʰ **T39.311** **Poisoning by propionic acid derivatives, accidental (unintentional)**

     7 √7ᵗʰ **T39.312** **Poisoning by propionic acid derivatives, intentional self-harm** HCC

     √7ᵗʰ **T39.313** **Poisoning by propionic acid derivatives, assault**

     √7ᵗʰ **T39.314** **Poisoning by propionic acid derivatives, undetermined**

     √7ᵗʰ **T39.315** Adverse effect **of propionic acid derivatives**

     √7ᵗʰ **T39.316** Underdosing **of propionic acid derivatives**

   √6ᵗʰ **T39.39** **Poisoning by, adverse effect of and underdosing of other nonsteroidal anti-inflammatory drugs [NSAID]**

     √7ᵗʰ **T39.391** **Poisoning by other nonsteroidal anti-inflammatory drugs [NSAID], accidental (unintentional)**

       Poisoning by other nonsteroidal anti-inflammatory drugs NOS

     7 √7ᵗʰ **T39.392** **Poisoning by other nonsteroidal anti-inflammatory drugs [NSAID], intentional self-harm** HCC

     √7ᵗʰ **T39.393** **Poisoning by other nonsteroidal anti-inflammatory drugs [NSAID], assault**

     √7ᵗʰ **T39.394** **Poisoning by other nonsteroidal anti-inflammatory drugs [NSAID], undetermined**

     √7ᵗʰ **T39.395** Adverse effect **of other nonsteroidal anti-inflammatory drugs [NSAID]**

     √7ᵗʰ **T39.396** Underdosing **of other nonsteroidal anti-inflammatory drugs [NSAID]**

√5ᵗʰ **T39.4** **Poisoning by, adverse effect of and underdosing of antirheumatics, not elsewhere classified**

   EXCLUDES 1   *poisoning by, adverse effect of and underdosing of glucocorticoids (T38.0-)*
       poisoning by, adverse effect of and underdosing of salicylates (T39.0-)

   √6ᵗʰ **T39.4X** **Poisoning by, adverse effect of and underdosing of antirheumatics, not elsewhere classified**

     √7ᵗʰ **T39.4X1** **Poisoning by antirheumatics, not elsewhere classified, accidental (unintentional)**

       Poisoning by antirheumatics, not elsewhere classified NOS

     7 √7ᵗʰ **T39.4X2** **Poisoning by antirheumatics, not elsewhere classified, intentional self-harm** HCC

     √7ᵗʰ **T39.4X3** **Poisoning by antirheumatics, not elsewhere classified, assault**

     √7ᵗʰ **T39.4X4** **Poisoning by antirheumatics, not elsewhere classified, undetermined**

     √7ᵗʰ **T39.4X5** Adverse effect **of antirheumatics, not elsewhere classified**

     √7ᵗʰ **T39.4X6** Underdosing **of antirheumatics, not elsewhere classified**

√5ᵗʰ **T39.8 Poisoning by, adverse effect of and underdosing of other nonopioid analgesics and antipyretics, not elsewhere classified**

　√6ᵗʰ **T39.8X Poisoning by, adverse effect of and underdosing of other nonopioid analgesics and antipyretics, not elsewhere classified**

　　√7ᵗʰ **T39.8X1 Poisoning by other nonopioid analgesics and antipyretics, not elsewhere classified, accidental (unintentional)**
　　　　Poisoning by other nonopioid analgesics and antipyretics, not elsewhere classified NOS

　　7 √7ᵗʰ **T39.8X2 Poisoning by other nonopioid analgesics and antipyretics, not elsewhere classified, intentional self-harm** `HCC`

　　√7ᵗʰ **T39.8X3 Poisoning by other nonopioid analgesics and antipyretics, not elsewhere classified, assault**

　　√7ᵗʰ **T39.8X4 Poisoning by other nonopioid analgesics and antipyretics, not elsewhere classified, undetermined**

　　√7ᵗʰ **T39.8X5 Adverse effect of other nonopioid analgesics and antipyretics, not elsewhere classified**

　　√7ᵗʰ **T39.8X6 Underdosing of other nonopioid analgesics and antipyretics, not elsewhere classified**

√5ᵗʰ **T39.9 Poisoning by, adverse effect of and underdosing of unspecified nonopioid analgesic, antipyretic and antirheumatic**

　√x7ᵗʰ **T39.91 Poisoning by unspecified nonopioid analgesic, antipyretic and antirheumatic, accidental (unintentional)**
　　　Poisoning by nonopioid analgesic, antipyretic and antirheumatic NOS

　7 √x7ᵗʰ **T39.92 Poisoning by unspecified nonopioid analgesic, antipyretic and antirheumatic, intentional self-harm** `HCC`

　√x7ᵗʰ **T39.93 Poisoning by unspecified nonopioid analgesic, antipyretic and antirheumatic, assault**

　√x7ᵗʰ **T39.94 Poisoning by unspecified nonopioid analgesic, antipyretic and antirheumatic, undetermined**

　√x7ᵗʰ **T39.95 Adverse effect of unspecified nonopioid analgesic, antipyretic and antirheumatic**

　√x7ᵗʰ **T39.96 Underdosing of unspecified nonopioid analgesic, antipyretic and antirheumatic**

√4ᵗʰ **T40 Poisoning by, adverse effect of and underdosing of narcotics and psychodysleptics [hallucinogens]**

　`EXCLUDES 2` drug dependence and related mental and behavioral disorders due to psychoactive substance use (F10.-F19.-)

　The appropriate 7th character is to be added to each code from category T40.
　A initial encounter
　D subsequent encounter
　S sequela

√5ᵗʰ **T40.0 Poisoning by, adverse effect of and underdosing of opium**

　√6ᵗʰ **T40.0X Poisoning by, adverse effect of and underdosing of opium**

　　6 √7ᵗʰ **T40.0X1 Poisoning by opium, accidental (unintentional)** `HCC`
　　　　Poisoning by opium NOS

　　7 √7ᵗʰ **T40.0X2 Poisoning by opium, intentional self-harm** `HCC`

　　√7ᵗʰ **T40.0X3 Poisoning by opium, assault**

　　6 √7ᵗʰ **T40.0X4 Poisoning by opium, undetermined** `HCC`

　　√7ᵗʰ **T40.0X5 Adverse effect of opium**

　　√7ᵗʰ **T40.0X6 Underdosing of opium**

√5ᵗʰ **T40.1 Poisoning by and adverse effect of heroin**

　√6ᵗʰ **T40.1X Poisoning by and adverse effect of heroin**

　　6 √7ᵗʰ **T40.1X1 Poisoning by heroin, accidental (unintentional)** `HCC`
　　　　Poisoning by heroin NOS

　　7 √7ᵗʰ **T40.1X2 Poisoning by heroin, intentional self-harm** `HCC`

　　√7ᵗʰ **T40.1X3 Poisoning by heroin, assault**

　　6 √7ᵗʰ **T40.1X4 Poisoning by heroin, undetermined** `HCC`

√5ᵗʰ **T40.2 Poisoning by, adverse effect of and underdosing of other opioids**

　√6ᵗʰ **T40.2X Poisoning by, adverse effect of and underdosing of other opioids**

　　6 √7ᵗʰ **T40.2X1 Poisoning by other opioids, accidental (unintentional)** `HCC`
　　　　Poisoning by other opioids NOS

　　7 √7ᵗʰ **T40.2X2 Poisoning by other opioids, intentional self-harm** `HCC`

　　√7ᵗʰ **T40.2X3 Poisoning by other opioids, assault**

　　6 √7ᵗʰ **T40.2X4 Poisoning by other opioids, undetermined** `HCC`

　　√7ᵗʰ **T40.2X5 Adverse effect of other opioids**
　　　　AHA: 2020,2Q,24

　　√7ᵗʰ **T40.2X6 Underdosing of other opioids**

√5ᵗʰ **T40.3 Poisoning by, adverse effect of and underdosing of methadone**

　√6ᵗʰ **T40.3X Poisoning by, adverse effect of and underdosing of methadone**

　　6 √7ᵗʰ **T40.3X1 Poisoning by methadone, accidental (unintentional)** `HCC`
　　　　Poisoning by methadone NOS

　　7 √7ᵗʰ **T40.3X2 Poisoning by methadone, intentional self-harm** `HCC`

　　√7ᵗʰ **T40.3X3 Poisoning by methadone, assault**

　　6 √7ᵗʰ **T40.3X4 Poisoning by methadone, undetermined** `HCC`

　　√7ᵗʰ **T40.3X5 Adverse effect of methadone**

　　√7ᵗʰ **T40.3X6 Underdosing of methadone**

√5ᵗʰ **T40.4 Poisoning by, adverse effect of and underdosing of other synthetic narcotics**

　~~T40.4X Poisoning by, adverse effect of and underdosing of other synthetic narcotics~~

　　~~T40.4X1 Poisoning by other synthetic narcotics, accidental (unintentional)~~

　　~~T40.4X2 Poisoning by other synthetic narcotics, intentional self-harm~~

　　~~T40.4X3 Poisoning by other synthetic narcotics, assault~~

　　~~T40.4X4 Poisoning by other synthetic narcotics, undetermined~~

　　~~T40.4X5 Adverse effect of other synthetic narcotics~~

　　~~T40.4X6 Underdosing of other synthetic narcotics~~

　√6ᵗʰ **T40.41 Poisoning by, adverse effect of and underdosing of fentanyl or fentanyl analogs**

　　√7ᵗʰ **T40.411 Poisoning by fentanyl or fentanyl analogs, accidental (unintentional)**

　　√7ᵗʰ **T40.412 Poisoning by fentanyl or fentanyl analogs, intentional self-harm**

　　√7ᵗʰ **T40.413 Poisoning by fentanyl or fentanyl analogs, assault**

　　√7ᵗʰ **T40.414 Poisoning by fentanyl or fentanyl analogs, undetermined**

　　√7ᵗʰ **T40.415 Adverse effect of fentanyl or fentanyl analogs**

　　√7ᵗʰ **T40.416 Underdosing of fentanyl or fentanyl analogs**

　√6ᵗʰ **T40.42 Poisoning by, adverse effect of and underdosing of tramadol**

　　√7ᵗʰ **T40.421 Poisoning by tramadol, accidental (unintentional)**

　　√7ᵗʰ **T40.422 Poisoning by tramadol, intentional self-harm**

　　√7ᵗʰ **T40.423 Poisoning by tramadol, assault**

　　√7ᵗʰ **T40.424 Poisoning by tramadol, undetermined**

　　√7ᵗʰ **T40.425 Adverse effect of tramadol**

　　√7ᵗʰ **T40.426 Underdosing of tramadol**

　√6ᵗʰ **T40.49 Poisoning by, adverse effect of and underdosing of other synthetic narcotics**

　　√7ᵗʰ **T40.491 Poisoning by other synthetic narcotics, accidental (unintentional)**

　　√7ᵗʰ **T40.492 Poisoning by other synthetic narcotics, intentional self-harm**

　　√7ᵗʰ **T40.493 Poisoning by other synthetic narcotics, assault**

　　√7ᵗʰ **T40.494 Poisoning by other synthetic narcotics, undetermined**

　　√7ᵗʰ **T40.495 Adverse effect of other synthetic narcotics**

● ✓7ᵗʰ **T40.496** Underdosing of other synthetic narcotics

✓5ᵗʰ **T40.5** Poisoning by, adverse effect of and underdosing of cocaine

　✓6ᵗʰ **T40.5X** Poisoning by, adverse effect of and underdosing of cocaine

　　6 ✓7ᵗʰ **T40.5X1** Poisoning by cocaine, accidental (unintentional) HCC
　　　　Poisoning by cocaine NOS
　　　　AHA: 2016,2Q,8

　　7 ✓7ᵗʰ **T40.5X2** Poisoning by cocaine, intentional self-harm HCC

　　✓7ᵗʰ **T40.5X3** Poisoning by cocaine, assault

　　6 ✓7ᵗʰ **T40.5X4** Poisoning by cocaine, undetermined HCC

　　✓7ᵗʰ **T40.5X5** Adverse effect of cocaine

　　✓7ᵗʰ **T40.5X6** Underdosing of cocaine

✓5ᵗʰ **T40.6** Poisoning by, adverse effect of and underdosing of other and unspecified narcotics

　✓6ᵗʰ **T40.60** Poisoning by, adverse effect of and underdosing of unspecified narcotics

　　6 ✓7ᵗʰ **T40.601** Poisoning by unspecified narcotics, accidental (unintentional) HCC
　　　　Poisoning by narcotics NOS

　　7 ✓7ᵗʰ **T40.602** Poisoning by unspecified narcotics, intentional self-harm HCC

　　✓7ᵗʰ **T40.603** Poisoning by unspecified narcotics, assault

　　6 ✓7ᵗʰ **T40.604** Poisoning by unspecified narcotics, undetermined HCC

　　✓7ᵗʰ **T40.605** Adverse effect of unspecified narcotics

　　✓7ᵗʰ **T40.606** Underdosing of unspecified narcotics

　✓6ᵗʰ **T40.69** Poisoning by, adverse effect of and underdosing of other narcotics

　　6 ✓7ᵗʰ **T40.691** Poisoning by other narcotics, accidental (unintentional) HCC
　　　　Poisoning by other narcotics NOS

　　7 ✓7ᵗʰ **T40.692** Poisoning by other narcotics, intentional self-harm HCC

　　✓7ᵗʰ **T40.693** Poisoning by other narcotics, assault

　　6 ✓7ᵗʰ **T40.694** Poisoning by other narcotics, undetermined HCC

　　✓7ᵗʰ **T40.695** Adverse effect of other narcotics

　　✓7ᵗʰ **T40.696** Underdosing of other narcotics

✓5ᵗʰ **T40.7** Poisoning by, adverse effect of and underdosing of cannabis (derivatives)

　✓6ᵗʰ **T40.7X** Poisoning by, adverse effect of and underdosing of cannabis (derivatives)

　　✓7ᵗʰ **T40.7X1** Poisoning by cannabis (derivatives), accidental (unintentional)
　　　　Poisoning by cannabis NOS
　　　　AHA: 2020,1Q,8

　　7 ✓7ᵗʰ **T40.7X2** Poisoning by cannabis (derivatives), intentional self-harm HCC

　　✓7ᵗʰ **T40.7X3** Poisoning by cannabis (derivatives), assault

　　✓7ᵗʰ **T40.7X4** Poisoning by cannabis (derivatives), undetermined

　　✓7ᵗʰ **T40.7X5** Adverse effect of cannabis (derivatives)

　　✓7ᵗʰ **T40.7X6** Underdosing of cannabis (derivatives)

✓5ᵗʰ **T40.8** Poisoning by and adverse effect of lysergide [LSD]

　✓6ᵗʰ **T40.8X** Poisoning by and adverse effect of lysergide [LSD]

　　6 ✓7ᵗʰ **T40.8X1** Poisoning by lysergide [LSD], accidental (unintentional) HCC
　　　　Poisoning by lysergide [LSD] NOS

　　7 ✓7ᵗʰ **T40.8X2** Poisoning by lysergide [LSD], intentional self-harm HCC

　　✓7ᵗʰ **T40.8X3** Poisoning by lysergide [LSD], assault

　　6 ✓7ᵗʰ **T40.8X4** Poisoning by lysergide [LSD], undetermined HCC

✓5ᵗʰ **T40.9** Poisoning by, adverse effect of and underdosing of other and unspecified psychodysleptics [hallucinogens]

　✓6ᵗʰ **T40.90** Poisoning by, adverse effect of and underdosing of unspecified psychodysleptics [hallucinogens]

　　6 ✓7ᵗʰ **T40.901** Poisoning by unspecified psychodysleptics [hallucinogens], accidental (unintentional) HCC

　　7 ✓7ᵗʰ **T40.902** Poisoning by unspecified psychodysleptics [hallucinogens], intentional self-harm HCC

　　✓7ᵗʰ **T40.903** Poisoning by unspecified psychodysleptics [hallucinogens], assault

　　6 ✓7ᵗʰ **T40.904** Poisoning by unspecified psychodysleptics [hallucinogens], undetermined HCC

　　✓7ᵗʰ **T40.905** Adverse effect of unspecified psychodysleptics [hallucinogens]

　　✓7ᵗʰ **T40.906** Underdosing of unspecified psychodysleptics [hallucinogens]

　✓6ᵗʰ **T40.99** Poisoning by, adverse effect of and underdosing of other psychodysleptics [hallucinogens]

　　6 ✓7ᵗʰ **T40.991** Poisoning by other psychodysleptics [hallucinogens], accidental (unintentional) HCC
　　　　Poisoning by other psychodysleptics [hallucinogens] NOS

　　7 ✓7ᵗʰ **T40.992** Poisoning by other psychodysleptics [hallucinogens], intentional self-harm HCC

　　✓7ᵗʰ **T40.993** Poisoning by other psychodysleptics [hallucinogens], assault

　　6 ✓7ᵗʰ **T40.994** Poisoning by other psychodysleptics [hallucinogens], undetermined HCC

　　✓7ᵗʰ **T40.995** Adverse effect of other psychodysleptics [hallucinogens]

　　✓7ᵗʰ **T40.996** Underdosing of other psychodysleptics [hallucinogens]

✓4ᵗʰ **T41** Poisoning by, adverse effect of and underdosing of anesthetics and therapeutic gases

　EXCLUDES 1 benzodiazepines (T42.4-)
　　　　cocaine (T40.5-)
　　　　complications of anesthesia during labor and delivery (O74.-)
　　　　complications of anesthesia during pregnancy (O29.-)
　　　　complications of anesthesia during the puerperium (O89.-)
　　　　opioids (T40.0-T40.2-)

The appropriate 7th character is to be added to each code from category T41.
A　initial encounter
D　subsequent encounter
S　sequela

✓5ᵗʰ **T41.0** Poisoning by, adverse effect of and underdosing of inhaled anesthetics

　EXCLUDES 1 oxygen (T41.5-)

　✓6ᵗʰ **T41.0X** Poisoning by, adverse effect of and underdosing of inhaled anesthetics

　　✓7ᵗʰ **T41.0X1** Poisoning by inhaled anesthetics, accidental (unintentional)
　　　　Poisoning by inhaled anesthetics NOS

　　7 ✓7ᵗʰ **T41.0X2** Poisoning by inhaled anesthetics, intentional self-harm HCC

　　✓7ᵗʰ **T41.0X3** Poisoning by inhaled anesthetics, assault

　　✓7ᵗʰ **T41.0X4** Poisoning by inhaled anesthetics, undetermined

　　✓7ᵗʰ **T41.0X5** Adverse effect of inhaled anesthetics

　　✓7ᵗʰ **T41.0X6** Underdosing of inhaled anesthetics

✓5ᵗʰ **T41.1** Poisoning by, adverse effect of and underdosing of intravenous anesthetics

Poisoning by, adverse effect of and underdosing of thiobarbiturates

　✓6ᵗʰ **T41.1X** Poisoning by, adverse effect of and underdosing of intravenous anesthetics

　　✓7ᵗʰ **T41.1X1** Poisoning by intravenous anesthetics, accidental (unintentional)
　　　　Poisoning by intravenous anesthetics NOS

　　7 ✓7ᵗʰ **T41.1X2** Poisoning by intravenous anesthetics, intentional self-harm HCC

　　✓7ᵗʰ **T41.1X3** Poisoning by intravenous anesthetics, assault

　　✓7ᵗʰ **T41.1X4** Poisoning by intravenous anesthetics, undetermined

　　✓7ᵗʰ **T41.1X5** Adverse effect of intravenous anesthetics

　　✓7ᵗʰ **T41.1X6** Underdosing of intravenous anesthetics

✓ Additional Character Required　✓7ᵗʰ Placeholder　Unacceptable PDx　Questionable PDx　Manifestation　Unspecified Dx　H1-H14 HAC　HCC CMS-HCC Dx　HIV HIV Dx

ICD-10-CM 2021　　　　　　　　　　　　　　　　　　　　　　　　　　　　　　　　　　　　　　　1115

√5ᵗʰ **T41.2** **Poisoning by, adverse effect of and underdosing of other and unspecified general anesthetics**

√6ᵗʰ **T41.20** **Poisoning by, adverse effect of and underdosing of unspecified general anesthetics**

√7ᵗʰ **T41.201** **Poisoning by unspecified general anesthetics, accidental (unintentional)**
Poisoning by general anesthetics NOS

7 √7ᵗʰ **T41.202** **Poisoning by unspecified general anesthetics, intentional self-harm** HCC

√7ᵗʰ **T41.203** **Poisoning by unspecified general anesthetics, assault**

√7ᵗʰ **T41.204** **Poisoning by unspecified general anesthetics, undetermined**

√7ᵗʰ **T41.205** **Adverse effect of unspecified general anesthetics**
AHA: 2016,4Q,73

√7ᵗʰ **T41.206** **Underdosing of unspecified general anesthetics**

√6ᵗʰ **T41.29** **Poisoning by, adverse effect of and underdosing of other general anesthetics**

√7ᵗʰ **T41.291** **Poisoning by other general anesthetics, accidental (unintentional)**
Poisoning by other general anesthetics NOS

7 √7ᵗʰ **T41.292** **Poisoning by other general anesthetics, intentional self-harm** HCC

√7ᵗʰ **T41.293** **Poisoning by other general anesthetics, assault**

√7ᵗʰ **T41.294** **Poisoning by other general anesthetics, undetermined**

√7ᵗʰ **T41.295** **Adverse effect of other general anesthetics**

√7ᵗʰ **T41.296** **Underdosing of other general anesthetics**

√5ᵗʰ **T41.3** **Poisoning by, adverse effect of and underdosing of local anesthetics**
Cocaine (topical)

EXCLUDES 2 poisoning by cocaine used as a central nervous system stimulant (T40.5X1-T40.5X4)

√6ᵗʰ **T41.3X** **Poisoning by, adverse effect of and underdosing of local anesthetics**

√7ᵗʰ **T41.3X1** **Poisoning by local anesthetics, accidental (unintentional)**
Poisoning by local anesthetics NOS

7 √7ᵗʰ **T41.3X2** **Poisoning by local anesthetics, intentional self-harm** HCC

√7ᵗʰ **T41.3X3** **Poisoning by local anesthetics, assault**

√7ᵗʰ **T41.3X4** **Poisoning by local anesthetics, undetermined**

√7ᵗʰ **T41.3X5** **Adverse effect of local anesthetics**

√7ᵗʰ **T41.3X6** **Underdosing of local anesthetics**

√5ᵗʰ **T41.4** **Poisoning by, adverse effect of and underdosing of unspecified anesthetic**

√x7ᵗʰ **T41.41** **Poisoning by unspecified anesthetic, accidental (unintentional)**
Poisoning by anesthetic NOS

7 √x7ᵗʰ **T41.42** **Poisoning by unspecified anesthetic, intentional self-harm** HCC

√x7ᵗʰ **T41.43** **Poisoning by unspecified anesthetic, assault**

√x7ᵗʰ **T41.44** **Poisoning by unspecified anesthetic, undetermined**

√x7ᵗʰ **T41.45** **Adverse effect of unspecified anesthetic**

√x7ᵗʰ **T41.46** **Underdosing of unspecified anesthetics**

√5ᵗʰ **T41.5** **Poisoning by, adverse effect of and underdosing of therapeutic gases**

√6ᵗʰ **T41.5X** **Poisoning by, adverse effect of and underdosing of therapeutic gases**

√7ᵗʰ **T41.5X1** **Poisoning by therapeutic gases, accidental (unintentional)**
Poisoning by therapeutic gases NOS

7 √7ᵗʰ **T41.5X2** **Poisoning by therapeutic gases, intentional self-harm** HCC

√7ᵗʰ **T41.5X3** **Poisoning by therapeutic gases, assault**

√7ᵗʰ **T41.5X4** **Poisoning by therapeutic gases, undetermined**

√7ᵗʰ **T41.5X5** **Adverse effect of therapeutic gases**

√7ᵗʰ **T41.5X6** **Underdosing of therapeutic gases**

√4ᵗʰ **T42** **Poisoning by, adverse effect of and underdosing of antiepileptic, sedative- hypnotic and antiparkinsonism drugs**

EXCLUDES 2 drug dependence and related mental and behavioral disorders due to psychoactive substance use (F10.- – F19.-)

The appropriate 7th character is to be added to each code from category T42.
A initial encounter
D subsequent encounter
S sequela

√5ᵗʰ **T42.0** **Poisoning by, adverse effect of and underdosing of hydantoin derivatives**

√6ᵗʰ **T42.0X** **Poisoning by, adverse effect of and underdosing of hydantoin derivatives**

√7ᵗʰ **T42.0X1** **Poisoning by hydantoin derivatives, accidental (unintentional)**
Poisoning by hydantoin derivatives NOS

7 √7ᵗʰ **T42.0X2** **Poisoning by hydantoin derivatives, intentional self-harm** HCC

√7ᵗʰ **T42.0X3** **Poisoning by hydantoin derivatives, assault**

√7ᵗʰ **T42.0X4** **Poisoning by hydantoin derivatives, undetermined**

√7ᵗʰ **T42.0X5** **Adverse effect of hydantoin derivatives**

√7ᵗʰ **T42.0X6** **Underdosing of hydantoin derivatives**

√5ᵗʰ **T42.1** **Poisoning by, adverse effect of and underdosing of iminostilbenes**
Poisoning by, adverse effect of and underdosing of carbamazepine

√6ᵗʰ **T42.1X** **Poisoning by, adverse effect of and underdosing of iminostilbenes**

√7ᵗʰ **T42.1X1** **Poisoning by iminostilbenes, accidental (unintentional)**
Poisoning by iminostilbenes NOS

7 √7ᵗʰ **T42.1X2** **Poisoning by iminostilbenes, intentional self-harm** HCC

√7ᵗʰ **T42.1X3** **Poisoning by iminostilbenes, assault**

√7ᵗʰ **T42.1X4** **Poisoning by iminostilbenes, undetermined**

√7ᵗʰ **T42.1X5** **Adverse effect of iminostilbenes**

√7ᵗʰ **T42.1X6** **Underdosing of iminostilbenes**

√5ᵗʰ **T42.2** **Poisoning by, adverse effect of and underdosing of succinimides and oxazolidinediones**

√6ᵗʰ **T42.2X** **Poisoning by, adverse effect of and underdosing of succinimides and oxazolidinediones**

√7ᵗʰ **T42.2X1** **Poisoning by succinimides and oxazolidinediones, accidental (unintentional)**
Poisoning by succinimides and oxazolidinediones NOS

7 √7ᵗʰ **T42.2X2** **Poisoning by succinimides and oxazolidinediones, intentional self-harm** HCC

√7ᵗʰ **T42.2X3** **Poisoning by succinimides and oxazolidinediones, assault**

√7ᵗʰ **T42.2X4** **Poisoning by succinimides and oxazolidinediones, undetermined**

√7ᵗʰ **T42.2X5** **Adverse effect of succinimides and oxazolidinediones**

√7ᵗʰ **T42.2X6** **Underdosing of succinimides and oxazolidinediones**

√5ᵗʰ **T42.3** **Poisoning by, adverse effect of and underdosing of barbiturates**

EXCLUDES 1 poisoning by, adverse effect of and underdosing of thiobarbiturates (T41.1-)

√6ᵗʰ **T42.3X** **Poisoning by, adverse effect of and underdosing of barbiturates**

√7ᵗʰ **T42.3X1** **Poisoning by barbiturates, accidental (unintentional)**
Poisoning by barbiturates NOS

7 √7ᵗʰ **T42.3X2** **Poisoning by barbiturates, intentional self-harm** HCC

√7ᵗʰ **T42.3X3** **Poisoning by barbiturates, assault**

√7ᵗʰ **T42.3X4** **Poisoning by barbiturates, undetermined**

√7ᵗʰ **T42.3X5** **Adverse effect of barbiturates**

√7ᵗʰ **T42.3X6** **Underdosing of barbiturates**

✓5ᵗʰ **T42.4** **Poisoning by, adverse effect of and underdosing of benzodiazepines**

    ✓6ᵗʰ **T42.4X** **Poisoning by, adverse effect of and underdosing of** benzodiazepines

        ✓7ᵗʰ **T42.4X1** **Poisoning by benzodiazepines,** accidental **(unintentional)**
            Poisoning by benzodiazepines NOS

        ⁷ ✓7ᵗʰ **T42.4X2** **Poisoning by benzodiazepines,** intentional self-harm   HCC

        ✓7ᵗʰ **T42.4X3** **Poisoning by benzodiazepines,** assault

        ✓7ᵗʰ **T42.4X4** **Poisoning by benzodiazepines,** undetermined

        ✓7ᵗʰ **T42.4X5** Adverse effect **of benzodiazepines**

        ✓7ᵗʰ **T42.4X6** Underdosing **of benzodiazepines**

✓5ᵗʰ **T42.5** **Poisoning by, adverse effect of and underdosing of mixed antiepileptics**

    ✓6ᵗʰ **T42.5X** **Poisoning by, adverse effect of and underdosing of** antiepileptics

        ✓7ᵗʰ **T42.5X1** **Poisoning by mixed antiepileptics,** accidental **(unintentional)**
            Poisoning by mixed antiepileptics NOS

        ⁷ ✓7ᵗʰ **T42.5X2** **Poisoning by mixed antiepileptics,** intentional self-harm   HCC

        ✓7ᵗʰ **T42.5X3** **Poisoning by mixed antiepileptics,** assault

        ✓7ᵗʰ **T42.5X4** **Poisoning by mixed antiepileptics,** undetermined

        ✓7ᵗʰ **T42.5X5** Adverse effect **of mixed antiepileptics**

        ✓7ᵗʰ **T42.5X6** Underdosing **of mixed antiepileptics**

✓5ᵗʰ **T42.6** **Poisoning by, adverse effect of and underdosing of other antiepileptic and sedative-hypnotic drugs**

    Poisoning by, adverse effect of and underdosing of methaqualone

    Poisoning by, adverse effect of and underdosing of valproic acid

    EXCLUDES 1   *poisoning by, adverse effect of and underdosing of carbamazepine (T42.1-)*

    ✓6ᵗʰ **T42.6X** **Poisoning by, adverse effect of and underdosing of other antiepileptic and sedative-hypnotic drugs**

        ✓7ᵗʰ **T42.6X1** **Poisoning by other antiepileptic and sedative-hypnotic drugs,** accidental **(unintentional)**
            Poisoning by other antiepileptic and sedative-hypnotic drugs NOS

        ⁷ ✓7ᵗʰ **T42.6X2** **Poisoning by other antiepileptic and sedative-hypnotic drugs,** intentional self-harm   HCC

        ✓7ᵗʰ **T42.6X3** **Poisoning by other antiepileptic and sedative-hypnotic drugs,** assault

        ✓7ᵗʰ **T42.6X4** **Poisoning by other antiepileptic and sedative-hypnotic drugs,** undetermined

        ✓7ᵗʰ **T42.6X5** Adverse effect **of other antiepileptic and sedative-hypnotic drugs**

        ✓7ᵗʰ **T42.6X6** Underdosing **of other antiepileptic and sedative-hypnotic drugs**

✓5ᵗʰ **T42.7** **Poisoning by, adverse effect of and underdosing of unspecified antiepileptic and sedative-hypnotic drugs**

    ✓x7ᵗʰ **T42.71** **Poisoning by unspecified antiepileptic and sedative-hypnotic drugs,** accidental **(unintentional)**
        Poisoning by antiepileptic and sedative-hypnotic drugs NOS

    ⁷ ✓x7ᵗʰ **T42.72** **Poisoning by unspecified antiepileptic and sedative-hypnotic drugs,** intentional self-harm   HCC

    ✓x7ᵗʰ **T42.73** **Poisoning by unspecified antiepileptic and sedative-hypnotic drugs,** assault

    ✓x7ᵗʰ **T42.74** **Poisoning by unspecified antiepileptic and sedative-hypnotic drugs,** undetermined

    ✓x7ᵗʰ **T42.75** Adverse effect **of unspecified antiepileptic and sedative-hypnotic drugs**

    ✓x7ᵗʰ **T42.76** Underdosing **of unspecified antiepileptic and sedative-hypnotic drugs**

✓5ᵗʰ **T42.8** **Poisoning by, adverse effect of and underdosing of antiparkinsonism drugs and other central muscle-tone depressants**

    Poisoning by, adverse effect of and underdosing of amantadine

    ✓6ᵗʰ **T42.8X** **Poisoning by, adverse effect of and underdosing of** antiparkinsonism drugs and other central muscle-tone depressants

        ✓7ᵗʰ **T42.8X1** **Poisoning by antiparkinsonism drugs and other central muscle-tone depressants,** accidental **(unintentional)**
            Poisoning by antiparkinsonism drugs and other central muscle-tone depressants NOS

        ⁷ ✓7ᵗʰ **T42.8X2** **Poisoning by antiparkinsonism drugs and other central muscle-tone depressants,** intentional self-harm   HCC

        ✓7ᵗʰ **T42.8X3** **Poisoning by antiparkinsonism drugs and other central muscle-tone depressants,** assault

        ✓7ᵗʰ **T42.8X4** **Poisoning by antiparkinsonism drugs and other central muscle-tone depressants,** undetermined

        ✓7ᵗʰ **T42.8X5** Adverse effect **of antiparkinsonism drugs and other central muscle-tone depressants**

        ✓7ᵗʰ **T42.8X6** Underdosing **of antiparkinsonism drugs and other central muscle-tone depressants**

✓4ᵗʰ **T43** **Poisoning by, adverse effect of and underdosing of psychotropic drugs, not elsewhere classified**

    EXCLUDES 1   *appetite depressants (T50.5-)*
            barbiturates (T42.3-)
            benzodiazepines (T42.4-)
            methaqualone (T42.6-)
            psychodysleptics [hallucinogens] (T40.7-T40.9-)

    EXCLUDES 2   *drug dependence and related mental and behavioral disorders due to psychoactive substance use (F10.- – F19.-)*

    The appropriate 7th character is to be added to each code from category T43.
    A   initial encounter
    D   subsequent encounter
    S   sequela

    ✓5ᵗʰ **T43.0** **Poisoning by, adverse effect of and underdosing of tricyclic and tetracyclic antidepressants**

        ✓6ᵗʰ **T43.01** **Poisoning by, adverse effect of and underdosing of** tricyclic antidepressants

            ✓7ᵗʰ **T43.011** **Poisoning by tricyclic antidepressants,** accidental **(unintentional)**
                Poisoning by tricyclic antidepressants NOS

            ⁷ ✓7ᵗʰ **T43.012** **Poisoning by tricyclic antidepressants,** intentional self-harm   HCC

            ✓7ᵗʰ **T43.013** **Poisoning by tricyclic antidepressants,** assault

            ✓7ᵗʰ **T43.014** **Poisoning by tricyclic antidepressants,** undetermined

            ✓7ᵗʰ **T43.015** Adverse effect **of tricyclic antidepressants**

            ✓7ᵗʰ **T43.016** Underdosing **of tricyclic antidepressants**

        ✓6ᵗʰ **T43.02** **Poisoning by, adverse effect of and underdosing of** tetracyclic antidepressants

            ✓7ᵗʰ **T43.021** **Poisoning by tetracyclic antidepressants,** accidental **(unintentional)**
                Poisoning by tetracyclic antidepressants NOS

            ⁷ ✓7ᵗʰ **T43.022** **Poisoning by tetracyclic antidepressants,** intentional self-harm   HCC

            ✓7ᵗʰ **T43.023** **Poisoning by tetracyclic antidepressants,** assault

            ✓7ᵗʰ **T43.024** **Poisoning by tetracyclic antidepressants,** undetermined

            ✓7ᵗʰ **T43.025** Adverse effect **of tetracyclic antidepressants**

            ✓7ᵗʰ **T43.026** Underdosing **of tetracyclic antidepressants**

✓ Additional Character Required   ✓x7ᵗʰ Placeholder   Unacceptable PDx   Questionable PDx   Manifestation   Unspecified Dx   H1-H4 HAC   HCC CMS-HCC Dx   HIV HIV Dx

ICD-10-CM 2021   1117

✓5th **T43.1** **Poisoning by, adverse effect of and underdosing of monoamine-oxidase-inhibitor antidepressants**

  ✓6th **T43.1X** **Poisoning by, adverse effect of and underdosing of** monoamine-oxidase-inhibitor antidepressants

    ✓7th **T43.1X1** **Poisoning by monoamine-oxidase-inhibitor antidepressants, accidental (unintentional)**
         Poisoning by monoamine-oxidase-inhibitor antidepressants NOS

    7 ✓7th **T43.1X2** **Poisoning by monoamine-oxidase-inhibitor antidepressants, intentional self-harm**   HCC

    ✓7th **T43.1X3** **Poisoning by monoamine-oxidase-inhibitor antidepressants, assault**

    ✓7th **T43.1X4** **Poisoning by monoamine-oxidase-inhibitor antidepressants, undetermined**

    ✓7th **T43.1X5** **Adverse effect of monoamine-oxidase-inhibitor antidepressants**

    ✓7th **T43.1X6** **Underdosing of monoamine-oxidase-inhibitor antidepressants**

✓5th **T43.2** **Poisoning by, adverse effect of and underdosing of other and unspecified antidepressants**

  ✓6th **T43.20** **Poisoning by, adverse effect of and underdosing of unspecified antidepressants**

    ✓7th **T43.201** **Poisoning by unspecified antidepressants, accidental (unintentional)**
         Poisoning by antidepressants NOS

    7 ✓7th **T43.202** **Poisoning by unspecified antidepressants, intentional self-harm**   HCC

    ✓7th **T43.203** **Poisoning by unspecified antidepressants, assault**

    ✓7th **T43.204** **Poisoning by unspecified antidepressants, undetermined**

    ✓7th **T43.205** **Adverse effect of unspecified antidepressants**
         Antidepressant discontinuation syndrome

    ✓7th **T43.206** **Underdosing of unspecified antidepressants**

  ✓6th **T43.21** **Poisoning by, adverse effect of and underdosing of** selective serotonin and norepinephrine reuptake inhibitors
     Poisoning by, adverse effect of and underdosing of SSNRI antidepressants

    ✓7th **T43.211** **Poisoning by selective serotonin and norepinephrine reuptake inhibitors, accidental (unintentional)**

    7 ✓7th **T43.212** **Poisoning by selective serotonin and norepinephrine reuptake inhibitors, intentional self-harm**   HCC

    ✓7th **T43.213** **Poisoning by selective serotonin and norepinephrine reuptake inhibitors, assault**

    ✓7th **T43.214** **Poisoning by selective serotonin and norepinephrine reuptake inhibitors, undetermined**

    ✓7th **T43.215** **Adverse effect of selective serotonin and norepinephrine reuptake inhibitors**

    ✓7th **T43.216** **Underdosing of selective serotonin and norepinephrine reuptake inhibitors**

  ✓6th **T43.22** **Poisoning by, adverse effect of and underdosing of** selective serotonin reuptake inhibitors
     Poisoning by, adverse effect of and underdosing of SSRI antidepressants

    ✓7th **T43.221** **Poisoning by selective serotonin reuptake inhibitors, accidental (unintentional)**

    7 ✓7th **T43.222** **Poisoning by selective serotonin reuptake inhibitors, intentional self-harm**   HCC

    ✓7th **T43.223** **Poisoning by selective serotonin reuptake inhibitors, assault**

    ✓7th **T43.224** **Poisoning by selective serotonin reuptake inhibitors, undetermined**

    ✓7th **T43.225** **Adverse effect of selective serotonin reuptake inhibitors**

    ✓7th **T43.226** **Underdosing of selective serotonin reuptake inhibitors**

  ✓6th **T43.29** **Poisoning by, adverse effect of and underdosing of other antidepressants**

    ✓7th **T43.291** **Poisoning by other antidepressants, accidental (unintentional)**
         Poisoning by other antidepressants NOS

    7 ✓7th **T43.292** **Poisoning by other antidepressants, intentional self-harm**   HCC

    ✓7th **T43.293** **Poisoning by other antidepressants, assault**

    ✓7th **T43.294** **Poisoning by other antidepressants, undetermined**

    ✓7th **T43.295** **Adverse effect of other antidepressants**

    ✓7th **T43.296** **Underdosing of other antidepressants**

✓5th **T43.3** **Poisoning by, adverse effect of and underdosing of phenothiazine antipsychotics and neuroleptics**

  ✓6th **T43.3X** **Poisoning by, adverse effect of and underdosing of** phenothiazine antipsychotics and neuroleptics

    ✓7th **T43.3X1** **Poisoning by phenothiazine antipsychotics and neuroleptics, accidental (unintentional)**
         Poisoning by phenothiazine antipsychotics and neuroleptics NOS

    7 ✓7th **T43.3X2** **Poisoning by phenothiazine antipsychotics and neuroleptics, intentional self-harm**   HCC

    ✓7th **T43.3X3** **Poisoning by phenothiazine antipsychotics and neuroleptics, assault**

    ✓7th **T43.3X4** **Poisoning by phenothiazine antipsychotics and neuroleptics, undetermined**

    ✓7th **T43.3X5** **Adverse effect of phenothiazine antipsychotics and neuroleptics**

    ✓7th **T43.3X6** **Underdosing of phenothiazine antipsychotics and neuroleptics**

✓5th **T43.4** **Poisoning by, adverse effect of and underdosing of butyrophenone and thiothixene neuroleptics**

  ✓6th **T43.4X** **Poisoning by, adverse effect of and underdosing of** butyrophenone and thiothixene neuroleptics

    ✓7th **T43.4X1** **Poisoning by butyrophenone and thiothixene neuroleptics, accidental (unintentional)**
         Poisoning by butyrophenone and thiothixene neuroleptics NOS

    7 ✓7th **T43.4X2** **Poisoning by butyrophenone and thiothixene neuroleptics, intentional self-harm**   HCC

    ✓7th **T43.4X3** **Poisoning by butyrophenone and thiothixene neuroleptics, assault**

    ✓7th **T43.4X4** **Poisoning by butyrophenone and thiothixene neuroleptics, undetermined**

    ✓7th **T43.4X5** **Adverse effect of butyrophenone and thiothixene neuroleptics**

    ✓7th **T43.4X6** **Underdosing of butyrophenone and thiothixene neuroleptics**

✓5th **T43.5** **Poisoning by, adverse effect of and underdosing of other and unspecified antipsychotics and neuroleptics**

     EXCLUDES 1   *poisoning by, adverse effect of and underdosing of rauwolfia (T46.5-)*

  ✓6th **T43.50** **Poisoning by, adverse effect of and underdosing of unspecified antipsychotics and neuroleptics**

    ✓7th **T43.501** **Poisoning by unspecified antipsychotics and neuroleptics, accidental (unintentional)**
         Poisoning by antipsychotics and neuroleptics NOS

    7 ✓7th **T43.502** **Poisoning by unspecified antipsychotics and neuroleptics, intentional self-harm**   HCC

    ✓7th **T43.503** **Poisoning by unspecified antipsychotics and neuroleptics, assault**

    ✓7th **T43.504** **Poisoning by unspecified antipsychotics and neuroleptics, undetermined**

    ✓7th **T43.505** **Adverse effect of unspecified antipsychotics and neuroleptics**

    ✓7th **T43.506** **Underdosing of unspecified antipsychotics and neuroleptics**

N Newborn: 0   P Pediatric: 0-17   M Maternity: 9-64   A Adult: 15-124   MCC Major Complication/Comorbidity   CC Complication/Comorbidity   SW Severe Wound Dx

1118   ICD-10-CM 2021

✓6th **T43.59** **Poisoning by, adverse effect of and underdosing of other antipsychotics and neuroleptics**
AHA: 2017,1Q,40

     ✓7th **T43.591** **Poisoning by other antipsychotics and neuroleptics, accidental (unintentional)**
Poisoning by other antipsychotics and neuroleptics NOS

     7 ✓7th **T43.592** **Poisoning by other antipsychotics and neuroleptics, intentional self-harm** HCC

     ✓7th **T43.593** **Poisoning by other antipsychotics and neuroleptics, assault**

     ✓7th **T43.594** **Poisoning by other antipsychotics and neuroleptics, undetermined**

     ✓7th **T43.595** **Adverse effect of other antipsychotics and neuroleptics**

     ✓7th **T43.596** **Underdosing of other antipsychotics and neuroleptics**

✓5th **T43.6** **Poisoning by, adverse effect of and underdosing of psychostimulants**
EXCLUDES 1   poisoning by, adverse effect of and underdosing of cocaine (T40.5-)

     ✓6th **T43.60** **Poisoning by, adverse effect of and underdosing of unspecified psychostimulant**

       6 ✓7th **T43.601** **Poisoning by unspecified psychostimulants, accidental (unintentional)** HCC
Poisoning by psychostimulants NOS

       7 ✓7th **T43.602** **Poisoning by unspecified psychostimulants, intentional self-harm** HCC

       ✓7th **T43.603** **Poisoning by unspecified psychostimulants, assault**

       6 ✓7th **T43.604** **Poisoning by unspecified psychostimulants, undetermined** HCC

       ✓7th **T43.605** **Adverse effect of unspecified psychostimulants**

       ✓7th **T43.606** **Underdosing of unspecified psychostimulants**

     ✓6th **T43.61** **Poisoning by, adverse effect of and underdosing of caffeine**

       6 ✓7th **T43.611** **Poisoning by caffeine, accidental (unintentional)** HCC
Poisoning by caffeine NOS

       7 ✓7th **T43.612** **Poisoning by caffeine, intentional self-harm** HCC

       ✓7th **T43.613** **Poisoning by caffeine, assault**

       6 ✓7th **T43.614** **Poisoning by caffeine, undetermined** HCC

       ✓7th **T43.615** **Adverse effect of caffeine**

       ✓7th **T43.616** **Underdosing of caffeine**

     ✓6th **T43.62** **Poisoning by, adverse effect of and underdosing of amphetamines**
Poisoning by, adverse effect of and underdosing of methamphetamines

       6 ✓7th **T43.621** **Poisoning by amphetamines, accidental (unintentional)** HCC
Poisoning by amphetamines NOS

       7 ✓7th **T43.622** **Poisoning by amphetamines, intentional self-harm** HCC

       ✓7th **T43.623** **Poisoning by amphetamines, assault**

       6 ✓7th **T43.624** **Poisoning by amphetamines, undetermined** HCC

       ✓7th **T43.625** **Adverse effect of amphetamines**

       ✓7th **T43.626** **Underdosing of amphetamines**

     ✓6th **T43.63** **Poisoning by, adverse effect of and underdosing of methylphenidate**

       6 ✓7th **T43.631** **Poisoning by methylphenidate, accidental (unintentional)** HCC
Poisoning by methylphenidate NOS

       7 ✓7th **T43.632** **Poisoning by methylphenidate, intentional self-harm** HCC

       ✓7th **T43.633** **Poisoning by methylphenidate, assault**

       6 ✓7th **T43.634** **Poisoning by methylphenidate, undetermined** HCC

       ✓7th **T43.635** **Adverse effect of methylphenidate**

       ✓7th **T43.636** **Underdosing of methylphenidate**

     ✓6th **T43.64** **Poisoning by ecstasy**
Poisoning by MDMA
Poisoning by 3,4-methylenedioxymethamphetamine
AHA: 2018,4Q,30-31

       6 ✓7th **T43.641** **Poisoning by ecstasy, accidental (unintentional)** HCC
Poisoning by ecstasy NOS

       7 ✓7th **T43.642** **Poisoning by ecstasy, intentional self-harm** HCC

       ✓7th **T43.643** **Poisoning by ecstasy, assault**

       6 ✓7th **T43.644** **Poisoning by ecstasy, undetermined** HCC

     ✓6th **T43.69** **Poisoning by, adverse effect of and underdosing of other psychostimulants**

       6 ✓7th **T43.691** **Poisoning by other psychostimulants, accidental (unintentional)** HCC
Poisoning by other psychostimulants NOS

       7 ✓7th **T43.692** **Poisoning by other psychostimulants, intentional self-harm** HCC

       ✓7th **T43.693** **Poisoning by other psychostimulants, assault**

       6 ✓7th **T43.694** **Poisoning by other psychostimulants, undetermined** HCC

       ✓7th **T43.695** **Adverse effect of other psychostimulants**

       ✓7th **T43.696** **Underdosing of other psychostimulants**

✓5th **T43.8** **Poisoning by, adverse effect of and underdosing of other psychotropic drugs**

     ✓6th **T43.8X** **Poisoning by, adverse effect of and underdosing of other psychotropic drugs**

       ✓7th **T43.8X1** **Poisoning by other psychotropic drugs, accidental (unintentional)**
Poisoning by other psychotropic drugs NOS

       7 ✓7th **T43.8X2** **Poisoning by other psychotropic drugs, intentional self-harm** HCC

       ✓7th **T43.8X3** **Poisoning by other psychotropic drugs, assault**

       ✓7th **T43.8X4** **Poisoning by other psychotropic drugs, undetermined**

       ✓7th **T43.8X5** **Adverse effect of other psychotropic drugs**

       ✓7th **T43.8X6** **Underdosing of other psychotropic drugs**

✓5th **T43.9** **Poisoning by, adverse effect of and underdosing of unspecified psychotropic drug**

     ✓x7th **T43.91** **Poisoning by unspecified psychotropic drug, accidental (unintentional)**
Poisoning by psychotropic drug NOS

     7 ✓x7th **T43.92** **Poisoning by unspecified psychotropic drug, intentional self-harm** HCC

     ✓x7th **T43.93** **Poisoning by unspecified psychotropic drug, assault**

     ✓x7th **T43.94** **Poisoning by unspecified psychotropic drug, undetermined**

     ✓x7th **T43.95** **Adverse effect of unspecified psychotropic drug**

     ✓x7th **T43.96** **Underdosing of unspecified psychotropic drug**

✓4th **T44** **Poisoning by, adverse effect of and underdosing of drugs primarily affecting the autonomic nervous system**

The appropriate 7th character is to be added to each code from category T44.
A   initial encounter
D   subsequent encounter
S   sequela

✓5th **T44.0** **Poisoning by, adverse effect of and underdosing of anticholinesterase agents**

     ✓6th **T44.0X** **Poisoning by, adverse effect of and underdosing of anticholinesterase agents**

       ✓7th **T44.0X1** **Poisoning by anticholinesterase agents, accidental (unintentional)**
Poisoning by anticholinesterase agents NOS

       7 ✓7th **T44.0X2** **Poisoning by anticholinesterase agents, intentional self-harm** HCC

       ✓7th **T44.0X3** **Poisoning by anticholinesterase agents, assault**

       ✓7th **T44.0X4** **Poisoning by anticholinesterase agents, undetermined**

       ✓7th **T44.0X5** **Adverse effect of anticholinesterase agents**

       ✓7th **T44.0X6** **Underdosing of anticholinesterase agents**

√5ᵗʰ **T44.1** Poisoning by, adverse effect of and underdosing of other parasympathomimetics [cholinergics]

√6ᵗʰ **T44.1X** Poisoning by, adverse effect of and underdosing of other parasympathomimetics [cholinergics]

√7ᵗʰ **T44.1X1** Poisoning by other parasympathomimetics [cholinergics], accidental (unintentional)

Poisoning by other parasympathomimetics [cholinergics] NOS

7 √7ᵗʰ **T44.1X2** Poisoning by other parasympathomimetics [cholinergics], intentional self-harm　　HCC

√7ᵗʰ **T44.1X3** Poisoning by other parasympathomimetics [cholinergics], assault

√7ᵗʰ **T44.1X4** Poisoning by other parasympathomimetics [cholinergics], undetermined

√7ᵗʰ **T44.1X5** Adverse effect of other parasympathomimetics [cholinergics]

√7ᵗʰ **T44.1X6** Underdosing of other parasympathomimetics [cholinergics]

√5ᵗʰ **T44.2** Poisoning by, adverse effect of and underdosing of ganglionic blocking drugs

√6ᵗʰ **T44.2X** Poisoning by, adverse effect of and underdosing of ganglionic blocking drugs

√7ᵗʰ **T44.2X1** Poisoning by ganglionic blocking drugs, accidental (unintentional)

Poisoning by ganglionic blocking drugs NOS

7 √7ᵗʰ **T44.2X2** Poisoning by ganglionic blocking drugs, intentional self-harm　　HCC

√7ᵗʰ **T44.2X3** Poisoning by ganglionic blocking drugs, assault

√7ᵗʰ **T44.2X4** Poisoning by ganglionic blocking drugs, undetermined

√7ᵗʰ **T44.2X5** Adverse effect of ganglionic blocking drugs

√7ᵗʰ **T44.2X6** Underdosing of ganglionic blocking drugs

√5ᵗʰ **T44.3** Poisoning by, adverse effect of and underdosing of other parasympatholytics [anticholinergics and antimuscarinics] and spasmolytics

Poisoning by, adverse effect of and underdosing of papaverine

√6ᵗʰ **T44.3X** Poisoning by, adverse effect of and underdosing of other parasympatholytics [anticholinergics and antimuscarinics] and spasmolytics

√7ᵗʰ **T44.3X1** Poisoning by other parasympatholytics [anticholinergics and antimuscarinics] and spasmolytics, accidental (unintentional)

Poisoning by other parasympatholytics [anticholinergics and antimuscarinics] and spasmolytics NOS

7 √7ᵗʰ **T44.3X2** Poisoning by other parasympatholytics [anticholinergics and antimuscarinics] and spasmolytics, intentional self-harm　　HCC

√7ᵗʰ **T44.3X3** Poisoning by other parasympatholytics [anticholinergics and antimuscarinics] and spasmolytics, assault

√7ᵗʰ **T44.3X4** Poisoning by other parasympatholytics [anticholinergics and antimuscarinics] and spasmolytics, undetermined

√7ᵗʰ **T44.3X5** Adverse effect of other parasympatholytics [anticholinergics and antimuscarinics] and spasmolytics

√7ᵗʰ **T44.3X6** Underdosing of other parasympatholytics [anticholinergics and antimuscarinics] and spasmolytics

√5ᵗʰ **T44.4** Poisoning by, adverse effect of and underdosing of predominantly alpha-adrenoreceptor agonists

Poisoning by, adverse effect of and underdosing of metaraminol

√6ᵗʰ **T44.4X** Poisoning by, adverse effect of and underdosing of predominantly alpha-adrenoreceptor agonists

√7ᵗʰ **T44.4X1** Poisoning by predominantly alpha-adrenoreceptor agonists, accidental (unintentional)

Poisoning by predominantly alpha-adrenoreceptor agonists NOS

7 √7ᵗʰ **T44.4X2** Poisoning by predominantly alpha-adrenoreceptor agonists, intentional self-harm　　HCC

√7ᵗʰ **T44.4X3** Poisoning by predominantly alpha-adrenoreceptor agonists, assault

√7ᵗʰ **T44.4X4** Poisoning by predominantly alpha-adrenoreceptor agonists, undetermined

√7ᵗʰ **T44.4X5** Adverse effect of predominantly alpha-adrenoreceptor agonists

√7ᵗʰ **T44.4X6** Underdosing of predominantly alpha-adrenoreceptor agonists

√5ᵗʰ **T44.5** Poisoning by, adverse effect of and underdosing of predominantly beta-adrenoreceptor agonists

EXCLUDES1　poisoning by, adverse effect of and underdosing of beta-adrenoreceptor agonists used in asthma therapy (T48.6-)

√6ᵗʰ **T44.5X** Poisoning by, adverse effect of and underdosing of predominantly beta-adrenoreceptor agonists

√7ᵗʰ **T44.5X1** Poisoning by predominantly beta-adrenoreceptor agonists, accidental (unintentional)

Poisoning by predominantly beta-adrenoreceptor agonists NOS

7 √7ᵗʰ **T44.5X2** Poisoning by predominantly beta-adrenoreceptor agonists, intentional self-harm　　HCC

√7ᵗʰ **T44.5X3** Poisoning by predominantly beta-adrenoreceptor agonists, assault

√7ᵗʰ **T44.5X4** Poisoning by predominantly beta-adrenoreceptor agonists, undetermined

√7ᵗʰ **T44.5X5** Adverse effect of predominantly beta-adrenoreceptor agonists

√7ᵗʰ **T44.5X6** Underdosing of predominantly beta-adrenoreceptor agonists

√5ᵗʰ **T44.6** Poisoning by, adverse effect of and underdosing of alpha-adrenoreceptor antagonists

EXCLUDES1　poisoning by, adverse effect of and underdosing of ergot alkaloids (T48.0)

√6ᵗʰ **T44.6X** Poisoning by, adverse effect of and underdosing of alpha-adrenoreceptor antagonists

√7ᵗʰ **T44.6X1** Poisoning by alpha-adrenoreceptor antagonists, accidental (unintentional)

Poisoning by alpha-adrenoreceptor antagonists NOS

7 √7ᵗʰ **T44.6X2** Poisoning by alpha-adrenoreceptor antagonists, intentional self-harm　　HCC

√7ᵗʰ **T44.6X3** Poisoning by alpha-adrenoreceptor antagonists, assault

√7ᵗʰ **T44.6X4** Poisoning by alpha-adrenoreceptor antagonists, undetermined

√7ᵗʰ **T44.6X5** Adverse effect of alpha-adrenoreceptor antagonists

√7ᵗʰ **T44.6X6** Underdosing of alpha-adrenoreceptor antagonists

√5ᵗʰ **T44.7** Poisoning by, adverse effect of and underdosing of beta-adrenoreceptor antagonists

√6ᵗʰ **T44.7X** Poisoning by, adverse effect of and underdosing of beta-adrenoreceptor antagonists

√7ᵗʰ **T44.7X1** Poisoning by beta-adrenoreceptor antagonists, accidental (unintentional)

Poisoning by beta-adrenoreceptor antagonists NOS

7 √7ᵗʰ **T44.7X2** Poisoning by beta-adrenoreceptor antagonists, intentional self-harm　　HCC

√7ᵗʰ **T44.7X3** Poisoning by beta-adrenoreceptor antagonists, assault

√7ᵗʰ **T44.7X4** Poisoning by beta-adrenoreceptor antagonists, undetermined

√7ᵗʰ **T44.7X5** Adverse effect of beta-adrenoreceptor antagonists

√7ᵗʰ **T44.7X6** Underdosing of beta-adrenoreceptor antagonists

N Newborn: 0　P Pediatric: 0-17　M Maternity: 9-64　A Adult: 15-124　MCC Major Complication/Comorbidity　CC Complication/Comorbidity　SW Severe Wound Dx

1120

ICD-10-CM 2021

√5ᵗʰ **T44.8** **Poisoning by, adverse effect of and underdosing of centrally-acting and adrenergic-neuron- blocking agents**

    EXCLUDES 1   *poisoning by, adverse effect of and underdosing of clonidine (T46.5)*

      poisoning by, adverse effect of and underdosing of guanethidine (T46.5)

    √6ᵗʰ **T44.8X** **Poisoning by, adverse effect of and underdosing of** centrally-acting and adrenergic- neuron-blocking agents

      √7ᵗʰ **T44.8X1** **Poisoning by centrally-acting and adrenergic-neuron-blocking agents,** accidental **(unintentional)**

        Poisoning by centrally-acting and adrenergic-neuron-blocking agents NOS

      7 √7ᵗʰ **T44.8X2** **Poisoning by centrally-acting and adrenergic-neuron-blocking agents,** intentional self-harm   HCC

      √7ᵗʰ **T44.8X3** **Poisoning by centrally-acting and adrenergic-neuron-blocking agents,** assault

      √7ᵗʰ **T44.8X4** **Poisoning by centrally-acting and adrenergic-neuron-blocking agents,** undetermined

      √7ᵗʰ **T44.8X5** Adverse effect **of centrally-acting and adrenergic-neuron-blocking agents**

      √7ᵗʰ **T44.8X6** Underdosing **of centrally-acting and adrenergic-neuron-blocking agents**

√5ᵗʰ **T44.9** **Poisoning by, adverse effect of and underdosing of other and unspecified drugs primarily affecting the autonomic nervous system**

    Poisoning by, adverse effect of and underdosing of drug stimulating both alpha and beta-adrenoreceptors

    √6ᵗʰ **T44.90** **Poisoning by, adverse effect of and underdosing of unspecified drugs primarily affecting the autonomic nervous system**

      √7ᵗʰ **T44.901** **Poisoning by unspecified drugs primarily affecting the autonomic nervous system,** accidental **(unintentional)**

        Poisoning by unspecified drugs primarily affecting the autonomic nervous system NOS

      7 √7ᵗʰ **T44.902** **Poisoning by unspecified drugs primarily affecting the autonomic nervous system,** intentional self-harm   HCC

      √7ᵗʰ **T44.903** **Poisoning by unspecified drugs primarily affecting the autonomic nervous system,** assault

      √7ᵗʰ **T44.904** **Poisoning by unspecified drugs primarily affecting the autonomic nervous system,** undetermined

      √7ᵗʰ **T44.905** Adverse effect **of unspecified drugs primarily affecting the autonomic nervous system**

      √7ᵗʰ **T44.906** Underdosing **of unspecified drugs primarily affecting the autonomic nervous system**

    √6ᵗʰ **T44.99** **Poisoning by, adverse effect of and underdosing of other drugs primarily affecting the autonomic nervous system**

      √7ᵗʰ **T44.991** **Poisoning by other drug primarily affecting the autonomic nervous system,** accidental **(unintentional)**

        Poisoning by other drugs primarily affecting the autonomic nervous system NOS

      7 √7ᵗʰ **T44.992** **Poisoning by other drug primarily affecting the autonomic nervous system,** intentional self-harm   HCC

      √7ᵗʰ **T44.993** **Poisoning by other drug primarily affecting the autonomic nervous system,** assault

      √7ᵗʰ **T44.994** **Poisoning by other drug primarily affecting the autonomic nervous system,** undetermined

      √7ᵗʰ **T44.995** Adverse effect **of other drug primarily affecting the autonomic nervous system**

      √7ᵗʰ **T44.996** Underdosing **of other drug primarily affecting the autonomic nervous system**

√4ᵗʰ **T45** **Poisoning by, adverse effect of and underdosing of primarily systemic and hematological agents, not elsewhere classified**

    The appropriate 7th character is to be added to each code from category T45.
    A   initial encounter
    D   subsequent encounter
    S   sequela

  √5ᵗʰ **T45.0** **Poisoning by, adverse effect of and underdosing of antiallergic and antiemetic drugs**

    EXCLUDES 1   *poisoning by, adverse effect of and underdosing of phenothiazine-based neuroleptics (T43.3)*

    √6ᵗʰ **T45.0X** **Poisoning by, adverse effect of and underdosing of** antiallergic and antiemetic drugs

      √7ᵗʰ **T45.0X1** **Poisoning by antiallergic and antiemetic drugs,** accidental **(unintentional)**

        Poisoning by antiallergic and antiemetic drugs NOS

      7 √7ᵗʰ **T45.0X2** **Poisoning by antiallergic and antiemetic drugs,** intentional self-harm   HCC

      √7ᵗʰ **T45.0X3** **Poisoning by antiallergic and antiemetic drugs,** assault

      √7ᵗʰ **T45.0X4** **Poisoning by antiallergic and antiemetic drugs,** undetermined

      √7ᵗʰ **T45.0X5** Adverse effect **of antiallergic and antiemetic drugs**

      √7ᵗʰ **T45.0X6** Underdosing **of antiallergic and antiemetic drugs**

  √5ᵗʰ **T45.1** **Poisoning by, adverse effect of and underdosing of antineoplastic and immunosuppressive drugs**

    EXCLUDES 1   *poisoning by, adverse effect of and underdosing of tamoxifen (T38.6)*

    AHA: 2019,1Q,17,20; 2014,4Q,22

    √6ᵗʰ **T45.1X** **Poisoning by, adverse effect of and underdosing of** antineoplastic and immunosuppressive drugs

      √7ᵗʰ **T45.1X1** **Poisoning by antineoplastic and immunosuppressive drugs,** accidental **(unintentional)**

        Poisoning by antineoplastic and immunosuppressive drugs NOS

      7 √7ᵗʰ **T45.1X2** **Poisoning by antineoplastic and immunosuppressive drugs,** intentional self-harm   HCC

      √7ᵗʰ **T45.1X3** **Poisoning by antineoplastic and immunosuppressive drugs,** assault

      √7ᵗʰ **T45.1X4** **Poisoning by antineoplastic and immunosuppressive drugs,** undetermined

      √7ᵗʰ **T45.1X5** Adverse effect **of antineoplastic and immunosuppressive drugs**

        AHA: 2019,2Q,24,28

      √7ᵗʰ **T45.1X6** Underdosing **of antineoplastic and immunosuppressive drugs**

  √5ᵗʰ **T45.2** **Poisoning by, adverse effect of and underdosing of vitamins**

    EXCLUDES 2   *poisoning by, adverse effect of and underdosing of iron (T45.4)*

      poisoning by, adverse effect of and underdosing of nicotinic acid (derivatives) (T46.7)

      poisoning by, adverse effect of and underdosing of vitamin K (T45.7)

    √6ᵗʰ **T45.2X** **Poisoning by, adverse effect of and underdosing of** vitamins

      √7ᵗʰ **T45.2X1** **Poisoning by vitamins,** accidental **(unintentional)**

        Poisoning by vitamins NOS

      7 √7ᵗʰ **T45.2X2** **Poisoning by vitamins,** intentional self-harm   HCC

      √7ᵗʰ **T45.2X3** **Poisoning by vitamins,** assault

      √7ᵗʰ **T45.2X4** **Poisoning by vitamins,** undetermined

      √7ᵗʰ **T45.2X5** Adverse effect **of vitamins**

      √7ᵗʰ **T45.2X6** Underdosing **of vitamins**

        EXCLUDES 1   *vitamin deficiencies (E50-E56)*

  √5ᵗʰ **T45.3** **Poisoning by, adverse effect of and underdosing of enzymes**

    √6ᵗʰ **T45.3X** **Poisoning by, adverse effect of and underdosing of** enzymes

      √7ᵗʰ **T45.3X1** **Poisoning by enzymes,** accidental **(unintentional)**

        Poisoning by enzymes NOS

      7 √7ᵗʰ **T45.3X2** **Poisoning by enzymes,** intentional self-harm   HCC

✔ Additional Character Required   √x7ᵗʰ Placeholder   Unacceptable PDx   Questionable PDx   Manifestation   Unspecified Dx   H1-H14 HAC   HCC CMS-HCC Dx   HIV HIV Dx

ICD-10-CM 2021   1121

√7ᵗʰ **T45.3X3** **Poisoning by enzymes,** assault

√7ᵗʰ **T45.3X4** **Poisoning by enzymes,** undetermined

√7ᵗʰ **T45.3X5** **Adverse effect** of enzymes

√7ᵗʰ **T45.3X6** **Underdosing** of enzymes

√5ᵗʰ **T45.4** **Poisoning by, adverse effect of and underdosing of iron and its compounds**

√6ᵗʰ **T45.4X** **Poisoning by, adverse effect of and underdosing of iron and its compounds**

√7ᵗʰ **T45.4X1** **Poisoning by iron and its compounds,** accidental (unintentional)
Poisoning by iron and its compounds NOS

7 √7ᵗʰ **T45.4X2** **Poisoning by iron and its compounds,** intentional self-harm ᴴᶜᶜ

√7ᵗʰ **T45.4X3** **Poisoning by iron and its compounds,** assault

√7ᵗʰ **T45.4X4** **Poisoning by iron and its compounds,** undetermined

√7ᵗʰ **T45.4X5** **Adverse effect** of iron and its compounds

√7ᵗʰ **T45.4X6** **Underdosing** of iron and its compounds
EXCLUDES 1 iron deficiency (E61.1)

√5ᵗʰ **T45.5** **Poisoning by, adverse effect of and underdosing of anticoagulants and antithrombotic drugs**

√6ᵗʰ **T45.51** **Poisoning by, adverse effect of and underdosing of anticoagulants**

√7ᵗʰ **T45.511** **Poisoning by anticoagulants,** accidental (unintentional)
Poisoning by anticoagulants NOS

7 √7ᵗʰ **T45.512** **Poisoning by anticoagulants,** intentional self-harm ᴴᶜᶜ

√7ᵗʰ **T45.513** **Poisoning by anticoagulants,** assault

√7ᵗʰ **T45.514** **Poisoning by anticoagulants,** undetermined

√7ᵗʰ **T45.515** **Adverse effect** of anticoagulants
AHA: 2016,1Q,14; 2013,2Q,34

√7ᵗʰ **T45.516** **Underdosing** of anticoagulants

√6ᵗʰ **T45.52** **Poisoning by, adverse effect of and underdosing of antithrombotic drugs**
Poisoning by, adverse effect of and underdosing of antiplatelet drugs
EXCLUDES 2 poisoning by, adverse effect of and underdosing of aspirin (T39.0l-)
poisoning by, adverse effect of and underdosing of acetylsalicylic acid (T39.0l-)

√7ᵗʰ **T45.521** **Poisoning by antithrombotic drugs,** accidental (unintentional)
Poisoning by antithrombotic drug NOS

7 √7ᵗʰ **T45.522** **Poisoning by antithrombotic drugs,** intentional self-harm ᴴᶜᶜ

√7ᵗʰ **T45.523** **Poisoning by antithrombotic drugs,** assault

√7ᵗʰ **T45.524** **Poisoning by antithrombotic drugs,** undetermined

√7ᵗʰ **T45.525** **Adverse effect** of antithrombotic drugs
AHA: 2016,1Q,15

√7ᵗʰ **T45.526** **Underdosing** of antithrombotic drugs

√5ᵗʰ **T45.6** **Poisoning by, adverse effect of and underdosing of fibrinolysis-affecting drugs**

√6ᵗʰ **T45.60** **Poisoning by, adverse effect of and underdosing of unspecified fibrinolysis-affecting drugs**

√7ᵗʰ **T45.601** **Poisoning by unspecified fibrinolysis-affecting drugs,** accidental (unintentional)
Poisoning by fibrinolysis-affecting drug NOS

7 √7ᵗʰ **T45.602** **Poisoning by unspecified fibrinolysis-affecting drugs,** intentional self-harm ᴴᶜᶜ

√7ᵗʰ **T45.603** **Poisoning by unspecified fibrinolysis-affecting drugs,** assault

√7ᵗʰ **T45.604** **Poisoning by unspecified fibrinolysis-affecting drugs,** undetermined

√7ᵗʰ **T45.605** **Adverse effect** of unspecified fibrinolysis-affecting drugs

√7ᵗʰ **T45.606** **Underdosing** of unspecified fibrinolysis-affecting drugs

√6ᵗʰ **T45.61** **Poisoning by, adverse effect of and underdosing of thrombolytic drugs**

√7ᵗʰ **T45.611** **Poisoning by thrombolytic drug,** accidental (unintentional)
Poisoning by thrombolytic drug NOS

7 √7ᵗʰ **T45.612** **Poisoning by thrombolytic drug,** intentional self-harm ᴴᶜᶜ

√7ᵗʰ **T45.613** **Poisoning by thrombolytic drug,** assault

√7ᵗʰ **T45.614** **Poisoning by thrombolytic drug,** undetermined

√7ᵗʰ **T45.615** **Adverse effect** of thrombolytic drugs
AHA: 2017,2Q,9

√7ᵗʰ **T45.616** **Underdosing** of thrombolytic drugs

√6ᵗʰ **T45.62** **Poisoning by, adverse effect of and underdosing of hemostatic drugs**

√7ᵗʰ **T45.621** **Poisoning by hemostatic drug,** accidental (unintentional)
Poisoning by hemostatic drug NOS

7 √7ᵗʰ **T45.622** **Poisoning by hemostatic drug,** intentional self-harm ᴴᶜᶜ

√7ᵗʰ **T45.623** **Poisoning by hemostatic drug,** assault

√7ᵗʰ **T45.624** **Poisoning by hemostatic drug,** undetermined

√7ᵗʰ **T45.625** **Adverse effect** of hemostatic drug

√7ᵗʰ **T45.626** **Underdosing** of hemostatic drugs

√6ᵗʰ **T45.69** **Poisoning by, adverse effect of and underdosing of other fibrinolysis-affecting drugs**

√7ᵗʰ **T45.691** **Poisoning by other fibrinolysis-affecting drugs,** accidental (unintentional)
Poisoning by other fibrinolysis-affecting drug NOS

7 √7ᵗʰ **T45.692** **Poisoning by other fibrinolysis-affecting drugs,** intentional self-harm ᴴᶜᶜ

√7ᵗʰ **T45.693** **Poisoning by other fibrinolysis-affecting drugs,** assault

√7ᵗʰ **T45.694** **Poisoning by other fibrinolysis-affecting drugs,** undetermined

√7ᵗʰ **T45.695** **Adverse effect** of other fibrinolysis-affecting drugs

√7ᵗʰ **T45.696** **Underdosing** of other fibrinolysis-affecting drugs

√5ᵗʰ **T45.7** **Poisoning by, adverse effect of and underdosing of anticoagulant antagonists, vitamin K and other coagulants**

√6ᵗʰ **T45.7X** **Poisoning by, adverse effect of and underdosing of anticoagulant antagonists, vitamin K and other coagulants**

√7ᵗʰ **T45.7X1** **Poisoning by anticoagulant antagonists, vitamin K and other coagulants,** accidental (unintentional)
Poisoning by anticoagulant antagonists, vitamin K and other coagulants NOS

7 √7ᵗʰ **T45.7X2** **Poisoning by anticoagulant antagonists, vitamin K and other coagulants,** intentional self-harm ᴴᶜᶜ

√7ᵗʰ **T45.7X3** **Poisoning by anticoagulant antagonists, vitamin K and other coagulants,** assault

√7ᵗʰ **T45.7X4** **Poisoning by anticoagulant antagonists, vitamin K and other coagulants,** undetermined

√7ᵗʰ **T45.7X5** **Adverse effect** of anticoagulant antagonists, vitamin K and other coagulants

√7ᵗʰ **T45.7X6** **Underdosing** of anticoagulant antagonist, vitamin K and other coagulants
EXCLUDES 1 vitamin K deficiency (E56.1)

N Newborn: 0 **P** Pediatric: 0-17 **M** Maternity: 9-64 **A** Adult: 15-124 **MCC** Major Complication/Comorbidity **CC** Complication/Comorbidity **SW** Severe Wound Dx

1122 ICD-10-CM 2021

√5ᵗʰ **T45.8 Poisoning by, adverse effect of and underdosing of other primarily systemic and hematological agents**

Poisoning by, adverse effect of and underdosing of liver preparations and other antianemic agents

Poisoning by, adverse effect of and underdosing of natural blood and blood products

Poisoning by, adverse effect of and underdosing of plasma substitute

EXCLUDES 2   poisoning by, adverse effect of and underdosing of immunoglobulin (T50.Z1)

poisoning by, adverse effect of and underdosing of iron (T45.4)

transfusion reactions (T80.-)

√6ᵗʰ **T45.8X Poisoning by, adverse effect of and underdosing of other primarily systemic and hematological agents**

√7ᵗʰ **T45.8X1 Poisoning by other primarily systemic and hematological agents, accidental (unintentional)**

Poisoning by other primarily systemic and hematological agents NOS

7 √7ᵗʰ **T45.8X2 Poisoning by other primarily systemic and hematological agents, intentional self-harm** HCC

√7ᵗʰ **T45.8X3 Poisoning by other primarily systemic and hematological agents, assault**

√7ᵗʰ **T45.8X4 Poisoning by other primarily systemic and hematological agents, undetermined**

√7ᵗʰ **T45.8X5 Adverse effect of other primarily systemic and hematological agents**

AHA: 2016,4Q,42

√7ᵗʰ **T45.8X6 Underdosing of other primarily systemic and hematological agents**

√5ᵗʰ **T45.9 Poisoning by, adverse effect of and underdosing of unspecified primarily systemic and hematological agent**

√x7ᵗʰ **T45.91 Poisoning by unspecified primarily systemic and hematological agent, accidental (unintentional)**

Poisoning by primarily systemic and hematological agent NOS

7 √x7ᵗʰ **T45.92 Poisoning by unspecified primarily systemic and hematological agent, intentional self-harm** HCC

√x7ᵗʰ **T45.93 Poisoning by unspecified primarily systemic and hematological agent, assault**

√x7ᵗʰ **T45.94 Poisoning by unspecified primarily systemic and hematological agent, undetermined**

√x7ᵗʰ **T45.95 Adverse effect of unspecified primarily systemic and hematological agent**

√x7ᵗʰ **T45.96 Underdosing of unspecified primarily systemic and hematological agent**

√4ᵗʰ **T46 Poisoning by, adverse effect of and underdosing of agents primarily affecting the cardiovascular system**

EXCLUDES 1   poisoning by, adverse effect of and underdosing of metaraminol (T44.4)

The appropriate 7th character is to be added to each code from category T46.
A   initial encounter
D   subsequent encounter
S   sequela

√5ᵗʰ **T46.0 Poisoning by, adverse effect of and underdosing of cardiac-stimulant glycosides and drugs of similar action**

√6ᵗʰ **T46.0X Poisoning by, adverse effect of and underdosing of cardiac-stimulant glycosides and drugs of similar action**

√7ᵗʰ **T46.0X1 Poisoning by cardiac-stimulant glycosides and drugs of similar action, accidental (unintentional)**

Poisoning by cardiac-stimulant glycosides and drugs of similar action NOS

7 √7ᵗʰ **T46.0X2 Poisoning by cardiac-stimulant glycosides and drugs of similar action, intentional self-harm** HCC

√7ᵗʰ **T46.0X3 Poisoning by cardiac-stimulant glycosides and drugs of similar action, assault**

√7ᵗʰ **T46.0X4 Poisoning by cardiac-stimulant glycosides and drugs of similar action, undetermined**

√7ᵗʰ **T46.0X5 Adverse effect of cardiac-stimulant glycosides and drugs of similar action**

√7ᵗʰ **T46.0X6 Underdosing of cardiac-stimulant glycosides and drugs of similar action**

√5ᵗʰ **T46.1 Poisoning by, adverse effect of and underdosing of calcium-channel blockers**

√6ᵗʰ **T46.1X Poisoning by, adverse effect of and underdosing of calcium-channel blockers**

√7ᵗʰ **T46.1X1 Poisoning by calcium-channel blockers, accidental (unintentional)**

Poisoning by calcium-channel blockers NOS

7 √7ᵗʰ **T46.1X2 Poisoning by calcium-channel blockers, intentional self-harm** HCC

√7ᵗʰ **T46.1X3 Poisoning by calcium-channel blockers, assault**

√7ᵗʰ **T46.1X4 Poisoning by calcium-channel blockers, undetermined**

√7ᵗʰ **T46.1X5 Adverse effect of calcium-channel blockers**

√7ᵗʰ **T46.1X6 Underdosing of calcium-channel blockers**

√5ᵗʰ **T46.2 Poisoning by, adverse effect of and underdosing of other antidysrhythmic drugs, not elsewhere classified**

EXCLUDES 1   poisoning by, adverse effect of and underdosing of beta-adrenoreceptor antagonists (T44.7-)

√6ᵗʰ **T46.2X Poisoning by, adverse effect of and underdosing of other antidysrhythmic drugs**

√7ᵗʰ **T46.2X1 Poisoning by other antidysrhythmic drugs, accidental (unintentional)**

Poisoning by other antidysrhythmic drugs NOS

7 √7ᵗʰ **T46.2X2 Poisoning by other antidysrhythmic drugs, intentional self-harm** HCC

√7ᵗʰ **T46.2X3 Poisoning by other antidysrhythmic drugs, assault**

√7ᵗʰ **T46.2X4 Poisoning by other antidysrhythmic drugs, undetermined**

√7ᵗʰ **T46.2X5 Adverse effect of other antidysrhythmic drugs**

√7ᵗʰ **T46.2X6 Underdosing of other antidysrhythmic drugs**

√5ᵗʰ **T46.3 Poisoning by, adverse effect of and underdosing of coronary vasodilators**

Poisoning by, adverse effect of and underdosing of dipyridamole

EXCLUDES 1   poisoning by, adverse effect of and underdosing of calcium-channel blockers (T46.1)

√6ᵗʰ **T46.3X Poisoning by, adverse effect of and underdosing of coronary vasodilators**

√7ᵗʰ **T46.3X1 Poisoning by coronary vasodilators, accidental (unintentional)**

Poisoning by coronary vasodilators NOS

7 √7ᵗʰ **T46.3X2 Poisoning by coronary vasodilators, intentional self-harm** HCC

√7ᵗʰ **T46.3X3 Poisoning by coronary vasodilators, assault**

√7ᵗʰ **T46.3X4 Poisoning by coronary vasodilators, undetermined**

√7ᵗʰ **T46.3X5 Adverse effect of coronary vasodilators**

√7ᵗʰ **T46.3X6 Underdosing of coronary vasodilators**

√5ᵗʰ **T46.4 Poisoning by, adverse effect of and underdosing of angiotensin-converting-enzyme inhibitors**

√6ᵗʰ **T46.4X Poisoning by, adverse effect of and underdosing of angiotensin-converting-enzyme inhibitors**

√7ᵗʰ **T46.4X1 Poisoning by angiotensin-converting-enzyme inhibitors, accidental (unintentional)**

Poisoning by angiotensin-converting-enzyme inhibitors NOS

7 √7ᵗʰ **T46.4X2 Poisoning by angiotensin-converting-enzyme inhibitors, intentional self-harm** HCC

√7ᵗʰ **T46.4X3 Poisoning by angiotensin-converting-enzyme inhibitors, assault**

√7ᵗʰ **T46.4X4 Poisoning by angiotensin-converting-enzyme inhibitors, undetermined**

√7ᵗʰ **T46.4X5 Adverse effect of angiotensin-converting-enzyme inhibitors**

√7ᵗʰ **T46.4X6 Underdosing of angiotensin-converting-enzyme inhibitors**

☑ Additional Character Required   √x7ᵗʰ Placeholder   Unacceptable PDx   Questionable PDx   Manifestation   Unspecified Dx   H1-H4 HAC   HCC CMS-HCC Dx   HIV HIV Dx

ICD-10-CM 2021   1123

√5ᵗʰ **T46.5** **Poisoning by, adverse effect of and underdosing of other antihypertensive drugs**

     EXCLUDES 2   *poisoning by, adverse effect of and underdosing of beta-adrenoreceptor antagonists (T44.7)*
           poisoning by, adverse effect of and underdosing of calcium-channel blockers (T46.1)
           poisoning by, adverse effect of and underdosing of diuretics (T50.0-T50.2)

   √6ᵗʰ **T46.5X** **Poisoning by, adverse effect of and underdosing of other antihypertensive drugs**

       √7ᵗʰ **T46.5X1** **Poisoning by other antihypertensive drugs, accidental (unintentional)**
           Poisoning by other antihypertensive drugs NOS

       7 √7ᵗʰ **T46.5X2** **Poisoning by other antihypertensive drugs, intentional self-harm**   HCC

       √7ᵗʰ **T46.5X3** **Poisoning by other antihypertensive drugs, assault**

       √7ᵗʰ **T46.5X4** **Poisoning by other antihypertensive drugs, undetermined**

       √7ᵗʰ **T46.5X5** **Adverse effect of other antihypertensive drugs**

       √7ᵗʰ **T46.5X6** **Underdosing of other antihypertensive drugs**

√5ᵗʰ **T46.6** **Poisoning by, adverse effect of and underdosing of antihyperlipidemic and antiarteriosclerotic drugs**

   √6ᵗʰ **T46.6X** **Poisoning by, adverse effect of and underdosing of antihyperlipidemic and antiarteriosclerotic drugs**

       √7ᵗʰ **T46.6X1** **Poisoning by antihyperlipidemic and antiarteriosclerotic drugs, accidental (unintentional)**
           Poisoning by antihyperlipidemic and antiarteriosclerotic drugs NOS

       7 √7ᵗʰ **T46.6X2** **Poisoning by antihyperlipidemic and antiarteriosclerotic drugs, intentional self-harm**   HCC

       √7ᵗʰ **T46.6X3** **Poisoning by antihyperlipidemic and antiarteriosclerotic drugs, assault**

       √7ᵗʰ **T46.6X4** **Poisoning by antihyperlipidemic and antiarteriosclerotic drugs, undetermined**

       √7ᵗʰ **T46.6X5** **Adverse effect of antihyperlipidemic and antiarteriosclerotic drugs**

       √7ᵗʰ **T46.6X6** **Underdosing of antihyperlipidemic and antiarteriosclerotic drugs**

√5ᵗʰ **T46.7** **Poisoning by, adverse effect of and underdosing of peripheral vasodilators**

     Poisoning by, adverse effect of and underdosing of nicotinic acid (derivatives)

     EXCLUDES 1   *poisoning by, adverse effect of and underdosing of papaverine (T44.3)*

   √6ᵗʰ **T46.7X** **Poisoning by, adverse effect of and underdosing of peripheral vasodilators**

       √7ᵗʰ **T46.7X1** **Poisoning by peripheral vasodilators, accidental (unintentional)**
           Poisoning by peripheral vasodilators NOS

       7 √7ᵗʰ **T46.7X2** **Poisoning by peripheral vasodilators, intentional self-harm**   HCC

       √7ᵗʰ **T46.7X3** **Poisoning by peripheral vasodilators, assault**

       √7ᵗʰ **T46.7X4** **Poisoning by peripheral vasodilators, undetermined**

       √7ᵗʰ **T46.7X5** **Adverse effect of peripheral vasodilators**

       √7ᵗʰ **T46.7X6** **Underdosing of peripheral vasodilators**

√5ᵗʰ **T46.8** **Poisoning by, adverse effect of and underdosing of antivaricose drugs, including sclerosing agents**

   √6ᵗʰ **T46.8X** **Poisoning by, adverse effect of and underdosing of antivaricose drugs, including sclerosing agents**

       √7ᵗʰ **T46.8X1** **Poisoning by antivaricose drugs, including sclerosing agents, accidental (unintentional)**
           Poisoning by antivaricose drugs, including sclerosing agents NOS

       7 √7ᵗʰ **T46.8X2** **Poisoning by antivaricose drugs, including sclerosing agents, intentional self-harm**   HCC

       √7ᵗʰ **T46.8X3** **Poisoning by antivaricose drugs, including sclerosing agents, assault**

       √7ᵗʰ **T46.8X4** **Poisoning by antivaricose drugs, including sclerosing agents, undetermined**

       √7ᵗʰ **T46.8X5** **Adverse effect of antivaricose drugs, including sclerosing agents**

       √7ᵗʰ **T46.8X6** **Underdosing of antivaricose drugs, including sclerosing agents**

√5ᵗʰ **T46.9** **Poisoning by, adverse effect of and underdosing of other and unspecified agents primarily affecting the cardiovascular system**

   √6ᵗʰ **T46.90** **Poisoning by, adverse effect of and underdosing of unspecified agents primarily affecting the cardiovascular system**

       √7ᵗʰ **T46.901** **Poisoning by unspecified agents primarily affecting the cardiovascular system, accidental (unintentional)**

       7 √7ᵗʰ **T46.902** **Poisoning by unspecified agents primarily affecting the cardiovascular system, intentional self-harm**   HCC

       √7ᵗʰ **T46.903** **Poisoning by unspecified agents primarily affecting the cardiovascular system, assault**

       √7ᵗʰ **T46.904** **Poisoning by unspecified agents primarily affecting the cardiovascular system, undetermined**

       √7ᵗʰ **T46.905** **Adverse effect of unspecified agents primarily affecting the cardiovascular system**

       √7ᵗʰ **T46.906** **Underdosing of unspecified agents primarily affecting the cardiovascular system**

   √6ᵗʰ **T46.99** **Poisoning by, adverse effect of and underdosing of other agents primarily affecting the cardiovascular system**

       √7ᵗʰ **T46.991** **Poisoning by other agents primarily affecting the cardiovascular system, accidental (unintentional)**

       7 √7ᵗʰ **T46.992** **Poisoning by other agents primarily affecting the cardiovascular system, intentional self-harm**   HCC

       √7ᵗʰ **T46.993** **Poisoning by other agents primarily affecting the cardiovascular system, assault**

       √7ᵗʰ **T46.994** **Poisoning by other agents primarily affecting the cardiovascular system, undetermined**

       √7ᵗʰ **T46.995** **Adverse effect of other agents primarily affecting the cardiovascular system**

       √7ᵗʰ **T46.996** **Underdosing of other agents primarily affecting the cardiovascular system**

√4ᵗʰ **T47** **Poisoning by, adverse effect of and underdosing of agents primarily affecting the gastrointestinal system**

     The appropriate 7th character is to be added to each code from category T47.
     A   initial encounter
     D   subsequent encounter
     S   sequela

√5ᵗʰ **T47.0** **Poisoning by, adverse effect of and underdosing of histamine H2-receptor blockers**

   √6ᵗʰ **T47.0X** **Poisoning by, adverse effect of and underdosing of histamine H2-receptor blockers**

       √7ᵗʰ **T47.0X1** **Poisoning by histamine H2-receptor blockers, accidental (unintentional)**
           Poisoning by histamine H2-receptor blockers NOS

       7 √7ᵗʰ **T47.0X2** **Poisoning by histamine H2-receptor blockers, intentional self-harm**   HCC

       √7ᵗʰ **T47.0X3** **Poisoning by histamine H2-receptor blockers, assault**

       √7ᵗʰ **T47.0X4** **Poisoning by histamine H2-receptor blockers, undetermined**

       √7ᵗʰ **T47.0X5** **Adverse effect of histamine H2-receptor blockers**

       √7ᵗʰ **T47.0X6** **Underdosing of histamine H2-receptor blockers**

√5ᵗʰ **T47.1** **Poisoning by, adverse effect of and underdosing of other antacids and anti-gastric-secretion drugs**

   √6ᵗʰ **T47.1X** **Poisoning by, adverse effect of and underdosing of other antacids and anti-gastric-secretion drugs**

       √7ᵗʰ **T47.1X1** **Poisoning by other antacids and anti-gastric-secretion drugs, accidental (unintentional)**
           Poisoning by other antacids and anti-gastric-secretion drugs NOS

       7 √7ᵗʰ **T47.1X2** **Poisoning by other antacids and anti-gastric-secretion drugs, intentional self-harm**   HCC

√7ᵗʰ **T47.1X3** **Poisoning by other antacids and anti-gastric-secretion drugs**, assault

√7ᵗʰ **T47.1X4** **Poisoning by other antacids and anti-gastric-secretion drugs, undetermined**

√7ᵗʰ **T47.1X5** Adverse effect **of other antacids and anti-gastric-secretion drugs**

√7ᵗʰ **T47.1X6** Underdosing **of other antacids and anti-gastric-secretion drugs**

√5ᵗʰ **T47.2** **Poisoning by, adverse effect of and underdosing of stimulant laxatives**

√6ᵗʰ **T47.2X** **Poisoning by, adverse effect of and underdosing of** stimulant laxatives

√7ᵗʰ **T47.2X1** **Poisoning by stimulant laxatives,** accidental **(unintentional)**
Poisoning by stimulant laxatives NOS

7 √7ᵗʰ **T47.2X2** **Poisoning by stimulant laxatives,** intentional self-harm   HCC

√7ᵗʰ **T47.2X3** **Poisoning by stimulant laxatives,** assault

√7ᵗʰ **T47.2X4** **Poisoning by stimulant laxatives, undetermined**

√7ᵗʰ **T47.2X5** Adverse effect **of stimulant laxatives**

√7ᵗʰ **T47.2X6** Underdosing **of stimulant laxatives**

√5ᵗʰ **T47.3** **Poisoning by, adverse effect of and underdosing of saline and osmotic laxatives**

√6ᵗʰ **T47.3X** **Poisoning by and adverse effect of** saline and osmotic laxatives

√7ᵗʰ **T47.3X1** **Poisoning by saline and osmotic laxatives,** accidental **(unintentional)**
Poisoning by saline and osmotic laxatives NOS

7 √7ᵗʰ **T47.3X2** **Poisoning by saline and osmotic laxatives, intentional self-harm**   HCC

√7ᵗʰ **T47.3X3** **Poisoning by saline and osmotic laxatives,** assault

√7ᵗʰ **T47.3X4** **Poisoning by saline and osmotic laxatives, undetermined**

√7ᵗʰ **T47.3X5** Adverse effect **of saline and osmotic laxatives**

√7ᵗʰ **T47.3X6** Underdosing **of saline and osmotic laxatives**

√5ᵗʰ **T47.4** **Poisoning by, adverse effect of and underdosing of other laxatives**

√6ᵗʰ **T47.4X** **Poisoning by, adverse effect of and underdosing of other laxatives**

√7ᵗʰ **T47.4X1** **Poisoning by other laxatives,** accidental **(unintentional)**
Poisoning by other laxatives NOS

7 √7ᵗʰ **T47.4X2** **Poisoning by other laxatives,** intentional self-harm   HCC

√7ᵗʰ **T47.4X3** **Poisoning by other laxatives,** assault

√7ᵗʰ **T47.4X4** **Poisoning by other laxatives, undetermined**

√7ᵗʰ **T47.4X5** Adverse effect **of other laxatives**

√7ᵗʰ **T47.4X6** Underdosing **of other laxatives**

√5ᵗʰ **T47.5** **Poisoning by, adverse effect of and underdosing of digestants**

√6ᵗʰ **T47.5X** **Poisoning by, adverse effect of and underdosing of** digestants

√7ᵗʰ **T47.5X1** **Poisoning by digestants,** accidental **(unintentional)**
Poisoning by digestants NOS

7 √7ᵗʰ **T47.5X2** **Poisoning by digestants,** intentional self-harm   HCC

√7ᵗʰ **T47.5X3** **Poisoning by digestants,** assault

√7ᵗʰ **T47.5X4** **Poisoning by digestants,** undetermined

√7ᵗʰ **T47.5X5** Adverse effect **of digestants**

√7ᵗʰ **T47.5X6** Underdosing **of digestants**

√5ᵗʰ **T47.6** **Poisoning by, adverse effect of and underdosing of antidiarrheal drugs**

EXCLUDES 2   *poisoning by, adverse effect of and underdosing of systemic antibiotics and other anti-infectives (T36-T37)*

√6ᵗʰ **T47.6X** **Poisoning by, adverse effect of and underdosing of** antidiarrheal drugs

√7ᵗʰ **T47.6X1** **Poisoning by antidiarrheal drugs,** accidental **(unintentional)**
Poisoning by antidiarrheal drugs NOS

7 √7ᵗʰ **T47.6X2** **Poisoning by antidiarrheal drugs, intentional self-harm**   HCC

√7ᵗʰ **T47.6X3** **Poisoning by antidiarrheal drugs,** assault

√7ᵗʰ **T47.6X4** **Poisoning by antidiarrheal drugs, undetermined**

√7ᵗʰ **T47.6X5** Adverse effect **of antidiarrheal drugs**

√7ᵗʰ **T47.6X6** Underdosing **of antidiarrheal drugs**

√5ᵗʰ **T47.7** **Poisoning by, adverse effect of and underdosing of emetics**

√6ᵗʰ **T47.7X** **Poisoning by, adverse effect of and underdosing of** emetics

√7ᵗʰ **T47.7X1** **Poisoning by emetics,** accidental **(unintentional)**
Poisoning by emetics NOS

7 √7ᵗʰ **T47.7X2** **Poisoning by emetics,** intentional self-harm   HCC

√7ᵗʰ **T47.7X3** **Poisoning by emetics,** assault

√7ᵗʰ **T47.7X4** **Poisoning by emetics,** undetermined

√7ᵗʰ **T47.7X5** Adverse effect **of emetics**

√7ᵗʰ **T47.7X6** Underdosing **of emetics**

√5ᵗʰ **T47.8** **Poisoning by, adverse effect of and underdosing of other agents primarily affecting gastrointestinal system**

√6ᵗʰ **T47.8X** **Poisoning by, adverse effect of and underdosing of other agents primarily affecting gastrointestinal system**

√7ᵗʰ **T47.8X1** **Poisoning by other agents primarily affecting gastrointestinal system,** accidental **(unintentional)**
Poisoning by other agents primarily affecting gastrointestinal system NOS

7 √7ᵗʰ **T47.8X2** **Poisoning by other agents primarily affecting gastrointestinal system,** intentional self-harm   HCC

√7ᵗʰ **T47.8X3** **Poisoning by other agents primarily affecting gastrointestinal system,** assault

√7ᵗʰ **T47.8X4** **Poisoning by other agents primarily affecting gastrointestinal system, undetermined**

√7ᵗʰ **T47.8X5** Adverse effect **of other agents primarily affecting gastrointestinal system**

√7ᵗʰ **T47.8X6** Underdosing **of other agents primarily affecting gastrointestinal system**

√5ᵗʰ **T47.9** **Poisoning by, adverse effect of and underdosing of unspecified agents primarily affecting the gastrointestinal system**

√×7ᵗʰ **T47.91** **Poisoning by unspecified agents primarily affecting the gastrointestinal system,** accidental **(unintentional)**
Poisoning by agents primarily affecting the gastrointestinal system NOS

7 √×7ᵗʰ **T47.92** **Poisoning by unspecified agents primarily affecting the gastrointestinal system,** intentional self-harm   HCC

√×7ᵗʰ **T47.93** **Poisoning by unspecified agents primarily affecting the gastrointestinal system,** assault

√×7ᵗʰ **T47.94** **Poisoning by unspecified agents primarily affecting the gastrointestinal system,** undetermined

√×7ᵗʰ **T47.95** Adverse effect **of unspecified agents primarily affecting the gastrointestinal system**

√×7ᵗʰ **T47.96** Underdosing **of unspecified agents primarily affecting the gastrointestinal system**

√4ᵗʰ **T48** **Poisoning by, adverse effect of and underdosing of agents primarily acting on smooth and skeletal muscles and the respiratory system**

The appropriate 7th character is to be added to each code from category T48.
A   initial encounter
D   subsequent encounter
S   sequela

√5ᵗʰ **T48.0** **Poisoning by, adverse effect of and underdosing of oxytocic drugs**

EXCLUDES 1   *poisoning by, adverse effect of and underdosing of estrogens, progestogens and antagonists (T38.4-T38.6)*

√6ᵗʰ **T48.0X** **Poisoning by, adverse effect of and underdosing of** oxytocic drugs

√7ᵗʰ **T48.0X1** **Poisoning by oxytocic drugs,** accidental **(unintentional)**
Poisoning by oxytocic drugs NOS

7 √7ᵗʰ **T48.0X2** **Poisoning by oxytocic drugs,** intentional self-harm   HCC

√7ᵗʰ **T48.0X3** **Poisoning by oxytocic drugs,** assault

☑ Additional Character Required   √×7ᵗʰ Placeholder   Unacceptable PDx   Questionable PDx   Manifestation   Unspecified Dx   H1-H4 HAC   HCC CMS-HCC Dx   HIV HIV Dx

ICD-10-CM 2021   1125

✓7th **T48.0X4** **Poisoning by oxytocic drugs, undetermined**

✓7th **T48.0X5** **Adverse effect of oxytocic drugs**

✓7th **T48.0X6** **Underdosing of oxytocic drugs**

✓5th **T48.1** **Poisoning by, adverse effect of and underdosing of skeletal muscle relaxants [neuromuscular blocking agents]**

   ✓6th **T48.1X** **Poisoning by, adverse effect of and underdosing of skeletal muscle relaxants [neuromuscular blocking agents]**

      ✓7th **T48.1X1** **Poisoning by skeletal muscle relaxants [neuromuscular blocking agents], accidental (unintentional)**

         Poisoning by skeletal muscle relaxants [neuromuscular blocking agents] NOS

     7 ✓7th **T48.1X2** **Poisoning by skeletal muscle relaxants [neuromuscular blocking agents], intentional self-harm**   HCC

      ✓7th **T48.1X3** **Poisoning by skeletal muscle relaxants [neuromuscular blocking agents], assault**

      ✓7th **T48.1X4** **Poisoning by skeletal muscle relaxants [neuromuscular blocking agents], undetermined**

      ✓7th **T48.1X5** **Adverse effect of skeletal muscle relaxants [neuromuscular blocking agents]**

      ✓7th **T48.1X6** **Underdosing of skeletal muscle relaxants [neuromuscular blocking agents]**

✓5th **T48.2** **Poisoning by, adverse effect of and underdosing of other and unspecified drugs acting on muscles**

   ✓6th **T48.20** **Poisoning by, adverse effect of and underdosing of unspecified drugs acting on muscles**

      ✓7th **T48.201** **Poisoning by unspecified drugs acting on muscles, accidental (unintentional)**

         Poisoning by unspecified drugs acting on muscles NOS

     7 ✓7th **T48.202** **Poisoning by unspecified drugs acting on muscles, intentional self-harm**   HCC

      ✓7th **T48.203** **Poisoning by unspecified drugs acting on muscles, assault**

      ✓7th **T48.204** **Poisoning by unspecified drugs acting on muscles, undetermined**

      ✓7th **T48.205** **Adverse effect of unspecified drugs acting on muscles**

      ✓7th **T48.206** **Underdosing of unspecified drugs acting on muscles**

   ✓6th **T48.29** **Poisoning by, adverse effect of and underdosing of other drugs acting on muscles**

      ✓7th **T48.291** **Poisoning by other drugs acting on muscles, accidental (unintentional)**

         Poisoning by other drugs acting on muscles NOS

     7 ✓7th **T48.292** **Poisoning by other drugs acting on muscles, intentional self-harm**   HCC

      ✓7th **T48.293** **Poisoning by other drugs acting on muscles, assault**

      ✓7th **T48.294** **Poisoning by other drugs acting on muscles, undetermined**

      ✓7th **T48.295** **Adverse effect of other drugs acting on muscles**

      ✓7th **T48.296** **Underdosing of other drugs acting on muscles**

✓5th **T48.3** **Poisoning by, adverse effect of and underdosing of antitussives**

   ✓6th **T48.3X** **Poisoning by, adverse effect of and underdosing of antitussives**

      ✓7th **T48.3X1** **Poisoning by antitussives, accidental (unintentional)**

         Poisoning by antitussives NOS

     7 ✓7th **T48.3X2** **Poisoning by antitussives, intentional self-harm**   HCC

      ✓7th **T48.3X3** **Poisoning by antitussives, assault**

      ✓7th **T48.3X4** **Poisoning by antitussives, undetermined**

      ✓7th **T48.3X5** **Adverse effect of antitussives**

      ✓7th **T48.3X6** **Underdosing of antitussives**

✓5th **T48.4** **Poisoning by, adverse effect of and underdosing of expectorants**

   ✓6th **T48.4X** **Poisoning by, adverse effect of and underdosing of expectorants**

      ✓7th **T48.4X1** **Poisoning by expectorants, accidental (unintentional)**

         Poisoning by expectorants NOS

     7 ✓7th **T48.4X2** **Poisoning by expectorants, intentional self-harm**   HCC

      ✓7th **T48.4X3** **Poisoning by expectorants, assault**

      ✓7th **T48.4X4** **Poisoning by expectorants, undetermined**

      ✓7th **T48.4X5** **Adverse effect of expectorants**

      ✓7th **T48.4X6** **Underdosing of expectorants**

✓5th **T48.5** **Poisoning by, adverse effect of and underdosing of other anti-common-cold drugs**

   Poisoning by, adverse effect of and underdosing of decongestants

   EXCLUDES 2   poisoning by, adverse effect of and underdosing of antipyretics, NEC (T39.9-)

        poisoning by, adverse effect of and underdosing of non-steroidal antiinflammatory drugs (T39.3-)

        poisoning by, adverse effect of and underdosing of salicylates (T39.0-)

   ✓6th **T48.5X** **Poisoning by, adverse effect of and underdosing of other anti-common-cold drugs**

      ✓7th **T48.5X1** **Poisoning by other anti-common-cold drugs, accidental (unintentional)**

         Poisoning by other anti-common-cold drugs NOS

     7 ✓7th **T48.5X2** **Poisoning by other anti-common-cold drugs, intentional self-harm**   HCC

      ✓7th **T48.5X3** **Poisoning by other anti-common-cold drugs, assault**

      ✓7th **T48.5X4** **Poisoning by other anti-common-cold drugs, undetermined**

      ✓7th **T48.5X5** **Adverse effect of other anti-common-cold drugs**

      ✓7th **T48.5X6** **Underdosing of other anti-common-cold drugs**

✓5th **T48.6** **Poisoning by, adverse effect of and underdosing of antiasthmatics, not elsewhere classified**

   Poisoning by, adverse effect of and underdosing of beta-adrenoreceptor agonists used in asthma therapy

   EXCLUDES 1   poisoning by, adverse effect of and underdosing of anterior pituitary [adenohypophyseal] hormones (T38.8)

        poisoning by, adverse effect of and underdosing of beta-adrenoreceptor agonists not used in asthma therapy (T44.5)

   ✓6th **T48.6X** **Poisoning by, adverse effect of and underdosing of antiasthmatics**

      ✓7th **T48.6X1** **Poisoning by antiasthmatics, accidental (unintentional)**

         Poisoning by antiasthmatics NOS

     7 ✓7th **T48.6X2** **Poisoning by antiasthmatics, intentional self-harm**   HCC

      ✓7th **T48.6X3** **Poisoning by antiasthmatics, assault**

      ✓7th **T48.6X4** **Poisoning by antiasthmatics, undetermined**

      ✓7th **T48.6X5** **Adverse effect of antiasthmatics**

      ✓7th **T48.6X6** **Underdosing of antiasthmatics**

✓5th **T48.9** **Poisoning by, adverse effect of and underdosing of other and unspecified agents primarily acting on the respiratory system**

   ✓6th **T48.90** **Poisoning by, adverse effect of and underdosing of unspecified agents primarily acting on the respiratory system**

      ✓7th **T48.901** **Poisoning by unspecified agents primarily acting on the respiratory system, accidental (unintentional)**

     7 ✓7th **T48.902** **Poisoning by unspecified agents primarily acting on the respiratory system, intentional self-harm**   HCC

      ✓7th **T48.903** **Poisoning by unspecified agents primarily acting on the respiratory system, assault**

      ✓7th **T48.904** **Poisoning by unspecified agents primarily acting on the respiratory system, undetermined**

N Newborn: 0   **P** Pediatric: 0-17   **M** Maternity: 9-64   **A** Adult: 15-124   **MCC** Major Complication/Comorbidity   **CC** Complication/Comorbidity   **SW** Severe Wound Dx

1126   ICD-10-CM 2021

√7ᵗʰ **T48.905** Adverse effect of unspecified agents primarily acting on the respiratory system

√7ᵗʰ **T48.906** Underdosing of unspecified agents primarily acting on the respiratory system

√6ᵗʰ **T48.99** Poisoning by, adverse effect of and underdosing of other agents primarily acting on the respiratory system

     √7ᵗʰ **T48.991** Poisoning by other agents primarily acting on the respiratory system, accidental (unintentional)

     7 √7ᵗʰ **T48.992** Poisoning by other agents primarily acting on the respiratory system, intentional self-harm   HCC

     √7ᵗʰ **T48.993** Poisoning by other agents primarily acting on the respiratory system, assault

     √7ᵗʰ **T48.994** Poisoning by other agents primarily acting on the respiratory system, undetermined

     √7ᵗʰ **T48.995** Adverse effect of other agents primarily acting on the respiratory system

     √7ᵗʰ **T48.996** Underdosing of other agents primarily acting on the respiratory system

√4ᵗʰ **T49** **Poisoning by, adverse effect of and underdosing of topical agents primarily affecting skin and mucous membrane and by ophthalmological, otorhinolaryngological and dental drugs**

     INCLUDES   poisoning by, adverse effect of and underdosing of glucocorticoids, topically used

> The appropriate 7th character is to be added to each code from category T49.
> A   initial encounter
> D   subsequent encounter
> S   sequela

√5ᵗʰ **T49.0** Poisoning by, adverse effect of and underdosing of local antifungal, anti-infective and anti-inflammatory drugs

   √6ᵗʰ **T49.0X** Poisoning by, adverse effect of and underdosing of local antifungal, anti-infective and anti-inflammatory drugs

     √7ᵗʰ **T49.0X1** Poisoning by local antifungal, anti-infective and anti-inflammatory drugs, accidental (unintentional)
       Poisoning by local antifungal, anti-infective and anti-inflammatory drugs NOS

     7 √7ᵗʰ **T49.0X2** Poisoning by local antifungal, anti-infective and anti-inflammatory drugs, intentional self-harm   HCC

     √7ᵗʰ **T49.0X3** Poisoning by local antifungal, anti-infective and anti-inflammatory drugs, assault

     √7ᵗʰ **T49.0X4** Poisoning by local antifungal, anti-infective and anti-inflammatory drugs, undetermined

     √7ᵗʰ **T49.0X5** Adverse effect of local antifungal, anti-infective and anti-inflammatory drugs

     √7ᵗʰ **T49.0X6** Underdosing of local antifungal, anti-infective and anti-inflammatory drugs

√5ᵗʰ **T49.1** Poisoning by, adverse effect of and underdosing of antipruritics

   √6ᵗʰ **T49.1X** Poisoning by, adverse effect of and underdosing of antipruritics

     √7ᵗʰ **T49.1X1** Poisoning by antipruritics, accidental (unintentional)
       Poisoning by antipruritics NOS

     7 √7ᵗʰ **T49.1X2** Poisoning by antipruritics, intentional self-harm   HCC

     √7ᵗʰ **T49.1X3** Poisoning by antipruritics, assault

     √7ᵗʰ **T49.1X4** Poisoning by antipruritics, undetermined

     √7ᵗʰ **T49.1X5** Adverse effect of antipruritics

     √7ᵗʰ **T49.1X6** Underdosing of antipruritics

√5ᵗʰ **T49.2** Poisoning by, adverse effect of and underdosing of local astringents and local detergents

   √6ᵗʰ **T49.2X** Poisoning by, adverse effect of and underdosing of local astringents and local detergents

     √7ᵗʰ **T49.2X1** Poisoning by local astringents and local detergents, accidental (unintentional)
       Poisoning by local astringents and local detergents NOS

     7 √7ᵗʰ **T49.2X2** Poisoning by local astringents and local detergents, intentional self-harm   HCC

     √7ᵗʰ **T49.2X3** Poisoning by local astringents and local detergents, assault

     √7ᵗʰ **T49.2X4** Poisoning by local astringents and local detergents, undetermined

     √7ᵗʰ **T49.2X5** Adverse effect of local astringents and local detergents

     √7ᵗʰ **T49.2X6** Underdosing of local astringents and local detergents

√5ᵗʰ **T49.3** Poisoning by, adverse effect of and underdosing of emollients, demulcents and protectants

   √6ᵗʰ **T49.3X** Poisoning by, adverse effect of and underdosing of emollients, demulcents and protectants

     √7ᵗʰ **T49.3X1** Poisoning by emollients, demulcents and protectants, accidental (unintentional)
       Poisoning by emollients, demulcents and protectants NOS

     7 √7ᵗʰ **T49.3X2** Poisoning by emollients, demulcents and protectants, intentional self-harm   HCC

     √7ᵗʰ **T49.3X3** Poisoning by emollients, demulcents and protectants, assault

     √7ᵗʰ **T49.3X4** Poisoning by emollients, demulcents and protectants, undetermined

     √7ᵗʰ **T49.3X5** Adverse effect of emollients, demulcents and protectants

     √7ᵗʰ **T49.3X6** Underdosing of emollients, demulcents and protectants

√5ᵗʰ **T49.4** Poisoning by, adverse effect of and underdosing of keratolytics, keratoplastics, and other hair treatment drugs and preparations

   √6ᵗʰ **T49.4X** Poisoning by, adverse effect of and underdosing of keratolytics, keratoplastics, and other hair treatment drugs and preparations

     √7ᵗʰ **T49.4X1** Poisoning by keratolytics, keratoplastics, and other hair treatment drugs and preparations, accidental (unintentional)
       Poisoning by keratolytics, keratoplastics, and other hair treatment drugs and preparations NOS

     7 √7ᵗʰ **T49.4X2** Poisoning by keratolytics, keratoplastics, and other hair treatment drugs and preparations, intentional self-harm   HCC

     √7ᵗʰ **T49.4X3** Poisoning by keratolytics, keratoplastics, and other hair treatment drugs and preparations, assault

     √7ᵗʰ **T49.4X4** Poisoning by keratolytics, keratoplastics, and other hair treatment drugs and preparations, undetermined

     √7ᵗʰ **T49.4X5** Adverse effect of keratolytics, keratoplastics, and other hair treatment drugs and preparations

     √7ᵗʰ **T49.4X6** Underdosing of keratolytics, keratoplastics, and other hair treatment drugs and preparations

√5ᵗʰ **T49.5** Poisoning by, adverse effect of and underdosing of ophthalmological drugs and preparations

   √6ᵗʰ **T49.5X** Poisoning by, adverse effect of and underdosing of ophthalmological drugs and preparations

     √7ᵗʰ **T49.5X1** Poisoning by ophthalmological drugs and preparations, accidental (unintentional)
       Poisoning by ophthalmological drugs and preparations NOS

     7 √7ᵗʰ **T49.5X2** Poisoning by ophthalmological drugs and preparations, intentional self-harm   HCC

     √7ᵗʰ **T49.5X3** Poisoning by ophthalmological drugs and preparations, assault

     √7ᵗʰ **T49.5X4** Poisoning by ophthalmological drugs and preparations, undetermined

     √7ᵗʰ **T49.5X5** Adverse effect of ophthalmological drugs and preparations

     √7ᵗʰ **T49.5X6** Underdosing of ophthalmological drugs and preparations

√5ᵗʰ **T49.6** Poisoning by, adverse effect of and underdosing of otorhinolaryngological drugs and preparations

   √6ᵗʰ **T49.6X** Poisoning by, adverse effect of and underdosing of otorhinolaryngological drugs and preparations

     √7ᵗʰ **T49.6X1** Poisoning by otorhinolaryngological drugs and preparations, accidental (unintentional)
       Poisoning by otorhinolaryngological drugs and preparations NOS

☑ Additional Character Required   √x7ᵗʰ Placeholder   Unacceptable PDx   Questionable PDx   Manifestation   Unspecified Dx   H1-H18 HAC   HCC CMS-HCC Dx   HIV HIV Dx

ICD-10-CM 2021   1127

7 √7ᵗʰ **T49.6X2** **Poisoning by otorhinolaryngological drugs and preparations, intentional self-harm** HCC

√7ᵗʰ **T49.6X3** **Poisoning by otorhinolaryngological drugs and preparations, assault**

√7ᵗʰ **T49.6X4** **Poisoning by otorhinolaryngological drugs and preparations, undetermined**

√7ᵗʰ **T49.6X5** **Adverse effect of otorhinolaryngological drugs and preparations**

√7ᵗʰ **T49.6X6** **Underdosing of otorhinolaryngological drugs and preparations**

√5ᵗʰ **T49.7** **Poisoning by, adverse effect of and underdosing of dental drugs, topically applied**

√6ᵗʰ **T49.7X** **Poisoning by, adverse effect of and underdosing of dental drugs, topically applied**

√7ᵗʰ **T49.7X1** **Poisoning by dental drugs, topically applied, accidental (unintentional)**
Poisoning by dental drugs, topically applied NOS

7 √7ᵗʰ **T49.7X2** **Poisoning by dental drugs, topically applied, intentional self-harm** HCC

√7ᵗʰ **T49.7X3** **Poisoning by dental drugs, topically applied, assault**

√7ᵗʰ **T49.7X4** **Poisoning by dental drugs, topically applied, undetermined**

√7ᵗʰ **T49.7X5** **Adverse effect of dental drugs, topically applied**

√7ᵗʰ **T49.7X6** **Underdosing of dental drugs, topically applied**

√5ᵗʰ **T49.8** **Poisoning by, adverse effect of and underdosing of other topical agents**
Poisoning by, adverse effect of and underdosing of spermicides

√6ᵗʰ **T49.8X** **Poisoning by, adverse effect of and underdosing of other topical agents**

√7ᵗʰ **T49.8X1** **Poisoning by other topical agents, accidental (unintentional)**
Poisoning by other topical agents NOS

7 √7ᵗʰ **T49.8X2** **Poisoning by other topical agents, intentional self-harm** HCC

√7ᵗʰ **T49.8X3** **Poisoning by other topical agents, assault**

√7ᵗʰ **T49.8X4** **Poisoning by other topical agents, undetermined**

√7ᵗʰ **T49.8X5** **Adverse effect of other topical agents**

√7ᵗʰ **T49.8X6** **Underdosing of other topical agents**

√5ᵗʰ **T49.9** **Poisoning by, adverse effect of and underdosing of unspecified topical agent**

√x7ᵗʰ **T49.91** **Poisoning by unspecified topical agent, accidental (unintentional)**

7 √x7ᵗʰ **T49.92** **Poisoning by unspecified topical agent, intentional self-harm** HCC

√x7ᵗʰ **T49.93** **Poisoning by unspecified topical agent, assault**

√x7ᵗʰ **T49.94** **Poisoning by unspecified topical agent, undetermined**

√x7ᵗʰ **T49.95** **Adverse effect of unspecified topical agent**

√x7ᵗʰ **T49.96** **Underdosing of unspecified topical agent**

√4ᵗʰ **T50** **Poisoning by, adverse effect of and underdosing of diuretics and other and unspecified drugs, medicaments and biological substances**

The appropriate 7th character is to be added to each code from category T50.
A   initial encounter
D   subsequent encounter
S   sequela

√5ᵗʰ **T50.0** **Poisoning by, adverse effect of and underdosing of mineralocorticoids and their antagonists**

√6ᵗʰ **T50.0X** **Poisoning by, adverse effect of and underdosing of mineralocorticoids and their antagonists**

√7ᵗʰ **T50.0X1** **Poisoning by mineralocorticoids and their antagonists, accidental (unintentional)**
Poisoning by mineralocorticoids and their antagonists NOS

7 √7ᵗʰ **T50.0X2** **Poisoning by mineralocorticoids and their antagonists, intentional self-harm** HCC

√7ᵗʰ **T50.0X3** **Poisoning by mineralocorticoids and their antagonists, assault**

√7ᵗʰ **T50.0X4** **Poisoning by mineralocorticoids and their antagonists, undetermined**

√7ᵗʰ **T50.0X5** **Adverse effect of mineralocorticoids and their antagonists**

√7ᵗʰ **T50.0X6** **Underdosing of mineralocorticoids and their antagonists**

√5ᵗʰ **T50.1** **Poisoning by, adverse effect of and underdosing of loop [high-ceiling] diuretics**

√6ᵗʰ **T50.1X** **Poisoning by, adverse effect of and underdosing of loop [high-ceiling] diuretics**

√7ᵗʰ **T50.1X1** **Poisoning by loop [high-ceiling] diuretics, accidental (unintentional)**
Poisoning by loop [high-ceiling] diuretics NOS

7 √7ᵗʰ **T50.1X2** **Poisoning by loop [high-ceiling] diuretics, intentional self-harm** HCC

√7ᵗʰ **T50.1X3** **Poisoning by loop [high-ceiling] diuretics, assault**

√7ᵗʰ **T50.1X4** **Poisoning by loop [high-ceiling] diuretics, undetermined**

√7ᵗʰ **T50.1X5** **Adverse effect of loop [high-ceiling] diuretics**

√7ᵗʰ **T50.1X6** **Underdosing of loop [high-ceiling] diuretics**

√5ᵗʰ **T50.2** **Poisoning by, adverse effect of and underdosing of carbonic-anhydrase inhibitors, benzothiadiazides and other diuretics**
Poisoning by, adverse effect of and underdosing of acetazolamide

√6ᵗʰ **T50.2X** **Poisoning by, adverse effect of and underdosing of carbonic-anhydrase inhibitors, benzothiadiazides and other diuretics**

√7ᵗʰ **T50.2X1** **Poisoning by carbonic-anhydrase inhibitors, benzothiadiazides and other diuretics, accidental (unintentional)**
Poisoning by carbonic-anhydrase inhibitors, benzothiadiazides and other diuretics NOS

7 √7ᵗʰ **T50.2X2** **Poisoning by carbonic-anhydrase inhibitors, benzothiadiazides and other diuretics, intentional self-harm** HCC

√7ᵗʰ **T50.2X3** **Poisoning by carbonic-anhydrase inhibitors, benzothiadiazides and other diuretics, assault**

√7ᵗʰ **T50.2X4** **Poisoning by carbonic-anhydrase inhibitors, benzothiadiazides and other diuretics, undetermined**

√7ᵗʰ **T50.2X5** **Adverse effect of carbonic-anhydrase inhibitors, benzothiadiazides and other diuretics**

√7ᵗʰ **T50.2X6** **Underdosing of carbonic-anhydrase inhibitors, benzothiadiazides and other diuretics**

√5ᵗʰ **T50.3** **Poisoning by, adverse effect of and underdosing of electrolytic, caloric and water-balance agents**
Poisoning by, adverse effect of and underdosing of oral rehydration salts

√6ᵗʰ **T50.3X** **Poisoning by, adverse effect of and underdosing of electrolytic, caloric and water-balance agents**

√7ᵗʰ **T50.3X1** **Poisoning by electrolytic, caloric and water-balance agents, accidental (unintentional)**
Poisoning by electrolytic, caloric and water-balance agents NOS

7 √7ᵗʰ **T50.3X2** **Poisoning by electrolytic, caloric and water-balance agents, intentional self-harm** HCC

√7ᵗʰ **T50.3X3** **Poisoning by electrolytic, caloric and water-balance agents, assault**

√7ᵗʰ **T50.3X4** **Poisoning by electrolytic, caloric and water-balance agents, undetermined**

√7ᵗʰ **T50.3X5** **Adverse effect of electrolytic, caloric and water-balance agents**

√7ᵗʰ **T50.3X6** **Underdosing of electrolytic, caloric and water-balance agents**

√5ᵗʰ **T50.4** **Poisoning by, adverse effect of and underdosing of drugs affecting uric acid metabolism**

√6ᵗʰ **T50.4X** **Poisoning by, adverse effect of and underdosing of drugs affecting uric acid metabolism**

√7ᵗʰ **T50.4X1** **Poisoning by drugs affecting uric acid metabolism, accidental (unintentional)**
Poisoning by drugs affecting uric acid metabolism NOS

7 √7ᵗʰ **T50.4X2** **Poisoning by drugs affecting uric acid metabolism, intentional self-harm** HCC

√7ᵗʰ **T50.4X3** **Poisoning by drugs affecting uric acid metabolism, assault**

    ✓7ᵗʰ **T50.4X4** **Poisoning by drugs affecting uric acid metabolism, undetermined**

    ✓7ᵗʰ **T50.4X5** Adverse effect **of drugs affecting uric acid metabolism**

    ✓7ᵗʰ **T50.4X6** Underdosing **of drugs affecting uric acid metabolism**

✓5ᵗʰ **T50.5** **Poisoning by, adverse effect of and underdosing of appetite depressants**

  ✓6ᵗʰ **T50.5X** **Poisoning by, adverse effect of and underdosing of** appetite depressants

    ✓7ᵗʰ **T50.5X1** **Poisoning by appetite depressants, accidental (unintentional)**
        Poisoning by appetite depressants NOS

    7 ✓7ᵗʰ **T50.5X2** **Poisoning by appetite depressants, intentional self-harm** HCC

    ✓7ᵗʰ **T50.5X3** **Poisoning by appetite depressants, assault**

    ✓7ᵗʰ **T50.5X4** **Poisoning by appetite depressants, undetermined**

    ✓7ᵗʰ **T50.5X5** Adverse effect **of appetite depressants**

    ✓7ᵗʰ **T50.5X6** Underdosing **of appetite depressants**

✓5ᵗʰ **T50.6** **Poisoning by, adverse effect of and underdosing of antidotes and chelating agents**
    Poisoning by, adverse effect of and underdosing of alcohol deterrents

  ✓6ᵗʰ **T50.6X** **Poisoning by, adverse effect of and underdosing of** antidotes and chelating agents

    ✓7ᵗʰ **T50.6X1** **Poisoning by antidotes and chelating agents, accidental (unintentional)**
        Poisoning by antidotes and chelating agents NOS

    7 ✓7ᵗʰ **T50.6X2** **Poisoning by antidotes and chelating agents, intentional self-harm** HCC

    ✓7ᵗʰ **T50.6X3** **Poisoning by antidotes and chelating agents, assault**

    ✓7ᵗʰ **T50.6X4** **Poisoning by antidotes and chelating agents, undetermined**

    ✓7ᵗʰ **T50.6X5** Adverse effect **of antidotes and chelating agents**

    ✓7ᵗʰ **T50.6X6** Underdosing **of antidotes and chelating agents**

✓5ᵗʰ **T50.7** **Poisoning by, adverse effect of and underdosing of analeptics and opioid receptor antagonists**

  ✓6ᵗʰ **T50.7X** **Poisoning by, adverse effect of and underdosing of** analeptics and opioid receptor antagonists

    ✓7ᵗʰ **T50.7X1** **Poisoning by analeptics and opioid receptor antagonists, accidental (unintentional)**
        Poisoning by analeptics and opioid receptor antagonists NOS

    7 ✓7ᵗʰ **T50.7X2** **Poisoning by analeptics and opioid receptor antagonists, intentional self-harm** HCC

    ✓7ᵗʰ **T50.7X3** **Poisoning by analeptics and opioid receptor antagonists, assault**

    ✓7ᵗʰ **T50.7X4** **Poisoning by analeptics and opioid receptor antagonists, undetermined**

    ✓7ᵗʰ **T50.7X5** Adverse effect **of analeptics and opioid receptor antagonists**

    ✓7ᵗʰ **T50.7X6** Underdosing **of analeptics and opioid receptor antagonists**

✓5ᵗʰ **T50.8** **Poisoning by, adverse effect of and underdosing of diagnostic agents**

  ✓6ᵗʰ **T50.8X** **Poisoning by, adverse effect of and underdosing of** diagnostic agents

    ✓7ᵗʰ **T50.8X1** **Poisoning by diagnostic agents, accidental (unintentional)**
        Poisoning by diagnostic agents NOS

    7 ✓7ᵗʰ **T50.8X2** **Poisoning by diagnostic agents, intentional self-harm** HCC

    ✓7ᵗʰ **T50.8X3** **Poisoning by diagnostic agents, assault**

    ✓7ᵗʰ **T50.8X4** **Poisoning by diagnostic agents, undetermined**

    ✓7ᵗʰ **T50.8X5** Adverse effect **of diagnostic agents**

    ✓7ᵗʰ **T50.8X6** Underdosing **of diagnostic agents**

✓5ᵗʰ **T50.A** **Poisoning by, adverse effect of and underdosing of bacterial vaccines**

  ✓6ᵗʰ **T50.A1** **Poisoning by, adverse effect of and underdosing of** pertussis vaccine, including combinations with a pertussis component

    ✓7ᵗʰ **T50.A11** **Poisoning by pertussis vaccine, including combinations with a pertussis component, accidental (unintentional)**

    7 ✓7ᵗʰ **T50.A12** **Poisoning by pertussis vaccine, including combinations with a pertussis component, intentional self-harm** HCC

    ✓7ᵗʰ **T50.A13** **Poisoning by pertussis vaccine, including combinations with a pertussis component, assault**

    ✓7ᵗʰ **T50.A14** **Poisoning by pertussis vaccine, including combinations with a pertussis component, undetermined**

    ✓7ᵗʰ **T50.A15** Adverse effect **of pertussis vaccine, including combinations with a pertussis component**

    ✓7ᵗʰ **T50.A16** Underdosing **of pertussis vaccine, including combinations with a pertussis component**

  ✓6ᵗʰ **T50.A2** **Poisoning by, adverse effect of and underdosing of** mixed bacterial vaccines without a pertussis component

    ✓7ᵗʰ **T50.A21** **Poisoning by mixed bacterial vaccines without a pertussis component, accidental (unintentional)**

    7 ✓7ᵗʰ **T50.A22** **Poisoning by mixed bacterial vaccines without a pertussis component, intentional self-harm** HCC

    ✓7ᵗʰ **T50.A23** **Poisoning by mixed bacterial vaccines without a pertussis component, assault**

    ✓7ᵗʰ **T50.A24** **Poisoning by mixed bacterial vaccines without a pertussis component, undetermined**

    ✓7ᵗʰ **T50.A25** Adverse effect **of mixed bacterial vaccines without a pertussis component**

    ✓7ᵗʰ **T50.A26** Underdosing **of mixed bacterial vaccines without a pertussis component**

  ✓6ᵗʰ **T50.A9** **Poisoning by, adverse effect of and underdosing of other bacterial vaccines**

    ✓7ᵗʰ **T50.A91** **Poisoning by other bacterial vaccines, accidental (unintentional)**

    7 ✓7ᵗʰ **T50.A92** **Poisoning by other bacterial vaccines, intentional self-harm** HCC

    ✓7ᵗʰ **T50.A93** **Poisoning by other bacterial vaccines, assault**

    ✓7ᵗʰ **T50.A94** **Poisoning by other bacterial vaccines, undetermined**

    ✓7ᵗʰ **T50.A95** Adverse effect **of other bacterial vaccines**

    ✓7ᵗʰ **T50.A96** Underdosing **of other bacterial vaccines**

✓5ᵗʰ **T50.B** **Poisoning by, adverse effect of and underdosing of viral vaccines**

  ✓6ᵗʰ **T50.B1** **Poisoning by, adverse effect of and underdosing of** smallpox vaccines

    ✓7ᵗʰ **T50.B11** **Poisoning by smallpox vaccines, accidental (unintentional)**

    7 ✓7ᵗʰ **T50.B12** **Poisoning by smallpox vaccines, intentional self-harm** HCC

    ✓7ᵗʰ **T50.B13** **Poisoning by smallpox vaccines, assault**

    ✓7ᵗʰ **T50.B14** **Poisoning by smallpox vaccines, undetermined**

    ✓7ᵗʰ **T50.B15** Adverse effect **of smallpox vaccines**

    ✓7ᵗʰ **T50.B16** Underdosing **of smallpox vaccines**

  ✓6ᵗʰ **T50.B9** **Poisoning by, adverse effect of and underdosing of other viral vaccines**

    ✓7ᵗʰ **T50.B91** **Poisoning by other viral vaccines, accidental (unintentional)**

  ✓6ᵗʰ **T50.90** **Poisoning by, adverse effect of and underdosing of unspecified drugs, medicaments and biological substances**

    7 ✓7ᵗʰ **T50.B92** **Poisoning by other viral vaccines, intentional self-harm** HCC

    ✓7ᵗʰ **T50.B93** **Poisoning by other viral vaccines, assault**

    ✓7ᵗʰ **T50.B94** **Poisoning by other viral vaccines, undetermined**

    ✓7ᵗʰ **T50.B95** Adverse effect **of other viral vaccines**

    ✓7ᵗʰ **T50.B96** Underdosing **of other viral vaccines**

☑ Additional Character Required   ✓x7ᵗʰ Placeholder   Unacceptable PDx   Questionable PDx   Manifestation   Unspecified Dx   H1-H4 HAC   HCC CMS-HCC Dx   HIV HIV Dx

ICD-10-CM 2021   1129

√5ᵗʰ **T50.Z** **Poisoning by, adverse effect of and underdosing of other vaccines and biological substances**

  √6ᵗʰ **T50.Z1** **Poisoning by, adverse effect of and underdosing of immunoglobulin**

    √7ᵗʰ **T50.Z11** **Poisoning by immunoglobulin, accidental (unintentional)**

    ⁷ √7ᵗʰ **T50.Z12** **Poisoning by immunoglobulin, intentional self-harm**   HCC

    √7ᵗʰ **T50.Z13** **Poisoning by immunoglobulin, assault**

    √7ᵗʰ **T50.Z14** **Poisoning by immunoglobulin, undetermined**

    √7ᵗʰ **T50.Z15** Adverse effect **of immunoglobulin**

    √7ᵗʰ **T50.Z16** Underdosing **of immunoglobulin**

  √6ᵗʰ **T50.Z9** **Poisoning by, adverse effect of and underdosing of other vaccines and biological substances**

    √7ᵗʰ **T50.Z91** **Poisoning by other vaccines and biological substances, accidental (unintentional)**

    ⁷ √7ᵗʰ **T50.Z92** **Poisoning by other vaccines and biological substances, intentional self-harm**   HCC

    √7ᵗʰ **T50.Z93** **Poisoning by other vaccines and biological substances, assault**

    √7ᵗʰ **T50.Z94** **Poisoning by other vaccines and biological substances, undetermined**

    √7ᵗʰ **T50.Z95** Adverse effect **of other vaccines and biological substances**

      AHA: 2020,1Q,18

    √7ᵗʰ **T50.Z96** Underdosing **of other vaccines and biological substances**

√5ᵗʰ **T50.9** **Poisoning by, adverse effect of and underdosing of other and unspecified drugs, medicaments and biological substances**

    √7ᵗʰ **T50.901** **Poisoning by unspecified drugs, medicaments and biological substances, accidental (unintentional)**

    ⁷ √7ᵗʰ **T50.902** **Poisoning by unspecified drugs, medicaments and biological substances, intentional self-harm**   HCC

    √7ᵗʰ **T50.903** **Poisoning by unspecified drugs, medicaments and biological substances, assault**

    √7ᵗʰ **T50.904** **Poisoning by unspecified drugs, medicaments and biological substances, undetermined**

    √7ᵗʰ **T50.905** Adverse effect **of unspecified drugs, medicaments and biological substances**

    √7ᵗʰ **T50.906** Underdosing **of unspecified drugs, medicaments and biological substances**

  √6ᵗʰ **T50.91** **Poisoning by, adverse effect of and underdosing of multiple unspecified drugs, medicaments and biological substances**

    Multiple drug ingestion NOS

    Code also any specific drugs, medicaments and biological substances

    √7ᵗʰ **T50.911** **Poisoning by multiple unspecified drugs, medicaments and biological substances, accidental (unintentional)**

    ⁷ √7ᵗʰ **T50.912** **Poisoning by multiple unspecified drugs, medicaments and biological substances, intentional self-harm**   HCC

    √7ᵗʰ **T50.913** **Poisoning by multiple unspecified drugs, medicaments and biological substances, assault**

    √7ᵗʰ **T50.914** **Poisoning by multiple unspecified drugs, medicaments and biological substances, undetermined**

    √7ᵗʰ **T50.915** Adverse effect **of multiple unspecified drugs, medicaments and biological substances**

    √7ᵗʰ **T50.916** Underdosing **of multiple unspecified drugs, medicaments and biological substances**

  √6ᵗʰ **T50.99** **Poisoning by, adverse effect of and underdosing of other drugs, medicaments and biological substances**

    √7ᵗʰ **T50.991** **Poisoning by other drugs, medicaments and biological substances, accidental (unintentional)**

    ⁷ √7ᵗʰ **T50.992** **Poisoning by other drugs, medicaments and biological substances, intentional self-harm**   HCC

    √7ᵗʰ **T50.993** **Poisoning by other drugs, medicaments and biological substances, assault**

    √7ᵗʰ **T50.994** **Poisoning by other drugs, medicaments and biological substances, undetermined**

    √7ᵗʰ **T50.995** Adverse effect **of other drugs, medicaments and biological substances**

    √7ᵗʰ **T50.996** Underdosing **of other drugs, medicaments and biological substances**

Toxic effects of substances chiefly nonmedicinal as to source (T51-T65)

NOTE   When no intent is indicated code to accidental. Undetermined intent is only for use when there is specific documentation in the record that the intent of the toxic effect cannot be determined.

Use additional code(s) for all associated manifestations of toxic effect, such as:
personal history of foreign body fully removed (Z87.821)
respiratory conditions due to external agents (J60-J70)
to identify any retained foreign body, if applicable (Z18.-)

EXCLUDES 1   contact with and (suspected) exposure to toxic substances (Z77.-)

AHA: 2017,1Q,39-40

√4ᵗʰ **T51** **Toxic effect of alcohol**

> The appropriate 7th character is to be added to each code from category T51.
> A   initial encounter
> D   subsequent encounter
> S   sequela

√5ᵗʰ **T51.0** **Toxic effect of ethanol**

  Toxic effect of ethyl alcohol

  EXCLUDES 2   acute alcohol intoxication or "hangover" effects (F10.129, F10.229, F10.929)
    drunkenness (F10.129, F10.229, F10.929)
    pathological alcohol intoxication (F10.129, F10.229, F10.929)

  √6ᵗʰ **T51.0X** **Toxic effect of ethanol**

    ⁶ √7ᵗʰ **T51.0X1** **Toxic effect of ethanol, accidental (unintentional)**   HCC
      Toxic effect of ethanol NOS

    ⁷ √7ᵗʰ **T51.0X2** **Toxic effect of ethanol, intentional self-harm**   HCC

    √7ᵗʰ **T51.0X3** **Toxic effect of ethanol, assault**

    ⁶ √7ᵗʰ **T51.0X4** **Toxic effect of ethanol, undetermined**   HCC

√5ᵗʰ **T51.1** **Toxic effect of methanol**

  Toxic effect of methyl alcohol

  √6ᵗʰ **T51.1X** **Toxic effect of methanol**

    √7ᵗʰ **T51.1X1** **Toxic effect of methanol, accidental (unintentional)**
      Toxic effect of methanol NOS

    ⁷ √7ᵗʰ **T51.1X2** **Toxic effect of methanol, intentional self-harm**   HCC

    √7ᵗʰ **T51.1X3** **Toxic effect of methanol, assault**

    √7ᵗʰ **T51.1X4** **Toxic effect of methanol, undetermined**

√5ᵗʰ **T51.2** **Toxic effect of 2-Propanol**

  Toxic effect of isopropyl alcohol

  √6ᵗʰ **T51.2X** **Toxic effect of 2-Propanol**

    √7ᵗʰ **T51.2X1** **Toxic effect of 2-Propanol, accidental (unintentional)**
      Toxic effect of 2-Propanol NOS

    ⁷ √7ᵗʰ **T51.2X2** **Toxic effect of 2-Propanol, intentional self-harm**   HCC

    √7ᵗʰ **T51.2X3** **Toxic effect of 2-Propanol, assault**

    √7ᵗʰ **T51.2X4** **Toxic effect of 2-Propanol, undetermined**

√5ᵗʰ **T51.3** **Toxic effect of fusel oil**

  Toxic effect of amyl alcohol
  Toxic effect of butyl [1-butanol] alcohol
  Toxic effect of propyl [1-propanol] alcohol

  √6ᵗʰ **T51.3X** **Toxic effect of fusel oil**

    √7ᵗʰ **T51.3X1** **Toxic effect of fusel oil, accidental (unintentional)**
      Toxic effect of fusel oil NOS

    ⁷ √7ᵗʰ **T51.3X2** **Toxic effect of fusel oil, intentional self-harm**   HCC

    √7ᵗʰ **T51.3X3** **Toxic effect of fusel oil, assault**

    √7ᵗʰ **T51.3X4** **Toxic effect of fusel oil, undetermined**

N Newborn: 0   P Pediatric: 0-17   M Maternity: 9-64   A Adult: 15-124   MCC Major Complication/Comorbidity   CC Complication/Comorbidity   SW Severe Wound Dx

1130   ICD-10-CM 2021

√5ᵗʰ **T51.8 Toxic effect of other alcohols**

   √6ᵗʰ **T51.8X Toxic effect of other alcohols**

      √7ᵗʰ **T51.8X1 Toxic effect of other alcohols, accidental (unintentional)**
          Toxic effect of other alcohols NOS

     7 √7ᵗʰ **T51.8X2 Toxic effect of other alcohols, intentional self-harm**   HCC

      √7ᵗʰ **T51.8X3 Toxic effect of other alcohols, assault**

      √7ᵗʰ **T51.8X4 Toxic effect of other alcohols, undetermined**

√5ᵗʰ **T51.9 Toxic effect of unspecified alcohol**

  √x7ᵗʰ **T51.91 Toxic effect of unspecified alcohol, accidental (unintentional)**

  7 √x7ᵗʰ **T51.92 Toxic effect of unspecified alcohol, intentional self-harm**   HCC

  √x7ᵗʰ **T51.93 Toxic effect of unspecified alcohol, assault**

  √x7ᵗʰ **T51.94 Toxic effect of unspecified alcohol, undetermined**

√4ᵗʰ **T52 Toxic effect of organic solvents**

  EXCLUDES 1   *halogen derivatives of aliphatic and aromatic hydrocarbons (T53.-)*

> The appropriate 7th character is to be added to each code from category T52.
> A   initial encounter
> D   subsequent encounter
> S   sequela

  √5ᵗʰ **T52.0 Toxic effects of petroleum products**
     Toxic effects of ether petroleum
     Toxic effects of gasoline [petrol]
     Toxic effects of kerosene [paraffin oil]
     Toxic effects of naphtha petroleum
     Toxic effects of paraffin wax
     Toxic effects of spirit petroleum

   √6ᵗʰ **T52.0X Toxic effects of petroleum products**

      √7ᵗʰ **T52.0X1 Toxic effect of petroleum products, accidental (unintentional)**
          Toxic effects of petroleum products NOS

     7 √7ᵗʰ **T52.0X2 Toxic effect of petroleum products, intentional self-harm**   HCC

      √7ᵗʰ **T52.0X3 Toxic effect of petroleum products, assault**

      √7ᵗʰ **T52.0X4 Toxic effect of petroleum products, undetermined**

  √5ᵗʰ **T52.1 Toxic effects of benzene**

    EXCLUDES 1   *homologues of benzene (T52.2)*
          nitroderivatives and aminoderivatives of benzene and its homologues (T65.3)

   √6ᵗʰ **T52.1X Toxic effects of benzene**

      √7ᵗʰ **T52.1X1 Toxic effect of benzene, accidental (unintentional)**
          Toxic effects of benzene NOS

     7 √7ᵗʰ **T52.1X2 Toxic effect of benzene, intentional self-harm**   HCC

      √7ᵗʰ **T52.1X3 Toxic effect of benzene, assault**

      √7ᵗʰ **T52.1X4 Toxic effect of benzene, undetermined**

  √5ᵗʰ **T52.2 Toxic effects of homologues of benzene**
     Toxic effects of toluene [methylbenzene]
     Toxic effects of xylene [dimethylbenzene]

   √6ᵗʰ **T52.2X Toxic effects of homologues of benzene**

      √7ᵗʰ **T52.2X1 Toxic effect of homologues of benzene, accidental (unintentional)**
          Toxic effects of homologues of benzene NOS

     7 √7ᵗʰ **T52.2X2 Toxic effect of homologues of benzene, intentional self-harm**   HCC

      √7ᵗʰ **T52.2X3 Toxic effect of homologues of benzene, assault**

      √7ᵗʰ **T52.2X4 Toxic effect of homologues of benzene, undetermined**

  √5ᵗʰ **T52.3 Toxic effects of glycols**

   √6ᵗʰ **T52.3X Toxic effects of glycols**

      √7ᵗʰ **T52.3X1 Toxic effect of glycols, accidental (unintentional)**
          Toxic effects of glycols NOS

     7 √7ᵗʰ **T52.3X2 Toxic effect of glycols, intentional self-harm**   HCC

      √7ᵗʰ **T52.3X3 Toxic effect of glycols, assault**

      √7ᵗʰ **T52.3X4 Toxic effect of glycols, undetermined**

√5ᵗʰ **T52.4 Toxic effects of ketones**

   √6ᵗʰ **T52.4X Toxic effects of ketones**

      √7ᵗʰ **T52.4X1 Toxic effect of ketones, accidental (unintentional)**
          Toxic effects of ketones NOS

     7 √7ᵗʰ **T52.4X2 Toxic effect of ketones, intentional self-harm**   HCC

      √7ᵗʰ **T52.4X3 Toxic effect of ketones, assault**

      √7ᵗʰ **T52.4X4 Toxic effect of ketones, undetermined**

√5ᵗʰ **T52.8 Toxic effects of other organic solvents**

   √6ᵗʰ **T52.8X Toxic effects of other organic solvents**

      √7ᵗʰ **T52.8X1 Toxic effect of other organic solvents, accidental (unintentional)**
          Toxic effects of other organic solvents NOS

     7 √7ᵗʰ **T52.8X2 Toxic effect of other organic solvents, intentional self-harm**   HCC

      √7ᵗʰ **T52.8X3 Toxic effect of other organic solvents, assault**

      √7ᵗʰ **T52.8X4 Toxic effect of other organic solvents, undetermined**

√5ᵗʰ **T52.9 Toxic effects of unspecified organic solvent**

  √x7ᵗʰ **T52.91 Toxic effect of unspecified organic solvent, accidental (unintentional)**

  7 √x7ᵗʰ **T52.92 Toxic effect of unspecified organic solvent, intentional self-harm**   HCC

  √x7ᵗʰ **T52.93 Toxic effect of unspecified organic solvent, assault**

  √x7ᵗʰ **T52.94 Toxic effect of unspecified organic solvent, undetermined**

√4ᵗʰ **T53 Toxic effect of halogen derivatives of aliphatic and aromatic hydrocarbons**

> The appropriate 7th character is to be added to each code from category T53.
> A   initial encounter
> D   subsequent encounter
> S   sequela

  √5ᵗʰ **T53.0 Toxic effects of carbon tetrachloride**
     Toxic effects of tetrachloromethane

   √6ᵗʰ **T53.0X Toxic effects of carbon tetrachloride**

      √7ᵗʰ **T53.0X1 Toxic effect of carbon tetrachloride, accidental (unintentional)**
          Toxic effects of carbon tetrachloride NOS

     7 √7ᵗʰ **T53.0X2 Toxic effect of carbon tetrachloride, intentional self-harm**   HCC

      √7ᵗʰ **T53.0X3 Toxic effect of carbon tetrachloride, assault**

      √7ᵗʰ **T53.0X4 Toxic effect of carbon tetrachloride, undetermined**

  √5ᵗʰ **T53.1 Toxic effects of chloroform**
     Toxic effects of trichloromethane

   √6ᵗʰ **T53.1X Toxic effects of chloroform**

      √7ᵗʰ **T53.1X1 Toxic effect of chloroform, accidental (unintentional)**
          Toxic effects of chloroform NOS

     7 √7ᵗʰ **T53.1X2 Toxic effect of chloroform, intentional self-harm**   HCC

      √7ᵗʰ **T53.1X3 Toxic effect of chloroform, assault**

      √7ᵗʰ **T53.1X4 Toxic effect of chloroform, undetermined**

  √5ᵗʰ **T53.2 Toxic effects of trichloroethylene**
     Toxic effects of trichloroethene

   √6ᵗʰ **T53.2X Toxic effects of trichloroethylene**

      √7ᵗʰ **T53.2X1 Toxic effect of trichloroethylene, accidental (unintentional)**
          Toxic effects of trichloroethylene NOS

     7 √7ᵗʰ **T53.2X2 Toxic effect of trichloroethylene, intentional self-harm**   HCC

      √7ᵗʰ **T53.2X3 Toxic effect of trichloroethylene, assault**

      √7ᵗʰ **T53.2X4 Toxic effect of trichloroethylene, undetermined**

☑ Additional Character Required   √x7ᵗʰ Placeholder   Unacceptable PDx   Questionable PDx   Manifestation   Unspecified Dx   H1-H14 HAC   HCC CMS-HCC Dx   HIV HIV Dx

√5th **T53.3** **Toxic effects of tetrachloroethylene**
Toxic effects of perchloroethylene
Toxic effect of tetrachloroethene

   √6th **T53.3X** **Toxic effects of** tetrachloroethylene

     √7th **T53.3X1** **Toxic effect of tetrachloroethylene, accidental (unintentional)**
Toxic effects of tetrachloroethylene NOS

     7 √7th **T53.3X2** **Toxic effect of tetrachloroethylene, intentional self-harm** HCC

     √7th **T53.3X3** **Toxic effect of tetrachloroethylene, assault**

     √7th **T53.3X4** **Toxic effect of tetrachloroethylene, undetermined**

√5th **T53.4** **Toxic effects of dichloromethane**
Toxic effects of methylene chloride

   √6th **T53.4X** **Toxic effects of** dichloromethane

     √7th **T53.4X1** **Toxic effect of dichloromethane, accidental (unintentional)**
Toxic effects of dichloromethane NOS

     7 √7th **T53.4X2** **Toxic effect of dichloromethane, intentional self-harm** HCC

     √7th **T53.4X3** **Toxic effect of dichloromethane, assault**

     √7th **T53.4X4** **Toxic effect of dichloromethane, undetermined**

√5th **T53.5** **Toxic effects of chlorofluorocarbons**

   √6th **T53.5X** **Toxic effects of** chlorofluorocarbons

     √7th **T53.5X1** **Toxic effect of chlorofluorocarbons, accidental (unintentional)**
Toxic effects of chlorofluorocarbons NOS

     7 √7th **T53.5X2** **Toxic effect of chlorofluorocarbons, intentional self-harm** HCC

     √7th **T53.5X3** **Toxic effect of chlorofluorocarbons, assault**

     √7th **T53.5X4** **Toxic effect of chlorofluorocarbons, undetermined**

√5th **T53.6** **Toxic effects of other halogen derivatives of aliphatic hydrocarbons**

   √6th **T53.6X** **Toxic effects of** other halogen derivatives of aliphatic hydrocarbons

     √7th **T53.6X1** **Toxic effect of other halogen derivatives of aliphatic hydrocarbons, accidental (unintentional)**
Toxic effects of other halogen derivatives of aliphatic hydrocarbons NOS

     7 √7th **T53.6X2** **Toxic effect of other halogen derivatives of aliphatic hydrocarbons, intentional self-harm** HCC

     √7th **T53.6X3** **Toxic effect of other halogen derivatives of aliphatic hydrocarbons, assault**

     √7th **T53.6X4** **Toxic effect of other halogen derivatives of aliphatic hydrocarbons, undetermined**

√5th **T53.7** **Toxic effects of other halogen derivatives of aromatic hydrocarbons**

   √6th **T53.7X** **Toxic effects of** other halogen derivatives of aromatic hydrocarbons

     √7th **T53.7X1** **Toxic effect of other halogen derivatives of aromatic hydrocarbons, accidental (unintentional)**
Toxic effects of other halogen derivatives of aromatic hydrocarbons NOS

     7 √7th **T53.7X2** **Toxic effect of other halogen derivatives of aromatic hydrocarbons, intentional self-harm** HCC

     √7th **T53.7X3** **Toxic effect of other halogen derivatives of aromatic hydrocarbons, assault**

     √7th **T53.7X4** **Toxic effect of other halogen derivatives of aromatic hydrocarbons, undetermined**

√5th **T53.9** **Toxic effects of unspecified halogen derivatives of aliphatic and aromatic hydrocarbons**

   √x7th **T53.91** **Toxic effect of unspecified halogen derivatives of aliphatic and aromatic hydrocarbons, accidental (unintentional)**

   7 √x7th **T53.92** **Toxic effect of unspecified halogen derivatives of aliphatic and aromatic hydrocarbons, intentional self-harm** HCC

   √x7th **T53.93** **Toxic effect of unspecified halogen derivatives of aliphatic and aromatic hydrocarbons, assault**

   √x7th **T53.94** **Toxic effect of unspecified halogen derivatives of aliphatic and aromatic hydrocarbons, undetermined**

√4th **T54** **Toxic effect of corrosive substances**

> The appropriate 7th character is to be added to each code from category T54.
> A   initial encounter
> D   subsequent encounter
> S   sequela

√5th **T54.0** **Toxic effects of phenol and phenol homologues**

   √6th **T54.0X** **Toxic effects of** phenol and phenol homologues

     √7th **T54.0X1** **Toxic effect of phenol and phenol homologues, accidental (unintentional)**
Toxic effects of phenol and phenol homologues NOS

     7 √7th **T54.0X2** **Toxic effect of phenol and phenol homologues, intentional self-harm** HCC

     √7th **T54.0X3** **Toxic effect of phenol and phenol homologues, assault**

     √7th **T54.0X4** **Toxic effect of phenol and phenol homologues, undetermined**

√5th **T54.1** **Toxic effects of other corrosive organic compounds**

   √6th **T54.1X** **Toxic effects of other corrosive organic compounds**

     √7th **T54.1X1** **Toxic effect of other corrosive organic compounds, accidental (unintentional)**
Toxic effects of other corrosive organic compounds NOS

     7 √7th **T54.1X2** **Toxic effect of other corrosive organic compounds, intentional self-harm** HCC

     √7th **T54.1X3** **Toxic effect of other corrosive organic compounds, assault**

     √7th **T54.1X4** **Toxic effect of other corrosive organic compounds, undetermined**

√5th **T54.2** **Toxic effects of corrosive acids and acid-like substances**
Toxic effects of hydrochloric acid
Toxic effects of sulfuric acid

   √6th **T54.2X** **Toxic effects of** corrosive acids and acid-like substances

     √7th **T54.2X1** **Toxic effect of corrosive acids and acid-like substances, accidental (unintentional)**
Toxic effects of corrosive acids and acid-like substances NOS

     7 √7th **T54.2X2** **Toxic effect of corrosive acids and acid-like substances, intentional self-harm** HCC

     √7th **T54.2X3** **Toxic effect of corrosive acids and acid-like substances, assault**

     √7th **T54.2X4** **Toxic effect of corrosive acids and acid-like substances, undetermined**

√5th **T54.3** **Toxic effects of corrosive alkalis and alkali-like substances**
Toxic effects of potassium hydroxide
Toxic effects of sodium hydroxide

   √6th **T54.3X** **Toxic effects of** corrosive alkalis and alkali-like substances

     √7th **T54.3X1** **Toxic effect of corrosive alkalis and alkali-like substances, accidental (unintentional)**
Toxic effects of corrosive alkalis and alkali-like substances NOS

     7 √7th **T54.3X2** **Toxic effect of corrosive alkalis and alkali-like substances, intentional self-harm** HCC

     √7th **T54.3X3** **Toxic effect of corrosive alkalis and alkali-like substances, assault**

     √7th **T54.3X4** **Toxic effect of corrosive alkalis and alkali-like substances, undetermined**

√5th **T54.9** **Toxic effects of unspecified corrosive substance**

   √x7th **T54.91** **Toxic effect of unspecified corrosive substance, accidental (unintentional)**

   7 √x7th **T54.92** **Toxic effect of unspecified corrosive substance, intentional self-harm** HCC

   √x7th **T54.93** **Toxic effect of unspecified corrosive substance, assault**

   √x7th **T54.94** **Toxic effect of unspecified corrosive substance, undetermined**

N Newborn: 0   P Pediatric: 0-17   M Maternity: 9-64   A Adult: 15-124   MCC Major Complication/Comorbidity   CC Complication/Comorbidity   SW Severe Wound Dx

1132   ICD-10-CM 2021

√4ᵗʰ **T55 Toxic effect of soaps and detergents**

> The appropriate 7th character is to be added to each code from category T55.
> A   initial encounter
> D   subsequent encounter
> S   sequela

√5ᵗʰ **T55.0 Toxic effect of soaps**

√6ᵗʰ **T55.0X Toxic effect of** soaps

√7ᵗʰ **T55.0X1 Toxic effect of soaps, accidental (unintentional)**
Toxic effect of soaps NOS

⁷ √7ᵗʰ **T55.0X2 Toxic effect of soaps, intentional self-harm** HCC

√7ᵗʰ **T55.0X3 Toxic effect of soaps, assault**

√7ᵗʰ **T55.0X4 Toxic effect of soaps, undetermined**

√5ᵗʰ **T55.1 Toxic effect of detergents**

√6ᵗʰ **T55.1X Toxic effect of** detergents

√7ᵗʰ **T55.1X1 Toxic effect of detergents, accidental (unintentional)**
Toxic effect of detergents NOS

⁷ √7ᵗʰ **T55.1X2 Toxic effect of detergents, intentional self-harm** HCC

√7ᵗʰ **T55.1X3 Toxic effect of detergents, assault**

√7ᵗʰ **T55.1X4 Toxic effect of detergents, undetermined**

√4ᵗʰ **T56 Toxic effect of metals**

> INCLUDES   toxic effects of fumes and vapors of metals
> toxic effects of metals from all sources, except medicinal substances
> Use additional code to identify any retained metal foreign body, if applicable (Z18.0-, T18.1-)
> EXCLUDES 1   *arsenic and its compounds (T57.0)*
> *manganese and its compounds (T57.2)*

> The appropriate 7th character is to be added to each code from category T56.
> A   initial encounter
> D   subsequent encounter
> S   sequela

√5ᵗʰ **T56.0 Toxic effects of lead and its compounds**

√6ᵗʰ **T56.0X Toxic effects of** lead **and its compounds**

√7ᵗʰ **T56.0X1 Toxic effect of lead and its compounds, accidental (unintentional)**
Toxic effects of lead and its compounds NOS

⁷ √7ᵗʰ **T56.0X2 Toxic effect of lead and its compounds, intentional self-harm** HCC

√7ᵗʰ **T56.0X3 Toxic effect of lead and its compounds, assault**

√7ᵗʰ **T56.0X4 Toxic effect of lead and its compounds, undetermined**

√5ᵗʰ **T56.1 Toxic effects of mercury and its compounds**

√6ᵗʰ **T56.1X Toxic effects of** mercury **and its compounds**

√7ᵗʰ **T56.1X1 Toxic effect of mercury and its compounds, accidental (unintentional)**
Toxic effects of mercury and its compounds NOS

⁷ √7ᵗʰ **T56.1X2 Toxic effect of mercury and its compounds, intentional self-harm** HCC

√7ᵗʰ **T56.1X3 Toxic effect of mercury and its compounds, assault**

√7ᵗʰ **T56.1X4 Toxic effect of mercury and its compounds, undetermined**

√5ᵗʰ **T56.2 Toxic effects of chromium and its compounds**

√6ᵗʰ **T56.2X Toxic effects of** chromium **and its compounds**

√7ᵗʰ **T56.2X1 Toxic effect of chromium and its compounds, accidental (unintentional)**
Toxic effects of chromium and its compounds NOS

⁷ √7ᵗʰ **T56.2X2 Toxic effect of chromium and its compounds, intentional self-harm** HCC

√7ᵗʰ **T56.2X3 Toxic effect of chromium and its compounds, assault**

√7ᵗʰ **T56.2X4 Toxic effect of chromium and its compounds, undetermined**

√5ᵗʰ **T56.3 Toxic effects of cadmium and its compounds**

√6ᵗʰ **T56.3X Toxic effects of** cadmium **and its compounds**

√7ᵗʰ **T56.3X1 Toxic effect of cadmium and its compounds, accidental (unintentional)**
Toxic effects of cadmium and its compounds NOS

⁷ √7ᵗʰ **T56.3X2 Toxic effect of cadmium and its compounds, intentional self-harm** HCC

√7ᵗʰ **T56.3X3 Toxic effect of cadmium and its compounds, assault**

√7ᵗʰ **T56.3X4 Toxic effect of cadmium and its compounds, undetermined**

√5ᵗʰ **T56.4 Toxic effects of copper and its compounds**

√6ᵗʰ **T56.4X Toxic effects of** copper **and its compounds**

√7ᵗʰ **T56.4X1 Toxic effect of copper and its compounds, accidental (unintentional)**
Toxic effects of copper and its compounds NOS

⁷ √7ᵗʰ **T56.4X2 Toxic effect of copper and its compounds, intentional self-harm** HCC

√7ᵗʰ **T56.4X3 Toxic effect of copper and its compounds, assault**

√7ᵗʰ **T56.4X4 Toxic effect of copper and its compounds, undetermined**

√5ᵗʰ **T56.5 Toxic effects of zinc and its compounds**

√6ᵗʰ **T56.5X Toxic effects of** zinc **and its compounds**

√7ᵗʰ **T56.5X1 Toxic effect of zinc and its compounds, accidental (unintentional)**
Toxic effects of zinc and its compounds NOS

⁷ √7ᵗʰ **T56.5X2 Toxic effect of zinc and its compounds, intentional self-harm** HCC

√7ᵗʰ **T56.5X3 Toxic effect of zinc and its compounds, assault**

√7ᵗʰ **T56.5X4 Toxic effect of zinc and its compounds, undetermined**

√5ᵗʰ **T56.6 Toxic effects of tin and its compounds**

√6ᵗʰ **T56.6X Toxic effects of** tin **and its compounds**

√7ᵗʰ **T56.6X1 Toxic effect of tin and its compounds, accidental (unintentional)**
Toxic effect of tin and its compounds NOS

⁷ √7ᵗʰ **T56.6X2 Toxic effect of tin and its compounds, intentional self-harm** HCC

√7ᵗʰ **T56.6X3 Toxic effect of tin and its compounds, assault**

√7ᵗʰ **T56.6X4 Toxic effect of tin and its compounds, undetermined**

√5ᵗʰ **T56.7 Toxic effects of beryllium and its compounds**

√6ᵗʰ **T56.7X Toxic effects of** beryllium **and its compounds**

√7ᵗʰ **T56.7X1 Toxic effect of beryllium and its compounds, accidental (unintentional)**
Toxic effect of beryllium and its compounds NOS

⁷ √7ᵗʰ **T56.7X2 Toxic effect of beryllium and its compounds, intentional self-harm** HCC

√7ᵗʰ **T56.7X3 Toxic effect of beryllium and its compounds, assault**

√7ᵗʰ **T56.7X4 Toxic effect of beryllium and its compounds, undetermined**

√5ᵗʰ **T56.8 Toxic effects of other metals**

√6ᵗʰ **T56.81 Toxic effect of** thallium

√7ᵗʰ **T56.811 Toxic effect of thallium, accidental (unintentional)**
Toxic effect of thallium NOS

⁷ √7ᵗʰ **T56.812 Toxic effect of thallium, intentional self-harm** HCC

√7ᵗʰ **T56.813 Toxic effect of thallium, assault**

√7ᵗʰ **T56.814 Toxic effect of thallium, undetermined**

√6ᵗʰ **T56.89 Toxic effects of other metals**

√7ᵗʰ **T56.891 Toxic effect of other metals, accidental (unintentional)**
Toxic effects of other metals NOS

⁷ √7ᵗʰ **T56.892 Toxic effect of other metals, intentional self-harm** HCC

√7ᵗʰ **T56.893 Toxic effect of other metals, assault**

√7ᵗʰ **T56.894 Toxic effect of other metals, undetermined**

☑ Additional Character Required   √x7ᵗʰ Placeholder   Unacceptable PDx   Questionable PDx   Manifestation   Unspecified Dx   H1 - H14 HAC   HCC CMS-HCC Dx   HIV HIV Dx

ICD-10-CM 2021   1133

√5ᵗʰ **T56.9 Toxic effects of unspecified metal**

    √x7ᵗʰ **T56.91 Toxic effect of unspecified metal, accidental (unintentional)**

    7 √x7ᵗʰ **T56.92 Toxic effect of unspecified metal, intentional self-harm** ᴴᶜᶜ

    √x7ᵗʰ **T56.93 Toxic effect of unspecified metal, assault**

    √x7ᵗʰ **T56.94 Toxic effect of unspecified metal, undetermined**

√4ᵗʰ **T57 Toxic effect of other inorganic substances**

> The appropriate 7th character is to be added to each code from category T57.
> A initial encounter
> D subsequent encounter
> S sequela

  √5ᵗʰ **T57.0 Toxic effect of arsenic and its compounds**

    √6ᵗʰ **T57.0X Toxic effect of arsenic and its compounds**

      √7ᵗʰ **T57.0X1 Toxic effect of arsenic and its compounds, accidental (unintentional)**
         Toxic effect of arsenic and its compounds NOS

      7 √7ᵗʰ **T57.0X2 Toxic effect of arsenic and its compounds, intentional self-harm** ᴴᶜᶜ

      √7ᵗʰ **T57.0X3 Toxic effect of arsenic and its compounds, assault**

      √7ᵗʰ **T57.0X4 Toxic effect of arsenic and its compounds, undetermined**

  √5ᵗʰ **T57.1 Toxic effect of phosphorus and its compounds**

    EXCLUDES 1   *organophosphate insecticides (T60.0)*

    √6ᵗʰ **T57.1X Toxic effect of phosphorus and its compounds**

      √7ᵗʰ **T57.1X1 Toxic effect of phosphorus and its compounds, accidental (unintentional)**
         Toxic effect of phosphorus and its compounds NOS

      7 √7ᵗʰ **T57.1X2 Toxic effect of phosphorus and its compounds, intentional self-harm** ᴴᶜᶜ

      √7ᵗʰ **T57.1X3 Toxic effect of phosphorus and its compounds, assault**

      √7ᵗʰ **T57.1X4 Toxic effect of phosphorus and its compounds, undetermined**

  √5ᵗʰ **T57.2 Toxic effect of manganese and its compounds**

    √6ᵗʰ **T57.2X Toxic effect of manganese and its compounds**

      √7ᵗʰ **T57.2X1 Toxic effect of manganese and its compounds, accidental (unintentional)**
         Toxic effect of manganese and its compounds NOS

      7 √7ᵗʰ **T57.2X2 Toxic effect of manganese and its compounds, intentional self-harm** ᴴᶜᶜ

      √7ᵗʰ **T57.2X3 Toxic effect of manganese and its compounds, assault**

      √7ᵗʰ **T57.2X4 Toxic effect of manganese and its compounds, undetermined**

  √5ᵗʰ **T57.3 Toxic effect of hydrogen cyanide**

    √6ᵗʰ **T57.3X Toxic effect of hydrogen cyanide**

      √7ᵗʰ **T57.3X1 Toxic effect of hydrogen cyanide, accidental (unintentional)**
         Toxic effect of hydrogen cyanide NOS

      7 √7ᵗʰ **T57.3X2 Toxic effect of hydrogen cyanide, intentional self-harm** ᴴᶜᶜ

      √7ᵗʰ **T57.3X3 Toxic effect of hydrogen cyanide, assault**

      √7ᵗʰ **T57.3X4 Toxic effect of hydrogen cyanide, undetermined**

  √5ᵗʰ **T57.8 Toxic effect of other specified inorganic substances**

    √6ᵗʰ **T57.8X Toxic effect of other specified inorganic substances**

      √7ᵗʰ **T57.8X1 Toxic effect of other specified inorganic substances, accidental (unintentional)**
         Toxic effect of other specified inorganic substances NOS

      7 √7ᵗʰ **T57.8X2 Toxic effect of other specified inorganic substances, intentional self-harm** ᴴᶜᶜ

      √7ᵗʰ **T57.8X3 Toxic effect of other specified inorganic substances, assault**

      √7ᵗʰ **T57.8X4 Toxic effect of other specified inorganic substances, undetermined**

  √5ᵗʰ **T57.9 Toxic effect of unspecified inorganic substance**

    √x7ᵗʰ **T57.91 Toxic effect of unspecified inorganic substance, accidental (unintentional)**

7 √x7ᵗʰ **T57.92 Toxic effect of unspecified inorganic substance, intentional self-harm** ᴴᶜᶜ

  √x7ᵗʰ **T57.93 Toxic effect of unspecified inorganic substance, assault**

  √x7ᵗʰ **T57.94 Toxic effect of unspecified inorganic substance, undetermined**

√4ᵗʰ **T58 Toxic effect of carbon monoxide**

> INCLUDES   asphyxiation from carbon monoxide
>   toxic effect of carbon monoxide from all sources

> The appropriate 7th character is to be added to each code from category T58.
> A initial encounter
> D subsequent encounter
> S sequela

  √5ᵗʰ **T58.0 Toxic effect of carbon monoxide from motor vehicle exhaust**
    Toxic effect of exhaust gas from gas engine
    Toxic effect of exhaust gas from motor pump

    √x7ᵗʰ **T58.01 Toxic effect of carbon monoxide from motor vehicle exhaust, accidental (unintentional)**

    7 √x7ᵗʰ **T58.02 Toxic effect of carbon monoxide from motor vehicle exhaust, intentional self-harm** ᴴᶜᶜ

    √x7ᵗʰ **T58.03 Toxic effect of carbon monoxide from motor vehicle exhaust, assault**

    √x7ᵗʰ **T58.04 Toxic effect of carbon monoxide from motor vehicle exhaust, undetermined**

  √5ᵗʰ **T58.1 Toxic effect of carbon monoxide from utility gas**
    Toxic effect of acetylene
    Toxic effect of gas NOS used for lighting, heating, cooking
    Toxic effect of water gas

    √x7ᵗʰ **T58.11 Toxic effect of carbon monoxide from utility gas, accidental (unintentional)**

    7 √x7ᵗʰ **T58.12 Toxic effect of carbon monoxide from utility gas, intentional self-harm** ᴴᶜᶜ

    √x7ᵗʰ **T58.13 Toxic effect of carbon monoxide from utility gas, assault**

    √x7ᵗʰ **T58.14 Toxic effect of carbon monoxide from utility gas, undetermined**

  √5ᵗʰ **T58.2 Toxic effect of carbon monoxide from incomplete combustion of other domestic fuels**
    Toxic effect of carbon monoxide from incomplete combustion of coal, coke, kerosene, wood

    √6ᵗʰ **T58.2X Toxic effect of carbon monoxide from incomplete combustion of other domestic fuels**

      √7ᵗʰ **T58.2X1 Toxic effect of carbon monoxide from incomplete combustion of other domestic fuels, accidental (unintentional)**

      7 √7ᵗʰ **T58.2X2 Toxic effect of carbon monoxide from incomplete combustion of other domestic fuels, intentional self-harm** ᴴᶜᶜ

      √7ᵗʰ **T58.2X3 Toxic effect of carbon monoxide from incomplete combustion of other domestic fuels, assault**

      √7ᵗʰ **T58.2X4 Toxic effect of carbon monoxide from incomplete combustion of other domestic fuels, undetermined**

  √5ᵗʰ **T58.8 Toxic effect of carbon monoxide from other source**
    Toxic effect of carbon monoxide from blast furnace gas
    Toxic effect of carbon monoxide from fuels in industrial use
    Toxic effect of carbon monoxide from kiln vapor

    √6ᵗʰ **T58.8X Toxic effect of carbon monoxide from other source**

      √7ᵗʰ **T58.8X1 Toxic effect of carbon monoxide from other source, accidental (unintentional)**

      7 √7ᵗʰ **T58.8X2 Toxic effect of carbon monoxide from other source, intentional self-harm** ᴴᶜᶜ

      √7ᵗʰ **T58.8X3 Toxic effect of carbon monoxide from other source, assault**

      √7ᵗʰ **T58.8X4 Toxic effect of carbon monoxide from other source, undetermined**

  √5ᵗʰ **T58.9 Toxic effect of carbon monoxide from unspecified source**

    √x7ᵗʰ **T58.91 Toxic effect of carbon monoxide from unspecified source, accidental (unintentional)**

    7 √x7ᵗʰ **T58.92 Toxic effect of carbon monoxide from unspecified source, intentional self-harm** ᴴᶜᶜ

    √x7ᵗʰ **T58.93 Toxic effect of carbon monoxide from unspecified source, assault**

    √x7ᵗʰ **T58.94 Toxic effect of carbon monoxide from unspecified source, undetermined**

N Newborn: 0   P Pediatric: 0-17   M Maternity: 9-64   A Adult: 15-124   MCC Major Complication/Comorbidity   CC Complication/Comorbidity   SW Severe Wound Dx

1134   ICD-10-CM 2021

✓4ᵗʰ T59 Toxic effect of other gases, fumes and vapors

INCLUDES   aerosol propellants

EXCLUDES 1   chlorofluorocarbons (T53.5)

The appropriate 7th character is to be added to each code from category T59.
A   initial encounter
D   subsequent encounter
S   sequela

✓5ᵗʰ T59.0 Toxic effect of nitrogen oxides

✓6ᵗʰ T59.0X Toxic effect of nitrogen oxides

✓7ᵗʰ T59.0X1 Toxic effect of nitrogen oxides, accidental (unintentional)
Toxic effect of nitrogen oxides NOS

7 ✓7ᵗʰ T59.0X2 Toxic effect of nitrogen oxides, intentional self-harm   HCC

✓7ᵗʰ T59.0X3 Toxic effect of nitrogen oxides, assault

✓7ᵗʰ T59.0X4 Toxic effect of nitrogen oxides, undetermined

✓5ᵗʰ T59.1 Toxic effect of sulfur dioxide

✓6ᵗʰ T59.1X Toxic effect of sulfur dioxide

✓7ᵗʰ T59.1X1 Toxic effect of sulfur dioxide, accidental (unintentional)
Toxic effect of sulfur dioxide NOS

7 ✓7ᵗʰ T59.1X2 Toxic effect of sulfur dioxide, intentional self-harm   HCC

✓7ᵗʰ T59.1X3 Toxic effect of sulfur dioxide, assault

✓7ᵗʰ T59.1X4 Toxic effect of sulfur dioxide, undetermined

✓5ᵗʰ T59.2 Toxic effect of formaldehyde

✓6ᵗʰ T59.2X Toxic effect of formaldehyde

✓7ᵗʰ T59.2X1 Toxic effect of formaldehyde, accidental (unintentional)
Toxic effect of formaldehyde NOS

7 ✓7ᵗʰ T59.2X2 Toxic effect of formaldehyde, intentional self-harm   HCC

✓7ᵗʰ T59.2X3 Toxic effect of formaldehyde, assault

✓7ᵗʰ T59.2X4 Toxic effect of formaldehyde, undetermined

✓5ᵗʰ T59.3 Toxic effect of lacrimogenic gas

Toxic effect of tear gas

✓6ᵗʰ T59.3X Toxic effect of lacrimogenic gas

✓7ᵗʰ T59.3X1 Toxic effect of lacrimogenic gas, accidental (unintentional)
Toxic effect of lacrimogenic gas NOS

7 ✓7ᵗʰ T59.3X2 Toxic effect of lacrimogenic gas, intentional self-harm   HCC

✓7ᵗʰ T59.3X3 Toxic effect of lacrimogenic gas, assault

✓7ᵗʰ T59.3X4 Toxic effect of lacrimogenic gas, undetermined

✓5ᵗʰ T59.4 Toxic effect of chlorine gas

✓6ᵗʰ T59.4X Toxic effect of chlorine gas

✓7ᵗʰ T59.4X1 Toxic effect of chlorine gas, accidental (unintentional)
Toxic effect of chlorine gas NOS

7 ✓7ᵗʰ T59.4X2 Toxic effect of chlorine gas, intentional self-harm   HCC

✓7ᵗʰ T59.4X3 Toxic effect of chlorine gas, assault

✓7ᵗʰ T59.4X4 Toxic effect of chlorine gas, undetermined

✓5ᵗʰ T59.5 Toxic effect of fluorine gas and hydrogen fluoride

✓6ᵗʰ T59.5X Toxic effect of fluorine gas and hydrogen fluoride

✓7ᵗʰ T59.5X1 Toxic effect of fluorine gas and hydrogen fluoride, accidental (unintentional)
Toxic effect of fluorine gas and hydrogen fluoride NOS

7 ✓7ᵗʰ T59.5X2 Toxic effect of fluorine gas and hydrogen fluoride, intentional self-harm   HCC

✓7ᵗʰ T59.5X3 Toxic effect of fluorine gas and hydrogen fluoride, assault

✓7ᵗʰ T59.5X4 Toxic effect of fluorine gas and hydrogen fluoride, undetermined

✓5ᵗʰ T59.6 Toxic effect of hydrogen sulfide

✓6ᵗʰ T59.6X Toxic effect of hydrogen sulfide

✓7ᵗʰ T59.6X1 Toxic effect of hydrogen sulfide, accidental (unintentional)
Toxic effect of hydrogen sulfide NOS

7 ✓7ᵗʰ T59.6X2 Toxic effect of hydrogen sulfide, intentional self-harm   HCC

✓7ᵗʰ T59.6X3 Toxic effect of hydrogen sulfide, assault

✓7ᵗʰ T59.6X4 Toxic effect of hydrogen sulfide, undetermined

✓5ᵗʰ T59.7 Toxic effect of carbon dioxide

✓6ᵗʰ T59.7X Toxic effect of carbon dioxide

✓7ᵗʰ T59.7X1 Toxic effect of carbon dioxide, accidental (unintentional)
Toxic effect of carbon dioxide NOS

7 ✓7ᵗʰ T59.7X2 Toxic effect of carbon dioxide, intentional self-harm   HCC

✓7ᵗʰ T59.7X3 Toxic effect of carbon dioxide, assault

✓7ᵗʰ T59.7X4 Toxic effect of carbon dioxide, undetermined

✓5ᵗʰ T59.8 Toxic effect of other specified gases, fumes and vapors

✓6ᵗʰ T59.81 Toxic effect of smoke

Smoke inhalation

EXCLUDES 2   toxic effect of cigarette (tobacco) smoke (T65.22-)

✓7ᵗʰ T59.811 Toxic effect of smoke, accidental (unintentional)
Toxic effect of smoke NOS
AHA: 2013,4Q,121

7 ✓7ᵗʰ T59.812 Toxic effect of smoke, intentional self-harm   HCC

✓7ᵗʰ T59.813 Toxic effect of smoke, assault

✓7ᵗʰ T59.814 Toxic effect of smoke, undetermined

✓6ᵗʰ T59.89 Toxic effect of other specified gases, fumes and vapors

✓7ᵗʰ T59.891 Toxic effect of other specified gases, fumes and vapors, accidental (unintentional)

7 ✓7ᵗʰ T59.892 Toxic effect of other specified gases, fumes and vapors, intentional self-harm   HCC

✓7ᵗʰ T59.893 Toxic effect of other specified gases, fumes and vapors, assault

✓7ᵗʰ T59.894 Toxic effect of other specified gases, fumes and vapors, undetermined

✓5ᵗʰ T59.9 Toxic effect of unspecified gases, fumes and vapors

✓x7ᵗʰ T59.91 Toxic effect of unspecified gases, fumes and vapors, accidental (unintentional)

7 ✓x7ᵗʰ T59.92 Toxic effect of unspecified gases, fumes and vapors, intentional self-harm   HCC

✓x7ᵗʰ T59.93 Toxic effect of unspecified gases, fumes and vapors, assault

✓x7ᵗʰ T59.94 Toxic effect of unspecified gases, fumes and vapors, undetermined

✓4ᵗʰ T60 Toxic effect of pesticides

INCLUDES   toxic effect of wood preservatives

The appropriate 7th character is to be added to each code from category T60.
A   initial encounter
D   subsequent encounter
S   sequela

✓5ᵗʰ T60.0 Toxic effect of organophosphate and carbamate insecticides

✓6ᵗʰ T60.0X Toxic effect of organophosphate and carbamate insecticides

✓7ᵗʰ T60.0X1 Toxic effect of organophosphate and carbamate insecticides, accidental (unintentional)
Toxic effect of organophosphate and carbamate insecticides NOS

7 ✓7ᵗʰ T60.0X2 Toxic effect of organophosphate and carbamate insecticides, intentional self-harm   HCC

✓7ᵗʰ T60.0X3 Toxic effect of organophosphate and carbamate insecticides, assault

✓7ᵗʰ T60.0X4 Toxic effect of organophosphate and carbamate insecticides, undetermined

√5th **T60.1** **Toxic effect of halogenated insecticides**
> EXCLUDES 1   *chlorinated hydrocarbon (T53.-)*

     √6th **T60.1X** **Toxic effect of** halogenated insecticides

         √7th **T60.1X1** **Toxic effect of halogenated insecticides, accidental (unintentional)**
> Toxic effect of halogenated insecticides NOS

         7 √7th **T60.1X2** **Toxic effect of halogenated insecticides, intentional self-harm**   HCC

         √7th **T60.1X3** **Toxic effect of halogenated insecticides, assault**

         √7th **T60.1X4** **Toxic effect of halogenated insecticides, undetermined**

√5th **T60.2** **Toxic effect of other insecticides**

     √6th **T60.2X** **Toxic effect of** other insecticides

         √7th **T60.2X1** **Toxic effect of other insecticides, accidental (unintentional)**
> Toxic effect of other insecticides NOS

         7 √7th **T60.2X2** **Toxic effect of other insecticides, intentional self-harm**   HCC

         √7th **T60.2X3** **Toxic effect of other insecticides, assault**

         √7th **T60.2X4** **Toxic effect of other insecticides, undetermined**

√5th **T60.3** **Toxic effect of herbicides and fungicides**

     √6th **T60.3X** **Toxic effect of** herbicides and fungicides

         √7th **T60.3X1** **Toxic effect of herbicides and fungicides, accidental (unintentional)**
> Toxic effect of herbicides and fungicides NOS

         7 √7th **T60.3X2** **Toxic effect of herbicides and fungicides, intentional self-harm**   HCC

         √7th **T60.3X3** **Toxic effect of herbicides and fungicides, assault**

         √7th **T60.3X4** **Toxic effect of herbicides and fungicides, undetermined**

√5th **T60.4** **Toxic effect of rodenticides**
> EXCLUDES 1   *strychnine and its salts (T65.1)*
> *thallium (T56.81-)*

     √6th **T60.4X** **Toxic effect of** rodenticides

         √7th **T60.4X1** **Toxic effect of rodenticides, accidental (unintentional)**
> Toxic effect of rodenticides NOS

         7 √7th **T60.4X2** **Toxic effect of rodenticides, intentional self-harm**   HCC

         √7th **T60.4X3** **Toxic effect of rodenticides, assault**

         √7th **T60.4X4** **Toxic effect of rodenticides, undetermined**

√5th **T60.8** **Toxic effect of other pesticides**

     √6th **T60.8X** **Toxic effect of other pesticides**

         √7th **T60.8X1** **Toxic effect of other pesticides,** accidental **(unintentional)**
> Toxic effect of other pesticides NOS

         7 √7th **T60.8X2** **Toxic effect of other pesticides, intentional self-harm**   HCC

         √7th **T60.8X3** **Toxic effect of other pesticides,** assault

         √7th **T60.8X4** **Toxic effect of other pesticides, undetermined**

√5th **T60.9** **Toxic effect of unspecified pesticide**

     √x7th **T60.91** **Toxic effect of unspecified pesticide,** accidental **(unintentional)**

     7 √x7th **T60.92** **Toxic effect of unspecified pesticide, intentional self-harm**   HCC

     √x7th **T60.93** **Toxic effect of unspecified pesticide,** assault

     √x7th **T60.94** **Toxic effect of unspecified pesticide,** undetermined

√4th **T61** **Toxic effect of noxious substances eaten as seafood**
> EXCLUDES 1   *allergic reaction to food, such as:*
>   *anaphylactic reaction or shock due to adverse food reaction (T78.0-)*
>   *bacterial foodborne intoxications (A05.-)*
>   *dermatitis (L23.6, L25.4, L27.2)*
>   *food protein-induced enterocolitis syndrome (K52.21)*
>   *food protein-induced enteropathy (K52.22)*
>   *gastroenteritis (noninfective) (K52.29)*
> *toxic effect of aflatoxin and other mycotoxins (T64)*
> *toxic effect of cyanides (T65.0-)*
> *toxic effect of harmful algae bloom (T65.82-)*
> *toxic effect of hydrogen cyanide (T57.3-)*
> *toxic effect of mercury (T56.1-)*
> *toxic effect of red tide (T65.82-)*

> The appropriate 7th character is to be added to each code from category T61.
> A   initial encounter
> D   subsequent encounter
> S   sequela

√5th **T61.0** **Ciguatera fish poisoning**

     √x7th **T61.01** **Ciguatera fish poisoning,** accidental **(unintentional)**

     7 √x7th **T61.02** **Ciguatera fish poisoning, intentional self-harm**   HCC

     √x7th **T61.03** **Ciguatera fish poisoning,** assault

     √x7th **T61.04** **Ciguatera fish poisoning,** undetermined

√5th **T61.1** **Scombroid fish poisoning**
> Histamine-like syndrome

     √x7th **T61.11** **Scombroid fish poisoning,** accidental **(unintentional)**

     7 √x7th **T61.12** **Scombroid fish poisoning, intentional self-harm**   HCC

     √x7th **T61.13** **Scombroid fish poisoning,** assault

     √x7th **T61.14** **Scombroid fish poisoning,** undetermined

√5th **T61.7** **Other fish and shellfish poisoning**

     √6th **T61.77** **Other fish poisoning**

         √7th **T61.771** **Other fish poisoning,** accidental **(unintentional)**

         7 √7th **T61.772** **Other fish poisoning, intentional self-harm**   HCC

         √7th **T61.773** **Other fish poisoning,** assault

         √7th **T61.774** **Other fish poisoning,** undetermined

     √6th **T61.78** **Other** shellfish **poisoning**

         √7th **T61.781** **Other shellfish poisoning,** accidental **(unintentional)**

         7 √7th **T61.782** **Other shellfish poisoning, intentional self-harm**   HCC

         √7th **T61.783** **Other shellfish poisoning,** assault

         √7th **T61.784** **Other shellfish poisoning,** undetermined

√5th **T61.8** **Toxic effect of other seafood**

     √6th **T61.8X** **Toxic effect of other seafood**

         √7th **T61.8X1** **Toxic effect of other seafood,** accidental **(unintentional)**

         7 √7th **T61.8X2** **Toxic effect of other seafood,** intentional **self-harm**   HCC

         √7th **T61.8X3** **Toxic effect of other seafood,** assault

         √7th **T61.8X4** **Toxic effect of other seafood, undetermined**

√5th **T61.9** **Toxic effect of unspecified seafood**

     √x7th **T61.91** **Toxic effect of unspecified seafood,** accidental **(unintentional)**

     7 √x7th **T61.92** **Toxic effect of unspecified seafood, intentional self-harm**   HCC

     √x7th **T61.93** **Toxic effect of unspecified seafood,** assault

     √x7th **T61.94** **Toxic effect of unspecified seafood,** undetermined

N Newborn: 0   P Pediatric: 0-17   M Maternity: 9-64   A Adult: 15-124   MCC Major Complication/Comorbidity   CC Complication/Comorbidity   SW Severe Wound Dx

1136   ICD-10-CM 2021

✓4ᵗʰ **T62 Toxic effect of other noxious substances eaten as food**

> **EXCLUDES 1**   allergic reaction to food, such as:
> anaphylactic shock (reaction) due to adverse food reaction (T78.0-)
> bacterial food borne intoxications (A05.-)
> dermatitis (L23.6, L25.4, L27.2)
> food protein-induced enterocolitis syndrome (K52.21)
> food protein-induced enteropathy (K52.22)
> gastroenteritis (noninfective) (K52.29)
> toxic effect of aflatoxin and other mycotoxins (T64)
> toxic effect of cyanides (T65.0-)
> toxic effect of hydrogen cyanide (T57.3-)
> toxic effect of mercury (T56.1-)

> The appropriate 7th character is to be added to each code from category T62.
> A   initial encounter
> D   subsequent encounter
> S   sequela

✓5ᵗʰ **T62.0 Toxic effect of ingested mushrooms**

✓6ᵗʰ   **T62.0X Toxic effect of ingested mushrooms**

✓7ᵗʰ   **T62.0X1 Toxic effect of ingested mushrooms, accidental (unintentional)**
    Toxic effect of ingested mushrooms NOS

⁷ ✓7ᵗʰ   **T62.0X2 Toxic effect of ingested mushrooms, intentional self-harm**   HCC

✓7ᵗʰ   **T62.0X3 Toxic effect of ingested mushrooms, assault**

✓7ᵗʰ   **T62.0X4 Toxic effect of ingested mushrooms, undetermined**

✓5ᵗʰ **T62.1 Toxic effect of ingested berries**

✓6ᵗʰ   **T62.1X Toxic effect of ingested berries**

✓7ᵗʰ   **T62.1X1 Toxic effect of ingested berries, accidental (unintentional)**
    Toxic effect of ingested berries NOS

⁷ ✓7ᵗʰ   **T62.1X2 Toxic effect of ingested berries, intentional self-harm**   HCC

✓7ᵗʰ   **T62.1X3 Toxic effect of ingested berries, assault**

✓7ᵗʰ   **T62.1X4 Toxic effect of ingested berries, undetermined**

✓5ᵗʰ **T62.2 Toxic effect of other ingested (parts of) plant(s)**

✓6ᵗʰ   **T62.2X Toxic effect of other ingested (parts of) plant(s)**

✓7ᵗʰ   **T62.2X1 Toxic effect of other ingested (parts of) plant(s), accidental (unintentional)**
    Toxic effect of other ingested (parts of) plant(s) NOS

⁷ ✓7ᵗʰ   **T62.2X2 Toxic effect of other ingested (parts of) plant(s), intentional self-harm**   HCC

✓7ᵗʰ   **T62.2X3 Toxic effect of other ingested (parts of) plant(s), assault**

✓7ᵗʰ   **T62.2X4 Toxic effect of other ingested (parts of) plant(s), undetermined**

✓5ᵗʰ **T62.8 Toxic effect of other specified noxious substances eaten as food**

✓6ᵗʰ   **T62.8X Toxic effect of other specified noxious substances eaten as food**

✓7ᵗʰ   **T62.8X1 Toxic effect of other specified noxious substances eaten as food, accidental (unintentional)**
    Toxic effect of other specified noxious substances eaten as food NOS

⁷ ✓7ᵗʰ   **T62.8X2 Toxic effect of other specified noxious substances eaten as food, intentional self-harm**   HCC

✓7ᵗʰ   **T62.8X3 Toxic effect of other specified noxious substances eaten as food, assault**

✓7ᵗʰ   **T62.8X4 Toxic effect of other specified noxious substances eaten as food, undetermined**

✓5ᵗʰ **T62.9 Toxic effect of unspecified noxious substance eaten as food**

✓×7ᵗʰ   **T62.91 Toxic effect of unspecified noxious substance eaten as food, accidental (unintentional)**
    Toxic effect of unspecified noxious substance eaten as food NOS

⁷ ✓×7ᵗʰ   **T62.92 Toxic effect of unspecified noxious substance eaten as food, intentional self-harm**   HCC

✓×7ᵗʰ   **T62.93 Toxic effect of unspecified noxious substance eaten as food, assault**

✓×7ᵗʰ   **T62.94 Toxic effect of unspecified noxious substance eaten as food, undetermined**

✓4ᵗʰ **T63 Toxic effect of contact with venomous animals and plants**

> **INCLUDES**   bite or touch of venomous animal
> pricked or stuck by thorn or leaf
> **EXCLUDES 2**   ingestion of toxic animal or plant (T61.-, T62.-)

> The appropriate 7th character is to be added to each code from category T63.
> A   initial encounter
> D   subsequent encounter
> S   sequela

✓5ᵗʰ **T63.0 Toxic effect of snake venom**

✓6ᵗʰ   **T63.00 Toxic effect of unspecified snake venom**

✓7ᵗʰ   **T63.001 Toxic effect of unspecified snake venom, accidental (unintentional)**
    Toxic effect of unspecified snake venom NOS

⁷ ✓7ᵗʰ   **T63.002 Toxic effect of unspecified snake venom, intentional self-harm**   HCC

✓7ᵗʰ   **T63.003 Toxic effect of unspecified snake venom, assault**

✓7ᵗʰ   **T63.004 Toxic effect of unspecified snake venom, undetermined**

✓6ᵗʰ   **T63.01 Toxic effect of rattlesnake venom**

✓7ᵗʰ   **T63.011 Toxic effect of rattlesnake venom, accidental (unintentional)**
    Toxic effect of rattlesnake venom NOS

⁷ ✓7ᵗʰ   **T63.012 Toxic effect of rattlesnake venom, intentional self-harm**   HCC

✓7ᵗʰ   **T63.013 Toxic effect of rattlesnake venom, assault**

✓7ᵗʰ   **T63.014 Toxic effect of rattlesnake venom, undetermined**

✓6ᵗʰ   **T63.02 Toxic effect of coral snake venom**

✓7ᵗʰ   **T63.021 Toxic effect of coral snake venom, accidental (unintentional)**
    Toxic effect of coral snake venom NOS

⁷ ✓7ᵗʰ   **T63.022 Toxic effect of coral snake venom, intentional self-harm**   HCC

✓7ᵗʰ   **T63.023 Toxic effect of coral snake venom, assault**

✓7ᵗʰ   **T63.024 Toxic effect of coral snake venom, undetermined**

✓6ᵗʰ   **T63.03 Toxic effect of taipan venom**

✓7ᵗʰ   **T63.031 Toxic effect of taipan venom, accidental (unintentional)**
    Toxic effect of taipan venom NOS

⁷ ✓7ᵗʰ   **T63.032 Toxic effect of taipan venom, intentional self-harm**   HCC

✓7ᵗʰ   **T63.033 Toxic effect of taipan venom, assault**

✓7ᵗʰ   **T63.034 Toxic effect of taipan venom, undetermined**

✓6ᵗʰ   **T63.04 Toxic effect of cobra venom**

✓7ᵗʰ   **T63.041 Toxic effect of cobra venom, accidental (unintentional)**
    Toxic effect of cobra venom NOS

⁷ ✓7ᵗʰ   **T63.042 Toxic effect of cobra venom, intentional self-harm**   HCC

✓7ᵗʰ   **T63.043 Toxic effect of cobra venom, assault**

✓7ᵗʰ   **T63.044 Toxic effect of cobra venom, undetermined**

✓6ᵗʰ   **T63.06 Toxic effect of venom of other North and South American snake**

✓7ᵗʰ   **T63.061 Toxic effect of venom of other North and South American snake, accidental (unintentional)**
    Toxic effect of venom of other North and South American snake NOS

⁷ ✓7ᵗʰ   **T63.062 Toxic effect of venom of other North and South American snake, intentional self-harm**   HCC

✓7ᵗʰ   **T63.063 Toxic effect of venom of other North and South American snake, assault**

✓7ᵗʰ   **T63.064 Toxic effect of venom of other North and South American snake, undetermined**

✓6ᵗʰ   **T63.07 Toxic effect of venom of other Australian snake**

✓7ᵗʰ   **T63.071 Toxic effect of venom of other Australian snake, accidental (unintentional)**
    Toxic effect of venom of other Australian snake NOS

⁷ ✓7ᵗʰ   **T63.072 Toxic effect of venom of other Australian snake, intentional self-harm**   HCC

✓7ᵗʰ **T63.073 Toxic effect of venom of other Australian snake, assault**

✓7ᵗʰ **T63.074 Toxic effect of venom of other Australian snake, undetermined**

✓6ᵗʰ **T63.08 Toxic effect of venom of other African and Asian snake**

    ✓7ᵗʰ **T63.081 Toxic effect of venom of other African and Asian snake, accidental (unintentional)**
        Toxic effect of venom of other African and Asian snake NOS

    ⁷ ✓7ᵗʰ **T63.082 Toxic effect of venom of other African and Asian snake, intentional self-harm** HCC

    ✓7ᵗʰ **T63.083 Toxic effect of venom of other African and Asian snake, assault**

    ✓7ᵗʰ **T63.084 Toxic effect of venom of other African and Asian snake, undetermined**

✓6ᵗʰ **T63.09 Toxic effect of venom of other snake**

    ✓7ᵗʰ **T63.091 Toxic effect of venom of other snake, accidental (unintentional)**
        Toxic effect of venom of other snake NOS

    ⁷ ✓7ᵗʰ **T63.092 Toxic effect of venom of other snake, intentional self-harm** HCC

    ✓7ᵗʰ **T63.093 Toxic effect of venom of other snake, assault**

    ✓7ᵗʰ **T63.094 Toxic effect of venom of other snake, undetermined**

✓5ᵗʰ **T63.1 Toxic effect of venom of other reptiles**

  ✓6ᵗʰ **T63.11 Toxic effect of venom of gila monster**

    ✓7ᵗʰ **T63.111 Toxic effect of venom of gila monster, accidental (unintentional)**
        Toxic effect of venom of gila monster NOS

    ⁷ ✓7ᵗʰ **T63.112 Toxic effect of venom of gila monster, intentional self-harm** HCC

    ✓7ᵗʰ **T63.113 Toxic effect of venom of gila monster, assault**

    ✓7ᵗʰ **T63.114 Toxic effect of venom of gila monster, undetermined**

  ✓6ᵗʰ **T63.12 Toxic effect of venom of other venomous lizard**

    ✓7ᵗʰ **T63.121 Toxic effect of venom of other venomous lizard, accidental (unintentional)**
        Toxic effect of venom of other venomous lizard NOS

    ⁷ ✓7ᵗʰ **T63.122 Toxic effect of venom of other venomous lizard, intentional self-harm** HCC

    ✓7ᵗʰ **T63.123 Toxic effect of venom of other venomous lizard, assault**

    ✓7ᵗʰ **T63.124 Toxic effect of venom of other venomous lizard, undetermined**

  ✓6ᵗʰ **T63.19 Toxic effect of venom of other reptiles**

    ✓7ᵗʰ **T63.191 Toxic effect of venom of other reptiles, accidental (unintentional)**
        Toxic effect of venom of other reptiles NOS

    ⁷ ✓7ᵗʰ **T63.192 Toxic effect of venom of other reptiles, intentional self-harm** HCC

    ✓7ᵗʰ **T63.193 Toxic effect of venom of other reptiles, assault**

    ✓7ᵗʰ **T63.194 Toxic effect of venom of other reptiles, undetermined**

✓5ᵗʰ **T63.2 Toxic effect of venom of scorpion**

  ✓6ᵗʰ **T63.2X Toxic effect of venom of scorpion**

    ✓7ᵗʰ **T63.2X1 Toxic effect of venom of scorpion, accidental (unintentional)**
        Toxic effect of venom of scorpion NOS

    ⁷ ✓7ᵗʰ **T63.2X2 Toxic effect of venom of scorpion, intentional self-harm** HCC

    ✓7ᵗʰ **T63.2X3 Toxic effect of venom of scorpion, assault**

    ✓7ᵗʰ **T63.2X4 Toxic effect of venom of scorpion, undetermined**

✓5ᵗʰ **T63.3 Toxic effect of venom of spider**

  ✓6ᵗʰ **T63.30 Toxic effect of unspecified spider venom**

    ✓7ᵗʰ **T63.301 Toxic effect of unspecified spider venom, accidental (unintentional)**

    ⁷ ✓7ᵗʰ **T63.302 Toxic effect of unspecified spider venom, intentional self-harm** HCC

    ✓7ᵗʰ **T63.303 Toxic effect of unspecified spider venom, assault**

    ✓7ᵗʰ **T63.304 Toxic effect of unspecified spider venom, undetermined**

✓6ᵗʰ **T63.31 Toxic effect of venom of black widow spider**

    ✓7ᵗʰ **T63.311 Toxic effect of venom of black widow spider, accidental (unintentional)**

    ⁷ ✓7ᵗʰ **T63.312 Toxic effect of venom of black widow spider, intentional self-harm** HCC

    ✓7ᵗʰ **T63.313 Toxic effect of venom of black widow spider, assault**

    ✓7ᵗʰ **T63.314 Toxic effect of venom of black widow spider, undetermined**

✓6ᵗʰ **T63.32 Toxic effect of venom of tarantula**

    ✓7ᵗʰ **T63.321 Toxic effect of venom of tarantula, accidental (unintentional)**

    ⁷ ✓7ᵗʰ **T63.322 Toxic effect of venom of tarantula, intentional self-harm** HCC

    ✓7ᵗʰ **T63.323 Toxic effect of venom of tarantula, assault**

    ✓7ᵗʰ **T63.324 Toxic effect of venom of tarantula, undetermined**

✓6ᵗʰ **T63.33 Toxic effect of venom of brown recluse spider**

    ✓7ᵗʰ **T63.331 Toxic effect of venom of brown recluse spider, accidental (unintentional)**

    ⁷ ✓7ᵗʰ **T63.332 Toxic effect of venom of brown recluse spider, intentional self-harm** HCC

    ✓7ᵗʰ **T63.333 Toxic effect of venom of brown recluse spider, assault**

    ✓7ᵗʰ **T63.334 Toxic effect of venom of brown recluse spider, undetermined**

✓6ᵗʰ **T63.39 Toxic effect of venom of other spider**

    ✓7ᵗʰ **T63.391 Toxic effect of venom of other spider, accidental (unintentional)**

    ⁷ ✓7ᵗʰ **T63.392 Toxic effect of venom of other spider, intentional self-harm** HCC

    ✓7ᵗʰ **T63.393 Toxic effect of venom of other spider, assault**

    ✓7ᵗʰ **T63.394 Toxic effect of venom of other spider, undetermined**

✓5ᵗʰ **T63.4 Toxic effect of venom of other arthropods**

  ✓6ᵗʰ **T63.41 Toxic effect of venom of centipedes and venomous millipedes**

    ✓7ᵗʰ **T63.411 Toxic effect of venom of centipedes and venomous millipedes, accidental (unintentional)**

    ⁷ ✓7ᵗʰ **T63.412 Toxic effect of venom of centipedes and venomous millipedes, intentional self-harm** HCC

    ✓7ᵗʰ **T63.413 Toxic effect of venom of centipedes and venomous millipedes, assault**

    ✓7ᵗʰ **T63.414 Toxic effect of venom of centipedes and venomous millipedes, undetermined**

✓6ᵗʰ **T63.42 Toxic effect of venom of ants**

    ✓7ᵗʰ **T63.421 Toxic effect of venom of ants, accidental (unintentional)**

    ⁷ ✓7ᵗʰ **T63.422 Toxic effect of venom of ants, intentional self-harm** HCC

    ✓7ᵗʰ **T63.423 Toxic effect of venom of ants, assault**

    ✓7ᵗʰ **T63.424 Toxic effect of venom of ants, undetermined**

✓6ᵗʰ **T63.43 Toxic effect of venom of caterpillars**

    ✓7ᵗʰ **T63.431 Toxic effect of venom of caterpillars, accidental (unintentional)**

    ⁷ ✓7ᵗʰ **T63.432 Toxic effect of venom of caterpillars, intentional self-harm** HCC

    ✓7ᵗʰ **T63.433 Toxic effect of venom of caterpillars, assault**

    ✓7ᵗʰ **T63.434 Toxic effect of venom of caterpillars, undetermined**

✓6ᵗʰ **T63.44 Toxic effect of venom of bees**

    ✓7ᵗʰ **T63.441 Toxic effect of venom of bees, accidental (unintentional)**

    ⁷ ✓7ᵗʰ **T63.442 Toxic effect of venom of bees, intentional self-harm** HCC

    ✓7ᵗʰ **T63.443 Toxic effect of venom of bees, assault**

    ✓7ᵗʰ **T63.444 Toxic effect of venom of bees, undetermined**

✓6ᵗʰ **T63.45 Toxic effect of venom of hornets**

    ✓7ᵗʰ **T63.451 Toxic effect of venom of hornets, accidental (unintentional)**

    ⁷ ✓7ᵗʰ **T63.452 Toxic effect of venom of hornets, intentional self-harm** HCC

    ✓7ᵗʰ **T63.453 Toxic effect of venom of hornets, assault**

Ⓝ Newborn: 0   Ⓟ Pediatric: 0-17   Ⓜ Maternity: 9-64   Ⓐ Adult: 15-124   **MCC** Major Complication/Comorbidity   **CC** Complication/Comorbidity   **SW** Severe Wound Dx

1138   ICD-10-CM 2021

√7ᵗʰ **T63.454** **Toxic effect of venom of hornets, undetermined**

√6ᵗʰ **T63.46** **Toxic effect of venom of** wasps

Toxic effect of yellow jacket

√7ᵗʰ **T63.461** **Toxic effect of venom of wasps,** accidental **(unintentional)**

⁷ √7ᵗʰ **T63.462** **Toxic effect of venom of wasps, intentional self-harm**   HCC

√7ᵗʰ **T63.463** **Toxic effect of venom of wasps,** assault

√7ᵗʰ **T63.464** **Toxic effect of venom of wasps, undetermined**

√6ᵗʰ **T63.48** **Toxic effect of venom of other arthropod**

√7ᵗʰ **T63.481** **Toxic effect of venom of other arthropod,** accidental **(unintentional)**

⁷ √7ᵗʰ **T63.482** **Toxic effect of venom of other arthropod, intentional self-harm**   HCC

√7ᵗʰ **T63.483** **Toxic effect of venom of other arthropod,** assault

√7ᵗʰ **T63.484** **Toxic effect of venom of other arthropod, undetermined**

√5ᵗʰ **T63.5** **Toxic effect of contact with** venomous fish

EXCLUDES 2   poisoning by ingestion of fish (T61.-)

√6ᵗʰ **T63.51** **Toxic effect of contact with** stingray

√7ᵗʰ **T63.511** **Toxic effect of contact with stingray,** accidental **(unintentional)**

⁷ √7ᵗʰ **T63.512** **Toxic effect of contact with stingray, intentional self-harm**   HCC

√7ᵗʰ **T63.513** **Toxic effect of contact with stingray,** assault

√7ᵗʰ **T63.514** **Toxic effect of contact with stingray, undetermined**

√6ᵗʰ **T63.59** **Toxic effect of contact with other venomous fish**

√7ᵗʰ **T63.591** **Toxic effect of contact with other venomous fish,** accidental **(unintentional)**

⁷ √7ᵗʰ **T63.592** **Toxic effect of contact with other venomous fish, intentional self-harm**   HCC

√7ᵗʰ **T63.593** **Toxic effect of contact with other venomous fish,** assault

√7ᵗʰ **T63.594** **Toxic effect of contact with other venomous fish, undetermined**

√5ᵗʰ **T63.6** **Toxic effect of contact with other** venomous marine animals

EXCLUDES 1   sea-snake venom (T63.09)

EXCLUDES 2   poisoning by ingestion of shellfish (T61.78-)

√6ᵗʰ **T63.61** **Toxic effect of contact with** Portugese Man-o-war

Toxic effect of contact with bluebottle

√7ᵗʰ **T63.611** **Toxic effect of contact with Portugese Man-o-war,** accidental **(unintentional)**

⁷ √7ᵗʰ **T63.612** **Toxic effect of contact with Portugese Man-o-war, intentional self-harm**   HCC

√7ᵗʰ **T63.613** **Toxic effect of contact with Portugese Man-o-war,** assault

√7ᵗʰ **T63.614** **Toxic effect of contact with Portugese Man-o-war,** undetermined

√6ᵗʰ **T63.62** **Toxic effect of contact with other jellyfish**

√7ᵗʰ **T63.621** **Toxic effect of contact with other jellyfish,** accidental **(unintentional)**

⁷ √7ᵗʰ **T63.622** **Toxic effect of contact with other jellyfish, intentional self-harm**   HCC

√7ᵗʰ **T63.623** **Toxic effect of contact with other jellyfish,** assault

√7ᵗʰ **T63.624** **Toxic effect of contact with other jellyfish, undetermined**

√6ᵗʰ **T63.63** **Toxic effect of contact with** sea anemone

√7ᵗʰ **T63.631** **Toxic effect of contact with sea anemone,** accidental **(unintentional)**

⁷ √7ᵗʰ **T63.632** **Toxic effect of contact with sea anemone, intentional self-harm**   HCC

√7ᵗʰ **T63.633** **Toxic effect of contact with sea anemone,** assault

√7ᵗʰ **T63.634** **Toxic effect of contact with sea anemone, undetermined**

√6ᵗʰ **T63.69** **Toxic effect of contact with other venomous marine animals**

√7ᵗʰ **T63.691** **Toxic effect of contact with other venomous marine animals,** accidental **(unintentional)**

⁷ √7ᵗʰ **T63.692** **Toxic effect of contact with other venomous marine animals, intentional self-harm**   HCC

√7ᵗʰ **T63.693** **Toxic effect of contact with other venomous marine animals,** assault

√7ᵗʰ **T63.694** **Toxic effect of contact with other venomous marine animals,** undetermined

√5ᵗʰ **T63.7** **Toxic effect of contact with** venomous plant

√6ᵗʰ **T63.71** **Toxic effect of contact with venomous** marine plant

√7ᵗʰ **T63.711** **Toxic effect of contact with venomous marine plant,** accidental **(unintentional)**

⁷ √7ᵗʰ **T63.712** **Toxic effect of contact with venomous marine plant, intentional self-harm**   HCC

√7ᵗʰ **T63.713** **Toxic effect of contact with venomous marine plant,** assault

√7ᵗʰ **T63.714** **Toxic effect of contact with venomous marine plant, undetermined**

√6ᵗʰ **T63.79** **Toxic effect of contact with other venomous plant**

√7ᵗʰ **T63.791** **Toxic effect of contact with other venomous plant,** accidental **(unintentional)**

⁷ √7ᵗʰ **T63.792** **Toxic effect of contact with other venomous plant, intentional self-harm**   HCC

√7ᵗʰ **T63.793** **Toxic effect of contact with other venomous plant,** assault

√7ᵗʰ **T63.794** **Toxic effect of contact with other venomous plant, undetermined**

√5ᵗʰ **T63.8** **Toxic effect of contact with other venomous animals**

√6ᵗʰ **T63.81** **Toxic effect of contact with venomous** frog

EXCLUDES 1   contact with nonvenomous frog (W62.0)

√7ᵗʰ **T63.811** **Toxic effect of contact with venomous frog,** accidental **(unintentional)**

⁷ √7ᵗʰ **T63.812** **Toxic effect of contact with venomous frog, intentional self-harm**   HCC

√7ᵗʰ **T63.813** **Toxic effect of contact with venomous frog,** assault

√7ᵗʰ **T63.814** **Toxic effect of contact with venomous frog, undetermined**

√6ᵗʰ **T63.82** **Toxic effect of contact with venomous** toad

EXCLUDES 1   contact with nonvenomous toad (W62.1)

√7ᵗʰ **T63.821** **Toxic effect of contact with venomous toad,** accidental **(unintentional)**

⁷ √7ᵗʰ **T63.822** **Toxic effect of contact with venomous toad, intentional self-harm**   HCC

√7ᵗʰ **T63.823** **Toxic effect of contact with venomous toad,** assault

√7ᵗʰ **T63.824** **Toxic effect of contact with venomous toad, undetermined**

√6ᵗʰ **T63.83** **Toxic effect of contact with other venomous amphibian**

EXCLUDES 1   contact with nonvenomous amphibian (W62.9)

√7ᵗʰ **T63.831** **Toxic effect of contact with other venomous amphibian,** accidental **(unintentional)**

⁷ √7ᵗʰ **T63.832** **Toxic effect of contact with other venomous amphibian, intentional self-harm**   HCC

√7ᵗʰ **T63.833** **Toxic effect of contact with other venomous amphibian,** assault

√7ᵗʰ **T63.834** **Toxic effect of contact with other venomous amphibian, undetermined**

√6ᵗʰ **T63.89** **Toxic effect of contact with other venomous animals**

√7ᵗʰ **T63.891** **Toxic effect of contact with other venomous animals,** accidental **(unintentional)**

⁷ √7ᵗʰ **T63.892** **Toxic effect of contact with other venomous animals, intentional self-harm**   HCC

√7ᵗʰ **T63.893** **Toxic effect of contact with other venomous animals,** assault

√7ᵗʰ **T63.894** **Toxic effect of contact with other venomous animals, undetermined**

√5ᵗʰ **T63.9** **Toxic effect of contact with unspecified venomous animal**

√x7ᵗʰ **T63.91** **Toxic effect of contact with unspecified venomous animal,** accidental **(unintentional)**

⁷ √x7ᵗʰ **T63.92** **Toxic effect of contact with unspecified venomous animal,** intentional self-harm   HCC

√x7ᵗʰ **T63.93** **Toxic effect of contact with unspecified venomous animal,** assault

√x7ᵗʰ **T63.94** **Toxic effect of contact with unspecified venomous animal, undetermined**

✔ Additional Character Required   √x7ᵗʰ Placeholder   Unacceptable PDx   Questionable PDx   Manifestation   Unspecified Dx   H1-H14 HAC   HCC CMS-HCC Dx   HIV HIV Dx

ICD-10-CM 2021   1139

√4ᵗʰ **T64 Toxic effect of aflatoxin and other mycotoxin food contaminants**

> The appropriate 7th character is to be added to each code from category T64.
> A   initial encounter
> D   subsequent encounter
> S   sequela

√5ᵗʰ **T64.0 Toxic effect of** aflatoxin

   √x7ᵗʰ **T64.01 Toxic effect of aflatoxin, accidental (unintentional)**

   7 √x7ᵗʰ **T64.02 Toxic effect of aflatoxin, intentional self-harm**   HCC

   √x7ᵗʰ **T64.03 Toxic effect of aflatoxin, assault**

   √x7ᵗʰ **T64.04 Toxic effect of aflatoxin, undetermined**

√5ᵗʰ **T64.8 Toxic effect of other mycotoxin food contaminants**

   √x7ᵗʰ **T64.81 Toxic effect of other mycotoxin food contaminants, accidental (unintentional)**

   7 √x7ᵗʰ **T64.82 Toxic effect of other mycotoxin food contaminants, intentional self-harm**   HCC

   √x7ᵗʰ **T64.83 Toxic effect of other mycotoxin food contaminants, assault**

   √x7ᵗʰ **T64.84 Toxic effect of other mycotoxin food contaminants, undetermined**

√4ᵗʰ **T65 Toxic effect of other and unspecified substances**

> The appropriate 7th character is to be added to each code from category T65.
> A   initial encounter
> D   subsequent encounter
> S   sequela

√5ᵗʰ **T65.0 Toxic effect of cyanides**

   EXCLUDES 1   *hydrogen cyanide (T57.3-)*

   √6ᵗʰ **T65.0X Toxic effect of** cyanides

     √7ᵗʰ **T65.0X1 Toxic effect of cyanides, accidental (unintentional)**
       Toxic effect of cyanides NOS

     7 √7ᵗʰ **T65.0X2 Toxic effect of cyanides, intentional self-harm**   HCC

     √7ᵗʰ **T65.0X3 Toxic effect of cyanides, assault**

     √7ᵗʰ **T65.0X4 Toxic effect of cyanides, undetermined**

√5ᵗʰ **T65.1 Toxic effect of strychnine and its salts**

   √6ᵗʰ **T65.1X Toxic effect of** strychnine and its salts

     √7ᵗʰ **T65.1X1 Toxic effect of strychnine and its salts, accidental (unintentional)**
       Toxic effect of strychnine and its salts NOS

     7 √7ᵗʰ **T65.1X2 Toxic effect of strychnine and its salts, intentional self-harm**   HCC

     √7ᵗʰ **T65.1X3 Toxic effect of strychnine and its salts, assault**

     √7ᵗʰ **T65.1X4 Toxic effect of strychnine and its salts, undetermined**

√5ᵗʰ **T65.2 Toxic effect of tobacco and nicotine**

   EXCLUDES 2   *nicotine dependence (F17.-)*

   √6ᵗʰ **T65.21 Toxic effect of** chewing tobacco

     √7ᵗʰ **T65.211 Toxic effect of chewing tobacco, accidental (unintentional)**
       Toxic effect of chewing tobacco NOS

     7 √7ᵗʰ **T65.212 Toxic effect of chewing tobacco, intentional self-harm**   HCC

     √7ᵗʰ **T65.213 Toxic effect of chewing tobacco, assault**

     √7ᵗʰ **T65.214 Toxic effect of chewing tobacco, undetermined**

   √6ᵗʰ **T65.22 Toxic effect of** tobacco cigarettes

     Toxic effect of tobacco smoke
     Use additional code for exposure to second hand tobacco smoke (Z57.31, Z77.22)

     √7ᵗʰ **T65.221 Toxic effect of tobacco cigarettes, accidental (unintentional)**
       Toxic effect of tobacco cigarettes NOS

     7 √7ᵗʰ **T65.222 Toxic effect of tobacco cigarettes, intentional self-harm**   HCC

     √7ᵗʰ **T65.223 Toxic effect of tobacco cigarettes, assault**

     √7ᵗʰ **T65.224 Toxic effect of tobacco cigarettes, undetermined**

   √6ᵗʰ **T65.29 Toxic effect of other tobacco and nicotine**

     √7ᵗʰ **T65.291 Toxic effect of other tobacco and nicotine, accidental (unintentional)**
       Toxic effect of other tobacco and nicotine NOS

     7 √7ᵗʰ **T65.292 Toxic effect of other tobacco and nicotine, intentional self-harm**   HCC

     √7ᵗʰ **T65.293 Toxic effect of other tobacco and nicotine, assault**

     √7ᵗʰ **T65.294 Toxic effect of other tobacco and nicotine, undetermined**

√5ᵗʰ **T65.3 Toxic effect of nitroderivatives and aminoderivatives of benzene and its homologues**

   Toxic effect of anilin [benzenamine]
   Toxic effect of nitrobenzene
   Toxic effect of trinitrotoluene

   √6ᵗʰ **T65.3X Toxic effect of** nitroderivatives and aminoderivatives of benzene and its homologues

     √7ᵗʰ **T65.3X1 Toxic effect of nitroderivatives and aminoderivatives of benzene and its homologues, accidental (unintentional)**
       Toxic effect of nitroderivatives and aminoderivatives of benzene and its homologues NOS

     7 √7ᵗʰ **T65.3X2 Toxic effect of nitroderivatives and aminoderivatives of benzene and its homologues, intentional self-harm**   HCC

     √7ᵗʰ **T65.3X3 Toxic effect of nitroderivatives and aminoderivatives of benzene and its homologues, assault**

     √7ᵗʰ **T65.3X4 Toxic effect of nitroderivatives and aminoderivatives of benzene and its homologues, undetermined**

√5ᵗʰ **T65.4 Toxic effect of carbon disulfide**

   √6ᵗʰ **T65.4X Toxic effect of** carbon disulfide

     √7ᵗʰ **T65.4X1 Toxic effect of carbon disulfide, accidental (unintentional)**
       Toxic effect of carbon disulfide NOS

     7 √7ᵗʰ **T65.4X2 Toxic effect of carbon disulfide, intentional self-harm**   HCC

     √7ᵗʰ **T65.4X3 Toxic effect of carbon disulfide, assault**

     √7ᵗʰ **T65.4X4 Toxic effect of carbon disulfide, undetermined**

√5ᵗʰ **T65.5 Toxic effect of nitroglycerin and other nitric acids and esters**

   Toxic effect of 1,2,3-Propanetriol trinitrate

   √6ᵗʰ **T65.5X Toxic effect of** nitroglycerin and other nitric acids and esters

     √7ᵗʰ **T65.5X1 Toxic effect of nitroglycerin and other nitric acids and esters, accidental (unintentional)**
       Toxic effect of nitroglycerin and other nitric acids and esters NOS

     7 √7ᵗʰ **T65.5X2 Toxic effect of nitroglycerin and other nitric acids and esters, intentional self-harm**   HCC

     √7ᵗʰ **T65.5X3 Toxic effect of nitroglycerin and other nitric acids and esters, assault**

     √7ᵗʰ **T65.5X4 Toxic effect of nitroglycerin and other nitric acids and esters, undetermined**

√5ᵗʰ **T65.6 Toxic effect of paints and dyes, not elsewhere classified**

   √6ᵗʰ **T65.6X Toxic effect of** paints and dyes, not elsewhere classified

     √7ᵗʰ **T65.6X1 Toxic effect of paints and dyes, not elsewhere classified, accidental (unintentional)**
       Toxic effect of paints and dyes NOS

     7 √7ᵗʰ **T65.6X2 Toxic effect of paints and dyes, not elsewhere classified, intentional self-harm**   HCC

     √7ᵗʰ **T65.6X3 Toxic effect of paints and dyes, not elsewhere classified, assault**

     √7ᵗʰ **T65.6X4 Toxic effect of paints and dyes, not elsewhere classified, undetermined**

√5ᵗʰ **T65.8 Toxic effect of other specified substances**

   √6ᵗʰ **T65.81 Toxic effect of** latex

     √7ᵗʰ **T65.811 Toxic effect of latex, accidental (unintentional)**
       Toxic effect of latex NOS

N Newborn: 0   P Pediatric: 0-17   M Maternity: 9-64   A Adult: 15-124   MCC Major Complication/Comorbidity   CC Complication/Comorbidity   SW Severe Wound Dx

1140   ICD-10-CM 2021

7 ✓7ᵗʰ **T65.812** **Toxic effect of latex, intentional self-harm** HCC

✓7ᵗʰ **T65.813** **Toxic effect of latex, assault**

✓7ᵗʰ **T65.814** **Toxic effect of latex, undetermined**

✓6ᵗʰ **T65.82** **Toxic effect of harmful algae and algae toxins**

Toxic effect of (harmful) algae bloom NOS
Toxic effect of blue-green algae bloom
Toxic effect of brown tide
Toxic effect of cyanobacteria bloom
Toxic effect of Florida red tide
Toxic effect of pfiesteria piscicida
Toxic effect of red tide

✓7ᵗʰ **T65.821** **Toxic effect of harmful algae and algae toxins, accidental (unintentional)**
Toxic effect of harmful algae and algae toxins NOS

7 ✓7ᵗʰ **T65.822** **Toxic effect of harmful algae and algae toxins, intentional self-harm** HCC

✓7ᵗʰ **T65.823** **Toxic effect of harmful algae and algae toxins, assault**

✓7ᵗʰ **T65.824** **Toxic effect of harmful algae and algae toxins, undetermined**

✓6ᵗʰ **T65.83** **Toxic effect of fiberglass**

✓7ᵗʰ **T65.831** **Toxic effect of fiberglass, accidental (unintentional)**
Toxic effect of fiberglass NOS

7 ✓7ᵗʰ **T65.832** **Toxic effect of fiberglass, intentional self-harm** HCC

✓7ᵗʰ **T65.833** **Toxic effect of fiberglass, assault**

✓7ᵗʰ **T65.834** **Toxic effect of fiberglass, undetermined**

✓6ᵗʰ **T65.89** **Toxic effect of other specified substances**

✓7ᵗʰ **T65.891** **Toxic effect of other specified substances, accidental (unintentional)**
Toxic effect of other specified substances NOS
AHA: 2018,1Q,5

7 ✓7ᵗʰ **T65.892** **Toxic effect of other specified substances, intentional self-harm** HCC

✓7ᵗʰ **T65.893** **Toxic effect of other specified substances, assault**

✓7ᵗʰ **T65.894** **Toxic effect of other specified substances, undetermined**

✓5ᵗʰ **T65.9** **Toxic effect of unspecified substance**

✓x7ᵗʰ **T65.91** **Toxic effect of unspecified substance, accidental (unintentional)**
Poisoning NOS

7 ✓x7ᵗʰ **T65.92** **Toxic effect of unspecified substance, intentional self-harm** HCC

✓x7ᵗʰ **T65.93** **Toxic effect of unspecified substance, assault**

✓x7ᵗʰ **T65.94** **Toxic effect of unspecified substance, undetermined**

Other and unspecified effects of external causes (T66-T78)

✓x7ᵗʰ **T66** **Radiation sickness, unspecified**

EXCLUDES 1   *specified adverse effects of radiation, such as:*
burns (T20-T31)
leukemia (C91-C95)
radiation gastroenteritis and colitis (K52.0)
radiation pneumonitis (J70.0)
radiation related disorders of the skin and subcutaneous tissue (L55-L59)
radiation sunburn (L55.-)

The appropriate 7th character is to be added to code T66.
A   initial encounter
D   subsequent encounter
S   sequela

✓4ᵗʰ **T67** **Effects of heat and light**

EXCLUDES 1   *erythema [dermatitis] ab igne (L59.0)*
malignant hyperpyrexia due to anesthesia (T88.3)
radiation-related disorders of the skin and subcutaneous tissue (L55-L59)

EXCLUDES 2   *burns (T20-T31)*
sunburn (L55.-)
sweat disorder due to heat (L74-L75)

The appropriate 7th character is to be added to each code from category T67.
A   initial encounter
D   subsequent encounter
S   sequela

✓5ᵗʰ **T67.0** **Heatstroke and sunstroke**

Use additional code(s) to identify any associated complications of heatstroke, such as:
coma and stupor (R40.-)
rhabdomyolysis (M62.82)
systemic inflammatory response syndrome (R65.1-)
AHA: 2019,4Q,17-18
DEF: Headache, vertigo, cramps, and elevated body temperature due to prolonged exposure to high environmental temperatures that requires emergency intervention.

✓x7ᵗʰ **T67.01** **Heatstroke and sunstroke** CC H5
Heat apoplexy
Heat pyrexia
Siriasis
Thermoplegia

✓x7ᵗʰ **T67.02** **Exertional heatstroke** CC H5

✓x7ᵗʰ **T67.09** **Other heatstroke and sunstroke** CC H5

✓x7ᵗʰ **T67.1** **Heat syncope**
Heat collapse

✓x7ᵗʰ **T67.2** **Heat cramp**

✓x7ᵗʰ **T67.3** **Heat exhaustion, anhydrotic**
Heat prostration due to water depletion
EXCLUDES 1   *heat exhaustion due to salt depletion (T67.4)*

✓x7ᵗʰ **T67.4** **Heat exhaustion due to salt depletion**
Heat prostration due to salt (and water) depletion

✓x7ᵗʰ **T67.5** **Heat exhaustion, unspecified**
Heat prostration NOS

✓x7ᵗʰ **T67.6** **Heat fatigue, transient**

✓x7ᵗʰ **T67.7** **Heat edema**

✓x7ᵗʰ **T67.8** **Other effects of heat and light**

✓x7ᵗʰ **T67.9** **Effect of heat and light, unspecified**

✓x7ᵗʰ **T68** **Hypothermia**

Accidental hypothermia
Hypothermia NOS
Use additional code to identify source of exposure:
exposure to excessive cold of man-made origin (W93)
exposure to excessive cold of natural origin (X31)
EXCLUDES 1   *hypothermia following anesthesia (T88.51)*
hypothermia not associated with low environmental temperature (R68.0)
hypothermia of newborn (P80.-)
EXCLUDES 2   *frostbite (T33-T34)*

The appropriate 7th character is to be added to code T68.
A   initial encounter
D   subsequent encounter
S   sequela

✓4ᵗʰ **T69** **Other effects of reduced temperature**

Use additional code to identify source of exposure:
exposure to excessive cold of man-made origin (W93)
exposure to excessive cold of natural origin (X31)
EXCLUDES 2   *frostbite (T33-T34)*

The appropriate 7th character is to be added to each code from category T69.
A   initial encounter
D   subsequent encounter
S   sequela

✓5ᵗʰ **T69.0** **Immersion hand and foot**

✓6ᵗʰ **T69.01** **Immersion hand**

✓7ᵗʰ **T69.011** **Immersion hand, right hand**

√7ᵗʰ **T69.012** Immersion hand, left hand

√7ᵗʰ **T69.019** Immersion hand, unspecified hand

√6ᵗʰ **T69.02** **Immersion foot**
Trench foot

√7ᵗʰ **T69.021** Immersion foot, right foot   CC H5

√7ᵗʰ **T69.022** Immersion foot, left foot   CC H5

√7ᵗʰ **T69.029** Immersion foot, unspecified foot   CC H5

√x7ᵗʰ **T69.1** **Chilblains**
DEF: Red, swollen, itchy skin primarily affecting the fingers and toes, nose and ears, and legs. Chilblains follows damp-cold exposure, and can also be associated with pruritus and a burning feeling.

√x7ᵗʰ **T69.8** **Other specified effects of reduced temperature**

√x7ᵗʰ **T69.9** **Effect of reduced temperature, unspecified**

√4ᵗʰ **T70** **Effects of air pressure and water pressure**

The appropriate 7th character is to be added to each code from category T70.
A   initial encounter
D   subsequent encounter
S   sequela

√x7ᵗʰ **T70.0** **Otitic barotrauma**
Aero-otitis media
Effects of change in ambient atmospheric pressure or water pressure on ears

√x7ᵗʰ **T70.1** **Sinus barotrauma**
Aerosinusitis
Effects of change in ambient atmospheric pressure on sinuses

√5ᵗʰ **T70.2** **Other and unspecified effects of high altitude**
EXCLUDES 2   polycythemia due to high altitude (D75.1)

√x7ᵗʰ **T70.20** **Unspecified effects of high altitude**

√x7ᵗʰ **T70.29** **Other effects of high altitude**
Alpine sickness
Anoxia due to high altitude
Barotrauma NOS
Hypobaropathy
Mountain sickness

√x7ᵗʰ **T70.3** **Caisson disease [decompression sickness]**   CC H5
Compressed-air disease
Diver's palsy or paralysis
DEF: Rapid reduction in air pressure while breathing compressed air. Symptoms include skin lesions, joint pains, and respiratory and neurological problems.

√x7ᵗʰ **T70.4** **Effects of high-pressure fluids**
Hydraulic jet injection (industrial)
Pneumatic jet injection (industrial)
Traumatic jet injection (industrial)

√x7ᵗʰ **T70.8** **Other effects of air pressure and water pressure**

√x7ᵗʰ **T70.9** **Effect of air pressure and water pressure, unspecified**

√4ᵗʰ **T71** **Asphyxiation**
Mechanical suffocation
Traumatic suffocation
EXCLUDES 1   acute respiratory distress (syndrome) (J80)
anoxia due to high altitude (T70.2)
asphyxia NOS (R09.01)
asphyxia from carbon monoxide (T58.-)
asphyxia from inhalation of food or foreign body (T17.-)
asphyxia from other gases, fumes and vapors (T59.-)
respiratory distress (syndrome) in newborn (P22.-)

The appropriate 7th character is to be added to each code from category T71.
A   initial encounter
D   subsequent encounter
S   sequela

√5ᵗʰ **T71.1** **Asphyxiation due to mechanical threat to breathing**
Suffocation due to mechanical threat to breathing

√6ᵗʰ **T71.11** **Asphyxiation due to smothering under pillow**

√7ᵗʰ **T71.111** Asphyxiation due to smothering under pillow, accidental   CC H5
Asphyxiation due to smothering under pillow NOS

7 √7ᵗʰ **T71.112** Asphyxiation due to smothering under pillow, intentional self-harm   CC H5 MCC

√7ᵗʰ **T71.113** Asphyxiation due to smothering under pillow, assault   CC H5

√7ᵗʰ **T71.114** Asphyxiation due to smothering under pillow, undetermined   CC H5

√6ᵗʰ **T71.12** **Asphyxiation due to plastic bag**

√7ᵗʰ **T71.121** Asphyxiation due to plastic bag, accidental   CC H5
Asphyxiation due to plastic bag NOS

7 √7ᵗʰ **T71.122** Asphyxiation due to plastic bag, intentional self-harm   CC H5 MCC

√7ᵗʰ **T71.123** Asphyxiation due to plastic bag, assault   CC H5

√7ᵗʰ **T71.124** Asphyxiation due to plastic bag, undetermined   CC H5

√6ᵗʰ **T71.13** **Asphyxiation due to being trapped in bed linens**

√7ᵗʰ **T71.131** Asphyxiation due to being trapped in bed linens, accidental   CC H5
Asphyxiation due to being trapped in bed linens NOS

7 √7ᵗʰ **T71.132** Asphyxiation due to being trapped in bed linens, intentional self-harm   CC H5 MCC

√7ᵗʰ **T71.133** Asphyxiation due to being trapped in bed linens, assault   CC H5

√7ᵗʰ **T71.134** Asphyxiation due to being trapped in bed linens, undetermined   CC H5

√6ᵗʰ **T71.14** **Asphyxiation due to smothering under another person's body (in bed)**

√7ᵗʰ **T71.141** Asphyxiation due to smothering under another person's body (in bed), accidental   CC H5
Asphyxiation due to smothering under another person's body (in bed) NOS

√7ᵗʰ **T71.143** Asphyxiation due to smothering under another person's body (in bed), assault   CC H5

√7ᵗʰ **T71.144** Asphyxiation due to smothering under another person's body (in bed), undetermined   CC H5

√6ᵗʰ **T71.15** **Asphyxiation due to smothering in furniture**

√7ᵗʰ **T71.151** Asphyxiation due to smothering in furniture, accidental   CC H5
Asphyxiation due to smothering in furniture NOS

7 √7ᵗʰ **T71.152** Asphyxiation due to smothering in furniture, intentional self-harm   CC H5 MCC

√7ᵗʰ **T71.153** Asphyxiation due to smothering in furniture, assault   CC H5

√7ᵗʰ **T71.154** Asphyxiation due to smothering in furniture, undetermined   CC H5

√6ᵗʰ **T71.16** **Asphyxiation due to hanging**
Hanging by window shade cord
Use additional code for any associated injuries, such as:
crushing injury of neck (S17.-)
fracture of cervical vertebrae (S12.0-S12.2-)
open wound of neck (S11.-)

√7ᵗʰ **T71.161** Asphyxiation due to hanging, accidental   CC H5
Asphyxiation due to hanging NOS
Hanging NOS

7 √7ᵗʰ **T71.162** Asphyxiation due to hanging, intentional self-harm   CC H5 MCC

√7ᵗʰ **T71.163** Asphyxiation due to hanging, assault   CC H5

√7ᵗʰ **T71.164** Asphyxiation due to hanging, undetermined   CC H5

√6ᵗʰ **T71.19** **Asphyxiation due to mechanical threat to breathing due to other causes**

√7ᵗʰ **T71.191** Asphyxiation due to mechanical threat to breathing due to other causes, accidental   CC H5
Asphyxiation due to other causes NOS

7 √7ᵗʰ **T71.192** Asphyxiation due to mechanical threat to breathing due to other causes, intentional self-harm   CC H5 MCC

☑7ᵗʰ **T71.193** **Asphyxiation due to mechanical threat to breathing due to other causes,** assault   CC H5

☑7ᵗʰ **T71.194** **Asphyxiation due to mechanical threat to breathing due to other causes,** undetermined   CC H5

☑5ᵗʰ **T71.2** **Asphyxiation due to** systemic oxygen deficiency due to low oxygen content in ambient air

Suffocation due to systemic oxygen deficiency due to low oxygen content in ambient air

☑x7ᵗʰ **T71.20** **Asphyxiation due to systemic oxygen deficiency due to low oxygen content in ambient air due to unspecified cause**   CC H5

☑x7ᵗʰ **T71.21** **Asphyxiation due to** cave-in or falling earth   CC H5

Use additional code for any associated cataclysm (X34-X38)

☑6ᵗʰ **T71.22** **Asphyxiation due to** being trapped in a car trunk

☑7ᵗʰ **T71.221** **Asphyxiation due to being trapped in a car trunk,** accidental   CC

7 ☑7ᵗʰ **T71.222** **Asphyxiation due to being trapped in a car trunk,** intentional self-harm   CC HCC

☑7ᵗʰ **T71.223** **Asphyxiation due to being trapped in a car trunk,** assault   CC

☑7ᵗʰ **T71.224** **Asphyxiation due to being trapped in a car trunk,** undetermined   CC

☑6ᵗʰ **T71.23** **Asphyxiation due to being** trapped in a (discarded) refrigerator

☑7ᵗʰ **T71.231** **Asphyxiation due to being trapped in a (discarded) refrigerator,** accidental   CC

7 ☑7ᵗʰ **T71.232** **Asphyxiation due to being trapped in a (discarded) refrigerator,** intentional self-harm   CC HCC

☑7ᵗʰ **T71.233** **Asphyxiation due to being trapped in a (discarded) refrigerator,** assault   CC

☑7ᵗʰ **T71.234** **Asphyxiation due to being trapped in a (discarded) refrigerator,** undetermined   CC

☑x7ᵗʰ **T71.29** **Asphyxiation due to being trapped in other low oxygen environment**   CC H5

☑x7ᵗʰ **T71.9** **Asphyxiation due to unspecified cause**   CC H5

Suffocation (by strangulation) due to unspecified cause

Suffocation NOS

Systemic oxygen deficiency due to low oxygen content in ambient air due to unspecified cause

Systemic oxygen deficiency due to mechanical threat to breathing due to unspecified cause

Traumatic asphyxia NOS

☑4ᵗʰ **T73** **Effects of other deprivation**

The appropriate 7th character is to be added to each code from category T73.
A   initial encounter
D   subsequent encounter
S   sequela

☑x7ᵗʰ **T73.0** **Starvation**

Deprivation of food

☑x7ᵗʰ **T73.1** **Deprivation of water**

☑x7ᵗʰ **T73.2** **Exhaustion due to exposure**

☑x7ᵗʰ **T73.3** **Exhaustion due to excessive exertion**

Exhaustion due to overexertion

☑x7ᵗʰ **T73.8** **Other effects of deprivation**

☑x7ᵗʰ **T73.9** **Effect of deprivation, unspecified**

☑4ᵗʰ **T74** **Adult and child abuse, neglect and other maltreatment,** confirmed

Use additional code, if applicable, to identify any associated current injury

Use additional external cause code to identify perpetrator, if known (Y07.-)

EXCLUDES 1   abuse and maltreatment in pregnancy (O9A.3-, O9A.4-, O9A.5-)

adult and child maltreatment, suspected (T76.-)

The appropriate 7th character is to be added to each code from category T74.
A   initial encounter
D   subsequent encounter
S   sequela

☑5ᵗʰ **T74.0** **Neglect or abandonment, confirmed**

☑x7ᵗʰ **T74.01** Adult **neglect or abandonment, confirmed**   CC A

☑x7ᵗʰ **T74.02** Child **neglect or abandonment, confirmed**   CC P

☑5ᵗʰ **T74.1** **Physical abuse, confirmed**

EXCLUDES 2   sexual abuse (T74.2-)

☑x7ᵗʰ **T74.11** Adult **physical abuse, confirmed**   CC A

☑x7ᵗʰ **T74.12** Child **physical abuse, confirmed**   CC P

EXCLUDES 2   shaken infant syndrome (T74.4)

☑5ᵗʰ **T74.2** **Sexual abuse, confirmed**

Rape, confirmed
Sexual assault, confirmed

☑x7ᵗʰ **T74.21** Adult **sexual abuse, confirmed**   CC A

☑x7ᵗʰ **T74.22** Child **sexual abuse, confirmed**   CC P

☑5ᵗʰ **T74.3** **Psychological abuse, confirmed**

Bullying and intimidation, confirmed
Intimidation through social media, confirmed

☑x7ᵗʰ **T74.31** Adult **psychological abuse, confirmed**   A

☑x7ᵗʰ **T74.32** Child **psychological abuse, confirmed**   CC P

☑x7ᵗʰ **T74.4** **Shaken infant syndrome**   CC P

☑5ᵗʰ **T74.5** **Forced sexual exploitation, confirmed**

AHA: 2018,4Q,32-33,65

☑x7ᵗʰ **T74.51** Adult **forced sexual exploitation, confirmed**   CC A

☑x7ᵗʰ **T74.52** Child **sexual exploitation, confirmed**   CC P

☑5ᵗʰ **T74.6** **Forced labor exploitation, confirmed**

AHA: 2018,4Q,32-33,65

☑x7ᵗʰ **T74.61** Adult **forced labor exploitation, confirmed**   CC A

☑x7ᵗʰ **T74.62** Child **forced labor exploitation, confirmed**   CC P

☑5ᵗʰ **T74.9** **Unspecified maltreatment, confirmed**

☑x7ᵗʰ **T74.91** **Unspecified** adult **maltreatment, confirmed**   CC A

☑x7ᵗʰ **T74.92** **Unspecified** child **maltreatment, confirmed**   CC P

☑4ᵗʰ **T75** **Other and unspecified effects of other external causes**

EXCLUDES 1   adverse effects NEC (T78.-)
EXCLUDES 2   burns (electric) (T20-T31)

The appropriate 7th character is to be added to each code from category T75.
A   initial encounter
D   subsequent encounter
S   sequela

☑5ᵗʰ **T75.0** **Effects of lightning**

Struck by lightning

☑x7ᵗʰ **T75.00** **Unspecified effects of lightning**

Struck by lightning NOS

☑x7ᵗʰ **T75.01** **Shock due to being struck by lightning**

☑x7ᵗʰ **T75.09** **Other effects of lightning**

Use additional code for other effects of lightning

☑x7ᵗʰ **T75.1** **Unspecified effects of drowning and nonfatal submersion**   CC H5

Immersion

EXCLUDES 1   specified effects of drowning — code to effects

☑5ᵗʰ **T75.2** **Effects of vibration**

☑x7ᵗʰ **T75.20** **Unspecified effects of vibration**

☑x7ᵗʰ **T75.21** **Pneumatic hammer syndrome**

☑x7ᵗʰ **T75.22** **Traumatic vasospastic syndrome**

√x7ᵗʰ **T75.23 Vertigo from infrasound**
    EXCLUDES 1   vertigo NOS (R42)

√x7ᵗʰ **T75.29 Other effects of vibration**

√x7ᵗʰ **T75.3 Motion sickness**
    Airsickness
    Seasickness
    Travel sickness
    Use additional external cause code to identify vehicle or type
      of motion (Y92.81-, Y93.5-)

√x7ᵗʰ **T75.4 Electrocution**
    Shock from electric current
    Shock from electroshock gun (taser)

√5ᵗʰ **T75.8 Other specified effects of external causes**

    √x7ᵗʰ **T75.81 Effects of abnormal gravitation [G] forces**

    √x7ᵗʰ **T75.82 Effects of weightlessness**

    √x7ᵗʰ **T75.89 Other specified effects of external causes**

√4ᵗʰ **T76 Adult and child abuse, neglect and other maltreatment, suspected**
    Use additional code, if applicable, to identify any associated current
      injury
    EXCLUDES 1   adult and child maltreatment, confirmed (T74.-)
        suspected abuse and maltreatment in pregnancy (O9A.3-,
          O9A.4-, O9A.5-)
        suspected adult physical abuse, ruled out (Z04.71)
        suspected adult sexual abuse, ruled out (Z04.41)
        suspected child physical abuse, ruled out (Z04.72)
        suspected child sexual abuse, ruled out (Z04.42)

    AHA: 2018,4Q,72

    The appropriate 7th character is to be added to each code from
    category T76.
    A   initial encounter
    D   subsequent encounter
    S   sequela

√5ᵗʰ **T76.0 Neglect or abandonment, suspected**

    √x7ᵗʰ **T76.01 Adult neglect or abandonment, suspected** cc A

    √x7ᵗʰ **T76.02 Child neglect or abandonment, suspected** cc P

√5ᵗʰ **T76.1 Physical abuse, suspected**

    √x7ᵗʰ **T76.11 Adult physical abuse, suspected** cc A

    √x7ᵗʰ **T76.12 Child physical abuse, suspected** cc P
        AHA: 2019,2Q,12

√5ᵗʰ **T76.2 Sexual abuse, suspected**
    Rape, suspected
    EXCLUDES 1   alleged abuse, ruled out (Z04.7)

    √x7ᵗʰ **T76.21 Adult sexual abuse, suspected** cc A

    √x7ᵗʰ **T76.22 Child sexual abuse, suspected** cc P

√5ᵗʰ **T76.3 Psychological abuse, suspected**
    Bullying and intimidation, suspected
    Intimidation through social media, suspected

    √x7ᵗʰ **T76.31 Adult psychological abuse, suspected** A

    √x7ᵗʰ **T76.32 Child psychological abuse, suspected** cc P

√5ᵗʰ **T76.5 Forced sexual exploitation, suspected**
    AHA: 2018,4Q,32-33,65

    √x7ᵗʰ **T76.51 Adult forced sexual exploitation,
        suspected** cc A

    √x7ᵗʰ **T76.52 Child sexual exploitation, suspected** cc P

√5ᵗʰ **T76.6 Forced labor exploitation, suspected**
    AHA: 2018,4Q,32-33,65

    √x7ᵗʰ **T76.61 Adult forced labor exploitation, suspected** cc A

    √x7ᵗʰ **T76.62 Child forced labor exploitation, suspected** cc P

√5ᵗʰ **T76.9 Unspecified maltreatment, suspected**

    √x7ᵗʰ **T76.91 Unspecified adult maltreatment,
        suspected** cc A

    √x7ᵗʰ **T76.92 Unspecified child maltreatment, suspected** cc P

√4ᵗʰ **T78 Adverse effects, not elsewhere classified**
    EXCLUDES 2   complications of surgical and medical care NEC (T80-T88)

    The appropriate 7th character is to be added to each code from
    category T78.
    A   initial encounter
    D   subsequent encounter
    S   sequela

√5ᵗʰ **T78.0 Anaphylactic reaction due to food**
    Anaphylactic reaction due to adverse food reaction
    Anaphylactic shock or reaction due to nonpoisonous foods
    Anaphylactoid reaction due to food

    √x7ᵗʰ **T78.00 Anaphylactic reaction due to unspecified
        food** cc

    √x7ᵗʰ **T78.01 Anaphylactic reaction due to peanuts** cc

    √x7ᵗʰ **T78.02 Anaphylactic reaction due to shellfish
        (crustaceans)** cc

    √x7ᵗʰ **T78.03 Anaphylactic reaction due to other fish**

    √x7ᵗʰ **T78.04 Anaphylactic reaction due to fruits and
        vegetables** cc

    √x7ᵗʰ **T78.05 Anaphylactic reaction due to tree nuts and
        seeds** cc
        EXCLUDES 2   anaphylactic reaction due to peanuts
          (T78.01)

    √x7ᵗʰ **T78.06 Anaphylactic reaction due to food additives** cc

    √x7ᵗʰ **T78.07 Anaphylactic reaction due to milk and dairy
        products** cc

    √x7ᵗʰ **T78.08 Anaphylactic reaction due to eggs** cc

    √x7ᵗʰ **T78.09 Anaphylactic reaction due to other food
        products** cc

√x7ᵗʰ **T78.1 Other adverse food reactions, not elsewhere classified**
    Use additional code to identify the type of reaction, if applicable
    EXCLUDES 1   anaphylactic reaction or shock due to adverse food
          reaction (T78.0-)
        anaphylactic reaction due to food (T78.0-)
        bacterial food borne intoxications (A05.-)
    EXCLUDES 2   allergic and dietetic gastroenteritis and colitis
          (K52.29)
        allergic rhinitis due to food (J30.5)
        dermatitis due to food in contact with skin (L23.6,
          L24.6, L25.4)
        dermatitis due to ingested food (L27.2)
        food protein-induced enterocolitis syndrome (K52.21)
        food protein-induced enteropathy (K52.22)

√x7ᵗʰ **T78.2 Anaphylactic shock, unspecified** cc
    Allergic shock
    Anaphylactic reaction
    Anaphylaxis
    EXCLUDES 1   anaphylactic reaction or shock due to adverse effect
          of correct medicinal substance properly
          administered (T88.6)
        anaphylactic reaction or shock due to adverse food
          reaction (T78.0-)
        anaphylactic reaction or shock due to serum (T80.5-)

√x7ᵗʰ **T78.3 Angioneurotic edema**
    Allergic angioedema
    Giant urticaria
    Quincke's edema
    EXCLUDES 1   serum urticaria (T80.6-)
        urticaria (L50.-)

√5ᵗʰ **T78.4 Other and unspecified allergy**
    EXCLUDES 1   specified types of allergic reaction such as:
        allergic diarrhea (K52.29)
        allergic gastroenteritis and colitis (K52.29)
        dermatitis (L23-L25, L27.-)
        food protein-induced enterocolitis syndrome
          (K52.21)
        food protein-induced enteropathy (K52.22)
        hay fever (J30.1)

    √x7ᵗʰ **T78.40 Allergy, unspecified**
        Allergic reaction NOS
        Hypersensitivity NOS

    √x7ᵗʰ **T78.41 Arthus phenomenon**
        Arthus reaction

    √x7ᵗʰ **T78.49 Other allergy**

N Newborn: 0   P Pediatric: 0-17   M Maternity: 9-64   A Adult: 15-124   MCC Major Complication/Comorbidity   cc Complication/Comorbidity   SW Severe Wound Dx

1144   ICD-10-CM 2021

√x7ʰ **T78.8**   **Other adverse effects, not elsewhere classified**

Certain early complications of trauma (T79)

√4ʰ **T79**   **Certain early complications of trauma, not elsewhere classified**

> EXCLUDES 2   acute respiratory distress syndrome (J80)
> complications occurring during or following medical
>   procedures (T80-T88)
> complications of surgical and medical care NEC (T80-T88)
> newborn respiratory distress syndrome (P22.0)

> The appropriate 7th character is to be added to each code from
> category T79.
> A   initial encounter
> D   subsequent encounter
> S   sequela

6 √x7ʰ **T79.0**   **Air embolism (traumatic)**   MCC HCC

> EXCLUDES 1   air embolism complicating abortion or ectopic or
>   molar pregnancy (O00-O07, O08.2)
> air embolism complicating pregnancy, childbirth and
>   the puerperium (O88.0)
> air embolism following infusion, transfusion, and
>   therapeutic injection (T80.0)
> air embolism following procedure NEC (T81.7-)

> **DEF:** Arterial or venous obstruction due to the introduction of air
> bubbles into the blood vessels following surgery or trauma.

6 √x7ʰ **T79.1**   **Fat embolism (traumatic)**   MCC HCC

> EXCLUDES 1   fat embolism complicating:
>   abortion or ectopic or molar pregnancy (O00-O07,
>   O08.2)
>   pregnancy, childbirth and the puerperium (O88.8)

> **DEF:** Arterial blockage due to the entrance of fat into the
> circulatory system after a fracture of the large bones or
> administration of corticosteroids.

6 √x7ʰ **T79.2**   **Traumatic secondary and recurrent hemorrhage and
seroma**   CC HCC

6 √x7ʰ **T79.4**   **Traumatic shock**   MCC HCC

> Shock (immediate) (delayed) following injury

> EXCLUDES 1   anaphylactic shock due to adverse food reaction
>   (T78.0-)
> anaphylactic shock due to correct medicinal
>   substance properly administered (T88.6)
> anaphylactic shock due to serum (T80.5-)
> anaphylactic shock NOS (T78.2)
> anesthetic shock (T88.2)
> electric shock (T75.4)
> nontraumatic shock NEC (R57.-)
> obstetric shock (O75.1)
> postprocedural shock (T81.1-)
> septic shock (R65.21)
> shock complicating abortion or ectopic or molar
>   pregnancy (O00-O07, O08.3)
> shock due to lightning (T75.01)
> shock NOS (R57.9)

6 √x7ʰ **T79.5**   **Traumatic anuria**   MCC HCC

> Crush syndrome
> Renal failure following crushing

6 √x7ʰ **T79.6**   **Traumatic ischemia of muscle**   HCC

> Traumatic rhabdomyolysis
> Volkmann's ischemic contracture

> EXCLUDES 2   anterior tibial syndrome (M76.8)
> compartment syndrome (traumatic) (T79.A-)
> nontraumatic ischemia of muscle (M62.2-)

> **AHA:** 2019,2Q,12

6 √x7ʰ **T79.7**   **Traumatic subcutaneous emphysema**   CC HCC

> EXCLUDES 1   ~~emphysema NOS (J43)~~
> ~~emphysema (subcutaneous) resulting from a~~
> ~~procedure (T81.82)~~

> EXCLUDES 2   ▶emphysema NOS (J43)◀
> ▶emphysema (subcutaneous) resulting from a
>   procedure (T81.82)◀

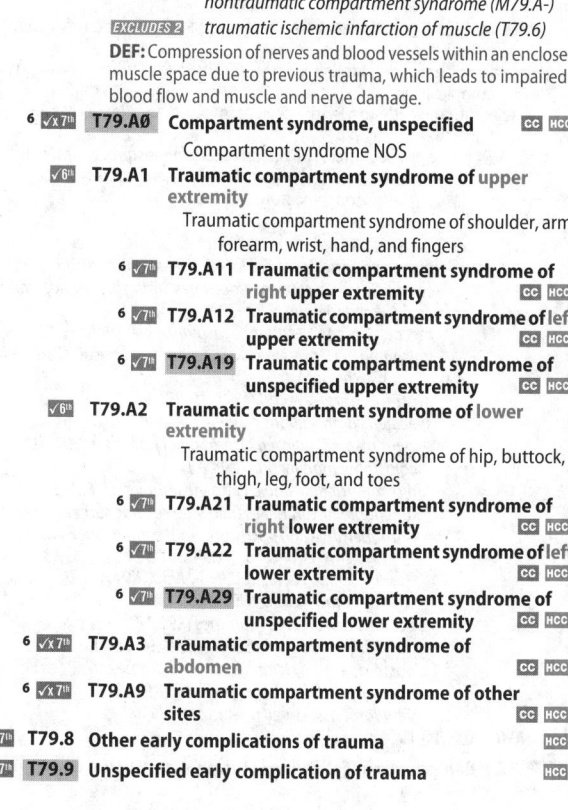

√5ʰ **T79.A**   **Traumatic compartment syndrome**

> EXCLUDES 1   fibromyalgia (M79.7)
> nontraumatic compartment syndrome (M79.A-)

> EXCLUDES 2   traumatic ischemic infarction of muscle (T79.6)

> **DEF:** Compression of nerves and blood vessels within an enclosed
> muscle space due to previous trauma, which leads to impaired
> blood flow and muscle and nerve damage.

6 √x7ʰ **T79.A0**   **Compartment syndrome, unspecified**   CC HCC

> Compartment syndrome NOS

√6ʰ **T79.A1**   **Traumatic compartment syndrome of upper
extremity**

> Traumatic compartment syndrome of shoulder, arm,
> forearm, wrist, hand, and fingers

6 √7ʰ **T79.A11**   **Traumatic compartment syndrome of
right upper extremity**   CC HCC

6 √7ʰ **T79.A12**   **Traumatic compartment syndrome of left
upper extremity**   CC HCC

6 √7ʰ **T79.A19**   **Traumatic compartment syndrome of
unspecified upper extremity**   CC HCC

√6ʰ **T79.A2**   **Traumatic compartment syndrome of lower
extremity**

> Traumatic compartment syndrome of hip, buttock,
> thigh, leg, foot, and toes

6 √7ʰ **T79.A21**   **Traumatic compartment syndrome of
right lower extremity**   CC HCC

6 √7ʰ **T79.A22**   **Traumatic compartment syndrome of left
lower extremity**   CC HCC

6 √7ʰ **T79.A29**   **Traumatic compartment syndrome of
unspecified lower extremity**   CC HCC

6 √x7ʰ **T79.A3**   **Traumatic compartment syndrome of
abdomen**   CC HCC

6 √x7ʰ **T79.A9**   **Traumatic compartment syndrome of other
sites**   CC HCC

6 √x7ʰ **T79.8**   **Other early complications of trauma**   HCC

6 √x7ʰ **T79.9**   **Unspecified early complication of trauma**   HCC

☑ Additional Character Required   √x7ʰ Placeholder   Unacceptable PDx   Questionable PDx   Manifestation   Unspecified Dx   H1-H14 HAC   HCC CMS-HCC Dx   HIV HIV Dx

ICD-10-CM 2021   1145

Complications of surgical and medical care, not elsewhere classified (T80-T88)

Use additional code for adverse effect, if applicable, to identify drug (T36-T50 with fifth or sixth character 5)

Use additional code(s) to identify the specified condition resulting from the complication

Use additional code to identify devices involved and details of circumstances (Y62-Y82)

EXCLUDES 2 *any encounters with medical care for postprocedural conditions in which no complications are present, such as:*
artificial opening status (Z93.-)
closure of external stoma (Z43.-)
fitting and adjustment of external prosthetic device (Z44.-)
burns and corrosions from local applications and irradiation (T20-T32)
complications of surgical procedures during pregnancy, childbirth and the puerperium (O00-O9A)
mechanical complication of respirator [ventilator] (J95.850)
poisoning and toxic effects of drugs and chemicals (T36-T65 with fifth or sixth character 1-4 or 6)
postprocedural fever (R50.82)
specified complications classified elsewhere, such as:
cerebrospinal fluid leak from spinal puncture (G97.0)
colostomy malfunction (K94.0-)
disorders of fluid and electrolyte imbalance (E86-E87)
functional disturbances following cardiac surgery (I97.0-I97.1)
intraoperative and postprocedural complications of specified body systems (D78.-, E36.-, E89.-, G97.3-, G97.4, H59.3-, H59.-, H95.2-, H95.3, I97.4-, I97.5, J95.6-, J95.7, K91.6-, L76.-, M96.-, N99.-)
ostomy complications (J95.0-, K94.-, N99.5-)
postgastric surgery syndromes (K91.1)
postlaminectomy syndrome NEC (M96.1)
postmastectomy lymphedema syndrome (I97.2)
postsurgical blind-loop syndrome (K91.2)
ventilator associated pneumonia (J95.851)

AHA: 2015,1Q,15

✓4ᵗʰ **T80** **Complications following infusion, transfusion and therapeutic injection**

INCLUDES complications following perfusion

EXCLUDES 2 *bone marrow transplant rejection (T86.01)*
febrile nonhemolytic transfusion reaction (R50.84)
fluid overload due to transfusion (E87.71)
posttransfusion purpura (D69.51)
transfusion associated circulatory overload (TACO) (E87.71)
transfusion (red blood cell) associated hemochromatosis (E83.111)
transfusion related acute lung injury (TRALI) (J95.84)

The appropriate 7th character is to be added to each code from category T80.
A   initial encounter
D   subsequent encounter
S   sequela

✓x7ᵗʰ **T80.0** **Air embolism following infusion, transfusion and therapeutic injection** MCC H2

✓x7ᵗʰ **T80.1** **Vascular complications following infusion, transfusion and therapeutic injection** CC
Use additional code to identify the vascular complication

EXCLUDES 2 *extravasation of vesicant agent (T80.81-)*
infiltration of vesicant agent (T80.81-)
postprocedural vascular complications (T81.7-)
vascular complications specified as due to prosthetic devices, implants and grafts (T82.8-, T83.8-, T84.8-, T85.8-)

✓5ᵗʰ **T80.2** **Infections following infusion, transfusion and therapeutic injection**
Use additional code to identify the specific infection, such as: sepsis (A41.9)
Use additional code (R65.2-) to identify severe sepsis, if applicable

EXCLUDES 2 *infections specified as due to prosthetic devices, implants and grafts (T82.6-T82.7, T83.5-T83.6, T84.5-T84.7, T85.7)*
postprocedural infections (T81.4-)

AHA: 2018,4Q,62

✓6ᵗʰ **T80.21** **Infection due to central venous catheter**
Infection due to pulmonary artery catheter (Swan-Ganz catheter)
AHA: 2019,1Q,13-14
TIP: Only centrally placed catheters are captured with this subcategory. Infections resulting from catheters that are not central lines, including those used for hemodialysis, should be coded to T82.7-.

✓7ᵗʰ **T80.211** **Bloodstream infection due to central venous catheter** CC H7
Catheter-related bloodstream infection (CRBSI) NOS
Central line-associated bloodstream infection (CLABSI)
Bloodstream infection due to Hickman catheter
Bloodstream infection due to peripherally inserted central catheter (PICC)
Bloodstream infection due to portacath (port-a-cath)
Bloodstream infection due to pulmonary artery catheter
Bloodstream infection due to triple lumen catheter
Bloodstream infection due to umbilical venous catheter
AHA: 2019,1Q,13,14; 2018,4Q,89

✓7ᵗʰ **T80.212** **Local infection due to central venous catheter** CC H7
Exit or insertion site infection
Local infection due to Hickman catheter
Local infection due to peripherally inserted central catheter (PICC)
Local infection due to portacath (port-a-cath)
Local infection due to pulmonary artery catheter
Local infection due to triple lumen catheter
Local infection due to umbilical venous catheter
Port or reservoir infection
Tunnel infection

✓7ᵗʰ **T80.218** **Other infection due to central venous catheter** CC H7
Other central line-associated infection
Other infection due to Hickman catheter
Other infection due to peripherally inserted central catheter (PICC)
Other infection due to portacath (port-a-cath)
Other infection due to pulmonary artery catheter
Other infection due to triple lumen catheter
Other infection due to umbilical venous catheter

√7ᵗʰ **T80.219 Unspecified infection due to central venous catheter** `CC` `H7`

    Central line-associated infection NOS

    Unspecified infection due to Hickman catheter

    Unspecified infection due to peripherally inserted central catheter (PICC)

    Unspecified infection due to portacath (port-a-cath)

    Unspecified infection due to pulmonary artery catheter

    Unspecified infection due to triple lumen catheter

    Unspecified infection due to umbilical venous catheter

√x7ᵗʰ **T80.22 Acute infection following transfusion, infusion, or injection of blood and blood products** `CC`

√x7ᵗʰ **T80.29 Infection following other infusion, transfusion and therapeutic injection** `CC`

√5ᵗʰ **T80.3 ABO incompatibility reaction due to transfusion of blood or blood products**

    EXCLUDES 1   *minor blood group antigens reactions (Duffy) (E) (K) (Kell) (Kidd) (Lewis) (M) (N) (P) (S) (T80.A-)*

√x7ᵗʰ **T80.30 ABO incompatibility reaction due to transfusion of blood or blood products, unspecified** `CC` `H3`

    ABO incompatibility blood transfusion NOS

    Reaction to ABO incompatibility from transfusion NOS

√6ᵗʰ **T80.31 ABO incompatibility with hemolytic transfusion reaction**

    √7ᵗʰ **T80.310 ABO incompatibility with acute hemolytic transfusion reaction** `CC` `H3`

        ABO incompatibility with hemolytic transfusion reaction less than 24 hours after transfusion

        Acute hemolytic transfusion reaction (AHTR) due to ABO incompatibility

    √7ᵗʰ **T80.311 ABO incompatibility with delayed hemolytic transfusion reaction** `CC` `H3`

        ABO incompatibility with hemolytic transfusion reaction 24 hours or more after transfusion

        Delayed hemolytic transfusion reaction (DHTR) due to ABO incompatibility

    √7ᵗʰ **T80.319 ABO incompatibility with hemolytic transfusion reaction, unspecified** `CC` `H3`

        ABO incompatibility with hemolytic transfusion reaction at unspecified time after transfusion

        Hemolytic transfusion reaction (HTR) due to ABO incompatibility NOS

√x7ᵗʰ **T80.39 Other ABO incompatibility reaction due to transfusion of blood or blood products** `CC` `H3`

    Delayed serologic transfusion reaction (DSTR) from ABO incompatibility

    Other ABO incompatible blood transfusion

    Other reaction to ABO incompatible blood transfusion

√5ᵗʰ **T80.4 Rh incompatibility reaction due to transfusion of blood or blood products**

    Reaction due to incompatibility of Rh antigens (C) (c) (D) (E) (e)

√x7ᵗʰ **T80.40 Rh incompatibility reaction due to transfusion of blood or blood products, unspecified** `CC`

    Reaction due to Rh factor in transfusion NOS

    Rh incompatible blood transfusion NOS

√6ᵗʰ **T80.41 Rh incompatibility with hemolytic transfusion reaction**

    √7ᵗʰ **T80.410 Rh incompatibility with acute hemolytic transfusion reaction** `CC`

        Acute hemolytic transfusion reaction (AHTR) due to Rh incompatibility

        Rh incompatibility with hemolytic transfusion reaction less than 24 hours after transfusion

√7ᵗʰ **T80.411 Rh incompatibility with delayed hemolytic transfusion reaction** `CC`

    Delayed hemolytic transfusion reaction (DHTR) due to Rh incompatibility

    Rh incompatibility with hemolytic transfusion reaction 24 hours or more after transfusion

√7ᵗʰ **T80.419 Rh incompatibility with hemolytic transfusion reaction, unspecified** `CC`

    Rh incompatibility with hemolytic transfusion reaction at unspecified time after transfusion

    Hemolytic transfusion reaction (HTR) due to Rh incompatibility NOS

√x7ᵗʰ **T80.49 Other Rh incompatibility reaction due to transfusion of blood or blood products** `CC`

    Delayed serologic transfusion reaction (DSTR) from Rh incompatibility

    Other reaction to Rh incompatible blood transfusion

√5ᵗʰ **T80.A Non-ABO incompatibility reaction due to transfusion of blood or blood products**

    Reaction due to incompatibility of minor antigens (Duffy) (Kell) (Kidd) (Lewis) (M) (N) (P) (S)

√x7ᵗʰ **T80.A0 Non-ABO incompatibility reaction due to transfusion of blood or blood products, unspecified** `CC`

    Non-ABO antigen incompatibility reaction from transfusion NOS

√6ᵗʰ **T80.A1 Non-ABO incompatibility with hemolytic transfusion reaction**

    √7ᵗʰ **T80.A10 Non-ABO incompatibility with acute hemolytic transfusion reaction** `CC`

        Acute hemolytic transfusion reaction (AHTR) due to non-ABO incompatibility

        Non-ABO incompatibility with hemolytic transfusion reaction less than 24 hours after transfusion

    √7ᵗʰ **T80.A11 Non-ABO incompatibility with delayed hemolytic transfusion reaction** `CC`

        Delayed hemolytic transfusion reaction (DHTR) due to non-ABO incompatibility

        Non-ABO incompatibility with hemolytic transfusion reaction 24 or more hours after transfusion

    √7ᵗʰ **T80.A19 Non-ABO incompatibility with hemolytic transfusion reaction, unspecified** `CC`

        Hemolytic transfusion reaction (HTR) due to non-ABO incompatibility NOS

        Non-ABO incompatibility with hemolytic transfusion reaction at unspecified time after transfusion

√x7ᵗʰ **T80.A9 Other non-ABO incompatibility reaction due to transfusion of blood or blood products** `CC`

    Delayed serologic transfusion reaction (DSTR) from non-ABO incompatibility

    Other reaction to non-ABO incompatible blood transfusion

√5ᵗʰ **T80.5 Anaphylactic reaction due to serum**

    Allergic shock due to serum

    Anaphylactic shock due to serum

    Anaphylactoid reaction due to serum

    Anaphylaxis due to serum

    EXCLUDES 1   *ABO incompatibility reaction due to transfusion of blood or blood products (T80.3-)*

        allergic reaction or shock NOS (T78.2)

        anaphylactic reaction or shock NOS (T78.2)

        anaphylactic reaction or shock due to adverse effect of correct medicinal substance properly administered (T88.6)

        other serum reaction (T80.6-)

    DEF: Life-threatening hypersensitivity to a foreign serum causing respiratory distress, vascular collapse, and shock.

√x7ᵗʰ **T80.51 Anaphylactic reaction due to administration of blood and blood products** `CC`

√x7ᵗʰ **T80.52 Anaphylactic reaction due to vaccination** `CC`

√x7ᵗʰ **T80.59 Anaphylactic reaction due to other serum** `CC`

☑ Additional Character Required   √x7ᵗʰ Placeholder   Unacceptable PDx   Questionable PDx   Manifestation   Unspecified Dx   H1 - H14 HAC   HCC CMS-HCC Dx   HIV HIV Dx

ICD-10-CM 2021   1147

✓5ᵗʰ **T80.6 Other serum reactions**

    Intoxication by serum

    Protein sickness

    Serum rash

    Serum sickness

    Serum urticaria

    EXCLUDES 2   *serum hepatitis (B16-B19)*

    DEF: Serum sickness: Hypersensitivity to a foreign serum that causes fever, hives, swelling, and lymphadenopathy.

    ✓x 7ᵗʰ **T80.61 Other serum reaction due to administration of blood and blood products**   CC

    ✓x 7ᵗʰ **T80.62 Other serum reaction due to vaccination**   CC

    ✓x 7ᵗʰ **T80.69 Other serum reaction due to other serum**   CC

        Code also, if applicable, arthropathy in hypersensitivity reactions classified elsewhere (M36.4)

✓5ᵗʰ **T80.8 Other complications following infusion, transfusion and therapeutic injection**

    ✓6ᵗʰ **T80.81 Extravasation of vesicant agent**

        Infiltration of vesicant agent

        ✓7ᵗʰ **T80.810 Extravasation of vesicant antineoplastic chemotherapy**   CC

            Infiltration of vesicant antineoplastic chemotherapy

        ✓7ᵗʰ **T80.818 Extravasation of other vesicant agent**   CC

            Infiltration of other vesicant agent

    ✓x 7ᵗʰ **T80.89 Other complications following infusion, transfusion and therapeutic injection**

        Delayed serologic transfusion reaction (DSTR), unspecified incompatibility

        Use additional code to identify graft-versus-host reaction, if applicable, (D89.81-)

✓5ᵗʰ **T80.9 Unspecified complication following infusion, transfusion and therapeutic injection**

    ✓x 7ᵗʰ **T80.90 Unspecified complication following infusion and therapeutic injection**

    ✓6ᵗʰ **T80.91 Hemolytic transfusion reaction, unspecified incompatibility**

        EXCLUDES 1   *ABO incompatibility with hemolytic transfusion reaction (T80.31-)*

            non-ABO incompatibility with hemolytic transfusion reaction (T80.A1-)

            Rh incompatibility with hemolytic transfusion reaction (T80.41-)

        ✓7ᵗʰ **T80.910 Acute hemolytic transfusion reaction, unspecified incompatibility**   CC

        ✓7ᵗʰ **T80.911 Delayed hemolytic transfusion reaction, unspecified incompatibility**   CC

        ✓7ᵗʰ **T80.919 Hemolytic transfusion reaction, unspecified incompatibility, unspecified as acute or delayed**   CC

            Hemolytic transfusion reaction NOS

    ✓x 7ᵗʰ **T80.92 Unspecified transfusion reaction**

        Transfusion reaction NOS

✓4ᵗʰ **T81 Complications of procedures, not elsewhere classified**

    Use additional code for adverse effect, if applicable, to identify drug (T36-T50 with fifth or sixth character 5)

    EXCLUDES 2   *complications following immunization (T88.0-T88.1)*

        complications following infusion, transfusion and therapeutic injection (T80.-)

        complications of transplanted organs and tissue (T86.-)

        specified complications classified elsewhere, such as:

        complication of prosthetic devices, implants and grafts (T82-T85)

        dermatitis due to drugs and medicaments (L23.3, L24.4, L25.1, L27.0-L27.1)

        endosseous dental implant failure (M27.6-)

        floppy iris syndrome (IFIS) (intraoperative) (H21.81)

        intraoperative and postprocedural complications of specific body system (D78.-, E36.-, E89.-, G97.3-, G97.4, H59.3-, H59.-, H95.2-, H95.3, I97.4-, I97.5, J95, K91.-, L76.-, M96.-, N99.-)

        ostomy complications (J95.0-, K94.-, N99.5-)

        plateau iris syndrome (post-iridectomy) (postprocedural) H21.82

        poisoning and toxic effects of drugs and chemicals (T36-T65 with fifth or sixth character 1-4 or 6)

    AHA: 2019,2Q,21

    The appropriate 7th character is to be added to each code from category T81.

    A   initial encounter

    D   subsequent encounter

    S   sequela

✓5ᵗʰ **T81.1 Postprocedural shock**

    Shock during or resulting from a procedure, not elsewhere classified

    EXCLUDES 1   *anaphylactic shock due to correct substance properly administered (T88.6)*

        anaphylactic shock due to serum (T80.5-)

        anaphylactic shock NOS (T78.2)

        anesthetic shock (T88.2)

        electric shock (T75.4)

        obstetric shock (O75.1)

        septic shock (R65.21)

        shock following abortion or ectopic or molar pregnancy (O00-O07, O08.3)

        traumatic shock (T79.4)

    ✓x 7ᵗʰ **T81.10 Postprocedural shock unspecified**   CC

        Collapse NOS during or resulting from a procedure, not elsewhere classified

        Postprocedural failure of peripheral circulation

        Postprocedural shock NOS

    6 ✓x 7ᵗʰ **T81.11 Postprocedural cardiogenic shock**   MCC HCC

    6 ✓x 7ᵗʰ **T81.12 Postprocedural septic shock**   MCC HCC

        Postprocedural endotoxic shock resulting from a procedure, not elsewhere classified

        Postprocedural gram-negative shock resulting from a procedure, not elsewhere classified

        Code first underlying infection

        Use additional code, to identify any associated acute organ dysfunction, if applicable

        AHA: 2018,4Q,63

    ✓x 7ᵗʰ **T81.19 Other postprocedural shock**   MCC

        Postprocedural hypovolemic shock

✓5ᵗʰ **T81.3 Disruption of wound, not elsewhere classified**

    Disruption of any suture materials or other closure methods

    EXCLUDES 1   *breakdown (mechanical) of permanent sutures (T85.612)*

        displacement of permanent sutures (T85.622)

        disruption of cesarean delivery wound (O90.0)

        disruption of perineal obstetric wound (O90.1)

        mechanical complication of permanent sutures NEC (T85.692)

    AHA: 2014,1Q,23

    ✓x 7ᵗʰ **T81.30 Disruption of wound, unspecified**   CC SW

        Disruption of wound NOS

N Newborn: 0   P Pediatric: 0-17   M Maternity: 9-64   A Adult: 15-124   MCC Major Complication/Comorbidity   CC Complication/Comorbidity   SW Severe Wound Dx

1148   ICD-10-CM 2021

√x7ᵗʰ **T81.31** **Disruption of** external operation (surgical) **wound, not elsewhere classified** `CC` `SW`
   Dehiscence of operation wound NOS
   Disruption of operation wound NOS
   Disruption or dehiscence of closure of cornea
   Disruption or dehiscence of closure of mucosa
   Disruption or dehiscence of closure of skin and
      subcutaneous tissue
   Full-thickness skin disruption or dehiscence
   Superficial disruption or dehiscence of operation
      wound
   `EXCLUDES 1` *dehiscence of amputation stump (T87.81)*

√x7ᵗʰ **T81.32** **Disruption of** internal operation (surgical) **wound, not elsewhere classified** `CC` `SW`
   Deep disruption or dehiscence of operation wound
      NOS
   Disruption or dehiscence of closure of internal organ
      or other internal tissue
   Disruption or dehiscence of closure of muscle or
      muscle flap
   Disruption or dehiscence of closure of ribs or rib cage
   Disruption or dehiscence of closure of skull or
      craniotomy
   Disruption or dehiscence of closure of sternum or
      sternotomy
   Disruption or dehiscence of closure of tendon or
      ligament
   Disruption or dehiscence of closure of superficial or
      muscular fascia
   AHA: 2020,2Q,22; 2017,3Q,4

√x7ᵗʰ **T81.33** **Disruption of** traumatic injury **wound** repair `CC`
   Disruption or dehiscence of closure of traumatic
      laceration (external) (internal)

√5ᵗʰ **T81.4** **Infection following a procedure**
   Wound abscess following a procedure
   Use additional code to identify infection
   Use additional code (R65.2-) to identify severe sepsis, if
      applicable
   `EXCLUDES 2` *bleb associated endophthalmitis (H59.4-)*
      infection due to infusion, transfusion and therapeutic
         injection (T80.2-)
      infection due to prosthetic devices, implants and
         grafts (T82.6-T82.7, T83.5-T83.6, T84.5-T84.7,
         T85.7)
      obstetric surgical wound infection (O86.0-)
      postprocedural fever NOS (R50.82)
      postprocedural retroperitoneal abscess (K68.11)
   AHA: 2018,4Q,33-34,62; 2014,1Q,23

√x7ᵗʰ **T81.40** **Infection following a procedure, unspecified** `CC` `H11` `H12` `H13`

√x7ᵗʰ **T81.41** **Infection following a procedure,** superficial incisional surgical site `CC` `H11` `H12` `H13`
   Subcutaneous abscess following a procedure
   Stitch abscess following a procedure

√x7ᵗʰ **T81.42** **Infection following a procedure,** deep incisional surgical site `CC` `H11` `H12` `H13`
   Intra-muscular abscess following a procedure

√x7ᵗʰ **T81.43** **Infection following a procedure,** organ and space surgical site `CC` `H11` `H12` `H13`
   Intra-abdominal abscess following a procedure
   Subphrenic abscess following a procedure

6 √x7ᵗʰ **T81.44** **Sepsis following a procedure** `CC` `H11` `H12` `H13` `HCC`
   Use additional code to identify the sepsis

√x7ᵗʰ **T81.49** **Infection following a procedure, other surgical site** `CC` `H11` `H12` `H13`

√5ᵗʰ **T81.5** **Complications of** foreign body accidentally left in body following procedure
   AHA: 2014,4Q,24

√6ᵗʰ **T81.50** **Unspecified complication of foreign body accidentally left in body following procedure**
   √7ᵗʰ **T81.500** Unspecified complication of foreign body
      accidentally left in body following
      surgical operation `CC` `H1`
   √7ᵗʰ **T81.501** Unspecified complication of foreign body
      accidentally left in body following
      infusion or transfusion `CC` `H1`

√7ᵗʰ **T81.502** Unspecified complication of foreign body
   accidentally left in body following kidney
   dialysis `CC` `H1` `HCC`

√7ᵗʰ **T81.503** Unspecified complication of foreign body
   accidentally left in body following
   injection or immunization `CC` `H1`

√7ᵗʰ **T81.504** Unspecified complication of foreign body
   accidentally left in body following
   endoscopic examination `CC` `H1`

√7ᵗʰ **T81.505** Unspecified complication of foreign body
   accidentally left in body following heart
   catheterization `CC` `H1`

√7ᵗʰ **T81.506** Unspecified complication of foreign body
   accidentally left in body following
   aspiration, puncture or other
   catheterization `CC` `H1`

√7ᵗʰ **T81.507** Unspecified complication of foreign body
   accidentally left in body following
   removal of catheter or packing `CC` `H1`

√7ᵗʰ **T81.508** Unspecified complication of foreign body
   accidentally left in body following other
   procedure `CC` `H1`

√7ᵗʰ **T81.509** Unspecified complication of foreign body
   accidentally left in body following
   unspecified procedure `CC` `H1`

√6ᵗʰ **T81.51** **Adhesions** due to foreign body accidentally left in body following procedure
   √7ᵗʰ **T81.510** **Adhesions due to foreign body**
      accidentally left in body following
      surgical operation `CC` `H1`
   √7ᵗʰ **T81.511** **Adhesions due to foreign body**
      accidentally left in body following
      infusion or transfusion `CC` `H1`
   √7ᵗʰ **T81.512** **Adhesions due to foreign body**
      accidentally left in body following kidney
      dialysis `CC` `H1` `HCC`
   √7ᵗʰ **T81.513** **Adhesions due to foreign body**
      accidentally left in body following
      injection or immunization `CC` `H1`
   √7ᵗʰ **T81.514** **Adhesions due to foreign body**
      accidentally left in body following
      endoscopic examination `CC` `H1`
   √7ᵗʰ **T81.515** **Adhesions due to foreign body**
      accidentally left in body following heart
      catheterization `CC` `H1`
   √7ᵗʰ **T81.516** **Adhesions due to foreign body**
      accidentally left in body following
      aspiration, puncture or other
      catheterization `CC` `H1`
   √7ᵗʰ **T81.517** **Adhesions due to foreign body**
      accidentally left in body following
      removal of catheter or packing `CC` `H1`
   √7ᵗʰ **T81.518** **Adhesions due to foreign body**
      accidentally left in body following other
      procedure `CC` `H1`
   √7ᵗʰ **T81.519** **Adhesions due to foreign body**
      accidentally left in body following
      unspecified procedure `CC` `H1`

√6ᵗʰ **T81.52** **Obstruction** due to foreign body accidentally left in body following procedure
   √7ᵗʰ **T81.520** **Obstruction due to foreign body**
      accidentally left in body following
      surgical operation `CC` `H1`
   √7ᵗʰ **T81.521** **Obstruction due to foreign body**
      accidentally left in body following
      infusion or transfusion `CC` `H1`
   √7ᵗʰ **T81.522** **Obstruction due to foreign body**
      accidentally left in body following kidney
      dialysis `CC` `H1` `HCC`
   √7ᵗʰ **T81.523** **Obstruction due to foreign body**
      accidentally left in body following
      injection or immunization `CC` `H1`
   √7ᵗʰ **T81.524** **Obstruction due to foreign body**
      accidentally left in body following
      endoscopic examination `CC` `H1`
   √7ᵗʰ **T81.525** **Obstruction due to foreign body**
      accidentally left in body following heart
      catheterization `CC` `H1`
   √7ᵗʰ **T81.526** **Obstruction due to foreign body**
      accidentally left in body following
      aspiration, puncture or other
      catheterization `CC` `H1`

√7ᵗʰ **T81.527 Obstruction due to foreign body accidentally left in body following removal of catheter or packing** CC H1

√7ᵗʰ **T81.528 Obstruction due to foreign body accidentally left in body following other procedure** CC H1

√7ᵗʰ **T81.529 Obstruction due to foreign body accidentally left in body following unspecified procedure** CC H1

√6ᵗʰ **T81.53 Perforation due to foreign body accidentally left in body following procedure**

√7ᵗʰ **T81.530 Perforation due to foreign body accidentally left in body following surgical operation** CC H1

√7ᵗʰ **T81.531 Perforation due to foreign body accidentally left in body following infusion or transfusion** CC H1

√7ᵗʰ **T81.532 Perforation due to foreign body accidentally left in body following kidney dialysis** CC H1 HCC

√7ᵗʰ **T81.533 Perforation due to foreign body accidentally left in body following injection or immunization** CC H1

√7ᵗʰ **T81.534 Perforation due to foreign body accidentally left in body following endoscopic examination** CC H1

√7ᵗʰ **T81.535 Perforation due to foreign body accidentally left in body following heart catheterization** CC H1

√7ᵗʰ **T81.536 Perforation due to foreign body accidentally left in body following aspiration, puncture or other catheterization** CC H1

√7ᵗʰ **T81.537 Perforation due to foreign body accidentally left in body following removal of catheter or packing** CC H1

√7ᵗʰ **T81.538 Perforation due to foreign body accidentally left in body following other procedure** CC H1

√7ᵗʰ **T81.539 Perforation due to foreign body accidentally left in body following unspecified procedure** CC H1

√6ᵗʰ **T81.59 Other complications of foreign body accidentally left in body following procedure**

EXCLUDES 2 *obstruction or perforation due to prosthetic devices and implants intentionally left in body (T82.0-T82.5, T83.0-T83.4, T83.7, T84.0-T84.4, T85.0-T85.6)*

√7ᵗʰ **T81.590 Other complications of foreign body accidentally left in body following surgical operation** CC H1

√7ᵗʰ **T81.591 Other complications of foreign body accidentally left in body following infusion or transfusion** CC H1

√7ᵗʰ **T81.592 Other complications of foreign body accidentally left in body following kidney dialysis** CC H1 HCC

√7ᵗʰ **T81.593 Other complications of foreign body accidentally left in body following injection or immunization** CC H1

√7ᵗʰ **T81.594 Other complications of foreign body accidentally left in body following endoscopic examination** CC H1

√7ᵗʰ **T81.595 Other complications of foreign body accidentally left in body following heart catheterization** CC H1

√7ᵗʰ **T81.596 Other complications of foreign body accidentally left in body following aspiration, puncture or other catheterization** CC H1

√7ᵗʰ **T81.597 Other complications of foreign body accidentally left in body following removal of catheter or packing** CC H1

√7ᵗʰ **T81.598 Other complications of foreign body accidentally left in body following other procedure** CC H1

√7ᵗʰ **T81.599 Other complications of foreign body accidentally left in body following unspecified procedure** CC H1

√5ᵗʰ **T81.6 Acute reaction to foreign substance accidentally left during a procedure**

EXCLUDES 2 *complications of foreign body accidentally left in body cavity or operation wound following procedure (T81.5-)*

√x7ᵗʰ **T81.60 Unspecified acute reaction to foreign substance accidentally left during a procedure** CC H1

√x7ᵗʰ **T81.61 Aseptic peritonitis due to foreign substance accidentally left during a procedure** CC H1
Chemical peritonitis

√x7ᵗʰ **T81.69 Other acute reaction to foreign substance accidentally left during a procedure** CC H1

√5ᵗʰ **T81.7 Vascular complications following a procedure, not elsewhere classified**
Air embolism following procedure NEC
Phlebitis or thrombophlebitis resulting from a procedure

EXCLUDES 1 *embolism complicating abortion or ectopic or molar pregnancy (O00-O07, O08.2)*
embolism complicating pregnancy, childbirth and the puerperium (O88.-)
traumatic embolism (T79.0)

EXCLUDES 2 *embolism due to prosthetic devices, implants and grafts (T82.8-, T83.81, T84.8-, T85.81-)*
embolism following infusion, transfusion and therapeutic injection (T80.0)

AHA: 2019,2Q,22

√6ᵗʰ **T81.71 Complication of artery following a procedure, not elsewhere classified**

√7ᵗʰ **T81.710 Complication of mesenteric artery following a procedure, not elsewhere classified** CC

√7ᵗʰ **T81.711 Complication of renal artery following a procedure, not elsewhere classified** CC

√7ᵗʰ **T81.718 Complication of other artery following a procedure, not elsewhere classified** CC
AHA: 2019,2Q,21-22

√7ᵗʰ **T81.719 Complication of unspecified artery following a procedure, not elsewhere classified** CC

√x7ᵗʰ **T81.72 Complication of vein following a procedure, not elsewhere classified** CC

√5ᵗʰ **T81.8 Other complications of procedures, not elsewhere classified**

EXCLUDES 2 *hypothermia following anesthesia (T88.51)*
malignant hyperpyrexia due to anesthesia (T88.3)

√x7ᵗʰ **T81.81 Complication of inhalation therapy**

√x7ᵗʰ **T81.82 Emphysema (subcutaneous) resulting from a procedure**

√x7ᵗʰ **T81.83 Persistent postprocedural fistula** CC SW
AHA: 2017,3Q,3-4

√x7ᵗʰ **T81.89 Other complications of procedures, not elsewhere classified** SW
Use additional code to specify complication, such as:
postprocedural delirium (F05)
AHA: 2014,1Q,23

√x7ᵗʰ **T81.9 Unspecified complication of procedure**

√4ᵗʰ **T82 Complications of cardiac and vascular prosthetic devices, implants and grafts**

EXCLUDES 2 *failure and rejection of transplanted organs and tissue (T86.-)*

The appropriate 7th character is to be added to each code from category T82.
A initial encounter
D subsequent encounter
S sequela

√5ᵗʰ **T82.0 Mechanical complication of heart valve prosthesis**
Mechanical complication of artificial heart valve

EXCLUDES 1 *mechanical complication of biological heart valve graft (T82.22-)*

√x7ᵗʰ **T82.01 Breakdown (mechanical) of heart valve prosthesis** CC

√x7ᵗʰ **T82.02 Displacement of heart valve prosthesis** CC
Malposition of heart valve prosthesis

√x7ᵗʰ **T82.03 Leakage of heart valve prosthesis** CC

√x7ᵗʰ **T82.09** **Other mechanical complication of heart valve prosthesis** `CC`
- Obstruction (mechanical) of heart valve prosthesis
- Perforation of heart valve prosthesis
- Protrusion of heart valve prosthesis

√5ᵗʰ **T82.1** **Mechanical complication of** cardiac electronic device

√6ᵗʰ **T82.11** Breakdown (mechanical) of cardiac electronic device

√7ᵗʰ **T82.110** **Breakdown (mechanical) of cardiac** electrode `CC`

√7ᵗʰ **T82.111** **Breakdown (mechanical) of cardiac** pulse generator (battery) `CC`

√7ᵗʰ **T82.118** **Breakdown (mechanical) of other cardiac** electronic device `CC`

√7ᵗʰ **T82.119** **Breakdown (mechanical) of unspecified** cardiac electronic device `CC`

√6ᵗʰ **T82.12** Displacement of cardiac electronic device
- Malposition of cardiac electronic device

√7ᵗʰ **T82.120** **Displacement of** cardiac electrode `CC`

√7ᵗʰ **T82.121** **Displacement of cardiac** pulse generator (battery) `CC`

√7ᵗʰ **T82.128** **Displacement of other cardiac electronic** device `CC`

√7ᵗʰ **T82.129** **Displacement of unspecified cardiac** electronic device `CC`

√6ᵗʰ **T82.19** Other mechanical complication of cardiac electronic device
- Leakage of cardiac electronic device
- Obstruction of cardiac electronic device
- Perforation of cardiac electronic device
- Protrusion of cardiac electronic device

√7ᵗʰ **T82.190** **Other mechanical complication of** cardiac electrode `CC`

√7ᵗʰ **T82.191** **Other mechanical complication of cardiac** pulse generator (battery) `CC`

√7ᵗʰ **T82.198** **Other mechanical complication of other cardiac electronic device** `CC`

√7ᵗʰ **T82.199** **Other mechanical complication of unspecified cardiac device** `CC`

√5ᵗʰ **T82.2** **Mechanical complication of coronary artery bypass graft and biological heart valve graft**
> `EXCLUDES 1` *mechanical complication of artificial heart valve prosthesis (T82.0-)*

√6ᵗʰ **T82.21** Mechanical complication of coronary artery bypass graft

√7ᵗʰ **T82.211** Breakdown (mechanical) of coronary artery bypass graft `CC`

√7ᵗʰ **T82.212** Displacement of coronary artery bypass graft `CC`
- Malposition of coronary artery bypass graft

√7ᵗʰ **T82.213** Leakage of coronary artery bypass graft `CC`

√7ᵗʰ **T82.218** **Other mechanical complication of coronary artery bypass graft** `CC`
- Obstruction, mechanical of coronary artery bypass graft
- Perforation of coronary artery bypass graft
- Protrusion of coronary artery bypass graft

√6ᵗʰ **T82.22** Mechanical complication of biological heart valve graft

√7ᵗʰ **T82.221** Breakdown (mechanical) of biological heart valve graft `CC`

√7ᵗʰ **T82.222** Displacement of biological heart valve graft `CC`
- Malposition of biological heart valve graft

√7ᵗʰ **T82.223** Leakage of biological heart valve graft `CC`

√7ᵗʰ **T82.228** **Other mechanical complication of biological heart valve graft** `CC`
- Obstruction of biological heart valve graft
- Perforation of biological heart valve graft
- Protrusion of biological heart valve graft

√5ᵗʰ **T82.3** **Mechanical complication of other vascular grafts**

√6ᵗʰ **T82.31** Breakdown (mechanical) of other vascular grafts

6 √7ᵗʰ **T82.310** Breakdown (mechanical) of aortic (bifurcation) graft (replacement) `CC` `HCC`

6 √7ᵗʰ **T82.311** Breakdown (mechanical) of carotid arterial graft (bypass) `CC` `HCC`

6 √7ᵗʰ **T82.312** Breakdown (mechanical) of femoral arterial graft (bypass) `CC` `HCC`

6 √7ᵗʰ **T82.318** Breakdown (mechanical) of other vascular grafts `CC` `HCC`

6 √7ᵗʰ **T82.319** Breakdown (mechanical) of unspecified vascular grafts `CC` `HCC`

√6ᵗʰ **T82.32** Displacement of other vascular grafts
- Malposition of other vascular grafts

6 √7ᵗʰ **T82.320** Displacement of aortic (bifurcation) graft (replacement) `CC` `HCC`

6 √7ᵗʰ **T82.321** Displacement of carotid arterial graft (bypass) `CC` `HCC`

6 √7ᵗʰ **T82.322** Displacement of femoral arterial graft (bypass) `CC` `HCC`

6 √7ᵗʰ **T82.328** Displacement of other vascular grafts `CC` `HCC`

6 √7ᵗʰ **T82.329** Displacement of unspecified vascular grafts `CC` `HCC`

√6ᵗʰ **T82.33** Leakage of other vascular grafts

6 √7ᵗʰ **T82.330** Leakage of aortic (bifurcation) graft (replacement) `CC` `HCC`

6 √7ᵗʰ **T82.331** Leakage of carotid arterial graft (bypass) `CC` `HCC`

6 √7ᵗʰ **T82.332** Leakage of femoral arterial graft (bypass) `CC` `HCC`

6 √7ᵗʰ **T82.338** Leakage of other vascular grafts `CC` `HCC`

6 √7ᵗʰ **T82.339** Leakage of unspecified vascular graft `CC` `HCC`

√6ᵗʰ **T82.39** Other mechanical complication of other vascular grafts
- Obstruction (mechanical) of other vascular grafts
- Perforation of other vascular grafts
- Protrusion of other vascular grafts

6 √7ᵗʰ **T82.390** Other mechanical complication of aortic (bifurcation) graft (replacement) `CC` `HCC`

6 √7ᵗʰ **T82.391** Other mechanical complication of carotid arterial graft (bypass) `CC` `HCC`

6 √7ᵗʰ **T82.392** Other mechanical complication of femoral arterial graft (bypass) `CC` `HCC`

6 √7ᵗʰ **T82.398** Other mechanical complication of other vascular grafts `CC` `HCC`

6 √7ᵗʰ **T82.399** Other mechanical complication of unspecified vascular grafts `CC` `HCC`

√5ᵗʰ **T82.4** **Mechanical complication of** vascular dialysis catheter
- Mechanical complication of hemodialysis catheter
> `EXCLUDES 1` *mechanical complication of intraperitoneal dialysis catheter (T85.62)*

√x7ᵗʰ **T82.41** Breakdown (mechanical) of vascular dialysis catheter `CC` `HCC`

√x7ᵗʰ **T82.42** Displacement of vascular dialysis catheter `CC` `HCC`
- Malposition of vascular dialysis catheter

√x7ᵗʰ **T82.43** Leakage of vascular dialysis catheter `CC` `HCC`

√x7ᵗʰ **T82.49** **Other complication of vascular dialysis catheter** `CC` `HCC`
- Obstruction (mechanical) of vascular dialysis catheter
- Perforation of vascular dialysis catheter
- Protrusion of vascular dialysis catheter

√5ᵗʰ **T82.5** **Mechanical complication of other cardiac and vascular devices and implants**
> `EXCLUDES 2` *mechanical complication of epidural and subdural infusion catheter (T85.61)*

√6ᵗʰ **T82.51** Breakdown (mechanical) of other cardiac and vascular devices and implants

6 √7ᵗʰ **T82.510** Breakdown (mechanical) of surgically created arteriovenous fistula `CC` `HCC`

6 √7ᵗʰ **T82.511** Breakdown (mechanical) of surgically created arteriovenous shunt `CC` `HCC`

√7ᵗʰ **T82.512** Breakdown (mechanical) of artificial heart `CC`

6 √7ᵗʰ **T82.513** Breakdown (mechanical) of balloon (counterpulsation) device `CC` `HCC`

6 √7ᵗʰ **T82.514** Breakdown (mechanical) of infusion catheter `CC` `HCC`

6 √7ᵗʰ **T82.515** Breakdown (mechanical) of umbrella device `CC` `HCC`

☑ Additional Character Required   √x7ᵗʰ Placeholder   Unacceptable PDx   Questionable PDx   Manifestation   Unspecified Dx   `H1`-`H14` HAC   `HCC` CMS-HCC Dx   `HIV` HIV Dx

ICD-10-CM 2021   1151

6 √7ᵗʰ **T82.518 Breakdown (mechanical) of other cardiac and vascular devices and implants** cc HCC

√7ᵗʰ **T82.519 Breakdown (mechanical) of unspecified cardiac and vascular devices and implants** cc

√6ᵗʰ **T82.52 Displacement of other cardiac and vascular devices and implants**

Malposition of other cardiac and vascular devices and implants

6 √7ᵗʰ **T82.520 Displacement of surgically created arteriovenous fistula** cc HCC

6 √7ᵗʰ **T82.521 Displacement of surgically created arteriovenous shunt** cc HCC

√7ᵗʰ **T82.522 Displacement of artificial heart** cc

6 √7ᵗʰ **T82.523 Displacement of balloon (counterpulsation) device** cc HCC

6 √7ᵗʰ **T82.524 Displacement of infusion catheter** cc HCC

AHA: 2020,2Q,21; 2019,3Q,15

6 √7ᵗʰ **T82.525 Displacement of umbrella device** cc HCC

6 √7ᵗʰ **T82.528 Displacement of other cardiac and vascular devices and implants** cc HCC

√7ᵗʰ **T82.529 Displacement of unspecified cardiac and vascular devices and implants** cc

√6ᵗʰ **T82.53 Leakage of other cardiac and vascular devices and implants**

6 √7ᵗʰ **T82.530 Leakage of surgically created arteriovenous fistula** cc HCC

6 √7ᵗʰ **T82.531 Leakage of surgically created arteriovenous shunt** cc HCC

√7ᵗʰ **T82.532 Leakage of artificial heart** cc

6 √7ᵗʰ **T82.533 Leakage of balloon (counterpulsation) device** cc HCC

6 √7ᵗʰ **T82.534 Leakage of infusion catheter** cc HCC

6 √7ᵗʰ **T82.535 Leakage of umbrella device** cc HCC

6 √7ᵗʰ **T82.538 Leakage of other cardiac and vascular devices and implants** cc HCC

√7ᵗʰ **T82.539 Leakage of unspecified cardiac and vascular devices and implants** cc

√6ᵗʰ **T82.59 Other mechanical complication of other cardiac and vascular devices and implants**

Obstruction (mechanical) of other cardiac and vascular devices and implants

Perforation of other cardiac and vascular devices and implants

Protrusion of other cardiac and vascular devices and implants

6 √7ᵗʰ **T82.590 Other mechanical complication of surgically created arteriovenous fistula** cc HCC

6 √7ᵗʰ **T82.591 Other mechanical complication of surgically created arteriovenous shunt** cc HCC

√7ᵗʰ **T82.592 Other mechanical complication of artificial heart** cc

6 √7ᵗʰ **T82.593 Other mechanical complication of balloon (counterpulsation) device** cc HCC

6 √7ᵗʰ **T82.594 Other mechanical complication of infusion catheter** cc HCC

6 √7ᵗʰ **T82.595 Other mechanical complication of umbrella device** cc HCC

6 √7ᵗʰ **T82.598 Other mechanical complication of other cardiac and vascular devices and implants** cc HCC

√7ᵗʰ **T82.599 Other mechanical complication of unspecified cardiac and vascular devices and implants** cc

6 √x7ᵗʰ **T82.6 Infection and inflammatory reaction due to cardiac valve prosthesis** cc H13 HCC

Use additional code to identify infection

6 √x7ᵗʰ **T82.7 Infection and inflammatory reaction due to other cardiac and vascular devices, implants and grafts** cc H13 HCC

Use additional code to identify infection

AHA: 2019,1Q,13-14

TIP: Assign this code for infections and/or cellulitis resulting from catheters that are not centrally placed (e.g., midline catheters).

√5ᵗʰ **T82.8 Other specified complications of cardiac and vascular prosthetic devices, implants and grafts**

AHA: 2016,4Q,70

√6ᵗʰ **T82.81 Embolism due to cardiac and vascular prosthetic devices, implants and grafts**

√7ᵗʰ **T82.817 Embolism due to cardiac prosthetic devices, implants and grafts** cc

6 √7ᵗʰ **T82.818 Embolism due to vascular prosthetic devices, implants and grafts** cc HCC

√6ᵗʰ **T82.82 Fibrosis due to cardiac and vascular prosthetic devices, implants and grafts**

√7ᵗʰ **T82.827 Fibrosis due to cardiac prosthetic devices, implants and grafts** cc

6 √7ᵗʰ **T82.828 Fibrosis due vascular prosthetic devices, implants and grafts** cc HCC

√6ᵗʰ **T82.83 Hemorrhage due to cardiac and vascular prosthetic devices, implants and grafts**

√7ᵗʰ **T82.837 Hemorrhage due to cardiac prosthetic devices, implants and grafts** cc

6 √7ᵗʰ **T82.838 Hemorrhage due to vascular prosthetic devices, implants and grafts** cc HCC

√6ᵗʰ **T82.84 Pain due to cardiac and vascular prosthetic devices, implants and grafts**

√7ᵗʰ **T82.847 Pain due to cardiac prosthetic devices, implants and grafts** cc

6 √7ᵗʰ **T82.848 Pain due to vascular prosthetic devices, implants and grafts** cc HCC

√6ᵗʰ **T82.85 Stenosis due to cardiac and vascular prosthetic devices, implants and grafts**

√7ᵗʰ **T82.855 Stenosis of coronary artery stent** cc

In-stent stenosis (restenosis) of coronary artery stent

Restenosis of coronary artery stent

6 √7ᵗʰ **T82.856 Stenosis of peripheral vascular stent** cc HCC

In-stent stenosis (restenosis) of peripheral vascular stent

Restenosis of peripheral vascular stent

√7ᵗʰ **T82.857 Stenosis of other cardiac prosthetic devices, implants and grafts** cc

6 √7ᵗʰ **T82.858 Stenosis of other vascular prosthetic devices, implants and grafts** cc HCC

√6ᵗʰ **T82.86 Thrombosis of cardiac and vascular prosthetic devices, implants and grafts**

√7ᵗʰ **T82.867 Thrombosis due to cardiac prosthetic devices, implants and grafts** cc

6 √7ᵗʰ **T82.868 Thrombosis due to vascular prosthetic devices, implants and grafts** cc HCC

√6ᵗʰ **T82.89 Other specified complication of cardiac and vascular prosthetic devices, implants and grafts**

√7ᵗʰ **T82.897 Other specified complication of cardiac prosthetic devices, implants and grafts** cc

AHA: 2019,2Q,33

6 √7ᵗʰ **T82.898 Other specified complication of vascular prosthetic devices, implants and grafts** cc HCC

√x7ᵗʰ **T82.9 Unspecified complication of cardiac and vascular prosthetic device, implant and graft** cc

√4ᵗʰ **T83 Complications of genitourinary prosthetic devices, implants and grafts**

EXCLUDES 2 failure and rejection of transplanted organs and tissue (T86.-)

AHA: 2016,4Q,70-71

The appropriate 7th character is to be added to each code from category T83.
A   initial encounter
D   subsequent encounter
S   sequela

√5ᵗʰ **T83.0 Mechanical complication of urinary catheter**

EXCLUDES 2 complications of stoma of urinary tract (N99.5-)

√6ᵗʰ **T83.01 Breakdown (mechanical) of urinary catheter**

6 √7ᵗʰ **T83.010 Breakdown (mechanical) of cystostomy catheter** cc HCC

6 √7ᵗʰ **T83.011 Breakdown (mechanical) of indwelling urethral catheter** HCC

6 √7ᵗʰ **T83.012 Breakdown (mechanical) of nephrostomy catheter** HCC

N Newborn: 0   P Pediatric: 0-17   M Maternity: 9-64   A Adult: 15-124   MCC Major Complication/Comorbidity   CC Complication/Comorbidity   SW Severe Wound Dx

1152   ICD-10-CM 2021

6 ✓7ᵗʰ **T83.018 Breakdown (mechanical) of other urinary catheter** HCC
- Breakdown (mechanical) of Hopkins catheter
- Breakdown (mechanical) of ileostomy catheter
- Breakdown (mechanical) urostomy catheter

✓6ᵗʰ **T83.02 Displacement of urinary catheter**
- Malposition of urinary catheter

6 ✓7ᵗʰ **T83.020 Displacement of cystostomy catheter** CC HCC

6 ✓7ᵗʰ **T83.021 Displacement of indwelling urethral catheter** HCC

6 ✓7ᵗʰ **T83.022 Displacement of nephrostomy catheter** HCC

6 ✓7ᵗʰ **T83.028 Displacement of other urinary catheter** HCC
- Displacement of Hopkins catheter
- Displacement of ileostomy catheter
- Displacement of urostomy catheter

✓6ᵗʰ **T83.03 Leakage of urinary catheter**

6 ✓7ᵗʰ **T83.030 Leakage of cystostomy catheter** CC HCC

6 ✓7ᵗʰ **T83.031 Leakage of indwelling urethral catheter** HCC

6 ✓7ᵗʰ **T83.032 Leakage of nephrostomy catheter** HCC

6 ✓7ᵗʰ **T83.038 Leakage of other urinary catheter** HCC
- Leakage of Hopkins catheter
- Leakage of ileostomy catheter
- Leakage of urostomy catheter

✓6ᵗʰ **T83.09 Other mechanical complication of urinary catheter**
- Obstruction (mechanical) of urinary catheter
- Perforation of urinary catheter
- Protrusion of urinary catheter

6 ✓7ᵗʰ **T83.090 Other mechanical complication of cystostomy catheter** CC HCC

6 ✓7ᵗʰ **T83.091 Other mechanical complication of indwelling urethral catheter** HCC

6 ✓7ᵗʰ **T83.092 Other mechanical complication of nephrostomy catheter** HCC

6 ✓7ᵗʰ **T83.098 Other mechanical complication of other urinary catheter** HCC
- Other mechanical complication of Hopkins catheter
- Other mechanical complication of ileostomy catheter
- Other mechanical complication of urostomy catheter

✓5ᵗʰ **T83.1 Mechanical complication of other urinary devices and implants**

✓6ᵗʰ **T83.11 Breakdown (mechanical) of other urinary devices and implants**

6 ✓7ᵗʰ **T83.110 Breakdown (mechanical) of urinary electronic stimulator device** CC HCC
- *EXCLUDES 2*   *breakdown (mechanical) of electrode (lead) for sacral nerve neurostimulator (T85.111)*
- *breakdown (mechanical) of implanted electronic sacral neurostimulator, pulse generator or receiver (T85.113)*

6 ✓7ᵗʰ **T83.111 Breakdown (mechanical) of implanted urinary sphincter** CC HCC

6 ✓7ᵗʰ **T83.112 Breakdown (mechanical) of indwelling ureteral stent** CC HCC

6 ✓7ᵗʰ **T83.113 Breakdown (mechanical) of other urinary stents** CC HCC
- Breakdown (mechanical) of ileal conduit stent
- Breakdown (mechanical) of nephroureteral stent

6 ✓7ᵗʰ **T83.118 Breakdown (mechanical) of other urinary devices and implants** CC HCC

✓6ᵗʰ **T83.12 Displacement of other urinary devices and implants**
- Malposition of other urinary devices and implants

6 ✓7ᵗʰ **T83.120 Displacement of urinary electronic stimulator device** CC HCC
- *EXCLUDES 2*   *displacement of electrode (lead) for sacral nerve neurostimulator (T85.121)*
- *displacement of implanted electronic sacral neurostimulator, pulse generator or receiver (T85.123)*

6 ✓7ᵗʰ **T83.121 Displacement of implanted urinary sphincter** CC HCC

6 ✓7ᵗʰ **T83.122 Displacement of indwelling ureteral stent** CC HCC

6 ✓7ᵗʰ **T83.123 Displacement of other urinary stents** CC HCC
- Displacement of ileal conduit stent
- Displacement of nephroureteral stent

6 ✓7ᵗʰ **T83.128 Displacement of other urinary devices and implants** CC HCC

✓6ᵗʰ **T83.19 Other mechanical complication of other urinary devices and implants**
- Leakage of other urinary devices and implants
- Obstruction (mechanical) of other urinary devices and implants
- Perforation of other urinary devices and implants
- Protrusion of other urinary devices and implants

6 ✓7ᵗʰ **T83.190 Other mechanical complication of urinary electronic stimulator device** CC HCC
- *EXCLUDES 2*   *other mechanical complication of electrode (lead) for sacral nerve neurostimulator (T85.191)*
- *other mechanical complication of implanted electronic sacral neurostimulator, pulse generator or receiver (T85.193)*

6 ✓7ᵗʰ **T83.191 Other mechanical complication of implanted urinary sphincter** CC HCC

6 ✓7ᵗʰ **T83.192 Other mechanical complication of indwelling ureteral stent** CC HCC

6 ✓7ᵗʰ **T83.193 Other mechanical complication of other urinary stent** CC HCC
- Other mechanical complication of ileal conduit stent
- Other mechanical complication of nephroureteral stent

6 ✓7ᵗʰ **T83.198 Other mechanical complication of other urinary devices and implants** CC HCC

✓5ᵗʰ **T83.2 Mechanical complication of graft of urinary organ**

6 ✓ₓ7ᵗʰ **T83.21 Breakdown (mechanical) of graft of urinary organ** CC HCC

6 ✓ₓ7ᵗʰ **T83.22 Displacement of graft of urinary organ** CC HCC
- Malposition of graft of urinary organ

6 ✓ₓ7ᵗʰ **T83.23 Leakage of graft of urinary organ** CC HCC

6 ✓ₓ7ᵗʰ **T83.24 Erosion of graft of urinary organ** CC HCC

6 ✓ₓ7ᵗʰ **T83.25 Exposure of graft of urinary organ** CC HCC

6 ✓ₓ7ᵗʰ **T83.29 Other mechanical complication of graft of urinary organ** CC HCC
- Obstruction (mechanical) of graft of urinary organ
- Perforation of graft of urinary organ
- Protrusion of graft of urinary organ

✓5ᵗʰ **T83.3 Mechanical complication of intrauterine contraceptive device**

✓ₓ7ᵗʰ **T83.31 Breakdown (mechanical) of intrauterine contraceptive device** ♀

✓ₓ7ᵗʰ **T83.32 Displacement of intrauterine contraceptive device** ♀
- Malposition of intrauterine contraceptive device
- Missing string of intrauterine contraceptive device
- **AHA:** 2018,1Q,5

☑ Additional Character Required   ✓ₓ7ᵗʰ Placeholder   Unacceptable PDx   Questionable PDx   Manifestation   Unspecified Dx   H1 - H14 HAC   HCC CMS-HCC Dx   HIV HIV Dx

ICD-10-CM 2021   1153

√x7ᵗʰ **T83.39 Other mechanical complication of intrauterine contraceptive device** ♀

     Leakage of intrauterine contraceptive device

     Obstruction (mechanical) of intrauterine contraceptive device

     Perforation of intrauterine contraceptive device

     Protrusion of intrauterine contraceptive device

√5ᵗʰ **T83.4 Mechanical complication of other prosthetic devices, implants and grafts of genital tract**

   √6ᵗʰ **T83.41 Breakdown (mechanical) of other prosthetic devices, implants and grafts of genital tract**

     6 √7ᵗʰ **T83.410 Breakdown (mechanical) of implanted penile prosthesis** CC HCC ♂

       Breakdown (mechanical) of penile prosthesis cylinder

       Breakdown (mechanical) of penile prosthesis pump

       Breakdown (mechanical) of penile prosthesis reservoir

     6 √7ᵗʰ **T83.411 Breakdown (mechanical) of implanted testicular prosthesis** CC HCC

     6 √7ᵗʰ **T83.418 Breakdown (mechanical) of other prosthetic devices, implants and grafts of genital tract** CC HCC

   √6ᵗʰ **T83.42 Displacement of other prosthetic devices, implants and grafts of genital tract**

     Malposition of other prosthetic devices, implants and grafts of genital tract

     6 √7ᵗʰ **T83.420 Displacement of implanted penile prosthesis** CC HCC ♂

       Displacement of penile prosthesis cylinder

       Displacement of penile prosthesis pump

       Displacement of penile prosthesis reservoir

     6 √7ᵗʰ **T83.421 Displacement of implanted testicular prosthesis** CC HCC

     6 √7ᵗʰ **T83.428 Displacement of other prosthetic devices, implants and grafts of genital tract** CC HCC

       AHA: 2018,1Q,5

   √6ᵗʰ **T83.49 Other mechanical complication of other prosthetic devices, implants and grafts of genital tract**

     Leakage of other prosthetic devices, implants and grafts of genital tract

     Obstruction, mechanical of other prosthetic devices, implants and grafts of genital tract

     Perforation of other prosthetic devices, implants and grafts of genital tract

     Protrusion of other prosthetic devices, implants and grafts of genital tract

     6 √7ᵗʰ **T83.490 Other mechanical complication of implanted penile prosthesis** CC HCC ♂

       Other mechanical complication of penile prosthesis cylinder

       Other mechanical complication of penile prosthesis pump

       Other mechanical complication of penile prosthesis reservoir

     6 √7ᵗʰ **T83.491 Other mechanical complication of implanted testicular prosthesis** CC HCC

     6 √7ᵗʰ **T83.498 Other mechanical complication of other prosthetic devices, implants and grafts of genital tract** CC HCC

√5ᵗʰ **T83.5 Infection and inflammatory reaction due to prosthetic device, implant and graft in urinary system**

     Use additional code to identify infection

   √6ᵗʰ **T83.51 Infection and inflammatory reaction due to urinary catheter**

     EXCLUDES 2   complications of stoma of urinary tract (N99.5-)

     AHA: 2019,3Q,17

     6 √7ᵗʰ **T83.510 Infection and inflammatory reaction due to cystostomy catheter** CC HCC

     6 √7ᵗʰ **T83.511 Infection and inflammatory reaction due to indwelling urethral catheter** CC H6 HCC

     6 √7ᵗʰ **T83.512 Infection and inflammatory reaction due to nephrostomy catheter** CC HCC

     6 √7ᵗʰ **T83.518 Infection and inflammatory reaction due to other urinary catheter** CC H6 HCC

       Infection and inflammatory reaction due to Hopkins catheter

       Infection and inflammatory reaction due to ileostomy catheter

       Infection and inflammatory reaction due to urostomy catheter

   √6ᵗʰ **T83.59 Infection and inflammatory reaction due to prosthetic device, implant and graft in urinary system**

     6 √7ᵗʰ **T83.590 Infection and inflammatory reaction due to implanted urinary neurostimulation device** CC HCC

       EXCLUDES 2   infection and inflammatory reaction due to electrode lead of sacral nerve neurostimulator (T85.732)

         infection and inflammatory reaction due to pulse generator or receiver of sacral nerve neurostimulator (T85.734)

     6 √7ᵗʰ **T83.591 Infection and inflammatory reaction due to implanted urinary sphincter** CC HCC

     6 √7ᵗʰ **T83.592 Infection and inflammatory reaction due to indwelling ureteral stent** CC HCC

     6 √7ᵗʰ **T83.593 Infection and inflammatory reaction due to other urinary stents** CC HCC

       Infection and inflammatory reaction due to ileal conduit stents

       Infection and inflammatory reaction due to nephroureteral stent

     6 √7ᵗʰ **T83.598 Infection and inflammatory reaction due to other prosthetic device, implant and graft in urinary system** CC HCC

√5ᵗʰ **T83.6 Infection and inflammatory reaction due to prosthetic device, implant and graft in genital tract**

     Use additional code to identify infection

   6 √x7ᵗʰ **T83.61 Infection and inflammatory reaction due to implanted penile prosthesis** CC HCC

     Infection and inflammatory reaction due to penile prosthesis cylinder

     Infection and inflammatory reaction due to penile prosthesis pump

     Infection and inflammatory reaction due to penile prosthesis reservoir

   6 √x7ᵗʰ **T83.62 Infection and inflammatory reaction due to implanted testicular prosthesis** CC HCC

   6 √x7ᵗʰ **T83.69 Infection and inflammatory reaction due to other prosthetic device, implant and graft in genital tract** CC HCC

√5ᵗʰ **T83.7 Complications due to implanted mesh and other prosthetic materials**

   √6ᵗʰ **T83.71 Erosion of implanted mesh and other prosthetic materials**

     6 √7ᵗʰ **T83.711 Erosion of implanted vaginal mesh to surrounding organ or tissue** HCC ♀

       Erosion of implanted vaginal mesh into pelvic floor muscles

     6 √7ᵗʰ **T83.712 Erosion of implanted urethral mesh to surrounding organ or tissue** CC HCC

       Erosion of implanted female urethral sling

       Erosion of implanted male urethral sling

       Erosion of implanted urethral mesh into pelvic floor muscles

     6 √7ᵗʰ **T83.713 Erosion of implanted urethral bulking agent to surrounding organ or tissue** CC HCC

     6 √7ᵗʰ **T83.714 Erosion of implanted ureteral bulking agent to surrounding organ or tissue** CC HCC

     6 √7ᵗʰ **T83.718 Erosion of other implanted mesh to organ or tissue** CC HCC

     6 √7ᵗʰ **T83.719 Erosion of other prosthetic materials to surrounding organ or tissue** CC HCC

N Newborn: 0   P Pediatric: 0-17   M Maternity: 9-64   A Adult: 15-124   MCC Major Complication/Comorbidity   CC Complication/Comorbidity   SW Severe Wound Dx

1154   ICD-10-CM 2021

√6ᵗʰ **T83.72** Exposure of implanted mesh and other prosthetic materials into surrounding organ or tissue
Extrusion of implanted mesh

    6 √7ᵗʰ **T83.721** Exposure of implanted vaginal mesh into vagina   HCC ♀
       Exposure of implanted vaginal mesh through vaginal wall

    6 √7ᵗʰ **T83.722** Exposure of implanted urethral mesh into urethra   CC HCC
       Exposure of implanted female urethral sling
       Exposure of implanted male urethral sling
       Exposure of implanted urethral mesh through urethral wall

    6 √7ᵗʰ **T83.723** Exposure of implanted urethral bulking agent into urethra   CC HCC

    6 √7ᵗʰ **T83.724** Exposure of implanted ureteral bulking agent into ureter   CC HCC

    6 √7ᵗʰ **T83.728** Exposure of other implanted mesh into organ or tissue

    6 √7ᵗʰ **T83.729** Exposure of other prosthetic materials into organ or tissue   CC HCC

6 √x7ᵗʰ **T83.79** Other specified complications due to other genitourinary prosthetic materials   CC HCC

√5ᵗʰ **T83.8** Other specified complications of genitourinary prosthetic devices, implants and grafts

    6 √x7ᵗʰ **T83.81** Embolism due to genitourinary prosthetic devices, implants and grafts   CC HCC

    6 √x7ᵗʰ **T83.82** Fibrosis due to genitourinary prosthetic devices, implants and grafts   CC HCC

    6 √x7ᵗʰ **T83.83** Hemorrhage due to genitourinary prosthetic devices, implants and grafts   CC HCC

    6 √x7ᵗʰ **T83.84** Pain due to genitourinary prosthetic devices, implants and grafts   CC HCC

    6 √x7ᵗʰ **T83.85** Stenosis due to genitourinary prosthetic devices, implants and grafts   CC HCC

    6 √x7ᵗʰ **T83.86** Thrombosis due to genitourinary prosthetic devices, implants and grafts   CC HCC

    6 √x7ᵗʰ **T83.89** Other specified complication of genitourinary prosthetic devices, implants and grafts   CC HCC

6 √x7ᵗʰ **T83.9** Unspecified complication of genitourinary prosthetic device, implant and graft   CC HCC

√4ᵗʰ **T84** Complications of internal orthopedic prosthetic devices, implants and grafts

    EXCLUDES 2   failure and rejection of transplanted organs and tissues (T86.-)
          fracture of bone following insertion of orthopedic implant, joint prosthesis or bone plate (M96.6)

The appropriate 7th character is to be added to each code from category T84.
A   initial encounter
D   subsequent encounter
S   sequela

√5ᵗʰ **T84.0** Mechanical complication of internal joint prosthesis

    √6ᵗʰ **T84.01** Broken internal joint prosthesis
       Breakage (fracture) of prosthetic joint
       Broken prosthetic joint implant
         EXCLUDES 1   periprosthetic joint implant fracture ►(M97.-)◄
       AHA: 2016,4Q,42

    6 √7ᵗʰ **T84.010** Broken internal right hip prosthesis   CC HCC
    6 √7ᵗʰ **T84.011** Broken internal left hip prosthesis   CC HCC
    6 √7ᵗʰ **T84.012** Broken internal right knee prosthesis   CC HCC
    6 √7ᵗʰ **T84.013** Broken internal left knee prosthesis   CC HCC
    6 √7ᵗʰ **T84.018** Broken internal joint prosthesis, other site   CC HCC
       Use additional code to identify the joint (Z96.6-)
    6 √7ᵗʰ **T84.019** Broken internal joint prosthesis, unspecified site   CC HCC

√6ᵗʰ **T84.02** Dislocation of internal joint prosthesis
       Instability of internal joint prosthesis
       Subluxation of internal joint prosthesis
       AHA: 2019,2Q,27

    6 √7ᵗʰ **T84.020** Dislocation of internal right hip prosthesis   CC HCC
    6 √7ᵗʰ **T84.021** Dislocation of internal left hip prosthesis   CC HCC
    6 √7ᵗʰ **T84.022** Instability of internal right knee prosthesis   CC HCC
    6 √7ᵗʰ **T84.023** Instability of internal left knee prosthesis   CC HCC
    6 √7ᵗʰ **T84.028** Dislocation of other internal joint prosthesis
       Use additional code to identify the joint (Z96.6-)
    6 √7ᵗʰ **T84.029** Dislocation of unspecified internal joint prosthesis   CC HCC

√6ᵗʰ **T84.03** Mechanical loosening of internal prosthetic joint
       Aseptic loosening of prosthetic joint

    6 √7ᵗʰ **T84.030** Mechanical loosening of internal right hip prosthetic joint   CC HCC
    6 √7ᵗʰ **T84.031** Mechanical loosening of internal left hip prosthetic joint   CC HCC
    6 √7ᵗʰ **T84.032** Mechanical loosening of internal right knee prosthetic joint   CC HCC
    6 √7ᵗʰ **T84.033** Mechanical loosening of internal left knee prosthetic joint   CC HCC
    6 √7ᵗʰ **T84.038** Mechanical loosening of other internal prosthetic joint   CC HCC
       Use additional code to identify the joint (Z96.6-)
    6 √7ᵗʰ **T84.039** Mechanical loosening of unspecified internal prosthetic joint   CC HCC

√6ᵗʰ **T84.05** Periprosthetic osteolysis of internal prosthetic joint
       Use additional code to identify major osseous defect, if applicable (M89.7-)

    6 √7ᵗʰ **T84.050** Periprosthetic osteolysis of internal prosthetic right hip joint   CC HCC
    6 √7ᵗʰ **T84.051** Periprosthetic osteolysis of internal prosthetic left hip joint   CC HCC
    6 √7ᵗʰ **T84.052** Periprosthetic osteolysis of internal prosthetic right knee joint   CC HCC
    6 √7ᵗʰ **T84.053** Periprosthetic osteolysis of internal prosthetic left knee joint   CC HCC
    6 √7ᵗʰ **T84.058** Periprosthetic osteolysis of other internal prosthetic joint   CC HCC
       Use additional code to identify the joint (Z96.6-)
    6 √7ᵗʰ **T84.059** Periprosthetic osteolysis of unspecified internal prosthetic joint   CC HCC

√6ᵗʰ **T84.06** Wear of articular bearing surface of internal prosthetic joint

    6 √7ᵗʰ **T84.060** Wear of articular bearing surface of internal prosthetic right hip joint   CC HCC
    6 √7ᵗʰ **T84.061** Wear of articular bearing surface of internal prosthetic left hip joint   CC HCC
    6 √7ᵗʰ **T84.062** Wear of articular bearing surface of internal prosthetic right knee joint   CC HCC
    6 √7ᵗʰ **T84.063** Wear of articular bearing surface of internal prosthetic left knee joint   CC HCC
    6 √7ᵗʰ **T84.068** Wear of articular bearing surface of other internal prosthetic joint   CC HCC
       Use additional code to identify the joint (Z96.6-)
    6 √7ᵗʰ **T84.069** Wear of articular bearing surface of unspecified internal prosthetic joint   CC HCC

√6ᵗʰ **T84.09** Other mechanical complication of internal joint prosthesis
       Prosthetic joint implant failure NOS
       AHA: 2019,1Q,20

    6 √7ᵗʰ **T84.090** Other mechanical complication of internal right hip prosthesis   CC HCC
    6 √7ᵗʰ **T84.091** Other mechanical complication of internal left hip prosthesis   CC HCC

Chapter 19. Injury, Poisoning and Certain Other Consequences of External Causes

6 √7ᵗʰ **T84.092 Other mechanical complication of internal** right knee prosthesis   CC HCC

6 √7ᵗʰ **T84.093 Other mechanical complication of internal** left knee prosthesis   CC HCC

6 √7ᵗʰ **T84.098 Other mechanical complication of other internal joint prosthesis**   CC HCC

Use additional code to identify the joint (Z96.6-)

6 √7ᵗʰ **T84.099 Other mechanical complication of unspecified internal joint prosthesis**   CC HCC

√5ᵗʰ **T84.1 Mechanical complication of** internal fixation device **of bones of limb**

EXCLUDES 2   *mechanical complication of internal fixation device of bones of feet (T84.2-)*

mechanical complication of internal fixation device of bones of fingers (T84.2-)

mechanical complication of internal fixation device of bones of hands (T84.2-)

mechanical complication of internal fixation device of bones of toes (T84.2-)

√6ᵗʰ **T84.11 Breakdown (mechanical) of internal fixation device of bones of limb**

6 √7ᵗʰ **T84.110 Breakdown (mechanical) of internal fixation device of** right humerus   CC HCC

6 √7ᵗʰ **T84.111 Breakdown (mechanical) of internal fixation device of** left humerus   CC HCC

6 √7ᵗʰ **T84.112 Breakdown (mechanical) of internal fixation device of bone of** right forearm

6 √7ᵗʰ **T84.113 Breakdown (mechanical) of internal fixation device of bone of** left forearm   CC HCC

6 √7ᵗʰ **T84.114 Breakdown (mechanical) of internal fixation device of** right femur   CC HCC

6 √7ᵗʰ **T84.115 Breakdown (mechanical) of internal fixation device of** left femur   CC HCC

6 √7ᵗʰ **T84.116 Breakdown (mechanical) of internal fixation device of bone of** right lower leg   CC HCC

6 √7ᵗʰ **T84.117 Breakdown (mechanical) of internal fixation device of bone of** left lower leg   CC HCC

6 √7ᵗʰ **T84.119 Breakdown (mechanical) of internal fixation device of unspecified bone of limb**   CC HCC

√6ᵗʰ **T84.12 Displacement of internal fixation device of bones of limb**

Malposition of internal fixation device of bones of limb

6 √7ᵗʰ **T84.120 Displacement of internal fixation device of** right humerus   CC HCC

6 √7ᵗʰ **T84.121 Displacement of internal fixation device of** left humerus   CC HCC

6 √7ᵗʰ **T84.122 Displacement of internal fixation device of bone of** right forearm   CC HCC

6 √7ᵗʰ **T84.123 Displacement of internal fixation device of bone of** left forearm   CC HCC

6 √7ᵗʰ **T84.124 Displacement of internal fixation device of** right femur   CC HCC

6 √7ᵗʰ **T84.125 Displacement of internal fixation device of** left femur   CC HCC

6 √7ᵗʰ **T84.126 Displacement of internal fixation device of bone of** right lower leg   CC HCC

6 √7ᵗʰ **T84.127 Displacement of internal fixation device of bone of** left lower leg   CC HCC

6 √7ᵗʰ **T84.129 Displacement of internal fixation device of unspecified bone of limb**   CC HCC

√6ᵗʰ **T84.19 Other mechanical complication of internal fixation device of bones of limb**

Obstruction (mechanical) of internal fixation device of bones of limb

Perforation of internal fixation device of bones of limb

Protrusion of internal fixation device of bones of limb

6 √7ᵗʰ **T84.190 Other mechanical complication of internal fixation device of** right humerus   CC HCC

6 √7ᵗʰ **T84.191 Other mechanical complication of internal fixation device of** left humerus   CC HCC

6 √7ᵗʰ **T84.192 Other mechanical complication of internal fixation device of bone of** right forearm   CC HCC

6 √7ᵗʰ **T84.193 Other mechanical complication of internal fixation device of bone of** left forearm   CC HCC

6 √7ᵗʰ **T84.194 Other mechanical complication of internal fixation device of** right femur   CC HCC

6 √7ᵗʰ **T84.195 Other mechanical complication of internal fixation device of** left femur   CC HCC

6 √7ᵗʰ **T84.196 Other mechanical complication of internal fixation device of bone of** right lower leg   CC HCC

6 √7ᵗʰ **T84.197 Other mechanical complication of internal fixation device of bone of** left lower leg   CC HCC

6 √7ᵗʰ **T84.199 Other mechanical complication of internal fixation device of unspecified bone of limb**   CC HCC

√5ᵗʰ **T84.2 Mechanical complication of** internal fixation device **of other bones**

√6ᵗʰ **T84.21 Breakdown (mechanical) of internal fixation device of other bones**

6 √7ᵗʰ **T84.210 Breakdown (mechanical) of internal fixation device of bones of** hand and fingers   CC HCC

6 √7ᵗʰ **T84.213 Breakdown (mechanical) of internal fixation device of bones of** foot and toes   CC HCC

6 √7ᵗʰ **T84.216 Breakdown (mechanical) of internal fixation device of** vertebrae   CC HCC

6 √7ᵗʰ **T84.218 Breakdown (mechanical) of internal fixation device of other bones**   CC HCC

√6ᵗʰ **T84.22 Displacement of internal fixation device of other bones**

Malposition of internal fixation device of other bones

6 √7ᵗʰ **T84.220 Displacement of internal fixation device of bones of** hand and fingers   CC HCC

6 √7ᵗʰ **T84.223 Displacement of internal fixation device of bones of** foot and toes   CC HCC

6 √7ᵗʰ **T84.226 Displacement of internal fixation device of** vertebrae   CC HCC

6 √7ᵗʰ **T84.228 Displacement of internal fixation device of other bones**   CC HCC

√6ᵗʰ **T84.29 Other mechanical complication of internal fixation device of other bones**

Obstruction (mechanical) of internal fixation device of other bones

Perforation of internal fixation device of other bones

Protrusion of internal fixation device of other bones

6 √7ᵗʰ **T84.290 Other mechanical complication of internal fixation device of bones of** hand and fingers   CC HCC

6 √7ᵗʰ **T84.293 Other mechanical complication of internal fixation device of bones of** foot and toes   CC HCC

6 √7ᵗʰ **T84.296 Other mechanical complication of internal fixation device of** vertebrae   CC HCC

6 √7ᵗʰ **T84.298 Other mechanical complication of internal fixation device of other bones**   CC HCC

√5ᵗʰ **T84.3 Mechanical complication of other bone devices, implants and grafts**

EXCLUDES 2   *other complications of bone graft (T86.83-)*

√6ᵗʰ **T84.31 Breakdown (mechanical) of other bone devices, implants and grafts**

6 √7ᵗʰ **T84.310 Breakdown (mechanical) of** electronic bone stimulator   CC HCC

6 √7ᵗʰ **T84.318 Breakdown (mechanical) of other bone devices, implants and grafts**   CC HCC

√6ᵗʰ **T84.32 Displacement of other bone devices, implants and grafts**

Malposition of other bone devices, implants and grafts

6 √7ᵗʰ **T84.320 Displacement of** electronic bone stimulator   CC HCC

N Newborn: 0   P Pediatric: 0-17   M Maternity: 9-64   A Adult: 15-124   MCC Major Complication/Comorbidity   CC Complication/Comorbidity   SW Severe Wound Dx

1156   ICD-10-CM 2021

6 √7ᵗʰ **T84.328 Displacement of other bone devices, implants and grafts** `CC` `HCC`
   AHA: 2014,4Q, 28

√6ᵗʰ **T84.39 Other mechanical complication of other bone devices, implants and grafts**
   Obstruction (mechanical) of other bone devices, implants and grafts
   Perforation of other bone devices, implants and grafts
   Protrusion of other bone devices, implants and grafts

6 √7ᵗʰ **T84.390 Other mechanical complication of electronic bone stimulator** `CC` `HCC`

6 √7ᵗʰ **T84.398 Other mechanical complication of other bone devices, implants and grafts** `CC` `HCC`

√5ᵗʰ **T84.4 Mechanical complication of other internal orthopedic devices, implants and grafts**

√6ᵗʰ **T84.41 Breakdown (mechanical) of other internal orthopedic devices, implants and grafts**

6 √7ᵗʰ **T84.410 Breakdown (mechanical) of muscle and tendon graft** `CC` `HCC`

6 √7ᵗʰ **T84.418 Breakdown (mechanical) of other internal orthopedic devices, implants and grafts** `CC` `HCC`

√6ᵗʰ **T84.42 Displacement of other internal orthopedic devices, implants and grafts**
   Malposition of other internal orthopedic devices, implants and grafts

6 √7ᵗʰ **T84.420 Displacement of muscle and tendon graft** `CC` `HCC`

6 √7ᵗʰ **T84.428 Displacement of other internal orthopedic devices, implants and grafts** `CC` `HCC`

√6ᵗʰ **T84.49 Other mechanical complication of other internal orthopedic devices, implants and grafts**
   Mechanical complication of other internal orthopedic devices, implants and grafts NOS
   Obstruction (mechanical) of other internal orthopedic devices, implants and grafts
   Perforation of other internal orthopedic devices, implants and grafts
   Protrusion of other internal orthopedic devices, implants and grafts

6 √7ᵗʰ **T84.490 Other mechanical complication of muscle and tendon graft** `CC` `HCC`

6 √7ᵗʰ **T84.498 Other mechanical complication of other internal orthopedic devices, implants and grafts** `CC` `HCC`

√5ᵗʰ **T84.5 Infection and inflammatory reaction due to internal joint prosthesis**
   Use additional code to identify infection
   AHA: 2019,3Q,16; 2015,1Q,16

6 √x7ᵗʰ **T84.50 Infection and inflammatory reaction due to unspecified internal joint prosthesis** `CC` `HCC`

6 √x7ᵗʰ **T84.51 Infection and inflammatory reaction due to internal right hip prosthesis** `CC` `HCC`

6 √x7ᵗʰ **T84.52 Infection and inflammatory reaction due to internal left hip prosthesis** `CC` `HCC`

6 √x7ᵗʰ **T84.53 Infection and inflammatory reaction due to internal right knee prosthesis** `CC` `HCC`

6 √x7ᵗʰ **T84.54 Infection and inflammatory reaction due to internal left knee prosthesis** `CC` `HCC`

6 √x7ᵗʰ **T84.59 Infection and inflammatory reaction due to other internal joint prosthesis** `CC` `HCC`

√5ᵗʰ **T84.6 Infection and inflammatory reaction due to internal fixation device**
   Use additional code to identify infection

6 √x7ᵗʰ **T84.60 Infection and inflammatory reaction due to internal fixation device of unspecified site** `CC` `H12` `HCC`

√6ᵗʰ **T84.61 Infection and inflammatory reaction due to internal fixation device of arm**

6 √7ᵗʰ **T84.610 Infection and inflammatory reaction due to internal fixation device of right humerus** `CC` `H12` `HCC`

6 √7ᵗʰ **T84.611 Infection and inflammatory reaction due to internal fixation device of left humerus** `CC` `H12` `HCC`

6 √7ᵗʰ **T84.612 Infection and inflammatory reaction due to internal fixation device of right radius** `CC` `H12` `HCC`

6 √7ᵗʰ **T84.613 Infection and inflammatory reaction due to internal fixation device of left radius** `CC` `H12` `HCC`

6 √7ᵗʰ **T84.614 Infection and inflammatory reaction due to internal fixation device of right ulna** `CC` `H12` `HCC`

6 √7ᵗʰ **T84.615 Infection and inflammatory reaction due to internal fixation device of left ulna** `CC` `H12` `HCC`

6 √7ᵗʰ **T84.619 Infection and inflammatory reaction due to internal fixation device of unspecified bone of arm** `CC` `H12` `HCC`

√6ᵗʰ **T84.62 Infection and inflammatory reaction due to internal fixation device of leg**

6 √7ᵗʰ **T84.620 Infection and inflammatory reaction due to internal fixation device of right femur** `CC` `HCC`

6 √7ᵗʰ **T84.621 Infection and inflammatory reaction due to internal fixation device of left femur** `CC` `HCC`

6 √7ᵗʰ **T84.622 Infection and inflammatory reaction due to internal fixation device of right tibia** `CC` `HCC`

6 √7ᵗʰ **T84.623 Infection and inflammatory reaction due to internal fixation device of left tibia** `CC` `HCC`

6 √7ᵗʰ **T84.624 Infection and inflammatory reaction due to internal fixation device of right fibula** `CC` `HCC`

6 √7ᵗʰ **T84.625 Infection and inflammatory reaction due to internal fixation device of left fibula** `CC` `HCC`

6 √7ᵗʰ **T84.629 Infection and inflammatory reaction due to internal fixation device of unspecified bone of leg** `CC` `HCC`

6 √x7ᵗʰ **T84.63 Infection and inflammatory reaction due to internal fixation device of spine** `CC` `H12` `HCC`

6 √x7ᵗʰ **T84.69 Infection and inflammatory reaction due to internal fixation device of other site** `CC` `H12` `HCC`

6 √x7ᵗʰ **T84.7 Infection and inflammatory reaction due to other internal orthopedic prosthetic devices, implants and grafts** `CC` `H12` `HCC`
   Use additional code to identify infection

√5ᵗʰ **T84.8 Other specified complications of internal orthopedic prosthetic devices, implants and grafts**

6 √x7ᵗʰ **T84.81 Embolism due to internal orthopedic prosthetic devices, implants and grafts** `CC` `HCC`

6 √x7ᵗʰ **T84.82 Fibrosis due to internal orthopedic prosthetic devices, implants and grafts** `CC` `HCC`

6 √x7ᵗʰ **T84.83 Hemorrhage due to internal orthopedic prosthetic devices, implants and grafts** `CC` `HCC`

6 √x7ᵗʰ **T84.84 Pain due to internal orthopedic prosthetic devices, implants and grafts** `CC` `HCC`

6 √x7ᵗʰ **T84.85 Stenosis due to internal orthopedic prosthetic devices, implants and grafts** `CC` `HCC`

6 √x7ᵗʰ **T84.86 Thrombosis due to internal orthopedic prosthetic devices, implants and grafts** `CC` `HCC`

6 √x7ᵗʰ **T84.89 Other specified complication of internal orthopedic prosthetic devices, implants and grafts** `CC` `HCC`

6 √x7ᵗʰ **T84.9 Unspecified complication of internal orthopedic prosthetic device, implant and graft** `CC` `HCC`

√4ᵗʰ **T85 Complications of other internal prosthetic devices, implants and grafts**
   EXCLUDES 2   *failure and rejection of transplanted organs and tissue (T86.-)*
   AHA: 2016,4Q,71-72

   The appropriate 7th character is to be added to each code from category T85.
   A   initial encounter
   D   subsequent encounter
   S   sequela

√5ᵗʰ **T85.0 Mechanical complication of ventricular intracranial (communicating) shunt**

6 √x7ᵗʰ **T85.01 Breakdown (mechanical) of ventricular intracranial (communicating) shunt** `CC` `HCC`

6 √x7ᵗʰ **T85.02 Displacement of ventricular intracranial (communicating) shunt** `CC` `HCC`
   Malposition of ventricular intracranial (communicating) shunt

6 √x7ᵗʰ **T85.03 Leakage of ventricular intracranial (communicating) shunt** `CC` `HCC`

Chapter 19. Injury, Poisoning and Certain Other Consequences of External Causes

6 ✓x7ᵗʰ **T85.09** **Other mechanical complication of ventricular intracranial (communicating) shunt** CC HCC

Obstruction (mechanical) of ventricular intracranial (communicating) shunt

Perforation of ventricular intracranial (communicating) shunt

Protrusion of ventricular intracranial (communicating) shunt

✓5ᵗʰ **T85.1** **Mechanical complication of implanted electronic stimulator of nervous system**

  ✓6ᵗʰ **T85.11** **Breakdown (mechanical) of implanted electronic stimulator of nervous system**

    6 ✓7ᵗʰ **T85.110** **Breakdown (mechanical) of implanted electronic neurostimulator of brain electrode (lead)** CC HCC

    6 ✓7ᵗʰ **T85.111** **Breakdown (mechanical) of implanted electronic neurostimulator of peripheral nerve electrode (lead)** CC HCC

Breakdown of electrode (lead) for cranial nerve neurostimulators

Breakdown of electrode (lead) for gastric neurostimulator

Breakdown of electrode (lead) for sacral nerve neurostimulator

Breakdown of electrode (lead) for vagal nerve neurostimulators

    6 ✓7ᵗʰ **T85.112** **Breakdown (mechanical) of implanted electronic neurostimulator of spinal cord electrode (lead)** CC HCC

    6 ✓7ᵗʰ **T85.113** **Breakdown (mechanical) of implanted electronic neurostimulator, generator** CC HCC

Breakdown (mechanical) of implanted electronic neurostimulator generator, brain, peripheral, gastric, spinal

Breakdown (mechanical) of implanted electronic sacral neurostimulator, pulse generator or receiver

    6 ✓7ᵗʰ **T85.118** **Breakdown (mechanical) of other implanted electronic stimulator of nervous system** CC HCC

  ✓6ᵗʰ **T85.12** **Displacement of implanted electronic stimulator of nervous system**

Malposition of implanted electronic stimulator of nervous system

    6 ✓7ᵗʰ **T85.120** **Displacement of implanted electronic neurostimulator of brain electrode (lead)** CC HCC

    6 ✓7ᵗʰ **T85.121** **Displacement of implanted electronic neurostimulator of peripheral nerve electrode (lead)** CC HCC

Displacement of electrode (lead) for cranial nerve neurostimulators

Displacement of electrode (lead) for gastric neurostimulator

Displacement of electrode (lead) for sacral nerve neurostimulator

Displacement of electrode (lead) for vagal nerve neurostimulators

    6 ✓7ᵗʰ **T85.122** **Displacement of implanted electronic neurostimulator of spinal cord electrode (lead)** CC HCC

    6 ✓7ᵗʰ **T85.123** **Displacement of implanted electronic neurostimulator, generator** CC HCC

Displacement of implanted electronic neurostimulator generator, brain, peripheral, gastric, spinal

Displacement of implanted electronic sacral neurostimulator, pulse generator or receiver

    6 ✓7ᵗʰ **T85.128** **Displacement of other implanted electronic stimulator of nervous system** CC HCC

✓6ᵗʰ **T85.19** **Other mechanical complication of implanted electronic stimulator of nervous system**

Leakage of implanted electronic stimulator of nervous system

Obstruction (mechanical) of implanted electronic stimulator of nervous system

Perforation of implanted electronic stimulator of nervous system

Protrusion of implanted electronic stimulator of nervous system

  6 ✓7ᵗʰ **T85.190** **Other mechanical complication of implanted electronic neurostimulator of brain electrode (lead)** CC HCC

  6 ✓7ᵗʰ **T85.191** **Other mechanical complication of implanted electronic neurostimulator of peripheral nerve electrode (lead)** CC HCC

Other mechanical complication of electrode (lead) for cranial nerve neurostimulators

Other mechanical complication of electrode (lead) for gastric neurostimulator

Other mechanical complication of electrode (lead) for sacral nerve neurostimulator

Other mechanical complication of electrode (lead) for vagal nerve neurostimulators

  6 ✓7ᵗʰ **T85.192** **Other mechanical complication of implanted electronic neurostimulator of spinal cord electrode (lead)** CC HCC

  6 ✓7ᵗʰ **T85.193** **Other mechanical complication of implanted electronic neurostimulator, generator** CC HCC

Other mechanical complication of implanted electronic neurostimulator generator, brain, peripheral, gastric, spinal

Other mechanical complication of implanted electronic sacral neurostimulator, pulse generator or receiver

  6 ✓7ᵗʰ **T85.199** **Other mechanical complication of other implanted electronic stimulator of nervous system** CC HCC

✓5ᵗʰ **T85.2** **Mechanical complication of intraocular lens**

  ✓x7ᵗʰ **T85.21** **Breakdown (mechanical) of intraocular lens** CC

  ✓x7ᵗʰ **T85.22** **Displacement of intraocular lens** CC

Malposition of intraocular lens

  ✓x7ᵗʰ **T85.29** **Other mechanical complication of intraocular lens** CC

Obstruction (mechanical) of intraocular lens

Perforation of intraocular lens

Protrusion of intraocular lens

✓5ᵗʰ **T85.3** **Mechanical complication of other ocular prosthetic devices, implants and grafts**

EXCLUDES 2   other complications of corneal graft (T86.84-)

  ✓6ᵗʰ **T85.31** **Breakdown (mechanical) of other ocular prosthetic devices, implants and grafts**

    ✓7ᵗʰ **T85.310** **Breakdown (mechanical) of prosthetic orbit of right eye** CC

    ✓7ᵗʰ **T85.311** **Breakdown (mechanical) of prosthetic orbit of left eye** CC

    ✓7ᵗʰ **T85.318** **Breakdown (mechanical) of other ocular prosthetic devices, implants and grafts**

  ✓6ᵗʰ **T85.32** **Displacement of other ocular prosthetic devices, implants and grafts**

Malposition of other ocular prosthetic devices, implants and grafts

    ✓7ᵗʰ **T85.320** **Displacement of prosthetic orbit of right eye** CC

    ✓7ᵗʰ **T85.321** **Displacement of prosthetic orbit of left eye** CC

    ✓7ᵗʰ **T85.328** **Displacement of other ocular prosthetic devices, implants and grafts**

N Newborn: 0   P Pediatric: 0-17   M Maternity: 9-64   A Adult: 15-124   MCC Major Complication/Comorbidity   CC Complication/Comorbidity   SW Severe Wound Dx

1158   ICD-10-CM 2021

√6ᵗʰ **T85.39 Other mechanical complication of other ocular prosthetic devices, implants and grafts**
> Obstruction (mechanical) of other ocular prosthetic devices, implants and grafts
> Perforation of other ocular prosthetic devices, implants and grafts
> Protrusion of other ocular prosthetic devices, implants and grafts

√7ᵗʰ **T85.390 Other mechanical complication of prosthetic orbit of** right eye   `CC`

√7ᵗʰ **T85.391 Other mechanical complication of prosthetic orbit of** left eye   `CC`

√7ᵗʰ **T85.398 Other mechanical complication of other ocular prosthetic devices, implants and grafts**

√5ᵗʰ **T85.4 Mechanical complication of** breast prosthesis and implant

√x7ᵗʰ **T85.41 Breakdown (mechanical) of breast prosthesis and implant**   `CC`

√x7ᵗʰ **T85.42 Displacement of breast prosthesis and implant**   `CC`
> Malposition of breast prosthesis and implant

√x7ᵗʰ **T85.43 Leakage of breast prosthesis and implant**   `CC`

√x7ᵗʰ **T85.44 Capsular contracture of breast implant**   `CC`

√x7ᵗʰ **T85.49 Other mechanical complication of breast prosthesis and implant**   `CC`
> Obstruction (mechanical) of breast prosthesis and implant
> Perforation of breast prosthesis and implant
> Protrusion of breast prosthesis and implant

√5ᵗʰ **T85.5 Mechanical complication of** gastrointestinal prosthetic devices, implants and grafts

√6ᵗʰ **T85.51 Breakdown (mechanical) of gastrointestinal prosthetic devices, implants and grafts**

√7ᵗʰ **T85.510 Breakdown (mechanical) of** bile duct prosthesis   `CC`

√7ᵗʰ **T85.511 Breakdown (mechanical) of** esophageal anti-reflux device   `CC`

√7ᵗʰ **T85.518 Breakdown (mechanical) of other gastrointestinal prosthetic devices, implants and grafts**   `CC`

√6ᵗʰ **T85.52 Displacement of gastrointestinal prosthetic devices, implants and grafts**
> Malposition of gastrointestinal prosthetic devices, implants and grafts

√7ᵗʰ **T85.520 Displacement of** bile duct prosthesis   `CC`

√7ᵗʰ **T85.521 Displacement of** esophageal anti-reflux device   `CC`

√7ᵗʰ **T85.528 Displacement of other gastrointestinal prosthetic devices, implants and grafts**   `CC`

√6ᵗʰ **T85.59 Other mechanical complication of gastrointestinal prosthetic devices, implants and**
> Obstruction, mechanical of gastrointestinal prosthetic devices, implants and grafts
> Perforation of gastrointestinal prosthetic devices, implants and grafts
> Protrusion of gastrointestinal prosthetic devices, implants and grafts

√7ᵗʰ **T85.590 Other mechanical complication of** bile duct prosthesis   `CC`

√7ᵗʰ **T85.591 Other mechanical complication of** esophageal anti-reflux device   `CC`

√7ᵗʰ **T85.598 Other mechanical complication of other gastrointestinal prosthetic devices, implants and grafts**   `CC`

√5ᵗʰ **T85.6 Mechanical complication of other specified internal and external prosthetic devices, implants and grafts**

√6ᵗʰ **T85.61 Breakdown (mechanical) of other specified internal prosthetic devices, implants and grafts**

√7ᵗʰ **T85.610 Breakdown (mechanical) of** cranial or spinal infusion catheter   `CC`
> Breakdown (mechanical) of epidural infusion catheter
> Breakdown (mechanical) of intrathecal infusion catheter
> Breakdown (mechanical) of subarachnoid infusion catheter
> Breakdown (mechanical) of subdural infusion catheter

√7ᵗʰ **T85.611 Breakdown (mechanical) of** intraperitoneal dialysis catheter   `CC` `HCC`
>> *EXCLUDES 1*   mechanical complication of vascular dialysis catheter (T82.4-)

√7ᵗʰ **T85.612 Breakdown (mechanical) of** permanent sutures   `CC`
>> *EXCLUDES 1*   mechanical complication of permanent (wire) suture used in bone repair (T84.1-T84.2)

√7ᵗʰ **T85.613 Breakdown (mechanical) of** artificial skin graft and decellularized allodermis   `CC`
> Failure of artificial skin graft and decellularized allodermis
> Non-adherence of artificial skin graft and decellularized allodermis
> Poor incorporation of artificial skin graft and decellularized allodermis
> Shearing of artificial skin graft and decellularized allodermis

√7ᵗʰ **T85.614 Breakdown (mechanical) of** insulin pump   `CC`

6 √7ᵗʰ **T85.615 Breakdown (mechanical) of other nervous system device, implant or graft**   `CC` `HCC`
> Breakdown (mechanical) of intrathecal infusion pump

√7ᵗʰ **T85.618 Breakdown (mechanical) of other specified internal prosthetic devices, implants and grafts**   `CC`

√6ᵗʰ **T85.62 Displacement of other specified internal prosthetic devices, implants and grafts**
> Malposition of other specified internal prosthetic devices, implants and grafts

√7ᵗʰ **T85.620 Displacement of** cranial or spinal infusion catheter   `CC`
> Displacement of epidural infusion catheter
> Displacement of intrathecal infusion catheter
> Displacement of subarachnoid infusion catheter
> Displacement of subdural infusion catheter

√7ᵗʰ **T85.621 Displacement of** intraperitoneal dialysis catheter   `CC` `HCC`
>> *EXCLUDES 1*   mechanical complication of vascular dialysis catheter (T82.4-)

√7ᵗʰ **T85.622 Displacement of** permanent sutures   `CC`
>> *EXCLUDES 1*   mechanical complication of permanent (wire) suture used in bone repair (T84.1-T84.2)

√7ᵗʰ **T85.623 Displacement of** artificial skin graft and decellularized allodermis   `CC`
> Dislodgement of artificial skin graft and decellularized allodermis

√7ᵗʰ **T85.624 Displacement of** insulin pump   `CC`

6 √7ᵗʰ **T85.625 Displacement of other nervous system device, implant or graft**   `CC` `HCC`
> Displacement of intrathecal infusion pump

√7ᵗʰ **T85.628 Displacement of other specified internal prosthetic devices, implants and grafts**   `CC`

✔ Additional Character Required   √x7ᵗʰ Placeholder   Unacceptable PDx   Questionable PDx   Manifestation   Unspecified Dx   H1-H14 HAC   HCC CMS-HCC Dx   HIV HIV Dx

ICD-10-CM 2021   1159

√6ᵗʰ **T85.63 Leakage of other specified internal prosthetic devices, implants and grafts**

√7ᵗʰ **T85.630 Leakage of cranial or spinal infusion catheter** CC

Leakage of epidural infusion catheter

Leakage of intrathecal infusion catheter infusion catheter

Leakage of subdural infusion catheter

Leakage of subarachnoid infusion catheter

√7ᵗʰ **T85.631 Leakage of intraperitoneal dialysis catheter** CC HCC

EXCLUDES 1   *mechanical complication of vascular dialysis catheter (T82.4)*

√7ᵗʰ **T85.633 Leakage of insulin pump** CC

6 √7ᵗʰ **T85.635 Leakage of other nervous system device, implant or graft** CC HCC

Leakage of intrathecal infusion pump

√7ᵗʰ **T85.638 Leakage of other specified internal prosthetic devices, implants and grafts** CC

√6ᵗʰ **T85.69 Other mechanical complication of other specified internal prosthetic devices, implants and grafts**

Obstruction, mechanical of other specified internal prosthetic devices, implants and grafts

Perforation of other specified internal prosthetic devices, implants and grafts

Protrusion of other specified internal prosthetic devices, implants and grafts

√7ᵗʰ **T85.690 Other mechanical complication of cranial or spinal infusion catheter** CC

Other mechanical complication of epidural infusion catheter

Other mechanical complication of intrathecal infusion catheter

Other mechanical complication of subarachnoid infusion catheter

Other mechanical complication of subdural infusion catheter

√7ᵗʰ **T85.691 Other mechanical complication of intraperitoneal dialysis catheter** CC HCC

EXCLUDES 1   *mechanical complication of vascular dialysis catheter (T82.4)*

√7ᵗʰ **T85.692 Other mechanical complication of permanent sutures** CC

EXCLUDES 1   *mechanical complication of permanent (wire) suture used in bone repair (T84.1-T84.2)*

√7ᵗʰ **T85.693 Other mechanical complication of artificial skin graft and decellularized allodermis** CC

√7ᵗʰ **T85.694 Other mechanical complication of insulin pump** CC

6 √7ᵗʰ **T85.695 Other mechanical complication of other nervous system device, implant or graft** CC HCC

Other mechanical complication of intrathecal infusion pump

√7ᵗʰ **T85.698 Other mechanical complication of other specified internal prosthetic devices, implants and grafts** CC

Mechanical complication of nonabsorbable surgical material NOS

√5ᵗʰ **T85.7 Infection and inflammatory reaction due to other internal prosthetic devices, implants and grafts**

Use additional code to identify infection

√x7ᵗʰ **T85.71 Infection and inflammatory reaction due to peritoneal dialysis catheter** CC HCC

6 √x7ᵗʰ **T85.72 Infection and inflammatory reaction due to insulin pump** CC HCC

√6ᵗʰ **T85.73 Infection and inflammatory reaction due to nervous system devices, implants and graft**

6 √7ᵗʰ **T85.730 Infection and inflammatory reaction due to ventricular intracranial (communicating) shunt** CC HCC

6 √7ᵗʰ **T85.731 Infection and inflammatory reaction due to implanted electronic neurostimulator of brain, electrode (lead)** CC HCC

6 √7ᵗʰ **T85.732 Infection and inflammatory reaction due to implanted electronic neurostimulator of peripheral nerve, electrode (lead)** CC HCC

Infection and inflammatory reaction due to electrode (lead) for cranial nerve neurostimulators

Infection and inflammatory reaction due to electrode (lead) for gastric neurostimulator

Infection and inflammatory reaction due to electrode (lead) for sacral nerve neurostimulator

Infection and inflammatory reaction due to electrode (lead) for vagal nerve neurostimulators

6 √7ᵗʰ **T85.733 Infection and inflammatory reaction due to implanted electronic neurostimulator of spinal cord, electrode (lead)** CC HCC

6 √7ᵗʰ **T85.734 Infection and inflammatory reaction due to implanted electronic neurostimulator, generator** CC HCC

Generator pocket infection

6 √7ᵗʰ **T85.735 Infection and inflammatory reaction due to cranial or spinal infusion catheter** CC HCC

Infection and inflammatory reaction due to epidural catheter

Infection and inflammatory reaction due to intrathecal infusion catheter

Infection and inflammatory reaction due to subarachnoid catheter

Infection and inflammatory reaction due to subdural catheter

6 √7ᵗʰ **T85.738 Infection and inflammatory reaction due to other nervous system device, implant or graft** CC HCC

Infection and inflammatory reaction due to intrathecal infusion pump

6 √x7ᵗʰ **T85.79 Infection and inflammatory reaction due to other internal prosthetic devices, implants and grafts** CC HCC

√5ᵗʰ **T85.8 Other specified complications of internal prosthetic devices, implants and grafts, not elsewhere classified**

√6ᵗʰ **T85.81 Embolism due to internal prosthetic devices, implants and grafts, not elsewhere classified**

5,6 √7ᵗʰ **T85.810 Embolism due to nervous system prosthetic devices, implants and grafts** CC HCC

√7ᵗʰ **T85.818 Embolism due to other internal prosthetic devices, implants and grafts**

√6ᵗʰ **T85.82 Fibrosis due to internal prosthetic devices, implants and grafts, not elsewhere classified**

5,6 √7ᵗʰ **T85.820 Fibrosis due to nervous system prosthetic devices, implants and grafts** CC HCC

√7ᵗʰ **T85.828 Fibrosis due to other internal prosthetic devices, implants and grafts**

√6ᵗʰ **T85.83 Hemorrhage due to internal prosthetic devices, implants and grafts, not elsewhere classified**

5,6 √7ᵗʰ **T85.830 Hemorrhage due to nervous system prosthetic devices, implants and grafts** CC HCC

√7ᵗʰ **T85.838 Hemorrhage due to other internal prosthetic devices, implants and grafts**

√6ᵗʰ **T85.84 Pain due to internal prosthetic devices, implants and grafts, not elsewhere classified**

5,6 √7ᵗʰ **T85.840 Pain due to nervous system prosthetic devices, implants and grafts** CC HCC

√7ᵗʰ **T85.848 Pain due to other internal prosthetic devices, implants and grafts**

√6ᵗʰ **T85.85 Stenosis due to internal prosthetic devices, implants and grafts, not elsewhere classified**

5,6 √7ᵗʰ **T85.850 Stenosis due to nervous system prosthetic devices, implants and grafts** CC HCC

√7ᵗʰ **T85.858 Stenosis due to other internal prosthetic devices, implants and grafts**

N Newborn: 0   P Pediatric: 0-17   M Maternity: 9-64   A Adult: 15-124   MCC Major Complication/Comorbidity   CC Complication/Comorbidity   SW Severe Wound Dx

1160   ICD-10-CM 2021

√6ᵗʰ **T85.86** Thrombosis due to internal prosthetic devices, implants and grafts, not elsewhere classified

5,6 √7ᵗʰ **T85.860** Thrombosis due to nervous system prosthetic devices, implants and grafts `CC` `HCC`

√7ᵗʰ **T85.868** Thrombosis due to other internal prosthetic devices, implants and grafts

√6ᵗʰ **T85.89** Other specified complication of internal prosthetic devices, implants and grafts, not elsewhere classified

Erosion or breakdown of subcutaneous device pocket

5,6 √7ᵗʰ **T85.890** Other specified complication of nervous system prosthetic devices, implants and grafts `CC` `HCC`

√7ᵗʰ **T85.898** Other specified complication of other internal prosthetic devices, implants and grafts

√x 7ᵗʰ **T85.9** Unspecified complication of internal prosthetic device, implant and graft

Complication of internal prosthetic device, implant and graft NOS

√4ᵗʰ **T86** Complications of transplanted organs and tissue

Use additional code to identify other transplant complications, such as:
graft-versus-host disease (D89.81-)
malignancy associated with organ transplant (C80.2)
post-transplant lymphoproliferative disorders (PTLD) (D47.Z1)
AHA: 2020,1Q,18

√5ᵗʰ **T86.0** Complications of bone marrow transplant

T86.00 Unspecified complication of bone marrow transplant `CC` `HCC`

T86.01 Bone marrow transplant rejection `CC` `HCC`

T86.02 Bone marrow transplant failure `CC` `HCC`

T86.03 Bone marrow transplant infection `CC` `HCC`

T86.09 Other complications of bone marrow transplant

√5ᵗʰ **T86.1** Complications of kidney transplant

T86.10 Unspecified complication of kidney transplant `CC`

T86.11 Kidney transplant rejection `CC`

T86.12 Kidney transplant failure `CC`
AHA: 2013,1Q,24

T86.13 Kidney transplant infection `CC`
Use additional code to specify infection

T86.19 Other complication of kidney transplant `CC`
AHA: 2019,2Q,7

√5ᵗʰ **T86.2** Complications of heart transplant

EXCLUDES 1 complication of:
artificial heart device (T82.5)
heart-lung transplant (T86.3)

T86.20 Unspecified complication of heart transplant `CC` `HCC`

T86.21 Heart transplant rejection `CC` `HCC`

T86.22 Heart transplant failure `CC` `HCC`

T86.23 Heart transplant infection `CC` `HCC`
Use additional code to specify infection

√6ᵗʰ **T86.29** Other complications of heart transplant

T86.290 Cardiac allograft vasculopathy `CC` `HCC`
EXCLUDES 1 atherosclerosis of coronary arteries (I25.75-, I25.76-, I25.81-)

T86.298 Other complications of heart transplant `CC` `HCC`

√5ᵗʰ **T86.3** Complications of heart-lung transplant

T86.30 Unspecified complication of heart-lung transplant `CC` `HCC`

T86.31 Heart-lung transplant rejection `CC` `HCC`

T86.32 Heart-lung transplant failure `CC` `HCC`

T86.33 Heart-lung transplant infection `CC` `HCC`
Use additional code to specify infection

T86.39 Other complications of heart-lung transplant `CC` `HCC`

√5ᵗʰ **T86.4** Complications of liver transplant

T86.40 Unspecified complication of liver transplant `CC` `HCC`

T86.41 Liver transplant rejection `CC` `HCC`

T86.42 Liver transplant failure `CC` `HCC`

T86.43 Liver transplant infection `CC` `HCC`
Use additional code to identify infection, such as:
cytomegalovirus (CMV) infection (B25.-)

T86.49 Other complications of liver transplant `CC` `HCC`

T86.5 Complications of stem cell transplant `CC` `HCC`
Complications from stem cells from peripheral blood
Complications from stem cells from umbilical cord

√5ᵗʰ **T86.8** Complications of other transplanted organs and tissues

√6ᵗʰ **T86.81** Complications of lung transplant

EXCLUDES 1 complication of heart-lung transplant (T86.3-)

T86.810 Lung transplant rejection `CC` `HCC`

T86.811 Lung transplant failure `CC` `HCC`

T86.812 Lung transplant infection `CC` `HCC`
Use additional code to specify infection

T86.818 Other complications of lung transplant `CC` `HCC`
AHA: 2019,2Q,6

T86.819 Unspecified complication of lung transplant `CC` `HCC`

√6ᵗʰ **T86.82** Complications of skin graft (allograft) (autograft)

EXCLUDES 2 complication of artificial skin graft (T85.693)

T86.820 Skin graft (allograft) rejection `CC`

T86.821 Skin graft (allograft) (autograft) failure `CC`

T86.822 Skin graft (allograft) (autograft) infection `CC`
Use additional code to specify infection

T86.828 Other complications of skin graft (allograft) (autograft) `CC`

T86.829 Unspecified complication of skin graft (allograft) (autograft) `CC`

√6ᵗʰ **T86.83** Complications of bone graft

EXCLUDES 2 mechanical complications of bone graft (T84.3-)

T86.830 Bone graft rejection `CC`

T86.831 Bone graft failure `CC`

T86.832 Bone graft infection `CC`
Use additional code to specify infection

T86.838 Other complications of bone graft `CC`

T86.839 Unspecified complication of bone graft `CC`

√6ᵗʰ **T86.84** Complications of corneal transplant

EXCLUDES 2 mechanical complications of corneal graft (T85.3-)

√7ᵗʰ **T86.840** Corneal transplant rejection

T86.8401 Corneal transplant rejection, right eye `CC`

T86.8402 Corneal transplant rejection, left eye `CC`

T86.8403 Corneal transplant rejection, bilateral `CC`

T86.8409 Corneal transplant rejection, unspecified eye `CC`

√7ᵗʰ **T86.841** Corneal transplant failure

T86.8411 Corneal transplant failure, right eye `CC`

T86.8412 Corneal transplant failure, left eye `CC`

T86.8413 Corneal transplant failure, bilateral `CC`

T86.8419 Corneal transplant failure, unspecified eye `CC`

√7ᵗʰ **T86.842** Corneal transplant infection
Use additional code to specify infection

T86.8421 Corneal transplant infection, right eye `CC`

T86.8422 Corneal transplant infection, left eye `CC`

T86.8423 Corneal transplant infection, bilateral `CC`

T86.8429 Corneal transplant infection, unspecified eye `CC`

√7ᵗʰ **T86.848** Other complications of corneal transplant

T86.8481 Other complications of corneal transplant, right eye `CC`

-     **T86.8482 Other complications of corneal transplant, left eye** `CC`
-     **T86.8483 Other complications of corneal transplant, bilateral** `CC`
-     **T86.8489 Other complications of corneal transplant, unspecified eye** `CC`
- ▲   ✓7ᵗʰ **T86.849 Unspecified complication of corneal transplant**
-     **T86.8491 Unspecified complication of corneal transplant, right eye** `CC`
-     **T86.8492 Unspecified complication of corneal transplant, left eye** `CC`
-     **T86.8493 Unspecified complication of corneal transplant, bilateral** `CC`
-     **T86.8499 Unspecified complication of corneal transplant, unspecified eye** `CC`

✓6ᵗʰ **T86.85 Complication of intestine transplant**

    T86.850 Intestine transplant rejection `CC` `HCC`
    T86.851 Intestine transplant failure `CC` `HCC`
    T86.852 Intestine transplant infection `CC` `HCC`
       Use additional code to specify infection
    T86.858 Other complications of intestine transplant `CC` `HCC`
    T86.859 Unspecified complication of intestine transplant `CC` `HCC`

✓6ᵗʰ **T86.89 Complications of other transplanted tissue**

    Transplant failure or rejection of pancreas
    AHA: 2020,1Q,18
    T86.890 Other transplanted tissue rejection `CC`
    T86.891 Other transplanted tissue failure `CC`
    T86.892 Other transplanted tissue infection `CC`
       Use additional code to specify infection
    T86.898 Other complications of other transplanted tissue `CC`
    T86.899 Unspecified complication of other transplanted tissue `CC`

✓5ᵗʰ **T86.9 Complication of unspecified transplanted organ and tissue**

    T86.90 Unspecified complication of unspecified transplanted organ and tissue `CC`
    T86.91 Unspecified transplanted organ and tissue rejection `CC`
    T86.92 Unspecified transplanted organ and tissue failure `CC`
    T86.93 Unspecified transplanted organ and tissue infection `CC`
       Use additional code to specify infection
    T86.99 Other complications of unspecified transplanted organ and tissue `CC`

✓4ᵗʰ **T87 Complications peculiar to reattachment and amputation**

✓5ᵗʰ **T87.0 Complications of reattached (part of) upper extremity**

   ✓6ᵗʰ **T87.0X Complications of reattached (part of) upper extremity**
      T87.0X1 Complications of reattached (part of) right upper extremity `CC` `HCC`
      T87.0X2 Complications of reattached (part of) left upper extremity `CC` `HCC`
      T87.0X9 Complications of reattached (part of) unspecified upper extremity `CC` `HCC`

✓5ᵗʰ **T87.1 Complications of reattached (part of) lower extremity**

   ✓6ᵗʰ **T87.1X Complications of reattached (part of) lower extremity**
      T87.1X1 Complications of reattached (part of) right lower extremity `CC` `HCC`
      T87.1X2 Complications of reattached (part of) left lower extremity `CC` `HCC`
      T87.1X9 Complications of reattached (part of) unspecified lower extremity `CC` `HCC`

   T87.2 Complications of other reattached body part `CC` `HCC`

✓5ᵗʰ **T87.3 Neuroma of amputation stump**

    DEF: Non-neoplastic tumor generated at the proximal end of severed, partially transected, or injured nerve following amputation.
    T87.30 Neuroma of amputation stump, unspecified extremity `HCC`

    T87.31 Neuroma of amputation stump, right upper extremity `HCC`
    T87.32 Neuroma of amputation stump, left upper extremity `HCC`
    T87.33 Neuroma of amputation stump, right lower extremity `HCC`
    T87.34 Neuroma of amputation stump, left lower extremity `HCC`

✓5ᵗʰ **T87.4 Infection of amputation stump**

    T87.40 Infection of amputation stump, unspecified extremity `CC` `HCC`
    T87.41 Infection of amputation stump, right upper extremity `CC` `HCC`
    T87.42 Infection of amputation stump, left upper extremity `CC` `HCC`
    T87.43 Infection of amputation stump, right lower extremity `CC` `HCC`
    T87.44 Infection of amputation stump, left lower extremity `CC` `HCC`

✓5ᵗʰ **T87.5 Necrosis of amputation stump**

    T87.50 Necrosis of amputation stump, unspecified extremity `HCC`
    T87.51 Necrosis of amputation stump, right upper extremity `HCC`
    T87.52 Necrosis of amputation stump, left upper extremity `HCC`
    T87.53 Necrosis of amputation stump, right lower extremity `HCC`
    T87.54 Necrosis of amputation stump, left lower extremity `HCC`

✓5ᵗʰ **T87.8 Other complications of amputation stump**

    T87.81 Dehiscence of amputation stump `HCC`
    T87.89 Other complications of amputation stump `HCC`
       Amputation stump contracture
       Amputation stump contracture of next proximal joint
       Amputation stump flexion
       Amputation stump edema
       Amputation stump hematoma
       EXCLUDES 2   *phantom limb syndrome (G54.6-G54.7)*

   T87.9 Unspecified complications of amputation stump `HCC`

✓4ᵗʰ **T88 Other complications of surgical and medical care, not elsewhere classified**

    EXCLUDES 2   *complication following infusion, transfusion and therapeutic injection (T80.-)*
       complication following procedure NEC (T81.-)
       complications of anesthesia in labor and delivery (O74.-)
       complications of anesthesia in pregnancy (O29.-)
       complications of anesthesia in puerperium (O89.-)
       complications of devices, implants and grafts (T82-T85)
       complications of obstetric surgery and procedure (O75.4)
       dermatitis due to drugs and medicaments (L23.3, L24.4, L25.1, L27.0-L27.1)
       poisoning and toxic effects of drugs and chemicals (T36-T65 with fifth or sixth character 1-4 or 6)
       specified complications classified elsewhere

    The appropriate 7th character is to be added to each code from category T88.
    A   initial encounter
    D   subsequent encounter
    S   sequela

✓x7ᵗʰ **T88.0 Infection following immunization** `CC`

    Sepsis following immunization
    AHA: 2018,4Q,62-63

✓x7ᵗʰ **T88.1 Other complications following immunization, not elsewhere classified** `CC`

    Generalized vaccinia
    Rash following immunization
    EXCLUDES 1   *vaccinia not from vaccine (B08.011)*
    EXCLUDES 2   *anaphylactic shock due to serum (T80.5-)*
       other serum reactions (T80.6-)
       postimmunization arthropathy (M02.2)
       postimmunization encephalitis (G04.02)
       postimmunization fever (R50.83)

N Newborn: 0   P Pediatric: 0-17   M Maternity: 9-64   A Adult: 15-124   MCC Major Complication/Comorbidity   CC Complication/Comorbidity   SW Severe Wound Dx

1162   ICD-10-CM 2021

√x 7ᵗʰ **T88.2** **Shock due to anesthesia**   `CC`

    Use additional code for adverse effect, if applicable, to identify drug (T41.- with fifth or sixth character 5)

      EXCLUDES 1   *complications of anesthesia (in):*
             labor and delivery (O74.-)
             postprocedural shock NOS (T81.1-)
             pregnancy (O29.-)
             puerperium (O89.-)

√x 7ᵗʰ **T88.3** **Malignant hyperthermia due to anesthesia**   `CC`

    Use additional code for adverse effect, if applicable, to identify drug (T41.- with fifth or sixth character 5)

√x 7ᵗʰ **T88.4** **Failed or difficult intubation**

√ 5ᵗʰ **T88.5** **Other complications of anesthesia**

    Use additional code for adverse effect, if applicable, to identify drug (T41.- with fifth or sixth character 5)

    √x 7ᵗʰ **T88.51** **Hypothermia following anesthesia**

    √x 7ᵗʰ **T88.52** **Failed moderate sedation during procedure**

        Failed conscious sedation during procedure
        EXCLUDES 2   *personal history of failed moderate sedation (Z92.83)*

    √x 7ᵗʰ **T88.53** **Unintended awareness under general anesthesia during procedure**

        EXCLUDES 2   *personal history of unintended awareness under general anesthesia (Z92.84)*

        AHA: 2016,4Q,72-73

    √x 7ᵗʰ **T88.59** **Other complications of anesthesia**

√x 7ᵗʰ **T88.6** **Anaphylactic reaction due to adverse effect of correct drug or medicament properly administered**   `CC`

    Anaphylactic shock due to adverse effect of correct drug or medicament properly administered

    Anaphylactoid reaction NOS

    Use additional code for adverse effect, if applicable, to identify drug (T36-T50 with fifth or sixth character 5)

      EXCLUDES 1   *anaphylactic reaction due to serum (T80.5-)*
             anaphylactic shock or reaction due to adverse food reaction (T78.0-)

    AHA: 2020,1Q,18

√x 7ᵗʰ **T88.7** **Unspecified adverse effect of drug or medicament**

    Drug hypersensitivity NOS

    Drug reaction NOS

    Use additional code for adverse effect, if applicable, to identify drug (T36-T50 with fifth or sixth character 5)

      EXCLUDES 1   *specified adverse effects of drugs and medicaments (A00-R94 and T80-T88.6, T88.8)*

√x 7ᵗʰ **T88.8** **Other specified complications of surgical and medical care, not elsewhere classified**

    Use additional code to identify the complication

√x 7ᵗʰ **T88.9** **Complication of surgical and medical care, unspecified**

☑ Additional Character Required   √x 7ᵗʰ Placeholder   Unacceptable PDx   Questionable PDx   Manifestation   Unspecified Dx   `H1`-`H14` HAC   `HCC` CMS-HCC Dx   `HIV` HIV Dx

ICD-10-CM 2021   **1163**

Chapter 20. External Causes of Morbidity (V00–Y99)

Chapter-specific Guidelines with Coding Examples

The chapter-specific guidelines from the ICD-10-CM Official Guidelines for Coding and Reporting have been provided below. Along with these guidelines are coding examples, contained in the shaded boxes, that have been developed to help illustrate the coding and/or sequencing guidance found in these guidelines.

The external causes of morbidity codes should never be sequenced as the first-listed or principal diagnosis.

External cause codes are intended to provide data for injury research and evaluation of injury prevention strategies. These codes capture how the injury or health condition happened (cause), the intent (unintentional or accidental; or intentional, such as suicide or assault), the place where the event occurred the activity of the patient at the time of the event, and the person's status (e.g., civilian, military).

There is no national requirement for mandatory ICD-10-CM external cause code reporting. Unless a provider is subject to a state-based external cause code reporting mandate or these codes are required by a particular payer, reporting of ICD-10-CM codes in Chapter 20, External Causes of Morbidity, is not required. In the absence of a mandatory reporting requirement, providers are encouraged to voluntarily report external cause codes, as they provide valuable data for injury research and evaluation of injury prevention strategies.

a. General external cause coding guidelines

1) Used with any code in the range of A00.0–T88.9, Z00–Z99

An external cause code may be used with any code in the range of A00.0–T88.9, Z00–Z99, classification that represents a health condition due to an external cause. Though they are most applicable to injuries, they are also valid for use with such things as infections or diseases due to an external source, and other health conditions, such as a heart attack that occurs during strenuous physical activity.

> Actinic reticuloid due to tanning bed use
>
> **L57.1**   **Actinic reticuloid**
>
> **W89.1XXA**   **Exposure to tanning bed, initial encounter**
>
> *Explanation:* An external cause code may be used with any code in the range of A00.0–T88.9, Z00–Z99, classifications that describe health conditions due to an external cause. Code W89.1 Exposure to tanning bed requires a seventh character of A to report this initial encounter, with a placeholder X for the fifth and sixth characters.

2) External cause code used for length of treatment

Assign the external cause code, with the appropriate 7th character (initial encounter, subsequent encounter or sequela) for each encounter for which the injury or condition is being treated.

Most categories in chapter 20 have a 7th character requirement for each applicable code. Most categories in this chapter have three 7th character values: A, initial encounter, D, subsequent encounter and S, sequela. While the patient may be seen by a new or different provider over the course of treatment for an injury or condition, assignment of the 7th character for external cause should match the 7th character of the code assigned for the associated injury or condition for the encounter.

3) Use the full range of external cause codes

Use the full range of external cause codes to completely describe the cause, the intent, the place of occurrence, and if applicable, the activity of the patient at the time of the event, and the patient's status, for all injuries, and other health conditions due to an external cause.

4) Assign as many external cause codes as necessary

Assign as many external cause codes as necessary to fully explain each cause. If only one external cause code can be recorded, assign the code most related to the principal diagnosis.

5) The selection of the appropriate external cause code

The selection of the appropriate external cause code is guided by the Alphabetic Index of External Causes and by Inclusion and Exclusion notes in the Tabular List.

6) External cause code can never be a principal diagnosis

An external cause code can never be a principal (first-listed) diagnosis.

7) Combination external cause codes

Certain of the external cause codes are combination codes that identify sequential events that result in an injury, such as a fall which results in striking against an object. The injury may be due to either event or both.

The combination external cause code used should correspond to the sequence of events regardless of which caused the most serious injury.

> Toddler tripped and fell while walking and struck his head on an end table, sustaining a scalp contusion
>
> **S00.03XA**   **Contusion of scalp, initial encounter**
>
> **W01.190A**   **Fall on same level from slipping, tripping and stumbling with subsequent striking against furniture, initial encounter**
>
> *Explanation:* Combination external cause codes identify sequential events that result in an injury, such as a fall resulting in striking against an object. The injury may be due to either or both events.

8) No external cause code needed in certain circumstances

No external cause code from Chapter 20 is needed if the external cause and intent are included in a code from another chapter (e.g. T36.0X1-Poisoning by penicillins, accidental (unintentional)).

b. Place of occurrence guideline

Codes from category Y92, Place of occurrence of the external cause, are secondary codes for use after other external cause codes to identify the location of the patient at the time of injury or other condition.

Generally, a place of occurrence code is assigned only once, at the initial encounter for treatment. However, in the rare instance that a new injury occurs during hospitalization, an additional place of occurrence code may be assigned. No 7th characters are used for Y92.

Do not use place of occurrence code Y92.9 if the place is not stated or is not applicable.

> A farmer was working in his barn and sustained a foot contusion when the horse stepped on his left foot
>
> **S90.32XA**   **Contusion of left foot, initial encounter**
>
> **W55.19XA**   **Other contact with horse, initial encounter**
>
> **Y92.71**   **Barn as the place of occurrence of the external cause**
>
> *Explanation:* A place-of-occurrence code from category Y92 is assigned at the initial encounter to identify the location of the patient at the time the injury occurred.

c. Activity code

Assign a code from category Y93, Activity code, to describe the activity of the patient at the time the injury or other health condition occurred.

An activity code is used only once, at the initial encounter for treatment. Only one code from Y93 should be recorded on a medical record.

The activity codes are not applicable to poisonings, adverse effects, misadventures or sequela.

Do not assign Y93.9, Unspecified activity, if the activity is not stated.

A code from category Y93 is appropriate for use with external cause and intent codes if identifying the activity provides additional information about the event.

> Ranch hand who was grooming a horse sustained a foot contusion when the horse stepped on his left foot
>
> **S90.32XA**   **Contusion of left foot, initial encounter**
>
> **W55.19XA**   **Other contact with horse, initial encounter**
>
> **Y93.K3**   **Activity, grooming and shearing an animal**
>
> *Explanation:* One activity code from category Y93 is assigned at the initial encounter only to describe the activity of the patient at the time the injury occurred.

d. Place of occurrence, activity, and status codes used with other external cause code

When applicable, place of occurrence, activity, and external cause status codes are sequenced after the main external cause code(s). Regardless of the number of external cause codes assigned, generally there should be only one place of occurrence code, one activity code, and one external cause status code assigned to an encounter. However, in the rare instance that a new injury occurs during hospitalization, an additional place of occurrence code may be assigned.

Chapter 20. External Causes of Morbidity

e. If the reporting format limits the number of external cause codes

If the reporting format limits the number of external cause codes that can be used in reporting clinical data, report the code for the cause/intent most related to the principal diagnosis. If the format permits capture of additional external cause codes, the cause/intent, including medical misadventures, of the additional events should be reported rather than the codes for place, activity, or external status.

f. Multiple external cause coding guidelines

More than one external cause code is required to fully describe the external cause of an illness or injury. The assignment of external cause codes should be sequenced in the following priority:

If two or more events cause separate injuries, an external cause code should be assigned for each cause. The first-listed external cause code will be selected in the following order:

External codes for child and adult abuse take priority over all other external cause codes.

See Section I.C.19., Child and Adult abuse guidelines.

External cause codes for terrorism events take priority over all other external cause codes except child and adult abuse.

External cause codes for cataclysmic events take priority over all other external cause codes except child and adult abuse and terrorism.

External cause codes for transport accidents take priority over all other external cause codes except cataclysmic events, child and adult abuse and terrorism.

Activity and external cause status codes are assigned following all causal (intent) external cause codes.

The first-listed external cause code should correspond to the cause of the most serious diagnosis due to an assault, accident, or self-harm, following the order of hierarchy listed above..

30-year-old man accidentally discharged his hunting rifle, sustaining an open gunshot wound to the right thigh, which caused him to fall down the stairs, resulting in closed displaced comminuted fracture of his left radial shaft

S71.131A	**Puncture wound without foreign body, right thigh, initial encounter**
W33.02XA	**Accidental discharge of hunting rifle, initial encounter**
S52.352A	**Displaced comminuted fracture of shaft of radius, left arm, initial encounter for closed fracture**
W10.9XXA	**Fall (on) (from) unspecified stairs and steps, initial encounter**

Explanation: If two or more events cause separate injuries, an external cause code should be assigned for each cause.

---

g. Child and adult abuse guideline

Adult and child abuse, neglect and maltreatment are classified as assault. Any of the assault codes may be used to indicate the external cause of any injury resulting from the confirmed abuse.

For confirmed cases of abuse, neglect and maltreatment, when the perpetrator is known, a code from Y07, Perpetrator of maltreatment and neglect, should accompany any other assault codes.

See Section I.C.19. Adult and child abuse, neglect and other maltreatment

h. Unknown or undetermined intent guideline

If the intent (accident, self-harm, assault) of the cause of an injury or other condition is unknown or unspecified, code the intent as accidental intent. All transport accident categories assume accidental intent.

1) Use of undetermined intent

External cause codes for events of undetermined intent are only for use if the documentation in the record specifies that the intent cannot be determined.

i. Sequelae (late effects) of external cause guidelines

1) Sequelae external cause codes

Sequela are reported using the external cause code with the 7th character "S" for sequela. These codes should be used with any report of a late effect or sequela resulting from a previous injury.

See Section I.B.10 Sequela (Late Effects)

2) Sequela external cause code with a related current injury

A sequela external cause code should never be used with a related current nature of injury code.

3) Use of sequela external cause codes for subsequent visits

Use a late effect external cause code for subsequent visits when a late effect of the initial injury is being treated. Do not use a late effect external cause code for subsequent visits for follow-up care (e.g., to assess healing, to receive rehabilitative therapy) of the injury when no late effect of the injury has been documented.

j. Terrorism guidelines

1) Cause of injury identified by the Federal Government (FBI) as terrorism

When the cause of an injury is identified by the Federal Government (FBI) as terrorism, the first-listed external cause code should be a code from category Y38, Terrorism. The definition of terrorism employed by the FBI is found at the inclusion note at the beginning of category Y38. Use additional code for place of occurrence (Y92.-). More than one Y38 code may be assigned if the injury is the result of more than one mechanism of terrorism.

2) Cause of an injury is suspected to be the result of terrorism

When the cause of an injury is suspected to be the result of terrorism a code from category Y38 should not be assigned. Suspected cases should be classified as assault.

3) Code Y38.9, Terrorism, secondary effects

Assign code Y38.9, Terrorism, secondary effects, for conditions occurring subsequent to the terrorist event. This code should not be assigned for conditions that are due to the initial terrorist act.

It is acceptable to assign code Y38.9 with another code from Y38 if there is an injury due to the initial terrorist event and an injury that is a subsequent result of the terrorist event.

k. External cause status

A code from category Y99, External cause status, should be assigned whenever any other external cause code is assigned for an encounter, including an Activity code, except for the events noted below. Assign a code from category Y99, External cause status, to indicate the work status of the person at the time the event occurred. The status code indicates whether the event occurred during military activity, whether a non-military person was at work, whether an individual including a student or volunteer was involved in a non-work activity at the time of the causal event.

A code from Y99, External cause status, should be assigned, when applicable, with other external cause codes, such as transport accidents and falls. The external cause status codes are not applicable to poisonings, adverse effects, misadventures or late effects.

Do not assign a code from category Y99 if no other external cause codes (cause, activity) are applicable for the encounter.

An external cause status code is used only once, at the initial encounter for treatment. Only one code from Y99 should be recorded on a medical record.

Do not assign code Y99.9, Unspecified external cause status, if the status is not stated.

Chapter 20. External Causes of Morbidity (V00-Y99)

NOTE This chapter permits the classification of environmental events and circumstances as the cause of injury, and other adverse effects. Where a code from this section is applicable, it is intended that it shall be used secondary to a code from another chapter of the Classification indicating the nature of the condition. Most often, the condition will be classifiable to Chapter 19, Injury, poisoning and certain other consequences of external causes (S00-T88). Other conditions that may be stated to be due to external causes are classified in Chapters I to XVIII. For these conditions, codes from Chapter 20 should be used to provide additional information as to the cause of the condition.

AHA: 2018,4Q,58-60

This chapter contains the following blocks:

V00-X58	Accidents
V00-V99	Transport accidents
V00-V09	Pedestrian injured in transport accident
V10-V19	Pedal cycle rider injured in transport accident
V20-V29	Motorcycle rider injured in transport accident
V30-V39	Occupant of three-wheeled motor vehicle injured in transport accident
V40-V49	Car occupant injured in transport accident
V50-V59	Occupant of pick-up truck or van injured in transport accident
V60-V69	Occupant of heavy transport vehicle injured in transport accident
V70-V79	Bus occupant injured in transport accident
V80-V89	Other land transport accidents
V90-V94	Water transport accidents
V95-V97	Air and space transport accidents
V98-V99	Other and unspecified transport accidents
W00-X58	Other external causes of accidental injury
W00-W19	Slipping, tripping, stumbling and falls
W20-W49	Exposure to inanimate mechanical forces
W50-W64	Exposure to animate mechanical forces
W65-W74	Accidental non-transport drowning and submersion
W85-W99	Exposure to electric current, radiation and extreme ambient air temperature and pressure
X00-X08	Exposure to smoke, fire and flames
X10-X19	Contact with heat and hot substances
X30-X39	Exposure to forces of nature
X50	Overexertion and strenuous or repetitive movements
X52-X58	Accidental exposure to other specified factors
X71-X83	Intentional self-harm
X92-Y09	Assault
Y21-Y33	Event of undetermined intent
Y35-Y38	Legal intervention, operations of war, military operations, and terrorism
Y62-Y84	Complications of medical and surgical care
Y62-Y69	Misadventures to patients during surgical and medical care
Y70-Y82	Medical devices associated with adverse incidents in diagnostic and therapeutic use
Y83-Y84	Surgical and other medical procedures as the cause of abnormal reaction of the patient, or of later complication, without mention of misadventure at the time of the procedure
Y90-Y99	Supplementary factors related to causes of morbidity classified elsewhere

ACCIDENTS (V00-X58)

AHA: 2018,2Q,7-8

Transport accidents (V00-V99)

NOTE This section is structured in 12 groups. Those relating to land transport accidents (V00-V89) reflect the victim's mode of transport and are subdivided to identify the victim's 'counterpart' or the type of event. The vehicle of which the injured person is an occupant is identified in the first two characters since it is seen as the most important factor to identify for prevention purposes. A transport accident is one in which the vehicle involved must be moving or running or in use for transport purposes at the time of the accident.

Use additional code to identify:
  airbag injury (W22.1)
  type of street or road (Y92.4-)
  use of cellular telephone and other electronic equipment at the time of the transport accident (Y93.C-)
EXCLUDES 1 agricultural vehicles in stationary use or maintenance (W31.-)
  assault by crashing of motor vehicle (Y03.-)
  automobile or motor cycle in stationary use or maintenance — code to type of accident
  crashing of motor vehicle, undetermined intent (Y32)
  intentional self-harm by crashing of motor vehicle (X82)
EXCLUDES 2 transport accidents due to cataclysm (X34-X38)
NOTE Definitions related to transport accidents:
  (a) A transport accident (V00-V99) is any accident involving a device designed primarily for, or used at the time primarily for, conveying persons or good from one place to another.

(b) A public highway [trafficway] or street is the entire width between property lines (or other boundary lines) of land open to the public as a matter of right or custom for purposes of moving persons or property from one place to another. A roadway is that part of the public highway designed, improved and customarily used for vehicular traffic.

(c) A traffic accident is any vehicle accident occurring on the public highway [i.e. originating on, terminating on, or involving a vehicle partially on the highway]. A vehicle accident is assumed to have occurred on the public highway unless another place is specified, except in the case of accidents involving only off-road motor vehicles, which are classified as nontraffic accidents unless the contrary is stated.

(d) A nontraffic accident is any vehicle accident that occurs entirely in any place other than a public highway.

(e) A pedestrian is any person involved in an accident who was not at the time of the accident riding in or on a motor vehicle, railway train, streetcar or animal-drawn or other vehicle, or on a pedal cycle or animal. This includes, a person changing a tire, working on a parked car, or a person on foot. It also includes the user of a pedestrian conveyance such as a baby stroller, ice-skates, skis, sled, roller skates, a skateboard, nonmotorized or motorized wheelchair, motorized mobility scooter, or nonmotorized scooter.

(f) A driver is an occupant of a transport vehicle who is operating or intending to operate it.

(g) A passenger is any occupant of a transport vehicle other than the driver, except a person traveling on the outside of the vehicle.

(h) A person on the outside of a vehicle is any person being transported by a vehicle but not occupying the space normally reserved for the driver or passengers, or the space intended for the transport of property. This includes a person travelling on the bodywork, bumper, fender, roof, running board or step of a vehicle, as well as, hanging on the outside of the vehicle.

(i) A pedal cycle is any land transport vehicle operated solely by nonmotorized pedals including a bicycle or tricycle.

(j) A pedal cyclist is any person riding a pedal cycle or in a sidecar or trailer attached to a pedal cycle.

(k) A motorcycle is a two-wheeled motor vehicle with one or two riding saddles and sometimes with a third wheel for the support of a sidecar. The sidecar is considered part of the motorcycle. This includes a moped, motor scooter, or motorized bicycle.

(l) A motorcycle rider is any person riding a motorcycle or in a sidecar or trailer attached to the motorcycle.

(m) A three-wheeled motor vehicle is a motorized tricycle designed primarily for on-road use. This includes a motor-driven tricycle, a motorized rickshaw, or a three-wheeled motor car.

(n) A car [automobile] is a four-wheeled motor vehicle designed primarily for carrying up to 7 persons. A trailer being towed by the car is considered part of the car. It does not include a van or minivan — see definition (o).

(o) A pick-up truck or van is a four or six-wheeled motor vehicle designed for carrying passengers as well as property or cargo weighing less than the local limit for classification as a heavy goods vehicle, and not requiring a special driver's license. This includes a minivan and a sport-utility vehicle (SUV).

(p) A heavy transport vehicle is a motor vehicle designed primarily for carrying property, meeting local criteria for classification as a heavy goods vehicle in terms of weight and requiring a special driver's license.

(q) A bus (coach) is a motor vehicle designed or adapted primarily for carrying more than 10 passengers, and requiring a special driver's license.

(r) A railway train or railway vehicle is any device, with or without freight or passenger cars couple to it, designed for traffic on a railway track. This includes subterranean (subways) or elevated trains.

(s) A streetcar, is a device designed and used primarily for transporting passengers within a municipality, running on rails, usually subject to normal traffic control signals, and operated principally on a right-of-way that forms part of the roadway. This includes a tram or trolley that runs on rails. A trailer being towed by a streetcar is considered part of the streetcar.

(t) A special vehicle mainly used on industrial premises is a motor vehicle designed primarily for use within the buildings and premises of industrial or commercial establishments. This includes battery-powered airport passenger vehicles or baggage/mail trucks, forklifts, coal-cars in a coal mine, logging cars and trucks used in mines or quarries.

(u) A special vehicle mainly used in agriculture is a motor vehicle designed specifically for use in farming and agriculture (horticulture), to work the land, tend and harvest crops and transport materials on the farm. This includes harvesters, farm machinery and tractor and trailers.

(v) A special construction vehicle is a motor vehicle designed specifically for use on construction and demolition sites. This includes bulldozers, diggers, earth levellers, dump trucks, backhoes, front-end loaders, pavers, and mechanical shovels.

(w) A special all-terrain vehicle is a motor vehicle of special design to enable it to negotiate over rough or soft terrain, snow or sand. Examples of special design are high construction, special wheels and tires, tracks, and support on a cushion of air. This includes snow mobiles, All-terrain vehicles (ATV), and dune buggies. It does not include passenger vehicle designated as Sport Utility Vehicles. (SUV)

(x) A watercraft is any device designed for transporting passengers or goods on water. This includes motor or sailboats, ships, and hovercraft.

(y) An aircraft is any device for transporting passengers or goods in the air. This includes hot-air balloons, gliders, helicopters and airplanes.

(z) A military vehicle is any motorized vehicle operating on a public roadway owned by the military and being operated by a member of the military.

Pedestrian injured in transport accident (V00-V09)

INCLUDES   person changing tire on transport vehicle
person examining engine of vehicle broken down in (on side of) road

EXCLUDES 1   *fall due to non-transport collision with other person (W03)*
pedestrian on foot falling (slipping) on ice and snow (W00.-)
struck or bumped by another person (W51)

The appropriate 7th character is to be added to each code from categories V00-V09.
A   initial encounter
D   subsequent encounter
S   sequela

✓4ᵗʰ **V00   Pedestrian conveyance accident**

Use additional place of occurrence and activity external cause codes, if known (Y92.-, Y93.-)

EXCLUDES 1   *collision with another person without fall (W51)*
fall due to person on foot colliding with another person on foot (W03)
fall from non-moving wheelchair, nonmotorized scooter and motorized mobility scooter without collision (W05.-)
pedestrian (conveyance) collision with other land transport vehicle (V01-V09)
pedestrian on foot falling (slipping) on ice and snow (W00.-)

✓5ᵗʰ **V00.0   Pedestrian on foot injured in collision with pedestrian conveyance**

✓x7ᵗʰ **V00.01   Pedestrian on foot injured in collision with roller-skater**

✓x7ᵗʰ **V00.02   Pedestrian on foot injured in collision with skateboarder**

● ✓6ᵗʰ **V00.03   Pedestrian on foot injured in collision with standing micro-mobility pedestrian conveyance**

● ✓7ᵗʰ **V00.031   Pedestrian on foot injured in collision with rider of** standing electric scooter

● ✓7ᵗʰ **V00.038   Pedestrian on foot injured in collision with rider of other standing micro-mobility pedestrian conveyance**

Pedestrian on foot injured in collision with rider of hoverboard
Pedestrian on foot injured in collision with rider of segway

✓x7ᵗʰ **V00.09   Pedestrian on foot injured in collision with other pedestrian conveyance**

✓5ᵗʰ **V00.1   Rolling-type pedestrian conveyance accident**

EXCLUDES 1   *accident with baby stroller (V00.82-)*
accident with motorized mobility scooter (V00.83-)
accident with wheelchair (powered) (V00.81-)

✓6ᵗʰ **V00.11   In-line roller-skate accident**

✓7ᵗʰ **V00.111   Fall from in-line roller-skates**

✓7ᵗʰ **V00.112   In-line roller-skater colliding with stationary object**

✓7ᵗʰ **V00.118   Other in-line roller-skate accident**

EXCLUDES 1   *roller-skater collision with other land transport vehicle (V01-V09 with 5th character 1)*

✓6ᵗʰ **V00.12   Non-in-line roller-skate accident**

✓7ᵗʰ **V00.121   Fall from non-in-line roller-skates**

✓7ᵗʰ **V00.122   Non-in-line roller-skater colliding with stationary object**

✓7ᵗʰ **V00.128   Other non-in-line roller-skating accident**

EXCLUDES 1   *roller-skater collision with other land transport vehicle (V01-V09 with 5th character 1)*

✓6ᵗʰ **V00.13   Skateboard accident**

✓7ᵗʰ **V00.131   Fall from skateboard**

✓7ᵗʰ **V00.132   Skateboarder colliding with stationary object**

✓7ᵗʰ **V00.138   Other skateboard accident**

EXCLUDES 1   *skateboarder collision with other land transport vehicle (V01-V09 with 5th character 2)*

✓6ᵗʰ **V00.14   Scooter (nonmotorized) accident**

EXCLUDES 1   *motor scooter accident (V20-V29)*

✓7ᵗʰ **V00.141   Fall from scooter (nonmotorized)**

✓7ᵗʰ **V00.142   Scooter (nonmotorized) colliding with stationary object**

✓7ᵗʰ **V00.148   Other scooter (nonmotorized) accident**

EXCLUDES 1   *scooter (nonmotorized) collision with other land transport vehicle (V01-V09 with fifth character 9)*

✓6ᵗʰ **V00.15   Heelies accident**

Rolling shoe
Wheeled shoe
Wheelies accident

✓7ᵗʰ **V00.151   Fall from heelies**

✓7ᵗʰ **V00.152   Heelies colliding with stationary object**

✓7ᵗʰ **V00.158   Other heelies accident**

✓6ᵗʰ **V00.18   Accident on other rolling-type pedestrian conveyance**

✓7ᵗʰ **V00.181   Fall from other rolling-type pedestrian conveyance**

✓7ᵗʰ **V00.182   Pedestrian on other rolling-type pedestrian conveyance colliding with stationary object**

✓7ᵗʰ **V00.188   Other accident on other rolling-type pedestrian conveyance**

✓5ᵗʰ **V00.2   Gliding-type pedestrian conveyance accident**

✓6ᵗʰ **V00.21   Ice-skates accident**

✓7ᵗʰ **V00.211   Fall from ice-skates**

✓7ᵗʰ **V00.212   Ice-skater colliding with stationary object**

✓7ᵗʰ **V00.218   Other ice-skates accident**

EXCLUDES 1   *ice-skater collision with other land transport vehicle (V01-V09 with 5th character 9)*

✓6ᵗʰ **V00.22   Sled accident**

✓7ᵗʰ **V00.221   Fall from sled**

✓7ᵗʰ **V00.222   Sledder colliding with stationary object**

✓7ᵗʰ **V00.228   Other sled accident**

EXCLUDES 1   *sled collision with other land transport vehicle (V01-V09 with 5th character 9)*

✓6ᵗʰ **V00.28   Other gliding-type pedestrian conveyance accident**

✓7ᵗʰ **V00.281   Fall from other gliding-type pedestrian conveyance**

✓7ᵗʰ **V00.282   Pedestrian on other gliding-type pedestrian conveyance colliding with stationary object**

√7ᵗʰ **V00.288 Other accident on other gliding-type pedestrian conveyance**
> EXCLUDES 1   *gliding-type pedestrian conveyance collision with other land transport vehicle (V01-V09 with 5th character 9)*

√5ᵗʰ **V00.3 Flat-bottomed pedestrian conveyance accident**

√6ᵗʰ **V00.31 Snowboard accident**

√7ᵗʰ **V00.311 Fall from snowboard**

√7ᵗʰ **V00.312 Snowboarder colliding with stationary object**

√7ᵗʰ **V00.318 Other snowboard accident**
> EXCLUDES 1   *snowboarder collision with other land transport vehicle (V01-V09 with 5th character 9)*

√6ᵗʰ **V00.32 Snow-ski accident**

√7ᵗʰ **V00.321 Fall from snow-skis**

√7ᵗʰ **V00.322 Snow-skier colliding with stationary object**

√7ᵗʰ **V00.328 Other snow-ski accident**
> EXCLUDES 1   *snow-skier collision with other land transport vehicle (V01-V09 with 5th character 9)*

√6ᵗʰ **V00.38 Other flat-bottomed pedestrian conveyance accident**

√7ᵗʰ **V00.381 Fall from other flat-bottomed conveyance**

√7ᵗʰ **V00.382 Pedestrian on other flat-bottomed pedestrian conveyance colliding with stationary object**

√7ᵗʰ **V00.388 Other accident on other flat-bottomed pedestrian conveyance**

√5ᵗʰ **V00.8 Accident on other pedestrian conveyance**

√6ᵗʰ **V00.81 Accident with wheelchair (powered)**

√7ᵗʰ **V00.811 Fall from moving wheelchair (powered)**
> EXCLUDES 1   *fall from non-moving wheelchair (W05.0)*

√7ᵗʰ **V00.812 Wheelchair (powered) colliding with stationary object**

√7ᵗʰ **V00.818 Other accident with wheelchair (powered)**

√6ᵗʰ **V00.82 Accident with baby stroller**

√7ᵗʰ **V00.821 Fall from baby stroller**

√7ᵗʰ **V00.822 Baby stroller colliding with stationary object**

√7ᵗʰ **V00.828 Other accident with baby stroller**

√6ᵗʰ **V00.83 Accident with motorized mobility scooter**

√7ᵗʰ **V00.831 Fall from motorized mobility scooter**
> EXCLUDES 1   *fall from non-moving motorized mobility scooter (W05.2)*

√7ᵗʰ **V00.832 Motorized mobility scooter colliding with stationary object**

√7ᵗʰ **V00.838 Other accident with motorized mobility scooter**

● √6ᵗʰ **V00.84 Accident with standing micro-mobility pedestrian conveyance**

● √7ᵗʰ **V00.841 Fall from standing electric scooter**

● √7ᵗʰ **V00.842 Pedestrian on standing electric scooter colliding with stationary object**

● √7ᵗʰ **V00.848 Other accident with standing micro-mobility pedestrian conveyance**
Accident with hoverboard
Accident with segway

√6ᵗʰ **V00.89 Accident on other pedestrian conveyance**

√7ᵗʰ **V00.891 Fall from other pedestrian conveyance**

√7ᵗʰ **V00.892 Pedestrian on other pedestrian conveyance colliding with stationary object**

√7ᵗʰ **V00.898 Other accident on other pedestrian conveyance**
> EXCLUDES 1   *other pedestrian (conveyance) collision with other land transport vehicle (V01-V09 with 5th character 9)*

√4ᵗʰ **V01 Pedestrian injured in collision with pedal cycle**

√5ᵗʰ **V01.0 Pedestrian injured in collision with pedal cycle in nontraffic accident**

√x7ᵗʰ **V01.00 Pedestrian on foot injured in collision with pedal cycle in nontraffic accident**
Pedestrian NOS injured in collision with pedal cycle in nontraffic accident

√x7ᵗʰ **V01.01 Pedestrian on roller-skates injured in collision with pedal cycle in nontraffic accident**

√x7ᵗʰ **V01.02 Pedestrian on skateboard injured in collision with pedal cycle in nontraffic accident**

● √6ᵗʰ **V01.03 Pedestrian on standing micro-mobility pedestrian conveyance injured in collision with pedal cycle in nontraffic accident**

● √7ᵗʰ **V01.031 Pedestrian on standing electric scooter injured in collision with pedal cycle in nontraffic accident**

● √7ᵗʰ **V01.038 Pedestrian on other standing micro-mobility pedestrian conveyance injured in collision with pedal cycle in nontraffic accident**
Pedestrian on hoverboard injured in collision with pedal cycle in nontraffic accident
Pedestrian on segway injured in collision with pedal cycle in nontraffic accident

√x7ᵗʰ **V01.09 Pedestrian with other conveyance injured in collision with pedal cycle in nontraffic accident**
Pedestrian with baby stroller injured in collision with pedal cycle in nontraffic accident
Pedestrian on ice-skates injured in collision with pedal cycle in nontraffic accident
Pedestrian on nonmotorized scooter injured in collision with pedal cycle in nontraffic accident
Pedestrian on sled injured in collision with pedal cycle in nontraffic accident
Pedestrian on snowboard injured in collision with pedal cycle in nontraffic accident
Pedestrian on snow-skis injured in collision with pedal cycle in nontraffic accident
Pedestrian in wheelchair (powered) injured in collision with pedal cycle in nontraffic accident
Pedestrian in motorized mobility scooter injured in collision with pedal cycle in nontraffic accident

√5ᵗʰ **V01.1 Pedestrian injured in collision with pedal cycle in traffic accident**

√x7ᵗʰ **V01.10 Pedestrian on foot injured in collision with pedal cycle in traffic accident**
Pedestrian NOS injured in collision with pedal cycle in traffic accident

√x7ᵗʰ **V01.11 Pedestrian on roller-skates injured in collision with pedal cycle in traffic accident**

√x7ᵗʰ **V01.12 Pedestrian on skateboard injured in collision with pedal cycle in traffic accident**

● √6ᵗʰ **V01.13 Pedestrian on standing micro-mobility pedestrian conveyance injured in collision with pedal cycle in traffic accident**

● √7ᵗʰ **V01.131 Pedestrian on standing electric scooter injured in collision with pedal cycle in traffic accident**

● √7ᵗʰ **V01.138 Pedestrian on other standing micro-mobility pedestrian conveyance injured in collision with pedal cycle in traffic accident**
Pedestrian on hoverboard injured in collision with pedal cycle in traffic accident
Pedestrian on segway injured in collision with pedal cycle in traffic accident

---

✔Additional Char Req   √x7ᵗʰ Placeholder   Unacceptable PDx   Questionable PDx   Wrong Procedure   Manifestation   Unspecified Dx   H1-H14 HAC   HCC CMS-HCC Dx   HIV HIV Dx

ICD-10-CM 2021   1169

√x7ᵗʰ **V01.19 Pedestrian with other conveyance injured in collision with pedal cycle in traffic accident**
Pedestrian with baby stroller injured in collision with pedal cycle in traffic accident
Pedestrian on ice-skates injured in collision with pedal cycle in traffic accident
Pedestrian on nonmotorized scooter injured in collision with pedal cycle in traffic accident
Pedestrian on sled injured in collision with pedal cycle in traffic accident
Pedestrian on snowboard injured in collision with pedal cycle in traffic accident
Pedestrian on snow-skis injured in collision with pedal cycle in traffic accident
Pedestrian in wheelchair (powered) injured in collision with pedal cycle in traffic accident
Pedestrian in motorized mobility scooter injured in collision with pedal cycle in traffic accident

√5ᵗʰ **V01.9 Pedestrian injured in collision with pedal cycle, unspecified whether traffic or nontraffic accident**

√x7ᵗʰ **V01.90 Pedestrian on foot injured in collision with pedal cycle, unspecified whether traffic or nontraffic accident**
Pedestrian NOS injured in collision with pedal cycle, unspecified whether traffic or nontraffic accident

√x7ᵗʰ **V01.91 Pedestrian on roller-skates injured in collision with pedal cycle, unspecified whether traffic or nontraffic accident**

√x7ᵗʰ **V01.92 Pedestrian on skateboard injured in collision with pedal cycle, unspecified whether traffic or nontraffic accident**

● √6ᵗʰ **V01.93 Pedestrian on standing micro-mobility pedestrian conveyance injured in collision with pedal cycle, unspecified whether traffic or nontraffic accident**

● √7ᵗʰ **V01.931 Pedestrian on standing electric scooter injured in collision with pedal cycle, unspecified whether traffic or nontraffic accident**

● √7ᵗʰ **V01.938 Pedestrian on other standing micro-mobility pedestrian conveyance injured in collision with pedal cycle, unspecified whether traffic or nontraffic accident**
Pedestrian on hoverboard injured in collision with pedal cycle, unspecified whether traffic or nontraffic accident
Pedestrian on segway injured in collision with pedal cycle, unspecified whether traffic or nontraffic accident

√x7ᵗʰ **V01.99 Pedestrian with other conveyance injured in collision with pedal cycle, unspecified whether traffic or nontraffic accident**
Pedestrian with baby stroller injured in collision with pedal cycle, unspecified whether traffic or nontraffic accident
Pedestrian on ice-skates injured in collision with pedal cycle unspecified, whether traffic or nontraffic accident
Pedestrian on nonmotorized scooter injured in collision with pedal cycle, unspecified whether traffic or nontraffic accident
Pedestrian on sled injured in collision with pedal cycle unspecified, whether traffic or nontraffic accident
Pedestrian on snowboard injured in collision with pedal cycle, unspecified whether traffic or nontraffic accident
Pedestrian on snow-skis injured in collision with pedal cycle, unspecified whether traffic or nontraffic accident
Pedestrian in wheelchair (powered) injured in collision with pedal cycle, unspecified whether traffic or nontraffic accident
Pedestrian in motorized mobility scooter injured in collision with pedal cycle, unspecified whether traffic or nontraffic accident

√4ᵗʰ **V02 Pedestrian injured in collision with two- or three-wheeled motor vehicle**

√5ᵗʰ **V02.0 Pedestrian injured in collision with two- or three-wheeled motor vehicle in nontraffic accident**

√x7ᵗʰ **V02.00 Pedestrian on foot injured in collision with two- or three-wheeled motor vehicle in nontraffic accident**
Pedestrian NOS injured in collision with two- or three-wheeled motor vehicle in nontraffic accident

√x7ᵗʰ **V02.01 Pedestrian on roller-skates injured in collision with two- or three-wheeled motor vehicle in nontraffic accident**

√x7ᵗʰ **V02.02 Pedestrian on skateboard injured in collision with two- or three-wheeled motor vehicle in nontraffic accident**

● √6ᵗʰ **V02.03 Pedestrian on standing micro-mobility pedestrian conveyance injured in collision with two- or three-wheeled motor vehicle in nontraffic accident**

● √7ᵗʰ **V02.031 Pedestrian on standing electric scooter injured in collision with two- or three-wheeled motor vehicle in nontraffic accident**

● √7ᵗʰ **V02.038 Pedestrian on other standing micro-mobility pedestrian conveyance injured in collision with two- or three-wheeled motor vehicle in nontraffic accident**
Pedestrian on hoverboard injured in collision with two-or three wheeled motor vehicle in nontraffic accident
Pedestrian on segway injured in collision with two- or three-wheeled motor vehicle in nontraffic accident

√x7ᵗʰ **V02.09 Pedestrian with other conveyance injured in collision with two- or three-wheeled motor vehicle in nontraffic accident**
Pedestrian with baby stroller injured in collision with two- or three-wheeled motor vehicle in nontraffic accident
Pedestrian on ice-skates injured in collision with two- or three-wheeled motor vehicle in nontraffic accident
Pedestrian on nonmotorized scooter injured in collision with two- or three-wheeled motor vehicle in nontraffic accident
Pedestrian on sled injured in collision with two- or three-wheeled motor vehicle in nontraffic accident
Pedestrian on snowboard injured in collision with two- or three-wheeled motor vehicle in nontraffic accident
Pedestrian on snow-skis injured in collision with two- or three-wheeled motor vehicle in nontraffic accident
Pedestrian in wheelchair (powered) injured in collision with two- or three-wheeled motor vehicle in nontraffic accident
Pedestrian in motorized mobility scooter injured in collision with two- or three-wheeled motor vehicle in nontraffic accident

√5ᵗʰ **V02.1 Pedestrian injured in collision with two- or three-wheeled motor vehicle in traffic accident**

√x7ᵗʰ **V02.10 Pedestrian on foot injured in collision with two- or three-wheeled motor vehicle in traffic accident**
Pedestrian NOS injured in collision with two- or three-wheeled motor vehicle in traffic accident

√x7ᵗʰ **V02.11 Pedestrian on roller-skates injured in collision with two- or three-wheeled motor vehicle in traffic accident**

√x7ᵗʰ **V02.12 Pedestrian on skateboard injured in collision with two- or three-wheeled motor vehicle in traffic accident**

● √6ᵗʰ **V02.13 Pedestrian on standing micro-mobility pedestrian conveyance injured in collision with two- or three-wheeled motor vehicle in traffic accident**

● √7ᵗʰ **V02.131 Pedestrian on standing electric scooter injured in collision with two- or three-wheeled motor vehicle in traffic accident**

✓7th **V02.138 Pedestrian on other standing micro-mobility pedestrian conveyance injured in collision with two- or three-wheeled motor vehicle in traffic accident**
  Pedestrian on hoverboard injured in collision with two-or three wheeled motor vehicle in traffic accident
  Pedestrian on segway injured in collision with two- or three-wheeled motor vehicle in traffic accident

✓x7th **V02.19 Pedestrian with other conveyance injured in collision with two- or three-wheeled motor vehicle in traffic accident**
  Pedestrian with baby stroller injured in collision with two- or three-wheeled motor vehicle in traffic accident
  Pedestrian on ice-skates injured in collision with two- or three-wheeled motor vehicle in traffic accident
  Pedestrian on nonmotorized scooter injured in collision with two- or three-wheeled motor vehicle in traffic accident
  Pedestrian on sled injured in collision with two- or three-wheeled motor vehicle in traffic accident
  Pedestrian on snowboard injured in collision with two- or three-wheeled motor vehicle in traffic accident
  Pedestrian on snow-skis injured in collision with two- or three-wheeled motor vehicle in traffic accident
  Pedestrian in wheelchair (powered) injured in collision with two- or three-wheeled motor vehicle in traffic accident
  Pedestrian in motorized mobility scooter injured in collision with two- or three-wheeled motor vehicle in traffic accident

✓5th **V02.9 Pedestrian injured in collision with two- or three-wheeled motor vehicle, unspecified whether traffic or nontraffic accident**

✓x7th **V02.90 Pedestrian on foot injured in collision with two- or three-wheeled motor vehicle, unspecified whether traffic or nontraffic accident**
  Pedestrian NOS injured in collision with two- or three-wheeled motor vehicle, unspecified whether traffic or nontraffic accident

✓x7th **V02.91 Pedestrian on roller-skates injured in collision with two- or three-wheeled motor vehicle, unspecified whether traffic or nontraffic accident**

✓x7th **V02.92 Pedestrian on skateboard injured in collision with two- or three-wheeled motor vehicle, unspecified whether traffic or nontraffic accident**

✓6th **V02.93 Pedestrian on standing micro-mobility pedestrian conveyance injured in collision with two- or three-wheeled motor vehicle, unspecified whether traffic or nontraffic accident**

✓7th **V02.931 Pedestrian on standing electric scooter injured in collision with two- or three wheeled motor vehicle, unspecified whether traffic or nontraffic accident**

✓7th **V02.938 Pedestrian on other standing micro-mobility pedestrian conveyance injured in collision with two- or three wheeled motor vehicle, unspecified whether traffic or nontraffic accident**
  Pedestrian on hoverboard injured in collision with two-three-wheeled motor vehicle, unspecified whether traffic or nontraffic accident
  Pedestrian on segway injured in collision with two- or three wheeled motor vehicle, unspecified whether traffic or nontraffic accident

✓x7th **V02.99 Pedestrian with other conveyance injured in collision with two- or three-wheeled motor vehicle, unspecified whether traffic or nontraffic accident**
  Pedestrian with baby stroller injured in collision with two- or three-wheeled motor vehicle, unspecified whether traffic or nontraffic accident
  Pedestrian on ice-skates injured in collision with two- or three-wheeled motor vehicle, unspecified whether traffic or nontraffic accident
  Pedestrian on nonmotorized scooter injured in collision with two- or three-wheeled motor vehicle, unspecified whether traffic or nontraffic accident
  Pedestrian on sled injured in collision with two- or three-wheeled motor vehicle, unspecified whether traffic or nontraffic accident
  Pedestrian on snowboard injured in collision with two- or three-wheeled motor vehicle, unspecified whether traffic or nontraffic accident
  Pedestrian on snow-skis injured in collision with two- or three-wheeled motor vehicle, unspecified whether traffic or nontraffic accident
  Pedestrian in wheelchair (powered) injured in collision with two- or three-wheeled motor vehicle, unspecified whether traffic or nontraffic accident
  Pedestrian in motorized mobility scooter injured in collision with two- or three wheeled motor vehicle, unspecified whether traffic or nontraffic accident

✓4th **V03 Pedestrian injured in collision with car, pick-up truck or van**

✓5th **V03.0 Pedestrian injured in collision with car, pick-up truck or van in nontraffic accident**

✓7th **V03.00 Pedestrian on foot injured in collision with car, pick-up truck or van in nontraffic accident**
  Pedestrian NOS injured in collision with car, pick-up truck or van in nontraffic accident

✓7th **V03.01 Pedestrian on roller-skates injured in collision with car, pick-up truck or van in nontraffic accident**

✓7th **V03.02 Pedestrian on skateboard injured in collision with car, pick-up truck or van in nontraffic accident**

✓6th **V03.03 Pedestrian on standing micro-mobility pedestrian conveyance injured in collision with car, pick-up or van in nontraffic accident**

✓7th **V03.031 Pedestrian on standing electric scooter injured in collision with car, pick-up or van in nontraffic accident**

✓7th **V03.038 Pedestrian on other standing micro-mobility pedestrian conveyance injured in collision with car, pick-up or van in nontraffic accident**
  Pedestrian on hoverboard injured in collision with car, pick-up or van in nontraffic accident
  Pedestrian on segway injured in collision with car, pick-up or van in nontraffic accident

✓x7th **V03.09 Pedestrian with other conveyance injured in collision with car, pick-up truck or van in nontraffic accident**
  Pedestrian with baby stroller injured in collision with car, pick-up truck or van in nontraffic accident
  Pedestrian on ice-skates injured in collision with car, pick-up truck or van in nontraffic accident
  Pedestrian on nonmotorized scooter injured in collision with car, pick-up truck or van in nontraffic accident
  Pedestrian on sled injured in collision with car, pick-up truck or van in nontraffic accident
  Pedestrian on snowboard injured in collision with car, pick-up truck or van in nontraffic accident
  Pedestrian on snow-skis injured in collision with car, pick-up truck or van in nontraffic accident
  Pedestrian in wheelchair (powered) injured in collision with car, pick-up truck or van in nontraffic accident
  Pedestrian in motorized mobility scooter injured in collision with car, pick-up truck or van in nontraffic accident

✅ Additional Char Req   ✓x7th Placeholder   Unacceptable PDx   Questionable PDx   Wrong Procedure   Manifestation   Unspecified Dx   H1-H14 HAC   HCC CMS-HCC Dx   HIV HIV Dx

ICD-10-CM 2021   1171

V02.138–V03.09

Chapter 20. External Causes of Morbidity

√5ᵗʰ **V03.1** **Pedestrian injured in collision with car, pick-up truck or van in traffic accident**

√x7ᵗʰ **V03.10** **Pedestrian** on foot **injured in collision with car, pick-up truck or van in traffic accident**
Pedestrian NOS injured in collision with car, pick-up truck or van in traffic accident

√x7ᵗʰ **V03.11** **Pedestrian** on roller-skates **injured in collision with car, pick-up truck or van in traffic accident**

√x7ᵗʰ **V03.12** **Pedestrian** on skateboard **injured in collision with car, pick-up truck or van in traffic accident**

● √6ᵗʰ **V03.13** **Pedestrian on standing micro-mobility pedestrian conveyance injured in collision with car, pick-up or van in traffic accident**

● √7ᵗʰ **V03.131** **Pedestrian** on standing electric scooter **injured in collision with car, pick-up or van in traffic accident**

● √7ᵗʰ **V03.138** **Pedestrian on other standing micro-mobility pedestrian conveyance injured in collision with car, pick-up or van in traffic accident**
Pedestrian on hoverboard injured in collision with car, pick-up or van in traffic accident
Pedestrian on segway injured in collision with car, pick-up or van in traffic accident

√x7ᵗʰ **V03.19** **Pedestrian with other conveyance injured in collision with car, pick-up truck or van in traffic accident**
Pedestrian with baby stroller injured in collision with car, pick-up truck or van in traffic accident
Pedestrian on ice-skates injured in collision with car, pick-up truck or van in traffic accident
Pedestrian on nonmotorized scooter injured in collision with car, pick-up truck or van in nontraffic accident
Pedestrian on sled injured in collision with car, pick-up truck or van in traffic accident
Pedestrian on snowboard injured in collision with car, pick-up truck or van in traffic accident
Pedestrian on snow-skis injured in collision with car, pick-up truck or van in traffic accident
Pedestrian in wheelchair (powered) injured in collision with car, pick-up truck or van in traffic accident
Pedestrian in motorized mobility scooter injured in collision with car, pick-up truck or van in nontraffic accident

√5ᵗʰ **V03.9** **Pedestrian injured in collision with car, pick-up truck or van, unspecified whether traffic or nontraffic accident**

√x7ᵗʰ **V03.90** **Pedestrian** on foot **injured in collision with car, pick-up truck or van, unspecified whether traffic or nontraffic accident**
Pedestrian NOS injured in collision with car, pick-up truck or van, unspecified whether traffic or nontraffic accident

√x7ᵗʰ **V03.91** **Pedestrian** on roller-skates **injured in collision with car, pick-up truck or van, unspecified whether traffic or nontraffic accident**

√x7ᵗʰ **V03.92** **Pedestrian** on skateboard **injured in collision with car, pick-up truck or van, unspecified whether traffic or nontraffic accident**

● √6ᵗʰ **V03.93** **Pedestrian on standing micro-mobility pedestrian conveyance injured in collision with car, pick-up or van, unspecified whether traffic or nontraffic accident**

● √7ᵗʰ **V03.931** **Pedestrian** on standing electric scooter **injured in collision with car, pick-up or van, unspecified whether traffic or nontraffic accident**

● √7ᵗʰ **V03.938** **Pedestrian on other standing micro-mobility pedestrian conveyance injured in collision with car, pick-up or van, unspecified whether traffic or nontraffic accident**
Pedestrian on hoverboard injured in collision with car, pick-up or van, unspecified whether traffic or nontraffic accident
Pedestrian on segway injured in collision with car, pick-up or van, unspecified whether traffic or nontraffic accident

√7ᵗʰ **V03.99** **Pedestrian with other conveyance injured in collision with car, pick-up truck or van, unspecified whether traffic or nontraffic accident**
Pedestrian with baby stroller injured in collision with car, pick-up truck or van, unspecified whether traffic or nontraffic accident
Pedestrian on ice-skates injured in collision with car, pick-up truck or van, unspecified whether traffic or nontraffic accident
Pedestrian on nonmotorized scooter injured in collision with car, pick-up truck or van, unspecified whether traffic or nontraffic accident
Pedestrian on sled injured in collision with car, pick-up truck or van in nontraffic accident
Pedestrian on snowboard injured in collision with car, pick-up truck or van, unspecified whether traffic or nontraffic accident
Pedestrian on snow-skis injured in collision with car, pick-up truck or van, unspecified whether traffic or nontraffic accident
Pedestrian in wheelchair (powered) injured in collision with car, pick-up truck or van, unspecified whether traffic or nontraffic accident
Pedestrian in motorized mobility scooter injured in collision with car, pick-up truck or van, unspecified whether traffic or nontraffic accident

√4ᵗʰ **V04** **Pedestrian injured in collision with heavy transport vehicle or bus**

EXCLUDES 1   *pedestrian injured in collision with military vehicle (V09.01, V09.21)*

√5ᵗʰ **V04.0** **Pedestrian injured in collision with heavy transport vehicle or bus** in nontraffic accident

√x7ᵗʰ **V04.00** **Pedestrian** on foot **injured in collision with heavy transport vehicle or bus in nontraffic accident**
Pedestrian NOS injured in collision with heavy transport vehicle or bus in nontraffic accident

√x7ᵗʰ **V04.01** **Pedestrian** on roller-skates **injured in collision with heavy transport vehicle or bus in nontraffic accident**

√x7ᵗʰ **V04.02** **Pedestrian** on skateboard **injured in collision with heavy transport vehicle or bus in nontraffic accident**

● √6ᵗʰ **V04.03** **Pedestrian on standing micro-mobility pedestrian conveyance injured in collision with heavy transport vehicle or bus in nontraffic accident**

● √7ᵗʰ **V04.031** **Pedestrian** on standing electric scooter **injured in collision with heavy transport vehicle or bus in nontraffic accident**

● √7ᵗʰ **V04.038** **Pedestrian on other standing micro-mobility pedestrian conveyance injured in collision with heavy transport vehicle or bus in nontraffic accident**
Pedestrian on hoverboard injured in collision with heavy transport vehicle or bus in nontraffic accident
Pedestrian on segway injured in collision with heavy transport vehicle or bus in nontraffic accident

√x7ᵗʰ **V04.09** **Pedestrian with other conveyance injured in collision with heavy transport vehicle or bus in nontraffic accident**

Pedestrian with baby stroller injured in collision with heavy transport vehicle or bus in nontraffic accident

Pedestrian on ice-skates injured in collision with heavy transport vehicle or bus in nontraffic accident

Pedestrian on nonmotorized scooter injured in collision with heavy transport vehicle or bus in nontraffic accident

Pedestrian on sled injured in collision with heavy transport vehicle or bus in nontraffic accident

Pedestrian on snowboard injured in collision with heavy transport vehicle or bus in nontraffic accident

Pedestrian on snow-skis injured in collision with heavy transport vehicle or bus in nontraffic accident

Pedestrian in wheelchair (powered) injured in collision with heavy transport vehicle or bus in nontraffic accident

Pedestrian in motorized mobility scooter injured in collision with heavy transport vehicle or bus in nontraffic accident

√5ᵗʰ **V04.1** **Pedestrian injured in collision with heavy transport vehicle or bus in traffic accident**

√x7ᵗʰ **V04.10** **Pedestrian on foot injured in collision with heavy transport vehicle or bus in traffic accident**

Pedestrian NOS injured in collision with heavy transport vehicle or bus in traffic accident

√x7ᵗʰ **V04.11** **Pedestrian on roller-skates injured in collision with heavy transport vehicle or bus in traffic accident**

√x7ᵗʰ **V04.12** **Pedestrian on skateboard injured in collision with heavy transport vehicle or bus in traffic accident**

● √6ᵗʰ **V04.13** **Pedestrian on standing micro-mobility pedestrian conveyance injured in collision with heavy transport vehicle or bus in traffic accident**

● √7ᵗʰ **V04.131** **Pedestrian on standing electric scooter injured in collision with heavy transport vehicle or bus in traffic accident**

● √7ᵗʰ **V04.138** **Pedestrian on other standing micro-mobility pedestrian conveyance injured in collision with heavy transport vehicle or bus in traffic accident**

Pedestrian on hoverboard injured in collision with heavy transport vehicle or bus in traffic accident

Pedestrian on segway injured in collision with heavy transport vehicle or bus in traffic accident

√x7ᵗʰ **V04.19** **Pedestrian with other conveyance injured in collision with heavy transport vehicle or bus in traffic accident**

Pedestrian with baby stroller injured in collision with heavy transport vehicle or bus in traffic accident

Pedestrian on ice-skates injured in collision with heavy transport vehicle or bus in traffic accident

Pedestrian on nonmotorized scooter injured in collision with heavy transport vehicle or bus in traffic accident

Pedestrian on sled injured in collision with heavy transport vehicle or bus in traffic accident

Pedestrian on snowboard injured in collision with heavy transport vehicle or bus in traffic accident

Pedestrian on snow-skis injured in collision with heavy transport vehicle or bus in traffic accident

Pedestrian in wheelchair (powered) injured in collision with heavy transport vehicle or bus in traffic accident

Pedestrian in motorized mobility scooter injured in collision with heavy transport vehicle or bus in traffic accident

√5ᵗʰ **V04.9** **Pedestrian injured in collision with heavy transport vehicle or bus, unspecified whether traffic or nontraffic accident**

√x7ᵗʰ **V04.90** **Pedestrian on foot injured in collision with heavy transport vehicle or bus, unspecified whether traffic or nontraffic accident**

Pedestrian NOS injured in collision with heavy transport vehicle or bus, unspecified whether traffic or nontraffic accident

√x7ᵗʰ **V04.91** **Pedestrian on roller-skates injured in collision with heavy transport vehicle or bus, unspecified whether traffic or nontraffic accident**

√x7ᵗʰ **V04.92** **Pedestrian on skateboard injured in collision with heavy transport vehicle or bus, unspecified whether traffic or nontraffic accident**

● √6ᵗʰ **V04.93** **Pedestrian on standing micro-mobility pedestrian conveyance injured in collision with heavy transport vehicle or bus, unspecified whether traffic or nontraffic accident**

● √7ᵗʰ **V04.931** **Pedestrian on standing electric scooter injured in collision with heavy transport vehicle or bus, unspecified whether traffic or nontraffic accident**

● √7ᵗʰ **V04.938** **Pedestrian on other standing micro-mobility pedestrian conveyance injured in collision with heavy transport vehicle or bus, unspecified whether traffic or nontraffic accident**

Pedestrian on hoverboard injured in collision with heavy transport vehicle or bus, unspecified whether traffic or nontraffic accident

Pedestrian on segway injured in collision with heavy transport vehicle or bus, unspecified whether traffic or nontraffic accident

√x7ᵗʰ **V04.99** **Pedestrian with other conveyance injured in collision with heavy transport vehicle or bus, unspecified whether traffic or nontraffic accident**

Pedestrian with baby stroller injured in collision with heavy transport vehicle or bus, unspecified whether traffic or nontraffic accident

Pedestrian on ice-skates injured in collision with heavy transport vehicle or bus, unspecified whether traffic or nontraffic accident

Pedestrian on nonmotorized scooter injured in collision with heavy transport vehicle or bus, unspecified whether traffic or nontraffic accident

Pedestrian on sled injured in collision with heavy transport vehicle or bus, unspecified whether traffic or nontraffic accident

Pedestrian on snowboard injured in collision with heavy transport vehicle or bus, unspecified whether traffic or nontraffic accident

Pedestrian on snow-skis injured in collision with heavy transport vehicle or bus, unspecified whether traffic or nontraffic accident

Pedestrian in wheelchair (powered) injured in collision with heavy transport vehicle or bus, unspecified whether traffic or nontraffic accident

Pedestrian in motorized mobility scooter injured in collision with heavy transport vehicle or bus, unspecified whether traffic or nontraffic accident

√4ᵗʰ **V05** **Pedestrian injured in collision with railway train or railway vehicle**

√5ᵗʰ **V05.0** **Pedestrian injured in collision with railway train or railway vehicle in nontraffic accident**

√x7ᵗʰ **V05.00** **Pedestrian on foot injured in collision with railway train or railway vehicle in nontraffic accident**

Pedestrian NOS injured in collision with railway train or railway vehicle in nontraffic accident

√x7ᵗʰ **V05.01** **Pedestrian on roller-skates injured in collision with railway train or railway vehicle in nontraffic accident**

√x7ᵗʰ **V05.02** **Pedestrian on skateboard injured in collision with railway train or railway vehicle in nontraffic accident**

● √6ᵗʰ **V05.03** **Pedestrian on standing micro-mobility pedestrian conveyance injured in collision with railway train or railway vehicle in nontraffic accident**

● √7ᵗʰ **V05.031** **Pedestrian on standing electric scooter injured in collision with railway train or railway vehicle in nontraffic accident**

☑ Additional Char Req   √x7ᵗʰ Placeholder   Unacceptable PDx   Questionable PDx   Wrong Procedure   Manifestation   Unspecified Dx   H1-H14 HAC   HCC CMS-HCC Dx   HIV HIV Dx

ICD-10-CM 2021   1173

Chapter 20. External Causes of Morbidity

- ✓7ᵗʰ **V05.038** **Pedestrian on other standing micro-mobility pedestrian conveyance injured in collision with railway train or railway vehicle in nontraffic accident**
  - Pedestrian on hoverboard injured in collision with railway train or railway vehicle in nontraffic accident
  - Pedestrian on segway injured in collision with railway train or railway vehicle in nontraffic accident

✓x7ᵗʰ **V05.09** **Pedestrian with other conveyance injured in collision with railway train or railway vehicle in nontraffic accident**
  - Pedestrian with baby stroller injured in collision with railway train or railway vehicle in nontraffic accident
  - Pedestrian on ice-skates injured in collision with railway train or railway vehicle in nontraffic accident
  - Pedestrian on nonmotorized scooter injured in collision with railway train or railway vehicle in nontraffic accident
  - Pedestrian on sled injured in collision with railway train or railway vehicle in nontraffic accident
  - Pedestrian on snowboard injured in collision with railway train or railway vehicle in nontraffic accident
  - Pedestrian on snow-skis injured in collision with railway train or railway vehicle in nontraffic accident
  - Pedestrian in wheelchair (powered) injured in collision with railway train or railway vehicle in nontraffic accident
  - Pedestrian in motorized mobility scooter injured in collision with railway train or railway vehicle in nontraffic accident

✓5ᵗʰ **V05.1** **Pedestrian injured in collision with railway train or railway vehicle in traffic accident**

✓x7ᵗʰ **V05.10** **Pedestrian on foot injured in collision with railway train or railway vehicle in traffic accident**
  - Pedestrian NOS injured in collision with railway train or railway vehicle in traffic accident

✓x7ᵗʰ **V05.11** **Pedestrian on roller-skates injured in collision with railway train or railway vehicle in traffic accident**

✓x7ᵗʰ **V05.12** **Pedestrian on skateboard injured in collision with railway train or railway vehicle in traffic accident**

- ✓6ᵗʰ **V05.13** **Pedestrian on standing micro-mobility pedestrian conveyance injured in collision with railway train or railway vehicle in traffic accident**
- ✓7ᵗʰ **V05.131** **Pedestrian on standing electric scooter injured in collision with railway train or railway vehicle in traffic accident**
- ✓7ᵗʰ **V05.138** **Pedestrian on other standing micro-mobility pedestrian conveyance injured in collision with railway train or railway vehicle in traffic accident**
  - Pedestrian on hoverboard injured in collision with railway train or railway vehicle in traffic accident
  - Pedestrian on segway injured in collision with railway train or railway vehicle in traffic accident

✓x7ᵗʰ **V05.19** **Pedestrian with other conveyance injured in collision with railway train or railway vehicle in traffic accident**
  - Pedestrian with baby stroller injured in collision with railway train or railway vehicle in traffic accident
  - Pedestrian on ice-skates injured in collision with railway train or railway vehicle in traffic accident
  - Pedestrian on nonmotorized scooter injured in collision with railway train or railway vehicle in traffic accident
  - Pedestrian on sled injured in collision with railway train or railway vehicle in traffic accident
  - Pedestrian on snowboard injured in collision with railway train or railway vehicle in traffic accident
  - Pedestrian on snow-skis injured in collision with railway train or railway vehicle in traffic accident
  - Pedestrian in wheelchair (powered) injured in collision with railway train or railway vehicle in traffic accident
  - Pedestrian in motorized mobility scooter injured in collision with railway train or railway vehicle in traffic accident

✓5ᵗʰ **V05.9** **Pedestrian injured in collision with railway train or railway vehicle, unspecified whether traffic or nontraffic accident**

✓x7ᵗʰ **V05.90** **Pedestrian on foot injured in collision with railway train or railway vehicle, unspecified whether traffic or nontraffic accident**
  - Pedestrian NOS injured in collision with railway train or railway vehicle, unspecified whether traffic or nontraffic accident

✓x7ᵗʰ **V05.91** **Pedestrian on roller-skates injured in collision with railway train or railway vehicle, unspecified whether traffic or nontraffic accident**

✓x7ᵗʰ **V05.92** **Pedestrian on skateboard injured in collision with railway train or railway vehicle, unspecified whether traffic or nontraffic accident**

✓6ᵗʰ **V05.93** **Pedestrian on standing micro-mobility pedestrian conveyance injured in collision with railway train or railway vehicle, unspecified whether traffic or nontraffic accident**

- ✓7ᵗʰ **V05.931** **Pedestrian on standing electric scooter injured in collision with railway train or railway vehicle, unspecified whether traffic or nontraffic accident**

- ✓7ᵗʰ **V05.938** **Pedestrian on other standing micro-mobility pedestrian conveyance injured in collision with railway train or railway vehicle, unspecified whether traffic or nontraffic accident**
  - Pedestrian on hoverboard injured in collision with railway train or railway vehicle, unspecified whether traffic or nontraffic accident
  - Pedestrian on segway injured in collision with railway train or railway vehicle, unspecified whether traffic or nontraffic accident

√x 7th **V05.99** **Pedestrian with other conveyance injured in collision with railway train or railway vehicle, unspecified whether traffic or nontraffic accident**
Pedestrian with baby stroller injured in collision with railway train or railway vehicle, unspecified whether traffic or nontraffic
Pedestrian on ice-skates injured in collision with railway train or railway vehicle, unspecified whether traffic or nontraffic
Pedestrian on nonmotorized scooter injured in collision with railway train or railway vehicle, unspecified whether traffic or nontraffic
Pedestrian on sled injured in collision with railway train or railway vehicle, unspecified whether traffic or nontraffic
Pedestrian on snowboard injured in collision with railway train or railway vehicle, unspecified whether traffic or nontraffic
Pedestrian on snow-skis injured in collision with railway train or railway vehicle, unspecified whether traffic or nontraffic
Pedestrian in wheelchair (powered) injured in collision with railway train or railway vehicle, unspecified whether traffic or nontraffic
Pedestrian in motorized mobility scooter injured in collision with railway train or railway vehicle, unspecified whether traffic or nontraffic

√4th **V06** **Pedestrian injured in collision with other nonmotor vehicle**
INCLUDES collision with animal-drawn vehicle, animal being ridden, nonpowered streetcar
EXCLUDES 1 pedestrian injured in collision with pedestrian conveyance (V00.0-)

√5th **V06.0** **Pedestrian injured in collision with other nonmotor vehicle in nontraffic accident**
√x 7th **V06.00** **Pedestrian on foot injured in collision with other nonmotor vehicle in nontraffic accident**
Pedestrian NOS injured in collision with nonmotor vehicle in nontraffic accident
√x 7th **V06.01** **Pedestrian on roller-skates injured in collision with other nonmotor vehicle in nontraffic accident**
√x 7th **V06.02** **Pedestrian on skateboard injured in collision with other nonmotor vehicle in nontraffic accident**
● √6th **V06.03** **Pedestrian on standing micro-mobility pedestrian conveyance injured in collision with other nonmotor vehicle in nontraffic accident**
● √7th **V06.031** **Pedestrian on standing electric scooter injured in collision with other nonmotor vehicle in nontraffic accident**
● √7th **V06.038** **Pedestrian on other standing micro-mobility pedestrian conveyance injured in collision with other nonmotor vehicle in nontraffic accident**
Pedestrian on hoverboard injured in collision with other nonmotor vehicle in nontraffic accident
Pedestrian on segway injured in collision with other nonmotor vehicle in nontraffic accident

√x 7th **V06.09** **Pedestrian with other conveyance injured in collision with other nonmotor vehicle in nontraffic accident**
Pedestrian with baby stroller injured in collision with other nonmotor vehicle in nontraffic accident
Pedestrian on ice-skates injured in collision with other nonmotor vehicle in nontraffic accident
Pedestrian on nonmotorized scooter injured in collision with other nonmotor vehicle in nontraffic accident
Pedestrian on sled injured in collision with other nonmotor vehicle in nontraffic accident
Pedestrian on snowboard injured in collision with other nonmotor vehicle in nontraffic accident
Pedestrian on snow-skis injured in collision with other nonmotor vehicle in nontraffic accident
Pedestrian in wheelchair (powered) injured in collision with other nonmotor vehicle in nontraffic accident
Pedestrian in motorized mobility scooter injured in collision with other nonmotor vehicle in nontraffic accident

√5th **V06.1** **Pedestrian injured in collision with other nonmotor vehicle in traffic accident**
√x 7th **V06.10** **Pedestrian on foot injured in collision with other nonmotor vehicle in traffic accident**
Pedestrian NOS injured in collision with other nonmotor vehicle in traffic accident
√x 7th **V06.11** **Pedestrian on roller-skates injured in collision with other nonmotor vehicle in traffic accident**
√x 7th **V06.12** **Pedestrian on skateboard injured in collision with other nonmotor vehicle in traffic accident**
● √6th **V06.13** **Pedestrian on standing micro-mobility pedestrian conveyance injured in collision with other nonmotor vehicle in traffic accident**
● √7th **V06.131** **Pedestrian on standing electric scooter injured in collision with other nonmotor vehicle in traffic accident**
● √7th **V06.138** **Pedestrian on other standing micro-mobility pedestrian conveyance injured in collision with other nonmotor vehicle in traffic accident**
Pedestrian on hoverboard injured in collision with other nonmotor vehicle in traffic accident
Pedestrian on segway injured in collision with other nonmotor vehicle in traffic accident

√x 7th **V06.19** **Pedestrian with other conveyance injured in collision with other nonmotor vehicle in traffic accident**
Pedestrian with baby stroller injured in collision with other nonmotor vehicle in nontraffic accident
Pedestrian on ice-skates injured in collision with other nonmotor vehicle in traffic accident
Pedestrian on nonmotorized scooter injured in collision with other nonmotor vehicle in traffic accident
Pedestrian on sled injured in collision with other nonmotor vehicle in traffic accident
Pedestrian on snowboard injured in collision with other nonmotor vehicle in traffic accident
Pedestrian on snow-skis injured in collision with other nonmotor vehicle in traffic accident
Pedestrian in wheelchair (powered) injured in collision with other nonmotor vehicle in traffic accident
Pedestrian in motorized mobility scooter injured in collision with other nonmotor vehicle in traffic accident

√5th **V06.9** **Pedestrian injured in collision with other nonmotor vehicle, unspecified whether traffic or nontraffic accident**
√x 7th **V06.90** **Pedestrian on foot injured in collision with other nonmotor vehicle, unspecified whether traffic or nontraffic accident**
Pedestrian NOS injured in collision with other nonmotor vehicle, unspecified whether traffic or nontraffic accident
√x 7th **V06.91** **Pedestrian on roller-skates injured in collision with other nonmotor vehicle, unspecified whether traffic or nontraffic accident**

☑7ᵗʰ **V06.92** Pedestrian on skateboard injured in collision with other nonmotor vehicle, unspecified whether traffic or nontraffic accident

● ☑6ᵗʰ **V06.93** Pedestrian on standing micro-mobility pedestrian conveyance injured in collision with other nonmotor vehicle, unspecified whether traffic or nontraffic accident

● ☑7ᵗʰ **V06.931** Pedestrian on standing electric scooter injured in collision with other nonmotor vehicle, unspecified whether traffic or nontraffic accident

● ☑7ᵗʰ **V06.938** Pedestrian on other standing micro-mobility pedestrian conveyance injured in collision with other nonmotor vehicle, unspecified whether traffic or nontraffic accident

Pedestrian on hoverboard injured in collision with other nonmotor, unspecified whether traffic or nontraffic accident

Pedestrian on segway injured in collision with other nonmotor vehicle, unspecified whether traffic or nontraffic accident

☑7ᵗʰ **V06.99** Pedestrian with other conveyance injured in collision with other nonmotor vehicle, unspecified whether traffic or nontraffic accident

Pedestrian with baby stroller injured in collision with other nonmotor vehicle, unspecified whether traffic or nontraffic accident

Pedestrian on ice-skates injured in collision with other nonmotor vehicle, unspecified whether traffic or nontraffic accident

Pedestrian on nonmotorized scooter injured in collision with other nonmotor vehicle, unspecified whether traffic or nontraffic accident

Pedestrian on sled injured in collision with other nonmotor vehicle, unspecified whether traffic or nontraffic accident

Pedestrian on snowboard injured in collision with other nonmotor vehicle, unspecified whether traffic or nontraffic accident

Pedestrian on snow-skis injured in collision with other nonmotor vehicle, unspecified whether traffic or nontraffic accident

Pedestrian in wheelchair (powered) injured in collision with other nonmotor vehicle, unspecified whether traffic or nontraffic accident

Pedestrian in motorized mobility scooter injured in collision with other nonmotorized vehicle, unspecified whether traffic or nontraffic accident

☑4ᵗʰ **V09** Pedestrian injured in other and unspecified transport accidents

☑6ᵗʰ **V09.0** Pedestrian injured in nontraffic accident involving other and unspecified motor vehicles

☑7ᵗʰ **V09.00** Pedestrian injured in nontraffic accident involving unspecified motor vehicles

☑7ᵗʰ **V09.01** Pedestrian injured in nontraffic accident involving military vehicle

☑7ᵗʰ **V09.09** Pedestrian injured in nontraffic accident involving other motor vehicles

Pedestrian injured in nontraffic accident by special vehicle

☑7ᵗʰ **V09.1** Pedestrian injured in unspecified nontraffic accident

☑5ᵗʰ **V09.2** Pedestrian injured in traffic accident involving other and unspecified motor vehicles

☑7ᵗʰ **V09.20** Pedestrian injured in traffic accident involving unspecified motor vehicles

☑7ᵗʰ **V09.21** Pedestrian injured in traffic accident involving military vehicle

☑7ᵗʰ **V09.29** Pedestrian injured in traffic accident involving other motor vehicles

☑7ᵗʰ **V09.3** Pedestrian injured in unspecified traffic accident

☑7ᵗʰ **V09.9** Pedestrian injured in unspecified transport accident

Pedal cycle rider injured in transport accident (V10-V19)

INCLUDES   any non-motorized vehicle, excluding an animal-drawn vehicle, or a sidecar or trailer attached to the pedal cycle

EXCLUDES 2   *rupture of pedal cycle tire (W37.0)*

The appropriate 7th character is to be added to each code from categories V10-V19.
A   initial encounter
D   subsequent encounter
S   sequela

☑4ᵗʰ **V10** Pedal cycle rider injured in collision with pedestrian or animal

EXCLUDES 1   *pedal cycle rider collision with animal-drawn vehicle or animal being ridden (V16.-)*

☑x7ᵗʰ **V10.0** Pedal cycle driver injured in collision with pedestrian or animal in nontraffic accident

☑x7ᵗʰ **V10.1** Pedal cycle passenger injured in collision with pedestrian or animal in nontraffic accident

☑x7ᵗʰ **V10.2** Unspecified pedal cyclist injured in collision with pedestrian or animal in nontraffic accident

☑x7ᵗʰ **V10.3** Person boarding or alighting a pedal cycle injured in collision with pedestrian or animal

☑x7ᵗʰ **V10.4** Pedal cycle driver injured in collision with pedestrian or animal in traffic accident

☑x7ᵗʰ **V10.5** Pedal cycle passenger injured in collision with pedestrian or animal in traffic accident

☑x7ᵗʰ **V10.9** Unspecified pedal cyclist injured in collision with pedestrian or animal in traffic accident

☑4ᵗʰ **V11** Pedal cycle rider injured in collision with other pedal cycle

☑x7ᵗʰ **V11.0** Pedal cycle driver injured in collision with other pedal cycle in nontraffic accident

☑x7ᵗʰ **V11.1** Pedal cycle passenger injured in collision with other pedal cycle in nontraffic accident

☑x7ᵗʰ **V11.2** Unspecified pedal cyclist injured in collision with other pedal cycle in nontraffic accident

☑x7ᵗʰ **V11.3** Person boarding or alighting a pedal cycle injured in collision with other pedal cycle

☑x7ᵗʰ **V11.4** Pedal cycle driver injured in collision with other pedal cycle in traffic accident

☑x7ᵗʰ **V11.5** Pedal cycle passenger injured in collision with other pedal cycle in traffic accident

☑x7ᵗʰ **V11.9** Unspecified pedal cyclist injured in collision with other pedal cycle in traffic accident

☑4ᵗʰ **V12** Pedal cycle rider injured in collision with two- or three-wheeled motor vehicle

☑x7ᵗʰ **V12.0** Pedal cycle driver injured in collision with two- or three-wheeled motor vehicle in nontraffic accident

☑x7ᵗʰ **V12.1** Pedal cycle passenger injured in collision with two- or three-wheeled motor vehicle in nontraffic accident

☑x7ᵗʰ **V12.2** Unspecified pedal cyclist injured in collision with two- or three-wheeled motor vehicle in nontraffic accident

☑x7ᵗʰ **V12.3** Person boarding or alighting a pedal cycle injured in collision with two- or three-wheeled motor vehicle

☑x7ᵗʰ **V12.4** Pedal cycle driver injured in collision with two- or three-wheeled motor vehicle in traffic accident

☑x7ᵗʰ **V12.5** Pedal cycle passenger injured in collision with two- or three-wheeled motor vehicle in traffic accident

☑x7ᵗʰ **V12.9** Unspecified pedal cyclist injured in collision with two- or three-wheeled motor vehicle in traffic accident

☑4ᵗʰ **V13** Pedal cycle rider injured in collision with car, pick-up truck or van

☑x7ᵗʰ **V13.0** Pedal cycle driver injured in collision with car, pick-up truck or van in nontraffic accident

☑x7ᵗʰ **V13.1** Pedal cycle passenger injured in collision with car, pick-up truck or van in nontraffic accident

☑x7ᵗʰ **V13.2** Unspecified pedal cyclist injured in collision with car, pick-up truck or van in nontraffic accident

☑x7ᵗʰ **V13.3** Person boarding or alighting a pedal cycle injured in collision with car, pick-up truck or van

☑x7ᵗʰ **V13.4** Pedal cycle driver injured in collision with car, pick-up truck or van in traffic accident

☑x7ᵗʰ **V13.5** Pedal cycle passenger injured in collision with car, pick-up truck or van in traffic accident

☑x7ᵗʰ **V13.9** Unspecified pedal cyclist injured in collision with car, pick-up truck or van in traffic accident

☑4ᵗʰ **V14** Pedal cycle rider injured in collision with heavy transport vehicle or bus

EXCLUDES 1   *pedal cycle rider injured in collision with military vehicle (V19.81)*

☑x7ᵗʰ **V14.0** Pedal cycle driver injured in collision with heavy transport vehicle or bus in nontraffic accident

---

√x7th **V14.1** Pedal cycle passenger injured in collision with heavy transport vehicle or bus in nontraffic accident

√x7th **V14.2** Unspecified pedal cyclist injured in collision with heavy transport vehicle or bus in nontraffic accident

√x7th **V14.3** Person boarding or alighting a pedal cycle injured in collision with heavy transport vehicle or bus

√x7th **V14.4** Pedal cycle driver injured in collision with heavy transport vehicle or bus in traffic accident

√x7th **V14.5** Pedal cycle passenger injured in collision with heavy transport vehicle or bus in traffic accident

√x7th **V14.9** Unspecified pedal cyclist injured in collision with heavy transport vehicle or bus in traffic accident

√4th **V15** Pedal cycle rider injured in collision with railway train or railway vehicle

√x7th **V15.0** Pedal cycle driver injured in collision with railway train or railway vehicle in nontraffic accident

√x7th **V15.1** Pedal cycle passenger injured in collision with railway train or railway vehicle in nontraffic accident

√x7th **V15.2** Unspecified pedal cyclist injured in collision with railway train or railway vehicle in nontraffic accident

√x7th **V15.3** Person boarding or alighting a pedal cycle injured in collision with railway train or railway vehicle

√x7th **V15.4** Pedal cycle driver injured in collision with railway train or railway vehicle in traffic accident

√x7th **V15.5** Pedal cycle passenger injured in collision with railway train or railway vehicle in traffic accident

√x7th **V15.9** Unspecified pedal cyclist injured in collision with railway train or railway vehicle in traffic accident

√4th **V16** Pedal cycle rider injured in collision with other nonmotor vehicle

> INCLUDES   collision with animal-drawn vehicle, animal being ridden, streetcar

√x7th **V16.0** Pedal cycle driver injured in collision with other nonmotor vehicle in nontraffic accident

√x7th **V16.1** Pedal cycle passenger injured in collision with other nonmotor vehicle in nontraffic accident

√x7th **V16.2** Unspecified pedal cyclist injured in collision with other nonmotor vehicle in nontraffic accident

√x7th **V16.3** Person boarding or alighting a pedal cycle injured in collision with other nonmotor vehicle in nontraffic accident

√x7th **V16.4** Pedal cycle driver injured in collision with other nonmotor vehicle in traffic accident

√x7th **V16.5** Pedal cycle passenger injured in collision with other nonmotor vehicle in traffic accident

√x7th **V16.9** Unspecified pedal cyclist injured in collision with other nonmotor vehicle in traffic accident

√4th **V17** Pedal cycle rider injured in collision with fixed or stationary object

√x7th **V17.0** Pedal cycle driver injured in collision with fixed or stationary object in nontraffic accident

√x7th **V17.1** Pedal cycle passenger injured in collision with fixed or stationary object in nontraffic accident

√x7th **V17.2** Unspecified pedal cyclist injured in collision with fixed or stationary object in nontraffic accident

√x7th **V17.3** Person boarding or alighting a pedal cycle injured in collision with fixed or stationary object

√x7th **V17.4** Pedal cycle driver injured in collision with fixed or stationary object in traffic accident

√x7th **V17.5** Pedal cycle passenger injured in collision with fixed or stationary object in traffic accident

√x7th **V17.9** Unspecified pedal cyclist injured in collision with fixed or stationary object in traffic accident

√4th **V18** Pedal cycle rider injured in noncollision transport accident

> INCLUDES   fall or thrown from pedal cycle (without antecedent collision)
> overturning pedal cycle NOS
> overturning pedal cycle without collision

√x7th **V18.0** Pedal cycle driver injured in noncollision transport accident in nontraffic accident

√x7th **V18.1** Pedal cycle passenger injured in noncollision transport accident in nontraffic accident

√x7th **V18.2** Unspecified pedal cyclist injured in noncollision transport accident in nontraffic accident

√x7th **V18.3** Person boarding or alighting a pedal cycle injured in noncollision transport accident

√x7th **V18.4** Pedal cycle driver injured in noncollision transport accident in traffic accident

√x7th **V18.5** Pedal cycle passenger injured in noncollision transport accident in traffic accident

√x7th **V18.9** Unspecified pedal cyclist injured in noncollision transport accident in traffic accident

√4th **V19** Pedal cycle rider injured in other and unspecified transport accidents

√5th **V19.0** Pedal cycle driver injured in collision with other and unspecified motor vehicles in nontraffic accident

√x7th **V19.00** Pedal cycle driver injured in collision with unspecified motor vehicles in nontraffic accident

√x7th **V19.09** Pedal cycle driver injured in collision with other motor vehicles in nontraffic accident

√5th **V19.1** Pedal cycle passenger injured in collision with other and unspecified motor vehicles in nontraffic accident

√x7th **V19.10** Pedal cycle passenger injured in collision with unspecified motor vehicles in nontraffic accident

√x7th **V19.19** Pedal cycle passenger injured in collision with other motor vehicles in nontraffic accident

√5th **V19.2** Unspecified pedal cyclist injured in collision with other and unspecified motor vehicles in nontraffic accident

√x7th **V19.20** Unspecified pedal cyclist injured in collision with unspecified motor vehicles in nontraffic accident
> Pedal cycle collision NOS, nontraffic

√x7th **V19.29** Unspecified pedal cyclist injured in collision with other motor vehicles in nontraffic accident

√x7th **V19.3** Pedal cyclist (driver) (passenger) injured in unspecified nontraffic accident
> Pedal cycle accident NOS, nontraffic
> Pedal cyclist injured in nontraffic accident NOS

√5th **V19.4** Pedal cycle driver injured in collision with other and unspecified motor vehicles in traffic accident

√x7th **V19.40** Pedal cycle driver injured in collision with unspecified motor vehicles in traffic accident

√x7th **V19.49** Pedal cycle driver injured in collision with other motor vehicles in traffic accident

√5th **V19.5** Pedal cycle passenger injured in collision with other and unspecified motor vehicles in traffic accident

√x7th **V19.50** Pedal cycle passenger injured in collision with unspecified motor vehicles in traffic accident

√x7th **V19.59** Pedal cycle passenger injured in collision with other motor vehicles in traffic accident

√5th **V19.6** Unspecified pedal cyclist injured in collision with other and unspecified motor vehicles in traffic accident

√x7th **V19.60** Unspecified pedal cyclist injured in collision with unspecified motor vehicles in traffic accident
> Pedal cycle collision NOS (traffic)

√x7th **V19.69** Unspecified pedal cyclist injured in collision with other motor vehicles in traffic accident

√5th **V19.8** Pedal cyclist (driver) (passenger) injured in other specified transport accidents

√x7th **V19.81** Pedal cyclist (driver) (passenger) injured in transport accident with military vehicle

√x7th **V19.88** Pedal cyclist (driver) (passenger) injured in other specified transport accidents

√x7th **V19.9** Pedal cyclist (driver) (passenger) injured in unspecified traffic accident
> Pedal cycle accident NOS

Motorcycle rider injured in transport accident (V20-V29)

> INCLUDES   moped
> motorcycle with sidecar
> motorized bicycle
> motor scooter
>
> EXCLUDES 1   *three-wheeled motor vehicle (V30-V39)*

The appropriate 7th character is to be added to each code from categories V20-V29.
A   initial encounter
D   subsequent encounter
S   sequela

√4th **V20** Motorcycle rider injured in collision with pedestrian or animal

> EXCLUDES 1   *motorcycle rider collision with animal-drawn vehicle or animal being ridden (V26.-)*

√x7th **V20.0** Motorcycle driver injured in collision with pedestrian or animal in nontraffic accident

√x7th **V20.1** Motorcycle passenger injured in collision with pedestrian or animal in nontraffic accident

√x7th **V20.2** Unspecified motorcycle rider injured in collision with pedestrian or animal in nontraffic accident

√x7th **V20.3** Person boarding or alighting a motorcycle injured in collision with pedestrian or animal

√x7th **V20.4** Motorcycle driver injured in collision with pedestrian or animal in traffic accident

√x7th **V20.5** Motorcycle passenger injured in collision with pedestrian or animal in traffic accident

✔ Additional Char Req   √x7th Placeholder   Unacceptable PDx   Questionable PDx   Wrong Procedure   Manifestation   Unspecified Dx   H1-H14 HAC   HCC CMS-HCC Dx   HIV HIV Dx

ICD-10-CM 2021   1177

√x7th **V20.9** **Unspecified motorcycle rider injured in collision with pedestrian or animal** in traffic accident

√4th **V21** **Motorcycle rider injured in collision with pedal cycle**

√x7th **V21.0** Motorcycle driver injured in collision with pedal cycle in nontraffic accident

√x7th **V21.1** Motorcycle passenger injured in collision with pedal cycle in nontraffic accident

√x7th **V21.2** Unspecified motorcycle rider injured in collision with pedal cycle in nontraffic accident

√x7th **V21.3** Person boarding or alighting a motorcycle injured in collision with pedal cycle

√x7th **V21.4** Motorcycle driver injured in collision with pedal cycle in traffic accident

√x7th **V21.5** Motorcycle passenger injured in collision with pedal cycle in traffic accident

√x7th **V21.9** Unspecified motorcycle rider injured in collision with pedal cycle in traffic accident

√4th **V22** **Motorcycle rider injured in collision with two- or three-wheeled motor vehicle**

√x7th **V22.0** Motorcycle driver injured in collision with two- or three-wheeled motor vehicle in nontraffic accident

√x7th **V22.1** Motorcycle passenger injured in collision with two- or three-wheeled motor vehicle in nontraffic accident

√x7th **V22.2** Unspecified motorcycle rider injured in collision with two- or three-wheeled motor vehicle in nontraffic accident

√x7th **V22.3** Person boarding or alighting a motorcycle injured in collision with two- or three-wheeled motor vehicle

√x7th **V22.4** Motorcycle driver injured in collision with two- or three-wheeled motor vehicle in traffic accident

√x7th **V22.5** Motorcycle passenger injured in collision with two- or three-wheeled motor vehicle in traffic accident

√x7th **V22.9** Unspecified motorcycle rider injured in collision with two- or three-wheeled motor vehicle in traffic accident

√4th **V23** **Motorcycle rider injured in collision with car, pick-up truck or van**

√x7th **V23.0** Motorcycle driver injured in collision with car, pick-up truck or van in nontraffic accident

√x7th **V23.1** Motorcycle passenger injured in collision with car, pick-up truck or van in nontraffic accident

√x7th **V23.2** Unspecified motorcycle rider injured in collision with car, pick-up truck or van in nontraffic accident

√x7th **V23.3** Person boarding or alighting a motorcycle injured in collision with car, pick-up truck or van

√x7th **V23.4** Motorcycle driver injured in collision with car, pick-up truck or van in traffic accident

√x7th **V23.5** Motorcycle passenger injured in collision with car, pick-up truck or van in traffic accident

√x7th **V23.9** Unspecified motorcycle rider injured in collision with car, pick-up truck or van in traffic accident

√4th **V24** **Motorcycle rider injured in collision with heavy transport vehicle or bus**

> EXCLUDES 1 | motorcycle rider injured in collision with military vehicle (V29.81)

√x7th **V24.0** Motorcycle driver injured in collision with heavy transport vehicle or bus in nontraffic accident

√x7th **V24.1** Motorcycle passenger injured in collision with heavy transport vehicle or bus in nontraffic accident

√x7th **V24.2** Unspecified motorcycle rider injured in collision with heavy transport vehicle or bus in nontraffic accident

√x7th **V24.3** Person boarding or alighting a motorcycle injured in collision with heavy transport vehicle or bus

√x7th **V24.4** Motorcycle driver injured in collision with heavy transport vehicle or bus in traffic accident

√x7th **V24.5** Motorcycle passenger injured in collision with heavy transport vehicle or bus in traffic accident

√x7th **V24.9** Unspecified motorcycle rider injured in collision with heavy transport vehicle or bus in traffic accident

√4th **V25** **Motorcycle rider injured in collision with railway train or railway vehicle**

√x7th **V25.0** Motorcycle driver injured in collision with railway train or railway vehicle in nontraffic accident

√x7th **V25.1** Motorcycle passenger injured in collision with railway train or railway vehicle in nontraffic accident

√x7th **V25.2** Unspecified motorcycle rider injured in collision with railway train or railway vehicle in nontraffic accident

√x7th **V25.3** Person boarding or alighting a motorcycle injured in collision with railway train or railway vehicle

√x7th **V25.4** Motorcycle driver injured in collision with railway train or railway vehicle in traffic accident

√x7th **V25.5** Motorcycle passenger injured in collision with railway train or railway vehicle in traffic accident

√x7th **V25.9** Unspecified motorcycle rider injured in collision with railway train or railway vehicle in traffic accident

√4th **V26** **Motorcycle rider injured in collision with other nonmotor vehicle**

> INCLUDES | collision with animal-drawn vehicle, animal being ridden, streetcar

√x7th **V26.0** Motorcycle driver injured in collision with other nonmotor vehicle in nontraffic accident

√x7th **V26.1** Motorcycle passenger injured in collision with other nonmotor vehicle in nontraffic accident

√x7th **V26.2** Unspecified motorcycle rider injured in collision with other nonmotor vehicle in nontraffic accident

√x7th **V26.3** Person boarding or alighting a motorcycle injured in collision with other nonmotor vehicle

√x7th **V26.4** Motorcycle driver injured in collision with other nonmotor vehicle in traffic accident

√x7th **V26.5** Motorcycle passenger injured in collision with other nonmotor vehicle in traffic accident

√x7th **V26.9** Unspecified motorcycle rider injured in collision with other nonmotor vehicle in traffic accident

√4th **V27** **Motorcycle rider injured in collision with fixed or stationary object**

√x7th **V27.0** Motorcycle driver injured in collision with fixed or stationary object in nontraffic accident

√x7th **V27.1** Motorcycle passenger injured in collision with fixed or stationary object in nontraffic accident

√x7th **V27.2** Unspecified motorcycle rider injured in collision with fixed or stationary object in nontraffic accident

√x7th **V27.3** Person boarding or alighting a motorcycle injured in collision with fixed or stationary object

√x7th **V27.4** Motorcycle driver injured in collision with fixed or stationary object in traffic accident

√x7th **V27.5** Motorcycle passenger injured in collision with fixed or stationary object in traffic accident

√x7th **V27.9** Unspecified motorcycle rider injured in collision with fixed or stationary object in traffic accident

√4th **V28** **Motorcycle rider injured in noncollision transport accident**

> INCLUDES | fall or thrown from motorcycle (without antecedent collision)
> overturning motorcycle NOS
> overturning motorcycle without collision

√x7th **V28.0** Motorcycle driver injured in noncollision transport accident in nontraffic accident

√x7th **V28.1** Motorcycle passenger injured in noncollision transport accident in nontraffic accident

√x7th **V28.2** Unspecified motorcycle rider injured in noncollision transport accident in nontraffic accident

√x7th **V28.3** Person boarding or alighting a motorcycle injured in noncollision transport accident

√x7th **V28.4** Motorcycle driver injured in noncollision transport accident in traffic accident

√x7th **V28.5** Motorcycle passenger injured in noncollision transport accident in traffic accident

√x7th **V28.9** Unspecified motorcycle rider injured in noncollision transport accident in traffic accident

√4th **V29** **Motorcycle rider injured in other and unspecified transport accidents**

√5th **V29.0** Motorcycle driver injured in collision with other and unspecified motor vehicles in nontraffic accident

√x7th **V29.00** Motorcycle driver injured in collision with unspecified motor vehicles in nontraffic accident

√x7th **V29.09** Motorcycle driver injured in collision with other motor vehicles in nontraffic accident

√5th **V29.1** Motorcycle passenger injured in collision with other and unspecified motor vehicles in nontraffic accident

√x7th **V29.10** Motorcycle passenger injured in collision with unspecified motor vehicles in nontraffic accident

√x7th **V29.19** Motorcycle passenger injured in collision with other motor vehicles in nontraffic accident

√5th **V29.2** Unspecified motorcycle rider injured in collision with other and unspecified motor vehicles in nontraffic accident

√x7th **V29.20** Unspecified motorcycle rider injured in collision with unspecified motor vehicles in nontraffic accident

Motorcycle collision NOS, nontraffic

√x7th **V29.29** Unspecified motorcycle rider injured in collision with other motor vehicles in nontraffic accident

✓x7ᵗʰ V29.3 Motorcycle rider (driver) (passenger) injured in unspecified nontraffic accident
    Motorcycle accident NOS, nontraffic
    Motorcycle rider injured in nontraffic accident NOS

✓5ᵗʰ V29.4 Motorcycle driver injured in collision with other and unspecified motor vehicles in traffic accident

    ✓x7ᵗʰ V29.40 Motorcycle driver injured in collision with unspecified motor vehicles in traffic accident

    ✓x7ᵗʰ V29.49 Motorcycle driver injured in collision with other motor vehicles in traffic accident

✓5ᵗʰ V29.5 Motorcycle passenger injured in collision with other and unspecified motor vehicles in traffic accident

    ✓x7ᵗʰ V29.50 Motorcycle passenger injured in collision with unspecified motor vehicles in traffic accident

    ✓x7ᵗʰ V29.59 Motorcycle passenger injured in collision with other motor vehicles in traffic accident

✓5ᵗʰ V29.6 Unspecified motorcycle rider injured in collision with other and unspecified motor vehicles in traffic accident

    ✓x7ᵗʰ V29.60 Unspecified motorcycle rider injured in collision with unspecified motor vehicles in traffic accident
        Motorcycle collision NOS (traffic)

    ✓x7ᵗʰ V29.69 Unspecified motorcycle rider injured in collision with other motor vehicles in traffic accident

✓5ᵗʰ V29.8 Motorcycle rider (driver) (passenger) injured in other specified transport accidents

    ✓x7ᵗʰ V29.81 Motorcycle rider (driver) (passenger) injured in transport accident with military vehicle

    ✓x7ᵗʰ V29.88 Motorcycle rider (driver) (passenger) injured in other specified transport accidents

✓x7ᵗʰ V29.9 Motorcycle rider (driver) (passenger) injured in unspecified traffic accident
    Motorcycle accident NOS

Occupant of three-wheeled motor vehicle injured in transport accident (V30-V39)

INCLUDES   motorized tricycle
              motorized rickshaw
              three-wheeled motor car
EXCLUDES 1   *all-terrain vehicles (V86.-)*
              motorcycle with sidecar (V20-V29)
              vehicle designed primarily for off-road use (V86.-)

The appropriate 7th character is to be added to each code from categories V30-V39.
A   initial encounter
D   subsequent encounter
S   sequela

✓4ᵗʰ V30 Occupant of three-wheeled motor vehicle injured in collision with pedestrian or animal
    EXCLUDES 1   *three-wheeled motor vehicle collision with animal-drawn vehicle or animal being ridden (V36.-)*

    ✓x7ᵗʰ V30.0 Driver of three-wheeled motor vehicle injured in collision with pedestrian or animal in nontraffic accident

    ✓x7ᵗʰ V30.1 Passenger in three-wheeled motor vehicle injured in collision with pedestrian or animal in nontraffic accident

    ✓x7ᵗʰ V30.2 Person on outside of three-wheeled motor vehicle injured in collision with pedestrian or animal in nontraffic accident

    ✓x7ᵗʰ V30.3 Unspecified occupant of three-wheeled motor vehicle injured in collision with pedestrian or animal in nontraffic accident

    ✓x7ᵗʰ V30.4 Person boarding or alighting a three-wheeled motor vehicle injured in collision with pedestrian or animal

    ✓x7ᵗʰ V30.5 Driver of three-wheeled motor vehicle injured in collision with pedestrian or animal in traffic accident

    ✓x7ᵗʰ V30.6 Passenger in three-wheeled motor vehicle injured in collision with pedestrian or animal in traffic accident

    ✓x7ᵗʰ V30.7 Person on outside of three-wheeled motor vehicle injured in collision with pedestrian or animal in traffic accident

    ✓x7ᵗʰ V30.9 Unspecified occupant of three-wheeled motor vehicle injured in collision with pedestrian or animal in traffic accident

✓4ᵗʰ V31 Occupant of three-wheeled motor vehicle injured in collision with pedal cycle

    ✓x7ᵗʰ V31.0 Driver of three-wheeled motor vehicle injured in collision with pedal cycle in nontraffic accident

    ✓x7ᵗʰ V31.1 Passenger in three-wheeled motor vehicle injured in collision with pedal cycle in nontraffic accident

    ✓x7ᵗʰ V31.2 Person on outside of three-wheeled motor vehicle injured in collision with pedal cycle in nontraffic accident

    ✓x7ᵗʰ V31.3 Unspecified occupant of three-wheeled motor vehicle injured in collision with pedal cycle in nontraffic accident

    ✓x7ᵗʰ V31.4 Person boarding or alighting a three-wheeled motor vehicle injured in collision with pedal cycle

    ✓x7ᵗʰ V31.5 Driver of three-wheeled motor vehicle injured in collision with pedal cycle in traffic accident

    ✓x7ᵗʰ V31.6 Passenger in three-wheeled motor vehicle injured in collision with pedal cycle in traffic accident

    ✓x7ᵗʰ V31.7 Person on outside of three-wheeled motor vehicle injured in collision with pedal cycle in traffic accident

    ✓x7ᵗʰ V31.9 Unspecified occupant of three-wheeled motor vehicle injured in collision with pedal cycle in traffic accident

✓4ᵗʰ V32 Occupant of three-wheeled motor vehicle injured in collision with two- or three-wheeled motor vehicle

    ✓x7ᵗʰ V32.0 Driver of three-wheeled motor vehicle injured in collision with two- or three-wheeled motor vehicle in nontraffic accident

    ✓x7ᵗʰ V32.1 Passenger in three-wheeled motor vehicle injured in collision with two- or three-wheeled motor vehicle in nontraffic accident

    ✓x7ᵗʰ V32.2 Person on outside of three-wheeled motor vehicle injured in collision with two- or three-wheeled motor vehicle in nontraffic accident

    ✓x7ᵗʰ V32.3 Unspecified occupant of three-wheeled motor vehicle injured in collision with two- or three-wheeled motor vehicle in nontraffic accident

    ✓x7ᵗʰ V32.4 Person boarding or alighting a three-wheeled motor vehicle injured in collision with two- or three-wheeled motor vehicle

    ✓x7ᵗʰ V32.5 Driver of three-wheeled motor vehicle injured in collision with two- or three-wheeled motor vehicle in traffic accident

    ✓x7ᵗʰ V32.6 Passenger in three-wheeled motor vehicle injured in collision with two- or three-wheeled motor vehicle in traffic accident

    ✓x7ᵗʰ V32.7 Person on outside of three-wheeled motor vehicle injured in collision with two- or three-wheeled motor vehicle in traffic accident

    ✓x7ᵗʰ V32.9 Unspecified occupant of three-wheeled motor vehicle injured in collision with two- or three-wheeled motor vehicle in traffic accident

✓4ᵗʰ V33 Occupant of three-wheeled motor vehicle injured in collision with car, pick-up truck or van

    ✓x7ᵗʰ V33.0 Driver of three-wheeled motor vehicle injured in collision with car, pick-up truck or van in nontraffic accident

    ✓x7ᵗʰ V33.1 Passenger in three-wheeled motor vehicle injured in collision with car, pick-up truck or van in nontraffic accident

    ✓x7ᵗʰ V33.2 Person on outside of three-wheeled motor vehicle injured in collision with car, pick-up truck or van in nontraffic accident

    ✓x7ᵗʰ V33.3 Unspecified occupant of three-wheeled motor vehicle injured in collision with car, pick-up truck or van in nontraffic accident

    ✓x7ᵗʰ V33.4 Person boarding or alighting a three-wheeled motor vehicle injured in collision with car, pick-up truck or van

    ✓x7ᵗʰ V33.5 Driver of three-wheeled motor vehicle injured in collision with car, pick-up truck or van in traffic accident

    ✓x7ᵗʰ V33.6 Passenger in three-wheeled motor vehicle injured in collision with car, pick-up truck or van in traffic accident

    ✓x7ᵗʰ V33.7 Person on outside of three-wheeled motor vehicle injured in collision with car, pick-up truck or van in traffic accident

    ✓x7ᵗʰ V33.9 Unspecified occupant of three-wheeled motor vehicle injured in collision with car, pick-up truck or van in traffic accident

✓4ᵗʰ V34 Occupant of three-wheeled motor vehicle injured in collision with heavy transport vehicle or bus
    EXCLUDES 1   *occupant of three-wheeled motor vehicle injured in collision with military vehicle (V39.81)*

    ✓x7ᵗʰ V34.0 Driver of three-wheeled motor vehicle injured in collision with heavy transport vehicle or bus in nontraffic accident

    ✓x7ᵗʰ V34.1 Passenger in three-wheeled motor vehicle injured in collision with heavy transport vehicle or bus in nontraffic accident

    ✓x7ᵗʰ V34.2 Person on outside of three-wheeled motor vehicle injured in collision with heavy transport vehicle or bus in nontraffic accident

    ✓x7ᵗʰ V34.3 Unspecified occupant of three-wheeled motor vehicle injured in collision with heavy transport vehicle or bus in nontraffic accident

    ✓x7ᵗʰ V34.4 Person boarding or alighting a three-wheeled motor vehicle injured in collision with heavy transport vehicle or bus

    ✓x7ᵗʰ V34.5 Driver of three-wheeled motor vehicle injured in collision with heavy transport vehicle or bus in traffic accident

    ✓x7ᵗʰ V34.6 Passenger in three-wheeled motor vehicle injured in collision with heavy transport vehicle or bus in traffic accident

    ✓x7ᵗʰ V34.7 Person on outside of three-wheeled motor vehicle injured in collision with heavy transport vehicle or bus in traffic accident

    ✓x7ᵗʰ V34.9 Unspecified occupant of three-wheeled motor vehicle injured in collision with heavy transport vehicle or bus in traffic accident

Chapter 20. External Causes of Morbidity

V35–V39.89

✓4ᵗʰ **V35** **Occupant of three-wheeled motor vehicle injured in collision with railway train or railway vehicle**

✓x7ᵗʰ **V35.0** Driver of three-wheeled motor vehicle injured in collision with railway train or railway vehicle in nontraffic accident

✓x7ᵗʰ **V35.1** Passenger in three-wheeled motor vehicle injured in collision with railway train or railway vehicle in nontraffic accident

✓x7ᵗʰ **V35.2** Person on outside of three-wheeled motor vehicle injured in collision with railway train or railway vehicle in nontraffic accident

✓x7ᵗʰ **V35.3** Unspecified occupant of three-wheeled motor vehicle injured in collision with railway train or railway vehicle in nontraffic accident

✓x7ᵗʰ **V35.4** Person boarding or alighting a three-wheeled motor vehicle injured in collision with railway train or railway vehicle

✓x7ᵗʰ **V35.5** Driver of three-wheeled motor vehicle injured in collision with railway train or railway vehicle in traffic accident

✓x7ᵗʰ **V35.6** Passenger in three-wheeled motor vehicle injured in collision with railway train or railway vehicle in traffic accident

✓x7ᵗʰ **V35.7** Person on outside of three-wheeled motor vehicle injured in collision with railway train or railway vehicle in traffic accident

✓x7ᵗʰ **V35.9** Unspecified occupant of three-wheeled motor vehicle injured in collision with railway train or railway vehicle in traffic accident

✓4ᵗʰ **V36** **Occupant of three-wheeled motor vehicle injured in collision with other nonmotor vehicle**

     INCLUDES   collision with animal-drawn vehicle, animal being ridden, streetcar

✓x7ᵗʰ **V36.0** Driver of three-wheeled motor vehicle injured in collision with other nonmotor vehicle in nontraffic accident

✓x7ᵗʰ **V36.1** Passenger in three-wheeled motor vehicle injured in collision with other nonmotor vehicle in nontraffic accident

✓x7ᵗʰ **V36.2** Person on outside of three-wheeled motor vehicle injured in collision with other nonmotor vehicle in nontraffic accident

✓x7ᵗʰ **V36.3** Unspecified occupant of three-wheeled motor vehicle injured in collision with other nonmotor vehicle in nontraffic accident

✓x7ᵗʰ **V36.4** Person boarding or alighting a three-wheeled motor vehicle injured in collision with other nonmotor vehicle

✓x7ᵗʰ **V36.5** Driver of three-wheeled motor vehicle injured in collision with other nonmotor vehicle in traffic accident

✓x7ᵗʰ **V36.6** Passenger in three-wheeled motor vehicle injured in collision with other nonmotor vehicle in traffic accident

✓x7ᵗʰ **V36.7** Person on outside of three-wheeled motor vehicle injured in collision with other nonmotor vehicle in traffic accident

✓x7ᵗʰ **V36.9** Unspecified occupant of three-wheeled motor vehicle injured in collision with other nonmotor vehicle in traffic accident

✓4ᵗʰ **V37** **Occupant of three-wheeled motor vehicle injured in collision with fixed or stationary object**

✓x7ᵗʰ **V37.0** Driver of three-wheeled motor vehicle injured in collision with fixed or stationary object in nontraffic accident

✓x7ᵗʰ **V37.1** Passenger in three-wheeled motor vehicle injured in collision with fixed or stationary object in nontraffic accident

✓x7ᵗʰ **V37.2** Person on outside of three-wheeled motor vehicle injured in in collision with fixed or stationary object in nontraffic accident

✓x7ᵗʰ **V37.3** Unspecified occupant of three-wheeled motor vehicle injured in collision with fixed or stationary object in nontraffic accident

✓x7ᵗʰ **V37.4** Person boarding or alighting a three-wheeled motor vehicle injured in collision with fixed or stationary object

✓x7ᵗʰ **V37.5** Driver of three-wheeled motor vehicle injured in collision with fixed or stationary object in traffic accident

✓x7ᵗʰ **V37.6** Passenger in three-wheeled motor vehicle injured in collision with fixed or stationary object in traffic accident

✓x7ᵗʰ **V37.7** Person on outside of three-wheeled motor vehicle injured in collision with fixed or stationary object in traffic accident

✓x7ᵗʰ **V37.9** Unspecified occupant of three-wheeled motor vehicle injured in collision with fixed or stationary object in traffic accident

✓4ᵗʰ **V38** **Occupant of three-wheeled motor vehicle injured in noncollision transport accident**

     INCLUDES   fall or thrown from three-wheeled motor vehicle
overturning of three-wheeled motor vehicle NOS
overturning of three-wheeled motor vehicle without collision

✓x7ᵗʰ **V38.0** Driver of three-wheeled motor vehicle injured in noncollision transport accident in nontraffic accident

✓x7ᵗʰ **V38.1** Passenger in three-wheeled motor vehicle injured in noncollision transport accident in nontraffic accident

✓x7ᵗʰ **V38.2** Person on outside of three-wheeled motor vehicle injured in noncollision transport accident in nontraffic accident

✓x7ᵗʰ **V38.3** Unspecified occupant of three-wheeled motor vehicle injured in noncollision transport accident in nontraffic accident

✓x7ᵗʰ **V38.4** Person boarding or alighting a three-wheeled motor vehicle injured in noncollision transport accident

✓x7ᵗʰ **V38.5** Driver of three-wheeled motor vehicle injured in noncollision transport accident in traffic accident

✓x7ᵗʰ **V38.6** Passenger in three-wheeled motor vehicle injured in noncollision transport accident in traffic accident

✓x7ᵗʰ **V38.7** Person on outside of three-wheeled motor vehicle injured in noncollision transport accident in traffic accident

✓x7ᵗʰ **V38.9** Unspecified occupant of three-wheeled motor vehicle injured in noncollision transport accident in traffic accident

✓4ᵗʰ **V39** **Occupant of three-wheeled motor vehicle injured in other and unspecified transport accidents**

✓5ᵗʰ **V39.0** Driver of three-wheeled motor vehicle injured in collision with other and unspecified motor vehicles in nontraffic accident

✓x7ᵗʰ **V39.00** Driver of three-wheeled motor vehicle injured in collision with unspecified motor vehicles in nontraffic accident

✓x7ᵗʰ **V39.09** Driver of three-wheeled motor vehicle injured in collision with other motor vehicles in nontraffic accident

✓5ᵗʰ **V39.1** Passenger in three-wheeled motor vehicle injured in collision with other and unspecified motor vehicles in nontraffic accident

✓x7ᵗʰ **V39.10** Passenger in three-wheeled motor vehicle injured in collision with unspecified motor vehicles in nontraffic accident

✓x7ᵗʰ **V39.19** Passenger in three-wheeled motor vehicle injured in collision with other motor vehicles in nontraffic accident

✓5ᵗʰ **V39.2** Unspecified occupant of three-wheeled motor vehicle injured in collision with other and unspecified motor vehicles in nontraffic accident

✓x7ᵗʰ **V39.20** Unspecified occupant of three-wheeled motor vehicle injured in collision with unspecified motor vehicles in nontraffic accident
Collision NOS involving three-wheeled motor vehicle, nontraffic

✓x7ᵗʰ **V39.29** Unspecified occupant of three-wheeled motor vehicle injured in collision with other motor vehicles in nontraffic accident

✓x7ᵗʰ **V39.3** Occupant (driver) (passenger) of three-wheeled motor vehicle injured in unspecified nontraffic accident
Accident NOS involving three-wheeled motor vehicle, nontraffic
Occupant of three-wheeled motor vehicle injured in nontraffic accident NOS

✓5ᵗʰ **V39.4** Driver of three-wheeled motor vehicle injured in collision with other and unspecified motor vehicles in traffic accident

✓x7ᵗʰ **V39.40** Driver of three-wheeled motor vehicle injured in collision with unspecified motor vehicles in traffic accident

✓x7ᵗʰ **V39.49** Driver of three-wheeled motor vehicle injured in collision with other motor vehicles in traffic accident

✓5ᵗʰ **V39.5** Passenger in three-wheeled motor vehicle injured in collision with other and unspecified motor vehicles in traffic accident

✓x7ᵗʰ **V39.50** Passenger in three-wheeled motor vehicle injured in collision with unspecified motor vehicles in traffic accident

✓x7ᵗʰ **V39.59** Passenger in three-wheeled motor vehicle injured in collision with other motor vehicles in traffic accident

✓5ᵗʰ **V39.6** Unspecified occupant of three-wheeled motor vehicle injured in collision with other and unspecified motor vehicles in traffic accident

✓x7ᵗʰ **V39.60** Unspecified occupant of three-wheeled motor vehicle injured in collision with unspecified motor vehicles in traffic accident
Collision NOS involving three-wheeled motor vehicle (traffic)

✓x7ᵗʰ **V39.69** Unspecified occupant of three-wheeled motor vehicle injured in collision with other motor vehicles in traffic accident

✓5ᵗʰ **V39.8** Occupant (driver) (passenger) of three-wheeled motor vehicle injured in other specified transport accidents

✓x7ᵗʰ **V39.81** Occupant (driver) (passenger) of three-wheeled motor vehicle injured in transport accident with military vehicle

✓x7ᵗʰ **V39.89** Occupant (driver) (passenger) of three-wheeled motor vehicle injured in other specified transport accidents

---

N Newborn: 0   **P** Pediatric: 0-17   **M** Maternity: 9-64   **A** Adult: 15-124   **MCC** Major Complication/Comorbidity   **CC** Complication/Comorbidity   **SW** Severe Wound Dx

1180   ICD-10-CM 2021

☑️x7ᵗʰ V39.9   **Occupant (driver) (passenger) of three-wheeled motor vehicle injured in unspecified traffic accident**
    Accident NOS involving three-wheeled motor vehicle

Car occupant injured in transport accident (V40-V49)

> **INCLUDES**   a four-wheeled motor vehicle designed primarily for carrying passengers
> automobile (pulling a trailer or camper)
>
> **EXCLUDES 1**   *bus (V50-V59)*
> *minibus (V50-V59)*
> *minivan (V50-V59)*
> *motorcoach (V70-V79)*
> *pick-up truck (V50-V59)*
> *sport utility vehicle (SUV) (V50-V59)*

> The appropriate 7th character is to be added to each code from categories V40-V49.
> A   initial encounter
> D   subsequent encounter
> S   sequela

☑️4ᵗʰ V40   **Car occupant injured in collision with pedestrian or animal**

> **EXCLUDES 1**   *car collision with animal-drawn vehicle or animal being ridden (V46.-)*

☑️x7ᵗʰ V40.0   **Car driver injured in collision with pedestrian or animal in nontraffic accident**

☑️x7ᵗʰ V40.1   **Car passenger injured in collision with pedestrian or animal in nontraffic accident**

☑️x7ᵗʰ V40.2   **Person on outside of car injured in collision with pedestrian or animal in nontraffic accident**

☑️x7ᵗʰ V40.3   **Unspecified car occupant injured in collision with pedestrian or animal in nontraffic accident**

☑️x7ᵗʰ V40.4   **Person boarding or alighting a car injured in collision with pedestrian or animal**

☑️x7ᵗʰ V40.5   **Car driver injured in collision with pedestrian or animal in traffic accident**

☑️x7ᵗʰ V40.6   **Car passenger injured in collision with pedestrian or animal in traffic accident**

☑️x7ᵗʰ V40.7   **Person on outside of car injured in collision with pedestrian or animal in traffic accident**

☑️x7ᵗʰ V40.9   **Unspecified car occupant injured in collision with pedestrian or animal in traffic accident**

☑️4ᵗʰ V41   **Car occupant injured in collision with pedal cycle**

☑️x7ᵗʰ V41.0   **Car driver injured in collision with pedal cycle in nontraffic accident**

☑️x7ᵗʰ V41.1   **Car passenger injured in collision with pedal cycle in nontraffic accident**

☑️x7ᵗʰ V41.2   **Person on outside of car injured in collision with pedal cycle in nontraffic accident**

☑️x7ᵗʰ V41.3   **Unspecified car occupant injured in collision with pedal cycle in nontraffic accident**

☑️x7ᵗʰ V41.4   **Person boarding or alighting a car injured in collision with pedal cycle**

☑️x7ᵗʰ V41.5   **Car driver injured in collision with pedal cycle in traffic accident**

☑️x7ᵗʰ V41.6   **Car passenger injured in collision with pedal cycle in traffic accident**

☑️x7ᵗʰ V41.7   **Person on outside of car injured in collision with pedal cycle in traffic accident**

☑️x7ᵗʰ V41.9   **Unspecified car occupant injured in collision with pedal cycle in traffic accident**

☑️4ᵗʰ V42   **Car occupant injured in collision with two- or three-wheeled motor vehicle**

☑️x7ᵗʰ V42.0   **Car driver injured in collision with two- or three-wheeled motor vehicle in nontraffic accident**

☑️x7ᵗʰ V42.1   **Car passenger injured in collision with two- or three-wheeled motor vehicle in nontraffic accident**

☑️x7ᵗʰ V42.2   **Person on outside of car injured in collision with two- or three-wheeled motor vehicle in nontraffic accident**

☑️x7ᵗʰ V42.3   **Unspecified car occupant injured in collision with two- or three-wheeled motor vehicle in nontraffic accident**

☑️x7ᵗʰ V42.4   **Person boarding or alighting a car injured in collision with two- or three-wheeled motor vehicle**

☑️x7ᵗʰ V42.5   **Car driver injured in collision with two- or three-wheeled motor vehicle in traffic accident**

☑️x7ᵗʰ V42.6   **Car passenger injured in collision with two- or three-wheeled motor vehicle in traffic accident**

☑️x7ᵗʰ V42.7   **Person on outside of car injured in collision with two- or three-wheeled motor vehicle in traffic accident**

☑️x7ᵗʰ V42.9   **Unspecified car occupant injured in collision with two- or three-wheeled motor vehicle in traffic accident**

☑️4ᵗʰ V43   **Car occupant injured in collision with car, pick-up truck or van**

☑️5ᵗʰ V43.0   **Car driver injured in collision with car, pick-up truck or van in nontraffic accident**

☑️x7ᵗʰ V43.01   **Car driver injured in collision with sport utility vehicle in nontraffic accident**

☑️x7ᵗʰ V43.02   **Car driver injured in collision with other type car in nontraffic accident**

☑️x7ᵗʰ V43.03   **Car driver injured in collision with pick-up truck in nontraffic accident**

☑️x7ᵗʰ V43.04   **Car driver injured in collision with van in nontraffic accident**

☑️5ᵗʰ V43.1   **Car passenger injured in collision with car, pick-up truck or van in nontraffic accident**

☑️x7ᵗʰ V43.11   **Car passenger injured in collision with sport utility vehicle in nontraffic accident**

☑️x7ᵗʰ V43.12   **Car passenger injured in collision with other type car in nontraffic accident**

☑️x7ᵗʰ V43.13   **Car passenger injured in collision with pick-up truck in nontraffic accident**

☑️x7ᵗʰ V43.14   **Car passenger injured in collision with van in nontraffic accident**

☑️5ᵗʰ V43.2   **Person on outside of car injured in collision with car, pick-up truck or van in nontraffic accident**

☑️x7ᵗʰ V43.21   **Person on outside of car injured in collision with sport utility vehicle in nontraffic accident**

☑️x7ᵗʰ V43.22   **Person on outside of car injured in collision with other type car in nontraffic accident**

☑️x7ᵗʰ V43.23   **Person on outside of car injured in collision with pick-up truck in nontraffic accident**

☑️x7ᵗʰ V43.24   **Person on outside of car injured in collision with van in nontraffic accident**

☑️5ᵗʰ V43.3   **Unspecified car occupant injured in collision with car, pick-up truck or van in nontraffic accident**

☑️x7ᵗʰ V43.31   **Unspecified car occupant injured in collision with sport utility vehicle in nontraffic accident**

☑️x7ᵗʰ V43.32   **Unspecified car occupant injured in collision with other type car in nontraffic accident**

☑️x7ᵗʰ V43.33   **Unspecified car occupant injured in collision with pick-up truck in nontraffic accident**

☑️x7ᵗʰ V43.34   **Unspecified car occupant injured in collision with van in nontraffic accident**

☑️5ᵗʰ V43.4   **Person boarding or alighting a car injured in collision with car, pick-up truck or van**

☑️x7ᵗʰ V43.41   **Person boarding or alighting a car injured in collision with sport utility vehicle**

☑️x7ᵗʰ V43.42   **Person boarding or alighting a car injured in collision with other type car**

☑️x7ᵗʰ V43.43   **Person boarding or alighting a car injured in collision with pick-up truck**

☑️x7ᵗʰ V43.44   **Person boarding or alighting a car injured in collision with van**

☑️5ᵗʰ V43.5   **Car driver injured in collision with car, pick-up truck or van in traffic accident**

☑️x7ᵗʰ V43.51   **Car driver injured in collision with sport utility vehicle in traffic accident**

☑️x7ᵗʰ V43.52   **Car driver injured in collision with other type car in traffic accident**

☑️x7ᵗʰ V43.53   **Car driver injured in collision with pick-up truck in traffic accident**

☑️x7ᵗʰ V43.54   **Car driver injured in collision with van in traffic accident**

☑️5ᵗʰ V43.6   **Car passenger injured in collision with car, pick-up truck or van in traffic accident**

☑️x7ᵗʰ V43.61   **Car passenger injured in collision with sport utility vehicle in traffic accident**

☑️x7ᵗʰ V43.62   **Car passenger injured in collision with other type car in traffic accident**

☑️x7ᵗʰ V43.63   **Car passenger injured in collision with pick-up truck in traffic accident**

☑️x7ᵗʰ V43.64   **Car passenger injured in collision with van in traffic accident**

☑️5ᵗʰ V43.7   **Person on outside of car injured in collision with car, pick-up truck or van in traffic accident**

☑️x7ᵗʰ V43.71   **Person on outside of car injured in collision with sport utility vehicle in traffic accident**

☑️x7ᵗʰ V43.72   **Person on outside of car injured in collision with other type car in traffic accident**

☑️x7ᵗʰ V43.73   **Person on outside of car injured in collision with pick-up truck in traffic accident**

☑️x7ᵗʰ V43.74   **Person on outside of car injured in collision with van in traffic accident**

☑️ Additional Char Req   ☑️x7ᵗʰ Placeholder   Unacceptable PDx   Questionable PDx   Wrong Procedure   Manifestation   Unspecified Dx   H1-H4 HAC   HCC CMS-HCC Dx   HIV HIV Dx

ICD-10-CM 2021   1181

√5ᵗʰ **V43.9** **Unspecified car occupant injured in collision with car, pick-up truck or van** in traffic accident

√x7ᵗʰ **V43.91** **Unspecified car occupant injured in collision with sport utility vehicle** in traffic accident

√x7ᵗʰ **V43.92** **Unspecified car occupant injured in collision with other type car** in traffic accident

√x7ᵗʰ **V43.93** **Unspecified car occupant injured in collision with pick-up truck** in traffic accident

√x7ᵗʰ **V43.94** **Unspecified car occupant injured in collision with van** in traffic accident

√4ᵗʰ **V44** **Car occupant injured in collision with heavy transport vehicle or bus**

EXCLUDES 1   *car occupant injured in collision with military vehicle (V49.81)*

√x7ᵗʰ **V44.0** **Car driver** injured in collision with heavy transport vehicle or bus in nontraffic accident

√x7ᵗʰ **V44.1** **Car passenger** injured in collision with heavy transport vehicle or bus in nontraffic accident

√x7ᵗʰ **V44.2** **Person on outside** of car injured in collision with heavy transport vehicle or bus in nontraffic accident

√x7ᵗʰ **V44.3** **Unspecified car occupant** injured in collision with heavy transport vehicle or bus in nontraffic accident

√x7ᵗʰ **V44.4** **Person boarding or alighting** a car injured in collision with heavy transport vehicle or bus

√x7ᵗʰ **V44.5** **Car driver** injured in collision with heavy transport vehicle or bus in traffic accident

√x7ᵗʰ **V44.6** **Car passenger** injured in collision with heavy transport vehicle or bus in traffic accident

√x7ᵗʰ **V44.7** **Person on outside** of car injured in collision with heavy transport vehicle or bus in traffic accident

√x7ᵗʰ **V44.9** **Unspecified car occupant** injured in collision with heavy transport vehicle or bus in traffic accident

√4ᵗʰ **V45** **Car occupant injured in collision with railway train or railway vehicle**

√x7ᵗʰ **V45.0** **Car driver** injured in collision with railway train or railway vehicle in nontraffic accident

√x7ᵗʰ **V45.1** **Car passenger** injured in collision with railway train or railway vehicle in nontraffic accident

√x7ᵗʰ **V45.2** **Person on outside** of car injured in collision with railway train or railway vehicle in nontraffic accident

√x7ᵗʰ **V45.3** **Unspecified car occupant** injured in collision with railway train or railway vehicle in nontraffic accident

√x7ᵗʰ **V45.4** **Person boarding or alighting** a car injured in collision with railway train or railway vehicle

√x7ᵗʰ **V45.5** **Car driver** injured in collision with railway train or railway vehicle in traffic accident

√x7ᵗʰ **V45.6** **Car passenger** injured in collision with railway train or railway vehicle in traffic accident

√x7ᵗʰ **V45.7** **Person on outside** of car injured in collision with railway train or railway vehicle in traffic accident

√x7ᵗʰ **V45.9** **Unspecified car occupant** injured in collision with railway train or railway vehicle in traffic accident

√4ᵗʰ **V46** **Car occupant injured in collision with other nonmotor vehicle**

INCLUDES   collision with animal-drawn vehicle, animal being ridden, streetcar

√x7ᵗʰ **V46.0** **Car driver** injured in collision with other nonmotor vehicle in nontraffic accident

√x7ᵗʰ **V46.1** **Car passenger** injured in collision with other nonmotor vehicle in nontraffic accident

√x7ᵗʰ **V46.2** **Person on outside** of car injured in collision with other nonmotor vehicle in nontraffic accident

√x7ᵗʰ **V46.3** **Unspecified car occupant** injured in collision with other nonmotor vehicle in nontraffic accident

√x7ᵗʰ **V46.4** **Person boarding or alighting** a car injured in collision with other nonmotor vehicle

√x7ᵗʰ **V46.5** **Car driver** injured in collision with other nonmotor vehicle in traffic accident

√x7ᵗʰ **V46.6** **Car passenger** injured in collision with other nonmotor vehicle in traffic accident

√x7ᵗʰ **V46.7** **Person on outside** of car injured in collision with other nonmotor vehicle in traffic accident

√x7ᵗʰ **V46.9** **Unspecified car occupant** injured in collision with other nonmotor vehicle in traffic accident

√4ᵗʰ **V47** **Car occupant injured in collision with fixed or stationary object**

AHA: 2016,4Q,73

√x7ᵗʰ **V47.0** **Car driver** injured in collision with fixed or stationary object in nontraffic accident

√x7ᵗʰ **V47.1** **Car passenger** injured in collision with fixed or stationary object in nontraffic accident

√x7ᵗʰ **V47.2** **Person on outside** of car injured in collision with fixed or stationary object in nontraffic accident

√x7ᵗʰ **V47.3** **Unspecified car occupant** injured in collision with fixed or stationary object in nontraffic accident

√x7ᵗʰ **V47.4** **Person boarding or alighting** a car injured in collision with fixed or stationary object

√x7ᵗʰ **V47.5** **Car driver** injured in collision with fixed or stationary object in traffic accident

√x7ᵗʰ **V47.6** **Car passenger** injured in collision with fixed or stationary object in traffic accident

√x7ᵗʰ **V47.7** **Person on outside** of car injured in collision with fixed or stationary object in traffic accident

√x7ᵗʰ **V47.9** **Unspecified car occupant** injured in collision with fixed or stationary object in traffic accident

√4ᵗʰ **V48** **Car occupant injured in noncollision transport accident**

INCLUDES   overturning car NOS
overturning car without collision

√x7ᵗʰ **V48.0** **Car driver** injured in noncollision transport accident in nontraffic accident

√x7ᵗʰ **V48.1** **Car passenger** injured in noncollision transport accident in nontraffic accident

√x7ᵗʰ **V48.2** **Person on outside** of car injured in noncollision transport accident in nontraffic accident

√x7ᵗʰ **V48.3** **Unspecified car occupant** injured in noncollision transport accident in nontraffic accident

√x7ᵗʰ **V48.4** **Person boarding or alighting** a car injured in noncollision transport accident

√x7ᵗʰ **V48.5** **Car driver** injured in noncollision transport accident in traffic accident

√x7ᵗʰ **V48.6** **Car passenger** injured in noncollision transport accident in traffic accident

√x7ᵗʰ **V48.7** **Person on outside** of car injured in noncollision transport accident in traffic accident

√x7ᵗʰ **V48.9** **Unspecified car occupant** injured in noncollision transport accident in traffic accident

√4ᵗʰ **V49** **Car occupant injured in other and unspecified transport accidents**

√5ᵗʰ **V49.0** **Driver** injured in collision with other and unspecified motor vehicles in nontraffic accident

√x7ᵗʰ **V49.00** **Driver injured in collision with unspecified motor vehicles in nontraffic accident**

√x7ᵗʰ **V49.09** **Driver injured in collision with other motor vehicles in nontraffic accident**

√5ᵗʰ **V49.1** **Passenger** injured in collision with other and unspecified motor vehicles in nontraffic accident

√x7ᵗʰ **V49.10** **Passenger injured in collision with unspecified motor vehicles in nontraffic accident**

√x7ᵗʰ **V49.19** **Passenger injured in collision with other motor vehicles in nontraffic accident**

√5ᵗʰ **V49.2** **Unspecified car occupant** injured in collision with other and unspecified motor vehicles in nontraffic accident

√x7ᵗʰ **V49.20** **Unspecified car occupant injured in collision with unspecified motor vehicles in nontraffic accident**
Car collision NOS, nontraffic

√x7ᵗʰ **V49.29** **Unspecified car occupant injured in collision with other motor vehicles in nontraffic accident**

√x7ᵗʰ **V49.3** **Car occupant (driver) (passenger) injured in unspecified nontraffic accident**
Car accident NOS, nontraffic
Car occupant injured in nontraffic accident NOS

√5ᵗʰ **V49.4** **Driver** injured in collision with other and unspecified motor vehicles in traffic accident

√x7ᵗʰ **V49.40** **Driver injured in collision with unspecified motor vehicles in traffic accident**

√x7ᵗʰ **V49.49** **Driver injured in collision with other motor vehicles in traffic accident**

√5ᵗʰ **V49.5** **Passenger** injured in collision with other and unspecified motor vehicles in traffic accident

√x7ᵗʰ **V49.50** **Passenger injured in collision with unspecified motor vehicles in traffic accident**

√x7ᵗʰ **V49.59** **Passenger injured in collision with other motor vehicles in traffic accident**

√5ᵗʰ **V49.6** **Unspecified car occupant** injured in collision with other and unspecified motor vehicles in traffic accident

√x7ᵗʰ **V49.60** **Unspecified car occupant injured in collision with unspecified motor vehicles in traffic accident**
Car collision NOS (traffic)

√x7ᵗʰ **V49.69** **Unspecified car occupant injured in collision with other motor vehicles in traffic accident**

√5ᵗʰ **V49.8** **Car occupant (driver) (passenger) injured in other specified transport accidents**

√x7ᵗʰ **V49.81** **Car occupant (driver) (passenger) injured in transport accident with military vehicle**

√x7ᵗʰ **V49.88**   **Car occupant (driver) (passenger) injured in other specified transport accidents**

√x7ᵗʰ **V49.9**   **Car occupant (driver) (passenger) injured in unspecified traffic accident**
     Car accident NOS

Occupant of pick-up truck or van injured in transport accident (V50-V59)

INCLUDES   a four or six wheel motor vehicle designed primarily for carrying passengers and property but weighing less than the local limit for classification as a heavy goods vehicle
     minibus
     minivan
     sport utility vehicle (SUV)
     truck
     van

EXCLUDES 1   *heavy transport vehicle (V60-V69)*

The appropriate 7th character is to be added to each code from categories V50-V59.
A   initial encounter
D   subsequent encounter
S   sequela

√4ᵗʰ **V50**   **Occupant of pick-up truck or van injured in collision with pedestrian or animal**
     EXCLUDES 1   *pick-up truck or van collision with animal-drawn vehicle or animal being ridden (V56.-)*

√x7ᵗʰ **V50.0**   Driver of pick-up truck or van injured in collision with pedestrian or animal in nontraffic accident

√x7ᵗʰ **V50.1**   Passenger in pick-up truck or van injured in collision with pedestrian or animal in nontraffic accident

√x7ᵗʰ **V50.2**   Person on outside of pick-up truck or van injured in collision with pedestrian or animal in nontraffic accident

√x7ᵗʰ **V50.3**   Unspecified occupant of pick-up truck or van injured in collision with pedestrian or animal in nontraffic accident

√x7ᵗʰ **V50.4**   Person boarding or alighting a pick-up truck or van injured in collision with pedestrian or animal

√x7ᵗʰ **V50.5**   Driver of pick-up truck or van injured in collision with pedestrian or animal in traffic accident

√x7ᵗʰ **V50.6**   Passenger in pick-up truck or van injured in collision with pedestrian or animal in traffic accident

√x7ᵗʰ **V50.7**   Person on outside of pick-up truck or van injured in collision with pedestrian or animal in traffic accident

√x7ᵗʰ **V50.9**   Unspecified occupant of pick-up truck or van injured in collision with pedestrian or animal in traffic accident

√4ᵗʰ **V51**   **Occupant of pick-up truck or van injured in collision with pedal cycle**

√x7ᵗʰ **V51.0**   Driver of pick-up truck or van injured in collision with pedal cycle in nontraffic accident

√x7ᵗʰ **V51.1**   Passenger in pick-up truck or van injured in collision with pedal cycle in nontraffic accident

√x7ᵗʰ **V51.2**   Person on outside of pick-up truck or van injured in collision with pedal cycle in nontraffic accident

√x7ᵗʰ **V51.3**   Unspecified occupant of pick-up truck or van injured in collision with pedal cycle in nontraffic accident

√x7ᵗʰ **V51.4**   Person boarding or alighting a pick-up truck or van injured in collision with pedal cycle

√x7ᵗʰ **V51.5**   Driver of pick-up truck or van injured in collision with pedal cycle in traffic accident

√x7ᵗʰ **V51.6**   Passenger in pick-up truck or van injured in collision with pedal cycle in traffic accident

√x7ᵗʰ **V51.7**   Person on outside of pick-up truck or van injured in collision with pedal cycle in traffic accident

√x7ᵗʰ **V51.9**   Unspecified occupant of pick-up truck or van injured in collision with pedal cycle in traffic accident

√4ᵗʰ **V52**   **Occupant of pick-up truck or van injured in collision with two- or three-wheeled motor vehicle**

√x7ᵗʰ **V52.0**   Driver of pick-up truck or van injured in collision with two- or three-wheeled motor vehicle in nontraffic accident

√x7ᵗʰ **V52.1**   Passenger in pick-up truck or van injured in collision with two- or three-wheeled motor vehicle in nontraffic accident

√x7ᵗʰ **V52.2**   Person on outside of pick-up truck or van injured in collision with two- or three-wheeled motor vehicle in nontraffic accident

√x7ᵗʰ **V52.3**   Unspecified occupant of pick-up truck or van injured in collision with two- or three-wheeled motor vehicle in nontraffic accident

√x7ᵗʰ **V52.4**   Person boarding or alighting a pick-up truck or van injured in collision with two- or three-wheeled motor vehicle

√x7ᵗʰ **V52.5**   Driver of pick-up truck or van injured in collision with two- or three-wheeled motor vehicle in traffic accident

√x7ᵗʰ **V52.6**   Passenger in pick-up truck or van injured in collision with two- or three-wheeled motor vehicle in traffic accident

√x7ᵗʰ **V52.7**   Person on outside of pick-up truck or van injured in collision with two- or three-wheeled motor vehicle in traffic accident

√x7ᵗʰ **V52.9**   Unspecified occupant of pick-up truck or van injured in collision with two- or three-wheeled motor vehicle in traffic accident

√4ᵗʰ **V53**   **Occupant of pick-up truck or van injured in collision with car, pick-up truck or van**

√x7ᵗʰ **V53.0**   Driver of pick-up truck or van injured in collision with car, pick-up truck or van in nontraffic accident

√x7ᵗʰ **V53.1**   Passenger in pick-up truck or van injured in collision with car, pick-up truck or van in nontraffic accident

√x7ᵗʰ **V53.2**   Person on outside of pick-up truck or van injured in collision with car, pick-up truck or van in nontraffic accident

√x7ᵗʰ **V53.3**   Unspecified occupant of pick-up truck or van injured in collision with car, pick-up truck or van in nontraffic accident

√x7ᵗʰ **V53.4**   Person boarding or alighting a pick-up truck or van injured in collision with car, pick-up truck or van

√x7ᵗʰ **V53.5**   Driver of pick-up truck or van injured in collision with car, pick-up truck or van in traffic accident

√x7ᵗʰ **V53.6**   Passenger in pick-up truck or van injured in collision with car, pick-up truck or van in traffic accident

√x7ᵗʰ **V53.7**   Person on outside of pick-up truck or van injured in collision with car, pick-up truck or van in traffic accident

√x7ᵗʰ **V53.9**   Unspecified occupant of pick-up truck or van injured in collision with car, pick-up truck or van in traffic accident

√4ᵗʰ **V54**   **Occupant of pick-up truck or van injured in collision with heavy transport vehicle or bus**
     EXCLUDES 1   *occupant of pick-up truck or van injured in collision with military vehicle (V59.81)*

√x7ᵗʰ **V54.0**   Driver of pick-up truck or van injured in collision with heavy transport vehicle or bus in nontraffic accident

√x7ᵗʰ **V54.1**   Passenger in pick-up truck or van injured in collision with heavy transport vehicle or bus in nontraffic accident

√x7ᵗʰ **V54.2**   Person on outside of pick-up truck or van injured in collision with heavy transport vehicle or bus in nontraffic accident

√x7ᵗʰ **V54.3**   Unspecified occupant of pick-up truck or van injured in collision with heavy transport vehicle or bus in nontraffic accident

√x7ᵗʰ **V54.4**   Person boarding or alighting a pick-up truck or van injured in collision with heavy transport vehicle or bus

√x7ᵗʰ **V54.5**   Driver of pick-up truck or van injured in collision with heavy transport vehicle or bus in traffic accident

√x7ᵗʰ **V54.6**   Passenger in pick-up truck or van injured in collision with heavy transport vehicle or bus in traffic accident

√x7ᵗʰ **V54.7**   Person on outside of pick-up truck or van injured in collision with heavy transport vehicle or bus in traffic accident

√x7ᵗʰ **V54.9**   Unspecified occupant of pick-up truck or van injured in collision with heavy transport vehicle or bus in traffic accident

√4ᵗʰ **V55**   **Occupant of pick-up truck or van injured in collision with railway train or railway vehicle**

√x7ᵗʰ **V55.0**   Driver of pick-up truck or van injured in collision with railway train or railway vehicle in nontraffic accident

√x7ᵗʰ **V55.1**   Passenger in pick-up truck or van injured in collision with railway train or railway vehicle in nontraffic accident

√x7ᵗʰ **V55.2**   Person on outside of pick-up truck or van injured in collision with railway train or railway vehicle in nontraffic accident

√x7ᵗʰ **V55.3**   Unspecified occupant of pick-up truck or van injured in collision with railway train or railway vehicle in nontraffic accident

√x7ᵗʰ **V55.4**   Person boarding or alighting a pick-up truck or van injured in collision with railway train or railway vehicle

√x7ᵗʰ **V55.5**   Driver of pick-up truck or van injured in collision with railway train or railway vehicle in traffic accident

√x7ᵗʰ **V55.6**   Passenger in pick-up truck or van injured in collision with railway train or railway vehicle in traffic accident

√x7ᵗʰ **V55.7**   Person on outside of pick-up truck or van injured in collision with railway train or railway vehicle in traffic accident

√x7ᵗʰ **V55.9**   Unspecified occupant of pick-up truck or van injured in collision with railway train or railway vehicle in traffic accident

√4ᵗʰ **V56**   **Occupant of pick-up truck or van injured in collision with other nonmotor vehicle**
     INCLUDES   collision with animal-drawn vehicle, animal being ridden, streetcar

√x7ᵗʰ **V56.0**   Driver of pick-up truck or van injured in collision with other nonmotor vehicle in nontraffic accident

√x7ᵗʰ **V56.1**   Passenger in pick-up truck or van injured in collision with other nonmotor vehicle in nontraffic accident

---

☑ Additional Char Req   √x7ᵗʰ Placeholder   Unacceptable PDx   Questionable PDx   Wrong Procedure   Manifestation   Unspecified Dx   H1-H14 HAC   HCC CMS-HCC Dx   HIV HIV Dx

√x7ᵗʰ **V56.2** Person on outside of pick-up truck or van injured in collision with other nonmotor vehicle in nontraffic accident

√x7ᵗʰ **V56.3** Unspecified occupant of pick-up truck or van injured in collision with other nonmotor vehicle in nontraffic accident

√x7ᵗʰ **V56.4** Person boarding or alighting a pick-up truck or van injured in collision with other nonmotor vehicle

√x7ᵗʰ **V56.5** Driver of pick-up truck or van injured in collision with other nonmotor vehicle in traffic accident

√x7ᵗʰ **V56.6** Passenger in pick-up truck or van injured in collision with other nonmotor vehicle in traffic accident

√x7ᵗʰ **V56.7** Person on outside of pick-up truck or van injured in collision with other nonmotor vehicle in traffic accident

√x7ᵗʰ **V56.9** Unspecified occupant of pick-up truck or van injured in collision with other nonmotor vehicle in traffic accident

√4ᵗʰ **V57** Occupant of pick-up truck or van injured in collision with fixed or stationary object

√x7ᵗʰ **V57.0** Driver of pick-up truck or van injured in collision with fixed or stationary object in nontraffic accident

√x7ᵗʰ **V57.1** Passenger in pick-up truck or van injured in collision with fixed or stationary object in nontraffic accident

√x7ᵗʰ **V57.2** Person on outside of pick-up truck or van injured in collision with fixed or stationary object in nontraffic accident

√x7ᵗʰ **V57.3** Unspecified occupant of pick-up truck or van injured in collision with fixed or stationary object in nontraffic accident

√x7ᵗʰ **V57.4** Person boarding or alighting a pick-up truck or van injured in collision with fixed or stationary object

√x7ᵗʰ **V57.5** Driver of pick-up truck or van injured in collision with fixed or stationary object in traffic accident

√x7ᵗʰ **V57.6** Passenger in pick-up truck or van injured in collision with fixed or stationary object in traffic accident

√x7ᵗʰ **V57.7** Person on outside of pick-up truck or van injured in collision with fixed or stationary object in traffic accident

√x7ᵗʰ **V57.9** Unspecified occupant of pick-up truck or van injured in collision with fixed or stationary object in traffic accident

√4ᵗʰ **V58** Occupant of pick-up truck or van injured in noncollision transport accident

     INCLUDES   overturning pick-up truck or van NOS
              overturning pick-up truck or van without collision

√x7ᵗʰ **V58.0** Driver of pick-up truck or van injured in noncollision transport accident in nontraffic accident

√x7ᵗʰ **V58.1** Passenger in pick-up truck or van injured in noncollision transport accident in nontraffic accident

√x7ᵗʰ **V58.2** Person on outside of pick-up truck or van injured in noncollision transport accident in nontraffic accident

√x7ᵗʰ **V58.3** Unspecified occupant of pick-up truck or van injured in noncollision transport accident in nontraffic accident

√x7ᵗʰ **V58.4** Person boarding or alighting a pick-up truck or van injured in noncollision transport accident

√x7ᵗʰ **V58.5** Driver of pick-up truck or van injured in noncollision transport accident in traffic accident

√x7ᵗʰ **V58.6** Passenger in pick-up truck or van injured in noncollision transport accident in traffic accident

√x7ᵗʰ **V58.7** Person on outside of pick-up truck or van injured in noncollision transport accident in traffic accident

√x7ᵗʰ **V58.9** Unspecified occupant of pick-up truck or van injured in noncollision transport accident in traffic accident

√4ᵗʰ **V59** Occupant of pick-up truck or van injured in other and unspecified transport accidents

√5ᵗʰ **V59.0** Driver of pick-up truck or van injured in collision with other and unspecified motor vehicles in nontraffic accident

√x7ᵗʰ **V59.00** Driver of pick-up truck or van injured in collision with unspecified motor vehicles in nontraffic accident

√x7ᵗʰ **V59.09** Driver of pick-up truck or van injured in collision with other motor vehicles in nontraffic accident

√5ᵗʰ **V59.1** Passenger in pick-up truck or van injured in collision with other and unspecified motor vehicles in nontraffic accident

√x7ᵗʰ **V59.10** Passenger in pick-up truck or van injured in collision with unspecified motor vehicles in nontraffic accident

√x7ᵗʰ **V59.19** Passenger in pick-up truck or van injured in collision with other motor vehicles in nontraffic accident

√5ᵗʰ **V59.2** Unspecified occupant of pick-up truck or van injured in collision with other and unspecified motor vehicles in nontraffic accident

√x7ᵗʰ **V59.20** Unspecified occupant of pick-up truck or van injured in collision with unspecified motor vehicles in nontraffic accident

         Collision NOS involving pick-up truck or van, nontraffic

√x7ᵗʰ **V59.29** Unspecified occupant of pick-up truck or van injured in collision with other motor vehicles in nontraffic accident

√x7ᵗʰ **V59.3** Occupant (driver) (passenger) of pick-up truck or van injured in unspecified nontraffic accident

         Accident NOS involving pick-up truck or van, nontraffic
         Occupant of pick-up truck or van injured in nontraffic accident NOS

√5ᵗʰ **V59.4** Driver of pick-up truck or van injured in collision with other and unspecified motor vehicles in traffic accident

√x7ᵗʰ **V59.40** Driver of pick-up truck or van injured in collision with unspecified motor vehicles in traffic accident

√x7ᵗʰ **V59.49** Driver of pick-up truck or van injured in collision with other motor vehicles in traffic accident

√5ᵗʰ **V59.5** Passenger in pick-up truck or van injured in collision with other and unspecified motor vehicles in traffic accident

√x7ᵗʰ **V59.50** Passenger in pick-up truck or van injured in collision with unspecified motor vehicles in traffic accident

√x7ᵗʰ **V59.59** Passenger in pick-up truck or van injured in collision with other motor vehicles in traffic accident

√5ᵗʰ **V59.6** Unspecified occupant of pick-up truck or van injured in collision with other and unspecified motor vehicles in traffic accident

√x7ᵗʰ **V59.60** Unspecified occupant of pick-up truck or van injured in collision with unspecified motor vehicles in traffic accident

         Collision NOS involving pick-up truck or van (traffic)

√x7ᵗʰ **V59.69** Unspecified occupant of pick-up truck or van injured in collision with other motor vehicles in traffic accident

√5ᵗʰ **V59.8** Occupant (driver) (passenger) of pick-up truck or van injured in other specified transport accidents

√x7ᵗʰ **V59.81** Occupant (driver) (passenger) of pick-up truck or van injured in transport accident with military vehicle

√x7ᵗʰ **V59.88** Occupant (driver) (passenger) of pick-up truck or van injured in other specified transport accidents

√x7ᵗʰ **V59.9** Occupant (driver) (passenger) of pick-up truck or van injured in unspecified traffic accident

         Accident NOS involving pick-up truck or van

Occupant of heavy transport vehicle injured in transport accident (V60-V69)

INCLUDES   18 wheeler
           armored car
           panel truck
EXCLUDES 1   *bus*
           motorcoach

The appropriate 7th character is to be added to each code from categories V60-V69.
A   initial encounter
D   subsequent encounter
S   sequela

√4ᵗʰ **V60** Occupant of heavy transport vehicle injured in collision with pedestrian or animal

     EXCLUDES 1   *heavy transport vehicle collision with animal-drawn vehicle or animal being ridden (V66.-)*

√x7ᵗʰ **V60.0** Driver of heavy transport vehicle injured in collision with pedestrian or animal in nontraffic accident

√x7ᵗʰ **V60.1** Passenger in heavy transport vehicle injured in collision with pedestrian or animal in nontraffic accident

√x7ᵗʰ **V60.2** Person on outside of heavy transport vehicle injured in collision with pedestrian or animal in nontraffic accident

√x7ᵗʰ **V60.3** Unspecified occupant of heavy transport vehicle injured in collision with pedestrian or animal in nontraffic accident

√x7ᵗʰ **V60.4** Person boarding or alighting a heavy transport vehicle injured in collision with pedestrian or animal

√x7ᵗʰ **V60.5** Driver of heavy transport vehicle injured in collision with pedestrian or animal in traffic accident

√x7ᵗʰ **V60.6** Passenger in heavy transport vehicle injured in collision with pedestrian or animal in traffic accident

√x7ᵗʰ **V60.7** Person on outside of heavy transport vehicle injured in collision with pedestrian or animal in traffic accident

√x7ᵗʰ **V60.9** Unspecified occupant of heavy transport vehicle injured in collision with pedestrian or animal in traffic accident

√4ᵗʰ **V61** Occupant of heavy transport vehicle injured in collision with pedal cycle

√x7ᵗʰ **V61.0** Driver of heavy transport vehicle injured in collision with pedal cycle in nontraffic accident

√x7ᵗʰ **V61.1** Passenger in heavy transport vehicle injured in collision with pedal cycle in nontraffic accident

√x7ᵗʰ **V61.2** Person on outside of heavy transport vehicle injured in collision with pedal cycle in nontraffic accident

√x7ᵗʰ **V61.3** Unspecified occupant of heavy transport vehicle injured in collision with pedal cycle in nontraffic accident

√x7ᵗʰ **V61.4** Person boarding or alighting a heavy transport vehicle injured in collision with pedal cycle while boarding or alighting

√x7ᵗʰ **V61.5** Driver of heavy transport vehicle injured in collision with pedal cycle in traffic accident

√x7ᵗʰ **V61.6** Passenger in heavy transport vehicle injured in collision with pedal cycle in traffic accident

√x7ᵗʰ **V61.7** Person on outside of heavy transport vehicle injured in collision with pedal cycle in traffic accident

√x7ᵗʰ **V61.9** Unspecified occupant of heavy transport vehicle injured in collision with pedal cycle in traffic accident

√4ᵗʰ **V62** Occupant of heavy transport vehicle injured in collision with two- or three-wheeled motor vehicle

√x7ᵗʰ **V62.0** Driver of heavy transport vehicle injured in collision with two- or three-wheeled motor vehicle in nontraffic accident

√x7ᵗʰ **V62.1** Passenger in heavy transport vehicle injured in collision with two- or three-wheeled motor vehicle in nontraffic accident

√x7ᵗʰ **V62.2** Person on outside of heavy transport vehicle injured in collision with two- or three-wheeled motor vehicle in nontraffic accident

√x7ᵗʰ **V62.3** Unspecified occupant of heavy transport vehicle injured in collision with two- or three-wheeled motor vehicle in nontraffic accident

√x7ᵗʰ **V62.4** Person boarding or alighting a heavy transport vehicle injured in collision with two- or three-wheeled motor vehicle

√x7ᵗʰ **V62.5** Driver of heavy transport vehicle injured in collision with two- or three-wheeled motor vehicle in traffic accident

√x7ᵗʰ **V62.6** Passenger in heavy transport vehicle injured in collision with two- or three-wheeled motor vehicle in traffic accident

√x7ᵗʰ **V62.7** Person on outside of heavy transport vehicle injured in collision with two- or three-wheeled motor vehicle in traffic accident

√x7ᵗʰ **V62.9** Unspecified occupant of heavy transport vehicle injured in collision with two- or three-wheeled motor vehicle in traffic accident

√4ᵗʰ **V63** Occupant of heavy transport vehicle injured in collision with car, pick-up truck or van

√x7ᵗʰ **V63.0** Driver of heavy transport vehicle injured in collision with car, pick-up truck or van in nontraffic accident

√x7ᵗʰ **V63.1** Passenger in heavy transport vehicle injured in collision with car, pick-up truck or van in nontraffic accident

√x7ᵗʰ **V63.2** Person on outside of heavy transport vehicle injured in collision with car, pick-up truck or van in nontraffic accident

√x7ᵗʰ **V63.3** Unspecified occupant of heavy transport vehicle injured in collision with car, pick-up truck or van in nontraffic accident

√x7ᵗʰ **V63.4** Person boarding or alighting a heavy transport vehicle injured in collision with car, pick-up truck or van

√x7ᵗʰ **V63.5** Driver of heavy transport vehicle injured in collision with car, pick-up truck or van in traffic accident

√x7ᵗʰ **V63.6** Passenger in heavy transport vehicle injured in collision with car, pick-up truck or van in traffic accident

√x7ᵗʰ **V63.7** Person on outside of heavy transport vehicle injured in collision with car, pick-up truck or van in traffic accident

√x7ᵗʰ **V63.9** Unspecified occupant of heavy transport vehicle injured in collision with car, pick-up truck or van in traffic accident

√4ᵗʰ **V64** Occupant of heavy transport vehicle injured in collision with heavy transport vehicle or bus

    EXCLUDES 1   occupant of heavy transport vehicle injured in collision with military vehicle (V69.81)

√x7ᵗʰ **V64.0** Driver of heavy transport vehicle injured in collision with heavy transport vehicle or bus in nontraffic accident

√x7ᵗʰ **V64.1** Passenger in heavy transport vehicle injured in collision with heavy transport vehicle or bus in nontraffic accident

√x7ᵗʰ **V64.2** Person on outside of heavy transport vehicle injured in collision with heavy transport vehicle or bus in nontraffic accident

√x7ᵗʰ **V64.3** Unspecified occupant of heavy transport vehicle injured in collision with heavy transport vehicle or bus in nontraffic accident

√x7ᵗʰ **V64.4** Person boarding or alighting a heavy transport vehicle injured in collision with heavy transport vehicle or bus while boarding or alighting

√x7ᵗʰ **V64.5** Driver of heavy transport vehicle injured in collision with heavy transport vehicle or bus in traffic accident

√x7ᵗʰ **V64.6** Passenger in heavy transport vehicle injured in collision with heavy transport vehicle or bus in traffic accident

√x7ᵗʰ **V64.7** Person on outside of heavy transport vehicle injured in collision with heavy transport vehicle or bus in traffic accident

√x7ᵗʰ **V64.9** Unspecified occupant of heavy transport vehicle injured in collision with heavy transport vehicle or bus in traffic accident

√4ᵗʰ **V65** Occupant of heavy transport vehicle injured in collision with railway train or railway vehicle

√x7ᵗʰ **V65.0** Driver of heavy transport vehicle injured in collision with railway train or railway vehicle in nontraffic accident

√x7ᵗʰ **V65.1** Passenger in heavy transport vehicle injured in collision with railway train or railway vehicle in nontraffic accident

√x7ᵗʰ **V65.2** Person on outside of heavy transport vehicle injured in collision with railway train or railway vehicle in nontraffic accident

√x7ᵗʰ **V65.3** Unspecified occupant of heavy transport vehicle injured in collision with railway train or railway vehicle in nontraffic accident

√x7ᵗʰ **V65.4** Person boarding or alighting a heavy transport vehicle injured in collision with railway train or railway vehicle

√x7ᵗʰ **V65.5** Driver of heavy transport vehicle injured in collision with railway train or railway vehicle in traffic accident

√x7ᵗʰ **V65.6** Passenger in heavy transport vehicle injured in collision with railway train or railway vehicle in traffic accident

√x7ᵗʰ **V65.7** Person on outside of heavy transport vehicle injured in collision with railway train or railway vehicle in traffic accident

√x7ᵗʰ **V65.9** Unspecified occupant of heavy transport vehicle injured in collision with railway train or railway vehicle in traffic accident

√4ᵗʰ **V66** Occupant of heavy transport vehicle injured in collision with other nonmotor vehicle

    INCLUDES   collision with animal-drawn vehicle, animal being ridden, streetcar

√x7ᵗʰ **V66.0** Driver of heavy transport vehicle injured in collision with other nonmotor vehicle in nontraffic accident

√x7ᵗʰ **V66.1** Passenger in heavy transport vehicle injured in collision with other nonmotor vehicle in nontraffic accident

√x7ᵗʰ **V66.2** Person on outside of heavy transport vehicle injured in collision with other nonmotor vehicle in nontraffic accident

√x7ᵗʰ **V66.3** Unspecified occupant of heavy transport vehicle injured in collision with other nonmotor vehicle in nontraffic accident

√x7ᵗʰ **V66.4** Person boarding or alighting a heavy transport vehicle injured in collision with other nonmotor vehicle

√x7ᵗʰ **V66.5** Driver of heavy transport vehicle injured in collision with other nonmotor vehicle in traffic accident

√x7ᵗʰ **V66.6** Passenger in heavy transport vehicle injured in collision with other nonmotor vehicle in traffic accident

√x7ᵗʰ **V66.7** Person on outside of heavy transport vehicle injured in collision with other nonmotor vehicle in traffic accident

√x7ᵗʰ **V66.9** Unspecified occupant of heavy transport vehicle injured in collision with other nonmotor vehicle in traffic accident

√4ᵗʰ **V67** Occupant of heavy transport vehicle injured in collision with fixed or stationary object

√x7ᵗʰ **V67.0** Driver of heavy transport vehicle injured in collision with fixed or stationary object in nontraffic accident

√x7ᵗʰ **V67.1** Passenger in heavy transport vehicle injured in collision with fixed or stationary object in nontraffic accident

√x7ᵗʰ **V67.2** Person on outside of heavy transport vehicle injured in collision with fixed or stationary object in nontraffic accident

√x7ᵗʰ **V67.3** Unspecified occupant of heavy transport vehicle injured in collision with fixed or stationary object in nontraffic accident

√x7ᵗʰ **V67.4** Person boarding or alighting a heavy transport vehicle injured in collision with fixed or stationary object

√x7ᵗʰ **V67.5** Driver of heavy transport vehicle injured in collision with fixed or stationary object in traffic accident

√x7ᵗʰ **V67.6** Passenger in heavy transport vehicle injured in collision with fixed or stationary object in traffic accident

√x7ᵗʰ **V67.7** Person on outside of heavy transport vehicle injured in collision with fixed or stationary object in traffic accident

√x7ᵗʰ **V67.9** Unspecified occupant of heavy transport vehicle injured in collision with fixed or stationary object in traffic accident

√4ᵗʰ **V68** Occupant of heavy transport vehicle injured in noncollision transport accident

    INCLUDES   overturning heavy transport vehicle NOS

                      overturning heavy transport vehicle without collision

√x7ᵗʰ **V68.0** Driver of heavy transport vehicle injured in noncollision transport accident in nontraffic accident

√x7ᵗʰ **V68.1** Passenger in heavy transport vehicle injured in noncollision transport accident in nontraffic accident

---

☑ Additional Char Req   √x7ᵗʰ Placeholder   Unacceptable PDx   Questionable PDx   Wrong Procedure   Manifestation   Unspecified Dx   **H1**-**H14** HAC   **HCC** CMS-HCC Dx   **HIV** HIV Dx

√x7ᵗʰ **V68.2** Person on outside of heavy transport vehicle injured in noncollision transport accident in nontraffic accident

√x7ᵗʰ **V68.3** Unspecified occupant of heavy transport vehicle injured in noncollision transport accident in nontraffic accident

√x7ᵗʰ **V68.4** Person boarding or alighting a heavy transport vehicle injured in noncollision transport accident

√x7ᵗʰ **V68.5** Driver of heavy transport vehicle injured in noncollision transport accident in traffic accident

√x7ᵗʰ **V68.6** Passenger in heavy transport vehicle injured in noncollision transport accident in traffic accident

√x7ᵗʰ **V68.7** Person on outside of heavy transport vehicle injured in noncollision transport accident in traffic accident

√x7ᵗʰ **V68.9** Unspecified occupant of heavy transport vehicle injured in noncollision transport accident in traffic accident

√4ᵗʰ **V69** Occupant of heavy transport vehicle injured in other and unspecified transport accidents

√5ᵗʰ **V69.0** Driver of heavy transport vehicle injured in collision with other and unspecified motor vehicles in nontraffic accident

√x7ᵗʰ **V69.00** Driver of heavy transport vehicle injured in collision with unspecified motor vehicles in nontraffic accident

√x7ᵗʰ **V69.09** Driver of heavy transport vehicle injured in collision with other motor vehicles in nontraffic accident

√5ᵗʰ **V69.1** Passenger in heavy transport vehicle injured in collision with other and unspecified motor vehicles in nontraffic accident

√x7ᵗʰ **V69.10** Passenger in heavy transport vehicle injured in collision with unspecified motor vehicles in nontraffic accident

√x7ᵗʰ **V69.19** Passenger in heavy transport vehicle injured in collision with other motor vehicles in nontraffic accident

√5ᵗʰ **V69.2** Unspecified occupant of heavy transport vehicle injured in collision with other and unspecified motor vehicles in nontraffic accident

√x7ᵗʰ **V69.20** Unspecified occupant of heavy transport vehicle injured in collision with unspecified motor vehicles in nontraffic accident

Collision NOS involving heavy transport vehicle, nontraffic

√x7ᵗʰ **V69.29** Unspecified occupant of heavy transport vehicle injured in collision with other motor vehicles in nontraffic accident

√x7ᵗʰ **V69.3** Occupant (driver) (passenger) of heavy transport vehicle injured in unspecified nontraffic accident

Accident NOS involving heavy transport vehicle, nontraffic
Occupant of heavy transport vehicle injured in nontraffic accident NOS

√5ᵗʰ **V69.4** Driver of heavy transport vehicle injured in collision with other and unspecified motor vehicles in traffic accident

√x7ᵗʰ **V69.40** Driver of heavy transport vehicle injured in collision with unspecified motor vehicles in traffic accident

√x7ᵗʰ **V69.49** Driver of heavy transport vehicle injured in collision with other motor vehicles in traffic accident

√5ᵗʰ **V69.5** Passenger in heavy transport vehicle injured in collision with other and unspecified motor vehicles in traffic accident

√x7ᵗʰ **V69.50** Passenger in heavy transport vehicle injured in collision with unspecified motor vehicles in traffic accident

√x7ᵗʰ **V69.59** Passenger in heavy transport vehicle injured in collision with other motor vehicles in traffic accident

√5ᵗʰ **V69.6** Unspecified occupant of heavy transport vehicle injured in collision with other and unspecified motor vehicles in traffic accident

√x7ᵗʰ **V69.60** Unspecified occupant of heavy transport vehicle injured in collision with unspecified motor vehicles in traffic accident

Collision NOS involving heavy transport vehicle (traffic)

√x7ᵗʰ **V69.69** Unspecified occupant of heavy transport vehicle injured in collision with other motor vehicles in traffic accident

√5ᵗʰ **V69.8** Occupant (driver) (passenger) of heavy transport vehicle injured in other specified transport accidents

√x7ᵗʰ **V69.81** Occupant (driver) (passenger) of heavy transport vehicle injured in transport accidents with military vehicle

√x7ᵗʰ **V69.88** Occupant (driver) (passenger) of heavy transport vehicle injured in other specified transport accidents

√x7ᵗʰ **V69.9** Occupant (driver) (passenger) of heavy transport vehicle injured in unspecified traffic accident

Accident NOS involving heavy transport vehicle

Bus occupant injured in transport accident (V70-V79)

| INCLUDES | motorcoach |
| EXCLUDES 1 | minibus (V50-V59) |

The appropriate 7th character is to be added to each code from categories V70-V79.
A   initial encounter
D   subsequent encounter
S   sequela

√4ᵗʰ **V70** Bus occupant injured in collision with pedestrian or animal

EXCLUDES 1   *bus collision with animal-drawn vehicle or animal being ridden (V76.-)*

√x7ᵗʰ **V70.0** Driver of bus injured in collision with pedestrian or animal in nontraffic accident

√x7ᵗʰ **V70.1** Passenger on bus injured in collision with pedestrian or animal in nontraffic accident

√x7ᵗʰ **V70.2** Person on outside of bus injured in collision with pedestrian or animal in nontraffic accident

√x7ᵗʰ **V70.3** Unspecified occupant of bus injured in collision with pedestrian or animal in nontraffic accident

√x7ᵗʰ **V70.4** Person boarding or alighting from bus injured in collision with pedestrian or animal

√x7ᵗʰ **V70.5** Driver of bus injured in collision with pedestrian or animal in traffic accident

√x7ᵗʰ **V70.6** Passenger on bus injured in collision with pedestrian or animal in traffic accident

√x7ᵗʰ **V70.7** Person on outside of bus injured in collision with pedestrian or animal in traffic accident

√x7ᵗʰ **V70.9** Unspecified occupant of bus injured in collision with pedestrian or animal in traffic accident

√4ᵗʰ **V71** Bus occupant injured in collision with pedal cycle

√x7ᵗʰ **V71.0** Driver of bus injured in collision with pedal cycle in nontraffic accident

√x7ᵗʰ **V71.1** Passenger on bus injured in collision with pedal cycle in nontraffic accident

√x7ᵗʰ **V71.2** Person on outside of bus injured in collision with pedal cycle in nontraffic accident

√x7ᵗʰ **V71.3** Unspecified occupant of bus injured in collision with pedal cycle in nontraffic accident

√x7ᵗʰ **V71.4** Person boarding or alighting from bus injured in collision with pedal cycle

√x7ᵗʰ **V71.5** Driver of bus injured in collision with pedal cycle in traffic accident

√x7ᵗʰ **V71.6** Passenger on bus injured in collision with pedal cycle in traffic accident

√x7ᵗʰ **V71.7** Person on outside of bus injured in collision with pedal cycle in traffic accident

√x7ᵗʰ **V71.9** Unspecified occupant of bus injured in collision with pedal cycle in traffic accident

√4ᵗʰ **V72** Bus occupant injured in collision with two- or three-wheeled motor vehicle

√x7ᵗʰ **V72.0** Driver of bus injured in collision with two- or three-wheeled motor vehicle in nontraffic accident

√x7ᵗʰ **V72.1** Passenger on bus injured in collision with two- or three-wheeled motor vehicle in nontraffic accident

√x7ᵗʰ **V72.2** Person on outside of bus injured in collision with two- or three-wheeled motor vehicle in nontraffic accident

√x7ᵗʰ **V72.3** Unspecified occupant of bus injured in collision with two- or three-wheeled motor vehicle in nontraffic accident

√x7ᵗʰ **V72.4** Person boarding or alighting from bus injured in collision with two- or three-wheeled motor vehicle

√x7ᵗʰ **V72.5** Driver of bus injured in collision with two- or three-wheeled motor vehicle in traffic accident

√x7ᵗʰ **V72.6** Passenger on bus injured in collision with two- or three-wheeled motor vehicle in traffic accident

√x7ᵗʰ **V72.7** Person on outside of bus injured in collision with two- or three-wheeled motor vehicle in traffic accident

√x7ᵗʰ **V72.9** Unspecified occupant of bus injured in collision with two- or three-wheeled motor vehicle in traffic accident

√4ᵗʰ **V73** Bus occupant injured in collision with car, pick-up truck or van

√x7ᵗʰ **V73.0** Driver of bus injured in collision with car, pick-up truck or van in nontraffic accident

√x7ᵗʰ **V73.1** Passenger on bus injured in collision with car, pick-up truck or van in nontraffic accident

√x7ᵗʰ **V73.2** Person on outside of bus injured in collision with car, pick-up truck or van in nontraffic accident

N Newborn: 0   **P** Pediatric: 0-17   **M** Maternity: 9-64   **A** Adult: 15-124   **MCC** Major Complication/Comorbidity   **CC** Complication/Comorbidity   **SW** Severe Wound Dx

1186   ICD-10-CM 2021

√x7ᵗʰ **V73.3** Unspecified occupant of bus injured in collision with car, pick-up truck or van in nontraffic accident

√x7ᵗʰ **V73.4** Person boarding or alighting from bus injured in collision with car, pick-up truck or van

√x7ᵗʰ **V73.5** Driver of bus injured in collision with car, pick-up truck or van in traffic accident

√x7ᵗʰ **V73.6** Passenger on bus injured in collision with car, pick-up truck or van in traffic accident

√x7ᵗʰ **V73.7** Person on outside of bus injured in collision with car, pick-up truck or van in traffic accident

√x7ᵗʰ **V73.9** Unspecified occupant of bus injured in collision with car, pick-up truck or van in traffic accident

√4ᵗʰ **V74** **Bus occupant injured in collision with heavy transport vehicle or bus**

     EXCLUDES 1   *bus occupant injured in collision with military vehicle (V79.81)*

√x7ᵗʰ **V74.0** Driver of bus injured in collision with heavy transport vehicle or bus in nontraffic accident

√x7ᵗʰ **V74.1** Passenger on bus injured in collision with heavy transport vehicle or bus in nontraffic accident

√x7ᵗʰ **V74.2** Person on outside of bus injured in collision with heavy transport vehicle or bus in nontraffic accident

√x7ᵗʰ **V74.3** Unspecified occupant of bus injured in collision with heavy transport vehicle or bus in nontraffic accident

√x7ᵗʰ **V74.4** Person boarding or alighting from bus injured in collision with heavy transport vehicle or bus

√x7ᵗʰ **V74.5** Driver of bus injured in collision with heavy transport vehicle or bus in traffic accident

√x7ᵗʰ **V74.6** Passenger on bus injured in collision with heavy transport vehicle or bus in traffic accident

√x7ᵗʰ **V74.7** Person on outside of bus injured in collision with heavy transport vehicle or bus in traffic accident

√x7ᵗʰ **V74.9** Unspecified occupant of bus injured in collision with heavy transport vehicle or bus in traffic accident

√4ᵗʰ **V75** **Bus occupant injured in collision with railway train or railway vehicle**

√x7ᵗʰ **V75.0** Driver of bus injured in collision with railway train or railway vehicle in nontraffic accident

√x7ᵗʰ **V75.1** Passenger on bus injured in collision with railway train or railway vehicle in nontraffic accident

√x7ᵗʰ **V75.2** Person on outside of bus injured in collision with railway train or railway vehicle in nontraffic accident

√x7ᵗʰ **V75.3** Unspecified occupant of bus injured in collision with railway train or railway vehicle in nontraffic accident

√x7ᵗʰ **V75.4** Person boarding or alighting from bus injured in collision with railway train or railway vehicle

√x7ᵗʰ **V75.5** Driver of bus injured in collision with railway train or railway vehicle in traffic accident

√x7ᵗʰ **V75.6** Passenger on bus injured in collision with railway train or railway vehicle in traffic accident

√x7ᵗʰ **V75.7** Person on outside of bus injured in collision with railway train or railway vehicle in traffic accident

√x7ᵗʰ **V75.9** Unspecified occupant of bus injured in collision with railway train or railway vehicle in traffic accident

√4ᵗʰ **V76** **Bus occupant injured in collision with other nonmotor vehicle**

     INCLUDES   collision with animal-drawn vehicle, animal being ridden, streetcar

√x7ᵗʰ **V76.0** Driver of bus injured in collision with other nonmotor vehicle in nontraffic accident

√x7ᵗʰ **V76.1** Passenger on bus injured in collision with other nonmotor vehicle in nontraffic accident

√x7ᵗʰ **V76.2** Person on outside of bus injured in collision with other nonmotor vehicle in nontraffic accident

√x7ᵗʰ **V76.3** Unspecified occupant of bus injured in collision with other nonmotor vehicle in nontraffic accident

√x7ᵗʰ **V76.4** Person boarding or alighting from bus injured in collision with other nonmotor vehicle

√x7ᵗʰ **V76.5** Driver of bus injured in collision with other nonmotor vehicle in traffic accident

√x7ᵗʰ **V76.6** Passenger on bus injured in collision with other nonmotor vehicle in traffic accident

√x7ᵗʰ **V76.7** Person on outside of bus injured in collision with other nonmotor vehicle in traffic accident

√x7ᵗʰ **V76.9** Unspecified occupant of bus injured in collision with other nonmotor vehicle in traffic accident

√4ᵗʰ **V77** **Bus occupant injured in collision with fixed or stationary object**

√x7ᵗʰ **V77.0** Driver of bus injured in collision with fixed or stationary object in nontraffic accident

√x7ᵗʰ **V77.1** Passenger on bus injured in collision with fixed or stationary object in nontraffic accident

√x7ᵗʰ **V77.2** Person on outside of bus injured in collision with fixed or stationary object in nontraffic accident

√x7ᵗʰ **V77.3** Unspecified occupant of bus injured in collision with fixed or stationary object in nontraffic accident

√x7ᵗʰ **V77.4** Person boarding or alighting from bus injured in collision with fixed or stationary object

√x7ᵗʰ **V77.5** Driver of bus injured in collision with fixed or stationary object in traffic accident

√x7ᵗʰ **V77.6** Passenger on bus injured in collision with fixed or stationary object in traffic accident

√x7ᵗʰ **V77.7** Person on outside of bus injured in collision with fixed or stationary object in traffic accident

√x7ᵗʰ **V77.9** Unspecified occupant of bus injured in collision with fixed or stationary object in traffic accident

√4ᵗʰ **V78** **Bus occupant injured in noncollision transport accident**

     INCLUDES   overturning bus NOS

                       overturning bus without collision

√x7ᵗʰ **V78.0** Driver of bus injured in noncollision transport accident in nontraffic accident

√x7ᵗʰ **V78.1** Passenger on bus injured in noncollision transport accident in nontraffic accident

√x7ᵗʰ **V78.2** Person on outside of bus injured in noncollision transport accident in nontraffic accident

√x7ᵗʰ **V78.3** Unspecified occupant of bus injured in noncollision transport accident in nontraffic accident

√x7ᵗʰ **V78.4** Person boarding or alighting from bus injured in noncollision transport accident

√x7ᵗʰ **V78.5** Driver of bus injured in noncollision transport accident in traffic accident

√x7ᵗʰ **V78.6** Passenger on bus injured in noncollision transport accident in traffic accident

√x7ᵗʰ **V78.7** Person on outside of bus injured in noncollision transport accident in traffic accident

√x7ᵗʰ **V78.9** Unspecified occupant of bus injured in noncollision transport accident in traffic accident

√4ᵗʰ **V79** **Bus occupant injured in other and unspecified transport accidents**

√5ᵗʰ **V79.0** Driver of bus injured in collision with other and unspecified motor vehicles in nontraffic accident

    √x7ᵗʰ **V79.00** Driver of bus injured in collision with unspecified motor vehicles in nontraffic accident

    √x7ᵗʰ **V79.09** Driver of bus injured in collision with other motor vehicles in nontraffic accident

√5ᵗʰ **V79.1** Passenger on bus injured in collision with other and unspecified motor vehicles in nontraffic accident

    √x7ᵗʰ **V79.10** Passenger on bus injured in collision with unspecified motor vehicles in nontraffic accident

    √x7ᵗʰ **V79.19** Passenger on bus injured in collision with other motor vehicles in nontraffic accident

√5ᵗʰ **V79.2** Unspecified bus occupant injured in collision with other and unspecified motor vehicles in nontraffic accident

    √x7ᵗʰ **V79.20** Unspecified bus occupant injured in collision with unspecified motor vehicles in nontraffic accident

         Bus collision NOS, nontraffic

    √x7ᵗʰ **V79.29** Unspecified bus occupant injured in collision with other motor vehicles in nontraffic accident

√x7ᵗʰ **V79.3** Bus occupant (driver) (passenger) injured in unspecified nontraffic accident

       Bus accident NOS, nontraffic

       Bus occupant injured in nontraffic accident NOS

√5ᵗʰ **V79.4** Driver of bus injured in collision with other and unspecified motor vehicles in traffic accident

    √x7ᵗʰ **V79.40** Driver of bus injured in collision with unspecified motor vehicles in traffic accident

    √x7ᵗʰ **V79.49** Driver of bus injured in collision with other motor vehicles in traffic accident

√5ᵗʰ **V79.5** Passenger on bus injured in collision with other and unspecified motor vehicles in traffic accident

    √x7ᵗʰ **V79.50** Passenger on bus injured in collision with unspecified motor vehicles in traffic accident

    √x7ᵗʰ **V79.59** Passenger on bus injured in collision with other motor vehicles in traffic accident

√5ᵗʰ **V79.6** Unspecified bus occupant injured in collision with other and unspecified motor vehicles in traffic accident

    √x7ᵗʰ **V79.60** Unspecified bus occupant injured in collision with unspecified motor vehicles in traffic accident

         Bus collision NOS (traffic)

    √x7ᵗʰ **V79.69** Unspecified bus occupant injured in collision with other motor vehicles in traffic accident

✔ Additional Char Req   √x7ᵗʰ Placeholder   Unacceptable PDx   Questionable PDx   Wrong Procedure   Manifestation   Unspecified Dx   H1-H14 HAC   HCC CMS-HCC Dx   HIV HIV Dx

ICD-10-CM 2021   1187

√5ᵗʰ **V79.8** Bus occupant (driver) (passenger) injured in other specified transport accidents

√x7ᵗʰ **V79.81** Bus occupant (driver) (passenger) injured in transport accidents with military vehicle

√x7ᵗʰ **V79.88** Bus occupant (driver) (passenger) injured in other specified transport accidents

√x7ᵗʰ **V79.9** Bus occupant (driver) (passenger) injured in unspecified traffic accident

Bus accident NOS

Other land transport accidents (V80–V89)

The appropriate 7th character is to be added to each code from categories V80-V89.
A   initial encounter
D   subsequent encounter
S   sequela

√4ᵗʰ **V80** Animal-rider or occupant of animal-drawn vehicle injured in transport accident

√5ᵗʰ **V80.0** Animal-rider or occupant of animal drawn vehicle injured by fall from or being thrown from animal or animal-drawn vehicle in noncollision accident

√6ᵗʰ **V80.01** Animal-rider injured by fall from or being thrown from animal in noncollision accident

√7ᵗʰ **V80.010** Animal-rider injured by fall from or being thrown from horse in noncollision accident

√7ᵗʰ **V80.018** Animal-rider injured by fall from or being thrown from other animal in noncollision accident

√x7ᵗʰ **V80.02** Occupant of animal-drawn vehicle injured by fall from or being thrown from animal-drawn vehicle in noncollision accident

Overturning animal-drawn vehicle NOS
Overturning animal-drawn vehicle without collision

√5ᵗʰ **V80.1** Animal-rider or occupant of animal-drawn vehicle injured in collision with pedestrian or animal

EXCLUDES 1   animal-rider or animal-drawn vehicle collision with animal-drawn vehicle or animal being ridden (V80.7)

√x7ᵗʰ **V80.11** Animal-rider injured in collision with pedestrian or animal

√x7ᵗʰ **V80.12** Occupant of animal-drawn vehicle injured in collision with pedestrian or animal

√5ᵗʰ **V80.2** Animal-rider or occupant of animal-drawn vehicle injured in collision with pedal cycle

√x7ᵗʰ **V80.21** Animal-rider injured in collision with pedal cycle

√x7ᵗʰ **V80.22** Occupant of animal-drawn vehicle injured in collision with pedal cycle

√5ᵗʰ **V80.3** Animal-rider or occupant of animal-drawn vehicle injured in collision with two- or three-wheeled motor vehicle

√x7ᵗʰ **V80.31** Animal-rider injured in collision with two- or three-wheeled motor vehicle

√x7ᵗʰ **V80.32** Occupant of animal-drawn vehicle injured in collision with two- or three-wheeled motor vehicle

√5ᵗʰ **V80.4** Animal-rider or occupant of animal-drawn vehicle injured in collision with car, pick-up truck, van, heavy transport vehicle or bus

EXCLUDES 1   animal-rider injured in collision with military vehicle (V80.910)
occupant of animal-drawn vehicle injured in collision with military vehicle (V80.920)

√x7ᵗʰ **V80.41** Animal-rider injured in collision with car, pick-up truck, van, heavy transport vehicle or bus

√x7ᵗʰ **V80.42** Occupant of animal-drawn vehicle injured in collision with car, pick-up truck, van, heavy transport vehicle or bus

√5ᵗʰ **V80.5** Animal-rider or occupant of animal-drawn vehicle injured in collision with other specified motor vehicle

√x7ᵗʰ **V80.51** Animal-rider injured in collision with other specified motor vehicle

√x7ᵗʰ **V80.52** Occupant of animal-drawn vehicle injured in collision with other specified motor vehicle

√5ᵗʰ **V80.6** Animal-rider or occupant of animal-drawn vehicle injured in collision with railway train or railway vehicle

√x7ᵗʰ **V80.61** Animal-rider injured in collision with railway train or railway vehicle

√x7ᵗʰ **V80.62** Occupant of animal-drawn vehicle injured in collision with railway train or railway vehicle

√5ᵗʰ **V80.7** Animal-rider or occupant of animal-drawn vehicle injured in collision with other nonmotor vehicles

√6ᵗʰ **V80.71** Animal-rider or occupant of animal-drawn vehicle injured in collision with animal being ridden

√7ᵗʰ **V80.710** Animal-rider injured in collision with other animal being ridden

√7ᵗʰ **V80.711** Occupant of animal-drawn vehicle injured in collision with animal being ridden

√6ᵗʰ **V80.72** Animal-rider or occupant of animal-drawn vehicle injured in collision with other animal-drawn vehicle

√7ᵗʰ **V80.720** Animal-rider injured in collision with animal-drawn vehicle

√7ᵗʰ **V80.721** Occupant of animal-drawn vehicle injured in collision with other animal-drawn vehicle

√6ᵗʰ **V80.73** Animal-rider or occupant of animal-drawn vehicle injured in collision with streetcar

√7ᵗʰ **V80.730** Animal-rider injured in collision with streetcar

√7ᵗʰ **V80.731** Occupant of animal-drawn vehicle injured in collision with streetcar

√6ᵗʰ **V80.79** Animal-rider or occupant of animal-drawn vehicle injured in collision with other nonmotor vehicles

√7ᵗʰ **V80.790** Animal-rider injured in collision with other nonmotor vehicles

√7ᵗʰ **V80.791** Occupant of animal-drawn vehicle injured in collision with other nonmotor vehicles

√5ᵗʰ **V80.8** Animal-rider or occupant of animal-drawn vehicle injured in collision with fixed or stationary object

√x7ᵗʰ **V80.81** Animal-rider injured in collision with fixed or stationary object

√x7ᵗʰ **V80.82** Occupant of animal-drawn vehicle injured in collision with fixed or stationary object

√5ᵗʰ **V80.9** Animal-rider or occupant of animal-drawn vehicle injured in other and unspecified transport accidents

√6ᵗʰ **V80.91** Animal-rider injured in other and unspecified transport accidents

√7ᵗʰ **V80.910** Animal-rider injured in transport accident with military vehicle

√7ᵗʰ **V80.918** Animal-rider injured in other transport accident

√7ᵗʰ **V80.919** Animal-rider injured in unspecified transport accident

Animal rider accident NOS

√6ᵗʰ **V80.92** Occupant of animal-drawn vehicle injured in other and unspecified transport accidents

√7ᵗʰ **V80.920** Occupant of animal-drawn vehicle injured in transport accident with military vehicle

√7ᵗʰ **V80.928** Occupant of animal-drawn vehicle injured in other transport accident

√7ᵗʰ **V80.929** Occupant of animal-drawn vehicle injured in unspecified transport accident

Animal-drawn vehicle accident NOS

√4ᵗʰ **V81** Occupant of railway train or railway vehicle injured in transport accident

INCLUDES   derailment of railway train or railway vehicle
person on outside of train

EXCLUDES 1   streetcar (V82.-)

√x7ᵗʰ **V81.0** Occupant of railway train or railway vehicle injured in collision with motor vehicle in nontraffic accident

EXCLUDES 1   occupant of railway train or railway vehicle injured due to collision with military vehicle (V81.83)

√x7ᵗʰ **V81.1** Occupant of railway train or railway vehicle injured in collision with motor vehicle in traffic accident

EXCLUDES 1   occupant of railway train or railway vehicle injured due to collision with military vehicle (V81.83)

√x7ᵗʰ **V81.2** Occupant of railway train or railway vehicle injured in collision with or hit by rolling stock

√x7ᵗʰ **V81.3** Occupant of railway train or railway vehicle injured in collision with other object

Railway collision NOS

√x7ᵗʰ **V81.4** Person injured while boarding or alighting from railway train or railway vehicle

√x7ᵗʰ **V81.5** Occupant of railway train or railway vehicle injured by fall in railway train or railway vehicle

√x7ᵗʰ **V81.6** Occupant of railway train or railway vehicle injured by fall from railway train or railway vehicle

√x7ᵗʰ **V81.7** Occupant of railway train or railway vehicle injured in derailment without antecedent collision

✓5ᵗʰ **V81.8** **Occupant of railway train or railway vehicle injured in other specified railway accidents**

     ✓x7ᵗʰ **V81.81** Occupant of railway train or railway vehicle injured due to explosion or fire on train

     ✓x7ᵗʰ **V81.82** Occupant of railway train or railway vehicle injured due to object falling onto train

         Occupant of railway train or railway vehicle injured due to falling earth onto train

         Occupant of railway train or railway vehicle injured due to falling rocks onto train

         Occupant of railway train or railway vehicle injured due to falling snow onto train

         Occupant of railway train or railway vehicle injured due to falling trees onto train

     ✓x7ᵗʰ **V81.83** Occupant of railway train or railway vehicle injured due to collision with military vehicle

     ✓x7ᵗʰ **V81.89** Occupant of railway train or railway vehicle injured due to other specified railway accident

✓x7ᵗʰ **V81.9** **Occupant of railway train or railway vehicle injured in unspecified railway accident**

     Railway accident NOS

✓4ᵗʰ **V82** **Occupant of powered streetcar injured in transport accident**

     INCLUDES   interurban electric car

         person on outside of streetcar

         tram (car)

         trolley (car)

     EXCLUDES 1   *bus (V70-V79)*

         motorcoach (V70-V79)

         nonpowered streetcar (V76.-)

         train (V81.-)

✓x7ᵗʰ **V82.0** **Occupant of streetcar injured in collision with motor vehicle in nontraffic accident**

✓x7ᵗʰ **V82.1** **Occupant of streetcar injured in collision with motor vehicle in traffic accident**

✓x7ᵗʰ **V82.2** **Occupant of streetcar injured in collision with or hit by rolling stock**

✓x7ᵗʰ **V82.3** **Occupant of streetcar injured in collision with other object**

     EXCLUDES 1   *collision with animal-drawn vehicle or animal being ridden (V82.8)*

✓x7ᵗʰ **V82.4** **Person injured while boarding or alighting from streetcar**

✓x7ᵗʰ **V82.5** **Occupant of streetcar injured by fall in streetcar**

     EXCLUDES 1   *fall in streetcar:*

         while boarding or alighting (V82.4)

         with antecedent collision (V82.0-V82.3)

✓x7ᵗʰ **V82.6** **Occupant of streetcar injured by fall from streetcar**

     EXCLUDES 1   *fall from streetcar:*

         while boarding or alighting (V82.4)

         with antecedent collision (V82.0-V82.3)

✓x7ᵗʰ **V82.7** **Occupant of streetcar injured in derailment without antecedent collision**

     EXCLUDES 1   *occupant of streetcar injured in derailment with antecedent collision (V82.0-V82.3)*

✓x7ᵗʰ **V82.8** **Occupant of streetcar injured in other specified transport accidents**

     Streetcar collision with military vehicle

     Streetcar collision with train or nonmotor vehicles

✓x7ᵗʰ **V82.9** **Occupant of streetcar injured in unspecified traffic accident**

     Streetcar accident NOS

✓4ᵗʰ **V83** **Occupant of special vehicle mainly used on industrial premises injured in transport accident**

     INCLUDES   battery-powered airport passenger vehicle

         battery-powered truck (baggage) (mail)

         coal-car in mine

         forklift (truck)

         logging car

         self-propelled industrial truck

         station baggage truck (powered)

         tram, truck, or tub (powered) in mine or quarry

     EXCLUDES 1   *special construction vehicles (V85.-)*

         special industrial vehicle in stationary use or maintenance (W31.-)

✓x7ᵗʰ **V83.0** **Driver of special industrial vehicle injured in traffic accident**

✓x7ᵗʰ **V83.1** **Passenger of special industrial vehicle injured in traffic accident**

✓x7ᵗʰ **V83.2** **Person on outside of special industrial vehicle injured in traffic accident**

✓x7ᵗʰ **V83.3** **Unspecified occupant of special industrial vehicle injured in traffic accident**

✓x7ᵗʰ **V83.4** **Person injured while boarding or alighting from special industrial vehicle**

✓x7ᵗʰ **V83.5** **Driver of special industrial vehicle injured in nontraffic accident**

✓x7ᵗʰ **V83.6** **Passenger of special industrial vehicle injured in nontraffic accident**

✓x7ᵗʰ **V83.7** **Person on outside of special industrial vehicle injured in nontraffic accident**

✓x7ᵗʰ **V83.9** **Unspecified occupant of special industrial vehicle injured in nontraffic accident**

     Special-industrial-vehicle accident NOS

✓4ᵗʰ **V84** **Occupant of special vehicle mainly used in agriculture injured in transport accident**

     INCLUDES   self-propelled farm machinery

         tractor (and trailer)

     EXCLUDES 1   *animal-powered farm machinery accident (W30.8-)*

         contact with combine harvester (W30.0)

         special agricultural vehicle in stationary use or maintenance (W30.-)

✓x7ᵗʰ **V84.0** **Driver of special agricultural vehicle injured in traffic accident**

✓x7ᵗʰ **V84.1** **Passenger of special agricultural vehicle injured in traffic accident**

✓x7ᵗʰ **V84.2** **Person on outside of special agricultural vehicle injured in traffic accident**

✓x7ᵗʰ **V84.3** **Unspecified occupant of special agricultural vehicle injured in traffic accident**

✓x7ᵗʰ **V84.4** **Person injured while boarding or alighting from special agricultural vehicle**

✓x7ᵗʰ **V84.5** **Driver of special agricultural vehicle injured in nontraffic accident**

✓x7ᵗʰ **V84.6** **Passenger of special agricultural vehicle injured in nontraffic accident**

✓x7ᵗʰ **V84.7** **Person on outside of special agricultural vehicle injured in nontraffic accident**

✓x7ᵗʰ **V84.9** **Unspecified occupant of special agricultural vehicle injured in nontraffic accident**

     Special-agricultural vehicle accident NOS

✓4ᵗʰ **V85** **Occupant of special construction vehicle injured in transport accident**

     INCLUDES   bulldozer

         digger

         dump truck

         earth-leveller

         mechanical shovel

         road-roller

     EXCLUDES 1   *special industrial vehicle (V83.-)*

         special construction vehicle in stationary use or maintenance (W31.-)

✓x7ᵗʰ **V85.0** **Driver of special construction vehicle injured in traffic accident**

✓x7ᵗʰ **V85.1** **Passenger of special construction vehicle injured in traffic accident**

✓x7ᵗʰ **V85.2** **Person on outside of special construction vehicle injured in traffic accident**

✓x7ᵗʰ **V85.3** **Unspecified occupant of special construction vehicle injured in traffic accident**

✓x7ᵗʰ **V85.4** **Person injured while boarding or alighting from special construction vehicle**

✓x7ᵗʰ **V85.5** **Driver of special construction vehicle injured in nontraffic accident**

✓x7ᵗʰ **V85.6** **Passenger of special construction vehicle injured in nontraffic accident**

✓x7ᵗʰ **V85.7** **Person on outside of special construction vehicle injured in nontraffic accident**

✓x7ᵗʰ **V85.9** **Unspecified occupant of special construction vehicle injured in nontraffic accident**

     Special-construction-vehicle accident NOS

✔ Additional Char Req   ✓x7ᵗʰ Placeholder   Unacceptable PDx   Questionable PDx   Wrong Procedure   Manifestation   Unspecified Dx   H1-H14 HAC   HCC CMS-HCC Dx   HIV HIV Dx

ICD-10-CM 2021   1189

√4ᵗʰ V86 Occupant of special all-terrain or other off-road motor vehicle, injured in transport accident

> EXCLUDES 1   special all-terrain vehicle in stationary use or maintenance (W31.-)
>
> sport-utility vehicle (V50-V59)
>
> three-wheeled motor vehicle designed for on-road use (V30-V39)

> AHA: 2017,4Q,26

√5ᵗʰ V86.0 Driver of special all-terrain or other off-road motor vehicle injured in traffic accident

- √x7ᵗʰ **V86.01** Driver of ambulance or fire engine injured in traffic accident
- √x7ᵗʰ **V86.02** Driver of snowmobile injured in traffic accident
- √x7ᵗʰ **V86.03** Driver of dune buggy injured in traffic accident
- √x7ᵗʰ **V86.04** Driver of military vehicle injured in traffic accident
- √x7ᵗʰ **V86.05** Driver of 3- or 4- wheeled all-terrain vehicle (ATV) injured in traffic accident
- √x7ᵗʰ **V86.06** Driver of dirt bike or motor/cross bike injured in traffic accident
- √x7ᵗʰ **V86.09** Driver of other special all-terrain or other off-road motor vehicle injured in traffic accident
  - Driver of go cart injured in traffic accident
  - Driver of golf cart injured in traffic accident

√5ᵗʰ V86.1 Passenger of special all-terrain or other off-road motor vehicle injured in traffic accident

- √x7ᵗʰ **V86.11** Passenger of ambulance or fire engine injured in traffic accident
- √x7ᵗʰ **V86.12** Passenger of snowmobile injured in traffic accident
- √x7ᵗʰ **V86.13** Passenger of dune buggy injured in traffic accident
- √x7ᵗʰ **V86.14** Passenger of military vehicle injured in traffic accident
- √x7ᵗʰ **V86.15** Passenger of 3- or 4- wheeled all-terrain vehicle (ATV) injured in traffic accident
- √x7ᵗʰ **V86.16** Passenger of dirt bike or motor/cross bike injured in traffic accident
- √x7ᵗʰ **V86.19** Passenger of other special all-terrain or other off-road motor vehicle injured in traffic accident
  - Passenger of go cart injured in traffic accident
  - Passenger of golf cart injured in traffic accident

√5ᵗʰ V86.2 Person on outside of special all-terrain or other off-road motor vehicle injured in traffic accident

- √x7ᵗʰ **V86.21** Person on outside of ambulance or fire engine injured in traffic accident
- √x7ᵗʰ **V86.22** Person on outside of snowmobile injured in traffic accident
- √x7ᵗʰ **V86.23** Person on outside of dune buggy injured in traffic accident
- √x7ᵗʰ **V86.24** Person on outside of military vehicle injured in traffic accident
- √x7ᵗʰ **V86.25** Person on outside of 3- or 4- wheeled all-terrain vehicle (ATV) injured in traffic accident
- √x7ᵗʰ **V86.26** Person on outside of dirt bike or motor/cross bike injured in traffic accident
- √x7ᵗʰ **V86.29** Person on outside of other special all-terrain or other off-road motor vehicle injured in traffic accident
  - Person on outside of go cart in traffic accident
  - Person on outside of golf cart injured in traffic accident

√5ᵗʰ V86.3 Unspecified occupant of special all-terrain or other off-road motor vehicle injured in traffic accident

- √x7ᵗʰ **V86.31** Unspecified occupant of ambulance or fire engine injured in traffic accident
- √x7ᵗʰ **V86.32** Unspecified occupant of snowmobile injured in traffic accident
- √x7ᵗʰ **V86.33** Unspecified occupant of dune buggy injured in traffic accident
- √x7ᵗʰ **V86.34** Unspecified occupant of military vehicle injured in traffic accident
- √x7ᵗʰ **V86.35** Unspecified occupant of 3- or 4- wheeled all-terrain vehicle (ATV) injured in traffic accident
- √x7ᵗʰ **V86.36** Unspecified occupant of dirt bike or motor/cross bike injured in traffic accident

- √x7ᵗʰ **V86.39** Unspecified occupant of other special all-terrain or other off-road motor vehicle injured in traffic accident
  - Unspecified occupant of go cart injured in traffic accident
  - Unspecified occupant of golf cart injured in traffic accident

√5ᵗʰ V86.4 Person injured while boarding or alighting from special all-terrain or other off-road motor vehicle

- √x7ᵗʰ **V86.41** Person injured while boarding or alighting from ambulance or fire engine
- √x7ᵗʰ **V86.42** Person injured while boarding or alighting from snowmobile
- √x7ᵗʰ **V86.43** Person injured while boarding or alighting from dune buggy
- √x7ᵗʰ **V86.44** Person injured while boarding or alighting from military vehicle
- √x7ᵗʰ **V86.45** Person injured while boarding or alighting from a 3- or 4- wheeled all-terrain vehicle (ATV)
- √x7ᵗʰ **V86.46** Person injured while boarding or alighting from a dirt bike or motor/cross bike
- √x7ᵗʰ **V86.49** Person injured while boarding or alighting from other special all-terrain or other off-road motor vehicle
  - Person injured while boarding or alighting from go cart
  - Person injured while boarding or alighting from golf cart

√5ᵗʰ V86.5 Driver of special all-terrain or other off-road motor vehicle injured in nontraffic accident

- √x7ᵗʰ **V86.51** Driver of ambulance or fire engine injured in nontraffic accident
- √x7ᵗʰ **V86.52** Driver of snowmobile injured in nontraffic accident
- √x7ᵗʰ **V86.53** Driver of dune buggy injured in nontraffic accident
- √x7ᵗʰ **V86.54** Driver of military vehicle injured in nontraffic accident
- √x7ᵗʰ **V86.55** Driver of 3- or 4- wheeled all-terrain vehicle (ATV) injured in nontraffic accident
- √x7ᵗʰ **V86.56** Driver of dirt bike or motor/cross bike injured in nontraffic accident
- √x7ᵗʰ **V86.59** Driver of other special all-terrain or other off-road motor vehicle injured in nontraffic accident
  - Driver of go cart injured in nontraffic accident
  - Driver of golf cart injured in nontraffic accident

√5ᵗʰ V86.6 Passenger of special all-terrain or other off-road motor vehicle injured in nontraffic accident

- √x7ᵗʰ **V86.61** Passenger of ambulance or fire engine injured in nontraffic accident
- √x7ᵗʰ **V86.62** Passenger of snowmobile injured in nontraffic accident
- √x7ᵗʰ **V86.63** Passenger of dune buggy injured in nontraffic accident
- √x7ᵗʰ **V86.64** Passenger of military vehicle injured in nontraffic accident
- √x7ᵗʰ **V86.65** Passenger of 3- or 4- wheeled all-terrain vehicle (ATV) injured in nontraffic accident
- √x7ᵗʰ **V86.66** Passenger of dirt bike or motor/cross bike injured in nontraffic accident
- √x7ᵗʰ **V86.69** Passenger of other special all-terrain or other off-road motor vehicle injured in nontraffic accident
  - Passenger of go cart injured in nontraffic accident
  - Passenger of golf cart injured in nontraffic accident

√5ᵗʰ V86.7 Person on outside of special all-terrain or other off-road motor vehicle injured in nontraffic accident

- √x7ᵗʰ **V86.71** Person on outside of ambulance or fire engine injured in nontraffic accident
- √x7ᵗʰ **V86.72** Person on outside of snowmobile injured in nontraffic accident
- √x7ᵗʰ **V86.73** Person on outside of dune buggy injured in nontraffic accident
- √x7ᵗʰ **V86.74** Person on outside of military vehicle injured in nontraffic accident
- √x7ᵗʰ **V86.75** Person on outside of 3- or 4- wheeled all-terrain vehicle (ATV) injured in nontraffic accident
- √x7ᵗʰ **V86.76** Person on outside of dirt bike or motor/cross bike injured in nontraffic accident

N Newborn: 0   P Pediatric: 0-17   M Maternity: 9-64   A Adult: 15-124   MCC Major Complication/Comorbidity   CC Complication/Comorbidity   SW Severe Wound Dx

1190   ICD-10-CM 2021

✓x7ᵗʰ **V86.79** **Person on outside of other special all-terrain or other off-road motor vehicles injured in nontraffic accident**

Person on outside of go cart injured in nontraffic accident

Person on outside of golf cart injured in nontraffic accident

✓5ᵗʰ **V86.9** **Unspecified occupant of special all-terrain or other off-road motor vehicle injured in nontraffic accident**

✓x7ᵗʰ **V86.91** **Unspecified occupant of ambulance or fire engine injured in nontraffic accident**

✓x7ᵗʰ **V86.92** **Unspecified occupant of snowmobile injured in nontraffic accident**

✓x7ᵗʰ **V86.93** **Unspecified occupant of dune buggy injured in nontraffic accident**

✓x7ᵗʰ **V86.94** **Unspecified occupant of military vehicle injured in nontraffic accident**

✓x7ᵗʰ **V86.95** **Unspecified occupant of 3- or 4- wheeled all-terrain vehicle (ATV) injured in nontraffic accident**

✓x7ᵗʰ **V86.96** **Unspecified occupant of dirt bike or motor/cross bike injured in nontraffic accident**

✓x7ᵗʰ **V86.99** **Unspecified occupant of other special all-terrain or other off-road motor vehicle injured in nontraffic accident**

Off-road motor-vehicle accident NOS

Other motor-vehicle accident NOS

Unspecified occupant of go cart injured in nontraffic accident

Unspecified occupant of golf cart injured in nontraffic accident

✓4ᵗʰ **V87** **Traffic accident of specified type but victim's mode of transport unknown**

EXCLUDES 1　collision involving:

pedal cycle (V10-V19)

pedestrian (V01-V09)

✓x7ᵗʰ **V87.0** **Person injured in collision between car and two- or three-wheeled powered vehicle (traffic)**

✓x7ᵗʰ **V87.1** **Person injured in collision between other motor vehicle and two- or three-wheeled motor vehicle (traffic)**

✓x7ᵗʰ **V87.2** **Person injured in collision between car and pick-up truck or van (traffic)**

✓x7ᵗʰ **V87.3** **Person injured in collision between car and bus (traffic)**

✓x7ᵗʰ **V87.4** **Person injured in collision between car and heavy transport vehicle (traffic)**

✓x7ᵗʰ **V87.5** **Person injured in collision between heavy transport vehicle and bus (traffic)**

✓x7ᵗʰ **V87.6** **Person injured in collision between railway train or railway vehicle and car (traffic)**

✓x7ᵗʰ **V87.7** **Person injured in collision between other specified motor vehicles (traffic)**

✓x7ᵗʰ **V87.8** **Person injured in other specified noncollision transport accidents involving motor vehicle (traffic)**

✓x7ᵗʰ **V87.9** **Person injured in other specified (collision)(noncollision) transport accidents involving nonmotor vehicle (traffic)**

✓4ᵗʰ **V88** **Nontraffic accident of specified type but victim's mode of transport unknown**

EXCLUDES 1　collision involving:

pedal cycle (V10-V19)

pedestrian (V01-V09)

✓x7ᵗʰ **V88.0** **Person injured in collision between car and two- or three-wheeled motor vehicle, nontraffic**

✓x7ᵗʰ **V88.1** **Person injured in collision between other motor vehicle and two- or three-wheeled motor vehicle, nontraffic**

✓x7ᵗʰ **V88.2** **Person injured in collision between car and pick-up truck or van, nontraffic**

✓x7ᵗʰ **V88.3** **Person injured in collision between car and bus, nontraffic**

✓x7ᵗʰ **V88.4** **Person injured in collision between car and heavy transport vehicle, nontraffic**

✓x7ᵗʰ **V88.5** **Person injured in collision between heavy transport vehicle and bus, nontraffic**

✓x7ᵗʰ **V88.6** **Person injured in collision between railway train or railway vehicle and car, nontraffic**

✓x7ᵗʰ **V88.7** **Person injured in collision between other specified motor vehicle, nontraffic**

✓x7ᵗʰ **V88.8** **Person injured in other specified noncollision transport accidents involving motor vehicle, nontraffic**

✓x7ᵗʰ **V88.9** **Person injured in other specified (collision)(noncollision) transport accidents involving nonmotor vehicle, nontraffic**

✓4ᵗʰ **V89** **Motor- or nonmotor-vehicle accident, type of vehicle unspecified**

✓x7ᵗʰ **V89.0** **Person injured in unspecified motor-vehicle accident, nontraffic**

Motor-vehicle accident NOS, nontraffic

✓x7ᵗʰ **V89.1** **Person injured in unspecified nonmotor-vehicle accident, nontraffic**

Nonmotor-vehicle accident NOS (nontraffic)

✓x7ᵗʰ **V89.2** **Person injured in unspecified motor-vehicle accident, traffic**

Motor-vehicle accident [MVA] NOS

Road (traffic) accident [RTA] NOS

✓x7ᵗʰ **V89.3** **Person injured in unspecified nonmotor-vehicle accident, traffic**

Nonmotor-vehicle traffic accident NOS

✓x7ᵗʰ **V89.9** **Person injured in unspecified vehicle accident**

Collision NOS

Water transport accidents (V90-V94)

The appropriate 7th character is to be added to each code from categories V90-V94.

A　initial encounter

D　subsequent encounter

S　sequela

✓4ᵗʰ **V90** **Drowning and submersion due to accident to watercraft**

EXCLUDES 1　civilian water transport accident involving military watercraft (V94.81-)

fall into water not from watercraft (W16.-)

military watercraft accident in military or war operations (Y36.0-, Y37.0-)

water-transport-related drowning or submersion without accident to watercraft (V92.-)

✓5ᵗʰ **V90.0** **Drowning and submersion due to watercraft overturning**

✓x7ᵗʰ **V90.00** **Drowning and submersion due to merchant ship overturning**

✓x7ᵗʰ **V90.01** **Drowning and submersion due to passenger ship overturning**

Drowning and submersion due to Ferry-boat overturning

Drowning and submersion due to Liner overturning

✓x7ᵗʰ **V90.02** **Drowning and submersion due to fishing boat overturning**

✓x7ᵗʰ **V90.03** **Drowning and submersion due to other powered watercraft overturning**

Drowning and submersion due to Hovercraft (on open water) overturning

Drowning and submersion due to Jet ski overturning

✓x7ᵗʰ **V90.04** **Drowning and submersion due to sailboat overturning**

✓x7ᵗʰ **V90.05** **Drowning and submersion due to canoe or kayak overturning**

✓x7ᵗʰ **V90.06** **Drowning and submersion due to (nonpowered) inflatable craft overturning**

✓x7ᵗʰ **V90.08** **Drowning and submersion due to other unpowered watercraft overturning**

Drowning and submersion due to windsurfer overturning

✓x7ᵗʰ **V90.09** **Drowning and submersion due to unspecified watercraft overturning**

Drowning and submersion due to boat NOS overturning

Drowning and submersion due to ship NOS overturning

Drowning and submersion due to watercraft NOS overturning

✓5ᵗʰ **V90.1** **Drowning and submersion due to watercraft sinking**

✓x7ᵗʰ **V90.10** **Drowning and submersion due to merchant ship sinking**

✓x7ᵗʰ **V90.11** **Drowning and submersion due to passenger ship sinking**

Drowning and submersion due to Ferry-boat sinking

Drowning and submersion due to Liner sinking

✓x7ᵗʰ **V90.12** **Drowning and submersion due to fishing boat sinking**

✓x7ᵗʰ **V90.13** **Drowning and submersion due to other powered watercraft sinking**

Drowning and submersion due to Hovercraft (on open water) sinking

Drowning and submersion due to Jet ski sinking

✓x7ᵗʰ **V90.14** **Drowning and submersion due to sailboat sinking**

✓ Additional Char Req　✓x7ᵗʰ Placeholder　Unacceptable PDx　Questionable PDx　Wrong Procedure　Manifestation　Unspecified Dx　H1-H14 HAC　HCC CMS-HCC Dx　HIV HIV Dx

ICD-10-CM 2021　　　　　　　　1191

√x7ᵗʰ **V90.15** **Drowning and submersion due to** canoe or kayak **sinking**

√x7ᵗʰ **V90.16** **Drowning and submersion due to (nonpowered)** inflatable craft **sinking**

√x7ᵗʰ **V90.18** **Drowning and submersion due to other** unpowered watercraft **sinking**

√x7ᵗʰ **V90.19** **Drowning and submersion due to unspecified watercraft sinking**

    Drowning and submersion due to boat NOS sinking

    Drowning and submersion due to ship NOS sinking

    Drowning and submersion due to watercraft NOS sinking

√5ᵗʰ **V90.2** **Drowning and submersion due to** falling or jumping from burning watercraft

√x7ᵗʰ **V90.20** **Drowning and submersion due to falling or jumping from burning** merchant ship

√x7ᵗʰ **V90.21** **Drowning and submersion due to falling or jumping from burning** passenger ship

    Drowning and submersion due to falling or jumping from burning Ferry-boat

    Drowning and submersion due to falling or jumping from burning Liner

√x7ᵗʰ **V90.22** **Drowning and submersion due to falling or jumping from burning** fishing boat

√x7ᵗʰ **V90.23** **Drowning and submersion due to falling or jumping from other burning** powered **watercraft**

    Drowning and submersion due to falling and jumping from burning Hovercraft (on open water)

    Drowning and submersion due to falling and jumping from burning Jet ski

√x7ᵗʰ **V90.24** **Drowning and submersion due to falling or jumping from burning** sailboat

√x7ᵗʰ **V90.25** **Drowning and submersion due to falling or jumping from burning** canoe or kayak

√x7ᵗʰ **V90.26** **Drowning and submersion due to falling or jumping from burning (nonpowered)** inflatable craft

√x7ᵗʰ **V90.27** **Drowning and submersion due to falling or jumping from burning** water-skis

√x7ᵗʰ **V90.28** **Drowning and submersion due to falling or jumping from other burning** unpowered **watercraft**

    Drowning and submersion due to falling and jumping from burning surf-board

    Drowning and submersion due to falling and jumping from burning windsurfer

√x7ᵗʰ **V90.29** **Drowning and submersion due to falling or jumping from unspecified burning watercraft**

    Drowning and submersion due to falling or jumping from burning boat NOS

    Drowning and submersion due to falling or jumping from burning ship NOS

    Drowning and submersion due to falling or jumping from burning watercraft NOS

√5ᵗʰ **V90.3** **Drowning and submersion due to** falling or jumping from crushed watercraft

√x7ᵗʰ **V90.30** **Drowning and submersion due to falling or jumping from crushed** merchant ship

√x7ᵗʰ **V90.31** **Drowning and submersion due to falling or jumping from crushed** passenger ship

    Drowning and submersion due to falling and jumping from crushed Ferry boat

    Drowning and submersion due to falling and jumping from crushed Liner

√x7ᵗʰ **V90.32** **Drowning and submersion due to falling or jumping from crushed** fishing boat

√x7ᵗʰ **V90.33** **Drowning and submersion due to falling or jumping from other crushed** powered **watercraft**

    Drowning and submersion due to falling and jumping from crushed Hovercraft

    Drowning and submersion due to falling and jumping from crushed Jet ski

√x7ᵗʰ **V90.34** **Drowning and submersion due to falling or jumping from crushed** sailboat

√x7ᵗʰ **V90.35** **Drowning and submersion due to falling or jumping from crushed** canoe or kayak

√x7ᵗʰ **V90.36** **Drowning and submersion due to falling or jumping from crushed (nonpowered)** inflatable craft

√x7ᵗʰ **V90.37** **Drowning and submersion due to falling or jumping from crushed** water-skis

√x7ᵗʰ **V90.38** **Drowning and submersion due to falling or jumping from other crushed** unpowered **watercraft**

    Drowning and submersion due to falling and jumping from crushed surf-board

    Drowning and submersion due to falling and jumping from crushed windsurfer

√x7ᵗʰ **V90.39** **Drowning and submersion due to falling or jumping from crushed unspecified watercraft**

    Drowning and submersion due to falling and jumping from crushed boat NOS

    Drowning and submersion due to falling and jumping from crushed ship NOS

    Drowning and submersion due to falling and jumping from crushed watercraft NOS

√5ᵗʰ **V90.8** **Drowning and submersion due to other accident to watercraft**

√x7ᵗʰ **V90.80** **Drowning and submersion due to other accident to** merchant ship

√x7ᵗʰ **V90.81** **Drowning and submersion due to other accident to** passenger ship

    Drowning and submersion due to other accident to Ferry-boat

    Drowning and submersion due to other accident to Liner

√x7ᵗʰ **V90.82** **Drowning and submersion due to other accident to** fishing boat

√x7ᵗʰ **V90.83** **Drowning and submersion due to other accident to other** powered **watercraft**

    Drowning and submersion due to other accident to Hovercraft (on open water)

    Drowning and submersion due to other accident to Jet ski

√x7ᵗʰ **V90.84** **Drowning and submersion due to other accident to** sailboat

√x7ᵗʰ **V90.85** **Drowning and submersion due to other accident to** canoe or kayak

√x7ᵗʰ **V90.86** **Drowning and submersion due to other accident to (nonpowered)** inflatable craft

√x7ᵗʰ **V90.87** **Drowning and submersion due to other accident to** water-skis

√x7ᵗʰ **V90.88** **Drowning and submersion due to other accident to other** unpowered **watercraft**

    Drowning and submersion due to other accident to surf-board

    Drowning and submersion due to other accident to windsurfer

√x7ᵗʰ **V90.89** **Drowning and submersion due to other accident to unspecified watercraft**

    Drowning and submersion due to other accident to boat NOS

    Drowning and submersion due to other accident to ship NOS

    Drowning and submersion due to other accident to watercraft NOS

√4ᵗʰ **V91** **Other injury due to accident to watercraft**

    INCLUDES   any injury except drowning and submersion as a result of an accident to watercraft

    EXCLUDES 1   civilian water transport accident involving military watercraft (V94.81-)

         military watercraft accident in military or war operations (Y36, Y37.-)

    EXCLUDES 2   drowning and submersion due to accident to watercraft (V90.-)

√5ᵗʰ **V91.0** **Burn due to watercraft on fire**

    EXCLUDES 1   burn from localized fire or explosion on board ship without accident to watercraft (V93.-)

√x7ᵗʰ **V91.00** **Burn due to** merchant ship **on fire**

√x7ᵗʰ **V91.01** **Burn due to** passenger ship **on fire**

    Burn due to Ferry-boat on fire

    Burn due to Liner on fire

√x7ᵗʰ **V91.02** **Burn due to** fishing boat **on fire**

√x7ᵗʰ **V91.03** **Burn due to other** powered **watercraft on fire**

    Burn due to Hovercraft (on open water) on fire

    Burn due to Jet ski on fire

√x7ᵗʰ **V91.04** **Burn due to** sailboat **on fire**

√x7ᵗʰ **V91.05** **Burn due to** canoe or kayak **on fire**

√x7ᵗʰ **V91.06** **Burn due to (nonpowered)** inflatable craft **on fire**

N Newborn: 0   P Pediatric: 0-17   M Maternity: 9-64   A Adult: 15-124   MCC Major Complication/Comorbidity   CC Complication/Comorbidity   SW Severe Wound Dx

1192   ICD-10-CM 2021

✔7ᵗʰ **V91.07** **Burn due to water-skis on fire**

✔7ᵗʰ **V91.08** **Burn due to other unpowered watercraft on fire**

✔7ᵗʰ **V91.09** **Burn due to unspecified watercraft on fire**
  Burn due to boat NOS on fire
  Burn due to ship NOS on fire
  Burn due to watercraft NOS on fire

✔5ᵗʰ **V91.1** **Crushed between watercraft and other watercraft or other object due to collision**
  Crushed by lifeboat after abandoning ship in a collision
  NOTE Select the specified type of watercraft that the victim was on at the time of the collision

✔x7ᵗʰ **V91.10** **Crushed between merchant ship and other watercraft or other object due to collision**

✔x7ᵗʰ **V91.11** **Crushed between passenger ship and other watercraft or other object due to collision**
  Crushed between Ferry-boat and other watercraft or other object due to collision
  Crushed between Liner and other watercraft or other object due to collision

✔x7ᵗʰ **V91.12** **Crushed between fishing boat and other watercraft or other object due to collision**

✔x7ᵗʰ **V91.13** **Crushed between other powered watercraft and other watercraft or other object due to collision**
  Crushed between Hovercraft (on open water) and other watercraft or other object due to collision
  Crushed between Jet ski and other watercraft or other object due to collision

✔x7ᵗʰ **V91.14** **Crushed between sailboat and other watercraft or other object due to collision**

✔x7ᵗʰ **V91.15** **Crushed between canoe or kayak and other watercraft or other object due to collision**

✔x7ᵗʰ **V91.16** **Crushed between (nonpowered) inflatable craft and other watercraft or other object due to collision**

✔x7ᵗʰ **V91.18** **Crushed between other unpowered watercraft and other watercraft or other object due to collision**
  Crushed between surfboard and other watercraft or other object due to collision
  Crushed between windsurfer and other watercraft or other object due to collision

✔x7ᵗʰ **V91.19** **Crushed between unspecified watercraft and other watercraft or other object due to collision**
  Crushed between boat NOS and other watercraft or other object due to collision
  Crushed between ship NOS and other watercraft or other object due to collision
  Crushed between watercraft NOS and other watercraft or other object due to collision

✔5ᵗʰ **V91.2** **Fall due to collision between watercraft and other watercraft or other object**
  Fall while remaining on watercraft after collision
  NOTE Select the specified type of watercraft that the victim was on at the time of the collision
  EXCLUDES 1 crushed between watercraft and other watercraft and other object due to collision (V91.1-)
  drowning and submersion due to falling from crushed watercraft (V90.3-)

✔x7ᵗʰ **V91.20** **Fall due to collision between merchant ship and other watercraft or other object**

✔x7ᵗʰ **V91.21** **Fall due to collision between passenger ship and other watercraft or other object**
  Fall due to collision between Ferry-boat and other watercraft or other object
  Fall due to collision between Liner and other watercraft or other object

✔x7ᵗʰ **V91.22** **Fall due to collision between fishing boat and other watercraft or other object**

✔x7ᵗʰ **V91.23** **Fall due to collision between other powered watercraft and other watercraft or other object**
  Fall due to collision between Hovercraft (on open water) and other watercraft or other object
  Fall due to collision between Jet ski and other watercraft or other object

✔x7ᵗʰ **V91.24** **Fall due to collision between sailboat and other watercraft or other object**

✔x7ᵗʰ **V91.25** **Fall due to collision between canoe or kayak and other watercraft or other object**

✔x7ᵗʰ **V91.26** **Fall due to collision between (nonpowered) inflatable craft and other watercraft or other object**

✔x7ᵗʰ **V91.29** **Fall due to collision between unspecified watercraft and other watercraft or other object**
  Fall due to collision between boat NOS and other watercraft or other object
  Fall due to collision between ship NOS and other watercraft or other object
  Fall due to collision between watercraft NOS and other watercraft or other object

✔5ᵗʰ **V91.3** **Hit or struck by falling object due to accident to watercraft**
  Hit or struck by falling object (part of damaged watercraft or other object) after falling or jumping from damaged watercraft
  EXCLUDES 2 drowning or submersion due to fall or jumping from damaged watercraft (V90.2-, V90.3-)

✔x7ᵗʰ **V91.30** **Hit or struck by falling object due to accident to merchant ship**

✔x7ᵗʰ **V91.31** **Hit or struck by falling object due to accident to passenger ship**
  Hit or struck by falling object due to accident to Ferry-boat
  Hit or struck by falling object due to accident to Liner

✔x7ᵗʰ **V91.32** **Hit or struck by falling object due to accident to fishing boat**

✔x7ᵗʰ **V91.33** **Hit or struck by falling object due to accident to other powered watercraft**
  Hit or struck by falling object due to accident to Hovercraft (on open water)
  Hit or struck by falling object due to accident to Jet ski

✔x7ᵗʰ **V91.34** **Hit or struck by falling object due to accident to sailboat**

✔x7ᵗʰ **V91.35** **Hit or struck by falling object due to accident to canoe or kayak**

✔x7ᵗʰ **V91.36** **Hit or struck by falling object due to accident to (nonpowered) inflatable craft**

✔x7ᵗʰ **V91.37** **Hit or struck by falling object due to accident to water-skis**
  Hit by water-skis after jumping off of waterskis

✔x7ᵗʰ **V91.38** **Hit or struck by falling object due to accident to other unpowered watercraft**
  Hit or struck by surf-board after falling off damaged surf-board
  Hit or struck by object after falling off damaged windsurfer

✔x7ᵗʰ **V91.39** **Hit or struck by falling object due to accident to unspecified watercraft**
  Hit or struck by falling object due to accident to boat NOS
  Hit or struck by falling object due to accident to ship NOS
  Hit or struck by falling object due to accident to watercraft NOS

✔5ᵗʰ **V91.8** **Other injury due to other accident to watercraft**

✔x7ᵗʰ **V91.80** **Other injury due to other accident to merchant ship**

✔x7ᵗʰ **V91.81** **Other injury due to other accident to passenger ship**
  Other injury due to other accident to Ferry-boat
  Other injury due to other accident to Liner

✔x7ᵗʰ **V91.82** **Other injury due to other accident to fishing boat**

✔x7ᵗʰ **V91.83** **Other injury due to other accident to other powered watercraft**
  Other injury due to other accident to Hovercraft (on open water)
  Other injury due to other accident to Jet ski

✔x7ᵗʰ **V91.84** **Other injury due to other accident to sailboat**

✔x7ᵗʰ **V91.85** **Other injury due to other accident to canoe or kayak**

✔x7ᵗʰ **V91.86** **Other injury due to other accident to (nonpowered) inflatable craft**

✔x7ᵗʰ **V91.87** **Other injury due to other accident to water-skis**

✔x7ᵗʰ **V91.88** **Other injury due to other accident to other unpowered watercraft**
  Other injury due to other accident to surf-board
  Other injury due to other accident to windsurfer

✓7th **V91.89** Other injury due to other accident to unspecified watercraft

Other injury due to other accident to boat NOS

Other injury due to other accident to ship NOS

Other injury due to other accident to watercraft NOS

✓4th **V92** **Drowning and submersion due to accident on board watercraft, without accident to watercraft**

EXCLUDES 1   civilian water transport accident involving military watercraft (V94.81-)

drowning or submersion due to accident to watercraft (V90-V91)

drowning or submersion of diver who voluntarily jumps from boat not involved in an accident (W16.711, W16.721)

fall into water without watercraft (W16.-)

military watercraft accident in military or war operations (Y36, Y37)

✓5th **V92.0** **Drowning and submersion due to fall off watercraft**

Drowning and submersion due to fall from gangplank of watercraft

Drowning and submersion due to fall overboard watercraft

EXCLUDES 2   hitting head on object or bottom of body of water due to fall from watercraft (V94.0-)

✓7th **V92.00** **Drowning and submersion due to fall off merchant ship**

✓7th **V92.01** **Drowning and submersion due to fall off passenger ship**

Drowning and submersion due to fall off Ferry-boat

Drowning and submersion due to fall off Liner

✓7th **V92.02** **Drowning and submersion due to fall off fishing boat**

✓7th **V92.03** **Drowning and submersion due to fall off other powered watercraft**

Drowning and submersion due to fall off Hovercraft (on open water)

Drowning and submersion due to fall off Jet ski

✓7th **V92.04** **Drowning and submersion due to fall off sailboat**

✓7th **V92.05** **Drowning and submersion due to fall off canoe or kayak**

✓7th **V92.06** **Drowning and submersion due to fall off (nonpowered) inflatable craft**

✓7th **V92.07** **Drowning and submersion due to fall off water-skis**

EXCLUDES 1   drowning and submersion due to falling off burning water-skis (V90.27)

drowning and submersion due to falling off crushed water-skis (V90.37)

hit by boat while water-skiing NOS (V94.X)

✓7th **V92.08** **Drowning and submersion due to fall off other unpowered watercraft**

Drowning and submersion due to fall off surf-board

Drowning and submersion due to fall off windsurfer

EXCLUDES 1   drowning and submersion due to fall off burning unpowered watercraft (V90.28)

drowning and submersion due to fall off crushed unpowered watercraft (V90.38)

drowning and submersion due to fall off damaged unpowered watercraft (V90.88)

drowning and submersion due to rider of nonpowered watercraft being hit by other watercraft (V94.-)

other injury due to rider of nonpowered watercraft being hit by other watercraft (V94.-)

✓7th **V92.09** **Drowning and submersion due to fall off unspecified watercraft**

Drowning and submersion due to fall off boat NOS

Drowning and submersion due to fall off ship

Drowning and submersion due to fall off watercraft NOS

✓5th **V92.1** **Drowning and submersion due to being thrown overboard by motion of watercraft**

EXCLUDES 1   drowning and submersion due to fall off surf-board (V92.08)

drowning and submersion due to fall off water-skis (V92.07)

drowning and submersion due to fall off windsurfer (V92.08)

✓7th **V92.10** **Drowning and submersion due to being thrown overboard by motion of merchant ship**

✓7th **V92.11** **Drowning and submersion due to being thrown overboard by motion of passenger ship**

Drowning and submersion due to being thrown overboard by motion of Ferry-boat

Drowning and submersion due to being thrown overboard by motion of Liner

✓7th **V92.12** **Drowning and submersion due to being thrown overboard by motion of fishing boat**

✓7th **V92.13** **Drowning and submersion due to being thrown overboard by motion of other powered watercraft**

Drowning and submersion due to being thrown overboard by motion of Hovercraft

✓7th **V92.14** **Drowning and submersion due to being thrown overboard by motion of sailboat**

✓7th **V92.15** **Drowning and submersion due to being thrown overboard by motion of canoe or kayak**

✓7th **V92.16** **Drowning and submersion due to being thrown overboard by motion of (nonpowered) inflatable craft**

✓7th **V92.19** **Drowning and submersion due to being thrown overboard by motion of unspecified watercraft**

Drowning and submersion due to being thrown overboard by motion of boat NOS

Drowning and submersion due to being thrown overboard by motion of ship NOS

Drowning and submersion due to being thrown overboard by motion of watercraft NOS

✓5th **V92.2** **Drowning and submersion due to being washed overboard from watercraft**

Code first any associated cataclysm (X37.0-)

✓7th **V92.20** **Drowning and submersion due to being washed overboard from merchant ship**

✓7th **V92.21** **Drowning and submersion due to being washed overboard from passenger ship**

Drowning and submersion due to being washed overboard from Ferry-boat

Drowning and submersion due to being washed overboard from Liner

✓7th **V92.22** **Drowning and submersion due to being washed overboard from fishing boat**

✓7th **V92.23** **Drowning and submersion due to being washed overboard from other powered watercraft**

Drowning and submersion due to being washed overboard from Hovercraft (on open water)

Drowning and submersion due to being washed overboard from Jet ski

✓7th **V92.24** **Drowning and submersion due to being washed overboard from sailboat**

✓7th **V92.25** **Drowning and submersion due to being washed overboard from canoe or kayak**

✓7th **V92.26** **Drowning and submersion due to being washed overboard from (nonpowered) inflatable craft**

✓7th **V92.27** **Drowning and submersion due to being washed overboard from water-skis**

EXCLUDES 1   drowning and submersion due to fall off water-skis (V92.07)

✓7th **V92.28** **Drowning and submersion due to being washed overboard from other unpowered watercraft**

Drowning and submersion due to being washed overboard from surf-board

Drowning and submersion due to being washed overboard from windsurfer

N Newborn: 0   P Pediatric: 0-17   M Maternity: 9-64   A Adult: 15-124   MCC Major Complication/Comorbidity   CC Complication/Comorbidity   SW Severe Wound Dx

1194   ICD-10-CM 2021

√x7ᵗʰ **V92.29** **Drowning and submersion due to being washed overboard from unspecified watercraft**
     Drowning and submersion due to being washed overboard from boat NOS
     Drowning and submersion due to being washed overboard from ship NOS
     Drowning and submersion due to being washed overboard from watercraft NOS

√4ᵗʰ **V93** **Other injury due to accident on board watercraft, without accident to watercraft**
     EXCLUDES 1   *civilian water transport accident involving military watercraft (V94.81-)*
         other injury due to accident to watercraft (V91.-)
         military watercraft accident in military or war operations (Y36, Y37.-)
     EXCLUDES 2   *drowning and submersion due to accident on board watercraft, without accident to watercraft (V92.-)*

√5ᵗʰ **V93.0** **Burn due to localized fire on board watercraft**
     EXCLUDES 1   *burn due to watercraft on fire (V91.0-)*

√x7ᵗʰ **V93.00** **Burn due to localized fire on board** merchant vessel

√x7ᵗʰ **V93.01** **Burn due to localized fire on board** passenger vessel
     Burn due to localized fire on board Ferry-boat
     Burn due to localized fire on board Liner

√x7ᵗʰ **V93.02** **Burn due to localized fire on board** fishing boat

√x7ᵗʰ **V93.03** **Burn due to localized fire on board other** powered watercraft
     Burn due to localized fire on board Hovercraft
     Burn due to localized fire on board Jet ski

√x7ᵗʰ **V93.04** **Burn due to localized fire on board** sailboat

√x7ᵗʰ **V93.09** **Burn due to localized fire on board unspecified watercraft**
     Burn due to localized fire on board boat NOS
     Burn due to localized fire on board ship NOS
     Burn due to localized fire on board watercraft NOS

√5ᵗʰ **V93.1** **Other burn on board watercraft**
     Burn due to source other than fire on board watercraft
     EXCLUDES 1   *burn due to watercraft on fire (V91.0-)*

√x7ᵗʰ **V93.10** **Other burn on board** merchant vessel

√x7ᵗʰ **V93.11** **Other burn on board** passenger vessel
     Other burn on board Ferry-boat
     Other burn on board Liner

√x7ᵗʰ **V93.12** **Other burn on board** fishing boat

√x7ᵗʰ **V93.13** **Other burn on board other** powered watercraft
     Other burn on board Hovercraft
     Other burn on board Jet ski

√x7ᵗʰ **V93.14** **Other burn on board** sailboat

√x7ᵗʰ **V93.19** **Other burn on board unspecified watercraft**
     Other burn on board boat NOS
     Other burn on board ship NOS
     Other burn on board watercraft NOS

√5ᵗʰ **V93.2** **Heat exposure on board watercraft**
     EXCLUDES 1   *exposure to man-made heat not aboard watercraft (W92)*
         exposure to natural heat while on board watercraft (X30)
         exposure to sunlight while on board watercraft (X32)
     EXCLUDES 2   *burn due to fire on board watercraft (V93.0-)*

√x7ᵗʰ **V93.20** **Heat exposure on board** merchant ship

√x7ᵗʰ **V93.21** **Heat exposure on board** passenger ship
     Heat exposure on board Ferry-boat
     Heat exposure on board Liner

√x7ᵗʰ **V93.22** **Heat exposure on board** fishing boat

√x7ᵗʰ **V93.23** **Heat exposure on board other** powered watercraft
     Heat exposure on board hovercraft

√x7ᵗʰ **V93.24** **Heat exposure on board** sailboat

√x7ᵗʰ **V93.29** **Heat exposure on board unspecified watercraft**
     Heat exposure on board boat NOS
     Heat exposure on board ship NOS
     Heat exposure on board watercraft NOS

√5ᵗʰ **V93.3** **Fall on board watercraft**
     EXCLUDES 1   *fall due to collision of watercraft (V91.2-)*

√x7ᵗʰ **V93.30** **Fall on board** merchant ship

√x7ᵗʰ **V93.31** **Fall on board** passenger ship
     Fall on board Ferry-boat
     Fall on board Liner

√x7ᵗʰ **V93.32** **Fall on board** fishing boat

√x7ᵗʰ **V93.33** **Fall on board other** powered watercraft
     Fall on board Hovercraft (on open water)
     Fall on board Jet ski

√x7ᵗʰ **V93.34** **Fall on board** sailboat

√x7ᵗʰ **V93.35** **Fall on board** canoe or kayak

√x7ᵗʰ **V93.36** **Fall on board (nonpowered)** inflatable craft

√x7ᵗʰ **V93.38** **Fall on board other** unpowered watercraft

√x7ᵗʰ **V93.39** **Fall on board unspecified watercraft**
     Fall on board boat NOS
     Fall on board ship NOS
     Fall on board watercraft NOS

√5ᵗʰ **V93.4** **Struck by falling object on board watercraft**
     Hit by falling object on board watercraft
     EXCLUDES 1   *struck by falling object due to accident to watercraft (V91.3)*

√x7ᵗʰ **V93.40** **Struck by falling object on** merchant ship

√x7ᵗʰ **V93.41** **Struck by falling object on** passenger ship
     Struck by falling object on Ferry-boat
     Struck by falling object on Liner

√x7ᵗʰ **V93.42** **Struck by falling object on** fishing boat

√x7ᵗʰ **V93.43** **Struck by falling object on other** powered watercraft
     Struck by falling object on Hovercraft

√x7ᵗʰ **V93.44** **Struck by falling object on** sailboat

√x7ᵗʰ **V93.48** **Struck by falling object on other** unpowered watercraft

√x7ᵗʰ **V93.49** **Struck by falling object on unspecified watercraft**

√5ᵗʰ **V93.5** **Explosion on board watercraft**
     Boiler explosion on steamship
     EXCLUDES 2   *fire on board watercraft (V93.0-)*

√x7ᵗʰ **V93.50** **Explosion on board** merchant ship

√x7ᵗʰ **V93.51** **Explosion on board** passenger ship
     Explosion on board Ferry-boat
     Explosion on board Liner

√x7ᵗʰ **V93.52** **Explosion on board** fishing boat

√x7ᵗʰ **V93.53** **Explosion on board other** powered watercraft
     Explosion on board Hovercraft
     Explosion on board Jet ski

√x7ᵗʰ **V93.54** **Explosion on board** sailboat

√x7ᵗʰ **V93.59** **Explosion on board unspecified watercraft**
     Explosion on board boat NOS
     Explosion on board ship NOS
     Explosion on board watercraft NOS

√5ᵗʰ **V93.6** **Machinery accident on board watercraft**
     EXCLUDES 1   *machinery explosion on board watercraft (V93.4-)*
         machinery fire on board watercraft (V93.0-)

√x7ᵗʰ **V93.60** **Machinery accident on board** merchant ship

√x7ᵗʰ **V93.61** **Machinery accident on board** passenger ship
     Machinery accident on board Ferry-boat
     Machinery accident on board Liner

√x7ᵗʰ **V93.62** **Machinery accident on board** fishing boat

√x7ᵗʰ **V93.63** **Machinery accident on board other** powered watercraft
     Machinery accident on board Hovercraft

√x7ᵗʰ **V93.64** **Machinery accident on board** sailboat

√x7ᵗʰ **V93.69** **Machinery accident on board unspecified watercraft**
     Machinery accident on board boat NOS
     Machinery accident on board ship NOS
     Machinery accident on board watercraft NOS

√5ᵗʰ **V93.8** **Other injury due to other accident on board watercraft**
     Accidental poisoning by gases or fumes on watercraft

√x7ᵗʰ **V93.80** **Other injury due to other accident on board** merchant ship

√x7ʰ **V93.81** **Other injury due to other accident on board** **passenger ship**
Other injury due to other accident on board Ferry-boat
Other injury due to other accident on board Liner

√x7ʰ **V93.82** **Other injury due to other accident on board** **fishing** **boat**

√x7ʰ **V93.83** **Other injury due to other accident on board other** **powered** **watercraft**
Other injury due to other accident on board Hovercraft
Other injury due to other accident on board Jet ski

√x7ʰ **V93.84** **Other injury due to other accident on board** **sailboat**

√x7ʰ **V93.85** **Other injury due to other accident on board** **canoe** **or kayak**

√x7ʰ **V93.86** **Other injury due to other accident on board** **(nonpowered)** **inflatable craft**

√x7ʰ **V93.87** **Other injury due to other accident on board** **water-skis**
Hit or struck by object while waterskiing

√x7ʰ **V93.88** **Other injury due to other accident on board other** **unpowered** **watercraft**
Hit or struck by object while surfing
Hit or struck by object while on board windsurfer

√x7ʰ **V93.89** **Other injury due to other accident on board** **unspecified watercraft**
Other injury due to other accident on board boat NOS
Other injury due to other accident on board ship NOS
Other injury due to other accident on board watercraft NOS

√4ʰ **V94** **Other and unspecified water transport accidents**

EXCLUDES 1 *military watercraft accidents in military or war operations (Y36, Y37)*

√x7ʰ **V94.0** **Hitting object or bottom of body of water due to fall from watercraft**

EXCLUDES 2 *drowning and submersion due to fall from watercraft (V92.0-)*

√5ʰ **V94.1** **Bather struck by watercraft**
Swimmer hit by watercraft

√x7ʰ **V94.11** **Bather struck by** **powered** **watercraft**

√x7ʰ **V94.12** **Bather struck by** **nonpowered** **watercraft**

√5ʰ **V94.2** **Rider of nonpowered watercraft struck by other watercraft**

√x7ʰ **V94.21** **Rider of nonpowered watercraft struck by other** **nonpowered** **watercraft**
Canoer hit by other nonpowered watercraft
Surfer hit by other nonpowered watercraft
Windsurfer hit by other nonpowered watercraft

√x7ʰ **V94.22** **Rider of nonpowered watercraft struck by** **powered** **watercraft**
Canoer hit by motorboat
Surfer hit by motorboat
Windsurfer hit by motorboat

√5ʰ **V94.3** **Injury to rider of (inflatable) watercraft being pulled behind other watercraft**

√x7ʰ **V94.31** **Injury to rider of (inflatable)** **recreational** **watercraft being pulled behind other watercraft**
Injury to rider of inner-tube pulled behind motor boat

√x7ʰ **V94.32** **Injury to rider of** **non-recreational** **watercraft being pulled behind other watercraft**
Injury to occupant of dingy being pulled behind boat or ship
Injury to occupant of life-raft being pulled behind boat or ship

√x7ʰ **V94.4** **Injury to barefoot water-skier**
Injury to person being pulled behind boat or ship

√5ʰ **V94.8** **Other water transport accident**

√6ʰ **V94.81** **Water transport accident involving military watercraft**

√7ʰ **V94.810** **Civilian watercraft involved in water transport accident with military watercraft**
Passenger on civilian watercraft injured due to accident with military watercraft

√7ʰ **V94.811** **Civilian in water injured by military watercraft**

√7ʰ **V94.818** **Other water transport accident involving military watercraft**

√x7ʰ **V94.89** **Other water transport accident**

√x7ʰ **V94.9** **Unspecified water transport accident**
Water transport accident NOS

Air and space transport accidents (V95-V97)

EXCLUDES 1 *military aircraft accidents in military or war operations (Y36, Y37)*

The appropriate 7th character is to be added to each code from categories V95-V97.
A   initial encounter
D   subsequent encounter
S   sequela

√4ʰ **V95** **Accident to powered aircraft causing injury to occupant**

√5ʰ **V95.0** **Helicopter** **accident injuring occupant**

√x7ʰ **V95.00** **Unspecified helicopter accident injuring occupant**

√x7ʰ **V95.01** **Helicopter** **crash** **injuring occupant**

√x7ʰ **V95.02** **Forced landing** **of helicopter injuring occupant**

√x7ʰ **V95.03** **Helicopter** **collision** **injuring occupant**
Helicopter collision with any object, fixed, movable or moving

√x7ʰ **V95.04** **Helicopter** **fire** **injuring occupant**

√x7ʰ **V95.05** **Helicopter** **explosion** **injuring occupant**

√x7ʰ **V95.09** **Other helicopter accident injuring occupant**

√5ʰ **V95.1** **Ultralight, microlight or powered-glider** **accident injuring occupant**

√x7ʰ **V95.10** **Unspecified ultralight, microlight or powered-glider accident injuring occupant**

√x7ʰ **V95.11** **Ultralight, microlight or powered-glider** **crash** **injuring occupant**

√x7ʰ **V95.12** **Forced landing** **of ultralight, microlight or powered-glider injuring occupant**

√x7ʰ **V95.13** **Ultralight, microlight or powered-glider** **collision** **injuring occupant**
Ultralight, microlight or powered-glider collision with any object, fixed, movable or moving

√x7ʰ **V95.14** **Ultralight, microlight or powered-glider** **fire** **injuring occupant**

√x7ʰ **V95.15** **Ultralight, microlight or powered-glider** **explosion** **injuring occupant**

√x7ʰ **V95.19** **Other ultralight, microlight or powered-glider accident injuring occupant**

√5ʰ **V95.2** **Other private fixed-wing aircraft accident injuring occupant**

√x7ʰ **V95.20** **Unspecified accident to other private fixed-wing aircraft, injuring occupant**

√x7ʰ **V95.21** **Other private fixed-wing aircraft crash injuring occupant**

√x7ʰ **V95.22** **Forced landing** **of other private fixed-wing aircraft injuring occupant**

√x7ʰ **V95.23** **Other private fixed-wing aircraft** **collision** **injuring occupant**
Other private fixed-wing aircraft collision with any object, fixed, movable or moving

√x7ʰ **V95.24** **Other private fixed-wing aircraft** **fire** **injuring occupant**

√x7ʰ **V95.25** **Other private fixed-wing aircraft** **explosion** **injuring occupant**

√x7ʰ **V95.29** **Other accident to other private fixed-wing aircraft injuring occupant**

√5ʰ **V95.3** **Commercial fixed-wing** **aircraft accident injuring occupant**

√x7ʰ **V95.30** **Unspecified accident to commercial fixed-wing aircraft injuring occupant**

√x7ʰ **V95.31** **Commercial fixed-wing aircraft** **crash** **injuring occupant**

√x7ʰ **V95.32** **Forced landing** **of commercial fixed-wing aircraft injuring occupant**

√x7ʰ **V95.33** **Commercial fixed-wing aircraft** **collision** **injuring occupant**
Commercial fixed-wing aircraft collision with any object, fixed, movable or moving

√x7ʰ **V95.34** **Commercial fixed-wing aircraft** **fire** **injuring occupant**

√x7ʰ **V95.35** **Commercial fixed-wing aircraft** **explosion** **injuring occupant**

√x7ʰ **V95.39** **Other accident to commercial fixed-wing aircraft injuring occupant**

√5ʰ **V95.4** **Spacecraft** **accident injuring occupant**

√x7ʰ **V95.40** **Unspecified spacecraft accident injuring occupant**

√x7ʰ **V95.41** **Spacecraft** **crash** **injuring occupant**

Chapter 20. External Causes of Morbidity

√x7ᵗʰ	**V95.42**	**Forced landing** of spacecraft injuring occupant
√x7ᵗʰ	**V95.43**	**Spacecraft collision** injuring occupant
		Spacecraft collision with any object, fixed, moveable or moving
√x7ᵗʰ	**V95.44**	**Spacecraft fire** injuring occupant
√x7ᵗʰ	**V95.45**	**Spacecraft explosion** injuring occupant
√x7ᵗʰ	**V95.49**	**Other spacecraft accident** injuring occupant
√x7ᵗʰ	**V95.8**	**Other powered aircraft accidents** injuring occupant
√x7ᵗʰ	**V95.9**	**Unspecified aircraft accident** injuring occupant
		Aircraft accident NOS
		Air transport accident NOS

√4ᵗʰ **V96** **Accident to nonpowered aircraft causing injury to occupant**

√5ᵗʰ **V96.0** **Balloon** accident injuring occupant

√x7ᵗʰ	**V96.00**	**Unspecified balloon accident** injuring occupant
√x7ᵗʰ	**V96.01**	**Balloon crash** injuring occupant
√x7ᵗʰ	**V96.02**	**Forced landing** of balloon injuring occupant
√x7ᵗʰ	**V96.03**	**Balloon collision** injuring occupant
		Balloon collision with any object, fixed, moveable or moving
√x7ᵗʰ	**V96.04**	**Balloon fire** injuring occupant
√x7ᵗʰ	**V96.05**	**Balloon explosion** injuring occupant
√x7ᵗʰ	**V96.09**	**Other balloon accident** injuring occupant

√5ᵗʰ **V96.1** **Hang-glider** accident injuring occupant

√x7ᵗʰ	**V96.10**	**Unspecified hang-glider accident** injuring occupant
√x7ᵗʰ	**V96.11**	**Hang-glider crash** injuring occupant
√x7ᵗʰ	**V96.12**	**Forced landing** of hang-glider injuring occupant
√x7ᵗʰ	**V96.13**	**Hang-glider collision** injuring occupant
		Hang-glider collision with any object, fixed, moveable or moving
√x7ᵗʰ	**V96.14**	**Hang-glider fire** injuring occupant
√x7ᵗʰ	**V96.15**	**Hang-glider explosion** injuring occupant
√x7ᵗʰ	**V96.19**	**Other hang-glider accident** injuring occupant

√5ᵗʰ **V96.2** **Glider (nonpowered)** accident injuring occupant

√x7ᵗʰ	**V96.20**	**Unspecified glider (nonpowered) accident** injuring occupant
√x7ᵗʰ	**V96.21**	**Glider (nonpowered) crash** injuring occupant
√x7ᵗʰ	**V96.22**	**Forced landing** of glider (nonpowered) injuring occupant
√x7ᵗʰ	**V96.23**	**Glider (nonpowered) collision** injuring occupant
		Glider (nonpowered) collision with any object, fixed, moveable or moving
√x7ᵗʰ	**V96.24**	**Glider (nonpowered) fire** injuring occupant
√x7ᵗʰ	**V96.25**	**Glider (nonpowered) explosion** injuring occupant
√x7ᵗʰ	**V96.29**	**Other glider (nonpowered) accident** injuring occupant
√x7ᵗʰ	**V96.8**	**Other nonpowered-aircraft accidents** injuring occupant
		Kite carrying a person accident injuring occupant
√x7ᵗʰ	**V96.9**	**Unspecified nonpowered-aircraft accident** injuring occupant
		Nonpowered-aircraft accident NOS

√4ᵗʰ **V97** **Other specified air transport accidents**

√x7ᵗʰ	**V97.0**	**Occupant of aircraft injured in other specified air transport accidents**
		Fall in, on or from aircraft in air transport accident
	EXCLUDES 1	accident while boarding or alighting aircraft (V97.1)
√x7ᵗʰ	**V97.1**	**Person injured while boarding or alighting from aircraft**

√5ᵗʰ **V97.2** **Parachutist accident**

√x7ᵗʰ	**V97.21**	**Parachutist entangled in object**
		Parachutist landing in tree
√x7ᵗʰ	**V97.22**	**Parachutist injured on landing**
√x7ᵗʰ	**V97.29**	**Other parachutist accident**

√5ᵗʰ **V97.3** **Person on ground injured in air transport accident**

√x7ᵗʰ	**V97.31**	**Hit by object falling from aircraft**
		Hit by crashing aircraft
		Injured by aircraft hitting house
		Injured by aircraft hitting car
√x7ᵗʰ	**V97.32**	**Injured by rotating propeller**
√x7ᵗʰ	**V97.33**	**Sucked into jet engine**
√x7ᵗʰ	**V97.39**	**Other injury to person on ground due to air transport accident**

√5ᵗʰ **V97.8** **Other air transport accidents, not elsewhere classified**

	EXCLUDES 1	aircraft accident NOS (V95.9)
		exposure to changes in air pressure during ascent or descent (W94.-)

√6ᵗʰ **V97.81** **Air transport accident involving military aircraft**

√7ᵗʰ	**V97.810**	**Civilian aircraft involved in air transport accident with military aircraft**
		Passenger in civilian aircraft injured due to accident with military aircraft
√7ᵗʰ	**V97.811**	**Civilian injured by military aircraft**
√7ᵗʰ	**V97.818**	**Other air transport accident involving military aircraft**
√x7ᵗʰ	**V97.89**	**Other air transport accidents, not elsewhere classified**
		Injury from machinery on aircraft

Other and unspecified transport accidents (V98-V99)

EXCLUDES 1	vehicle accident, type of vehicle unspecified (V89.-)

The appropriate 7th character is to be added to each code from categories V98-V99.
A   initial encounter
D   subsequent encounter
S   sequela

√4ᵗʰ **V98** **Other specified transport accidents**

√x7ᵗʰ	**V98.0**	**Accident to, on or involving cable-car, not on rails**
		Caught or dragged by cable-car, not on rails
		Fall or jump from cable-car, not on rails
		Object thrown from or in cable-car, not on rails
√x7ᵗʰ	**V98.1**	**Accident to, on or involving land-yacht**
√x7ᵗʰ	**V98.2**	**Accident to, on or involving ice yacht**
√x7ᵗʰ	**V98.3**	**Accident to, on or involving ski lift**
		Accident to, on or involving ski chair-lift
		Accident to, on or involving ski-lift with gondola
√x7ᵗʰ	**V98.8**	**Other specified transport accidents**

√x7ᵗʰ **V99** **Unspecified transport accident**

OTHER EXTERNAL CAUSES OF ACCIDENTAL INJURY (W00-X58)

Slipping, tripping, stumbling and falls (W00-W19)

EXCLUDES 1	assault involving a fall (Y01-Y02)
	fall from animal (V80.-)
	fall (in) (from) machinery (in operation) (W28-W31)
	fall (in) (from) transport vehicle (V01-V99)
	intentional self-harm involving a fall (X80-X81)
EXCLUDES 2	at risk for fall (history of fall) Z91.81
	fall (in) (from) burning building (X00.-)
	fall into fire (X00-X04, X08)

The appropriate 7th character is to be added to each code from categories W00-W19.
A   initial encounter
D   subsequent encounter
S   sequela

√4ᵗʰ **W00** **Fall due to ice and snow**

	INCLUDES	pedestrian on foot falling (slipping) on ice and snow
	EXCLUDES 1	fall on (from) ice and snow involving pedestrian conveyance (V00.-)
		fall from stairs and steps not due to ice and snow (W10.-)
	AHA: 2016,2Q,4	
√x7ᵗʰ	**W00.0**	**Fall on same level due to ice and snow**
√x7ᵗʰ	**W00.1**	**Fall from stairs and steps due to ice and snow**
√x7ᵗʰ	**W00.2**	**Other fall from one level to another due to ice and snow**
√x7ᵗʰ	**W00.9**	**Unspecified fall due to ice and snow**

☑ Additional Char Req   √x7ᵗʰ Placeholder   Unacceptable PDx   Questionable PDx   Wrong Procedure   Manifestation   Unspecified Dx   **H1-H14** HAC   **HCC** CMS-HCC Dx   **HIV** HIV Dx

ICD-10-CM 2021   **1197**

✓4ᵗʰ **W01 Fall on same level from slipping, tripping and stumbling**
- INCLUDES   fall on moving sidewalk
- EXCLUDES 1   *fall due to bumping (striking) against object (W18.0-)*
  - *fall in shower or bathtub (W18.2-)*
  - *fall on same level NOS (W18.30)*
  - *fall on same level from slipping, tripping and stumbling due to ice or snow (W00.0)*
  - *fall off or from toilet (W18.1-)*
  - *slipping, tripping and stumbling NOS (W18.40)*
  - *slipping, tripping and stumbling without falling (W18.4-)*

✓7ᵗʰ **W01.0 Fall on same level from slipping, tripping and stumbling without subsequent striking against object**
- Falling over animal

✓5ᵗʰ **W01.1 Fall on same level from slipping, tripping and stumbling with subsequent striking against object**

     ✓7ᵗʰ **W01.10 Fall on same level from slipping, tripping and stumbling with subsequent striking against unspecified object**

     ✓6ᵗʰ **W01.11 Fall on same level from slipping, tripping and stumbling with subsequent striking against sharp object**

         ✓7ᵗʰ **W01.110 Fall on same level from slipping, tripping and stumbling with subsequent striking against sharp glass**

         ✓7ᵗʰ **W01.111 Fall on same level from slipping, tripping and stumbling with subsequent striking against power tool or machine**

         ✓7ᵗʰ **W01.118 Fall on same level from slipping, tripping and stumbling with subsequent striking against other sharp object**

         ✓7ᵗʰ **W01.119 Fall on same level from slipping, tripping and stumbling with subsequent striking against unspecified sharp object**

     ✓6ᵗʰ **W01.19 Fall on same level from slipping, tripping and stumbling with subsequent striking against other object**

         ✓7ᵗʰ **W01.190 Fall on same level from slipping, tripping and stumbling with subsequent striking against furniture**

         ✓7ᵗʰ **W01.198 Fall on same level from slipping, tripping and stumbling with subsequent striking against other object**

✓x7ᵗʰ **W03 Other fall on same level due to collision with another person**
- Fall due to non-transport collision with other person
- EXCLUDES 1   *collision with another person without fall (W51)*
  - *crushed or pushed by a crowd or human stampede (W52)*
  - *fall involving pedestrian conveyance (V00-V09)*
  - *fall due to ice or snow (W00)*
  - *fall on same level NOS (W18.30)*
- **AHA:** 2012,4Q,108

✓x7ᵗʰ **W04 Fall while being carried or supported by other persons**
- Accidentally dropped while being carried

✓4ᵗʰ **W05 Fall from non-moving wheelchair, nonmotorized scooter and motorized mobility scooter**
- EXCLUDES 1   *fall from moving wheelchair (powered) (V00.811)*
  - *fall from moving motorized mobility scooter (V00.831)*
  - *fall from nonmotorized scooter (V00.141)*

✓x7ᵗʰ **W05.0 Fall from non-moving wheelchair**
- **AHA:** 2019,2Q,27

✓x7ᵗʰ **W05.1 Fall from non-moving nonmotorized scooter**

✓x7ᵗʰ **W05.2 Fall from non-moving motorized mobility scooter**

✓x7ᵗʰ **W06 Fall from bed**

✓x7ᵗʰ **W07 Fall from chair**

✓x7ᵗʰ **W08 Fall from other furniture**

✓4ᵗʰ **W09 Fall on and from playground equipment**
- EXCLUDES 1   *fall involving recreational machinery (W31)*

✓x7ᵗʰ **W09.0 Fall on or from playground slide**

✓x7ᵗʰ **W09.1 Fall from playground swing**

✓x7ᵗʰ **W09.2 Fall on or from jungle gym**

✓x7ᵗʰ **W09.8 Fall on or from other playground equipment**

✓4ᵗʰ **W10 Fall on and from stairs and steps**
- EXCLUDES 1   *Fall from stairs and steps due to ice and snow (W00.1)*

✓x7ᵗʰ **W10.0 Fall (on)(from) escalator**

✓x7ᵗʰ **W10.1 Fall (on)(from) sidewalk curb**

✓x7ᵗʰ **W10.2 Fall (on)(from) incline**
- Fall (on) (from) ramp

✓x7ᵗʰ **W10.8 Fall (on)(from) other stairs and steps**

✓x7ᵗʰ **W10.9 Fall (on)(from) unspecified stairs and steps**

✓x7ᵗʰ **W11 Fall on and from ladder**

✓x7ᵗʰ **W12 Fall on and from scaffolding**

✓4ᵗʰ **W13 Fall from, out of or through building or structure**

✓x7ᵗʰ **W13.0 Fall from, out of or through balcony**
- Fall from, out of or through railing

✓x7ᵗʰ **W13.1 Fall from, out of or through bridge**

✓x7ᵗʰ **W13.2 Fall from, out of or through roof**

✓x7ᵗʰ **W13.3 Fall through floor**

✓x7ᵗʰ **W13.4 Fall from, out of or through window**
- EXCLUDES 2   *fall with subsequent striking against sharp glass (W01.110)*

✓x7ᵗʰ **W13.8 Fall from, out of or through other building or structure**
- Fall from, out of or through viaduct
- Fall from, out of or through wall
- Fall from, out of or through flag-pole

✓x7ᵗʰ **W13.9 Fall from, out of or through building, not otherwise specified**
- EXCLUDES 1   *collapse of a building or structure (W20.-)*
  - *fall or jump from burning building or structure (X00.-)*

✓x7ᵗʰ **W14 Fall from tree**

✓x7ᵗʰ **W15 Fall from cliff**

✓4ᵗʰ **W16 Fall, jump or diving into water**
- EXCLUDES 1   *accidental non-watercraft drowning and submersion not involving fall (W65-W74)*
  - *effects of air pressure from diving (W94.-)*
  - *fall into water from watercraft (V90-V94)*
  - *hitting an object or against bottom when falling from watercraft (V94.0)*
- EXCLUDES 2   *striking or hitting diving board (W21.4)*

✓5ᵗʰ **W16.0 Fall into swimming pool**
- Fall into swimming pool NOS
- EXCLUDES 1   *fall into empty swimming pool (W17.3)*

     ✓6ᵗʰ **W16.01 Fall into swimming pool striking water surface**

         ✓7ᵗʰ **W16.011 Fall into swimming pool striking water surface causing drowning and submersion**
- EXCLUDES 1   *drowning and submersion while in swimming pool without fall (W67)*

         ✓7ᵗʰ **W16.012 Fall into swimming pool striking water surface causing other injury**

     ✓6ᵗʰ **W16.02 Fall into swimming pool striking bottom**

         ✓7ᵗʰ **W16.021 Fall into swimming pool striking bottom causing drowning and submersion**
- EXCLUDES 1   *drowning and submersion while in swimming pool without fall (W67)*

         ✓7ᵗʰ **W16.022 Fall into swimming pool striking bottom causing other injury**

     ✓6ᵗʰ **W16.03 Fall into swimming pool striking wall**

         ✓7ᵗʰ **W16.031 Fall into swimming pool striking wall causing drowning and submersion**
- EXCLUDES 1   *drowning and submersion while in swimming pool without fall (W67)*

         ✓7ᵗʰ **W16.032 Fall into swimming pool striking wall causing other injury**

√5ᵗʰ **W16.1 Fall into** natural body of water
    Fall into lake
    Fall into open sea
    Fall into river
    Fall into stream
  √6ᵗʰ **W16.11 Fall into natural body of water** striking water surface
    √7ᵗʰ **W16.111 Fall into natural body of water striking water surface causing** drowning and submersion
      EXCLUDES 1   *drowning and submersion while in natural body of water without fall (W69)*
    √7ᵗʰ **W16.112 Fall into natural body of water striking water surface causing other injury**
  √6ᵗʰ **W16.12 Fall into natural body of water** striking bottom
    √7ᵗʰ **W16.121 Fall into natural body of water striking bottom causing** drowning and submersion
      EXCLUDES 1   *drowning and submersion while in natural body of water without fall (W69)*
    √7ᵗʰ **W16.122 Fall into natural body of water striking bottom causing other injury**
  √6ᵗʰ **W16.13 Fall into natural body of water** striking side
    √7ᵗʰ **W16.131 Fall into natural body of water striking side causing** drowning and submersion
      EXCLUDES 1   *drowning and submersion while in natural body of water without fall (W69)*
    √7ᵗʰ **W16.132 Fall into natural body of water striking side causing other injury**
√5ᵗʰ **W16.2 Fall in (into) filled** bathtub or bucket of water
  √6ᵗʰ **W16.21 Fall in (into)** filled bathtub
    EXCLUDES 1   *fall into empty bathtub (W18.2)*
    √7ᵗʰ **W16.211 Fall in (into) filled bathtub causing** drowning and submersion
      EXCLUDES 1   *drowning and submersion while in filled bathtub without fall (W65)*
    √7ᵗʰ **W16.212 Fall in (into) filled bathtub causing other injury**
  √6ᵗʰ **W16.22 Fall in (into)** bucket of water
    √7ᵗʰ **W16.221 Fall in (into) bucket of water causing** drowning and submersion
    √7ᵗʰ **W16.222 Fall in (into) bucket of water causing other injury**
√5ᵗʰ **W16.3 Fall into other water**
    Fall into fountain
    Fall into reservoir
  √6ᵗʰ **W16.31 Fall into other water** striking water surface
    √7ᵗʰ **W16.311 Fall into other water striking water surface causing** drowning and submersion
      EXCLUDES 1   *drowning and submersion while in other water without fall (W73)*
    √7ᵗʰ **W16.312 Fall into other water striking water surface causing other injury**
  √6ᵗʰ **W16.32 Fall into other water** striking bottom
    √7ᵗʰ **W16.321 Fall into other water striking bottom causing** drowning and submersion
      EXCLUDES 1   *drowning and submersion while in other water without fall (W73)*
    √7ᵗʰ **W16.322 Fall into other water striking bottom causing other injury**
  √6ᵗʰ **W16.33 Fall into other water** striking wall
    √7ᵗʰ **W16.331 Fall into other water striking wall causing** drowning and submersion
      EXCLUDES 1   *drowning and submersion while in other water without fall (W73)*
    √7ᵗʰ **W16.332 Fall into other water striking wall causing other injury**
√5ᵗʰ **W16.4 Fall into unspecified water**
  √x7ᵗʰ **W16.41 Fall into unspecified water causing** drowning and submersion

√x7ᵗʰ **W16.42 Fall into unspecified water causing other injury**
√5ᵗʰ **W16.5 Jumping or diving into** swimming pool
  √6ᵗʰ **W16.51 Jumping or diving into swimming pool** striking water surface
    √7ᵗʰ **W16.511 Jumping or diving into swimming pool striking water surface causing** drowning and submersion
      EXCLUDES 1   *drowning and submersion while in swimming pool without jumping or diving (W67)*
    √7ᵗʰ **W16.512 Jumping or diving into swimming pool striking water surface causing other injury**
  √6ᵗʰ **W16.52 Jumping or diving into swimming pool** striking bottom
    √7ᵗʰ **W16.521 Jumping or diving into swimming pool striking bottom causing** drowning and submersion
      EXCLUDES 1   *drowning and submersion while in swimming pool without jumping or diving (W67)*
    √7ᵗʰ **W16.522 Jumping or diving into swimming pool striking bottom causing other injury**
  √6ᵗʰ **W16.53 Jumping or diving into swimming pool** striking wall
    √7ᵗʰ **W16.531 Jumping or diving into swimming pool striking wall causing** drowning and submersion
      EXCLUDES 1   *drowning and submersion while in swimming pool without jumping or diving (W67)*
    √7ᵗʰ **W16.532 Jumping or diving into swimming pool striking wall causing other injury**
√5ᵗʰ **W16.6 Jumping or diving into** natural body of water
    Jumping or diving into lake
    Jumping or diving into open sea
    Jumping or diving into river
    Jumping or diving into stream
  √6ᵗʰ **W16.61 Jumping or diving into natural body of water** striking water surface
    √7ᵗʰ **W16.611 Jumping or diving into natural body of water striking water surface causing** drowning and submersion
      EXCLUDES 1   *drowning and submersion while in natural body of water without jumping or diving (W69)*
    √7ᵗʰ **W16.612 Jumping or diving into natural body of water striking water surface causing other injury**
  √6ᵗʰ **W16.62 Jumping or diving into natural body of water** striking bottom
    √7ᵗʰ **W16.621 Jumping or diving into natural body of water striking bottom causing** drowning and submersion
      EXCLUDES 1   *drowning and submersion while in natural body of water without jumping or diving (W69)*
    √7ᵗʰ **W16.622 Jumping or diving into natural body of water striking bottom causing other injury**
√5ᵗʰ **W16.7 Jumping or diving** from boat
    EXCLUDES 1   *fall from boat into water — see watercraft accident (V90-V94)*
  √6ᵗʰ **W16.71 Jumping or diving from boat** striking water surface
    √7ᵗʰ **W16.711 Jumping or diving from boat striking water surface causing** drowning and submersion
    √7ᵗʰ **W16.712 Jumping or diving from boat striking water surface causing other injury**
  √6ᵗʰ **W16.72 Jumping or diving from boat** striking bottom
    √7ᵗʰ **W16.721 Jumping or diving from boat striking bottom causing** drowning and submersion
    √7ᵗʰ **W16.722 Jumping or diving from boat striking bottom causing other injury**

✓5ᵗʰ **W16.8** **Jumping or diving into other water**
- Jumping or diving into fountain
- Jumping or diving into reservoir

✓6ᵗʰ **W16.81** **Jumping or diving into other water striking water surface**

✓7ᵗʰ **W16.811** **Jumping or diving into other water striking water surface causing** drowning and submersion

     EXCLUDES 1   *drowning and submersion while in other water without jumping or diving (W73)*

✓7ᵗʰ **W16.812** **Jumping or diving into other water striking water surface causing other injury**

✓6ᵗʰ **W16.82** **Jumping or diving into other water striking bottom**

✓7ᵗʰ **W16.821** **Jumping or diving into other water striking bottom causing** drowning and submersion

     EXCLUDES 1   *drowning and submersion while in other water without jumping or diving (W73)*

✓7ᵗʰ **W16.822** **Jumping or diving into other water striking bottom causing other injury**

✓6ᵗʰ **W16.83** **Jumping or diving into other water striking wall**

✓7ᵗʰ **W16.831** **Jumping or diving into other water striking wall causing** drowning and submersion

     EXCLUDES 1   *drowning and submersion while in other water without jumping or diving (W73)*

✓7ᵗʰ **W16.832** **Jumping or diving into other water striking wall causing other injury**

✓5ᵗʰ **W16.9** **Jumping or diving into unspecified water**

✓7ᵗʰ **W16.91** **Jumping or diving into unspecified water causing** drowning and submersion

✓7ᵗʰ **W16.92** **Jumping or diving into unspecified water causing other injury**

✓4ᵗʰ **W17** **Other fall from one level to another**

✓7ᵗʰ **W17.0** **Fall into well**

✓7ᵗʰ **W17.1** **Fall into storm drain or manhole**

✓7ᵗʰ **W17.2** **Fall into hole**
- Fall into pit

✓7ᵗʰ **W17.3** **Fall into empty swimming pool**

     EXCLUDES 1   *fall into filled swimming pool (W16.0-)*

✓7ᵗʰ **W17.4** **Fall from dock**

✓5ᵗʰ **W17.8** **Other fall from one level to another**

✓7ᵗʰ **W17.81** **Fall down embankment (hill)**

✓7ᵗʰ **W17.82** **Fall from (out of) grocery cart**
- Fall due to grocery cart tipping over

✓7ᵗʰ **W17.89** **Other fall from one level to another**
- Fall from cherry picker
- Fall from lifting device
- Fall from mobile elevated work platform [MEWP]
- Fall from sky lift
- **AHA:** 2015,2Q,6

✓4ᵗʰ **W18** **Other slipping, tripping and stumbling and falls**

✓5ᵗʰ **W18.0** **Fall due to bumping against object**
- Striking against object with subsequent fall

     EXCLUDES 1   *fall on same level due to slipping, tripping, or stumbling with subsequent striking against object (W01.1-)*

✓7ᵗʰ **W18.00** **Striking against unspecified object with subsequent fall**

✓7ᵗʰ **W18.01** **Striking against** sports equipment **with subsequent fall**

✓7ᵗʰ **W18.02** **Striking against** glass **with subsequent fall**

✓7ᵗʰ **W18.09** **Striking against other object with subsequent fall**

✓5ᵗʰ **W18.1** **Fall from or off toilet**

✓7ᵗʰ **W18.11** **Fall from or off toilet** without subsequent striking against object
- Fall from (off) toilet NOS

✓7ᵗʰ **W18.12** **Fall from or off toilet** with subsequent striking against object

✓7ᵗʰ **W18.2** **Fall in (into) shower or empty bathtub**

     EXCLUDES 1   *fall in full bathtub causing drowning or submersion (W16.21-)*

✓5ᵗʰ **W18.3** **Other and unspecified fall on same level**

✓7ᵗʰ **W18.30** **Fall on same level, unspecified**

✓7ᵗʰ **W18.31** **Fall on same level due to stepping on an object**
- Fall on same level due to stepping on an animal

     EXCLUDES 1   *slipping, tripping and stumbling without fall due to stepping on animal (W18.41)*

✓7ᵗʰ **W18.39** **Other fall on same level**

✓5ᵗʰ **W18.4** **Slipping, tripping and stumbling without falling**

     EXCLUDES 1   *collision with another person without fall (W51)*

✓7ᵗʰ **W18.40** **Slipping, tripping and stumbling without falling, unspecified**

✓7ᵗʰ **W18.41** **Slipping, tripping and stumbling without falling due to** stepping on object
- Slipping, tripping and stumbling without falling due to stepping on animal

     EXCLUDES 1   *slipping, tripping and stumbling with fall due to stepping on animal (W18.31)*

✓7ᵗʰ **W18.42** **Slipping, tripping and stumbling without falling due to** stepping into hole or opening

✓7ᵗʰ **W18.43** **Slipping, tripping and stumbling without falling due to** stepping from one level to another

✓7ᵗʰ **W18.49** **Other slipping, tripping and stumbling without falling**

✓7ᵗʰ **W19** **Unspecified fall**
- Accidental fall NOS
- **AHA:** 2012,4Q,95

Exposure to inanimate mechanical forces (W20-W49)

     EXCLUDES 1   *assault (X92-Y09)*
        contact or collision with animals or persons (W50-W64)
        exposure to inanimate mechanical forces involving military or war operations (Y36.-, Y37.-)
        intentional self-harm (X71-X83)

The appropriate 7th character is to be added to each code from categories W20-W49.
A   initial encounter
D   subsequent encounter
S   sequela

✓4ᵗʰ **W20** **Struck by thrown, projected or falling object**
- Code first any associated:
- cataclysm (X34-X39)
- lightning strike (T75.00)

     EXCLUDES 1   *falling object in machinery accident (W24, W28-W31)*
        falling object in transport accident (V01-V99)
        object set in motion by explosion (W35-W40)
        object set in motion by firearm (W32-W34)
        struck by thrown sports equipment (W21.-)

✓7ᵗʰ **W20.0** **Struck by falling object in cave-in**

     EXCLUDES 2   *asphyxiation due to cave-in (T71.21)*

✓7ᵗʰ **W20.1** **Struck by object due to collapse of building**

     EXCLUDES 1   *struck by object due to collapse of burning building (X00.2, X02.2)*

✓7ᵗʰ **W20.8** **Other cause of strike by thrown, projected or falling object**

     EXCLUDES 1   *struck by thrown sports equipment (W21.-)*

✓4ᵗʰ **W21** **Striking against or struck by sports equipment**

     EXCLUDES 1   *assault with sports equipment (Y08.0-)*
        striking against or struck by sports equipment with subsequent fall (W18.01)

✓5ᵗʰ **W21.0** **Struck by** hit or thrown ball

✓7ᵗʰ **W21.00** **Struck by hit or thrown ball, unspecified type**

✓7ᵗʰ **W21.01** **Struck by football**

✓7ᵗʰ **W21.02** **Struck by soccer ball**

✓7ᵗʰ **W21.03** **Struck by baseball**

✓7ᵗʰ **W21.04** **Struck by golf ball**

✓7ᵗʰ **W21.05** **Struck by basketball**

✓7ᵗʰ **W21.06** **Struck by volleyball**

✓7ᵗʰ **W21.07** **Struck by softball**

☑x7ᵗʰ W21.09 **Struck by** other hit or thrown ball

☑5ᵗʰ W21.1 **Struck by** bat, racquet or club

   ☑x7ᵗʰ W21.11 **Struck by** baseball bat

   ☑x7ᵗʰ W21.12 **Struck by** tennis racquet

   ☑x7ᵗʰ W21.13 **Struck by** golf club

   ☑x7ᵗʰ W21.19 **Struck by** other bat, racquet or club

☑5ᵗʰ W21.2 **Struck by** hockey stick or puck

   ☑6ᵗʰ W21.21 **Struck by** hockey stick

      ☑7ᵗʰ W21.210 **Struck by** ice hockey stick

      ☑7ᵗʰ W21.211 **Struck by** field hockey stick

   ☑6ᵗʰ W21.22 **Struck by** hockey puck

      ☑7ᵗʰ W21.220 **Struck by** ice hockey puck

      ☑7ᵗʰ W21.221 **Struck by** field hockey puck

☑5ᵗʰ W21.3 **Struck by** sports foot wear

   ☑x7ᵗʰ W21.31 **Struck by** shoe cleats

      Stepped on by shoe cleats

   ☑x7ᵗʰ W21.32 **Struck by** skate blades

      Skated over by skate blades

   ☑x7ᵗʰ W21.39 **Struck by** other sports foot wear

☑x7ᵗʰ W21.4 **Striking against** diving board

      Use additional code for subsequent falling into water, if applicable (W16.-)

☑5ᵗʰ W21.8 **Striking against or struck by** other sports equipment

   ☑x7ᵗʰ W21.81 **Striking against or struck by** football helmet

   ☑x7ᵗʰ W21.89 **Striking against or struck by** other sports equipment

☑x7ᵗʰ W21.9 **Striking against or struck by** unspecified sports equipment

☑4ᵗʰ **W22** **Striking against or struck by other objects**

   EXCLUDES 1 striking against or struck by object with subsequent fall (W18.09)

☑5ᵗʰ W22.0 **Striking against** stationary object

   EXCLUDES 1 striking against stationary sports equipment (W21.8)

   ☑x7ᵗʰ W22.01 **Walked into** wall

   ☑x7ᵗʰ W22.02 **Walked into** lamppost

   ☑x7ᵗʰ W22.03 **Walked into** furniture

   ☑6ᵗʰ W22.04 **Striking against** wall of swimming pool

      ☑7ᵗʰ W22.041 **Striking against** wall of swimming pool causing drowning and submersion

         EXCLUDES 1 drowning and submersion while swimming without striking against wall (W67)

      ☑7ᵗʰ W22.042 **Striking against** wall of swimming pool causing other injury

   ☑x7ᵗʰ W22.09 **Striking against** other stationary object

☑5ᵗʰ W22.1 **Striking against or struck by** automobile airbag

   ☑x7ᵗʰ W22.10 **Striking against or struck by** unspecified automobile airbag

   ☑x7ᵗʰ W22.11 **Striking against or struck by** driver side automobile airbag

   ☑x7ᵗʰ W22.12 **Striking against or struck by** front passenger side automobile airbag

   ☑x7ᵗʰ W22.19 **Striking against or struck by** other automobile airbag

☑x7ᵗʰ W22.8 **Striking against or struck by** other objects

      Striking against or struck by object NOS

   EXCLUDES 1 struck by thrown, projected or falling object (W20.-)

☑4ᵗʰ **W23** **Caught, crushed, jammed or pinched in or between objects**

   EXCLUDES 1 injury caused by cutting or piercing instruments (W25-W27)

        injury caused by firearms malfunction (W32.1, W33.1-, W34.1-)

        injury caused by lifting and transmission devices (W24.-)

        injury caused by machinery (W28-W31)

        injury caused by nonpowered hand tools (W27.-)

        injury caused by transport vehicle being used as a means of transportation (V01-V99)

        injury caused by struck by thrown, projected or falling object (W20.-)

☑x7ᵗʰ W23.0 **Caught, crushed, jammed, or pinched between** moving objects

☑x7ᵗʰ W23.1 **Caught, crushed, jammed, or pinched between** stationary objects

☑4ᵗʰ **W24** **Contact with lifting and transmission devices, not elsewhere classified**

   EXCLUDES 1 transport accidents (V01-V99)

☑x7ᵗʰ W24.0 **Contact with** lifting devices, not elsewhere classified

      Contact with chain hoist

      Contact with drive belt

      Contact with pulley (block)

☑x7ᵗʰ W24.1 **Contact with** transmission devices, not elsewhere classified

      Contact with transmission belt or cable

☑x7ᵗʰ **W25** **Contact with sharp glass**

   Code first any associated:

      injury due to flying glass from explosion or firearm discharge (W32-W40)

      transport accident (V00-V99)

   EXCLUDES 1 fall on same level due to slipping, tripping and stumbling with subsequent striking against sharp glass (W01.110)

        striking against sharp glass with subsequent fall (W18.02)

   EXCLUDES 2 glass embedded in skin (W45)

☑4ᵗʰ **W26** **Contact with other sharp objects**

   EXCLUDES 2 sharp object(s) embedded in skin (W45)

   AHA: 2016,4Q,73

☑x7ᵗʰ W26.0 **Contact with** knife

   EXCLUDES 1 contact with electric knife (W29.1)

☑x7ᵗʰ W26.1 **Contact with** sword or dagger

☑x7ᵗʰ W26.2 **Contact with** edge of stiff paper

      Paper cut

☑x7ᵗʰ W26.8 **Contact with** other sharp object(s), not elsewhere classified

      Contact with tin can lid

☑x7ᵗʰ W26.9 **Contact with** unspecified sharp object(s)

☑4ᵗʰ **W27** **Contact with nonpowered hand tool**

☑x7ᵗʰ W27.0 **Contact with** workbench tool

      Contact with auger

      Contact with axe

      Contact with chisel

      Contact with handsaw

      Contact with screwdriver

☑x7ᵗʰ W27.1 **Contact with** garden tool

      Contact with hoe

      Contact with nonpowered lawn mower

      Contact with pitchfork

      Contact with rake

☑x7ᵗʰ W27.2 **Contact with** scissors

☑x7ᵗʰ W27.3 **Contact with** needle (sewing)

   EXCLUDES 1 contact with hypodermic needle (W46.-)

☑x7ᵗʰ W27.4 **Contact with** kitchen utensil

      Contact with fork

      Contact with ice-pick

      Contact with can-opener NOS

☑x7ᵗʰ W27.5 **Contact with** paper-cutter

☑x7ᵗʰ W27.8 **Contact with** other nonpowered hand tool

      Contact with nonpowered sewing machine

      Contact with shovel

☑x7ᵗʰ **W28** **Contact with powered lawn mower**

   Powered lawn mower (commercial) (residential)

   EXCLUDES 1 contact with nonpowered lawn mower (W27.1)

   EXCLUDES 2 exposure to electric current (W86.-)

☑4ᵗʰ **W29** **Contact with other powered hand tools and household machinery**

   EXCLUDES 1 contact with commercial machinery (W31.82)

        contact with hot household appliance (X15)

        contact with nonpowered hand tool (W27.-)

        exposure to electric current (W86)

☑x7ᵗʰ W29.0 **Contact with** powered kitchen appliance

      Contact with blender

      Contact with can-opener

      Contact with garbage disposal

      Contact with mixer

☑x7ᵗʰ W29.1 **Contact with** electric knife

Chapter 20. External Causes of Morbidity

W29.2 Contact with other powered household machinery
Contact with electric fan
Contact with powered dryer (clothes) (powered) (spin)
Contact with washing-machine
Contact with sewing machine

W29.3 Contact with powered garden and outdoor hand tools and machinery
Contact with chainsaw
Contact with edger
Contact with garden cultivator (tiller)
Contact with hedge trimmer
Contact with other powered garden tool
EXCLUDES 1 *contact with powered lawn mower (W28)*

W29.4 Contact with nail gun

W29.8 Contact with other powered hand tools and household machinery
Contact with do-it-yourself tool NOS

W30 Contact with agricultural machinery
INCLUDES animal-powered farm machine
EXCLUDES 1 *agricultural transport vehicle accident (V01-V99)*
explosion of grain store (W40.8)
exposure to electric current (W86.-)

W30.0 Contact with combine harvester
Contact with reaper
Contact with thresher

W30.1 Contact with power take-off devices (PTO)

W30.2 Contact with hay derrick

W30.3 Contact with grain storage elevator
EXCLUDES 1 *explosion of grain store (W40.8)*

W30.8 Contact with other specified agricultural machinery

W30.81 Contact with agricultural transport vehicle in stationary use
Contact with agricultural transport vehicle under repair, not on public roadway
EXCLUDES 1 *agricultural transport vehicle accident (V01-V99)*

W30.89 Contact with other specified agricultural machinery

W30.9 Contact with unspecified agricultural machinery
Contact with farm machinery NOS

W31 Contact with other and unspecified machinery
EXCLUDES 1 *contact with agricultural machinery (W30.-)*
contact with machinery in transport under own power or being towed by a vehicle (V01-V99)
exposure to electric current (W86)

W31.0 Contact with mining and earth-drilling machinery
Contact with bore or drill (land) (seabed)
Contact with shaft hoist
Contact with shaft lift
Contact with undercutter

W31.1 Contact with metalworking machines
Contact with abrasive wheel
Contact with forging machine
Contact with lathe
Contact with mechanical shears
Contact with metal drilling machine
Contact with milling machine
Contact with power press
Contact with rolling-mill
Contact with metal sawing machine

W31.2 Contact with powered woodworking and forming machines
Contact with band saw
Contact with bench saw
Contact with circular saw
Contact with molding machine
Contact with overhead plane
Contact with powered saw
Contact with radial saw
Contact with sander
EXCLUDES 1 *nonpowered woodworking tools (W27.0)*

W31.3 Contact with prime movers
Contact with gas turbine
Contact with internal combustion engine
Contact with steam engine
Contact with water driven turbine

W31.8 Contact with other specified machinery

W31.81 Contact with recreational machinery
Contact with roller coaster

W31.82 Contact with other commercial machinery
Contact with commercial electric fan
Contact with commercial kitchen appliances
Contact with commercial powered dryer (clothes) (powered) (spin)
Contact with commercial washing-machine
Contact with commercial sewing machine
EXCLUDES 1 *contact with household machinery (W29.-)*
contact with powered lawn mower (W28)

W31.83 Contact with special construction vehicle in stationary use
Contact with special construction vehicle under repair, not on public roadway
EXCLUDES 1 *special construction vehicle accident (V01-V99)*

W31.89 Contact with other specified machinery

W31.9 Contact with unspecified machinery
Contact with machinery NOS

W32 Accidental handgun discharge and malfunction
INCLUDES accidental discharge and malfunction of gun for single hand use
accidental discharge and malfunction of pistol
accidental discharge and malfunction of revolver
handgun discharge and malfunction NOS
EXCLUDES 1 *accidental airgun discharge and malfunction (W34.010, W34.110)*
accidental BB gun discharge and malfunction (W34.010, W34.110)
accidental pellet gun discharge and malfunction (W34.010, W34.110)
accidental shotgun discharge and malfunction (W33.01, W33.11)
assault by handgun discharge (X93)
handgun discharge involving legal intervention (Y35.0-)
handgun discharge involving military or war operations (Y36.4-)
intentional self-harm by handgun discharge (X72)
Very pistol discharge and malfunction (W34.09, W34.19)

W32.0 Accidental handgun discharge

W32.1 Accidental handgun malfunction
Injury due to explosion of handgun (parts)
Injury due to malfunction of mechanism or component of handgun
Injury due to recoil of handgun
Powder burn from handgun

W33 Accidental rifle, shotgun and larger firearm discharge and malfunction
INCLUDES rifle, shotgun and larger firearm discharge and malfunction NOS
EXCLUDES 1 *accidental airgun discharge and malfunction (W34.010, W34.110)*
accidental BB gun discharge and malfunction (W34.010, W34.110)
accidental handgun discharge and malfunction (W32.-)
accidental pellet gun discharge and malfunction (W34.010, W34.110)
assault by rifle, shotgun and larger firearm discharge (X94)
firearm discharge involving legal intervention (Y35.0-)
firearm discharge involving military or war operations (Y36.4-)
intentional self-harm by rifle, shotgun and larger firearm discharge (X73)

W33.0 Accidental rifle, shotgun and larger firearm discharge

W33.00 Accidental discharge of unspecified larger firearm
Discharge of unspecified larger firearm NOS

√x7ᵗʰ **W33.01 Accidental discharge of** shotgun
     Discharge of shotgun NOS

√x7ᵗʰ **W33.02 Accidental discharge of** hunting rifle
     Discharge of hunting rifle NOS

√x7ᵗʰ **W33.03 Accidental discharge of** machine gun
     Discharge of machine gun NOS

√x7ᵗʰ **W33.09 Accidental discharge of other larger firearm**
     Discharge of other larger firearm NOS

√5ᵗʰ **W33.1 Accidental rifle, shotgun and larger firearm** malfunction
     Injury due to explosion of rifle, shotgun and larger firearm (parts)
     Injury due to malfunction of mechanism or component of rifle, shotgun and larger firearm
     Injury due to piercing, cutting, crushing or pinching due to (by) slide trigger mechanism, scope or other gun part
     Injury due to recoil of rifle, shotgun and larger firearm
     Powder burn from rifle, shotgun and larger firearm

√x7ᵗʰ **W33.10 Accidental malfunction of unspecified larger firearm**
     Malfunction of unspecified larger firearm NOS

√x7ᵗʰ **W33.11 Accidental malfunction of** shotgun
     Malfunction of shotgun NOS

√x7ᵗʰ **W33.12 Accidental malfunction of** hunting rifle
     Malfunction of hunting rifle NOS

√x7ᵗʰ **W33.13 Accidental malfunction of** machine gun
     Malfunction of machine gun NOS

√x7ᵗʰ **W33.19 Accidental malfunction of other larger firearm**
     Malfunction of other larger firearm NOS

√4ᵗʰ **W34 Accidental discharge and malfunction from other and unspecified firearms and guns**

√5ᵗʰ **W34.0 Accidental** discharge **from other and unspecified firearms and guns**

√x6ᵗʰ **W34.00 Accidental discharge from unspecified firearms or gun**
     Discharge from firearm NOS
     Gunshot wound NOS
     Shot NOS

√6ᵗʰ **W34.01 Accidental discharge of** gas, air or spring-operated **guns**

√7ᵗʰ **W34.010 Accidental discharge of** airgun
     Accidental discharge of BB gun
     Accidental discharge of pellet gun

√7ᵗʰ **W34.011 Accidental discharge of** paintball gun
     Accidental injury due to paintball discharge

√7ᵗʰ **W34.018 Accidental discharge of other gas, air or spring-operated gun**

√x7ᵗʰ **W34.09 Accidental discharge from other specified firearms**
     Accidental discharge from Very pistol [flare]

√5ᵗʰ **W34.1 Accidental** malfunction **from other and unspecified firearms and guns**

√x7ᵗʰ **W34.10 Accidental malfunction from unspecified firearms or gun**
     Firearm malfunction NOS

√6ᵗʰ **W34.11 Accidental malfunction of** gas, air or spring-operated **guns**

√7ᵗʰ **W34.110 Accidental malfunction of** airgun
     Accidental malfunction of BB gun
     Accidental malfunction of pellet gun

√7ᵗʰ **W34.111 Accidental malfunction of** paintball gun
     Accidental injury due to paintball gun malfunction

√7ᵗʰ **W34.118 Accidental malfunction of other gas, air or spring-operated gun**

√x7ᵗʰ **W34.19 Accidental malfunction from other specified firearms**
     Accidental malfunction from Very pistol [flare]

√x7ᵗʰ **W35 Explosion and rupture of** boiler
     EXCLUDES 1   explosion and rupture of boiler on watercraft (V93.4)

√4ᵗʰ **W36 Explosion and rupture of** gas cylinder

√x7ᵗʰ **W36.1 Explosion and rupture of** aerosol can

√x7ᵗʰ **W36.2 Explosion and rupture of** air tank

√x7ᵗʰ **W36.3 Explosion and rupture of** pressurized-gas tank

√x7ᵗʰ **W36.8 Explosion and rupture of other gas cylinder**

√x7ᵗʰ **W36.9 Explosion and rupture of unspecified gas cylinder**

√4ᵗʰ **W37 Explosion and rupture of** pressurized tire, pipe or hose

√x7ᵗʰ **W37.0 Explosion of** bicycle tire

√x7ᵗʰ **W37.8 Explosion and rupture of other pressurized tire, pipe or hose**

√x7ᵗʰ **W38 Explosion and rupture of other specified** pressurized devices

√4ᵗʰ **W39 Discharge of** firework

√4ᵗʰ **W40 Explosion of other materials**
     EXCLUDES 1   assault by explosive material (X96)
       explosion involving legal intervention (Y35.1-)
       explosion involving military or war operations (Y36.0-, Y36.2-)
       intentional self-harm by explosive material (X75)

√x7ᵗʰ **W40.0 Explosion of** blasting material
     Explosion of blasting cap
     Explosion of detonator
     Explosion of dynamite
     Explosion of explosive (any) used in blasting operations

√x7ᵗʰ **W40.1 Explosion of** explosive gases
     Explosion of acetylene
     Explosion of butane
     Explosion of coal gas
     Explosion in mine NOS
     Explosion of explosive gas
     Explosion of fire damp
     Explosion of gasoline fumes
     Explosion of methane
     Explosion of propane

√x7ᵗʰ **W40.8 Explosion of other specified explosive materials**
     Explosion in dump NOS
     Explosion in factory NOS
     Explosion in grain store
     Explosion in munitions
     EXCLUDES 1   explosion involving legal intervention (Y35.1-)
       explosion involving military or war operations (Y36.0-, Y36.2-)

√x7ᵗʰ **W40.9 Explosion of unspecified explosive materials**
     Explosion NOS

√4ᵗʰ **W42 Exposure to noise**

√x7ᵗʰ **W42.0 Exposure to supersonic waves**

√x7ᵗʰ **W42.9 Exposure to other noise**
     Exposure to sound waves NOS

√4ᵗʰ **W45 Foreign body or object entering through skin**
     INCLUDES   foreign body or object embedded in skin
       nail embedded in skin
     EXCLUDES 2   contact with hand tools (nonpowered) (powered) (W27-W29)
       contact with other sharp objects (W26.-)
       contact with sharp glass (W25.-)
       struck by objects (W20-W22)

√x7ᵗʰ **W45.0 Nail entering through skin**

√x7ᵗʰ **W45.8 Other foreign body or object entering through skin**
     Splinter in skin NOS

√4ᵗʰ **W46 Contact with hypodermic needle**

√x7ᵗʰ **W46.0 Contact with hypodermic needle**
     Hypodermic needle stick NOS

√x7ᵗʰ **W46.1 Contact with** contaminated **hypodermic needle**

√4ᵗʰ **W49 Exposure to other inanimate mechanical forces**
     INCLUDES   exposure to abnormal gravitational [G] forces
       exposure to inanimate mechanical forces NEC
     EXCLUDES 1   exposure to inanimate mechanical forces involving military or war operations (Y36.-, Y37.-)

√5ᵗʰ **W49.0 Item causing** external constriction

√x7ᵗʰ **W49.01 Hair causing external constriction**

√x7ᵗʰ **W49.02 String or thread causing external constriction**

√x7ᵗʰ **W49.03 Rubber band causing external constriction**

√x7ᵗʰ **W49.04 Ring or other jewelry causing external constriction**

√x7ᵗʰ **W49.09 Other specified item causing external constriction**

√x7ᵗʰ **W49.9 Exposure to other inanimate mechanical forces**

Exposure to animate mechanical forces (W5Ø-W64)

EXCLUDES 1 　toxic effect of contact with venomous animals and plants (T63.-)

The appropriate 7th character is to be added to each code from categories W50-W64.
A　initial encounter
D　subsequent encounter
S　sequela

✓4ᵗʰ **W50　Accidental hit, strike, kick, twist, bite or scratch by another person**

　　INCLUDES 　hit, strike, kick, twist, bite, or scratch by another person NOS

　　EXCLUDES 1 　assault by bodily force (Y04)
　　　　　　struck by objects (W20-W22)

✓x7ᵗʰ **W50.Ø　Accidental hit or strike by another person**
　　Hit or strike by another person NOS

✓x7ᵗʰ **W50.1　Accidental kick by another person**
　　Kick by another person NOS

✓x7ᵗʰ **W50.2　Accidental twist by another person**
　　Twist by another person NOS

✓x7ᵗʰ **W50.3　Accidental bite by another person**
　　Human bite
　　Bite by another person NOS

✓x7ᵗʰ **W50.4　Accidental scratch by another person**
　　Scratch by another person NOS

✓x7ᵗʰ **W51　Accidental striking against or bumped into by another person**

　　EXCLUDES 1 　assault by striking against or bumping into by another person (Y04.2)
　　　　　　fall due to collision with another person (W03)

✓x7ᵗʰ **W52　Crushed, pushed or stepped on by crowd or human stampede**
　　Crushed, pushed or stepped on by crowd or human stampede with or without fall

✓4ᵗʰ **W53　Contact with rodent**
　　INCLUDES 　contact with saliva, feces or urine of rodent

　✓5ᵗʰ **W53.Ø　Contact with mouse**
　　✓x7ᵗʰ **W53.Ø1　Bitten by mouse**
　　✓x7ᵗʰ **W53.Ø9　Other contact with mouse**

　✓5ᵗʰ **W53.1　Contact with rat**
　　✓x7ᵗʰ **W53.11　Bitten by rat**
　　✓x7ᵗʰ **W53.19　Other contact with rat**

　✓5ᵗʰ **W53.2　Contact with squirrel**
　　✓x7ᵗʰ **W53.21　Bitten by squirrel**
　　✓x7ᵗʰ **W53.29　Other contact with squirrel**

　✓5ᵗʰ **W53.8　Contact with other rodent**
　　✓x7ᵗʰ **W53.81　Bitten by other rodent**
　　✓x7ᵗʰ **W53.89　Other contact with other rodent**

✓4ᵗʰ **W54　Contact with dog**
　　INCLUDES 　contact with saliva, feces or urine of dog

✓x7ᵗʰ **W54.Ø　Bitten by dog**

✓x7ᵗʰ **W54.1　Struck by dog**
　　Knocked over by dog

✓x7ᵗʰ **W54.8　Other contact with dog**

✓4ᵗʰ **W55　Contact with other mammals**
　　INCLUDES 　contact with saliva, feces or urine of mammal
　　EXCLUDES 1 　animal being ridden — see transport accidents
　　　　　　bitten or struck by dog (W54)
　　　　　　bitten or struck by rodent (W53.-)
　　　　　　contact with marine mammals (W56.-)

　✓5ᵗʰ **W55.Ø　Contact with cat**
　　✓x7ᵗʰ **W55.Ø1　Bitten by cat**
　　✓x7ᵗʰ **W55.Ø3　Scratched by cat**
　　✓x7ᵗʰ **W55.Ø9　Other contact with cat**

　✓5ᵗʰ **W55.1　Contact with horse**
　　✓x7ᵗʰ **W55.11　Bitten by horse**
　　✓x7ᵗʰ **W55.12　Struck by horse**
　　✓x7ᵗʰ **W55.19　Other contact with horse**

　✓5ᵗʰ **W55.2　Contact with cow**
　　Contact with bull
　　✓x7ᵗʰ **W55.21　Bitten by cow**

　　✓x7ᵗʰ **W55.22　Struck by cow**
　　　Gored by bull
　　✓x7ᵗʰ **W55.29　Other contact with cow**

　✓5ᵗʰ **W55.3　Contact with other hoof stock**
　　Contact with goats
　　Contact with sheep
　　✓x7ᵗʰ **W55.31　Bitten by other hoof stock**
　　✓x7ᵗʰ **W55.32　Struck by other hoof stock**
　　　Gored by goat
　　　Gored by ram
　　✓x7ᵗʰ **W55.39　Other contact with other hoof stock**

　✓5ᵗʰ **W55.4　Contact with pig**
　　✓x7ᵗʰ **W55.41　Bitten by pig**
　　✓x7ᵗʰ **W55.42　Struck by pig**
　　✓x7ᵗʰ **W55.49　Other contact with pig**

　✓5ᵗʰ **W55.5　Contact with raccoon**
　　✓x7ᵗʰ **W55.51　Bitten by raccoon**
　　✓x7ᵗʰ **W55.52　Struck by raccoon**
　　✓x7ᵗʰ **W55.59　Other contact with raccoon**

　✓5ᵗʰ **W55.8　Contact with other mammals**
　　✓x7ᵗʰ **W55.81　Bitten by other mammals**
　　✓x7ᵗʰ **W55.82　Struck by other mammals**
　　✓x7ᵗʰ **W55.89　Other contact with other mammals**

✓4ᵗʰ **W56　Contact with nonvenomous marine animal**
　　EXCLUDES 1 　contact with venomous marine animal (T63.-)

　✓5ᵗʰ **W56.Ø　Contact with dolphin**
　　✓x7ᵗʰ **W56.Ø1　Bitten by dolphin**
　　✓x7ᵗʰ **W56.Ø2　Struck by dolphin**
　　✓x7ᵗʰ **W56.Ø9　Other contact with dolphin**

　✓5ᵗʰ **W56.1　Contact with sea lion**
　　✓x7ᵗʰ **W56.11　Bitten by sea lion**
　　✓x7ᵗʰ **W56.12　Struck by sea lion**
　　✓x7ᵗʰ **W56.19　Other contact with sea lion**

　✓5ᵗʰ **W56.2　Contact with orca**
　　Contact with killer whale
　　✓x7ᵗʰ **W56.21　Bitten by orca**
　　✓x7ᵗʰ **W56.22　Struck by orca**
　　✓x7ᵗʰ **W56.29　Other contact with orca**

　✓5ᵗʰ **W56.3　Contact with other marine mammals**
　　✓x7ᵗʰ **W56.31　Bitten by other marine mammals**
　　✓x7ᵗʰ **W56.32　Struck by other marine mammals**
　　✓x7ᵗʰ **W56.39　Other contact with other marine mammals**

　✓5ᵗʰ **W56.4　Contact with shark**
　　✓x7ᵗʰ **W56.41　Bitten by shark**
　　✓x7ᵗʰ **W56.42　Struck by shark**
　　✓x7ᵗʰ **W56.49　Other contact with shark**

　✓5ᵗʰ **W56.5　Contact with other fish**
　　✓x7ᵗʰ **W56.51　Bitten by other fish**
　　✓x7ᵗʰ **W56.52　Struck by other fish**
　　✓x7ᵗʰ **W56.59　Other contact with other fish**

　✓5ᵗʰ **W56.8　Contact with other nonvenomous marine animals**
　　✓x7ᵗʰ **W56.81　Bitten by other nonvenomous marine animals**
　　✓x7ᵗʰ **W56.82　Struck by other nonvenomous marine animals**
　　✓x7ᵗʰ **W56.89　Other contact with other nonvenomous marine animals**

✓x7ᵗʰ **W57　Bitten or stung by nonvenomous insect and other nonvenomous arthropods**
　　EXCLUDES 1 　contact with venomous insects and arthropods (T63.2-, T63.3-, T63.4-)

✓4ᵗʰ **W58　Contact with crocodile or alligator**

　✓5ᵗʰ **W58.Ø　Contact with alligator**
　　✓x7ᵗʰ **W58.Ø1　Bitten by alligator**
　　✓x7ᵗʰ **W58.Ø2　Struck by alligator**
　　✓x7ᵗʰ **W58.Ø3　Crushed by alligator**
　　✓x7ᵗʰ **W58.Ø9　Other contact with alligator**

N Newborn: 0　　P Pediatric: 0-17　　M Maternity: 9-64　　A Adult: 15-124　　MCC Major Complication/Comorbidity　　CC Complication/Comorbidity　　SW Severe Wound Dx

1204　　　　　　ICD-10-CM 2021

√5ᵗʰ **W58.1 Contact with** crocodile

    √x7ᵗʰ   **W58.11   Bitten** by crocodile

    √x7ᵗʰ   **W58.12   Struck** by crocodile

    √x7ᵗʰ   **W58.13   Crushed** by crocodile

    √x7ᵗʰ   **W58.19   Other contact** with crocodile

√4ᵗʰ **W59 Contact with other nonvenomous reptiles**

     EXCLUDES 1   *contact with venomous reptile (T63.0-, T63.1-)*

   √5ᵗʰ **W59.0 Contact with** nonvenomous lizards

    √x7ᵗʰ   **W59.01   Bitten** by nonvenomous lizards

    √x7ᵗʰ   **W59.02   Struck** by nonvenomous lizards

    √x7ᵗʰ   **W59.09   Other contact** with nonvenomous lizards

       Exposure to nonvenomous lizards

   √5ᵗʰ **W59.1 Contact with** nonvenomous snakes

    √x7ᵗʰ   **W59.11   Bitten** by nonvenomous snake

    √x7ᵗʰ   **W59.12   Struck** by nonvenomous snake

    √x7ᵗʰ   **W59.13   Crushed** by nonvenomous snake

    √x7ᵗʰ   **W59.19   Other contact** with nonvenomous snake

   √5ᵗʰ **W59.2 Contact with** turtles

     EXCLUDES 1   *contact with tortoises (W59.8-)*

    √x7ᵗʰ   **W59.21   Bitten** by turtle

    √x7ᵗʰ   **W59.22   Struck** by turtle

    √x7ᵗʰ   **W59.29   Other contact** with turtle

       Exposure to turtles

   √5ᵗʰ **W59.8 Contact with other** nonvenomous reptiles

    √x7ᵗʰ   **W59.81   Bitten** by other nonvenomous reptiles

    √x7ᵗʰ   **W59.82   Struck** by other nonvenomous reptiles

    √x7ᵗʰ   **W59.83   Crushed** by other nonvenomous reptiles

    √x7ᵗʰ   **W59.89   Other contact** with other nonvenomous reptiles

√x7ᵗʰ **W60 Contact with nonvenomous plant thorns and spines and sharp leaves**

     EXCLUDES 1   *contact with venomous plants (T63.7-)*

√4ᵗʰ **W61 Contact with birds (domestic) (wild)**

     INCLUDES   contact with excreta of birds

   √5ᵗʰ **W61.0 Contact with** parrot

    √x7ᵗʰ   **W61.01   Bitten** by parrot

    √x7ᵗʰ   **W61.02   Struck** by parrot

    √x7ᵗʰ   **W61.09   Other contact** with parrot

       Exposure to parrots

   √5ᵗʰ **W61.1 Contact with** macaw

    √x7ᵗʰ   **W61.11   Bitten** by macaw

    √x7ᵗʰ   **W61.12   Struck** by macaw

    √x7ᵗʰ   **W61.19   Other contact** with macaw

       Exposure to macaws

   √5ᵗʰ **W61.2 Contact with other** psittacines

    √x7ᵗʰ   **W61.21   Bitten** by other psittacines

    √x7ᵗʰ   **W61.22   Struck** by other psittacines

    √x7ᵗʰ   **W61.29   Other contact** with other psittacines

       Exposure to other psittacines

   √5ᵗʰ **W61.3 Contact with** chicken

    √x7ᵗʰ   **W61.32   Struck** by chicken

    √x7ᵗʰ   **W61.33   Pecked** by chicken

    √x7ᵗʰ   **W61.39   Other contact** with chicken

       Exposure to chickens

   √5ᵗʰ **W61.4 Contact with** turkey

    √x7ᵗʰ   **W61.42   Struck** by turkey

    √x7ᵗʰ   **W61.43   Pecked** by turkey

    √x7ᵗʰ   **W61.49   Other contact** with turkey

   √5ᵗʰ **W61.5 Contact with** goose

    √x7ᵗʰ   **W61.51   Bitten** by goose

    √x7ᵗʰ   **W61.52   Struck** by goose

    √x7ᵗʰ   **W61.59   Other contact** with goose

   √5ᵗʰ **W61.6 Contact with** duck

    √x7ᵗʰ   **W61.61   Bitten** by duck

    √x7ᵗʰ   **W61.62   Struck** by duck

    √x7ᵗʰ   **W61.69   Other contact** with duck

√5ᵗʰ **W61.9 Contact with other birds**

    √x7ᵗʰ   **W61.91   Bitten** by other birds

    √x7ᵗʰ   **W61.92   Struck** by other birds

    √x7ᵗʰ   **W61.99   Other contact** with other birds

       Contact with bird NOS

√4ᵗʰ **W62 Contact with nonvenomous amphibians**

     EXCLUDES 1   *contact with venomous amphibians (T63.81-R63.83)*

√x7ᵗʰ **W62.0 Contact with nonvenomous** frogs

√x7ᵗʰ **W62.1 Contact with nonvenomous** toads

√x7ᵗʰ **W62.9 Contact with other nonvenomous amphibians**

√x7ᵗʰ **W64 Exposure to other animate mechanical forces**

     INCLUDES   exposure to nonvenomous animal NOS

     EXCLUDES 1   *contact with venomous animal (T63.-)*

Accidental non-transport drowning and submersion (W65-W74)

     EXCLUDES 1   *accidental drowning and submersion due to fall into water (W16.-)*
                 accidental drowning and submersion due to water transport accident (V90.-, V92.-)

     EXCLUDES 2   *accidental drowning and submersion due to cataclysm (X34-X39)*

The appropriate 7th character is to be added to each code from categories W65-W74.
A   initial encounter
D   subsequent encounter
S   sequela

√x7ᵗʰ **W65 Accidental drowning and submersion while in** bath-tub

     EXCLUDES 1   *accidental drowning and submersion due to fall in (into) bathtub (W16.211)*

√x7ᵗʰ **W67 Accidental drowning and submersion while in** swimming-pool

     EXCLUDES 1   *accidental drowning and submersion due to fall into swimming pool (W16.011, W16.021, W16.031)*
                 accidental drowning and submersion due to striking into wall of swimming pool (W22.041)

√x7ᵗʰ **W69 Accidental drowning and submersion while in** natural water

   Accidental drowning and submersion while in lake
   Accidental drowning and submersion while in open sea
   Accidental drowning and submersion while in river
   Accidental drowning and submersion while in stream

     EXCLUDES 1   *accidental drowning and submersion due to fall into natural body of water (W16.111, W16.121, W16.131)*

√x7ᵗʰ **W73 Other specified cause of accidental non-transport drowning and submersion**

   Accidental drowning and submersion while in quenching tank
   Accidental drowning and submersion while in reservoir

     EXCLUDES 1   *accidental drowning and submersion due to fall into other water (W16.311, W16.321, W16.331)*

√x7ᵗʰ **W74 Unspecified cause of accidental drowning and submersion**

   Drowning NOS

Exposure to electric current, radiation and extreme ambient air temperature and pressure (W85-W99)

     EXCLUDES 1   *exposure to:*
         failure in dosage of radiation or temperature during surgical and medical care (Y63.2-Y63.5)
         lightning (T75.0-)
         natural cold (X31)
         natural heat (X30)
         natural radiation NOS (X39)
         radiological procedure and radiotherapy (Y84.2)
         sunlight (X32)

AHA: 2018,2Q,7-8

The appropriate 7th character is to be added to each code from categories W85-W99.
A   initial encounter
D   subsequent encounter
S   sequela

√x7ᵗʰ **W85 Exposure to electric transmission lines**

   Broken power line

√4ᵗʰ **W86 Exposure to other specified electric current**

√x7ᵗʰ **W86.0 Exposure to domestic wiring and appliances**

✓ Additional Char Req   √x7ᵗʰ Placeholder   Unacceptable PDx   Questionable PDx   Wrong Procedure   Manifestation   Unspecified Dx   H1-H14 HAC   HCC CMS-HCC Dx   HIV HIV Dx

ICD-10-CM 2021   1205

√x7th **W86.1** **Exposure to industrial wiring, appliances and electrical machinery**
> Exposure to conductors
> Exposure to control apparatus
> Exposure to electrical equipment and machinery
> Exposure to transformers

√x7th **W86.8** **Exposure to other electric current**
> Exposure to wiring and appliances in or on farm (not farmhouse)
> Exposure to wiring and appliances outdoors
> Exposure to wiring and appliances in or on public building
> Exposure to wiring and appliances in or on residential institutions
> Exposure to wiring and appliances in or on schools

√4th **W88** **Exposure to ionizing radiation**
> EXCLUDES 1   *exposure to sunlight (X32)*

√x7th **W88.0** **Exposure to X-rays**

√x7th **W88.1** **Exposure to radioactive isotopes**

√x7th **W88.8** **Exposure to other ionizing radiation**

√4th **W89** **Exposure to man-made visible and ultraviolet light**
> INCLUDES   exposure to welding light (arc)
> EXCLUDES 1   *exposure to sunlight (X32)*
> EXCLUDES 2   ▶*exposure to sunlight (X32)*◀

√x7th **W89.0** **Exposure to welding light (arc)**

√x7th **W89.1** **Exposure to tanning bed**

√x7th **W89.8** **Exposure to other man-made visible and ultraviolet light**

√x7th **W89.9** **Exposure to unspecified man-made visible and ultraviolet light**

√4th **W90** **Exposure to other nonionizing radiation**
> EXCLUDES 1   *exposure to sunlight (X32)*
> EXCLUDES 2   ▶*exposure to sunlight (X32)*◀
> AHA: 2019,1Q,21

√x7th **W90.0** **Exposure to radiofrequency**

√x7th **W90.1** **Exposure to infrared radiation**

√x7th **W90.2** **Exposure to laser radiation**

√x7th **W90.8** **Exposure to other nonionizing radiation**

√x7th **W92** **Exposure to excessive heat of man-made origin**

√4th **W93** **Exposure to excessive cold of man-made origin**

√5th **W93.0** **Contact with or inhalation of dry ice**

√x7th **W93.01** **Contact with dry ice**

√x7th **W93.02** **Inhalation of dry ice**

√5th **W93.1** **Contact with or inhalation of liquid air**

√x7th **W93.11** **Contact with liquid air**
> Contact with liquid hydrogen
> Contact with liquid nitrogen

√x7th **W93.12** **Inhalation of liquid air**
> Inhalation of liquid hydrogen
> Inhalation of liquid nitrogen

√x7th **W93.2** **Prolonged exposure in deep freeze unit or refrigerator**

√x7th **W93.8** **Exposure to other excessive cold of man-made origin**

√4th **W94** **Exposure to high and low air pressure and changes in air pressure**

√x7th **W94.0** **Exposure to prolonged high air pressure**

√5th **W94.1** **Exposure to prolonged low air pressure**

√x7th **W94.11** **Exposure to residence or prolonged visit at high altitude**

√x7th **W94.12** **Exposure to other prolonged low air pressure**

√5th **W94.2** **Exposure to rapid changes in air pressure during ascent**

√x7th **W94.21** **Exposure to reduction in atmospheric pressure while surfacing from deep-water diving**

√x7th **W94.22** **Exposure to reduction in atmospheric pressure while surfacing from underground**

√x7th **W94.23** **Exposure to sudden change in air pressure in aircraft during ascent**

√x7th **W94.29** **Exposure to other rapid changes in air pressure during ascent**

√5th **W94.3** **Exposure to rapid changes in air pressure during descent**

√x7th **W94.31** **Exposure to sudden change in air pressure in aircraft during descent**

√x7th **W94.32** **Exposure to high air pressure from rapid descent in water**

√x7th **W94.39** **Exposure to other rapid changes in air pressure during descent**

√x7th **W99** **Exposure to other man-made environmental factors**

Exposure to smoke, fire and flames (X00-X08)

EXCLUDES 1   *arson (X97)*
EXCLUDES 2   *explosions (W35-W40)*
> *lightning (T75.0-)*
> *transport accident (V01-V99)*
AHA: 2018,2Q,7-8

The appropriate 7th character is to be added to each code from categories X00-X08.
A   initial encounter
D   subsequent encounter
S   sequela

√4th **X00** **Exposure to uncontrolled fire in building or structure**
> INCLUDES   conflagration in building or structure
> Code first any associated cataclysm
> EXCLUDES 2   *exposure to ignition or melting of nightwear (X05)*
>   *exposure to ignition or melting of other clothing and apparel (X06.-)*
>   *exposure to other specified smoke, fire and flames (X08.-)*
> AHA: 2016,2Q,5

√x7th **X00.0** **Exposure to flames in uncontrolled fire in building or structure**

√x7th **X00.1** **Exposure to smoke in uncontrolled fire in building or structure**

√x7th **X00.2** **Injury due to collapse of burning building or structure in uncontrolled fire**
> EXCLUDES 1   *injury due to collapse of building not on fire (W20.1)*

√x7th **X00.3** **Fall from burning building or structure in uncontrolled fire**

√x7th **X00.4** **Hit by object from burning building or structure in uncontrolled fire**
> AHA: 2016,2Q,4

√x7th **X00.5** **Jump from burning building or structure in uncontrolled fire**

√x7th **X00.8** **Other exposure to uncontrolled fire in building or structure**

√4th **X01** **Exposure to uncontrolled fire, not in building or structure**
> INCLUDES   exposure to forest fire

√x7th **X01.0** **Exposure to flames in uncontrolled fire, not in building or structure**

√x7th **X01.1** **Exposure to smoke in uncontrolled fire, not in building or structure**

√x7th **X01.3** **Fall due to uncontrolled fire, not in building or structure**

√x7th **X01.4** **Hit by object due to uncontrolled fire, not in building or structure**

√x7th **X01.8** **Other exposure to uncontrolled fire, not in building or structure**

√4th **X02** **Exposure to controlled fire in building or structure**
> INCLUDES   exposure to fire in fireplace
>   exposure to fire in stove

√x7th **X02.0** **Exposure to flames in controlled fire in building or structure**

√x7th **X02.1** **Exposure to smoke in controlled fire in building or structure**

√x7th **X02.2** **Injury due to collapse of burning building or structure in controlled fire**
> EXCLUDES 1   *injury due to collapse of building not on fire (W20.1)*

√x7th **X02.3** **Fall from burning building or structure in controlled fire**

√x7th **X02.4** **Hit by object from burning building or structure in controlled fire**

√x7th **X02.5** **Jump from burning building or structure in controlled fire**

√x7th **X02.8** **Other exposure to controlled fire in building or structure**

√4th **X03** **Exposure to controlled fire, not in building or structure**
> INCLUDES   exposure to bon fire
>   exposure to camp-fire
>   exposure to trash fire

√x7th **X03.0** **Exposure to flames in controlled fire, not in building or structure**

√x7th **X03.1** **Exposure to smoke in controlled fire, not in building or structure**

√x7th **X03.3** **Fall due to controlled fire, not in building or structure**

√x7th **X03.4** **Hit by object due to controlled fire, not in building or structure**

√x7th **X03.8** **Other exposure to controlled fire, not in building or structure**

✓x7ᵗʰ **X04　Exposure to ignition of highly flammable material**
　　Exposure to ignition of gasoline
　　Exposure to ignition of kerosene
　　Exposure to ignition of petrol
　　　EXCLUDES 2　　exposure to ignition or melting of nightwear (X05)
　　　　　　　　exposure to ignition or melting of other clothing and apparel (X06)
　　AHA: 2016,2Q,4

✓x7ᵗʰ **X05　Exposure to ignition or melting of nightwear**
　　　EXCLUDES 2　　exposure to uncontrolled fire in building or structure (X00.-)
　　　　　　　　exposure to uncontrolled fire, not in building or structure (X01.-)
　　　　　　　　exposure to controlled fire in building or structure (X02.-)
　　　　　　　　exposure to controlled fire, not in building or structure (X03.-)
　　　　　　　　exposure to ignition of highly flammable materials (X04.-)

✓4ᵗʰ **X06　Exposure to ignition or melting of other clothing and apparel**
　　　EXCLUDES 2　　exposure to uncontrolled fire in building or structure (X00.-)
　　　　　　　　exposure to uncontrolled fire, not in building or structure (X01.-)
　　　　　　　　exposure to controlled fire in building or structure (X02.-)
　　　　　　　　exposure to controlled fire, not in building or structure (X03.-)
　　　　　　　　exposure to ignition of highly flammable materials (X04.-)

　✓x7ᵗʰ **X06.0　Exposure to ignition of plastic jewelry**
　✓x7ᵗʰ **X06.1　Exposure to melting of plastic jewelry**
　✓x7ᵗʰ **X06.2　Exposure to ignition of other clothing and apparel**
　✓x7ᵗʰ **X06.3　Exposure to melting of other clothing and apparel**

✓4ᵗʰ **X08　Exposure to other specified smoke, fire and flames**
　✓5ᵗʰ **X08.0　Exposure to bed fire**
　　　Exposure to mattress fire
　　✓x7ᵗʰ **X08.00　Exposure to bed fire due to unspecified burning material**
　　✓x7ᵗʰ **X08.01　Exposure to bed fire due to burning cigarette**
　　✓x7ᵗʰ **X08.09　Exposure to bed fire due to other burning material**
　✓5ᵗʰ **X08.1　Exposure to sofa fire**
　　✓x7ᵗʰ **X08.10　Exposure to sofa fire due to unspecified burning material**
　　✓x7ᵗʰ **X08.11　Exposure to sofa fire due to burning cigarette**
　　✓x7ᵗʰ **X08.19　Exposure to sofa fire due to other burning material**
　✓5ᵗʰ **X08.2　Exposure to other furniture fire**
　　✓x7ᵗʰ **X08.20　Exposure to other furniture fire due to unspecified burning material**
　　✓x7ᵗʰ **X08.21　Exposure to other furniture fire due to burning cigarette**
　　✓x7ᵗʰ **X08.29　Exposure to other furniture fire due to other burning material**
　✓x7ᵗʰ **X08.8　Exposure to other specified smoke, fire and flames**

Contact with heat and hot substances (X10-X19)

　EXCLUDES 1　　exposure to excessive natural heat (X30)
　　　　　　exposure to fire and flames (X00-X08)
AHA: 2018,2Q,7-8

The appropriate 7th character is to be added to each code from categories X10-X19.
A　initial encounter
D　subsequent encounter
S　sequela

✓4ᵗʰ **X10　Contact with hot drinks, food, fats and cooking oils**
　✓x7ᵗʰ **X10.0　Contact with hot drinks**
　✓x7ᵗʰ **X10.1　Contact with hot food**
　✓x7ᵗʰ **X10.2　Contact with fats and cooking oils**

✓4ᵗʰ **X11　Contact with hot tap-water**
　　INCLUDES　　contact with boiling tap-water
　　　　　　contact with boiling water NOS
　　EXCLUDES 1　　contact with water heated on stove (X12)
　✓x7ᵗʰ **X11.0　Contact with hot water in bath or tub**
　　　EXCLUDES 1　　contact with running hot water in bath or tub (X11.1)
　✓x7ᵗʰ **X11.1　Contact with running hot water**
　　　Contact with hot water running out of hose
　　　Contact with hot water running out of tap

✓x7ᵗʰ **X11.8　Contact with other hot tap-water**
　　Contact with hot water in bucket
　　Contact with hot tap-water NOS

✓x7ᵗʰ **X12　Contact with other hot fluids**
　　Contact with water heated on stove
　　　EXCLUDES 1　　hot (liquid) metals (X18)

✓4ᵗʰ **X13　Contact with steam and other hot vapors**
　✓x7ᵗʰ **X13.0　Inhalation of steam and other hot vapors**
　✓x7ᵗʰ **X13.1　Other contact with steam and other hot vapors**

✓4ᵗʰ **X14　Contact with hot air and other hot gases**
　✓x7ᵗʰ **X14.0　Inhalation of hot air and gases**
　✓x7ᵗʰ **X14.1　Other contact with hot air and other hot gases**

✓4ᵗʰ **X15　Contact with hot household appliances**
　　　EXCLUDES 1　　contact with heating appliances (X16)
　　　　　　　　contact with powered household appliances (W29.-)
　　　　　　　　exposure to controlled fire in building or structure due to household appliance (X02.8)
　　　　　　　　exposure to household appliances electrical current (W86.0)
　✓x7ᵗʰ **X15.0　Contact with hot stove (kitchen)**
　✓x7ᵗʰ **X15.1　Contact with hot toaster**
　✓x7ᵗʰ **X15.2　Contact with hotplate**
　✓x7ᵗʰ **X15.3　Contact with hot saucepan or skillet**
　✓x7ᵗʰ **X15.8　Contact with other hot household appliances**
　　　Contact with cooker
　　　Contact with kettle
　　　Contact with light bulbs

✓x7ᵗʰ **X16　Contact with hot heating appliances, radiators and pipes**
　　　EXCLUDES 1　　contact with powered appliances (W29.-)
　　　　　　　　exposure to controlled fire in building or structure due to appliance (X02.8)
　　　　　　　　exposure to industrial appliances electrical current (W86.1)

✓x7ᵗʰ **X17　Contact with hot engines, machinery and tools**
　　　EXCLUDES 1　　contact with hot heating appliances, radiators and pipes (X16)
　　　　　　　　contact with hot household appliances (X15)

✓x7ᵗʰ **X18　Contact with other hot metals**
　　Contact with liquid metal

✓x7ᵗʰ **X19　Contact with other heat and hot substances**
　　　EXCLUDES 1　　objects that are not normally hot, e.g., an object made hot by a house fire (X00-X08)

Exposure to forces of nature (X30-X39)

AHA: 2018,2Q,7-8

The appropriate 7th character is to be added to each code from categories X30-X39.
A　initial encounter
D　subsequent encounter
S　sequela

✓x7ᵗʰ **X30　Exposure to excessive natural heat**
　　Exposure to excessive heat as the cause of sunstroke
　　Exposure to heat NOS
　　　EXCLUDES 1　　excessive heat of man-made origin (W92)
　　　　　　　　exposure to man-made radiation (W89)
　　　　　　　　exposure to sunlight (X32)
　　　　　　　　exposure to tanning bed (W89)

✓x7ᵗʰ **X31　Exposure to excessive natural cold**
　　Excessive cold as the cause of chilblains NOS
　　Excessive cold as the cause of immersion foot or hand
　　Exposure to cold NOS
　　Exposure to weather conditions
　　　EXCLUDES 1　　cold of man-made origin (W93.-)
　　　　　　　　contact with or inhalation of dry ice (W93.-)
　　　　　　　　contact with or inhalation of liquefied gas (W93.-)

✓x7ᵗʰ **X32　Exposure to sunlight**
　　　EXCLUDES 1　　man-made radiation (tanning bed) (W89)
　　　EXCLUDES 2　　radiation-related disorders of the skin and subcutaneous tissue (L55-L59)

✓ Additional Char Req　✓x7ᵗʰ Placeholder　Unacceptable PDx　Questionable PDx　Wrong Procedure　Manifestation　Unspecified Dx　H1-H14 HAC　HCC CMS-HCC Dx　HIV HIV Dx

√x7ᵗʰ **X34 Earthquake**

> EXCLUDES 2 *tidal wave (tsunami) due to earthquake (X37.41)*

√x7ᵗʰ **X35 Volcanic eruption**

> EXCLUDES 2 *tidal wave (tsunami) due to volcanic eruption (X37.41)*

√4ᵗʰ **X36 Avalanche, landslide and other earth movements**

> INCLUDES victim of mudslide of cataclysmic nature
> EXCLUDES 1 *earthquake (X34)*
> EXCLUDES 2 *transport accident involving collision with avalanche or landslide not in motion (V01-V99)*

> √x7ᵗʰ **X36.0 Collapse of dam or man-made structure causing earth movement**
>
> √x7ᵗʰ **X36.1 Avalanche, landslide, or mudslide**

√4ᵗʰ **X37 Cataclysmic storm**

> √x7ᵗʰ **X37.0 Hurricane**
>
> > Storm surge
> > Typhoon
>
> √x7ᵗʰ **X37.1 Tornado**
>
> > Cyclone
> > Twister
>
> √x7ᵗʰ **X37.2 Blizzard (snow)(ice)**
>
> √x7ᵗʰ **X37.3 Dust storm**
>
> √5ᵗʰ **X37.4 Tidalwave**
>
> > √x7ᵗʰ **X37.41 Tidal wave due to earthquake or volcanic eruption**
> > > Tidal wave NOS
> > > Tsunami
> >
> > √x7ᵗʰ **X37.42 Tidal wave due to storm**
> >
> > √x7ᵗʰ **X37.43 Tidal wave due to landslide**
>
> √x7ᵗʰ **X37.8 Other cataclysmic storms**
>
> > Cloudburst
> > Torrential rain
> > EXCLUDES 2 *flood (X38)*
>
> √x7ᵗʰ **X37.9 Unspecified cataclysmic storm**
>
> > Storm NOS
> > EXCLUDES 1 *collapse of dam or man-made structure causing earth movement (X36.0)*

√x7ᵗʰ **X38 Flood**

> Flood arising from remote storm
> Flood of cataclysmic nature arising from melting snow
> Flood resulting directly from storm
> EXCLUDES 1 *collapse of dam or man-made structure causing earth movement (X36.0)*
> *tidal wave NOS (X37.41)*
> *tidal wave caused by storm (X37.42)*

√4ᵗʰ · **X39 Exposure to other forces of nature**

> √5ᵗʰ **X39.0 Exposure to natural radiation**
>
> > EXCLUDES 1 *contact with and (suspected) exposure to radon and other naturally occurring radiation (Z77.123)*
> > *exposure to man-made radiation (W88-W90)*
> > *exposure to sunlight (X32)*
> >
> > √x7ᵗʰ **X39.01 Exposure to radon**
> >
> > √x7ᵗʰ **X39.08 Exposure to other natural radiation**
>
> √x7ᵗʰ **X39.8 Other exposure to forces of nature**

Overexertion and strenuous or repetitive movements (X50)

√4ᵗʰ **X50 Overexertion and strenuous or repetitive movements**

> AHA: 2018,2Q,7-8; 2016,4Q,73-74
>
> The appropriate 7th character is to be added to each code from category X50.
> A initial encounter
> D subsequent encounter
> S sequela

> √x7ᵗʰ **X50.0 Overexertion from strenuous movement or load**
>
> > Lifting heavy objects
> > Lifting weights

√x7ᵗʰ **X50.1 Overexertion from prolonged static or awkward postures**

> Prolonged bending
> Prolonged kneeling
> Prolonged reaching
> Prolonged sitting
> Prolonged standing
> Prolonged twisting
> Static bending
> Static kneeling
> Static reaching
> Static sitting
> Static standing
> Static twisting

√x7ᵗʰ **X50.3 Overexertion from repetitive movements**

> Use of hand as hammer
> EXCLUDES 2 *overuse from prolonged static or awkward postures (X50.1)*

√x7ᵗʰ **X50.9 Other and unspecified overexertion or strenuous movements or postures**

> Contact pressure
> Contact stress

Accidental exposure to other specified factors (X52-X58)

AHA: 2018,2Q,7-8

The appropriate 7th character is to be added to each code from categories X52-X58.
A initial encounter
D subsequent encounter
S sequela

√x7ᵗʰ **X52 Prolonged stay in weightless environment**

> Weightlessness in spacecraft (simulator)

√x7ᵗʰ **X58 Exposure to other specified factors**

> Accident NOS
> Exposure NOS

Intentional self-harm (X71-X83)

Purposely self-inflicted injury
Suicide (attempted)

The appropriate 7th character is to be added to each code from categories X71-X83.
A initial encounter
D subsequent encounter
S sequela

√4ᵗʰ **X71 Intentional self-harm by drowning and submersion**

> √x7ᵗʰ **X71.0 Intentional self-harm by drowning and submersion while in bathtub** HCC
>
> √x7ᵗʰ **X71.1 Intentional self-harm by drowning and submersion while in swimming pool** HCC
>
> √x7ᵗʰ **X71.2 Intentional self-harm by drowning and submersion after jump into swimming pool** HCC
>
> √x7ᵗʰ **X71.3 Intentional self-harm by drowning and submersion in natural water** HCC
>
> √x7ᵗʰ **X71.8 Other intentional self-harm by drowning and submersion** HCC
>
> √x7ᵗʰ **X71.9 Intentional self-harm by drowning and submersion, unspecified** HCC

√x7ᵗʰ **X72 Intentional self-harm by handgun discharge** HCC

> Intentional self-harm by gun for single hand use
> Intentional self-harm by pistol
> Intentional self-harm by revolver
> EXCLUDES 1 *Very pistol (X74.8)*

√4ᵗʰ **X73 Intentional self-harm by rifle, shotgun and larger firearm discharge**

> EXCLUDES 1 *airgun (X74.01)*

> √x7ᵗʰ **X73.0 Intentional self-harm by shotgun discharge** HCC
>
> √x7ᵗʰ **X73.1 Intentional self-harm by hunting rifle discharge** HCC
>
> √x7ᵗʰ **X73.2 Intentional self-harm by machine gun discharge** HCC
>
> √x7ᵗʰ **X73.8 Intentional self-harm by other larger firearm discharge** HCC
>
> √x7ᵗʰ **X73.9 Intentional self-harm by unspecified larger firearm discharge** HCC

☑4ᵗʰ **X74 Intentional self-harm by other and unspecified firearm and gun discharge**

    ☑5ᵗʰ **X74.0 Intentional self-harm by** gas, air or spring-operated guns

        √x7ᵗʰ **X74.01 Intentional self-harm by** airgun   HCC
                Intentional self-harm by BB gun discharge
                Intentional self-harm by pellet gun discharge

        √x7ᵗʰ **X74.02 Intentional self-harm by** paintball gun   HCC

        √x7ᵗʰ **X74.09 Intentional self-harm by other gas, air or spring-operated gun**   HCC

    √x7ᵗʰ **X74.8 Intentional self-harm by other firearm discharge**   HCC
        Intentional self-harm by Very pistol [flare] discharge

    √x7ᵗʰ **X74.9 Intentional self-harm by unspecified firearm discharge**   HCC

√x7ᵗʰ **X75 Intentional self-harm by explosive material**   HCC

√x7ᵗʰ **X76 Intentional self-harm by smoke, fire and flames**   HCC

☑4ᵗʰ **X77 Intentional self-harm by steam, hot vapors and hot objects**

    √x7ᵗʰ **X77.0 Intentional self-harm by** steam or hot vapors   HCC

    √x7ᵗʰ **X77.1 Intentional self-harm by hot** tap water   HCC

    √x7ᵗʰ **X77.2 Intentional self-harm by other hot fluids**   HCC

    √x7ᵗʰ **X77.3 Intentional self-harm by hot** household appliances   HCC

    √x7ᵗʰ **X77.8 Intentional self-harm by other hot objects**   HCC

    √x7ᵗʰ **X77.9 Intentional self-harm by unspecified hot objects**   HCC

☑4ᵗʰ **X78 Intentional self-harm by sharp object**

    √x7ᵗʰ **X78.0 Intentional self-harm by sharp** glass   HCC

    √x7ᵗʰ **X78.1 Intentional self-harm by** knife   HCC

    √x7ᵗʰ **X78.2 Intentional self-harm by** sword or dagger   HCC

    √x7ᵗʰ **X78.8 Intentional self-harm by other sharp object**   HCC

    √x7ᵗʰ **X78.9 Intentional self-harm by unspecified sharp object**   HCC

√x7ᵗʰ **X79 Intentional self-harm by blunt object**   HCC

√x7ᵗʰ **X80 Intentional self-harm by jumping from a high place**   HCC
    Intentional fall from one level to another

☑4ᵗʰ **X81 Intentional self-harm by jumping or lying in front of moving object**

    √x7ᵗʰ **X81.0 Intentional self-harm by jumping or lying in front of** motor vehicle   HCC

    √x7ᵗʰ **X81.1 Intentional self-harm by jumping or lying in front of (subway) train**   HCC

    √x7ᵗʰ **X81.8 Intentional self-harm by jumping or lying in front of other moving object**   HCC

☑4ᵗʰ **X82 Intentional self-harm by crashing of motor vehicle**

    √x7ᵗʰ **X82.0 Intentional collision of motor vehicle with other motor vehicle**   HCC

    √x7ᵗʰ **X82.1 Intentional collision of motor vehicle with** train   HCC

    √x7ᵗʰ **X82.2 Intentional collision of motor vehicle with** tree   HCC

    √x7ᵗʰ **X82.8 Other intentional self-harm by crashing of motor vehicle**   HCC

☑4ᵗʰ **X83 Intentional self-harm by other specified means**

    EXCLUDES 1   *intentional self-harm by poisoning or contact with toxic substance — see Table of Drugs and Chemicals*

    √x7ᵗʰ **X83.0 Intentional self-harm by** crashing of aircraft   HCC

    √x7ᵗʰ **X83.1 Intentional self-harm by** electrocution   HCC

    √x7ᵗʰ **X83.2 Intentional self-harm by** exposure to extremes of cold   HCC

    √x7ᵗʰ **X83.8 Intentional self-harm by other specified means**   HCC

Assault (X92-Y09)

INCLUDES   homicide
               injuries inflicted by another person with intent to injure or kill, by any means

EXCLUDES 1   *injuries due to legal intervention (Y35.-)*
               injuries due to operations of war (Y36.-)
               injuries due to terrorism (Y38.-)

The appropriate 7th character is to be added to each code from categories X92-Y04 and Y08.
A   initial encounter
D   subsequent encounter
S   sequela

☑4ᵗʰ **X92 Assault by drowning and submersion**

    √x7ᵗʰ **X92.0 Assault by drowning and submersion while in** bathtub

    √x7ᵗʰ **X92.1 Assault by drowning and submersion while in** swimming pool

    √x7ᵗʰ **X92.2 Assault by drowning and submersion** after push into swimming pool

    √x7ᵗʰ **X92.3 Assault by drowning and submersion** in natural water

    √x7ᵗʰ **X92.8 Other assault by drowning and submersion** HCC

    √x7ᵗʰ **X92.9 Assault by drowning and submersion, unspecified**

√x7ᵗʰ **X93 Assault by** handgun **discharge**
    Assault by discharge of gun for single hand use
    Assault by discharge of pistol
    Assault by discharge of revolver
    EXCLUDES 1   *Very pistol (X95.8)*

☑4ᵗʰ **X94 Assault by rifle, shotgun and larger firearm discharge**

    EXCLUDES 1   *airgun (X95.01)*

    √x7ᵗʰ **X94.0 Assault by** shotgun

    √x7ᵗʰ **X94.1 Assault by** hunting rifle

    √x7ᵗʰ **X94.2 Assault by** machine gun

    √x7ᵗʰ **X94.8 Assault by other larger firearm discharge**

    √x7ᵗʰ **X94.9 Assault by unspecified larger firearm discharge**

☑4ᵗʰ **X95 Assault by other and unspecified firearm and gun discharge**

    ☑5ᵗʰ **X95.0 Assault by** gas, air or spring-operated **guns**

        √x7ᵗʰ **X95.01 Assault by** airgun **discharge**
                Assault by BB gun discharge
                Assault by pellet gun discharge

        √x7ᵗʰ **X95.02 Assault by** paintball gun **discharge**

        √x7ᵗʰ **X95.09 Assault by other gas, air or spring-operated gun**

    √x7ᵗʰ **X95.8 Assault by other firearm discharge**
        Assault by Very pistol [flare] discharge

    √x7ᵗʰ **X95.9 Assault by unspecified firearm discharge**

☑4ᵗʰ **X96 Assault by explosive material**

    EXCLUDES 1   *incendiary device (X97)*
               terrorism involving explosive material (Y38.2-)

    √x7ᵗʰ **X96.0 Assault by** antipersonnel **bomb**

        EXCLUDES 1   *antipersonnel bomb use in military or war (Y36.2-)*

    √x7ᵗʰ **X96.1 Assault by** gasoline **bomb**

    √x7ᵗʰ **X96.2 Assault by** letter **bomb**

    √x7ᵗʰ **X96.3 Assault by** fertilizer **bomb**

    √x7ᵗʰ **X96.4 Assault by** pipe **bomb**

    √x7ᵗʰ **X96.8 Assault by other specified explosive**

    √x7ᵗʰ **X96.9 Assault by unspecified explosive**

√x7ᵗʰ **X97 Assault by smoke, fire and flames**
    Assault by arson
    Assault by cigarettes
    Assault by incendiary device

☑4ᵗʰ **X98 Assault by steam, hot vapors and hot objects**

    √x7ᵗʰ **X98.0 Assault by** steam or hot vapors

    √x7ᵗʰ **X98.1 Assault by hot** tap water

    √x7ᵗʰ **X98.2 Assault by hot fluids**

    √x7ᵗʰ **X98.3 Assault by hot** household appliances

    √x7ᵗʰ **X98.8 Assault by other hot** objects

    √x7ᵗʰ **X98.9 Assault by unspecified hot objects**

☑4ᵗʰ **X99 Assault by sharp object**

    EXCLUDES 1   *assault by strike by sports equipment (Y08.0-)*

    √x7ᵗʰ **X99.0 Assault by sharp** glass

    √x7ᵗʰ **X99.1 Assault by** knife

    √x7ᵗʰ **X99.2 Assault by** sword or dagger

    √x7ᵗʰ **X99.8 Assault by other sharp object**

    √x7ᵗʰ **X99.9 Assault by unspecified sharp object**
        Assault by stabbing NOS

√x7ᵗʰ **Y00 Assault by blunt object**
    EXCLUDES 1   *assault by strike by sports equipment (Y08.0-)*

√x7ᵗʰ **Y01 Assault by pushing from high place**

☑4ᵗʰ **Y02 Assault by pushing or placing victim in front of moving object**

    √x7ᵗʰ **Y02.0 Assault by pushing or placing victim in front of** motor vehicle

    √x7ᵗʰ **Y02.1 Assault by pushing or placing victim in front of (subway) train**

☑ Additional Char Req   √x7ᵗʰ Placeholder   Unacceptable PDx   Questionable PDx   Wrong Procedure   Manifestation   Unspecified Dx   H1-H14 HAC   HCC CMS-HCC Dx   HIV HIV Dx

ICD-10-CM 2021   1209

Chapter 20. External Causes of Morbidity

Y02.8–Y21.1

☑x7ᵗʰ **Y02.8**   **Assault by pushing or placing victim in front of other moving object**

☑4ᵗʰ **Y03**   **Assault by crashing of motor vehicle**

☑x7ᵗʰ **Y03.0**   **Assault by being hit or run over by motor vehicle**

☑x7ᵗʰ **Y03.8**   **Other assault by crashing of motor vehicle**

☑4ᵗʰ **Y04**   **Assault by bodily force**

    EXCLUDES 1   *assault by:*
        submersion (X92.-)
        use of weapon (X93-X95, X99, Y00)

☑x7ᵗʰ **Y04.0**   **Assault by unarmed brawl or fight**

☑x7ᵗʰ **Y04.1**   **Assault by human bite**

☑x7ᵗʰ **Y04.2**   **Assault by strike against or bumped into by another person**

☑x7ᵗʰ **Y04.8**   **Assault by other bodily force**
        Assault by bodily force NOS

☑4ᵗʰ **Y07**   **Perpetrator of assault, maltreatment and neglect**

    NOTE   Codes from this category are for use only in cases of confirmed abuse (T74.-).
        Selection of the correct perpetrator code is based on the relationship between the perpetrator and the victim

    INCLUDES   perpetrator of abandonment
        perpetrator of emotional neglect
        perpetrator of mental cruelty
        perpetrator of physical abuse
        perpetrator of physical neglect
        perpetrator of sexual abuse
        perpetrator of torture

☑5ᵗʰ **Y07.0**   **Spouse or partner, perpetrator of maltreatment and neglect**
        Spouse or partner, perpetrator of maltreatment and neglect against spouse or partner

    Y07.01   **Husband, perpetrator of maltreatment and neglect**

    Y07.02   **Wife, perpetrator of maltreatment and neglect**

    Y07.03   **Male partner, perpetrator of maltreatment and neglect**

    Y07.04   **Female partner, perpetrator of maltreatment and neglect**

☑5ᵗʰ **Y07.1**   **Parent (adoptive) (biological), perpetrator of maltreatment and neglect**

    Y07.11   **Biological father, perpetrator of maltreatment and neglect**

    Y07.12   **Biological mother, perpetrator of maltreatment and neglect**

    Y07.13   **Adoptive father, perpetrator of maltreatment and neglect**

    Y07.14   **Adoptive mother, perpetrator of maltreatment and neglect**

☑5ᵗʰ **Y07.4**   **Other family member, perpetrator of maltreatment and neglect**

  ☑6ᵗʰ **Y07.41**   **Sibling, perpetrator of maltreatment and neglect**

      EXCLUDES 1   *stepsibling, perpetrator of maltreatment and neglect (Y07.435, Y07.436)*

    Y07.410   **Brother, perpetrator of maltreatment and neglect**

    Y07.411   **Sister, perpetrator of maltreatment and neglect**

  ☑6ᵗʰ **Y07.42**   **Foster parent, perpetrator of maltreatment and neglect**

    Y07.420   **Foster father, perpetrator of maltreatment and neglect**

    Y07.421   **Foster mother, perpetrator of maltreatment and neglect**

  ☑6ᵗʰ **Y07.43**   **Stepparent or stepsibling, perpetrator of maltreatment and neglect**

    Y07.430   **Stepfather, perpetrator of maltreatment and neglect**

    Y07.432   **Male friend of parent (co-residing in household), perpetrator of maltreatment and neglect**

    Y07.433   **Stepmother, perpetrator of maltreatment and neglect**

    Y07.434   **Female friend of parent (co-residing in household), perpetrator of maltreatment and neglect**

    Y07.435   **Stepbrother, perpetrator or maltreatment and neglect**

    Y07.436   **Stepsister, perpetrator of maltreatment and neglect**

  ☑6ᵗʰ **Y07.49**   **Other family member, perpetrator of maltreatment and neglect**

    Y07.490   **Male cousin, perpetrator of maltreatment and neglect**

    Y07.491   **Female cousin, perpetrator of maltreatment and neglect**

    Y07.499   **Other family member, perpetrator of maltreatment and neglect**

☑5ᵗʰ **Y07.5**   **Non-family member, perpetrator of maltreatment and neglect**

    Y07.50   **Unspecified non-family member, perpetrator of maltreatment and neglect**

  ☑6ᵗʰ **Y07.51**   **Daycare provider, perpetrator of maltreatment and neglect**

    Y07.510   **At-home childcare provider, perpetrator of maltreatment and neglect**

    Y07.511   **Daycare center childcare provider, perpetrator of maltreatment and neglect**

    Y07.512   **At-home adultcare provider, perpetrator of maltreatment and neglect**

    Y07.513   **Adultcare center provider, perpetrator of maltreatment and neglect**

    Y07.519   **Unspecified daycare provider, perpetrator of maltreatment and neglect**

  ☑6ᵗʰ **Y07.52**   **Healthcare provider, perpetrator of maltreatment and neglect**

    Y07.521   **Mental health provider, perpetrator of maltreatment and neglect**

    Y07.528   **Other therapist or healthcare provider, perpetrator of maltreatment and neglect**
        Nurse perpetrator of maltreatment and neglect
        Occupational therapist perpetrator of maltreatment and neglect
        Physical therapist perpetrator of maltreatment and neglect
        Speech therapist perpetrator of maltreatment and neglect

    Y07.529   **Unspecified healthcare provider, perpetrator of maltreatment and neglect**

    Y07.53   **Teacher or instructor, perpetrator of maltreatment and neglect**
        Coach, perpetrator of maltreatment and neglect

    Y07.59   **Other non-family member, perpetrator of maltreatment and neglect**

  Y07.6   **Multiple perpetrators of maltreatment and neglect**
    AHA: 2018,4Q,32

  Y07.9   **Unspecified perpetrator of maltreatment and neglect**

☑4ᵗʰ **Y08**   **Assault by other specified means**

☑5ᵗʰ **Y08.0**   **Assault by strike by sport equipment**

  ☑x7ᵗʰ **Y08.01**   **Assault by strike by hockey stick**

  ☑x7ᵗʰ **Y08.02**   **Assault by strike by baseball bat**

  ☑x7ᵗʰ **Y08.09**   **Assault by strike by other specified type of sport equipment**

☑5ᵗʰ **Y08.8**   **Assault by other specified means**

  ☑x7ᵗʰ **Y08.81**   **Assault by crashing of aircraft**

  ☑x7ᵗʰ **Y08.89**   **Assault by other specified means**

Y09   **Assault by unspecified means**
    Assassination (attempted) NOS
    Homicide (attempted) NOS
    Manslaughter (attempted) NOS
    Murder (attempted) NOS

Event of undetermined intent (Y21-Y33)

Undetermined intent is only for use when there is specific documentation in the record that the intent of the injury cannot be determined. If no such documentation is present, code to accidental (unintentional).

The appropriate 7th character is to be added to each code from categories Y21-Y33.
A   initial encounter
D   subsequent encounter
S   sequela

☑4ᵗʰ **Y21**   **Drowning and submersion, undetermined intent**

☑x7ᵗʰ **Y21.0**   **Drowning and submersion while in bathtub, undetermined intent**

☑x7ᵗʰ **Y21.1**   **Drowning and submersion after fall into bathtub, undetermined intent**

N Newborn: 0   P Pediatric: 0-17   M Maternity: 9-64   A Adult: 15-124   MCC Major Complication/Comorbidity   CC Complication/Comorbidity   SW Severe Wound Dx

1210   ICD-10-CM 2021

✓x7ᵗʰ **Y21.2 Drowning and submersion** while in swimming pool, undetermined intent

✓x7ᵗʰ **Y21.3 Drowning and submersion** after fall into swimming pool, undetermined intent

✓x7ᵗʰ **Y21.4 Drowning and submersion** in natural water, **undetermined intent**

✓x7ᵗʰ **Y21.8 Other drowning and submersion, undetermined intent**

✓x7ᵗʰ **Y21.9 Unspecified drowning and submersion, undetermined intent**

✓x7ᵗʰ **Y22 Handgun discharge, undetermined intent**

Discharge of gun for single hand use, undetermined intent
Discharge of pistol, undetermined intent
Discharge of revolver, undetermined intent
EXCLUDES 2 Very pistol (Y24.8)

✓4ᵗʰ **Y23 Rifle, shotgun and larger firearm discharge, undetermined intent**
EXCLUDES 2 airgun (Y24.0)

✓x7ᵗʰ **Y23.0 Shotgun discharge, undetermined intent**

✓x7ᵗʰ **Y23.1 Hunting rifle discharge, undetermined intent**

✓x7ᵗʰ **Y23.2 Military firearm discharge, undetermined intent**

✓x7ᵗʰ **Y23.3 Machine gun discharge, undetermined intent**

✓x7ᵗʰ **Y23.8 Other larger firearm discharge, undetermined intent**

✓x7ᵗʰ **Y23.9 Unspecified larger firearm discharge, undetermined intent**

✓4ᵗʰ **Y24 Other and unspecified firearm discharge, undetermined intent**

✓x7ᵗʰ **Y24.0 Airgun discharge, undetermined intent**
BB gun discharge, undetermined intent
Pellet gun discharge, undetermined intent

✓x7ᵗʰ **Y24.8 Other firearm discharge, undetermined intent**
Paintball gun discharge, undetermined intent
Very pistol [flare] discharge, undetermined intent

✓x7ᵗʰ **Y24.9 Unspecified firearm discharge, undetermined intent**

✓x7ᵗʰ **Y25 Contact with explosive material, undetermined intent**

✓x7ᵗʰ **Y26 Exposure to smoke, fire and flames, undetermined intent**

✓4ᵗʰ **Y27 Contact with steam, hot vapors and hot objects, undetermined intent**

✓x7ᵗʰ **Y27.0 Contact with steam and hot vapors, undetermined intent**

✓x7ᵗʰ **Y27.1 Contact with hot tap water, undetermined intent**

✓x7ᵗʰ **Y27.2 Contact with hot fluids, undetermined intent**

✓x7ᵗʰ **Y27.3 Contact with hot household appliance, undetermined intent**

✓x7ᵗʰ **Y27.8 Contact with other hot objects, undetermined intent**

✓x7ᵗʰ **Y27.9 Contact with unspecified hot objects, undetermined intent**

✓4ᵗʰ **Y28 Contact with sharp object, undetermined intent**

✓x7ᵗʰ **Y28.0 Contact with sharp glass, undetermined intent**

✓x7ᵗʰ **Y28.1 Contact with knife, undetermined intent**

✓x7ᵗʰ **Y28.2 Contact with sword or dagger, undetermined intent**

✓x7ᵗʰ **Y28.8 Contact with other sharp object, undetermined intent**

✓x7ᵗʰ **Y28.9 Contact with unspecified sharp object, undetermined intent**

✓x7ᵗʰ **Y29 Contact with blunt object, undetermined intent**

✓x7ᵗʰ **Y30 Falling, jumping or pushed from a high place, undetermined intent**
Victim falling from one level to another, undetermined intent

✓x7ᵗʰ **Y31 Falling, lying or running before or into moving object, undetermined intent**

✓x7ᵗʰ **Y32 Crashing of motor vehicle, undetermined intent**

✓x7ᵗʰ **Y33 Other specified events, undetermined intent**

Legal intervention, operations of war, military operations, and terrorism (Y35-Y38)

The appropriate 7th character is to be added to each code from categories Y35-Y38.
A initial encounter
D subsequent encounter
S sequela

✓4ᵗʰ **Y35 Legal intervention**

INCLUDES any injury sustained as a result of an encounter with any law enforcement official, serving in any capacity at the time of the encounter, whether on-duty or off-duty. Includes injury to law enforcement official, suspect and bystander

AHA: 2019,4Q,18-19

✓5ᵗʰ **Y35.0 Legal intervention involving firearm discharge**

✓6ᵗʰ **Y35.00 Legal intervention involving unspecified firearm discharge**
Legal intervention involving gunshot wound
Legal intervention involving shot NOS

✓7ᵗʰ **Y35.001 Legal intervention involving unspecified firearm discharge, law enforcement official injured**

✓7ᵗʰ **Y35.002 Legal intervention involving unspecified firearm discharge, bystander injured**

✓7ᵗʰ **Y35.003 Legal intervention involving unspecified firearm discharge, suspect injured**

✓7ᵗʰ **Y35.009 Legal intervention involving unspecified firearm discharge, unspecified person injured**

✓6ᵗʰ **Y35.01 Legal intervention involving injury by machine gun**

✓7ᵗʰ **Y35.011 Legal intervention involving injury by machine gun, law enforcement official injured**

✓7ᵗʰ **Y35.012 Legal intervention involving injury by machine gun, bystander injured**

✓7ᵗʰ **Y35.013 Legal intervention involving injury by machine gun, suspect injured**

✓7ᵗʰ **Y35.019 Legal intervention involving injury by machine gun, unspecified person injured**

✓6ᵗʰ **Y35.02 Legal intervention involving injury by handgun**

✓7ᵗʰ **Y35.021 Legal intervention involving injury by handgun, law enforcement official injured**

✓7ᵗʰ **Y35.022 Legal intervention involving injury by handgun, bystander injured**

✓7ᵗʰ **Y35.023 Legal intervention involving injury by handgun, suspect injured**

✓7ᵗʰ **Y35.029 Legal intervention involving injury by handgun, unspecified person injured**

✓6ᵗʰ **Y35.03 Legal intervention involving injury by rifle pellet**

✓7ᵗʰ **Y35.031 Legal intervention involving injury by rifle pellet, law enforcement official injured**

✓7ᵗʰ **Y35.032 Legal intervention involving injury by rifle pellet, bystander injured**

✓7ᵗʰ **Y35.033 Legal intervention involving injury by rifle pellet, suspect injured**

✓7ᵗʰ **Y35.039 Legal intervention involving injury by rifle pellet, unspecified person injured**

✓6ᵗʰ **Y35.04 Legal intervention involving injury by rubber bullet**

✓7ᵗʰ **Y35.041 Legal intervention involving injury by rubber bullet, law enforcement official injured**

✓7ᵗʰ **Y35.042 Legal intervention involving injury by rubber bullet, bystander injured**

✓7ᵗʰ **Y35.043 Legal intervention involving injury by rubber bullet, suspect injured**

✓7ᵗʰ **Y35.049 Legal intervention involving injury by rubber bullet, unspecified person injured**

✓6ᵗʰ **Y35.09 Legal intervention involving other firearm discharge**

✓7ᵗʰ **Y35.091 Legal intervention involving other firearm discharge, law enforcement official injured**

✓7ᵗʰ **Y35.092 Legal intervention involving other firearm discharge, bystander injured**

✓7ᵗʰ **Y35.093 Legal intervention involving other firearm discharge, suspect injured**

√7ᵗʰ **Y35.099** Legal intervention involving other firearm discharge, unspecified person injured

√5ᵗʰ **Y35.1** Legal intervention involving explosives

√6ᵗʰ **Y35.10** Legal intervention involving unspecified explosives

√7ᵗʰ **Y35.101** Legal intervention involving unspecified explosives, law enforcement official injured

√7ᵗʰ **Y35.102** Legal intervention involving unspecified explosives, bystander injured

√7ᵗʰ **Y35.103** Legal intervention involving unspecified explosives, suspect injured

√7ᵗʰ **Y35.109** Legal intervention involving unspecified explosives, unspecified person injured

√6ᵗʰ **Y35.11** Legal intervention involving injury by dynamite

√7ᵗʰ **Y35.111** Legal intervention involving injury by dynamite, law enforcement official injured

√7ᵗʰ **Y35.112** Legal intervention involving injury by dynamite, bystander injured

√7ᵗʰ **Y35.113** Legal intervention involving injury by dynamite, suspect injured

√7ᵗʰ **Y35.119** Legal intervention involving injury by dynamite, unspecified person injured

√6ᵗʰ **Y35.12** Legal intervention involving injury by explosive shell

√7ᵗʰ **Y35.121** Legal intervention involving injury by explosive shell, law enforcement official injured

√7ᵗʰ **Y35.122** Legal intervention involving injury by explosive shell, bystander injured

√7ᵗʰ **Y35.123** Legal intervention involving injury by explosive shell, suspect injured

√7ᵗʰ **Y35.129** Legal intervention involving injury by explosive shell, unspecified person injured

√6ᵗʰ **Y35.19** Legal intervention involving other explosives

Legal intervention involving injury by grenade
Legal intervention involving injury by mortar bomb

√7ᵗʰ **Y35.191** Legal intervention involving other explosives, law enforcement official injured

√7ᵗʰ **Y35.192** Legal intervention involving other explosives, bystander injured

√7ᵗʰ **Y35.193** Legal intervention involving other explosives, suspect injured

√7ᵗʰ **Y35.199** Legal intervention involving other explosives, unspecified person injured

√5ᵗʰ **Y35.2** Legal intervention involving gas

Legal intervention involving asphyxiation by gas
Legal intervention involving poisoning by gas

√6ᵗʰ **Y35.20** Legal intervention involving unspecified gas

√7ᵗʰ **Y35.201** Legal intervention involving unspecified gas, law enforcement official injured

√7ᵗʰ **Y35.202** Legal intervention involving unspecified gas, bystander injured

√7ᵗʰ **Y35.203** Legal intervention involving unspecified gas, suspect injured

√7ᵗʰ **Y35.209** Legal intervention involving unspecified gas, unspecified person injured

√6ᵗʰ **Y35.21** Legal intervention involving injury by tear gas

√7ᵗʰ **Y35.211** Legal intervention involving injury by tear gas, law enforcement official injured

√7ᵗʰ **Y35.212** Legal intervention involving injury by tear gas, bystander injured

√7ᵗʰ **Y35.213** Legal intervention involving injury by tear gas, suspect injured

√7ᵗʰ **Y35.219** Legal intervention involving injury by tear gas, unspecified person injured

√6ᵗʰ **Y35.29** Legal intervention involving other gas

√7ᵗʰ **Y35.291** Legal intervention involving other gas, law enforcement official injured

√7ᵗʰ **Y35.292** Legal intervention involving other gas, bystander injured

√7ᵗʰ **Y35.293** Legal intervention involving other gas, suspect injured

√7ᵗʰ **Y35.299** Legal intervention involving other gas, unspecified person injured

√5ᵗʰ **Y35.3** Legal intervention involving blunt objects

Legal intervention involving being hit or struck by blunt object

√6ᵗʰ **Y35.30** Legal intervention involving unspecified blunt objects

√7ᵗʰ **Y35.301** Legal intervention involving unspecified blunt objects, law enforcement official injured

√7ᵗʰ **Y35.302** Legal intervention involving unspecified blunt objects, bystander injured

√7ᵗʰ **Y35.303** Legal intervention involving unspecified blunt objects, suspect injured

√7ᵗʰ **Y35.309** Legal intervention involving unspecified blunt objects, unspecified person injured

√6ᵗʰ **Y35.31** Legal intervention involving baton

√7ᵗʰ **Y35.311** Legal intervention involving baton, law enforcement official injured

√7ᵗʰ **Y35.312** Legal intervention involving baton, bystander injured

√7ᵗʰ **Y35.313** Legal intervention involving baton, suspect injured

√7ᵗʰ **Y35.319** Legal intervention involving baton, unspecified person injured

√6ᵗʰ **Y35.39** Legal intervention involving other blunt objects

√7ᵗʰ **Y35.391** Legal intervention involving other blunt objects, law enforcement official injured

√7ᵗʰ **Y35.392** Legal intervention involving other blunt objects, bystander injured

√7ᵗʰ **Y35.393** Legal intervention involving other blunt objects, suspect injured

√7ᵗʰ **Y35.399** Legal intervention involving other blunt objects, unspecified person injured

√5ᵗʰ **Y35.4** Legal intervention involving sharp objects

Legal intervention involving being cut by sharp objects
Legal intervention involving being stabbed by sharp objects

√6ᵗʰ **Y35.40** Legal intervention involving unspecified sharp objects

√7ᵗʰ **Y35.401** Legal intervention involving unspecified sharp objects, law enforcement official injured

√7ᵗʰ **Y35.402** Legal intervention involving unspecified sharp objects, bystander injured

√7ᵗʰ **Y35.403** Legal intervention involving unspecified sharp objects, suspect injured

√7ᵗʰ **Y35.409** Legal intervention involving unspecified sharp objects, unspecified person injured

√6ᵗʰ **Y35.41** Legal intervention involving bayonet

√7ᵗʰ **Y35.411** Legal intervention involving bayonet, law enforcement official injured

√7ᵗʰ **Y35.412** Legal intervention involving bayonet, bystander injured

√7ᵗʰ **Y35.413** Legal intervention involving bayonet, suspect injured

√7ᵗʰ **Y35.419** Legal intervention involving bayonet, unspecified person injured

√6ᵗʰ **Y35.49** Legal intervention involving other sharp objects

√7ᵗʰ **Y35.491** Legal intervention involving other sharp objects, law enforcement official injured

√7ᵗʰ **Y35.492** Legal intervention involving other sharp objects, bystander injured

√7ᵗʰ **Y35.493** Legal intervention involving other sharp objects, suspect injured

√7ᵗʰ **Y35.499** Legal intervention involving other sharp objects, unspecified person injured

√5ᵗʰ **Y35.8** Legal intervention involving other specified means

AHA: 2019,4Q,19

√6ᵗʰ **Y35.81** Legal intervention involving manhandling

√7ᵗʰ **Y35.811** Legal intervention involving manhandling, law enforcement official injured

√7ᵗʰ **Y35.812** Legal intervention involving manhandling, bystander injured

√7ᵗʰ **Y35.813** Legal intervention involving manhandling, suspect injured

√7ᵗʰ **Y35.819** Legal intervention involving manhandling, unspecified person injured

√6ᵗʰ **Y35.83** **Legal intervention involving a** conducted energy device

     Electroshock device (taser)

     Stun gun

     √7ᵗʰ **Y35.831** **Legal intervention involving a conducted energy device,** law enforcement official **injured**

     √7ᵗʰ **Y35.832** **Legal intervention involving a conducted energy device,** bystander **injured**

     √7ᵗʰ **Y35.833** **Legal intervention involving a conducted energy device,** suspect **injured**

     √7ᵗʰ **Y35.839** **Legal intervention involving a conducted energy device, unspecified person injured**

√6ᵗʰ **Y35.89** **Legal intervention involving other specified means**

     √7ᵗʰ **Y35.891** **Legal intervention involving other specified means,** law enforcement official **injured**

     √7ᵗʰ **Y35.892** **Legal intervention involving other specified means,** bystander **injured**

     √7ᵗʰ **Y35.893** **Legal intervention involving other specified means,** suspect **injured**

         AHA: 2018,1Q,5

√5ᵗʰ **Y35.9** **Legal intervention, means unspecified**

     √x7ᵗʰ **Y35.91** **Legal intervention, means unspecified,** law enforcement official **injured**

     √x7ᵗʰ **Y35.92** **Legal intervention, means unspecified,** bystander **injured**

     √x7ᵗʰ **Y35.93** **Legal intervention, means unspecified,** suspect **injured**

     √x7ᵗʰ **Y35.99** **Legal intervention, means unspecified, unspecified person injured**

√4ᵗʰ **Y36** **Operations of war**

     INCLUDES   injuries to military personnel and civilians caused by war, civil insurrection, and peacekeeping missions

     EXCLUDES 1   *injury to military personnel occurring during peacetime military operations (Y37.-)*

         military vehicles involved in transport accidents with non-military vehicle during peacetime (V09.01, V09.21, V19.81, V29.81, V39.81, V49.81, V59.81, V69.81, V79.81)

     AHA: 2014,3Q,4

√5ᵗʰ **Y36.0** **War operations involving** explosion of marine weapons

     √6ᵗʰ **Y36.00** **War operations involving explosion of unspecified marine weapon**

         War operations involving underwater blast NOS

         √7ᵗʰ **Y36.000** **War operations involving explosion of unspecified marine weapon,** military personnel

         √7ᵗʰ **Y36.001** **War operations involving explosion of unspecified marine weapon,** civilian

     √6ᵗʰ **Y36.01** **War operations involving explosion of** depth-charge

         √7ᵗʰ **Y36.010** **War operations involving explosion of depth-charge,** military personnel

         √7ᵗʰ **Y36.011** **War operations involving explosion of depth-charge,** civilian

     √6ᵗʰ **Y36.02** **War operations involving explosion of** marine mine

         War operations involving explosion of marine mine, at sea or in harbor

         √7ᵗʰ **Y36.020** **War operations involving explosion of marine mine,** military personnel

         √7ᵗʰ **Y36.021** **War operations involving explosion of marine mine,** civilian

     √6ᵗʰ **Y36.03** **War operations involving explosion of** sea-based artillery shell

         √7ᵗʰ **Y36.030** **War operations involving explosion of sea-based artillery shell,** military personnel

         √7ᵗʰ **Y36.031** **War operations involving explosion of sea-based artillery shell,** civilian

     √6ᵗʰ **Y36.04** **War operations involving explosion of** torpedo

         √7ᵗʰ **Y36.040** **War operations involving explosion of torpedo,** military personnel

         √7ᵗʰ **Y36.041** **War operations involving explosion of torpedo,** civilian

     √6ᵗʰ **Y36.05** **War operations involving** accidental detonation of onboard marine weapons

         √7ᵗʰ **Y36.050** **War operations involving accidental detonation of onboard marine weapons,** military personnel

         √7ᵗʰ **Y36.051** **War operations involving accidental detonation of onboard marine weapons,** civilian

√6ᵗʰ **Y36.09** **War operations involving explosion of other marine weapons**

     √7ᵗʰ **Y36.090** **War operations involving explosion of other marine weapons,** military personnel

     √7ᵗʰ **Y36.091** **War operations involving explosion of other marine weapons,** civilian

√5ᵗʰ **Y36.1** **War operations involving** destruction of aircraft

     √6ᵗʰ **Y36.10** **War operations involving unspecified destruction of aircraft**

         √7ᵗʰ **Y36.100** **War operations involving unspecified destruction of aircraft,** military personnel

         √7ᵗʰ **Y36.101** **War operations involving unspecified destruction of aircraft,** civilian

     √6ᵗʰ **Y36.11** **War operations involving destruction of aircraft due to** enemy fire or explosives

         War operations involving destruction of aircraft due to air to air missile

         War operations involving destruction of aircraft due to explosive placed on aircraft

         War operations involving destruction of aircraft due to rocket propelled grenade [RPG]

         War operations involving destruction of aircraft due to small arms fire

         War operations involving destruction of aircraft due to surface to air missile

         √7ᵗʰ **Y36.110** **War operations involving destruction of aircraft due to enemy fire or explosives,** military personnel

         √7ᵗʰ **Y36.111** **War operations involving destruction of aircraft due to enemy fire or explosives,** civilian

     √6ᵗʰ **Y36.12** **War operations involving destruction of aircraft due to** collision with other aircraft

         √7ᵗʰ **Y36.120** **War operations involving destruction of aircraft due to collision with other aircraft,** military personnel

         √7ᵗʰ **Y36.121** **War operations involving destruction of aircraft due to collision with other aircraft,** civilian

     √6ᵗʰ **Y36.13** **War operations involving destruction of aircraft due to** onboard fire

         √7ᵗʰ **Y36.130** **War operations involving destruction of aircraft due to onboard fire,** military personnel

         √7ᵗʰ **Y36.131** **War operations involving destruction of aircraft due to onboard fire,** civilian

     √6ᵗʰ **Y36.14** **War operations involving destruction of aircraft due to** accidental detonation of onboard munitions and explosives

         √7ᵗʰ **Y36.140** **War operations involving destruction of aircraft due to accidental detonation of onboard munitions and explosives,** military personnel

         √7ᵗʰ **Y36.141** **War operations involving destruction of aircraft due to accidental detonation of onboard munitions and explosives,** civilian

     √6ᵗʰ **Y36.19** **War operations involving other destruction of aircraft**

         √7ᵗʰ **Y36.190** **War operations involving other destruction of aircraft,** military personnel

         √7ᵗʰ **Y36.191** **War operations involving other destruction of aircraft,** civilian

√ Additional Char Req   √x7ᵗʰ Placeholder   Unacceptable PDx   Questionable PDx   Wrong Procedure   Manifestation   Unspecified Dx   H1-H14 HAC   HCC CMS-HCC Dx   HIV HIV Dx

ICD-10-CM 2021   1213

Y35.83–Y36.191

☑5ᵗʰ **Y36.2　War operations involving other explosions and fragments**

> EXCLUDES 1　*war operations involving explosion of aircraft (Y36.1-)*
> *war operations involving explosion of marine weapons (Y36.0-)*
> *war operations involving explosion of nuclear weapons (Y36.5-)*
> *war operations involving explosion occurring after cessation of hostilities (Y36.8-)*

☑6ᵗʰ **Y36.20　War operations involving unspecified explosion and fragments**

> War operations involving air blast NOS
> War operations involving blast NOS
> War operations involving blast fragments NOS
> War operations involving blast wave NOS
> War operations involving blast wind NOS
> War operations involving explosion NOS
> War operations involving explosion of bomb NOS

☑7ᵗʰ **Y36.200　War operations involving unspecified explosion and fragments, military personnel**

☑7ᵗʰ **Y36.201　War operations involving unspecified explosion and fragments, civilian**

☑6ᵗʰ **Y36.21　War operations involving explosion of aerial bomb**

☑7ᵗʰ **Y36.210　War operations involving explosion of aerial bomb, military personnel**

☑7ᵗʰ **Y36.211　War operations involving explosion of aerial bomb, civilian**

☑6ᵗʰ **Y36.22　War operations involving explosion of guided missile**

☑7ᵗʰ **Y36.220　War operations involving explosion of guided missile, military personnel**

☑7ᵗʰ **Y36.221　War operations involving explosion of guided missile, civilian**

☑6ᵗʰ **Y36.23　War operations involving explosion of improvised explosive device [IED]**

> War operations involving explosion of person-borne improvised explosive device [IED]
> War operations involving explosion of vehicle-borne improvised explosive device [IED]
> War operations involving explosion of roadside improvised explosive device [IED]

☑7ᵗʰ **Y36.230　War operations involving explosion of improvised explosive device [IED], military personnel**

☑7ᵗʰ **Y36.231　War operations involving explosion of improvised explosive device [IED], civilian**

☑6ᵗʰ **Y36.24　War operations involving explosion due to accidental detonation and discharge of own munitions or munitions launch device**

☑7ᵗʰ **Y36.240　War operations involving explosion due to accidental detonation and discharge of own munitions or munitions launch device, military personnel**

☑7ᵗʰ **Y36.241　War operations involving explosion due to accidental detonation and discharge of own munitions or munitions launch device, civilian**

☑6ᵗʰ **Y36.25　War operations involving fragments from munitions**

☑7ᵗʰ **Y36.250　War operations involving fragments from munitions, military personnel**

☑7ᵗʰ **Y36.251　War operations involving fragments from munitions, civilian**

☑6ᵗʰ **Y36.26　War operations involving fragments of improvised explosive device [IED]**

> War operations involving fragments of person-borne improvised explosive device [IED]
> War operations involving fragments of vehicle-borne improvised explosive device [IED]
> War operations involving fragments of roadside improvised explosive device [IED]

☑7ᵗʰ **Y36.260　War operations involving fragments of improvised explosive device [IED], military personnel**

☑7ᵗʰ **Y36.261　War operations involving fragments of improvised explosive device [IED], civilian**

☑6ᵗʰ **Y36.27　War operations involving fragments from weapons**

☑7ᵗʰ **Y36.270　War operations involving fragments from weapons, military personnel**

☑7ᵗʰ **Y36.271　War operations involving fragments from weapons, civilian**

☑6ᵗʰ **Y36.29　War operations involving other explosions and fragments**

> War operations involving explosion of grenade
> War operations involving explosions of land mine
> War operations involving shrapnel NOS

☑7ᵗʰ **Y36.290　War operations involving other explosions and fragments, military personnel**

☑7ᵗʰ **Y36.291　War operations involving other explosions and fragments, civilian**

☑5ᵗʰ **Y36.3　War operations involving fires, conflagrations and hot substances**

> War operations involving smoke, fumes, and heat from fires, conflagrations and hot substances

> EXCLUDES 1　*war operations involving fires and conflagrations aboard military aircraft (Y36.1-)*
> *war operations involving fires and conflagrations aboard military watercraft (Y36.0-)*
> *war operations involving fires and conflagrations caused indirectly by conventional weapons (Y36.2-)*
> *war operations involving fires and thermal effects of nuclear weapons (Y36.53-)*

☑6ᵗʰ **Y36.30　War operations involving unspecified fire, conflagration and hot substance**

☑7ᵗʰ **Y36.300　War operations involving unspecified fire, conflagration and hot substance, military personnel**

☑7ᵗʰ **Y36.301　War operations involving unspecified fire, conflagration and hot substance, civilian**

☑6ᵗʰ **Y36.31　War operations involving gasoline bomb**

> War operations involving incendiary bomb
> War operations involving petrol bomb

☑7ᵗʰ **Y36.310　War operations involving gasoline bomb, military personnel**

☑7ᵗʰ **Y36.311　War operations involving gasoline bomb, civilian**

☑6ᵗʰ **Y36.32　War operations involving incendiary bullet**

☑7ᵗʰ **Y36.320　War operations involving incendiary bullet, military personnel**

☑7ᵗʰ **Y36.321　War operations involving incendiary bullet, civilian**

☑6ᵗʰ **Y36.33　War operations involving flamethrower**

☑7ᵗʰ **Y36.330　War operations involving flamethrower, military personnel**

☑7ᵗʰ **Y36.331　War operations involving flamethrower, civilian**

☑6ᵗʰ **Y36.39　War operations involving other fires, conflagrations and hot substances**

☑7ᵗʰ **Y36.390　War operations involving other fires, conflagrations and hot substances, military personnel**

☑7ᵗʰ **Y36.391　War operations involving other fires, conflagrations and hot substances, civilian**

☑5ᵗʰ **Y36.4　War operations involving firearm discharge and other forms of conventional warfare**

☑6ᵗʰ **Y36.41　War operations involving rubber bullets**

☑7ᵗʰ **Y36.410　War operations involving rubber bullets, military personnel**

☑7ᵗʰ **Y36.411　War operations involving rubber bullets, civilian**

☑6ᵗʰ **Y36.42　War operations involving firearms pellets**

☑7ᵗʰ **Y36.420　War operations involving firearms pellets, military personnel**

☑7ᵗʰ **Y36.421　War operations involving firearms pellets, civilian**

☑6ᵗʰ **Y36.43　War operations involving other firearms discharge**

> War operations involving bullets NOS

> EXCLUDES 1　*war operations involving munitions fragments (Y36.25-)*
> *war operations involving incendiary bullets (Y36.32-)*

☑7ᵗʰ **Y36.430　War operations involving other firearms discharge, military personnel**

☑7ᵗʰ **Y36.431　War operations involving other firearms discharge, civilian**

Ⓝ Newborn: 0　Ⓟ Pediatric: 0-17　Ⓜ Maternity: 9-64　Ⓐ Adult: 15-124　ᴹᶜᶜ Major Complication/Comorbidity　ᶜᶜ Complication/Comorbidity　ˢᵂ Severe Wound Dx

1214　　　　　　　　　　　　　　　　　　　　　　　　　　　　　　　　　　　　ICD-10-CM 2021

√6ᵗʰ **Y36.44** **War operations involving** unarmed hand to hand combat

> EXCLUDES 1   *war operations involving combat using blunt or piercing object (Y36.45-)*
> *war operations involving intentional restriction of air and airway (Y36.46-)*
> *war operations involving unintentional restriction of air and airway (Y36.47-)*

√7ᵗʰ **Y36.440** **War operations involving unarmed hand to hand combat,** military personnel

√7ᵗʰ **Y36.441** **War operations involving unarmed hand to hand combat,** civilian

√6ᵗʰ **Y36.45** **War operations involving combat using** blunt or piercing object

√7ᵗʰ **Y36.450** **War operations involving combat using blunt or piercing object,** military personnel

√7ᵗʰ **Y36.451** **War operations involving combat using blunt or piercing object,** civilian

√6ᵗʰ **Y36.46** **War operations involving** intentional restriction of air and airway

√7ᵗʰ **Y36.460** **War operations involving intentional restriction of air and airway,** military personnel

√7ᵗʰ **Y36.461** **War operations involving intentional restriction of air and airway,** civilian

√6ᵗʰ **Y36.47** **War operations involving** unintentional restriction of air and airway

√7ᵗʰ **Y36.470** **War operations involving unintentional restriction of air and airway,** military personnel

√7ᵗʰ **Y36.471** **War operations involving unintentional restriction of air and airway,** civilian

√6ᵗʰ **Y36.49** **War operations involving other forms of conventional warfare**

√7ᵗʰ **Y36.490** **War operations involving other forms of conventional warfare,** military personnel

√7ᵗʰ **Y36.491** **War operations involving other forms of conventional warfare,** civilian

√5ᵗʰ **Y36.5** **War operations involving** nuclear weapons

> War operations involving dirty bomb NOS

√6ᵗʰ **Y36.50** **War operations involving unspecified effect of nuclear weapon**

√7ᵗʰ **Y36.500** **War operations involving unspecified effect of nuclear weapon,** military personnel

√7ᵗʰ **Y36.501** **War operations involving unspecified effect of nuclear weapon,** civilian

√6ᵗʰ **Y36.51** **War operations involving** direct blast **effect of nuclear weapon**

> War operations involving blast pressure of nuclear weapon

√7ᵗʰ **Y36.510** **War operations involving direct blast effect of nuclear weapon,** military personnel

√7ᵗʰ **Y36.511** **War operations involving direct blast effect of nuclear weapon,** civilian

√6ᵗʰ **Y36.52** **War operations involving** indirect blast **effect of nuclear weapon**

> War operations involving being thrown by blast of nuclear weapon
> War operations involving being struck or crushed by blast debris of nuclear weapon

√7ᵗʰ **Y36.520** **War operations involving indirect blast effect of nuclear weapon,** military personnel

√7ᵗʰ **Y36.521** **War operations involving indirect blast effect of nuclear weapon,** civilian

√6ᵗʰ **Y36.53** **War operations involving** thermal radiation **effect of nuclear weapon**

> War operations involving direct heat from nuclear weapon
> War operation involving fireball effects from nuclear weapon

√7ᵗʰ **Y36.530** **War operations involving thermal radiation effect of nuclear weapon,** military personnel

√7ᵗʰ **Y36.531** **War operations involving thermal radiation effect of nuclear weapon,** civilian

√6ᵗʰ **Y36.54** **War operation involving** nuclear radiation **effects of nuclear weapon**

> War operation involving acute radiation exposure from nuclear weapon
> War operation involving exposure to immediate ionizing radiation from nuclear weapon
> War operation involving fallout exposure from nuclear weapon
> War operation involving secondary effects of nuclear weapons

√7ᵗʰ **Y36.540** **War operation involving nuclear radiation effects of nuclear weapon,** military personnel

√7ᵗʰ **Y36.541** **War operation involving nuclear radiation effects of nuclear weapon,** civilian

√6ᵗʰ **Y36.59** **War operation involving other effects of nuclear weapons**

√7ᵗʰ **Y36.590** **War operation involving other effects of nuclear weapons,** military personnel

√7ᵗʰ **Y36.591** **War operation involving other effects of nuclear weapons,** civilian

√5ᵗʰ **Y36.6** **War operations involving biological weapons**

√6ᵗʰ **Y36.6X** **War operations involving** biological weapons

√7ᵗʰ **Y36.6X0** **War operations involving biological weapons,** military personnel

√7ᵗʰ **Y36.6X1** **War operations involving biological weapons,** civilian

√5ᵗʰ **Y36.7** **War operations involving chemical weapons and other forms of unconventional warfare**

> EXCLUDES 1   *war operations involving incendiary devices (Y36.3-, Y36.5-)*

√6ᵗʰ **Y36.7X** **War operations involving** chemical weapons and other forms of unconventional warfare

√7ᵗʰ **Y36.7X0** **War operations involving chemical weapons and other forms of unconventional warfare,** military personnel

√7ᵗʰ **Y36.7X1** **War operations involving chemical weapons and other forms of unconventional warfare,** civilian

√5ᵗʰ **Y36.8** **War operations occurring** after cessation of hostilities

> War operations classifiable to categories Y36.0-Y36.8 but occurring after cessation of hostilities

√6ᵗʰ **Y36.81** **Explosion of** mine **placed during war operations but exploding after cessation of hostilities**

√7ᵗʰ **Y36.810** **Explosion of mine placed during war operations but exploding after cessation of hostilities,** military personnel

√7ᵗʰ **Y36.811** **Explosion of mine placed during war operations but exploding after cessation of hostilities,** civilian

√6ᵗʰ **Y36.82** **Explosion of** bomb **placed during war operations but exploding after cessation of hostilities**

√7ᵗʰ **Y36.820** **Explosion of bomb placed during war operations but exploding after cessation of hostilities,** military personnel

√7ᵗʰ **Y36.821** **Explosion of bomb placed during war operations but exploding after cessation of hostilities,** civilian

√6ᵗʰ **Y36.88** **Other war operations occurring after cessation of hostilities**

√7ᵗʰ **Y36.880** **Other war operations occurring after cessation of hostilities,** military personnel

√7ᵗʰ **Y36.881** **Other war operations occurring after cessation of hostilities,** civilian

√6ᵗʰ **Y36.89** **Unspecified war operations occurring after cessation of hostilities**

√7ᵗʰ **Y36.890** **Unspecified war operations occurring after cessation of hostilities,** military personnel

√7ᵗʰ **Y36.891** **Unspecified war operations occurring after cessation of hostilities,** civilian

√5ᵗʰ **Y36.9** **Other and unspecified war operations**

√x7ᵗʰ **Y36.90** **War operations, unspecified**

√x7ᵗʰ **Y36.91** **War operations involving unspecified** weapon of mass destruction **[WMD]**

√x7ᵗʰ **Y36.92** **War operations involving** friendly fire

☑ Additional Char Req   √x7ᵗʰ Placeholder   Unacceptable PDx   Questionable PDx   Wrong Procedure   Manifestation   Unspecified Dx   H1-H4 HAC   HCC CMS-HCC Dx   HIV HIV Dx

ICD-10-CM 2021   **1215**

✓4ᵗʰ **Y37** **Military operations**

> INCLUDES   injuries to military personnel and civilians occurring during peacetime on military property and during routine military exercises and operations
>
> EXCLUDES 1   *military aircraft involved in aircraft accident with civilian aircraft (V97.81-)*
>
> *military vehicles involved in transport accident with civilian vehicle (VØ9.Ø1, VØ9.21, V19.81, V29.81, V39.81, V49.81, V59.81, V69.81, V79.81)*
>
> *military watercraft involved in water transport accident with civilian watercraft (V94.81-)*
>
> *war operations (Y36.-)*

✓5ᵗʰ **Y37.Ø** **Military operations involving** explosion of marine weapons

  ✓6ᵗʰ **Y37.ØØ** **Military operations involving explosion of unspecified marine weapon**

    Military operations involving underwater blast NOS

    ✓7ᵗʰ **Y37.ØØØ** **Military operations involving explosion of unspecified marine weapon, military personnel**

    ✓7ᵗʰ **Y37.ØØ1** **Military operations involving explosion of unspecified marine weapon, civilian**

  ✓6ᵗʰ **Y37.Ø1** **Military operations involving explosion of depth-charge**

    ✓7ᵗʰ **Y37.Ø1Ø** **Military operations involving explosion of depth-charge, military personnel**

    ✓7ᵗʰ **Y37.Ø11** **Military operations involving explosion of depth-charge, civilian**

  ✓6ᵗʰ **Y37.Ø2** **Military operations involving explosion of marine mine**

    Military operations involving explosion of marine mine, at sea or in harbor

    ✓7ᵗʰ **Y37.Ø2Ø** **Military operations involving explosion of marine mine, military personnel**

    ✓7ᵗʰ **Y37.Ø21** **Military operations involving explosion of marine mine, civilian**

  ✓6ᵗʰ **Y37.Ø3** **Military operations involving explosion of sea-based artillery shell**

    ✓7ᵗʰ **Y37.Ø3Ø** **Military operations involving explosion of sea-based artillery shell, military personnel**

    ✓7ᵗʰ **Y37.Ø31** **Military operations involving explosion of sea-based artillery shell, civilian**

  ✓6ᵗʰ **Y37.Ø4** **Military operations involving explosion of torpedo**

    ✓7ᵗʰ **Y37.Ø4Ø** **Military operations involving explosion of torpedo, military personnel**

    ✓7ᵗʰ **Y37.Ø41** **Military operations involving explosion of torpedo, civilian**

  ✓6ᵗʰ **Y37.Ø5** **Military operations involving accidental detonation of onboard marine weapons**

    ✓7ᵗʰ **Y37.Ø5Ø** **Military operations involving accidental detonation of onboard marine weapons, military personnel**

    ✓7ᵗʰ **Y37.Ø51** **Military operations involving accidental detonation of onboard marine weapons, civilian**

  ✓6ᵗʰ **Y37.Ø9** **Military operations involving explosion of other marine weapons**

    ✓7ᵗʰ **Y37.Ø9Ø** **Military operations involving explosion of other marine weapons, military personnel**

    ✓7ᵗʰ **Y37.Ø91** **Military operations involving explosion of other marine weapons, civilian**

✓5ᵗʰ **Y37.1** **Military operations involving** destruction of aircraft

  ✓6ᵗʰ **Y37.1Ø** **Military operations involving unspecified destruction of aircraft**

    ✓7ᵗʰ **Y37.1ØØ** **Military operations involving unspecified destruction of aircraft, military personnel**

    ✓7ᵗʰ **Y37.1Ø1** **Military operations involving unspecified destruction of aircraft, civilian**

  ✓6ᵗʰ **Y37.11** **Military operations involving destruction of aircraft due to enemy fire or explosives**

    Military operations involving destruction of aircraft due to air to air missile

    Military operations involving destruction of aircraft due to explosive placed on aircraft

    Military operations involving destruction of aircraft due to rocket propelled grenade [RPG]

    Military operations involving destruction of aircraft due to small arms fire

    Military operations involving destruction of aircraft due to surface to air missile

    ✓7ᵗʰ **Y37.11Ø** **Military operations involving destruction of aircraft due to enemy fire or explosives, military personnel**

    ✓7ᵗʰ **Y37.111** **Military operations involving destruction of aircraft due to enemy fire or explosives, civilian**

  ✓6ᵗʰ **Y37.12** **Military operations involving destruction of aircraft due to collision with other aircraft**

    ✓7ᵗʰ **Y37.12Ø** **Military operations involving destruction of aircraft due to collision with other aircraft, military personnel**

    ✓7ᵗʰ **Y37.121** **Military operations involving destruction of aircraft due to collision with other aircraft, civilian**

  ✓6ᵗʰ **Y37.13** **Military operations involving destruction of aircraft due to onboard fire**

    ✓7ᵗʰ **Y37.13Ø** **Military operations involving destruction of aircraft due to onboard fire, military personnel**

    ✓7ᵗʰ **Y37.131** **Military operations involving destruction of aircraft due to onboard fire, civilian**

  ✓6ᵗʰ **Y37.14** **Military operations involving destruction of aircraft due to** accidental detonation of onboard munitions and explosives

    ✓7ᵗʰ **Y37.14Ø** **Military operations involving destruction of aircraft due to accidental detonation of onboard munitions and explosives, military personnel**

    ✓7ᵗʰ **Y37.141** **Military operations involving destruction of aircraft due to accidental detonation of onboard munitions and explosives, civilian**

  ✓6ᵗʰ **Y37.19** **Military operations involving other destruction of aircraft**

    ✓7ᵗʰ **Y37.19Ø** **Military operations involving other destruction of aircraft, military personnel**

    ✓7ᵗʰ **Y37.191** **Military operations involving other destruction of aircraft, civilian**

✓5ᵗʰ **Y37.2** **Military operations involving** other explosions and fragments

> EXCLUDES 1   *military operations involving explosion of aircraft (Y37.1-)*
>
> *military operations involving explosion of marine weapons (Y37.Ø-)*
>
> *military operations involving explosion of nuclear weapons (Y37.5-)*

  ✓6ᵗʰ **Y37.2Ø** **Military operations involving unspecified explosion and fragments**

    Military operations involving air blast NOS

    Military operations involving blast NOS

    Military operations involving blast fragments NOS

    Military operations involving blast wave NOS

    Military operations involving blast wind NOS

    Military operations involving explosion NOS

    Military operations involving explosion of bomb NOS

    ✓7ᵗʰ **Y37.2ØØ** **Military operations involving unspecified explosion and fragments, military personnel**

    ✓7ᵗʰ **Y37.2Ø1** **Military operations involving unspecified explosion and fragments, civilian**

  ✓6ᵗʰ **Y37.21** **Military operations involving explosion of aerial bomb**

    ✓7ᵗʰ **Y37.21Ø** **Military operations involving explosion of aerial bomb, military personnel**

    ✓7ᵗʰ **Y37.211** **Military operations involving explosion of aerial bomb, civilian**

  ✓6ᵗʰ **Y37.22** **Military operations involving explosion of guided missile**

    ✓7ᵗʰ **Y37.22Ø** **Military operations involving explosion of guided missile, military personnel**

N Newborn: 0   P Pediatric: 0-17   M Maternity: 9-64   A Adult: 15-124   MCC Major Complication/Comorbidity   CC Complication/Comorbidity   SW Severe Wound Dx

1216   ICD-10-CM 2021

✓7ᵗʰ **Y37.221** **Military operations involving explosion of guided missile, civilian**

✓6ᵗʰ **Y37.23** **Military operations involving explosion of improvised explosive device [IED]**

Military operations involving explosion of person-borne improvised explosive device [IED]

Military operations involving explosion of vehicle-borne improvised explosive device [IED]

Military operations involving explosion of roadside improvised explosive device [IED]

✓7ᵗʰ **Y37.230** **Military operations involving explosion of improvised explosive device [IED], military personnel**

✓7ᵗʰ **Y37.231** **Military operations involving explosion of improvised explosive device [IED], civilian**

✓6ᵗʰ **Y37.24** **Military operations involving explosion due to accidental detonation and discharge of own munitions or munitions launch device**

✓7ᵗʰ **Y37.240** **Military operations involving explosion due to accidental detonation and discharge of own munitions or munitions launch device, military personnel**

✓7ᵗʰ **Y37.241** **Military operations involving explosion due to accidental detonation and discharge of own munitions or munitions launch device, civilian**

✓6ᵗʰ **Y37.25** **Military operations involving fragments from munitions**

✓7ᵗʰ **Y37.250** **Military operations involving fragments from munitions, military personnel**

✓7ᵗʰ **Y37.251** **Military operations involving fragments from munitions, civilian**

✓6ᵗʰ **Y37.26** **Military operations involving fragments of improvised explosive device [IED]**

Military operations involving fragments of person-borne improvised explosive device [IED]

Military operations involving fragments of vehicle-borne improvised explosive device [IED]

Military operations involving fragments of roadside improvised explosive device [IED]

✓7ᵗʰ **Y37.260** **Military operations involving fragments of improvised explosive device [IED], military personnel**

✓7ᵗʰ **Y37.261** **Military operations involving fragments of improvised explosive device [IED], civilian**

✓6ᵗʰ **Y37.27** **Military operations involving fragments from weapons**

✓7ᵗʰ **Y37.270** **Military operations involving fragments from weapons, military personnel**

✓7ᵗʰ **Y37.271** **Military operations involving fragments from weapons, civilian**

✓6ᵗʰ **Y37.29** **Military operations involving other explosions and fragments**

Military operations involving explosion of grenade

Military operations involving explosions of land mine

Military operations involving shrapnel NOS

✓7ᵗʰ **Y37.290** **Military operations involving other explosions and fragments, military personnel**

✓7ᵗʰ **Y37.291** **Military operations involving other explosions and fragments, civilian**

✓5ᵗʰ **Y37.3** **Military operations involving fires, conflagrations and hot substances**

Military operations involving smoke, fumes, and heat from fires, conflagrations and hot substances

EXCLUDES 1   *military operations involving fires and conflagrations aboard military aircraft (Y37.1-)*

military operations involving fires and conflagrations aboard military watercraft (Y37.0-)

military operations involving fires and conflagrations caused indirectly by conventional weapons (Y37.2-)

military operations involving fires and thermal effects of nuclear weapons (Y36.53-)

✓6ᵗʰ **Y37.30** **Military operations involving unspecified fire, conflagration and hot substance**

✓7ᵗʰ **Y37.300** **Military operations involving unspecified fire, conflagration and hot substance, military personnel**

✓7ᵗʰ **Y37.301** **Military operations involving unspecified fire, conflagration and hot substance, civilian**

✓6ᵗʰ **Y37.31** **Military operations involving gasoline bomb**

Military operations involving incendiary bomb

Military operations involving petrol bomb

✓7ᵗʰ **Y37.310** **Military operations involving gasoline bomb, military personnel**

✓7ᵗʰ **Y37.311** **Military operations involving gasoline bomb, civilian**

✓6ᵗʰ **Y37.32** **Military operations involving incendiary bullet**

✓7ᵗʰ **Y37.320** **Military operations involving incendiary bullet, military personnel**

✓7ᵗʰ **Y37.321** **Military operations involving incendiary bullet, civilian**

✓6ᵗʰ **Y37.33** **Military operations involving flamethrower**

✓7ᵗʰ **Y37.330** **Military operations involving flamethrower, military personnel**

✓7ᵗʰ **Y37.331** **Military operations involving flamethrower, civilian**

✓6ᵗʰ **Y37.39** **Military operations involving other fires, conflagrations and hot substances**

✓7ᵗʰ **Y37.390** **Military operations involving other fires, conflagrations and hot substances, military personnel**

✓7ᵗʰ **Y37.391** **Military operations involving other fires, conflagrations and hot substances, civilian**

✓5ᵗʰ **Y37.4** **Military operations involving firearm discharge and other forms of conventional warfare**

✓6ᵗʰ **Y37.41** **Military operations involving rubber bullets**

✓7ᵗʰ **Y37.410** **Military operations involving rubber bullets, military personnel**

✓7ᵗʰ **Y37.411** **Military operations involving rubber bullets, civilian**

✓6ᵗʰ **Y37.42** **Military operations involving firearms pellets**

✓7ᵗʰ **Y37.420** **Military operations involving firearms pellets, military personnel**

✓7ᵗʰ **Y37.421** **Military operations involving firearms pellets, civilian**

✓6ᵗʰ **Y37.43** **Military operations involving other firearms discharge**

Military operations involving bullets NOS

EXCLUDES 1   *military operations involving munitions fragments (Y37.25-)*

military operations involving incendiary bullets (Y37.32-)

✓7ᵗʰ **Y37.430** **Military operations involving other firearms discharge, military personnel**

✓7ᵗʰ **Y37.431** **Military operations involving other firearms discharge, civilian**

✓6ᵗʰ **Y37.44** **Military operations involving unarmed hand to hand combat**

EXCLUDES 1   *military operations involving combat using blunt or piercing object (Y37.45-)*

military operations involving intentional restriction of air and airway (Y37.46-)

military operations involving unintentional restriction of air and airway (Y37.47-)

✓7ᵗʰ **Y37.440** **Military operations involving unarmed hand to hand combat, military personnel**

✓7ᵗʰ **Y37.441** **Military operations involving unarmed hand to hand combat, civilian**

✓6ᵗʰ **Y37.45** **Military operations involving combat using blunt or piercing object**

✓7ᵗʰ **Y37.450** **Military operations involving combat using blunt or piercing object, military personnel**

✓7ᵗʰ **Y37.451** **Military operations involving combat using blunt or piercing object, civilian**

✓6ᵗʰ **Y37.46** **Military operations involving intentional restriction of air and airway**

✓7ᵗʰ **Y37.460** **Military operations involving intentional restriction of air and airway, military personnel**

✓7ᵗʰ **Y37.461** **Military operations involving intentional restriction of air and airway, civilian**

✓ Additional Char Req   ✓×7ᵗʰ Placeholder   Unacceptable PDx   Questionable PDx   Wrong Procedure   Manifestation   Unspecified Dx   H1-H14 HAC   HCC CMS-HCC Dx   HIV HIV Dx

✓6ᵗʰ **Y37.47** **Military operations involving** unintentional restriction of air and airway
    ✓7ᵗʰ **Y37.470** **Military operations involving unintentional restriction of air and airway,** military personnel
    ✓7ᵗʰ **Y37.471** **Military operations involving unintentional restriction of air and airway,** civilian

✓6ᵗʰ **Y37.49** **Military operations involving other forms of conventional warfare**
    ✓7ᵗʰ **Y37.490** **Military operations involving other forms of conventional warfare,** military personnel
    ✓7ᵗʰ **Y37.491** **Military operations involving other forms of conventional warfare,** civilian

✓5ᵗʰ **Y37.5** **Military operations involving** nuclear weapons

Military operation involving dirty bomb NOS

✓6ᵗʰ **Y37.50** **Military operations involving unspecified effect of nuclear weapon**
    ✓7ᵗʰ **Y37.500** **Military operations involving unspecified effect of nuclear weapon,** military personnel
    ✓7ᵗʰ **Y37.501** **Military operations involving unspecified effect of nuclear weapon,** civilian

✓6ᵗʰ **Y37.51** **Military operations involving** direct blast effect of nuclear weapon

Military operations involving blast pressure of nuclear weapon
    ✓7ᵗʰ **Y37.510** **Military operations involving direct blast effect of nuclear weapon,** military personnel
    ✓7ᵗʰ **Y37.511** **Military operations involving direct blast effect of nuclear weapon,** civilian

✓6ᵗʰ **Y37.52** **Military operations involving** indirect blast effect of nuclear weapon

Military operations involving being thrown by blast of nuclear weapon

Military operations involving being struck or crushed by blast debris of nuclear weapon
    ✓7ᵗʰ **Y37.520** **Military operations involving indirect blast effect of nuclear weapon,** military personnel
    ✓7ᵗʰ **Y37.521** **Military operations involving indirect blast effect of nuclear weapon,** civilian

✓6ᵗʰ **Y37.53** **Military operations involving** thermal radiation effect of nuclear weapon

Military operations involving direct heat from nuclear weapon

Military operation involving fireball effects from nuclear weapon
    ✓7ᵗʰ **Y37.530** **Military operations involving thermal radiation effect of nuclear weapon,** military personnel
    ✓7ᵗʰ **Y37.531** **Military operations involving thermal radiation effect of nuclear weapon,** civilian

✓6ᵗʰ **Y37.54** **Military operation involving** nuclear radiation effects of nuclear weapon

Military operation involving acute radiation exposure from nuclear weapon

Military operation involving exposure to immediate ionizing radiation from nuclear weapon

Military operation involving fallout exposure from nuclear weapon

Military operation involving secondary effects of nuclear weapons
    ✓7ᵗʰ **Y37.540** **Military operation involving nuclear radiation effects of nuclear weapon,** military personnel
    ✓7ᵗʰ **Y37.541** **Military operation involving nuclear radiation effects of nuclear weapon,** civilian

✓6ᵗʰ **Y37.59** **Military operation involving other effects of nuclear weapons**
    ✓7ᵗʰ **Y37.590** **Military operation involving other effects of nuclear weapons,** military personnel
    ✓7ᵗʰ **Y37.591** **Military operation involving other effects of nuclear weapons,** civilian

✓5ᵗʰ **Y37.6** **Military operations involving** biological weapons

✓6ᵗʰ **Y37.6X** **Military operations involving biological weapons**
    ✓7ᵗʰ **Y37.6X0** **Military operations involving biological weapons,** military personnel

    ✓7ᵗʰ **Y37.6X1** **Military operations involving biological weapons,** civilian

✓5ᵗʰ **Y37.7** **Military operations involving chemical weapons and other forms of unconventional warfare**

    EXCLUDES 1   *military operations involving incendiary devices (Y36.3-, Y36.5-)*

✓6ᵗʰ **Y37.7X** **Military operations involving** chemical weapons and other forms of unconventional warfare
    ✓7ᵗʰ **Y37.7X0** **Military operations involving chemical weapons and other forms of unconventional warfare,** military personnel
    ✓7ᵗʰ **Y37.7X1** **Military operations involving chemical weapons and other forms of unconventional warfare,** civilian

✓5ᵗʰ **Y37.9** **Other and unspecified military operations**

    ✓x7ᵗʰ **Y37.90** **Military operations, unspecified**

    ✓x7ᵗʰ **Y37.91** **Military operations involving unspecified** weapon of mass destruction [WMD]

    ✓x7ᵗʰ **Y37.92** **Military operations involving** friendly fire

✓4ᵗʰ **Y38** **Terrorism**

NOTE   These codes are for use to identify injuries resulting from the unlawful use of force or violence against persons or property to intimidate or coerce a Government, the civilian population, or any segment thereof, in furtherance of political or social objective

Use additional code for place of occurrence (Y92.-)

✓5ᵗʰ **Y38.0** **Terrorism involving explosion of marine weapons**

Terrorism involving depth-charge
Terrorism involving marine mine
Terrorism involving mine NOS, at sea or in harbor
Terrorism involving sea-based artillery shell
Terrorism involving torpedo
Terrorism involving underwater blast

✓6ᵗʰ **Y38.0X** **Terrorism involving explosion of** marine weapons
    ✓7ᵗʰ **Y38.0X1** **Terrorism involving explosion of marine weapons, public safety official injured**
    ✓7ᵗʰ **Y38.0X2** **Terrorism involving explosion of marine weapons, civilian injured**
    ✓7ᵗʰ **Y38.0X3** **Terrorism involving explosion of marine weapons, terrorist injured**

✓5ᵗʰ **Y38.1** **Terrorism involving destruction of aircraft**

Terrorism involving aircraft burned
Terrorism involving aircraft exploded
Terrorism involving aircraft being shot down
Terrorism involving aircraft used as a weapon

✓6ᵗʰ **Y38.1X** **Terrorism involving** destruction of aircraft
    ✓7ᵗʰ **Y38.1X1** **Terrorism involving destruction of aircraft, public safety official injured**
    ✓7ᵗʰ **Y38.1X2** **Terrorism involving destruction of aircraft, civilian injured**
    ✓7ᵗʰ **Y38.1X3** **Terrorism involving destruction of aircraft, terrorist injured**

✓5ᵗʰ **Y38.2** **Terrorism involving other explosions and fragments**

Terrorism involving antipersonnel (fragments) bomb
Terrorism involving blast NOS
Terrorism involving explosion NOS
Terrorism involving explosion of breech block
Terrorism involving explosion of cannon block
Terrorism involving explosion (fragments) of artillery shell
Terrorism involving explosion (fragments) of bomb
Terrorism involving explosion (fragments) of grenade
Terrorism involving explosion (fragments) of guided missile
Terrorism involving explosion (fragments) of land mine
Terrorism involving explosion of mortar bomb
Terrorism involving explosion of munitions
Terrorism involving explosion (fragments) of rocket
Terrorism involving explosion (fragments) of shell
Terrorism involving shrapnel
Terrorism involving mine NOS, on land

    EXCLUDES 1   *terrorism involving explosion of nuclear weapon (Y38.5)*

       terrorism involving suicide bomber (Y38.81)

✓6ᵗʰ **Y38.2X** **Terrorism involving other explosions and fragments**
    ✓7ᵗʰ **Y38.2X1** **Terrorism involving other explosions and fragments, public safety official injured**

N Newborn: 0   P Pediatric: 0-17   M Maternity: 9-64   A Adult: 15-124   MCC Major Complication/Comorbidity   CC Complication/Comorbidity   SW Severe Wound Dx

1218   ICD-10-CM 2021

√7ᵗʰ **Y38.2X2** **Terrorism involving other explosions and fragments, civilian injured**

√7ᵗʰ **Y38.2X3** **Terrorism involving other explosions and fragments, terrorist injured**

√5ᵗʰ **Y38.3** **Terrorism involving fires, conflagration and hot substances**

Terrorism involving conflagration NOS

Terrorism involving fire NOS

Terrorism involving petrol bomb

EXCLUDES 1 *terrorism involving fire or heat of nuclear weapon (Y38.5)*

√6ᵗʰ **Y38.3X** **Terrorism involving fires, conflagration and hot substances**

√7ᵗʰ **Y38.3X1** **Terrorism involving fires, conflagration and hot substances, public safety official injured**

√7ᵗʰ **Y38.3X2** **Terrorism involving fires, conflagration and hot substances, civilian injured**

√7ᵗʰ **Y38.3X3** **Terrorism involving fires, conflagration and hot substances, terrorist injured**

√5ᵗʰ **Y38.4** **Terrorism involving firearms**

Terrorism involving carbine bullet

Terrorism involving machine gun bullet

Terrorism involving pellets (shotgun)

Terrorism involving pistol bullet

Terrorism involving rifle bullet

Terrorism involving rubber (rifle) bullet

√6ᵗʰ **Y38.4X** **Terrorism involving firearms**

√7ᵗʰ **Y38.4X1** **Terrorism involving firearms, public safety official injured**

√7ᵗʰ **Y38.4X2** **Terrorism involving firearms, civilian injured**

√7ᵗʰ **Y38.4X3** **Terrorism involving firearms, terrorist injured**

√5ᵗʰ **Y38.5** **Terrorism involving nuclear weapons**

Terrorism involving blast effects of nuclear weapon

Terrorism involving exposure to ionizing radiation from nuclear weapon

Terrorism involving fireball effect of nuclear weapon

Terrorism involving heat from nuclear weapon

√6ᵗʰ **Y38.5X** **Terrorism involving nuclear weapons**

√7ᵗʰ **Y38.5X1** **Terrorism involving nuclear weapons, public safety official injured**

√7ᵗʰ **Y38.5X2** **Terrorism involving nuclear weapons, civilian injured**

√7ᵗʰ **Y38.5X3** **Terrorism involving nuclear weapons, terrorist injured**

√5ᵗʰ **Y38.6** **Terrorism involving biological weapons**

Terrorism involving anthrax

Terrorism involving cholera

Terrorism involving smallpox

√6ᵗʰ **Y38.6X** **Terrorism involving biological weapons**

√7ᵗʰ **Y38.6X1** **Terrorism involving biological weapons, public safety official injured**

√7ᵗʰ **Y38.6X2** **Terrorism involving biological weapons, civilian injured**

√7ᵗʰ **Y38.6X3** **Terrorism involving biological weapons, terrorist injured**

√5ᵗʰ **Y38.7** **Terrorism involving chemical weapons**

Terrorism involving gases, fumes, chemicals

Terrorism involving hydrogen cyanide

Terrorism involving phosgene

Terrorism involving sarin

√6ᵗʰ **Y38.7X** **Terrorism involving chemical weapons**

√7ᵗʰ **Y38.7X1** **Terrorism involving chemical weapons, public safety official injured**

√7ᵗʰ **Y38.7X2** **Terrorism involving chemical weapons, civilian injured**

√7ᵗʰ **Y38.7X3** **Terrorism involving chemical weapons, terrorist injured**

√5ᵗʰ **Y38.8** **Terrorism involving other and unspecified means**

√x7ᵗʰ **Y38.80** **Terrorism involving unspecified means**

Terrorism NOS

√6ᵗʰ **Y38.81** **Terrorism involving suicide bomber**

√7ᵗʰ **Y38.811** **Terrorism involving suicide bomber, public safety official injured**

√7ᵗʰ **Y38.812** **Terrorism involving suicide bomber, civilian injured**

√6ᵗʰ **Y38.89** **Terrorism involving other means**

Terrorism involving drowning and submersion

Terrorism involving lasers

Terrorism involving piercing or stabbing instruments

√7ᵗʰ **Y38.891** **Terrorism involving other means, public safety official injured**

√7ᵗʰ **Y38.892** **Terrorism involving other means, civilian injured**

√7ᵗʰ **Y38.893** **Terrorism involving other means, terrorist injured**

√5ᵗʰ **Y38.9** **Terrorism, secondary effects**

NOTE This code is for use to identify conditions occurring subsequent to a terrorist attack not those that are due to the initial terrorist attack

√6ᵗʰ **Y38.9X** **Terrorism, secondary effects**

√7ᵗʰ **Y38.9X1** **Terrorism, secondary effects, public safety official injured**

√7ᵗʰ **Y38.9X2** **Terrorism, secondary effects, civilian injured**

COMPLICATIONS OF MEDICAL AND SURGICAL CARE (Y62-Y84)

INCLUDES complications of medical devices

surgical and medical procedures as the cause of abnormal reaction of the patient, or of later complication, without mention of misadventure at the time of the procedure

Misadventures to patients during surgical and medical care (Y62-Y69)

EXCLUDES 1 *surgical and medical procedures as the cause of abnormal reaction of the patient, without mention of misadventure at the time of the procedure (Y83-Y84)*

EXCLUDES 2 *breakdown or malfunctioning of medical device (during procedure) (after implantation) (ongoing use) (Y70-Y82)*

√4ᵗʰ **Y62** **Failure of sterile precautions during surgical and medical care**

Y62.0 **Failure of sterile precautions during surgical operation**

Y62.1 **Failure of sterile precautions during infusion or transfusion**

Y62.2 **Failure of sterile precautions during kidney dialysis and other perfusion** HCC

Y62.3 **Failure of sterile precautions during injection or immunization**

Y62.4 **Failure of sterile precautions during endoscopic examination**

Y62.5 **Failure of sterile precautions during heart catheterization**

Y62.6 **Failure of sterile precautions during aspiration, puncture and other catheterization**

Y62.8 **Failure of sterile precautions during other surgical and medical care**

Y62.9 **Failure of sterile precautions during unspecified surgical and medical care**

√4ᵗʰ **Y63** **Failure in dosage during surgical and medical care**

EXCLUDES 2 *accidental overdose of drug or wrong drug given in error (T36-T50)*

Y63.0 **Excessive amount of blood or other fluid given during transfusion or infusion**

Y63.1 **Incorrect dilution of fluid used during infusion**

Y63.2 **Overdose of radiation given during therapy**

Y63.3 **Inadvertent exposure of patient to radiation during medical care**

Y63.4 **Failure in dosage in electroshock or insulin-shock therapy**

Y63.5 **Inappropriate temperature in local application and packing**

Y63.6 **Underdosing and nonadministration of necessary drug, medicament or biological substance**

AHA: 2018,4Q,72

Y63.8 **Failure in dosage during other surgical and medical care**

AHA: 2018,4Q,72

Y63.9 **Failure in dosage during unspecified surgical and medical care**

AHA: 2018,4Q,72

√4ᵗʰ **Y64** **Contaminated medical or biological substances**

Y64.0 **Contaminated medical or biological substance, transfused or infused**

Y64.1 **Contaminated medical or biological substance, injected or used for immunization**

Y64.8 **Contaminated medical or biological substance administered by other means**

✅ Additional Char Req   ✅x7ᵗʰ Placeholder   Unacceptable PDx   Questionable PDx   Wrong Procedure   Manifestation   Unspecified Dx   H1-H14 HAC   HCC CMS-HCC Dx   HIV HIV Dx

ICD-10-CM 2021   **1219**

Y64.9 **Contaminated medical or biological substance administered by unspecified means**
Administered contaminated medical or biological substance NOS

✓4ᵗʰ **Y65** **Other misadventures during surgical and medical care**

Y65.0 **Mismatched blood in transfusion**

Y65.1 **Wrong fluid used in infusion**

Y65.2 **Failure in suture or ligature during surgical operation**

Y65.3 **Endotracheal tube wrongly placed during anesthetic procedure**

Y65.4 **Failure to introduce or to remove other tube or instrument**

✓5ᵗʰ **Y65.5** **Performance of wrong procedure (operation)**

Y65.51 **Performance of wrong procedure (operation) on correct patient**
Wrong device implanted into correct surgical site
EXCLUDES 1 *performance of correct procedure (operation) on wrong side or body part (Y65.53)*

Y65.52 **Performance of procedure (operation) on patient not scheduled for surgery**
Performance of procedure (operation) intended for another patient
Performance of procedure (operation) on wrong patient

Y65.53 **Performance of correct procedure (operation) on wrong side or body part**
Performance of correct procedure (operation) on wrong side
Performance of correct procedure (operation) on wrong site

Y65.8 **Other specified misadventures during surgical and medical care**
AHA: 2019,2Q,23-24

Y66 **Nonadministration of surgical and medical care**
Premature cessation of surgical and medical care
EXCLUDES 1 *DNR status (Z66)*
palliative care (Z51.5)

Y69 **Unspecified misadventure during surgical and medical care**

Medical devices associated with adverse incidents in diagnostic and therapeutic use (Y70-Y82)

INCLUDES breakdown or malfunction of medical devices (during use) (after implantation) (ongoing use)
EXCLUDES 2 *later complications following use of medical devices without breakdown or malfunctioning of device (Y83-Y84)*
misadventure to patients during surgical and medical care, classifiable to (Y62-Y69)
surgical and other medical procedures as the cause of abnormal reaction of the patient, or of later complication, without mention of misadventure at the time of the procedure (Y83-Y84)

✓4ᵗʰ **Y70** **Anesthesiology devices associated with adverse incidents**

Y70.0 **Diagnostic and monitoring anesthesiology devices associated with adverse incidents**

Y70.1 **Therapeutic (nonsurgical) and rehabilitative anesthesiology devices associated with adverse incidents**

Y70.2 **Prosthetic and other implants, materials and accessory anesthesiology devices associated with adverse incidents**

Y70.3 **Surgical instruments, materials and anesthesiology devices (including sutures) associated with adverse incidents**

Y70.8 **Miscellaneous anesthesiology devices associated with adverse incidents, not elsewhere classified**

✓4ᵗʰ **Y71** **Cardiovascular devices associated with adverse incidents**

Y71.0 **Diagnostic and monitoring cardiovascular devices associated with adverse incidents**

Y71.1 **Therapeutic (nonsurgical) and rehabilitative cardiovascular devices associated with adverse incidents**

Y71.2 **Prosthetic and other implants, materials and accessory cardiovascular devices associated with adverse incidents**

Y71.3 **Surgical instruments, materials and cardiovascular devices (including sutures) associated with adverse incidents**

Y71.8 **Miscellaneous cardiovascular devices associated with adverse incidents, not elsewhere classified**

✓4ᵗʰ **Y72** **Otorhinolaryngological devices associated with adverse incidents**

Y72.0 **Diagnostic and monitoring otorhinolaryngological devices associated with adverse incidents**

Y72.1 **Therapeutic (nonsurgical) and rehabilitative otorhinolaryngological devices associated with adverse incidents**

Y72.2 **Prosthetic and other implants, materials and accessory otorhinolaryngological devices associated with adverse incidents**

Y72.3 **Surgical instruments, materials and otorhinolaryngological devices (including sutures) associated with adverse incidents**

Y72.8 **Miscellaneous otorhinolaryngological devices associated with adverse incidents, not elsewhere classified**

✓4ᵗʰ **Y73** **Gastroenterology and urology devices associated with adverse incidents**

Y73.0 **Diagnostic and monitoring gastroenterology and urology devices associated with adverse incidents**

Y73.1 **Therapeutic (nonsurgical) and rehabilitative gastroenterology and urology devices associated with adverse incidents**

Y73.2 **Prosthetic and other implants, materials and accessory gastroenterology and urology devices associated with adverse incidents**

Y73.3 **Surgical instruments, materials and gastroenterology and urology devices (including sutures) associated with adverse incidents**

Y73.8 **Miscellaneous gastroenterology and urology devices associated with adverse incidents, not elsewhere classified**

✓4ᵗʰ **Y74** **General hospital and personal-use devices associated with adverse incidents**

Y74.0 **Diagnostic and monitoring general hospital and personal-use devices associated with adverse incidents**

Y74.1 **Therapeutic (nonsurgical) and rehabilitative general hospital and personal-use devices associated with adverse incidents**

Y74.2 **Prosthetic and other implants, materials and accessory general hospital and personal-use devices associated with adverse incidents**

Y74.3 **Surgical instruments, materials and general hospital and personal-use devices (including sutures) associated with adverse incidents**

Y74.8 **Miscellaneous general hospital and personal-use devices associated with adverse incidents, not elsewhere classified**

✓4ᵗʰ **Y75** **Neurological devices associated with adverse incidents**

Y75.0 **Diagnostic and monitoring neurological devices associated with adverse incidents**

Y75.1 **Therapeutic (nonsurgical) and rehabilitative neurological devices associated with adverse incidents**

Y75.2 **Prosthetic and other implants, materials and neurological devices associated with adverse incidents**

Y75.3 **Surgical instruments, materials and neurological devices (including sutures) associated with adverse incidents**

Y75.8 **Miscellaneous neurological devices associated with adverse incidents, not elsewhere classified**

✓4ᵗʰ **Y76** **Obstetric and gynecological devices associated with adverse incidents**

Y76.0 **Diagnostic and monitoring obstetric and gynecological devices associated with adverse incidents** ♀

Y76.1 **Therapeutic (nonsurgical) and rehabilitative obstetric and gynecological devices associated with adverse incidents** ♀

Y76.2 **Prosthetic and other implants, materials and accessory obstetric and gynecological devices associated with adverse incidents** ♀

Y76.3 **Surgical instruments, materials and obstetric and gynecological devices (including sutures) associated with adverse incidents** ♀

Y76.8 **Miscellaneous obstetric and gynecological devices associated with adverse incidents, not elsewhere classified** ♀

✓4ᵗʰ **Y77** **Ophthalmic devices associated with adverse incidents**

Y77.0 **Diagnostic and monitoring ophthalmic devices associated with adverse incidents**

▲ ✓5ᵗʰ **Y77.1** **Therapeutic (nonsurgical) and rehabilitative ophthalmic devices associated with adverse incidents**

● **Y77.11** **Contact lens associated with adverse incidents**
Rigid gas permeable contact lens associated with adverse incidents
Soft (hydrophilic) contact lens associated with adverse incidents

● **Y77.19** **Other therapeutic (nonsurgical) and rehabilitative ophthalmic devices associated with adverse incidents**

Y77.2 **Prosthetic and other implants, materials and accessory ophthalmic devices associated with adverse incidents**

Y77.3 **Surgical instruments, materials and ophthalmic devices (including sutures) associated with adverse incidents**

Y77.8 **Miscellaneous ophthalmic devices associated with adverse incidents, not elsewhere classified**

N Newborn: 0   P Pediatric: 0-17   M Maternity: 9-64   A Adult: 15-124   MCC Major Complication/Comorbidity   CC Complication/Comorbidity   SW Severe Wound Dx

1220   ICD-10-CM 2021

✓4ᵗʰ **Y78** Radiological **devices associated with adverse incidents**

    Y78.0 Diagnostic and monitoring radiological devices associated with adverse incidents

    Y78.1 Therapeutic (nonsurgical) and rehabilitative radiological devices associated with adverse incidents

    Y78.2 Prosthetic and other implants, **materials and accessory** radiological **devices associated with adverse incidents**

    Y78.3 Surgical instruments, **materials and radiological devices (including sutures) associated with adverse incidents**

    Y78.8 Miscellaneous radiological devices associated with adverse incidents, not elsewhere classified

✓4ᵗʰ **Y79** Orthopedic **devices associated with adverse incidents**

    Y79.0 Diagnostic and monitoring orthopedic devices associated with adverse incidents

    Y79.1 Therapeutic (nonsurgical) and rehabilitative orthopedic devices associated with adverse incidents

    Y79.2 Prosthetic and other implants, **materials and accessory** orthopedic **devices associated with adverse incidents**

    Y79.3 Surgical instruments, **materials and orthopedic devices (including sutures) associated with adverse incidents**

    Y79.8 Miscellaneous orthopedic devices associated with adverse incidents, not elsewhere classified

✓4ᵗʰ **Y80** Physical medicine **devices associated with adverse incidents**

    Y80.0 Diagnostic and monitoring physical medicine devices associated with adverse incidents

    Y80.1 Therapeutic (nonsurgical) and rehabilitative physical medicine devices associated with adverse incidents

    Y80.2 Prosthetic and other implants, **materials and accessory** physical medicine **devices associated with adverse incidents**

    Y80.3 Surgical instruments, **materials and physical medicine devices (including sutures) associated with adverse incidents**

    Y80.8 Miscellaneous physical medicine devices associated with adverse incidents, not elsewhere classified

✓4ᵗʰ **Y81** General- and plastic-surgery **devices associated with adverse incidents**

    Y81.0 Diagnostic and monitoring general- and plastic-surgery devices associated with adverse incidents

    Y81.1 Therapeutic (nonsurgical) and rehabilitative general- and plastic-surgery devices associated with adverse incidents

    Y81.2 Prosthetic and other implants, **materials and accessory** general- and plastic-surgery **devices associated with adverse incidents**

    Y81.3 Surgical instruments, **materials and general- and plastic-surgery devices (including sutures) associated with adverse incidents**

    Y81.8 Miscellaneous general- and plastic-surgery devices associated with adverse incidents, not elsewhere classified

✓4ᵗʰ **Y82** Other and unspecified medical devices associated with adverse incidents

    Y82.8 Other medical devices associated with adverse incidents

    Y82.9 Unspecified medical devices associated with adverse incidents

Surgical and other medical procedures as the cause of abnormal reaction of the patient, or of later complication, without mention of misadventure at the time of the procedure (Y83-Y84)

    EXCLUDES 1   misadventures to patients during surgical and medical care, classifiable to (Y62-Y69)

    EXCLUDES 2   breakdown or malfunctioning of medical device (during procedure) (after implantation) (ongoing use) (Y70-Y82)

✓4ᵗʰ **Y83** Surgical operation **and other** surgical procedures **as the cause of abnormal reaction of the patient, or of later complication, without mention of misadventure at the time of the procedure**

    Y83.0 Surgical operation with transplant of whole organ as the cause of abnormal reaction of the patient, or of later complication, without mention of misadventure at the time of the procedure

    Y83.1 Surgical operation with implant of artificial internal device as the cause of abnormal reaction of the patient, or of later complication, without mention of misadventure at the time of the procedure

    Y83.2 Surgical operation with anastomosis, bypass or graft as the cause of abnormal reaction of the patient, or of later complication, without mention of misadventure at the time of the procedure

    Y83.3 Surgical operation with formation of external stoma as the cause of abnormal reaction of the patient, or of later complication, without mention of misadventure at the time of the procedure

    Y83.4 Other reconstructive surgery as the cause of abnormal reaction of the patient, or of later complication, without mention of misadventure at the time of the procedure

    Y83.5 Amputation of limb(s) as the cause of abnormal reaction of the patient, or of later complication, without mention of misadventure at the time of the procedure

    Y83.6 Removal of other organ (partial) (total) as the cause of abnormal reaction of the patient, or of later complication, without mention of misadventure at the time of the procedure

    Y83.8 Other surgical procedures as the cause of abnormal reaction of the patient, or of later complication, without mention of misadventure at the time of the procedure

    Y83.9 Surgical procedure, unspecified as the cause of abnormal reaction of the patient, or of later complication, without mention of misadventure at the time of the procedure

✓4ᵗʰ **Y84** Other medical procedures as the cause of abnormal reaction of the patient, or of later complication, without mention of misadventure at the time of the procedure

    Y84.0 Cardiac catheterization as the cause of abnormal reaction of the patient, or of later complication, without mention of misadventure at the time of the procedure

    Y84.1 Kidney dialysis as the cause of abnormal reaction of the patient, or of later complication, without mention of misadventure at the time of the procedure

    Y84.2 Radiological procedure and radiotherapy as the cause of abnormal reaction of the patient, or of later complication, without mention of misadventure at the time of the procedure
        AHA: 2019,1Q,21; 2017,1Q,33

    Y84.3 Shock therapy as the cause of abnormal reaction of the patient, or of later complication, without mention of misadventure at the time of the procedure

    Y84.4 Aspiration of fluid as the cause of abnormal reaction of the patient, or of later complication, without mention of misadventure at the time of the procedure

    Y84.5 Insertion of gastric or duodenal sound as the cause of abnormal reaction of the patient, or of later complication, without mention of misadventure at the time of the procedure

    Y84.6 Urinary catheterization as the cause of abnormal reaction of the patient, or of later complication, without mention of misadventure at the time of the procedure

    Y84.7 Blood-sampling as the cause of abnormal reaction of the patient, or of later complication, without mention of misadventure at the time of the procedure

    Y84.8 Other medical procedures as the cause of abnormal reaction of the patient, or of later complication, without mention of misadventure at the time of the procedure
        AHA: 2014,4Q,24

    Y84.9 Medical procedure, unspecified as the cause of abnormal reaction of the patient, or of later complication, without mention of misadventure at the time of the procedure

Supplementary factors related to causes of morbidity classified elsewhere (Y90-Y99)

    NOTE   These categories may be used to provide supplementary information concerning causes of morbidity. They are not to be used for single-condition coding.

✓4ᵗʰ **Y90** Evidence of alcohol involvement determined by blood alcohol level

    Code first any associated alcohol related disorders (F10)

    Y90.0 Blood alcohol level of less than 20 mg/100 ml

    Y90.1 Blood alcohol level of 20-39 mg/100 ml

    Y90.2 Blood alcohol level of 40-59 mg/100 ml

    Y90.3 Blood alcohol level of 60-79 mg/100 ml

    Y90.4 Blood alcohol level of 80-99 mg/100 ml

    Y90.5 Blood alcohol level of 100-119 mg/100 ml

    Y90.6 Blood alcohol level of 120-199 mg/100 ml

    Y90.7 Blood alcohol level of 200-239 mg/100 ml

    Y90.8 Blood alcohol level of 240 mg/100 ml or more

    Y90.9 Presence of alcohol in blood, level not specified

✓ Additional Char Req   ✓x7ᵗʰ Placeholder   Unacceptable PDx   Questionable PDx   Wrong Procedure   Manifestation   Unspecified Dx   H1 - H14 HAC   HCC CMS-HCC Dx   HIV HIV Dx

ICD-10-CM 2021   1221

√4ᵗʰ **Y92** **Place of occurrence of the external cause**

The following category is for use, when relevant, to identify the place of occurrence of the external cause. Use in conjunction with an activity code.

Place of occurrence should be recorded only at the initial encounter for treatment

√5ᵗʰ **Y92.0** Non-institutional (private) residence as the place of occurrence of the external cause

EXCLUDES 1 *abandoned or derelict house (Y92.89)*

home under construction but not yet occupied (Y92.6-)

institutional place of residence (Y92.1-)

√6ᵗʰ **Y92.00** **Unspecified non-institutional (private) residence as the place of occurrence of the external cause**

▲ **Y92.000** Kitchen of unspecified non-institutional (private) residence as the place of occurrence of the external cause

Y92.001 Dining room of unspecified non-institutional (private) residence as the place of occurrence of the external cause

Y92.002 Bathroom of unspecified non-institutional (private) residence as the place of occurrence of the external cause

Y92.003 Bedroom of unspecified non-institutional (private) residence as the place of occurrence of the external cause

Y92.007 Garden or yard of unspecified non-institutional (private) residence as the place of occurrence of the external cause

Y92.008 Other place in unspecified non-institutional (private) residence as the place of occurrence of the external cause

Y92.009 Unspecified place in unspecified non-institutional (private) residence as the place of occurrence of the external cause

Home (NOS) as the place of occurrence of the external cause

√6ᵗʰ **Y92.01** **Single-family non-institutional (private) house as the place of occurrence of the external cause**

Farmhouse as the place of occurrence of the external cause

EXCLUDES 1 *barn (Y92.71)*

chicken coop or hen house (Y92.72)

farm field (Y92.73)

orchard (Y92.74)

single family mobile home or trailer (Y92.02-)

slaughter house (Y92.86)

Y92.010 Kitchen of single-family (private) house as the place of occurrence of the external cause

Y92.011 Dining room of single-family (private) house as the place of occurrence of the external cause

Y92.012 Bathroom of single-family (private) house as the place of occurrence of the external cause

Y92.013 Bedroom of single-family (private) house as the place of occurrence of the external cause

Y92.014 Private driveway to single-family (private) house as the place of occurrence of the external cause

Y92.015 Private garage of single-family (private) house as the place of occurrence of the external cause

Y92.016 Swimming-pool in single-family (private) house or garden as the place of occurrence of the external cause

Y92.017 Garden or yard in single-family (private) house as the place of occurrence of the external cause

Y92.018 Other place in single-family (private) house as the place of occurrence of the external cause

Y92.019 Unspecified place in single-family (private) house as the place of occurrence of the external cause

√6ᵗʰ **Y92.02** Mobile home as the place of occurrence of the external cause

Y92.020 Kitchen in mobile home as the place of occurrence of the external cause

Y92.021 Dining room in mobile home as the place of occurrence of the external cause

Y92.022 Bathroom in mobile home as the place of occurrence of the external cause

Y92.023 Bedroom in mobile home as the place of occurrence of the external cause

Y92.024 Driveway of mobile home as the place of occurrence of the external cause

Y92.025 Garage of mobile home as the place of occurrence of the external cause

Y92.026 Swimming-pool of mobile home as the place of occurrence of the external cause

Y92.027 Garden or yard of mobile home as the place of occurrence of the external cause

Y92.028 Other place in mobile home as the place of occurrence of the external cause

Y92.029 Unspecified place in mobile home as the place of occurrence of the external cause

√6ᵗʰ **Y92.03** Apartment as the place of occurrence of the external cause

Condominium as the place of occurrence of the external cause

Co-op apartment as the place of occurrence of the external cause

Y92.030 Kitchen in apartment as the place of occurrence of the external cause

Y92.031 Bathroom in apartment as the place of occurrence of the external cause

Y92.032 Bedroom in apartment as the place of occurrence of the external cause

Y92.038 Other place in apartment as the place of occurrence of the external cause

Y92.039 Unspecified place in apartment as the place of occurrence of the external cause

√6ᵗʰ **Y92.04** Boarding-house as the place of occurrence of the external cause

Y92.040 Kitchen in boarding-house as the place of occurrence of the external cause

Y92.041 Bathroom in boarding-house as the place of occurrence of the external cause

Y92.042 Bedroom in boarding-house as the place of occurrence of the external cause

Y92.043 Driveway of boarding-house as the place of occurrence of the external cause

Y92.044 Garage of boarding-house as the place of occurrence of the external cause

Y92.045 Swimming-pool of boarding-house as the place of occurrence of the external cause

Y92.046 Garden or yard of boarding-house as the place of occurrence of the external cause

Y92.048 Other place in boarding-house as the place of occurrence of the external cause

Y92.049 Unspecified place in boarding-house as the place of occurrence of the external cause

√6ᵗʰ **Y92.09** Other non-institutional residence as the place of occurrence of the external cause

AHA: 2017,2Q,10

Y92.090 Kitchen in other non-institutional residence as the place of occurrence of the external cause

Y92.091 Bathroom in other non-institutional residence as the place of occurrence of the external cause

Y92.092 Bedroom in other non-institutional residence as the place of occurrence of the external cause

Y92.093 Driveway of other non-institutional residence as the place of occurrence of the external cause

Y92.094 Garage of other non-institutional residence as the place of occurrence of the external cause

Y92.095 Swimming-pool of other non-institutional residence as the place of occurrence of the external cause

Y92.096 Garden or yard of other non-institutional residence as the place of occurrence of the external cause

N Newborn: 0 P Pediatric: 0-17 M Maternity: 9-64 A Adult: 15-124 MCC Major Complication/Comorbidity CC Complication/Comorbidity SW Severe Wound Dx

1222

ICD-10-CM 2021

Chapter 20. External Causes of Morbidity

Y92.Ø98 Other place in other non-institutional residence as the place of occurrence of the external cause

Y92.Ø99 Unspecified place in other non-institutional residence as the place of occurrence of the external cause

✓5ᵗʰ **Y92.1** Institutional (nonprivate) residence as the place of occurrence of the external cause

Y92.1Ø Unspecified residential institution as the place of occurrence of the external cause

✓6ᵗʰ **Y92.11** Children's home and orphanage as the place of occurrence of the external cause

Y92.11Ø Kitchen in children's home and orphanage as the place of occurrence of the external cause

Y92.111 Bathroom in children's home and orphanage as the place of occurrence of the external cause

Y92.112 Bedroom in children's home and orphanage as the place of occurrence of the external cause

Y92.113 Driveway of children's home and orphanage as the place of occurrence of the external cause

Y92.114 Garage of children's home and orphanage as the place of occurrence of the external cause

Y92.115 Swimming-pool of children's home and orphanage as the place of occurrence of the external cause

Y92.116 Garden or yard of children's home and orphanage as the place of occurrence of the external cause

Y92.118 Other place in children's home and orphanage as the place of occurrence of the external cause

Y92.119 Unspecified place in children's home and orphanage as the place of occurrence of the external cause

✓6ᵗʰ **Y92.12** Nursing home as the place of occurrence of the external cause

Home for the sick as the place of occurrence of the external cause

Hospice as the place of occurrence of the external cause

AHA: 2017,2Q,10

Y92.12Ø Kitchen in nursing home as the place of occurrence of the external cause

Y92.121 Bathroom in nursing home as the place of occurrence of the external cause

Y92.122 Bedroom in nursing home as the place of occurrence of the external cause

Y92.123 Driveway of nursing home as the place of occurrence of the external cause

Y92.124 Garage of nursing home as the place of occurrence of the external cause

Y92.125 Swimming-pool of nursing home as the place of occurrence of the external cause

Y92.126 Garden or yard of nursing home as the place of occurrence of the external cause

Y92.128 Other place in nursing home as the place of occurrence of the external cause

Y92.129 Unspecified place in nursing home as the place of occurrence of the external cause

✓6ᵗʰ **Y92.13** Military base as the place of occurrence of the external cause

EXCLUDES 1   military training grounds (Y92.84)

Y92.13Ø Kitchen on military base as the place of occurrence of the external cause

Y92.131 Mess hall on military base as the place of occurrence of the external cause

Y92.133 Barracks on military base as the place of occurrence of the external cause

Y92.135 Garage on military base as the place of occurrence of the external cause

Y92.136 Swimming-pool on military base as the place of occurrence of the external cause

Y92.137 Garden or yard on military base as the place of occurrence of the external cause

Y92.138 Other place on military base as the place of occurrence of the external cause

Y92.139 Unspecified place military base as the place of occurrence of the external cause

✓6ᵗʰ **Y92.14** Prison as the place of occurrence of the external cause

Y92.14Ø Kitchen in prison as the place of occurrence of the external cause

Y92.141 Dining room in prison as the place of occurrence of the external cause

Y92.142 Bathroom in prison as the place of occurrence of the external cause

Y92.143 Cell of prison as the place of occurrence of the external cause

Y92.146 Swimming-pool of prison as the place of occurrence of the external cause

Y92.147 Courtyard of prison as the place of occurrence of the external cause

Y92.148 Other place in prison as the place of occurrence of the external cause

Y92.149 Unspecified place in prison as the place of occurrence of the external cause

✓6ᵗʰ **Y92.15** Reform school as the place of occurrence of the external cause

Y92.15Ø Kitchen in reform school as the place of occurrence of the external cause

Y92.151 Dining room in reform school as the place of occurrence of the external cause

Y92.152 Bathroom in reform school as the place of occurrence of the external cause

Y92.153 Bedroom in reform school as the place of occurrence of the external cause

Y92.154 Driveway of reform school as the place of occurrence of the external cause

Y92.155 Garage of reform school as the place of occurrence of the external cause

Y92.156 Swimming-pool of reform school as the place of occurrence of the external cause

Y92.157 Garden or yard of reform school as the place of occurrence of the external cause

Y92.158 Other place in reform school as the place of occurrence of the external cause

Y92.159 Unspecified place in reform school as the place of occurrence of the external cause

✓6ᵗʰ **Y92.16** School dormitory as the place of occurrence of the external cause

EXCLUDES 1   reform school as the place of occurrence of the external cause (Y92.15-)

school buildings and grounds as the place of occurrence of the external cause (Y92.2-)

school sports and athletic areas as the place of occurrence of the external cause (Y92.3-)

Y92.16Ø Kitchen in school dormitory as the place of occurrence of the external cause

Y92.161 Dining room in school dormitory as the place of occurrence of the external cause

Y92.162 Bathroom in school dormitory as the place of occurrence of the external cause

Y92.163 Bedroom in school dormitory as the place of occurrence of the external cause

Y92.168 Other place in school dormitory as the place of occurrence of the external cause

Y92.169 Unspecified place in school dormitory as the place of occurrence of the external cause

✓6ᵗʰ **Y92.19** Other specified residential institution as the place of occurrence of the external cause

AHA: 2017,2Q,10

Y92.19Ø Kitchen in other specified residential institution as the place of occurrence of the external cause

Y92.191 Dining room in other specified residential institution as the place of occurrence of the external cause

Y92.192 Bathroom in other specified residential institution as the place of occurrence of the external cause

Y92.193 Bedroom in other specified residential institution as the place of occurrence of the external cause

Y92.194 Driveway of other specified residential institution as the place of occurrence of the external cause

✓ Additional Char Req   ✓x7ᵗʰ Placeholder   Unacceptable PDx   Questionable PDx   Wrong Procedure   Manifestation   Unspecified Dx   H1-H14 HAC   HCC CMS-HCC Dx   HIV HIV Dx

ICD-10-CM 2021   1223

Y92.195 Garage of other specified residential institution as the place of occurrence of the external cause

Y92.196 Pool of other specified residential institution as the place of occurrence of the external cause

Y92.197 Garden or yard of other specified residential institution as the place of occurrence of the external cause

Y92.198 Other place in other specified residential institution as the place of occurrence of the external cause

Y92.199 Unspecified place in other specified residential institution as the place of occurrence of the external cause

✓5ᵗʰ **Y92.2 School, other institution and public administrative area** as the place of occurrence of the external cause

Building and adjacent grounds used by the general public or by a particular group of the public

EXCLUDES 1   *building under construction as the place of occurrence of the external cause (Y92.6)*

residential institution as the place of occurrence of the external cause (Y92.1)

school dormitory as the place of occurrence of the external cause (Y92.16-)

sports and athletics area of schools as the place of occurrence of the external cause (Y92.3-)

✓6ᵗʰ **Y92.21 School (private) (public) (state)** as the place of occurrence of the external cause

Y92.210 Daycare center as the place of occurrence of the external cause

Y92.211 Elementary school as the place of occurrence of the external cause

Kindergarten as the place of occurrence of the external cause

Y92.212 Middle school as the place of occurrence of the external cause

Y92.213 High school as the place of occurrence of the external cause

AHA: 2012,4Q,108

Y92.214 College as the place of occurrence of the external cause

University as the place of occurrence of the external cause

Y92.215 Trade school as the place of occurrence of the external cause

Y92.218 Other school as the place of occurrence of the external cause

Y92.219 Unspecified school as the place of occurrence of the external cause

Y92.22 Religious institution as the place of occurrence of the external cause

Church as the place of occurrence of the external cause

Mosque as the place of occurrence of the external cause

Synagogue as the place of occurrence of the external cause

✓6ᵗʰ **Y92.23 Hospital** as the place of occurrence of the external cause

EXCLUDES 1   *ambulatory (outpatient) health services establishments (Y92.53-)*

home for the sick as the place of occurrence of the external cause (Y92.12-)

hospice as the place of occurrence of the external cause (Y92.12-)

nursing home as the place of occurrence of the external cause (Y92.12-)

Y92.230 Patient room in hospital as the place of occurrence of the external cause

Y92.231 Patient bathroom in hospital as the place of occurrence of the external cause

Y92.232 Corridor of hospital as the place of occurrence of the external cause

Y92.233 Cafeteria of hospital as the place of occurrence of the external cause

Y92.234 Operating room of hospital as the place of occurrence of the external cause

Y92.238 Other place in hospital as the place of occurrence of the external cause

Y92.239 Unspecified place in hospital as the place of occurrence of the external cause

✓6ᵗʰ **Y92.24 Public administrative building** as the place of occurrence of the external cause

Y92.240 Courthouse as the place of occurrence of the external cause

Y92.241 Library as the place of occurrence of the external cause

Y92.242 Post office as the place of occurrence of the external cause

Y92.243 City hall as the place of occurrence of the external cause

Y92.248 Other public administrative building as the place of occurrence of the external cause

✓6ᵗʰ **Y92.25 Cultural building** as the place of occurrence of the external cause

Y92.250 Art Gallery as the place of occurrence of the external cause

Y92.251 Museum as the place of occurrence of the external cause

Y92.252 Music hall as the place of occurrence of the external cause

Y92.253 Opera house as the place of occurrence of the external cause

Y92.254 Theater (live) as the place of occurrence of the external cause

Y92.258 Other cultural public building as the place of occurrence of the external cause

Y92.26 Movie house or cinema as the place of occurrence of the external cause

Y92.29 Other specified public building as the place of occurrence of the external cause

Assembly hall as the place of occurrence of the external cause

Clubhouse as the place of occurrence of the external cause

✓5ᵗʰ **Y92.3 Sports and athletics area** as the place of occurrence of the external cause

✓6ᵗʰ **Y92.31 Athletic court** as the place of occurrence of the external cause

EXCLUDES 1   *tennis court in private home or garden (Y92.09)*

Y92.310 Basketball court as the place of occurrence of the external cause

Y92.311 Squash court as the place of occurrence of the external cause

Y92.312 Tennis court as the place of occurrence of the external cause

Y92.318 Other athletic court as the place of occurrence of the external cause

✓6ᵗʰ **Y92.32 Athletic field** as the place of occurrence of the external cause

Y92.320 Baseball field as the place of occurrence of the external cause

Y92.321 Football field as the place of occurrence of the external cause

Y92.322 Soccer field as the place of occurrence of the external cause

Y92.328 Other athletic field as the place of occurrence of the external cause

Cricket field as the place of occurrence of the external cause

Hockey field as the place of occurrence of the external cause

✓6ᵗʰ **Y92.33 Skating rink** as the place of occurrence of the external cause

Y92.330 Ice skating rink (indoor) (outdoor) as the place of occurrence of the external cause

Y92.331 Roller skating rink as the place of occurrence of the external cause

Y92.34 Swimming pool (public) as the place of occurrence of the external cause

EXCLUDES 1   *swimming pool in private home or garden (Y92.016)*

N Newborn: 0   P Pediatric: 0-17   M Maternity: 9-64   A Adult: 15-124   MCC Major Complication/Comorbidity   CC Complication/Comorbidity   SW Severe Wound Dx

1224   ICD-10-CM 2021

Y92.39   **Other specified sports and athletic area as the place of occurrence of the external cause**

Golf-course as the place of occurrence of the external cause

Gymnasium as the place of occurrence of the external cause

Riding-school as the place of occurrence of the external cause

Stadium as the place of occurrence of the external cause

✓5ᵗʰ **Y92.4**   **Street, highway and other paved roadways as the place of occurrence of the external cause**

EXCLUDES 1   *private driveway of residence (Y92.014, Y92.024, Y92.043, Y92.093, Y92.113, Y92.123, Y92.154, Y92.194)*

✓6ᵗʰ **Y92.41**   **Street and highway as the place of occurrence of the external cause**

Y92.410   **Unspecified street and highway as the place of occurrence of the external cause**

Road NOS as the place of occurrence of the external cause

Y92.411   **Interstate highway as the place of occurrence of the external cause**

Freeway as the place of occurrence of the external cause

Motorway as the place of occurrence of the external cause

Y92.412   **Parkway as the place of occurrence of the external cause**

Y92.413   **State road as the place of occurrence of the external cause**

Y92.414   **Local residential or business street as the place of occurrence of the external cause**

Y92.415   **Exit ramp or entrance ramp of street or highway as the place of occurrence of the external cause**

✓6ᵗʰ **Y92.48**   **Other paved roadways as the place of occurrence of the external cause**

Y92.480   **Sidewalk as the place of occurrence of the external cause**

Y92.481   **Parking lot as the place of occurrence of the external cause**

Y92.482   **Bike path as the place of occurrence of the external cause**

Y92.488   **Other paved roadways as the place of occurrence of the external cause**

✓5ᵗʰ **Y92.5**   **Trade and service area as the place of occurrence of the external cause**

EXCLUDES 1   *garage in private home (Y92.015)*

schools and other public administration buildings (Y92.2-)

✓6ᵗʰ **Y92.51**   **Private commercial establishments as the place of occurrence of the external cause**

Y92.510   **Bank as the place of occurrence of the external cause**

Y92.511   **Restaurant or café as the place of occurrence of the external cause**

Y92.512   **Supermarket, store or market as the place of occurrence of the external cause**

Y92.513   **Shop (commercial) as the place of occurrence of the external cause**

✓6ᵗʰ **Y92.52**   **Service areas as the place of occurrence of the external cause**

Y92.520   **Airport as the place of occurrence of the external cause**

Y92.521   **Bus station as the place of occurrence of the external cause**

Y92.522   **Railway station as the place of occurrence of the external cause**

Y92.523   **Highway rest stop as the place of occurrence of the external cause**

Y92.524   **Gas station as the place of occurrence of the external cause**

Petroleum station as the place of occurrence of the external cause

Service station as the place of occurrence of the external cause

✓6ᵗʰ **Y92.53**   **Ambulatory health services establishments as the place of occurrence of the external cause**

Y92.530   **Ambulatory surgery center as the place of occurrence of the external cause**

Outpatient surgery center, including that connected with a hospital as the place of occurrence of the external cause

Same day surgery center, including that connected with a hospital as the place of occurrence of the external cause

Y92.531   **Health care provider office as the place of occurrence of the external cause**

Physician office as the place of occurrence of the external cause

Y92.532   **Urgent care center as the place of occurrence of the external cause**

Y92.538   **Other ambulatory health services establishments as the place of occurrence of the external cause**

AHA: 2019,1Q,21

Y92.59   **Other trade areas as the place of occurrence of the external cause**

Office building as the place of occurrence of the external cause

Casino as the place of occurrence of the external cause

Garage (commercial) as the place of occurrence of the external cause

Hotel as the place of occurrence of the external cause

Radio or television station as the place of occurrence of the external cause

Shopping mall as the place of occurrence of the external cause

Warehouse as the place of occurrence of the external cause

✓5ᵗʰ **Y92.6**   **Industrial and construction area as the place of occurrence of the external cause**

Y92.61   **Building [any] under construction as the place of occurrence of the external cause**

Y92.62   **Dock or shipyard as the place of occurrence of the external cause**

Dockyard as the place of occurrence of the external cause

Dry dock as the place of occurrence of the external cause

Shipyard as the place of occurrence of the external cause

Y92.63   **Factory as the place of occurrence of the external cause**

Factory building as the place of occurrence of the external cause

Factory premises as the place of occurrence of the external cause

Industrial yard as the place of occurrence of the external cause

Y92.64   **Mine or pit as the place of occurrence of the external cause**

Mine as the place of occurrence of the external cause

Y92.65   **Oil rig as the place of occurrence of the external cause**

Pit (coal) (gravel) (sand) as the place of occurrence of the external cause

Y92.69   **Other specified industrial and construction area as the place of occurrence of the external cause**

Gasworks as the place of occurrence of the external cause

Power-station (coal) (nuclear) (oil) as the place of occurrence of the external cause

Tunnel under construction as the place of occurrence of the external cause

Workshop as the place of occurrence of the external cause

✓5ᵗʰ **Y92.7**   **Farm as the place of occurrence of the external cause**

Ranch as the place of occurrence of the external cause

EXCLUDES 1   *farmhouse and home premises of farm (Y92.01-)*

Y92.71   **Barn as the place of occurrence of the external cause**

☑ Additional Char Req   ✓x7ᵗʰ Placeholder   Unacceptable PDx   Questionable PDx   Wrong Procedure   Manifestation   Unspecified Dx   H1-H14 HAC   HCC CMS-HCC Dx   HIV HIV Dx

ICD-10-CM 2021   **1225**

Y92.72 Chicken coop as the place of occurrence of the external cause

Hen house as the place of occurrence of the external cause

Y92.73 Farm field as the place of occurrence of the external cause

Y92.74 Orchard as the place of occurrence of the external cause

Y92.79 Other farm location as the place of occurrence of the external cause

✓5ᵗʰ **Y92.8 Other places** as the place of occurrence of the external cause

✓6ᵗʰ **Y92.81 Transport vehicle** as the place of occurrence of the external cause

EXCLUDES 1 *transport accidents (V00-V99)*

Y92.810 Car as the place of occurrence of the external cause

Y92.811 Bus as the place of occurrence of the external cause

Y92.812 Truck as the place of occurrence of the external cause

Y92.813 Airplane as the place of occurrence of the external cause

Y92.814 Boat as the place of occurrence of the external cause

Y92.815 Train as the place of occurrence of the external cause

Y92.816 Subway car as the place of occurrence of the external cause

Y92.818 Other transport vehicle as the place of occurrence of the external cause

✓6ᵗʰ **Y92.82 Wilderness area**

Y92.820 Desert as the place of occurrence of the external cause

Y92.821 Forest as the place of occurrence of the external cause

Y92.828 Other wilderness area as the place of occurrence of the external cause

Swamp as the place of occurrence of the external cause

Mountain as the place of occurrence of the external cause

Marsh as the place of occurrence of the external cause

Prairie as the place of occurrence of the external cause

✓6ᵗʰ **Y92.83 Recreation area** as the place of occurrence of the external cause

Y92.830 Public park as the place of occurrence of the external cause

Y92.831 Amusement park as the place of occurrence of the external cause

Y92.832 Beach as the place of occurrence of the external cause

Seashore as the place of occurrence of the external cause

Y92.833 Campsite as the place of occurrence of the external cause

Y92.834 Zoological garden (Zoo) as the place of occurrence of the external cause

Y92.838 Other recreation area as the place of occurrence of the external cause

Y92.84 Military training ground as the place of occurrence of the external cause

Y92.85 Railroad track as the place of occurrence of the external cause

Y92.86 Slaughter house as the place of occurrence of the external cause

Y92.89 Other specified places as the place of occurrence of the external cause

Derelict house as the place of occurrence of the external cause

Y92.9 Unspecified place or not applicable

✓4ᵗʰ **Y93 Activity codes**

NOTE   Category Y93 is provided for use to indicate the activity of the person seeking healthcare for an injury or health condition, such as a heart attack while shoveling snow, which resulted from, or was contributed to, by the activity. These codes are appropriate for use for both acute injuries, such as those from chapter 19, and conditions that are due to the long-term, cumulative effects of an activity, such as those from chapter 13. They are also appropriate for use with external cause codes for cause and intent if identifying the activity provides additional information on the event. These codes should be used in conjunction with codes for external cause status (Y99) and place of occurrence (Y92).

This section contains the following broad activity categories:

Y93.0	Activities involving walking and running
Y93.1	Activities involving water and water craft
Y93.2	Activities involving ice and snow
Y93.3	Activities involving climbing, rappelling, and jumping off
Y93.4	Activities involving dancing and other rhythmic movement
Y93.5	Activities involving other sports and athletics played individually
Y93.6	Activities involving other sports and athletics played as a team or group
Y93.7	Activities involving other specified sports and athletics
Y93.A	Activities involving other cardiorespiratory exercise
Y93.B	Activities involving other muscle strengthening exercises
Y93.C	Activities involving computer technology and electronic devices
Y93.D	Activities involving arts and handcrafts
Y93.E	Activities involving personal hygiene and interior property and clothing maintenance
Y93.F	Activities involving caregiving
Y93.G	Activities involving food preparation, cooking and grilling
Y93.H	Activities involving exterior property and land maintenance, building and construction
Y93.I	Activities involving roller coasters and other types of external motion
Y93.J	Activities involving playing musical instrument
Y93.K	Activities involving animal care
Y93.8	Activities, other specified
Y93.9	Activity, unspecified

✓5ᵗʰ **Y93.0 Activities involving walking and running**

EXCLUDES 1 *activity, walking an animal (Y93.K1)*

activity, walking or running on a treadmill (Y93.A1)

Y93.01 Activity, walking, marching and hiking

Activity, walking, marching and hiking on level or elevated terrain

EXCLUDES 1 *activity, mountain climbing (Y93.31)*

Y93.02 Activity, running

✓5ᵗʰ **Y93.1 Activities involving water and water craft**

EXCLUDES 1 *activities involving ice (Y93.2-)*

Y93.11 Activity, swimming

Y93.12 Activity, springboard and platform diving

Y93.13 Activity, water polo

Y93.14 Activity, water aerobics and water exercise

Y93.15 Activity, underwater diving and snorkeling

Activity, SCUBA diving

Y93.16 Activity, rowing, canoeing, kayaking, rafting and tubing

Activity, canoeing, kayaking, rafting and tubing in calm and turbulent water

Y93.17 Activity, water skiing and wake boarding

Y93.18 Activity, surfing, windsurfing and boogie boarding

Activity, water sliding

Y93.19 Activity, other involving water and watercraft

Activity involving water NOS

Activity, parasailing

Activity, water survival training and testing

N Newborn: 0   **P** Pediatric: 0-17   **M** Maternity: 9-64   **A** Adult: 15-124   **MCC** Major Complication/Comorbidity   **CC** Complication/Comorbidity   **SW** Severe Wound Dx

1226   ICD-10-CM 2021

✓5ᵗʰ **Y93.2　Activities involving ice and snow**

　　　EXCLUDES 1　*activity, shoveling ice and snow (Y93.H1)*

　Y93.21　Activity, ice skating
　　　Activity, figure skating (singles) (pairs)
　　　Activity, ice dancing
　　　EXCLUDES 1　*activity, ice hockey (Y93.22)*

　Y93.22　Activity, ice hockey

　Y93.23　Activity, snow (alpine) (downhill) skiing, snowboarding, sledding, tobogganing and snow tubing
　　　EXCLUDES 1　*activity, cross country skiing (Y93.24)*

　Y93.24　Activity, cross country skiing
　　　Activity, nordic skiing

　Y93.29　Activity, other involving ice and snow
　　　Activity involving ice and snow NOS

✓5ᵗʰ **Y93.3　Activities involving climbing, rappelling and jumping off**

　　　EXCLUDES 1　*activity, hiking on level or elevated terrain (Y93.Ø1)*
　　　　　　　　　activity, jumping rope (Y93.56)
　　　　　　　　　activity, trampoline jumping (Y93.44)

　Y93.31　Activity, mountain climbing, rock climbing and wall climbing

　Y93.32　Activity, rappelling

　Y93.33　Activity, BASE jumping
　　　Activity, Building, Antenna, Span, Earth jumping

　Y93.34　Activity, bungee jumping

　Y93.35　Activity, hang gliding

　Y93.39　Activity, other involving climbing, rappelling and jumping off

✓5ᵗʰ **Y93.4　Activities involving dancing and other rhythmic movement**

　　　EXCLUDES 1　*activity, martial arts (Y93.75)*

　Y93.41　Activity, dancing
　　　AHA: 2012,4Q,108

　Y93.42　Activity, yoga

　Y93.43　Activity, gymnastics
　　　Activity, rhythmic gymnastics
　　　EXCLUDES 1　*activity, trampolining (Y93.44)*

　Y93.44　Activity, trampolining

　Y93.45　Activity, cheerleading

　Y93.49　Activity, other involving dancing and other rhythmic movements

✓5ᵗʰ **Y93.5　Activities involving other sports and athletics played individually**

　　　EXCLUDES 1　*activity, dancing (Y93.41)*
　　　　　　　　　activity, gymnastic (Y93.43)
　　　　　　　　　activity, trampolining (Y93.44)
　　　　　　　　　activity, yoga (Y93.42)

　Y93.51　Activity, roller skating (inline) and skateboarding

　Y93.52　Activity, horseback riding

　Y93.53　Activity, golf

　Y93.54　Activity, bowling

　Y93.55　Activity, bike riding

　Y93.56　Activity, jumping rope

　Y93.57　Activity, non-running track and field events
　　　EXCLUDES 1　*activity, running (any form) (Y93.Ø2)*

　Y93.59　Activity, other involving other sports and athletics played individually
　　　EXCLUDES 1　*activities involving climbing, rappelling, and jumping (Y93.3-)*
　　　　　　　　　activities involving ice and snow (Y93.2-)
　　　　　　　　　activities involving walking and running (Y93.Ø-)
　　　　　　　　　activities involving water and watercraft (Y93.1-)

✓5ᵗʰ **Y93.6　Activities involving other sports and athletics played as a team or group**

　　　EXCLUDES 1　*activity, ice hockey (Y93.22)*
　　　　　　　　　activity, water polo (Y93.13)

　Y93.61　Activity, American tackle football
　　　Activity, football NOS

　Y93.62　Activity, American flag or touch football

　Y93.63　Activity, rugby

　Y93.64　Activity, baseball
　　　Activity, softball

　Y93.65　Activity, lacrosse and field hockey

　Y93.66　Activity, soccer

　Y93.67　Activity, basketball

　Y93.68　Activity, volleyball (beach) (court)

　Y93.6A　Activity, physical games generally associated with school recess, summer camp and children
　　　Activity, capture the flag
　　　Activity, dodge ball
　　　Activity, four square
　　　Activity, kickball

　Y93.69　Activity, other involving other sports and athletics played as a team or group
　　　Activity, cricket

✓5ᵗʰ **Y93.7　Activities involving other specified sports and athletics**

　Y93.71　Activity, boxing

　Y93.72　Activity, wrestling

　Y93.73　Activity, racquet and hand sports
　　　Activity, handball
　　　Activity, racquetball
　　　Activity, squash
　　　Activity, tennis

　Y93.74　Activity, frisbee
　　　Activity, ultimate frisbee

　Y93.75　Activity, martial arts
　　　Activity, combatives

　Y93.79　Activity, other specified sports and athletics
　　　EXCLUDES 1　*sports and athletics activities specified in categories Y93.Ø-Y93.6*

✓5ᵗʰ **Y93.A　Activities involving other cardiorespiratory exercise**

　　　Activities involving physical training

　Y93.A1　Activity, exercise machines primarily for cardiorespiratory conditioning
　　　Activity, elliptical and stepper machines
　　　Activity, stationary bike
　　　Activity, treadmill

　Y93.A2　Activity, calisthenics
　　　Activity, jumping jacks
　　　Activity, warm up and cool down

　Y93.A3　Activity, aerobic and step exercise

　Y93.A4　Activity, circuit training

　Y93.A5　Activity, obstacle course
　　　Activity, challenge course
　　　Activity, confidence course

　Y93.A6　Activity, grass drills
　　　Activity, guerilla drills

　Y93.A9　Activity, other involving cardiorespiratory exercise
　　　EXCLUDES 1　*activities involving cardiorespiratory exercise specified in categories Y93.Ø-Y93.7*

✓5ᵗʰ **Y93.B　Activities involving other muscle strengthening exercises**

　Y93.B1　Activity, exercise machines primarily for muscle strengthening

　Y93.B2　Activity, push-ups, pull-ups, sit-ups

　Y93.B3　Activity, free weights
　　　Activity, barbells
　　　Activity, dumbbells

　Y93.B4　Activity, pilates

　Y93.B9　Activity, other involving muscle strengthening exercises
　　　EXCLUDES 1　*activities involving muscle strengthening specified in categories Y93.Ø-Y93.A*

✓5ᵗʰ **Y93.C　Activities involving computer technology and electronic devices**

　　　EXCLUDES 1　*activity, electronic musical keyboard or instruments (Y93.J-)*

　Y93.C1　Activity, computer keyboarding
　　　Activity, electronic game playing using keyboard or other stationary device

　Y93.C2　Activity, hand held interactive electronic device
　　　Activity, cellular telephone and communication device
　　　Activity, electronic game playing using interactive device
　　　EXCLUDES 1　*activity, electronic game playing using keyboard or other stationary device (Y93.C1)*

　Y93.C9　Activity, other involving computer technology and electronic devices

✓5ᵗʰ **Y93.D　Activities involving arts and handcrafts**

　　　EXCLUDES 1　*activities involving playing musical instrument (Y93.J-)*

　Y93.D1　Activity, knitting and crocheting

Y93.D2   **Activity,** sewing

Y93.D3   **Activity,** furniture building and finishing
         Activity, furniture repair

Y93.D9   **Activity, other involving arts and handcrafts**

✓5ᵗʰ **Y93.E**   **Activities involving personal hygiene and interior property and clothing maintenance**

> EXCLUDES 1   *activities involving cooking and grilling (Y93.G-)*
> *activities involving exterior property and land maintenance, building and construction (Y93.H-)*
> *activities involving caregiving (Y93.F-)*
> *activity, dishwashing (Y93.G1)*
> *activity, food preparation (Y93.G1)*
> *activity, gardening (Y93.H2)*

Y93.E1   **Activity, personal bathing and showering**

Y93.E2   **Activity,** laundry

Y93.E3   **Activity,** vacuuming

Y93.E4   **Activity,** ironing

Y93.E5   **Activity,** floor mopping and cleaning

Y93.E6   **Activity,** residential relocation
         Activity, packing up and unpacking involved in moving to a new residence

Y93.E8   **Activity, other personal hygiene**

Y93.E9   **Activity, other interior property and clothing maintenance**

✓5ᵗʰ **Y93.F**   **Activities involving** caregiving

         Activity involving the provider of caregiving

Y93.F1   **Activity, caregiving,** bathing

Y93.F2   **Activity, caregiving,** lifting

Y93.F9   **Activity, other caregiving**

✓5ᵗʰ **Y93.G**   **Activities involving food preparation, cooking and grilling**

Y93.G1   **Activity,** food preparation and clean up
         Activity, dishwashing

Y93.G2   **Activity,** grilling and smoking food

Y93.G3   **Activity,** cooking and baking
         Activity, use of stove, oven and microwave oven

Y93.G9   **Activity, other involving cooking and grilling**

✓5ᵗʰ **Y93.H**   **Activities involving exterior property and land maintenance, building and construction**

Y93.H1   **Activity,** digging, shoveling and raking
         Activity, dirt digging
         Activity, raking leaves
         Activity, snow shoveling

Y93.H2   **Activity,** gardening and landscaping
         Activity, pruning, trimming shrubs, weeding

Y93.H3   **Activity,** building and construction

Y93.H9   **Activity, other involving exterior property and land maintenance, building and construction**

✓5ᵗʰ **Y93.I**   **Activities involving roller coasters and other types of external motion**

Y93.I1   **Activity,** rollercoaster riding

Y93.I9   **Activity, other involving external motion**

✓5ᵗʰ **Y93.J**   **Activities involving playing musical instrument**

         Activity involving playing electric musical instrument

Y93.J1   **Activity,** piano **playing**
         Activity, musical keyboard (electronic) playing

Y93.J2   **Activity,** drum and other percussion instrument **playing**

Y93.J3   **Activity,** string instrument **playing**

Y93.J4   **Activity,** winds and brass instrument **playing**

✓5ᵗʰ **Y93.K**   **Activities involving animal care**

> EXCLUDES 1   *activity, horseback riding (Y93.52)*

Y93.K1   **Activity,** walking **an animal**

Y93.K2   **Activity,** milking **an animal**

Y93.K3   **Activity,** grooming and shearing **an animal**

Y93.K9   **Activity, other involving animal care**

✓5ᵗʰ **Y93.8**   **Activities, other specified**

Y93.81   **Activity,** refereeing **a sports activity**

Y93.82   **Activity,** spectator **at an event**

Y93.83   **Activity,** rough housing and horseplay

Y93.84   **Activity,** sleeping

Y93.85   **Activity,** choking game
         Activity, blackout game
         Activity, fainting game
         Activity, pass out game
         AHA: 2016,4Q,74-76

Y93.89   **Activity, other specified**

Y93.9   **Activity, unspecified**

Y95   Nosocomial condition
    AHA: 2013,4Q,119

✓4ᵗʰ **Y99   External cause status**

> NOTE   A single code from category Y99 should be used in conjunction with the external cause code(s) assigned to a record to indicate the status of the person at the time the event occurred.

Y99.0   **Civilian activity done for income or pay**
         Civilian activity done for financial or other compensation

> EXCLUDES 1   *military activity (Y99.1)*
> *volunteer activity (Y99.2)*

Y99.1   **Military activity**

> EXCLUDES 1   *activity of off duty military personnel (Y99.8)*

Y99.2   **Volunteer activity**

> EXCLUDES 1   *activity of child or other family member assisting in compensated work of other family member (Y99.8)*

Y99.8   **Other external cause status**
         Activity NEC
         Activity of child or other family member assisting in compensated work of other family member
         Hobby not done for income
         Leisure activity
         Off-duty activity of military personnel
         Recreation or sport not for income or while a student
         Student activity

> EXCLUDES 1   *civilian activity done for income or compensation (Y99.0)*
> *military activity (Y99.1)*

AHA: 2012,4Q,108

Y99.9   **Unspecified external cause status**

Chapter 21. Factors Influencing Health Status and Contact with Health Services (Z00–Z99)

Chapter-specific Guidelines with Coding Examples

The chapter-specific guidelines from the ICD-10-CM Official Guidelines for Coding and Reporting have been provided below. Along with these guidelines are coding examples, contained in the shaded boxes, that have been developed to help illustrate the coding and/or sequencing guidance found in these guidelines.

Note: The chapter-specific guidelines provide additional information about the use of Z codes for specified encounters.

a. Use of Z Codes in any healthcare setting

Z codes are for use in any healthcare setting. Z codes may be used as either a first-listed (principal diagnosis code in the inpatient setting) or secondary code, depending on the circumstances of the encounter. Certain Z codes may only be used as first-listed or principal diagnosis.

> Patient with middle lobe lung cancer admitted for initiation of chemotherapy
>
> **Z51.11**   **Encounter for antineoplastic chemotherapy**
>
> **C34.2**   **Malignant neoplasm of middle lobe, bronchus or lung**
>
> *Explanation:* A Z code can be used as first-listed in this situation based on guidelines in this chapter as well as chapter 2, "Neoplasms."

b. Z Codes indicate a reason for an encounter

Z codes are not procedure codes. A corresponding procedure code must accompany a Z code to describe any procedure performed.

c. Categories of Z Codes

1) Contact/exposure

Category Z20 indicates contact with, and suspected exposure to, communicable diseases. These codes are for patients who are suspected to have been exposed to **a disease** by close personal contact with an infected individual or are in an area where a disease is epidemic.

Category Z77, Other contact with and (suspected) exposures hazardous to health, indicates contact with and suspected exposures hazardous to health.

Contact/exposure codes may be used as a first-listed code to explain an encounter for testing, or, more commonly, as a secondary code to identify a potential risk.

2) Inoculations and vaccinations

Code Z23 is for encounters for inoculations and vaccinations. It indicates that a patient is being seen to receive a prophylactic inoculation against a disease. Procedure codes are required to identify the actual administration of the injection and the type(s) of immunizations given. Code Z23 may be used as a secondary code if the inoculation is given as a routine part of preventive health care, such as a well-baby visit.

3) Status

Status codes indicate that a patient is either a carrier of a disease or has the sequelae or residual of a past disease or condition. This includes such things as the presence of prosthetic or mechanical devices resulting from past treatment. A status code is informative, because the status may affect the course of treatment and its outcome. A status code is distinct from a history code. The history code indicates that the patient no longer has the condition.

A status code should not be used with a diagnosis code from one of the body system chapters, if the diagnosis code includes the information provided by the status code. For example, code Z94.1, Heart transplant status, should not be used with a code from subcategory T86.2, Complications of heart transplant. The status code does not provide additional information. The complication code indicates that the patient is a heart transplant patient.

For encounters for weaning from a mechanical ventilator, assign a code from subcategory J96.1, Chronic respiratory failure, followed by code Z99.11, Dependence on respirator [ventilator] status.

The status Z codes/categories are:

Z14   Genetic carrier

      Genetic carrier status indicates that a person carries a gene, associated with a particular disease, which may be passed to offspring who may develop that disease. The person does not have the disease and is not at risk of developing the disease.

Z15   Genetic susceptibility to disease

      Genetic susceptibility indicates that a person has a gene that increases the risk of that person developing the disease.

      Codes from category Z15 should not be used as principal or first-listed codes. If the patient has the condition to which he/she is susceptible, and that condition is the reason for the encounter, the code for the current condition should be sequenced first. If the patient is being seen for follow-up after completed treatment for this condition, and the condition no longer exists, a follow-up code should be sequenced first, followed by the appropriate personal history and genetic susceptibility codes. If the purpose of the encounter is genetic counseling associated with procreative management, code Z31.5, Encounter for genetic counseling, should be assigned as the first-listed code, followed by a code from category Z15. Additional codes should be assigned for any applicable family or personal history.

Z16   Resistance to antimicrobial drugs

      This code indicates that a patient has a condition that is resistant to antimicrobial drug treatment. Sequence the infection code first.

> Penicillin resistant streptococcus pneumoniae meningitis
>
> **G00.1**   **Pneumococcal meningitis**
>
> **Z16.11**   **Resistance to penicillins**
>
> *Explanation:* The status Z code is used to describe the presence of a drug-resistant organism that most likely altered how the meningitis was treated.

Z17   Estrogen receptor status

Z18   Retained foreign body fragments

Z19   Hormone sensitivity malignancy status

Z21   Asymptomatic HIV infection status

      This code indicates that a patient has tested positive for HIV but has manifested no signs or symptoms of the disease.

Z22   Carrier of infectious disease

      Carrier status indicates that a person harbors the specific organisms of a disease without manifest symptoms and is capable of transmitting the infection.

Z28.3   Underimmunization status

Z33.1   Pregnant state, incidental

      This code is a secondary code only for use when the pregnancy is in no way complicating the reason for visit. Otherwise, a code from the obstetric chapter is required.

Z66   Do not resuscitate

      This code may be used when it is documented by the provider that a patient is on do not resuscitate status at any time during the stay.

Z67   Blood type

Z68   Body mass index (BMI)

      BMI codes should only be assigned when there is an associated, reportable diagnosis (such as obesity). Do not assign BMI codes during pregnancy.

      See Section I.B.14 for BMI documentation by clinicians other than the patient's provider.

Z74.01   Bed confinement status

Z76.82   Awaiting organ transplant status

Z78   Other specified health status

      Code Z78.1, Physical restraint status, may be used when it is documented by the provider that a patient has been put in restraints during the current encounter. Please note that this code should not be reported when it is documented by the provider that a patient is temporarily restrained during a procedure.

Z79 Long-term (current) drug therapy

Codes from this category indicate a patient's continuous use of a prescribed drug (including such things as aspirin therapy) for the long-term treatment of a condition or for prophylactic use. It is not for use for patients who have addictions to drugs. This subcategory is not for use of medications for detoxification or maintenance programs to prevent withdrawal symptoms (e.g., methadone maintenance for opiate dependence). Assign the appropriate code for the drug **use, abuse, or** dependence instead.

Assign a code from Z79 if the patient is receiving a medication for an extended period as a prophylactic measure (such as for the prevention of deep vein thrombosis) or as treatment of a chronic condition (such as arthritis) or a disease requiring a lengthy course of treatment (such as cancer). Do not assign a code from category Z79 for medication being administered for a brief period of time to treat an acute illness or injury (such as a course of antibiotics to treat acute bronchitis).

Z88 Allergy status to drugs, medicaments and biological substances

Except: Z88.9, Allergy status to unspecified drugs, medicaments and biological substances status

Z89 Acquired absence of limb

Z90 Acquired absence of organs, not elsewhere classified

Z91.0- Allergy status, other than to drugs and biological substances

Z92.82 Status post administration of tPA (rtPA) in a different facility within the last 24 hours prior to admission to a current facility

Assign code Z92.82, Status post administration of tPA (rtPA) in a different facility within the last 24 hours prior to admission to current facility, as a secondary diagnosis when a patient is received by transfer into a facility and documentation indicates they were administered tissue plasminogen activator (tPA) within the last 24 hours prior to admission to the current facility.

This guideline applies even if the patient is still receiving the tPA at the time they are received into the current facility.

The appropriate code for the condition for which the tPA was administered (such as cerebrovascular disease or myocardial infarction) should be assigned first.

Code Z92.82 is only applicable to the receiving facility record and not to the transferring facility record.

Z93 Artificial opening status

Z94 Transplanted organ and tissue status

Z95 Presence of cardiac and vascular implants and grafts

Z96 Presence of other functional implants

Z97 Presence of other devices

Z98 Other postprocedural states

Assign code Z98.85, Transplanted organ removal status, to indicate that a transplanted organ has been previously removed. This code should not be assigned for the encounter in which the transplanted organ is removed. The complication necessitating removal of the transplant organ should be assigned for that encounter.

See section I.C19. for information on the coding of organ transplant complications.

Z99 Dependence on enabling machines and devices, not elsewhere classified

Note: Categories Z89-Z90 and Z93-Z99 are for use only if there are no complications or malfunctions of the organ or tissue replaced, the amputation site or the equipment on which the patient is dependent.

4) History (of)

There are two types of history Z codes, personal and family. Personal history codes explain a patient's past medical condition that no longer exists and is not receiving any treatment, but that has the potential for recurrence, and therefore may require continued monitoring.

Family history codes are for use when a patient has a family member(s) who has had a particular disease that causes the patient to be at higher risk of also contracting the disease.

Personal history codes may be used in conjunction with follow-up codes and family history codes may be used in conjunction with screening codes to explain the need for a test or procedure. History codes are also acceptable on any medical record regardless of the reason for visit. A history of an illness, even if no longer present, is important information that may alter the type of treatment ordered.

The history Z code categories are:

Z80 Family history of primary malignant neoplasm

Z81 Family history of mental and behavioral disorders

Z82 Family history of certain disabilities and chronic diseases (leading to disablement)

Z83 Family history of other specific disorders

Z84 Family history of other conditions

Z85 Personal history of malignant neoplasm

Z86 Personal history of certain other diseases

Z87 Personal history of other diseases and conditions

Z91.4- Personal history of psychological trauma, not elsewhere classified

Z91.5 Personal history of self-harm

Z91.81 History of falling

Z91.82 Personal history of military deployment

Z92 Personal history of medical treatment

Except: Z92.0, Personal history of contraception

Except: Z92.82, Status post administration of tPA (rtPA) in a different facility within the last 24 hours prior to admission to a current facility

---

Patient has chronic lymphocytic leukemia for which the patient had previous chemotherapy and is now in remission

C91.11 **Chronic lymphocytic leukemia of B-cell type in remission**

Z92.21 **Personal history of antineoplastic chemotherapy**

Explanation: The personal history Z code is used to describe a secondary (supplementary) diagnosis to identify that this patient has had chemotherapy in the past.

---

5) Screening

Screening is the testing for disease or disease precursors in seemingly well individuals so that early detection and treatment can be provided for those who test positive for the disease (e.g., screening mammogram).

The testing of a person to rule out or confirm a suspected diagnosis because the patient has some sign or symptom is a diagnostic examination, not a screening. In these cases, the sign or symptom is used to explain the reason for the test.

A screening code may be a first-listed code if the reason for the visit is specifically the screening exam. It may also be used as an additional code if the screening is done during an office visit for other health problems. A screening code is not necessary if the screening is inherent to a routine examination, such as a pap smear done during a routine pelvic examination.

Should a condition be discovered during the screening then the code for the condition may be assigned as an additional diagnosis.

The Z code indicates that a screening exam is planned. A procedure code is required to confirm that the screening was performed.

The screening Z codes/categories:

Z11 Encounter for screening for infectious and parasitic diseases

Z12 Encounter for screening for malignant neoplasms

Z13 Encounter for screening for other diseases and disorders

Except: Z13.9, Encounter for screening, unspecified

Z36 Encounter for antenatal screening for mother

6) Observation

There are three observation Z code categories. They are for use in very limited circumstances when a person is being observed for a suspected condition that is ruled out. The observation codes are not for use if an injury or illness or any signs or symptoms related to the suspected condition are present. In such cases the diagnosis/symptom code is used with the corresponding external cause code.

The observation codes are **primarily** to be used as a principal/**first-listed** diagnosis. **An observation code may be assigned as a secondary diagnosis code when the patient is being observed for a condition that is ruled out and is unrelated to the principal/first-listed diagnosis (e.g., patient presents for treatment following injuries sustained in a motor vehicle accident and is also observed for suspected COVID-19 infection that is subsequently ruled out). Also,** when the principal diagnosis is required to be a code from category Z38, Liveborn infants according to place of birth and type of delivery, **then** a code from category Z05, Encounter for observation and evaluation of newborn for suspected diseases and conditions ruled out, is sequenced after the Z38 code. Additional codes may be used in addition to the observation code, but only if they are unrelated to the suspected condition being observed.

Codes from subcategory Z03.7, Encounter for suspected maternal and fetal conditions ruled out, may either be used as a first-listed or as an additional code assignment depending on the case. They are for use in very limited circumstances on a maternal record when an encounter is for a suspected maternal or fetal condition that is ruled out during that encounter (for example, a maternal or fetal condition may be suspected due to an abnormal test result). These codes should not be used when the condition is confirmed. In those cases, the confirmed condition should be coded. In addition, these codes are not for use if an illness or any signs or symptoms related to the suspected condition or problem are present. In such cases the diagnosis/symptom code is used.

Additional codes may be used in addition to the code from subcategory Z03.7, but only if they are unrelated to the suspected condition being evaluated.

Codes from subcategory Z03.7 may not be used for encounters for antenatal screening of mother. *See Section I.C.21. Screening.*

For encounters for suspected fetal condition that are inconclusive following testing and evaluation, assign the appropriate code from category O35, O36, O40 or O41.

The observation Z code categories:

Z03	Encounter for medical observation for suspected diseases and conditions ruled out
Z04	Encounter for examination and observation for other reasons Except: Z04.9, Encounter for examination and observation for unspecified reason
Z05	Encounter for observation and evaluation of newborn for suspected diseases and conditions ruled out

> Upon initial examination, a heart murmur was heard in a newborn infant delivered vaginally in the hospital; however, after further observation, any serious cardiac conditions were ruled out.
>
> **Z38.00   Single liveborn infant, delivered vaginally**
>
> **Z05.0   Observation and evaluation of newborn for suspected cardiac condition ruled out**
>
> *Explanation:* Normally an observation code is used as the principal diagnosis except when the patient is a newborn. A code from category Z38 Liveborn infants according to place of birth and type of delivery code would be sequenced first, followed by the encounter for observation and evaluation of newborn for suspected diseases and conditions ruled out.

7) Aftercare

Aftercare visit codes cover situations when the initial treatment of a disease has been performed and the patient requires continued care during the healing or recovery phase, or for the long-term consequences of the disease. The aftercare Z code should not be used if treatment is directed at a current, acute disease. The diagnosis code is to be used in these cases. Exceptions to this rule are codes Z51.0, Encounter for antineoplastic radiation therapy, and codes from subcategory Z51.1, Encounter for antineoplastic chemotherapy and immunotherapy. These codes are to be first listed, followed by the diagnosis code when a patient's encounter is solely to receive radiation therapy, chemotherapy, or immunotherapy for the treatment of a neoplasm. If the reason for the encounter is more than one type of antineoplastic therapy, code Z51.0 and a code from subcategory Z51.1 may be assigned together, in which case one of these codes would be reported as a secondary diagnosis.

The aftercare Z codes should also not be used for aftercare for injuries. For aftercare of an injury, assign the acute injury code with the appropriate 7th character (for subsequent encounter).

The aftercare codes are generally first listed to explain the specific reason for the encounter. An aftercare code may be used as an additional code when some type of aftercare is provided in addition to the reason for admission and no diagnosis code is applicable. An example of this would be the closure of a colostomy during an encounter for treatment of another condition.

Aftercare codes should be used in conjunction with other aftercare codes or diagnosis codes to provide better detail on the specifics of an aftercare encounter visit, unless otherwise directed by the classification. The sequencing of multiple aftercare codes depends on the circumstances of the encounter.

Certain aftercare Z code categories need a secondary diagnosis code to describe the resolving condition or sequelae. For others, the condition is included in the code title.

Additional Z code aftercare category terms include fitting and adjustment, and attention to artificial openings.

Status Z codes may be used with aftercare Z codes to indicate the nature of the aftercare. For example code Z95.1, Presence of aortocoronary bypass graft, may be used with code Z48.812, Encounter for surgical aftercare following surgery on the circulatory system, to indicate the surgery for which the aftercare is being performed. A status code should not be used when the aftercare code indicates the type of status, such as using Z43.0, Encounter for attention to tracheostomy, with Z93.0, Tracheostomy status.

The aftercare Z category/codes:

Z42	Encounter for plastic and reconstructive surgery following medical procedure or healed injury
Z43	Encounter for attention to artificial openings
Z44	Encounter for fitting and adjustment of external prosthetic device
Z45	Encounter for adjustment and management of implanted device
Z46	Encounter for fitting and adjustment of other devices
Z47	Orthopedic aftercare
Z48	Encounter for other postprocedural aftercare
Z49	Encounter for care involving renal dialysis
Z51	Encounter for other aftercare and medical care

8) Follow-up

The follow-up codes are used to explain continuing surveillance following completed treatment of a disease, condition, or injury. They imply that the condition has been fully treated and no longer exists. They should not be confused with aftercare codes, or injury codes with a 7th character for subsequent encounter, that explain ongoing care of a healing condition or its sequelae. Follow-up codes may be used in conjunction with history codes to provide the full picture of the healed condition and its treatment. The follow-up code is sequenced first, followed by the history code.

A follow-up code may be used to explain multiple visits. Should a condition be found to have recurred on the follow-up visit, then the diagnosis code for the condition should be assigned in place of the follow-up code.

The follow-up Z code categories:

Z08	Encounter for follow-up examination after completed treatment for malignant neoplasm
Z09	Encounter for follow-up examination after completed treatment for conditions other than malignant neoplasm
Z39	Encounter for maternal postpartum care and examination

9) Donor

Codes in category Z52, Donors of organs and tissues, are used for living individuals who are donating blood or other body tissue. These codes are only for individuals donating for others, not for self-donations. They are not used to identify cadaveric donations.

10) Counseling

Counseling Z codes are used when a patient or family member receives assistance in the aftermath of an illness or injury, or when support is required in coping with family or social problems.

The counseling Z codes/categories:

Z30.0-	Encounter for general counseling and advice on contraception
Z31.5	Encounter for procreative genetic counseling
Z31.6-	Encounter for general counseling and advice on procreation
Z32.2	Encounter for childbirth instruction
Z32.3	Encounter for childcare instruction
Z69	Encounter for mental health services for victim and perpetrator of abuse
Z70	Counseling related to sexual attitude, behavior and orientation
Z71	Persons encountering health services for other counseling and medical advice, not elsewhere classified **Note:** Code Z71.84, Encounter for health counseling related to travel, is to be used for health risk and safety counseling for future travel purposes.
Z76.81	Expectant mother prebirth pediatrician visit

11) Encounters for obstetrical and reproductive services

See Section I.C.15. Pregnancy, Childbirth, and the Puerperium, for further instruction on the use of these codes.

Z codes for pregnancy are for use in those circumstances when none of the problems or complications included in the codes from the Obstetrics chapter exist (a routine prenatal visit or postpartum care). Codes in category Z34, Encounter for supervision of normal pregnancy, are always first listed and are not to be used with any other code from the OB chapter.

Codes in category Z3A, Weeks of gestation, may be assigned to provide additional information about the pregnancy. Category Z3A codes should not be assigned for pregnancies with abortive outcomes (categories O00-O08), elective termination of pregnancy (code Z33.2), nor for postpartum conditions, as category Z3A is not applicable to these conditions. The date of the admission should be used to determine weeks of gestation for inpatient admissions that encompass more than one gestational week.

The outcome of delivery, category Z37, should be included on all maternal delivery records. It is always a secondary code. Codes in category Z37 should not be used on the newborn record.

Z codes for family planning (contraceptive) or procreative management and counseling should be included on an obstetric record either during the pregnancy or the postpartum stage, if applicable.

Z codes/categories for obstetrical and reproductive services:

Z30	Encounter for contraceptive management
Z31	Encounter for procreative management
Z32.2	Encounter for childbirth instruction
Z32.3	Encounter for childcare instruction
Z33	Pregnant state
Z34	Encounter for supervision of normal pregnancy
Z36	Encounter for antenatal screening of mother
Z3A	Weeks of gestation
Z37	Outcome of delivery
Z39	Encounter for maternal postpartum care and examination
Z76.81	Expectant mother prebirth pediatrician visit

12) Newborns and infants

See Section I.C.16. Newborn (Perinatal) Guidelines, for further instruction on the use of these codes.

Newborn Z codes/categories:

Z76.1	Encounter for health supervision and care of foundling
Z00.1-	Encounter for routine child health examination
Z38	Liveborn infants according to place of birth and type of delivery

13) Routine and administrative examinations

The Z codes allow for the description of encounters for routine examinations, such as, a general check-up, or, examinations for administrative purposes, such as, a pre-employment physical. The codes are not to be used if the examination is for diagnosis of a suspected condition or for treatment purposes. In such cases the diagnosis code is used. During a routine exam, should a diagnosis or condition be discovered, it should be coded as an additional code. Pre-existing and chronic conditions and history codes may also be included as additional codes as long as the examination is for administrative purposes and not focused on any particular condition.

Some of the codes for routine health examinations distinguish between "with" and "without" abnormal findings. Code assignment depends on the information that is known at the time the encounter is being coded. For example, if no abnormal findings were found during the examination, but the encounter is being coded before test results are back, it is acceptable to assign the code for "without abnormal findings." When assigning a code for "with abnormal findings," additional code(s) should be assigned to identify the specific abnormal finding(s).

Pre-operative examination and pre-procedural laboratory examination Z codes are for use only in those situations when a patient is being cleared for a procedure or surgery and no treatment is given.

The Z codes/categories for routine and administrative examinations:

Z00	Encounter for general examination without complaint, suspected or reported diagnosis
Z01	Encounter for other special examination without complaint, suspected or reported diagnosis
Z02	Encounter for administrative examination
	Except: Z02.9, Encounter for administrative examinations, unspecified
Z32.0-	Encounter for pregnancy test

14) Miscellaneous Z codes

The miscellaneous Z codes capture a number of other health care encounters that do not fall into one of the other categories. Certain of these codes identify the reason for the encounter; others are for use as additional codes that provide useful information on circumstances that may affect a patient's care and treatment.

Prophylactic organ removal

For encounters specifically for prophylactic removal of an organ (such as prophylactic removal of breasts due to a genetic susceptibility to cancer or a family history of cancer), the principal or first-listed code should be a code from category Z40, Encounter for prophylactic surgery, followed by the appropriate codes to identify the associated risk factor (such as genetic susceptibility or family history).

If the patient has a malignancy of one site and is having prophylactic removal at another site to prevent either a new primary malignancy or metastatic disease, a code for the malignancy should also be assigned in addition to a code from subcategory Z40.0, Encounter for prophylactic surgery for risk factors related to malignant neoplasms. A Z40.0 code should not be assigned if the patient is having organ removal for treatment of a malignancy, such as the removal of the testes for the treatment of prostate cancer.

> Female patient with cancer in lower inner quadrant of right breast and positive BRCA 1 noted on testing is admitted for mastectomy of right breast and prophylactic removal of left breast
>
> **C50.311** **Malignant neoplasm of lower-inner quadrant of right female breast**
>
> **Z40.01** **Encounter for prophylactic removal of breast**
>
> **Z15.01** **Genetic susceptibility to malignant neoplasm of breast**
>
> *Explanation:* Removal of the current neoplastic disease in the right breast was the focus of treatment for this admission and is sequenced first. The removal of the left breast was not required to treat a current disease process but as a means of prevention. The two Z codes are informational; they capture the reason behind the removal of what is currently a healthy left breast.

Miscellaneous Z codes/categories:

Z28	Immunization not carried out
	Except: Z28.3, Underimmunization status
Z29	Encounter for other prophylactic measures
Z40	Encounter for prophylactic surgery
Z41	Encounter for procedures for purposes other than remedying health state
	Except: Z41.9, Encounter for procedure for purposes other than remedying health state, unspecified
Z53	Persons encountering health services for specific procedures and treatment, not carried out
Z55	Problems related to education and literacy
Z56	Problems related to employment and unemployment
Z57	Occupational exposure to risk factors
Z58	Problems related to physical environment
Z59	Problems related to housing and economic circumstances
Z60	Problems related to social environment
Z62	Problems related to upbringing
Z63	Other problems related to primary support group, including family circumstances
Z64	Problems related to certain psychosocial circumstances
Z65	Problems related to other psychosocial circumstances
Z72	Problems related to lifestyle
	Note: These codes should be assigned only when the documentation specifies that the patient has an associated problem
Z73	Problems related to life management difficulty
Z74	Problems related to care provider dependency
	Except: Z74.01, Bed confinement status
Z75	Problems related to medical facilities and other health care
Z76.0	Encounter for issue of repeat prescription
Z76.3	Healthy person accompanying sick person
Z76.4	Other boarder to healthcare facility
Z76.5	Malingerer [conscious simulation]
Z91.1-	Patient's noncompliance with medical treatment and regimen
Z91.83	Wandering in diseases classified elsewhere
Z91.84-	Oral health risk factors
Z91.89	Other specified personal risk factors, not elsewhere classified

See Section I.B.14 for Z55-Z65 Persons with potential health hazards related to socioeconomic and psychosocial circumstances, documentation by clinicians other than the patient's provider

15) Nonspecific Z codes

Certain Z codes are so non-specific, or potentially redundant with other codes in the classification, that there can be little justification for their use in the inpatient setting. Their use in the outpatient setting should be limited to those instances when there is no further documentation to permit more precise coding. Otherwise, any sign or symptom or any other reason for visit that is captured in another code should be used.

Nonspecific Z codes/categories:

Z02.9	Encounter for administrative examinations, unspecified
Z04.9	Encounter for examination and observation for unspecified reason
Z13.9	Encounter for screening, unspecified
Z41.9	Encounter for procedure for purposes other than remedying health state, unspecified
Z52.9	Donor of unspecified organ or tissue
Z86.59	Personal history of other mental and behavioral disorders
Z88.9	Allergy status to unspecified drugs, medicaments and biological substances status
Z92.0	Personal history of contraception

16) Z codes that may only be principal/first-listed diagnosis

The following Z codes/categories may only be reported as the principal/first-listed diagnosis, except when there are multiple encounters on the same day and the medical records for the encounters are combined:

Z00	Encounter for general examination without complaint, suspected or reported diagnosis
	Except: Z00.6
Z01	Encounter for other special examination without complaint, suspected or reported diagnosis
Z02	Encounter for administrative examination

Z04	Encounter for examination and observation for other reasons
Z33.2	Encounter for elective termination of pregnancy
Z31.81	Encounter for male factor infertility in female patient
Z31.83	Encounter for assisted reproductive fertility procedure cycle
Z31.84	Encounter for fertility preservation procedure
Z34	Encounter for supervision of normal pregnancy
Z39	Encounter for maternal postpartum care and examination
Z38	Liveborn infants according to place of birth and type of delivery
Z40	Encounter for prophylactic surgery
Z42	Encounter for plastic and reconstructive surgery following medical procedure or healed injury
Z51.0	Encounter for antineoplastic radiation therapy
Z51.1-	Encounter for antineoplastic chemotherapy and immunotherapy
Z52	Donors of organs and tissues
	Except: Z52.9, Donor of unspecified organ or tissue
Z76.1	Encounter for health supervision and care of foundling
Z76.2	Encounter for health supervision and care of other healthy infant and child
Z99.12	Encounter for respirator [ventilator] dependence during power failure

Chapter 21. Factors Influencing Health Status and Contact With Health Services (Z00-Z99)

NOTE   Z codes represent reasons for encounters. A corresponding procedure code must accompany a Z code if a procedure is performed. Categories Z00-Z99 are provided for occasions when circumstances other than a disease, injury or external cause classifiable to categories A00-Y89 are recorded as "diagnoses" or "problems." This can arise in two main ways:

(a) When a person who may or may not be sick encounters the health services for some specific purpose, such as to receive limited care or service for a current condition, to donate an organ or tissue, to receive prophylactic vaccination (immunization), or to discuss a problem which is in itself not a disease or injury.

(b) When some circumstance or problem is present which influences the person's health status but is not in itself a current illness or injury.

AHA: 2018,4Q,60-61

This chapter contains the following blocks:

Z00-Z13	Persons encountering health services for examinations
Z14-Z15	Genetic carrier and genetic susceptibility to disease
Z16	Resistance to antimicrobial drugs
Z17	Estrogen receptor status
Z18	Retained foreign body fragments
Z19	Hormone sensitivity malignancy status
Z20-Z29	Persons with potential health hazards related to communicable diseases
Z30-Z39	Persons encountering health services in circumstances related to reproduction
Z40-Z53	Encounters for other specific health care
Z55-Z65	Persons with potential health hazards related to socioeconomic and psychosocial circumstances
Z66	Do not resuscitate status
Z67	Blood type
Z68	Body mass index (BMI)
Z69-Z76	Persons encountering health services in other circumstances
Z77-Z99	Persons with potential health hazards related to family and personal history and certain conditions influencing health status

Persons encountering health services for examinations (Z00-Z13)

NOTE   Nonspecific abnormal findings disclosed at the time of these examinations are classified to categories R70-R94.

EXCLUDES 1   *examinations related to pregnancy and reproduction (Z30-Z36, Z39.-)*

√4ᵗʰ **Z00**   **Encounter for general examination without complaint, suspected or reported diagnosis**

> **EXCLUDES 1**   *encounter for examination for administrative purposes (Z02.-)*
> **EXCLUDES 2**   *encounter for pre-procedural examinations (Z01.81-)*
> *special screening examinations (Z11-Z13)*
> **AHA:** 2017,4Q,95

√5ᵗʰ **Z00.0**   **Encounter for general adult medical examination**

> Encounter for adult periodic examination (annual) (physical) and any associated laboratory and radiologic examinations
>
> > **EXCLUDES 1**   *encounter for examination of sign or symptom — code to sign or symptom*
> > *general health check-up of infant or child (Z00.12.-)*

> **Z00.00**   **Encounter for general adult medical examination without abnormal findings**   **A**
> > Encounter for adult health check-up NOS
> > **AHA:** 2016,1Q,36

> **Z00.01**   **Encounter for general adult medical examination with abnormal findings**   **A**
> > Use additional code to identify abnormal findings
> > **AHA:** 2016,1Q,35-36

√5ᵗʰ **Z00.1**   **Encounter for newborn, infant and child health examinations**

> √6ᵗʰ **Z00.11**   **Newborn health examination**
> > Health check for child under 29 days old
> > Use additional code to identify any abnormal findings
> > > **EXCLUDES 1**   *health check for child over 28 days old (Z00.12.-)*

> > **Z00.110**   **Health examination for newborn under 8 days old**   **N**
> > > Health check for newborn under 8 days old

> > **Z00.111**   **Health examination for newborn 8 to 28 days old**   **N**
> > > Health check for newborn 8 to 28 days old
> > > Newborn weight check

√6ᵗʰ **Z00.12**   **Encounter for routine child health examination**

> Health check (routine) for child over 28 days old
> Immunizations appropriate for age
> Routine developmental screening of infant or child
> Routine vison and hearing testing
>
> > **EXCLUDES 1**   *health check for child under 29 days old (Z00.11-)*
> > *health supervision of foundling or other healthy infant or child (Z76.1-Z76.2)*
> > *newborn health examination (Z00.11-)*
> > **AHA:** 2018,4Q,36

> **Z00.121**   **Encounter for routine child health examination with abnormal findings**   **P**
> > Use additional code to identify abnormal findings
> > **AHA:** 2016,1Q,34-35

> **Z00.129**   **Encounter for routine child health examination without abnormal findings**   **P**
> > Encounter for routine child health examination NOS
> > **AHA:** 2016,1Q,34

Z00.2   **Encounter for examination for period of rapid growth in childhood**   **P**

Z00.3   **Encounter for examination for adolescent development state**   **P**
> Encounter for puberty development state

Z00.5   **Encounter for examination of potential donor of organ and tissue**

Z00.6   **Encounter for examination for normal comparison and control in clinical research program**
> Examination of participant or control in clinical research program

√5ᵗʰ **Z00.7**   **Encounter for examination for period of delayed growth in childhood**

> **Z00.70**   **Encounter for examination for period of delayed growth in childhood without abnormal findings**   **P**

> **Z00.71**   **Encounter for examination for period of delayed growth in childhood with abnormal findings**   **P**
> > Use additional code to identify abnormal findings

Z00.8   **Encounter for other general examination**
> Encounter for health examination in population surveys

√4ᵗʰ **Z01**   **Encounter for other special examination without complaint, suspected or reported diagnosis**

> **INCLUDES**   routine examination of specific system

> **NOTE**   Codes from category Z01 represent the reason for the encounter. A separate procedure code is required to identify any examinations or procedures performed

> **EXCLUDES 1**   *encounter for examination for administrative purposes (Z02.-)*
> *encounter for examination for suspected conditions, proven not to exist (Z03.-)*
> *encounter for laboratory and radiologic examinations as a component of general medical examinations (Z00.0-)*
> *encounter for laboratory, radiologic and imaging examinations for sign(s) and symptom(s) — code to the sign(s) or symptom(s)*
> **EXCLUDES 2**   *screening examinations (Z11-Z13)*

√5ᵗʰ **Z01.0**   **Encounter for examination of eyes and vision**

> **EXCLUDES 1**   *examination for driving license (Z02.4)*

> **Z01.00**   **Encounter for examination of eyes and vision without abnormal findings**
> > Encounter for examination of eyes and vision NOS

> **Z01.01**   **Encounter for examination of eyes and vision with abnormal findings**
> > Use additional code to identify abnormal findings
> > **AHA:** 2016,4Q,21

N Newborn: 0   **P** Pediatric: 0-17   **M** Maternity: 9-64   **A** Adult: 15-124   **MCC** Major Complication/Comorbidity   **CC** Complication/Comorbidity   **SW** Severe Wound Dx

1234   ICD-10-CM 2021

✓6ᵗʰ Z01.02 Encounter for examination of eyes and vision following failed vision screening
> EXCLUDES 1   *examination for examination of eyes and vision with abnormal findings (Z01.01)*
> *examination for examination of eyes and vision without abnormal findings (Z01.00)*

AHA: 2019,4Q,20

Z01.020 Encounter for examination of eyes and vision following failed vision screening without abnormal findings

Z01.021 Encounter for examination of eyes and vision following failed vision screening with abnormal findings
> Use additional code to identify abnormal findings

✓5ᵗʰ Z01.1 Encounter for examination of ears and hearing

Z01.10 Encounter for examination of ears and hearing without abnormal findings
> Encounter for examination of ears and hearing NOS
> AHA: 2016,4Q,24

✓6ᵗʰ Z01.11 Encounter for examination of ears and hearing with abnormal findings
> AHA: 2016,3Q,17-18

Z01.110 Encounter for hearing examination following failed hearing screening

Z01.118 Encounter for examination of ears and hearing with other abnormal findings
> Use additional code to identify abnormal findings

Z01.12 Encounter for hearing conservation and treatment

✓5ᵗʰ Z01.2 Encounter for dental examination and cleaning

Z01.20 Encounter for dental examination and cleaning without abnormal findings
> Encounter for dental examination and cleaning NOS

Z01.21 Encounter for dental examination and cleaning with abnormal findings
> Use additional code to identify abnormal findings

✓5ᵗʰ Z01.3 Encounter for examination of blood pressure

Z01.30 Encounter for examination of blood pressure without abnormal findings
> Encounter for examination of blood pressure NOS

Z01.31 Encounter for examination of blood pressure with abnormal findings
> Use additional code to identify abnormal findings

✓5ᵗʰ Z01.4 Encounter for gynecological examination
> EXCLUDES 2   *pregnancy examination or test (Z32.0-)*
> *routine examination for contraceptive maintenance (Z30.4-)*

✓6ᵗʰ Z01.41 Encounter for routine gynecological examination
> Encounter for general gynecological examination with or without cervical smear
> Encounter for gynecological examination (general) (routine) NOS
> Encounter for pelvic examination (annual) (periodic)
> Use additional code:
> for screening for human papillomavirus, if applicable, (Z11.51)
> for screening vaginal pap smear, if applicable (Z12.72)
> to identify acquired absence of uterus, if applicable (Z90.71-)
> EXCLUDES 1   *gynecologic examination status-post hysterectomy for malignant condition (Z08)*
> *screening cervical pap smear not a part of a routine gynecological examination (Z12.4)*

Z01.411 Encounter for gynecological examination (general) (routine) with abnormal findings ♀
> Use additional code to identify abnormal findings

Z01.419 Encounter for gynecological examination (general) (routine) without abnormal findings ♀

Z01.42 Encounter for cervical smear to confirm findings of recent normal smear following initial abnormal smear ♀

✓5ᵗʰ Z01.8 Encounter for other specified special examinations

✓6ᵗʰ Z01.81 Encounter for preprocedural examinations
> Encounter for preoperative examinations
> Encounter for radiological and imaging examinations as part of preprocedural examination

Z01.810 Encounter for preprocedural cardiovascular examination

Z01.811 Encounter for preprocedural respiratory examination

Z01.812 Encounter for preprocedural laboratory examination
> Blood and urine tests prior to treatment or procedure

Z01.818 Encounter for other preprocedural examination
> Encounter for preprocedural examination NOS
> Encounter for examinations prior to antineoplastic chemotherapy

Z01.82 Encounter for allergy testing
> EXCLUDES 1   *encounter for antibody response examination (Z01.84)*

Z01.83 Encounter for blood typing
> Encounter for Rh typing

Z01.84 Encounter for antibody response examination
> Encounter for immunity status testing
> EXCLUDES 1   *encounter for allergy testing (Z01.82)*
> AHA: 2020,2Q,11

Z01.89 Encounter for other specified special examinations

✓4ᵗʰ Z02 Encounter for administrative examination

Z02.0 Encounter for examination for admission to educational institution
> Encounter for examination for admission to preschool (education)
> Encounter for examination for re-admission to school following illness or medical treatment

Z02.1 Encounter for pre-employment examination

Z02.2 Encounter for examination for admission to residential institution
> EXCLUDES 1   *examination for admission to prison (Z02.89)*

Z02.3 Encounter for examination for recruitment to armed forces

Z02.4 Encounter for examination for driving license

Z02.5 Encounter for examination for participation in sport
> EXCLUDES 1   *blood-alcohol and blood-drug test (Z02.83)*

Z02.6 Encounter for examination for insurance purposes

✓5ᵗʰ Z02.7 Encounter for issue of medical certificate
> EXCLUDES 1   *encounter for general medical examination (Z00-Z01, Z02.0-Z02.6, Z02.8-Z02.9)*

Z02.71 Encounter for disability determination
> Encounter for issue of medical certificate of incapacity
> Encounter for issue of medical certificate of invalidity

Z02.79 Encounter for issue of other medical certificate

✓5ᵗʰ Z02.8 Encounter for other administrative examinations

Z02.81 Encounter for paternity testing

Z02.82 Encounter for adoption services

Z02.83 Encounter for blood-alcohol and blood-drug test
> Use additional code for findings of alcohol or drugs in blood (R78.-)

Z02.89 Encounter for other administrative examinations
> Encounter for examination for admission to prison
> Encounter for examination for admission to summer camp
> Encounter for immigration examination
> Encounter for naturalization examination
> Encounter for premarital examination
> EXCLUDES 1   *health supervision of foundling or other healthy infant or child (Z76.1-Z76.2)*

Z02.9 Encounter for administrative examinations, unspecified

Chapter 21. Factors Influencing Health Status and Contact With Health Services

✓4ᵗʰ **Z03 Encounter for** medical observation **for suspected diseases and conditions ruled out**

This category is to be used when a person without a diagnosis is suspected of having an abnormal condition, without signs or symptoms, which requires study, but after examination and observation, is ruled out. This category is also for use for administrative and legal observation status.

EXCLUDES 1 contact with and (suspected) exposures hazardous to health (Z77.-)

encounter for observation and evaluation of newborn for suspected diseases and conditions ruled out (Z05.-)

person with feared complaint in whom no diagnosis is made (Z71.1)

signs or symptoms under study — code to signs or symptoms

AHA: 2020,2Q,8; 2018,2Q,7-8; 2017,4Q,27

Z03.6 Encounter for observation for suspected toxic effect from ingested substance **ruled out**

Encounter for observation for suspected adverse effect from drug

Encounter for observation for suspected poisoning

✓5ᵗʰ **Z03.7 Encounter for suspected** maternal and fetal conditions **ruled out**

Encounter for suspected maternal and fetal conditions not found

EXCLUDES 1 known or suspected fetal anomalies affecting management of mother, not ruled out (O26.-, O35.-, O36.-, O40.-, O41.-)

Z03.71 Encounter for suspected problem with amniotic cavity and membrane **ruled out**   Ⓜ ♀

Encounter for suspected oligohydramnios ruled out

Encounter for suspected polyhydramnios ruled out

Z03.72 Encounter for suspected placental problem **ruled out**   Ⓜ ♀

Z03.73 Encounter for suspected fetal anomaly **ruled out**   Ⓜ ♀

Z03.74 Encounter for suspected problem with fetal growth **ruled out**   Ⓜ ♀

Z03.75 Encounter for suspected cervical shortening **ruled out**   Ⓜ ♀

Z03.79 Encounter for other suspected maternal and fetal conditions ruled out   Ⓜ ♀

✓5ᵗʰ **Z03.8 Encounter for** observation **for other suspected diseases and conditions ruled out**

✓6ᵗʰ **Z03.81 Encounter for observation for suspected** exposure to biological agents **ruled out**

Z03.810 Encounter for observation for suspected exposure to anthrax **ruled out**

Z03.818 Encounter for observation for suspected exposure to other biological agents ruled out

AHA: 2020,2Q,8; 2020,1Q,34-36

TIP: Assign for cases in which there is concern for possible exposure to COVID-19 that is ruled out after evaluation.

● ✓6ᵗʰ **Z03.82 Encounter for observation for suspected** foreign body **ruled out**

EXCLUDES 1 retained foreign body (Z18.-)

retained foreign body in eyelid (H02.81)

residual foreign body in soft tissue (M79.5)

EXCLUDES 2 confirmed foreign body ingestion or aspiration including:

foreign body in alimentary tract (T18)

foreign body in ear (T16)

foreign body on external eye (T15)

foreign body in respiratory tract (T17)

● **Z03.821 Encounter for observation for suspected** ingested **foreign body ruled out**

● **Z03.822 Encounter for observation for suspected** aspirated (inhaled) **foreign body ruled out**

● **Z03.823 Encounter for observation for suspected** inserted (injected) **foreign body ruled out**

Encounter for observation for suspected inserted (injected) foreign body in eye ruled out

Encounter for observation for suspected inserted (injected) foreign body in orifice ruled out

Encounter for observation for suspected inserted (injected) foreign body in skin ruled out

Z03.89 Encounter for observation for other suspected diseases and conditions ruled out

✓4ᵗʰ **Z04 Encounter for examination and observation for other reasons**

INCLUDES encounter for examination for medicolegal reasons

This category is to be used when a person without a diagnosis is suspected of having an abnormal condition, without signs or symptoms, which requires study, but after examination and observation, is ruled-out. This category is also for use for administrative and legal observation status.

AHA: 2018,2Q,7-8

Z04.1 Encounter for examination and observation following transport accident

EXCLUDES 1 encounter for examination and observation following work accident (Z04.2)

AHA: 2019,2Q,11; 2018,2Q,8

Z04.2 Encounter for examination and observation following work accident

Z04.3 Encounter for examination and observation following other accident

✓5ᵗʰ **Z04.4 Encounter for examination and observation following** alleged rape

Encounter for examination and observation of victim following alleged rape

Encounter for examination and observation of victim following alleged sexual abuse

Z04.41 Encounter for examination and observation following alleged adult rape   Ⓐ

Suspected adult rape, ruled out

Suspected adult sexual abuse, ruled out

Z04.42 Encounter for examination and observation following alleged child rape   Ⓟ

Suspected child rape, ruled out

Suspected child sexual abuse, ruled out

Z04.6 Encounter for general psychiatric examination, requested by authority

✓5ᵗʰ **Z04.7 Encounter for examination and observation following** alleged physical abuse

Z04.71 Encounter for examination and observation following alleged adult physical abuse   Ⓐ

Suspected adult physical abuse, ruled out

EXCLUDES 1 confirmed case of adult physical abuse (T74.-)

encounter for examination and observation following alleged adult sexual abuse (Z04.41)

suspected case of adult physical abuse, not ruled out (T76.-)

Z04.72 Encounter for examination and observation following alleged child physical abuse   Ⓟ

Suspected child physical abuse, ruled out

EXCLUDES 1 confirmed case of child physical abuse (T74.-)

encounter for examination and observation following alleged child sexual abuse (Z04.42)

suspected case of child physical abuse, not ruled out (T76.-)

✓5ᵗʰ **Z04.8 Encounter for examination and observation for** other specified reasons

Encounter for examination and observation for request for expert evidence

AHA: 2018,4Q,32,35,72

Z04.81 Encounter for examination and observation of victim following forced sexual exploitation

Z04.82 Encounter for examination and observation of victim following forced labor exploitation

Z04.89 Encounter for examination and observation for other specified reasons

Ⓝ Newborn: 0   Ⓟ Pediatric: 0-17   Ⓜ Maternity: 9-64   Ⓐ Adult: 15-124   �ⒸⒸ Major Complication/Comorbidity   ⒸⒸ Complication/Comorbidity   Ⓢⓦ Severe Wound Dx

1236   ICD-10-CM 2021

Z04.9 Encounter for examination and observation for unspecified reason

Encounter for observation NOS

☑4ᵗʰ **Z05** Encounter for observation and evaluation of newborn for suspected diseases and conditions ruled out

This category is to be used for newborns, within the neonatal period (the first 28 days of life), who are suspected of having an abnormal condition, but without signs or symptoms, and which, after examination and observation, is ruled out.

AHA: 2017,4Q,27; 2016,4Q,77

Z05.0 Observation and evaluation of newborn for suspected cardiac condition ruled out   N

Z05.1 Observation and evaluation of newborn for suspected infectious condition ruled out

AHA: 2019,2Q,10

Z05.2 Observation and evaluation of newborn for suspected neurological condition ruled out   N

Z05.3 Observation and evaluation of newborn for suspected respiratory condition ruled out   N

☑5ᵗʰ **Z05.4** Observation and evaluation of newborn for suspected genetic, metabolic or immunologic condition ruled out

Z05.41 Observation and evaluation of newborn for suspected genetic condition ruled out   N

AHA: 2016,4Q,55

Z05.42 Observation and evaluation of newborn for suspected metabolic condition ruled out   N

Z05.43 Observation and evaluation of newborn for suspected immunologic condition ruled out   N

Z05.5 Observation and evaluation of newborn for suspected gastrointestinal condition ruled out   N

Z05.6 Observation and evaluation of newborn for suspected genitourinary condition ruled out   N

☑5ᵗʰ **Z05.7** Observation and evaluation of newborn for suspected skin, subcutaneous, musculoskeletal and connective tissue condition ruled out

Z05.71 Observation and evaluation of newborn for suspected skin and subcutaneous tissue condition ruled out   N

Z05.72 Observation and evaluation of newborn for suspected musculoskeletal condition ruled out   N

Z05.73 Observation and evaluation of newborn for suspected connective tissue condition ruled out   N

Z05.8 Observation and evaluation of newborn for other specified suspected condition ruled out   N

Z05.9 Observation and evaluation of newborn for unspecified suspected condition ruled out   N

Z08 Encounter for follow-up examination after completed treatment for malignant neoplasm

Medical surveillance following completed treatment

Use additional code to identify any acquired absence of organs (Z90.-)

Use additional code to identify the personal history of malignant neoplasm (Z85.-)

EXCLUDES 1   aftercare following medical care (Z43-Z49, Z51)

Z09 Encounter for follow-up examination after completed treatment for conditions other than malignant neoplasm

Medical surveillance following completed treatment

Use additional code to identify any applicable history of disease code (Z86.-. Z87.-)

EXCLUDES 1   aftercare following medical care (Z43-Z49, Z51)
              surveillance of contraception (Z30.4-)
              surveillance of prosthetic and other medical devices (Z44-Z46)

AHA: 2020,2Q,10; 2017,1Q,9; 2015,1Q,8

☑4ᵗʰ **Z11** Encounter for screening for infectious and parasitic diseases

Screening is the testing for disease or disease precursors in asymptomatic individuals so that early detection and treatment can be provided for those who test positive for the disease.

EXCLUDES 1   encounter for diagnostic examination — code to sign or symptom

Z11.0 Encounter for screening for intestinal infectious diseases

Z11.1 Encounter for screening for respiratory tuberculosis

Encounter for screening for active tuberculosis disease

Z11.2 Encounter for screening for other bacterial diseases

Z11.3 Encounter for screening for infections with a predominantly sexual mode of transmission

EXCLUDES 2   encounter for screening for human immunodeficiency virus [HIV] (Z11.4)
              encounter for screening for human papillomavirus (Z11.51)

Z11.4 Encounter for screening for human immunodeficiency virus [HIV]

☑5ᵗʰ **Z11.5** Encounter for screening for other viral diseases

EXCLUDES 2   encounter for screening for viral intestinal disease (Z11.0)

Z11.51 Encounter for screening for human papillomavirus (HPV)

Z11.59 Encounter for screening for other viral diseases

Z11.6 Encounter for screening for other protozoal diseases and helminthiases

EXCLUDES 2   encounter for screening for protozoal intestinal disease (Z11.0)

Z11.7 Encounter for testing for latent tuberculosis infection

AHA: 2019,4Q,20

Z11.8 Encounter for screening for other infectious and parasitic diseases

Encounter for screening for chlamydia
Encounter for screening for rickettsial
Encounter for screening for spirochetal
Encounter for screening for mycoses

Z11.9 Encounter for screening for infectious and parasitic diseases, unspecified

☑4ᵗʰ **Z12** Encounter for screening for malignant neoplasms

Screening is the testing for disease or disease precursors in asymptomatic individuals so that early detection and treatment can be provided for those who test positive for the disease.

Use additional code to identify any family history of malignant neoplasm (Z80.-)

EXCLUDES 1   encounter for diagnostic examination — code to sign or symptom

Z12.0 Encounter for screening for malignant neoplasm of stomach

☑5ᵗʰ **Z12.1** Encounter for screening for malignant neoplasm of intestinal tract

AHA: 2017,1Q,8,9

Z12.10 Encounter for screening for malignant neoplasm of intestinal tract, unspecified

Z12.11 Encounter for screening for malignant neoplasm of colon

Encounter for screening colonoscopy NOS

AHA: 2019,1Q,32-33; 2018,1Q,6

Z12.12 Encounter for screening for malignant neoplasm of rectum

AHA: 2018,1Q,6

Z12.13 Encounter for screening for malignant neoplasm of small intestine

Z12.2 Encounter for screening for malignant neoplasm of respiratory organs

☑5ᵗʰ **Z12.3** Encounter for screening for malignant neoplasm of breast

Z12.31 Encounter for screening mammogram for malignant neoplasm of breast

EXCLUDES 1   inconclusive mammogram (R92.2)

AHA: 2015,1Q,24

Z12.39 Encounter for other screening for malignant neoplasm of breast

Z12.4 Encounter for screening for malignant neoplasm of cervix   ♀

Encounter for screening pap smear for malignant neoplasm of cervix

EXCLUDES 1   when screening is part of general gynecological examination (Z01.4-)

EXCLUDES 2   encounter for screening for human papillomavirus (Z11.51)

Z12.5 Encounter for screening for malignant neoplasm of prostate   ♂

Z12.6 Encounter for screening for malignant neoplasm of bladder

☑5ᵗʰ **Z12.7** Encounter for screening for malignant neoplasm of other genitourinary organs

Z12.71 Encounter for screening for malignant neoplasm of testis   ♂

☑ Additional Character Required   ☑ᴀᵀᵗʰ Placeholder   Unacceptable PDx   Questionable PDx   Manifestation   Unspecified Dx   H1-H14 HAC   HCC CMS-HCC Dx   HIV HIV Dx

ICD-10-CM 2021   **1237**

Z12.72 **Encounter for screening for malignant neoplasm of vagina** ♀

Vaginal pap smear status-post hysterectomy for non-malignant condition

Use additional code to identify acquired absence of uterus (Z90.71-)

EXCLUDES 1   *vaginal pap smear status-post hysterectomy for malignant conditions (ZØ8)*

Z12.73 **Encounter for screening for malignant neoplasm of ovary** ♀

Z12.79 **Encounter for screening for malignant neoplasm of other genitourinary organs**

√5ᵗʰ **Z12.8** **Encounter for screening for malignant neoplasm of other sites**

Z12.81 **Encounter for screening for malignant neoplasm of oral cavity**

Z12.82 **Encounter for screening for malignant neoplasm of nervous system**

Z12.83 **Encounter for screening for malignant neoplasm of skin**

Z12.89 **Encounter for screening for malignant neoplasm of other sites**

Z12.9 **Encounter for screening for malignant neoplasm, site unspecified**

√4ᵗʰ **Z13** **Encounter for screening for other diseases and disorders**

Screening is the testing for disease or disease precursors in asymptomatic individuals so that early detection and treatment can be provided for those who test positive for the disease.

EXCLUDES 1   *encounter for diagnostic examination — code to sign or symptom*

Z13.Ø **Encounter for screening for diseases of the blood and blood-forming organs and certain disorders involving the immune mechanism**

Z13.1 **Encounter for screening for diabetes mellitus**

√5ᵗʰ **Z13.2** **Encounter for screening for nutritional, metabolic and other endocrine disorders**

Z13.21 **Encounter for screening for nutritional disorder**

√6ᵗʰ **Z13.22** **Encounter for screening for metabolic disorder**

Z13.22Ø **Encounter for screening for lipoid disorders**

Encounter for screening for cholesterol level

Encounter for screening for hypercholesterolemia

Encounter for screening for hyperlipidemia

Z13.228 **Encounter for screening for other metabolic disorders**

Z13.29 **Encounter for screening for other suspected endocrine disorder**

EXCLUDES 1   *encounter for screening for diabetes mellitus (Z13.1)*

√5ᵗʰ **Z13.3** **Encounter for screening examination for mental health and behavioral disorders**

AHA: 2018,4Q,35-36

Z13.3Ø **Encounter for screening examination for mental health and behavioral disorders, unspecified**

Z13.31 **Encounter for screening for depression**

Encounter for screening for depression, adult

Encounter for screening for depression for child or adolescent

Z13.32 **Encounter for screening for maternal depression** ♀

Encounter for screening for perinatal depression

Z13.39 **Encounter for screening examination for other mental health and behavioral disorders**

Encounter for screening for alcoholism

Encounter for screening for intellectual disabilities

√5ᵗʰ **Z13.4** **Encounter for screening for certain developmental disorders in childhood**

Encounter for development testing of infant or child

Encounter for screening for developmental handicaps in early childhood

EXCLUDES 2   *encounter for routine child health examination (ZØØ.12-)*

AHA: 2018,4Q,36

Z13.4Ø **Encounter for screening for unspecified developmental delays**

Z13.41 **Encounter for autism screening**

Z13.42 **Encounter for screening for global developmental delays (milestones)**

Encounter for screening for developmental handicaps in early childhood

Z13.49 **Encounter for screening for other developmental delays**

Z13.5 **Encounter for screening for eye and ear disorders**

EXCLUDES 2   *encounter for general hearing examination (ZØ1.1-)*
encounter for general vision examination (ZØ1.Ø-)

AHA: 2016,3Q,17

Z13.6 **Encounter for screening for cardiovascular disorders**

√5ᵗʰ **Z13.7** **Encounter for screening for genetic and chromosomal anomalies**

EXCLUDES 1   *genetic testing for procreative management (Z31.4-)*

Z13.71 **Encounter for nonprocreative screening for genetic disease carrier status**

Z13.79 **Encounter for other screening for genetic and chromosomal anomalies**

√5ᵗʰ **Z13.8** **Encounter for screening for other specified diseases and disorders**

EXCLUDES 2   *screening for malignant neoplasms (Z12.-)*

√6ᵗʰ **Z13.81** **Encounter for screening for digestive system disorders**

Z13.81Ø **Encounter for screening for upper gastrointestinal disorder**

Z13.811 **Encounter for screening for lower gastrointestinal disorder**

EXCLUDES 1   *encounter for screening for intestinal infectious disease (Z11.Ø)*

Z13.818 **Encounter for screening for other digestive system disorders**

√6ᵗʰ **Z13.82** **Encounter for screening for musculoskeletal disorder**

Z13.82Ø **Encounter for screening for osteoporosis**

Z13.828 **Encounter for screening for other musculoskeletal disorder**

Z13.83 **Encounter for screening for respiratory disorder NEC**

EXCLUDES 1   *encounter for screening for respiratory tuberculosis (Z11.1)*

Z13.84 **Encounter for screening for dental disorders**

√6ᵗʰ **Z13.85** **Encounter for screening for nervous system disorders**

Z13.85Ø **Encounter for screening for traumatic brain injury**

Z13.858 **Encounter for screening for other nervous system disorders**

Z13.88 **Encounter for screening for disorder due to exposure to contaminants**

EXCLUDES 1   *those exposed to contaminants without suspected disorders (Z57.-, Z77.-)*

Z13.89 **Encounter for screening for other disorder**

Encounter for screening for genitourinary disorders

Z13.9 **Encounter for screening, unspecified**

Genetic carrier and genetic susceptibility to disease (Z14-Z15)

√4ᵗʰ **Z14** **Genetic carrier**

DEF: Individuals carrying a gene mutation associated with a certain disease that typically do not develop the disease but are able to pass the mutated genes to offspring.

√5ᵗʰ **Z14.Ø** **Hemophilia A carrier**

Z14.Ø1 **Asymptomatic hemophilia A carrier**

Z14.Ø2 **Symptomatic hemophilia A carrier**

Z14.1 **Cystic fibrosis carrier**

Z14.8 **Genetic carrier of other disease**

√4ᵗʰ **Z15** **Genetic susceptibility to disease**

INCLUDES   confirmed abnormal gene

Use additional code, if applicable, for any associated family history of the disease (Z80-Z84)

EXCLUDES 1   *chromosomal anomalies (Q90-Q99)*

√5ᵗʰ **Z15.Ø** **Genetic susceptibility to malignant neoplasm**

Code first, if applicable, any current malignant neoplasm (CØØ-C75, C81-C96)

Use additional code, if applicable, for any personal history of malignant neoplasm (Z85.-)

Z15.Ø1 **Genetic susceptibility to malignant neoplasm of breast**

N Newborn: 0   P Pediatric: 0-17   M Maternity: 9-64   A Adult: 15-124   MCC Major Complication/Comorbidity   CC Complication/Comorbidity   SW Severe Wound Dx

1238   ICD-10-CM 2021

Z15.02   Genetic susceptibility to malignant neoplasm of ovary ♀

Z15.03   Genetic susceptibility to malignant neoplasm of prostate ♂

Z15.04   Genetic susceptibility to malignant neoplasm of endometrium ♀

Z15.09   Genetic susceptibility to other malignant neoplasm

√5ᵗʰ **Z15.8**   Genetic susceptibility to other disease

Z15.81   Genetic susceptibility to multiple endocrine neoplasia [MEN]

EXCLUDES 1   multiple endocrine neoplasia [MEN] syndromes (E31.2-)

DEF: Group of conditions in which several endocrine glands grow excessively (such as in adenomatous hyperplasia) and/or develop benign or malignant tumors. Tumors and hyperplasia associated with MEN often produce excess hormones, which impede normal physiology. There is no comprehensive cure known for MEN syndrome. Treatment is directed at the hyperplasia or tumors in each individual gland. Tumors are usually surgically removed and oral medications or hormonal injections are used to correct hormone imbalances.

Z15.89   Genetic susceptibility to other disease

Resistance to antimicrobial drugs (Z16)

√4ᵗʰ **Z16**   Resistance to antimicrobial drugs

NOTE   The codes in this category are provided for use as additional codes to identify the resistance and non-responsiveness of a condition to antimicrobial drugs.

Code first the infection

EXCLUDES 1   Methicillin resistant Staphylococcus aureus infection (A49.02)
Methicillin resistant Staphylococcus aureus pneumonia (J15.212)
sepsis due to Methicillin resistant Staphylococcus aureus (A41.02)

√5ᵗʰ **Z16.1**   Resistance to beta lactam antibiotics

Z16.10   Resistance to unspecified beta lactam antibiotics   cc

Z16.11   Resistance to penicillins   cc
Resistance to amoxicillin
Resistance to ampicillin

Z16.12   Extended spectrum beta lactamase (ESBL) resistance   cc
EXCLUDES 2   Methicillin resistant Staphylococcus aureus infection in diseases classified elsewhere (B95.62)

Z16.19   Resistance to other specified beta lactam antibiotics   cc
Resistance to cephalosporins

√5ᵗʰ **Z16.2**   Resistance to other antibiotics

Z16.20   Resistance to unspecified antibiotic   cc
Resistance to antibiotics NOS

Z16.21   Resistance to vancomycin   cc

Z16.22   Resistance to vancomycin related antibiotics   cc

Z16.23   Resistance to quinolones and fluoroquinolones   cc

Z16.24   Resistance to multiple antibiotics   cc

Z16.29   Resistance to other single specified antibiotic   cc
Resistance to aminoglycosides
Resistance to macrolides
Resistance to sulfonamides
Resistance to tetracyclines

√5ᵗʰ **Z16.3**   Resistance to other antimicrobial drugs

EXCLUDES 1   resistance to antibiotics (Z16.1-, Z16.2-)

Z16.30   Resistance to unspecified antimicrobial drugs   cc
Drug resistance NOS

Z16.31   Resistance to antiparasitic drug(s)   cc
Resistance to quinine and related compounds

Z16.32   Resistance to antifungal drug(s)   cc

Z16.33   Resistance to antiviral drug(s)   cc

√6ᵗʰ **Z16.34**   Resistance to antimycobacterial drug(s)
Resistance to tuberculostatics

Z16.341   Resistance to single antimycobacterial drug   cc
Resistance to antimycobacterial drug NOS

Z16.342   Resistance to multiple antimycobacterial drugs   cc

Z16.35   Resistance to multiple antimicrobial drugs   cc
EXCLUDES 1   resistance to multiple antibiotics only (Z16.24)

Z16.39   Resistance to other specified antimicrobial drug   cc

Estrogen receptor status (Z17)

√4ᵗʰ **Z17**   Estrogen receptor status
Code first malignant neoplasm of breast (C50.-)
DEF: Receptor status of breast cancer cells for the hormone estrogen that is used to help determine treatment and evaluate prognosis. ER+ breast cancer responds to hormone therapies while ER- breast cancer does not.

Z17.0   Estrogen receptor positive status [ER+]

Z17.1   Estrogen receptor negative status [ER-]

Retained foreign body fragments (Z18)

√4ᵗʰ **Z18**   Retained foreign body fragments

INCLUDES   embedded fragment (status)
embedded splinter (status)
retained foreign body status

EXCLUDES 1   artificial joint prosthesis status (Z96.6-)
foreign body accidentally left during a procedure (T81.5-)
foreign body entering through orifice (T15-T19)
in situ cardiac device (Z95.-)
organ or tissue replaced by means other than transplant (Z96.-, Z97.-)
organ or tissue replaced by transplant (Z94.-)
personal history of retained foreign body fully removed Z87.821
superficial foreign body (non-embedded splinter) — code to superficial foreign body, by site

DEF: Embedded or retained fragment, splinter, or foreign body, natural or synthetic that can cause infection.

√5ᵗʰ **Z18.0**   Retained radioactive fragments

Z18.01   Retained depleted uranium fragments

Z18.09   Other retained radioactive fragments
Other retained depleted isotope fragments
Retained nontherapeutic radioactive fragments

√5ᵗʰ **Z18.1**   Retained metal fragments

EXCLUDES 1   retained radioactive metal fragments (Z18.01-Z18.09)

Z18.10   Retained metal fragments, unspecified
Retained metal fragment NOS

Z18.11   Retained magnetic metal fragments

Z18.12   Retained nonmagnetic metal fragments

Z18.2   Retained plastic fragments
Acrylics fragments
Diethylhexyl phthalates fragments
Isocyanate fragments

√5ᵗʰ **Z18.3**   Retained organic fragments

Z18.31   Retained animal quills or spines

Z18.32   Retained tooth

Z18.33   Retained wood fragments

Z18.39   Other retained organic fragments

√5ᵗʰ **Z18.8**   Other specified retained foreign body

Z18.81   Retained glass fragments

Z18.83   Retained stone or crystalline fragments
Retained concrete or cement fragments

Z18.89   Other specified retained foreign body fragments

Z18.9   Retained foreign body fragments, unspecified material

Hormone sensitivity malignancy status (Z19)

√4ᵗʰ **Z19**   Hormone sensitivity malignancy status
Code first malignant neoplasm — see Table of Neoplasms, by site, malignant
AHA: 2016,4Q,76

Z19.1   Hormone sensitive malignancy status

☑ Additional Character Required   √x7ᵗʰ Placeholder   Unacceptable PDx   Questionable PDx   Manifestation   Unspecified Dx   H1-H14 HAC   HCC CMS-HCC Dx   HIV HIV Dx

ICD-10-CM 2021   1239

Chapter 21. Factors Influencing Health Status and Contact With Health Services

Z19.2   **Hormone resistant malignancy status**
Castrate resistant prostate malignancy status

Persons with potential health hazards related to communicable diseases (Z20-Z29)

✓4ᵗʰ **Z20**   **Contact with and (suspected) exposure to communicable diseases**
    EXCLUDES 1   carrier of infectious disease (Z22.-)
            diagnosed current infectious or parasitic disease — see Alphabetic Index
    EXCLUDES 2   personal history of infectious and parasitic diseases (Z86.1-)

✓5ᵗʰ **Z20.0**   **Contact with and (suspected) exposure to intestinal infectious diseases**
    Z20.01   **Contact with and (suspected) exposure to intestinal infectious diseases due to Escherichia coli (E. coli)**
    Z20.09   **Contact with and (suspected) exposure to other intestinal infectious diseases**

Z20.1   **Contact with and (suspected) exposure to tuberculosis**
Z20.2   **Contact with and (suspected) exposure to infections with a predominantly sexual mode of transmission**
Z20.3   **Contact with and (suspected) exposure to rabies**
Z20.4   **Contact with and (suspected) exposure to rubella**
Z20.5   **Contact with and (suspected) exposure to viral hepatitis**
Z20.6   **Contact with and (suspected) exposure to human immunodeficiency virus [HIV]**
    EXCLUDES 1   asymptomatic human immunodeficiency virus [HIV] HIV infection status (Z21)

Z20.7   **Contact with and (suspected) exposure to pediculosis, acariasis and other infestations**

✓5ᵗʰ **Z20.8**   **Contact with and (suspected) exposure to other communicable diseases**
    ✓6ᵗʰ **Z20.81**   **Contact with and (suspected) exposure to other bacterial communicable diseases**
       Z20.810   **Contact with and (suspected) exposure to anthrax**
       Z20.811   **Contact with and (suspected) exposure to meningococcus**
       Z20.818   **Contact with and (suspected) exposure to other bacterial communicable diseases**
          AHA: 2019,2Q,10
    ✓6ᵗʰ **Z20.82**   **Contact with and (suspected) exposure to other viral communicable diseases**
       Z20.820   **Contact with and (suspected) exposure to varicella**
       Z20.821   **Contact with and (suspected) exposure to Zika virus**
          AHA: 2018,4Q,35,64
       Z20.828   **Contact with and (suspected) exposure to other viral communicable diseases**
          AHA: 2020,2Q,4,8; 2020,1Q,34-36
          TIP: Assign for cases in which there is actual exposure to someone who is confirmed or suspected (not ruled out) to have COVID-19 and the exposed individual either tests negative or the test results are unknown. If the exposed individual tests positive for the COVID-19 virus, assign U07.1.

    Z20.89   **Contact with and (suspected) exposure to other communicable diseases**

Z20.9   **Contact with and (suspected) exposure to unspecified communicable disease**

Z21   **Asymptomatic human immunodeficiency virus [HIV] infection status**   HCC
HIV positive NOS
Code first human immunodeficiency virus [HIV] disease complicating pregnancy, childbirth and the puerperium, if applicable (O98.7-)
    EXCLUDES 1   acquired immunodeficiency syndrome (B20)
            contact with human immunodeficiency virus [HIV] (Z20.6)
            exposure to human immunodeficiency virus [HIV] (Z20.6)
            human immunodeficiency virus [HIV] disease (B20)
            inconclusive laboratory evidence of human immunodeficiency virus [HIV] (R75)
AHA: 2019,1Q,8-11
DEF: Phase of human immunodeficiency virus (HIV) infection with no clinical symptoms. This phase may last for 10 years or more.

✓4ᵗʰ **Z22**   **Carrier of infectious disease**
    INCLUDES   colonization status
           suspected carrier
    EXCLUDES 2   carrier of viral hepatitis (B18.-)

Z22.0   **Carrier of typhoid**
Z22.1   **Carrier of other intestinal infectious diseases**
Z22.2   **Carrier of diphtheria**
✓5ᵗʰ **Z22.3**   **Carrier of other specified bacterial diseases**
    Z22.31   **Carrier of bacterial disease due to meningococci**
    ✓6ᵗʰ **Z22.32**   **Carrier of bacterial disease due to staphylococci**
       Z22.321   **Carrier or suspected carrier of Methicillin susceptible Staphylococcus aureus**
          MSSA colonization
       Z22.322   **Carrier or suspected carrier of Methicillin resistant Staphylococcus aureus**
          MRSA colonization
          DEF: Carriers (colonization) of methicillin resistant Staphylococcus aureus (MRSA) have MRSA on their skin or in their body but do not exhibit signs of infection. These individuals are able to pass MRSA on to others who may develop an infection.

    ✓6ᵗʰ **Z22.33**   **Carrier of bacterial disease due to streptococci**
       Z22.330   **Carrier of Group B streptococcus**
          EXCLUDES 1   carrier of streptococcus group B (GBS) complicating pregnancy, childbirth and the puerperium (O99.82-)
       Z22.338   **Carrier of other streptococcus**
    Z22.39   **Carrier of other specified bacterial diseases**

Z22.4   **Carrier of infections with a predominantly sexual mode of transmission**
Z22.6   **Carrier of human T-lymphotropic virus type-1 [HTLV-1] infection**
Z22.7   **Latent tuberculosis**
Latent tuberculosis infection (LTBI)
    EXCLUDES 1   nonspecific reaction to cell mediated immunity measurement of gamma interferon antigen response without active tuberculosis (R76.12)
            nonspecific reaction to tuberculin skin test without active tuberculosis (R76.11)
AHA: 2019,4Q,19

Z22.8   **Carrier of other infectious diseases**
Z22.9   **Carrier of infectious disease, unspecified**

Z23   **Encounter for immunization**
Code first any routine childhood examination
    NOTE   Procedure codes are required to identify the types of immunizations given

✓4ᵗʰ **Z28**   **Immunization not carried out and underimmunization status**
    INCLUDES   vaccination not carried out

✓5ᵗʰ **Z28.0**   **Immunization not carried out because of contraindication**
    DEF: Contraindication: Situation where a drug, surgery, or other procedure may negatively affect or cause harm to a patient.
    Z28.01   **Immunization not carried out because of acute illness of patient**
    Z28.02   **Immunization not carried out because of chronic illness or condition of patient**
    Z28.03   **Immunization not carried out because of immune compromised state of patient**
    Z28.04   **Immunization not carried out because of patient allergy to vaccine or component**
    Z28.09   **Immunization not carried out because of other contraindication**

Z28.1   **Immunization not carried out because of patient decision for reasons of belief or group pressure**
Immunization not carried out because of religious belief

✓5ᵗʰ **Z28.2**   **Immunization not carried out because of patient decision for other and unspecified reason**
    Z28.20   **Immunization not carried out because of patient decision for unspecified reason**
    Z28.21   **Immunization not carried out because of patient refusal**
    Z28.29   **Immunization not carried out because of patient decision for other reason**

Z28.3   **Underimmunization status**
     Delinquent immunization status
     Lapsed immunization schedule status

√5ᵗʰ **Z28.8**   **Immunization not carried out for other reason**

     Z28.81   **Immunization not carried out due to patient having had the disease**

     Z28.82   **Immunization not carried out because of caregiver refusal**
         Immunization not carried out because of guardian refusal
         Immunization not carried out because of parent refusal
         EXCLUDES 1   *immunization not carried out because of caregiver refusal because of religious belief (Z28.1)*

     Z28.83   **Immunization not carried out due to unavailability of vaccine**
         Delay in delivery of vaccine
         Lack of availability of vaccine
         Manufacturer delay of vaccine
         AHA: 2018,4Q,36

     Z28.89   **Immunization not carried out for other reason**

     Z28.9   **Immunization not carried out for unspecified reason**

√4ᵗʰ **Z29**   **Encounter for other prophylactic measures**
     EXCLUDES 1   *desensitization to allergens (Z51.6)*
                     prophylactic surgery (Z40.-)
     AHA: 2016,4Q,78-79

√5ᵗʰ **Z29.1**   **Encounter for prophylactic immunotherapy**
     Encounter for administration of immunoglobulin

     Z29.11   **Encounter for prophylactic immunotherapy for respiratory syncytial virus (RSV)**

     Z29.12   **Encounter for prophylactic antivenin**

     Z29.13   **Encounter for prophylactic Rho(D) immune globulin**
         AHA: 2019,3Q,5

     Z29.14   **Encounter for prophylactic rabies immune globin**

     Z29.3   **Encounter for prophylactic fluoride administration**

     Z29.8   **Encounter for other specified prophylactic measures**

     Z29.9   **Encounter for prophylactic measures, unspecified**

Persons encountering health services in circumstances related to reproduction (Z30-Z39)

√4ᵗʰ **Z30**   **Encounter for contraceptive management**
     AHA: 2016,4Q,78
     DEF: Contraceptive management to prevent pregnancy. Methods include oral medications, intrauterine devices, and surgical procedures for males and females (sterilization).

√5ᵗʰ **Z30.0**   **Encounter for general counseling and advice on contraception**

     √6ᵗʰ **Z30.01**   **Encounter for initial prescription of contraceptives**
         EXCLUDES 1   *encounter for surveillance of contraceptives (Z30.4-)*

         Z30.011   **Encounter for initial prescription of contraceptive pills** ♀

         Z30.012   **Encounter for prescription of emergency contraception** ♀
             Encounter for postcoital contraception

         Z30.013   **Encounter for initial prescription of injectable contraceptive** ♀

         Z30.014   **Encounter for initial prescription of intrauterine contraceptive device** ♀
             EXCLUDES 1   *encounter for insertion of intrauterine contraceptive device (Z30.430, Z30.432)*

         Z30.015   **Encounter for initial prescription of vaginal ring hormonal contraceptive** ♀

         Z30.016   **Encounter for initial prescription of transdermal patch hormonal contraceptive device**

         Z30.017   **Encounter for initial prescription of implantable subdermal contraceptive**

         Z30.018   **Encounter for initial prescription of other contraceptives** ♀
             Encounter for initial prescription of barrier contraception
             Encounter for initial prescription of diaphragm

         Z30.019   **Encounter for initial prescription of contraceptives, unspecified** ♀

     Z30.02   **Counseling and instruction in natural family planning to avoid pregnancy**

     Z30.09   **Encounter for other general counseling and advice on contraception**
         Encounter for family planning advice NOS

Z30.2   **Encounter for sterilization**

√5ᵗʰ **Z30.4**   **Encounter for surveillance of contraceptives**

     Z30.40   **Encounter for surveillance of contraceptives, unspecified**

     Z30.41   **Encounter for surveillance of contraceptive pills** ♀
         Encounter for repeat prescription for contraceptive pill

     Z30.42   **Encounter for surveillance of injectable contraceptive** ♀

     √6ᵗʰ **Z30.43**   **Encounter for surveillance of intrauterine contraceptive device**

         Z30.430   **Encounter for insertion of intrauterine contraceptive device** ♀

         Z30.431   **Encounter for routine checking of intrauterine contraceptive device** ♀

         Z30.432   **Encounter for removal of intrauterine contraceptive device** ♀

         Z30.433   **Encounter for removal and reinsertion of intrauterine contraceptive device** ♀
             Encounter for replacement of intrauterine contraceptive device

     Z30.44   **Encounter for surveillance of vaginal ring hormonal contraceptive device**

     Z30.45   **Encounter for surveillance of transdermal patch hormonal contraceptive device**

     Z30.46   **Encounter for surveillance of implantable subdermal contraceptive** ♀
         Encounter for checking, reinsertion or removal of implantable subdermal contraceptive

     Z30.49   **Encounter for surveillance of other contraceptives** ♀
         Encounter for surveillance of barrier contraception
         Encounter for surveillance of diaphragm

Z30.8   **Encounter for other contraceptive management**
     Encounter for postvasectomy sperm count
     Encounter for routine examination for contraceptive maintenance
     EXCLUDES 1   *sperm count following sterilization reversal (Z31.42)*
                  sperm count for fertility testing (Z31.41)

Z30.9   **Encounter for contraceptive management, unspecified**

√4ᵗʰ **Z31**   **Encounter for procreative management**
     EXCLUDES 1   *complications associated with artificial fertilization (N98.-)*
                  female infertility (N97.-)
                  male infertility (N46.-)

Z31.0   **Encounter for reversal of previous sterilization**

√5ᵗʰ **Z31.4**   **Encounter for procreative investigation and testing**
     EXCLUDES 1   *postvasectomy sperm count (Z30.8)*

     Z31.41   **Encounter for fertility testing**
         Encounter for fallopian tube patency testing
         Encounter for sperm count for fertility testing

     Z31.42   **Aftercare following sterilization reversal**
         Sperm count following sterilization reversal

     √6ᵗʰ **Z31.43**   **Encounter for genetic testing of female for procreative management**
         Use additional code for recurrent pregnancy loss, if applicable (N96, O26.2-)
         EXCLUDES 1   *nonprocreative genetic testing (Z13.7-)*

         Z31.430   **Encounter of female for testing for genetic disease carrier status for procreative management** ♀

         Z31.438   **Encounter for other genetic testing of female for procreative management** ♀

√6ᵗʰ **Z31.44 Encounter for genetic testing of** male **for procreative management**
> EXCLUDES 1   nonprocreative genetic testing (Z13.7-)

     Z31.440 Encounter of male for testing for genetic disease carrier status for procreative management ♂

     Z31.441 Encounter for testing of male partner of patient with recurrent pregnancy loss Ⓐ ♂

     Z31.448 Encounter for other genetic testing of male for procreative management Ⓐ ♂

   Z31.49 Encounter for other procreative investigation and testing

Z31.5 Encounter for procreative genetic counseling
> AHA: 2017,4Q,27

√5ᵗʰ **Z31.6 Encounter for general counseling and advice on procreation**

   Z31.61 Procreative counseling and advice using natural family planning

   Z31.62 Encounter for fertility preservation counseling
Encounter for fertility preservation counseling prior to cancer therapy
Encounter for fertility preservation counseling prior to surgical removal of gonads

   Z31.69 Encounter for other general counseling and advice on procreation

Z31.7 Encounter for procreative management and counseling for gestational carrier ♀
> EXCLUDES 1   pregnant state, gestational carrier (Z33.3)

> AHA: 2016,4Q,78

√5ᵗʰ **Z31.8 Encounter for other procreative management**

   Z31.81 Encounter for male factor infertility in female patient ♀

   Z31.82 Encounter for Rh incompatibility status ♀
> AHA: 2015,3Q,40; 2014,4Q,17

   Z31.83 Encounter for assisted reproductive fertility procedure cycle ♀
Patient undergoing in vitro fertilization cycle
Use additional code to identify the type of infertility
> EXCLUDES 1   pre-cycle diagnosis and testing — code to reason for encounter

   Z31.84 Encounter for fertility preservation procedure
Encounter for fertility preservation procedure prior to cancer therapy
Encounter for fertility preservation procedure prior to surgical removal of gonads

   Z31.89 Encounter for other procreative management

Z31.9 Encounter for procreative management, unspecified

√4ᵗʰ **Z32 Encounter for pregnancy test and childbirth and childcare instruction**

√5ᵗʰ **Z32.0 Encounter for pregnancy test**

   Z32.00 Encounter for pregnancy test, result unknown ♀
Encounter for pregnancy test NOS

   Z32.01 Encounter for pregnancy test, result positive Ⓜ ♀

   Z32.02 Encounter for pregnancy test, result negative ♀

Z32.2 Encounter for childbirth instruction

Z32.3 Encounter for childcare instruction
Encounter for prenatal or postpartum childcare instruction

√4ᵗʰ **Z33 Pregnant state**

Z33.1 Pregnant state, incidental Ⓜ ♀
▶Pregnancy NOS◀
Pregnant state NOS
> EXCLUDES 1   complications of pregnancy (O00-O9A)
>   pregnant state, gestational carrier (Z33.3)

Z33.2 Encounter for elective termination of pregnancy Ⓜ ♀
> EXCLUDES 1   early fetal death with retention of dead fetus (O02.1)
>   late fetal death (O36.4)
>   spontaneous abortion (O03)

> TIP: Do not assign a code from category Z3A with this code.

Z33.3 Pregnant state, gestational carrier Ⓜ ♀
> EXCLUDES 1   encounter for procreative management and counseling for gestational carrier (Z31.7)

> AHA: 2016,4Q,78

√4ᵗʰ **Z34 Encounter for supervision of normal pregnancy**
> EXCLUDES 1   any complication of pregnancy (O00-O9A)
>   encounter for pregnancy test (Z32.0-)
>   encounter for supervision of high risk pregnancy (O09.-)

> AHA: 2019,3Q,5; 2014,4Q,17

√5ᵗʰ **Z34.0 Encounter for supervision of normal first pregnancy**

   Z34.00 Encounter for supervision of normal first pregnancy, unspecified trimester Ⓜ ♀

   Z34.01 Encounter for supervision of normal first pregnancy, first trimester Ⓜ ♀

   Z34.02 Encounter for supervision of normal first pregnancy, second trimester Ⓜ ♀

   Z34.03 Encounter for supervision of normal first pregnancy, third trimester Ⓜ ♀

√5ᵗʰ **Z34.8 Encounter for supervision of other normal pregnancy**

   Z34.80 Encounter for supervision of other normal pregnancy, unspecified trimester Ⓜ ♀

   Z34.81 Encounter for supervision of other normal pregnancy, first trimester Ⓜ ♀

   Z34.82 Encounter for supervision of other normal pregnancy, second trimester Ⓜ ♀

   Z34.83 Encounter for supervision of other normal pregnancy, third trimester Ⓜ ♀

√5ᵗʰ **Z34.9 Encounter for supervision of normal pregnancy, unspecified**

   Z34.90 Encounter for supervision of normal pregnancy, unspecified, unspecified trimester Ⓜ ♀

   Z34.91 Encounter for supervision of normal pregnancy, unspecified, first trimester Ⓜ ♀

   Z34.92 Encounter for supervision of normal pregnancy, unspecified, second trimester Ⓜ ♀

   Z34.93 Encounter for supervision of normal pregnancy, unspecified, third trimester Ⓜ ♀

√4ᵗʰ **Z36 Encounter for antenatal screening of mother**
> INCLUDES   encounter for placental sample (taken vaginally)
>   screening is the testing for disease or disease precursors in asymptomatic individuals so that early detection and treatment can be provided for those who test positive for the disease.

> EXCLUDES 1   diagnostic examination — code to sign or symptom
>   encounter for suspected maternal and fetal conditions ruled out (Z03.7-)
>   suspected fetal condition affecting management of pregnancy — code to condition in Chapter 15

> EXCLUDES 2   abnormal findings on antenatal screening of mother (O28.-)
>   genetic counseling and testing (Z31.43-, Z31.5)
>   routine prenatal care (Z34)

> AHA: 2017,4Q,28

Z36.0 Encounter for antenatal screening for chromosomal anomalies Ⓜ ♀

Z36.1 Encounter for antenatal screening for raised alphafetoprotein level Ⓜ ♀
Encounter for antenatal screening for elevated maternal serum alphafetoprotein level
DEF: High levels of alpha-fetoprotein (AFP) that may indicate a possibility of spina bifida and other neural tube defects, anencephaly, or omphalocele in the fetus.

Z36.2 Encounter for other antenatal screening follow-up Ⓜ ♀
Non-visualized anatomy on a previous scan

Z36.3 Encounter for antenatal screening for malformations Ⓜ ♀
Screening for a suspected anomaly

Z36.4 Encounter for antenatal screening for fetal growth retardation Ⓜ ♀
Intrauterine growth restriction (IUGR)/small-for-dates

Z36.5 Encounter for antenatal screening for isoimmunization Ⓜ ♀

√5ᵗʰ **Z36.8 Encounter for other antenatal screening**

   Z36.81 Encounter for antenatal screening for hydrops fetalis Ⓜ ♀
DEF: Hydrops fetalis: Abnormal accumulation of fluid in two or more parts of the fetus, such as ascites, effusion of the pleural or pericardial tissues, or edema.

   Z36.82 Encounter for antenatal screening for nuchal translucency Ⓜ ♀

   Z36.83 Encounter for fetal screening for congenital cardiac abnormalities Ⓜ ♀

   Z36.84 Encounter for antenatal screening for fetal lung maturity Ⓜ ♀

Ⓝ Newborn: 0   Ⓟ Pediatric: 0-17   Ⓜ Maternity: 9-64   Ⓐ Adult: 15-124   MCC Major Complication/Comorbidity   CC Complication/Comorbidity   SW Severe Wound Dx

1242   ICD-10-CM 2021

Z36.85   **Encounter for antenatal screening for** Streptococcus B   Ⓜ♀

Z36.86   **Encounter for antenatal screening for** cervical length   Ⓜ♀
    Screening for risk of pre-term labor

Z36.87   **Encounter for antenatal screening for** uncertain dates   Ⓜ♀

Z36.88   **Encounter for antenatal screening for** fetal macrosomia   Ⓜ♀
    Screening for large-for-dates

Z36.89   **Encounter for other specified antenatal screening**   Ⓜ♀

Z36.8A   **Encounter for antenatal screening for other genetic defects**   Ⓜ♀

Z36.9   **Encounter for antenatal screening, unspecified**   Ⓜ♀

✓4ᵗʰ **Z3A**   **Weeks of gestation**

> NOTE   Codes from category Z3A are for use, only on the maternal record, to indicate the weeks of gestation of the pregnancy, if known.

Code first complications of pregnancy, childbirth and the puerperium (O09-O9A)
AHA: 2019,2Q,11; 2016,2Q,34; 2014,3Q,17; 2014,2Q,9; 2013,2Q,33
TIP: Do not assign a code from this category with codes from categories O00-O08 or code Z33.2.

✓5ᵗʰ **Z3A.0**   **Weeks of gestation of pregnancy,** unspecified or less than 10 weeks

    Z3A.00   **Weeks of gestation of pregnancy** not specified   Ⓜ♀

    Z3A.01   Less than 8 weeks **gestation of pregnancy**   Ⓜ♀

    Z3A.08   8 weeks **gestation of pregnancy**   Ⓜ♀

    Z3A.09   9 weeks **gestation of pregnancy**   Ⓜ♀

✓5ᵗʰ **Z3A.1**   **Weeks of gestation of pregnancy, weeks** 10-19

    Z3A.10   10 weeks **gestation of pregnancy**   Ⓜ♀

    Z3A.11   11 weeks **gestation of pregnancy**   Ⓜ♀

    Z3A.12   12 weeks **gestation of pregnancy**   Ⓜ♀

    Z3A.13   13 weeks **gestation of pregnancy**   Ⓜ♀

    Z3A.14   14 weeks **gestation of pregnancy**   Ⓜ♀

    Z3A.15   15 weeks **gestation of pregnancy**   Ⓜ♀

    Z3A.16   16 weeks **gestation of pregnancy**   Ⓜ♀

    Z3A.17   17 weeks **gestation of pregnancy**   Ⓜ♀

    Z3A.18   18 weeks **gestation of pregnancy**   Ⓜ♀

    Z3A.19   19 weeks **gestation of pregnancy**   Ⓜ♀

✓5ᵗʰ **Z3A.2**   **Weeks of gestation of pregnancy, weeks** 20-29

    Z3A.20   20 weeks **gestation of pregnancy**   Ⓜ♀

    Z3A.21   21 weeks **gestation of pregnancy**   Ⓜ♀

    Z3A.22   22 weeks **gestation of pregnancy**   Ⓜ♀

    Z3A.23   23 weeks **gestation of pregnancy**   Ⓜ♀

    Z3A.24   24 weeks **gestation of pregnancy**   Ⓜ♀

    Z3A.25   25 weeks **gestation of pregnancy**   Ⓜ♀

    Z3A.26   26 weeks **gestation of pregnancy**   Ⓜ♀

    Z3A.27   27 weeks **gestation of pregnancy**   Ⓜ♀

    Z3A.28   28 weeks **gestation of pregnancy**   Ⓜ♀

    Z3A.29   29 weeks **gestation of pregnancy**   Ⓜ♀

✓5ᵗʰ **Z3A.3**   **Weeks of gestation of pregnancy, weeks** 30-39

    Z3A.30   30 weeks **gestation of pregnancy**   Ⓜ♀

    Z3A.31   31 weeks **gestation of pregnancy**   Ⓜ♀

    Z3A.32   32 weeks **gestation of pregnancy**   Ⓜ♀

    Z3A.33   33 weeks **gestation of pregnancy**   Ⓜ♀

    Z3A.34   34 weeks **gestation of pregnancy**   Ⓜ♀

    Z3A.35   35 weeks **gestation of pregnancy**   Ⓜ♀

    Z3A.36   36 weeks **gestation of pregnancy**   Ⓜ♀

    Z3A.37   37 weeks **gestation of pregnancy**   Ⓜ♀

    Z3A.38   38 weeks **gestation of pregnancy**   Ⓜ♀

    Z3A.39   39 weeks **gestation of pregnancy**   Ⓜ♀

✓5ᵗʰ **Z3A.4**   **Weeks of gestation of pregnancy, weeks** 40 or greater
    AHA: 2014,4Q,23

    Z3A.40   40 weeks **gestation of pregnancy**   Ⓜ♀

    Z3A.41   41 weeks **gestation of pregnancy**   Ⓜ♀

    Z3A.42   42 weeks **gestation of pregnancy**   Ⓜ♀

    Z3A.49   Greater than 42 weeks **gestation of pregnancy**   Ⓜ♀

✓4ᵗʰ **Z37**   **Outcome of delivery**

This category is intended for use as an additional code to identify the outcome of delivery on the mother's record. It is not for use on the newborn record.

> **EXCLUDES 1**   stillbirth (P95)

Z37.0   **Single live birth**   Ⓜ♀
    AHA: 2016,2Q,34; 2014,2Q,9

Z37.1   **Single stillbirth**   Ⓜ♀

Z37.2   **Twins, both liveborn**   Ⓜ♀

Z37.3   **Twins, one liveborn and one stillborn**   Ⓜ♀

Z37.4   **Twins, both stillborn**   Ⓜ♀

✓5ᵗʰ **Z37.5**   **Other multiple births, all liveborn**

    Z37.50   **Multiple births, unspecified, all liveborn**   Ⓜ♀

    Z37.51   **Triplets, all liveborn**   Ⓜ♀

    Z37.52   **Quadruplets, all liveborn**   Ⓜ♀

    Z37.53   **Quintuplets, all liveborn**   Ⓜ♀

    Z37.54   **Sextuplets, all liveborn**   Ⓜ♀

    Z37.59   **Other multiple births, all liveborn**   Ⓜ♀

✓5ᵗʰ **Z37.6**   **Other multiple births, some liveborn**

    Z37.60   **Multiple births, unspecified, some liveborn**   Ⓜ♀

    Z37.61   **Triplets, some liveborn**   Ⓜ♀

    Z37.62   **Quadruplets, some liveborn**   Ⓜ♀

    Z37.63   **Quintuplets, some liveborn**   Ⓜ♀

    Z37.64   **Sextuplets, some liveborn**   Ⓜ♀

    Z37.69   **Other multiple births, some liveborn**   Ⓜ♀

Z37.7   **Other multiple births, all stillborn**   Ⓜ♀

Z37.9   **Outcome of delivery, unspecified**   Ⓜ♀
    Multiple birth NOS
    Single birth NOS

✓4ᵗʰ **Z38**   **Liveborn infants according to place of birth and type of delivery**

This category is for use as the principal code on the initial record of a newborn baby. It is to be used for the initial birth record only. It is not to be used on the mother's record.
AHA: 2020,2Q,13; 2017,2Q,5-7; 2016,3Q,18; 2015,2Q,15

✓5ᵗʰ **Z38.0**   **Single liveborn infant,** born in hospital

    Single liveborn infant, born in birthing center or other health care facility

    Z38.00   **Single liveborn infant,** delivered vaginally   Ⓝ

    Z38.01   **Single liveborn infant,** delivered by cesarean   Ⓝ

Z38.1   **Single liveborn infant,** born outside hospital   Ⓝ

Z38.2   **Single liveborn infant, unspecified as to place of birth**   Ⓝ
    Single liveborn infant NOS

✓5ᵗʰ **Z38.3**   **Twin liveborn infant,** born in hospital

    Z38.30   **Twin liveborn infant,** delivered vaginally   Ⓝ

    Z38.31   **Twin liveborn infant,** delivered by cesarean   Ⓝ

Z38.4   **Twin liveborn infant,** born outside hospital   Ⓝ

Z38.5   **Twin liveborn infant, unspecified as to place of birth**   Ⓝ

✓5ᵗʰ **Z38.6**   **Other multiple liveborn infant, born in hospital**

    Z38.61   **Triplet liveborn infant,** delivered vaginally   Ⓝ

    Z38.62   **Triplet liveborn infant,** delivered by cesarean   Ⓝ

    Z38.63   **Quadruplet liveborn infant,** delivered vaginally   Ⓝ

    Z38.64   **Quadruplet liveborn infant,** delivered by cesarean   Ⓝ

    Z38.65   **Quintuplet liveborn infant,** delivered vaginally   Ⓝ

    Z38.66   **Quintuplet liveborn infant,** delivered by cesarean   Ⓝ

    Z38.68   **Other multiple liveborn infant,** delivered vaginally   Ⓝ

    Z38.69   **Other multiple liveborn infant,** delivered by cesarean   Ⓝ

Z38.7   **Other multiple liveborn infant,** born outside hospital   Ⓝ

Z38.8   **Other multiple liveborn infant, unspecified as to place of birth**   Ⓝ

✓4ᵗʰ **Z39**   **Encounter for maternal postpartum care and examination**

Z39.0   **Encounter for care and examination of mother** immediately after delivery   Ⓜ♀

    Care and observation in uncomplicated cases when the delivery occurs outside a healthcare facility

> **EXCLUDES 1**   care for postpartum complication — see Alphabetic Index

Chapter 21. Factors Influencing Health Status and Contact With Health Services

Z39.1 **Encounter for care and examination of lactating mother**   Ⓜ ♀
Encounter for supervision of lactation
EXCLUDES 1   disorders of lactation (O92.-)

Z39.2 **Encounter for routine postpartum follow-up**   Ⓜ ♀

Encounters for other specific health care (Z40-Z53)

Categories Z40-Z53 are intended for use to indicate a reason for care. They may be used for patients who have already been treated for a disease or injury, but who are receiving aftercare or prophylactic care, or care to consolidate the treatment, or to deal with a residual state

EXCLUDES 2   *follow-up examination for medical surveillance after treatment (Z08-Z09)*

✓4ᵗʰ **Z40** **Encounter for prophylactic surgery**
EXCLUDES 1   organ donations (Z52.-)
    therapeutic organ removal — code to condition
DEF: Agent or treatment measure intended to prevent or ward off a disease condition.

✓5ᵗʰ **Z40.0** **Encounter for prophylactic surgery for risk factors related to malignant neoplasms**
Admission for prophylactic organ removal
Use additional code to identify risk factor
AHA: 2017,4Q,28-29

    Z40.00 **Encounter for prophylactic removal of unspecified organ**

    Z40.01 **Encounter for prophylactic removal of breast**

    Z40.02 **Encounter for prophylactic removal of ovary(s)** ♀
       Encounter for prophylactic removal of ovary(s) and fallopian tube(s)

    Z40.03 **Encounter for prophylactic removal of fallopian tube(s)** ♀

    Z40.09 **Encounter for prophylactic removal of other organ**

    Z40.8 **Encounter for other prophylactic surgery**

    Z40.9 **Encounter for prophylactic surgery, unspecified**

✓4ᵗʰ **Z41** **Encounter for procedures for purposes other than remedying health state**

    Z41.1 **Encounter for cosmetic surgery**
Encounter for cosmetic breast implant
Encounter for cosmetic procedure
EXCLUDES 1   *encounter for plastic and reconstructive surgery following medical procedure or healed injury (Z42.-)*
      encounter for post-mastectomy breast implantation (Z42.1)

    Z41.2 **Encounter for routine and ritual male circumcision** ♂
AHA: 2018,3Q,15
TIP: Do not report this code when circumcision is performed during the birth admission.

    Z41.3 **Encounter for ear piercing**

    Z41.8 **Encounter for other procedures for purposes other than remedying health state**

    Z41.9 **Encounter for procedure for purposes other than remedying health state, unspecified**

✓4ᵗʰ **Z42** **Encounter for plastic and reconstructive surgery following medical procedure or healed injury**
EXCLUDES 1   *encounter for cosmetic plastic surgery (Z41.1)*
      encounter for plastic surgery for treatment of current injury — code to relevent injury

    Z42.1 **Encounter for breast reconstruction following mastectomy**   Ⓐ
EXCLUDES 1   *deformity and disproportion of reconstructed breast (N65.1-)*

    Z42.8 **Encounter for other plastic and reconstructive surgery following medical procedure or healed injury**
AHA: 2017,1Q,42

✓4ᵗʰ **Z43** **Encounter for attention to artificial openings**
INCLUDES   closure of artificial openings
      passage of sounds or bougies through artificial openings
      reforming artificial openings
      removal of catheter from artificial openings
      toilet or cleansing of artificial openings
EXCLUDES 1   *complications of external stoma (J95.0-, K94.-, N99.5-)*
EXCLUDES 2   *fitting and adjustment of prosthetic and other devices (Z44-Z46)*
AHA: 2019,2Q,33

    Z43.0 **Encounter for attention to tracheostomy**   HCC

    Z43.1 **Encounter for attention to gastrostomy**   CC HCC
EXCLUDES 2   *artificial opening status only, without need for care (Z93.-)*

    Z43.2 **Encounter for attention to ileostomy**   HCC

    Z43.3 **Encounter for attention to colostomy**   HCC

    Z43.4 **Encounter for attention to other artificial openings of digestive tract**   HCC

    Z43.5 **Encounter for attention to cystostomy**   HCC

    Z43.6 **Encounter for attention to other artificial openings of urinary tract**   HCC
Encounter for attention to nephrostomy
Encounter for attention to ureterostomy
Encounter for attention to urethrostomy

    Z43.7 **Encounter for attention to artificial vagina**

    Z43.8 **Encounter for attention to other artificial openings**   HCC

    Z43.9 **Encounter for attention to unspecified artificial opening**   HCC

✓4ᵗʰ **Z44** **Encounter for fitting and adjustment of external prosthetic device**
INCLUDES   removal or replacement of external prosthetic device
EXCLUDES 1   *malfunction or other complications of device — see Alphabetical Index*
      presence of prosthetic device (Z97.-)

✓5ᵗʰ **Z44.0** **Encounter for fitting and adjustment of artificial arm**

   ✓6ᵗʰ **Z44.00** **Encounter for fitting and adjustment of unspecified artificial arm**

    Z44.001 **Encounter for fitting and adjustment of unspecified right artificial arm**

    Z44.002 **Encounter for fitting and adjustment of unspecified left artificial arm**

    Z44.009 **Encounter for fitting and adjustment of unspecified artificial arm, unspecified arm**

   ✓6ᵗʰ **Z44.01** **Encounter for fitting and adjustment of complete artificial arm**

    Z44.011 **Encounter for fitting and adjustment of complete right artificial arm**

    Z44.012 **Encounter for fitting and adjustment of complete left artificial arm**

    Z44.019 **Encounter for fitting and adjustment of complete artificial arm, unspecified arm**

   ✓6ᵗʰ **Z44.02** **Encounter for fitting and adjustment of partial artificial arm**

    Z44.021 **Encounter for fitting and adjustment of partial artificial right arm**

    Z44.022 **Encounter for fitting and adjustment of partial artificial left arm**

    Z44.029 **Encounter for fitting and adjustment of partial artificial arm, unspecified arm**

✓5ᵗʰ **Z44.1** **Encounter for fitting and adjustment of artificial leg**

   ✓6ᵗʰ **Z44.10** **Encounter for fitting and adjustment of unspecified artificial leg**

    Z44.101 **Encounter for fitting and adjustment of unspecified right artificial leg**   HCC

    Z44.102 **Encounter for fitting and adjustment of unspecified left artificial leg**   HCC

    Z44.109 **Encounter for fitting and adjustment of unspecified artificial leg, unspecified leg**   HCC

   ✓6ᵗʰ **Z44.11** **Encounter for fitting and adjustment of complete artificial leg**

    Z44.111 **Encounter for fitting and adjustment of complete right artificial leg**   HCC

    Z44.112 **Encounter for fitting and adjustment of complete left artificial leg**   HCC

    Z44.119 **Encounter for fitting and adjustment of complete artificial leg, unspecified leg**   HCC

   ✓6ᵗʰ **Z44.12** **Encounter for fitting and adjustment of partial artificial leg**

    Z44.121 **Encounter for fitting and adjustment of partial artificial right leg**   HCC

    Z44.122 **Encounter for fitting and adjustment of partial artificial left leg**   HCC

    Z44.129 **Encounter for fitting and adjustment of partial artificial leg, unspecified leg**   HCC

☑5ᵗʰ **Z44.2** **Encounter for fitting and adjustment of** artificial eye

EXCLUDES 1   *mechanical complication of ocular prosthesis (T85.3)*

Z44.20 **Encounter for fitting and adjustment of artificial eye, unspecified**

Z44.21 **Encounter for fitting and adjustment of artificial** right **eye**

Z44.22 **Encounter for fitting and adjustment of artificial** left **eye**

☑5ᵗʰ **Z44.3** **Encounter for fitting and adjustment of** external breast prosthesis

EXCLUDES 1   *complications of breast implant (T85.4-)*

encounter for adjustment or removal of breast implant (Z45.81-)

encounter for initial breast implant insertion for cosmetic breast augmentation (Z41.1)

encounter for breast reconstruction following mastectomy (Z42.1)

Z44.30 **Encounter for fitting and adjustment of external breast prosthesis, unspecified breast**

Z44.31 **Encounter for fitting and adjustment of external** right **breast prosthesis**

Z44.32 **Encounter for fitting and adjustment of external** left **breast prosthesis**

Z44.8 **Encounter for fitting and adjustment of other external prosthetic devices**

Z44.9 **Encounter for fitting and adjustment of unspecified external prosthetic device**

☑4ᵗʰ **Z45** **Encounter for adjustment and management of implanted device**

INCLUDES   removal or replacement of implanted device

EXCLUDES 1   *malfunction or other complications of device — see Alphabetical Index*

EXCLUDES 2   *encounter for fitting and adjustment of non-implanted device (Z46.-)*

☑5ᵗʰ **Z45.0** **Encounter for adjustment and management of** cardiac device

☑6ᵗʰ **Z45.01** **Encounter for adjustment and management of cardiac** pacemaker

Encounter for adjustment and management of cardiac resynchronization therapy pacemaker (CRT-P)

EXCLUDES 1   *encounter for adjustment and management of automatic implantable cardiac defibrillator with synchronous cardiac pacemaker (Z45.02)*

TIP: Assign an additional code for the condition the pacemaker is controlling (e.g., sick sinus syndrome). Even though the pacemaker controls the heart rate, it does not cure the sick sinus syndrome; it is still present and a reportable chronic condition.

Z45.010 **Encounter for checking and testing of cardiac pacemaker** pulse generator **[battery]**

Encounter for replacing cardiac pacemaker pulse generator [battery]

Z45.018 **Encounter for adjustment and management of other part of cardiac pacemaker**

EXCLUDES 1   *presence of other part of cardiac pacemaker (Z95.0)*

EXCLUDES 2   *presence of prosthetic and other devices (Z95.1-Z95.5, Z95.811-Z97)*

Z45.02 **Encounter for adjustment and management of** automatic implantable cardiac defibrillator

Encounter for adjustment and management of automatic implantable cardiac defibrillator with synchronous cardiac pacemaker

Encounter for adjustment and management of cardiac resynchronization therapy defibrillator (CRT-D)

Z45.09 **Encounter for adjustment and management of other cardiac device**

Z45.1 **Encounter for adjustment and management of** infusion pump

Z45.2 **Encounter for adjustment and management of** vascular access device

Encounter for adjustment and management of vascular catheters

EXCLUDES 1   *encounter for adjustment and management of renal dialysis catheter (Z49.01)*

AHA: 2020,2Q,21; 2018,3Q,20

☑5ᵗʰ **Z45.3** **Encounter for adjustment and management of implanted** devices of the special senses

Z45.31 **Encounter for adjustment and management of implanted** visual substitution device

☑6ᵗʰ **Z45.32** **Encounter for adjustment and management of implanted** hearing device

EXCLUDES 1   *encounter for fitting and adjustment of hearing aide (Z46.1)*

Z45.320 **Encounter for adjustment and management of** bone conduction **device**

Z45.321 **Encounter for adjustment and management of** cochlear **device**

Z45.328 **Encounter for adjustment and management of other implanted hearing device**

☑5ᵗʰ **Z45.4** **Encounter for adjustment and management of implanted** nervous system device

Z45.41 **Encounter for adjustment and management of** cerebrospinal fluid drainage **device**

Encounter for adjustment and management of cerebral ventricular (communicating) shunt

Z45.42 **Encounter for adjustment and management of** neurostimulator

Encounter for adjustment and management of brain neurostimulator

Encounter for adjustment and management of gastric neurostimulator

Encounter for adjustment and management of peripheral nerve neurostimulator

Encounter for adjustment and management of sacral nerve neurostimulator

Encounter for adjustment and management of spinal cord neurostimulator

Encounter for adjustment and management of vagus nerve neurostimulator

Z45.49 **Encounter for adjustment and management of other implanted nervous system device**

AHA: 2014,3Q,19

☑5ᵗʰ **Z45.8** **Encounter for adjustment and management of other implanted devices**

☑6ᵗʰ **Z45.81** **Encounter for adjustment or** removal of breast implant

Encounter for elective implant exchange (different material) (different size)

Encounter removal of tissue expander with or without synchronous insertion of permanent implant

EXCLUDES 1   *complications of breast implant (T85.4-)*

encounter for initial breast implant insertion for cosmetic breast augmentation (Z41.1)

encounter for breast reconstruction following mastectomy (Z42.1)

Z45.811 **Encounter for adjustment or removal of** right **breast implant**

Z45.812 **Encounter for adjustment or removal of** left **breast implant**

Z45.819 **Encounter for adjustment or removal of unspecified breast implant**

Z45.82 **Encounter for** adjustment or removal of myringotomy device **(stent) (tube)**

Z45.89 **Encounter for adjustment and management of other implanted devices**

AHA: 2014,4Q,26-28

Z45.9 **Encounter for adjustment and management of unspecified implanted device**

☑ Additional Character Required   ☑x7ᵗʰ Placeholder   Unacceptable PDx   Questionable PDx   Manifestation   Unspecified Dx   H1-H14 HAC   HCC CMS-HCC Dx   HIV HIV Dx

ICD-10-CM 2021   1245

Chapter 21. Factors Influencing Health Status and Contact With Health Services

✓4ᵗʰ **Z46 Encounter for fitting and adjustment of other devices**

INCLUDES   removal or replacement of other device

EXCLUDES 1   malfunction or other complications of device — see Alphabetical Index

EXCLUDES 2   encounter for fitting and management of implanted devices (Z45.-)

issue of repeat prescription only (Z76.Ø)

presence of prosthetic and other devices (Z95-Z97)

Z46.Ø Encounter for fitting and adjustment of spectacles and contact lenses

Z46.1 Encounter for fitting and adjustment of hearing aid

EXCLUDES 1   encounter for adjustment and management of implanted hearing device (Z45.32-)

Z46.2 Encounter for fitting and adjustment of other devices related to nervous system and special senses

EXCLUDES 2   encounter for adjustment and management of implanted nervous system device (Z45.4-)

encounter for adjustment and management of implanted visual substitution device (Z45.31)

Z46.3 Encounter for fitting and adjustment of dental prosthetic device

Encounter for fitting and adjustment of dentures

Z46.4 Encounter for fitting and adjustment of orthodontic device

✓5ᵗʰ **Z46.5 Encounter for fitting and adjustment of other gastrointestinal appliance and device**

EXCLUDES 1   encounter for attention to artificial openings of digestive tract (Z43.1-Z43.4)

Z46.51 Encounter for fitting and adjustment of gastric lap band

Z46.59 Encounter for fitting and adjustment of other gastrointestinal appliance and device

Z46.6 Encounter for fitting and adjustment of urinary device

EXCLUDES 2   attention to artificial openings of urinary tract (Z43.5, Z43.6)

✓5ᵗʰ **Z46.8 Encounter for fitting and adjustment of other specified devices**

Z46.81 Encounter for fitting and adjustment of insulin pump

Encounter for insulin pump instruction and training

Encounter for insulin pump titration

Z46.82 Encounter for fitting and adjustment of non-vascular catheter

Z46.89 Encounter for fitting and adjustment of other specified devices

Encounter for fitting and adjustment of wheelchair

Z46.9 Encounter for fitting and adjustment of unspecified device

✓4ᵗʰ **Z47 Orthopedic aftercare**

EXCLUDES 1   aftercare for healing fracture — code to fracture with 7th character D

Z47.1 Aftercare following joint replacement surgery

Use additional code to identify the joint (Z96.6-)

AHA: 2020,1Q,23

Z47.2 Encounter for removal of internal fixation device

EXCLUDES 1   encounter for adjustment of internal fixation device for fracture treatment — code to fracture with appropriate 7th character

encounter for removal of external fixation device — code to fracture with 7th character D

infection or inflammatory reaction to internal fixation device (T84.6-)

mechanical complication of internal fixation device (T84.1-)

✓5ᵗʰ **Z47.3 Aftercare following explantation of joint prosthesis**

Aftercare following explantation of joint prosthesis, staged procedure

Encounter for joint prosthesis insertion following prior explantation of joint prosthesis

AHA: 2020,1Q,23; 2015,1Q,16

Z47.31 Aftercare following explantation of shoulder joint prosthesis

EXCLUDES 1   acquired absence of shoulder joint following prior explantation of shoulder joint prosthesis (Z89.23-)

shoulder joint prosthesis explantation status (Z89.23-)

Z47.32 Aftercare following explantation of hip joint prosthesis

EXCLUDES 1   acquired absence of hip joint following prior explantation of hip joint prosthesis (Z89.62-)

hip joint prosthesis explantation status (Z89.62-)

Z47.33 Aftercare following explantation of knee joint prosthesis

EXCLUDES 1   acquired absence of knee joint following prior explantation of knee prosthesis (Z89.52-)

knee joint prosthesis explantation status (Z89.52-)

✓5ᵗʰ **Z47.8 Encounter for other orthopedic aftercare**

Z47.81 Encounter for orthopedic aftercare following surgical amputation

Use additional code to identify the limb amputated (Z89.-)

Z47.82 Encounter for orthopedic aftercare following scoliosis surgery

Z47.89 Encounter for other orthopedic aftercare

AHA: 2015,1Q,8

✓4ᵗʰ **Z48 Encounter for other postprocedural aftercare**

EXCLUDES 1   encounter for aftercare following injury — code to Injury, by site, with appropriate 7th character for subsequent encounter

encounter for follow-up examination after completed treatment (ZØ8-ZØ9)

EXCLUDES 2   encounter for attention to artificial openings (Z43.-)

encounter for fitting and adjustment of prosthetic and other devices (Z44-Z46)

AHA: 2015,4Q,38; 2015,1Q,6-7

✓5ᵗʰ **Z48.Ø Encounter for attention to dressings, sutures and drains**

EXCLUDES 1   encounter for planned postprocedural wound closure (Z48.1)

Z48.ØØ Encounter for change or removal of nonsurgical wound dressing

Encounter for change or removal of wound dressing NOS

Z48.Ø1 Encounter for change or removal of surgical wound dressing

AHA: 2019,2Q,33

Z48.Ø2 Encounter for removal of sutures

Encounter for removal of staples

Z48.Ø3 Encounter for change or removal of drains

AHA: 2019,2Q,33

Z48.1 Encounter for planned postprocedural wound closure

EXCLUDES 1   encounter for attention to dressings and sutures (Z48.Ø-)

✓5ᵗʰ **Z48.2 Encounter for aftercare following organ transplant**

Z48.21 Encounter for aftercare following heart transplant   CC   HCC

Z48.22 Encounter for aftercare following kidney transplant   CC

Z48.23 Encounter for aftercare following liver transplant   CC   HCC

Z48.24 Encounter for aftercare following lung transplant   CC   HCC

✓6ᵗʰ **Z48.28 Encounter for aftercare following multiple organ transplant**

Z48.28Ø Encounter for aftercare following heart-lung transplant   CC   HCC

Z48.288 Encounter for aftercare following multiple organ transplant

✓6ᵗʰ **Z48.29 Encounter for aftercare following other organ transplant**

Z48.29Ø Encounter for aftercare following bone marrow transplant   CC   HCC

Z48.298 Encounter for aftercare following other organ transplant

Z48.3 Aftercare following surgery for neoplasm

Use additional code to identify the neoplasm

N Newborn: 0   P Pediatric: 0-17   M Maternity: 9-64   A Adult: 15-124   MCC Major Complication/Comorbidity   CC Complication/Comorbidity   SW Severe Wound Dx

1246   ICD-10-CM 2021

✓5th Z48.8 Encounter for other specified postprocedural aftercare

   ✓6th **Z48.81 Encounter for surgical aftercare following surgery on specified body systems**

         These codes identify the body system requiring aftercare. They are for use in conjunction with other aftercare codes to fully explain the aftercare encounter. The condition treated should also be coded if still present.

         EXCLUDES 1   *aftercare for injury — code the injury with 7th character D*
                    aftercare following surgery for neoplasm (Z48.3)

         EXCLUDES 2   *aftercare following organ transplant (Z48.2-)*
                    orthopedic aftercare (Z47.-)

         AHA: 2015,4Q,38

         Z48.810 Encounter for surgical aftercare following surgery on the sense organs

         Z48.811 Encounter for surgical aftercare following surgery on the nervous system
                 EXCLUDES 2   *encounter for surgical aftercare following surgery on the sense organs (Z48.810)*

         Z48.812 Encounter for surgical aftercare following surgery on the circulatory system
                 AHA: 2012,4Q,96

         Z48.813 Encounter for surgical aftercare following surgery on the respiratory system
                 AHA: 2019,2Q,33

         Z48.814 Encounter for surgical aftercare following surgery on the teeth or oral cavity

         Z48.815 Encounter for surgical aftercare following surgery on the digestive system

         Z48.816 Encounter for surgical aftercare following surgery on the genitourinary system
                 EXCLUDES 1   *encounter for aftercare following sterilization reversal (Z31.42)*

         Z48.817 Encounter for surgical aftercare following surgery on the skin and subcutaneous tissue

         Z48.89 Encounter for other specified surgical aftercare

✓4th Z49 Encounter for care involving renal dialysis

    Code also associated end stage renal disease (N18.6)

   ✓5th **Z49.0 Preparatory care for renal dialysis**

         Encounter for dialysis instruction and training

         Z49.01 Encounter for fitting and adjustment of extracorporeal dialysis catheter HCC
                 Removal or replacement of renal dialysis catheter
                 Toilet or cleansing of renal dialysis catheter

         Z49.02 Encounter for fitting and adjustment of peritoneal dialysis catheter HCC

   ✓5th **Z49.3 Encounter for adequacy testing for dialysis**

         Z49.31 Encounter for adequacy testing for hemodialysis HCC

         Z49.32 Encounter for adequacy testing for peritoneal dialysis HCC
                 Encounter for peritoneal equilibration test

✓4th Z51 Encounter for other aftercare and medical care

    Code also condition requiring care
    EXCLUDES 1   *follow-up examination after treatment (Z08-Z09)*

    Z51.0 Encounter for antineoplastic radiation therapy
         AHA: 2017,4Q,103
         TIP: Do not assign when admission is for insertion/implantation of radioactive elements. Assign a code for the malignancy instead. Any complications related to the radioactive elements should be assigned as secondary diagnoses.

   ✓5th **Z51.1 Encounter for antineoplastic chemotherapy and immunotherapy**
         EXCLUDES 2   *encounter for chemotherapy and immunotherapy for nonneoplastic condition — code to condition*

         Z51.11 Encounter for antineoplastic chemotherapy
                 AHA: 2015,3Q,19

         Z51.12 Encounter for antineoplastic immunotherapy

    Z51.5 Encounter for palliative care
         AHA: 2017,1Q,48

    Z51.6 Encounter for desensitization to allergens
         AHA: 2016,4Q,77

   ✓5th **Z51.8 Encounter for other specified aftercare**
         EXCLUDES 1   *holiday relief care (Z75.5)*

         Z51.81 Encounter for therapeutic drug level monitoring
                 Code also any long-term (current) drug therapy (Z79.-)
                 EXCLUDES 1   *encounter for blood-drug test for administrative or medicolegal reasons (Z02.83)*
                 DEF: Drug monitoring: Measurement of the level of a specific drug in the body or measurement of a specific function to assess effectiveness of a drug.

         Z51.89 Encounter for other specified aftercare
                 AHA: 2012,4Q,95-97

✓4th Z52 Donors of organs and tissues

    INCLUDES   autologous and other living donors
    EXCLUDES 1   *cadaveric donor - omit code*
                 examination of potential donor (Z00.5)
    AHA: 2012,4Q,99

   ✓5th **Z52.0 Blood donor**

        ✓6th **Z52.00 Unspecified blood donor**
                 Z52.000 Unspecified donor, whole blood
                 Z52.001 Unspecified donor, stem cells
                 Z52.008 Unspecified donor, other blood

        ✓6th **Z52.01 Autologous blood donor**
                 Z52.010 Autologous donor, whole blood
                 Z52.011 Autologous donor, stem cells
                 Z52.018 Autologous donor, other blood

        ✓6th **Z52.09 Other blood donor**
                 Volunteer donor
                 Z52.090 Other blood donor, whole blood
                 Z52.091 Other blood donor, stem cells
                 Z52.098 Other blood donor, other blood

   ✓5th **Z52.1 Skin donor**
         Z52.10 Skin donor, unspecified
         Z52.11 Skin donor, autologous
         Z52.19 Skin donor, other

   ✓5th **Z52.2 Bone donor**
         Z52.20 Bone donor, unspecified
         Z52.21 Bone donor, autologous
         Z52.29 Bone donor, other

    Z52.3 Bone marrow donor

    Z52.4 Kidney donor

    Z52.5 Cornea donor

    Z52.6 Liver donor

   ✓5th **Z52.8 Donor of other specified organs or tissues**

        ✓6th **Z52.81 Egg (Oocyte) donor**
                 Z52.810 Egg (Oocyte) donor under age 35, anonymous recipient ♀
                      Egg donor under age 35 NOS
                 Z52.811 Egg (Oocyte) donor under age 35, designated recipient ♀
                 Z52.812 Egg (Oocyte) donor age 35 and over, anonymous recipient ♀
                      Egg donor age 35 and over NOS
                 Z52.813 Egg (Oocyte) donor age 35 and over, designated recipient ♀
                 Z52.819 Egg (Oocyte) donor unspecified ♀

         Z52.89 Donor of other specified organs or tissues

    Z52.9 Donor of unspecified organ or tissue
         Donor NOS

✓4th Z53 Persons encountering health services for specific procedures and treatment, not carried out

   ✓5th **Z53.0 Procedure and treatment not carried out because of contraindication**
         Z53.01 Procedure and treatment not carried out due to patient smoking
         Z53.09 Procedure and treatment not carried out because of other contraindication

    Z53.1 Procedure and treatment not carried out because of patient's decision for reasons of belief and group pressure

   ✓5th **Z53.2 Procedure and treatment not carried out because of patient's decision for other and unspecified reasons**
         Z53.20 Procedure and treatment not carried out because of patient's decision for unspecified reasons

---

✓ Additional Character Required   ✓x7th Placeholder   Unacceptable PDx   Questionable PDx   Manifestation   Unspecified Dx   H1-H14 HAC   HCC CMS-HCC Dx   HIV HIV Dx

Z53.21 **Procedure and treatment not carried out due to patient** leaving prior to being seen by health care provider

Z53.29 **Procedure and treatment not carried out because of patient's decision for other reasons**

✓5ᵗʰ Z53.3 **Procedure converted to open procedure**
    AHA: 2016,4Q,79

Z53.31 **Laparoscopic surgical procedure converted to open procedure**

Z53.32 **Thoracoscopic surgical procedure converted to open procedure**

Z53.33 **Arthroscopic surgical procedure converted to open procedure**

Z53.39 **Other specified procedure converted to open procedure**

Z53.8 **Procedure and treatment not carried out for other reasons**

Z53.9 **Procedure and treatment not carried out, unspecified reason**

Persons with potential health hazards related to socioeconomic and psychosocial circumstances (Z55-Z65)

AHA: 2019,4Q,66; 2018,4Q,58,73; 2018,1Q,18
TIP: Codes from this code block can be assigned based on documentation from clinicians other than the diagnosing provider.

✓4ᵗʰ Z55 **Problems related to education and literacy**
    EXCLUDES 1   disorders of psychological development (F80-F89)

Z55.0 **Illiteracy and low-level literacy**

Z55.1 **Schooling unavailable and unattainable**

Z55.2 **Failed school examinations**

Z55.3 **Underachievement in school**

Z55.4 **Educational maladjustment and discord with teachers and classmates**

Z55.8 **Other problems related to education and literacy**
    Problems related to inadequate teaching

Z55.9 **Problems related to education and literacy, unspecified**
    Academic problems NOS

✓4ᵗʰ Z56 **Problems related to employment and unemployment**
    EXCLUDES 2   occupational exposure to risk factors (Z57.-)
         problems related to housing and economic circumstances (Z59.-)

Z56.0 **Unemployment, unspecified**

Z56.1 **Change of job**   A

Z56.2 **Threat of job loss**

Z56.3 **Stressful work schedule**

Z56.4 **Discord with boss and workmates**

Z56.5 **Uncongenial work environment**
    Difficult conditions at work

Z56.6 **Other physical and mental strain related to work**

✓5ᵗʰ Z56.8 **Other problems related to employment**

Z56.81 **Sexual harassment on the job**

Z56.82 **Military deployment status**
    Individual (civilian or military) currently deployed in theater or in support of military war, peacekeeping and humanitarian operations

Z56.89 **Other problems related to employment**

Z56.9 **Unspecified problems related to employment**
    Occupational problems NOS

✓4ᵗʰ Z57 **Occupational exposure to risk factors**

Z57.0 **Occupational exposure to noise**

Z57.1 **Occupational exposure to radiation**

Z57.2 **Occupational exposure to dust**

✓5ᵗʰ Z57.3 **Occupational exposure to other air contaminants**

Z57.31 **Occupational exposure to environmental tobacco smoke**
    EXCLUDES 2   exposure to environmental tobacco smoke (Z77.22)

Z57.39 **Occupational exposure to other air contaminants**

Z57.4 **Occupational exposure to toxic agents in agriculture**
    Occupational exposure to solids, liquids, gases or vapors in agriculture

Z57.5 **Occupational exposure to toxic agents in other industries**
    Occupational exposure to solids, liquids, gases or vapors in other industries

Z57.6 **Occupational exposure to extreme temperature**

Z57.7 **Occupational exposure to vibration**

Z57.8 **Occupational exposure to other risk factors**

Z57.9 **Occupational exposure to unspecified risk factor**

✓4ᵗʰ Z59 **Problems related to housing and economic circumstances**
    EXCLUDES 2   problems related to upbringing (Z62.-)

Z59.0 **Homelessness**

Z59.1 **Inadequate housing**
    Lack of heating
    Restriction of space
    Technical defects in home preventing adequate care
    Unsatisfactory surroundings
    EXCLUDES 1   problems related to the natural and physical environment (Z77.1-)

Z59.2 **Discord with neighbors, lodgers and landlord**

Z59.3 **Problems related to living in residential institution**
    Boarding-school resident
    EXCLUDES 1   institutional upbringing (Z62.2)

Z59.4 **Lack of adequate food and safe drinking water**
    Inadequate drinking water supply
    EXCLUDES 1   effects of hunger (T73.0)
         inappropriate diet or eating habits (Z72.4)
         malnutrition (E40-E46)

Z59.5 **Extreme poverty**

Z59.6 **Low income**

Z59.7 **Insufficient social insurance and welfare support**

Z59.8 **Other problems related to housing and economic circumstances**
    Foreclosure on loan
    Isolated dwelling
    Problems with creditors

Z59.9 **Problem related to housing and economic circumstances, unspecified**

✓4ᵗʰ Z60 **Problems related to social environment**

Z60.0 **Problems of adjustment to life-cycle transitions**
    Empty nest syndrome
    Phase of life problem
    Problem with adjustment to retirement [pension]

Z60.2 **Problems related to living alone**

Z60.3 **Acculturation difficulty**
    Problem with migration
    Problem with social transplantation
    DEF: Problem adapting to a different culture or environment not based on any coexisting mental disorder.

Z60.4 **Social exclusion and rejection**
    Exclusion and rejection on the basis of personal characteristics, such as unusual physical appearance, illness or behavior.
    EXCLUDES 1   target of adverse discrimination such as for racial or religious reasons (Z60.5)

Z60.5 **Target of (perceived) adverse discrimination and persecution**
    EXCLUDES 1   social exclusion and rejection (Z60.4)

Z60.8 **Other problems related to social environment**

Z60.9 **Problem related to social environment, unspecified**

✓4ᵗʰ Z62 **Problems related to upbringing**
    INCLUDES   current and past negative life events in childhood
         current and past problems of a child related to upbringing
    EXCLUDES 2   maltreatment syndrome (T74.-)
         problems related to housing and economic circumstances (Z59.-)

Z62.0 **Inadequate parental supervision and control**

Z62.1 **Parental overprotection**

✓5ᵗʰ Z62.2 **Upbringing away from parents**
    EXCLUDES 1   problems with boarding school (Z59.3)

Z62.21 **Child in welfare custody**   P
    Child in care of non-parental family member
    Child in foster care
    EXCLUDES 2   problem for parent due to child in welfare custody (Z63.5)

Z62.22 **Institutional upbringing**
    Child living in orphanage or group home

Z62.29 **Other upbringing away from parents**

Z62.3 **Hostility towards and scapegoating of child**   P

Z62.6 **Inappropriate (excessive) parental pressure**

✓5ʰ Z62.8 Other specified problems related to upbringing

     ✓6ʰ Z62.81 Personal history of abuse in childhood

         Z62.810 Personal history of physical and sexual abuse in childhood

             EXCLUDES 1   current child physical abuse (T74.12, T76.12)

                 current child sexual abuse (T74.22, T76.22)

         Z62.811 Personal history of psychological abuse in childhood

             EXCLUDES 1   current child psychological abuse (T74.32, T76.32)

         Z62.812 Personal history of neglect in childhood

             EXCLUDES 1   current child neglect (T74.02, T76.02)

         Z62.813 Personal history of forced labor or sexual exploitation in childhood

             AHA: 2018,4Q,32,35

         Z62.819 Personal history of unspecified abuse in childhood

             EXCLUDES 1   current child abuse NOS (T74.92, T76.92)

     ✓6ʰ Z62.82 Parent-child conflict

         Z62.820 Parent-biological child conflict

             Parent-child problem NOS

         Z62.821 Parent-adopted child conflict

         Z62.822 Parent-foster child conflict

     ✓6ʰ Z62.89 Other specified problems related to upbringing

         Z62.890 Parent-child estrangement NEC

         Z62.891 Sibling rivalry

         Z62.898 Other specified problems related to upbringing

Z62.9 Problem related to upbringing, unspecified

✓4ʰ Z63 Other problems related to primary support group, including family circumstances

     EXCLUDES 2   maltreatment syndrome (T74.-, T76)

               parent-child problems (Z62.-)

               problems related to negative life events in childhood (Z62.-)

               problems related to upbringing (Z62.-)

Z63.0 Problems in relationship with spouse or partner

     Relationship distress with spouse or intimate partner

     EXCLUDES 1   counseling for spousal or partner abuse problems (Z69.1)

               counseling related to sexual attitude, behavior, and orientation (Z70.-)

Z63.1 Problems in relationship with in-laws

✓5ʰ Z63.3 Absence of family member

     EXCLUDES 1   absence of family member due to disappearance and death (Z63.4)

               absence of family member due to separation and divorce (Z63.5)

     Z63.31 Absence of family member due to military deployment

         Individual or family affected by other family member being on military deployment

         EXCLUDES 1   family disruption due to return of family member from military deployment (Z63.71)

     Z63.32 Other absence of family member

Z63.4 Disappearance and death of family member

     Assumed death of family member

     Bereavement

     AHA: 2014,1Q,25

Z63.5 Disruption of family by separation and divorce

     Marital estrangement

Z63.6 Dependent relative needing care at home

✓5ʰ Z63.7 Other stressful life events affecting family and household

     Z63.71 Stress on family due to return of family member from military deployment

         Individual or family affected by family member having returned from military deployment (current or past conflict)

     Z63.72 Alcoholism and drug addiction in family

     Z63.79 Other stressful life events affecting family and household

         Anxiety (normal) about sick person in family

         Health problems within family

         Ill or disturbed family member

         Isolated family

Z63.8 Other specified problems related to primary support group

     Family discord NOS

     Family estrangement NOS

     High expressed emotional level within family

     Inadequate family support NOS

     Inadequate or distorted communication within family

Z63.9 Problem related to primary support group, unspecified

     Relationship disorder NOS

✓4ʰ Z64 Problems related to certain psychosocial circumstances

     Z64.0 Problems related to unwanted pregnancy   ♀

     Z64.1 Problems related to multiparity   ♀

     Z64.4 Discord with counselors

         Discord with probation officer

         Discord with social worker

✓4ʰ Z65 Problems related to other psychosocial circumstances

     Z65.0 Conviction in civil and criminal proceedings without imprisonment

     Z65.1 Imprisonment and other incarceration

     Z65.2 Problems related to release from prison

     Z65.3 Problems related to other legal circumstances

         Arrest

         Child custody or support proceedings

         Litigation

         Prosecution

     Z65.4 Victim of crime and terrorism

         Victim of torture

     Z65.5 Exposure to disaster, war and other hostilities

         EXCLUDES 1   target of perceived discrimination or persecution (Z60.5)

     Z65.8 Other specified problems related to psychosocial circumstances

         Religious or spiritual problem

     Z65.9 Problem related to unspecified psychosocial circumstances

Do not resuscitate status (Z66)

Z66 Do not resuscitate

     DNR status

     DEF: Medical order written by a physician that instructs others not to perform cardiopulmonary resuscitation (CPR), intubation, or advanced life support (ACLS). It prevents unnecessary invasive treatment to prolong life should breathing stop or cardiac arrest occur.

Blood type (Z67)

✓4ʰ Z67 Blood type

     AHA: 2015,3Q,40

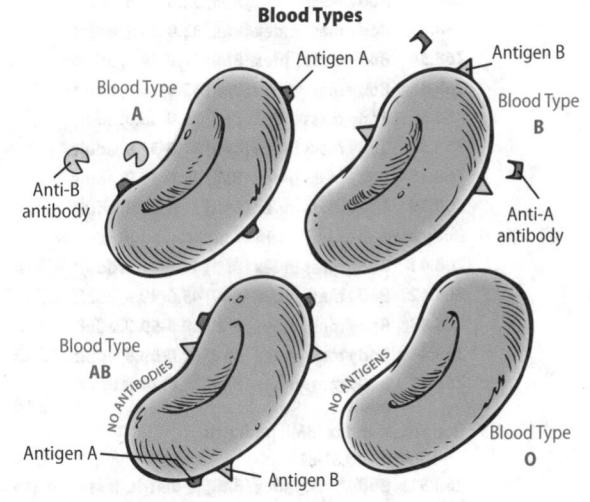

Blood Types

Blood Type A — Antigen A — Anti-B antibody

Blood Type B — Antigen B — Anti-A antibody

Blood Type AB — NO ANTIBODIES — Antigen A — Antigen B

Blood Type O — NO ANTIGENS

✓5ʰ Z67.1 Type A blood

     Z67.10 Type A blood, Rh positive

☑ Additional Character Required   ✓x7ʰ Placeholder   Unacceptable PDx   Questionable PDx   Manifestation   Unspecified Dx   H1-H14 HAC   HCC CMS-HCC Dx   HIV HIV Dx

ICD-10-CM 2021   1249

Z67.11 **Type A blood,** Rh negative

✓5ᵗʰ Z67.2 **Type B** blood

Z67.20 **Type B blood,** Rh positive
Z67.21 **Type B blood,** Rh negative

✓5ᵗʰ Z67.3 **Type AB** blood

Z67.30 **Type AB blood,** Rh positive
Z67.31 **Type AB blood,** Rh negative

✓5ᵗʰ Z67.4 **Type O** blood

Z67.40 **Type O blood,** Rh positive
Z67.41 **Type O blood,** Rh negative

✓5ᵗʰ Z67.9 **Unspecified blood type**

Z67.90 **Unspecified blood type,** Rh positive
Z67.91 **Unspecified blood type,** Rh negative

Body mass index [BMI] (Z68)

✓4ᵗʰ Z68 **Body mass index [BMI]**

Kilograms per meters squared

NOTE BMI adult codes are for use for persons 20 years of age or older

BMI pediatric codes are for use for persons 2-19 years of age.

These percentiles are based on the growth charts published by the Centers for Disease Control and Prevention (CDC)

AHA: 2019,4Q,19,57; 2018,4Q,73,77-83; 2017,1Q,39
DEF: Index used to help determine whether an individual is underweight, a healthy weight, overweight, or obese.
TIP: A BMI code may be assigned to support an associated condition based on medical record documentation from clinicians who are not the patient's provider.
TIP: Do not assign when used in association with fluctuations in body fluid during an encounter, such as fluid overload or fluid retention.
TIP: In order to assign a BMI code, the associated condition must meet the definition of a reportable diagnosis for nonoutpatient encounters, per section III of the *ICD-10-CM Official Guidelines for Coding and Reporting*.

▲ Z68.1 **Body mass index [BMI]** 19.9 or less, **adult** 〔CC〕〔A〕

▲ ✓5ᵗʰ Z68.2 **Body mass index [BMI]** 20-29, **adult**

▲ Z68.20 **Body mass index [BMI]** 20.0-20.9, **adult** 〔A〕
▲ Z68.21 **Body mass index [BMI]** 21.0-21.9, **adult** 〔A〕
▲ Z68.22 **Body mass index [BMI]** 22.0-22.9, **adult** 〔A〕
▲ Z68.23 **Body mass index [BMI]** 23.0-23.9, **adult** 〔A〕
▲ Z68.24 **Body mass index [BMI]** 24.0-24.9, **adult** 〔A〕
▲ Z68.25 **Body mass index [BMI]** 25.0-25.9, **adult** 〔A〕
▲ Z68.26 **Body mass index [BMI]** 26.0-26.9, **adult** 〔A〕
▲ Z68.27 **Body mass index [BMI]** 27.0-27.9, **adult** 〔A〕
▲ Z68.28 **Body mass index [BMI]** 28.0-28.9, **adult** 〔A〕
▲ Z68.29 **Body mass index [BMI]** 29.0-29.9, **adult** 〔A〕

▲ ✓5ᵗʰ Z68.3 **Body mass index [BMI]** 30-39, **adult**

▲ Z68.30 **Body mass index [BMI]** 30.0-30.9, **adult** 〔A〕
▲ Z68.31 **Body mass index [BMI]** 31.0-31.9, **adult** 〔A〕
▲ Z68.32 **Body mass index [BMI]** 32.0-32.9, **adult** 〔A〕
▲ Z68.33 **Body mass index [BMI]** 33.0-33.9, **adult** 〔A〕
▲ Z68.34 **Body mass index [BMI]** 34.0-34.9, **adult** 〔A〕
▲ Z68.35 **Body mass index [BMI]** 35.0-35.9, **adult** 〔A〕
▲ Z68.36 **Body mass index [BMI]** 36.0-36.9, **adult** 〔A〕
▲ Z68.37 **Body mass index [BMI]** 37.0-37.9, **adult** 〔A〕
▲ Z68.38 **Body mass index [BMI]** 38.0-38.9, **adult** 〔A〕
▲ Z68.39 **Body mass index [BMI]** 39.0-39.9, **adult** 〔A〕

▲ ✓5ᵗʰ Z68.4 **Body mass index [BMI]** 40 or greater, **adult**

▲ Z68.41 **Body mass index [BMI]** 40.0-44.9, **adult** 〔CC〕〔HCC〕〔A〕
▲ Z68.42 **Body mass index [BMI]** 45.0-49.9, **adult** 〔CC〕〔HCC〕〔A〕
▲ Z68.43 **Body mass index [BMI]** 50.0-59.9, **adult** 〔CC〕〔HCC〕〔A〕
▲ Z68.44 **Body mass index [BMI]** 60.0-69.9, **adult** 〔CC〕〔HCC〕〔A〕
▲ Z68.45 **Body mass index [BMI]** 70 or greater, **adult** 〔CC〕〔HCC〕〔A〕

▲ ✓5ᵗʰ Z68.5 **Body mass index [BMI]** pediatric

AHA: 2018,4Q,81-82

▲ Z68.51 **Body mass index [BMI]** pediatric, less than 5th percentile for age

▲ Z68.52 **Body mass index [BMI]** pediatric, 5th percentile to less than 85th percentile for age

▲ Z68.53 **Body mass index [BMI]** pediatric, 85th percentile to less than 95th percentile for age

▲ Z68.54 **Body mass index [BMI]** pediatric, greater than or equal to 95th percentile for age

Persons encountering health services in other circumstances (Z69-Z76)

✓4ᵗʰ Z69 **Encounter for mental health services for victim and perpetrator of abuse**

INCLUDES counseling for victims and perpetrators of abuse

✓5ᵗʰ Z69.0 **Encounter for mental health services for child abuse problems**

✓6ᵗʰ Z69.01 **Encounter for mental health services for** parental child abuse

Z69.010 **Encounter for mental health services for** victim of **parental child abuse** 〔P〕
Encounter for mental health services for victim of child abuse by parent
Encounter for mental health services for victim of child neglect by parent
Encounter for mental health services for victim of child psychological abuse by parent
Encounter for mental health services for victim of child sexual abuse by parent

Z69.011 **Encounter for mental health services for** perpetrator of **parental child abuse**
Encounter for mental health services for perpetrator of parental child neglect
Encounter for mental health services for perpetrator of parental child psychological abuse
Encounter for mental health services for perpetrator of parental child sexual abuse
EXCLUDES 1 *encounter for mental health services for non-parental child abuse (Z69.02-)*

✓6ᵗʰ Z69.02 **Encounter for mental health services for** non-parental child abuse

Z69.020 **Encounter for mental health services for** victim of **non-parental child abuse** 〔P〕
Encounter for mental health services for victim of non-parental child neglect
Encounter for mental health services for victim of non-parental child psychological abuse
Encounter for mental health services for victim of non-parental child sexual abuse

Z69.021 **Encounter for mental health services for** perpetrator of **non-parental child abuse**
Encounter for mental health services for perpetrator of non-parental child neglect
Encounter for mental health services for perpetrator of non-parental child psychological abuse
Encounter for mental health services for perpetrator of non-parental child sexual abuse

✓5ᵗʰ Z69.1 **Encounter for mental health services for** spousal or partner abuse **problems**

Z69.11 **Encounter for mental health services for** victim of **spousal or partner abuse**
Encounter for mental health services for victim of spouse or partner neglect
Encounter for mental health services for victim of spouse or partner psychological abuse
Encounter for mental health services for victim of spouse or partner violence, physical

---

〔N〕 Newborn: 0 〔P〕 Pediatric: 0-17 〔M〕 Maternity: 9-64 〔A〕 Adult: 15-124 〔MCC〕 Major Complication/Comorbidity 〔CC〕 Complication/Comorbidity 〔SW〕 Severe Wound Dx

Z69.12   **Encounter for mental health services for perpetrator of spousal or partner abuse**
Encounter for mental health services for perpetrator of spouse or partner neglect
Encounter for mental health services for perpetrator of spouse or partner psychological abuse
Encounter for mental health services for perpetrator of spouse or partner violence, physical
Encounter for mental health services for perpetrator of spouse or partner violence, sexual

√5ᵗʰ Z69.8   **Encounter for mental health services for victim or perpetrator of other abuse**

Z69.81   **Encounter for mental health services for victim of other abuse**
Encounter for mental health services for victim of non-spousal adult abuse
Encounter for mental health services for victim of spouse or partner violence, sexual
Encounter for rape victim counseling

Z69.82   **Encounter for mental health services for perpetrator of other abuse**
Encounter for mental health services for perpetrator of non-spousal adult abuse

√4ᵗʰ **Z70   Counseling related to sexual attitude, behavior and orientation**

INCLUDES   encounter for mental health services for sexual attitude, behavior and orientation

EXCLUDES 2   contraceptive or procreative counseling (Z30-Z31)

Z70.0   **Counseling related to sexual attitude**

Z70.1   **Counseling related to patient's sexual behavior and orientation**
Patient concerned regarding impotence
Patient concerned regarding non-responsiveness
Patient concerned regarding promiscuity
Patient concerned regarding sexual orientation

Z70.2   **Counseling related to sexual behavior and orientation of third party**
Advice sought regarding sexual behavior and orientation of child
Advice sought regarding sexual behavior and orientation of partner
Advice sought regarding sexual behavior and orientation of spouse

Z70.3   **Counseling related to combined concerns regarding sexual attitude, behavior and orientation**

Z70.8   **Other sex counseling**
Encounter for sex education

Z70.9   **Sex counseling, unspecified**

√4ᵗʰ **Z71   Persons encountering health services for other counseling and medical advice, not elsewhere classified**

EXCLUDES 2   contraceptive or procreation counseling (Z30-Z31)
sex counseling (Z70.-)

Z71.0   **Person encountering health services to consult on behalf of another person**
Person encountering health services to seek advice or treatment for non-attending third party

EXCLUDES 2   anxiety (normal) about sick person in family (Z63.7)
expectant (adoptive) parent(s) pre-birth pediatrician visit (Z76.81)

Z71.1   **Person with feared health complaint in whom no diagnosis is made**
Person encountering health services with feared condition which was not demonstrated
Person encountering health services in which problem was normal state
"Worried well"

EXCLUDES 1   medical observation for suspected diseases and conditions proven not to exist (Z03.-)

Z71.2   **Person consulting for explanation of examination or test findings**

Z71.3   **Dietary counseling and surveillance**
Use additional code for any associated underlying medical condition
Use additional code to identify body mass index (BMI), if known (Z68.-)

√5ᵗʰ Z71.4   **Alcohol abuse counseling and surveillance**
Use additional code for alcohol abuse or dependence (F10.-)

Z71.41   **Alcohol abuse counseling and surveillance of alcoholic**

Z71.42   **Counseling for family member of alcoholic**
Counseling for significant other, partner, or friend of alcoholic

√5ᵗʰ Z71.5   **Drug abuse counseling and surveillance**
Use additional code for drug abuse or dependence (F11-F16, F18-F19)

Z71.51   **Drug abuse counseling and surveillance of drug abuser**

Z71.52   **Counseling for family member of drug abuser**
Counseling for significant other, partner, or friend of drug abuser

Z71.6   **Tobacco abuse counseling**
Use additional code for nicotine dependence (F17.-)

Z71.7   **Human immunodeficiency virus [HIV] counseling**

√5ᵗʰ Z71.8   **Other specified counseling**

EXCLUDES 2   counseling for contraception (Z30.0-)

AHA: 2017,4Q,27

Z71.81   **Spiritual or religious counseling**

Z71.82   **Exercise counseling**

Z71.83   **Encounter for nonprocreative genetic counseling**

EXCLUDES 1   counseling for procreative genetics (Z31.5)
counseling for procreative management (Z31.6)

Z71.84   **Encounter for health counseling related to travel**
Encounter for health risk and safety counseling for (international) travel
Code also, if applicable, encounter for immunization (Z23)

EXCLUDES 2   encounter for administrative examination (Z02.-)
encounter for other special examination without complaint, suspected or reported diagnosis (Z01.-)

AHA: 2019,4Q,20,57

Z71.89   **Other specified counseling**

Z71.9   **Counseling, unspecified**
Encounter for medical advice NOS

√4ᵗʰ **Z72   Problems related to lifestyle**

EXCLUDES 2   problems related to life-management difficulty (Z73.-)
problems related to socioeconomic and psychosocial circumstances (Z55-Z65)

Z72.0   **Tobacco use**
Tobacco use NOS

EXCLUDES 1   history of tobacco dependence (Z87.891)
nicotine dependence (F17.2-)
tobacco dependence (F17.2-)
tobacco use during pregnancy (O99.33-)

Z72.3   **Lack of physical exercise**

Z72.4   **Inappropriate diet and eating habits**

EXCLUDES 1   behavioral eating disorders of infancy or childhood (F98.2-F98.3)
eating disorders (F50.-)
lack of adequate food (Z59.4)
malnutrition and other nutritional deficiencies (E40-E64)

√5ᵗʰ Z72.5   **High risk sexual behavior**
Promiscuity

EXCLUDES 1   paraphilias (F65)

Z72.51   **High risk heterosexual behavior**

Z72.52   **High risk homosexual behavior**

Z72.53   **High risk bisexual behavior**

Z72.6   **Gambling and betting**

EXCLUDES 1   compulsive or pathological gambling (F63.0)

☑5ᵗʰ **Z72.8 Other problems related to lifestyle**

  ☑6ᵗʰ **Z72.81 Antisocial behavior**

    EXCLUDES 1 *conduct disorders (F91.-)*

    Z72.810 Child and adolescent antisocial behavior ℗

      Antisocial behavior (child) (adolescent) without manifest psychiatric disorder

      Delinquency NOS

      Group delinquency

      Offenses in the context of gang membership

      Stealing in company with others

      Truancy from school

    Z72.811 Adult antisocial behavior Ⓐ

      Adult antisocial behavior without manifest psychiatric disorder

  ☑6ᵗʰ **Z72.82 Problems related to sleep**

    Z72.820 Sleep deprivation

      Lack of adequate sleep

      EXCLUDES 1 *insomnia (G47.0-)*

    Z72.821 Inadequate sleep hygiene

      Bad sleep habits

      Irregular sleep habits

      Unhealthy sleep wake schedule

      EXCLUDES 1 *insomnia (F51.0-, G47.0-)*

  Z72.89 Other problems related to lifestyle

    Self-damaging behavior

Z72.9 Problem related to lifestyle, unspecified

☑4ᵗʰ **Z73 Problems related to life management difficulty**

  EXCLUDES 2 *problems related to socioeconomic and psychosocial circumstances (Z55-Z65)*

  DEF: State of emotional, mental, and physical exhaustion causing difficulties in managing personal, school, or work circumstances. It is usually due to prolonged stress or poor interpersonal relationship skills or parenting skills.

  Z73.0 Burn-out

  Z73.1 Type A behavior pattern

  Z73.2 Lack of relaxation and leisure

  Z73.3 Stress, not elsewhere classified

    Physical and mental strain NOS

    EXCLUDES 1 *stress related to employment or unemployment (Z56.-)*

  Z73.4 Inadequate social skills, not elsewhere classified

  Z73.5 Social role conflict, not elsewhere classified

  Z73.6 Limitation of activities due to disability

    EXCLUDES 1 *care-provider dependency (Z74.-)*

  ☑5ᵗʰ **Z73.8 Other problems related to life management difficulty**

    ☑6ᵗʰ **Z73.81 Behavioral insomnia of childhood**

      DEF: Behaviors on the part of the child or caregivers that cause negative compliance with a child's sleep schedule resulting in lack of adequate sleep.

      Z73.810 Behavioral insomnia of childhood, sleep-onset association type ℗

      Z73.811 Behavioral insomnia of childhood, limit setting type ℗

      Z73.812 Behavioral insomnia of childhood, combined type ℗

      Z73.819 Behavioral insomnia of childhood, unspecified type ℗

    Z73.82 Dual sensory impairment

    Z73.89 Other problems related to life management difficulty

  Z73.9 Problem related to life management difficulty, unspecified

☑4ᵗʰ **Z74 Problems related to care provider dependency**

  EXCLUDES 2 *dependence on enabling machines or devices NEC (Z99.-)*

  ☑5ᵗʰ **Z74.0 Reduced mobility**

    Z74.01 Bed confinement status

      Bedridden

    Z74.09 Other reduced mobility

      Chair ridden

      Reduced mobility NOS

      EXCLUDES 2 *wheelchair dependence (Z99.3)*

  Z74.1 Need for assistance with personal care

  Z74.2 Need for assistance at home and no other household member able to render care

  Z74.3 Need for continuous supervision

Z74.8 Other problems related to care provider dependency

Z74.9 Problem related to care provider dependency, unspecified

☑4ᵗʰ **Z75 Problems related to medical facilities and other health care**

  Z75.0 Medical services not available in home

    EXCLUDES 1 *no other household member able to render care (Z74.2)*

  Z75.1 Person awaiting admission to adequate facility elsewhere

  Z75.2 Other waiting period for investigation and treatment

  Z75.3 Unavailability and inaccessibility of health-care facilities

    EXCLUDES 1 *bed unavailable (Z75.1)*

  Z75.4 Unavailability and inaccessibility of other helping agencies

  Z75.5 Holiday relief care

  Z75.8 Other problems related to medical facilities and other health care

  Z75.9 Unspecified problem related to medical facilities and other health care

☑4ᵗʰ **Z76 Persons encountering health services in other circumstances**

  Z76.0 Encounter for issue of repeat prescription

    Encounter for issue of repeat prescription for appliance

    Encounter for issue of repeat prescription for medicaments

    Encounter for issue of repeat prescription for spectacles

    EXCLUDES 2 *issue of medical certificate (Z02.7)*

    repeat prescription for contraceptive (Z30.4-)

  Z76.1 Encounter for health supervision and care of foundling

  Z76.2 Encounter for health supervision and care of other healthy infant and child ℗

    Encounter for medical or nursing care or supervision of healthy infant under circumstances such as adverse socioeconomic conditions at home

    Encounter for medical or nursing care or supervision of healthy infant under circumstances such as awaiting foster or adoptive placement

    Encounter for medical or nursing care or supervision of healthy infant under circumstances such as maternal illness

    Encounter for medical or nursing care or supervision of healthy infant under circumstances such as number of children at home preventing or interfering with normal care

  Z76.3 Healthy person accompanying sick person

  Z76.4 Other boarder to healthcare facility

    EXCLUDES 1 *homelessness (Z59.0)*

  Z76.5 Malingerer [conscious simulation]

    Person feigning illness (with obvious motivation)

    EXCLUDES 1 *factitious disorder (F68.1-, F68.A)*

    peregrinating patient (F68.1-)

    DEF: Act of intentionally exaggerating an illness or disability in order to receive personal gain or to avoid punishment or responsibility.

  ☑5ᵗʰ **Z76.8 Persons encountering health services in other specified circumstances**

    Z76.81 Expectant parent(s) prebirth pediatrician visit

      Pre-adoption pediatrician visit for adoptive parent(s)

    Z76.82 Awaiting organ transplant status

      Patient waiting for organ availability

    Z76.89 Persons encountering health services in other specified circumstances

      Persons encountering health services NOS

      AHA: 2014,2Q,10

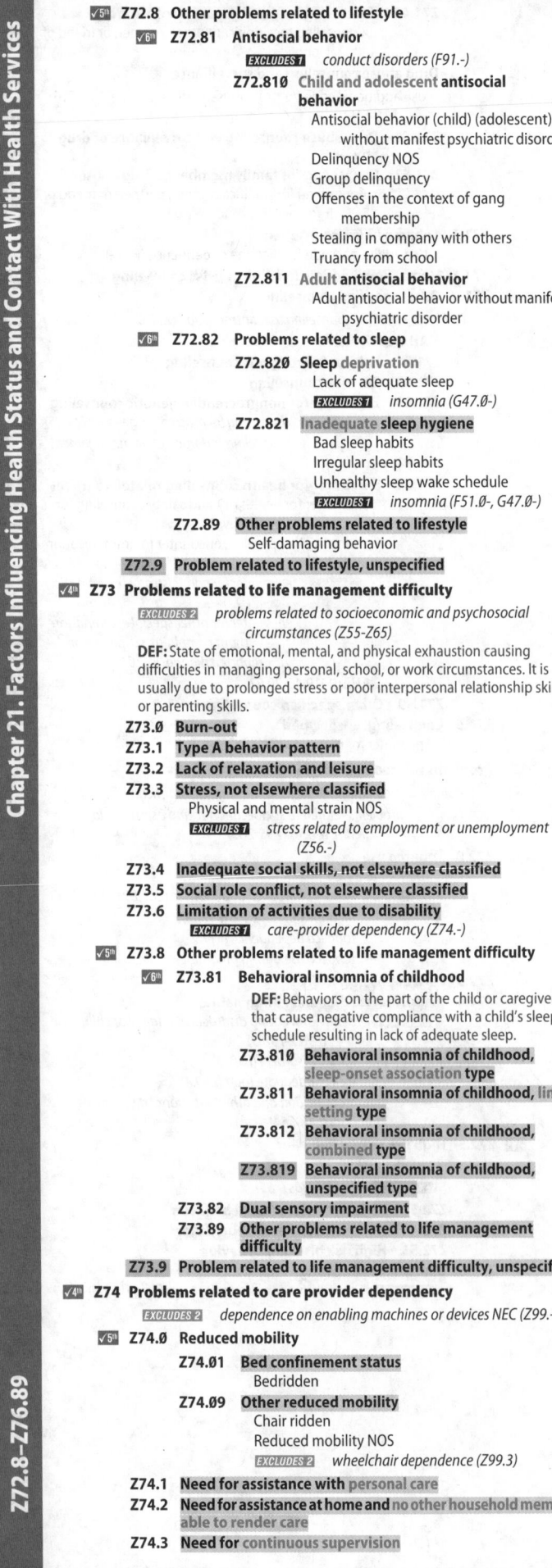

Ⓝ Newborn: 0   ℗ Pediatric: 0-17   Ⓜ Maternity: 9-64   Ⓐ Adult: 15-124   **MCC** Major Complication/Comorbidity   **CC** Complication/Comorbidity   **SW** Severe Wound Dx

1252   ICD-10-CM 2021

Persons with potential health hazards related to family and personal history and certain conditions influencing health status (Z77-Z99)

Code also any follow-up examination (Z08-Z09)

☑4ᵗʰ **Z77 Other contact with and (suspected) exposures hazardous to health**

    INCLUDES   contact with and (suspected) exposures to potential hazards to health

    EXCLUDES 2   *contact with and (suspected) exposure to communicable diseases (Z20.-)*

      exposure to (parental) (environmental) tobacco smoke in the perinatal period (P96.81)

      newborn affected by noxious substances transmitted via placenta or breast milk (P04.-)

      occupational exposure to risk factors (Z57.-)

      retained foreign body (Z18.-)

      retained foreign body fully removed (Z87.821)

      toxic effects of substances chiefly nonmedicinal as to source (T51-T65)

☑5ᵗʰ **Z77.0 Contact with and (suspected) exposure to hazardous, chiefly nonmedicinal, chemicals**

    ☑6ᵗʰ **Z77.01 Contact with and (suspected) exposure to hazardous metals**

      Z77.010 Contact with and (suspected) exposure to arsenic

      Z77.011 Contact with and (suspected) exposure to lead

      Z77.012 Contact with and (suspected) exposure to uranium

        EXCLUDES 1   *retained depleted uranium fragments (Z18.01)*

      Z77.018 Contact with and (suspected) exposure to other hazardous metals

        Contact with and (suspected) exposure to chromium compounds

        Contact with and (suspected) exposure to nickel dust

    ☑6ᵗʰ **Z77.02 Contact with and (suspected) exposure to hazardous aromatic compounds**

      Z77.020 Contact with and (suspected) exposure to aromatic amines

      Z77.021 Contact with and (suspected) exposure to benzene

      Z77.028 Contact with and (suspected) exposure to other hazardous aromatic compounds

        Aromatic dyes NOS

        Polycyclic aromatic hydrocarbons

    ☑6ᵗʰ **Z77.09 Contact with and (suspected) exposure to other hazardous, chiefly nonmedicinal, chemicals**

      Z77.090 Contact with and (suspected) exposure to asbestos

      Z77.098 Contact with and (suspected) exposure to other hazardous, chiefly nonmedicinal, chemicals

        Dyes NOS

☑5ᵗʰ **Z77.1 Contact with and (suspected) exposure to environmental pollution and hazards in the physical environment**

    ☑6ᵗʰ **Z77.11 Contact with and (suspected) exposure to environmental pollution**

      Z77.110 Contact with and (suspected) exposure to air pollution

      Z77.111 Contact with and (suspected) exposure to water pollution

      Z77.112 Contact with and (suspected) exposure to soil pollution

      Z77.118 Contact with and (suspected) exposure to other environmental pollution

    ☑6ᵗʰ **Z77.12 Contact with and (suspected) exposure to hazards in the physical environment**

      Z77.120 Contact with and (suspected) exposure to mold (toxic)

      Z77.121 Contact with and (suspected) exposure to harmful algae and algae toxins

        Contact with and (suspected) exposure to (harmful) algae bloom NOS

        Contact with and (suspected) exposure to blue-green algae bloom

        Contact with and (suspected) exposure to brown tide

        Contact with and (suspected) exposure to cyanobacteria bloom

        Contact with and (suspected) exposure to Florida red tide

        Contact with and (suspected) exposure to pfiesteria piscicida

        Contact with and (suspected) exposure to red tide

      Z77.122 Contact with and (suspected) exposure to noise

      Z77.123 Contact with and (suspected) exposure to radon and other naturally occurring radiation

        EXCLUDES 2   *radiation exposure as the cause of a confirmed condition (W88-W90, X39.0-)*

          radiation sickness NOS (T66)

      Z77.128 Contact with and (suspected) exposure to other hazards in the physical environment

☑5ᵗʰ **Z77.2 Contact with and (suspected) exposure to other hazardous substances**

    Z77.21 Contact with and (suspected) exposure to potentially hazardous body fluids

    Z77.22 Contact with and (suspected) exposure to environmental tobacco smoke (acute) (chronic)

      Exposure to second hand tobacco smoke (acute) (chronic)

      Passive smoking (acute) (chronic)

      EXCLUDES 1   *nicotine dependence (F17.-)*

        tobacco use (Z72.0)

      EXCLUDES 2   *occupational exposure to environmental tobacco smoke (Z57.31)*

    Z77.29 Contact with and (suspected) exposure to other hazardous substances

      AHA: 2016,2Q,33

    Z77.9 Other contact with and (suspected) exposures hazardous to health

☑4ᵗʰ **Z78 Other specified health status**

    EXCLUDES 2   *asymptomatic human immunodeficiency virus [HIV] infection status (Z21)*

      postprocedural status (Z93-Z99)

      sex reassignment status (Z87.890)

    Z78.0 Asymptomatic menopausal state   A ♀

      Menopausal state NOS

      Postmenopausal status NOS

      EXCLUDES 2   *symptomatic menopausal state (N95.1)*

    Z78.1 Physical restraint status

      EXCLUDES 1   *physical restraint due to a procedure — omit code*

      DEF: Application of mechanical restraining devices or manual restraints to limit physical mobility of a patient.

    Z78.9 Other specified health status

☑4ᵗʰ **Z79 Long term (current) drug therapy**

    INCLUDES   long term (current) drug use for prophylactic purposes

    Code also any therapeutic drug level monitoring (Z51.81)

    EXCLUDES 2   *drug abuse and dependence (F11-F19)*

      drug use complicating pregnancy, childbirth, and the puerperium (O99.32-)

      ~~*long term (current) use of oral antidiabetic drugs (Z79.84)*~~

      ~~*long term (current) use of oral hypoglycemic drugs (Z79.84)*~~

    ☑5ᵗʰ **Z79.0 Long term (current) use of anticoagulants and antithrombotics/antiplatelets**

      EXCLUDES 2   *long term (current) use of aspirin (Z79.82)*

      Z79.01 Long term (current) use of anticoagulants

        AHA: 2020,2Q,20

      Z79.02 Long term (current) use of antithrombotics/antiplatelets

☑ Additional Character Required   ☑7ᵗʰ Placeholder   Unacceptable PDx   Questionable PDx   Manifestation   Unspecified Dx   H1 - H14 HAC   HCC CMS-HCC Dx   HIV HIV Dx

ICD-10-CM 2021   **1253**

Z79.1 **Long term (current) use of** non-steroidal anti-inflammatories (NSAID)
> EXCLUDES 2   *long term (current) use of aspirin (Z79.82)*

Z79.2 **Long term (current) use of** antibiotics

Z79.3 **Long term (current) use of** hormonal contraceptives
Long term (current) use of birth control pill or patch

Z79.4 **Long term (current) use of** insulin   HCC
> EXCLUDES 1   ▶*long term (current) use of oral antidiabetic drugs (Z79.84)*◀
> ▶*long term (current) use of oral hypoglycemic drugs (Z79.84)*◀

TIP: When both long-term (current) insulin and long-term (current) oral hypoglycemic use is documented, assign only a code for the long-term insulin use.

✓5ᵗʰ **Z79.5** **Long term (current) use of steroids**

     Z79.51 **Long term (current) use of** inhaled steroids
     Z79.52 **Long term (current) use of** systemic steroids

✓5ᵗʰ **Z79.8** **Other long term (current) drug therapy**

     ✓6ᵗʰ **Z79.81** **Long term (current) use of agents affecting estrogen receptors and estrogen levels**
Code first, if applicable:
malignant neoplasm of breast (C50.-)
malignant neoplasm of prostate (C61)
Use additional code, if applicable, to identify:
estrogen receptor positive status (Z17.0)
family history of breast cancer (Z80.3)
genetic susceptibility to malignant neoplasm (cancer) (Z15.0-)
personal history of breast cancer (Z85.3)
personal history of prostate cancer (Z85.46)
postmenopausal status (Z78.0)
> EXCLUDES 1   *hormone replacement therapy (Z79.890)*

       Z79.810 **Long term (current) use of selective estrogen receptor modulators (SERMs)**
Long term (current) use of raloxifene (Evista)
Long term (current) use of tamoxifen (Nolvadex)
Long term (current) use of toremifene (Fareston)

       Z79.811 **Long term (current) use of** aromatase inhibitors
Long term (current) use of anastrozole (Arimidex)
Long term (current) use of exemestane (Aromasin)
Long term (current) use of letrozole (Femara)

       Z79.818 **Long term (current) use of other agents affecting estrogen receptors and estrogen levels**
Long term (current) use of estrogen receptor downregulators
Long term (current) use of fulvestrant (Faslodex)
Long term (current) use of gonadotropin-releasing hormone (GnRH) agonist
Long term (current) use of goserelin acetate (Zoladex)
Long term (current) use of leuprolide acetate (leuprorelin) (Lupron)
Long term (current) use of megestrol acetate (Megace)

     Z79.82 **Long term (current) use of** aspirin

     Z79.83 **Long term (current) use of** bisphosphonates
AHA: 2016,4Q,42

     Z79.84 **Long term (current) use of** oral hypoglycemic drugs
Long term (current) use of oral antidiabetic drugs
> EXCLUDES 2   *long term (current) use of insulin (Z79.4)*

AHA: 2016,4Q,76
TIP: When both long-term (current) insulin and long-term (current) oral hypoglycemic use is documented, assign only code Z79.4 for the long-term insulin use.

     ✓6ᵗʰ **Z79.89** **Other long term (current) drug therapy**

       Z79.890 Hormone replacement therapy

Z79.891 **Long term (current) use of** opiate analgesic
Long term (current) use of methadone for pain management
> EXCLUDES 1   *methadone use NOS (F11.9-)*
> *use of methodone for treatment of heroin addiction (F11.2-)*

Z79.899 **Other long term (current) drug therapy**
AHA: 2020,2Q,14; 2015,4Q,34; 2015,3Q,21

✓4ᵗʰ **Z80** **Family history of primary malignant neoplasm**

     Z80.0 **Family history of malignant neoplasm of** digestive organs
Conditions classifiable to C15-C26
AHA: 2018,1Q,6

     Z80.1 **Family history of malignant neoplasm of** trachea, bronchus and lung
Conditions classifiable to C33-C34

     Z80.2 **Family history of malignant neoplasm of other respiratory and intrathoracic organs**
Conditions classifiable to C30-C32, C37-C39

     Z80.3 **Family history of malignant neoplasm of** breast
Conditions classifiable to C50.-

     ✓5ᵗʰ **Z80.4** **Family history of malignant neoplasm of genital organs**
Conditions classifiable to C51-C63

       Z80.41 **Family history of malignant neoplasm of** ovary
       Z80.42 **Family history of malignant neoplasm of** prostate
       Z80.43 **Family history of malignant neoplasm of** testis
       Z80.49 **Family history of malignant neoplasm of other genital organs**

     ✓5ᵗʰ **Z80.5** **Family history of malignant neoplasm of urinary tract**
Conditions classifiable to C64-C68

       Z80.51 **Family history of malignant neoplasm of** kidney
       Z80.52 **Family history of malignant neoplasm of** bladder
       Z80.59 **Family history of malignant neoplasm of other urinary tract organ**

     Z80.6 **Family history of** leukemia
Conditions classifiable to C91-C95

     Z80.7 **Family history of other malignant neoplasms of** lymphoid, hematopoietic and related tissues
Conditions classifiable to C81-C90, C96.-

     Z80.8 **Family history of malignant neoplasm of other organs or systems**
Conditions classifiable to C00-C14, C40-C49, C69-C79

     Z80.9 **Family history of malignant neoplasm, unspecified**
Conditions classifiable to C80.1

✓4ᵗʰ **Z81** **Family history of mental and behavioral disorders**

     Z81.0 **Family history of** intellectual disabilities
Conditions classifiable to F70-F79

     Z81.1 **Family history of** alcohol abuse and dependence
Conditions classifiable to F10.-

     Z81.2 **Family history of** tobacco abuse and dependence
Conditions classifiable to F17.-

     Z81.3 **Family history of other psychoactive substance abuse and dependence**
Conditions classifiable to F11-F16, F18-F19

     Z81.4 **Family history of other substance abuse and dependence**
Conditions classifiable to F55

     Z81.8 **Family history of other mental and behavioral disorders**
Conditions classifiable elsewhere in F01-F99

✓4ᵗʰ **Z82** **Family history of certain disabilities and chronic diseases (leading to disablement)**

     Z82.0 **Family history of** epilepsy **and other diseases of the nervous system**
Conditions classifiable to G00-G99

     Z82.1 **Family history of** blindness and visual loss
Conditions classifiable to H54.-

     Z82.2 **Family history of** deafness and hearing loss
Conditions classifiable to H90-H91

     Z82.3 **Family history of** stroke
Conditions classifiable to I60-I64

     ✓5ᵗʰ **Z82.4** **Family history of ischemic heart disease and other diseases of the circulatory system**
Conditions classifiable to I00-I52, I65-I99

       Z82.41 **Family history of** sudden cardiac death
       Z82.49 **Family history of** ischemic heart disease **and other diseases of the circulatory system**

N Newborn: 0   P Pediatric: 0-17   M Maternity: 9-64   A Adult: 15-124   MCC Major Complication/Comorbidity   CC Complication/Comorbidity   SW Severe Wound Dx

1254   ICD-10-CM 2021

Z82.5   **Family history of** asthma **and other chronic lower respiratory diseases**
     Conditions classifiable to J40-J47
     EXCLUDES 2   *family history of other diseases of the respiratory system (Z83.6)*

✓5ᵗʰ Z82.6   **Family history of arthritis and other diseases of the musculoskeletal system and connective tissue**
     Conditions classifiable to M00-M99

     Z82.61   **Family history of** arthritis
     Z82.62   **Family history of** osteoporosis
     Z82.69   **Family history of other diseases of the musculoskeletal system and connective tissue**

✓6ᵗʰ Z82.7   **Family history of congenital malformations, deformations and chromosomal abnormalities**
     Conditions classifiable to Q00-Q99

     Z82.71   **Family history of** polycystic kidney
     Z82.79   **Family history of other congenital malformations, deformations and chromosomal abnormalities**

Z82.8   **Family history of other disabilities and chronic diseases leading to disablement, not elsewhere classified**

✓4ᵗʰ Z83   **Family history of other specific disorders**
     EXCLUDES 2   *contact with and (suspected) exposure to communicable disease in the family (Z20.-)*

Z83.0   **Family history of** human immunodeficiency virus **[HIV] disease**
     Conditions classifiable to B20

Z83.1   **Family history of other infectious and parasitic diseases**
     Conditions classifiable to A00-B19, B25-B94, B99

Z83.2   **Family history of diseases of the** blood and blood-forming organs **and certain disorders involving the immune mechanism**
     Conditions classifiable to D50-D89

Z83.3   **Family history of** diabetes mellitus
     Conditions classifiable to E08-E13

✓5ᵗʰ Z83.4   **Family history of other endocrine, nutritional and metabolic diseases**
     Conditions classifiable to E00-E07, E15-E88

     Z83.41   **Family history of** multiple endocrine neoplasia [MEN] syndrome
     Z83.42   **Family history of** familial hypercholesterolemia
         AHA: 2016,4Q,77
     ✓6ᵗʰ Z83.43   **Family history of other disorder of lipoprotein metabolism and other lipidemias**
         AHA: 2018,4Q,6,35
         Z83.430   **Family history of** elevated lipoprotein(a)
             Family history of elevated Lp(a)
         Z83.438   **Family history of other disorder of lipoprotein metabolism and other lipidemia**
             Family history of familial combined hyperlipidemia
     Z83.49   **Family history of other endocrine, nutritional and metabolic diseases**

✓5ᵗʰ Z83.5   **Family history of eye and ear disorders**

     ✓6ᵗʰ Z83.51   **Family history of** eye **disorders**
         Conditions classifiable to H00-H53, H55-H59
         EXCLUDES 2   *family history of blindness and visual loss (Z82.1)*
         Z83.511   **Family history of** glaucoma
         Z83.518   **Family history of other specified eye disorder**
     Z83.52   **Family history of** ear **disorders**
         Conditions classifiable to H60-H83, H92-H95
         EXCLUDES 2   *family history of deafness and hearing loss (Z82.2)*

Z83.6   **Family history of other diseases of the** respiratory system
     Conditions classifiable to J00-J39, J60-J99
     EXCLUDES 2   *family history of asthma and other chronic lower respiratory diseases (Z82.5)*

✓5ᵗʰ Z83.7   **Family history of diseases of the digestive system**
     Conditions classifiable to K00-K93

     Z83.71   **Family history of** colonic polyps
         EXCLUDES 2   *family history of malignant neoplasm of digestive organs (Z80.0)*
     Z83.79   **Family history of other diseases of the digestive system**

✓4ᵗʰ Z84   **Family history of other conditions**

Z84.0   **Family history of diseases of the** skin and subcutaneous tissue
     Conditions classifiable to L00-L99

Z84.1   **Family history of disorders of** kidney and ureter
     Conditions classifiable to N00-N29

Z84.2   **Family history of other diseases of the** genitourinary system
     Conditions classifiable to N30-N99

Z84.3   **Family history of** consanguinity

✓5ᵗʰ Z84.8   **Family history of other specified conditions**

     Z84.81   **Family history of carrier of** genetic disease
     Z84.82   **Family history of** sudden infant death syndrome
         Family history of SIDS
         AHA: 2016,4Q,77
     Z84.89   **Family history of other specified conditions**

✓4ᵗʰ Z85   **Personal history of malignant neoplasm**
     Code first any follow-up examination after treatment of malignant neoplasm (Z08)
     Use additional code to identify:
         alcohol use and dependence (F10.-)
         exposure to environmental tobacco smoke (Z77.22)
         history of tobacco dependence (Z87.891)
         occupational exposure to environmental tobacco smoke (Z57.31)
         tobacco dependence (F17.-)
         tobacco use (Z72.0)
     EXCLUDES 2   *personal history of benign neoplasm (Z86.01-)*
                 personal history of carcinoma-in-situ (Z86.00-)
     AHA: 2018,4Q,64

✓5ᵗʰ Z85.0   **Personal history of malignant neoplasm of** digestive organs
     AHA: 2017,1Q,9

     Z85.00   **Personal history of malignant neoplasm of unspecified digestive organ**
     Z85.01   **Personal history of malignant neoplasm of** esophagus
         Conditions classifiable to C15
     ✓6ᵗʰ Z85.02   **Personal history of malignant neoplasm of** stomach
         Z85.020   **Personal history of malignant** carcinoid tumor **of stomach**
             Conditions classifiable to C7A.092
         Z85.028   **Personal history of other malignant neoplasm of stomach**
             Conditions classifiable to C16
     ✓6ᵗʰ Z85.03   **Personal history of malignant neoplasm of** large intestine
         Z85.030   **Personal history of malignant** carcinoid tumor **of large intestine**
             Conditions classifiable to C7A.022-C7A.025, C7A.029
         Z85.038   **Personal history of other malignant neoplasm of large intestine**
             Conditions classifiable to C18
     ✓6ᵗʰ Z85.04   **Personal history of malignant neoplasm of** rectum, rectosigmoid junction, and anus
         Z85.040   **Personal history of malignant** carcinoid tumor **of rectum**
             Conditions classifiable to C7A.026
         Z85.048   **Personal history of other malignant neoplasm of rectum, rectosigmoid junction, and anus**
             Conditions classifiable to C19-C21
     Z85.05   **Personal history of malignant neoplasm of** liver
         Conditions classifiable to C22
     ✓6ᵗʰ Z85.06   **Personal history of malignant neoplasm of** small intestine
         Z85.060   **Personal history of malignant** carcinoid tumor **of small intestine**
             Conditions classifiable to C7A.01-
         Z85.068   **Personal history of other malignant neoplasm of small intestine**
             Conditions classifiable to C17
     Z85.07   **Personal history of malignant neoplasm of** pancreas
         Conditions classifiable to C25
     Z85.09   **Personal history of malignant neoplasm of other digestive organs**

☑ Additional Character Required   ✓x7ᵗʰ Placeholder   Unacceptable PDx   Questionable PDx   Manifestation   Unspecified Dx   H1-H14 HAC   HCC CMS-HCC Dx   HIV HIV Dx

Chapter 21. Factors Influencing Health Status and Contact With Health Services

☑5ᵗʰ **Z85.1** Personal history of malignant neoplasm of trachea, bronchus and lung

  ☑6ᵗʰ **Z85.11** Personal history of malignant neoplasm of bronchus and lung

    Z85.110 Personal history of malignant carcinoid tumor of bronchus and lung
      Conditions classifiable to C7A.090

    Z85.118 Personal history of other malignant neoplasm of bronchus and lung
      Conditions classifiable to C34

  Z85.12 Personal history of malignant neoplasm of trachea
    Conditions classifiable to C33

☑5ᵗʰ **Z85.2** Personal history of malignant neoplasm of other respiratory and intrathoracic organs

  Z85.20 Personal history of malignant neoplasm of unspecified respiratory organ

  Z85.21 Personal history of malignant neoplasm of larynx
    Conditions classifiable to C32

  Z85.22 Personal history of malignant neoplasm of nasal cavities, middle ear, and accessory sinuses
    Conditions classifiable to C30-C31

  ☑6ᵗʰ **Z85.23** Personal history of malignant neoplasm of thymus

    Z85.230 Personal history of malignant carcinoid tumor of thymus
      Conditions classifiable to C7A.091

    Z85.238 Personal history of other malignant neoplasm of thymus
      Conditions classifiable to C37

  Z85.29 Personal history of malignant neoplasm of other respiratory and intrathoracic organs

Z85.3 Personal history of malignant neoplasm of breast
  Conditions classifiable to C50.-

☑5ᵗʰ **Z85.4** Personal history of malignant neoplasm of genital organs
  Conditions classifiable to C51-C63

  Z85.40 Personal history of malignant neoplasm of unspecified female genital organ ♀

  Z85.41 Personal history of malignant neoplasm of cervix uteri ♀

  Z85.42 Personal history of malignant neoplasm of other parts of uterus ♀

  Z85.43 Personal history of malignant neoplasm of ovary ♀

  Z85.44 Personal history of malignant neoplasm of other female genital organs ♀

  Z85.45 Personal history of malignant neoplasm of unspecified male genital organ ♂

  Z85.46 Personal history of malignant neoplasm of prostate ♂

  Z85.47 Personal history of malignant neoplasm of testis ♂

  Z85.48 Personal history of malignant neoplasm of epididymis ♂

  Z85.49 Personal history of malignant neoplasm of other male genital organs ♂

☑5ᵗʰ **Z85.5** Personal history of malignant neoplasm of urinary tract
  Conditions classifiable to C64-C68

  Z85.50 Personal history of malignant neoplasm of unspecified urinary tract organ

  Z85.51 Personal history of malignant neoplasm of bladder

  ☑6ᵗʰ **Z85.52** Personal history of malignant neoplasm of kidney
    EXCLUDES 1   personal history of malignant neoplasm of renal pelvis (Z85.53)

    Z85.520 Personal history of malignant carcinoid tumor of kidney
      Conditions classifiable to C7A.093

    Z85.528 Personal history of other malignant neoplasm of kidney
      Conditions classifiable to C64

  Z85.53 Personal history of malignant neoplasm of renal pelvis

  Z85.54 Personal history of malignant neoplasm of ureter

  Z85.59 Personal history of malignant neoplasm of other urinary tract organ

Z85.6 Personal history of leukemia
  Conditions classifiable to C91-C95
  EXCLUDES 1   leukemia in remission C91.0-C95.9 with 5th character 1

☑5ᵗʰ **Z85.7** Personal history of other malignant neoplasms of lymphoid, hematopoietic and related tissues

  Z85.71 Personal history of Hodgkin lymphoma
    Conditions classifiable to C81

  Z85.72 Personal history of non-Hodgkin lymphomas
    Conditions classifiable to C82-C85

  Z85.79 Personal history of other malignant neoplasm of lymphoid, hematopoietic and related tissues
    Conditions classifiable to C88-C90, C96
    EXCLUDES 1   multiple myeloma in remission (C90.01)
      plasma cell leukemia in remission (C90.11)
      plasmacytoma in remission (C90.21)

☑5ᵗʰ **Z85.8** Personal history of malignant neoplasms of other organs and systems
  Conditions classifiable to C00-C14, C40-C49, C69-C75, C7A.098, C76-C79

  ☑6ᵗʰ **Z85.81** Personal history of malignant neoplasm of lip, oral cavity, and pharynx
    ►Conditions classifiable to C00-C14◄

    Z85.810 Personal history of malignant neoplasm of tongue

    Z85.818 Personal history of malignant neoplasm of other sites of lip, oral cavity, and pharynx

    Z85.819 Personal history of malignant neoplasm of unspecified site of lip, oral cavity, and pharynx

  ☑6ᵗʰ **Z85.82** Personal history of malignant neoplasm of skin

    Z85.820 Personal history of malignant melanoma of skin
      Conditions classifiable to C43

    Z85.821 Personal history of Merkel cell carcinoma
      Conditions classifiable to C4A

    Z85.828 Personal history of other malignant neoplasm of skin
      Conditions classifiable to C44

  ☑6ᵗʰ **Z85.83** Personal history of malignant neoplasm of bone and soft tissue
    ►Conditions classifiable to C40-C41; C45-C49◄

    Z85.830 Personal history of malignant neoplasm of bone

    Z85.831 Personal history of malignant neoplasm of soft tissue
      EXCLUDES 2   personal history of malignant neoplasm of skin (Z85.82-)

  ☑6ᵗʰ **Z85.84** Personal history of malignant neoplasm of eye and nervous tissue
    ►Conditions classifiable to C69-C72◄

    Z85.840 Personal history of malignant neoplasm of eye

    Z85.841 Personal history of malignant neoplasm of brain

    Z85.848 Personal history of malignant neoplasm of other parts of nervous tissue

  ☑6ᵗʰ **Z85.85** Personal history of malignant neoplasm of endocrine glands
    ►Conditions classifiable to C73-C75◄

    Z85.850 Personal history of malignant neoplasm of thyroid

    Z85.858 Personal history of malignant neoplasm of other endocrine glands

  Z85.89 Personal history of malignant neoplasm of other organs and systems
    ►Conditions classifiable to C7A.098, C76, C77-C79◄

Z85.9 Personal history of malignant neoplasm, unspecified
  Conditions classifiable to C7A.00, C80.1

☑4ᵗʰ **Z86** Personal history of certain other diseases
  Code first any follow-up examination after treatment (Z09)

☑5ᵗʰ **Z86.0** Personal history of in-situ and benign neoplasms and neoplasms of uncertain behavior
  EXCLUDES 2   personal history of malignant neoplasms (Z85.-)
  AHA: 2017,1Q,9

  ☑6ᵗʰ **Z86.00** Personal history of in-situ neoplasm
    Conditions classifiable to D00-D09
    AHA: 2019,4Q,20

    Z86.000 Personal history of in-situ neoplasm of breast
      Conditions classifiable to D05

Z86.001 Personal history of in-situ neoplasm of cervix uteri ♀
- Conditions classifiable to D06
- Personal history of cervical intraepithelial neoplasia III [CIN III]

Z86.002 Personal history of in-situ neoplasm of other and unspecified genital organs
- Conditions classifiable to D07
- Personal history of high-grade prostatic intraepithelial neoplasia III [HGPIN III]
- Personal history of vaginal intraepithelial neoplasia III [VAIN III]
- Personal history of vulvar intraepithelial neoplasia III [VIN III]

Z86.003 Personal history of in-situ neoplasm of oral cavity, esophagus and stomach
- Conditions classifiable to D00

Z86.004 Personal history of in-situ neoplasm of other and unspecified digestive organs
- Conditions classifiable to D01
- Personal history of anal intraepithelial neoplasia (AIN III)

Z86.005 Personal history of in-situ neoplasm of middle ear and respiratory system
- Conditions classifiable to D02

Z86.006 Personal history of melanoma in-situ
- Conditions classifiable to D03
  - EXCLUDES 2   sites other than skin — code to personal history of in-situ neoplasm of the site

Z86.007 Personal history of in-situ neoplasm of skin
- Conditions classifiable to D04
- Personal history of carcinoma in situ of skin

Z86.008 Personal history of in-situ neoplasm of other site
- Conditions classifiable to D09

√6ᵗʰ **Z86.01** Personal history of benign neoplasm

Z86.010 Personal history of colonic polyps
- AHA: 2017,1Q,14

Z86.011 Personal history of benign neoplasm of the brain

Z86.012 Personal history of benign carcinoid tumor

Z86.018 Personal history of other benign neoplasm
- AHA: 2017,1Q,14

Z86.03 Personal history of neoplasm of uncertain behavior

√5ᵗʰ **Z86.1** Personal history of infectious and parasitic diseases
- Conditions classifiable to A00-B89, B99
  - EXCLUDES 1   personal history of infectious diseases specific to a body system
  - sequelae of infectious and parasitic diseases (B90-B94)

Z86.11 Personal history of tuberculosis

Z86.12 Personal history of poliomyelitis

Z86.13 Personal history of malaria

Z86.14 Personal history of Methicillin resistant Staphylococcus aureus infection
- Personal history of MRSA infection

Z86.15 Personal history of latent tuberculosis infection

Z86.19 Personal history of other infectious and parasitic diseases
- AHA: 2020,2Q,10,12

Z86.2 Personal history of diseases of the blood and blood-forming organs and certain disorders involving the immune mechanism
- Conditions classifiable to D50-D89

√5ᵗʰ **Z86.3** Personal history of endocrine, nutritional and metabolic diseases
- Conditions classifiable to E00-E88

Z86.31 Personal history of diabetic foot ulcer
- EXCLUDES 2   current diabetic foot ulcer (E08.621, E09.621, E10.621, E11.621, E13.621)

Z86.32 Personal history of gestational diabetes ♀
- Personal history of conditions classifiable to O24.4-
  - EXCLUDES 1   gestational diabetes mellitus in current pregnancy (O24.4-)

Z86.39 Personal history of other endocrine, nutritional and metabolic disease
- AHA: 2020,1Q,12

√5ᵗʰ **Z86.5** Personal history of mental and behavioral disorders
- Conditions classifiable to F40-F59

Z86.51 Personal history of combat and operational stress reaction   Ⓐ

Z86.59 Personal history of other mental and behavioral disorders

√5ᵗʰ **Z86.6** Personal history of diseases of the nervous system and sense organs
- Conditions classifiable to G00-G99, H00-H95

Z86.61 Personal history of infections of the central nervous system
- Personal history of encephalitis
- Personal history of meningitis

Z86.69 Personal history of other diseases of the nervous system and sense organs
- AHA: 2016,4Q,24

√5ᵗʰ **Z86.7** Personal history of diseases of the circulatory system
- Conditions classifiable to I00-I99
  - EXCLUDES 2   old myocardial infarction (I25.2)
  - personal history of anaphylactic shock (Z87.892)
  - postmyocardial infarction syndrome (I24.1)

√6ᵗʰ **Z86.71** Personal history of venous thrombosis and embolism

Z86.711 Personal history of pulmonary embolism

Z86.718 Personal history of other venous thrombosis and embolism
- AHA: 2020,2Q,20

Z86.72 Personal history of thrombophlebitis

Z86.73 Personal history of transient ischemic attack (TIA), and cerebral infarction without residual deficits
- Personal history of prolonged reversible ischemic neurological deficit (PRIND)
- Personal history of stroke NOS without residual deficits
  - EXCLUDES 1   personal history of traumatic brain injury (Z87.820)
  - sequelae of cerebrovascular disease (I69.-)
- AHA: 2012,4Q,92

Z86.74 Personal history of sudden cardiac arrest
- Personal history of sudden cardiac death successfully resuscitated

Z86.79 Personal history of other diseases of the circulatory system
- AHA: 2020,1Q,12

√4ᵗʰ **Z87** Personal history of other diseases and conditions
- Code first any follow-up examination after treatment (Z09)

√5ᵗʰ **Z87.0** Personal history of diseases of the respiratory system
- Conditions classifiable to J00-J99

Z87.01 Personal history of pneumonia (recurrent)

Z87.09 Personal history of other diseases of the respiratory system

√5ᵗʰ **Z87.1** Personal history of diseases of the digestive system
- Conditions classifiable to K00-K93

Z87.11 Personal history of peptic ulcer disease

Z87.19 Personal history of other diseases of the digestive system
- AHA: 2017,1Q,14

Z87.2 Personal history of diseases of the skin and subcutaneous tissue
- Conditions classifiable to L00-L99
  - EXCLUDES 2   personal history of diabetic foot ulcer (Z86.31)

✔ Additional Character Required   ✔x7ᵗʰ Placeholder   Unacceptable PDx   Questionable PDx   Manifestation   Unspecified Dx   H1-H10 HAC   HCC CMS-HCC Dx   HIV HIV Dx

ICD-10-CM 2021   1257

√5ᵗʰ **Z87.3** **Personal history of diseases of the musculoskeletal system and connective tissue**
Conditions classifiable to M00-M99
> EXCLUDES 2   *personal history of (healed) traumatic fracture (Z87.81)*

√6ᵗʰ **Z87.31** **Personal history of (healed) nontraumatic fracture**

Z87.310 **Personal history of (healed) osteoporosis fracture**
Personal history of (healed) fragility fracture
Personal history of (healed) collapsed vertebra due to osteoporosis
TIP: Assign for history of osteoporosis fractures that have resolved, even when a code from category M80 indicating current osteoporosis fracture is also reported.

Z87.311 **Personal history of (healed) other pathological fracture**
Personal history of (healed) collapsed vertebra NOS
> EXCLUDES 2   *personal history of osteoporosis fracture (Z87.310)*

Z87.312 **Personal history of (healed) stress fracture**
Personal history of (healed) fatigue fracture

Z87.39 **Personal history of other diseases of the musculoskeletal system and connective tissue**

√5ᵗʰ **Z87.4** **Personal history of diseases of the genitourinary system**
Conditions classifiable to N00-N99

√6ᵗʰ **Z87.41** **Personal history of dysplasia of the female genital tract**
> EXCLUDES 1   *personal history of intraepithelial neoplasia III of female genital tract (Z86.001, Z86.008)*
> *personal history of malignant neoplasm of female genital tract (Z85.40-Z85.44)*

Z87.410 **Personal history of cervical dysplasia** ♀

Z87.411 **Personal history of vaginal dysplasia** ♀

Z87.412 **Personal history of vulvar dysplasia** ♀

Z87.42 **Personal history of other diseases of the female genital tract** ♀

√6ᵗʰ **Z87.43** **Personal history of diseases of the male genital organs**

Z87.430 **Personal history of prostatic dysplasia** ♂
> EXCLUDES 1   *personal history of malignant neoplasm of prostate (Z85.46)*

Z87.438 **Personal history of other diseases of male genital organs** ♂

√6ᵗʰ **Z87.44** **Personal history of diseases of the urinary system**
> EXCLUDES 1   *personal history of malignant neoplasm of cervix uteri (Z85.41)*

Z87.440 **Personal history of urinary (tract) infections**

Z87.441 **Personal history of nephrotic syndrome**

Z87.442 **Personal history of urinary calculi**
Personal history of kidney stones

Z87.448 **Personal history of other diseases of urinary system**

√5ᵗʰ **Z87.5** **Personal history of complications of pregnancy, childbirth and the puerperium**
Conditions classifiable to O00-O9A
> EXCLUDES 2   *recurrent pregnancy loss (N96)*

Z87.51 **Personal history of pre-term labor** ♀
> EXCLUDES 1   *current pregnancy with history of pre-term labor (O09.21-)*

Z87.59 **Personal history of other complications of pregnancy, childbirth and the puerperium** ♀
Personal history of trophoblastic disease

√5ᵗʰ **Z87.7** **Personal history of (corrected) congenital malformations**
Conditions classifiable to Q00-Q89 that have been repaired or corrected
> EXCLUDES 1   *congenital malformations that have been partially corrected or repair but which still require medical treatment — code to condition*
> EXCLUDES 2   *other postprocedural states (Z98.-)*
> *personal history of medical treatment (Z92.-)*
> *presence of cardiac and vascular implants and grafts (Z95.-)*
> *presence of other devices (Z97.-)*
> *presence of other functional implants (Z96.-)*
> *transplanted organ and tissue status (Z94.-)*

√6ᵗʰ **Z87.71** **Personal history of (corrected) congenital malformations of genitourinary system**

Z87.710 **Personal history of (corrected) hypospadias** ♂

Z87.718 **Personal history of other specified (corrected) congenital malformations of genitourinary system**

√6ᵗʰ **Z87.72** **Personal history of (corrected) congenital malformations of nervous system and sense organs**

Z87.720 **Personal history of (corrected) congenital malformations of eye**

Z87.721 **Personal history of (corrected) congenital malformations of ear**

Z87.728 **Personal history of other specified (corrected) congenital malformations of nervous system and sense organs**

√6ᵗʰ **Z87.73** **Personal history of (corrected) congenital malformations of digestive system**

Z87.730 **Personal history of (corrected) cleft lip and palate**

Z87.738 **Personal history of other specified (corrected) congenital malformations of digestive system**

Z87.74 **Personal history of (corrected) congenital malformations of heart and circulatory system**

Z87.75 **Personal history of (corrected) congenital malformations of respiratory system**

Z87.76 **Personal history of (corrected) congenital malformations of integument, limbs and musculoskeletal system**

√6ᵗʰ **Z87.79** **Personal history of other (corrected) congenital malformations**

Z87.790 **Personal history of (corrected) congenital malformations of face and neck**

Z87.798 **Personal history of other (corrected) congenital malformations**

√5ᵗʰ **Z87.8** **Personal history of other specified conditions**
> EXCLUDES 2   *personal history of self harm (Z91.5)*

Z87.81 **Personal history of (healed) traumatic fracture**
> EXCLUDES 2   *personal history of (healed) nontraumatic fracture (Z87.31-)*

√6ᵗʰ **Z87.82** **Personal history of other (healed) physical injury and trauma**
Conditions classifiable to S00-T88, except traumatic fractures

Z87.820 **Personal history of traumatic brain injury**
> EXCLUDES 1   *personal history of transient ischemic attack (TIA), and cerebral infarction without residual deficits (Z86.73)*

Z87.821 **Personal history of retained foreign body fully removed**

Z87.828 **Personal history of other (healed) physical injury and trauma**

√6ᵗʰ **Z87.89** **Personal history of other specified conditions**

Z87.890 **Personal history of sex reassignment**

Z87.891 **Personal history of nicotine dependence**
> EXCLUDES 1   *current nicotine dependence (F17.2-)*

AHA: 2017,2Q,27

Z87.892   **Personal history of** anaphylaxis
Code also allergy status such as:
     allergy status to drugs, medicaments and
        biological substances (Z88.-)
     allergy status, other than to drugs and
        biological substances (Z91.0-)

Z87.898   **Personal history of other specified conditions**
     AHA: 2013,1Q,21

√4ᵗʰ **Z88**   **Allergy status to drugs, medicaments and biological substances**
     EXCLUDES 2   *allergy status, other than to drugs and biological substances (Z91.0-)*
     AHA: 2015,3Q,23

     Z88.0   **Allergy status to** penicillin
▲   **Z88.1**   **Allergy status to other antibiotic agents**
▲   **Z88.2**   **Allergy status to** sulfonamides
▲   **Z88.3**   **Allergy status to other anti-infective agents**
▲   **Z88.4**   **Allergy status to** anesthetic **agent**
▲   **Z88.5**   **Allergy status to** narcotic **agent**
▲   **Z88.6**   **Allergy status to** analgesic **agent**
▲   **Z88.7**   **Allergy status to** serum and vaccine
▲   **Z88.8**   **Allergy status to other drugs, medicaments and biological substances**
▲   **Z88.9**   **Allergy status to unspecified drugs, medicaments and biological substances**

√4ᵗʰ **Z89**   **Acquired absence of limb**
     INCLUDES   amputation status
                  postprocedural loss of limb
                  post-traumatic loss of limb
     EXCLUDES 1   *acquired deformities of limbs (M20-M21)*
                  congenital absence of limbs (Q71-Q73)

     √5ᵗʰ **Z89.0**   **Acquired absence of** thumb and other finger(s)
         √6ᵗʰ **Z89.01**   **Acquired absence of** thumb
             Z89.011   **Acquired absence of** right **thumb**
             Z89.012   **Acquired absence of** left **thumb**
             Z89.019   **Acquired absence of unspecified thumb**
         √6ᵗʰ **Z89.02**   **Acquired absence of other** finger(s)
             EXCLUDES 2   *acquired absence of thumb (Z89.01-)*
             Z89.021   **Acquired absence of** right **finger(s)**
             Z89.022   **Acquired absence of** left **finger(s)**
             Z89.029   **Acquired absence of unspecified finger(s)**

     √5ᵗʰ **Z89.1**   **Acquired absence of** hand and wrist
         √6ᵗʰ **Z89.11**   **Acquired absence of** hand
             Z89.111   **Acquired absence of** right **hand**
             Z89.112   **Acquired absence of** left **hand**
             Z89.119   **Acquired absence of unspecified hand**
         √6ᵗʰ **Z89.12**   **Acquired absence of** wrist
             Disarticulation at wrist
             Z89.121   **Acquired absence of** right **wrist**
             Z89.122   **Acquired absence of** left **wrist**
             Z89.129   **Acquired absence of unspecified wrist**

     √5ᵗʰ **Z89.2**   **Acquired absence of** upper limb above wrist
         √6ᵗʰ **Z89.20**   **Acquired absence of upper limb, unspecified level**
             Z89.201   **Acquired absence of** right **upper limb, unspecified level**
             Z89.202   **Acquired absence of** left **upper limb, unspecified level**
             Z89.209   **Acquired absence of unspecified upper limb, unspecified level**
                Acquired absence of arm NOS
         √6ᵗʰ **Z89.21**   **Acquired absence of** upper limb below elbow
             Z89.211   **Acquired absence of** right **upper limb below elbow**
             Z89.212   **Acquired absence of** left **upper limb below elbow**
             Z89.219   **Acquired absence of unspecified upper limb below elbow**
         √6ᵗʰ **Z89.22**   **Acquired absence of** upper limb above elbow
             Disarticulation at elbow
             Z89.221   **Acquired absence of** right **upper limb above elbow**
             Z89.222   **Acquired absence of** left **upper limb above elbow**
             Z89.229   **Acquired absence of unspecified upper limb above elbow**

√6ᵗʰ **Z89.23**   **Acquired absence of** shoulder
     Acquired absence of shoulder joint following explantation of shoulder joint prosthesis, with or without presence of antibiotic-impregnated cement spacer
     Z89.231   **Acquired absence of** right **shoulder**
     Z89.232   **Acquired absence of** left **shoulder**
     Z89.239   **Acquired absence of unspecified shoulder**

√5ᵗʰ **Z89.4**   **Acquired absence of** toe(s), foot, and ankle
     √6ᵗʰ **Z89.41**   **Acquired absence of** great toe
         Z89.411   **Acquired absence of** right great toe   HCC
         Z89.412   **Acquired absence of** left great toe   HCC
         Z89.419   **Acquired absence of unspecified great toe**   HCC
     √6ᵗʰ **Z89.42**   **Acquired absence of other** toe(s)
         EXCLUDES 2   *acquired absence of great toe (Z89.41-)*
         Z89.421   **Acquired absence of other** right **toe(s)**   HCC
         Z89.422   **Acquired absence of other** left **toe(s)**   HCC
         Z89.429   **Acquired absence of other toe(s), unspecified side**   HCC
     √6ᵗʰ **Z89.43**   **Acquired absence of** foot
         Z89.431   **Acquired absence of** right foot   HCC
         Z89.432   **Acquired absence of** left foot   HCC
         Z89.439   **Acquired absence of unspecified foot**   HCC
     √6ᵗʰ **Z89.44**   **Acquired absence of** ankle
         Disarticulation of ankle
         Z89.441   **Acquired absence of** right **ankle**   HCC
         Z89.442   **Acquired absence of** left **ankle**   HCC
         Z89.449   **Acquired absence of unspecified ankle**   HCC

√5ᵗʰ **Z89.5**   **Acquired absence of leg below knee**
     √6ᵗʰ **Z89.51**   **Acquired absence of** leg below knee
         Z89.511   **Acquired absence of** right **leg below knee**   HCC
         Z89.512   **Acquired absence of** left **leg below knee**   HCC
         Z89.519   **Acquired absence of unspecified leg below knee**   HCC
     √6ᵗʰ **Z89.52**   **Acquired absence of** knee
         Acquired absence of knee joint following explantation of knee joint prosthesis, with or without presence of antibiotic-impregnated cement spacer
         Z89.521   **Acquired absence of** right **knee**
         Z89.522   **Acquired absence of** left **knee**
         Z89.529   **Acquired absence of unspecified knee**

√5ᵗʰ **Z89.6**   **Acquired absence of leg above knee**
     √6ᵗʰ **Z89.61**   **Acquired absence of** leg above knee
         Acquired absence of leg NOS
         Disarticulation at knee
         Z89.611   **Acquired absence of** right **leg above knee**   HCC
         Z89.612   **Acquired absence of** left **leg above knee**   HCC
         Z89.619   **Acquired absence of unspecified leg above knee**   HCC
     √6ᵗʰ **Z89.62**   **Acquired absence of** hip
         Acquired absence of hip joint following explantation of hip joint prosthesis, with or without presence of antibiotic-impregnated cement spacer
         Disarticulation at hip
         Z89.621   **Acquired absence of** right **hip joint**
         Z89.622   **Acquired absence of** left **hip joint**
         Z89.629   **Acquired absence of unspecified hip joint**
     Z89.9   **Acquired absence of limb, unspecified**

√4ᵗʰ **Z90**   **Acquired absence of organs, not elsewhere classified**
     INCLUDES   postprocedural or post-traumatic loss of body part NEC
     EXCLUDES 1   *congenital absence — see Alphabetical Index*
     EXCLUDES 2   *postprocedural absence of endocrine glands (E89.-)*
     √5ᵗʰ **Z90.0**   **Acquired absence of part of** head and neck
         Z90.01   **Acquired absence of** eye
         Z90.02   **Acquired absence of** larynx

✔ Additional Character Required   √x7ᵗʰ Placeholder   Unacceptable PDx   Questionable PDx   Manifestation   Unspecified Dx   H1-H4 HAC   HCC CMS-HCC Dx   HIV HIV Dx

ICD-10-CM 2021   1259

Z90.09   **Acquired absence of other part of head and neck**
Acquired absence of nose
   EXCLUDES 2   *teeth (K08.1)*

✓5ᵗʰ **Z90.1**   **Acquired absence of breast and nipple**

Z90.10   **Acquired absence of unspecified breast and nipple**
Z90.11   **Acquired absence of right breast and nipple**
Z90.12   **Acquired absence of left breast and nipple**
Z90.13   **Acquired absence of bilateral breasts and nipples**

Z90.2   **Acquired absence of lung [part of]**

Z90.3   **Acquired absence of stomach [part of]**

✓5ᵗʰ **Z90.4**   **Acquired absence of other specified parts of digestive tract**

✓6ᵗʰ **Z90.41**   **Acquired absence of pancreas**
Code also exocrine pancreatic insufficiency (K86.81)
Use additional code to identify any associated:
   diabetes mellitus, postpancreatectomy (E13.-)
   insulin use (Z79.4)

Z90.410   **Acquired total absence of pancreas**
Acquired absence of pancreas NOS
Z90.411   **Acquired partial absence of pancreas**

Z90.49   **Acquired absence of other specified parts of digestive tract**

Z90.5   **Acquired absence of kidney**

Z90.6   **Acquired absence of other parts of urinary tract**
Acquired absence of bladder

✓5ᵗʰ **Z90.7**   **Acquired absence of genital organ(s)**
   EXCLUDES 1   *personal history of sex reassignment (Z87.890)*
   EXCLUDES 2   *female genital mutilation status (N90.81-)*

✓6ᵗʰ **Z90.71**   **Acquired absence of cervix and uterus**

Z90.710   **Acquired absence of both cervix and uterus**   ♀
Acquired absence of uterus NOS
Status post total hysterectomy
Z90.711   **Acquired absence of uterus with remaining cervical stump**   ♀
Status post partial hysterectomy with remaining cervical stump
Z90.712   **Acquired absence of cervix with remaining uterus**   ♀

✓6ᵗʰ **Z90.72**   **Acquired absence of ovaries**

Z90.721   **Acquired absence of ovaries, unilateral**   ♀
Z90.722   **Acquired absence of ovaries, bilateral**   ♀

Z90.79   **Acquired absence of other genital organ(s)**

✓5ᵗʰ **Z90.8**   **Acquired absence of other organs**

Z90.81   **Acquired absence of spleen**
Z90.89   **Acquired absence of other organs**

✓4ᵗʰ **Z91**   **Personal risk factors, not elsewhere classified**
   EXCLUDES 2   *contact with and (suspected) exposures hazardous to health (Z77.-)*
exposure to pollution and other problems related to physical environment (Z77.1-)
female genital mutilation status (N90.81-)
personal history of physical injury and trauma (Z87.81, Z87.82-)
occupational exposure to risk factors (Z57.-)

✓5ᵗʰ **Z91.0**   **Allergy status, other than to drugs and biological substances**
   EXCLUDES 2   *allergy status to drugs, medicaments, and biological substances (Z88.-)*

✓6ᵗʰ **Z91.01**   **Food allergy status**
   EXCLUDES 2   *food additives allergy status (Z91.02)*

Z91.010   **Allergy to peanuts**
Z91.011   **Allergy to milk products**
   EXCLUDES 1   *lactose intolerance (E73.-)*
Z91.012   **Allergy to eggs**
Z91.013   **Allergy to seafood**
Allergy to shellfish
Allergy to octopus or squid ink
Z91.018   **Allergy to other foods**
Allergy to nuts other than peanuts

Z91.02   **Food additives allergy status**

✓6ᵗʰ **Z91.03**   **Insect allergy status**

Z91.030   **Bee allergy status**
Z91.038   **Other insect allergy status**

✓6ᵗʰ **Z91.04**   **Nonmedicinal substance allergy status**

Z91.040   **Latex allergy status**
Latex sensitivity status
Z91.041   **Radiographic dye allergy status**
Allergy status to contrast media used for diagnostic X-ray procedure
Z91.048   **Other nonmedicinal substance allergy status**

Z91.09   **Other allergy status, other than to drugs and biological substances**

✓5ᵗʰ **Z91.1**   **Patient's noncompliance with medical treatment and regimen**

Z91.11   **Patient's noncompliance with dietary regimen**

✓6ᵗʰ **Z91.12**   **Patient's intentional underdosing of medication regimen**
Code first underdosing of medication (T36-T50) with fifth or sixth character 6
   EXCLUDES 1   *adverse effect of prescribed drug taken as directed — code to adverse effect*
poisoning (overdose) — code to poisoning
   AHA: 2018,4Q,72

Z91.120   **Patient's intentional underdosing of medication regimen due to financial hardship**
Z91.128   **Patient's intentional underdosing of medication regimen for other reason**

✓6ᵗʰ **Z91.13**   **Patient's unintentional underdosing of medication regimen**
Code first underdosing of medication (T36-T50) with fifth or sixth character 6
   EXCLUDES 1   *adverse effect of prescribed drug taken as directed — code to adverse effect*
poisoning (overdose) — code to poisoning
   AHA: 2018,4Q,72

Z91.130   **Patient's unintentional underdosing of medication regimen due to age-related debility**
Z91.138   **Patient's unintentional underdosing of medication regimen for other reason**

Z91.14   **Patient's other noncompliance with medication regimen**
Patient's underdosing of medication NOS
   AHA: 2018,4Q,72

Z91.15   **Patient's noncompliance with renal dialysis**   HCC

Z91.19   **Patient's noncompliance with other medical treatment and regimen**
Nonadherence to medical treatment

✓5ᵗʰ **Z91.4**   **Personal history of psychological trauma, not elsewhere classified**

✓6ᵗʰ **Z91.41**   **Personal history of adult abuse**
   EXCLUDES 2   *personal history of abuse in childhood (Z62.81-)*

Z91.410   **Personal history of adult physical and sexual abuse**   A
   EXCLUDES 1   *current adult physical abuse (T74.11, T76.11)*
current adult sexual abuse (T74.21, T76.11)
Z91.411   **Personal history of adult psychological abuse**   A
Z91.412   **Personal history of adult neglect**   A
   EXCLUDES 1   *current adult neglect (T74.01, T76.01)*
Z91.419   **Personal history of unspecified adult abuse**   A

Z91.42   **Personal history of forced labor or sexual exploitation**
   AHA: 2018,4Q,32,35

Z91.49   **Other personal history of psychological trauma, not elsewhere classified**

Z91.5   **Personal history of self-harm**
Personal history of parasuicide
Personal history of self-poisoning
Personal history of suicide attempt

✓5ᵗʰ **Z91.8**   **Other specified personal risk factors, not elsewhere classified**

Z91.81   **History of falling**
At risk for falling

N Newborn: 0   P Pediatric: 0-17   M Maternity: 9-64   A Adult: 15-124   MCC Major Complication/Comorbidity   CC Complication/Comorbidity   SW Severe Wound Dx

1260   ICD-10-CM 2021

Z91.82   **Personal history of military deployment**   `A`
Individual (civilian or military) with past history of military war, peacekeeping and humanitarian deployment (current or past conflict)
Returned from military deployment

Z91.83   *Wandering in diseases classified elsewhere*
Code first underlying disorder such as:
Alzheimer's disease (G30.-)
autism or pervasive developmental disorder (F84.-)
intellectual disabilities (F70-F79)
unspecified dementia with behavioral disturbance (F03.9-)

✓6th **Z91.84**   **Oral health risk factors**
AHA: 2017,4Q,29

     Z91.841   **Risk for dental caries, low**
     Z91.842   **Risk for dental caries, moderate**
     Z91.843   **Risk for dental caries, high**
     Z91.849   **Unspecified risk for dental caries**

Z91.89   **Other specified personal risk factors, not elsewhere classified**
AHA: 2017,1Q,45

✓4th **Z92**   **Personal history of medical treatment**
EXCLUDES 2   postprocedural states (Z98.-)

Z92.0   **Personal history of contraception**
EXCLUDES 1   counseling or management of current contraceptive practices (Z30.-)
long term (current) use of contraception (Z79.3)
presence of (intrauterine) contraceptive device (Z97.5)

✓5th **Z92.2**   **Personal history of drug therapy**
EXCLUDES 2   long term (current) drug therapy (Z79.-)

     Z92.21   **Personal history of antineoplastic chemotherapy**
     Z92.22   **Personal history of monoclonal drug therapy**
     Z92.23   **Personal history of estrogen therapy**
✓6th   **Z92.24**   **Personal history of steroid therapy**

         Z92.240   **Personal history of inhaled steroid therapy**
         Z92.241   **Personal history of systemic steroid therapy**
            Personal history of steroid therapy NOS

     Z92.25   **Personal history of immunosupression therapy**
       EXCLUDES 2   personal history of steroid therapy (Z92.24)

     Z92.29   **Personal history of other drug therapy**

Z92.3   **Personal history of irradiation**
Personal history of exposure to therapeutic radiation
EXCLUDES 1   exposure to radiation in the physical environment (Z77.12)
occupational exposure to radiation (Z57.1)

✓5th **Z92.8**   **Personal history of other medical treatment**

     Z92.81   **Personal history of extracorporeal membrane oxygenation (ECMO)**
     Z92.82   **Status post administration of tPA (rtPA) in a different facility within the last 24 hours prior to admission to current facility**
Code first condition requiring tPA administration, such as:
acute cerebral infarction (I63.-)
acute myocardial infarction (I21.-, I22.-)
AHA: 2013,4Q,124

     Z92.83   **Personal history of failed moderate sedation**
Personal history of failed conscious sedation
EXCLUDES 2   failed moderate sedation during procedure (T88.52)

     Z92.84   **Personal history of unintended awareness under general anesthesia**
EXCLUDES 2   unintended awareness under general anesthesia during procedure (T88.53)
AHA: 2016,4Q,72-73,77

     Z92.89   **Personal history of other medical treatment**
AHA: 2020,1Q,18

✓4th **Z93**   **Artificial opening status**
EXCLUDES 1   artificial openings requiring attention or management (Z43.-)
complications of external stoma (J95.0-, K94.-, N99.5-)

Z93.0   **Tracheostomy status**   `HCC`
AHA: 2013,4Q,129

Z93.1   **Gastrostomy status**   `HCC`

Z93.2   **Ileostomy status**   `HCC`
Z93.3   **Colostomy status**   `HCC`
Z93.4   **Other artificial openings of gastrointestinal tract status**   `HCC`

✓5th **Z93.5**   **Cystostomy status**

     Z93.50   **Unspecified cystostomy status**   `HCC`
     Z93.51   **Cutaneous-vesicostomy status**   `HCC`
     Z93.52   **Appendico-vesicostomy status**   `HCC`
     Z93.59   **Other cystostomy status**   `HCC`

Z93.6   **Other artificial openings of urinary tract status**   `HCC`
Nephrostomy status
Ureterostomy status
Urethrostomy status

Z93.8   **Other artificial opening status**   `HCC`
Z93.9   **Artificial opening status, unspecified**   `HCC`

✓4th **Z94**   **Transplanted organ and tissue status**
`INCLUDES`   organ or tissue replaced by heterogenous or homogenous transplant
EXCLUDES 1   complications of transplanted organ or tissue — see Alphabetical Index
EXCLUDES 2   presence of vascular grafts (Z95.-)

Z94.0   **Kidney transplant status**   `CC`
Z94.1   **Heart transplant status**   `CC` `HCC`
EXCLUDES 1   artificial heart status (Z95.812)
heart-valve replacement status (Z95.2-Z95.4)

Z94.2   **Lung transplant status**   `CC` `HCC`
Z94.3   **Heart and lungs transplant status**   `CC` `HCC`
Z94.4   **Liver transplant status**   `CC` `HCC`
Z94.5   **Skin transplant status**
Autogenous skin transplant status
Z94.6   **Bone transplant status**
Z94.7   **Corneal transplant status**

✓5th **Z94.8**   **Other transplanted organ and tissue status**

     Z94.81   **Bone marrow transplant status**   `CC` `HCC`
     Z94.82   **Intestine transplant status**   `CC` `HCC`
     Z94.83   **Pancreas transplant status**   `CC` `HCC`
     Z94.84   **Stem cells transplant status**   `CC` `HCC`
     Z94.89   **Other transplanted organ and tissue status**

Z94.9   **Transplanted organ and tissue status, unspecified**

✓4th **Z95**   **Presence of cardiac and vascular implants and grafts**
EXCLUDES 2   complications of cardiac and vascular devices, implants and grafts (T82.-)

Z95.0   **Presence of cardiac pacemaker**
Presence of cardiac resynchronization therapy (CRT-P) pacemaker
EXCLUDES 1   adjustment or management of cardiac device (Z45.0-)
adjustment or management of cardiac pacemaker (Z45.0)
presence of automatic (implantable) cardiac defibrillator with synchronous cardiac pacemaker (Z95.810)
AHA: 2019,1Q,33
TIP: Assign an additional code for the condition the pacemaker is controlling (e.g., sick sinus syndrome). Even though the pacemaker controls the heart rate, it does not cure the sick sinus syndrome; it is still present and a reportable chronic condition.

Z95.1   **Presence of aortocoronary bypass graft**
Presence of coronary artery bypass graft
Z95.2   **Presence of prosthetic heart valve**
Presence of heart valve NOS
Z95.3   **Presence of xenogenic heart valve**
Z95.4   **Presence of other heart-valve replacement**
Z95.5   **Presence of coronary angioplasty implant and graft**
EXCLUDES 1   coronary angioplasty status without implant and graft (Z98.61)

✓ Additional Character Required   ✓x7th Placeholder   Unacceptable PDx   Questionable PDx   Manifestation   Unspecified Dx   H1-H14 HAC   HCC CMS-HCC Dx   HIV HIV Dx

ICD-10-CM 2021   1261

Chapter 21. Factors Influencing Health Status and Contact With Health Services

✓5ᵗʰ **Z95.8 Presence of other cardiac and vascular implants and grafts**

    ✓6ᵗʰ **Z95.81 Presence of other cardiac implants and grafts**

        Z95.810 Presence of automatic (implantable) cardiac defibrillator

            Presence of automatic (implantable) cardiac defibrillator with synchronous cardiac pacemaker

            Presence of cardiac resynchronization therapy defibrillator (CRT-D)

            Presence of cardioverter-defibrillator (ICD)

        Z95.811 Presence of heart assist device CC HCC

        Z95.812 Presence of fully implantable artificial heart CC HCC

        Z95.818 Presence of other cardiac implants and grafts

    ✓6ᵗʰ **Z95.82 Presence of other vascular implants and grafts**

        Z95.820 Peripheral vascular angioplasty status with implants and grafts

            EXCLUDES 1   peripheral vascular angioplasty without implant and graft (Z98.62)

        Z95.828 Presence of other vascular implants and grafts

            Presence of intravascular prosthesis NEC

Z95.9 Presence of cardiac and vascular implant and graft, unspecified

✓4ᵗʰ **Z96 Presence of other functional implants**

    EXCLUDES 2   complications of internal prosthetic devices, implants and grafts (T82-T85)

                fitting and adjustment of prosthetic and other devices (Z44-Z46)

    Z96.0 Presence of urogenital implants

    Z96.1 Presence of intraocular lens

        Presence of pseudophakia

    ✓5ᵗʰ **Z96.2 Presence of otological and audiological implants**

        Z96.20 Presence of otological and audiological implant, unspecified

        Z96.21 Cochlear implant status

        Z96.22 Myringotomy tube(s) status

        Z96.29 Presence of other otological and audiological implants

            Presence of bone-conduction hearing device

            Presence of eustachian tube stent

            Stapes replacement

    Z96.3 Presence of artificial larynx

    ✓5ᵗʰ **Z96.4 Presence of endocrine implants**

        Z96.41 Presence of insulin pump (external) (internal)

        Z96.49 Presence of other endocrine implants

    Z96.5 Presence of tooth-root and mandibular implants

    ✓5ᵗʰ **Z96.6 Presence of orthopedic joint implants**

        AHA: 2019,3Q,16

        Z96.60 Presence of unspecified orthopedic joint implant

    ✓6ᵗʰ **Z96.61 Presence of artificial shoulder joint**

        Z96.611 Presence of right artificial shoulder joint

        Z96.612 Presence of left artificial shoulder joint

        Z96.619 Presence of unspecified artificial shoulder joint

    ✓6ᵗʰ **Z96.62 Presence of artificial elbow joint**

        Z96.621 Presence of right artificial elbow joint

        Z96.622 Presence of left artificial elbow joint

        Z96.629 Presence of unspecified artificial elbow joint

    ✓6ᵗʰ **Z96.63 Presence of artificial wrist joint**

        Z96.631 Presence of right artificial wrist joint

        Z96.632 Presence of left artificial wrist joint

        Z96.639 Presence of unspecified artificial wrist joint

    ✓6ᵗʰ **Z96.64 Presence of artificial hip joint**

        Hip-joint replacement (partial) (total)

        Z96.641 Presence of right artificial hip joint

        Z96.642 Presence of left artificial hip joint

        Z96.643 Presence of artificial hip joint, bilateral

        Z96.649 Presence of unspecified artificial hip joint

    ✓6ᵗʰ **Z96.65 Presence of artificial knee joint**

        Z96.651 Presence of right artificial knee joint

        Z96.652 Presence of left artificial knee joint

        Z96.653 Presence of artificial knee joint, bilateral

        Z96.659 Presence of unspecified artificial knee joint

    ✓6ᵗʰ **Z96.66 Presence of artificial ankle joint**

        Z96.661 Presence of right artificial ankle joint

        Z96.662 Presence of left artificial ankle joint

        Z96.669 Presence of unspecified artificial ankle joint

    ✓6ᵗʰ **Z96.69 Presence of other orthopedic joint implants**

        Z96.691 Finger-joint replacement of right hand

        Z96.692 Finger-joint replacement of left hand

        Z96.693 Finger-joint replacement, bilateral

        Z96.698 Presence of other orthopedic joint implants

    Z96.7 Presence of other bone and tendon implants

        Presence of skull plate

    ✓5ᵗʰ **Z96.8 Presence of other specified functional implants**

        Z96.81 Presence of artificial skin

        Z96.82 Presence of neurostimulator

            Presence of brain neurostimulator

            Presence of gastric neurostimulator

            Presence of peripheral nerve neurostimulator

            Presence of sacral nerve neurostimulator

            Presence of spinal cord neurostimulator

            Presence of vagus nerve neurostimulator

            AHA: 2019,4Q,19

        Z96.89 Presence of other specified functional implants

    Z96.9 Presence of functional implant, unspecified

✓4ᵗʰ **Z97 Presence of other devices**

    EXCLUDES 1   complications of internal prosthetic devices, implants and grafts (T82-T85)

    EXCLUDES 2   fitting and adjustment of prosthetic and other devices (Z44-Z46)

                presence of cerebrospinal fluid drainage device (Z98.2)

    Z97.0 Presence of artificial eye

    ✓5ᵗʰ **Z97.1 Presence of artificial limb (complete) (partial)**

        Z97.10 Presence of artificial limb (complete) (partial), unspecified

        Z97.11 Presence of artificial right arm (complete) (partial)

        Z97.12 Presence of artificial left arm (complete) (partial)

        Z97.13 Presence of artificial right leg (complete) (partial)

        Z97.14 Presence of artificial left leg (complete) (partial)

        Z97.15 Presence of artificial arms, bilateral (complete) (partial)

        Z97.16 Presence of artificial legs, bilateral (complete) (partial)

    Z97.2 Presence of dental prosthetic device (complete) (partial)

        Presence of dentures (complete) (partial)

    Z97.3 Presence of spectacles and contact lenses

    Z97.4 Presence of external hearing-aid

    Z97.5 Presence of (intrauterine) contraceptive device ♀

        EXCLUDES 1   checking, reinsertion or removal of implantable subdermal contraceptive (Z30.46)

                checking, reinsertion or removal of intrauterine contraceptive device (Z30.43-)

    Z97.8 Presence of other specified devices

✓4ᵗʰ **Z98 Other postprocedural states**

    EXCLUDES 2   aftercare (Z43-Z49, Z51)

                follow-up medical care (Z08-Z09)

                postprocedural complication — see Alphabetical Index

    Z98.0 Intestinal bypass and anastomosis status

        EXCLUDES 2   bariatric surgery status (Z98.84)

                gastric bypass status (Z98.84)

                obesity surgery status (Z98.84)

    Z98.1 Arthrodesis status

    Z98.2 Presence of cerebrospinal fluid drainage device

        Presence of CSF shunt

    Z98.3 Post therapeutic collapse of lung status

        Code first underlying disease

    ✓5ᵗʰ **Z98.4 Cataract extraction status**

        Use additional code to identify intraocular lens implant status (Z96.1)

        EXCLUDES 1   aphakia (H27.0)

        Z98.41 Cataract extraction status, right eye

        Z98.42 Cataract extraction status, left eye

N Newborn: 0   P Pediatric: 0-17   M Maternity: 9-64   A Adult: 15-124   MCC Major Complication/Comorbidity   CC Complication/Comorbidity   SW Severe Wound Dx

1262   ICD-10-CM 2021

Z98.49   **Cataract extraction status, unspecified eye**

√5ᵗʰ **Z98.5**   **Sterilization status**
> *EXCLUDES 1*   *female infertility (N97.-)*
> *male infertility (N46.-)*

Z98.51   **Tubal ligation status**   ♀
Z98.52   **Vasectomy status**   Ⓐ ♂

√5ᵗʰ **Z98.6**   **Angioplasty status**

Z98.61   **Coronary angioplasty status**
> *EXCLUDES 1*   *coronary angioplasty status with implant and graft (Z95.5)*

Z98.62   **Peripheral vascular angioplasty status**
> *EXCLUDES 1*   *peripheral vascular angioplasty status with implant and graft (Z95.820)*

√5ᵗʰ **Z98.8**   **Other specified postprocedural states**

√6ᵗʰ **Z98.81**   **Dental procedure status**

Z98.810   **Dental sealant status**
Z98.811   **Dental restoration status**
> Dental crown status
> Dental fillings status

Z98.818   **Other dental procedure status**

Z98.82   **Breast implant status**
> *EXCLUDES 1*   *breast implant removal status (Z98.86)*

Z98.83   **Filtering (vitreous) bleb after glaucoma surgery status**
> *EXCLUDES 1*   *inflammation (infection) of postprocedural bleb (H59.4-)*

Z98.84   **Bariatric surgery status**
> Gastric banding status
> Gastric bypass status for obesity
> Obesity surgery status
> *EXCLUDES 1*   *bariatric surgery status complicating pregnancy, childbirth, or the puerperium (O99.84)*
> *EXCLUDES 2*   *intestinal bypass and anastomosis status (Z98.0)*
> **AHA:** 2020,1Q,12

Z98.85   **Transplanted organ removal status**
> Transplanted organ previously removed due to complication, failure, rejection or infection
> *EXCLUDES 1*   *encounter for removal of transplanted organ — code to complication of transplanted organ (T86.-)*

Z98.86   **Personal history of breast implant removal**

√6ᵗʰ **Z98.87**   **Personal history of in utero procedure**

Z98.870   **Personal history of in utero procedure during pregnancy**   ♀
> *EXCLUDES 2*   *complications from in utero procedure for current pregnancy (O35.7)*
> *supervision of current pregnancy with history of in utero procedure during previous pregnancy (O09.82-)*

Z98.871   **Personal history of in utero procedure while a fetus**

√6ᵗʰ **Z98.89**   **Other specified postprocedural states**

Z98.890   **Other specified postprocedural states**
> Personal history of surgery, not elsewhere classified

Z98.891   **History of uterine scar from previous surgery**   ♀
> *EXCLUDES 1*   *maternal care due to uterine scar from previous surgery (O34.2-)*
> **AHA:** 2016,4Q,51-52,76

√4ᵗʰ **Z99**   **Dependence on enabling machines and devices, not elsewhere classified**
> *EXCLUDES 1*   *cardiac pacemaker status (Z95.0)*
> **AHA:** 2020,1Q,11

Z99.0   **Dependence on aspirator**

√5ᵗʰ **Z99.1**   **Dependence on respirator**
> Dependence on ventilator

Z99.11   **Dependence on respirator [ventilator] status**   CC HCC
> **AHA:** 2015,1Q,21

Z99.12   **Encounter for respirator [ventilator] dependence during power failure**   CC HCC
> *EXCLUDES 1*   *mechanical complication of respirator [ventilator] (J95.850)*

Z99.2   **Dependence on renal dialysis**   HCC
> Hemodialysis status
> Peritoneal dialysis status
> Presence of arteriovenous shunt for dialysis
> Renal dialysis status NOS
> *EXCLUDES 1*   *encounter for fitting and adjustment of dialysis catheter (Z49.0-)*
> *EXCLUDES 2*   *noncompliance with renal dialysis (Z91.15)*
> **AHA:** 2016,1Q,12; 2013,4Q,125

Z99.3   **Dependence on wheelchair**
> Wheelchair confinement status
> Code first cause of dependence, such as:
>   muscular dystrophy (G71.0-)
>   obesity (E66.-)

√5ᵗʰ **Z99.8**   **Dependence on other enabling machines and devices**

Z99.81   **Dependence on supplemental oxygen**
> Dependence on long-term oxygen
> **AHA:** 2013,4Q,129

Z99.89   **Dependence on other enabling machines and devices**
> Dependence on machine or device NOS
> **AHA:** 2020,1Q,11

✅ Additional Character Required   ✗ʷᵗʰ Placeholder   Unacceptable PDx   Questionable PDx   Manifestation   Unspecified Dx   H1-H14 HAC   HCC CMS-HCC Dx   HIV HIV Dx

ICD-10-CM 2021   1263

Chapter 21. Factors Influencing Health Status and Contact With Health Services

Z98.49–Z99.89

Chapter 22. Codes for Special Purposes (U00–U85)

Chapter-specific Guidelines with Coding Examples

     U07.0   Vaping-related disorder (see Section I.C.10.e., Vaping-related disorders)

     U07.1   COVID-19 (see Section I.C.1.g.1., COVID-19 infection)

Chapter 22. Codes for Special Purposes (U00-U85)

This chapter contains the following blocks:

U00-U49   Provisional assignment of new diseases of uncertain etiology or emergency use

Provisional assignment of new diseases of uncertain etiology or emergency use (U00-U49)

✓4ᵗʰ **U07**   **Emergency use of U07**

●   **U07.0**   **Vaping-related disorder**

Dabbing related lung damage

Dabbing related lung injury

E-cigarette, or vaping, product use associated lung injury [EVALI]

Electronic cigarette related lung damage

Electronic cigarette related lung injury

Use additional code, to identify manifestations, such as:

    abdominal pain (R10.84)

    acute respiratory distress syndrome (J80)

    diarrhea (R19.7)

    drug-induced interstitial lung disorder (J70.4)

    lipoid pneumonia (J69.1)

    weight loss (R63.4)

DEF: Respiratory illness or injury caused by harmful aerosolized substances and chemicals produced by electronic cigarettes, vapes, e-pipes, and other battery-powered vaping devices. Symptoms may include shortness of breath and fever, while some patients experience severe, sometimes fatal, lung damage. *Synonyms: e-cigarette and vaping product use-associated lung injury, EVALI.*

●   **U07.1**   **COVID-19**   `HIV` `MCC`

Use additional code to identify pneumonia or other manifestations

`EXCLUDES 1`   *coronavirus infection, unspecified (B34.2)*

          coronavirus as the cause of diseases classified elsewhere (B97.2-)

          pneumonia due to SARS-associated coronavirus (J12.81)

AHA: 2020,2Q,3-13

DEF: First diagnosed in December 2019 in China, coronavirus disease 2019 (COVID-19) is a respiratory infection caused by a newly identified (novel) virus not previously seen in humans, known as severe acute respiratory syndrome coronavirus 2 (SARS-CoV-2). Symptoms of this lower respiratory illness include fever, dry cough, and tiredness that may progress to include difficulty breathing. Older patients and those with high blood pressure, heart problems, and diabetes are more likely to develop serious symptoms of the illness. *Synonyms: 2019 novel coronavirus, 2019-nCoV, coronavirus, SARS-CoV-2, Wuhan coronavirus.*

TIP: Only a confirmed diagnosis of COVID-19 can be coded to U07.1; a positive COVID-19 test result or documentation by the provider that the disease is confirmed is sufficient.

TIP: Assign for asymptomatic individuals who test positive for COVID-19. Even though asymptomatic, the individual is considered to have the COVID-19 infection due to the positive test result.

TIP: Assign appropriate codes for presenting signs/symptoms associated with COVID-19 (cough, fever, shortness of breath), instead of U07.1, if a definitive diagnosis has not been established.

| N Newborn: 0 | P Pediatric: 0-17 | M Maternity: 9-64 | A Adult: 15-124 | MCC Major Complication/Comorbidity | CC Complication/Comorbidity | SW Severe Wound Dx |

1266   ICD-10-CM 2021

Code	Description
A09	Infectious gastroenteritis and colitis, unspecified
A33	Tetanus neonatorum
A34	Obstetrical tetanus
A35	Other tetanus
A46	Erysipelas
A55	Chlamydial lymphogranuloma (venereum)
A57	Chancroid
A58	Granuloma inguinale
A64	Unspecified sexually transmitted disease
A65	Nonvenereal syphilis
A70	Chlamydia psittaci infections
A78	Q fever
A86	Unspecified viral encephalitis
A89	Unspecified viral infection of central nervous system
A90	Dengue fever [classical dengue]
A91	Dengue hemorrhagic fever
A94	Unspecified arthropod-borne viral fever
A99	Unspecified viral hemorrhagic fever
B03	Smallpox
B04	Monkeypox
B09	Unspecified viral infection characterized by skin and mucous membrane lesions
B20	Human immunodeficiency virus [HIV] disease
B49	Unspecified mycosis
B54	Unspecified malaria
B59	Pneumocystosis
B64	Unspecified protozoal disease
B72	Dracunculiasis
B75	Trichinellosis
B79	Trichuriasis
B80	Enterobiasis
B86	Scabies
B89	Unspecified parasitic disease
B91	Sequelae of poliomyelitis
B92	Sequelae of leprosy
C01	Malignant neoplasm of base of tongue
C07	Malignant neoplasm of parotid gland
C12	Malignant neoplasm of pyriform sinus
C19	Malignant neoplasm of rectosigmoid junction
C20	Malignant neoplasm of rectum
C23	Malignant neoplasm of gallbladder
C33	Malignant neoplasm of trachea
C37	Malignant neoplasm of thymus
C52	Malignant neoplasm of vagina
C55	Malignant neoplasm of uterus, part unspecified
C58	Malignant neoplasm of placenta
C61	Malignant neoplasm of prostate
C73	Malignant neoplasm of thyroid gland
D34	Benign neoplasm of thyroid gland
D45	Polycythemia vera
D62	Acute posthemorrhagic anemia
D65	Disseminated intravascular coagulation [defibrination A syndrome]
D66	Hereditary factor VIII deficiency
D67	Hereditary factor IX deficiency
D71	Functional disorders of polymorphonuclear neutrophils
D77	Other disorders of blood and blood-forming organs in diseases classified elsewhere
E02	Subclinical iodine-deficiency hypothyroidism
E15	Nondiabetic hypoglycemic coma
E35	Disorders of endocrine glands in diseases classified elsewhere
E40	Kwashiorkor
E41	Nutritional marasmus
E42	Marasmic kwashiorkor
E43	Unspecified severe protein-calorie malnutrition
E45	Retarded development following protein-calorie malnutrition
E46	Unspecified protein-calorie malnutrition
E52	Niacin deficiency [pellagra]
E54	Ascorbic acid deficiency
E58	Dietary calcium deficiency
E59	Dietary selenium deficiency
E60	Dietary zinc deficiency
E65	Localized adiposity
E68	Sequelae of hyperalimentation
F04	Amnestic disorder due to known physiological condition
F05	Delirium due to known physiological condition
F09	Unspecified mental disorder due to known physiological condition
F21	Schizotypal disorder
F22	Delusional disorders
F23	Brief psychotic disorder
F24	Shared psychotic disorder
F28	Other psychotic disorder not due to a substance or known physiological condition
F29	Unspecified psychosis not due to a substance or known physiological condition
F39	Unspecified mood [affective] disorder
F54	Psychological and behavioral factors associated with disorders or diseases classified elsewhere
F59	Unspecified behavioral syndromes associated with physiological disturbances and physical factors
F66	Other sexual disorders
F69	Unspecified disorder of adult personality and behavior
F70	Mild intellectual disabilities
F71	Moderate intellectual disabilities
F72	Severe intellectual disabilities
F73	Profound intellectual disabilities
F78	Other intellectual disabilities
F79	Unspecified intellectual disabilities
F82	Specific developmental disorder of motor function
F88	Other disorders of psychological development
F89	Unspecified disorder of psychological development
F99	Mental disorder, not otherwise specified
G01	Meningitis in bacterial diseases classified elsewhere
G02	Meningitis in other infectious and parasitic diseases classified elsewhere
G07	Intracranial and intraspinal abscess and granuloma in diseases classified elsewhere
G08	Intracranial and intraspinal phlebitis and thrombophlebitis
G09	Sequelae of inflammatory diseases of central nervous system
G10	Huntington's disease
G14	Postpolio syndrome
G20	Parkinson's disease
G26	Extrapyramidal and movement disorders in diseases classified elsewhere
G35	Multiple sclerosis
G53	Cranial nerve disorders in diseases classified elsewhere
G55	Nerve root and plexus compressions in diseases classified elsewhere
G59	Mononeuropathy in diseases classified elsewhere
G63	Polyneuropathy in diseases classified elsewhere
G64	Other disorders of peripheral nervous system
G92	Toxic encephalopathy
G94	Other disorders of brain in diseases classified elsewhere
H22	Disorders of iris and ciliary body in diseases classified elsewhere
H28	Cataract in diseases classified elsewhere
H32	Chorioretinal disorders in diseases classified elsewhere
H36	Retinal disorders in diseases classified elsewhere
H42	Glaucoma in diseases classified elsewhere
I00	Rheumatic fever without heart involvement
I10	Essential (primary) hypertension
I32	Pericarditis in diseases classified elsewhere
I38	Endocarditis, valve unspecified

I39	Endocarditis and heart valve disorders in diseases classified elsewhere	N37	Urethral disorders in diseases classified elsewhere
I41	Myocarditis in diseases classified elsewhere	N51	Disorders of male genital organs in diseases classified elsewhere
I43	Cardiomyopathy in diseases classified elsewhere	N62	Hypertrophy of breast
I52	Other heart disorders in diseases classified elsewhere	N72	Inflammatory disease of cervix uteri
I76	Septic arterial embolism	N74	Female pelvic inflammatory disorders in diseases classified elsewhere
I81	Portal vein thrombosis	N86	Erosion and ectropion of cervix uteri
I96	Gangrene, not elsewhere classified	N96	Recurrent pregnancy loss
J00	Acute nasopharyngitis (common cold)	O68	Labor and delivery complicated by abnormality of fetal acid-base balance
J13	Pneumonia due to Streptococcus pneumoniae	O76	Abnormality in fetal heart rate and rhythm complicating labor and delivery
J14	Pneumonia due to Hemophilus influenzae	O80	Encounter for full-term uncomplicated delivery
J17	Pneumonia in diseases classified elsewhere	O82	Encounter for cesarean delivery without indication
J22	Unspecified acute lower respiratory infection	O85	Puerperal sepsis
J36	Peritonsillar abscess	O94	Sequelae of complication of pregnancy, childbirth, and the puerperium
J40	Bronchitis, not specified as acute or chronic	P09	Abnormal findings on neonatal screening
J42	Unspecified chronic bronchitis	P53	Hemorrhagic disease of newborn
J60	Coalworker's pneumoconiosis	P60	Disseminated intravascular coagulation of newborn
J61	Pneumoconiosis due to asbestos and other mineral fibers	P84	Other problems with newborn
J64	Unspecified pneumoconiosis	P90	Convulsions of newborn
J65	Pneumoconiosis associated with tuberculosis	P95	Stillbirth
J80	Acute respiratory distress syndrome	Q02	Microcephaly
J90	Pleural effusion, not elsewhere classified	R05	Cough
J99	Respiratory disorders in diseases classified elsewhere	R12	Heartburn
K23	Disorders of esophagus in diseases classified elsewhere	R17	Unspecified jaundice
K30	Functional dyspepsia	R21	Rash and other nonspecific skin eruption
K36	Other appendicitis	R32	Unspecified urinary incontinence
K37	Unspecified appendicitis	R34	Anuria and oliguria
K67	Disorders of peritoneum in infectious diseases classified elsewhere	R37	Sexual dysfunction, unspecified
K77	Liver disorders in diseases classified elsewhere	R42	Dizziness and giddiness
K87	Disorders of gallbladder, biliary tract and pancreas in diseases classified elsewhere	R52	Pain, unspecified
L00	Staphylococcal scalded skin syndrome	R54	Age-related physical debility
L14	Bullous disorders in diseases classified elsewhere	R55	Syncope and collapse
L22	Diaper dermatitis	R58	Hemorrhage, not elsewhere classified
L26	Exfoliative dermatitis	R61	Generalized hyperhidrosis
L42	Pityriasis rosea	R64	Cachexia
L45	Papulosquamous disorders in diseases classified elsewhere	R69	Illness, unspecified
L52	Erythema nodosum	R75	Inconclusive laboratory evidence of human immunodeficiency virus [HIV]
L54	Erythema in diseases classified elsewhere	R81	Glycosuria
L62	Nail disorders in diseases classified elsewhere	R99	Ill-defined and unknown cause of mortality
L80	Vitiligo	Y09	Assault by unspecified means
L83	Acanthosis nigricans	Y66	Nonadministration of surgical and medical care
L84	Corns and callosities	Y69	Unspecified misadventure during surgical and medical care
L86	Keratoderma in diseases classified elsewhere	Y95	Nosocomial condition
L88	Pyoderma gangrenosum	Z08	Encounter for follow-up examination after completed treatment for malignant neoplasm
L99	Other disorders of skin and subcutaneous tissue in diseases classified elsewhere	Z09	Encounter for follow-up examination after completed treatment for conditions other than malignant neoplasm
N08	Glomerular disorders in diseases classified elsewhere	Z21	Asymptomatic human immunodeficiency virus [HIV] infection status
N10	Acute tubulo-interstitial nephritis	Z23	Encounter for immunization
N12	Tubulo-interstitial nephritis, not specified as acute or chronic	Z66	Do not resuscitate
N16	Renal tubulo-interstitial disorders in diseases classified elsewhere		
N19	Unspecified kidney failure		
N22	Calculus of urinary tract in diseases classified elsewhere		
N23	Unspecified renal colic		
N29	Other disorders of kidney and ureter in diseases classified elsewhere		
N33	Bladder disorders in diseases classified elsewhere		

Appendix B: Pharmacology List 2021

This section enables the coder to quickly review drugs, drug actions, and indications that are often associated with overlooked or undocumented diagnoses. The coder should review the patient's medication record and know what condition the physician is treating with the prescribed medication based on documentation in the medical record. When documentation is lacking, the coder can reference this section to locate the drug, determine the drug action, confirm drug indications, and when necessary query the physician. When applicable, some of the drugs provided in this resource have also been mapped to their appropriate Z code for long-term drug use.

Drug	Z Code	Drug Action/Classification	Indications
Abilify [aripiprazole]		Antipsychotic	Depression, bipolar disorder, schizophrenia, autism symptoms
Acarbose [acarbose]	Z79.84	Oral hypoglycemic	Diabetes mellitus
Accupril [quinapril hydrochloride]		ACE inhibitor	Congestive heart failure; hypertension
Acetaminophen with codeine [acetaminophen/codeine phosphate]	Z79.891	Analgesic, narcotic	Pain, moderate to severe
Actemra [tocilizumab]		Antirheumatic	Rheumatoid arthritis
Actimmune [interferon gamma-1b]	Z79.899	Antineoplastic interferons; antiviral interferons	Chronic granulomatous disease; malignant osteopetrosis
Activella [estradiol/norethindrone acetate]	Z79.890	Estrogen therapy	Menopause symptoms; vaginal and vulvar atrophy; osteoporosis prevention
Actonel [risedronate sodium]	Z79.83	Bisphosphonate	Decrease in bone loss in multiple myeloma patients; Paget's disease; hyperparathyroidism; osteoporosis
Actoplus Met [metformin hydrochloride/pioglitazone hydrochloride]	Z79.84	Oral hypoglycemic	Diabetes mellitus
Actos [pioglitazone hydrochloride]	Z79.84	Oral hypoglycemic	Diabetes mellitus
Aczone [dapsone]		Acne agent, topical	Acne vulgaris
Adalat CC [nifedipine]		Calcium channel blocker	Vasospastic angina; chronic stable angina; hypertension
Adderall XR [amphetamine aspartate and sulfate/dextroamphetamine saccharate and sulfate]		CNS stimulant	Attention deficit hyperactivity disorder (ADHD)
Admelog [insulin lispro]	Z79.4	Insulin	Diabetes mellitus
Advair [fluticasone propionate/salmeterol xinafoate]	Z79.51	Corticosteroid – inhaled; antiasthmatic	Prophylaxis and treatment of asthma and COPD
Advil [ibuprofen]	Z79.1	Nonsteroidal anti-inflammatory drug (NSAID)	Pain or fever relief
Afrezza [human insulin recombinant]	Z79.4	Insulin – inhaled	Diabetes mellitus
Aggrastat [tirofiban hydrochloride]	Z79.02	Antiplatelet	Unstable angina; heart attacks
Aggrenox [aspirin/dipyridamole]	Z79.02	Antiplatelet	Lessening of the chance of heart attack or stroke
Aimovig [erenumab-aooe]		Antimigraine	Migraine headache
AirDuo RespiClick [fluticasone propionate/salmeterol xinafoate]	Z79.51	Corticosteroid – inhaled; antiasthmatic	Asthma
Aklief [trifarotene]		Acne agent, topical	Acne vulgaris
Aldactone [spironolactone]		Cardiovascular agent; antihypertensive agent; diuretic; electrolytic and renal agent	Severe heart failure; ascites associated with cirrhosis; hypokalemia
Aleve [naproxen sodium]	Z79.1	Nonsteroidal anti-inflammatory drug (NSAID)	Reduction of temporary aches and pains
Allegra allergy [fexofenadine hydrochloride]		Antihistamine	Seasonal allergic rhinitis
Allopurinol [allopurinol]		Antigout	Gouty arthritis, renal calculus, hyperuricemia, hyperuricemia secondary to leukemia, hyperuricemia secondary to lymphoma
Alora [estradiol]	Z79.890	Estrogen therapy	Menopause symptoms
Alphagan P [brimonidine tartrate]		Antiglaucoma agent (ophthalmic); antihypertensive, ocular	Open angle glaucoma or another condition in which pressure in the eye is too high (ocular hypertension)
Alprazolam [alprazolam]		Antianxiety; sedative/hypnotic	
Altabax [retapamulin]	Z79.2	Antibiotic, topical	Skin infections
Altace [ramipril]		ACE inhibitor	Congestive heart failure; hypertension
Altavera [ethinyl estradiol/levonorgestrel]	Z79.3	Contraceptive	Prevention of pregnancy
Alvesco [ciclesonide]	Z79.51	Corticosteroid – inhaled; antiasthmatic	Prophylaxis and treatment of asthma

Appendix B: Pharmacology List 2021

Drug	Z Code	Drug Action/Classification	Indications
Alyacen [ethinyl estradiol/norethindrone]	Z79.3	Contraceptive	Prevention of pregnancy
Amaryl [glimepiride]	Z79.84	Oral hypoglycemic	Diabetes mellitus
Ambien [zolpidem tartrate]		CNS depressant; anxiolytic/sedative/hypnotic	Insomnia
Amikacin [amikacin sulfate]	Z79.2	Antibiotic	Gram-negative bacterial infections such as Pseudomonas, Escherichia coli (E. coli), Proteus, Klebsiella-Enterobacter-Serratia
Amitriptyline HCl [amitriptyline hydrochloride]		Antidepressant	Depression
Amoxicillin [amoxicillin]	Z79.2	Antibiotic	Treatment of infections with a broad spectrum of bactericidal activity against many gram-positive and gram-negative micro-organisms; otitis media, gonorrhea, skin, respiratory, gastrointestinal, and genitourinary infections
Ampicillin [ampicillin sodium]	Z79.2	Antibiotic	Bacterial infections
Ampyra [dalfampridine]		Potassium channel blocker	Improvement in walking in patients with multiple sclerosis
Amrix [cyclobenzaprine hydrochloride]		Muscle relaxant	Adjunct to rest and physical therapy for muscle spasms
Anaprox DS [naproxen sodium]	Z79.1	Nonsteroidal anti-inflammatory drug (NSAID)	Pain, inflammation or fever relief
Anastrozole [anastrozole]	Z79.811	Aromatase inhibitor	Postmenopausal breast cancer
Ancef [cefazolin sodium]	Z79.2	Antibiotic	Respiratory tract infections due to Streptococcus pneumoniae, Klebsiella species, Haemophilus influenzae (H. influenzae), Staphylococcus aureus, and group A betahemolytic streptococci; urinary tract infections due to E. coli, Proteus mirabilis, Klebsiella species and some strains of Enterobacter and enterococci; skin and skin structure infections, biliary tract infections, bone and joint infections, genital infections, septicemia, and endocarditis
Androderm [testosterone]	Z79.890	Testosterone therapy – topical	Primary hypogonadism, hypogonadotropic hypogonadism
AndroGel [testosterone]	Z79.890	Testosterone therapy – topical	Primary hypogonadism, hypogonadotropic hypogonadism
Angeliq [drospirenone/estradiol]	Z79.890	Estrogen therapy	Menopause symptoms
Angiomax [bivalirudin]	Z79.01	Anticoagulant	Prevention of blood clots
Antabuse [disulfiram]		Alcohol treatment	Alcoholism
Antineoplastic/chemotherapy	Z79.899	Antineoplastic	Cancer
Apidra [insulin glulisine recombinant]	Z79.4	Insulin	Diabetes mellitus
Aranelle [ethinyl estradiol/norethindrone]	Z79.3	Contraceptive	Prevention of pregnancy; acne
Aranesp [darbepoetin alfa]		Erythropoiesis-stimulating agent (ESA)	Treatment of lower than normal blood cells (anemia) from disorders such as CKD and neoplasms
Argatroban [argatroban]	Z79.01	Anticoagulant	Prophylaxis and treatment of venous thrombosis in thrombocytopenia patients
Aricept [donepezil hydrochloride]		Acetylcholinesterase/cholinesterase inhibitors	Symptoms of mild to moderate Alzheimer's disease; can improve thinking ability in some patients
Arimidex [anastrozole]	Z79.811	Aromatase inhibitor	Postmenopausal breast cancer
Aristospan [triamcinolone hexacetonide]	Z79.52	Corticosteroid	Severe inflammation
Arixtra [fondaparinux sodium]	Z79.01	Anticoagulant	Venous thrombosis and pulmonary embolism
Arnuity Ellipta [fluticasone furoate]	Z79.51	Corticosteroid – inhaled; antiasthmatic	Prophylaxis and treatment of asthma
Aromasin [exemestane]	Z79.811	Aromatase inhibitor	Postmenopausal breast cancer
Arthrotec [diclofenac sodium/misoprostol]	Z79.1	Nonsteroidal anti-inflammatory drug (NSAID)-prostaglandin combo	Treatment of patients with arthritis who may develop stomach ulcers from taking nonsteroidal anti-inflammatory drugs (NSAIDs) alone; used to help relieve some symptoms of arthritis, such as inflammation, swelling, stiffness, and joint pain
Asacol HD [mesalamine]		Anti-inflammatory	Ulcerative colitis
Ashlyna [ethinyl estradiol/levonorgestrel]	Z79.3	Contraceptive	Prevention of pregnancy
Asmanex [mometasone furoate]	Z79.51	Corticosteroid – inhaled; antiasthmatic	Prophylaxis and treatment of asthma
Astagraf XL [tacrolimus]	Z79.899	Immunosuppressant	Prophylaxis of organ transplant rejection
Atelvia [risedronate sodium]	Z79.83	Bisphosphonate	Prevention of thinning of the bones (osteoporosis)

Drug	Z Code	Drug Action/Classification	Indications
Atenolol [atenolol]		Beta blocker	Angina pectoris; hypertension; acute myocardial infarction
Ativan [lorazepam]		Antianxiety; sedative/hypnotic	Anxiety disorder associated with depressive symptoms; controls tension, agitation, irritability, and insomnia
Atripla [efavirenz/emtricitabine/tenofovir disoproxil fumarate]	Z79.899	Antiviral	HIV
Atrovent HFA [ipratropium bromide]		Antiasthmatic/bronchodilator	Chronic bronchitis, emphysema; bronchial asthma
Augmentin [amoxicillin/clavulanate potassium]	Z79.2	Antibiotic	Middle ear, lower respiratory, sinus, skin and skin structures, and urinary tract infections
Avandia [rosiglitazone maleate]	Z79.84	Oral hypoglycemic	Diabetes mellitus
Avapro [irbesartan]		Antihypertensive	Hypertension
Avelox [moxifloxacin hydrochloride]	Z79.2	Antibiotic	Bacterial infections, specifically pneumonia; skin; intra-abdominal; plague; acute sinusitis; acute chronic bronchitis
Aviane-28 [ethinyl estradiol/levonorgestrel]	Z79.3	Contraceptive	Prevention of pregnancy
Avonex [interferon beta-1a]	Z79.899	Antiviral	Treatment of relapsing multiple sclerosis
Axid AR [nizatidine]		Histamine H2-receptor antagonist	Acid/peptic disorder; gastroesophageal reflux; duodenal, gastric, and peptic ulcers
Ayvakit [avapritinib]		Multikinase inhibitor	Unresectable or metastatic gastrointestinal stromal tumor (GIST)
Azactam [aztreonam]	Z79.2	Antibiotic	Severe bacterial infections
Azithromycin [azithromycin]	Z79.2	Antibiotic	Bacterial infections
Bactrim [sulfamethoxazole/trimethoprim]	Z79.2	Antibiotic	Treatment of urinary tract infections, acute otitis media, acute exacerbation of chronic bronchitis, shigellosis, and pneumocystis carinii
Balziva-28 [ethinyl estradiol/norethindrone]	Z79.3	Contraceptive	Prevention of pregnancy
Basaglar [insulin glargine]	Z79.4	Insulin	Diabetes mellitus
Bayer [acetylsalicylic acid]	Z79.82	Aspirin	Prophylaxis and treatment of heart attacks, angina or strokes; reduction of fever, pain and inflammation
Beconase AQ [beclomethasone dipropionate monohydrate]	Z79.899	Corticosteroid – intranasal	Perennial and seasonal allergies; vasomotor rhinitis
Bekyree [desogestrel/ethinyl estradiol]	Z79.3	Contraceptive	Prevention of pregnancy
Betaseron [interferon beta-1b]	Z79.899	Antiviral	Treatment of relapsing multiple sclerosis
Betoptic [betaxolol hydrochloride]		Beta blocker; ophthalmic glaucoma agent	Lowering of intraocular pressure; also used for treatment of ocular hypertension and chronic open-angle glaucoma
Bevyxxa	Z79.01	Anticoagulant	Prophylaxis of venous thromboembolism
Beyaz [drospirenone/ethinyl estradiol/levomefolate calcium]	Z79.3	Contraceptive	Prevention of pregnancy; acne
Biaxin XL [clarithromycin]	Z79.2	Antibiotic	Acid/peptic disorder or ulcer, acute exacerbation chronic bronchitis, human immunodeficiency virus, lower and upper respiratory tract infection, sinus infection, prophylaxis mycobacterium avium complex, pharyngitis, pneumonia, tonsillitis
Bijuva [estradiol/progesterone]	Z79.890	Estrogen/progesterone therapy	Menopausal symptoms
Biltricide [praziquantel]		Antiparasitic	Infections from Schistosoma species and liver flukes
Binosto [alendronate sodium]	Z79.83	Bisphosphonate	Prevention of thinning of the bones (osteoporosis)
Boniva [ibandronate sodium]	Z79.83	Bisphosphonate	Prevention of thinning of the bones (osteoporosis)
Breo Ellipta [fluticasone furoate/vilanterol trifenatate]	Z79.51	Corticosteroid – inhaled; anitasthmatic	Maintenance treatment of asthma and COPD
Brevicon 28-day [ethinyl estradiol/norethindrone]	Z79.3	Contraceptive	Prevention of pregnancy; acne
Briellyn [ethinyl estradiol/norethindrone]	Z79.3	Contraceptive	Prevention of pregnancy
Brilinta [ticagrelor]	Z79.02	Antiplatelet	Unstable angina; heart attacks; prevention of blood clots
Brisdelle [paroxetine]		Selective serotonin reuptake inhibitor (SSRI)	Vasomotor symptoms related to menopause
Buprenex [buprenorphine hydrochloride]	Z79.891	Analgesic, narcotic	Moderate to severe pain

Drug	Z Code	Drug Action/Classification	Indications
Buprenorphine HCl and Naloxone HCl [buprenorphine hydrochloride/naloxone hydrochloride]	Z79.891	Analgesic, narcotic	Moderate to severe pain
Buspirone HCl [buspirone hydrochloride]		Antianxiety	Generalized anxiety disorder
Butorphanol tartrate [butorphanol tartrate]	Z79.891	Analgesic, narcotic	Moderate to severe postsurgical pain
Butrans [buprenorphine]	Z79.891	Analgesic, narcotic	Chronic pain
Byetta [exenatide]	Z79.899	Antidiabetic – noninsulin injectable	Diabetes mellitus
Calan [verapamil hydrochloride]		Calcium channel blocker	Angina pectoris at rest and chronic stable, arrhythmia, atrial fibrillation, atrial flutter, paroxysmal supraventricular tachycardia, ventricular arrhythmia, Hypertension
Caldolor [ibuprofen]	Z79.1	Nonsteroidal anti-inflammatory drug (NSAID)	Pain or fever relief
Cambia [diclofenac potassium]	Z79.1	Nonsteroidal anti-inflammatory drug (NSAID)	Migraine headaches
Camila [norethindrone]	Z79.3	Contraceptive	Prevention of pregnancy; menstrual disorders
Caplyta [lumateperone]		Antipsychotic	Schizophrenia
Cardizem CD [diltiazem hydrochloride]		Calcium channel blocker	Chronic stable angina, atrial fibrillation, atrial flutter, hypertension, paroxysmal supraventricular tachycardia
Cardura [doxazosin mesylate]		Antihypertensive	Benign prostatic hyperplasia; hypertension
Catapres [clonidine hydrochloride]		Antihypertensive	Hypertension
Cefprozil [cefprozil]	Z79.2	Antibiotic	Acute exacerbation and chronic bronchitis, lower respiratory tract infection, upper respiratory tract infection, pharyngitis, tonsillitis
Ceftriaxone [ceftriaxone sodium]	Z79.2	Antibiotic	Bacterial infections
Celebrex [celecoxib]	Z79.1	Nonsteroidal anti-inflammatory drug (NSAID)	Relief of some symptoms caused by arthritis, such as inflammation, swelling, stiffness, and joint pain
Celestone Soluspan [betamethasone acetate/betamethasone sodium phosphate]	Z79.52	Corticosteroid; antiasthmatic	Asthma; severe inflammation
Celexa [citalopram hydrobromide]		Antidepressant	Depression
Cellcept [mycophenolate mofetil]	Z79.899	Immunosuppressant	Prophylaxis of organ transplant rejection
Centany [mupirocin]	Z79.2	Antibiotic	Skin infections
Cephalexin [cephalexin]	Z79.2	Antibiotic	Bacterial infections
Chantix [varenicline tartrate]		Smoking cessation aid	Nicotine addiction, smoking
Cimduo [lamivudine/tenofovir disoproxil fumarate]	Z79.899	Antiviral	HIV
Cipro [ciprofloxacin hydrochloride]	Z79.2	Antibiotic	Cystitis, infectious diarrhea, gonorrhea, bone and joint infection, gastrointestinal tract infection, lower and upper respiratory tract infection, sinus infection, urinary tract infection, nosocomial pneumonia, chronic prostatitis
Ciprofloxacin [ciprofloxacin]	Z79.2	Antibiotic	Bacterial infections
Clarithromycin [clarithromycin]	Z79.2	Antibiotic	Skin and respiratory bacterial infections
Claritin [loratadine]		Antihistamine	Seasonal allergic rhinitis; chronic idiopathic urticaria
Cleocin [clindamycin phosphate]	Z79.2	Antibiotic	Bacterial infections
Climara [estradiol]	Z79.890	Estrogen therapy	Osteoporosis prevention and to treat menopausal symptoms; vaginal and vulvar atrophy; hypoestrogenism; ovarian failure
Clindamycin [clindamycin phosphate]	Z79.2	Antibiotic	Bacterial infections
Clonazepam [clonazepam]		Anticonvulsant	Absence, akinetic and myoclonic epilepsy, Lennox-Gastaut syndrome
Clonidine HCl [clonidine hydrochloride]		Antihypertensive	Hypertension
Clopidogrel bisulfate [clopidogrel bisulfate]	Z79.02	Antiplatelet	Unstable angina; heart attacks; prevention of blood clots
Codeine [codeine sulfate]	Z79.891	Analgesic, narcotic	Mild to moderate pain
Cogentin [benztropine mesylate]		Antiparkinsonism	Parkinson's disease
Colace [docusate sodium]		Gastrointestinal agent; laxative, stool softener	Constipation

Drug	Z Code	Drug Action/Classification	Indications
Colocort [hydrocortisone]	Z79.52	Corticosteroid	Inflammation of the colon
CombiPatch [ethinyl estradiol/norethindrone acetate]	Z79.890	Estrogen therapy	Menopause symptoms; vaginal and vulvar atrophy; osteoporosis prevention
Combivent respimat [ipratropium bromide/albuterol sulfate]		Antiasthmatic/bronchodilator	Chronic bronchitis, emphysema; bronchial asthma
Compro [prochlorperazine]		Antiemetic; antipsychotic	Nausea, vomiting, and manic phase of bipolar syndrome or schizophrenia
Conjupri [levamlodipine maleate]		Antihypertensive	Hypertension
Copaxone [glatiramer acetate]		Immunostimulant	Treatment of relapsing multiple sclerosis
Coreg [carvedilol]		Beta blocker	Hypertension; chronic heart failure; left ventricular dysfunction following myocardial infarction
Coreg CR [carvedilol phosphate]		Beta blocker	Hypertension; chronic heart failure; left ventricular dysfunction following myocardial infarction
Cortef [hydrocortisone]	Z79.52	Corticosteroid	Severe inflammation
Cortenema [hydrocortisone]	Z79.52	Corticosteroid	Inflammation of the colon
Cortifoam [hydrocortisone acetate]	Z79.52	Corticosteroid	Colon and rectum inflammation
Cortisone acetate [cortisone acetate]	Z79.52	Corticosteroid	Inflammation
Cortisporin [hydrocortisone acetate/neomycin sulfate/polymyxin B sulfate]		Topical anti-infective, topical steroid	Dermatosis
Cosentyx [secukinumab]	Z79.899	Immunosuppressant	Plaque psoriasis; psoriatic arthritis; ankylosing spondylitis
Coumadin [warfarin sodium]	Z79.01	Anticoagulant	Prophylaxis and treatment of venous thrombosis, treatment of atrial fibrillation with embolization (pulmonary embolism), arrhythmias, myocardial infarction, and stroke prevention
Cozaar [losartan potassium]		Antihypertensive	Hypertension
Crestor [rosuvastatin calcium]		HMG-CoA reductase inhibitor (statin)	Hypercholesterolemia; hyperlipidemia; hyperproteinemia
Crixivan [indinavir sulfate]	Z79.899	Antiviral	HIV, asymptomatic HIV
Cryselle [ethinyl estradiol/norgestrel]	Z79.3	Contraceptive	Prevention of pregnancy
Cubicin [daptomycin]	Z79.2	Antibiotic	Bacterial skin infections; Staphylococcus aureus bloodstream infections
Cyclafem [ethinyl estradiol/norethindrone]	Z79.3	Contraceptive	Prevention of pregnancy
Cyclessa [desogestrel/ethinyl estradiol]	Z79.3	Contraceptive	Prevention of pregnancy
Cyclosporine [cyclosporine]	Z79.899	Immunosuppressant	Prophylaxis of organ transplant rejection
Cyltezo [adalimumab-abdm]	Z79.899	Antirheumatic	Rheumatoid arthritis; juvenile idiopathic arthritis; psoriatic arthritis; Crohn's disease; ulcerative colitis; plaque psoriasis
Cymbalta [duloxetine hydrochloride]		Antidepressant, serotonin and norepinephrine reuptake inhibitor (SNRI)	Major depressive disorder; general anxiety disorder; fibromyalgia; diabetic peripheral neuropathy; chronic musculoskeletal pain
Cytomel [liothyronine sodium]		Thyroid hormone	Hypothyroidism or prevention of euthyroid goiters
Daptomycin [daptomycin]	Z79.2	Antibiotic	Skin and underlying tissue bacterial infections
Dasetta [ethinyl estradiol/norethindrone]	Z79.3	Contraceptive	Prevention of pregnancy
Daypro [oxaprozin]	Z79.1	Nonsteroidal anti-inflammatory drug (NSAID)	Osteoarthritis and rheumatoid arthritis
Daysee [ethinyl estradiol/levonorgestrel]	Z79.3	Contraceptive	Prevention of pregnancy
Delestrogen [estradiol valerate]	Z79.890	Estrogen therapy	Menopause symptoms
Demerol [meperidine hydrochloride]	Z79.891	Analgesic, narcotic	Moderate to severe pain
Depakote [divalproex sodium]		Anticonvulsant	Bipolar affective disorder; complex absence, complex partial and mixed pattern epilepsy; migraine headache
Depo-Medrol [methylprednisolone acetate]	Z79.52	Corticosteroid	Arthritis; joint disorders
Depo-Provera [medroxyprogesterone acetate]	Z79.3, Z79.890	Antineoplastic; contraceptive; progestin	Amenorrhea; carcinoma, endometrium, adjunct; carcinoma, renal; Prevention of pregnancy; hemorrhage
Depo-SubQ Provera [medroxyprogesterone acetate]	Z79.3	Contraceptive	Prevention of pregnancy; menstrual disorder pain

Drug	Z Code	Drug Action/Classification	Indications
Descovy [emtricitabine/tenofovir alafenamide]	Z79.899	Antiretroviral	HIV
Desogestrel; Ethinyl [desogestrel/ethinyl estradiol]	Z79.3	Contraceptive	Prevention of pregnancy
Detrol [tolterodine tartrate]		Muscarinic receptor antagonist	Overactive bladders in patients with urinary frequency, urgency, or urge incontinence
Dexamethasone Intensol [dexamethasone]	Z79.52	Corticosteroid	Arthritis; allergic disorders; breathing disorders; lupus
Dexilant [dexlansoprazole]		Proton pump inhibitor	Healing of erosive esophagitis; relieve of heartburn; treatment of non-erosive gastroesophageal reflux disease
Diaβeta [glyburide]	Z79.84	Oral hypoglycemic	Diabetes mellitus
Diclegis [doxylamine succinate/pyridoxine hydrochloride]		Antiemetic	Nausea/vomiting in pregnancy
Dificid [fidaxomicin]	Z79.2	Antibiotic	Clostridium difficile
Diflucan [fluconazole]		Antifungal	Oropharyngeal and esophageal candidiasis and cryptococcal meningitis in AIDS patients
Digoxin [digoxin]		Cardiotonic glycoside	Heart failure, atrial flutter, atrial fibrillation, and supraventricular tachycardia
Dilantin [phenytoin sodium]		Anticonvulsant	Grand mal and psychomotor seizures
Dilaudid [hydromorphone hydrochloride]	Z79.891	Analgesic, narcotic	Moderate to severe pain
Diovan [valsartan]		Antihypertensive	Hypertension
Diskets [methadone hydrochloride]		Opioid agonist	Treatment of opioid addiction
Divigel [estradiol]	Z79.890	Estrogen therapy – topical	Menopause symptoms
Dolophine HCl [methadone hydrochloride]	Z79.891	Analgesic, narcotic; opioid agonist	Pain; treatment of opioid addiction
Doxycycline [doxycycline]	Z79.2	Antibiotic	Bacterial infections; acne
Duavee [bazedoxifene acetate/conjugated estrogens]	Z79.890	Estrogen therapy	Menopause symptoms; osteoporosis prevention
Duetact [glimepiride/pioglitazone hydrochloride]	Z79.84	Oral hypoglycemic	Diabetes mellitus
Duexis [famotidine/ibuprofen]	Z79.1	Nonsteroidal anti-inflammatory drug (NSAID)	Symptomatic treatment of osteoarthritis and rheumatoid arthritis; reduce risk of ulcers
Dulera [formoterol fumarate/mometasone furoate]	Z79.51	Corticosteroid – inhaled; antiasthmatic	Prophylaxis and treatment of asthma
Duragesic [fentanyl]	Z79.891	Analgesic, narcotic	Chronic pain
Duramorph PF [morphine sulfate]	Z79.891	Analgesic, narcotic	Moderate to severe pain
Durlaza [aspirin]	Z79.82	Aspirin	Prevention of heart attack, stroke, angina
Dynacin [minocycline hydrochloride]	Z79.2	Antibiotic	Severe acne treatment
E.E.S. [erythromycin ethylsuccinate]	Z79.2	Antibiotic	Bacterial infections
Effexor XR [venlafaxine hydrochloride]		Antidepressant, serotonin and norepinephrine reuptake inhibitors (SNRIs)	Major depressive disorder; social anxiety disorder; panic disorder
Effient [prasugrel hydrochloride]	Z79.02	Antiplatelet	Lessening of the chance of heart attack or stroke
Elestrin [estradiol]	Z79.890	Estrogen therapy	Menopause symptoms
Eligard [leuprolide acetate]	Z79.818	Agents affecting estrogen receptors and estrogen levels	Palliative treatment of prostate cancer symptoms
Elinest [norgestrel/ethinyl estradiol]	Z79.3	Contraceptive	Prevention of pregnancy
Eliquis [apixaban]	Z79.01	Anticoagulant	Venous thrombosis
Emoquette [ethinyl estradiol/desogestrel]	Z79.3	Contraceptive	Prevention of pregnancy
Emtriva [emtricitabine]	Z79.899	Antiretroviral	HIV
Enbrel [etanercept]	Z79.899	Antirheumatic	Rheumatoid arthritis; polyarticular juvenile idiopathic arthritis; psoriatic arthritis; ankylosing spondylitis, plaque psoriasis
Enpresse-28 [ethinyl estradiol/levonorgestrel]	Z79.3	Contraceptive	Prevention of pregnancy

Drug	Z Code	Drug Action/Classification	Indications
Enskyce [desogestrel/ethinyl estradiol]	Z79.3	Contraceptive	Prevention of pregnancy
Entocort EC [budesonide]	Z79.52	Corticosteroid	Crohn's disease; ulcerative colitis
Entresto [sacubitril/valsartan]		Angiotensin II receptor blocker; neprilysin inhibitor	Chronic heart failure
Entyvio [vedolizumab]	Z79.899	Immunosuppressant	Ulcerative colitis; Crohn's disease
Envarsus XR [tacrolimus]	Z79.899	Immunosuppressant	Prophylaxis of organ transplant rejection
Epinephrine [epinephrine]		Bronchodilator, cardiotonic	Most commonly, relief of distress due to bronchospasm and restoration of cardiac rhythm in cardiac arrest
Epivir, Epivir-HBV [lamivudine]	Z79.899	Antiretroviral	HIV, hepatitis B (HBV), asymptomatic HIV
Erelzi [etanercept-szzs]	Z79.899	Antirheumatic	Rheumatoid arthritis; polyarticular juvenile idiopathic arthritis; psoriatic arthritis; ankylosing spondylitis, plaque psoriasis
Errin [norethindrone]	Z79.3	Contraceptive	Prevention of pregnancy
Ertapenem [ertapenem sodium]	Z79.2	Antibiotic	Stomach, urinary tract, pelvis, skin and lung infections
ERYC [erythromycin]	Z79.2	Antibiotic	Respiratory tract infections
Erygel [erythromycin]	Z79.2	Antibiotic, topical	Bacterial skin infections
EryPed [erythromycin ethylsuccinate]	Z79.2	Antibiotic	Bacterial infections; rheumatic fever attacks
Ery-Tab [erythromycin]	Z79.2	Antibiotic	Bacterial infections
Erythrocin [erythromycin lactobionate]	Z79.2	Antibiotic	Bacterial infections
Erythromycin [erythromycin]	Z79.2	Antibiotic	Respiratory tract infections
Estarylla [ethinyl estradiol/norgestimate]	Z79.3	Contraceptive	Prevention of pregnancy
Estrace [estradiol]	Z79.890	Estrogen therapy	Vaginal cream for treatment of vaginal and vulvar atrophy
EstroGel [estradiol]	Z79.890	Estrogen therapy – topical	Menopause symptoms
Estrostep Fe [ethinyl estradiol/norethindrone acetate]	Z79.3	Contraceptive	Prevention of pregnancy
Evista [raloxifene hydrochloride]	Z79.810	Selective estrogen receptor modulator (SERM)	Prevention of thinning of the bones (osteoporosis) only in postmenopausal women
Exemestane [exemestane]	Z79.811	Aromatase inhibitor	Postmenopausal breast cancer
Factive [gemifloxacin mesylate]	Z79.2	Antibiotic	Bacterial lung infections
Falmina [ethinyl estradiol/levonorgestrel]	Z79.3	Contraceptive	Prevention of pregnancy
Fareston [toremifene citrate]	Z79.810	Selective estrogen receptor modulator (SERM)	Treatment of metastatic breast cancer in postmenopausal women
Farxiga [dapagliflozin propanediol]	Z79.84	Oral hypoglycemic	Diabetes mellitus
Faslodex [fulvestrant]	Z79.818	Agents affecting estrogen receptors and estrogen levels	Hormone-related breast cancer; metastatic breast cancer
Feldene [piroxicam]	Z79.1	Nonsteroidal anti-inflammatory drug (NSAID)	Treatment of pain and inflammation due to arthritis
Femara [letrozole]	Z79.811	Aromatase inhibitor	Postmenopausal breast cancer
Femhrt [ethinyl estradiol/norethindrone acetate]	Z79.3, Z79.890	Contraceptive; estrogen therapy	Prevention of pregnancy; menopause symptoms; osteoporosis prevention
Femring [estradiol acetate]	Z79.890	Estrogen therapy	Osteoporosis prevention and to treat menopausal symptoms; hypoestrogenism; ovarian failure
Fentanyl citrate [fentanyl citrate]	Z79.891	Analgesic, narcotic	Postprocedural or chronic pain
Fentora [fentanyl citrate]	Z79.891	Analgesic, narcotic	Breakthrough cancer pain
Fetroja [cefiderocol]	Z79.2	Antibiotic	Complicated urinary tract infections; pyelonephritis
Fiasp [insulin aspart]	Z79.4	Insulin	Diabetes mellitus
Fioricet with codeine [acetaminophen/butalbital/caffeine/codeine phosphate]	Z79.891	Analgesic, narcotic	Tension headaches
Firmagon [degarelix]	Z79.890	Hormone therapy	Prostate cancer
Flagyl [metronidazole]	Z79.2	Antibiotic	Bacterial infections
Flavoxate HCl [flavoxate hydrochloride]		Urinary tract spasmolytic	Relief of dysuria, urgency, nocturia, suprapubic pain, frequency, and incontinence associated with cystitis, prostatitis, urethritis, and urethrocystitis/urethrotrigonitis

Drug	Z Code	Drug Action/Classification	Indications
Flomax [tamsulosin hydrochloride]		Antiadrenergic	Benign prostatic hyperplasia
Flonase allergy relief [fluticasone propionate]	Z79.899	Corticosteroid – intranasal	Perennial and seasonal allergic rhinitis
Flovent HFA [fluticasone propionate]	Z79.51	Corticosteroid – inhaled; antiasthmatic	Asthma
Fortaz [ceftazidime]	Z79.2	Antibiotic	Pneumonia and lower respiratory infections
Fosamax [alendronate sodium]	Z79.83	Bisphosphonate	Osteoporosis; Paget's disease
Fosinopril sodium [fosinopril sodium]		ACE inhibitor	Hypertension
Fosrenol [lanthanum carbonate]		Phosphate binder	End-stage renal disease (ESRD)
Fragmin [dalteparin sodium]	Z79.Ø1	Anticoagulant	Prophylaxis and treatment of blood clots
Gengraf [cyclosporine]	Z79.899	Immunosuppressant	Prophylaxis of organ transplant rejection
Gentamicin sulfate [gentamicin sulfate]	Z79.2	Antibiotic	Severe bacterial infections
Gildagia [ethinyl estradiol/norethindrone]	Z79.3	Contraceptive	Prevention of pregnancy
Gildess [ethinyl estradiol/norethindrone acetate]	Z79.3	Contraceptive	Prevention of pregnancy
Glimepiride [glimepiride]	Z79.84	Oral hypoglycemic	Diabetes mellitus
Glucotrol [glipizide]	Z79.84	Oral hypoglycemic	Diabetes mellitus
Glumetza [metformin hydrochloride]	Z79.84	Oral hypoglycemic	Diabetes mellitus
Glyburide (micronized) [glyburide]	Z79.84	Oral hypoglycemic	Diabetes mellitus
Glynase [glyburide]	Z79.84	Oral hypoglycemic	Diabetes mellitus
Glyset [miglitol]	Z79.84	Oral hypoglycemic	Diabetes mellitus
Harvoni [ledipasvir/sofosbuvir]	Z79.899	Antiviral	Chronic hepatitis C
Heparin sodium [heparin sodium]	Z79.Ø1	Anticoagulant	Prophylaxis and treatment of venous thrombosis, pulmonary embolism; prevention of cerebral thrombosis, and treatment of consumptive coagulopathies
Humalog [insulin lispro recombinant]	Z79.4	Insulin	Diabetes mellitus
Humira [adalimumab]	Z79.899	Antirheumatic	Rheumatoid arthritis; juvenile idiopathic arthritis; psoriatic arthritis; Crohn's disease; ulcerative colitis; plaque psoriasis; hidradenitis suppurativa; uveitis
Humulin R [insulin recombinant]	Z79.4	Insulin	Diabetes mellitus
Hydrochlorothiazide [hydrochlorothiazide]		Diuretic; antihypertensive	Management of hypertension and in adjunctive therapy for edema associated with congestive heart failure; hepatic cirrhosis; corticosteroid, and estrogen therapy
Hydrocodone [acetaminophen/hydrocodone bitartrate]	Z79.891	Analgesic, narcotic	Moderate to severe pain
Hydrocodone bitartrate and acetaminophen [acetaminophen/ hydrocodone bitartrate]	Z79.891	Analgesic, narcotic	Pain, moderate to severe
Hydrocortisone [hydrocortisone]	Z79.52	Corticosteroid	Addison's disease; arthritis; immune disorders; allergies; breathing problems
Hydromorphone HCl [hydromorphone hydrochloride]	Z79.891	Analgesic, narcotic	Moderate to severe pain
Hyrimoz [adalimumab-adaz]	Z79.899	Antirheumatic	Rheumatoid arthritis; juvenile idiopathic arthritis; psoriatic arthritis; Crohn's disease; ulcerative colitis; plaque psoriasis
Hyzaar [hydrochlorothiazide/ losartan potassium]		Antihypertensive	Hypertension
Ibsrela [tenapanor hydrochloride]		NHE-3 inhibitor	Irritable bowel syndrome with constipation (IBS-C)
Ibuprofen [ibuprofen]	Z79.1	Nonsteroidal anti-inflammatory drug (NSAID)	Pain or fever relief
Imitrex [sumatriptan succinate]		Antimigraine	Migraine headache
Imuran [azathioprine]	Z79.899	Immunosuppressant	Rheumatoid arthritis
Inderal [propranolol hydrochloride]		Beta blocker	Angina pectoris; hypertension; cardiac arrhythmias
Indocin [indomethacin]	Z79.1	Nonsteroidal anti-inflammatory drug (NSAID)	Treatment of pain and inflammation

Drug	Z Code	Drug Action/Classification	Indications
Integrilin [eptifibatide]	Z79.02	Antiplatelet	Unstable angina; heart attacks; prevention of blood clots
Intron A [interferon alfa 2-b]	Z79.899	Antineoplastic interferons; antiviral interferons	Cancer; hepatitis
Introvale [levonorgestrel/ethinyl estradiol]	Z79.3	Contraceptive	Prevention of pregnancy
Invanz [ertapeneum sodium]	Z79.2	Antibiotic	Stomach, urinary tract, pelvis, skin and lung infections
Invokamet [canagliflozin/metformin hydrochloride]	Z79.84	Oral hypoglycemic	Diabetes mellitus
Invokana [canagliflozin]	Z79.84	Oral hypoglycemic	Diabetes mellitus
Isoniazid [isoniazid]	Z79.2	Antibiotic	Tuberculosis
Isopto carpine [pilocarpine hydrochloride]		Cholinergic parasympathomimetic agent	Reduction of intraocular pressure in open-angle glaucoma or ocular hypertension; management of acute angle-closure glaucoma
Isordil [isosorbide dinitrate]		Smooth muscle relaxant	Acute anginal attacks
Isturisa [osilodrostat]		Cortisol synthesis inhibitor	Cushing's disease in adults
Isuprel [isoproterenol hydrochloride]		Adrenergic agent	Bronchodilator for asthma, chronic pulmonary emphysema, bronchitis, and other conditions accompanied by bronchospasm; can be used in cardiogenic shock cases
Jantoven [warfarin sodium]	Z79.01	Anticoagulant	Prophylaxis and treatment of venous thrombosis, pulmonary embolism; prevention of cerebral thrombosis, and treatment of consumptive coagulopathies
Janumet [metformin hydrochloride/sitagliptin phosphate]	Z79.84	Oral hypoglycemic	Diabetes mellitus
Januvia [sitagliptin phosphate]	Z79.84	Oral hypoglycemic	Diabetes mellitus
Jencycla [norethindrone]	Z79.3	Contraceptive	Prevention of pregnancy
Jentadueto [linagliptin/metformin hydrochloride]]	Z79.84	Oral hypoglycemic	Diabetes mellitus
Junel [ethinyl estradiol/norethindrone acetate]	Z79.3	Contraceptive	Prevention of pregnancy
Kadian [morphine sulfate]	Z79.891	Analgesic, narcotic	Moderate to severe pain
Kariva [desogestrel/ethinyl estradiol]	Z79.3	Contraceptive	Prevention of pregnancy
Katerzia [amlodipine benzoate]		Antihypertensive	Hypertension; coronary artery disease (CAD); chronic stable angina; prinzmetal's angina; variant angina
Kazano [alogliptin benzoate/metformin hydrochloride]	Z79.84	Oral hypoglycemic	Diabetes mellitus
Keflex [cephalexin]	Z79.2	Antibiotic	Bone, middle ear, skin and skin structures, upper respiratory tract and urinary tract infections; acute prostatitis
Kelnor [ethynodiol diacetate/ethinyl estradiol]	Z79.3	Contraceptive	Prevention of pregnancy
Kenalog-10; Kenalog-40 [triamcinolone acetonide]	Z79.52	Corticosteroid	Gouty arthritis; bursitis; tenosynovitis; epicondylitis; rheumatoid arthritis; synovitis; osteoarthritis
Keytruda [pembrolizumab]	Z79.899	Antineoplastic	Cancer
Kimidess [ethinyl estradiol/desogestrel]	Z79.3	Contraceptive	Prevention of pregnancy
Klaron [sulfacetamide sodium]	Z79.2	Antibiotic, topical	Acne vulgaris
Klonopin [clonazepam]		Anticonvulsant; CNS depressant	Epilepsy; seizures; panic disorder
Klor-Con [potassium chloride]		Replaces potassium and maintains potassium level	Hypokalemia
Kombiglyze [metformin hydrochloride/saxagliptin hydrochloride]	Z79.84	Oral hypoglycemic	Diabetes mellitus
K-Tab [potassium chloride]		Replaces potassium and maintains potassium level	Hypokalemia
Kurvelo [ethinyl estradiol/levonorgestrel]	Z79.3	Contraceptive	Prevention of pregnancy; menstrual disorders
Kyleena [levonorgestrel]	Z79.3	Contraceptive	Prevention of pregnancy
Lamisil [terbinafine hydrochloride]		Antifungal	Tinea cruris (jock itch), T. pedis (athlete's foot), T. corporis (ringworm)

Drug	Z Code	Drug Action/Classification	Indications
Lanoxin [digoxin]		Cardiotonic glycoside	Congestive heart failure
Lantus [insulin glargine recombinant]	Z79.4	Insulin	Diabetes mellitus
Larin [ethinyl estradiol/norethindrone acetate]	Z79.3	Contraceptive	Prevention of pregnancy
Lasix [furosemide]		Antihypertensive; diuretic	Management of edema associated with congestive heart failure, renal disease, including nephrotic syndrome and hypertension
Lazanda [fentanyl citrate]	Z79.891	Analgesics, narcotic	Breakthrough cancer pain
Lescol XL [fluvastatin sodium]		HMG-CoA reductase inhibitor (statin)	Hypercholesterolemia; hyperlipidemia; hyperlipoproteinemia
Lessina-28 [ethinyl estradiol/levonorgestrel]	Z79.3	Contraceptive	Prevention of pregnancy
Letrozole [letrozole]	Z79.811	Aromatase inhibitor	Postmenopausal breast cancer
Levemir [insulin detemir recombinant]	Z79.4	Insulin	Diabetes mellitus
Levonest [levonorgestrel/ethinyl estradiol]	Z79.3	Contraceptive	Prevention of pregnancy; menstrual disorders; acne
Levora [levonorgestrel/ethinyl estradiol]	Z79.3	Contraceptive	Prevention of pregnancy
Levothroid [levothyroxine sodium]		Thyroid hormone	Hypothyroidism
Levoxyl [levothyroxine sodium]		Thyroid hormone	Euthyroid goiter; hypothyroidism
Lexapro [escitalopram oxalate]		Antidepressant, selective serotonin reuptake inhibitor (SSRI)	Depression; anxiety
Lialda [mesalamine]		Anti-inflammatory	Ulcerative colitis
Librium [chlordiazepoxide hydrochloride]		Antianxiety	Acute withdrawal symptoms, especially from alcohol, or for other anxiety-producing conditions
Lidocaine HCl [lidocaine hydrochloride]		Antiarrhythmic	Management of ventricular arrhythmias or during cardiac manipulation, such as cardiac surgery
Liletta [levonorgestrel]	Z79.3	Contraceptive	Intrauterine device to Prevention of pregnancy
Lincocin [lincocin hydrochloride]	Z79.2	Antibiotic	Severe bacterial infections
Lipitor [atorvastatin calcium]		HMG-CoA reductase inhibitor (statin)	Hypercholesterolemia; hyperlipidemia; hyperproteinemia
Lithium carbonate [lithium carbonate]		Antimanic	Control of manic episodes in bipolar disorders
Lo Loestrin Fe [ethinyl estradiol/norethindrone acetate]	Z79.3	Contraceptive	Prevention of pregnancy
Locoid [hydrocotisone butyrate]	Z79.52	Corticosteroid – topical	Atopic dermatitis; other dermatoses
Loestrin [ethinyl estradiol/norethindrone acetate]	Z79.3	Contraceptive	Prevention of pregnancy
Lomotil [diphenoxylate hydrochloride/atropine sulfate]		Antidiarrheal	Symptoms of chronic and functional diarrhea
Lopid [gemfibrozil]		Lipid regulating agent	Hypercholesterolemia, hyperlipidemia, hyperlipoproteinemia, hypertriglyceridemia
Lopressor [metoprolol tartrate]		Beta blocker	Angina pectoris; hypertension; acute myocardial infarction
Lorazepam [lorazepam]		Antianxiety; sedative/hypnotic	Anxiety disorder associated with depressive symptoms; controls tension, agitation, irritability, and insomnia
Loryna [drospirenone/ethinyl estradiol]	Z79.3	Contraceptive	Prevention of pregnancy
LoSeasonique [ethinyl estradiol/levonorgestrel]	Z79.3	Contraceptive	Prevention of pregnancy
Lotensin [benazepril hydrochloride]		ACE inhibitor	Hypertension
Lotrel [amlodipine besylate/benazepril hydrochloride]		Antihypertensive	Hypertension
Lotrisone [clotrimazole/ betamethasone dipropionate]		Antifungal-corticosteroid	Relief of redness, swelling, itching, and other discomfort of fungus infections
Lovastatin [lovastatin]		HMG-CoA reductase inhibitor (statin)	Hypercholesterolemia; hyperlipidemia; hyperlipoproteinemia
Lovenox [enoxaparin sodium]	Z79.01	Anticoagulant	Prophylaxis and treatment of venous thrombosis and pulmonary embolism
Low-Ogestrel-28 [norgestrel/ethinyl estradiol]	Z79.3	Contraceptive	Prevention of pregnancy
Lupron Depot [leuprolide acetate]	Z79.818	Agents affecting estrogen receptors and estrogen levels	Endometriosis symptoms; uterine fibroids

Drug	Z Code	Drug Action/Classification	Indications
Macrobid [nitrofuantoin]	Z79.2	Antibiotic	Urinary tract infections
Macrodantin [nitrofurantoin]	Z79.2	Antibiotic	Urinary tract infections
Marlissa [ethinyl estradiol/levonorgestrel]	Z79.3	Contraceptive	Prevention of pregnancy
Maxipime [cefepime hydrochloride]	Z79.2	Antibiotic	Bacterial infections
Meclizine hydrochloride [meclizine hydrochloride]		Antihistamine	Nausea and vomiting, and dizziness associated with motion sickness
Medrol [methylprednisolone]	Z79.52	Corticosteroid	Endocrine, rheumatic, hematologic disorders; collagen, dermatological, ophthalmic, respiratory, neoplastic, gastrointestinal, nervous system disorders; allergic and edematous states
Mefoxin [cefoxitin sodium]	Z79.2	Antibiotic	Bacterial infections
Megace ES [megestrol acetate]	Z79.818	Agents affecting estrogen receptors and estrogen levels	Endometrial or advanced breast cancers; weight loss due to AIDS
Menest [esteriefied estrogens]	Z79.890	Estrogen therapy	Menopause symptoms; ovarian failure
Menostar [estradiol]	Z79.890	Estrogen therapy	Menopause symptoms; osteoporosis prevention
Mepron [atovaquone]	Z79.2	Antibiotic	Pneumonia due to penumocystis jiroveci
Merrem [meropenem]	Z79.2	Antibiotic	Bacterial infections of skin or stomach; bacterial meningitis
Metformin [metformin hydrochloride]	Z79.84	Oral hypoglycemic	Diabetes mellitus
Methadone HCl [methadone hydrochloride]	Z79.891	Analgesic, narcotic; opioid agonist	Pain; treatment of opioid addiction
Methadose [methadone hydrochloride]	Z79.891	Analgesic, narcotic	Acute and chronic pain
Methergine [methylergonovine maleate]		Oxytocic agent	Routine management of postpartum hemorrhage after delivery of placenta
Methylprednisolone [methylprednisolone]	Z79.52	Corticosteroid	Inflammatory disorders
Metronidazole [metronidazole]	Z79.2	Antibiotic	Bacterial infections
Miacalcin [calcitonin salmon]		Calcitonin; a peptide hormone	Hypercalcemia, osteoporosis, postmenopausal symptoms, Paget's disease
Microgestin [ethinyl estradiol/norethindrone acetate]	Z79.3	Contraceptive	Prevention of pregnancy
Minastrin [ethinyl estradiol/norethindrone acetate]	Z79.3	Contraceptive	Prevention of pregnancy
Minivelle [estradiol]	Z79.890	Estrogen therapy	Menopause symptoms; osteoporosis prevention
Minocin [minocycline hydrochloride]	Z79.2	Antibiotic	Bacterial infections; acne
Mirena [levonorgestrel]	Z79.3	Contraceptive	Intrauterine device for prevention of pregnancy; menstrual disorders
Mobic [meloxicam]	Z79.1	Nonsteroidal anti-inflammatory drug (NSAID)	Treatment of pain and inflammation due to osteoarthritis and rheumatoid arthritis
Monoclonal antibodies	Z79.899	Monoclonal antibodies	Cancer; prophylaxis of organ transplant rejection
Monodox [doxycycline]	Z79.2	Antibiotic	Bacterial infections; acne
Monoket [isosorbide mononitrate]		Antianginal; coronary vasodilator, nitrate	Angina pectoris
Mono-Linyah [norgestimate/ethinyl estradiol]	Z79.3	Contraceptive	Prevention of pregnancy; menstrual disorders; acne
Monurol [fosfomycin tromethamine]	Z79.2	Antibiotic	Bacterial bladder infections
Morphabond ER [morphine sulfate]	Z79.891	Analgesics, narcotic	Pain
Morphine sulfate [morphine sulfate]	Z79.891	Analgesic, narcotic	Moderate to severe pain
Motrin IB [ibuprofen]	Z79.1	Nonsteroidal anti-inflammatory drug (NSAID)	Pain or fever relief
MS Contin [morphine sulfate]	Z79.891	Analgesic, narcotic	Moderate to severe pain
Multaq [dronedarone hydrochloride]		Cardiac rhythm regulator	Treatment of patients with recent episodes of atrial fibrillation or atrial flutter
Mycobutin [rifabutin]	Z79.2	Antibiotic	Mycobacterium avium complex (MAC) prophylactic in HIV patients
Mytesi [crofelemer]		Antidiarrheal	Diarrhea occurring in HIV/AIDs patient's on anti-retroviral therapy
Myzilra [ethinyl estradiol/levonorgestrel]	Z79.3	Contraceptive	Prevention of pregnancy

Drug	Z Code	Drug Action/Classification	Indications
Nabumetone [nabumetone]	Z79.1	Nonsteroidal anti-inflammatory drug (NSAID)	Osteoarthritis and rheumatoid arthritis
Nalfon [fenoprofen calcium]	Z79.1	Nonsteroidal anti-inflammatory drug (NSAID)	Pain or inflammation relief
Namzaric [memantine/donepezil hydrochlroides]		Acetylcholinesterase/cholinesterase inhibitors	Dementia due to Alzheimer's
Naprelan [naproxen sodium]	Z79.1	Nonsteroidal anti-inflammatory drug (NSAID)	Pain or inflammation relief
Naprosyn [naproxen]	Z79.1	Nonsteroidal anti-inflammatory drug (NSAID)	Rheumatoid, gouty arthritis and osteoarthritis; ankylosing spondylitis; bursitis; dysmenorrhea; pain, mild to moderate; tendonitis
Natazia [estradiol valerate/dienogest]	Z79.3	Contraceptive	Prevention of pregnancy; menstrual disorders
Nebupent [pentamidine isethionate]	Z79.2	Antibiotic	Severe bacterial lung infection in high risk patients with HIV
Nefazodone HCl [nefazodone hydrochloride]		Antidepressant	Depression
Nembutal sodium [pentobarbital sodium]		Sedative/hypnotic	Adjunct medication in diagnostic procedures or for emergency use with convulsive disorders
NeoProfen [ibuprofen lysine]	Z79.1	Nonsteroidal anti-inflammatory drug (NSAID)	Pain or fever relief
Neoral [cyclosporine]	Z79.899	Immunosuppressant	Prophylaxis of organ transplant rejection
Neurontin [gabapentin]		Anticonvulsant	Epilepsy, partial
Nexium [esomeprazole magnesium]		Proton pump inhibitor	Gastroesophageal reflux disease (GERD), erosive esophagitis
Nexplanon [etonogestrel]	Z79.3	Contraceptive	Implantable device used for prevention of pregnancy
Nitrofurantoin [nitrofurantoin]	Z79.2	Antibiotic	Bacterial urinary tract infections
Nitropress [sodium nitroprusside]		Vasodilator	Potent, rapid action in reducing blood pressure in hypertensive crisis or for controlling bleeding during anesthesia by producing controlled hypotension
Nitrostat [nitroglycerin]		Muscle relaxant; antianginal; antihypertensive; coronary vasodilator	Prophylaxis and treatment of angina pectoris; heart failure associated with myocardial infarction; hypertension, perioperative; surgery, adjunct
Norco [acetaminophen/hydrocodone bitartrate]	Z79.891	Analgesic, narcotic	Moderate to severe pain
Norinyl [mestranol/norethisterone]	Z79.3	Contraceptive	Prevention of pregnancy
Norpace [disopyramide phosphate]		Antiarrhythmic	Coronary artery disease, for prevention, recurrence and control of unifocal, multifocal, and paired PVCs
Nor-QD [norethindrone]	Z79.3	Contraceptive	Prevention of pregnancy
Nortrel [ethinyl estradiol/norethindrone]	Z79.3	Contraceptive	Prevention of pregnancy
Norvasc [amlodipine besylate]		Antihypertensive	Hypertension; coronary artery disease (CAD); chronic stable angina; prinzmetal's angina; variant angina
Novolin [insulin recombinant]	Z79.4	Insulin	Diabetes mellitus
Novolog [insulin aspart recombinant]	Z79.4	Insulin	Diabetes mellitus
Nucynta [tapentadol hydrochloride]	Z79.891	Analgesic, narcotic	Moderate to severe pain
NuvaRing [etonogestrel/ethinyl estradiol]	Z79.3	Contraceptive	Vaginal ring to Prevention of pregnancy
Ogestrel [norgestrel/ethinyl estradiol]	Z79.3	Contraceptive	Prevention of pregnancy
Onglyza [saxagliptin hydrochloride]	Z79.84	Oral hypoglycemic	Diabetes mellitus
Oracea [doxycycline]	Z79.2	Antibiotic	Rosacea
Orapred ODT [prednisolone sodium phosphate]	Z79.52	Corticosteroid	Inflammatory disorders
Orbactiv [oritavancin diphosphate]	Z79.2	Antibiotic	Bacterial skin infections
Orencia [abatacept]	Z79.899	Antirheumatic	Rheumatoid arthritis; polyarticular juvenile idiopathic arthritis; psoriatic arthritis
Orilissa [elagolix]	Z79.890	Hormone therapy	Pain associated with endometriosis
Orphenadrine citrate [orphenadrine citrate]		Muscle relaxant	Acute spasms, tension, and post-trauma cases

Drug	Z Code	Drug Action/Classification	Indications
Orsythia [ethinyl estradiol/levonorgestrel]	Z79.3	Contraceptive	Prevention of pregnancy
Ortho-Novum [norethindrone/ethinyl estradiol]	Z79.3	Contraceptive	Prevention of pregnancy
Ortho-Tri-Cyclen [ethinyl estradiol/norgestimate]	Z79.3	Contraceptive	Prevention of pregnancy
Oseni [alogliptin benzoate/pioglitazone hydrochloride]	Z79.84	Oral hypoglycemic	Diabetes mellitus
Osphena [ospemifene]	Z79.810, Z79.890	Selective estrogen receptor modulator (SERM)	Postmenopausal dyspareunia due to vaginal atrophy; osteoporosis prevention and treatment of menopausal symptoms
Otezla [apremilast]	Z79.899	Antirheumatic	Psoriatic arthritis; plaque psoriasis
Oxazepam [oxazepam]		Antianxiety	Anxiety, tension, and alcohol withdrawal
Oxbryta [voxelotor]		Hemoglobin S polymerization inhibitor	Sickle cell disease
Oxycodone HCl [oxycodone hydrochloride]	Z79.891	Analgesic, narcotic	Moderate to severe pain
OxyContin [oxycodone hydrochloride]	Z79.891	Analgesic, narcotic	Moderate to severe pain
Ozempic [semaglutide]	Z79.899	Antidiabetic – noninsulin injectable	Diabetes mellitus
Paxil [paroxetine hydrochloride]		Antidepressant	Anxiety with panic disorder and depression; obsessive-compulsive disorder
PediaPred [prednisolone sodium phosphate]	Z79.52	Corticosteroid	Inflammatory disorders
Pegintron [peginterferon alfa-2b]	Z79.899	Antiviral	Hepatitis C
Penicillin-VK [penicillin V potassium]	Z79.2	Antibiotic	Chorea, prevention; endocarditis, prevention, secondary to tooth extraction; erysipelas; infections of the skin and skin structures, upper respiratory tract; rheumatic fever, prophylaxis; scarlet fever; Vincent's gingivitis; Vincent's pharyngitis
Pentam [pentamidine isethionate]	Z79.2	Antibiotic	Severe bacterial lung infections
Pepcid [famotidine]		Histamine H2-receptor inhibitor	Acid/peptic disorder; adenoma, secretory; gastroesophageal reflux; duodenal and gastric ulcer; Zollinger-Ellison syndrome
Percocet [oxycodone hydrochloride/acetaminophen]	Z79.891	Analgesic, narcotic	Pain, moderate to severe
Persantine [dipyridamole]	Z79.02	Antiplatelet	Therapy for chronic angina pectoris, preventing clots post heart valve surgery
Pfizerpen [penicillin g potassium]	Z79.2	Antibiotic	Severe bacterial infections
Phenobarbital [phenobarbital sodium]		Anticonvulsant	Grand mal epilepsy
Philith [ethinyl estradiol/norethindrone]	Z79.3	Contraceptive	Prevention of pregnancy
Pimtrea [desogestrel/ethinyl estradiol]	Z79.3	Contraceptive	Prevention of pregnancy
Piqray [alpelisib]		Kinase inhibitor	Postmenopausal advanced or metastatic breast cancer that is HR positive, HER2 negative
Pirmella [ethinyl estradiol/norethindrone]	Z79.3	Contraceptive	Prevention of pregnancy
Pitocin [oxytocin]		Uterotonic	Induction or stimulation of labor at term
Plan B One-Step [levonorgestrel]	Z79.3	Contraceptive	Prevention of pregnancy
Plavix [clopidogrel bisulfate]	Z79.02	Antiplatelet	Lessening of the chance of heart attack or stroke
Ponstel [mefenamic acid]	Z79.1	Nonsteroidal anti-inflammatory drug (NSAID)	Treatment of pain
Portia-28 [ethinyl estradiol/levonorgestrel]	Z79.3	Contraceptive	Prevention of pregnancy
Pradaxa [dabigatran etexilate mesylate]	Z79.01	Anticoagulant	Prophylaxis and treatment of blood clots in patients with atrial fibrillation
Prasugrel [prasugrel hydrocloride]	Z79.02	Antiplatelet	Lessening the chance of heart attack or stroke
Pravachol [pravastatin sodium]		HMG-CoA reductase inhibitor (statin)	Hypercholesterolemia; hyperlipidemia; hyperlipoproteinemia
Prednisolone [prednisolone]	Z79.52	Corticosteroid	Inflammatory disorders
Prednisone [prednisone]	Z79.52	Corticosteroid	Used for its immunosuppressant effects and for relief of inflammation; used in arthritis, polymyositis and other systemic diseases

Drug	Z Code	Drug Action/Classification	Indications
Pregnyl [chorionic gonadotropin]		Gonadotropic hormone	Prepubertal cryptorchidism; hypogonadism; corpus luteum insufficiency and infertility
Prelone [prednisolone]	Z79.52	Corticosteroid	Inflammatory disorders
Prempro [conjugated estrogens/medroxyprogesterone acetate]	Z79.890	Estrogen/progesterone therapy	Menopause; osteoporosis; atrophic vaginitis
Prevacid [lansoprazole]		Proton pump inhibitor	Acid/peptic disorder, erosive esophagitis, duodenal ulcer, Zollinger-Ellison syndrome
Previfem [ethinyl estradiol/norgestimate]	Z79.3	Contraceptive	Prevention of pregnancy
Prezcobix [darunavir/cobicistat]	Z79.899	Antiviral	HIV
Prezista [darunavir ethanolate]	Z79.899	Antiviral	HIV
Priftin [rifapentine]	Z79.2	Antibiotic	Tuberculosis
Prilosec [omeprazole magnesium]		Proton pump inhibitor	Acid/peptic disorder; endocrine adenoma; erosive esophagitis; systemic mastocytosis; gastroesophageal reflux; duodenal, peptic and gastric ulcer; Zollinger-Ellison syndrome
Primaxin [cilastatin sodium/imipenem]	Z79.2	Antibiotic	Skin, stomach, female reproductive organs or lower respiratory tract infections
Prinivil [lisinopril]		ACE inhibitor	Congestive heart failure; hypertension
Pristiq [desvenlafaxine]		Antidepressant; serotonin and norepinephrine reuptake inhibitor (SNRI)	Major depressive disorder
Procardia [nifedipine]		Calcium channel blocker	Management of vasospastic angina and chronic stable angina, hypertension
Prograf [tacrolimus]	Z79.899	Immunosuppressant	Prophylaxis of organ transplant rejection
Prolia [denosumab]	Z79.899	Monoclonal antibody	Treatment and prevention of bone resorption and prevention of bone fracture
Promethazine hydrochloride [promethazine hydrochloride]		Anesthesia, adjunct to; antiemetic; antihistamine; antitussive/expectorant; sedative/hypnotic; vertigo/motion sickness/vomiting	Anesthesia; adjunct; angioedema; conjunctivitis; dermographism; hypersensitivity, motion sickness; pain; perennial, seasonal, and allergic rhinitis; sedation, obstetrical; urticaria
Protonix [pantoprazole]		Proton pump inhibitor	Short-term treatment and maintenance therapy of erosive esophagitis associated with gastroesophageal reflux disease (GERD)
Protopic [tacrolimus]	Z79.899	Immunosuppressant	Atomic dermatitis (eczema)
Proventil-HFA [albuterol sulfate]		Antiasthmatic/bronchodilator	Asthma
Provera [medroxyprogesterone acetate]	Z79.3, Z79.890	Antineoplastic; contraceptive; progestin	Amenorrhea; carcinoma, endometrium, adjunct; carcinoma, renal; Prevention of pregnancy; hemorrhage
Prozac [fluoxetine hydrochloride]		Selective serotonin reuptake inhibitor (SSRI)	Bulimia nervosa; depression; obsessive-compulsive disorder
Pulmicort [budesonide]	Z79.51	Corticosteroid – inhaled; antiasthmatic	Prophylaxis and treatment of asthma
Qnasl [beclomethasone dipropionate]	Z79.899	Corticosteroid – intranasal	Perennial and seasonal allergies; vasomotor rhinitis
Qtern [dapagliflozin propanediol/saxagliptin hydrochloride]	Z79.84	Oral hypoglycemic	Diabetes mellitus
Quartette [levonorgestrel/ethinyl estradiol]	Z79.3	Contraceptive	Prevention of pregnancy
Quasense [ethinyl estradiol/levonorgestrel]	Z79.3	Contraceptive	Prevention of pregnancy
Quinidine gluconate [quinidine gluconate]		Antiarrhythmic	Management of cardiac arrhythmias
Qvar Redihaler [beclomethasone dipropionate]	Z79.51	Corticosteroid – inhaled; antiasthmatic	Prophylaxis and treatment of asthma
Raloxifene HCl [raloxifene hydrochloride]	Z79.810	Selective estrogen receptor modulator (SERM)	Prevention of thinning of the bones (osteoporosis) only in postmenopausal women
Rapaflo [silodosin]		Antiadrenergic	Benign prostatic hyperplasia
Rapamune [sirolimus]	Z79.899	Immunosuppressant	Prophylaxis of organ transplant rejection
Rayos [prednisone]	Z79.52	Corticosteroid; antiasthmatic	Arthritis; blood disorders; allergies; asthma
Rebetol [ribavirin]	Z79.899	Antiviral	Chronic hepatitis C
Rebif [interferon beta-1a]	Z79.899	Antiviral	Treatment of relapsing multiple sclerosis

Drug	Z Code	Drug Action/Classification	Indications
Reclast [zoledronic acid]	Z79.83	Bisphosphonate	Prevention of thinning of the bones (osteoporosis); Paget's disease; bone cancer
Relenza [zanamivir]		Antiviral	Treat and prevent influenza A and B
Renvela [sevelamer carbonate]		Phosphate binder	Chronic kidney disease (CKD) on dialysis
Repaglinide [repaglinide]	Z79.84	Oral hypoglycemic	Diabetes mellitus
Reprexain [hydrocodone bitartrate/ibuprofen]	Z79.891	Analgesic, narcotic; nonsteroidal anti-inflammatory drug (NSAID)	Pain, inflammation or fever relief
Restasis [cyclosporine ophthalmic emulsion]		Anti-inflammatory, ophthalmic	Ocular inflammation due to keratoconjunctivitis sicca
Restoril [temazepam]		Sedative/hypnotic	Insomnia
Retrovir [zidovudine]	Z79.899	Antiretroviral	Indicated in symptomatic HIV infection
Reyvow [lasmiditan]		Serotonin 1F receptor agonist	Migraine with or without aura
Rifadin [rifampin]	Z79.2	Antibiotic	Tuberculosis
Rimactane [rifampin]	Z79.2	Antibiotic	Tuberculosis
Rinvoq [upadacitinib]	Z79.899	Antirheumatic	Rheumatoid arthritis
Riomet [metformin hydrochloride]	Z79.84	Oral hypoglycemic	Diabetes mellitus
Risperdal [risperidone]		Antipsychotic/antimanic	Schizophrenia; bipolar I disorder
Ritalin [methylphenidate hydrochloride]		CNS stimulant	Depression; hyperkinetic activity in children
Roxicet [oxycodone hydrochloride/acetaminophen]	Z79.891	Analgesic, narcotic	Pain, moderate to severe
Roxicodone [oxycodone hydrochloride]	Z79.891	Analgesic, narcotic	Pain relief
Rybelsus [semaglutide]	Z79.84	Oral hypoglycemic	Diabetes mellitus
Sabril [vigabatrin]		Anticonvulsant	Refractory complex partial seizures
Safyral [drospirenone/ethinyl estradiol/levomefolate calcium]	Z79.3	Contraceptive	Prevention of pregnancy
Sandimmune [cyclosporine]	Z79.899	Immunosuppressant	Prophylaxis of organ transplant rejection
Sarafem [fluoxetine hydrochloride]		Selective serotonin reuptake inhibitor (SSRI)	Premenstrual dysphoric disorder (PMDD)
Savaysa [edoxaban tosylate]	Z79.01	Anticoagulant	Prophylaxis and treatment of venous thrombosis, pulmonary embolism; prevention of blood clots due to atrial fibrillation
Seasonale [levonorgestrel/ethinyl estradiol]	Z79.3	Contraceptive	Prevention of pregnancy
Seasonique [ethinyl estradiol/levonorgestrel]	Z79.3	Contraceptive	Prevention of pregnancy
Selfemra [fluoxetine hydrochloride]		Selective serotonin reuptake inhibitor (SSRI)	Premenstrual dysphoric disorder (PMDD)
Septra [sulfamethoxazole trimethoprim]	Z79.2	Antibiotic	Urinary tract infections, acute otitis media, acute exacerbations of chronic bronchitis, and shigellosis
Serevent [salmeterol xinafoate]		Bronchodilator	Asthma
Seromycin [cycloserine]	Z79.2	Antibiotic	Tuberculosis; urinary tract infections
Seroquel XR [quetiapine fumarate]		Antipsychotic	Schizophrenia; bipolar disorder; major depressive disorder
Setlakin [ethinyl estradiol/levonorgestrel]	Z79.3	Contraceptive	Prevention of pregnancy
Silvadene [silver sulfadiazine]	Z79.2	Antibiotic, topical	Wound sepsis due to second/third degree burns
Simulect [basiliximab]	Z79.899	Immunosuppressant	Prophylaxis of organ transplant rejection
Sinemet [carbidopa/levodopa]		Antiparkinsonism	Parkinson's disease
Singulair [montelukast sodium]		Antiasthmatic	Asthma; exercise-induced bronchoconstriction; perennial and seasonal allergic rhinitis
Sirolimus [sirolimus]	Z79.899	Immunosuppressant	Prophylaxis of organ transplant rejection
Sitagliptin [sitagliptin/metformin hydrochloride]	Z79.84	Oral hypoglycemic	Diabetes mellitus
Sivextro [tedizolid phosphate]	Z79.2	Antibiotic	Skin infections including MRSA
Skyla [levonorgestrel]	Z79.3	Contraceptive	Intrauterine device to Prevention of pregnancy
Soliqua [insulin glargine/lixisenatide]	Z79.4	Insulin	Diabetes mellitus
Solodyn [minocycline hydrochloride]	Z79.2	Antibiotic	Bacterial infections

Drug	Z Code	Drug Action/Classification	Indications
Soltamox [tamoxifen citrate]	Z79.810	Selective estrogen receptor modulator (SERM)	Breast cancer
Solu-Cortef [hydrocortisone sodium succinate]	Z79.52	Corticosteroid; antiasthmatic	Asthma; severe inflammation; allergic reactions
Solu-Medrol [methylprednisolone sodium succinate]	Z79.52	Corticosteroid	Anti-inflammatory and antiallergenic for shock and ulcerative colitis
Spiriva [tiotropium bromide]		Antiasthmatic/bronchodilator	Chronic obstructive pulmonary disease (COPD); asthma
Sprintec [norgestimate/ethinyl estradiol]	Z79.3	Contraceptive	Prevention of pregnancy
Strattera [atomexetine hydrochloride]		CNS stimulant	Attention deficit hyperactivity disorder (ADHD)
Streptomycin sulfate [streptomycin sulfate]	Z79.2	Antibiotic	Severe bacterial infections
Sublimaze preservative free [fentanyl citrate]	Z79.891	Analgesic, narcotic	Pain relief
Supprelin LA [histrelin acetate]	Z79.818	Agents affecting estrogen receptors and estrogen levels	Precocious puberty
Suprax [cefixime]	Z79.2	Antibiotic	Bacterial infections
Sustiva [efavirenz]	Z79.899	Antiviral	HIV/AIDs
Syeda [drospirenone/ethinyl estradiol]	Z79.3	Contraceptive	Prevention of pregnancy
Sylatron [peginterferon alfa-2b]	Z79.899	Antineoplastic interferons; antiviral interferons	Prevention of recurrent malignant melanoma
Symbicort [budesonide/formoterol fumarate dihydrate]	Z79.51	Corticosteroid – inhaled; antiasthmatic	Prophylaxis and treatment of asthma and COPD
Symbyax [olanzapine/fluoxetine]		Antidepressant	Acute depressive episodes associated with bipolar I disorder; treatment resistant depression
Symtuza [darunavir/cobicistat/emtricitabine/tenofovir alafenamide]	Z79.899	Antiretroviral	HIV
Synarel [nafarelin acetate]	Z79.818	Agents affecting estrogen receptors and estrogen levels	Endometriosis symptoms; precocious puberty
Synercid [dalfopristin/quinupristin]	Z79.2	Antibiotic	Severe blood infections
Synjardy [empagliflozin/metformin hydrochloride]	Z79.84	Oral hypoglycemic	Diabetes mellitus
Synthroid [levothyroxine sodium]		Thyroid hormone	Hypothyroidism
Tacrolimus [tacrolimus]	Z79.899	Immunosuppressant	Prophylaxis of organ transplant rejection
Talicia [omeprazole magnesium/amoxicillin/rifabutin]	Z79.2	Combination antibiotic	Helicobacter pylori infection
Tamiflu [oseltamivir phosphate]		Antiviral	Treatment and prevention of influenza A and B
Tamoxifen citrate [tamoxifen citrate]	Z79.810	Selective estrogen receptor modulator (SERM)	Metastatic breast cancer in postmenopausal women
Tazicef [ceftazidime]	Z79.2	Antibiotic	Confirmed or suspected bacterial infections
Teflaro [ceftaroline fosamil]	Z79.2	Antibiotic	Bacterial skin infections; pneumonia
Tegretol [carbamazepine]		Anticonvulsant; analgesic	Epilepsy, especially with complex symptomatology; specific analgesic for trigeminal neuralgia
Tenormin [atenolol]		Beta blocker	Angina pectoris; hypertension; acute myocardial infarction
Terazosin HCl [terazosin hydrochloride]		Antiadrenergic	Benign prostatic hypertrophy; hypertension
Testim [testosterone]	Z79.890	Testosterone therapy – topical	Primary hypogonadism; hypogonadotropic hypogonadism
Tetracycline HCl [tetracycline hydrochloride]	Z79.2	Antibiotic	Bacterial infections
Tiazac [diltiazem hydrochloride]		Calcium channel blocker	Chronic stable angina, atrial fibrillation, atrial flutter, hypertension, paroxysmal supraventricular tachycardia
Tivorbex [indomethacin]	Z79.1	Nonsteroidal anti-inflammatory drug (NSAID)	Treatment of pain, inflammation and joint stiffness
Tobradex [tobramycin/dexamethasone]		Aminoglycoside ocular anti-infective; anti-inflammatory	Infectious conjunctivitis; dermatosis, corticosteroid-responsive with secondary infection; foreign body in eye; corneal inflammation; uveitis

Drug	Z Code	Drug Action/Classification	Indications
Tobramycin [dexamethasone/tobramycin]	Z79.2	Antibiotic	Bacterial eye infections
Topamax [topiramate]		Anticonvulsant	Epilepsy; primary generalized tonic-clonic seizures; seizures associated with Lennox-Gastaut syndrome; migraine headache
Toprol-XL [metoprolol succinate]		Beta blocker	Angina pectoris; hypertension
Toremifene citrate [toremifene citrate]	Z79.810	Selective estrogen receptor modulator (SERM)	Metastatic breast cancer in postmenopausal women
Torisel [temsirolimus]	Z79.899	Antineoplastic	Renal cell carcinoma
Toujeo Solostar [insulin glargine recombinant]	Z79.4	Insulin	Diabetes mellitus
Tradjenta [linagliptin]	Z79.84	Oral hypoglycemic	Diabetes mellitus
Trazodone HCl [trazodone hydrochloride]		Antidepressant	Depression
Trelegy Ellipta [fluticasone furoate/umeclidinium bromide/vilanterol trifenatate]	Z79.51	Corticosteroid – inhaled; anitasthmatic	COPD
Trelstar [triptorelin pamoate]	Z79.818	Agents affecting estrogen receptors and estrogen levels	Palliative treatment of prostate cancer symptoms
Tresiba [insulin degludec]	Z79.4	Insulin	Diabetes mellitus
Triamterene and hydrochlorothiazide [triamterene/ hydrochlorothiazide]		Antihypertensive; diuretic	Edema; hypertension
Tri-Estarylla [ethinyl estradiol/norgestimate]	Z79.3	Contraceptive	Prevention of pregnancy; acne
Trijardy XR [empagliflozin/linagliptin/metformin hydrochloride]	Z79.84	Oral hypoglycemic	Diabetes mellitus
Tri-Legest [ethinyl estradiol/norethindrone acetate]	Z79.3	Contraceptive	Prevention of pregnancy
Tri-Linyah [ethinyl estradiol/norgestimate]	Z79.3	Contraceptive	Prevention of pregnancy
Tri-Lo-Estarylla [ethinyl estradiol/norgestimate]	Z79.3	Contraceptive	Prevention of pregnancy
Tri-Lo-Sprintec [ethinyl estradiol/norgestimate]	Z79.3	Contraceptive	Prevention of pregnancy
Trimethoprim [trimethoprim]	Z79.2	Antibiotic	Acute exacerbation chronic bronchitis; travelers' diarrhea; infections of the middle, lower respiratory tract, and urinary tract; pneumonia, pneumocystis; shigellosis
Tri-Norinyl 28-day [ethinyl estradiol/norethindrone]	Z79.3	Contraceptive	Prevention of pregnancy
Tri-Previfem [ethinyl estradiol/norgestimate]	Z79.3	Contraceptive	Prevention of pregnancy
Triptodur [triptorelin]	Z79.818	Agents affecting estrogen receptors and estrogen levels	Precocious puberty
Tri-Sprintec [ethinyl estradiol/norgestimate]	Z79.3	Contraceptive	Prevention of pregnancy; acne
Trivora-28 [ethinyl estradiol/ levonorgestrel]	Z79.3	Contraceptive	Prevention of pregnancy
Trokendi XR [topiramate]		Anticonvulsant	Epilepsy; primary generalized tonic-clonic seizures; seizures associated with Lennox-Gastaut syndrome; migraine headache
Trulicity [dulaglutide]	Z79.899	Antidiabetic – noninsulin injectable	Diabetes mellitus
Truvada [emtricitabine/ tenofovir disoproxil fumarate]	Z79.899	Antiviral	Treatment and prevention of HIV
Turalio [pexidartinib]		Kinase inhibitor	Symptomatic tenosynovial giant cell tumor
Tygacil [tigecycline]	Z79.2	Antibiotic	Bacterial skin or digestive system infections; pneumonia
Tylenol with codeine [acetaminophen/codeine phosphate]	Z79.891	Analgesic, narcotic	Pain and cough
Ubrelvy [ubrogepant]		Antimigraine	Migraine with or without aura
Ultram [tramadol hydrochloride]	Z79.891	Analgesic, non-narcotic (opiate, narcotic-like)	Moderate to severe pain

Drug	Z Code	Drug Action/Classification	Indications
Unasyn [ampicillin sodium/sulbactam sodium]	Z79.2	Antibiotic	Bacterial infections
Vabomere [meropenem; vaborbactam]	Z79.2	Antibiotic	Complicated urinary tract infections; pyelonephritis
Vagifem [estradiol]	Z79.890	Estrogen therapy	Menopause symptoms
Valium [diazepam]		Antianxiety; muscle relaxant; anticonvulsant	Anxiety, tension, withdrawal from alcohol, muscle spasms and anticonvulsant therapy; epilepsy, generalized tonic-clonic; status epilepticus; stiff-man syndrome; tetanus
Vancocin HCl [vancomycin hydrochloride]	Z79.2	Antibiotic	Severe bacterial infections
Vancomycin HCl [vancomycin hydrochloride]	Z79.2	Antibiotic	Severe bacterial infections
Vantas [histrelin acetate]	Z79.818	Agents affecting estrogen receptors and estrogen levels	Palliative treatment of prostate cancer symptoms
Vasotec [enalaprilat maleate]		ACE inhibitor	Congestive heart failure; hypertension
Velivet [desogestrel/ethinyl estradiol]	Z79.3	Contraceptive	Prevention of pregnancy
Venlafaxine HCl [venlafaxine hydrochloride]		Antidepressant, serotonin and norepinephrine reuptake inhibitor (SNRI)	Major depressive disorder; social anxiety disorder; panic disorder
Ventolin HFA [albuterol sulfate]		Antiasthmatic/bronchodilator	Asthma
Verapamil HCL [verapamil hydrochloride]		Calcium channel blocker	Angina pectoris, chronic stable angina, atrial fibrillation, atrial flutter, paroxysmal supraventricular tachycardia, ventricular arrhythmia, hypertension
Viagra [sildenafil citrate]		Phosphodiesterase-5 (PDE5) inhibitor	Erectile dysfunction
Vibativ [telavancin hydrochloride]	Z79.2	Antibiotic	Pneumonia; severe bacterial skin infections
Vibramycin [doxycycline calcium]	Z79.2	Antibiotic	Bacterial infections
Victoza [liraglutide]	Z79.899	Antidiabetic – noninsulin injectable	Diabetes mellitus
Vienva [ethinyl estradiol/levonorgestrel]	Z79.3	Contraceptive	Prevention of pregnancy
Viorele [desogestrel/ethinyl estradiol]	Z79.3	Contraceptive	Prevention of pregnancy
Virazole [ribavirin]	Z79.899	Antiviral	Respiratory syncytial virus (RSV)
Viread [tenofovir disoproxil fumarate]	Z79.899	Antiviral	HIV; chronic hepatitis B
Vistaril [hydroxyzine pamoate]		Antianxiety; antiemetic	Treatment of nausea and vomiting, for reducing narcotic requirement in surgery and as tranquilizer for tension, anxiety, or agitation states
Vivelle [estradiol]	Z79.890	Estrogen therapy	Menopause symptoms; osteoporosis prevention
Voltaren [diclofenac sodium]	Z79.1	Nonsteroidal anti-inflammatory drug (NSAID)	Treatment of pain, inflammation and joint stiffness due to arthritis
Vumerity [diroximel fumarate]		Immunostimulant	Relapsing forms of multiple sclerosis (MS)
Vytorin [ezetimibe/simvastatin]		HMG-CoA reductase inhibitor (statin); cholesterol absorption inhibitor	Hyperlipidemia; hypercholesterolemia
Wakix [pitolisant hydrochloride]		CNS stimulant	Narcolepsy
Warfarin [warfarin sodium]	Z79.01	Anticoagulant	Prophylaxis and treatment of venous thrombosis, treatment of atrial fibrillation with embolization (pulmonary embolism), arrhythmias, myocardial infarction, and stroke prevention
Wellbutrin SR, Wellbutrin XL [bupropion hydrochloride]		Antidepressant	Depression
Wera [ethinyl estradiol/norethindrone]	Z79.3	Contraceptive	Prevention of pregnancy
Xalatan [latanoprost]		Prostaglandin F2α analogue	Glaucoma, open-angle; ocular hypertension
Xanax, Xanax XR [alprazolam]		Antianxiety; sedative/hypnotic	Anxiety disorders with panic disorder and depression
Xarelto [rivaraxaban]	Z79.01	Anticoagulant	Prophylaxis and treatment of venous thrombosis, pulmonary embolism; prevention of blood clots due to atrial fibrillation
Xeljanz [tofacitinib citrate]	Z79.899	Antirheumatic	Rheumatoid arthritis; psoriatic arthritis
Xenleta [lefamulin acetate]	Z79.2	Antibiotic	Community-acquired bacterial pneumonia
Xgeva [denosumab]	Z79.899	Monoclonal antibody	Treatment and prevention of bone resorption and prevention of bone fracture
Xifaxan [rifaximin]	Z79.2	Antibiotic	E. coli diarrhea

Drug	Z Code	Drug Action/Classification	Indications
Xigduo [dapagliflozin propanediol/metformin hydrochloride]	Z79.84	Oral hypoglycemic	Diabetes mellitus
Xpovio [selinexor]	Z79.899	Antineoplastic	Multiple myeloma in adults
Xultophy [insulin degludec/liraglutide]	Z79.4	Insulin	Diabetes mellitus
Xyrem [sodium oxybate]		CNS depressant; anxiolytic/sedative/hypnotic	Cataplexy and/or excessive daytime sleepiness in narcolepsy
Xyzal [levocetirizine dihydrochloride]		Antihistamine	Perennial allergic rhinitis; chronic idiopathic urticaria
Yasmin [drospirenone/ethinyl estradiol]	Z79.3	Contraceptive	Prevention of pregnancy
Yaz [drospirenone/ethinyl estradiol]	Z79.3	Contraceptive	Prevention of pregnancy; menstrual disorders
Zantac [ranitidine hydrochloride]		Histamine H2-receptors inhibitor	Acid/peptic disorder, erosive esophagitis, gastrointestinal hypersecretion, mastocytosis, gastroesophageal reflux, peptic ulcer, Zollinger-Ellison syndrome
Zerbaxa [ceftolozane sulfate/tazobactam sodium]	Z79.2	Antibiotic	Complicated urinary tract and intra-abdominal infections
Zestoretic [lisinopril/hydrochlorothiazide]		ACE inhibitor	Congestive heart failure; hypertension
Zestril [lisinopril]		ACE inhibitor	Congestive heart failure; hypertension
Zetia [exetimibe]		Antihyperlipidemic	Hypercholesterolemia; sitosterolemia
Ziac [bisoprolol fumarate/hydrochlorothiazide]		Antihypertensive	Hypertension
Zinacef [cefuroxime sodium]	Z79.2	Antibiotic	Bacterial infections
Zipsor [diclofenac potassium]	Z79.1	Nonsteroidal anti-inflammatory drug (NSAID)	Pain and inflammation relief
Zithromax [azithromycin]	Z79.2	Antibiotic	Infections of the cervix, lower respiratory tract, skin and skin structures, urethra, nongonococcal; mycobacterium avium complex; pharyngitis, streptococcal pneumonia; tonsillitis
Zocor [simvastatin]		HMG-CoA reductase inhibitor (statin)	Hypercholesterolemia; hyperlipidemia; hyperlipoproteinemia; hypertriglyceridemia
Zoladex [goserelin acetate]	Z79.818	Agents affecting estrogen receptors and estrogen levels	Palliative treatment of prostate cancer and breast cancer symptoms; endometriosis
Zoloft [sertraline hydrochloride]		Antidepressant	Anxiety with panic disorder and depression; obsessive-compulsive disorder
Zometa [zoledronic acid]	Z79.83	Bisphosphonate	Multiple myeloma; Paget's disease
Zorvolex [diclofenac]	Z79.1	Nonsteroidal anti-inflammatory drug (NSAID)	Pain, inflammation or fever relief
Zosyn [piperacillin sodium/tazobactam sodium]	Z79.2	Antibiotic	Bacterial infections
Zovia [ethynodiol diacetate/ethinyl estradiol]	Z79.3	Contraceptive	Prevention of pregnancy
Zovirax [acyclovir]		Antiviral	Genital herpes and herpes zoster infections
Zubsolv [buprenorphine/naloxone]		Opioid agonist	Treatment of opioid addiction
Zyban [bupropion hydrochloride]		Smoking cessation aid	Nicotine addiction, smoking
Zyflo [zileuton]		Antiasthmatic	Asthma
Zyloprim [allopurinol]		Antigout	Gouty arthritis, renal calculus, hyperuricemia, hyperuricemia secondary to leukemia, hyperuricemia secondary to lymphoma
Zyprexa [olanzapine]		Antipsychotic/antimanic	Psychotic disorders; schizophrenia
Zyrtec allergy [cetirizine hydrochloride]		Antihistamine	Perennial and seasonal allergic rhinitis; chronic urticaria
Zyvox [linezolid]	Z79.2	Antibiotic	Severe bacterial infections

Appendix C: Z Codes for Long-Term Drug Use with Associated Drugs

This resource correlates the Z codes that are used to identify current long-term drug use with a list of drugs that are typically categorized to that class of drug. These lists are not all-inclusive, providing only the more commonly used drugs.

Z79.Ø1 **Long term (current) use of anticoagulants**
Angiomax
Argatroban
Arixtra
Bevyxxa
Coumadin
Eliquis
Fragmin
Heparin
Jantoven
Lovenox
Pradaxa
Savaysa
Warfarin
Xarelto

Z79.Ø2 **Long term (current) use of antithrombotics/antiplatelets**
Aggrastat
Aggrenox
Brilinta
Clopidogrel bisulfate
Effient
Integrilin
Persantine
Plavix
Prasugrel

Z79.1 **Long term (current) use of non-steroidal anti-inflammatories (NSAID)**
Advil
Aleve
Anaprox DS
Arthrotec
Caldolor
Cambia
Celebrex
Daypro
Duexis
Feldene
Ibuprofen
Indocin
Mobic
Motrin IB
Nabumetone
Nalfon
Naprelan
Naprosyn
NeoProfen
Ponstel
Tivorbex
Voltaren
Zipsor
Zorvolex

Z79.2 **Long term (current) use of antibiotics**
Altabax
Amikacin
Amoxicillin
Ampicillin
Ancef
Augmentin
Avelox
Azactam
Azithromycin

Bactrim
Biaxin XL
Cefprozil
Ceftriaxone
Centany
Cephalexin
Cipro
Ciprofloxacin
Clarithromycin
Cleocin
Clindamycin
Cubicin
Daptomycin
Dificid
Doxycycline
Dynacin
E.E.S.
Ertapenem
ERYC
Erygel
EryPed
Ery-Tab
Erythrocin
Erythromycin
Factive
Fetroja
Flagyl
Fortaz
Gentamicin sulfate
Invanz
Isoniazid
Keflex
Klaron
Lincocin
Macrobid
Macrodantin
Maxipime
Mefoxin
Mepron
Merrem
Metronidazole
Minocin
Monodox
Monurol
Mycobutin
Nebupent
Nitrofurantoin
Oracea
Orbactiv
Penicillin-VK
Pentam
Pfizerpen
Priftin
Primaxin
Rifadin
Rimactane
Septra
Seromycin
Silvadene
Sivextro
Solodyn
Streptomycin sulfate
Suprax
Synercid

Talicia
Tazicef
Teflaro
Tetracycline HCl
Tobramycin
Trimethoprim
Tygacil
Unasyn
Vabomere
Vancocin HCl
Vancomycin HCl
Vibativ
Vibramycin
Xenleta
Xifaxan
Zerbaxa
Zinacef
Zithromax
Zosyn
Zyvox

Z79.3 **Long term (current) use of hormonal contraceptives**
Altavera
Alyacen
Aranelle
Ashlyna
Aviane-28
Balziva-28
Bekyree
Beyaz
Brevicon 28-day
Briellyn
Camila
Cryselle
Cyclafem
Cyclessa
Dasetta
Daysee
Depo-Provera
Depo-SubQ Provera
Desogestrel:
    Ethinyl
Elinest
Emoquette
Enpresse-28
Enskyce
Errin
Estarylla
Estrostep Fe
Falmina
Femhrt
Gildagia
Gildess
Introvale
Jencycla
Junel
Kariva
Kelnor
Kimidess
Kurvelo
Kyleena
Larin
Lessina-28
Levonest

Levora
Liletta
Lo Loestrin Fe
Loestrin
Loryna
LoSeasonique
Low-Ogestrel-28
Marlissa
Microgestin
Minastrin
Mirena
Mono-Linyah
Myzilra
Natazia
Nexplanon
Norinyl
Nor-QD
Nortrel
NuvaRing
Ogestrel
Orsythia
Ortho-Novum
Ortho-Tri-Cyclen-28
Philith
Pimtrea
Pirmella
Plan B One-Step
Portia-28
Previfem
Provera
Quartette
Quasense
Safyral
Seasonale
Seasonique
Setlakin
Skyla
Sprintec
Syeda
Tri-Estarylla
Tri-Legest
Tri-Linyah
Tri-Lo-Estarylla
Tri-Lo-Sprintec
Tri-Norinyl 28-day
Tri-Previfem
Tri-Sprintec
Trivora-28
Velivet
Vienva
Viorele
Wera
Yasmin
Yaz
Zovia

Z79.4   Long term (current) use of insulin
Admelog
Afrezza
Apidra
Basaglar
Fiasp
Humalog
Humulin R
Lantus
Levemir
Novolin
Novolog

Soliqua
Toujeo Solostar
Tresiba
Xultophy

Z79.51   Long term (current) use of inhaled steroids
Advair
Airduo Respiclick
Alvesco
Arnuity Ellipta
Asmanex
Breo Ellipta
Dulera
Flovent
Pulmicort
Qvar Redihaler
Symbicort
Trelegy Ellipta

Z79.52   Long term (current) use of systemic steroids
Aristospan
Celestone Soluspan
Colocort
Cortef
Cortenema
Cortifoam
Cortisone acetate
Depo-Medrol
Dexamethasone Intensol
Entocort EC
Hydrocortisone
Kenalog-10
Kenalog-40
Locoid
Medrol
Methylprednisolone
Orapred ODT
PediaPred
Prednisolone
Prednisone
Prelone
Rayos
Solu-Cortef
Solu-Medrol

Z79.810 Long term (current) use of selective estrogen receptor modulators (SERMs)
Evista
Fareston
Osphena
Raloxifene HCl
Soltamox
Tamoxifen Citrate
Toremifene Citrate

Z79.811 Long term (current) use of aromatase inhibitors
Anastrozole
Arimidex
Aromasin
Exemestane
Femara
Letrozole

Z79.818 Long term (current) use of other agents affecting estrogen receptors and estrogen levels
Eligard
Faslodex

Lupron Depot
Megace ES
Supprelin LA
Synarel
Trelstar
Triptodur
Vantas
Zoladex

Z79.82   Long term (current) use of aspirin
Bayer
Durlaza

Z79.83   Long term (current) use of bisphosphonates
Actonel
Atelvia
Binosto
Boniva
Fosamax
Reclast
Zometa

Z79.84   Long term (current) use of oral hypoglycemic drugs
Acarbose
Actoplus Met
Actos
Amaryl
Avandia
DiaBeta
Duetact
Farxiga
Glimepiride
Glucotrol
Glumetza
Glyburide
Glynase
Glyset
Invokamet
Invokana
Janumet
Januvia
Jentadueto
Kazano
Kombiglyze
Metformin
Onglyza
Oseni
Qtern
Repaglinide
Riomet
Rybelsus
Sitagliptin
Synjardy
Tradjenta
Trijardy XR
Xigduo

Z79.890 Hormone replacement therapy
Activella
Alora
Androderm
AndroGel
Angeliq
Bijuva
Climara
CombiPatch
Delestrogen
Depo-Provera
Divigel

Duavee
Elestrin
Estrace
EstroGel
Femhrt
Femring
Firmagon
Menest
Menostar
Minivelle
Orlissa
Osphena
Prempro
Provera
Testim
Vagifem
Vivelle

Z79.891 Long term (current) use of opiate analgesic

Acetaminophen with codeine
Buprenex
Buprenorphine HCl and Naloxone HCl
Butorphanol tartrate
Butrans
Codeine
Demerol
Dilaudid
Dolophine HCl
Duragesic
Duramorph PF
Fentanyl Citrate
Fentora
Fioricet with codeine
Hydrocodone
Hydrocodone bitartrate and acetaminophen
Hydromorphone HCl
Kadian
Lazanda
Methadone HCl

Methadose
Morphabond ER
Morphine Sulfate
MS Contin
Norco
Nucynta
Oxycodone HCl
OxyContin
Percocet
Reprexain
Roxicet
Roxicodone
Sublimaze Preservative Free
Tylenol with codeine
Ultram

Z79.899 Other long term (current) drug therapy

Actimmune
Antineoplastic/chemotherapy
Astagraf XL
Atripla
Avonex
Beconase AQ
Betaseron
Byetta
Cellcept
Cimduo
Cosentyx
Crixivan
Cyclosporine
Cyltezo
Descovy
Emtriva
Enbrel
Entyvio
Envarsus XR
Epivir
Erelzi
Flonase
Gengraf

Harvoni
Humira
Hyrimoz
Imuran
Intron A
Keytruda
Monoclonal antibodies
Neoral
Orencia
Otezla
Ozempic
Pegintron
Prezcobix
Prezista
Prograf
Prolia
Protopic
Qnasl
Rapamune
Rebetol
Rebif
Retrovir
Rinvoq
Sandimmune
Simulect
Sirolimus
Sustiva
Sylatron
Symtuza
Tacrolimus
Torisel
Trulicity
Truvada
Victoza
Virazole
Viread
Xeljanz
Xgeva
Xpovio

Appendix D: Major Complication and Comorbidity (MCC) Code List

Note: The following is a comprehensive list of ICD-10-CM codes designated as MCCs in the tabular section of this manual. Codes listed in this resource and identified as MCCs in the tabular section reflect the most current information that was available at the time of publication. Because the fiscal 2021 IPPS final rule was not available at the time this book was printed, the ICD-10-CM codes designated as MCCs are based on the proposed, version 38, MS-DRG Grouper software and Definitions Manual files published with the fiscal 2021 IPPS proposed rule.

For the most current list of MCC designations based on the final version of the MS-DRG Grouper software and MS-DRG Definitions Manual files, Optum360 has provided an easily searchable data file that can be accessed at the following:

https://www.optum360coding.com/ProductUpdates/
Title: "2021 ICD-10-CM for Hospital IPPS Data File"
Password: Hospital21

A02.1	A41.59	B25.2	D60.9	G04.02	I26.90	I63.019	I63.442	J12.0
A02.21	A41.81	B26.1	D61.1	G04.2	I26.92	I63.02	I63.443	J12.1
A02.22	A41.89	B26.2	D61.2	G04.30	I26.93	I63.031	I63.449	J12.2
A06.4	A41.9	B37.1	D61.3	G04.31	I26.94	I63.032	I63.49	J12.3
A06.5	A42.7	B37.5	D61.810	G04.32	I26.99	I63.033	I63.50	J12.81
A06.6	A48.0	B37.6	D61.811	G04.39	I33.0	I63.039	I63.511	J12.89
A17.0	A48.1	B37.7	D61.89	G04.81	I33.9	I63.09	I63.512	J12.9
A17.1	A48.3	B38.4	D65	G04.89	I40.0	I63.10	I63.513	J13
A17.81	A50.41	B39.0	D66	G04.90	I40.1	I63.111	I63.519	J14
A17.82	A50.42	B39.1	D67	G04.91	I40.8	I63.112	I63.521	J15.0
A17.83	A51.41	B39.2	E03.5	G05.3	I40.9	I63.113	I63.522	J15.1
A17.89	A52.13	B44.0	E05.01	G05.4	I41	I63.119	I63.523	J15.20
A18.31	A52.14	B45.1	E05.11	G06.0	I46.2	I63.12	I63.529	J15.211
A19.0	A54.81	B46.0	E05.21	G06.1	I46.8	I63.131	I63.531	J15.212
A19.1	A54.86	B46.1	E05.31	G06.2	I46.9	I63.132	I63.532	J15.29
A19.2	A80.0	B46.2	E05.41	G07	I49.01	I63.133	I63.533	J15.3
A19.8	A80.1	B46.3	E05.81	G08	I49.02	I63.139	I63.539	J15.4
A19.9	A80.2	B46.4	E05.91	G21.0	I50.21	I63.19	I63.541	J15.5
A20.0	A80.30	B46.5	E08.00	G37.4	I50.23	I63.20	I63.542	J15.6
A20.1	A80.39	B46.8	E08.01	G40.301	I50.31	I63.211	I63.543	J15.7
A20.2	A83.0	B46.9	E08.10	G40.311	I50.33	I63.212	I63.549	J15.8
A20.3	A83.1	B50.9	E08.11	G40.319	I50.41	I63.213	I63.59	J15.9
A20.7	A83.2	B58.2	E08.641	G70.01	I50.43	I63.219	I63.6	J16.0
A20.8	A83.3	B58.3	E09.00	G80.0	I51.1	I63.22	I63.81	J16.8
A20.9	A83.4	B58.81	E09.01	G82.50	I51.2	I63.231	I63.89	J17
A22.1	A83.5	B59	E09.10	G82.51	I60.00	I63.232	I63.9	J18.0
A22.7	A83.6	B77.81	E09.11	G82.52	I60.01	I63.233	I67.0	J18.1
A26.7	A83.8	D57.00	E09.641	G82.53	I60.02	I63.239	I67.83	J18.8
A27.81	A83.9	D57.01	E10.10	G82.54	I60.10	I63.29	I71.00	J18.9
A32.7	A84.0	D57.02	E10.11	G83.5	I60.11	I63.30	I71.01	J68.1
A33	A84.1	D57.03	E10.641	G92	I60.12	I63.311	I71.02	J69.0
A35	A84.81	D57.09	E11.00	G93.41	I60.2	I63.312	I71.03	J69.1
A37.01	A84.89	D57.211	E11.01	G93.5	I60.30	I63.313	I71.1	J69.8
A37.11	A84.9	D57.212	E11.10	G93.6	I60.31	I63.319	I71.3	J80
A37.81	A85.2	D57.213	E11.11	G93.7	I60.32	I63.321	I71.5	J81.0
A37.91	A92.30	D57.218	E11.641	G93.82	I60.4	I63.322	I71.8	J84.81
A39.0	A92.31	D57.219	E13.00	G95.11	I60.50	I63.323	I74.01	J84.83
A39.1	A92.32	D57.411	E13.01	G95.19	I60.51	I63.329	I77.70	J84.841
A39.2	A92.39	D57.412	E13.10	I21.01	I60.52	I63.331	I77.71	J84.842
A39.3	B00.3	D57.413	E13.11	I21.02	I60.6	I63.332	I77.72	J84.843
A39.4	B00.4	D57.418	E13.641	I21.09	I60.7	I63.333	I77.73	J84.848
A39.50	B00.7	D57.419	E40	I21.11	I60.8	I63.339	I77.74	J85.0
A39.51	B00.82	D57.431	E41	I21.19	I60.9	I63.341	I77.75	J85.1
A39.52	B01.11	D57.432	E42	I21.21	I61.0	I63.342	I77.76	J85.2
A39.53	B01.12	D57.433	E43	I21.29	I61.1	I63.343	I77.77	J85.3
A39.81	B01.2	D57.438	E84.0	I21.3	I61.2	I63.349	I77.79	J86.0
A40.0	B02.1	D57.439	E84.11	I21.4	I61.3	I63.39	I81	J86.9
A40.1	B02.24	D57.451	E88.3	I21.9	I61.4	I63.40	I82.0	J93.0
A40.3	B05.0	D57.452	G00.0	I21.A1	I61.5	I63.411	I82.220	J95.1
A40.8	B05.2	D57.453	G00.1	I21.A9	I61.6	I63.412	I82.221	J95.2
A40.9	B06.01	D57.458	G00.2	I22.0	I61.8	I63.413	I85.01	J95.3
A41.01	B10.01	D57.459	G00.3	I22.1	I61.9	I63.419	I85.11	J95.821
A41.02	B10.09	D57.811	G00.8	I22.2	I62.00	I63.421	J04.11	J95.822
A41.1	B15.0	D57.812	G00.9	I22.8	I62.01	I63.422	J04.31	J96.00
A41.2	B16.0	D57.813	G01	I22.9	I62.02	I63.423	J05.11	J96.01
A41.3	B16.2	D57.818	G02	I23.4	I62.03	I63.429	J09.X1	J96.02
A41.4	B17.11	D57.819	G03.0	I23.5	I62.1	I63.431	J10.00	J96.20
A41.50	B19.0	D59.3	G03.8	I25.42	I63.00	I63.432	J10.01	J96.21
A41.51	B19.11	D60.0	G03.9	I26.01	I63.011	I63.433	J10.08	J96.22
A41.52	B19.21	D60.1	G04.00	I26.02	I63.012	I63.439	J11.00	J96.90
A41.53	B25.0	D60.8	G04.01	I26.09	I63.013	I63.441	J11.08	J96.91

Appendix D: Major Complication and Comorbidity (MCC) Code List

J96.92	K55.061	L89.123	O04.82	O41.1419	O60.22X0	P25.0	P91.63	R40.2310
J98.51	K55.062	L89.124	O07.2	O41.1420	O60.22X1	P25.1	P91.821	R40.2311
J98.59	K55.069	L89.133	O07.31	O41.1421	O60.22X2	P25.2	P91.822	R40.2312
K20.81	K55.21	L89.134	O07.32	O41.1422	O60.22X3	P25.3	P91.823	R40.2313
K20.91	K55.30	L89.143	O08.2	O41.1423	O60.22X4	P25.8	P91.829	R40.2314
K21.01	K55.31	L89.144	O08.3	O41.1424	O60.22X5	P26.0	P92.01	R40.2320
K22.11	K55.32	L89.153	O08.4	O41.1425	O60.22X9	P26.1	Q00.0	R40.2321
K22.3	K55.33	L89.154	O10.42	O41.1429	O60.23X0	P26.8	Q00.1	R40.2322
K22.6	K56.2	L89.203	O11.1	O41.1430	O60.23X1	P26.9	Q00.2	R40.2323
K25.0	K57.01	L89.204	O11.2	O41.1431	O60.23X2	P27.0	Q04.0	R40.2324
K25.1	K57.11	L89.213	O11.3	O41.1432	O60.23X3	P27.1	Q04.1	R40.2340
K25.2	K57.13	L89.214	O14.12	O41.1433	O60.23X4	P27.8	Q04.2	R40.2341
K25.4	K57.21	L89.223	O14.13	O41.1434	O60.23X5	P27.9	Q04.3	R40.2342
K25.5	K57.31	L89.224	O14.22	O41.1435	O60.23X9	P28.5	Q20.0	R40.2343
K25.6	K57.33	L89.303	O14.23	O41.1439	O67.0	P28.81	Q20.1	R40.2344
K26.0	K57.41	L89.304	O15.02	O44.11	O71.02	P29.30	Q20.2	R53.2
K26.1	K57.51	L89.313	O15.03	O44.12	O71.03	P29.38	Q20.3	R57.0
K26.2	K57.53	L89.314	O15.1	O44.13	O71.1	P29.81	Q20.4	R57.1
K26.4	K57.81	L89.323	O15.2	O44.31	O75.1	P35.1	Q21.3	R57.8
K26.5	K57.91	L89.324	O22.31	O44.32	O75.3	P35.2	Q22.0	R65.11
K26.6	K57.93	L89.43	O22.32	O44.33	O85	P35.3	Q22.4	R65.20
K27.0	K63.1	L89.44	O22.33	O44.51	O86.04	P35.4	Q22.5	R65.21
K27.1	K63.81	L89.503	O24.02	O44.52	O86.81	P35.8	Q22.6	S02.0XXB
K27.2	K65.0	L89.504	O24.12	O44.53	O86.89	P35.9	Q22.8	S02.101B
K27.4	K65.1	L89.513	O24.32	O45.001	O87.1	P36.0	Q22.9	S02.102B
K27.5	K65.2	L89.514	O24.82	O45.002	O88.011	P36.10	Q23.4	S02.109B
K27.6	K65.3	L89.523	O34.31	O45.003	O88.012	P36.19	Q24.2	S02.110B
K28.0	K65.8	L89.524	O34.32	O45.011	O88.013	P36.2	Q24.4	S02.111B
K28.1	K65.9	L89.603	O34.33	O45.012	O88.02	P36.30	Q24.6	S02.112B
K28.2	K66.1	L89.604	O41.1010	O45.013	O88.03	P36.39	Q25.5	S02.113B
K28.4	K67	L89.613	O41.1011	O45.021	O88.111	P36.4	Q25.6	S02.118B
K28.5	K68.12	L89.614	O41.1012	O45.022	O88.112	P36.5	Q25.71	S02.119B
K28.6	K68.19	L89.623	O41.1013	O45.023	O88.113	P36.8	Q25.72	S02.11AB
K29.01	K68.9	L89.624	O41.1014	O45.091	O88.12	P36.9	Q25.79	S02.11BB
K29.21	K70.41	L89.813	O41.1015	O45.092	O88.13	P37.0	Q28.2	S02.11CB
K29.31	K71.11	L89.814	O41.1019	O45.093	O88.211	P37.1	Q28.3	S02.11DB
K29.41	K72.00	L89.893	O41.1020	O45.8X1	O88.212	P37.2	Q33.2	S02.11EB
K29.51	K72.01	L89.894	O41.1021	O45.8X2	O88.213	P37.3	Q33.3	S02.11FB
K29.61	K72.11	L89.93	O41.1022	O45.8X3	O88.22	P37.4	Q33.6	S02.11GB
K29.71	K72.91	L89.94	O41.1023	O45.91	O88.23	P37.8	Q39.0	S02.11HB
K29.81	K75.0	M31.1	O41.1024	O45.92	O88.311	P37.9	Q39.1	S02.121B
K29.91	K75.1	M72.6	O41.1025	O45.93	O88.312	P52.21	Q39.2	S02.122B
K31.811	K76.2	N00.0	O41.1029	O46.001	O88.313	P52.22	Q39.3	S02.129B
K31.82	K76.3	N00.1	O41.1030	O46.002	O88.32	P52.4	Q39.4	S02.19XB
K35.21	K76.7	N00.2	O41.1031	O46.003	O88.33	P52.5	Q44.2	S02.91XB
K35.32	K80.67	N00.3	O41.1032	O46.011	O88.811	P52.6	Q44.3	S06.1X0A
K35.33	K82.2	N00.4	O41.1033	O46.012	O88.812	P52.8	Q79.0	S06.1X1A
K40.10	K83.1	N00.5	O41.1034	O46.013	O88.813	P52.9	Q79.1	S06.1X2A
K40.11	K83.2	N00.6	O41.1035	O46.021	O88.82	P54.1	Q79.2	S06.1X3A
K40.40	K85.00	N00.7	O41.1039	O46.022	O88.83	P54.2	Q79.3	S06.1X4A
K40.41	K85.01	N00.8	O41.1210	O46.023	O90.3	P54.3	Q79.4	S06.1X5A
K41.10	K85.02	N00.9	O41.1211	O46.091	O90.4	P56.0	Q79.51	S06.1X6A
K41.11	K85.10	N00.A	O41.1212	O46.092	O99.42	P56.90	Q79.59	S06.1X7A
K41.40	K85.11	N01.0	O41.1213	O46.093	P10.0	P56.99	Q89.4	S06.1X8A
K41.41	K85.12	N01.1	O41.1214	O60.02	P10.1	P57.0	Q93.81	S06.1X9A
K42.1	K85.20	N01.2	O41.1215	O60.03	P10.3	P57.8	R09.2	S06.2X6A
K43.1	K85.21	N01.3	O41.1219	O60.12X0	P10.4	P57.9	R40.20	S06.2X7A
K43.4	K85.22	N01.4	O41.1220	O60.12X1	P10.8	P59.1	R40.2110	S06.2X8A
K43.7	K85.30	N01.5	O41.1221	O60.12X2	P10.9	P59.20	R40.2111	S06.306A
K44.1	K85.31	N01.6	O41.1222	O60.12X3	P11.0	P59.29	R40.2112	S06.307A
K45.1	K85.32	N01.7	O41.1223	O60.12X4	P11.2	P60	R40.2113	S06.308A
K46.1	K85.80	N01.8	O41.1224	O60.12X5	P11.9	P61.0	R40.2114	S06.310A
K55.011	K85.81	N01.9	O41.1225	O60.12X9	P22.0	P61.5	R40.2120	S06.311A
K55.012	K85.82	N01.A	O41.1229	O60.13X0	P23.0	P74.0	R40.2121	S06.312A
K55.019	K85.90	N15.1	O41.1230	O60.13X1	P23.1	P77.1	R40.2122	S06.313A
K55.021	K85.91	N17.0	O41.1231	O60.13X2	P23.2	P77.2	R40.2123	S06.314A
K55.022	K85.92	N17.1	O41.1232	O60.13X3	P23.3	P77.3	R40.2124	S06.315A
K55.029	L89.003	N17.2	O41.1233	O60.13X4	P23.4	P77.9	R40.2210	S06.316A
K55.031	L89.004	N18.6	O41.1234	O60.13X5	P23.5	P78.0	R40.2211	S06.317A
K55.032	L89.013	N73.3	O41.1235	O60.13X9	P23.6	P83.2	R40.2212	S06.318A
K55.039	L89.014	O03.2	O41.1239	O60.14X0	P23.8	P90	R40.2213	S06.319A
K55.041	L89.023	O03.31	O41.1410	O60.14X1	P23.9	P91.0	R40.2214	S06.320A
K55.042	L89.024	O03.32	O41.1411	O60.14X2	P24.01	P91.1	R40.2220	S06.321A
K55.049	L89.103	O03.81	O41.1412	O60.14X3	P24.11	P91.2	R40.2221	S06.322A
K55.051	L89.104	O03.82	O41.1413	O60.14X4	P24.21	P91.3	R40.2222	S06.323A
K55.052	L89.113	O04.7	O41.1414	O60.14X5	P24.31	P91.4	R40.2223	S06.324A
K55.059	L89.114	O04.81	O41.1415	O60.14X9	P24.81	P91.5	R40.2224	S06.325A

S06.326A	S06.6X5A	S12.400B	S21.301A	S22.081B	S25.419A	S31.650A	S32.412B	S32.475A
S06.327A	S06.6X6A	S12.401B	S21.302A	S22.082B	S25.421A	S31.651A	S32.413A	S32.475B
S06.328A	S06.6X7A	S12.430B	S21.309A	S22.088B	S25.422A	S31.652A	S32.413B	S32.476A
S06.329A	S06.6X8A	S12.431B	S21.311A	S22.089B	S25.429A	S31.653A	S32.414A	S32.476B
S06.330A	S06.6X9A	S12.44XB	S21.312A	S22.20XB	S25.491A	S31.654A	S32.414B	S32.481A
S06.331A	S06.816A	S12.450B	S21.319A	S22.21XB	S25.492A	S31.655A	S32.415A	S32.481B
S06.332A	S06.817A	S12.451B	S21.321A	S22.22XB	S25.499A	S31.659A	S32.415B	S32.482A
S06.333A	S06.818A	S12.490B	S21.322A	S22.23XB	S26.020A	S32.000B	S32.416A	S32.482B
S06.334A	S06.826A	S12.491B	S21.329A	S22.24XB	S26.021A	S32.001B	S32.416B	S32.483A
S06.335A	S06.827A	S12.500B	S21.331A	S22.31XB	S26.022A	S32.002B	S32.421A	S32.483B
S06.336A	S06.828A	S12.501B	S21.332A	S22.32XB	S26.12XA	S32.008B	S32.421B	S32.484A
S06.337A	S06.896A	S12.530B	S21.339A	S22.39XB	S26.92XA	S32.009B	S32.422A	S32.484B
S06.338A	S06.897A	S12.531B	S21.341A	S22.41XB	S27.1XXA	S32.010B	S32.422B	S32.485A
S06.339A	S06.898A	S12.54XB	S21.342A	S22.42XB	S27.2XXA	S32.011B	S32.423A	S32.485B
S06.340A	S06.9X6A	S12.550B	S21.349A	S22.43XB	S27.331A	S32.012B	S32.423B	S32.486A
S06.341A	S06.9X7A	S12.551B	S21.351A	S22.49XB	S27.332A	S32.018B	S32.424A	S32.486B
S06.342A	S06.9X8A	S12.590B	S21.352A	S22.5XXA	S27.339A	S32.019B	S32.424B	S32.491A
S06.343A	S11.011A	S12.591B	S21.359A	S22.5XXB	S27.401A	S32.020B	S32.425A	S32.491B
S06.344A	S11.012A	S12.600B	S21.401A	S22.9XXB	S27.402A	S32.021B	S32.425B	S32.492A
S06.345A	S11.013A	S12.601B	S21.402A	S24.0XXA	S27.409A	S32.022B	S32.426A	S32.492B
S06.346A	S11.014A	S12.630B	S21.409A	S24.101A	S27.411A	S32.028B	S32.426B	S32.499A
S06.347A	S11.015A	S12.631B	S21.411A	S24.102A	S27.412A	S32.029B	S32.431A	S32.499B
S06.348A	S11.019A	S12.64XB	S21.412A	S24.103A	S27.419A	S32.030B	S32.431B	S32.501B
S06.349A	S11.021A	S12.650B	S21.419A	S24.104A	S27.421A	S32.031B	S32.432A	S32.502B
S06.350A	S11.022A	S12.651B	S21.421A	S24.111A	S27.422A	S32.032B	S32.432B	S32.509B
S06.351A	S11.023A	S12.690B	S21.422A	S24.112A	S27.429A	S32.038B	S32.433A	S32.511B
S06.352A	S11.024A	S12.691B	S21.429A	S24.113A	S27.431A	S32.039B	S32.433B	S32.512B
S06.353A	S11.025A	S12.8XXA	S21.431A	S24.114A	S27.432A	S32.040B	S32.434A	S32.519B
S06.354A	S11.029A	S14.0XXA	S21.432A	S24.131A	S27.439A	S32.041B	S32.434B	S32.591B
S06.355A	S11.031A	S14.101A	S21.439A	S24.132A	S27.491A	S32.042B	S32.435A	S32.592B
S06.356A	S11.032A	S14.102A	S21.441A	S24.133A	S27.492A	S32.048B	S32.435B	S32.599B
S06.357A	S11.033A	S14.103A	S21.442A	S24.134A	S27.499A	S32.049B	S32.436A	S32.601B
S06.358A	S11.034A	S14.104A	S21.449A	S24.141A	S27.812A	S32.050B	S32.436B	S32.602B
S06.359A	S11.035A	S14.105A	S21.451A	S24.142A	S27.813A	S32.051B	S32.441A	S32.609B
S06.360A	S11.039A	S14.106A	S21.452A	S24.143A	S27.818A	S32.052B	S32.441B	S32.611B
S06.361A	S12.000B	S14.107A	S21.459A	S24.144A	S27.819A	S32.058B	S32.442A	S32.612B
S06.362A	S12.001B	S14.108A	S22.000B	S24.151A	S31.001A	S32.059B	S32.442B	S32.613B
S06.363A	S12.01XB	S14.111A	S22.001B	S24.152A	S31.011A	S32.10XB	S32.443A	S32.614B
S06.364A	S12.02XB	S14.112A	S22.002B	S24.153A	S31.021A	S32.110B	S32.443B	S32.615B
S06.365A	S12.030B	S14.113A	S22.008B	S24.154A	S31.031A	S32.111B	S32.444A	S32.616B
S06.366A	S12.031B	S14.114A	S22.009B	S25.00XA	S31.041A	S32.112B	S32.444B	S32.691B
S06.367A	S12.040B	S14.115A	S22.010B	S25.01XA	S31.051A	S32.119B	S32.445A	S32.692B
S06.368A	S12.041B	S14.116A	S22.011B	S25.02XA	S31.600A	S32.120B	S32.445B	S32.699B
S06.369A	S12.090B	S14.117A	S22.012B	S25.09XA	S31.601A	S32.121B	S32.446A	S32.810B
S06.370A	S12.091B	S14.118A	S22.018B	S25.101A	S31.602A	S32.122B	S32.446B	S32.811B
S06.376A	S12.100B	S14.121A	S22.019B	S25.102A	S31.603A	S32.129B	S32.451A	S32.82XB
S06.377A	S12.101B	S14.122A	S22.020B	S25.109A	S31.604A	S32.130B	S32.451B	S32.89XB
S06.378A	S12.110B	S14.123A	S22.021B	S25.111A	S31.605A	S32.131B	S32.452A	S32.9XXB
S06.380A	S12.111B	S14.124A	S22.022B	S25.112A	S31.609A	S32.132B	S32.452B	S34.01XA
S06.386A	S12.112B	S14.125A	S22.028B	S25.119A	S31.610A	S32.139B	S32.453A	S34.02XA
S06.387A	S12.120B	S14.126A	S22.029B	S25.121A	S31.611A	S32.14XB	S32.453B	S34.101A
S06.388A	S12.121B	S14.127A	S22.030B	S25.122A	S31.612A	S32.15XB	S32.454A	S34.102A
S06.4X0A	S12.130B	S14.128A	S22.031B	S25.129A	S31.613A	S32.16XB	S32.454B	S34.103A
S06.4X1A	S12.131B	S14.131A	S22.032B	S25.191A	S31.614A	S32.17XB	S32.455A	S34.104A
S06.4X2A	S12.14XB	S14.132A	S22.038B	S25.192A	S31.615A	S32.19XB	S32.455B	S34.105A
S06.4X3A	S12.150B	S14.133A	S22.039B	S25.199A	S31.619A	S32.2XXB	S32.456A	S34.109A
S06.4X4A	S12.151B	S14.134A	S22.040B	S25.20XA	S31.620A	S32.301B	S32.456B	S34.111A
S06.4X5A	S12.190B	S14.135A	S22.041B	S25.21XA	S31.621A	S32.302B	S32.461A	S34.112A
S06.4X6A	S12.191B	S14.136A	S22.042B	S25.22XA	S31.622A	S32.309B	S32.461B	S34.113A
S06.4X7A	S12.200B	S14.137A	S22.048B	S25.29XA	S31.623A	S32.311B	S32.462A	S34.114A
S06.4X8A	S12.201B	S14.138A	S22.049B	S25.301A	S31.624A	S32.312B	S32.462B	S34.115A
S06.4X9A	S12.230B	S14.141A	S22.050B	S25.302A	S31.625A	S32.313B	S32.463A	S34.119A
S06.5X0A	S12.231B	S14.142A	S22.051B	S25.309A	S31.629A	S32.314B	S32.463B	S34.121A
S06.5X1A	S12.24XB	S14.143A	S22.052B	S25.311A	S31.630A	S32.315B	S32.464A	S34.122A
S06.5X2A	S12.250B	S14.144A	S22.058B	S25.312A	S31.631A	S32.316B	S32.464B	S34.123A
S06.5X3A	S12.251B	S14.145A	S22.059B	S25.319A	S31.632A	S32.391B	S32.465A	S34.124A
S06.5X4A	S12.290B	S14.146A	S22.060B	S25.321A	S31.633A	S32.392B	S32.465B	S34.125A
S06.5X5A	S12.291B	S14.147A	S22.061B	S25.322A	S31.634A	S32.399B	S32.466A	S34.129A
S06.5X6A	S12.300B	S14.148A	S22.062B	S25.329A	S31.635A	S32.401A	S32.466B	S34.131A
S06.5X7A	S12.301B	S14.151A	S22.068B	S25.391A	S31.639A	S32.401B	S32.471A	S34.132A
S06.5X8A	S12.330B	S14.152A	S22.069B	S25.392A	S31.640A	S32.402A	S32.471B	S34.139A
S06.5X9A	S12.331B	S14.153A	S22.070B	S25.399A	S31.641A	S32.402B	S32.472A	S34.3XXA
S06.6X0A	S12.34XB	S14.154A	S22.071B	S25.401A	S31.642A	S32.409A	S32.472B	S35.00XA
S06.6X1A	S12.350B	S14.155A	S22.072B	S25.402A	S31.643A	S32.409B	S32.473A	S35.01XA
S06.6X2A	S12.351B	S14.156A	S22.078B	S25.409A	S31.644A	S32.411A	S32.473B	S35.02XA
S06.6X3A	S12.390B	S14.157A	S22.079B	S25.411A	S31.645A	S32.411B	S32.474A	S35.09XA
S06.6X4A	S12.391B	S14.158A	S22.080B	S25.412A	S31.649A	S32.412A	S32.474B	S35.10XA

S35.11XA	S42.222B	S42.424B	S52.033C	S52.226B	S52.322C	S52.502B	S52.90XC	S72.051A
S35.12XA	S42.223B	S42.425B	S52.034B	S52.226C	S52.323B	S52.502C	S52.91XB	S72.051B
S35.19XA	S42.224B	S42.426B	S52.034C	S52.231B	S52.323C	S52.509B	S52.91XC	S72.051C
S35.211A	S42.225B	S42.431B	S52.035B	S52.231C	S52.324B	S52.509C	S52.92XB	S72.052A
S35.212A	S42.226B	S42.432B	S52.035C	S52.232B	S52.324C	S52.511B	S52.92XC	S72.052B
S35.218A	S42.231B	S42.433B	S52.036B	S52.232C	S52.325B	S52.511C	S72.001A	S72.052C
S35.219A	S42.232B	S42.434B	S52.036C	S52.233B	S52.325C	S52.512B	S72.001B	S72.059A
S35.221A	S42.239B	S42.435B	S52.041B	S52.233C	S52.326B	S52.512C	S72.001C	S72.059B
S35.222A	S42.241B	S42.436B	S52.041C	S52.234B	S52.326C	S52.513B	S72.002A	S72.059C
S35.228A	S42.242B	S42.441B	S52.042B	S52.234C	S52.331B	S52.513C	S72.002B	S72.061A
S35.229A	S42.249B	S42.442B	S52.042C	S52.235B	S52.331C	S52.514B	S72.002C	S72.061B
S35.231A	S42.251B	S42.443B	S52.043B	S52.235C	S52.332B	S52.514C	S72.009A	S72.061C
S35.232A	S42.252B	S42.444B	S52.043C	S52.236B	S52.332C	S52.515B	S72.009B	S72.062A
S35.238A	S42.253B	S42.445B	S52.044B	S52.236C	S52.333B	S52.515C	S72.009C	S72.062B
S35.239A	S42.254B	S42.446B	S52.044C	S52.241B	S52.333C	S52.516B	S72.011A	S72.062C
S35.291A	S42.255B	S42.447B	S52.045B	S52.241C	S52.334B	S52.516C	S72.011B	S72.063A
S35.292A	S42.256B	S42.448B	S52.045C	S52.242B	S52.334C	S52.531B	S72.011C	S72.063B
S35.298A	S42.261B	S42.449B	S52.046B	S52.242C	S52.335B	S52.531C	S72.012A	S72.064A
S35.299A	S42.262B	S42.451B	S52.046C	S52.243B	S52.335C	S52.532B	S72.012B	S72.064B
S35.311A	S42.263B	S42.452B	S52.091B	S52.243C	S52.336B	S52.532C	S72.012C	S72.064C
S35.318A	S42.264B	S42.453B	S52.091C	S52.244B	S52.336C	S52.539B	S72.019A	S72.065A
S35.319A	S42.265B	S42.454B	S52.092B	S52.244C	S52.341B	S52.539C	S72.019B	S72.065B
S35.321A	S42.266B	S42.455B	S52.092C	S52.245B	S52.341C	S52.541B	S72.019C	S72.065C
S35.328A	S42.291B	S42.456B	S52.099B	S52.245C	S52.342B	S52.541C	S72.021A	S72.066A
S35.329A	S42.292B	S42.461B	S52.099C	S52.246B	S52.342C	S52.542B	S72.021B	S72.066B
S35.331A	S42.293B	S42.462B	S52.101B	S52.246C	S52.343B	S52.542C	S72.021C	S72.066C
S35.338A	S42.294B	S42.463B	S52.101C	S52.251B	S52.343C	S52.549B	S72.022A	S72.091A
S35.339A	S42.295B	S42.464B	S52.102B	S52.251C	S52.344B	S52.549C	S72.022B	S72.091B
S35.341A	S42.296B	S42.465B	S52.102C	S52.252B	S52.344C	S52.551B	S72.022C	S72.091C
S35.348A	S42.301B	S42.466B	S52.109B	S52.252C	S52.345B	S52.551C	S72.023A	S72.092A
S35.349A	S42.302B	S42.471B	S52.109C	S52.253B	S52.345C	S52.552B	S72.023B	S72.092B
S35.401A	S42.309B	S42.472B	S52.121B	S52.253C	S52.346B	S52.552C	S72.023C	S72.092C
S35.402A	S42.321B	S42.473B	S52.121C	S52.254B	S52.346C	S52.559B	S72.024A	S72.099A
S35.403A	S42.322B	S42.474B	S52.122B	S52.254C	S52.351B	S52.559C	S72.024B	S72.099B
S35.404A	S42.323B	S42.475B	S52.122C	S52.255B	S52.351C	S52.561B	S72.024C	S72.099C
S35.405A	S42.324B	S42.476B	S52.123B	S52.255C	S52.352B	S52.561C	S72.025A	S72.101A
S35.406A	S42.325B	S42.491B	S52.123C	S52.256B	S52.352C	S52.562B	S72.025B	S72.101B
S35.411A	S42.326B	S42.492B	S52.124B	S52.256C	S52.353B	S52.562C	S72.025C	S72.101C
S35.412A	S42.331B	S42.493B	S52.124C	S52.261B	S52.353C	S52.569B	S72.026A	S72.102A
S35.413A	S42.332B	S42.494B	S52.125B	S52.261C	S52.354B	S52.569C	S72.026B	S72.102B
S35.414A	S42.333B	S42.495B	S52.125C	S52.262B	S52.354C	S52.571B	S72.026C	S72.102C
S35.415A	S42.334B	S42.496B	S52.126B	S52.262C	S52.355B	S52.571C	S72.031A	S72.109A
S35.416A	S42.335B	S42.90XB	S52.126C	S52.263B	S52.355C	S52.572B	S72.031B	S72.109B
S35.491A	S42.336B	S42.91XB	S52.131B	S52.263C	S52.356B	S52.572C	S72.031C	S72.109C
S35.492A	S42.341B	S42.92XB	S52.131C	S52.264B	S52.356C	S52.579B	S72.032A	S72.111A
S35.493A	S42.342B	S45.001A	S52.132B	S52.264C	S52.361B	S52.579C	S72.032B	S72.111B
S35.494A	S42.343B	S45.002A	S52.132C	S52.265B	S52.361C	S52.591B	S72.032C	S72.111C
S35.495A	S42.344B	S45.009A	S52.133B	S52.265C	S52.362B	S52.591C	S72.033A	S72.112A
S35.496A	S42.345B	S45.011A	S52.133C	S52.266B	S52.362C	S52.592B	S72.033B	S72.112B
S35.50XA	S42.346B	S45.012A	S52.134B	S52.266C	S52.363B	S52.592C	S72.033C	S72.112C
S35.511A	S42.351B	S45.019A	S52.134C	S52.271B	S52.363C	S52.599B	S72.034A	S72.113A
S35.512A	S42.352B	S45.091A	S52.135B	S52.271C	S52.364B	S52.599C	S72.034B	S72.113B
S35.513A	S42.353B	S45.092A	S52.135C	S52.272B	S52.364C	S52.601B	S72.034C	S72.113C
S35.514A	S42.354B	S45.099A	S52.136B	S52.272C	S52.365B	S52.601C	S72.035A	S72.114A
S35.515A	S42.355B	S52.001B	S52.136C	S52.279B	S52.365C	S52.602B	S72.035B	S72.114B
S35.516A	S42.356B	S52.001C	S52.181B	S52.279C	S52.366B	S52.602C	S72.035C	S72.114C
S35.59XA	S42.361B	S52.002B	S52.181C	S52.281B	S52.366C	S52.609B	S72.036A	S72.115A
S36.031A	S42.362B	S52.002C	S52.182B	S52.281C	S52.371B	S52.609C	S72.036B	S72.115B
S36.032A	S42.363B	S52.009B	S52.182C	S52.282B	S52.371C	S52.611B	S72.036C	S72.115C
S36.115A	S42.364B	S52.009C	S52.189B	S52.282C	S52.372B	S52.611C	S72.041A	S72.116A
S36.116A	S42.365B	S52.021B	S52.189C	S52.283B	S52.372C	S52.612B	S72.041B	S72.116B
S37.061A	S42.366B	S52.021C	S52.201B	S52.283C	S52.379B	S52.612C	S72.041C	S72.116C
S37.062A	S42.391B	S52.022B	S52.201C	S52.291B	S52.379C	S52.613B	S72.042A	S72.121A
S37.069A	S42.392B	S52.022C	S52.202B	S52.291C	S52.381B	S52.613C	S72.042B	S72.121B
S37.091A	S42.399B	S52.023B	S52.202C	S52.292B	S52.381C	S52.614B	S72.042C	S72.121C
S37.092A	S42.401B	S52.023C	S52.209B	S52.292C	S52.382B	S52.614C	S72.043A	S72.122A
S37.099A	S42.402B	S52.024B	S52.209C	S52.299B	S52.382C	S52.615B	S72.043B	S72.122B
S42.201B	S42.409B	S52.024C	S52.221B	S52.299C	S52.389B	S52.615C	S72.043C	S72.122C
S42.202B	S42.411B	S52.025B	S52.221C	S52.301B	S52.389C	S52.616B	S72.044A	S72.123A
S42.209B	S42.412B	S52.025C	S52.222B	S52.301C	S52.391B	S52.616C	S72.044B	S72.123B
S42.211B	S42.413B	S52.026B	S52.222C	S52.302B	S52.391C	S52.691B	S72.044C	S72.123C
S42.212B	S42.414B	S52.026C	S52.223B	S52.302C	S52.392B	S52.691C	S72.045A	S72.124A
S42.213B	S42.415B	S52.031B	S52.223C	S52.309B	S52.392C	S52.692B	S72.045B	S72.124B
S42.214B	S42.416B	S52.031C	S52.224B	S52.309C	S52.399B	S52.692C	S72.045C	S72.124C
S42.215B	S42.421B	S52.032B	S52.224C	S52.321B	S52.399C	S52.699B	S72.046A	S72.125A
S42.216B	S42.422B	S52.032C	S52.225B	S52.321C	S52.501B	S52.699C	S72.046B	S72.125B
S42.221B	S42.423B	S52.033B	S52.225C	S52.322B	S52.501C	S52.90XB	S72.046C	

S72.125C	S72.323A	S72.363B	S72.446C	S79.001A	S82.156B	S82.266C	S82.491B	T31.85
S72.126A	S72.323B	S72.363C	S72.451B	S79.002A	S82.156C	S82.291B	S82.491C	T31.86
S72.126B	S72.323C	S72.364A	S72.451C	S79.009A	S82.191B	S82.291C	S82.492B	T31.87
S72.126C	S72.324A	S72.364B	S72.452B	S79.011A	S82.191C	S82.292B	S82.492C	T31.88
S72.131A	S72.324B	S72.364C	S72.452C	S79.012A	S82.192B	S82.292C	S82.499B	T31.91
S72.131B	S72.324C	S72.365A	S72.453B	S79.019A	S82.192C	S82.299B	S82.499C	T31.92
S72.131C	S72.325A	S72.365B	S72.453C	S79.091A	S82.199B	S82.299C	S82.831B	T31.93
S72.132A	S72.325B	S72.365C	S72.454B	S79.092A	S82.199C	S82.401B	S82.831C	T31.94
S72.132B	S72.325C	S72.366A	S72.454C	S79.099A	S82.201B	S82.401C	S82.832B	T31.95
S72.132C	S72.326A	S72.366B	S72.455B	S82.101B	S82.201C	S82.402B	S82.832C	T31.96
S72.133A	S72.326B	S72.366C	S72.455C	S82.101C	S82.202B	S82.402C	S82.839B	T31.97
S72.133B	S72.326C	S72.391A	S72.456B	S82.102B	S82.202C	S82.409B	S82.839C	T31.98
S72.133C	S72.331A	S72.391B	S72.456C	S82.102C	S82.209B	S82.409C	S82.861B	T31.99
S72.134A	S72.331B	S72.391C	S72.461B	S82.109B	S82.209C	S82.421B	S82.861C	T32.21
S72.134B	S72.331C	S72.392A	S72.461C	S82.109C	S82.221B	S82.421C	S82.862B	T32.22
S72.134C	S72.332A	S72.392B	S72.462B	S82.111B	S82.221C	S82.422B	S82.862C	T32.31
S72.135A	S72.332B	S72.392C	S72.462C	S82.111C	S82.222B	S82.422C	S82.863B	T32.32
S72.135B	S72.332C	S72.399A	S72.463B	S82.112B	S82.222C	S82.423B	S82.863C	T32.33
S72.135C	S72.333A	S72.399B	S72.463C	S82.112C	S82.223B	S82.423C	S82.864B	T32.41
S72.136A	S72.333B	S72.399C	S72.464B	S82.113B	S82.223C	S82.424B	S82.864C	T32.42
S72.136B	S72.333C	S72.401B	S72.464C	S82.113C	S82.224B	S82.424C	S82.865B	T32.43
S72.136C	S72.334A	S72.401C	S72.465B	S82.114B	S82.224C	S82.425B	S82.865C	T32.44
S72.141A	S72.334B	S72.402B	S72.465C	S82.114C	S82.225B	S82.425C	S82.866B	T32.51
S72.141B	S72.334C	S72.402C	S72.466B	S82.115B	S82.225C	S82.426B	S82.866C	T32.52
S72.141C	S72.335A	S72.409B	S72.466C	S82.115C	S82.226B	S82.426C	S85.001A	T32.53
S72.142A	S72.335B	S72.409C	S72.491B	S82.116B	S82.226C	S82.431B	S85.002A	T32.54
S72.142B	S72.335C	S72.411B	S72.491C	S82.116C	S82.231B	S82.431C	S85.009A	T32.55
S72.142C	S72.336A	S72.411C	S72.492B	S82.121B	S82.231C	S82.432B	S85.011A	T32.61
S72.143A	S72.336B	S72.412B	S72.492C	S82.121C	S82.232B	S82.432C	S85.012A	T32.62
S72.143B	S72.336C	S72.412C	S72.499B	S82.122B	S82.232C	S82.433B	S85.019A	T32.63
S72.143C	S72.341A	S72.413B	S72.499C	S82.122C	S82.233B	S82.433C	S85.091A	T32.64
S72.144A	S72.341B	S72.413C	S72.8X1A	S82.123B	S82.233C	S82.434B	S85.092A	T32.65
S72.144B	S72.341C	S72.414B	S72.8X1B	S82.123C	S82.234B	S82.434C	S85.099A	T32.66
S72.144C	S72.342A	S72.414C	S72.8X1C	S82.124B	S82.234C	S82.435B	S85.501A	T32.71
S72.145A	S72.342B	S72.415B	S72.8X2A	S82.124C	S82.235B	S82.435C	S85.502A	T32.72
S72.145B	S72.342C	S72.415C	S72.8X2B	S82.125B	S82.235C	S82.436B	S85.509A	T32.73
S72.145C	S72.343A	S72.416B	S72.8X2C	S82.125C	S82.236B	S82.436C	S85.511A	T32.74
S72.146A	S72.343B	S72.416C	S72.8X9A	S82.126B	S82.236C	S82.441B	S85.512A	T32.75
S72.146B	S72.343C	S72.421B	S72.8X9B	S82.126C	S82.241B	S82.441C	S85.519A	T32.76
S72.146C	S72.344A	S72.421C	S72.8X9C	S82.131B	S82.241C	S82.442B	S85.591A	T32.77
S72.21XA	S72.344B	S72.422B	S72.90XA	S82.131C	S82.242B	S82.442C	S85.592A	T32.81
S72.21XB	S72.344C	S72.422C	S72.90XB	S82.132B	S82.242C	S82.443B	S85.599A	T32.82
S72.21XC	S72.345A	S72.423B	S72.90XC	S82.132C	S82.243B	S82.443C	T31.21	T32.83
S72.22XA	S72.345B	S72.423C	S72.91XA	S82.133B	S82.243C	S82.444B	T31.22	T32.84
S72.22XB	S72.345C	S72.424B	S72.91XB	S82.133C	S82.244B	S82.444C	T31.31	T32.85
S72.22XC	S72.346A	S72.424C	S72.91XC	S82.134B	S82.244C	S82.445B	T31.32	T32.86
S72.23XA	S72.346B	S72.425B	S72.92XA	S82.134C	S82.245B	S82.445C	T31.33	T32.87
S72.23XB	S72.346C	S72.425C	S72.92XB	S82.135B	S82.245C	S82.446B	T31.41	T32.88
S72.23XC	S72.351A	S72.426B	S72.92XC	S82.135C	S82.246B	S82.446C	T31.42	T32.91
S72.24XA	S72.351B	S72.426C	S75.001A	S82.136B	S82.246C	S82.451B	T31.43	T32.92
S72.24XB	S72.351C	S72.431B	S75.002A	S82.136C	S82.251B	S82.451C	T31.44	T32.93
S72.24XC	S72.352A	S72.431C	S75.009A	S82.141B	S82.251C	S82.452B	T31.51	T32.94
S72.25XA	S72.352B	S72.432B	S75.011A	S82.141C	S82.252B	S82.452C	T31.52	T32.95
S72.25XB	S72.352C	S72.432C	S75.012A	S82.142B	S82.252C	S82.453B	T31.53	T32.96
S72.25XC	S72.353A	S72.433B	S75.019A	S82.142C	S82.253B	S82.453C	T31.54	T32.97
S72.26XA	S72.353B	S72.433C	S75.021A	S82.143B	S82.253C	S82.454B	T31.55	T32.98
S72.26XB	S72.353C	S72.434B	S75.022A	S82.143C	S82.254B	S82.454C	T31.61	T32.99
S72.26XC	S72.354A	S72.434C	S75.029A	S82.144B	S82.254C	S82.455B	T31.62	T79.0XXA
S72.301A	S72.354B	S72.435B	S75.091A	S82.144C	S82.255B	S82.455C	T31.63	T79.1XXA
S72.301B	S72.354C	S72.435C	S75.092A	S82.145B	S82.255C	S82.456B	T31.64	T79.4XXA
S72.301C	S72.355A	S72.436B	S75.099A	S82.145C	S82.256B	S82.456C	T31.65	T79.5XXA
S72.302A	S72.355B	S72.436C	S75.101A	S82.146B	S82.256C	S82.461B	T31.66	T80.0XXA
S72.302B	S72.355C	S72.441B	S75.102A	S82.146C	S82.261B	S82.461C	T31.71	T81.11XA
S72.302C	S72.356A	S72.441C	S75.109A	S82.151B	S82.261C	S82.462B	T31.72	T81.12XA
S72.309A	S72.356B	S72.442B	S75.111A	S82.151C	S82.262B	S82.462C	T31.73	T81.19XA
S72.309B	S72.356C	S72.442C	S75.112A	S82.152B	S82.262C	S82.463B	T31.74	U07.1
S72.309C	S72.361A	S72.443B	S75.119A	S82.152C	S82.263B	S82.463C	T31.75	
S72.321A	S72.361B	S72.443C	S75.121A	S82.153B	S82.263C	S82.464B	T31.76	
S72.321B	S72.361C	S72.444B	S75.122A	S82.153C	S82.264B	S82.464C	T31.77	
S72.321C	S72.362A	S72.444C	S75.129A	S82.154B	S82.264C	S82.465B	T31.81	
S72.322A	S72.362B	S72.445B	S75.191A	S82.154C	S82.265B	S82.465C	T31.82	
S72.322B	S72.362C	S72.445C	S75.192A	S82.155B	S82.265C	S82.466B	T31.83	
S72.322C	S72.363A	S72.446B	S75.199A	S82.155C	S82.266B	S82.466C	T31.84	

Appendix E: Complication and Comorbidity (CC) Code List

Note: The following is a comprehensive list of ICD-10-CM codes designated as CCs in the tabular section of this manual. Codes listed in this resource and identified as CCs in the tabular section reflect the most current information that was available at the time of publication. Because the fiscal 2021 IPPS final rule was not available at the time this book was printed, the ICD-10-CM codes designated as CCs are based on the proposed, version 38, MS-DRG Grouper software and Definitions Manual files published with the fiscal 2021 IPPS proposed rule.

For the most current list of CC designations based on the final version of the MS-DRG Grouper software and MS-DRG Definitions Manual files, Optum360 has provided an easily searchable data file that can be accessed at the following:

https://www.optum360coding.com/ProductUpdates/
Title: "2021 ICD-10-CM for Hospital IPPS Data File"
Password: Hospital21

A00.0	A15.0	A27.89	A43.1	A52.3	A78	B00.52	B26.89	B51.9
A00.1	A15.4	A27.9	A43.8	A52.71	A79.0	B00.53	B33.1	B52.0
A00.9	A15.5	A28.0	A43.9	A52.72	A79.1	B00.59	B33.20	B52.8
A01.00	A15.6	A28.1	A44.0	A52.73	A79.81	B00.81	B33.21	B52.9
A01.01	A15.7	A28.2	A44.1	A52.74	A79.89	B00.89	B33.22	B53.0
A01.02	A15.8	A28.8	A44.8	A52.75	A79.9	B01.0	B33.23	B53.1
A01.03	A15.9	A28.9	A44.9	A52.76	A81.00	B01.81	B33.4	B53.8
A01.04	A17.9	A30.0	A48.51	A52.77	A81.01	B01.89	B34.3	B54
A01.05	A18.01	A30.1	A48.52	A52.78	A81.09	B01.9	B37.0	B55.0
A01.09	A18.02	A30.2	A50.01	A52.79	A81.1	B02.0	B37.41	B55.1
A01.1	A18.03	A30.3	A50.02	A54.00	A81.2	B02.21	B37.49	B55.2
A01.2	A18.09	A30.4	A50.03	A54.01	A81.81	B02.22	B37.81	B55.9
A01.3	A18.10	A30.5	A50.04	A54.02	A81.82	B02.23	B37.82	B56.0
A01.4	A18.11	A30.8	A50.05	A54.03	A81.83	B02.29	B37.83	B56.1
A02.0	A18.12	A30.9	A50.06	A54.09	A81.89	B02.30	B37.84	B56.9
A02.23	A18.13	A31.0	A50.07	A54.1	A81.9	B02.31	B37.89	B57.0
A02.24	A18.14	A31.1	A50.08	A54.21	A82.0	B02.32	B38.0	B57.1
A02.25	A18.15	A31.2	A50.09	A54.22	A82.1	B02.33	B38.1	B57.2
A02.29	A18.16	A31.8	A50.2	A54.23	A82.9	B02.34	B38.2	B57.30
A02.8	A18.17	A31.9	A50.30	A54.24	A85.0	B02.39	B38.3	B57.31
A02.9	A18.18	A32.0	A50.31	A54.29	A85.1	B02.7	B38.7	B57.32
A03.0	A18.2	A32.11	A50.32	A54.30	A85.8	B02.8	B38.81	B57.39
A04.0	A18.32	A32.12	A50.39	A54.31	A86	B03	B38.89	B57.40
A04.1	A18.39	A32.81	A50.40	A54.32	A87.0	B04	B38.9	B57.41
A04.2	A18.4	A32.82	A50.43	A54.33	A87.1	B05.1	B39.3	B57.42
A04.3	A18.50	A32.89	A50.44	A54.39	A87.2	B05.4	B40.0	B57.49
A04.4	A18.51	A32.9	A50.45	A54.40	A87.8	B05.81	B40.1	B57.5
A04.5	A18.52	A34	A50.49	A54.41	A87.9	B05.89	B40.2	B58.00
A04.6	A18.53	A36.0	A50.51	A54.42	A88.0	B06.00	B40.3	B58.01
A04.71	A18.54	A36.1	A50.52	A54.43	A88.8	B06.02	B40.7	B58.09
A04.72	A18.59	A36.2	A50.53	A54.49	A89	B06.09	B40.81	B58.1
A04.8	A18.6	A36.3	A50.54	A54.82	A90	B06.81	B40.89	B58.82
A04.9	A18.7	A36.81	A50.55	A54.83	A91	B06.82	B40.9	B58.83
A05.0	A18.81	A36.82	A50.56	A54.84	A92.0	B06.89	B41.0	B58.89
A05.1	A18.82	A36.83	A50.57	A54.85	A92.1	B08.3	B41.7	B58.9
A05.2	A18.83	A36.84	A50.59	A54.89	A92.2	B08.71	B41.8	B60.00
A05.3	A18.84	A36.85	A51.31	A54.9	A92.4	B15.9	B41.9	B60.01
A05.4	A18.85	A36.86	A51.32	A68.0	A92.5	B16.1	B44.1	B60.02
A05.5	A18.89	A36.89	A51.39	A68.1	A92.8	B16.9	B44.2	B60.03
A05.8	A21.0	A36.9	A51.42	A68.9	A92.9	B17.0	B44.7	B60.09
A06.0	A21.1	A37.00	A51.43	A69.1	A93.0	B17.10	B44.81	B60.10
A06.1	A21.2	A37.10	A51.44	A69.20	A93.1	B17.2	B44.89	B60.19
A06.2	A21.3	A37.80	A51.45	A69.21	A93.2	B17.8	B44.9	B60.2
A06.3	A21.7	A37.90	A51.46	A69.22	A93.8	B17.9	B45.0	B65.0
A06.81	A21.8	A38.0	A51.49	A69.23	A94	B18.0	B45.2	B65.1
A06.82	A21.9	A38.1	A52.00	A69.29	A95.0	B18.1	B45.3	B65.2
A06.89	A22.0	A38.8	A52.01	A70	A95.1	B18.8	B45.7	B65.3
A07.1	A22.2	A38.9	A52.02	A75.0	A95.9	B18.9	B45.8	B65.8
A07.2	A22.8	A39.82	A52.03	A75.1	A96.0	B19.10	B45.9	B65.9
A07.3	A22.9	A39.83	A52.04	A75.2	A96.1	B19.9	B47.0	B66.0
A07.4	A23.8	A39.84	A52.05	A75.3	A96.8	B20	B47.1	B66.1
A07.8	A23.9	A39.89	A52.06	A75.9	A96.9	B25.1	B47.9	B66.2
A07.9	A24.0	A39.9	A52.09	A77.0	A98.0	B25.8	B48.2	B66.3
A08.0	A24.1	A42.0	A52.10	A77.1	A98.1	B25.9	B48.3	B66.4
A08.11	A24.2	A42.1	A52.11	A77.2	A98.2	B26.0	B48.4	B66.5
A08.19	A24.3	A42.2	A52.12	A77.3	A98.5	B26.3	B48.8	B66.8
A08.2	A24.9	A42.81	A52.15	A77.40	A98.8	B26.81	B49	B67.0
A08.31	A25.0	A42.82	A52.16	A77.41	A99	B26.82	B50.0	B67.1
A08.32	A25.1	A42.89	A52.17	A77.49	B00.2	B26.83	B50.8	B67.2
A08.39	A25.9	A42.9	A52.19	A77.8	B00.50	B26.84	B51.0	B67.31
A09	A27.0	A43.0	A52.2	A77.9	B00.51	B26.85	B51.8	B67.32

Appendix E: Complication and Comorbidity (CC) Code List

B67.39	C17.8	C40.82	C70.1	C79.60	C81.36	C82.43	C83.50	C84.67
B67.4	C17.9	C40.90	C70.9	C79.61	C81.37	C82.44	C83.51	C84.68
B67.5	C18.0	C40.91	C71.0	C79.62	C81.38	C82.45	C83.52	C84.69
B67.61	C18.1	C40.92	C71.1	C79.70	C81.39	C82.46	C83.53	C84.70
B67.69	C18.2	C41.0	C71.2	C79.71	C81.40	C82.47	C83.54	C84.71
B67.7	C18.3	C41.1	C71.3	C79.72	C81.41	C82.48	C83.55	C84.72
B67.8	C18.4	C41.2	C71.4	C79.81	C81.42	C82.49	C83.56	C84.73
B67.90	C18.5	C41.3	C71.5	C79.82	C81.43	C82.50	C83.57	C84.74
B67.99	C18.6	C41.4	C71.6	C79.89	C81.44	C82.51	C83.58	C84.75
B68.0	C18.7	C41.9	C71.7	C79.9	C81.45	C82.52	C83.59	C84.76
B68.1	C18.8	C45.0	C71.8	C7A.00	C81.46	C82.53	C83.70	C84.77
B68.9	C18.9	C45.1	C71.9	C7A.010	C81.47	C82.54	C83.71	C84.78
B69.0	C19	C45.2	C72.0	C7A.011	C81.48	C82.55	C83.72	C84.79
B69.1	C20	C46.0	C72.1	C7A.012	C81.49	C82.56	C83.73	C84.90
B69.81	C21.0	C46.1	C72.20	C7A.019	C81.70	C82.57	C83.74	C84.91
B69.89	C21.1	C46.2	C72.21	C7A.020	C81.71	C82.58	C83.75	C84.92
B69.9	C21.2	C46.3	C72.30	C7A.021	C81.72	C82.59	C83.76	C84.93
B70.0	C21.8	C46.4	C72.31	C7A.022	C81.73	C82.60	C83.77	C84.94
B70.1	C22.0	C46.50	C72.32	C7A.023	C81.74	C82.61	C83.78	C84.95
B71.0	C22.1	C46.51	C72.40	C7A.024	C81.75	C82.62	C83.79	C84.96
B71.1	C22.2	C46.52	C72.41	C7A.025	C81.76	C82.63	C83.80	C84.97
B71.8	C22.3	C46.7	C72.42	C7A.026	C81.77	C82.64	C83.81	C84.98
B72	C22.4	C46.9	C72.50	C7A.029	C81.78	C82.65	C83.82	C84.99
B73.00	C22.7	C47.0	C72.59	C7A.090	C81.79	C82.66	C83.83	C84.A0
B73.01	C22.8	C47.10	C72.9	C7A.091	C81.90	C82.67	C83.84	C84.A1
B73.02	C22.9	C47.11	C74.00	C7A.092	C81.91	C82.68	C83.85	C84.A2
B73.09	C23	C47.12	C74.01	C7A.093	C81.92	C82.69	C83.86	C84.A3
B73.1	C24.0	C47.20	C74.02	C7A.094	C81.93	C82.80	C83.87	C84.A4
B74.0	C24.1	C47.21	C74.10	C7A.095	C81.94	C82.81	C83.88	C84.A5
B74.1	C24.8	C47.22	C74.11	C7A.096	C81.95	C82.82	C83.89	C84.A6
B74.2	C24.9	C47.3	C74.12	C7A.098	C81.96	C82.83	C83.90	C84.A7
B74.3	C25.0	C47.4	C74.90	C7A.1	C81.97	C82.84	C83.91	C84.A8
B74.4	C25.1	C47.5	C74.91	C7A.8	C81.98	C82.85	C83.92	C84.A9
B74.8	C25.2	C47.6	C74.92	C7B.01	C81.99	C82.86	C83.93	C84.Z0
B74.9	C25.3	C47.8	C75.0	C7B.02	C82.00	C82.87	C83.94	C84.Z1
B75	C25.4	C47.9	C75.1	C7B.03	C82.01	C82.88	C83.95	C84.Z2
B76.0	C25.7	C48.0	C75.2	C7B.04	C82.02	C82.89	C83.96	C84.Z3
B76.1	C25.8	C48.1	C75.3	C7B.09	C82.03	C82.90	C83.97	C84.Z4
B76.8	C25.9	C48.2	C75.4	C7B.8	C82.04	C82.91	C83.98	C84.Z5
B76.9	C33	C48.8	C75.5	C80.0	C82.05	C82.92	C83.99	C84.Z6
B77.0	C34.00	C49.0	C75.8	C80.2	C82.06	C82.93	C84.00	C84.Z7
B77.89	C34.01	C49.10	C75.9	C81.00	C82.07	C82.94	C84.01	C84.Z8
B77.9	C34.02	C49.11	C77.0	C81.01	C82.08	C82.95	C84.02	C84.Z9
B78.0	C34.10	C49.12	C77.1	C81.02	C82.09	C82.96	C84.03	C85.10
B78.7	C34.11	C49.20	C77.2	C81.03	C82.10	C82.97	C84.04	C85.11
B78.9	C34.12	C49.21	C77.3	C81.04	C82.11	C82.98	C84.05	C85.12
B79	C34.2	C49.22	C77.4	C81.05	C82.12	C82.99	C84.06	C85.13
B80	C34.30	C49.3	C77.5	C81.06	C82.13	C83.00	C84.07	C85.14
B81.0	C34.31	C49.4	C77.8	C81.07	C82.14	C83.01	C84.08	C85.15
B81.1	C34.32	C49.5	C77.9	C81.08	C82.15	C83.02	C84.09	C85.16
B81.2	C34.80	C49.6	C78.00	C81.09	C82.16	C83.03	C84.10	C85.17
B81.3	C34.81	C49.8	C78.01	C81.10	C82.17	C83.04	C84.11	C85.18
B81.4	C34.82	C49.9	C78.02	C81.11	C82.18	C83.05	C84.12	C85.19
B81.8	C34.90	C49.A0	C78.1	C81.12	C82.19	C83.06	C84.13	C85.20
B82.0	C34.91	C49.A1	C78.2	C81.13	C82.20	C83.07	C84.14	C85.21
B97.21	C34.92	C49.A2	C78.30	C81.14	C82.21	C83.08	C84.15	C85.22
B97.33	C37	C49.A3	C78.39	C81.15	C82.22	C83.09	C84.16	C85.23
B97.34	C38.0	C49.A4	C78.4	C81.16	C82.23	C83.10	C84.17	C85.24
B97.35	C38.1	C49.A5	C78.5	C81.17	C82.24	C83.11	C84.18	C85.25
C15.3	C38.2	C49.A9	C78.6	C81.18	C82.25	C83.12	C84.19	C85.26
C15.4	C38.3	C56.1	C78.7	C81.19	C82.26	C83.13	C84.40	C85.27
C15.5	C38.4	C56.2	C78.80	C81.20	C82.27	C83.14	C84.41	C85.28
C15.8	C38.8	C56.9	C78.89	C81.21	C82.28	C83.15	C84.42	C85.29
C15.9	C40.00	C64.1	C79.00	C81.22	C82.29	C83.16	C84.43	C85.80
C16.0	C40.01	C64.2	C79.01	C81.23	C82.30	C83.17	C84.44	C85.81
C16.1	C40.02	C64.9	C79.02	C81.24	C82.31	C83.18	C84.45	C85.82
C16.2	C40.10	C65.1	C79.10	C81.25	C82.32	C83.19	C84.46	C85.83
C16.3	C40.11	C65.2	C79.11	C81.26	C82.33	C83.30	C84.47	C85.84
C16.4	C40.12	C65.9	C79.19	C81.27	C82.34	C83.31	C84.48	C85.85
C16.5	C40.20	C66.1	C79.2	C81.28	C82.35	C83.32	C84.49	C85.86
C16.6	C40.21	C66.2	C79.31	C81.29	C82.36	C83.33	C84.60	C85.87
C16.8	C40.22	C66.9	C79.32	C81.30	C82.37	C83.34	C84.61	C85.88
C16.9	C40.30	C68.0	C79.40	C81.31	C82.38	C83.35	C84.62	C85.89
C17.0	C40.31	C68.1	C79.49	C81.32	C82.39	C83.36	C84.63	C85.90
C17.1	C40.32	C68.8	C79.51	C81.33	C82.40	C83.37	C84.64	C85.91
C17.2	C40.80	C68.9	C79.52	C81.34	C82.41	C83.38	C84.65	C85.92
C17.3	C40.81	C70.0	C79.52	C81.35	C82.42	C83.39	C84.66	C85.93

C85.94	C92.62	D59.13	D83.2	E70.41	E75.01	F10.14	F13.280	F18.259
C85.95	C92.90	D59.19	D83.8	E70.49	E75.02	F10.151	F13.281	F18.27
C85.96	C92.91	D59.2	D83.9	E70.5	E75.09	F10.159	F13.282	F18.280
C85.97	C92.92	D59.4	D84.81	E70.81	E75.10	F10.180	F13.288	F18.288
C85.98	C92.A0	D59.9	D84.821	E70.89	E75.11	F10.181	F13.921	F18.921
C85.99	C92.A1	D61.01	D84.822	E70.9	E75.19	F10.188	F13.930	F18.950
C86.0	C92.A2	D61.09	D84.89	E71.0	E75.23	F10.19	F13.931	F18.951
C86.1	C92.Z0	D61.818	D84.9	E71.110	E75.25	F10.221	F13.932	F18.97
C86.2	C92.Z1	D61.82	D89.810	E71.111	E75.26	F10.231	F13.939	F19.121
C86.3	C92.Z2	D61.9	D89.811	E71.118	E75.29	F10.232	F13.950	F19.130
C86.4	C93.00	D62	D89.812	E71.120	E75.4	F10.239	F13.951	F19.131
C86.5	C93.01	D68.0	D89.813	E71.121	E76.01	F10.24	F13.97	F19.132
C86.6	C93.02	D68.1	E06.0	E71.128	E76.02	F10.251	F14.121	F19.139
C88.2	C93.10	D68.2	E08.52	E71.19	E76.03	F10.259	F14.13	F19.150
C88.3	C93.11	D68.311	E09.52	E71.2	E76.1	F10.27	F14.150	F19.151
C88.4	C93.12	D68.312	E10.52	E71.310	E76.210	F10.280	F14.151	F19.17
C88.8	C93.30	D68.318	E11.52	E71.311	E76.211	F10.281	F14.20	F19.20
C88.9	C93.31	D68.32	E13.52	E71.312	E76.219	F10.288	F14.221	F19.221
C90.00	C93.32	D68.4	E15	E71.313	E76.22	F10.29	F14.222	F19.222
C90.01	C93.90	D68.51	E22.1	E71.314	E76.29	F10.921	F14.229	F19.230
C90.02	C93.91	D68.52	E22.2	E71.318	E76.3	F10.930	F14.23	F19.231
C90.10	C93.92	D68.59	E22.8	E71.32	E76.8	F10.931	F14.250	F19.232
C90.11	C93.Z0	D68.61	E22.9	E71.39	E76.9	F10.932	F14.251	F19.239
C90.12	C93.Z1	D68.62	E23.0	E71.50	E78.71	F10.939	F14.259	F19.250
C90.20	C93.Z2	D68.69	E23.2	E71.510	E78.72	F10.94	F14.280	F19.251
C90.21	C94.00	D68.8	E24.0	E71.511	E79.1	F10.951	F14.281	F19.259
C90.22	C94.01	D68.9	E24.2	E71.518	E79.2	F10.959	F14.282	F19.26
C90.30	C94.02	D69.0	E24.3	E71.520	E79.8	F10.980	F14.288	F19.27
C90.31	C94.20	D69.3	E24.4	E71.521	E79.9	F10.981	F14.921	F19.280
C90.32	C94.21	D69.41	E24.8	E71.522	E80.0	F10.988	F14.93	F19.281
C91.00	C94.22	D69.42	E24.9	E71.528	E80.1	F10.99	F14.950	F19.282
C91.01	C94.30	D74.0	E27.0	E71.529	E80.20	F11.121	F14.951	F19.288
C91.02	C94.31	D74.8	E27.1	E71.53	E80.21	F11.13	F15.121	F19.921
C91.10	C94.32	D74.9	E27.2	E71.540	E80.29	F11.150	F15.13	F19.930
C91.11	C94.40	D75.81	E27.3	E71.541	E80.3	F11.151	F15.150	F19.931
C91.12	C94.41	D76.1	E27.40	E71.542	E84.19	F11.20	F15.151	F19.932
C91.30	C94.42	D76.2	E27.49	E71.548	E84.8	F11.221	F15.20	F19.939
C91.31	C94.6	D76.3	E27.5	E72.00	E84.9	F11.222	F15.221	F19.950
C91.32	C94.80	D78.01	E32.1	E72.01	E85.0	F11.23	F15.222	F19.951
C91.40	C94.81	D78.02	E34.0	E72.02	E85.1	F11.250	F15.23	F19.97
C91.41	C94.82	D78.11	E36.01	E72.03	E85.2	F11.251	F15.250	F20.0
C91.42	C95.00	D78.12	E36.02	E72.04	E85.3	F11.259	F15.251	F20.1
C91.50	C95.01	D78.21	E36.11	E72.09	E85.4	F11.281	F15.259	F20.2
C91.51	C95.02	D78.22	E36.12	E72.10	E85.81	F11.282	F15.280	F20.5
C91.52	C95.10	D78.31	E44.0	E72.11	E85.82	F11.288	F15.281	F20.81
C91.60	C95.11	D78.32	E44.1	E72.12	E85.89	F11.921	F15.282	F20.89
C91.61	C95.12	D78.33	E45	E72.19	E85.9	F11.93	F15.288	F23
C91.62	C95.90	D78.34	E46	E72.20	E87.0	F11.950	F15.921	F30.10
C91.90	C95.91	D78.81	E51.11	E72.21	E87.1	F11.951	F15.93	F30.11
C91.91	C95.92	D78.89	E51.12	E72.22	E87.2	F12.121	F15.950	F30.12
C91.92	C96.0	D80.0	E51.2	E72.23	E87.3	F12.150	F15.951	F30.13
C91.A0	C96.20	D80.1	E51.8	E72.29	E87.4	F12.151	F16.121	F30.2
C91.A1	C96.21	D80.2	E51.9	E72.3	E88.02	F12.221	F16.150	F30.9
C91.A2	C96.22	D80.3	E53.0	E72.4	E88.40	F12.250	F16.151	F31.0
C91.Z0	C96.29	D80.4	E55.0	E72.50	E88.41	F12.251	F16.20	F31.10
C91.Z1	C96.4	D80.5	E64.0	E72.51	E88.42	F12.921	F16.221	F31.11
C91.Z2	C96.5	D80.6	E66.2	E72.52	E88.49	F12.950	F16.250	F31.12
C92.00	C96.6	D80.7	E70.0	E72.53	E89.1	F12.951	F16.251	F31.13
C92.01	C96.9	D80.8	E70.1	E72.59	E89.6	F13.121	F16.259	F31.2
C92.02	C96.A	D80.9	E70.20	E72.81	E89.810	F13.130	F16.280	F31.30
C92.10	C96.Z	D81.0	E70.21	E72.89	E89.811	F13.131	F16.283	F31.31
C92.11	D46.22	D81.1	E70.29	E72.9	E89.820	F13.132	F16.288	F31.32
C92.12	D46.C	D81.2	E70.30	E74.00	E89.821	F13.139	F16.921	F31.4
C92.20	D47.01	D81.30	E70.310	E74.01	E89.822	F13.150	F16.950	F31.5
C92.21	D47.02	D81.31	E70.311	E74.02	E89.823	F13.151	F16.951	F31.60
C92.22	D47.09	D81.32	E70.318	E74.03	E89.89	F13.20	F17.203	F31.61
C92.30	D47.1	D81.39	E70.319	E74.04	F01.51	F13.221	F17.213	F31.62
C92.31	D47.9	D81.4	E70.320	E74.09	F02.81	F13.230	F17.223	F31.63
C92.32	D47.Z1	D81.5	E70.321	E74.20	F03.91	F13.231	F17.293	F31.64
C92.40	D47.Z2	D81.6	E70.328	E74.21	F05	F13.232	F18.121	F31.81
C92.41	D47.Z9	D81.7	E70.329	E74.29	F06.0	F13.239	F18.150	F31.89
C92.42	D58.8	D81.89	E70.330	E74.4	F06.2	F13.250	F18.151	F32.0
C92.50	D58.9	D81.9	E70.331	E74.810	F10.121	F13.251	F18.17	F32.1
C92.51	D59.0	D82.0	E70.338	E74.818	F10.130	F13.259	F18.20	F32.2
C92.52	D59.10	D82.1	E70.339	E74.819	F10.131	F13.26	F18.221	F32.3
C92.60	D59.11	D83.0	E70.39	E74.89	F10.132	F13.27	F18.250	F33.0
C92.61	D59.12	D83.1	E70.40	E75.00	F10.139		F18.251	F33.1

Appendix E: Complication and Comorbidity (CC) Code List

F33.2	G37.8	G81.03	H05.032	H33.8	H46.8	H59.339	I24.1	I49.2
F33.3	G37.9	G81.04	H05.033	H34.00	H46.9	H59.341	I24.8	I50.1
F33.40	G40.001	G81.10	H05.039	H34.01	H47.10	H59.342	I24.9	I50.20
F33.8	G40.009	G81.11	H20.00	H34.02	H47.11	H59.343	I25.110	I50.22
F33.9	G40.011	G81.12	H20.011	H34.03	H47.41	H59.349	I25.3	I50.30
F34.81	G40.019	G81.13	H20.012	H34.10	H47.42	H59.351	I25.700	I50.32
F34.89	G40.101	G81.14	H20.013	H34.11	H47.43	H59.352	I25.710	I50.40
F34.9	G40.109	G81.90	H20.019	H34.12	H47.49	H59.353	I25.711	I50.42
F50.00	G40.111	G81.91	H20.021	H34.13	H47.511	H59.359	I25.718	I51.0
F50.01	G40.119	G81.92	H20.022	H34.211	H47.512	H59.361	I25.719	I51.81
F50.02	G40.201	G81.93	H20.023	H34.212	H47.519	H59.362	I25.720	I62.9
F50.2	G40.209	G81.94	H20.029	H34.213	H47.521	H59.363	I25.721	I67.3
F68.10	G40.211	G82.20	H20.031	H34.219	H47.522	H59.369	I25.728	I67.4
F68.12	G40.219	G82.21	H20.032	H34.231	H47.529	H59.811	I25.729	I67.5
F68.A	G40.411	G82.22	H20.033	H34.232	H47.531	H59.812	I25.730	I67.6
F72	G40.419	G83.0	H20.039	H34.233	H47.532	H59.813	I25.731	I67.7
F73	G40.501	G83.4	H20.9	H34.239	H47.539	H59.819	I25.738	I67.81
F84.0	G40.509	G90.3	H21.331	H34.8110	H47.621	H59.88	I25.739	I67.82
F84.2	G40.801	G90.50	H21.332	H34.8111	H47.622	H59.89	I25.750	I67.841
F84.3	G40.802	G90.511	H21.333	H34.8112	H47.629	H60.20	I25.751	I67.848
F84.5	G40.803	G90.512	H21.339	H34.8120	H47.631	H60.21	I25.758	I67.850
F84.8	G40.804	G90.513	H30.101	H34.8121	H47.632	H60.22	I25.759	I67.858
F84.9	G40.811	G90.519	H30.102	H34.8122	H47.639	H60.23	I25.760	I67.89
G03.1	G40.812	G90.521	H30.103	H34.8130	H47.641	H70.001	I25.761	I68.2
G03.2	G40.813	G90.522	H30.109	H34.8131	H47.642	H70.002	I25.768	I69.051
G04.1	G40.814	G90.523	H30.111	H34.8132	H47.649	H70.003	I25.769	I69.052
G10	G40.821	G90.529	H30.112	H34.8190	H49.811	H70.009	I25.790	I69.053
G11.0	G40.822	G90.59	H30.113	H34.8191	H49.812	H70.011	I25.791	I69.054
G11.10	G40.823	G91.0	H30.119	H34.8192	H49.813	H70.012	I25.798	I69.059
G11.11	G40.824	G91.1	H30.121	H34.9	H49.819	H70.013	I25.799	I69.151
G11.19	G40.833	G91.2	H30.122	H35.70	H53.121	H70.019	I25.810	I69.152
G11.2	G40.834	G91.3	H30.123	H35.721	H53.122	H70.091	I25.811	I69.153
G11.3	G40.89	G91.8	H30.129	H35.722	H53.123	H70.092	I25.812	I69.154
G11.4	G40.911	G91.9	H30.131	H35.723	H53.129	H70.093	I27.0	I69.159
G11.8	G40.919	G93.1	H30.132	H35.729	H53.131	H70.099	I27.1	I69.251
G11.9	G40.A11	G93.40	H30.133	H35.731	H53.132	H95.21	I27.82	I69.252
G12.0	G40.A19	G93.49	H30.139	H35.732	H53.133	H95.22	I28.0	I69.253
G12.1	G40.B01	G95.0	H30.141	H35.733	H53.139	H95.31	I28.1	I69.254
G12.20	G40.B09	G95.20	H30.142	H35.739	H59.011	H95.32	I30.0	I69.259
G12.21	G40.B11	G95.29	H30.143	H35.82	H59.012	H95.41	I30.1	I69.351
G12.22	G40.B19	G95.81	H30.149	H40.211	H59.013	H95.42	I30.8	I69.352
G12.23	G43.601	G95.89	H30.891	H40.212	H59.019	H95.51	I30.9	I69.353
G12.24	G43.609	G95.9	H30.892	H40.213	H59.031	H95.52	I31.0	I69.354
G12.25	G43.611	G96.00	H30.893	H40.219	H59.032	H95.53	I31.1	I69.359
G12.29	G43.619	G96.01	H30.899	H44.001	H59.033	H95.54	I31.2	I69.851
G12.8	G45.0	G96.02	H30.90	H44.002	H59.039	H95.811	I31.3	I69.852
G12.9	G45.1	G96.08	H30.91	H44.003	H59.091	H95.812	I31.4	I69.853
G21.11	G45.2	G96.09	H30.92	H44.009	H59.092	H95.813	I31.8	I69.854
G21.19	G45.3	G96.11	H30.93	H44.011	H59.093	H95.819	I31.9	I69.859
G21.2	G45.8	G97.0	H31.321	H44.012	H59.099	H95.88	I32	I69.951
G21.3	G45.9	G97.2	H31.322	H44.013	H59.111	H95.89	I38	I69.952
G21.8	G46.0	G97.31	H31.323	H44.019	H59.112	I01.0	I39	I69.953
G21.9	G46.1	G97.32	H31.329	H44.021	H59.113	I01.1	I42.0	I69.954
G23.0	G46.2	G97.41	H31.401	H44.022	H59.119	I01.2	I42.1	I69.959
G23.1	G60.1	G97.48	H31.402	H44.023	H59.121	I01.8	I42.2	I70.261
G23.2	G61.0	G97.49	H31.403	H44.029	H59.122	I01.9	I42.3	I70.262
G23.8	G61.81	G97.51	H31.409	H44.111	H59.123	I02.0	I42.4	I70.263
G23.9	G62.81	G97.52	H31.411	H44.112	H59.129	I02.9	I42.5	I70.268
G24.02	G70.80	G97.61	H31.412	H44.113	H59.211	I09.0	I42.6	I70.269
G24.09	G70.81	G97.62	H31.413	H44.119	H59.212	I09.2	I42.7	I70.331
G24.2	G71.20	G97.63	H31.419	H44.121	H59.213	I09.81	I42.8	I70.332
G24.8	G71.21	G97.64	H31.421	H44.122	H59.219	I12.0	I42.9	I70.333
G25.82	G71.220	G97.81	H31.422	H44.123	H59.221	I13.0	I43	I70.334
G25.9	G71.228	G97.82	H31.423	H44.129	H59.222	I13.11	I44.2	I70.338
G31.81	G71.29	G97.83	H31.429	H44.131	H59.223	I13.2	I45.2	I70.339
G31.82	G72.0	G97.84	H33.121	H44.132	H59.229	I16.1	I45.3	I70.341
G32.0	G72.1	G99.0	H33.122	H44.133	H59.311	I16.9	I45.89	I70.342
G32.81	G72.2	G99.2	H33.123	H44.139	H59.312	I20.0	I47.0	I70.343
G36.0	G72.81	H05.011	H33.129	H44.19	H59.313	I20.1	I47.1	I70.344
G36.1	G73.1	H05.012	H33.20	H46.00	H59.319	I23.0	I47.2	I70.348
G36.8	G73.3	H05.013	H33.21	H46.01	H59.321	I23.1	I48.11	I70.349
G36.9	G80.1	H05.019	H33.22	H46.02	H59.322	I23.2	I48.19	I70.361
G37.0	G80.2	H05.021	H33.23	H46.03	H59.323	I23.3	I48.20	I70.362
G37.1	G80.3	H05.022	H33.40	H46.10	H59.329	I23.7	I48.21	I70.363
G37.2	G81.00	H05.023	H33.41	H46.11	H59.331	I23.8	I48.3	I70.368
G37.3	G81.01	H05.029	H33.42	H46.12	H59.332	I24.0	I48.4	I70.369
G37.5	G81.02	H05.031	H33.43	H46.13	H59.333		I48.92	I70.431

I70.432	I74.8	I82.499	I82.A11	I97.51	J94.0	K50.10	K56.3	K83.01
I70.433	I74.9	I82.4Y1	I82.A12	I97.52	J94.2	K50.111	K56.49	K83.09
I70.434	I75.011	I82.4Y2	I82.A13	I97.610	J94.8	K50.112	K56.50	K83.3
I70.438	I75.012	I82.4Y3	I82.A19	I97.611	J95.00	K50.113	K56.51	K86.0
I70.439	I75.013	I82.4Y9	I82.A21	I97.618	J95.01	K50.114	K56.52	K86.1
I70.441	I75.019	I82.4Z1	I82.A22	I97.620	J95.02	K50.118	K56.600	K86.2
I70.442	I75.021	I82.4Z2	I82.A23	I97.621	J95.03	K50.119	K56.601	K86.3
I70.443	I75.022	I82.4Z3	I82.A29	I97.622	J95.04	K50.80	K56.609	K90.1
I70.444	I75.023	I82.4Z9	I82.B11	I97.630	J95.09	K50.811	K56.690	K90.2
I70.448	I75.029	I82.501	I82.B12	I97.631	J95.4	K50.812	K56.691	K90.3
I70.449	I75.81	I82.502	I82.B13	I97.638	J95.5	K50.813	K56.699	K90.41
I70.461	I76	I82.503	I82.B19	I97.640	J95.61	K50.814	K56.7	K90.49
I70.462	I77.2	I82.509	I82.B21	I97.641	J95.62	K50.818	K57.00	K90.81
I70.463	I77.4	I82.511	I82.B22	I97.648	J95.71	K50.819	K57.12	K90.89
I70.468	I77.5	I82.512	I82.B23	I97.710	J95.72	K50.90	K57.20	K90.9
I70.469	I80.10	I82.513	I82.B29	I97.711	J95.811	K50.911	K57.32	K91.2
I70.531	I80.11	I82.519	I82.C11	I97.790	J95.812	K50.912	K57.40	K91.30
I70.532	I80.12	I82.521	I82.C12	I97.791	J95.830	K50.913	K57.52	K91.31
I70.533	I80.13	I82.522	I82.C13	I97.810	J95.831	K50.914	K57.80	K91.32
I70.534	I80.201	I82.523	I82.C19	I97.811	J95.84	K50.918	K57.92	K91.61
I70.538	I80.202	I82.529	I82.C21	I97.820	J95.850	K50.919	K59.2	K91.62
I70.539	I80.203	I82.531	I82.C22	I97.821	J95.851	K51.00	K59.31	K91.71
I70.541	I80.209	I82.532	I82.C23	I97.88	J95.859	K51.011	K59.39	K91.72
I70.542	I80.211	I82.533	I82.C29	I97.89	J95.860	K51.012	K61.0	K91.81
I70.543	I80.212	I82.539	I83.201	J05.10	J95.861	K51.013	K61.1	K91.82
I70.544	I80.213	I82.541	I83.202	J18.2	J95.862	K51.014	K61.2	K91.83
I70.548	I80.219	I82.542	I83.203	J21.0	J95.863	K51.018	K61.4	K91.840
I70.549	I80.221	I82.543	I83.204	J21.1	J95.88	K51.019	K62.5	K91.841
I70.561	I80.222	I82.549	I83.205	J21.8	J95.89	K51.20	K62.6	K91.850
I70.562	I80.223	I82.551	I83.208	J21.9	J96.10	K51.211	K63.0	K91.858
I70.563	I80.229	I82.552	I83.209	J36	J96.11	K51.212	K63.2	K91.86
I70.568	I80.231	I82.553	I83.211	J39.0	J96.12	K51.213	K63.3	K91.870
I70.569	I80.232	I82.559	I83.212	J39.1	J98.11	K51.214	K65.4	K91.871
I70.631	I80.233	I82.591	I83.213	J44.0	J98.19	K51.218	K68.11	K91.872
I70.632	I80.239	I82.592	I83.214	J44.1	K04.01	K51.219	K76.6	K91.873
I70.633	I80.241	I82.593	I83.215	J45.21	K04.02	K51.30	K77	K91.89
I70.634	I80.242	I82.599	I83.218	J45.22	K04.4	K51.311	K80.00	K92.0
I70.638	I80.243	I82.5Y1	I83.219	J45.31	K11.3	K51.312	K80.01	K92.1
I70.639	I80.249	I82.5Y2	I83.221	J45.32	K11.4	K51.313	K80.10	K92.2
I70.641	I80.291	I82.5Y3	I83.222	J45.41	K12.2	K51.314	K80.11	K92.81
I70.642	I80.292	I82.5Y9	I83.223	J45.42	K22.10	K51.318	K80.12	K94.01
I70.643	I80.293	I82.5Z1	I83.224	J45.51	K25.3	K51.319	K80.13	K94.02
I70.644	I80.299	I82.5Z2	I83.225	J45.52	K26.3	K51.40	K80.18	K94.03
I70.648	I82.1	I82.5Z3	I83.228	J45.901	K27.3	K51.411	K80.19	K94.09
I70.649	I82.210	I82.5Z9	I83.229	J45.902	K28.3	K51.412	K80.21	K94.11
I70.661	I82.211	I82.601	I85.00	J47.0	K31.0	K51.413	K80.30	K94.12
I70.662	I82.290	I82.602	I85.10	J47.1	K31.1	K51.414	K80.31	K94.13
I70.663	I82.291	I82.603	I87.011	J67.7	K31.5	K51.418	K80.32	K94.19
I70.668	I82.3	I82.609	I87.012	J67.8	K31.6	K51.419	K80.33	K94.22
I70.669	I82.401	I82.611	I87.013	J67.9	K35.20	K51.50	K80.34	K94.23
I70.731	I82.402	I82.612	I87.019	J68.0	K35.30	K51.511	K80.35	K94.30
I70.732	I82.403	I82.613	I87.031	J70.0	K35.80	K51.512	K80.36	K94.31
I70.733	I82.409	I82.619	I87.032	J70.1	K35.890	K51.513	K80.37	K94.32
I70.734	I82.411	I82.621	I87.033	J81.1	K35.891	K51.514	K80.40	K94.33
I70.738	I82.412	I82.622	I87.039	J82.81	K40.00	K51.518	K80.41	K94.39
I70.739	I82.413	I82.623	I87.1	J82.82	K40.01	K51.519	K80.42	K95.01
I70.741	I82.419	I82.629	I87.311	J82.83	K40.30	K51.80	K80.43	K95.09
I70.742	I82.421	I82.701	I87.312	J82.89	K40.31	K51.811	K80.44	K95.81
I70.743	I82.422	I82.702	I87.313	J84.01	K41.00	K51.812	K80.45	K95.89
I70.744	I82.423	I82.703	I87.319	J84.02	K41.01	K51.813	K80.46	L02.01
I70.748	I82.429	I82.709	I87.331	J84.03	K41.30	K51.814	K80.47	L02.11
I70.749	I82.431	I82.711	I87.332	J84.09	K41.31	K51.818	K80.51	L02.211
I70.761	I82.432	I82.712	I87.333	J84.114	K42.0	K51.819	K80.60	L02.212
I70.762	I82.433	I82.713	I87.339	J84.116	K43.0	K51.90	K80.61	L02.213
I70.763	I82.439	I82.719	I96	J84.117	K43.3	K51.911	K80.62	L02.214
I70.768	I82.441	I82.721	I97.110	J84.2	K43.6	K51.912	K80.63	L02.215
I70.769	I82.442	I82.722	I97.111	J84.82	K44.0	K51.913	K80.64	L02.216
I70.92	I82.443	I82.723	I97.120	J84.9	K45.0	K51.914	K80.65	L02.219
I73.01	I82.449	I82.729	I97.121	J90	K46.0	K51.918	K80.66	L02.31
I74.09	I82.451	I82.811	I97.130	J91.0	K50.00	K51.919	K80.71	L02.411
I74.10	I82.452	I82.812	I97.131	J91.8	K50.011	K52.0	K80.81	L02.412
I74.11	I82.453	I82.813	I97.190	J93.11	K50.012	K52.1	K81.0	L02.413
I74.19	I82.459	I82.819	I97.191	J93.12	K50.013	K55.1	K81.2	L02.414
I74.2	I82.491	I82.890	I97.410	J93.81	K50.014	K55.8	K82.0	L02.415
I74.3	I82.492	I82.891	I97.411	J93.82	K50.018	K55.9	K82.1	L02.416
I74.4	I82.493	I82.90	I97.418	J93.83	K50.019	K56.0	K82.3	L02.419
I74.5		I82.91	I97.42	J93.9		K56.1	K82.A2	L02.511

Appendix E: Complication and Comorbidity (CC) Code List

L02.512	L53.0	L97.318	L97.913	M00.222	M02.139	M05.452	M46.20	M60.031
L02.519	L53.1	L97.319	L97.914	M00.229	M02.141	M05.459	M46.21	M60.032
L02.611	L53.2	L97.321	L97.915	M00.231	M02.142	M05.461	M46.22	M60.039
L02.612	L53.3	L97.322	L97.916	M00.232	M02.149	M05.462	M46.23	M60.041
L02.619	L76.01	L97.323	L97.918	M00.239	M02.151	M05.469	M46.24	M60.042
L02.811	L76.02	L97.324	L97.919	M00.241	M02.152	M05.471	M46.25	M60.043
L02.818	L76.11	L97.325	L97.921	M00.242	M02.159	M05.472	M46.26	M60.044
L02.91	L76.12	L97.326	L97.922	M00.249	M02.161	M05.479	M46.27	M60.045
L03.111	L76.21	L97.328	L97.923	M00.251	M02.162	M05.49	M46.28	M60.046
L03.112	L76.22	L97.329	L97.924	M00.252	M02.169	M25.00	M46.30	M60.051
L03.113	L76.31	L97.401	L97.925	M00.259	M02.171	M25.011	M46.31	M60.052
L03.114	L76.32	L97.402	L97.926	M00.261	M02.172	M25.012	M46.32	M60.059
L03.115	L76.33	L97.403	L97.928	M00.262	M02.179	M25.019	M46.33	M60.061
L03.116	L76.34	L97.404	L97.929	M00.269	M02.18	M25.021	M46.34	M60.062
L03.119	L88	L97.405	L98.3	M00.271	M02.19	M25.022	M46.35	M60.069
L03.121	L97.101	L97.406	L98.415	M00.272	M02.311	M25.029	M46.36	M60.070
L03.122	L97.102	L97.408	L98.416	M00.279	M02.312	M25.031	M46.37	M60.071
L03.123	L97.103	L97.409	L98.418	M00.28	M02.319	M25.032	M46.38	M60.072
L03.124	L97.104	L97.411	L98.425	M00.29	M02.321	M25.039	M46.39	M60.073
L03.125	L97.105	L97.412	L98.426	M00.80	M02.322	M25.041	M47.011	M60.074
L03.126	L97.106	L97.413	L98.428	M00.811	M02.329	M25.042	M47.012	M60.075
L03.129	L97.108	L97.414	L98.495	M00.812	M02.331	M25.049	M47.013	M60.076
L03.211	L97.109	L97.415	L98.496	M00.819	M02.332	M25.051	M47.014	M60.077
L03.212	L97.111	L97.416	L98.498	M00.821	M02.339	M25.052	M47.015	M60.078
L03.213	L97.112	L97.418	M00.00	M00.822	M02.341	M25.059	M47.016	M60.08
L03.221	L97.113	L97.419	M00.011	M00.829	M02.342	M25.061	M47.019	M60.09
L03.222	L97.114	L97.421	M00.012	M00.831	M02.349	M25.062	M47.021	M62.82
L03.311	L97.115	L97.422	M00.019	M00.832	M02.351	M25.069	M47.022	M79.A11
L03.312	L97.116	L97.423	M00.021	M00.839	M02.352	M25.071	M47.029	M79.A12
L03.313	L97.118	L97.424	M00.022	M00.841	M02.359	M25.072	M47.10	M79.A19
L03.314	L97.119	L97.425	M00.029	M00.842	M02.361	M25.073	M47.11	M79.A21
L03.315	L97.121	L97.426	M00.031	M00.849	M02.362	M25.074	M47.12	M79.A22
L03.316	L97.122	L97.428	M00.032	M00.851	M02.369	M25.075	M47.13	M79.A29
L03.317	L97.123	L97.429	M00.039	M00.852	M02.371	M25.076	M47.14	M79.A3
L03.319	L97.124	L97.505	M00.041	M00.859	M02.372	M25.08	M47.15	M79.A9
L03.321	L97.125	L97.506	M00.042	M00.861	M02.379	M30.0	M47.16	M80.00XA
L03.322	L97.126	L97.508	M00.049	M00.862	M02.38	M30.1	M48.30	M80.00XK
L03.323	L97.128	L97.515	M00.051	M00.869	M02.39	M30.2	M48.31	M80.00XP
L03.324	L97.129	L97.516	M00.052	M00.871	M02.80	M30.3	M48.32	M80.011A
L03.325	L97.201	L97.518	M00.059	M00.872	M02.811	M30.8	M48.33	M80.011K
L03.326	L97.202	L97.525	M00.061	M00.879	M02.812	M31.0	M48.34	M80.011P
L03.327	L97.203	L97.526	M00.062	M00.88	M02.819	M31.2	M48.35	M80.012A
L03.329	L97.204	L97.528	M00.069	M00.89	M02.821	M31.30	M48.36	M80.012K
L03.811	L97.205	L97.801	M00.071	M00.9	M02.822	M31.31	M48.37	M80.012P
L03.818	L97.206	L97.802	M00.072	M01.X0	M02.829	M31.4	M48.38	M80.019A
L03.891	L97.208	L97.803	M00.079	M01.X11	M02.831	M31.7	M48.50XA	M80.019K
L03.898	L97.209	L97.804	M00.08	M01.X12	M02.832	M31.8	M48.51XA	M80.019P
L03.90	L97.211	L97.805	M00.09	M01.X19	M02.839	M31.9	M48.52XA	M80.021A
L03.91	L97.212	L97.806	M00.10	M01.X21	M02.841	M32.11	M48.53XA	M80.021K
L05.01	L97.213	L97.808	M00.111	M01.X22	M02.842	M32.12	M48.54XA	M80.021P
L05.02	L97.214	L97.809	M00.112	M01.X29	M02.849	M33.00	M48.55XA	M80.022A
L08.1	L97.215	L97.811	M00.119	M01.X31	M02.851	M33.01	M48.56XA	M80.022K
L10.0	L97.216	L97.812	M00.121	M01.X32	M02.852	M33.02	M48.57XA	M80.022P
L10.1	L97.218	L97.813	M00.122	M01.X39	M02.859	M33.03	M48.58XA	M80.029A
L10.2	L97.219	L97.814	M00.129	M01.X41	M02.861	M33.09	M50.00	M80.029K
L10.3	L97.221	L97.815	M00.131	M01.X42	M02.862	M33.10	M50.01	M80.029P
L10.4	L97.222	L97.816	M00.132	M01.X49	M02.869	M33.11	M50.020	M80.031A
L10.5	L97.223	L97.818	M00.139	M01.X51	M02.871	M33.12	M50.021	M80.031K
L10.81	L97.224	L97.819	M00.141	M01.X52	M02.872	M33.13	M50.022	M80.031P
L10.89	L97.225	L97.821	M00.142	M01.X59	M02.879	M33.19	M50.023	M80.032A
L10.9	L97.226	L97.822	M00.149	M01.X61	M02.88	M33.20	M50.03	M80.032K
L12.0	L97.228	L97.823	M00.151	M01.X62	M02.89	M33.21	M51.04	M80.032P
L12.30	L97.229	L97.824	M00.152	M01.X69	M05.40	M33.22	M51.05	M80.039A
L12.31	L97.301	L97.825	M00.159	M01.X71	M05.411	M33.29	M51.06	M80.039K
L12.35	L97.302	L97.826	M00.161	M01.X72	M05.412	M33.90	M60.000	M80.039P
L12.8	L97.303	L97.828	M00.162	M01.X79	M05.419	M33.91	M60.001	M80.041A
L12.9	L97.304	L97.829	M00.169	M01.X8	M05.421	M33.92	M60.002	M80.041K
L49.3	L97.305	L97.901	M00.171	M01.X9	M05.422	M33.93	M60.003	M80.041P
L49.4	L97.306	L97.902	M00.172	M02.10	M05.429	M33.99	M60.004	M80.042A
L49.5	L97.308	L97.903	M00.179	M02.111	M05.431	M34.81	M60.005	M80.042K
L49.6	L97.309	L97.904	M00.18	M02.112	M05.432	M34.82	M60.009	M80.042P
L49.7	L97.311	L97.905	M00.19	M02.119	M05.439	M35.03	M60.011	M80.049A
L49.8	L97.312	L97.906	M00.20	M02.121	M05.441	M35.1	M60.019	M80.049K
L49.9	L97.313	L97.908	M00.211	M02.122	M05.442	M35.2	M60.021	M80.049P
L51.1	L97.314	L97.909	M00.212	M02.129	M05.449	M35.5	M60.022	M80.051A
L51.2	L97.315	L97.911	M00.219	M02.131	M05.451	M35.8	M60.029	M80.051K
L51.3	L97.316	L97.912	M00.221	M02.132	M05.451	M36.0		M80.051P

M80.052A	M80.859P	M84.364K	M84.446P	M84.522K	M84.58XA	M84.669P	M86.111	M86.429
M80.052K	M80.861A	M84.364P	M84.451A	M84.522P	M84.58XK	M84.671A	M86.112	M86.431
M80.052P	M80.861K	M84.369K	M84.451K	M84.529K	M84.58XP	M84.671K	M86.119	M86.432
M80.059A	M80.861P	M84.369P	M84.451P	M84.529P	M84.60XA	M84.671P	M86.121	M86.439
M80.059K	M80.862A	M84.371K	M84.452A	M84.531A	M84.60XK	M84.672A	M86.122	M86.441
M80.059P	M80.862K	M84.371P	M84.452K	M84.531K	M84.60XP	M84.672K	M86.129	M86.442
M80.061A	M80.862P	M84.372K	M84.452P	M84.531P	M84.611A	M84.672P	M86.131	M86.449
M80.061K	M80.869A	M84.372P	M84.453A	M84.532A	M84.611K	M84.673A	M86.132	M86.451
M80.061P	M80.869K	M84.373K	M84.453K	M84.532K	M84.611P	M84.673K	M86.139	M86.452
M80.062A	M80.869P	M84.373P	M84.453P	M84.532P	M84.612A	M84.674A	M86.141	M86.459
M80.062K	M80.871A	M84.374K	M84.454A	M84.533A	M84.612K	M84.674K	M86.142	M86.461
M80.069A	M80.871K	M84.374P	M84.454K	M84.533K	M84.612P	M84.674P	M86.149	M86.462
M80.069K	M80.871P	M84.375K	M84.454P	M84.533P	M84.619A	M84.675A	M86.151	M86.469
M80.069P	M80.872A	M84.375P	M84.459A	M84.534A	M84.619K	M84.675K	M86.152	M86.471
M80.071A	M80.872K	M84.376K	M84.459K	M84.534K	M84.619P	M84.675P	M86.159	M86.472
M80.071K	M80.872P	M84.376P	M84.459P	M84.534P	M84.621A	M84.676A	M86.161	M86.479
M80.071P	M80.879A	M84.377K	M84.461A	M84.539A	M84.621K	M84.676K	M86.162	M86.48
M80.072A	M80.879K	M84.377P	M84.461K	M84.539K	M84.621P	M84.676P	M86.169	M86.49
M80.072K	M80.879P	M84.378K	M84.461P	M84.539P	M84.622A	M84.68XA	M86.171	M86.50
M80.072P	M80.88XA	M84.378P	M84.462A	M84.541A	M84.622K	M84.68XK	M86.172	M86.511
M80.079A	M80.88XK	M84.379K	M84.462K	M84.541K	M84.622P	M84.68XP	M86.179	M86.512
M80.079K	M80.88XP	M84.379P	M84.462P	M84.541P	M84.629A	M84.750A	M86.18	M86.519
M80.079P	M80.8AXA	M84.38XK	M84.463A	M84.542A	M84.629K	M84.750K	M86.19	M86.521
M80.08XA	M80.8AXK	M84.38XP	M84.463K	M84.542K	M84.629P	M84.750P	M86.20	M86.522
M80.08XK	M80.8AXP	M84.40XA	M84.463P	M84.542P	M84.631A	M84.751A	M86.211	M86.529
M80.08XP	M84.30XK	M84.40XK	M84.464A	M84.549A	M84.631K	M84.751K	M86.212	M86.531
M80.0AXA	M84.30XP	M84.40XP	M84.464K	M84.549K	M84.631P	M84.751P	M86.219	M86.532
M80.0AXK	M84.311K	M84.411A	M84.464P	M84.549P	M84.632A	M84.752A	M86.221	M86.539
M80.0AXP	M84.311P	M84.411K	M84.469A	M84.550K	M84.632K	M84.752K	M86.222	M86.541
M80.80XA	M84.312K	M84.411P	M84.469K	M84.550P	M84.632P	M84.752P	M86.229	M86.542
M80.80XK	M84.312P	M84.412A	M84.469P	M84.551A	M84.633A	M84.753A	M86.231	M86.549
M80.80XP	M84.319K	M84.412K	M84.471A	M84.551K	M84.633K	M84.753K	M86.232	M86.551
M80.811A	M84.319P	M84.412P	M84.471K	M84.551P	M84.633P	M84.753P	M86.239	M86.552
M80.811K	M84.321K	M84.419A	M84.471P	M84.552A	M84.634A	M84.754A	M86.241	M86.559
M80.811P	M84.321P	M84.419K	M84.472A	M84.552K	M84.634K	M84.754K	M86.242	M86.561
M80.812A	M84.322K	M84.419P	M84.472K	M84.552P	M84.634P	M84.754P	M86.249	M86.562
M80.812K	M84.322P	M84.421A	M84.472P	M84.553A	M84.639A	M84.755A	M86.251	M86.569
M80.812P	M84.329K	M84.421K	M84.473A	M84.553K	M84.639K	M84.755K	M86.252	M86.571
M80.819A	M84.329P	M84.421P	M84.473K	M84.553P	M84.639P	M84.755P	M86.259	M86.572
M80.819K	M84.331K	M84.422A	M84.473P	M84.559A	M84.641A	M84.756A	M86.261	M86.579
M80.819P	M84.331P	M84.422K	M84.474A	M84.559K	M84.641K	M84.756K	M86.262	M86.58
M80.821A	M84.332K	M84.422P	M84.474K	M84.559P	M84.642A	M84.756P	M86.269	M86.59
M80.821K	M84.332P	M84.429A	M84.474P	M84.561A	M84.642K	M84.757A	M86.271	M86.60
M80.821P	M84.333K	M84.429K	M84.475A	M84.561K	M84.642P	M84.757K	M86.272	M86.611
M80.822A	M84.333P	M84.429P	M84.475K	M84.561P	M84.649A	M84.757P	M86.279	M86.612
M80.822K	M84.334K	M84.431A	M84.475P	M84.562A	M84.649K	M84.758A	M86.28	M86.619
M80.822P	M84.334P	M84.431K	M84.476A	M84.562K	M84.649P	M84.758K	M86.29	M86.621
M80.829A	M84.339K	M84.431P	M84.476K	M84.562P	M84.650A	M84.758P	M86.30	M86.622
M80.829K	M84.339P	M84.432A	M84.476P	M84.563A	M84.650K	M84.759A	M86.311	M86.629
M80.829P	M84.341K	M84.432K	M84.477A	M84.563K	M84.650P	M84.759K	M86.312	M86.631
M80.831A	M84.341P	M84.432P	M84.477K	M84.563P	M84.651A	M84.759P	M86.319	M86.632
M80.831K	M84.342K	M84.433A	M84.477P	M84.564A	M84.651K	M86.00	M86.321	M86.639
M80.831P	M84.342P	M84.433K	M84.478A	M84.564K	M84.651P	M86.011	M86.322	M86.641
M80.832A	M84.343K	M84.433P	M84.478K	M84.564P	M84.652A	M86.012	M86.329	M86.642
M80.832K	M84.343P	M84.434A	M84.478P	M84.569A	M84.652K	M86.019	M86.331	M86.649
M80.832P	M84.344K	M84.434K	M84.479A	M84.569K	M84.652P	M86.021	M86.332	M86.651
M80.839A	M84.344P	M84.434P	M84.479K	M84.569P	M84.653A	M86.022	M86.339	M86.652
M80.839K	M84.345K	M84.439A	M84.479P	M84.571A	M84.653K	M86.029	M86.341	M86.659
M80.839P	M84.345P	M84.439K	M84.48XA	M84.571K	M84.653P	M86.031	M86.342	M86.661
M80.841A	M84.346K	M84.439P	M84.48XK	M84.571P	M84.659A	M86.032	M86.349	M86.662
M80.841K	M84.346P	M84.441A	M84.48XP	M84.572A	M84.659K	M86.039	M86.351	M86.669
M80.841P	M84.350K	M84.441K	M84.50XA	M84.572K	M84.659P	M86.041	M86.352	M86.671
M80.842A	M84.350P	M84.441P	M84.50XK	M84.572P	M84.661A	M86.042	M86.359	M86.672
M80.842K	M84.351K	M84.442A	M84.50XP	M84.573A	M84.661K	M86.049	M86.361	M86.679
M80.842P	M84.351P	M84.442K	M84.511A	M84.573K	M84.661P	M86.051	M86.362	M86.68
M80.849A	M84.352K	M84.442P	M84.511K	M84.573P	M84.662A	M86.052	M86.369	M86.69
M80.849K	M84.352P	M84.443A	M84.511P	M84.574A	M84.662K	M86.059	M86.371	M86.8X0
M80.849P	M84.353K	M84.443K	M84.512A	M84.574K	M84.662P	M86.061	M86.372	M86.8X1
M80.851A	M84.353P	M84.443P	M84.512K	M84.574P	M84.663A	M86.062	M86.379	M86.8X2
M80.851K	M84.359K	M84.444A	M84.512P	M84.575A	M84.663K	M86.069	M86.38	M86.8X3
M80.851P	M84.359P	M84.444K	M84.519A	M84.575K	M84.663P	M86.071	M86.39	M86.8X4
M80.852A	M84.361K	M84.444P	M84.519K	M84.575P	M84.664A	M86.072	M86.40	M86.8X5
M80.852K	M84.361P	M84.445A	M84.519P	M84.576A	M84.664K	M86.079	M86.411	M86.8X6
M80.852P	M84.362K	M84.445K	M84.521A	M84.576K	M84.664P	M86.08	M86.412	M86.8X7
M80.859A	M84.362P	M84.445P	M84.521K	M84.576P	M84.669A	M86.09	M86.419	M86.8X8
M80.859K	M84.363K	M84.446A	M84.521P		M84.669K	M86.10	M86.421	M86.8X9
	M84.363P	M84.446K	M84.522A				M86.422	M86.9

M87.00	M87.173	M87.352	M90.552	N04.4	N76.4	O04.84	O23.21	O30.221
M87.011	M87.174	M87.353	M90.559	N04.5	N76.81	O04.85	O23.22	O30.222
M87.012	M87.175	M87.361	M90.561	N04.6	N82.0	O04.86	O23.23	O30.223
M87.019	M87.176	M87.362	M90.562	N04.7	N82.1	O04.87	O23.31	O30.231
M87.021	M87.177	M87.363	M90.569	N04.8	N82.2	O04.88	O23.32	O30.232
M87.022	M87.178	M87.364	M90.571	N04.9	N82.3	O04.89	O23.33	O30.233
M87.029	M87.179	M87.365	M90.572	N04.A	N82.4	O07.0	O23.41	O30.291
M87.031	M87.180	M87.366	M90.579	N05.2	N82.5	O07.1	O23.42	O30.292
M87.032	M87.188	M87.371	M90.58	N05.3	N82.8	O07.30	O23.43	O30.293
M87.033	M87.19	M87.372	M90.59	N05.4	N82.9	O07.33	O23.511	O30.801
M87.034	M87.20	M87.373	M96.0	N05.5	N83.511	O07.34	O23.512	O30.802
M87.035	M87.211	M87.374	M96.621	N05.A	N83.512	O07.35	O23.513	O30.803
M87.036	M87.212	M87.375	M96.622	N06.2	N83.519	O07.36	O23.521	O30.811
M87.037	M87.219	M87.376	M96.629	N06.3	N83.521	O07.37	O23.522	O30.812
M87.038	M87.221	M87.377	M96.631	N06.4	N83.522	O07.38	O23.523	O30.813
M87.039	M87.222	M87.378	M96.632	N06.5	N83.529	O07.39	O23.591	O30.821
M87.041	M87.229	M87.379	M96.639	N06.A	N83.53	O08.0	O23.592	O30.822
M87.042	M87.231	M87.38	M96.65	N07.2	N98.0	O08.1	O23.593	O30.823
M87.043	M87.232	M87.39	M96.661	N07.3	N98.1	O08.5	O23.91	O30.831
M87.044	M87.233	M87.80	M96.662	N07.4	N98.2	O08.6	O23.92	O30.832
M87.045	M87.234	M87.811	M96.669	N07.5	N98.3	O08.7	O23.93	O30.833
M87.046	M87.235	M87.812	M96.671	N07.A	N98.8	O08.81	O24.011	O30.891
M87.050	M87.236	M87.819	M96.672	N10	N98.9	O08.82	O24.012	O30.892
M87.051	M87.237	M87.821	M96.679	N11.1	N99.510	O08.83	O24.013	O30.893
M87.052	M87.238	M87.822	M96.69	N11.8	N99.511	O08.89	O24.019	O31.8X10
M87.059	M87.239	M87.829	M96.810	N11.9	N99.512	O08.9	O24.03	O31.8X11
M87.061	M87.241	M87.831	M96.811	N12	N99.518	O10.011	O24.111	O31.8X12
M87.062	M87.242	M87.832	M96.820	N13.0	N99.61	O10.012	O24.112	O31.8X13
M87.063	M87.243	M87.833	M96.821	N13.1	N99.62	O10.013	O24.113	O31.8X14
M87.064	M87.244	M87.834	M96.830	N13.2	N99.71	O10.02	O24.119	O31.8X15
M87.065	M87.245	M87.835	M96.831	N13.30	N99.72	O10.411	O24.13	O31.8X19
M87.066	M87.246	M87.836	M96.840	N13.39	N99.820	O10.412	O24.311	O31.8X20
M87.071	M87.250	M87.837	M96.841	N13.4	N99.821	O10.413	O24.312	O31.8X21
M87.072	M87.251	M87.838	M96.842	N13.6	N99.840	O10.43	O24.313	O31.8X22
M87.073	M87.252	M87.839	M96.843	N13.8	N99.841	O10.911	O24.319	O31.8X23
M87.074	M87.256	M87.841	M96.89	N17.8	N99.842	O10.912	O24.33	O31.8X24
M87.075	M87.261	M87.842	M97.01XA	N17.9	N99.843	O10.913	O24.811	O31.8X25
M87.076	M87.262	M87.843	M97.02XA	N18.4	O00.00	O10.92	O24.812	O31.8X29
M87.077	M87.263	M87.844	M97.11XA	N18.5	O00.01	O12.11	O24.813	O31.8X30
M87.078	M87.264	M87.845	M97.12XA	N20.1	O00.101	O12.12	O24.819	O31.8X31
M87.079	M87.265	M87.849	M97.21XA	N20.2	O00.102	O12.13	O24.83	O31.8X32
M87.08	M87.266	M87.850	M97.22XA	N25.1	O00.109	O12.21	O24.911	O31.8X33
M87.09	M87.271	M87.851	M97.31XA	N25.81	O00.111	O12.22	O24.912	O31.8X34
M87.10	M87.272	M87.852	M97.32XA	N28.0	O00.112	O12.23	O24.913	O31.8X35
M87.111	M87.273	M87.859	M97.41XA	N28.84	O00.119	O14.02	O24.919	O31.8X39
M87.112	M87.274	M87.861	M97.42XA	N28.85	O00.201	O14.03	O24.93	O33.0
M87.119	M87.275	M87.862	M97.8XXA	N28.86	O00.202	O14.92	O26.611	O36.0110
M87.121	M87.276	M87.863	M97.9XXA	N30.00	O00.209	O14.93	O26.612	O36.0111
M87.122	M87.277	M87.864	M99.10	N30.01	O00.211	O16.1	O26.613	O36.0112
M87.129	M87.278	M87.865	M99.11	N30.40	O00.212	O16.2	O26.62	O36.0113
M87.131	M87.279	M87.869	M99.18	N30.41	O00.219	O16.3	O26.831	O36.0114
M87.132	M87.28	M87.871	N02.0	N32.1	O00.80	O20.0	O26.832	O36.0115
M87.133	M87.29	M87.872	N02.1	N32.2	O00.81	O20.9	O26.833	O36.0119
M87.134	M87.30	M87.873	N02.2	N34.0	O00.90	O22.20	O26.872	O36.0120
M87.135	M87.311	M87.874	N02.3	N36.0	O00.91	O22.21	O26.873	O36.0121
M87.136	M87.312	M87.875	N02.4	N39.0	O03.0	O22.22	O26.879	O36.0122
M87.137	M87.319	M87.876	N02.5	N41.0	O03.30	O22.23	O30.101	O36.0123
M87.138	M87.321	M87.877	N02.6	N41.2	O03.33	O22.30	O30.102	O36.0124
M87.139	M87.322	M87.878	N02.7	N43.1	O03.34	O22.40	O30.103	O36.0125
M87.141	M87.329	M87.879	N02.8	N44.00	O03.35	O22.41	O30.111	O36.0129
M87.142	M87.331	M87.88	N02.9	N44.01	O03.36	O22.42	O30.112	O36.0130
M87.143	M87.332	M87.89	N02.A	N44.02	O03.37	O22.43	O30.113	O36.0131
M87.144	M87.333	M87.9	N03.0	N44.03	O03.38	O22.50	O30.121	O36.0132
M87.145	M87.334	M90.50	N03.1	N44.04	O03.39	O22.51	O30.122	O36.0133
M87.146	M87.335	M90.511	N03.2	N45.4	O03.5	O22.52	O30.123	O36.0134
M87.150	M87.336	M90.519	N03.3	N48.30	O03.7	O22.53	O30.131	O36.0135
M87.151	M87.337	M90.521	N03.4	N48.31	O03.80	O22.8X1	O30.132	O36.0139
M87.152	M87.338	M90.522	N03.5	N48.32	O03.83	O22.8X2	O30.133	O36.0910
M87.159	M87.339	M90.529	N03.6	N48.33	O03.84	O22.8X3	O30.191	O36.0911
M87.161	M87.341	M90.531	N03.7	N48.39	O03.85	O22.8X9	O30.192	O36.0912
M87.162	M87.342	M90.532	N03.8	N70.01	O03.86	O22.90	O30.193	O36.0913
M87.163	M87.343	M90.539	N03.9	N70.02	O03.87	O23.01	O30.201	O36.0914
M87.164	M87.344	M90.541	N03.A	N70.03	O03.88	O23.02	O30.202	O36.0915
M87.165	M87.345	M90.542	N04.0	N71.0	O03.89	O23.03	O30.203	O36.0919
M87.166	M87.346	M90.549	N04.1	N73.0	O04.5	O23.11	O30.211	O36.0920
M87.171	M87.350	M90.551	N04.2	N73.4	O04.80	O23.12	O30.212	O36.0921
M87.172	M87.351	M90.551	N04.3	N75.1	O04.83	O23.13	O30.213	O36.0922

O36.0923	O71.6	O99.322	Q04.8	Q42.2	Q79.62	S02.101K	S02.40FB	S02.670K
O36.0924	O71.7	O99.323	Q05.0	Q42.3	Q79.63	S02.102A	S02.40FK	S02.671A
O36.0925	O72.0	O99.324	Q05.1	Q42.8	Q79.69	S02.102K	S02.411A	S02.671B
O36.0929	O72.1	O99.325	Q05.2	Q42.9	Q85.1	S02.109A	S02.411B	S02.671K
O36.0930	O72.2	O99.354	Q05.3	Q43.1	Q85.8	S02.109K	S02.411K	S02.672A
O36.0931	O75.2	O99.355	Q05.4	Q43.2	Q85.9	S02.110A	S02.412A	S02.672B
O36.0932	O86.11	O99.411	Q07.02	Q43.3	Q87.11	S02.110K	S02.412B	S02.672K
O36.0933	O86.12	O99.412	Q07.03	Q43.4	Q87.19	S02.111A	S02.412K	S02.69XA
O36.0934	O86.13	O99.413	Q20.5	Q43.5	Q87.2	S02.111K	S02.413A	S02.69XB
O36.0935	O86.19	O99.43	Q21.0	Q43.6	Q87.3	S02.112A	S02.413B	S02.69XK
O36.0939	O86.20	O99.830	Q21.1	Q43.7	Q87.40	S02.112K	S02.413K	S02.80XA
O36.4XX0	O86.21	O99.834	Q21.2	Q43.8	Q87.410	S02.113A	S02.42XA	S02.80XB
O36.4XX1	O86.22	O99.835	Q22.1	Q43.9	Q87.418	S02.113K	S02.42XB	S02.80XK
O36.4XX2	O86.29	P10.2	Q22.2	Q44.0	Q87.42	S02.118A	S02.42XK	S02.81XA
O36.4XX3	O86.4	P12.2	Q22.3	Q44.1	Q87.43	S02.118K	S02.5XXB	S02.81XB
O36.4XX4	O87.0	P28.0	Q23.0	Q44.4	Q87.5	S02.119A	S02.600A	S02.81XK
O36.4XX5	O87.2	P28.10	Q23.1	Q44.5	Q87.81	S02.119K	S02.600B	S02.82XA
O36.4XX9	O87.3	P28.11	Q23.2	Q44.6	Q87.82	S02.11AA	S02.600K	S02.82XB
O41.01X0	O87.8	P28.19	Q23.3	Q44.7	Q87.89	S02.11AK	S02.601A	S02.82XK
O41.01X1	O88.319	P28.2	Q24.0	Q45.0	Q89.01	S02.11BA	S02.601B	S02.831A
O41.01X2	O98.011	P28.3	Q24.1	Q45.1	Q89.09	S02.11BK	S02.601K	S02.831B
O41.01X3	O98.012	P28.4	Q24.3	Q45.2	Q89.3	S02.11CA	S02.602A	S02.831K
O41.01X4	O98.013	P35.0	Q24.5	Q45.3	Q89.7	S02.11CK	S02.602B	S02.832A
O41.01X5	O98.02	P38.1	Q25.0	Q60.0	Q89.8	S02.11DA	S02.602K	S02.832B
O41.01X9	O98.03	P38.9	Q25.1	Q60.1	Q91.0	S02.11DK	S02.609A	S02.832K
O41.02X0	O98.111	P39.0	Q25.21	Q60.2	Q91.1	S02.11EA	S02.609B	S02.839A
O41.02X1	O98.112	P39.2	Q25.29	Q60.3	Q91.2	S02.11EK	S02.609K	S02.839B
O41.02X2	O98.113	P39.3	Q25.3	Q60.4	Q91.3	S02.11FA	S02.610A	S02.839K
O41.02X3	O98.12	P39.4	Q25.40	Q60.5	Q91.4	S02.11FK	S02.610B	S02.841A
O41.02X4	O98.13	P39.8	Q25.41	Q60.6	Q91.5	S02.11GA	S02.610K	S02.841B
O41.02X5	O98.211	P39.9	Q25.42	Q61.00	Q91.6	S02.11GK	S02.611A	S02.841K
O41.02X9	O98.212	P52.0	Q25.43	Q61.01	Q91.7	S02.11HA	S02.611B	S02.842A
O41.03X0	O98.213	P52.1	Q25.44	Q61.02	Q93.3	S02.11HK	S02.611K	S02.842B
O41.03X1	O98.22	P52.3	Q25.45	Q61.11	Q93.4	S02.121A	S02.612A	S02.842K
O41.03X2	O98.23	P53	Q25.46	Q61.19	Q93.51	S02.121K	S02.612B	S02.849A
O41.03X3	O98.311	P54.4	Q25.47	Q61.2	Q93.59	S02.122A	S02.612K	S02.849B
O41.03X4	O98.312	P61.2	Q25.48	Q61.3	Q93.7	S02.122K	S02.620A	S02.849K
O41.03X5	O98.313	P61.3	Q25.49	Q61.4	Q93.82	S02.129A	S02.620B	S02.85XA
O41.03X9	O98.32	P61.4	Q25.8	Q61.5	Q93.88	S02.129K	S02.620K	S02.85XB
O44.01	O98.33	P61.6	Q25.9	Q61.8	Q93.89	S02.19XA	S02.621A	S02.85XK
O44.02	O98.411	P70.2	Q26.0	Q61.9	Q93.9	S02.19XK	S02.621B	S02.91XA
O44.03	O98.412	P70.8	Q26.1	Q62.0	R04.2	S02.2XXB	S02.621K	S02.91XK
O44.21	O98.413	P71.0	Q26.2	Q62.10	R04.81	S02.2XXK	S02.622A	S02.92XA
O44.22	O98.42	P71.1	Q26.3	Q62.11	R04.89	S02.30XA	S02.622B	S02.92XB
O44.23	O98.43	P71.2	Q26.4	Q62.12	R04.9	S02.30XB	S02.622K	S02.92XK
O44.41	O98.511	P71.3	Q26.8	Q62.2	R06.3	S02.30XK	S02.630A	S04.011A
O44.42	O98.512	P71.4	Q26.9	Q62.31	R09.01	S02.31XA	S02.630B	S04.012A
O44.43	O98.513	P71.8	Q27.30	Q62.32	R17	S02.31XB	S02.630K	S04.019A
O47.02	O98.52	P71.9	Q27.4	Q62.39	R18.0	S02.31XK	S02.631A	S04.02XA
O47.03	O98.53	P72.0	Q28.0	Q64.10	R18.8	S02.32XA	S02.631B	S04.031A
O47.1	O98.611	P72.1	Q28.1	Q64.11	R29.0	S02.32XB	S02.631K	S04.032A
O60.10X0	O98.612	P72.2	Q28.8	Q64.12	R29.1	S02.32XK	S02.632A	S04.039A
O60.10X1	O98.613	P72.8	Q28.9	Q64.19	R29.5	S02.400A	S02.632B	S04.041A
O60.10X2	O98.62	P74.41	Q31.1	Q64.2	R39.0	S02.400B	S02.632K	S04.042A
O60.10X3	O98.63	P74.5	Q31.2	Q64.31	R40.3	S02.400K	S02.640A	S04.049A
O60.10X4	O98.711	P74.6	Q31.3	Q64.32	R41.4	S02.401A	S02.640B	S04.10XA
O60.10X5	O98.712	P74.8	Q31.5	Q64.33	R44.0	S02.401B	S02.640K	S04.11XA
O60.10X9	O98.713	P76.1	Q31.8	Q64.39	R44.2	S02.401K	S02.641A	S04.12XA
O60.20X0	O98.72	P83.0	Q31.9	Q67.5	R44.3	S02.402A	S02.641B	S04.20XA
O60.20X1	O98.73	P83.30	Q32.0	Q67.8	R45.851	S02.402B	S02.641K	S04.21XA
O60.20X2	O98.811	P83.39	Q32.1	Q68.1	R47.01	S02.402K	S02.642A	S04.22XA
O60.20X3	O98.812	P91.60	Q32.2	Q74.3	R56.00	S02.40AA	S02.642B	S04.30XA
O60.20X4	O98.813	P91.61	Q32.3	Q76.3	R56.01	S02.40AB	S02.642K	S04.31XA
O60.20X5	O98.82	P91.62	Q32.4	Q76.425	R56.1	S02.40AK	S02.650A	S04.32XA
O60.20X9	O98.83	P93.0	Q33.0	Q76.426	R57.9	S02.40BA	S02.650B	S04.40XA
O63.9	O98.911	P93.8	Q33.4	Q76.427	R64	S02.40BB	S02.650K	S04.41XA
O68	O98.912	P94.0	Q39.5	Q76.428	R65.10	S02.40BK	S02.651A	S04.42XA
O70.20	O98.913	P96.1	Q39.6	Q76.429	R71.0	S02.40CA	S02.651B	S04.50XA
O70.21	O98.92	P96.2	Q39.8	Q76.6	R78.81	S02.40CB	S02.651K	S04.51XA
O70.22	O98.93	Q01.0	Q39.9	Q76.7	R82.0	S02.40CK	S02.652A	S04.52XA
O70.23	O99.111	Q01.1	Q41.0	Q76.8	R82.1	S02.40DA	S02.652B	S04.60XA
O70.3	O99.112	Q01.2	Q41.1	Q76.9	S01.101A	S02.40DB	S02.652K	S04.61XA
O70.4	O99.113	Q01.8	Q41.2	Q77.2	S01.102A	S02.40DK	S02.66XA	S04.62XA
O71.2	O99.119	Q01.9	Q41.8	Q78.0	S01.109A	S02.40EA	S02.66XB	S04.70XA
O71.3	O99.12	Q04.4	Q41.9	Q78.2	S02.0XXA	S02.40EB	S02.66XK	S04.71XA
O71.4	O99.13	Q04.5	Q42.0	Q79.60	S02.0XXK	S02.40EK	S02.670A	S04.72XA
O71.5	O99.321	Q04.6	Q42.1	Q79.61	S02.101A	S02.40FA	S02.670B	S04.811A

Appendix E: Complication and Comorbidity (CC) Code List

S04.812A	S07.1XXA	S12.200A	S12.630K	S15.321A	S22.041A	S25.509A	S32.018A	S32.17XK
S04.819A	S07.8XXA	S12.200K	S12.631A	S15.322A	S22.041K	S25.511A	S32.018K	S32.19XA
S04.891A	S07.9XXA	S12.201A	S12.631K	S15.329A	S22.042A	S25.512A	S32.019A	S32.19XK
S04.892A	S09.0XXA	S12.201K	S12.64XA	S15.391A	S22.042K	S25.519A	S32.019K	S32.2XXA
S04.899A	S09.20XA	S12.230A	S12.64XK	S15.392A	S22.048A	S25.591A	S32.020A	S32.2XXK
S04.9XXA	S09.21XA	S12.230K	S12.650A	S15.399A	S22.048K	S25.592A	S32.020K	S32.301A
S05.20XA	S09.22XA	S12.231A	S12.650K	S15.8XXA	S22.049A	S25.599A	S32.021A	S32.301K
S05.21XA	S09.301A	S12.231K	S12.651A	S15.9XXA	S22.049K	S25.801A	S32.021K	S32.302A
S05.22XA	S09.302A	S12.24XA	S12.651K	S17.0XXA	S22.050A	S25.802A	S32.022A	S32.302K
S05.30XA	S09.309A	S12.24XK	S12.690A	S17.8XXA	S22.050K	S25.809A	S32.022K	S32.309A
S05.31XA	S09.311A	S12.250A	S12.690K	S17.9XXA	S22.051A	S25.811A	S32.028A	S32.309K
S05.32XA	S09.312A	S12.250K	S12.691A	S21.101A	S22.051K	S25.812A	S32.028K	S32.311A
S05.40XA	S09.313A	S12.251A	S12.691K	S21.102A	S22.052A	S25.819A	S32.029A	S32.311K
S05.41XA	S09.319A	S12.251K	S12.9XXA	S21.109A	S22.052K	S25.891A	S32.029K	S32.312A
S05.42XA	S09.391A	S12.290A	S13.0XXA	S21.111A	S22.058A	S25.892A	S32.030A	S32.312K
S05.50XA	S09.392A	S12.290K	S13.100A	S21.112A	S22.058K	S25.899A	S32.030K	S32.313A
S05.51XA	S09.399A	S12.291A	S13.101A	S21.119A	S22.059A	S25.90XA	S32.031A	S32.313K
S05.52XA	S11.10XA	S12.291K	S13.110A	S21.121A	S22.059K	S25.91XA	S32.031K	S32.314A
S05.70XA	S11.11XA	S12.300A	S13.111A	S21.122A	S22.060A	S25.99XA	S32.032A	S32.314K
S05.71XA	S11.12XA	S12.300K	S13.120A	S21.129A	S22.060K	S26.00XA	S32.032K	S32.315A
S05.72XA	S11.13XA	S12.301A	S13.121A	S21.131A	S22.061A	S26.01XA	S32.038A	S32.315K
S05.8X1A	S11.14XA	S12.301K	S13.130A	S21.132A	S22.061K	S26.09XA	S32.038K	S32.316A
S05.8X2A	S11.15XA	S12.330A	S13.131A	S21.139A	S22.062A	S26.10XA	S32.039A	S32.316K
S05.8X9A	S11.20XA	S12.330K	S13.140A	S21.141A	S22.062K	S26.11XA	S32.039K	S32.391A
S05.91XA	S11.21XA	S12.331A	S13.141A	S21.142A	S22.068A	S26.12XA	S32.040A	S32.391K
S05.92XA	S11.22XA	S12.331K	S13.150A	S21.149A	S22.068K	S26.19XA	S32.040K	S32.392A
S06.0X1A	S11.23XA	S12.34XA	S13.151A	S21.151A	S22.069A	S26.90XA	S32.041A	S32.392K
S06.0X9A	S11.24XA	S12.34XK	S13.160A	S21.152A	S22.069K	S26.91XA	S32.041K	S32.399A
S06.2X1A	S11.25XA	S12.350A	S13.161A	S21.159A	S22.070A	S26.99XA	S32.042A	S32.399K
S06.2X2A	S12.000A	S12.350K	S13.170A	S21.90XA	S22.070K	S27.0XXA	S32.042K	S32.401K
S06.2X3A	S12.000K	S12.351A	S13.171A	S21.91XA	S22.071A	S27.301A	S32.048A	S32.402K
S06.2X4A	S12.001A	S12.351K	S13.180A	S21.92XA	S22.071K	S27.302A	S32.048K	S32.409K
S06.2X5A	S12.001K	S12.390A	S13.181A	S21.93XA	S22.072A	S27.309A	S32.049A	S32.411K
S06.2X9A	S12.01XA	S12.390K	S13.20XA	S21.94XA	S22.072K	S27.311A	S32.049K	S32.412K
S06.301A	S12.01XK	S12.391A	S13.29XA	S21.95XA	S22.078A	S27.312A	S32.050A	S32.413K
S06.302A	S12.02XA	S12.391K	S15.001A	S22.000A	S22.078K	S27.319A	S32.050K	S32.414K
S06.303A	S12.02XK	S12.400A	S15.002A	S22.000K	S22.079A	S27.321A	S32.051A	S32.415K
S06.304A	S12.030A	S12.400K	S15.009A	S22.001A	S22.079K	S27.322A	S32.051K	S32.416K
S06.305A	S12.030K	S12.401A	S15.011A	S22.001K	S22.080A	S27.329A	S32.052A	S32.421K
S06.309A	S12.031A	S12.401K	S15.012A	S22.002A	S22.080K	S27.391A	S32.052K	S32.422K
S06.371A	S12.031K	S12.430A	S15.019A	S22.002K	S22.081A	S27.392A	S32.058A	S32.423K
S06.372A	S12.040A	S12.430K	S15.021A	S22.008A	S22.081K	S27.399A	S32.058K	S32.424K
S06.373A	S12.040K	S12.431A	S15.022A	S22.008K	S22.082A	S27.50XA	S32.059A	S32.425K
S06.374A	S12.041A	S12.431K	S15.029A	S22.009A	S22.082K	S27.51XA	S32.059K	S32.426K
S06.375A	S12.041K	S12.44XA	S15.091A	S22.009K	S22.088A	S27.52XA	S32.10XA	S32.431K
S06.379A	S12.090A	S12.44XK	S15.092A	S22.010A	S22.088K	S27.53XA	S32.10XK	S32.432K
S06.381A	S12.090K	S12.450A	S15.099A	S22.010K	S22.089A	S27.59XA	S32.110A	S32.433K
S06.382A	S12.091A	S12.450K	S15.101A	S22.011A	S22.089K	S27.60XA	S32.110K	S32.434K
S06.383A	S12.091K	S12.451A	S15.102A	S22.011K	S22.20XA	S27.63XA	S32.111A	S32.435K
S06.384A	S12.100A	S12.451K	S15.109A	S22.012A	S22.20XK	S27.69XA	S32.111K	S32.436K
S06.385A	S12.100K	S12.490A	S15.111A	S22.012K	S22.21XA	S27.802A	S32.112A	S32.441K
S06.389A	S12.101A	S12.490K	S15.112A	S22.018A	S22.21XK	S27.803A	S32.112K	S32.442K
S06.811A	S12.101K	S12.491A	S15.119A	S22.018K	S22.22XA	S27.809A	S32.119A	S32.443K
S06.812A	S12.110A	S12.491K	S15.121A	S22.019A	S22.22XK	S27.892A	S32.119K	S32.444K
S06.813A	S12.110K	S12.500A	S15.122A	S22.019K	S22.23XA	S27.893A	S32.120A	S32.445K
S06.814A	S12.111A	S12.500K	S15.129A	S22.020A	S22.23XK	S27.898A	S32.120K	S32.446K
S06.815A	S12.111K	S12.501A	S15.191A	S22.020K	S22.24XA	S27.899A	S32.121A	S32.451K
S06.819A	S12.112A	S12.501K	S15.192A	S22.021A	S22.24XK	S27.9XXA	S32.121K	S32.452K
S06.821A	S12.112K	S12.530A	S15.199A	S22.021K	S22.31XA	S28.1XXA	S32.122A	S32.453K
S06.822A	S12.120A	S12.530K	S15.201A	S22.022A	S22.31XK	S29.021A	S32.122K	S32.454K
S06.823A	S12.120K	S12.531A	S15.202A	S22.022K	S22.32XA	S29.029A	S32.129A	S32.455K
S06.824A	S12.121A	S12.531K	S15.209A	S22.028A	S22.32XK	S32.000A	S32.129K	S32.456K
S06.825A	S12.121K	S12.54XA	S15.211A	S22.028K	S22.39XA	S32.000K	S32.130A	S32.461K
S06.829A	S12.130A	S12.54XK	S15.212A	S22.029A	S22.39XK	S32.001A	S32.130K	S32.462K
S06.891A	S12.130K	S12.550A	S15.219A	S22.029K	S22.41XA	S32.001K	S32.131A	S32.463K
S06.892A	S12.131A	S12.550K	S15.221A	S22.030A	S22.41XK	S32.002A	S32.131K	S32.464K
S06.893A	S12.131K	S12.551A	S15.222A	S22.030K	S22.42XA	S32.002K	S32.132A	S32.465K
S06.894A	S12.14XA	S12.551K	S15.229A	S22.031A	S22.42XK	S32.008A	S32.132K	S32.466K
S06.895A	S12.14XK	S12.590A	S15.291A	S22.031K	S22.43XA	S32.008K	S32.139A	S32.471K
S06.899A	S12.150A	S12.590K	S15.292A	S22.032A	S22.43XK	S32.009A	S32.139K	S32.472K
S06.9X1A	S12.150K	S12.591A	S15.299A	S22.032K	S22.49XA	S32.009K	S32.14XA	S32.473K
S06.9X2A	S12.151A	S12.591K	S15.301A	S22.038A	S22.49XK	S32.010A	S32.14XK	S32.474K
S06.9X3A	S12.151K	S12.600A	S15.302A	S22.038K	S22.5XXA	S32.010K	S32.15XA	S32.475K
S06.9X4A	S12.190A	S12.600K	S15.309A	S22.039A	S22.9XXA	S32.011A	S32.15XK	S32.476K
S06.9X5A	S12.190K	S12.601A	S15.311A	S22.039K	S22.9XXK	S32.011K	S32.16XA	S32.481K
S06.9X9A	S12.191A	S12.601K	S15.312A	S22.040A	S25.501A	S32.012A	S32.16XK	S32.482K
S07.0XXA	S12.191K	S12.630A	S15.319A	S22.040K	S25.502A	S32.012K	S32.17XA	S32.483K

S32.484K	S36.112A	S36.532A	S42.009K	S42.112B	S42.153P	S42.242K	S42.311A	S42.355P
S32.485K	S36.113A	S36.533A	S42.009P	S42.112K	S42.154B	S42.242P	S42.311K	S42.356A
S32.486K	S36.114A	S36.538A	S42.011B	S42.112P	S42.154K	S42.249A	S42.311P	S42.356K
S32.491K	S36.118A	S36.539A	S42.011K	S42.113B	S42.154P	S42.249K	S42.312A	S42.356P
S32.492K	S36.119A	S36.590A	S42.011P	S42.113K	S42.155B	S42.249P	S42.312K	S42.361A
S32.499K	S36.122A	S36.591A	S42.012B	S42.113P	S42.155K	S42.251A	S42.312P	S42.361K
S32.501A	S36.123A	S36.592A	S42.012K	S42.114B	S42.155P	S42.251K	S42.319A	S42.361P
S32.501K	S36.128A	S36.593A	S42.012P	S42.114K	S42.156B	S42.251P	S42.319K	S42.362A
S32.502A	S36.129A	S36.598A	S42.013B	S42.114P	S42.156K	S42.252A	S42.319P	S42.362K
S32.502K	S36.13XA	S36.599A	S42.013K	S42.115B	S42.156P	S42.252K	S42.321A	S42.362P
S32.509A	S36.200A	S36.60XA	S42.013P	S42.115K	S42.191B	S42.252P	S42.321K	S42.363A
S32.509K	S36.201A	S36.61XA	S42.014B	S42.115P	S42.191K	S42.253A	S42.321P	S42.363K
S32.511A	S36.202A	S36.62XA	S42.014K	S42.116B	S42.191P	S42.253K	S42.322A	S42.363P
S32.511K	S36.209A	S36.63XA	S42.014P	S42.116K	S42.192B	S42.253P	S42.322K	S42.364A
S32.512A	S36.220A	S36.69XA	S42.015B	S42.116P	S42.192K	S42.254A	S42.322P	S42.364K
S32.512K	S36.221A	S36.81XA	S42.015K	S42.121B	S42.192P	S42.254K	S42.323A	S42.364P
S32.519A	S36.222A	S36.892A	S42.015P	S42.121K	S42.199B	S42.254P	S42.323K	S42.365A
S32.519K	S36.229A	S36.893A	S42.016B	S42.121P	S42.199K	S42.255A	S42.323P	S42.365K
S32.591A	S36.230A	S36.898A	S42.016K	S42.122B	S42.199P	S42.255K	S42.324A	S42.365P
S32.591K	S36.231A	S36.899A	S42.016P	S42.122K	S42.201A	S42.255P	S42.324K	S42.366A
S32.592A	S36.232A	S36.90XA	S42.017B	S42.122P	S42.201K	S42.256A	S42.324P	S42.366K
S32.592K	S36.239A	S36.92XA	S42.017K	S42.123B	S42.201P	S42.256K	S42.325A	S42.366P
S32.599A	S36.240A	S36.93XA	S42.017P	S42.123K	S42.202A	S42.256P	S42.325K	S42.391A
S32.599K	S36.241A	S36.99XA	S42.018B	S42.123P	S42.202K	S42.261A	S42.325P	S42.391K
S32.601A	S36.242A	S37.001A	S42.018K	S42.124B	S42.202P	S42.261K	S42.326A	S42.391P
S32.601K	S36.249A	S37.002A	S42.018P	S42.124K	S42.209A	S42.261P	S42.326K	S42.392A
S32.602A	S36.250A	S37.009A	S42.019B	S42.124P	S42.209K	S42.262A	S42.326P	S42.392K
S32.602K	S36.251A	S37.011A	S42.019K	S42.125B	S42.209P	S42.262K	S42.331A	S42.392P
S32.609A	S36.252A	S37.012A	S42.019P	S42.125K	S42.211A	S42.262P	S42.331K	S42.399A
S32.609K	S36.259A	S37.019A	S42.021B	S42.125P	S42.211K	S42.263A	S42.331P	S42.399K
S32.611A	S36.260A	S37.021A	S42.021K	S42.126B	S42.211P	S42.263K	S42.332A	S42.399P
S32.611K	S36.261A	S37.022A	S42.021P	S42.126K	S42.212A	S42.263P	S42.332K	S42.401A
S32.612A	S36.262A	S37.029A	S42.022B	S42.126P	S42.212K	S42.264A	S42.332P	S42.401K
S32.612K	S36.269A	S37.031A	S42.022K	S42.131B	S42.213A	S42.264K	S42.333A	S42.401P
S32.613A	S36.290A	S37.032A	S42.022P	S42.131K	S42.213K	S42.264P	S42.333K	S42.402A
S32.613K	S36.291A	S37.039A	S42.023B	S42.131P	S42.213P	S42.265A	S42.333P	S42.402K
S32.614A	S36.292A	S37.041A	S42.023K	S42.132B	S42.214A	S42.265K	S42.334A	S42.402P
S32.614K	S36.299A	S37.042A	S42.023P	S42.132K	S42.214K	S42.265P	S42.334K	S42.409A
S32.615A	S36.30XA	S37.049A	S42.024B	S42.132P	S42.214P	S42.266A	S42.334P	S42.409K
S32.615K	S36.32XA	S37.051A	S42.024K	S42.133B	S42.215A	S42.266K	S42.335A	S42.409P
S32.616A	S36.33XA	S37.052A	S42.024P	S42.133K	S42.215K	S42.266P	S42.335K	S42.411A
S32.616K	S36.39XA	S37.059A	S42.025B	S42.133P	S42.215P	S42.271A	S42.335P	S42.411K
S32.691A	S36.400A	S37.10XA	S42.025K	S42.134B	S42.216A	S42.271K	S42.336A	S42.411P
S32.691K	S36.408A	S37.12XA	S42.025P	S42.134K	S42.216K	S42.271P	S42.336K	S42.412A
S32.692A	S36.409A	S37.13XA	S42.026B	S42.134P	S42.216P	S42.272A	S42.336P	S42.412K
S32.692K	S36.410A	S37.19XA	S42.026K	S42.135B	S42.221A	S42.272K	S42.341A	S42.412P
S32.699A	S36.418A	S37.20XA	S42.026P	S42.135K	S42.221K	S42.272P	S42.341K	S42.413A
S32.699K	S36.419A	S37.22XA	S42.031B	S42.135P	S42.221P	S42.279A	S42.341P	S42.413K
S32.810A	S36.420A	S37.23XA	S42.031K	S42.136B	S42.222A	S42.279K	S42.342A	S42.413P
S32.810K	S36.428A	S37.29XA	S42.031P	S42.136K	S42.222K	S42.279P	S42.342K	S42.414A
S32.811A	S36.429A	S37.30XA	S42.032B	S42.136P	S42.222P	S42.291A	S42.342P	S42.414K
S32.811K	S36.430A	S37.32XA	S42.032K	S42.141B	S42.223A	S42.291K	S42.343A	S42.414P
S32.82XA	S36.438A	S37.33XA	S42.032P	S42.141K	S42.223K	S42.291P	S42.343K	S42.415A
S32.82XK	S36.439A	S37.39XA	S42.033B	S42.141P	S42.223P	S42.292A	S42.343P	S42.415K
S32.89XA	S36.490A	S37.60XA	S42.033K	S42.142B	S42.224A	S42.292K	S42.344A	S42.415P
S32.89XK	S36.498A	S37.62XA	S42.033P	S42.142K	S42.224K	S42.292P	S42.344K	S42.416A
S32.9XXA	S36.499A	S37.63XA	S42.034B	S42.142P	S42.224P	S42.293A	S42.344P	S42.416K
S32.9XXK	S36.500A	S37.69XA	S42.034K	S42.143B	S42.225A	S42.293K	S42.345A	S42.416P
S35.531A	S36.501A	S37.812A	S42.034P	S42.143K	S42.225K	S42.293P	S42.345K	S42.421A
S35.532A	S36.502A	S37.813A	S42.035B	S42.143P	S42.225P	S42.294A	S42.345P	S42.421K
S35.533A	S36.503A	S37.818A	S42.035K	S42.144B	S42.226A	S42.294K	S42.346A	S42.421P
S35.534A	S36.508A	S37.819A	S42.035P	S42.144K	S42.226K	S42.294P	S42.346K	S42.422A
S35.535A	S36.509A	S37.892A	S42.036B	S42.144P	S42.226P	S42.295A	S42.346P	S42.422K
S35.536A	S36.510A	S37.893A	S42.036K	S42.145B	S42.231A	S42.295K	S42.351A	S42.422P
S35.8X1A	S36.511A	S37.898A	S42.036P	S42.145K	S42.231K	S42.295P	S42.351K	S42.423A
S35.8X8A	S36.512A	S37.899A	S42.101B	S42.145P	S42.231P	S42.296A	S42.351P	S42.423K
S35.8X9A	S36.513A	S37.90XA	S42.101K	S42.146B	S42.232A	S42.296K	S42.352A	S42.423P
S35.90XA	S36.518A	S37.92XA	S42.101P	S42.146K	S42.232K	S42.296P	S42.352K	S42.424A
S35.91XA	S36.519A	S37.93XA	S42.102B	S42.146P	S42.232P	S42.301A	S42.352P	S42.424K
S35.99XA	S36.520A	S37.99XA	S42.102K	S42.151B	S42.239A	S42.301K	S42.353A	S42.424P
S36.00XA	S36.521A	S42.001B	S42.102P	S42.151K	S42.239K	S42.301P	S42.353K	S42.425A
S36.020A	S36.522A	S42.001K	S42.109B	S42.151P	S42.239P	S42.302A	S42.353P	S42.425K
S36.021A	S36.523A	S42.001P	S42.109K	S42.152B	S42.241A	S42.302K	S42.354A	S42.425P
S36.029A	S36.528A	S42.002B	S42.109P	S42.152K	S42.241K	S42.302P	S42.354K	S42.426A
S36.030A	S36.529A	S42.002K	S42.111B	S42.152P	S42.242A	S42.309A	S42.354P	S42.426K
S36.039A	S36.530A	S42.002P	S42.111K	S42.153B	S42.242A	S42.309K	S42.355A	S42.426P
S36.09XA	S36.531A	S42.009B	S42.111P	S42.153K		S42.309P	S42.355K	S42.431A

Appendix E: Complication and Comorbidity (CC) Code List

S42.431K	S42.466A	S45.109A	S48.922A	S49.122A	S52.023R	S52.044Q	S52.124K	S52.201Q
S42.431P	S42.466K	S45.111A	S48.929A	S49.122K	S52.024K	S52.044R	S52.124M	S52.201R
S42.432A	S42.466P	S45.112A	S49.001A	S49.122P	S52.024M	S52.045K	S52.124N	S52.202A
S42.432K	S42.471A	S45.119A	S49.001K	S49.129A	S52.024N	S52.045M	S52.124P	S52.202K
S42.432P	S42.471K	S45.191A	S49.001P	S49.129K	S52.024P	S52.045N	S52.124Q	S52.202M
S42.433A	S42.471P	S45.192A	S49.002A	S49.129P	S52.024Q	S52.045P	S52.124R	S52.202N
S42.433K	S42.472A	S45.199A	S49.002K	S49.131A	S52.024R	S52.045Q	S52.125K	S52.202P
S42.433P	S42.472K	S45.201A	S49.002P	S49.131K	S52.025K	S52.045R	S52.125M	S52.202Q
S42.434A	S42.472P	S45.202A	S49.009A	S49.131P	S52.025M	S52.046K	S52.125N	S52.202R
S42.434K	S42.473A	S45.209A	S49.009K	S49.132A	S52.025N	S52.046M	S52.125P	S52.209A
S42.434P	S42.473K	S45.211A	S49.009P	S49.132K	S52.025P	S52.046N	S52.125R	S52.209K
S42.435A	S42.473P	S45.212A	S49.011A	S49.132P	S52.025Q	S52.046P	S52.126K	S52.209M
S42.435K	S42.474A	S45.219A	S49.011K	S49.139A	S52.025R	S52.046Q	S52.126M	S52.209N
S42.435P	S42.474K	S45.291A	S49.011P	S49.139K	S52.026K	S52.046R	S52.126N	S52.209P
S42.436A	S42.474P	S45.292A	S49.012A	S49.139P	S52.026M	S52.091K	S52.126P	S52.209Q
S42.436K	S42.475A	S45.299A	S49.012K	S49.141A	S52.026N	S52.091M	S52.126Q	S52.209R
S42.436P	S42.475K	S45.301A	S49.012P	S49.141K	S52.026P	S52.091N	S52.126R	S52.211A
S42.441A	S42.475P	S45.302A	S49.019A	S49.141P	S52.026Q	S52.091P	S52.131K	S52.211K
S42.441K	S42.476A	S45.309A	S49.019K	S49.142A	S52.026R	S52.091R	S52.131M	S52.211P
S42.441P	S42.476K	S45.311A	S49.019P	S49.142K	S52.031K	S52.092K	S52.131N	S52.212A
S42.442A	S42.476P	S45.312A	S49.021A	S49.142P	S52.031M	S52.092M	S52.131P	S52.212K
S42.442K	S42.481A	S45.319A	S49.021K	S49.149A	S52.031N	S52.092N	S52.131Q	S52.212P
S42.442P	S42.481K	S45.391A	S49.021P	S49.149K	S52.031P	S52.092P	S52.131R	S52.219A
S42.443A	S42.481P	S45.392A	S49.022A	S49.149P	S52.031Q	S52.092Q	S52.132K	S52.219K
S42.443K	S42.482A	S45.399A	S49.022K	S49.191A	S52.031R	S52.092R	S52.132M	S52.219P
S42.443P	S42.482K	S45.801A	S49.022P	S49.191K	S52.032K	S52.099K	S52.132N	S52.221A
S42.444A	S42.482P	S45.802A	S49.029A	S49.191P	S52.032M	S52.099M	S52.132P	S52.221K
S42.444K	S42.489A	S45.809A	S49.029K	S49.192A	S52.032N	S52.099N	S52.132Q	S52.221M
S42.444P	S42.489K	S45.811A	S49.029P	S49.192K	S52.032P	S52.099P	S52.132R	S52.221N
S42.445A	S42.489P	S45.812A	S49.031A	S49.192P	S52.032Q	S52.099Q	S52.133K	S52.221P
S42.445K	S42.491A	S45.819A	S49.031K	S49.199A	S52.032R	S52.099R	S52.133M	S52.221Q
S42.445P	S42.491K	S45.891A	S49.031P	S49.199K	S52.033M	S52.101K	S52.133N	S52.221R
S42.446A	S42.491P	S45.892A	S49.032A	S49.199P	S52.033N	S52.101M	S52.133P	S52.222A
S42.446K	S42.492A	S45.899A	S49.032K	S52.001K	S52.033P	S52.101N	S52.133Q	S52.222K
S42.446P	S42.492K	S45.901A	S49.032P	S52.001M	S52.033Q	S52.101P	S52.133R	S52.222M
S42.447A	S42.492P	S45.902A	S49.039A	S52.001N	S52.033R	S52.101Q	S52.134K	S52.222N
S42.447K	S42.493A	S45.909A	S49.039K	S52.001P	S52.034K	S52.101R	S52.134M	S52.222P
S42.447P	S42.493K	S45.911A	S49.039P	S52.001Q	S52.034M	S52.102K	S52.134N	S52.222Q
S42.448A	S42.493P	S45.912A	S49.041A	S52.001R	S52.034N	S52.102M	S52.134P	S52.222R
S42.448K	S42.494A	S45.919A	S49.041K	S52.002K	S52.034P	S52.102N	S52.134Q	S52.223A
S42.448P	S42.494K	S45.991A	S49.041P	S52.002M	S52.034Q	S52.102P	S52.134R	S52.223K
S42.449A	S42.494P	S45.992A	S49.042A	S52.002N	S52.034R	S52.102Q	S52.135K	S52.223M
S42.449K	S42.495A	S45.999A	S49.042K	S52.002P	S52.035K	S52.102R	S52.135M	S52.223N
S42.449P	S42.495K	S46.021A	S49.042P	S52.002Q	S52.035M	S52.109K	S52.135N	S52.223P
S42.451A	S42.495P	S46.022A	S49.049A	S52.002R	S52.035P	S52.109M	S52.135P	S52.223Q
S42.451K	S42.496A	S46.029A	S49.049K	S52.009K	S52.035Q	S52.109N	S52.135Q	S52.223R
S42.451P	S42.496K	S46.121A	S49.049P	S52.009M	S52.035R	S52.109P	S52.135R	S52.224A
S42.452A	S42.496P	S46.122A	S49.091A	S52.009N	S52.036K	S52.109Q	S52.136K	S52.224K
S42.452K	S42.90XA	S46.129A	S49.091K	S52.009P	S52.036M	S52.109R	S52.136M	S52.224M
S42.452P	S42.90XK	S46.221A	S49.091P	S52.009Q	S52.036N	S52.111A	S52.136N	S52.224N
S42.453A	S42.90XP	S46.222A	S49.092A	S52.009R	S52.036P	S52.111K	S52.136P	S52.224P
S42.453K	S42.91XA	S46.229A	S49.092K	S52.011A	S52.036Q	S52.111P	S52.136Q	S52.224Q
S42.453P	S42.91XK	S46.321A	S49.092P	S52.011K	S52.036R	S52.112A	S52.136R	S52.224R
S42.454A	S42.91XP	S46.322A	S49.099A	S52.011P	S52.041K	S52.112K	S52.181K	S52.225A
S42.454K	S42.92XA	S46.329A	S49.099K	S52.012A	S52.041M	S52.112P	S52.181M	S52.225K
S42.454P	S42.92XK	S46.821A	S49.099P	S52.012K	S52.041N	S52.119A	S52.181N	S52.225M
S42.455A	S42.92XP	S46.822A	S49.101A	S52.012P	S52.041P	S52.119K	S52.181P	S52.225N
S42.455K	S43.201A	S46.829A	S49.101K	S52.019A	S52.041Q	S52.119P	S52.181Q	S52.225P
S42.455P	S43.202A	S46.921A	S49.101P	S52.019K	S52.041R	S52.121K	S52.181R	S52.225Q
S42.456A	S43.203A	S46.922A	S49.102A	S52.019P	S52.041Q	S52.121M	S52.182K	S52.225R
S42.456K	S43.204A	S46.929A	S49.102K	S52.021K	S52.042K	S52.121N	S52.182M	S52.226A
S42.456P	S43.205A	S48.011A	S49.102P	S52.021M	S52.042M	S52.121P	S52.182N	S52.226K
S42.461A	S43.206A	S48.012A	S49.109A	S52.021N	S52.042N	S52.121Q	S52.182P	S52.226M
S42.461K	S43.211A	S48.019A	S49.109K	S52.021P	S52.042P	S52.121R	S52.182Q	S52.226N
S42.461P	S43.212A	S48.021A	S49.109P	S52.021Q	S52.042Q	S52.122K	S52.182R	S52.226P
S42.462A	S43.213A	S48.022A	S49.111A	S52.021R	S52.042R	S52.122M	S52.189K	S52.226Q
S42.462K	S43.214A	S48.029A	S49.111K	S52.022K	S52.043K	S52.122N	S52.189M	S52.226R
S42.462P	S43.215A	S48.111A	S49.111P	S52.022M	S52.043M	S52.122P	S52.189N	S52.231A
S42.463A	S43.216A	S48.112A	S49.112A	S52.022N	S52.043N	S52.122Q	S52.189P	S52.231K
S42.463K	S43.221A	S48.119A	S49.112K	S52.022P	S52.043P	S52.122R	S52.189Q	S52.231M
S42.463P	S43.222A	S48.121A	S49.112P	S52.022Q	S52.043Q	S52.123K	S52.189R	S52.231N
S42.464A	S43.223A	S48.122A	S49.119A	S52.022R	S52.043R	S52.123M	S52.201A	S52.231P
S42.464K	S43.224A	S48.129A	S49.119K	S52.023K	S52.044K	S52.123N	S52.201K	S52.231Q
S42.464P	S43.225A	S48.911A	S49.119P	S52.023M	S52.044M	S52.123P	S52.201M	S52.231R
S42.465A	S43.226A	S48.912A	S49.121A	S52.023N	S52.044N	S52.123Q	S52.201N	S52.232A
S42.465K	S45.101A	S48.919A	S49.121K	S52.023P	S52.044P	S52.123R	S52.201P	S52.232K
S42.465P	S45.102A	S48.921A	S49.121P	S52.023Q	S52.044R			S52.232M

S52.232N	S52.251N	S52.266N	S52.302R	S52.333P	S52.352P	S52.371P	S52.509P	S52.541M
S52.232P	S52.251P	S52.266P	S52.309A	S52.333Q	S52.352Q	S52.371Q	S52.509Q	S52.541N
S52.232Q	S52.251Q	S52.266Q	S52.309K	S52.333R	S52.352R	S52.371R	S52.509R	S52.541P
S52.232R	S52.251R	S52.266R	S52.309M	S52.334A	S52.353A	S52.372A	S52.511A	S52.541Q
S52.233A	S52.252A	S52.271K	S52.309N	S52.334K	S52.353K	S52.372K	S52.511K	S52.541R
S52.233K	S52.252K	S52.271M	S52.309P	S52.334M	S52.353M	S52.372M	S52.511M	S52.542A
S52.233M	S52.252M	S52.271N	S52.309Q	S52.334N	S52.353N	S52.372N	S52.511N	S52.542K
S52.233N	S52.252N	S52.271P	S52.309R	S52.334P	S52.353P	S52.372P	S52.511P	S52.542M
S52.233P	S52.252P	S52.271Q	S52.311A	S52.334Q	S52.353Q	S52.372Q	S52.511Q	S52.542N
S52.233Q	S52.252Q	S52.271R	S52.311K	S52.334R	S52.353R	S52.372R	S52.511R	S52.542P
S52.233R	S52.252R	S52.272K	S52.311N	S52.335A	S52.354A	S52.379A	S52.512A	S52.542Q
S52.234A	S52.253A	S52.272M	S52.312A	S52.335K	S52.354K	S52.379K	S52.512K	S52.542R
S52.234K	S52.253K	S52.272N	S52.312K	S52.335M	S52.354M	S52.379M	S52.512M	S52.549A
S52.234M	S52.253M	S52.272P	S52.312P	S52.335N	S52.354N	S52.379N	S52.512N	S52.549K
S52.234N	S52.253N	S52.272Q	S52.319A	S52.335P	S52.354P	S52.379P	S52.512P	S52.549M
S52.234P	S52.253P	S52.272R	S52.319K	S52.335Q	S52.354Q	S52.379Q	S52.512Q	S52.549N
S52.234Q	S52.253Q	S52.279K	S52.319P	S52.335R	S52.354R	S52.379R	S52.512R	S52.549P
S52.234R	S52.253R	S52.279M	S52.321A	S52.336A	S52.355A	S52.381A	S52.512R	S52.549Q
S52.235A	S52.254A	S52.279N	S52.321K	S52.336K	S52.355K	S52.381K	S52.513A	S52.549R
S52.235K	S52.254K	S52.279P	S52.321M	S52.336M	S52.355M	S52.381M	S52.513K	S52.551A
S52.235M	S52.254M	S52.279Q	S52.321N	S52.336N	S52.355N	S52.381N	S52.513M	S52.551K
S52.235N	S52.254N	S52.279R	S52.321P	S52.336P	S52.355P	S52.381P	S52.513N	S52.551M
S52.235P	S52.254P	S52.281A	S52.321Q	S52.336Q	S52.355Q	S52.381Q	S52.513P	S52.551N
S52.235Q	S52.254Q	S52.281K	S52.321R	S52.336R	S52.355R	S52.381R	S52.513Q	S52.551P
S52.235R	S52.254R	S52.281M	S52.322A	S52.341A	S52.356A	S52.382A	S52.513R	S52.551Q
S52.236A	S52.255A	S52.281N	S52.322K	S52.341K	S52.356K	S52.382K	S52.514A	S52.551R
S52.236K	S52.255K	S52.281P	S52.322M	S52.341M	S52.356M	S52.382M	S52.514K	S52.552A
S52.236M	S52.255M	S52.281Q	S52.322N	S52.341N	S52.356N	S52.382N	S52.514M	S52.552K
S52.236N	S52.255N	S52.281R	S52.322P	S52.341P	S52.356P	S52.382P	S52.514N	S52.552M
S52.236P	S52.255P	S52.282A	S52.322Q	S52.341Q	S52.356Q	S52.382Q	S52.514P	S52.552N
S52.236Q	S52.255Q	S52.282K	S52.322R	S52.341R	S52.356R	S52.382R	S52.514Q	S52.552P
S52.236R	S52.255R	S52.282M	S52.323A	S52.342A	S52.361A	S52.389A	S52.514R	S52.552Q
S52.241A	S52.256A	S52.282N	S52.323K	S52.342K	S52.361K	S52.389K	S52.515A	S52.552R
S52.241K	S52.256K	S52.282P	S52.323M	S52.342M	S52.361M	S52.389M	S52.515K	S52.559A
S52.241M	S52.256M	S52.282Q	S52.323N	S52.342N	S52.361N	S52.389N	S52.515M	S52.559K
S52.241N	S52.256N	S52.282R	S52.323P	S52.342P	S52.361P	S52.389P	S52.515N	S52.559M
S52.241P	S52.256P	S52.283A	S52.323Q	S52.342Q	S52.361Q	S52.389Q	S52.515P	S52.559N
S52.241Q	S52.256Q	S52.283K	S52.323R	S52.342R	S52.361R	S52.389R	S52.515Q	S52.559P
S52.241R	S52.256R	S52.283M	S52.324A	S52.343A	S52.362A	S52.391A	S52.515R	S52.559Q
S52.242A	S52.261A	S52.283N	S52.324K	S52.343K	S52.362K	S52.391K	S52.516A	S52.559R
S52.242K	S52.261K	S52.283P	S52.324M	S52.343M	S52.362M	S52.391M	S52.516K	S52.561A
S52.242M	S52.261M	S52.283Q	S52.324N	S52.343N	S52.362N	S52.391N	S52.516M	S52.561K
S52.242N	S52.261N	S52.283R	S52.324P	S52.343P	S52.362P	S52.391P	S52.516N	S52.561M
S52.242P	S52.261P	S52.291A	S52.324Q	S52.343Q	S52.362Q	S52.391Q	S52.516P	S52.561N
S52.242Q	S52.261Q	S52.291K	S52.324R	S52.343R	S52.362R	S52.391R	S52.516Q	S52.561P
S52.242R	S52.261R	S52.291M	S52.325A	S52.344A	S52.363A	S52.392A	S52.516R	S52.561Q
S52.243A	S52.262A	S52.291N	S52.325K	S52.344K	S52.363K	S52.392K	S52.521A	S52.561R
S52.243K	S52.262K	S52.291P	S52.325M	S52.344M	S52.363M	S52.392M	S52.521K	S52.562A
S52.243M	S52.262M	S52.291Q	S52.325N	S52.344N	S52.363N	S52.392N	S52.521P	S52.562K
S52.243N	S52.262N	S52.291R	S52.325P	S52.344P	S52.363P	S52.392P	S52.522A	S52.562M
S52.243P	S52.262P	S52.292A	S52.325Q	S52.344Q	S52.363Q	S52.392Q	S52.522K	S52.562N
S52.243Q	S52.262Q	S52.292K	S52.325R	S52.344R	S52.363R	S52.392R	S52.522P	S52.562P
S52.243R	S52.262R	S52.292M	S52.326A	S52.345A	S52.364A	S52.399A	S52.529A	S52.562Q
S52.244A	S52.263A	S52.292N	S52.326K	S52.345K	S52.364K	S52.399K	S52.529K	S52.562R
S52.244K	S52.263K	S52.292P	S52.326M	S52.345M	S52.364M	S52.399M	S52.529P	S52.569A
S52.244M	S52.263M	S52.292Q	S52.326N	S52.345N	S52.364N	S52.399N	S52.531A	S52.569K
S52.244N	S52.263N	S52.292R	S52.326P	S52.345P	S52.364P	S52.399P	S52.531K	S52.569M
S52.244P	S52.263P	S52.299A	S52.326Q	S52.345Q	S52.364Q	S52.399Q	S52.531M	S52.569N
S52.244Q	S52.263Q	S52.299K	S52.326R	S52.345R	S52.364R	S52.399R	S52.531N	S52.569P
S52.244R	S52.263R	S52.299M	S52.331A	S52.346A	S52.365A	S52.501A	S52.531P	S52.569Q
S52.245A	S52.264A	S52.299N	S52.331K	S52.346K	S52.365K	S52.501K	S52.531Q	S52.569R
S52.245K	S52.264K	S52.299P	S52.331M	S52.346M	S52.365M	S52.501M	S52.531R	S52.571A
S52.245M	S52.264M	S52.299Q	S52.331N	S52.346N	S52.365N	S52.501N	S52.532A	S52.571K
S52.245N	S52.264N	S52.299R	S52.331P	S52.346P	S52.365P	S52.501P	S52.532K	S52.571M
S52.245P	S52.264P	S52.301A	S52.331Q	S52.346Q	S52.365Q	S52.501Q	S52.532M	S52.571N
S52.245Q	S52.264Q	S52.301K	S52.331R	S52.346R	S52.365R	S52.501R	S52.532N	S52.571P
S52.245R	S52.264R	S52.301M	S52.332A	S52.351A	S52.366A	S52.502A	S52.532P	S52.571Q
S52.246A	S52.265A	S52.301N	S52.332K	S52.351K	S52.366K	S52.502K	S52.532Q	S52.571R
S52.246K	S52.265K	S52.301P	S52.332M	S52.351M	S52.366M	S52.502M	S52.532R	S52.572A
S52.246M	S52.265M	S52.301Q	S52.332N	S52.351N	S52.366N	S52.502N	S52.539A	S52.572K
S52.246N	S52.265N	S52.301R	S52.332P	S52.351P	S52.366P	S52.502P	S52.539K	S52.572M
S52.246P	S52.265P	S52.302A	S52.332Q	S52.351Q	S52.366Q	S52.502Q	S52.539M	S52.572N
S52.246Q	S52.265Q	S52.302K	S52.332R	S52.351R	S52.366R	S52.502R	S52.539N	S52.572P
S52.246R	S52.265R	S52.302M	S52.333A	S52.352A	S52.371A	S52.509A	S52.539P	S52.572Q
S52.251A	S52.266A	S52.302N	S52.333K	S52.352K	S52.371K	S52.509K	S52.539Q	S52.572R
S52.251K	S52.266K	S52.302P	S52.333M	S52.352M	S52.371M	S52.509M	S52.539R	S52.579A
S52.251M	S52.266M	S52.302Q	S52.333N	S52.352N	S52.371N	S52.509N	S52.541A	S52.579K

Appendix E: Complication and Comorbidity (CC) Code List

S52.579M	S52.615M	S55.119A	S58.122A	S59.122P	S62.001P	S62.113K	S62.155B	S62.213P
S52.579N	S52.615N	S55.191A	S58.129A	S59.129K	S62.002B	S62.113P	S62.155K	S62.221B
S52.579P	S52.615P	S55.192A	S58.911A	S59.129P	S62.002K	S62.114B	S62.155P	S62.221K
S52.579Q	S52.615Q	S55.199A	S58.912A	S59.131K	S62.002P	S62.114K	S62.156B	S62.221P
S52.579R	S52.615R	S55.201A	S58.919A	S59.131P	S62.009B	S62.114P	S62.156K	S62.222B
S52.591A	S52.616A	S55.202A	S58.921A	S59.132K	S62.009K	S62.115B	S62.156P	S62.222K
S52.591K	S52.616K	S55.209A	S58.922A	S59.132P	S62.009P	S62.115K	S62.161B	S62.222P
S52.591M	S52.616M	S55.211A	S58.929A	S59.139K	S62.011B	S62.115P	S62.161K	S62.223B
S52.591N	S52.616N	S55.212A	S59.001A	S59.139P	S62.011K	S62.116B	S62.161P	S62.223K
S52.591P	S52.616P	S55.219A	S59.001K	S59.141K	S62.011P	S62.116K	S62.162B	S62.223P
S52.591Q	S52.616Q	S55.291A	S59.001P	S59.141P	S62.012B	S62.116P	S62.162K	S62.224B
S52.591R	S52.616R	S55.292A	S59.002A	S59.142K	S62.012K	S62.121B	S62.162P	S62.224K
S52.592A	S52.621A	S55.299A	S59.002K	S59.142P	S62.012P	S62.121K	S62.163B	S62.224P
S52.592K	S52.621K	S55.801A	S59.002P	S59.149K	S62.013B	S62.121P	S62.163K	S62.225B
S52.592M	S52.621P	S55.802A	S59.009A	S59.149P	S62.013K	S62.122B	S62.163P	S62.225K
S52.592N	S52.622A	S55.809A	S59.009K	S59.191K	S62.013P	S62.122K	S62.164B	S62.225P
S52.592P	S52.622K	S55.811A	S59.009P	S59.191P	S62.014B	S62.122P	S62.164K	S62.226B
S52.592Q	S52.622P	S55.812A	S59.011A	S59.192K	S62.014K	S62.123B	S62.164P	S62.226K
S52.592R	S52.629A	S55.819A	S59.011K	S59.192P	S62.014P	S62.123K	S62.165B	S62.226P
S52.599A	S52.629K	S55.891A	S59.011P	S59.199K	S62.015B	S62.123P	S62.165K	S62.231B
S52.599K	S52.629P	S55.892A	S59.012A	S59.199P	S62.015K	S62.124B	S62.165P	S62.231K
S52.599M	S52.691A	S55.899A	S59.012K	S59.201A	S62.015P	S62.124K	S62.166B	S62.231P
S52.599N	S52.691K	S55.901A	S59.012P	S59.201K	S62.016B	S62.124P	S62.166K	S62.232B
S52.599P	S52.691M	S55.902A	S59.019A	S59.201P	S62.016K	S62.125B	S62.166P	S62.232K
S52.599Q	S52.691N	S55.909A	S59.019K	S59.202A	S62.016P	S62.125K	S62.171B	S62.232P
S52.599R	S52.691P	S55.911A	S59.019P	S59.202K	S62.021B	S62.125P	S62.171K	S62.233B
S52.601A	S52.691Q	S55.912A	S59.021A	S59.202P	S62.021K	S62.126B	S62.171P	S62.233K
S52.601K	S52.691R	S55.919A	S59.021K	S59.209A	S62.021P	S62.126K	S62.172B	S62.233P
S52.601M	S52.692A	S55.991A	S59.021P	S59.209K	S62.022B	S62.126P	S62.172K	S62.234B
S52.601N	S52.692K	S55.992A	S59.022A	S59.209P	S62.022K	S62.131B	S62.172P	S62.234K
S52.601P	S52.692M	S55.999A	S59.022K	S59.211A	S62.022P	S62.131K	S62.173B	S62.234P
S52.601Q	S52.692N	S56.021A	S59.022P	S59.211K	S62.023B	S62.131P	S62.173K	S62.235B
S52.601R	S52.692P	S56.022A	S59.029A	S59.211P	S62.023K	S62.132B	S62.173P	S62.235K
S52.602A	S52.692Q	S56.029A	S59.029K	S59.212A	S62.023P	S62.132K	S62.174B	S62.235P
S52.602K	S52.692R	S56.121A	S59.029P	S59.212K	S62.024B	S62.132P	S62.174K	S62.236B
S52.602M	S52.699A	S56.122A	S59.031A	S59.212P	S62.024K	S62.133B	S62.174P	S62.236K
S52.602N	S52.699K	S56.123A	S59.031K	S59.219A	S62.024P	S62.133K	S62.175B	S62.236P
S52.602P	S52.699M	S56.124A	S59.031P	S59.219K	S62.025B	S62.133P	S62.175K	S62.241B
S52.602Q	S52.699N	S56.125A	S59.032A	S59.219P	S62.025K	S62.134B	S62.175P	S62.241K
S52.602R	S52.699P	S56.126A	S59.032K	S59.221A	S62.025P	S62.134K	S62.176B	S62.241P
S52.609A	S52.699Q	S56.127A	S59.032P	S59.221K	S62.026B	S62.134P	S62.176K	S62.242B
S52.609K	S52.699R	S56.128A	S59.039A	S59.221P	S62.026K	S62.135B	S62.176P	S62.242K
S52.609M	S52.90XA	S56.129A	S59.039K	S59.222A	S62.026P	S62.135K	S62.181B	S62.242P
S52.609N	S52.90XK	S56.221A	S59.039P	S59.222K	S62.031B	S62.135P	S62.181K	S62.243B
S52.609P	S52.90XM	S56.222A	S59.041A	S59.222P	S62.031K	S62.136B	S62.181P	S62.243K
S52.609Q	S52.90XN	S56.229A	S59.041K	S59.229A	S62.031P	S62.136K	S62.182B	S62.243P
S52.609R	S52.90XP	S56.321A	S59.041P	S59.229K	S62.032B	S62.136P	S62.182K	S62.244B
S52.611A	S52.90XQ	S56.322A	S59.042A	S59.229P	S62.032K	S62.141B	S62.182P	S62.244K
S52.611K	S52.90XR	S56.329A	S59.042K	S59.231A	S62.032P	S62.141K	S62.183B	S62.244P
S52.611M	S52.91XA	S56.421A	S59.042P	S59.231K	S62.033B	S62.141P	S62.183K	S62.245B
S52.611N	S52.91XK	S56.422A	S59.049A	S59.231P	S62.033K	S62.142B	S62.183P	S62.245K
S52.611P	S52.91XM	S56.423A	S59.049K	S59.232A	S62.033P	S62.142K	S62.184B	S62.245P
S52.611Q	S52.91XN	S56.424A	S59.049P	S59.232K	S62.034B	S62.142P	S62.184K	S62.246B
S52.611R	S52.91XP	S56.425A	S59.091A	S59.232P	S62.034K	S62.143B	S62.184P	S62.246K
S52.612A	S52.91XQ	S56.426A	S59.091K	S59.239A	S62.034P	S62.143K	S62.185B	S62.246P
S52.612K	S52.91XR	S56.427A	S59.091P	S59.239K	S62.035B	S62.143P	S62.185K	S62.251B
S52.612M	S52.92XA	S56.428A	S59.092A	S59.239P	S62.035K	S62.144B	S62.185P	S62.251K
S52.612N	S52.92XK	S56.429A	S59.092K	S59.241A	S62.035P	S62.144K	S62.186B	S62.251P
S52.612P	S52.92XM	S56.521A	S59.092P	S59.241K	S62.036B	S62.144P	S62.186K	S62.252B
S52.612Q	S52.92XN	S56.522A	S59.099A	S59.241P	S62.036K	S62.145B	S62.186P	S62.252K
S52.612R	S52.92XP	S56.529A	S59.099K	S59.242A	S62.036P	S62.145K	S62.201B	S62.252P
S52.613A	S52.92XQ	S56.821A	S59.099P	S59.242K	S62.101B	S62.145P	S62.201K	S62.253B
S52.613K	S52.92XR	S56.822A	S59.101K	S59.242P	S62.101K	S62.146B	S62.201P	S62.253K
S52.613M	S55.001A	S56.829A	S59.101P	S59.249A	S62.101P	S62.146K	S62.202B	S62.253P
S52.613N	S55.002A	S56.921A	S59.102K	S59.249K	S62.102B	S62.146P	S62.202K	S62.254B
S52.613P	S55.009A	S56.922A	S59.102P	S59.249P	S62.102K	S62.151B	S62.202P	S62.254K
S52.613Q	S55.011A	S56.929A	S59.109K	S59.291A	S62.102P	S62.151K	S62.209B	S62.254P
S52.613R	S55.012A	S58.011A	S59.109P	S59.291K	S62.109B	S62.151P	S62.209K	S62.255B
S52.614A	S55.019A	S58.012A	S59.111K	S59.291P	S62.109K	S62.152B	S62.209P	S62.255K
S52.614K	S55.091A	S58.019A	S59.111P	S59.292A	S62.109P	S62.152K	S62.211B	S62.255P
S52.614M	S55.092A	S58.021A	S59.112K	S59.292K	S62.111B	S62.152P	S62.211K	S62.256B
S52.614N	S55.099A	S58.022A	S59.112P	S59.292P	S62.111K	S62.153B	S62.211P	S62.256K
S52.614P	S55.101A	S58.029A	S59.119K	S59.299A	S62.111P	S62.153K	S62.212B	S62.256P
S52.614Q	S55.102A	S58.111A	S59.119P	S59.299K	S62.112B	S62.153P	S62.212K	S62.291B
S52.614R	S55.109A	S58.112A	S59.121K	S59.299P	S62.112K	S62.154B	S62.212P	S62.291K
S52.615A	S55.111A	S58.119A	S59.121P	S62.001B	S62.112P	S62.154K	S62.213B	S62.291P
S52.615K	S55.112A	S58.121A	S59.122K	S62.001K	S62.113B	S62.154P	S62.213K	S62.292B

S62.292K	S62.324B	S62.349P	S62.395K	S62.606B	S62.631P	S62.657K	S65.311A	S66.222A
S62.292P	S62.324K	S62.350B	S62.395P	S62.606K	S62.632B	S62.657P	S65.312A	S66.229A
S62.299B	S62.324P	S62.350K	S62.396B	S62.606P	S62.632K	S62.658B	S65.319A	S66.320A
S62.299K	S62.325B	S62.350P	S62.396K	S62.607B	S62.632P	S62.658K	S65.391A	S66.321A
S62.299P	S62.325K	S62.351B	S62.396P	S62.607K	S62.633B	S62.658P	S65.392A	S66.322A
S62.300B	S62.325P	S62.351K	S62.397B	S62.607P	S62.633K	S62.659B	S65.399A	S66.323A
S62.300K	S62.326B	S62.351P	S62.397K	S62.608B	S62.633P	S62.659K	S65.401A	S66.324A
S62.300P	S62.326K	S62.352B	S62.397P	S62.608K	S62.634B	S62.659P	S65.402A	S66.325A
S62.301B	S62.326P	S62.352K	S62.398B	S62.608P	S62.634K	S62.660B	S65.409A	S66.326A
S62.301K	S62.327B	S62.352P	S62.398K	S62.609B	S62.634P	S62.660K	S65.411A	S66.327A
S62.301P	S62.327K	S62.353B	S62.398P	S62.609K	S62.635B	S62.660P	S65.412A	S66.328A
S62.302B	S62.327P	S62.353K	S62.399B	S62.609P	S62.635K	S62.661B	S65.419A	S66.329A
S62.302K	S62.328B	S62.353P	S62.399K	S62.610B	S62.635P	S62.661K	S65.491A	S66.421A
S62.302P	S62.328K	S62.354B	S62.399P	S62.610K	S62.636B	S62.661P	S65.492A	S66.422A
S62.303B	S62.328P	S62.354K	S62.501B	S62.610P	S62.636K	S62.662B	S65.499A	S66.429A
S62.303K	S62.329B	S62.354P	S62.501K	S62.611B	S62.636P	S62.662K	S65.500A	S66.520A
S62.303P	S62.329K	S62.355B	S62.501P	S62.611K	S62.637B	S62.662P	S65.501A	S66.521A
S62.304B	S62.329P	S62.355K	S62.502B	S62.611P	S62.637K	S62.663B	S65.502A	S66.522A
S62.304K	S62.330B	S62.355P	S62.502K	S62.612B	S62.637P	S62.663K	S65.503A	S66.523A
S62.304P	S62.330K	S62.356B	S62.502P	S62.612K	S62.638B	S62.663P	S65.504A	S66.524A
S62.305B	S62.330P	S62.356K	S62.509B	S62.612P	S62.638K	S62.664B	S65.505A	S66.525A
S62.305K	S62.331B	S62.356P	S62.509K	S62.613B	S62.638P	S62.664K	S65.506A	S66.526A
S62.305P	S62.331K	S62.357B	S62.509P	S62.613K	S62.639B	S62.664P	S65.507A	S66.527A
S62.306B	S62.331P	S62.357K	S62.511B	S62.613P	S62.639K	S62.665B	S65.508A	S66.528A
S62.306K	S62.332B	S62.357P	S62.511K	S62.614B	S62.639P	S62.665K	S65.509A	S66.529A
S62.306P	S62.332K	S62.358B	S62.511P	S62.614K	S62.640B	S62.665P	S65.510A	S66.821A
S62.307B	S62.332P	S62.358K	S62.512B	S62.614P	S62.640K	S62.666B	S65.511A	S66.822A
S62.307K	S62.333B	S62.358P	S62.512K	S62.615B	S62.640P	S62.666K	S65.512A	S66.829A
S62.307P	S62.333K	S62.359B	S62.512P	S62.615K	S62.641B	S62.666P	S65.513A	S66.921A
S62.308B	S62.333P	S62.359K	S62.513B	S62.615P	S62.641K	S62.667B	S65.514A	S66.922A
S62.308K	S62.334B	S62.359P	S62.513K	S62.616B	S62.641P	S62.667K	S65.515A	S66.929A
S62.308P	S62.334K	S62.360B	S62.513P	S62.616K	S62.642B	S62.667P	S65.516A	S68.411A
S62.309B	S62.334P	S62.360K	S62.514B	S62.616P	S62.642K	S62.668B	S65.517A	S68.412A
S62.309K	S62.335B	S62.360P	S62.514K	S62.617B	S62.642P	S62.668K	S65.518A	S68.419A
S62.309P	S62.335K	S62.361B	S62.514P	S62.617K	S62.643B	S62.668P	S65.519A	S68.421A
S62.310B	S62.335P	S62.361K	S62.515B	S62.617P	S62.643K	S62.669B	S65.590A	S68.422A
S62.310K	S62.336B	S62.361P	S62.515K	S62.618B	S62.643P	S62.669K	S65.591A	S68.429A
S62.310P	S62.336K	S62.362B	S62.515P	S62.618K	S62.644B	S62.669P	S65.592A	S68.711A
S62.311B	S62.336P	S62.362K	S62.516B	S62.618P	S62.644K	S62.90XB	S65.593A	S68.712A
S62.311K	S62.337B	S62.362P	S62.516K	S62.619B	S62.644P	S62.90XK	S65.594A	S68.719A
S62.311P	S62.337K	S62.363B	S62.516P	S62.619K	S62.645B	S62.90XP	S65.595A	S68.721A
S62.312B	S62.337P	S62.363K	S62.521B	S62.619P	S62.645K	S62.91XB	S65.596A	S68.722A
S62.312K	S62.338B	S62.363P	S62.521K	S62.620B	S62.645P	S62.91XK	S65.597A	S68.729A
S62.312P	S62.338K	S62.364B	S62.521P	S62.620K	S62.646B	S62.91XP	S65.598A	S72.001K
S62.313B	S62.338P	S62.364K	S62.522B	S62.620P	S62.646K	S62.92XB	S65.599A	S72.001M
S62.313K	S62.339B	S62.364P	S62.522K	S62.621B	S62.646P	S62.92XK	S65.801A	S72.001N
S62.313P	S62.339K	S62.365B	S62.522P	S62.621K	S62.647B	S62.92XP	S65.802A	S72.001P
S62.314B	S62.339P	S62.365K	S62.523B	S62.621P	S62.647K	S65.001A	S65.809A	S72.001Q
S62.314K	S62.340B	S62.365P	S62.523K	S62.622B	S62.647P	S65.002A	S65.811A	S72.001R
S62.314P	S62.340K	S62.366B	S62.523P	S62.622K	S62.648B	S65.009A	S65.812A	S72.002K
S62.315B	S62.340P	S62.366K	S62.524B	S62.622P	S62.648K	S65.011A	S65.819A	S72.002M
S62.315K	S62.341B	S62.366P	S62.524K	S62.623B	S62.648P	S65.012A	S65.891A	S72.002N
S62.315P	S62.341K	S62.367B	S62.524P	S62.623K	S62.649B	S65.019A	S65.892A	S72.002P
S62.316B	S62.341P	S62.367K	S62.525B	S62.623P	S62.649K	S65.091A	S65.899A	S72.002Q
S62.316K	S62.342B	S62.367P	S62.525K	S62.624B	S62.649P	S65.092A	S65.901A	S72.002R
S62.316P	S62.342K	S62.368B	S62.525P	S62.624K	S62.650B	S65.099A	S65.902A	S72.009K
S62.317B	S62.342P	S62.368K	S62.526B	S62.624P	S62.650K	S65.101A	S65.909A	S72.009M
S62.317K	S62.343B	S62.368P	S62.526K	S62.625B	S62.650P	S65.102A	S65.911A	S72.009N
S62.317P	S62.343K	S62.369B	S62.526P	S62.625K	S62.651B	S65.109A	S65.912A	S72.009P
S62.318B	S62.343P	S62.369K	S62.600B	S62.625P	S62.651K	S65.111A	S65.919A	S72.009Q
S62.318K	S62.344B	S62.369P	S62.600K	S62.626B	S62.651P	S65.112A	S65.991A	S72.009R
S62.318P	S62.344K	S62.390B	S62.600P	S62.626K	S62.652B	S65.119A	S65.992A	S72.011K
S62.319B	S62.344P	S62.390K	S62.601B	S62.626P	S62.652K	S65.191A	S65.999A	S72.011M
S62.319K	S62.345B	S62.390P	S62.601K	S62.627B	S62.652P	S65.192A	S66.021A	S72.011N
S62.319P	S62.345K	S62.391B	S62.601P	S62.627K	S62.653B	S65.199A	S66.022A	S72.011P
S62.320B	S62.345P	S62.391K	S62.602B	S62.627P	S62.653K	S65.201A	S66.029A	S72.011Q
S62.320K	S62.346B	S62.391P	S62.602K	S62.628B	S62.653P	S65.202A	S66.120A	S72.011R
S62.320P	S62.346K	S62.392B	S62.602P	S62.628K	S62.654B	S65.209A	S66.121A	S72.012K
S62.321B	S62.346P	S62.392K	S62.603B	S62.628P	S62.654K	S65.211A	S66.122A	S72.012M
S62.321K	S62.347B	S62.392P	S62.603K	S62.629B	S62.654P	S65.212A	S66.123A	S72.012N
S62.321P	S62.347K	S62.393B	S62.603P	S62.629K	S62.655B	S65.219A	S66.124A	S72.012P
S62.322B	S62.347P	S62.393K	S62.604B	S62.629P	S62.655K	S65.291A	S66.125A	S72.012Q
S62.322K	S62.348B	S62.393P	S62.604K	S62.630B	S62.655P	S65.292A	S66.126A	S72.012R
S62.322P	S62.348K	S62.394B	S62.604P	S62.630K	S62.656B	S65.299A	S66.127A	S72.019K
S62.323B	S62.348P	S62.394K	S62.605B	S62.630P	S62.656K	S65.301A	S66.128A	S72.019M
S62.323K	S62.349B	S62.394P	S62.605K	S62.631B	S62.656P	S65.302A	S66.129A	S72.019N
S62.323P	S62.349K	S62.395B	S62.605P	S62.631K	S62.657B	S65.309A	S66.221A	S72.019P

Appendix E: Complication and Comorbidity (CC) Code List

S72.019Q	S72.041P	S72.065N	S72.116M	S72.141K	S72.301R	S72.335Q	S72.356P	S72.409R
S72.019R	S72.041Q	S72.065P	S72.116N	S72.141M	S72.302K	S72.335R	S72.356Q	S72.411A
S72.021K	S72.041R	S72.065Q	S72.116P	S72.141N	S72.302M	S72.336K	S72.356R	S72.411K
S72.021M	S72.042K	S72.065R	S72.116Q	S72.141P	S72.302N	S72.336M	S72.361K	S72.411M
S72.021N	S72.042M	S72.066K	S72.116R	S72.141Q	S72.302P	S72.336N	S72.361M	S72.411N
S72.021P	S72.042P	S72.066M	S72.121K	S72.141R	S72.302Q	S72.336P	S72.361N	S72.411P
S72.021Q	S72.042Q	S72.066N	S72.121M	S72.142K	S72.302R	S72.336Q	S72.361P	S72.411Q
S72.021R	S72.042R	S72.066P	S72.121N	S72.142M	S72.309K	S72.336R	S72.361Q	S72.411R
S72.022K	S72.043K	S72.066Q	S72.121P	S72.142N	S72.309M	S72.341K	S72.361R	S72.412A
S72.022M	S72.043M	S72.066R	S72.121Q	S72.142P	S72.309N	S72.341M	S72.362K	S72.412K
S72.022N	S72.043N	S72.091K	S72.121R	S72.142Q	S72.309P	S72.341N	S72.362M	S72.412M
S72.022P	S72.043P	S72.091M	S72.122K	S72.142R	S72.309Q	S72.341P	S72.362N	S72.412P
S72.022Q	S72.043Q	S72.091N	S72.122M	S72.143K	S72.309R	S72.341Q	S72.362P	S72.412Q
S72.022R	S72.043R	S72.091P	S72.122N	S72.143M	S72.321K	S72.341R	S72.362Q	S72.412R
S72.023K	S72.044K	S72.091Q	S72.122P	S72.143N	S72.321M	S72.342K	S72.362R	S72.413A
S72.023M	S72.044M	S72.091R	S72.122Q	S72.143P	S72.321N	S72.342M	S72.363K	S72.413K
S72.023N	S72.044N	S72.092K	S72.122R	S72.143Q	S72.321P	S72.342N	S72.363M	S72.413M
S72.023P	S72.044P	S72.092M	S72.123K	S72.143R	S72.321Q	S72.342P	S72.363N	S72.413N
S72.023Q	S72.044Q	S72.092N	S72.123M	S72.144K	S72.321R	S72.342Q	S72.363P	S72.413P
S72.023R	S72.044R	S72.092P	S72.123N	S72.144M	S72.322K	S72.342R	S72.363Q	S72.413Q
S72.024K	S72.045K	S72.092Q	S72.123P	S72.144N	S72.322M	S72.343K	S72.363R	S72.413R
S72.024M	S72.045M	S72.092R	S72.123Q	S72.144P	S72.322N	S72.343M	S72.364K	S72.414A
S72.024N	S72.045N	S72.099K	S72.123R	S72.144Q	S72.322P	S72.343N	S72.364M	S72.414K
S72.024P	S72.045P	S72.099M	S72.124K	S72.144R	S72.322Q	S72.343P	S72.364N	S72.414M
S72.024Q	S72.045Q	S72.099N	S72.124M	S72.145K	S72.322R	S72.343Q	S72.364P	S72.414N
S72.024R	S72.045R	S72.099P	S72.124N	S72.145M	S72.323K	S72.343R	S72.364Q	S72.414P
S72.025K	S72.046K	S72.099Q	S72.124P	S72.145N	S72.323M	S72.344K	S72.364R	S72.414Q
S72.025M	S72.046M	S72.099R	S72.124Q	S72.145P	S72.323N	S72.344M	S72.365K	S72.414R
S72.025N	S72.046N	S72.101K	S72.124R	S72.145Q	S72.323P	S72.344N	S72.365M	S72.415A
S72.025P	S72.046P	S72.101M	S72.125K	S72.145R	S72.323Q	S72.344P	S72.365N	S72.415K
S72.025Q	S72.046Q	S72.101N	S72.125M	S72.146K	S72.323R	S72.344Q	S72.365P	S72.415N
S72.025R	S72.046R	S72.101P	S72.125N	S72.146M	S72.324K	S72.344R	S72.365Q	S72.415P
S72.026K	S72.051K	S72.101Q	S72.125P	S72.146N	S72.324N	S72.345K	S72.365R	S72.415Q
S72.026M	S72.051M	S72.101R	S72.125Q	S72.146P	S72.324P	S72.345M	S72.366K	S72.415R
S72.026N	S72.051N	S72.102K	S72.125R	S72.146Q	S72.324Q	S72.345N	S72.366M	S72.416A
S72.026P	S72.051P	S72.102M	S72.126K	S72.146R	S72.324R	S72.345P	S72.366N	S72.416K
S72.026Q	S72.051Q	S72.102N	S72.126M	S72.21XK	S72.325K	S72.345Q	S72.366P	S72.416M
S72.026R	S72.051R	S72.102P	S72.126N	S72.21XM	S72.325M	S72.345R	S72.366Q	S72.416P
S72.031K	S72.052K	S72.102Q	S72.126P	S72.21XN	S72.325N	S72.346K	S72.366R	S72.416Q
S72.031M	S72.052M	S72.102R	S72.126Q	S72.21XP	S72.325P	S72.346M	S72.391K	S72.416R
S72.031N	S72.052N	S72.109K	S72.126R	S72.21XQ	S72.325Q	S72.346N	S72.391M	S72.421A
S72.031P	S72.052P	S72.109M	S72.131K	S72.21XR	S72.325R	S72.346P	S72.391N	S72.421K
S72.031Q	S72.052Q	S72.109N	S72.131M	S72.22XK	S72.326K	S72.346Q	S72.391P	S72.421M
S72.031R	S72.052R	S72.109P	S72.131N	S72.22XM	S72.326M	S72.346R	S72.391Q	S72.421N
S72.032K	S72.059K	S72.109Q	S72.131P	S72.22XN	S72.326N	S72.351K	S72.391R	S72.421P
S72.032M	S72.059M	S72.109R	S72.131Q	S72.22XP	S72.326P	S72.351M	S72.392K	S72.421Q
S72.032N	S72.059N	S72.111K	S72.131R	S72.22XQ	S72.326Q	S72.351N	S72.392M	S72.421R
S72.032P	S72.059P	S72.111M	S72.132K	S72.22XR	S72.326R	S72.351P	S72.392N	S72.422A
S72.032Q	S72.059Q	S72.111N	S72.132M	S72.23XK	S72.331K	S72.351Q	S72.392P	S72.422K
S72.032R	S72.059R	S72.111P	S72.132N	S72.23XM	S72.331M	S72.351R	S72.392Q	S72.422M
S72.033K	S72.061K	S72.111Q	S72.132P	S72.23XN	S72.331N	S72.352K	S72.399K	S72.422N
S72.033M	S72.061M	S72.111R	S72.132Q	S72.23XP	S72.331P	S72.352M	S72.399M	S72.422P
S72.033N	S72.061N	S72.112K	S72.132R	S72.23XQ	S72.331Q	S72.352N	S72.399N	S72.422Q
S72.033P	S72.061P	S72.112M	S72.133K	S72.23XR	S72.331R	S72.352P	S72.399P	S72.422R
S72.033Q	S72.061Q	S72.112N	S72.133M	S72.24XK	S72.332K	S72.352Q	S72.399Q	S72.423A
S72.033R	S72.061R	S72.112P	S72.133N	S72.24XM	S72.332M	S72.352R	S72.399R	S72.423K
S72.034K	S72.062K	S72.112Q	S72.133P	S72.24XN	S72.332N	S72.353K	S72.401A	S72.423M
S72.034M	S72.062M	S72.112R	S72.133Q	S72.24XP	S72.332P	S72.353M	S72.401K	S72.423N
S72.034N	S72.062N	S72.113K	S72.133R	S72.24XQ	S72.332Q	S72.353N	S72.401M	S72.423P
S72.034P	S72.062P	S72.113M	S72.134K	S72.24XR	S72.332R	S72.353P	S72.401N	S72.423Q
S72.034Q	S72.062Q	S72.113N	S72.134M	S72.25XK	S72.333K	S72.353Q	S72.401P	S72.423R
S72.034R	S72.062R	S72.113P	S72.134N	S72.25XM	S72.333M	S72.353R	S72.401Q	S72.424A
S72.035K	S72.063K	S72.113Q	S72.134P	S72.25XN	S72.333N	S72.354K	S72.401R	S72.424K
S72.035M	S72.063M	S72.113R	S72.134Q	S72.25XP	S72.333P	S72.354M	S72.402A	S72.424M
S72.035N	S72.063N	S72.114K	S72.134R	S72.25XQ	S72.333Q	S72.354N	S72.402K	S72.424N
S72.035P	S72.063P	S72.114M	S72.135K	S72.25XR	S72.333R	S72.354P	S72.402M	S72.424P
S72.035Q	S72.063Q	S72.114N	S72.135M	S72.26XK	S72.334K	S72.354Q	S72.402N	S72.424Q
S72.035R	S72.063R	S72.114P	S72.135N	S72.26XM	S72.334M	S72.354R	S72.402P	S72.424R
S72.036K	S72.064K	S72.114Q	S72.135P	S72.26XN	S72.334N	S72.355K	S72.402Q	S72.425A
S72.036M	S72.064M	S72.114R	S72.135Q	S72.26XP	S72.334P	S72.355M	S72.402R	S72.425K
S72.036N	S72.064N	S72.115K	S72.135R	S72.26XQ	S72.334Q	S72.355N	S72.409A	S72.425N
S72.036P	S72.064P	S72.115M	S72.136K	S72.26XR	S72.334R	S72.355P	S72.409K	S72.425P
S72.036Q	S72.064Q	S72.115N	S72.136M	S72.301K	S72.335K	S72.355Q	S72.409M	S72.425Q
S72.036R	S72.064R	S72.115P	S72.136N	S72.301M	S72.335M	S72.355R	S72.409N	
S72.041K	S72.065K	S72.115Q	S72.136P	S72.301N	S72.335N	S72.356K	S72.409P	
S72.041M	S72.065M	S72.115R	S72.136Q	S72.301P	S72.335P	S72.356M	S72.409Q	
S72.041N		S72.116K	S72.136R	S72.301Q		S72.356N		

S72.425R	S72.444R	S72.463R	S72.91XM	S76.221A	S79.122P	S82.013B	S82.025P	S82.042C
S72.426A	S72.445A	S72.464A	S72.91XN	S76.222A	S79.129A	S82.013C	S82.025Q	S82.042K
S72.426K	S72.445K	S72.464K	S72.91XP	S76.229A	S79.129K	S82.013K	S82.025R	S82.042M
S72.426M	S72.445M	S72.464M	S72.91XQ	S76.321A	S79.129P	S82.013M	S82.026A	S82.042N
S72.426N	S72.445N	S72.464N	S72.91XR	S76.322A	S79.131A	S82.013N	S82.026B	S82.042P
S72.426P	S72.445P	S72.464P	S72.92XK	S76.329A	S79.131K	S82.013P	S82.026C	S82.042Q
S72.426Q	S72.445Q	S72.464Q	S72.92XM	S76.821A	S79.131P	S82.013Q	S82.026K	S82.042R
S72.426R	S72.445R	S72.464R	S72.92XN	S76.822A	S79.132A	S82.013R	S82.026M	S82.043A
S72.431A	S72.446A	S72.465A	S72.92XP	S76.829A	S79.132K	S82.014A	S82.026N	S82.043B
S72.431K	S72.446K	S72.465K	S72.92XQ	S76.921A	S79.132P	S82.014B	S82.026P	S82.043C
S72.431M	S72.446M	S72.465M	S72.92XR	S76.922A	S79.139A	S82.014C	S82.026Q	S82.043M
S72.431N	S72.446N	S72.465N	S73.001A	S76.929A	S79.139K	S82.014K	S82.031A	S82.043N
S72.431P	S72.446P	S72.465P	S73.002A	S77.00XA	S79.139P	S82.014M	S82.031B	S82.043P
S72.431Q	S72.446Q	S72.465Q	S73.003A	S77.01XA	S79.141A	S82.014N	S82.031C	S82.043Q
S72.431R	S72.446R	S72.465R	S73.004A	S77.02XA	S79.141K	S82.014P	S82.031K	S82.043R
S72.432A	S72.451A	S72.466A	S73.005A	S77.10XA	S79.141P	S82.014Q	S82.031M	S82.044A
S72.432K	S72.451K	S72.466K	S73.006A	S77.11XA	S79.142A	S82.014R	S82.031N	S82.044B
S72.432M	S72.451M	S72.466M	S73.011A	S77.12XA	S79.142K	S82.015A	S82.031P	S82.044C
S72.432N	S72.451N	S72.466N	S73.012A	S78.011A	S79.142P	S82.015B	S82.031Q	S82.044K
S72.432P	S72.451P	S72.466P	S73.013A	S78.012A	S79.149A	S82.015C	S82.031R	S82.044M
S72.432Q	S72.451Q	S72.466Q	S73.014A	S78.019A	S79.149K	S82.015K	S82.032A	S82.044N
S72.432R	S72.451R	S72.466R	S73.015A	S78.021A	S79.149P	S82.015M	S82.032B	S82.044P
S72.433A	S72.452A	S72.471A	S73.016A	S78.022A	S79.191A	S82.015N	S82.032C	S82.044Q
S72.433K	S72.452K	S72.471K	S73.021A	S78.029A	S79.191K	S82.015P	S82.032K	S82.044R
S72.433M	S72.452M	S72.471P	S73.022A	S78.111A	S79.191P	S82.015Q	S82.032M	S82.045A
S72.433N	S72.452N	S72.472A	S73.023A	S78.112A	S79.192A	S82.015R	S82.032N	S82.045B
S72.433P	S72.452P	S72.472K	S73.024A	S78.119A	S79.192K	S82.016A	S82.032P	S82.045C
S72.433Q	S72.452Q	S72.472P	S73.025A	S78.121A	S79.192P	S82.016B	S82.032Q	S82.045K
S72.433R	S72.452R	S72.479A	S73.026A	S78.122A	S79.199A	S82.016C	S82.032R	S82.045M
S72.434A	S72.453A	S72.479K	S73.031A	S78.129A	S79.199K	S82.016K	S82.033A	S82.045N
S72.434K	S72.453K	S72.479P	S73.032A	S78.911A	S79.199P	S82.016M	S82.033B	S82.045P
S72.434M	S72.453M	S72.491A	S73.033A	S78.912A	S82.001A	S82.016N	S82.033C	S82.045Q
S72.434N	S72.453N	S72.491K	S73.034A	S78.919A	S82.001B	S82.016P	S82.033K	S82.045R
S72.434P	S72.453P	S72.491M	S73.035A	S78.921A	S82.001C	S82.016Q	S82.033M	S82.046A
S72.434Q	S72.453Q	S72.491N	S73.036A	S78.922A	S82.001K	S82.016R	S82.033N	S82.046B
S72.434R	S72.453R	S72.491P	S73.041A	S78.929A	S82.001M	S82.021A	S82.033P	S82.046C
S72.435A	S72.454A	S72.491Q	S73.042A	S79.001K	S82.001N	S82.021B	S82.033Q	S82.046K
S72.435K	S72.454K	S72.491R	S73.043A	S79.001P	S82.001P	S82.021C	S82.033R	S82.046M
S72.435M	S72.454M	S72.492A	S73.044A	S79.002K	S82.001Q	S82.021K	S82.034A	S82.046N
S72.435N	S72.454N	S72.492K	S73.045A	S79.002P	S82.001R	S82.021M	S82.034B	S82.046P
S72.435P	S72.454P	S72.492M	S73.046A	S79.009K	S82.002A	S82.021N	S82.034C	S82.046Q
S72.435Q	S72.454Q	S72.492N	S75.201A	S79.009P	S82.002B	S82.021P	S82.034K	S82.046R
S72.435R	S72.454R	S72.492P	S75.202A	S79.011K	S82.002C	S82.021Q	S82.034M	S82.091A
S72.436A	S72.455A	S72.492Q	S75.209A	S79.011P	S82.002K	S82.021R	S82.034N	S82.091B
S72.436K	S72.455K	S72.492R	S75.211A	S79.012K	S82.002M	S82.022A	S82.034P	S82.091C
S72.436M	S72.455M	S72.499A	S75.212A	S79.012P	S82.002N	S82.022B	S82.034Q	S82.091K
S72.436N	S72.455N	S72.499K	S75.219A	S79.019K	S82.002P	S82.022C	S82.034R	S82.091M
S72.436P	S72.455P	S72.499M	S75.221A	S79.019P	S82.002Q	S82.022K	S82.035A	S82.091N
S72.436Q	S72.455Q	S72.499N	S75.222A	S79.091K	S82.002R	S82.022M	S82.035B	S82.091P
S72.436R	S72.455R	S72.499P	S75.229A	S79.091P	S82.009A	S82.022N	S82.035C	S82.091Q
S72.441A	S72.456A	S72.499Q	S75.291A	S79.092K	S82.009B	S82.022P	S82.035K	S82.091R
S72.441K	S72.456K	S72.499R	S75.292A	S79.092P	S82.009C	S82.022Q	S82.035M	S82.092A
S72.441M	S72.456M	S72.8X1K	S75.299A	S79.099K	S82.009K	S82.022R	S82.035N	S82.092B
S72.441N	S72.456N	S72.8X1M	S75.801A	S79.099P	S82.009M	S82.023A	S82.035P	S82.092C
S72.441P	S72.456P	S72.8X1N	S75.802A	S79.101A	S82.009N	S82.023B	S82.035Q	S82.092K
S72.441Q	S72.456Q	S72.8X1P	S75.809A	S79.101K	S82.009P	S82.023C	S82.035R	S82.092M
S72.441R	S72.456R	S72.8X1Q	S75.811A	S79.101P	S82.009Q	S82.023K	S82.036A	S82.092N
S72.442A	S72.461A	S72.8X1R	S75.812A	S79.102A	S82.009R	S82.023M	S82.036B	S82.092P
S72.442K	S72.461K	S72.8X2K	S75.819A	S79.102K	S82.011A	S82.023N	S82.036C	S82.092Q
S72.442M	S72.461M	S72.8X2M	S75.891A	S79.102P	S82.011B	S82.023P	S82.036K	S82.092R
S72.442N	S72.461N	S72.8X2N	S75.892A	S79.109A	S82.011C	S82.023Q	S82.036M	S82.099A
S72.442P	S72.461P	S72.8X2P	S75.899A	S79.109K	S82.011K	S82.023R	S82.036N	S82.099B
S72.442Q	S72.461Q	S72.8X2Q	S75.901A	S79.109P	S82.011M	S82.024A	S82.036P	S82.099C
S72.442R	S72.461R	S72.8X2R	S75.902A	S79.111A	S82.011N	S82.024B	S82.036Q	S82.099K
S72.443A	S72.462A	S72.8X9K	S75.909A	S79.111K	S82.011P	S82.024C	S82.036R	S82.099M
S72.443K	S72.462K	S72.8X9M	S75.911A	S79.111P	S82.011Q	S82.024K	S82.041A	S82.099N
S72.443M	S72.462M	S72.8X9N	S75.912A	S79.112A	S82.011R	S82.024M	S82.041B	S82.099P
S72.443N	S72.462N	S72.8X9P	S75.919A	S79.112K	S82.012A	S82.024N	S82.041C	S82.099Q
S72.443P	S72.462P	S72.8X9Q	S75.991A	S79.112P	S82.012B	S82.024P	S82.041K	S82.099R
S72.443Q	S72.462Q	S72.8X9R	S75.992A	S79.119A	S82.012C	S82.024Q	S82.041M	S82.101A
S72.443R	S72.462R	S72.90XK	S75.999A	S79.119K	S82.012K	S82.024R	S82.041N	S82.101K
S72.444A	S72.463A	S72.90XM	S76.021A	S79.119P	S82.012M	S82.025A	S82.041P	S82.101M
S72.444K	S72.463K	S72.90XN	S76.022A	S79.121A	S82.012N	S82.025B	S82.041R	S82.101N
S72.444M	S72.463M	S72.90XP	S76.029A	S79.121K	S82.012P	S82.025C	S82.041Q	S82.101P
S72.444N	S72.463N	S72.90XQ	S76.121A	S79.121P	S82.012Q	S82.025K	S82.041R	S82.101Q
S72.444P	S72.463P	S72.90XR	S76.122A	S79.122A	S82.012R	S82.025M	S82.042A	S82.101R
S72.444Q	S72.463Q	S72.91XK	S76.129A	S79.122K	S82.013A	S82.025N	S82.042B	

S82.102A	S82.124A	S82.143A	S82.169K	S82.225Q	S82.244Q	S82.263Q	S82.391B	S82.426R
S82.102K	S82.124K	S82.143K	S82.169P	S82.225R	S82.244R	S82.263R	S82.391C	S82.431K
S82.102M	S82.124M	S82.143M	S82.191A	S82.226A	S82.245A	S82.264A	S82.391K	S82.431M
S82.102N	S82.124N	S82.143N	S82.191K	S82.226K	S82.245K	S82.264K	S82.391M	S82.431N
S82.102P	S82.124P	S82.143P	S82.191M	S82.226M	S82.245M	S82.264M	S82.391N	S82.431P
S82.102Q	S82.124Q	S82.143Q	S82.191N	S82.226N	S82.245N	S82.264N	S82.391P	S82.431Q
S82.102R	S82.124R	S82.143R	S82.191P	S82.226P	S82.245P	S82.264P	S82.391Q	S82.431R
S82.109A	S82.125A	S82.144A	S82.191Q	S82.226Q	S82.245Q	S82.264Q	S82.391R	S82.432K
S82.109K	S82.125K	S82.144K	S82.191R	S82.226R	S82.245R	S82.264R	S82.392B	S82.432M
S82.109M	S82.125M	S82.144M	S82.192A	S82.231A	S82.246A	S82.265A	S82.392C	S82.432N
S82.109N	S82.125N	S82.144N	S82.192K	S82.231K	S82.246K	S82.265K	S82.392K	S82.432P
S82.109P	S82.125P	S82.144P	S82.192M	S82.231M	S82.246M	S82.265M	S82.392M	S82.432Q
S82.109Q	S82.125Q	S82.144Q	S82.192N	S82.231N	S82.246N	S82.265N	S82.392N	S82.432R
S82.109R	S82.125R	S82.144R	S82.192P	S82.231P	S82.246P	S82.265P	S82.392P	S82.433K
S82.111A	S82.126A	S82.145A	S82.192Q	S82.231Q	S82.246Q	S82.265Q	S82.392Q	S82.433M
S82.111K	S82.126K	S82.145K	S82.192R	S82.231R	S82.246R	S82.265R	S82.392R	S82.433N
S82.111M	S82.126M	S82.145M	S82.199A	S82.232A	S82.251A	S82.266A	S82.399B	S82.433P
S82.111N	S82.126N	S82.145N	S82.199K	S82.232K	S82.251K	S82.266K	S82.399C	S82.433Q
S82.111P	S82.126P	S82.145P	S82.199M	S82.232M	S82.251M	S82.266M	S82.399K	S82.433R
S82.111Q	S82.126Q	S82.145Q	S82.199N	S82.232N	S82.251N	S82.266N	S82.399M	S82.434K
S82.111R	S82.126R	S82.145R	S82.199P	S82.232P	S82.251P	S82.266P	S82.399N	S82.434M
S82.112A	S82.131A	S82.146A	S82.199Q	S82.232Q	S82.251Q	S82.266Q	S82.399P	S82.434N
S82.112K	S82.131K	S82.146K	S82.199R	S82.232R	S82.251R	S82.266R	S82.399Q	S82.434P
S82.112M	S82.131M	S82.146M	S82.201A	S82.233A	S82.252A	S82.291A	S82.399R	S82.434Q
S82.112N	S82.131N	S82.146N	S82.201K	S82.233K	S82.252K	S82.291K	S82.401K	S82.434R
S82.112P	S82.131P	S82.146P	S82.201M	S82.233M	S82.252M	S82.291M	S82.401N	S82.435K
S82.112Q	S82.131Q	S82.146Q	S82.201N	S82.233N	S82.252N	S82.291N	S82.401P	S82.435M
S82.112R	S82.131R	S82.146R	S82.201P	S82.233P	S82.252P	S82.291P	S82.401Q	S82.435N
S82.113A	S82.132A	S82.151A	S82.201Q	S82.233Q	S82.252Q	S82.291Q	S82.401R	S82.435P
S82.113K	S82.132K	S82.151K	S82.201R	S82.233R	S82.252R	S82.291R	S82.402K	S82.435Q
S82.113M	S82.132M	S82.151M	S82.202A	S82.234A	S82.253A	S82.292A	S82.402M	S82.435R
S82.113N	S82.132N	S82.151N	S82.202K	S82.234K	S82.253K	S82.292K	S82.402N	S82.436K
S82.113P	S82.132P	S82.151P	S82.202M	S82.234M	S82.253M	S82.292M	S82.402P	S82.436M
S82.113Q	S82.132Q	S82.151Q	S82.202N	S82.234N	S82.253N	S82.292N	S82.402Q	S82.436N
S82.113R	S82.132R	S82.151R	S82.202P	S82.234P	S82.253P	S82.292P	S82.402R	S82.436P
S82.114A	S82.133A	S82.152A	S82.202Q	S82.234Q	S82.253Q	S82.292Q	S82.409K	S82.436Q
S82.114K	S82.133K	S82.152K	S82.202R	S82.234R	S82.253R	S82.292R	S82.409M	S82.436R
S82.114M	S82.133M	S82.152M	S82.209A	S82.235A	S82.254A	S82.299A	S82.409N	S82.441K
S82.114N	S82.133N	S82.152N	S82.209K	S82.235K	S82.254K	S82.299K	S82.409P	S82.441M
S82.114P	S82.133P	S82.152P	S82.209M	S82.235M	S82.254M	S82.299M	S82.409Q	S82.441N
S82.114Q	S82.133Q	S82.152Q	S82.209N	S82.235N	S82.254N	S82.299N	S82.409R	S82.441P
S82.114R	S82.133R	S82.152R	S82.209P	S82.235P	S82.254P	S82.299P	S82.421K	S82.441Q
S82.115A	S82.134A	S82.153A	S82.209Q	S82.235Q	S82.254Q	S82.299Q	S82.421M	S82.441R
S82.115K	S82.134K	S82.153K	S82.209R	S82.235R	S82.254R	S82.299R	S82.421N	S82.442K
S82.115M	S82.134M	S82.153M	S82.221A	S82.236A	S82.255A	S82.301B	S82.421P	S82.442M
S82.115N	S82.134N	S82.153N	S82.221K	S82.236K	S82.255K	S82.301C	S82.421Q	S82.442N
S82.115P	S82.134P	S82.153P	S82.221M	S82.236M	S82.255M	S82.301K	S82.421R	S82.442P
S82.115Q	S82.134Q	S82.153Q	S82.221N	S82.236N	S82.255N	S82.301M	S82.422K	S82.442Q
S82.115R	S82.134R	S82.153R	S82.221P	S82.236P	S82.255P	S82.301N	S82.422M	S82.442R
S82.116A	S82.135A	S82.154A	S82.221Q	S82.236Q	S82.255Q	S82.301P	S82.422N	S82.443K
S82.116K	S82.135K	S82.154K	S82.221R	S82.236R	S82.255R	S82.301Q	S82.422P	S82.443M
S82.116M	S82.135M	S82.154M	S82.222A	S82.241A	S82.256A	S82.301R	S82.422Q	S82.443N
S82.116N	S82.135N	S82.154N	S82.222K	S82.241K	S82.256K	S82.302B	S82.422R	S82.443P
S82.116P	S82.135P	S82.154P	S82.222M	S82.241M	S82.256M	S82.302C	S82.423K	S82.443Q
S82.116Q	S82.135Q	S82.154Q	S82.222N	S82.241N	S82.256N	S82.302K	S82.423M	S82.443R
S82.116R	S82.135R	S82.154R	S82.222P	S82.241P	S82.256P	S82.302M	S82.423N	S82.444K
S82.121A	S82.136A	S82.155A	S82.222Q	S82.241Q	S82.256Q	S82.302N	S82.423P	S82.444M
S82.121K	S82.136K	S82.155K	S82.222R	S82.241R	S82.256R	S82.302P	S82.423Q	S82.444N
S82.121M	S82.136M	S82.155M	S82.223A	S82.242A	S82.261A	S82.302Q	S82.423R	S82.444P
S82.121N	S82.136N	S82.155N	S82.223K	S82.242K	S82.261K	S82.302R	S82.424K	S82.444Q
S82.121P	S82.136P	S82.155P	S82.223M	S82.242M	S82.261M	S82.309B	S82.424M	S82.444R
S82.121Q	S82.136Q	S82.155Q	S82.223N	S82.242N	S82.261N	S82.309C	S82.424N	S82.445K
S82.121R	S82.136R	S82.155R	S82.223P	S82.242P	S82.261P	S82.309K	S82.424P	S82.445M
S82.122A	S82.141A	S82.156A	S82.223Q	S82.242Q	S82.261Q	S82.309M	S82.424Q	S82.445N
S82.122K	S82.141K	S82.156K	S82.223R	S82.242R	S82.261R	S82.309N	S82.424R	S82.445P
S82.122M	S82.141M	S82.156M	S82.224A	S82.243A	S82.262A	S82.309P	S82.425K	S82.445Q
S82.122N	S82.141N	S82.156N	S82.224K	S82.243K	S82.262K	S82.309Q	S82.425M	S82.445R
S82.122P	S82.141P	S82.156P	S82.224M	S82.243M	S82.262M	S82.309R	S82.425N	S82.446K
S82.122Q	S82.141Q	S82.156Q	S82.224N	S82.243N	S82.262N	S82.311A	S82.425P	S82.446M
S82.122R	S82.141R	S82.156R	S82.224P	S82.243P	S82.262P	S82.311K	S82.425Q	S82.446N
S82.123A	S82.142A	S82.161A	S82.224Q	S82.243Q	S82.262Q	S82.311P	S82.425R	S82.446P
S82.123K	S82.142K	S82.161K	S82.224R	S82.243R	S82.262R	S82.312A	S82.426K	S82.446Q
S82.123M	S82.142M	S82.161P	S82.225A	S82.244A	S82.263A	S82.312K	S82.426M	S82.446R
S82.123N	S82.142N	S82.162A	S82.225K	S82.244K	S82.263K	S82.312P	S82.426N	S82.451K
S82.123P	S82.142P	S82.162K	S82.225M	S82.244M	S82.263M	S82.319A	S82.426P	S82.451N
S82.123Q	S82.142Q	S82.162P	S82.225N	S82.244N	S82.263N	S82.319K	S82.426Q	S82.451P
S82.123R	S82.142R	S82.169A	S82.225P	S82.244P	S82.263P	S82.319P		

S82.451Q	S82.492P	S82.63XN	S82.843M	S82.861K	S82.876C	S85.172A	S88.121A	S89.122K
S82.451R	S82.492Q	S82.63XP	S82.843N	S82.861M	S82.876K	S85.179A	S88.122A	S89.122P
S82.452K	S82.492R	S82.63XQ	S82.843P	S82.861N	S82.876M	S85.181A	S88.129A	S89.129K
S82.452M	S82.499K	S82.63XR	S82.843Q	S82.861P	S82.876N	S85.182A	S88.911A	S89.129P
S82.452N	S82.499M	S82.64XB	S82.843R	S82.861Q	S82.876P	S85.189A	S88.912A	S89.131K
S82.452P	S82.499N	S82.64XC	S82.844B	S82.861R	S82.876Q	S85.201A	S88.919A	S89.131P
S82.452Q	S82.499P	S82.64XK	S82.844C	S82.862K	S82.876R	S85.202A	S88.921A	S89.132K
S82.452R	S82.499Q	S82.64XM	S82.844K	S82.862M	S82.891B	S85.209A	S88.922A	S89.132P
S82.453K	S82.499R	S82.64XN	S82.844M	S82.862N	S82.891C	S85.211A	S88.929A	S89.139K
S82.453M	S82.51XB	S82.64XP	S82.844N	S82.862Q	S82.891K	S85.212A	S89.001A	S89.139P
S82.453N	S82.51XC	S82.64XQ	S82.844P	S82.862R	S82.891M	S85.219A	S89.001K	S89.141K
S82.453P	S82.51XK	S82.64XR	S82.844Q	S82.862R	S82.891N	S85.291A	S89.001P	S89.141P
S82.453Q	S82.51XM	S82.65XB	S82.844R	S82.863K	S82.891P	S85.292A	S89.002A	S89.142K
S82.453R	S82.51XN	S82.65XC	S82.845B	S82.863M	S82.891Q	S85.299A	S89.002K	S89.142P
S82.454K	S82.51XP	S82.65XK	S82.845C	S82.863N	S82.891R	S85.301A	S89.002P	S89.149K
S82.454M	S82.51XQ	S82.65XM	S82.845K	S82.863P	S82.892B	S85.302A	S89.009A	S89.149P
S82.454N	S82.51XR	S82.65XN	S82.845M	S82.863Q	S82.892C	S85.309A	S89.009K	S89.191K
S82.454P	S82.52XB	S82.65XP	S82.845N	S82.863R	S82.892K	S85.311A	S89.009P	S89.191P
S82.454Q	S82.52XC	S82.65XQ	S82.845P	S82.864K	S82.892M	S85.312A	S89.011A	S89.192K
S82.454R	S82.52XK	S82.65XR	S82.845Q	S82.864M	S82.892N	S85.319A	S89.011K	S89.192P
S82.455K	S82.52XM	S82.66XB	S82.845R	S82.864N	S82.892P	S85.391A	S89.011P	S89.199K
S82.455M	S82.52XN	S82.66XC	S82.846B	S82.864P	S82.892Q	S85.392A	S89.012A	S89.199P
S82.455N	S82.52XP	S82.66XK	S82.846C	S82.864Q	S82.892R	S85.399A	S89.012K	S89.201K
S82.455P	S82.52XQ	S82.66XM	S82.846K	S82.864R	S82.899B	S85.401A	S89.012P	S89.201P
S82.455Q	S82.52XR	S82.66XN	S82.846M	S82.865K	S82.899C	S85.402A	S89.019A	S89.202K
S82.455R	S82.53XB	S82.66XP	S82.846N	S82.865M	S82.899K	S85.409A	S89.019K	S89.202P
S82.456K	S82.53XC	S82.66XQ	S82.846P	S82.865N	S82.899M	S85.411A	S89.019P	S89.209K
S82.456M	S82.53XK	S82.66XR	S82.846Q	S82.865P	S82.899N	S85.412A	S89.021A	S89.209P
S82.456N	S82.53XM	S82.811K	S82.846R	S82.865Q	S82.899P	S85.419A	S89.021K	S89.211K
S82.456P	S82.53XN	S82.811P	S82.851B	S82.865R	S82.899Q	S85.491A	S89.021P	S89.211P
S82.456Q	S82.53XP	S82.812K	S82.851C	S82.866K	S82.899R	S85.492A	S89.022A	S89.212K
S82.456R	S82.53XQ	S82.812P	S82.851K	S82.866M	S82.90XB	S85.499A	S89.022K	S89.212P
S82.461K	S82.53XR	S82.819K	S82.851M	S82.866N	S82.90XC	S85.801A	S89.022P	S89.219K
S82.461M	S82.54XB	S82.819P	S82.851N	S82.866P	S82.90XK	S85.802A	S89.029A	S89.219P
S82.461N	S82.54XC	S82.821K	S82.851P	S82.866Q	S82.90XM	S85.809A	S89.029K	S89.221K
S82.461P	S82.54XK	S82.821P	S82.851Q	S82.866R	S82.90XN	S85.811A	S89.029P	S89.221P
S82.461Q	S82.54XM	S82.822K	S82.851R	S82.871B	S82.90XP	S85.812A	S89.031A	S89.222K
S82.461R	S82.54XN	S82.822P	S82.852B	S82.871C	S82.90XQ	S85.819A	S89.031K	S89.222P
S82.462K	S82.54XP	S82.829K	S82.852C	S82.871K	S82.90XR	S85.891A	S89.031P	S89.229K
S82.462M	S82.54XQ	S82.829P	S82.852K	S82.871M	S82.91XB	S85.892A	S89.032A	S89.229P
S82.462N	S82.54XR	S82.831K	S82.852M	S82.871N	S82.91XC	S85.899A	S89.032K	S89.291K
S82.462P	S82.55XB	S82.831M	S82.852N	S82.871P	S82.91XK	S85.901A	S89.032P	S89.291P
S82.462Q	S82.55XC	S82.831N	S82.852P	S82.871Q	S82.91XM	S85.902A	S89.039A	S89.292K
S82.462R	S82.55XK	S82.831P	S82.852Q	S82.871R	S82.91XN	S85.909A	S89.039K	S89.292P
S82.463K	S82.55XM	S82.831Q	S82.852R	S82.872B	S82.91XP	S85.911A	S89.039P	S89.299K
S82.463M	S82.55XN	S82.831R	S82.853B	S82.872C	S82.91XQ	S85.912A	S89.041A	S89.299P
S82.463N	S82.55XP	S82.832K	S82.853C	S82.872K	S82.91XR	S85.919A	S89.041K	S89.301K
S82.463P	S82.55XQ	S82.832M	S82.853K	S82.872M	S82.92XB	S85.991A	S89.041P	S89.301P
S82.463Q	S82.55XR	S82.832N	S82.853M	S82.872N	S82.92XC	S85.992A	S89.042A	S89.302K
S82.463R	S82.56XB	S82.832P	S82.853N	S82.872P	S82.92XK	S85.999A	S89.042K	S89.302P
S82.464K	S82.56XC	S82.832Q	S82.853P	S82.872Q	S82.92XM	S86.021A	S89.042P	S89.309K
S82.464M	S82.56XK	S82.832R	S82.853Q	S82.872R	S82.92XN	S86.022A	S89.049A	S89.309P
S82.464N	S82.56XM	S82.839K	S82.853R	S82.873B	S82.92XP	S86.029A	S89.049K	S89.311K
S82.464P	S82.56XN	S82.839M	S82.854B	S82.873C	S82.92XQ	S86.121A	S89.049P	S89.311P
S82.464Q	S82.56XP	S82.839N	S82.854C	S82.873K	S82.92XR	S86.122A	S89.091A	S89.312K
S82.464R	S82.56XQ	S82.839P	S82.854K	S82.873M	S85.101A	S86.129A	S89.091K	S89.312P
S82.465K	S82.56XR	S82.839Q	S82.854M	S82.873N	S85.102A	S86.221A	S89.091P	S89.319K
S82.465M	S82.61XB	S82.839R	S82.854N	S82.873P	S85.109A	S86.222A	S89.092A	S89.319P
S82.465N	S82.61XC	S82.841B	S82.854P	S82.873Q	S85.111A	S86.229A	S89.092K	S89.321K
S82.465P	S82.61XK	S82.841C	S82.854Q	S82.873R	S85.112A	S86.321A	S89.092P	S89.321P
S82.465Q	S82.61XM	S82.841K	S82.854R	S82.874B	S85.119A	S86.322A	S89.099A	S89.322K
S82.465R	S82.61XN	S82.841M	S82.855B	S82.874C	S85.121A	S86.329A	S89.099K	S89.322P
S82.466K	S82.61XP	S82.841N	S82.855C	S82.874K	S85.122A	S86.821A	S89.099P	S89.329K
S82.466M	S82.61XQ	S82.841P	S82.855K	S82.874M	S85.129A	S86.822A	S89.101K	S89.329P
S82.466N	S82.61XR	S82.841Q	S82.855M	S82.874N	S85.131A	S86.829A	S89.101P	S89.391K
S82.466P	S82.62XB	S82.841R	S82.855N	S82.874P	S85.132A	S86.921A	S89.102K	S89.391P
S82.466Q	S82.62XC	S82.842B	S82.855P	S82.874Q	S85.139A	S86.922A	S89.102P	S89.392K
S82.466R	S82.62XK	S82.842C	S82.855Q	S82.874R	S85.141A	S86.929A	S89.109K	S89.392P
S82.491K	S82.62XM	S82.842K	S82.855R	S82.875B	S85.142A	S88.011A	S89.109P	S89.399K
S82.491M	S82.62XN	S82.842M	S82.856B	S82.875C	S85.149A	S88.012A	S89.111K	S89.399P
S82.491N	S82.62XP	S82.842N	S82.856C	S82.875K	S85.151A	S88.019A	S89.111P	S92.001B
S82.491P	S82.62XQ	S82.842P	S82.856K	S82.875M	S85.152A	S88.021A	S89.112K	S92.001K
S82.491Q	S82.62XR	S82.842Q	S82.856M	S82.875N	S85.159A	S88.022A	S89.112P	S92.001P
S82.491R	S82.63XB	S82.842R	S82.856N	S82.875P	S85.161A	S88.029A	S89.119K	S92.002B
S82.492K	S82.63XC	S82.843B	S82.856P	S82.875Q	S85.162A	S88.111A	S89.119P	S92.002K
S82.492M	S82.63XK	S82.843C	S82.856Q	S82.875R	S85.169A	S88.112A	S89.121K	S92.002P
S82.492N	S82.63XM	S82.843K	S82.856R	S82.876B	S85.171A	S88.119A	S89.121P	S92.009B

Appendix E: Complication and Comorbidity (CC) Code List

S92.009K	S92.052B	S92.126P	S92.212K	S92.254B	S92.342P	S92.503K	S95.011A	T17.410A
S92.009P	S92.052K	S92.131B	S92.212P	S92.254K	S92.343B	S92.503P	S95.012A	T17.418A
S92.011B	S92.052P	S92.131K	S92.213B	S92.254P	S92.343K	S92.504K	S95.019A	T17.420A
S92.011K	S92.053B	S92.131P	S92.213K	S92.255B	S92.343P	S92.504P	S95.091A	T17.428A
S92.011P	S92.053K	S92.132B	S92.213P	S92.255K	S92.344B	S92.505K	S95.092A	T17.490A
S92.012B	S92.053P	S92.132K	S92.214B	S92.255P	S92.344K	S92.505P	S95.099A	T17.498A
S92.012K	S92.054B	S92.132P	S92.214K	S92.256B	S92.344P	S92.506K	S95.101A	T17.500A
S92.012P	S92.054K	S92.133B	S92.214P	S92.256K	S92.345B	S92.506P	S95.102A	T17.508A
S92.013B	S92.054P	S92.133K	S92.215B	S92.256P	S92.345K	S92.511K	S95.109A	T17.510A
S92.013K	S92.055B	S92.133P	S92.215K	S92.301B	S92.345P	S92.511P	S95.111A	T17.518A
S92.013P	S92.055K	S92.134B	S92.215P	S92.301K	S92.346B	S92.512K	S95.112A	T17.520A
S92.014B	S92.055P	S92.134K	S92.216B	S92.301P	S92.346K	S92.512P	S95.119A	T17.528A
S92.014K	S92.056B	S92.134P	S92.216K	S92.302B	S92.346P	S92.513K	S95.191A	T17.590A
S92.014P	S92.056K	S92.135B	S92.216P	S92.302K	S92.351B	S92.513P	S95.192A	T17.598A
S92.015B	S92.056P	S92.135K	S92.221B	S92.302P	S92.351K	S92.514K	S95.199A	T17.800A
S92.015K	S92.061B	S92.135P	S92.221K	S92.309B	S92.351P	S92.514P	S95.201A	T17.808A
S92.015P	S92.061K	S92.136B	S92.221P	S92.309K	S92.352B	S92.515K	S95.202A	T17.810A
S92.016B	S92.061P	S92.136K	S92.222B	S92.309P	S92.352K	S92.515P	S95.209A	T17.818A
S92.016K	S92.062B	S92.136P	S92.222K	S92.311B	S92.352P	S92.516K	S95.211A	T17.820A
S92.016P	S92.062K	S92.141B	S92.222P	S92.311P	S92.353B	S92.516P	S95.212A	T17.828A
S92.021B	S92.062P	S92.141K	S92.223B	S92.312B	S92.353K	S92.521K	S95.219A	T17.890A
S92.021K	S92.063B	S92.141P	S92.223K	S92.312K	S92.353P	S92.521P	S95.291A	T17.898A
S92.021P	S92.063K	S92.142B	S92.223P	S92.312P	S92.354B	S92.522K	S95.292A	T20.30XA
S92.022B	S92.063P	S92.142K	S92.224B	S92.313B	S92.354K	S92.522P	S95.299A	T20.311A
S92.022K	S92.064B	S92.142P	S92.224K	S92.313K	S92.354P	S92.523K	S95.801A	T20.312A
S92.022P	S92.064K	S92.143B	S92.224P	S92.313P	S92.355B	S92.523P	S95.802A	T20.319A
S92.023B	S92.064P	S92.143K	S92.225B	S92.314B	S92.355K	S92.524K	S95.809A	T20.32XA
S92.023K	S92.065B	S92.143P	S92.225K	S92.314K	S92.355P	S92.524P	S95.811A	T20.33XA
S92.023P	S92.065K	S92.144B	S92.225P	S92.314P	S92.356B	S92.525K	S95.812A	T20.34XA
S92.024B	S92.065P	S92.144K	S92.226B	S92.315B	S92.356K	S92.525P	S95.819A	T20.35XA
S92.024K	S92.066B	S92.144P	S92.226K	S92.315K	S92.356P	S92.526K	S95.891A	T20.36XA
S92.024P	S92.066K	S92.145B	S92.226P	S92.315P	S92.401K	S92.526P	S95.892A	T20.37XA
S92.025B	S92.066P	S92.145K	S92.231B	S92.316B	S92.401P	S92.531K	S95.899A	T20.39XA
S92.025K	S92.101B	S92.145P	S92.231K	S92.316K	S92.402K	S92.531P	S95.901A	T20.70XA
S92.025P	S92.101K	S92.146B	S92.231P	S92.316P	S92.402P	S92.532K	S95.902A	T20.711A
S92.026B	S92.101P	S92.146K	S92.232B	S92.321B	S92.403K	S92.532P	S95.909A	T20.712A
S92.026K	S92.102B	S92.146P	S92.232K	S92.321K	S92.403P	S92.533K	S95.911A	T20.719A
S92.026P	S92.102K	S92.151B	S92.232P	S92.321P	S92.404K	S92.533P	S95.912A	T20.72XA
S92.031B	S92.102P	S92.151K	S92.233B	S92.322B	S92.404P	S92.534K	S95.919A	T20.73XA
S92.031K	S92.109B	S92.151P	S92.233K	S92.322K	S92.405K	S92.534P	S95.991A	T20.74XA
S92.031P	S92.109K	S92.152B	S92.233P	S92.322P	S92.405P	S92.535K	S95.992A	T20.75XA
S92.032B	S92.109P	S92.152K	S92.234B	S92.323B	S92.406K	S92.535P	S95.999A	T20.76XA
S92.032K	S92.111B	S92.152P	S92.234K	S92.323K	S92.406P	S92.536K	S96.021A	T20.77XA
S92.032P	S92.111K	S92.153B	S92.234P	S92.323P	S92.411K	S92.536P	S96.022A	T20.79XA
S92.033B	S92.111P	S92.153K	S92.235B	S92.324B	S92.411P	S92.591K	S96.029A	T21.30XA
S92.033K	S92.112B	S92.153P	S92.235K	S92.324K	S92.412K	S92.591P	S96.121A	T21.31XA
S92.033P	S92.112K	S92.154B	S92.235P	S92.324P	S92.412P	S92.592K	S96.122A	T21.32XA
S92.034B	S92.112P	S92.154K	S92.236B	S92.325B	S92.413K	S92.592P	S96.129A	T21.33XA
S92.034K	S92.113B	S92.154P	S92.236K	S92.325K	S92.413P	S92.599K	S96.221A	T21.34XA
S92.034P	S92.113K	S92.155B	S92.236P	S92.325P	S92.414K	S92.599P	S96.222A	T21.35XA
S92.035B	S92.113P	S92.155K	S92.241B	S92.326B	S92.414P	S92.811B	S96.229A	T21.36XA
S92.035K	S92.114B	S92.155P	S92.241K	S92.326K	S92.415K	S92.811K	S96.821A	T21.37XA
S92.035P	S92.114K	S92.156B	S92.241P	S92.326P	S92.415P	S92.811P	S96.822A	T21.39XA
S92.036B	S92.114P	S92.156K	S92.242B	S92.331B	S92.416K	S92.812B	S96.829A	T21.70XA
S92.036K	S92.115B	S92.156P	S92.242K	S92.331K	S92.416P	S92.812K	S96.921A	T21.71XA
S92.036P	S92.115K	S92.191B	S92.242P	S92.331P	S92.421K	S92.812P	S96.922A	T21.72XA
S92.041B	S92.115P	S92.191K	S92.243B	S92.332B	S92.421P	S92.819B	S96.929A	T21.73XA
S92.041K	S92.116B	S92.191P	S92.243K	S92.332K	S92.422K	S92.819K	S98.011A	T21.74XA
S92.041P	S92.116K	S92.192B	S92.243P	S92.332P	S92.422P	S92.819P	S98.012A	T21.75XA
S92.042B	S92.116P	S92.192K	S92.244B	S92.333B	S92.423K	S92.901B	S98.019A	T21.76XA
S92.042K	S92.121B	S92.192P	S92.244K	S92.333K	S92.423P	S92.901K	S98.021A	T21.77XA
S92.042P	S92.121K	S92.199B	S92.244P	S92.333P	S92.424K	S92.901P	S98.022A	T21.79XA
S92.043B	S92.121P	S92.199K	S92.245B	S92.334B	S92.424P	S92.902B	S98.029A	T22.30XA
S92.043K	S92.122B	S92.199P	S92.245K	S92.334K	S92.425K	S92.902K	S98.311A	T22.311A
S92.043P	S92.122K	S92.201B	S92.245P	S92.334P	S92.425P	S92.902P	S98.312A	T22.312A
S92.044B	S92.122P	S92.201K	S92.246B	S92.335B	S92.426K	S92.909B	S98.319A	T22.319A
S92.044K	S92.123B	S92.201P	S92.246K	S92.335K	S92.426P	S92.909P	S98.321A	T22.321A
S92.044P	S92.123K	S92.202B	S92.246P	S92.335P	S92.491K	S92.911K	S98.322A	T22.322A
S92.045B	S92.123P	S92.202K	S92.251B	S92.336B	S92.491P	S92.911P	S98.329A	T22.329A
S92.045K	S92.124B	S92.202P	S92.251K	S92.336K	S92.492K	S92.912K	S98.911A	T22.331A
S92.045P	S92.124K	S92.209B	S92.251P	S92.336P	S92.492P	S92.912P	S98.912A	T22.332A
S92.046B	S92.124P	S92.209K	S92.252B	S92.341B	S92.499K	S92.919K	S98.919A	T22.339A
S92.046K	S92.125B	S92.209P	S92.252K	S92.341K	S92.499P	S92.919P	S98.921A	T22.341A
S92.046P	S92.125K	S92.211B	S92.252P	S92.341P	S92.501K	S95.001A	S98.922A	T22.342A
S92.051B	S92.125P	S92.211K	S92.253B	S92.342B	S92.501P	S95.002A	S98.929A	T22.349A
S92.051K	S92.126B	S92.211P	S92.253K	S92.342K	S92.502K	S95.009A	T17.400A	T22.351A
S92.051P	S92.126K	S92.212B	S92.253P		S92.502P		T17.408A	T22.352A

T22.359A	T23.771A	T28.7XXA	T34.539A	T74.92XA	T81.42XA	T82.198A	T82.856A	T84.018A
T22.361A	T23.772A	T31.10	T34.60XA	T75.1XXA	T81.43XA	T82.199A	T82.857A	T84.019A
T22.362A	T23.779A	T31.11	T34.61XA	T76.01XA	T81.44XA	T82.211A	T82.858A	T84.020A
T22.369A	T23.791A	T31.20	T34.62XA	T76.02XA	T81.49XA	T82.212A	T82.867A	T84.021A
T22.391A	T23.792A	T31.30	T34.70XA	T76.11XA	T81.500A	T82.213A	T82.868A	T84.022A
T22.392A	T23.799A	T31.40	T34.71XA	T76.12XA	T81.501A	T82.218A	T82.897A	T84.023A
T22.399A	T24.301A	T31.50	T34.72XA	T76.21XA	T81.502A	T82.221A	T82.898A	T84.028A
T22.70XA	T24.302A	T31.60	T34.811A	T76.22XA	T81.503A	T82.222A	T82.9XXA	T84.029A
T22.711A	T24.309A	T31.70	T34.812A	T76.32XA	T81.504A	T82.223A	T83.010A	T84.030A
T22.712A	T24.311A	T31.80	T34.819A	T76.51XA	T81.505A	T82.228A	T83.020A	T84.031A
T22.719A	T24.312A	T31.90	T34.821A	T76.52XA	T81.506A	T82.310A	T83.030A	T84.032A
T22.721A	T24.319A	T32.10	T34.822A	T76.61XA	T81.507A	T82.311A	T83.090A	T84.033A
T22.722A	T24.321A	T32.11	T34.829A	T76.62XA	T81.508A	T82.312A	T83.110A	T84.038A
T22.729A	T24.322A	T32.20	T34.831A	T76.91XA	T81.509A	T82.318A	T83.111A	T84.039A
T22.731A	T24.329A	T32.30	T34.832A	T76.92XA	T81.510A	T82.319A	T83.112A	T84.050A
T22.732A	T24.331A	T32.40	T34.839A	T78.00XA	T81.511A	T82.320A	T83.113A	T84.051A
T22.739A	T24.332A	T32.50	T34.90XA	T78.01XA	T81.512A	T82.321A	T83.118A	T84.052A
T22.741A	T24.339A	T32.60	T34.99XA	T78.02XA	T81.513A	T82.322A	T83.120A	T84.053A
T22.742A	T24.391A	T32.70	T67.01XA	T78.03XA	T81.514A	T82.328A	T83.121A	T84.058A
T22.749A	T24.392A	T32.80	T67.02XA	T78.04XA	T81.515A	T82.329A	T83.122A	T84.059A
T22.751A	T24.399A	T32.90	T67.09XA	T78.05XA	T81.516A	T82.330A	T83.123A	T84.060A
T22.752A	T24.701A	T33.011A	T69.021A	T78.06XA	T81.517A	T82.331A	T83.128A	T84.061A
T22.759A	T24.702A	T33.012A	T69.022A	T78.07XA	T81.518A	T82.332A	T83.190A	T84.062A
T22.761A	T24.709A	T33.019A	T69.029A	T78.08XA	T81.519A	T82.338A	T83.191A	T84.063A
T22.762A	T24.711A	T33.02XA	T70.3XXA	T78.09XA	T81.520A	T82.339A	T83.192A	T84.068A
T22.769A	T24.712A	T33.09XA	T71.111A	T78.2XXA	T81.521A	T82.390A	T83.193A	T84.069A
T22.791A	T24.719A	T33.1XXA	T71.112A	T79.2XXA	T81.522A	T82.391A	T83.198A	T84.090A
T22.792A	T24.721A	T33.2XXA	T71.113A	T79.7XXA	T81.523A	T82.392A	T83.21XA	T84.091A
T22.799A	T24.722A	T33.3XXA	T71.114A	T79.A0XA	T81.524A	T82.398A	T83.22XA	T84.092A
T23.301A	T24.729A	T33.40XA	T71.121A	T79.A11A	T81.525A	T82.399A	T83.23XA	T84.093A
T23.302A	T24.731A	T33.41XA	T71.122A	T79.A12A	T81.526A	T82.41XA	T83.24XA	T84.098A
T23.309A	T24.732A	T33.42XA	T71.123A	T79.A19A	T81.527A	T82.42XA	T83.25XA	T84.099A
T23.311A	T24.739A	T33.511A	T71.124A	T79.A21A	T81.528A	T82.43XA	T83.29XA	T84.110A
T23.312A	T24.791A	T33.512A	T71.131A	T79.A22A	T81.529A	T82.49XA	T83.410A	T84.111A
T23.319A	T24.792A	T33.519A	T71.132A	T79.A29A	T81.530A	T82.510A	T83.411A	T84.112A
T23.321A	T24.799A	T33.521A	T71.133A	T79.A3XA	T81.531A	T82.511A	T83.418A	T84.113A
T23.322A	T25.311A	T33.522A	T71.134A	T79.A9XA	T81.532A	T82.512A	T83.420A	T84.114A
T23.329A	T25.312A	T33.529A	T71.141A	T80.1XXA	T81.533A	T82.513A	T83.421A	T84.115A
T23.331A	T25.319A	T33.531A	T71.143A	T80.211A	T81.534A	T82.514A	T83.428A	T84.116A
T23.332A	T25.321A	T33.532A	T71.144A	T80.212A	T81.535A	T82.515A	T83.490A	T84.117A
T23.339A	T25.322A	T33.539A	T71.151A	T80.218A	T81.536A	T82.518A	T83.491A	T84.119A
T23.341A	T25.329A	T33.60XA	T71.152A	T80.219A	T81.537A	T82.519A	T83.498A	T84.120A
T23.342A	T25.331A	T33.61XA	T71.153A	T80.22XA	T81.538A	T82.520A	T83.510A	T84.121A
T23.349A	T25.332A	T33.62XA	T71.154A	T80.29XA	T81.539A	T82.521A	T83.511A	T84.122A
T23.351A	T25.339A	T33.70XA	T71.161A	T80.30XA	T81.590A	T82.522A	T83.512A	T84.123A
T23.352A	T25.391A	T33.71XA	T71.162A	T80.310A	T81.591A	T82.523A	T83.518A	T84.124A
T23.359A	T25.392A	T33.72XA	T71.163A	T80.311A	T81.592A	T82.524A	T83.590A	T84.125A
T23.361A	T25.399A	T33.811A	T71.164A	T80.319A	T81.593A	T82.525A	T83.591A	T84.126A
T23.362A	T25.711A	T33.812A	T71.191A	T80.39XA	T81.594A	T82.528A	T83.592A	T84.127A
T23.369A	T25.712A	T33.819A	T71.192A	T80.40XA	T81.595A	T82.529A	T83.593A	T84.129A
T23.371A	T25.719A	T33.821A	T71.193A	T80.410A	T81.596A	T82.530A	T83.598A	T84.190A
T23.372A	T25.721A	T33.822A	T71.194A	T80.411A	T81.597A	T82.531A	T83.61XA	T84.191A
T23.379A	T25.722A	T33.829A	T71.20XA	T80.419A	T81.598A	T82.532A	T83.62XA	T84.192A
T23.391A	T25.729A	T33.831A	T71.21XA	T80.49XA	T81.599A	T82.533A	T83.69XA	T84.193A
T23.392A	T25.731A	T33.832A	T71.221A	T80.51XA	T81.60XA	T82.534A	T83.712A	T84.194A
T23.399A	T25.732A	T33.839A	T71.222A	T80.52XA	T81.61XA	T82.535A	T83.713A	T84.195A
T23.701A	T25.739A	T33.90XA	T71.223A	T80.59XA	T81.69XA	T82.538A	T83.714A	T84.196A
T23.702A	T25.791A	T33.99XA	T71.224A	T80.61XA	T81.710A	T82.539A	T83.718A	T84.197A
T23.709A	T25.792A	T34.011A	T71.231A	T80.62XA	T81.711A	T82.590A	T83.719A	T84.199A
T23.711A	T25.799A	T34.012A	T71.232A	T80.69XA	T81.718A	T82.591A	T83.722A	T84.210A
T23.712A	T26.20XA	T34.019A	T71.233A	T80.810A	T81.719A	T82.592A	T83.723A	T84.213A
T23.719A	T26.21XA	T34.02XA	T71.234A	T80.818A	T81.72XA	T82.593A	T83.724A	T84.216A
T23.721A	T26.22XA	T34.09XA	T71.29XA	T80.910A	T81.83XA	T82.594A	T83.728A	T84.218A
T23.722A	T26.70XA	T34.1XXA	T71.9XXA	T80.911A	T82.01XA	T82.595A	T83.729A	T84.220A
T23.729A	T26.71XA	T34.2XXA	T74.01XA	T80.919A	T82.02XA	T82.598A	T83.79XA	T84.223A
T23.731A	T26.72XA	T34.3XXA	T74.02XA	T80.A0XA	T82.03XA	T82.599A	T83.81XA	T84.226A
T23.732A	T27.0XXA	T34.40XA	T74.11XA	T80.A10A	T82.09XA	T82.6XXA	T83.82XA	T84.228A
T23.739A	T27.1XXA	T34.41XA	T74.12XA	T80.A11A	T82.110A	T82.7XXA	T83.83XA	T84.290A
T23.741A	T27.2XXA	T34.42XA	T74.21XA	T80.A19A	T82.111A	T82.817A	T83.84XA	T84.293A
T23.742A	T27.3XXA	T34.511A	T74.22XA	T80.A9XA	T82.118A	T82.818A	T83.85XA	T84.296A
T23.749A	T27.4XXA	T34.512A	T74.32XA	T81.10XA	T82.119A	T82.827A	T83.86XA	T84.298A
T23.751A	T27.5XXA	T34.519A	T74.4XXA	T81.30XA	T82.120A	T82.828A	T83.89XA	T84.310A
T23.752A	T27.6XXA	T34.521A	T74.51XA	T81.31XA	T82.121A	T82.837A	T83.9XXA	T84.318A
T23.759A	T27.7XXA	T34.522A	T74.52XA	T81.32XA	T82.128A	T82.838A	T84.010A	T84.320A
T23.761A	T28.1XXA	T34.529A	T74.61XA	T81.33XA	T82.129A	T82.847A	T84.011A	T84.328A
T23.762A	T28.2XXA	T34.531A	T74.62XA	T81.40XA	T82.190A	T82.848A	T84.012A	T84.390A
T23.769A	T28.6XXA	T34.532A	T74.91XA	T81.41XA	T82.191A	T82.855A	T84.013A	T84.398A

T84.410A	T84.82XA	T85.320A	T85.628A	T85.850A	T86.49	T86.8483	T87.43	Z48.290
T84.418A	T84.83XA	T85.321A	T85.630A	T85.850D	T86.5	T86.8489	T87.44	Z68.1
T84.420A	T84.84XA	T85.390A	T85.631A	T85.860A	T86.810	T86.8491	T88.0XXA	Z68.41
T84.428A	T84.85XA	T85.391A	T85.633A	T85.860D	T86.811	T86.8492	T88.1XXA	Z68.42
T84.490A	T84.86XA	T85.41XA	T85.635A	T85.890A	T86.812	T86.8493	T88.2XXA	Z68.43
T84.498A	T84.89XA	T85.42XA	T85.638A	T85.890D	T86.818	T86.8499	T88.3XXA	Z68.44
T84.50XA	T84.9XXA	T85.43XA	T85.690A	T86.00	T86.819	T86.850	T88.6XXA	Z68.45
T84.51XA	T85.01XA	T85.44XA	T85.691A	T86.01	T86.820	T86.851	Z16.10	Z94.0
T84.52XA	T85.02XA	T85.49XA	T85.692A	T86.02	T86.821	T86.852	Z16.11	Z94.1
T84.53XA	T85.03XA	T85.510A	T85.693A	T86.03	T86.822	T86.858	Z16.12	Z94.2
T84.54XA	T85.09XA	T85.511A	T85.694A	T86.09	T86.828	T86.859	Z16.19	Z94.3
T84.59XA	T85.110A	T85.518A	T85.695A	T86.10	T86.829	T86.890	Z16.20	Z94.4
T84.60XA	T85.111A	T85.520A	T85.698A	T86.11	T86.830	T86.891	Z16.21	Z94.81
T84.610A	T85.112A	T85.521A	T85.71XA	T86.12	T86.831	T86.892	Z16.22	Z94.82
T84.611A	T85.113A	T85.528A	T85.72XA	T86.13	T86.832	T86.898	Z16.23	Z94.83
T84.612A	T85.118A	T85.590A	T85.730A	T86.19	T86.838	T86.899	Z16.24	Z94.84
T84.613A	T85.120A	T85.591A	T85.731A	T86.20	T86.839	T86.90	Z16.29	Z95.811
T84.614A	T85.121A	T85.598A	T85.732A	T86.21	T86.8401	T86.91	Z16.30	Z95.812
T84.615A	T85.122A	T85.610A	T85.733A	T86.22	T86.8402	T86.92	Z16.31	Z99.11
T84.619A	T85.123A	T85.611A	T85.734A	T86.23	T86.8403	T86.93	Z16.32	Z99.12
T84.620A	T85.128A	T85.612A	T85.735A	T86.290	T86.8409	T86.99	Z16.33	
T84.621A	T85.190A	T85.613A	T85.738A	T86.298	T86.8411	T87.0X1	Z16.341	
T84.622A	T85.191A	T85.614A	T85.79XA	T86.30	T86.8412	T87.0X2	Z16.342	
T84.623A	T85.192A	T85.615A	T85.810A	T86.31	T86.8413	T87.0X9	Z16.35	
T84.624A	T85.193A	T85.618A	T85.810D	T86.32	T86.8419	T87.1X1	Z16.39	
T84.625A	T85.199A	T85.620A	T85.820A	T86.33	T86.8421	T87.1X2	Z43.1	
T84.629A	T85.21XA	T85.621A	T85.820D	T86.39	T86.8422	T87.1X9	Z48.21	
T84.63XA	T85.22XA	T85.622A	T85.830A	T86.40	T86.8423	T87.2	Z48.22	
T84.69XA	T85.29XA	T85.623A	T85.830D	T86.41	T86.8429	T87.40	Z48.23	
T84.7XXA	T85.310A	T85.624A	T85.840A	T86.42	T86.8481	T87.41	Z48.24	
T84.81XA	T85.311A	T85.625A	T85.840D	T86.43	T86.8482	T87.42	Z48.280	

Present-on-admission (POA) indicators are required on all diagnoses and external cause-of-injury codes for all inpatient acute care hospital discharges, according to the requirement outlined in the Deficit Reduction Act of 2005, section 5001(c). The only exception is for a select group of codes that have been designated as exempt from the POA regulations. Certain facilities are also exempt from this reporting requirement and include the following:

- Critical access hospitals
- Long-term care hospitals
- Cancer hospitals
- Inpatient psychiatric hospitals
- Inpatient rehabilitation facilities
- Veterans Administration/Department of Defense Hospitals
- Children's inpatient facilities

The POA indicator guidelines are not intended to replace the official *ICD-10-CM Official Guidelines for Coding and Reporting*. Nor will the POA guidelines supersede the Uniform Hospital Discharge Data Set (UHDDS) definition of principal diagnosis, defined as the condition established after study to be chiefly responsible for occasioning the admission of the patient to the hospital. The definition of "additional diagnoses" also remains the same. Coders must report all conditions that coexist at the time of admission, develop subsequently, or that affect the treatment received and/or the length of stay. This significantly affects assignment of the POA indicators. Because the POA indicator should accurately reflect the patient's conditions upon admission, review of POA guidelines as well as the *ICD-10-CM Official Guidelines for Coding and Reporting* is required.

The following is a summary of the POA guidelines:

- A POA condition is defined not only as one that is clearly present at the time of admission, but also one that was clearly present but not diagnosed until after the time of admission.

- Present on admission is defined as present at the time the order for an inpatient admission is made, whether or not the patient's episode of care originated in the emergency department, ambulatory surgery area, or other outpatient area. Conditions that develop during an outpatient encounter are considered present on admission.

- A POA indicator is assigned to the principal diagnosis, secondary diagnoses, and the external cause-of-injury codes.

- The POA guidelines are not intended to replace any of the other *ICD-10-CM Official Guidelines for Coding and Reporting*.

- The intent of the POA guidelines is not to determine whether or not a condition should be coded, but rather how to apply the POA indicator.

The following reporting options, with definitions, should be used to indicate whether a condition was POA:

Y   Yes: Present at the time of inpatient admission
N   No: Not present at the time of inpatient admission
U   Unknown: Documentation is insufficient to determine if condition is present at the time of inpatient admission
W   Clinically undetermined: Provider is unable to clinically determine whether condition was or was not present at the time of inpatient admission

Unreported/not used—(exempt from POA reporting)—Most ICD-10-CM codes require the assignment of a POA indicator. However, there are some diagnoses that are considered exempt from the POA reporting. For these exempt conditions the POA field should be left blank.

Note: *A data file of all POA exempt codes can be accessed at the following: http://www.optum360coding.com/ProductUpdates/ Title: "2021 ICD-10-CM for Hospitals POA Exemption Data File" Password: Hospital21*

Timeframe for POA identification and documentation

There is no timeframe during the encounter in which a condition must be diagnosed to be considered present on admission. In many cases, it is not clinically possible for the provider to determine a definitive diagnosis until well into the admission, after labs, imaging, and other tests have been performed and results examined. In these cases the condition is still considered to be present on admission, indicated with Y.

Examples

- A patient was admitted for diagnostic work-up for cachexia. The final diagnosis was malignant neoplasm of lung with metastasis.

   Assign Y in the POA field for the malignant neoplasm, which was clearly present on admission, although it was not diagnosed until after the admission occurred.

- A patient with severe cough and difficulty breathing was diagnosed during his hospitalization to have lung cancer.

   Assign Y in the POA field for the lung cancer. Even though the cancer was not diagnosed until after admission, it is a chronic condition that was clearly present before the patient's admission.

- A urine culture was obtained on admission. The provider documented urinary tract infection when the culture results became available a few days later.

   Assign Y to the urinary tract infection since the diagnosis is based on test results from a specimen obtained on admission. It may not be possible for a provider to make a definitive diagnosis for a period of time after admission. There is no required timeframe as to when a provider must identify or document a condition for it to be considered present on admission.

Condition is on the "Exempt from Reporting" list

The POA field is left blank for codes excluded from POA reporting.

Examples

- A patient was admitted for inpatient surgery on a burn contracture from scar tissue from a burn five years ago.

   Assign Y for the principal condition of the scar; however, the secondary code for the specifics of the burn injury with a seventh character for sequela is left blank since it is excluded from POA reporting.

- A patient was admitted to inpatient for a PEG tube insertion because of residual dysphagia due to a recent CVA.

   No POA indicator is assigned for the dysphagia following a CVA. Codes under I69.- are defined as sequela of cerebrovascular disease and are exempt from POA reporting.

- A patient was admitted to inpatient for corrective surgery for a malunion of a closed femur fracture.

   No POA indicator is assigned for the malunion of a closed fracture because the seventh character for malunion of fractures is considered a subsequent encounter and is exempt from POA reporting.

- A patient was admitted for breast reconstruction following mastectomy.

   The POA indicator field is left blank as this Z code is exempt from POA reporting.

- A patient was admitted for changing the battery in his AICD as it is at the end of its useful life.

   The POA indicator field is left blank as this Z code is exempt from POA reporting.

POA explicitly documented

If the provider explicitly documents a condition as being present on admission or not present on admission, assign the appropriate Y or N POA indicator based on that documentation. If there is conflicting documentation by different providers, query the attending physician.

Examples

- Even though sepsis is not diagnosed in the ED, the discharge summary states that the patient presented with sepsis at the time of admission.

   The provider explicitly stated that the sepsis was present on admission and therefore the Y POA indicator should be used.

- The patient was admitted with chills and cough and two days later diagnosed with pneumonia. The discharge summary documents that the pneumonia was not present on admission.

   Although the patient showed some symptoms of pneumonia on admission, the provider may have clinical evidence (e.g., chest x-rays, cultures) that indicates that pneumonia did not develop until after admission. Since this was explicitly stated in the discharge summary, the appropriate POA indicator is N.

- A consult note states that a patient came in with renal failure while the discharge summary states that the renal failure was not present on admission.

  When in doubt and there is conflicting documentation, query the attending physician.

Conditions diagnosed prior to inpatient admission

Conditions that were diagnosed prior to admission—for example, chronic conditions such as hypertension, diabetes, and asthma—are assigned the POA indicator of Y. A tip to help establish that a condition was POA is to check the patient's medication history for drugs that are routinely prescribed for these types of chronic conditions.

Examples

- The history and physical states that the patient has a history of hypertension and seizure disorder, and it is noted that the patient is currently on Atenolol and Dilantin.

  The hypertension and seizure disorder existed prior to admission; therefore, the appropriate POA indicator is Y. Verification that the patient is on long-term use of Atenolol and Dilantin can help solidify that these conditions are currently being treated.

- A 56-year-old male was admitted as an inpatient for multi-trauma wounds. Because the patient was unconscious on admission, his medical history was unknown. A progress note two days into the stay noted that the patient was on Metformin for history of type 2 diabetes.

  The timeframe of the diagnosis is irrelevant to POA. Even though it was not discovered until two days into the encounter that the patient had a history of DM2, the DM2 was still present prior to this admission and would be identified as such with the Y POA indicator.

- A patient was admitted to an inpatient facility from the ED. The admitting provider indicated that the patient had a current history of lung cancer and chronic kidney disease.

  Both of these conditions are indicated with Y, present on admission.

- During the course of an eight-day inpatient stay with surgery, a patient was diagnosed postoperatively with hypertension and discharged on Metoprolol.

  The hypertension was not diagnosed prior to admission and would be reported with an N POA indicator.

Conditions diagnosed during the admission but clearly present before admission

The POA indicator Y is assigned for conditions that clearly presented with applicable signs and symptoms but may have not been definitively diagnosed until later on, or even at the end of the encounter. Even if the presenting diagnosis was documented on admission as suspected, possible, or rule out, or written as a differential diagnosis and later confirmed, it is still considered present on admission.

Examples

- A patient was admitted with jaundice, fatigue, and mental confusion. Differential diagnosis on admission lists possible liver failure. The definitive diagnosis of liver failure is not made until two days after admission.

  Assign Y to the liver failure since the symptoms were present on admission and the differential diagnosis listed "possible" liver failure on admission even though the final diagnosis was two days later.

- An aid worker recently returned from Afghanistan presents to the ED with hematemesis, chest pain, and fever. Patient is put into inpatient isolation with suspected TB documented on the H & P. TB is confirmed the next day.

  The POA indicator Y is assigned because, even though the TB was only "suspected" on admission, it was confirmed the next day.

Condition develops during outpatient encounter prior to inpatient admission

Assign Y for any condition that develops during an outpatient encounter such as same-day surgery, observation, or extended recovery prior to a written order for inpatient admission. This also pertains to conditions that develop in

facilities such as transitional care units, skilled nursing homes, long-term care, hospice, or rehabilitation facilities with the patient transferring to inpatient hospital admission.

Examples

- A patient underwent outpatient surgery. During the recovery period, the patient developed atrial fibrillation and was subsequently admitted to the hospital as an inpatient.

  Assign Y on the POA field for the atrial fibrillation since it developed prior to a written order for inpatient admission.

- A patient was treated in observation and while in observation fell out of bed and broke a hip. The patient was subsequently admitted as an inpatient to treat the hip fracture.

  Assign Y on the POA field for the hip fracture since it developed prior to a written order for inpatient admission.

- An elderly patient underwent outpatient surgery with plans to go home after the surgery. In recovery, the patient developed shortness of breath, chest pain, and fever. A sputum sample was taken, and the surgeon decided to admit the patient to inpatient. The next day the patient was diagnosed with staphylococcal pneumonia based on sputum results and admitting chest x-ray.

  Assign Y to the staphylococcal pneumonia even though it was not diagnosed until the day following the admission. Even though the patient had undergone outpatient surgery, the sputum sample, signs, and symptoms were evident prior to the inpatient admission.

Documentation does not indicate whether condition was present on admission

If the documentation in the medical record is unclear as to the presence of a condition on admission, assign a U for unknown. This should be used sparingly and, if possible, the physician should be queried for further clarification.

Example

- A wheelchair-bound patient was admitted in respiratory failure from a long-term care facility to an inpatient hospital with severe aspiration pneumonia. A progress note three days into the admission listed a pressure ulcer stage 2 on the lower back.

  Assign U for the stage 2 pressure ulcer if unknown whether it was present on admission. Since the patient was wheelchair-bound and critically ill on admission, it is possible that the ulcer was present and not immediately addressed. The admitting physician can be queried to clarify, or a U is assigned if that is not possible.

Documentation states it cannot be determined whether the condition was or was not present on admission

A W is assigned when the documentation states that it cannot be clinically determined whether the condition was POA or not.

Examples

- An elderly patient was admitted with multi-trauma injuries from a motor vehicle accident. Two days into the admission, a urinary tract infection was diagnosed. No labs or urine cultures had been taken on admission as focus was stabilization from traumatic wounds. Documentation from the provider in a progress note stated that it was not clinically possible to determine whether the UTI was present on admission.

  Assign W for the UTI as it was specifically stated that it was not clinically possible to determine whether it was present on admission.

- A patient was admitted with high fever and pneumonia. The patient rapidly deteriorated and became septic. The discharge diagnosis listed sepsis and pneumonia. The documentation was unclear as to whether the sepsis was present on admission or developed shortly after admission.

  Query the physician as to whether the sepsis was present on admission, developed shortly after admission, or it cannot be clinically determined as to whether it was or was not present on admission.

Chronic condition with acute exacerbation during the admission

If a single code identifies only the chronic condition and not the acute exacerbation, assign Y. For instance, when there is no code for the acute exacerbation of a chronic condition as in acute exacerbation of chronic leukemia, the Y is assigned for the chronic leukemia.

For a single combination code that identifies both the chronic and acute exacerbation, see the combination code instructions.

Example

- Documentation on admission stated that the patient had chronic myelomonocytic leukemia. A progress note three days into the stay stated that the patient had, since admission, developed an acute exacerbation of his myelomonocytic leukemia.

  There is no code for an acute exacerbation of chronic myelomonocytic leukemia; therefore, assign Y since the chronic leukemia (either not specified as in remission, or in relapse) is represented by a single code and was present on admission.

Acute and chronic conditions

Assign Y to acute conditions present on admission and N to acute conditions not present at the time of admission.

Assign Y to conditions specified as chronic, even though they may not be diagnosed until after admission.

See the POA guideline "Codes that contain multiple clinical concepts" for a single code that identifies both the acute and chronic condition.

Examples

- A patient was admitted to the hospital for coronary artery bypass surgery. Postoperatively he developed a pulmonary embolism.

  Assign N in the POA field for the pulmonary embolism. This is an acute condition that was not present on admission.

- A patient admitted with sepsis due to pneumonia with acute respiratory failure, developed acute renal failure on day three.

  Assign Y for the sepsis, pneumonia, and acute respiratory failure, which were all acute conditions, present on admission. Assign N for the acute renal failure; even though it is an acute condition, it was not present until after the patient was admitted.

- A patient admitted with hypoglycemia, weakness, confusion, and slurred speech was diagnosed the next day with type 2 diabetes.

  Assign Y to the type 2 diabetes since it is a chronic condition that was present on admission, even though it was not diagnosed until the next day.

Codes that contain multiple clinical concepts

If at least one of the clinical concepts included in a code was not present on admission, assign N. If all the clinical concepts included in a code are present on admission, assign Y.

Examples

- Patient has history of gastrojejunal ulcer which started bleeding two days into the encounter.

  Assign a POA indicator of N to chronic gastrojejunal ulcer with bleeding; although the gastrojejunal ulcer is a chronic condition that was present at the time of admission, the bleeding did not occur until after the admission.

- A patient with chronic diastolic heart failure decompensated after admission.

  Assign N to the code for acute on chronic diastolic (congestive) heart failure. Although the heart failure was present on admission, the acute decompensation of the failure was not.

- A patient with viral hepatitis B progressed to hepatic coma after admission.

  Assign N for the viral hepatitis B with hepatic coma because a condition described by part of the code description did not develop until after admission.

- A patient with known systolic congestive heart failure was admitted to the hospital with decompensated systolic heart failure.

  Assign Y in the POA field for the acute on chronic systolic (congestive) heart failure as both the chronic and acute parts of the condition were present on admission.

Assign Y for infection codes that include the organism if the infection was present on admission even though the culture results are not available until after admission.

Example

- A patient was septic on admission with blood, sputum, and urine cultures taken. Two days later, *E. coli* was determined to be the causal organism.

  Assign Y even though the test results were not confirmed until after admission.

Conditions documented as possible, probable, suspected, or rule out at the time of discharge or conditions documented as impending or threatened at the time of discharge

If the final diagnosis contains language identifying a condition as possible, probable, suspected, or rule out, or as an impending or threatened diagnosis but the diagnosis is based on signs and symptoms that were present on admission, the POA indicator is Y. If those signs and symptoms were not present on admission, the appropriate POA indicator is N.

Examples

- A patient underwent inpatient surgery, after which the patient developed fever and was treated aggressively. The physician's final diagnosis documented "possible postoperative infection following surgery."

  Assign N on the POA field for the postoperative infection since final diagnoses that contain the terms "possible," "probable," "suspected," or "rule out" and that are based on symptoms or clinical findings that were not present on admission should be reported as N.

- A patient with prior cardiac intervention history was admitted with chest pain. After two days, the chest pain diminished with no underlying cause found. The discharge summary stated, "Suspected costochondritis or coronary artery spasm. Pain resolved. Follow up at regular cardiology office visit."

  Since the chest pain was present on admission, both suspected conditions of costochondritis and coronary artery spasm are represented by the POA indicator of Y.

- A patient was admitted with a known history of coronary atherosclerosis, status post myocardial infarction five years ago, and was then admitted for treatment of impending myocardial infarction. The patient was transferred to a larger facility with a cath lab. The final diagnosis was documented as "impending myocardial infarction."

  Assign Y to the impending myocardial infarction because the condition is present on admission.

Same diagnosis code for two or more conditions

When two or more separate conditions are classified to the same diagnosis code in the same encounter, assign Y if all conditions represented by the single code were present on admission and N if any of the conditions were not present on admission.

Examples

- A patient was admitted with diabetes type 2 with ketoacidosis.

  Assign Y since both the diabetes and ketoacidosis were present on admission.

- A patient involved in a car accident was admitted with hemorrhage to the abdomen secondary to the trauma; shortly after being admitted the patient also developed a seroma as a result of the trauma.

  The secondary traumatic hemorrhage was present on admission, and the traumatic seroma did not develop until after admission. Both of these conditions are classified to one code, but because both conditions were not present when the patient was admitted, a POA of N should be assigned.

Obstetrical conditions

The POA assignment for obstetrical conditions is not affected by whether the patient delivers during the encounter but rather by whether the pregnancy complication was or was not present at the time of admission. If two or more conditions are classified to a single code, all conditions represented by that single code must be present on admission to correctly assign a Y. If all conditions are not present at the time of admission, the appropriate POA indicator is N. Several obstetrics codes are listed in the POA exclusion list; for obstetrics codes that are not on the exclusion list, all applicable POA guidelines apply.

Examples

- A female patient was admitted to the hospital and underwent a normal delivery.

  Leave the "present on admission" (POA) field blank. Code O80 Normal delivery, is on the "exempt from reporting" list.
- A patient was admitted in late pregnancy due to excessive vomiting and dehydration. During admission, the patient went into premature labor.

  Assign Y for the excessive vomiting and the dehydration. Assign N for the premature labor.
- A patient was admitted in active labor. During the stay, a breast abscess was noted when the mother attempted to breastfeed. The provider was unable to clinically determine whether the abscess was present on admission.

  Assign W for the breast abscess since the provider was unable to clinically determine whether the abscess was present on admission.
- A patient was admitted in active labor. After 12 hours of labor, it was noted that the infant was in fetal distress, and a cesarean section was performed.

  Assign N for the fetal distress even if it is used for the principal diagnosis, since it did not develop until later in the admission. In obstetrics cases, the principal diagnosis may have a POA indicator of N.

Perinatal and congenital conditions

Newborns are not considered admitted until after birth; therefore all conditions that develop in utero, occur during delivery, or are present at birth are represented by the POA indicator Y. Any conditions that develop after birth and admission are represented by N.

All congenital conditions and anomalies not found in chapter 17 should have a POA indicator of Y assigned. Chapter 17 codes in categories Q00–Q99 are exempt from POA reporting. All congenital conditions, regardless of the coding chapter to which they are assigned, are considered present on admission.

Examples

- A single liveborn infant was delivered in the hospital via cesarean section. The physician documented fetal bradycardia during labor as the final diagnosis in the newborn record.

  Assign Y because the bradycardia developed prior to the newborn admission (birth).
- A newborn developed diarrhea, which was believed to be due to the hospital baby formula.

  Assign N because the diarrhea developed after admission.
- A newborn was diagnosed with cephalhematoma due to birth injury.

  Assign Y because the injury occurred during delivery.
- A newborn was diagnosed with congenital pneumonia.

  Assign Y for the congenital pneumonia. Congenital conditions from chapter 16 are always considered present on admission and require the POA indicator.
- A newborn was diagnosed with congenital hydrocephalus.

  There should be no POA indicator assigned. This condition is coded in chapter 17 and is excluded from POA reporting.
- A 10-year-old boy was admitted for complications of spina bifida with hydrocephalus.

  No POA indicator is assigned. This condition is coded in chapter 17 and is excluded from POA reporting.

External cause and injury codes

If an injury or poisoning occurred prior to or at the time of admission and the seventh character indicates an initial encounter or active treatment, the code for the injury/poisoning is reported with POA indicator Y. Injury and poisoning codes S00–T88 with the seventh character indicating subsequent or sequela

are exempt from POA indicators since, in order to be a subsequent or sequela encounter, the condition must have occurred before the admission. Many of the external causes of morbidity codes from chapters V, W, and X are also exempt from POA reporting when the seventh character of S or D, representing subsequent or sequela encounters, are used.

Coders should be extremely careful in assigning the appropriate POA indicator if a patient suffers an injury while an inpatient. For example, if a patient falls from the hospital bed and fractures a hip, the codes representing that injury (along with the appropriate initial-encounter seventh character) should be assigned N for the corresponding POA indicator.

Examples

- A 12-year-old was admitted for treatment of fractured arm from falling out of a tree house.

  The injury itself and the cause of the injury are both assigned a Y POA indicator.
  Note: *The injury code and external cause code POA indicators should always match.*
- A patient admitted for pneumonia sustained a laceration of the right arm after falling and hitting his arm against a cart in the hospital room, requiring stitches.

  Assign N for the laceration for the right arm because it was not present on admission. The external cause code POA indicator should also be N.
- A patient was admitted for manipulation of a knee contracture due to a scar from a burn injury 10 years ago.

  Assign Y for the code for the scar, but leave blank the POA indicator for the burn injury with the seventh character of S for sequela. Sequela and subsequent-encounter codes in chapter 19 are exempt from POA reporting.

Appendix G: Hospital Acquired Conditions

Hospital-acquired conditions (HACs) are conditions considered reasonably preventable through the application of evidence-based guidelines. These conditions, in and of themselves, are either a complication or comorbidity (CC) or major complication or comorbidity (MCC) that as a secondary diagnosis will move the MS-DRG assignment from a lower-paying MS-DRG to a higher-paying MS-DRG. However, if these conditions are not present on admission (meaning they developed during the hospital stay), the CC or MCC designation is nullified and the case will not group to the higher-paying MS-DRG based solely upon the reporting of the HAC code.

HACs are grouped into 14 categories. ICD-10-CM codes in the tabular section of this book that are grouped to one of these HAC categories are identified by an icon specific to that category. As many of these HACs are conditional, this resource provides any additional stipulations that may be required before the code can be considered a HAC. For example, code I26.02 has an 🔟 indicating it falls in the HAC 10 category for Deep Vein Thrombosis (DVT) or Pulmonary Embolism (PE) with Total Knee or Hip Replacement. However I26.02 is not, by itself, a HAC there must also be a specific ICD-10-PCS code, such as 0SR9019 Replacement of Right Hip Joint with Metal Synthetic Substitute, Cemented, Open Approach, applied in order for I26.02 to act as a HAC.

Note: The resource used to compile this list is based on the proposed, version 38, MS-DRG Grouper software and Definitions Manual files published with the fiscal 2021 IPPS proposed rule. The final, version 38, MS-DRG Grouper files and MS-DRG Definitions Manual files can be found at the following: https://www.cms.gov/Medicare/Medicare-Fee-for-Service-Payment/AcuteInpatientPPS/IPPS-Regulations-and-Notices.html.

HAC 01: Foreign Object Retained After Surgery
Secondary diagnosis not POA:

T81.500A
T81.501A
T81.502A
T81.503A
T81.504A
T81.505A
T81.506A
T81.507A
T81.508A
T81.509A
T81.510A
T81.511A
T81.512A
T81.513A
T81.514A
T81.515A
T81.516A
T81.517A
T81.518A
T81.519A
T81.520A
T81.521A
T81.522A
T81.523A
T81.524A
T81.525A
T81.526A
T81.527A
T81.528A
T81.529A
T81.530A
T81.531A
T81.532A
T81.533A
T81.534A
T81.535A
T81.536A
T81.537A
T81.538A
T81.539A
T81.590A
T81.591A
T81.592A
T81.593A
T81.594A
T81.595A
T81.596A
T81.597A
T81.598A
T81.599A
T81.60XA
T81.61XA
T81.69XA

HAC 02: Air Embolism
Secondary diagnosis not POA:

T80.0XXA

HAC 03: Blood Incompatibility
Secondary diagnosis not POA:

T80.30XA
T80.310A
T80.311A
T80.319A
T80.39XA

HAC 04: Stage III and IV Pressure Ulcers
Secondary diagnosis not POA:

L89.003
L89.004
L89.013
L89.014
L89.023
L89.024
L89.103
L89.104
L89.113
L89.114
L89.123
L89.124
L89.133
L89.134
L89.143
L89.144
L89.153
L89.154
L89.203
L89.204
L89.213
L89.214
L89.223
L89.224
L89.303
L89.304
L89.313
L89.314
L89.323
L89.324
L89.43
L89.44
L89.503
L89.504
L89.513
L89.514
L89.523
L89.524

L89.603
L89.604
L89.613
L89.614
L89.623
L89.624
L89.813
L89.814
L89.893
L89.894
L89.93
L89.94

HAC 05: Falls and Trauma
Secondary diagnosis not POA:

M99.10
M99.11
M99.18
S02.0XXA
S02.0XXB
S02.101A
S02.101B
S02.102A
S02.102B
S02.109A
S02.109B
S02.110A
S02.110B
S02.111A
S02.111B
S02.112A
S02.112B
S02.113A
S02.113B
S02.118A
S02.118B
S02.119A
S02.119B
S02.11AA
S02.11AB
S02.11BA
S02.11BB
S02.11CA
S02.11CB
S02.11DA
S02.11DB
S02.11EA
S02.11EB
S02.11FA
S02.11FB
S02.11GA
S02.11GB
S02.11HA
S02.11HB
S02.121A

S02.121B
S02.122A
S02.122B
S02.129A
S02.129B
S02.19XA
S02.19XB
S02.2XXB
S02.30XA
S02.30XB
S02.31XA
S02.31XB
S02.32XA
S02.32XB
S02.400A
S02.400B
S02.401A
S02.401B
S02.402A
S02.402B
S02.40AA
S02.40AB
S02.40BA
S02.40BB
S02.40CA
S02.40CB
S02.40DA
S02.40DB
S02.40EA
S02.40EB
S02.40FA
S02.40FB
S02.411A
S02.411B
S02.412A
S02.412B
S02.413A
S02.413B
S02.42XA
S02.42XB
S02.600A
S02.600B
S02.601A
S02.601B
S02.602A
S02.602B
S02.609A
S02.609B
S02.610A
S02.610B
S02.611A
S02.611B
S02.612A
S02.612B
S02.620A
S02.620B
S02.621A

S02.621B
S02.622A
S02.622B
S02.630A
S02.630B
S02.631A
S02.631B
S02.632A
S02.632B
S02.640A
S02.640B
S02.641A
S02.641B
S02.642A
S02.642B
S02.650A
S02.650B
S02.651A
S02.651B
S02.652A
S02.652B
S02.66XA
S02.66XB
S02.670A
S02.670B
S02.671A
S02.671B
S02.672A
S02.672B
S02.69XA
S02.69XB
S02.80XA
S02.80XB
S02.81XA
S02.81XB
S02.82XA
S02.82XB
S02.831A
S02.831B
S02.832A
S02.832B
S02.839A
S02.839B
S02.841A
S02.841B
S02.842A
S02.842B
S02.849A
S02.849B
S02.85XA
S02.85XB
S02.91XA
S02.91XB
S02.92XA
S02.92XB
S06.0X1A
S06.0X9A

S06.1X1A
S06.1X2A
S06.1X3A
S06.1X4A
S06.1X5A
S06.1X6A
S06.1X7A
S06.1X8A
S06.1X9A
S06.2X1A
S06.2X2A
S06.2X3A
S06.2X4A
S06.2X5A
S06.2X6A
S06.2X7A
S06.2X8A
S06.2X9A
S06.301A
S06.302A
S06.303A
S06.304A
S06.305A
S06.306A
S06.307A
S06.308A
S06.309A
S06.310A
S06.311A
S06.312A
S06.313A
S06.314A
S06.315A
S06.316A
S06.317A
S06.318A
S06.319A
S06.320A
S06.321A
S06.322A
S06.323A
S06.324A
S06.325A
S06.326A
S06.327A
S06.328A
S06.329A
S06.330A
S06.331A
S06.332A
S06.333A
S06.334A
S06.335A
S06.336A
S06.337A
S06.338A
S06.339A

HAC 05: Falls and Trauma (continued)

S06.340A	S06.6X5A	S12.121A	S12.531B	S14.135A	S22.062A
S06.341A	S06.6X6A	S12.121B	S12.54XA	S14.136A	S22.062B
S06.342A	S06.6X7A	S12.130A	S12.54XB	S14.137A	S22.068A
S06.343A	S06.6X8A	S12.130B	S12.550A	S14.151A	S22.068B
S06.344A	S06.6X9A	S12.131A	S12.550B	S14.152A	S22.069A
S06.345A	S06.811A	S12.131B	S12.551A	S14.153A	S22.069B
S06.346A	S06.812A	S12.14XA	S12.551B	S14.154A	S22.070A
S06.347A	S06.813A	S12.14XB	S12.590A	S14.155A	S22.070B
S06.348A	S06.814A	S12.150A	S12.590B	S14.156A	S22.071A
S06.349A	S06.815A	S12.150B	S12.591A	S14.157A	S22.071B
S06.350A	S06.816A	S12.151A	S12.591B	S17.0XXA	S22.072A
S06.351A	S06.817A	S12.151B	S12.600A	S17.8XXA	S22.072B
S06.352A	S06.818A	S12.190A	S12.600B	S17.9XXA	S22.078A
S06.353A	S06.819A	S12.190B	S12.601A	S22.000A	S22.078B
S06.354A	S06.821A	S12.191A	S12.601B	S22.000B	S22.079A
S06.355A	S06.822A	S12.191B	S12.630A	S22.001A	S22.079B
S06.356A	S06.823A	S12.200A	S12.630B	S22.001B	S22.080A
S06.357A	S06.824A	S12.200B	S12.631A	S22.002A	S22.080B
S06.358A	S06.825A	S12.201A	S12.631B	S22.002B	S22.081A
S06.359A	S06.826A	S12.201B	S12.64XA	S22.008A	S22.081B
S06.360A	S06.827A	S12.230A	S12.64XB	S22.008B	S22.082A
S06.361A	S06.828A	S12.230B	S12.650A	S22.009A	S22.082B
S06.362A	S06.829A	S12.231A	S12.650B	S22.009B	S22.088A
S06.363A	S06.891A	S12.231B	S12.651A	S22.010A	S22.088B
S06.364A	S06.892A	S12.24XA	S12.651B	S22.010B	S22.089A
S06.365A	S06.893A	S12.24XB	S12.690A	S22.011A	S22.089B
S06.366A	S06.894A	S12.250A	S12.690B	S22.011B	S22.20XA
S06.367A	S06.895A	S12.250B	S12.691A	S22.012A	S22.20XB
S06.368A	S06.896A	S12.251A	S12.691B	S22.012B	S22.21XA
S06.369A	S06.897A	S12.251B	S12.8XXA	S22.018A	S22.21XB
S06.370A	S06.898A	S12.290A	S12.9XXA	S22.018B	S22.22XA
S06.371A	S06.899A	S12.290B	S13.0XXA	S22.019A	S22.22XB
S06.372A	S06.9X1A	S12.291A	S13.100A	S22.019B	S22.23XA
S06.373A	S06.9X2A	S12.291B	S13.101A	S22.020A	S22.23XB
S06.374A	S06.9X3A	S12.300A	S13.110A	S22.020B	S22.24XA
S06.375A	S06.9X4A	S12.300B	S13.111A	S22.021A	S22.24XB
S06.376A	S06.9X5A	S12.301A	S13.120A	S22.021B	S22.31XA
S06.377A	S06.9X6A	S12.301B	S13.121A	S22.022A	S22.31XB
S06.378A	S06.9X7A	S12.330A	S13.130A	S22.022B	S22.32XA
S06.379A	S06.9X8A	S12.330B	S13.131A	S22.028A	S22.32XB
S06.380A	S06.9X9A	S12.331A	S13.140A	S22.028B	S22.39XA
S06.381A	S07.0XXA	S12.331B	S13.141A	S22.029A	S22.39XB
S06.382A	S07.1XXA	S12.34XA	S13.150A	S22.029B	S22.41XA
S06.383A	S07.8XXA	S12.34XB	S13.151A	S22.030A	S22.41XB
S06.384A	S07.9XXA	S12.350A	S13.160A	S22.030B	S22.42XA
S06.385A	S12.000A	S12.350B	S13.161A	S22.031A	S22.42XB
S06.386A	S12.000B	S12.351A	S13.170A	S22.031B	S22.43XA
S06.387A	S12.001A	S12.351B	S13.171A	S22.032A	S22.43XB
S06.388A	S12.001B	S12.390A	S13.180A	S22.032B	S22.49XA
S06.389A	S12.01XA	S12.390B	S13.181A	S22.038A	S22.49XB
S06.4X0A	S12.01XB	S12.391A	S13.20XA	S22.038B	S22.5XXA
S06.4X1A	S12.02XA	S12.391B	S13.29XA	S22.039A	S22.5XXB
S06.4X2A	S12.02XB	S12.400A	S14.101A	S22.039B	S22.9XXA
S06.4X3A	S12.030A	S12.400B	S14.102A	S22.040A	S22.9XXB
S06.4X4A	S12.030B	S12.401A	S14.103A	S22.040B	S24.101A
S06.4X5A	S12.031A	S12.401B	S14.104A	S22.041A	S24.102A
S06.4X6A	S12.031B	S12.430A	S14.105A	S22.041B	S24.103A
S06.4X7A	S12.040A	S12.430B	S14.106A	S22.042A	S24.104A
S06.4X8A	S12.040B	S12.431A	S14.107A	S22.042B	S24.111A
S06.4X9A	S12.041A	S12.431B	S14.111A	S22.048A	S24.112A
S06.5X0A	S12.041B	S12.44XA	S14.112A	S22.048B	S24.113A
S06.5X1A	S12.090A	S12.44XB	S14.113A	S22.049A	S24.114A
S06.5X2A	S12.090B	S12.450A	S14.114A	S22.049B	S24.131A
S06.5X3A	S12.091A	S12.450B	S14.115A	S22.050A	S24.132A
S06.5X4A	S12.091B	S12.451A	S14.116A	S22.050B	S24.133A
S06.5X5A	S12.100A	S12.451B	S14.117A	S22.051A	S24.134A
S06.5X6A	S12.100B	S12.490A	S14.121A	S22.051B	S24.151A
S06.5X7A	S12.101A	S12.490B	S14.122A	S22.052A	S24.152A
S06.5X8A	S12.101B	S12.491A	S14.123A	S22.052B	S24.153A
S06.5X9A	S12.110A	S12.491B	S14.124A	S22.058A	S24.154A
S06.6X0A	S12.110B	S12.500A	S14.125A	S22.058B	S32.000A
S06.6X1A	S12.111A	S12.500B	S14.126A	S22.059A	S32.000B
S06.6X2A	S12.111B	S12.501A	S14.127A	S22.059B	S32.001A
S06.6X3A	S12.112A	S12.501B	S14.131A	S22.060A	S32.001B
S06.6X4A	S12.112B	S12.530A	S14.132A	S22.060B	S32.002A
	S12.120A	S12.530B	S14.133A	S22.061A	S32.002B
	S12.120B	S12.531A	S14.134A	S22.061B	S32.008A

HAC 05: Falls and Trauma (continued)

S32.008B	S32.132A	S32.434B	S32.511A	S42.017B	S42.225A
S32.009A	S32.132B	S32.435A	S32.511B	S42.018B	S42.225B
S32.009B	S32.139A	S32.435B	S32.512A	S42.019B	S42.226B
S32.010A	S32.139B	S32.436A	S32.512B	S42.021B	S42.231A
S32.010B	S32.14XA	S32.436B	S32.519A	S42.022B	S42.231B
S32.011A	S32.14XB	S32.441A	S32.519B	S42.023B	S42.232A
S32.011B	S32.15XA	S32.441B	S32.591A	S42.024B	S42.232B
S32.012A	S32.15XB	S32.442A	S32.591B	S42.025B	S42.239A
S32.012B	S32.16XA	S32.442B	S32.592A	S42.026B	S42.239B
S32.018A	S32.16XB	S32.443A	S32.592B	S42.031B	S42.241A
S32.018B	S32.17XA	S32.443B	S32.599A	S42.032B	S42.241B
S32.019A	S32.17XB	S32.444A	S32.599B	S42.033B	S42.242A
S32.019B	S32.19XA	S32.444B	S32.601A	S42.034B	S42.242B
S32.020A	S32.19XB	S32.445A	S32.601B	S42.035B	S42.249A
S32.020B	S32.2XXA	S32.445B	S32.602A	S42.036B	S42.249B
S32.021A	S32.2XXB	S32.446A	S32.602B	S42.101B	S42.251A
S32.021B	S32.301A	S32.446B	S32.609A	S42.102B	S42.251B
S32.022A	S32.301B	S32.451A	S32.609B	S42.109B	S42.252A
S32.022B	S32.302A	S32.451B	S32.611A	S42.111B	S42.252B
S32.028A	S32.302B	S32.452A	S32.611B	S42.112B	S42.253A
S32.028B	S32.309A	S32.452B	S32.612A	S42.113B	S42.253B
S32.029A	S32.309B	S32.453A	S32.612B	S42.114B	S42.254A
S32.029B	S32.311A	S32.453B	S32.613A	S42.115B	S42.254B
S32.030A	S32.311B	S32.454A	S32.613B	S42.116B	S42.255A
S32.030B	S32.312A	S32.454B	S32.614A	S42.121B	S42.255B
S32.031A	S32.312B	S32.455A	S32.614B	S42.122B	S42.256A
S32.031B	S32.313A	S32.455B	S32.615A	S42.123B	S42.256B
S32.032A	S32.313B	S32.456A	S32.615B	S42.124B	S42.261A
S32.032B	S32.314A	S32.456B	S32.616A	S42.125B	S42.261B
S32.038A	S32.314B	S32.461A	S32.616B	S42.126B	S42.262A
S32.038B	S32.315A	S32.461B	S32.691A	S42.131B	S42.262B
S32.039A	S32.315B	S32.462A	S32.691B	S42.132B	S42.263A
S32.039B	S32.316A	S32.462B	S32.692A	S42.133B	S42.263B
S32.040A	S32.316B	S32.463A	S32.692B	S42.134B	S42.264A
S32.040B	S32.391A	S32.463B	S32.699A	S42.135B	S42.264B
S32.041A	S32.391B	S32.464A	S32.699B	S42.136B	S42.265A
S32.041B	S32.392A	S32.464B	S32.810A	S42.141B	S42.265B
S32.042A	S32.392B	S32.465A	S32.810B	S42.142B	S42.266A
S32.042B	S32.399A	S32.465B	S32.811A	S42.143B	S42.266B
S32.048A	S32.399B	S32.466A	S32.811B	S42.144B	S42.271A
S32.048B	S32.401A	S32.466B	S32.82XA	S42.145B	S42.272A
S32.049A	S32.401B	S32.471A	S32.82XB	S42.146B	S42.279A
S32.049B	S32.402A	S32.471B	S32.89XA	S42.151B	S42.291A
S32.050A	S32.402B	S32.472A	S32.89XB	S42.152B	S42.291B
S32.050B	S32.409A	S32.472B	S32.9XXA	S42.153B	S42.292A
S32.051A	S32.409B	S32.473A	S32.9XXB	S42.154B	S42.292B
S32.051B	S32.411A	S32.473B	S34.101A	S42.155B	S42.293A
S32.052A	S32.411B	S32.474A	S34.102A	S42.156B	S42.293B
S32.052B	S32.412A	S32.474B	S34.103A	S42.191B	S42.294A
S32.058A	S32.412B	S32.475A	S34.104A	S42.192B	S42.294B
S32.058B	S32.413A	S32.475B	S34.105A	S42.199B	S42.295A
S32.059A	S32.413B	S32.476A	S34.109A	S42.201A	S42.295B
S32.059B	S32.414A	S32.476B	S34.111A	S42.201B	S42.296A
S32.10XA	S32.414B	S32.481A	S34.112A	S42.202A	S42.296B
S32.10XB	S32.415A	S32.481B	S34.113A	S42.202B	S42.301A
S32.110A	S32.415B	S32.482A	S34.114A	S42.209A	S42.301B
S32.110B	S32.416A	S32.482B	S34.115A	S42.209B	S42.302A
S32.111A	S32.416B	S32.483A	S34.119A	S42.211A	S42.302B
S32.111B	S32.421A	S32.483B	S34.121A	S42.211B	S42.309A
S32.112A	S32.421B	S32.484A	S34.122A	S42.212A	S42.309B
S32.112B	S32.422A	S32.484B	S34.123A	S42.212B	S42.311A
S32.119A	S32.422B	S32.485A	S34.124A	S42.213A	S42.312A
S32.119B	S32.423A	S32.485B	S34.125A	S42.213B	S42.319A
S32.120A	S32.423B	S32.486A	S34.129A	S42.214A	S42.321A
S32.120B	S32.424A	S32.486B	S34.131A	S42.214B	S42.321B
S32.121A	S32.424B	S32.491A	S34.132A	S42.215A	S42.322A
S32.121B	S32.425A	S32.491B	S34.139A	S42.215B	S42.322B
S32.122A	S32.425B	S32.492A	S34.3XXA	S42.216A	S42.323A
S32.122B	S32.426A	S32.492B	S42.001B	S42.216B	S42.323B
S32.129A	S32.426B	S32.499A	S42.002B	S42.221A	S42.324A
S32.129B	S32.431A	S32.499B	S42.009B	S42.221B	S42.324B
S32.130A	S32.431B	S32.501A	S42.011B	S42.222A	S42.325A
S32.130B	S32.432A	S32.501B	S42.012B	S42.222B	S42.325B
S32.131A	S32.432B	S32.502A	S42.013B	S42.223A	S42.326A
S32.131B	S32.433A	S32.502B	S42.014B	S42.223B	S42.326B
	S32.433B	S32.509A	S42.015B	S42.224A	S42.331A
	S32.434A	S32.509B	S42.016B	S42.224B	

HAC 05: Falls and Trauma (continued)

S42.331B	S42.423A	S42.491A	S52.009C	S52.136B	S52.252A
S42.332A	S42.423B	S42.491B	S52.011A	S52.136C	S52.252B
S42.332B	S42.424A	S42.492A	S52.012A	S52.181B	S52.252C
S42.333A	S42.424B	S42.492B	S52.019A	S52.181C	S52.253A
S42.333B	S42.425A	S42.493A	S52.021B	S52.182B	S52.253B
S42.334A	S42.425B	S42.493B	S52.021C	S52.182C	S52.253C
S42.334B	S42.426A	S42.494A	S52.022B	S52.189B	S52.254A
S42.335A	S42.426B	S42.494B	S52.022C	S52.189C	S52.254B
S42.335B	S42.431A	S42.495A	S52.023B	S52.201A	S52.254C
S42.336A	S42.431B	S42.495B	S52.023C	S52.201B	S52.255A
S42.336B	S42.432A	S42.496A	S52.024B	S52.201C	S52.255B
S42.341A	S42.432B	S42.496B	S52.024C	S52.202A	S52.255C
S42.341B	S42.433A	S42.90XA	S52.025B	S52.202B	S52.256A
S42.342A	S42.433B	S42.90XB	S52.025C	S52.202C	S52.256B
S42.342B	S42.434A	S42.91XA	S52.026B	S52.209A	S52.256C
S42.343A	S42.434B	S42.91XB	S52.026C	S52.209B	S52.261A
S42.343B	S42.435A	S42.92XA	S52.031B	S52.209C	S52.261B
S42.344A	S42.435B	S42.92XB	S52.031C	S52.211A	S52.261C
S42.344B	S42.436A	S43.201A	S52.032B	S52.212A	S52.262A
S42.345A	S42.436B	S43.202A	S52.032C	S52.219A	S52.262B
S42.345B	S42.441A	S43.203A	S52.033B	S52.221A	S52.262C
S42.346A	S42.441B	S43.204A	S52.033C	S52.221B	S52.263A
S42.346B	S42.442A	S43.205A	S52.034B	S52.221C	S52.263B
S42.351A	S42.442B	S43.206A	S52.034C	S52.222A	S52.263C
S42.351B	S42.443A	S43.211A	S52.035B	S52.222B	S52.264A
S42.352A	S42.443B	S43.212A	S52.035C	S52.222C	S52.264B
S42.352B	S42.444A	S43.213A	S52.036B	S52.223A	S52.264C
S42.353A	S42.444B	S43.214A	S52.036C	S52.223B	S52.265A
S42.353B	S42.445A	S43.215A	S52.041B	S52.223C	S52.265B
S42.354A	S42.445B	S43.216A	S52.041C	S52.224A	S52.265C
S42.354B	S42.446A	S43.221A	S52.042B	S52.224B	S52.266A
S42.355A	S42.446B	S43.222A	S52.042C	S52.224C	S52.266B
S42.355B	S42.447A	S43.223A	S52.043B	S52.225A	S52.266C
S42.356A	S42.447B	S43.224A	S52.043C	S52.225B	S52.271B
S42.356B	S42.448A	S43.225A	S52.044B	S52.225C	S52.271C
S42.361A	S42.448B	S43.226A	S52.044C	S52.226A	S52.272B
S42.361B	S42.449A	S49.001A	S52.045B	S52.226B	S52.272C
S42.362A	S42.449B	S49.002A	S52.045C	S52.226C	S52.279B
S42.362B	S42.451A	S49.009A	S52.046B	S52.231A	S52.279C
S42.363A	S42.451B	S49.011A	S52.046C	S52.231B	S52.281A
S42.363B	S42.452A	S49.012A	S52.091B	S52.231C	S52.281B
S42.364A	S42.452B	S49.019A	S52.091C	S52.232A	S52.281C
S42.364B	S42.453A	S49.021A	S52.092B	S52.232B	S52.282A
S42.365A	S42.453B	S49.022A	S52.092C	S52.232C	S52.282B
S42.365B	S42.454A	S49.029A	S52.099B	S52.233A	S52.282C
S42.366A	S42.454B	S49.031A	S52.099C	S52.233B	S52.283A
S42.366B	S42.455A	S49.032A	S52.101B	S52.233C	S52.283B
S42.391A	S42.455B	S49.039A	S52.101C	S52.234A	S52.283C
S42.391B	S42.456A	S49.041A	S52.102B	S52.234B	S52.291A
S42.392A	S42.456B	S49.042A	S52.102C	S52.234C	S52.291B
S42.392B	S42.461A	S49.049A	S52.109B	S52.235A	S52.291C
S42.399A	S42.461B	S49.091A	S52.109C	S52.235B	S52.292A
S42.399B	S42.462A	S49.092A	S52.111A	S52.235C	S52.292B
S42.401A	S42.462B	S49.099A	S52.112A	S52.236A	S52.292C
S42.401B	S42.463A	S49.101A	S52.119A	S52.236B	S52.299A
S42.402A	S42.463B	S49.102A	S52.121B	S52.236C	S52.299B
S42.402B	S42.464A	S49.109A	S52.121C	S52.241A	S52.299C
S42.409A	S42.464B	S49.111A	S52.122B	S52.241B	S52.301A
S42.409B	S42.465A	S49.112A	S52.122C	S52.241C	S52.301B
S42.411A	S42.465B	S49.119A	S52.123B	S52.242A	S52.301C
S42.411B	S42.466A	S49.121A	S52.123C	S52.242B	S52.302A
S42.412A	S42.466B	S49.122A	S52.124B	S52.242C	S52.302B
S42.412B	S42.471A	S49.129A	S52.124C	S52.243A	S52.302C
S42.413A	S42.471B	S49.131A	S52.125B	S52.243B	S52.309A
S42.413B	S42.472A	S49.132A	S52.125C	S52.243C	S52.309B
S42.414A	S42.472B	S49.139A	S52.126B	S52.244A	S52.309C
S42.414B	S42.473A	S49.141A	S52.126C	S52.244B	S52.311A
S42.415A	S42.473B	S49.142A	S52.131B	S52.244C	S52.312A
S42.415B	S42.474A	S49.149A	S52.131C	S52.245A	S52.319A
S42.416A	S42.474B	S49.191A	S52.132B	S52.245B	S52.321A
S42.416B	S42.475A	S49.192A	S52.132C	S52.245C	S52.321B
S42.421A	S42.475B	S49.199A	S52.133B	S52.246A	S52.321C
S42.421B	S42.476A	S52.001B	S52.133C	S52.246B	S52.322A
S42.422A	S42.476B	S52.001C	S52.134B	S52.246C	S52.322B
S42.422B	S42.481A	S52.002B	S52.134C	S52.251A	S52.322C
	S42.482A	S52.002C	S52.135B	S52.251B	S52.323A
	S42.489A	S52.009B	S52.135C	S52.251C	S52.323B

HAC 05: Falls and Trauma (continued)

S52.323C	S52.364C	S52.542B	S52.699A	S62.116B	S62.301B
S52.324A	S52.365A	S52.542C	S52.699B	S62.121B	S62.302B
S52.324B	S52.365B	S52.549A	S52.699C	S62.122B	S62.303B
S52.324C	S52.365C	S52.549B	S52.90XA	S62.123B	S62.304B
S52.325A	S52.366A	S52.549C	S52.90XB	S62.124B	S62.305B
S52.325B	S52.366B	S52.551A	S52.90XC	S62.125B	S62.306B
S52.325C	S52.366C	S52.551B	S52.91XA	S62.126B	S62.307B
S52.326A	S52.371A	S52.551C	S52.91XB	S62.131B	S62.308B
S52.326B	S52.371B	S52.552A	S52.91XC	S62.132B	S62.309B
S52.326C	S52.371C	S52.552B	S52.92XA	S62.133B	S62.310B
S52.331A	S52.372A	S52.552C	S52.92XB	S62.134B	S62.311B
S52.331B	S52.372B	S52.559A	S52.92XC	S62.135B	S62.312B
S52.331C	S52.372C	S52.559B	S59.001A	S62.136B	S62.313B
S52.332A	S52.379A	S52.559C	S59.002A	S62.141B	S62.314B
S52.332B	S52.379B	S52.561A	S59.009A	S62.142B	S62.315B
S52.332C	S52.379C	S52.561B	S59.011A	S62.143B	S62.316B
S52.333A	S52.381A	S52.561C	S59.012A	S62.144B	S62.317B
S52.333B	S52.381B	S52.562A	S59.019A	S62.145B	S62.318B
S52.333C	S52.381C	S52.562B	S59.021A	S62.146B	S62.319B
S52.334A	S52.382A	S52.562C	S59.022A	S62.151B	S62.320B
S52.334B	S52.382B	S52.569A	S59.029A	S62.152B	S62.321B
S52.334C	S52.382C	S52.569B	S59.031A	S62.153B	S62.322B
S52.335A	S52.389A	S52.569C	S59.032A	S62.154B	S62.323B
S52.335B	S52.389B	S52.571A	S59.039A	S62.155B	S62.324B
S52.335C	S52.389C	S52.571B	S59.041A	S62.156B	S62.325B
S52.336A	S52.391A	S52.571C	S59.042A	S62.161B	S62.326B
S52.336B	S52.391B	S52.572A	S59.049A	S62.162B	S62.327B
S52.336C	S52.391C	S52.572B	S59.091A	S62.163B	S62.328B
S52.341A	S52.392A	S52.572C	S59.092A	S62.164B	S62.329B
S52.341B	S52.392B	S52.579A	S59.099A	S62.165B	S62.330B
S52.341C	S52.392C	S52.579B	S59.201A	S62.166B	S62.331B
S52.342A	S52.399A	S52.579C	S59.202A	S62.171B	S62.332B
S52.342B	S52.399B	S52.591A	S59.209A	S62.172B	S62.333B
S52.342C	S52.399C	S52.591B	S59.211A	S62.173B	S62.334B
S52.343A	S52.501A	S52.591C	S59.212A	S62.174B	S62.335B
S52.343B	S52.501B	S52.592A	S59.219A	S62.175B	S62.336B
S52.343C	S52.501C	S52.592B	S59.221A	S62.176B	S62.337B
S52.344A	S52.502A	S52.592C	S59.222A	S62.181B	S62.338B
S52.344B	S52.502B	S52.599A	S59.229A	S62.182B	S62.339B
S52.344C	S52.502C	S52.599B	S59.231A	S62.183B	S62.340B
S52.345A	S52.509A	S52.599C	S59.232A	S62.184B	S62.341B
S52.345B	S52.509B	S52.601B	S59.239A	S62.185B	S62.342B
S52.345C	S52.509C	S52.601C	S59.241A	S62.186B	S62.343B
S52.346A	S52.511A	S52.602A	S59.242A	S62.201B	S62.344B
S52.346B	S52.511B	S52.602B	S59.249A	S62.202B	S62.345B
S52.346C	S52.511C	S52.602C	S59.291A	S62.209B	S62.346B
S52.351A	S52.512A	S52.609A	S59.292A	S62.211B	S62.347B
S52.351B	S52.512B	S52.609B	S59.299A	S62.212B	S62.348B
S52.351C	S52.512C	S52.609C	S62.001B	S62.213B	S62.349B
S52.352A	S52.513A	S52.611A	S62.002B	S62.221B	S62.350B
S52.352B	S52.513B	S52.611B	S62.009B	S62.222B	S62.351B
S52.352C	S52.513C	S52.611C	S62.011B	S62.223B	S62.352B
S52.353A	S52.514A	S52.612A	S62.012B	S62.224B	S62.353B
S52.353B	S52.514B	S52.612B	S62.013B	S62.225B	S62.354B
S52.353C	S52.514C	S52.612C	S62.014B	S62.226B	S62.355B
S52.354A	S52.515A	S52.613A	S62.015B	S62.231B	S62.356B
S52.354B	S52.515B	S52.613B	S62.016B	S62.232B	S62.357B
S52.354C	S52.515C	S52.613C	S62.021B	S62.233B	S62.358B
S52.355A	S52.516A	S52.614A	S62.022B	S62.234B	S62.359B
S52.355B	S52.516B	S52.614B	S62.023B	S62.235B	S62.360B
S52.355C	S52.516C	S52.614C	S62.024B	S62.236B	S62.361B
S52.356A	S52.521A	S52.615A	S62.025B	S62.241B	S62.362B
S52.356B	S52.522A	S52.615B	S62.026B	S62.242B	S62.363B
S52.356C	S52.529A	S52.615C	S62.031B	S62.243B	S62.364B
S52.361A	S52.531A	S52.616A	S62.032B	S62.244B	S62.365B
S52.361B	S52.531B	S52.616B	S62.033B	S62.245B	S62.366B
S52.361C	S52.531C	S52.616C	S62.034B	S62.246B	S62.367B
S52.362A	S52.532A	S52.621A	S62.035B	S62.251B	S62.368B
S52.362B	S52.532B	S52.622A	S62.036B	S62.252B	S62.369B
S52.362C	S52.532C	S52.629A	S62.101B	S62.253B	S62.390B
S52.363A	S52.539A	S52.691A	S62.102B	S62.254B	S62.391B
S52.363B	S52.539B	S52.691B	S62.109B	S62.255B	S62.392B
S52.363C	S52.539C	S52.691C	S62.111B	S62.256B	S62.393B
S52.364A	S52.541A	S52.692A	S62.112B	S62.291B	S62.394B
S52.364B	S52.541B	S52.692B	S62.113B	S62.292B	S62.395B
	S52.541C	S52.692C	S62.114B	S62.299B	S62.396B
	S52.542A		S62.115B	S62.300B	S62.397B

HAC 05: Falls and Trauma (continued)

S62.398B	S62.658B	S72.043C	S72.122B	S72.321A	S72.362C
S62.399B	S62.659B	S72.044A	S72.122C	S72.321B	S72.363A
S62.501B	S62.660B	S72.044C	S72.123A	S72.321C	S72.363B
S62.502B	S62.661B	S72.045A	S72.123B	S72.322A	S72.363C
S62.509B	S62.662B	S72.045B	S72.123C	S72.322B	S72.364A
S62.511B	S62.663B	S72.045C	S72.124A	S72.322C	S72.364B
S62.512B	S62.664B	S72.046A	S72.124B	S72.323A	S72.364C
S62.513B	S62.665B	S72.046B	S72.124C	S72.323B	S72.365A
S62.514B	S62.666B	S72.046C	S72.125A	S72.323C	S72.365B
S62.515B	S62.667B	S72.051A	S72.125B	S72.324A	S72.365C
S62.516B	S62.668B	S72.051B	S72.125C	S72.324B	S72.366A
S62.521B	S62.669B	S72.051C	S72.126A	S72.324C	S72.366B
S62.522B	S62.90XB	S72.052A	S72.126B	S72.325A	S72.366C
S62.523B	S62.91XB	S72.052B	S72.126C	S72.325B	S72.391A
S62.524B	S62.92XB	S72.052C	S72.131A	S72.325C	S72.391B
S62.525B	S72.001A	S72.059A	S72.131B	S72.326A	S72.391C
S62.526B	S72.001B	S72.059B	S72.131C	S72.326B	S72.392A
S62.600B	S72.001C	S72.059C	S72.132A	S72.326C	S72.392B
S62.601B	S72.002A	S72.061A	S72.132B	S72.331A	S72.392C
S62.602B	S72.002B	S72.061B	S72.132C	S72.331B	S72.399A
S62.603B	S72.002C	S72.061C	S72.133A	S72.331C	S72.399B
S62.604B	S72.009A	S72.062A	S72.133B	S72.332A	S72.399C
S62.605B	S72.009B	S72.062B	S72.133C	S72.332B	S72.401A
S62.606B	S72.009C	S72.062C	S72.134A	S72.332C	S72.401B
S62.607B	S72.011A	S72.063A	S72.134B	S72.333A	S72.401C
S62.608B	S72.011B	S72.063B	S72.134C	S72.333B	S72.402A
S62.609B	S72.011C	S72.063C	S72.135A	S72.333C	S72.402B
S62.610B	S72.012A	S72.064A	S72.135B	S72.334A	S72.402C
S62.611B	S72.012B	S72.064B	S72.135C	S72.334B	S72.409A
S62.612B	S72.012C	S72.064C	S72.136A	S72.334C	S72.409B
S62.613B	S72.019A	S72.065A	S72.136B	S72.335A	S72.409C
S62.614B	S72.019B	S72.065B	S72.136C	S72.335B	S72.411A
S62.615B	S72.019C	S72.065C	S72.141A	S72.335C	S72.411B
S62.616B	S72.021A	S72.066A	S72.141B	S72.336A	S72.411C
S62.617B	S72.021B	S72.066B	S72.141C	S72.336B	S72.412A
S62.618B	S72.021C	S72.066C	S72.142A	S72.336C	S72.412B
S62.619B	S72.022A	S72.091A	S72.142B	S72.341A	S72.412C
S62.620B	S72.022B	S72.091B	S72.142C	S72.341B	S72.413A
S62.621B	S72.022C	S72.091C	S72.143A	S72.341C	S72.413B
S62.622B	S72.023A	S72.092A	S72.143B	S72.342A	S72.413C
S62.623B	S72.023B	S72.092B	S72.143C	S72.342B	S72.414A
S62.624B	S72.023C	S72.092C	S72.144A	S72.342C	S72.414B
S62.625B	S72.024A	S72.099A	S72.144B	S72.343A	S72.414C
S62.626B	S72.024B	S72.099B	S72.144C	S72.343B	S72.415A
S62.627B	S72.024C	S72.099C	S72.145A	S72.343C	S72.415B
S62.628B	S72.025A	S72.101A	S72.145B	S72.344A	S72.415C
S62.629B	S72.025B	S72.101B	S72.145C	S72.344B	S72.416A
S62.630B	S72.025C	S72.101C	S72.146A	S72.344C	S72.416B
S62.631B	S72.026A	S72.102A	S72.146B	S72.345A	S72.416C
S62.632B	S72.026B	S72.102B	S72.146C	S72.345B	S72.421A
S62.633B	S72.026C	S72.102C	S72.21XA	S72.345C	S72.421B
S62.634B	S72.031A	S72.109A	S72.21XB	S72.346A	S72.421C
S62.635B	S72.031B	S72.109B	S72.21XC	S72.346B	S72.422A
S62.636B	S72.031C	S72.109C	S72.22XA	S72.346C	S72.422B
S62.637B	S72.032A	S72.111A	S72.22XB	S72.351A	S72.422C
S62.638B	S72.032B	S72.111B	S72.22XC	S72.351B	S72.423A
S62.639B	S72.032C	S72.111C	S72.23XA	S72.351C	S72.423B
S62.640B	S72.033A	S72.112A	S72.23XB	S72.352A	S72.423C
S62.641B	S72.033B	S72.112B	S72.23XC	S72.352B	S72.424A
S62.642B	S72.033C	S72.112C	S72.24XA	S72.352C	S72.424B
S62.643B	S72.034A	S72.113A	S72.24XB	S72.353A	S72.424C
S62.644B	S72.034B	S72.113B	S72.24XC	S72.353B	S72.425A
S62.645B	S72.034C	S72.113C	S72.25XA	S72.353C	S72.425B
S62.646B	S72.035A	S72.114A	S72.25XB	S72.354A	S72.425C
S62.647B	S72.035B	S72.114B	S72.25XC	S72.354B	S72.426A
S62.648B	S72.035C	S72.114C	S72.26XA	S72.354C	S72.426B
S62.649B	S72.036A	S72.115A	S72.26XB	S72.355A	S72.426C
S62.650B	S72.036B	S72.115B	S72.26XC	S72.355B	S72.431A
S62.651B	S72.036C	S72.115C	S72.301A	S72.355C	S72.431B
S62.652B	S72.041A	S72.116A	S72.301B	S72.356A	S72.431C
S62.653B	S72.041B	S72.116B	S72.301C	S72.356B	S72.432A
S62.654B	S72.041C	S72.116C	S72.302A	S72.356C	S72.432B
S62.655B	S72.042A	S72.121A	S72.302B	S72.361A	S72.432C
S62.656B	S72.042B	S72.121B	S72.302C	S72.361B	S72.433A
S62.657B	S72.042C	S72.121C	S72.309A	S72.361C	S72.433B
	S72.043A	S72.122A	S72.309B	S72.362A	S72.433C
	S72.043B		S72.309C	S72.362B	S72.434A

HAC 05: Falls and Trauma (continued)

S72.434B	S72.8X1B	S79.191A	S82.044C	S82.136B	S82.231A
S72.434C	S72.8X1C	S79.192A	S82.045A	S82.136C	S82.231B
S72.435A	S72.8X2A	S79.199A	S82.045B	S82.141A	S82.231C
S72.435B	S72.8X2B	S82.001A	S82.045C	S82.141B	S82.232B
S72.435C	S72.8X2C	S82.001B	S82.046A	S82.141C	S82.232C
S72.436A	S72.8X9A	S82.001C	S82.046B	S82.142A	S82.233A
S72.436B	S72.8X9B	S82.002A	S82.046C	S82.142B	S82.233B
S72.436C	S72.8X9C	S82.002B	S82.091A	S82.142C	S82.233C
S72.441A	S72.90XA	S82.002C	S82.091B	S82.143A	S82.234A
S72.441B	S72.90XB	S82.009A	S82.091C	S82.143B	S82.234B
S72.441C	S72.90XC	S82.009B	S82.092A	S82.143C	S82.234C
S72.442A	S72.91XA	S82.009C	S82.092B	S82.144A	S82.235A
S72.442B	S72.91XB	S82.011A	S82.092C	S82.144B	S82.235B
S72.442C	S72.91XC	S82.011B	S82.099A	S82.144C	S82.235C
S72.443A	S72.92XA	S82.011C	S82.099B	S82.145A	S82.236A
S72.443B	S72.92XB	S82.012A	S82.099C	S82.145B	S82.236B
S72.443C	S72.92XC	S82.012B	S82.101A	S82.145C	S82.236C
S72.444A	S73.001A	S82.012C	S82.101B	S82.146A	S82.241A
S72.444B	S73.002A	S82.013A	S82.101C	S82.146B	S82.241B
S72.444C	S73.003A	S82.013B	S82.102A	S82.146C	S82.241C
S72.445A	S73.004A	S82.013C	S82.102B	S82.151A	S82.242A
S72.445B	S73.005A	S82.014A	S82.102C	S82.151B	S82.242B
S72.445C	S73.006A	S82.014B	S82.109A	S82.151C	S82.242C
S72.446A	S73.011A	S82.014C	S82.109B	S82.152A	S82.243A
S72.446B	S73.012A	S82.015A	S82.109C	S82.152B	S82.243B
S72.446C	S73.013A	S82.015B	S82.111A	S82.152C	S82.243C
S72.451A	S73.014A	S82.015C	S82.111B	S82.153A	S82.244A
S72.451B	S73.015A	S82.016A	S82.111C	S82.153B	S82.244B
S72.451C	S73.016A	S82.016B	S82.112A	S82.153C	S82.244C
S72.452A	S73.021A	S82.016C	S82.112B	S82.154A	S82.245A
S72.452B	S73.022A	S82.021A	S82.112C	S82.154B	S82.245B
S72.452C	S73.023A	S82.021B	S82.113A	S82.154C	S82.245C
S72.453A	S73.024A	S82.021C	S82.113B	S82.155A	S82.246A
S72.453B	S73.025A	S82.022A	S82.113C	S82.155B	S82.246B
S72.453C	S73.026A	S82.022B	S82.114A	S82.155C	S82.246C
S72.454A	S73.031A	S82.022C	S82.114B	S82.156A	S82.251A
S72.454B	S73.032A	S82.023A	S82.114C	S82.156B	S82.251B
S72.454C	S73.033A	S82.023B	S82.115A	S82.156C	S82.251C
S72.455A	S73.034A	S82.023C	S82.115B	S82.161A	S82.252A
S72.455B	S73.035A	S82.024A	S82.115C	S82.162A	S82.252B
S72.455C	S73.036A	S82.024B	S82.116A	S82.169A	S82.252C
S72.456A	S73.041A	S82.024C	S82.116B	S82.191A	S82.253A
S72.456B	S73.042A	S82.025A	S82.116C	S82.191B	S82.253B
S72.456C	S73.043A	S82.025B	S82.121A	S82.191C	S82.253C
S72.461A	S73.044A	S82.025C	S82.121B	S82.192A	S82.254A
S72.461B	S73.045A	S82.026A	S82.121C	S82.192B	S82.254B
S72.461C	S73.046A	S82.026B	S82.122A	S82.192C	S82.254C
S72.462A	S77.00XA	S82.026C	S82.122B	S82.199A	S82.255A
S72.462B	S77.01XA	S82.031A	S82.122C	S82.199B	S82.255B
S72.462C	S77.02XA	S82.031B	S82.123A	S82.199C	S82.255C
S72.463A	S77.10XA	S82.031C	S82.123B	S82.201A	S82.256A
S72.463B	S77.11XA	S82.032A	S82.123C	S82.201B	S82.256B
S72.463C	S77.12XA	S82.032B	S82.124A	S82.201C	S82.256C
S72.464A	S79.001A	S82.032C	S82.124B	S82.202A	S82.261A
S72.464B	S79.002A	S82.033A	S82.124C	S82.202B	S82.261B
S72.464C	S79.009A	S82.033B	S82.125A	S82.202C	S82.261C
S72.465A	S79.011A	S82.033C	S82.125B	S82.209A	S82.262A
S72.465B	S79.012A	S82.034A	S82.125C	S82.209B	S82.262B
S72.465C	S79.019A	S82.034B	S82.126A	S82.209C	S82.262C
S72.466A	S79.091A	S82.034C	S82.126B	S82.221A	S82.263A
S72.466B	S79.092A	S82.035A	S82.126C	S82.221B	S82.263B
S72.466C	S79.099A	S82.035B	S82.131A	S82.221C	S82.263C
S72.471A	S79.101A	S82.035C	S82.131B	S82.222A	S82.264A
S72.472A	S79.102A	S82.036A	S82.131C	S82.222B	S82.264B
S72.479A	S79.109A	S82.036B	S82.132A	S82.222C	S82.264C
S72.491A	S79.111A	S82.036C	S82.132B	S82.223A	S82.265A
S72.491B	S79.112A	S82.041A	S82.132C	S82.223B	S82.265B
S72.491C	S79.119A	S82.041B	S82.133A	S82.223C	S82.265C
S72.492A	S79.121A	S82.041C	S82.133B	S82.224A	S82.266A
S72.492B	S79.122A	S82.042A	S82.133C	S82.224B	S82.266B
S72.492C	S79.129A	S82.042B	S82.134A	S82.224C	S82.266C
S72.499A	S79.131A	S82.042C	S82.134B	S82.225A	S82.291A
S72.499B	S79.132A	S82.043A	S82.134C	S82.225B	S82.291B
S72.499C	S79.139A	S82.043B	S82.135A	S82.225C	S82.291C
S72.8X1A	S79.141A	S82.043C	S82.135B	S82.226A	S82.292A
	S79.142A	S82.044A	S82.135C	S82.226B	S82.292B
	S79.149A	S82.044B	S82.136A	S82.226C	

Appendix G: Hospital Acquired Conditions

HAC 05: Falls and Trauma (continued)					
S82.292C	S82.462B	S82.864C	S92.054B	S92.256B	T21.76XA
S82.299A	S82.462C	S82.865B	S92.055B	S92.301B	T21.77XA
S82.299B	S82.463B	S82.865C	S92.056B	S92.302B	T21.79XA
S82.299C	S82.463C	S82.866B	S92.061B	S92.309B	T22.30XA
S82.301B	S82.464B	S82.866C	S92.062B	S92.311B	T22.311A
S82.301C	S82.464C	S82.871B	S92.063B	S92.312B	T22.312A
S82.302B	S82.465B	S82.871C	S92.064B	S92.313B	T22.319A
S82.302C	S82.465C	S82.872B	S92.065B	S92.314B	T22.321A
S82.309B	S82.466B	S82.872C	S92.066B	S92.315B	T22.329A
S82.309C	S82.466C	S82.873B	S92.101B	S92.316B	T22.331A
S82.311A	S82.491B	S82.873C	S92.102B	S92.321B	T22.332A
S82.312A	S82.491C	S82.874B	S92.109B	S92.322B	T22.339A
S82.319A	S82.492B	S82.874C	S92.111B	S92.323B	T22.341A
S82.391B	S82.492C	S82.875B	S92.112B	S92.324B	T22.342A
S82.391C	S82.499B	S82.875C	S92.113B	S92.325B	T22.349A
S82.392B	S82.499C	S82.876B	S92.114B	S92.326B	T22.351A
S82.392C	S82.51XB	S82.876C	S92.115B	S92.331B	T22.352A
S82.399B	S82.51XC	S82.891B	S92.116B	S92.332B	T22.359A
S82.399C	S82.52XB	S82.891C	S92.121B	S92.333B	T22.361A
S82.401B	S82.52XC	S82.892B	S92.122B	S92.334B	T22.362A
S82.401C	S82.53XB	S82.892C	S92.123B	S92.335B	T22.369A
S82.402B	S82.53XC	S82.899B	S92.124B	S92.336B	T22.391A
S82.402C	S82.54XB	S82.899C	S92.125B	S92.341B	T22.392A
S82.409B	S82.54XC	S82.90XB	S92.126B	S92.342B	T22.399A
S82.409C	S82.55XB	S82.90XC	S92.131B	S92.343B	T22.70XA
S82.421B	S82.55XC	S82.91XB	S92.132B	S92.344B	T22.711A
S82.421C	S82.56XB	S82.91XC	S92.133B	S92.345B	T22.712A
S82.422B	S82.56XC	S82.92XB	S92.134B	S92.346B	T22.719A
S82.422C	S82.61XB	S82.92XC	S92.135B	S92.351B	T22.721A
S82.423B	S82.61XC	S89.001A	S92.136B	S92.352B	T22.722A
S82.423C	S82.62XB	S89.002A	S92.141B	S92.353B	T22.729A
S82.424B	S82.62XC	S89.009A	S92.142B	S92.354B	T22.731A
S82.424C	S82.63XB	S89.011A	S92.143B	S92.355B	T22.732A
S82.425B	S82.63XC	S89.012A	S92.144B	S92.356B	T22.739A
S82.425C	S82.64XB	S89.019A	S92.145B	S92.811B	T22.741A
S82.426B	S82.64XC	S89.021A	S92.146B	S92.812B	T22.742A
S82.426C	S82.65XB	S89.022A	S92.151B	S92.819B	T22.749A
S82.431B	S82.65XC	S89.029A	S92.152B	S92.901B	T22.751A
S82.431C	S82.66XB	S89.031A	S92.153B	S92.902B	T22.752A
S82.432B	S82.66XC	S89.032A	S92.154B	S92.909B	T22.759A
S82.432C	S82.831B	S89.039A	S92.155B	T20.30XA	T22.761A
S82.433B	S82.831C	S89.041A	S92.156B	T20.311A	T22.762A
S82.433C	S82.832B	S89.042A	S92.191B	T20.312A	T22.769A
S82.434B	S82.832C	S89.049A	S92.192B	T20.319A	T22.791A
S82.434C	S82.839B	S89.091A	S92.199B	T20.32XA	T22.792A
S82.435B	S82.839C	S89.092A	S92.201B	T20.33XA	T22.799A
S82.435C	S82.841B	S89.099A	S92.202B	T20.34XA	T23.301A
S82.436B	S82.841C	S92.001B	S92.209B	T20.35XA	T23.302A
S82.436C	S82.842B	S92.002B	S92.211B	T20.36XA	T23.309A
S82.441B	S82.842C	S92.009B	S92.212B	T20.37XA	T23.311A
S82.441C	S82.843B	S92.011B	S92.213B	T20.39XA	T23.312A
S82.442B	S82.843C	S92.012B	S92.214B	T20.70XA	T23.319A
S82.442C	S82.844B	S92.013B	S92.215B	T20.711A	T23.321A
S82.443B	S82.844C	S92.014B	S92.216B	T20.712A	T23.322A
S82.443C	S82.845B	S92.015B	S92.221B	T20.719A	T23.329A
S82.444B	S82.845C	S92.016B	S92.222B	T20.72XA	T23.331A
S82.444C	S82.846B	S92.021B	S92.223B	T20.73XA	T23.332A
S82.445B	S82.846C	S92.022B	S92.224B	T20.74XA	T23.339A
S82.445C	S82.851B	S92.023B	S92.225B	T20.75XA	T23.341A
S82.446B	S82.851C	S92.024B	S92.226B	T20.76XA	T23.342A
S82.446C	S82.852B	S92.025B	S92.231B	T20.77XA	T23.349A
S82.451B	S82.852C	S92.026B	S92.232B	T20.79XA	T23.351A
S82.451C	S82.853B	S92.031B	S92.233B	T21.30XA	T23.352A
S82.452B	S82.853C	S92.032B	S92.234B	T21.31XA	T23.359A
S82.452C	S82.854B	S92.033B	S92.235B	T21.32XA	T23.361A
S82.453B	S82.854C	S92.034B	S92.236B	T21.33XA	T23.362A
S82.453C	S82.855B	S92.035B	S92.241B	T21.34XA	T23.369A
S82.454B	S82.855C	S92.036B	S92.242B	T21.35XA	T23.371A
S82.454C	S82.856B	S92.041B	S92.243B	T21.36XA	T23.372A
S82.455B	S82.856C	S92.042B	S92.244B	T21.37XA	T23.379A
S82.455C	S82.861B	S92.043B	S92.245B	T21.39XA	T23.391A
S82.456B	S82.861C	S92.044B	S92.246B	T21.70XA	T23.392A
S82.456C	S82.862B	S92.045B	S92.251B	T21.71XA	T23.399A
S82.461B	S82.862C	S92.046B	S92.252B	T21.72XA	T23.701A
S82.461C	S82.863B	S92.051B	S92.253B	T21.73XA	T23.702A
	S82.863C	S92.052B	S92.254B	T21.74XA	T23.709A
	S82.864B	S92.053B	S92.255B	T21.75XA	

HAC 05: Falls and Trauma (continued)

T23.711A	T25.322A	T31.62	T32.71	T33.839A	T71.143A
T23.712A	T25.329A	T31.63	T32.72	T33.90XA	T71.144A
T23.719A	T25.331A	T31.64	T32.73	T33.99XA	T71.151A
T23.721A	T25.332A	T31.65	T32.74	T34.011A	T71.152A
T23.722A	T25.339A	T31.66	T32.75	T34.012A	T71.153A
T23.729A	T25.391A	T31.70	T32.76	T34.019A	T71.154A
T23.731A	T25.392A	T31.71	T32.77	T34.02XA	T71.161A
T23.732A	T25.399A	T31.72	T32.80	T34.09XA	T71.162A
T23.739A	T25.711A	T31.73	T32.81	T34.1XXA	T71.163A
T23.741A	T25.712A	T31.74	T32.82	T34.2XXA	T71.164A
T23.742A	T25.719A	T31.75	T32.83	T34.3XXA	T71.191A
T23.749A	T25.721A	T31.76	T32.84	T34.40XA	T71.192A
T23.751A	T25.722A	T31.77	T32.85	T34.41XA	T71.193A
T23.752A	T25.729A	T31.80	T32.86	T34.42XA	T71.194A
T23.759A	T25.731A	T31.81	T32.87	T34.511A	T71.20XA
T23.761A	T25.732A	T31.82	T32.88	T34.512A	T71.21XA
T23.762A	T25.739A	T31.83	T32.90	T34.519A	T71.29XA
T23.769A	T25.791A	T31.84	T32.91	T34.521A	T71.9XXA
T23.771A	T25.792A	T31.85	T32.92	T34.522A	T75.1XXA
T23.772A	T25.799A	T31.86	T32.93	T34.529A	
T23.779A	T26.20XA	T31.87	T32.94	T34.531A	**HAC 06: Catheter Associated Urinary Tract Infection (UTI)**
T23.791A	T26.21XA	T31.88	T32.95	T34.532A	
T23.792A	T26.22XA	T31.90	T32.96	T34.539A	
T23.799A	T26.70XA	T31.91	T32.97	T34.60XA	Secondary diagnosis not POA:
T24.301A	T26.71XA	T31.92	T32.98	T34.61XA	
T24.302A	T26.72XA	T31.93	T32.99	T34.62XA	T83.511A
T24.309A	T27.0XXA	T31.94	T33.011A	T34.70XA	T83.518A
T24.311A	T27.1XXA	T31.95	T33.012A	T34.71XA	
T24.312A	T27.2XXA	T31.96	T33.019A	T34.72XA	**With or Without**
T24.319A	T27.3XXA	T31.97	T33.02XA	T34.811A	Secondary diagnosis (also not POA) of:
T24.321A	T27.4XXA	T31.98	T33.09XA	T34.812A	
T24.322A	T27.5XXA	T31.99	T33.1XXA	T34.819A	B37.41
T24.329A	T27.6XXA	T32.10	T33.2XXA	T34.821A	B37.49
T24.331A	T27.7XXA	T32.11	T33.3XXA	T34.822A	N10
T24.332A	T28.1XXA	T32.20	T33.40XA	T34.829A	N11.9
T24.339A	T28.2XXA	T32.21	T33.41XA	T34.831A	N12
T24.391A	T28.6XXA	T32.22	T33.42XA	T34.832A	N13.6
T24.392A	T28.7XXA	T32.30	T33.511A	T34.839A	N15.1
T24.399A	T31.10	T32.31	T33.512A	T34.90XA	N28.84
T24.701A	T31.11	T32.32	T33.519A	T34.99XA	N28.85
T24.702A	T31.20	T32.33	T33.521A	T67.01XA	N28.86
T24.709A	T31.21	T32.40	T33.522A	T67.02XA	N30.00
T24.711A	T31.22	T32.41	T33.529A	T67.09XA	N30.01
T24.712A	T31.30	T32.42	T33.531A	T69.021A	N34.0
T24.719A	T31.31	T32.43	T33.532A	T69.022A	N39.0
T24.721A	T31.32	T32.44	T33.539A	T69.029A	
T24.722A	T31.33	T32.50	T33.60XA	T70.3XXA	**HAC 07: Vascular Catheter Associated Infection**
T24.729A	T31.40	T32.51	T33.61XA	T71.111A	
T24.731A	T31.41	T32.52	T33.62XA	T71.112A	
T24.732A	T31.42	T32.53	T33.70XA	T71.113A	Secondary diagnosis not POA:
T24.739A	T31.43	T32.54	T33.71XA	T71.114A	
T24.791A	T31.44	T32.55	T33.72XA	T71.121A	T80.211A
T24.792A	T31.50	T32.60	T33.811A	T71.122A	T80.212A
T24.799A	T31.51	T32.61	T33.812A	T71.123A	T80.218A
T25.311A	T31.52	T32.62	T33.819A	T71.124A	T80.219A
T25.312A	T31.53	T32.63	T33.821A	T71.131A	
T25.319A	T31.54	T32.64	T33.822A	T71.132A	
T25.321A	T31.55	T32.65	T33.829A	T71.133A	
	T31.60	T32.66	T33.831A	T71.134A	
	T31.61	T32.70	T33.832A	T71.141A	

HAC 08: Surgical Site Infection of Mediastinitis after Coronary Bypass Graft (CABG)

Secondary diagnosis not POA:
  J98.51
  J98.59

AND

Any of the following procedures:

0210083 Bypass Coronary Artery, One Artery from Coronary Artery with Zooplastic Tissue, Open Approach

0210088 Bypass Coronary Artery, One Artery from Right Internal Mammary with Zooplastic Tissue, Open Approach

0210089 Bypass Coronary Artery, One Artery from Left Internal Mammary with Zooplastic Tissue, Open Approach

021008C Bypass Coronary Artery, One Artery from Thoracic Artery with Zooplastic Tissue, Open Approach

021008F Bypass Coronary Artery, One Artery from Abdominal Artery with Zooplastic Tissue, Open Approach

021008W Bypass Coronary Artery, One Artery from Aorta with Zooplastic Tissue, Open Approach

0210093 Bypass Coronary Artery, One Artery from Coronary Artery with Autologous Venous Tissue, Open Approach

0210098 Bypass Coronary Artery, One Artery from Right Internal Mammary with Autologous Venous Tissue, Open Approach

0210099 Bypass Coronary Artery, One Artery from Left Internal Mammary with Autologous Venous Tissue, Open Approach

021009C Bypass Coronary Artery, One Artery from Thoracic Artery with Autologous Venous Tissue, Open Approach

021009F Bypass Coronary Artery, One Artery from Abdominal Artery with Autologous Venous Tissue, Open Approach

021009W Bypass Coronary Artery, One Artery from Aorta with Autologous Venous Tissue, Open Approach

02100A3 Bypass Coronary Artery, One Artery from Coronary Artery with Autologous Arterial Tissue, Open Approach

02100A8 Bypass Coronary Artery, One Artery from Right Internal Mammary with Autologous Arterial Tissue, Open Approach

02100A9 Bypass Coronary Artery, One Artery from Left Internal Mammary with Autologous Arterial Tissue, Open Approach

02100AC Bypass Coronary Artery, One Artery from Thoracic Artery with Autologous Arterial Tissue, Open Approach

02100AF Bypass Coronary Artery, One Artery from Abdominal Artery with Autologous Arterial Tissue, Open Approach

02100AW Bypass Coronary Artery, One Artery from Aorta with Autologous Arterial Tissue, Open Approach

02100J3 Bypass Coronary Artery, One Artery from Coronary Artery with Synthetic Substitute, Open Approach

02100J8 Bypass Coronary Artery, One Artery from Right Internal Mammary with Synthetic Substitute, Open Approach

02100J9 Bypass Coronary Artery, One Artery from Left Internal Mammary with Synthetic Substitute, Open Approach

02100JC Bypass Coronary Artery, One Artery from Thoracic Artery with Synthetic Substitute, Open Approach

02100JF Bypass Coronary Artery, One Artery from Abdominal Artery with Synthetic Substitute, Open Approach

02100JW Bypass Coronary Artery, One Artery from Aorta with Synthetic Substitute, Open Approach

02100K3 Bypass Coronary Artery, One Artery from Coronary Artery with Nonautologous Tissue Substitute, Open Approach

02100K8 Bypass Coronary Artery, One Artery from Right Internal Mammary with Nonautologous Tissue Substitute, Open Approach

02100K9 Bypass Coronary Artery, One Artery from Left Internal Mammary with Nonautologous Tissue Substitute, Open Approach

02100KC Bypass Coronary Artery, One Artery from Thoracic Artery with Nonautologous Tissue Substitute, Open Approach

02100KF Bypass Coronary Artery, One Artery from Abdominal Artery with Nonautologous Tissue Substitute, Open Approach

02100KW Bypass Coronary Artery, One Artery from Aorta with Nonautologous Tissue Substitute, Open Approach

02100Z3 Bypass Coronary Artery, One Artery from Coronary Artery, Open Approach

02100Z8 Bypass Coronary Artery, One Artery from Right Internal Mammary, Open Approach

02100Z9 Bypass Coronary Artery, One Artery from Left Internal Mammary, Open Approach

02100ZC Bypass Coronary Artery, One Artery from Thoracic Artery, Open Approach

02100ZF Bypass Coronary Artery, One Artery from Abdominal Artery, Open Approach

0210483 Bypass Coronary Artery, One Artery from Coronary Artery with Zooplastic Tissue, Percutaneous Endoscopic Approach

0210488 Bypass Coronary Artery, One Artery from Right Internal Mammary with Zooplastic Tissue, Percutaneous Endoscopic Approach

0210489 Bypass Coronary Artery, One Artery from Left Internal Mammary with Zooplastic Tissue, Percutaneous Endoscopic Approach

021048C Bypass Coronary Artery, One Artery from Thoracic Artery with Zooplastic Tissue, Percutaneous Endoscopic Approach

021048F Bypass Coronary Artery, One Artery from Abdominal Artery with Zooplastic Tissue, Percutaneous Endoscopic Approach

021048W Bypass Coronary Artery, One Artery from Aorta with Zooplastic Tissue, Percutaneous Endoscopic Approach

0210493 Bypass Coronary Artery, One Artery from Coronary Artery with Autologous Venous Tissue, Percutaneous Endoscopic Approach

0210498 Bypass Coronary Artery, One Artery from Right Internal Mammary with Autologous Venous Tissue, Percutaneous Endoscopic Approach

0210499 Bypass Coronary Artery, One Artery from Left Internal Mammary with Autologous Venous Tissue, Percutaneous Endoscopic Approach

021049C Bypass Coronary Artery, One Artery from Thoracic Artery with Autologous Venous Tissue, Percutaneous Endoscopic Approach

021049F Bypass Coronary Artery, One Artery from Abdominal Artery with Autologous Venous Tissue, Percutaneous Endoscopic Approach

021049W Bypass Coronary Artery, One Artery from Aorta with Autologous Venous Tissue, Percutaneous Endoscopic Approach

02104A3 Bypass Coronary Artery, One Artery from Coronary Artery with Autologous Arterial Tissue, Percutaneous Endoscopic Approach

02104A8 Bypass Coronary Artery, One Artery from Right Internal Mammary with Autologous Arterial Tissue, Percutaneous Endoscopic Approach

02104A9 Bypass Coronary Artery, One Artery from Left Internal Mammary with Autologous Arterial Tissue, Percutaneous Endoscopic Approach

02104AC Bypass Coronary Artery, One Artery from Thoracic Artery with Autologous Arterial Tissue, Percutaneous Endoscopic Approach

02104AF Bypass Coronary Artery, One Artery from Abdominal Artery with Autologous Arterial Tissue, Percutaneous Endoscopic Approach

02104AW Bypass Coronary Artery, One Artery from Aorta with Autologous Arterial Tissue, Percutaneous Endoscopic Approach

02104J3 Bypass Coronary Artery, One Artery from Coronary Artery with Synthetic Substitute, Percutaneous Endoscopic Approach

02104J8 Bypass Coronary Artery, One Artery from Right Internal Mammary with Synthetic Substitute, Percutaneous Endoscopic Approach

02104J9 Bypass Coronary Artery, One Artery from Left Internal Mammary with Synthetic Substitute, Percutaneous Endoscopic Approach

02104JC Bypass Coronary Artery, One Artery from Thoracic Artery with Synthetic Substitute, Percutaneous Endoscopic Approach

02104JF Bypass Coronary Artery, One Artery from Abdominal Artery with Synthetic Substitute, Percutaneous Endoscopic Approach

02104JW Bypass Coronary Artery, One Artery from Aorta with Synthetic Substitute, Percutaneous Endoscopic Approach

02104K3 Bypass Coronary Artery, One Artery from Coronary Artery with Nonautologous Tissue Substitute, Percutaneous Endoscopic Approach

02104K8 Bypass Coronary Artery, One Artery from Right Internal Mammary with Nonautologous Tissue Substitute, Percutaneous Endoscopic Approach

02104K9 Bypass Coronary Artery, One Artery from Left Internal Mammary with Nonautologous Tissue Substitute, Percutaneous Endoscopic Approach

02104KC Bypass Coronary Artery, One Artery from Thoracic Artery with Nonautologous Tissue Substitute, Percutaneous Endoscopic Approach

02104KF Bypass Coronary Artery, One Artery from Abdominal Artery with Nonautologous Tissue Substitute, Percutaneous Endoscopic Approach

02104KW Bypass Coronary Artery, One Artery from Aorta with Nonautologous Tissue Substitute, Percutaneous Endoscopic Approach

02104Z3 Bypass Coronary Artery, One Artery from Coronary Artery, Percutaneous Endoscopic Approach

HAC 08: Surgical Artery Infection of Mediastinitis after Coronary Bypass Graft (CABG) (continued)

02104Z8 Bypass Coronary Artery, One Artery from Right Internal Mammary, Percutaneous Endoscopic Approach

02104Z9 Bypass Coronary Artery, One Artery from Left Internal Mammary, Percutaneous Endoscopic Approach

02104ZC Bypass Coronary Artery, One Artery from Thoracic Artery, Percutaneous Endoscopic Approach

02104ZF Bypass Coronary Artery, One Artery from Abdominal Artery, Percutaneous Endoscopic Approach

0211083 Bypass Coronary Artery, Two Arteries from Coronary Artery with Zooplastic Tissue, Open Approach

0211088 Bypass Coronary Artery, Two Arteries from Right Internal Mammary with Zooplastic Tissue, Open Approach

0211089 Bypass Coronary Artery, Two Arteries from Left Internal Mammary with Zooplastic Tissue, Open Approach

021108C Bypass Coronary Artery, Two Arteries from Thoracic Artery with Zooplastic Tissue, Open Approach

021108F Bypass Coronary Artery, Two Arteries from Abdominal Artery with Zooplastic Tissue, Open Approach

021108W Bypass Coronary Artery, Two Arteries from Aorta with Zooplastic Tissue, Open Approach

0211093 Bypass Coronary Artery, Two Arteries from Coronary Artery with Autologous Venous Tissue, Open Approach

0211098 Bypass Coronary Artery, Two Arteries from Right Internal Mammary with Autologous Venous Tissue, Open Approach

0211099 Bypass Coronary Artery, Two Arteries from Left Internal Mammary with Autologous Venous Tissue, Open Approach

021109C Bypass Coronary Artery, Two Arteries from Thoracic Artery with Autologous Venous Tissue, Open Approach

021109F Bypass Coronary Artery, Two Arteries from Abdominal Artery with Autologous Venous Tissue, Open Approach

021109W Bypass Coronary Artery, Two Arteries from Aorta with Autologous Venous Tissue, Open Approach

02110A3 Bypass Coronary Artery, Two Arteries from Coronary Artery with Autologous Arterial Tissue, Open Approach

02110A8 Bypass Coronary Artery, Two Arteries from Right Internal Mammary with Autologous Arterial Tissue, Open Approach

02110A9 Bypass Coronary Artery, Two Arteries from Left Internal Mammary with Autologous Arterial Tissue, Open Approach

02110AC Bypass Coronary Artery, Two Arteries from Thoracic Artery with Autologous Arterial Tissue, Open Approach

02110AF Bypass Coronary Artery, Two Arteries from Abdominal Artery with Autologous Arterial Tissue, Open Approach

02110AW Bypass Coronary Artery, Two Arteries from Aorta with Autologous Arterial Tissue, Open Approach

02110J3 Bypass Coronary Artery, Two Arteries from Coronary Artery with Synthetic Substitute, Open Approach

02110J8 Bypass Coronary Artery, Two Arteries from Right Internal Mammary with Synthetic Substitute, Open Approach

02110J9 Bypass Coronary Artery, Two Arteries from Left Internal Mammary with Synthetic Substitute, Open Approach

02110JC Bypass Coronary Artery, Two Arteries from Thoracic Artery with Synthetic Substitute, Open Approach

02110JF Bypass Coronary Artery, Two Arteries from Abdominal Artery with Synthetic Substitute, Open Approach

02110JW Bypass Coronary Artery, Two Arteries from Aorta with Synthetic Substitute, Open Approach

02110K3 Bypass Coronary Artery, Two Arteries from Coronary Artery with Nonautologous Tissue Substitute, Open Approach

02110K8 Bypass Coronary Artery, Two Arteries from Right Internal Mammary with Nonautologous Tissue Substitute, Open Approach

02110K9 Bypass Coronary Artery, Two Arteries from Left Internal Mammary with Nonautologous Tissue Substitute, Open Approach

02110KC Bypass Coronary Artery, Two Arteries from Thoracic Artery with Nonautologous Tissue Substitute, Open Approach

02110KF Bypass Coronary Artery, Two Arteries from Abdominal Artery with Nonautologous Tissue Substitute, Open Approach

02110KW Bypass Coronary Artery, Two Arteries from Aorta with Nonautologous Tissue Substitute, Open Approach

02110Z3 Bypass Coronary Artery, Two Arteries from Coronary Artery, Open Approach

02110Z8 Bypass Coronary Artery, Two Arteries from Right Internal Mammary, Open Approach

02110Z9 Bypass Coronary Artery, Two Arteries from Left Internal Mammary, Open Approach

02110ZC Bypass Coronary Artery, Two Arteries from Thoracic Artery, Open Approach

02110ZF Bypass Coronary Artery, Two Arteries from Abdominal Artery, Open Approach

0211483 Bypass Coronary Artery, Two Arteries from Coronary Artery with Zooplastic Tissue, Percutaneous Endoscopic Approach

0211488 Bypass Coronary Artery, Two Arteries from Right Internal Mammary with Zooplastic Tissue, Percutaneous Endoscopic Approach

0211489 Bypass Coronary Artery, Two Arteries from Left Internal Mammary with Zooplastic Tissue, Percutaneous Endoscopic Approach

021148C Bypass Coronary Artery, Two Arteries from Thoracic Artery with Zooplastic Tissue, Percutaneous Endoscopic Approach

021148F Bypass Coronary Artery, Two Arteries from Abdominal Artery with Zooplastic Tissue, Percutaneous Endoscopic Approach

021148W Bypass Coronary Artery, Two Arteries from Aorta with Zooplastic Tissue, Percutaneous Endoscopic Approach

0211493 Bypass Coronary Artery, Two Arteries from Coronary Artery with Autologous Venous Tissue, Percutaneous Endoscopic Approach

0211498 Bypass Coronary Artery, Two Arteries from Right Internal Mammary with Autologous Venous Tissue, Percutaneous Endoscopic Approach

0211499 Bypass Coronary Artery, Two Arteries from Left Internal Mammary with Autologous Venous Tissue, Percutaneous Endoscopic Approach

021149C Bypass Coronary Artery, Two Arteries from Thoracic Artery with Autologous Venous Tissue, Percutaneous Endoscopic Approach

021149F Bypass Coronary Artery, Two Arteries from Abdominal Artery with Autologous Venous Tissue, Percutaneous Endoscopic Approach

021149W Bypass Coronary Artery, Two Arteries from Aorta with Autologous Venous Tissue, Percutaneous Endoscopic Approach

02114A3 Bypass Coronary Artery, Two Arteries from Coronary Artery with Autologous Arterial Tissue, Percutaneous Endoscopic Approach

02114A8 Bypass Coronary Artery, Two Arteries from Right Internal Mammary with Autologous Arterial Tissue, Percutaneous Endoscopic Approach

02114A9 Bypass Coronary Artery, Two Arteries from Left Internal Mammary with Autologous Arterial Tissue, Percutaneous Endoscopic Approach

02114AC Bypass Coronary Artery, Two Arteries from Thoracic Artery with Autologous Arterial Tissue, Percutaneous Endoscopic Approach

02114AF Bypass Coronary Artery, Two Arteries from Abdominal Artery with Autologous Arterial Tissue, Percutaneous Endoscopic Approach

02114AW Bypass Coronary Artery, Two Arteries from Aorta with Autologous Arterial Tissue, Percutaneous Endoscopic Approach

02114J3 Bypass Coronary Artery, Two Arteries from Coronary Artery with Synthetic Substitute, Percutaneous Endoscopic Approach

02114J8 Bypass Coronary Artery, Two Arteries from Right Internal Mammary with Synthetic Substitute, Percutaneous Endoscopic Approach

02114J9 Bypass Coronary Artery, Two Arteries from Left Internal Mammary with Synthetic Substitute, Percutaneous Endoscopic Approach

02114JC Bypass Coronary Artery, Two Arteries from Thoracic Artery with Synthetic Substitute, Percutaneous Endoscopic Approach

02114JF Bypass Coronary Artery, Two Arteries from Abdominal Artery with Synthetic Substitute, Percutaneous Endoscopic Approach

02114JW Bypass Coronary Artery, Two Arteries from Aorta with Synthetic Substitute, Percutaneous Endoscopic Approach

02114K3 Bypass Coronary Artery, Two Arteries from Coronary Artery with Nonautologous Tissue Substitute, Percutaneous Endoscopic Approach

02114K8 Bypass Coronary Artery, Two Arteries from Right Internal Mammary with Nonautologous Tissue Substitute, Percutaneous Endoscopic Approach

HAC 08: Surgical Site Infection of Mediastinitis after Coronary Bypass Graft (CABG) (continued)

02114K9 Bypass Coronary Artery, Two Arteries from Left Internal Mammary with Nonautologous Tissue Substitute, Percutaneous Endoscopic Approach

02114KC Bypass Coronary Artery, Two Arteries from Thoracic Artery with Nonautologous Tissue Substitute, Percutaneous Endoscopic Approach

02114KF Bypass Coronary Artery, Two Arteries from Abdominal Artery with Nonautologous Tissue Substitute, Percutaneous Endoscopic Approach

02114KW Bypass Coronary Artery, Two Arteries from Aorta with Nonautologous Tissue Substitute, Percutaneous Endoscopic Approach

02114Z3 Bypass Coronary Artery, Two Arteries from Coronary Artery, Percutaneous Endoscopic Approach

02114Z8 Bypass Coronary Artery, Two Arteries from Right Internal Mammary, Percutaneous Endoscopic Approach

02114Z9 Bypass Coronary Artery, Two Arteries from Left Internal Mammary, Percutaneous Endoscopic Approach

02114ZC Bypass Coronary Artery, Two Arteries from Thoracic Artery, Percutaneous Endoscopic Approach

02114ZF Bypass Coronary Artery, Two Arteries from Abdominal Artery, Percutaneous Endoscopic Approach

0212083 Bypass Coronary Artery, Three Arteries from Coronary Artery with Zooplastic Tissue, Open Approach

0212088 Bypass Coronary Artery, Three Arteries from Right Internal Mammary with Zooplastic Tissue, Open Approach

0212089 Bypass Coronary Artery, Three Arteries from Left Internal Mammary with Zooplastic Tissue, Open Approach

021208C Bypass Coronary Artery, Three Arteries from Thoracic Artery with Zooplastic Tissue, Open Approach

021208F Bypass Coronary Artery, Three Arteries from Abdominal Artery with Zooplastic Tissue, Open Approach

021208W Bypass Coronary Artery, Three Arteries from Aorta with Zooplastic Tissue, Open Approach

0212093 Bypass Coronary Artery, Three Arteries from Coronary Artery with Autologous Venous Tissue, Open Approach

0212098 Bypass Coronary Artery, Three Arteries from Right Internal Mammary with Autologous Venous Tissue, Open Approach

0212099 Bypass Coronary Artery, Three Arteries from Left Internal Mammary with Autologous Venous Tissue, Open Approach

021209C Bypass Coronary Artery, Three Arteries from Thoracic Artery with Autologous Venous Tissue, Open Approach

021209F Bypass Coronary Artery, Three Arteries from Abdominal Artery with Autologous Venous Tissue, Open Approach

021209W Bypass Coronary Artery, Three Arteries from Aorta with Autologous Venous Tissue, Open Approach

02120A3 Bypass Coronary Artery, Three Arteries from Coronary Artery with Autologous Arterial Tissue, Open Approach

02120A8 Bypass Coronary Artery, Three Arteries from Right Internal Mammary with Autologous Arterial Tissue, Open Approach

02120A9 Bypass Coronary Artery, Three Arteries from Left Internal Mammary with Autologous Arterial Tissue, Open Approach

02120AC Bypass Coronary Artery, Three Arteries from Thoracic Artery with Autologous Arterial Tissue, Open Approach

02120AF Bypass Coronary Artery, Three Arteries from Abdominal Artery with Autologous Arterial Tissue, Open Approach

02120AW Bypass Coronary Artery, Three Arteries from Aorta with Autologous Arterial Tissue, Open Approach

02120J3 Bypass Coronary Artery, Three Arteries from Coronary Artery with Synthetic Substitute, Open Approach

02120J8 Bypass Coronary Artery, Three Arteries from Right Internal Mammary with Synthetic Substitute, Open Approach

02120J9 Bypass Coronary Artery, Three Arteries from Left Internal Mammary with Synthetic Substitute, Open Approach

02120JC Bypass Coronary Artery, Three Arteries from Thoracic Artery with Synthetic Substitute, Open Approach

02120JF Bypass Coronary Artery, Three Arteries from Abdominal Artery with Synthetic Substitute, Open Approach

02120JW Bypass Coronary Artery, Three Arteries from Aorta with Synthetic Substitute, Open Approach

02120K3 Bypass Coronary Artery, Three Arteries from Coronary Artery with Nonautologous Tissue Substitute, Open Approach

02120K8 Bypass Coronary Artery, Three Arteries from Right Internal Mammary with Nonautologous Tissue Substitute, Open Approach

02120K9 Bypass Coronary Artery, Three Arteries from Left Internal Mammary with Nonautologous Tissue Substitute, Open Approach

02120KC Bypass Coronary Artery, Three Arteries from Thoracic Artery with Nonautologous Tissue Substitute, Open Approach

02120KF Bypass Coronary Artery, Three Arteries from Abdominal Artery with Nonautologous Tissue Substitute, Open Approach

02120KW Bypass Coronary Artery, Three Arteries from Aorta with Nonautologous Tissue Substitute, Open Approach

02120Z3 Bypass Coronary Artery, Three Arteries from Coronary Artery, Open Approach

02120Z8 Bypass Coronary Artery, Three Arteries from Right Internal Mammary, Open Approach

02120Z9 Bypass Coronary Artery, Three Arteries from Left Internal Mammary, Open Approach

02120ZC Bypass Coronary Artery, Three Arteries from Thoracic Artery, Open Approach

02120ZF Bypass Coronary Artery, Three Arteries from Abdominal Artery, Open Approach

0212483 Bypass Coronary Artery, Three Arteries from Coronary Artery with Zooplastic Tissue, Percutaneous Endoscopic Approach

0212488 Bypass Coronary Artery, Three Arteries from Right Internal Mammary with Zooplastic Tissue, Percutaneous Endoscopic Approach

0212489 Bypass Coronary Artery, Three Arteries from Left Internal Mammary with Zooplastic Tissue, Percutaneous Endoscopic Approach

021248C Bypass Coronary Artery, Three Arteries from Thoracic Artery with Zooplastic Tissue, Percutaneous Endoscopic Approach

021248F Bypass Coronary Artery, Three Arteries from Abdominal Artery with Zooplastic Tissue, Percutaneous Endoscopic Approach

021248W Bypass Coronary Artery, Three Arteries from Aorta with Zooplastic Tissue, Percutaneous Endoscopic Approach

0212493 Bypass Coronary Artery, Three Arteries from Coronary Artery with Autologous Venous Tissue, Percutaneous Endoscopic Approach

0212498 Bypass Coronary Artery, Three Arteries from Right Internal Mammary with Autologous Venous Tissue, Percutaneous Endoscopic Approach

0212499 Bypass Coronary Artery, Three Arteries from Left Internal Mammary with Autologous Venous Tissue, Percutaneous Endoscopic Approach

021249C Bypass Coronary Artery, Three Arteries from Thoracic Artery with Autologous Venous Tissue, Percutaneous Endoscopic Approach

021249F Bypass Coronary Artery, Three Arteries from Abdominal Artery with Autologous Venous Tissue, Percutaneous Endoscopic Approach

021249W Bypass Coronary Artery, Three Arteries from Aorta with Autologous Venous Tissue, Percutaneous Endoscopic Approach

02124A3 Bypass Coronary Artery, Three Arteries from Coronary Artery with Autologous Arterial Tissue, Percutaneous Endoscopic Approach

02124A8 Bypass Coronary Artery, Three Arteries from Right Internal Mammary with Autologous Arterial Tissue, Percutaneous Endoscopic Approach

02124A9 Bypass Coronary Artery, Three Arteries from Left Internal Mammary with Autologous Arterial Tissue, Percutaneous Endoscopic Approach

02124AC Bypass Coronary Artery, Three Arteries from Thoracic Artery with Autologous Arterial Tissue, Percutaneous Endoscopic Approach

02124AF Bypass Coronary Artery, Three Arteries from Abdominal Artery with Autologous Arterial Tissue, Percutaneous Endoscopic Approach

02124AW Bypass Coronary Artery, Three Arteries from Aorta with Autologous Arterial Tissue, Percutaneous Endoscopic Approach

02124J3 Bypass Coronary Artery, Three Arteries from Coronary Artery with Synthetic Substitute, Percutaneous Endoscopic Approach

02124J8 Bypass Coronary Artery, Three Arteries from Right Internal Mammary with Synthetic Substitute, Percutaneous Endoscopic Approach

HAC 08: Surgical Site Infection of Mediastinitis after Coronary Bypass Graft (CABG) (continued)

02124J9   Bypass Coronary Artery, Three Arteries from Left Internal Mammary with Synthetic Substitute, Percutaneous Endoscopic Approach

02124JC   Bypass Coronary Artery, Three Arteries from Thoracic Artery with Synthetic Substitute, Percutaneous Endoscopic Approach

02124JF   Bypass Coronary Artery, Three Arteries from Abdominal Artery with Synthetic Substitute, Percutaneous Endoscopic Approach

02124JW   Bypass Coronary Artery, Three Arteries from Aorta with Synthetic Substitute, Percutaneous Endoscopic Approach

02124K3   Bypass Coronary Artery, Three Arteries from Coronary Artery with Nonautologous Tissue Substitute, Percutaneous Endoscopic Approach

02124K8   Bypass Coronary Artery, Three Arteries from Right Internal Mammary with Nonautologous Tissue Substitute, Percutaneous Endoscopic Approach

02124K9   Bypass Coronary Artery, Three Arteries from Left Internal Mammary with Nonautologous Tissue Substitute, Percutaneous Endoscopic Approach

02124KC   Bypass Coronary Artery, Three Arteries from Thoracic Artery with Nonautologous Tissue Substitute, Percutaneous Endoscopic Approach

02124KF   Bypass Coronary Artery, Three Arteries from Abdominal Artery with Nonautologous Tissue Substitute, Percutaneous Endoscopic Approach

02124KW   Bypass Coronary Artery, Three Arteries from Aorta with Nonautologous Tissue Substitute, Percutaneous Endoscopic Approach

02124Z3   Bypass Coronary Artery, Three Arteries from Coronary Artery, Percutaneous Endoscopic Approach

02124Z8   Bypass Coronary Artery, Three Arteries from Right Internal Mammary, Percutaneous Endoscopic Approach

02124Z9   Bypass Coronary Artery, Three Arteries from Left Internal Mammary, Percutaneous Endoscopic Approach

02124ZC   Bypass Coronary Artery, Three Arteries from Thoracic Artery, Percutaneous Endoscopic Approach

02124ZF   Bypass Coronary Artery, Three Arteries from Abdominal Artery, Percutaneous Endoscopic Approach

0213083   Bypass Coronary Artery, Four or More Arteries from Coronary Artery with Zooplastic Tissue, Open Approach

0213088   Bypass Coronary Artery, Four or More Arteries from Right Internal Mammary with Zooplastic Tissue, Open Approach

0213089   Bypass Coronary Artery, Four or More Arteries from Left Internal Mammary with Zooplastic Tissue, Open Approach

021308C   Bypass Coronary Artery, Four or More Arteries from Thoracic Artery with Zooplastic Tissue, Open Approach

021308F   Bypass Coronary Artery, Four or More Arteries from Abdominal Artery with Zooplastic Tissue, Open Approach

021308W   Bypass Coronary Artery, Four or More Arteries from Aorta with Zooplastic Tissue, Open Approach

0213093   Bypass Coronary Artery, Four or More Arteries from Coronary Artery with Autologous Venous Tissue, Open Approach

0213098   Bypass Coronary Artery, Four or More Arteries from Right Internal Mammary with Autologous Venous Tissue, Open Approach

0213099   Bypass Coronary Artery, Four or More Arteries from Left Internal Mammary with Autologous Venous Tissue, Open Approach

021309C   Bypass Coronary Artery, Four or More Arteries from Thoracic Artery with Autologous Venous Tissue, Open Approach

021309F   Bypass Coronary Artery, Four or More Arteries from Abdominal Artery with Autologous Venous Tissue, Open Approach

021309W   Bypass Coronary Artery, Four or More Arteries from Aorta with Autologous Venous Tissue, Open Approach

02130A3   Bypass Coronary Artery, Four or More Arteries from Coronary Artery with Autologous Arterial Tissue, Open Approach

02130A8   Bypass Coronary Artery, Four or More Arteries from Right Internal Mammary with Autologous Arterial Tissue, Open Approach

02130A9   Bypass Coronary Artery, Four or More Arteries from Left Internal Mammary with Autologous Arterial Tissue, Open Approach

02130AC   Bypass Coronary Artery, Four or More Arteries from Thoracic Artery with Autologous Arterial Tissue, Open Approach

02130AF   Bypass Coronary Artery, Four or More Arteries from Abdominal Artery with Autologous Arterial Tissue, Open Approach

02130AW   Bypass Coronary Artery, Four or More Arteries from Aorta with Autologous Arterial Tissue, Open Approach

02130J3   Bypass Coronary Artery, Four or More Arteries from Coronary Artery with Synthetic Substitute, Open Approach

02130J8   Bypass Coronary Artery, Four or More Arteries from Right Internal Mammary with Synthetic Substitute, Open Approach

02130J9   Bypass Coronary Artery, Four or More Arteries from Left Internal Mammary with Synthetic Substitute, Open Approach

02130JC   Bypass Coronary Artery, Four or More Arteries from Thoracic Artery with Synthetic Substitute, Open Approach

02130JF   Bypass Coronary Artery, Four or More Arteries from Abdominal Artery with Synthetic Substitute, Open Approach

02130JW   Bypass Coronary Artery, Four or More Arteries from Aorta with Synthetic Substitute, Open Approach

02130K3   Bypass Coronary Artery, Four or More Arteries from Coronary Artery with Nonautologous Tissue Substitute, Open Approach

02130K8   Bypass Coronary Artery, Four or More Arteries from Right Internal Mammary with Nonautologous Tissue Substitute, Open Approach

02130K9   Bypass Coronary Artery, Four or More Arteries from Left Internal Mammary with Nonautologous Tissue Substitute, Open Approach

02130KC   Bypass Coronary Artery, Four or More Arteries from Thoracic Artery with Nonautologous Tissue Substitute, Open Approach

02130KF   Bypass Coronary Artery, Four or More Arteries from Abdominal Artery with Nonautologous Tissue Substitute, Open Approach

02130KW   Bypass Coronary Artery, Four or More Arteries from Aorta with Nonautologous Tissue Substitute, Open Approach

02130Z3   Bypass Coronary Artery, Four or More Arteries from Coronary Artery, Open Approach

02130Z8   Bypass Coronary Artery, Four or More Arteries from Right Internal Mammary, Open Approach

02130Z9   Bypass Coronary Artery, Four or More Arteries from Left Internal Mammary, Open Approach

02130ZC   Bypass Coronary Artery, Four or More Arteries from Thoracic Artery, Open Approach

02130ZF   Bypass Coronary Artery, Four or More Arteries from Abdominal Artery, Open Approach

0213483   Bypass Coronary Artery, Four or More Arteries from Coronary Artery with Zooplastic Tissue, Percutaneous Endoscopic Approach

0213488   Bypass Coronary Artery, Four or More Arteries from Right Internal Mammary with Zooplastic Tissue, Percutaneous Endoscopic Approach

0213489   Bypass Coronary Artery, Four or More Arteries from Left Internal Mammary with Zooplastic Tissue, Percutaneous Endoscopic Approach

021348C   Bypass Coronary Artery, Four or More Arteries from Thoracic Artery with Zooplastic Tissue, Percutaneous Endoscopic Approach

021348F   Bypass Coronary Artery, Four or More Arteries from Abdominal Artery with Zooplastic Tissue, Percutaneous Endoscopic Approach

021348W   Bypass Coronary Artery, Four or More Arteries from Aorta with Zooplastic Tissue, Percutaneous Endoscopic Approach

0213493   Bypass Coronary Artery, Four or More Arteries from Coronary Artery with Autologous Venous Tissue, Percutaneous Endoscopic Approach

0213498   Bypass Coronary Artery, Four or More Arteries from Right Internal Mammary with Autologous Venous Tissue, Percutaneous Endoscopic Approach

0213499   Bypass Coronary Artery, Four or More Arteries from Left Internal Mammary with Autologous Venous Tissue, Percutaneous Endoscopic Approach

021349C   Bypass Coronary Artery, Four or More Arteries from Thoracic Artery with Autologous Venous Tissue, Percutaneous Endoscopic Approach

021349F   Bypass Coronary Artery, Four or More Arteries from Abdominal Artery with Autologous Venous Tissue, Percutaneous Endoscopic Approach

021349W   Bypass Coronary Artery, Four or More Arteries from Aorta with Autologous Venous Tissue, Percutaneous Endoscopic Approach

HAC 08: Surgical Site Infection of Mediastinitis after Coronary Bypass Graft (CABG) (continued)

02134A3 Bypass Coronary Artery, Four or More Arteries from Coronary Artery with Autologous Arterial Tissue, Percutaneous Endoscopic Approach

02134A8 Bypass Coronary Artery, Four or More Arteries from Right Internal Mammary with Autologous Arterial Tissue, Percutaneous Endoscopic Approach

02134A9 Bypass Coronary Artery, Four or More Arteries from Left Internal Mammary with Autologous Arterial Tissue, Percutaneous Endoscopic Approach

02134AC Bypass Coronary Artery, Four or More Arteries from Thoracic Artery with Autologous Arterial Tissue, Percutaneous Endoscopic Approach

02134AF Bypass Coronary Artery, Four or More Arteries from Abdominal Artery with Autologous Arterial Tissue, Percutaneous Endoscopic Approach

02134AW Bypass Coronary Artery, Four or More Arteries from Aorta with Autologous Arterial Tissue, Percutaneous Endoscopic Approach

02134J3 Bypass Coronary Artery, Four or More Arteries from Coronary Artery with Synthetic Substitute, Percutaneous Endoscopic Approach

02134J8 Bypass Coronary Artery, Four or More Arteries from Right Internal Mammary with Synthetic Substitute, Percutaneous Endoscopic Approach

02134J9 Bypass Coronary Artery, Four or More Arteries from Left Internal Mammary with Synthetic Substitute, Percutaneous Endoscopic Approach

02134JC Bypass Coronary Artery, Four or More Arteries from Thoracic Artery with Synthetic Substitute, Percutaneous Endoscopic Approach

02134JF Bypass Coronary Artery, Four or More Arteries from Abdominal Artery with Synthetic Substitute, Percutaneous Endoscopic Approach

02134JW Bypass Coronary Artery, Four or More Arteries from Aorta with Synthetic Substitute, Percutaneous Endoscopic Approach

02134K3 Bypass Coronary Artery, Four or More Arteries from Coronary Artery with Nonautologous Tissue Substitute, Percutaneous Endoscopic Approach

02134K8 Bypass Coronary Artery, Four or More Arteries from Right Internal Mammary with Nonautologous Tissue Substitute, Percutaneous Endoscopic Approach

02134K9 Bypass Coronary Artery, Four or More Arteries from Left Internal Mammary with Nonautologous Tissue Substitute, Percutaneous Endoscopic Approach

02134KC Bypass Coronary Artery, Four or More Arteries from Thoracic Artery with Nonautologous Tissue Substitute, Percutaneous Endoscopic Approach

02134KF Bypass Coronary Artery, Four or More Arteries from Abdominal Artery with Nonautologous Tissue Substitute, Percutaneous Endoscopic Approach

02134KW Bypass Coronary Artery, Four or More Arteries from Aorta with Nonautologous Tissue Substitute, Percutaneous Endoscopic Approach

02134Z3 Bypass Coronary Artery, Four or More Arteries from Coronary Artery, Percutaneous Endoscopic Approach

02134Z8 Bypass Coronary Artery, Four or More Arteries from Right Internal Mammary, Percutaneous Endoscopic Approach

02134Z9 Bypass Coronary Artery, Four or More Arteries from Left Internal Mammary, Percutaneous Endoscopic Approach

02134ZC Bypass Coronary Artery, Four or More Arteries from Thoracic Artery, Percutaneous Endoscopic Approach

02134ZF Bypass Coronary Artery, Four or More Arteries from Abdominal Artery, Percutaneous Endoscopic Approach

HAC 09: Manifestations of Poor Glycemic Control

Secondary diagnosis not POA:

E08.00
E08.01
E08.10
E09.00
E09.01
E09.10
E10.10
E11.00
E11.01
E13.00
E13.01
E13.10
E15

HAC 10: Deep Vein Thrombosis (DVT) or Pulmonary Embolism (PE) with Total Knee or Hip Replacement

Secondary diagnosis not POA:

I26.02
I26.09
I26.92
I26.93
I26.94
I26.99
I82.401
I82.402
I82.403
I82.409
I82.411
I82.412
I82.413
I82.419
I82.421
I82.422
I82.423
I82.429
I82.431
I82.432
I82.433
I82.439
I82.441
I82.442
I82.443
I82.449
I82.451
I82.452
I82.453
I82.459
I82.491
I82.492
I82.493
I82.499
I82.4Y1
I82.4Y2
I82.4Y3
I82.4Y9
I82.4Z1
I82.4Z2
I82.4Z3
I82.4Z9

AND

Any of the following procedures:

0SR9019 Replacement of Right Hip Joint with Metal Synthetic Substitute, Cemented, Open Approach

0SR901A Replacement of Right Hip Joint with Metal Synthetic Substitute, Uncemented, Open Approach

0SR901Z Replacement of Right Hip Joint with Metal Synthetic Substitute, Open Approach

0SR9029 Replacement of Right Hip Joint with Metal on Polyethylene Synthetic Substitute, Cemented, Open Approach

0SR902A Replacement of Right Hip Joint with Metal on Polyethylene Synthetic Substitute, Uncemented, Open Approach

0SR902Z Replacement of Right Hip Joint with Metal on Polyethylene Synthetic Substitute, Open Approach

0SR9039 Replacement of Right Hip Joint with Ceramic Synthetic Substitute, Cemented, Open Approach

0SR903A Replacement of Right Hip Joint with Ceramic Synthetic Substitute, Uncemented, Open Approach

0SR903Z Replacement of Right Hip Joint with Ceramic Synthetic Substitute, Open Approach

0SR9049 Replacement of Right Hip Joint with Ceramic on Polyethylene Synthetic Substitute, Cemented, Open Approach

0SR904A Replacement of Right Hip Joint with Ceramic on Polyethylene Synthetic Substitute, Uncemented, Open Approach

0SR904Z Replacement of Right Hip Joint with Ceramic on Polyethylene Synthetic Substitute, Open Approach

0SR9069 Replacement of Right Hip Joint with Oxidized Zirconium on Polyethylene Synthetic Substitute, Cemented, Open Approach

0SR906A Replacement of Right Hip Joint with Oxidized Zirconium on Polyethylene Synthetic Substitute, Uncemented, Open Approach

0SR906Z Replacement of Right Hip Joint with Oxidized Zirconium on Polyethylene Synthetic Substitute, Open Approach

0SR907Z Replacement of Right Hip Joint with Autologous Tissue Substitute, Open Approach

0SR90EZ Replacement of Right Hip Joint with Articulating Spacer, Open Approach

0SR90J9 Replacement of Right Hip Joint with Synthetic Substitute, Cemented, Open Approach

0SR90JA Replacement of Right Hip Joint with Synthetic Substitute, Uncemented, Open Approach

0SR90JZ Replacement of Right Hip Joint with Synthetic Substitute, Open Approach

0SR90KZ Replacement of Right Hip Joint with Nonautologous Tissue Substitute, Open Approach

0SRA009 Replacement of Right Hip Joint, Acetabular Surface with Polyethylene Synthetic Substitute, Cemented, Open Approach

0SRA00A Replacement of Right Hip Joint, Acetabular Surface with Polyethylene Synthetic Substitute, Uncemented, Open Approach

0SRA00Z Replacement of Right Hip Joint, Acetabular Surface with Polyethylene Synthetic Substitute, Open Approach

HAC 10: Deep Vein Thrombosis (DVT) or Pulmonary Embolism (PE) with Total Knee or Hip Replacement (continued)

ØSRAØ19 Replacement of Right Hip Joint, Acetabular Surface with Metal Synthetic Substitute, Cemented, Open Approach

ØSRAØ1A Replacement of Right Hip Joint, Acetabular Surface with Metal Synthetic Substitute, Uncemented, Open Approach

ØSRAØ1Z Replacement of Right Hip Joint, Acetabular Surface with Metal Synthetic Substitute, Open Approach

ØSRAØ39 Replacement of Right Hip Joint, Acetabular Surface with Ceramic Synthetic Substitute, Cemented, Open Approach

ØSRAØ3A Replacement of Right Hip Joint, Acetabular Surface with Ceramic Synthetic Substitute, Uncemented, Open Approach

ØSRAØ3Z Replacement of Right Hip Joint, Acetabular Surface with Ceramic Synthetic Substitute, Open Approach

ØSRAØ7Z Replacement of Right Hip Joint, Acetabular Surface with Autologous Tissue Substitute, Open Approach

ØSRAØJ9 Replacement of Right Hip Joint, Acetabular Surface with Synthetic Substitute, Cemented, Open Approach

ØSRAØJA Replacement of Right Hip Joint, Acetabular Surface with Synthetic Substitute, Uncemented, Open Approach

ØSRAØJZ Replacement of Right Hip Joint, Acetabular Surface with Synthetic Substitute, Open Approach

ØSRAØKZ Replacement of Right Hip Joint, Acetabular Surface with Nonautologous Tissue Substitute, Open Approach

ØSRBØ19 Replacement of Left Hip Joint with Metal Synthetic Substitute, Cemented, Open Approach

ØSRBØ1A Replacement of Left Hip Joint with Metal Synthetic Substitute, Uncemented, Open Approach

ØSRBØ1Z Replacement of Left Hip Joint with Metal Synthetic Substitute, Open Approach

ØSRBØ29 Replacement of Left Hip Joint with Metal on Polyethylene Synthetic Substitute, Cemented, Open Approach

ØSRBØ2A Replacement of Left Hip Joint with Metal on Polyethylene Synthetic Substitute, Uncemented, Open Approach

ØSRBØ2Z Replacement of Left Hip Joint with Metal on Polyethylene Synthetic Substitute, Open Approach

ØSRBØ39 Replacement of Left Hip Joint with Ceramic Synthetic Substitute, Cemented, Open Approach

ØSRBØ3A Replacement of Left Hip Joint with Ceramic Synthetic Substitute, Uncemented, Open Approach

ØSRBØ3Z Replacement of Left Hip Joint with Ceramic Synthetic Substitute, Open Approach

ØSRBØ49 Replacement of Left Hip Joint with Ceramic on Polyethylene Synthetic Substitute, Cemented, Open Approach

ØSRBØ4A Replacement of Left Hip Joint with Ceramic on Polyethylene Synthetic Substitute, Uncemented, Open Approach

ØSRBØ4Z Replacement of Left Hip Joint with Ceramic on Polyethylene Synthetic Substitute, Open Approach

ØSRBØ69 Replacement of Left Hip Joint with Oxidized Zirconium on Polyethylene Synthetic Substitute, Cemented, Open Approach

ØSRBØ6A Replacement of Left Hip Joint with Oxidized Zirconium on Polyethylene Synthetic Substitute, Uncemented, Open Approach

ØSRBØ6Z Replacement of Left Hip Joint with Oxidized Zirconium on Polyethylene Synthetic Substitute, Open Approach

ØSRBØ7Z Replacement of Left Hip Joint with Autologous Tissue Substitute, Open Approach

ØSRBØEZ Replacement of Left Hip Joint with Articulating Spacer, Open Approach

ØSRBØJ9 Replacement of Left Hip Joint with Synthetic Substitute, Cemented, Open Approach

ØSRBØJA Replacement of Left Hip Joint with Synthetic Substitute, Uncemented, Open Approach

ØSRBØJZ Replacement of Left Hip Joint with Synthetic Substitute, Open Approach

ØSRBØKZ Replacement of Left Hip Joint with Nonautologous Tissue Substitute, Open Approach

ØSRCØ69 Replacement of Right Knee Joint with Oxidized Zirconium on Polyethylene Synthetic Substitute, Cemented, Open Approach

ØSRCØ6A Replacement of Right Knee Joint with Oxidized Zirconium on Polyethylene Synthetic Substitute, Uncemented, Open Approach

ØSRCØ6Z Replacement of Right Knee Joint with Oxidized Zirconium on Polyethylene Synthetic Substitute, Open Approach

ØSRCØ7Z Replacement of Right Knee Joint with Autologous Tissue Substitute, Open Approach

ØSRCØEZ Replacement of Right Knee Joint with Articulating Spacer, Open Approach

ØSRCØJ9 Replacement of Right Knee Joint with Synthetic Substitute, Cemented, Open Approach

ØSRCØJA Replacement of Right Knee Joint with Synthetic Substitute, Uncemented, Open Approach

ØSRCØJZ Replacement of Right Knee Joint with Synthetic Substitute, Open Approach

ØSRCØKZ Replacement of Right Knee Joint with Nonautologous Tissue Substitute, Open Approach

ØSRCØL9 Replacement of Right Knee Joint with Medial Unicondylar Synthetic Substitute, Cemented, Open Approach

ØSRCØLA Replacement of Right Knee Joint with Medial Unicondylar Synthetic Substitute, Uncemented, Open Approach

ØSRCØLZ Replacement of Right Knee Joint with Medial Unicondylar Synthetic Substitute, Open Approach

ØSRCØM9 Replacement of Right Knee Joint with Lateral Unicondylar Synthetic Substitute, Cemented, Open Approach

ØSRCØMA Replacement of Right Knee Joint with Lateral Unicondylar Synthetic Substitute, Uncemented, Open Approach

ØSRCØMZ Replacement of Right Knee Joint with Lateral Unicondylar Synthetic Substitute, Open Approach

ØSRCØN9 Replacement of Right Knee Joint with Patellofemoral Synthetic Substitute, Cemented, Open Approach

ØSRCØNA Replacement of Right Knee Joint with Patellofemoral Synthetic Substitute, Uncemented, Open Approach

ØSRCØNZ Replacement of Right Knee Joint with Patellofemoral Synthetic Substitute, Open Approach

ØSRDØ69 Replacement of Left Knee Joint with Oxidized Zirconium on Polyethylene Synthetic Substitute, Cemented, Open Approach

ØSRDØ6A Replacement of Left Knee Joint with Oxidized Zirconium on Polyethylene Synthetic Substitute, Uncemented, Open Approach

ØSRDØ6Z Replacement of Left Knee Joint with Oxidized Zirconium on Polyethylene Synthetic Substitute, Open Approach

ØSRDØ7Z Replacement of Left Knee Joint with Autologous Tissue Substitute, Open Approach

ØSRDØEZ Replacement of Left Knee Joint with Articulating Spacer, Open Approach

ØSRDØJ9 Replacement of Left Knee Joint with Synthetic Substitute, Cemented, Open Approach

ØSRDØJA Replacement of Left Knee Joint with Synthetic Substitute, Uncemented, Open Approach

ØSRDØJZ Replacement of Left Knee Joint with Synthetic Substitute, Open Approach

ØSRDØKZ Replacement of Left Knee Joint with Nonautologous Tissue Substitute, Open Approach

ØSRDØL9 Replacement of Left Knee Joint with Medial Unicondylar Synthetic Substitute, Cemented, Open Approach

ØSRDØLA Replacement of Left Knee Joint with Medial Unicondylar Synthetic Substitute, Uncemented, Open Approach

ØSRDØLZ Replacement of Left Knee Joint with Medial Unicondylar Synthetic Substitute, Open Approach

ØSRDØM9 Replacement of Left Knee Joint with Lateral Unicondylar Synthetic Substitute, Cemented, Open Approach

ØSRDØMA Replacement of Left Knee Joint with Lateral Unicondylar Synthetic Substitute, Uncemented, Open Approach

ØSRDØMZ Replacement of Left Knee Joint with Lateral Unicondylar Synthetic Substitute, Open Approach

ØSRDØN9 Replacement of Left Knee Joint with Patellofemoral Synthetic Substitute, Cemented, Open Approach

ØSRDØNA Replacement of Left Knee Joint with Patellofemoral Synthetic Substitute, Uncemented, Open Approach

ØSRDØNZ Replacement of Left Knee Joint with Patellofemoral Synthetic Substitute, Open Approach

ØSREØØ9 Replacement of Left Hip Joint, Acetabular Surface with Polyethylene Synthetic Substitute, Cemented, Open Approach

ØSREØØA Replacement of Left Hip Joint, Acetabular Surface with Polyethylene Synthetic Substitute, Uncemented, Open Approach

ØSREØØZ Replacement of Left Hip Joint, Acetabular Surface with Polyethylene Synthetic Substitute, Open Approach

ØSREØ19 Replacement of Left Hip Joint, Acetabular Surface with Metal Synthetic Substitute, Cemented, Open Approach

ØSREØ1A Replacement of Left Hip Joint, Acetabular Surface with Metal Synthetic Substitute, Uncemented, Open Approach

ØSREØ1Z Replacement of Left Hip Joint, Acetabular Surface with Metal Synthetic Substitute, Open Approach

ØSREØ39 Replacement of Left Hip Joint, Acetabular Surface with Ceramic Synthetic Substitute, Cemented, Open Approach

HAC 10: Deep Vein Thrombosis (DVT) or Pulmonary Embolism (PE) with Total Knee or Hip Replacement (continued)

ØSRE03A Replacement of Left Hip Joint, Acetabular Surface with Ceramic Synthetic Substitute, Uncemented, Open Approach

ØSRE03Z Replacement of Left Hip Joint, Acetabular Surface with Ceramic Synthetic Substitute, Open Approach

ØSRE07Z Replacement of Left Hip Joint, Acetabular Surface with Autologous Tissue Substitute, Open Approach

ØSRE0J9 Replacement of Left Hip Joint, Acetabular Surface with Synthetic Substitute, Cemented, Open Approach

ØSRE0JA Replacement of Left Hip Joint, Acetabular Surface with Synthetic Substitute, Uncemented, Open Approach

ØSRE0JZ Replacement of Left Hip Joint, Acetabular Surface with Synthetic Substitute, Open Approach

ØSRE0KZ Replacement of Left Hip Joint, Acetabular Surface with Nonautologous Tissue Substitute, Open Approach

ØSRR019 Replacement of Right Hip Joint, Femoral Surface with Metal Synthetic Substitute, Cemented, Open Approach

ØSRR01A Replacement of Right Hip Joint, Femoral Surface with Metal Synthetic Substitute, Uncemented, Open Approach

ØSRR01Z Replacement of Right Hip Joint, Femoral Surface with Metal Synthetic Substitute, Open Approach

ØSRR039 Replacement of Right Hip Joint, Femoral Surface with Ceramic Synthetic Substitute, Cemented, Open Approach

ØSRR03A Replacement of Right Hip Joint, Femoral Surface with Ceramic Synthetic Substitute, Uncemented, Open Approach

ØSRR03Z Replacement of Right Hip Joint, Femoral Surface with Ceramic Synthetic Substitute, Open Approach

ØSRR07Z Replacement of Right Hip Joint, Femoral Surface with Autologous Tissue Substitute, Open Approach

ØSRR0J9 Replacement of Right Hip Joint, Femoral Surface with Synthetic Substitute, Cemented, Open Approach

ØSRR0JA Replacement of Right Hip Joint, Femoral Surface with Synthetic Substitute, Uncemented, Open Approach

ØSRR0JZ Replacement of Right Hip Joint, Femoral Surface with Synthetic Substitute, Open Approach

ØSRR0KZ Replacement of Right Hip Joint, Femoral Surface with Nonautologous Tissue Substitute, Open Approach

ØSRS019 Replacement of Left Hip Joint, Femoral Surface with Metal Synthetic Substitute, Cemented, Open Approach

ØSRS01A Replacement of Left Hip Joint, Femoral Surface with Metal Synthetic Substitute, Uncemented, Open Approach

ØSRS01Z Replacement of Left Hip Joint, Femoral Surface with Metal Synthetic Substitute, Open Approach

ØSRS039 Replacement of Left Hip Joint, Femoral Surface with Ceramic Synthetic Substitute, Cemented, Open Approach

ØSRS03A Replacement of Left Hip Joint, Femoral Surface with Ceramic Synthetic Substitute, Uncemented, Open Approach

ØSRS03Z Replacement of Left Hip Joint, Femoral Surface with Ceramic Synthetic Substitute, Open Approach

ØSRS07Z Replacement of Left Hip Joint, Femoral Surface with Autologous Tissue Substitute, Open Approach

ØSRS0J9 Replacement of Left Hip Joint, Femoral Surface with Synthetic Substitute, Cemented, Open Approach

ØSRS0JA Replacement of Left Hip Joint, Femoral Surface with Synthetic Substitute, Uncemented, Open Approach

ØSRS0JZ Replacement of Left Hip Joint, Femoral Surface with Synthetic Substitute, Open Approach

ØSRS0KZ Replacement of Left Hip Joint, Femoral Surface with Nonautologous Tissue Substitute, Open Approach

ØSRT07Z Replacement of Right Knee Joint, Femoral Surface with Autologous Tissue Substitute, Open Approach

ØSRT0J9 Replacement of Right Knee Joint, Femoral Surface with Synthetic Substitute, Cemented, Open Approach

ØSRT0JA Replacement of Right Knee Joint, Femoral Surface with Synthetic Substitute, Uncemented, Open Approach

ØSRT0JZ Replacement of Right Knee Joint, Femoral Surface with Synthetic Substitute, Open Approach

ØSRT0KZ Replacement of Right Knee Joint, Femoral Surface with Nonautologous Tissue Substitute, Open Approach

ØSRU07Z Replacement of Left Knee Joint, Femoral Surface with Autologous Tissue Substitute, Open Approach

ØSRU0J9 Replacement of Left Knee Joint, Femoral Surface with Synthetic Substitute, Cemented, Open Approach

ØSRU0JA Replacement of Left Knee Joint, Femoral Surface with Synthetic Substitute, Uncemented, Open Approach

ØSRU0JZ Replacement of Left Knee Joint, Femoral Surface with Synthetic Substitute, Open Approach

ØSRU0KZ Replacement of Left Knee Joint, Femoral Surface with Nonautologous Tissue Substitute, Open Approach

ØSRV07Z Replacement of Right Knee Joint, Tibial Surface with Autologous Tissue Substitute, Open Approach

ØSRV0J9 Replacement of Right Knee Joint, Tibial Surface with Synthetic Substitute, Cemented, Open Approach

ØSRV0JA Replacement of Right Knee Joint, Tibial Surface with Synthetic Substitute, Uncemented, Open Approach

ØSRV0JZ Replacement of Right Knee Joint, Tibial Surface with Synthetic Substitute, Open Approach

ØSRV0KZ Replacement of Right Knee Joint, Tibial Surface with Nonautologous Tissue Substitute, Open Approach

ØSRW07Z Replacement of Left Knee Joint, Tibial Surface with Autologous Tissue Substitute, Open Approach

ØSRW0J9 Replacement of Left Knee Joint, Tibial Surface with Synthetic Substitute, Cemented, Open Approach

ØSRW0JA Replacement of Left Knee Joint, Tibial Surface with Synthetic Substitute, Uncemented, Open Approach

ØSRW0JZ Replacement of Left Knee Joint, Tibial Surface with Synthetic Substitute, Open Approach

ØSRW0KZ Replacement of Left Knee Joint, Tibial Surface with Nonautologous Tissue Substitute, Open Approach

ØSU90BZ Supplement Right Hip Joint with Resurfacing Device, Open Approach

ØSUA0BZ Supplement Right Hip Joint, Acetabular Surface with Resurfacing Device, Open Approach

ØSUB0BZ Supplement Left Hip Joint with Resurfacing Device, Open Approach

ØSUE0BZ Supplement Left Hip Joint, Acetabular Surface with Resurfacing Device, Open Approach

ØSUR0BZ Supplement Right Hip Joint, Femoral Surface with Resurfacing Device, Open Approach

ØSUS0BZ Supplement Left Hip Joint, Femoral Surface with Resurfacing Device, Open Approach

HAC 11: Surgical Site Infection—Bariatric Surgery

Principal diagnosis of:
E66.01

AND

Secondary diagnosis not POA:
K68.11
K95.01
K95.81
T81.40XA
T81.41XA
T81.42XA
T81.43XA
T81.44XA
T81.49XA

AND

Any of the following procedures:

ØD16079 Bypass Stomach to Duodenum with Autologous Tissue Substitute, Open Approach

ØD1607A Bypass Stomach to Jejunum with Autologous Tissue Substitute, Open Approach

ØD1607B Bypass Stomach to Ileum with Autologous Tissue Substitute, Open Approach

ØD1607L Bypass Stomach to Transverse Colon with Autologous Tissue Substitute, Open Approach

ØD160J9 Bypass Stomach to Duodenum with Synthetic Substitute, Open Approach

ØD160JA Bypass Stomach to Jejunum with Synthetic Substitute, Open Approach

ØD160JB Bypass Stomach to Ileum with Synthetic Substitute, Open Approach

ØD160JL Bypass Stomach to Transverse Colon with Synthetic Substitute, Open Approach

ØD160K9 Bypass Stomach to Duodenum with Nonautologous Tissue Substitute, Open Approach

ØD160KA Bypass Stomach to Jejunum with Nonautologous Tissue Substitute, Open Approach

ØD160KB Bypass Stomach to Ileum with Nonautologous Tissue Substitute, Open Approach

ØD160KL Bypass Stomach to Transverse Colon with Nonautologous Tissue Substitute, Open Approach

ØD160Z9 Bypass Stomach to Duodenum, Open Approach

ØD160ZA Bypass Stomach to Jejunum, Open Approach

ØD160ZB Bypass Stomach to Ileum, Open Approach

ØD160ZL Bypass Stomach to Transverse Colon, Open Approach

ØD16479 Bypass Stomach to Duodenum with Autologous Tissue Substitute, Percutaneous Endoscopic Approach

HAC 11: Surgical Site Infection—Bariatric Surgery (continued)

ØD1647A Bypass Stomach to Jejunum with Autologous Tissue Substitute, Percutaneous Endoscopic Approach

ØD1647B Bypass Stomach to Ileum with Autologous Tissue Substitute, Percutaneous Endoscopic Approach

ØD1647L Bypass Stomach to Transverse Colon with Autologous Tissue Substitute, Percutaneous Endoscopic Approach

ØD164J9 Bypass Stomach to Duodenum with Synthetic Substitute, Percutaneous Endoscopic Approach

ØD164JA Bypass Stomach to Jejunum with Synthetic Substitute, Percutaneous Endoscopic Approach

ØD164JB Bypass Stomach to Ileum with Synthetic Substitute, Percutaneous Endoscopic Approach

ØD164JL Bypass Stomach to Transverse Colon with Synthetic Substitute, Percutaneous Endoscopic Approach

ØD164K9 Bypass Stomach to Duodenum with Nonautologous Tissue Substitute, Percutaneous Endoscopic Approach

ØD164KA Bypass Stomach to Jejunum with Nonautologous Tissue Substitute, Percutaneous Endoscopic Approach

ØD164KB Bypass Stomach to Ileum with Nonautologous Tissue Substitute, Percutaneous Endoscopic Approach

ØD164KL Bypass Stomach to Transverse Colon with Nonautologous Tissue Substitute, Percutaneous Endoscopic Approach

ØD164Z9 Bypass Stomach to Duodenum, Percutaneous Endoscopic Approach

ØD164ZA Bypass Stomach to Jejunum, Percutaneous Endoscopic Approach

ØD164ZB Bypass Stomach to Ileum, Percutaneous Endoscopic Approach

ØD164ZL Bypass Stomach to Transverse Colon, Percutaneous Endoscopic Approach

ØD16879 Bypass Stomach to Duodenum with Autologous Tissue Substitute, Via Natural or Artificial Opening Endoscopic

ØD1687A Bypass Stomach to Jejunum with Autologous Tissue Substitute, Via Natural or Artificial Opening Endoscopic

ØD1687B Bypass Stomach to Ileum with Autologous Tissue Substitute, Via Natural or Artificial Opening Endoscopic

ØD1687L Bypass Stomach to Transverse Colon with Autologous Tissue Substitute, Via Natural or Artificial Opening Endoscopic

ØD168J9 Bypass Stomach to Duodenum with Synthetic Substitute, Via Natural or Artificial Opening Endoscopic

ØD168JA Bypass Stomach to Jejunum with Synthetic Substitute, Via Natural or Artificial Opening Endoscopic

ØD168JB Bypass Stomach to Ileum with Synthetic Substitute, Via Natural or Artificial Opening Endoscopic

ØD168JL Bypass Stomach to Transverse Colon with Synthetic Substitute, Via Natural or Artificial Opening Endoscopic

ØD168K9 Bypass Stomach to Duodenum with Nonautologous Tissue Substitute, Via Natural or Artificial Opening Endoscopic

ØD168KA Bypass Stomach to Jejunum with Nonautologous Tissue Substitute, Via Natural or Artificial Opening Endoscopic

ØD168KB Bypass Stomach to Ileum with Nonautologous Tissue Substitute, Via Natural or Artificial Opening Endoscopic

ØD168KL Bypass Stomach to Transverse Colon with Nonautologous Tissue Substitute, Via Natural or Artificial Opening Endoscopic

ØD168Z9 Bypass Stomach to Duodenum, Via Natural or Artificial Opening Endoscopic

ØD168ZA Bypass Stomach to Jejunum, Via Natural or Artificial Opening Endoscopic

ØD168ZB Bypass Stomach to Ileum, Via Natural or Artificial Opening Endoscopic

ØD168ZL Bypass Stomach to Transverse Colon, Via Natural or Artificial Opening Endoscopic

ØDV64CZ Restriction of Stomach with Extraluminal Device, Percutaneous Endoscopic Approach

HAC 12: Surgical Site Infection—Certain Orthopedic Procedures of the Spine, Shoulder, and Elbow

Secondary diagnosis not POA:

K68.11
T81.40XA
T81.41XA
T81.42XA
T81.43XA
T81.44XA
T81.49XA
T84.60XA
T84.610A
T84.611A
T84.612A
T84.613A
T84.614A
T84.615A
T84.619A
T84.63XA
T84.69XA
T84.7XXA

AND

Any of the following procedures:

ØRG0070 Fusion of Occipital-cervical Joint with Autologous Tissue Substitute, Anterior Approach, Anterior Column, Open Approach

ØRG0071 Fusion of Occipital-cervical Joint with Autologous Tissue Substitute, Posterior Approach, Posterior Column, Open Approach

ØRG007J Fusion of Occipital-cervical Joint with Autologous Tissue Substitute, Posterior Approach, Anterior Column, Open Approach

ØRG00A0 Fusion of Occipital-cervical Joint with Interbody Fusion Device, Anterior Approach, Anterior Column, Open Approach

ØRG00AJ Fusion of Occipital-cervical Joint with Interbody Fusion Device, Posterior Approach, Anterior Column, Open Approach

ØRG00J0 Fusion of Occipital-cervical Joint with Synthetic Substitute, Anterior Approach, Anterior Column, Open Approach

ØRG00J1 Fusion of Occipital-cervical Joint with Synthetic Substitute, Posterior Approach, Posterior Column, Open Approach

ØRG00JJ Fusion of Occipital-cervical Joint with Synthetic Substitute, Posterior Approach, Anterior Column, Open Approach

ØRG00K0 Fusion of Occipital-cervical Joint with Nonautologous Tissue Substitute, Anterior Approach, Anterior Column, Open Approach

ØRG00K1 Fusion of Occipital-cervical Joint with Nonautologous Tissue Substitute, Posterior Approach, Posterior Column, Open Approach

ØRG00KJ Fusion of Occipital-cervical Joint with Nonautologous Tissue Substitute, Posterior Approach, Anterior Column, Open Approach

ØRG0370 Fusion of Occipital-cervical Joint with Autologous Tissue Substitute, Anterior Approach, Anterior Column, Percutaneous Approach

ØRG0371 Fusion of Occipital-cervical Joint with Autologous Tissue Substitute, Posterior Approach, Posterior Column, Percutaneous Approach

ØRG037J Fusion of Occipital-cervical Joint with Autologous Tissue Substitute, Posterior Approach, Anterior Column, Percutaneous Approach

ØRG03A0 Fusion of Occipital-cervical Joint with Interbody Fusion Device, Anterior Approach, Anterior Column, Percutaneous Approach

ØRG03AJ Fusion of Occipital-cervical Joint with Interbody Fusion Device, Posterior Approach, Anterior Column, Percutaneous Approach

ØRG03J0 Fusion of Occipital-cervical Joint with Synthetic Substitute, Anterior Approach, Anterior Column, Percutaneous Approach

ØRG03J1 Fusion of Occipital-cervical Joint with Synthetic Substitute, Posterior Approach, Posterior Column, Percutaneous Approach

ØRG03JJ Fusion of Occipital-cervical Joint with Synthetic Substitute, Posterior Approach, Anterior Column, Percutaneous Approach

ØRG03K0 Fusion of Occipital-cervical Joint with Nonautologous Tissue Substitute, Anterior Approach, Anterior Column, Percutaneous Approach

ØRG03K1 Fusion of Occipital-cervical Joint with Nonautologous Tissue Substitute, Posterior Approach, Posterior Column, Percutaneous Approach

ØRG03KJ Fusion of Occipital-cervical Joint with Nonautologous Tissue Substitute, Posterior Approach, Anterior Column, Percutaneous Approach

ØRG0470 Fusion of Occipital-cervical Joint with Autologous Tissue Substitute, Anterior Approach, Anterior Column, Percutaneous Endoscopic Approach

ØRG0471 Fusion of Occipital-cervical Joint with Autologous Tissue Substitute, Posterior Approach, Posterior Column, Percutaneous Endoscopic Approach

ØRG047J Fusion of Occipital-cervical Joint with Autologous Tissue Substitute, Posterior Approach, Anterior Column, Percutaneous Endoscopic Approach

ØRG04A0 Fusion of Occipital-cervical Joint with Interbody Fusion Device, Anterior Approach, Anterior Column, Percutaneous Endoscopic Approach

ØRG04AJ Fusion of Occipital-cervical Joint with Interbody Fusion Device, Posterior Approach, Anterior Column, Percutaneous Endoscopic Approach

ØRG04J0 Fusion of Occipital-cervical Joint with Synthetic Substitute, Anterior Approach, Anterior Column, Percutaneous Endoscopic Approach

ØRG04J1 Fusion of Occipital-cervical Joint with Synthetic Substitute, Posterior Approach, Posterior Column, Percutaneous Endoscopic Approach

HAC 12: Surgical Site Infection—Certain Orthopedic Procedures of the Spine, Shoulder, and Elbow (continued)

ØRG04JJ Fusion of Occipital-cervical Joint with Synthetic Substitute, Posterior Approach, Anterior Column, Percutaneous Endoscopic Approach

ØRG04KØ Fusion of Occipital-cervical Joint with Nonautologous Tissue Substitute, Anterior Approach, Anterior Column, Percutaneous Endoscopic Approach

ØRG04K1 Fusion of Occipital-cervical Joint with Nonautologous Tissue Substitute, Posterior Approach, Posterior Column, Percutaneous Endoscopic Approach

ØRG04KJ Fusion of Occipital-cervical Joint with Nonautologous Tissue Substitute, Posterior Approach, Anterior Column, Percutaneous Endoscopic Approach

ØRG1Ø7Ø Fusion of Cervical Vertebral Joint with Autologous Tissue Substitute, Anterior Approach, Anterior Column, Open Approach

ØRG1Ø71 Fusion of Cervical Vertebral Joint with Autologous Tissue Substitute, Posterior Approach, Posterior Column, Open Approach

ØRG1Ø7J Fusion of Cervical Vertebral Joint with Autologous Tissue Substitute, Posterior Approach, Anterior Column, Open Approach

ØRG1ØAØ Fusion of Cervical Vertebral Joint with Interbody Fusion Device, Anterior Approach, Anterior Column, Open Approach

ØRG1ØAJ Fusion of Cervical Vertebral Joint with Interbody Fusion Device, Posterior Approach, Anterior Column, Open Approach

ØRG1ØJØ Fusion of Cervical Vertebral Joint with Synthetic Substitute, Anterior Approach, Anterior Column, Open Approach

ØRG1ØJ1 Fusion of Cervical Vertebral Joint with Synthetic Substitute, Posterior Approach, Posterior Column, Open Approach

ØRG1ØJJ Fusion of Cervical Vertebral Joint with Synthetic Substitute, Posterior Approach, Anterior Column, Open Approach

ØRG1ØKØ Fusion of Cervical Vertebral Joint with Nonautologous Tissue Substitute, Anterior Approach, Anterior Column, Open Approach

ØRG1ØK1 Fusion of Cervical Vertebral Joint with Nonautologous Tissue Substitute, Posterior Approach, Posterior Column, Open Approach

ØRG1ØKJ Fusion of Cervical Vertebral Joint with Nonautologous Tissue Substitute, Posterior Approach, Anterior Column, Open Approach

ØRG137Ø Fusion of Cervical Vertebral Joint with Autologous Tissue Substitute, Anterior Approach, Anterior Column, Percutaneous Approach

ØRG1371 Fusion of Cervical Vertebral Joint with Autologous Tissue Substitute, Posterior Approach, Posterior Column, Percutaneous Approach

ØRG137J Fusion of Cervical Vertebral Joint with Autologous Tissue Substitute, Posterior Approach, Anterior Column, Percutaneous Approach

ØRG13AØ Fusion of Cervical Vertebral Joint with Interbody Fusion Device, Anterior Approach, Anterior Column, Percutaneous Approach

ØRG13AJ Fusion of Cervical Vertebral Joint with Interbody Fusion Device, Posterior Approach, Anterior Column, Percutaneous Approach

ØRG13JØ Fusion of Cervical Vertebral Joint with Synthetic Substitute, Anterior Approach, Anterior Column, Percutaneous Approach

ØRG13J1 Fusion of Cervical Vertebral Joint with Synthetic Substitute, Posterior Approach, Posterior Column, Percutaneous Approach

ØRG13JJ Fusion of Cervical Vertebral Joint with Synthetic Substitute, Posterior Approach, Anterior Column, Percutaneous Approach

ØRG13KØ Fusion of Cervical Vertebral Joint with Nonautologous Tissue Substitute, Anterior Approach, Anterior Column, Percutaneous Approach

ØRG13K1 Fusion of Cervical Vertebral Joint with Nonautologous Tissue Substitute, Posterior Approach, Posterior Column, Percutaneous Approach

ØRG13KJ Fusion of Cervical Vertebral Joint with Nonautologous Tissue Substitute, Posterior Approach, Anterior Column, Percutaneous Approach

ØRG147Ø Fusion of Cervical Vertebral Joint with Autologous Tissue Substitute, Anterior Approach, Anterior Column, Percutaneous Endoscopic Approach

ØRG1471 Fusion of Cervical Vertebral Joint with Autologous Tissue Substitute, Posterior Approach, Posterior Column, Percutaneous Endoscopic Approach

ØRG147J Fusion of Cervical Vertebral Joint with Autologous Tissue Substitute, Posterior Approach, Anterior Column, Percutaneous Endoscopic Approach

ØRG14AØ Fusion of Cervical Vertebral Joint with Interbody Fusion Device, Anterior Approach, Anterior Column, Percutaneous Endoscopic Approach

ØRG14AJ Fusion of Cervical Vertebral Joint with Interbody Fusion Device, Posterior Approach, Anterior Column, Percutaneous Endoscopic Approach

ØRG14JØ Fusion of Cervical Vertebral Joint with Synthetic Substitute, Anterior Approach, Anterior Column, Percutaneous Endoscopic Approach

ØRG14J1 Fusion of Cervical Vertebral Joint with Synthetic Substitute, Posterior Approach, Posterior Column, Percutaneous Endoscopic Approach

ØRG14JJ Fusion of Cervical Vertebral Joint with Synthetic Substitute, Posterior Approach, Anterior Column, Percutaneous Endoscopic Approach

ØRG14KØ Fusion of Cervical Vertebral Joint with Nonautologous Tissue Substitute, Anterior Approach, Anterior Column, Percutaneous Endoscopic Approach

ØRG14K1 Fusion of Cervical Vertebral Joint with Nonautologous Tissue Substitute, Posterior Approach, Posterior Column, Percutaneous Endoscopic Approach

ØRG14KJ Fusion of Cervical Vertebral Joint with Nonautologous Tissue Substitute, Posterior Approach, Anterior Column, Percutaneous Endoscopic Approach

ØRG2Ø7Ø Fusion of 2 or more Cervical Vertebral Joints with Autologous Tissue Substitute, Anterior Approach, Anterior Column, Open Approach

ØRG2Ø71 Fusion of 2 or more Cervical Vertebral Joints with Autologous Tissue Substitute, Posterior Approach, Posterior Column, Open Approach

ØRG2Ø7J Fusion of 2 or more Cervical Vertebral Joints with Autologous Tissue Substitute, Posterior Approach, Anterior Column, Open Approach

ØRG2ØAØ Fusion of 2 or more Cervical Vertebral Joints with Interbody Fusion Device, Anterior Approach, Anterior Column, Open Approach

ØRG2ØAJ Fusion of 2 or more Cervical Vertebral Joints with Interbody Fusion Device, Posterior Approach, Anterior Column, Open Approach

ØRG2ØJØ Fusion of 2 or more Cervical Vertebral Joints with Synthetic Substitute, Anterior Approach, Anterior Column, Open Approach

ØRG2ØJ1 Fusion of 2 or more Cervical Vertebral Joints with Synthetic Substitute, Posterior Approach, Posterior Column, Open Approach

ØRG2ØJJ Fusion of 2 or more Cervical Vertebral Joints with Synthetic Substitute, Posterior Approach, Anterior Column, Open Approach

ØRG2ØKØ Fusion of 2 or more Cervical Vertebral Joints with Nonautologous Tissue Substitute, Anterior Approach, Anterior Column, Open Approach

ØRG2ØK1 Fusion of 2 or more Cervical Vertebral Joints with Nonautologous Tissue Substitute, Posterior Approach, Posterior Column, Open Approach

ØRG2ØKJ Fusion of 2 or more Cervical Vertebral Joints with Nonautologous Tissue Substitute, Posterior Approach, Anterior Column, Open Approach

ØRG237Ø Fusion of 2 or more Cervical Vertebral Joints with Autologous Tissue Substitute, Anterior Approach, Anterior Column, Percutaneous Approach

ØRG2371 Fusion of 2 or more Cervical Vertebral Joints with Autologous Tissue Substitute, Posterior Approach, Posterior Column, Percutaneous Approach

ØRG237J Fusion of 2 or more Cervical Vertebral Joints with Autologous Tissue Substitute, Posterior Approach, Anterior Column, Percutaneous Approach

ØRG23AØ Fusion of 2 or more Cervical Vertebral Joints with Interbody Fusion Device, Anterior Approach, Anterior Column, Percutaneous Approach

ØRG23AJ Fusion of 2 or more Cervical Vertebral Joints with Interbody Fusion Device, Posterior Approach, Anterior Column, Percutaneous Approach

ØRG23JØ Fusion of 2 or more Cervical Vertebral Joints with Synthetic Substitute, Anterior Approach, Anterior Column, Percutaneous Approach

ØRG23J1 Fusion of 2 or more Cervical Vertebral Joints with Synthetic Substitute, Posterior Approach, Posterior Column, Percutaneous Approach

ØRG23JJ Fusion of 2 or more Cervical Vertebral Joints with Synthetic Substitute, Posterior Approach, Anterior Column, Percutaneous Approach

ØRG23KØ Fusion of 2 or more Cervical Vertebral Joints with Nonautologous Tissue Substitute, Anterior Approach, Anterior Column, Percutaneous Approach

HAC 12: Surgical Site Infection— Certain Orthopedic Procedures of the Spine, Shoulder, and Elbow (continued)

ØRG23K1 Fusion of 2 or more Cervical Vertebral Joints with Nonautologous Tissue Substitute, Posterior Approach, Posterior Column, Percutaneous Approach

ØRG23KJ Fusion of 2 or more Cervical Vertebral Joints with Nonautologous Tissue Substitute, Posterior Approach, Anterior Column, Percutaneous Approach

ØRG247Ø Fusion of 2 or more Cervical Vertebral Joints with Autologous Tissue Substitute, Anterior Approach, Anterior Column, Percutaneous Endoscopic Approach

ØRG2471 Fusion of 2 or more Cervical Vertebral Joints with Autologous Tissue Substitute, Posterior Approach, Posterior Column, Percutaneous Endoscopic Approach

ØRG247J Fusion of 2 or more Cervical Vertebral Joints with Autologous Tissue Substitute, Posterior Approach, Anterior Column, Percutaneous Endoscopic Approach

ØRG24AØ Fusion of 2 or more Cervical Vertebral Joints with Interbody Fusion Device, Anterior Approach, Anterior Column, Percutaneous Endoscopic Approach

ØRG24AJ Fusion of 2 or more Cervical Vertebral Joints with Interbody Fusion Device, Posterior Approach, Anterior Column, Percutaneous Endoscopic Approach

ØRG24JØ Fusion of 2 or more Cervical Vertebral Joints with Synthetic Substitute, Anterior Approach, Anterior Column, Percutaneous Endoscopic Approach

ØRG24J1 Fusion of 2 or more Cervical Vertebral Joints with Synthetic Substitute, Posterior Approach, Posterior Column, Percutaneous Endoscopic Approach

ØRG24JJ Fusion of 2 or more Cervical Vertebral Joints with Synthetic Substitute, Posterior Approach, Anterior Column, Percutaneous Endoscopic Approach

ØRG24KØ Fusion of 2 or more Cervical Vertebral Joints with Nonautologous Tissue Substitute, Anterior Approach, Anterior Column, Percutaneous Endoscopic Approach

ØRG24K1 Fusion of 2 or more Cervical Vertebral Joints with Nonautologous Tissue Substitute, Posterior Approach, Posterior Column, Percutaneous Endoscopic Approach

ØRG24KJ Fusion of 2 or more Cervical Vertebral Joints with Nonautologous Tissue Substitute, Posterior Approach, Anterior Column, Percutaneous Endoscopic Approach

ØRG4Ø7Ø Fusion of Cervicothoracic Vertebral Joint with Autologous Tissue Substitute, Anterior Approach, Anterior Column, Open Approach

ØRG4Ø71 Fusion of Cervicothoracic Vertebral Joint with Autologous Tissue Substitute, Posterior Approach, Posterior Column, Open Approach

ØRG4Ø7J Fusion of Cervicothoracic Vertebral Joint with Autologous Tissue Substitute, Posterior Approach, Anterior Column, Open Approach

ØRG4ØAØ Fusion of Cervicothoracic Vertebral Joint with Interbody Fusion Device, Anterior Approach, Anterior Column, Open Approach

ØRG4ØAJ Fusion of Cervicothoracic Vertebral Joint with Interbody Fusion Device, Posterior Approach, Anterior Column, Open Approach

ØRG4ØJØ Fusion of Cervicothoracic Vertebral Joint with Synthetic Substitute, Anterior Approach, Anterior Column, Open Approach

ØRG4ØJ1 Fusion of Cervicothoracic Vertebral Joint with Synthetic Substitute, Posterior Approach, Posterior Column, Open Approach

ØRG4ØJJ Fusion of Cervicothoracic Vertebral Joint with Synthetic Substitute, Posterior Approach, Anterior Column, Open Approach

ØRG4ØKØ Fusion of Cervicothoracic Vertebral Joint with Nonautologous Tissue Substitute, Anterior Approach, Anterior Column, Open Approach

ØRG4ØK1 Fusion of Cervicothoracic Vertebral Joint with Nonautologous Tissue Substitute, Posterior Approach, Posterior Column, Open Approach

ØRG4ØKJ Fusion of Cervicothoracic Vertebral Joint with Nonautologous Tissue Substitute, Posterior Approach, Anterior Column, Open Approach

ØRG437Ø Fusion of Cervicothoracic Vertebral Joint with Autologous Tissue Substitute, Anterior Approach, Anterior Column, Percutaneous Approach

ØRG4371 Fusion of Cervicothoracic Vertebral Joint with Autologous Tissue Substitute, Posterior Approach, Posterior Column, Percutaneous Approach

ØRG437J Fusion of Cervicothoracic Vertebral Joint with Autologous Tissue Substitute, Posterior Approach, Anterior Column, Percutaneous Approach

ØRG43AØ Fusion of Cervicothoracic Vertebral Joint with Interbody Fusion Device, Anterior Approach, Anterior Column, Percutaneous Approach

ØRG43AJ Fusion of Cervicothoracic Vertebral Joint with Interbody Fusion Device, Posterior Approach, Anterior Column, Percutaneous Approach

ØRG43JØ Fusion of Cervicothoracic Vertebral Joint with Synthetic Substitute, Anterior Approach, Anterior Column, Percutaneous Approach

ØRG43J1 Fusion of Cervicothoracic Vertebral Joint with Synthetic Substitute, Posterior Approach, Posterior Column, Percutaneous Approach

ØRG43JJ Fusion of Cervicothoracic Vertebral Joint with Synthetic Substitute, Posterior Approach, Anterior Column, Percutaneous Approach

ØRG43KØ Fusion of Cervicothoracic Vertebral Joint with Nonautologous Tissue Substitute, Anterior Approach, Anterior Column, Percutaneous Approach

ØRG43K1 Fusion of Cervicothoracic Vertebral Joint with Nonautologous Tissue Substitute, Posterior Approach, Posterior Column, Percutaneous Approach

ØRG43KJ Fusion of Cervicothoracic Vertebral Joint with Nonautologous Tissue Substitute, Posterior Approach, Anterior Column, Percutaneous Approach

ØRG447Ø Fusion of Cervicothoracic Vertebral Joint with Autologous Tissue Substitute, Anterior Approach, Anterior Column, Percutaneous Endoscopic Approach

ØRG4471 Fusion of Cervicothoracic Vertebral Joint with Autologous Tissue Substitute, Posterior Approach, Posterior Column, Percutaneous Endoscopic Approach

ØRG447J Fusion of Cervicothoracic Vertebral Joint with Autologous Tissue Substitute, Posterior Approach, Anterior Column, Percutaneous Endoscopic Approach

ØRG44AØ Fusion of Cervicothoracic Vertebral Joint with Interbody Fusion Device, Anterior Approach, Anterior Column, Percutaneous Endoscopic Approach

ØRG44AJ Fusion of Cervicothoracic Vertebral Joint with Interbody Fusion Device, Posterior Approach, Anterior Column, Percutaneous Endoscopic Approach

ØRG44JØ Fusion of Cervicothoracic Vertebral Joint with Synthetic Substitute, Anterior Approach, Anterior Column, Percutaneous Endoscopic Approach

ØRG44J1 Fusion of Cervicothoracic Vertebral Joint with Synthetic Substitute, Posterior Approach, Posterior Column, Percutaneous Endoscopic Approach

ØRG44JJ Fusion of Cervicothoracic Vertebral Joint with Synthetic Substitute, Posterior Approach, Anterior Column, Percutaneous Endoscopic Approach

ØRG44KØ Fusion of Cervicothoracic Vertebral Joint with Nonautologous Tissue Substitute, Anterior Approach, Anterior Column, Percutaneous Endoscopic Approach

ØRG44K1 Fusion of Cervicothoracic Vertebral Joint with Nonautologous Tissue Substitute, Posterior Approach, Posterior Column, Percutaneous Endoscopic Approach

ØRG44KJ Fusion of Cervicothoracic Vertebral Joint with Nonautologous Tissue Substitute, Posterior Approach, Anterior Column, Percutaneous Endoscopic Approach

ØRG6Ø7Ø Fusion of Thoracic Vertebral Joint with Autologous Tissue Substitute, Anterior Approach, Anterior Column, Open Approach

ØRG6Ø71 Fusion of Thoracic Vertebral Joint with Autologous Tissue Substitute, Posterior Approach, Posterior Column, Open Approach

ØRG6Ø7J Fusion of Thoracic Vertebral Joint with Autologous Tissue Substitute, Posterior Approach, Anterior Column, Open Approach

ØRG6ØAØ Fusion of Thoracic Vertebral Joint with Interbody Fusion Device, Anterior Approach, Anterior Column, Open Approach

ØRG6ØAJ Fusion of Thoracic Vertebral Joint with Interbody Fusion Device, Posterior Approach, Anterior Column, Open Approach

ØRG6ØJØ Fusion of Thoracic Vertebral Joint with Synthetic Substitute, Anterior Approach, Anterior Column, Open Approach

ØRG6ØJ1 Fusion of Thoracic Vertebral Joint with Synthetic Substitute, Posterior Approach, Posterior Column, Open Approach

ØRG6ØJJ Fusion of Thoracic Vertebral Joint with Synthetic Substitute, Posterior Approach, Anterior Column, Open Approach

ØRG6ØKØ Fusion of Thoracic Vertebral Joint with Nonautologous Tissue Substitute, Anterior Approach, Anterior Column, Open Approach

ØRG6ØK1 Fusion of Thoracic Vertebral Joint with Nonautologous Tissue Substitute, Posterior Hopproach, Posterior Column, Open Approach

HAC 12: Surgical Site Infection—Certain Orthopedic Procedures of the Spine, Shoulder, and Elbow (continued)

ØRG60KJ   Fusion of Thoracic Vertebral Joint with Nonautologous Tissue Substitute, Posterior Approach, Anterior Column, Open Approach

ØRG637Ø   Fusion of Thoracic Vertebral Joint with Autologous Tissue Substitute, Anterior Approach, Anterior Column, Percutaneous Approach

ØRG6371   Fusion of Thoracic Vertebral Joint with Autologous Tissue Substitute, Posterior Approach, Posterior Column, Percutaneous Approach

ØRG637J   Fusion of Thoracic Vertebral Joint with Autologous Tissue Substitute, Posterior Approach, Anterior Column, Percutaneous Approach

ØRG63AØ   Fusion of Thoracic Vertebral Joint with Interbody Fusion Device, Anterior Approach, Anterior Column, Percutaneous Approach

ØRG63AJ   Fusion of Thoracic Vertebral Joint with Interbody Fusion Device, Posterior Approach, Anterior Column, Percutaneous Approach

ØRG63JØ   Fusion of Thoracic Vertebral Joint with Synthetic Substitute, Anterior Approach, Anterior Column, Percutaneous Approach

ØRG63J1   Fusion of Thoracic Vertebral Joint with Synthetic Substitute, Posterior Approach, Posterior Column, Percutaneous Approach

ØRG63JJ   Fusion of Thoracic Vertebral Joint with Synthetic Substitute, Posterior Approach, Anterior Column, Percutaneous Approach

ØRG63KØ   Fusion of Thoracic Vertebral Joint with Nonautologous Tissue Substitute, Anterior Approach, Anterior Column, Percutaneous Approach

ØRG63K1   Fusion of Thoracic Vertebral Joint with Nonautologous Tissue Substitute, Posterior Approach, Posterior Column, Percutaneous Approach

ØRG63KJ   Fusion of Thoracic Vertebral Joint with Nonautologous Tissue Substitute, Posterior Approach, Anterior Column, Percutaneous Approach

ØRG647Ø   Fusion of Thoracic Vertebral Joint with Autologous Tissue Substitute, Anterior Approach, Anterior Column, Percutaneous Endoscopic Approach

ØRG6471   Fusion of Thoracic Vertebral Joint with Autologous Tissue Substitute, Posterior Approach, Posterior Column, Percutaneous Endoscopic Approach

ØRG647J   Fusion of Thoracic Vertebral Joint with Autologous Tissue Substitute, Posterior Approach, Anterior Column, Percutaneous Endoscopic Approach

ØRG64AØ   Fusion of Thoracic Vertebral Joint with Interbody Fusion Device, Anterior Approach, Anterior Column, Percutaneous Endoscopic Approach

ØRG64AJ   Fusion of Thoracic Vertebral Joint with Interbody Fusion Device, Posterior Approach, Anterior Column, Percutaneous Endoscopic Approach

ØRG64JØ   Fusion of Thoracic Vertebral Joint with Synthetic Substitute, Anterior Approach, Anterior Column, Percutaneous Endoscopic Approach

ØRG64J1   Fusion of Thoracic Vertebral Joint with Synthetic Substitute, Posterior Approach, Posterior Column, Percutaneous Endoscopic Approach

ØRG64JJ   Fusion of Thoracic Vertebral Joint with Synthetic Substitute, Posterior Approach, Anterior Column, Percutaneous Endoscopic Approach

ØRG64KØ   Fusion of Thoracic Vertebral Joint with Nonautologous Tissue Substitute, Anterior Approach, Anterior Column, Percutaneous Endoscopic Approach

ØRG64K1   Fusion of Thoracic Vertebral Joint with Nonautologous Tissue Substitute, Posterior Approach, Posterior Column, Percutaneous Endoscopic Approach

ØRG64KJ   Fusion of Thoracic Vertebral Joint with Nonautologous Tissue Substitute, Posterior Approach, Anterior Column, Percutaneous Endoscopic Approach

ØRG7Ø7Ø   Fusion of 2 to 7 Thoracic Vertebral Joints with Autologous Tissue Substitute, Anterior Approach, Anterior Column, Open Approach

ØRG7Ø71   Fusion of 2 to 7 Thoracic Vertebral Joints with Autologous Tissue Substitute, Posterior Approach, Posterior Column, Open Approach

ØRG7Ø7J   Fusion of 2 to 7 Thoracic Vertebral Joints with Autologous Tissue Substitute, Posterior Approach, Anterior Column, Open Approach

ØRG7ØAØ   Fusion of 2 to 7 Thoracic Vertebral Joints with Interbody Fusion Device, Anterior Approach, Anterior Column, Open Approach

ØRG7ØAJ   Fusion of 2 to 7 Thoracic Vertebral Joints with Interbody Fusion Device, Posterior Approach, Anterior Column, Open Approach

ØRG7ØJØ   Fusion of 2 to 7 Thoracic Vertebral Joints with Synthetic Substitute, Anterior Approach, Anterior Column, Open Approach

ØRG7ØJ1   Fusion of 2 to 7 Thoracic Vertebral Joints with Synthetic Substitute, Posterior Approach, Posterior Column, Open Approach

ØRG7ØJJ   Fusion of 2 to 7 Thoracic Vertebral Joints with Synthetic Substitute, Posterior Approach, Anterior Column, Open Approach

ØRG7ØKØ   Fusion of 2 to 7 Thoracic Vertebral Joints with Nonautologous Tissue Substitute, Anterior Approach, Anterior Column, Open Approach

ØRG7ØK1   Fusion of 2 to 7 Thoracic Vertebral Joints with Nonautologous Tissue Substitute, Posterior Approach, Posterior Column, Open Approach

ØRG7ØKJ   Fusion of 2 to 7 Thoracic Vertebral Joints with Nonautologous Tissue Substitute, Posterior Approach, Anterior Column, Open Approach

ØRG737Ø   Fusion of 2 to 7 Thoracic Vertebral Joints with Autologous Tissue Substitute, Anterior Approach, Anterior Column, Percutaneous Approach

ØRG7371   Fusion of 2 to 7 Thoracic Vertebral Joints with Autologous Tissue Substitute, Posterior Approach, Posterior Column, Percutaneous Approach

ØRG737J   Fusion of 2 to 7 Thoracic Vertebral Joints with Autologous Tissue Substitute, Posterior Approach, Anterior Column, Percutaneous Approach

ØRG73AØ   Fusion of 2 to 7 Thoracic Vertebral Joints with Interbody Fusion Device, Anterior Approach, Anterior Column, Percutaneous Approach

ØRG73AJ   Fusion of 2 to 7 Thoracic Vertebral Joints with Interbody Fusion Device, Posterior Approach, Anterior Column, Percutaneous Approach

ØRG73JØ   Fusion of 2 to 7 Thoracic Vertebral Joints with Synthetic Substitute, Anterior Approach, Anterior Column, Percutaneous Approach

ØRG73J1   Fusion of 2 to 7 Thoracic Vertebral Joints with Synthetic Substitute, Posterior Approach, Posterior Column, Percutaneous Approach

ØRG73JJ   Fusion of 2 to 7 Thoracic Vertebral Joints with Synthetic Substitute, Posterior Approach, Anterior Column, Percutaneous Approach

ØRG73KØ   Fusion of 2 to 7 Thoracic Vertebral Joints with Nonautologous Tissue Substitute, Anterior Approach, Anterior Column, Percutaneous Approach

ØRG73K1   Fusion of 2 to 7 Thoracic Vertebral Joints with Nonautologous Tissue Substitute, Posterior Approach, Posterior Column, Percutaneous Approach

ØRG73KJ   Fusion of 2 to 7 Thoracic Vertebral Joints with Nonautologous Tissue Substitute, Posterior Approach, Anterior Column, Percutaneous Approach

ØRG747Ø   Fusion of 2 to 7 Thoracic Vertebral Joints with Autologous Tissue Substitute, Anterior Approach, Anterior Column, Percutaneous Endoscopic Approach

ØRG7471   Fusion of 2 to 7 Thoracic Vertebral Joints with Autologous Tissue Substitute, Posterior Approach, Posterior Column, Percutaneous Endoscopic Approach

ØRG747J   Fusion of 2 to 7 Thoracic Vertebral Joints with Autologous Tissue Substitute, Posterior Approach, Anterior Column, Percutaneous Endoscopic Approach

ØRG74AØ   Fusion of 2 to 7 Thoracic Vertebral Joints with Interbody Fusion Device, Anterior Approach, Anterior Column, Percutaneous Endoscopic Approach

ØRG74AJ   Fusion of 2 to 7 Thoracic Vertebral Joints with Interbody Fusion Device, Posterior Approach, Anterior Column, Percutaneous Endoscopic Approach

ØRG74JØ   Fusion of 2 to 7 Thoracic Vertebral Joints with Synthetic Substitute, Anterior Approach, Anterior Column, Percutaneous Endoscopic Approach

ØRG74J1   Fusion of 2 to 7 Thoracic Vertebral Joints with Synthetic Substitute, Posterior Approach, Posterior Column, Percutaneous Endoscopic Approach

ØRG74JJ   Fusion of 2 to 7 Thoracic Vertebral Joints with Synthetic Substitute, Posterior Approach, Anterior Column, Percutaneous Endoscopic Approach

ØRG74KØ   Fusion of 2 to 7 Thoracic Vertebral Joints with Nonautologous Tissue Substitute, Anterior Approach, Anterior Column, Percutaneous Endoscopic Approach

ØRG74K1   Fusion of 2 to 7 Thoracic Vertebral Joints with Nonautologous Tissue Substitute, Posterior Approach, Posterior Column, Percutaneous Endoscopic Approach

ØRG74KJ   Fusion of 2 to 7 Thoracic Vertebral Joints with Nonautologous Tissue Substitute, Posterior Approach, Anterior Column, Percutaneous Endoscopic Approach

HAC 12: Surgical Site Infection—Certain Orthopedic Procedures of the Spine, Shoulder, and Elbow (continued)

ØRG8070 Fusion of 8 or More Thoracic Vertebral Joints with Autologous Tissue Substitute, Anterior Approach, Anterior Column, Open Approach

ØRG8071 Fusion of 8 or More Thoracic Vertebral Joints with Autologous Tissue Substitute, Posterior Approach, Posterior Column, Open Approach

ØRG807J Fusion of 8 or More Thoracic Vertebral Joints with Autologous Tissue Substitute, Posterior Approach, Anterior Column, Open Approach

ØRG80A0 Fusion of 8 or More Thoracic Vertebral Joints with Interbody Fusion Device, Anterior Approach, Anterior Column, Open Approach

ØRG80AJ Fusion of 8 or More Thoracic Vertebral Joints with Interbody Fusion Device, Posterior Approach, Anterior Column, Open Approach

ØRG80J0 Fusion of 8 or More Thoracic Vertebral Joints with Synthetic Substitute, Anterior Approach, Anterior Column, Open Approach

ØRG80J1 Fusion of 8 or More Thoracic Vertebral Joints with Synthetic Substitute, Posterior Approach, Posterior Column, Open Approach

ØRG80JJ Fusion of 8 or More Thoracic Vertebral Joints with Synthetic Substitute, Posterior Approach, Anterior Column, Open Approach

ØRG80K0 Fusion of 8 or More Thoracic Vertebral Joints with Nonautologous Tissue Substitute, Anterior Approach, Anterior Column, Open Approach

ØRG80K1 Fusion of 8 or More Thoracic Vertebral Joints with Nonautologous Tissue Substitute, Posterior Approach, Posterior Column, Open Approach

ØRG80KJ Fusion of 8 or More Thoracic Vertebral Joints with Nonautologous Tissue Substitute, Posterior Approach, Anterior Column, Open Approach

ØRG8370 Fusion of 8 or More Thoracic Vertebral Joints with Autologous Tissue Substitute, Anterior Approach, Anterior Column, Percutaneous Approach

ØRG8371 Fusion of 8 or More Thoracic Vertebral Joints with Autologous Tissue Substitute, Posterior Approach, Posterior Column, Percutaneous Approach

ØRG837J Fusion of 8 or More Thoracic Vertebral Joints with Autologous Tissue Substitute, Posterior Approach, Anterior Column, Percutaneous Approach

ØRG83A0 Fusion of 8 or More Thoracic Vertebral Joints with Interbody Fusion Device, Anterior Approach, Anterior Column, Percutaneous Approach

ØRG83AJ Fusion of 8 or More Thoracic Vertebral Joints with Interbody Fusion Device, Posterior Approach, Anterior Column, Percutaneous Approach

ØRG83J0 Fusion of 8 or More Thoracic Vertebral Joints with Synthetic Substitute, Anterior Approach, Anterior Column, Percutaneous Approach

ØRG83J1 Fusion of 8 or More Thoracic Vertebral Joints with Synthetic Substitute, Posterior Approach, Posterior Column, Percutaneous Approach

ØRG83JJ Fusion of 8 or More Thoracic Vertebral Joints with Synthetic Substitute, Posterior Approach, Anterior Column, Percutaneous Approach

ØRG83K0 Fusion of 8 or More Thoracic Vertebral Joints with Nonautologous Tissue Substitute, Anterior Approach, Anterior Column, Percutaneous Approach

ØRG83K1 Fusion of 8 or More Thoracic Vertebral Joints with Nonautologous Tissue Substitute, Posterior Approach, Posterior Column, Percutaneous Approach

ØRG83KJ Fusion of 8 or More Thoracic Vertebral Joints with Nonautologous Tissue Substitute, Posterior Approach, Anterior Column, Percutaneous Approach

ØRG8470 Fusion of 8 or More Thoracic Vertebral Joints with Autologous Tissue Substitute, Anterior Approach, Anterior Column, Percutaneous Endoscopic Approach

ØRG8471 Fusion of 8 or More Thoracic Vertebral Joints with Autologous Tissue Substitute, Posterior Approach, Posterior Column, Percutaneous Endoscopic Approach

ØRG847J Fusion of 8 or More Thoracic Vertebral Joints with Autologous Tissue Substitute, Posterior Approach, Anterior Column, Percutaneous Endoscopic Approach

ØRG84A0 Fusion of 8 or More Thoracic Vertebral Joints with Interbody Fusion Device, Anterior Approach, Anterior Column, Percutaneous Endoscopic Approach

ØRG84AJ Fusion of 8 or More Thoracic Vertebral Joints with Interbody Fusion Device, Posterior Approach, Anterior Column, Percutaneous Endoscopic Approach

ØRG84J0 Fusion of 8 or More Thoracic Vertebral Joints with Synthetic Substitute, Anterior Approach, Anterior Column, Percutaneous Endoscopic Approach

ØRG84J1 Fusion of 8 or More Thoracic Vertebral Joints with Synthetic Substitute, Posterior Approach, Posterior Column, Percutaneous Endoscopic Approach

ØRG84JJ Fusion of 8 or More Thoracic Vertebral Joints with Synthetic Substitute, Posterior Approach, Anterior Column, Percutaneous Endoscopic Approach

ØRG84K0 Fusion of 8 or More Thoracic Vertebral Joints with Nonautologous Tissue Substitute, Anterior Approach, Anterior Column, Percutaneous Endoscopic Approach

ØRG84K1 Fusion of 8 or More Thoracic Vertebral Joints with Nonautologous Tissue Substitute, Posterior Approach, Posterior Column, Percutaneous Endoscopic Approach

ØRG84KJ Fusion of 8 or More Thoracic Vertebral Joints with Nonautologous Tissue Substitute, Posterior Approach, Anterior Column, Percutaneous Endoscopic Approach

ØRGA070 Fusion of Thoracolumbar Vertebral Joint with Autologous Tissue Substitute, Anterior Approach, Anterior Column, Open Approach

ØRGA071 Fusion of Thoracolumbar Vertebral Joint with Autologous Tissue Substitute, Posterior Approach, Posterior Column, Open Approach

ØRGA07J Fusion of Thoracolumbar Vertebral Joint with Autologous Tissue Substitute, Posterior Approach, Anterior Column, Open Approach

ØRGA0A0 Fusion of Thoracolumbar Vertebral Joint with Interbody Fusion Device, Anterior Approach, Anterior Column, Open Approach

ØRGA0AJ Fusion of Thoracolumbar Vertebral Joint with Interbody Fusion Device, Posterior Approach, Anterior Column, Open Approach

ØRGA0J0 Fusion of Thoracolumbar Vertebral Joint with Synthetic Substitute, Anterior Approach, Anterior Column, Open Approach

ØRGA0J1 Fusion of Thoracolumbar Vertebral Joint with Synthetic Substitute, Posterior Approach, Posterior Column, Open Approach

ØRGA0JJ Fusion of Thoracolumbar Vertebral Joint with Synthetic Substitute, Posterior Approach, Anterior Column, Open Approach

ØRGA0K0 Fusion of Thoracolumbar Vertebral Joint with Nonautologous Tissue Substitute, Anterior Approach, Anterior Column, Open Approach

ØRGA0K1 Fusion of Thoracolumbar Vertebral Joint with Nonautologous Tissue Substitute, Posterior Approach, Posterior Column, Open Approach

ØRGA0KJ Fusion of Thoracolumbar Vertebral Joint with Nonautologous Tissue Substitute, Posterior Approach, Anterior Column, Open Approach

ØRGA370 Fusion of Thoracolumbar Vertebral Joint with Autologous Tissue Substitute, Anterior Approach, Anterior Column, Percutaneous Approach

ØRGA371 Fusion of Thoracolumbar Vertebral Joint with Autologous Tissue Substitute, Posterior Approach, Posterior Column, Percutaneous Approach

ØRGA37J Fusion of Thoracolumbar Vertebral Joint with Autologous Tissue Substitute, Posterior Approach, Anterior Column, Percutaneous Approach

ØRGA3A0 Fusion of Thoracolumbar Vertebral Joint with Interbody Fusion Device, Anterior Approach, Anterior Column, Percutaneous Approach

ØRGA3AJ Fusion of Thoracolumbar Vertebral Joint with Interbody Fusion Device, Posterior Approach, Anterior Column, Percutaneous Approach

ØRGA3J0 Fusion of Thoracolumbar Vertebral Joint with Synthetic Substitute, Anterior Approach, Anterior Column, Percutaneous Approach

ØRGA3J1 Fusion of Thoracolumbar Vertebral Joint with Synthetic Substitute, Posterior Approach, Posterior Column, Percutaneous Approach

ØRGA3JJ Fusion of Thoracolumbar Vertebral Joint with Synthetic Substitute, Posterior Approach, Anterior Column, Percutaneous Approach

ØRGA3K0 Fusion of Thoracolumbar Vertebral Joint with Nonautologous Tissue Substitute, Anterior Approach, Anterior Column, Percutaneous Approach

ØRGA3K1 Fusion of Thoracolumbar Vertebral Joint with Nonautologous Tissue Substitute, Posterior Approach, Posterior Column, Percutaneous Approach

ØRGA3KJ Fusion of Thoracolumbar Vertebral Joint with Nonautologous Tissue Substitute, Posterior Approach, Anterior Column, Percutaneous Approach

HAC 12: Surgical Site Infection—Certain Orthopedic Procedures of the Spine, Shoulder, and Elbow (continued)

ØRGA47Ø   Fusion of Thoracolumbar Vertebral Joint with Autologous Tissue Substitute, Anterior Approach, Anterior Column, Percutaneous Endoscopic Approach

ØRGA471   Fusion of Thoracolumbar Vertebral Joint with Autologous Tissue Substitute, Posterior Approach, Posterior Column, Percutaneous Endoscopic Approach

ØRGA47J   Fusion of Thoracolumbar Vertebral Joint with Autologous Tissue Substitute, Posterior Approach, Anterior Column, Percutaneous Endoscopic Approach

ØRGA4AØ   Fusion of Thoracolumbar Vertebral Joint with Interbody Fusion Device, Anterior Approach, Anterior Column, Percutaneous Endoscopic Approach

ØRGA4AJ   Fusion of Thoracolumbar Vertebral Joint with Interbody Fusion Device, Posterior Approach, Anterior Column, Percutaneous Endoscopic Approach

ØRGA4JØ   Fusion of Thoracolumbar Vertebral Joint with Synthetic Substitute, Anterior Approach, Anterior Column, Percutaneous Endoscopic Approach

ØRGA4J1   Fusion of Thoracolumbar Vertebral Joint with Synthetic Substitute, Posterior Approach, Posterior Column, Percutaneous Endoscopic Approach

ØRGA4JJ   Fusion of Thoracolumbar Vertebral Joint with Synthetic Substitute, Posterior Approach, Anterior Column, Percutaneous Endoscopic Approach

ØRGA4KØ   Fusion of Thoracolumbar Vertebral Joint with Nonautologous Tissue Substitute, Anterior Approach, Anterior Column, Percutaneous Endoscopic Approach

ØRGA4K1   Fusion of Thoracolumbar Vertebral Joint with Nonautologous Tissue Substitute, Posterior Approach, Posterior Column, Percutaneous Endoscopic Approach

ØRGA4KJ   Fusion of Thoracolumbar Vertebral Joint with Nonautologous Tissue Substitute, Posterior Approach, Anterior Column, Percutaneous Endoscopic Approach

ØRGE04Z   Fusion of Right Sternoclavicular Joint with Internal Fixation Device, Open Approach

ØRGE07Z   Fusion of Right Sternoclavicular Joint with Autologous Tissue Substitute, Open Approach

ØRGE0JZ   Fusion of Right Sternoclavicular Joint with Synthetic Substitute, Open Approach

ØRGE0KZ   Fusion of Right Sternoclavicular Joint with Nonautologous Tissue Substitute, Open Approach

ØRGE34Z   Fusion of Right Sternoclavicular Joint with Internal Fixation Device, Percutaneous Approach

ØRGE37Z   Fusion of Right Sternoclavicular Joint with Autologous Tissue Substitute, Percutaneous Approach

ØRGE3JZ   Fusion of Right Sternoclavicular Joint with Synthetic Substitute, Percutaneous Approach

ØRGE3KZ   Fusion of Right Sternoclavicular Joint with Nonautologous Tissue Substitute, Percutaneous Approach

ØRGE44Z   Fusion of Right Sternoclavicular Joint with Internal Fixation Device, Percutaneous Endoscopic Approach

ØRGE47Z   Fusion of Right Sternoclavicular Joint with Autologous Tissue Substitute, Percutaneous Endoscopic Approach

ØRGE4JZ   Fusion of Right Sternoclavicular Joint with Synthetic Substitute, Percutaneous Endoscopic Approach

ØRGE4KZ   Fusion of Right Sternoclavicular Joint with Nonautologous Tissue Substitute, Percutaneous Endoscopic Approach

ØRGF04Z   Fusion of Left Sternoclavicular Joint with Internal Fixation Device, Open Approach

ØRGF07Z   Fusion of Left Sternoclavicular Joint with Autologous Tissue Substitute, Open Approach

ØRGF0JZ   Fusion of Left Sternoclavicular Joint with Synthetic Substitute, Open Approach

ØRGF0KZ   Fusion of Left Sternoclavicular Joint with Nonautologous Tissue Substitute, Open Approach

ØRGF34Z   Fusion of Left Sternoclavicular Joint with Internal Fixation Device, Percutaneous Approach

ØRGF37Z   Fusion of Left Sternoclavicular Joint with Autologous Tissue Substitute, Percutaneous Approach

ØRGF3JZ   Fusion of Left Sternoclavicular Joint with Synthetic Substitute, Percutaneous Approach

ØRGF3KZ   Fusion of Left Sternoclavicular Joint with Nonautologous Tissue Substitute, Percutaneous Approach

ØRGF44Z   Fusion of Left Sternoclavicular Joint with Internal Fixation Device, Percutaneous Endoscopic Approach

ØRGF47Z   Fusion of Left Sternoclavicular Joint with Autologous Tissue Substitute, Percutaneous Endoscopic Approach

ØRGF4JZ   Fusion of Left Sternoclavicular Joint with Synthetic Substitute, Percutaneous Endoscopic Approach

ØRGF4KZ   Fusion of Left Sternoclavicular Joint with Nonautologous Tissue Substitute, Percutaneous Endoscopic Approach

ØRGG04Z   Fusion of Right Acromioclavicular Joint with Internal Fixation Device, Open Approach

ØRGG07Z   Fusion of Right Acromioclavicular Joint with Autologous Tissue Substitute, Open Approach

ØRGG0JZ   Fusion of Right Acromioclavicular Joint with Synthetic Substitute, Open Approach

ØRGG0KZ   Fusion of Right Acromioclavicular Joint with Nonautologous Tissue Substitute, Open Approach

ØRGG34Z   Fusion of Right Acromioclavicular Joint with Internal Fixation Device, Percutaneous Approach

ØRGG37Z   Fusion of Right Acromioclavicular Joint with Autologous Tissue Substitute, Percutaneous Approach

ØRGG3JZ   Fusion of Right Acromioclavicular Joint with Synthetic Substitute, Percutaneous Approach

ØRGG3KZ   Fusion of Right Acromioclavicular Joint with Nonautologous Tissue Substitute, Percutaneous Approach

ØRGG44Z   Fusion of Right Acromioclavicular Joint with Internal Fixation Device, Percutaneous Endoscopic Approach

ØRGG47Z   Fusion of Right Acromioclavicular Joint with Autologous Tissue Substitute, Percutaneous Endoscopic Approach

ØRGG4JZ   Fusion of Right Acromioclavicular Joint with Synthetic Substitute, Percutaneous Endoscopic Approach

ØRGG4KZ   Fusion of Right Acromioclavicular Joint with Nonautologous Tissue Substitute, Percutaneous Endoscopic Approach

ØRGH04Z   Fusion of Left Acromioclavicular Joint with Internal Fixation Device, Open Approach

ØRGH07Z   Fusion of Left Acromioclavicular Joint with Autologous Tissue Substitute, Open Approach

ØRGH0JZ   Fusion of Left Acromioclavicular Joint with Synthetic Substitute, Open Approach

ØRGH0KZ   Fusion of Left Acromioclavicular Joint with Nonautologous Tissue Substitute, Open Approach

ØRGH34Z   Fusion of Left Acromioclavicular Joint with Internal Fixation Device, Percutaneous Approach

ØRGH37Z   Fusion of Left Acromioclavicular Joint with Autologous Tissue Substitute, Percutaneous Approach

ØRGH3JZ   Fusion of Left Acromioclavicular Joint with Synthetic Substitute, Percutaneous Approach

ØRGH3KZ   Fusion of Left Acromioclavicular Joint with Nonautologous Tissue Substitute, Percutaneous Approach

ØRGH44Z   Fusion of Left Acromioclavicular Joint with Internal Fixation Device, Percutaneous Endoscopic Approach

ØRGH47Z   Fusion of Left Acromioclavicular Joint with Autologous Tissue Substitute, Percutaneous Endoscopic Approach

ØRGH4JZ   Fusion of Left Acromioclavicular Joint with Synthetic Substitute, Percutaneous Endoscopic Approach

ØRGH4KZ   Fusion of Left Acromioclavicular Joint with Nonautologous Tissue Substitute, Percutaneous Endoscopic Approach

ØRGJ04Z   Fusion of Right Shoulder Joint with Internal Fixation Device, Open Approach

ØRGJ07Z   Fusion of Right Shoulder Joint with Autologous Tissue Substitute, Open Approach

ØRGJ0JZ   Fusion of Right Shoulder Joint with Synthetic Substitute, Open Approach

ØRGJ0KZ   Fusion of Right Shoulder Joint with Nonautologous Tissue Substitute, Open Approach

ØRGJ34Z   Fusion of Right Shoulder Joint with Internal Fixation Device, Percutaneous Approach

ØRGJ37Z   Fusion of Right Shoulder Joint with Autologous Tissue Substitute, Percutaneous Approach

ØRGJ3JZ   Fusion of Right Shoulder Joint with Synthetic Substitute, Percutaneous Approach

ØRGJ3KZ   Fusion of Right Shoulder Joint with Nonautologous Tissue Substitute, Percutaneous Approach

ØRGJ44Z   Fusion of Right Shoulder Joint with Internal Fixation Device, Percutaneous Endoscopic Approach

ØRGJ47Z   Fusion of Right Shoulder Joint with Autologous Tissue Substitute, Percutaneous Endoscopic Approach

ØRGJ4JZ   Fusion of Right Shoulder Joint with Synthetic Substitute, Percutaneous Endoscopic Approach

ØRGJ4KZ   Fusion of Right Shoulder Joint with Nonautologous Tissue Substitute, Percutaneous Endoscopic Approach

ØRGK04Z   Fusion of Left Shoulder Joint with Internal Fixation Device, Open Approach

ØRGK07Z   Fusion of Left Shoulder Joint with Autologous Tissue Substitute, Open Approach

ØRGK0JZ   Fusion of Left Shoulder Joint with Synthetic Substitute, Open Approach

HAC 12: Surgical Site Infection—Certain Orthopedic Procedures of the Spine, Shoulder, and Elbow (continued)

ØRGKØKZ   Fusion of Left Shoulder Joint with Nonautologous Tissue Substitute, Open Approach

ØRGK34Z   Fusion of Left Shoulder Joint with Internal Fixation Device, Percutaneous Approach

ØRGK37Z   Fusion of Left Shoulder Joint with Autologous Tissue Substitute, Percutaneous Approach

ØRGK3JZ   Fusion of Left Shoulder Joint with Synthetic Substitute, Percutaneous Approach

ØRGK3KZ   Fusion of Left Shoulder Joint with Nonautologous Tissue Substitute, Percutaneous Approach

ØRGK44Z   Fusion of Left Shoulder Joint with Internal Fixation Device, Percutaneous Endoscopic Approach

ØRGK47Z   Fusion of Left Shoulder Joint with Autologous Tissue Substitute, Percutaneous Endoscopic Approach

ØRGK4JZ   Fusion of Left Shoulder Joint with Synthetic Substitute, Percutaneous Endoscopic Approach

ØRGK4KZ   Fusion of Left Shoulder Joint with Nonautologous Tissue Substitute, Percutaneous Endoscopic Approach

ØRGLØ4Z   Fusion of Right Elbow Joint with Internal Fixation Device, Open Approach

ØRGLØ5Z   Fusion of Right Elbow Joint with External Fixation Device, Open Approach

ØRGLØ7Z   Fusion of Right Elbow Joint with Autologous Tissue Substitute, Open Approach

ØRGLØJZ   Fusion of Right Elbow Joint with Synthetic Substitute, Open Approach

ØRGLØKZ   Fusion of Right Elbow Joint with Nonautologous Tissue Substitute, Open Approach

ØRGL34Z   Fusion of Right Elbow Joint with Internal Fixation Device, Percutaneous Approach

ØRGL35Z   Fusion of Right Elbow Joint with External Fixation Device, Percutaneous Approach

ØRGL37Z   Fusion of Right Elbow Joint with Autologous Tissue Substitute, Percutaneous Approach

ØRGL3JZ   Fusion of Right Elbow Joint with Synthetic Substitute, Percutaneous Approach

ØRGL3KZ   Fusion of Right Elbow Joint with Nonautologous Tissue Substitute, Percutaneous Approach

ØRGL44Z   Fusion of Right Elbow Joint with Internal Fixation Device, Percutaneous Endoscopic Approach

ØRGL45Z   Fusion of Right Elbow Joint with External Fixation Device, Percutaneous Endoscopic Approach

ØRGL47Z   Fusion of Right Elbow Joint with Autologous Tissue Substitute, Percutaneous Endoscopic Approach

ØRGL4JZ   Fusion of Right Elbow Joint with Synthetic Substitute, Percutaneous Endoscopic Approach

ØRGL4KZ   Fusion of Right Elbow Joint with Nonautologous Tissue Substitute, Percutaneous Endoscopic Approach

ØRGMØ4Z   Fusion of Left Elbow Joint with Internal Fixation Device, Open Approach

ØRGMØ5Z   Fusion of Left Elbow Joint with External Fixation Device, Open Approach

ØRGMØ7Z   Fusion of Left Elbow Joint with Autologous Tissue Substitute, Open Approach

ØRGMØJZ   Fusion of Left Elbow Joint with Synthetic Substitute, Open Approach

ØRGMØKZ   Fusion of Left Elbow Joint with Nonautologous Tissue Substitute, Open Approach

ØRGM34Z   Fusion of Left Elbow Joint with Internal Fixation Device, Percutaneous Approach

ØRGM35Z   Fusion of Left Elbow Joint with External Fixation Device, Percutaneous Approach

ØRGM37Z   Fusion of Left Elbow Joint with Autologous Tissue Substitute, Percutaneous Approach

ØRGM3JZ   Fusion of Left Elbow Joint with Synthetic Substitute, Percutaneous Approach

ØRGM3KZ   Fusion of Left Elbow Joint with Nonautologous Tissue Substitute, Percutaneous Approach

ØRGM44Z   Fusion of Left Elbow Joint with Internal Fixation Device, Percutaneous Endoscopic Approach

ØRGM45Z   Fusion of Left Elbow Joint with External Fixation Device, Percutaneous Endoscopic Approach

ØRGM47Z   Fusion of Left Elbow Joint with Autologous Tissue Substitute, Percutaneous Endoscopic Approach

ØRGM4JZ   Fusion of Left Elbow Joint with Synthetic Substitute, Percutaneous Endoscopic Approach

ØRGM4KZ   Fusion of Left Elbow Joint with Nonautologous Tissue Substitute, Percutaneous Endoscopic Approach

ØRQEØZZ   Repair Right Sternoclavicular Joint, Open Approach

ØRQE3ZZ   Repair Right Sternoclavicular Joint, Percutaneous Approach

ØRQE4ZZ   Repair Right Sternoclavicular Joint, Percutaneous Endoscopic Approach

ØRQEXZZ   Repair Right Sternoclavicular Joint, External Approach

ØRQFØZZ   Repair Left Sternoclavicular Joint, Open Approach

ØRQF3ZZ   Repair Left Sternoclavicular Joint, Percutaneous Approach

ØRQF4ZZ   Repair Left Sternoclavicular Joint, Percutaneous Endoscopic Approach

ØRQFXZZ   Repair Left Sternoclavicular Joint, External Approach

ØRQGØZZ   Repair Right Acromioclavicular Joint, Open Approach

ØRQG3ZZ   Repair Right Acromioclavicular Joint, Percutaneous Approach

ØRQG4ZZ   Repair Right Acromioclavicular Joint, Percutaneous Endoscopic Approach

ØRQGXZZ   Repair Right Acromioclavicular Joint, External Approach

ØRQHØZZ   Repair Left Acromioclavicular Joint, Open Approach

ØRQH3ZZ   Repair Left Acromioclavicular Joint, Percutaneous Approach

ØRQH4ZZ   Repair Left Acromioclavicular Joint, Percutaneous Endoscopic Approach

ØRQHXZZ   Repair Left Acromioclavicular Joint, External Approach

ØRQJØZZ   Repair Right Shoulder Joint, Open Approach

ØRQJ3ZZ   Repair Right Shoulder Joint, Percutaneous Approach

ØRQJ4ZZ   Repair Right Shoulder Joint, Percutaneous Endoscopic Approach

ØRQJXZZ   Repair Right Shoulder Joint, External Approach

ØRQKØZZ   Repair Left Shoulder Joint, Open Approach

ØRQK3ZZ   Repair Left Shoulder Joint, Percutaneous Approach

ØRQK4ZZ   Repair Left Shoulder Joint, Percutaneous Endoscopic Approach

ØRQKXZZ   Repair Left Shoulder Joint, External Approach

ØRQLØZZ   Repair Right Elbow Joint, Open Approach

ØRQL3ZZ   Repair Right Elbow Joint, Percutaneous Approach

ØRQL4ZZ   Repair Right Elbow Joint, Percutaneous Endoscopic Approach

ØRQLXZZ   Repair Right Elbow Joint, External Approach

ØRQMØZZ   Repair Left Elbow Joint, Open Approach

ØRQM3ZZ   Repair Left Elbow Joint, Percutaneous Approach

ØRQM4ZZ   Repair Left Elbow Joint, Percutaneous Endoscopic Approach

ØRQMXZZ   Repair Left Elbow Joint, External Approach

ØRUEØ7Z   Supplement Right Sternoclavicular Joint with Autologous Tissue Substitute, Open Approach

ØRUEØJZ   Supplement Right Sternoclavicular Joint with Synthetic Substitute, Open Approach

ØRUEØKZ   Supplement Right Sternoclavicular Joint with Nonautologous Tissue Substitute, Open Approach

ØRUE37Z   Supplement Right Sternoclavicular Joint with Autologous Tissue Substitute, Percutaneous Approach

ØRUE3JZ   Supplement Right Sternoclavicular Joint with Synthetic Substitute, Percutaneous Approach

ØRUE3KZ   Supplement Right Sternoclavicular Joint with Nonautologous Tissue Substitute, Percutaneous Approach

ØRUE47Z   Supplement Right Sternoclavicular Joint with Autologous Tissue Substitute, Percutaneous Endoscopic Approach

ØRUE4JZ   Supplement Right Sternoclavicular Joint with Synthetic Substitute, Percutaneous Endoscopic Approach

ØRUE4KZ   Supplement Right Sternoclavicular Joint with Nonautologous Tissue Substitute, Percutaneous Endoscopic Approach

ØRUFØ7Z   Supplement Left Sternoclavicular Joint with Autologous Tissue Substitute, Open Approach

ØRUFØJZ   Supplement Left Sternoclavicular Joint with Synthetic Substitute, Open Approach

ØRUFØKZ   Supplement Left Sternoclavicular Joint with Nonautologous Tissue Substitute, Open Approach

ØRUF37Z   Supplement Left Sternoclavicular Joint with Autologous Tissue Substitute, Percutaneous Approach

ØRUF3JZ   Supplement Left Sternoclavicular Joint with Synthetic Substitute, Percutaneous Approach

ØRUF3KZ   Supplement Left Sternoclavicular Joint with Nonautologous Tissue Substitute, Percutaneous Approach

ØRUF47Z   Supplement Left Sternoclavicular Joint with Autologous Tissue Substitute, Percutaneous Endoscopic Approach

ØRUF4JZ   Supplement Left Sternoclavicular Joint with Synthetic Substitute, Percutaneous Endoscopic Approach

ØRUF4KZ   Supplement Left Sternoclavicular Joint with Nonautologous Tissue Substitute, Percutaneous Endoscopic Approach

ØRUGØ7Z   Supplement Right Acromioclavicular Joint with Autologous Tissue Substitute, Open Approach

HAC 12: Surgical Site Infection—Certain Orthopedic Procedures of the Spine, Shoulder, and Elbow (continued)

ØRUGØJZ Supplement Right Acromioclavicular Joint with Synthetic Substitute, Open Approach

ØRUGØKZ Supplement Right Acromioclavicular Joint with Nonautologous Tissue Substitute, Open Approach

ØRUG37Z Supplement Right Acromioclavicular Joint with Autologous Tissue Substitute, Percutaneous Approach

ØRUG3JZ Supplement Right Acromioclavicular Joint with Synthetic Substitute, Percutaneous Approach

ØRUG3KZ Supplement Right Acromioclavicular Joint with Nonautologous Tissue Substitute, Percutaneous Approach

ØRUG47Z Supplement Right Acromioclavicular Joint with Autologous Tissue Substitute, Percutaneous Endoscopic Approach

ØRUG4JZ Supplement Right Acromioclavicular Joint with Synthetic Substitute, Percutaneous Endoscopic Approach

ØRUG4KZ Supplement Right Acromioclavicular Joint with Nonautologous Tissue Substitute, Percutaneous Endoscopic Approach

ØRUH07Z Supplement Left Acromioclavicular Joint with Autologous Tissue Substitute, Open Approach

ØRUHØJZ Supplement Left Acromioclavicular Joint with Synthetic Substitute, Open Approach

ØRUHØKZ Supplement Left Acromioclavicular Joint with Nonautologous Tissue Substitute, Open Approach

ØRUH37Z Supplement Left Acromioclavicular Joint with Autologous Tissue Substitute, Percutaneous Approach

ØRUH3JZ Supplement Left Acromioclavicular Joint with Synthetic Substitute, Percutaneous Approach

ØRUH3KZ Supplement Left Acromioclavicular Joint with Nonautologous Tissue Substitute, Percutaneous Approach

ØRUH47Z Supplement Left Acromioclavicular Joint with Autologous Tissue Substitute, Percutaneous Endoscopic Approach

ØRUH4JZ Supplement Left Acromioclavicular Joint with Synthetic Substitute, Percutaneous Endoscopic Approach

ØRUH4KZ Supplement Left Acromioclavicular Joint with Nonautologous Tissue Substitute, Percutaneous Endoscopic Approach

ØRUJ07Z Supplement Right Shoulder Joint with Autologous Tissue Substitute, Open Approach

ØRUJØJZ Supplement Right Shoulder Joint with Synthetic Substitute, Open Approach

ØRUJØKZ Supplement Right Shoulder Joint with Nonautologous Tissue Substitute, Open Approach

ØRUJ37Z Supplement Right Shoulder Joint with Autologous Tissue Substitute, Percutaneous Approach

ØRUJ3JZ Supplement Right Shoulder Joint with Synthetic Substitute, Percutaneous Approach

ØRUJ3KZ Supplement Right Shoulder Joint with Nonautologous Tissue Substitute, Percutaneous Approach

ØRUJ47Z Supplement Right Shoulder Joint with Autologous Tissue Substitute, Percutaneous Endoscopic Approach

ØRUJ4JZ Supplement Right Shoulder Joint with Synthetic Substitute, Percutaneous Endoscopic Approach

ØRUJ4KZ Supplement Right Shoulder Joint with Nonautologous Tissue Substitute, Percutaneous Endoscopic Approach

ØRUK07Z Supplement Left Shoulder Joint with Autologous Tissue Substitute, Open Approach

ØRUKØJZ Supplement Left Shoulder Joint with Synthetic Substitute, Open Approach

ØRUKØKZ Supplement Left Shoulder Joint with Nonautologous Tissue Substitute, Open Approach

ØRUK37Z Supplement Left Shoulder Joint with Autologous Tissue Substitute, Percutaneous Approach

ØRUK3JZ Supplement Left Shoulder Joint with Synthetic Substitute, Percutaneous Approach

ØRUK3KZ Supplement Left Shoulder Joint with Nonautologous Tissue Substitute, Percutaneous Approach

ØRUK47Z Supplement Left Shoulder Joint with Autologous Tissue Substitute, Percutaneous Endoscopic Approach

ØRUK4JZ Supplement Left Shoulder Joint with Synthetic Substitute, Percutaneous Endoscopic Approach

ØRUK4KZ Supplement Left Shoulder Joint with Nonautologous Tissue Substitute, Percutaneous Endoscopic Approach

ØRUL07Z Supplement Right Elbow Joint with Autologous Tissue Substitute, Open Approach

ØRULØJZ Supplement Right Elbow Joint with Synthetic Substitute, Open Approach

ØRULØKZ Supplement Right Elbow Joint with Nonautologous Tissue Substitute, Open Approach

ØRUL37Z Supplement Right Elbow Joint with Autologous Tissue Substitute, Percutaneous Approach

ØRUL3JZ Supplement Right Elbow Joint with Synthetic Substitute, Percutaneous Approach

ØRUL3KZ Supplement Right Elbow Joint with Nonautologous Tissue Substitute, Percutaneous Approach

ØRUL47Z Supplement Right Elbow Joint with Autologous Tissue Substitute, Percutaneous Endoscopic Approach

ØRUL4JZ Supplement Right Elbow Joint with Synthetic Substitute, Percutaneous Endoscopic Approach

ØRUL4KZ Supplement Right Elbow Joint with Nonautologous Tissue Substitute, Percutaneous Endoscopic Approach

ØRUM07Z Supplement Left Elbow Joint with Autologous Tissue Substitute, Open Approach

ØRUMØJZ Supplement Left Elbow Joint with Synthetic Substitute, Open Approach

ØRUMØKZ Supplement Left Elbow Joint with Nonautologous Tissue Substitute, Open Approach

ØRUM37Z Supplement Left Elbow Joint with Autologous Tissue Substitute, Percutaneous Approach

ØRUM3JZ Supplement Left Elbow Joint with Synthetic Substitute, Percutaneous Approach

ØRUM3KZ Supplement Left Elbow Joint with Nonautologous Tissue Substitute, Percutaneous Approach

ØRUM47Z Supplement Left Elbow Joint with Autologous Tissue Substitute, Percutaneous Endoscopic Approach

ØRUM4JZ Supplement Left Elbow Joint with Synthetic Substitute, Percutaneous Endoscopic Approach

ØRUM4KZ Supplement Left Elbow Joint with Nonautologous Tissue Substitute, Percutaneous Endoscopic Approach

ØSG0070 Fusion of Lumbar Vertebral Joint with Autologous Tissue Substitute, Anterior Approach, Anterior Column, Open Approach

ØSG0071 Fusion of Lumbar Vertebral Joint with Autologous Tissue Substitute, Posterior Approach, Posterior Column, Open Approach

ØSG007J Fusion of Lumbar Vertebral Joint with Autologous Tissue Substitute, Posterior Approach, Anterior Column, Open Approach

ØSG00A0 Fusion of Lumbar Vertebral Joint with Interbody Fusion Device, Anterior Approach, Anterior Column, Open Approach

ØSG00AJ Fusion of Lumbar Vertebral Joint with Interbody Fusion Device, Posterior Approach, Anterior Column, Open Approach

ØSG00J0 Fusion of Lumbar Vertebral Joint with Synthetic Substitute, Anterior Approach, Anterior Column, Open Approach

ØSG00J1 Fusion of Lumbar Vertebral Joint with Synthetic Substitute, Posterior Approach, Posterior Column, Open Approach

ØSG00JJ Fusion of Lumbar Vertebral Joint with Synthetic Substitute, Posterior Approach, Anterior Column, Open Approach

ØSG00K0 Fusion of Lumbar Vertebral Joint with Nonautologous Tissue Substitute, Anterior Approach, Anterior Column, Open Approach

ØSG00K1 Fusion of Lumbar Vertebral Joint with Nonautologous Tissue Substitute, Posterior Approach, Posterior Column, Open Approach

ØSG00KJ Fusion of Lumbar Vertebral Joint with Nonautologous Tissue Substitute, Posterior Approach, Anterior Column, Open Approach

ØSG0370 Fusion of Lumbar Vertebral Joint with Autologous Tissue Substitute, Anterior Approach, Anterior Column, Percutaneous Approach

ØSG0371 Fusion of Lumbar Vertebral Joint with Autologous Tissue Substitute, Posterior Approach, Posterior Column, Percutaneous Approach

ØSG037J Fusion of Lumbar Vertebral Joint with Autologous Tissue Substitute, Posterior Approach, Anterior Column, Percutaneous Approach

ØSG03A0 Fusion of Lumbar Vertebral Joint with Interbody Fusion Device, Anterior Approach, Anterior Column, Percutaneous Approach

ØSG03AJ Fusion of Lumbar Vertebral Joint with Interbody Fusion Device, Posterior Approach, Anterior Column, Percutaneous Approach

ØSG03J0 Fusion of Lumbar Vertebral Joint with Synthetic Substitute, Anterior Approach, Anterior Column, Percutaneous Approach

HAC 12: Surgical Site Infection—Certain Orthopedic Procedures of the Spine, Shoulder, and Elbow (continued)

ØSG03J1 Fusion of Lumbar Vertebral Joint with Synthetic Substitute, Posterior Approach, Posterior Column, Percutaneous Approach

ØSG03JJ Fusion of Lumbar Vertebral Joint with Synthetic Substitute, Posterior Approach, Anterior Column, Percutaneous Approach

ØSG03KØ Fusion of Lumbar Vertebral Joint with Nonautologous Tissue Substitute, Anterior Approach, Anterior Column, Percutaneous Approach

ØSG03K1 Fusion of Lumbar Vertebral Joint with Nonautologous Tissue Substitute, Posterior Approach, Posterior Column, Percutaneous Approach

ØSG03KJ Fusion of Lumbar Vertebral Joint with Nonautologous Tissue Substitute, Posterior Approach, Anterior Column, Percutaneous Approach

ØSG047Ø Fusion of Lumbar Vertebral Joint with Autologous Tissue Substitute, Anterior Approach, Anterior Column, Percutaneous Endoscopic Approach

ØSG0471 Fusion of Lumbar Vertebral Joint with Autologous Tissue Substitute, Posterior Approach, Posterior Column, Percutaneous Endoscopic Approach

ØSG047J Fusion of Lumbar Vertebral Joint with Autologous Tissue Substitute, Posterior Approach, Anterior Column, Percutaneous Endoscopic Approach

ØSG04AØ Fusion of Lumbar Vertebral Joint with Interbody Fusion Device, Anterior Approach, Anterior Column, Percutaneous Endoscopic Approach

ØSG04AJ Fusion of Lumbar Vertebral Joint with Interbody Fusion Device, Posterior Approach, Anterior Column, Percutaneous Endoscopic Approach

ØSG04JØ Fusion of Lumbar Vertebral Joint with Synthetic Substitute, Anterior Approach, Anterior Column, Percutaneous Endoscopic Approach

ØSG04J1 Fusion of Lumbar Vertebral Joint with Synthetic Substitute, Posterior Approach, Posterior Column, Percutaneous Endoscopic Approach

ØSG04JJ Fusion of Lumbar Vertebral Joint with Synthetic Substitute, Posterior Approach, Anterior Column, Percutaneous Endoscopic Approach

ØSG04KØ Fusion of Lumbar Vertebral Joint with Nonautologous Tissue Substitute, Anterior Approach, Anterior Column, Percutaneous Endoscopic Approach

ØSG04K1 Fusion of Lumbar Vertebral Joint with Nonautologous Tissue Substitute, Posterior Approach, Posterior Column, Percutaneous Endoscopic Approach

ØSG04KJ Fusion of Lumbar Vertebral Joint with Nonautologous Tissue Substitute, Posterior Approach, Anterior Column, Percutaneous Endoscopic Approach

ØSG107Ø Fusion of 2 or More Lumbar Vertebral Joints with Autologous Tissue Substitute, Anterior Approach, Anterior Column, Open Approach

ØSG1071 Fusion of 2 or More Lumbar Vertebral Joints with Autologous Tissue Substitute, Posterior Approach, Posterior Column, Open Approach

ØSG107J Fusion of 2 or More Lumbar Vertebral Joints with Autologous Tissue Substitute, Posterior Approach, Anterior Column, Open Approach

ØSG10AØ Fusion of 2 or More Lumbar Vertebral Joints with Interbody Fusion Device, Anterior Approach, Anterior Column, Open Approach

ØSG10AJ Fusion of 2 or More Lumbar Vertebral Joints with Interbody Fusion Device, Posterior Approach, Anterior Column, Open Approach

ØSG10JØ Fusion of 2 or More Lumbar Vertebral Joints with Synthetic Substitute, Anterior Approach, Anterior Column, Open Approach

ØSG10J1 Fusion of 2 or More Lumbar Vertebral Joints with Synthetic Substitute, Posterior Approach, Posterior Column, Open Approach

ØSG10JJ Fusion of 2 or More Lumbar Vertebral Joints with Synthetic Substitute, Posterior Approach, Anterior Column, Open Approach

ØSG10KØ Fusion of 2 or More Lumbar Vertebral Joints with Nonautologous Tissue Substitute, Anterior Approach, Anterior Column, Open Approach

ØSG10K1 Fusion of 2 or More Lumbar Vertebral Joints with Nonautologous Tissue Substitute, Posterior Approach, Posterior Column, Open Approach

ØSG10KJ Fusion of 2 or More Lumbar Vertebral Joints with Nonautologous Tissue Substitute, Posterior Approach, Anterior Column, Open Approach

ØSG137Ø Fusion of 2 or More Lumbar Vertebral Joints with Autologous Tissue Substitute, Anterior Approach, Anterior Column, Percutaneous Approach

ØSG1371 Fusion of 2 or More Lumbar Vertebral Joints with Autologous Tissue Substitute, Posterior Approach, Posterior Column, Percutaneous Approach

ØSG137J Fusion of 2 or More Lumbar Vertebral Joints with Autologous Tissue Substitute, Posterior Approach, Anterior Column, Percutaneous Approach

ØSG13AØ Fusion of 2 or More Lumbar Vertebral Joints with Interbody Fusion Device, Anterior Approach, Anterior Column, Percutaneous Approach

ØSG13AJ Fusion of 2 or More Lumbar Vertebral Joints with Interbody Fusion Device, Posterior Approach, Anterior Column, Percutaneous Approach

ØSG13JØ Fusion of 2 or More Lumbar Vertebral Joints with Synthetic Substitute, Anterior Approach, Anterior Column, Percutaneous Approach

ØSG13J1 Fusion of 2 or More Lumbar Vertebral Joints with Synthetic Substitute, Posterior Approach, Posterior Column, Percutaneous Approach

ØSG13JJ Fusion of 2 or More Lumbar Vertebral Joints with Synthetic Substitute, Posterior Approach, Anterior Column, Percutaneous Approach

ØSG13KØ Fusion of 2 or More Lumbar Vertebral Joints with Nonautologous Tissue Substitute, Anterior Approach, Anterior Column, Percutaneous Approach

ØSG13K1 Fusion of 2 or More Lumbar Vertebral Joints with Nonautologous Tissue Substitute, Posterior Approach, Posterior Column, Percutaneous Approach

ØSG13KJ Fusion of 2 or More Lumbar Vertebral Joints with Nonautologous Tissue Substitute, Posterior Approach, Anterior Column, Percutaneous Approach

ØSG147Ø Fusion of 2 or More Lumbar Vertebral Joints with Autologous Tissue Substitute, Anterior Approach, Anterior Column, Percutaneous Endoscopic Approach

ØSG1471 Fusion of 2 or More Lumbar Vertebral Joints with Autologous Tissue Substitute, Posterior Approach, Posterior Column, Percutaneous Endoscopic Approach

ØSG147J Fusion of 2 or More Lumbar Vertebral Joints with Autologous Tissue Substitute, Posterior Approach, Anterior Column, Percutaneous Endoscopic Approach

ØSG14AØ Fusion of 2 or More Lumbar Vertebral Joints with Interbody Fusion Device, Anterior Approach, Anterior Column, Percutaneous Endoscopic Approach

ØSG14AJ Fusion of 2 or More Lumbar Vertebral Joints with Interbody Fusion Device, Posterior Approach, Anterior Column, Percutaneous Endoscopic Approach

ØSG14JØ Fusion of 2 or More Lumbar Vertebral Joints with Synthetic Substitute, Anterior Approach, Anterior Column, Percutaneous Endoscopic Approach

ØSG14J1 Fusion of 2 or More Lumbar Vertebral Joints with Synthetic Substitute, Posterior Approach, Posterior Column, Percutaneous Endoscopic Approach

ØSG14JJ Fusion of 2 or More Lumbar Vertebral Joints with Synthetic Substitute, Posterior Approach, Anterior Column, Percutaneous Endoscopic Approach

ØSG14KØ Fusion of 2 or More Lumbar Vertebral Joints with Nonautologous Tissue Substitute, Anterior Approach, Anterior Column, Percutaneous Endoscopic Approach

ØSG14K1 Fusion of 2 or More Lumbar Vertebral Joints with Nonautologous Tissue Substitute, Posterior Approach, Posterior Column, Percutaneous Endoscopic Approach

ØSG14KJ Fusion of 2 or More Lumbar Vertebral Joints with Nonautologous Tissue Substitute, Posterior Approach, Anterior Column, Percutaneous Endoscopic Approach

ØSG307Ø Fusion of Lumbosacral Joint with Autologous Tissue Substitute, Anterior Approach, Anterior Column, Open Approach

ØSG3071 Fusion of Lumbosacral Joint with Autologous Tissue Substitute, Posterior Approach, Posterior Column, Open Approach

ØSG307J Fusion of Lumbosacral Joint with Autologous Tissue Substitute, Posterior Approach, Anterior Column, Open Approach

ØSG30AØ Fusion of Lumbosacral Joint with Interbody Fusion Device, Anterior Approach, Anterior Column, Open Approach

ØSG30AJ Fusion of Lumbosacral Joint with Interbody Fusion Device, Posterior Approach, Anterior Column, Open Approach

ØSG30JØ Fusion of Lumbosacral Joint with Synthetic Substitute, Anterior Approach, Anterior Column, Open Approach

ØSG30J1 Fusion of Lumbosacral Joint with Synthetic Substitute, Posterior Approach, Posterior Column, Open Approach

HAC 12: Surgical Site Infection—Certain Orthopedic Procedures of the Spine, Shoulder, and Elbow (continued)

ØSG30JJ   Fusion of Lumbosacral Joint with Synthetic Substitute, Posterior Approach, Anterior Column, Open Approach

ØSG30KØ   Fusion of Lumbosacral Joint with Nonautologous Tissue Substitute, Anterior Approach, Anterior Column, Open Approach

ØSG30K1   Fusion of Lumbosacral Joint with Nonautologous Tissue Substitute, Posterior Approach, Posterior Column, Open Approach

ØSG30KJ   Fusion of Lumbosacral Joint with Nonautologous Tissue Substitute, Posterior Approach, Anterior Column, Open Approach

ØSG337Ø   Fusion of Lumbosacral Joint with Autologous Tissue Substitute, Anterior Approach, Anterior Column, Percutaneous Approach

ØSG3371   Fusion of Lumbosacral Joint with Autologous Tissue Substitute, Posterior Approach, Posterior Column, Percutaneous Approach

ØSG337J   Fusion of Lumbosacral Joint with Autologous Tissue Substitute, Posterior Approach, Anterior Column, Percutaneous Approach

ØSG33AØ   Fusion of Lumbosacral Joint with Interbody Fusion Device, Anterior Approach, Anterior Column, Percutaneous Approach

ØSG33AJ   Fusion of Lumbosacral Joint with Interbody Fusion Device, Posterior Approach, Anterior Column, Percutaneous Approach

ØSG33JØ   Fusion of Lumbosacral Joint with Synthetic Substitute, Anterior Approach, Anterior Column, Percutaneous Approach

ØSG33J1   Fusion of Lumbosacral Joint with Synthetic Substitute, Posterior Approach, Posterior Column, Percutaneous Approach

ØSG33JJ   Fusion of Lumbosacral Joint with Synthetic Substitute, Posterior Approach, Anterior Column, Percutaneous Approach

ØSG33KØ   Fusion of Lumbosacral Joint with Nonautologous Tissue Substitute, Anterior Approach, Anterior Column, Percutaneous Approach

ØSG33K1   Fusion of Lumbosacral Joint with Nonautologous Tissue Substitute, Posterior Approach, Posterior Column, Percutaneous Approach

ØSG33KJ   Fusion of Lumbosacral Joint with Nonautologous Tissue Substitute, Posterior Approach, Anterior Column, Percutaneous Approach

ØSG347Ø   Fusion of Lumbosacral Joint with Autologous Tissue Substitute, Anterior Approach, Anterior Column, Percutaneous Endoscopic Approach

ØSG3471   Fusion of Lumbosacral Joint with Autologous Tissue Substitute, Posterior Approach, Posterior Column, Percutaneous Endoscopic Approach

ØSG347J   Fusion of Lumbosacral Joint with Autologous Tissue Substitute, Posterior Approach, Anterior Column, Percutaneous Endoscopic Approach

ØSG34AØ   Fusion of Lumbosacral Joint with Interbody Fusion Device, Anterior Approach, Anterior Column, Percutaneous Endoscopic Approach

ØSG34AJ   Fusion of Lumbosacral Joint with Interbody Fusion Device, Posterior Approach, Anterior Column, Percutaneous Endoscopic Approach

ØSG34JØ   Fusion of Lumbosacral Joint with Synthetic Substitute, Anterior Approach, Anterior Column, Percutaneous Endoscopic Approach

ØSG34J1   Fusion of Lumbosacral Joint with Synthetic Substitute, Posterior Approach, Posterior Column, Percutaneous Endoscopic Approach

ØSG34JJ   Fusion of Lumbosacral Joint with Synthetic Substitute, Posterior Approach, Anterior Column, Percutaneous Endoscopic Approach

ØSG34KØ   Fusion of Lumbosacral Joint with Nonautologous Tissue Substitute, Anterior Approach, Anterior Column, Percutaneous Endoscopic Approach

ØSG34K1   Fusion of Lumbosacral Joint with Nonautologous Tissue Substitute, Posterior Approach, Posterior Column, Percutaneous Endoscopic Approach

ØSG34KJ   Fusion of Lumbosacral Joint with Nonautologous Tissue Substitute, Posterior Approach, Anterior Column, Percutaneous Endoscopic Approach

ØSG704Z   Fusion of Right Sacroiliac Joint with Internal Fixation Device, Open Approach

ØSG707Z   Fusion of Right Sacroiliac Joint with Autologous Tissue Substitute, Open Approach

ØSG70JZ   Fusion of Right Sacroiliac Joint with Synthetic Substitute, Open Approach

ØSG70KZ   Fusion of Right Sacroiliac Joint with Nonautologous Tissue Substitute, Open Approach

ØSG734Z   Fusion of Right Sacroiliac Joint with Internal Fixation Device, Percutaneous Approach

ØSG737Z   Fusion of Right Sacroiliac Joint with Autologous Tissue Substitute, Percutaneous Approach

ØSG73JZ   Fusion of Right Sacroiliac Joint with Synthetic Substitute, Percutaneous Approach

ØSG73KZ   Fusion of Right Sacroiliac Joint with Nonautologous Tissue Substitute, Percutaneous Approach

ØSG744Z   Fusion of Right Sacroiliac Joint with Internal Fixation Device, Percutaneous Endoscopic Approach

ØSG747Z   Fusion of Right Sacroiliac Joint with Autologous Tissue Substitute, Percutaneous Endoscopic Approach

ØSG74JZ   Fusion of Right Sacroiliac Joint with Synthetic Substitute, Percutaneous Endoscopic Approach

ØSG74KZ   Fusion of Right Sacroiliac Joint with Nonautologous Tissue Substitute, Percutaneous Endoscopic Approach

ØSG804Z   Fusion of Left Sacroiliac Joint with Internal Fixation Device, Open Approach

ØSG807Z   Fusion of Left Sacroiliac Joint with Autologous Tissue Substitute, Open Approach

ØSG80JZ   Fusion of Left Sacroiliac Joint with Synthetic Substitute, Open Approach

ØSG80KZ   Fusion of Left Sacroiliac Joint with Nonautologous Tissue Substitute, Open Approach

ØSG834Z   Fusion of Left Sacroiliac Joint with Internal Fixation Device, Percutaneous Approach

ØSG837Z   Fusion of Left Sacroiliac Joint with Autologous Tissue Substitute, Percutaneous Approach

ØSG83JZ   Fusion of Left Sacroiliac Joint with Synthetic Substitute, Percutaneous Approach

ØSG83KZ   Fusion of Left Sacroiliac Joint with Nonautologous Tissue Substitute, Percutaneous Approach

ØSG844Z   Fusion of Left Sacroiliac Joint with Internal Fixation Device, Percutaneous Endoscopic Approach

ØSG847Z   Fusion of Left Sacroiliac Joint with Autologous Tissue Substitute, Percutaneous Endoscopic Approach

ØSG84JZ   Fusion of Left Sacroiliac Joint with Synthetic Substitute, Percutaneous Endoscopic Approach

ØSG84KZ   Fusion of Left Sacroiliac Joint with Nonautologous Tissue Substitute, Percutaneous Endoscopic Approach

XRG0092   Fusion of Occipital-cervical Joint using Nanotextured Surface Interbody Fusion Device, Open Approach, New Technology Group 2

XRG00F3   Fusion of Occipital-cervical Joint using Radiolucent Porous Interbody Fusion Device, Open Approach, New Technology Group 3

XRG1092   Fusion of Cervical Vertebral Joint using Nanotextured Surface Interbody Fusion Device, Open Approach, New Technology Group 2

XRG10F3   Fusion of Cervical Vertebral Joint using Radiolucent Porous Interbody Fusion Device, Open Approach, New Technology Group 3

XRG2092   Fusion of 2 or more Cervical Vertebral Joints using Nanotextured Surface Interbody Fusion Device, Open Approach, New Technology Group 2

XRG20F3   Fusion of 2 or more Cervical Vertebral Joints using Radiolucent Porous Interbody Fusion Device, Open Approach, New Technology Group 3

XRG4092   Fusion of Cervicothoracic Vertebral Joint using Nanotextured Surface Interbody Fusion Device, Open Approach, New Technology Group 2

XRG40F3   Fusion of Cervicothoracic Vertebral Joint using Radiolucent Porous Interbody Fusion Device, Open Approach, New Technology Group 3

XRG6092   Fusion of Thoracic Vertebral Joint using Nanotextured Surface Interbody Fusion Device, Open Approach, New Technology Group 2

XRG60F3   Fusion of Thoracic Vertebral Joint using Radiolucent Porous Interbody Fusion Device, Open Approach, New Technology Group 3

XRG7092   Fusion of 2 to 7 Thoracic Vertebral Joints using Nanotextured Surface Interbody Fusion Device, Open Approach, New Technology Group 2

XRG70F3   Fusion of 2 to 7 Thoracic Vertebral Joints using Radiolucent Porous Interbody Fusion Device, Open Approach, New Technology Group 3

XRG8092   Fusion of 8 or more Thoracic Vertebral Joints using Nanotextured Surface Interbody Fusion Device, Open Approach, New Technology Group 2

HAC 12: Surgical Site Infection—Certain Orthopedic Procedures of the Spine, Shoulder, and Elbow (continued)

XRG80F3 Fusion of 8 or more Thoracic Vertebral Joints using Radiolucent Porous Interbody Fusion Device, Open Approach, New Technology Group 3

XRGA092 Fusion of Thoracolumbar Vertebral Joint using Nanotextured Surface Interbody Fusion Device, Open Approach, New Technology Group 2

XRGA0F3 Fusion of Thoracolumbar Vertebral Joint using Radiolucent Porous Interbody Fusion Device, Open Approach, New Technology Group 3

XRGB092 Fusion of Lumbar Vertebral Joint using Nanotextured Surface Interbody Fusion Device, Open Approach, New Technology Group 2

XRGB0F3 Fusion of Lumbar Vertebral Joint using Radiolucent Porous Interbody Fusion Device, Open Approach, New Technology Group 3

XRGC092 Fusion of 2 or more Lumbar Vertebral Joints using Nanotextured Surface Interbody Fusion Device, Open Approach, New Technology Group 2

XRGC0F3 Fusion of 2 or more Lumbar Vertebral Joints using Radiolucent Porous Interbody Fusion Device, Open Approach, New Technology Group 3

XRGD092 Fusion of Lumbosacral Joint using Nanotextured Surface Interbody Fusion Device, Open Approach, New Technology Group 2

XRGD0F3 Fusion of Lumbosacral Joint using Radiolucent Porous Interbody Fusion Device, Open Approach, New Technology Group 3

HAC 13: Surgical Site Infection (SSI) Following Cardiac Implantable Electronic Device (CIED) Procedures

Secondary diagnosis not POA:

K68.11
T81.40XA
T81.41XA
T81.42XA
T81.43XA
T81.44XA
T81.49XA
T82.6XXA
T82.7XXA

AND

Any of the following procedures:

02H43JZ Insertion of Pacemaker Lead into Coronary Vein, Percutaneous Approach

02H43KZ Insertion of Defibrillator Lead into Coronary Vein, Percutaneous Approach

02H43MZ Insertion of Cardiac Lead into Coronary Vein, Percutaneous Approach

02H63JZ Insertion of Pacemaker Lead into Right Atrium, Percutaneous Approach

02H63MZ Insertion of Cardiac Lead into Right Atrium, Percutaneous Approach

02H73JZ Insertion of Pacemaker Lead into Left Atrium, Percutaneous Approach

02H73MZ Insertion of Cardiac Lead into Left Atrium, Percutaneous Approach

02HK3JZ Insertion of Pacemaker Lead into Right Ventricle, Percutaneous Approach

02HL3JZ Insertion of Pacemaker Lead into Left Ventricle, Percutaneous Approach

02HN0JZ Insertion of Pacemaker Lead into Pericardium, Open Approach

02HN0MZ Insertion of Cardiac Lead into Pericardium, Open Approach

02HN3JZ Insertion of Pacemaker Lead into Pericardium, Percutaneous Approach

02HN3MZ Insertion of Cardiac Lead into Pericardium, Percutaneous Approach

02HN4JZ Insertion of Pacemaker Lead into Pericardium, Percutaneous Endoscopic Approach

02HN4MZ Insertion of Cardiac Lead into Pericardium, Percutaneous Endoscopic Approach

02PA0MZ Removal of Cardiac Lead from Heart, Open Approach

02PA3MZ Removal of Cardiac Lead from Heart, Percutaneous Approach

02PA4MZ Removal of Cardiac Lead from Heart, Percutaneous Endoscopic Approach

02PAXMZ Removal of Cardiac Lead from Heart, External Approach

02WA0MZ Revision of Cardiac Lead in Heart, Open Approach

02WA3MZ Revision of Cardiac Lead in Heart, Percutaneous Approach

02WA4MZ Revision of Cardiac Lead in Heart, Percutaneous Endoscopic Approach

0JH604Z Insertion of Pacemaker, Single Chamber into Chest Subcutaneous Tissue and Fascia, Open Approach

0JH605Z Insertion of Pacemaker, Single Chamber Rate Responsive into Chest Subcutaneous Tissue and Fascia, Open Approach

0JH606Z Insertion of Pacemaker, Dual Chamber into Chest Subcutaneous Tissue and Fascia, Open Approach

0JH607Z Insertion of Cardiac Resynchronization Pacemaker Pulse Generator into Chest Subcutaneous Tissue and Fascia, Open Approach

0JH608Z Insertion of Defibrillator Generator into Chest Subcutaneous Tissue and Fascia, Open Approach

0JH609Z Insertion of Cardiac Resynchronization Defibrillator Pulse Generator into Chest Subcutaneous Tissue and Fascia, Open Approach

0JH60PZ Insertion of Cardiac Rhythm Related Device into Chest Subcutaneous Tissue and Fascia, Open Approach

0JH634Z Insertion of Pacemaker, Single Chamber into Chest Subcutaneous Tissue and Fascia, Percutaneous Approach

0JH635Z Insertion of Pacemaker, Single Chamber Rate Responsive into Chest Subcutaneous Tissue and Fascia, Percutaneous Approach

0JH636Z Insertion of Pacemaker, Dual Chamber into Chest Subcutaneous Tissue and Fascia, Percutaneous Approach

0JH637Z Insertion of Cardiac Resynchronization Pacemaker Pulse Generator into Chest Subcutaneous Tissue and Fascia, Percutaneous Approach

0JH638Z Insertion of Defibrillator Generator into Chest Subcutaneous Tissue and Fascia, Percutaneous Approach

0JH639Z Insertion of Cardiac Resynchronization Defibrillator Pulse Generator into Chest Subcutaneous Tissue and Fascia, Percutaneous Approach

0JH63PZ Insertion of Cardiac Rhythm Related Device into Chest Subcutaneous Tissue and Fascia, Percutaneous Approach

0JH804Z Insertion of Pacemaker, Single Chamber into Abdomen Subcutaneous Tissue and Fascia, Open Approach

0JH805Z Insertion of Pacemaker, Single Chamber Rate Responsive into Abdomen Subcutaneous Tissue and Fascia, Open Approach

0JH806Z Insertion of Pacemaker, Dual Chamber into Abdomen Subcutaneous Tissue and Fascia, Open Approach

0JH807Z Insertion of Cardiac Resynchronization Pacemaker Pulse Generator into Abdomen Subcutaneous Tissue and Fascia, Open Approach

0JH808Z Insertion of Defibrillator Generator into Abdomen Subcutaneous Tissue and Fascia, Open Approach

0JH809Z Insertion of Cardiac Resynchronization Defibrillator Pulse Generator into Abdomen Subcutaneous Tissue and Fascia, Open Approach

0JH80PZ Insertion of Cardiac Rhythm Related Device into Abdomen Subcutaneous Tissue and Fascia, Open Approach

0JH834Z Insertion of Pacemaker, Single Chamber into Abdomen Subcutaneous Tissue and Fascia, Percutaneous Approach

0JH835Z Insertion of Pacemaker, Single Chamber Rate Responsive into Abdomen Subcutaneous Tissue and Fascia, Percutaneous Approach

0JH836Z Insertion of Pacemaker, Dual Chamber into Abdomen Subcutaneous Tissue and Fascia, Percutaneous Approach

0JH837Z Insertion of Cardiac Resynchronization Pacemaker Pulse Generator into Abdomen Subcutaneous Tissue and Fascia, Percutaneous Approach

0JH838Z Insertion of Defibrillator Generator into Abdomen Subcutaneous Tissue and Fascia, Percutaneous Approach

0JH839Z Insertion of Cardiac Resynchronization Defibrillator Pulse Generator into Abdomen Subcutaneous Tissue and Fascia, Percutaneous Approach

0JH83PZ Insertion of Cardiac Rhythm Related Device into Abdomen Subcutaneous Tissue and Fascia, Percutaneous Approach

0JPT0FZ Removal of Subcutaneous Defibrillator Lead from Trunk Subcutaneous Tissue and Fascia, Open Approach

0JPT0PZ Removal of Cardiac Rhythm Related Device from Trunk Subcutaneous Tissue and Fascia, Open Approach

0JPT3FZ Removal of Subcutaneous Defibrillator Lead from Trunk Subcutaneous Tissue and Fascia, Percutaneous Approach

0JPT3PZ Removal of Cardiac Rhythm Related Device from Trunk Subcutaneous Tissue and Fascia, Percutaneous Approach

0JWT0FZ Revision of Subcutaneous Defibrillator Lead in Trunk Subcutaneous Tissue and Fascia, Open Approach

0JWT0PZ Revision of Cardiac Rhythm Related Device in Trunk Subcutaneous Tissue and Fascia, Open Approach

0JWT3FZ Revision of Subcutaneous Defibrillator Lead in Trunk Subcutaneous Tissue and Fascia, Percutaneous Approach

0JWT3PZ Revision of Cardiac Rhythm Related Device in Trunk Subcutaneous Tissue and Fascia, Percutaneous Approach

HAC 14: Iatrogenic Pneumothorax with Venous Catheterization

Secondary diagnosis not POA:

J95.811

AND

Any of the following procedures:

02H633Z Insertion of Infusion Device into Right Atrium, Percutaneous Approach

02HK33Z Insertion of Infusion Device into Right Ventricle, Percutaneous Approach

02HS33Z Insertion of Infusion Device into Right Pulmonary Vein, Percutaneous Approach

02HS43Z Insertion of Infusion Device into Right Pulmonary Vein, Percutaneous Endoscopic Approach

02HT33Z Insertion of Infusion Device into Left Pulmonary Vein, Percutaneous Approach

02HT43Z Insertion of Infusion Device into Left Pulmonary Vein, Percutaneous Endoscopic Approach

02HV33Z Insertion of Infusion Device into Superior Vena Cava, Percutaneous Approach

02HV43Z Insertion of Infusion Device into Superior Vena Cava, Percutaneous Endoscopic Approach

05H033Z Insertion of Infusion Device into Azygos Vein, Percutaneous Approach

05H043Z Insertion of Infusion Device into Azygos Vein, Percutaneous Endoscopic Approach

05H133Z Insertion of Infusion Device into Hemiazygos Vein, Percutaneous Approach

05H143Z Insertion of Infusion Device into Hemiazygos Vein, Percutaneous Endoscopic Approach

05H333Z Insertion of Infusion Device into Right Innominate Vein, Percutaneous Approach

05H343Z Insertion of Infusion Device into Right Innominate Vein, Percutaneous Endoscopic Approach

05H433Z Insertion of Infusion Device into Left Innominate Vein, Percutaneous Approach

05H443Z Insertion of Infusion Device into Left Innominate Vein, Percutaneous Endoscopic Approach

05H533Z Insertion of Infusion Device into Right Subclavian Vein, Percutaneous Approach

05H543Z Insertion of Infusion Device into Right Subclavian Vein, Percutaneous Endoscopic Approach

05H633Z Insertion of Infusion Device into Left Subclavian Vein, Percutaneous Approach

05H643Z Insertion of Infusion Device into Left Subclavian Vein, Percutaneous Endoscopic Approach

05HM33Z Insertion of Infusion Device into Right Internal Jugular Vein, Percutaneous Approach

05HN33Z Insertion of Infusion Device into Left Internal Jugular Vein, Percutaneous Approach

05HP33Z Insertion of Infusion Device into Right External Jugular Vein, Percutaneous Approach

05HQ33Z Insertion of Infusion Device into Left External Jugular Vein, Percutaneous Approach

0JH63XZ Insertion of Vascular Access Device into Chest Subcutaneous Tissue and Fascia, Percutaneous Approach

Appendix H: Centers for Medicare & Medicaid Services Hierarchical Condition Categories (CMS-HCC)

In the 1970s, Medicare began demonstration projects that contracted with health maintenance organizations (HMOs) to provide care for Medicare beneficiaries in exchange for prospective payments. In 1985, this project changed from demonstration status to a regular part of the Medicare program, Medicare Part C. The Balanced Budget Act (BBA) of 1997 named Medicare's Part C managed care program Medicare+Choice, and the Medicare Modernization Act (MMA) of 2003 again renamed it to Medicare Advantage (MA).

Medicare is one of the world's largest health insurance programs, and about one-third of the beneficiaries on Medicare are enrolled in a MA private health care plan. Due to the great variance in the health status of Medicare beneficiaries, risk adjustment provides a means of adequately compensating those plans with large numbers of seriously ill patients while not overburdening other plans that have healthier individuals. Medicare Advantage (MA) plans have been using the Hierarchical Condition Category (HCC) risk adjustment model since 2004.

The Risk Adjustment Model

The primary purpose of a risk adjustment model is to predict (on average) the future health care costs for specific consortiums enrolled in Medicare Advantage (MA) health plans. CMS is then able to provide capitation payments to these private health plans. Capitation payments are an incentive for health plans to enroll not only healthier individuals but those with chronic conditions or who are more seriously ill by removing some of the financial burden.

The MA risk adjustment model uses HCCs to assess the disease burden of its enrollees. HCC diagnostic groupings were created after examining claims data so that enrollees with similar disease processes, and consequently similar health care expenditures, could be pooled into a larger data set in which an average expenditure rate could be determined. The medical conditions included in HCC categories are those that were determined to most predictably affect the health status and health care costs of any individual. Several important principles to the risk adjustment model and the development of the HCC categories include but are not limited to:

1. The HCC diagnostic categories should be clinically meaningful.

   - Diagnostic categories are well-defined.

   - Clinically specific diseases or medical conditions are grouped to each category.

2. The HCC diagnostic categories should predict medical expenditures.

   - The diagnoses grouped to a specific category should have as close to the same cost burden not only in the current year but also in the future.

3. The HCC diagnostic categories should have adequate sample sizes and discretionary categories excluded to be as accurate and stable in their estimate of costs as possible.

   - A diagnostic category that groups extremely rare diseases or conditions would not be reliably effective in determining current or future costs.

   - Codes that are not credible as cost predictors or may be subject to coding variation should be excluded, when possible.

4. The HCC diagnostic categories should be both hierarchical and additive.

   - Hierarchical measurement is used within a specific disease process.

   - Disease processes that are unrelated to each other are measured additively.

5. The diagnostic classification should encourage specificity and should not reward coding proliferation.

   - More diagnosis codes and vague diagnosis codes do not equal greater disease burden.

More than 10,000 ICD-10-CM diagnosis codes map to 86 HCCs in the current risk adjustment model. Diagnoses are excluded from mapping when they do not predict future cost or are vague or variable in diagnosis, coding, or treatment, such as symptoms or osteoarthritis. Also excluded are diagnosis codes from laboratories, radiology, and home health claims.

Risk Adjustment Factors

The CMS-HCC risk adjustment model uses "risk adjustment factors" to calculate a risk score for each member. This score summarizes that particular patient's expected cost of care relative to other members'. Each member's risk score is based on demographic and health status information and is calculated as the sum of these demographic and health factors weighted by their estimated marginal contributions to total risk. The model also takes into account where the patient resides (community or institutional), Medicaid eligibility (full or partial benefits), the patient's Medicare enrollment status (new or established), age, disability status, whether the patient is frail or has end-stage renal disease (ESRD), and even prescription drug use.

No procedure codes, ICD-10-PCS or CPT, are included in the MA risk adjustment model. The model relies solely on diagnostic and demographic data. Not all ICD-10-CM diagnoses map to an HCC, and there is no specific code sequencing involved. The CMS-HCC model is additive as well as hierarchical. The additive functionality allows a patient to have more than one HCC category assigned, providing a more complete clinical picture and prediction of resource consumption. The hierarchical aspect of the model provides a means of ranking diagnoses that are similar in disease process, by severity. The hierarchy of the condition categories ensures the patient's conditions are classified to the most severe condition within the related group. Less severe conditions within a particular hierarchy are superseded by more severe diagnoses within the same group. The hierarchy and additive relationship permits this model to characterize the person's illness level within each disease process, while still allowing the effects of unrelated disease processes to be counted in the patient's overall score.

Certain combinations of coexisting diagnoses for an individual can increase medical costs. The CMS-HCC model adjusts for these higher costs by the addition of "disease interaction" factors. For each patient, multiple HCCs assigned, along with demographic and disease interaction factors, are used to calculate a single, combined risk adjustment factor (RAF). The RAF score for an individual member represents all of the HCCs that have been submitted from all sources for that member to CMS during the course of an entire calendar year.

There are separate CMS-HCC models for new enrollees and continuing enrollees. The new enrollee model uses demographic factors only, such as age, sex, and disability status, and is used when the enrollee has less than 12 months of medical history. The community model accounts for age, sex, original reason for Medicare entitlement (age or disability), Medicaid eligibility, and clinical conditions as measured by HCCs. In the second step, expected costs are adjusted for outliers based on the member's risk score and whether the patient has ESRD.

Demographic data (age, sex, eligibility) as well as health status (diagnoses codes submitted on claims to CMS) of an MA population are used to determine the reimbursement to the health plan to care for their members.

CMS considers a RAF score of 1.0 as the benchmark to indicate the score of the average healthy patient with the same demographic and diagnostic factors. These patients are expected to use average or lower-than-average resources. When the RAF score is higher than 1.0, CMS considers the patient to be sicker than the average patient with the same criteria and expects greater-than-average resource utilization.

A low RAF score may accurately indicate a healthier patient, but it may also falsely indicate a healthier patient due to incomplete or inaccurate coding, incomplete or insufficient record documentation, or patients who fail to complete an annual assessment.

A high RAF score may accurately indicate a sicker patient, or it may be falsely inflated from overcoding due to diagnoses that are reported but not documented, or from copying and pasting from previous encounters or problem lists of resolved conditions.

Documentation Requirements

Payment is made per HCC category (not per diagnosis code). No matter how many times in the year the diagnosis codes are reported, a single payment is made to the MA plan each year. Each year the list of HCCs and the RAF for each patient is "reset." This means the annual health assessment is extremely important, and adequate documentation is critical. Accurate risk adjustment payment relies on complete medical record documentation and diagnosis coding. CMS requires that all applicable diagnosis codes be reported and that all diagnoses be reported to the highest level of specificity and that these be substantiated by the medical record.

CMS's Guiding Principle:

The risk adjustment diagnosis must be based on clinical medical record documentation from a face-to-face encounter, coded according to the *ICD-10-CM Guidelines for Coding and Reporting*; assigned based on dates of service within the data collection period, submitted to the MA organization from an appropriate risk adjustment provider type and an appropriate risk adjustment physician data source.

A "face-to-face" health service encounter between a patient and healthcare provider describes an encounter between the patient and the provider (MD, DO), including qualified nonphysician practitioners (NPP) (e.g. nurse practitioner or physician's assistant), which is face-to-face with the patient. CMS provides a current listing of acceptable physician specialty types for risk adjustment data submission within the 2012 Regional Technical Assistance Participant Guide. The only exception to the face-to-face encounter requirement is pathology services (professional component only). Currently, CMS does not provide a listing of all services that are considered face-to-face visits for risk adjustment data, but does provide guidance on what types of services are not acceptable for risk adjustment in the Participant Guide. For example, diagnostic radiology does not qualify because diagnostic radiologists typically do not document confirmed diagnoses. Other examples of services that are not acceptable include diagnostic reports that have not been interpreted, such as laboratory reports.

It is essential that the medical record documentation show evidence by provider authentication that the direct face-to-face service was personally furnished by the physician or qualified NPP. Examples of these services include office visits, hospital visits, preoperative anesthesia assessment, and surgical and invasive procedures.

Risk adjustment relies on annual health information. Each enrollee is assigned an individual risk score based on the health status information obtained from the diagnosis codes on the claims. The CMS-HCC model relies on ICD-10-CM coding specificity for accurate risk adjustment by using the most specific code available that is substantiated by the documentation in the medical record. Providers should fully document and accurately code the evaluation and management of all severe and chronic conditions to ensure a full, complete, and accurate clinical record of the patient's condition and reflect the work involved in caring for the patient, particularly those with complex and challenging health issues. All conditions affecting the treatment or management of the patient's health should be documented at least once a year, as applicable to care provided, to accurately describe the true complexity and severity of the patient's health. If the diagnosis coding on the claim is not accurate or complete, the claim may indicate that the provider did much less medical decision-making, evaluation, and management than was actually performed.

Documentation to support or validate risk adjustment conditions may be found anywhere in the note for the face-to-face encounter. It is important to ensure that the note accurately reflects all chronic conditions that affect the health and care of the patient. Each encounter must be unique and reflect only that visit as it occurred. Insufficient documentation influences the assignment of diagnosis codes and directly affects the patient's risk score.

Documentation should properly validate all reported conditions. Each page of progress notes should be properly authenticated and include the patient's name and the date.

Providers should document each clinical diagnosis to the highest degree of specificity per encounter, including all complications and/or manifestations, including clear links to causal conditions. Only confirmed conditions should be documented—no rule-out conditions or abnormal findings without clinical significance. All known conditions, including chronic conditions, that affect the care and treatment of the patient at least once per year should be noted.

Providers should specifically document the condition and clinical significance, and any pertinent changes, using terminology such as decreased, increased, worsening, improving, or unchanged, or abnormal findings.

Documentation Tips

- Document all cause-and-effect relationships.
- Report the most specific diagnosis code available that is supported by the documentation.
- Include all current diagnoses as part of the current medical decision-making, and document for every visit.
- Identify diagnoses that are current or chronic problems rather than a past medical history or previous resolved condition.
- Document history of heart attack, status codes, etc., that affect the patient's care as "history of" or "PMH" when they no longer exist or are not current conditions.
- Ensure each progress note has the date, signature, and credentials/specialty.
- Document the thought processes used to assess each condition.
- Know high revenue HCCs that are often undiagnosed or undercoded.
- Avoid "unspecified" codes.

- Ensure the codes reported are accurate.
- Ensure each encounter is billed.
- Review rejection reports, and audit reports to assess risks.

Audits

Because reimbursement is by patient, rather than based on an average of the entire population, and is based upon documentation, there is the potential for upcoding. Audits are conducted by the MA plan and CMS recovery auditors.

Initial Validation Audit (IVA)

CMS requires that the MA plan validate HCCs. This is usually performed by an independent auditor working with the plan or a contracted vendor to validate the MA plan's data submitted to CMS.

The MA plan submits the one best medical record that supports each HCC identified for the beneficiary.

Risk Adjustment Data Validation Audit

Risk adjustment data validation (RADV) audits were introduced in 2011 and updated for 2015. They are performed by CMS to validate the integrity and accuracy of risk-adjusted payments by verifying that the diagnosis codes the MA plans submit are supported by the medical record documentation for a member.

MA plans can be selected by CMS for RADV audits annually and if chosen are required to submit their members' medical records to CMS. Providers are required to assist the MA plan by providing the medical record documentation included in the audit. Even though each diagnosis needs to be reported only once in a calendar year, during a RADV audit up to five dates of service may be submitted to support any one HCC.

To be validated, medical record documentation must meet certain criteria and standards. Even if the diagnosis is documented and coded correctly, any deficiency in the documentation can make the encounter and the HCC invalid. Diagnoses that cannot be validated are considered payment errors. The results of the audit are communicated to the MA plan, which then communicates these results to the provider. Under- and overpayments are subject to payment adjustment. The results of RADV audits can be extrapolated over the MA plan population to calculate potential payment errors and overpayments/ recoupments. Regulations include a RADV appeal process, a document dispute process, and a procedure for obtaining physician-signature attestations.

The following items are reviewed during the validation process:

- The record is for the correct enrollee.
- The record is from the correct calendar year for the payment year being audited.
- The record is legible.
- The date of service is present on the records and is for a face-to-face visit.
- The record is from a valid provider type.
- Valid credentials and/or a valid physician specialty are documented on the record.
- The record contains a signature from an acceptable type of physician.
- There is a diagnosis on the record.
- The diagnosis supports an HCC.
- The diagnosis supports the submitted HCC.

Mitigate audit risk by coding each reportable diagnosis each time it meets reporting guidelines. Audit regularly to assess areas of risk and in need of improvement and to capture conditions documented but not coded. Check for additional qualifying HCCs. Ensure claims are submitted and that corrected claims are submitted when indicated. There are three claims submission deadlines: January, March, and September. CMS adjusts each member's risk score twice a year, with the final reconciliation in August of the year after the plan year.

If providers emphasize correct coding and documentation and perform internal audits to determine where the risks are and prepare for audits, incorrect payment is less likely.

For additional information on risk adjustment coding, see Optum360's *Risk Adjustment Coding and HCC Guide*.

Appendix I: Long-term Care Hospital Prospective Payment System Overview

Information in this appendix is based on the Centers for Medicare and Medicaid Services (CMS) FY 2021 long-term care hospital prospective payment system (LTCH PPS) proposed rule published in the *Federal Register,* volume 85, number 104, May 29, 2020 ("Hospital Inpatient Prospective Payment Systems for Acute Care Hospitals and the Long-Term Care Hospital Prospective Payment System and Proposed Policy Changes and Fiscal Year 2021 Rates").

Classification As a Long-term Care Hospital

Under the regulations at § 412.23(e)(1), to qualify to be paid under the long-term care hospital prospective payment system (LTCH PPS), a hospital must have a provider agreement with Medicare. Furthermore, § 412.23(e)(2)(i), which implements section 1886(d)(1)(B)(iv) of the Social Security Act, requires that a hospital have an average Medicare inpatient length of stay of greater than 25 days to be paid under the LTCH PPS. In accordance with section 1206(a)(3) of the Pathway for SGR Reform Act of 2013 (Pub. L. 113–67), as amended by section 15007 of Public Law 114–255, CMS amended the regulations to specify that Medicare Advantage plans' and site-neutral payment rate discharges are excluded from the calculation of the average length of stay for all LTCHs, for discharges occurring in cost reporting period beginning on or after October 1, 2015.

The following hospitals are paid under special payment provisions, as described in § 412.22(c) and, therefore, are not subject to the LTCH PPS rules:

- Veterans Administration hospitals

- Hospitals that are reimbursed under state cost control systems approved under 42 CFR part 403

- Hospitals that are reimbursed in accordance with demonstration projects authorized under section 402(a) of the Social Security Amendments of 1967 (Pub. L. 90-248) (42 U.S.C. 1395b-1), section 222(a) of the Social Security Amendments of 1972 (Pub. L. 92-603) (42 U.S.C. 1395b-1 (note)) (statewide all-payer systems, subject to the rate-of-increase test at section 1814(b) of the Act), or section 3201 of the Patient Protection and Affordable Care Act (Pub. L. 111-148 (42 U.S.C. 1315a))

- Nonparticipating hospitals furnishing emergency services to Medicare beneficiaries

Proposed Medicare Severity Long-Term Care Diagnosis-Related Group Classification and Relative Weights for FY 2021

Background

Section 123 of the BBRA required that the secretary of the Department of Health and Human Services implement a PPS for LTCHs to replace the cost-based payment system under TEFRA. Section 307(b)(1) of the BIPA modified the requirements of section 123 of the BBRA by requiring that the HHS secretary examine the feasibility and impact of basing payment under the LTCH PPS on the use of existing (or refined) hospital DRGs that have been modified to account for different resource use of LTCH patients.

When the LTCH PPS was implemented for cost reporting periods beginning on or after October 1, 2002, CMS adopted the same DRG patient classification system used at that time under the IPPS. As a component of the LTCH PPS, CMS referred to this patient classification system as the "long-term care diagnosis-related groups (LTCH-DRGs)." Although the patient classification system used under both the LTCH PPS and the IPPS are the same, the relative weights are different. The established relative weight methodology and data used under the LTCH PPS result in relative weights under the LTCH PPS that reflect the differences in patient resource use of LTCH patients, consistent with section 123(a)(1) of the BBRA (Pub. L. 106-113).

As part of CMS' efforts to better recognize severity of illness among patients, in the FY 2008 IPPS final rule with comment period (72 FR 47130), the MS-DRGs and the Medicare severity LTCH-DRGs (MS-LTC-DRGs) were adopted under the IPPS and the LTCH PPS, respectively, effective beginning October 1, 2007 (FY 2008). (CMS noted, in that same final rule, that it revised the regulations at § 412.503 to specify that for LTCH discharges occurring on or after October 1, 2007, when applying the provisions of 42 CFR part 412, subpart O, applicable to LTCHs for policy descriptions and payment calculations, all references to LTC-DRGs would be considered a reference to MS-LTC-DRGs.)

The MS-DRG classifications are updated annually. There are currently 761 MS-DRG groupings. For FY 2021, there would be 767 MS-DRG groupings based on the proposed changes. Consistent with section 123 of the BBRA, as amended by section 307(b)(1) of the BIPA, and § 412.515 of the regulations, CMS used information derived from LTCH PPS patient records to classify LTCH discharges into distinct MS-LTC-DRGs based on clinical characteristics and estimated resource needs. Then CMS assigned an appropriate weight to the MS-LTC-DRGs to account for the difference in resource use by patients exhibiting the case complexity and multiple medical problems characteristic of LTCHs.

For FY 2021, CMS is proposing to continue to use existing methodology to determine the MS-LTC-DRG relative weights. As previously established when CMS implemented the dual-rate LTCH PPS payment structure codified under § 412.522, which began in FY 2016, CMS is proposing that the annual recalibration of the MS-LTC-DRG relative weights be determined: (1) using only data from available LTCH PPS claims that (1) would have qualified for payment under the new LTCH PPS standard federal payment rate if that rate had been in effect at the time of discharge when claims data from time periods before the dual-rate LTCH PPS payment structure applies are used to calculate the relative weights; and (2) qualify for payment under the new LTCH PPS standard federal payment rate when claims data from time periods after the dual-rate LTCH PPS payment structure applies are used to calculate the relative weights (80 FR 49624). That is, under the current methodology, MS-LTC-DRG relative weight calculations do not use data from cases paid at the site-neutral payment rate under § 412.522(c)(1) or data from cases that would have been paid at the site-neutral payment rate if the dual-rate LTCH PPS payment structure had been in effect at the time of that discharge. In addition, for FY 2021, CMS is proposing to continue to exclude the data from all-inclusive rate providers and LTCHs paid in accordance with demonstration projects, as well as any Medicare Advantage claims from the MS-LTC-DRG relative weight calculations.

Furthermore, for FY 2021, in using data from applicable LTCH cases to establish MS-LTC-DRG relative weights, CMS is proposing to continue to establish low-volume MS-LTC-DRGs (that is, MS-LTC-DRGs with less than 25 cases) using existing quintile methodology in determining the MS-LTC-DRG relative weights because LTCHs do not typically treat the full range of diagnoses as do acute care hospitals. Therefore, for purposes of determining the relative weights for the large number of low-volume MS-LTC-DRGs, CMS grouped all of the low-volume MS-LTC-DRGs into five quintiles based on average charges per discharge. Then, under the existing methodology, CMS accounted for adjustments made to LTCH PPS standard federal payments for short-stay outlier (SSO) cases (that is, cases for which the covered length of stay at the LTCH is less than or equal to five-sixths of the geometric average length of stay for the MS-LTC-DRG), and adjustments made to account for nonmonotonically increasing weights, when necessary. The methodology is premised on more severe cases under the MS-LTC-DRG system requiring greater expenditure of medical care resources and higher average charges such that, in the severity levels within a base MS-LTC-DRG, the relative weights should increase monotonically with severity from the lowest to highest severity level.

Patient Classifications into MS-LTC-DRGs

The MS-DRGs (used under the IPPS) and the MS-LTC-DRGs (used under the LTCH PPS) are based on the CMS DRG structure. As noted previously in this section, CMS refers to the DRGs under the LTCH PPS as MS-LTC-DRGs although they are structurally identical to the MS-DRGs used under the IPPS. The MS-DRGs are organized into 25 major diagnostic categories (MDCs), most of which are based on a particular organ system of the body; the remainder involve multiple organ systems (such as MDC 22 Burns). Within most MDCs, cases are then divided into surgical DRGs and medical DRGs. Surgical DRGs are assigned based on a surgical hierarchy that orders operating room (O.R.) procedures or groups of O.R. procedures by resource intensity. The GROUPER software program does not recognize all ICD-10-PCS procedure codes as procedures affecting DRG assignment. That is, procedures that are not surgical (for example, EKGs), or minor surgical procedures (for example, a biopsy of skin and subcutaneous tissue (procedure code 0JBH3ZX)) do not affect the MS-LTC-DRG assignment based on their presence on the claim.

Generally, under the LTCH PPS, a Medicare payment is made at a predetermined specific rate for each discharge that varies based on the MS-LTC-DRG to which a beneficiary's discharge is assigned. Cases are classified into MS-LTC-DRGs for payment based on the following six data elements:

- Principal diagnosis

- Additional or secondary diagnoses

- Surgical procedures

- Age
- Sex
- Discharge status of the patient

The Health Information Portability and Accountability Act (HIPAA) requires covered entities to use the applicable medical data code set requirements when conducting HIPAA transactions (45 CFR 162.1000). Currently, upon the discharge of the patient, the LTCH must assign appropriate diagnosis and procedure codes from the most current version of ICD-10-CM for diagnosis coding and ICD-10-PCS for inpatient hospital procedure coding, both of which were required to be implemented October 1, 2015 (45 CFR 162.1002(c)(2) and (3)).

To create the MS-DRGs (and by extension, the MS-LTC-DRGs), base DRGs were subdivided according to the presence of specific secondary diagnoses designated as complications or comorbidities (CCs) into one, two, or three levels of severity, depending on the impact of the CCs on resources used for those cases. Specifically, there are sets of MS-DRGs that are split into two or three subgroups based on the presence or absence of a CC or a major complication or comorbidity (MCC).

Medicare administrative contractors (MAC) enter the clinical and demographic information submitted by LTCHs into their claims processing systems and subject this information to a series of automated screening processes called the Medicare Code Editor (MCE). These screens are designed to identify cases that require further review before being assigned into a MS-LTC-DRG. During this process, certain cases are selected for further explanation (74 FR 43949).

After screening through the MCE, each claim is classified into the appropriate MS-LTC-DRG by the Medicare LTCH Grouper software on the basis of diagnosis and procedure codes and other demographic information (age, sex, and discharge status). The Grouper software used under the LTCH PPS is the same software program used under the IPPS. Following the MS-LTC-DRG assignment, the MAC determines the prospective payment amount by using the Medicare Pricer program, which accounts for hospital-specific adjustments. Under the LTCH PPS, CMS provided an opportunity for LTCHs to review the MS-LTC-DRG assignments made by the MAC and to submit additional information within a specified timeframe as provided in § 412.513(c).

The Grouper software is used both to classify past cases to measure relative hospital resource consumption to establish the MS-LTC-DRG relative weights and to classify current cases for purposes of determining payment. The records for all Medicare hospital inpatient discharges are maintained in the MedPAR file. The data in this file are used to evaluate possible MS-DRG and MS-LTC-DRG classification changes and to recalibrate the MS-DRG and MS-LTC-DRG relative weights during the annual update under both the IPPS (§ 412.60(e)) and the LTCH PPS (§ 412.517), respectively.

Proposed Changes to the MS-LTC-DRGs for FY 2021

As specified by § 412.517(a), which require that the MS-LTC-DRG classifications and relative weights be updated annually, and consistent with our historical practice of using the same patient classification system under the LTCH PPS as is used under the IPPS, in FY 2021 proposed rule, CMS is proposing to update the MS-LTC-DRG classifications effective October 1, 2020 through September 30, 2021 (FY 2021), consistent with the proposed changes to specific MS-DRG classifications.

Accordingly, the proposed MS-LTC-DRGs for FY 2021 will be the same as the MS-DRGs that are being used under the IPPS for FY 2021. In addition, because the proposed MS-LTC-DRGs for FY 2021 are the same as the proposed MS-DRGs for FY 2021, the other proposed changes that affect MS-DRG (and by extension MS-LTC-DRG) assignments under proposed GROUPER Version 38, including the proposed changes to the MCE software and the ICD-10-CM/PCS coding system, also are applicable under the LTCH PPS for FY 2021.

Development of the Proposed MS-LTC-DRG Relative Weights for FY 2021

CMS is proposing to continue to use current methodology to determine the MS-LTC-DRG relative weights for FY 2021, including the continued application of established policies related to the hospital-specific relative value methodology, the treatment of severity levels in the MS-LTC-DRGs, low-volume and no-volume MS-LTC-DRGs, adjustments for nonmonotonicity, the steps for calculating the MS-LTC-DRG relative weights with a budget neutrality factor, and only using data from applicable LTCH cases (which includes the policy of using only cases that would meet the criteria for exclusion from the site-neutral payment rate [or, for discharges occurring prior to the implementation of the dual-rate LTCH PPS payment structure, would have met the criteria for exclusion had those criteria been in effect at the time of the discharge]).

Data

For FY 2021 IPPS/LTCH PPS proposed rule, consistent with proposals regarding the calculation of the proposed MS-LTC-DRG relative weights for FY 2021, CMS obtained total charges from FY 2019 Medicare LTCH claims data from the December 2019 update of the FY 2019 MedPAR file, which are the best available data at this time, and is proposing to use version 38 of the Grouper to classify LTCH cases. Consistent with historical practice, CMS is proposing that if more recent data become available, that data would be used, with the finalized version 38 of the Grouper, in establishing the FY 2021 MS-LTC-DRG relative weights in the final rule.

To calculate the proposed FY 2021 MS-LTC-DRG relative weights under the dual-rate LTCH PPS payment structure, CMS is proposing to continue to use applicable LTCH data, which includes the policy of using only cases that meet the criteria for exclusion from the site-neutral payment rate (or would have met the criteria had they been in effect at the time of the discharge) (80 FR 49624). Specifically, CMS began by first evaluating the LTCH claims data in the December 2019 update of the FY 2019 MedPAR file to determine which LTCH cases would meet the criteria for exclusion from the site-neutral payment rate under § 412.522(b) or had the dual-rate LTCH PPS payment structure applied to those cases at the time of discharge. CMS identified the FY 2019 LTCH cases that were not assigned to MS-LTC-DRGs 876, 880, 881, 882, 883, 884, 885, 886, 887, 894, 895, 896, 897, 945, and 946, which identify LTCH cases that do not have a principal diagnosis relating to a psychiatric diagnosis or to rehabilitation and for which one of the following is true:

- The admission to the LTCH was "immediately preceded" by discharge from a subsection (d) hospital and the immediately preceding stay in that subsection (d) hospital included at least three days in an intensive care unit (ICU), as defined under the ICU criterion.

- The admission to the LTCH was "immediately preceded" by discharge from a subsection (d) hospital and the claim for the LTCH discharge includes the applicable procedure code that indicates at least 96 hours of ventilator services were provided during the LTCH stay, as defined under the ventilator criterion. Claims data from the FY 2019 MedPAR file that reported ICD-10-PCS procedure code 5A1955Z were used to identify cases involving at least 96 hours of ventilator services in accordance with the ventilator criterion. (CMS notes that, for purposes of developing the MS-LTC-DRG relative weights, it has previously addressed the treatment of cases that would have been excluded from the site-neutral payment rate under the statutory provisions that provided for temporary exception from the site-neutral payment rate under the LTCH PPS for certain spinal cord specialty hospitals or for certain severe wound care discharges from certain LTCHs provided by sections 15009 and 15010 of Pub. L. 114-255, respectively. This temporary exception from the site-neutral payment rate for certain spinal cord specialty hospitals is effective for discharges in cost reporting periods beginning during FYs 2018 and 2019, and the temporary exception from the site-neutral payment rate for certain severe wound care discharges from certain LTCHs was effective for a discharge in cost reporting period beginning during FY 2018. These statutory provisions will no longer be in effect for any discharges occurring in FY 2021 [that is, an LTCH with a cost reporting period that begins on the last day of FY 2019, on September 30, 2019, would end on September 29, 2020, the day before the start of FY 2021 on October 1, 2020]. Therefore, CMS says it no longer needs to address the treatment of these cases for purposes of developing the MS-LTC-DRG relative weights for FY 2021 and subsequent years.)

Furthermore, consistent with historical methodology, CMS excluded any claims in the resulting data set that were submitted by LTCHs that were all-inclusive rate providers and LTCHs that are paid in accordance with demonstration projects authorized under section 402(a) of Pub. L. 90-248 or section 222(a) of Pub. L. 92-603. In addition, consistent with historical practice and policies, CMS excluded any Medicare Advantage (Part C) claims in the resulting data. Such claims were identified based on the presence of a GHO Paid indicator value of "1" in the MedPAR files. The claims that remained after these three trims (that is, the applicable LTCH data) were then used to calculate the MS-LTC-DRG relative weights for FY 2021.

In summary, in general, CMS identified the claims data used in developing the proposed FY 2021 MS-LTC-DRG relative weights in this proposed rule, by trimming claims data that were paid the site-neutral payment rate or would have been paid the site-neutral payment rate had the dual-payment-rate structure been in effect. Finally, CMS proposes to trim the claims data of all-inclusive rate providers reported in the December 2019 update of the FY 2019 MedPAR file and any Medicare Advantage claims data. There were no data from any LTCHs that are paid in accordance with a demonstration project reported in the December 2019 update of the FY 2019 MedPAR file, but, had there been any, CMS would have trimmed the claims data from those LTCHs as well, in accordance with established policy. CMS is proposing to use the remaining data (that is, the applicable LTCH data) to calculate the relative weights for FY 2021.

Steps for Determining the Proposed FY 2021 MS-LTC-DRG Relative Weights

CMS is proposing to continue to use its current methodology to determine the proposed FY 2021 MS-LTC-DRG relative weights. To determine the proposed relative weights, CMS is proposing to group applicable LTCH cases to the appropriate proposed MS-LTC-DRG, while taking into account the proposed low-volume quintiles (as described previously) and cross-walked proposed no-volume MS-LTC-DRGs. After establishing the appropriate proposed MS-LTC-DRG (or proposed low-volume quintile), CMS is proposing to calculate the proposed FY 2021 relative weights in several steps.

Step 1 Remove cases with a length of stay of seven days or less and statistical outliers

Step 2 Remove statistical outliers

Step 3 Adjust charges for the effects of short-stay outliers (SSO)

Step 4 Calculate the proposed FY 2021 MS-LTC-DRG relative weights on an iterative basis.

Step 5 Determine a proposed FY 2021 relative weight for MS-LTC-DRGs with no applicable LTCH cases

Step 6 Adjust the proposed FY 2021 MS-LTC-DRG relative weights to account for nonmonotonically increasing relative weights

Step 7Calculate the proposed FY 2021 MS-LTC-DRG reclassification and recalibration budget neutrality factor

Accordingly, in determining the proposed FY 2021 MS-LTC-DRG relative weights in this proposed rule, consistent with existing methodology, the agency is proposing to apply a normalization factor of 1.25878 and a budget neutrality factor of 0.9993445. Table 11, which is available via the internet on the CMS website, lists the proposed MS-LTC-DRGs and their respective proposed relative weights, geometric mean length of stay, and five-sixths of the geometric mean length of stay (used to identify SSO cases under § 412.529(a)) for FY 2021.

Proposed Changes to the LTCH PPS Payment Rates and Other Changes to the LTCH PPS for FY 2021

Overview

The basic methodology for determining LTCH PPS standard federal payment rates is currently set forth at 42 CFR 412.515 through 412.533 and 412.535. In this section, CMS discusses the factors it is proposing to use to update the LTCH PPS standard federal payment rate for FY 2021, that is, effective for LTCH discharges occurring on or after October 1, 2020, through September 30, 2021. Under the dual-rate LTCH PPS payment structure required by statute, beginning with discharges in cost reporting periods beginning in FY 2016, only LTCH discharges that meet the criteria for exclusion from the site-neutral payment rate are paid based on the LTCH PPS standard federal payment rate specified at § 412.523.

Before the dual-payment-rate system was implemented in FY 2016, all LTCH discharges were paid similarly to those now exempt from the site-neutral payment rate. That legacy payment rate was called the standard federal rate.

In this FY 2021 IPPS/LTCH PPS proposed rule, CMS presents proposals related to the annual update to the LTCH PPS standard federal payment rate for FY 2021. It is also proposing to adjust the LTCH PPS standard federal payment rate to account for the estimated effect of the changes to the area wage level for FY 2021 on estimated aggregate LTCH PPS payments, in accordance with § 412.523(d)(4). In addition, as discussed in the FY 2019 IPPS/LTCH PPS final rule (83 FR 41532 through 41537), CMS has eliminated the 25 percent threshold policy in a budget-neutral manner. The budget neutrality requirements are codified in the regulations at § 412.523(d)(6). Under these regulations, a temporary, one-time factor is applied to the standard federal payment rate in FY 2019 and FY 2020, and a permanent, one-time factor in FY 2021. These factors as established in the correction to the FY 2019 IPPS/LTCH PPS final rule (83 FR 41536) area as follows:

- For FY 2019, a temporary, one-time factor of 0.990878
- For FY 2020, a temporary, one-time factor of 0.990737
- For FY 2021 and subsequent years, a permanent, one-time factor of 0.991249

Therefore, in determining the FY 2021 LTCH PPS standard federal payment rate, CMS is proposing to:

- Remove the temporary, one-time factor of 0.990737 for the estimated cost of elimination of the 25-percent threshold policy in FY 2020 by applying a factor of (1/0.990737)
- Apply a permanent, one-time factor of 0.991249 for the estimated cost of the elimination of the 25-percent threshold policy in FY 2021

Proposed Annual Update to the LTCH PPS Standard Federal Payment Rate for FY 2021

CMS has used an estimated market basket increase to update the LTCH PPS. As previously noted, for FY 2021 CMS is proposing to rebase and revise the 2013-based LTCH market basket to reflect a 2017 base year. The proposed 2017-based LTCH market basket is primarily based on the Medicare cost report data submitted by LTCHs and, therefore, specifically reflects the cost structures of only LTCHs. CMS is proposing to use data from cost reports beginning in FY 2017 because these data are the latest available complete data at the time of rulemaking for purposes of calculating cost weights for the market basket. CMS believes that the proposed 2017-based LTCH market basket appropriately reflects the cost structure of LTCHs. CMS is proposing to use the proposed 2017-based LTCH market basket to update the LTCH PPS standard federal payment rate for FY 2021.

Section 1886(m)(3)(A) of the Social Security Act provides that, beginning in FY 2010, any annual update to the LTCH PPS standard federal payment rate is reduced by the adjustments specified in clauses (i) and (ii) of subparagraph (A). Clause (i) of section 1886(m)(3)(A) of the act provides for a reduction, for FY 2012 and each subsequent rate year, by the productivity adjustment described in section 1886(b)(3)(B)(xi)(II) of the act (that is, "the multifactor productivity [MFP] adjustment"). Clause (ii) of section 1886(m)(3)(A) of the act provided for a reduction, for each of FYs 2010 through 2019, by the "other adjustment" described in section 1886(m)(4)(F) of the act; therefore, it is not applicable for FY 2021.

Section 1886(m)(3)(B) of the act provides that the application of paragraph (3) of section 1886(m) of the act may result in the annual update being less than zero for a rate year and may result in payment rates for a rate year being less than such payment rates for the preceding rate year.

Appendix J: Long-Term Care Hospital Quality Reporting Program

Information in this appendix is based on:

Centers for Medicare and Medicaid Services (CMS) FY 2021 long-term care hospital prospective payment system (LTCH PPS) proposed rule published in the *Federal Register*, volume 85, number 104, May 29, 2020 ("Hospital Inpatient Prospective Payment Systems for Acute Care Hospitals and the Long-Term Care Hospital Prospective Payment System and Proposed Policy Changes and Fiscal Year 2021 Rates").

LTCH Quality Reporting Program (QRP)

https://www.cms.gov/Medicare/Quality-Initiatives-Patient-Assessment-Instruments/LTCH-Quality-Reporting

Patient Protection and Affordable Care Act (ACA) of 2010, Section 3004(a)

https://www.gpo.gov/fdsys/pkg/PLAW-111publ148/pdf/PLAW-111publ148.pdf

Improving Medicare Post-Acute Care Transformation Act of 2014 (IMPACT Act), Section 1899B

https://www.gpo.gov/fdsys/pkg/PLAW-113publ185/pdf/PLAW-113publ185.pdf

https://www.cms.gov/Medicare/Quality-Initiatives-Patient-Assessment-Instruments/Post-Acute-Care-Quality-Initiatives/IMPACT-Act-of-2014/IMPACT-Act-of-2014-Data-Standardization-and-Cross-Setting-Measures

LTCH QRP Overview

The LTCH QRP creates LTCH quality reporting requirements, as mandated by section 3004(a) of the ACA. Every year, by October 1, CMS publishes the quality measures LTCHs must report.

The IMPACT act added section 1899B to the SSA and requires the reporting of standardized patient assessment data regarding quality measures and standardized patient assessment data elements (SPADE). It requires the submission of data pertaining to quality measure, resource use, and other domains. Using standardized quality measures and standardized data, the intent of the IMPACT Act, among other obligations, is to allow for the exchange of standardized and interoperable data among post-acute providers and other providers. The IMPACT Act intends for standardized post-acute care data to improve Medicare beneficiary outcomes through shared decision-making, care coordination, and enhanced discharge planning.

For FY 2014 and each subsequent year, if an LTCH fails to submit the required quality data, the LTCH will be subject to a 2 percentage point reduction in the annual payment update. CMS strongly encourages submitting quality data prior to the deadline to allow LTCH providers an opportunity to review their data submissions for completeness and accuracy and to address any submission issues.

LTCH Continuity Assessment Record and Evaluation Data Set

The LTCH Continuity Assessment Record and Evaluation (CARE) Data Set is applicable to all patients receiving inpatient services in a facility certified as a hospital and designated as an LTCH under the Medicare program. These hospitals are certified as acute-care hospitals that treat patients requiring extended hospital-level care, typically following initial treatment at a general acute-care hospital. If a hospital is classified as an LTCH, for purposes of Medicare payments (as denoted by the last four digits of its six-digit CMS Certification Number [CCN] in the range of 2000–2299), it is subject to the requirements of the LTCH QRP. It is not applicable to patients receiving services in LTCH units that are not designated as LTCHs under the Medicare program. Data collection using the LTCH CARE Data Set is applicable regardless of patient's age, diagnosis, length of stay, or payment/payer source. Data collected must be submitted in the time frame, manner, and form established by CMS for the LTCH QRP.

Effective July 1, 2018, the data collection instrument for these measures is the LTCH CARE Data Set version 4.00.

Effective October 1, 2020, the data collection instrument for these measures is the LTCH CARE Data Set version 5.00.

Note: CMS is delaying the release of LTCH CARE Data Set version 5.00 needed to support the Transfer of Health (TOH) Information Quality Measures in order to provide maximum flexibilities for providers of LTCHs to respond to the COVID-19 pubic health emergency (PHE).

The release of updated versions of the LTCH CARE Data Set will be delayed until October 1st of the year that is at least one full fiscal year after the end of the COVID-19 PHE. For example, if the COVID-19 PHE ends on September 20, 2020, LTCHs will be required to begin collecting data using the updated versions of the item sets beginning with patients discharged on October 1, 2021.

Standardized Patient Assessment Data Elements

The IMPACT Act required CMS to develop, implement, and maintain standardized patient assessment data elements (SPADE) for post-acute care (PAC) settings. The four PAC settings specified in the IMPACT Act are home health agencies (HHAs), inpatient rehabilitation facilities (IRFs), long-term care hospitals (LTCHs), and skilled nursing facilities (SNFs). The goals of implementing cross-setting SPADEs are to facilitate care coordination, interoperability, and improve Medicare beneficiary outcomes.

The IMPACT Act further required that the assessment instruments be modified to include core data elements on health assessment categories and that such data be standardized and interoperable. Implementation of a core set of standardized assessment items across PAC settings has important implications for Medicare beneficiaries, families, providers, and policymakers.

For FY 2019 and each subsequent year, LTCHs must report standardized patient assessment data, required under section 1899B(b)(1) of the Social Security Act. Section 1899B(b)(1)(B) of the act defines standardized patient assessment data as data required for at least the quality measures described in section 1899B(c)(1) of the act and that is with respect to the following categories:

1. Functional status
2. Cognitive function
3. Special services, treatments, and interventions
4. Medical conditions and comorbidities
5. Impairments
6. Other categories deemed necessary and appropriate by the secretary of the Department of Health and Human Services

In FY 2020 IPPS/LTCH PPS final rule, CMS adopted the first five categories listed above in addition to a new category. Each category and their respective data elements are outlined in the following table.

Category	Data Elements
Functional Status	Car transfer
	Walking 10 feet on uneven surfaces
	1-step (curb)
	4 steps
	12 steps
	Picking up object
Cognitive Function	Brief interview for mental status (BIMS)
	Confusion assessment method (CAM)
	Patient health questionnaire — 2 to 9 (PHQ-2 to 9)
Special Services, Treatments, and Interventions	Chemotherapy (IV, oral, other)
	Radiation
	Oxygen therapy (intermittent, continuous, high-concentration oxygen delivery system)
	Suctioning (scheduled, as needed)
	Tracheostomy care
	Noninvasive mechanical ventilator (bilevel positive airway pressure [BiPAP]; continuous positive airway pressure [CPAP])
	Invasive mechanical ventilator
	IV medications (antibiotics, anticoagulation, vasoactive medications, other)
	Transfusions
	Dialysis (hemodialysis, peritoneal dialysis)
	IV access (peripheral IV, midline, central line)
	Parenteral/IV feeding
	Feeding tube
	Mechanically altered diet
	Therapeutic diet
	High-risk drug classes: use and indication
Medical Conditions and Comorbidities	Pain interference (pain effect on sleep, pain interference with therapy activities, and pain interference with day-to-day activities)

Category	Data Elements
Impairments	Hearing
	Vision
Social Determinants of Health (SDOH)	Race
	Ethnicity
	Preferred language
	Interpreter services
	Health literacy
	Transportation
	Social isolation

For the first program year in which measures or standardized patient assessment data are adopted, LTCHs will be required to report data only on patients who are admitted and discharged during the last quarter (October 1 to December 31) of the calendar year that applies to the program year. For subsequent program years, LTCHs will be required to report data on patients who are admitted and discharged during the 12-month calendar year that applies to the program year.

Note: CMS is delaying the release of new or revised SPADEs in order to provide maximum flexibilities for providers of LTCHs to respond to the COVID-19 pubic health emergency (PHE).

The release of new or revised SPADEs will be delayed until October 1st of the year that is at least one full fiscal year after the end of the COVID-19 PHE. For example, if the COVID-19 PHE ends on September 20, 2020, LTCHs will be required to begin collecting data beginning with patients discharged on October 1, 2021.

Quality Measures Currently Adopted for the FY 2022 LTCH QRP

The LTCH QRP currently has 17 measures for the FY 2022 program year, which are outlined in the following table:

Quality Measures Currently Adopted for the FY 2022 LTCH QRP	
LTCH CARE Data Set	
Short Name	**Measure Name & Data Source**
Pressure Ulcer/Injury	Changes in Skin Integrity Post-Acute Care: Pressure Ulcer/Injury
Application of Falls	Application of Percent of Residents Experiencing One or More Falls with Major Injury (Long Stay) (NQF #0674)
Functional Assessment	Percent of Long-Term Care Hospital (LTCH) Patients with an Admission and Discharge Functional Assessment and a Care Plan That Addresses Function (NQF #2631)
Application of Functional Assessment	Application of Percent of Long-Term Care Hospital (LTCH) Patients with an Admission and Discharge Functional Assessment and a Care Plan That Addresses Function (NQF #2631)
Change in Mobility	Functional Outcome Measure: Change in Mobility Among Long-Term Care Hospital (LTCH) Patients Requiring Ventilator Support (NQF #2632)
DRR	Drug Regimen Review Conducted With Follow-Up for Identified Issues—Post Acute Care (PAC) Long-Term Care Hospital (LTCH) Quality Reporting Program (QRP)
Compliance with SBT	Compliance with Spontaneous Breathing Trial (SBT) by Day 2 of the LTCH Stay
Ventilator Liberation	Ventilator Liberation Rate
TOH* – Provider	Transfer of Health Information to the Provider Post-Acute Care
TOH* – Patient	Transfer of Health Information to the Patient Post-Acute Care

Quality Measures Currently Adopted for the FY 2022 LTCH QRP	
NHSN	
CAUTI	National Healthcare Safety Network (NHSN) Catheter-Associated Urinary Tract Infection (CAUTI) Outcome Measure (NQF #0138)
CLABSI	National Healthcare Safety Network (NHSN) Central Line-Associated Bloodstream Infection (CLABSI) Outcome Measure (NQF #0139)
CDI	National Healthcare Safety Network (NHSN) Facility-wide Inpatient Hospital-onset *Clostridium difficile* Infection (CDI) Outcome Measure (NQF #1717)
HCP Influenza Vaccine	Influenza Vaccination Coverage among Healthcare Personnel (NQF #0431)
Claims-based	
MSPB LTCH	Medicare Spending Per Beneficiary (MSPB)—Post Acute Care (PAC) Long-Term Care Hospital (LTCH) Quality Reporting Program (QRP)
DTC	Discharge to Community—Post Acute Care (PAC) Long-Term Care Hospital (LTCH) Quality Reporting Program (QRP)
PPR	Potentially Preventable 30-Day Post-Discharge Readmission Measure for Long-Term Care Hospital (LTCH) Quality Reporting Program (QRP)

* Transfer of Health Information

Form, Manner, and Timing of Data Submission Under the LTCH QRP

Under the current CMS policy, LTCHs report data on LTCH QRP assessment-based measures and standardized patient assessment data by reporting the designated data elements for each applicable patient on the LTCH CARE Data Set patient assessment instrument and then submitting the completed instruments to CMS using the Quality Improvement and Evaluation System (QIES) Assessment and Submission Processing (ASAP) system. Data on LTCH QRP measures that are also collected by the CDC for other purposes are reported by LTCHs to the CDC through the NHSN, and the CDC then transmits the relevant data to CMS. Readers are referred to the FY 2018 IPPS/LTCH PPS final rule (82 FR 38454 through 38456) for the data collection and submission timeframes that were finalized for the LTCH QRP.

In the FY 2020 IPPS/LTCH PPS final rule, CMS finalized their proposal to move the implementation date of any new version of the LTCH CARE Data Set from April to October, beginning October 1, 2020. This would give LTCHs an additional six months (April-October) to update their systems so that they can comply with the new reporting requirements.

Appendix K: Severe Wound Diagnosis Codes by Category

The following lists the ICD-10-CM codes describing severe wound diagnoses. CMS allows for a temporary exception for certain wound care discharges from the site-neutral payment rate for certain long-term care hospitals (LTCHs). This exception applies to discharges occurring during FY2018 (that is, for cost reporting period beginning on or after October 1, 2017, and on or before September 30, 2018) from LTCHs that are grandfathered hospitals-within-hospitals (HwHs) (that is, hospitals that are described under § 412.23(e)(2)(i) that meet the criteria of § 412.22(f)) when the individual discharged "has a severe wound." Based upon the FY 2018 IPPS/LTCH final rule classification, the definition of "severe wound" has been refined to include only five categories (stage 3 wound, stage 4 wound, unstageable wound, nonhealing surgical wound, and fistula) and exclusions are limited to discharges that both meet the definition of a severe wound and are additionally grouped to certain specified MS-LTC-DRGs.

Note: An updated ICD-10-CM list was not available at the time this publication was printed and therefore does not reflect any FY 2021 code changes. An updated list of severe wound codes, effective October 1, 2020, can be found at: https://www.cms.gov/Medicare/Medicare-Fee-for-Service-Payment/LongTermCareHospitalPPS/download.html.

Stage 3 Wound

L89.003	L89.123	L89.213	L89.43	L89.613	L97.112	L97.124	L97.922
L89.013	L89.133	L89.223	L89.503	L89.623	L97.113	L97.912	L97.923
L89.023	L89.143	L89.303	L89.513	L89.813	L97.114	L97.913	L97.924
L89.103	L89.153	L89.313	L89.523	L89.893	L97.122	L97.914	
L89.113	L89.203	L89.323	L89.603	L89.93	L97.123	L97.921	

Stage 4 Wound

L89.004	L89.104	L89.134	L89.204	L89.304	L89.44	L89.524	L89.624	L89.94
L89.014	L89.114	L89.144	L89.214	L89.314	L89.504	L89.604	L89.814	
L89.024	L89.124	L89.154	L89.224	L89.324	L89.514	L89.614	L89.894	

Unstageable Wound

L89.000	T20.319D	T20.72XA	T21.34XS	T21.77XD	T22.341A	T22.399S	T22.742D	T23.302A
L89.010	T20.319S	T20.72XD	T21.35XA	T21.77XS	T22.341D	T22.70XA	T22.742S	T23.302D
L89.020	T20.32XA	T20.72XS	T21.35XD	T21.79XA	T22.341S	T22.70XD	T22.749A	T23.302S
L89.100	T20.32XD	T20.73XA	T21.35XS	T21.79XD	T22.342A	T22.70XS	T22.749D	T23.309A
L89.110	T20.32XS	T20.73XD	T21.36XA	T21.79XS	T22.342D	T22.711A	T22.749S	T23.309D
L89.120	T20.33XA	T20.73XS	T21.36XD	T22.30XA	T22.342S	T22.711D	T22.751A	T23.309S
L89.130	T20.33XD	T20.74XA	T21.36XS	T22.30XD	T22.349A	T22.711S	T22.751D	T23.311A
L89.140	T20.33XS	T20.74XD	T21.37XA	T22.30XS	T22.349D	T22.712A	T22.751S	T23.311D
L89.150	T20.34XA	T20.74XS	T21.37XD	T22.311A	T22.349S	T22.712D	T22.752A	T23.311S
L89.200	T20.34XD	T20.75XA	T21.37XS	T22.311D	T22.351A	T22.712S	T22.752D	T23.312A
L89.210	T20.34XS	T20.75XD	T21.39XA	T22.311S	T22.351D	T22.719A	T22.752S	T23.312D
L89.220	T20.35XA	T20.75XS	T21.39XD	T22.312A	T22.351S	T22.719D	T22.759A	T23.312S
L89.300	T20.35XD	T20.76XA	T21.39XS	T22.312D	T22.352A	T22.719S	T22.759D	T23.319A
L89.310	T20.35XS	T20.76XD	T21.70XA	T22.312S	T22.352D	T22.721A	T22.759S	T23.319D
L89.320	T20.36XA	T20.76XS	T21.70XD	T22.319A	T22.352S	T22.721D	T22.761A	T23.319S
L89.45	T20.36XD	T20.77XA	T21.70XS	T22.319D	T22.359A	T22.721S	T22.761D	T23.321A
L89.500	T20.36XS	T20.77XD	T21.71XA	T22.319S	T22.359D	T22.722A	T22.761S	T23.321D
L89.510	T20.37XA	T20.77XS	T21.71XD	T22.321A	T22.359S	T22.722D	T22.762A	T23.321S
L89.520	T20.37XD	T20.79XA	T21.71XS	T22.321D	T22.361A	T22.722S	T22.762D	T23.322A
L89.600	T20.37XS	T20.79XD	T21.72XA	T22.321S	T22.361D	T22.729A	T22.762S	T23.322D
L89.610	T20.39XA	T20.79XS	T21.72XD	T22.322A	T22.361S	T22.729D	T22.769A	T23.322S
L89.620	T20.39XD	T21.30XA	T21.72XS	T22.322D	T22.362A	T22.729S	T22.769D	T23.329A
L89.810	T20.39XS	T21.30XD	T21.73XA	T22.322S	T22.362D	T22.731A	T22.769S	T23.329D
L89.890	T20.70XA	T21.30XS	T21.73XD	T22.329A	T22.362S	T22.731D	T22.791A	T23.329S
L89.95	T20.70XD	T21.31XA	T21.73XS	T22.329D	T22.369A	T22.731S	T22.791D	T23.331A
T20.30XA	T20.70XS	T21.31XD	T21.74XA	T22.329S	T22.369D	T22.732A	T22.791S	T23.331D
T20.30XD	T20.711A	T21.31XS	T21.74XD	T22.331A	T22.369S	T22.732D	T22.792A	T23.331S
T20.30XS	T20.711D	T21.32XA	T21.74XS	T22.331D	T22.391A	T22.732S	T22.792D	T23.332A
T20.311A	T20.711S	T21.32XD	T21.75XA	T22.331S	T22.391D	T22.739A	T22.792S	T23.332D
T20.311D	T20.712A	T21.32XS	T21.75XD	T22.332A	T22.391S	T22.739D	T22.799A	T23.332S
T20.311S	T20.712D	T21.33XA	T21.75XS	T22.332D	T22.392A	T22.739S	T22.799D	T23.339A
T20.312A	T20.712S	T21.33XD	T21.76XA	T22.332S	T22.392D	T22.741A	T22.799S	T23.339D
T20.312D	T20.719A	T21.33XS	T21.76XD	T22.339A	T22.392S	T22.741D	T23.301A	T23.339S
T20.312S	T20.719D	T21.34XA	T21.76XS	T22.339D	T22.399A	T22.741S	T23.301D	T23.341A
T20.319A	T20.719S	T21.34XD	T21.77XA	T22.339S	T22.399D	T22.742A	T23.301S	T23.341D

Appendix K: Severe Wound Diagnosis Codes by Category

Unstageable Wound (continued)

T23.341S	T23.379D	T23.722A	T23.759S	T24.302D	T24.391A	T24.729A	T25.321S	T25.719D
T23.342A	T23.379S	T23.722D	T23.761A	T24.302S	T24.391D	T24.729D	T25.322A	T25.719S
T23.342D	T23.391A	T23.722S	T23.761D	T24.309A	T24.391S	T24.729S	T25.322D	T25.721A
T23.342S	T23.391D	T23.729A	T23.761S	T24.309D	T24.392A	T24.731A	T25.322S	T25.721D
T23.349A	T23.391S	T23.729D	T23.762A	T24.309S	T24.392D	T24.731D	T25.329A	T25.721S
T23.349D	T23.392A	T23.729S	T23.762D	T24.311A	T24.392S	T24.731S	T25.329D	T25.722A
T23.349S	T23.392D	T23.731A	T23.762S	T24.311D	T24.399A	T24.732A	T25.329S	T25.722D
T23.351A	T23.392S	T23.731D	T23.769A	T24.311S	T24.399D	T24.732D	T25.331A	T25.722S
T23.351D	T23.399A	T23.731S	T23.769D	T24.312A	T24.701A	T24.732S	T25.331D	T25.729A
T23.351S	T23.399D	T23.732A	T23.769S	T24.312D	T24.701D	T24.739A	T25.331S	T25.729D
T23.352A	T23.399S	T23.732D	T23.771A	T24.312S	T24.701S	T24.739D	T25.332A	T25.729S
T23.352D	T23.701A	T23.732S	T23.771D	T24.319A	T24.702A	T24.739S	T25.332D	T25.731A
T23.352S	T23.701D	T23.739A	T23.771S	T24.319D	T24.702D	T24.791A	T25.332S	T25.731D
T23.359A	T23.701S	T23.739D	T23.772A	T24.319S	T24.702S	T24.791D	T25.339A	T25.731S
T23.359D	T23.702A	T23.739S	T23.772D	T24.321A	T24.709A	T24.791S	T25.339D	T25.732A
T23.359S	T23.702D	T23.741A	T23.772S	T24.321D	T24.709D	T24.792A	T25.339S	T25.732D
T23.361A	T23.702S	T23.741D	T23.779A	T24.321S	T24.709S	T24.792D	T25.391A	T25.732S
T23.361D	T23.709A	T23.741S	T23.779D	T24.322A	T24.711A	T24.792S	T25.391D	T25.739A
T23.361S	T23.709D	T23.742A	T23.779S	T24.322D	T24.711D	T24.799A	T25.391S	T25.739D
T23.362A	T23.709S	T23.742D	T23.791A	T24.322S	T24.711S	T24.799D	T25.392A	T25.739S
T23.362D	T23.711A	T23.742S	T23.791D	T24.329A	T24.712A	T24.799S	T25.392D	T25.791A
T23.362S	T23.711D	T23.749A	T23.791S	T24.329D	T24.712D	T25.311A	T25.392S	T25.791D
T23.369A	T23.711S	T23.749D	T23.792A	T24.329S	T24.712S	T25.311D	T25.399A	T25.791S
T23.369D	T23.712A	T23.749S	T23.792D	T24.331A	T24.719A	T25.311S	T25.399D	T25.792A
T23.369S	T23.712D	T23.751A	T23.792S	T24.331D	T24.719D	T25.312A	T25.399S	T25.792D
T23.371A	T23.712S	T23.751D	T23.799A	T24.331S	T24.719S	T25.312D	T25.711A	T25.792S
T23.371D	T23.719A	T23.751S	T23.799D	T24.332A	T24.721A	T25.312S	T25.711D	T25.799A
T23.371S	T23.719D	T23.752A	T23.799S	T24.332D	T24.721D	T25.319A	T25.711S	T25.799D
T23.372A	T23.719S	T23.752D	T24.301A	T24.332S	T24.721S	T25.319D	T25.712A	T25.799S
T23.372D	T23.721A	T23.752S	T24.301D	T24.339A	T24.722A	T25.319S	T25.712D	
T23.372S	T23.721D	T23.759A	T24.301S	T24.339D	T24.722D	T25.321A	T25.712S	
T23.379A	T23.721S	T23.759D	T24.302A	T24.339S	T24.722S	T25.321D	T25.719A	

Non-Healing Surgical Wound

L97.102	L97.214	L97.313	L97.412	L97.504	L97.803	L97.902	L98.424	T81.32XA
L97.103	L97.222	L97.314	L97.413	L97.512	L97.804	L97.903	L98.492	T81.32XD
L97.104	L97.223	L97.322	L97.414	L97.513	L97.812	L97.904	L98.493	T81.89XA
L97.202	L97.224	L97.323	L97.422	L97.514	L97.813	L98.412	L98.494	T81.89XD
L97.203	L97.302	L97.324	L97.423	L97.522	L97.814	L98.413	T81.30XA	
L97.204	L97.303	L97.402	L97.424	L97.523	L97.822	L98.414	T81.30XD	
L97.212	L97.304	L97.403	L97.502	L97.524	L97.823	L98.422	T81.31XA	
L97.213	L97.312	L97.404	L97.503	L97.802	L97.824	L98.423	T81.31XD	

Fistula* (which includes osteomyelitis)

H04.611	H83.12	K50.113	K51.813	L05.92	M25.131	M25.159	M25.175	Q18.1
H04.612	H83.13	K50.813	K51.913	M25.10	M25.132	M25.161	M25.176	T81.83XA
H04.613	H83.19	K50.913	K60.3	M25.111	M25.139	M25.162	M25.18	T81.83XD
H04.619	J86.0	K51.013	K60.4	M25.112	M25.141	M25.169	N82.0	T81.83XS
H70.811	K04.6	K51.213	K60.5	M25.119	M25.142	M25.171	N82.2	
H70.812	K11.4	K51.313	K63.2	M25.121	M25.149	M25.172	N82.3	
H70.813	K31.6	K51.413	L05.01	M25.122	M25.151	M25.173	N82.4	
H70.819	K50.013	K51.513	L05.02	M25.129	M25.152	M25.174	N82.5	

Illustrations

Chapter 3. Diseases of the Blood and Blood-forming Organs and Certain Disorders Involving the Immune Mechanism (D50–D89)

Red Blood Cells

White Blood Cell

Platelet

Coagulation

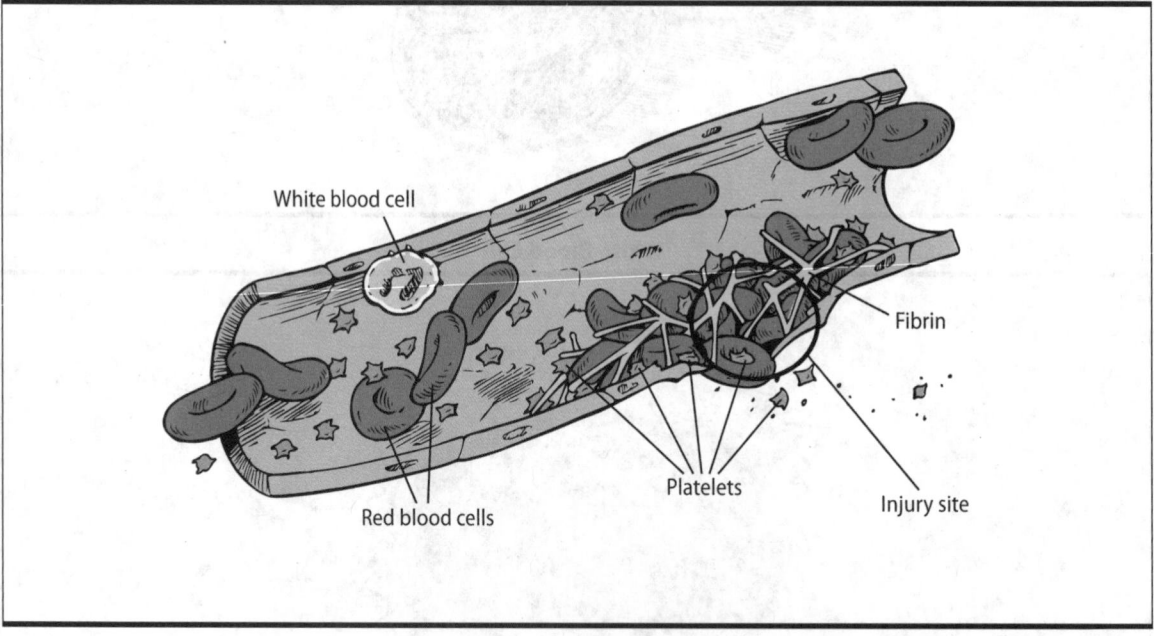

Spleen Anatomical Location and External Structures

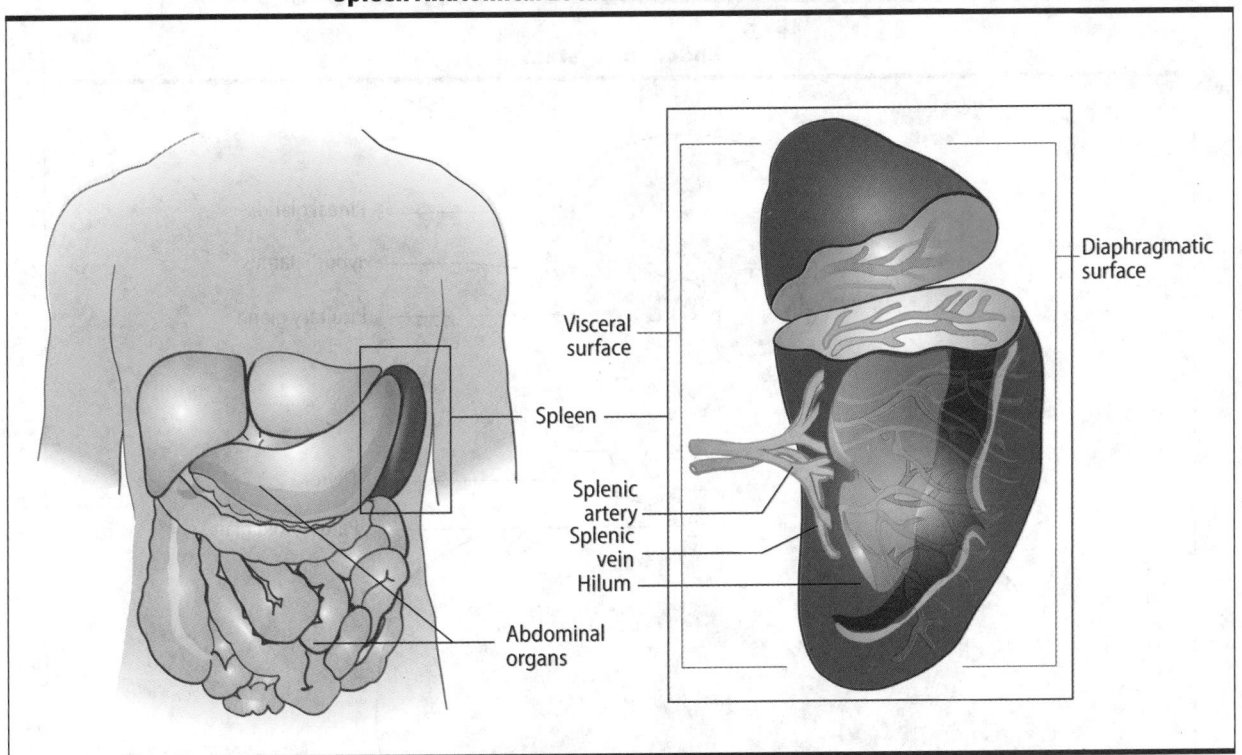

Visceral surface

Spleen

Splenic artery

Splenic vein

Hilum

Abdominal organs

Diaphragmatic surface

Spleen Interior Structures

Capsule

Trabecula

Vascular sinusoid

White pulp

Red pulp

Splenic artery

Splenic vein

Chapter 4. Endocrine, Nutritional and Metabolic Diseases (E00–E89)

Endocrine System

Thyroid

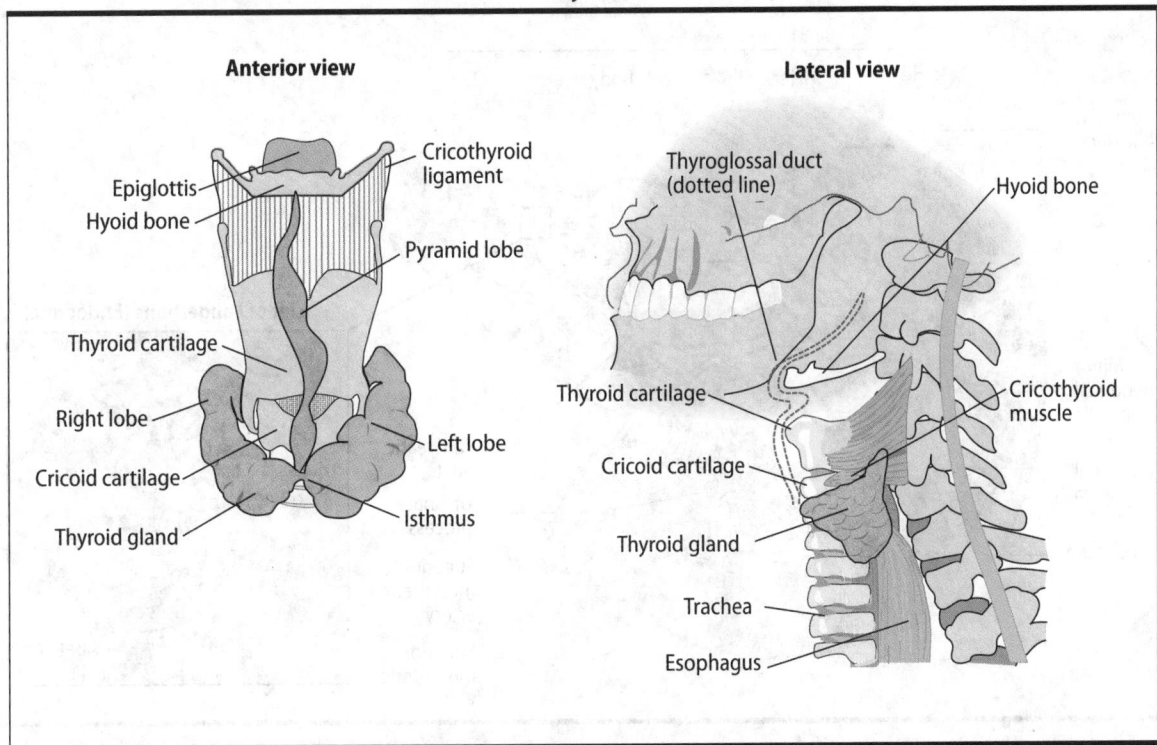

Thyroid and Parathyroid Glands

Pancreas

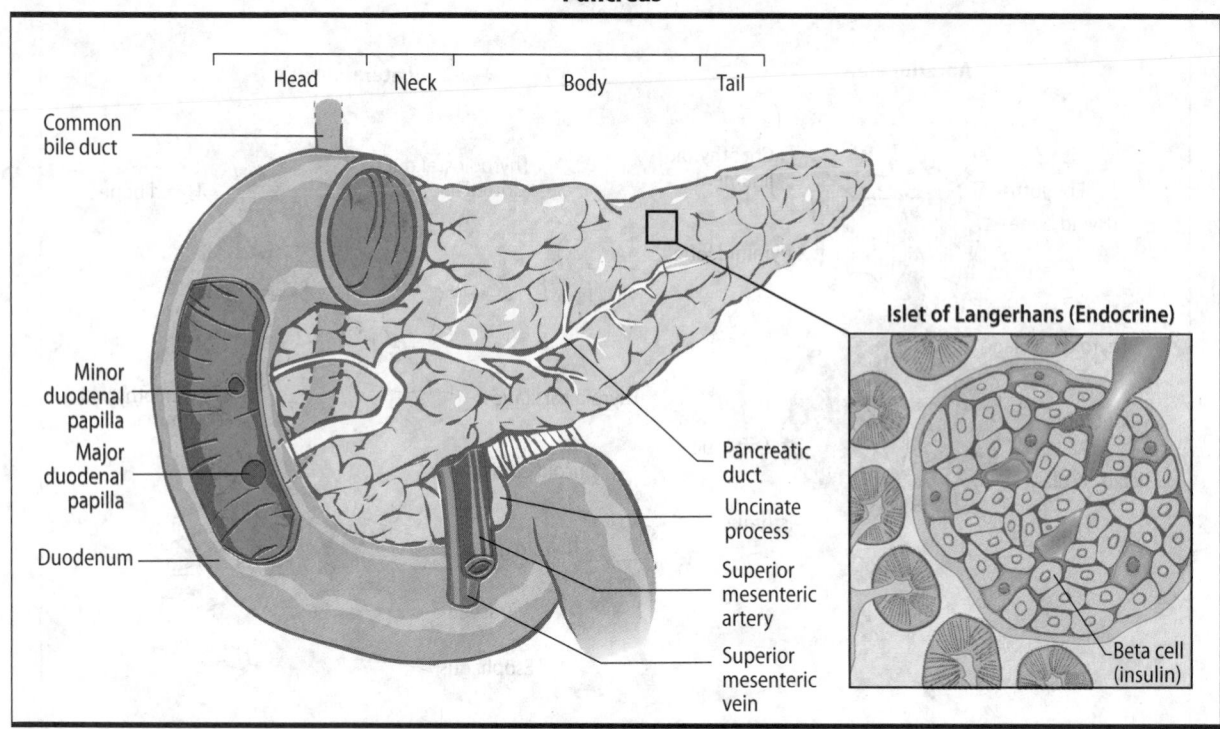

Islet of Langerhans (Endocrine)

Beta cell (insulin)

Head   Neck   Body   Tail

Common bile duct

Minor duodenal papilla

Major duodenal papilla

Duodenum

Pancreatic duct

Uncinate process

Superior mesenteric artery

Superior mesenteric vein

Anatomy of the Adrenal Gland

Adrenal glands

Kidney

Capsule

Cortex

Medulla

Structure of an Ovary

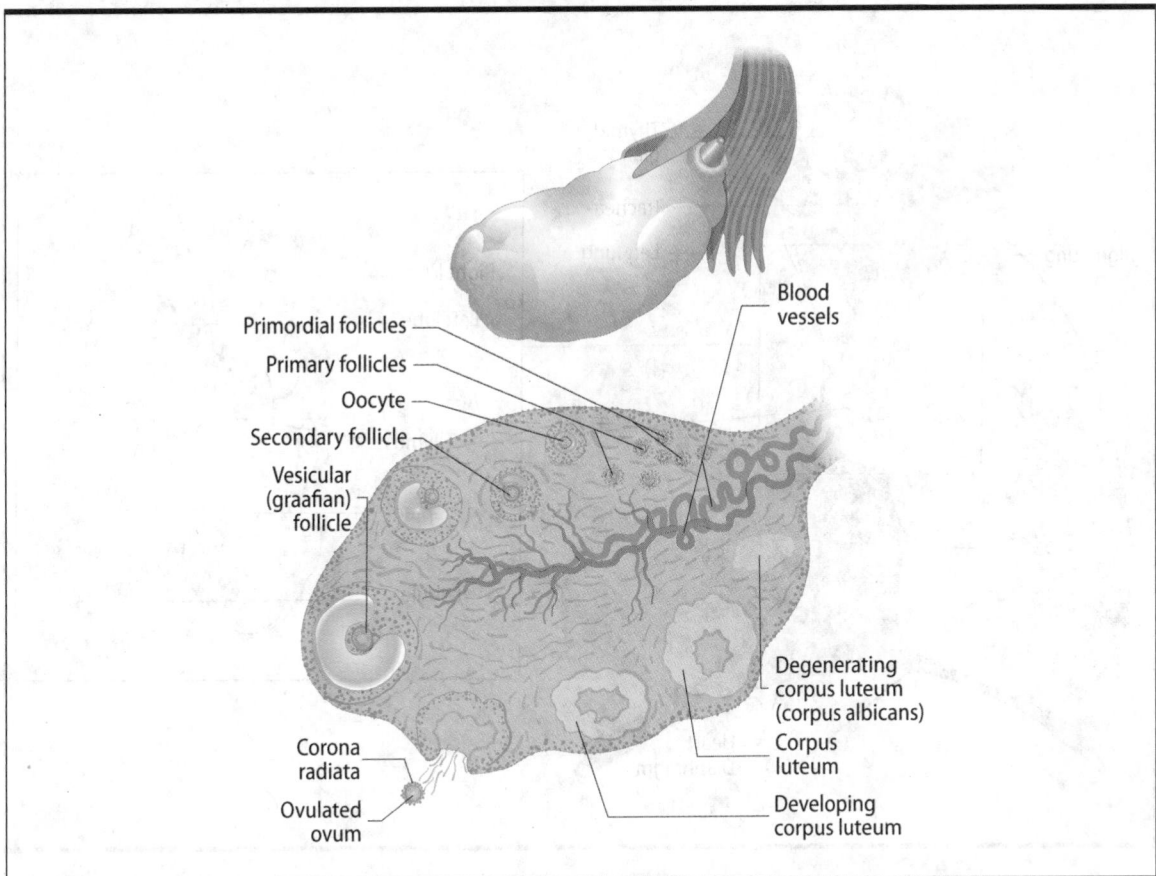

Testis and Associated Structures

Thymus

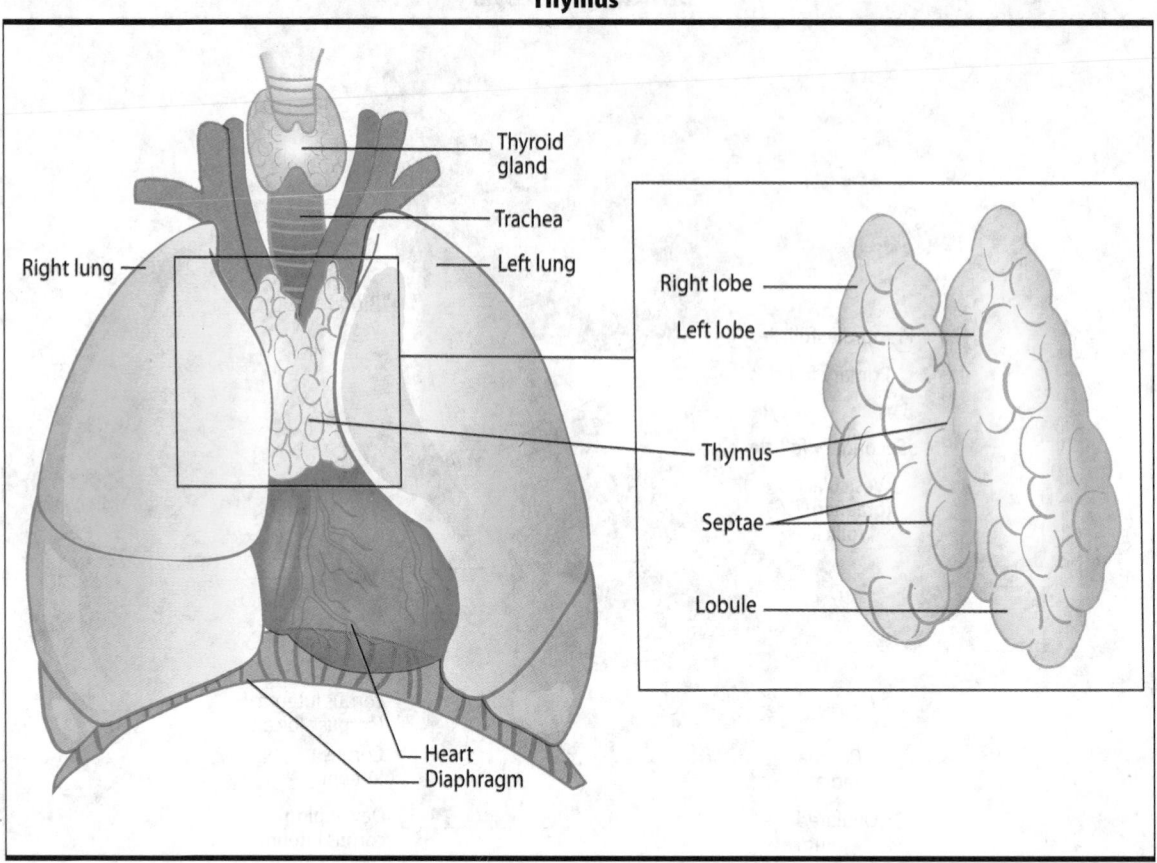

Chapter 6. Diseases of the Nervous System (GØØ–G99)

Brain

Cranial Nerves

Peripheral Nervous System

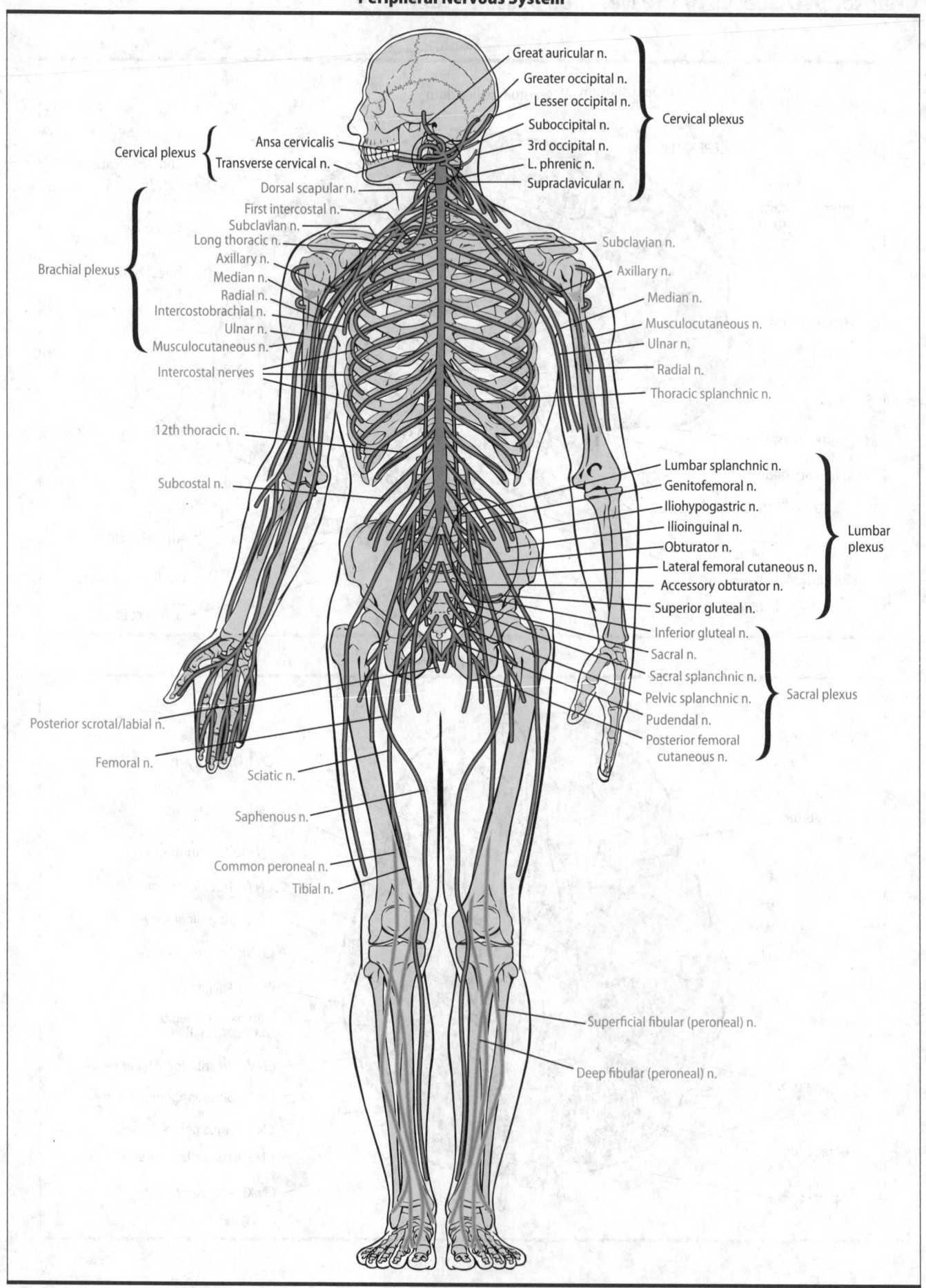

Spinal Cord and Spinal Nerves

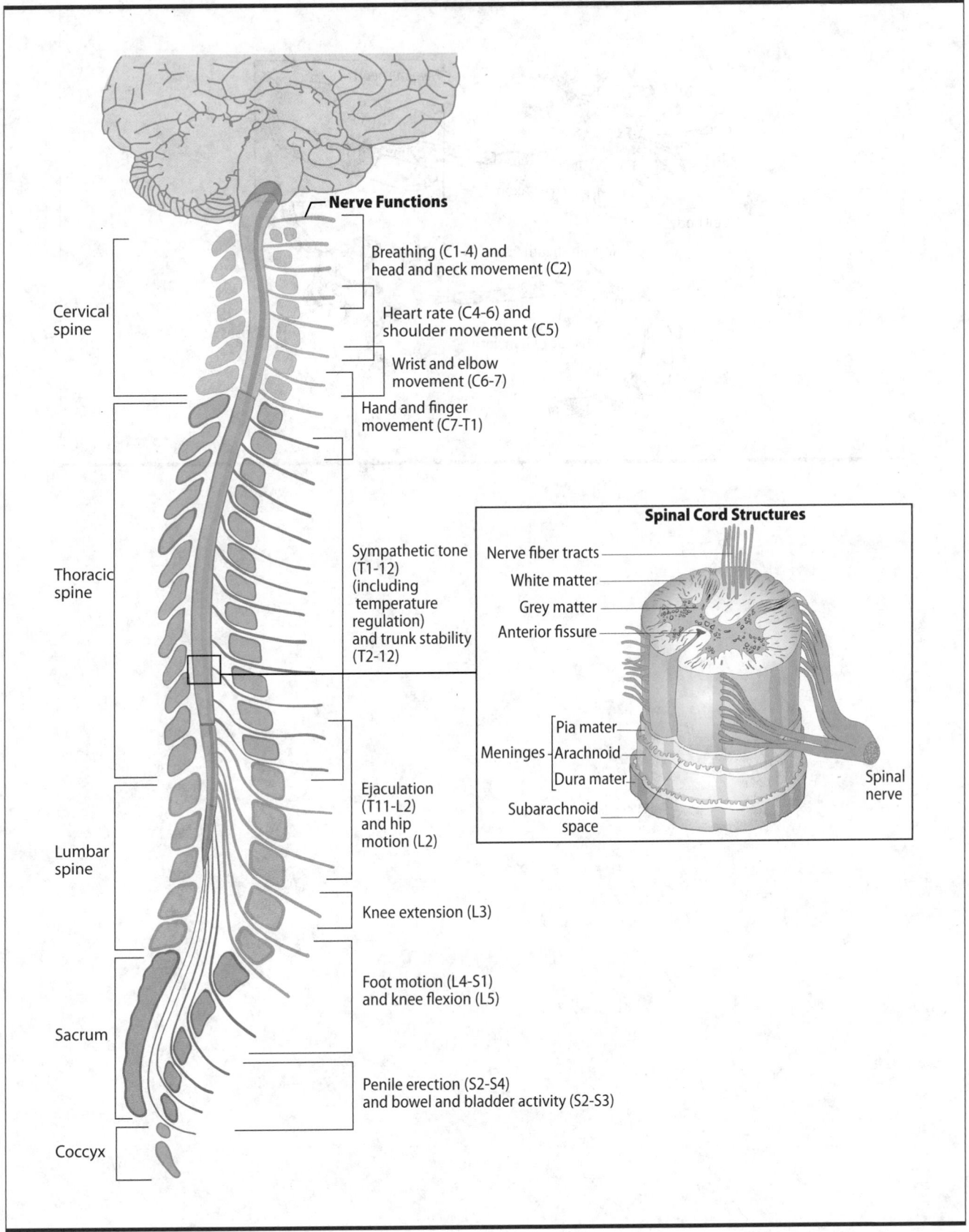

Nerve Functions

Breathing (C1-4) and head and neck movement (C2)

Heart rate (C4-6) and shoulder movement (C5)

Wrist and elbow movement (C6-7)

Hand and finger movement (C7-T1)

Cervical spine

Thoracic spine

Sympathetic tone (T1-12) (including temperature regulation) and trunk stability (T2-12)

Ejaculation (T11-L2) and hip motion (L2)

Lumbar spine

Knee extension (L3)

Foot motion (L4-S1) and knee flexion (L5)

Sacrum

Penile erection (S2-S4) and bowel and bladder activity (S2-S3)

Coccyx

Spinal Cord Structures

Nerve fiber tracts
White matter
Grey matter
Anterior fissure

Meninges — Pia mater / Arachnoid / Dura mater

Subarachnoid space

Spinal nerve

Nerve Cell

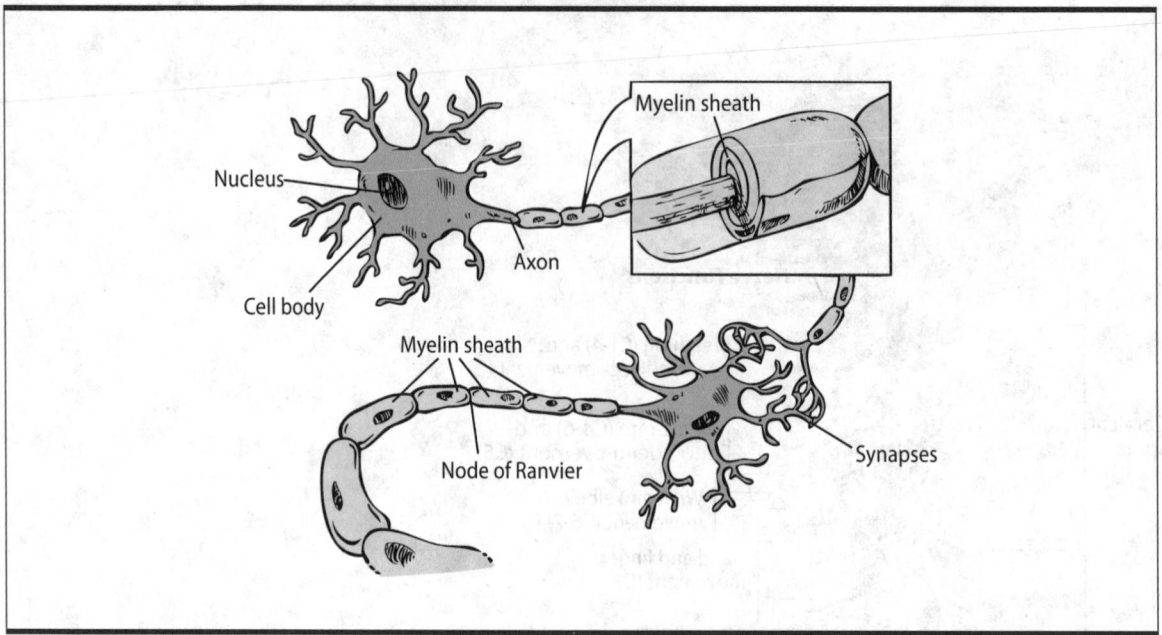

Chapter 7. Diseases of the Eye and Adnexa (HØØ–H59)

Eye

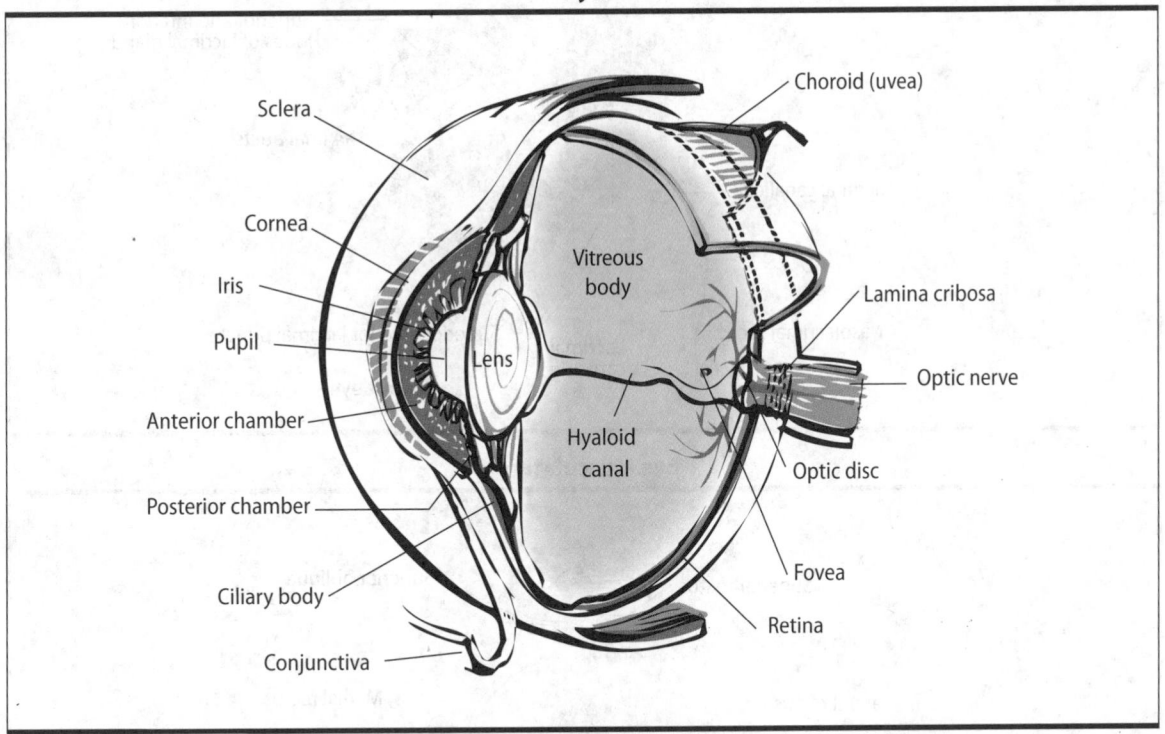

Posterior Pole of Globe/Flow of Aqueous Humor

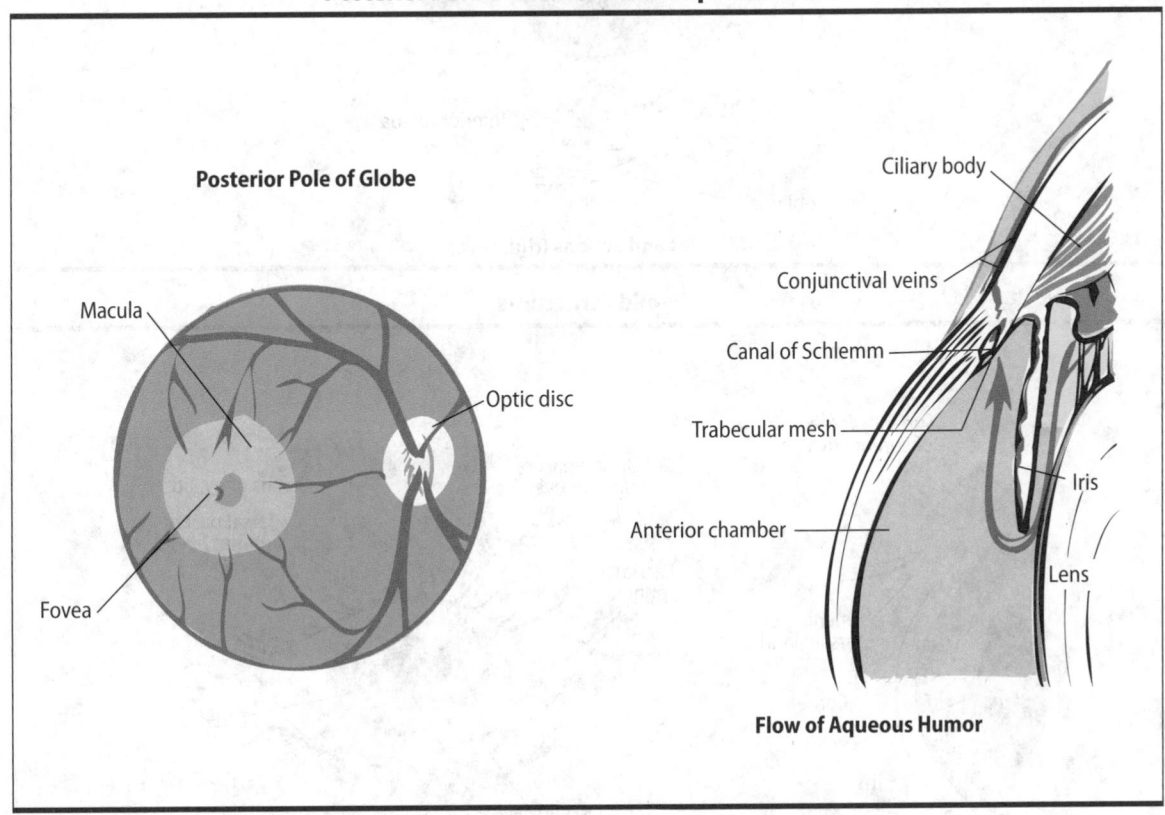

Posterior Pole of Globe

Flow of Aqueous Humor

Lacrimal System

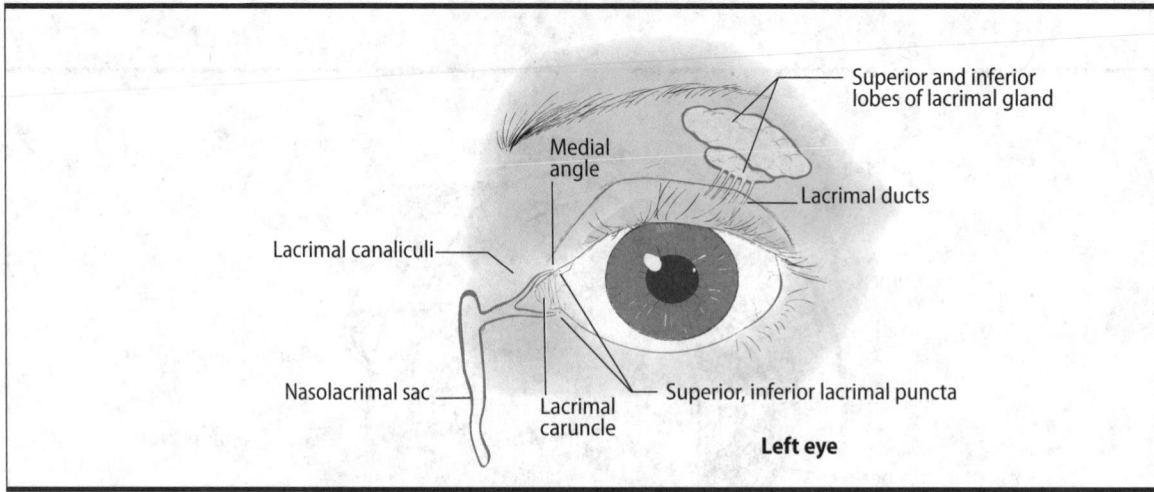

Superior and inferior lobes of lacrimal gland

Medial angle

Lacrimal ducts

Lacrimal canaliculi

Nasolacrimal sac

Lacrimal caruncle

Superior, inferior lacrimal puncta

Left eye

Eye Musculature

Superior rectus

Superior oblique

Lateral rectus

Medial rectus

Inferior rectus

Inferior oblique

Muscles and actions (right eye)

Eyelid Structures

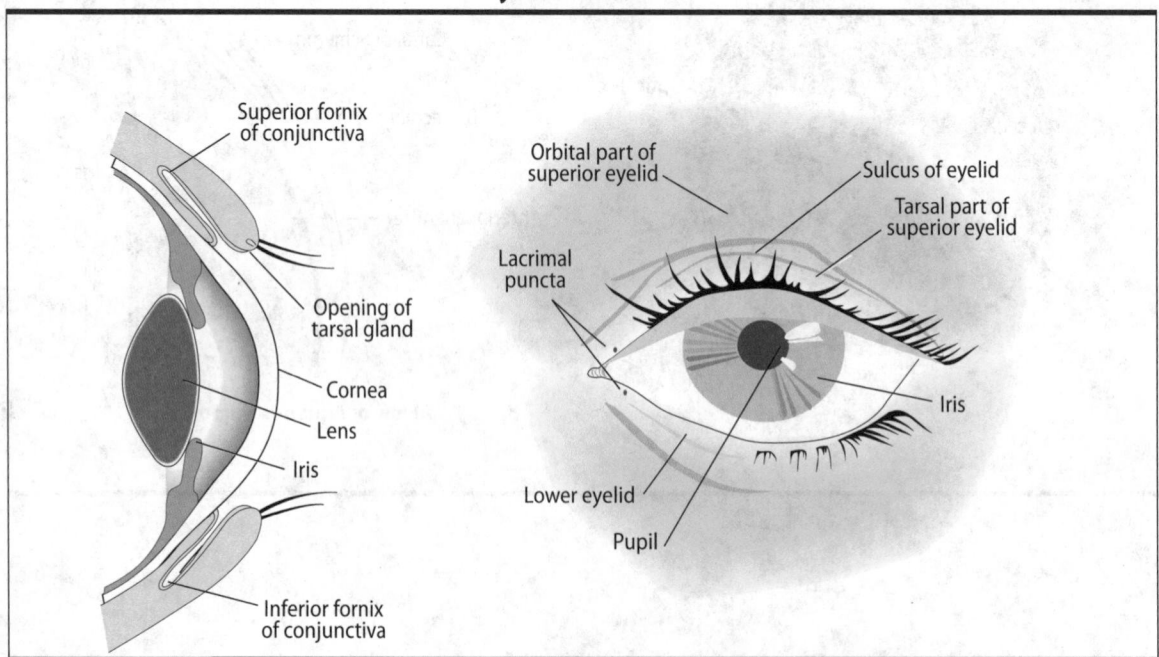

Superior fornix of conjunctiva

Opening of tarsal gland

Cornea

Lens

Iris

Inferior fornix of conjunctiva

Orbital part of superior eyelid

Sulcus of eyelid

Tarsal part of superior eyelid

Lacrimal puncta

Lower eyelid

Pupil

Iris

Chapter 8. Diseases of the Ear and Mastoid Process (H60–H95)

Ear Anatomy

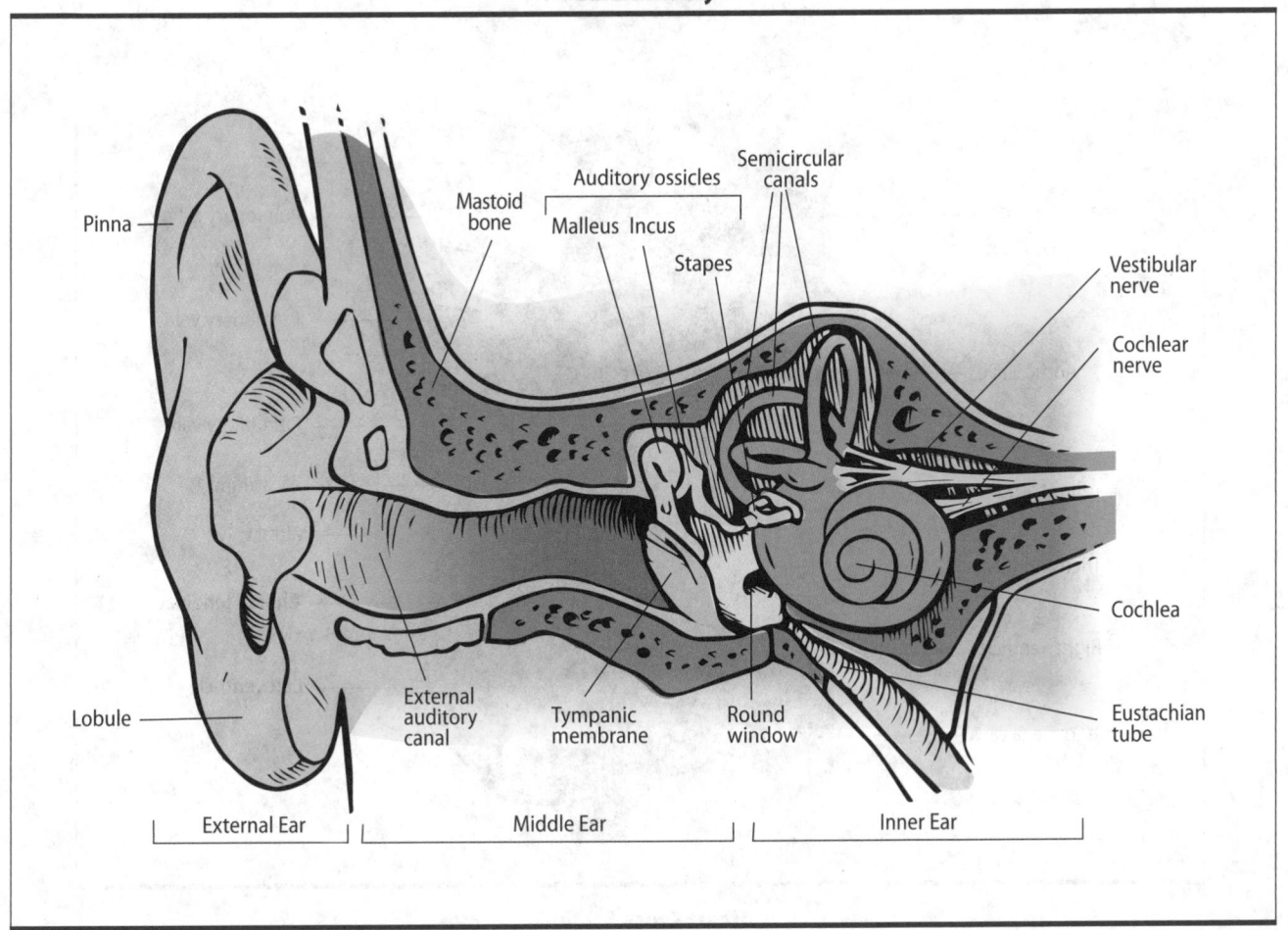

Chapter 9. Diseases of the Circulatory System (I00–I99)

Anatomy of the Heart

Heart Cross Section

Heart Valves

Schematic shows valves of the heart as blood is pumped out.
The septum is the wall dividing the left and right ventricles.
The papillary muscles and chordae tendineae (above right)
function to open and close the atrioventricular valves

Side view of a mitral valve leaflet

Overhead view of aortic (left)
and pulmonary valves while closed

Heart Conduction System

Coronary Arteries

Arteries

Veins

Superficial temporal v.

Vertebral v.

Internal jugular v.

External jugular v.

Subclavian v.

Innominate v.

Azygos v.

Axillary v.

Hemiazygos v.

Brachial v.

Cephalic v.

Basilic v.

Inferior vena cava

Esophageal v.

Common hepatic v.

L. gastric v.

Portal v.

R. gastric v.

Splenic v.

Renal v.

R. colic v.

Inferior mesenteric v.

Superior mesenteric v.

Radial v.

L. colic v.

Ulnar v.

Common iliac v.

Internal iliac v. (Hypogastric v.)

External iliac v.

Internal pudendal v.

Rectal venous plexus

Femoral v.

Greater saphenous v.

Popliteal v.

Lesser saphenous v.

Anterior tibial v.

Lesser saphenous v.

Posterior tibial v.

Greater saphenous v.

Internal Carotid and Vertebral Arteries and Branches

Side View

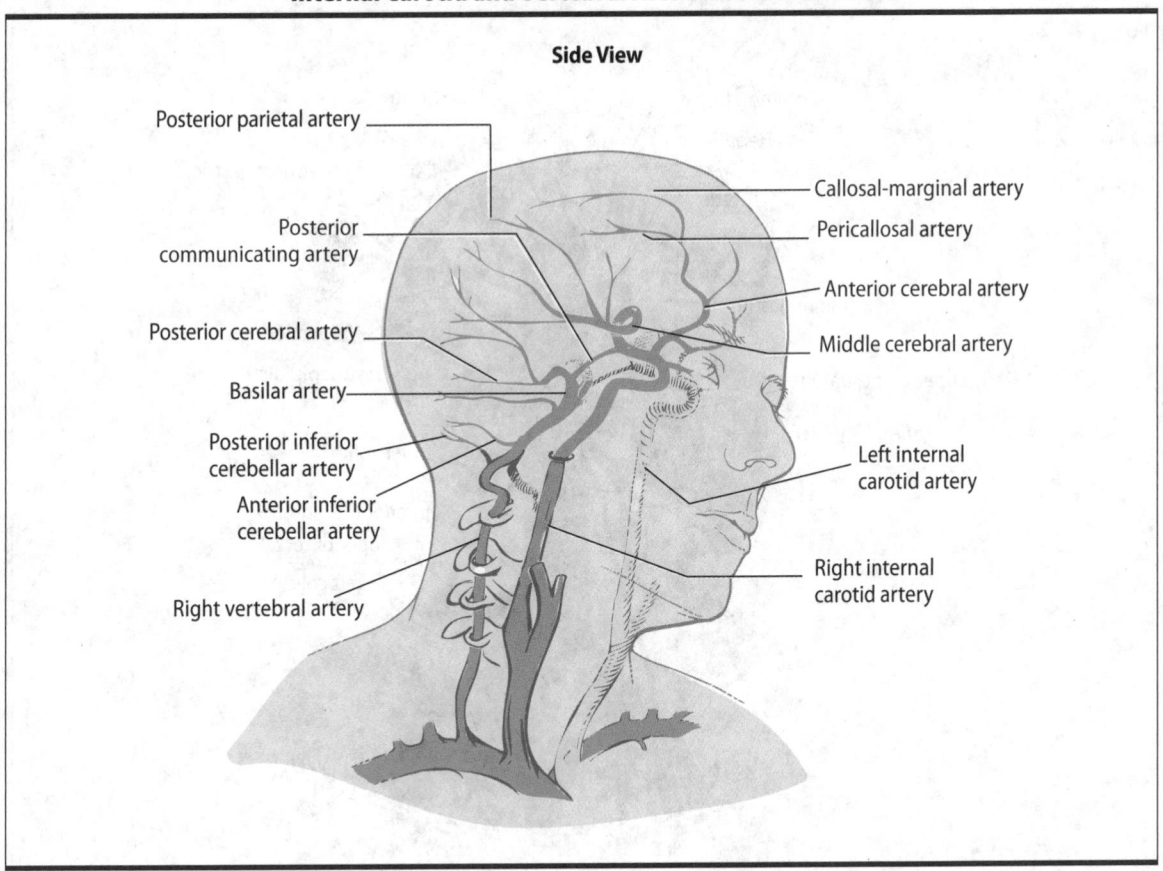

External Carotid Artery and Branches

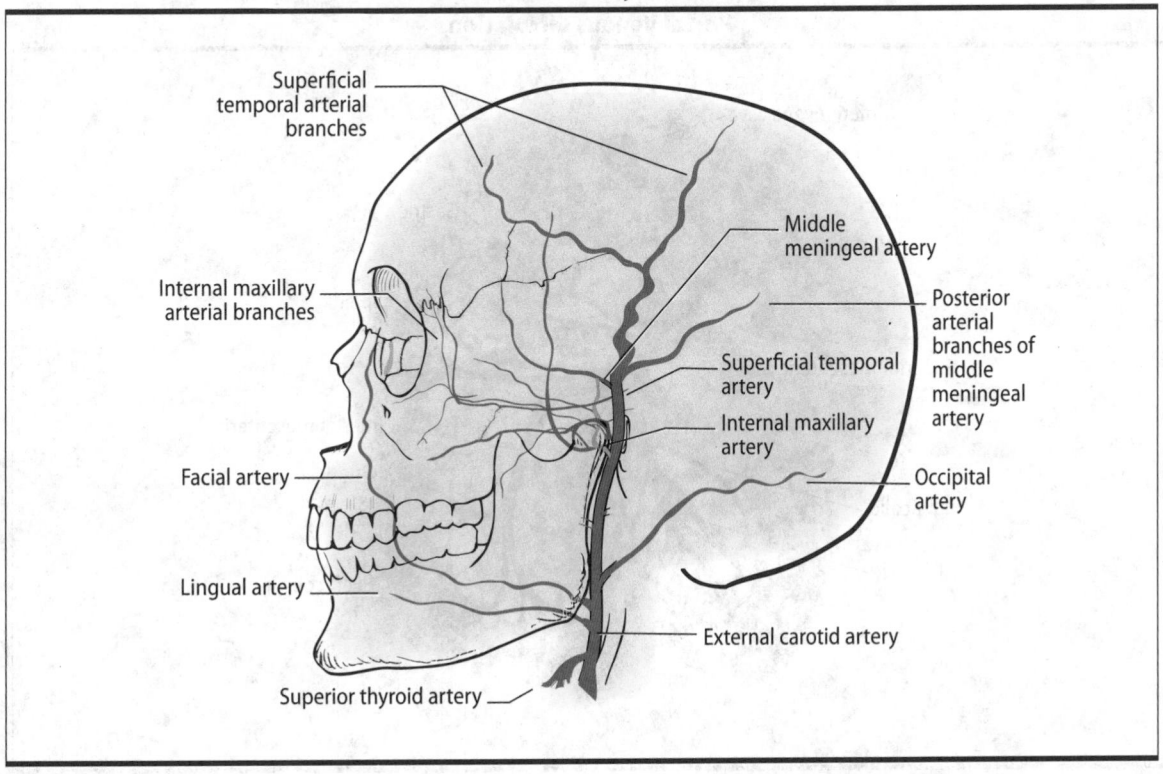

Branches of Abdominal Aorta

Portal Venous Circulation

Lymphatic System

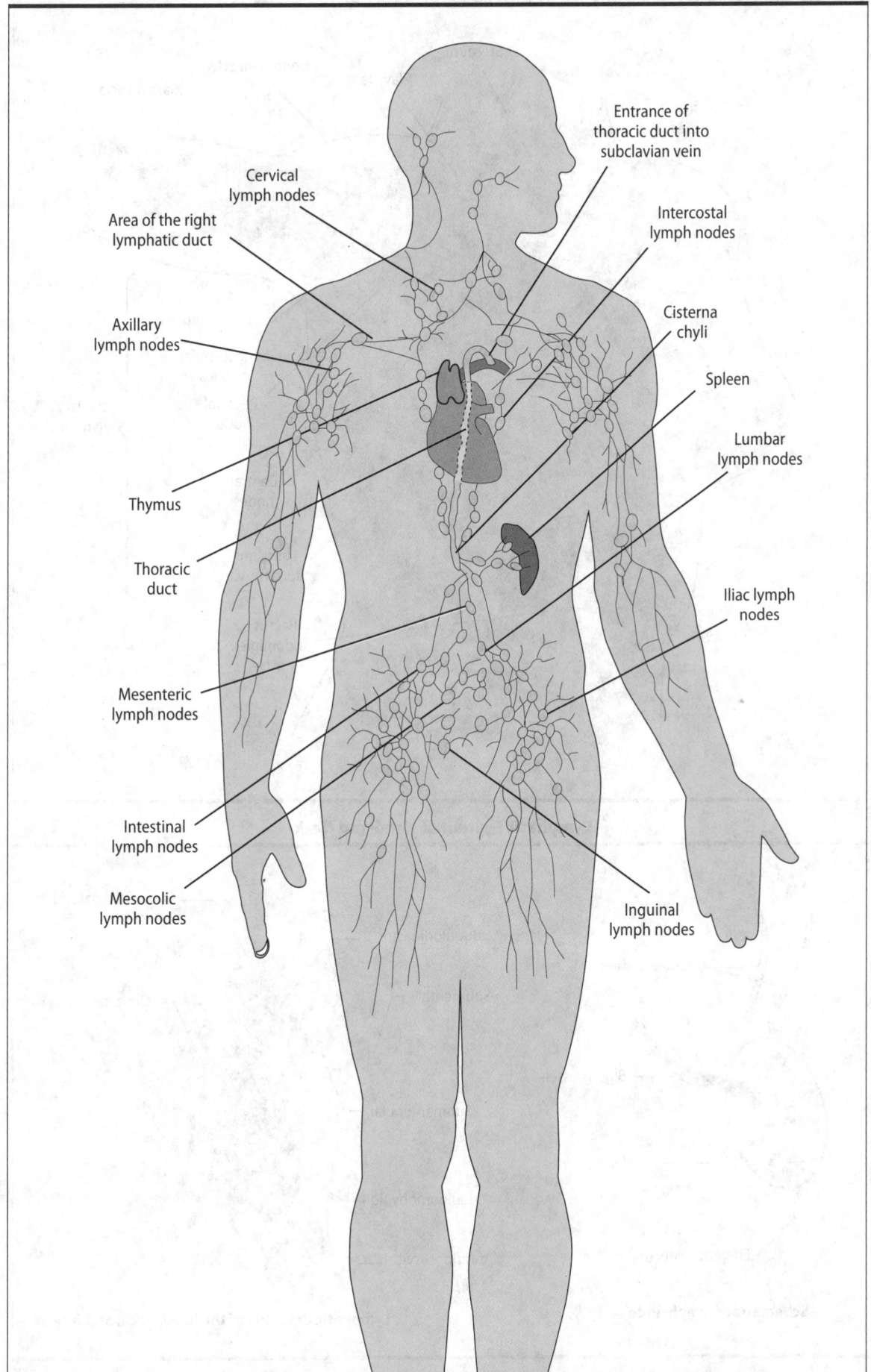

Axillary Lymph Nodes

Parasternal nodes

Sternum

Clavicle

Deltoid muscle

Brachialis muscle

Lateral nodes

Subscapular nodes

Pectoral nodes

Axillary lymph nodes

Central nodes

Latissimus dorsi muscle

Rectus abdominis muscle

Lymphatic System of Head and Neck

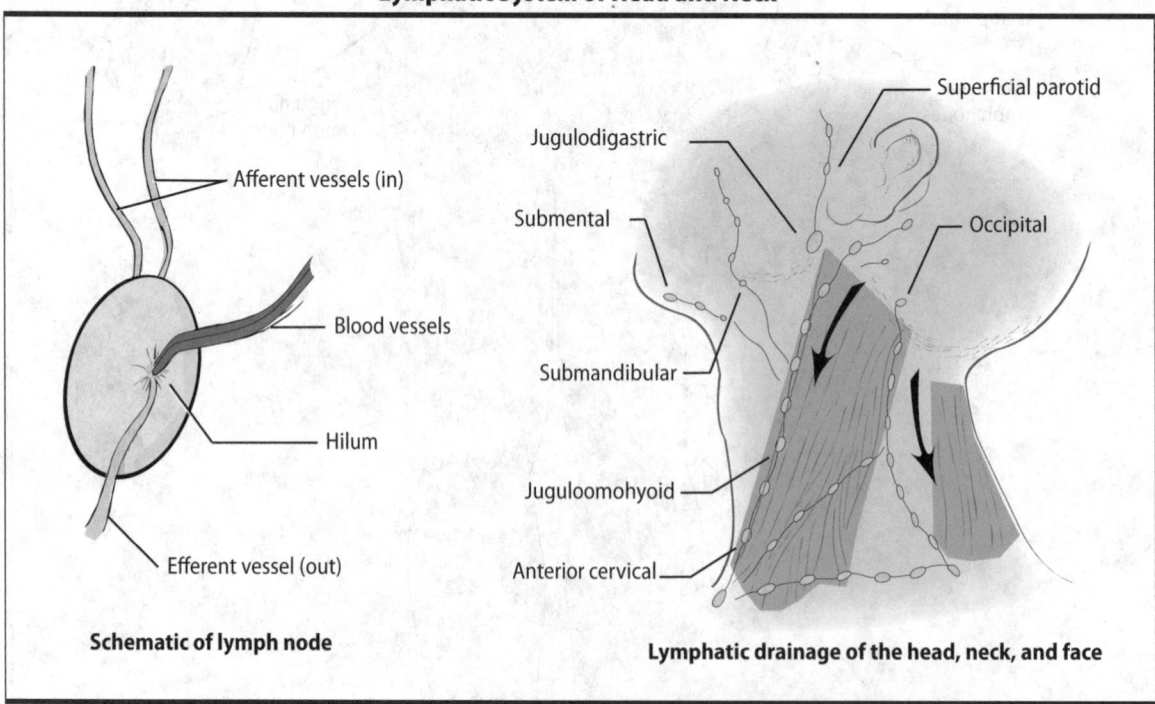

Afferent vessels (in)

Blood vessels

Hilum

Efferent vessel (out)

Schematic of lymph node

Jugulodigastric

Submental

Superficial parotid

Occipital

Submandibular

Juguloomohyoid

Anterior cervical

Lymphatic drainage of the head, neck, and face

Lymphatic Capillaries

Schematic of lymphatic capillaries

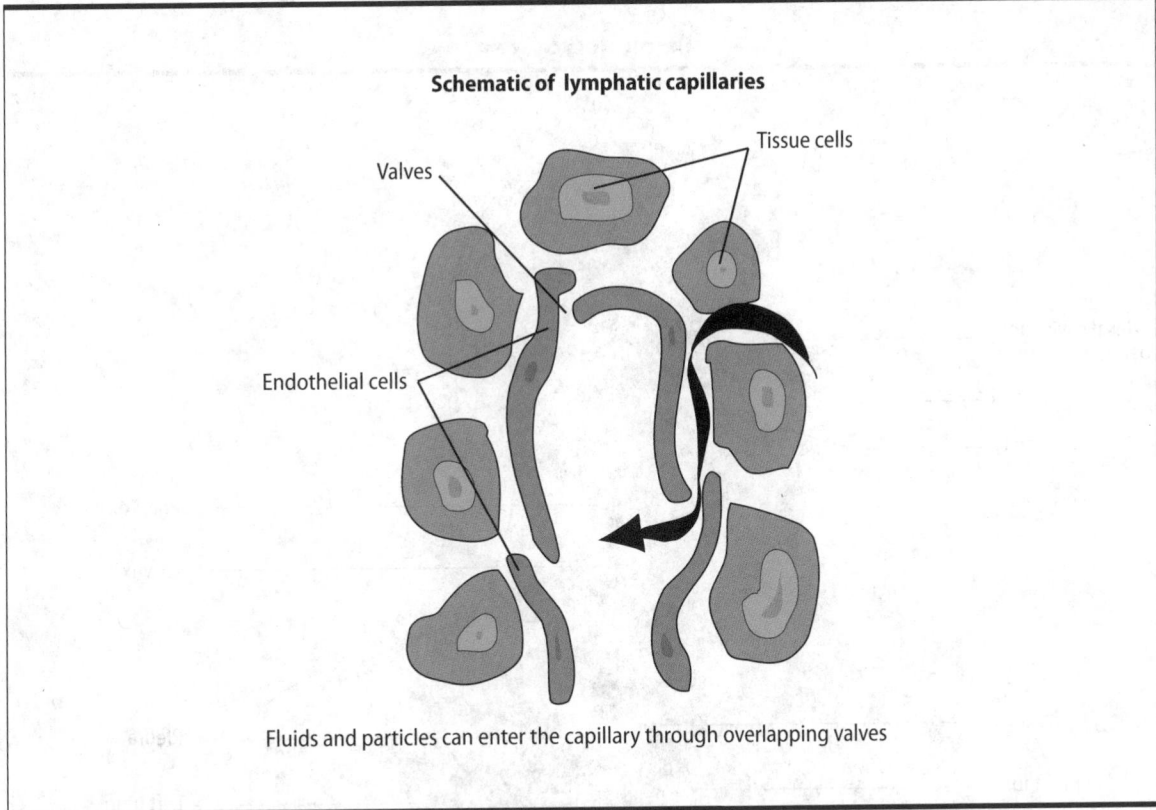

Tissue cells

Valves

Endothelial cells

Fluids and particles can enter the capillary through overlapping valves

Lymphatic Drainage

Lymphatic drainage of the colon follows blood supply

Middle colic nodes

Paracolic nodes

Left colic nodes

Ascending colon

Cecum

Rectum

Chapter 10. Diseases of the Respiratory System (J00–J99)

Respiratory System

Nasal cavity and paranasal sinuses

Nostril

Oral cavity

Pharynx

Larynx

Trachea

Pleura

Right lung

Left lung

Carina of trachea

Right main / primary bronchus

Left main/ primary bronchus

Secondary (lobar) bronchi

Tertiary (segmental) bronchi

Bronchioles

Alveoli

Diaphragm

Upper Respiratory System

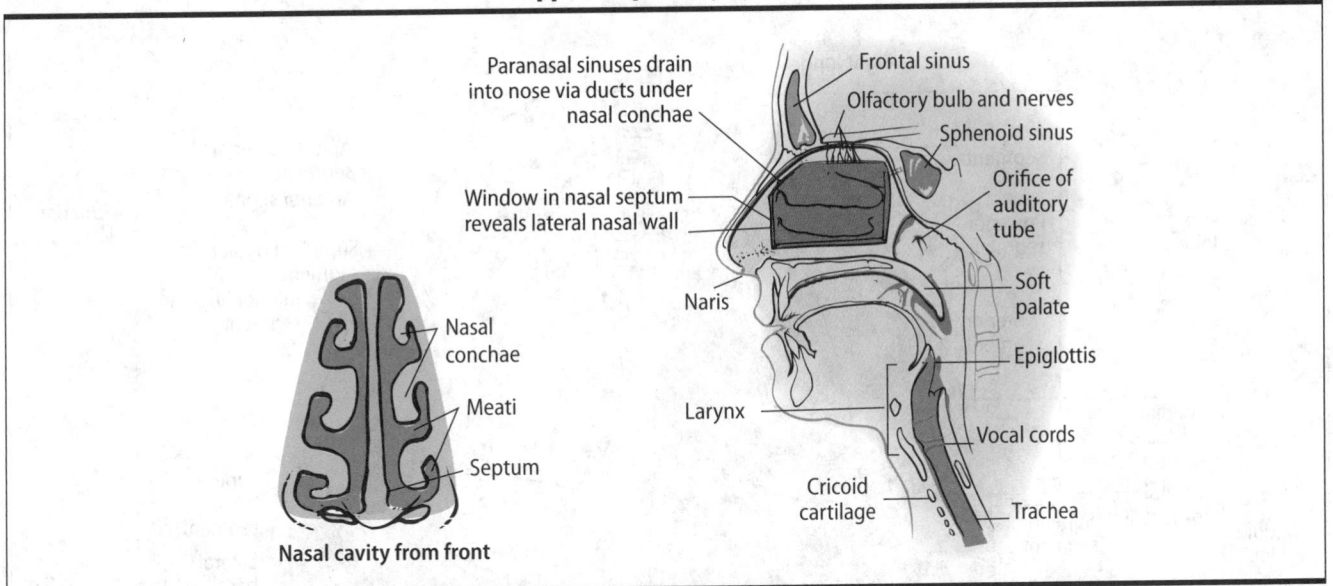

Paranasal sinuses drain into nose via ducts under nasal conchae

Window in nasal septum reveals lateral nasal wall

Naris

Larynx

Cricoid cartilage

Frontal sinus

Olfactory bulb and nerves

Sphenoid sinus

Orifice of auditory tube

Soft palate

Epiglottis

Vocal cords

Trachea

Nasal conchae

Meati

Septum

Nasal cavity from front

Lower Respiratory System

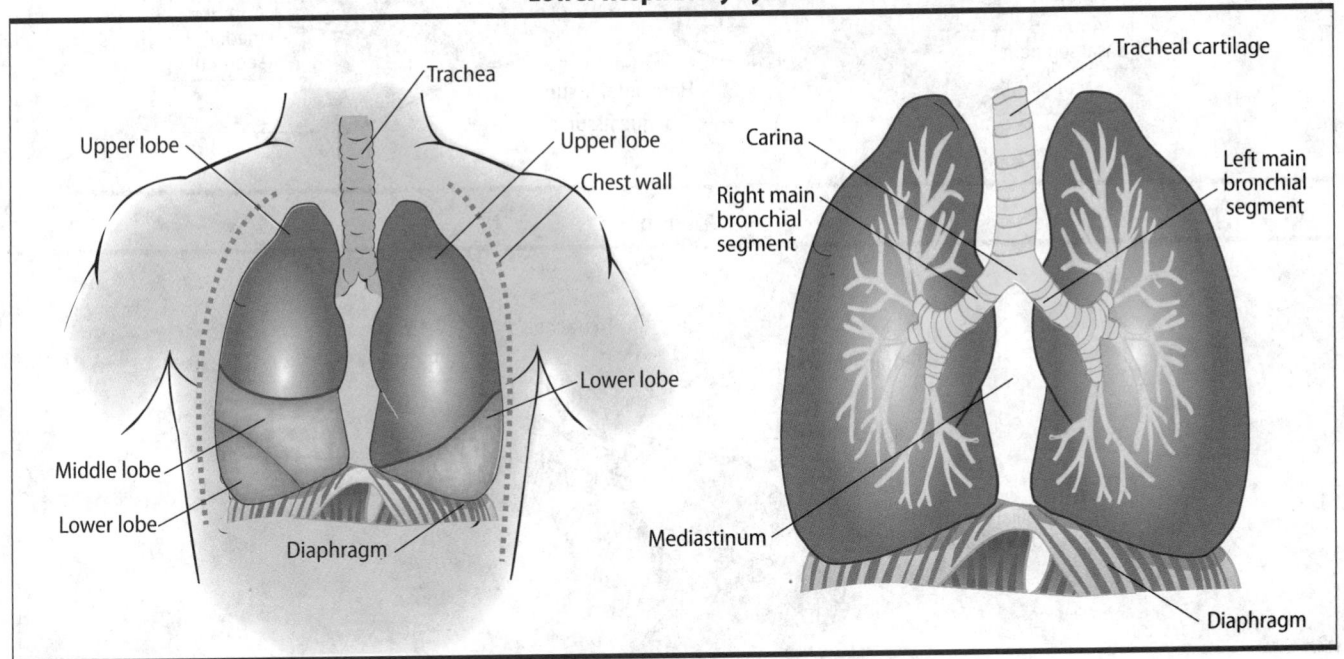

Upper lobe

Trachea

Upper lobe

Chest wall

Lower lobe

Middle lobe

Lower lobe

Diaphragm

Tracheal cartilage

Carina

Right main bronchial segment

Left main bronchial segment

Mediastinum

Diaphragm

Paranasal Sinuses

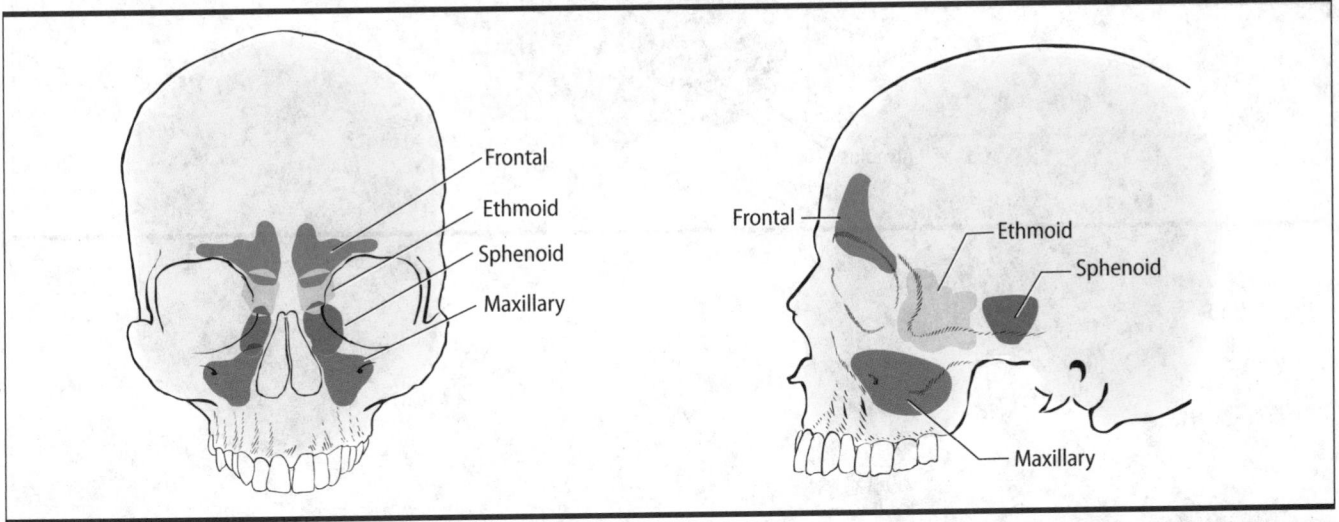

Frontal

Ethmoid

Sphenoid

Maxillary

Frontal

Ethmoid

Sphenoid

Maxillary

Lung Segments

Right lung

Left lung

Apical segment

Apical-posterior segment

Anterior segment

Superior lobe

Superior lobe

Posterior segment

Superior lingular segment

Inferior lingular segment

Anterior segment

Medial basal segment

Lateral segment

Superior basal segment

Middle lobe

Superior segment

Lateral basal segment

Inferior lobe

Posterior basal segment

Inferior lobe

Anterior basal segment

Anterior medial segment

Horizontal fissure

Oblique fissures

Alveoli

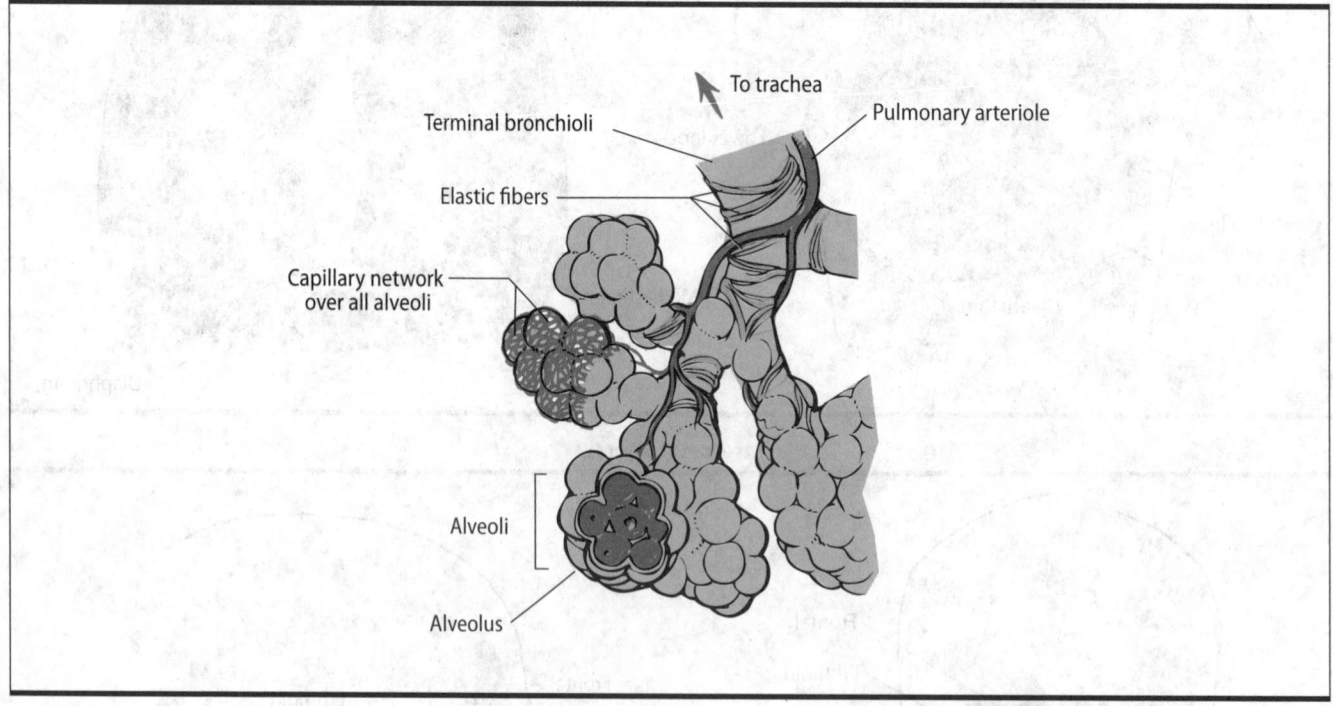

To trachea

Terminal bronchioli

Pulmonary arteriole

Elastic fibers

Capillary network over all alveoli

Alveoli

Alveolus

Chapter 11. Diseases of the Digestive System (KØØ–K95)

Digestive System

Omentum and Mesentery

Peritoneum and Retroperitoneum

Chapter 12. Diseases of the Skin and Subcutaneous Tissue (LØØ–L99)

Nail Anatomy

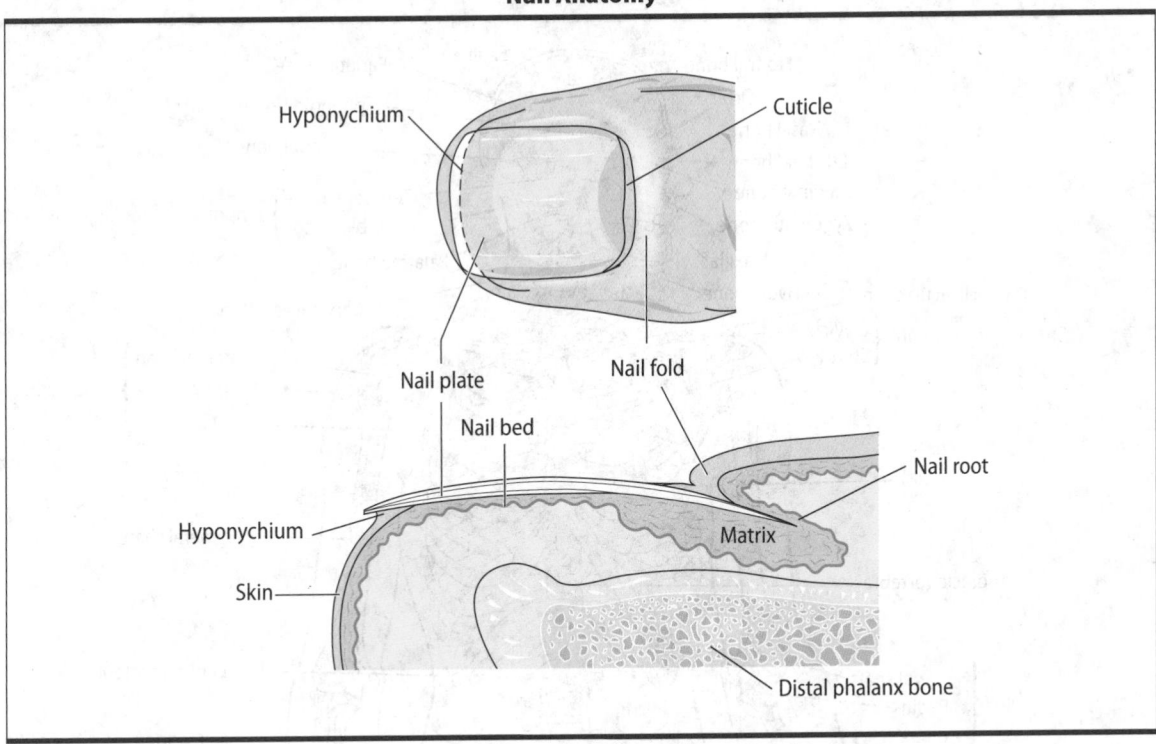

Skin and Subcutaneous Tissue

Chapter 13. Diseases of the Musculoskeletal System and Connective Tissue (M00–M99)

Bones and Joints

Shoulder Anterior View

Shoulder Posterior View

Elbow Anterior View

Elbow Posterior View

Hand

Hip Anterior View

Hip Posterior View

Knee Anterior View

Knee Posterior View

Foot

Muscles

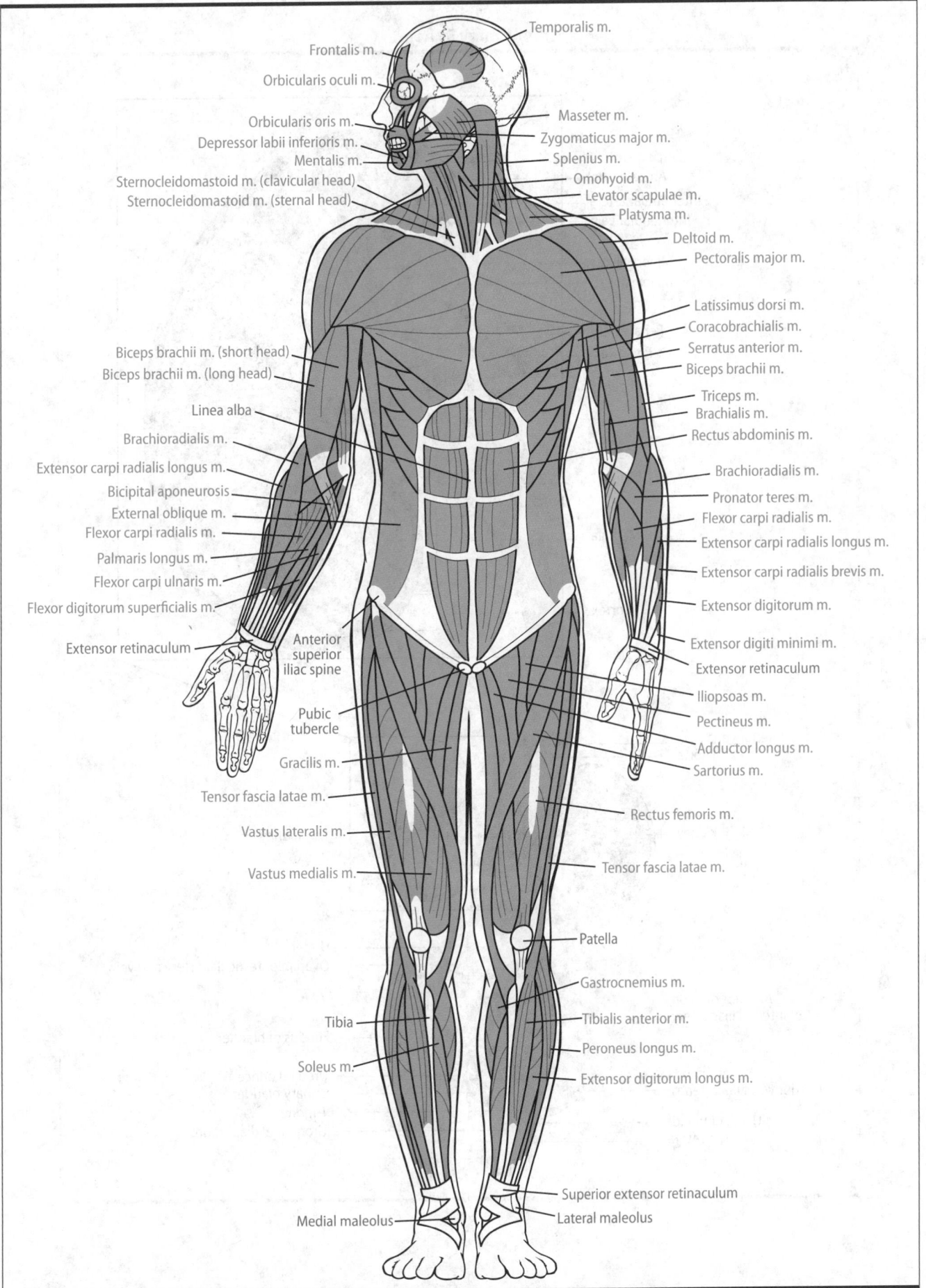

Chapter 14. Diseases of the Genitourinary System (NØØ–N99)

Urinary System

Male Genitourinary System

Female Internal Genitalia

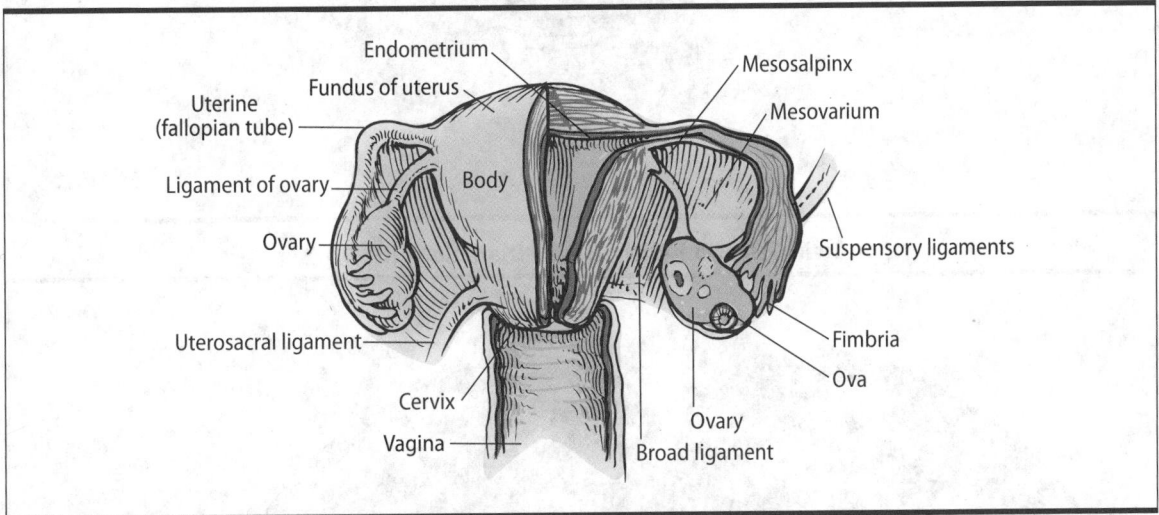

Female Genitourinary Tract Lateral View

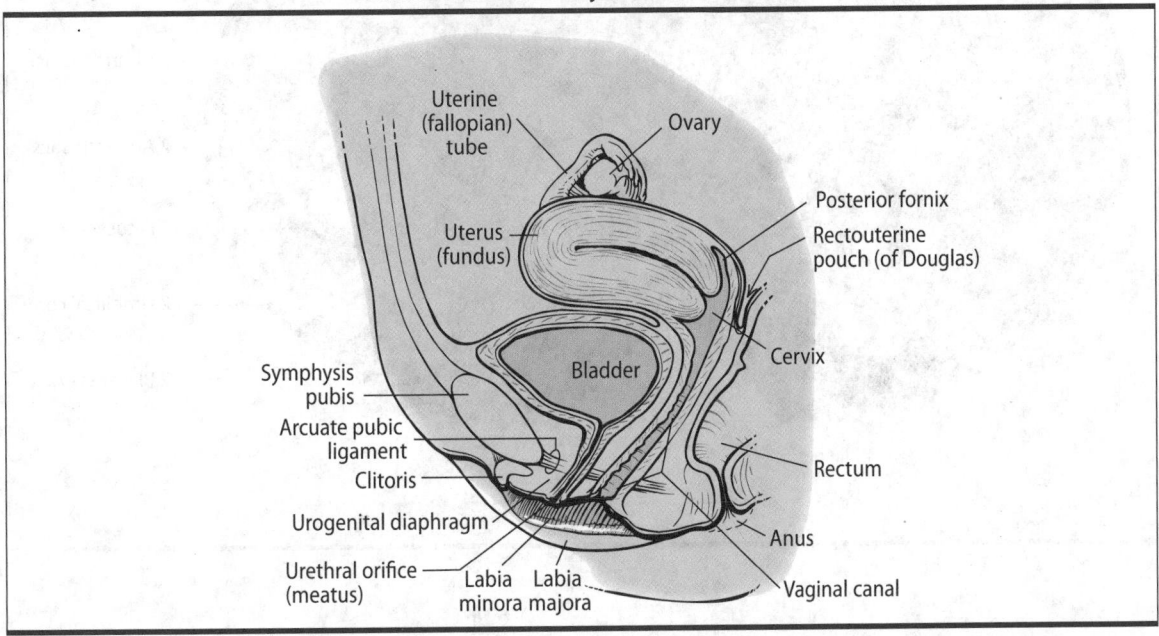

Chapter 15. Pregnancy, Childbirth and the Puerperium (O00–O9A)

Term Pregnancy – Single Gestation

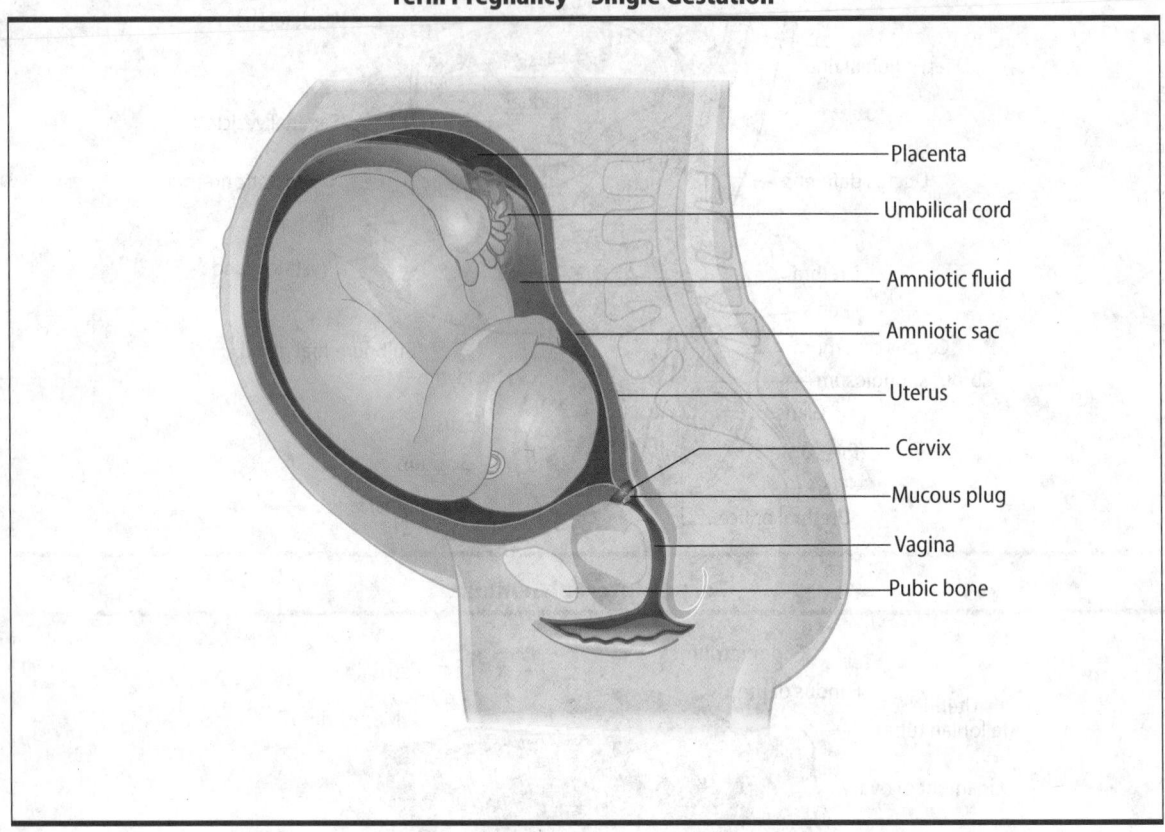

Placenta

Umbilical cord

Amniotic fluid

Amniotic sac

Uterus

Cervix

Mucous plug

Vagina

Pubic bone

Twin Gestation–Dichorionic–Diamniotic (DI-DI)

2 Chorionic sacs

2 Amniotic sacs

2 Fetuses

2 Umbilical cords

2 Placentas

Twin Gestation–Monochorionic–Diamniotic (MO-DI)

1 Chorionic sac

2 Amniotic sacs

2 Fetuses

2 Umbilical cords

1 Placenta

Twin Gestation–Monochorionic–Monoamniotic (MO-MO)

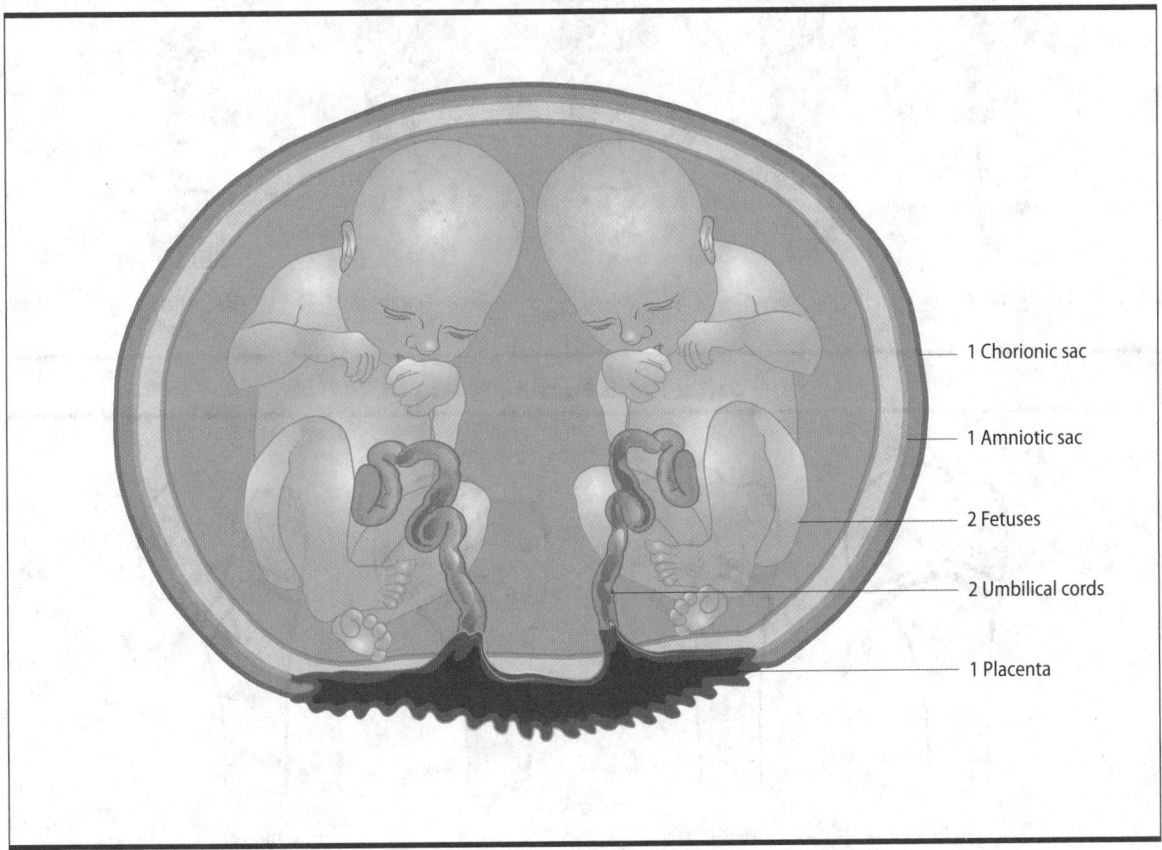

1 Chorionic sac

1 Amniotic sac

2 Fetuses

2 Umbilical cords

1 Placenta

Chapter 19. Injury, Poisoning and Certain Other Consequences of External Causes (S00–T88)

Types of Fractures

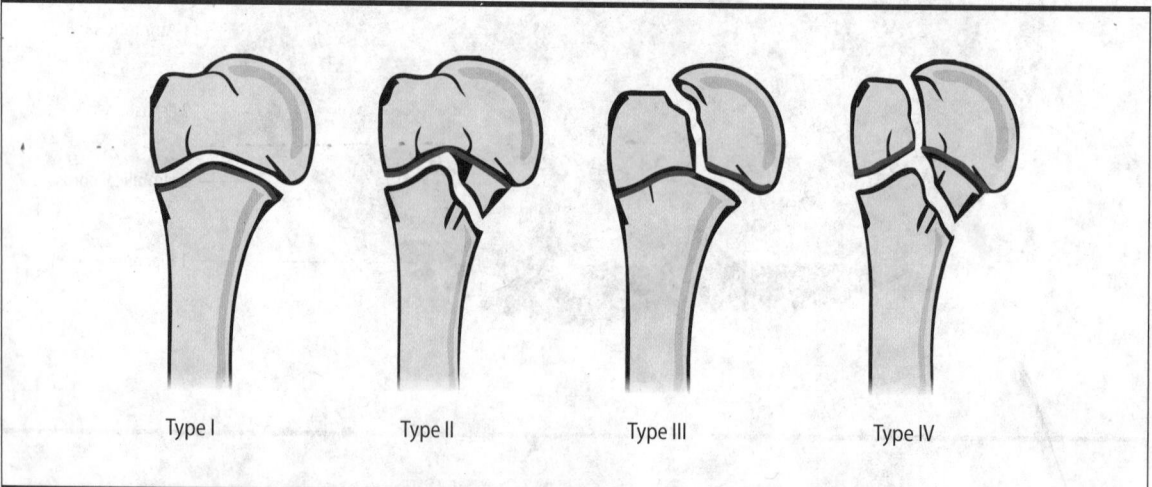

Normal | Transverse | Open/Compound | Oblique | Oblique displaced

Comminuted | Segmental | Avulsed | Spiral | Greenstick

Salter-Harris Fracture Types

Type I | Type II | Type III | Type IV